AMA

AMERICAN MEDICAL
ASSOCIATION

ICD
10-CM
2018

The Complete Official
Codebook

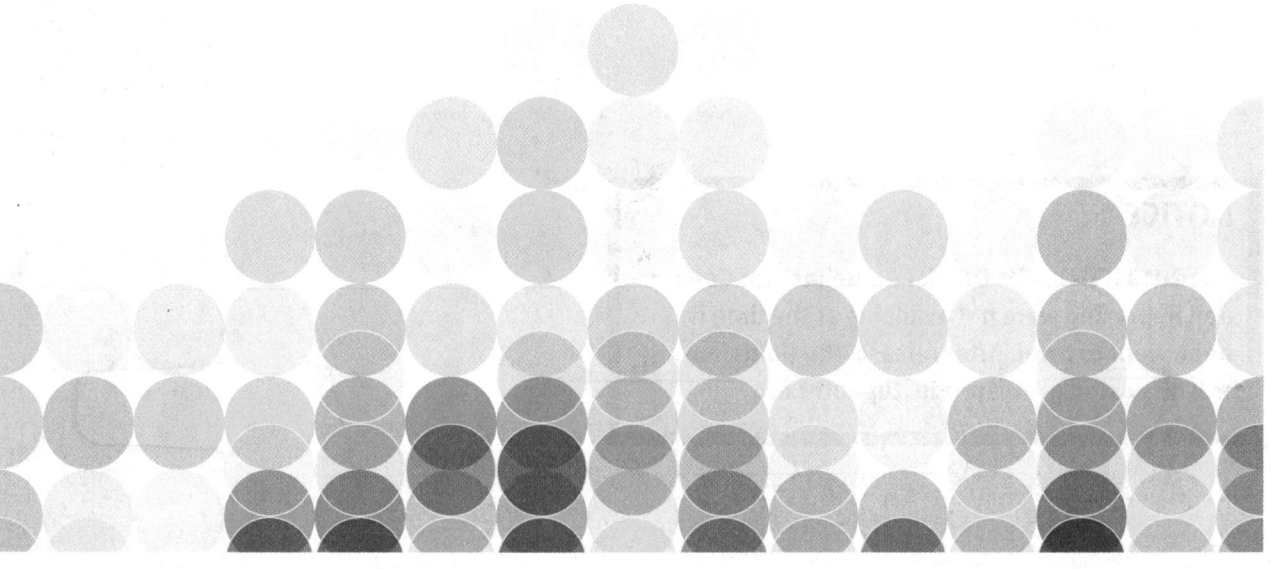

Publisher's Notice

The *ICD-10-CM: The Complete Official Codebook* is designed to be an accurate and authoritative source regarding coding and every reasonable effort has been made to ensure accuracy and completeness of the content. However, the AMA makes no guarantee, warranty, or representation that this publication is accurate, complete or without errors. It is understood that the AMA is not rendering any legal or other professional services or advice in this publication and that the AMA bears no liability for any results or consequences that may arise from the use of this book.

Our Commitment to Accuracy

The AMA is committed to producing accurate and reliable materials.

AMA product updates, errata, and addenda can be found at amaproductupdates.org.

To report corrections, please call the AMA Unified Service Center at (800) 621-8335.

To purchase additional copies, contact the American Medical Association at 800 621-8335 or visit the AMA store at amastore.com. Refer to product number OP201418.

Acknowledgments

Lauri Gray, RHIT, CPC, AHIMA-approved ICD-10-CM/PCS Trainer, *Product Manager*
Karen Schmidt, BSN, *Technical Director*
Anita Schmidt, BS, RHIT, AHIMA-approved ICD-10-CM/PCS Trainer, *Clinical Technical Editor*
Leanne Patterson, CPC, *Clinical Technical Editor*
Anne Kenney, BA, MBA, CCA, CCS, *Clinical Technical Editor*
Karen Krawzik, RHIT, CCS, AHIMA-approved ICD-10-CM/PCS Trainer, *Clinical Technical Editor*
Peggy Willard, CCS, AHIMA-approved ICD-10-CM/PCS Trainer, *Clinical Technical Editor*
Dr. Vikas Kumar, BHMS, CPC, CPC-H, *Clinical Technical Editor*
Stacy Perry, *Manager, Desktop Publishing*
Lisa Singley, *Project Manager*
Tracy Betzler, *Senior Desktop Publishing Specialist*
Hope M. Dunn, *Senior Desktop Publishing Specialist*
Katie Russell, *Desktop Publishing Specialist*
Kate Holden, *Editor*

NOTICE

The 2018 ICD-10-CM Official Guidelines for Coding and Reporting were not available at the time this book went to print. After release, the Guidelines will be posted at amaproductupdates.org

---

Anita Schmidt, BS, RHIT, AHIMA-approved ICD-10-CM/PCS Trainer

Ms. Schmidt has expertise in Level I Adult and Pediatric Trauma hospital coding, specializing in ICD-9-CM, ICD-10-CM/PCS, DRG, and CPT coding. Her experience includes analysis of medical record documentation, assignment of ICD-10-CM and PCS codes, DRG validation, as well as CPT code assignments for same-day surgery cases. She has conducted coding training and auditing, including DRG validation, conducted electronic health record training, and worked with clinical documentation specialists to identify documentation needs and potential areas for physician education. Most recently she has been developing content for resource and educational products related to ICD-10-CM and ICD-10-PCS. Ms. Schmidt is an AHIMA-approved ICD-10-CM/PCS trainer, and is an active member of the American Health Information Management Association (AHIMA) and the Minnesota Health Information Management Association (MHIMA).

Leanne Patterson, CPC

Ms. Patterson has more than 10 years of experience in the health care profession. She has an extensive background in professional component coding, with expertise in E/M coding and auditing, and HIPAA compliance. Her experience includes general surgery coding, serving as director of compliance, conducting chart-to-claim audits and physician education. She has been responsible for coding and denial management in large multispecialty physician practices, and most recently served as a practice manager where she supervised implementation of a new EHR system. Ms. Patterson is credentialed by the American Academy of Professional Coders (AAPC) as a Certified Professional Coder (CPC).

Contents

Preface iii
    ICD-10-CM Official Preface iii
    Characteristics of ICD-10-CM iii

What's New for 2018 iv
    Official Updates iv

Introduction vii
    History of ICD-10-CM vii

How to Use ICD-10-CM: The Complete Official
Codebook 2018 viii
    Use of Official Sources viii
    Steps to Correct Coding viii
    Organization viii
        Introduction viii
        Official ICD-10-CM Conventions and Guidelines........ viii
        Alphabetic Index to Diseases viii
        Neoplasm Table viii
        Table of Drugs and Chemicals viii
        Index to External Causes viii
        Tabular List of Diseases viii
        Appendixes.. ix
        Illustrations ix

Overview of ICD-10-CM Official Conventions x
    Format x
    Punctuation x
    Abbreviations x
        NEC x
        NOS x
    Typeface x
    General Notes x
        Includes Notes x
        Inclusion Terms.. x
        Excludes Notes x
        Note xi
        Default Codes... xi
        Syndromes... xi
        And xi
        With xi
        See and See Also xi
        Instructional Notes Used in the Tabular List xi
        Code Assignment and Clinical Criteria xi

Additional Annotations xii
    Code-Level Notations xii
        Italics xii
        Color Coding/Symbols xii
        Other Code-Level Notations................................ xiii
    Chapter-Level Notations xiii
        Chapter-Specific Guidelines with Coding Examples xiii
        Muscle and Tendon Table.................................... xiii
    Index Notations xiv
        Following References xiv

ICD-10-CM Official Guidelines for Coding
and Reporting .... Coding Guidelines–1

ICD-10-CM Index to Diseases and Injuries 1

ICD-10-CM Neoplasm Table 331

ICD-10-CM Table of Drugs and Chemicals 349

ICD-10-CM Index to External Causes 397

ICD-10-CM Tabular List of Diseases and Injuries 433
    Chapter 1.   Certain Infectious and Parasitic Diseases
                   (A00-B99) 433
    Chapter 2.   Neoplasms (C00-D49) 457
    Chapter 3.   Diseases of the Blood and Blood-forming Organs
                   and Certain Disorders Involving the Immune
                   Mechanism (D50-D89) 495
    Chapter 4.   Endocrine, Nutritional and Metabolic Diseases
                   (E00-E89) 505
    Chapter 5.   Mental, Behavioral, and Neurodevelopmental
                   Disorders (F01-F99) 525
    Chapter 6.   Diseases of the Nervous System (G00-G99) 549
    Chapter 7.   Diseases of the Eye and Adnexa (H00-H59) 569
    Chapter 8.   Diseases of the Ear and Mastoid Process
                   (H60-H95) 605
    Chapter 9.   Diseases of the Circulatory System (I00-I99) 617
    Chapter 10.   Diseases of the Respiratory System (J00-J99) 657
    Chapter 11.   Diseases of the Digestive System (K00-K95) 671
    Chapter 12.   Diseases of the Skin and Subcutaneous Tissue
                   (L00-L99) 693
    Chapter 13.   Diseases of the Musculoskeletal System and
                   Connective Tissue (M00-M99) 713
    Chapter 14.   Diseases of the Genitourinary System
                   (N00-N99) 801
    Chapter 15.   Pregnancy, Childbirth, and the Puerperium
                   (O00-O9A) 819
    Chapter 16.   Certain Conditions Originating in the Perinatal
                   Period (P00-P96) 857
    Chapter 17.   Congenital Malformations, Deformations and
                   Chromosomal Abnormalities (Q00-Q99) 869
    Chapter 18.   Symptoms, Signs and Abnormal Clinical and
                   Laboratory Findings, Not Elsewhere
                   Classified (R00-R99) 887
    Chapter 19.   Injury, Poisoning and Certain Other Consequences
                   of External Causes (S00-T88) 907
    Chapter 20.   External Causes of Morbidity (V00-Y99)................ 1113
    Chapter 21.   Factors Influencing Health Status and Contact
                   With Health Services (Z00-Z99) 1175

Appendixes Appendixes-1
    Appendix A: 10 Steps to Correct Coding Appendixes–1
    Appendix B: Valid 3-character ICD-10-CM Codes.......Appendixes–3
    Appendix C: Pharmacology List 2018................Appendixes–5
    Appendix D: Z Codes for Long-Term Drug Use with
                   Associated Drugs Appendixes–23
    Appendix E: Z Codes Only as Principal/First-Listed
                   Diagnosis Appendixes–27
    Appendix F: Centers for Medicare & Medicaid Services
                   Hierarchical Condition Categories
                   (CMS-HCC) Appendixes–29

Illustrations Illustrations–1

Chapter 3.   Diseases of the Blood and Blood-forming
              Organs and Certain Disorders Involving
              the Immune Mechanism (D50–D89) Illustrations–1

              Red Blood Cells Illustrations–1
              White Blood Cell Illustrations–1
              Platelet Illustrations–2
              Coagulation Illustrations–2
              Spleen Anatomical Location and
              External Structures Illustrations–3
              Spleen Interior Structures Illustrations–3

Chapter 4.   Endocrine, Nutritional and Metabolic
              Diseases (E00–E89) Illustrations–4

              Endocrine System Illustrations–4
              Thyroid Illustrations–5
              Thyroid and Parathyroid Glands Illustrations–5
              Pancreas Illustrations–6
              Anatomy of the Adrenal Gland Illustrations–6
              Structure of an Ovary Illustrations–7
              Testis and Associated Structures Illustrations–7
              Thymus Illustrations–8

Chapter 6.   Diseases of the Nervous System
              (G00–G99) Illustrations–9

              Brain Illustrations–9
              Cranial Nerves Illustrations–9
              Peripheral Nervous System Illustrations–10
              Spinal Cord and Spinal Nerves Illustrations–11
              Nerve Cell Illustrations–12

Chapter 7.   Diseases of the Eye and Adnexa
              (H00–H59) Illustrations–13

              Eye Illustrations–13
              Posterior Pole of Globe/Flow of
              Aqueous Humor Illustrations–13
              Lacrimal System Illustrations–14
              Eye Musculature Illustrations–14
              Eyelid Structures Illustrations–15

Chapter 8.   Diseases of the Ear and Mastoid
              Process (H60–H95) Illustrations–16

              Ear Anatomy Illustrations–16

Chapter 9.   Diseases of the Circulatory
              System (I00–I99) Illustrations–17

              Anatomy of the Heart Illustrations–17
              Heart Cross Section Illustrations–17
              Heart Valves......................... Illustrations–18
              Heart Conduction System Illustrations–18
              Coronary Arteries Illustrations–19
              Arteries............................. Illustrations–20
              Veins Illustrations–21
              Internal Carotid and Vertebral
              Arteries and Branches Illustrations–22
              External Carotid Artery and
              Branches Illustrations–22
              Branches of Abdominal Aorta Illustrations–23
              Portal Venous Circulation Illustrations–23
              Lymphatic System Illustrations–24
              Axillary Lymph Nodes Illustrations–25
              Lymphatic System of Head and
              Neck Illustrations–25
              Lymphatic Capillaries Illustrations–26
              Lymphatic Drainage Illustrations–26

Chapter 10.   Diseases of the Respiratory
              System (J00–J99) Illustrations–27

              Respiratory System Illustrations–27
              Upper Respiratory System Illustrations–28
              Lower Respiratory System Illustrations–28
              Paranasal Sinuses Illustrations–28
              Lung Segments Illustrations–29
              Alveoli Illustrations–29

Chapter 11.   Diseases of the Digestive System
              (K00–K95) Illustrations–30

              Digestive System Illustrations–30
              Omentum and Mesentery Illustrations–31
              Peritoneum and Retroperitoneum Illustrations–31

Chapter 12.   Diseases of the Skin and Subcutaneous
              Tissue (L00–L99) Illustrations–32

              Nail Anatomy Illustrations–32
              Skin and Subcutaneous Tissue Illustrations–33

Chapter 13.   Diseases of the Musculoskeletal
              System and Connective Tissue
              (M00–M99) Illustrations–34

              Bones and Joints Illustrations–34
              Shoulder Anterior View Illustrations–35
              Shoulder Posterior View Illustrations–35
              Elbow Anterior View Illustrations–35
              Elbow Posterior View Illustrations–36
              Hand Illustrations–36
              Hip Anterior View Illustrations–37
              Hip Posterior View Illustrations–37
              Knee Anterior View Illustrations–37
              Knee Posterior View Illustrations–38
              Foot Illustrations–38
              Muscles Illustrations–39

Chapter 14.   Diseases of the Genitourinary
              System (N00–N99) Illustrations–40

              Urinary System Illustrations–40
              Male Genitourinary System Illustrations–41
              Female Internal Genitalia Illustrations–41
              Female Genitourinary Tract
              Lateral View Illustrations–42

Chapter 15.   Pregnancy, Childbirth, and the
              Puerperium (O00–O9A) Illustrations–43

              Term Pregnancy – Single
              Gestation Illustrations–43
              Twin Gestation–Dichorionic–
              Diamniotic (DI-DI) Illustrations–43
              Twin Gestation–Monochorionic–
              Diamniotic (MO-DI) .... Illustrations– 44
              Twin Gestation–Monochorionic–
              Monoamniotic (MO-MO) Illustrations–44

Chapter 19.   Injury, Poisoning and Certain Other
              Consequences of External Causes
              (S00–T88) Illustrations–45

              Types of Fractures................... Illustrations–45
              Salter-Harris Fracture Types......... Illustrations–45

Preface

ICD-10-CM Official Preface

This FY 2018 update of the International Statistical Classification of Diseases and Related Health Problems, 10th revision, Clinical Modification (ICD-10-CM) is being published by the United States government in recognition of its responsibility to promulgate this classification throughout the United States for morbidity coding. The International Statistical Classification of Diseases and Related Health Problems, 10th Revision (ICD-10), published by the World Health Organization (WHO), is the foundation of ICD-10-CM. ICD-10 continues to be the classification used in cause-of-death coding in the United States. The ICD-10-CM is comparable with the ICD-10. The WHO Collaborating Center for the Family of International Classifications in North America, housed at the Centers for Disease Control and Prevention's National Center for Health Statistics (NCHS), has responsibility for the implementation of ICD and other WHO-FIC classifications and serves as a liaison with the WHO, fulfilling international obligations for comparable classifications and the national health data needs of the United States. The historical background of ICD and ICD-10 can be found in the Introduction to the International Classification of Diseases and Related Health Problems (ICD-10), 2010, World Health Organization, Geneva, Switzerland.

ICD-10-CM is the United States' clinical modification of the World Health Organization's ICD-10. The term "clinical" is used to emphasize the modification's intent: to serve as a useful tool in the area of classification of morbidity data for indexing of health records, medical care review, and ambulatory and other health care programs, as well as for basic health statistics. To describe the clinical picture of the patient the codes must be more precise than those needed only for statistical groupings and trend analysis.

Characteristics of ICD-10-CM

ICD-10-CM far exceeds its predecessors in the number of concepts and codes provided. The disease classification has been expanded to include health-related conditions and to provide greater specificity at the sixth and seventh character level. The sixth and seventh characters are not optional and are intended for use in recording the information documented in the clinical record.

ICD-10-CM extensions, interpretations, modifications, addenda, or errata other than those approved by the Centers for Disease Control and Prevention are not to be considered official and should not be utilized. Continuous maintenance of the ICD-10- CM is the responsibility of the aforementioned agencies. However, because the ICD-10- CM represents the best in contemporary thinking of clinicians, nosologists, epidemiologists, and statisticians from both public and private sectors, when future modifications are considered, advice will be sought from all stakeholders.

All official authorized addenda since the last complete update (October 1, 2017) have been included in this revision. For more detailed information please see the complete official authorized addenda to ICD-10-CM, including the "ICD-10-CM Official Guidelines for Coding and Reporting," and a description of the ICD-10-CM updating and maintenance process.

What's New for 2018

Official Updates

The National Center for Health Statistics (NCHS), a section of the Centers for Disease Control and Prevention (CDC), is the agency charged with maintaining and updating ICD-10-CM. The 2018 official addendum was posted to the Centers for Medicare and Medicaid Services (CMS) website on June 13, 2017, identifying the changes to the ICD-10-CM code set for fiscal 2018. A summary of changes is provided below:

- 360 new codes added

- 226 code descriptions revised

- 34 codes changed from valid to invalid

Note: Validity changes are the result of new codes being added to the classification, changing a previously valid code to an invalid code, creating a new subcategory.

A04.7	Enterocolitis due to Clostridium difficile
C96.2	Malignant mast cell tumor
D47.0	Histiocytic and mast cell tumors of uncertain behavior
E85.8	Other amyloidosis
H54.0	Blindness, both eyes
H54.11	Blindness, right eye, low vision left eye
H54.12	Blindness, left eye, low vision right eye
H54.2	Low vision, both eyes
H54.41	Blindness, right eye, normal vision left eye
H54.42	Blindness, left eye, normal vision right eye
H54.51	Low vision, right eye, normal vision left eye
H54.52	Low vision, left eye, normal vision right eye
I27.2	Other secondary pulmonary hypertension
K06.0	Gingival recession
K56.5	Intestinal adhesions [bands] with obstruction (postprocedural) (postinfection)
K56.60	Unspecified intestinal obstruction
K56.69	Other intestinal obstruction
K91.3	Postprocedural intestinal obstruction
M48.06	Spinal stenosis, lumbar region
N63	Unspecified lump in breast
O00.10	Tubal pregnancy without intrauterine pregnancy
O00.11	Tubal pregnancy with intrauterine pregnancy
O00.20	Ovarian pregnancy without intrauterine pregnancy
O00.21	Ovarian pregnancy with intrauterine pregnancy
P29.3	Persistent fetal circulation
P83.8	Other specified conditions of integument specific to newborn
P91.8	Other specified disturbances of cerebral status of newborn
Q53.11	Abdominal testis, unilateral
Q53.21	Abdominal testis, bilateral
T07	Unspecified multiple injuries
T14.8	Other injury of unspecified body region
T14.90	Injury, unspecified
T14.91	Suicide attempt
Z36	Encounter for antenatal screening of mother

- 122 codes deleted from the classification

S06.1X7D	Traumatic cerebral edema with loss of consciousness of any duration with death due to brain injury prior to regaining consciousness, subsequent encounter
S06.1X7S	Traumatic cerebral edema with loss of consciousness of any duration with death due to brain injury prior to regaining consciousness, sequela
S06.1X8D	Traumatic cerebral edema with loss of consciousness of any duration with death due to other cause prior to regaining consciousness, subsequent encounter
S06.1X8S	Traumatic cerebral edema with loss of consciousness of any duration with death due to other cause prior to regaining consciousness, sequela
S06.2X7D	Diffuse traumatic brain injury with loss of consciousness of any duration with death due to brain injury prior to regaining consciousness, subsequent encounter
S06.2X7S	Diffuse traumatic brain injury with loss of consciousness of any duration with death due to brain injury prior to regaining consciousness, sequela
S06.2X8D	Diffuse traumatic brain injury with loss of consciousness of any duration with death due to other cause prior to regaining consciousness, subsequent encounter
S06.2X8S	Diffuse traumatic brain injury with loss of consciousness of any duration with death due to other cause prior to regaining consciousness, sequela
S06.307D	Unspecified focal traumatic brain injury with loss of consciousness of any duration with death due to brain injury prior to regaining consciousness, subsequent encounter
S06.307S	Unspecified focal traumatic brain injury with loss of consciousness of any duration with death due to brain injury prior to regaining consciousness, sequela
S06.308D	Unspecified focal traumatic brain injury with loss of consciousness of any duration with death due to other cause prior to regaining consciousness, subsequent encounter
S06.308S	Unspecified focal traumatic brain injury with loss of consciousness of any duration with death due to other cause prior to regaining consciousness, sequela
S06.317D	Contusion and laceration of right cerebrum with loss of consciousness of any duration with death due to brain injury prior to regaining consciousness, subsequent encounter
S06.317S	Contusion and laceration of right cerebrum with loss of consciousness of any duration with death due to brain injury prior to regaining consciousness, sequela
S06.318D	Contusion and laceration of right cerebrum with loss of consciousness of any duration with death due to other cause prior to regaining consciousness, subsequent encounter
S06.318S	Contusion and laceration of right cerebrum with loss of consciousness of any duration with death due to other cause prior to regaining consciousness, sequela
S06.327D	Contusion and laceration of left cerebrum with loss of consciousness of any duration with death due to brain injury prior to regaining consciousness, subsequent encounter
S06.327S	Contusion and laceration of left cerebrum with loss of consciousness of any duration with death due to brain injury prior to regaining consciousness, sequela
S06.328D	Contusion and laceration of left cerebrum with loss of consciousness of any duration with death due to other cause prior to regaining consciousness, subsequent encounter
S06.328S	Contusion and laceration of left cerebrum with loss of consciousness of any duration with death due to other cause prior to regaining consciousness, sequela
S06.337D	Contusion and laceration of cerebrum, unspecified, with loss of consciousness of any duration with death due to brain injury prior to regaining consciousness, subsequent encounter
S06.337S	Contusion and laceration of cerebrum, unspecified, with loss of consciousness of any duration with death due to brain injury prior to regaining consciousness, sequela
S06.338D	Contusion and laceration of cerebrum, unspecified, with loss of consciousness of any duration with death due to other cause prior to regaining consciousness, subsequent encounter
S06.338S	Contusion and laceration of cerebrum, unspecified, with loss of consciousness of any duration with death due to other cause prior to regaining consciousness, sequela
S06.347D	Traumatic hemorrhage of right cerebrum with loss of consciousness of any duration with death due to brain injury prior to regaining consciousness, subsequent encounter

S06.347S   Traumatic hemorrhage of right cerebrum with loss of consciousness of any duration with death due to brain injury prior to regaining consciousness, sequela

S06.348D   Traumatic hemorrhage of right cerebrum with loss of consciousness of any duration with death due to other cause prior to regaining consciousness, subsequent encounter

S06.348S   Traumatic hemorrhage of right cerebrum with loss of consciousness of any duration with death due to other cause prior to regaining consciousness, sequela

S06.357D   Traumatic hemorrhage of left cerebrum with loss of consciousness of any duration with death due to brain injury prior to regaining consciousness, subsequent encounter

S06.357S   Traumatic hemorrhage of left cerebrum with loss of consciousness of any duration with death due to brain injury prior to regaining consciousness, sequela

S06.358D   Traumatic hemorrhage of left cerebrum with loss of consciousness of any duration with death due to other cause prior to regaining consciousness, subsequent encounter

S06.358S   Traumatic hemorrhage of left cerebrum with loss of consciousness of any duration with death due to other cause prior to regaining consciousness, sequela

S06.367D   Traumatic hemorrhage of cerebrum, unspecified, with loss of consciousness of any duration with death due to brain injury prior to regaining consciousness, subsequent encounter

S06.367S   Traumatic hemorrhage of cerebrum, unspecified, with loss of consciousness of any duration with death due to brain injury prior to regaining consciousness, sequela

S06.368D   Traumatic hemorrhage of cerebrum, unspecified, with loss of consciousness of any duration with death due to other cause prior to regaining consciousness, subsequent encounter

S06.368S   Traumatic hemorrhage of cerebrum, unspecified, with loss of consciousness of any duration with death due to other cause prior to regaining consciousness, sequela

S06.377D   Contusion, laceration, and hemorrhage of cerebellum with loss of consciousness of any duration with death due to brain injury prior to regaining consciousness, subsequent encounter

S06.377S   Contusion, laceration, and hemorrhage of cerebellum with loss of consciousness of any duration with death due to brain injury prior to regaining consciousness, sequela

S06.378D   Contusion, laceration, and hemorrhage of cerebellum with loss of consciousness of any duration with death due to other cause prior to regaining consciousness, subsequent encounter

S06.378S   Contusion, laceration, and hemorrhage of cerebellum with loss of consciousness of any duration with death due to other cause prior to regaining consciousness, sequela

S06.387D   Contusion, laceration, and hemorrhage of brainstem with loss of consciousness of any duration with death due to brain injury prior to regaining consciousness, subsequent encounter

S06.387S   Contusion, laceration, and hemorrhage of brainstem with loss of consciousness of any duration with death due to brain injury prior to regaining consciousness, sequela

S06.388D   Contusion, laceration, and hemorrhage of brainstem with loss of consciousness of any duration with death due to other cause prior to regaining consciousness, subsequent encounter

S06.388S   Contusion, laceration, and hemorrhage of brainstem with loss of consciousness of any duration with death due to other cause prior to regaining consciousness, sequela

S06.4X7D   Epidural hemorrhage with loss of consciousness of any duration with death due to brain injury prior to regaining consciousness, subsequent encounter

S06.4X7S   Epidural hemorrhage with loss of consciousness of any duration with death due to brain injury prior to regaining consciousness, sequela

S06.4X8D   Epidural hemorrhage with loss of consciousness of any duration with death due to other causes prior to regaining consciousness, subsequent encounter

S06.4X8S   Epidural hemorrhage with loss of consciousness of any duration with death due to other causes prior to regaining consciousness, sequela

S06.5X7D   Traumatic subdural hemorrhage with loss of consciousness of any duration with death due to brain injury before regaining consciousness, subsequent encounter

S06.5X7S   Traumatic subdural hemorrhage with loss of consciousness of any duration with death due to brain injury before regaining consciousness, sequela

S06.5X8D   Traumatic subdural hemorrhage with loss of consciousness of any duration with death due to other cause before regaining consciousness, subsequent encounter

S06.5X8S   Traumatic subdural hemorrhage with loss of consciousness of any duration with death due to other cause before regaining consciousness, sequela

S06.6X7D   Traumatic subarachnoid hemorrhage with loss of consciousness of any duration with death due to brain injury prior to regaining consciousness, subsequent encounter

S06.6X7S   Traumatic subarachnoid hemorrhage with loss of consciousness of any duration with death due to brain injury prior to regaining consciousness, sequela

S06.6X8D   Traumatic subarachnoid hemorrhage with loss of consciousness of any duration with death due to other cause prior to regaining consciousness, subsequent encounter

S06.6X8S   Traumatic subarachnoid hemorrhage with loss of consciousness of any duration with death due to other cause prior to regaining consciousness, sequela

S06.817D   Injury of right internal carotid artery, intracranial portion, not elsewhere classified with loss of consciousness of any duration with death due to brain injury prior to regaining consciousness, subsequent encounter

S06.817S   Injury of right internal carotid artery, intracranial portion, not elsewhere classified with loss of consciousness of any duration with death due to brain injury prior to regaining consciousness, sequela

S06.818D   Injury of right internal carotid artery, intracranial portion, not elsewhere classified with loss of consciousness of any duration with death due to other cause prior to regaining consciousness, subsequent encounter

S06.818S   Injury of right internal carotid artery, intracranial portion, not elsewhere classified with loss of consciousness of any duration with death due to other cause prior to regaining consciousness, sequela

S06.827D   Injury of left internal carotid artery, intracranial portion, not elsewhere classified with loss of consciousness of any duration with death due to brain injury prior to regaining consciousness, subsequent encounter

S06.827S   Injury of left internal carotid artery, intracranial portion, not elsewhere classified with loss of consciousness of any duration with death due to brain injury prior to regaining consciousness, sequela

S06.828D   Injury of left internal carotid artery, intracranial portion, not elsewhere classified with loss of consciousness of any duration with death due to other cause prior to regaining consciousness, subsequent encounter

S06.828S   Injury of left internal carotid artery, intracranial portion, not elsewhere classified with loss of consciousness of any duration with death due to other cause prior to regaining consciousness, sequela

S06.897D   Other specified intracranial injury with loss of consciousness of any duration with death due to brain injury prior to regaining consciousness, subsequent encounter

S06.897S   Other specified intracranial injury with loss of consciousness of any duration with death due to brain injury prior to regaining consciousness, sequela

S06.898D   Other specified intracranial injury with loss of consciousness of any duration with death due to other cause prior to regaining consciousness, subsequent encounter

S06.898S   Other specified intracranial injury with loss of consciousness of any duration with death due to other cause prior to regaining consciousness, sequela

S06.9X7D   Unspecified intracranial injury with loss of consciousness of any duration with death due to brain injury prior to regaining consciousness, subsequent encounter

S06.9X7S	Unspecified intracranial injury with loss of consciousness of any duration with death due to brain injury prior to regaining consciousness, sequela
S06.9X8D	Unspecified intracranial injury with loss of consciousness of any duration with death due to other cause prior to regaining consciousness, subsequent encounter
S06.9X8S	Unspecified intracranial injury with loss of consciousness of any duration with death due to other cause prior to regaining consciousness, sequela
S63.13	Subluxation and dislocation of proximal interphalangeal joint of thumb
S63.131	Subluxation of proximal interphalangeal joint of right thumb
S63.131A	Subluxation of proximal interphalangeal joint of right thumb, initial encounter
S63.131D	Subluxation of proximal interphalangeal joint of right thumb, subsequent encounter
S63.131S	Subluxation of proximal interphalangeal joint of right thumb, sequela
S63.132	Subluxation of proximal interphalangeal joint of left thumb
S63.132A	Subluxation of proximal interphalangeal joint of left thumb, initial encounter
S63.132D	Subluxation of proximal interphalangeal joint of left thumb, subsequent encounter
S63.132S	Subluxation of proximal interphalangeal joint of left thumb, sequela
S63.133	Subluxation of proximal interphalangeal joint of unspecified thumb
S63.133A	Subluxation of proximal interphalangeal joint of unspecified thumb, initial encounter
S63.133D	Subluxation of proximal interphalangeal joint of unspecified thumb, subsequent encounter
S63.133S	Subluxation of proximal interphalangeal joint of unspecified thumb, sequela
S63.134	Dislocation of proximal interphalangeal joint of right thumb
S63.134A	Dislocation of proximal interphalangeal joint of right thumb, initial encounter
S63.134D	Dislocation of proximal interphalangeal joint of right thumb, subsequent encounter
S63.134S	Dislocation of proximal interphalangeal joint of right thumb, sequela
S63.135	Dislocation of proximal interphalangeal joint of left thumb
S63.135A	Dislocation of proximal interphalangeal joint of left thumb, initial encounter
S63.135D	Dislocation of proximal interphalangeal joint of left thumb, subsequent encounter
S63.135S	Dislocation of proximal interphalangeal joint of left thumb, sequela
S63.136	Dislocation of proximal interphalangeal joint of unspecified thumb
S63.136A	Dislocation of proximal interphalangeal joint of unspecified thumb, initial encounter

S63.136D	Dislocation of proximal interphalangeal joint of unspecified thumb, subsequent encounter
S63.136S	Dislocation of proximal interphalangeal joint of unspecified thumb, sequela
S63.14	Subluxation and dislocation of distal interphalangeal joint of thumb
S63.141	Subluxation of distal interphalangeal joint of right thumb
S63.141A	Subluxation of distal interphalangeal joint of right thumb, initial encounter
S63.141D	Subluxation of distal interphalangeal joint of right thumb, subsequent encounter
S63.141S	Subluxation of distal interphalangeal joint of right thumb, sequela
S63.142	Subluxation of distal interphalangeal joint of left thumb
S63.142A	Subluxation of distal interphalangeal joint of left thumb, initial encounter
S63.142D	Subluxation of distal interphalangeal joint of left thumb, subsequent encounter
S63.142S	Subluxation of distal interphalangeal joint of left thumb, sequela
S63.143	Subluxation of distal interphalangeal joint of unspecified thumb
S63.143A	Subluxation of distal interphalangeal joint of unspecified thumb, initial encounter
S63.143D	Subluxation of distal interphalangeal joint of unspecified thumb, subsequent encounter
S63.143S	Subluxation of distal interphalangeal joint of unspecified thumb, sequela
S63.144	Dislocation of distal interphalangeal joint of right thumb
S63.144A	Dislocation of distal interphalangeal joint of right thumb, initial encounter
S63.144D	Dislocation of distal interphalangeal joint of right thumb, subsequent encounter
S63.144S	Dislocation of distal interphalangeal joint of right thumb, sequela
S63.145	Dislocation of distal interphalangeal joint of left thumb
S63.145A	Dislocation of distal interphalangeal joint of left thumb, initial encounter
S63.145D	Dislocation of distal interphalangeal joint of left thumb, subsequent encounter
S63.145S	Dislocation of distal interphalangeal joint of left thumb, sequela
S63.146	Dislocation of distal interphalangeal joint of unspecified thumb
S63.146A	Dislocation of distal interphalangeal joint of unspecified thumb, initial encounter
S63.146D	Dislocation of distal interphalangeal joint of unspecified thumb, subsequent encounter
S63.146S	Dislocation of distal interphalangeal joint of unspecified thumb, sequela

Introduction

History of ICD-10-CM

The ICD-10-CM classification system was developed by the National Center for Health Statistics (NCHS) as a clinical modification to the ICD-10 system developed by the World Health Organization (WHO), primarily as a unique system for use in the United States for morbidity and mortality reporting. Although ICD-10 replaced ICD-9 for use in coding and classifying mortality data from death certificates beginning January 1, 1999, ICD-10-CM implementation was postponed many years until legislation to replace ICD-9-CM, volumes 1 and 2, with ICD-10-CM was approved.

ICD-10 is the copyrighted product of the World Health Organization (WHO), which has authorized the development of a clinical modification (CM) of ICD-10 for use in the United States. However, all modifications to the ICD-10 must conform to WHO conventions for ICD. The development of ICD-10-CM included comprehensive evaluation by a Technical Advisory Panel and extensive consultation with physician groups, clinical coders, and other industry experts.

The ICD-10-CM draft and crosswalk between ICD-9-CM and ICD-10-CM were made available on the Centers for Medicare and Medicaid Services (CMS) website for public comment. The initial public comment period extended from December 1997 through February 1998. A field test for ICD-10-CM was conducted in the summer of 2003 jointly by the American Hospital Association (AHA) and the American Health Information Management Association (AHIMA). Public comments and suggestions were reviewed and additional modifications to ICD-10-CM were made. Revisions were made to ICD-10-CM based on the established update process for ICD-10-CM (the ICD-10-CM Coordination and Maintenance Committee) and the World Health Organization's ICD-10 (the Update and Revision Committee).

These revisions to ICD-10-CM have included:

- Information relevant to ambulatory and managed care encounters

- Expanded injury codes

- Creation of combination diagnosis/symptom codes to reduce the number of codes needed to fully describe a condition

- The addition of 6th and 7th character classifications

- Incorporation of common 4th and 5th character classifications

- Classifications specific to laterality

- Classification refinement for increased data granularity

This new structure allows for further expansion than was possible with the ICD-9-CM classification system.

The Department of Health and Human Services (HHS) published the final rule regarding the adoption of both ICD-10-CM and ICD-10-PCS in the January 16, 2009, *Federal Register* (45 CFR part 162 [CMS—0013—F]). The initial compliance date for implementation of ICD-10-CM and ICD-10-PCS as a replacement for ICD-9-CM was set at October 1, 2013. On April 17, 2012, the Department of Health and Human Services (HHS) released a notice to postpone the date by which certain health care entities have to comply with International Classification of Diseases, 10th Revision diagnosis and procedure codes (ICD-10). The compliance date for implementation of ICD-10-CM and ICD-10-PCS as a replacement for ICD-9-CM was changed to October 1, 2014. On April 1, 2014, Congress enacted the Protecting Access to Medicare Act of 2014, which contained a provision to delay the implementation of ICD-10-CM/PCS by at least one year, prohibiting the Department of Health and Human Services (HHS) from adopting the ICD-10-CM/PCS code sets as the mandatory standard until October 1, 2015. Eventually, the ICD-10-CM/PCS code sets were implemented in entirety on October 1, 2015, and volumes 1 and 2 of ICD-9-CM were retired.

ICD-10-CM: The Complete Official Code Set

ICD-10-CM: The Complete Official Code Set 2018 edition includes many of the enhancements described below in direct response to requests from our subscribers. Users will find many of the conventions, icons, color bars, and other enhancements familiar since many of these features are similar to the hallmark color coding and symbols of our ICD-9-CM code books.

As you review the content, you will find the following:

- Exclusive feature — Check Placeholder Alert symbol, indicating the need for one or more "filler" X character assignments in the 5th and/or 6th character position, in order to appropriately assign a required character in the 7th character position

- Exclusive feature — Key word differentiation by the use of a green font that highlights the differentiating terms in similar code descriptions in a given category

- Exclusive color coding, symbols, and footnotes that alert coders to coding and reimbursement issues, including the majority of the Medicare code edits

- Exclusive feature — Exclusive *following* references and Check Additional Character symbol in the indexes. The *following* references help coders locate those alphanumeric codes that are out of sequence in the tabular section.

- Exclusive feature — Exclusive shaded guides in the index that help users easily follow the indent levels for the subterms under a main term

- Illustrations throughout the tabular list and at the back of the book that feature anatomy and terminology included in the ICD-10-CM classification system

- Exclusive feature — Detailed Muscle/Tendon tables that correspond to codes in chapters 13 and 19

- The complete ICD-10-CM Official Guidelines for Coding and Reporting, published by the U.S. Department of Health and Human Services and approved by the cooperating parties (American Health Information Management Association, National Center for Health Statistics, Centers for Medicare and Medicaid Services, American Hospital Association)

- Exclusive feature — Official chapter-specific guidelines with coding examples at the beginning of each chapter

- All the official ICD-10-CM codes, indexes, notes, footnotes, and symbols

- Icons and definitions to differentiate between the two types of Excludes notes

- Check 4th, 5th, 6th, and 7th character symbols that identify codes that require the addition of a 4th, 5th, 6th, or 7th character for code specificity and validity

- Color coding and symbol legend at the bottom of each page

Please review "How to Use *ICD-10-CM: The Complete Official Codebook*" in this section to learn about the features that will help you assign and report correct codes, ensuring appropriate reimbursement.

How to Use ICD-10-CM: The Complete Official Codebook 2018

This International Classification of Diseases, 10th Revision, Clinical Modification (ICD-10-CM) is being published by the United States Government in recognition of its responsibility to promulgate this classification throughout the United States for morbidity coding. This code book represents an adaptation of ICD-10 that was created specifically for use in the United States. Revisions to ICD-10-CM will be made based on the established update process for ICD-10-CM (the ICD-10-CM Coordination and Maintenance Committee) and the World Health Organization's ICD-10 (the Update and Revision Committee).

Use of Official Sources

The *ICD-10-CM: The Complete Official Codebook* contains the official U.S. Department of Health and Human Services, Tenth Revision, Clinical Modification, ICD-10-CM codes, effective for the current year.

Much of the color coding and many of the symbols that identify coding and reimbursement issues are derived from official federal government sources, including the Integrated Outpatient Code Editor (IOCE), version 18.2.

For the most current IOCE documents please refer to the following: https://www.cms.gov/Medicare/Coding/OutpatientCodeEdit/OCEQtrReleaseSpecs.html.

Steps to Correct Coding

1. Before beginning to use this code book, review section I.A., "Conventions for the ICD-10-CM," and section I.B., "General Coding Guidelines," of the ICD-10-CM Official Guidelines for Coding and Reporting.

2. Look up the main term in the alphabetic index and scan the subterm entries as appropriate. Review continued lines and additional subterms that may appear in the next column or on the next page.

3. Note all parenthetical terms (nonessential modifiers) that help in code selection but do not affect code assignment. Shaded vertical guidelines in the index are provided to help determine the indentation level for each subterm in relation to the main terms.

4. Pay close attention to the following instructions in the index:

    – "See," "see also," and "see category" cross-references

    – "With"/"without" notes

    – "Omit code" notes

    – "Due to" subterms

    – Other instructions found in note boxes, such as "code by site"

    – *Following* references and Check Additional Character symbol in the indexes. The *following* references help coders locate those alphanumeric codes that are out of sequence in the tabular section.

5. Do not code from the alphabetic index without verifying the accuracy of the code in the tabular list. Locate the code in the alphanumerically arranged tabular list.

6. To determine the appropriateness of the code selection and proper coding, read all instructional material:

    – "Includes" and both types of "Excludes" notes

    – "Use additional code" and "code first underlying disease" instructions

    – "Code also"

    – 4th, 5th, and 6th character requirements and 7th character extension requirements

    – Age and sex symbols

7. Consult the official ICD-10-CM guidelines, which govern the use of specific codes. These guidelines provide both general and chapter-specific coding guidance.

8. Confirm and assign the correct code.

Organization

This book is organized in the following manner:

Introduction
The introductory material in this book includes the ICD-10-CM Official Preface, the history of ICD-10-CM as well as an overview of the classification system.

Official ICD-10-CM Conventions and Guidelines
This section provides an explanation of the conventions and guidelines regulating the appropriate assignment and reporting of ICD-10-CM codes. This coding guidance is presented by the National Center for Health Statistics (NCHS), a governmental agency of the Centers for Disease Control and Prevention (CDC), within the United States Department of Health and Human Services (DHHS). **Note: The 2018 *ICD-10-CM Official Guidelines for Coding and Reporting* were not available at the time this book went to print. Updated guidelines will be posted at amaproductupdates.org.**

Alphabetic Index to Diseases
The Alphabetic Index to Diseases is arranged in alphabetic order by disease — by specific illness, injury, eponym, abbreviation, or other descriptive diagnostic term. The Index also lists diagnostic terms for other reasons for encounters with health care professionals.

Neoplasm Table
The Neoplasm Table provides the proper code based upon histology of the neoplasm and site.

Table of Drugs and Chemicals
The Table of Drugs and Chemicals lists the drug and the specific codes that identify the drug and the intent. No additional external cause of injury and poisoning code is assigned in ICD-10-CM.

Index to External Causes
The Alphabetic Index to External Causes of Injuries is arranged in alphabetic order by main term indicating the event.

Tabular List of Diseases
ICD-10-CM codes and descriptors are arranged numerically within the tabular list of diseases within 21 separate chapters according to body system or nature of injury and disease. Classifications that were previously considered supplemental to ICD-9-CM (e.g., V codes and E codes) are incorporated into the tabular listing of ICD-10-CM as individual chapters. Chapters 20, "External Causes of Morbidity," and 21, "Factors Influencing Health Status and Contact with Health Services," include chapter-specific guidelines.

Appendixes

The additional resources described below have been included as appendixes for the *ICD-10-CM: The Complete Official Codebook*. These resources further instruct the professional coder on the appropriate application of the ICD-10-CM code set.

Appendix A: 10 Steps to Correct Coding

This step-by-step tutorial walks the coder through the process of locating the correct code in the alphabetic index and verifying it in the tabular section while following applicable conventions and guidelines. Detailed examples are provided and explained along with advice for proper sequencing.

Appendix B: Valid 3-character ICD-10-CM Codes

The user may consult this table to confirm that no further specificity, such as the use of 4th, 5th, 6th, or 7th characters or placeholders (X), is necessary. All ICD-10-CM codes that are valid at the three-character level are listed.

Appendix C: Pharmacology List 2018

This reference is provided to assist in accurate coding of drug classifications for adverse effects and poisonings, in addition to alerting the coder of potential chronic conditions in a patient record by identifying various medications used and their actions. This list is not all-inclusive but discusses many commonly used drugs.

Appendix D: Z Codes for Long-Term Drug Use with Associated Drugs

This resource correlates Z codes that are used to identify current long-term drug use with a list of drugs that are typically categorized to that class of drug.

Note: These tables are not all-inclusive but list some of the more commonly used drugs.

Appendix E: Z Codes Only as Principal/First-Listed Diagnosis

Chapter 21, "Factors Influencing Health Status and Contact with Health Services," provides codes to deal with encounters for circumstances other than a disease or injury. Many of these codes may be reported *only* as the principal/first-listed diagnosis. This resource lists all of these codes in one table for quick and easy reference to ensure accurate reporting.

Appendix F: Centers for Medicare & Medicaid Services Hierarchical Condition Categories (CMS-HCC)

This resource provides the framework behind the Centers for Medicare and Medicaid Services' (CMS) Medicare Advantage (MA) program, a risk-adjustment model developed as a means of compensating health care plans with large numbers of Medicare Part C beneficiaries. It includes a brief synopsis of the evolution of the program from its inception; insight into the various elements needed to predict risk, including the principles used to develop the hierarchical condition categories (HCCs), which make up one of the fundamental components of the risk-adjustment model. This appendix also outlines the audit process used to ensure the accuracy of payments made to MA plans.

Illustrations

This section includes illustrations of normal anatomy with ICD-10-CM specific terminology.

Overview of ICD-10-CM Official Conventions

This is an overview of the ICD-10-CM official conventions, which are general rules for using the classification system, independent of the guidelines. The official conventions and instructions of the classification, which take precedence over the guidelines, are incorporated within the alphabetic index and tabular list as instructional notes and are applicable regardless of the health care setting. For the full version of the official conventions, see the ICD-10-CM Official Guidelines for Coding and Reporting, section I.A., which is included in this book.

Format

ICD-10-CM is divided into two main parts: the index, an alphabetical list of terms and their corresponding code, and the tabular list, a sequential, alphanumeric list of codes divided into chapters based on body system or condition. The index contains the Index to Diseases and Injuries (main index) and the Index to External Causes of Injury. Also included in the main index is the Neoplasm Table and a Table of Drugs and Chemicals.

The tabular list contains categories, subcategories, and valid codes. ICD-10-CM is an alphanumeric classification system. The 1st character of a three-character category is a letter. The 2nd and 3rd characters may be numbers or alpha characters. A three-character category without further subclassification is equivalent to a valid three-character code. Subcategories are either four or five characters. Subcategory characters include either letters or numbers. Codes may be three, four, five, six, or seven characters in length, in which each level of subdivision after a category is a subcategory. The final level of subdivision is a valid code. The final character in a code may be either a letter or a number.

The ICD-10-CM uses the letter "X" as a placeholder. A placeholder "X" is used as a 5th character placeholder at certain six-character codes to allow for future expansion, without disturbing the 6th character structure. For instance, an initial encounter for accidental poisoning by penicillin is coded to T36.0X1A. The "X" in the 5th character position is a placeholder, or filler character.

Similarly, certain categories have applicable 7th character extensions. In these cases, the 7th character extension is required for all codes within the category, or as otherwise instructed in the tabular list notations. 7th character extensions must always be the last character in the data field. If a code is not a full six characters in length, a dummy placeholder "X" must be used to fill in the empty characters when a 7th character extension is required.

Punctuation

[ ]   In the tabular list, brackets are used to enclose synonyms, alternative wording, or explanatory phrases. In the index, brackets are used to identify manifestation codes.

( )   Parentheses are used in both the index and tabular list to enclose nonessential modifiers; supplementary words that may be present or absent in the statement of a disease or procedure without affecting the code number to which it is assigned.

:   Colons are used in the tabular list after an incomplete term that needs one or more of the modifiers following the colon to make it assignable to a given category.

Abbreviations

NEC

The abbreviation NEC, "Not elsewhere classifiable" represents "other specified" in the ICD-10-CM. An index entry that states NEC directs the coder to an "other specified" code in the tabular list. Codes titled "Other"

or "Other specified" in the tabular list (usually a code with a 4th or 6th character 8 and 5th character 9) are for use when the information in the medical record provides detail for which a specific code does not exist.

NOS

The abbreviation NOS, "Not otherwise specified," in the tabular list may be interpreted as "unspecified." Codes in the tabular list with "Unspecified" in the title (usually a code with a 4th or 6th character 9 and 5th character Ø) are for use when the information in the medical record is insufficient to assign a more specific code.

Typeface

Boldface

Boldface type is used for main term entries in the alphabetic index, and all codes and descriptions in the tabular list.

General Notes

The following conventions and notes appear only in the tabular list of diseases:

Includes Notes

The word INCLUDES appears immediately under certain categories to further define, clarify, or give examples of the content of a code category.

Inclusion Terms

Lists of inclusion terms are included under certain codes. These terms indicate some of the conditions for which that code number may be used. Inclusion terms may be synonyms with the code title, or, in the case of "other specified" codes, the terms may also provide a list of various conditions included within a classification code. The inclusion terms are not exhaustive. The index may provide additional terms that may also be assigned to a given code.

Excludes Notes

ICD-10-CM has two types of excludes notes. Each note has a different definition for use. However, they are similar in that they both indicate that codes excluded from each other are independent of each other.

Excludes 1

An EXCLUDES1 note is a "pure" excludes. It means "NOT CODED HERE!" An Excludes 1 note indicates mutually exclusive codes: two conditions that cannot be reported together. For example, a congenital form of a disease may not be reported with the acquired form of the same condition. The code excluded should never be reported with the applicable codes listed above the excludes notation.

An exception to the Excludes 1 definition is when the two conditions are unrelated to each other. If it is not clear whether the two conditions involving an Excludes 1 note are related or not, query the provider. For example, code F45.8 Other somatoform disorders, has an Excludes 1 note for "sleep related teeth grinding (G47.63)" because "teeth grinding" is an inclusion term under F45.8. Only one of these two codes should be assigned for teeth grinding. However psychogenic dysmenorrhea is also an inclusion term under F45.8, and a patient could have both this condition and sleep-related teeth grinding. In this case, the two conditions are clearly unrelated to each other, so it would be appropriate to report F45.8 and G47.63 together.

Excludes 2

An EXCLUDES2 note means "NOT INCLUDED HERE." An Excludes 2 note indicates that although the excluded condition is not part of the condition it is excluded from, a patient may have both conditions at the same time. Therefore, when an Excludes 2 note appears under a code, it may be acceptable to use both the code and the excluded code together if supported by the medical documentation.

Note

NOTE The term "NOTE" appears as an icon and precedes the instructional information. These notes function as alerts to highlight coding instructions within the text.

Default Codes

In the index, the default code is the code listed next to the main term. The default code represents the condition most commonly associated with the main term. This code may be assigned when documentation does not facilitate reporting a more specific code. Alternatively, it may provide an unspecified code for the condition.

Syndromes

Follow the alphabetic index guidance when coding syndromes. In the absence of index guidance, assign codes for the documented manifestations of the syndrome.

And

When the term "and" is used in a narrative statement or code title it may be interpreted as "and/or."

With

The word "with" should be interpreted to mean "associated with" or "due to" when it appears in a code title, the Alphabetic Index, or an instructional note in the Tabular List. The classification presumes a causal relationship between the two conditions linked by these terms in the Alphabetic Index or Tabular List. These conditions should be coded as related even in the absence of provider documentation explicitly linking them, unless the documentation clearly states the conditions are unrelated. For conditions not specifically linked by these relational terms in the classification, provider documentation must link the conditions in order to code them as related. The word "with" in the Alphabetic Index is sequenced immediately following the main term, not in alphabetical order.

See and See Also

When the instruction "See" follows a main term in the alphabetic index, it indicates that another term must be referenced in order to locate the correct code. The instructional note "See also" simply provides alternative terms that may be useful in determining the correct code but is not necessary to follow if the main term supplies the appropriate code.

Instructional Notes Used in the Tabular List

In the tabular section, the following instructional notes appear in red type for emphasis:

Code First/Use additional code:

These instructional notes provide sequencing instruction. They may appear independently of each other or to designate certain etiology/manifestation paired codes. These instructions signal the coder that an additional code should be reported to provide a more complete picture of that diagnosis.

In etiology/manifestation coding, ICD-10-CM requires the underlying condition to be sequenced first, followed by the manifestation. In these situations, codes with "In diseases classified elsewhere" in the code description are never permitted as a first-listed or principal diagnosis code and must be sequenced following the underlying condition code.

Code Also:

A "code also" note alerts the coder that more than one code may be required to fully describe the condition. Code sequencing is discretionary. Factors that may determine sequencing include severity and reason for the encounter.

Code Assignment and Clinical Criteria

Diagnosis code assignment must be based on the provider's diagnostic statement that the condition exists and is not based on clinical criteria the provider used to establish the diagnosis. Conflicting documentation must be queried.

Additional Annotations

Code-Level Notations

The tabular section of ICD-10-CM has various colors, symbols, and other tabular annotations that may help in code selection, provide clinical or coding information, or alert the coder to reimbursement issues affected by the diagnosis code assignment. Some codes may have more than one annotation. For quick reference to the meanings of the colors and symbols, look at the color/symbol legend at the bottom of each page in the tabular list.

Italics

Italicized type is used for all exclusion notes and to identify manifestation codes, those codes that should not be reported as first-listed (principal) diagnoses.

Color Coding/Symbols

New Code

This ● icon identifies the codes that are new to the classification system for the current year. The new code icon is to the left of the code.

Revised Code Title

This ▲ icon to the left of a code alerts the user to a change in that code's title. This change may be as simple as adding or removing punctuation, which may or may not change the intent of the code, to adding or removing specific terms from a code description that completely alter the circumstances in which the code would be used.

Revised Text

The revised text ▶◀ "bow ties" alert the user to changes in parenthetical notes for the current year. Revised text may include the following:

- A change in a current parenthetical description

- A change in the code(s) associated with a current parenthetical note

- A change in how a current parenthetical note is classified (e.g., an Excludes 1 note that changes to an Excludes 2 note)

- Addition of a new parenthetical note(s) to a code

Deleted Text

Strikethrough on code description(s) and/or code note(s) indicates a deletion from the classification for the current year. For example:

☑4ᵗʰ **N25 Disorders resulting from impaired renal tubular function**
      ~~EXCLUDES 1   metabolic disorders classifiable to E70-E88~~

The strikethrough over the Excludes 1 note indicates that this note was deleted from the classification and is no longer applicable to codes in category N25.

☑7ᵗʰ ~~**S63.131 Subluxation of proximal interphalangeal joint of right thumb**~~

The strikethrough over the code and the code description indicates that all codes in subcategory S63.131 (S63.131A, S63.131D, and S63.131S) have been deleted from the classification.

Additional Characters Required

☑4ᵗʰ This symbol indicates that the code requires a 4th character.

☑5ᵗʰ This symbol indicates that the code requires a 5th character.

☑6ᵗʰ This symbol indicates that the code requires a 6th character.

☑7ᵗʰ This symbol indicates that the code requires a 7th character.

☑x7ᵗʰ This symbol indicates that the code requires a 7th character following the placeholder "X." Codes with fewer than six characters that require a 7th character must contain placeholder "X" to fill in the empty character(s).

Key Word

Green font is used throughout the Tabular List of Diseases to differentiate the key words that appear in similar code descriptions in a given category or subcategory.

For example, refer to the list of codes below from category C7A:

C7A.020   Malignant carcinoid tumor of the **appendix**

C7A.021   Malignant carcinoid tumor of the **cecum**

C7A.022   Malignant carcinoid tumor of the **ascending colon**

C7A.023   Malignant carcinoid tumor of the **transverse colon**

C7A.024   Malignant carcinoid tumor of the **descending colon**

C7A.025   Malignant carcinoid tumor of the **sigmoid colon**

C7A.026   Malignant carcinoid tumor of the **rectum**

C7A.029   Malignant carcinoid tumor of the large intestine, unspecified portion

The portion of the code description that appears in **green font** in the tabular list assists the coder in quickly identifying the key terms and in identifying the correct code. This convention is especially useful when the codes describe laterality, such as the following codes from subcategory H40.22:

H40.221   Chronic angle-closure glaucoma, **right** eye

H40.222   Chronic angle-closure glaucoma, **left** eye

H40.223   Chronic angle-closure glaucoma, **bilateral**

H40.229   Chronic angle-closure glaucoma, unspecified eye

The key word convention is used only in those categories in which there are multiple codes with very similar descriptions with only a few words that differentiate them.

Medicare Code Edits

Medicare Administrative Contractors and many payers use Medicare code edits to check the coding accuracy on claims. The coding edit information in this manual reflects those edits used for outpatient institutional providers, which also include hospitals that are subject to the outpatient prospective payment system (OPPS). These edits have been updated to reflect changes in the Integrated Outpatient Code Editor (IOCE), version 18.2.

Manifestation Code

These codes appear in italic type, with a ***blue color bar*** over the title. A manifestation code cannot be reported as a first-listed or principal diagnosis. By definition, a manifestation code represents a demonstration of some aspect of an underlying disease, which is separately classifiable. In the alphabetic index, these codes are listed as the secondary code in brackets. The underlying disease code is listed first.

Age and Sex Edit

The age and sex edits below are used to detect inconsistencies between the patient's age and/or sex and the patient's diagnosis. The following edit symbols appear in the tabular list to the right of the code description.

Newborn Age: 0   N

These diagnoses are intended for newborns and neonates and the patient's age must be 0 years.

Pediatric Age: 0-17   P

> These diagnoses are intended for children and the patient's age must be between 0 and 17 years.

Maternity Age: 12-55   M

> These diagnoses are intended for childbearing patients between the age of 12 and 55 years.

Adult Age: 15-124   A

> These diagnoses are intended for patients between the age of 15 and 124 years.

Male diagnosis only   ♂

Female diagnosis only   ♀

Medicare Advantage Risk Adjustment Edits

Medicare Advantage plans provided as part of the Medicare Part C program use a risk-adjustment model to plan for future healthcare costs of Medicare Part C participants. The risk-adjustment model measures disease burden by assigning certain ICD-10-CM diagnosis codes to hierarchical condition categories (HCC). The HCC information in this manual has been updated to reflect the CMS-HCC model category for v22 of the CMS-HCC risk-adjustment software.

HCC   HCC

This symbol indicates that the condition is considered a CMS-HCC diagnosis. All HCC conditions that are appropriately documented are used in the risk-adjustment model for Medicare Advantage to provide a means of comparing quality of care across Medicare Part C participants as well as predict future healthcare costs.

The HCC icon appears to the right of the code description.

Other Code-Level Notations

Unspecified Code   ▽

Use these codes when neither the diagnostic statement nor the documentation provides enough information to assign a more specific diagnosis code. These codes may be stated as "Unspecified" or "Not otherwise specified (NOS)."

Note: Do not assign these codes when a more specific diagnosis has been determined.

PDx Symbol   PDx

This symbol identifies a Z code that generally is for use as a first-listed (or principal) diagnosis only but may be used as an additional diagnosis if the patient has more than one encounter on the same day or there is more than one reason for the encounter.

The instructions for Z code use contained in the ICD-10-CM official coding guidelines identify those Z codes that can be used only as a PDx. All other Z codes may either be SDx or PDx, depending upon circumstances of the encounter, by meeting the definition of first-listed or principal diagnosis, and by following any specific Z code guidelines in section I.C.21 a-c. The responsibility of those assigning the Z codes as PDx is to make sure the circumstances of the encounter meet the definition of first-listed or principal diagnosis, follow all coding instructions, and follow the Z code specific guidelines. Optum360 does not include any SDx edit since there is no official source for it and the Z code use is determined by circumstances of the encounter.

Note: Please note that the symbols indicating the Z code "principal or first-listed only" designation and the Z codes that may be principal or first-listed diagnoses included in the official coding guidelines [section I.C.21.c.16] are consistent with reporting guidelines for health care encounters *excluding acute care inpatient admissions.* These Z code edits are often in conflict with the inpatient prospective payment system (IPPS) edits. For example, code Z34.90 Encounter for supervision of normal pregnancy, unspecified, unspecified trimester, may be an appropriate primary reason for an outpatient encounter. However, supervision for a normal pregnancy is not an acceptable principal diagnosis or reason for an inpatient admission and will have an unacceptable principal diagnosis edit under the inpatient prospective payment system (IPPS).

AHA:

This symbol precedes official citations from AHA's *Coding Clinic for ICD-10-CM/PCS.* Similar to the parenthetical notes, AHA references are placed in a hierarchical pattern at the chapter, code block, category, subcategory, or valid code level. This means that the information found in the reference applies to one or more codes depending on where the citation is placed.

The citations appear in purple type and are listed with the most current citation first. *Coding Clinic* citations included in this edition have been updated through second quarter 2017.

DEF:

This symbol precedes a definition of a condition or disease.

The definition appears in purple type directly under the code.

TIP:

This symbol precedes coding advice that is not readily available within the tabular section of ICD-10-CM. It may relate official coding guidelines, indexing nuances, or advice garnered from AHA's *Coding Clinic for ICD-10-CM/PCS.*

The tip appears in purple type directly under the code.

Footnotes

All footnotes are identified by a numerical superscript that appears to the upper left of the code. For example:

> [1] ✓x 7ᵗʰ **M48.50 Collapsed vertebra, not elsewhere classified,** HCC
> **site unspecified**

The footnote 1 indicates "HCC with 7th character indicating initial encounter." This means that a collapsed vertebra would be considered an HCC only when the 7th character represents an initial encounter, such as 7th character A, B, or C, depending on the category.

The following list identifies the meaning of each footnote number in the Tabular List of Diseases:

1   These codes are considered an HCC when reported with a 7th character indicating an initial encounter (7th character A, B, or C).

2   These codes are considered an HCC when reported with a 7th character indicating an initial encounter (7th character A or B) OR sequela.

3   These codes are considered an HCC when reported with a 7th character indicating sequela.

Chapter-Level Notations

Chapter-Specific Guidelines with Coding Examples

Each chapter begins with the Official Guidelines for Coding and Reporting specific to that chapter, where provided. Coding examples illustrate the coding and/or sequencing guidance in these guidelines.

Muscle and Tendon Table

ICD-10-CM categorizes certain muscles and tendons in the upper and lower extremities by their action (e.g., extension or flexion) as well as their anatomical location. The Muscle/Tendon table is provided at the beginning of chapter 13 and chapter 19 to help users when code selection depends on the action of the muscle and/or tendon.

Note: This table is not all-inclusive, and proper code assignment should be based on the provider's documentation.

Index Notations

▽ Subterms under main terms may continue to next column or page. This warning statement is a reminder to always check for additional subterms and information that may continue onto the next page or column before making a final selection.

Following References

The index includes *following* references to assist in locating "out-of-sequence" codes in the tabular list. "Out-of-sequence" codes contain an alphabetic character (letter) in the 3rd or 4th character position. These codes are placed according to the classification rules — the placement of the codes according to condition — not according to alphabetic or numeric sequencing rules.

Examples:

Carcinoma (malignant) (*see also,* Neoplasm, by site, malignant)
    neuroendocrine (*see also* Tumor, neuroendocrine)
        high grade, any site C7A.1 (*following* C75)
        poorly differentiated, any site C7A.1 (*following* C75)

In the tabular rubric, C7A is included after rubric C75 and before C76.

Gout, chronic (*see also* Gout, gouty) M1A.9
    drug-induced M1A.20 (*following* M08)
        ankle M1A.27-(*following* M08)
        elbow M1A.22-(*following* M08)

In the tabular rubric, M1A is included after rubric M08 and before M10.

ICD-10-CM Official Guidelines for Coding and Reporting

Note: The 2017 *ICD-10-CM Official Guidelines for Coding and Reporting* have been included as the 2018 guidelines were not available at the time of printing. As soon as the 2018 guidelines become available a downloadable PDF version will be posted to our website. You will also receive a booklet containing the updated 2018 ICD-10-CM guidelines in a separate shipment.

Narrative changes appear in **bold** text

Items underlined have been moved within the guidelines since the FY 2017 version

Italics are used to indicate revisions to heading changes

The Centers for Medicare and Medicaid Services (CMS) and the National Center for Health Statistics (NCHS), two departments within the U.S. Federal Government's Department of Health and Human Services (DHHS) provide the following guidelines for coding and reporting using the International Classification of Diseases, 10th Revision, Clinical Modification (ICD-10-CM). These guidelines should be used as a companion document to the official version of the ICD-10-CM as published on the NCHS website. The ICD-10-CM is a morbidity classification published by the United States for classifying diagnoses and reason for visits in all health care settings. The ICD-10-CM is based on the ICD-10, the statistical classification of disease published by the World Health Organization (WHO).

These guidelines have been approved by the four organizations that make up the Cooperating Parties for the ICD-10-CM: the American Hospital Association (AHA), the American Health Information Management Association (AHIMA), CMS, and NCHS.

These guidelines are a set of rules that have been developed to accompany and complement the official conventions and instructions provided within the ICD-10-CM itself. The instructions and conventions of the classification take precedence over guidelines. These guidelines are based on the coding and sequencing instructions in the Tabular List and Alphabetic Index of ICD-10-CM, but provide additional instruction. Adherence to these guidelines when assigning ICD-10-CM diagnosis codes is required under the Health Insurance Portability and Accountability Act (HIPAA). The diagnosis codes (Tabular List and Alphabetic Index) have been adopted under HIPAA for all healthcare settings. A joint effort between the healthcare provider and the coder is essential to achieve complete and accurate documentation, code assignment, and reporting of diagnoses and procedures. These guidelines have been developed to assist both the healthcare provider and the coder in identifying those diagnoses that are to be reported. The importance of consistent, complete documentation in the medical record cannot be overemphasized. Without such documentation accurate coding cannot be achieved. The entire record should be reviewed to determine the specific reason for the encounter and the conditions treated.

The term encounter is used for all settings, including hospital admissions. In the context of these guidelines, the term provider is used throughout the guidelines to mean physician or any qualified health care practitioner who is legally accountable for establishing the patient's diagnosis. Only this set of guidelines, approved by the Cooperating Parties, is official.

The guidelines are organized into sections. Section I includes the structure and conventions of the classification and general guidelines that apply to the entire classification, and chapter-specific guidelines that correspond to the chapters as they are arranged in the classification. Section II includes guidelines for selection of principal diagnosis for non-outpatient settings. Section III includes guidelines for reporting additional diagnoses in non-outpatient settings. Section IV is for outpatient coding and reporting. It is necessary to review all sections of the guidelines to fully understand all of the rules and instructions needed to code properly.

Section I. Conventions, general coding guidelines and chapter specific guidelines 3

A. Conventions for the ICD-10-CM 3
  1. The Alphabetic Index and Tabular List 3
  2. Format and Structure: 3
  3. Use of codes for reporting purposes 3
  4. Placeholder character 3
  5. 7th Characters 3
  6. Abbreviations 3
    a. Alphabetic Index abbreviations 3
    b. Tabular List abbreviations 3
  7. Punctuation 3
  8. Use of "and". 3
  9. Other and Unspecified codes 3
    a. "Other" codes 3
    b. "Unspecified" codes 3
  10. Includes Notes 3
  11. Inclusion terms 3
  12. Excludes Notes 4
    a. Excludes1 4
    b. Excludes2 4
  13. Etiology/manifestation convention ("code first", "use additional code" and "in diseases classified elsewhere" notes) 4
  14. "And" 4
  15. "With" 4
  16. "See" and "See Also" 4
  17. "Code also" note 4
  18. Default codes 4
  19. Code assignment and Clinical Criteria 4

B. General Coding Guidelines 4
  1. Locating a code in the ICD-10-CM 4
  2. Level of Detail in Coding 4
  3. Code or codes from A00.0 through T88.9, Z00-Z99.8 5
  4. Signs and symptoms 5
  5. Conditions that are an integral part of a disease process 5
  6. Conditions that are not an integral part of a disease process 5
  7. Multiple coding for a single condition 5
  8. Acute and Chronic Conditions 5
  9. Combination Code 5
  10. Sequela (Late Effects) 5
  11. Impending or Threatened Condition 5
  12. Reporting Same Diagnosis Code More than Once 5
  13. Laterality 5
  14. Documentation for BMI, Depth of Non-pressure ulcers, Pressure Ulcer Stages, Coma Scale, and NIH Stroke Scale 6
  15. Syndromes 6
  16. Documentation of Complications of Care 6
  17. Borderline Diagnosis 6
  18. Use of Sign/Symptom/Unspecified Codes 6

C. Chapter Specific Coding Guidelines 6
  1. Chapter 1: Certain Infectious and Parasitic Diseases (A00-B99) 6
    a. Human Immunodeficiency Virus (HIV) Infections 6
    b. Infectious agents as the cause of diseases classified to other chapters 7
    c. Infections resistant to antibiotics 7
    d. Sepsis, Severe Sepsis, and Septic Shock 7
    e. Methicillin Resistant *Staphylococcus aureus* (MRSA) Conditions 8
    f. Zika virus infections 8
  2. Chapter 2: Neoplasms (C00-D49) 9
    a. Treatment directed at the malignancy 9
    b. Treatment of secondary site 9
    c. Coding and sequencing of complications 9
    d. Primary malignancy previously excised 9
    e. Admissions/Encounters involving chemotherapy, immunotherapy and radiation therapy 9
    f. Admission/encounter to determine extent of malignancy 10
    g. Symptoms, signs, and abnormal findings listed in Chapter 18 associated with neoplasms 10
    h. Admission/encounter for pain control/management 10
    i. Malignancy in two or more noncontiguous sites 10
    j. Disseminated malignant neoplasm, unspecified 10
    k. Malignant neoplasm without specification of site 10
    l. Sequencing of neoplasm codes 10
    m. Current malignancy versus personal history of malignancy 10
    n. Leukemia, Multiple Myeloma, and Malignant Plasma Cell Neoplasms in remission versus personal history 10
    o. Aftercare following surgery for neoplasm 10
    p. Follow-up care for completed treatment of a malignancy 10
    q. Prophylactic organ removal for prevention of malignancy 10
    r. Malignant neoplasm associated with transplanted organ 10
  3. Chapter 3: Disease of the blood and blood-forming organs and certain disorders involving the immune mechanism (D50-D89) 10
  4. Chapter 4: Endocrine, Nutritional, and Metabolic Diseases (E00-E89) 11
    a. Diabetes mellitus 11

5. Chapter 5: Mental, Behavioral and Neurodevelopmental disorders (F01-F99) 11
   a. Pain disorders related to psychological factors 11
   b. Mental and behavioral disorders due to psychoactive substance use 11
6. Chapter 6: Diseases of the Nervous System (G00-G99) 12
   a. Dominant/nondominant side 12
   b. Pain - Category G89 12
7. Chapter 7: Diseases of the Eye and Adnexa (H00-H59) 13
   a. Glaucoma 13
8. Chapter 8: Diseases of the Ear and Mastoid Process (H60-H95) 13
9. Chapter 9: Diseases of the Circulatory System (I00-I99) 13
   a. Hypertension 13
   b. Atherosclerotic Coronary Artery Disease and Angina 14
   c. Intraoperative and Postprocedural Cerebrovascular Accident 14
   d. Sequelae of Cerebrovascular Disease 14
   e. Acute myocardial infarction (AMI) 14
10. Chapter 10: Diseases of the Respiratory System (J00-J99) 14
   a. Chronic Obstructive Pulmonary Disease [COPD] and Asthma 14
   b. Acute Respiratory Failure 15
   c. Influenza due to certain identified influenza viruses 15
   d. Ventilator associated Pneumonia 15
11. Chapter 11: Diseases of the Digestive System (K00-K95) 15
12. Chapter 12: Diseases of the Skin and Subcutaneous Tissue (L00-L99) 15
   a. Pressure ulcer stage codes 15
13. Chapter 13: Diseases of the Musculoskeletal System and Connective Tissue (M00-M99) 16
   a. Site and laterality 16
   b. Acute traumatic versus chronic or recurrent musculoskeletal conditions 16
   c. Coding of Pathologic Fractures 16
   d. Osteoporosis 16
14. Chapter 14: Diseases of Genitourinary System (N00-N99) 16
   a. Chronic kidney disease 16
15. Chapter 15: Pregnancy, Childbirth, and the Puerperium (O00-O9A) 16
   a. General Rules for Obstetric Cases 16
   b. Selection of OB Principal or First-listed Diagnosis 17
   c. Pre-existing conditions versus conditions due to the pregnancy 17
   d. Pre-existing hypertension in pregnancy 17
   e. Fetal Conditions Affecting the Management of the Mother 17
   f. HIV Infection in Pregnancy, Childbirth and the Puerperium 18
   g. Diabetes mellitus in pregnancy 18
   h. Long term use of insulin and oral hypoglycemics 18
   i. Gestational (pregnancy induced) diabetes 18
   j. Sepsis and septic shock complicating abortion, pregnancy, childbirth and the puerperium 18
   k. Puerperal sepsis 18
   l. Alcohol and tobacco use during pregnancy, childbirth and the puerperium 18
   m. Poisoning, toxic effects, adverse effects and underdosing in a pregnant patient 18
   n. Normal Delivery, Code O80 18
   o. The Peripartum and Postpartum Periods 18
   p. Code O94, Sequelae of complication of pregnancy, childbirth, and the puerperium 19
   q. *Termination of Pregnancy and Spontaneous abortions* 19
   r. Abuse in a pregnant patient 19
16. Chapter 16: Certain Conditions Originating in the Perinatal Period (P00-P96) 19
   a. General Perinatal Rules 19
   b. Observation and Evaluation of Newborns for Suspected Conditions not Found 19
   c. Coding Additional Perinatal Diagnoses 20
   d. Prematurity and Fetal Growth Retardation 20
   e. Low birth weight and immaturity status 20
   f. Bacterial Sepsis of Newborn 20
   g. Stillbirth 20
17. Chapter 17: Congenital malformations, deformations, and chromosomal abnormalities (Q00-Q99) 20

18. Chapter 18: Symptoms, signs, and abnormal clinical and laboratory findings, not elsewhere classified (R00-R99) 20
   a. Use of symptom codes 20
   b. Use of a symptom code with a definitive diagnosis code 20
   c. Combination codes that include symptoms 20
   d. Repeated falls 20
   e. Coma scale 20
   f. Functional quadriplegia 20
   g. SIRS due to Non-Infectious Process 21
   h. Death NOS 21
   i. NIHSS Stroke Scale 21
19. Chapter 19: Injury, poisoning, and certain other consequences of external causes (S00-T88) 21
   a. Application of 7th Characters in Chapter 19 21
   b. Coding of Injuries 21
   c. Coding of Traumatic Fractures 21
   d. Coding of Burns and Corrosions 22
   e. Adverse Effects, Poisoning, Underdosing and Toxic Effects 22
   f. Adult and child abuse, neglect and other maltreatment 23
   g. Complications of care 23
20. Chapter 20: External Causes of Morbidity (V00-Y99) 24
   a. General External Cause Coding Guidelines 24
   b. Place of Occurrence Guideline 24
   c. Activity Code 24
   d. Place of Occurrence, Activity, and Status Codes Used with other External Cause Code 24
   e. If the Reporting Format Limits the Number of External Cause Codes 24
   f. Multiple External Cause Coding Guidelines 24
   g. Child and Adult Abuse Guideline 25
   h. Unknown or Undetermined Intent Guideline 25
   i. Sequelae (Late Effects) of External Cause Guidelines 25
   j. Terrorism Guidelines 25
   k. External cause status 25
21. Chapter 21: Factors influencing health status and contact with health services (Z00-Z99) 25
   a. Use of Z codes in any healthcare setting 25
   b. Z Codes indicate a reason for an encounter 25
   c. Categories of Z Codes 25

Section II. Selection of Principal Diagnosis **30**
  A. Codes for symptoms, signs, and ill-defined conditions 30
  B. Two or more interrelated conditions, each potentially meeting the definition for principal diagnosis. 30
  C. Two or more diagnoses that equally meet the definition for principal diagnosis 31
  D. Two or more comparative or contrasting conditions 31
  E. A symptom(s) followed by contrasting/comparative diagnoses 31
  F. Original treatment plan not carried out 31
  G. Complications of surgery and other medical care 31
  H. Uncertain Diagnosis 31
  I. Admission from Observation Unit 31
    1. Admission Following Medical Observation 31
    2. Admission Following Post-Operative Observation 31
  J. Admission from Outpatient Surgery 31
  K. Admissions/Encounters for Rehabilitation 31

Section III. Reporting Additional Diagnoses **31**
  A. Previous conditions 31
  B. Abnormal findings 31
  C. Uncertain Diagnosis 32

Section IV. Diagnostic Coding and Reporting Guidelines for Outpatient Services **32**
  A. Selection of first-listed condition 32
    1. Outpatient Surgery 32
    2. Observation Stay 32
  B. Codes from A00.0 through T88.9, Z00-Z99 32
  C. Accurate reporting of ICD-10-CM diagnosis codes 32
  D. Codes that describe symptoms and signs 32
  E. Encounters for circumstances other than a disease or injury 32
  F. Level of Detail in Coding 32
    1. ICD-10-CM codes with 3, 4, 5, 6 or 7 characters 32
    2. Use of full number of characters required for a code 32

G. ICD-10-CM code for the diagnosis, condition, problem, or other reason for encounter/visit 32
H. Uncertain diagnosis 32
I. Chronic diseases 32
J. Code all documented conditions that coexist 32
K. Patients receiving diagnostic services only 33
L. Patients receiving therapeutic services only 33
M. Patients receiving preoperative evaluations only 33
N. Ambulatory surgery 33
O. Routine outpatient prenatal visits 33
P. Encounters for general medical examinations with abnormal findings.. 33
Q. Encounters for routine health screenings............................ 33

Appendix I. Present on Admission Reporting Guidelines 33

Section I. Conventions, general coding guidelines and chapter specific guidelines

The conventions, general guidelines and chapter-specific guidelines are applicable to all health care settings unless otherwise indicated. The conventions and instructions of the classification take precedence over guidelines.

A. Conventions for the ICD-10-CM

The conventions for the ICD-10-CM are the general rules for use of the classification independent of the guidelines. These conventions are incorporated within the Alphabetic Index and Tabular List of the ICD-10-CM as instructional notes.

1. **The Alphabetic Index and Tabular List**
   The ICD-10-CM is divided into the Alphabetic Index, an alphabetical list of terms and their corresponding code, and the Tabular List, a structured list of codes divided into chapters based on body system or condition. The Alphabetic Index consists of the following parts: the Index of Diseases and Injury, the Index of External Causes of Injury, the Table of Neoplasms and the Table of Drugs and Chemicals.

   See Section I.C2. General guidelines

   See Section I.C.19. Adverse effects, poisoning, underdosing and toxic effects

2. **Format and Structure:**
   The ICD-10-CM Tabular List contains categories, subcategories and codes. Characters for categories, subcategories and codes may be either a letter or a number. All categories are 3 characters. A three-character category that has no further subdivision is equivalent to a code. Subcategories are either 4 or 5 characters. Codes may be 3, 4, 5, 6 or 7 characters. That is, each level of subdivision after a category is a subcategory. The final level of subdivision is a code. Codes that have applicable 7th characters are still referred to as codes, not subcategories. A code that has an applicable 7th character is considered invalid without the 7th character.

   The ICD-10-CM uses an indented format for ease in reference.

3. **Use of codes for reporting purposes**
   For reporting purposes only codes are permissible, not categories or subcategories, and any applicable 7th character is required.

4. **Placeholder character**
   The ICD-10-CM utilizes a placeholder character "X". The "X" is used as a placeholder at certain codes to allow for future expansion. An example of this is at the poisoning, adverse effect and underdosing codes, categories T36-T50.

   Where a placeholder exists, the X must be used in order for the code to be considered a valid code.

5. **7th Characters**
   Certain ICD-10-CM categories have applicable 7th characters. The applicable 7th character is required for all codes within the category, or as the notes in the Tabular List instruct. The 7th character must always be the 7th character in the data field. If a code that requires a 7th character is not 6 characters, a placeholder X must be used to fill in the empty characters.

6. **Abbreviations**
   a. **Alphabetic Index abbreviations**
      NEC   "Not elsewhere classifiable"

This abbreviation in the Alphabetic Index represents "other specified." When a specific code is not available for a condition, the Alphabetic Index directs the coder to the "other specified" code in the Tabular List.

      NOS   "Not otherwise specified"
This abbreviation is the equivalent of unspecified.

   b. **Tabular List abbreviations**
      NEC   "Not elsewhere classifiable"
This abbreviation in the Tabular List represents "other specified". When a specific code is not available for a condition, the Tabular List includes an NEC entry under a code to identify the code as the "other specified" code.

      NOS   "Not otherwise specified"
This abbreviation is the equivalent of unspecified.

7. **Punctuation**
   [ ]   Brackets are used in the Tabular List to enclose synonyms, alternative wording or explanatory phrases. Brackets are used in the Alphabetic Index to identify manifestation codes.

   ( )   Parentheses are used in both the Alphabetic Index and Tabular List to enclose supplementary words that may be present or absent in the statement of a disease or procedure without affecting the code number to which it is assigned. The terms within the parentheses are referred to as nonessential modifiers. The nonessential modifiers in the Alphabetic Index to Diseases apply to subterms following a main term except when a nonessential modifier and a subentry are mutually exclusive, the subentry takes precedence. For example, in the ICD-10-CM Alphabetic Index under the main term Enteritis, "acute" is a nonessential modifier and "chronic" is a subentry. In this case, the nonessential modifier "acute" does not apply to the subentry "chronic".

   :   Colons are used in the Tabular List after an incomplete term which needs one or more of the modifiers following the colon to make it assignable to a given category.

8. **Use of "and".**
   See Section I.A.14. Use of the term "And"

9. **Other and Unspecified codes**
   a. **"Other" codes**
      Codes titled "other" or "other specified" are for use when the information in the medical record provides detail for which a specific code does not exist. Alphabetic Index entries with NEC in the line designate "other" codes in the Tabular List. These Alphabetic Index entries represent specific disease entities for which no specific code exists so the term is included within an "other" code.

   b. **"Unspecified" codes**
      Codes titled "unspecified" are for use when the information in the medical record is insufficient to assign a more specific code. For those categories for which an unspecified code is not provided, the "other specified" code may represent both other and unspecified.

      See Section I.B.18 Use of Signs/Symptom/Unspecified Codes

10. **Includes Notes**
    This note appears immediately under a three character code title to further define, or give examples of, the content of the category.

11. **Inclusion terms**
    List of terms is included under some codes. These terms are the conditions for which that code is to be used. The terms may be synonyms of the code title, or, in the case of "other specified" codes, the terms are a list of the various conditions assigned to that code. The inclusion terms are not necessarily exhaustive. Additional terms found only in the Alphabetic Index may also be assigned to a code.

12. **Excludes Notes**
    The ICD-10-CM has two types of excludes notes. Each type of note has a different definition for use but they are all similar in that they indicate that codes excluded from each other are independent of each other.

    a. **Excludes1**
       A type 1 Excludes note is a pure excludes note. It means "NOT CODED HERE!" An Excludes1 note indicates that the code excluded should never be used at the same time as the code above the Excludes1 note. An Excludes1 is used when two conditions cannot occur together, such as a congenital form versus an acquired form of the same condition.

An exception to the Excludes1 definition is the circumstance when the two conditions are unrelated to each other. If it is not clear whether the two conditions involving an Excludes1 note are related or not, query the provider. For example, code F45.8, Other somatoform disorders, has an Excludes1 note for "sleep related teeth grinding (G47.63)," because "teeth grinding" is an inclusion term under F45.8. Only one of these two codes should be assigned for teeth grinding. However psychogenic dysmenorrhea is also an inclusion term under F45.8, and a patient could have both this condition and sleep related teeth grinding. In this case, the two conditions are clearly unrelated to each other, and so it would be appropriate to report F45.8 and G47.63 together.

b.   Excludes2

A type 2 Excludes note represents "Not included here." An excludes2 note indicates that the condition excluded is not part of the condition represented by the code, but a patient may have both conditions at the same time. When an Excludes2 note appears under a code, it is acceptable to use both the code and the excluded code together, when appropriate.

13. Etiology/manifestation convention ("code first", "use additional code" and "in diseases classified elsewhere" notes)

Certain conditions have both an underlying etiology and multiple body system manifestations due to the underlying etiology. For such conditions, the ICD-10-CM has a coding convention that requires the underlying condition be sequenced first, if applicable, followed by the manifestation. Wherever such a combination exists, there is a "use additional code" note at the etiology code, and a "code first" note at the manifestation code. These instructional notes indicate the proper sequencing order of the codes, etiology followed by manifestation.

In most cases the manifestation codes will have in the code title, "in diseases classified elsewhere." Codes with this title are a component of the etiology/ manifestation convention. The code title indicates that it is a manifestation code. "In diseases classified elsewhere" codes are never permitted to be used as first-listed or principal diagnosis codes. They must be used in conjunction with an underlying condition code and they must be listed following the underlying condition. See category F02, Dementia in other diseases classified elsewhere, for an example of this convention.

There are manifestation codes that do not have "in diseases classified elsewhere" in the title. For such codes, there is a "use additional code" note at the etiology code and a "code first" note at the manifestation code, and the rules for sequencing apply.

In addition to the notes in the Tabular List, these conditions also have a specific Alphabetic Index entry structure. In the Alphabetic Index both conditions are listed together with the etiology code first followed by the manifestation codes in brackets. The code in brackets is always to be sequenced second.

An example of the etiology/manifestation convention is dementia in Parkinson's disease. In the Alphabetic Index, code G20 is listed first, followed by code F02.80 or F02.81 in brackets. Code G20 represents the underlying etiology, Parkinson's disease, and must be sequenced first, whereas codes F02.80 and F02.81 represent the manifestation of dementia in diseases classified elsewhere, with or without behavioral disturbance.

"Code first" and "Use additional code" notes are also used as sequencing rules in the classification for certain codes that are not part of an etiology/ manifestation combination.

See Section I.B.7. Multiple coding for a single condition.

14. "And"

The word "and" should be interpreted to mean either "and" or "or" when it appears in a title.

For example, cases of "tuberculosis of bones", "tuberculosis of joints" and "tuberculosis of bones and joints" are classified to subcategory A18.0, Tuberculosis of bones and joints.

15. "With"

The word "with" should be interpreted to mean "associated with" or "due to" when it appears in a code title, the Alphabetic Index, or an instructional note in the Tabular List. The classification presumes a causal relationship between the two conditions linked by these terms in the Alphabetic Index or Tabular List. These conditions should be coded as related even in the absence of provider documentation explicitly linking

them, unless the documentation clearly states the conditions are unrelated. For conditions not specifically linked by these relational terms in the classification, provider documentation must link the conditions in order to code them as related. The word "with" in the Alphabetic Index is sequenced immediately following the main term, not in alphabetical order.

16. "See" and "See Also"

The "see" instruction following a main term in the Alphabetic Index indicates that another term should be referenced. It is necessary to go to the main term referenced with the "see" note to locate the correct code.

A "see also" instruction following a main term in the Alphabetic Index instructs that there is another main term that may also be referenced that may provide additional Alphabetic Index entries that may be useful. It is not necessary to follow the "see also" note when the original main term provides the necessary code.

17. "Code also" note

A "code also" note instructs that two codes may be required to fully describe a condition, but this note does not provide sequencing direction.

18. Default codes

A code listed next to a main term in the ICD-10-CM Alphabetic Index is referred to as a default code. The default code represents that condition that is most commonly associated with the main term, or is the unspecified code for the condition. If a condition is documented in a medical record (for example, appendicitis) without any additional information, such as acute or chronic, the default code should be assigned.

19. Code assignment and Clinical Criteria

The assignment of a diagnosis code is based on the provider's diagnostic statement that the condition exists. The provider's statement that the patient has a particular condition is sufficient. Code assignment is not based on clinical criteria used by the provider to establish the diagnosis.

B. General Coding Guidelines

1.   Locating a code in the ICD-10-CM

To select a code in the classification that corresponds to a diagnosis or reason for visit documented in a medical record, first locate the term in the Alphabetic Index, and then verify the code in the Tabular List. Read and be guided by instructional notations that appear in both the Alphabetic Index and the Tabular List.

It is essential to use both the Alphabetic Index and Tabular List when locating and assigning a code. The Alphabetic Index does not always provide the full code. Selection of the full code, including laterality and any applicable 7th character can only be done in the Tabular List. A dash (-) at the end of an Alphabetic Index entry indicates that additional characters are required. Even if a dash is not included at the Alphabetic Index entry, it is necessary to refer to the Tabular List to verify that no 7th character is required.

2.   Level of Detail in Coding

Diagnosis codes are to be used and reported at their highest number of characters available.

ICD-10-CM diagnosis codes are composed of codes with 3, 4, 5, 6 or 7 characters. Codes with three characters are included in ICD-10-CM as the heading of a category of codes that may be further subdivided by the use of fourth and/or fifth characters and/or sixth characters, which provide greater detail.

A three-character code is to be used only if it is not further subdivided. A code is invalid if it has not been coded to the full number of characters required for that code, including the 7th character, if applicable.

3.   Code or codes from A00.0 through T88.9, Z00-Z99.8

The appropriate code or codes from A00.0 through T88.9, Z00-Z99.8 must be used to identify diagnoses, symptoms, conditions, problems, complaints or other reason(s) for the encounter/visit.

4.   Signs and symptoms

Codes that describe symptoms and signs, as opposed to diagnoses, are acceptable for reporting purposes when a related definitive diagnosis has not been established (confirmed) by the provider. Chapter 18 of ICD-10-CM, Symptoms, Signs, and Abnormal Clinical and Laboratory Findings, Not Elsewhere Classified (codes R00.0 - R99) contains many, but not all, codes for symptoms.

See Section I.B.18 Use of Signs/Symptom/Unspecified Codes

5. Conditions that are an integral part of a disease process
Signs and symptoms that are associated routinely with a disease process should not be assigned as additional codes, unless otherwise instructed by the classification.

6. Conditions that are not an integral part of a disease process
Additional signs and symptoms that may not be associated routinely with a disease process should be coded when present.

7. Multiple coding for a single condition
In addition to the etiology/manifestation convention that requires two codes to fully describe a single condition that affects multiple body systems, there are other single conditions that also require more than one code. "Use additional code" notes are found in the Tabular List at codes that are not part of an etiology/manifestation pair where a secondary code is useful to fully describe a condition. The sequencing rule is the same as the etiology/manifestation pair, "use additional code" indicates that a secondary code should be added.

For example, for bacterial infections that are not included in chapter 1, a secondary code from category B95, Streptococcus, Staphylococcus, and Enterococcus, as the cause of diseases classified elsewhere, or B96, Other bacterial agents as the cause of diseases classified elsewhere, may be required to identify the bacterial organism causing the infection. A "use additional code" note will normally be found at the infectious disease code, indicating a need for the organism code to be added as a secondary code.

"Code first" notes are also under certain codes that are not specifically manifestation codes but may be due to an underlying cause. When there is a "code first" note and an underlying condition is present, the underlying condition should be sequenced first.

"Code, if applicable, any causal condition first" notes indicate that this code may be assigned as a principal diagnosis when the causal condition is unknown or not applicable. If a causal condition is known, then the code for that condition should be sequenced as the principal or first-listed diagnosis.

Multiple codes may be needed for sequela, complication codes and obstetric codes to more fully describe a condition. See the specific guidelines for these conditions for further instruction.

8. Acute and Chronic Conditions
If the same condition is described as both acute (subacute) and chronic, and separate subentries exist in the Alphabetic Index at the same indentation level, code both and sequence the acute (subacute) code first.

9. Combination Code
A combination code is a single code used to classify:
Two diagnoses, or
A diagnosis with an associated secondary process (manifestation)
A diagnosis with an associated complication

Combination codes are identified by referring to subterm entries in the Alphabetic Index and by reading the inclusion and exclusion notes in the Tabular List.

Assign only the combination code when that code fully identifies the diagnostic conditions involved or when the Alphabetic Index so directs. Multiple coding should not be used when the classification provides a combination code that clearly identifies all of the elements documented in the diagnosis. When the combination code lacks necessary specificity in describing the manifestation or complication, an additional code should be used as a secondary code.

10. Sequela (Late Effects)
A sequela is the residual effect (condition produced) after the acute phase of an illness or injury has terminated. There is no time limit on when a sequela code can be used. The residual may be apparent early, such as in cerebral infarction, or it may occur months or years later, such as that due to a previous injury. Examples of sequela include: scar formation resulting from a burn, deviated septum due to a nasal fracture, and infertility due to tubal occlusion from old tuberculosis. Coding of sequela generally requires two codes sequenced in the following order: the condition or nature of the sequela is sequenced first. The sequela code is sequenced second.

An exception to the above guidelines are those instances where the code for the sequela is followed by a manifestation code identified in the Tabular List and title, or the sequela code has been expanded (at the fourth, fifth or sixth character levels) to include the manifestation(s). The code for the acute phase of an illness or injury that led to the sequela is never used with a code for the late effect.

See Section I.C.9. Sequelae of cerebrovascular disease

See Section I.C.15. Sequelae of complication of pregnancy, childbirth and the puerperium

See Section I.C.19. Application of 7th characters for Chapter 19

11. Impending or Threatened Condition
Code any condition described at the time of discharge as "impending" or "threatened" as follows:

If it did occur, code as confirmed diagnosis.
If it did not occur, reference the Alphabetic Index to determine if the condition has a subentry term for "impending" or "threatened" and also reference main term entries for "Impending" and for "Threatened."
If the subterms are listed, assign the given code.
If the subterms are not listed, code the existing underlying condition(s) and not the condition described as impending or threatened.

12. Reporting Same Diagnosis Code more than Once
Each unique ICD-10-CM diagnosis code may be reported only once for an encounter. This applies to bilateral conditions when there are no distinct codes identifying laterality or two different conditions classified to the same ICD-10-CM diagnosis code.

13. Laterality
Some ICD-10-CM codes indicate laterality, specifying whether the condition occurs on the left, right or is bilateral. If no bilateral code is provided and the condition is bilateral, assign separate codes for both the left and right side. If the side is not identified in the medical record, assign the code for the unspecified side.

When a patient has a bilateral condition and each side is treated during separate encounters, assign the "bilateral" code (as the condition still exists on both sides), including for the encounter to treat the first side. For the second encounter for treatment after one side has previously been treated and the condition no longer exists on that side, assign the appropriate unilateral code for the side where the condition still exists (e.g., cataract surgery performed on each eye in separate encounters). The bilateral code would not be assigned for the subsequent encounter, as the patient no longer has the condition in the previously-treated site. If the treatment on the first side did not completely resolve the condition, then the bilateral code would still be appropriate.

14. Documentation for BMI, Depth of Non-pressure ulcers, Pressure Ulcer Stages, Coma Scale, and NIH Stroke Scale
For the Body Mass Index (BMI), depth of non-pressure chronic ulcers, pressure ulcer stage, coma scale, and NIH stroke scale (NIHSS) codes, code assignment may be based on medical record documentation from clinicians who are not the patient's provider (i.e., physician or other qualified healthcare practitioner legally accountable for establishing the patient's diagnosis), since this information is typically documented by other clinicians involved in the care of the patient (e.g., a dietitian often documents the BMI, a nurse often documents the pressure ulcer stages, and an emergency medical technician often documents the coma scale). However, the associated diagnosis (such as overweight, obesity, acute stroke, or pressure ulcer) must be documented by the patient's provider. If there is conflicting medical record documentation, either from the same clinician or different clinicians, the patient's attending provider should be queried for clarification.

The BMI, coma scale, and NIHSS codes should only be reported as secondary diagnoses.

15. Syndromes
Follow the Alphabetic Index guidance when coding syndromes. In the absence of Alphabetic Index guidance, assign codes for the documented manifestations of the syndrome. Additional codes for manifestations that are not an integral part of the disease process may also be assigned when the condition does not have a unique code.

16. Documentation of Complications of Care
Code assignment is based on the provider's documentation of the relationship between the condition and the care or procedure, unless otherwise instructed by the classification. The guideline extends to any complications of care, regardless of the chapter the code is located in. It is important to note that not all conditions that occur during or following medical care or surgery are classified as complications. There must be a cause-and-effect relationship between the care provided and

the condition, and an indication in the documentation that it is a complication. Query the provider for clarification, if the complication is not clearly documented.

17. Borderline Diagnosis

If the provider documents a "borderline" diagnosis at the time of discharge, the diagnosis is coded as confirmed, unless the classification provides a specific entry (e.g., borderline diabetes). If a borderline condition has a specific index entry in ICD-10-CM, it should be coded as such. Since borderline conditions are not uncertain diagnoses, no distinction is made between the care setting (inpatient versus outpatient). Whenever the documentation is unclear regarding a borderline condition, coders are encouraged to query for clarification.

18. Use of Sign/Symptom/Unspecified Codes

Sign/symptom and "unspecified" codes have acceptable, even necessary, uses. While specific diagnosis codes should be reported when they are supported by the available medical record documentation and clinical knowledge of the patient's health condition, there are instances when signs/symptoms or unspecified codes are the best choices for accurately reflecting the healthcare encounter. Each healthcare encounter should be coded to the level of certainty known for that encounter.

If a definitive diagnosis has not been established by the end of the encounter, it is appropriate to report codes for sign(s) and/or symptom(s) in lieu of a definitive diagnosis. When sufficient clinical information isn't known or available about a particular health condition to assign a more specific code, it is acceptable to report the appropriate "unspecified" code (e.g., a diagnosis of pneumonia has been determined, but not the specific type). Unspecified codes should be reported when they are the codes that most accurately reflect what is known about the patient's condition at the time of that particular encounter. It would be inappropriate to select a specific code that is not supported by the medical record documentation or conduct medically unnecessary diagnostic testing in order to determine a more specific code.

C. Chapter-Specific Coding Guidelines

In addition to general coding guidelines, there are guidelines for specific diagnoses and/or conditions in the classification. Unless otherwise indicated, these guidelines apply to all health care settings. Please refer to Section II for guidelines on the selection of principal diagnosis.

1. **Chapter 1: Certain Infectious and Parasitic Diseases (A00-B99)**
   a. **Human Immunodeficiency Virus (HIV) Infections**

   1) **Code only confirmed cases**

      Code only confirmed cases of HIV infection/illness. This is an exception to the hospital inpatient guideline Section II, H.

      In this context, "confirmation" does not require documentation of positive serology or culture for HIV; the provider's diagnostic statement that the patient is HIV positive, or has an HIV-related illness is sufficient.

   2) **Selection and sequencing of HIV codes**

      (a) **Patient admitted for HIV-related condition**

         If a patient is admitted for an HIV-related condition, the principal diagnosis should be B20, Human immunodeficiency virus [HIV] disease followed by additional diagnosis codes for all reported HIV-related conditions.

      (b) **Patient with HIV disease admitted for unrelated condition**

         If a patient with HIV disease is admitted for an unrelated condition (such as a traumatic injury), the code for the unrelated condition (e.g., the nature of injury code) should be the principal diagnosis. Other diagnoses would be B20 followed by additional diagnosis codes for all reported HIV-related conditions.

      (c) **Whether the patient is newly diagnosed**

         Whether the patient is newly diagnosed or has had previous admissions/encounters for HIV conditions is irrelevant to the sequencing decision.

      (d) **Asymptomatic human immunodeficiency virus**

         Z21, Asymptomatic human immunodeficiency virus [HIV] infection status, is to be applied when the patient without any documentation of symptoms is listed as being "HIV

positive," "known HIV," "HIV test positive," or similar terminology. Do not use this code if the term "AIDS" is used or if the patient is treated for any HIV-related illness or is described as having any condition(s) resulting from his/her HIV positive status; use B20 in these cases.

(e) **Patients with inconclusive HIV serology**

Patients with inconclusive HIV serology, but no definitive diagnosis or manifestations of the illness, may be assigned code R75, Inconclusive laboratory evidence of human immunodeficiency virus [HIV].

(f) **Previously diagnosed HIV-related illness**

Patients with any known prior diagnosis of an HIV-related illness should be coded to B20. Once a patient has developed an HIV-related illness, the patient should always be assigned code B20 on every subsequent admission/encounter. Patients previously diagnosed with any HIV illness (B20) should never be assigned to R75 or Z21, Asymptomatic human immunodeficiency virus [HIV] infection status.

(g) **HIV Infection in Pregnancy, Childbirth and the Puerperium**

During pregnancy, childbirth or the puerperium, a patient admitted (or presenting for a health care encounter) because of an HIV-related illness should receive a principal diagnosis code of O98.7-, Human immunodeficiency [HIV] disease complicating pregnancy, childbirth and the puerperium, followed by B20 and the code(s) for the HIV-related illness(es). Codes from Chapter 15 always take sequencing priority.

Patients with asymptomatic HIV infection status admitted (or presenting for a health care encounter) during pregnancy, childbirth, or the puerperium should receive codes of O98.7- and Z21.

(h) **Encounters for testing for HIV**

If a patient is being seen to determine his/her HIV status, use code Z11.4, Encounter for screening for human immunodeficiency virus [HIV]. Use additional codes for any associated high risk behavior.

If a patient with signs or symptoms is being seen for HIV testing, code the signs and symptoms. An additional counseling code Z71.7, Human immunodeficiency virus [HIV] counseling, may be used if counseling is provided during the encounter for the test.

When a patient returns to be informed of his/her HIV test results and the test result is negative, use code Z71.7, Human immunodeficiency virus [HIV] counseling.

If the results are positive, see previous guidelines and assign codes as appropriate.

b. **Infectious agents as the cause of diseases classified to other chapters**

Certain infections are classified in chapters other than Chapter 1 and no organism is identified as part of the infection code. In these instances, it is necessary to use an additional code from Chapter 1 to identify the organism. A code from category B95, Streptococcus, Staphylococcus, and Enterococcus as the cause of diseases classified to other chapters, B96, Other bacterial agents as the cause of diseases classified to other chapters, or B97, Viral agents as the cause of diseases classified to other chapters, is to be used as an additional code to identify the organism. An instructional note will be found at the infection code advising that an additional organism code is required.

c. **Infections resistant to antibiotics**

Many bacterial infections are resistant to current antibiotics. It is necessary to identify all infections documented as antibiotic resistant. Assign a code from category Z16, Resistance to antimicrobial drugs, following the infection code only if the infection code does not identify drug resistance.

d. Sepsis, Severe Sepsis, and Septic Shock

1) Coding of Sepsis and Severe Sepsis

(a) Sepsis

For a diagnosis of sepsis, assign the appropriate code for the underlying systemic infection. If the type of infection or causal organism is not further specified, assign code A41.9, Sepsis, unspecified organism.

A code from subcategory R65.2, Severe sepsis, should not be assigned unless severe sepsis or an associated acute organ dysfunction is documented.

(i) Negative or inconclusive blood cultures and sepsis

Negative or inconclusive blood cultures do not preclude a diagnosis of sepsis in patients with clinical evidence of the condition; however, the provider should be queried.

(ii) Urosepsis

The term urosepsis is a nonspecific term. It is not to be considered synonymous with sepsis. It has no default code in the Alphabetic Index. Should a provider use this term, he/she must be queried for clarification.

(iii) Sepsis with organ dysfunction

If a patient has sepsis and associated acute organ dysfunction or multiple organ dysfunction (MOD), follow the instructions for coding severe sepsis.

(iv) Acute organ dysfunction that is not clearly associated with the sepsis

If a patient has sepsis and an acute organ dysfunction, but the medical record documentation indicates that the acute organ dysfunction is related to a medical condition other than the sepsis, do not assign a code from subcategory R65.2, Severe sepsis. An acute organ dysfunction must be associated with the sepsis in order to assign the severe sepsis code. If the documentation is not clear as to whether an acute organ dysfunction is related to the sepsis or another medical condition, query the provider.

(b) Severe sepsis

The coding of severe sepsis requires a minimum of 2 codes: first a code for the underlying systemic infection, followed by a code from subcategory R65.2, Severe sepsis. If the causal organism is not documented, assign code A41.9, Sepsis, unspecified organism, for the infection. Additional code(s) for the associated acute organ dysfunction are also required.

Due to the complex nature of severe sepsis, some cases may require querying the provider prior to assignment of the codes.

2) Septic shock

(a) Septic shock generally refers to circulatory failure associated with severe sepsis, and therefore, it represents a type of acute organ dysfunction.

For cases of septic shock, the code for the systemic infection should be sequenced first, followed by code R65.21, Severe sepsis with septic shock or code T81.12, Postprocedural septic shock. Any additional codes for the other acute organ dysfunctions should also be assigned. As noted in the sequencing instructions in the Tabular List, the code for septic shock cannot be assigned as a principal diagnosis.

3) Sequencing of severe sepsis

If severe sepsis is present on admission, and meets the definition of principal diagnosis, the underlying systemic infection should be assigned as principal diagnosis followed by the appropriate code from subcategory R65.2 as required by the sequencing rules in the Tabular List. A code from subcategory R65.2 can never be assigned as a principal diagnosis.

When severe sepsis develops during an encounter (it was not present on admission), the underlying systemic infection and

the appropriate code from subcategory R65.2 should be assigned as secondary diagnoses.

Severe sepsis may be present on admission, but the diagnosis may not be confirmed until sometime after admission. If the documentation is not clear whether severe sepsis was present on admission, the provider should be queried.

4) Sepsis and severe sepsis with a localized infection

If the reason for admission is both sepsis or severe sepsis and a localized infection, such as pneumonia or cellulitis, a code(s) for the underlying systemic infection should be assigned first and the code for the localized infection should be assigned as a secondary diagnosis. If the patient has severe sepsis, a code from subcategory R65.2 should also be assigned as a secondary diagnosis. If the patient is admitted with a localized infection, such as pneumonia, and sepsis/severe sepsis doesn't develop until after admission, the localized infection should be assigned first, followed by the appropriate sepsis/severe sepsis codes.

5) Sepsis due to a postprocedural infection

(a) Documentation of causal relationship

As with all postprocedural complications, code assignment is based on the provider's documentation of the relationship between the infection and the procedure.

(b) Sepsis due to a postprocedural infection

For such cases, the postprocedural infection code, such as T80.2, Infections following infusion, transfusion, and therapeutic injection, T81.4, Infection following a procedure, T88.0, Infection following immunization, or O86.0, Infection of obstetric surgical wound, should be coded first, followed by the code for the specific infection. If the patient has severe sepsis, the appropriate code from subcategory R65.2 should also be assigned with the additional code(s) for any acute organ dysfunction.

(c) Postprocedural infection and postprocedural septic shock

In cases where a postprocedural infection has occurred and has resulted in severe sepsis the code for the precipitating complication such as code T81.4, Infection following a procedure, or O86.0, Infection of obstetrical surgical wound should be coded first followed by code R65.20, Severe sepsis without septic shock. A code for the systemic infection should also be assigned.

If a postprocedural infection has resulted in postprocedural septic shock, the code for the precipitating complication such as code T81.4, Infection following a procedure, or O86.0, Infection of obstetrical surgical wound should be coded first followed by code T81.12-, Postprocedural septic shock. A code for the systemic infection should also be assigned.

6) Sepsis and severe sepsis associated with a noninfectious process (condition)

In some cases a noninfectious process (condition), such as trauma, may lead to an infection which can result in sepsis or severe sepsis. If sepsis or severe sepsis is documented as associated with a noninfectious condition, such as a burn or serious injury, and this condition meets the definition for principal diagnosis, the code for the noninfectious condition should be sequenced first, followed by the code for the resulting infection. If severe sepsis is present, a code from subcategory R65.2 should also be assigned with any associated organ dysfunction(s) codes. It is not necessary to assign a code from subcategory R65.1, Systemic inflammatory response syndrome (SIRS) of non-infectious origin, for these cases.

If the infection meets the definition of principal diagnosis, it should be sequenced before the non-infectious condition. When both the associated non-infectious condition and the infection meet the definition of principal diagnosis, either may be assigned as principal diagnosis.

Only one code from category R65, Symptoms and signs specifically associated with systemic inflammation and infection, should be assigned. Therefore, when a non-infectious condition leads to an infection resulting in severe sepsis, assign the appropriate code from subcategory R65.2, Severe sepsis. Do not additionally assign a code from subcategory R65.1, Systemic inflammatory response syndrome (SIRS) of non-infectious origin.

See Section I.C.18. SIRS due to non-infectious process

7) Sepsis and septic shock complicating abortion, pregnancy, childbirth, and the puerperium
See Section I.C.15. Sepsis and septic shock complicating abortion, pregnancy, childbirth and the puerperium

8) Newborn sepsis
See Section I.C.16. f. Bacterial sepsis of Newborn

e. Methicillin Resistant *Staphylococcus aureus* (MRSA) Conditions
1) Selection and sequencing of MRSA codes
(a) Combination codes for MRSA infection
When a patient is diagnosed with an infection that is due to methicillin resistant *Staphylococcus aureus* (MRSA), and that infection has a combination code that includes the causal organism (e.g., sepsis, pneumonia) assign the appropriate combination code for the condition (e.g., code A41.02, Sepsis due to Methicillin resistant Staphylococcus aureus or code J15.212, Pneumonia due to Methicillin resistant Staphylococcus aureus). Do not assign code B95.62, Methicillin resistant Staphylococcus aureus infection as the cause of diseases classified elsewhere, as an additional code, because the combination code includes the type of infection and the MRSA organism. Do not assign a code from subcategory Z16.11, Resistance to penicillins, as an additional diagnosis.

See Section C.1. for instructions on coding and sequencing of sepsis and severe sepsis.

(b) Other codes for MRSA infection
When there is documentation of a current infection (e.g., wound infection, stitch abscess, urinary tract infection) due to MRSA, and that infection does not have a combination code that includes the causal organism, assign the appropriate code to identify the condition along with code B95.62, Methicillin resistant Staphylococcus aureus infection as the cause of diseases classified elsewhere for the MRSA infection. Do not assign a code from subcategory Z16.11, Resistance to penicillins.

(c) Methicillin susceptible Staphylococcus aureus (MSSA) and MRSA colonization
The condition or state of being colonized or carrying MSSA or MRSA is called colonization or carriage, while an individual person is described as being colonized or being a carrier. Colonization means that MSSA or MSRA is present on or in the body without necessarily causing illness. A positive MRSA colonization test might be documented by the provider as "MRSA screen positive" or "MRSA nasal swab positive".

Assign code Z22.322, Carrier or suspected carrier of Methicillin resistant Staphylococcus aureus, for patients documented as having MRSA colonization. Assign code Z22.321, Carrier or suspected carrier of Methicillin susceptible Staphylococcus aureus, for patient documented as having MSSA colonization. Colonization is not necessarily indicative of a disease process or as the cause of a specific condition the patient may have unless documented as such by the provider.

(d) MRSA colonization and infection
If a patient is documented as having both MRSA colonization and infection during a hospital admission, code Z22.322, Carrier or suspected carrier of Methicillin resistant Staphylococcus aureus, and a code for the MRSA infection may both be assigned.

f. Zika virus infections
1) Code only confirmed cases
Code only a confirmed diagnosis of Zika virus (A92.5, Zika virus disease) as documented by the provider. This is an exception to the hospital inpatient guideline Section II, H.

In this context, "confirmation" does not require documentation of the type of test performed; the physician's diagnostic statement that the condition is confirmed is sufficient. This code should be assigned regardless of the stated mode of transmission.

If the provider documents "suspected", "possible" or "probable" Zika, do not assign code A92.5. Assign a code(s) explaining the reason for encounter (such as fever, rash, or joint pain) or Z20.828, Contact with and (suspected) exposure to other viral communicable diseases.

2. Chapter 2: Neoplasms (C00-D49)
General guidelines
Chapter 2 of the ICD-10-CM contains the codes for most benign and all malignant neoplasms. Certain benign neoplasms, such as prostatic adenomas, may be found in the specific body system chapters. To properly code a neoplasm it is necessary to determine from the record if the neoplasm is benign, in-situ, malignant, or of uncertain histologic behavior. If malignant, any secondary (metastatic) sites should also be determined.

Primary malignant neoplasms overlapping site boundaries

A primary malignant neoplasm that overlaps two or more contiguous (next to each other) sites should be classified to the subcategory/code .8 ('overlapping lesion'), unless the combination is specifically indexed elsewhere. For multiple neoplasms of the same site that are not contiguous such as tumors in different quadrants of the same breast, codes for each site should be assigned.

Malignant neoplasm of ectopic tissue

Malignant neoplasms of ectopic tissue are to be coded to the site of origin mentioned, e.g., ectopic pancreatic malignant neoplasms involving the stomach are coded to pancreas, unspecified (C25.9).

The neoplasm table in the Alphabetic Index should be referenced first. However, if the histological term is documented, that term should be referenced first, rather than going immediately to the Neoplasm Table, in order to determine which column in the Neoplasm Table is appropriate. For example, if the documentation indicates "adenoma," refer to the term in the Alphabetic Index to review the entries under this term and the instructional note to "see also neoplasm, by site, benign." The table provides the proper code based on the type of neoplasm and the site. It is important to select the proper column in the table that corresponds to the type of neoplasm. The Tabular List should then be referenced to verify that the correct code has been selected from the table and that a more specific site code does not exist.

See Section I.C.21. Factors influencing health status and contact with health services, Status, for information regarding Z15.0, codes for genetic susceptibility to cancer.

a. Treatment directed at the malignancy
If the treatment is directed at the malignancy, designate the malignancy as the principal diagnosis.

The only exception to this guideline is if a patient admission/encounter is solely for the administration of chemotherapy, immunotherapy or radiation therapy, assign the appropriate Z51.-- code as the first-listed or principal diagnosis, and the diagnosis or problem for which the service is being performed as a secondary diagnosis.

b. Treatment of secondary site
When a patient is admitted because of a primary neoplasm with metastasis and treatment is directed toward the secondary site only, the secondary neoplasm is designated as the principal diagnosis even though the primary malignancy is still present.

c. Coding and sequencing of complications
Coding and sequencing of complications associated with the malignancies or with the therapy thereof are subject to the following guidelines:

1) Anemia associated with malignancy
When admission/encounter is for management of an anemia associated with the malignancy, and the treatment is only for anemia, the appropriate code for the malignancy is sequenced as the principal or first-listed diagnosis followed by the appropriate code for the anemia (such as code D63.0, Anemia in neoplastic disease).

2) **Anemia associated with chemotherapy, immunotherapy and radiation therapy**

When the admission/encounter is for management of an anemia associated with an adverse effect of the administration of chemotherapy or immunotherapy and the only treatment is for the anemia, the anemia code is sequenced first followed by the appropriate codes for the neoplasm and the adverse effect (T45.1X5, Adverse effect of antineoplastic and immunosuppressive drugs).

When the admission/encounter is for management of an anemia associated with an adverse effect of radiotherapy, the anemia code should be sequenced first, followed by the appropriate neoplasm code and code Y84.2, Radiological procedure and radiotherapy as the cause of abnormal reaction of the patient, or of later complication, without mention of misadventure at the time of the procedure.

3) **Management of dehydration due to the malignancy**

When the admission/encounter is for management of dehydration due to the malignancy and only the dehydration is being treated (intravenous rehydration), the dehydration is sequenced first, followed by the code(s) for the malignancy.

4) **Treatment of a complication resulting from a surgical procedure**

When the admission/encounter is for treatment of a complication resulting from a surgical procedure, designate the complication as the principal or first-listed diagnosis if treatment is directed at resolving the complication.

d. **Primary malignancy previously excised**

When a primary malignancy has been previously excised or eradicated from its site and there is no further treatment directed to that site and there is no evidence of any existing primary malignancy, a code from category Z85, Personal history of malignant neoplasm, should be used to indicate the former site of the malignancy. Any mention of extension, invasion, or metastasis to another site is coded as a secondary malignant neoplasm to that site. The secondary site may be the principal or first-listed with the Z85 code used as a secondary code.

e. **Admissions/Encounters involving chemotherapy, immunotherapy and radiation therapy**

1) **Episode of care involves surgical removal of neoplasm**

When an episode of care involves the surgical removal of a neoplasm, primary or secondary site, followed by adjunct chemotherapy or radiation treatment during the same episode of care, the code for the neoplasm should be assigned as principal or first-listed diagnosis.

2) **Patient admission/encounter solely for administration of chemotherapy, immunotherapy and radiation therapy**

If a patient admission/encounter is solely for the administration of chemotherapy, immunotherapy or radiation therapy assign code Z51.0, Encounter for antineoplastic radiation therapy, or Z51.11, Encounter for antineoplastic chemotherapy, or Z51.12, Encounter for antineoplastic immunotherapy as the first-listed or principal diagnosis. If a patient receives more than one of these therapies during the same admission more than one of these codes may be assigned, in any sequence.

The malignancy for which the therapy is being administered should be assigned as a secondary diagnosis.

3) **Patient admitted for radiation therapy, chemotherapy or immunotherapy and develops complications**

When a patient is admitted for the purpose of radiotherapy, immunotherapy or chemotherapy and develops complications such as uncontrolled nausea and vomiting or dehydration, the principal or first-listed diagnosis is Z51.0, Encounter for antineoplastic radiation therapy, or Z51.11, Encounter for antineoplastic chemotherapy, or Z51.12, Encounter for antineoplastic immunotherapy followed by any codes for the complications.

f. **Admission/encounter to determine extent of malignancy**

When the reason for admission/encounter is to determine the extent of the malignancy, or for a procedure such as paracentesis or thoracentesis, the primary malignancy or appropriate metastatic site is designated as the principal or first-listed diagnosis, even though chemotherapy or radiotherapy is administered.

g. **Symptoms, signs, and abnormal findings listed in Chapter 18 associated with neoplasms**

Symptoms, signs, and ill-defined conditions listed in Chapter 18 characteristic of, or associated with, an existing primary or secondary site malignancy cannot be used to replace the malignancy as principal or first-listed diagnosis, regardless of the number of admissions or encounters for treatment and care of the neoplasm.

See section I.C.21. Factors influencing health status and contact with health services, Encounter for prophylactic organ removal.

h. **Admission/encounter for pain control/management**

See Section I.C.6. for information on coding admission/encounter for pain control/management.

i. **Malignancy in two or more noncontiguous sites**

A patient may have more than one malignant tumor in the same organ. These tumors may represent different primaries or metastatic disease, depending on the site. Should the documentation be unclear, the provider should be queried as to the status of each tumor so that the correct codes can be assigned.

j. **Disseminated malignant neoplasm, unspecified**

Code C80.0, Disseminated malignant neoplasm, unspecified, is for use only in those cases where the patient has advanced metastatic disease and no known primary or secondary sites are specified. It should not be used in place of assigning codes for the primary site and all known secondary sites.

k. **Malignant neoplasm without specification of site**

Code C80.1, Malignant (primary) neoplasm, unspecified, equates to Cancer, unspecified. This code should only be used when no determination can be made as to the primary site of a malignancy. This code should rarely be used in the inpatient setting.

l. **Sequencing of neoplasm codes**

1) **Encounter for treatment of primary malignancy**

If the reason for the encounter is for treatment of a primary malignancy, assign the malignancy as the principal/first-listed diagnosis. The primary site is to be sequenced first, followed by any metastatic sites.

2) **Encounter for treatment of secondary malignancy**

When an encounter is for a primary malignancy with metastasis and treatment is directed toward the metastatic (secondary) site(s) only, the metastatic site(s) is designated as the principal/first-listed diagnosis. The primary malignancy is coded as an additional code.

3) **Malignant neoplasm in a pregnant patient**

When a pregnant woman has a malignant neoplasm, a code from subcategory O9A.1-, Malignant neoplasm complicating pregnancy, childbirth, and the puerperium, should be sequenced first, followed by the appropriate code from Chapter 2 to indicate the type of neoplasm.

4) **Encounter for complication associated with a neoplasm**

When an encounter is for management of a complication associated with a neoplasm, such as dehydration, and the treatment is only for the complication, the complication is coded first, followed by the appropriate code(s) for the neoplasm.

The exception to this guideline is anemia. When the admission/encounter is for management of an anemia associated with the malignancy, and the treatment is only for anemia, the appropriate code for the malignancy is sequenced as the principal or first-listed diagnosis followed by code D63.0, Anemia in neoplastic disease.

5) **Complication from surgical procedure for treatment of a neoplasm**

When an encounter is for treatment of a complication resulting from a surgical procedure performed for the treatment of the neoplasm, designate the complication as the principal/first-listed diagnosis. See guideline regarding the coding of a current malignancy versus personal history to determine if the code for the neoplasm should also be assigned.

6) Pathologic fracture due to a neoplasm

When an encounter is for a pathological fracture due to a neoplasm, and the focus of treatment is the fracture, a code from subcategory M84.5, Pathological fracture in neoplastic disease, should be sequenced first, followed by the code for the neoplasm.

If the focus of treatment is the neoplasm with an associated pathological fracture, the neoplasm code should be sequenced first, followed by a code from M84.5 for the pathological fracture.

m. Current malignancy versus personal history of malignancy

When a primary malignancy has been excised but further treatment, such as an additional surgery for the malignancy, radiation therapy or chemotherapy is directed to that site, the primary malignancy code should be used until treatment is completed.

When a primary malignancy has been previously excised or eradicated from its site, there is no further treatment (of the malignancy) directed to that site, and there is no evidence of any existing primary malignancy, a code from category Z85, Personal history of malignant neoplasm, should be used to indicate the former site of the malignancy.

See Section I.C.21. Factors influencing health status and contact with health services, History (of)

n. Leukemia, Multiple Myeloma, and Malignant Plasma Cell Neoplasms in remission versus personal history

The categories for leukemia, and category C90, Multiple myeloma and malignant plasma cell neoplasms, have codes indicating whether or not the leukemia has achieved remission. There are also codes Z85.6, Personal history of leukemia, and Z85.79, Personal history of other malignant neoplasms of lymphoid, hematopoietic and related tissues. If the documentation is unclear as to whether the leukemia has achieved remission, the provider should be queried.

See Section I.C.21. Factors influencing health status and contact with health services, History (of)

o. Aftercare following surgery for neoplasm

See Section I.C.21. Factors influencing health status and contact with health services, Aftercare

p. Follow-up care for completed treatment of a malignancy

See Section I.C.21. Factors influencing health status and contact with health services, Follow-up

q. Prophylactic organ removal for prevention of malignancy

See Section I.C. 21, Factors influencing health status and contact with health services, Prophylactic organ removal

r. Malignant neoplasm associated with transplanted organ

A malignant neoplasm of a transplanted organ should be coded as a transplant complication. Assign first the appropriate code from category T86.-, Complications of transplanted organs and tissue, followed by code C80.2, Malignant neoplasm associated with transplanted organ. Use an additional code for the specific malignancy.

3. Chapter 3: Disease of the blood and blood-forming organs and certain disorders involving the immune mechanism (D50-D89)

Reserved for future guideline expansion

4. Chapter 4: Endocrine, Nutritional, and Metabolic Diseases (E00-E89)

a. Diabetes mellitus

The diabetes mellitus codes are combination codes that include the type of diabetes mellitus, the body system affected, and the complications affecting that body system. As many codes within a particular category as are necessary to describe all of the complications of the disease may be used. They should be sequenced based on the reason for a particular encounter. Assign as many codes from categories E08 – E13 as needed to identify all of the associated conditions that the patient has.

1) Type of diabetes

The age of a patient is not the sole determining factor, though most type 1 diabetics develop the condition before reaching puberty. For this reason type 1 diabetes mellitus is also referred to as juvenile diabetes.

2) Type of diabetes mellitus not documented

If the type of diabetes mellitus is not documented in the medical record the default is E11.-, Type 2 diabetes mellitus.

3) Diabetes mellitus and the use of insulin and oral hypoglycemics

If the documentation in a medical record does not indicate the type of diabetes but does indicate that the patient uses insulin, code E11, Type 2 diabetes mellitus, should be assigned. Code Z79.4, Long-term (current) use of insulin, or Z79.84, Long term (current) use of oral hypoglycemic drugs, should also be assigned to indicate that the patient uses insulin or hypoglycemic drugs. Code Z79.4 should not be assigned if insulin is given temporarily to bring a type 2 patient's blood sugar under control during an encounter.

4) Diabetes mellitus in pregnancy and gestational diabetes

See Section I.C.15. Diabetes mellitus in pregnancy.

See Section I.C.15. Gestational (pregnancy induced) diabetes

5) Complications due to insulin pump malfunction

(a) Underdose of insulin due to insulin pump failure

An underdose of insulin due to an insulin pump failure should be assigned to a code from subcategory T85.6, Mechanical complication of other specified internal and external prosthetic devices, implants and grafts, that specifies the type of pump malfunction, as the principal or first-listed code, followed by code T38.3X6-, Underdosing of insulin and oral hypoglycemic [antidiabetic] drugs. Additional codes for the type of diabetes mellitus and any associated complications due to the underdosing should also be assigned.

(b) Overdose of insulin due to insulin pump failure

The principal or first-listed code for an encounter due to an insulin pump malfunction resulting in an overdose of insulin, should also be T85.6-, Mechanical complication of other specified internal and external prosthetic devices, implants and grafts, followed by code T38.3X1-, Poisoning by insulin and oral hypoglycemic [antidiabetic] drugs, accidental (unintentional).

6) Secondary diabetes mellitus

Codes under categories E08, Diabetes mellitus due to underlying condition, E09, Drug or chemical induced diabetes mellitus, and E13, Other specified diabetes mellitus, identify complications/manifestations associated with secondary diabetes mellitus. Secondary diabetes is always caused by another condition or event (e.g., cystic fibrosis, malignant neoplasm of pancreas, pancreatectomy, adverse effect of drug, or poisoning).

(a) Secondary diabetes mellitus and the use of insulin or hypoglycemic drugs

For patients who routinely use insulin or hypoglycemic drugs, code Z79.4, Long-term (current) use of insulin, or Z79.84, Long term (current) use of oral hypoglycemic drugs should also be assigned. Code Z79.4 should not be assigned if insulin is given temporarily to bring a patient's blood sugar under control during an encounter.

(b) Assigning and sequencing secondary diabetes codes and its causes

The sequencing of the secondary diabetes codes in relationship to codes for the cause of the diabetes is based on the Tabular List instructions for categories E08, E09 and E13.

(i) Secondary diabetes mellitus due to pancreatectomy

For postpancreatectomy diabetes mellitus (lack of insulin due to the surgical removal of all or part of the pancreas), assign code E89.1, Postprocedural hypoinsulinemia. Assign a code from category E13 and a code from subcategory Z90.41-, Acquired absence of pancreas, as additional codes.

(ii) Secondary diabetes due to drugs

Secondary diabetes may be caused by an adverse effect of correctly administered medications, poisoning or sequela of poisoning.

See section I.C.19.e for coding of adverse effects and poisoning, and section I.C.20 for external cause code reporting.

5. **Chapter 5: Mental, Behavioral and Neurodevelopmental disorders (F01-F99)**

a. **Pain disorders related to psychological factors**

Assign code F45.41, for pain that is exclusively related to psychological disorders. As indicated by the Excludes 1 note under category G89, a code from category G89 should not be assigned with code F45.41.

Code F45.42, Pain disorders with related psychological factors, should be used with a code from category G89, Pain, not elsewhere classified, if there is documentation of a psychological component for a patient with acute or chronic pain.

See Section I.C.6. Pain

b. **Mental and behavioral disorders due to psychoactive substance use**

1) **In Remission**

Selection of codes for "in remission" for categories F10-F19, Mental and behavioral disorders due to psychoactive substance use (categories F10-F19 with -.21) requires the provider's clinical judgment. The appropriate codes for "in remission" are assigned only on the basis of provider documentation (as defined in the Official Guidelines for Coding and Reporting).

2) **Psychoactive Substance Use, Abuse And Dependence**

When the provider documentation refers to use, abuse and dependence of the same substance (e.g. alcohol, opioid, cannabis, etc.), only one code should be assigned to identify the pattern of use based on the following hierarchy:

- If both use and abuse are documented, assign only the code for abuse
- If both abuse and dependence are documented, assign only the code for dependence
- If use, abuse and dependence are all documented, assign only the code for dependence
- If both use and dependence are documented, assign only the code for dependence.

3) **Psychoactive Substance Use**

As with all other diagnoses, the codes for psychoactive substance use (F10.9-, F11.9-, F12.9-, F13.9-, F14.9-, F15.9-, F16.9-) should only be assigned based on provider documentation and when they meet the definition of a reportable diagnosis (see Section III, Reporting Additional Diagnoses). The codes are to be used only when the psychoactive substance use is associated with a mental or behavioral disorder, and such a relationship is documented by the provider.

6. **Chapter 6: Diseases of the Nervous System (G00-G99)**

a. **Dominant/nondominant side**

Codes from category G81, Hemiplegia and hemiparesis, and subcategories G83.1, Monoplegia of lower limb, G83.2, Monoplegia of upper limb, and G83.3, Monoplegia, unspecified, identify whether the dominant or nondominant side is affected. Should the affected side be documented, but not specified as dominant or nondominant, and the classification system does not indicate a default, code selection is as follows:

- For ambidextrous patients, the default should be dominant.
- If the left side is affected, the default is non-dominant.
- If the right side is affected, the default is dominant.

b. **Pain - Category G89**

1) **General coding information**

Codes in category G89, Pain, not elsewhere classified, may be used in conjunction with codes from other categories and chapters to provide more detail about acute or chronic pain and neoplasm-related pain, unless otherwise indicated below.

If the pain is not specified as acute or chronic, post-thoracotomy, postprocedural, or neoplasm-related, do not assign codes from category G89.

A code from category G89 should not be assigned if the underlying (definitive) diagnosis is known, unless the reason for the encounter is pain control/ management and not management of the underlying condition.

When an admission or encounter is for a procedure aimed at treating the underlying condition (e.g., spinal fusion, kyphoplasty), a code for the underlying condition (e.g., vertebral fracture, spinal stenosis) should be assigned as the principal diagnosis. No code from category G89 should be assigned.

(a) **Category G89 Codes as Principal or First-Listed Diagnosis**

Category G89 codes are acceptable as principal diagnosis or the first-listed code:

- When pain control or pain management is the reason for the admission/encounter (e.g., a patient with displaced intervertebral disc, nerve impingement and severe back pain presents for injection of steroid into the spinal canal). The underlying cause of the pain should be reported as an additional diagnosis, if known.

- When a patient is admitted for the insertion of a neurostimulator for pain control, assign the appropriate pain code as the principal or first-listed diagnosis. When an admission or encounter is for a procedure aimed at treating the underlying condition and a neurostimulator is inserted for pain control during the same admission/encounter, a code for the underlying condition should be assigned as the principal diagnosis and the appropriate pain code should be assigned as a secondary diagnosis.

(b) **Use of Category G89 Codes in Conjunction with Site Specific Pain Codes**

(i) **Assigning Category G89 and Site-Specific Pain Codes**

Codes from category G89 may be used in conjunction with codes that identify the site of pain (including codes from chapter 18) if the category G89 code provides additional information. For example, if the code describes the site of the pain, but does not fully describe whether the pain is acute or chronic, then both codes should be assigned.

(ii) **Sequencing of Category G89 Codes with Site-Specific Pain Codes**

The sequencing of category G89 codes with site-specific pain codes (including chapter 18 codes), is dependent on the circumstances of the encounter/admission as follows:

- If the encounter is for pain control or pain management, assign the code from category G89 followed by the code identifying the specific site of pain (e.g., encounter for pain management for acute neck pain from trauma is assigned code G89.11, Acute pain due to trauma, followed by code M54.2, Cervicalgia, to identify the site of pain).

- If the encounter is for any other reason except pain control or pain management, and a related definitive diagnosis has not been established (confirmed) by the provider, assign the code for the specific site of pain first, followed by the appropriate code from category G89.

2) **Pain due to devices, implants and grafts**

See Section I.C.19. Pain due to medical devices

3) **Postoperative Pain**

The provider's documentation should be used to guide the coding of postoperative pain, as well as *Section III. Reporting Additional Diagnoses* and *Section IV. Diagnostic Coding and Reporting in the Outpatient Setting.*

The default for post-thoracotomy and other postoperative pain not specified as acute or chronic is the code for the acute form.

Routine or expected postoperative pain immediately after surgery should not be coded.

(a) Postoperative pain not associated with specific postoperative complication
Postoperative pain not associated with a specific postoperative complication is assigned to the appropriate postoperative pain code in category G89.

(b) Postoperative pain associated with specific postoperative complication
Postoperative pain associated with a specific postoperative complication (such as painful wire sutures) is assigned to the appropriate code(s) found in Chapter 19, Injury, poisoning, and certain other consequences of external causes. If appropriate, use additional code(s) from category G89 to identify acute or chronic pain (G89.18 or G89.28).

4) Chronic pain
Chronic pain is classified to subcategory G89.2. There is no time frame defining when pain becomes chronic pain. The provider's documentation should be used to guide use of these codes.

5) Neoplasm Related Pain
Code G89.3 is assigned to pain documented as being related, associated or due to cancer, primary or secondary malignancy, or tumor. This code is assigned regardless of whether the pain is acute or chronic.

This code may be assigned as the principal or first-listed code when the stated reason for the admission/encounter is documented as pain control/pain management. The underlying neoplasm should be reported as an additional diagnosis.

When the reason for the admission/encounter is management of the neoplasm and the pain associated with the neoplasm is also documented, code G89.3 may be assigned as an additional diagnosis. It is not necessary to assign an additional code for the site of the pain.

See Section I.C.2 for instructions on the sequencing of neoplasms for all other stated reasons for the admission/encounter (except for pain control/pain management).

6) Chronic pain syndrome
Central pain syndrome (G89.0) and chronic pain syndrome (G89.4) are different than the term "chronic pain," and therefore codes should only be used when the provider has specifically documented this condition.

See Section I.C.5. Pain disorders related to psychological factors

7. Chapter 7: Diseases of the Eye and Adnexa (H00-H59)
a. Glaucoma
1) Assigning Glaucoma Codes
Assign as many codes from category H40, Glaucoma, as needed to identify the type of glaucoma, the affected eye, and the glaucoma stage.

2) Bilateral glaucoma with same type and stage
When a patient has bilateral glaucoma and both eyes are documented as being the same type and stage, and there is a code for bilateral glaucoma, report only the code for the type of glaucoma, bilateral, with the seventh character for the stage.

When a patient has bilateral glaucoma and both eyes are documented as being the same type and stage, and the classification does not provide a code for bilateral glaucoma (i.e. subcategories H40.10, H40.11 and H40.20) report only one code for the type of glaucoma with the appropriate seventh character for the stage.

3) Bilateral glaucoma stage with different types or stages
When a patient has bilateral glaucoma and each eye is documented as having a different type or stage, and the classification distinguishes laterality, assign the appropriate code for each eye rather than the code for bilateral glaucoma.

When a patient has bilateral glaucoma and each eye is documented as having a different type, and the classification does not distinguish laterality (i.e. subcategories H40.10, H40.11 and H40.20), assign one code for each type of glaucoma with the appropriate seventh character for the stage.

When a patient has bilateral glaucoma and each eye is documented as having the same type, but different stage, and the classification does not distinguish laterality (i.e. subcategories H40.10, H40.11 and H40.20), assign a code for the type of glaucoma for each eye with the seventh character for the specific glaucoma stage documented for each eye.

4) Patient admitted with glaucoma and stage evolves during the admission
If a patient is admitted with glaucoma and the stage progresses during the admission, assign the code for highest stage documented.

5) Indeterminate stage glaucoma
Assignment of the seventh character "4" for "indeterminate stage" should be based on the clinical documentation. The seventh character "4" is used for glaucomas whose stage cannot be clinically determined. This seventh character should not be confused with the seventh character "0", unspecified, which should be assigned when there is no documentation regarding the stage of the glaucoma.

8. Chapter 8: Diseases of the Ear and Mastoid Process (H60-H95)
Reserved for future guideline expansion

9. Chapter 9: Diseases of the Circulatory System (I00-I99)
a. Hypertension
The classification presumes a causal relationship between hypertension and heart involvement and between hypertension and kidney involvement, as the two conditions are linked by the term "with" in the Alphabetic Index. These conditions should be coded as related even in the absence of provider documentation explicitly linking them, unless the documentation clearly states the conditions are unrelated.

For hypertension and conditions not specifically linked by relational terms such as "with," "associated with" or "due to" in the classification, provider documentation must link the conditions in order to code them as related.

1) Hypertension with Heart Disease
Hypertension with heart conditions classified to I50.- or I51.4-I51.9, are assigned to a code from category I11, Hypertensive heart disease. Use an additional code from category I50, Heart failure, to identify the type of heart failure in those patients with heart failure.

The same heart conditions (I50.-, I51.4-I51.9) with hypertension are coded separately if the provider has specifically documented a different cause. Sequence according to the circumstances of the admission/encounter.

2) Hypertensive Chronic Kidney Disease
Assign codes from category I12, Hypertensive chronic kidney disease, when both hypertension and a condition classifiable to category N18, Chronic kidney disease (CKD), are present. CKD should not be coded as hypertensive if the physician has specifically documented a different cause.

The appropriate code from category N18 should be used as a secondary code with a code from category I12 to identify the stage of chronic kidney disease.

See Section I.C.14. Chronic kidney disease.

If a patient has hypertensive chronic kidney disease and acute renal failure, an additional code for the acute renal failure is required.

3) Hypertensive Heart and Chronic Kidney Disease
Assign codes from combination category I13, Hypertensive heart and chronic kidney disease, when there is hypertension with both heart and kidney involvement. If heart failure is present, assign an additional code from category I50 to identify the type of heart failure.

The appropriate code from category N18, Chronic kidney disease, should be used as a secondary code with a code from category I13 to identify the stage of chronic kidney disease.

See Section I.C.14. Chronic kidney disease.

The codes in category I13, Hypertensive heart and chronic kidney disease, are combination codes that include hypertension, heart disease and chronic kidney disease. The

Includes note at I13 specifies that the conditions included at I11 and I12 are included together in I13. If a patient has hypertension, heart disease and chronic kidney disease, then a code from I13 should be used, not individual codes for hypertension, heart disease and chronic kidney disease, or codes from I11 or I12.

For patients with both acute renal failure and chronic kidney disease, an additional code for acute renal failure is required.

4) Hypertensive Cerebrovascular Disease
For hypertensive cerebrovascular disease, first assign the appropriate code from categories I60-I69, followed by the appropriate hypertension code.

5) Hypertensive Retinopathy
Subcategory H35.0, Background retinopathy and retinal vascular changes, should be used with a code from category I10 – I15, Hypertensive disease to include the systemic hypertension. The sequencing is based on the reason for the encounter.

6) Hypertension, Secondary
Secondary hypertension is due to an underlying condition. Two codes are required: one to identify the underlying etiology and one from category I15 to identify the hypertension. Sequencing of codes is determined by the reason for admission/encounter.

7) Hypertension, Transient
Assign code R03.0, Elevated blood pressure reading without diagnosis of hypertension, unless patient has an established diagnosis of hypertension. Assign code O13.-, Gestational [pregnancy-induced] hypertension without significant proteinuria, or O14.-, Pre-eclampsia, for transient hypertension of pregnancy.

8) Hypertension, Controlled
This diagnostic statement usually refers to an existing state of hypertension under control by therapy. Assign the appropriate code from categories I10-I15, Hypertensive diseases.

9) Hypertension, Uncontrolled
Uncontrolled hypertension may refer to untreated hypertension or hypertension not responding to current therapeutic regimen. In either case, assign the appropriate code from categories I10-I15, Hypertensive diseases.

10) Hypertensive Crisis
Assign a code from category I16, Hypertensive crisis, for documented hypertensive urgency, hypertensive emergency or unspecified hypertensive crisis. Code also any identified hypertensive disease (I10-I15). The sequencing is based on the reason for the encounter.

b. Atherosclerotic Coronary Artery Disease and Angina
ICD-10-CM has combination codes for atherosclerotic heart disease with angina pectoris. The subcategories for these codes are I25.11, Atherosclerotic heart disease of native coronary artery with angina pectoris and I25.7, Atherosclerosis of coronary artery bypass graft(s) and coronary artery of transplanted heart with angina pectoris.

When using one of these combination codes it is not necessary to use an additional code for angina pectoris. A causal relationship can be assumed in a patient with both atherosclerosis and angina pectoris, unless the documentation indicates the angina is due to something other than the atherosclerosis.

If a patient with coronary artery disease is admitted due to an acute myocardial infarction (AMI), the AMI should be sequenced before the coronary artery disease.

See Section I.C.9. Acute myocardial infarction (AMI)

c. Intraoperative and Postprocedural Cerebrovascular Accident
Medical record documentation should clearly specify the cause-and-effect relationship between the medical intervention and the cerebrovascular accident in order to assign a code for intraoperative or postprocedural cerebrovascular accident.

Proper code assignment depends on whether it was an infarction or hemorrhage and whether it occurred intraoperatively or postoperatively. If it was a cerebral hemorrhage, code assignment depends on the type of procedure performed.

d. Sequelae of Cerebrovascular Disease

1) Category I69, Sequelae of Cerebrovascular disease
Category I69 is used to indicate conditions classifiable to categories I60-I67 as the causes of sequela (neurologic deficits), themselves classified elsewhere. These "late effects" include neurologic deficits that persist after initial onset of conditions classifiable to categories I60-I67. The neurologic deficits caused by cerebrovascular disease may be present from the onset or may arise at any time after the onset of the condition classifiable to categories I60-I67.

Codes from category I69, Sequelae of cerebrovascular disease, that specify hemiplegia, hemiparesis and monoplegia identify whether the dominant or nondominant side is affected. Should the affected side be documented, but not specified as dominant or nondominant, and the classification system does not indicate a default, code selection is as follows:

- For ambidextrous patients, the default should be dominant.
- If the left side is affected, the default is non-dominant.
- If the right side is affected, the default is dominant.

2) Codes from category I69 with codes from I60-I67
Codes from category I69 may be assigned on a health care record with codes from I60-I67, if the patient has a current cerebrovascular disease and deficits from an old cerebrovascular disease.

3) Codes from category I69 and Personal history of transient ischemic attack (TIA) and cerebral infarction (Z86.73)
Codes from category I69 should not be assigned if the patient does not have neurologic deficits.

See Section I.C.21. 4. History (of) for use of personal history codes

e. Acute myocardial infarction (AMI)

1) ST elevation myocardial infarction (STEMI) and non ST elevation myocardial infarction (NSTEMI)
The ICD-10-CM codes for acute myocardial infarction (AMI) identify the site, such as anterolateral wall or true posterior wall. Subcategories I21.0-I21.2 and code I21.3 are used for ST elevation myocardial infarction (STEMI). Code I21.4, Non-ST elevation (NSTEMI) myocardial infarction, is used for non ST elevation myocardial infarction (NSTEMI) and nontransmural MIs.

If NSTEMI evolves to STEMI, assign the STEMI code. If STEMI converts to NSTEMI due to thrombolytic therapy, it is still coded as STEMI.

For encounters occurring while the myocardial infarction is equal to, or less than, four weeks old, including transfers to another acute setting or a postacute setting, and the myocardial infarction meets the definition for "other diagnoses" (see Section III, Reporting Additional Diagnoses), codes from category I21 may continue to be reported. For encounters after the 4 week time frame and the patient is still receiving care related to the myocardial infarction, the appropriate aftercare code should be assigned, rather than a code from category I21. For old or healed myocardial infarctions not requiring further care, code I25.2, Old myocardial infarction, may be assigned.

2) Acute myocardial infarction, unspecified
Code I21.3, ST elevation (STEMI) myocardial infarction of unspecified site, is the default for unspecified acute myocardial infarction. If only STEMI or transmural MI without the site is documented, assign code I21.3.

3) AMI documented as nontransmural or subendocardial but site provided
If an AMI is documented as nontransmural or subendocardial, but the site is provided, it is still coded as a subendocardial AMI.

See Section I.C.21.3 for information on coding status post administration of tPA in a different facility within the last 24 hours.

4) Subsequent acute myocardial infarction
A code from category I22, Subsequent ST elevation (STEMI) and non ST elevation (NSTEMI) myocardial infarction, is to be used when a patient who has suffered an AMI has a new AMI within the 4 week time frame of the initial AMI. A code from category I22 must be used in conjunction with a code from category I21.

The sequencing of the I22 and I21 codes depends on the circumstances of the encounter.

10. **Chapter 10: Diseases of the Respiratory System (J00-J99)**
   a. **Chronic Obstructive Pulmonary Disease [COPD] and Asthma**
      1) **Acute exacerbation of chronic obstructive bronchitis and asthma**
      The codes in categories J44 and J45 distinguish between uncomplicated cases and those in acute exacerbation. An acute exacerbation is a worsening or a decompensation of a chronic condition. An acute exacerbation is not equivalent to an infection superimposed on a chronic condition, though an exacerbation may be triggered by an infection.

   b. **Acute Respiratory Failure**
      1) **Acute respiratory failure as principal diagnosis**
      A code from subcategory J96.0, Acute respiratory failure, or subcategory J96.2, Acute and chronic respiratory failure, may be assigned as a principal diagnosis when it is the condition established after study to be chiefly responsible for occasioning the admission to the hospital, and the selection is supported by the Alphabetic Index and Tabular List. However, chapter-specific coding guidelines (such as obstetrics, poisoning, HIV, newborn) that provide sequencing direction take precedence.

      2) **Acute respiratory failure as secondary diagnosis**
      Respiratory failure may be listed as a secondary diagnosis if it occurs after admission, or if it is present on admission, but does not meet the definition of principal diagnosis.

      3) **Sequencing of acute respiratory failure and another acute condition**
      When a patient is admitted with respiratory failure and another acute condition, (e.g., myocardial infarction, cerebrovascular accident, aspiration pneumonia), the principal diagnosis will not be the same in every situation. This applies whether the other acute condition is a respiratory or nonrespiratory condition. Selection of the principal diagnosis will be dependent on the circumstances of admission. If both the respiratory failure and the other acute condition are equally responsible for occasioning the admission to the hospital, and there are no chapter-specific sequencing rules, the guideline regarding two or more diagnoses that equally meet the definition for principal diagnosis *(Section II, C.)* may be applied in these situations.

      If the documentation is not clear as to whether acute respiratory failure and another condition are equally responsible for occasioning the admission, query the provider for clarification.

   c. **Influenza due to certain identified influenza viruses**
   Code only confirmed cases of influenza due to certain identified influenza viruses (category J09), and due to other identified influenza virus (category J10). This is an exception to the hospital inpatient guideline Section II, H. (Uncertain Diagnosis).

   In this context, "confirmation" does not require documentation of positive laboratory testing specific for avian or other novel influenza A or other identified influenza virus. However, coding should be based on the provider's diagnostic statement that the patient has avian influenza, or other novel influenza A, for category J09, or has another particular identified strain of influenza, such as H1N1 or H3N2, but not identified as novel or variant, for category J10.

   If the provider records "suspected" or "possible" or "probable" avian influenza, or novel influenza, or other identified influenza, then the appropriate influenza code from category J11, Influenza due to unidentified influenza virus, should be assigned. A code from category J09, Influenza due to certain identified influenza viruses, should not be assigned nor should a code from category J10, Influenza due to other identified influenza virus.

   d. **Ventilator associated Pneumonia**
      1) **Documentation of Ventilator associated Pneumonia**
      As with all procedural or postprocedural complications, code assignment is based on the provider's documentation of the relationship between the condition and the procedure.

      Code J95.851, Ventilator associated pneumonia, should be assigned only when the provider has documented ventilator associated pneumonia (VAP). An additional code to identify the organism (e.g., Pseudomonas aeruginosa, code B96.5) should also be assigned. Do not assign an additional code from categories J12-J18 to identify the type of pneumonia.

      Code J95.851 should not be assigned for cases where the patient has pneumonia and is on a mechanical ventilator and the provider has not specifically stated that the pneumonia is ventilator-associated pneumonia. If the documentation is unclear as to whether the patient has a pneumonia that is a complication attributable to the mechanical ventilator, query the provider.

      2) **Ventilator associated Pneumonia Develops after Admission**
      A patient may be admitted with one type of pneumonia (e.g., code J13, Pneumonia due to Streptococcus pneumonia) and subsequently develop VAP. In this instance, the principal diagnosis would be the appropriate code from categories J12-J18 for the pneumonia diagnosed at the time of admission. Code J95.851, Ventilator associated pneumonia, would be assigned as an additional diagnosis when the provider has also documented the presence of ventilator associated pneumonia.

11. **Chapter 11: Diseases of the Digestive System (K00-K95)**
   Reserved for future guideline expansion

12. **Chapter 12: Diseases of the Skin and Subcutaneous Tissue (L00-L99)**
   a. **Pressure ulcer stage codes**
      1) **Pressure ulcer stages**
      Codes from category L89, Pressure ulcer, identify the site of the pressure ulcer as well as the stage of the ulcer.

      The ICD-10-CM classifies pressure ulcer stages based on severity, which is designated by stages 1-4, unspecified stage and unstageable.

      Assign as many codes from category L89 as needed to identify all the pressure ulcers the patient has, if applicable.

      2) **Unstageable pressure ulcers**
      Assignment of the code for unstageable pressure ulcer (L89.--0) should be based on the clinical documentation. These codes are used for pressure ulcers whose stage cannot be clinically determined (e.g., the ulcer is covered by eschar or has been treated with a skin or muscle graft) and pressure ulcers that are documented as deep tissue injury but not documented as due to trauma. This code should not be confused with the codes for unspecified stage (L89.--9). When there is no documentation regarding the stage of the pressure ulcer, assign the appropriate code for unspecified stage (L89.--9).

      3) **Documented pressure ulcer stage**
      Assignment of the pressure ulcer stage code should be guided by clinical documentation of the stage or documentation of the terms found in the Alphabetic Index. For clinical terms describing the stage that are not found in the Alphabetic Index, and there is no documentation of the stage, the provider should be queried.

      4) **Patients admitted with pressure ulcers documented as healed**
      No code is assigned if the documentation states that the pressure ulcer is completely healed.

      5) **Patients admitted with pressure ulcers documented as healing**
      Pressure ulcers described as healing should be assigned the appropriate pressure ulcer stage code based on the documentation in the medical record. If the documentation does not provide information about the stage of the healing pressure ulcer, assign the appropriate code for unspecified stage.

      If the documentation is unclear as to whether the patient has a current (new) pressure ulcer or if the patient is being treated for a healing pressure ulcer, query the provider.

      For ulcers that were present on admission but healed at the time of discharge, assign the code for the site and stage of the pressure ulcer at the time of admission.

6) Patient admitted with pressure ulcer evolving into another stage during the admission

If a patient is admitted with a pressure ulcer at one stage and it progresses to a higher stage, two separate codes should be assigned: one code for the site and stage of the ulcer on admission and a second code for the same ulcer site and the highest stage reported during the stay.

13. Chapter 13: Diseases of the Musculoskeletal System and Connective Tissue (M00-M99)

a. Site and laterality

Most of the codes within Chapter 13 have site and laterality designations. The site represents the bone, joint or the muscle involved. For some conditions where more than one bone, joint or muscle is usually involved, such as osteoarthritis, there is a "multiple sites" code available. For categories where no multiple site code is provided and more than one bone, joint or muscle is involved, multiple codes should be used to indicate the different sites involved.

1) Bone versus joint

For certain conditions, the bone may be affected at the upper or lower end, (e.g., avascular necrosis of bone, M87, Osteoporosis, M80, M81). Though the portion of the bone affected may be at the joint, the site designation will be the bone, not the joint.

b. Acute traumatic versus chronic or recurrent musculoskeletal conditions

Many musculoskeletal conditions are a result of previous injury or trauma to a site, or are recurrent conditions. Bone, joint or muscle conditions that are the result of a healed injury are usually found in chapter 13. Recurrent bone, joint or muscle conditions are also usually found in chapter 13. Any current, acute injury should be coded to the appropriate injury code from chapter 19. Chronic or recurrent conditions should generally be coded with a code from chapter 13. If it is difficult to determine from the documentation in the record which code is best to describe a condition, query the provider.

c. Coding of Pathologic Fractures

7th character A is for use as long as the patient is receiving active treatment for the fracture. While the patient may be seen by a new or different provider over the course of treatment for a pathological fracture, assignment of the 7th character is based on whether the patient is undergoing active treatment and not whether the provider is seeing the patient for the first time.

7th character D is to be used for encounters after the patient has completed active treatment. The other 7th characters, listed under each subcategory in the Tabular List, are to be used for subsequent encounters for routine care of fractures during the healing and recovery phase as well as treatment of problems associated with the healing, such as malunions, nonunions, and sequelae.

Care for complications of surgical treatment for fracture repairs during the healing or recovery phase should be coded with the appropriate complication codes.

See Section I.C.19. Coding of traumatic fractures.

d. Osteoporosis

Osteoporosis is a systemic condition, meaning that all bones of the musculoskeletal system are affected. Therefore, site is not a component of the codes under category M81, Osteoporosis without current pathological fracture. The site codes under category M80, Osteoporosis with current pathological fracture, identify the site of the fracture, not the osteoporosis.

1) Osteoporosis without pathological fracture

Category M81, Osteoporosis without current pathological fracture, is for use for patients with osteoporosis who do not currently have a pathologic fracture due to the osteoporosis, even if they have had a fracture in the past. For patients with a history of osteoporosis fractures, status code Z87.310, Personal history of (healed) osteoporosis fracture, should follow the code from M81.

2) Osteoporosis with current pathological fracture

Category M80, Osteoporosis with current pathological fracture, is for patients who have a current pathologic fracture at the time of an encounter. The codes under M80 identify the site of the fracture. A code from category M80, not a traumatic fracture

code, should be used for any patient with known osteoporosis who suffers a fracture, even if the patient had a minor fall or trauma, if that fall or trauma would not usually break a normal, healthy bone.

14. Chapter 14: Diseases of Genitourinary System (N00-N99)

a. Chronic kidney disease

1) Stages of chronic kidney disease (CKD)

The ICD-10-CM classifies CKD based on severity. The severity of CKD is designated by stages 1-5. Stage 2, code N18.2, equates to mild CKD; stage 3, code N18.3, equates to moderate CKD; and stage 4, code N18.4, equates to severe CKD. Code N18.6, End stage renal disease (ESRD), is assigned when the provider has documented end-stage-renal disease (ESRD).

If both a stage of CKD and ESRD are documented, assign code N18.6 only.

2) Chronic kidney disease and kidney transplant status

Patients who have undergone kidney transplant may still have some form of chronic kidney disease (CKD) because the kidney transplant may not fully restore kidney function. Therefore, the presence of CKD alone does not constitute a transplant complication. Assign the appropriate N18 code for the patient's stage of CKD and code Z94.0, Kidney transplant status. If a transplant complication such as failure or rejection or other transplant complication is documented, see section I.C.19.g for information on coding complications of a kidney transplant. If the documentation is unclear as to whether the patient has a complication of the transplant, query the provider.

3) Chronic kidney disease with other conditions

Patients with CKD may also suffer from other serious conditions, most commonly diabetes mellitus and hypertension. The sequencing of the CKD code in relationship to codes for other contributing conditions is based on the conventions in the Tabular List.

See I.C.9. Hypertensive chronic kidney disease.

See I.C.19. Chronic kidney disease and kidney transplant complications.

15. Chapter 15: Pregnancy, Childbirth, and the Puerperium (O00-O9A)

a. General Rules for Obstetric Cases

1) Codes from chapter 15 and sequencing priority

Obstetric cases require codes from chapter 15, codes in the range O00-O9A, Pregnancy, Childbirth, and the Puerperium. Chapter 15 codes have sequencing priority over codes from other chapters. Additional codes from other chapters may be used in conjunction with chapter 15 codes to further specify conditions. Should the provider document that the pregnancy is incidental to the encounter, then code Z33.1, Pregnant state, incidental, should be used in place of any chapter 15 codes. It is the provider's responsibility to state that the condition being treated is not affecting the pregnancy.

2) Chapter 15 codes used only on the maternal record

Chapter 15 codes are to be used only on the maternal record, never on the record of the newborn.

3) Final character for trimester

The majority of codes in Chapter 15 have a final character indicating the trimester of pregnancy. The timeframes for the trimesters are indicated at the beginning of the chapter. If trimester is not a component of a code, it is because the condition always occurs in a specific trimester, or the concept of trimester of pregnancy is not applicable. Certain codes have characters for only certain trimesters because the condition does not occur in all trimesters, but it may occur in more than just one. Assignment of the final character for trimester should be based on the provider's documentation of the trimester (or number of weeks) for the current admission/encounter. This applies to the assignment of trimester for pre-existing conditions as well as those that develop during or are due to the pregnancy. The provider's documentation of the number of weeks may be used to assign the appropriate code identifying the trimester.

Whenever delivery occurs during the current admission, and there is an "in childbirth" option for the obstetric complication being coded, the "in childbirth" code should be assigned.

4) Selection of trimester for inpatient admissions that encompass more than one trimester

In instances when a patient is admitted to a hospital for complications of pregnancy during one trimester and remains in the hospital into a subsequent trimester, the trimester character for the antepartum complication code should be assigned on the basis of the trimester when the complication developed, not the trimester of the discharge. If the condition developed prior to the current admission/encounter or represents a pre-existing condition, the trimester character for the trimester at the time of the admission/encounter should be assigned.

5) Unspecified trimester

Each category that includes codes for trimester has a code for "unspecified trimester." The "unspecified trimester" code should rarely be used, such as when the documentation in the record is insufficient to determine the trimester and it is not possible to obtain clarification.

6) 7th character for Fetus Identification

Where applicable, a 7th character is to be assigned for certain categories (O31, O32, O33.3 - O33.6, O35, O36, O40, O41, O60.1, O60.2, O64, and O69) to identify the fetus for which the complication code applies.

Assign 7th character "Ø":

- For single gestations
- When the documentation in the record is insufficient to determine the fetus affected and it is not possible to obtain clarification.
- When it is not possible to clinically determine which fetus is affected.

b. Selection of OB Principal or First-listed Diagnosis

1) Routine outpatient prenatal visits

For routine outpatient prenatal visits when no complications are present, a code from category Z34, Encounter for supervision of normal pregnancy, should be used as the first-listed diagnosis. These codes should not be used in conjunction with chapter 15 codes.

2) Supervision of High-Risk Pregnancy

Codes from category O09, Supervision of high-risk pregnancy, are intended for use only during the prenatal period. For complications during the labor or delivery episode as a result of a high-risk pregnancy, assign the applicable complication codes from Chapter 15. If there are no complications during the labor or delivery episode, assign code O80, Encounter for full-term uncomplicated delivery.

For routine prenatal outpatient visits for patients with high-risk pregnancies, a code from category O09, Supervision of high-risk pregnancy, should be used as the first-listed diagnosis. Secondary chapter 15 codes may be used in conjunction with these codes if appropriate.

3) Episodes when no delivery occurs

In episodes when no delivery occurs, the principal diagnosis should correspond to the principal complication of the pregnancy which necessitated the encounter. Should more than one complication exist, all of which are treated or monitored, any of the complications codes may be sequenced first.

4) When a delivery occurs

When an obstetric patient is admitted and delivers during that admission, the condition that prompted the admission should be sequenced as the principal diagnosis. If multiple conditions prompted the admission, sequence the one most related to the delivery as the principal diagnosis. A code for any complication of the delivery should be assigned as an additional diagnosis. In cases of cesarean delivery, if the patient was admitted with a condition that resulted in the performance of a cesarean procedure, that condition should be selected as the principal diagnosis. If the reason for the admission was unrelated to the condition resulting in the cesarean delivery, the condition related to the reason for the admission should be selected as the principal diagnosis.

5) Outcome of delivery

A code from category Z37, Outcome of delivery, should be included on every maternal record when a delivery has occurred. These codes are not to be used on subsequent records or on the newborn record.

c. Pre-existing conditions versus conditions due to the pregnancy

Certain categories in Chapter 15 distinguish between conditions of the mother that existed prior to pregnancy (pre-existing) and those that are a direct result of pregnancy. When assigning codes from Chapter 15, it is important to assess if a condition was pre-existing prior to pregnancy or developed during or due to the pregnancy in order to assign the correct code.

Categories that do not distinguish between pre-existing and pregnancy-related conditions may be used for either. It is acceptable to use codes specifically for the puerperium with codes complicating pregnancy and childbirth if a condition arises postpartum during the delivery encounter.

d. Pre-existing hypertension in pregnancy

Category O10, Pre-existing hypertension complicating pregnancy, childbirth and the puerperium, includes codes for hypertensive heart and hypertensive chronic kidney disease. When assigning one of the O10 codes that includes hypertensive heart disease or hypertensive chronic kidney disease, it is necessary to add a secondary code from the appropriate hypertension category to specify the type of heart failure or chronic kidney disease.

See Section I.C.9. Hypertension.

e. Fetal Conditions Affecting the Management of the Mother

1) Codes from categories O35 and O36

Codes from categories O35, Maternal care for known or suspected fetal abnormality and damage, and O36, Maternal care for other fetal problems, are assigned only when the fetal condition is actually responsible for modifying the management of the mother, i.e., by requiring diagnostic studies, additional observation, special care, or termination of pregnancy. The fact that the fetal condition exists does not justify assigning a code from this series to the mother's record.

2) In utero surgery

In cases when surgery is performed on the fetus, a diagnosis code from category O35, Maternal care for known or suspected fetal abnormality and damage, should be assigned identifying the fetal condition. Assign the appropriate procedure code for the procedure performed.

No code from Chapter 16, the perinatal codes, should be used on the mother's record to identify fetal conditions. Surgery performed in utero on a fetus is still to be coded as an obstetric encounter.

f. HIV Infection in Pregnancy, Childbirth and the Puerperium

During pregnancy, childbirth or the puerperium, a patient admitted because of an HIV-related illness should receive a principal diagnosis from subcategory O98.7-, Human immunodeficiency [HIV] disease complicating pregnancy, childbirth and the puerperium, followed by the code(s) for the HIV-related illness(es).

Patients with asymptomatic HIV infection status admitted during pregnancy, childbirth, or the puerperium should receive codes of O98.7- and Z21, Asymptomatic human immunodeficiency virus [HIV] infection status.

g. Diabetes mellitus in pregnancy

Diabetes mellitus is a significant complicating factor in pregnancy. Pregnant women who are diabetic should be assigned a code from category O24, Diabetes mellitus in pregnancy, childbirth, and the puerperium, first, followed by the appropriate diabetes code(s) (E08-E13) from Chapter 4.

h. Long term use of insulin and oral hypoglycemics

Code Z79.4, Long-term (current) use of insulin, or code Z79.84, Long-term (current) use of oral hypoglycemic drugs, should also be assigned if the diabetes mellitus is being treated with insulin or oral medications. If the patient is treated with both oral medications and insulin, only the code for insulin-controlled should be assigned.

i. **Gestational (pregnancy induced) diabetes**

Gestational (pregnancy induced) diabetes can occur during the second and third trimester of pregnancy in women who were not diabetic prior to pregnancy. Gestational diabetes can cause complications in the pregnancy similar to those of pre-existing diabetes mellitus. It also puts the woman at greater risk of developing diabetes after the pregnancy. Codes for gestational diabetes are in subcategory O24.4, Gestational diabetes mellitus. No other code from category O24, Diabetes mellitus in pregnancy, childbirth, and the puerperium, should be used with a code from O24.4.

The codes under subcategory O24.4 include diet controlled, insulin controlled, and controlled by oral hypoglycemic drugs. If a patient with gestational diabetes is treated with both diet and insulin, only the code for insulin-controlled is required. If a patient with gestational diabetes is treated with both diet and oral hypoglycemic medications, only the code for "controlled by oral hypoglycemic drugs" is required. Code Z79.4, Long-term (current) use of insulin or code Z79.84, Long-term (current) use of oral hypoglycemic drugs, should not be assigned with codes from subcategory O24.4.

An abnormal glucose tolerance in pregnancy is assigned a code from subcategory O99.81, Abnormal glucose complicating pregnancy, childbirth, and the puerperium.

j. **Sepsis and septic shock complicating abortion, pregnancy, childbirth and the puerperium**

When assigning a chapter 15 code for sepsis complicating abortion, pregnancy, childbirth, and the puerperium, a code for the specific type of infection should be assigned as an additional diagnosis. If severe sepsis is present, a code from subcategory R65.2, Severe sepsis, and code(s) for associated organ dysfunction(s) should also be assigned as additional diagnoses.

k. **Puerperal sepsis**

Code O85, Puerperal sepsis, should be assigned with a secondary code to identify the causal organism (e.g., for a bacterial infection, assign a code from category B95-B96, Bacterial infections in conditions classified elsewhere). A code from category A40, Streptococcal sepsis, or A41, Other sepsis, should not be used for puerperal sepsis. If applicable, use additional codes to identify severe sepsis (R65.2-) and any associated acute organ dysfunction.

l. **Alcohol and tobacco use during pregnancy, childbirth and the puerperium**

1) **Alcohol use during pregnancy, childbirth and the puerperium**

Codes under subcategory O99.31, Alcohol use complicating pregnancy, childbirth, and the puerperium, should be assigned for any pregnancy case when a mother uses alcohol during the pregnancy or postpartum. A secondary code from category F10, Alcohol related disorders, should also be assigned to identify manifestations of the alcohol use.

2) **Tobacco use during pregnancy, childbirth and the puerperium**

Codes under subcategory O99.33, Smoking (tobacco) complicating pregnancy, childbirth, and the puerperium, should be assigned for any pregnancy case when a mother uses any type of tobacco product during the pregnancy or postpartum. A secondary code from category F17, Nicotine dependence, should also be assigned to identify the type of nicotine dependence.

m. **Poisoning, toxic effects, adverse effects and underdosing in a pregnant patient**

A code from subcategory O9A.2, Injury, poisoning and certain other consequences of external causes complicating pregnancy, childbirth, and the puerperium, should be sequenced first, followed by the appropriate injury, poisoning, toxic effect, adverse effect or underdosing code, and then the additional code(s) that specifies the condition caused by the poisoning, toxic effect, adverse effect or underdosing.

See Section I.C.19. Adverse effects, poisoning, underdosing and toxic effects.

n. **Normal Delivery, Code O80**

1) **Encounter for full term uncomplicated delivery**

Code O80 should be assigned when a woman is admitted for a full-term normal delivery and delivers a single, healthy infant without any complications antepartum, during the delivery, or postpartum during the delivery episode. Code O80 is always a principal diagnosis. It is not to be used if any other code from chapter 15 is needed to describe a current complication of the antenatal, delivery, or perinatal period. Additional codes from other chapters may be used with code O80 if they are not related to or are in any way complicating the pregnancy.

2) **Uncomplicated delivery with resolved antepartum complication**

Code O80 may be used if the patient had a complication at some point during the pregnancy, but the complication is not present at the time of the admission for delivery.

3) **Outcome of delivery for O80**

Z37.0, Single live birth, is the only outcome of delivery code appropriate for use with O80.

o. **The Peripartum and Postpartum Periods**

1) **Peripartum and Postpartum periods**

The postpartum period begins immediately after delivery and continues for six weeks following delivery. The peripartum period is defined as the last month of pregnancy to five months postpartum.

2) **Peripartum and postpartum complication**

A postpartum complication is any complication occurring within the six-week period.

3) **Pregnancy-related complications after 6 week period**

Chapter 15 codes may also be used to describe pregnancy-related complications after the peripartum or postpartum period if the provider documents that a condition is pregnancy related.

4) **Admission for routine postpartum care following delivery outside hospital**

When the mother delivers outside the hospital prior to admission and is admitted for routine postpartum care and no complications are noted, code Z39.0, Encounter for care and examination of mother immediately after delivery, should be assigned as the principal diagnosis.

5) **Pregnancy associated cardiomyopathy**

Pregnancy associated cardiomyopathy, code O90.3, is unique in that it may be diagnosed in the third trimester of pregnancy but may continue to progress months after delivery. For this reason, it is referred to as peripartum cardiomyopathy. Code O90.3 is only for use when the cardiomyopathy develops as a result of pregnancy in a woman who did not have pre-existing heart disease.

p. **Code O94, Sequelae of complication of pregnancy, childbirth, and the puerperium**

1) **Code O94**

Code O94, Sequelae of complication of pregnancy, childbirth, and the puerperium, is for use in those cases when an initial complication of a pregnancy develops a sequelae requiring care or treatment at a future date.

2) **After the initial postpartum period**

This code may be used at any time after the initial postpartum period.

3) **Sequencing of Code O94**

This code, like all sequela codes, is to be sequenced following the code describing the sequelae of the complication.

q. **Termination of Pregnancy and Spontaneous abortions**

1) **Abortion with Liveborn Fetus**

When an attempted termination of pregnancy results in a liveborn fetus, assign code Z33.2, Encounter for elective termination of pregnancy and a code from category Z37, Outcome of Delivery.

2) **Retained Products of Conception following an abortion**

Subsequent encounters for retained products of conception following a spontaneous abortion or elective termination of pregnancy are assigned the appropriate code from category

OØ3, Spontaneous abortion, or codes OØ7.4, Failed attempted termination of pregnancy without complication and codes Z33.2, Encounter for elective termination of pregnancy. This advice is appropriate even when the patient was discharged previously with a discharge diagnosis of complete abortion.

3) Complications leading to abortion
Codes from Chapter 15 may be used as additional codes to identify any documented complications of the pregnancy in conjunction with codes in categories in OØ7 and OØ8.

r. Abuse in a pregnant patient
For suspected or confirmed cases of abuse of a pregnant patient, a code(s) from subcategories O9A.3, Physical abuse complicating pregnancy, childbirth, and the puerperium, O9A.4, Sexual abuse complicating pregnancy, childbirth, and the puerperium, and O9A.5, Psychological abuse complicating pregnancy, childbirth, and the puerperium, should be sequenced first, followed by the appropriate codes (if applicable) to identify any associated current injury due to physical abuse, sexual abuse, and the perpetrator of abuse.

See Section I.C.19. Adult and child abuse, neglect and other maltreatment.

16. Chapter 16: Certain Conditions Originating in the Perinatal Period (PØØ-P96)
For coding and reporting purposes the perinatal period is defined as before birth through the 28th day following birth. The following guidelines are provided for reporting purposes.

a. General Perinatal Rules
1) Use of Chapter 16 Codes
Codes in this chapter are never for use on the maternal record. Codes from Chapter 15, the obstetric chapter, are never permitted on the newborn record. Chapter 16 codes may be used throughout the life of the patient if the condition is still present.

2) Principal Diagnosis for Birth Record
When coding the birth episode in a newborn record, assign a code from category Z38, Liveborn infants according to place of birth and type of delivery, as the principal diagnosis. A code from category Z38 is assigned only once, to a newborn at the time of birth. If a newborn is transferred to another institution, a code from category Z38 should not be used at the receiving hospital.

A code from category Z38 is used only on the newborn record, not on the mother's record.

3) Use of Codes from other Chapters with Codes from Chapter 16
Codes from other chapters may be used with codes from chapter 16 if the codes from the other chapters provide more specific detail. Codes for signs and symptoms may be assigned when a definitive diagnosis has not been established. If the reason for the encounter is a perinatal condition, the code from chapter 16 should be sequenced first.

4) Use of Chapter 16 Codes after the Perinatal Period
Should a condition originate in the perinatal period, and continue throughout the life of the patient, the perinatal code should continue to be used regardless of the patient's age.

5) Birth process or community acquired conditions
If a newborn has a condition that may be either due to the birth process or community acquired and the documentation does not indicate which it is, the default is due to the birth process and the code from Chapter 16 should be used. If the condition is community-acquired, a code from Chapter 16 should not be assigned.

6) Code all clinically significant conditions
All clinically significant conditions noted on routine newborn examination should be coded. A condition is clinically significant if it requires:

- clinical evaluation; or
- therapeutic treatment; or
- diagnostic procedures; or
- extended length of hospital stay; or
- increased nursing care and/or monitoring; or
- has implications for future health care needs

Note: The perinatal guidelines listed above are the same as the general coding guidelines for "additional diagnoses", except for the final point regarding implications for future health care needs. Codes should be assigned for conditions that have been specified by the provider as having implications for future health care needs.

b. Observation and Evaluation of Newborns for Suspected Conditions not Found
1)
Assign a code from category Z05, Observation and evaluation of newborns and infants for suspected conditions ruled out, to identify those instances when a healthy newborn is evaluated for a suspected condition that is determined after study not to be present. Do not use a code from category Z05 when the patient has identified signs or symptoms of a suspected problem; in such cases code the sign or symptom.

2)
A code from category Z05 may also be assigned as a principal or first-listed code for readmissions or encounters when the code from category Z38 code no longer applies. Codes from category Z05 are for use only for healthy newborns and infants for which no condition after study is found to be present.

3) Z05 on a birth record
A code from category Z05 is to be used as a secondary code after the code from category Z38, Liveborn infants according to place of birth and type of delivery.

c. Coding Additional Perinatal Diagnoses
1) Assigning codes for conditions that require treatment
Assign codes for conditions that require treatment or further investigation, prolong the length of stay, or require resource utilization.

2) Codes for conditions specified as having implications for future health care needs
Assign codes for conditions that have been specified by the provider as having implications for future health care needs.

Note: This guideline should not be used for adult patients.

d. Prematurity and Fetal Growth Retardation
Providers utilize different criteria in determining prematurity. A code for prematurity should not be assigned unless it is documented. Assignment of codes in categories PØ5, Disorders of newborn related to slow fetal growth and fetal malnutrition, and PØ7, Disorders of newborn related to short gestation and low birth weight, not elsewhere classified, should be based on the recorded birth weight and estimated gestational age. Codes from category PØ5 should not be assigned with codes from category PØ7.

When both birth weight and gestational age are available, two codes from category PØ7 should be assigned, with the code for birth weight sequenced before the code for gestational age.

e. Low birth weight and immaturity status
Codes from category PØ7, Disorders of newborn related to short gestation and low birth weight, not elsewhere classified, are for use for a child or adult who was premature or had a low birth weight as a newborn and this is affecting the patient's current health status.

See Section I.C.21. Factors influencing health status and contact with health services, Status.

f. Bacterial Sepsis of Newborn
Category P36, Bacterial sepsis of newborn, includes congenital sepsis. If a perinate is documented as having sepsis without documentation of congenital or community acquired, the default is congenital and a code from category P36 should be assigned. If the P36 code includes the causal organism, an additional code from category B95, Streptococcus, Staphylococcus, and Enterococcus as the cause of diseases classified elsewhere, or B96, Other bacterial agents as the cause of diseases classified elsewhere, should not be assigned. If the P36 code does not include the causal organism, assign an additional code from category B96. If applicable, use additional codes to identify severe sepsis (R65.2-) and any associated acute organ dysfunction.

g. **Stillbirth**
Code P95, Stillbirth, is only for use in institutions that maintain separate records for stillbirths. No other code should be used with P95. Code P95 should not be used on the mother's record.

17. **Chapter 17: Congenital malformations, deformations, and chromosomal abnormalities (Q00-Q99)**
Assign an appropriate code(s) from categories Q00-Q99, Congenital malformations, deformations, and chromosomal abnormalities when a malformation/deformation or chromosomal abnormality is documented. A malformation/deformation/or chromosomal abnormality may be the principal/first-listed diagnosis on a record or a secondary diagnosis.

When a malformation/deformation or chromosomal abnormality does not have a unique code assignment, assign additional code(s) for any manifestations that may be present.

When the code assignment specifically identifies the malformation/deformation or chromosomal abnormality, manifestations that are an inherent component of the anomaly should not be coded separately. Additional codes should be assigned for manifestations that are not an inherent component.

Codes from Chapter 17 may be used throughout the life of the patient. If a congenital malformation or deformity has been corrected, a personal history code should be used to identify the history of the malformation or deformity. Although present at birth, malformation/deformation/or chromosomal abnormality may not be identified until later in life. Whenever the condition is diagnosed by the physician, it is appropriate to assign a code from codes Q00-Q99.For the birth admission, the appropriate code from category Z38, Liveborn infants, according to place of birth and type of delivery, should be sequenced as the principal diagnosis, followed by any congenital anomaly codes, Q00- Q99.

18. **Chapter 18: Symptoms, signs, and abnormal clinical and laboratory findings, not elsewhere classified (R00-R99)**
Chapter 18 includes symptoms, signs, abnormal results of clinical or other investigative procedures, and ill-defined conditions regarding which no diagnosis classifiable elsewhere is recorded. Signs and symptoms that point to a specific diagnosis have been assigned to a category in other chapters of the classification.

a. **Use of symptom codes**
Codes that describe symptoms and signs are acceptable for reporting purposes when a related definitive diagnosis has not been established (confirmed) by the provider.

b. **Use of a symptom code with a definitive diagnosis code**
Codes for signs and symptoms may be reported in addition to a related definitive diagnosis when the sign or symptom is not routinely associated with that diagnosis, such as the various signs and symptoms associated with complex syndromes. The definitive diagnosis code should be sequenced before the symptom code.

Signs or symptoms that are associated routinely with a disease process should not be assigned as additional codes, unless otherwise instructed by the classification.

c. **Combination codes that include symptoms**
ICD-10-CM contains a number of combination codes that identify both the definitive diagnosis and common symptoms of that diagnosis. When using one of these combination codes, an additional code should not be assigned for the symptom.

d. **Repeated falls**
Code R29.6, Repeated falls, is for use for encounters when a patient has recently fallen and the reason for the fall is being investigated.

Code Z91.81, History of falling, is for use when a patient has fallen in the past and is at risk for future falls. When appropriate, both codes R29.6 and Z91.81 may be assigned together.

e. **Coma scale**
The coma scale codes (R40.2-) can be used in conjunction with traumatic brain injury codes, acute cerebrovascular disease or sequelae of cerebrovascular disease codes. These codes are primarily for use by trauma registries, but they may be used in any setting where this information is collected. The coma scale may also be used to assess the status of the central nervous system for other non-trauma conditions, such as monitoring patients in the intensive care unit regardless of medical condition. The coma scale codes should be sequenced after the diagnosis code(s).

These codes, one from each subcategory, are needed to complete the scale. The 7th character indicates when the scale was recorded. The 7th character should match for all three codes.

At a minimum, report the initial score documented on presentation at your facility. This may be a score from the emergency medicine technician (EMT) or in the emergency department. If desired, a facility may choose to capture multiple coma scale scores.

Assign code R40.24, Glasgow coma scale, total score, when only the total score is documented in the medical record and not the individual score(s).

f. **Functional quadriplegia**
Functional quadriplegia (code R53.2) is the lack of ability to use one's limbs or to ambulate due to extreme debility. It is not associated with neurologic deficit or injury, and code R53.2 should not be used for cases of neurologic quadriplegia. It should only be assigned if functional quadriplegia is specifically documented in the medical record.

g. **SIRS due to Non-Infectious Process**
The systemic inflammatory response syndrome (SIRS) can develop as a result of certain non-infectious disease processes, such as trauma, malignant neoplasm, or pancreatitis. When SIRS is documented with a noninfectious condition, and no subsequent infection is documented, the code for the underlying condition, such as an injury, should be assigned, followed by code R65.10, Systemic inflammatory response syndrome (SIRS) of non-infectious origin without acute organ dysfunction, or code R65.11, Systemic inflammatory response syndrome (SIRS) of non-infectious origin with acute organ dysfunction. If an associated acute organ dysfunction is documented, the appropriate code(s) for the specific type of organ dysfunction(s) should be assigned in addition to code R65.11. If acute organ dysfunction is documented, but it cannot be determined if the acute organ dysfunction is associated with SIRS or due to another condition (e.g., directly due to the trauma), the provider should be queried.

h. **Death NOS**
Code R99, Ill-defined and unknown cause of mortality, is only for use in the very limited circumstance when a patient who has already died is brought into an emergency department or other healthcare facility and is pronounced dead upon arrival. It does not represent the discharge disposition of death.

i. **NIHSS Stroke Scale**
The NIH stroke scale (NIHSS) codes (R29.7- -) can be used in conjunction with acute stroke codes (I63) to identify the patient's neurological status and the severity of the stroke. The stroke scale codes should be sequenced after the acute stroke diagnosis code(s).

At a minimum, report the initial score documented. If desired, a facility may choose to capture multiple stroke scale scores.

See Section I.B.14. for information concerning the medical record documentation that may be used for assignment of the NIHSS codes.

19. **Chapter 19: Injury, poisoning, and certain other consequences of external causes (S00-T88)**
a. **Application of 7th Characters in Chapter 19**
Most categories in chapter 19 have a 7th character requirement for each applicable code. Most categories in this chapter have three 7th character values (with the exception of fractures): A, initial encounter, D, subsequent encounter and S, sequela. Categories for traumatic fractures have additional 7th character values. While the patient may be seen by a new or different provider over the course of treatment for an injury, assignment of the 7th character is based on whether the patient is undergoing active treatment and not whether the provider is seeing the patient for the first time.

For complication codes, active treatment refers to treatment for the condition described by the code, even though it may be related to an earlier precipitating problem. For example, code T84.50XA, Infection and inflammatory reaction due to unspecified internal joint prosthesis, initial encounter, is used when active treatment is provided for the infection, even though the condition relates to the prosthetic device, implant or graft that was placed at a previous encounter.

7th character "A", initial encounter is used for each encounter where the patient is receiving active treatment for the condition.

7th character "D" subsequent encounter is used for encounters after the patient has completed active treatment of the condition and is receiving routine care for the condition during the healing or recovery phase.

The aftercare Z codes should not be used for aftercare for conditions such as injuries or poisonings, where 7th characters are provided to identify subsequent care. For example, for aftercare of an injury, assign the acute injury code with the 7th character "D" (subsequent encounter).

7th character "S", sequela, is for use for complications or conditions that arise as a direct result of a condition, such as scar formation after a burn. The scars are sequelae of the burn. When using 7th character "S", it is necessary to use both the injury code that precipitated the sequela and the code for the sequela itself. The "S" is added only to the injury code, not the sequela code. The 7th character "S" identifies the injury responsible for the sequela. The specific type of sequela (e.g. scar) is sequenced first, followed by the injury code.

See Section I.B.10 Sequelae, (Late Effects)

b.   Coding of Injuries

When coding injuries, assign separate codes for each injury unless a combination code is provided, in which case the combination code is assigned. Code T07, Unspecified multiple injuries should not be assigned in the inpatient setting unless information for a more specific code is not available. Traumatic injury codes (S00-T14.9) are not to be used for normal, healing surgical wounds or to identify complications of surgical wounds.

The code for the most serious injury, as determined by the provider and the focus of treatment, is sequenced first.

1)   Superficial injuries

Superficial injuries such as abrasions or contusions are not coded when associated with more severe injuries of the same site.

2)   Primary injury with damage to nerves/blood vessels

When a primary injury results in minor damage to peripheral nerves or blood vessels, the primary injury is sequenced first with additional code(s) for injuries to nerves and spinal cord (such as category S04), and/or injury to blood vessels (such as category S15). When the primary injury is to the blood vessels or nerves, that injury should be sequenced first.

c.   Coding of Traumatic Fractures

The principles of multiple coding of injuries should be followed in coding fractures. Fractures of specified sites are coded individually by site in accordance with both the provisions within categories S02, S12, S22, S32, S42, S49, S52, S59, S62, S72, S79, S82, S89, S92 and the level of detail furnished by medical record content.

A fracture not indicated as open or closed should be coded to closed. A fracture not indicated whether displaced or not displaced should be coded to displaced.

More specific guidelines are as follows:

1)   Initial vs. Subsequent Encounter for Fractures

Traumatic fractures are coded using the appropriate 7th character for initial encounter (A, B, C) for each encounter where the patient is receiving active treatment for the fracture. The appropriate 7th character for initial encounter should also be assigned for a patient who delayed seeking treatment for the fracture or nonunion.

Fractures are coded using the appropriate 7th character for subsequent care for encounters after the patient has completed active treatment of the fracture and is receiving routine care for the fracture during the healing or recovery phase.

Care for complications of surgical treatment for fracture repairs during the healing or recovery phase should be coded with the appropriate complication codes.

Care of complications of fractures, such as malunion and nonunion, should be reported with the appropriate 7th character for subsequent care with nonunion (K, M, N,) or subsequent care with malunion (P, Q, R).

Malunion/nonunion: The appropriate 7th character for initial encounter should also be assigned for a patient who delayed seeking treatment for the fracture or nonunion.

The open fracture designations in the assignment of the 7th character for fractures of the forearm, femur and lower leg, including ankle are based on the Gustilo open fracture classification. When the Gustilo classification type is not specified for an open fracture, the 7th character for open fracture type I or II should be assigned (B, E, H, M, Q).

A code from category M80, not a traumatic fracture code, should be used for any patient with known osteoporosis who suffers a fracture, even if the patient had a minor fall or trauma, if that fall or trauma would not usually break a normal, healthy bone.

See Section I.C.13. Osteoporosis.

The aftercare Z codes should not be used for aftercare for traumatic fractures. For aftercare of a traumatic fracture, assign the acute fracture code with the appropriate 7th character.

2)   Multiple fractures sequencing

Multiple fractures are sequenced in accordance with the severity of the fracture.

d.   Coding of Burns and Corrosions

The ICD-10-CM makes a distinction between burns and corrosions. The burn codes are for thermal burns, except sunburns, that come from a heat source, such as a fire or hot appliance. The burn codes are also for burns resulting from electricity and radiation. Corrosions are burns due to chemicals. The guidelines are the same for burns and corrosions.

Current burns (T20-T25) are classified by depth, extent and by agent (X code). Burns are classified by depth as first degree (erythema), second degree (blistering), and third degree (full-thickness involvement). Burns of the eye and internal organs (T26-T28) are classified by site, but not by degree.

1)   Sequencing of burn and related condition codes

Sequence first the code that reflects the highest degree of burn when more than one burn is present.

a.   When the reason for the admission or encounter is for treatment of external multiple burns, sequence first the code that reflects the burn of the highest degree.

b.   When a patient has both internal and external burns, the circumstances of admission govern the selection of the principal diagnosis or first-listed diagnosis.

c.   When a patient is admitted for burn injuries and other related conditions such as smoke inhalation and/or respiratory failure, the circumstances of admission govern the selection of the principal or first-listed diagnosis.

2)   Burns of the same local site

Classify burns of the same local site (three-character category level, T20-T28) but of different degrees to the subcategory identifying the highest degree recorded in the diagnosis.

3)   Non-healing burns

Non-healing burns are coded as acute burns.

Necrosis of burned skin should be coded as a non-healed burn.

4)   Infected Burn

For any documented infected burn site, use an additional code for the infection.

5)   Assign separate codes for each burn site

When coding burns, assign separate codes for each burn site. Category T30, Burn and corrosion, body region unspecified is extremely vague and should rarely be used.

6)   Burns and Corrosions Classified According to Extent of Body Surface Involved

Assign codes from category T31, Burns classified according to extent of body surface involved, or T32, Corrosions classified according to extent of body surface involved, when the site of the burn is not specified or when there is a need for additional data. It is advisable to use category T31 as additional coding when needed to provide data for evaluating burn mortality, such as that needed by burn units. It is also advisable to use category T31 as an additional code for reporting purposes when there is mention of a third-degree burn involving 2Ø percent or more of the body surface.

Categories T31 and T32 are based on the classic "rule of nines" in estimating body surface involved: head and neck are assigned nine percent, each arm nine percent, each leg 18 percent, the anterior trunk 18 percent, posterior trunk 18 percent, and genitalia one percent. Providers may change these percentage assignments where necessary to accommodate infants and children who have proportionately larger heads than adults, and patients who have large buttocks, thighs, or abdomen that involve burns.

7) Encounters for treatment of sequela of burns
Encounters for the treatment of the late effects of burns or corrosions (i.e., scars or joint contractures) should be coded with a burn or corrosion code with the 7th character "S" for sequela.

8) Sequelae with a late effect code and current burn
When appropriate, both a code for a current burn or corrosion with 7th character "A" or "D" and a burn or corrosion code with 7th character "S" may be assigned on the same record (when both a current burn and sequelae of an old burn exist). Burns and corrosions do not heal at the same rate and a current healing wound may still exist with sequela of a healed burn or corrosion.

See Section I.B.10 Sequela (Late Effects)

9) Use of an external cause code with burns and corrosions
An external cause code should be used with burns and corrosions to identify the source and intent of the burn, as well as the place where it occurred.

e. Adverse Effects, Poisoning, Underdosing and Toxic Effects
Codes in categories T36-T65 are combination codes that include the substance that was taken as well as the intent. No additional external cause code is required for poisonings, toxic effects, adverse effects and underdosing codes.

1) Do not code directly from the Table of Drugs
Do not code directly from the Table of Drugs and Chemicals. Always refer back to the Tabular List.

2) Use as many codes as necessary to describe
Use as many codes as necessary to describe completely all drugs, medicinal or biological substances.

3) If the same code would describe the causative agent
If the same code would describe the causative agent for more than one adverse reaction, poisoning, toxic effect or underdosing, assign the code only once.

4) If two or more drugs, medicinal or biological substances
If two or more drugs, medicinal or biological substances are reported, code each individually unless a combination code is listed in the Table of Drugs and Chemicals.

5) The occurrence of drug toxicity is classified in ICD-10-CM as follows:
(a) Adverse Effect
When coding an adverse effect of a drug that has been correctly prescribed and properly administered, assign the appropriate code for the nature of the adverse effect followed by the appropriate code for the adverse effect of the drug (T36-T5Ø). The code for the drug should have a 5th or 6th character "5" (for example T36.ØX5-) Examples of the nature of an adverse effect are tachycardia, delirium, gastrointestinal hemorrhaging, vomiting, hypokalemia, hepatitis, renal failure, or respiratory failure.

(b) Poisoning
When coding a poisoning or reaction to the improper use of a medication (e.g., overdose, wrong substance given or taken in error, wrong route of administration), first assign the appropriate code from categories T36-T5Ø. The poisoning codes have an associated intent as their 5th or 6th character (accidental, intentional self-harm, assault and undetermined. If the intent of the poisoning is unknown or unspecified, code the intent as accidental intent. The

undetermined intent is only for use if the documentation in the record specifies that the intent cannot be determined. Use additional code(s) for all manifestations of poisonings.

If there is also a diagnosis of abuse or dependence of the substance, the abuse or dependence is assigned as an additional code.

Examples of poisoning include:

(i) Error was made in drug prescription

Errors made in drug prescription or in the administration of the drug by provider, nurse, patient, or other person.

(ii) Overdose of a drug intentionally taken

If an overdose of a drug was intentionally taken or administered and resulted in drug toxicity, it would be coded as a poisoning.

(iii) Nonprescribed drug taken with correctly prescribed and properly administered drug

If a nonprescribed drug or medicinal agent was taken in combination with a correctly prescribed and properly administered drug, any drug toxicity or other reaction resulting from the interaction of the two drugs would be classified as a poisoning.

(iv) Interaction of drug(s) and alcohol

When a reaction results from the interaction of a drug(s) and alcohol, this would be classified as poisoning.

See Section I.C.4. if poisoning is the result of insulin pump malfunctions.

(c) Underdosing
Underdosing refers to taking less of a medication than is prescribed by a provider or a manufacturer's instruction. For underdosing, assign the code from categories T36-T5Ø (fifth or sixth character "6").

Codes for underdosing should never be assigned as principal or first-listed codes. If a patient has a relapse or exacerbation of the medical condition for which the drug is prescribed because of the reduction in dose, then the medical condition itself should be coded.

Noncompliance (Z91.12-, Z91.13-) or complication of care (Y63.6-Y63.9) codes are to be used with an underdosing code to indicate intent, if known.

(d) Toxic Effects
When a harmful substance is ingested or comes in contact with a person, this is classified as a toxic effect. The toxic effect codes are in categories T51-T65.

Toxic effect codes have an associated intent: accidental, intentional self-harm, assault and undetermined.

f. Adult and child abuse, neglect and other maltreatment
Sequence first the appropriate code from categories T74.- (Adult and child abuse, neglect and other maltreatment, confirmed) or T76.- (Adult and child abuse, neglect and other maltreatment, suspected) for abuse, neglect and other maltreatment, followed by any accompanying mental health or injury code(s).

If the documentation in the medical record states abuse or neglect it is coded as confirmed (T74.-). It is coded as suspected if it is documented as suspected (T76.-).

For cases of confirmed abuse or neglect an external cause code from the assault section (X92-YØ9) should be added to identify the cause of any physical injuries. A perpetrator code (YØ7) should be added when the perpetrator of the abuse is known. For suspected cases of abuse or neglect, do not report external cause or perpetrator code.

If a suspected case of abuse, neglect or mistreatment is ruled out during an encounter code ZØ4.71, Encounter for examination and observation following alleged physical adult abuse, ruled out, or code ZØ4.72, Encounter for examination and observation following alleged child physical abuse, ruled out, should be used, not a code from T76.

If a suspected case of alleged rape or sexual abuse is ruled out during an encounter code Z04.41, Encounter for examination and observation following alleged adult rape or code Z04.42, Encounter for examination and observation following alleged child rape, should be used, not a code from T76.

See Section I.C.15. Abuse in a pregnant patient.

g. **Complications of care**

1) **General guidelines for complications of care**

(a) **Documentation of complications of care**
See Section I.B.16. for information on documentation of complications of care.

2) **Pain due to medical devices**
Pain associated with devices, implants or grafts left in a surgical site (for example painful hip prosthesis) is assigned to the appropriate code(s) found in Chapter 19, Injury, poisoning, and certain other consequences of external causes. Specific codes for pain due to medical devices are found in the T code section of the ICD-10-CM. Use additional code(s) from category G89 to identify acute or chronic pain due to presence of the device, implant or graft (G89.18 or G89.28).

3) **Transplant complications**

(a) **Transplant complications other than kidney**
Codes under category T86, Complications of transplanted organs and tissues, are for use for both complications and rejection of transplanted organs. A transplant complication code is only assigned if the complication affects the function of the transplanted organ. Two codes are required to fully describe a transplant complication: the appropriate code from category T86 and a secondary code that identifies the complication.

Pre-existing conditions or conditions that develop after the transplant are not coded as complications unless they affect the function of the transplanted organs.

See I.C.21. for transplant organ removal status

See I.C.2. for malignant neoplasm associated with transplanted organ.

(b) **Kidney transplant complications**
Patients who have undergone kidney transplant may still have some form of chronic kidney disease (CKD) because the kidney transplant may not fully restore kidney function. Code T86.1- should be assigned for documented complications of a kidney transplant, such as transplant failure or rejection or other transplant complication. Code T86.1- should not be assigned for post kidney transplant patients who have chronic kidney (CKD) unless a transplant complication such as transplant failure or rejection is documented. If the documentation is unclear as to whether the patient has a complication of the transplant, query the provider.

Conditions that affect the function of the transplanted kidney, other than CKD, should be assigned a code from subcategory T86.1, Complications of transplanted organ, Kidney, and a secondary code that identifies the complication.

For patients with CKD following a kidney transplant, but who do not have a complication such as failure or rejection, *see section I.C.14. Chronic kidney disease and kidney transplant status.*

4) **Complication codes that include the external cause**
As with certain other T codes, some of the complications of care codes have the external cause included in the code. The code includes the nature of the complication as well as the type of procedure that caused the complication. No external cause code indicating the type of procedure is necessary for these codes.

5) **Complications of care codes within the body system chapters**
Intraoperative and postprocedural complication codes are found within the body system chapters with codes specific to the organs and structures of that body system. These codes

should be sequenced first, followed by a code(s) for the specific complication, if applicable.

20. **Chapter 20: External Causes of Morbidity (V00-Y99)**
The external causes of morbidity codes should never be sequenced as the first-listed or principal diagnosis.

External cause codes are intended to provide data for injury research and evaluation of injury prevention strategies. These codes capture how the injury or health condition happened (cause), the intent (unintentional or accidental; or intentional, such as suicide or assault), the place where the event occurred the activity of the patient at the time of the event, and the person's status (e.g., civilian, military).

There is no national requirement for mandatory ICD-10-CM external cause code reporting. Unless a provider is subject to a state-based external cause code reporting mandate or these codes are required by a particular payer, reporting of ICD-10-CM codes in Chapter 20, External Causes of Morbidity, is not required. In the absence of a mandatory reporting requirement, providers are encouraged to voluntarily report external cause codes, as they provide valuable data for injury research and evaluation of injury prevention strategies.

a. **General External Cause Coding Guidelines**

1) **Used with any code in the range of A00.0-T88.9, Z00-Z99**
An external cause code may be used with any code in the range of A00.0-T88.9, Z00-Z99, classification that is a health condition due to an external cause. Though they are most applicable to injuries, they are also valid for use with such things as infections or diseases due to an external source, and other health conditions, such as a heart attack that occurs during strenuous physical activity.

2) **External cause code used for length of treatment**
Assign the external cause code, with the appropriate 7th character (initial encounter, subsequent encounter or sequela) for each encounter for which the injury or condition is being treated.

Most categories in chapter 20 have a 7th character requirement for each applicable code. Most categories in this chapter have three 7th character values: A, initial encounter, D, subsequent encounter and S, sequela. While the patient may be seen by a new or different provider over the course of treatment for an injury or condition, assignment of the 7th character for external cause should match the 7th character of the code assigned for the associated injury or condition for the encounter.

3) **Use the full range of external cause codes**
Use the full range of external cause codes to completely describe the cause, the intent, the place of occurrence, and if applicable, the activity of the patient at the time of the event, and the patient's status, for all injuries, and other health conditions due to an external cause.

4) **Assign as many external cause codes as necessary**
Assign as many external cause codes as necessary to fully explain each cause. If only one external code can be recorded, assign the code most related to the principal diagnosis.

5) **The selection of the appropriate external cause code**
The selection of the appropriate external cause code is guided by the Alphabetic Index of External Causes and by Inclusion and Exclusion notes in the Tabular List.

6) **External cause code can never be a principal diagnosis**
An external cause code can never be a principal (first-listed) diagnosis.

7) **Combination external cause codes**
Certain of the external cause codes are combination codes that identify sequential events that result in an injury, such as a fall which results in striking against an object. The injury may be due to either event or both. The combination external cause code used should correspond to the sequence of events regardless of which caused the most serious injury.

8) **No external cause code needed in certain circumstances**
No external cause code from Chapter 20 is needed if the external cause and intent are included in a code from another chapter (e.g. T36.0X1- Poisoning by penicillins, accidental (unintentional)).

b. Place of Occurrence Guideline

Codes from category Y92, Place of occurrence of the external cause, are secondary codes for use after other external cause codes to identify the location of the patient at the time of injury or other condition.

Generally, a place of occurrence code is assigned only once, at the initial encounter for treatment. However, in the rare instance that a new injury occurs during hospitalization, an additional place of occurrence code may be assigned. No 7th characters are used for Y92.

Do not use place of occurrence code Y92.9 if the place is not stated or is not applicable.

c. Activity Code

Assign a code from category Y93, Activity code, to describe the activity of the patient at the time the injury or other health condition occurred.

An activity code is used only once, at the initial encounter for treatment. Only one code from Y93 should be recorded on a medical record.

The activity codes are not applicable to poisonings, adverse effects, misadventures or sequela.

Do not assign Y93.9, Unspecified activity, if the activity is not stated.

A code from category Y93 is appropriate for use with external cause and intent codes if identifying the activity provides additional information about the event.

d. Place of Occurrence, Activity, and Status Codes Used with other External Cause Code

When applicable, place of occurrence, activity, and external cause status codes are sequenced after the main external cause code(s). Regardless of the number of external cause codes assigned, generally there should be only one place of occurrence code, one activity code, and one external cause status code assigned to an encounter. However, in the rare instance that a new injury occurs during hospitalization, an additional place of occurrence code may be assigned.

e. If the Reporting Format Limits the Number of External Cause Codes

If the reporting format limits the number of external cause codes that can be used in reporting clinical data, report the code for the cause/intent most related to the principal diagnosis. If the format permits capture of additional external cause codes, the cause/intent, including medical misadventures, of the additional events should be reported rather than the codes for place, activity, or external status.

f. Multiple External Cause Coding Guidelines

More than one external cause code is required to fully describe the external cause of an illness or injury. The assignment of external cause codes should be sequenced in the following priority:

If two or more events cause separate injuries, an external cause code should be assigned for each cause. The first-listed external cause code will be selected in the following order:

External codes for child and adult abuse take priority over all other external cause codes.

See Section I.C.19., Child and Adult abuse guidelines.

External cause codes for terrorism events take priority over all other external cause codes except child and adult abuse.

External cause codes for cataclysmic events take priority over all other external cause codes except child and adult abuse and terrorism.

External cause codes for transport accidents take priority over all other external cause codes except cataclysmic events, child and adult abuse and terrorism.

Activity and external cause status codes are assigned following all causal (intent) external cause codes.

The first-listed external cause code should correspond to the cause of the most serious diagnosis due to an assault, accident, or self-harm, following the order of hierarchy listed above.

g. Child and Adult Abuse Guideline

Adult and child abuse, neglect and maltreatment are classified as assault. Any of the assault codes may be used to indicate the external cause of any injury resulting from the confirmed abuse.

For confirmed cases of abuse, neglect and maltreatment, when the perpetrator is known, a code from Y07, Perpetrator of maltreatment and neglect, should accompany any other assault codes.

See Section I.C.19. Adult and child abuse, neglect and other maltreatment

h. Unknown or Undetermined Intent Guideline

If the intent (accident, self-harm, assault) of the cause of an injury or other condition is unknown or unspecified, code the intent as accidental intent. All transport accident categories assume accidental intent.

1) Use of undetermined intent

External cause codes for events of undetermined intent are only for use if the documentation in the record specifies that the intent cannot be determined.

i. Sequelae (Late Effects) of External Cause Guidelines

1) Sequelae external cause codes

Sequela are reported using the external cause code with the 7th character "S" for sequela. These codes should be used with any report of a late effect or sequela resulting from a previous injury.

See Section I.B.10 Sequela (Late Effects)

2) Sequela external cause code with a related current injury

A sequela external cause code should never be used with a related current nature of injury code.

3) Use of sequela external cause codes for subsequent visits

Use a late effect external cause code for subsequent visits when a late effect of the initial injury is being treated. Do not use a late effect external cause code for subsequent visits for follow-up care (e.g., to assess healing, to receive rehabilitative therapy) of the injury when no late effect of the injury has been documented.

j. Terrorism Guidelines

1) Cause of injury identified by the Federal Government (FBI) as terrorism

When the cause of an injury is identified by the Federal Government (FBI) as terrorism, the first-listed external cause code should be a code from category Y38, Terrorism. The definition of terrorism employed by the FBI is found at the inclusion note at the beginning of category Y38. Use additional code for place of occurrence (Y92.-). More than one Y38 code may be assigned if the injury is the result of more than one mechanism of terrorism.

2) Cause of an injury is suspected to be the result of terrorism

When the cause of an injury is suspected to be the result of terrorism a code from category Y38 should not be assigned. Suspected cases should be classified as assault.

3) Code Y38.9, Terrorism, secondary effects

Assign code Y38.9, Terrorism, secondary effects, for conditions occurring subsequent to the terrorist event. This code should not be assigned for conditions that are due to the initial terrorist act.

It is acceptable to assign code Y38.9 with another code from Y38 if there is an injury due to the initial terrorist event and an injury that is a subsequent result of the terrorist event.

k. External cause status

A code from category Y99, External cause status, should be assigned whenever any other external cause code is assigned for an encounter, including an Activity code, except for the events noted below. Assign a code from category Y99, External cause status, to indicate the work status of the person at the time the event occurred. The status code indicates whether the event occurred during military activity, whether a non-military person was at work, whether an individual including a student or volunteer was involved in a non-work activity at the time of the causal event.

A code from Y99, External cause status, should be assigned, when applicable, with other external cause codes, such as transport accidents and falls. The external cause status codes are not applicable to poisonings, adverse effects, misadventures or late effects.

Do not assign a code from category Y99 if no other external cause codes (cause, activity) are applicable for the encounter.

An external cause status code is used only once, at the initial encounter for treatment. Only one code from Y99 should be recorded on a medical record.

Do not assign code Y99.9, Unspecified external cause status, if the status is not stated.

21. **Chapter 21: Factors influencing health status and contact with health services (Z00-Z99)**
Note: The chapter specific guidelines provide additional information about the use of Z codes for specified encounters.

a. **Use of Z codes in any healthcare setting**
Z codes are for use in any healthcare setting. Z codes may be used as either a first-listed (principal diagnosis code in the inpatient setting) or secondary code, depending on the circumstances of the encounter. Certain Z codes may only be used as first-listed or principal diagnosis.

b. **Z Codes indicate a reason for an encounter**
Z codes are not procedure codes. A corresponding procedure code must accompany a Z code to describe any procedure performed.

c. **Categories of Z Codes**
1) **Contact/Exposure**
Category Z20 indicates contact with, and suspected exposure to, communicable diseases. These codes are for patients who do not show any sign or symptom of a disease but are suspected to have been exposed to it by close personal contact with an infected individual or are in an area where a disease is epidemic.

Category Z77, Other contact with and (suspected) exposures hazardous to health, indicates contact with and suspected exposures hazardous to health.

Contact/exposure codes may be used as a first-listed code to explain an encounter for testing, or, more commonly, as a secondary code to identify a potential risk.

2) **Inoculations and vaccinations**
Code Z23 is for encounters for inoculations and vaccinations. It indicates that a patient is being seen to receive a prophylactic inoculation against a disease. Procedure codes are required to identify the actual administration of the injection and the type(s) of immunizations given. Code Z23 may be used as a secondary code if the inoculation is given as a routine part of preventive health care, such as a well-baby visit.

3) **Status**
Status codes indicate that a patient is either a carrier of a disease or has the sequelae or residual of a past disease or condition. This includes such things as the presence of prosthetic or mechanical devices resulting from past treatment. A status code is informative, because the status may affect the course of treatment and its outcome. A status code is distinct from a history code. The history code indicates that the patient no longer has the condition.

A status code should not be used with a diagnosis code from one of the body system chapters, if the diagnosis code includes the information provided by the status code. For example, code Z94.1, Heart transplant status, should not be used with a code from subcategory T86.2, Complications of heart transplant. The status code does not provide additional information. The complication code indicates that the patient is a heart transplant patient.

For encounters for weaning from a mechanical ventilator, assign a code from subcategory J96.1, Chronic respiratory failure, followed by code Z99.11, Dependence on respirator [ventilator] status.

The status Z codes/categories are:

Z14 Genetic carrier
Genetic carrier status indicates that a person carries a gene, associated with a particular disease, which may be passed to offspring who may develop that disease. The person does not have the disease and is not at risk of developing the disease.

Z15 Genetic susceptibility to disease
Genetic susceptibility indicates that a person has a gene that increases the risk of that person developing the disease.

Codes from category Z15 should not be used as principal or first-listed codes. If the patient has the condition to which he/she is susceptible, and that condition is the reason for the encounter, the code for the current condition should be sequenced first. If the patient is being seen for follow-up after completed treatment for this condition, and the condition no longer exists, a follow-up code should be sequenced first, followed by the appropriate personal history and genetic susceptibility codes. If the purpose of the encounter is genetic counseling associated with procreative management, code Z31.5, Encounter for genetic counseling, should be assigned as the first-listed code, followed by a code from category Z15. Additional codes should be assigned for any applicable family or personal history.

Z16 Resistance to antimicrobial drugs
This code indicates that a patient has a condition that is resistant to antimicrobial drug treatment. Sequence the infection code first.

Z17 Estrogen receptor status

Z18 Retained foreign body fragments

Z19 Hormone sensitivity malignancy status

Z21 Asymptomatic HIV infection status
This code indicates that a patient has tested positive for HIV but has manifested no signs or symptoms of the disease.

Z22 Carrier of infectious disease
Carrier status indicates that a person harbors the specific organisms of a disease without manifest symptoms and is capable of transmitting the infection.

Z28.3 Underimmunization status

Z33.1 Pregnant state, incidental
This code is a secondary code only for use when the pregnancy is in no way complicating the reason for visit. Otherwise, a code from the obstetric chapter is required.

Z66 Do not resuscitate
This code may be used when it is documented by the provider that a patient is on do not resuscitate status at any time during the stay.

Z67 Blood type

Z68 Body mass index (BMI)
As with all other secondary diagnosis codes, the BMI codes should only be assigned when they meet the definition of a reportable diagnosis (see Section III, Reporting Additional Diagnoses).

Z74.01 Bed confinement status

Z76.82 Awaiting organ transplant status

Z78 Other specified health status
Code Z78.1, Physical restraint status, may be used when it is documented by the provider that a patient has been put in restraints during the current encounter. Please note that this code should not be reported when it is documented by the provider that a patient is temporarily restrained during a procedure.

Z79   Long-term (current) drug therapy

Codes from this category indicate a patient's continuous use of a prescribed drug (including such things as aspirin therapy) for the long-term treatment of a condition or for prophylactic use. It is not for use for patients who have addictions to drugs. This subcategory is not for use of medications for detoxification or maintenance programs to prevent withdrawal symptoms in patients with drug dependence (e.g., methadone maintenance for opiate dependence). Assign the appropriate code for the drug dependence instead.

Assign a code from Z79 if the patient is receiving a medication for an extended period as a prophylactic measure (such as for the prevention of deep vein thrombosis) or as treatment of a chronic condition (such as arthritis) or a disease requiring a lengthy course of treatment (such as cancer). Do not assign a code from category Z79 for medication being administered for a brief period of time to treat an acute illness or injury (such as a course of antibiotics to treat acute bronchitis).

Z88   Allergy status to drugs, medicaments and biological substances

Except: Z88.9, Allergy status to unspecified drugs, medicaments and biological substances status

Z89   Acquired absence of limb

Z90   Acquired absence of organs, not elsewhere classified

Z91.0-   Allergy status, other than to drugs and biological substances

Z92.82   Status post administration of tPA (rtPA) in a different facility within the last 24 hours prior to admission to a current facility

Assign code Z92.82, Status post administration of tPA (rtPA) in a different facility within the last 24 hours prior to admission to current facility, as a secondary diagnosis when a patient is received by transfer into a facility and documentation indicates they were administered tissue plasminogen activator (tPA) within the last 24 hours prior to admission to the current facility.

This guideline applies even if the patient is still receiving the tPA at the time they are received into the current facility.

The appropriate code for the condition for which the tPA was administered (such as cerebrovascular disease or myocardial infarction) should be assigned first.

Code Z92.82 is only applicable to the receiving facility record and not to the transferring facility record.

Z93   Artificial opening status

Z94   Transplanted organ and tissue status

Z95   Presence of cardiac and vascular implants and grafts

Z96   Presence of other functional implants

Z97   Presence of other devices

Z98   Other postprocedural states

Assign code Z98.85, Transplanted organ removal status, to indicate that a transplanted organ has been previously removed. This code should not be assigned for the encounter in which the transplanted organ is removed. The complication necessitating removal of the transplant organ should be assigned for that encounter.

See section I.C19. for information on the coding of organ transplant complications.

Z99   Dependence on enabling machines and devices, not elsewhere classified

Note: Categories Z89-Z90 and Z93-Z99 are for use only if there are no complications or malfunctions of the organ or tissue replaced, the amputation site or the equipment on which the patient is dependent.

4)   **History (of)**

There are two types of history Z codes, personal and family. Personal history codes explain a patient's past medical condition that no longer exists and is not receiving any treatment, but that has the potential for recurrence, and therefore may require continued monitoring.

Family history codes are for use when a patient has a family member(s) who has had a particular disease that causes the patient to be at higher risk of also contracting the disease.

Personal history codes may be used in conjunction with follow-up codes and family history codes may be used in conjunction with screening codes to explain the need for a test or procedure. History codes are also acceptable on any medical record regardless of the reason for visit. A history of an illness, even if no longer present, is important information that may alter the type of treatment ordered.

The history Z code categories are:

Z80   Family history of primary malignant neoplasm

Z81   Family history of mental and behavioral disorders

Z82   Family history of certain disabilities and chronic diseases (leading to disablement)

Z83   Family history of other specific disorders

Z84   Family history of other conditions

Z85   Personal history of malignant neoplasm

Z86   Personal history of certain other diseases

Z87   Personal history of other diseases and conditions

Z91.4-   Personal history of psychological trauma, not elsewhere classified

Z91.5   Personal history of self-harm

Z91.8-   Other specified personal risk factors, not elsewhere classified

Exception: Z91.83, Wandering in diseases classified elsewhere

Z92   Personal history of medical treatment

Except: Z92.0, Personal history of contraception

Except: Z92.82, Status post administration of tPA (rtPA) in a different facility within the last 24 hours prior to admission to a current facility

5)   **Screening**

Screening is the testing for disease or disease precursors in seemingly well individuals so that early detection and treatment can be provided for those who test positive for the disease (e.g., screening mammogram).

The testing of a person to rule out or confirm a suspected diagnosis because the patient has some sign or symptom is a diagnostic examination, not a screening. In these cases, the sign or symptom is used to explain the reason for the test.

A screening code may be a first-listed code if the reason for the visit is specifically the screening exam. It may also be used as an additional code if the screening is done during an office visit for other health problems. A screening code is not necessary if the screening is inherent to a routine examination, such as a pap smear done during a routine pelvic examination.

Should a condition be discovered during the screening then the code for the condition may be assigned as an additional diagnosis.

The Z code indicates that a screening exam is planned. A procedure code is required to confirm that the screening was performed.

The screening Z codes/categories:

Z11   Encounter for screening for infectious and parasitic diseases

Z12   Encounter for screening for malignant neoplasms

Z13   Encounter for screening for other diseases and disorders

Except: Z13.9, Encounter for screening, unspecified

Z36   Encounter for antenatal screening for mother

6) Observation

There are three observation Z code categories. They are for use in very limited circumstances when a person is being observed for a suspected condition that is ruled out. The observation codes are not for use if an injury or illness or any signs or symptoms related to the suspected condition are present. In such cases the diagnosis/symptom code is used with the corresponding external cause code.

The observation codes are to be used as principal diagnosis only. The only exception to this is when the principal diagnosis is required to be a code from category Z38, Liveborn infants according to place of birth and type of delivery. Then a code from category Z05, Encounter for observation and evaluation of newborn for suspected diseases and conditions ruled out, is sequenced after the Z38 code. Additional codes may be used in addition to the observation code, but only if they are unrelated to the suspected condition being observed.

Codes from subcategory Z03.7, Encounter for suspected maternal and fetal conditions ruled out, may either be used as a first-listed or as an additional code assignment depending on the case. They are for use in very limited circumstances on a maternal record when an encounter is for a suspected maternal or fetal condition that is ruled out during that encounter (for example, a maternal or fetal condition may be suspected due to an abnormal test result). These codes should not be used when the condition is confirmed. In those cases, the confirmed condition should be coded. In addition, these codes are not for use if an illness or any signs or symptoms related to the suspected condition or problem are present. In such cases the diagnosis/symptom code is used.

Additional codes may be used in addition to the code from subcategory Z03.7, but only if they are unrelated to the suspected condition being evaluated.

Codes from subcategory Z03.7 may not be used for encounters for antenatal screening of mother. *See Section I.C.21. Screening.*

For encounters for suspected fetal condition that are inconclusive following testing and evaluation, assign the appropriate code from category O35, O36, O40 or O41.

The observation Z code categories:

Z03   Encounter for medical observation for suspected diseases and conditions ruled out

Z04   Encounter for examination and observation for other reasons

Except: Z04.9, Encounter for examination and observation for unspecified reason

Z05   Encounter for observation and evaluation of newborn for suspected diseases and conditions ruled out

7) Aftercare

Aftercare visit codes cover situations when the initial treatment of a disease has been performed and the patient requires continued care during the healing or recovery phase, or for the long-term consequences of the disease. The aftercare Z code should not be used if treatment is directed at a current, acute disease. The diagnosis code is to be used in these cases. Exceptions to this rule are codes Z51.0, Encounter for antineoplastic radiation therapy, and codes from subcategory Z51.1, Encounter for antineoplastic chemotherapy and immunotherapy. These codes are to be first-listed, followed by the diagnosis code when a patient's encounter is solely to receive radiation therapy, chemotherapy, or immunotherapy for the treatment of a neoplasm. If the reason for the encounter is more than one type of antineoplastic therapy, code Z51.0 and a code from subcategory Z51.1 may be assigned together, in which case one of these codes would be reported as a secondary diagnosis.

The aftercare Z codes should also not be used for aftercare for injuries. For aftercare of an injury, assign the acute injury code with the appropriate 7th character (for subsequent encounter).

The aftercare codes are generally first-listed to explain the specific reason for the encounter. An aftercare code may be used as an additional code when some type of aftercare is provided in addition to the reason for admission and no diagnosis code is applicable. An example of this would be the closure of a colostomy during an encounter for treatment of another condition.

Aftercare codes should be used in conjunction with other aftercare codes or diagnosis codes to provide better detail on the specifics of an aftercare encounter visit, unless otherwise directed by the classification. Should a patient receive multiple types of antineoplastic therapy during the same encounter, code Z51.0, Encounter for antineoplastic radiation therapy, and codes from subcategory Z51.1, Encounter for antineoplastic chemotherapy and immunotherapy, may be used together on a record. The sequencing of multiple aftercare codes depends on the circumstances of the encounter.

Certain aftercare Z code categories need a secondary diagnosis code to describe the resolving condition or sequelae. For others, the condition is included in the code title.

Additional Z code aftercare category terms include fitting and adjustment, and attention to artificial openings.

Status Z codes may be used with aftercare Z codes to indicate the nature of the aftercare. For example code Z95.1, Presence of aortocoronary bypass graft, may be used with code Z48.812, Encounter for surgical aftercare following surgery on the circulatory system, to indicate the surgery for which the aftercare is being performed. A status code should not be used when the aftercare code indicates the type of status, such as using Z43.0, Encounter for attention to tracheostomy, with Z93.0, Tracheostomy status.

The aftercare Z category/codes:

Z42   Encounter for plastic and reconstructive surgery following medical procedure or healed injury

Z43   Encounter for attention to artificial openings

Z44   Encounter for fitting and adjustment of external prosthetic device

Z45   Encounter for adjustment and management of implanted device

Z46   Encounter for fitting and adjustment of other devices

Z47   Orthopedic aftercare

Z48   Encounter for other postprocedural aftercare

Z49   Encounter for care involving renal dialysis

Z51   Encounter for other aftercare and medical care

8) Follow-up

The follow-up codes are used to explain continuing surveillance following completed treatment of a disease, condition, or injury. They imply that the condition has been fully treated and no longer exists. They should not be confused with aftercare codes, or injury codes with a 7th character for subsequent encounter, that explain ongoing care of a healing condition or its sequelae. Follow-up codes may be used in conjunction with history codes to provide the full picture of the healed condition and its treatment. The follow-up code is sequenced first, followed by the history code.

A follow-up code may be used to explain multiple visits. Should a condition be found to have recurred on the follow-up visit, then the diagnosis code for the condition should be assigned in place of the follow-up code.

The follow-up Z code categories:

Z08   Encounter for follow-up examination after completed treatment for malignant neoplasm

Z09   Encounter for follow-up examination after completed treatment for conditions other than malignant neoplasm

Z39   Encounter for maternal postpartum care and examination

9) Donor

Codes in category Z52, Donors of organs and tissues, are used for living individuals who are donating blood or other body tissue. These codes are only for individuals donating for others, not for self-donations. They are not used to identify cadaveric donations.

10) Counseling

Counseling Z codes are used when a patient or family member receives assistance in the aftermath of an illness or injury, or when support is required in coping with family or social problems. They are not used in conjunction with a diagnosis code when the counseling component of care is considered integral to standard treatment.

The counseling Z codes/categories:

Z30.0- Encounter for general counseling and advice on contraception

Z31.5 Encounter for genetic counseling

Z31.6- Encounter for general counseling and advice on procreation

Z32.2 Encounter for childbirth instruction

Z32.3 Encounter for childcare instruction

Z69 Encounter for mental health services for victim and perpetrator of abuse

Z70 Counseling related to sexual attitude, behavior and orientation

Z71 Persons encountering health services for other counseling and medical advice, not elsewhere classified

Z76.81 Expectant mother prebirth pediatrician visit

11) Encounters for Obstetrical and Reproductive Services

See Section I.C.15. Pregnancy, Childbirth, and the Puerperium, for further instruction on the use of these codes.

Z codes for pregnancy are for use in those circumstances when none of the problems or complications included in the codes from the Obstetrics chapter exist (a routine prenatal visit or postpartum care). Codes in category Z34, Encounter for supervision of normal pregnancy, are always first-listed and are not to be used with any other code from the OB chapter.

Codes in category Z3A, Weeks of gestation, may be assigned to provide additional information about the pregnancy. Category Z3A codes should not be assigned for pregnancies with abortive outcomes (categories O00-O08), elective termination of pregnancy (code Z33.32), nor for postpartum conditions, as category Z3A is not applicable to these conditions. The date of the admission should be used to determine weeks of gestation for inpatient admissions that encompass more than one gestational week.

The outcome of delivery, category Z37, should be included on all maternal delivery records. It is always a secondary code. Codes in category Z37 should not be used on the newborn record.

Z codes for family planning (contraceptive) or procreative management and counseling should be included on an obstetric record either during the pregnancy or the postpartum stage, if applicable.

Z codes/categories for obstetrical and reproductive services:

Z30 Encounter for contraceptive management

Z31 Encounter for procreative management

Z32.2 Encounter for childbirth instruction

Z32.3 Encounter for childcare instruction

Z33 Pregnant state

Z34 Encounter for supervision of normal pregnancy

Z36 Encounter for antenatal screening of mother

Z3A Weeks of gestation

Z37 Outcome of delivery

Z39 Encounter for maternal postpartum care and examination

Z76.81 Expectant mother prebirth pediatrician visit

12) Newborns and Infants

See Section I.C.16. Newborn (Perinatal) Guidelines, for further instruction on the use of these codes.

Newborn Z codes/categories:

Z76.1 Encounter for health supervision and care of foundling

Z00.1- Encounter for routine child health examination

Z38 Liveborn infants according to place of birth and type of delivery

13) Routine and administrative examinations

The Z codes allow for the description of encounters for routine examinations, such as, a general check-up, or, examinations for administrative purposes, such as, a pre-employment physical. The codes are not to be used if the examination is for diagnosis of a suspected condition or for treatment purposes. In such cases the diagnosis code is used. During a routine exam, should a diagnosis or condition be discovered, it should be coded as an additional code. Pre-existing and chronic conditions and history codes may also be included as additional codes as long as the examination is for administrative purposes and not focused on any particular condition.

Some of the codes for routine health examinations distinguish between "with" and "without" abnormal findings. Code assignment depends on the information that is known at the time the encounter is being coded. For example, if no abnormal findings were found during the examination, but the encounter is being coded before test results are back, it is acceptable to assign the code for "without abnormal findings." When assigning a code for "with abnormal findings," additional code(s) should be assigned to identify the specific abnormal finding(s).

Pre-operative examination and pre-procedural laboratory examination Z codes are for use only in those situations when a patient is being cleared for a procedure or surgery and no treatment is given.

The Z codes/categories for routine and administrative examinations:

Z00 Encounter for general examination without complaint, suspected or reported diagnosis

Z01 Encounter for other special examination without complaint, suspected or reported diagnosis

Z02 Encounter for administrative examination

     Except: Z02.9, Encounter for administrative examinations, unspecified

Z32.0- Encounter for pregnancy test

14) Miscellaneous Z codes

The miscellaneous Z codes capture a number of other health care encounters that do not fall into one of the other categories. Certain of these codes identify the reason for the encounter; others are for use as additional codes that provide useful information on circumstances that may affect a patient's care and treatment.

Prophylactic Organ Removal

For encounters specifically for prophylactic removal of an organ (such as prophylactic removal of breasts due to a genetic susceptibility to cancer or a family history of cancer), the principal or first-listed code should be a code from category Z40, Encounter for prophylactic surgery, followed by the appropriate codes to identify the associated risk factor (such as genetic susceptibility or family history).

If the patient has a malignancy of one site and is having prophylactic removal at another site to prevent either a new primary malignancy or metastatic disease, a code for the malignancy should also be assigned in addition to a code from subcategory Z40.0, Encounter for prophylactic surgery for risk factors related to malignant neoplasms. A Z40.0 code should not be assigned if the patient is having organ removal for treatment of a malignancy, such as the removal of the testes for the treatment of prostate cancer.

Miscellaneous Z codes/categories:

Z28 Immunization not carried out

Except: Z28.3, Underimmunization status

Z29 Encounter for other prophylactic measures

Z40 Encounter for prophylactic surgery

Z41 Encounter for procedures for purposes other than remedying health state

Except: Z41.9, Encounter for procedure for purposes other than remedying health state, unspecified

Z53 Persons encountering health services for specific procedures and treatment, not carried out

Z55 Problems related to education and literacy

Z56 Problems related to employment and unemployment

Z57 Occupational exposure to risk factors

Z58 Problems related to physical environment

Z59 Problems related to housing and economic circumstances

Z60 Problems related to social environment

Z62 Problems related to upbringing

Z63 Other problems related to primary support group, including family circumstances

Z64 Problems related to certain psychosocial circumstances

Z65 Problems related to other psychosocial circumstances

Z72 Problems related to lifestyle

Note: These codes should be assigned only when the documentation specifies that the patient has an associated problem

Z73 Problems related to life management difficulty

Z74 Problems related to care provider dependency

Except: Z74.01, Bed confinement status

Z75 Problems related to medical facilities and other health care

Z76.0 Encounter for issue of repeat prescription

Z76.3 Healthy person accompanying sick person

Z76.4 Other boarder to healthcare facility

Z76.5 Malingerer [conscious simulation]

Z91.1- Patient's noncompliance with medical treatment and regimen

Z91.83 Wandering in diseases classified elsewhere

Z91.89 Other specified personal risk factors, not elsewhere classified

15) Nonspecific Z codes

Certain Z codes are so non-specific, or potentially redundant with other codes in the classification, that there can be little justification for their use in the inpatient setting. Their use in the outpatient setting should be limited to those instances when there is no further documentation to permit more precise coding. Otherwise, any sign or symptom or any other reason for visit that is captured in another code should be used.

Nonspecific Z codes/categories:

Z02.9 Encounter for administrative examinations, unspecified

Z04.9 Encounter for examination and observation for unspecified reason

Z13.9 Encounter for screening, unspecified

Z41.9 Encounter for procedure for purposes other than remedying health state, unspecified

Z52.9 Donor of unspecified organ or tissue

Z86.59 Personal history of other mental and behavioral disorders

Z88.9 Allergy status to unspecified drugs, medicaments and biological substances status

Z92.0 Personal history of contraception

16) Z Codes That May Only be Principal/First-Listed Diagnosis

The following Z codes/categories may only be reported as the principal/first-listed diagnosis, except when there are multiple encounters on the same day and the medical records for the encounters are combined:

Z00 Encounter for general examination without complaint, suspected or reported diagnosis

Except: Z00.6

Z01 Encounter for other special examination without complaint, suspected or reported diagnosis

Z02 Encounter for administrative examination

Z03 Encounter for medical observation for suspected diseases and conditions ruled out

Z04 Encounter for examination and observation for other reasons

Z33.2 Encounter for elective termination of pregnancy

Z31.81 Encounter for male factor infertility in female patient

Z31.83 Encounter for assisted reproductive fertility procedure cycle

Z31.84 Encounter for fertility preservation procedure

Z34 Encounter for supervision of normal pregnancy

Z39 Encounter for maternal postpartum care and examination

Z38 Liveborn infants according to place of birth and type of delivery

Z42 Encounter for plastic and reconstructive surgery following medical procedure or healed injury

Z51.0 Encounter for antineoplastic radiation therapy

Z51.1- Encounter for antineoplastic chemotherapy and immunotherapy

Z52 Donors of organs and tissues

Except: Z52.9, Donor of unspecified organ or tissue

Z76.1 Encounter for health supervision and care of foundling

Z76.2 Encounter for health supervision and care of other healthy infant and child

Z99.12 Encounter for respirator [ventilator] dependence during power failure

Section II. Selection of Principal Diagnosis

The circumstances of inpatient admission always govern the selection of principal diagnosis. The principal diagnosis is defined in the Uniform Hospital Discharge Data Set (UHDDS) as "that condition established after study to be chiefly responsible for occasioning the admission of the patient to the hospital for care."

The UHDDS definitions are used by hospitals to report inpatient data elements in a standardized manner. These data elements and their definitions can be found in the July 31, 1985, Federal Register (Vol. 50, No, 147), pp. 31038-40.

Since that time the application of the UHDDS definitions has been expanded to include all non-outpatient settings (acute care, short term, long term care and psychiatric hospitals; home health agencies; rehab facilities; nursing homes, etc). The UHDDS definitions also apply to hospice services (all levels of care).

In determining principal diagnosis, coding conventions in the ICD-10-CM, the Tabular List and Alphabetic Index take precedence over these official coding guidelines.

(See Section I.A., Conventions for the ICD-10-CM)

The importance of consistent, complete documentation in the medical record cannot be overemphasized. Without such documentation the application of all coding guidelines is a difficult, if not impossible, task.

A. Codes for symptoms, signs, and ill-defined conditions

Codes for symptoms, signs, and ill-defined conditions from Chapter 18 are not to be used as principal diagnosis when a related definitive diagnosis has been established.

B. **Two or more interrelated conditions, each potentially meeting the definition for principal diagnosis.**

When there are two or more interrelated conditions (such as diseases in the same ICD-10-CM chapter or manifestations characteristically associated with a certain disease) potentially meeting the definition of principal diagnosis, either condition may be sequenced first, unless the circumstances of the admission, the therapy provided, the Tabular List, or the Alphabetic Index indicate otherwise.

C. **Two or more diagnoses that equally meet the definition for principal diagnosis**

In the unusual instance when two or more diagnoses equally meet the criteria for principal diagnosis as determined by the circumstances of admission, diagnostic workup and/or therapy provided, and the Alphabetic Index, Tabular List, or another coding guidelines does not provide sequencing direction, any one of the diagnoses may be sequenced first.

D. **Two or more comparative or contrasting conditions**

In those rare instances when two or more contrasting or comparative diagnoses are documented as "either/or" (or similar terminology), they are coded as if the diagnoses were confirmed and the diagnoses are sequenced according to the circumstances of the admission. If no further determination can be made as to which diagnosis should be principal, either diagnosis may be sequenced first.

E. **A symptom(s) followed by contrasting/comparative diagnoses**

GUIDELINE HAS BEEN DELETED EFFECTIVE OCTOBER 1, 2014

F. **Original treatment plan not carried out**

Sequence as the principal diagnosis the condition, which after study occasioned the admission to the hospital, even though treatment may not have been carried out due to unforeseen circumstances.

G. **Complications of surgery and other medical care**

When the admission is for treatment of a complication resulting from surgery or other medical care, the complication code is sequenced as the principal diagnosis. If the complication is classified to the T80-T88 series and the code lacks the necessary specificity in describing the complication, an additional code for the specific complication should be assigned.

H. **Uncertain Diagnosis**

If the diagnosis documented at the time of discharge is qualified as "probable", "suspected", "likely", "questionable", "possible", or "still to be ruled out", or other similar terms indicating uncertainty, code the condition as if it existed or was established. The bases for these guidelines are the diagnostic workup, arrangements for further workup or observation, and initial therapeutic approach that correspond most closely with the established diagnosis.

Note: This guideline is applicable only to inpatient admissions to short-term, acute, long-term care and psychiatric hospitals.

I. **Admission from Observation Unit**

1. **Admission Following Medical Observation**

When a patient is admitted to an observation unit for a medical condition, which either worsens or does not improve, and is subsequently admitted as an inpatient of the same hospital for this same medical condition, the principal diagnosis would be the medical condition which led to the hospital admission.

2. **Admission Following Post-Operative Observation**

When a patient is admitted to an observation unit to monitor a condition (or complication) that develops following outpatient surgery, and then is subsequently admitted as an inpatient of the same hospital, hospitals should apply the Uniform Hospital Discharge Data Set (UHDDS) definition of principal diagnosis as "that condition established after study to be chiefly responsible for occasioning the admission of the patient to the hospital for care."

J. **Admission from Outpatient Surgery**

When a patient receives surgery in the hospital's outpatient surgery department and is subsequently admitted for continuing inpatient care at the same hospital, the following guidelines should be followed in selecting the principal diagnosis for the inpatient admission:

- If the reason for the inpatient admission is a complication, assign the complication as the principal diagnosis.

- If no complication, or other condition, is documented as the reason for the inpatient admission, assign the reason for the outpatient surgery as the principal diagnosis.

- If the reason for the inpatient admission is another condition unrelated to the surgery, assign the unrelated condition as the principal diagnosis.

K. **Admissions/Encounters for Rehabilitation**

When the purpose for the admission/encounter is rehabilitation, sequence first the code for the condition for which the service is being performed. For example, for an admission/encounter for rehabilitation for right-sided dominant hemiplegia following a cerebrovascular infarction, report code I69.351, Hemiplegia and hemiparesis following cerebral infarction affecting right dominant side, as the first-listed or principal diagnosis. If the condition for which the rehabilitation service is no longer present, report the appropriate aftercare code as the first-listed or principal diagnosis. For example, if a patient with severe degenerative osteoarthritis of the hip, underwent hip replacement and the current encounter/admission is for rehabilitation, report code Z47.1, Aftercare following joint replacement surgery, as the first-listed or principal diagnosis.

See Section I.C.21.c.7, Factors influencing health states and contact with health services, Aftercare.

Section III. Reporting Additional Diagnoses

GENERAL RULES FOR OTHER (ADDITIONAL) DIAGNOSES

For reporting purposes the definition for "other diagnoses" is interpreted as additional conditions that affect patient care in terms of requiring:

clinical evaluation; or

therapeutic treatment; or

diagnostic procedures; or

extended length of hospital stay; or

increased nursing care and/or monitoring.

The UHDDS item #11-b defines Other Diagnoses as "all conditions that coexist at the time of admission, that develop subsequently, or that affect the treatment received and/or the length of stay. Diagnoses that relate to an earlier episode which have no bearing on the current hospital stay are to be excluded." UHDDS definitions apply to inpatients in acute care, short-term, long term care and psychiatric hospital setting. The UHDDS definitions are used by acute care short-term hospitals to report inpatient data elements in a standardized manner. These data elements and their definitions can be found in the July 31, 1985, Federal Register (Vol. 50, No, 147), pp. 31038-40.

Since that time the application of the UHDDS definitions has been expanded to include all non-outpatient settings (acute care, short term, long term care and psychiatric hospitals; home health agencies; rehab facilities; nursing homes, etc). The UHDDS definitions also apply to hospice services (all levels of care).

The following guidelines are to be applied in designating "other diagnoses" when neither the Alphabetic Index nor the Tabular List in ICD-10-CM provide direction. The listing of the diagnoses in the patient record is the responsibility of the attending provider.

A. **Previous conditions**

If the provider has included a diagnosis in the final diagnostic statement, such as the discharge summary or the face sheet, it should ordinarily be coded. Some providers include in the diagnostic statement resolved conditions or diagnoses and status-post procedures from previous admission that have no bearing on the current stay. Such conditions are not to be reported and are coded only if required by hospital policy.

However, history codes (categories Z80-Z87) may be used as secondary codes if the historical condition or family history has an impact on current care or influences treatment.

B. **Abnormal findings**

Abnormal findings (laboratory, x-ray, pathologic, and other diagnostic results) are not coded and reported unless the provider indicates their clinical significance. If the findings are outside the normal range and the attending provider has ordered other tests to evaluate the condition or prescribed treatment, it is appropriate to ask the provider whether the abnormal finding should be added.

Please note: This differs from the coding practices in the outpatient setting for coding encounters for diagnostic tests that have been interpreted by a provider.

C. Uncertain Diagnosis

If the diagnosis documented at the time of discharge is qualified as "probable", "suspected", "likely", "questionable", "possible", or "still to be ruled out" or other similar terms indicating uncertainty, code the condition as if it existed or was established. The bases for these guidelines are the diagnostic workup, arrangements for further workup or observation, and initial therapeutic approach that correspond most closely with the established diagnosis.

Note: This guideline is applicable only to inpatient admissions to short-term, acute, long-term care and psychiatric hospitals.

Section IV. Diagnostic Coding and Reporting Guidelines for Outpatient Services

These coding guidelines for outpatient diagnoses have been approved for use by hospitals/ providers in coding and reporting hospital-based outpatient services and provider-based office visits. Guidelines in Section I, Conventions, general coding guidelines and chapter-specific guidelines, should also be applied for outpatient services and office visits.

Information about the use of certain abbreviations, punctuation, symbols, and other conventions used in the ICD-10-CM Tabular List (code numbers and titles), can be found in Section IA of these guidelines, under "Conventions Used in the Tabular List." Section I.B. contains general guidelines that apply to the entire classification. Section I.C. contains chapter-specific guidelines that correspond to the chapters as they are arranged in the classification. Information about the correct sequence to use in finding a code is also described in Section I.

The terms encounter and visit are often used interchangeably in describing outpatient service contacts and, therefore, appear together in these guidelines without distinguishing one from the other.

Though the conventions and general guidelines apply to all settings, coding guidelines for outpatient and provider reporting of diagnoses will vary in a number of instances from those for inpatient diagnoses, recognizing that:

> The Uniform Hospital Discharge Data Set (UHDDS) definition of principal diagnosis does not apply to hospital-based outpatient services and provider-based office visits.
>
> Coding guidelines for inconclusive diagnoses (probable, suspected, rule out, etc.) were developed for inpatient reporting and do not apply to outpatients.

A. Selection of first-listed condition

In the outpatient setting, the term first-listed diagnosis is used in lieu of principal diagnosis.

In determining the first-listed diagnosis the coding conventions of ICD-10-CM, as well as the general and disease specific guidelines take precedence over the outpatient guidelines.

Diagnoses often are not established at the time of the initial encounter/visit. It may take two or more visits before the diagnosis is confirmed.

The most critical rule involves beginning the search for the correct code assignment through the Alphabetic Index. Never begin searching initially in the Tabular List as this will lead to coding errors.

1. Outpatient Surgery

When a patient presents for outpatient surgery (same day surgery), code the reason for the surgery as the first-listed diagnosis (reason for the encounter), even if the surgery is not performed due to a contraindication.

2. Observation Stay

When a patient is admitted for observation for a medical condition, assign a code for the medical condition as the first-listed diagnosis.

When a patient presents for outpatient surgery and develops complications requiring admission to observation, code the reason for the surgery as the first reported diagnosis (reason for the encounter), followed by codes for the complications as secondary diagnoses.

B. Codes from A00.0 through T88.9, Z00-Z99

The appropriate code(s) from A00.0 through T88.9, Z00-Z99 must be used to identify diagnoses, symptoms, conditions, problems, complaints, or other reason(s) for the encounter/visit.

C. Accurate reporting of ICD-10-CM diagnosis codes

For accurate reporting of ICD-10-CM diagnosis codes, the documentation should describe the patient's condition, using terminology which includes specific diagnoses as well as symptoms, problems, or reasons for the encounter. There are ICD-10-CM codes to describe all of these.

D. Codes that describe symptoms and signs

Codes that describe symptoms and signs, as opposed to diagnoses, are acceptable for reporting purposes when a diagnosis has not been established (confirmed) by the provider. Chapter 18 of ICD-10-CM, Symptoms, Signs, and Abnormal Clinical and Laboratory Findings Not Elsewhere Classified (codes R00-R99) contain many, but not all codes for symptoms.

E. Encounters for circumstances other than a disease or injury

ICD-10-CM provides codes to deal with encounters for circumstances other than a disease or injury. The Factors Influencing Health Status and Contact with Health Services codes (Z00-Z99) are provided to deal with occasions when circumstances other than a disease or injury are recorded as diagnosis or problems.

See Section I.C.21. Factors influencing health status and contact with health services.

F. Level of Detail in Coding

1. ICD-10-CM codes with 3, 4, 5, 6 or 7 characters

ICD-10-CM is composed of codes with 3, 4, 5, 6 or 7 characters. Codes with three characters are included in ICD-10-CM as the heading of a category of codes that may be further subdivided by the use of fourth, fifth, sixth or seventh characters to provide greater specificity.

2. Use of full number of characters required for a code

A three-character code is to be used only if it is not further subdivided. A code is invalid if it has not been coded to the full number of characters required for that code, including the 7th character, if applicable.

G. ICD-10-CM code for the diagnosis, condition, problem, or other reason for encounter/visit

List first the ICD-10-CM code for the diagnosis, condition, problem, or other reason for encounter/visit shown in the medical record to be chiefly responsible for the services provided. List additional codes that describe any coexisting conditions. In some cases the first-listed diagnosis may be a symptom when a diagnosis has not been established (confirmed) by the physician.

H. Uncertain diagnosis

Do not code diagnoses documented as "probable", "suspected," "questionable," "rule out," or "working diagnosis" or other similar terms indicating uncertainty. Rather, code the condition(s) to the highest degree of certainty for that encounter/visit, such as symptoms, signs, abnormal test results, or other reason for the visit.

Please note: This differs from the coding practices used by short-term, acute care, long-term care and psychiatric hospitals.

I. Chronic diseases

Chronic diseases treated on an ongoing basis may be coded and reported as many times as the patient receives treatment and care for the condition(s)

J. Code all documented conditions that coexist

Code all documented conditions that coexist at the time of the encounter/visit, and require or affect patient care treatment or management. Do not code conditions that were previously treated and no longer exist. However, history codes (categories Z80-Z87) may be used as secondary codes if the historical condition or family history has an impact on current care or influences treatment.

K. Patients receiving diagnostic services only

For patients receiving diagnostic services only during an encounter/visit, sequence first the diagnosis, condition, problem, or other reason for encounter/visit shown in the medical record to be chiefly responsible for the outpatient services provided during the encounter/visit. Codes for other diagnoses (e.g., chronic conditions) may be sequenced as additional diagnoses.

For encounters for routine laboratory/radiology testing in the absence of any signs, symptoms, or associated diagnosis, assign Z01.89, Encounter for other specified special examinations. If routine testing is performed during the same encounter as a test to evaluate a sign, symptom, or diagnosis, it is appropriate to assign both the Z code and the code describing the reason for the non-routine test.

For outpatient encounters for diagnostic tests that have been interpreted by a physician, and the final report is available at the time of coding, code any confirmed or definitive diagnosis(es) documented in the interpretation. Do not code related signs and symptoms as additional diagnoses.

Please note: This differs from the coding practice in the hospital inpatient setting regarding abnormal findings on test results.

L. Patients receiving therapeutic services only

For patients receiving therapeutic services only during an encounter/visit, sequence first the diagnosis, condition, problem, or other reason for encounter/visit shown in the medical record to be chiefly responsible for the outpatient services provided during the encounter/visit. Codes for other diagnoses (e.g., chronic conditions) may be sequenced as additional diagnoses.

The only exception to this rule is that when the primary reason for the admission/encounter is chemotherapy or radiation therapy, the appropriate Z code for the service is listed first, and the diagnosis or problem for which the service is being performed listed second.

M. Patients receiving preoperative evaluations only

For patients receiving preoperative evaluations only, sequence first a code from subcategory Z01.81, Encounter for pre-procedural examinations, to describe the pre-op consultations. Assign a code for the condition to describe the reason for the surgery as an additional diagnosis. Code also any findings related to the pre-op evaluation.

N. Ambulatory surgery

For ambulatory surgery, code the diagnosis for which the surgery was performed. If the postoperative diagnosis is known to be different from the preoperative diagnosis at the time the diagnosis is confirmed, select the postoperative diagnosis for coding, since it is the most definitive.

O. Routine outpatient prenatal visits

See Section I.C.15. Routine outpatient prenatal visits.

P. Encounters for general medical examinations with abnormal findings

The subcategories for encounters for general medical examinations, Z00.0-, provide codes for with and without abnormal findings. Should a general medical examination result in an abnormal finding, the code for general medical examination with abnormal finding should be assigned as the first-listed diagnosis. An examination with abnormal findings refers to a condition/diagnosis that is newly identified or a change in severity of a chronic condition (such as uncontrolled hypertension, or an acute exacerbation of chronic obstructive pulmonary disease) during a routine physical examination. A secondary code for the abnormal finding should also be coded.

Q. Encounters for routine health screenings

See Section I.C.21. Factors influencing health status and contact with health services, Screening

Appendix I. Present on Admission Reporting Guidelines

Introduction

These guidelines are to be used as a supplement to the *ICD-10-CM Official Guidelines for Coding and Reporting* to facilitate the assignment of the Present on Admission (POA) indicator for each diagnosis and external cause of injury code reported on claim forms (UB-04 and 837 Institutional).

These guidelines are not intended to replace any guidelines in the main body of the *ICD-10-CM Official Guidelines for Coding and Reporting*. The POA guidelines are not intended to provide guidance on when a condition should be coded, but rather, how to apply the POA indicator to the final set of diagnosis codes that have been assigned in accordance with Sections I, II, and III of the official coding guidelines. Subsequent to the assignment of the ICD-10-CM codes, the POA indicator should then be assigned to those conditions that have been coded.

As stated in the Introduction to the ICD-10-CM Official Guidelines for Coding and Reporting, a joint effort between the healthcare provider and the coder is essential to achieve complete and accurate documentation, code assignment, and reporting of diagnoses and procedures. The importance of consistent, complete documentation in the medical record cannot be overemphasized.

Medical record documentation from any provider involved in the care and treatment of the patient may be used to support the determination of whether a condition was present on admission or not. In the context of the official coding guidelines, the term "provider" means a physician or any qualified healthcare practitioner who is legally accountable for establishing the patient's diagnosis.

These guidelines are not a substitute for the provider's clinical judgment as to the determination of whether a condition was/was not present on admission. The provider should be queried regarding issues related to the linking of signs/symptoms, timing of test results, and the timing of findings.

Please see the CDC website for the detailed list of ICD-10-CM codes that do not require the use of a POA indicator (ftp://ftp.cdc.gov/pub/Health_Statistics/NCHS/Publications/ICD10CM/2017/). The conditions on this exempt list represent categories and/or codes for circumstances regarding the healthcare encounter or factors influencing health status that do not represent a current disease or injury or are always present on admission.

General Reporting Requirements

All claims involving inpatient admissions to general acute care hospitals or other facilities that are subject to a law or regulation mandating collection of present on admission information.

Present on admission is defined as present at the time the order for inpatient admission occurs -- conditions that develop during an outpatient encounter, including emergency department, observation, or outpatient surgery, are considered as present on admission.

POA indicator is assigned to principal and secondary diagnoses (as defined in Section II of the Official Guidelines for Coding and Reporting) and the external cause of injury codes.

Issues related to inconsistent, missing, conflicting or unclear documentation must still be resolved by the provider.

If a condition would not be coded and reported based on UHDDS definitions and current official coding guidelines, then the POA indicator would not be reported.

Reporting Options

    Y - Yes

    N - No

    U - Unknown

    W – Clinically undetermined

    Unreported/Not used – (Exempt from POA reporting)

Reporting Definitions

    Y = present at the time of inpatient admission

    N = not present at the time of inpatient admission

    U = documentation is insufficient to determine if condition is present on admission

    W = provider is unable to clinically determine whether condition was present on admission or not

Timeframe for POA Identification and Documentation

There is no required timeframe as to when a provider (per the definition of "provider" used in these guidelines) must identify or document a condition to be present on admission. In some clinical situations, it may not be possible for a provider to make a definitive diagnosis (or a condition may not be recognized or reported by the patient) for a period of time after admission. In some cases it may be several days before the provider arrives at a definitive diagnosis. This does not mean that the condition was not present on admission. Determination of whether the condition was present on admission or not will be based on the applicable POA guideline as identified in this document, or on the provider's best clinical judgment.

If at the time of code assignment the documentation is unclear as to whether a condition was present on admission or not, it is appropriate to query the provider for clarification.

Assigning the POA Indicator

Condition is on the "Exempt from Reporting" list

Leave the "present on admission" field blank if the condition is on the list of ICD-10-CM codes for which this field is not applicable. This is the only circumstance in which the field may be left blank.

POA Explicitly Documented

Assign Y for any condition the provider explicitly documents as being present on admission.

Assign N for any condition the provider explicitly documents as not present at the time of admission.

Conditions diagnosed prior to inpatient admission

Assign "Y" for conditions that were diagnosed prior to admission (example: hypertension, diabetes mellitus, asthma)

Conditions diagnosed during the admission but clearly present before admission

Assign "Y" for conditions diagnosed during the admission that were clearly present but not diagnosed until after admission occurred.

Diagnoses subsequently confirmed after admission are considered present on admission if at the time of admission they are documented as suspected, possible, rule out, differential diagnosis, or constitute an underlying cause of a symptom that is present at the time of admission.

Condition develops during outpatient encounter prior to inpatient admission

Assign Y for any condition that develops during an outpatient encounter prior to a written order for inpatient admission.

Documentation does not indicate whether condition was present on admission

Assign "U" when the medical record documentation is unclear as to whether the condition was present on admission. "U" should not be routinely assigned and used only in very limited circumstances. Coders are encouraged to query the providers when the documentation is unclear.

Documentation states that it cannot be determined whether the condition was or was not present on admission

Assign "W" when the medical record documentation indicates that it cannot be clinically determined whether or not the condition was present on admission.

Chronic condition with acute exacerbation during the admission

If a single code identifies both the chronic condition and the acute exacerbation, see POA guidelines pertaining to codes that contain multiple clinical concepts.

If a single code only identifies the chronic condition and not the acute exacerbation (e.g., acute exacerbation of chronic leukemia), assign "Y."

Conditions documented as possible, probable, suspected, or rule out at the time of discharge

If the final diagnosis contains a possible, probable, suspected, or rule out diagnosis, and this diagnosis was based on signs, symptoms or clinical findings suspected at the time of inpatient admission, assign "Y."

If the final diagnosis contains a possible, probable, suspected, or rule out diagnosis, and this diagnosis was based on signs, symptoms or clinical findings that were not present on admission, assign "N".

Conditions documented as impending or threatened at the time of discharge

If the final diagnosis contains an impending or threatened diagnosis, and this diagnosis is based on symptoms or clinical findings that were present on admission, assign "Y".

If the final diagnosis contains an impending or threatened diagnosis, and this diagnosis is based on symptoms or clinical findings that were not present on admission, assign "N".

Acute and Chronic Conditions

Assign "Y" for acute conditions that are present at time of admission and N for acute conditions that are not present at time of admission.

Assign "Y" for chronic conditions, even though the condition may not be diagnosed until after admission.

If a single code identifies both an acute and chronic condition, see the POA guidelines for codes that contain multiple clinical concepts.

Codes That Contain Multiple Clinical Concepts

Assign "N" if at least one of the clinical concepts included in the code was not present on admission (e.g., COPD with acute exacerbation and the exacerbation was not present on admission; gastric ulcer that does not start bleeding until after admission; asthma patient develops status asthmaticus after admission).

Assign "Y" if all of the clinical concepts included in the code were present on admission (e.g., duodenal ulcer that perforates prior to admission).

For infection codes that include the causal organism, assign "Y" if the infection (or signs of the infection) were present on admission, even though the culture results may not be known until after admission (e.g., patient is admitted with pneumonia and the provider documents Pseudomonas as the causal organism a few days later).

Same Diagnosis Code for Two or More Conditions

When the same ICD-10-CM diagnosis code applies to two or more conditions during the same encounter (e.g. two separate conditions classified to the same ICD-10-CM diagnosis code):

Assign "Y" if all conditions represented by the single ICD-10-CM code were present on admission (e.g. bilateral unspecified age-related cataracts).

Assign "N" if any of the conditions represented by the single ICD-10-CM code was not present on admission (e.g. traumatic secondary and recurrent hemorrhage and seroma is assigned to a single code T79.2, but only one of the conditions was present on admission).

Obstetrical conditions

Whether or not the patient delivers during the current hospitalization does not affect assignment of the POA indicator. The determining factor for POA assignment is whether the pregnancy complication or obstetrical condition described by the code was present at the time of admission or not.

If the pregnancy complication or obstetrical condition was present on admission (e.g., patient admitted in preterm labor), assign "Y".

If the pregnancy complication or obstetrical condition was not present on admission (e.g., 2nd degree laceration during delivery, postpartum hemorrhage that occurred during current hospitalization, fetal distress develops after admission), assign "N".

If the obstetrical code includes more than one diagnosis and any of the diagnoses identified by the code were not present on admission assign "N".

(e.g., Category O11, Pre-existing hypertension with pre-eclampsia)

Perinatal conditions

Newborns are not considered to be admitted until after birth. Therefore, any condition present at birth or that developed in utero is considered present at admission and should be assigned "Y". This includes conditions that occur during delivery (e.g., injury during delivery, meconium aspiration, exposure to streptococcus B in the vaginal canal).

Congenital conditions and anomalies

Assign "Y" for congenital conditions and anomalies except for categories Q00-Q99, Congenital anomalies, which are on the exempt list. Congenital conditions are always considered present on admission.

External cause of injury codes

Assign "Y" for any external cause code representing an external cause of morbidity that occurred prior to inpatient admission (e.g., patient fell out of bed at home, patient fell out of bed in emergency room prior to admission)

Assign "N" for any external cause code representing an external cause of morbidity that occurred during inpatient hospitalization (e.g., patient fell out of hospital bed during hospital stay, patient experienced an adverse reaction to a medication administered after inpatient admission)

A

Aarskog's syndrome Q87.1
Abandonment — *see* Maltreatment
Abasia (-astasia) (hysterical) F44.4
Abderhalden-Kaufmann-Lignac syndrome (cystinosis) E72.04
Abdomen, abdominal (*see also* condition)
  acute R10.0
  angina K55.1
  muscle deficiency syndrome Q79.4
Abdominalgia — *see* Pain, abdominal
Abduction contracture, hip or other joint — *see* Contraction, joint
Aberrant (congenital) (*see also* Malposition, congenital)
  adrenal gland Q89.1
  artery (peripheral) Q27.8
    basilar NEC Q28.1
    cerebral Q28.3
    coronary Q24.5
    digestive system Q27.8
    eye Q15.8
    lower limb Q27.8
    precerebral Q28.1
    pulmonary Q25.79
    renal Q27.2
    retina Q14.1
    specified site NEC Q27.8
    subclavian Q27.8
    upper limb Q27.8
    vertebral Q28.1
  breast Q83.8
  endocrine gland NEC Q89.2
  hepatic duct Q44.5
  pancreas Q45.3
  parathyroid gland Q89.2
  pituitary gland Q89.2
  sebaceous glands, mucous membrane, mouth, congenital Q38.6
  spleen Q89.09
  subclavian artery Q27.8
  thymus (gland) Q89.2
  thyroid gland Q89.2
  vein (peripheral) NEC Q27.8
    cerebral Q28.3
    digestive system Q27.8
    lower limb Q27.8
    precerebral Q28.1
    specified site NEC Q27.8
    upper limb Q27.8
Aberration
  distantial — *see* Disturbance, visual
  mental F99
Abetalipoproteinemia E78.6
Abiotrophy R68.89
Ablatio, ablation
  retinae — *see* Detachment, retina
Ablepharia, ablepharon Q10.3
Abnormal, abnormality, abnormalities (*see also* Anomaly)
  acid-base balance (mixed) E87.4
  albumin R77.0
  alphafetoprotein R77.2
  alveolar ridge K08.9
  anatomical relationship Q89.9
  apertures, congenital, diaphragm Q79.1
  auditory perception H93.29- ☑
    diplacusis — *see* Diplacusis
    hyperacusis — *see* Hyperacusis
    recruitment — *see* Recruitment, auditory
    threshold shift — *see* Shift, auditory threshold
  autosomes Q99.9
    fragile site Q95.5
  basal metabolic rate R94.8
  biosynthesis, testicular androgen E29.1
  bleeding time R79.1
  blood level (of)
    cobalt R79.0
    copper R79.0
    iron R79.0
    lithium R78.89
    magnesium R79.0

Abnormal, abnormality, abnormalities — *continued*
  blood level — *continued*
    mineral NEC R79.0
    zinc R79.0
  blood pressure
    elevated R03.0
    low reading (nonspecific) R03.1
  blood sugar R73.09
  blood-gas level R79.81
  bowel sounds R19.15
    absent R19.11
    hyperactive R19.12
  brain scan R94.02
  breathing R06.9
  caloric test R94.138
  cerebrospinal fluid R83.9
    cytology R83.6
    drug level R83.2
    enzyme level R83.0
    hormones R83.1
    immunology R83.4
    microbiology R83.5
    nonmedicinal level R83.3
    specified type NEC R83.8
  chemistry, blood R79.9
    C-reactive protein R79.82
    drugs — *see* Findings, abnormal, in blood
    gas level R79.81
    minerals R79.0
    pancytopenia D61.818
    PTT R79.1
    specified NEC R79.89
    toxins — *see* Findings, abnormal, in blood
  chest sounds (friction) (rales) R09.89
  chromosome, chromosomal Q99.9
    with more than three X chromosomes, female Q97.1
    analysis result R89.8
      bronchial washings R84.8
      cerebrospinal fluid R83.8
      cervix uteri NEC R87.89
      nasal secretions R84.8
      nipple discharge R89.8
      peritoneal fluid R85.89
      pleural fluid R84.8
      prostatic secretions R86.8
      saliva R85.89
      seminal fluid R86.8
      sputum R84.8
      synovial fluid R89.8
      throat scrapings R84.8
      vagina R87.89
      vulva R87.89
      wound secretions R89.8
    dicentric replacement Q93.2
    ring replacement Q93.2
    sex Q99.8
      female phenotype Q97.9
        specified NEC Q97.8
      male phenotype Q98.9
        specified NEC Q98.8
      structural male Q98.6
    specified NEC Q99.8
  clinical findings NEC R68.89
  coagulation D68.9
    newborn, transient P61.6
    profile R79.1
    time R79.1
  communication — *see* Fistula
  conjunctiva, vascular H11.41- ☑
  coronary artery Q24.5
  cortisol-binding globulin E27.8
  course, eustachian tube Q17.8
  creatinine clearance R94.4
  cytology
    anus R85.619
      atypical squamous cells cannot exclude high grade squamous intraepithelial lesion (ASC-H) R85.611
      atypical squamous cells of undetermined significance (ASC-US) R85.610
      cytologic evidence of malignancy R85.614

Abnormal, abnormality, abnormalities — *continued*
  cytology — *continued*
    anus — *continued*
      high grade squamous intraepithelial lesion (HGSIL) R85.613
      human papillomavirus (HPV) DNA test
        high risk positive R85.81
        low risk postive R85.82
      inadequate smear R85.615
      low grade squamous intraepithelial lesion (LGSIL) R85.612
      satisfactory anal smear but lacking transformation zone R85.616
      specified NEC R85.618
      unsatisfactory smear R85.615
    female genital organs — *see* Abnormal, Papanicolaou (smear)
  dark adaptation curve H53.61
  dentofacial NEC — *see* Anomaly, dentofacial
  development, developmental Q89.9
    central nervous system Q07.9
  diagnostic imaging
    abdomen, abdominal region NEC R93.5
    biliary tract R93.2
    bladder R93.41
    breast R92.8
    central nervous system NEC R90.89
    cerebrovascular NEC R90.89
    coronary circulation R93.1
    digestive tract NEC R93.3
    gastrointestinal (tract) R93.3
    genitourinary organs R93.8
    head R93.0
    heart R93.1
    intrathoracic organ NEC R93.8
    kidney R93.42- ☑
    limbs R93.6
    liver R93.2
    lung (field) R91.8
    musculoskeletal system NEC R93.7
    renal pelvis R93.41
    retroperitoneum R93.5
    site specified NEC R93.8
    skin and subcutaneous tissue R93.8
    skull R93.0
    ureter R93.41
    urinary organs specified NEC R93.49
  direction, teeth, fully erupted M26.30
  ear ossicles, acquired NEC H74.39- ☑
    ankylosis — *see* Ankylosis, ear ossicles
    discontinuity — *see* Discontinuity, ossicles, ear
    partial loss — *see* Loss, ossicles, ear (partial)
  Ebstein Q22.5
  echocardiogram R93.1
  echoencephalogram R90.81
  echogram — *see* Abnormal, diagnostic imaging
  electrocardiogram [ECG] [EKG] R94.31
  electroencephalogram [EEG] R94.01
  electrolyte — *see* Imbalance, electrolyte
  electromyogram [EMG] R94.131
  electro-oculogram [EOG] R94.110
  electrophysiological intracardiac studies R94.39
  electroretinogram [ERG] R94.111
  erythrocytes
    congenital, with perinatal jaundice D58.9
  feces (color) (contents) (mucus) R19.5
  finding — *see* Findings, abnormal, without diagnosis
  fluid
    amniotic — *see* Abnormal, specimen, specified
    cerebrospinal — *see* Abnormal, cerebrospinal fluid
    peritoneal — *see* Abnormal, specimen, digestive organs
    pleural — *see* Abnormal, specimen, respiratory organs
    synovial — *see* Abnormal, specimen, specified
    thorax (bronchial washings) (pleural fluid) — *see* Abnormal, specimen, respiratory organs
    vaginal — *see* Abnormal, specimen, female genital organs
  form
    teeth K00.2
    uterus — *see* Anomaly, uterus

▼ Subterms under main terms may continue to next column or page ☑ Additional Character Required — Refer to the Tabular List for Character Selection 1

Aarskog's syndrome — Abnormal, abnormality, abnormalities

Abnormal, abnormality, abnormalities — *continued*

function studies
- auditory R94.120
- bladder R94.8
- brain R94.09
- cardiovascular R94.30
- ear R94.128
- endocrine NEC R94.7
- eye NEC R94.118
- kidney R94.4
- liver R94.5
- nervous system
  - central NEC R94.09
  - peripheral NEC R94.138
- pancreas R94.8
- placenta R94.8
- pulmonary R94.2
- special senses NEC R94.128
- spleen R94.8
- thyroid R94.6
- vestibular R94.121

gait — *see* Gait
- hysterical F44.4

gastrin secretion E16.4

globulin R77.1
- cortisol-binding E27.8
- thyroid-binding E07.89

glomerular, minor (*see also* N00-N07 with fourth character .0) N05.0

glucagon secretion E16.3

glucose tolerance (test) (non-fasting) R73.09

gravitational (G) forces or states (effect of) T75.81 ☑

hair (color) (shaft) L67.9
- specified NEC L67.8

hard tissue formation in pulp (dental) K04.3

head movement R25.0

heart
- rate R00.9
  - specified NEC R00.8
- shadow R93.1
- sounds NEC R01.2

hemoglobin (disease) (*see also* Disease, hemoglobin) D58.2
- trait — *see* Trait, hemoglobin, abnormal

histology NEC R89.7

immunological findings R89.4
- in serum R76.9
  - specified NEC R76.8

increase in appetite R63.2

involuntary movement — *see* Abnormal, movement, involuntary

jaw closure M26.51

karyotype R89.8

kidney function test R94.4

knee jerk R29.2

leukocyte (cell) (differential) NEC D72.9

liver function test R94.5

loss of
- height R29.890
- weight R63.4

mammogram NEC R92.8
- calcification (calculus) R92.1
- microcalcification R92.0

Mantoux test R76.11

movement (disorder) (*see also* Disorder, movement)
- head R25.0
- involuntary R25.9
  - fasciculation R25.3
  - of head R25.0
  - spasm R25.2
  - specified type NEC R25.8
  - tremor R25.1

myoglobin (Aberdeen) (Annapolis) R89.7

neonatal screening P09

oculomotor study R94.113

palmar creases Q82.8

Papanicolaou (smear)
- anus R85.619
  - atypical squamous cells cannot exclude high grade squamous intraepithelial lesion (ASC-H) R85.611
  - atypical squamous cells of undetermined significance (ASC-US) R85.610
  - cytologic evidence of malignancy R85.614
  - high grade squamous intraepithelial lesion (HGSIL) R85.613
  - human papillomavirus (HPV) DNA test
    - high risk positive R85.81

Abnormal, abnormality, abnormalities — *continued*

Papanicolaou — *continued*
- anus — *continued*
  - human papillomavirus DNA test — *continued*
    - low risk postive R85.82
  - inadequate smear R85.615
  - low grade squamous intraepithelial lesion (LGSIL) R85.612
  - satisfactory anal smear but lacking transformation zone R85.616
  - specified NEC R85.618
  - unsatisfactory smear R85.615
- bronchial washings R84.6
- cerebrospinal fluid R83.6
- cervix R87.619
  - atypical squamous cells cannot exclude high grade squamous intraepithelial lesion (ASC-H) R87.611
  - atypical squamous cells of undetermined significance (ASC-US) R87.610
  - cytologic evidence of malignancy R87.614
  - high grade squamous intraepithelial lesion (HGSIL) R87.613
  - inadequate smear R87.615
  - low grade squamous intraepithelial lesion (LGSIL) R87.612
  - non-atypical endometrial cells R87.618
  - satisfactory cervical smear but lacking transformation zone R87.616
  - specified NEC R87.618
  - thin preparaton R87.619
  - unsatisfactory smear R87.615
- nasal secretions R84.6
- nipple discharge R89.6
- peritoneal fluid R85.69
- pleural fluid R84.6
- prostatic secretions R86.6
- saliva R85.69
- seminal fluid R86.6
- sites NEC R89.6
- sputum R84.6
- synovial fluid R89.6
- throat scrapings R84.6
- vagina R87.629
  - atypical squamous cells cannot exclude high grade squamous intraepithelial lesion (ASC-H) R87.621
  - atypical squamous cells of undetermined significance (ASC-US) R87.620
  - cytologic evidence of malignancy R87.624
  - high grade squamous intraepithelial lesion (HGSIL) R87.623
  - inadequate smear R87.625
  - low grade squamous intraepithelial lesion (LGSIL) R87.622
  - specified NEC R87.628
  - thin preparation R87.629
  - unsatisfactory smear R87.625
- vulva R87.69
- wound secretions R89.6

partial thromboplastin time (PTT) R79.1

pelvis (bony) — *see* Deformity, pelvis

percussion, chest (tympany) R09.89

periods (grossly) — *see* Menstruation

phonocardiogram R94.39

plantar reflex R29.2

plasma
- protein R77.9
  - specified NEC R77.8
- viscosity R70.1

pleural (folds) Q34.0

posture R29.3

product of conception O02.9
- specified type NEC O02.89

prothrombin time (PT) R79.1

pulmonary
- artery, congenital Q25.79
- function, newborn P28.89
- test results R94.2

pulsations in neck R00.2

pupillary H21.56- ☑
- function (reaction) (reflex) — *see* Anomaly, pupil, function

radiological examination — *see* Abnormal, diagnostic imaging

red blood cell(s) (morphology) (volume) R71.8

reflex — *see* Reflex

Abnormal, abnormality, abnormalities — *continued*

renal function test R94.4

response to nerve stimulation R94.130

retinal correspondence H53.31

retinal function study R94.111

rhythm, heart (*see also* Arrhythmia)

saliva — *see* Abnormal, specimen, digestive organs

scan
- kidney R94.4
- liver R93.2
- thyroid R94.6

secretion
- gastrin E16.4
- glucagon E16.3

semen, seminal fluid — *see* Abnormal, specimen, male genital organs

serum level (of)
- acid phosphatase R74.8
- alkaline phosphatase R74.8
- amylase R74.8
- enzymes R74.9
  - specified NEC R74.8
- lipase R74.8
- triacylglycerol lipase R74.8

shape
- gravid uterus — *see* Anomaly, uterus

sinus venosus Q21.1

size, tooth, teeth K00.2

spacing, tooth, teeth, fully erupted M26.30

specimen
- digestive organs (peritoneal fluid) (saliva) R85.9
  - cytology R85.69
  - drug level R85.2
  - enzyme level R85.0
  - histology R85.7
  - hormones R85.1
  - immunology R85.4
  - microbiology R85.5
  - nonmedicinal level R85.3
  - specified type NEC R85.89
- female genital organs (secretions) (smears) R87.9
  - cytology R87.69
    - cervix R87.619
      - human papillomavirus (HPV) DNA test
        - high risk positive R87.810
        - low risk positive R87.820
      - inadequate (unsatisfactory) smear R87.615
      - non-atypical endometrial cells R87.618
      - specified NEC R87.618
    - vagina R87.629
      - human papillomavirus (HPV) DNA test
        - high risk positive R87.811
        - low risk positive R87.821
      - inadequate (unsatisfactory) smear R87.625
    - vulva R87.69
  - drug level R87.2
  - enzyme level R87.0
  - histological R87.7
  - hormones R87.1
  - immunology R87.4
  - microbiology R87.5
  - nonmedicinal level R87.3
  - specified type NEC R87.89
- male genital organs (prostatic secretions) (semen) R86.9
  - cytology R86.6
  - drug level R86.2
  - enzyme level R86.0
  - histological R86.7
  - hormones R86.1
  - immunology R86.4
  - microbiology R86.5
  - nonmedicinal level R86.3
  - specified type NEC R86.8
- nipple discharge — *see* Abnormal, specimen, specified
- respiratory organs (bronchial washings) (nasal secretions) (pleural fluid) (sputum) R84.9
  - cytology R84.6
  - drug level R84.2
  - enzyme level R84.0
  - histology R84.7
  - hormones R84.1
  - immunology R84.4
  - microbiology R84.5
  - nonmedicinal level R84.3

☑ **Additional Character Required — Refer to the Tabular List for Character Selection** ▽ **Subterms under main terms may continue to next column or page**

Abnormal, abnormality, abnormalities — *continued*
  specimen — *continued*
    respiratory organs — *continued*
      specified type NEC R84.8
    specified organ, system and tissue NOS R89.9
      cytology R89.6
      drug level R89.2
      enzyme level R89.0
      histology R89.7
      hormones R89.1
      immunology R89.4
      microbiology R89.5
      nonmedicinal level R89.3
      specified type NEC R89.8
    synovial fluid — *see* Abnormal, specimen, specified
    thorax (bronchial washings) (pleural fluids) — *see* Abnormal, specimen, respiratory organs
    vagina (secretion) (smear) R87.629
    vulva (secretion) (smear) R87.69
    wound secretion — *see* Abnormal, specimen, specified
  spermatozoa — *see* Abnormal, specimen, male genital organs
  sputum (amount) (color) (odor) R09.3
  stool (color) (contents) (mucus) R19.5
    bloody K92.1
    guaiac positive R19.5
  synchondrosis Q78.8
  thermography (*see also* Abnormal, diagnostic imaging) R93.8
  thyroid-binding globulin E07.89
  tooth, teeth (form) (size) K00.2
  toxicology (findings) R78.9
  transport protein E88.09
  tumor marker NEC R97.8
  ultrasound results — *see* Abnormal, diagnostic imaging
  umbilical cord complicating delivery O69.9 ☑
  urination NEC R39.198
  urine (constituents) R82.90
    bile R82.2
    cytological examination R82.8
    drugs R82.5
    fat R82.0
    glucose R81
    heavy metals R82.6
    hemoglobin R82.3
    histological examination R82.8
    ketones R82.4
    microbiological examination (culture) R82.79
    myoglobin R82.1
    positive culture R82.79
    protein — *see* Proteinuria
    specified substance NEC R82.99
      chromoabnormality NEC R82.91
    substances nonmedical R82.6
  uterine hemorrhage — *see* Hemorrhage, uterus
  vectorcardiogram R94.39
  visually evoked potential (VEP) R94.112
  white blood cells D72.9
    specified NEC D72.89
  X-ray examination — *see* Abnormal, diagnostic imaging
Abnormity (any organ or part) — *see* Anomaly
Abocclusion M26.29
  hemolytic disease (newborn) P55.1
  incompatibility reaction ABO — *see* Complication(s), transfusion, incompatibility reaction, ABO
Abolition, language R48.8
Aborter, habitual or recurrent — *see* Loss (of), pregnancy, recurrent
Abortion (complete) (spontaneous) O03.9
  with
    retained products of conception — *see* Abortion, incomplete
  attempted (elective) (failed) O07.4
    complicated by O07.30
      afibrinogenemia O07.1
      cardiac arrest O07.36
      chemical damage of pelvic organ(s) O07.34
      circulatory collapse O07.31
      cystitis O07.38
      defibrination syndrome O07.1
      electrolyte imbalance O07.33
      embolism (air) (amniotic fluid) (blood clot) (fat) (pulmonary) (septic) (soap) O07.2
      endometritis O07.0

Abortion — *continued*
  attempted — *continued*
    complicated by — *continued*
      genital tract and pelvic infection O07.0
      hemolysis O07.1
      hemorrhage (delayed) (excessive) O07.1
      infection
        genital tract or pelvic O07.0
        urinary tract tract O07.38
      intravascular coagulation O07.1
      laceration of pelvic organ(s) O07.34
      metabolic disorder O07.33
      oliguria O07.32
      oophoritis O07.0
      parametritis O07.0
      pelvic peritonitis O07.0
      perforation of pelvic organ(s) O07.34
      renal failure or shutdown O07.32
      salpingitis or salpingo-oophoritis O07.0
      sepsis O07.37
      shock O07.31
      specified condition NEC O07.39
      tubular necrosis (renal) O07.32
      uremia O07.32
      urinary tract infection O07.38
      venous complication NEC O07.35
        embolism (air) (amniotic fluid) (blood clot) (fat) (pulmonary) (septic) (soap) O07.2
  complicated (by) (following) O03.80
    afibrinogenemia O03.6
    cardiac arrest O03.86
    chemical damage of pelvic organ(s) O03.84
    circulatory collapse O03.81
    cystitis O03.88
    defibrination syndrome O03.6
    electrolyte imbalance O03.83
    embolism (air) (amniotic fluid) (blood clot) (fat) (pulmonary) (septic) (soap) O03.7
    endometritis O03.5
    genital tract and pelvic infection O03.5
    hemolysis O03.6
    hemorrhage (delayed) (excessive) O03.6
    infection
      genital tract or pelvic O03.5
      urinary tract O03.88
    intravascular coagulation O03.6
    laceration of pelvic organ(s) O03.84
    metabolic disorder O03.83
    oliguria O03.82
    oophoritis O03.5
    parametritis O03.5
    pelvic peritonitis O03.5
    perforation of pelvic organ(s) O03.84
    renal failure or shutdown O03.82
    salpingitis or salpingo-oophoritis O03.5
    sepsis O03.87
    shock O03.81
    specified condition NEC O03.89
    tubular necrosis (renal) O03.82
    uremia O03.82
    urinary tract infection O03.88
    venous complication NEC O03.85
      embolism (air) (amniotic fluid) (blood clot) (fat) (pulmonary) (septic) (soap) O03.7
  failed — *see* Abortion, attempted
  habitual or recurrent N96
    with current abortion — *see* categories O03-O04
    without current pregnancy N96
    care in current pregnancy O26.2- ☑
  incomplete (spontaneous) O03.4
    complicated (by) (following) O03.30
      afibrinogenemia O03.1
      cardiac arrest O03.36
      chemical damage of pelvic organ(s) O03.34
      circulatory collapse O03.31
      cystitis O03.38
      defibrination syndrome O03.1
      electrolyte imbalance O03.33
      embolism (air) (amniotic fluid) (blood clot) (fat) (pulmonary) (septic) (soap) O03.2
      endometritis O03.0
      genital tract and pelvic infection O03.0
      hemolysis O03.1
      hemorrhage (delayed) (excessive) O03.1
      infection
        genital tract or pelvic O03.0
        urinary tract O03.38
      intravascular coagulation O03.1
      laceration of pelvic organ(s) O03.34

Abortion — *continued*
  incomplete — *continued*
    complicated — *continued*
      metabolic disorder O03.33
      oliguria O03.32
      oophoritis O03.0
      parametritis O03.0
      pelvic peritonitis O03.0
      perforation of pelvic organ(s) O03.34
      renal failure or shutdown O03.32
      salpingitis or salpingo-oophoritis O03.0
      sepsis O03.37
      shock O03.31
      specified condition NEC O03.39
      tubular necrosis (renal) O03.32
      uremia O03.32
      urinary infection O03.38
      venous complication NEC O03.35
        embolism (air) (amniotic fluid) (blood clot) (fat) (pulmonary) (septic) (soap) O03.2
  induced (encounter for) Z33.2
    complicated by O04.80
      afibrinogenemia O04.6
      cardiac arrest O04.86
      chemical damage of pelvic organ(s) O04.84
      circulatory collapse O04.81
      cystitis O04.88
      defibrination syndrome O04.6
      electrolyte imbalance O04.83
      embolism (air) (amniotic fluid) (blood clot) (fat) (pulmonary) (septic) (soap) O04.7
      endometritis O04.5
      genital tract and pelvic infection O04.5
      hemolysis O04.6
      hemorrhage (delayed) (excessive) O04.6
      infection
        genital tract or pelvic O04.5
        urinary tract O04.88
      intravascular coagulation O04.6
      laceration of pelvic organ(s) O04.84
      metabolic disorder O04.83
      oliguria O04.82
      oophoritis O04.5
      parametritis O04.5
      pelvic peritonitis O04.5
      perforation of pelvic organ(s) O04.84
      renal failure or shutdown O04.82
      salpingitis or salpingo-oophoritis O04.5
      sepsis O04.87
      shock O04.81
      specified condition NEC O04.89
      tubular necrosis (renal) O04.82
      uremia O04.82
      urinary tract infection O04.88
      venous complication NEC O04.85
        embolism (air) (amniotic fluid) (blood clot) (fat) (pulmonary) (septic) (soap) O04.7
  missed O02.1
  spontaneous — *see* Abortion (complete) (spontaneous)
    threatened O20.0
  threatened (spontaneous) O20.0
  tubal O00.10- ☑
    with intrauterine pregnancy O00.11- ☑
Abortus fever A23.1
Aboulomania F60.7
Abrami's disease D59.8
Abramov-Fiedler myocarditis (acute isolated myocarditis) I40.1
Abrasion T14.8 ☑
  abdomen, abdominal (wall) S30.811 ☑
  alveolar process S00.512 ☑
  ankle S90.51- ☑
  antecubital space — *see* Abrasion, elbow
  anus S30.817 ☑
  arm (upper) S40.81- ☑
  auditory canal — *see* Abrasion, ear
  auricle — *see* Abrasion, ear
  axilla — *see* Abrasion, arm
  back, lower S30.810 ☑
  breast S20.11- ☑
  brow S00.81 ☑
  buttock S30.810 ☑
  calf — *see* Abrasion, leg
  canthus — *see* Abrasion, eyelid
  cheek S00.81 ☑
    internal S00.512 ☑
  chest wall — *see* Abrasion, thorax

Abrasion — continued
  chin S00.81 ☑
  clitoris S30.814 ☑
  cornea S05.0- ☑
  costal region — see Abrasion, thorax
  dental K03.1
  digit(s)
    foot — see Abrasion, toe
    hand — see Abrasion, finger
  ear S00.41- ☑
  elbow S50.31- ☑
  epididymis S30.813 ☑
  epigastric region S30.811 ☑
  epiglottis S10.11 ☑
  esophagus (thoracic) S27.818 ☑
    cervical S10.11 ☑
  eyebrow — see Abrasion, eyelid
  eyelid S00.21- ☑
  face S00.81 ☑
  finger(s) S60.41- ☑
    index S60.41- ☑
    little S60.41- ☑
    middle S60.41- ☑
    ring S60.41- ☑
  flank S30.811 ☑
  foot (except toe(s) alone) S90.81- ☑
    toe — see Abrasion, toe
  forearm S50.81- ☑
    elbow only — see Abrasion, elbow
  forehead S00.81 ☑
  genital organs, external
    female S30.816 ☑
    male S30.815 ☑
  groin S30.811 ☑
  gum S00.512 ☑
  hand S60.51- ☑
  head S00.91 ☑
    ear — see Abrasion, ear
    eyelid — see Abrasion, eyelid
    lip S00.511 ☑
    nose S00.31 ☑
    oral cavity S00.512 ☑
    scalp S00.01 ☑
    specified site NEC S00.81 ☑
  heel — see Abrasion, foot
  hip S70.21- ☑
  inguinal region S30.811 ☑
  interscapular region S20.419 ☑
  jaw S00.81 ☑
  knee S80.21- ☑
  labium (majus) (minus) S30.814 ☑
  larynx S10.11 ☑
  leg (lower) S80.81- ☑
    knee — see Abrasion, knee
    upper — see Abrasion, thigh
  lip S00.511 ☑
  lower back S30.810 ☑
  lumbar region S30.810 ☑
  malar region S00.81 ☑
  mammary — see Abrasion, breast
  mastoid region S00.81 ☑
  mouth S00.512 ☑
  nail
    finger — see Abrasion, finger
    toe — see Abrasion, toe
  nape S10.81 ☑
  nasal S00.31 ☑
  neck S10.91 ☑
    specified site NEC S10.81 ☑
    throat S10.11 ☑
  nose S00.31 ☑
  occipital region S00.01 ☑
  oral cavity S00.512 ☑
  orbital region — see Abrasion, eyelid
  palate S00.512 ☑
  palm — see Abrasion, hand
  parietal region S00.01 ☑
  pelvis S30.810 ☑
  penis S30.812 ☑
  perineum
    female S30.814 ☑
    male S30.810 ☑
  periocular area — see Abrasion, eyelid
  phalanges
    finger — see Abrasion, finger
    toe — see Abrasion, toe

Abrasion — continued
  pharynx S10.11 ☑
  pinna — see Abrasion, ear
  popliteal space — see Abrasion, knee
  prepuce S30.812 ☑
  pubic region S30.810 ☑
  pudendum
    female S30.816 ☑
    male S30.815 ☑
  sacral region S30.810 ☑
  scalp S00.01 ☑
  scapular region — see Abrasion, shoulder
  scrotum S30.813 ☑
  shin — see Abrasion, leg
  shoulder S40.21- ☑
  skin NEC T14.8 ☑
  sternal region S20.319 ☑
  submaxillary region S00.81 ☑
  submental region S00.81 ☑
  subungual
    finger(s) — see Abrasion, finger
    toe(s) — see Abrasion, toe
  supraclavicular fossa S10.81 ☑
  supraorbital S00.81 ☑
  temple S00.81 ☑
  temporal region S00.81 ☑
  testis S30.813 ☑
  thigh S70.31- ☑
  thorax, thoracic (wall) S20.91 ☑
    back S20.41- ☑
    front S20.31- ☑
  throat S10.11 ☑
  thumb S60.31- ☑
  toe(s) (lesser) S90.416 ☑
    great S90.41- ☑
  tongue S00.512 ☑
  tooth, teeth (dentifrice) (habitual) (hard tissues) (occupational) (ritual) (traditional) K03.1
  trachea S10.11 ☑
  tunica vaginalis S30.813 ☑
  tympanum, tympanic membrane — see Abrasion, ear
  uvula S00.512 ☑
  vagina S30.814 ☑
  vocal cords S10.11 ☑
  vulva S30.814 ☑
  wrist S60.81- ☑
Abrism — see Poisoning, food, noxious, plant
Abruptio placentae O45.9- ☑
  with
    afibrinogenemia O45.01- ☑
    coagulation defect O45.00- ☑
      specified NEC O45.09- ☑
    disseminated intravascular coagulation O45.02- ☑
    hypofibrinogenemia O45.01- ☑
  specified NEC O45.8- ☑
Abruption, placenta — see Abruptio placentae
Abscess (connective tissue) (embolic) (fistulous) (infective) (metastatic) (multiple) (pernicious) (pyogenic) (septic) L02.91
  with
    diverticular disease (intestine) K57.80
      with bleeding K57.81
      large intestine K57.20
        with
          bleeding K57.21
          small intestine K57.40
            with bleeding K57.41
      small intestine K57.00
        with
          bleeding K57.01
          large intestine K57.40
            with bleeding K57.41
    lymphangitis — code by site under Abscess
  abdomen, abdominal
    cavity K65.1
    wall L02.211
  abdominopelvic K65.1
  accessory sinus — see Sinusitis
  adrenal (capsule) (gland) E27.8
  alveolar K04.7
    with sinus K04.6
  amebic A06.4
    brain (and liver or lung abscess) A06.6
    genitourinary tract A06.82
    liver (without mention of brain or lung abscess) A06.4

Abscess — continued
  amebic — continued
    lung (and liver) (without mention of brain abscess) A06.5
      specified site NEC A06.89
      spleen A06.89
  anerobic A48.0
  ankle — see Abscess, lower limb
  anorectal K61.2
  antecubital space — see Abscess, upper limb
  antrum (chronic) (Highmore) — see Sinusitis, maxillary
  anus K61.0
  apical (tooth) K04.7
    with sinus (alveolar) K04.6
  appendix K35.3
  areola (acute) (chronic) (nonpuerperal) N61.1
    puerperal, postpartum or gestational — see Infection, nipple
  arm (any part) — see Abscess, upper limb
  artery (wall) I77.89
  atheromatous I77.2
  auricle, ear — see Abscess, ear, external
  axilla (region) L02.41- ☑
    lymph gland or node L04.2
  back (any part, except buttock) L02.212
  Bartholin's gland N75.1
    with
      abortion — see Abortion, by type complicated by, sepsis
      ectopic or molar pregnancy O08.0
    following ectopic or molar pregnancy O08.0
  Bezold's — see Mastoiditis, acute
  bilharziasis B65.1
  bladder (wall) — see Cystitis, specified type NEC
  bone (subperiosteal) (see also Osteomyelitis, specified type NEC)
    accessory sinus (chronic) — see Sinusitis
    chronic or old — see Osteomyelitis, chronic
    jaw (lower) (upper) M27.2
    mastoid — see Mastoiditis, acute, subperiosteal
    petrous — see Petrositis
    spinal (tuberculous) A18.01
      nontuberculous — see Osteomyelitis, vertebra
  bowel K63.0
  brain (any part) (cystic) (otogenic) G06.0
    amebic (with abscess of any other site) A06.6
    gonococcal A54.82
    pheomycotic (chromomycotic) B43.1
    tuberculous A17.81
  breast (acute) (chronic) (nonpuerperal) N61.1
    newborn P39.0
    puerperal, postpartum, gestational — see Mastitis, obstetric, purulent
  broad ligament N73.2
    acute N73.0
    chronic N73.1
  Brodie's (localized) (chronic) M86.8X- ☑
  bronchi J98.09
  buccal cavity K12.2
  bulbourethral gland N34.0
  bursa M71.00
    ankle M71.07- ☑
    elbow M71.02- ☑
    foot M71.07- ☑
    hand M71.04- ☑
    hip M71.05- ☑
    knee M71.06- ☑
    multiple sites M71.09
    pharyngeal J39.1
    shoulder M71.01- ☑
    specified site NEC M71.08
    wrist M71.03- ☑
  buttock L02.31
  canthus — see Blepharoconjunctivitis
  cartilage — see Disorder, cartilage, specified type NEC
  cecum K35.3
  cerebellum, cerebellar G06.0
    sequelae G09
  cerebral (embolic) G06.0
    sequelae G09
  cervical (meaning neck) L02.11
    lymph gland or node L04.0
  cervix (stump) (uteri) — see Cervicitis
  cheek (external) L02.01
    inner K12.2
  chest J86.9
    with fistula J86.0
    wall L02.213

4

☑ **Additional Character Required** — Refer to the Tabular List for Character Selection   ☷ **Subterms under main terms may continue to next column or page**

Abscess — *continued*
chin L02.01
choroid — *see* Inflammation, chorioretinal
circumtonsillar J36
cold (lung) (tuberculous) (*see also* Tuberculosis, abscess, lung)
    articular — *see* Tuberculosis, joint
colon (wall) K63.0
colostomy K94.02
conjunctiva — *see* Conjunctivitis, acute
cornea H16.31- ☑
corpus
    cavernosum N48.21
    luteum — *see* Oophoritis
Cowper's gland N34.0
cranium G06.0
cul-de-sac (Douglas') (posterior) — *see* Peritonitis, pelvic, female
cutaneous — *see* Abscess, by site
dental K04.7
    with sinus (alveolar) K04.6
dentoalveolar K04.7
    with sinus K04.6
diaphragm, diaphragmatic K65.1
Douglas' cul-de-sac or pouch — *see* Peritonitis, pelvic, female
Dubois A50.59
ear (middle) (*see also* Otitis, media, suppurative)
    acute — *see* Otitis, media, suppurative, acute
    external H60.0- ☑
entamebic — *see* Abscess, amebic
enterostomy K94.12
epididymis N45.4
epidural G06.2
    brain G06.0
    spinal cord G06.1
epiglottis J38.7
epiploon, epiploic K65.1
erysipelatous — *see* Erysipelas
esophagus K20.8
ethmoid (bone) (chronic) (sinus) J32.2
external auditory canal — *see* Abscess, ear, external
extradural G06.2
    brain G06.0
      sequelae G09
    spinal cord G06.1
extraperitoneal K68.19
eye — *see* Endophthalmitis, purulent
eyelid H00.03- ☑
face (any part, except ear, eye and nose) L02.01
fallopian tube — *see* Salpingitis
fascia M72.8
fauces J39.1
fecal K63.0
femoral (region) — *see* Abscess, lower limb
filaria, filarial — *see* Infestation, filarial
finger (any) (*see also* Abscess, hand)
    nail — *see* Cellulitis, finger
foot L02.61- ☑
forehead L02.01
frontal sinus (chronic) J32.1
gallbladder K81.0
genital organ or tract
    female (external) N76.4
    male N49.9
      multiple sites N49.8
      specified NEC N49.8
gestational mammary O91.11- ☑
gestational subareolar O91.11- ☑
gingival — *see* Peridontitis, aggressive, localized
gland, glandular (lymph) (acute) — *see* Lymphadenitis, acute
gluteal (region) L02.31
gonorrheal — *see* Gonococcus
groin L02.214
gum — *see* Peridontitis, aggressive, localized
hand L02.51- ☑
head NEC L02.811
    face (any part, except ear, eye and nose) L02.01
heart — *see* Carditis
heel — *see* Abscess, foot
helminthic — *see* Infestation, helminth
hepatic (cholangitic) (hematogenic) (lymphogenic) (pylephlebitic) K75.0
    amebic A06.4
hip (region) — *see* Abscess, lower limb
ileocecal K35.3
ileostomy (bud) K94.12

Abscess — *continued*
iliac (region) L02.214
    fossa K35.3
infraclavicular (fossa) — *see* Abscess, upper limb
inguinal (region) L02.214
    lymph gland or node L04.1
intestine, intestinal NEC K63.0
    rectal K61.1
intra-abdominal (*see also* Abscess, peritoneum) K65.1
    postprocedural T81.4 ☑
      retroperitoneal K68.11
intracranial G06.0
intramammary — *see* Abscess, breast
intraorbital — *see* Abscess, orbit
intraperitoneal K65.1
intrasphincteric (anus) K61.4
intraspinal G06.1
intratonsillar J36
ischiorectal (fossa) K61.3
jaw (bone) (lower) (upper) M27.2
joint — *see* Arthritis, pyogenic or pyemic
    spine (tuberculous) A18.01
      nontuberculous — *see* Spondylopathy, infective
kidney N15.1
    with calculus N20.0
      with hydronephrosis N13.6
    puerperal (postpartum) O86.21
knee (*see also* Abscess, lower limb)
    joint M00.9
labium (majus) (minus) N76.4
lacrimal
    caruncle — *see* Inflammation, lacrimal, passages, acute
    gland — *see* Dacryoadenitis
    passages (duct) (sac) — *see* Inflammation, lacrimal, passages, acute
lacunar N34.0
larynx J38.7
lateral (alveolar) K04.7
    with sinus K04.6
leg (any part) — *see* Abscess, lower limb
lens H27.8
lingual K14.0
    tonsil J36
lip K13.0
Littre's gland N34.0
liver (cholangitic) (hematogenic) (lymphogenic) (pylephlebitic) (pyogenic) K75.0
    amebic (due to Entamoeba histolytica) (dysenteric) (tropical) A06.4
      with
        brain abscess (and liver or lung abscess) A06.6
        lung abscess A06.5
loin (region) L02.211
lower limb L02.41- ☑
lumbar (tuberculous) A18.01
    nontuberculous L02.212
lung (miliary) (putrid) J85.2
    with pneumonia J85.1
      due to specified organism (see Pneumonia, in (due to))
    amebic (with liver abscess) A06.5
      with
        brain abscess A06.6
        pneumonia A06.5
lymph, lymphatic, gland or node (acute) (*see also* Lymphadenitis, acute)
    mesentery I88.0
malar M27.2
mammary gland — *see* Abscess, breast
marginal, anus K61.0
mastoid — *see* Mastoiditis, acute
maxilla, maxillary M27.2
    molar (tooth) K04.7
      with sinus K04.6
    premolar K04.7
    sinus (chronic) J32.0
mediastinum J85.3
meibomian gland — *see* Hordeolum
meninges G06.2
mesentery, mesenteric K65.1
mesosalpinx — *see* Salpingitis
mons pubis L02.215
mouth (floor) K12.2
muscle — *see* Myositis, infective
myocardium I40.0

Abscess — *continued*
nabothian (follicle) — *see* Cervicitis
nasal J32.9
nasopharyngeal J39.1
navel L02.216
    newborn P38.9
      with mild hemorrhage P38.1
      without hemorrhage P38.9
neck (region) L02.11
    lymph gland or node L04.0
nephritic — *see* Abscess, kidney
nipple N61.1
    associated with
      lactation — *see* Pregnancy, complicated by
      pregnancy — *see* Pregnancy, complicated by
nose (external) (fossa) (septum) J34.0
    sinus (chronic) — *see* Sinusitis
omentum K65.1
operative wound T81.4 ☑
orbit, orbital — *see* Cellulitis, orbit
otogenic G06.0
ovary, ovarian (corpus luteum) — *see* Oophoritis
oviduct — *see* Oophoritis
palate (soft) K12.2
    hard M27.2
palmar (space) — *see* Abscess, hand
pancreas (duct) — *see* Pancreatitis, acute
parafrenal N48.21
parametric, parametrium N73.2
    acute N73.0
    chronic N73.1
paranephric N15.1
parapancreatic — *see* Pancreatitis, acute
parapharyngeal J39.0
pararectal K61.1
parasinus — *see* Sinusitis
parauterine (*see also* Disease, pelvis, inflammatory) N73.2
paravaginal — *see* Vaginitis
parietal region (scalp) L02.811
parodontal — *see* Peridontitis, aggressive, localized
parotid (duct) (gland) K11.3
    region K12.2
pectoral (region) L02.213
pelvis, pelvic
    female — *see* Disease, pelvis, inflammatory
    male, peritoneal K65.1
penis N48.21
    gonococcal (accessory gland) (periurethral) A54.1
perianal N48.21
periapical K04.7
    with sinus (alveolar) K04.6
periappendicular K35.3
pericardial I30.1
pericecal K35.3
pericemental — *see* Peridontitis, aggressive, localized
pericholecystic — *see* Cholecystitis, acute
pericoronal — *see* Peridontitis, aggressive, localized
peridental — *see* Peridontitis, aggressive, localized
perimetric (*see also* Disease, pelvis, inflammatory) N73.2
perinephric, perinephritic — *see* Abscess, kidney
perineum, perineal (superficial) L02.215
    urethra N34.0
periodontal (parietal) — *see* Peridontitis, aggressive, localized
    apical K04.7
periosteum, periosteal (*see also* Osteomyelitis, specified type NEC)
    with osteomyelitis (*see also* Osteomyelitis, specified type NEC)
      acute — *see* Osteomyelitis, acute
      chronic — *see* Osteomyelitis, chronic
peripharyngeal J39.0
peripleuritic J86.9
    with fistula J86.0
periprostatic N41.2
perirectal K61.1
perirenal (tissue) — *see* Abscess, kidney
perisinuous (nose) — *see* Sinusitis
peritoneum, peritoneal (perforated) (ruptured) K65.1
    with appendicitis K35.3
    pelvic
      female — *see* Peritonitis, pelvic, female
      male K65.1
    postoperative T81.4 ☑
    puerperal, postpartum, childbirth O85
    tuberculous A18.31

Abscess — *continued*
 peritonsillar J36
 perityphlic K35.3
 periureteral N28.89
 periurethral N34.0
  gonococcal (accessory gland) (periurethral) A54.1
 periuterine (*see also* Disease, pelvis, inflammatory) N73.2
 perivesical — *see* Cystitis, specified type NEC
 petrous bone — *see* Petrositis
 phagedenic NOS L02.91
  chancroid A57
 pharynx, pharyngeal (lateral) J39.1
 pilonidal L05.01
 pituitary (gland) E23.6
 pleura J86.9
  with fistula J86.0
 popliteal — *see* Abscess, lower limb
 postcecal K35.3
 postlaryngeal J38.7
 postnasal J34.0
 postoperative (any site) T81.4 ☑
  retroperitoneal K68.11
 postpharyngeal J39.0
 posttonsillar J36
 post-typhoid A01.09
 pouch of Douglas — *see* Peritonitis, pelvic, female
 premammary — *see* Abscess, breast
 prepatellar — *see* Abscess, lower limb
 prostate N41.2
  gonococcal (acute) (chronic) A54.22
 psoas muscle K68.12
 puerperal — *code by* site under Puerperal, abscess
 pulmonary — *see* Abscess, lung
 pulp, pulpal (dental) K04.01
  irreversible K04.02
  reversible K04.01
 rectovaginal septum K63.0
 rectovesical — *see* Cystitis, specified type NEC
 rectum K61.1
 renal — *see* Abscess, kidney
 retina — *see* Inflammation, chorioretinal
 retrobulbar — *see* Abscess, orbit
 retrocecal K65.1
 retrolaryngeal J38.7
 retromammary — *see* Abscess, breast
 retroperitoneal NEC K68.19
  postprocedural K68.11
 retropharyngeal J39.0
 retrouterine — *see* Peritonitis, pelvic, female
 retrovesical — *see* Cystitis, specified type NEC
 root, tooth K04.7
  with sinus (alveolar) K04.6
 round ligament (*see also* Disease, pelvis, inflammatory) N73.2
 rupture (spontaneous) NOS L02.91
 sacrum (tuberculous) A18.01
  nontuberculous M46.28
 salivary (duct) (gland) K11.3
 scalp (any part) L02.811
 scapular — *see* Osteomyelitis, specified type NEC
 sclera — *see* Scleritis
 scrofulous (tuberculous) A18.2
 scrotum N49.2
 seminal vesicle N49.0
 septal, dental K04.7
  with sinus (alveolar) K04.6
 serous — *see* Periostitis
 shoulder (region) — *see* Abscess, upper limb
 sigmoid K63.0
 sinus (accessory) (chronic) (nasal) (*see also* Sinusitis)
  intracranial venous (any) G06.0
 Skene's duct or gland N34.0
 skin — *see* Abscess, by site
 specified site NEC L02.818
 spermatic cord N49.1
 sphenoidal (sinus) (chronic) J32.3
 spinal cord (any part) (staphylococcal) G06.1
  tuberculous A17.81
 spine (column) (tuberculous) A18.01
  epidural G06.1
  nontuberculous — *see* Osteomyelitis, vertebra
 spleen D73.3
  amebic A06.89
 stitch T81.4 ☑
 subarachnoid G06.2
  brain G06.0
  spinal cord G06.1

Abscess — *continued*
 subareolar — *see* Abscess, breast
 subcecal K35.3
 subcutaneous (*see also* Abscess, by site)
  pheomycotic (chromomycotic) B43.2
 subdiaphragmatic K65.1
 subdural G06.2
  brain G06.0
   sequelae G09
  spinal cord G06.1
 subgaleal L02.811
 subhepatic K65.1
 sublingual K12.2
  gland K11.3
 submammary — *see* Abscess, breast
 submandibular (region) (space) (triangle) K12.2
  gland K11.3
 submaxillary (region) L02.01
  gland K11.3
 submental L02.01
  gland K11.3
 subperiosteal — *see* Osteomyelitis, specified type NEC
 subphrenic K65.1
  postoperative T81.4 ☑
 suburethral N34.0
 sudoriparous L75.8
 supraclavicular (fossa) — *see* Abscess, upper limb
 suprapelvic, acute N73.0
 suprarenal (capsule) (gland) E27.8
 sweat gland L74.8
 tear duct — *see* Inflammation, lacrimal, passages, acute
 temple L02.01
 temporal region L02.01
 temporosphenoidal G06.0
 tendon (sheath) M65.00
  ankle M65.07- ☑
  foot M65.07- ☑
  forearm M65.03- ☑
  hand M65.04- ☑
  lower leg M65.06- ☑
  pelvic region M65.05- ☑
  shoulder region M65.01- ☑
  specified site NEC M65.08
  thigh M65.05- ☑
  upper arm M65.02- ☑
 testis N45.4
 thigh — *see* Abscess, lower limb
 thorax J86.9
  with fistula J86.0
 throat J39.1
 thumb (*see also* Abscess, hand)
  nail — *see* Cellulitis, finger
 thymus E32.1
 thyroid (gland) E06.0
 toe (any) (*see also* Abscess, foot)
  nail — *see* Cellulitis, toe
 tongue (staphylococcal) K14.0
 tonsil(s) (lingual) J36
 tonsillopharyngeal J36
 tooth, teeth (root) K04.7
  with sinus (alveolar) K04.6
  supporting structures NEC — *see* Peridontitis, aggressive, localized
 trachea J39.8
 trunk L02.219
  abdominal wall L02.211
  back L02.212
  chest wall L02.213
  groin L02.214
  perineum L02.215
  umbilicus L02.216
 tubal — *see* Salpingitis
 tuberculous — *see* Tuberculosis, abscess
 tubo-ovarian — *see* Salpingo-oophoritis
 tunica vaginalis N49.1
 umbilicus L02.216
 upper
  limb L02.41- ☑
  respiratory J39.8
 urethral (gland) N34.0
 urinary N34.0
 uterus, uterine (wall) (*see also* Endometritis)
  ligament (*see also* Disease, pelvis, inflammatory) N73.2
  neck — *see* Cervicitis
 uvula K12.2
 vagina (wall) — *see* Vaginitis

Abscess — *continued*
 vaginorectal — *see* Vaginitis
 vas deferens N49.1
 vermiform appendix K35.3
 vertebra (column) (tuberculous) A18.01
  nontuberculous — *see* Osteomyelitis, vertebra
 vesical — *see* Cystitis, specified type NEC
 vesico-uterine pouch — *see* Peritonitis, pelvic, female
 vitreous (humor) — *see* Endophthalmitis, purulent
 vocal cord J38.3
 von Bezold's — *see* Mastoiditis, acute
 vulva N76.4
 vulvovaginal gland N75.1
 web space — *see* Abscess, hand
 wound T81.4 ☑
 wrist — *see* Abscess, upper limb
Absence (of) (organ or part) (complete or partial)
 adrenal (gland) (congenital) Q89.1
  acquired E89.6
 albumin in blood E88.09
 alimentary tract (congenital) Q45.8
  upper Q40.8
 alveolar process (acquired) — *see* Anomaly, alveolar
 ankle (acquired) Z89.44- ☑
 anus (congenital) Q42.3
  with fistula Q42.2
 aorta (congenital) Q25.41
 appendix, congenital Q42.8
 arm (acquired) Z89.20- ☑
  above elbow Z89.22- ☑
   congenital (with hand present) — *see* Agenesis, arm, with hand present
   and hand — *see* Agenesis, forearm, and hand
  below elbow Z89.21- ☑
   congenital (with hand present) — *see* Agenesis, arm, with hand present
   and hand — *see* Agenesis, forearm, and hand
  congenital — *see* Defect, reduction, upper limb
  shoulder (following explantation of shoulder joint prosthesis) (joint) (with or without presence of antibiotic-impregnated cement spacer) Z89.23- ☑
   congenital (with hand present) — *see* Agenesis, arm, with hand present
 artery (congenital) (peripheral) Q27.8
  brain Q28.3
  coronary Q24.5
  pulmonary Q25.79
  specified NEC Q27.8
  umbilical Q27.0
 atrial septum (congenital) Q21.1
 auditory canal (congenital) (external) Q16.1
 auricle (ear), congenital Q16.0
 bile, biliary duct, congenital Q44.5
 bladder (acquired) Z90.6
  congenital Q64.5
 bowel sounds R19.11
 brain Q00.0
  part of Q04.3
 breast(s) (and nipple(s)) (acquired) Z90.1- ☑
  congenital Q83.8
 broad ligament Q50.6
 bronchus (congenital) Q32.4
 canaliculus lacrimalis, congenital Q10.4
 cerebellum (vermis) Q04.3
 cervix (acquired) (with uterus) Z90.710
  with remaining uterus Z90.712
  congenital Q51.5
 chin (congenital) Q18.8
 cilia (congenital) Q10.3
  acquired — *see* Madarosis
 clitoris (congenital) Q52.6
 coccyx, congenital Q76.49
 cold sense R20.8
 congenital
  lumen — *see* Atresia
  organ or site NEC — *see* Agenesis
  septum — *see* Imperfect, closure
 corpus callosum Q04.0
 cricoid cartilage, congenital Q31.8
 diaphragm (with hernia), congenital Q79.1
 digestive organ(s) or tract, congenital Q45.8
  acquired NEC Z90.49
  upper Q40.8
 ductus arteriosus Q28.8
 duodenum (acquired) Z90.49

Absence — *continued*
  duodenum — *continued*
    congenital Q41.0
  ear, congenital Q16.9
    acquired H93.8- ☑
    auricle Q16.0
    external Q16.0
    inner Q16.5
    lobe, lobule Q17.8
    middle, except ossicles Q16.4
      ossicles Q16.3
    ossicles Q16.3
  ejaculatory duct (congenital) Q55.4
  endocrine gland (congenital) NEC Q89.2
    acquired E89.89
  epididymis (congenital) Q55.4
    acquired Z90.79
  epiglottis, congenital Q31.8
  esophagus (congenital) Q39.8
    acquired (partial) Z90.49
  eustachian tube (congenital) Q16.2
  extremity (acquired) Z89.9
    congenital Q73.8
    knee (following explantation of knee joint prosthe-
        sis) (joint) (with or without presence of an-
        tibiotic-impregnated cement spacer)
        Z89.52- ☑
    lower (above knee) Z89.619
      below knee Z89.51- ☑
    upper — *see* Absence, arm
  eye (acquired) Z90.01
    congenital Q11.1
    muscle (congenital) Q10.3
  eyeball (acquired) Z90.01
  eyelid (fold) (congenital) Q10.3
    acquired Z90.01
  face, specified part NEC Q18.8
  fallopian tube(s) (acquired) Z90.79
    congenital Q50.6
  family member (causing problem in home) NEC (*see
        also* Disruption, family) Z63.32
  femur, congenital — *see* Defect, reduction, lower limb,
        longitudinal, femur
  fibrinogen (congenital) D68.2
    acquired D65
  finger(s) (acquired) Z89.02- ☑
    congenital — *see* Agenesis, hand
  foot (acquired) Z89.43- ☑
    congenital — *see* Agenesis, foot
  forearm (acquired) — *see* Absence, arm, below elbow
  gallbladder (acquired) Z90.49
    congenital Q44.0
  gamma globulin in blood D80.1
    hereditary D80.0
  genital organs
    acquired (female) (male) Z90.79
    female, congenital Q52.8
      external Q52.71
      internal NEC Q52.8
    male, congenital Q55.8
  genitourinary organs, congenital NEC
    female Q52.8
    male Q55.8
  globe (acquired) Z90.01
    congenital Q11.1
  glottis, congenital Q31.8
  hand and wrist (acquired) Z89.11- ☑
    congenital — *see* Agenesis, hand
  head, part (acquired) NEC Z90.09
  heat sense R20.8
  hip (following explantation of hip joint prosthesis)
        (joint) (with or without presence of antibiotic-
        impregnated cement spacer) Z89.62- ☑
  hymen (congenital) Q52.4
  ileum (acquired) Z90.49
    congenital Q41.2
  immunoglobulin, isolated NEC D80.3
    IgA D80.2
    IgG D80.3
    IgM D80.4
  incus (acquired) — *see* Loss, ossicles, ear
    congenital Q16.3
  inner ear, congenital Q16.5
  intestine (acquired) (small) Z90.49
    congenital Q41.9
      specified NEC Q41.8
    large Z90.49
      congenital Q42.9

Absence — *continued*
  intestine — *continued*
    large — *continued*
      congenital — *continued*
        specified NEC Q42.8
  iris, congenital Q13.1
  jejunum (acquired) Z90.49
    congenital Q41.1
  joint
    acquired
      hip (following explantation of hip joint prosthe-
          sis) (with or without presence of antibiot-
          ic-impregnated cement spacer)
          Z89.62- ☑
      knee (following explantation of knee joint
          prosthesis) (with or without presence of
          antibiotic-impregnated cement spacer)
          Z89.52- ☑
      shoulder (following explantation of shoulder
          joint prosthesis) (with or without pres-
          ence of antibiotic-impregnated cement
          spacer) Z89.23- ☑
    congenital NEC Q74.8
  kidney(s) (acquired) Z90.5
    congenital Q60.2
      bilateral Q60.1
      unilateral Q60.0
  knee (following explantation of knee joint prosthesis)
        (joint) (with or without presence of antibiotic-
        impregnated cement spacer) Z89.52- ☑
  labyrinth, membranous Q16.5
  larynx (congenital) Q31.8
    acquired Z90.02
  leg (acquired) (above knee) Z89.61- ☑
    below knee (acquired) Z89.51- ☑
    congenital — *see* Defect, reduction, lower limb
  lens (acquired) (*see also* Aphakia)
    congenital Q12.3
    post cataract extraction Z98.4- ☑
  limb (acquired) — *see* Absence, extremity
  lip Q38.6
  liver (congenital) Q44.7
  lung (fissure) (lobe) (bilateral) (unilateral) (congenital)
        Q33.3
    acquired (any part) Z90.2
  menstruation — *see* Amenorrhea
  muscle (congenital) (pectoral) Q79.8
    ocular Q10.3
  neck, part Q18.8
  neutrophil — *see* Agranulocytosis
  nipple(s) (with breast(s)) (acquired) Z90.1- ☑
    congenital Q83.2
  nose (congenital) Q30.1
    acquired Z90.09
  organ
    of Corti, congenital Q16.5
    or site, congenital NEC Q89.8
      acquired NEC Z90.89
  osseous meatus (ear) Q16.4
  ovary (acquired)
    bilateral Z90.722
    congenital
      bilateral Q50.02
      unilateral Q50.01
    unilateral Z90.721
  oviduct (acquired)
    bilateral Z90.722
    congenital Q50.6
    unilateral Z90.721
  pancreas (congenital) Q45.0
    acquired Z90.410
      complete Z90.410
      partial Z90.411
      total Z90.410
  parathyroid gland (acquired) E89.2
    congenital Q89.2
  patella, congenital Q74.1
  penis (congenital) Q55.5
    acquired Z90.79
  pericardium (congenital) Q24.8
  pituitary gland (congenital) Q89.2
    acquired E89.3
  prostate (acquired) Z90.79
    congenital Q55.4
  pulmonary valve Q22.0
  punctum lacrimale (congenital) Q10.4
  radius, congenital — *see* Defect, reduction, upper limb,
        longitudinal, radius

Absence — *continued*
  rectum (congenital) Q42.1
    with fistula Q42.0
    acquired Z90.49
  respiratory organ NOS Q34.9
  rib (acquired) Z90.89
    congenital Q76.6
  sacrum, congenital Q76.49
  salivary gland(s), congenital Q38.4
  scrotum, congenital Q55.29
  seminal vesicles (congenital) Q55.4
    acquired Z90.79
  septum
    atrial (congenital) Q21.1
    between aorta and pulmonary artery Q21.4
    ventricular (congenital) Q20.4
  sex chromosome
    female phenotype Q97.8
    male phenotype Q98.8
  skull bone (congenital) Q75.8
    with
      anencephaly Q00.0
      encephalocele — *see* Encephalocele
      hydrocephalus Q03.9
        with spina bifida — *see* Spina bifida, by site,
            with hydrocephalus
      microcephaly Q02
  spermatic cord, congenital Q55.4
  spine, congenital Q76.49
  spleen (congenital) Q89.01
    acquired Z90.81
  sternum, congenital Q76.7
  stomach (acquired) (partial) Z90.3
    congenital Q40.2
  superior vena cava, congenital Q26.8
  teeth, tooth (congenital) K00.0
    acquired (complete) K08.109
      class I K08.101
      class II K08.102
      class III K08.103
      class IV K08.104
      due to
        caries K08.139
          class I K08.131
          class II K08.132
          class III K08.133
          class IV K08.134
        periodontal disease K08.129
          class I K08.121
          class II K08.122
          class III K08.123
          class IV K08.124
        specified NEC K08.199
          class I K08.191
          class II K08.192
          class III K08.193
          class IV K08.194
        trauma K08.119
          class I K08.111
          class II K08.112
          class III K08.113
          class IV K08.114
      partial K08.409
        class I K08.401
        class II K08.402
        class III K08.403
        class IV K08.404
        due to
          caries K08.439
            class I K08.431
            class II K08.432
            class III K08.433
            class IV K08.434
          periodontal disease K08.429
            class I K08.421
            class II K08.422
            class III K08.423
            class IV K08.424
          specified NEC K08.499
            class I K08.491
            class II K08.492
            class III K08.493
            class IV K08.494
          trauma K08.419
            class I K08.411
            class II K08.412
            class III K08.413
            class IV K08.414
  tendon (congenital) Q79.8

Index

Absence — Absence

Index

Absence — Abuse

Absence — *continued*
testis (congenital) Q55.0
acquired Z90.79
thumb (acquired) Z89.01- ☑
congenital — *see* Agenesis, hand
thymus gland Q89.2
thyroid (gland) (acquired) E89.0
cartilage, congenital Q31.8
congenital E03.1
toe(s) (acquired) Z89.42- ☑
with foot — *see* Absence, foot and ankle
congenital — *see* Agenesis, foot
great Z89.41- ☑
tongue, congenital Q38.3
trachea (cartilage), congenital Q32.1
transverse aortic arch, congenital Q25.49
tricuspid valve Q22.4
umbilical artery, congenital Q27.0
upper arm and forearm with hand present, congenital
— *see* Agenesis, arm, with hand present
ureter (congenital) Q62.4
acquired Z90.6
urethra, congenital Q64.5
uterus (acquired) Z90.710
with cervix Z90.710
with remaining cervical stump Z90.711
congenital Q51.0
uvula, congenital Q38.5
vagina, congenital Q52.0
vas deferens (congenital) Q55.4
acquired Z90.79
vein (peripheral) congenital NEC Q27.8
cerebral Q28.3
digestive system Q27.8
great Q26.8
lower limb Q27.8
portal Q26.5
precerebral Q28.1
specified site NEC Q27.8
upper limb Q27.8
vena cava (inferior) (superior), congenital Q26.8
ventricular septum Q20.4
vertebra, congenital Q76.49
vulva, congenital Q52.71
wrist (acquired) Z89.12- ☑
Absorbent system disease I87.8
Absorption
carbohydrate, disturbance K90.49
chemical — *see* Table of Drugs and Chemicals
through placenta (newborn) P04.9
environmental substance P04.6
nutritional substance P04.5
obstetric anesthetic or analgesic drug P04.0
drug NEC — *see* Table of Drugs and Chemicals
addictive
through placenta (newborn) P04.49
cocaine P04.41
medicinal
through placenta (newborn) P04.1
through placenta (newborn) P04.1
obstetric anesthetic or analgesic drug P04.0
fat, disturbance K90.49
pancreatic K90.3
noxious substance — *see* Table of Drugs and Chemicals
protein, disturbance K90.49
starch, disturbance K90.49
toxic substance — *see* Table of Drugs and Chemicals
uremic — *see* Uremia
Abstinence symptoms, syndrome
alcohol F10.239
with delirium F10.231
cocaine F14.23
neonatal P96.1
nicotine — *see* Dependence, drug, nicotine, with, withdrawal
opioid F11.93
with dependence F11.23
psychoactive NEC F19.939
with
delirium F19.931
dependence F19.239
with
delirium F19.231
perceptual disturbance F19.232
uncomplicated F19.230
perceptual disturbance F19.932
uncomplicated F19.930

Abstinence symptoms, syndrome — *continued*
sedative F13.939
with
delirium F13.931
dependence F13.239
with
delirium F13.231
perceptual disturbance F13.232
uncomplicated F13.230
perceptual disturbance F13.932
uncomplicated F13.930
stimulant NEC F15.93
with dependence F15.23
Abulia R68.89
Abulomania F60.7
Abuse
adult — *see* Maltreatment, adult
as reason for
couple seeking advice (including offender)
Z63.0
alcohol (non-dependent) F10.10
with
anxiety disorder F10.180
intoxication F10.129
with delirium F10.121
uncomplicated F10.120
mood disorder F10.14
other specified disorder F10.188
psychosis F10.159
delusions F10.150
hallucinations F10.151
sexual dysfunction F10.181
sleep disorder F10.182
unspecified disorder F10.19
counseling and surveillance Z71.41
in remission (early) (sustained) F10.11
amphetamine (or related substance) — *see* Abuse,
drug, stimulant NEC
analgesics (non-prescribed) (over the counter) F55.8
antacids F55.0
antidepressants — *see* Abuse, drug, psychoactive NEC
anxiolytic — *see* Abuse, drug, sedative
barbiturates — *see* Abuse, drug, sedative
caffeine — *see* Abuse, drug, stimulant NEC
cannabis, cannabinoids — *see* Abuse, drug, cannabis
child — *see* Maltreatment, child
cocaine — *see* Abuse, drug, cocaine
drug NEC (non-dependent) F19.10
with sleep disorder F19.182
amphetamine type — *see* Abuse, drug, stimulant
NEC
analgesics (non-prescribed) (over the counter)
F55.8
antacids F55.0
antidepressants — *see* Abuse, drug, psychoactive
NEC
anxiolytics — *see* Abuse, drug, sedative
barbiturates — *see* Abuse, drug, sedative
caffeine — *see* Abuse, drug, stimulant NEC
cannabis F12.10
with
anxiety disorder F12.180
intoxication F12.129
with
delirium F12.121
perceptual disturbance F12.122
uncomplicated F12.120
other specified disorder F12.188
psychosis F12.159
delusions F12.150
hallucinations F12.151
unspecified disorder F12.19
in remission (early) (sustained) F12.11
cocaine F14.10
with
anxiety disorder F14.180
intoxication F14.129
with
delirium F14.121
perceptual disturbance F14.122
uncomplicated F14.120
mood disorder F14.14
other specified disorder F14.188
psychosis F14.159
delusions F14.150
hallucinations F14.151
sexual dysfunction F14.181
sleep disorder F14.182

Abuse — *continued*
drug — *continued*
cocaine — *continued*
with — *continued*
unspecified disorder F14.19
in remission (early) (sustained) F14.11
counseling and surveillance Z71.51
hallucinogen F16.10
with
anxiety disorder F16.180
flashbacks F16.183
intoxication F16.129
with
delirium F16.121
perceptual disturbance F16.122
uncomplicated F16.120
mood disorder F16.14
other specified disorder F16.188
perception disorder, persisting F16.183
psychosis F16.159
delusions F16.150
hallucinations F16.151
unspecified disorder F16.19
in remission (early) (sustained) F16.11
hashish — *see* Abuse, drug, cannabis
herbal or folk remedies F55.1
hormones F55.3
hypnotics — *see* Abuse, drug, sedative
in remission (early) (sustained) F19.11
inhalant F18.10
with
anxiety disorder F18.180
dementia, persisting F18.17
intoxication F18.129
with delirium F18.121
uncomplicated F18.120
mood disorder F18.14
other specified disorder F18.188
psychosis F18.159
delusions F18.150
hallucinations F18.151
unspecified disorder F18.19
in remission (early) (sustained) F18.11
laxatives F55.2
LSD — *see* Abuse, drug, hallucinogen
marihuana — *see* Abuse, drug, cannabis
morphine type (opioids) — *see* Abuse, drug, opioid
opioid F11.10
with
intoxication F11.129
with
delirium F11.121
perceptual disturbance F11.122
uncomplicated F11.120
mood disorder F11.14
other specified disorder F11.188
psychosis F11.159
delusions F11.150
hallucinations F11.151
sexual dysfunction F11.181
sleep disorder F11.182
unspecified disorder F11.19
in remission (early) (sustained) F11.11
PCP (phencyclidine) (or related substance) — *see*
Abuse, drug, hallucinogen
psychoactive NEC F19.10
with
amnestic disorder F19.16
anxiety disorder F19.180
dementia F19.17
intoxication F19.129
with
delirium F19.121
perceptual disturbance F19.122
uncomplicated F19.120
mood disorder F19.14
other specified disorder F19.188
psychosis F19.159
delusions F19.150
hallucinations F19.151
sexual dysfunction F19.181
sleep disorder F19.182
unspecified disorder F19.19
sedative, hypnotic or anxiolytic F13.10
with
anxiety disorder F13.180
intoxication F13.129
with delirium F13.121
uncomplicated F13.120

Abuse — *continued*
  drug — *continued*
    sedative, hypnotic or anxiolytic — *continued*
      with — *continued*
        mood disorder F13.14
        other specified disorder F13.188
        psychosis F13.159
          delusions F13.150
          hallucinations F13.151
        sexual dysfunction F13.181
        sleep disorder F13.182
        unspecified disorder F13.19
      in remission (early) (sustained) F13.11
    solvent — *see* Abuse, drug, inhalant
    steroids F55.3
    stimulant NEC F15.10
      with
        anxiety disorder F15.180
        intoxication F15.129
          with
            delirium F15.121
            perceptual disturbance F15.122
          uncomplicated F15.120
        mood disorder F15.14
        other specified disorder F15.188
        psychosis F15.159
          delusions F15.150
          hallucinations F15.151
        sexual dysfunction F15.181
        sleep disorder F15.182
        unspecified disorder F15.19
      in remission (early) (sustained) F15.11
    tranquilizers — *see* Abuse, drug, sedative
    vitamins F55.4
  hallucinogens — *see* Abuse, drug, hallucinogen
  hashish — *see* Abuse, drug, cannabis
  herbal or folk remedies F55.1
  hormones F55.3
  hypnotic — *see* Abuse, drug, sedative
  inhalant — *see* Abuse, drug, inhalant
  laxatives F55.2
  LSD — *see* Abuse, drug, hallucinogen
  marihuana — *see* Abuse, drug, cannabis
  morphine type (opioids) — *see* Abuse, drug, opioid
  non-psychoactive substance NEC F55.8
    antacids F55.0
    folk remedies F55.1
    herbal remedies F55.1
    hormones F55.3
    laxatives F55.2
    steroids F55.3
    vitamins F55.4
  opioids — *see* Abuse, drug, opioid
  PCP (phencyclidine) (or related substance) — *see* Abuse, drug, hallucinogen
  physical (adult) (child) — *see* Maltreatment
  psychoactive substance — *see* Abuse, drug, psychoactive NEC
  psychological (adult) (child) — *see* Maltreatment
  sedative — *see* Abuse, drug, sedative
  sexual — *see* Maltreatment
  solvent — *see* Abuse, drug, inhalant
  steroids F55.3
  vitamins F55.4
Acalculia R48.8
  developmental F81.2
Acanthamebiasis (with) B60.10
  conjunctiva B60.12
  keratoconjunctivitis B60.13
  meningoencephalitis B60.11
  other specified B60.19
Acanthocephaliasis B83.8
Acanthocheilonemiasis B74.4
Acanthocytosis E78.6
Acantholysis L11.9
Acanthosis (acquired) (nigricans) L83
  benign Q82.8
  congenital Q82.8
  seborrheic L82.1
    inflamed L82.0
  tongue K14.3
Acapnia E87.3
Acarbia E87.2
Acardia, acardius Q89.8
Acardiacus amorphus Q89.8
Acardiotrophia I51.4
Acariasis B88.0
  scabies B86

Acarodermatitis (urticarioides) B88.0
Acarophobia F40.218
Acatalasemia, acatalasia E80.3
Acathisia (drug induced) G25.71
Accelerated atrioventricular conduction I45.6
Accentuation of personality traits (type A) Z73.1
Accessory (congenital)
  adrenal gland Q89.1
  anus Q43.4
  appendix Q43.4
  atrioventricular conduction I45.6
  auditory ossicles Q16.3
  auricle (ear) Q17.0
  biliary duct or passage Q44.5
  bladder Q64.79
  blood vessels NEC Q27.9
    coronary Q24.5
  bone NEC Q79.8
  breast tissue, axilla Q83.1
  carpal bones Q74.0
  cecum Q43.4
  chromosome(s) NEC (nonsex) Q92.9
    with complex rearrangements NEC Q92.5
      seen only at prometaphase Q92.8
    13 — *see* Trisomy, 13
    18 — *see* Trisomy, 18
    21 — *see* Trisomy, 21
    partial Q92.9
    sex
      female phenotype Q97.8
  coronary artery Q24.5
  cusp(s), heart valve NEC Q24.8
    pulmonary Q22.3
  cystic duct Q44.5
  digit(s) Q69.9
  ear (auricle) (lobe) Q17.0
  endocrine gland NEC Q89.2
  eye muscle Q10.3
  eyelid Q10.3
  face bone(s) Q75.8
  fallopian tube (fimbria) (ostium) Q50.6
  finger(s) Q69.0
  foreskin N47.8
  frontonasal process Q75.8
  gallbladder Q44.1
  genital organ(s)
    female Q52.8
      external Q52.79
      internal NEC Q52.8
    male Q55.8
  genitourinary organs NEC Q89.8
    female Q52.8
    male Q55.8
  hallux Q69.2
  heart Q24.8
    valve NEC Q24.8
      pulmonary Q22.3
  hepatic ducts Q44.5
  hymen Q52.4
  intestine (large) (small) Q43.4
  kidney Q63.0
  lacrimal canal Q10.6
  leaflet, heart valve NEC Q24.8
  ligament, broad Q50.6
  liver Q44.7
    duct Q44.5
  lobule (ear) Q17.0
  lung (lobe) Q33.1
  muscle Q79.8
  navicular of carpus Q74.0
  nervous system, part NEC Q07.8
  nipple Q83.3
  nose Q30.8
  organ or site not listed — *see* Anomaly, by site
  ovary Q50.31
  oviduct Q50.6
  pancreas Q45.3
  parathyroid gland Q89.2
  parotid gland (and duct) Q38.4
  pituitary gland Q89.2
  preauricular appendage Q17.0
  prepuce N47.8
  renal arteries (multiple) Q27.2
  rib Q76.6
    cervical Q76.5
  roots (teeth) K00.2
  salivary gland Q38.4
  sesamoid bones Q74.8

Accessory — *continued*
  sesamoid bones — *continued*
    foot Q74.2
    hand Q74.0
  skin tags Q82.8
  spleen Q89.09
  sternum Q76.7
  submaxillary gland Q38.4
  tarsal bones Q74.2
  teeth, tooth K00.1
  tendon Q79.8
  thumb Q69.1
  thymus gland Q89.2
  thyroid gland Q89.2
  toes Q69.2
  tongue Q38.3
  tooth, teeth K00.1
  tragus Q17.0
  ureter Q62.5
  urethra Q64.79
  urinary organ or tract NEC Q64.8
  uterus Q51.2
  vagina Q52.10
  valve, heart NEC Q24.8
    pulmonary Q22.3
  vertebra Q76.49
  vocal cords Q31.8
  vulva Q52.79
Accident
  birth — *see* Birth, injury
  cardiac — *see* Infarct, myocardium
  cerebral I63.9
  cerebrovascular (embolic) (ischemic) (thrombotic) I63.9
    aborted I63.9
    hemorrhagic — *see* Hemorrhage, intracranial, intracerebral
    old (without sequelae) Z86.73
      with sequelae (of) — *see* Sequelae, infarction, cerebral
  coronary — *see* Infarct, myocardium
  craniovascular I63.9
  vascular, brain I63.9
Accidental — *see* condition
Accommodation (disorder) (*see also* condition)
  hysterical paralysis of F44.89
  insufficiency of H52.4
  paresis — *see* Paresis, of accommodation
  spasm — *see* Spasm, of accommodation
Accouchement — *see* Delivery
Accreta placenta O43.21- ☑
Accretio cordis (nonrheumatic) I31.0
Accretions, tooth, teeth K03.6
Acculturation difficulty Z60.3
Accumulation secretion, prostate N42.89
Acephalia, acephalism, acephalus, acephaly Q00.0
Acephalobrachia monster Q89.8
Acephalochirus monster Q89.8
Acephalogaster Q89.8
Acephalostomus monster Q89.8
Acephalothorax Q89.8
Acerophobia F40.298
Acetonemia R79.89
  in Type 1 diabetes E10.10
    with coma E10.11
Acetonuria R82.4
Achalasia (cardia) (esophagus) K22.0
  congenital Q39.5
  pylorus Q40.0
  sphincteral NEC K59.8
Ache(s) — *see* Pain
Acheilia Q38.6
Achillobursitis — *see* Tendinitis, Achilles
Achillodynia — *see* Tendinitis, Achilles
Achlorhydria, achlorhydric (neurogenic) K31.83
  anemia D50.8
  diarrhea K31.83
  psychogenic F45.8
  secondary to vagotomy K91.1
Achluophobia F40.228
Acholia K82.8
Acholuric jaundice (familial) (splenomegalic) (*see also* Spherocytosis)
  acquired D59.8
Achondrogenesis Q77.0
Achondroplasia (osteosclerosis congenita) Q77.4
Achroma, cutis L80

Index

Achromat — Adenocarcinoma

Achromat (ism), achromatopsia (acquired) (congenital) H53.51
Achromia, congenital — see Albinism
Achromia parasitica B36.0
Achylia gastrica K31.89
  psychogenic F45.8
Acid
  burn — see Corrosion
  deficiency
    amide nicotinic E52
    ascorbic E54
    folic E53.8
    nicotinic E52
    pantothenic E53.8
  intoxication E87.2
  peptic disease K30
  phosphatase deficiency E83.39
  stomach K30
    psychogenic F45.8
Acidemia E87.2
  argininosuccinic E72.22
  isovaleric E71.110
  metabolic (newborn) P19.9
    first noted before onset of labor P19.0
    first noted during labor P19.1
    noted at birth P19.2
  methylmalonic E71.120
  pipecolic E72.3
  propionic E71.121
Acidity, gastric (high) K30
  psychogenic F45.8
Acidocytopenia — see Agranulocytosis
Acidocytosis D72.1
Acidopenia — see Agranulocytosis
Acidosis (lactic) (respiratory) E87.2
  in Type 1 diabetes E10.10
    with coma E10.11
  kidney, tubular N25.89
  lactic E87.2
  metabolic NEC E87.2
    with respiratory acidosis E87.4
    late, of newborn P74.0
  mixed metabolic and respiratory, newborn P84
  newborn P84
  renal (hyperchloremic) (tubular) N25.89
  respiratory E87.2
    complicated by
      metabolic
        acidosis E87.4
        alkalosis E87.4
Aciduria
  argininosuccinic E72.22
  glutaric (type I) E72.3
    type II E71.313
    type III E71.5- ☑
  orotic (congenital) (hereditary) (pyrimidine deficiency) E79.8
    anemia D53.0
Acladiosis (skin) B36.0
Aclasis, diaphyseal Q78.6
Acleistocardia Q21.1
Aclusion — see Anomaly, dentofacial, malocclusion
Acne L70.9
  artificialis L70.8
  atrophica L70.2
  cachecticorum (Hebra) L70.8
  conglobata L70.1
  cystic L70.0
  decalvans L66.2
  excoriée (des jeunes filles) L70.5
  frontalis L70.2
  indurata L70.0
  infantile L70.4
  keloid L73.0
  lupoid L70.2
  necrotic, necrotica (miliaris) L70.2
  neonatal L70.4
  nodular L70.0
  occupational L70.8
  picker's L70.5
  pustular L70.0
  rodens L70.2
  rosacea L71.9
  specified NEC L70.8
  tropica L70.3
  varioliformis L70.2
  vulgaris L70.0
Acnitis (primary) A18.4

Acosta's disease T70.29 ☑
Acoustic — see condition
Acousticophobia F40.298
Acquired (see also condition)
  immunodeficiency syndrome (AIDS) B20
Acrania Q00.0
Acroangiodermatitis I78.9
Acroasphyxia, chronic I73.89
Acrobystitis N47.7
Acrocephalopolysyndactyly Q87.0
Acrocephalosyndactyly Q87.0
Acrocephaly Q75.0
Acrochondrohyperplasia — see Syndrome, Marfan's
Acrocyanosis I73.8 ☑
  newborn P28.2
    meaning transient blue hands and feet — omit code
Acrodermatitis L30.8
  atrophicans (chronica) L90.4
  continua (Hallopeau) L40.2
  enteropathica (hereditary) E83.2
  Hallopeau's L40.2
  infantile papular L44.4
  perstans L40.2
  pustulosa continua L40.2
  recalcitrant pustular L40.2
Acrodynia — see Poisoning, mercury
Acromegaly, acromegalia E22.0
Acromelalgia I73.81
Acromicria, acromikria Q79.8
Acronyx L60.0
Acropachy, thyroid — see Thyrotoxicosis
Acroparesthesia (simple) (vasomotor) I73.89
Acropathy, thyroid — see Thyrotoxicosis
Acrophobia F40.241
Acroposthitis N47.7
Acroscleriasis, acroscleroderma, acrosclerosis — see Sclerosis, systemic
Acrosphacelus I96
Acrospiroma, eccrine — see Neoplasm, skin, benign
Acrostealgia — see Osteochondropathy
Acrotrophodynia — see Immersion
ACTH ectopic syndrome E24.3
Actinic — see condition
Actinobacillosis, actinobacillus A28.8
  mallei A24.0
  muris A25.1
Actinomyces israelii (infection) — see Actinomycosis
Actinomycetoma (foot) B47.1
Actinomycosis, actinomycotic A42.9
  with pneumonia A42.0
  abdominal A42.1
  cervicofacial A42.2
  cutaneous A42.89
  gastrointestinal A42.1
  pulmonary A42.0
  sepsis A42.7
  specified site NEC A42.89
Actinoneuritis G62.82
Action, heart
  disorder I49.9
  irregular I49.9
    psychogenic F45.8
Activated protein C resistance D68.51
Activation
  mast cell (disorder) (syndrome) D89.40
    idiopathic D89.42
    monoclonal D89.41
    secondary D89.43
    specified type NEC D89.49
Active — see condition
Acute (see also condition)
  abdomen R10.0
  gallbladder — see Cholecystitis, acute
Acyanotic heart disease (congenital) Q24.9
Acystia Q64.5
Adair-Dighton syndrome (brittle bones and blue sclera, deafness) Q78.0
Adamantinoblastoma — see Ameloblastoma
Adamantinoma (see also Cyst, calcifying odontogenic)
  long bones C40.90
    lower limb C40.2- ☑
    upper limb C40.0- ☑
  malignant C41.1
    jaw (bone) (lower) C41.1
      upper C41.0
  tibial C40.2- ☑

Adamantoblastoma — see Ameloblastoma
Adams-Stokes (-Morgagni) disease or syndrome I45.9
Adaption reaction — see Disorder, adjustment
Addiction (see also Dependence) F19.20
  alcohol, alcoholic (ethyl) (methyl) (wood) (without remission) F10.20
    with remission F10.21
  drug — see Dependence, drug
  ethyl alcohol (without remission) F10.20
    with remission F10.21
  heroin — see Dependence, drug, opioid
  methyl alcohol (without remission) F10.20
    with remission F10.21
  methylated spirit (without remission) F10.20
    with remission F10.21
  morphine (-like substances) — see Dependence, drug, opioid
  nicotine — see Dependence, drug, nicotine
  opium and opioids — see Dependence, drug, opioid
  tobacco — see Dependence, drug, nicotine
Addison-Biermer anemia (pernicious) D51.0
Addisonian crisis E27.2
Addison's
  anemia (pernicious) D51.0
  disease (bronze) or syndrome E27.1
    tuberculous A18.7
  keloid L94.0
Addison-Schilder complex E71.528
Additional (see also Accessory)
  chromosome(s) Q99.8
    21 — see Trisomy, 21
    sex — see Abnormal, chromosome, sex
Adduction contracture, hip or other joint — see Contraction, joint
Adenitis (see also Lymphadenitis)
  acute, unspecified site L04.9
  axillary I88.9
    acute L04.2
    chronic or subacute I88.1
  Bartholin's gland N75.8
  bulbourethral gland — see Urethritis
  cervical I88.9
    acute L04.0
    chronic or subacute I88.1
  chancroid (Hemophilus ducreyi) A57
  chronic, unspecified site I88.1
  Cowper's gland — see Urethritis
  due to Pasteurella multocida (P. septica) A28.0
  epidemic, acute B27.09
  gangrenous L04.9
  gonorrheal NEC A54.89
  groin I88.9
    acute L04.1
    chronic or subacute I88.1
  infectious (acute) (epidemic) B27.09
  inguinal I88.9
    acute L04.1
    chronic or subacute I88.1
  lymph gland or node, except mesenteric I88.9
    acute — see Lymphadenitis, acute
    chronic or subacute I88.1
  mesenteric (acute) (chronic) (nonspecific) (subacute) I88.0
  parotid gland (suppurative) — see Sialoadenitis
  salivary gland (any) (suppurative) — see Sialoadenitis
  scrofulous (tuberculous) A18.2
  Skene's duct or gland — see Urethritis
  strumous, tuberculous A18.2
  subacute, unspecified site I88.1
  sublingual gland (suppurative) — see Sialoadenitis
  submandibular gland (suppurative) — see Sialoadenitis
  submaxillary gland (suppurative) — see Sialoadenitis
  tuberculous — see Tuberculosis, lymph gland
  urethral gland — see Urethritis
  Wharton's duct (suppurative) — see Sialoadenitis
Adenoacanthoma — see Neoplasm, malignant, by site
Adenoameloblastoma — see Cyst, calcifying odontogenic
Adenocarcinoid (tumor) — see Neoplasm, malignant, by site
Adenocarcinoma (see also Neoplasm, malignant, by site)
  acidophil
    specified site — see Neoplasm, malignant, by site
    unspecified site C75.1
  adrenal cortical C74.0- ☑
  alveolar — see Neoplasm, lung, malignant

☑ Additional Character Required — Refer to the Tabular List for Character Selection   ▽ Subterms under main terms may continue to next column or page

Adenocarcinoma — *continued*
  apocrine
    breast — *see* Neoplasm, breast, malignant
    in situ
      breast D05.8- ☑
      specified site NEC — *see* Neoplasm, skin, in situ
      unspecified site D04.9
    specified site NEC — *see* Neoplasm, skin, malignant
    unspecified site C44.99
  basal cell
    specified site — *see* Neoplasm, skin, malignant
    unspecified site C08.9
  basophil
    specified site — *see* Neoplasm, malignant, by site
    unspecified site C75.1
  bile duct type C22.1
    liver C22.1
    specified site NEC — *see* Neoplasm, malignant, by site
    unspecified site C22.1
  bronchiolar — *see* Neoplasm, lung, malignant
  bronchioloalveolar — *see* Neoplasm, lung, malignant
  ceruminous C44.29- ☑
  cervix, in situ (*see also* Carcinoma, cervix uteri, in situ) D06.9
  chromophobe
    specified site — *see* Neoplasm, malignant, by site
    unspecified site C75.1
  diffuse type
    specified site — *see* Neoplasm, malignant, by site
    unspecified site C16.9
  duct
    infiltrating
      with Paget's disease — *see* Neoplasm, breast, malignant
      specified site — *see* Neoplasm, malignant, by site
      unspecified site (female) C50.91- ☑
        male C50.92- ☑
    specified site — *see* Neoplasm, malignant, by site
    unspecified site
      female C56.9
      male C61
  eosinophil
    specified site — *see* Neoplasm, malignant, by site
    unspecified site C75.1
  follicular
    with papillary C73
    moderately differentiated C73
    specified site — *see* Neoplasm, malignant, by site
    trabecular C73
    unspecified site C73
    well differentiated C73
  Hurthle cell C73
  in
    adenomatous
      polyposis coli C18.9
  infiltrating duct
    with Paget's disease — *see* Neoplasm, breast, malignant
    specified site — *see* Neoplasm, by site, malignant
    unspecified site (female) C50.91- ☑
      male C50.92- ☑
  inflammatory
    specified site — *see* Neoplasm, by site, malignant
    unspecified site (female) C50.91- ☑
      male C50.92- ☑
  intestinal type
    specified site — *see* Neoplasm, by site, malignant
    unspecified site C16.9
  intracystic papillary
  intraductal
    breast D05.1- ☑
    noninfiltrating
      breast D05.1- ☑
      papillary
        with invasion
          specified site — *see* Neoplasm, by site, malignant
          unspecified site (female) C50.91- ☑
            male C50.92- ☑
        breast D05.1- ☑
        specified site NEC — *see* Neoplasm, in situ, by site
        unspecified site D05.1- ☑
      specified site NEC — *see* Neoplasm, in situ, by site

Adenocarcinoma — *continued*
  intraductal — *continued*
    noninfiltrating — *continued*
      unspecified site D05.1- ☑
      papillary
        with invasion
          specified site — *see* Neoplasm, malignant, by site
          unspecified site (female) C50.91- ☑
            male C50.92- ☑
        breast D05.1- ☑
        specified site — *see* Neoplasm, in situ, by site
        unspecified site D05.1- ☑
    specified site NEC — *see* Neoplasm, in situ, by site
    unspecified site D05.1- ☑
  islet cell
    with exocrine, mixed
      specified site — *see* Neoplasm, malignant, by site
      unspecified site C25.9
    pancreas C25.4
    specified site NEC — *see* Neoplasm, malignant, by site
    unspecified site C25.4
  lobular
    in situ
      breast D05.0- ☑
      specified site NEC — *see* Neoplasm, in situ, by site
      unspecified site D05.0- ☑
    specified site — *see* Neoplasm, malignant, by site
    unspecified site (female) C50.91- ☑
      male C50.92- ☑
  mucoid (*see also* Neoplasm, malignant, by site)
    cell
      specified site — *see* Neoplasm, malignant, by site
      unspecified site C75.1
  nonencapsulated sclerosing C73
  papillary
    with follicular C73
    follicular variant C73
    intraductal (noninfiltrating)
      with invasion
        specified site — *see* Neoplasm, malignant, by site
        unspecified site (female) C50.91- ☑
          male C50.92- ☑
      breast D05.1- ☑
      specified site NEC — *see* Neoplasm, in situ, by site
      unspecified site D05.1- ☑
    serous
      specified site — *see* Neoplasm, malignant, by site
      unspecified site C56.9
  papillocystic
    specified site — *see* Neoplasm, malignant, by site
    unspecified site C56.9
  pseudomucinous
    specified site — *see* Neoplasm, malignant, by site
    unspecified site C56.9
  renal cell C64-
  sebaceous — *see* Neoplasm, skin, malignant
  serous (*see also* Neoplasm, malignant, by site)
    papillary
      specified site — *see* Neoplasm, malignant, by site
      unspecified site C56.9
  sweat gland — *see* Neoplasm, skin, malignant
  water-clear cell C75.0
Adenocarcinoma-in-situ (*see also* Neoplasm, in situ, by site)
  breast D05.9- ☑
Adenofibroma
  clear cell — *see* Neoplasm, benign, by site
  endometrioid D27.9
    borderline malignancy D39.10
    malignant C56- ☑
  mucinous
    specified site — *see* Neoplasm, benign, by site
    unspecified site D27.9
  papillary
    specified site — *see* Neoplasm, benign, by site
    unspecified site D27.9
  prostate — *see* Enlargement, enlarged, prostate

Adenofibroma — *continued*
  serous
    specified site — *see* Neoplasm, benign, by site
    unspecified site D27.9
  specified site — *see* Neoplasm, benign, by site
  unspecified site D27.9
Adenofibrosis
  breast — *see* Fibroadenosis, breast
  endometrioid N80.0
Adenoiditis (chronic) J35.02
  with tonsillitis J35.03
  acute J03.90
    recurrent J03.91
    specified organism NEC J03.80
      recurrent J03.81
    staphylococcal J03.80
      recurrent J03.81
    streptococcal J03.00
      recurrent J03.01
Adenoids — *see* condition
Adenolipoma — *see* Neoplasm, benign, by site
Adenolipomatosis, Launois-Bensaude E88.89
Adenolymphoma
  specified site — *see* Neoplasm, benign, by site
  unspecified site D11.9
Adenoma (*see also* Neoplasm, benign, by site)
  acidophil
    specified site — *see* Neoplasm, benign, by site
    unspecified site D35.2
  acidophil-basophil, mixed
    specified site — *see* Neoplasm, benign, by site
    unspecified site D35.2
  adrenal (cortical) D35.00
    clear cell D35.00
    compact cell D35.00
    glomerulosa cell D35.00
    heavily pigmented variant D35.00
    mixed cell D35.00
  alpha-cell
    pancreas D13.7
    specified site NEC — *see* Neoplasm, benign, by site
    unspecified site D13.7
  alveolar D14.30
  apocrine
    breast D24- ☑
    specified site NEC — *see* Neoplasm, skin, benign, by site
    unspecified site D23.9
  basal cell D11.9
  basophil
    specified site — *see* Neoplasm, benign, by site
    unspecified site D35.2
  basophil-acidophil, mixed
    specified site — *see* Neoplasm, benign, by site
    unspecified site D35.2
  beta-cell
    pancreas D13.7
    specified site NEC — *see* Neoplasm, benign, by site
    unspecified site D13.7
  bile duct D13.4
    common D13.5
    extrahepatic D13.5
    intrahepatic D13.4
    specified site NEC — *see* Neoplasm, benign, by site
    unspecified site D13.4
  black D35.00
  bronchial D38.1
    cylindroid type — *see* Neoplasm, lung, malignant
  ceruminous D23.2- ☑
  chief cell D35.1
  chromophobe
    specified site — *see* Neoplasm, benign, by site
    unspecified site D35.2
  colloid
    specified site — *see* Neoplasm, benign, by site
    unspecified site D34
  duct
  eccrine, papillary — *see* Neoplasm, skin, benign
  endocrine, multiple
    single specified site — *see* Neoplasm, uncertain behavior, by site
    two or more specified sites D44- ☑
    unspecified site D44.9
  endometrioid (*see also* Neoplasm, benign)
    borderline malignancy — *see* Neoplasm, uncertain behavior, by site
  eosinophil
    specified site — *see* Neoplasm, benign, by site

Adenoma — *continued*
  eosinophil — *continued*
    unspecified site D35.2
  fetal
    specified site — *see* Neoplasm, benign, by site
    unspecified site D34
  follicular
    specified site — *see* Neoplasm, benign, by site
    unspecified site D34
  hepatocellular D13.4
  Hurthle cell D34
  islet cell
    pancreas D13.7
    specified site NEC — *see* Neoplasm, benign, by site
    unspecified site D13.7
  liver cell D13.4
  macrofollicular
    specified site — *see* Neoplasm, benign, by site
    unspecified site D34
  malignant, malignum — *see* Neoplasm, malignant, by site
  microcystic
    pancreas D13.6
    specified site NEC — *see* Neoplasm, benign, by site
    unspecified site D13.6
  microfollicular
    specified site — *see* Neoplasm, benign, by site
    unspecified site D34
  mucoid cell
    specified site — *see* Neoplasm, benign, by site
    unspecified site D35.2
  multiple endocrine
    single specified site — *see* Neoplasm, uncertain behavior, by site
    two or more specified sites D44- ☑
    unspecified site D44.9
  nipple D24- ☑
  papillary (*see also* Neoplasm, benign, by site)
    eccrine — *see* Neoplasm, skin, benign, by site
  Pick's tubular
    specified site — *see* Neoplasm, benign, by site
    unspecified site
      female D27.9
      male D29.20
  pleomorphic
    carcinoma in — *see* Neoplasm, salivary gland, malignant
      specified site — *see* Neoplasm, malignant, by site
      unspecified site C08.9
  polypoid (*see also* Neoplasm, benign)
    adenocarcinoma in — *see* Neoplasm, malignant, by site
    adenocarcinoma in situ — *see* Neoplasm, in situ, by site
  prostate — *see* Neoplasm, benign, prostate
  rete cell D29.20
  sebaceous — *see* Neoplasm, skin, benign
  Sertoli cell
    specified site — *see* Neoplasm, benign, by site
    unspecified site
      female D27.9
      male D29.20
  skin appendage — *see* Neoplasm, skin, benign
  sudoriferous gland — *see* Neoplasm, skin, benign
  sweat gland — *see* Neoplasm, skin, benign
  testicular
    specified site — *see* Neoplasm, benign, by site
    unspecified site
      female D27.9
      male D29.20
  tubular (*see also* Neoplasm, benign, by site)
    adenocarcinoma in — *see* Neoplasm, malignant, by site
    adenocarcinoma in situ — *see* Neoplasm, in situ, by site
    Pick's
      specified site — *see* Neoplasm, benign, by site
      unspecified site
        female D27.9
        male D29.20
  tubulovillous (*see also* Neoplasm, benign, by site)
    adenocarcinoma in — *see* Neoplasm, malignant, by site
    adenocarcinoma in situ — *see* Neoplasm, in situ, by site
  villous — *see* Neoplasm, uncertain behavior, by site

Adenoma — *continued*
  villous — *see* Neoplasm, uncertain behavior, by site — *continued*
    adenocarcinoma in — *see* Neoplasm, malignant, by site
    adenocarcinoma in situ — *see* Neoplasm, in situ, by site
  water-clear cell D35.1
Adenomatosis
  endocrine (multiple) E31.20
    single specified site — *see* Neoplasm, uncertain behavior, by site
  erosive of nipple D24- ☑
  pluriendocrine — *see* Adenomatosis, endocrine
  pulmonary D38.1
    malignant — *see* Neoplasm, lung, malignant
  specified site — *see* Neoplasm, benign, by site
  unspecified site D12.6
Adenomatous
  goiter (nontoxic) E04.9
    with hyperthyroidism — *see* Hyperthyroidism, with, goiter, nodular
    toxic — *see* Hyperthyroidism, with, goiter, nodular
Adenomyoma (*see also* Neoplasm, benign, by site)
  prostate — *see* Enlarged, prostate
Adenomyometritis N80.0
Adenomyosis N80.0
Adenopathy (lymph gland) R59.9
  generalized R59.1
  inguinal R59.0
  localized R59.0
  mediastinal R59.0
  mesentery R59.0
  syphilitic (secondary) A51.49
  tracheobronchial R59.0
    tuberculous A15.4
      primary (progressive) A15.7
  tuberculous (*see also* Tuberculosis, lymph gland)
    tracheobronchial A15.4
      primary (progressive) A15.7
Adenosalpingitis — *see* Salpingitis
Adenosarcoma — *see* Neoplasm, malignant, by site
Adenosclerosis I88.8
Adenosis (sclerosing) breast — *see* Fibroadenosis, breast
Adenovirus, as cause of disease classified elsewhere B97.0
Adentia (complete) (partial) — *see* Absence, teeth
Adherent (*see also* Adhesions)
  labia (minora) N90.89
  pericardium (nonrheumatic) I31.0
    rheumatic I09.2
  placenta (with hemorrhage) O72.0
    without hemorrhage O73.0
  prepuce, newborn N47.0
  scar (skin) L90.5
  tendon in scar L90.5
Adhesions, adhesive (postinfective) K66.0
  with intestinal obstruction K56.50
    complete K56.52
    incomplete K56.51
    partial K56.51
  abdominal (wall) — *see* Adhesions, peritoneum
  appendix K38.8
  bile duct (common) (hepatic) K83.8
  bladder (sphincter) N32.89
  bowel — *see* Adhesions, peritoneum
  cardiac I31.0
    rheumatic I09.2
  cecum — *see* Adhesions, peritoneum
  cervicovaginal N88.1
    congenital Q52.8
    postpartal O90.89
      old N88.1
  cervix N88.1
  ciliary body NEC — *see* Adhesions, iris
  clitoris N90.89
  colon — *see* Adhesions, peritoneum
  common duct K83.8
  congenital (*see also* Anomaly, by site)
    fingers — *see* Syndactylism, complex, fingers
    omental, anomalous Q43.3
    peritoneal Q43.3
    tongue (to gum or roof of mouth) Q38.3
  conjunctiva (acquired) H11.21- ☑
    congenital Q15.8
  cystic duct K82.8
  diaphragm — *see* Adhesions, peritoneum
  due to foreign body — *see* Foreign body

Adhesions, adhesive — *continued*
  duodenum — *see* Adhesions, peritoneum
  ear
    middle H74.1- ☑
  epididymis N50.89
  epidural — *see* Adhesions, meninges
  epiglottis J38.7
  eyelid H02.59
  female pelvis N73.6
  gallbladder K82.8
  globe H44.89
  heart I31.0
    rheumatic I09.2
  ileocecal (coil) — *see* Adhesions, peritoneum
  ileum — *see* Adhesions, peritoneum
  intestine (*see also* Adhesions, peritoneum)
    with obstruction K56.50
      complete K56.52
      incomplete K56.51
      partial K56.51
  intra-abdominal — *see* Adhesions, peritoneum
  iris H21.50- ☑
    anterior H21.51- ☑
    goniosynechiae H21.52- ☑
    posterior H21.54- ☑
    to corneal graft T85.898 ☑
  joint — *see* Ankylosis
    knee M23.8X ☑
    temporomandibular M26.61- ☑
  labium (majus) (minus), congenital Q52.5
  liver — *see* Adhesions, peritoneum
  lung J98.4
  mediastinum J98.59
  meninges (cerebral) (spinal) G96.12
    congenital Q07.8
    tuberculous (cerebral) (spinal) A17.0
  mesenteric — *see* Adhesions, peritoneum
  nasal (septum) (to turbinates) J34.89
  ocular muscle — *see* Strabismus, mechanical
  omentum — *see* Adhesions, peritoneum
  ovary N73.6
    congenital (to cecum, kidney or omentum) Q50.39
  paraovarian N73.6
  pelvic (peritoneal)
    female N73.6
      postprocedural N99.4
    male — *see* Adhesions, peritoneum
    postpartal (old) N73.6
    tuberculous A18.17
  penis to scrotum (congenital) Q55.8
  periappendiceal (*see also* Adhesions, peritoneum)
  pericardium (nonrheumatic) I31.0
    focal I31.8
    rheumatic I09.2
    tuberculous A18.84
  pericholecystic K82.8
  perigastric — *see* Adhesions, peritoneum
  periovarian N73.6
  periprostatic N42.89
  perirectal — *see* Adhesions, peritoneum
  perirenal N28.89
  peritoneum, peritoneal (postinfective)
    with obstruction (intestinal) K56.50
      complete K56.52
      incomplete K56.51
      partial K56.51
    congenital Q43.3
    pelvic, female N73.6
      postprocedural N99.4
    postpartal, pelvic N73.6
    postprocedural K66.0
    to uterus N73.6
  peritubal N73.6
  periureteral N28.89
  periuterine N73.6
  perivesical N32.89
  perivesicular (seminal vesicle) N50.89
  pleura, pleuritic J94.8
    tuberculous NEC A15.6
  pleuropericardial J94.8
  postoperative (gastrointestinal tract) K66.0
    with obstruction (*see also* Obstruction, intestine, postoperative) K91.30
    due to foreign body accidentally left in wound — *see* Foreign body, accidentally left during a procedure
    pelvic peritoneal N99.4
    urethra — *see* Stricture, urethra, postprocedural

☑ **Additional Character Required** — Refer to the Tabular List for Character Selection   ▽ Subterms under main terms may continue to next column or page

Adhesions, adhesive — *continued*
  postoperative — *continued*
    vagina N99.2
  postpartal, old (vulva or perineum) N90.89
  preputial, prepuce N47.5
  pulmonary J98.4
  pylorus — *see* Adhesions, peritoneum
  sciatic nerve — *see* Lesion, nerve, sciatic
  seminal vesicle N50.89
  shoulder (joint) — *see* Capsulitis, adhesive
  sigmoid flexure — *see* Adhesions, peritoneum
  spermatic cord (acquired) N50.89
    congenital Q55.4
  spinal canal G96.12
  stomach — *see* Adhesions, peritoneum
  subscapular — *see* Capsulitis, adhesive
  temporomandibular M26.61- ☑
  tendinitis (*see also* Tenosynovitis, specified type NEC)
    shoulder — *see* Capsulitis, adhesive
  testis N44.8
  tongue, congenital (to gum or roof of mouth) Q38.3
    acquired K14.8
  trachea J39.8
  tubo-ovarian N73.6
  tunica vaginalis N44.8
  uterus N73.6
    internal N85.6
    to abdominal wall N73.6
  vagina (chronic) N89.5
    postoperative N99.2
  vitreomacular H43.82- ☑
  vitreous H43.89
  vulva N90.89
Adiaspiromycosis B48.8
Adie (-Holmes) **pupil or syndrome** — *see* Anomaly,
    pupil, function, tonic pupil
Adiponecrosis neonatorum P83.88
Adiposis (*see also* Obesity)
  cerebralis E23.6
  dolorosa E88.2
Adiposity (*see also* Obesity)
  heart — *see* Degeneration, myocardial
  localized E65
Adiposogenital dystrophy E23.6
Adjustment
  disorder — *see* Disorder, adjustment
  implanted device — *see* Encounter (for), adjustment
    (of)
  prosthesis, external — *see* Fitting
  reaction — *see* Disorder, adjustment
Administration of tPA (rtPA) in a different facility within
    the last 24 hours prior to admission to current facil-
    ity Z92.82
Admission (for) (*see also* Encounter (for))
  adjustment (of)
    artificial
      arm Z44.00- ☑
        complete Z44.01- ☑
        partial Z44.02- ☑
      eye Z44.2 ☑
      leg Z44.10- ☑
        complete Z44.11- ☑
        partial Z44.12- ☑
    brain neuropacemaker Z46.2
      implanted Z45.42
    breast
      implant Z45.81 ☑
      prosthesis (external) Z44.3 ☑
    colostomy belt Z46.89
    contact lenses Z46.0
    cystostomy device Z46.6
    dental prosthesis Z46.3
    device NEC
      abdominal Z46.89
      implanted Z45.89
        cardiac Z45.09
          defibrillator (with synchronous cardiace
            pacemaker) Z45.02
          pacemaker (cardiac resynchronization
            therapy (CRT-P)) Z45.018
          pulse generator Z45.010
          resynchronization therapy defibrillator
            (CRT-D) Z45.02
        hearing device Z45.328
          bone conduction Z45.320
          cochlear Z45.321
        infusion pump Z45.1
        nervous system Z45.49

Admission — *continued*
  adjustment — *continued*
    device — *continued*
      implanted — *continued*
        nervous system — *continued*
          CSF drainage Z45.41
          hearing device — *see* Admission, adjust-
            ment, device, implanted, hearing
            device
          neuropacemaker Z45.42
          visual substitution Z45.31
        specified NEC Z45.89
        vascular access Z45.2
        visual substitution Z45.31
      nervous system Z46.2
        implanted — *see* Admission, adjustment,
          device, implanted, nervous system
      orthodontic Z46.4
      prosthetic Z44.9
        arm — *see* Admission, adjustment, artificial,
          arm
        breast Z44.3 ☑
        dental Z46.3
        eye Z44.2 ☑
        leg — *see* Admission, adjustment, artificial,
          leg
        specified type NEC Z44.8
      substitution
        auditory Z46.2
          implanted — *see* Admission, adjust-
            ment, device, implanted, hearing
            device
        nervous system Z46.2
          implanted — *see* Admission, adjust-
            ment, device, implanted, nervous
            system
        visual Z46.2
          implanted Z45.31
    urinary Z46.6
    hearing aid Z46.1
      implanted — *see* Admission, adjustment, de-
        vice, implanted, hearing device
    ileostomy device Z46.89
    intestinal appliance or device NEC Z46.89
    neuropacemaker (brain) (peripheral nerve) (spinal
      cord) Z46.2
      implanted Z45.42
    orthodontic device Z46.4
    orthopedic (brace) (cast) (device) (shoes) Z46.89
    pacemaker (cardiac resynchronization therapy
      (CRT-P))
      cardiac Z45.018
        pulse generator Z45.010
      nervous system Z46.2
        implanted Z45.42
    portacath (port-a-cath) Z45.2
    prosthesis Z44.9
      arm — *see* Admission, adjustment, artificial,
        arm
      breast Z44.3 ☑
      dental Z46.3
      eye Z44.2 ☑
      leg — *see* Admission, adjustment, artificial, leg
      specified NEC Z44.8
    spectacles Z46.0
  aftercare (*see also* Aftercare) Z51.89
    postpartum
      immediately after delivery Z39.0
      routine follow-up Z39.2
    radiation therapy (antineoplastic) Z51.0
  attention to artificial opening (of) Z43.9
    artificial vagina Z43.7
    colostomy Z43.3
    cystostomy Z43.5
    enterostomy Z43.4
    gastrostomy Z43.1
    ileostomy Z43.2
    jejunostomy Z43.4
    nephrostomy Z43.6
    specified site NEC Z43.8
      intestinal tract Z43.4
      urinary tract Z43.6
    tracheostomy Z43.0
    ureterostomy Z43.6
    urethrostomy Z43.6
  breast augmentation or reduction Z41.1
  breast reconstruction following mastectomy Z42.1

Admission — *continued*
  change of
    dressing (nonsurgical) Z48.00
      neuropacemaker device (brain) (peripheral nerve)
        (spinal cord) Z46.2
        implanted Z45.42
      surgical dressing Z48.01
  circumcision, ritual or routine (in absence of diagnosis)
    Z41.2
  clinical research investigation (control) (normal com-
    parison) (participant) Z00.6
  contraceptive management Z30.9
  cosmetic surgery NEC Z41.1
  counseling (*see also* Counseling)
    dietary Z71.3
    gestational carrier Z31.7
    HIV Z71.7
    human immunodeficiency virus Z71.7
    nonattending third party Z71.0
    procreative management NEC Z31.69
  delivery, full-term, uncomplicated O80
    cesarean, without indication O82
  desensitization to allergens Z51.6
  dietary surveillance and counseling Z71.3
  ear piercing Z41.3
  examination at health care facility (adult) (*see also*
    Examination) Z00.00
    with abnormal findings Z00.01
    clinical research investigation (control) (normal
      comparison) (participant) Z00.6
    dental Z01.20
      with abnormal findings Z01.21
    donor (potential) Z00.5
    ear Z01.10
      with abnormal findings NEC Z01.118
    eye Z01.00
      with abnormal findings Z01.01
    general, specified reason NEC Z00.8
    hearing Z01.10
      with abnormal findings NEC Z01.118
    postpartum checkup Z39.2
    psychiatric (general) Z00.8
      requested by authority Z04.6
    vision Z01.00
      with abnormal findings Z01.01
  fitting (of)
    artificial
      arm — *see* Admission, adjustment, artificial,
        arm
      eye Z44.2 ☑
      leg — *see* Admission, adjustment, artificial, leg
    brain neuropacemaker Z46.2
      implanted Z45.42
    breast prosthesis (external) Z44.3 ☑
    colostomy belt Z46.89
    contact lenses Z46.0
    cystostomy device Z46.6
    dental prosthesis Z46.3
    dentures Z46.3
    device NEC
      abdominal Z46.89
      nervous system Z46.2
        implanted — *see* Admission, adjustment,
          device, implanted, nervous system
      orthodontic Z46.4
      prosthetic Z44.9
        breast Z44.3 ☑
        dental Z46.3
        eye Z44.2 ☑
      substitution
        auditory Z46.2
          implanted — *see* Admission, adjust-
            ment, device, implanted, hearing
            device
        nervous system Z46.2
          implanted — *see* Admission, adjust-
            ment, device, implanted, nervous
            system
        visual Z46.2
          implanted Z45.31
    hearing aid Z46.1
    ileostomy device Z46.89
    intestinal appliance or device NEC Z46.89
    neuropacemaker (brain) (peripheral nerve) (spinal
      cord) Z46.2
      implanted Z45.42
    orthodontic device Z46.4
    orthopedic device (brace) (cast) (shoes) Z46.89

Admission — *continued*
  fitting — *continued*
    prosthesis Z44.9
      arm — *see* Admission, adjustment, artificial, arm
      breast Z44.3 ☑
      dental Z46.3
      eye Z44.2 ☑
      leg — *see* Admission, adjustment, artificial, leg
      specified type NEC Z44.8
    spectacles Z46.0
  follow-up examination Z09
  intrauterine device management Z30.431
    initial prescription Z30.014
  mental health evaluation Z00.8
    requested by authority Z04.6
  observation — *see* Observation
  Papanicolaou smear, cervix Z12.4
    for suspected malignant neoplasm Z12.4
  plastic and reconstructive surgery following medical procedure or healed injury NEC Z42.8
  plastic surgery, cosmetic NEC Z41.1
  postpartum observation
    immediately after delivery Z39.0
    routine follow-up Z39.2
  poststerilization (for restoration) Z31.0
    aftercare Z31.42
  procreative management Z31.9
  prophylactic (measure) — (*see also* Encounter, prophylactic measures)
    organ removal Z40.00
      breast Z40.01
      fallopian tube(s) Z40.03
        with ovary(s) Z40.02
      ovary(s) Z40.02
      specified organ NEC Z40.09
      testes Z40.09
    vaccination Z23
  psychiatric examination (general) Z00.8
    requested by authority Z04.6
  radiation therapy (antineoplastic) Z51.0
  reconstructive surgery following medical procedure or healed injury NEC Z42.8
  removal of
    cystostomy catheter Z43.5
    drains Z48.03
    dressing (nonsurgical) Z48.00
    implantable subdermal contraceptive Z30.46
    intrauterine contraceptive device Z30.432
    neuropacemaker (brain) (peripheral nerve) (spinal cord) Z46.2
      implanted Z45.42
    staples Z48.02
    surgical dressing Z48.01
    sutures Z48.02
    ureteral stent Z46.6
  respirator [ventilator] use during power failure Z99.12
  restoration of organ continuity (poststerilization) Z31.0
    aftercare Z31.42
  sensitivity test (*see also* Test, skin)
    allergy NEC Z01.82
    Mantoux Z11.1
  tuboplasty following previous sterilization Z31.0
    aftercare Z31.42
  vasoplasty following previous sterilization Z31.0
    aftercare Z31.42
  vision examination Z01.00
    with abnormal findings Z01.01
  waiting period for admission to other facility Z75.1
Adnexitis (suppurative) — *see* Salpingo-oophoritis
Adolescent X-linked adrenoleukodystrophy E71.521
Adrenal (gland) — *see* condition
Adrenalism, tuberculous A18.7
Adrenalitis, adrenitis E27.8
  autoimmune E27.1
  meningococcal, hemorrhagic A39.1
Adrenarche, premature E27.0
Adrenocortical syndrome — *see* Cushing's, syndrome
Adrenogenital syndrome E25.9
  acquired E25.8
  congenital E25.0
  salt loss E25.0
Adrenogenitalism, congenital E25.0
Adrenoleukodystrophy E71.529
  neonatal E71.511
  X-linked E71.529
    Addison only phenotype E71.528
    Addison-Schilder E71.528

Adrenoleukodystrophy — *continued*
  X-linked — *continued*
    adolescent E71.521
    adrenomyeloneuropathy E71.522
    childhood cerebral E71.520
    other specified E71.528
Adrenomyeloneuropathy E71.522
Adventitious bursa — *see* Bursopathy, specified type NEC
Adverse effect — *see* Table of Drugs and Chemicals, categories T36-T50, with 6th character 5
Advice — *see* Counseling
Adynamia (episodica) (hereditary) (periodic) G72.3
Aeration lung imperfect, newborn — *see* Atelectasis
Aerobullosis T70.3 ☑
Aerocele — *see* Embolism, air
Aerodermectasia
  subcutaneous (traumatic) T79.7 ☑
Aerodontalgia T70.29 ☑
Aeroembolism T70.3 ☑
Aerogenes capsulatus infection A48.0
Aero-otitis media T70.0 ☑
Aerophagy, aerophagia (psychogenic) F45.8
Aerophobia F40.228
Aerosinusitis T70.1 ☑
Aerotitis T70.0 ☑
Affection — *see* Disease
Afibrinogenemia (*see also* Defect, coagulation) D68.8
  acquired D65
  congenital D68.2
  following ectopic or molar pregnancy O08.1
  in abortion — *see* Abortion, by type, complicated by, afibrinogenemia
  puerperal O72.3
African
  sleeping sickness B56.9
  tick fever A68.1
  trypanosomiasis B56.9
    gambian B56.0
    rhodesian B56.1
Aftercare (*see also* Care) Z51.89
  following surgery (for) (on)
    amputation Z47.81
    attention to
      drains Z48.03
      dressings (nonsurgical) Z48.00
        surgical Z48.01
      sutures Z48.02
    circulatory system Z48.812
    delayed (planned) wound closure Z48.1
    digestive system Z48.815
    explantation of joint prosthesis (staged procedure)
      hip Z47.32
      knee Z47.33
      shoulder Z47.31
    genitourinary system Z48.816
    joint replacement Z47.1
    neoplasm Z48.3
    nervous system Z48.811
    oral cavity Z48.814
    organ transplant
      bone marrow Z48.290
      heart Z48.21
      heart-lung Z48.280
      kidney Z48.22
      liver Z48.23
      lung Z48.24
      multiple organs NEC Z48.288
      specified NEC Z48.298
    orthopedic NEC Z47.89
    planned wound closure Z48.1
    removal of internal fixation device Z47.2
    respiratory system Z48.813
    scoliosis Z47.82
    sense organs Z48.810
    skin and subcutaneous tissue Z48.817
    specified body system
      circulatory Z48.812
      digestive Z48.815
      genitourinary Z48.816
      nervous Z48.811
      oral cavity Z48.814
      respiratory Z48.813
      sense organs Z48.810
      skin and subcutaneous tissue Z48.817
      teeth Z48.814
    specified NEC Z48.89
    spinal Z47.89

Aftercare — *continued*
  following surgery — *continued*
    teeth Z48.814
  fracture — *code to* fracture with seventh character D
  involving
    removal of
      drains Z48.03
      dressings (nonsurgical) Z48.00
      staples Z48.02
      surgical dressings Z48.01
      sutures Z48.02
    neuropacemaker (brain) (peripheral nerve) (spinal cord) Z46.2
      implanted Z45.42
    orthopedic NEC Z47.89
    postprocedural — *see* Aftercare, following surgery
After-cataract — *see* Cataract, secondary
Agalactia (primary) O92.3
  elective, secondary or therapeutic O92.5
Agammaglobulinemia (acquired (secondary) (nonfamilial) D80.1
  with
    immunoglobulin-bearing B-lymphocytes D80.1
    lymphopenia D81.9
  autosomal recessive (Swiss type) D80.0
  Bruton's X-linked D80.0
  common variable (CVAgamma) D80.1
  congenital sex-linked D80.0
  hereditary D80.0
  lymphopenic D81.9
  Swiss type (autosomal recessive) D80.0
  X-linked (with growth hormone deficiency) (Bruton) D80.0
Aganglionosis (bowel) (colon) Q43.1
Age (old) — *see* Senility
Agenesis
  adrenal (gland) Q89.1
  alimentary tract (complete) (partial) NEC Q45.8
    upper Q40.8
  anus, anal (canal) Q42.3
    with fistula Q42.2
  aorta Q25.41
  appendix Q42.8
  arm (complete) Q71.0- ☑
    with hand present Q71.1- ☑
  artery (peripheral) Q27.9
    brain Q28.3
    coronary Q24.5
    pulmonary Q25.79
    specified NEC Q27.8
    umbilical Q27.0
  auditory (canal) (external) Q16.1
  auricle (ear) Q16.0
  bile duct or passage Q44.5
  bladder Q64.5
  bone Q79.9
  brain Q00.0
    part of Q04.3
  breast (with nipple present) Q83.8
    with absent nipple Q83.0
  bronchus Q32.4
  canaliculus lacrimalis Q10.4
  carpus — *see* Agenesis, hand
  cartilage Q79.9
  cecum Q42.8
  cerebellum Q04.3
  cervix Q51.5
  chin Q18.8
  cilia Q10.3
  circulatory system, part NOS Q28.9
  clavicle Q74.0
  clitoris Q52.6
  coccyx Q76.49
  colon Q42.9
    specified NEC Q42.8
  corpus callosum Q04.0
  cricoid cartilage Q31.8
  diaphragm (with hernia) Q79.1
  digestive organ(s) or tract (complete) (partial) NEC Q45.8
    upper Q40.8
  ductus arteriosus Q28.8
  duodenum Q41.0
  ear Q16.9
    auricle Q16.0
    lobe Q17.8
  ejaculatory duct Q55.4
  endocrine (gland) NEC Q89.2

☑ **Additional Character Required — Refer to the Tabular List for Character Selection**   ▽ **Subterms under main terms may continue to next column or page**

Agenesis — *continued*
  epiglottis Q31.8
  esophagus Q39.8
  eustachian tube Q16.2
  eye Q11.1
    adnexa Q15.8
  eyelid (fold) Q10.3
  face
    bones NEC Q75.8
    specified part NEC Q18.8
  fallopian tube Q50.6
  femur — *see* Defect, reduction, lower limb, longitudinal, femur
  fibula — *see* Defect, reduction, lower limb, longitudinal, fibula
  finger (complete) (partial) — *see* Agenesis, hand
  foot (and toes) (complete) (partial) Q72.3- ☑
  forearm (with hand present) — *see* Agenesis, arm, with hand present
    and hand Q71.2- ☑
  gallbladder Q44.0
  gastric Q40.2
  genitalia, genital (organ(s))
    female Q52.8
      external Q52.71
      internal NEC Q52.8
    male Q55.8
  glottis Q31.8
  hair Q84.0
  hand (and fingers) (complete) (partial) Q71.3- ☑
  heart Q24.8
    valve NEC Q24.8
      pulmonary Q22.0
  hepatic Q44.7
  humerus — *see* Defect, reduction, upper limb
  hymen Q52.4
  ileum Q41.2
  incus Q16.3
  intestine (small) Q41.9
    large Q42.9
      specified NEC Q42.8
  iris (dilator fibers) Q13.1
  jaw M26.09
  jejunum Q41.1
  kidney(s) (partial) Q60.2
    bilateral Q60.1
    unilateral Q60.0
  labium (majus) (minus) Q52.71
  labyrinth, membranous Q16.5
  lacrimal apparatus Q10.4
  larynx Q31.8
  leg (complete) Q72.0- ☑
    with foot present Q72.1- ☑
    lower leg (with foot present) — *see* Agenesis, leg, with foot present
      and foot Q72.2- ☑
  lens Q12.3
  limb (complete) Q73.0
    lower — *see* Agenesis, leg
    upper — *see* Agenesis, arm
  lip Q38.0
  liver Q44.7
  lung (fissure) (lobe) (bilateral) (unilateral) Q33.3
  mandible, maxilla M26.09
  metacarpus — *see* Agenesis, hand
  metatarsus — *see* Agenesis, foot
  muscle Q79.8
    eyelid Q10.3
    ocular Q15.8
  musculoskeletal system NEC Q79.8
  nail(s) Q84.3
  neck, part Q18.8
  nerve Q07.8
  nervous system, part NEC Q07.8
  nipple Q83.2
  nose Q30.1
  nuclear Q07.8
  organ
    of Corti Q16.5
    or site not listed — *see* Anomaly, by site
  osseous meatus (ear) Q16.1
  ovary
    bilateral Q50.02
    unilateral Q50.01
  oviduct Q50.6
  pancreas Q45.0
  parathyroid (gland) Q89.2
  parotid gland(s) Q38.4

Agenesis — *continued*
  patella Q74.1
  pelvic girdle (complete) (partial) Q74.2
  penis Q55.5
  pericardium Q24.8
  pituitary (gland) Q89.2
  prostate Q55.4
  punctum lacrimale Q10.4
  radioulnar — *see* Defect, reduction, upper limb
  radius — *see* Defect, reduction, upper limb, longitudinal, radius
  rectum Q42.1
    with fistula Q42.0
  renal Q60.2
    bilateral Q60.1
    unilateral Q60.0
  respiratory organ NEC Q34.8
  rib Q76.6
  roof of orbit Q75.8
  round ligament Q52.8
  sacrum Q76.49
  salivary gland Q38.4
  scapula Q74.0
  scrotum Q55.29
  seminal vesicles Q55.4
  septum
    atrial Q21.1
    between aorta and pulmonary artery Q21.4
    ventricular Q20.4
  shoulder girdle (complete) (partial) Q74.0
  skull (bone) Q75.8
    with
      anencephaly Q00.0
      encephalocele — *see* Encephalocele
      hydrocephalus Q03.9
        with spina bifida — *See* Spina bifida, by site, with hydrocephalus
      microcephaly Q02
  spermatic cord Q55.4
  spinal cord Q06.0
  spine Q76.49
  spleen Q89.01
  sternum Q76.7
  stomach Q40.2
  submaxillary gland(s) (congenital) Q38.4
  tarsus — *see* Agenesis, foot
  tendon Q79.8
  testicle Q55.0
  thymus (gland) Q89.2
  thyroid (gland) E03.1
    cartilage Q31.8
  tibia — *see* Defect, reduction, lower limb, longitudinal, tibia
  tibiofibular — *see* Defect, reduction, lower limb, specified type NEC
  toe (and foot) (complete) (partial) — *see* Agenesis, foot
  tongue Q38.3
  trachea (cartilage) Q32.1
  ulna — *see* Defect, reduction, upper limb, longitudinal, ulna
  upper limb — *see* Agenesis, arm
  ureter Q62.4
  urethra Q64.5
  urinary tract NEC Q64.8
  uterus Q51.0
  uvula Q38.5
  vagina Q52.0
  vas deferens Q55.4
  vein(s) (peripheral) Q27.9
    brain Q28.3
    great NEC Q26.8
    portal Q26.5
  vena cava (inferior) (superior) Q26.8
  vermis of cerebellum Q04.3
  vertebra Q76.49
  vulva Q52.71
Ageusia R43.2
Agitated — *see* condition
Agitation R45.1
Aglossia (congenital) Q38.3
Aglossia-adactylia syndrome Q87.0
Aglycogenosis E74.00
Agnosia (body image) (other senses) (tactile) R48.1
  developmental F88
  verbal R48.1
    auditory R48.1
      developmental F80.2

Agnosia — *continued*
  verbal — *continued*
    developmental F80.2
  visual (object) R48.3
Agoraphobia F40.00
  with panic disorder F40.01
  without panic disorder F40.02
Agrammatism R48.8
Agranulocytopenia — *see* Agranulocytosis
Agranulocytosis (chronic) (cyclical) (genetic) (infantile) (periodic) (pernicious) (*see also* Neutropenia) D70.9
  congenital D70.0
  cytoreductive cancer chemotherapy sequela D70.1
  drug-induced D70.2
    due to cytoreductive cancer chemotherapy D70.1
  due to infection D70.3
  secondary D70.4
    drug-induced D70.2
    due to cytoreductive cancer chemotherapy D70.1
Agraphia (absolute) R48.8
  with alexia R48.0
  developmental F81.81
Ague (dumb) — *see* Malaria
Agyria Q04.3
Ahumada-del Castillo syndrome E23.0
Aichomophobia F40.298
AIDS (related complex) B20
Ailment heart — *see* Disease, heart
Ailurophobia F40.218
AIN — *see* Neoplasia, intraepithelial, anal
Ainhum (disease) L94.6
AIPHI (acute idiopathic pulmonary hemorrhage in infants (over 28 days old)) R04.81
Air
  anterior mediastinum J98.2
  compressed, disease T70.3 ☑
  conditioner lung or pneumonitis J67.7
  embolism (artery) (cerebral) (any site) T79.0 ☑
    with ectopic or molar pregnancy O08.2
    due to implanted device NEC — *see* Complications, by site and type, specified NEC
    following
      abortion — *see* Abortion by type, complicated by, embolism
      ectopic or molar pregnancy O08.2
      infusion, therapeutic injection or transfusion T80.0 ☑
    in pregnancy, childbirth or puerperium — *see* Embolism, obstetric
    traumatic T79.0 ☑
  hunger, psychogenic F45.8
  rarefied, effects of — *see* Effect, adverse, high altitude
  sickness T75.3 ☑
Airplane sickness T75.3 ☑
Akathisia (drug-induced) (treatment-induced) G25.71
  neuroleptic induced (acute) G25.71
  tardive G25.71
Akinesia R29.898
Akinetic mutism R41.89
Akureyri's disease G93.3
Alactasia, congenital E73.0
Alagille's syndrome Q44.7
Alastrim B03
Albers-Schönberg syndrome Q78.2
Albert's syndrome — *see* Tendinitis, Achilles
Albinism, albino E70.30
  with hematologic abnormality E70.339
    Chédiak-Higashi syndrome E70.330
    Hermansky-Pudlak syndrome E70.331
    other specified E70.338
  I E70.320
  II E70.321
  ocular E70.319
    autosomal recessive E70.311
    other specified E70.318
    X-linked E70.310
  oculocutaneous E70.329
    other specified E70.328
    tyrosinase (ty) negative E70.320
    tyrosinase (ty) positive E70.321
  other specified E70.39
Albinismus E70.30
Albright (-McCune)(-Sternberg) syndrome Q78.1
Albuminous — *see* condition
Albuminuria, albuminuric (acute) (chronic) (subacute) (*see also* Proteinuria) R80.9

Albuminuria, albuminuric — *continued*
  complicating pregnancy — *see* Proteinuria, gestational
    with
        gestational hypertension — *see* Pre-eclampsia
        pre-existing hypertension — *see* Hypertension,
            complicating pregnancy, pre-existing,
            with, pre-eclampsia
    gestational — *see* Proteinuria, gestational
        with
            gestational hypertension — *see* Pre-eclampsia
            pre-existing hypertension — *see* Hypertension,
                complicating pregnancy, pre-existing,
                with, pre-eclampsia
  orthostatic R80.2
  postural R80.2
  pre-eclamptic — *see* Pre-eclampsia
  scarlatinal A38.8
Albuminurophobia F40.298
Alcaptonuria E70.29
Alcohol, alcoholic, alcohol-induced
  addiction (without remission) F10.20
    with remission F10.21
  amnestic disorder, persisting F10.96
    with dependence F10.26
  anxiety disorder F10.980
  bipolar and related disorder F10.94
  brain syndrome, chronic F10.97
    with dependence F10.27
  cardiopathy I42.6
  counseling and surveillance Z71.41
    family member Z71.42
  delirium (acute) (tremens) (withdrawal) F10.231
    with intoxication F10.921
      in
          abuse F10.121
          dependence F10.221
  dementia F10.97
    with dependence F10.27
  depressive disorder F10.94
  deterioration F10.97
    with dependence F10.27
  hallucinosis (acute) F10.951
    in
        abuse F10.151
        dependence F10.251
  insanity F10.959
  intoxication (acute) (without dependence) F10.129
    with
        delirium F10.121
        dependence F10.229
            with delirium F10.221
            uncomplicated F10.220
    uncomplicated F10.120
  jealousy F10.988
  Korsakoff's, Korsakov's, Korsakow's F10.26
  liver K70.9
    acute — *see* Disease, liver, alcoholic, hepatitis
  major neurocognitive disorder, amnestic-confabulatory type F10.96
  major neurocognitive disorder, nonamnestic-confabulatory type F10.97
  mania (acute) (chronic) F10.959
  mild neurocognitive disorder F10.988
  paranoia, paranoid (type) psychosis F10.950
  pellagra E52
  poisoning, accidental (acute) NEC — *see* Table of Drugs and Chemicals, alcohol, poisoning
  psychosis — *see* Psychosis, alcoholic
  psychotic disorder F10.959
  sexual dysfunction F10.981
  sleep disorder F10.982
  withdrawal (without convulsions) F10.239
    with delirium F10.231
Alcoholism (chronic) (without remission) F10.20
  with
      psychosis — *see* Psychosis, alcoholic
      remission F10.21
  Korsakov's F10.96
    with dependence F10.26
Alder (-Reilly) **anomaly or syndrome** (leukocyte granulation) D72.0
Aldosteronism E26.9
  familial (type I) E26.02
  glucocorticoid-remediable E26.02
  primary (due to) (bilateral) adrenal hyperplasia E26.09
  primary NEC E26.09
  secondary E26.1
  specified NEC E26.89

Aldosteronoma D44.10
Aldrich (-Wiskott) **syndrome** (eczema-thrombocytopenia) D82.0
Alektorophobia F40.218
Aleppo boil B55.1
Aleukemic — *see* condition
Aleukia
  congenital D70.0
  hemorrhagica D61.9
    congenital D61.09
  splenica D73.1
Alexia R48.0
  developmental F81.0
  secondary to organic lesion R48.0
Algoneurodystrophy M89.00
  ankle M89.07- ☑
  foot M89.07- ☑
  forearm M89.03- ☑
  hand M89.04- ☑
  lower leg M89.06- ☑
  multiple sites M89.0- ☑
  shoulder M89.01- ☑
  specified site NEC M89.08
  thigh M89.05- ☑
  upper arm M89.02- ☑
Algophobia F40.298
Alienation, mental — *see* Psychosis
Alkalemia E87.3
Alkalosis E87.3
  metabolic E87.3
    with respiratory acidosis E87.4
  respiratory E87.3
Alkaptonuria E70.29
Allen-Masters syndrome N83.8
Allergy, allergic (reaction) (to) T78.40 ☑
  air-borne substance NEC (rhinitis) J30.89
  alveolitis (extrinsic) J67.9
    due to
        Aspergillus clavatus J67.4
        Cryptostroma corticale J67.6
        organisms (fungal, thermophilic actinomycete) growing in ventilation (air conditioning) systems J67.7
    specified type NEC J67.8
  anaphylactic reaction or shock T78.2 ☑
  angioneurotic edema T78.3 ☑
  animal (dander) (epidermal) (hair) (rhinitis) J30.81
  bee sting (anaphylactic shock) — *see* Toxicity, venom, arthropod, bee
  biological — *see* Allergy, drug
  colitis (*see also* Colitis, allergic) K52.29
  dander (animal) (rhinitis) J30.81
  dandruff (rhinitis) J30.81
  dental restorative material (existing) K08.55
  dermatitis — *see* Dermatitis, contact, allergic
  diathesis — *see* History, allergy
  drug, medicament & biological (any) (external) (internal) T78.40 ☑
    correct substance properly administered — *see* Table of Drugs and Chemicals, by drug, adverse effect
    wrong substance given or taken NEC (by accident) — *see* Table of Drugs and Chemicals, by drug, poisoning
  due to pollen J30.1
  dust (house) (stock) (rhinitis) J30.89
    with asthma — *see* Asthma, allergic extrinsic
  eczema — *see* Dermatitis, contact, allergic
  epidermal (animal) (rhinitis) J30.81
  feathers (rhinitis) J30.89
  food (any) (ingested) NEC T78.1 ☑
    anaphylactic shock — *see* Shock, anaphylactic, due to food
    dermatitis — *see* Dermatitis, due to, food
    dietary counseling and surveillance Z71.3
    in contact with skin L23.6
    rhinitis J30.5
    status (without reaction) Z91.018
        eggs Z91.012
        milk products Z91.011
        peanuts Z91.010
        seafood Z91.013
        specified NEC Z91.018
  gastrointestinal — *see also* specific type of allergic reaction
    meaning colitis (*see also* Colitis, allergic) K52.29

Allergy, allergic — *continued*
  gastrointestinal — *see also* specific type of allergic reaction — *continued*
      meaning gastroenteritis (*see also* Gastroenteritis, allergic) K52.29
      meaning other adverse food reaction not elsewhere classified T78.1 ☑
  grain J30.1
  grass (hay fever) (pollen) J30.1
    asthma — *see* Asthma, allergic extrinsic
  hair (animal) (rhinitis) J30.81
  history (of) — *see* History, allergy
  horse serum — *see* Allergy, serum
  inhalant (rhinitis) J30.89
    pollen J30.1
  kapok (rhinitis) J30.89
  medicine — *see* Allergy, drug
  milk protein (*see also* Allergy, food) Z91.011
    anaphylactic reaction T78.07 ☑
    dermatitis L27.2
    enterocolitis syndrome K52.21
    enteropathy K52.22
    gastroenteritis K52.29
    gastroesophageal reflux (*see also* Reaction, adverse, food) K21.9
        with esophagitis K21.0
    proctocolitis K52.82
  nasal, seasonal due to pollen J30.1
  pneumonia J82
  pollen (any) (hay fever) J30.1
    asthma — *see* Asthma, allergic extrinsic
  primrose J30.1
  primula J30.1
  proctocolitis K52.82
  purpura D69.0
  ragweed (hay fever) (pollen) J30.1
    asthma — *see* Asthma, allergic extrinsic
  rose (pollen) J30.1
  seasonal NEC J30.2
  Senecio jacobae (pollen) J30.1
  serum (*see also* Reaction, serum) T80.69 ☑
    anaphylactic shock T80.59 ☑
  shock (anaphylactic) T78.2 ☑
    due to
        administration of blood and blood products T80.51 ☑
        adverse effect of correct medicinal substance properly administered T88.6 ☑
        immunization T80.52 ☑
        serum NEC T80.59 ☑
        vaccination T80.52 ☑
  specific NEC T78.49 ☑
  tree (any) (hay fever) (pollen) J30.1
    asthma — *see* Asthma, allergic extrinsic
  upper respiratory J30.9
  urticaria L50.0
  vaccine — *see* Allergy, serum
  wheat — *see* Allergy, food
Allescheriasis B48.2
Alligator skin disease Q80.9
Allocheiria, allochiria R20.8
Almeida's disease — *see* Paracoccidioidomycosis
Alopecia (hereditaria) (seborrheica) L65.9
  androgenic L64.9
    drug-induced L64.0
    specified NEC L64.8
  areata L63.9
    ophiasis L63.2
    specified NEC L63.8
    totalis L63.0
    universalis L63.1
  cicatricial L66.9
    specified NEC L66.8
  circumscripta L63.9
  congenital, congenitalis Q84.0
  due to cytotoxic drugs NEC L65.8
  mucinosa L65.2
  postinfective NEC L65.8
  postpartum L65.0
  premature L64.8
  specific (syphilitic) A51.32
  specified NEC L65.8
  syphilitic (secondary) A51.32
  totalis (capitis) L63.0
  universalis (entire body) L63.1
  X-ray L58.1
Alpers' disease G31.81
Alpine sickness T70.29 ☑

☑ **Additional Character Required — Refer to the Tabular List for Character Selection**   ▽ **Subterms under main terms may continue to next column or page**

Alport syndrome Q87.81
ALTE (apparent life threatening event) **in newborn and infant** R68.13
Alteration (of), **Altered**
  awareness
    transient R40.4
    unintended under general anesthesia, during procedure T88.53 ☑
  mental status R41.82
  pattern of family relationships affecting child Z62.898
  sensation
    following
      cerebrovascular disease I69.998
        cerebral infarction I69.398
        intracerebral hemorrhage I69.198
        nontraumatic intracranial hemorrhage NEC I69.298
        specified disease NEC I69.898
        subarachnoid hemorrhage I69.098
Alternating — *see* condition
Altitude, high (effects) — *see* Effect, adverse, high altitude
Aluminosis (of lung) J63.0
Alveolitis
  allergic (extrinsic) — *see* Pneumonitis, hypersensitivity
  due to
    Aspergillus clavatus J67.4
    Cryptostroma corticale J67.6
  fibrosing (cryptogenic) (idiopathic) J84.112
  jaw M27.3
  sicca dolorosa M27.3
Alveolus, alveolar — *see* condition
Alymphocytosis D72.810
  thymic (with immunodeficiency) D82.1
Alymphoplasia, thymic D82.1
Alzheimer's disease or sclerosis — *see* Disease, Alzheimer's
Amastia (with nipple present) Q83.8
  with absent nipple Q83.0
Amathophobia F40.228
Amaurosis (acquired) (congenital) (*see also* Blindness)
  fugax G45.3
  hysterical F44.6
  Leber's congenital H35.50
  uremic — *see* Uremia
Amaurotic idiocy (infantile) (juvenile) (late) E75.4
Amaxophobia F40.248
Ambiguous genitalia Q56.4
Amblyopia (congenital) (ex anopsia) (partial) (suppression) H53.00-
  anisometropic — *see* Amblyopia, refractive
  deprivation H53.01- ☑
  hysterical F44.6
  nocturnal (*see also* Blindness, night)
    vitamin A deficiency E50.5
  refractive H53.02- ☑
  strabismic H53.03- ☑
  suspect H53.04- ☑
  tobacco H53.8
  toxic NEC H53.8
  uremic — *see* Uremia
Ameba, amebic (histolytica) (*see also* Amebiasis)
  abscess (liver) A06.4
Amebiasis A06.9
  with abscess — *see* Abscess, amebic
  acute A06.0
  chronic (intestine) A06.1
    with abscess — *see* Abscess, amebic
  cutaneous A06.7
  cutis A06.7
  cystitis A06.81
  genitourinary tract NEC A06.82
  hepatic — *see* Abscess, liver, amebic
  intestine A06.0
  nondysenteric colitis A06.2
  skin A06.7
  specified site NEC A06.89
Ameboma (of intestine) A06.3
Amelia Q73.0
  lower limb — *see* Agenesis, leg
  upper limb — *see* Agenesis, arm
Ameloblastoma (*see also* Cyst, calcifying odontogenic)
  long bones C40.9- ☑
    lower limb C40.2- ☑
    upper limb C40.0- ☑
  malignant C41.1
    jaw (bone) (lower) C41.1

Ameloblastoma — *continued*
  malignant — *continued*
    jaw — *continued*
      upper C41.0
  tibial C40.2- ☑
Amelogenesis imperfecta K00.5
  nonhereditaria (segmentalis) K00.4
Amenorrhea N91.2
  hyperhormonal E28.8
  primary N91.0
  secondary N91.1
Amentia — *see* Disability, intellectual
  Meynert's (nonalcoholic) F04
American
  leishmaniasis B55.2
  mountain tick fever A93.2
Ametropia — *see* Disorder, refraction
AMH (asymptomatic microscopic hematuria) R31.21
Amianthosis J61
Amimia R48.8
Amino-acid disorder E72.9
  anemia D53.0
Aminoacidopathy E72.9
Aminoaciduria E72.9
Amnesia R41.3
  anterograde R41.1
  auditory R48.8
  dissociative F44.0
    with dissociative fugue F44.1
  hysterical F44.0
  postictal in epilepsy — *see* Epilepsy
  psychogenic F44.0
  retrograde R41.2
  transient global G45.4
Amnes(t)ic syndrome (post-traumatic) F04
  induced by
    alcohol F10.96
      with dependence F10.26
    psychoactive NEC F19.96
      with
        abuse F19.16
        dependence F19.26
    sedative F13.96
      with dependence F13.26
Amnion, amniotic — *see* condition
Amnionitis — *see* Pregnancy, complicated by
Amok F68.8
Amoral traits F60.89
Amphetamine (or other stimulant) -**induced**
  anxiety disorder F15.980
  bipolar and related disorder F15.94
  delirium F15.921
  depressive disorder F15.94
  obsessive-compulsive and related disorder F15.988
  psychotic disorder F15.959
  sexual dysfunction F15.981
  sleep disorder F15.982
  stimulant withdrawal F15.23
Ampulla
  lower esophagus K22.8
  phrenic K22.8
Amputation (*see also* Absence, by site, acquired)
  neuroma (postoperative) (traumatic) — *see* Complications, amputation stump, neuroma
  stump (surgical)
    abnormal, painful, or with complication (late) — *see* Complications, amputation stump
    healed or old NOS Z89.9
  traumatic (complete) (partial)
    arm (upper) (complete) S48.91- ☑
      at
        elbow S58.01- ☑
          partial S58.02- ☑
        shoulder joint (complete) S48.01- ☑
          partial S48.02- ☑
      between
        elbow and wrist (complete) S58.11- ☑
          partial S58.12- ☑
        shoulder and elbow (complete) S48.11- ☑
          partial S48.12- ☑
      partial S48.92- ☑
    breast (complete) S28.21- ☑
      partial S28.22- ☑
    clitoris (complete) S38.211 ☑
      partial S38.212
    ear (complete) S08.11- ☑
      partial S08.12- ☑

Amputation — *continued*
  traumatic — *continued*
    finger (complete) (metacarpophalangeal)
      S68.11- ☑
      index S68.11- ☑
      little S68.11- ☑
      middle S68.11- ☑
      partial S68.12- ☑
        index S68.12- ☑
        little S68.12- ☑
        middle S68.12- ☑
        ring S68.12- ☑
      ring S68.11- ☑
      thumb — *see* Amputation, traumatic, thumb
      transphalangeal (complete) S68.61- ☑
        index S68.61- ☑
        little S68.61- ☑
        middle S68.61- ☑
        partial S68.62- ☑
          index S68.62- ☑
          little S68.62- ☑
          middle S68.62- ☑
          ring S68.62- ☑
        ring S68.61- ☑
    foot (complete) S98.91- ☑
      at ankle level S98.01- ☑
        partial S98.02- ☑
      midfoot S98.31- ☑
        partial S98.32- ☑
      partial S98.92- ☑
    forearm (complete) S58.91- ☑
      at elbow level (complete) S58.01- ☑
        partial S58.02- ☑
      between elbow and wrist (complete) S58.11- ☑
        partial S58.12- ☑
      partial S58.92- ☑
    genital organ(s) (external)
      female (complete) S38.211 ☑
        partial S38.212 ☑
      male
        penis (complete) S38.221 ☑
          partial S38.222 ☑
        scrotum (complete) S38.231 ☑
          partial S38.232 ☑
        testes (complete) S38.231 ☑
          partial S38.232 ☑
    hand (complete) (wrist level) S68.41- ☑
      finger(s) alone — *see* Amputation, traumatic, finger
      partial S68.42- ☑
      thumb alone — *see* Amputation, traumatic, thumb
      transmetacarpal (complete) S68.71- ☑
        partial S68.72- ☑
    head
      ear — *see* Amputation, traumatic, ear
      nose (partial) S08.812 ☑
        complete S08.811 ☑
      part S08.89 ☑
        scalp S08.0 ☑
    hip (and thigh) (complete) S78.91- ☑
      at hip joint (complete) S78.01- ☑
        partial S78.02- ☑
      between hip and knee (complete) S78.11- ☑
        partial S78.12- ☑
      partial S78.92- ☑
    labium (majus) (minus) (complete) S38.21- ☑
      partial S38.21- ☑
    leg (lower) S88.91- ☑
      at knee level S88.01- ☑
        partial S88.02- ☑
      between knee and ankle S88.11- ☑
        partial S88.12- ☑
      partial S88.92- ☑
    nose (partial) S08.812 ☑
      complete S08.811 ☑
    penis (complete) S38.221 ☑
      partial S38.222 ☑
    scrotum (complete) S38.231 ☑
      partial S38.232 ☑
    shoulder — *see* Amputation, traumatic, arm
      at shoulder joint — *see* Amputation, traumatic, arm, at shoulder joint
    testes (complete) S38.231 ☑
      partial S38.232 ☑
    thigh — *see* Amputation, traumatic, hip

Amputation — *continued*
traumatic — *continued*
thorax, part of S28.1 ☑
breast — *see* Amputation, traumatic, breast
thumb (complete) (metacarpophalangeal)
S68.01- ☑
partial S68.02- ☑
transphalangeal (complete) S68.51- ☑
partial S68.52- ☑
toe (lesser) S98.13- ☑
great S98.11- ☑
partial S98.12- ☑
more than one S98.21- ☑
partial S98.22- ☑
partial S98.14- ☑
vulva (complete) S38.211 ☑
partial S38.212 ☑
Amputee (bilateral) (old) Z89.9
Amsterdam dwarfism Q87.1
Amusia R48.8
developmental F80.89
Amyelencephalus, amyelencephaly Q00.0
Amyelia Q06.0
Amygdalitis — *see* Tonsillitis
Amygdalolith J35.8
Amyloid heart (disease) E85.4 [I43]
Amyloidosis (generalized) (primary) E85.9
with lung involvement E85.4 [J99]
familial E85.2
genetic E85.2
heart E85.4 [I43]
hemodialysis-associated E85.3
light chain (AL) E85.81
liver E85.4 [K77]
localized E85.4
neuropathic heredofamilial E85.1
non-neuropathic heredofamilial E85.0
organ limited E85.4
Portuguese E85.1
pulmonary E85.4 [J99]
secondary systemic E85.3
senile systemic (SSA) E85.82
skin (lichen) (macular) E85.4 [L99]
specified NEC E85.89
subglottic E85.4 [J99]
wild-type transthyretin-related (ATTR) E85.82
Amylopectinosis (brancher enzyme deficiency) E74.03
Amylophagia — *see* Pica
Amyoplasia congenita Q79.8
Amyotonia M62.89
congenita G70.2
Amyotrophia, amyotrophy, amyotrophic G71.8
congenita Q79.8
diabetic — *see* Diabetes, amyotrophy
lateral sclerosis G12.21
neuralgic G54.5
spinal progressive G12.25
Anacidity, gastric K31.83
psychogenic F45.8
Anaerosis of newborn P28.89
Analbuminemia E88.09
Analgesia — *see* Anesthesia
Analphalipoproteinemia E78.6
Anaphylactic
purpura D69.0
shock or reaction — *see* Shock, anaphylactic
Anaphylactoid shock or reaction — *see* Shock, anaphylactic
Anaphylactoid syndrome of pregnancy O88.01- ☑
Anaphylaxis — *see* Shock, anaphylactic
Anaplasia cervix (*see also* Dysplasia, cervix) N87.9
Anaplasmosis, human A77.49
Anarthria R47.1
Anasarca R60.1
cardiac — *see* Failure, heart, congestive
lung J18.2
newborn P83.2
nutritional E43
pulmonary J18.2
renal N04.9
Anastomosis
aneurysmal — *see* Aneurysm
arteriovenous ruptured brain I60.8
intestinal K63.89
complicated NEC K91.89
involving urinary tract N99.89
retinal and choroidal vessels (congenital) Q14.8

Anatomical narrow angle H40.03- ☑
Ancylostoma, ancylostomiasis (braziliense) (caninum) (ceylanicum) (duodenale) B76.0
Necator americanus B76.1
Andersen's disease (glycogen storage) E74.09
Anderson-Fabry disease E75.21
Andes disease T70.29
Andrews' disease (bacterid) L08.89
Androblastoma
benign
specified site — *see* Neoplasm, benign, by site
unspecified site
female D27.9
male D29.20
malignant
specified site — *see* Neoplasm, malignant, by site
unspecified site
female C56.9
male C62.90
specified site — *see* Neoplasm, uncertain behavior, by site
tubular
with lipid storage
specified site — *see* Neoplasm, benign, by site
unspecified site
female D27.9
male D29.20
specified site — *see* Neoplasm, benign, by site
unspecified site
female D27.9
male D29.20
unspecified site
female D39.10
male D40.10
Androgen insensitivity syndrome (*see also* Syndrome, androgen insensitivity) E34.50
Androgen resistance syndrome (*see also* Syndrome, androgen insensitivity) E34.50
Android pelvis Q74.2
with disproportion (fetopelvic) O33.3 ☑
causing obstructed labor O65.3
Androphobia F40.290
Anectasis, pulmonary (newborn) — *see* Atelectasis
Anemia (essential) (general) (hemoglobin deficiency) (infantile) (primary) (profound) D64.9
with (due to) (in)
disorder of
anaerobic glycolysis D55.2
pentose phosphate pathway D55.1
koilonychia D50.9
achlorhydric D50.8
achrestic D53.1
Addison (-Biermer) (pernicious) D51.0
agranulocytic — *see* Agranulocytosis
amino-acid-deficiency D53.0
aplastic D61.9
congenital D61.09
drug-induced D61.1
due to
drugs D61.1
external agents NEC D61.2
infection D61.2
radiation D61.2
idiopathic D61.3
red cell (pure) D60.9
chronic D60.0
congenital D61.01
specified type NEC D60.8
transient D60.1
specified type NEC D61.89
toxic D61.2
aregenerative
congenital D61.09
asiderotic D50.9
atypical (primary) D64.9
Baghdad spring D55.0
Balantidium coli A07.0
Biermer's (pernicious) D51.0
blood loss (chronic) D50.0
acute D62
bothriocephalus B70.0 [D63.8]
brickmaker's B76.9 [D63.8]
cerebral I67.89
childhood D58.9
chlorotic D50.8
chronic
blood loss D50.0
hemolytic D58.9

Anemia — *continued*
chronic — *continued*
hemolytic — *continued*
idiopathic D59.9
simple D53.9
chronica congenita aregenerativa D61.09
combined system disease NEC D51.0 [G32.0]
due to dietary vitamin B12 deficiency D51.3 [G32.0]
complicating pregnancy, childbirth or puerperium — *see* Pregnancy, complicated by (management affected by), anemia
congenital P61.4
aplastic D61.09
due to isoimmunization NOS P55.9
dyserythropoietic, dyshematopoietic D64.4
following fetal blood loss P61.3
Heinz body D58.2
hereditary hemolytic NOS D58.9
pernicious D51.0
spherocytic D58.0
Cooley's (erythroblastic) D56.1
cytogenic D51.0
deficiency D53.9
6-PGD D55.1
2, 3 diphosphoglycurate mutase D55.2
2, 3 PG D55.2
6 phosphogluconate dehydrogenase D55.1
amino-acid D53.0
combined B12 and folate D53.1
enzyme D55.9
drug-induced (hemolytic) D59.2
glucose-6-phosphate dehydrogenase (G6PD) D55.0
glycolytic D55.2
nucleotide metabolism D55.3
related to hexose monophosphate (HMP) shunt pathway NEC D55.1
specified type NEC D55.8
erythrocytic glutathione D55.1
folate D52.9
dietary D52.0
drug-induced D52.1
folic acid D52.9
dietary D52.0
drug-induced D52.1
G SH D55.1
G6PD D55.0
GGS-R D55.1
glucose-6-phosphate dehydrogenase D55.0
glutathione reductase D55.1
glyceraldehyde phosphate dehydrogenase D55.2
hexokinase D55.2
iron D50.9
secondary to blood loss (chronic) D50.0
nutritional D53.9
with
poor iron absorption D50.8
specified deficiency NEC D53.8
phosphofructo-aldolase D55.2
phosphoglycerate kinase D55.2
PK D55.2
protein D53.0
pyruvate kinase D55.2
transcobalamin II D51.2
triose-phosphate isomerase D55.2
vitamin B12 NOS D51.9
dietary D51.3
due to
intrinsic factor deficiency D51.0
selective vitamin B12 malabsorption with proteinuria D51.1
pernicious D51.0
specified type NEC D51.8
Diamond-Blackfan (congenital hypoplastic) D61.01
dibothriocephalus B70.0 [D63.8]
dimorphic D53.1
diphasic D53.1
Diphyllobothrium (Dibothriocephalus) B70.0 [D63.8]
due to (in) (with)
antineoplastic chemotherapy D64.81
blood loss (chronic) D50.0
acute D62
chemotherapy, antineoplastic D64.81
chronic disease classified elsewhere NEC D63.8
chronic kidney disease D63.1
deficiency
amino-acid D53.0
copper D53.8
folate (folic acid) D52.9

☑ **Additional Character Required** — Refer to the Tabular List for Character Selection   ▽ **Subterms under main terms may continue to next column or page**

Anemia — *continued*
  due to — *continued*
    deficiency — *continued*
      folate — *continued*
        dietary D52.0
        drug-induced D52.1
      molybdenum D53.8
      protein D53.0
      zinc D53.8
    dietary vitamin B12 deficiency D51.3
    disorder of
      glutathione metabolism D55.1
      nucleotide metabolism D55.3
    drug — *see* Anemia, by type (*see also* Table of Drugs and Chemicals)
    end stage renal disease D63.1
    enzyme disorder D55.9
    fetal blood loss P61.3
    fish tapeworm (D.latum) infestation B70.0 [D63.8]
    hemorrhage (chronic) D50.0
      acute D62
    impaired absorption D50.9
    loss of blood (chronic) D50.0
      acute D62
    myxedema E03.9 [D63.8]
    Necator americanus B76.1 [D63.8]
    prematurity P61.2
    selective vitamin B12 malabsorption with proteinuria D51.1
    transcobalamin II deficiency D51.2
  Dyke-Young type (secondary) (symptomatic) D59.1
  dyserythropoietic (congenital) D64.4
  dyshematopoietic (congenital) D64.4
  Egyptian B76.9 [D63.8]
  elliptocytosis — *see* Elliptocytosis
  enzyme-deficiency, drug-induced D59.2
  epidemic (*see also* Ancylostomiasis) B76.9 [D63.8]
  erythroblastic
    familial D56.1
    newborn (*see also* Disease, hemolytic) P55.9
    of childhood D56.1
  erythrocytic glutathione deficiency D55.1
  erythropoietin-resistant anemia (EPO resistant anemia) D63.1
  Faber's (achlorhydric anemia) D50.9
  factitious (self-induced blood letting) D50.0
  familial erythroblastic D56.1
  Fanconi's (congenital pancytopenia) D61.09
  favism D55.0
  fish tapeworm (D. latum) infestation B70.0 [D63.8]
  folate (folic acid) deficiency D52.9
  glucose-6-phosphate dehydrogenase (G6PD) deficiency D55.0
  glutathione-reductase deficiency D55.1
  goat's milk D52.0
  granulocytic — *see* Agranulocytosis
  Heinz body, congenital D58.2
  hemolytic D58.9
    acquired D59.9
      with hemoglobinuria NEC D59.6
      autoimmune NEC D59.1
      infectious D59.4
      specified type NEC D59.8
      toxic D59.4
    acute D59.9
      due to enzyme deficiency specified type NEC D55.8
      Lederer's D59.1
    autoimmune D59.1
      drug-induced D59.0
    chronic D58.9
      idiopathic D59.9
    cold type (secondary) (symptomatic) D59.1
    congenital (spherocytic) — *see* Spherocytosis
    due to
      cardiac conditions D59.4
      drugs (nonautoimmune) D59.2
        autoimmune D59.0
      enzyme disorder D55.9
        drug-induced D59.2
      presence of shunt or other internal prosthetic device D59.4
    familial D58.9
    hereditary D58.9
      due to enzyme disorder D55.9
        specified type NEC D55.8
      specified type NEC D58.8
    idiopathic (chronic) D59.9
    mechanical D59.4

Anemia — *continued*
  hemolytic — *continued*
    microangiopathic D59.4
    nonautoimmune D59.4
      drug-induced D59.2
    nonspherocytic
      congenital or hereditary NEC D55.8
        glucose-6-phosphate dehydrogenase deficiency D55.0
        pyruvate kinase deficiency D55.2
        type
          I D55.1
          II D55.2
      type
        I D55.1
        II D55.2
    secondary D59.4
      autoimmune D59.1
    specified (hereditary) type NEC D58.8
    Stransky-Regala type (*see also* Hemoglobinopathy) D58.8
    symptomatic D59.4
      autoimmune D59.1
    toxic D59.4
    warm type (secondary) (symptomatic) D59.1
  hemorrhagic (chronic) D50.0
    acute D62
  Herrick's D57.1
  hexokinase deficiency D55.2
  hookworm B76.9 [D63.8]
  hypochromic (idiopathic) (microcytic) (normoblastic) D50.9
    due to blood loss (chronic) D50.0
      acute D62
    familial sex-linked D64.0
    pyridoxine-responsive D64.3
    sideroblastic, sex-linked D64.0
  hypoplasia, red blood cells D61.9
    congenital or familial D61.01
  hypoplastic (idiopathic) D61.9
    congenital or familial (of childhood) D61.01
  hypoproliferative (refractive) D61.9
  idiopathic D64.9
    aplastic D61.3
    hemolytic, chronic D59.9
  in (due to) (with)
    chronic kidney disease D63.1
    end stage renal disease D63.1
    failure, kidney (renal) D63.1
    neoplastic disease (*see also* Neoplasm) D63.0
  intertropical (*see also* Ancylostomiasis) D63.8
  iron deficiency D50.9
    secondary to blood loss (chronic) D50.0
      acute D62
    specified type NEC D50.8
  Joseph-Diamond-Blackfan (congenital hypoplastic) D61.01
  Lederer's (hemolytic) D59.1
  leukoerythroblastic D61.82
  macrocytic D53.9
    nutritional D52.0
    tropical D52.8
  malarial (*see also* Malaria) B54 [D63.8]
  malignant (progressive) D51.0
  malnutrition D53.9
  marsh (*see also* Malaria) B54 [D63.8]
  Mediterranean (with other hemoglobinopathy) D56.9
  megaloblastic D53.1
    combined B12 and folate deficiency D53.1
    hereditary D51.1
    nutritional D52.0
    orotic aciduria D53.0
    refractory D53.1
    specified type NEC D53.1
  megalocytic D53.1
  microcytic (hypochromic) D50.9
    due to blood loss (chronic) D50.0
      acute D62
    familial D56.8
  microdrepanocytosis D57.40
  microelliptopoikilocytic (Rietti-Greppi- Micheli) D56.9
  miner's B76.9 [D63.8]
  myelodysplastic D46.9
  myelofibrosis D75.81
  myelogenous D64.89
  myelopathic D64.89
  myelophthisic D61.82
  myeloproliferative D47.Z9 (*following* D47.4)
  newborn P61.4

Anemia — *continued*
  newborn — *continued*
    due to
      ABO (antibodies, isoimmunization, maternal/fetal incompatibility) P55.1
      Rh (antibodies, isoimmunization, maternal/fetal incompatibility) P55.0
    following fetal blood loss P61.3
    posthemorrhagic (fetal) P61.3
  nonspherocytic hemolytic — *see* Anemia, hemolytic, nonspherocytic
  normocytic (infectional) D64.9
    due to blood loss (chronic) D50.0
      acute D62
    myelophthisic D61.82
  nutritional (deficiency) D53.9
    with
      poor iron absorption D50.8
      specified deficiency NEC D53.8
    megaloblastic D52.0
  of prematurity P61.2
  orotaciduric (congenital) (hereditary) D53.0
  osteosclerotic D64.89
  ovalocytosis (hereditary) — *see* Elliptocytosis
  paludal (*see also* Malaria) B54 [D63.8]
  pernicious (congenital) (malignant) (progressive) D51.0
  pleochromic D64.89
    of sprue D52.8
  posthemorrhagic (chronic) D50.0
    acute D62
    newborn P61.3
  postoperative (postprocedural)
    due to (acute) blood loss D62
      chronic blood loss D50.0
    specified NEC D64.9
  postpartum O90.81
  pressure D64.89
  progressive D64.9
    malignant D51.0
    pernicious D51.0
  protein-deficiency D53.0
  pseudoleukemica infantum D64.89
  pure red cell D60.9
    congenital D61.01
  pyridoxine-responsive D64.3
  pyruvate kinase deficiency D55.2
  refractory D46.4
    with
      excess of blasts D46.20
        1 (RAEB 1) D46.21
        2 (RAEB 2) D46.22
        in transformation (RAEB T) — *see* Leukemia, acute myeloblastic
      hemochromatosis D46.1
      sideroblasts (ring) (RARS) D46.1
    without ring sideroblasts, so stated D46.0
    without sideroblasts without excess of blasts D46.0
    megaloblastic D53.1
    sideroblastic D46.1
    sideropenic D50.9
  Rietti-Greppi-Micheli D56.9
  scorbutic D53.2
  secondary to
    blood loss (chronic) D50.0
      acute D62
    hemorrhage (chronic) D50.0
      acute D62
  semiplastic D61.89
  sickle-cell — *see* Disease, sickle-cell
  sideroblastic D64.3
    hereditary D64.0
    hypochromic, sex-linked D64.0
    pyridoxine-responsive NEC D64.3
    refractory D46.1
    secondary (due to)
      disease D64.1
      drugs and toxins D64.2
    specified type NEC D64.3
  sideropenic (refractory) D50.9
    due to blood loss (chronic) D50.0
      acute D62
  simple chronic D53.9
  specified type NEC D64.89
  spherocytic (hereditary) — *see* Spherocytosis
  splenic D64.89
  splenomegalic D64.89
  stomatocytosis D58.8
  syphilitic (acquired) (late) A52.79 [D63.8]
  target cell D64.89

Subterms under main terms may continue to next column or page   ☑ Additional Character Required — Refer to the Tabular List for Character Selection   **19**

Anemia — Anemia

Anemia — *continued*
thalassemia D56.9
thrombocytopenic — *see* Thrombocytopenia
toxic D61.2
tropical B76.9 [D63.8]
macrocytic D52.8
tuberculous A18.89 [D63.8]
vegan D51.3
vitamin
B6-responsive D64.3
B12 deficiency (dietary) pernicious D51.0
von Jaksch's D64.89
Witts' (achlorhydric anemia) D50.8
Anemophobia F40.228
Anencephalus, anencephaly Q00.0
Anergasia — *see* Psychosis, organic
Anesthesia, anesthetic R20.0
complication or reaction NEC (*see also* Complications, anesthesia) T88.59 ☑
due to
correct substance properly administered — *see* Table of Drugs and Chemicals, by drug, adverse effect
overdose or wrong substance given — *see* Table of Drugs and Chemicals, by drug, poisoning
unintended awareness under general anesthesia during procedure T88.53 ☑
personal history of Z92.84
cornea H18.81- ☑
dissociative F44.6
functional (hysterical) F44.6
hyperesthetic, thalamic G89.0
hysterical F44.6
local skin lesion R20.0
sexual (psychogenic) F52.1
shock (due to) T88.2 ☑
skin R20.0
testicular N50.9
Anetoderma (maculosum) (of) L90.8
Jadassohn-Pellizzari L90.2
Schweniger-Buzzi L90.1
Aneurin deficiency E51.9
Aneurysm (anastomotic) (artery) (cirsoid) (diffuse) (false) (fusiform) (multiple) (saccular) I72.9
abdominal (aorta) I71.4
ruptured I71.3
syphilitic A52.01
aorta, aortic (nonsyphilitic) I71.9
abdominal I71.4
ruptured I71.3
arch I71.2
ruptured I71.1
arteriosclerotic I71.9
ruptured I71.8
ascending I71.2
ruptured I71.1
congenital Q25.43
descending I71.9
abdominal I71.4
ruptured I71.3
ruptured I71.8
thoracic I71.2
ruptured I71.1
root Q25.43
ruptured I71.8
sinus, congenital Q25.43
syphilitic A52.01
thoracic I71.2
ruptured I71.1
thoracoabdominal I71.6
ruptured I71.5
thorax, thoracic (arch) I71.2
ruptured I71.1
transverse I71.2
ruptured I71.1
valve (heart) (*see also* Endocarditis, aortic) I35.8
arteriosclerotic I72.9
cerebral I67.1
ruptured — *see* Hemorrhage, intracranial, subarachnoid
arteriovenous (congenital) (*see also* Malformation, arteriovenous)
acquired I77.0
brain I67.1
coronary I25.41
pulmonary I28.0
brain Q28.2

Aneurysm — *continued*
arteriovenous (*see also* Malformation, arteriovenous) — *continued*
brain — *continued*
ruptured I60.8
peripheral — *see* Malformation, arteriovenous, peripheral
precerebral vessels Q28.0
specified site NEC (*see also* Malformation, arteriovenous)
acquired I77.0
basal — *see* Aneurysm, brain
basilar (trunk) I72.5
berry (congenital) (nonruptured) I67.1
ruptured I60.7
brain I67.1
arteriosclerotic I67.1
ruptured — *see* Hemorrhage, intracranial, subarachnoid
arteriovenous (congenital) (nonruptured) Q28.2
acquired I67.1
ruptured I60.8
ruptured I60.8
berry (congenital) (nonruptured) I67.1
ruptured (*see also* Hemorrhage, intracranial, subarachnoid) I60.7
congenital Q28.3
ruptured I60.7
meninges I67.1
ruptured I60.8
miliary (congenital) (nonruptured) I67.1
ruptured (*see also* Hemorrhage, intracranial, subarachnoid) I60.7
mycotic I33.0
ruptured — *see* Hemorrhage, intracranial, subarachnoid
syphilitic (hemorrhage) A52.05
cardiac (false) (*see also* Aneurysm, heart) I25.3
carotid artery (common) (external) I72.0
internal (intracranial) I67.1
extracranial portion I72.0
ruptured into brain I60.0- ☑
syphilitic A52.09
intracranial A52.05
cavernous sinus I67.1
arteriovenous (congenital) (nonruptured) Q28.3
ruptured I60.8
celiac I72.8
central nervous system, syphilitic A52.05
cerebral — *see* Aneurysm, brain
chest — *see* Aneurysm, thorax
circle of Willis I67.1
congenital Q28.3
ruptured I60.6
ruptured I60.6
common iliac artery I72.3
congenital (peripheral) Q27.8
aorta (root) (sinus) Q25.43
brain Q28.3
ruptured I60.7
coronary Q24.5
digestive system Q27.8
lower limb Q27.8
pulmonary Q25.79
retina Q14.1
specified site NEC Q27.8
upper limb Q27.8
conjunctiva — *see* Abnormality, conjunctiva, vascular
conus arteriosus — *see* Aneurysm, heart
coronary (arteriosclerotic) (artery) I25.41
arteriovenous, congenital Q24.5
congenital Q24.5
ruptured — *see* Infarct, myocardium
syphilitic A52.06
vein I25.89
cylindroid (aorta) I71.9
ruptured I71.8
syphilitic A52.01
ductus arteriosus Q25.0
endocardial, infective (any valve) I33.0
femoral (artery) (ruptured) I72.4
gastroduodenal I72.8
gastroepiploic I72.8
heart (wall) (chronic or with a stated duration of over 4 weeks) I25.3
valve — *see* Endocarditis
hepatic I72.8
iliac (common) (artery) (ruptured) I72.3

Aneurysm — *continued*
infective I72.9
endocardial (any valve) I33.0
innominate (nonsyphilitic) I72.8
syphilitic A52.09
interauricular septum — *see* Aneurysm, heart
interventricular septum — *see* Aneurysm, heart
intrathoracic (nonsyphilitic) I71.2
ruptured I71.1
syphilitic A52.01
lower limb I72.4
lung (pulmonary artery) I28.1
mediastinal (nonsyphilitic) I72.8
syphilitic A52.09
miliary (congenital) I67.1
ruptured — *see* Hemorrhage, intracerebral, subarachnoid, intracranial
mitral (heart) (valve) I34.8
mural — *see* Aneurysm, heart
mycotic I72.9
endocardial (any valve) I33.0
ruptured, brain — *see* Hemorrhage, intracerebral, subarachnoid
myocardium — *see* Aneurysm, heart
neck I72.0
pancreaticoduodenal I72.8
patent ductus arteriosus Q25.0
peripheral NEC I72.8
congenital Q27.8
digestive system Q27.8
lower limb Q27.8
specified site NEC Q27.8
upper limb Q27.8
popliteal (artery) (ruptured) I72.4
precerebral
congenital (nonruptured) Q28.1
specified site, NEC I72.5
pulmonary I28.1
arteriovenous Q25.72
acquired I28.0
syphilitic A52.09
valve (heart) — *see* Endocarditis, pulmonary
racemose (peripheral) I72.9
congenital — *see* Aneurysm, congenital
radial I72.1
Rasmussen NEC A15.0
renal (artery) I72.2
retina (*see also* Disorder, retina, microaneurysms)
congenital Q14.1
diabetic — *see* Diabetes, microaneurysms, retinal
sinus of Valsalva Q25.49
specified NEC I72.8
spinal (cord) I72.8
syphilitic (hemorrhage) A52.09
splenic I72.8
subclavian (artery) (ruptured) I72.8
syphilitic A52.09
superior mesenteric I72.8
syphilitic (aorta) A52.01
central nervous system A52.05
congenital (late) A50.54 [I79.0]
spine, spinal A52.09
thoracoabdominal (aorta) I71.6
ruptured I71.5
syphilitic A52.01
thorax, thoracic (aorta) (arch) (nonsyphilitic) I71.2
ruptured I71.1
syphilitic A52.01
traumatic (complication) (early), specified site — *see* Injury, blood vessel
tricuspid (heart) (valve) I07.8
ulnar I72.1
upper limb (ruptured) I72.1
valve, valvular — *see* Endocarditis
venous (*see also* Varix) I86.8
congenital Q27.8
digestive system Q27.8
lower limb Q27.8
specified site NEC Q27.8
upper limb Q27.8
ventricle — *see* Aneurysm, heart
vertebral artery I72.6
visceral NEC I72.8
Angelman syndrome Q93.5
Anger R45.4
Angiectasis, angiectopia I99.8
Angiitis I77.6
allergic granulomatous M30.1

20

☑ **Additional Character Required** — Refer to the Tabular List for Character Selection   ▽ Subterms under main terms may continue to next column or page

Anemia — Angiitis

Angiitis — continued
  hypersensitivity M31.0
  necrotizing M31.9
    specified NEC M31.8
  nervous system, granulomatous I67.7
Angina (attack) (cardiac) (chest) (heart) (pectoris) (syndrome) (vasomotor) I20.9
  with
    atherosclerotic heart disease — see Arteriosclerosis, coronary (artery),
    documented spasm I20.1
  abdominal K55.1
  accelerated — see Angina, unstable
  agranulocytic — see Agranulocytosis
  angiospastic — see Angina, with documented spasm
  aphthous B08.5
  crescendo — see Angina, unstable
  croupous J05.0
  cruris I73.9
  de novo effort — see Angina, unstable
  diphtheritic, membranous A36.0
  equivalent I20.8
  exudative, chronic J37.0
  following acute myocardial infarction I23.7
  gangrenous diphtheritic A36.0
  intestinal K55.1
  Ludovici K12.2
  Ludwig's K12.2
  malignant diphtheritic A36.0
  membranous J05.0
    diphtheritic A36.0
    Vincent's A69.1
  mesenteric K55.1
  monocytic — see Mononucleosis, infectious
  of effort — see Angina, specified NEC
  phlegmonous J36
    diphtheritic A36.0
  post-infarctional I23.7
  pre-infarctional — see Angina, unstable
  Prinzmetal — see Angina, with documented spasm
  progressive — see Angina, unstable
  pseudomembranous A69.1
  pultaceous, diphtheritic A36.0
  spasm-induced — see Angina, with documented spasm
  specified NEC I20.8
  stable I20.8
  stenocardia — see Angina, specified NEC
  stridulous, diphtheritic A36.2
  tonsil J36
  trachealis J05.0
  unstable I20.0
  variant — see Angina, with documented spasm
  Vincent's A69.1
  worsening effort — see Angina, unstable
Angioblastoma — see Neoplasm, connective tissue, uncertain behavior
Angiocholecystitis — see Cholecystitis, acute
Angiocholitis (see also Cholecystitis, acute) K83.0
Angiodysgenesis spinalis G95.19
Angiodysplasia (cecum) (colon) K55.20
  with bleeding K55.21
  duodenum (and stomach) K31.819
    with bleeding K31.811
  stomach (and duodenum) K31.819
    with bleeding K31.811
Angioedema (allergic) (any site) (with urticaria) T78.3 ☑
  hereditary D84.1
Angioendothelioma — see Neoplasm, uncertain behavior, by site
  benign D18.00
    intra-abdominal D18.03
    intracranial D18.02
    skin D18.01
    specified site NEC D18.09
  bone — see Neoplasm, bone, malignant
  Ewing's — see Neoplasm, bone, malignant
Angioendotheliomatosis C85.8- ☑
Angiofibroma (see also Neoplasm, benign, by site)
  juvenile
    specified site — see Neoplasm, benign, by site
    unspecified site D10.6
Angiohemophilia (A) (B) D68.0
Angioid streaks (choroid) (macula) (retina) H35.33
Angiokeratoma — see Neoplasm, skin, benign
  corporis diffusum E75.21
Angioleiomyoma — see Neoplasm, connective tissue, benign

Angiolipoma (see also Lipoma)
  infiltrating — see Lipoma
Angioma (see also Hemangioma, by site)
  capillary I78.1
  hemorrhagicum hereditaria I78.0
  intra-abdominal D18.03
  intracranial D18.02
  malignant — see Neoplasm, connective tissue, malignant
  plexiform D18.00
    intra-abdominal D18.03
    intracranial D18.02
    skin D18.01
    specified site NEC D18.09
  senile I78.1
  serpiginosum L81.7
  skin D18.01
  specified site NEC D18.09
  spider I78.1
  stellate I78.1
  venous Q28.3
Angiomatosis Q82.8
  bacillary A79.89
  encephalotrigeminal Q85.8
  hemorrhagic familial I78.0
  hereditary familial I78.0
  liver K76.4
Angiomyolipoma — see Lipoma
Angiomyoliposarcoma — see Neoplasm, connective tissue, malignant
Angiomyoma — see Neoplasm, connective tissue, benign
Angiomyosarcoma — see Neoplasm, connective tissue, malignant
Angiomyxoma — see Neoplasm, connective tissue, uncertain behavior
Angioneurosis F45.8
Angioneurotic edema (allergic) (any site) (with urticaria) T78.3 ☑
  hereditary D84.1
Angiopathia, angiopathy I99.9
  cerebral I67.9
    amyloid E85.4 [I68.0]
  diabetic (peripheral) — see Diabetes, angiopathy
  peripheral I73.9
    diabetic — see Diabetes, angiopathy
    specified type NEC I73.89
  retinae syphilitica A52.05
  retinalis (juvenilis)
    diabetic — see Diabetes, retinopathy
    proliferative — see Retinopathy, proliferative
Angiosarcoma (see also Neoplasm, connective tissue, malignant)
  liver C22.3
Angiosclerosis — see Arteriosclerosis
Angiospasm (peripheral) (traumatic) (vessel) I73.9
  brachial plexus G54.0
  cerebral G45.9
  cervical plexus G54.2
  nerve
    arm — see Mononeuropathy, upper limb
      axillary G54.0
      median — see Lesion, nerve, median
      ulnar — see Lesion, nerve, ulnar
    axillary G54.0
    leg — see Mononeuropathy, lower limb
    median — see Lesion, nerve, median
    plantar — see Lesion, nerve, plantar
    ulnar — see Lesion, nerve, ulnar
Angiospastic disease or edema I73.9
Angiostrongyliasis
  due to
    Parastrongylus
      cantonensis B83.2
      costaricensis B81.3
  intestinal B81.3
Anguillulosis — see Strongyloidiasis
Angulation
  cecum — see Obstruction, intestine
  coccyx (acquired) (see also subcategory) M43.8 ☑
    congenital NEC Q76.49
  femur (acquired) (see also Deformity, limb, specified type NEC, thigh)
    congenital Q74.2
  intestine (large) (small) — see Obstruction, intestine
  sacrum (acquired) (see also subcategory) M43.8 ☑
    congenital NEC Q76.49
  sigmoid (flexure) — see Obstruction, intestine

Angulation — continued
  spine — see Dorsopathy, deforming, specified NEC
  tibia (acquired) (see also Deformity, limb, specified type NEC, lower leg)
    congenital Q74.2
  ureter N13.5
    with infection N13.6
  wrist (acquired) (see also Deformity, limb, specified type NEC, forearm)
    congenital Q74.0
Angulus infectiosus (lips) K13.0
Anhedonia R45.84
  sexual F52.0
Anhidrosis L74.4
Anhydration E86.0
Anhydremia E86.0
Anidrosis L74.4
Aniridia (congenital) Q13.1
Anisakiasis (infection) (infestation) B81.0
Anisakis larvae infestation B81.0
Aniseikonia H52.32
Anisocoria (pupil) H57.02
  congenital Q13.2
Anisocytosis R71.8
Anisometropia (congenital) H52.31
Ankle — see condition
Ankyloblepharon (eyelid) (acquired) (see also Blepharophimosis)
  filiforme (adnatum) (congenital) Q10.3
  total Q10.3
Ankyloglossia Q38.1
Ankylosis (fibrous) (osseous) (joint) M24.60
  ankle M24.67- ☑
  arthrodesis status Z98.1
  cricoarytenoid (cartilage) (joint) (larynx) J38.7
  dental K03.5
  ear ossicles H74.31- ☑
  elbow M24.62- ☑
  foot M24.67- ☑
  hand M24.64- ☑
  hip M24.65- ☑
  incostapedial joint (infectional) — see Ankylosis, ear ossicles
  jaw (temporomandibular) M26.61- ☑
  knee M24.66- ☑
  lumbosacral (joint) M43.27
  postoperative (status) Z98.1
  produced by surgical fusion, status Z98.1
  sacro-iliac (joint) M43.28
  shoulder M24.61- ☑
  spine (joint) (see also Fusion, spine)
    spondylitic — see Spondylitis, ankylosing
  surgical Z98.1
  temporomandibular M26.61- ☑
  tooth, teeth (hard tissues) K03.5
  wrist M24.63- ☑
Ankylostoma — see Ancylostoma
Ankylostomiasis — see Ancylostomiasis
Ankylurethria — see Stricture, urethra
Annular (see also condition)
  detachment, cervix N88.8
  organ or site, congenital NEC — see Distortion
  pancreas (congenital) Q45.1
Anodontia (complete) (partial) (vera) K00.0
  acquired K08.10 ☑
Anomaly, anomalous (congenital) (unspecified type) Q89.9
  abdominal wall NEC Q79.59
  acoustic nerve Q07.8
  adrenal (gland) Q89.1
  Alder (-Reilly) (leukocyte granulation) D72.0
  alimentary tract Q45.9
    upper Q40.9
  alveolar M26.70
    hyperplasia M26.79
      mandibular M26.72
      maxillary M26.71
    hypoplasia M26.79
      mandibular M26.74
      maxillary M26.73
    ridge (process) M26.79
    specified NEC M26.79
  ankle (joint) Q74.2
  anus Q43.9
  aorta (arch) NEC Q25.40
    coarctation (preductal) (postductal) Q25.1
  aortic cusp or valve Q23.9

Anomaly, anomalous — continued
appendix Q43.8
apple peel syndrome Q41.1
aqueduct of Sylvius Q03.0
    with spina bifida — see Spina bifida, with hydro-
        cephalus
arm Q74.0
arteriovenous NEC
    coronary Q24.5
    gastrointestinal Q27.33
        acquired — see Angiodysplasia
artery (peripheral) Q27.9
    basilar NEC Q28.1
    cerebral Q28.3
    coronary Q24.5
    digestive system Q27.8
    eye Q15.8
    great Q25.9
        specified NEC Q25.8
    lower limb Q27.8
    peripheral Q27.9
        specified NEC Q27.8
    pulmonary NEC Q25.79
    renal Q27.2
    retina Q14.1
    specified site NEC Q27.8
    subclavian Q27.8
        origin Q25.48
    umbilical Q27.0
    upper limb Q27.8
    vertebral NEC Q28.1
aryteno-epiglottic folds Q31.8
atrial
    bands or folds Q20.8
    septa Q21.1
atrioventricular
    excitation I45.6
    septum Q21.0
auditory canal Q17.8
auricle
    ear Q17.8
        causing impairment of hearing Q16.9
    heart Q20.8
Axenfeld's Q15.0
back Q89.9
band
    atrial Q20.8
    heart Q24.8
    ventricular Q24.8
Bartholin's duct Q38.4
biliary duct or passage Q44.5
bladder Q64.70
    absence Q64.5
    diverticulum Q64.6
    exstrophy Q64.10
        cloacal Q64.12
        extroversion Q64.19
        specified type NEC Q64.19
        supravesical fissure Q64.11
    neck obstruction Q64.31
    specified type NEC Q64.79
bone Q79.9
    arm Q74.0
    face Q75.9
    leg Q74.2
    pelvic girdle Q74.2
    shoulder girdle Q74.0
    skull Q75.9
        with
            anencephaly Q00.0
            encephalocele — see Encephalocele
            hydrocephalus Q03.9
                with spina bifida — see Spina bifida, by
                    site, with hydrocephalus
            microcephaly Q02
brain (multiple) Q04.9
    vessel Q28.3
breast Q83.9
broad ligament Q50.6
bronchus Q32.4
bulbus cordis Q21.9
bursa Q79.9
canal of Nuck Q52.4
canthus Q10.3
capillary Q27.9
cardiac Q24.9
    chambers Q20.9
        specified NEC Q20.8
    septal closure Q21.9

Anomaly, anomalous — continued
cardiac — continued
    septal closure — continued
        specified NEC Q21.8
    valve NEC Q24.8
        pulmonary Q22.3
cardiovascular system Q28.8
carpus Q74.0
caruncle, lacrimal Q10.6
cascade stomach Q40.2
cauda equina Q06.3
cecum Q43.9
cerebral Q04.9
    vessels Q28.3
cervix Q51.9
Chédiak-Higashi (-Steinbrinck) (congenital gigantism
        of peroxidase granules) E70.330
cheek Q18.9
chest wall Q67.8
    bones Q76.9
chin Q18.9
chordae tendineae Q24.8
choroid Q14.3
    plexus Q07.8
chromosomes, chromosomal Q99.9
    D (1) — see condition, chromosome 13
    E (3) — see condition, chromosome 18
    G — see condition, chromosome 21
    sex
        female phenotype Q97.8
        gonadal dysgenesis (pure) Q99.1
        Klinefelter's Q98.4
        male phenotype Q98.9
        Turner's Q96.9
    specified NEC Q99.8
cilia Q10.3
circulatory system Q28.9
clavicle Q74.0
clitoris Q52.6
coccyx Q76.49
colon Q43.9
common duct Q44.5
communication
    coronary artery Q24.5
    left ventricle with right atrium Q21.0
concha (ear) Q17.3
connection
    portal vein Q26.5
    pulmonary venous Q26.4
        partial Q26.3
        total Q26.2
    renal artery with kidney Q27.2
cornea (shape) Q13.4
coronary artery or vein Q24.5
cranium — see Anomaly, skull
cricoid cartilage Q31.8
cystic duct Q44.5
dental
    alveolar — see Anomaly, alveolar
    arch relationship M26.20
        specified NEC M26.29
dentofacial M26.9
    alveolar — see Anomaly, alveolar
    dental arch relationship M26.20
        specified NEC M26.29
    functional M26.50
        specified NEC M26.59
    jaw size M26.00
        macrogenia M26.05
        mandibular
            hyperplasia M26.03
            hypoplasia M26.04
        maxillary
            hyperplasia M26.01
            hypoplasia M26.02
        microgenia M26.06
        specified type NEC M26.09
    jaw-cranial base relationship M26.10
        asymmetry M26.12
            maxillary M26.11
        specified type NEC M26.19
    malocclusion M26.4
        dental arch relationship NEC M26.29
        jaw size — see Anomaly, dentofacial, jaw size
        jaw-cranial base relationship — see Anomaly,
            dentofacial, jaw-cranial base relationship
    specified type NEC M26.89
    temporomandibular joint M26.60- ☑

Anomaly, anomalous — continued
dentofacial — continued
    temporomandibular joint — continued
        adhesions M26.61- ☑
        ankylosis M26.61- ☑
        arthralgia M26.62- ☑
        articular disc M26.63- ☑
        specified type NEC M26.69
    tooth position, fully erupted M26.30
    specified NEC M26.39
dermatoglyphic Q82.8
diaphragm (apertures) NEC Q79.1
digestive organ(s) or tract Q45.9
    lower Q43.9
    upper Q40.9
distance, interarch (excessive) (inadequate) M26.25
distribution, coronary artery Q24.5
ductus
    arteriosus Q25.0
    botalli Q25.0
duodenum Q43.9
dura (brain) Q04.9
    spinal cord Q06.9
ear (external) Q17.9
    causing impairment of hearing Q16.9
    inner Q16.5
    middle (causing impairment of hearing) Q16.4
        ossicles Q16.3
Ebstein's (heart) (tricuspid valve) Q22.5
ectodermal Q82.9
Eisenmenger's (ventricular septal defect) Q21.8
ejaculatory duct Q55.4
elbow Q74.0
endocrine gland NEC Q89.2
epididymis Q55.4
epiglottis Q31.8
esophagus Q39.9
eustachian tube Q17.8
eye Q15.9
    anterior segment Q13.9
        specified NEC Q13.89
    posterior segment Q14.9
        specified NEC Q14.8
    ptosis (eyelid) Q10.0
    specified NEC Q15.8
eyebrow Q18.8
eyelid Q10.3
    ptosis Q10.0
face Q18.9
    bone(s) Q75.9
fallopian tube Q50.6
fascia Q79.9
femur NEC Q74.2
fibula NEC Q74.2
finger Q74.0
fixation, intestine Q43.3
flexion (joint) NOS Q74.9
    hip or thigh Q65.89
foot NEC Q74.2
    varus (congenital) Q66.3
foramen
    Botalli Q21.1
    ovale Q21.1
forearm Q74.0
forehead Q75.8
form, teeth K00.2
fovea centralis Q14.1
frontal bone — see Anomaly, skull
gallbladder (position) (shape) (size) Q44.1
Gartner's duct Q52.4
gastrointestinal tract Q45.9
genitalia, genital organ(s) or system
    female Q52.9
        external Q52.70
        internal NOS Q52.9
    male Q55.9
        hydrocele P83.5
        specified NEC Q55.8
genitourinary NEC
    female Q52.9
    male Q55.9
Gerbode Q21.0
glottis Q31.8
granulation or granulocyte, genetic (constitutional)
        (leukocyte) D72.0
gum Q38.6
gyri Q07.9
hair Q84.2
hand Q74.0

☑ **Additional Character Required — Refer to the Tabular List for Character Selection**   ▽ Subterms under main terms may continue to next column or page

Anomaly, anomalous — *continued*
  hard tissue formation in pulp K04.3
  head — *see* Anomaly, skull
  heart Q24.9
    auricle Q20.8
    bands or folds Q24.8
    fibroelastosis cordis I42.4
    obstructive NEC Q22.6
    patent ductus arteriosus (Botalli) Q25.0
    septum Q21.9
      auricular Q21.1
      interatrial Q21.1
      interventricular Q21.0
        with pulmonary stenosis or atresia, dextra-
          position of aorta and hypertrophy of
          right ventricle Q21.3
      specified NEC Q21.8
      ventricular Q21.0
        with pulmonary stenosis or atresia, dextra-
          position of aorta and hypertrophy of
          right ventricle Q21.3
    tetralogy of Fallot Q21.3
    valve NEC Q24.8
      aortic
        bicuspid valve Q23.1
        insufficiency Q23.1
        stenosis Q23.0
          subaortic Q24.4
      mitral
        insufficiency Q23.3
        stenosis Q23.2
      pulmonary Q22.3
        atresia Q22.0
        insufficiency Q22.2
        stenosis Q22.1
          infundibular Q24.3
          subvalvular Q24.3
      tricuspid
        atresia Q22.4
        stenosis Q22.4
    ventricle Q20.8
  heel NEC Q74.2
  Hegglin's D72.0
  hemianencephaly Q00.0
  hemicephaly Q00.0
  hemicrania Q00.0
  hepatic duct Q44.5
  hip NEC Q74.2
  hourglass stomach Q40.2
  humerus Q74.0
  hydatid of Morgagni
    female Q50.5
    male (epididymal) Q55.4
      testicular Q55.29
  hymen Q52.4
  hypersegmentation of neutrophils, hereditary D72.0
  hypophyseal Q89.2
  ileocecal (coil) (valve) Q43.9
  ileum Q43.9
  ilium NEC Q74.2
  integument Q84.9
    specified NEC Q84.8
  interarch distance (excessive) (inadequate) M26.25
  intervertebral cartilage or disc Q76.49
  intestine (large) (small) Q43.9
    with anomalous adhesions, fixation or malrotation
      Q43.3
  iris Q13.2
  ischium NEC Q74.2
  jaw — *see* Anomaly, dentofacial
    alveolar — *see* Anomaly, alveolar
  jaw-cranial base relationship — *see* Anomaly, dento-
    facial, jaw-cranial base relationship
  jejunum Q43.8
  joint Q74.9
    specified NEC Q74.8
  Jordan's D72.0
  kidney(s) (calyx) (pelvis) Q63.9
    artery Q27.2
    specified NEC Q63.8
  Klippel-Feil (brevicollis) Q76.1
  knee Q74.1
  labium (majus) (minus) Q52.70
  labyrinth, membranous Q16.5
  lacrimal apparatus or duct Q10.6
  larynx, laryngeal (muscle) Q31.9
    web (bed) Q31.0
  lens Q12.9
  leukocytes, genetic D72.0

Anomaly, anomalous — *continued*
  leukocytes, genetic — *continued*
    granulation (constitutional) D72.0
  lid (fold) Q10.3
  ligament Q79.9
    broad Q50.6
    round Q52.8
  limb Q74.9
    lower NEC Q74.2
      reduction deformity — *see* Defect, reduction,
        lower limb
    upper Q74.0
  lip Q38.0
  liver Q44.7
    duct Q44.5
  lower limb NEC Q74.2
  lumbosacral (joint) (region) Q76.49
    kyphosis — *see* Kyphosis, congenital
    lordosis — *see* Lordosis, congenital
  lung (fissure) (lobe) Q33.9
  mandible — *see* Anomaly, dentofacial
  maxilla — *see* Anomaly, dentofacial
  May (-Hegglin) D72.0
  meatus urinarius NEC Q64.79
  meningeal bands or folds Q07.9
    constriction of Q07.8
    spinal Q06.9
  meninges Q07.9
    cerebral Q04.8
    spinal Q06.9
  meningocele Q05.9
  mesentery Q45.9
  metacarpus Q74.0
  metatarsus NEC Q74.2
  middle ear Q16.4
    ossicles Q16.3
  mitral (leaflets) (valve) Q23.9
    insufficiency Q23.3
    specified NEC Q23.8
    stenosis Q23.2
  mouth Q38.6
  Müllerian (*see also* Anomaly, by site)
    uterus NEC Q51.818
  multiple NEC Q89.7
  muscle Q79.9
    eyelid Q10.3
  musculoskeletal system, except limbs Q79.9
  myocardium Q24.8
  nail Q84.6
  narrowness, eyelid Q10.3
  nasal sinus (wall) Q30.8
  neck (any part) Q18.9
  nerve Q07.9
    acoustic Q07.8
    optic Q07.8
  nervous system (central) Q07.9
  nipple Q83.9
  nose, nasal (bones) (cartilage) (septum) (sinus) Q30.9
    specified NEC Q30.8
  ocular muscle Q15.8
  omphalomesenteric duct Q43.0
  opening, pulmonary veins Q26.4
  optic
    disc Q14.2
    nerve Q07.8
  opticociliary vessels Q13.2
  orbit (eye) Q10.7
  organ Q89.9
    of Corti Q16.5
  origin
    artery
      innominate Q25.8
      pulmonary Q25.79
      renal Q27.2
      subclavian Q25.48
  osseous meatus (ear) Q16.1
  ovary Q50.39
  oviduct Q50.6
  palate (hard) (soft) NEC Q38.5
  pancreas or pancreatic duct Q45.3
  papillary muscles Q24.8
  parathyroid gland Q89.2
  paraurethral ducts Q64.79
  parotid (gland) Q38.4
  patella Q74.1
  Pelger-Huët (hereditary hyposegmentation) D72.0
  pelvic girdle NEC Q74.2
  pelvis (bony) NEC Q74.2
    rachitic E64.3

Anomaly, anomalous — *continued*
  penis (glans) Q55.69
  pericardium Q24.8
  peripheral vascular system Q27.9
  Peter's Q13.4
  pharynx Q38.8
  pigmentation L81.9
    congenital Q82.8
  pituitary (gland) Q89.2
  pleural (folds) Q34.0
  portal vein Q26.5
    connection Q26.5
  position, tooth, teeth, fully erupted M26.30
    specified NEC M26.39
  precerebral vessel Q28.1
  prepuce Q55.69
  prostate Q55.4
  pulmonary Q33.9
    artery NEC Q25.79
    valve Q22.3
      atresia Q22.0
      insufficiency Q22.2
      specified type NEC Q22.3
      stenosis Q22.1
        infundibular Q24.3
        subvalvular Q24.3
    venous connection Q26.4
      partial Q26.3
      total Q26.2
  pupil Q13.2
    function H57.00
      anisocoria H57.02
      Argyll Robertson pupil H57.01
      miosis H57.03
      mydriasis H57.04
      specified type NEC H57.09
      tonic pupil H57.05- ☑
  pylorus Q40.3
  radius Q74.0
  rectum Q43.9
  reduction (extremity) (limb)
    femur (longitudinal) — *see* Defect, reduction,
      lower limb, longitudinal, femur
    fibula (longitudinal) — *see* Defect, reduction, lower
      limb, longitudinal, fibula
    lower limb — *see* Defect, reduction, lower limb
    radius (longitudinal) — *see* Defect, reduction, up-
      per limb, longitudinal, radius
    tibia (longitudinal) — *see* Defect, reduction, lower
      limb, longitudinal, tibia
    ulna (longitudinal) — *see* Defect, reduction, upper
      limb, longitudinal, ulna
    upper limb — *see* Defect, reduction, upper limb
  refraction — *see* Disorder, refraction
  renal Q63.9
    artery Q27.2
    pelvis Q63.9
      specified NEC Q63.8
  respiratory system Q34.9
    specified NEC Q34.8
  retina Q14.1
  rib Q76.6
    cervical Q76.5
  Rieger's Q13.81
  rotation — *see* Malrotation
    hip or thigh Q65.89
  round ligament Q52.8
  sacroiliac (joint) NEC Q74.2
  sacrum NEC Q76.49
    kyphosis — *see* Kyphosis, congenital
    lordosis — *see* Lordosis, congenital
  saddle nose, syphilitic A50.57
  salivary duct or gland Q38.4
  scapula Q74.0
  scrotum — *see* Malformation, testis and scrotum
  sebaceous gland Q82.9
  seminal vesicles Q55.4
  sense organs NEC Q07.8
  sex chromosomes NEC (*see also* Anomaly, chromo-
    somes)
    female phenotype Q97.8
    male phenotype Q98.9
  shoulder (girdle) (joint) Q74.0
  sigmoid (flexure) Q43.9
  simian crease Q82.8
  sinus of Valsalva Q25.49
  skeleton generalized Q78.9
  skin (appendage) Q82.9

Anomaly, anomalous — *continued*
  skull Q75.9
    with
      anencephaly Q00.0
      encephalocele — *see* Encephalocele
      hydrocephalus Q03.9
        with spina bifida — *see* Spina bifida, by site, with hydrocephalus
      microcephaly Q02
  specified organ or site NEC Q89.8
  spermatic cord Q55.4
  spine, spinal NEC Q76.49
    column NEC Q76.49
      kyphosis — *see* Kyphosis, congenital
      lordosis — *see* Lordosis, congenital
    cord Q06.9
    nerve root Q07.8
  spleen Q89.09
    agenesis Q89.01
  stenonian duct Q38.4
  sternum NEC Q76.7
  stomach Q40.3
  submaxillary gland Q38.4
  tarsus NEC Q74.2
  tendon Q79.9
  testis — *see* Malformation, testis and scrotum
  thigh NEC Q74.2
  thorax (wall) Q67.8
    bony Q76.9
  throat Q38.8
  thumb Q74.0
  thymus gland Q89.2
  thyroid (gland) Q89.2
    cartilage Q31.8
  tibia NEC Q74.2
    saber A50.56
  toe Q74.2
  tongue Q38.3
  tooth, teeth K00.9
    eruption K00.6
    position, fully erupted M26.30
    spacing, fully erupted M26.30
  trachea (cartilage) Q32.1
  tragus Q17.9
  tricuspid (leaflet) (valve) Q22.9
    atresia or stenosis Q22.4
    Ebstein's Q22.5
  Uhl's (hypoplasia of myocardium, right ventricle) Q24.8
  ulna Q74.0
  umbilical artery Q27.0
  union
    cricoid cartilage and thyroid cartilage Q31.8
    thyroid cartilage and hyoid bone Q31.8
    trachea with larynx Q31.8
  upper limb Q74.0
  urachus Q64.4
  ureter Q62.8
    obstructive NEC Q62.39
      cecoureterocele Q62.32
      orthotopic ureterocele Q62.31
  urethra Q64.70
    absence Q64.5
    double Q64.74
    fistula to rectum Q64.73
    obstructive Q64.39
      stricture Q64.32
    prolapse Q64.71
    specified type NEC Q64.79
  urinary tract Q64.9
  uterus Q51.9
    with only one functioning horn Q51.4
  uvula Q38.5
  vagina Q52.4
  valleculae Q31.8
  valve (heart) NEC Q24.8
    coronary sinus Q24.5
    inferior vena cava Q24.8
    pulmonary Q22.3
    sinus coronario Q24.5
    venae cavae inferioris Q24.8
  vas deferens Q55.4
  vascular Q27.9
    brain Q28.3
    ring Q25.45
  vein(s) (peripheral) Q27.9
    brain Q28.3
    cerebral Q28.3
    coronary Q24.5
    developmental Q28.3

Anomaly, anomalous — *continued*
  vein(s) — *continued*
    great Q26.9
      specified NEC Q26.8
  vena cava (inferior) (superior) Q26.9
  venous — *see* Anomaly, vein(s)
  venous return Q26.8
  ventricular
    bands or folds Q24.8
    septa Q21.0
  vertebra Q76.49
    kyphosis — *see* Kyphosis, congenital
    lordosis — *see* Lordosis, congenital
  vesicourethral orifice Q64.79
  vessel(s) Q27.9
    optic papilla Q14.2
    precerebral Q28.1
  vitelline duct Q43.0
  vitreous body or humor Q14.0
  vulva Q52.70
  wrist (joint) Q74.0
Anomia R48.8
Anonychia (congenital) Q84.3
  acquired L60.8
Anophthalmos, anophthalmus (congenital) (globe) Q11.1
  acquired Z90.01
Anopia, anopsia H53.46- ☑
  quadrant H53.46- ☑
Anorchia, anorchism, anorchidism Q55.0
Anorexia R63.0
  hysterical F44.89
  nervosa F50.00
    atypical F50.9
    binge-eating type F50.2
      with purging F50.02
    restricting type F50.01
Anorgasmy, psychogenic (female) F52.31
  male F52.32
Anosmia R43.0
  hysterical F44.6
  postinfectional J39.8
Anosognosia R41.89
Anosteoplasia Q78.9
Anovulatory cycle N97.0
Anoxemia R09.02
  newborn P84
Anoxia (pathological) R09.02
  altitude T70.29 ☑
  cerebral G93.1
    complicating
      anesthesia (general) (local) or other sedation T88.59 ☑
        in labor and delivery O74.3
        in pregnancy O29.21- ☑
        postpartum, puerperal O89.2
      delivery (cesarean) (instrumental) O75.4
    during a procedure G97.81
    newborn P84
    resulting from a procedure G97.82
  due to
    drowning T75.1 ☑
    high altitude T70.29 ☑
  heart — *see* Insufficiency, coronary
  intrauterine P84
  myocardial — *see* Insufficiency, coronary
  newborn P84
  spinal cord G95.11
  systemic (by suffocation) (low content in atmosphere) — *see* Asphyxia, traumatic
Anteflexion — *see* Anteversion
Antenatal
  care (normal pregnancy) Z34.90
  screening (encounter for) of mother (*see also* Encounter, antenatal screening) Z36.9
Antepartum — *see* condition
Anterior — *see* condition
Antero-occlusion M26.220
Anteversion
  cervix — *see* Anteversion, uterus
  femur (neck), congenital Q65.89
  uterus, uterine (cervix) (postinfectional) (postpartal, old) N85.4
    congenital Q51.818
    in pregnancy or childbirth — *see* Pregnancy, complicated by
Anthophobia F40.228
Anthracosilicosis J60

Anthracosis (lung) (occupational) J60
  lingua K14.3
Anthrax A22.9
  with pneumonia A22.1
  cerebral A22.8
  colitis A22.2
  cutaneous A22.0
  gastrointestinal A22.2
  inhalation A22.1
  intestinal A22.2
  meningitis A22.8
  pulmonary A22.1
  respiratory A22.1
  sepsis A22.7
  specified manifestation NEC A22.8
Anthropoid pelvis Q74.2
  with disproportion (fetopelvic) O33.0
Anthropophobia F40.10
  generalized F40.11
Antibodies, maternal (blood group) — *see* Isoimmunization, affecting management of pregnancy
  anti-D — *see* Isoimmunization, affecting management of pregnancy, Rh
  newborn P55.0
Antibody
  anticardiolipin R76.0
    with
      hemorrhagic disorder D68.312
      hypercoagulable state D68.61
  antiphosphatidylglycerol R76.0
    with
      hemorrhagic disorder D68.312
      hypercoagulable state D68.61
  antiphosphatidylinositol R76.0
    with
      hemorrhagic disorder D68.312
      hypercoagulable state D68.61
  antiphosphatidylserine R76.0
    with
      hemorrhagic disorder D68.312
      hypercoagulable state D68.61
  antiphospholipid R76.0
    with
      hemorrhagic disorder D68.312
      hypercoagulable state D68.61
Anticardiolipin syndrome D68.61
Anticoagulant, circulating (intrinsic) (*see also* Disorder, hemorrhagic) D68.318
  drug-induced (extrinsic) (*see also* Disorder, hemorrhagic) D68.32
  iatrogenic D68.32
Antidiuretic hormone syndrome E22.2
Antimonial cholera — *see* Poisoning, antimony
Antiphospholipid
  antibody
    with hemorrhagic disorder D68.312
    syndrome D68.61
Antisocial personality F60.2
Antithrombinemia — *see* Circulating anticoagulants
Antithromboplastinemia D68.318
Antithromboplastinogenemia D68.318
Antitoxin complication or reaction — *see* Complications, vaccination
Antlophobia F40.228
Antritis J32.0
  maxilla J32.0
    acute J01.00
      recurrent J01.01
  stomach K29.60
    with bleeding K29.61
Antrum, antral — *see* condition
Anuria R34
  calculous (impacted) (recurrent) (*see also* Calculus, urinary) N20.9
  following
    abortion — *see* Abortion by type complicated by, renal failure
    ectopic or molar pregnancy O08.4
  newborn P96.0
  postprocedural N99.0
  postrenal N13.8
  traumatic (following crushing) T79.5 ☑
Anus, anal — *see* condition
Anusitis K62.89
Anxiety F41.9
  depression F41.8
  episodic paroxysmal F41.0
  generalized F41.1

Anxiety — *continued*
　hysteria F41.8
　neurosis F41.1
　panic type F41.0
　reaction F41.1
　separation, abnormal (of childhood) F93.0
　specified NEC F41.8
　state F41.1
Aorta, aortic — *see* condition
Aortectasia — *see* Ectasia, aorta
　with aneurysm — *see* Aneurysm, aorta
Aortitis (nonsyphilitic) (calcific) I77.6
　arteriosclerotic I70.0
　Doehle-Heller A52.02
　luetic A52.02
　rheumatic — *see* Endocarditis, acute, rheumatic
　specific (syphilitic) A52.02
　syphilitic A52.02
　　congenital A50.54 [I79.1]
Apathetic thyroid storm — *see* Thyrotoxicosis
Apathy R45.3
Apeirophobia F40.228
Apepsia K30
　psychogenic F45.8
Aperistalsis, esophagus K22.0
Apertognathia M26.29
Apert's syndrome Q87.0
Aphagia R13.0
　psychogenic F50.9
Aphakia (acquired) (postoperative) H27.0- ☑
　congenital Q12.3
Aphasia (amnestic) (global) (nominal) (semantic) (syntactic) R47.01
　acquired, with epilepsy (Landau-Kleffner syndrome)
　　— *see* Epilepsy, specified NEC
　auditory (developmental) F80.2
　developmental (receptive type) F80.2
　　expressive type F80.1
　　Wernicke's F80.2
　following
　　cerebrovascular disease I69.920
　　　cerebral infarction I69.320
　　　intracerebral hemorrhage I69.120
　　　nontraumatic intracranial hemorrhage NEC
　　　　I69.220
　　　specified disease NEC I69.820
　　　subarachnoid hemorrhage I69.020
　primary progressive G31.01 [F02.80]
　　with behavioral disturbance G31.01 [F02.81]
　progressive isolated G31.01 [F02.80]
　　with behavioral disturbance G31.01 [F02.81]
　sensory F80.2
　syphilis, tertiary A52.19
　Wernicke's (developmental) F80.2
Aphonia (organic) R49.1
　hysterical F44.4
　psychogenic F44.4
Aphthae, aphthous (*see also* condition)
　Bednar's K12.0
　cachectic K14.0
　epizootic B08.8
　fever B08.8
　oral (recurrent) K12.0
　stomatitis (major) (minor) K12.0
　thrush B37.0
　ulcer (oral) (recurrent) K12.0
　　genital organ(s) NEC
　　　female N76.6
　　　male N50.89
　　larynx J38.7
Apical — *see* condition
Apiphobia F40.218
Aplasia (*see also* Agenesis)
　abdominal muscle syndrome Q79.4
　alveolar process (acquired) — *see* Anomaly, alveolar
　　congenital Q38.6
　aorta (congenital) Q25.41
　axialis extracorticalis (congenita) E75.29
　bone marrow (myeloid) D61.9
　　congenital D61.01
　brain Q00.0
　　part of Q04.3
　bronchus Q32.4
　cerebellum Q04.3
　cervix (congenital) Q51.5
　congenital pure red cell D61.01
　corpus callosum Q04.0

Aplasia — *continued*
　cutis congenita Q84.8
　erythrocyte congenital D61.01
　extracortical axial E75.29
　eye Q11.1
　fovea centralis (congenital) Q14.1
　gallbladder, congenital Q44.0
　iris Q13.1
　labyrinth, membranous Q16.5
　limb (congenital) Q73.8
　　lower — *see* Defect, reduction, lower limb
　　upper — *see* Agenesis, arm
　lung, congenital (bilateral) (unilateral) Q33.3
　pancreas Q45.0
　parathyroid-thymic D82.1
　Pelizaeus-Merzbacher E75.29
　penis Q55.5
　prostate Q55.4
　red cell (with thymoma) D60.9
　　acquired D60.9
　　　due to drugs D60.9
　　adult D60.9
　　chronic D60.0
　　congenital D61.01
　　constitutional D61.01
　　due to drugs D60.9
　　hereditary D61.01
　　of infants D61.01
　　primary D61.01
　　pure D61.01
　　　due to drugs D60.9
　　specified type NEC D60.8
　　transient D60.1
　round ligament Q52.8
　skin Q84.8
　spermatic cord Q55.4
　spleen Q89.01
　testicle Q55.0
　thymic, with immunodeficiency D82.1
　thyroid (congenital) (with myxedema) E03.1
　uterus Q51.0
　ventral horn cell Q06.1
Apnea, apneic (of) (spells) R06.81
　newborn NEC P28.4
　　obstructive P28.4
　　sleep (central) (obstructive) (primary) P28.3
　prematurity P28.4
　sleep G47.30
　　central (primary) G47.31
　　　idiopathic G47.31
　　　in conditions classified elsewhere G47.37
　　obstructive (adult) (pediatric) G47.33
　　　hypopnea G47.33
　　primary central G47.31
　　specified NEC G47.39
Apneumatosis, newborn P28.0
Apocrine metaplasia (breast) — *see* Dysplasia, mammary, specified type NEC
Apophysitis (bone) (*see also* Osteochondropathy)
　calcaneus M92.8
　juvenile M92.9
Apoplectiform convulsions (cerebral ischemia) I67.82
Apoplexia, apoplexy, apoplectic
　adrenal A39.1
　heart (auricle) (ventricle) — *see* Infarct, myocardium
　heat T67.0 ☑
　hemorrhagic (stroke) — *see* Hemorrhage, intracranial
　meninges, hemorrhagic — *see* Hemorrhage, intracranial, subarachnoid
　uremic N18.9 [I68.8]
Appearance
　bizarre R46.1
　specified NEC R46.89
　very low level of personal hygiene R46.0
Appendage
　epididymal (organ of Morgagni) Q55.4
　intestine (epiploic) Q43.8
　preauricular Q17.0
　testicular (organ of Morgagni) Q55.29
Appendicitis (pneumococcal) (retrocecal) K37
　with
　　perforation or rupture K35.2
　　peritoneal abscess K35.3
　　peritonitis NEC K35.3
　　　generalized (with perforation or rupture) K35.2
　　　localized (with perforation or rupture) K35.3
　acute (catarrhal) (fulminating) (gangrenous) (obstructive) (retrocecal) (suppurative) K35.80

Appendicitis — *continued*
　acute — *continued*
　　with
　　　peritoneal abscess K35.3
　　　peritonitis NEC K35.3
　　　　generalized (with perforation or rupture) K35.2
　　　　localized (with perforation or rupture) K35.3
　　　specified NEC K35.89
　amebic A06.89
　chronic (recurrent) K36
　exacerbation — *see* Appendicitis, acute
　gangrenous — *see* Appendicitis, acute
　healed (obliterative) K36
　interval K36
　neurogenic K36
　obstructive K36
　recurrent K36
　relapsing K36
　subacute (adhesive) K36
　subsiding K36
　suppurative — *see* Appendicitis, acute
　tuberculous A18.32
Appendicopathia oxyurica B80
Appendix, appendicular (*see also* condition)
　epididymis Q55.4
　Morgagni
　　female Q50.5
　　male (epididymal) Q55.4
　　　testicular Q55.29
　testis Q55.29
Appetite
　depraved — *see* Pica
　excessive R63.2
　lack or loss (*see also* Anorexia) R63.0
　　nonorganic origin F50.89
　　psychogenic F50.89
　perverted (hysterical) — *see* Pica
Apple peel syndrome Q41.1
Apprehension state F41.1
Apprehensiveness, abnormal F41.9
Approximal wear K03.0
Apraxia (classic) (ideational) (ideokinetic) (ideomotor) (motor) (verbal) R48.2
　following
　　cerebrovascular disease I69.990
　　　cerebral infarction I69.390
　　　intracerebral hemorrhage I69.190
　　　nontraumatic intracranial hemorrhage NEC
　　　　I69.290
　　　specified disease NEC I69.890
　　　subarachnoid hemorrhage I69.090
　oculomotor, congenital H51.8
Aptyalism K11.7
Apudoma — *see* Neoplasm, uncertain behavior, by site
Aqueous misdirection H40.83- ☑
Arabicum elephantiasis — *see* Infestation, filarial
Arachnitis — *see* Meningitis
Arachnodactyly — *see* Syndrome, Marfan's
Arachnoiditis (acute) (adhesive) (basal) (brain) (cerebrospinal) — *see* Meningitis
Arachnophobia F40.210
Arboencephalitis, Australian A83.4
Arborization block (heart) I45.5
ARC (AIDS-related complex) B20
Arch
　aortic Q25.49
　bovine Q25.49
Arches — *see* condition
Arcuate uterus Q51.810
Arcuatus uterus Q51.810
Arcus (cornea) senilis — *see* Degeneration, cornea, senile
Arc-welder's lung J63.4
Areflexia R29.2
Areola — *see* condition
Argentaffinoma (*see also* Neoplasm, uncertain behavior, by site)
　malignant — *see* Neoplasm, malignant, by site
　syndrome E34.0
Argininemia E72.21
Arginosuccinic aciduria E72.22
Argyll Robertson phenomenon, pupil or syndrome (syphilitic) A52.19
　atypical H57.09
　nonsyphilitic H57.09
Argyria, argyriasis
　conjunctival H11.13- ☑

Argyria, argyriasis — continued
  from drug or medicament — see Table of Drugs and
    Chemicals, by substance
Argyrosis, conjunctival H11.13- ☑
Arhinencephaly Q04.1
Ariboflavinosis E53.0
Arm — see condition
Arnold-Chiari disease, obstruction or syndrome (type
  II) Q07.00
  with
    hydrocephalus Q07.02
      with spina bifida Q07.03
    spina bifida Q07.01
      with hydrocephalus Q07.03
  type III — see Encephalocele
  type IV Q04.8
Aromatic amino-acid metabolism disorder E70.9
  specified NEC E70.8
Arousals, confusional G47.51
Arrest, arrested
  cardiac I46.9
    complicating
      abortion — see Abortion, by type, complicated
        by, cardiac arrest
      anesthesia (general) (local) or other sedation
        — see Table of Drugs and Chemicals, by
        drug
        in labor and delivery O74.2
        in pregnancy O29.11- ☑
        postpartum, puerperal O89.1
      delivery (cesarean) (instrumental) O75.4
    due to
      cardiac condition I46.2
      specified condition NEC I46.8
    intraoperative I97.71- ☑
    newborn P29.81
    personal history, successfully resuscitated Z86.74
    postprocedural I97.12- ☑
      obstetric procedure O75.4
  cardiorespiratory — see Arrest, cardiac
  circulatory — see Arrest, cardiac
  deep transverse O64.0 ☑
  development or growth
    bone — see Disorder, bone, development or
      growth
    child R62.50
    tracheal rings Q32.1
  epiphyseal
    complete
      femur M89.15- ☑
      humerus M89.12- ☑
      tibia M89.16- ☑
      ulna M89.13- ☑
    forearm M89.13- ☑
      specified NEC M89.13- ☑
      ulna — see Arrest, epiphyseal, by type, ulna
    lower leg M89.16- ☑
      specified NEC M89.168
      tibia — see Arrest, epiphyseal, by type, tibia
    partial
      femur M89.15- ☑
      humerus M89.12- ☑
      tibia M89.16- ☑
      ulna M89.13- ☑
    specified NEC M89.18
  granulopoiesis — see Agranulocytosis
  growth plate — see Arrest, epiphyseal
  heart — see Arrest, cardiac
  legal, anxiety concerning Z65.3
  physeal — see Arrest, epiphyseal
  respiratory R09.2
    newborn P28.81
  sinus I45.5
  spermatogenesis (complete) — see Azoospermia
    incomplete — see Oligospermia
  transverse (deep) O64.0 ☑
Arrhenoblastoma
  benign
    specified site — see Neoplasm, benign, by site
    unspecified site
      female D27.9
      male D29.20
  malignant
    specified site — see Neoplasm, malignant, by site
    unspecified site
      female C56.9
      male C62.90

Arrhenoblastoma — continued
  specified site — see Neoplasm, uncertain behavior,
    by site
  unspecified site
    female D39.10
    male D40.10
Arrhythmia (auricle) (cardiac) (juvenile) (nodal) (reflex)
  (sinus) (supraventricular) (transitory) (ventricle) I49.9
  block I45.9
  extrasystolic I49.49
  newborn
    bradycardia P29.12
    occurring before birth P03.819
      before onset of labor P03.810
      during labor P03.811
    tachycardia P29.11
  psychogenic F45.8
  specified NEC I49.8
  vagal R55
  ventricular re-entry I47.0
Arrillaga-Ayerza syndrome (pulmonary sclerosis with
  pulmonary hypertension) I27.0
Arsenical pigmentation L81.8
  from drug or medicament — see Table of Drugs and
    Chemicals
Arsenism — see Poisoning, arsenic
Arterial — see condition
Arteriofibrosis — see Arteriosclerosis
Arteriolar sclerosis — see Arteriosclerosis
Arteriolith — see Arteriosclerosis
Arteriolitis I77.6
  necrotizing, kidney I77.5
  renal — see Hypertension, kidney
Arteriolosclerosis — see Arteriosclerosis
Arterionephrosclerosis — see Hypertension, kidney
Arteriopathy I77.9
Arteriosclerosis, arteriosclerotic (diffuse) (obliterans)
  (of) (senile) (with calcification) I70.90
  aorta I70.0
  arteries of extremities — see Arteriosclerosis, extrem-
    ities
  brain I67.2
  bypass graft
    coronary — see Arteriosclerosis, coronary, bypass
      graft
    extremities — see Arteriosclerosis, extremities,
      bypass graft
  cardiac — see Disease, heart, ischemic, atherosclerotic
  cardiopathy — see Disease, heart, ischemic,
    atherosclerotic
  cardiorenal — see Hypertension, cardiorenal
  cardiovascular — see Disease, heart, ischemic,
    atherosclerotic
  carotid (see also Occlusion, artery, carotid) I65.2- ☑
  central nervous system I67.2
  cerebral I67.2
  cerebrovascular I67.2
  coronary (artery) I25.10
    bypass graft I25.810
      with
        angina pectoris I25.709
          with documented spasm I25.701
          specified type NEC I25.708
          unstable I25.700
        ischemic chest pain I25.709
      autologous artery I25.810
        with
          angina pectoris I25.729
            with documented spasm I25.721
            specified type I25.728
            unstable I25.720
          ischemic chest pain I25.729
      autologous vein I25.810
        with
          angina pectoris I25.719
            with documented spasm I25.711
            specified type I25.718
            unstable I25.710
          ischemic chest pain I25.719
      nonautologous biological I25.810
        with
          angina pectoris I25.739
            with documented spasm I25.731
            specified type I25.738
            unstable I25.730
          ischemic chest pain I25.739
      specified type NEC I25.810

Arteriosclerosis, arteriosclerotic — continued
  coronary — continued
    bypass graft — continued
      specified type — continued
        with
          angina pectoris I25.799
            with documented spasm I25.791
            specified type I25.798
            unstable I25.790
          ischemic chest pain I25.799
    due to
      calcified coronary lesion (severely) I25.84
      lipid rich plaque I25.83
    native vessel
      with
        angina pectoris I25.119
          with documented spasm I25.111
          specified type NEC I25.118
          unstable I25.110
        ischemic chest pain I25.119
    transplanted heart I25.811
      bypass graft I25.812
        with
          angina pectoris I25.769
           with documented spasm I25.761
           specified type I25.768
           unstable I25.760
        ischemic chest pain I25.769
      native coronary artery I25.811
        with
          angina pectoris I25.759
           with documented spasm I25.751
           specified type I25.758
           unstable I25.750
        ischemic chest pain I25.759
  extremities (native arteries) I70.209
    bypass graft I70.309
      autologous vein graft I70.409
        leg I70.409
          with
            gangrene (and intermittent claudica-
              tion, rest pain and ulcer)
              I70.469
            intermittent claudication I70.419
            rest pain (and intermittent claudica-
              tion) I70.429
        bilateral I70.403
          with
            gangrene (and intermittent clau-
              dication, rest pain and ul-
              cer) I70.463
            intermittent claudication I70.463
            rest pain (and intermittent claudi-
              cation) I70.423
          specified type NEC I70.493
        left I70.402
          with
            gangrene (and intermittent clau-
              dication, rest pain and ul-
              cer) I70.462
            intermittent claudication I70.412
            rest pain (and intermittent claudi-
              cation) I70.422
            ulceration (and intermittent
             claudication and rest pain)
             I70.449
             ankle I70.443
             calf I70.442
             foot site NEC I70.445
             heel I70.444
             lower leg NEC I70.448
             midfoot I70.444
             thigh I70.441
          specified type NEC I70.492
        right I70.401
          with
            gangrene (and intermittent clau-
              dication, rest pain and ul-
              cer) I70.461
            intermittent claudication I70.411
            rest pain (and intermittent claudi-
              cation) I70.421
            ulceration (and intermittent
             claudication and rest pain)
             I70.439
             ankle I70.433
             calf I70.432
             foot site NEC I70.435
             heel I70.434

☑ Additional Character Required — Refer to the Tabular List for Character Selection   ▽ Subterms under main terms may continue to next column or page

Arteriosclerosis, arteriosclerotic — *continued*
  extremities — *continued*
    bypass graft — *continued*
      autologous vein graft — *continued*
        leg — *continued*
          right — *continued*
            with — *continued*
              ulceration — *continued*
                lower leg NEC I70.438
                midfoot I70.434
                thigh I70.431
            specified type NEC I70.491
          specified type NEC I70.499
        specified NEC I70.408
          with
            gangrene (and intermittent claudication, rest pain and ulcer) I70.468
            intermittent claudication I70.418
            rest pain (and intermittent claudication) I70.428
            ulceration (and intermittent claudication and rest pain) I70.45
          specified type NEC I70.498
      leg I70.309
        with
          gangrene (and intermittent claudication, rest pain and ulcer) I70.369
          intermittent claudication I70.319
          rest pain (and intermittent claudication) I70.329
        bilateral I70.303
          with
            gangrene (and intermittent claudication, rest pain and ulcer) I70.363
            intermittent claudication I70.313
            rest pain (and intermittent claudication) I70.323
          specified type NEC I70.393
        left I70.302
          with
            gangrene (and intermittent claudication, rest pain and ulcer) I70.362
            intermittent claudication I70.312
            rest pain (and intermittent claudication) I70.322
            ulceration (and intermittent claudication and rest pain) I70.349
              ankle I70.343
              calf I70.342
              foot site NEC I70.345
              heel I70.344
              lower leg NEC I70.348
              midfoot I70.344
              thigh I70.341
          specified type NEC I70.392
        right I70.301
          with
            gangrene (and intermittent claudication, rest pain and ulcer) I70.361
            intermittent claudication I70.311
            rest pain (and intermittent claudication) I70.321
            ulceration (and intermittent claudication and rest pain I70.339
              ankle I70.333
              calf I70.332
              foot site NEC I70.335
              heel I70.334
              lower leg NEC I70.338
              midfoot I70.334
              thigh I70.331
          specified type NEC I70.391
      nonautologous biological graft I70.509
        leg I70.509
          with
            gangrene (and intermittent claudication, rest pain and ulcer) I70.569
            intermittent claudication I70.519
            rest pain (and intermittent claudication) I70.529
          bilateral I70.503

Arteriosclerosis, arteriosclerotic — *continued*
  extremities — *continued*
    bypass graft — *continued*
      nonautologous biological graft — *continued*
        leg — *continued*
          bilateral — *continued*
            with
              gangrene (and intermittent claudication, rest pain and ulcer) I70.563
              intermittent claudication I70.513
              rest pain (and intermittent claudication) I70.523
            specified type NEC I70.593
          left I70.502
            with
              gangrene (and intermittent claudication, rest pain and ulcer) I70.562
              intermittent claudication I70.512
              rest pain (and intermittent claudication) I70.522
              ulceration (and intermittent claudication and rest pain) I70.549
                ankle I70.543
                calf I70.542
                foot site NEC I70.545
                heel I70.544
                lower leg NEC I70.548
                midfoot I70.544
                thigh I70.541
            specified type NEC I70.592
          right I70.501
            with
              gangrene (and intermittent claudication, rest pain and ulcer) I70.561
              intermittent claudication I70.511
              rest pain (and intermittent claudication) I70.521
              ulceration (and intermittent claudication and rest pain) I70.539
                ankle I70.533
                calf I70.532
                foot site NEC I70.535
                heel I70.534
                lower leg NEC I70.538
                midfoot I70.534
                thigh I70.531
            specified type NEC I70.591
          specified type NEC I70.599
        specified NEC I70.508
          with
            gangrene (and intermittent claudication, rest pain and ulcer) I70.568
            intermittent claudication I70.518
            rest pain (and intermittent claudication) I70.528
            ulceration (and intermittent claudication and rest pain) I70.55
          specified type NEC I70.598
      nonbiological graft I70.609
        leg I70.609
          with
            gangrene (and intermittent claudication, rest pain and ulcer) I70.669
            intermittent claudication I70.619
            rest pain (and intermittent claudication) I70.629
          bilateral I70.603
            with
              gangrene (and intermittent claudication, rest pain and ulcer) I70.663
              intermittent claudication I70.613
              rest pain (and intermittent claudication) I70.623
            specified type NEC I70.693
          left I70.602
            with
              gangrene (and intermittent claudication, rest pain and ulcer) I70.662
              intermittent claudication I70.612

Arteriosclerosis, arteriosclerotic — *continued*
  extremities — *continued*
    bypass graft — *continued*
      nonbiological graft — *continued*
        leg — *continued*
          left — *continued*
            with — *continued*
              rest pain (and intermittent claudication) I70.622
              ulceration (and intermittent claudication and rest pain) I70.649
                ankle I70.643
                calf I70.642
                foot site NEC I70.645
                heel I70.644
                lower leg NEC I70.648
                midfoot I70.644
                thigh I70.641
            specified type NEC I70.692
          right I70.601
            with
              gangrene (and intermittent claudication, rest pain and ulcer) I70.661
              intermittent claudication I70.611
              rest pain (and intermittent claudication) I70.621
              ulceration (and intermittent claudication and rest pain) I70.639
                ankle I70.633
                calf I70.632
                foot site NEC I70.635
                heel I70.634
                lower leg NEC I70.638
                midfoot I70.634
                thigh I70.631
            specified type NEC I70.691
        specified NEC I70.608
          with
            gangrene (and intermittent claudication, rest pain and ulcer) I70.668
            intermittent claudication I70.618
            rest pain (and intermittent claudication) I70.628
            ulceration (and intermittent claudication and rest pain) I70.65
          specified type NEC I70.698
      specified graft NEC I70.709
        leg I70.709
          with
            gangrene (and intermittent claudication, rest pain and ulcer) I70.769
            intermittent claudication I70.719
            rest pain (and intermittent claudication) I70.729
          bilateral I70.703
            with
              gangrene (and intermittent claudication, rest pain and ulcer) I70.763
              intermittent claudication I70.713
              rest pain (and intermittent claudication) I70.723
            specified type NEC I70.793
          left I70.702
            with
              gangrene (and intermittent claudication, rest pain and ulcer) I70.762
              intermittent claudication I70.712
              rest pain (and intermittent claudication) I70.722
              ulceration (and intermittent claudication and rest pain) I70.749
                ankle I70.743
                calf I70.742
                foot site NEC I70.745
                heel I70.744
                lower leg NEC I70.748
                midfoot I70.744
                thigh I70.741
            specified type NEC I70.792
          right I70.701

Arteriosclerosis, arteriosclerotic — *continued*
extremities — *continued*
bypass graft — *continued*
specified graft — *continued*
leg — *continued*
right — *continued*
with
gangrene (and intermittent claudication, rest pain and ulcer) I70.761
intermittent claudication I70.711
rest pain (and intermittent claudication) I70.721
ulceration (and intermittent
claudication and rest pain)
I70.739
ankle I70.733
calf I70.732
foot site NEC I70.735
heel I70.734
lower leg NEC I70.738
midfoot I70.734
thigh I70.731
specified type NEC I70.791
specified type NEC I70.799
specified NEC I70.708
with
gangrene (and intermittent claudication, rest pain and ulcer)
I70.768
intermittent claudication I70.718
rest pain (and intermittent claudication) I70.728
ulceration (and intermittent claudication and rest pain) I70.75
specified type NEC I70.798
specified NEC I70.308
with
gangrene (and intermittent claudication,
rest pain and ulcer) I70.368
intermittent claudication I70.318
rest pain (and intermittent claudication)
I70.328
ulceration (and intermittent claudication
and rest pain) I70.35
specifiec type NEC I70.398
leg I70.209
with
gangrene (and intermittent claudication,
rest pain and ulcer) I70.269
intermittent claudication I70.219
rest pain (and intermittent claudication)
I70.229
bilateral I70.203
with
gangrene (and intermittent claudication,
rest pain and ulcer) I70.263
intermittent claudication I70.213
rest pain (and intermittent claudication)
I70.223
specified type NEC I70.293
left I70.202
with
gangrene (and intermittent claudication,
rest pain and ulcer) I70.262
intermittent claudication I70.212
rest pain (and intermittent claudication)
I70.222
ulceration (and intermittent claudication
and rest pain) I70.249
ankle I70.243
calf I70.242
foot site NEC I70.245
heel I70.244
lower leg NEC I70.248
midfoot I70.244
thigh I70.241
specified type NEC I70.292
right I70.201
with
gangrene (and intermittent claudication,
rest pain and ulcer) I70.261
intermittent claudication I70.211
rest pain (and intermittent claudication)
I70.221
ulceration (and intermittent claudication
and rest pain) I70.239
ankle I70.233
calf I70.232

Arteriosclerosis, arteriosclerotic — *continued*
extremities — *continued*
leg — *continued*
right — *continued*
with
ulceration — *continued*
foot site NEC I70.235
heel I70.234
lower leg NEC I70.238
midfoot I70.234
thigh I70.231
specified type NEC I70.291
specified type NEC I70.299
specified site NEC I70.208
with
gangrene (and intermittent claudication,
rest pain and ulcer) I70.268
intermittent claudication I70.218
rest pain (and intermittent claudication)
I70.228
ulceration (and intermittent claudication
and rest pain) I70.25
specified type NEC I70.298
generalized I70.91
heart (disease) — *see* Arteriosclerosis, coronary
(artery),
kidney — *see* Hypertension, kidney
medial — *see* Arteriosclerosis, extremities
mesenteric (artery) K55.1
Mönckeberg's — *see* Arteriosclerosis, extremities
myocarditis I51.4
peripheral (of extremities) — *see* Arteriosclerosis, extremities
pulmonary (idiopathic) I27.0
renal (arterioles) (*see also* Hypertension, kidney)
artery I70.1
retina (vascular) I70.8 [H35.0-] ☑
specified artery NEC I70.8
spinal (cord) G95.19
vertebral (artery) I67.2
Arteriospasm I73.9
Arteriovenous — *see* condition
Arteritis I77.6
allergic M31.0
aorta (nonsyphilitic) I77.6
syphilitic A52.02
aortic arch M31.4
brachiocephalic M31.4
brain I67.7
syphilitic A52.04
cerebral I67.7
in systemic lupus erythematosus M32.19
listerial A32.89
syphilitic A52.04
tuberculous A18.89
coronary (artery) I25.89
rheumatic I01.8
chronic I09.89
syphilitic A52.06
cranial (left) (right), giant cell M31.6
deformans — *see* Arteriosclerosis
giant cell NEC M31.6
with polymyalgia rheumatica M31.5
necrosing or necrotizing M31.9
specified NEC M31.8
nodosa M30.0
obliterans — *see* Arteriosclerosis
pulmonary I28.8
rheumatic — *see* Fever, rheumatic
senile — *see* Arteriosclerosis
suppurative I77.2
syphilitic (general) A52.09
brain A52.04
coronary A52.06
spinal A52.09
temporal, giant cell M31.6
young female aortic arch syndrome M31.4
Artery, arterial (*see also* condition)
abscess I77.89
single umbilical Q27.0
Arthralgia (allergic) (*see also* Pain, joint)
in caisson disease T70.3 ☑
temporomandibular M26.62- ☑
Arthritis, arthritic (acute) (chronic) (nonpyogenic)
(subacute) M19.90
allergic — *see* Arthritis, specified form NEC
ankylosing (crippling) (spine) (*see also* Spondylitis,
ankylosing)

Arthritis, arthritic — *continued*
ankylosing (*see also* Spondylitis, ankylosing) — *continued*
sites other than spine — *see* Arthritis, specified
form NEC
atrophic — *see* Osteoarthritis
spine — *see* Spondylitis, ankylosing
back — *see* Spondylopathy, inflammatory
blennorrhagic (gonococcal) A54.42
Charcot's — *see* Arthropathy, neuropathic
diabetic — *see* Diabetes, arthropathy, neuropathic
syringomyelic G95.0
chylous (filarial) (*see also* category M01) B74.9
climacteric (any site) NEC — *see* Arthritis, specified
form NEC
crystal (-induced) — *see* Arthritis, in, crystals
deformans — *see* Osteoarthritis
degenerative — *see* Osteoarthritis
due to or associated with
acromegaly E22.0
brucellosis — *see* Brucellosis
caisson disease T70.3 ☑
diabetes — *see* Diabetes, arthropathy
dracontiasis (*see also* category M01) B72
enteritis NEC
regional — *see* Enteritis, regional
erysipelas (*see also* category M01) A46
erythema
epidemic A25.1
nodosum L52
filariasis NOS B74.9
glanders A24.0
helminthiasis (*see also* category M01) B83.9
hemophilia D66 [M36.2]
Henoch- (Schönlein) purpura D69.0 [M36.4]
human parvovirus (*see also* category M01) B97.6
infectious disease NEC M01 ☑
leprosy (*see also* category M01) (*see also* Leprosy)
A30.9
Lyme disease A69.23
mycobacteria (*see also* category M01) A31.8
parasitic disease NEC (*see also* category M01) B89
paratyphoid fever (*see also* category M01) (*see also*
Fever, paratyphoid) A01.4
rat bite fever (*see also* category M01) A25.1
regional enteritis — *see* Enteritis, regional
respiratory disorder NOS J98.9
serum sickness (*see also* Reaction, serum) T80.69 ☑
syringomyelia G95.0
typhoid fever A01.04
epidemic erythema A25.1
febrile — *see* Fever, rheumatic
gonococcal A54.42
gouty (acute) — *see* Gout
in (due to)
acromegaly (*see also* subcategory M14.8-) E22.0
amyloidosis (*see also* subcategory M14.8-) E85.4
bacterial disease (*see also* subcategory M01) A49.9
Behçet's syndrome M35.2
caisson disease (*see also* subcategory M14.8-)
T70.3 ☑
coliform bacilli (Escherichia coli) — *see* Arthritis,
in, pyogenic organism NEC
crystals M11.9
dicalcium phosphate — *see* Arthritis, in, crystals, specified type NEC
hydroxyapatite M11.0- ☑
pyrophosphate — *see* Arthritis, in, crystals,
specified type NEC
specified type NEC M11.80
ankle M11.87- ☑
elbow M11.82- ☑
foot joint M11.87- ☑
hand joint M11.84- ☑
hip M11.85- ☑
knee M11.86- ☑
multiple sites M11.8- ☑
shoulder M11.81- ☑
vertebrae M11.88
wrist M11.83- ☑
dermatoarthritis, lipoid E78.81
dracontiasis (dracunculiasis) (*see also* category
M01) B72
endocrine disorder NEC (*see also* subcategory
M14.8-) E34.9
enteritis, infectious NEC (*see also* category M01)
A09

Arthritis, arthritic — *continued*
  in — *continued*
    enteritis, infectious (*see also* category M01) —
      continued
      specified organism NEC (*see also* category M01)
        A08.8
    erythema
      multiforme (*see also* subcategory M14.8-) L51.9
      nodosum (*see also* subcategory M14.8-) L52
    gout — *see* Gout
    helminthiasis NEC (*see also* category M01) B83.9
    hemochromatosis (*see also* subcategory M14.8-)
      E83.118
    hemoglobinopathy NEC D58.2 [M36.3]
    hemophilia NEC D66 [M36.2]
    Hemophilus influenzae M00.8- [B96.3]
    Henoch (-Schönlein) purpura D69.0 [M36.4]
    hyperparathyroidism NEC (*see also* subcategory
      M14.8-) E21.3
    hypersensitivity reaction NEC T78.49 ☑ [M36.4]
    hypogammaglobulinemia (*see also* subcategory
      M14.8-) D80.1
    hypothyroidism NEC (*see also* subcategory M14.8-)
      E03.9
    infection — *see* Arthritis, pyogenic or pyemic
      spine — *see* Spondylopathy, infective
    infectious disease NEC M01 ☑
    leprosy (*see also* category M01) A30.9
    leukemia NEC C95.9- ☑ [M36.1]
    lipoid dermatoarthritis E78.81
    Lyme disease A69.23
    Mediterranean fever, familial (*see also* subcategory
      M14.8-) M04.1
    Meningococcus A39.83
    metabolic disorder NEC (*see also* subcategory
      M14.8-) E88.9
    multiple myelomatosis C90.0- ☑ [M36.1]
    mumps B26.85
    mycosis NEC (*see also* category M01) B49
    myelomatosis (multiple) C90.0- ☑ [M36.1]
    neurological disorder NEC G98.0
    ochronosis (*see also* subcategory M14.8-) E70.29
    O'nyong-nyong (*see also* category M01) A92.1
    parasitic disease NEC (*see also* category M01) B89
    paratyphoid fever (*see also* category M01) A01.4
    Pseudomonas — *see* Arthritis, pyogenic, bacterial
      NEC
    psoriasis L40.50
    pyogenic organism NEC — *see* Arthritis, pyogenic,
      bacterial NEC
    Reiter's disease — *see* Reiter's disease
    respiratory disorder NEC (*see also* subcategory
      M14.8-) J98.9
    reticulosis, malignant (*see also* subcategory M14.8-
) C86.0
    rubella B06.82
    Salmonella (arizonae) (cholerae-suis) (enteritidis)
      (typhimurium) A02.23
    sarcoidosis D86.86
    specified bacteria NEC — *see* Arthritis, pyogenic,
      bacterial NEC
    sporotrichosis B42.82
    syringomyelia G95.0
    thalassemia NEC D56.9 [M36.3]
    tuberculosis — *see* Tuberculosis, arthritis
    typhoid fever A01.04
    urethritis, Reiter's — *see* Reiter's disease
    viral disease NEC (*see also* category M01) B34.9
  infectious or infective (*see also* Arthritis, pyogenic or
    pyemic)
    spine — *see* Spondylopathy, infective
  juvenile M08.90
    with systemic onset — *see* Still's disease
    ankle M08.97- ☑
    elbow M08.92- ☑
    foot joint M08.97- ☑
    hand joint M08.94- ☑
    hip M08.95- ☑
    knee M08.96- ☑
    multiple site M08.99
    pauciarticular M08.40
      ankle M08.47- ☑
      elbow M08.42- ☑
      foot joint M08.47- ☑
      hand joint M08.44- ☑
      hip M08.45- ☑
      knee M08.46- ☑

Arthritis, arthritic — *continued*
  juvenile — *continued*
    pauciarticular — *continued*
      shoulder M08.41- ☑
      vertebrae M08.48
      wrist M08.43- ☑
    psoriatic — *see* Arthritis, rheumatoid, juvenile
    rheumatoid — *see* Arthritis, rheumatoid, juvenile
    shoulder M08.91- ☑
    specified type NEC M08.80
      ankle M08.87- ☑
      elbow M08.82- ☑
      foot joint M08.87- ☑
      hand joint M08.84- ☑
      hip M08.85- ☑
      knee M08.86- ☑
      multiple site M08.89
      shoulder M08.81- ☑
      specified joint NEC M08.88
      vertebrae M08.88
      wrist M08.83- ☑
    wrist M08.93- ☑
  meaning osteoarthritis — *see* Osteoarthritis
  meningococcal A39.83
  menopausal (any site) NEC — *see* Arthritis, specified
    form NEC
  mutilans (psoriatic) L40.52
  mycotic NEC (*see also* category M01) B49
  neuropathic (Charcot) — *see* Arthropathy, neuropathic
    diabetic — *see* Diabetes, arthropathy, neuropathic
    nonsyphilitic NEC G98.0
    syringomyelic G95.0
  ochronotic (*see also* subcategory M14.8-) E70.29
  palindromic (any site) — *see* Rheumatism, palindromic
  pneumococcal M00.10
    ankle M00.17- ☑
    elbow M00.12- ☑
    foot joint — *see* Arthritis, pneumococcal, ankle
    hand joint M00.14- ☑
    hip M00.15- ☑
    knee M00.16- ☑
    multiple site M00.19
    shoulder M00.11- ☑
    vertebra M00.18
    wrist M00.13- ☑
  postdysenteric — *see* Arthropathy, postdysenteric
  postmeningococcal A39.84
  postrheumatic, chronic — *see* Arthropathy,
    postrheumatic, chronic
  primary progressive (*see also* Arthritis, specified form
    NEC)
    spine — *see* Spondylitis, ankylosing
  psoriatic L40.50
  purulent (any site except spine) — *see* Arthritis, pyo-
    genic or pyemic
    spine — *see* Spondylopathy, infective
  pyogenic or pyemic (any site except spine) M00.9
    bacterial NEC M00.80
      ankle M00.87- ☑
      elbow M00.82- ☑
      foot joint — *see* Arthritis, pyogenic, bacterial
        NEC, ankle
      hand joint M00.84- ☑
      hip M00.85- ☑
      knee M00.86- ☑
      multiple site M00.89
      shoulder M00.81- ☑
      vertebra M00.88
      wrist M00.83- ☑
    pneumococcal — *see* Arthritis, pneumococcal
    spine — *see* Spondylopathy, infective
    staphylococcal — *see* Arthritis, staphylococcal
    streptococcal — *see* Arthritis, streptococcal NEC
      pneumococcal — *see* Arthritis, pneumococcal
  reactive — *see* Reiter's disease
  rheumatic (*see also* Arthritis, rheumatoid)
    acute or subacute — *see* Fever, rheumatic
  rheumatoid M06.9
    with
      carditis — *see* Rheumatoid, carditis
      endocarditis — *see* Rheumatoid, carditis
      heart involvement NEC — *see* Rheumatoid,
        carditis
      lung involvement — *see* Rheumatoid, lung
      myocarditis — *see* Rheumatoid, carditis
      myopathy — *see* Rheumatoid, myopathy
      pericarditis — *see* Rheumatoid, carditis

Arthritis, arthritic — *continued*
  rheumatoid — *continued*
    with — *continued*
      polyneuropathy — *see* Rheumatoid, polyneu-
        ropathy
      rheumatoid factor — *see* Arthritis, rheumatoid,
        seropositive
      splenoadenomegaly and leukopenia — *see*
        Felty's syndrome
      vasculitis — *see* Rheumatoid, vasculitis
      visceral involvement NEC — *see* Rheumatoid,
        arthritis, with involvement of organs NEC
    juvenile (with or without rheumatoid factor)
      M08.00
      ankle M08.07- ☑
      elbow M08.02- ☑
      foot joint M08.07- ☑
      hand joint M08.04- ☑
      hip M08.05- ☑
      knee M08.06- ☑
      multiple site M08.09
      shoulder M08.01- ☑
      vertebra M08.08
      wrist M08.03- ☑
    seronegative M06.00
      ankle M06.07- ☑
      elbow M06.02- ☑
      foot joint M06.07- ☑
      hand joint M06.04- ☑
      hip M06.05- ☑
      knee M06.06- ☑
      multiple site M06.09
      shoulder M06.01- ☑
      vertebra M06.08
      wrist M06.03- ☑
    seropositive M05.9
      without organ involvement M05.70
        ankle M05.77- ☑
        elbow M05.72- ☑
        foot joint M05.77- ☑
        hand joint M05.74- ☑
        hip M05.75- ☑
        knee M05.76- ☑
        multiple sites M05.79
        shoulder M05.71- ☑
        vertebra — *see* Spondylitis, ankylosing
        wrist M05.73- ☑
      specified NEC M05.80
        ankle M05.87- ☑
        elbow M05.82- ☑
        foot joint M05.87- ☑
        hand joint M05.84- ☑
        hip M05.85- ☑
        knee M05.86- ☑
        multiple sites M05.89
        shoulder M05.81- ☑
        vertebra — *see* Spondylitis, ankylosing
        wrist M05.83- ☑
    specified type NEC M06.80
      ankle M06.87- ☑
      elbow M06.82- ☑
      foot joint M06.87- ☑
      hand joint M06.84- ☑
      hip M06.85- ☑
      knee M06.86- ☑
      multiple site M06.89
      shoulder M06.81- ☑
      vertebra M06.88
      wrist M06.83- ☑
    spine — *see* Spondylitis, ankylosing
  rubella B06.82
  scorbutic (*see also* subcategory M14.8-) E54
  senile or senescent — *see* Osteoarthritis
  septic (any site except spine) — *see* Arthritis, pyogenic
    or pyemic
    spine — *see* Spondylopathy, infective
  serum (nontherapeutic) (therapeutic) — *see*
    Arthropathy, postimmunization
  specified form NEC M13.80
    ankle M13.87- ☑
    elbow M13.82- ☑
    foot joint M13.87- ☑
    hand joint M13.84- ☑
    hip M13.85- ☑
    knee M13.86- ☑
    multiple site M13.89

Arthritis, arthritic — *continued*
  specified form — *continued*
    shoulder M13.81- ☑
    specified joint NEC M13.88
    wrist M13.83- ☑
  spine (*see also* Spondylopathy, inflammatory)
    infectious or infective NEC — *see* Spondylopathy, infective
    Marie-Strümpell — *see* Spondylitis, ankylosing
    pyogenic — *see* Spondylopathy, infective
    rheumatoid — *see* Spondylitis, ankylosing
    traumatic (old) — *see* Spondylopathy, traumatic
    tuberculous A18.01
  staphylococcal M00.00
    ankle M00.07- ☑
    elbow M00.02- ☑
    foot joint — *see* Arthritis, staphylococcal, ankle
    hand joint M00.04- ☑
    hip M00.05- ☑
    knee M00.06- ☑
    multiple site M00.09
    shoulder M00.01- ☑
    vertebra M00.08
    wrist M00.03- ☑
  streptococcal NEC M00.20
    ankle M00.27- ☑
    elbow M00.22- ☑
    foot joint — *see* Arthritis, streptococcal, ankle
    hand joint M00.24- ☑
    hip M00.25- ☑
    knee M00.26- ☑
    multiple site M00.29
    shoulder M00.21- ☑
    vertebra M00.28
    wrist M00.23- ☑
  suppurative — *see* Arthritis, pyogenic or pyemic
  syphilitic (late) A52.16
    congenital A50.55 [M12.80]
  syphilitica deformans (Charcot) A52.16
  temporomandibular M26.69
  toxic of menopause (any site) — *see* Arthritis, specified form NEC
  transient — *see* Arthropathy, specified form NEC
  traumatic (chronic) — *see* Arthropathy, traumatic
  tuberculous A18.02
    spine A18.01
  uratic — *see* Gout
  urethritica (Reiter's) — *see* Reiter's disease
  vertebral — *see* Spondylopathy, inflammatory
  villous (any site) — *see* Arthropathy, specified form NEC
Arthrocele — *see* Effusion, joint
Arthrodesis status Z98.1
Arthrodynia (*see also* Pain, joint)
Arthrodysplasia Q74.9
Arthrofibrosis, joint — *see* Ankylosis
Arthrogryposis (congenital) Q68.8
  multiplex congenita Q74.3
Arthrokatadysis M24.7
Arthropathy (*see also* Arthritis) M12.9
  Charcot's — *see* Arthropathy, neuropathic
    diabetic — *see* Diabetes, arthropathy, neuropathic
    syringomyelic G95.0
  cricoarytenoid J38.7
  crystal (-induced) — *see* Arthritis, in, crystals
  diabetic NEC — *see* Diabetes, arthropathy
  distal interphalangeal, psoriatic L40.51
  enteropathic M07.60
    ankle M07.67- ☑
    elbow M07.62- ☑
    foot joint M07.67- ☑
    hand joint M07.64- ☑
    hip M07.65- ☑
    knee M07.66- ☑
    multiple site M07.69
    shoulder M07.61- ☑
    vertebra M07.68
    wrist M07.63- ☑
  following intestinal bypass M02.00
    ankle M02.07- ☑
    elbow M02.02- ☑
    foot joint M02.07- ☑
    hand joint M02.04- ☑
    hip M02.05- ☑
    knee M02.06- ☑
    multiple site M02.09
    shoulder M02.01- ☑

Arthropathy — *continued*
  following intestinal bypass — *continued*
    vertebra M02.08
    wrist M02.03- ☑
  gouty (*see also* Gout)
    in (due to)
      Lesch-Nyhan syndrome E79.1 [M14.8-] ☑
      sickle-cell disorders D57- ☑ [M14.8-] ☑
  hemophilic NEC D66 [M36.2]
    in (due to)
      hyperparathyroidism NEC E21.3 [M14.8-] ☑
      metabolic disease NOS E88.9 [M14.8-] ☑
  in (due to)
    acromegaly E22.0 [M14.8-] ☑
    amyloidosis E85.4 [M14.8-] ☑
    blood disorder NOS D75.9 [M36.3]
    diabetes — *see* Diabetes, arthropathy
    endocrine disease NOS E34.9 [M14.8-] ☑
    erythema
      multiforme L51.9 [M14.8-] ☑
      nodosum L52 [M14.8-] ☑
    hemochromatosis E83.118 [M14.8-] ☑
    hemoglobinopathy NEC D58.2 [M36.3]
    hemophilia NEC D66 [M36.2]
    Henoch-Schönlein purpura D69.0 [M36.4]
    hyperthyroidism E05.90 [M14.8-] ☑
    hypothyroidism E03.9 [M14.8-] ☑
    infective endocarditis I33.0 [M12.80]
    leukemia NEC C95.9- ☑ [M36.1]
    malignant histiocytosis C96.A [M36.1]
    metabolic disease NOS E88.9 [M14.8-] ☑
    multiple myeloma C90.0- ☑ [M36.1]
    neoplastic disease NOS (*see also* Neoplasm) D49.9 [M36.1]
    nutritional deficiency (*see also* subcategory M14.8-) E63.9
    psoriasis NOS L40.50
    sarcoidosis D86.86
    syphilis (late) A52.77
      congenital A50.55 [M12.80]
    thyrotoxicosis (*see also* subcategory M14.8-) E05.90
    ulcerative colitis K51.90 [M07.60]
    viral hepatitis (postinfectious) NEC B19.9 [M12.80]
    Whipple's disease (*see also* subcategory M14.8-) K90.81
  Jaccoud — *see* Arthropathy, postrheumatic, chronic
  juvenile — *see* Arthritis, juvenile
    psoriatic L40.54
  mutilans (psoriatic) L40.52
  neuropathic (Charcot) M14.60
    ankle M14.67- ☑
    diabetic — *see* Diabetes, arthropathy, neuropathic
    elbow M14.62- ☑
    foot joint M14.67- ☑
    hand joint M14.64- ☑
    hip M14.65- ☑
    knee M14.66- ☑
    multiple site M14.69
    nonsyphilitic NEC G98.0
    shoulder M14.61- ☑
    syringomyelic G95.0
    vertebra M14.68
    wrist M14.63- ☑
  osteopulmonary — *see* Osteoarthropathy, hypertrophic, specified NEC
  postdysenteric M02.10
    ankle M02.17- ☑
    elbow M02.12- ☑
    foot joint M02.17- ☑
    hand joint M02.14- ☑
    hip M02.15- ☑
    knee M02.16- ☑
    multiple site M02.19
    shoulder M02.11- ☑
    vertebra M02.18
    wrist M02.13- ☑
  postimmunization M02.20
    ankle M02.27- ☑
    elbow M02.22- ☑
    foot joint M02.27- ☑
    hand joint M02.24- ☑
    hip M02.25- ☑
    knee M02.26- ☑
    multiple site M02.29
    shoulder M02.21- ☑
    vertebra M02.28
    wrist M02.23- ☑

Arthropathy — *continued*
  postinfectious NEC B99 ☑ [M12.80]
    in (due to)
      enteritis due to Yersinia enterocolitica A04.6 [M12.80]
      syphilis A52.77
      viral hepatitis NEC B19.9 [M12.80]
  postrheumatic, chronic (Jaccoud) M12.00
    ankle M12.07- ☑
    elbow M12.02- ☑
    foot joint M12.07- ☑
    hand joint M12.04- ☑
    hip M12.05- ☑
    knee M12.06- ☑
    multiple site M12.09
    shoulder M12.01- ☑
    specified joint NEC M12.08
    vertebrae M12.08
    wrist M12.03- ☑
  psoriatic NEC L40.59
    interphalangeal, distal L40.51
  reactive M02.9
    in (due to)
      infective endocarditis I33.0 [M02.9]
    specified type NEC M02.80
      ankle M02.87- ☑
      elbow M02.82- ☑
      foot joint M02.87- ☑
      hand joint M02.84- ☑
      hip M02.85- ☑
      knee M02.86- ☑
      multiple site M02.89
      shoulder M02.81- ☑
      vertebra M02.88
      wrist M02.83- ☑
  specified form NEC M12.80
    ankle M12.87- ☑
    elbow M12.82- ☑
    foot joint M12.87- ☑
    hand joint M12.84- ☑
    hip M12.85- ☑
    knee M12.86- ☑
    multiple site M12.89
    shoulder M12.81- ☑
    specified joint NEC M12.88
    vertebrae M12.88
    wrist M12.83- ☑
  syringomyelic G95.0
  tabes dorsalis A52.16
  tabetic A52.16
  transient — *see* Arthropathy, specified form NEC
  traumatic M12.50
    ankle M12.57- ☑
    elbow M12.52- ☑
    foot joint M12.57- ☑
    hand joint M12.54- ☑
    hip M12.55- ☑
    knee M12.56- ☑
    multiple site M12.59
    shoulder M12.51- ☑
    specified joint NEC M12.58
    vertebrae M12.58
    wrist M12.53- ☑
Arthropyosis — *see* Arthritis, pyogenic or pyemic
Arthrosis (deformans) (degenerative) (localized) (*see also* Osteoarthritis) M19.90
  spine — *see* Spondylosis
Arthus' phenomenon or reaction T78.41 ☑
  due to
    drug — *see* Table of Drugs and Chemicals, by drug
Articular — *see* condition
Articulation, reverse (teeth) M26.24
Artificial
  insemination complication — *see* Complications, artificial, fertilization
  opening status (functioning) (without complication) Z93.9
    anus (colostomy) Z93.3
    colostomy Z93.3
    cystostomy Z93.50
      appendico-vesicostomy Z93.52
      cutaneous Z93.51
      specified NEC Z93.59
    enterostomy Z93.4
    gastrostomy Z93.1
    ileostomy Z93.2
    intestinal tract NEC Z93.4

Artificial — *continued*
> opening status — *continued*
>> jejunostomy Z93.4
>> nephrostomy Z93.6
>> specified site NEC Z93.8
>> tracheostomy Z93.0
>> ureterostomy Z93.6
>> urethrostomy Z93.6
>> urinary tract NEC Z93.6
>> vagina Z93.8
>> vagina status Z93.8

Arytenoid — *see* condition

Asbestosis (occupational) J61

Ascariasis B77.9
> with
>> complications NEC B77.89
>> intestinal complications B77.0
>> pneumonia, pneumonitis B77.81

Ascaridosis, ascaridiasis — *see* Ascariasis

Ascaris (infection) (infestation) (lumbricoides) — *see* Ascariasis

Ascending — *see* condition

ASC-H (atypical squamous cells cannot exclude high grade squamous intraepithelial lesion on cytologic smear)
> anus R85.611
> cervix R87.611
> vagina R87.621

Aschoff's bodies — *see* Myocarditis, rheumatic

Ascites (abdominal) R18.8
> cardiac (*see also* Failure, heart, right) I50.810
> chylous (nonfilarial) I89.8
>> filarial — *see* Infestation, filarial
> due to
>> cirrhosis, alcoholic K70.31
>> hepatitis
>>> alcoholic K70.11
>>> chronic active K71.51
>> S. japonicum B65.2
> heart (*see also* Failure, heart, right) I50.810
> malignant R18.0
> pseudochylous R18.8
> syphilitic A52.74
> tuberculous A18.31

ASC-US (atypical squamous cells of undetermined significance on cytologic smear)
> anus R85.610
> cervix R87.610
> vagina R87.620

Aseptic — *see* condition

Asherman's syndrome N85.6

Asialia K11.7

Asiatic cholera — *see* Cholera

Asimultagnosia (simultanagnosia) R48.3

Askin's tumor — *see* Neoplasm, connective tissue, malignant

Asocial personality F60.2

Asomatognosia R41.4

Aspartylglucosaminuria E77.1

Asperger's disease or syndrome F84.5

Aspergilloma — *see* Aspergillosis

Aspergillosis (with pneumonia) B44.9
> bronchopulmonary, allergic B44.81
> disseminated B44.7
> generalized B44.7
> pulmonary NEC B44.1
>> allergic B44.81
>> invasive B44.0
> specified NEC B44.89
> tonsillar B44.2

Aspergillus (flavus) (fumigatus) (infection) (terreus) — *see* Aspergillosis

Aspermatogenesis — *see* Azoospermia

Aspermia (testis) — *see* Azoospermia

Asphyxia, asphyxiation (by) R09.01
> antenatal P84
> birth P84
> bunny bag — *see* Asphyxia, due to, mechanical threat to breathing, trapped in bed clothes
> crushing S28.0 ☑
> drowning T75.1 ☑
> gas, fumes, or vapor — *see* Table of Drugs and Chemicals
> inhalation — *see* Inhalation
> intrauterine P84
> local I73.00
>> with gangrene I73.01

Asphyxia, asphyxiation — *continued*
> mucus (*see also* Foreign body, respiratory tract, causing asphyxia)
> newborn P84
> pathological R09.01
> postnatal P84
>> mechanical — *see* Asphyxia, due to, mechanical threat to breathing
> prenatal P84
> reticularis R23.1
> strangulation — *see* Asphyxia, due to, mechanical threat to breathing
> submersion T75.1 ☑
> traumatic T71.9 ☑
>> due to
>>> crushed chest S28.0 ☑
>>> foreign body (in) — *see* Foreign body, respiratory tract, causing asphyxia
>>> low oxygen content of ambient air T71.20 ☑
>>>> due to
>>>>> being trapped in
>>>>>> low oxygen environment T71.29 ☑
>>>>>> in car trunk T71.221 ☑
>>>>>>> circumstances undetermined T71.224 ☑
>>>>>>> done with intent to harm by
>>>>>>>> another person T71.223 ☑
>>>>>>>> self T71.222 ☑
>>>>>> in refrigerator T71.231 ☑
>>>>>>> circumstances undetermined T71.234 ☑
>>>>>>> done with intent to harm by
>>>>>>>> another person T71.233 ☑
>>>>>>>> self T71.232 ☑
>>> cave-in T71.21 ☑
>> mechanical threat to breathing (accidental) T71.191 ☑
>>> circumstances undetermined T71.194 ☑
>>> done with intent to harm by
>>>> another person T71.193 ☑
>>>> self T71.192 ☑
>>> hanging T71.161 ☑
>>>> circumstances undetermined T71.164 ☑
>>>> done with intent to harm by
>>>>> another person T71.163 ☑
>>>>> self T71.162 ☑
>>> plastic bag T71.121 ☑
>>>> circumstances undetermined T71.124 ☑
>>>> done with intent to harm by
>>>>> another person T71.123 ☑
>>>>> self T71.122 ☑
>>> smothering
>>>> in furniture T71.151 ☑
>>>>> circumstances undetermined T71.154 ☑
>>>>> done with intent to harm by
>>>>>> another person T71.153 ☑
>>>>>> self T71.152 ☑
>>>> under
>>>>> another person's body T71.141 ☑
>>>>>> circumstances undetermined T71.144 ☑
>>>>>> done with intent to harm T71.143 ☑
>>>>> pillow T71.111 ☑
>>>>>> circumstances undetermined T71.114 ☑
>>>>>> done with intent to harm by
>>>>>>> another person T71.113 ☑
>>>>>>> self T71.112 ☑
>>>> trapped in bed clothes T71.131 ☑
>>>>> circumstances undetermined T71.134 ☑
>>>>> done with intent to harm by
>>>>>> another person T71.133 ☑
>>>>>> self T71.132 ☑
> vomiting, vomitus — *see* Foreign body, respiratory tract, causing asphyxia

Aspiration
> amniotic (clear) fluid (newborn) P24.10
>> with
>>> pneumonia (pneumonitis) P24.11
>>> respiratory symptoms P24.11
> blood
>> newborn (without respiratory symptoms) P24.20
>>> with
>>>> pneumonia (pneumonitis) P24.21
>>>> respiratory symptoms P24.21

Aspiration — *continued*
> blood — *continued*
>> specified age NEC — *see* Foreign body, respiratory tract
> bronchitis J69.0
> food or foreign body (with asphyxiation) — *see* Asphyxia, food
> liquor (amnii) (newborn) P24.10
>> with
>>> pneumonia (pneumonitis) P24.11
>>> respiratory symptoms P24.11
> meconium (newborn) (without respiratory symptoms) P24.00
>> with
>>> pneumonitis (pneumonitis) P24.01
>>> respiratory symptoms P24.01
> milk (newborn) (without respiratory symptoms) P24.30
>> with
>>> pneumonia (pneumonitis) P24.31
>>> respiratory symptoms P24.31
> specified age NEC — *see* Foreign body, respiratory tract
> mucus (*see also* Foreign body, by site, causing asphyxia)
>> newborn P24.10
>>> with
>>>> pneumonia (pneumonitis) P24.11
>>>> respiratory symptoms P24.11
>> neonatal P24.9
>>> specific NEC (without respiratory symptoms) P24.80
>>>> with
>>>>> pneumonia (pneumonitis) P24.81
>>>>> respiratory symptoms P24.81
>> newborn P24.9
>>> specific NEC (without respiratory symptoms) P24.80
>>>> with
>>>>> pneumonia (pneumonitis) P24.81
>>>>> respiratory symptoms P24.81
> pneumonia J69.0
> pneumonitis J69.0
> syndrome of newborn — *see* Aspiration, by substance, with pneumonia
> vernix caseosa (newborn) P24.80
>> with
>>> pneumonia (pneumonitis) P24.81
>>> respiratory symptoms P24.81
> vomitus (*see also* Foreign body, respiratory tract)
>> newborn (without respiratory symptoms) P24.30
>>> with
>>>> pneumonia (pneumonitis) P24.31
>>>> respiratory symptoms P24.31

Asplenia (congenital) Q89.01
> postsurgical Z90.81

Assam fever B55.0

Assault, sexual — *see* Maltreatment

Assmann's focus NEC A15.0

Astasia (-abasia) (hysterical) F44.4

Asteatosis cutis L85.3

Astereognosia, astereognosis R48.1

Asterixis R27.8
> in liver disease K71.3

Asteroid hyalitis — *see* Deposit, crystalline

Asthenia, asthenic R53.1
> cardiac (*see also* Failure, heart) I50.9
>> psychogenic F45.8
> cardiovascular (*see also* Failure, heart) I50.9
>> psychogenic F45.8
> heart (*see also* Failure, heart) I50.9
>> psychogenic F45.8
> hysterical F44.4
> myocardial (*see also* Failure, heart) I50.9
>> psychogenic F45.8
> nervous F48.8
> neurocirculatory F45.8
> neurotic F48.8
> psychogenic F48.8
> psychoneurotic F48.8
> psychophysiologic F48.8
> reaction (psychophysiologic) F48.8
> senile R54

Asthenopia (*see also* Discomfort, visual)
> hysterical F44.6
> psychogenic F44.6

Asthenospermia — *see* Abnormal, specimen, male genital organs

Asthma, asthmatic (bronchial) (catarrh) (spasmodic) J45.909

Asthma, asthmatic — continued
  with
    chronic obstructive bronchitis J44.9
      with
        acute lower respiratory infection J44.0
        exacerbation (acute) J44.1
    chronic obstructive pulmonary disease J44.9
      with
        acute lower respiratory infection J44.0
        exacerbation (acute) J44.1
    exacerbation (acute) J45.901
    hay fever — see Asthma, allergic extrinsic
    rhinitis, allergic — see Asthma, allergic extrinsic
    status asthmaticus J45.902
  allergic extrinsic J45.909
    with
      exacerbation (acute) J45.901
      status asthmaticus J45.902
  atopic — see Asthma, allergic extrinsic
  cardiac — see Failure, ventricular, left
  cardiobronchial I50.1
  childhood J45.909
    with
      exacerbation (acute) J45.901
      status asthmaticus J45.902
  chronic obstructive J44.9
    with
      acute lower respiratory infection J44.0
      exacerbation (acute) J44.1
  collier's J60
  cough variant J45.991
  detergent J69.8
  due to
    detergent J69.8
    inhalation of fumes J68.3
  eosinophilic J82
  extrinsic, allergic — see Asthma, allergic extrinsic
  grinder's J62.8
  hay — see Asthma, allergic extrinsic
  heart I50.1
  idiosyncratic — see Asthma, nonallergic
  intermittent (mild) J45.20
    with
      exacerbation (acute) J45.21
      status asthmaticus J45.22
  intrinsic, nonallergic — see Asthma, nonallergic
  Kopp's E32.8
  late-onset J45.909
    with
      exacerbation (acute) J45.901
      status asthmaticus J45.902
  mild intermittent J45.20
    with
      exacerbation (acute) J45.21
      status asthmaticus J45.22
  mild persistent J45.30
    with
      exacerbation (acute) J45.31
      status asthmaticus J45.32
  Millar's (laryngismus stridulus) J38.5
  miner's J60
  mixed J45.909
    with
      exacerbation (acute) J45.901
      status asthmaticus J45.902
  moderate persistent J45.40
    with
      exacerbation (acute) J45.41
      status asthmaticus J45.42
  nervous — see Asthma, nonallergic
  nonallergic (intrinsic) J45.909
    with
      exacerbation (acute) J45.901
      status asthmaticus J45.902
  persistent
    mild J45.30
      with
        exacerbation (acute) J45.31
        status asthmaticus J45.32
    moderate J45.40
      with
        exacerbation (acute) J45.41
        status asthmaticus J45.42
    severe J45.50
      with
        exacerbation (acute) J45.51
        status asthmaticus J45.52
  platinum J45.998

Asthma, asthmatic — continued
  pneumoconiotic NEC J64
  potter's J62.8
  predominantly allergic J45.909
  psychogenic F54
  pulmonary eosinophilic J82
  red cedar J67.8
  Rostan's I50.1
  sandblaster's J62.8
  sequoiosis J67.8
  severe persistent J45.50
    with
      exacerbation (acute) J45.51
      status asthmaticus J45.52
  specified NEC J45.998
  stonemason's J62.8
  thymic E32.8
  tuberculous — see Tuberculosis, pulmonary
  Wichmann's (laryngismus stridulus) J38.5
  wood J67.8
Astigmatism (compound) (congenital) H52.20- ☑
  irregular H52.21- ☑
  regular H52.22- ☑
Astraphobia F40.220
Astroblastoma
  specified site — see Neoplasm, malignant, by site
  unspecified site C71.9
Astrocytoma (cystic)
  anaplastic
    specified site — see Neoplasm, malignant, by site
    unspecified site C71.9
  fibrillary
    specified site — see Neoplasm, malignant, by site
    unspecified site C71.9
  fibrous
    specified site — see Neoplasm, malignant, by site
    unspecified site C71.9
  gemistocytic
    specified site — see Neoplasm, malignant, by site
    unspecified site C71.9
  juvenile
    specified site — see Neoplasm, malignant, by site
    unspecified site C71.9
  pilocytic
    specified site — see Neoplasm, malignant, by site
    unspecified site C71.9
  piloid
    specified site — see Neoplasm, malignant, by site
    unspecified site C71.9
  protoplasmic
    specified site — see Neoplasm, malignant, by site
    unspecified site C71.9
  specified site NEC — see Neoplasm, malignant, by site
  subependymal D43.2
    giant cell
      specified site — see Neoplasm, uncertain be-
        havior, by site
      unspecified site D43.2
    specified site — see Neoplasm, uncertain behavior,
      by site
    unspecified site D43.2
  unspecified site C71.9
Astroglioma
  specified site — see Neoplasm, malignant, by site
  unspecified site C71.9
Asymbolia R48.8
Asymmetry (see also Distortion)
  between native and reconstructed breast N65.1
  face Q67.0
  jaw (lower) — see Anomaly, dentofacial, jaw-cranial
    base relationship, asymmetry
Asynergia, asynergy R27.8
  ventricular I51.89
Asystole (heart) — see Arrest, cardiac
At risk
  for
    dental caries Z91.849
      high Z91.843
      low Z91.841
      moderate Z91.842
    falling Z91.81
Ataxia, ataxy, ataxic R27.0
  acute R27.8
  brain (hereditary) G11.9
  cerebellar (hereditary) G11.9
    with defective DNA repair G11.3
    alcoholic G31.2
    early-onset G11.1

Ataxia, ataxy, ataxic — continued
  cerebellar — continued
    in
      alcoholism G31.2
      myxedema E03.9 [G13.2]
      neoplastic disease (see also Neoplasm)
        D49.9 [G32.81]
      specified disease NEC G32.81
    late-onset (Marie's) G11.2
  cerebral (hereditary) G11.9
  congenital nonprogressive G11.0
  family, familial — see Ataxia, hereditary
  following
    cerebrovascular disease I69.993
      cerebral infarction I69.393
      intracerebral hemorrhage I69.193
      nontraumatic intracranial hemorrhage NEC
        I69.293
      specified disease NEC I69.893
      subarachnoid hemorrhage I69.093
  Friedreich's (heredofamilial) (cerebellar) (spinal) G11.1
  gait R26.0
    hysterical F44.4
  general R27.8
  gluten M35.9 [G32.81]
    with celiac disease K90.0 [G32.81]
  hereditary G11.9
    with neuropathy G60.2
    cerebellar — see Ataxia, cerebellar
    spastic G11.4
    specified NEC G11.8
    spinal (Friedreich's) G11.1
  heredofamilial — see Ataxia, hereditary
  Hunt's G11.1
  hysterical F44.4
  locomotor (progressive) (syphilitic) (partial) (spastic)
    A52.11
    diabetic — see Diabetes, ataxia
  Marie's (cerebellar) (heredofamilial) (late-onset) G11.2
  nonorganic origin F44.4
  nonprogressive, congenital G11.0
  psychogenic F44.4
  Roussy-Lévy G60.0
  Sanger-Brown's (hereditary) G11.2
  spastic hereditary G11.4
  spinal
    hereditary (Friedreich's) G11.1
    progressive (syphilitic) A52.11
  spinocerebellar, X-linked recessive G11.1
  telangiectasia (Louis-Bar) G11.3
Ataxia-telangiectasia (Louis-Bar) G11.3
Atelectasis (massive) (partial) (pressure) (pulmonary)
  J98.11
  newborn P28.10
    due to resorption P28.11
    partial P28.19
    primary P28.0
    secondary P28.19
  primary (newborn) P28.0
  tuberculous — see Tuberculosis, pulmonary
Atelocardia Q24.9
Atelomyelia Q06.1
Atheroembolism
  of
    extremities
      lower I75.02- ☑
      upper I75.01- ☑
    kidney I75.81
    specified NEC I75.89
Atheroma, atheromatous (see also Arteriosclerosis)
  I70.90
  aorta, aortic I70.0
    valve (see also Endocarditis, aortic) I35.8
  aorto-iliac I70.0
  artery — see Arteriosclerosis
  basilar (artery) I67.2
  carotid (artery) (common) (internal) I67.2
  cerebral (arteries) I67.2
  coronary (artery) I25.10
    with angina pectoris — see Arteriosclerosis, coro-
      nary (artery),
  degeneration — see Arteriosclerosis
  heart, cardiac — see Disease, heart, ischemic,
    atherosclerotic
  mitral (valve) I34.8
  myocardium, myocardial — see Disease, heart, is-
    chemic, atherosclerotic

Atheroma, atheromatous — *continued*
  pulmonary valve (heart) (*see also* Endocarditis, pulmonary) I37.8
  tricuspid (heart) (valve) I36.8
  valve, valvular — *see* Endocarditis
  vertebral (artery) I67.2
Atheromatosis — *see* Arteriosclerosis
Atherosclerosis (*see also* Arteriosclerosis)
  coronary
    artery I25.10
      with angina pectoris — *see* Arteriosclerosis, coronary (artery),
      due to
        calcified coronary lesion (severely) I25.84
        lipid rich plaque I25.83
    transplanted heart I25.811
      bypass graft I25.812
        with angina pectoris — *see* Arteriosclerosis, coronary (artery),
      native coronary artery I25.811
        with angina pectoris — *see* Arteriosclerosis, coronary (artery),
Athetosis (acquired) R25.8
  bilateral (congenital) G80.3
  congenital (bilateral) (double) G80.3
  double (congenital) G80.3
  unilateral R25.8
Athlete's
  foot B35.3
  heart I51.7
Athrepsia E41
Athyrea (acquired) (*see also* Hypothyroidism)
  congenital E03.1
Atonia, atony, atonic
  bladder (sphincter) (neurogenic) N31.2
  capillary I78.8
  cecum K59.8
    psychogenic F45.8
  colon — *see* Atony, intestine
  congenital P94.2
  esophagus K22.8
  intestine K59.8
    psychogenic F45.8
  stomach K31.89
    neurotic or psychogenic F45.8
  uterus (during labor) O62.2
    with hemorrhage (postpartum) O72.1
    postpartum (with hemorrhage) O72.1
      without hemorrhage O75.89
Atopy — *see* History, allergy
Atransferrinemia, congenital E88.09
Atresia, atretic
  alimentary organ or tract NEC Q45.8
    upper Q40.8
  ani, anus, anal (canal) Q42.3
    with fistula Q42.2
  aorta (ring) Q25.29
  aortic (orifice) (valve) Q23.0
    arch Q25.21
    congenital with hypoplasia of ascending aorta and defective development of left ventricle (with mitral stenosis) Q23.4
    in hypoplastic left heart syndrome Q23.4
  aqueduct of Sylvius Q03.0
    with spina bifida — *see* Spina bifida, with hydrocephalus
  artery NEC Q27.8
    cerebral Q28.3
    coronary Q24.5
    digestive system Q27.8
    eye Q15.8
    lower limb Q27.8
    pulmonary Q25.5
    specified site NEC Q27.8
    umbilical Q27.0
    upper limb Q27.8
  auditory canal (external) Q16.1
  bile duct (common) (congenital) (hepatic) Q44.2
    acquired — *see* Obstruction, bile duct
  bladder (neck) Q64.39
    obstruction Q64.31
  bronchus Q32.4
  cecum Q42.8
  cervix (acquired) N88.2
    congenital Q51.828
    in pregnancy or childbirth — *see* Anomaly, cervix, in pregnancy or childbirth
      causing obstructed labor O65.5

Atresia, atretic — *continued*
  choana Q30.0
  colon Q42.9
    specified NEC Q42.8
  common duct Q44.2
  cricoid cartilage Q31.8
  cystic duct Q44.2
    acquired K82.8
      with obstruction K82.0
  digestive organs NEC Q45.8
  duodenum Q41.0
  ear canal Q16.1
  ejaculatory duct Q55.4
  epiglottis Q31.8
  esophagus Q39.0
    with tracheoesophageal fistula Q39.1
  eustachian tube Q17.8
  fallopian tube (congenital) Q50.6
    acquired N97.1
  follicular cyst N83.0- ☑
  foramen of
    Luschka Q03.1
      with spina bifida — *see* Spina bifida, with hydrocephalus
    Magendie Q03.1
      with spina bifida — *see* Spina bifida, with hydrocephalus
  gallbladder Q44.1
  genital organ
    external
      female Q52.79
      male Q55.8
    internal
      female Q52.8
      male Q55.8
  glottis Q31.8
  gullet Q39.0
    with tracheoesophageal fistula Q39.1
  heart valve NEC Q24.8
    pulmonary Q22.0
    tricuspid Q22.4
  hymen Q52.3
    acquired (postinfective) N89.6
  ileum Q41.2
  intestine (small) Q41.9
    large Q42.9
      specified NEC Q42.8
  iris, filtration angle Q15.0
  jejunum Q41.1
  lacrimal apparatus Q10.4
  larynx Q31.8
  meatus urinarius Q64.33
  mitral valve Q23.2
    in hypoplastic left heart syndrome Q23.4
  nares (anterior) (posterior) Q30.0
  nasopharynx Q34.8
  nose, nostril Q30.0
    acquired J34.89
  organ or site NEC Q89.8
  osseous meatus (ear) Q16.1
  oviduct (congenital) Q50.6
    acquired N97.1
  parotid duct Q38.4
    acquired K11.8
  pulmonary (artery) Q25.5
    valve Q22.0
  pulmonic Q22.0
  pupil Q13.2
  rectum Q42.1
    with fistula Q42.0
  salivary duct Q38.4
    acquired K11.8
  sublingual duct Q38.4
    acquired K11.8
  submandibular duct Q38.4
    acquired K11.8
  submaxillary duct Q38.4
    acquired K11.8
  thyroid cartilage Q31.8
  trachea Q32.1
  tricuspid valve Q22.4
  ureter Q62.10
    pelvic junction Q62.11
    vesical orifice Q62.12
  ureteropelvic junction Q62.11
  ureterovesical orifice Q62.12
  urethra (valvular) Q64.39
    stricture Q64.32
  urinary tract NEC Q64.8

Atresia, atretic — *continued*
  uterus Q51.818
    acquired N85.8
  vagina (congenital) Q52.4
    acquired (postinfectional) (senile) N89.5
  vas deferens Q55.3
  vascular NEC Q27.8
    cerebral Q28.3
    digestive system Q27.8
    lower limb Q27.8
    specified site NEC Q27.8
    upper limb Q27.8
    vein NEC Q27.8
      digestive system Q27.8
      great Q26.8
      lower limb Q27.8
      portal Q26.5
      pulmonary Q26.4
        partial Q26.3
        total Q26.2
      specified site NEC Q27.8
      upper limb Q27.8
  vena cava (inferior) (superior) Q26.8
  vesicourethral orifice Q64.31
  vulva Q52.79
    acquired N90.5
Atrichia, atrichosis — *see* Alopecia
Atrophia (*see also* Atrophy)
  cutis senilis L90.8
    due to radiation L57.8
  gyrata of choroid and retina H31.23
  senilis R54
    dermatological L90.8
      due to radiation (nonionizing) (solar) L57.8
  unguium L60.3
    congenita Q84.6
Atrophie blanche (en plaque) (de Milian) L95.0
Atrophoderma, atrophodermia (of) L90.9
  diffusum (idiopathic) L90.4
  maculatum L90.8
    et striatum L90.8
      due to syphilis A52.79
    syphilitic A51.39
  neuriticum L90.8
  Pasini and Pierini L90.3
  pigmentosum Q82.1
  reticulatum symmetricum faciei L66.4
  senile L90.8
    due to radiation (nonionizing) (solar) L57.8
  vermiculata (cheeks) L66.4
Atrophy, atrophic (of)
  adrenal (capsule) (gland) E27.49
    primary (autoimmune) E27.1
  alveolar process or ridge (edentulous) K08.20
  anal sphincter (disuse) N81.84
  appendix K38.8
  arteriosclerotic — *see* Arteriosclerosis
  bile duct (common) (hepatic) K83.8
  bladder N32.89
    neurogenic N31.8
  blanche (en plaque) (of Milian) L95.0
  bone (senile) NEC (*see also* Disorder, bone, specified type NEC)
    due to
      tabes dorsalis (neurogenic) A52.11
  brain (cortex) (progressive) G31.9
    frontotemporal circumscribed G31.01 [F02.80]
      with behavioral disturbance G31.01 [F02.81]
    senile NEC G31.1
  breast N64.2
    obstetric — *see* Disorder, breast, specified type NEC
  buccal cavity K13.79
  cardiac — *see* Degeneration, myocardial
  cartilage (infectional) (joint) — *see* Disorder, cartilage, specified NEC
  cerebellar — *see* Atrophy, brain
  cerebral — *see* Atrophy, brain
  cervix (mucosa) (senile) (uteri) N88.8
    menopausal N95.8
  Charcot-Marie-Tooth G60.0
  choroid (central) (macular) (myopic) (retina) H31.10- ☑
    diffuse secondary H31.12- ☑
    gyrate H31.23
    senile H31.11- ☑
  ciliary body — *see* Atrophy, iris
  conjunctiva (senile) H11.89
  corpus cavernosum N48.89

Index

Atrophy, atrophic — continued
cortical — see Atrophy, brain
cystic duct K82.8
Déjérine-Thomas G23.8
disuse NEC — see Atrophy, muscle
Duchenne-Aran G12.21
ear H93.8- ☑
edentulous alveolar ridge K08.20
endometrium (senile) N85.8
   cervix N88.8
enteric K63.89
epididymis N50.89
eyeball — see Disorder, globe, degenerated condition, atrophy
eyelid (senile) — see Disorder, eyelid, degenerative
facial (skin) L90.9
fallopian tube (senile) N83.32- ☑
   with ovary N83.33- ☑
fascioscapulohumeral (Landouzy- Déjérine) G71.0
fatty, thymus (gland) E32.8
gallbladder K82.8
gastric K29.40
   with bleeding K29.41
gastrointestinal K63.89
glandular I89.8
globe H44.52- ☑
gum — see Recession, gingival
hair L67.8
heart (brown) — see Degeneration, myocardial
hemifacial Q67.4
   Romberg G51.8
infantile E41
   paralysis, acute — see Poliomyelitis, paralytic
intestine K63.89
iris (essential) (progressive) H21.26- ☑
   specified NEC H21.29
kidney (senile) (terminal) (see also Sclerosis, renal) N26.1
   congenital or infantile Q60.5
     bilateral Q60.4
     unilateral Q60.3
   hydronephrotic — see Hydronephrosis
lacrimal gland (primary) H04.14- ☑
   secondary H04.15- ☑
Landouzy-Déjérine G71.0
laryngitis, infective J37.0
larynx J38.7
Leber's optic (hereditary) H47.22
lip K13.0
liver (yellow) K72.90
   with coma K72.91
   acute, subacute K72.00
     with coma K72.01
   chronic K72.10
     with coma K72.11
lung (senile) J98.4
macular (dermatological) L90.8
   syphilitic, skin A51.39
     striated A52.79
mandible (edentulous) K08.20
   minimal K08.21
   moderate K08.22
   severe K08.23
maxilla K08.20
   minimal K08.24
   moderate K08.25
   severe K08.26
muscle, muscular (diffuse) (general) (idiopathic) (primary) M62.50
   ankle M62.57- ☑
   Duchenne-Aran G12.21
   foot M62.57- ☑
   forearm M62.53- ☑
   hand M62.54- ☑
   infantile spinal G12.0
   lower leg M62.56- ☑
   multiple sites M62.59
   myelopathic — see Atrophy, muscle, spinal
   myotonic G71.11
   neuritic G58.9
   neuropathic (peroneal) (progressive) G60.0
   pelvic (disuse) N81.84
   peroneal G60.0
   progressive (bulbar) G12.21
     adult G12.1
     infantile (spinal) G12.0
     spinal G12.25
       adult G12.1

Atrophy, atrophic — continued
muscle, muscular — continued
   progressive — continued
     spinal — continued
       infantile G12.0
   pseudohypertrophic G71.0
   shoulder region M62.51- ☑
   specified site NEC M62.58
   spinal G12.9
     adult form G12.1
     Aran-Duchenne G12.21
     childhood form, type II G12.1
     distal G12.1
     hereditary NEC G12.1
     infantile, type I (Werdnig-Hoffmann) G12.0
     juvenile form, type III (Kugelberg- Welander) G12.1
     progressive G12.25
     scapuloperoneal form G12.1
     specified NEC G12.8
   syphilitic A52.78
   thigh M62.55- ☑
   upper arm M62.52- ☑
myocardium — see Degeneration, myocardial
myometrium (senile) N85.8
   cervix N88.8
myopathic NEC — see Atrophy, muscle
myotonia G71.11
nail L60.3
nasopharynx J31.1
nerve (see also Disorder, nerve)
   abducens — see Strabismus, paralytic, sixth nerve
   accessory G52.8
   acoustic or auditory H93.3 ☑
   cranial G52.9
     eighth (auditory) H93.3 ☑
     eleventh (accessory) G52.8
     fifth (trigeminal) G50.8
     first (olfactory) G52.0
     fourth (trochlear) — see Strabismus, paralytic, fourth nerve
     second (optic) H47.20
     sixth (abducens) — see Strabismus, paralytic, sixth nerve
     tenth (pneumogastric) (vagus) G52.2
     third (oculomotor) — see Strabismus, paralytic, third nerve
     twelfth (hypoglossal) G52.3
   hypoglossal G52.3
   oculomotor — see Strabismus, paralytic, third nerve
   olfactory G52.0
   optic (papillomacular bundle)
     syphilitic (late) A52.15
       congenital A50.44
   pneumogastric G52.2
   trigeminal G50.8
   trochlear — see Strabismus, paralytic, fourth nerve
   vagus (pneumogastric) G52.2
neurogenic, bone, tabetic A52.11
nutritional E41
old age R54
olivopontocerebellar G23.8
optic (nerve) H47.20
   glaucomatous H47.23- ☑
   hereditary H47.22
   primary H47.21- ☑
   specified type NEC H47.29- ☑
   syphilitic (late) A52.15
     congenital A50.44
orbit H05.31- ☑
ovary (senile) N83.31- ☑
   with fallopian tube N83.33- ☑
oviduct (senile) — see Atrophy, fallopian tube
palsy, diffuse (progressive) G12.22
pancreas (duct) (senile) K86.89
parotid gland K11.0
pelvic muscle N81.84
penis N48.89
pharynx J39.2
pluriglandular E31.8
   autoimmune E31.0
polyarthritis M15.9
prostate N42.89
pseudohypertrophic (muscle) G71.0
renal (see also Sclerosis, renal) N26.1
retina, retinal (postinfectional) H35.89
rhinitis J31.0

Atrophy, atrophic — continued
salivary gland K11.0
scar L90.5
sclerosis, lobar (of brain) G31.09 [F02.80]
   with behavioral disturbance G31.09 [F02.81]
scrotum N50.89
seminal vesicle N50.89
senile R54
   due to radiation (nonionizing) (solar) L57.8
skin (patches) (spots) L90.9
   degenerative (senile) L90.8
   due to radiation (nonionizing) (solar) L57.8
   senile L90.8
spermatic cord N50.89
spinal (acute) (cord) G95.89
   muscular — see Atrophy, muscle, spinal
   paralysis G12.20
     acute — see Poliomyelitis, paralytic
     meaning progressive muscular atrophy G12.21
spine (column) — see Spondylopathy, specified NEC
spleen (senile) D73.0
stomach K29.40
   with bleeding K29.41
striate (skin) L90.6
   syphilitic A52.79
subcutaneous L90.9
sublingual gland K11.0
submandibular gland K11.0
submaxillary gland K11.0
Sudeck's — see Algoneurodystrophy
suprarenal (capsule) (gland) E27.49
   primary E27.1
systemic affecting central nervous system
   in
     myxedema E03.9 [G13.2]
     neoplastic disease (see also Neoplasm) D49.9 [G13.1]
     specified disease NEC G13.8
tarso-orbital fascia, congenital Q10.3
testis N50.0
thenar, partial — see Syndrome, carpal tunnel
thymus (fatty) E32.8
thyroid (gland) (acquired) E03.4
   with cretinism E03.1
   congenital (with myxedema) E03.1
tongue (senile) K14.8
   papillae K14.4
trachea J39.8
tunica vaginalis N50.89
turbinate J34.89
tympanic membrane (nonflaccid) H73.82- ☑
   flaccid H73.81- ☑
upper respiratory tract J39.8
uterus, uterine (senile) N85.8
   cervix N88.8
   due to radiation (intended effect) N85.8
     adverse effect or misadventure N99.89
vagina (senile) N95.2
vas deferens N50.89
vascular I99.8
vertebra (senile) — see Spondylopathy, specified NEC
vulva (senile) N90.5
Werdnig-Hoffmann G12.0
yellow — see Failure, hepatic

Attack, attacks
with alteration of consciousness (with automatisms) — see Epilepsy, localization-related, symptomatic, with complex partial seizures
without alteration of consciousness — see Epilepsy, localization-related, symptomatic, with simple partial seizures
Adams-Stokes I45.9
akinetic — see Epilepsy, generalized, specified NEC
angina — see Angina
atonic — see Epilepsy, generalized, specified NEC
benign shuddering G25.83
cataleptic — see Catalepsy
coronary — see Infarct, myocardium
cyanotic, newborn P28.2
drop NEC R55
epileptic — see Epilepsy
heart — see infarct, myocardium
hysterical F44.9
jacksonian — see Epilepsy, localization-related, symptomatic, with simple partial seizures
myocardium, myocardial — see Infarct, myocardium
myoclonic — see Epilepsy, generalized, specified NEC
panic F41.0

☑ Additional Character Required — Refer to the Tabular List for Character Selection   🔽 Subterms under main terms may continue to next column or page

Attack, attacks — *continued*
  psychomotor — *see* Epilepsy, localization-related,
    symptomatic, with complex partial seizures
  salaam — *see* Epilepsy, spasms
  schizophreniform, brief F23
  shuddering, benign G25.83
  Stokes-Adams I45.9
  syncope R55
  transient ischemic (TIA) G45.9
    specified NEC G45.8
  unconsciousness R55
    hysterical F44.89
  vasomotor R55
  vasovagal (paroxysmal) (idiopathic) R55
Attention (to)
  artificial
    opening (of) Z43.9
      digestive tract NEC Z43.4
        colon Z43.3
        ilium Z43.2
        stomach Z43.1
      specified NEC Z43.8
      trachea Z43.0
      urinary tract NEC Z43.6
        cystostomy Z43.5
        nephrostomy Z43.6
        ureterostomy Z43.6
        urethrostomy Z43.6
      vagina Z43.7
  colostomy Z43.3
  cystostomy Z43.5
  deficit disorder or syndrome F98.8
    with hyperactivity — *see* Disorder, attention-deficit
      hyperactivity
  gastrostomy Z43.1
  ileostomy Z43.2
  jejunostomy Z43.4
  nephrostomy Z43.6
  surgical dressings Z48.01
  sutures Z48.02
  tracheostomy Z43.0
  ureterostomy Z43.6
  urethrostomy Z43.6
Attrition
  gum — *see* Recession, gingival
  tooth, teeth (excessive) (hard tissues) K03.0
Atypical, atypism (*see also* condition)
  cells (on cytolgocial smear) (endocervical) (endometri-
    al) (glandular)
    cervix R87.619
    vagina R87.629
  cervical N87.9
  endometrium N85.9
    hyperplasia N85.00
  parenting situation Z62.9
Auditory — *see* condition
Aujeszky's disease B33.8
Aurantiasis, cutis E67.1
Auricle, auricular (*see also* condition)
  cervical Q18.2
Auriculotemporal syndrome G50.8
Austin Flint murmur (aortic insufficiency) I35.1
Australian
  Q fever A78
  X disease A83.4
Autism, autistic (childhood) (infantile) F84.0
  atypical F84.9
  spectrum disorder F84.0
Autodigestion R68.89
Autoerythrocyte sensitization (syndrome) D69.2
Autographism L50.3
Autoimmune
  disease (systemic) M35.9
  inhibitors to clotting factors D68.311
  lymphoproliferative syndrome [ALPS] D89.82
  thyroiditis E06.3
Autointoxication R68.89
Automatism G93.89
  with temporal sclerosis G93.81
  epileptic — *see* Epilepsy, localization-related, symp-
    tomatic, with complex partial seizures
  paroxysmal, idiopathic — *see* Epilepsy, localization-
    related, symptomatic, with complex partial
    seizures
Autonomic, autonomous
  bladder (neurogenic) N31.2
  hysteria seizure F44.5
Autosensitivity, erythrocyte D69.2

Autosensitization, cutaneous L30.2
Autosome — *see* condition by chromosome involved
Autotopagnosia R48.1
Autotoxemia R68.89
Autumn — *see* condition
Avellis' syndrome G46.8
Aversion
  oral R63.3
    newborn P92.- ☑
    nonorganic origin F98.2 ☑
  sexual F52.1
Aviator's
  disease or sickness — *see* Effect, adverse, high altitude
  ear T70.0 ☑
Avitaminosis (multiple) (*see also* Deficiency, vitamin)
  E56.9
  B E53.9
    with
      beriberi E51.11
      pellagra E52
  B2 E53.0
  B6 E53.1
  B12 E53.8
  D E55.9
    with rickets E55.0
  G E53.0
  K E56.1
  nicotinic acid E52
AVNRT (atrioventricular nodal re-entrant tachycardia)
  I47.1
AVRT (atrioventricular nodal re-entrant tachycardia) I47.1
Avulsion (traumatic)
  blood vessel — *see* Injury, blood vessel
  bone — *see* Fracture, by site
  cartilage (*see also* Dislocation, by site)
    symphyseal (inner), complicating delivery O71.6
  external site other than limb — *see* Wound, open, by
    site
  eye S05.7- ☑
  head (intracranial)
    external site NEC S08.89 ☑
    scalp S08.0 ☑
  internal organ or site — *see* Injury, by site
  joint (*see also* Dislocation, by site)
    capsule — *see* Sprain, by site
  kidney S37.06- ☑
  ligament — *see* Sprain, by site
  limb (*see also* Amputation, traumatic, by site)
    skin and subcutaneous tissue — *see* Wound, open,
      by site
  muscle — *see* Injury, muscle
  nerve (root) — *see* Injury, nerve
  scalp S08.0 ☑
  skin and subcutaneous tissue — *see* Wound, open, by
    site
  spleen S36.032 ☑
  symphyseal cartilage (inner), complicating delivery
    O71.6
  tendon — *see* Injury, muscle
  tooth S03.2 ☑
Awareness of heart beat R00.2
Axenfeld's
  anomaly or syndrome Q15.0
  degeneration (calcareous) Q13.4
Axilla, axillary (*see also* condition)
  breast Q83.1
Axonotmesis — *see* Injury, nerve
Ayerza's disease or syndrome (pulmonary artery sclerosis with pulmonary hypertension) I27.0
Azoospermia (organic) N46.01
  due to
    drug therapy N46.021
    efferent duct obstruction N46.023
    infection N46.022
    radiation N46.024
    specified cause NEC N46.029
    systemic disease N46.025
Azotemia R79.89
  meaning uremia N19
Aztec ear Q17.3
Azygos
  continuation inferior vena cava Q26.8
  lobe (lung) Q33.1

B

Baastrup's disease — *see* Kissing spine

Babesiosis B60.0
Babington's disease (familial hemorrhagic telangiecta-
  sia) I78.0
Babinski's syndrome A52.79
Baby
  crying constantly R68.11
  floppy (syndrome) P94.2
Bacillary — *see* condition
Bacilluria R82.71
Bacillus (*see also* Infection, bacillus)
  abortus infection A23.1
  anthracis infection A22.9
  coli infection (*see also* Escherichia coli) B96.20
  Flexner's A03.1
  mallei infection A24.0
  Shiga's A03.0
  suipestifer infection — *see* Infection, salmonella
Back — *see* condition
Backache (postural) M54.9
  sacroiliac M53.3
  specified NEC M54.89
Backflow — *see* Reflux
Backward reading (dyslexia) F81.0
Bacteremia R78.81
  with sepsis — *see* Sepsis
Bactericholia — *see* Cholecystitis, acute
Bacterid, bacteride (pustular) L40.3
Bacterium, bacteria, bacterial
  agent NEC, as cause of disease classified elsewhere
    B96.89
  in blood — *see* Bacteremia
  in urine — *see* Bacteriuria
Bacteriuria, bacteruria R82.71
  asymptomatic R82.71
Bacteroides
  fragilis, as cause of disease classified elsewhere B96.6
Bad
  heart — *see* Disease, heart
  trip
    due to drug abuse — *see* Abuse, drug, hallucino-
      gen
    due to drug dependence — *see* Dependence, drug,
      hallucinogen
Baelz's disease (cheilitis glandularis apostematosa) K13.0
Baerensprung's disease (eczema marginatum) B35.6
Bagasse disease or pneumonitis J67.1
Bagassosis J67.1
Baker's cyst — *see* Cyst, Baker's
Bakwin-Krida syndrome (metaphyseal dysplasia) Q78.5
Balancing side interference M26.56
Balanitis (circinata) (erosiva) (gangrenosa) (phagedenic)
  (vulgaris) N48.1
  amebic A06.82
  candidal B37.42
  due to Haemophilus ducreyi A57
  gonococcal (acute) (chronic) A54.09
  xerotica obliterans N48.0
Balanoposthitis N47.6
  gonococcal (acute) (chronic) A54.09
  ulcerative (specific) A63.8
Balanorrhagia — *see* Balanitis
Balantidiasis, balantidiosis A07.0
Bald tongue K14.4
Baldness (*see also* Alopecia)
  male-pattern — *see* Alopecia, androgenic
Balkan grippe A78
Balloon disease — *see* Effect, adverse, high altitude
Balo's disease (concentric sclerosis) G37.5
Bamberger-Marie disease — *see* Osteoarthropathy,
  hypertrophic, specified type NEC
Bancroft's filariasis B74.0
Band(s)
  adhesive — *see* Adhesions, peritoneum
  anomalous or congenital (*see also* Anomaly, by site)
    heart (atrial) (ventricular) Q24.8
    intestine Q43.3
    omentum Q43.3
  cervix N88.1
  constricting, congenital Q79.8
  gallbladder (congenital) Q44.1
  intestinal (adhesive) — *see* Adhesions, peritoneum
  obstructive
    intestine K56.50
      complete K56.52
      incomplete K56.51
      partial K56.51
    peritoneum K56.50

Band(s) — *continued*
  obstructive — *continued*
    peritoneum — *continued*
      complete K56.52
      incomplete K56.51
      partial K56.51
    periappendiceal, congenital Q43.3
    peritoneal (adhesive) — *see* Adhesions, peritoneum
    uterus N73.6
      internal N85.6
    vagina N89.5
Bandemia D72.825
Bandl's ring (contraction), complicating delivery O62.4
Bangkok hemorrhagic fever A91
Bang's disease (brucella abortus) A23.1
Bankruptcy, anxiety concerning Z59.8
Bannister's disease T78.3 ☑
  hereditary D84.1
Banti's disease or syndrome (with cirrhosis) (with portal hypertension) K76.6
Bar, median, prostate — *see* Enlargement, enlarged, prostate
Barcoo disease or rot — *see* Ulcer, skin
Barlow's disease E54
Barodontalgia T70.29 ☑
Baron Münchausen syndrome — *see* Disorder, factitious
Barosinusitis T70.1 ☑
Barotitis T70.0 ☑
Barotrauma T70.29 ☑
  odontalgia T70.29 ☑
  otitic T70.0 ☑
  sinus T70.1 ☑
Barraquer (-Simons) **disease or syndrome** (progressive lipodystrophy) E88.1
Barré-Guillain disease or syndrome G61.0
Barrel chest M95.4
Barré-Liéou syndrome (posterior cervical sympathetic) M53.0
Barrett's
  disease — *see* Barrett's, esophagus
  esophagus K22.70
    with dysplasia K22.719
      high grade K22.711
      low grade K22.710
    without dysplasia K22.70
  syndrome — *see* Barrett's, esophagus
  ulcer K22.10
    with bleeding K22.11
    without bleeding K22.10
Bársony (-Polgár) (-Teschendorf) **syndrome** (corkscrew esophagus) K22.4
Barth syndrome E78.71
Bartholinitis (suppurating) N75.8
  gonococcal (acute) (chronic) (with abscess) A54.1
Bartonellosis A44.9
  cutaneous A44.1
  mucocutaneous A44.1
  specified NEC A44.8
  systemic A44.0
Barton's fracture S52.56- ☑
Bartter's syndrome E26.81
Basal — *see* condition
Basan's (hidrotic) ectodermal dysplasia Q82.4
Baseball finger — *see* Dislocation, finger
Basedow's disease (exophthalmic goiter) — *see* Hyperthyroidism, with, goiter
Basic — *see* condition
Basilar — *see* condition
Bason's (hidrotic) ectodermal dysplasia Q82.4
Basopenia — *see* Agranulocytosis
Basophilia D72.824
Basophilism (cortico-adrenal) (Cushing's) (pituitary) E24.0
Bassen-Kornzweig disease or syndrome E78.6
Bat ear Q17.5
Bateman's
  disease B08.1
  purpura (senile) D69.2
Bathing cramp T75.1 ☑
Bathophobia F40.248
Batten (-Mayou) **disease** E75.4
  retina E75.4 [H36]
Batten-Steinert syndrome G71.11
Battered — *see* Maltreatment
Battey Mycobacterium infection A31.0
Battle exhaustion F43.0

Battledore placenta O43.19- ☑
Baumgarten-Cruveilhier cirrhosis, disease or syndrome K74.69
Bauxite fibrosis (of lung) J63.1
Bayle's disease (general paresis) A52.17
Bazin's disease (primary) (tuberculous) A18.4
Beach ear — *see* Swimmer's, ear
Beaded hair (congenital) Q84.1
Béal conjunctivitis or syndrome B30.2
Beard's disease (neurasthenia) F48.8
Beat(s)
  atrial, premature I49.1
  ectopic I49.49
  elbow — *see* Bursitis, elbow
  escaped, heart I49.49
  hand — *see* Bursitis, hand
  knee — *see* Bursitis, knee
  premature I49.40
    atrial I49.1
    auricular I49.1
    supraventricular I49.1
Beau's
  disease or syndrome — *see* Degeneration, myocardial
  lines (transverse furrows on fingernails) L60.4
Bechterev's syndrome — *see* Spondylitis, ankylosing
Becker's
  cardiomyopathy I42.8
  disease
    idiopathic mural endomyocardial disease I42.3
    myotonia congenita, recessive form G71.12
  dystrophy G71.0
  pigmented hairy nevus D22.5
Beck's syndrome (anterior spinal artery occlusion) I65.8
Beckwith-Wiedemann syndrome Q87.3
Bed confinement status Z74.01
Bed sore — *see* Ulcer, pressure, by site
Bedbug bite(s) — *see* Bite(s), by site, superficial, insect
Bedclothes, asphyxiation or suffocation by — *see* Asphyxia, traumatic, due to, mechanical, trapped
Bednar's
  aphthae K12.0
  tumor — *see* Neoplasm, malignant, by site
Bedridden Z74.01
Bedsore — *see* Ulcer, pressure, by site
Bedwetting — *see* Enuresis
Bee sting (with allergic or anaphylactic shock) — *see* Toxicity, venom, arthropod, bee
Beer drinker's heart (disease) I42.6
Begbie's disease (exophthalmic goiter) — *see* Hyperthyroidism, with, goiter
Behavior
  antisocial
    adult Z72.811
    child or adolescent Z72.810
  disorder, disturbance — *see* Disorder, conduct
  disruptive — *see* Disorder, conduct
  drug seeking Z76.5
  inexplicable R46.2
  marked evasiveness R46.5
  obsessive-compulsive R46.81
  overactivity R46.3
  poor responsiveness R46.4
  self-damaging (life-style) Z72.89
  sleep-incompatible Z72.821
  slowness R46.4
  specified NEC R46.89
  strange (and inexplicable) R46.2
  suspiciousness R46.5
  type A pattern Z73.1
  undue concern or preoccupation with stressful events R46.6
  verbosity and circumstantial detail obscuring reason for contact R46.7
Behçet's disease or syndrome M35.2
Behr's disease — *see* Degeneration, macula
Beigel's disease or morbus (white piedra) B36.2
Bejel A65
Bekhterev's syndrome — *see* Spondylitis, ankylosing
Belching — *see* Eructation
Bell's
  mania F30.8
  palsy, paralysis G51.0
    infant or newborn P11.3
  spasm G51.3
Bence Jones albuminuria or proteinuria NEC R80.3
Bends T70.3 ☑
Benedikt's paralysis or syndrome G46.3

Benign (*see also* condition)
  prostatic hyperplasia — *see* Hyperplasia, prostate
Bennett's fracture (displaced) S62.21- ☑
Benson's disease — *see* Deposit, crystalline
Bent
  back (hysterical) F44.4
  nose M95.0
    congenital Q67.4
Bereavement (uncomplicated) Z63.4
Bergeron's disease (hysterical chorea) F44.4
Berger's disease — *see* Nephropathy, IgA
Beriberi (dry) E51.11
  heart (disease) E51.12
  polyneuropathy E51.11
  wet E51.12
    involving circulatory system E51.11
Berlin's disease or edema (traumatic) S05.8X- ☑
Berlock (berloque) **dermatitis** L56.2
Bernard-Horner syndrome G90.2
Bernard-Soulier disease or thrombopathia D69.1
Bernhardt (-Roth) **disease** — *see* Mononeuropathy, lower limb, meralgia paresthetica
Bernheim's syndrome — *see* Failure, heart, right
Bertielliasis B71.8
Berylliosis (lung) J63.2
Besnier-Boeck (-Schaumann) **disease** — *see* Sarcoidosis
Besnier's
  lupus pernio D86.3
  prurigo L20.0
Bestiality F65.89
Best's disease H35.50
Betalipoproteinemia, broad or floating E78.2
Beta-mercaptolactate-cysteine disulfiduria E72.09
Betting and gambling Z72.6
  pathological (compulsive) F63.0
Bezoar T18.9 ☑
  intestine T18.3 ☑
  stomach T18.2 ☑
Bezold's abscess — *see* Mastoiditis, acute
Bianchi's syndrome R48.8
Bicornate or bicornis uterus Q51.3
  in pregnancy or childbirth O34.00
    causing obstructed labor O65.5
Bicuspid aortic valve Q23.1
Biedl-Bardet syndrome Q87.89
Bielschowsky (-Jansky) disease E75.4
Biermer's (pernicious) anemia or disease D51.0
Biett's disease L93.0
Bifid (congenital)
  apex, heart Q24.8
  clitoris Q52.6
  kidney Q63.8
  nose Q30.2
  patella Q74.1
  scrotum Q55.29
  toe NEC Q74.2
  tongue Q38.3
  ureter Q62.8
  uterus Q51.3
  uvula Q35.7
Biforis uterus (suprasimplex) Q51.3
Bifurcation (congenital)
  gallbladder Q44.1
  kidney pelvis Q63.8
  renal pelvis Q63.8
  rib Q76.6
  tongue, congenital Q38.3
  trachea Q32.1
  ureter Q62.8
  urethra Q64.74
  vertebra Q76.49
Big spleen syndrome D73.1
Bigeminal pulse R00.8
Bilateral — *see* condition
Bile
  duct — *see* condition
  pigments in urine R82.2
Bilharziasis (*see also* Schistosomiasis)
  chyluria B65.0
  cutaneous B65.3
  galactura B65.0
  hematochyluria B65.0
  intestinal B65.1
  lipemia B65.9
  lipuria B65.0
  oriental B65.2
  piarhemia B65.9

Bilharziasis — *continued*
  pulmonary NOS B65.9 [J99]
    pneumonia B65.9 [J17]
  tropical hematuria B65.0
  vesical B65.0
Biliary — *see* condition
Bilirubin metabolism disorder E80.7
  specified NEC E80.6
Bilirubinemia, familial nonhemolytic E80.4
Bilirubinuria R82.2
Biliuria R82.2
Bilocular stomach K31.2
Binswanger's disease I67.3
Biparta, bipartite
  carpal scaphoid Q74.0
  patella Q74.1
  vagina Q52.10
Bird
  face Q75.8
  fancier's disease or lung J67.2
Birth
  complications in mother — *see* Delivery, complicated
  compression during NOS P15.9
  defect — *see* Anomaly
  immature (less than 37 completed weeks) — *see* Preterm, newborn
    extremely (less than 28 completed weeks) — *see* Immaturity, extreme
  inattention, at or after — *see* Maltreatment, child, neglect
  injury NOS P15.9
    basal ganglia P11.1
    brachial plexus NEC P14.3
    brain (compression) (pressure) P11.2
    central nervous system NOS P11.9
    cerebellum P11.1
    cerebral hemorrhage P10.1
    external genitalia P15.5
    eye P15.3
    face P15.4
    fracture
      bone P13.9
        specified NEC P13.8
      clavicle P13.4
      femur P13.2
      humerus P13.3
      long bone, except femur P13.3
      radius and ulna P13.3
      skull P13.0
      spine P11.5
      tibia and fibula P13.3
    intracranial P11.2
      laceration or hemorrhage P10.9
        specified NEC P10.8
    intraventricular hemorrhage P10.2
    laceration
      brain P10.1
      by scalpel P15.8
      peripheral nerve P14.9
    liver P15.0
    meninges
      brain P11.1
      spinal cord P11.5
    nerve
      brachial plexus P14.3
      cranial NEC (except facial) P11.4
      facial P11.3
      peripheral P14.9
      phrenic (paralysis) P14.2
    paralysis
      facial nerve P11.3
      spinal P11.5
    penis P15.5
    rupture
      spinal cord P11.5
    scalp P12.9
    scalpel wound P15.8
    scrotum P15.5
    skull NEC P13.1
      fracture P13.0
    specified type NEC P15.8
    spinal cord P11.5
    spine P11.5
    spleen P15.1
    sternomastoid (hematoma) P15.2
    subarachnoid hemorrhage P10.3
    subcutaneous fat necrosis P15.6
    subdural hemorrhage P10.0

Birth — *continued*
  injury — *continued*
    tentorial tear P10.4
    testes P15.5
    vulva P15.5
  lack of care, at or after — *see* Maltreatment, child, neglect
  neglect, at or after — *see* Maltreatment, child, neglect
  palsy or paralysis, newborn, NOS (birth injury) P14.9
  premature (infant) — *see* Preterm, newborn
  shock, newborn P96.89
  trauma — *see* Birth, injury
  weight
    4000 grams to 4499 grams P08.1
    4500 grams or more P08.0
    low (2499 grams or less) — *see* Low, birthweight
      extremely (999 grams or less) — *see* Low, birthweight, extreme
Birthmark Q82.5
Birt-Hogg-Dube syndrome Q87.89
Bisalbuminemia E88.09
Biskra's button B55.1
Bite(s) (animal) (human)
  abdomen, abdominal
    wall S31.159 ✔
      with penetration into peritoneal cavity S31.659 ✔
      epigastric region S31.152 ✔
        with penetration into peritoneal cavity S31.652 ✔
      left
        lower quadrant S31.154 ✔
          with penetration into peritoneal cavity S31.654 ✔
        upper quadrant S31.151 ✔
          with penetration into peritoneal cavity S31.651 ✔
      periumbilic region S31.155 ✔
        with penetration into peritoneal cavity S31.655 ✔
      right
        lower quadrant S31.153 ✔
          with penetration into peritoneal cavity S31.653 ✔
        upper quadrant S31.150 ✔
          with penetration into peritoneal cavity S31.650 ✔
      superficial NEC S30.871 ✔
        insect S30.861 ✔
  alveolar (process) — *see* Bite, oral cavity
  amphibian (venomous) — *see* Venom, bite, amphibian
  animal (*see also* Bite, by site)
    venomous — *see* Venom
  ankle S91.05- ✔
    superficial NEC S90.57- ✔
      insect S90.56- ✔
  antecubital space — *see* Bite, elbow
  anus S31.835 ✔
    superficial NEC S30.877 ✔
      insect S30.867 ✔
  arm (upper) S41.15- ✔
    lower — *see* Bite, forearm
    superficial NEC S40.87- ✔
      insect S40.86- ✔
  arthropod NEC — *see* Venom, bite, arthropod
  auditory canal (external) (meatus) — *see* Bite, ear
  auricle, ear — *see* Bite, ear
  axilla — *see* Bite, arm
  back (*see also* Bite, thorax, back)
    lower S31.050 ✔
      with penetration into retroperitoneal space S31.051 ✔
      superficial NEC S30.870 ✔
        insect S30.860 ✔
  bedbug — *see* Bite(s), by site, superficial, insect
  breast S21.05- ✔
    superficial NEC S20.17- ✔
      insect S20.16- ✔
  brow — *see* Bite, head, specified site NEC
  buttock S31.805 ✔
    left S31.825 ✔
    right S31.815 ✔
    superficial NEC S30.870 ✔
      insect S30.860 ✔
  calf — *see* Bite, leg
  canaliculus lacrimalis — *see* Bite, eyelid

Bite(s) — *continued*
  canthus, eye — *see* Bite, eyelid
  centipede — *see* Toxicity, venom, arthropod, centipede
  cheek (external) S01.45- ✔
    internal — *see* Bite, oral cavity
    superficial NEC S00.87 ✔
      insect S00.86 ✔
  chest wall — *see* Bite, thorax
  chigger B88.0
  chin — *see* Bite, head, specified site NEC
  clitoris — *see* Bite, vulva
  costal region — *see* Bite, thorax
  digit(s)
    hand — *see* Bite, finger
    toe — *see* Bite, toe
  ear (canal) (external) S01.35- ✔
    superficial NEC S00.47- ✔
      insect S00.46- ✔
  elbow S51.05- ✔
    superficial NEC S50.37- ✔
      insect S50.36- ✔
  epididymis — *see* Bite, testis
  epigastric region — *see* Bite, abdomen
  epiglottis — *see* Bite, neck, specified site NEC
  esophagus, cervical S11.25 ✔
    superficial NEC S10.17 ✔
      insect S10.16 ✔
  eyebrow — *see* Bite, eyelid
  eyelid S01.15- ✔
    superficial NEC S00.27- ✔
      insect S00.26- ✔
  face NEC — *see* Bite, head, specified site NEC
  finger(s) S61.259 ✔
    with
      damage to nail S61.359 ✔
    index S61.258 ✔
      with
        damage to nail S61.358 ✔
      left S61.251 ✔
        with
          damage to nail S61.351 ✔
      right S61.250 ✔
        with
          damage to nail S61.350 ✔
      superficial NEC S60.478 ✔
        insect S60.46- ✔
    little S61.25- ✔
      with
        damage to nail S61.35- ✔
      superficial NEC S60.47- ✔
        insect S60.46- ✔
    middle S61.25- ✔
      with
        damage to nail S61.35- ✔
      superficial NEC S60.47- ✔
        insect S60.46- ✔
    ring S61.25- ✔
      with
        damage to nail S61.35- ✔
      superficial NEC S60.47- ✔
        insect S60.46- ✔
    superficial NEC S60.479 ✔
      insect S60.469 ✔
    thumb — *see* Bite, thumb
  flank — *see* Bite, abdomen, wall
  flea — *see* Bite, by site, superficial, insect
  foot (except toe(s) alone) S91.35- ✔
    superficial NEC S90.87- ✔
      insect S90.86- ✔
    toe — *see* Bite, toe
  forearm S51.85- ✔
    elbow only — *see* Bite, elbow
    superficial NEC S50.87- ✔
      insect S50.86- ✔
  forehead — *see* Bite, head, specified site NEC
  genital organs, external
    female S31.552 ✔
      superficial NEC S30.876 ✔
        insect S30.866 ✔
      vagina and vulva — *see* Bite, vulva
    male S31.551 ✔
      penis — *see* Bite, penis
      scrotum — *see* Bite, scrotum
      superficial NEC S30.875 ✔
        insect S30.865 ✔

Bite(s) — *continued*
  genital organs, external — *continued*
    male — *continued*
      testes — *see* Bite, testis
  groin — *see* Bite, abdomen, wall
  gum — *see* Bite, oral cavity
  hand S61.45- ☑
    finger — *see* Bite, finger
    superficial NEC S60.57- ☑
      insect S60.56- ☑
    thumb — *see* Bite, thumb
  head S01.95 ☑
    cheek — *see* Bite, cheek
    ear — *see* Bite, ear
    eyelid — *see* Bite, eyelid
    lip — *see* Bite, lip
    nose — *see* Bite, nose
    oral cavity — *see* Bite, oral cavity
    scalp — *see* Bite, scalp
    specified site NEC S01.85 ☑
      superficial NEC S00.87 ☑
        insect S00.86 ☑
    superficial NEC S00.97 ☑
      insect S00.96 ☑
    temporomandibular area — *see* Bite, cheek
  heel — *see* Bite, foot
  hip S71.05- ☑
    superficial NEC S70.27- ☑
      insect S70.26- ☑
  hymen S31.45 ☑
  hypochondrium — *see* Bite, abdomen, wall
  hypogastric region — *see* Bite, abdomen, wall
  inguinal region — *see* Bite, abdomen, wall
  insect — *see* Bite, by site, superficial, insect
  instep — *see* Bite, foot
  interscapular region — *see* Bite, thorax, back
  jaw — *see* Bite, head, specified site NEC
  knee S81.05- ☑
    superficial NEC S80.27- ☑
      insect S80.26- ☑
  labium (majus) (minus) — *see* Bite, vulva
  lacrimal duct — *see* Bite, eyelid
  larynx S11.015 ☑
    superficial NEC S10.17 ☑
      insect S10.16 ☑
  leg (lower) S81.85- ☑
    ankle — *see* Bite, ankle
    foot — *see* Bite, foot
    knee — *see* Bite, knee
    superficial NEC S80.87- ☑
      insect S80.86- ☑
    toe — *see* Bite, toe
    upper — *see* Bite, thigh
  lip S01.551 ☑
    superficial NEC S00.571 ☑
      insect S00.561 ☑
  lizard (venomous) — *see* Venom, bite, reptile
  loin — *see* Bite, abdomen, wall
  lower back — *see* Bite, back, lower
  lumbar region — *see* Bite, back, lower
  malar region — *see* Bite, head, specified site NEC
  mammary — *see* Bite, breast
  marine animals (venomous) — *see* Toxicity, venom, marine animal
  mastoid region — *see* Bite, head, specified site NEC
  mouth — *see* Bite, oral cavity
  nail
    finger — *see* Bite, finger
    toe — *see* Bite, toe
  nape — *see* Bite, neck, specified site NEC
  nasal (septum) (sinus) — *see* Bite, nose
  nasopharynx — *see* Bite, head, specified site NEC
  neck S11.95 ☑
    involving
      cervical esophagus — *see* Bite, esophagus, cervical
      larynx — *see* Bite, larynx
      pharynx — *see* Bite, pharynx
      thyroid gland S11.15 ☑
      trachea — *see* Bite, trachea
    specified site NEC S11.85 ☑
      superficial NEC S10.87 ☑
        insect S10.86 ☑
    superficial NEC S10.97 ☑
      insect S10.96 ☑
    throat S11.85 ☑

Bite(s) — *continued*
  neck — *continued*
    throat — *continued*
      superficial NEC S10.17 ☑
        insect S10.16 ☑
  nose (septum) (sinus) S01.25 ☑
    superficial NEC S00.37 ☑
      insect S00.36 ☑
  occipital region — *see* Bite, scalp
  oral cavity S01.552 ☑
    superficial NEC S00.572 ☑
      insect S00.562 ☑
  orbital region — *see* Bite, eyelid
  palate — *see* Bite, oral cavity
  palm — *see* Bite, hand
  parietal region — *see* Bite, scalp
  pelvis S31.050 ☑
    with penetration into retroperitoneal space S31.051 ☑
    superficial NEC S30.870 ☑
      insect S30.860 ☑
  penis S31.25 ☑
    superficial NEC S30.872 ☑
      insect S30.862 ☑
  perineum
    female — *see* Bite, vulva
    male — *see* Bite, pelvis
  periocular area (with or without lacrimal passages) — *see* Bite, eyelid
  phalanges
    finger — *see* Bite, finger
    toe — *see* Bite, toe
  pharynx S11.25 ☑
    superficial NEC S10.17 ☑
      insect S10.16 ☑
  pinna — *see* Bite, ear
  poisonous — *see* Venom
  popliteal space — *see* Bite, knee
  prepuce — *see* Bite, penis
  pubic region — *see* Bite, abdomen, wall
  rectovaginal septum — *see* Bite, vulva
  red bug B88.0
  reptile NEC (*see also* Venom, bite, reptile)
    nonvenomous — *see* Bite, by site
    snake — *see* Venom, bite, snake
  sacral region — *see* Bite, back, lower
  sacroiliac region — *see* Bite, back, lower
  salivary gland — *see* Bite, oral cavity
  scalp S01.05 ☑
    superficial NEC S00.07 ☑
      insect S00.06 ☑
  scapular region — *see* Bite, shoulder
  scrotum S31.35 ☑
    superficial NEC S30.873 ☑
      insect S30.863 ☑
  sea-snake (venomous) — *see* Toxicity, venom, snake, sea snake
  shin — *see* Bite, leg
  shoulder S41.05- ☑
    superficial NEC S40.27- ☑
      insect S40.26- ☑
  snake (*see also* Venom, bite, snake)
    nonvenomous — *see* Bite, by site
  spermatic cord — *see* Bite, testis
  spider (venomous) — *see* Toxicity, venom, spider
    nonvenomous — *see* Bite, by site, superficial, insect
  sternal region — *see* Bite, thorax, front
  submaxillary region — *see* Bite, head, specified site NEC
  submental region — *see* Bite, head, specified site NEC
  subungual
    finger(s) — *see* Bite, finger
    toe — *see* Bite, toe
  superficial — *see* Bite, by site, superficial
  supraclavicular fossa S11.85 ☑
  supraorbital — *see* Bite, head, specified site NEC
  temple, temporal region — *see* Bite, head, specified site NEC
  temporomandibular area — *see* Bite, cheek
  testis S31.35 ☑
    superficial NEC S30.873 ☑
      insect S30.863 ☑
  thigh S71.15- ☑
    superficial NEC S70.37- ☑
      insect S70.36- ☑
  thorax, thoracic (wall) S21.95 ☑

Bite(s) — *continued*
  thorax, thoracic — *continued*
    back S21.25- ☑
      with penetration into thoracic cavity S21.45- ☑
    breast — *see* Bite, breast
    front S21.15- ☑
      with penetration into thoracic cavity S21.35- ☑
    superficial NEC S20.97 ☑
      back S20.47- ☑
      front S20.37- ☑
      insect S20.96 ☑
        back S20.46- ☑
        front S20.36- ☑
  throat — *see* Bite, neck, throat
  thumb S61.05- ☑
    with
      damage to nail S61.15- ☑
    superficial NEC S60.37- ☑
      insect S60.36- ☑
  thyroid S11.15 ☑
    superficial NEC S10.87 ☑
      insect S10.86 ☑
  toe(s) S91.15- ☑
    with
      damage to nail S91.25- ☑
    great S91.15- ☑
      with
        damage to nail S91.25- ☑
    lesser S91.15- ☑
      with
        damage to nail S91.25- ☑
    superficial NEC S90.47- ☑
      great S90.47- ☑
      insect S90.46- ☑
        great S90.46- ☑
  tongue S01.552 ☑
  trachea S11.025 ☑
    superficial NEC S10.17 ☑
      insect S10.16 ☑
  tunica vaginalis — *see* Bite, testis
  tympanum, tympanic membrane — *see* Bite, ear
  umbilical region S31.155 ☑
  uvula — *see* Bite, oral cavity
  vagina — *see* Bite, vulva
  venomous — *see* Venom
  vocal cords S11.035 ☑
    superficial NEC S10.17 ☑
      insect S10.16 ☑
  vulva S31.45 ☑
    superficial NEC S30.874 ☑
      insect S30.864 ☑
  wrist S61.55- ☑
    superficial NEC S60.87- ☑
      insect S60.86- ☑
Biting, cheek or lip K13.1
Biventricular failure (heart) I50.82
Björck (-Thorson) **syndrome** (malignant carcinoid) E34.0
Black
  death A20.9
  eye S00.1- ☑
  hairy tongue K14.3
  heel (foot) S90.3- ☑
  lung (disease) J60
  palm (hand) S60.22- ☑
Blackfan-Diamond anemia or syndrome (congenital hypoplastic anemia) D61.01
Blackhead L70.0
Blackout R55
Bladder — *see* condition
Blast (air) (hydraulic) (immersion) (underwater)
  blindness S05.8X- ☑
  injury
    abdomen or thorax — *see* Injury, by site
    ear (acoustic nerve trauma) — *see* Injury, nerve, acoustic, specified type NEC
    syndrome NEC T70.8 ☑
Blastoma — *see* Neoplasm, malignant, by site
  pulmonary — *see* Neoplasm, lung, malignant
Blastomycosis, blastomycotic B40.9
  Brazilian — *see* Paracoccidioidomycosis
  cutaneous B40.3
  disseminated B40.7
  European — *see* Cryptococcosis
  generalized B40.7
  keloidal B48.0
  North American B40.9

Blastomycosis, blastomycotic — *continued*
　primary pulmonary B40.0
　pulmonary B40.2
　　acute B40.0
　　chronic B40.1
　skin B40.3
　South American — *see* Paracoccidioidomycosis
　specified NEC B40.89
Bleb(s) R23.8
　emphysematous (lung) (solitary) J43.9
　endophthalmitis H59.43
　filtering (vitreous), after glaucoma surgery Z98.83
　inflamed (infected), postprocedural H59.40
　　stage 1 H59.41
　　stage 2 H59.42
　　stage 3 H59.43
　lung (ruptured) J43.9
　　congenital — *see* Atelectasis
　　newborn P25.8
　subpleural (emphysematous) J43.9
Blebitis, postprocedural H59.40
　stage 1 H59.41
　stage 2 H59.42
　stage 3 H59.43
Bleeder (familial) (hereditary) — *see* Hemophilia
Bleeding (*see also* Hemorrhage)
　anal K62.5
　anovulatory N97.0
　atonic, following delivery O72.1
　capillary I78.8
　　puerperal O72.2
　contact (postcoital) N93.0
　due to uterine subinvolution N85.3
　ear — *see* Otorrhagia
　excessive, associated with menopausal onset N92.4
　familial — *see* Defect, coagulation
　following intercourse N93.0
　gastrointestinal K92.2
　hemorrhoids — *see* Hemorrhoids
　intermenstrual (regular) N92.3
　　irregular N92.1
　intraoperative — *see* Complication, intraoperative, hemorrhage
　irregular N92.6
　menopausal N92.4
　newborn, intraventricular — *see* Newborn, affected by, hemorrhage, intraventricular
　nipple N64.59
　nose R04.0
　ovulation N92.3
　postclimacteric N95.0
　postcoital N93.0
　postmenopausal N95.0
　postoperative — *see* Complication, postprocedural, hemorrhage
　preclimacteric N92.4
　pre-pubertal vaginal N93.1
　puberty (excessive, with onset of menstrual periods) N92.2
　rectum, rectal K62.5
　　newborn P54.2
　tendencies — *see* Defect, coagulation
　throat R04.1
　tooth socket (post-extraction) K91.840
　umbilical stump P51.9
　uterus, uterine NEC N93.9
　　climacteric N92.4
　　dysfunctional or functional N93.8
　　menopausal N92.4
　　preclimacteric or premenopausal N92.4
　　unrelated to menstrual cycle N93.9
　vagina, vaginal (abnormal) N93.9
　　dysfunctional or functional N93.8
　　newborn P54.6
　　pre-pubertal N93.1
　vicarious N94.89
Blennorrhagia, blennorrhagic — *see* Gonorrhea
Blennorrhea (acute) (chronic) (*see also* Gonorrhea)
　inclusion (neonatal) (newborn) P39.1
　lower genitourinary tract (gonococcal) A54.00
　neonatorum (gonococcal ophthalmia) A54.31
Blepharelosis — *see* Entropion
Blepharitis (angularis) (ciliaris) (eyelid) (marginal) (nonulcerative) H01.009
　herpes zoster B02.39
　left H01.006
　　lower H01.005
　　upper H01.004

Blepharitis — *continued*
　right H01.003
　　lower H01.002
　　upper H01.001
　squamous H01.029
　　left H01.026
　　　lower H01.025
　　　upper H01.024
　　right H01.023
　　　lower H01.022
　　　upper H01.021
　ulcerative H01.019
　　left H01.016
　　　lower H01.015
　　　upper H01.014
　　right H01.013
　　　lower H01.012
　　　upper H01.011
Blepharochalasis H02.30
　congenital Q10.0
　left H02.36
　　lower H02.35
　　upper H02.34
　right H02.33
　　lower H02.32
　　upper H02.31
Blepharoclonus H02.59
Blepharoconjunctivitis H10.50- ☑
　angular H10.52- ☑
　contact H10.53- ☑
　ligneous H10.51- ☑
Blepharophimosis (eyelid) H02.529
　congenital Q10.3
　left H02.526
　　lower H02.525
　　upper H02.524
　right H02.523
　　lower H02.522
　　upper H02.521
Blepharoptosis H02.40- ☑
　congenital Q10.0
　mechanical H02.41- ☑
　myogenic H02.42- ☑
　neurogenic H02.43- ☑
　paralytic H02.43- ☑
Blepharopyorrhea, gonococcal A54.39
Blepharospasm G24.5
　drug induced G24.01
Blighted ovum O02.0
Blind (*see also* Blindness)
　bronchus (congenital) Q32.4
　loop syndrome K90.2
　　congenital Q43.8
　sac, fallopian tube (congenital) Q50.6
　spot, enlarged — *see* Defect, visual field, localized, scotoma, blind spot area
　tract or tube, congenital NEC — *see* Atresia, by site
Blindness (acquired) (congenital) (both eyes) H54.0X- ☑
　blast S05.8X- ☑
　color — *see* Deficiency, color vision
　concussion S05.8X- ☑
　cortical H47.619
　　left brain H47.612
　　right brain H47.611
　day H53.11
　due to injury (current episode) S05.9- ☑
　　sequelae — *code to* injury with seventh character S
　eclipse (total) — *see* Retinopathy, solar
　emotional (hysterical) F44.6
　face H53.16
　hysterical F44.6
　legal (both eyes) (USA definition) H54.8
　mind R48.8
　night H53.60
　　abnormal dark adaptation curve H53.61
　　acquired H53.62
　　congenital H53.63
　　specified type NEC H53.69
　　vitamin A deficiency E50.5
　one eye (other eye normal) H54.40
　　left (normal vision on right) H54.42- ☑
　　　low vision on right H54.12- ☑
　　low vision, other eye H54.10
　　right (normal vision on left) H54.41- ☑
　　　low vision on left H54.11- ☑
　psychic R48.8
　river B73.01

Blindness — *continued*
　snow — *see* Photokeratitis
　sun, solar — *see* Retinopathy, solar
　transient — *see* Disturbance, vision, subjective, loss, transient
　traumatic (current episode) S05.9- ☑
　word (developmental) F81.0
　　acquired R48.0
　　secondary to organic lesion R48.0
Blister (nonthermal)
　abdominal wall S30.821 ☑
　alveolar process S00.522 ☑
　ankle S90.52- ☑
　antecubital space — *see* Blister, elbow
　anus S30.827 ☑
　arm (upper) S40.82- ☑
　auditory canal — *see* Blister, ear
　auricle — *see* Blister, ear
　axilla — *see* Blister, arm
　back, lower S30.820 ☑
　beetle dermatitis L24.89
　breast S20.12- ☑
　brow S00.82 ☑
　calf — *see* Blister, leg
　canthus — *see* Blister, eyelid
　cheek S00.82 ☑
　　internal S00.522 ☑
　chest wall — *see* Blister, thorax
　chin S00.82 ☑
　costal region — *see* Blister, thorax
　digit(s)
　　foot — *see* Blister, toe
　　hand — *see* Blister, finger
　due to burn — *see* Burn, by site, second degree
　ear S00.42- ☑
　elbow S50.32- ☑
　epiglottis S10.12 ☑
　esophagus, cervical S10.12 ☑
　eyebrow — *see* Blister, eyelid
　eyelid S00.22- ☑
　face S00.82 ☑
　fever B00.1
　finger(s) S60.429 ☑
　　index S60.42- ☑
　　little S60.42- ☑
　　middle S60.42- ☑
　　ring S60.42- ☑
　foot (except toe(s) alone) S90.82- ☑
　　toe — *see* Blister, toe
　forearm S50.82- ☑
　　elbow only — *see* Blister, elbow
　forehead S00.82 ☑
　fracture — *omit code*
　genital organ
　　female S30.826 ☑
　　male S30.825 ☑
　gum S00.522 ☑
　hand S60.52- ☑
　head S00.92 ☑
　　ear — *see* Blister, ear
　　eyelid — *see* Blister, eyelid
　　lip S00.521 ☑
　　nose S00.32 ☑
　　oral cavity S00.522 ☑
　　scalp S00.02 ☑
　　specified site NEC S00.82 ☑
　heel — *see* Blister, foot
　hip S70.22- ☑
　interscapular region S20.429 ☑
　jaw S00.82 ☑
　knee S80.22- ☑
　larynx S10.12 ☑
　leg (lower) S80.82- ☑
　　knee — *see* Blister, knee
　　upper — *see* Blister, thigh
　lip S00.521 ☑
　malar region S00.82 ☑
　mammary — *see* Blister, breast
　mastoid region S00.82 ☑
　mouth S00.522 ☑
　multiple, skin, nontraumatic R23.8
　nail
　　finger — *see* Blister, finger
　　toe — *see* Blister, toe
　nasal S00.32 ☑
　neck S10.92 ☑

Blister — *continued*
  neck — *continued*
    specified site NEC S10.82 ☑
      throat S10.12 ☑
  nose S00.32 ☑
  occipital region S00.02 ☑
  oral cavity S00.522 ☑
  orbital region — *see* Blister, eyelid
  palate S00.522 ☑
  palm — *see* Blister, hand
  parietal region S00.02 ☑
  pelvis S30.820 ☑
  penis S30.822 ☑
  periocular area — *see* Blister, eyelid
  phalanges
    finger — *see* Blister, finger
    toe — *see* Blister, toe
  pharynx S10.12 ☑
  pinna — *see* Blister, ear
  popliteal space — *see* Blister, knee
  scalp S00.02 ☑
  scapular region — *see* Blister, shoulder
  scrotum S30.823 ☑
  shin — *see* Blister, leg
  shoulder S40.22- ☑
  sternal region S20.329 ☑
  submaxillary region S00.82 ☑
  submental region S00.82 ☑
  subungual
    finger(s) — *see* Blister, finger
    toe(s) — *see* Blister, toe
  supraclavicular fossa S10.82 ☑
  supraorbital S00.82 ☑
  temple S00.82 ☑
  temporal region S00.82 ☑
  testis S30.823 ☑
  thermal — *see* Burn, second degree, by site
  thigh S70.32- ☑
  thorax, thoracic (wall) S20.92 ☑
    back S20.42- ☑
    front S20.32- ☑
  throat S10.12 ☑
  thumb S60.32- ☑
  toe(s) S90.42- ☑
    great S90.42- ☑
  tongue S00.522 ☑
  trachea S10.12 ☑
  tympanum, tympanic membrane — *see* Blister, ear
  upper arm — *see* Blister, arm (upper)
  uvula S00.522 ☑
  vagina S30.824 ☑
  vocal cords S10.12 ☑
  vulva S30.824 ☑
  wrist S60.82- ☑
Bloating R14.0
Bloch-Sulzberger disease or syndrome Q82.3
Block, blocked
  alveolocapillary J84.10
  arborization (heart) I45.5
  arrhythmic I45.9
  atrioventricular (incomplete) (partial) I44.30
    with atrioventricular dissociation I44.2
    complete I44.2
      congenital Q24.6
    congenital Q24.6
    first degree I44.0
    second degree (types I and II) I44.1
    specified NEC I44.39
    third degree I44.2
    types I and II I44.1
  auriculoventricular — *see* Block, atrioventricular
  bifascicular (cardiac) I45.2
  bundle-branch (complete) (false) (incomplete) I45.4
    bilateral I45.2
    left I44.7
      with right bundle branch block I45.2
      hemiblock I44.60
        anterior I44.4
        posterior I44.5
      incomplete I44.7
        with right bundle branch block I45.2
    right I45.10
      with
        left bundle branch block I45.2
        left fascicular block I45.2
      specified NEC I45.19
    Wilson's type I45.19

Block, blocked — *continued*
  cardiac I45.9
  conduction I45.9
    complete I44.2
  fascicular (left) I44.60
    anterior I44.4
    posterior I44.5
    right I45.0
    specified NEC I44.69
  foramen Magendie (acquired) G91.1
    congenital Q03.1
      with spina bifida — *see* Spina bifida, by site, with hydrocephalus
  heart I45.9
    bundle branch I45.4
      bilateral I45.2
    complete (atrioventricular) I44.2
    congenital Q24.6
    first degree (atrioventricular) I44.0
    second degree (atrioventricular) I44.1
    specified type NEC I45.5
    third degree (atrioventricular) I44.2
  hepatic vein I82.0
  intraventricular (nonspecific) I45.4
    bundle branch
      bilateral I45.2
  kidney N28.9
    postcystoscopic or postprocedural N99.0
  Mobitz (types I and II) I44.1
  myocardial — *see* Block, heart
  nodal I45.5
  organ or site, congenital NEC — *see* Atresia, by site
  portal (vein) I81
  second degree (types I and II) I44.1
  sinoatrial I45.5
  sinoauricular I45.5
  third degree I44.2
  trifascicular I45.3
  tubal N97.1
  vein NOS I82.90
  Wenckebach (types I and II) I44.1
Blockage — *see* Obstruction
Blocq's disease F44.4
Blood
  constituents, abnormal R78.9
  disease D75.9
  donor — *see* Donor, blood
  dyscrasia D75.9
    with
      abortion — *see* Abortion, by type, complicated by, hemorrhage
      ectopic pregnancy O08.1
      molar pregnancy O08.1
    following ectopic or molar pregnancy O08.1
    newborn P61.9
    puerperal, postpartum O72.3
  flukes NEC — *see* Schistosomiasis
  in
    feces K92.1
      occult R19.5
    urine — *see* Hematuria
  mole O02.0
  occult in feces R19.5
  pressure
    decreased, due to shock following injury T79.4 ☑
    examination only Z01.30
    fluctuating I99.8
    high — *see* Hypertension
      borderline R03.0
      incidental reading, without diagnosis of hypertension R03.0
    low (*see also* Hypotension)
      incidental reading, without diagnosis of hypotension R03.1
  spitting — *see* Hemoptysis
  staining cornea — *see* Pigmentation, cornea, stromal
  transfusion
    reaction or complication — *see* Complications, transfusion
  type
    A (Rh positive) Z67.10
      Rh negative Z67.11
    AB (Rh positive) Z67.30
      Rh negative Z67.31
    B (Rh positive) Z67.20
      Rh negative Z67.21
    O (Rh positive) Z67.40
      Rh negative Z67.41

Blood — *continued*
  type — *continued*
    Rh (positive) Z67.90
      negative Z67.91
  vessel rupture — *see* Hemorrhage
  vomiting — *see* Hematemesis
Blood-forming organs, disease D75.9
Bloodgood's disease — *see* Mastopathy, cystic
Bloom (-Machacek)(-Torre) **syndrome** Q82.8
Blount's disease or osteochondrosis — *see* Osteochondrosis, juvenile, tibia
Blue
  baby Q24.9
  diaper syndrome E72.09
  dome cyst (breast) — *see* Cyst, breast
  dot cataract Q12.0
  nevus D22.9
  sclera Q13.5
    with fragility of bone and deafness Q78.0
  toe syndrome I75.02- ☑
Blueness — *see* Cyanosis
Blues, postpartal O90.6
  baby O90.6
Blurring, visual H53.8
Blushing (abnormal) (excessive) R23.2
BMI — *see* Body, mass index
Boarder, hospital NEC Z76.4
  accompanying sick person Z76.3
  healthy infant or child Z76.2
    foundling Z76.1
Bockhart's impetigo L01.02
Bodechtel-Guttman disease (subacute sclerosing panencephalitis) A81.1
Boder-Sedgwick syndrome (ataxia-telangiectasia) G11.3
Body, bodies
  Aschoff's — *see* Myocarditis, rheumatic
  asteroid, vitreous — *see* Deposit, crystalline
  cytoid (retina) — *see* Occlusion, artery, retina
  drusen (degenerative) (macula) (retinal) (*see also* Degeneration, macula, drusen)
    optic disc — *see* Drusen, optic disc
  foreign — *see* Foreign body
  loose
    joint, except knee — *see* Loose, body, joint
      knee M23.4- ☑
    sheath, tendon — *see* Disorder, tendon, specified type NEC
  mass index (BMI)
    adult
      19.9 or less Z68.1
      20.0-20.9 Z68.20
      21.0-21.9 Z68.21
      22.0-22.9 Z68.22
      23.0-23.9 Z68.23
      24.0-24.9 Z68.24
      25.0-25.9 Z68.25
      26.0-26.9 Z68.26
      27.0-27.9 Z68.27
      28.0-28.9 Z68.28
      29.0-29.9 Z68.29
      30.0-30.9 Z68.30
      31.0-31.9 Z68.31
      32.0-32.9 Z68.32
      33.0-33.9 Z68.33
      34.0-34.9 Z68.34
      35.0-35.9 Z68.35
      36.0-36.9 Z68.36
      37.0-37.9 Z68.37
      38.0-38.9 Z68.38
      39.0-39.9 Z68.39
      40.0-44.9 Z68.41
      45.0-49.9 Z68.42
      50.0-59.9 Z68.43
      60.0-69.9 Z68.44
      70 and over Z68.45
    pediatric
      5th percentile to less than 85th percentile for age Z68.52
      85th percentile to less than 95th percentile for age Z68.53
      less than fifth percentile for age Z68.51
      greater than or equal to ninety-fifth percentile for age Z68.54
  Mooser's A75.2
  rice (*see also* Loose, body, joint)
    knee M23.4- ☑
  rocking F98.4

☑ **Additional Character Required — Refer to the Tabular List for Character Selection**   ▽ᴿᴱˣ **Subterms under main terms may continue to next column or page**

Boeck's
　disease or sarcoid — *see* Sarcoidosis
　lupoid (miliary) D86.3
Boerhaave's syndrome (spontaneous esophageal rupture) K22.3
Boggy
　cervix N88.8
　uterus N85.8
Boil (*see also* Furuncle, by site)
　Aleppo B55.1
　Baghdad B55.1
　Delhi B55.1
　lacrimal
　　gland — *see* Dacryoadenitis
　　passages (duct) (sac) — *see* Inflammation, lacrimal, passages, acute
　Natal B55.1
　orbit, orbital — *see* Abscess, orbit
　tropical B55.1
Bold hives — *see* Urticaria
Bombé, iris — *see* Membrane, pupillary
Bone — *see* condition
Bonnevie-Ullrich syndrome (*see also* Turner's syndrome) Q87.1
Bonnier's syndrome H81.8 ☑
Bonvale dam fever T73.3 ☑
Bony block of joint — *see* Ankylosis
BOOP (bronchiolitis obliterans organized pneumonia) J84.89
Borderline
　diabetes mellitus R73.03
　hypertension R03.0
　osteopenia M85.8- ☑
　pelvis, with obstruction during labor O65.1
　personality F60.3
Borna disease A83.9
Bornholm disease B33.0
Boston exanthem A88.0
Botalli, ductus (patent) (persistent) Q25.0
Bothriocephalus latus infestation B70.0
Botulism (foodborne intoxication) A05.1
　infant A48.51
　non-foodborne A48.52
　wound A48.52
Bouba — *see* Yaws
Bouchard's nodes (with arthropathy) M15.2
Bouffée délirante F23
Bouillaud's disease or syndrome (rheumatic heart disease) I01.9
Bourneville's disease Q85.1
Boutonniere deformity (finger) — *see* Deformity, finger, boutonniere
Bouveret (-Hoffmann) **syndrome** (paroxysmal tachycardia) I47.9
Bovine heart — *see* Hypertrophy, cardiac
Bowel — *see* condition
Bowen's
　dermatosis (precancerous) — *see* Neoplasm, skin, in situ
　disease — *see* Neoplasm, skin, in situ
　epithelioma — *see* Neoplasm, skin, in situ
　type
　　epidermoid carcinoma-in-situ — *see* Neoplasm, skin, in situ
　　intraepidermal squamous cell carcinoma — *see* Neoplasm, skin, in situ
Bowing
　femur (*see also* Deformity, limb, specified type NEC, thigh)
　　congenital Q68.3
　fibula (*see also* Deformity, limb, specified type NEC, lower leg)
　　congenital Q68.4
　forearm — *see* Deformity, limb, specified type NEC, forearm
　leg(s), long bones, congenital Q68.5
　radius — *see* Deformity, limb, specified type NEC, forearm
　tibia (*see also* Deformity, limb, specified type NEC, lower leg)
　　congenital Q68.4
Bowleg(s) (acquired) M21.16- ☑
　congenital Q68.5
　rachitic E64.3
Boyd's dysentery A03.2
Brachial — *see* condition
Brachycardia R00.1

Brachycephaly Q75.0
Bradley's disease A08.19
Bradyarrhythmia, cardiac I49.8
Bradycardia (sinoatrial) (sinus) (vagal) R00.1
　neonatal P29.12
　reflex G90.09
　tachycardia syndrome I49.5
Bradykinesia R25.8
Bradypnea R06.89
Bradytachycardia I49.5
Brailsford's disease or osteochondrosis — *see* Osteochondrosis, juvenile, radius
Brain (*see also* condition)
　death G93.82
　syndrome — *see* Syndrome, brain
Branched-chain amino-acid disorder E71.2
Branchial — *see* condition
　cartilage, congenital Q18.2
Branchiogenic remnant (in neck) Q18.0
Brandt's syndrome (acrodermatitis enteropathica) E83.2
Brash (water) R12
Bravais-jacksonian epilepsy — *see* Epilepsy, localization-related, symptomatic, with simple partial seizures
Braxton Hicks contractions — *see* False, labor
Brazilian leishmaniasis B55.2
BRBPR K62.5
Break, retina (without detachment) H33.30- ☑
　with retinal detachment — *see* Detachment, retina
　horseshoe tear H33.31- ☑
　multiple H33.33- ☑
　round hole H33.32- ☑
Breakdown
　device, graft or implant (*see also* Complications, by site and type, mechanical) T85.618 ☑
　　arterial graft NEC — *see* Complication, cardiovascular device, mechanical, vascular
　　breast (implant) T85.41 ☑
　　catheter NEC T85.618 ☑
　　　cystostomy T83.010 ☑
　　　dialysis (renal) T82.41 ☑
　　　　intraperitoneal T85.611 ☑
　　　Hopkins T83.018 ☑
　　　ileostomy T83.018 ☑
　　　infusion NEC T82.514 ☑
　　　　cranial T85.610- ☑
　　　　epidural T85.610 ☑
　　　　intrathecal T85.610 ☑
　　　　spinal T85.610 ☑
　　　　subarachnoid T85.610 ☑
　　　　subdural T85.610 ☑
　　　nephrostomy T83.012 ☑
　　　urethral indwelling T83.011 ☑
　　　urinary NEC T83.018 ☑
　　　urostomy T83.018 ☑
　　electronic (electrode) (pulse generator) (stimulator)
　　　bone T84.310 ☑
　　　cardiac T82.119 ☑
　　　　electrode T82.110 ☑
　　　　pulse generator T82.111 ☑
　　　　specified type NEC T82.118 ☑
　　　nervous system — *see* Complication, prosthetic device, mechanical, electronic nervous system stimulator
　　　urinary — *see* Complication, genitourinary, device, urinary, mechanical
　　fixation, internal (orthopedic) NEC — *see* Complication, fixation device, mechanical
　　gastrointestinal — *see* Complications, prosthetic device, mechanical, gastrointestinal device
　　genital NEC T83.418 ☑
　　　intrauterine contraceptive device T83.31 ☑
　　　penile prosthesis (cylinder) (implanted) (pump) (resevoir) T83.410 ☑
　　　testicular prosthesis T83.411 ☑
　　heart NEC — *see* Complication, cardiovascular device, mechanical
　　intrathecal infusion pump T85.615 ☑
　　joint prosthesis — *see* Complications..., joint prosthesis, internal, mechanical, by site
　　nervous system, specified device NEC T85.615 ☑
　　ocular NEC — *see* Complications, prosthetic device, mechanical, ocular device
　　orthopedic NEC — *see* Complication, orthopedic, device, mechanical
　　specified NEC T85.618 ☑

Breakdown — *continued*
　device, graft or implant (*see also* Complications, by site and type, mechanical) — *continued*
　　subcutaneous device pocket
　　　nervous system prosthetic device, implant, or graft T85.890 ☑
　　　other internal prosthetic device, implant, or graft T85.898 ☑
　　sutures, permanent T85.612 ☑
　　　used in bone repair — *see* Complications, fixation device, internal (orthopedic), mechanical
　　urinary NEC T83.118 ☑
　　　graft T83.21 ☑
　　　sphincter, implanted T83.111 ☑
　　　stent (ileal conduit) (nephroureteral) T83.113 ☑
　　　　ureteral indwelling T83.112 ☑
　　vascular NEC — *see* Complication, cardiovascular device, mechanical
　　ventricular intracranial shunt T85.01 ☑
　nervous F48.8
　perineum O90.1
　respirator J95.850
　　specified NEC J95.859
　ventilator J95.850
　　specified NEC J95.859
Breast (*see also* condition)
　buds E30.1
　　in newborn P96.89
　dense R92.2
　nodule (*see also* Lump, breast) N63.0
Breath
　foul R19.6
　holder, child R06.89
　holding spell R06.89
　shortness R06.02
Breathing
　labored — *see* Hyperventilation
　mouth R06.5
　　causing malocclusion M26.5 ☑
　periodic R06.3
　　high altitude G47.32
Breathlessness R06.81
Breda's disease — *see* Yaws
Breech presentation (mother) O32.1 ☑
　causing obstructed labor O64.1 ☑
　footling O32.8 ☑
　　causing obstructed labor O64.8 ☑
　incomplete O32.8 ☑
　　causing obstructed labor O64.8 ☑
Breisky's disease N90.4
Brennemann's syndrome I88.0
Brenner
　tumor (benign) D27.9
　　borderline malignancy D39.1- ☑
　　malignant C56 ☑
　　proliferating D39.1- ☑
Bretonneau's disease or angina A36.0
Breus' mole O02.0
Brevicollis Q76.49
Brickmakers' anemia B76.9 [D63.8]
Bridge, myocardial Q24.5
Bright red blood per rectum (BRBPR) K62.5
Bright's disease (*see also* Nephritis)
　arteriosclerotic — *see* Hypertension, kidney
Brill (-Zinsser) **disease** (recrudescent typhus) A75.1
　flea-borne A75.2
　louse-borne A75.1
Brill-Symmers' disease C82.90
Brion-Kayser disease — *see* Fever, parathyroid
Briquet's disorder or syndrome F45.0
Brissaud's
　infantilism or dwarfism E23.0
　motor-verbal tic F95.2
Brittle
　bones disease Q78.0
　nails L60.3
　　congenital Q84.6
Broad (*see also* condition)
　beta disease E78.2
　ligament laceration syndrome N83.8
Broad- or floating-betalipoproteinemia E78.2
Brock's syndrome (atelectasis due to enlarged lymph nodes) J98.19
Brocq-Duhring disease (dermatitis herpetiformis) L13.0
Brodie's abscess or disease M86.8X- ☑

Broken
arches (see also Deformity, limb, flat foot)
arm (meaning upper limb) — see Fracture, arm
back — see Fracture, vertebra
bone — see Fracture
implant or internal device — see Complications, by
    site and type, mechanical
leg (meaning lower limb) — see Fracture, leg
nose S02.2 ☑
tooth, teeth — see Fracture, tooth
Bromhidrosis, bromidrosis L75.0
Bromidism, bromism G92
chronic (dependence) F13.20
due to
    correct substance properly administered — see
        Table of Drugs and Chemicals, by drug, ad-
        verse effect
    overdose or wrong substance given or taken —
        see Table of Drugs and Chemicals, by drug,
        poisoning
Bromidrosiphobia F40.298
Bronchi, bronchial — see condition
Bronchiectasis (cylindrical) (diffuse) (fusiform) (localized)
    (saccular) J47.9
with
    acute
        bronchitis J47.0
        lower respiratory infection J47.0
    exacerbation (acute) J47.1
congenital Q33.4
tuberculous NEC — see Tuberculosis, pulmonary
Bronchiolectasis — see Bronchiectasis
Bronchiolitis (acute) (infective) (subacute) J21.9
with
    bronchospasm or obstruction J21.9
    influenza, flu or grippe — see Influenza, with, res-
        piratory manifestations NEC
chemical (chronic) J68.4
    acute J68.0
chronic (fibrosing) (obliterative) J44.9
due to
    external agent — see Bronchitis, acute, due to
    human metapneumovirus J21.1
    respiratory syncytial virus J21.0
    specified organism NEC J21.8
fibrosa obliterans J44.9
influenzal — see Influenza, with, respiratory manifes-
    tations NEC
obliterans J42
    with organizing pneumonia (BOOP) J84.89
obliterative (chronic) (subacute) J44.9
    due to chemicals, gases, fumes or vapors (inhala-
        tion) J68.4
    due to fumes or vapors J68.4
respiratory, interstitial lung disease J84.115
Bronchitis (diffuse) (fibrinous) (hypostatic) (infective)
    (membranous) J40
with
    influenza, flu or grippe — see Influenza, with, res-
        piratory manifestations NEC
    obstruction (airway) (lung) J44.9
    tracheitis (l5 years of age and above) J40
        acute or subacute J20.9
        chronic J42
        under l5 years of age J20.9
acute or subacute (with bronchospasm or obstruction)
    J20.9
with
    bronchiectasis J47.0
    chronic obstructive pulmonary disease J44.0
    chemical (due to gases, fumes or vapors) J68.0
    due to
        fumes or vapors J68.0
        Haemophilus influenzae J20.1
        Mycoplasma pneumoniae J20.0
        radiation J70.0
        specified organism NEC J20.8
        Streptococcus J20.2
        virus
            coxsackie J20.3
            echovirus J20.7
            parainfluenzae J20.4
            respiratory syncytial J20.5
            rhinovirus J20.6
        viral NEC J20.8
allergic (acute) J45.909
    with
        exacerbation (acute) J45.901

Bronchitis — continued
allergic — continued
    with — continued
        status asthmaticus J45.902
arachidic T17.528 ☑
aspiration (due to fumes or vapors) J68.0
asthmatic J45.9 ☑
    chronic J44.9
        with
            acute lower respiratory infection J44.0
            exacerbation (acute) J44.1
capillary — see Pneumonia, broncho
caseous (tuberculous) A15.5
Castellani's A69.8
catarrhal (l5 years of age and above) J40
    acute — see Bronchitis, acute
    chronic J41.0
    under l5 years of age J20.9
chemical (acute) (subacute) J68.0
    chronic J68.4
    due to fumes or vapors J68.0
        chronic J68.4
chronic J42
    with
        airways obstruction J44.9
        tracheitis (chronic) J42
    asthmatic (obstructive) J44.9
    catarrhal J41.0
    chemical (due to fumes or vapors) J68.4
    due to
        chemicals, gases, fumes or vapors (inhalation)
            J68.4
        radiation J70.1
        tobacco smoking J41.0
    emphysematous J44.9
    mucopurulent J41.1
    non-obstructive J41.0
    obliterans J44.9
    obstructive J44.9
    purulent J41.1
    simple J41.0
croupous — see Bronchitis, acute
due to gases, fumes or vapors (chemical) J68.0
emphysematous (obstructive) J44.9
exudative — see Bronchitis, acute
fetid J41.1
grippal — see Influenza, with, respiratory manifesta-
    tions NEC
in those under l5 years age — see Bronchitis, acute
    chronic — see Bronchitis, chronic
influenzal — see Influenza, with, respiratory manifes-
    tations NEC
mixed simple and mucopurulent J41.8
moulder's J62.8
mucopurulent (chronic) (recurrent) J41.1
    acute or subacute J20.9
    simple (mixed) J41.8
obliterans (chronic) J44.9
obstructive (chronic) (diffuse) J44.9
pituitous J41.1
pneumococcal, acute or subacute J20.2
pseudomembranous, acute or subacute — see Bron-
    chitis, acute
purulent (chronic) (recurrent) J41.1
    acute or subacute — see Bronchitis, acute
putrid J41.1
senile (chronic) J42
simple and mucopurulent (mixed) J41.8
smokers' J41.0
spirochetal NEC A69.8
subacute — see Bronchitis, acute
suppurative (chronic) J41.1
    acute or subacute — see Bronchitis, acute
tuberculous A15.5
under l5 years of age — see Bronchitis, acute
    chronic — see Bronchitis, chronic
viral NEC, acute or subacute (see also Bronchitis, acute)
    J20.8
Bronchoalveolitis J18.0
Bronchoaspergillosis B44.1
Bronchocele meaning goiter E04.0
Broncholithiasis J98.09
    tuberculous NEC A15.5
Bronchomalacia J98.09
    congenital Q32.2
Bronchomycosis NOS B49 [J99]
    candidal B37.1
Bronchopleuropneumonia — see Pneumonia, broncho

Bronchopneumonia — see Pneumonia, broncho
Bronchopneumonitis — see Pneumonia, broncho
Bronchopulmonary — see condition
Bronchopulmonitis — see Pneumonia, broncho
Bronchorrhagia (see Hemoptysis)
Bronchorrhea J98.09
    acute J20.9
    chronic (infective) (purulent) J42
Bronchospasm (acute) J98.01
    with
        bronchiolitis, acute J21.9
        bronchitis, acute (conditions in J20) — see Bronchi-
            tis, acute
    due to external agent — see condition, respiratory,
        acute, due to
    exercise induced J45.990
Bronchospirochetosis A69.8
    Castellani A69.8
Bronchostenosis J98.09
Bronchus — see condition
Brontophobia F40.220
Bronze baby syndrome P83.88
Brooke's tumor — see Neoplasm, skin, benign
Brown enamel of teeth (hereditary) K00.5
Brown's sheath syndrome H50.61- ☑
Brown-Séquard disease, paralysis or syndrome
    G83.81
Bruce sepsis A23.0
Brucellosis (infection) A23.9
    abortus A23.1
    canis A23.3
    dermatitis A23.9
    melitensis A23.0
    mixed A23.8
    sepsis A23.9
        melitensis A23.0
        specified NEC A23.8
    suis A23.2
Bruck-de Lange disease Q87.1
Bruck's disease — see Deformity, limb
BRUE (brief resolved unexplained event) R68.13
Brugsch's syndrome Q82.8
Bruise (skin surface intact) (see also Contusion)
    with
        open wound — see Wound, open
    internal organ — see Injury, by site
    newborn P54.5
    scalp, due to birth injury, newborn P12.3
    umbilical cord O69.5 ☑
Bruit (arterial) R09.89
    cardiac R01.1
Brush burn — see Abrasion, by site
Bruton's X-linked agammaglobulinemia D80.0
Bruxism
    psychogenic F45.8
    sleep related G47.63
Bubbly lung syndrome P27.0
Bubo I88.8
    blennorrhagic (gonococcal) A54.89
    chancroidal A57
    climatic A55
    due to Haemophilus ducreyi A57
    gonococcal A54.89
    indolent (nonspecific) I88.8
    inguinal (nonspecific) I88.8
        chancroidal A57
        climatic A55
        due to H. ducreyi A57
        infective I88.8
    scrofulous (tuberculous) A18.2
    soft chancre A57
    suppurating — see Lymphadenitis, acute
    syphilitic (primary) A51.0
        congenital A50.07
    tropical A55
    virulent (chancroidal) A57
Bubonic plague A20.0
Bubonocele — see Hernia, inguinal
Buccal — see condition
Buchanan's disease or osteochondrosis M91.0
Buchem's syndrome (hyperostosis corticalis) M85.2
Bucket-handle fracture or tear (semilunar cartilage)
    — see Tear, meniscus
Budd-Chiari syndrome (hepatic vein thrombosis) I82.0
Budgerigar fancier's disease or lung J67.2
Buds
    breast E30.1

Buds — *continued*
  breast — *continued*
    in newborn P96.89
Buerger's disease (thromboangiitis obliterans) I73.1
Bulbar — *see* condition
Bulbus cordis (left ventricle) (persistent) Q21.8
Bulimia (nervosa) F50.2
  atypical F50.9
  normal weight F50.9
Bulky
  stools R19.5
  uterus N85.2
Bulla (e) R23.8
  lung (emphysematous) (solitary) J43.9
    newborn P25.8
Bullet wound (*see also* Wound, open)
  fracture — *code as* Fracture, by site
  internal organ — *see* Injury, by site
Bundle
  branch block (complete) (false) (incomplete) — *see*
    Block, bundle-branch
  of His — *see* condition
Bunion M21.61- ☑
  tailor's M21.62- ☑
Bunionette M21.62- ☑
Buphthalmia, buphthalmos (congenital) Q15.0
Burdwan fever B55.0
Bürger-Grütz disease or syndrome E78.3
Buried
  penis (congenital) Q55.64
    acquired N48.83
  roots K08.3
Burke's syndrome K86.89
Burkitt
  cell leukemia C91.0- ☑
  lymphoma (malignant) C83.7- ☑
    small noncleaved, diffuse C83.7- ☑
    spleen C83.77
    undifferentiated C83.7- ☑
  tumor C83.7- ☑
  type
    acute lymphoblastic leukemia C91.0- ☑
    undifferentiated C83.7- ☑
Burn (electricity) (flame) (hot gas, liquid or hot object)
  (radiation) (steam) (thermal) T30.0
  abdomen, abdominal (muscle) (wall) T21.02 ☑
    first degree T21.12 ☑
    second degree T21.22 ☑
    third degree T21.32 ☑
  above elbow T22.039 ☑
    first degree T22.139 ☑
    left T22.032 ☑
      first degree T22.132 ☑
      second degree T22.232 ☑
      third degree T22.332 ☑
    right T22.031 ☑
      first degree T22.131 ☑
      second degree T22.231 ☑
      third degree T22.331 ☑
    second degree T22.239 ☑
    third degree T22.339 ☑
  acid (caustic) (external) (internal) — *see* Corrosion, by
    site
  alimentary tract NEC T28.2 ☑
    esophagus T28.1 ☑
    mouth T28.0 ☑
    pharynx T28.0 ☑
  alkaline (caustic) (external) (internal) — *see* Corrosion,
    by site
  ankle T25.019 ☑
    first degree T25.119 ☑
    left T25.012 ☑
      first degree T25.112 ☑
      second degree T25.212 ☑
      third degree T25.312 ☑
    multiple with foot — *see* Burn, lower, limb, multi-
      ple, ankle and foot
    right T25.011 ☑
      first degree T25.111 ☑
      second degree T25.211 ☑
      third degree T25.311 ☑
    second degree T25.219 ☑
    third degree T25.319 ☑
  anus — *see* Burn, buttock
  arm (lower) (upper) — *see* Burn, upper, limb
  axilla T22.049 ☑

Burn — *continued*
  axilla — *continued*
    first degree T22.149 ☑
    left T22.042 ☑
      first degree T22.142 ☑
      second degree T22.242 ☑
      third degree T22.342 ☑
    right T22.041 ☑
      first degree T22.141 ☑
      second degree T22.241 ☑
      third degree T22.341 ☑
    second degree T22.249 ☑
    third degree T22.349 ☑
  back (lower) T21.04 ☑
    first degree T21.14 ☑
    second degree T21.24 ☑
    third degree T21.34 ☑
    upper T21.03 ☑
      first degree T21.13 ☑
      second degree T21.23 ☑
      third degree T21.33 ☑
  blisters — *code as* Burn, second degree, by site
  breast(s) — *see* Burn, chest wall
  buttock(s) T21.05 ☑
    first degree T21.15 ☑
    second degree T21.25 ☑
    third degree T21.35 ☑
  calf T24.039 ☑
    first degree T24.139 ☑
    left T24.032 ☑
      first degree T24.132 ☑
      second degree T24.232 ☑
      third degree T24.332 ☑
    right T24.031 ☑
      first degree T24.131 ☑
      second degree T24.231 ☑
      third degree T24.331 ☑
    second degree T24.239 ☑
    third degree T24.339 ☑
  canthus (eye) — *see* Burn, eyelid
  caustic acid or alkaline — *see* Corrosion, by site
  cervix T28.3 ☑
  cheek T20.06 ☑
    first degree T20.16 ☑
    second degree T20.26 ☑
    third degree T20.36 ☑
  chemical (acids) (alkalines) (caustics) (external) (inter-
    nal) — *see* Corrosion, by site
  chest wall T21.01 ☑
    first degree T21.11 ☑
    second degree T21.21 ☑
    third degree T21.31 ☑
  chin T20.03 ☑
    first degree T20.13 ☑
    second degree T20.23 ☑
    third degree T20.33 ☑
  colon T28.2 ☑
  conjunctiva (and cornea) — *see* Burn, cornea
  cornea (and conjunctiva) T26.1- ☑
    chemical — *see* Corrosion, cornea
  corrosion (external) (internal) — *see* Corrosion, by site
  deep necrosis of underlying tissue — *code as* Burn,
    third degree, by site
  dorsum of hand T23.069 ☑
    first degree T23.169 ☑
    left T23.062 ☑
      first degree T23.162 ☑
      second degree T23.262 ☑
      third degree T23.362 ☑
    right T23.061 ☑
      first degree T23.161 ☑
      second degree T23.261 ☑
      third degree T23.361 ☑
    second degree T23.269 ☑
    third degree T23.369 ☑
  due to ingested chemical agent — *see* Corrosion, by
    site
  ear (auricle) (external) (canal) T20.01 ☑
    first degree T20.11 ☑
    second degree T20.21 ☑
    third degree T20.31 ☑
  elbow T22.029 ☑
    first degree T22.129 ☑
    left T22.022 ☑
      first degree T22.122 ☑
      second degree T22.222 ☑

Burn — *continued*
  elbow — *continued*
    left — *continued*
      third degree T22.322 ☑
    right T22.021 ☑
      first degree T22.121 ☑
      second degree T22.221 ☑
      third degree T22.321 ☑
    second degree T22.229 ☑
    third degree T22.329 ☑
  epidermal loss — *code as* Burn, second degree, by site
  erythema, erythematous — *code as* Burn, first degree,
    by site
  esophagus T28.1 ☑
  extent (percentage of body surface)
    less than 10 percent T31.0
    10-19 percent T31.10
      with 0-9 percent third degree burns T31.10
      with 10-19 percent third degree burns T31.11
    20-29 percent T31.20
      with 0-9 percent third degree burns T31.20
      with 10-19 percent third degree burns T31.21
      with 20-29 percent third degree burns T31.22
    30-39 percent T31.30
      with 0-9 percent third degree burns T31.30
      with 10-19 percent third degree burns T31.31
      with 20-29 percent third degree burns T31.32
      with 30-39 percent third degree burns T31.33
    40-49 percent T31.40
      with 0-9 percent third degree burns T31.40
      with 10-19 percent third degree burns T31.41
      with 20-29 percent third degree burns T31.42
      with 30-39 percent third degree burns T31.43
      with 40-49 percent third degree burns T31.44
    50-59 percent T31.50
      with 0-9 percent third degree burns T31.50
      with 10-19 percent third degree burns T31.51
      with 20-29 percent third degree burns T31.52
      with 30-39 percent third degree burns T31.53
      with 40-49 percent third degree burns T31.54
      with 50-59 percent third degree burns T31.55
    60-69 percent T31.60
      with 0-9 percent third degree burns T31.60
      with 10-19 percent third degree burns T31.61
      with 20-29 percent third degree burns T31.62
      with 30-39 percent third degree burns T31.63
      with 40-49 percent third degree burns T31.64
      with 50-59 percent third degree burns T31.65
      with 60-69 percent third degree burns T31.66
    70-79 percent T31.70
      with 0-9 percent third degree burns T31.70
      with 10-19 percent third degree burns T31.71
      with 20-29 percent third degree burns T31.72
      with 30-39 percent third degree burns T31.73
      with 40-49 percent third degree burns T31.74
      with 50-59 percent third degree burns T31.75
      with 60-69 percent third degree burns T31.76
      with 70-79 percent third degree burns T31.77
    80-89 percent T31.80
      with 0-9 percent third degree burns T31.80
      with 10-19 percent third degree burns T31.81
      with 20-29 percent third degree burns T31.82
      with 30-39 percent third degree burns T31.83
      with 40-49 percent third degree burns T31.84
      with 50-59 percent third degree burns T31.85
      with 60-69 percent third degree burns T31.86
      with 70-79 percent third degree burns T31.87
      with 80-89 percent third degree burns T31.88
    90 percent or more T31.90
      with 0-9 percent third degree burns T31.90
      with 10-19 percent third degree burns T31.91
      with 20-29 percent third degree burns T31.92
      with 30-39 percent third degree burns T31.93
      with 40-49 percent third degree burns T31.94
      with 50-59 percent third degree burns T31.95
      with 60-69 percent third degree burns T31.96
      with 70-79 percent third degree burns T31.97
      with 80-89 percent third degree burns T31.98
      with 90 percent or more third degree burns
        T31.99
  extremity — *see* Burn, limb
  eye(s) and adnexa T26.4- ☑
    with resulting rupture and destruction of eyeball
      T26.2- ☑
    conjunctival sac — *see* Burn, cornea
    cornea — *see* Burn, cornea
    lid — *see* Burn, eyelid
    periocular area — *see* Burn, eyelid

Burn — *continued*
- eye(s) and adnexa — *continued*
  - specified site NEC T26.3- ☑
- eyeball — *see* Burn, eye
- eyelid(s) T26.0- ☑
  - chemical — *see* Corrosion, eyelid
- face — *see* Burn, head
- finger T23.029 ☑
  - first degree T23.129 ☑
  - left T23.022 ☑
    - first degree T23.122 ☑
    - second degree T23.222 ☑
    - third degree T23.322 ☑
  - multiple sites (without thumb) T23.039 ☑
    - with thumb T23.049 ☑
      - first degree T23.149 ☑
      - left T23.042 ☑
        - first degree T23.142 ☑
        - second degree T23.242 ☑
        - third degree T23.342 ☑
      - right T23.041 ☑
        - first degree T23.141 ☑
        - second degree T23.241 ☑
        - third degree T23.341 ☑
      - second degree T23.249 ☑
      - third degree T23.349 ☑
    - first degree T23.139 ☑
    - left T23.032 ☑
      - first degree T23.132 ☑
      - second degree T23.232 ☑
      - third degree T23.332 ☑
    - right T23.031 ☑
      - first degree T23.131 ☑
      - second degree T23.231 ☑
      - third degree T23.331 ☑
    - second degree T23.239 ☑
    - third degree T23.339 ☑
  - right T23.021 ☑
    - first degree T23.121 ☑
    - second degree T23.221 ☑
    - third degree T23.321 ☑
  - second degree T23.229 ☑
  - third degree T23.329 ☑
- flank — *see* Burn, abdominal wall
- foot T25.029 ☑
  - first degree T25.129 ☑
  - left T25.022 ☑
    - first degree T25.122 ☑
    - second degree T25.222 ☑
    - third degree T25.322 ☑
  - multiple with ankle — *see* Burn, lower, limb, multiple, ankle and foot
  - right T25.021 ☑
    - first degree T25.121 ☑
    - second degree T25.221 ☑
    - third degree T25.321 ☑
  - second degree T25.229 ☑
  - third degree T25.329 ☑
- forearm T22.019 ☑
  - first degree T22.119 ☑
  - left T22.012 ☑
    - first degree T22.112 ☑
    - second degree T22.212 ☑
    - third degree T22.312 ☑
  - right T22.011 ☑
    - first degree T22.111 ☑
    - second degree T22.211 ☑
    - third degree T22.311 ☑
  - second degree T22.219 ☑
  - third degree T22.319 ☑
- forehead T20.06 ☑
  - first degree T20.16 ☑
  - second degree T20.26 ☑
  - third degree T20.36 ☑
- fourth degree — *code as* Burn, third degree, by site
- friction — *see* Burn, by site
- from swallowing caustic or corrosive substance NEC — *see* Corrosion, by site
- full thickness skin loss — *code as* Burn, third degree, by site
- gastrointestinal tract NEC T28.2 ☑
  - from swallowing caustic or corrosive substance T28.7 ☑
- genital organs
  - external
    - female T21.07 ☑

Burn — *continued*
- genital organs — *continued*
  - external — *continued*
    - female — *continued*
      - first degree T21.17 ☑
      - second degree T21.27 ☑
      - third degree T21.37 ☑
    - male T21.06 ☑
      - first degree T21.16 ☑
      - second degree T21.26 ☑
      - third degree T21.36 ☑
  - internal T28.3 ☑
    - from caustic or corrosive substance T28.8 ☑
- groin — *see* Burn, abdominal wall
- hand(s) T23.009 ☑
  - back — *see* Burn, dorsum of hand
  - finger — *see* Burn, finger
  - first degree T23.109 ☑
  - left T23.002 ☑
    - first degree T23.102 ☑
    - second degree T23.202 ☑
    - third degree T23.302 ☑
  - multiple sites with wrist T23.099 ☑
    - first degree T23.199 ☑
    - left T23.092 ☑
      - first degree T23.192 ☑
      - second degree T23.292 ☑
      - third degree T23.392 ☑
    - right T23.091 ☑
      - first degree T23.191 ☑
      - second degree T23.291 ☑
      - third degree T23.391 ☑
    - second degree T23.299 ☑
    - third degree T23.399 ☑
  - palm — *see* Burn, palm
  - right T23.001 ☑
    - first degree T23.101 ☑
    - second degree T23.201 ☑
    - third degree T23.301 ☑
  - second degree T23.209 ☑
  - third degree T23.309 ☑
  - thumb — *see* Burn, thumb
- head (and face) (and neck) T20.00 ☑
  - cheek — *see* Burn, cheek
  - chin — *see* Burn, chin
  - ear — *see* Burn, ear
  - eye(s) only — *see* Burn, eye
  - first degree T20.10 ☑
  - forehead — *see* Burn, forehead
  - lip — *see* Burn, lip
  - multiple sites T20.09 ☑
    - first degree T20.19 ☑
    - second degree T20.29 ☑
    - third degree T20.39 ☑
  - neck — *see* Burn, neck
  - nose — *see* Burn, nose
  - scalp — *see* Burn, scalp
  - second degree T20.20 ☑
  - third degree T20.30 ☑
- hip(s) — *see* Burn, thigh
- inhalation — *see* Burn, respiratory tract
  - caustic or corrosive substance (fumes) — *see* Corrosion, respiratory tract
- internal organ(s) T28.40 ☑
  - alimentary tract T28.2 ☑
    - esophagus T28.1 ☑
  - eardrum T28.41 ☑
  - esophagus T28.1 ☑
  - from caustic or corrosive substance (swallowing) NEC — *see* Corrosion, by site
  - genitourinary T28.3 ☑
  - mouth T28.0 ☑
  - pharynx T28.0 ☑
  - respiratory tract — *see* Burn, respiratory tract
  - specified organ NEC T28.49 ☑
- interscapular region — *see* Burn, back, upper
- intestine (large) (small) T28.2 ☑
- knee T24.029 ☑
  - first degree T24.129 ☑
  - left T24.022 ☑
    - first degree T24.122 ☑
    - second degree T24.222 ☑
    - third degree T24.322 ☑
  - right T24.021 ☑
    - first degree T24.121 ☑
    - second degree T24.221 ☑

Burn — *continued*
- knee — *continued*
  - right — *continued*
    - third degree T24.321 ☑
  - second degree T24.229 ☑
  - third degree T24.329 ☑
- labium (majus) (minus) — *see* Burn, genital organs, external, female
- lacrimal apparatus, duct, gland or sac — *see* Burn, eye, specified site NEC
- larynx T27.0 ☑
  - with lung T27.1 ☑
- leg(s) (lower) (upper) — *see* Burn, lower, limb
- lightning — *see* Burn, by site
- limb(s)
  - lower (except ankle or foot alone) — *see* Burn, lower, limb
  - upper — *see* Burn, upper limb
- lip(s) T20.02 ☑
  - first degree T20.12 ☑
  - second degree T20.22 ☑
  - third degree T20.32 ☑
- lower
  - back — *see* Burn, back
  - limb T24.009 ☑
    - ankle — *see* Burn, ankle
    - calf — *see* Burn, calf
    - first degree T24.109 ☑
    - foot — *see* Burn, foot
    - hip — *see* Burn, thigh
    - knee — *see* Burn, knee
    - left T24.002 ☑
      - first degree T24.102 ☑
      - second degree T24.202 ☑
      - third degree T24.302 ☑
    - multiple sites, except ankle and foot T24.099 ☑
      - ankle and foot T25.099 ☑
        - first degree T25.199 ☑
        - left T25.092 ☑
          - first degree T25.192 ☑
          - second degree T25.292 ☑
          - third degree T25.392 ☑
        - right T25.091 ☑
          - first degree T25.191 ☑
          - second degree T25.291 ☑
          - third degree T25.391 ☑
        - second degree T25.299 ☑
        - third degree T25.399 ☑
      - first degree T24.199 ☑
      - left T24.092 ☑
        - first degree T24.192 ☑
        - second degree T24.292 ☑
        - third degree T24.392 ☑
      - right T24.091 ☑
        - first degree T24.191 ☑
        - second degree T24.291 ☑
        - third degree T24.391 ☑
      - second degree T24.299 ☑
      - third degree T24.399 ☑
    - right T24.001 ☑
      - first degree T24.101 ☑
      - second degree T24.201 ☑
      - third degree T24.301 ☑
    - second degree T24.209 ☑
    - thigh — *see* Burn, thigh
    - third degree T24.309 ☑
    - toe — *see* Burn, toe
- lung (with larynx and trachea) T27.1 ☑
- mouth T28.0 ☑
- neck T20.07 ☑
  - first degree T20.17 ☑
  - second degree T20.27 ☑
  - third degree T20.37 ☑
- nose (septum) T20.04 ☑
  - first degree T20.14 ☑
  - second degree T20.24 ☑
  - third degree T20.34 ☑
- ocular adnexa — *see* Burn, eye
- orbit region — *see* Burn, eyelid
- palm T23.059 ☑
  - first degree T23.159 ☑
  - left T23.052 ☑
    - first degree T23.152 ☑
    - second degree T23.252 ☑
    - third degree T23.352 ☑
  - right T23.051 ☑

☑ Additional Character Required — Refer to the Tabular List for Character Selection   🔻 Subterms under main terms may continue to next column or page

Burn — *continued*
- palm — *continued*
  - right — *continued*
    - first degree T23.151 ☑
    - second degree T23.251 ☑
    - third degree T23.351 ☑
  - second degree T23.259 ☑
  - third degree T23.359 ☑
- partial thickness — *code as* Burn, unspecified degree, by site
- pelvis — *see* Burn, trunk
- penis — *see* Burn, genital organs, external, male
- perineum
  - female — *see* Burn, genital organs, external, female
  - male — *see* Burn, genital organs, external, male
- periocular area — *see* Burn, eyelid
- pharynx T28.0 ☑
- rectum T28.2 ☑
- respiratory tract T27.3 ☑
  - larynx — *see* Burn, larynx
  - specified part NEC T27.2 ☑
  - trachea — *see* Burn, trachea
- sac, lacrimal — *see* Burn, eye, specified site NEC
- scalp T20.05 ☑
  - first degree T20.15 ☑
  - second degree T20.25 ☑
  - third degree T20.35 ☑
- scapular region T22.069 ☑
  - first degree T22.169 ☑
  - left T22.062 ☑
    - first degree T22.162 ☑
    - second degree T22.262 ☑
    - third degree T22.362 ☑
  - right T22.061 ☑
    - first degree T22.161 ☑
    - second degree T22.261 ☑
    - third degree T22.361 ☑
  - second degree T22.269 ☑
  - third degree T22.369 ☑
- sclera — *see* Burn, eye, specified site NEC
- scrotum — *see* Burn, genital organs, external, male
- shoulder T22.059 ☑
  - first degree T22.159 ☑
  - left T22.052 ☑
    - first degree T22.152 ☑
    - second degree T22.252 ☑
    - third degree T22.352 ☑
  - right T22.051 ☑
    - first degree T22.151 ☑
    - second degree T22.251 ☑
    - third degree T22.351 ☑
  - second degree T22.259 ☑
  - third degree T22.359 ☑
- stomach T28.2 ☑
- temple — *see* Burn, head
- testis — *see* Burn, genital organs, external, male
- thigh T24.019 ☑
  - first degree T24.119 ☑
  - left T24.012 ☑
    - first degree T24.112 ☑
    - second degree T24.212 ☑
    - third degree T24.312 ☑
  - right T24.011 ☑
    - first degree T24.111 ☑
    - second degree T24.211 ☑
    - third degree T24.311 ☑
  - second degree T24.219 ☑
  - third degree T24.319 ☑
- thorax (external) — *see* Burn, trunk
- throat (meaning pharynx) T28.0 ☑
- thumb(s) T23.019 ☑
  - first degree T23.119 ☑
  - left T23.012 ☑
    - first degree T23.112 ☑
    - second degree T23.212 ☑
    - third degree T23.312 ☑
  - multiple sites with fingers T23.049 ☑
    - first degree T23.149 ☑
    - left T23.042 ☑
      - first degree T23.142 ☑
      - second degree T23.242 ☑
      - third degree T23.342 ☑
    - right T23.041 ☑
      - first degree T23.141 ☑
      - second degree T23.241 ☑
      - third degree T23.341 ☑

Burn — *continued*
- thumb(s) — *continued*
  - multiple sites with fingers — *continued*
    - second degree T23.249 ☑
    - third degree T23.349 ☑
  - right T23.011 ☑
    - first degree T23.111 ☑
    - second degree T23.211 ☑
    - third degree T23.311 ☑
  - second degree T23.219 ☑
  - third degree T23.319 ☑
- toe T25.039 ☑
  - first degree T25.139 ☑
  - left T25.032 ☑
    - first degree T25.132 ☑
    - second degree T25.232 ☑
    - third degree T25.332 ☑
  - right T25.031 ☑
    - first degree T25.131 ☑
    - second degree T25.231 ☑
    - third degree T25.331 ☑
  - second degree T25.239 ☑
  - third degree T25.339 ☑
- tongue T28.0 ☑
- tonsil(s) T28.0 ☑
- trachea T27.0 ☑
  - with lung T27.1 ☑
- trunk T21.00 ☑
  - abdominal wall — *see* Burn, abdominal wall
  - anus — *see* Burn, buttock
  - axilla — *see* Burn, upper limb
  - back — *see* Burn, back
  - breast — *see* Burn, chest wall
  - buttock — *see* Burn, buttock
  - chest wall — *see* Burn, chest wall
  - first degree T21.10 ☑
  - flank — *see* Burn, abdominal wall
  - genital
    - female — *see* Burn, genital organs, external, female
    - male — *see* Burn, genital organs, external, male
  - groin — *see* Burn, abdominal wall
  - interscapular region — *see* Burn, back, upper
  - labia — *see* Burn, genital organs, external, female
  - lower back — *see* Burn, back
  - penis — *see* Burn, genital organs, external, male
  - perineum
    - female — *see* Burn, genital organs, external, female
    - male — *see* Burn, genital organs, external, male
  - scapula region — *see* Burn, scapular region
  - scrotum — *see* Burn, genital organs, external, male
  - second degree T21.20 ☑
  - specified site NEC T21.09 ☑
    - first degree T21.19 ☑
    - second degree T21.29 ☑
    - third degree T21.39 ☑
  - testes — *see* Burn, genital organs, external, male
  - third degree T21.30 ☑
  - upper back — *see* Burn, back, upper
  - vulva — *see* Burn, genital organs, external, female
- unspecified site with extent of body surface involved specified
  - less than 10 percent T31.0
  - 10-19 percent (0-9 percent third degree) T31.10
    - with 10-19 percent third degree T31.11
  - 20-29 percent (0-9 percent third degree) T31.20
    - with
      - 10-19 percent third degree T31.21
      - 20-29 percent third degree T31.22
  - 30-39 percent (0-9 percent third degree) T31.30
    - with
      - 10-19 percent third degree T31.31
      - 20-29 percent third degree T31.32
      - 30-39 percent third degree T31.33
  - 40-49 percent (0-9 percent third degree) T31.40
    - with
      - 10-19 percent third degree T31.41
      - 20-29 percent third degree T31.42
      - 30-39 percent third degree T31.43
      - 40-49 percent third degree T31.44
  - 50-59 percent (0-9 percent third degree) T31.50
    - with
      - 10-19 percent third degree T31.51
      - 20-29 percent third degree T31.52
      - 30-39 percent third degree T31.53
      - 40-49 percent third degree T31.54

Burn — *continued*
- unspecified site with extent of body surface involved specified — *continued*
  - 50-59 percent — *continued*
    - with — *continued*
      - 50-59 percent third degree T31.55
  - 60-69 percent (0-9 percent third degree) T31.60
    - with
      - 10-19 percent third degree T31.61
      - 20-29 percent third degree T31.62
      - 30-39 percent third degree T31.63
      - 40-49 percent third degree T31.64
      - 50-59 percent third degree T31.65
      - 60-69 percent third degree T31.66
  - 70-79 percent (0-9 percent third degree) T31.70
    - with
      - 10-19 percent third degree T31.71
      - 20-29 percent third degree T31.72
      - 30-39 percent third degree T31.73
      - 40-49 percent third degree T31.74
      - 50-59 percent third degree T31.75
      - 60-69 percent third degree T31.76
      - 70-79 percent third degree T31.77
  - 80-89 percent (0-9 percent third degree) T31.80
    - with
      - 10-19 percent third degree T31.81
      - 20-29 percent third degree T31.82
      - 30-39 percent third degree T31.83
      - 40-49 percent third degree T31.84
      - 50-59 percent third degree T31.85
      - 60-69 percent third degree T31.86
      - 70-79 percent third degree T31.87
      - 80-89 percent third degree T31.88
  - 90 percent or more (0-9 percent third degree) T31.90
    - with
      - 10-19 percent third degree T31.91
      - 20-29 percent third degree T31.92
      - 30-39 percent third degree T31.93
      - 40-49 percent third degree T31.94
      - 50-59 percent third degree T31.95
      - 60-69 percent third degree T31.96
      - 70-79 percent third degree T31.97
      - 80-89 percent third degree T31.98
      - 90-99 percent third degree T31.99
- upper limb T22.00 ☑
  - above elbow — *see* Burn, above elbow
  - axilla — *see* Burn, axilla
  - elbow — *see* Burn, elbow
  - first degree T22.10 ☑
  - forearm — *see* Burn, forearm
  - hand — *see* Burn, hand
  - interscapular region — *see* Burn, back, upper
  - multiple sites T22.099 ☑
    - first degree T22.199 ☑
    - left T22.092 ☑
      - first degree T22.192 ☑
      - second degree T22.292 ☑
      - third degree T22.392 ☑
    - right T22.091 ☑
      - first degree T22.191 ☑
      - second degree T22.291 ☑
      - third degree T22.391 ☑
    - second degree T22.299 ☑
    - third degree T22.399 ☑
  - scapular region — *see* Burn, scapular region
  - second degree T22.20 ☑
  - shoulder — *see* Burn, shoulder
  - third degree T22.30 ☑
  - wrist — *see* Burn, wrist
- uterus T28.3 ☑
- vagina T28.3 ☑
- vulva — *see* Burn, genital organs, external, female
- wrist T23.079 ☑
  - first degree T23.179 ☑
  - left T23.072 ☑
    - first degree T23.172 ☑
    - second degree T23.272 ☑
    - third degree T23.372 ☑
  - multiple sites with hand T23.099 ☑
    - first degree T23.199 ☑
    - left T23.092 ☑
      - first degree T23.192 ☑
      - second degree T23.292 ☑
      - third degree T23.392 ☑
    - right T23.091 ☑
      - first degree T23.191 ☑

Burn — *continued*
  wrist — *continued*
    multiple sites with hand — *continued*
      right — *continued*
        second degree T23.291 ☑
          third degree T23.391 ☑
      second degree T23.299 ☑
        third degree T23.399 ☑
      right T23.071 ☑
        first degree T23.171 ☑
        second degree T23.271 ☑
        third degree T23.371 ☑
      second degree T23.279 ☑
      third degree T23.379 ☑
Burnett's syndrome E83.52
Burning
  feet syndrome E53.9
  sensation R20.8
  tongue K14.6
Burn-out (state) Z73.0
Burns' disease or osteochondrosis — *see* Osteochondrosis, juvenile, ulna
Bursa — *see* condition
Bursitis M71.9
  Achilles — *see* Tendinitis, Achilles
  adhesive — *see* Bursitis, specified NEC
  ankle — *see* Enthesopathy, lower limb, ankle, specified type NEC
  calcaneal — *see* Enthesopathy, foot, specified type NEC
  collateral ligament, tibial — *see* Bursitis, tibial collateral
  due to use, overuse, pressure (*see also* Disorder, soft tissue, due to use, specified type NEC)
    specified NEC — *see* Disorder, soft tissue, due to use, specified NEC
  Duplay's M75.0 ☑
  elbow NEC M70.3- ☑
    olecranon M70.2- ☑
  finger — *see* Disorder, soft tissue, due to use, specified type NEC, hand
  foot — *see* Enthesopathy, foot, specified type NEC
  gonococcal A54.49
  gouty — *see* Gout
  hand M70.1- ☑
  hip NEC M70.7- ☑
    trochanteric M70.6- ☑
  infective NEC M71.10
    abscess — *see* Abscess, bursa
    ankle M71.17- ☑
    elbow M71.12- ☑
    foot M71.17- ☑
    hand M71.14- ☑
    hip M71.15- ☑
    knee M71.16- ☑
    multiple sites M71.19
    shoulder M71.11- ☑
    specified site NEC M71.18
    wrist M71.13- ☑
  ischial — *see* Bursitis, hip
  knee NEC M70.5- ☑
    prepatellar M70.4- ☑
  occupational NEC (*see also* Disorder, soft tissue, due to, use)
  olecranon — *see* Bursitis, elbow, olecranon
  pharyngeal J39.1
  popliteal — *see* Bursitis, knee
  prepatellar M70.4- ☑
  radiohumeral M77.8
  rheumatoid M06.20
    ankle M06.27- ☑
    elbow M06.22- ☑
    foot joint M06.27- ☑
    hand joint M06.24- ☑
    hip M06.25- ☑
    knee M06.26- ☑
    multiple site M06.29
    shoulder M06.21- ☑
    vertebra M06.28
    wrist M06.23- ☑
  scapulohumeral — *see* Bursitis, shoulder
  semimembranous muscle (knee) — *see* Bursitis, knee
  shoulder M75.5- ☑
    adhesive — *see* Capsulitis, adhesive
  specified NEC M71.50
    ankle M71.57- ☑

Bursitis — *continued*
  specified — *continued*
    due to use, overuse or pressure — *see* Disorder, soft tissue, due to, use
    elbow M71.52- ☑
    foot M71.57- ☑
    hand M71.54- ☑
    hip M71.55- ☑
    knee M71.56- ☑
    shoulder — *see* Bursitis, shoulder
    specified site NEC M71.58
    tibial collateral M76.4- ☑
    wrist M71.53- ☑
  subacromial — *see* Bursitis, shoulder
  subcoracoid — *see* Bursitis, shoulder
  subdeltoid — *see* Bursitis, shoulder
  syphilitic A52.78
  Thornwaldt, Tornwaldt J39.2
  tibial collateral M76.4- ☑
  toe — *see* Enthesopathy, foot, specified type NEC
  trochanteric (area) — *see* Bursitis, hip, trochanteric
  wrist — *see* Bursitis, hand
Bursopathy M71.9
  specified type NEC M71.80
    ankle M71.87- ☑
    elbow M71.82- ☑
    foot M71.87- ☑
    hand M71.84- ☑
    hip M71.85- ☑
    knee M71.86- ☑
    multiple sites M71.89
    shoulder M71.81- ☑
    specified site NEC M71.88
    wrist M71.83- ☑
Burst stitches or sutures (complication of surgery) T81.31 ☑
  external operation wound T81.31 ☑
  internal operation wound T81.32 ☑
Buruli ulcer A31.1
Bury's disease L95.1
Buschke's
  disease B45.3
  scleredema — *see* Sclerosis, systemic
Busse-Buschke disease B45.3
Buttock — *see* condition
Button
  Biskra B55.1
  Delhi B55.1
  oriental B55.1
Buttonhole deformity (finger) — *see* Deformity, finger, boutonniere
Bwamba fever A92.8
Byssinosis J66.0
Bywaters' syndrome T79.5 ☑

C

Cachexia R64
  cancerous R64
  cardiac — *see* Disease, heart
  dehydration E86.0
  due to malnutrition R64
  exophthalmic — *see* Hyperthyroidism
  heart — *see* Disease, heart
  hypophyseal E23.0
  hypopituitary E23.0
  lead — *see* Poisoning, lead
  malignant R64
  marsh — *see* Malaria
  nervous F48.8
  old age R54
  paludal — *see* Malaria
  pituitary E23.0
  renal N28.9
  saturnine — *see* Poisoning, lead
  senile R54
  Simmonds' E23.0
  splenica D73.0
  strumipriva E03.4
  tuberculous NEC — *see* Tuberculosis
Café, au lait spots L81.3
Caffeine-induced
  anxiety disorder F15.980
  sleep disorder F15.982
Caffey's syndrome Q78.8
Caisson disease T70.3 ☑
Cake kidney Q63.1

Caked breast (puerperal, postpartum) O92.79
Calabar swelling B74.3
Calcaneal spur — *see* Spur, bone, calcaneal
Calcaneo-apophysitis M92.8
Calcareous — *see* condition
Calcicosis J62.8
Calciferol (vitamin D) deficiency E55.9
  with rickets E55.0
Calcification
  adrenal (capsule) (gland) E27.49
    tuberculous E35 [B90.8]
  aorta I70.0
  artery (annular) — *see* Arteriosclerosis
  auricle (ear) — *see* Disorder, pinna, specified type NEC
  basal ganglia G23.8
  bladder N32.89
    due to Schistosoma hematobium B65.0
  brain (cortex) — *see* Calcification, cerebral
  bronchus J98.09
  bursa M71.40
    ankle M71.47- ☑
    elbow M71.42- ☑
    foot M71.47- ☑
    hand M71.44- ☑
    hip M71.45- ☑
    knee M71.46- ☑
    multiple sites M71.49
    shoulder M75.3- ☑
    specified site NEC M71.48
    wrist M71.43- ☑
  cardiac — *see* Degeneration, myocardial
  cerebral (cortex) G93.89
    artery I67.2
  cervix (uteri) N88.8
  choroid plexus G93.89
  conjunctiva — *see* Concretion, conjunctiva
  corpora cavernosa (penis) N48.89
  cortex (brain) — *see* Calcification, cerebral
  dental pulp (nodular) K04.2
  dentinal papilla K00.4
  fallopian tube N83.8
  falx cerebri G96.19
  gallbladder K82.8
  general E83.59
  heart (*see also* Degeneration, myocardial)
    valve — *see* Endocarditis
  idiopathic infantile arterial (IIAC) Q28.8
  intervertebral cartilage or disc (postinfective) — *see* Disorder, disc, specified NEC
  intracranial — *see* Calcification, cerebral
  joint — *see* Disorder, joint, specified type NEC
  kidney N28.89
    tuberculous N29 [B90.1]
  larynx (senile) J38.7
  lens — *see* Cataract, specified NEC
  lung (active) (postinfectional) J98.4
    tuberculous B90.9
  lymph gland or node (postinfectional) I89.8
    tuberculous (*see also* Tuberculosis, lymph gland) B90.8
  mammographic R92.1
  massive (paraplegic) — *see* Myositis, ossificans, in, quadriplegia
  medial — *see* Arteriosclerosis, extremities
  meninges (cerebral) (spinal) G96.19
  metastatic E83.59
  Mönckeberg's — *see* Arteriosclerosis, extremities
  muscle M61.9
    due to burns — *see* Myositis, ossificans, in, burns
    paralytic — *see* Myositis, ossificans, in, quadriplegia
    specified type NEC M61.40
      ankle M61.47- ☑
      foot M61.47- ☑
      forearm M61.43- ☑
      hand M61.44- ☑
      lower leg M61.46- ☑
      multiple sites M61.49
      pelvic region M61.45- ☑
      shoulder region M61.41- ☑
      specified site NEC M61.48
      thigh M61.45- ☑
      upper arm M61.42- ☑
  myocardium, myocardial — *see* Degeneration, myocardial
  ovary N83.8
  pancreas K86.89
  penis N48.89

☑ Additional Character Required — Refer to the Tabular List for Character Selection   ▼ Subterms under main terms may continue to next column or page

Calcification — *continued*
- periarticular — *see* Disorder, joint, specified type NEC
- pericardium (*see also* Pericarditis) I31.1
- pineal gland E34.8
- pleura J94.8
  - postinfectional J94.8
  - tuberculous NEC B90.9
- pulpal (dental) (nodular) K04.2
- sclera H15.89
- spleen D73.89
- subcutaneous L94.2
- suprarenal (capsule) (gland) E27.49
- tendon (sheath) (*see also* Tenosynovitis, specified type NEC)
  - with bursitis, synovitis or tenosynovitis — *see* Tendinitis, calcific
- trachea J39.8
- ureter N28.89
- uterus N85.8
- vitreous — *see* Deposit, crystalline

Calcified — *see* Calcification

Calcinosis (interstitial) (tumoral) (universalis) E83.59
- with Raynaud's phenomenon, esophageal dysfunction, sclerodactyly, telangiectasia (CREST syndrome) M34.1
- circumscripta (skin) L94.2
- cutis L94.2

Calciphylaxis (*see also* Calcification, by site) E83.59

Calcium
- deposits — *see* Calcification, by site
- metabolism disorder E83.50
- salts or soaps in vitreous — *see* Deposit, crystalline

Calciuria R82.99

Calculi — *see* Calculus

Calculosis, intrahepatic — *see* Calculus, bile duct

Calculus, calculi, calculous
- ampulla of Vater — *see* Calculus, bile duct
- anuria (impacted) (recurrent) (*see also* Calculus, urinary) N20.9
- appendix K38.1
- bile duct (common) (hepatic) K80.50
  - with
    - calculus of gallbladder — *see* Calculus, gallbladder and bile duct
    - cholangitis K80.30
      - with
        - cholecystitis — *see* Calculus, bile duct, with cholecystitis
        - obstruction K80.31
      - acute K80.32
        - with
          - chronic cholangitis K80.36
            - with obstruction K80.37
          - obstruction K80.33
      - chronic K80.34
        - with
          - acute cholangitis K80.36
            - with obstruction K80.37
          - obstruction K80.35
    - cholecystitis (with cholangitis) K80.40
      - with obstruction K80.41
      - acute K80.42
        - with
          - chronic cholecystitis K80.46
            - with obstruction K80.47
          - obstruction K80.43
      - chronic K80.44
        - with
          - acute cholecystitis K80.46
            - with obstruction K80.47
          - obstruction K80.45
- biliary (*see also* Calculus, gallbladder)
  - specified NEC K80.80
    - with obstruction K80.81
- bilirubin, multiple — *see* Calculus, gallbladder
- bladder (encysted) (impacted) (urinary) (diverticulum) N21.0
- bronchus J98.09
- calyx (kidney) (renal) — *see* Calculus, kidney
- cholesterol (pure) (solitary) — *see* Calculus, gallbladder
- common duct (bile) — *see* Calculus, bile duct
- conjunctiva — *see* Concretion, conjunctiva
- cystic N21.0
  - duct — *see* Calculus, gallbladder
- dental (subgingival) (supragingival) K03.6
- diverticulum
  - bladder N21.0
  - kidney N20.0

Calculus, calculi, calculous — *continued*
- epididymis N50.89
- gallbladder K80.20
  - with
    - bile duct calculus — *see* Calculus, gallbladder and bile duct
    - cholecystitis K80.10
      - with obstruction K80.11
      - acute K80.00
        - with
          - chronic cholecystitis K80.12
            - with obstruction K80.13
          - obstruction K80.01
      - chronic K80.10
        - with
          - acute cholecystitis K80.12
            - with obstruction K80.13
          - obstruction K80.11
      - specified NEC K80.18
        - with obstruction K80.19
    - obstruction K80.21
- gallbladder and bile duct K80.70
  - with
    - cholecystitis K80.60
      - with obstruction K80.61
      - acute K80.62
        - with
          - chronic cholecystitis K80.66
            - with obstruction K80.67
          - obstruction K80.63
      - chronic K80.64
        - with
          - acute cholecystitis K80.66
            - with obstruction K80.67
          - obstruction K80.65
    - obstruction K80.71
- hepatic (duct) — *see* Calculus, bile duct
- ileal conduit N21.8
- intestinal (impaction) (obstruction) K56.49
- kidney (impacted) (multiple) (pelvis) (recurrent) (staghorn) N20.0
  - with calculus, ureter N20.2
  - congenital Q63.8
- lacrimal passages — *see* Dacryolith
- liver (impacted) — *see* Calculus, bile duct
- lung J98.4
- mammographic R92.1
- nephritic (impacted) (recurrent) — *see* Calculus, kidney
- nose J34.89
- pancreas (duct) K86.89
- parotid duct or gland K11.5
- pelvis, encysted — *see* Calculus, kidney
- prostate N42.0
- pulmonary J98.4
- pyelitis (impacted) (recurrent) N20.0
  - with hydronephrosis N13.2
- pyelonephritis (impacted) (recurrent) N20 ☑
  - with hydronephrosis N13.2
- renal (impacted) (recurrent) — *see* Calculus, kidney
- salivary (duct) (gland) K11.5
- seminal vesicle N50.89
- staghorn — *see* Calculus, kidney
- Stensen's duct K11.5
- stomach K31.89
- sublingual duct or gland K11.5
  - congenital Q38.4
- submandibular duct, gland or region K11.5
- submaxillary duct, gland or region K11.5
- suburethral N21.8
- tonsil J35.8
- tooth, teeth (subgingival) (supragingival) K03.6
- tunica vaginalis N50.89
- ureter (impacted) (recurrent) N20.1
  - with calculus, kidney N20.2
    - with hydronephrosis N13.2
      - with infection N13.6
- urethra (impacted) N21.1
- urinary (duct) (impacted) (passage) (tract) N20.9
  - with hydronephrosis N13.2
    - with infection N13.6
  - in (due to)
    - lower N21.9
      - specified NEC N21.8
- vagina N89.8
- vesical (impacted) N21.0
- Wharton's duct K11.5
- xanthine E79.8 [N22]

Caliectasis N28.89

Caliectasis N28.89

California
- disease B38.9
- encephalitis A83.5

Caligo cornea — *see* Opacity, cornea, central

Callositas, callosity (infected) L84

Callus (infected) L84
- bone — *see* Osteophyte
  - excessive, following fracture — *code as* Sequelae of fracture

CALME (childhood asymmetric labium majus enlargement) N90.61

Calorie deficiency or malnutrition (*see also* Malnutrition) E46

Calvé-Perthes disease — *see* Legg-Calvé-Perthes disease

Calvé's disease — *see* Osteochondrosis, juvenile, spine

Calvities — *see* Alopecia, androgenic

Cameroon fever — *see* Malaria

Camptocormia (hysterical) F44.4

Camurati-Engelmann syndrome Q78.3

Canal (*see also* condition)
- atrioventricular common Q21.2

Canaliculitis (lacrimal) (acute) (subacute) H04.33- ☑
- Actinomyces A42.89
- chronic H04.42- ☑

Canavan's disease E75.29

Canceled procedure (surgical) Z53.9
- because of
  - contraindication Z53.09
    - smoking Z53.01
  - left against medical advice (AMA) Z53.21
  - patient's decision Z53.20
    - for reasons of belief or group pressure Z53.1
    - specified reason NEC Z53.29
  - specified reason NEC Z53.8

Cancer (*see also* Neoplasm, by site, malignant)
- bile duct type liver C22.1
- blood — *see* Leukemia
- breast (*see also* Neoplasm, breast, malignant) C50.91- ☑
- hepatocellular C22.0
- lung (*see also* Neoplasm, lung, malignant) C34.90
- ovarian (*see also* Neoplasm ovary, malignant) C56.9
- unspecified site (primary) C80.1

Cancer (o)**phobia** F45.29

Cancerous — *see* Neoplasm, malignant, by site

Cancrum oris A69.0

Candidiasis, candidal B37.9
- balanitis B37.42
- bronchitis B37.1
- cheilitis B37.83
- congenital P37.5
- cystitis B37.41
- disseminated B37.7
- endocarditis B37.6
- enteritis B37.82
- esophagitis B37.81
- intertrigo B37.2
- lung B37.1
- meningitis B37.5
- mouth B37.0
- nails B37.2
- neonatal P37.5
- onychia B37.2
- oral B37.0
- osteomyelitis B37.89
- otitis externa B37.84
- paronychia B37.2
- perionyxis B37.2
- pneumonia B37.1
- proctitis B37.82
- pulmonary B37.1
- pyelonephritis B37.49
- sepsis B37.7
- skin B37.2
- specified site NEC B37.89
- stomatitis B37.0
- systemic B37.7
- urethritis B37.41
- urogenital site NEC B37.49
- vagina B37.3
- vulva B37.3
- vulvovaginitis B37.3

Candidid L30.2

Candidosis — *see* Candidiasis

Candiru infection or infestation B88.8

Canities (premature) L67.1

Canities — *continued*
congenital Q84.2
Canker (mouth) (sore) K12.0
rash A38.9
Cannabinosis J66.2
Cannabis induced
anxiety disorder F12.980
psychotic disorder F12.959
sleep disorder F12.988
Canton fever A75.9
Cantrell's syndrome Q87.89
Capillariasis (intestinal) B81.1
hepatic B83.8
Capillary — *see* condition
Caplan's syndrome — *see* Rheumatoid, lung
Capsule — *see* condition
Capsulitis (joint) (*see also* Enthesopathy)
adhesive (shoulder) M75.0- ☑
hepatic K65.8
labyrinthine — *see* Otosclerosis, specified NEC
thyroid E06.9
Caput
crepitus Q75.8
medusae I86.8
succedaneum P12.81
Car sickness T75.3 ☑
Carapata (disease) A68.0
Carate — *see* Pinta
Carbon lung J60
Carbuncle L02.93
abdominal wall L02.231
anus K61.0
auditory canal, external — *see* Abscess, ear, external
auricle ear — *see* Abscess, ear, external
axilla L02.43- ☑
back (any part) L02.232
breast N61.1
buttock L02.33
cheek (external) L02.03
chest wall L02.233
chin L02.03
corpus cavernosum N48.21
ear (any part) (external) (middle) — *see* Abscess, ear, external
external auditory canal — *see* Abscess, ear, external
eyelid — *see* Abscess, eyelid
face NEC L02.03
femoral (region) — *see* Carbuncle, lower limb
finger — *see* Carbuncle, hand
flank L02.231
foot L02.63- ☑
forehead L02.03
genital — *see* Abscess, genital
gluteal (region) L02.33
groin L02.234
hand L02.53- ☑
head NEC L02.831
heel — *see* Carbuncle, foot
hip — *see* Carbuncle, lower limb
kidney — *see* Abscess, kidney
knee — *see* Carbuncle, lower limb
labium (majus) (minus) N76.4
lacrimal
gland — *see* Dacryoadenitis
passages (duct) (sac) — *see* Inflammation, lacrimal, passages, acute
leg — *see* Carbuncle, lower limb
lower limb L02.43- ☑
malignant A22.0
navel L02.236
neck L02.13
nose (external) (septum) J34.0
orbit, orbital — *see* Abscess, orbit
palmar (space) — *see* Carbuncle, hand
partes posteriores L02.33
pectoral region L02.233
penis N48.21
perineum L02.235
pinna — *see* Abscess, ear, external
popliteal — *see* Carbuncle, lower limb
scalp L02.831
seminal vesicle N49.0
shoulder — *see* Carbuncle, upper limb
specified site NEC L02.838
temple (region) L02.03
thumb — *see* Carbuncle, hand
toe — *see* Carbuncle, foot

Carbuncle — *continued*
trunk L02.239
abdominal wall L02.231
back L02.232
chest wall L02.233
groin L02.234
perineum L02.235
umbilicus L02.236
umbilicus L02.236
upper limb L02.43- ☑
urethra N34.0
vulva N76.4
Carbunculus — *see* Carbuncle
Carcinoid (tumor) — *see* Tumor, carcinoid
Carcinoidosis E34.0
Carcinoma (malignant) (*see also* Neoplasm, by site, malignant)
acidophil
specified site — *see* Neoplasm, malignant, by site
unspecified site C75.1
acidophil-basophil, mixed
specified site — *see* Neoplasm, malignant, by site
unspecified site C75.1
adnexal (skin) — *see* Neoplasm, skin, malignant
adrenal cortical C74.0- ☑
alveolar — *see* Neoplasm, lung, malignant
cell — *see* Neoplasm, lung, malignant
ameloblastic C41.1
upper jaw (bone) C41.0
apocrine
breast — *see* Neoplasm, breast, malignant
specified site NEC — *see* Neoplasm, skin, malignant
unspecified site C44.99
basal cell (pigmented) (*see also* Neoplasm, skin, malignant) C44.91
fibro-epithelial — *see* Neoplasm, skin, malignant
morphea — *see* Neoplasm, skin, malignant
multicentric — *see* Neoplasm, skin, malignant
basaloid
basal-squamous cell, mixed — *see* Neoplasm, skin, malignant
basophil
specified site — *see* Neoplasm, malignant, by site
unspecified site C75.1
basophil-acidophil, mixed
specified site — *see* Neoplasm, malignant, by site
unspecified site C75.1
basosquamous — *see* Neoplasm, skin, malignant
bile duct
with hepatocellular, mixed C22.0
liver C22.1
specified site NEC — *see* Neoplasm, malignant, by site
unspecified site C22.1
branchial or branchiogenic C10.4
bronchial or bronchogenic — *see* Neoplasm, lung, malignant
bronchiolar — *see* Neoplasm, lung, malignant
bronchioloalveolar — *see* Neoplasm, lung, malignant
C cell
specified site — *see* Neoplasm, malignant, by site
unspecified site C73
ceruminous C44.29- ☑
cervix uteri
in situ D06.9
endocervix D06.0
exocervix D06.1
specified site NEC D06.7
chorionic
specified site — *see* Neoplasm, malignant, by site
unspecified site
female C58
male C62.90
chromophobe
specified site — *see* Neoplasm, malignant, by site
unspecified site C75.1
cloacogenic
specified site — *see* Neoplasm, malignant, by site
unspecified site C21.2
diffuse type
specified site — *see* Neoplasm, malignant, by site
unspecified site C16.9
duct (cell)
with Paget's disease — *see* Neoplasm, breast, malignant

Carcinoma — *continued*
duct — *continued*
infiltrating
with lobular carcinoma (in situ)
specified site — *see* Neoplasm, malignant, by site
unspecified site (female) C50.91- ☑
male C50.92- ☑
specified site — *see* Neoplasm, malignant, by site
unspecified site (female) C50.91- ☑
male C50.92- ☑
ductal
with lobular
specified site — *see* Neoplasm, malignant, by site
unspecified site (female) C50.91- ☑
male C50.92- ☑
ductular, infiltrating
specified site — *see* Neoplasm, malignant, by site
unspecified site (female) C50.91- ☑
male C50.92- ☑
embryonal
liver C22.7
endometrioid
specified site — *see* Neoplasm, malignant, by site
unspecified site
female C56.9
male C61
eosinophil
specified site — *see* Neoplasm, malignant, by site
unspecified site C75.1
epidermoid (*see also* Neoplasm, skin, malignant)
in situ, Bowen's type — *see* Neoplasm, skin, in situ
fibroepithelial, basal cell — *see* Neoplasm, skin, malignant
follicular
with papillary (mixed) C73
moderately differentiated C73
pure follicle C73
specified site — *see* Neoplasm, malignant, by site
trabecular C73
unspecified site C73
well differentiated C73
generalized, with unspecified primary site C80.0
glycogen-rich — *see* Neoplasm, breast, malignant
granulosa cell C56- ☑
hepatic cell C22.0
hepatocellular C22.0
with bile duct, mixed C22.0
fibrolamellar C22.0
hepatocholangiolitic C22.0
Hurthle cell C73
in
adenomatous
polyposis coli C18.9
pleomorphic adenoma — *see* Neoplasm, salivary glands, malignant
situ — *see* Carcinoma-in-situ
infiltrating
duct
with lobular
specified site — *see* Neoplasm, malignant, by site
unspecified site (female) C50.91- ☑
male C50.92- ☑
with Paget's disease — *see* Neoplasm, breast, malignant
specified site — *see* Neoplasm, malignant
unspecified site (female) C50.91- ☑
male C50.92- ☑
ductular
specified site — *see* Neoplasm, malignant
unspecified site (female) C50.91- ☑
male C50.92- ☑
lobular
specified site — *see* Neoplasm, malignant
unspecified site (female) C50.91- ☑
male C50.92- ☑
inflammatory
specified site — *see* Neoplasm, malignant
unspecified site (female) C50.91- ☑
male C50.92- ☑
intestinal type
specified site — *see* Neoplasm, malignant, by site
unspecified site C16.9

Carcinoma — *continued*
  intracystic
    noninfiltrating — *see* Neoplasm, in situ, by site
  intraductal (noninfiltrating)
    with Paget's disease — *see* Neoplasm, breast, malignant
    breast D05.1- ☑
    papillary
      with invasion
        specified site — *see* Neoplasm, malignant, by site
        unspecified site (female) C50.91- ☑
          male C50.92- ☑
      breast D05.1- ☑
      specified site NEC — *see* Neoplasm, in situ, by site
      unspecified site (female) D05.1- ☑
    specified site NEC — *see* Neoplasm, in situ, by site
    unspecified site (female) D05.1- ☑
  intraepidermal — *see* Neoplasm, in situ
    squamous cell, Bowen's type — *see* Neoplasm, skin, in situ
  intraepithelial — *see* Neoplasm, in situ, by site
    squamous cell — *see* Neoplasm, in situ, by site
  intraosseous C41.1
    upper jaw (bone) C41.0
  islet cell
    with exocrine, mixed
      specified site — *see* Neoplasm, malignant, by site
      unspecified site C25.9
    pancreas C25.4
    specified site NEC — *see* Neoplasm, malignant, by site
    unspecified site C25.4
  juvenile, breast — *see* Neoplasm, breast, malignant
  large cell
    small cell
      specified site — *see* Neoplasm, malignant, by site
      unspecified site C34.90
  Leydig cell (testis)
    specified site — *see* Neoplasm, malignant, by site
    unspecified site
      female C56.9
      male C62.90
  lipid-rich (female) C50.91- ☑
    male C50.92- ☑
  liver cell C22.0
  liver NEC C22.7
  lobular (infiltrating)
    with intraductal
      specified site — *see* Neoplasm, malignant, by site
      unspecified site (female) C50.91- ☑
        male C50.92- ☑
    noninfiltrating
      breast D05.0- ☑
      specified site NEC — *see* Neoplasm, in situ, by site
      unspecified site D05.0- ☑
    specified site — *see* Neoplasm, malignant, by site
    unspecified site (female) C50.91- ☑
      male C50.92- ☑
  medullary
    with
      amyloid stroma
        specified site — *see* Neoplasm, malignant, by site
        unspecified site C73
      lymphoid stroma
        specified site — *see* Neoplasm, malignant, by site
        unspecified site (female) C50.91- ☑
          male C50.92- ☑
  Merkel cell C4A.9 (*following* C43)
    anal margin C4A.51 (*following* C43)
    anal skin C4A.51 (*following* C43)
    canthus C4A.1- ☑ (*following* C43)
    ear and external auricular canal C4A.2- ☑ (*following* C43)
    external auricular canal C4A.2- ☑ (*following* C43)
    eyelid, including canthus C4A.1- ☑ (*following* C43)
    face C4A.30 (*following* C43)
      specified NEC C4A.39 (*following* C43)
    hip C4A.7- ☑ (*following* C43)
    lip C4A.0 (*following* C43)

Carcinoma — *continued*
  Merkel cell — *continued*
    lower limb, including hip C4A.7- ☑ (*following* C43)
    neck C4A.4 (*following* C43)
    nodal presentation C7B.1 (*following* C75)
    nose C4A.31 (*following* C43)
    overlapping sites C4A.8 (*following* C43)
    perianal skin C4A.51 (*following* C43)
    scalp C4A.4 (*following* C43)
    secondary C7B.1 (*following* C75)
    shoulder C4A.6- ☑ (*following* C43)
    skin of breast C4A.52 (*following* C43)
    trunk NEC C4A.59 (*following* C43)
    upper limb, including shoulder C4A.6- ☑ (*following* C43)
    visceral metastatic C7B.1 (*following* C75)
  metastatic — *see* Neoplasm, secondary, by site
  metatypical — *see* Neoplasm, skin, malignant
  morphea, basal cell — *see* Neoplasm, skin, malignant
  mucoid
    cell
      specified site — *see* Neoplasm, malignant, by site
      unspecified site C75.1
  neuroendocrine (*see also* Tumor, neuroendocrine)
    high grade, any site C7A.1 (*following* C75)
    poorly differentiated, any site C7A.1 (*following* C75)
  nonencapsulated sclerosing C73
  noninfiltrating
    intracystic — *see* Neoplasm, in situ, by site
    intraductal
      breast D05.1- ☑
      papillary
        breast D05.1- ☑
        specified site NEC — *see* Neoplasm, in situ, by site
        unspecified site D05.1- ☑
      specified site — *see* Neoplasm, in situ, by site
      unspecified site D05.1- ☑
    lobular
      breast D05.0- ☑
      specified site NEC — *see* Neoplasm, in situ, by site
      unspecified site (female) D05.0- ☑
  oat cell
    specified site — *see* Neoplasm, malignant, by site
    unspecified site C34.90
  odontogenic C41.1
    upper jaw (bone) C41.0
  papillary
    with follicular (mixed) C73
    follicular variant C73
    intraductal (noninfiltrating)
      with invasion
        specified site — *see* Neoplasm, malignant, by site
        unspecified site (female) C50.91- ☑
          male C50.92- ☑
      breast D05.1- ☑
      specified site NEC — *see* Neoplasm, in situ, by site
      unspecified site D05.1- ☑
    serous
      specified site — *see* Neoplasm, malignant, by site
    surface
      specified site — *see* Neoplasm, malignant, by site
      unspecified site C56.9
    unspecified site C56.9
  papillocystic
    specified site — *see* Neoplasm, malignant, by site
    unspecified site C56.9
  parafollicular cell
    specified site — *see* Neoplasm, malignant, by site
    unspecified site C73
  pilomatrix — *see* Neoplasm, skin, malignant
  pseudomucinous
    specified site — *see* Neoplasm, malignant, by site
    unspecified site C56.9
  renal cell C64- ☑
  Schmincke — *see* Neoplasm, nasopharynx, malignant
  Schneiderian
    specified site — *see* Neoplasm, malignant, by site
    unspecified site C30.0
  sebaceous — *see* Neoplasm, skin, malignant

Carcinoma — *continued*
  secondary (*see also* Neoplasm, secondary, by site)
    Merkel cell C7B.1 (*following* C75)
  secretory, breast — *see* Neoplasm, breast, malignant
  serous
    papillary
      specified site — *see* Neoplasm, malignant, by site
      unspecified site C56.9
    surface, papillary
      specified site — *see* Neoplasm, malignant, by site
      unspecified site C56.9
  Sertoli cell
    specified site — *see* Neoplasm, malignant, by site
    unspecified site C62.90
      female C56.9
      male C62.90
  skin appendage — *see* Neoplasm, skin, malignant
  small cell
    fusiform cell
      specified site — *see* Neoplasm, malignant, by site
      unspecified site C34.90
    intermediate cell
      specified site — *see* Neoplasm, malignant, by site
      unspecified site C34.90
    large cell
      specified site — *see* Neoplasm, malignant, by site
      unspecified site C34.90
  solid
    with amyloid stroma
      specified site — *see* Neoplasm, malignant, by site
      unspecified site C73
    microinvasive
      specified site — *see* Neoplasm, malignant, by site
      unspecified site C53.9
  sweat gland — *see* Neoplasm, skin, malignant
  theca cell C56.- ☑
  thymic C37
  unspecified site (primary) C80.1
  water-clear cell C75.0
Carcinoma-in-situ (*see also* Neoplasm, in situ, by site)
  breast NOS D05.9- ☑
    specified type NEC D05.8- ☑
  epidermoid (*see also* Neoplasm, in situ, by site)
    with questionable stromal invasion
      cervix D06.9
      specified site NEC — *see* Neoplasm, in situ, by site
      unspecified site D06.9
    Bowen's type — *see* Neoplasm, skin, in situ
  intraductal
    breast D05.1- ☑
    specified site NEC — *see* Neoplasm, in situ, by site
    unspecified site D05.1- ☑
  lobular
    with
      infiltrating duct
        breast (female) C50.91- ☑
          male C50.92- ☑
        specified site NEC — *see* Neoplasm, malignant
        unspecified site (female) C50.91- ☑
          male C50.92- ☑
      intraductal
        breast D05.8- ☑
        specified site NEC — *see* Neoplasm, in situ, by site
        unspecified site (female) D05.8- ☑
    breast D05.0- ☑
    specified site NEC — *see* Neoplasm, in situ, by site
    unspecified site D05.0- ☑
  squamous cell (*see also* Neoplasm, in situ, by site)
    with questionable stromal invasion
      cervix D06.9
      specified site NEC — *see* Neoplasm, in situ, by site
      unspecified site D06.9
Carcinomaphobia F45.29
Carcinomatosis C80.0
  peritonei C78.6

Carcinomatosis — *continued*
  unspecified site (primary) (secondary) C80.0
Carcinosarcoma — *see* Neoplasm, malignant, by site
  embryonal — *see* Neoplasm, malignant, by site
Cardia, cardial — *see* condition
Cardiac (*see also* condition)
  death, sudden — *see* Arrest, cardiac
  pacemaker
    in situ Z95.0
      management or adjustment Z45.018
  tamponade I31.4
Cardialgia — *see* Pain, precordial
Cardiectasis — *see* Hypertrophy, cardiac
Cardiochalasia K21.9
Cardiomalacia I51.5
Cardiomegalia glycogenica diffusa E74.02 [I43]
Cardiomegaly (*see also* Hypertrophy, cardiac)
  congenital Q24.8
  glycogen E74.02 [I43]
  idiopathic I51.7
Cardiomyoliposis I51.5
Cardiomyopathy (familial) (idiopathic) I42.9
  alcoholic I42.6
  amyloid E85.4 [I43]
    transthyretin-related (ATTR) familial E85.4
  arteriosclerotic — *see* Disease, heart, ischemic, atherosclerotic
  beriberi E51.12
  cobalt-beer I42.6
  congenital I42.4
  congestive I42.0
  constrictive NOS I42.5
  dilated I42.0
  due to
    alcohol I42.6
    beriberi E51.12
    cardiac glycogenosis E74.02 [I43]
    drugs I42.7
    external agents NEC I42.7
    Friedreich's ataxia G11.1
    myotonia atrophica G71.11 [I43]
    progressive muscular dystrophy G71.0 [I43]
  glycogen storage E74.02 [I43]
  hypertensive — *see* Hypertension, heart
  hypertrophic (nonobstructive) I42.2
    obstructive I42.1
      congenital Q24.8
  in
    Chagas' disease (chronic) B57.2
      acute B57.0
    sarcoidosis D86.85
  ischemic I25.5
  metabolic E88.9 [I43]
    thyrotoxic E05.90 [I43]
      with thyroid storm E05.91 [I43]
  newborn I42.8
    congenital I42.4
  nutritional E63.9 [I43]
    beriberi E51.12
  obscure of Africa I42.8
  peripartum O90.3
  postpartum O90.3
  restrictive NEC I42.5
  rheumatic I09.0
  secondary I42.9
  stress induced I51.81
  takotsubo I51.81
  thyrotoxic E05.90 [I43]
    with thyroid storm E05.91 [I43]
  toxic NEC I42.7
  transthyretin-related (ATTR) familial amyloid E85.4
  tuberculous A18.84
  viral B33.24
Cardionephritis — *see* Hypertension, cardiorenal
Cardionephropathy — *see* Hypertension, cardiorenal
Cardionephrosis — *see* Hypertension, cardiorenal
Cardiopathia nigra I27.0
Cardiopathy (*see also* Disease, heart) I51.9
  idiopathic I42.9
  mucopolysaccharidosis E76.3 [I52]
Cardiopericarditis — *see* Pericarditis
Cardiophobia F45.29
Cardiorenal — *see* condition
Cardiorrhexis — *see* Infarct, myocardium
Cardiosclerosis — *see* Disease, heart, ischemic, atherosclerotic
Cardiosis — *see* Disease, heart
Cardiospasm (esophagus) (reflex) (stomach) K22.0

Cardiospasm — *continued*
  congenital Q39.5
    with megaesophagus Q39.5
Cardiostenosis — *see* Disease, heart
Cardiosymphysis I31.0
Cardiovascular — *see* condition
Carditis (acute) (bacterial) (chronic) (subacute) I51.89
  meningococcal A39.50
  rheumatic — *see* Disease, heart, rheumatic
  rheumatoid — *see* Rheumatoid, carditis
  viral B33.20
Care (of) (for) (following)
  child (routine) Z76.2
  family member (handicapped) (sick)
    creating problem for family Z63.6
    provided away from home for holiday relief Z75.5
    unavailable, due to
      absence (person rendering care) (sufferer) Z74.2
      inability (any reason) of person rendering care Z74.2
  foundling Z76.1
  holiday relief Z75.5
  improper — *see* Maltreatment
  lack of (at or after birth) (infant) — *see* Maltreatment, child, neglect
  lactating mother Z39.1
  palliative Z51.5
  postpartum
    immediately after delivery Z39.0
    routine follow-up Z39.2
  respite Z75.5
  unavailable, due to
    absence of person rendering care Z74.2
    inability (any reason) of person rendering care Z74.2
  well-baby Z76.2
Caries
  bone NEC A18.03
  dental (dentino enamel junction) (early childhood) (of dentine) (pre-eruptive) (recurrent) (to the pulp) K02.9
    arrested (coronal) (root) K02.3
    chewing surface
      limited to enamel K02.51
      penetrating into dentin K02.52
      penetrating into pulp K02.53
    coronal surface
      chewing surface
        limited to enamel K02.51
        penetrating into dentin K02.52
        penetrating into pulp K02.53
      pit and fissure surface
        limited to enamel K02.51
        penetrating into dentin K02.52
        penetrating into pulp K02.53
      smooth surface
        limited to enamel K02.61
        penetrating into dentin K02.62
        penetrating into pulp K02.63
    pit and fissure surface
      limited to enamel K02.51
      penetrating into dentin K02.52
      penetrating into pulp K02.53
    primary, cervical origin K02.52
    root K02.7
    smooth surface
      limited to enamel K02.61
      penetrating into dentin K02.62
      penetrating into pulp K02.63
  external meatus — *see* Disorder, ear, external, specified type NEC
  hip (tuberculous) A18.02
  initial (tooth)
    chewing surface K02.51
    pit and fissure surface K02.51
    smooth surface K02.61
  knee (tuberculous) A18.02
  labyrinth H83.8 ☑
  limb NEC (tuberculous) A18.03
  mastoid process (chronic) — *see* Mastoiditis, chronic
    tuberculous A18.03
  middle ear H74.8 ☑
  nose (tuberculous) A18.03
  orbit (tuberculous) A18.03
  ossicles, ear — *see* Abnormal, ear ossicles
  petrous bone — *see* Petrositis
  root (dental) (tooth) K02.7
  sacrum (tuberculous) A18.01

Caries — *continued*
  spine, spinal (column) (tuberculous) A18.01
  syphilitic A52.77
    congenital (early) A50.02 [M90.80]
  tooth, teeth — *see* Caries, dental
  tuberculous A18.03
  vertebra (column) (tuberculous) A18.01
Carious teeth — *see* Caries, dental
Carneous mole O02.0
Carnitine insufficiency E71.40
Carotid body or sinus syndrome G90.01
Carotidynia G90.01
Carotinemia (dietary) E67.1
Carotinosis (cutis) (skin) E67.1
Carpal tunnel syndrome — *see* Syndrome, carpal tunnel
Carpenter's syndrome Q87.0
Carpopedal spasm — *see* Tetany
Carr-Barr-Plunkett syndrome Q97.1
Carrier (suspected) of
  amebiasis Z22.1
  bacterial disease NEC Z22.39
    diphtheria Z22.2
    intestinal infectious NEC Z22.1
      typhoid Z22.0
    meningococcal Z22.31
    sexually transmitted Z22.4
    specified NEC Z22.39
    staphylococcal (Methicillin susceptible) Z22.321
      Methicillin resistant Z22.322
    streptococcal Z22.338
      group B Z22.330
        complicating pregnancy or delivery O99.82- ☑
    typhoid Z22.0
  cholera Z22.1
  diphtheria Z22.2
  gastrointestinal pathogens NEC Z22.1
  genetic Z14.8
    cystic fibrosis Z14.1
    hemophilia A (asymptomatic) Z14.01
      symptomatic Z14.02
  gestational, pregnant Z33.1
  gonorrhea Z22.4
  HAA (hepatitis Australian-antigen) B18.8
  HB (c)(s)-AG B18.1
  hepatitis (viral) B18.9
    Australia-antigen (HAA) B18.8
    B surface antigen (HBsAg) B18.1
      with acute delta- (super)infection B17.0
    C B18.2
    specified NEC B18.8
  human T-cell lymphotropic virus type-1 (HTLV-1) infection Z22.6
  infectious organism Z22.9
    specified NEC Z22.8
  meningococci Z22.31
  Salmonella typhosa Z22.0
  serum hepatitis — *see* Carrier, hepatitis
  staphylococci (Methicillin susceptible) Z22.321
    Methicillin resistant Z22.322
  streptococci Z22.338
    group B Z22.330
      complicating pregnancy or delivery O99.82- ☑
  syphilis Z22.4
  typhoid Z22.0
  venereal disease NEC Z22.4
Carrion's disease A44.0
Carter's relapsing fever (Asiatic) A68.1
Cartilage — *see* condition
Caruncle (inflamed)
  conjunctiva (acute) — *see* Conjunctivitis, acute
  labium (majus) (minus) N90.89
  lacrimal — *see* Inflammation, lacrimal, passages
  myrtiform N89.8
  urethral (benign) N36.2
Cascade stomach K31.2
Caseation lymphatic gland (tuberculous) A18.2
Cassidy (-Scholte) syndrome (malignant carcinoid) E34.0
Castellani's disease A69.8
Castration, traumatic, male S38.231 ☑
Casts in urine R82.99
Cat
  cry syndrome Q93.4
  ear Q17.3
  eye syndrome Q92.8
Catabolism, senile R54
Catalepsy (hysterical) F44.2
  schizophrenic F20.2

Cataplexy (idiopathic) — *see* Narcolepsy
Cataract (cortical) (immature) (incipient) H26.9
 with
  neovascularization — *see* Cataract, complicated
 age-related — *see* Cataract, senile
 anterior
  and posterior axial embryonal Q12.0
  pyramidal Q12.0
 associated with
  galactosemia E74.21 [H28]
  myotonic disorders G71.19 [H28]
 blue Q12.0
 central Q12.0
 cerulean Q12.0
 complicated H26.20
  with
   neovascularization H26.21- ☑
   ocular disorder H26.22- ☑
  glaucomatous flecks H26.23- ☑
 congenital Q12.0
 coraliform Q12.0
 coronary Q12.0
 crystalline Q12.0
 diabetic — *see* Diabetes, cataract
 drug-induced H26.3- ☑
 due to
  ocular disorder — *see* Cataract, complicated
  radiation H26.8
 electric H26.8
 extraction status Z98.4- ☑
 glass-blower's H26.8
 heat ray H26.8
 heterochromic — *see* Cataract, complicated
 hypermature — *see* Cataract, senile, morgagnian type
 in (due to)
  chronic iridocyclitis — *see* Cataract, complicated
  diabetes — *see* Diabetes, cataract
  endocrine disease E34.9 [H28]
  eye disease — *see* Cataract, complicated
  hypoparathyroidism E20.9 [H28]
  malnutrition-dehydration E46 [H28]
  metabolic disease E88.9 [H28]
  myotonic disorders G71.19 [H28]
  nutritional disease E63.9 [H28]
 infantile — *see* Cataract, presenile
 irradiational — *see* Cataract, specified NEC
 juvenile — *see* Cataract, presenile
 malnutrition-dehydration E46 [H28]
 morgagnian — *see* Cataract, senile, morgagnian type
 myotonic G71.19 [H28]
 myxedema E03.9 [H28]
 nuclear
  embryonal Q12.0
  sclerosis — *see* Cataract, senile, nuclear
 presenile H26.00- ☑
  combined forms H26.06- ☑
  cortical H26.01- ☑
  lamellar — *see* Cataract, presenile, cortical
  nuclear H26.03- ☑
  specified NEC H26.09
  subcapsular polar (anterior) H26.04- ☑
   posterior H26.05- ☑
  zonular — *see* Cataract, presenile, cortical
 secondary H26.40
  Soemmering's ring H26.41- ☑
  specified NEC H26.49- ☑
  to eye disease — *see* Cataract, complicated
 senile H25.9
  brunescens — *see* Cataract, senile, nuclear
  combined forms H25.81- ☑
  coronary — *see* Cataract, senile, incipient
  cortical H25.01- ☑
  hypermature — *see* Cataract, senile, morgagnian
   type
  incipient (mature) (total) H25.09- ☑
   cortical — *see* Cataract, senile, cortical
   subcapsular — *see* Cataract, senile, subcapsular
  morgagnian type (hypermature) H25.2- ☑
  nuclear (sclerosis) H25.1- ☑
  polar subcapsular (anterior) (posterior) — *see*
   Cataract, senile, incipient
  punctate — *see* Cataract, senile, incipient
  specified NEC H25.89
  subcapsular polar (anterior) H25.03- ☑
   posterior H25.04- ☑
 snowflake — *see* Diabetes, cataract
 specified NEC H26.8

Cataract — *continued*
 toxic — *see* Cataract, drug-induced
 traumatic H26.10- ☑
  localized H26.11- ☑
  partially resolved H26.12- ☑
  total H26.13- ☑
 zonular (perinuclear) Q12.0
Cataracta (*see also* Cataract)
 brunescens — *see* Cataract, senile, nuclear
 centralis pulverulenta Q12.0
 cerulea Q12.0
 complicata — *see* Cataract, complicated
 congenita Q12.0
 coralliformis Q12.0
 coronaria Q12.0
 diabetic — *see* Diabetes, cataract
 membranacea
  accreta — *see* Cataract, secondary
  congenita Q12.0
 nigra — *see* Cataract, senile, nuclear
 sunflower — *see* Cataract, complicated
Catarrh, catarrhal (acute) (febrile) (infectious) (inflammation) (*see also* condition) J00
 bronchial — *see* Bronchitis
 chest — *see* Bronchitis
 chronic J31.0
 due to congenital syphilis A50.03
 enteric — *see* Enteritis
 eustachian H68.009
 fauces — *see* Pharyngitis
 gastrointestinal — *see* Enteritis
 gingivitis K05.00
  nonplaque induced K05.01
  plaque induced K05.00
 hay — *see* Fever, hay
 intestinal — *see* Enteritis
 larynx, chronic J37.0
 liver B15.9
  with hepatic coma B15.0
 lung — *see* Bronchitis
 middle ear, chronic — *see* Otitis, media, nonsuppurative, chronic, serous
 mouth K12.1
 nasal (chronic) — *see* Rhinitis
 nasobronchial J31.1
 nasopharyngeal (chronic) J31.1
  acute J00
 pulmonary — *see* Bronchitis
 spring (eye) (vernal) — *see* Conjunctivitis, acute, atopic
 summer (hay) — *see* Fever, hay
 throat J31.2
 tubotympanal (*see also* Otitis, media, nonsuppurative)
  chronic — *see* Otitis, media, nonsuppurative, chronic, serous
Catatonia (schizophrenic) F20.2
Catatonic
 disorder due to known physiologic condition F06.1
 schizophrenia F20.2
 stupor R40.1
Cat-scratch (*see also* Abrasion)
 disease or fever A28.1
Cauda equina — *see* condition
Cauliflower ear M95.1- ☑
Causalgia (upper limb) G56.4- ☑
 lower limb G57.7- ☑
Cause
 external, general effects T75.89 ☑
Caustic burn — *see* Corrosion, by site
Cavare's disease (familial periodic paralysis) G72.3
Cave-in, injury
 crushing (severe) — *see* Crush
 suffocation — *see* Asphyxia, traumatic, due to low oxygen, due to cave-in
Cavernitis (penis) N48.29
Cavernositis N48.29
Cavernous — *see* condition
Cavitation of lung (*see also* Tuberculosis, pulmonary)
 nontuberculous J98.4
Cavities, dental — *see* Caries, dental
Cavity
 lung — *see* Cavitation of lung
 optic papilla Q14.2
 pulmonary — *see* Cavitation of lung
Cavovarus foot, congenital Q66.1
Cavus foot (congenital) Q66.7
 acquired — *see* Deformity, limb, foot, specified NEC
Cazenave's disease L10.2

Cecitis K52.9
 with perforation, peritonitis, or rupture K65.8
Cecum — *see* condition
Celiac
 artery compression syndrome I77.4
 disease (with steatorrhea) K90.0
 infantilism K90.0
Cell(s), **cellular** (*see also* condition)
 in urine R82.99
Cellulitis (diffuse) (phlegmonous) (septic) (suppurative) L03.90
 abdominal wall L03.311
 anaerobic A48.0
 ankle — *see* Cellulitis, lower limb
 anus K61.0
 arm — *see* Cellulitis, upper limb
 auricle (ear) — *see* Cellulitis, ear
 axilla L03.11- ☑
 back (any part) L03.312
 breast (acute) (nonpuerperal) (subacute) N61.0
  nipple N61.0
 broad ligament
  acute N73.0
 buttock L03.317
 cervical (meaning neck) L03.221
 cervix (uteri) — *see* Cervicitis
 cheek (external) L03.211
  internal K12.2
 chest wall L03.313
 chronic L03.90
 clostridial A48.0
 corpus cavernosum N48.22
 digit
  finger — *see* Cellulitis, finger
  toe — *see* Cellulitis, toe
 Douglas' cul-de-sac or pouch
  acute N73.0
 drainage site (following operation) T81.4 ☑
 ear (external) H60.1- ☑
 eosinophilic (granulomatous) L98.3
 erysipelatous — *see* Erysipelas
 external auditory canal — *see* Cellulitis, ear
 eyelid — *see* Abscess, eyelid
 face NEC L03.211
 finger (intrathecal) (periosteal) (subcutaneous) (subcuticular) L03.01- ☑
 foot — *see* Cellulitis, lower limb
 gangrenous — *see* Gangrene
 genital organ NEC
  female (external) N76.4
  male N49.9
   multiple sites N49.8
   specified NEC N49.8
 gluteal (region) L03.317
 gonococcal A54.89
 groin L03.314
 hand — *see* Cellulitis, upper limb
 head NEC L03.811
  face (any part, except ear, eye and nose) L03.211
 heel — *see* Cellulitis, lower limb
 hip — *see* Cellulitis, lower limb
 jaw (region) L03.211
 knee — *see* Cellulitis, lower limb
 labium (majus) (minus) — *see* Vulvitis
 lacrimal passages — *see* Inflammation, lacrimal, passages
 larynx J38.7
 leg — *see* Cellulitis, lower limb
 lip K13.0
 lower limb L03.11- ☑
  toe — *see* Cellulitis, toe
 mouth (floor) K12.2
 multiple sites, so stated L03.90
 nasopharynx J39.1
 navel L03.316
  newborn P38.9
   with mild hemorrhage P38.1
   without hemorrhage P38.9
 neck (region) L03.221
 nipple (acute) (nonpuerperal) (subacute) N61.0
 nose (septum) (external) J34.0
 orbit, orbital H05.01- ☑
 palate (soft) K12.2
 pectoral (region) L03.313
 pelvis, pelvic (chronic)
  female (*see also* Disease, pelvis, inflammatory) N73.2
   acute N73.0

Cellulitis — *continued*
  pelvis, pelvic — *continued*
    following ectopic or molar pregnancy O08.0
      male K65.0
  penis N48.22
  perineal, perineum L03.315
  periorbital L03.213
  perirectal K61.1
  peritonsillar J36
  periurethral N34.0
  periuterine (*see also* Disease, pelvis, inflammatory)
    N73.2
    acute N73.0
  pharynx J39.1
  preseptal L03.213
  rectum K61.1
  retroperitoneal K68.9
  round ligament
    acute N73.0
  scalp (any part) L03.811
  scrotum N49.2
  seminal vesicle N49.0
  shoulder — *see* Cellulitis, upper limb
  specified site NEC L03.818
  submandibular (region) (space) (triangle) K12.2
    gland K11.3
  submaxillary (region) K12.2
    gland K11.3
  thigh — *see* Cellulitis, lower limb
  thumb (intrathecal) (periosteal) (subcutaneous) (sub-
    cuticular) — *see* Cellulitis, finger
  toe (intrathecal) (periosteal) (subcutaneous) (subcutic-
    ular) L03.03- ☑
  tonsil J36
  trunk L03.319
    abdominal wall L03.311
    back (any part) L03.312
    buttock L03.317
    chest wall L03.313
    groin L03.314
    perineal, perineum L03.315
    umbilicus L03.316
  tuberculous (primary) A18.4
  umbilicus L03.316
  upper limb L03.11- ☑
    axilla — *see* Cellulitis, axilla
    finger — *see* Cellulitis, finger
    thumb — *see* Cellulitis, finger
  vaccinal T88.0 ☑
  vocal cord J38.3
  vulva — *see* Vulvitis
  wrist — *see* Cellulitis, upper limb
Cementoblastoma, benign — *see* Cyst, calcifying
  odontogenic
Cementoma — *see* Cyst, calcifying odontogenic
Cementoperiostitis — *see* Periodontitis
Cementosis K03.4
Central auditory processing disorder H93.25
Central pain syndrome G89.0
Cephalematocele, cephal (o)hematocele
  newborn P52.8
    birth injury P10.8
  traumatic — *see* Hematoma, brain
Cephalematoma, cephalhematoma (calcified)
  newborn (birth injury) P12.0
  traumatic — *see* Hematoma, brain
Cephalgia, cephalalgia (*see also* Headache)
  histamine G44.009
    intractable G44.001
    not intractable G44.009
  trigeminal autonomic (TAC) NEC G44.099
    intractable G44.091
    not intractable G44.099
Cephalic — *see* condition
Cephalitis — *see* Encephalitis
Cephalocele — *see* Encephalocele
Cephalomenia N94.89
Cephalopelvic — *see* condition
Cerclage (with cervical incompetence) in pregnancy —
  see Incompetence, cervix, in pregnancy
Cerebellitis — *see* Encephalitis
Cerebellum, cerebellar — *see* condition
Cerebral — *see* condition
Cerebritis — *see* Encephalitis
Cerebro-hepato-renal syndrome Q87.89
Cerebromalacia — *see* Softening, brain
  sequelae of cerebrovascular disease I69.398
Cerebroside lipidosis E75.22

Cerebrospasticity (congenital) G80.1
Cerebrospinal — *see* condition
Cerebrum — *see* condition
Ceroid-lipofuscinosis, neuronal E75.4
Cerumen (accumulation) (impacted) H61.2- ☑
Cervical (*see also* condition)
  auricle Q18.2
  dysplasia in pregnancy — *see* Abnormal, cervix, in
    pregnancy or childbirth
  erosion in pregnancy — *see* Abnormal, cervix, in
    pregnancy or childbirth
  fibrosis in pregnancy — *see* Abnormal, cervix, in
    pregnancy or childbirth
  fusion syndrome Q76.1
  rib Q76.5
  shortening (complicating pregnancy) O26.87- ☑
Cervicalgia M54.2
Cervicitis (acute) (chronic) (nonvenereal) (senile (atrophic)) (subacute) (with ulceration) N72
  with
    abortion — *see* Abortion, by type complicated by
      genital tract and pelvic infection
    ectopic pregnancy O08.0
    molar pregnancy O08.0
  chlamydial A56.09
  gonococcal A54.03
  herpesviral A60.03
  puerperal (postpartum) O86.11
  syphilitic A52.76
  trichomonal A59.09
  tuberculous A18.16
Cervicocolpitis (emphysematosa) (see also Cervicitis)
  N72
Cervix — *see* condition
**Cesarean delivery, previous, affecting management
  of pregnancy** O34.219
  classical (vertical) scar O34.212
  low transverse scar O34.211
Céstan (-Chenais) paralysis or syndrome G46.3
Céstan-Raymond syndrome I65.8
Cestode infestation B71.9
  specified type NEC B71.8
Cestodiasis B71.9
Chabert's disease A22.9
Chacaleh E53.8
Chafing L30.4
Chagas' (-Mazza) disease (chronic) B57.2
  with
    cardiovascular involvement NEC B57.2
    digestive system involvement B57.30
      megacolon B57.32
      megaesophagus B57.31
      other specified B57.39
    megacolon B57.32
    megaesophagus B57.31
    myocarditis B57.2
    nervous system involvement B57.40
      meningitis B57.41
      meningoencephalitis B57.42
      other specified B57.49
    specified organ involvement NEC B57.5
  acute (with) B57.1
    cardiovascular NEC B57.0
    myocarditis B57.0
Chagres fever B50.9
Chairridden Z74.09
Chalasia (cardiac sphincter) K21.9
Chalazion H00.19
  left H00.16
    lower H00.15
    upper H00.14
  right H00.13
    lower H00.12
    upper H00.11
Chalcosis (*see also* Disorder, globe, degenerative, chalcosis)
  cornea — *see* Deposit, cornea
  crystalline lens — *see* Cataract, complicated
  retina H35.89
Chalicosis (pulmonum) J62.8
Chancre (any genital site) (hard) (hunterian) (mixed)
  (primary) (seronegative) (seropositive) (syphilitic)
  A51.0
  congenital A50.07
  conjunctiva NEC A51.2
  Ducrey's A57
  extragenital A51.2
  eyelid A51.2

Chancre — *continued*
  lip A51.2
  nipple A51.2
  Nisbet's A57
  of
    carate A67.0
    pinta A67.0
    yaws A66.0
  palate, soft A51.2
  phagedenic A57
  simple A57
  soft A57
    bubo A57
    palate A51.2
  urethra A51.0
  yaws A66.0
Chancroid (anus) (genital) (penis) (perineum) (rectum)
  (urethra) (vulva) A57
Chandler's disease (osteochondritis dissecans, hip) —
  see Osteochondritis, dissecans, hip
Change(s) (in) (of) (*see also* Removal)
  arteriosclerotic — *see* Arteriosclerosis
  bone (*see also* Disorder, bone)
    diabetic — *see* Diabetes, bone change
  bowel habit R19.4
  cardiorenal (vascular) — *see* Hypertension, cardiorenal
  cardiovascular — *see* Disease, cardiovascular
  circulatory I99.9
  cognitive (mild) (organic) R41.89
  color, tooth, teeth
    during formation K00.8
    posteruptive K03.7
  contraceptive device Z30.433
  corneal membrane H18.30
    Bowman's membrane fold or rupture H18.31- ☑
    Descemet's membrane
      fold H18.32- ☑
      rupture H18.33- ☑
  coronary — *see* Disease, heart, ischemic
  degenerative, spine or vertebra — *see* Spondylosis
  dental pulp, regressive K04.2
  dressing (nonsurgical) Z48.00
    surgical Z48.01
  heart — *see* Disease, heart
  hip joint — *see* Derangement, joint, hip
  hyperplastic larynx J38.7
  hypertrophic
    nasal sinus J34.89
    turbinate, nasal J34.3
    upper respiratory tract J39.8
  indwelling catheter Z46.6
  inflammatory (*see also* Inflammation)
    sacroiliac M46.1
  job, anxiety concerning Z56.1
  joint — *see* Derangement, joint
  life — *see* Menopause
  mental status R41.82
  minimal (glomerular) (*see also* N00-N07 with fourth
    character .0) N05.0
  myocardium, myocardial — *see* Degeneration, myocar-
    dial
  of life — *see* Menopause
  pacemaker Z45.018
    pulse generator Z45.010
  personality (enduring) F68.8
    due to (secondary to)
      general medical condition F07.0
    secondary (nonspecific) F60.89
  regressive, dental pulp K04.2
  renal — *see* Disease, renal
  retina H35.9
    myopic (*see also* Myopia, degenerative) H44.2- ☑
  sacroiliac joint M53.3
  senile (*see also* condition) R54
  sensory R20.8
  skin R23.9
    acute, due to ultraviolet radiation L56.9
      specified NEC L56.8
    chronic, due to nonionizing radiation L57.9
      specified NEC L57.8
    cyanosis R23.0
    flushing R23.2
    pallor R23.1
    petechiae R23.3
    specified change NEC R23.8
    swelling — *see* Mass, localized
    texture R23.4

Change(s) — *continued*
  trophic
    arm — *see* Mononeuropathy, upper limb
    leg — *see* Mononeuropathy, lower limb
  vascular I99.9
  vasomotor I73.9
  voice R49.9
    psychogenic F44.4
    specified NEC R49.8
Changing sleep-work schedule, affecting sleep G47.26
Changuinola fever A93.1
Chapping skin T69.8 ☑
Charcot-Marie-Tooth disease, paralysis or syndrome G60.0
Charcot's
  arthropathy — *see* Arthropathy, neuropathic
  cirrhosis K74.3
  disease (tabetic arthropathy) A52.16
  joint (disease) (tabetic) A52.16
    diabetic — *see* Diabetes, with, arthropathy
    syringomyelic G95.0
  syndrome (intermittent claudication) I73.9
CHARGE association Q89.8
Charley-horse (quadriceps) M62.831
  traumatic (quadriceps) S76.11- ☑
Charlouis' disease — *see* Yaws
Cheadle's disease E54
Checking (of)
  cardiac pacemaker (battery) (electrode(s)) Z45.018
    pulse generator Z45.010
  implantable subdermal contraceptive Z30.46
  intrauterine contraceptive device Z30.431
  wound Z48.0- ☑
    due to injury — code to Injury, by site, using appropriate seventh character for subsequent encounter
Check-up — *see* Examination
Chédiak-Higashi (-Steinbrinck) **syndrome** (congenital gigantism of peroxidase granules) E70.330
Cheek — *see* condition
Cheese itch B88.0
Cheese-washer's lung J67.8
Cheese-worker's lung J67.8
Cheilitis (acute) (angular) (catarrhal) (chronic) (exfoliative) (gangrenous) (glandular) (infectional) (suppurative) (ulcerative) (vesicular) K13.0
  actinic (due to sun) L56.8
    other than from sun L59.8
  candidal B37.83
Cheilodynia K13.0
Cheiloschisis — *see* Cleft, lip
Cheilosis (angular) K13.0
  with pellagra E52
  due to
    vitamin B2 (riboflavin) deficiency E53.0
Cheiromegaly M79.89
Cheiropompholyx L30.1
Cheloid — *see* Keloid
Chemical burn — *see* Corrosion, by site
Chemodectoma — *see* Paraganglioma, nonchromaffin
Chemosis, conjunctiva — *see* Edema, conjunctiva
Chemotherapy (session) (for)
  cancer Z51.11
  neoplasm Z51.11
Cherubism M27.8
Chest — *see* condition
Cheyne-Stokes breathing (respiration) R06.3
Chiari's
  disease or syndrome (hepatic vein thrombosis) I82.0
  malformation
    type I G93.5
    type II — *see* Spina bifida
    net Q24.8
Chicago disease B40.9
Chickenpox — *see* Varicella
Chiclero ulcer or sore B55.1
Chigger (infestation) B88.0
Chignon (disease) B36.8
  newborn (from vacuum extraction) (birth injury) P12.1
Chilaiditi's syndrome (subphrenic displacement, colon) Q43.3
Chilblain(s) (lupus) T69.1 ☑
Child
  custody dispute Z65.3
Childbirth — *see* Delivery

Childhood
  cerebral X-linked adrenoleukodystrophy E71.520
  period of rapid growth Z00.2
Chill(s) R68.83
  with fever R50.9
  without fever R68.83
  congestive in malarial regions B54
Chilomastigiasis A07.8
Chimera 46,XX/46,XY Q99.0
Chin — *see* condition
Chinese dysentery A03.9
Chionophobia F40.228
Chitral fever A93.1
Chlamydia, chlamydial A74.9
  cervicitis A56.09
  conjunctivitis A74.0
  cystitis A56.01
  endometritis A56.11
  epididymitis A56.19
  female
    pelvic inflammatory disease A56.11
    pelviperitonitis A56.11
  orchitis A56.19
  peritonitis A74.81
  pharyngitis A56.4
  proctitis A56.3
  psittaci (infection) A70
  salpingitis A56.11
  sexually-transmitted infection NEC A56.8
  specified NEC A74.89
  urethritis A56.01
  vulvovaginitis A56.02
Chlamydiosis — *see* Chlamydia
Chloasma (skin) (idiopathic) (symptomatic) L81.1
  eyelid H02.719
    hyperthyroid E05.90 [H02.719]
      with thyroid storm E05.91 [H02.719]
    left H02.716
      lower H02.715
      upper H02.714
    right H02.713
      lower H02.712
      upper H02.711
Chloroma C92.3- ☑
Chlorosis D50.9
  Egyptian B76.9 [D63.8]
  miner's B76.9 [D63.8]
Chlorotic anemia D50.8
Chocolate cyst (ovary) N80.1
Choked
  disc or disk — *see* Papilledema
  on food, phlegm, or vomitus NOS — *see* Foreign body, by site
  while vomiting NOS — *see* Foreign body, by site
Chokes (resulting from bends) T70.3 ☑
Choking sensation R09.89
Cholangiectasis K83.8
Cholangiocarcinoma
  with hepatocellular carcinoma, combined C22.0
  liver C22.1
  specified site NEC — *see* Neoplasm, malignant, by site
  unspecified site C22.1
Cholangiohepatitis K83.8
  due to fluke infestation B66.1
Cholangiohepatoma C22.0
Cholangiolitis (acute) (chronic) (extrahepatic) (gangrenous) (intrahepatic) K83.0
  paratyphoidal — *see* Fever, paratyphoid
  typhoidal A01.09
Cholangioma D13.4
  malignant — *see* Cholangiocarcinoma
Cholangitis (ascending) (primary) (recurrent) (sclerosing) (secondary) (stenosing) (suppurative) K83.0
  with calculus, bile duct — *see* Calculus, bile duct, with cholangitis
  chronic nonsuppurative destructive K74.3
Cholecystectasia K82.8
Cholecystitis K81.9
  with
    calculus, stones in
      bile duct (common) (hepatic) — *see* Calculus, bile duct, with cholecystitis
      cystic duct — *see* Calculus, gallbladder, with cholecystitis
      gallbladder — *see* Calculus, gallbladder, with cholecystitis
      choledocholithiasis — *see* Calculus, bile duct, with cholecystitis

Cholecystitis — *continued*
  with — *continued*
    cholelithiasis — *see* Calculus, gallbladder, with cholecystitis
  acute (emphysematous) (gangrenous) (suppurative) K81.0
    with
      calculus, stones in
        cystic duct — *see* Calculus, gallbladder, with cholecystitis, acute
        gallbladder — *see* Calculus, gallbladder, with cholecystitis, acute
        choledocholithiasis — *see* Calculus, bile duct, with cholecystitis, acute
        cholelithiasis — *see* Calculus, gallbladder, with cholecystitis, acute
    chronic cholecystitis K81.2
      with gallbladder calculus K80.12
        with obstruction K80.13
  chronic K81.1
    with acute cholecystitis K81.2
      with gallbladder calculus K80.12
        with obstruction K80.13
  emphysematous (acute) — *see* Cholecystitis, acute
  gangrenous — *see* Cholecystitis, acute
  paratyphoidal, current A01.4
  suppurative — *see* Cholecystitis, acute
  typhoidal A01.09
Cholecystolithiasis — *see* Calculus, gallbladder
Choledochitis (suppurative) K83.0
Choledocholith — *see* Calculus, bile duct
Choledocholithiasis (common duct) (hepatic duct) — *see* Calculus, bile duct
  cystic — *see* Calculus, gallbladder
  typhoidal A01.09
Cholelithiasis (cystic duct) (gallbladder) (impacted) (multiple) — *see* Calculus, gallbladder
  bile duct (common) (hepatic) — *see* Calculus, bile duct
  hepatic duct — *see* Calculus, bile duct
  specified NEC K80.80
    with obstruction K80.81
Cholemia (*see also* Jaundice)
  familial (simple) (congenital) E80.4
  Gilbert's E80.4
Choleperitoneum, choleperitonitis K65.3
Cholera (Asiatic) (epidemic) (malignant) A00.9
  antimonial — *see* Poisoning, antimony
  classical A00.0
  due to Vibrio cholerae 01 A00.9
    biovar cholerae A00.0
    biovar eltor A00.1
    el tor A00.1
  el tor A00.1
Cholerine — *see* Cholera
Cholestasis NEC K83.1
  with hepatocyte injury K71.0
  due to total parenteral nutrition (TPN) K76.89
  pure K71.0
Cholesteatoma (ear) (middle) (with reaction) H71.9- ☑
  attic H71.0- ☑
  external ear (canal) H60.4- ☑
  mastoid H71.2- ☑
  postmastoidectomy cavity (recurrent) — *see* Complications, postmastoidectomy, recurrent cholesteatoma
  recurrent (postmastoidectomy) — *see* Complications, postmastoidectomy, recurrent cholesteatoma
  tympanum H71.1- ☑
Cholesteatosis, diffuse H71.3- ☑
Cholesteremia E78.00
Cholesterin in vitreous — *see* Deposit, crystalline
Cholesterol
  deposit
    retina H35.89
    vitreous — *see* Deposit, crystalline
  elevated (high) E78.00
    with elevated (high) triglycerides E78.2
    screening for Z13.220
  imbibition of gallbladder K82.4
Cholesterolemia (essential) (pure) E78.00
  familial E78.01
  hereditary E78.01
Cholesterolosis, cholesterosis (gallbladder) K82.4
  cerebrotendinous E75.5
Cholocolic fistula K82.3
Choluria R82.2
Chondritis M94.8X9

Chondritis — continued
aurical H61.03- ☑
costal (Tietze's) M94.0
external ear H61.03- ☑
patella, posttraumatic — see Chondromalacia, patella
pinna H61.03- ☑
purulent M94.8X- ☑
tuberculous NEC A18.02
intervertebral A18.01
Chondroblastoma (see also Neoplasm, bone, benign)
malignant — see Neoplasm, bone, malignant
Chondrocalcinosis M11.20
ankle M11.27- ☑
elbow M11.22- ☑
familial M11.10
ankle M11.17- ☑
elbow M11.12- ☑
foot joint M11.17- ☑
hand joint M11.14- ☑
hip M11.15- ☑
knee M11.16- ☑
multiple site M11.19
shoulder M11.11- ☑
vertebrae M11.18
wrist M11.13- ☑
foot joint M11.27- ☑
hand joint M11.24- ☑
hip M11.25- ☑
knee M11.26- ☑
multiple site M11.29
shoulder M11.21- ☑
specified type NEC M11.20
ankle M11.27- ☑
elbow M11.22- ☑
foot joint M11.27- ☑
hand joint M11.24- ☑
hip M11.25- ☑
knee M11.26- ☑
multiple site M11.29
shoulder M11.21- ☑
vertebrae M11.28
wrist M11.23- ☑
vertebrae M11.28
wrist M11.23- ☑
Chondrodermatitis nodularis helicis or anthelicis
— see Perichondritis, ear
Chondrodysplasia Q78.9
with hemangioma Q78.4
calcificans congenita Q77.3
fetalis Q77.4
metaphyseal (Jansen's) (McKusick's) (Schmid's) Q78.8
punctata Q77.3
Chondrodystrophy, chondrodystrophia (familial)
(fetalis) (hypoplastic) Q78.9
calcificans congenita Q77.3
myotonic (congenital) G71.13
punctata Q77.3
Chondroectodermal dysplasia Q77.6
Chondrogenesis imperfecta Q77.4
Chondrolysis M94.35- ☑
Chondroma (see also Neoplasm, cartilage, benign)
juxtacortical — see Neoplasm, bone, benign
periosteal — see Neoplasm, bone, benign
Chondromalacia (systemic) M94.20
acromioclavicular joint M94.21- ☑
ankle M94.27- ☑
elbow M94.22- ☑
foot joint M94.27- ☑
glenohumeral joint M94.21- ☑
hand joint M94.24- ☑
hip M94.25- ☑
knee M94.26- ☑
patella M22.4- ☑
multiple sites M94.29
patella M22.4- ☑
rib M94.28
sacroiliac joint M94.259
shoulder M94.21- ☑
sternoclavicular joint M94.21- ☑
vertebral joint M94.28
wrist M94.23- ☑
Chondromatosis (see also Neoplasm, cartilage, uncertain
behavior)
internal Q78.4
Chondromyxosarcoma — see Neoplasm, cartilage,
malignant

Chondro-osteodysplasia (Morquio-Brailsford type)
E76.219
Chondro-osteodystrophy E76.29
Chondro-osteoma — see Neoplasm, bone, benign
Chondropathia tuberosa M94.0
Chondrosarcoma — see Neoplasm, cartilage, malignant
juxtacortical — see Neoplasm, bone, malignant
mesenchymal — see Neoplasm, connective tissue,
malignant
myxoid — see Neoplasm, cartilage, malignant
Chordee (nonvenereal) N48.89
congenital Q54.4
gonococcal A54.09
Chorditis (fibrinous) (nodosa) (tuberosa) J38.2
Chordoma — see Neoplasm, vertebral (column), malignant
Chorea (chronic) (gravis) (posthemiplegic) (senile)
(spasmodic) G25.5
with
heart involvement I02.0
active or acute (conditions in I01-) I02.0
rheumatic I02.9
with valvular disorder I02.0
rheumatic heart disease (chronic) (inactive)(quiescent) — code to rheumatic heart condition
involved
drug-induced G25.4
habit F95.8
hereditary G10
Huntington's G10
hysterical F44.4
minor I02.9
with heart involvement I02.0
progressive G25.5
hereditary G10
rheumatic (chronic) I02.9
with heart involvement I02.0
Sydenham's I02.9
with heart involvement — see Chorea, with
rheumatic heart disease
nonrheumatic G25.5
Choreoathetosis (paroxysmal) G25.5
Chorioadenoma (destruens) D39.2
Chorioamnionitis O41.12- ☑
Chorioangioma D26.7
Choriocarcinoma — see Neoplasm, malignant, by site
combined with
embryonal carcinoma — see Neoplasm, malignant,
by site
other germ cell elements — see Neoplasm, malignant, by site
teratoma — see Neoplasm, malignant, by site
specified site — see Neoplasm, malignant, by site
unspecified site
female C58
male C62.90
Chorioencephalitis (acute) (lymphocytic) (serous) A87.2
Chorioepithelioma — see Choriocarcinoma
Choriomeningitis (acute) (lymphocytic) (serous) A87.2
Chorionepithelioma — see Choriocarcinoma
Chorioretinitis (see also Inflammation, chorioretinal)
disseminated (see also Inflammation, chorioretinal,
disseminated)
in neurosyphilis A52.19
Egyptian B76.9 [D63.8]
focal (see also Inflammation, chorioretinal, focal)
histoplasmic B39.9 [H32]
in (due to)
histoplasmosis B39.9 [H32]
syphilis (secondary) A51.43
late A52.71
toxoplasmosis (acquired) B58.01
congenital (active) P37.1 [H32]
tuberculosis A18.53
juxtapapillary, juxtapapillaris — see Inflammation,
chorioretinal, focal, juxtapapillary
leprous A30.9 [H32]
miner's B76.9 [D63.8]
progressive myopia (degeneration) (see also Myopia,
degenerative) H44.2- ☑
syphilitic (secondary) A51.43
congenital (early) A50.01 [H32]
late A50.32
late A52.71
tuberculous A18.53
Chorioretinopathy, central serous H35.71- ☑
Choroid — see condition
Choroideremia H31.21

Choroiditis — see Chorioretinitis
Choroidopathy — see Disorder, choroid
Choroidoretinitis — see Chorioretinitis
Choroidoretinopathy, central serous — see Chori-
oretinopathy, central serous
Christian-Weber disease M35.6
Christmas disease D67
Chromaffinoma (see also Neoplasm, benign, by site)
malignant — see Neoplasm, malignant, by site
Chromatopsia — see Deficiency, color vision
Chromhidrosis, chromidrosis L75.1
Chromoblastomycosis — see Chromomycosis
Chromoconversion R82.91
Chromomycosis B43.9
brain abscess B43.1
cerebral B43.1
cutaneous B43.0
skin B43.0
specified NEC B43.8
subcutaneous abscess or cyst B43.2
Chromophytosis B36.0
Chromosome — see Anomaly, by chromosome involved
D (1) — see Anomaly, chromosome 13
E (3) — see Anomaly, chromosome 18
G — see Anomaly, chromosome 21
Chromotrichomycosis B36.8
Chronic — see condition
fracture — see Fracture, pathological
Churg-Strauss syndrome M30.1
Chyle cyst, mesentery I89.8
Chylocele (nonfilarial) I89.8
filarial (see also Infestation, filarial) B74.9 [N51]
tunica vaginalis N50.89
filarial (see also Infestation, filarial) B74.9 [N51]
Chylomicronemia (fasting) (with hyperprebetalipopro-
teinemia) E78.3
Chylopericardium I31.3
acute I30.9
Chylothorax (nonfilarial) I89.8
filarial (see also Infestation, filarial) B74.9 [J91.8]
Chylous — see condition
Chyluria (nonfilarial) R82.0
due to
bilharziasis B65.0
Brugia (malayi) B74.1
timori B74.2
schistosomiasis (bilharziasis) B65.0
Wuchereria (bancrofti) B74.0
filarial — see Infestation, filarial
Cicatricial (deformity) — see Cicatrix
Cicatrix (adherent) (contracted) (painful) (vicious) (see
also Scar) L90.5
adenoid (and tonsil) J35.8
alveolar process M26.79
anus K62.89
auricle — see Disorder, pinna, specified type NEC
bile duct (common) (hepatic) K83.8
bladder N32.89
bone — see Disorder, bone, specified type NEC
brain G93.89
cervix (postoperative) (postpartal) N88.1
common duct K83.8
cornea H17.9
tuberculous A18.59
duodenum (bulb), obstructive K31.5
esophagus K22.2
eyelid — see Disorder, eyelid function
hypopharynx J39.2
lacrimal passages — see Obstruction, lacrimal
larynx J38.7
lung J98.4
middle ear H74.8 ☑
mouth K13.79
muscle M62.89
with contracture — see Contraction, muscle NEC
nasopharynx J39.2
palate (soft) K13.79
penis N48.89
pharynx J39.2
prostate N42.89
rectum K62.89
retina — see Scar, chorioretinal
semilunar cartilage — see Derangement, meniscus
seminal vesicle N50.89
skin L90.5
infected L08.89
postinfective L90.5

☑ **Additional Character Required — Refer to the Tabular List for Character Selection**   ▽ Subterms under main terms may continue to next column or page

Cicatrix — *continued*
  skin — *continued*
    tuberculous B90.8
    specified site NEC L90.5
  throat J39.2
  tongue K14.8
  tonsil (and adenoid) J35.8
  trachea J39.8
  tuberculous NEC B90.9
  urethra N36.8
  uterus N85.8
  vagina N89.8
    postoperative N99.2
  vocal cord J38.3
  wrist, constricting (annular) L90.5
CIDP (chronic inflammatory demyelinating polyneuropathy) G61.81
CIN — *see* Neoplasia, intraepithelial, cervix
CINCA (chronic infantile neurological, cutaneous and articular syndrome) M04.2
Cinchonism — *see* Deafness, ototoxic
  correct substance properly administered — *see* Table of Drugs and Chemicals, by drug, adverse effect
  overdose or wrong substance given or taken — *see* Table of Drugs and Chemicals, by drug, poisoning
Circle of Willis — *see* condition
Circular — *see* condition
Circulating anticoagulants (*see also* Disorder, hemorrhagic) D68.318
  due to drugs (*see also* Disorder, hemorrhagic) D68.32
  following childbirth O72.3
Circulation
  collateral, any site I99.8
  defective (lower extremity) I99.9
    congenital Q28.9
  embryonic Q28.9
  failure (peripheral) R57.9
    newborn P29.89
  fetal, persistent P29.38
  heart, incomplete Q28.9
Circulatory system — *see* condition
Circulus senilis (cornea) — *see* Degeneration, cornea, senile
Circumcision (in absence of medical indication) (ritual) (routine) Z41.2
Circumscribed — *see* condition
Circumvallate placenta O43.11- ☑
Cirrhosis, cirrhotic (hepatic) (liver) K74.60
  alcoholic K70.30
    with ascites K70.31
  atrophic — *see* Cirrhosis, liver
  Baumgarten-Cruveilhier K74.69
  biliary (cholangiolitic) (cholangitic) (hypertrophic) (obstructive) (pericholangiolitic) K74.5
    due to
      Clonorchiasis B66.1
      flukes B66.3
    primary K74.3
    secondary K74.4
  cardiac (of liver) K76.1
  Charcot's K74.3
  cholangiolitic, cholangitic, cholostatic (primary) K74.3
  congestive K76.1
  Cruveilhier-Baumgarten K74.69
  cryptogenic (liver) K74.69
  due to
    hepatolenticular degeneration E83.01
    Wilson's disease E83.01
    xanthomatosis E78.2
  fatty K76.0
    alcoholic K70.0
  Hanot's (hypertrophic) K74.3
  hepatic — *see* Cirrhosis, liver
  hypertrophic K74.3
  Indian childhood K74.69
  kidney — *see* Sclerosis, renal
  Laennec's K70.30
    with ascites K70.31
    alcoholic K70.30
      with ascites K70.31
    nonalcoholic K74.69
  liver K74.60
    alcoholic K70.30
      with ascites K70.31
      fatty K70.0
    congenital P78.81
    syphilitic A52.74

Cirrhosis, cirrhotic — *continued*
  lung (chronic) J84.10
  macronodular K74.69
    alcoholic K70.30
      with ascites K70.31
  micronodular K74.69
    alcoholic K70.30
      with ascites K70.31
  mixed type K74.69
  monolobular K74.3
  nephritis — *see* Sclerosis, renal
  nutritional K74.69
    alcoholic K70.30
      with ascites K70.31
  obstructive — *see* Cirrhosis, biliary
  ovarian N83.8
  pancreas (duct) K86.89
  pigmentary E83.110
  portal K74.69
    alcoholic K70.30
      with ascites K70.31
  postnecrotic K74.69
    alcoholic K70.30
      with ascites K70.31
  pulmonary J84.10
  renal — *see* Sclerosis, renal
  spleen D73.2
  stasis K76.1
  Todd's K74.3
  unilobar K74.3
  xanthomatous (biliary) K74.5
    due to xanthomatosis (familial) (metabolic) (primary) E78.2
Cistern, subarachnoid R93.0
Citrullinemia E72.23
Citrullinuria E72.23
Civatte's disease or poikiloderma L57.3
Clam digger's itch B65.3
Clammy skin R23.1
Clap — *see* Gonorrhea
Clarke-Hadfield syndrome (pancreatic infantilism) K86.89
Clark's paralysis G80.9
Clastothrix L67.8
Claude Bernard-Horner syndrome G90.2
  traumatic — *see* Injury, nerve, cervical sympathetic
Claude's disease or syndrome G46.3
Claudicatio venosa intermittens I87.8
Claudication (intermittent) I73.9
  cerebral (artery) G45.9
  spinal cord (arteriosclerotic) G95.19
    syphilitic A52.09
  venous (axillary) I87.8
Claustrophobia F40.240
Clavus (infected) L84
Clawfoot (congenital) Q66.89
  acquired — *see* Deformity, limb, clawfoot
Clawhand (acquired) (*see also* Deformity, limb, clawhand)
  congenital Q68.1
Clawtoe (congenital) Q66.89
  acquired — *see* Deformity, toe, specified NEC
Clay eating — *see* Pica
Cleansing of artificial opening — *see* Attention to, artificial, opening
Cleft (congenital) — *see also* Imperfect, closure
  alveolar process M26.79
  branchial (persistent) Q18.2
    cyst Q18.0
      fistula Q18.0
      sinus Q18.0
  cricoid cartilage, posterior Q31.8
  cyst Q18.0
    fistula Q18.0
    sinus Q18.0
  foot Q72.7 ☑
  hand Q71.6 ☑
  lip (unilateral) Q36.9
    with cleft palate Q37.9
      hard Q37.1
        with soft Q37.5
      soft Q37.3
        with hard Q37.5
    bilateral Q36.0
      with cleft palate Q37.8
      hard Q37.0
        with soft Q37.4
      soft Q37.2
        with hard Q37.4

Cleft — *continued*
  lip — *continued*
    median Q36.1
  nose Q30.2
  palate Q35.9
    with cleft lip (unilateral) Q37.9
      bilateral Q37.8
    hard Q35.1
      with
        cleft lip (unilateral) Q37.1
          bilateral Q37.0
        soft Q35.5
          with cleft lip (unilateral) Q37.5
            bilateral Q37.4
    medial Q35.5
    soft Q35.3
      with
        cleft lip (unilateral) Q37.3
          bilateral Q37.2
        hard Q35.5
          with cleft lip (unilateral) Q37.5
            bilateral Q37.4
  penis Q55.69
  scrotum Q55.29
  thyroid cartilage Q31.8
  uvula Q35.7
Cleidocranial dysostosis Q74.0
Cleptomania F63.2
Clicking hip (newborn) R29.4
Climacteric (female) (*see also* Menopause)
  arthritis (any site) NEC — *see* Arthritis, specified form NEC
  depression (single episode) F32.89
    recurrent episode F33.8
  male (symptoms) (syndrome) NEC N50.89
  melancholia (single episode) F32.89
    recurrent episode F33.8
  paranoid state F22
  polyarthritis NEC — *see* Arthritis, specified form NEC
  symptoms (female) N95.1
Clinical research investigation (clinical trial) (control subject) (normal comparison) (participant) Z00.6
Clitoris — *see* condition
Cloaca (persistent) Q43.7
Clonorchiasis, clonorchis infection (liver) B66.1
Clonus R25.8
Closed bite M26.29
Clostridium (C.) **perfringens, as cause of disease classified elsewhere** B96.7
Closure
  congenital, nose Q30.0
  cranial sutures, premature Q75.0
  defective or imperfect NEC — *see* Imperfect, closure
  fistula, delayed — *see* Fistula
  foramen ovale, imperfect Q21.1
  hymen N89.6
  interauricular septum, defective Q21.1
  interventricular septum, defective Q21.0
  lacrimal duct (*see also* Stenosis, lacrimal, duct)
    congenital Q10.5
  nose (congenital) Q30.0
    acquired M95.0
  of artificial opening — *see* Attention to, artificial, opening
  vagina N89.5
  valve — *see* Endocarditis
  vulva N90.5
Clot (blood) (*see also* Embolism)
  artery (obstruction) (occlusion) — *see* Embolism
  bladder N32.89
  brain (intradural or extradural) — *see* Occlusion, artery, cerebral
  circulation I74.9
  heart (*see also* Infarct, myocardium)
    not resulting in infarction I51.3
  vein — *see* Thrombosis
Clouded state R40.1
  epileptic — *see* Epilepsy, specified NEC
  paroxysmal — *see* Epilepsy, specified NEC
Cloudy antrum, antra J32.0
Clouston's (hidrotic) **ectodermal dysplasia** Q82.4
Clubbed nail pachydermoperiostosis M89.40 [L62]
Clubbing of finger(s) (nails) R68.3
Clubfinger R68.3
  congenital Q68.1
Clubfoot (congenital) Q66.89
  acquired — *see* Deformity, limb, clubfoot
  equinovarus Q66.0

⬛ **Subterms under main terms may continue to next column or page**   ☑ **Additional Character Required — Refer to the Tabular List for Character Selection**   **55**

Cicatrix — Clubfoot

Clubfoot — *continued*
  paralytic — *see* Deformity, limb, clubfoot
Clubhand (congenital) (radial) Q71.4- ☑
  acquired — *see* Deformity, limb, clubhand
Clubnail R68.3
  congenital Q84.6
Clump, kidney Q63.1
Clumsiness, clumsy child syndrome F82
Cluttering F80.81
Clutton's joints A50.51 [M12.80]
Coagulation, intravascular (diffuse) (disseminated)
  (*see also* Defibrination syndrome)
  complicating abortion — *see* Abortion, by type, com-
    plicated by, intravascular coagulation
  following ectopic or molar pregnancy O08.1
Coagulopathy (*see also* Defect, coagulation)
  consumption D65
  intravascular D65
    newborn P60
Coalition
  calcaneo-scaphoid Q66.89
  tarsal Q66.89
Coalminer's
  elbow — *see* Bursitis, elbow, olecranon
  lung or pneumoconiosis J60
Coalworker's lung or pneumoconiosis J60
Coarctation
  aorta (preductal) (postductal) Q25.1
  pulmonary artery Q25.71
Coated tongue K14.3
Coats' disease (exudative retinopathy) — *see*
  Retinopathy, exudative
Cocaine-induced
  anxiety disorder F14.980
  bipolar and related disorder F14.94
  depressive disorder F14.94
  obsessive-compulsive and related disorder F14.988
  psychotic disorder F14.959
  sexual dysfunction F14.981
  sleep disorder F14.982
Cocainism — *see* Disorder, cocaine use
Coccidioidomycosis B38.9
  cutaneous B38.3
  disseminated B38.7
  generalized B38.7
  meninges B38.4
  prostate B38.81
  pulmonary B38.2
    acute B38.0
    chronic B38.1
  skin B38.3
  specified NEC B38.89
Coccidioidosis — *see* Coccidioidomycosis
Coccidiosis (intestinal) A07.3
Coccydynia, coccygodynia M53.3
Coccyx — *see* condition
Cochin-China diarrhea K90.1
Cockayne's syndrome Q87.1
Cocked up toe — *see* Deformity, toe, specified NEC
Cock's peculiar tumor L72.3
Codman's tumor — *see* Neoplasm, bone, benign
Coenurosis B71.8
Coffee-worker's lung J67.8
Cogan's syndrome H16.32- ☑
  oculomotor apraxia H51.8
Coitus, painful (female) N94.10
  male N53.12
  psychogenic F52.6
Cold J00
  with influenza, flu, or grippe — *see* Influenza, with,
    respiratory manifestations NEC
  agglutinin disease or hemoglobinuria (chronic) D59.1
  bronchial — *see* Bronchitis
  chest — *see* Bronchitis
  common (head) J00
  effects of T69.9 ☑
    specified effect NEC T69.8 ☑
  excessive, effects of T69.9 ☑
    specified effect NEC T69.8 ☑
  exhaustion from T69.8 ☑
  exposure to T69.9 ☑
    specified effect NEC T69.8 ☑
  head J00
  injury syndrome (newborn) P80.0
  on lung — *see* Bronchitis
  rose J30.1
  sensitivity, auto-immune D59.1

Cold — *continued*
  symptoms J00
  virus J00
Coldsore B00.1
Colibacillosis A49.8
  as the cause of other disease (*see also* Escherichia coli)
    B96.20
  generalized A41.50
Colic (bilious) (infantile) (intestinal) (recurrent) (spasmodic) R10.83
  abdomen R10.83
    psychogenic F45.8
  appendix, appendicular K38.8
  bile duct — *see* Calculus, bile duct
  biliary — *see* Calculus, bile duct
  common duct — *see* Calculus, bile duct
  cystic duct — *see* Calculus, gallbladder
  Devonshire NEC — *see* Poisoning, lead
  gallbladder — *see* Calculus, gallbladder
  gallstone — *see* Calculus, gallbladder
    gallbladder or cystic duct — *see* Calculus, gallblad-
      der
  hepatic (duct) — *see* Calculus, bile duct
  hysterical F45.8
  kidney N23
  lead NEC — *see* Poisoning, lead
  mucous K58.9
    with diarrhea K58.0
    psychogenic F54
  nephritic N23
  painter's NEC — *see* Poisoning, lead
  pancreas K86.89
  psychogenic F45.8
  renal N23
  saturnine NEC — *see* Poisoning, lead
  ureter N23
  urethral N36.8
    due to calculus N21.1
  uterus NEC N94.89
    menstrual — *see* Dysmenorrhea
  worm NOS B83.9
Colicystitis — *see* Cystitis
Colitis (acute) (catarrhal) (chronic) (noninfective) (hemorrhagic) (*see also* Enteritis) K52.9
  allergic K52.29
    with
      food protein-induced enterocolitis syndrome
        K52.21
      proctocolitis K52.82
  amebic (acute) (*see also* Amebiasis) A06.0
    nondysenteric A06.2
  anthrax A22.2
  bacillary — *see* Infection, Shigella
  balantidial A07.0
  Clostridium difficile
    not specified as recurrent A04.72
    recurrent A04.71
  coccidial A07.3
  collagenous K52.831
  cystica superficialis K52.89
  dietary counseling and surveillance (for) Z71.3
  dietetic (*see also* Colitis, allergic) K52.29
  drug-induced K52.1
  due to radiation K52.0
  eosinophilic K52.82
  food hypersensitivity (*see also* Colitis, allergic) K52.29
  giardial A07.1
  granulomatous — *see* Enteritis, regional, large intes-
    tine
  indeterminate, so stated K52.3
  infectious — *see* Enteritis, infectious
  ischemic K55.9
    acute (subacute) (*see also* Ischemia, intestine,
      acute) K55.039
    chronic K55.1
    due to mesenteric artery insufficiency K55.1
    fulminant (acute) (*see also* Ischemia, intestine,
      acute) K55.039
  left sided K51.50
    with
      abscess K51.514
      complication K51.519
        specified NEC K51.518
      fistula K51.513
      obstruction K51.512
      rectal bleeding K51.511
  lymphocytic K52.832

Colitis — *continued*
  membranous
    psychogenic F54
  microscopic K52.839
    specified NEC K52.838
  mucous — *see* Syndrome, irritable, bowel
    psychogenic F54
  noninfective K52.9
    specified NEC K52.89
  polyposa — *see* Polyp, colon, inflammatory
  protozoal A07.9
  pseudomembranous
    not specified as recurrent A04.72
    recurrent A04.71
  pseudomucinous — *see* Syndrome, irritable, bowel
  regional — *see* Enteritis, regional, large intestine
    infectious A09
  segmental — *see* Enteritis, regional, large intestine
  septic — *see* Enteritis, infectious
  spastic K58.9
    with diarrhea K58.0
    psychogenic F54
  staphylococcal A04.8
    foodborne A05.0
  subacute ischemic (*see also* Ischemia, intestine, acute)
    K55.039
  thromboulcerative (*see also* Ischemia, intestine, acute)
    K55.039
  toxic NEC K52.1
    due to Clostridium difficile
      not specified as recurrent A04.72
      recurrent A04.71
  transmural — *see* Enteritis, regional, large intestine
  trichomonal A07.8
  tuberculous (ulcerative) A18.32
  ulcerative (chronic) K51.90
    with
      complication K51.919
        abscess K51.914
        fistula K51.913
        obstruction K51.912
        rectal bleeding K51.911
        specified complication NEC K51.918
    enterocolitis — *see* Enterocolitis, ulcerative
    ileocolitis — *see* Ileocolitis, ulcerative
    mucosal proctocolitis — *see* Proctocolitis, mucosal
    proctitis — *see* Proctitis, ulcerative
    pseudopolyposis — *see* Polyp, colon, inflammatory
    psychogenic F54
    rectosigmoiditis — *see* Rectosigmoiditis, ulcerative
    specified type NEC K51.80
      with
        complication K51.819
          abscess K51.814
          fistula K51.813
          obstruction K51.812
          rectal bleeding K51.811
          specified complication NEC K51.818
Collagenosis, collagen disease (nonvascular) (vascular)
  M35.9
  cardiovascular I42.8
  reactive perforating L87.1
  specified NEC M35.8
Collapse R55
  adrenal E27.2
  cardiorespiratory R57.0
  cardiovascular R57.0
    newborn P29.89
  circulatory (peripheral) R57.9
    during or after labor and delivery O75.1
    following ectopic or molar pregnancy O08.3
    newborn P29.89
  during or
    after labor and delivery O75.1
    resulting from a procedure, not elsewhere classified
      T81.10 ☑
  external ear canal — *see* Stenosis, external ear canal
  general R55
  heart — *see* Disease, heart
  heat T67.1 ☑
  hysterical F44.89
  labyrinth, membranous (congenital) Q16.5
  lung (massive) (*see also* Atelectasis) J98.19
    pressure due to anesthesia (general) (local) or
      other sedation T88.2 ☑
      during labor and delivery O74.1
      in pregnancy O29.02- ☑
      postpartum, puerperal O89.09

Collapse — continued
  myocardial — see Disease, heart
  nervous F48.8
  neurocirculatory F45.8
  nose M95.0
  postoperative T81.10 ☑
  pulmonary (see also Atelectasis) J98.19
    newborn — see Atelectasis
  trachea J39.8
  tracheobronchial J98.09
  valvular — see Endocarditis
  vascular (peripheral) R57.9
    during or after labor and delivery O75.1
    following ectopic or molar pregnancy O08.3
    newborn P29.89
  vertebra M48.50- ☑
    cervical region M48.52- ☑
    cervicothoracic region M48.53- ☑
    in (due to)
      metastasis — see Collapse, vertebra, in, specified disease NEC
      osteoporosis (see also Osteoporosis) M80.88 ☑
        cervical region M80.88 ☑
        cervicothoracic region M80.88 ☑
        lumbar region M80.88 ☑
        lumbosacral region M80.88 ☑
        multiple sites M80.88 ☑
        occipito-atlanto-axial region M80.88 ☑
        sacrococcygeal region M80.88 ☑
        thoracic region M80.88 ☑
        thoracolumbar region M80.88 ☑
      specified disease NEC M48.50- ☑
        cervical region M48.52- ☑
        cervicothoracic region M48.53- ☑
        lumbar region M48.56- ☑
        lumbosacral region M48.57- ☑
        occipito-atlanto-axial region M48.51- ☑
        sacrococcygeal region M48.58- ☑
        thoracic region M48.54- ☑
        thoracolumbar region M48.55- ☑
    lumbar region M48.56- ☑
    lumbosacral region M48.57- ☑
    occipito-atlanto-axial region M48.51- ☑
    sacrococcygeal region M48.58- ☑
    thoracic region M48.54- ☑
    thoracolumbar region M48.55- ☑
Collateral (see also condition)
  circulation (venous) I87.8
  dilation, veins I87.8
Colles' fracture S52.53- ☑
Collet (-Sicard) syndrome G52.7
Collier's asthma or lung J60
Collodion baby Q80.2
Colloid nodule (of thyroid) (cystic) E04.1
Coloboma (iris) Q13.0
  eyelid Q10.3
  fundus Q14.8
  lens Q12.2
  optic disc (congenital) Q14.2
    acquired H47.31- ☑
Coloenteritis — see Enteritis
Colon — see condition
Colonization
  MRSA (Methicillin resistant Staphylococcus aureus) Z22.322
  MSSA (Methicillin susceptible Staphylococcus aureus) Z22.321
  status — see Carrier (suspected) of
Coloptosis K63.4
Color blindness — see Deficiency, color vision
Colostomy
  attention to Z43.3
  fitting or adjustment Z46.89
  malfunctioning K94.03
  status Z93.3
Colpitis (acute) — see Vaginitis
Colpocele N81.5
Colpocystitis — see Vaginitis
Colpospasm N94.2
Column, spinal, vertebral — see condition
Coma R40.20
  with
    motor response (none) R40.231 ☑
      abnormal extensor posturing to pain or noxious stimuli (< 2 years of age) R40.232 ☑
      abnormal flexure posturing to pain or noxious stimuli (0-5 years of age) R40.233 ☑

Coma — continued
  with — continued
    motor response — continued
      extensor posturing to pain or noxious stimuli (2-5 years of age) R40.232 ☑
      flexion/decorticate posturing (< 2 years of age) R40.233 ☑
      localizes pain (2-5 years of age) R40.235 ☑
      normal or spontaneous movement (< 2 years of age) R40.236 ☑
      obeys commands (2-5 years of age) R40.236 ☑
      withdraws from pain or noxious stimuli (0-5 years of age) R40.234 ☑
      withdraws to touch (< 2 years of age) R40.235 ☑
    opening of eyes (never) R40.211 ☑
      in response to
        pain R40.212 ☑
        sound R40.213 ☑
      spontaneous R40.214 ☑
    verbal response (none) R40.221 ☑
      confused conversation R40.224 ☑
      cooing or babbling or crying appropriately (< 2 years of age) R40.225 ☑
      inappropriate crying or screaming (< 2 years of age) R40.223 ☑
      inappropriate words (2-5 years of age) R40.224 ☑
      incomprehensible sounds (2-5 years of age) R40.222 ☑
      incomprehensible words R40.222 ☑
      irritable cries (< 2 years of age) R40.224 ☑
      moans/grunts to pain; restless (< 2 years old) R40.222 ☑
      oriented R40.225 ☑
      screaming (2-5 years of age) R40.223 ☑
      uses appropriate words (2-5 years of age) R40.225 ☑
  eclamptic — see Eclampsia
  epileptic — see Epilepsy
  Glasgow, scale score — see Glasgow coma scale
  hepatic — see Failure, hepatic, by type, with coma
  hyperglycemic (diabetic) — see Diabetes, by type, with hyperosmolarity, with coma
  hyperosmolar (diabetic) — see Diabetes, by type, with hyperosmolarity, with coma
  hypoglycemic (diabetic) — see Diabetes, by type, with hypoglycemia, with coma
    nondiabetic E15
  in diabetes — see Diabetes, coma
  insulin-induced — see Coma, hypoglycemic
  ketoacidotic (diabetic) — see Diabetes, by type, with ketoacidosis, with coma
  myxedematous E03.5
  newborn P91.5
  persistent vegetative state R40.3
  specified NEC, without documented Glasgow coma scale score, or with partial Glasgow coma scale score reported R40.244 ☑
Comatose — see Coma
Combat fatigue F43.0
Combined — see condition
Comedo, comedones (giant) L70.0
Comedocarcinoma (see also Neoplasm, breast, malignant)
  noninfiltrating
    breast D05.8- ☑
    specified site — see Neoplasm, in situ, by site
    unspecified site D05.8- ☑
Comedomastitis — see Ectasia, mammary duct
Comminuted fracture — code as Fracture, closed
Common
  arterial trunk Q20.0
  atrioventricular canal Q21.2
  atrium Q21.1
  cold (head) J00
  truncus (arteriosus) Q20.0
  variable immunodeficiency — see Immunodeficiency, common variable
  ventricle Q20.4
Commotio, commotion (current)
  brain — see Injury, intracranial, concussion
  cerebri — see Injury, intracranial, concussion
  retinae S05.8X- ☑
  spinal cord — see Injury, spinal cord, by region
  spinalis — see Injury, spinal cord, by region

Communication
  between
    base of aorta and pulmonary artery Q21.4
    left ventricle and right atrium Q20.5
    pericardial sac and pleural sac Q34.8
    pulmonary artery and pulmonary vein, congenital Q25.72
  congenital between uterus and digestive or urinary tract Q51.7
Compartment syndrome (deep) (posterior) (traumatic) T79.A0 ☑ (following T79.7)
  abdomen T79.A3 ☑ (following T79.7)
  lower extremity (hip, buttock, thigh, leg, foot, toes) T79.A2 ☑ (following T79.7)
  nontraumatic
    abdomen M79.A3 (following M79.7)
    lower extremity (hip, buttock, thigh, leg, foot, toes) M79.A2- ☑ (following M79.7)
    specified site NEC M79.A9 (following M79.7)
    upper extremity (shoulder, arm, forearm, wrist, hand, fingers) M79.A1- ☑ (following M79.7)
  specified site NEC T79.A9 ☑ (following T79.7)
  upper extremity (shoulder, arm, forearm, wrist, hand, fingers) T79.A1- ☑ (following T79.7)
Compensation
  failure — see Disease, heart
  neurosis, psychoneurosis — see Disorder, factitious
Complaint (see also Disease)
  bowel, functional K59.9
    psychogenic F45.8
  intestine, functional K59.9
    psychogenic F45.8
  kidney — see Disease, renal
  miners' J60
Complete — see condition
Complex
  Addison-Schilder E71.528
  cardiorenal — see Hypertension, cardiorenal
  Costen's M26.69
  disseminated mycobacterium avium- intracellulare (DMAC) A31.2
  Eisenmenger's (ventricular septal defect) I27.83
  hypersexual F52.8
  jumped process, spine — see Dislocation, vertebra
  primary, tuberculous A15.7
  Schilder-Addison E71.528
  subluxation (vertebral) M99.19
    abdomen M99.19
    acromioclavicular M99.17
    cervical region M99.11
    cervicothoracic M99.11
    costochondral M99.18
    costovertebral M99.18
    head region M99.10
    hip M99.15
    lower extremity M99.16
    lumbar region M99.13
    lumbosacral M99.13
    occipitocervical M99.10
    pelvic region M99.15
    pubic M99.15
    rib cage M99.18
    sacral region M99.14
    sacrococcygeal M99.14
    sacroiliac M99.14
    specified NEC M99.19
    sternochondral M99.18
    sternoclavicular M99.17
    thoracic region M99.12
    thoracolumbar M99.12
    upper extremity M99.17
  Taussig-Bing (transposition, aorta and overriding pulmonary artery) Q20.1
Complication(s) (from) (of)
  accidental puncture or laceration during a procedure (of) — see Complications, intraoperative (intraprocedural), puncture or laceration
  amputation stump (surgical) (late) NEC T87.9
    dehiscence T87.81
    infection or inflammation T87.40
      lower limb T87.4- ☑
      upper limb T87.4- ☑
    necrosis T87.50
      lower limb T87.5- ☑
      upper limb T87.5- ☑
    neuroma T87.30
      lower limb T87.3- ☑
      upper limb T87.3- ☑

⬇ Subterms under main terms may continue to next column or page   ☑ Additional Character Required — Refer to the Tabular List for Character Selection   57

Collapse — Complication

Complication(s) — *continued*

amputation stump — *continued*
    specified type NEC T87.89
anastomosis (and bypass) (*see also* Complications, prosthetic device or implant)
    intestinal (internal) NEC K91.89
        involving urinary tract N99.89
    urinary tract (involving intestinal tract) N99.89
    vascular — *see* Complications, cardiovascular device or implant
anesthesia, anesthetic (*see also* Anesthesia, complication) T88.59 ☑
    brain, postpartum, puerperal O89.2
    cardiac
        in
            labor and delivery O74.2
            pregnancy O29.19- ☑
        postpartum, puerperal O89.1
    central nervous system
        in
            labor and delivery O74.3
            pregnancy O29.29- ☑
        postpartum, puerperal O89.2
    difficult or failed intubation T88.4 ☑
        in pregnancy O29.6- ☑
    failed sedation (conscious) (moderate) during procedure T88.52 ☑
    general, unintended awareness during procedure T88.53 ☑
    hyperthermia, malignant T88.3 ☑
    hypothermia T88.51 ☑
    intubation failure T88.4 ☑
    malignant hyperthermia T88.3 ☑
    pulmonary
        in
            labor and delivery O74.1
            pregnancy NEC O29.09- ☑
        postpartum, puerperal O89.09
    shock T88.2 ☑
    spinal and epidural
        in
            labor and delivery NEC O74.6
                headache O74.5
            pregnancy NEC O29.5X- ☑
        postpartum, puerperal NEC O89.5
            headache O89.4
    unintended awareness under general anesthesia during procedure T88.53 ☑
anti-reflux device — *see* Complications, esophageal anti-reflux device
aortic (bifurcation) graft — *see* Complications, graft, vascular
aortocoronary (bypass) graft — *see* Complications, coronary artery (bypass) graft
aortofemoral (bypass) graft — *see* Complications, extremity artery (bypass) graft
arteriovenous
    fistula, surgically created T82.9 ☑
        embolism T82.818 ☑
        fibrosis T82.828 ☑
        hemorrhage T82.838 ☑
        infection or inflammation T82.7 ☑
        mechanical
            breakdown T82.510 ☑
            displacement T82.520 ☑
            leakage T82.530 ☑
            malposition T82.520 ☑
            obstruction T82.590 ☑
            perforation T82.590 ☑
            protrusion T82.590 ☑
        pain T82.848 ☑
        specified type NEC T82.898 ☑
        stenosis T82.858 ☑
        thrombosis T82.868 ☑
    shunt, surgically created T82.9 ☑
        embolism T82.818 ☑
        fibrosis T82.828 ☑
        hemorrhage T82.838 ☑
        infection or inflammation T82.7 ☑
        mechanical
            breakdown T82.511 ☑
            displacement T82.521 ☑
            leakage T82.531 ☑
            malposition T82.521 ☑
            obstruction T82.591 ☑
            perforation T82.591 ☑
            protrusion T82.591 ☑

Complication(s) — *continued*

arteriovenous — *continued*
    shunt, surgically created — *continued*
        pain T82.848 ☑
        specified type NEC T82.898 ☑
        stenosis T82.858 ☑
        thrombosis T82.868 ☑
arthroplasty — *see* Complications, joint prosthesis
artificial
    fertilization or insemination N98.9
        attempted introduction (of)
            embryo in embryo transfer N98.3
            ovum following in vitro fertilization N98.2
        hyperstimulation of ovaries N98.1
        infection N98.0
        specified NEC N98.8
    heart T82.9 ☑
        embolism T82.817 ☑
        fibrosis T82.827 ☑
        hemorrhage T82.837 ☑
        infection or inflammation T82.7 ☑
        mechanical
            breakdown T82.512 ☑
            displacement T82.522 ☑
            leakage T82.532 ☑
            malposition T82.522 ☑
            obstruction T82.592 ☑
            perforation T82.592 ☑
            protrusion T82.592 ☑
        pain T82.847 ☑
        specified type NEC T82.897 ☑
        stenosis T82.857 ☑
        thrombosis T82.867 ☑
    opening
        cecostomy — *see* Complications, colostomy
        colostomy — *see* Complications, colostomy
        cystostomy — *see* Complications, cystostomy
        enterostomy — *see* Complications, enterostomy
        gastrostomy — *see* Complications, gastrostomy
        ileostomy — *see* Complications, enterostomy
        jejunostomy — *see* Complications, enterostomy
        nephrostomy — *see* Complications, stoma, urinary tract
        tracheostomy — *see* Complications, tracheostomy
        ureterostomy — *see* Complications, stoma, urinary tract
        urethrostomy — *see* Complications, stoma, urinary tract
balloon implant or device
    gastrointestinal T85.9 ☑
        embolism T85.818 ☑
        fibrosis T85.828 ☑
        hemorrhage T85.838 ☑
        infection and inflammation T85.79 ☑
        pain T85.848 ☑
        specified type NEC T85.898 ☑
        stenosis T85.858 ☑
        thrombosis T85.868 ☑
    vascular (counterpulsation) T82.9 ☑
        embolism T82.818 ☑
        fibrosis T82.828 ☑
        hemorrhage T82.838 ☑
        infection or inflammation T82.7 ☑
        mechanical
            breakdown T82.513 ☑
            displacement T82.523 ☑
            leakage T82.533 ☑
            malposition T82.523 ☑
            obstruction T82.593 ☑
            perforation T82.593 ☑
            protrusion T82.593 ☑
        pain T82.848 ☑
        specified type NEC T82.898 ☑
        stenosis T82.858 ☑
        thrombosis T82.868 ☑
bariatric procedure
    gastric band procedure K95.09
        infection K95.01
    specified procedure NEC K95.89
        infection K95.81
bile duct implant (prosthetic) T85.9 ☑
    embolism T85.818 ☑
    fibrosis T85.828 ☑
    hemorrhage T85.838 ☑

Complication(s) — *continued*

bile duct implant — *continued*
    infection and inflammation T85.79 ☑
    mechanical
        breakdown T85.510 ☑
        displacement T85.520 ☑
        malfunction T85.510 ☑
        malposition T85.520 ☑
        obstruction T85.590 ☑
        perforation T85.590 ☑
        protrusion T85.590 ☑
        specified NEC T85.590 ☑
    pain T85.848 ☑
    specified type NEC T85.898 ☑
    stenosis T85.858 ☑
    thrombosis T85.868 ☑
bladder device (auxiliary) — *see* Complications, genitourinary, device or implant, urinary system
bleeding (postoperative) — *see* Complication, postoperative, hemorrhage
    intraoperative — *see* Complication, intraoperative, hemorrhage
blood vessel graft — *see* Complications, graft, vascular
bone
    device NEC T84.9 ☑
        embolism T84.81 ☑
        fibrosis T84.82 ☑
        hemorrhage T84.83 ☑
        infection or inflammation T84.7 ☑
        mechanical
            breakdown T84.318 ☑
            displacement T84.328 ☑
            malposition T84.328 ☑
            obstruction T84.398 ☑
            perforation T84.398 ☑
            protrusion T84.398 ☑
        pain T84.84 ☑
        specified type NEC T84.89 ☑
        stenosis T84.85 ☑
        thrombosis T84.86 ☑
    graft — *see* Complications, graft, bone
    growth stimulator (electrode) — *see* Complications, electronic stimulator device, bone
    marrow transplant — *see* Complications, transplant, bone, marrow
brain neurostimulator (electrode) — *see* Complications, electronic stimulator device, brain
breast implant (prosthetic) T85.9 ☑
    capsular contracture T85.44 ☑
    embolism T85.818 ☑
    fibrosis T85.828 ☑
    hemorrhage T85.838 ☑
    infection and inflammation T85.79 ☑
    mechanical
        breakdown T85.41 ☑
        displacement T85.42 ☑
        leakage T85.43 ☑
        malposition T85.42 ☑
        obstruction T85.49 ☑
        perforation T85.49 ☑
        protrusion T85.49 ☑
        specified NEC T85.49 ☑
    pain T85.848 ☑
    specified type NEC T85.898 ☑
    stenosis T85.858 ☑
    thrombosis T85.868 ☑
bypass (*see also* Complications, prosthetic device or implant)
    aortocoronary — *see* Complications, coronary artery (bypass) graft
    arterial (*see also* Complications, graft, vascular)
        extremity — *see* Complications, extremity artery (bypass) graft
cardiac (*see also* Disease, heart)
    device, implant or graft T82.9 ☑
        embolism T82.817 ☑
        fibrosis T82.827 ☑
        hemorrhage T82.837 ☑
        infection or inflammation T82.7 ☑
            valve prosthesis T82.6 ☑
        mechanical
            breakdown T82.519 ☑
                specified device NEC T82.518 ☑
            displacement T82.529 ☑
                specified device NEC T82.528 ☑
            leakage T82.539 ☑

Complication(s) — *continued*
  cardiac (*see also* Disease, heart) — *continued*
    device, implant or graft — *continued*
      mechanical — *continued*
        leakage — *continued*
          specified device NEC T82.538 ☑
        malposition T82.529 ☑
          specified device NEC T82.528 ☑
        obstruction T82.599 ☑
          specified device NEC T82.598 ☑
        perforation T82.599 ☑
          specified device NEC T82.598 ☑
        protrusion T82.599 ☑
          specified device NEC T82.598 ☑
      pain T82.847 ☑
      specified type NEC T82.897 ☑
      stenosis T82.857 ☑
      thrombosis T82.867 ☑
  cardiovascular device, graft or implant T82.9 ☑
    aortic graft — *see* Complications, graft, vascular
    arteriovenous
      fistula, artificial — *see* Complication, arteriovenous, fistula, surgically created
      shunt — *see* Complication, arteriovenous, shunt, surgically created
    artificial heart — *see* Complication, artificial, heart
    balloon (counterpulsation) device — *see* Complication, balloon implant, vascular
    carotid artery graft — *see* Complications, graft, vascular
    coronary bypass graft — *see* Complication, coronary artery (bypass) graft
    dialysis catheter (vascular) — *see* Complication, catheter, dialysis
    electronic T82.9 ☑
      electrode T82.9 ☑
        embolism T82.817 ☑
        fibrosis T82.827 ☑
        hemorrhage T82.837 ☑
        infection T82.7 ☑
        mechanical
          breakdown T82.110 ☑
          displacement T82.120 ☑
          leakage T82.190 ☑
          obstruction T82.190 ☑
          perforation T82.190 ☑
          protrusion T82.190 ☑
          specified type NEC T82.190 ☑
        pain T82.847 ☑
        specified NEC T82.897 ☑
        stenosis T82.857 ☑
        thrombosis T82.867 ☑
      embolism T82.817 ☑
      fibrosis T82.827 ☑
      hemorrhage T82.837 ☑
      infection T82.7 ☑
      mechanical
        breakdown T82.119 ☑
        displacement T82.129 ☑
        leakage T82.199 ☑
        obstruction T82.199 ☑
        perforation T82.199 ☑
        protrusion T82.199 ☑
        specified type NEC T82.199 ☑
      pain T82.847 ☑
      pulse generator T82.9 ☑
        embolism T82.817 ☑
        fibrosis T82.827 ☑
        hemorrhage T82.837 ☑
        infection T82.7 ☑
        mechanical
          breakdown T82.111 ☑
          displacement T82.121 ☑
          leakage T82.191 ☑
          obstruction T82.191 ☑
          perforation T82.191 ☑
          protrusion T82.191 ☑
          specified type NEC T82.191 ☑
        pain T82.847 ☑
        specified NEC T82.897 ☑
        stenosis T82.857 ☑
        thrombosis T82.867 ☑
      specified condition NEC T82.897 ☑
      specified device NEC T82.9 ☑
        embolism T82.817 ☑
        fibrosis T82.827 ☑

Complication(s) — *continued*
  cardiovascular device, graft or implant — *continued*
    electronic — *continued*
      specified device — *continued*
        hemorrhage T82.837 ☑
        infection T82.7 ☑
        mechanical
          breakdown T82.118 ☑
          displacement T82.128 ☑
          leakage T82.198 ☑
          obstruction T82.198 ☑
          perforation T82.198 ☑
          protrusion T82.198 ☑
          specified type NEC T82.198 ☑
        pain T82.847 ☑
        specified NEC T82.897 ☑
        stenosis T82.857 ☑
        thrombosis T82.867 ☑
      stenosis T82.857 ☑
      thrombosis T82.867 ☑
    extremity artery graft — *see* Complication, extremity artery (bypass) graft
    femoral artery graft — *see* Complication, extremity artery (bypass) graft
    heart
      transplant — *see* Complication, transplant, heart
      valve — *see* Complication, prosthetic device, heart valve
        graft — *see* Complication, heart, valve, graft
    heart-lung transplant — *see* Complication, transplant, heart, with lung
    infection or inflammation T82.7 ☑
    umbrella device — *see* Complication, umbrella device, vascular
    vascular graft (or anastomosis) — *see* Complication, graft, vascular
  carotid artery (bypass) graft — *see* Complications, graft, vascular
  catheter (device) NEC (*see also* Complications, prosthetic device or implant)
    cranial infusion
      infection and inflammation T85.735 ☑
      mechanical
        breakdown T85.610 ☑
        displacement T85.620 ☑
        leakage T85.630 ☑
        malfunction T85.690 ☑
        malposition T85.620 ☑
        obstruction T85.690 ☑
        perforation T85.690 ☑
        protrusion T85.690 ☑
        specified NEC T85.690 ☑
    cystostomy T83.9 ☑
      embolism T83.81 ☑
      fibrosis T83.82 ☑
      hemorrhage T83.83 ☑
      infection and inflammation T83.510 ☑
      mechanical
        breakdown T83.010 ☑
        displacement T83.020 ☑
        leakage T83.030 ☑
        malposition T83.020 ☑
        obstruction T83.090 ☑
        perforation T83.090 ☑
        protrusion T83.090 ☑
        specified NEC T83.090 ☑
      pain T83.84 ☑
      specified type NEC T83.89 ☑
      stenosis T83.85 ☑
      thrombosis T83.86 ☑
    dialysis (vascular) T82.9 ☑
      embolism T82.818 ☑
      fibrosis T82.828 ☑
      hemorrhage T82.838 ☑
      infection and inflammation T82.7 ☑
      intraperitoneal — *see* Complications, catheter, intraperitoneal
      mechanical
        breakdown T82.41 ☑
        displacement T82.42 ☑
        leakage T82.43 ☑
        malposition T82.42 ☑
        obstruction T82.49 ☑
        perforation T82.49 ☑

Complication(s) — *continued*
  catheter (*see also* Complications, prosthetic device or implant) — *continued*
    dialysis — *continued*
      mechanical — *continued*
        protrusion T82.49 ☑
      pain T82.848 ☑
      specified type NEC T82.898 ☑
      stenosis T82.858 ☑
      thrombosis T82.868 ☑
    epidural infusion T85.9 ☑
      embolism T85.810 ☑
      fibrosis T85.820 ☑
      hemorrhage T85.830 ☑
      infection and inflammation T85.735 ☑
      mechanical
        breakdown T85.610 ☑
        displacement T85.620 ☑
        leakage T85.630 ☑
        malfunction T85.610 ☑
        malposition T85.620 ☑
        obstruction T85.690 ☑
        perforation T85.690 ☑
        protrusion T85.690 ☑
        specified NEC T85.690 ☑
      pain T85.840 ☑
      specified type NEC T85.890 ☑
      stenosis T85.850 ☑
      thrombosis T85.860 ☑
    intraperitoneal dialysis T85.9 ☑
      embolism T85.818 ☑
      fibrosis T85.828 ☑
      hemorrhage T85.838 ☑
      infection and inflammation T85.71 ☑
      mechanical
        breakdown T85.611 ☑
        displacement T85.621 ☑
        leakage T85.631 ☑
        malfunction T85.611 ☑
        malposition T85.621 ☑
        obstruction T85.691 ☑
        perforation T85.691 ☑
        protrusion T85.691 ☑
        specified NEC T85.691 ☑
      pain T85.848 ☑
      specified type NEC T85.898 ☑
      stenosis T85.858 ☑
      thrombosis T85.868 ☑
    intrathecal infusion
      infection and inflammation T85.735 ☑
      mechanical
        breakdown T85.610 ☑
        displacement T85.620 ☑
        leakage T85.630 ☑
        malfunction T85.690 ☑
        malposition T85.620 ☑
        obstruction T85.690 ☑
        perforation T85.690 ☑
        protrusion T85.690 ☑
        specified NEC T85.690 ☑
    intravenous infusion T82.9 ☑
      embolism T82.818 ☑
      fibrosis T82.828 ☑
      hemorrhage T82.838 ☑
      infection or inflammation T82.7 ☑
      mechanical
        breakdown T82.514 ☑
        displacement T82.524 ☑
        leakage T82.534 ☑
        malposition T82.524 ☑
        obstruction T82.594 ☑
        perforation T82.594 ☑
        protrusion T82.594 ☑
      pain T82.848 ☑
      specified type NEC T82.898 ☑
      stenosis T82.858 ☑
      thrombosis T82.868 ☑
    spinal infusion
      infection and inflammation T85.735 ☑
      mechanical
        breakdown T85.610 ☑
        displacement T85.620 ☑
        leakage T85.630 ☑
        malfunction T85.690 ☑
        malposition T85.620 ☑
        obstruction T85.690 ☑

Complication(s) — *continued*
catheter (*see also* Complications, prosthetic device or implant) — *continued*
  spinal infusion — *continued*
    mechanical — *continued*
      perforation T85.690 ☑
      protrusion T85.690 ☑
      specified NEC T85.690 ☑
    subarachnoid infusion
      infection and inflammation T85.735 ☑
      mechanical
        breakdown T85.610 ☑
        displacement T85.620 ☑
        leakage T85.630 ☑
        malfunction T85.690 ☑
        malposition T85.620 ☑
        obstruction T85.690 ☑
        perforation T85.690 ☑
        protrusion T85.690 ☑
        specified NEC T85.690 ☑
    subdural infusion T85.9 ☑
      embolism T85.810 ☑
      fibrosis T85.820 ☑
      hemorrhage T85.830 ☑
      infection and inflammation T85.735 ☑
      mechanical
        breakdown T85.610 ☑
        displacement T85.620 ☑
        leakage T85.630 ☑
        malfunction T85.610 ☑
        malposition T85.620 ☑
        obstruction T85.690 ☑
        perforation T85.690 ☑
        protrusion T85.690 ☑
        specified NEC T85.690 ☑
      pain T85.840 ☑
      specified type NEC T85.890 ☑
      stenosis T85.850 ☑
      thrombosis T85.860 ☑
  urethral T83.9 ☑
    displacement T83.028 ☑
    embolism T83.81 ☑
    fibrosis T83.82 ☑
    hemorrhage T83.83 ☑
    indwelling
      breakdown T83.011 ☑
      displacement T83.021 ☑
      infection and inflammation T83.511 ☑
      leakage T83.031 ☑
      specified complication NEC T83.091 ☑
    infection and inflammation T83.511 ☑
    leakage T83.038 ☑
    malposition T83.028 ☑
    mechanical
      breakdown T83.011 ☑
    obstruction (mechanical) T83.091 ☑
    pain T83.84 ☑
    perforation T83.091 ☑
    protrusion T83.091 ☑
    specified type NEC T83.091 ☑
    stenosis T83.85 ☑
    thrombosis T83.86 ☑
  urinary NEC
    breakdown T83.018 ☑
    displacement T83.028 ☑
    infection and inflammation T83.518 ☑
    leakage T83.038 ☑
    specified complication NEC T83.098 ☑
cecostomy (stoma) — *see* Complications, colostomy
cesarean delivery wound NEC O90.89
  disruption O90.0
  hematoma O90.2
  infection (following delivery) O86.0
chemotherapy (antineoplastic) NEC T88.7 ☑
chin implant (prosthetic) — *see* Complication, prosthetic device or implant, specified NEC
circulatory system I99.8
  intraoperative I97.88
  postprocedural I97.89
    following cardiac surgery (*see also* Infarct, myocardium, associated with revascularization procedure) I97.19- ☑
      postcardiotomy syndrome I97.0
    hypertension I97.3
    lymphedema after mastectomy I97.2
    postcardiotomy syndrome I97.0

Complication(s) — *continued*
circulatory system — *continued*
  postprocedural — *continued*
    specified NEC I97.89
colostomy (stoma) K94.00
  hemorrhage K94.01
  infection K94.02
  malfunction K94.03
  mechanical K94.03
  specified complication NEC K94.09
contraceptive device, intrauterine — *see* Complications, intrauterine, contraceptive device
cord (umbilical) — *see* Complications, umbilical cord
corneal graft — *see* Complications, graft, cornea
coronary artery (bypass) graft T82.9
  atherosclerosis — *see* Arteriosclerosis, coronary (artery),
  embolism T82.818 ☑
  fibrosis T82.828 ☑
  hemorrhage T82.838 ☑
  infection and inflammation T82.7 ☑
  mechanical
    breakdown T82.211 ☑
    displacement T82.212 ☑
    leakage T82.213 ☑
    malposition T82.212 ☑
    obstruction T82.218 ☑
    perforation T82.218 ☑
    protrusion T82.218 ☑
    specified NEC T82.218 ☑
  pain T82.848 ☑
  specified type NEC T82.898 ☑
  stenosis T82.858 ☑
  thrombosis T82.868 ☑
counterpulsation device (balloon), intra- aortic — *see* Complications, balloon implant, vascular
cystostomy (stoma) N99.518
  catheter — *see* Complications, catheter, cystostomy
  hemorrhage N99.510
  infection N99.511
  malfunction N99.512
  specified type NEC N99.518
delivery (*see also* Complications, obstetric) O75.9
  procedure (instrumental) (manual) (surgical) O75.4
  specified NEC O75.89
dialysis (peritoneal) (renal) (*see also* Complications, infusion)
  catheter (vascular) — *see* Complication, catheter, dialysis
  peritoneal, intraperitoneal — *see* Complications, catheter, intraperitoneal
dorsal column (spinal) neurostimulator — *see* Complications, electronic stimulator device, spinal cord
drug NEC T88.7 ☑
ear procedure (*see also* Disorder, ear)
  intraoperative H95.88
    hematoma — *see* Complications, intraoperative, hemorrhage (hematoma) (of), ear
    hemorrhage — *see* Complications, intraoperative, hemorrhage (hematoma) (of), ear
    laceration — *see* Complications, intraoperative, puncture or laceration..., ear
    specified NEC H95.88
  postoperative H95.89
    external ear canal stenosis H95.81- ☑
    hematoma — *see* Complications, postprocedural, hematoma (of), ear
    hemorrhage — *see* Complications, postprocedural, hemorrhage (of), ear
    postmastoidectomy — *see* Complications, postmastoidectomy
    seroma — *see* Complications, postprocedural, seroma (of), mastoid process
    specified NEC H95.89
ectopic pregnancy O08.9
  damage to pelvic organs O08.6
  embolism O08.2
  genital infection O08.0
  hemorrhage (delayed) (excessive) O08.1
  metabolic disorder O08.5
  renal failure O08.4
  shock O08.3
  specified type NEC O08.8
  venous complication NEC O08.7

Complication(s) — *continued*
electronic stimulator device
  bladder (urinary) — *see* Complications, electronic stimulator device, urinary
  bone T84.9 ☑
    breakdown T84.310 ☑
    displacement T84.320 ☑
    embolism T84.81 ☑
    fibrosis T84.82 ☑
    hemorrhage T84.83 ☑
    infection or inflammation T84.7 ☑
    malfunction T84.310 ☑
    malposition T84.320 ☑
    mechanical NEC T84.390 ☑
    obstruction T84.390 ☑
    pain T84.84 ☑
    perforation T84.390 ☑
    protrusion T84.390 ☑
    specified type NEC T84.89 ☑
    stenosis T84.85 ☑
    thrombosis T84.86 ☑
  brain T85.9 ☑
    embolism T85.810 ☑
    fibrosis T85.820 ☑
    hemorrhage T85.830 ☑
    infection and inflammation T85.731 ☑
    mechanical
      breakdown T85.110 ☑
      displacement T85.120 ☑
      leakage T85.190 ☑
      malposition T85.120 ☑
      obstruction T85.190 ☑
      perforation T85.190 ☑
      protrusion T85.190 ☑
      specified NEC T85.190 ☑
    pain T85.840 ☑
    specified type NEC T85.890 ☑
    stenosis T85.850 ☑
    thrombosis T85.860 ☑
  cardiac (defibrillator) (pacemaker) — *see* Complications, cardiovascular device or implant, electronic
  generator (brain) (gastric) (peripheral) (sacral) (spinal)
    breakdown T85.113 ☑
    displacement T85.123 ☑
    leakage T85.193 ☑
    malposition T85.123 ☑
    obstruction T85.193 ☑
    perforation T85.193 ☑
    protrusion T85.193 ☑
    specified type NEC T85.193 ☑
  muscle T84.9 ☑
    breakdown T84.418 ☑
    displacement T84.428 ☑
    embolism T84.81 ☑
    fibrosis T84.82 ☑
    hemorrhage T84.83 ☑
    infection or inflammation T84.7 ☑
    mechanical NEC T84.498 ☑
    pain T84.84 ☑
    specified type NEC T84.89 ☑
    stenosis T84.85 ☑
    thrombosis T84.86 ☑
  nervous system T85.9 ☑
    brain — *see* Complications, electronic stimulator device, brain
    cranial nerve — *see* Complications, electronic stimulator device, peripheral nerve
    embolism T85.810 ☑
    fibrosis T85.820 ☑
    gastric nerve — *see* Complications, electronic stimulator device, peripheral nerve
    hemorrhage T85.830 ☑
    infection and inflammation T85.738 ☑
    mechanical
      breakdown T85.118 ☑
      displacement T85.128 ☑
      leakage T85.199 ☑
      malposition T85.128 ☑
      obstruction T85.199 ☑
      perforation T85.199 ☑
      protrusion T85.199 ☑
      specified NEC T85.199 ☑
    pain T85.840 ☑

☑ **Additional Character Required — Refer to the Tabular List for Character Selection**   ▽ Subterms under main terms may continue to next column or page

Complication(s) — *continued*
  electronic stimulator device — *continued*
    nervous system — *continued*
      peripheral nerve — *see* Complications, electronic stimulator device, peripheral nerve
      sacral nerve — *see* Complications, electronic stimulator device, peripheral nerve
      specified type NEC T85.890 ☑
      spinal cord — *see* Complications, electronic stimulator device, spinal cord
      stenosis T85.850 ☑
      thrombosis T85.860 ☑
      vagal nerve — *see* Complications, electronic stimulator device, peripheral nerve
    peripheral nerve T85.9 ☑
      embolism T85.810 ☑
      fibrosis T85.820 ☑
      hemorrhage T85.830 ☑
      infection and inflammation T85.732 ☑
      mechanical
        breakdown T85.111 ☑
        displacement T85.121 ☑
        leakage T85.191 ☑
        malposition T85.121 ☑
        obstruction T85.191 ☑
        perforation T85.191 ☑
        protrusion T85.191 ☑
        specified NEC T85.191 ☑
      pain T85.840 ☑
      specified type NEC T85.890 ☑
      stenosis T85.850 ☑
      thrombosis T85.860 ☑
    spinal cord T85.9 ☑
      embolism T85.810 ☑
      fibrosis T85.820 ☑
      hemorrhage T85.830 ☑
      infection and inflammation T85.733 ☑
      mechanical
        breakdown T85.112 ☑
        displacement T85.122 ☑
        leakage T85.192 ☑
        malposition T85.122 ☑
        obstruction T85.192 ☑
        perforation T85.192 ☑
        protrusion T85.192 ☑
        specified NEC T85.192 ☑
      pain T85.840 ☑
      specified type NEC T85.890 ☑
      stenosis T85.850 ☑
      thrombosis T85.860 ☑
    urinary T83.9 ☑
      embolism T83.81 ☑
      fibrosis T83.82 ☑
      hemorrhage T83.83 ☑
      infection and inflammation T83.598 ☑
      mechanical
        breakdown T83.110 ☑
        displacement T83.120 ☑
        malposition T83.120 ☑
        perforation T83.190 ☑
        protrusion T83.190 ☑
        specified NEC T83.190 ☑
      pain T83.84 ☑
      specified type NEC T83.89 ☑
      stenosis T83.85 ☑
      thrombosis T83.86 ☑
  electroshock therapy T88.9 ☑
    specified NEC T88.8 ☑
  endocrine E34.9
    postprocedural
      adrenal hypofunction E89.6
      hypoinsulinemia E89.1
      hypoparathyroidism E89.2
      hypopituitarism E89.3
      hypothyroidism E89.0
      ovarian failure E89.40
        asymptomatic E89.40
        symptomatic E89.41
      specified NEC E89.89
      testicular hypofunction E89.5
  endodontic treatment NEC M27.59
  enterostomy (stoma) K94.10
    hemorrhage K94.11
    infection K94.12
    malfunction K94.13
    mechanical K94.13

Complication(s) — *continued*
  enterostomy — *continued*
    specified complication NEC K94.19
  episiotomy, disruption O90.1
  esophageal anti-reflux device T85.9 ☑
    embolism T85.818 ☑
    fibrosis T85.828 ☑
    hemorrhage T85.838 ☑
    infection and inflammation T85.79 ☑
    mechanical
      breakdown T85.511 ☑
      displacement T85.521 ☑
      malfunction T85.511 ☑
      malposition T85.521 ☑
      obstruction T85.591 ☑
      perforation T85.591 ☑
      protrusion T85.591 ☑
      specified NEC T85.591 ☑
    pain T85.848 ☑
    specified type NEC T85.898 ☑
    stenosis T85.858 ☑
    thrombosis T85.868 ☑
  esophagostomy K94.30
    hemorrhage K94.31
    infection K94.32
    malfunction K94.33
    mechanical K94.33
    specified complication NEC K94.39
  extracorporeal circulation T80.90 ☑
  extremity artery (bypass) graft T82.9 ☑
    arteriosclerosis — *see* Arteriosclerosis, extremities, bypass graft
    embolism T82.818 ☑
    fibrosis T82.828 ☑
    hemorrhage T82.838 ☑
    infection and inflammation T82.7 ☑
    mechanical
      breakdown T82.318 ☑
        femoral artery T82.312 ☑
      displacement T82.328 ☑
        femoral artery T82.322 ☑
      leakage T82.338 ☑
        femoral artery T82.332 ☑
      malposition T82.328 ☑
        femoral artery T82.322 ☑
      obstruction T82.398 ☑
        femoral artery T82.392 ☑
      perforation T82.398 ☑
        femoral artery T82.392 ☑
      protrusion T82.398 ☑
        femoral artery T82.392 ☑
    pain T82.848 ☑
    specified type NEC T82.898 ☑
    stenosis T82.858 ☑
    thrombosis T82.868 ☑
  eye H57.9
    corneal graft — *see* Complications, graft, cornea
    implant (prosthetic) T85.9 ☑
      embolism T85.818 ☑
      fibrosis T85.828 ☑
      hemorrhage T85.838 ☑
      infection and inflammation T85.79 ☑
      mechanical
        breakdown T85.318 ☑
        displacement T85.328 ☑
        leakage T85.398 ☑
        malposition T85.328 ☑
        obstruction T85.398 ☑
        perforation T85.398 ☑
        protrusion T85.398 ☑
        specified NEC T85.398 ☑
      pain T85.848 ☑
      specified type NEC T85.898 ☑
      stenosis T85.858 ☑
      thrombosis T85.868 ☑
    intraocular lens — *see* Complications, intraocular lens
    orbital prosthesis — *see* Complications, orbital prosthesis
  female genital N94.9
    device, implant or graft NEC — *see* Complications, genitourinary, device or implant, genital tract
  femoral artery (bypass) graft — *see* Complication, extremity artery (bypass) graft
  fixation device, internal (orthopedic) T84.9 ☑
    infection and inflammation T84.60 ☑

Complication(s) — *continued*
  fixation device, internal — *continued*
    infection and inflammation — *continued*
      arm T84.61- ☑
        humerus T84.61- ☑
        radius T84.61- ☑
        ulna T84.61- ☑
      leg T84.629 ☑
        femur T84.62- ☑
        fibula T84.62- ☑
        tibia T84.62- ☑
      specified site NEC T84.89 ☑
      spine T84.63 ☑
    mechanical
      breakdown
        limb T84.119 ☑
          carpal T84.210 ☑
          femur T84.11- ☑
          fibula T84.11- ☑
          humerus T84.11- ☑
          metacarpal T84.210 ☑
          metatarsal T84.213 ☑
          phalanx
            foot T84.213 ☑
            hand T84.210 ☑
          radius T84.11- ☑
          tarsal T84.213 ☑
          tibia T84.11- ☑
          ulna T84.11- ☑
        specified bone NEC T84.218 ☑
        spine T84.216 ☑
      displacement
        limb T84.129 ☑
          carpal T84.220 ☑
          femur T84.12- ☑
          fibula T84.12- ☑
          humerus T84.12- ☑
          metacarpal T84.220 ☑
          metatarsal T84.223 ☑
          phalanx
            foot T84.223 ☑
            hand T84.220 ☑
          radius T84.12- ☑
          tarsal T84.223 ☑
          tibia T84.12- ☑
          ulna T84.12- ☑
        specified bone NEC T84.228 ☑
        spine T84.226 ☑
      malposition — *see* Complications, fixation device, internal, mechanical, displacement
      obstruction — *see* Complications, fixation device, internal, mechanical, specified type NEC
      perforation — *see* Complications, fixation device, internal, mechanical, specified type NEC
      protrusion — *see* Complications, fixation device, internal, mechanical, specified type NEC
      specified type NEC
        limb T84.199 ☑
          carpal T84.290 ☑
          femur T84.19- ☑
          fibula T84.19- ☑
          humerus T84.19- ☑
          metacarpal T84.290 ☑
          metatarsal T84.293 ☑
          phalanx
            foot T84.293 ☑
            hand T84.290 ☑
          radius T84.19- ☑
          tarsal T84.293 ☑
          tibia T84.19- ☑
          ulna T84.19- ☑
        specified bone NEC T84.298 ☑
        vertebra T84.296 ☑
    specified type NEC T84.89 ☑
      embolism T84.81 ☑
      fibrosis T84.82 ☑
      hemorrhage T84.83 ☑
      pain T84.84 ☑
      specified complication NEC T84.89 ☑
      stenosis T84.85 ☑
      thrombosis T84.86 ☑
  following
    acute myocardial infarction NEC I23.8

Complication(s) — *continued*
following — *continued*
  acute myocardial infarction — *continued*
    aneurysm (false) (of cardiac wall) (of heart wall) (ruptured) I23.3
    angina I23.7
    atrial
      septal defect I23.1
      thrombosis I23.6
    cardiac wall rupture I23.3
    chordae tendinae rupture I23.4
    defect
      septal
        atrial (heart) I23.1
        ventricular (heart) I23.2
    hemopericardium I23.0
    papillary muscle rupture I23.5
    rupture
      cardiac wall I23.3
        with hemopericardium I23.0
      chordae tendineae I23.4
      papillary muscle I23.5
    specified NEC I23.8
    thrombosis
      atrium I23.6
      auricular appendage I23.6
      ventricle (heart) I23.6
    ventricular
      septal defect I23.2
      thrombosis I23.6
  ectopic or molar pregnancy O08.9
    cardiac arrest O08.81
    sepsis O08.82
    specified type NEC O08.89
    urinary tract infection O08.83
  termination of pregnancy — *see* Abortion
gastrointestinal K92.9
  bile duct prosthesis — *see* Complications, bile duct implant
  esophageal anti-reflux device — *see* Complications, esophageal anti-reflux device
  postoperative
    colostomy — *see* Complications, colostomy
    dumping syndrome K91.1
    enterostomy — *see* Complications, enterostomy
    gastrostomy — *see* Complications, gastrostomy
    malabsorption NEC K91.2
    obstruction (*see also* Obstruction, intestine, postoperative) K91.30
    postcholecystectomy syndrome K91.5
    specified NEC K91.89
    vomiting after GI surgery K91.0
  prosthetic device or implant
    bile duct prosthesis — *see* Complications, bile duct implant
    esophageal anti-reflux device — *see* Complications, esophageal anti-reflux device
    specified type NEC
      embolism T85.818 ☑
      fibrosis T85.828 ☑
      hemorrhage T85.838 ☑
      mechanical
        breakdown T85.518 ☑
        displacement T85.528 ☑
        malfunction T85.518 ☑
        malposition T85.528 ☑
        obstruction T85.598 ☑
        perforation T85.598 ☑
        protrusion T85.598 ☑
        specified NEC T85.598 ☑
      pain T85.848 ☑
      specified complication NEC T85.898 ☑
      stenosis T85.858 ☑
      thrombosis T85.868 ☑
gastrostomy (stoma) K94.20
  hemorrhage K94.21
  infection K94.22
  malfunction K94.23
  mechanical K94.23
  specified complication NEC K94.29
genitourinary
  device or implant T83.9 ☑
    genital tract T83.9 ☑
      infection or inflammation T83.69 ☑
      intrauterine contraceptive device — *see* Complications, intrauterine, contraceptive device

Complication(s) — *continued*
genitourinary — *continued*
  device or implant — *continued*
    genital tract — *continued*
      mechanical — *see* Complications, by device, mechanical
      mesh — *see* Complications, mesh
      penile prosthesis — *see* Complications, prosthetic device, penile
      specified type NEC T83.89 ☑
        embolism T83.81 ☑
        fibrosis T83.82 ☑
        hemorrhage T83.83 ☑
        pain T83.84 ☑
        specified complication NEC T83.89 ☑
        stenosis T83.85 ☑
        thrombosis T83.86 ☑
      vaginal mesh — *see* Complications, mesh
    urinary system T83.9 ☑
      cystostomy catheter — *see* Complication, catheter, cystostomy
      electronic stimulator — *see* Complications, electronic stimulator device, urinary
      indwelling urethral catheter — *see* Complications, catheter, urethral, indwelling
      infection or inflammation T83.598 ☑
        indwelling urethral catheter T83.511 ☑
      kidney transplant — *see* Complication, transplant, kidney
      organ graft — *see* Complication, graft, urinary organ
      specified type NEC T83.89 ☑
        embolism T83.81 ☑
        fibrosis T83.82 ☑
        hemorrhage T83.83 ☑
        mechanical T83.198 ☑
          breakdown T83.118 ☑
          displacement T83.128 ☑
          malfunction T83.118 ☑
          malposition T83.128 ☑
          obstruction T83.198 ☑
          perforation T83.198 ☑
          protrusion T83.198 ☑
          specified NEC T83.198 ☑
      sphincter implant — *see* Complications, implant, urinary sphincter
      sphincter, implanted T83.191 ☑
      stent (ileal conduit) (nephroureteral) T83.193 ☑
      pain T83.84 ☑
      specified complication NEC T83.89 ☑
      stenosis T83.85 ☑
      thrombosis T83.86 ☑
      ureteral indwelling T83.192 ☑
  postprocedural
    pelvic peritoneal adhesions N99.4
    renal failure N99.0
    specified NEC N99.89
    stoma — *see* Complications, stoma, urinary tract
    urethral stricture — *see* Stricture, urethra, postprocedural
    vaginal
      adhesions N99.2
      vault prolapse N99.3
graft (bypass) (patch) (*see also* Complications, prosthetic device or implant)
  aorta — *see* Complications, graft, vascular
  arterial — *see* Complication, graft, vascular
  bone T86.839
    failure T86.831
    infection T86.832
    mechanical T84.318 ☑
      breakdown T84.318 ☑
      displacement T84.328 ☑
      protrusion T84.398 ☑
      specified type NEC T84.398 ☑
    rejection T86.830
    specified type NEC T86.838
  carotid artery — *see* Complications, graft, vascular
  cornea T86.849
    failure T86.841
    infection T86.842
    mechanical T85.398 ☑
      breakdown T85.318 ☑
      displacement T85.328 ☑
      protrusion T85.398 ☑

Complication(s) — *continued*
graft (*see also* Complications, prosthetic device or implant) — *continued*
  cornea — *continued*
    mechanical — *continued*
      specified type NEC T85.398 ☑
    rejection T86.840
    retroprosthetic membrane T85.398 ☑
    specified type NEC T86.848
  femoral artery (bypass) — *see* Complication, extremity artery (bypass) graft
  genital organ or tract — *see* Complications, genitourinary, device or implant, genital tract
  muscle T84.9 ☑
    breakdown T84.410 ☑
    displacement T84.420 ☑
    embolism T84.81 ☑
    fibrosis T84.82 ☑
    hemorrhage T84.83 ☑
    infection and inflammation T84.7 ☑
    mechanical NEC T84.490 ☑
    pain T84.84 ☑
    specified type NEC T84.89 ☑
    stenosis T84.85 ☑
    thrombosis T84.86 ☑
  nerve — *see* Complication, prosthetic device or implant, specified NEC
  skin — *see* Complications, prosthetic device or implant, skin graft
  tendon T84.9 ☑
    breakdown T84.410 ☑
    displacement T84.420 ☑
    embolism T84.81 ☑
    fibrosis T84.82 ☑
    hemorrhage T84.83 ☑
    infection and inflammation T84.7 ☑
    mechanical NEC T84.490 ☑
    pain T84.84 ☑
    specified type NEC T84.89 ☑
    stenosis T84.85 ☑
    thrombosis T84.86 ☑
  urinary organ T83.9 ☑
    embolism T83.81 ☑
    fibrosis T83.82 ☑
    hemorrhage T83.83 ☑
    infection and inflammation T83.598 ☑
      indwelling urethral catheter T83.511 ☑
    mechanical
      breakdown T83.21 ☑
      displacement T83.22 ☑
      erosion T83.24 ☑
      exposure T83.25 ☑
      leakage T83.23 ☑
      malposition T83.22 ☑
      obstruction T83.29 ☑
      perforation T83.29 ☑
      protrusion T83.29 ☑
      specified NEC T83.29 ☑
    pain T83.84 ☑
    specified type NEC T83.89 ☑
    stenosis T83.85 ☑
    thrombosis T83.86 ☑
  vascular T82.9 ☑
    embolism T82.818 ☑
    femoral artery — *see* Complication, extremity artery (bypass) graft
    fibrosis T82.828 ☑
    hemorrhage T82.838 ☑
    mechanical
      breakdown T82.319 ☑
        aorta (bifurcation) T82.310 ☑
        carotid artery T82.311 ☑
        specified vessel NEC T82.318 ☑
      displacement T82.329 ☑
        aorta (bifurcation) T82.320 ☑
        carotid artery T82.321 ☑
        specified vessel NEC T82.328 ☑
      leakage T82.339 ☑
        aorta (bifurcation) T82.330 ☑
        carotid artery T82.331 ☑
        specified vessel NEC T82.338 ☑
      malposition T82.329 ☑
        aorta (bifurcation) T82.320 ☑
        carotid artery T82.321 ☑
        specified vessel NEC T82.328 ☑
      obstruction T82.399 ☑

Complication(s) — *continued*
　graft (*see also* Complications, prosthetic device or implant) — *continued*
　　vascular — *continued*
　　　mechanical — *continued*
　　　　obstruction — *continued*
　　　　　aorta (bifurcation) T82.390 ☑
　　　　　carotid artery T82.391 ☑
　　　　　specified vessel NEC T82.398 ☑
　　　　perforation T82.399 ☑
　　　　　aorta (bifurcation) T82.390 ☑
　　　　　carotid artery T82.391 ☑
　　　　　specified vessel NEC T82.398 ☑
　　　　protrusion T82.399 ☑
　　　　　aorta (bifurcation) T82.390 ☑
　　　　　carotid artery T82.391 ☑
　　　　　specified vessel NEC T82.398 ☑
　　　　pain T82.848 ☑
　　　　specified complication NEC T82.898 ☑
　　　　stenosis T82.858 ☑
　　　　thrombosis T82.868 ☑
　heart I51.9
　　assist device
　　　infection and inflammation T82.7 ☑
　　following acute myocardial infarction — *see* Complications, following, acute myocardial infarction
　　postoperative — *see* Complications, circulatory system
　　transplant — *see* Complication, transplant, heart and lung(s) — *see* Complications, transplant, heart, with lung
　　valve
　　　graft (biological) T82.9 ☑
　　　　embolism T82.817 ☑
　　　　fibrosis T82.827 ☑
　　　　hemorrhage T82.837 ☑
　　　　infection and inflammation T82.7 ☑
　　　　mechanical T82.228 ☑
　　　　　breakdown T82.221 ☑
　　　　　displacement T82.222 ☑
　　　　　leakage T82.223 ☑
　　　　　malposition T82.222 ☑
　　　　　obstruction T82.228 ☑
　　　　　perforation T82.228 ☑
　　　　　protrusion T82.228 ☑
　　　　pain T82.847 ☑
　　　　specified type NEC T82.897 ☑
　　　　stenosis T82.857 ☑
　　　　thrombosis T82.867 ☑
　　　prosthesis T82.9 ☑
　　　　embolism T82.817 ☑
　　　　fibrosis T82.827 ☑
　　　　hemorrhage T82.837 ☑
　　　　infection or inflammation T82.6 ☑
　　　　mechanical T82.09 ☑
　　　　　breakdown T82.01 ☑
　　　　　displacement T82.02 ☑
　　　　　leakage T82.03 ☑
　　　　　malposition T82.02 ☑
　　　　　obstruction T82.09 ☑
　　　　　perforation T82.09 ☑
　　　　　protrusion T82.09 ☑
　　　　pain T82.847 ☑
　　　　specified type NEC T82.897 ☑
　　　　　mechanical T82.09 ☑
　　　　stenosis T82.857 ☑
　　　　thrombosis T82.867 ☑
　hematoma
　　intraoperative — *see* Complication, intraoperative, hemorrhage
　　postprocedural — *see* Complication, postprocedural, hematoma
　hemodialysis — *see* Complications, dialysis
　hemorrhage
　　intraoperative — *see* Complication, intraoperative, hemorrhage
　　postprocedural — *see* Complication, postprocedural, hemorrhage
　ileostomy (stoma) — *see* Complications, enterostomy
　immunization (procedure) — *see* Complications, vaccination
　implant (*see also* Complications, by site and type)
　　urinary sphincter T83.9 ☑
　　　embolism T83.81 ☑
　　　fibrosis T83.82 ☑

Complication(s) — *continued*
　implant (*see also* Complications, by site and type) — *continued*
　　urinary sphincter — *continued*
　　　hemorrhage T83.83 ☑
　　　infection and inflammation T83.591 ☑
　　　mechanical
　　　　breakdown T83.111 ☑
　　　　displacement T83.121 ☑
　　　　leakage T83.191 ☑
　　　　malposition T83.121 ☑
　　　　obstruction T83.191 ☑
　　　　perforation T83.191 ☑
　　　　protrusion T83.191 ☑
　　　　specified NEC T83.191 ☑
　　　pain T83.84 ☑
　　　specified type NEC T83.89 ☑
　　　stenosis T83.85 ☑
　　　thrombosis T83.86 ☑
　infusion (procedure) T80.90 ☑
　　air embolism T80.0 ☑
　　blood — *see* Complications, transfusion
　　catheter — *see* Complications, catheter
　　infection T80.29 ☑
　　pump — *see* Complications, cardiovascular, device or implant
　　sepsis T80.29 ☑
　　serum reaction (*see also* Reaction, serum) T80.69 ☑
　　　anaphylactic shock (*see also* Shock, anaphylactic) T80.59 ☑
　　specified type NEC T80.89 ☑
　inhalation therapy NEC T81.81 ☑
　injection (procedure) T80.90 ☑
　　drug reaction — *see* Reaction, drug
　　infection T80.29 ☑
　　sepsis T80.29 ☑
　　serum (prophylactic) (therapeutic) — *see* Complications, vaccination
　　specified type NEC T80.89 ☑
　　vaccine (any) — *see* Complications, vaccination
　inoculation (any) — *see* Complications, vaccination
　insulin pump
　　infection and inflammation T85.72 ☑
　　mechanical
　　　breakdown T85.614 ☑
　　　displacement T85.624 ☑
　　　leakage T85.633 ☑
　　　malposition T85.624 ☑
　　　obstruction T85.694 ☑
　　　perforation T85.694 ☑
　　　protrusion T85.694 ☑
　　　specified NEC T85.694 ☑
　intestinal pouch NEC K91.858
　intraocular lens (prosthetic) T85.9 ☑
　　embolism T85.818 ☑
　　fibrosis T85.828 ☑
　　hemorrhage T85.838 ☑
　　infection and inflammation T85.79 ☑
　　mechanical
　　　breakdown T85.21 ☑
　　　displacement T85.22 ☑
　　　malposition T85.22 ☑
　　　obstruction T85.29 ☑
　　　perforation T85.29 ☑
　　　protrusion T85.29 ☑
　　　specified NEC T85.29 ☑
　　pain T85.848 ☑
　　specified type NEC T85.898 ☑
　　stenosis T85.858 ☑
　　thrombosis T85.868 ☑
　intraoperative (intraprocedural)
　　cardiac arrest (*see also* Infarct, myocardium, associated with revascularization procedure)
　　　during cardiac surgery I97.710
　　　during other surgery I97.711
　　cardiac functional disturbance NEC (*see also* Infarct, myocardium, associated with revascularization procedure)
　　　during cardiac surgery I97.790
　　　during other surgery I97.791
　　hemorrhage (hematoma) (of)
　　　circulatory system organ or structure
　　　　during cardiac bypass I97.411
　　　　during cardiac catheterization I97.410
　　　　during other circulatory system procedure I97.418

Complication(s) — *continued*
　intraoperative — *continued*
　　hemorrhage — *continued*
　　　circulatory system organ or structure — *continued*
　　　　during other procedure I97.42
　　　digestive system organ
　　　　during procedure on digestive system K91.61
　　　　during procedure on other organ K91.62
　　　ear
　　　　during procedure on ear and mastoid process H95.21
　　　　during procedure on other organ H95.22
　　　endocrine system organ or structure
　　　　during procedure on endocrine system organ or structure E36.01
　　　　during procedure on other organ E36.02
　　　eye and adnexa
　　　　during ophthalmic procedure H59.11- ☑
　　　　during other procedure H59.12- ☑
　　　genitourinary organ or structure
　　　　during procedure on genitourinary organ or structure N99.61
　　　　during procedure on other organ N99.62
　　　mastoid process
　　　　during procedure on ear and mastoid process H95.21
　　　　during procedure on other organ H95.22
　　　musculoskeletal structure
　　　　during musculoskeletal surgery M96.810
　　　　during non-orthopedic surgery M96.811
　　　　during orthopedic surgery M96.810
　　　nervous system
　　　　during a nervous system procedure G97.31
　　　　during other procedure G97.32
　　　respiratory system
　　　　during other procedure J95.62
　　　　during procedure on respiratory system organ or structure J95.61
　　　skin and subcutaneous tissue
　　　　during a dermatologic procedure L76.01
　　　　during a procedure on other organ L76.02
　　　spleen
　　　　during a procedure on other organ D78.02
　　　　during a procedure on the spleen D78.01
　　puncture or laceration (accidental) (unintentional) (of)
　　　brain
　　　　during a nervous system procedure G97.48
　　　　during other procedure G97.49
　　　circulatory system organ or structure
　　　　during circulatory system procedure I97.51
　　　　during other procedure I97.52
　　　digestive system
　　　　during procedure on digestive system K91.71
　　　　during procedure on other organ K91.72
　　　ear
　　　　during procedure on ear and mastoid process H95.31
　　　　during procedure on other organ H95.32
　　　endocrine system organ or structure
　　　　during procedure on endocrine system organ or structure E36.11
　　　　during procedure on other organ E36.12
　　　eye and adnexa
　　　　during ophthalmic procedure H59.21- ☑
　　　　during other procedure H59.22- ☑
　　　genitourinary organ or structure
　　　　during procedure on genitourinary organ or structure N99.71
　　　　during procedure on other organ N99.72
　　　mastoid process
　　　　during procedure on ear and mastoid process H95.31
　　　　during procedure on other organ H95.32
　　　musculoskeletal structure
　　　　during musculoskeletal surgery M96.820
　　　　during non-orthopedic surgery M96.821
　　　　during orthopedic surgery M96.820
　　　nervous system
　　　　during a nervous system procedure G97.48
　　　　during other procedure G97.49
　　　respiratory system
　　　　during other procedure J95.72
　　　　during procedure on respiratory system organ or structure J95.71

Complication(s) — *continued*
  intraoperative — *continued*
    puncture or laceration — *continued*
      skin and subcutaneous tissue
        during a dermatologic procedure L76.11
        during a procedure on other organ L76.12
      spleen
        during a procedure on other organ D78.12
        during a procedure on the spleen D78.11
    specified NEC
      circulatory system I97.88
      digestive system K91.81
      ear H95.88
      endocrine system E36.8
      eye and adnexa H59.88
      genitourinary system N99.81
      mastoid process H95.88
      musculoskeletal structure M96.89
      nervous system G97.81
      respiratory system J95.88
      skin and subcutaneous tissue L76.81
      spleen D78.81
  intraperitoneal catheter (dialysis) (infusion) — *see* Complications, catheter, intraperitoneal
  intrathecal infusion pump
    infection and inflammation T85.738 ☑
    mechanical
      breakdown T85.615 ☑
      displacement T85.625 ☑
      leakage T85.635 ☑
      malfunction T85.695 ☑
      malposition T85.625 ☑
      obstruction T85.695 ☑
      perforation T85.695 ☑
      protrusion T85.695 ☑
      specified NEC T85.695 ☑
  intrauterine
    contraceptive device
      embolism T83.81 ☑
      fibrosis T83.82 ☑
      hemorrhage T83.83 ☑
      infection and inflammation T83.69 ☑
      mechanical
        breakdown T83.31 ☑
        displacement T83.32 ☑
        malposition T83.32 ☑
        obstruction T83.39 ☑
        perforation T83.39 ☑
        protrusion T83.39 ☑
        specified NEC T83.39 ☑
      pain T83.84 ☑
      specified type NEC T83.89 ☑
      stenosis T83.85 ☑
      thrombosis T83.86 ☑
    procedure (fetal), to newborn P96.5
  jejunostomy (stoma) — *see* Complications, enterostomy
  joint prosthesis, internal T84.9 ☑
    breakage (fracture) T84.01- ☑
    dislocation T84.02- ☑
    fracture T84.01- ☑
    infection or inflammation T84.50 ☑
      hip T84.5- ☑
      knee T84.5- ☑
      specified joint NEC T84.59 ☑
    instability T84.02- ☑
    malposition — *see* Complications, joint prosthesis, mechanical, displacement
    mechanical
      breakage, broken T84.01- ☑
      dislocation T84.02- ☑
      fracture T84.01- ☑
      instability T84.02- ☑
      leakage — *see* Complications, joint prosthesis, mechanical, specified NEC
      loosening T84.039 ☑
        hip T84.03- ☑
        knee T84.03- ☑
        specified joint NEC T84.038 ☑
      obstruction — *see* Complications, joint prosthesis, mechanical, specified NEC
      perforation — *see* Complications, joint prosthesis, mechanical, specified NEC
      osteolysis T84.059 ☑
        hip T84.05- ☑
        knee T84.05- ☑
        other specified joint T84.058 ☑

Complication(s) — *continued*
  joint prosthesis, internal — *continued*
    mechanical — *continued*
      protrusion — *see* Complications, joint prosthesis, mechanical, specified NEC
      specified complication NEC T84.099 ☑
        hip T84.09- ☑
        knee T84.09- ☑
        other specified joint T84.098 ☑
      subluxation T84.02- ☑
      wear of articular bearing surface T84.069 ☑
        hip T84.06- ☑
        knee T84.06- ☑
        other specified joint T84.068 ☑
    specified joint NEC T84.89 ☑
      embolism T84.81 ☑
      fibrosis T84.82 ☑
      hemorrhage T84.83 ☑
      pain T84.84 ☑
      specified complication NEC T84.89 ☑
      stenosis T84.85 ☑
      thrombosis T84.86 ☑
    subluxation T84.02- ☑
  kidney transplant — *see* Complications, transplant, kidney
  labor O75.9
    specified NEC O75.89
  liver transplant (immune or nonimmune) — *see* Complications, transplant, liver
  lumbar puncture G97.1
    cerebrospinal fluid leak G97.0
    headache or reaction G97.1
  lung transplant — *see* Complications, transplant, lung
    and heart — *see* Complications, transplant, lung, with heart
  male genital N50.9
    device, implant or graft — *see* Complications, genitourinary, device or implant, genital tract
    postprocedural or postoperative — *see* Complications, genitourinary, postprocedural
    specified NEC N99.89
  mastoid (process) procedure
    intraoperative H95.88
      hematoma — *see* Complications, intraoperative, hemorrhage (hematoma) (of), mastoid process
      hemorrhage — *see* Complications, intraoperative, hemorrhage (hematoma) (of), mastoid process
      laceration — *see* Complications, intraoperative, puncture or laceration, mastoid process
      specified NEC H95.88
    postmastoidectomy — *see* Complications, postmastoidectomy
    postoperative H95.89
      external ear canal stenosis H95.81 ☑
      hematoma — *see* Complications, postprocedural, hematoma (of), mastoid process
      hemorrhage — *see* Complications, postprocedural, hemorrhage (of), mastoid process
      postmastoidectomy — *see* Complications, postmastoidectomy
      seroma — *see* Complications, postprocedural, seroma (of), mastoid process
      specified NEC H95.89
  mastoidectomy cavity — *see* Complications, postmastoidectomy
  mechanical — *see* Complications, by site and type, mechanical
  medical procedures (*see also* Complication(s), intraoperative) T88.9 ☑
  metabolic E88.9
    postoperative E89.89
    specified NEC E89.89
  molar pregnancy NOS O08.9
    damage to pelvic organs O08.6
    embolism O08.2
    genital infection O08.0
    hemorrhage (delayed) (excessive) O08.1
    metabolic disorder O08.5
    renal failure O08.4
    shock O08.3
    specified type NEC O08.0
    venous complication NEC O08.7

Complication(s) — *continued*
  musculoskeletal system (*see also* Complication, intraoperative (intraprocedural), by site)
    device, implant or graft NEC — *see* Complications, orthopedic, device or implant
    internal fixation (nail) (plate) (rod) — *see* Complications, fixation device, internal
    joint prosthesis — *see* Complications, joint prosthesis
    post radiation M96.89
      kyphosis M96.2
      scoliosis M96.5
      specified complication NEC M96.89
    postoperative (postprocedural) M96.89
      with osteoporosis — *see* Osteoporosis
      fracture following insertion of device — *see* Fracture, following insertion of orthopedic implant, joint prosthesis or bone plate
      joint instability after prosthesis removal M96.89
      lordosis M96.4
      postlaminectomy syndrome NEC M96.1
        kyphosis M96.3
      pseudarthrosis M96.0
      specified complication NEC M96.89
  nephrostomy (stoma) — *see* Complications, stoma, urinary tract, external NEC
  nervous system G98.8
    central G96.9
    device, implant or graft (*see also* Complication, prosthetic device or implant, specified NEC)
      electronic stimulator (electrode(s)) — *see* Complications, electronic stimulator device
      specified NEC
        infection and inflammation T85.738 ☑
        mechanical T85.695 ☑
          breakdown T85.615 ☑
          displacement T85.625 ☑
          leakage T85.635 ☑
          malfunction T85.695 ☑
          malposition T85.625 ☑
          obstruction T85.695 ☑
          perforation T85.695 ☑
          protrusion T85.695 ☑
          specified NEC T85.695 ☑
      ventricular shunt — *see* Complications, ventricular shunt
    electronic stimulator (electrode(s)) — *see* Complications, electronic stimulator device
    postprocedural G97.82
      intracranial hypotension G97.2
      specified NEC G97.82
      spinal fluid leak G97.0
  newborn, due to intrauterine (fetal) procedure P96.5
  nonabsorbable (permanent) sutures — *see* Complication, sutures, permanent
  obstetric O75.9
    procedure (instrumental) (manual) (surgical)
      specified NEC O75.4
    specified NEC O75.89
    surgical wound NEC O90.89
      hematoma O90.2
      infection O86.0
  ocular lens implant — *see* Complications, intraocular lens
  ophthalmologic
    postprocedural bleb — *see* Blebitis
  orbital prosthesis T85.9 ☑
    embolism T85.818 ☑
    fibrosis T85.828 ☑
    hemorrhage T85.838 ☑
    infection and inflammation T85.79 ☑
    mechanical
      breakdown T85.31- ☑
      displacement T85.32- ☑
      malposition T85.32- ☑
      obstruction T85.39- ☑
      perforation T85.39- ☑
      protrusion T85.39- ☑
      specified NEC T85.39- ☑
    pain T85.848 ☑
    specified type NEC T85.898 ☑
    stenosis T85.858 ☑
    thrombosis T85.868 ☑
  organ or tissue transplant (partial) (total) — *see* Complications, transplant

Complication(s) — *continued*
  orthopedic (*see also* Disorder, soft tissue)
    device or implant T84.9 ☑
      bone
        device or implant — *see* Complication,
          bone, device NEC
        graft — *see* Complication, graft, bone
      breakdown T84.418 ☑
      displacement T84.428 ☑
      electronic bone stimulator — *see* Complica-
        tions, electronic stimulator device, bone
      embolism T84.81 ☑
      fibrosis T84.82 ☑
      fixation device — *see* Complication, fixation
        device, internal
      hemorrhage T84.83 ☑
      infection or inflammation T84.7 ☑
      joint prosthesis — *see* Complication, joint
        prosthesis, internal
      malfunction T84.418 ☑
      malposition T84.428 ☑
      mechanical NEC T84.498 ☑
      muscle graft — *see* Complications, graft, muscle
      obstruction T84.498 ☑
      pain T84.84 ☑
      perforation T84.498 ☑
      protrusion T84.498 ☑
      specified complication NEC T84.89 ☑
      stenosis T84.85 ☑
      tendon graft — *see* Complications, graft, ten-
        don
      thrombosis T84.86 ☑
    fracture (following insertion of device) — *see*
      Fracture, following insertion of orthopedic
      implant, joint prosthesis or bone plate
    postprocedural M96.89
      fracture — *see* Fracture, following insertion of
        orthopedic implant, joint prosthesis or
        bone plate
      postlaminectomy syndrome NEC M96.1
        kyphosis M96.3
        lordosis M96.4
      postradiation
        kyphosis M96.2
        scoliosis M96.5
      pseudarthrosis post-fusion M96.0
      specified type NEC M96.89
  pacemaker (cardiac) — *see* Complications, cardiovas-
    cular device or implant, electronic
  pancreas transplant — *see* Complications, transplant,
    pancreas
  penile prosthesis (implant) — *see* Complications,
    prosthetic device, penile
  perfusion NEC T80.90 ☑
  perineal repair (obstetrical) NEC O90.89
    disruption O90.1
    hematoma O90.2
    infection (following delivery) O86.0
  phototherapy T88.9 ☑
    specified NEC T88.8 ☑
  postmastoidectomy NEC H95.19- ☑
    cyst, mucosal H95.13- ☑
    granulation H95.12- ☑
    inflammation, chronic H95.11- ☑
    recurrent cholesteatoma H95.0- ☑
  postoperative — *see* Complications, postprocedural
    circulatory — *see* Complications, circulatory system
    ear — *see* Complications, ear
    endocrine — *see* Complications, endocrine
    eye — *see* Complications, eye
    lumbar puncture G97.1
      cerebrospinal fluid leak G97.0
    nervous system (central) (peripheral) — *see* Com-
      plications, nervous system
    respiratory system — *see* Complications, respirato-
      ry system
  postprocedural (*see also* Complications, surgical pro-
    cedure)
    cardiac arrest (*see also* Infarct, myocardium, associ-
      ated with revascularization procedure)
      following cardiac surgery I97.120
      following other surgery I97.121
    cardiac functional disturbance NEC (*see also* Infarct,
      myocardium, associated with revasculariza-
      tion procedure)
      following cardiac surgery I97.190

Complication(s) — *continued*
  postprocedural (*see also* Complications, surgical pro-
    cedure) — *continued*
    cardiac functional disturbance (*see also* Infarct,
      myocardium, associated with revasculariza-
      tion procedure) — *continued*
      following other surgery I97.191
    cardiac insufficiency
      following cardiac surgery I97.110
      following other surgery I97.111
    chorioretinal scars following retinal surgery
      H59.81- ☑
    following cataract surgery
      cataract (lens) fragments H59.02- ☑
      cystoid macular edema H59.03- ☑
      specified NEC H59.09- ☑
      vitreous (touch) syndrome H59.01- ☑
    heart failure
      following cardiac surgery I97.130
      following other surgery I97.131
    hematoma (of)
      circulatory system organ or structure
        following cardiac bypass I97.631
        following cardiac catheterization I97.630
        following other circulatory system proce-
          dure I97.638
        following other procedure I97.621
      digestive system
        following procedure on digestive system
          K91.870
        following procedure on other organ K91.871
      ear
        following other procedure H95.52
        following procedure on ear and mastoid
          process H95.51
      endocrine system
        following endocrine system procedure
          E89.820
        following other procedure E89.821
      eye and adnexa
        following ophthalmic procedure H59.33- ☑
        following other procedure H59.34- ☑
      genitourinary organ or structure
        following procedure on genitourinary organ
          or structure N99.840
        following procedure on other organ
          N99.841
      mastoid process
        following other procedure H95.52
        following procedure on ear and mastoid
          process H95.51
      musculoskeletal structure
        following musculoskeletal surgery M96.840
        following non-orthopedic surgery M96.841
        following orthopedic surgery M96.840
      nervous system
        following nervous system procedure G97.61
        following other procedure G97.62
      respiratory system
        following other procedure J95.861
        following procedure on respiratory system
          organ or structure J95.860
      skin and subcutaneous tissue
        following dermatologic procedure L76.31
        following procedure on other organ L76.32
      spleen
        following procedure on other organ D78.32
        following procedure on the spleen D78.31
    hemorrhage (of)
      circulatory system organ or structure
        following cardiac bypass I97.611
        following cardiac catheterization I97.610
        following other circulatory system proce-
          dure I97.618
        following other procedure I97.620
      digestive system
        following procedure on digestive system
          K91.840
        following procedure on other organ K91.841
      ear
        following other procedure H95.42
        following procedure on ear and mastoid
          process H95.41
      endocrine system
        following endocrine system procedure
          E89.810
        following other procedure E89.811

Complication(s) — *continued*
  postprocedural (*see also* Complications, surgical pro-
    cedure) — *continued*
    hemorrhage — *continued*
      eye and adnexa
        following ophthalmic procedure H59.31- ☑
        following other procedure H59.32- ☑
      genitourinary organ or structure
        following procedure on genitourinary organ
          or structure N99.820
        following procedure on other organ
          N99.821
      mastoid process
        following other procedure H95.42
        following procedure on ear and mastoid
          process H95.41
      musculoskeletal structure
        following musculoskeletal surgery M96.830
        following non-orthopedic surgery M96.831
        following orthopedic surgery M96.830
      nervous system
        following nervous system procedure G97.51
        following other procedure G97.52
      respiratory system
        following a respiratory system procedure
          J95.830
        following other procedure J95.831
      skin and subcutaneous tissue
        following a procedure on other organ
          L76.22
        following dermatologic procedure L76.21
      spleen
        following procedure on other organ D78.22
        following procedure on the spleen D78.21
    seroma (of)
      circulatory system organ or structure
        following cardiac bypass I97.641
        following cardiac catheterization I97.640
        following other circulatory system proce-
          dure I97.648
        following other procedure I97.622
      digestive system
        following procedure on digestive system
          K91.872
        following procedure on other organ K91.873
      ear
        following other procedure H95.54
        following procedure on ear and mastoid
          process H95.53
      endocrine system
        following endocrine system procedure
          E89.822
        following other procedure E89.823
      eye and adnexa
        following ophthalmic procedure H59.35- ☑
        following other procedure H59.36- ☑
      genitourinary organ or structure
        following procedure on genitourinary organ
          or structure N99.842
        following procedure on other organ
          N99.843
      mastoid process
        following other procedure H95.54
        following procedure on ear and mastoid
          process H95.53
      musculoskeletal structure
        following musculoskeletal surgery M96.842
        following non-orthopedic surgery M96.843
        following orthopedic surgery M96.842
      nervous system
        following nervous system procedure G97.63
        following other procedure G97.64
      respiratory system
        following other procedure J95.863
        following procedure on respiratory system
          organ or structure J95.862
      skin and subcutaneous tissue
        following dermatologic procedure L76.33
        following procedure on other organ L76.34
      spleen
        following procedure on other organ D78.34
        following procedure on the spleen D78.33
    specified NEC
      circulatory system I97.89
      digestive K91.89
      ear H95.89
      endocrine E89.89
      eye and adnexa H59.89
      genitourinary N99.89

Complication(s) — *continued*
  postprocedural (*see also* Complications, surgical procedure) — *continued*
    specified — *continued*
      mastoid process H95.89
      metabolic E89.89
      musculoskeletal structure M96.89
      nervous system G97.82
      respiratory system J95.89
      skin and subcutaneous tissue L76.82
      spleen D78.89
  pregnancy NEC — *see* Pregnancy, complicated by
  prosthetic device or implant T85.9 ☑
    bile duct — *see* Complications, bile duct implant
    breast — *see* Complications, breast implant
    bulking agent
      ureteral
        erosion T83.714 ☑
        exposure T83.724 ☑
      urethral
        erosion T83.713 ☑
        exposure T83.723 ☑
    cardiac and vascular NEC — *see* Complications, cardiovascular device or implant
    corneal transplant — *see* Complications, graft, cornea
    electronic nervous system stimulator — *see* Complications, electronic stimulator device
    epidural infusion catheter — *see* Complications, catheter, epidural
    esophageal anti-reflux device — *see* Complications, esophageal anti-reflux device
    genital organ or tract — *see* Complications, genitourinary, device or implant, genital tract
      specified NEC T83.79- ☑
    heart valve — *see* Complications, heart, valve, prosthesis
    infection or inflammation T85.79 ☑
      intestine transplant T86.892
      liver transplant T86.43
      lung transplant T86.812
      pancreas transplant T86.892
      skin graft T86.822
    intraocular lens — *see* Complications, intraocular lens
    intraperitoneal (dialysis) catheter — *see* Complications, catheter, intraperitoneal
    joint — *see* Complications, joint prosthesis, internal
    mechanical NEC T85.698 ☑
      dialysis catheter (vascular) (*see also* Complication, catheter, dialysis, mechanical)
        peritoneal — *see* Complication, catheter, intraperitoneal, mechanical
      gastrointestinal device T85.598 ☑
      ocular device T85.398 ☑
      subdural (infusion) catheter T85.690 ☑
      suture, permanent T85.692 ☑
        that for bone repair — *see* Complications, fixation device, internal (orthopedic), mechanical
      ventricular shunt
        breakdown T85.01 ☑
        displacement T85.02 ☑
        leakage T85.03 ☑
        malposition T85.02 ☑
        obstruction T85.09 ☑
        perforation T85.09 ☑
        protrusion T85.09 ☑
        specified NEC T85.09 ☑
    mesh
      erosion (to surrounding organ or tissue) T83.718 ☑
        urethral (into pelvic floor muscles) T83.712 ☑
        vaginal (into pelvic floor muscles) T83.711 ☑
      exposure (into surrounding organ or tissue) T83.728 ☑
        urethral (through urethral wall) T83.722 ☑
        vaginal (into vagina) (through vaginal wall) T83.721 ☑
    orbital — *see* Complications, orbital prosthesis
    penile T83.9 ☑
      embolism T83.81 ☑
      fibrosis T83.82 ☑
      hemorrhage T83.83 ☑
      infection and inflammation T83.61 ☑

Complication(s) — *continued*
  prosthetic device or implant — *continued*
    penile — *continued*
      mechanical
        breakdown T83.410 ☑
        displacement T83.420 ☑
        leakage T83.490 ☑
        malposition T83.420 ☑
        obstruction T83.490 ☑
        perforation T83.490 ☑
        protrusion T83.490 ☑
        specified NEC T83.490 ☑
      pain T83.84 ☑
      specified type NEC T83.89 ☑
      stenosis T83.85 ☑
      thrombosis T83.86 ☑
    prosthetic materials NEC
      erosion (to surrounding organ or tissue) T83.718 ☑
      exposure (into surrounding organ or tissue) T83.728 ☑
    skin graft T86.829
      artificial skin or decellularized allodermis
        embolism T85.818 ☑
        fibrosis T85.828 ☑
        hemorrhage T85.838 ☑
        infection and inflammation T85.79 ☑
        mechanical
          breakdown T85.613 ☑
          displacement T85.623 ☑
          malfunction T85.613 ☑
          malposition T85.623 ☑
          obstruction T85.693 ☑
          perforation T85.693 ☑
          protrusion T85.693 ☑
          specified NEC T85.693 ☑
        pain T85.848 ☑
        specified type NEC T85.898 ☑
        stenosis T85.858 ☑
        thrombosis T85.868 ☑
      failure T86.821
      infection T86.822
      rejection T86.820
      specified NEC T86.828
    sling
      urethral (female) (male)
        erosion T83.712 ☑
        exposure T83.722 ☑
    specified NEC T85.9 ☑
      embolism T85.818 ☑
      fibrosis T85.828 ☑
      hemorrhage T85.838 ☑
      infection and inflammation T85.79 ☑
      mechanical
        breakdown T85.618 ☑
        displacement T85.628 ☑
        leakage T85.638 ☑
        malfunction T85.618 ☑
        malposition T85.628 ☑
        obstruction T85.698 ☑
        perforation T85.698 ☑
        protrusion T85.698 ☑
        specified NEC T85.698 ☑
      pain T85.848 ☑
      specified type NEC T85.898 ☑
      stenosis T85.858 ☑
      thrombosis T85.868 ☑
    subdural infusion catheter — *see* Complications, catheter, subdural
    sutures — *see* Complications, sutures
    urinary organ or tract NEC — *see* Complications, genitourinary, device or implant, urinary system
    vascular — *see* Complications, cardiovascular device or implant
    ventricular shunt — *see* Complications, ventricular shunt (device)
  puerperium — *see* Puerperal
  puncture, spinal G97.1
    cerebrospinal fluid leak G97.0
    headache or reaction G97.1
  pyelogram N99.89
  radiation
    kyphosis M96.2
    scoliosis M96.5

Complication(s) — *continued*
  reattached
    extremity (infection) (rejection)
      lower T87.1X- ☑
      upper T87.0X- ☑
    specified body part NEC T87.2
  reconstructed breast
    asymmetry between native and reconstructed breast N65.1
    deformity N65.0
    disproportion between native and reconstructed breast N65.1
    excess tissue N65.0
    misshappen N65.0
  reimplant NEC (*see also* Complications, prosthetic device or implant)
    limb (infection) (rejection) — *see* Complications, reattached, extremity
    organ (partial) (total) — *see* Complications, transplant
    prosthetic device NEC — *see* Complications, prosthetic device
  renal N28.9
    allograft — *see* Complications, transplant, kidney
    dialysis — *see* Complications, dialysis
  respirator
    mechanical J95.850
      specified NEC J95.859
  respiratory system J98.9
    device, implant or graft — *see* Complication, prosthetic device or implant, specified NEC
    lung transplant — *see* Complications, prosthetic device or implant, lung transplant
    postoperative J95.89
      air leak J95.812
      Mendelson's syndrome (chemical pneumonitis) J95.4
      pneumothorax J95.811
      pulmonary insufficiency (acute) (after nonthoracic surgery) J95.2
        chronic J95.3
        following thoracic surgery J95.1
      respiratory failure (acute) J95.821
        acute and chronic J95.822
      specified NEC J95.89
      subglottic stenosis J95.5
      tracheostomy complication — *see* Complications, tracheostomy
    therapy T81.89 ☑
  sedation during labor and delivery O74.9
    cardiac O74.2
    central nervous system O74.3
    pulmonary NEC O74.1
  shunt (*see also* Complications, prosthetic device or implant)
    arteriovenous — *see* Complications, arteriovenous, shunt
    ventricular (communicating) — *see* Complications, ventricular shunt
  skin
    graft T86.829
      failure T86.821
      infection T86.822
      rejection T86.820
      specified type NEC T86.828
  spinal
    anesthesia — *see* Complications, anesthesia, spinal
    catheter (epidural) (subdural) — *see* Complications, catheter
    puncture or tap G97.1
      cerebrospinal fluid leak G97.0
      headache or reaction G97.1
  stent
    bile duct — *see* Complications, bile duct prosthesis
    ureteral indwelling
      breakdown T83.112 ☑
      displacement T83.122 ☑
      leakage T83.192 ☑
      malposition T83.122 ☑
      obstruction T83.192 ☑
      perforation T83.192 ☑
      protrusion T83.192 ☑
      specified NEC T83.192 ☑
    urinary NEC (ileal conduit) (nephroureteral) T83.193 ☑
      embolism T83.81 ☑
      fibrosis T83.82 ☑
      hemorrhage T83.83 ☑

☑ **Additional Character Required — Refer to the Tabular List for Character Selection**   ⩗ **Subterms under main terms may continue to next column or page**

Complication(s) — *continued*
  stent — *continued*
    urinary — *continued*
      infection and inflammation T83.593 ☑
      mechanical
        breakdown T83.113 ☑
        displacement T83.123 ☑
        leakage T83.193 ☑
        malposition T83.123 ☑
        obstruction T83.193 ☑
        perforation T83.193 ☑
        protrusion T83.193 ☑
        specified NEC T83.193 ☑
      pain T83.84 ☑
      specified type NEC T83.89 ☑
      stenosis T83.85 ☑
      thrombosis T83.86 ☑
    vascular
      end stent stenosis — *see* Restenosis, stent
      in stent stenosis — *see* Restenosis, stent
  stoma
    digestive tract
      colostomy — *see* Complications, colostomy
      enterostomy — *see* Complications, enterostomy
      esophagostomy — *see* Complications, esophagostomy
      gastrostomy — *see* Complications, gastrostomy
    urinary tract N99.528
      continent N99.538
        hemorrhage N99.530
        herniation N99.533
        infection N99.531
        malfunction N99.532
        specified type NEC N99.538
        stenosis N99.534
      cystostomy — *see* Complications, cystostomy
      external NOS N99.528
      hemorrhage N99.520
      herniation N99.523
      incontinent N99.528
        hemorrhage N99.520
        herniation N99.523
        infection N99.521
        malfunction N99.522
        specified type NEC N99.528
        stenosis N99.524
      infection N99.521
      malfunction N99.522
      specified type NEC N99.528
      stenosis N99.524
  stomach banding — *see* Complication(s), bariatric procedure
  stomach stapling — *see* Complication(s), bariatric procedure
  surgical material, nonabsorbable — *see* Complication, suture, permanent
  surgical procedure (on) T81.9 ☑
    amputation stump (late) — *see* Complications, amputation stump
    cardiac — *see* Complications, circulatory system
    cholesteatoma, recurrent — *see* Complications, postmastoidectomy, recurrent cholesteatoma
    circulatory (early) — *see* Complications, circulatory system
    digestive system — *see* Complications, gastrointestinal
    dumping syndrome (postgastrectomy) K91.1
    ear — *see* Complications, ear
    elephantiasis or lymphedema I97.89
      postmastectomy I97.2
    emphysema (surgical) T81.82 ☑
    endocrine — *see* Complications, endocrine
    eye — *see* Complications, eye
    fistula (persistent postoperative) T81.83 ☑
    foreign body inadvertently left in wound (sponge) (suture) (swab) — *see* Foreign body, accidentally left during a procedure
    gastrointestinal — *see* Complications, gastrointestinal
    genitourinary NEC N99.89
    hematoma
      intraoperative — *see* Complication, intraoperative, hemorrhage
      postprocedural — *see* Complication, postprocedural, hematoma

Complication(s) — *continued*
  surgical procedure — *continued*
    hemorrhage
      intraoperative — *see* Complication, intraoperative, hemorrhage
      postprocedural — *see* Complication, postprocedural, hemorrhage
    hepatic failure K91.82
    hyperglycemia (postpancreatectomy) E89.1
    hypoinsulinemia (postpancreatectomy) E89.1
    hypoparathyroidism (postparathyroidectomy) E89.2
    hypopituitarism (posthypophysectomy) E89.3
    hypothyroidism (post-thyroidectomy) E89.0
    intestinal obstruction (*see also* Obstruction, intestine, postoperative) K91.30
    intracranial hypotension following ventricular shunting (ventriculostomy) G97.2
    lymphedema I97.89
      postmastectomy I97.2
    malabsorption (postsurgical) NEC K91.2
      osteoporosis — *see* Osteoporosis, postsurgical malabsorption
    mastoidectomy cavity NEC — *see* Complications, postmastoidectomy
    metabolic E89.89
      specified NEC E89.89
    musculoskeletal — *see* Complications, musculoskeletal system
    nervous system (central) (peripheral) — *see* Complications, nervous system
    ovarian failure E89.40
      asymptomatic E89.40
      symptomatic E89.41
    peripheral vascular — *see* Complications, surgical procedure, vascular
    postcardiotomy syndrome I97.0
    postcholecystectomy syndrome K91.5
    postcommissurotomy syndrome I97.0
    postgastrectomy dumping syndrome K91.1
    postlaminectomy syndrome NEC M96.1
      kyphosis M96.3
    postmastectomy lymphedema syndrome I97.2
    postmastoidectomy cholesteatoma — *see* Complications, postmastoidectomy, recurrent cholesteatoma
    postvagotomy syndrome K91.1
    postvalvulotomy syndrome I97.0
    pulmonary insufficiency (acute) J95.2
      chronic J95.3
      following thoracic surgery J95.1
    reattached body part — *see* Complications, reattached
    respiratory — *see* Complications, respiratory system
    shock (hypovolemic) T81.19 ☑
    spleen (postoperative) D78.89
      intraoperative D78.81
    stitch abscess T81.4 ☑
    subglottic stenosis (postsurgical) J95.5
    testicular hypofunction E89.5
    transplant — *see* Complications, organ or tissue transplant
    urinary NEC N99.89
    vaginal vault prolapse (posthysterectomy) N99.3
    vascular (peripheral)
      artery T81.719 ☑
        mesenteric T81.710 ☑
        renal T81.711 ☑
        specified NEC T81.718 ☑
      vein T81.72 ☑
    wound infection T81.4 ☑
  suture, permanent (wire) NEC T85.9 ☑
    with repair of bone — *see* Complications, fixation device, internal
    embolism T85.818 ☑
    fibrosis T85.828 ☑
    hemorrhage T85.838 ☑
    infection and inflammation T85.79 ☑
    mechanical
      breakdown T85.612 ☑
      displacement T85.622 ☑
      malfunction T85.612 ☑
      malposition T85.622 ☑
      obstruction T85.692 ☑
      perforation T85.692 ☑
      protrusion T85.692 ☑

Complication(s) — *continued*
  suture, permanent — *continued*
    mechanical — *continued*
      specified NEC T85.692 ☑
    pain T85.848 ☑
    specified type NEC T85.898 ☑
    stenosis T85.858 ☑
    thrombosis T85.868 ☑
  tracheostomy J95.00
    granuloma J95.09
    hemorrhage J95.01
    infection J95.02
    malfunction J95.03
    mechanical J95.03
    obstruction J95.03
    specified type NEC J95.09
    tracheo-esophageal fistula J95.04
  transfusion (blood) (lymphocytes) (plasma) T80.92 ☑
    air embolism T80.0 ☑
    circulatory overload E87.71
    febrile nonhemolytic transfusion reaction R50.84
    hemochromatosis E83.111
    hemolysis T80.89 ☑
    hemolytic reaction (antigen unspecified) T80.919 ☑
    incompatibility reaction (antigen unspecified) T80.919 ☑
      ABO T80.30 ☑
        delayed serologic (DSTR) T80.39 ☑
        hemolytic transfusion reaction (HTR) (unspecified time after transfusion) T80.319 ☑
          acute (AHTR) (less than 24 hours after transfusion) T80.310 ☑
          delayed (DHTR) (24 hours or more after transfusion) T80.311 ☑
        specified NEC T80.39 ☑
      acute (antigen unspecified) T80.910 ☑
      delayed (antigen unspecified) T80.911 ☑
      delayed serologic (DSTR) T80.89 ☑
      non-ABO (minor antigens (Duffy) (Kell) (Kidd) (Lewis) (M) (N) (P) (S)) T80.A0 ☑ (*following* T80.4)
        delayed serologic (DSTR) T80.A9 ☑ (*following* T80.4)
        hemolytic transfusion reaction (HTR) (unspecified time after transfusion) T80.A19 ☑ (*following* T80.4)
          acute (AHTR) (less than 24 hours after transfusion) T80.A10 ☑ (*following* T80.4)
          delayed (DHTR) (24 hours or more after transfusion) T80.A11 ☑ (*following* T80.4)
        specified NEC T80.A9 ☑ (*following* T80.4)
      Rh (antigens (C) (c) (D) (E) (e)) (factor) T80.40 ☑
        delayed serologic (DSTR) T80.49 ☑
        hemolytic transfusion reaction (HTR) (unspecified time after transfusion) T80.419 ☑
          acute (AHTR) (less than 24 hours after transfusion) T80.410 ☑
          delayed (DHTR) (24 hours or more after transfusion) T80.411 ☑
        specified NEC T80.49 ☑
    infection T80.29 ☑
      acute T80.22- ☑
    reaction NEC T80.89 ☑
    sepsis T80.29 ☑
    shock T80.89 ☑
  transplant T86.90
    bone T86.839
      failure T86.831
      infection T86.832
      rejection T86.830
      specified type NEC T86.838
    bone marrow T86.00
      failure T86.02
      infection T86.03
      rejection T86.01
      specified type NEC T86.09
    cornea T86.849
      failure T86.841
      infection T86.842
      rejection T86.840
      specified type NEC T86.848
    failure T86.92

⚕ Subterms under main terms may continue to next column or page   ☑ Additional Character Required — Refer to the Tabular List for Character Selection   67

Complication — Complication

Complication(s) — *continued*
transplant — *continued*
  heart T86.20
    with lung T86.30
    cardiac allograft vasculopathy T86.290
      failure T86.32
      infection T86.33
      rejection T86.31
      specified type NEC T86.39
    failure T86.22
    infection T86.23
    rejection T86.21
    specified type NEC T86.298
  infection T86.93
  intestine T86.859
    failure T86.851
    infection T86.852
    rejection T86.850
    specified type NEC T86.858
  kidney T86.10
    failure T86.12
    infection T86.13
    rejection T86.11
    specified type NEC T86.19
  liver T86.40
    failure T86.42
    infection T86.43
    rejection T86.41
    specified type NEC T86.49
  lung T86.819
    with heart T86.30
      failure T86.32
      infection T86.33
      rejection T86.31
      specified type NEC T86.39
    failure T86.811
    infection T86.812
    rejection T86.810
    specified type NEC T86.818
  malignant neoplasm C80.2
  pancreas T86.899
    failure T86.891
    infection T86.892
    rejection T86.890
    specified type NEC T86.898
  peripheral blood stem cells T86.5
  post-transplant lymphoproliferative disorder
    (PTLD) D47.Z1 (*following* D47.4)
  rejection T86.91
  skin T86.829
    failure T86.821
    infection T86.822
    rejection T86.820
    specified type NEC T86.828
  specified
    tissue T86.899
      failure T86.891
      infection T86.892
      rejection T86.890
      specified type NEC T86.898
    type NEC T86.99
  stem cell (from peripheral blood) (from umbilical
    cord) T86.5
  umbilical cord stem cells T86.5
trauma (early) T79.9 ☑
  specified NEC T79.8 ☑
ultrasound therapy NEC T88.9 ☑
umbilical cord NEC
  complicating delivery O69.9 ☑
    specified NEC O69.89 ☑
umbrella device, vascular T82.9 ☑
  embolism T82.818 ☑
  fibrosis T82.828 ☑
  hemorrhage T82.838 ☑
  infection or inflammation T82.7 ☑
  mechanical
    breakdown T82.515 ☑
    displacement T82.525 ☑
    leakage T82.535 ☑
    malposition T82.525 ☑
    obstruction T82.595 ☑
    perforation T82.595 ☑
    protrusion T82.595 ☑
  pain T82.848 ☑
  specified type NEC T82.898 ☑
  stenosis T82.858 ☑
  thrombosis T82.868 ☑

Complication(s) — *continued*
urethral catheter — *see* Complications, catheter, urethral, indwelling
vaccination T88.1 ☑
  anaphylaxis NEC T80.52 ☑
  arthropathy — *see* Arthropathy, postimmunization
  cellulitis T88.0 ☑
  encephalitis or encephalomyelitis G04.02
  infection (general) (local) NEC T88.0 ☑
  meningitis G03.8
  myelitis G04.02
  protein sickness T80.62 ☑
  rash T88.1 ☑
  reaction (allergic) T88.1 ☑
    serum T80.62 ☑
  sepsis T88.0 ☑
  serum intoxication, sickness, rash, or other serum
    reaction NEC T80.62 ☑
  anaphylactic shock T80.52 ☑
  shock (allergic) (anaphylactic) T80.52 ☑
  vaccinia (generalized) (localized) T88.1 ☑
vas deferens device or implant — *see* Complications,
  genitourinary, device or implant, genital tract
vascular I99.9
  device or implant T82.9 ☑
    embolism T82.818 ☑
    fibrosis T82.828 ☑
    hemorrhage T82.838 ☑
    infection or inflammation T82.7 ☑
    mechanical
      breakdown T82.519 ☑
        specified device NEC T82.518 ☑
      displacement T82.529 ☑
        specified device NEC T82.528 ☑
      leakage T82.539 ☑
        specified device NEC T82.538 ☑
      malposition T82.529 ☑
        specified device NEC T82.528 ☑
      obstruction T82.599 ☑
        specified device NEC T82.598 ☑
      perforation T82.599 ☑
        specified device NEC T82.598 ☑
      protrusion T82.599 ☑
        specified device NEC T82.598 ☑
    pain T82.848 ☑
    specified type NEC T82.898 ☑
    stenosis T82.858 ☑
    thrombosis T82.868 ☑
  dialysis catheter — *see* Complication, catheter,
    dialysis
  following infusion, therapeutic injection or transfu-
    sion T80.1 ☑
  graft T82.9 ☑
    embolism T82.818 ☑
    fibrosis T82.828 ☑
    hemorrhage T82.838 ☑
    mechanical
      breakdown T82.319 ☑
        aorta (bifurcation) T82.310 ☑
        carotid artery T82.311 ☑
        specified vessel NEC T82.318 ☑
      displacement T82.329 ☑
        aorta (bifurcation) T82.320 ☑
        carotid artery T82.321 ☑
        specified vessel NEC T82.328 ☑
      leakage T82.339 ☑
        aorta (bifurcation) T82.330 ☑
        carotid artery T82.331 ☑
        specified vessel NEC T82.338 ☑
      malposition T82.329 ☑
        aorta (bifurcation) T82.320 ☑
        carotid artery T82.321 ☑
        specified vessel NEC T82.328 ☑
      obstruction T82.399 ☑
        aorta (bifurcation) T82.390 ☑
        carotid artery T82.391 ☑
        specified vessel NEC T82.398 ☑
      perforation T82.399 ☑
        aorta (bifurcation) T82.390 ☑
        carotid artery T82.391 ☑
        specified vessel NEC T82.398 ☑
      protrusion T82.399 ☑
        aorta (bifurcation) T82.390 ☑
        carotid artery T82.391 ☑
        specified vessel NEC T82.398 ☑
    pain T82.848 ☑

Complication(s) — *continued*
vascular — *continued*
  graft — *continued*
    specified complication NEC T82.898 ☑
    stenosis T82.858 ☑
    thrombosis T82.868 ☑
  postoperative — *see* Complications, postoperative,
    circulatory
vena cava device (filter) (sieve) (umbrella) — *see*
  Complications, umbrella device, vascular
ventilation therapy NEC T81.81 ☑
ventilator
  mechanical J95.850
    specified NEC J95.859
ventricular (communicating) shunt (device) T85.9 ☑
  embolism T85.810 ☑
  fibrosis T85.820 ☑
  hemorrhage T85.830 ☑
  infection and inflammation T85.730 ☑
  mechanical
    breakdown T85.01 ☑
    displacement T85.02 ☑
    leakage T85.03 ☑
    malposition T85.02 ☑
    obstruction T85.09 ☑
    perforation T85.09 ☑
    protrusion T85.09 ☑
    specified NEC T85.09 ☑
  pain T85.840 ☑
  specified type NEC T85.890 ☑
  stenosis T85.850 ☑
  thrombosis T85.860 ☑
wire suture, permanent (implanted) — *see* Complications, suture, permanent
Compressed air disease T70.3 ☑
Compression
  with injury — *code by* Nature of injury
  artery I77.1
    celiac, syndrome I77.4
  brachial plexus G54.0
  brain (stem) G93.5
    due to
      contusion (diffuse) — *see* Injury, intracranial,
        diffuse
        focal — *see* Injury, intracranial, focal
      injury NEC — *see* Injury, intracranial, diffuse
      traumatic — *see* Injury, intracranial, diffuse
  bronchus J98.09
  cauda equina G83.4
  celiac (artery) (axis) I77.4
  cerebral — *see* Compression, brain
  cervical plexus G54.2
  cord
    spinal — *see* Compression, spinal
    umbilical — *see* Compression, umbilical cord
  cranial nerve G52.9
    eighth H93.3 ☑
    eleventh G52.8
    fifth G50.8
    first G52.0
    fourth — *see* Strabismus, paralytic, fourth nerve
    ninth G52.1
    second — *see* Disorder, nerve, optic
    seventh G51.8
    sixth — *see* Strabismus, paralytic, sixth nerve
    tenth G52.2
    third — *see* Strabismus, paralytic, third nerve
    twelfth G52.3
  diver's squeeze T70.3 ☑
  during birth (newborn) P15.9
  esophagus K22.2
  eustachian tube — *see* Obstruction, eustachian tube,
    cartilaginous
  facies Q67.1
  fracture
    nontraumatic NOS — *see* Collapse, vertebra
    pathological — *see* Fracture, pathological
    traumatic — *see* Fracture, traumatic
  heart — *see* Disease, heart
  intestine — *see* Obstruction, intestine
  laryngeal nerve, recurrent G52.2
    with paralysis of vocal cords and larynx J38.00
      bilateral J38.02
      unilateral J38.01
  lumbosacral plexus G54.1
  lung J98.4
  lymphatic vessel I89.0

☑ **Additional Character Required** — Refer to the Tabular List for Character Selection   ⑄ Subterms under main terms may continue to next column or page

Compression — *continued*
 medulla — *see* Compression, brain
 nerve (*see also* Disorder, nerve) G58.9
  arm NEC — *see* Mononeuropathy, upper limb
  axillary G54.0
  cranial — *see* Compression, cranial nerve
  leg NEC — *see* Mononeuropathy, lower limb
  median (in carpal tunnel) — *see* Syndrome, carpal
    tunnel
  optic — *see* Disorder, nerve, optic
  plantar — *see* Lesion, nerve, plantar
  posterior tibial (in tarsal tunnel) — *see* Syndrome,
    tarsal tunnel
  root or plexus NOS (in) G54.9
   intervertebral disc disorder NEC — *see* Disorder,
     disc, with, radiculopathy
    with myelopathy — *see* Disorder, disc, with,
      myelopathy
   neoplastic disease (*see also* Neoplasm)
     D49.9 [G55]
   spondylosis — *see* Spondylosis, with radiculopa-
     thy
  sciatic (acute) — *see* Lesion, nerve, sciatic
  sympathetic G90.8
  traumatic — *see* Injury, nerve
  ulnar — *see* Lesion, nerve, ulnar
  upper extremity NEC — *see* Mononeuropathy,
    upper limb
 spinal (cord) G95.20
  by displacement of intervertebral disc NEC (*see also*
    Disorder, disc, with, myelopathy)
  nerve root NOS G54.9
   due to displacement of intervertebral disc NEC
     — *see* Disorder, disc, with, radiculopathy
    with myelopathy — *see* Disorder, disc, with,
      myelopathy
  specified NEC G95.29
  spondylogenic (cervical) (lumbar, lumbosacral)
    (thoracic) — *see* Spondylosis, with
    myelopathy NEC
  anterior — *see* Syndrome, anterior, spinal
    artery, compression
  traumatic — *see* Injury, spinal cord, by region
 subcostal nerve (syndrome) — *see* Mononeuropathy,
   upper limb, specified NEC
 sympathetic nerve NEC G90.8
 syndrome T79.5 ☑
 trachea J39.8
 ulnar nerve (by scar tissue) — *see* Lesion, nerve, ulnar
 umbilical cord
  complicating delivery O69.2 ☑
   cord around neck O69.1 ☑
   prolapse O69.0 ☑
   specified NEC O69.2 ☑
 ureter N13.5
 vein I87.1
 vena cava (inferior) (superior) I87.1
Compulsion, compulsive
 gambling F63.0
 neurosis F42.8
 personality F60.5
 states F42.8
 swearing F42.8
  in Gilles de la Tourette's syndrome F95.2
 tics and spasms F95.9
Concato's disease (pericardial polyserositis) A19.9
 nontubercular I31.1
 pleural — *see* Pleurisy, with effusion
Concavity chest wall M95.4
Concealed penis Q55.69
Concern (normal) **about sick person in family** Z63.6
Concrescence (teeth) K00.2
Concretio cordis I31.1
 rheumatic I09.2
Concretion (*see also* Calculus)
 appendicular K38.1
 canaliculus — *see* Dacryolith
 clitoris N90.89
 conjunctiva H11.12- ☑
 eyelid — *see* Disorder, eyelid, specified type NEC
 lacrimal passages — *see* Dacryolith
 prepuce (male) N47.8
 salivary gland (any) K11.5
 seminal vesicle N50.89
 tonsil J35.8
Concussion (brain) (cerebral) (current) S06.0X9 ☑

Concussion — *continued*
 with
  loss of consciousness of 30 minutes or less
    S06.0X1 ☑
  loss of consciousness of unspecified duration
    S06.0X9 ☑
  without loss of consciousness S06.0X0 ☑
 blast (air) (hydraulic) (immersion) (underwater)
  abdomen or thorax — *see* Injury, blast, by site
  ear with acoustic nerve injury — *see* Injury, nerve,
    acoustic, specified type NEC
 cauda equina S34.3 ☑
 conus medullaris S34.02 ☑
 ocular S05.8X- ☑
 spinal (cord)
  cervical S14.0 ☑
  lumbar S34.01 ☑
  sacral S34.02 ☑
  thoracic S24.0 ☑
 syndrome F07.81
Condition — *see* Disease
Conditions arising in the perinatal period — *see*
  Newborn, affected by
Conduct disorder — *see* Disorder, conduct
Condyloma A63.0
 acuminatum A63.0
 gonorrheal A54.09
 latum A51.31
 syphilitic A51.31
  congenital A50.07
 venereal, syphilitic A51.31
Conflagration (*see also* Burn)
 asphyxia (by inhalation of gases, fumes or vapors) (*see
  also* Table of Drugs and Chemicals) T59.9- ☑
Conflict (with) (*see also* Discord)
 family Z73.9
 marital Z63.0
  involving divorce or estrangement Z63.5
 parent-child Z62.820
  parent-adopted child Z62.821
  parent-biological child Z62.820
  parent-foster child Z62.822
 social role NEC Z73.5
Confluent — *see* condition
Confusion, confused R41.0
 epileptic F05
 mental state (psychogenic) F44.89
 psychogenic F44.89
 reactive (from emotional stress, psychological trauma)
   F44.89
Confusional arousals G47.51
Congelation T69.9 ☑
Congenital (*see also* condition)
 aortic septum Q25.49
 intrinsic factor deficiency D51.0
 malformation — *see* Anomaly
Congestion, congestive
 bladder N32.89
 bowel K63.89
 brain G93.89
 breast N64.59
 bronchial J98.09
 catarrhal J31.0
 chest R09.89
 chill, malarial — *see* Malaria
 circulatory NEC I99.8
 duodenum K31.89
 eye — *see* Hyperemia, conjunctiva
 facial, due to birth injury P15.4
 general R68.89
 glottis J37.0
 heart — *see* Failure, heart, congestive
 hepatic K76.1
 hypostatic (lung) — *see* Edema, lung
 intestine K63.89
 kidney N28.89
 labyrinth H83.8 ☑
 larynx J37.0
 liver K76.1
 lung R09.89
  active or acute — *see* Pneumonia
 malaria, malarial — *see* Malaria
 nasal R09.81
 nose R09.81
 orbit, orbital (*see also* Exophthalmos)
  inflammatory (chronic) — *see* Inflammation, orbit
 ovary N83.8

Congestion, congestive — *continued*
 pancreas K86.89
 pelvic, female N94.89
 pleural J94.8
 prostate (active) N42.1
 pulmonary — *see* Congestion, lung
 renal N28.89
 retina H35.81
 seminal vesicle N50.1
 spinal cord G95.19
 spleen (chronic) D73.2
 stomach K31.89
 trachea — *see* Tracheitis
 urethra N36.8
 uterus N85.8
  with subinvolution N85.3
 venous (passive) I87.8
 viscera R68.89
Congestive — *see* Congestion
Conical
 cervix (hypertrophic elongation) N88.4
 cornea — *see* Keratoconus
 teeth K00.2
Conjoined twins Q89.4
Conjugal maladjustment Z63.0
 involving divorce or estrangement Z63.5
Conjunctiva — *see* condition
Conjunctivitis (staphylococcal) (streptococcal) NOS
  H10.9
 Acanthamoeba B60.12
 acute H10.3- ☑
  atopic H10.1- ☑
  chemical (*see also* Corrosion, cornea) H10.21- ☑
  mucopurulent H10.02- ☑
   follicular H10.01- ☑
  pseudomembranous H10.22- ☑
  serous except viral H10.23- ☑
   viral — *see* Conjunctivitis, viral
  toxic H10.21- ☑
 adenoviral (acute) (follicular) B30.1
 allergic (acute) — *see* Conjunctivitis, acute, atopic
  chronic H10.45
   vernal H10.44
 anaphylactic — *see* Conjunctivitis, acute, atopic
 Apollo B30.3
 atopic (acute) — *see* Conjunctivitis, acute, atopic
 Béal's B30.2
 blennorrhagic (gonococcal) (neonatorum) A54.31
 chemical (acute) (*see also* Corrosion, cornea)
   H10.21- ☑
 chlamydial A74.0
  due to trachoma A71.1
  neonatal P39.1
 chronic (nodosa) (petrificans) (phlyctenular) H10.40- ☑
  allergic H10.45
   vernal H10.44
  follicular H10.43- ☑
  giant papillary H10.41- ☑
  simple H10.42- ☑
  vernal H10.44
 coxsackievirus 24 B30.3
 diphtheritic A36.86
 due to
  dust — *see* Conjunctivitis, acute, atopic
  filariasis B74.9
  mucocutaneous leishmaniasis B55.2
  enterovirus type 70 (hemorrhagic) B30.3
 epidemic (viral) B30.9
  hemorrhagic B30.3
 gonococcal (neonatorum) A54.31
 granular (trachomatous) A71.1
  sequelae (late effect) B94.0
 hemorrhagic (acute) (epidemic) B30.3
 herpes zoster B02.31
 in (due to)
  Acanthamoeba B60.12
  adenovirus (acute) (follicular) B30.1
  Chlamydia A74.0
  coxsackievirus 24 B30.3
  diphtheria A36.86
  enterovirus type 70 (hemorrhagic) B30.3
  filariasis B74.9
  gonococci A54.31
  herpes (simplex) virus B00.53
   zoster B02.31
  infectious disease NEC B99 ☑
  meningococci A39.89
  mucocutaneous leishmaniasis B55.2

Conjunctivitis — continued
- in — continued
  - rosacea L71.9
  - syphilis (late) A52.71
  - zoster B02.31
  - inclusion A74.0
  - infantile P39.1
    - gonococcal A54.31
  - Koch-Weeks' — see Conjunctivitis, acute, mucopurulent
  - light — see Conjunctivitis, acute, atopic
  - ligneous — see Blepharoconjunctivitis, ligneous
  - meningococcal A39.89
  - mucopurulent — see Conjunctivitis, acute, mucopurulent
  - neonatal P39.1
    - gonococcal A54.31
  - Newcastle B30.8
  - of Béal B30.2
  - parasitic
    - filariasis B74.9
    - mucocutaneous leishmaniasis B55.2
  - Parinaud's H10.89
  - petrificans H10.89
  - rosacea L71.9
  - specified NEC H10.89
  - swimming-pool B30.1
  - trachomatous A71.1
    - acute A71.0
    - sequelae (late effect) B94.0
  - traumatic NEC H10.89
  - tuberculous A18.59
  - tularemic A21.1
  - tularensis A21.1
  - viral B30.9
    - due to
      - adenovirus B30.1
      - enterovirus B30.3
    - specified NEC B30.8

Conjunctivochalasis H11.82- ☑
Connective tissue — see condition
Conn's syndrome E26.01
Conradi (-Hunermann) **disease** Q77.3
Consanguinity Z84.3
- counseling Z71.89

Conscious simulation (of illness) Z76.5
Consecutive — see condition
Consolidation lung (base) — see Pneumonia, lobar
Constipation (atonic) (neurogenic) (simple) (spastic) K59.00
- chronic K59.09
  - idiopathic K59.04
- drug-induced K59.03
- functional K59.04
- outlet dysfunction K59.02
- psychogenic F45.8
- slow transit K59.01
- specified NEC K59.09

Constitutional (see also condition)
- substandard F60.7

Constitutionally substandard F60.7
Constriction (see also Stricture)
- auditory canal — see Stenosis, external ear canal
- bronchial J98.09
- duodenum K31.5
- esophagus K22.2
- external
  - abdomen, abdominal (wall) S30.841 ☑
  - alveolar process S00.542 ☑
  - ankle S90.54- ☑
  - antecubital space — see Constriction, external, forearm
  - arm (upper) S40.84- ☑
  - auricle — see Constriction, external, ear
  - axilla — see Constriction, external, arm
  - back, lower S30.840 ☑
  - breast S20.14- ☑
  - brow S00.84 ☑
  - buttock S30.840 ☑
  - calf — see Constriction, external, leg
  - canthus — see Constriction, external, eyelid
  - cheek S00.84 ☑
    - internal S00.542 ☑
  - chest wall — see Constriction, external, thorax
  - chin S00.84 ☑
  - clitoris S30.844 ☑
  - costal region — see Constriction, external, thorax

Constriction — continued
- external — continued
  - digit(s)
    - foot — see Constriction, external, toe
    - hand — see Constriction, external, finger
  - ear S00.44- ☑
  - elbow S50.34- ☑
  - epididymis S30.843 ☑
  - epigastric region S30.841 ☑
  - esophagus, cervical S10.14 ☑
  - eyebrow — see Constriction, external, eyelid
  - eyelid S00.24- ☑
  - face S00.84 ☑
  - finger(s) S60.44- ☑
    - index S60.44- ☑
    - little S60.44- ☑
    - middle S60.44- ☑
    - ring S60.44- ☑
  - flank S30.841 ☑
  - foot (except toe(s) alone) S90.84- ☑
    - toe — see Constriction, external, toe
  - forearm S50.84- ☑
    - elbow only — see Constriction, external, elbow
  - forehead S00.84 ☑
  - genital organs, external
    - female S30.846 ☑
    - male S30.845 ☑
  - groin S30.841 ☑
  - gum S00.542 ☑
  - hand S60.54- ☑
  - head S00.94 ☑
    - ear — see Constriction, external, ear
    - eyelid — see Constriction, external, eyelid
    - lip S00.541 ☑
    - nose S00.34 ☑
    - oral cavity S00.542 ☑
    - scalp S00.04 ☑
    - specified site NEC S00.84 ☑
  - heel — see Constriction, external, foot
  - hip S70.24- ☑
  - inguinal region S30.841 ☑
  - interscapular region S20.449 ☑
  - jaw S00.84 ☑
  - knee S80.24- ☑
  - labium (majus) (minus) S30.844 ☑
  - larynx S10.14 ☑
  - leg (lower) S80.84- ☑
    - knee — see Constriction, external, knee
    - upper — see Constriction, external, thigh
  - lip S00.541 ☑
  - lower back S30.840 ☑
  - lumbar region S30.840 ☑
  - malar region S00.84 ☑
  - mammary — see Constriction, external, breast
  - mastoid region S00.84 ☑
  - mouth S00.542 ☑
  - nail
    - finger — see Constriction, external, finger
    - toe — see Constriction, external, toe
  - nasal S00.34 ☑
  - neck S10.94 ☑
    - specified site NEC S10.84 ☑
    - throat S10.14 ☑
  - nose S00.34 ☑
  - occipital region S00.04 ☑
  - oral cavity S00.542 ☑
  - orbital region — see Constriction, external, eyelid
  - palate S00.542 ☑
  - palm — see Constriction, external, hand
  - parietal region S00.04 ☑
  - pelvis S30.840 ☑
  - penis S30.842 ☑
  - perineum
    - female S30.844 ☑
    - male S30.840 ☑
  - periocular area — see Constriction, external, eyelid
  - phalanges
    - finger — see Constriction, external, finger
    - toe — see Constriction, external, toe
  - pharynx S10.14 ☑
  - pinna — see Constriction, external, ear
  - popliteal space — see Constriction, external, knee
  - prepuce S30.842 ☑
  - pubic region S30.840 ☑
  - pudendum
    - female S30.846 ☑

Constriction — continued
- external — continued
  - pudendum — continued
    - male S30.845 ☑
  - sacral region S30.840 ☑
  - scalp S00.04 ☑
  - scapular region — see Constriction, external, shoulder
  - scrotum S30.843 ☑
  - shin — see Constriction, external, leg
  - shoulder S40.24- ☑
  - sternal region S20.349 ☑
  - submaxillary region S00.84 ☑
  - submental region S00.84 ☑
  - subungual
    - finger(s) — see Constriction, external, finger
    - toe(s) — see Constriction, external, toe
  - supraclavicular fossa S10.84 ☑
  - supraorbital S00.84 ☑
  - temple S00.84 ☑
  - temporal region S00.84 ☑
  - testis S30.843 ☑
  - thigh S70.34- ☑
  - thorax, thoracic (wall) S20.94 ☑
    - back S20.44- ☑
    - front S20.34- ☑
  - throat S10.14 ☑
  - thumb S60.34- ☑
  - toe(s) (lesser) S90.44- ☑
    - great S90.44- ☑
  - tongue S00.542 ☑
  - trachea S10.14 ☑
  - tunica vaginalis S30.843 ☑
  - uvula S00.542 ☑
  - vagina S30.844 ☑
  - vulva S30.844 ☑
  - wrist S60.84- ☑
- gallbladder — see Obstruction, gallbladder
- intestine — see Obstruction, intestine
- larynx J38.6
  - congenital Q31.8
    - specified NEC Q31.8
    - subglottic Q31.1
- organ or site, congenital NEC — see Atresia, by site
- prepuce (acquired) (congenital) N47.1
- pylorus (adult hypertrophic) K31.1
  - congenital or infantile Q40.0
  - newborn Q40.0
- ring dystocia (uterus) O62.4
- spastic (see also Spasm)
  - ureter N13.5
- ureter N13.5
  - with infection N13.6
- urethra — see Stricture, urethra
- visual field (peripheral) (functional) — see Defect, visual field

Constrictive — see condition
Consultation
- without complaint or sickness Z71.9
  - feared complaint unfounded Z71.1
    - specified reason NEC Z71.89
- medical — see Counseling, medical
- religious Z71.81
- specified reason NEC Z71.89
- spiritual Z71.81

Consumption — see Tuberculosis
Contact (with) (see also Exposure (to))
- acariasis Z20.7
- AIDS virus Z20.6
- air pollution Z77.110
- algae and algae toxins Z77.121
- algae bloom Z77.121
- anthrax Z20.810
- aromatic amines Z77.020
- aromatic (hazardous) compounds NEC Z77.028
- aromatic dyes NOS Z77.028
- arsenic Z77.010
- asbestos Z77.090
- bacterial disease NEC Z20.818
- benzene Z77.021
- blue-green algae bloom Z77.121
- body fluids (potentially hazardous) Z77.21
- brown tide Z77.121
- chemicals (chiefly nonmedicinal) (hazardous) NEC Z77.098
- cholera Z20.09
- chromium compounds Z77.018

☑ **Additional Character Required** — Refer to the Tabular List for Character Selection   ☝ **Subterms under main terms may continue to next column or page**

Contact — *continued*
  communicable disease Z20.9
    bacterial NEC Z20.818
    specified NEC Z20.89
    viral NEC Z20.828
  cyanobacteria bloom Z77.121
  dyes Z77.098
  Escherichia coli (E. coli) Z20.01
  fiberglass — *see* Table of Drugs and Chemicals, fiber-glass
  German measles Z20.4
  gonorrhea Z20.2
  hazardous metals NEC Z77.018
  hazardous substances NEC Z77.29
  hazards in the physical environment NEC Z77.128
  hazards to health NEC Z77.9
  HIV Z20.6
  HTLV-III/LAV Z20.6
  human immunodeficiency virus (HIV) Z20.6
  infection Z20.9
    specified NEC Z20.89
  infestation (parasitic) NEC Z20.7
  intestinal infectious disease NEC Z20.09
    Escherichia coli (E. coli) Z20.01
  lead Z77.011
  meningococcus Z20.811
  mold (toxic) Z77.120
  nickel dust Z77.018
  noise Z77.122
  parasitic disease Z20.7
  pediculosis Z20.7
  pfiesteria piscicida Z77.121
  poliomyelitis Z20.89
  pollution
    air Z77.110
    environmental NEC Z77.118
    soil Z77.112
    water Z77.111
  polycyclic aromatic hydrocarbons Z77.028
  rabies Z20.3
  radiation, naturally occurring NEC Z77.123
  radon Z77.123
  red tide (Florida) Z77.121
  rubella Z20.4
  sexually-transmitted disease Z20.2
  smallpox (laboratory) Z20.89
  syphilis Z20.2
  tuberculosis Z20.1
  uranium Z77.012
  varicella Z20.820
  venereal disease Z20.2
  viral disease NEC Z20.828
  viral hepatitis Z20.5
  water pollution Z77.111
Contamination, food — *see* Intoxication, foodborne
Contraception, contraceptive
  advice Z30.09
  counseling Z30.09
  device (intrauterine) (in situ) Z97.5
    causing menorrhagia T83.83 ☑
    checking Z30.431
    complications — *see* Complications, intrauterine, contraceptive device
    in place Z97.5
    initial prescription Z30.014
    reinsertion Z30.433
    removal Z30.432
    replacement Z30.433
  emergency (postcoital) Z30.012
  initial prescription Z30.019
    barrier Z30.018
    diaphragm Z30.018
    injectable Z30.013
    intrauterine device Z30.014
    pills Z30.011
    postcoital (emergency) Z30.012
    specified type NEC Z30.018
    subdermal implantable Z30.017
    transdermal patch hormonal Z30.016
    vaginal ring hormonal Z30.015
  maintenance Z30.40
    barrier Z30.49
    diaphragm Z30.49
    examination Z30.8
    injectable Z30.42
    intrauterine device Z30.431
    pills Z30.41
    specified type NEC Z30.49
    subdermal implantable Z30.46

Contraception, contraceptive — *continued*
  maintenance — *continued*
    transdermal patch hormonal Z30.45
    vaginal ring hormonal Z30.44
  management Z30.9
    specified NEC Z30.8
  postcoital (emergency) Z30.012
  prescription Z30.019
    repeat Z30.40
  sterilization Z30.2
  surveillance (drug) — *see* Contraception, maintenance
Contraction(s), contracture, contracted
  Achilles tendon (*see also* Short, tendon, Achilles)
    congenital Q66.89
  amputation stump (surgical) (flexion) (late) (next proximal joint) T87.89
  anus K59.8
  bile duct (common) (hepatic) K83.8
  bladder N32.89
    neck or sphincter N32.0
  bowel, cecum, colon or intestine, any part — *see* Obstruction, intestine
  Braxton Hicks — *see* False, labor
  breast implant, capsular T85.44 ☑
  bronchial J98.09
  burn (old) — *see* Cicatrix
  cervix — *see* Stricture, cervix
  cicatricial — *see* Cicatrix
  conjunctiva, trachomatous, active A71.1
    sequelae (late effect) B94.0
  Dupuytren's M72.0
  eyelid — *see* Disorder, eyelid function
  fascia (lata) (postural) M72.8
    Dupuytren's M72.0
    palmar M72.0
    plantar M72.2
  finger NEC (*see also* Deformity, finger)
    congenital Q68.1
    joint — *see* Contraction, joint, hand
  flaccid — *see* Contraction, paralytic
  gallbladder K82.0
  heart valve — *see* Endocarditis
  hip — *see* Contraction, joint, hip
  hourglass
    bladder N32.89
      congenital Q64.79
    gallbladder K82.0
      congenital Q44.1
    stomach K31.89
      congenital Q40.2
      psychogenic F45.8
    uterus (complicating delivery) O62.4
  hysterical F44.4
  internal os — *see* Stricture, cervix
  joint (abduction) (acquired) (adduction) (flexion) (rotation) M24.50
    ankle M24.57- ☑
    congenital NEC Q68.8
      hip Q65.89
    elbow M24.52- ☑
    foot joint M24.57- ☑
    hand joint M24.54- ☑
    hip M24.55- ☑
      congenital Q65.89
    hysterical F44.4
    knee M24.56- ☑
    shoulder M24.51- ☑
    wrist M24.53- ☑
  kidney (granular) (secondary) N26.9
    congenital Q63.8
    hydronephritic — *see* Hydronephrosis
    Page N26.2
    pyelonephritic — *see* Pyelitis, chronic
    tuberculous A18.11
  ligament (*see also* Disorder, ligament)
    congenital Q79.8
  muscle (postinfective) (postural) NEC M62.40
    with contracture of joint — *see* Contraction, joint
    ankle M62.47- ☑
    congenital Q79.8
      sternocleidomastoid Q68.0
    extraocular — *see* Strabismus
    eye (extrinsic) — *see* Strabismus
    foot M62.47- ☑
    forearm M62.43- ☑
    hand M62.44- ☑
    hysterical F44.4

Contraction(s), contracture, contracted — *continued*
  muscle — *continued*
    ischemic (Volkmann's) T79.6 ☑
    lower leg M62.46- ☑
    multiple sites M62.49
    pelvic region M62.45- ☑
    posttraumatic — *see* Strabismus, paralytic
    psychogenic F45.8
      conversion reaction F44.4
    shoulder region M62.41- ☑
    specified site NEC M62.48
    thigh M62.45- ☑
    upper arm M62.42- ☑
  neck — *see* Torticollis
  ocular muscle — *see* Strabismus
  organ or site, congenital NEC — *see* Atresia, by site
  outlet (pelvis) — *see* Contraction, pelvis
  palmar fascia M72.0
  paralytic
    joint — *see* Contraction, joint
    muscle (*see also* Contraction, muscle NEC)
      ocular — *see* Strabismus, paralytic
  pelvis (acquired) (general) M95.5
    with disproportion (fetopelvic) O33.1
      causing obstructed labor O65.1
    inlet O33.2
    mid-cavity O33.3 ☑
    outlet O33.3 ☑
  plantar fascia M72.2
  premature
    atrium I49.1
    auriculoventricular I49.49
    heart I49.49
    junctional I49.2
    supraventricular I49.1
    ventricular I49.3
  prostate N42.89
  pylorus NEC (*see also* Pylorospasm)
    psychogenic F45.8
  rectum, rectal (sphincter) K59.8
  ring (Bandl's) (complicating delivery) O62.4
  scar — *see* Cicatrix
  spine — *see* Dorsopathy, deforming
  sternocleidomastoid (muscle), congenital Q68.0
  stomach K31.89
    hourglass K31.89
      congenital Q40.2
      psychogenic F45.8
    psychogenic F45.8
  tendon (sheath) M62.40
    with contracture of joint — *see* Contraction, joint
    Achilles — *see* Short, tendon, Achilles
    ankle M62.47- ☑
      Achilles — *see* Short, tendon, Achilles
    foot M62.47- ☑
    forearm M62.43- ☑
    hand M62.44- ☑
    lower leg M62.46- ☑
    multiple sites M62.49
    neck M62.48
    pelvic region M62.45- ☑
    shoulder region M62.41- ☑
    specified site NEC M62.48
    thigh M62.45- ☑
    thorax M62.48
    trunk M62.48
    upper arm M62.42- ☑
  toe — *see* Deformity, toe, specified NEC
  ureterovesical orifice (postinfectional) N13.5
    with infection N13.6
  urethra (*see also* Stricture, urethra)
    orifice N32.0
  uterus N85.8
    abnormal NEC O62.9
    clonic (complicating delivery) O62.4
    dyscoordinate (complicating delivery) O62.4
    hourglass (complicating delivery) O62.4
    hypertonic O62.4
    hypotonic NEC O62.2
    inadequate
      primary O62.0
      secondary O62.1
    incoordinate (complicating delivery) O62.4
    poor O62.2
    tetanic (complicating delivery) O62.4
  vagina (outlet) N89.5
  vesical N32.89

Contraction(s), contracture, contracted — *continued*
- vesical — *continued*
  - neck or urethral orifice N32.0
- visual field — *see* Defect, visual field, generalized
- Volkmann's (ischemic) T79.6 ☑
Contusion (skin surface intact) T14.8 ☑
- abdomen, abdominal (muscle) (wall) S30.1 ☑
- adnexa, eye NEC S05.8X- ☑
- adrenal gland S37.812 ☑
- alveolar process S00.532 ☑
- ankle S90.0- ☑
- antecubital space — *see* Contusion, forearm
- anus S30.3 ☑
- arm (upper) S40.02- ☑
  - lower (with elbow) — *see* Contusion, forearm
- auditory canal — *see* Contusion, ear
- auricle — *see* Contusion, ear
- axilla — *see* Contusion, arm, upper
- back (*see also* Contusion, thorax, back)
  - lower S30.0 ☑
- bile duct S36.13 ☑
- bladder S37.22 ☑
- bone NEC T14.8 ☑
- brain (diffuse) — *see* Injury, intracranial, diffuse
  - focal — *see* Injury, intracranial, focal
- brainstem S06.38- ☑
- breast S20.0- ☑
- broad ligament S37.892 ☑
- brow S00.83 ☑
- buttock S30.0 ☑
- canthus, eye S00.1- ☑
- cauda equina S34.3 ☑
- cerebellar, traumatic S06.37- ☑
- cerebral S06.33- ☑
  - left side S06.32- ☑
  - right side S06.31- ☑
- cheek S00.83 ☑
  - internal S00.532 ☑
- chest (wall) — *see* Contusion, thorax
- chin S00.83 ☑
- clitoris S30.23 ☑
- colon — *see* Injury, intestine, large, contusion
- common bile duct S36.13 ☑
- conjunctiva S05.1- ☑
  - with foreign body (in conjunctival sac) — *see* Foreign body, conjunctival sac
- conus medullaris (spine) S34.139 ☑
- cornea — *see* Contusion, eyeball
  - with foreign body — *see* Foreign body, cornea
- corpus cavernosum S30.21 ☑
- cortex (brain) (cerebral) — *see* Injury, intracranial, diffuse
  - focal — *see* Injury, intracranial, focal
- costal region — *see* Contusion, thorax
- cystic duct S36.13 ☑
- diaphragm S27.802 ☑
- duodenum S36.420 ☑
- ear S00.43- ☑
- elbow S50.0- ☑
  - with forearm — *see* Contusion, forearm
- epididymis S30.22 ☑
- epigastric region S30.1 ☑
- epiglottis S10.0 ☑
- esophagus (thoracic) S27.812 ☑
  - cervical S10.0 ☑
- eyeball S05.1- ☑
- eyebrow S00.1- ☑
- eyelid (and periocular area) S00.1- ☑
- face NEC S00.83 ☑
- fallopian tube S37.529 ☑
  - bilateral S37.522 ☑
  - unilateral S37.521 ☑
- femoral triangle S30.1 ☑
- finger(s) S60.00 ☑
  - with damage to nail (matrix) S60.10 ☑
  - index S60.02- ☑
    - with damage to nail S60.12- ☑
  - little S60.05- ☑
    - with damage to nail S60.15- ☑
  - middle S60.03- ☑
    - with damage to nail S60.13- ☑
  - ring S60.04- ☑
    - with damage to nail S60.14- ☑
  - thumb — *see* Contusion, thumb
- flank S30.1 ☑

Contusion — *continued*
- foot (except toe(s) alone) S90.3- ☑
  - toe — *see* Contusion, toe
- forearm S50.1- ☑
  - elbow only — *see* Contusion, elbow
- forehead S00.83 ☑
- gallbladder S36.122 ☑
- genital organs, external
  - female S30.202 ☑
  - male S30.201 ☑
- globe (eye) — *see* Contusion, eyeball
- groin S30.1 ☑
- gum S00.532 ☑
- hand S60.22- ☑
  - finger(s) — *see* Contusion, finger
  - wrist — *see* Contusion, wrist
- head S00.93 ☑
  - ear — *see* Contusion, ear
  - eyelid — *see* Contusion, eyelid
  - lip S00.531 ☑
  - nose S00.33 ☑
  - oral cavity S00.532 ☑
  - scalp S00.03 ☑
  - specified part NEC S00.83 ☑
- heart (*see also* Injury, heart) S26.91 ☑
- heel — *see* Contusion, foot
- hepatic duct S36.13 ☑
- hip S70.0- ☑
- ileum S36.428 ☑
- iliac region S30.1 ☑
- inguinal region S30.1 ☑
- interscapular region S20.229 ☑
- intra-abdominal organ S36.92 ☑
  - colon — *see* Injury, intestine, large, contusion
  - liver S36.112 ☑
  - pancreas — *see* Contusion, pancreas
  - rectum S36.62 ☑
  - small intestine — *see* Injury, intestine, small, contusion
  - specified organ NEC S36.892 ☑
  - spleen — *see* Contusion, spleen
  - stomach S36.32 ☑
- iris (eye) — *see* Contusion, eyeball
- jaw S00.83 ☑
- jejunum S36.428 ☑
- kidney S37.01- ☑
  - major (greater than 2 cm) S37.02- ☑
  - minor (less than 2 cm) S37.01- ☑
- knee S80.0- ☑
- labium (majus) (minus) S30.23 ☑
- lacrimal apparatus, gland or sac S05.8X- ☑
- larynx S10.0 ☑
- leg (lower) S80.1- ☑
  - knee — *see* Contusion, knee
- lens — *see* Contusion, eyeball
- lip S00.531 ☑
- liver S36.112 ☑
- lower back S30.0 ☑
- lumbar region S30.0 ☑
- lung S27.329 ☑
  - bilateral S27.322 ☑
  - unilateral S27.321 ☑
- malar region S00.83 ☑
- mastoid region S00.83 ☑
- membrane, brain — *see* Injury, intracranial, diffuse
  - focal — *see* Injury, intracranial, focal
- mesentery S36.892 ☑
- mesosalpinx S37.892 ☑
- mouth S00.532 ☑
- muscle — *see* Contusion, by site
- nail
  - finger — *see* Contusion, finger, with damage to nail
  - toe — *see* Contusion, toe, with damage to nail
- nasal S00.33 ☑
- neck S10.93 ☑
  - specified site NEC S10.83 ☑
  - throat S10.0 ☑
- nerve — *see* Injury, nerve
- newborn P54.5
- nose S00.33 ☑
- occipital
  - lobe (brain) — *see* Injury, intracranial, diffuse
    - focal — *see* Injury, intracranial, focal
  - region (scalp) S00.03 ☑
- orbit (region) (tissues) S05.1- ☑

Contusion — *continued*
- ovary S37.429 ☑
  - bilateral S37.422 ☑
  - unilateral S37.421 ☑
- palate S00.532 ☑
- pancreas S36.229 ☑
  - body S36.221 ☑
  - head S36.220 ☑
  - tail S36.222 ☑
- parietal
  - lobe (brain) — *see* Injury, intracranial, diffuse
    - focal — *see* Injury, intracranial, focal
  - region (scalp) S00.03 ☑
- pelvic organ S37.92 ☑
  - adrenal gland S37.812 ☑
  - bladder S37.22 ☑
  - fallopian tube — *see* Contusion, fallopian tube
  - kidney — *see* Contusion, kidney
  - ovary — *see* Contusion, ovary
  - prostate S37.822 ☑
  - specified organ NEC S37.892 ☑
  - ureter S37.12 ☑
  - urethra S37.32 ☑
  - uterus S37.62 ☑
- pelvis S30.0 ☑
- penis S30.21 ☑
- perineum
  - female S30.23 ☑
  - male S30.0 ☑
- periocular area S00.1- ☑
- peritoneum S36.81 ☑
- periurethral tissue — *see* Contusion, urethra
- pharynx S10.0 ☑
- pinna — *see* Contusion, ear
- popliteal space — *see* Contusion, knee
- prepuce S30.21 ☑
- prostate S37.822 ☑
- pubic region S30.1 ☑
- pudendum
  - female S30.202 ☑
  - male S30.201 ☑
- quadriceps femoris — *see* Contusion, thigh
- rectum S36.62 ☑
- retroperitoneum S36.892 ☑
- round ligament S37.892 ☑
- sacral region S30.0 ☑
- scalp S00.03 ☑
  - due to birth injury P12.3
- scapular region — *see* Contusion, shoulder
- sclera — *see* Contusion, eyeball
- scrotum S30.22 ☑
- seminal vesicle S37.892 ☑
- shoulder S40.01- ☑
- skin NEC T14.8 ☑
- small intestine — *see* Injury, intestine, small, contusion
- spermatic cord S30.22 ☑
- spinal cord — *see* Injury, spinal cord, by region
  - cauda equina S34.3 ☑
  - conus medullaris S34.139 ☑
- spleen S36.029 ☑
  - major S36.021 ☑
  - minor S36.020 ☑
- sternal region S20.219 ☑
- stomach S36.32 ☑
- subconjunctival S05.1- ☑
- subcutaneous NEC T14.8 ☑
- submaxillary region S00.83 ☑
- submental region S00.83 ☑
- subperiosteal NEC T14.8 ☑
- subungual
  - finger — *see* Contusion, finger, with damage to nail
  - toe — *see* Contusion, toe, with damage to nail
- supraclavicular fossa S10.83 ☑
- supraorbital S00.83 ☑
- suprarenal gland S37.812 ☑
- temple (region) S00.83 ☑
- temporal
  - lobe (brain) — *see* Injury, intracranial, diffuse
    - focal — *see* Injury, intracranial, focal
  - region S00.83 ☑
- testis S30.22 ☑
- thigh S70.1- ☑
- thorax (wall) S20.20 ☑
  - back S20.22- ☑
  - front S20.21- ☑

☑ **Additional Character Required** — Refer to the Tabular List for Character Selection

▽ **Subterms under main terms may continue to next column or page**

Contusion — *continued*
  throat S10.0 ☑
  thumb S60.01- ☑
    with damage to nail S60.11- ☑
  toe(s) (lesser) S90.12- ☑
    with damage to nail S90.22- ☑
    great S90.11- ☑
      with damage to nail S90.21- ☑
  tongue S00.532 ☑
  trachea (cervical) S10.0 ☑
    thoracic S27.52 ☑
  tunica vaginalis S30.22 ☑
  tympanum, tympanic membrane — *see* Contusion,
      ear
  ureter S37.12 ☑
  urethra S37.32 ☑
  urinary organ NEC S37.892 ☑
  uterus S37.62 ☑
  uvula S00.532 ☑
  vagina S30.23 ☑
  vas deferens S37.892 ☑
  vesical S37.22 ☑
  vocal cord(s) S10.0 ☑
  vulva S30.23 ☑
  wrist S60.21- ☑
Conus (congenital) (any type) Q14.8
  cornea — *see* Keratoconus
  medullaris syndrome G95.81
Conversion hysteria, neurosis or reaction F44.9
Converter, tuberculosis (test reaction) R76.11
Conviction (legal), **anxiety concerning** Z65.0
  with imprisonment Z65.1
Convulsions (idiopathic) (*see also* Seizure(s)) R56.9
  apoplectiform (cerebral ischemia) I67.82
  dissociative F44.5
  epileptic — *see* Epilepsy
  epileptiform, epileptoid — *see* Seizure, epileptiform
  ether (anesthetic) — *see* Table of Drugs and Chemicals,
      by drug
  febrile R56.00
    with status epilepticus G40.901
    complex R56.01
      with status epilepticus G40.901
    simple R56.00
  hysterical F44.5
  infantile P90
    epilepsy — *see* Epilepsy
  jacksonian — *see* Epilepsy, localization-related,
      symptomatic, with simple partial seizures
  myoclonic G25.3
  newborn P90
  obstetrical (nephritic) (uremic) — *see* Eclampsia
  paretic A52.17
  post traumatic R56.1
  psychomotor — *see* Epilepsy, localization-related,
      symptomatic, with complex partial seizures
  recurrent R56.9
  reflex R25.8
  scarlatinal A38.8
  tetanus, tetanic — *see* Tetanus
  thymic E32.8
Convulsive (*see also* Convulsions)
Cooley's anemia D56.1
Coolie itch B76.9
Cooper's
  disease — *see* Mastopathy, cystic
  hernia — *see* Hernia, abdomen, specified site NEC
Copra itch B88.0
Coprophagy F50.89
Coprophobia F40.298
Coproporphyria, hereditary E80.29
Cor
  biloculare Q20.8
  bovis, bovinum — *see* Hypertrophy, cardiac
  pulmonale (chronic) I27.81
    acute I26.09
  triatriatum, triatrium Q24.2
  triloculare Q20.8
    biatrium Q20.4
    biventriculare Q21.1
Corbus' disease (gangrenous balanitis) N48.1
Cord (*see also* condition)
  around neck
    complicating delivery O69.81 ☑
      with compression O69.1 ☑
  bladder G95.89
    tabetic A52.19

Cordis ectopia Q24.8
Corditis (spermatic) N49.1
Corectopia Q13.2
Cori's disease (glycogen storage) E74.03
Corkhandler's disease or lung J67.3
Corkscrew esophagus K22.4
Corkworker's disease or lung J67.3
Corn (infected) L84
Cornea (*see also* condition)
  donor Z52.5
  plana Q13.4
Cornelia de Lange syndrome Q87.1
Cornu cutaneum L85.8
Cornual gestation or pregnancy O00.80
  with intrauterine pregnancy O00.81
Coronary (artery) — *see* condition
Coronavirus, as cause of disease classified elsewhere
    B97.29
  SARS-associated B97.21
Corpora (*see also* condition)
  amylacea, prostate N42.89
  cavernosa — *see* condition
Corpulence — *see* Obesity
Corpus — *see* condition
Corrected transposition Q20.5
Corrosion (injury) (acid) (caustic) (chemical) (lime) (exter-
    nal) (internal) T30.4
  abdomen, abdominal (muscle) (wall) T21.42 ☑
    first degree T21.52 ☑
    second degree T21.62 ☑
    third degree T21.72 ☑
  above elbow T22.439 ☑
    first degree T22.539 ☑
    left T22.432 ☑
      first degree T22.532 ☑
      second degree T22.632 ☑
      third degree T22.732 ☑
    right T22.431 ☑
      first degree T22.531 ☑
      second degree T22.631 ☑
      third degree T22.731 ☑
    second degree T22.639 ☑
    third degree T22.739 ☑
  alimentary tract NEC T28.7 ☑
  ankle T25.419 ☑
    first degree T25.519 ☑
    left T25.412 ☑
      first degree T25.512 ☑
      second degree T25.612 ☑
      third degree T25.712 ☑
    multiple with foot — *see* Corrosion, lower, limb,
        multiple, ankle and foot
    right T25.411 ☑
      first degree T25.511 ☑
      second degree T25.611 ☑
      third degree T25.711 ☑
    second degree T25.619 ☑
    third degree T25.719 ☑
  anus — *see* Corrosion, buttock
  arm(s) (meaning upper limb(s)) — *see* Corrosion, upper
      limb
  axilla T22.449 ☑
    first degree T22.549 ☑
    left T22.442 ☑
      first degree T22.542 ☑
      second degree T22.642 ☑
      third degree T22.742 ☑
    right T22.441 ☑
      first degree T22.541 ☑
      second degree T22.641 ☑
      third degree T22.741 ☑
    second degree T22.649 ☑
    third degree T22.749 ☑
  back (lower) T21.44 ☑
    first degree T21.54 ☑
    second degree T21.64 ☑
    third degree T21.74 ☑
    upper T21.43 ☑
      first degree T21.53 ☑
      second degree T21.63 ☑
      third degree T21.73 ☑
  blisters — *code as* Corrosion, second degree, by site
  breast(s) — *see* Corrosion, chest wall
  buttock(s) T21.45 ☑
    first degree T21.55 ☑
    second degree T21.65 ☑

Corrosion — *continued*
  buttock(s) — *continued*
    third degree T21.75 ☑
  calf T24.439 ☑
    first degree T24.539 ☑
    left T24.432 ☑
      first degree T24.532 ☑
      second degree T24.632 ☑
      third degree T24.732 ☑
    right T24.431 ☑
      first degree T24.531 ☑
      second degree T24.631 ☑
      third degree T24.731 ☑
    second degree T24.639 ☑
    third degree T24.739 ☑
  canthus (eye) — *see* Corrosion, eyelid
  cervix T28.8 ☑
  cheek T20.46 ☑
    first degree T20.56 ☑
    second degree T20.66 ☑
    third degree T20.76 ☑
  chest wall T21.41 ☑
    first degree T21.51 ☑
    second degree T21.61 ☑
    third degree T21.71 ☑
  chin T20.43 ☑
    first degree T20.53 ☑
    second degree T20.63 ☑
    third degree T20.73 ☑
  colon T28.7 ☑
  conjunctiva (and cornea) — *see* Corrosion, cornea
  cornea (and conjunctiva) T26.6- ☑
  deep necrosis of underlying tissue — *code as* Corro-
      sion, third degree, by site
  dorsum of hand T23.469 ☑
    first degree T23.569 ☑
    left T23.462 ☑
      first degree T23.562 ☑
      second degree T23.662 ☑
      third degree T23.762 ☑
    right T23.461 ☑
      first degree T23.561 ☑
      second degree T23.661 ☑
      third degree T23.761 ☑
    second degree T23.669 ☑
    third degree T23.769 ☑
  ear (auricle) (external) (canal) T20.41 ☑
    drum T28.91 ☑
    first degree T20.51 ☑
    second degree T20.61 ☑
    third degree T20.71 ☑
  elbow T22.429 ☑
    first degree T22.529 ☑
    left T22.422 ☑
      first degree T22.522 ☑
      second degree T22.622 ☑
      third degree T22.722 ☑
    right T22.421 ☑
      first degree T22.521 ☑
      second degree T22.621 ☑
      third degree T22.721 ☑
    second degree T22.629 ☑
    third degree T22.729 ☑
  entire body — *see* Corrosion, multiple body regions
  epidermal loss — *code as* Corrosion, second degree,
      by site
  epiglottis T27.4 ☑
  erythema, erythematous — *code as* Corrosion, first
      degree, by site
  esophagus T28.6 ☑
  extent (percentage of body surface)
    less than 10 percent T32.0
    10-19 percent (0-9 percent third degree) T32.10
      with 10-19 percent third degree T32.11
    20-29 percent (0-9 percent third degree) T32.20
      with
        10-19 percent third degree T32.21
        20-29 percent third degree T32.22
    30-39 percent (0-9 percent third degree) T32.30
      with
        10-19 percent third degree T32.31
        20-29 percent third degree T32.32
        30-39 percent third degree T32.33
    40-49 percent (0-9 percent third degree) T32.40
      with
        10-19 percent third degree T32.41

Corrosion — continued
extent — continued
  40-49 percent — continued
    with — continued
      20-29 percent third degree T32.42
      30-39 percent third degree T32.43
      40-49 percent third degree T32.44
    50-59 percent (0-9 percent third degree) T32.50
      with
        10-19 percent third degree T32.51
        20-29 percent third degree T32.52
        30-39 percent third degree T32.53
        40-49 percent third degree T32.54
        50-59 percent third degree T32.55
    60-69 percent (0-9 percent third degree) T32.60
      with
        10-19 percent third degree T32.61
        20-29 percent third degree T32.62
        30-39 percent third degree T32.63
        40-49 percent third degree T32.64
        50-59 percent third degree T32.65
        60-69 percent third degree T32.66
    70-79 percent (0-9 percent third degree) T32.70
      with
        10-19 percent third degree T32.71
        20-29 percent third degree T32.72
        30-39 percent third degree T32.73
        40-49 percent third degree T32.74
        50-59 percent third degree T32.75
        60-69 percent third degree T32.76
        70-79 percent third degree T32.77
    80-89 percent (0-9 percent third degree) T32.80
      with
        10-19 percent third degree T32.81
        20-29 percent third degree T32.82
        30-39 percent third degree T32.83
        40-49 percent third degree T32.84
        50-59 percent third degree T32.85
        60-69 percent third degree T32.86
        70-79 percent third degree T32.87
        80-89 percent third degree T32.88
    90 percent or more (0-9 percent third degree) T32.90
      with
        10-19 percent third degree T32.91
        20-29 percent third degree T32.92
        30-39 percent third degree T32.93
        40-49 percent third degree T32.94
        50-59 percent third degree T32.95
        60-69 percent third degree T32.96
        70-79 percent third degree T32.97
        80-89 percent third degree T32.98
        90-99 percent third degree T32.99
  extremity — see Corrosion, limb
  eye(s) and adnexa T26.9- ☑
    with resulting rupture and destruction of eyeball T26.7- ☑
    conjunctival sac — see Corrosion, cornea
    cornea — see Corrosion, cornea
    lid — see Corrosion, eyelid
    periocular area — see Corrosion eyelid
    specified site NEC T26.8- ☑
  eyeball — see Corrosion, eye
  eyelid(s) T26.5- ☑
  face — see Corrosion, head
  finger T23.429 ☑
    first degree T23.529 ☑
    left T23.422 ☑
      first degree T23.522 ☑
      second degree T23.622 ☑
      third degree T23.722 ☑
    multiple sites (without thumb) T23.439 ☑
      with thumb T23.449 ☑
        first degree T23.549 ☑
        left T23.442 ☑
          first degree T23.542 ☑
          second degree T23.642 ☑
          third degree T23.742 ☑
        right T23.441 ☑
          first degree T23.541 ☑
          second degree T23.641 ☑
          third degree T23.741 ☑
        second degree T23.649 ☑
        third degree T23.749 ☑
      first degree T23.539 ☑
      left T23.432 ☑
        first degree T23.532 ☑

Corrosion — continued
finger — continued
  multiple sites — continued
    left — continued
      second degree T23.632 ☑
      third degree T23.732 ☑
    right T23.431 ☑
      first degree T23.531 ☑
      second degree T23.631 ☑
      third degree T23.731 ☑
    second degree T23.639 ☑
    third degree T23.739 ☑
  right T23.421 ☑
    first degree T23.521 ☑
    second degree T23.621 ☑
    third degree T23.721 ☑
  second degree T23.629 ☑
  third degree T23.729 ☑
flank — see Corrosion, abdomen
foot T25.429 ☑
  first degree T25.529 ☑
  left T25.422 ☑
    first degree T25.522 ☑
    second degree T25.622 ☑
    third degree T25.722 ☑
  multiple with ankle — see Corrosion, lower, limb, multiple, ankle and foot
  right T25.421 ☑
    first degree T25.521 ☑
    second degree T25.621 ☑
    third degree T25.721 ☑
  second degree T25.629 ☑
  third degree T25.729 ☑
forearm T22.419 ☑
  first degree T22.519 ☑
  left T22.412 ☑
    first degree T22.512 ☑
    second degree T22.612 ☑
    third degree T22.712 ☑
  right T22.411 ☑
    first degree T22.511 ☑
    second degree T22.611 ☑
    third degree T22.711 ☑
  second degree T22.619 ☑
  third degree T22.719 ☑
forehead T20.46 ☑
  first degree T20.56 ☑
  second degree T20.66 ☑
  third degree T20.76 ☑
fourth degree — code as Corrosion, third degree, by site
full thickness skin loss — code as Corrosion, third degree, by site
gastrointestinal tract NEC T28.7 ☑
genital organs
  external
    female T21.47 ☑
      first degree T21.57 ☑
      second degree T21.67 ☑
      third degree T21.77 ☑
    male T21.46 ☑
      first degree T21.56 ☑
      second degree T21.66 ☑
      third degree T21.76 ☑
  internal T28.8 ☑
groin — see Corrosion, abdominal wall
hand(s) T23.409 ☑
  back — see Corrosion, dorsum of hand
  finger — see Corrosion, finger
  first degree T23.509 ☑
  left T23.402 ☑
    first degree T23.502 ☑
    second degree T23.602 ☑
    third degree T23.702 ☑
  multiple sites with wrist T23.499 ☑
    first degree T23.599 ☑
    left T23.492 ☑
      first degree T23.592 ☑
      second degree T23.692 ☑
      third degree T23.792 ☑
    right T23.491 ☑
      first degree T23.591 ☑
      second degree T23.691 ☑
      third degree T23.791 ☑
    second degree T23.699 ☑
    third degree T23.799 ☑

Corrosion — continued
hand(s) — continued
  palm — see Corrosion, palm
  right T23.401 ☑
    first degree T23.501 ☑
    second degree T23.601 ☑
    third degree T23.701 ☑
  second degree T23.609 ☑
  third degree T23.709 ☑
  thumb — see Corrosion, thumb
head (and face) (and neck) T20.40 ☑
  cheek — see Corrosion, cheek
  chin — see Corrosion, chin
  ear — see Corrosion, ear
  eye(s) only — see Corrosion, eye
  first degree T20.50 ☑
  forehead — see Corrosion, forehead
  lip — see Corrosion, lip
  multiple sites T20.49 ☑
    first degree T20.59 ☑
    second degree T20.69 ☑
    third degree T20.79 ☑
  neck — see Corrosion, neck
  nose — see Corrosion, nose
  scalp — see Corrosion, scalp
  second degree T20.60 ☑
  third degree T20.70 ☑
hip(s) — see Corrosion, lower, limb
inhalation — see Corrosion, respiratory tract
internal organ(s) (see also Corrosion, by site) T28.90 ☑
  alimentary tract T28.7 ☑
    esophagus T28.6 ☑
  esophagus T28.6 ☑
  genitourinary T28.8 ☑
  mouth T28.5 ☑
  pharynx T28.5 ☑
  specified organ NEC T28.99 ☑
interscapular region — see Corrosion, back, upper
intestine (large) (small) T28.7 ☑
knee T24.429 ☑
  first degree T24.529 ☑
  left T24.422 ☑
    first degree T24.522 ☑
    second degree T24.622 ☑
    third degree T24.722 ☑
  right T24.421 ☑
    first degree T24.521 ☑
    second degree T24.621 ☑
    third degree T24.721 ☑
  second degree T24.629 ☑
  third degree T24.729 ☑
labium (majus) (minus) — see Corrosion, genital organs, external, female
lacrimal apparatus, duct, gland or sac — see Corrosion, eye, specified site NEC
larynx T27.4 ☑
  with lung T27.5 ☑
leg(s) (meaning lower limb(s)) — see Corrosion, lower limb
limb(s)
  lower — see Corrosion, lower, limb
  upper — see Corrosion, upper limb
lip T20.42 ☑
  first degree T20.52 ☑
  second degree T20.62 ☑
  third degree T20.72 ☑
lower
  back — see Corrosion, back
  limb T24.409 ☑
    ankle — see Corrosion, ankle
    calf — see Corrosion, calf
    first degree T24.509 ☑
    foot — see Corrosion, foot
    knee — see Corrosion, knee
    left T24.402 ☑
      first degree T24.502 ☑
      second degree T24.602 ☑
      third degree T24.702 ☑
    multiple sites, except ankle and foot T24.499 ☑
      ankle and foot T25.499 ☑
        first degree T25.599 ☑
        left T25.492 ☑
          first degree T25.592 ☑
          second degree T25.692 ☑
          third degree T25.792 ☑
        right T25.491 ☑

☑ Additional Character Required — Refer to the Tabular List for Character Selection   ▽ Subterms under main terms may continue to next column or page

Corrosion — *continued*
  lower — *continued*
    limb — *continued*
      multiple sites, except ankle and foot — *continued*
        ankle and foot — *continued*
          right — *continued*
            first degree T25.591 ☑
              second degree T25.691 ☑
                third degree T25.791 ☑
              second degree T25.699 ☑
                third degree T25.799 ☑
          first degree T24.599 ☑
            left T24.492 ☑
              first degree T24.592 ☑
              second degree T24.692 ☑
              third degree T24.792 ☑
            right T24.491 ☑
              first degree T24.591 ☑
              second degree T24.691 ☑
              third degree T24.791 ☑
            second degree T24.699 ☑
              third degree T24.799 ☑
          right T24.401 ☑
            first degree T24.501 ☑
            second degree T24.601 ☑
            third degree T24.701 ☑
          second degree T24.609 ☑
          thigh — *see* Corrosion, thigh
          third degree T24.709 ☑
  lung (with larynx and trachea) T27.5 ☑
  mouth T28.5 ☑
  neck T20.47 ☑
    first degree T20.57 ☑
    second degree T20.67 ☑
    third degree T20.77 ☑
  nose (septum) T20.44 ☑
    first degree T20.54 ☑
    second degree T20.64 ☑
    third degree T20.74 ☑
  ocular adnexa — *see* Corrosion, eye
  orbit region — *see* Corrosion, eyelid
  palm T23.459 ☑
    first degree T23.559 ☑
    left T23.452 ☑
      first degree T23.552 ☑
      second degree T23.652 ☑
      third degree T23.752 ☑
    right T23.451 ☑
      first degree T23.551 ☑
      second degree T23.651 ☑
      third degree T23.751 ☑
    second degree T23.659 ☑
    third degree T23.759 ☑
  partial thickness — *code as* Corrosion, unspecified
      degree, by site
  pelvis — *see* Corrosion, trunk
  penis — *see* Corrosion, genital organs, external, male
  perineum
    female — *see* Corrosion, genital organs, external,
        female
    male — *see* Corrosion, genital organs, external,
        male
  periocular area — *see* Corrosion, eyelid
  pharynx T28.5 ☑
  rectum T28.7 ☑
  respiratory tract T27.7 ☑
    larynx — *see* Corrosion, larynx
    specified part NEC T27.6 ☑
    trachea — *see* Corrosion, larynx
  sac, lacrimal — *see* Corrosion, eye, specified site NEC
  scalp T20.45 ☑
    first degree T20.55 ☑
    second degree T20.65 ☑
    third degree T20.75 ☑
  scapular region T22.469 ☑
    first degree T22.569 ☑
    left T22.462 ☑
      first degree T22.562 ☑
      second degree T22.662 ☑
      third degree T22.762 ☑
    right T22.461 ☑
      first degree T22.561 ☑
      second degree T22.661 ☑
      third degree T22.761 ☑
    second degree T22.669 ☑

Corrosion — *continued*
  scapular region — *continued*
    third degree T22.769 ☑
  sclera — *see* Corrosion, eye, specified site NEC
  scrotum — *see* Corrosion, genital organs, external,
      male
  shoulder T22.459 ☑
    first degree T22.559 ☑
    left T22.452 ☑
      first degree T22.552 ☑
      second degree T22.652 ☑
      third degree T22.752 ☑
    right T22.451 ☑
      first degree T22.551 ☑
      second degree T22.651 ☑
      third degree T22.751 ☑
    second degree T22.659 ☑
    third degree T22.759 ☑
  stomach T28.7 ☑
  temple — *see* Corrosion, head
  testis — *see* Corrosion, genital organs, external, male
  thigh T24.419 ☑
    first degree T24.519 ☑
    left T24.412 ☑
      first degree T24.512 ☑
      second degree T24.612 ☑
      third degree T24.712 ☑
    right T24.411 ☑
      first degree T24.511 ☑
      second degree T24.611 ☑
      third degree T24.711 ☑
    second degree T24.619 ☑
    third degree T24.719 ☑
  thorax (external) — *see* Corrosion, trunk
  throat (meaning pharynx) T28.5 ☑
  thumb(s) T23.419 ☑
    first degree T23.519 ☑
    left T23.412 ☑
      first degree T23.512 ☑
      second degree T23.612 ☑
      third degree T23.712 ☑
    multiple sites with fingers T23.449 ☑
      first degree T23.549 ☑
      left T23.442 ☑
        first degree T23.542 ☑
        second degree T23.642 ☑
        third degree T23.742 ☑
      right T23.441 ☑
        first degree T23.541 ☑
        second degree T23.641 ☑
        third degree T23.741 ☑
      second degree T23.649 ☑
      third degree T23.749 ☑
    right T23.411 ☑
      first degree T23.511 ☑
      second degree T23.611 ☑
      third degree T23.711 ☑
    second degree T23.619 ☑
    third degree T23.719 ☑
  toe T25.439 ☑
    first degree T25.539 ☑
    left T25.432 ☑
      first degree T25.532 ☑
      second degree T25.632 ☑
      third degree T25.732 ☑
    right T25.431 ☑
      first degree T25.531 ☑
      second degree T25.631 ☑
      third degree T25.731 ☑
    second degree T25.639 ☑
    third degree T25.739 ☑
  tongue T28.5 ☑
  tonsil(s) T28.5 ☑
  total body — *see* Corrosion, multiple body regions
  trachea T27.4 ☑
    with lung T27.5 ☑
  trunk T21.40 ☑
    abdominal wall — *see* Corrosion, abdominal wall
    anus — *see* Corrosion, buttock
    axilla — *see* Corrosion, upper limb
    back — *see* Corrosion, back
    breast — *see* Corrosion, chest wall
    buttock — *see* Corrosion, buttock
    chest wall — *see* Corrosion, chest wall
    first degree T21.50 ☑
    flank — *see* Corrosion, abdominal wall

Corrosion — *continued*
  trunk — *continued*
    genital
      female — *see* Corrosion, genital organs, exter-
          nal, female
      male — *see* Corrosion, genital organs, external,
          male
    groin — *see* Corrosion, abdominal wall
    interscapular region — *see* Corrosion, back, upper
    labia — *see* Corrosion, genital organs, external,
        female
    lower back — *see* Corrosion, back
    penis — *see* Corrosion, genital organs, external,
        male
    perineum
      female — *see* Corrosion, genital organs, exter-
          nal, female
      male — *see* Corrosion, genital organs, external,
          male
    scapular region — *see* Corrosion, upper limb
    scrotum — *see* Corrosion, genital organs, external,
        male
    second degree T21.60 ☑
    shoulder — *see* Corrosion, upper limb
    specified site NEC T21.49 ☑
      first degree T21.59 ☑
      second degree T21.69 ☑
      third degree T21.79 ☑
    testes — *see* Corrosion, genital organs, external,
        male
    third degree T21.70 ☑
    upper back — *see* Corrosion, back, upper
    vagina T28.8 ☑
    vulva — *see* Corrosion, genital organs, external,
        female
  unspecified site with extent of body surface involved
      specified
    less than 10 percent T32.0
    10-19 percent (0-9 percent third degree) T32.10
      with 10-19 percent third degree T32.11
    20-29 percent (0-9 percent third degree) T32.20
      with
        10-19 percent third degree T32.21
        20-29 percent third degree T32.22
    30-39 percent (0-9 percent third degree) T32.30
      with
        10-19 percent third degree T32.31
        20-29 percent third degree T32.32
        30-39 percent third degree T32.33
    40-49 percent (0-9 percent third degree) T32.40
      with
        10-19 percent third degree T32.41
        20-29 percent third degree T32.42
        30-39 percent third degree T32.43
        40-49 percent third degree T32.44
    50-59 percent (0-9 percent third degree) T32.50
      with
        10-19 percent third degree T32.51
        20-29 percent third degree T32.52
        30-39 percent third degree T32.53
        40-49 percent third degree T32.54
        50-59 percent third degree T32.55
    60-69 percent (0-9 percent third degree) T32.60
      with
        10-19 percent third degree T32.61
        20-29 percent third degree T32.62
        30-39 percent third degree T32.63
        40-49 percent third degree T32.64
        50-59 percent third degree T32.65
        60-69 percent third degree T32.66
    70-79 percent (0-9 percent third degree) T32.70
      with
        10-19 percent third degree T32.71
        20-29 percent third degree T32.72
        30-39 percent third degree T32.73
        40-49 percent third degree T32.74
        50-59 percent third degree T32.75
        60-69 percent third degree T32.76
        70-79 percent third degree T32.77
    80-89 percent (0-9 percent third degree) T32.80
      with
        10-19 percent third degree T32.81
        20-29 percent third degree T32.82
        30-39 percent third degree T32.83
        40-49 percent third degree T32.84
        50-59 percent third degree T32.85
        60-69 percent third degree T32.86
        70-79 percent third degree T32.87

Corrosion — *continued*
  unspecified site with extent of body surface involved specified — *continued*
    80-89 percent — *continued*
      with — *continued*
        80-89 percent third degree T32.88
    90 percent or more (0-9 percent third degree) T32.90
      with
        10-19 percent third degree T32.91
        20-29 percent third degree T32.92
        30-39 percent third degree T32.93
        40-49 percent third degree T32.94
        50-59 percent third degree T32.95
        60-69 percent third degree T32.96
        70-79 percent third degree T32.97
        80-89 percent third degree T32.98
        90-99 percent third degree T32.99
  upper limb (axilla) (scapular region) T22.40 ☑
    above elbow — *see* Corrosion, above elbow
    axilla — *see* Corrosion, axilla
    elbow — *see* Corrosion, elbow
    first degree T22.50 ☑
    forearm — *see* Corrosion, forearm
    hand — *see* Corrosion, hand
    interscapular region — *see* Corrosion, back, upper
    multiple sites T22.499 ☑
      first degree T22.599 ☑
      left T22.492 ☑
        first degree T22.592 ☑
        second degree T22.692 ☑
        third degree T22.792 ☑
      right T22.491 ☑
        first degree T22.591 ☑
        second degree T22.691 ☑
        third degree T22.791 ☑
      second degree T22.699 ☑
      third degree T22.799 ☑
    scapular region — *see* Corrosion, scapular region
    second degree T22.60 ☑
    shoulder — *see* Corrosion, shoulder
    third degree T22.70 ☑
    wrist — *see* Corrosion, hand
  uterus T28.8 ☑
  vagina T28.8 ☑
  vulva — *see* Corrosion, genital organs, external, female
  wrist T23.479 ☑
    first degree T23.579 ☑
    left T23.472 ☑
      first degree T23.572 ☑
      second degree T23.672 ☑
      third degree T23.772 ☑
    multiple sites with hand T23.499 ☑
      first degree T23.599 ☑
      left T23.492 ☑
        first degree T23.592 ☑
        second degree T23.692 ☑
        third degree T23.792 ☑
      right T23.491 ☑
        first degree T23.591 ☑
        second degree T23.691 ☑
        third degree T23.791 ☑
      second degree T23.699 ☑
      third degree T23.799 ☑
    right T23.471 ☑
      first degree T23.571 ☑
      second degree T23.671 ☑
      third degree T23.771 ☑
    second degree T23.679 ☑
    third degree T23.779 ☑
Corrosive burn — *see* Corrosion
Corsican fever — *see* Malaria
Cortical — *see* condition
Cortico-adrenal — *see* condition
Coryza (acute) J00
  with grippe or influenza — *see* Influenza, with, respiratory manifestations NEC
  syphilitic
    congenital (chronic) A50.05
Costen's syndrome or complex M26.69
Costiveness — *see* Constipation
Costochondritis M94.0
Cot death R99
Cotard's syndrome F22
Cotia virus B08.8
Cotton wool spots (retinal) H35.81

Cotungo's disease — *see* Sciatica
Cough (affected) (chronic) (epidemic) (nervous) R05
  with hemorrhage — *see* Hemoptysis
  bronchial R05
    with grippe or influenza — *see* Influenza, with, respiratory manifestations NEC
  functional F45.8
  hysterical F45.8
  laryngeal, spasmodic R05
  psychogenic F45.8
  smokers' J41.0
  tea taster's B49
Counseling (for) Z71.9
  abuse NEC
    perpetrator Z69.82
    victim Z69.81
  alcohol abuser Z71.41
    family Z71.42
  child abuse
    nonparental
      perpetrator Z69.021
      victim Z69.020
    parental
      perpetrator Z69.011
      victim Z69.010
  consanguinity Z71.89
  contraceptive Z30.09
  dietary Z71.3
  drug abuser Z71.51
    family member Z71.52
  exercise Z71.82
  family Z71.89
  fertility preservation (prior to cancer therapy) (prior to removal of gonads) Z31.62
  for non-attending third party Z71.0
    related to sexual behavior or orientation Z70.2
  genetic
    nonprocreative Z71.83
    procreative NEC Z31.5
  gestational carrier Z31.7
  health (advice) (education) (instruction) — *see* Counseling, medical
  human immunodeficiency virus (HIV) Z71.7
  impotence Z70.1
  insulin pump use Z46.81
  medical (for) Z71.9
    boarding school resident Z59.3
    consanguinity Z71.89
    feared complaint and no disease found Z71.1
    human immunodeficiency virus (HIV) Z71.7
    institutional resident Z59.3
    on behalf of another Z71.0
      related to sexual behavior or orientation Z70.2
    person living alone Z60.2
    specified reason NEC Z71.89
  natural family planning
    procreative Z31.61
    to avoid pregnancy Z30.02
  perpetrator (of)
    abuse NEC Z69.82
    child abuse
      non-parental Z69.021
      parental Z69.011
    rape NEC Z69.82
    spousal abuse Z69.12
  procreative NEC Z31.69
    fertility preservation (prior to cancer therapy) (prior to removal of gonads) Z31.62
    using natural family planning Z31.61
  promiscuity Z70.1
  rape victim Z69.81
  religious Z71.81
  sex, sexual (related to) Z70.9
    attitude(s) Z70.0
    behavior or orientation Z70.1
    combined concerns Z70.3
    non-responsiveness Z70.1
    on behalf of third party Z70.2
    specified reason NEC Z70.8
  specified reason NEC Z71.89
  spiritual Z71.81
  spousal abuse (perpetrator) Z69.12
    victim Z69.11
  substance abuse Z71.89
    alcohol Z71.41
    drug Z71.51
    tobacco Z71.6
  tobacco use Z71.6

Counseling — *continued*
  use (of)
    insulin pump Z46.81
  victim (of)
    abuse Z69.81
    child abuse
      by parent Z69.010
      non-parental Z69.020
    rape NEC Z69.81
Coupled rhythm R00.8
Couvelaire syndrome or uterus (complicating delivery) O45.8X- ☑
Cowperitis — *see* Urethritis
Cowper's gland — *see* condition
Cowpox B08.010
  due to vaccination T88.1 ☑
Coxa
  magna M91.4- ☑
  plana M91.2- ☑
  valga (acquired) (*see also* Deformity, limb, specified type NEC, thigh)
    congenital Q65.81
    sequelae (late effect) of rickets E64.3
  vara (acquired) (*see also* Deformity, limb, specified type NEC, thigh)
    congenital Q65.82
    sequelae (late effect) of rickets E64.3
Coxalgia, coxalgic (nontuberculous) (*see also* Pain, joint, hip)
  tuberculous A18.02
Coxitis — *see* Monoarthritis, hip
Coxsackie (virus) (infection) B34.1
  as cause of disease classified elsewhere B97.11
  carditis B33.20
  central nervous system NEC A88.8
  endocarditis B33.21
  enteritis A08.39
  meningitis (aseptic) A87.0
  myocarditis B33.22
  pericarditis B33.23
  pharyngitis B08.5
  pleurodynia B33.0
  specific disease NEC B33.8
Crabs, meaning pubic lice B85.3
Crack baby P04.41
Cracked nipple N64.0
  associated with
    lactation O92.13
    pregnancy O92.11- ☑
    puerperium O92.12
Cracked tooth K03.81
Cradle cap L21.0
Craft neurosis F48.8
Cramp(s) R25.2
  abdominal — *see* Pain, abdominal
  bathing T75.1 ☑
  colic R10.83
    psychogenic F45.8
  due to immersion T75.1 ☑
  fireman T67.2 ☑
  heat T67.2 ☑
  immersion T75.1 ☑
  intestinal — *see* Pain, abdominal
    psychogenic F45.8
  leg, sleep related G47.62
  limb (lower) (upper) NEC R25.2
    sleep related G47.62
  linotypist's F48.8
    organic G25.89
  muscle (limb) (general) R25.2
    due to immersion T75.1 ☑
    psychogenic F45.8
  occupational (hand) F48.8
    organic G25.89
  salt-depletion E87.1
  sleep related, leg G47.62
  stoker's T67.2 ☑
  swimmer's T75.1 ☑
  telegrapher's F48.8
    organic G25.89
  typist's F48.8
    organic G25.89
  uterus N94.89
    menstrual — *see* Dysmenorrhea
  writer's F48.8
    organic G25.89
Cranial — *see* condition

☑ Additional Character Required — Refer to the Tabular List for Character Selection   ▽ Subterms under main terms may continue to next column or page

Craniocleidodysostosis Q74.0
Craniofenestria (skull) Q75.8
Craniolacunia (skull) Q75.8
Craniopagus Q89.4
Craniopathy, metabolic M85.2
Craniopharyngeal — see condition
Craniopharyngioma D44.4
Craniorachischisis (totalis) Q00.1
Cranioschisis Q75.8
Craniostenosis Q75.0
Craniosynostosis Q75.0
Craniotabes (cause unknown) M83.8
　neonatal P96.3
　rachitic E64.3
　syphilitic A50.56
Cranium — see condition
Craw-craw — see Onchocerciasis
Creaking joint — see Derangement, joint, specified type
　　NEC
Creeping
　eruption B76.9
　palsy or paralysis G12.22
Crenated tongue K14.8
Creotoxism A05.9
Crepitus
　caput Q75.8
　joint — see Derangement, joint, specified type NEC
Crescent or conus choroid, congenital Q14.3
CREST syndrome M34.1
Cretin, cretinism (congenital) (endemic) (nongoitrous)
　　(sporadic) E00.9
　pelvis
　　with disproportion (fetopelvic) O33.0
　　　causing obstructed labor O65.0
　type
　　hypothyroid E00.1
　　mixed E00.2
　　myxedematous E00.1
　　neurological E00.0
Creutzfeldt-Jakob disease or syndrome (with demen-
　　tia) A81.00
　familial A81.09
　iatrogenic A81.09
　specified NEC A81.09
　sporadic A81.09
　variant (vCJD) A81.01
Crib death R99
Cribriform hymen Q52.3
Cri-du-chat syndrome Q93.4
Crigler-Najjar disease or syndrome E80.5
Crime, victim of Z65.4
Crimean hemorrhagic fever A98.0
Criminalism F60.2
Crisis
　abdomen R10.0
　acute reaction F43.0
　addisonian E27.2
　adrenal (cortical) E27.2
　celiac K90.0
　Dietl's N13.8
　emotional (see also Disorder, adjustment)
　　acute reaction to stress F43.0
　　specific to childhood and adolescence F93.8
　glaucomatocyclitic — see Glaucoma, secondary, in-
　　flammation
　heart — see Failure, heart
　nitritoid I95.2
　　correct substance properly administered — see
　　　Table of Drugs and Chemicals, by drug, ad-
　　　verse effect
　　overdose or wrong substance given or taken —
　　　see Table of Drugs and Chemicals, by drug,
　　　poisoning
　oculogyric H51.8
　　psychogenic F45.8
　Pel's (tabetic) A52.11
　psychosexual identity F64.2
　renal N28.0
　sickle-cell D57.00
　　with
　　　acute chest syndrome D57.01
　　　splenic sequestration D57.02
　state (acute reaction) F43.0
　tabetic A52.11
　thyroid — see Thyrotoxicosis with thyroid storm
　thyrotoxic — see Thyrotoxicosis with thyroid storm
Crocq's disease (acrocyanosis) I73.89

Crohn's disease — see Enteritis, regional
Crooked septum, nasal J34.2
Cross syndrome E70.328
Crossbite (anterior) (posterior) M26.24
Cross-eye — see Strabismus, convergent concomitant
Croup, croupous (catarrhal) (infectious) (inflammatory)
　　(nondiphtheritic) J05.0
　bronchial J20.9
　diphtheritic A36.2
　false J38.5
　spasmodic J38.5
　　diphtheritic A36.2
　stridulous J38.5
　　diphtheritic A36.2
Crouzon's disease Q75.1
Crowding, tooth, teeth, fully erupted M26.31
CRST syndrome M34.1
Cruchet's disease A85.8
Cruelty in children (see also Disorder, conduct)
Crural ulcer — see Ulcer, lower limb
Crush, crushed, crushing T14.8 ☑
　abdomen S38.1 ☑
　ankle S97.0- ☑
　arm (upper) (and shoulder) S47.- ☑
　axilla — see Crush, arm
　back, lower S38.1 ☑
　buttock S38.1 ☑
　cheek S07.0 ☑
　chest S28.0 ☑
　cranium S07.1 ☑
　ear S07.0 ☑
　elbow S57.0- ☑
　extremity
　　lower
　　　ankle — see Crush, ankle
　　　below knee — see Crush, leg
　　　foot — see Crush, foot
　　　hip — see Crush, hip
　　　knee — see Crush, knee
　　　thigh — see Crush, thigh
　　　toe — see Crush, toe
　　upper
　　　below elbow S67.9- ☑
　　　elbow — see Crush, elbow
　　　finger — see Crush, finger
　　　forearm — see Crush, forearm
　　　hand — see Crush, hand
　　　thumb — see Crush, thumb
　　　upper arm — see Crush, arm
　　　wrist — see Crush, wrist
　face S07.0 ☑
　finger(s) S67.1- ☑
　　with hand (and wrist) — see Crush, hand, specified
　　　site NEC
　　index S67.19- ☑
　　little S67.19- ☑
　　middle S67.19- ☑
　　ring S67.19- ☑
　　thumb — see Crush, thumb
　foot S97.8- ☑
　　toe — see Crush, toe
　forearm S57.8- ☑
　genitalia, external
　　female S38.002 ☑
　　　vagina S38.03 ☑
　　　vulva S38.03 ☑
　　male S38.001 ☑
　　　penis S38.01 ☑
　　　scrotum S38.02 ☑
　　　testis S38.02 ☑
　hand (except fingers alone) S67.2- ☑
　　with wrist S67.4- ☑
　head S07.9 ☑
　　specified NEC S07.8 ☑
　heel — see Crush, foot
　hip S77.0- ☑
　　with thigh S77.2- ☑
　internal organ (abdomen, chest, or pelvis) NEC
　　T14.8 ☑
　knee S87.0- ☑
　labium (majus) (minus) S38.03 ☑
　larynx S17.0 ☑
　leg (lower) S87.8- ☑
　　knee — see Crush, knee
　lip S07.0 ☑

Crush, crushed, crushing — continued
　lower
　　back S38.1 ☑
　　leg — see Crush, leg
　neck S17.9 ☑
　nerve — see Injury, nerve
　nose S07.0 ☑
　pelvis S38.1 ☑
　penis S38.01 ☑
　scalp S07.8 ☑
　scapular region — see Crush, arm
　scrotum S38.02 ☑
　severe, unspecified site T14.8 ☑
　shoulder (and upper arm) — see Crush, arm
　skull S07.1 ☑
　syndrome (complication of trauma) T79.5 ☑
　testis S38.02 ☑
　thigh S77.1- ☑
　　with hip S77.2- ☑
　throat S17.8 ☑
　thumb S67.0- ☑
　　with hand (and wrist) — see Crush, hand, specified
　　　site NEC
　toe(s) S97.10- ☑
　　great S97.11- ☑
　　lesser S97.12- ☑
　trachea S17.0 ☑
　vagina S38.03 ☑
　vulva S38.03 ☑
　wrist S67.3- ☑
　　with hand S67.4- ☑
Crusta lactea L21.0
Crusts R23.4
Crutch paralysis — see Injury, brachial plexus
Cruveilhier-Baumgarten cirrhosis, disease or syn-
　　drome K74.69
Cruveilhier's atrophy or disease G12.8
Crying (constant) (continuous) (excessive)
　child, adolescent, or adult R45.83
　infant (baby) (newborn) R68.11
Cryofibrinogenemia D89.2
Cryoglobulinemia (essential) (idiopathic) (mixed) (pri-
　　mary) (purpura) (secondary) (vasculitis) D89.1
　with lung involvement D89.1 [J99]
Cryptitis (anal) (rectal) K62.89
Cryptococcosis, cryptococcus (infection) (neoformans)
　　B45.9
　bone B45.3
　cerebral B45.1
　cutaneous B45.2
　disseminated B45.7
　generalized B45.7
　meningitis B45.1
　meningocerebralis B45.1
　osseous B45.3
　pulmonary B45.0
　skin B45.2
　specified NEC B45.8
Cryptopapillitis (anus) K62.89
Cryptophthalmos Q11.2
　syndrome Q87.0
Cryptorchid, cryptorchism, cryptorchidism Q53.9
　bilateral Q53.20
　　abdominal Q53.211
　　perineal Q53.22
　unilateral Q53.10
　　abdominal Q53.111
　　perineal Q53.12
Cryptosporidiosis A07.2
　hepatobiliary B88.8
　respiratory B88.8
Cryptostromosis J67.6
Crystalluria R82.99
Cubitus
　congenital Q68.8
　valgus (acquired) M21.0- ☑
　　congenital Q68.8
　　sequelae (late effect) of rickets E64.3
　varus (acquired) M21.1- ☑
　　congenital Q68.8
　　sequelae (late effect) of rickets E64.3
Cultural deprivation or shock Z60.3
Curling esophagus K22.4
Curling's ulcer — see Ulcer, peptic, acute
Curschmann (-Batten) (-Steinert) **disease or syndrome**
　　G71.11
Curse, Ondine's — see Apnea, sleep

Curvature

Curvature
- organ or site, congenital NEC — *see* Distortion
- penis (lateral) Q55.61
- Pott's (spinal) A18.01
- radius, idiopathic, progressive (congenital) Q74.0
- spine (acquired) (angular) (idiopathic) (incorrect) (postural) — *see* Dorsopathy, deforming
  - congenital Q67.5
  - due to or associated with
    - Charcot-Marie-Tooth disease (*see also* subcategory M49.8) G60.0
    - osteitis
      - deformans M88.88
      - fibrosa cystica (*see also* subcategory M49.8) E21.0
    - tuberculosis (Pott's curvature) A18.01
  - sequelae (late effect) of rickets E64.3
  - tuberculous A18.01

Cushingoid due to steroid therapy E24.2
- correct substance properly administered — *see* Table of Drugs and Chemicals, by drug, adverse effect
- overdose or wrong substance given or taken — *see* Table of Drugs and Chemicals, by drug, poisoning

Cushing's
- syndrome or disease E24.9
  - drug-induced E24.2
  - iatrogenic E24.2
  - pituitary-dependent E24.0
  - specified NEC E24.8
- ulcer — *see* Ulcer, peptic, acute

Cusp, Carabelli — *omit code*

Cut (external) (*see also* Laceration)
- muscle — *see* Injury, muscle

Cutaneous (*see also* condition)
- hemorrhage R23.3
- larva migrans B76.9

Cutis (*see also* condition)
- hyperelastica Q82.8
  - acquired L57.4
- laxa (hyperelastica) — *see* Dermatolysis
- marmorata R23.8
- osteosis L94.2
- pendula — *see* Dermatolysis
- rhomboidalis nuchae L57.2
- verticis gyrata Q82.8
  - acquired L91.8

Cyanosis R23.0
- due to
  - patent foramen botalli Q21.1
  - persistent foramen ovale Q21.1
- enterogenous D74.8
- paroxysmal digital — *see* Raynaud's disease
  - with gangrene I73.01
- retina, retinal H35.89

Cyanotic heart disease I24.9
- congenital Q24.9

Cycle
- anovulatory N97.0
- menstrual, irregular N92.6

Cyclencephaly Q04.9

Cyclical vomiting (*see also* Vomiting, cyclical) G43.A0 (*following* G43.7)
- psychogenic F50.89

Cyclitis (*see also* Iridocyclitis) H20.9
- chronic — *see* Iridocyclitis, chronic
- Fuchs' heterochromic H20.81- ☑
- granulomatous — *see* Iridocyclitis, chronic
- lens-induced — *see* Iridocyclitis, lens-induced
- posterior H30.2- ☑

Cycloid personality F34.0

Cyclophoria H50.54

Cyclopia, cyclops Q87.0

Cyclopism Q87.0

Cyclosporiasis A07.4

Cyclothymia F34.0

Cyclothymic personality F34.0

Cyclotropia H50.41- ☑

Cylindroma (*see also* Neoplasm, malignant, by site)
- eccrine dermal — *see* Neoplasm, skin, benign
- skin — *see* Neoplasm, skin, benign

Cylindruria R82.99

Cynanche
- diphtheritic A36.2
- tonsillaris J36

Cynophobia F40.218

Cynorexia R63.2

Cyphosis — *see* Kyphosis

Cyprus fever — *see* Brucellosis

Cyst (colloid) (mucous) (simple) (retention)
- adenoid (infected) J35.8
- adrenal gland E27.8
  - congenital Q89.1
- air, lung J98.4
- allantoic Q64.4
- alveolar process (jaw bone) M27.40
- amnion, amniotic O41.8X- ☑
- aneurysmal M27.49
- anterior
  - chamber (eye) — *see* Cyst, iris
  - nasopalatine K09.1
- antrum J34.1
- anus K62.89
- apical (tooth) (periodontal) K04.8
- appendix K38.8
- arachnoid, brain (acquired) G93.0
  - congenital Q04.6
- arytenoid J38.7
- Baker's M71.2- ☑
  - ruptured M66.0
  - tuberculous A18.02
- Bartholin's gland N75.0
- bile duct (common) (hepatic) K83.5
- bladder (multiple) (trigone) N32.89
- blue dome (breast) — *see* Cyst, breast
- bone (local) NEC M85.60
  - aneurysmal M85.50
    - ankle M85.57- ☑
    - foot M85.57- ☑
    - forearm M85.53- ☑
    - hand M85.54- ☑
    - jaw M27.49
    - lower leg M85.56- ☑
    - multiple site M85.59
    - neck M85.58
    - rib M85.58
    - shoulder M85.51- ☑
    - skull M85.58
    - specified site NEC M85.58
    - thigh M85.55- ☑
    - toe M85.57- ☑
    - upper arm M85.52- ☑
    - vertebra M85.58
  - solitary M85.40
    - ankle M85.47- ☑
    - fibula M85.46- ☑
    - foot M85.47- ☑
    - hand M85.44- ☑
    - humerus M85.42- ☑
    - jaw M27.49
    - neck M85.48
    - pelvis M85.45- ☑
    - radius M85.43- ☑
    - rib M85.48
    - shoulder M85.41- ☑
    - skull M85.48
    - specified site NEC M85.48
    - tibia M85.46- ☑
    - toe M85.47- ☑
    - ulna M85.43- ☑
    - vertebra M85.48
  - specified type NEC M85.60
    - ankle M85.67- ☑
    - foot M85.67- ☑
    - forearm M85.63- ☑
    - hand M85.64- ☑
    - jaw M27.40
      - developmental (nonodontogenic) K09.1
      - odontogenic K09.0
      - latent M27.0
    - lower leg M85.66- ☑
    - multiple site M85.69
    - neck M85.68
    - rib M85.68
    - shoulder M85.61- ☑
    - skull M85.68
    - specified site NEC M85.68
    - thigh M85.65- ☑
    - toe M85.67- ☑
    - upper arm M85.62- ☑
    - vertebra M85.68
- brain (acquired) G93.0
  - congenital Q04.6
  - hydatid B67.99 [G94]
- **Cyst** — *continued*
  - brain — *continued*
    - third ventricle (colloid), congenital Q04.6
  - branchial (cleft) Q18.0
  - branchiogenic Q18.0
  - breast (benign) (blue dome) (pedunculated) (solitary) N60.0- ☑
    - involution — *see* Dysplasia, mammary, specified type NEC
    - sebaceous — *see* Dysplasia, mammary, specified type NEC
  - broad ligament (benign) N83.8
  - bronchogenic (mediastinal) (sequestration) J98.4
    - congenital Q33.0
  - buccal K09.8
  - bulbourethral gland N36.8
  - bursa, bursal NEC M71.30
    - with rupture — *see* Rupture, synovium
    - ankle M71.37- ☑
    - elbow M71.32- ☑
    - foot M71.37- ☑
    - hand M71.34- ☑
    - hip M71.35- ☑
    - multiple sites M71.39
    - pharyngeal J39.2
    - popliteal space — *see* Cyst, Baker's
    - shoulder M71.31- ☑
    - specified site NEC M71.38
    - wrist M71.33- ☑
  - calcifying odontogenic D16.5
    - upper jaw (bone) (maxilla) D16.4
  - canal of Nuck (female) N94.89
    - congenital Q52.4
  - canthus — *see* Cyst, conjunctiva
  - carcinomatous — *see* Neoplasm, malignant, by site
  - cauda equina G95.89
  - celomic (pericardium) Q24.8
  - cerebellopontine (angle) — *see* Cyst, brain
  - cerebellum — *see* Cyst, brain
  - cerebral — *see* Cyst, brain
  - cervical lateral Q18.0
  - cervix NEC N88.8
    - embryonic Q51.6
    - nabothian N88.8
  - chiasmal optic NEC — *see* Disorder, optic, chiasm
  - chocolate (ovary) N80.1
  - choledochus, congenital Q44.4
  - chorion O41.8X- ☑
  - choroid plexus G93.0
  - ciliary body — *see* Cyst, iris
  - clitoris N90.7
  - colon K63.89
  - common (bile) duct K83.5
  - congenital NEC Q89.8
    - adrenal gland Q89.1
    - epiglottis Q31.8
    - esophagus Q39.8
    - fallopian tube Q50.4
    - kidney Q61.00
      - more than one (multiple) Q61.02
        - specified as polycystic Q61.3
          - adult type Q61.2
          - infantile type NEC Q61.19
            - collecting duct dilation Q61.11
      - solitary Q61.01
    - larynx Q31.8
    - liver Q44.6
    - lung Q33.0
    - mediastinum Q34.1
    - ovary Q50.1
    - oviduct Q50.4
    - periurethral (tissue) Q64.79
    - prepuce Q55.69
    - salivary gland (any) Q38.4
    - sublingual Q38.6
    - submaxillary gland Q38.6
    - thymus (gland) Q89.2
    - tongue Q38.3
    - ureterovesical orifice Q62.8
    - vulva Q52.79
  - conjunctiva H11.44- ☑
  - cornea H18.89- ☑
  - corpora quadrigemina G93.0
  - corpus
    - albicans N83.29- ☑
    - luteum (hemorrhagic) (ruptured) N83.1- ☑
  - Cowper's gland (benign) (infected) N36.8

☑ **Additional Character Required** — Refer to the Tabular List for Character Selection

🔺 **Subterms under main terms may continue to next column or page**

Cyst — *continued*
  cranial meninges G93.0
  craniobuccal pouch E23.6
  craniopharyngeal pouch E23.6
  cystic duct K82.8
  Cysticercus — *see* Cysticercosis
  Dandy-Walker Q03.1
    with spina bifida — *see* Spina bifida
  dental (root) K04.8
    developmental K09.0
    eruption K09.0
    primordial K09.0
  dentigerous (mandible) (maxilla) K09.0
  dermoid — *see* Neoplasm, benign, by site
    with malignant transformation C56.- ☑
    implantation
      external area or site (skin) NEC L72.0
      iris — *see* Cyst, iris, implantation
      vagina N89.8
      vulva N90.7
    mouth K09.8
    oral soft tissue K09.8
    sacrococcygeal — *see* Cyst, pilonidal
  developmental K09.1
    odontogenic K09.0
    oral region (nonodontogenic) K09.1
    ovary, ovarian Q50.1
  dura (cerebral) G93.0
    spinal G96.19
  ear (external) Q18.1
  echinococcal — *see* Echinococcus
  embryonic
    cervix uteri Q51.6
    fallopian tube Q50.4
    vagina Q52.4
  endometrium, endometrial (uterus) N85.8
    ectopic — *see* Endometriosis
  enterogenous Q43.8
  epidermal, epidermoid (inclusion) (*see also* Cyst, skin)
      L72.0
    mouth K09.8
    oral soft tissue K09.8
  epididymis N50.3
  epiglottis J38.7
  epiphysis cerebri E34.8
  epithelial (inclusion) L72.0
  epoophoron Q50.5
  eruption K09.0
  esophagus K22.8
  ethmoid sinus J34.1
  external female genital organs NEC N90.7
  eyelid (sebaceous) H02.829
    infected — *see* Hordeolum
    left H02.826
      lower H02.825
      upper H02.824
    right H02.823
      lower H02.822
      upper H02.821
  eye NEC H57.8
    congenital Q15.8
  fallopian tube N83.8
    congenital Q50.4
  fimbrial (twisted) Q50.4
  fissural (oral region) K09.1
  follicle (graafian) (hemorrhagic) N83.0- ☑
    nabothian N88.8
  follicular (atretic) (hemorrhagic) (ovarian) N83.0- ☑
    dentigerous K09.0
    odontogenic K09.0
    skin L72.9
      specified NEC L72.8
  frontal sinus J34.1
  gallbladder K82.8
  ganglion — *see* Ganglion
  Gartner's duct Q52.4
  gingiva K09.0
  gland of Moll — *see* Cyst, eyelid
  globulomaxillary K09.1
  graafian follicle (hemorrhagic) N83.0- ☑
  granulosal lutein (hemorrhagic) N83.1- ☑
  hemangiomatous D18.00
    intra-abdominal D18.03
    intracranial D18.02
    skin D18.01
    specified site NEC D18.09
  hemorrhagic M27.49
  hydatid (*see also* Echinococcus) B67.90

Cyst — *continued*
  hydatid (*see also* Echinococcus) — *continued*
    brain B67.99 [G94]
    liver (*see also* Cyst, liver, hydatid) B67.8
    lung NEC B67.99 [J99]
    Morgagni
      female Q50.5
      male (epididymal) Q55.4
        testicular Q55.29
    specified site NEC B67.99
  hymen N89.8
    embryonic Q52.4
  hypopharynx J39.2
  hypophysis, hypophyseal (duct) (recurrent) E23.6
    cerebri E23.6
  implantation (dermoid)
    external area or site (skin) NEC L72.0
    iris — *see* Cyst, iris, implantation
    vagina N89.8
    vulva N90.7
  incisive canal K09.1
  inclusion (epidermal) (epithelial) (epidermoid) (squa-
      mous) L72.0
    not of skin — *code under* Cyst, by site
  intestine (large) (small) K63.89
  intracranial — *see* Cyst, brain
  intraligamentous (*see also* Disorder, ligament)
    knee — *see* Derangement, knee
  intrasellar E23.6
  iris H21.309
    exudative H21.31- ☑
    idiopathic H21.30- ☑
    implantation H21.32- ☑
    parasitic H21.33- ☑
    pars plana (primary) H21.34- ☑
      exudative H21.35- ☑
  jaw (bone) M27.40
    aneurysmal M27.49
    developmental (odontogenic) K09.0
    fissural K09.1
    hemorrhagic M27.49
    traumatic M27.49
  joint NEC — *see* Disorder, joint, specified type NEC
  kidney (acquired) N28.1
    calyceal — *see* Hydronephrosis
    congenital Q61.00
    more than one (multiple) Q61.02
      specified as polycystic Q61.3
        adult type (autosomal dominant) Q61.2
        infantile type (autosomal recessive) NEC
          Q61.19
          collecting duct dilation Q61.11
    pyelogenic — *see* Hydronephrosis
    simple N28.1
    solitary (single) Q61.01
      acquired N28.1
  labium (majus) (minus) N90.7
    sebaceous N90.7
  lacrimal (*see also* Disorder, lacrimal system, specified
      NEC)
    gland H04.13- ☑
    passages or sac — *see* Disorder, lacrimal system,
      specified NEC
  larynx J38.7
  lateral periodontal K09.0
  lens H27.8
    congenital Q12.8
  lip (gland) K13.0
  liver (idiopathic) (simple) K76.89
    congenital Q44.6
    hydatid B67.8
      granulosus B67.0
      multilocularis B67.5
  lung J98.4
    congenital Q33.0
    giant bullous J43.9
  lutein N83.1- ☑
  lymphangiomatous D18.1
  lymphoepithelial, oral soft tissue K09.8
  macula — *see* Degeneration, macula, hole
  malignant — *see* Neoplasm, malignant, by site
  mammary gland — *see* Cyst, breast
  mandible M27.40
    dentigerous K09.0
    radicular K04.8
  maxilla M27.40
    dentigerous K09.0
    radicular K04.8

Cyst — *continued*
  medial, face and neck Q18.8
  median
    anterior maxillary K09.1
    palatal K09.1
  mediastinum, congenital Q34.1
  meibomian (gland) — *see* Chalazion
    infected — *see* Hordeolum
  membrane, brain G93.0
  meninges (cerebral) G93.0
    spinal G96.19
  meniscus, knee — *see* Derangement, knee, meniscus,
      cystic
  mesentery, mesenteric K66.8
    chyle I89.8
  mesonephric duct
    female Q50.5
    male Q55.4
  milk N64.89
  Morgagni (hydatid)
    female Q50.5
    male (epididymal) Q55.4
      testicular Q55.29
  mouth K09.8
  Müllerian duct Q50.4
    appendix testis Q55.29
    cervix Q51.6
    fallopian tube Q50.4
    female Q50.4
    male Q55.29
    prostatic utricle Q55.4
    vagina (embryonal) Q52.4
  multilocular (ovary) D39.10
    benign — *see* Neoplasm, benign, by site
  myometrium N85.8
  nabothian (follicle) (ruptured) N88.8
  nasoalveolar K09.1
  nasolabial K09.1
  nasopalatine (anterior) (duct) K09.1
  nasopharynx J39.2
  neoplastic — *see* Neoplasm, uncertain behavior, by
      site
    benign — *see* Neoplasm, benign, by site
  nervous system NEC G96.8
  neuroenteric (congenital) Q06.8
  nipple — *see* Cyst, breast
  nose (turbinates) J34.1
    sinus J34.1
  odontogenic, developmental K09.0
  omentum (lesser) K66.8
    congenital Q45.8
  ora serrata — *see* Cyst, retina, ora serrata
  oral
    region K09.9
      developmental (nonodontogenic) K09.1
      specified NEC K09.8
    soft tissue K09.9
      specified NEC K09.8
  orbit H05.81- ☑
  ovary, ovarian (twisted) N83.20- ☑
    adherent N83.20- ☑
    chocolate N80.1
    corpus
      albicans N83.29- ☑
      luteum (hemorrhagic) N83.1- ☑
    dermoid D27.9
    developmental Q50.1
    due to failure of involution NEC N83.20- ☑
    endometrial N80.1
    follicular (graafian) (hemorrhagic) N83.0- ☑
    hemorrhagic N83.20- ☑
    in pregnancy or childbirth O34.8- ☑
      with obstructed labor O65.5
    multilocular D39.10
    pseudomucinous D27.9
    retention N83.29- ☑
    serous N83.20- ☑
    specified NEC N83.29- ☑
    theca lutein (hemorrhagic) N83.1- ☑
    tuberculous A18.18
  oviduct N83.8
  palate (median) (fissural) K09.1
  palatine papilla (jaw) K09.1
  pancreas, pancreatic (hemorrhagic) (true) K86.2
    congenital Q45.2
    false K86.3
  paralabral
    hip M24.85- ☑

Cyst — continued
paralabral — continued
  shoulder S43.43- ☑
paramesonephric duct Q50.4
  female Q50.4
  male Q55.29
paranephric N28.1
paraphysis, cerebri, congenital Q04.6
parasitic B89
parathyroid (gland) E21.4
paratubal N83.8
paraurethral duct N36.8
paroophoron Q50.5
parotid gland K11.6
parovarian Q50.5
pelvis, female N94.89
  in pregnancy or childbirth O34.8- ☑
    causing obstructed labor O65.5
penis (sebaceous) N48.89
periapical K04.8
pericardial (congenital) Q24.8
  acquired (secondary) I31.8
pericoronal K09.0
periodontal K04.8
  lateral K09.0
peripelvic (lymphatic) N28.1
peritoneum K66.8
  chylous I89.8
periventricular, acquired, newborn P91.1
pharynx (wall) J39.2
pilar L72.11
pilonidal (infected) (rectum) L05.91
  with abscess L05.01
  malignant C44.59- ☑
pituitary (duct) (gland) E23.6
placenta O43.19- ☑
pleura J94.8
popliteal — see Cyst, Baker's
porencephalic Q04.6
  acquired G93.0
postanal (infected) — see Cyst, pilonidal
postmastoidectomy cavity (mucosal) — see Complications, postmastoidectomy, cyst
preauricular Q18.1
prepuce N47.4
  congenital Q55.69
primordial (jaw) K09.0
prostate N42.83
pseudomucinous (ovary) D27.9
pupillary, miotic H21.27- ☑
radicular (residual) K04.8
radiculodental K04.8
ranular K11.8
Rathke's pouch E23.6
rectum (epithelium) (mucous) K62.89
renal — see Cyst, kidney
residual (radicular) K04.8
retention (ovary) N83.29- ☑
  salivary gland K11.6
retina H33.19- ☑
  ora serrata H33.11- ☑
  parasitic H33.12- ☑
retroperitoneal K68.9
sacrococcygeal (dermoid) — see Cyst, pilonidal
salivary gland or duct (mucous extravasation or retention) K11.6
Sampson's N80.1
sclera H15.89
scrotum L72.9
  sebaceous L72.3
sebaceous (duct) (gland) L72.3
  breast — see Dysplasia, mammary, specified type NEC
  eyelid — see Cyst, eyelid
  genital organ NEC
    female N94.89
    male N50.89
  scrotum L72.3
semilunar cartilage (knee) (multiple) — see Derangement, knee, meniscus, cystic
seminal vesicle N50.89
serous (ovary) N83.20- ☑
sinus (accessory) (nasal) J34.1
Skene's gland N36.8
skin L72.9
  breast — see Dysplasia, mammary, specified type NEC
  epidermal, epidermoid L72.0

Cyst — continued
skin — continued
  epithelial L72.0
  eyelid — see Cyst, eyelid
  genital organ NEC
    female N90.7
    male N50.89
  inclusion L72.0
  scrotum L72.9
  sebaceous L72.3
  sweat gland or duct L74.8
solitary
  bone — see Cyst, bone, solitary
  jaw M27.40
  kidney N28.1
spermatic cord N50.89
sphenoid sinus J34.1
spinal meninges G96.19
spleen NEC D73.4
  congenital Q89.09
  hydatid (see also Echinococcus) B67.99 [D77]
Stafne's M27.0
subarachnoid intrasellar R93.0
subcutaneous, pheomycotic (chromomycotic) B43.2
subdural (cerebral) G93.0
  spinal cord G96.19
sublingual gland K11.6
submandibular gland K11.6
submaxillary gland K11.6
suburethral N36.8
suprarenal gland E27.8
suprasellar — see Cyst, brain
sweat gland or duct L74.8
synovial (see also Cyst, bursa)
  ruptured — see Rupture, synovium
tarsal — see Chalazion
tendon (sheath) — see Disorder, tendon, specified type NEC
testis N44.2
  tunica albuginea N44.1
theca lutein (ovary) N83.1- ☑
Thornwaldt's J39.2
thymus (gland) E32.8
thyroglossal duct (infected) (persistent) Q89.2
thyroid (gland) E04.1
thyrolingual duct (infected) (persistent) Q89.2
tongue K14.8
tonsil J35.8
tooth — see Cyst, dental
Tornwaldt's J39.2
trichilemmal (proliferating) L72.12
trichodermal L72.12
tubal (fallopian) N83.8
  inflammatory — see Salpingitis, chronic
tubo-ovarian N83.8
  inflammatory N70.13
tunica
  albuginea testis N44.1
  vaginalis N50.89
turbinate (nose) J34.1
Tyson's gland N48.89
urachus, congenital Q64.4
ureter N28.89
ureterovesical orifice N28.89
urethra, urethral (gland) N36.8
uterine ligament N83.8
uterus (body) (corpus) (recurrent) N85.8
  embryonic Q51.818
    cervix Q51.6
vagina, vaginal (implantation) (inclusion) (squamous cell) (wall) N89.8
  embryonic Q52.4
vallecula, vallecular (epiglottis) J38.7
vesical (orifice) N32.89
vitreous body H43.89
vulva (implantation) (inclusion) N90.7
  congenital Q52.79
  sebaceous gland N90.7
vulvovaginal gland N90.7
wolffian
  female Q50.5
  male Q55.4
Cystadenocarcinoma — see Neoplasm, malignant, by site
bile duct C22.1
endometrioid — see Neoplasm, malignant, by site
  specified site — see Neoplasm, malignant, by site

Cystadenocarcinoma — continued
endometrioid — see Neoplasm, malignant, by site — continued
  unspecified site
    female C56.9
    male C61
mucinous
  papillary
    specified site — see Neoplasm, malignant, by site
    unspecified site C56.9
  specified site — see Neoplasm, malignant, by site
  unspecified site C56.9
papillary
  mucinous
    specified site — see Neoplasm, malignant, by site
    unspecified site C56.9
  pseudomucinous
    specified site — see Neoplasm, malignant, by site
    unspecified site C56.9
  serous
    specified site — see Neoplasm, malignant, by site
    unspecified site C56.9
  specified site — see Neoplasm, malignant, by site
  unspecified site C56.9
pseudomucinous
  papillary
    specified site — see Neoplasm, malignant, by site
    unspecified site C56.9
  specified site — see Neoplasm, malignant, by site
  unspecified site C56.9
serous
  papillary
    specified site — see Neoplasm, malignant, by site
    unspecified site C56.9
  specified site — see Neoplasm, malignant, by site
  unspecified site C56.9
Cystadenofibroma
clear cell — see Neoplasm, benign, by site
endometrioid D27.9
  borderline malignancy D39.1- ☑
  malignant C56.- ☑
mucinous
  specified site — see Neoplasm, benign, by site
  unspecified site D27.9
serous
  specified site — see Neoplasm, benign, by site
  unspecified site D27.9
specified site — see Neoplasm, benign, by site
unspecified site D27.9
Cystadenoma (see also Neoplasm, benign, by site)
bile duct D13.4
endometrioid — see Neoplasm, benign, by site
  borderline malignancy — see Neoplasm, uncertain behavior, by site
malignant — see Neoplasm, malignant, by site
mucinous
  borderline malignancy
    ovary C56.- ☑
    specified site NEC — see Neoplasm, uncertain behavior, by site
    unspecified site C56.9
  papillary
    borderline malignancy
      ovary C56.- ☑
      specified site NEC — see Neoplasm, uncertain behavior, by site
      unspecified site C56.9
    specified site — see Neoplasm, benign, by site
    unspecified site D27.9
  specified site — see Neoplasm, benign, by site
  unspecified site D27.9
papillary
  borderline malignancy
    ovary C56.- ☑
    specified site NEC — see Neoplasm, uncertain behavior, by site
    unspecified site C56.9
  lymphomatosum
    specified site — see Neoplasm, benign, by site
    unspecified site D11.9

☑ **Additional Character Required** — Refer to the Tabular List for Character Selection   ⬇ Subterms under main terms may continue to next column or page

Cystadenoma — *continued*
  papillary — *continued*
    mucinous
      borderline malignancy
        ovary C56.- ☑
        specified site NEC — *see* Neoplasm, uncertain behavior, by site
        unspecified site C56.9
      specified site — *see* Neoplasm, benign, by site
      unspecified site D27.9
    pseudomucinous
      borderline malignancy
        ovary C56.- ☑
        specified site NEC — *see* Neoplasm, uncertain behavior, by site
        unspecified site C56.9
      specified site — *see* Neoplasm, benign, by site
      unspecified site D27.9
    serous
      borderline malignancy
        ovary C56.- ☑
        specified site NEC — *see* Neoplasm, uncertain behavior, by site
        unspecified site C56.9
      specified site — *see* Neoplasm, benign, by site
      unspecified site D27.9
    specified site — *see* Neoplasm, benign, by site
    unspecified site D27.9
  pseudomucinous
    borderline malignancy
      ovary C56.- ☑
      specified site NEC — *see* Neoplasm, uncertain behavior, by site
      unspecified site C56.9
    papillary
      borderline malignancy
        ovary C56.- ☑
        specified site NEC — *see* Neoplasm, uncertain behavior, by site
        unspecified site C56.9
      specified site — *see* Neoplasm, benign, by site
      unspecified site D27.9
    specified site — *see* Neoplasm, benign, by site
    unspecified site D27.9
  serous
    borderline malignancy
      ovary C56.- ☑
      specified site NEC — *see* Neoplasm, uncertain behavior, by site
      unspecified site C56.9
    papillary
      borderline malignancy
        ovary C56.- ☑
        specified site NEC — *see* Neoplasm, uncertain behavior, by site
        unspecified site C56.9
      specified site — *see* Neoplasm, benign, by site
      unspecified site D27.9
    specified site — *see* Neoplasm, benign, by site
    unspecified site D27.9

Cystathionine synthase deficiency E72.11
Cystathioninemia E72.19
Cystathioninuria E72.19
Cystic (*see also* condition)
  breast (chronic) — *see* Mastopathy, cystic
  corpora lutea (hemorrhagic) N83.1- ☑
  duct — *see* condition
  eyeball (congenital) Q11.0
  fibrosis — *see* Fibrosis, cystic
  kidney (congenital) Q61.9

Cystic — *continued*
  kidney — *continued*
    adult type Q61.2
    infantile type NEC Q61.19
      collecting duct dilatation Q61.11
    medullary Q61.5
  liver, congenital Q44.6
  lung disease J98.4
    congenital Q33.0
  mastitis, chronic — *see* Mastopathy, cystic
  medullary, kidney Q61.5
  meniscus — *see* Derangement, knee, meniscus, cystic
  ovary N83.20- ☑
Cysticercosis, cysticerciasis B69.9
  with
    epileptiform fits B69.0
    myositis B69.81
  brain B69.0
  central nervous system B69.0
  cerebral B69.0
  ocular B69.1
  specified NEC B69.89
Cysticercus cellulose infestation — *see* Cysticercosis
Cystinosis (malignant) E72.04
Cystinuria E72.01
Cystitis (exudative) (hemorrhagic) (septic) (suppurative) N30.90
  with
    fibrosis — *see* Cystitis, chronic, interstitial
    hematuria N30.91
    leukoplakia — *see* Cystitis, chronic, interstitial
    malakoplakia — *see* Cystitis, chronic, interstitial
    metaplasia — *see* Cystitis, chronic, interstitial
    prostatitis N41.3
  acute N30.00
    with hematuria N30.01
    of trigone N30.30
      with hematuria N30.31
  allergic — *see* Cystitis, specified type NEC
  amebic A06.81
  bilharzial B65.9 [N33]
  blennorrhagic (gonococcal) A54.01
  bullous — *see* Cystitis, specified type NEC
  calculous N21.0
  chlamydial A56.01
  chronic N30.20
    with hematuria N30.21
    interstitial N30.10
      with hematuria N30.11
    of trigone N30.30
      with hematuria N30.31
    specified NEC N30.20
      with hematuria N30.21
  cystic (a) — *see* Cystitis, specified type NEC
  diphtheritic A36.85
  echinococcal
    granulosus B67.39
    multilocularis B67.69
  emphysematous — *see* Cystitis, specified type NEC
  encysted — *see* Cystitis, specified type NEC
  eosinophilic — *see* Cystitis, specified type NEC
  follicular — *see* Cystitis, of trigone
  gangrenous — *see* Cystitis, specified type NEC
  glandularis — *see* Cystitis, specified type NEC
  gonococcal A54.01
  incrusted — *see* Cystitis, specified type NEC
  interstitial (chronic) — *see* Cystitis, chronic, interstitial
  irradiation N30.40
    with hematuria N30.41
  irritation — *see* Cystitis, specified type NEC

Cystitis — *continued*
  malignant — *see* Cystitis, specified type NEC
  of trigone N30.30
    with hematuria N30.31
  panmural — *see* Cystitis, chronic, interstitial
  polyposa — *see* Cystitis, specified type NEC
  prostatic N41.3
  puerperal (postpartum) O86.22
  radiation — *see* Cystitis, irradiation
  specified type NEC N30.80
    with hematuria N30.81
  subacute — *see* Cystitis, chronic
  submucous — *see* Cystitis, chronic, interstitial
  syphilitic (late) A52.76
  trichomonal A59.03
  tuberculous A18.12
  ulcerative — *see* Cystitis, chronic, interstitial
Cystocele (-urethrocele)
  female N81.10
    with prolapse of uterus — *see* Prolapse, uterus
    lateral N81.12
    midline N81.11
    paravaginal N81.12
  in pregnancy or childbirth O34.8- ☑
    causing obstructed labor O65.5
  male N32.89
Cystolithiasis N21.0
Cystoma (*see also* Neoplasm, benign, by site)
  endometrial, ovary N80.1
  mucinous
    specified site — *see* Neoplasm, benign, by site
    unspecified site D27.9
  serous
    specified site — *see* Neoplasm, benign, by site
    unspecified site D27.9
  simple (ovary) N83.29- ☑
Cystoplegia N31.2
Cystoptosis N32.89
Cystopyelitis — *see* Pyelonephritis
Cystorrhagia N32.89
Cystosarcoma phyllodes D48.6- ☑
  benign D24- ☑
  malignant — *see* Neoplasm, breast, malignant
Cystostomy
  attention to Z43.5
  complication — *see* Complications, cystostomy
  status Z93.50
    appendico-vesicostomy Z93.52
    cutaneous Z93.51
    specified NEC Z93.59
Cystourethritis — *see* Urethritis
Cystourethrocele (*see also* Cystocele)
  female N81.10
    with uterine prolapse — *see* Prolapse, uterus
    lateral N81.12
    midline N81.11
    paravaginal N81.12
  male N32.89
Cytomegalic inclusion disease
  congenital P35.1
Cytomegalovirus infection B25.9
Cytomycosis (reticuloendothelial) B39.4
Cytopenia D75.9
  refractory
    with multilineage dysplasia D46.A (*following* D46.2)
      and ring sideroblasts (RCMD RS) D46.B (*following* D46.2)
Czerny's disease (periodic hydrarthrosis of the knee) — *see* Effusion, joint, knee

D

Da Costa's syndrome F45.8
Daae (-Finsen) **disease** (epidemic pleurodynia) B33.Ø
Dabney's grip B33.Ø
Dacryoadenitis, dacryadenitis HØ4.ØØ- ✅
    acute HØ4.Ø1- ✅
    chronic HØ4.Ø2- ✅
Dacryocystitis HØ4.3Ø- ✅
    acute HØ4.32- ✅
    chronic HØ4.41- ✅
    neonatal P39.1
    phlegmonous HØ4.31- ✅
    syphilitic A52.71
        congenital (early) A5Ø.Ø1
    trachomatous, active A71.1
        sequelae (late effect) B94.Ø
Dacryocystoblenorrhea — *see* Inflammation, lacrimal, passages, chronic
Dacryocystocele — *see* Disorder, lacrimal system, changes
Dacryolith, dacryolithiasis HØ4.51- ✅
Dacryoma — *see* Disorder, lacrimal system, changes
Dacryopericystitis — *see* Dacryocystitis
Dacryops HØ4.11- ✅
Dacryostenosis (*see also* Stenosis, lacrimal)
    congenital Q1Ø.5
Dactylitis
    bone — *see* Osteomyelitis
    sickle-cell D57.ØØ
        Hb C D57.219
        Hb SS D57.ØØ
        specified NEC D57.819
    skin LØ8.9
    syphilitic A52.77
    tuberculous A18.Ø3
Dactylolysis spontanea (ainhum) L94.6
Dactylosymphysis Q7Ø.9
    fingers — *see* Syndactylism, complex, fingers
    toes — *see* Syndactylism, complex, toes
Damage
    arteriosclerotic — *see* Arteriosclerosis
    brain (nontraumatic) G93.9
        anoxic, hypoxic G93.1
            resulting from a procedure G97.82
        child NEC G8Ø.9
        due to birth injury P11.2
    cardiorenal (vascular) — *see* Hypertension, cardiorenal
    cerebral NEC — *see* Damage, brain
    coccyx, complicating delivery O71.6
    coronary — *see* Disease, heart, ischemic
    eye, birth injury P15.3
    liver (nontraumatic) K76.9
        alcoholic K7Ø.9
        due to drugs — *see* Disease, liver, toxic
        toxic — *see* Disease, liver, toxic
    medication T88.7 ✅
    pelvic
        joint or ligament, during delivery O71.6
        organ NEC
            during delivery O71.5
            following ectopic or molar pregnancy OØ8.6
    renal — *see* Disease, renal
    subendocardium, subendocardial — *see* Degeneration, myocardial
    vascular I99.9
Dana-Putnam syndrome (subacute combined sclerosis with pernicious anemia) — *see* Degeneration, combined
Danbolt (-Cross) **syndrome** (acrodermatitis enteropathica) E83.2
Dandruff L21.Ø
Dandy-Walker syndrome QØ3.1
    with spina bifida — *see* Spina bifida
Danlos' syndrome Q79.6
Darier (-White) **disease** (congenital) Q82.8
    meaning erythema annulare centrifugum L53.1
Darier-Roussy sarcoid D86.3
Darwin's tubercle Q17.8
Dawson's (inclusion body) **encephalitis** A81.1

De Beurmann (-Gougerot) **disease** B42.1
De la Tourette's syndrome F95.2
De Lange's syndrome Q87.1
De Morgan's spots (senile angiomas) I78.1
De Quervain's
    disease (tendon sheath) M65.4
    syndrome E34.51
    thyroiditis (subacute granulomatous thyroiditis) EØ6.1
De Toni-Fanconi (-Debré) **syndrome** E72.Ø9
    with cystinosis E72.Ø4
Dead
    fetus, retained (mother) O36.4 ✅
        early pregnancy OØ2.1
    labyrinth H83.2 ✅
    ovum, retained OØ2.Ø
Deaf nonspeaking NEC H91.3
Deafmutism (acquired) (congenital) NEC H91.3
    hysterical F44.6
    syphilitic, congenital (*see also* subcategory) H94.8 A5Ø.Ø9
Deafness (acquired) (complete) (hereditary) (partial) H91.9- ✅
    with blue sclera and fragility of bone Q78.Ø
    auditory fatigue — *see* Deafness, specified type NEC
    aviation T7Ø.Ø ✅
        nerve injury — *see* Injury, nerve, acoustic, specified type NEC
    boilermaker's H83.3 ✅
    central — *see* Deafness, sensorineural
    conductive H9Ø.2
        and sensorineural
            mixed H9Ø.8
                bilateral H9Ø.6
            bilateral H9Ø.Ø
            unilateral H9Ø.1- ✅
                with restricted hearing on the contralateral side H9Ø.A- ✅
    congenital H9Ø.5
        with blue sclera and fragility of bone Q78.Ø
    due to toxic agents — *see* Deafness, ototoxic
    emotional (hysterical) F44.6
    functional (hysterical) F44.6
    high frequency H91.9- ✅
    hysterical F44.6
    low frequency H91.9- ✅
    mental R48.8
    mixed conductive and sensorineural H9Ø.8
        bilateral H9Ø.6
        unilateral H9Ø.7- ✅
    nerve — *see* Deafness, sensorineural
    neural — *see* Deafness, sensorineural
    noise-induced (*see also* subcategory) H83.3 ✅
        nerve injury — *see* Injury, nerve, acoustic, specified type NEC
    nonspeaking H91.3
    ototoxic H91.Ø ✅
    perceptive — *see* Deafness, sensorineural
    psychogenic (hysterical) F44.6
    sensorineural H9Ø.5
        and conductive
            bilateral H9Ø.6
            mixed H9Ø.8
                bilateral H9Ø.6
            bilateral H9Ø.3
            unilateral H9Ø.4- ✅
                with restricted hearing on the contralateral side H9Ø.A- ✅
    sensory — *see* Deafness, sensorineural
    specified type NEC H91.8 ✅
    sudden (idiopathic) H91.2- ✅
    syphilitic A52.15
    transient ischemic H93.Ø1- ✅
    traumatic — *see* Injury, nerve, acoustic, specified type NEC
    word (developmental) H93.25
Death (cause unknown) (of) (unexplained) (unspecified cause) R99
    brain G93.82
    cardiac (sudden) (with successful resuscitation) — *code to* underlying disease
        family history of Z82.41
        personal history of Z86.74

Death — *continued*
    family member (assumed) Z63.4
Debility (chronic) (general) (nervous) R53.81
    congenital or neonatal NOS P96.9
    nervous R53.81
    old age R54
    senile R54
Débove's disease (splenomegaly) R16.1
Decalcification
    bone — *see* Osteoporosis
    teeth KØ3.89
Decapsulation, kidney N28.89
Decay
    dental — *see* Caries, dental
    senile R54
    tooth, teeth — *see* Caries, dental
Deciduitis (acute)
    following ectopic or molar pregnancy OØ8.Ø
Decline (general) — *see* Debility
    cognitive, age-associated R41.81
Decompensation
    cardiac (acute) (chronic) — *see* Disease, heart
    cardiovascular — *see* Disease, cardiovascular
    heart — *see* Disease, heart
    hepatic — *see* Failure, hepatic
    myocardial (acute) (chronic) — *see* Disease, heart
    respiratory J98.8
Decompression sickness T7Ø.3 ✅
Decrease (d)
    absolute neutrophile count — *see* Neutropenia
    blood
        platelets — *see* Thrombocytopenia
        pressure RØ3.1
            due to shock following
                injury T79.4 ✅
                operation T81.19 ✅
    estrogen E28.39
        postablative E89.4Ø
            asymptomatic E89.4Ø
            symptomatic E89.41
    fragility of erythrocytes D58.8
    function
        lipase (pancreatic) K9Ø.3
        ovary in hypopituitarism E23.Ø
        parenchyma of pancreas K86.89
        pituitary (gland) (anterior) (lobe) E23.Ø
            posterior (lobe) E23.Ø
    functional activity R68.89
    glucose R73.Ø9
    hematocrit R71.Ø
    hemoglobin R71.Ø
    leukocytes D72.819
        specified NEC D72.818
    libido R68.82
    lymphocytes D72.81Ø
    platelets D69.6
    respiration, due to shock following injury T79.4 ✅
    sexual desire R68.82
    tear secretion NEC — *see* Syndrome, dry eye
    tolerance
        fat K9Ø.49
        glucose R73.Ø9
        pancreatic K9Ø.3
        salt and water E87.8
    vision NEC H54.7
    white blood cell count D72.819
        specified NEC D72.818
Decubitus (ulcer) — *see* Ulcer, pressure, by site
    cervix N86
Deepening acetabulum — *see* Derangement, joint, specified type NEC, hip
Defect, defective Q89.9
    3-beta-hydroxysteroid dehydrogenase E25.Ø
    11-hydroxylase E25.Ø
    21-hydroxylase E25.Ø
    abdominal wall, congenital Q79.59
    antibody immunodeficiency D8Ø.9
    aorticopulmonary septum Q21.4
    atrial septal (ostium secundum type) Q21.1
        following acute myocardial infarction (current complication) I23.1
        ostium primum type Q21.2

Defect, defective — *continued*
 atrioventricular
  canal Q21.2
  septum Q21.2
 auricular septal Q21.1
 bilirubin excretion NEC E80.6
 biosynthesis, androgen (testicular) E29.1
 bulbar septum Q21.0
 catalase E80.3
 cell membrane receptor complex (CR3) D71
 circulation I99.9
  congenital Q28.9
  newborn Q28.9
 coagulation (factor) (*see also* Deficiency, factor) D68.9
  with
   ectopic pregnancy O08.1
   molar pregnancy O08.1
  acquired D68.4
  antepartum with hemorrhage — *see* Hemorrhage, antepartum, with coagulation defect
  due to
   liver disease D68.4
   vitamin K deficiency D68.4
  hereditary NEC D68.2
  intrapartum O67.0
  newborn, transient P61.6
  postpartum O99.13
   with hemorrhage O72.3
  specified type NEC D68.8
 complement system D84.1
 conduction (heart) I45.5
  bone — *see* Deafness, conductive
 congenital, organ or site not listed — *see* Anomaly, by site
 coronary sinus Q21.1
 cushion, endocardial Q21.2
 degradation, glycoprotein E77.1
 dental bridge, crown, fillings — *see* Defect, dental restoration
 dental restoration K08.50
  specified NEC K08.59
 dentin (hereditary) K00.5
 Descemet's membrane, congenital Q13.89
 developmental (*see also* Anomaly)
  cauda equina Q06.3
 diaphragm
  with elevation, eventration or hernia — *see* Hernia, diaphragm
  congenital Q79.1
   with hernia Q79.0
   gross (with hernia) Q79.0
 ectodermal, congenital Q82.9
 Eisenmenger's Q21.8
 enzyme
  catalase E80.3
  peroxidase E80.3
 esophagus, congenital Q39.9
 extensor retinaculum M62.89
 fibrin polymerization D68.2
 filling
  bladder R93.41
  kidney R93.42- ☑
  renal pelvis R93.41
  stomach R93.3
  ureter R93.41
  urinary organs, specified NEC R93.49
 Gerbode Q21.0
 glycoprotein degradation E77.1
 Hageman (factor) D68.2
 hearing — *see* Deafness
 high grade F70
 interatrial septal Q21.1
 interauricular septal Q21.1
 interventricular septal Q21.0
  with dextroposition of aorta, pulmonary stenosis and hypertrophy of right ventricle Q21.3
  in tetralogy of Fallot Q21.3
 learning (specific) — *see* Disorder, learning
 lymphocyte function antigen-1 (LFA-1) D84.0
 lysosomal enzyme, post-translational modification E77.0
 major osseous M89.70
  ankle M89.77- ☑
  carpus M89.74- ☑
  clavicle M89.71- ☑
  femur M89.75- ☑
  fibula M89.76- ☑
  fingers M89.74- ☑

Defect, defective — *continued*
 major osseous — *continued*
  foot M89.77- ☑
  forearm M89.73- ☑
  hand M89.74- ☑
  humerus M89.72- ☑
  lower leg M89.76- ☑
  metacarpus M89.74- ☑
  metatarsus M89.77- ☑
  multiple sites M89.79
  pelvic region M89.75- ☑
  pelvis M89.75- ☑
  radius M89.73- ☑
  scapula M89.71- ☑
  shoulder region M89.71- ☑
  specified NEC M89.78
  tarsus M89.77- ☑
  thigh M89.75- ☑
  tibia M89.76- ☑
  toes M89.77- ☑
  ulna M89.73- ☑
 mental — *see* Disability, intellectual
 modification, lysosomal enzymes, post-translational E77.0
 obstructive, congenital
  renal pelvis Q62.39
  ureter Q62.39
   atresia — *see* Atresia, ureter
   cecoureterocele Q62.32
   megaureter Q62.2
   orthotopic ureterocele Q62.31
 osseous, major M89.70
  ankle M89.77- ☑
  carpus M89.74- ☑
  clavicle M89.71- ☑
  femur M89.75- ☑
  fibula M89.76- ☑
  fingers M89.74- ☑
  foot M89.77- ☑
  forearm M89.73- ☑
  hand M89.74- ☑
  humerus M89.72- ☑
  lower leg M89.76- ☑
  metacarpus M89.74- ☑
  metatarsus M89.77- ☑
  multiple sites M89.9
  pelvic region M89.75- ☑
  pelvis M89.75- ☑
  radius M89.73- ☑
  scapula M89.71- ☑
  shoulder region M89.71- ☑
  specified NEC M89.78
  tarsus M89.77- ☑
  thigh M89.75- ☑
  tibia M89.76- ☑
  toes M89.77- ☑
  ulna M89.73- ☑
 osteochondral NEC (*see also* Deformity) M95.8
 ostium
  primum Q21.2
  secundum Q21.1
 peroxidase E80.3
 placental blood supply — *see* Insufficiency, placental
 platelets, qualitative D69.1
  constitutional D68.0
 postural NEC, spine — *see* Dorsopathy, deforming
 reduction
  limb Q73.8
   lower Q72.9- ☑
    absence — *see* Agenesis, leg
     foot — *see* Agenesis, foot
    longitudinal
     femur Q72.4- ☑
     fibula Q72.6- ☑
     tibia Q72.5- ☑
    specified type NEC Q72.89- ☑
    split foot Q72.7- ☑
   specified type NEC Q73.8
   upper Q71.9- ☑
    absence — *see* Agenesis, arm
     forearm — *see* Agenesis, forearm
     hand — *see* Agenesis, hand
    lobster-claw hand Q71.6- ☑
    longitudinal
     radius Q71.4- ☑
     ulna Q71.5- ☑

Defect, defective — *continued*
 reduction — *continued*
  limb — *continued*
   upper — *continued*
    specified type NEC Q71.89- ☑
 renal Q63.8
  obstructive Q62.39
 respiratory system, congenital Q34.9
 restoration, dental K08.50
  specified NEC K08.59
 retinal nerve bundle fibers H35.89
 septal (heart) NOS Q21.9
  acquired (atrial) (auricular) (ventricular) (old) I51.0
  atrial Q21.1
   concurrent with acute myocardial infarction — *see* Infarct, myocardium
   following acute myocardial infarction (current complication) I23.1
  ventricular (*see also* Defect, ventricular septal) Q21.0
 sinus venosus Q21.1
 speech R47.9
  developmental F80.9
  specified NEC R47.89
 Taussig-Bing (aortic transposition and overriding pulmonary artery) Q20.1
 teeth, wedge K03.1
 vascular (local) I99.9
  congenital Q27.9
 ventricular septal Q21.0
  concurrent with acute myocardial infarction — *see* Infarct, myocardium
  following acute myocardial infarction (current complication) I23.2
  in tetralogy of Fallot Q21.3
 vision NEC H54.7
 visual field H53.40
  bilateral
   heteronymous H53.47
   homonymous H53.46- ☑
  generalized contraction H53.48- ☑
  localized
   arcuate H53.43- ☑
   scotoma (central area) H53.41- ☑
    blind spot area H53.42- ☑
   sector H53.43- ☑
   specified type NEC H53.45- ☑
 voice R49.9
  specified NEC R49.8
 wedge, tooth, teeth (abrasion) K03.1
Deferentitis N49.1
 gonorrheal (acute) (chronic) A54.23
Defibrination (syndrome) D65
 antepartum — *see* Hemorrhage, antepartum, with coagulation defect, disseminated intravascular coagulation
 following ectopic or molar pregnancy O08.1
 intrapartum O67.0
 newborn P60
 postpartum O72.3
Deficiency, deficient
 3-beta hydroxysteroid dehydrogenase E25.0
 5-alpha reductase (with male pseudo-hermaphroditism) E29.1
 11-hydroxylase E25.0
 21-hydroxylase E25.0
 abdominal muscle syndrome Q79.4
 AC globulin (congenital) (hereditary) D68.2
  acquired D68.4
 accelerator globulin (Ac G) (blood) D68.2
 acid phosphatase E83.39
 activating factor (blood) D68.2
 adenosine deaminase (ADA) D81.3
 aldolase (hereditary) E74.19
 alpha-1-antitrypsin E88.01
 amino-acids E72.9
 anemia — *see* Anemia
 aneurin E51.9
 antibody with
  hyperimmunoglobulinemia D80.6
  near-normal immunoglobins D80.6
 antidiuretic hormone E23.2
 anti-hemophilic
  factor (A) D66
   B D67
   C D68.1
  globulin (AHG) NEC D66
 antithrombin (antithrombin III) D68.59

Deficiency, deficient — *continued*
- ascorbic acid E54
- attention (disorder) (syndrome) F98.8
  - with hyperactivity — *see* Disorder, attention-deficit hyperactivity
- autoprothrombin
  - C D68.2
  - I D68.2
  - II D67
- beta-glucuronidase E76.29
- biotin E53.8
- biotin-dependent carboxylase D81.819
- biotinidase D81.810
- brancher enzyme (amylopectinosis) E74.03
- C1 esterase inhibitor (C1-INH) D84.1
- calciferol E55.9
  - with
    - adult osteomalacia M83.8
    - rickets — *see* Rickets
- calcium (dietary) E58
- calorie, severe E43
  - with marasmus E41
    - and kwashiorkor E42
- cardiac — *see* Insufficiency, myocardial
- carnitine E71.40
  - due to
    - hemodialysis E71.43
    - inborn errors of metabolism E71.42
    - Valproic acid therapy E71.43
  - iatrogenic E71.43
  - muscle palmityltransferase E71.314
  - primary E71.41
  - secondary E71.448
- carotene E50.9
- central nervous system G96.8
- ceruloplasmin (Wilson) E83.01
- choline E53.8
- Christmas factor D67
- chromium E61.4
- clotting (blood) (*see also* Deficiency, coagulation factor) D68.9
- clotting factor NEC (hereditary) (*see also* Deficiency, factor) D68.2
- coagulation NOS D68.9
  - with
    - ectopic pregnancy O08.1
    - molar pregnancy O08.1
  - acquired (any) D68.4
  - antepartum hemorrhage — *see* Hemorrhage, antepartum, with coagulation defect
  - clotting factor NEC (*see also* Deficiency, factor) D68.2
  - due to
    - hyperprothrombinemia D68.4
    - liver disease D68.4
    - vitamin K deficiency D68.4
  - newborn, transient P61.6
  - postpartum O72.3
  - specified NEC D68.8
- cognitive F09
- color vision H53.50
  - achromatopsia H53.51
  - acquired H53.52
  - deuteranomaly H53.53
  - protanomaly H53.54
  - specified type NEC H53.59
  - tritanomaly H53.55
- combined glucocorticoid and mineralocorticoid E27.49
- contact factor D68.2
- copper (nutritional) E61.0
- corticoadrenal E27.40
  - primary E27.1
- craniofacial axis Q75.0
- cyanocobalamin E53.8
- debrancher enzyme (limit dextrinosis) E74.03
- dehydrogenase
  - long chain/very long chain acyl CoA E71.310
  - medium chain acyl CoA E71.311
  - short chain acyl CoA E71.312
- diet E63.9
- dihydropyrimidine dehydrogenase (DPD) E88.89
- disaccharidase E73.9
- edema — *see* Malnutrition, severe
- endocrine E34.9
- energy-supply — *see* Malnutrition
- enzymes, circulating NEC E88.09
- ergosterol E55.9

Deficiency, deficient — *continued*
- ergosterol — *continued*
  - with
    - adult osteomalacia M83.8
    - rickets — *see* Rickets
- essential fatty acid (EFA) E63.0
- factor (*see also* Deficiency, coagulation)
  - Hageman D68.2
  - I (congenital) (hereditary) D68.2
  - II (congenital) (hereditary) D68.2
  - IX (congenital) (functional) (hereditary) (with functional defect) D67
  - multiple (congenital) D68.8
    - acquired D68.4
  - V (congenital) (hereditary) D68.2
  - VII (congenital) (hereditary) D68.2
  - VIII (congenital) (functional) (hereditary) (with functional defect) D66
    - with vascular defect D68.0
  - X (congenital) (hereditary) D68.2
  - XI (congenital) (hereditary) D68.1
  - XII (congenital) (hereditary) D68.2
  - XIII (congenital) (hereditary) D68.2
- femoral, proximal focal (congenital) — *see* Defect, reduction, lower limb, longitudinal, femur
- fibrinase D68.2
- fibrinogen (congenital) (hereditary) D68.2
  - acquired D65
- fibrin-stabilizing factor (congenital) (hereditary) D68.2
  - acquired D68.4
- folate E53.8
- folic acid E53.8
- foreskin N47.3
- fructokinase E74.11
- fructose 1,6-diphosphatase E74.19
- fructose-1-phosphate aldolase E74.19
- galactokinase E74.29
- galactose-1-phosphate uridyl transferase E74.29
- gammaglobulin in blood D80.1
  - hereditary D80.0
- glass factor D68.2
- glucocorticoid E27.49
  - mineralocorticoid E27.49
- glucose-6-phosphatase E74.01
- glucose-6-phosphate dehydrogenase anemia D55.0
- glucuronyl transferase E80.5
- glycogen synthetase E74.09
- gonadotropin (isolated) E23.0
- growth hormone (idiopathic) (isolated) E23.0
- Hageman factor D68.2
- hemoglobin D64.9
- hepatophosphorylase E74.09
- homogentisate 1,2-dioxygenase E70.29
- hormone
  - anterior pituitary (partial) NEC E23.0
    - growth E23.0
  - growth (isolated) E23.0
  - pituitary E23.0
  - testicular E29.1
- hypoxanthine- (guanine)-phosphoribosyltransferase (HG- PRT) (total H-PRT) E79.1
- immunity D84.9
  - cell-mediated D84.8
    - with thrombocytopenia and eczema D82.0
  - combined D81.9
  - humoral D80.9
  - IgA (secretory) D80.2
  - IgG D80.3
  - IgM D80.4
- immuno — *see* Immunodeficiency
- immunoglobulin, selective
  - A (IgA) D80.2
  - G (IgG) (subclasses) D80.3
  - M (IgM) D80.4
- inositol (B complex) E53.8
- intrinsic
  - factor (congenital) D51.0
  - sphincter N36.42
    - with urethral hypermobility N36.43
- iodine E61.8
  - congenital syndrome — *see* Syndrome, iodine-deficiency, congenital
- iron E61.1
  - anemia D50.9
- kalium E87.6
- kappa-light chain D80.8
- labile factor (congenital) (hereditary) D68.2
  - acquired D68.4

Deficiency, deficient — *continued*
- lacrimal fluid (acquired) (*see also* Syndrome, dry eye)
  - congenital Q10.6
- lactase
  - congenital E73.0
  - secondary E73.1
- Laki-Lorand factor D68.2
- lecithin cholesterol acyltransferase E78.6
- lipocaic K86.89
- lipoprotein (familial) (high density) E78.6
- liver phosphorylase E74.09
- lysosomal alpha-1, 4 glucosidase E74.02
- magnesium E61.2
- major histocompatibility complex
  - class I D81.6
  - class II D81.7
- manganese E61.3
- menadione (vitamin K) E56.1
  - newborn P53
- mental (familial) (hereditary) — *see* Disability, intellectual
- methylenetetrahydrofolate reductase (MTHFR) E72.12
- mevalonate kinase M04.1
- mineralocorticoid E27.49
  - with glucocorticoid E27.49
- mineral NEC E61.8
- molybdenum (nutritional) E61.5
- moral F60.2
- multiple nutrient elements E61.7
- muscle
  - carnitine (palmityltransferase) E71.314
  - phosphofructokinase E74.09
- myoadenylate deaminase E79.2
- myocardial — *see* Insufficiency, myocardial
- myophosphorylase E74.04
- NADH diaphorase or reductase (congenital) D74.0
- NADH-methemoglobin reductase (congenital) D74.0
- natrium E87.1
- niacin (amide) (-tryptophan) E52
- nicotinamide E52
- nicotinic acid E52
- number of teeth — *see* Anodontia
- nutrient element E61.9
  - multiple E61.7
  - specified NEC E61.8
- nutrition, nutritional E63.9
  - sequelae — *see* Sequelae, nutritional deficiency
  - specified NEC E63.8
- of interleukin 1 receptor antagonist [DIRA] M04.8
- ornithine transcarbamylase E72.4
- ovarian E28.39
- oxygen — *see* Anoxia
- pantothenic acid E53.8
- parathyroid (gland) E20.9
- perineum (female) N81.89
- phenylalanine hydroxylase E70.1
- phosphoenolpyruvate carboxykinase E74.4
- phosphofructokinase E74.19
- phosphomannomutase E74.8
- phosphomannose isomerase E74.8
- phosphomannosyl mutase E74.8
- phosphorylase kinase, liver E74.09
- pituitary hormone (isolated) E23.0
- plasma thromboplastin
  - antecedent (PTA) D68.1
  - component (PTC) D67
- platelet NEC D69.1
  - constitutional D68.0
- polyglandular E31.8
  - autoimmune E31.0
- potassium (K) E87.6
- prepuce N47.3
- proaccelerin (congenital) (hereditary) D68.2
  - acquired D68.4
- proconvertin factor (congenital) (hereditary) D68.2
  - acquired D68.4
- protein (*see also* Malnutrition) E46
  - anemia D53.0
  - C D68.59
  - S D68.59
- prothrombin (congenital) (hereditary) D68.2
  - acquired D68.4
- Prower factor D68.2
- pseudocholinesterase E88.09
- PTA (plasma thromboplastin antecedent) D68.1
- PTC (plasma thromboplastin component) D67
- purine nucleoside phosphorylase (PNP) D81.5

☑ **Additional Character Required — Refer to the Tabular List for Character Selection**   ▽ **Subterms under main terms may continue to next column or page**

Deficiency, deficient — *continued*
  pyracin (alpha) (beta) E53.1
  pyridoxal E53.1
  pyridoxamine E53.1
  pyridoxine (derivatives) E53.1
  pyruvate
    carboxylase E74.4
    dehydrogenase E74.4
  riboflavin (vitamin B2) E53.0
  salt E87.1
  secretion
    ovary E28.39
    salivary gland (any) K11.7
    urine R34
  selenium (dietary) E59
  serum antitrypsin, familial E88.01
  short stature homeobox gene (SHOX)
    with
      dyschondrosteosis Q78.8
      short stature (idiopathic) E34.3
      Turner's syndrome Q96.9
  sodium (Na) E87.1
  SPCA (factor VII) D68.2
  sphincter, intrinsic N36.42
    with urethral hypermobility N36.43
  stable factor (congenital) (hereditary) D68.2
    acquired D68.4
  Stuart-Prower (factor X) D68.2
  sucrase E74.39
  sulfatase E75.29
  sulfite oxidase E72.19
  thiamin, thiaminic (chloride) E51.9
    beriberi (dry) E51.11
      wet E51.12
  thrombokinase D68.2
    newborn P53
  thyroid (gland) — *see* Hypothyroidism
  tocopherol E56.0
  tooth bud K00.0
  transcobalamine II (anemia) D51.2
  vanadium E61.6
  vascular I99.9
  vasopressin E23.2
  vertical ridge K06.8
  viosterol — *see* Deficiency, calciferol
  vitamin (multiple) NOS E56.9
    A E50.9
      with
        Bitot's spot (corneal) E50.1
        follicular keratosis E50.8
        keratomalacia E50.4
        manifestations NEC E50.8
        night blindness E50.5
        scar of cornea, xerophthalmic E50.6
        xeroderma E50.8
        xerophthalmia E50.7
        xerosis
          conjunctival E50.0
            and Bitot's spot E50.1
          cornea E50.2
            and ulceration E50.3
      sequelae E64.1
    B (complex) NOS E53.9
      with
        beriberi (dry) E51.11
          wet E51.12
        pellagra E52
    B1 NOS E51.9
      beriberi (dry) E51.11
        with circulatory system manifestations
          E51.11
        wet E51.12
    B2 (riboflavin) E53.0
    B6 E53.1
    B12 E53.8
    C E54
      sequelae E64.2
    D E55.9
      with
        adult osteomalacia M83.8
        rickets — *see* Rickets
      25-hydroxylase E83.32
    E E56.0
    folic acid E53.8
    G E53.0
    group B E53.9
      specified NEC E53.8
    H (biotin) E53.8
    K E56.1

Deficiency, deficient — *continued*
  vitamin — *continued*
    K — *continued*
      of newborn P53
    nicotinic E52
    P E56.8
    PP (pellagra-preventing) E52
    specified NEC E56.8
    thiamin E51.9
      beriberi — *see* Beriberi
  zinc, dietary E60
Deficit (*see also* Deficiency)
  attention and concentration R41.840
    disorder — *see* Attention, deficit
    following
      cerebral infarction I69.310
      cerebrovascular disease I69.910
        specified disease NEC I69.810
      nontraumatic
        intracerebral hemorrhage I69.110
        specified intracranial hemorrhage NEC
          I69.210
        subarachnoid hemorrhage I69.010
  cognitive
    communication R41.841
    emotional
      following
        cerebral infarction I69.315
        cerebrovascular disease I69.915
          specified disease NEC I69.815
        nontraumatic
          intracerebral hemorrhage I69.115
          specified intracranial hemorrhage NEC
            I69.215
          subarachnoid hemorrhage I69.015
    following
      cerebral infarction I69.319
      cerebrovascular disease I69.919
        specified disease NEC I69.819
      nontraumatic
        intracerebral hemorrhage I69.119
        specified intracranial hemorrhage NEC
          I69.219
        subarachnoid hemorrhage I69.019
    social
      following
        cerebral infarction I69.315
        cerebrovascular disease I69.915
          specified disease NEC I69.815
        nontraumatic
          intracerebral hemorrhage I69.115
          specified intracranial hemorrhage NEC
            I69.215
          subarachnoid hemorrhage I69.015
  cognitive NEC R41.89
    following
      cerebral infarction I69.318
      cerebrovascular disease I69.918
        specified disease NEC I69.818
      nontraumatic
        intracerebral hemorrhage I69.118
        specified intracranial hemorrhage NEC
          I69.218
        subarachnoid hemorrhage I69.018
  concentration R41.840
  executive function R41.844
    following
      cerebral infarction I69.314
      cerebrovascular disease I69.914
        specified disease NEC I69.814
      nontraumatic
        intracerebral hemorrhage I69.114
        specified intracranial hemorrhage NEC
          I69.214
        subarachnoid hemorrhage I69.014
  frontal lobe R41.844
    following
      cerebral infarction I69.314
      cerebrovascular disease I69.914
        specified disease NEC I69.814
      nontraumatic
        intracerebral hemorrhage I69.114
        specified intracranial hemorrhage NEC
          I69.214
        subarachnoid hemorrhage I69.014
  memory
    following
      cerebral infarction I69.311
      cerebrovascular disease I69.911

Deficit — *continued*
  memory — *continued*
    following — *continued*
      cerebrovascular disease — *continued*
        specified disease NEC I69.811
      nontraumatic
        intracerebral hemorrhage I69.111
        specified intracranial hemorrhage NEC
          I69.211
        subarachnoid hemorrhage I69.011
  neurologic NEC R29.818
    ischemic
      reversible (RIND) I63.9
      prolonged (PRIND) I63.9
  oxygen R09.02
  prolonged reversible ischemic neurologic (PRIND) I63.9
  psychomotor R41.843
    following
      cerebral infarction I69.313
      cerebrovascular disease I69.913
        specified disease NEC I69.813
      nontraumatic
        intracerebral hemorrhage I69.113
        specified intracranial hemorrhage NEC
          I69.213
        subarachnoid hemorrhage I69.013
  visuospatial R41.842
    following
      cerebral infarction I69.312
      cerebrovascular disease I69.912
        specified disease NEC I69.812
      nontraumatic
        intracerebral hemorrhage I69.112
        specified intracranial hemorrhage NEC
          I69.212
        subarachnoid hemorrhage I69.012
Deflection
  radius — *see* Deformity, limb, specified type NEC,
    forearm
  septum (acquired) (nasal) (nose) J34.2
  spine — *see* Curvature, spine
  turbinate (nose) J34.2
Defluvium
  capillorum — *see* Alopecia
  ciliorum — *see* Madarosis
  unguium L60.8
Deformity Q89.9
  abdomen, congenital Q89.9
  abdominal wall
    acquired M95.8
    congenital Q79.59
  acquired (unspecified site) M95.9
  adrenal gland Q89.1
  alimentary tract, congenital Q45.9
    upper Q40.9
  ankle (joint) (acquired) (*see also* Deformity, limb, lower
    leg)
    abduction — *see* Contraction, joint, ankle
    congenital Q68.8
    contraction — *see* Contraction, joint, ankle
    specified type NEC — *see* Deformity, limb, foot,
      specified NEC
  anus (acquired) K62.89
    congenital Q43.9
  aorta (arch) (congenital) Q25.40
    acquired I77.89
  aortic
    arch, acquired I77.89
    cusp or valve (congenital) Q23.8
      acquired (*see also* Endocarditis, aortic) I35.8
  arm (acquired) (upper) (*see also* Deformity, limb, upper
    arm)
    congenital Q68.8
    forearm — *see* Deformity, limb, forearm
  artery (congenital) (peripheral) NOS Q27.9
    acquired I77.89
    coronary (acquired) I25.9
      congenital Q24.5
    umbilical Q27.0
  atrial septal Q21.1
  auditory canal (external) (congenital) (*see also* Malfor-
    mation, ear, external)
    acquired — *see* Disorder, ear, external, specified
      type NEC
  auricle
    ear (congenital) (*see also* Malformation, ear, exter-
      nal)
      acquired — *see* Disorder, pinna, deformity

Deformity — *continued*
  back — *see* Dorsopathy, deforming
  bile duct (common) (congenital) (hepatic) Q44.5
    acquired K83.8
  biliary duct or passage (congenital) Q44.5
    acquired K83.8
  bladder (neck) (trigone) (sphincter) (acquired) N32.89
    congenital Q64.79
  bone (acquired) NOS M95.9
    congenital Q79.9
    turbinate M95.0
  brain (congenital) Q04.9
    acquired G93.89
    reduction Q04.3
  breast (acquired) N64.89
    congenital Q83.9
    reconstructed N65.0
  bronchus (congenital) Q32.4
    acquired NEC J98.09
  bursa, congenital Q79.9
  canaliculi (lacrimalis) (acquired) (*see also* Disorder,
      lacrimal system, changes)
    congenital Q10.6
  canthus, acquired — *see* Disorder, eyelid, specified
      type NEC
  capillary (acquired) I78.8
  cardiovascular system, congenital Q28.9
  caruncle, lacrimal (acquired) (*see also* Disorder, lacrimal
      system, changes)
    congenital Q10.6
  cascade, stomach K31.2
  cecum (congenital) Q43.9
    acquired K63.89
  cerebral, acquired G93.89
    congenital Q04.9
  cervix (uterus) (acquired) NEC N88.8
    congenital Q51.9
  cheek (acquired) M95.2
    congenital Q18.9
  chest (acquired) (wall) M95.4
    congenital Q67.8
    sequelae (late effect) of rickets E64.3
  chin (acquired) M95.2
    congenital Q18.9
  choroid (congenital) Q14.3
    acquired H31.8
    plexus Q07.8
      acquired G96.19
  cicatricial — *see* Cicatrix
  cilia, acquired — *see* Disorder, eyelid, specified type
      NEC
  clavicle (acquired) M95.8
    congenital Q68.8
  clitoris (congenital) Q52.6
    acquired N90.89
  clubfoot — *see* Clubfoot
  coccyx (acquired) — *see* subcategory M43.8 ☑
  colon (congenital) Q43.9
    acquired K63.89
  concha (ear), congenital (*see also* Malformation, ear,
      external)
    acquired — *see* Disorder, pinna, deformity
  cornea (acquired) H18.70
    congenital Q13.4
    descemetocele — *see* Descemetocele
    ectasia — *see* Ectasia, cornea
    specified NEC H18.79- ☑
    staphyloma — *see* Staphyloma, cornea
  coronary artery (acquired) I25.9
    congenital Q24.5
  cranium (acquired) — *see* Deformity, skull
  cricoid cartilage (congenital) Q31.8
    acquired J38.7
  cystic duct (congenital) Q44.5
    acquired K82.8
  Dandy-Walker Q03.1
    with spina bifida — *see* Spina bifida
  diaphragm (congenital) Q79.1
    acquired J98.6
  digestive organ NOS Q45.9
  ductus arteriosus Q25.0
  duodenal bulb K31.89
  duodenum (congenital) Q43.9
    acquired K31.89
  dura — *see* Deformity, meninges
  ear (acquired) (*see also* Disorder, pinna, deformity)
    congenital (external) Q17.9
      internal Q16.5

Deformity — *continued*
  ear (*see also* Disorder, pinna, deformity) — *contin-
      ued*
    congenital — *continued*
      middle Q16.4
        ossicles Q16.3
      ossicles Q16.3
  ectodermal (congenital) NEC Q84.9
  ejaculatory duct (congenital) Q55.4
    acquired N50.89
  elbow (joint) (acquired) (*see also* Deformity, limb, up-
      per arm)
    congenital Q68.8
    contraction — *see* Contraction, joint, elbow
  endocrine gland NEC Q89.2
  epididymis (congenital) Q55.4
    acquired N50.89
  epiglottis (congenital) Q31.8
    acquired J38.7
  esophagus (congenital) Q39.9
    acquired K22.8
  eustachian tube (congenital) NEC Q17.8
  eye, congenital Q15.9
  eyebrow (congenital) Q18.8
  eyelid (acquired) (*see also* Disorder, eyelid, specified
      type NEC)
    congenital Q10.3
  face (acquired) M95.2
    congenital Q18.9
  fallopian tube, acquired N83.8
  femur (acquired) — *see* Deformity, limb, specified type
      NEC, thigh
  fetal
    with fetopelvic disproportion O33.7 ☑
    causing obstructed labor O66.3
  finger (acquired) M20.00- ☑
    boutonniere M20.02- ☑
    congenital Q68.1
    flexion contracture — *see* Contraction, joint, hand
    mallet finger M20.01- ☑
    specified NEC M20.09- ☑
    swan-neck M20.03- ☑
  flexion (joint) (acquired) (*see also* Deformity, limb,
      flexion) M21.20
    congenital NOS Q74.9
      hip Q65.89
  foot (acquired) (*see also* Deformity, limb, lower leg)
    cavovarus (congenital) Q66.1
    congenital NOS Q66.9
      specified type NEC Q66.89
    specified type NEC — *see* Deformity, limb, foot,
        specified NEC
    valgus (congenital) Q66.6
      acquired — *see* Deformity, valgus, ankle
    varus (congenital) NEC Q66.3
      acquired — *see* Deformity, varus, ankle
  forearm (acquired) (*see also* Deformity, limb, forearm)
    congenital Q68.8
  forehead (acquired) M95.2
    congenital Q75.8
  frontal bone (acquired) M95.2
    congenital Q75.8
  gallbladder (congenital) Q44.1
    acquired K82.8
  gastrointestinal tract (congenital) NOS Q45.9
    acquired K63.89
  genitalia, genital organ(s) or system NEC
    female (congenital) Q52.9
      acquired N94.89
      external Q52.70
    male (congenital) Q55.9
      acquired N50.89
  globe (eye) (congenital) Q15.8
    acquired H44.89
  gum, acquired NEC K06.8
  hand (acquired) — *see* Deformity, limb, hand
    congenital Q68.1
  head (acquired) M95.2
    congenital Q75.8
  heart (congenital) Q24.9
    septum Q21.9
      auricular Q21.1
      ventricular Q21.0
    valve (congenital) NEC Q24.8
      acquired — *see* Endocarditis
  heel (acquired) — *see* Deformity, foot
  hepatic duct (congenital) Q44.5
    acquired K83.8

Deformity — *continued*
  hip (joint) (acquired) (*see also* Deformity, limb, thigh)
    congenital Q65.9
    due to (previous) juvenile osteochondrosis — *see*
        Coxa, plana
    flexion — *see* Contraction, joint, hip
  hourglass — *see* Contraction, hourglass
  humerus (acquired) M21.82- ☑
    congenital Q74.0
  hypophyseal (congenital) Q89.2
  ileocecal (coil) (valve) (acquired) K63.89
    congenital Q43.9
  ileum (congenital) Q43.9
    acquired K63.89
  ilium (acquired) M95.5
    congenital Q74.2
  integument (congenital) Q84.9
  intervertebral cartilage or disc (acquired) — *see* Disor-
      der, disc, specified NEC
  intestine (large) (small) (congenital) NOS Q43.9
    acquired K63.89
  intrinsic minus or plus (hand) — *see* Deformity, limb,
      specified type NEC, forearm
  iris (acquired) H21.89
    congenital Q13.2
  ischium (acquired) M95.5
    congenital Q74.2
  jaw (acquired) (congenital) M26.9
  joint (acquired) NEC M21.90
    congenital Q68.8
    elbow M21.92- ☑
    hand M21.94- ☑
    hip M21.95- ☑
    knee M21.96- ☑
    shoulder M21.92- ☑
    wrist M21.93- ☑
  kidney(s) (calyx) (pelvis) (congenital) Q63.9
    acquired N28.89
    artery (congenital) Q27.2
      acquired I77.89
  Klippel-Feil (brevicollis) Q76.1
  knee (acquired) NEC (*see also* Deformity, limb, lower
      leg)
    congenital Q68.2
  labium (majus) (minus) (congenital) Q52.79
    acquired N90.89
  lacrimal passages or duct (congenital) NEC Q10.6
    acquired — *see* Disorder, lacrimal system, changes
  larynx (muscle) (congenital) Q31.8
    acquired J38.7
    web (glottic) Q31.0
  leg (upper) (acquired) NEC (*see also* Deformity, limb,
      thigh)
    congenital Q68.8
    lower leg — *see* Deformity, limb, lower leg
  lens (acquired) H27.8
    congenital Q12.9
  lid (fold) (acquired) (*see also* Disorder, eyelid, specified
      type NEC)
    congenital Q10.3
  ligament (acquired) — *see* Disorder, ligament
    congenital Q79.9
  limb (acquired) M21.90
    clawfoot M21.53- ☑
    clawhand M21.51- ☑
    clubfoot M21.54- ☑
    clubhand M21.52- ☑
    congenital, except reduction deformity Q74.9
    flat foot M21.4- ☑
    flexion M21.20
      ankle M21.27- ☑
      elbow M21.22- ☑
      finger M21.24- ☑
      hip M21.25- ☑
      knee M21.26- ☑
      shoulder M21.21- ☑
      toe M21.27- ☑
      wrist M21.23- ☑
    foot
      claw — *see* Deformity, limb, clawfoot
      club — *see* Deformity, limb, clubfoot
      drop M21.37- ☑
      flat — *see* Deformity, limb, flat foot
      specified NEC M21.6X- ☑
    forearm M21.93- ☑
    hand M21.94- ☑
    lower leg M21.96- ☑

Deformity — *continued*
  limb — *continued*
    specified type NEC M21.80
      forearm M21.83- ☑
      lower leg M21.86- ☑
      thigh M21.85- ☑
      upper arm M21.82- ☑
    thigh M21.95- ☑
    unequal length M21.70
      short site is
        femur M21.75- ☑
        fibula M21.76- ☑
        humerus M21.72- ☑
        radius M21.73- ☑
        tibia M21.76- ☑
        ulna M21.73- ☑
    upper arm M21.92- ☑
    valgus — *see* Deformity, valgus
    varus — *see* Deformity, varus
    wrist drop M21.33- ☑
  lip (acquired) NEC K13.0
    congenital Q38.0
  liver (congenital) Q44.7
    acquired K76.89
  lumbosacral (congenital) (joint) (region) Q76.49
    acquired — *see* subcategory M43.8 ☑
    kyphosis — *see* Kyphosis, congenital
    lordosis — *see* Lordosis, congenital
  lung (congenital) Q33.9
    acquired J98.4
  lymphatic system, congenital Q89.9
  Madelung's (radius) Q74.0
  mandible (acquired) (congenital) M26.9
  maxilla (acquired) (congenital) M26.9
  meninges or membrane (congenital) Q07.9
    cerebral Q04.8
      acquired G96.19
    spinal cord (congenital) G96.19
      acquired G96.19
  metacarpus (acquired) — *see* Deformity, limb, forearm
    congenital Q74.0
  metatarsus (acquired) — *see* Deformity, foot
    congenital Q66.9
  middle ear (congenital) Q16.4
    ossicles Q16.3
  mitral (leaflets) (valve) I05.8
    parachute Q23.2
    stenosis, congenital Q23.2
  mouth (acquired) K13.79
    congenital Q38.6
  multiple, congenital NEC Q89.7
  muscle (acquired) M62.89
    congenital Q79.9
      sternocleidomastoid Q68.0
  musculoskeletal system (acquired) M95.9
    congenital Q79.9
    specified NEC M95.8
  nail (acquired) L60.8
    congenital Q84.6
  nasal — *see* Deformity, nose
  neck (acquired) M95.3
    congenital Q18.9
      sternocleidomastoid Q68.0
  nervous system (congenital) Q07.9
  nipple (congenital) Q83.9
    acquired N64.89
  nose (acquired) (cartilage) M95.0
    bone (turbinate) M95.0
    congenital Q30.9
      bent or squashed Q67.4
    saddle M95.0
      syphilitic A50.57
    septum (acquired) J34.2
      congenital Q30.8
    sinus (wall) (congenital) Q30.8
      acquired M95.0
    syphilitic (congenital) A50.57
      late A52.73
  ocular muscle (congenital) Q10.3
    acquired — *see* Strabismus, mechanical
  opticociliary vessels (congenital) Q13.2
  orbit (eye) (acquired) H05.30
    atrophy — *see* Atrophy, orbit
    congenital Q10.7
    due to
      bone disease NEC H05.32- ☑
      trauma or surgery H05.33- ☑
    enlargement — *see* Enlargement, orbit

Deformity — *continued*
  orbit — *continued*
    exostosis — *see* Exostosis, orbit
  organ of Corti (congenital) Q16.5
  ovary (congenital) Q50.39
    acquired N83.8
  oviduct, acquired N83.8
  palate (congenital) Q38.5
    acquired M27.8
    cleft (congenital) — *see* Cleft, palate
  pancreas (congenital) Q45.3
    acquired K86.89
  parathyroid (gland) Q89.2
  parotid (gland) (congenital) Q38.4
    acquired K11.8
  patella (acquired) — *see* Disorder, patella, specified
    NEC
  pelvis, pelvic (acquired) (bony) M95.5
    with disproportion (fetopelvic) O33.0
      causing obstructed labor O65.0
    congenital Q74.2
    rachitic sequelae (late effect) E64.3
  penis (glans) (congenital) Q55.69
    acquired N48.89
  pericardium (congenital) Q24.8
    acquired — *see* Pericarditis
  pharynx (congenital) Q38.8
    acquired J39.2
  pinna, acquired (*see also* Disorder, pinna, deformity)
    congenital Q17.9
  pituitary (congenital) Q89.2
  posture — *see* Dorsopathy, deforming
  prepuce (congenital) Q55.69
    acquired N47.8
  prostate (congenital) Q55.4
    acquired N42.89
  pupil (congenital) Q13.2
    acquired — *see* Abnormality, pupillary
  pylorus (congenital) Q40.3
    acquired K31.89
  rachitic (acquired), old or healed E64.3
  radius (acquired) (*see also* Deformity, limb, forearm)
    congenital Q68.8
  rectum (congenital) Q43.9
    acquired K62.89
  reduction (extremity) (limb), congenital (*see also* condition and site) Q73.8
    brain Q04.3
    lower — *see* Defect, reduction, lower limb
    upper — *see* Defect, reduction, upper limb
  renal — *see* Deformity, kidney
  respiratory system (congenital) Q34.9
  rib (acquired) M95.4
    congenital Q76.6
    cervical Q76.5
  rotation (joint) (acquired) — *see* Deformity, limb, specified site NEC
    congenital Q74.9
    hip — *see* Deformity, limb, specified type NEC, thigh
      congenital Q65.89
  sacroiliac joint (congenital) — *see* subcategory Q74.2
    acquired — *see* subcategory M43.8 ☑
  sacrum (acquired) — *see* subcategory M43.8 ☑
  saddle
    back — *see* Lordosis
    nose M95.0
      syphilitic A50.57
  salivary gland or duct (congenital) Q38.4
    acquired K11.8
  scapula (acquired) M95.8
    congenital Q68.8
  scrotum (congenital) (*see also* Malformation, testis and scrotum)
    acquired N50.89
  seminal vesicles (congenital) Q55.4
    acquired N50.89
  septum, nasal (acquired) J34.2
  shoulder (joint) (acquired) — *see* Deformity, limb, upper arm
    congenital Q74.0
    contraction — *see* Contraction, joint, shoulder
  sigmoid (flexure) (congenital) Q43.9
    acquired K63.89
  skin (congenital) Q82.9
  skull (acquired) M95.2
    congenital Q75.8

Deformity — *continued*
  skull — *continued*
    congenital — *continued*
      with
        anencephaly Q00.0
        encephalocele — *see* Encephalocele
        hydrocephalus Q03.9
          with spina bifida — *see* Spina bifida, by site, with hydrocephalus
        microcephaly Q02
  soft parts, organs or tissues (of pelvis)
    in pregnancy or childbirth NEC O34.8- ☑
      causing obstructed labor O65.5
  spermatic cord (congenital) Q55.4
    acquired N50.89
    torsion — *see* Torsion, spermatic cord
  spinal — *see* Dorsopathy, deforming
    column (acquired) — *see* Dorsopathy, deforming
      congenital Q67.5
    cord (congenital) Q06.9
      acquired G95.89
    nerve root (congenital) Q07.9
  spine (acquired) (*see also* Dorsopathy, deforming)
    congenital Q67.5
    rachitic E64.3
    specified NEC — *see* Dorsopathy, deforming, specified NEC
  spleen
    acquired D73.89
    congenital Q89.09
  Sprengel's (congenital) Q74.0
  sternocleidomastoid (muscle), congenital Q68.0
  sternum (acquired) M95.4
    congenital NEC Q76.7
  stomach (congenital) Q40.3
    acquired K31.89
  submandibular gland (congenital) Q38.4
  submaxillary gland (congenital) Q38.4
    acquired K11.8
  talipes — *see* Talipes
  testis (congenital) (*see also* Malformation, testis and scrotum)
    acquired N44.8
    torsion — *see* Torsion, testis
  thigh (acquired) (*see also* Deformity, limb, thigh)
    congenital NEC Q68.8
  thorax (acquired) (wall) M95.4
    congenital Q67.8
    sequelae of rickets E64.3
  thumb (acquired) (*see also* Deformity, finger)
    congenital NEC Q68.1
  thymus (tissue) (congenital) Q89.2
  thyroid (gland) (congenital) Q89.2
    cartilage Q31.8
      acquired J38.7
  tibia (acquired) (*see also* Deformity, limb, specified type NEC, lower leg)
    congenital NEC Q68.8
    saber (syphilitic) A50.56
  toe (acquired) M20.6- ☑
    congenital Q66.9
    hallux rigidus M20.2- ☑
    hallux valgus M20.1- ☑
    hallux varus M20.3- ☑
    hammer toe M20.4- ☑
    specified NEC M20.5X- ☑
  tongue (congenital) Q38.3
    acquired K14.8
  tooth, teeth K00.2
  trachea (rings) (congenital) Q32.1
    acquired J39.8
  transverse aortic arch (congenital) Q25.49
  tricuspid (leaflets) (valve) I07.8
    atresia or stenosis Q22.4
    Ebstein's Q22.5
  trunk (acquired) M95.8
    congenital Q89.9
  ulna (acquired) (*see also* Deformity, limb, forearm)
    congenital NEC Q68.8
  urachus, congenital Q64.4
  ureter (opening) (congenital) Q62.8
    acquired N28.89
  urethra (congenital) Q64.79
    acquired N36.8
  urinary tract (congenital) Q64.9
    urachus Q64.4
  uterus (congenital) Q51.9
    acquired N85.8

Deformity — *continued*
uvula (congenital) Q38.5
vagina (acquired) N89.8
congenital Q52.4
valgus NEC M21.00
ankle M21.07- ☑
elbow M21.02- ☑
hip M21.05- ☑
knee M21.06- ☑
valve, valvular (congenital) (heart) Q24.8
acquired — *see* Endocarditis
varus NEC M21.10
ankle M21.17- ☑
elbow M21.12- ☑
hip M21.15 ☑
knee M21.16- ☑
tibia — *see* Osteochondrosis, juvenile, tibia
vas deferens (congenital) Q55.4
acquired N50.89
vein (congenital) Q27.9
great Q26.9
vertebra — *see* Dorsopathy, deforming
vertical talus (congenital) Q66.80
left foot Q66.82
right foot Q66.81
vesicourethral orifice (acquired) N32.89
congenital NEC Q64.79
vessels of optic papilla (congenital) Q14.2
visual field (contraction) — *see* Defect, visual field
vitreous body, acquired H43.89
vulva (congenital) Q52.79
acquired N90.89
wrist (joint) (acquired) (*see also* Deformity, limb, forearm)
congenital Q68.8
contraction — *see* Contraction, joint, wrist
Degeneration, degenerative
adrenal (capsule) (fatty) (gland) (hyaline) (infectional)
E27.8
amyloid (*see also* Amyloidosis) E85.9
anterior cornua, spinal cord G12.29
anterior labral S43.49- ☑
aorta, aortic I70.0
fatty I77.89
aortic valve (heart) — *see* Endocarditis, aortic
arteriovascular — *see* Arteriosclerosis
artery, arterial (atheromatous) (calcareous) (*see also*
Arteriosclerosis)
cerebral, amyloid E85.4 [I68.0]
medial — *see* Arteriosclerosis, extremities
articular cartilage NEC — *see* Derangement, joint, articular cartilage, by site
atheromatous — *see* Arteriosclerosis
basal nuclei or ganglia G23.9
specified NEC G23.8
bone NEC — *see* Disorder, bone, specified type NEC
brachial plexus G54.0
brain (cortical) (progressive) G31.9
alcoholic G31.2
arteriosclerotic I67.2
childhood G31.9
specified NEC G31.89
cystic G31.89
congenital Q04.6
in
alcoholism G31.2
beriberi E51.2
cerebrovascular disease I67.9
congenital hydrocephalus Q03.9
with spina bifida (*see also* Spina bifida)
Fabry-Anderson disease E75.21
Gaucher's disease E75.22
Hunter's syndrome E76.1
lipidosis
cerebral E75.4
generalized E75.6
mucopolysaccharidosis — *see* Mucopolysaccharidosis
myxedema E03.9 [G32.89]
neoplastic disease (*see also* Neoplasm)
D49.6 [G32.89]
Niemann-Pick disease E75.249 [G32.89]
sphingolipidosis E75.3 [G32.89]
vitamin B12 deficiency E53.8 [G32.89]
senile NEC G31.1
breast N64.89
Bruch's membrane — *see* Degeneration, choroid
capillaries (fatty) I78.8

Degeneration, degenerative — *continued*
capillaries (fatty) I78.8
amyloid E85.89 [I79.8]
cardiac (*see also* Degeneration, myocardial)
valve, valvular — *see* Endocarditis
cardiorenal — *see* Hypertension, cardiorenal
cardiovascular (*see also* Disease, cardiovascular)
renal — *see* Hypertension, cardiorenal
cerebellar NOS G31.9
alcoholic G31.2
primary (hereditary) (sporadic) G11.9
cerebral — *see* Degeneration, brain
cerebrovascular I67.9
due to hypertension I67.4
cervical plexus G54.2
cervix N88.8
due to radiation (intended effect) N88.8
adverse effect or misadventure N99.89
chamber angle H21.21- ☑
changes, spine or vertebra — *see* Spondylosis
chorioretinal (*see also* Degeneration, choroid)
hereditary H31.20
choroid (colloid) (drusen) H31.10- ☑
atrophy — *see* Atrophy, choroidal
hereditary — *see* Dystrophy, choroidal, hereditary
ciliary body H21.22- ☑
cochlear — *see* subcategory H83.8 ☑
combined (spinal cord) (subacute) E53.8 [G32.0]
with anemia (pernicious) D51.0 [G32.0]
due to dietary vitamin B12 deficiency
D51.3 [G32.0]
in (due to)
vitamin B12 deficiency E53.8 [G32.0]
anemia D51.9 [G32.0]
conjunctiva H11.10
concretions — *see* Concretion, conjunctiva
deposits — *see* Deposit, conjunctiva
pigmentations — *see* Pigmentation, conjunctiva
pinguecula — *see* Pinguecula
xerosis — *see* Xerosis, conjunctiva
cornea H18.40
calcerous H18.43
band keratopathy H18.42- ☑
familial, hereditary — *see* Dystrophy, cornea
hyaline (of old scars) H18.49
keratomalacia — *see* Keratomalacia
nodular H18.45- ☑
peripheral H18.46- ☑
senile H18.41- ☑
specified type NEC H18.49
cortical (cerebellar) (parenchymatous) G31.89
alcoholic G31.2
diffuse, due to arteriopathy I67.2
corticobasal G31.85
cutis L98.8
amyloid E85.4 [L99]
dental pulp K04.2
disc disease — *see* Degeneration, intervertebral disc
NEC
dorsolateral (spinal cord) — *see* Degeneration, combined
extrapyramidal G25.9
eye, macular (*see also* Degeneration, macula)
congenital or hereditary — *see* Dystrophy, retina
facet joints — *see* Spondylosis
fatty
liver NEC K76.0
alcoholic K70.0
grey matter (brain) (Alpers') G31.81
heart (*see also* Degeneration, myocardial)
amyloid E85.4 [I43]
atheromatous — *see* Disease, heart, ischemic,
atherosclerotic
ischemic — *see* Disease, heart, ischemic
hepatolenticular (Wilson's) E83.01
hepatorenal K76.7
hyaline (diffuse) (generalized)
localized — *see* Degeneration, by site
infrapatellar fat pad M79.4
intervertebral disc NOS
with
myelopathy — *see* Disorder, disc, with,
myelopathy
radiculitis or radiculopathy — *see* Disorder, disc,
with, radiculopathy
cervical, cervicothoracic — *see* Disorder, disc, cervical, degeneration

Degeneration, degenerative — *continued*
intervertebral disc — *continued*
cervical, cervicothoracic — *see* Disorder, disc, cervical, degeneration — *continued*
with
myelopathy — *see* Disorder, disc, cervical,
with myelopathy
neuritis, radiculitis or radiculopathy — *see*
Disorder, disc, cervical, with neuritis
lumbar region M51.36
with
myelopathy M51.06
neuritis, radiculitis, radiculopathy or sciatica
M51.16
lumbosacral region M51.37
with
neuritis, radiculitis, radiculopathy or sciatica
M51.17
sacrococcygeal region M53.3
thoracic region M51.34
with
myelopathy M51.04
neuritis, radiculitis, radiculopathy M51.14
thoracolumbar region M51.35
with
myelopathy M51.05
neuritis, radiculitis, radiculopathy M51.15
intestine, amyloid E85.4
iris (pigmentary) H21.23- ☑
ischemic — *see* Ischemia
joint disease — *see* Osteoarthritis
kidney N28.89
amyloid E85.4 [N29]
cystic, congenital Q61.9
fatty N28.89
polycystic Q61.3
adult type (autosomal dominant) Q61.2
infantile type (autosomal recessive) NEC Q61.19
collecting duct dilatation Q61.11
Kuhnt-Junius (*see also* Degeneration, macula)
H35.32- ☑
lens — *see* Cataract
lenticular (familial) (progressive) (Wilson's) (with cirrhosis of liver) E83.01
liver (diffuse) NEC K76.89
amyloid E85.4 [K77]
cystic K76.89
congenital Q44.6
fatty NEC K76.0
alcoholic K70.0
hypertrophic K76.89
parenchymatous, acute or subacute K72.00
with coma K72.01
pigmentary K76.89
toxic (acute) K71.9
lung J98.4
lymph gland I89.8
hyaline I89.8
macula, macular (acquired) (age-related) (senile)
H35.30
angioid streaks H35.33
atrophic age-related H35.31- ☑
congenital or hereditary — *see* Dystrophy, retina
cystoid H35.35- ☑
drusen H35.36- ☑
dry age-related H35.31- ☑
exudative H35.32- ☑
hole H35.34- ☑
nonexudative H35.31- ☑
puckering H35.37- ☑
toxic H35.38- ☑
wet age-related H35.32- ☑
membranous labyrinth, congenital (causing impairment of hearing) Q16.5
meniscus — *see* Derangement, meniscus
mitral — *see* Insufficiency, mitral
Mönckeberg's — *see* Arteriosclerosis, extremities
motor centers, senile G31.1
multi-system G90.3
mural — *see* Degeneration, myocardial
muscle (fatty) (fibrous) (hyaline) (progressive) M62.89
heart — *see* Degeneration, myocardial
myelin, central nervous system G37.9
myocardial, myocardium (fatty) (hyaline) (senile) I51.5
with rheumatic fever (conditions in I00) I09.0
active, acute or subacute I01.2
with chorea I02.0
inactive or quiescent (with chorea) I09.0

☑ **Additional Character Required — Refer to the Tabular List for Character Selection** � Subterms under main terms may continue to next column or page

Degeneration, degenerative — *continued*
  myocardial, myocardium — *continued*
    hypertensive — *see* Hypertension, heart
    rheumatic — *see* Degeneration, myocardial, with
      rheumatic fever
    syphilitic A52.06
  nasal sinus (mucosa) J32.9
    frontal J32.1
    maxillary J32.0
  nerve — *see* Disorder, nerve
  nervous system G31.9
    alcoholic G31.2
    amyloid E85.4 [G99.8]
    autonomic G90.9
    fatty G31.89
    specified NEC G31.89
  nipple N64.89
  olivopontocerebellar (hereditary) (familial) G23.8
  osseous labyrinth — *see* subcategory H83.8 ☑
  ovary N83.8
    cystic N83.20- ☑
    microcystic N83.20- ☑
  pallidal pigmentary (progressive) G23.0
  pancreas K86.89
    tuberculous A18.83
  penis N48.89
  pigmentary (diffuse) (general)
    localized — *see* Degeneration, by site
    pallidal (progressive) G23.0
  pineal gland E34.8
  pituitary (gland) E23.6
  popliteal fat pad M79.4
  posterolateral (spinal cord) — *see* Degeneration,
    combined
  pulmonary valve (heart) I37.8
  pulp (tooth) K04.2
  pupillary margin H21.24- ☑
  renal — *see* Degeneration, kidney
  retina H35.9
    hereditary (cerebroretinal) (congenital) (juvenile)
      (macula) (peripheral) (pigmentary) — *see*
      Dystrophy, retina
    Kuhnt-Junius (*see also* Degeneration, macula)
      H35.32- ☑
    macula (cystic) (exudative) (hole) (nonexudative)
      (pseudohole) (senile) (toxic) — *see* Degener-
      ation, macula
    peripheral H35.40
      lattice H35.41- ☑
      microcystoid H35.42- ☑
      paving stone H35.43- ☑
      secondary
        pigmentary H35.45- ☑
        vitreoretinal H35.46- ☑
      senile reticular H35.44- ☑
    pigmentary (primary) (*see also* Dystrophy, retina)
      secondary — *see* Degeneration, retina, periph-
      eral, secondary
    posterior pole — *see* Degeneration, macula
  saccule, congenital (causing impairment of hearing)
    Q16.5
  senile R54
    brain G31.1
    cardiac, heart or myocardium — *see* Degeneration,
      myocardial
    motor centers G31.1
    vascular — *see* Arteriosclerosis
  sinus (cystic) (*see also* Sinusitis)
    polypoid J33.1
  skin L98.8
    amyloid E85.4 [L99]
    colloid L98.8
  spinal (cord) G31.89
    amyloid E85.4 [G32.89]
    combined (subacute) — *see* Degeneration, com-
      bined
    dorsolateral — *see* Degeneration, combined
    familial NEC G31.89
    fatty G31.89
    funicular — *see* Degeneration, combined
    posterolateral — *see* Degeneration, combined
    subacute combined — *see* Degeneration, com-
      bined
    tuberculous A17.81
  spleen D73.0
    amyloid E85.4 [D77]
  stomach K31.89
  striatonigral G23.2

Degeneration, degenerative — *continued*
  suprarenal (capsule) (gland) E27.8
  synovial membrane (pulpy) — *see* Disorder, synovium,
    specified type NEC
  tapetoretinal — *see* Dystrophy, retina
  thymus (gland) E32.8
    fatty E32.8
  thyroid (gland) E07.89
  tricuspid (heart) (valve) I07.9
  tuberculous NEC — *see* Tuberculosis
  turbinate J34.89
  uterus (cystic) N85.8
  vascular (senile) — *see* Arteriosclerosis
    hypertensive — *see* Hypertension
  vitreoretinal, secondary — *see* Degeneration, retina,
    peripheral, secondary, vitreoretinal
  vitreous (body) H43.81- ☑
  Wallerian — *see* Disorder, nerve
  Wilson's hepatolenticular E83.01
Deglutition
  paralysis R13.0
    hysterical F44.4
  pneumonia J69.0
Degos' disease I77.89
Dehiscence (of)
  amputation stump T87.81
  cesarean wound O90.0
  closure of
    cornea T81.31 ☑
    craniotomy T81.32 ☑
    fascia (muscular) (superficial) T81.32 ☑
    internal organ or tissue T81.32 ☑
    laceration (external) (internal) T81.33 ☑
    ligament T81.32 ☑
    mucosa T81.31 ☑
    muscle or muscle flap T81.32 ☑
    ribs or rib cage T81.32 ☑
    skin and subcutaneous tissue (full-thickness) (su-
      perficial) T81.31 ☑
    skull T81.32 ☑
    sternum (sternotomy) T81.32 ☑
    tendon T81.32 ☑
    traumatic laceration (external) (internal) T81.33 ☑
  episiotomy O90.1
  operation wound NEC T81.31 ☑
    external operation wound (superficial) T81.31 ☑
    internal operation wound (deep) T81.32 ☑
  perineal wound (postpartum) O90.1
  traumatic injury wound repair T81.33 ☑
  wound T81.30 ☑
    traumatic repair T81.33 ☑
Dehydration E86.0
  newborn P74.1
Déjérine-Roussy syndrome G89.0
Déjérine-Sottas disease or neuropathy (hypertrophic)
  G60.0
Déjérine-Thomas atrophy G23.8
Delay, delayed
  any plane in pelvis
    complicating delivery O66.9
  birth or delivery NOS O63.9
  closure, ductus arteriosus (Botalli) P29.38
  coagulation — *see* Defect, coagulation
  conduction (cardiac) (ventricular) I45.9
  delivery, second twin, triplet, etc O63.2
  development R62.50
    global F88
    intellectual (specific) F81.9
    language F80.9
      due to hearing loss F80.4
    learning F81.9
    pervasive F84.9
    physiological R62.50
      specified stage NEC R62.0
    reading F81.0
    sexual E30.0
    speech F80.9
      due to hearing loss F80.4
    spelling F81.81
  ejaculation F52.32
  gastric emptying K30
  menarche E30.0
  menstruation (cause unknown) N91.0
  milestone R62.0
  passage of meconium (newborn) P76.0
  primary respiration P28.9
  puberty (constitutional) E30.0

Delay, delayed — *continued*
  separation of umbilical cord P96.82
  sexual maturation, female E30.0
  sleep phase syndrome G47.21
  union, fracture — *see* Fracture, by site
  vaccination Z28.9
Deletion(s)
  autosome Q93.9
    identified by fluorescence in situ hybridization
      (FISH) Q93.89
    identified by in situ hybridization (ISH) Q93.89
  chromosome
    with complex rearrangements NEC Q93.7
    part of NEC Q93.5
    seen only at prometaphase Q93.89
    short arm
      22q11.2 Q93.81
      4 Q93.3
      5p Q93.4
    specified NEC Q93.89
  long arm chromosome 18 or 21 Q93.89
    with complex rearrangements NEC Q93.7
  microdeletions NEC Q93.88
Delhi boil or button B55.1
Delinquency (juvenile) (neurotic) F91.8
  group Z72.810
Delinquent immunization status Z28.3
Delirium, delirious (acute or subacute) (not alcohol- or
  drug-induced) (with dementia) R41.0
  alcoholic (acute) (tremens) (withdrawal) F10.921
    with intoxication F10.921
      in
        abuse F10.121
        dependence F10.221
  due to (secondary to)
    alcohol
      intoxication F10.921
        in
          abuse F10.121
          dependence F10.221
      withdrawal F10.231
    amphetamine intoxication F15.921
      in
        abuse F15.121
        dependence F15.221
    anxiolytic
      intoxication F13.921
        in
          abuse F13.121
          dependence F13.221
      withdrawal F13.231
    cannabis intoxication (acute) F12.921
      in
        abuse F12.121
        dependence F12.221
    cocaine intoxication (acute) F14.921
      in
        abuse F14.121
        dependence F14.221
    general medical condition F05
    hallucinogen intoxication F16.921
      in
        abuse F16.121
        dependence F16.221
    hypnotic
      intoxication F13.921
        in
          abuse F13.121
          dependence F13.221
      withdrawal F13.231
    inhalant intoxication (acute) F18.921
      in
        abuse F18.121
        dependence F18.221
    multiple etiologies F05
    opioid intoxication (acute) F11.921
      in
        abuse F11.121
        dependence F11.221
    other (or unknown) substance F19.921
    phencyclidine intoxication (acute) F16.921
      in
        abuse F16.121
        dependence F16.221
    psychoactive substance NEC intoxication (acute)
      F19.921
      in
        abuse F19.121
        dependence F19.221

Delirium, delirious — *continued*
  due to — *continued*
    sedative
      intoxication F13.921
        in
          abuse F13.121
          dependence F13.221
      withdrawal F13.231
    unknown etiology F05
  exhaustion F43.0
  hysterical F44.89
  postprocedural (postoperative) F05
  puerperal F05
  thyroid — *see* Thyrotoxicosis with thyroid storm
  traumatic — *see* Injury, intracranial
  tremens (alcohol-induced) F10.231
    sedative-induced F13.231
Delivery (childbirth) (labor)
  arrested active phase O62.1
  cesarean (for)
    without indication O82
    abnormal
      pelvis (bony) (deformity) (major) NEC with dis-
        proportion (fetopelvic) O33.0
        with obstructed labor O65.0
      presentation or position O32.9 ☑
    abruptio placentae (*see also* Abruptio placentae)
      O45.9- ☑
    acromion presentation O32.2 ☑
    atony, uterus O62.2
    breech presentation O32.1 ☑
      incomplete O32.8 ☑
    brow presentation O32.3 ☑
    cephalopelvic disproportion O33.9
    cerclage O34.3- ☑
    chin presentation O32.3 ☑
    cicatrix of cervix O34.4- ☑
    contracted pelvis (general)
      inlet O33.2
      outlet O33.3
    cord presentation or prolapse O69.0 ☑
    cystocele O34.8- ☑
    deformity (acquired) (congenital)
      pelvic organs or tissues NEC O34.8- ☑
      pelvis (bony) NEC O33.0
    disproportion NOS O33.9
    eclampsia — *see* Eclampsia
    face presentation O32.3 ☑
    failed
      forceps O66.5
      induction of labor O61.9
        instrumental O61.1
        mechanical O61.1
        medical O61.0
        specified NEC O61.8
        surgical O61.1
      trial of labor NOS O66.40
        following previous cesarean delivery O66.41
      vacuum extraction O66.5
      ventouse O66.5
    fetal-maternal hemorrhage O43.01- ☑
    hemorrhage (intrapartum) O67.9
      with coagulation defect O67.0
      specified cause NEC O67.8
    high head at term O32.4 ☑
    hydrocephalic fetus O33.6 ☑
    incarceration of uterus O34.51- ☑
    incoordinate uterine action O62.4
    increased size, fetus O33.5 ☑
    inertia, uterus O62.2
      primary O62.0
      secondary O62.1
    lateroversion, uterus O34.59- ☑
    mal lie O32.9 ☑
    malposition
      fetus O32.9 ☑
      pelvic organs or tissues NEC O34.8- ☑
      uterus NEC O34.59- ☑
    malpresentation NOS O32.9 ☑
    oblique presentation O32.2 ☑
    occurring after 37 completed weeks of gestation
      but before 39 completed weeks gestation
      due to (spontaneous) onset of labor O75.82
    oversize fetus O33.5 ☑
    pelvic tumor NEC O34.8- ☑
    placenta previa O44.0- ☑
      complete O44.0- ☑

Delivery — *continued*
  cesarean — *continued*
    placenta previa — *continued*
      complete — *continued*
        with hemorrhage O44.1- ☑
    placental insufficiency O36.51- ☑
    planned, occurring after 37 completed weeks of
      gestation but before 39 completed weeks
      gestation due to (spontaneous) onset of la-
      bor O75.82
    polyp, cervix O34.4- ☑
      causing obstructed labor O65.5
    poor dilatation, cervix O62.0
    pre-eclampsia O14.94
      mild O14.04
      moderate O14.04
      severe O14.14
        with hemolysis, elevated liver enzymes and
          low platelet count (HELLP) O14.24
    previous
      cesarean delivery O34.219
        classical (vertical) scar O34.212
        low transverse scar O34.211
      surgery (to)
        cervix O34.4- ☑
        gynecological NEC O34.8- ☑
        rectum O34.7- ☑
        uterus O34.29
        vagina O34.6- ☑
    prolapse
      arm or hand O32.2 ☑
      uterus O34.52- ☑
    prolonged labor NOS O63.9
    rectocele O34.8- ☑
    retroversion
      uterus O34.53- ☑
    rigid
      cervix O34.4- ☑
      pelvic floor O34.8- ☑
      perineum O34.7- ☑
      vagina O34.6- ☑
      vulva O34.7- ☑
    sacculation, pregnant uterus O34.59- ☑
    scar(s)
      cervix O34.4- ☑
      cesarean delivery O34.219
        classical (vertical) O34.212
        low transverse O34.211
      transmural uterine O34.29
      uterus O34.29
    Shirodkar suture in situ O34.3- ☑
    shoulder presentation O32.2 ☑
    stenosis or stricture, cervix O34.4- ☑
    streptococcus group B (GBS) carrier state O99.824
    transmural uterine scar O34.29
    transverse presentation or lie O32.2 ☑
    tumor, pelvic organs or tissues NEC O34.8- ☑
      cervix O34.4- ☑
    umbilical cord presentation or prolapse O69.0 ☑
  completely normal case O80
  complicated O75.9
    by
      abnormal, abnormality (of)
        forces of labor O62.9
          specified type NEC O62.8
        glucose O99.814
        uterine contractions NOS O62.9
      abruptio placentae (*see also* Abruptio placen-
        tae) O45.9- ☑
      abuse
        physical O9A.32 (*following* O99)
        psychological O9A.52 (*following* O99)
        sexual O9A.42 (*following* O99)
      adherent placenta O72.0
        without hemorrhage O73.0
      alcohol use O99.314
      anemia (pre-existing) O99.02
      anesthetic death O74.8
      annular detachment of cervix O71.3
      atony, uterus O62.2
      attempted vacuum extraction and forceps
        O66.5
      Bandl's ring O62.4
      bariatric surgery status O99.844
      biliary tract disorder O26.62
      bleeding — *see* Delivery, complicated by,
        hemorrhage
      blood disorder NEC O99.12

Delivery — *continued*
  complicated — *continued*
    by — *continued*
      cervical dystocia (hypotonic) O62.2
        primary O62.0
        secondary O62.1
      circulatory system disorder O99.42
      compression of cord (umbilical) NEC O69.2 ☑
      condition NEC O99.89
      contraction, contracted ring O62.4
      cord (umbilical)
        around neck
          with compression O69.1 ☑
          without compression O69.81 ☑
        bruising O69.5 ☑
        complication O69.9 ☑
          specified NEC O69.89 ☑
        compression NEC O69.2 ☑
        entanglement O69.2 ☑
          without compression O69.82 ☑
        hematoma O69.5 ☑
        presentation O69.0 ☑
        prolapse O69.0 ☑
        short O69.3 ☑
        thrombosis (vessels) O69.5 ☑
        vascular lesion O69.5 ☑
      Couvelaire uterus O45.8X- ☑
      damage to (injury to) NEC
        perineum O71.82
        periurethral tissue O71.82
        vulva O71.82
      delay following rupture of membranes (sponta-
        neous) — *see* Pregnancy, complicated
        by, premature rupture of membranes
      depressed fetal heart tones O76
      diabetes O24.92
        gestational O24.429
          diet controlled O24.420
          insulin controlled O24.424
          oral drug controlled (antidiabetic) (hypo-
            glycemic) O24.425
        pre-existing O24.32
          specified NEC O24.82
          type 1 O24.02
          type 2 O24.12
      diastasis recti (abdominis) O71.89
      dilatation
        bladder O66.8
        cervix incomplete, poor or slow O62.0
      disease NEC O99.89
      disruptio uteri — *see* Delivery, complicated by,
        rupture, uterus
      drug use O99.324
      dysfunction, uterus NOS O62.9
        hypertonic O62.4
        hypotonic O62.2
          primary O62.0
          secondary O62.1
        incoordinate O62.4
      eclampsia O15.1
      embolism (pulmonary) — *see* Embolism, obstet-
        ric
      endocrine, nutritional or metabolic disease NEC
        O99.284
      failed
        attempted vaginal birth after previous ce-
          sarean delivery O66.41
        induction of labor O61.9
          instrumental O61.1
          mechanical O61.1
          medical O61.0
          specified NEC O61.8
          surgical O61.1
        trial of labor O66.40
      female genital mutilation O65.5
      fetal
        abnormal acid-base balance O68
        acidemia O68
        acidosis O68
        alkalosis O68
        death, early O02.1
        deformity O66.3
        heart rate or rhythm (abnormal) (non-reas-
          suring) O76
        hypoxia O77.8
        stress O77.9
          due to drug administration O77.1
          electrocardiographic evidence of O77.8

☑ **Additional Character Required** — **Refer to the Tabular List for Character Selection**   ▽ **Subterms under main terms may continue to next column or page**

Delivery — *continued*
  complicated — *continued*
    by — *continued*
      fetal — *continued*
        stress — *continued*
          specified NEC O77.8
          ultrasound evidence of O77.8
      fever during labor O75.2
      gastric banding status O99.844
      gastric bypass status O99.844
      gastrointestinal disease NEC O99.62
      gestational
        diabetes O24.429
          diet controlled O24.420
          insulin (and diet) controlled O24.424
          oral drug controlled (antidiabetic) (hypo-
            glycemic) O24.425
        edema O12.04
          with proteinuria O12.24
        proteinuria O12.14
      gonorrhea O98.22
      hematoma O71.7
        ischial spine O71.7
        pelvic O71.7
        vagina O71.7
        vulva or perineum O71.7
      hemorrhage (uterine) O67.9
        associated with
          afibrinogenemia O67.0
          coagulation defect O67.0
          hyperfibrinolysis O67.0
          hypofibrinogenemia O67.0
        due to
          low implantation of placenta O44.5- ☑
          low-lying placenta O44.5- ☑
          placenta previa O44.1- ☑
            marginal O44.3- ☑
            partial O44.3- ☑
          premature separation of placenta (nor-
            mally implanted) (*see also* Abrup-
            tio placentae) O45.9- ☑
          retained placenta O72.0
          uterine leiomyoma O67.8
        placenta NEC O67.8
        postpartum NEC (atonic) (immediate) O72.1
          with retained or trapped placenta O72.0
          delayed O72.2
          secondary O72.2
          third stage O72.0
      hourglass contraction, uterus O62.4
      hypertension, hypertensive (pre-existing) —
        see Hypertension, complicated by, child-
        birth (labor)
      hypotension O26.5- ☑
      incomplete dilatation (cervix) O62.0
      incoordinate uterus contractions O62.4
      inertia, uterus O62.2
        during latent phase of labor O62.0
        primary O62.0
        secondary O62.1
      infection (maternal) O98.92
        carrier state NEC O99.834
        gonorrhea O98.22
        human immunodeficiency virus (HIV)
          O98.72
        sexually transmitted NEC O98.32
        specified NEC O98.82
        syphilis O98.12
        tuberculosis O98.02
        viral hepatitis O98.42
        viral NEC O98.52
      injury (to mother) (*see also* Delivery, complicat-
        ed, by, damage to) O71.9
      nonobstetric O9A.22 (*following* O99)
        caused by abuse — *see* Delivery, compli-
          cated by, abuse
      intrauterine fetal death, early O02.1
      inversion, uterus O71.2
      laceration (perineal) O70.9
        anus (sphincter) O70.4
          with third degree laceration (*see also*
            Delivery, complicated, by, lacera-
            tion, perineum, third degree)
            O70.20
            with mucosa O70.3
          without third degree laceration O70.2 ☑
        bladder (urinary) O71.5
        bowel O71.5

Delivery — *continued*
  complicated — *continued*
    by — *continued*
      laceration — *continued*
        cervix (uteri) O71.3
        fourchette O70.0
        hymen O70.0
        labia O70.0
        pelvic
          floor O70.1
          organ NEC O71.5
        perineum, perineal O70.9
          first degree O70.0
          fourth degree O70.3
          muscles O70.1
          second degree O70.1
          skin O70.0
          slight O70.0
          third degree O70.20
            with
              less than 50% of external anal
                sphincter (EAS) thickness
                torn (IIIa) O70.21
              both external anal sphincter (EAS)
                and internal anal sphincter
                (IAS) torn (IIIc) O70.23
              more than 50% of external anal
                sphincter (EAS) thickness
                torn (IIIb) O70.22
            IIIa O70.21
            IIIb O70.22
            IIIc O70.23
        peritoneum (pelvic) O71.5
        rectovaginal (septum) (without perineal
          laceration) O71.4
          with perineum (*see also* Delivery, compli-
            cated, by, laceration, perineum,
            third degree) O70.20
            with anal or rectal mucosa O70.3
        specified NEC O71.89
        sphincter ani — *see* Delivery, complicated,
          by, laceration, anus (sphincter)
        urethra O71.5
        uterus O71.81
          before labor O71.81
        vagina, vaginal (deep) (high) (without per-
          ineal laceration) O71.4
          with perineum O70.0
          muscles, with perineum O70.1
        vulva O70.0
      liver disorder O26.62
      malignancy O9A.12 (*following* O99)
      malnutrition O25.2
      malposition, malpresentation
        without obstruction (*see also* Delivery,
          complicated by, obstruction) O32.9 ☑
          breech O32.1 ☑
          compound O32.6 ☑
          face (brow) (chin) O32.3 ☑
          footling O32.8 ☑
          high head O32.4 ☑
          oblique O32.2 ☑
          specified NEC O32.8 ☑
          transverse O32.2 ☑
          unstable lie O32.0 ☑
        placenta O44.0- ☑
          with hemorrhage O44.1- ☑
        uterus or cervix O65.5
      meconium in amniotic fluid O77.0
      mental disorder NEC O99.344
      metrorrhexis — *see* Delivery, complicated by,
        rupture, uterus
      nervous system disorder O99.354
      obesity (pre-existing) O99.214
      obesity surgery status O99.844
      obstetric trauma O71.9
        specified NEC O71.89
      obstructed labor
        due to
          breech (complete) (frank) presentation
            O64.1 ☑
            incomplete O64.8 ☑
          brow presenation O64.3 ☑
          buttock presentation O64.1 ☑
          chin presentation O64.2 ☑
          compound presentation O64.5 ☑
          contracted pelvis O65.1
          deep transverse arrest O64.0 ☑

Delivery — *continued*
  complicated — *continued*
    by — *continued*
      obstructed labor — *continued*
        due to — *continued*
          deformed pelvis O65.0
          dystocia (fetal) O66.9
            due to
              conjoined twins O66.3
              fetal
                abnormality NEC O66.3
                ascites O66.3
                hydrops O66.3
                meningomyelocele O66.3
                sacral teratoma O66.3
                tumor O66.3
              hydrocephalic fetus O66.3
              shoulder O66.0
          face presentation O64.2 ☑
          fetopelvic disproportion O65.4
          footling presentation O64.8 ☑
          impacted shoulders O66.0
          incomplete rotation of fetal head
            O64.0 ☑
          large fetus O66.2
          locked twins O66.1
          malposition O64.9 ☑
            specified NEC O64.8 ☑
          malpresentation O64.9 ☑
            specified NEC O64.8 ☑
          multiple fetuses NEC O66.6
          pelvic
            abnormality (maternal) O65.9
              organ O65.5
              specified NEC O65.8
            contraction
              inlet O65.2
              mid-cavity O65.3
              outlet O65.3
          persistent (position)
            occipitoiliac O64.0 ☑
            occipitoposterior O64.0 ☑
            occipitosacral O64.0 ☑
            occipitotransverse O64.0 ☑
          prolapsed arm O64.4 ☑
          shoulder presentation O64.4 ☑
        specified NEC O66.8
      pathological retraction ring, uterus O62.4
      penetration, pregnant uterus by instrument
        O71.1
      perforation — *see* Delivery, complicated by,
        laceration
      placenta, placental
        ablatio (*see also* Abruptio placentae)
          O45.9- ☑
        abnormality O43.9- ☑
          specified NEC O43.89- ☑
        abruptio (*see also* Abruptio placentae)
          O45.9- ☑
        accreta O43.21- ☑
        adherent (with hemorrhage) O72.0
          without hemorrhage O73.0
        detachment (premature) (*see also* Abruptio
          placentae) O45.9- ☑
        disorder O43.9- ☑
          specified NEC O43.89- ☑
        hemorrhage NEC O67.8
        increta O43.22- ☑
        low (implantation) (lying) O44.4- ☑
          with hemorrhage O44.5- ☑
        malformation O43.10- ☑
        malposition O44.0- ☑
          without hemorrhage O44.1- ☑
        percreta O43.23- ☑
        previa (central) (complete) (lateral) (total)
          O44.0- ☑
          with hemorrhage O44.1- ☑
          marginal O44.2- ☑
            with hemorrhage O44.3- ☑
          partial O44.2- ☑
            with hemorrhage O44.3- ☑
        retained (with hemorrhage) O72.0
          without hemorrhage O73.0
        separation (premature) O45.9- ☑
          specified NEC O45.8X- ☑
        vicious insertion O44.1- ☑
      precipitate labor O62.3

Delivery — *continued*
  complicated — *continued*
    by — *continued*
      premature rupture, membranes (*see also* Pregnancy, complicated by, premature rupture of membranes) O42.90
      prolapse
        arm or hand O32.2 ☑
        cord (umbilical) O69.0 ☑
        foot or leg O32.8 ☑
        uterus O34.52- ☑
      prolonged labor O63.9
        first stage O63.0
        second stage O63.1
      protozoal disease (maternal) O98.62
      respiratory disease NEC O99.52
      retained membranes or portions of placenta O72.2
        without hemorrhage O73.1
      retarded birth O63.9
      retention of secundines (with hemorrhage) O72.0
        without hemorrhage O73.0
        partial O72.2
          without hemorrhage O73.1
      rupture
        bladder (urinary) O71.5
        cervix O71.3
        pelvic organ NEC O71.5
        urethra O71.5
        uterus (during or after labor) O71.1
          before labor O71.0- ☑
      separation, pubic bone (symphysis pubis) O71.6
      shock O75.1
      shoulder presentation O64.4 ☑
      skin disorder NEC O99.72
      spasm, cervix O62.4
      stenosis or stricture, cervix O65.5
      streptococcus group B (GBS) carrier state O99.824
      subluxation of symphysis (pubis) O26.72
      syphilis (maternal) O98.12
      tear — *see* Delivery, complicated by, laceration
      tetanic uterus O62.4
      trauma (obstetrical) (*see also* Delivery, complicated, by, damage to) O71.9
        non-obstetric O9A.22 (*following* O99)
        periurethral O71.82
        specified NEC O71.89
      tuberculosis (maternal) O98.02
      tumor, pelvic organs or tissues NEC O65.5
      umbilical cord around neck
        with compression O69.1 ☑
        without compression O69.81 ☑
      uterine inertia O62.2
        during latent phase of labor O62.0
        primary O62.0
        secondary O62.1
      vasa previa O69.4 ☑
      velamentous insertion of cord O43.12- ☑
    specified complication NEC O75.89
  delayed NOS O63.9
    following rupture of membranes
      artificial O75.5
    second twin, triplet, etc. O63.2
  forceps, low following failed vacuum extraction O66.5
  missed (at or near term) O36.4 ☑
  normal O80
  obstructed — *see* Delivery, complicated by, obstructed labor
  precipitate O62.3
  preterm (*see also* Pregnancy, complicated by, preterm labor) O60.10 ☑
  spontaneous O80
  term pregnancy NOS O80
  uncomplicated O80
  vaginal, following previous cesarean delivery O34.219
    classical (vertical) scar O34.212
    low transverse scar O34.211
Delusions (paranoid) — *see* Disorder, delusional
Dementia (degenerative (primary)) (old age) (persisting) F03.90
  with
    aggressive behavior F03.91
    behavioral disturbance F03.91
    combative behavior F03.91
    Lewy bodies G31.83 [F02.80]
      with behavioral disturbance G31.83 [F02.81]

Dementia — *continued*
  with — *continued*
    Parkinsonism G31.83 [F02.80]
      with behavioral disturbance G31.83 [F02.81]
    Parkinson's disease G20 [F02.80]
      with behavioral disturbance G20 [F02.81]
    violent behavior F03.91
  alcoholic F10.97
    with dependence F10.27
  Alzheimer's type — *see* Disease, Alzheimer's
  arteriosclerotic — *see* Dementia, vascular
  atypical, Alzheimer's type — *see* Disease, Alzheimer's, specified NEC
  congenital — *see* Disability, intellectual
  frontal (lobe) G31.09 [F02.80]
    with behavioral disturbance G31.09 [F02.81]
  frontotemporal G31.09 [F02.80]
    with behavioral disturbance G31.09 [F02.81]
    specified NEC G31.09 [F02.80]
      with behavioral disturbance G31.09 [F02.81]
  Huntington's disease or chorea G10
    with dementia G10 [F02.80]
  in (due to)
    with behavioral disturbance G31.83 [F02.81]
    alcohol F10.97
      with dependence F10.27
    Alzheimer's disease — *see* Disease, Alzheimer's
    arteriosclerotic brain disease — *see* Dementia, vascular
    cerebral lipidoses E75.- ☑ [F02.80]
      with behavioral disturbance E75.- ☑ [F02.81]
    Creutzfeldt-Jakob disease (*see also* Creutzfeldt-Jakob disease or syndrome (with dementia)) A81.00
    epilepsy G40.- ☑ [F02.80]
      with behavioral disturbance G40.- ☑ [F02.81]
    hepatolenticular degeneration E83.01 [F02.80]
      with behavioral disturbance E83.01 [F02.81]
    human immunodeficiency virus (HIV) disease B20 [F02.80]
      with behavioral disturbance B20 [F02.81]
    Huntington's disease or chorea G10 [F02.80]
      with behavioral disturbance G10 [F02.81]
    hypercalcemia E83.52 [F02.80]
      with behavioral disturbance E83.52 [F02.81]
    hypothyroidism, acquired E03.9 [F02.80]
      with behavioral disturbance E03.9 [F02.81]
      due to iodine deficiency E01.8 [F02.80]
        with behavioral disturbance E01.8 [F02.81]
    inhalants F18.97
      with dependence F18.27
    multiple
      etiologies F03 ☑
      sclerosis G35 [F02.80]
        with behavioral disturbance G35 [F02.81]
    neurosyphilis A52.17 [F02.80]
      with behavioral disturbance A52.17 [F02.81]
      juvenile A50.49 [F02.80]
        with behavioral disturbance A50.49 [F02.81]
    niacin deficiency E52 [F02.80]
      with behavioral disturbance E52 [F02.81]
    paralysis agitans G20 [F02.80]
      with behavioral disturbance G20 [F02.81]
    Parkinson's disease G20 [F02.80]
    pellagra E52 [F02.80]
      with behavioral disturbance E52 [F02.81]
    Pick's G31.01 [F02.80]
      with behavioral disturbance G31.01 [F02.81]
    polyarteritis nodosa M30.0 [F02.80]
      with behavioral disturbance M30.0 [F02.81]
    psychoactive drug F19.97
      with dependence F19.27
      inhalants F18.97
        with dependence F18.27
      sedatives, hypnotics or anxiolytics F13.97
        with dependence F13.27
    sedatives, hypnotics or anxiolytics F13.97
      with dependence F13.27
    systemic lupus erythematosus M32.- ☑ [F02.80]
      with behavioral disturbance M32.- ☑ [F02.81]
    trypanosomiasis
      African B56.9 [F02.80]
        with behavioral disturbance B56.9 [F02.81]
    unknown etiology F03 ☑
    vitamin B12 deficiency E53.8 [F02.80]
      with behavioral disturbance E53.8 [F02.81]
    volatile solvents F18.97
      with dependence F18.27

Dementia — *continued*
  infantile, infantilis F84.3
  Lewy body G31.83 [F02.80]
    with behavioral disturbance G31.83 [F02.81]
  multi-infarct — *see* Dementia, vascular
  paralytica, paralytic (syphilitic) A52.17 [F02.80]
    with behavioral disturbance A52.17 [F02.81]
    juvenilis A50.45
  paretic A52.17
  praecox — *see* Schizophrenia
  presenile F03 ☑
    Alzheimer's type — *see* Disease, Alzheimer's, early onset
  primary degenerative F03 ☑
  progressive, syphilitic A52.17
  senile F03 ☑
    with acute confusional state F05
    Alzheimer's type — *see* Disease, Alzheimer's, late onset
    depressed or paranoid type F03 ☑
  vascular (acute onset) (mixed) (multi-infarct) (subcortical) F01.50
    with behavioral disturbance F01.51
Demineralization, bone — *see* Osteoporosis
Demodex folliculorum (infestation) B88.0
Demophobia F40.248
Demoralization R45.3
Demyelination, demyelinization
  central nervous system G37.9
    specified NEC G37.8
  corpus callosum (central) G37.1
  disseminated, acute G36.9
    specified NEC G36.8
  global G35
  in optic neuritis G36.0
Dengue (classical) (fever) A90
  hemorrhagic A91
  sandfly A93.1
Dennie-Marfan syphilitic syndrome A50.45
Dens evaginatus, in dente or invaginatus K00.2
Dense breasts R92.2
Density
  increased, bone (disseminated) (generalized) (spotted) — *see* Disorder, bone, density and structure, specified type NEC
  lung (nodular) J98.4
Dental (*see also* condition)
  examination Z01.20
    with abnormal findings Z01.21
  restoration
    aesthetically inadequate or displeasing K08.56
    defective K08.50
      specified NEC K08.59
    failure of marginal integrity K08.51
    failure of periodontal anatomical integrity K08.54
Dentia praecox K00.6
Denticles (pulp) K04.2
Dentigerous cyst K09.0
Dentin
  irregular (in pulp) K04.3
  opalescent K00.5
  secondary (in pulp) K04.3
  sensitive K03.89
Dentinogenesis imperfecta K00.5
Dentinoma — *see* Cyst, calcifying odontogenic
Dentition (syndrome) K00.7
  delayed K00.6
  difficult K00.7
  precocious K00.6
  premature K00.6
  retarded K00.6
Dependence (on) (syndrome) F19.20
  with remission F19.21
  alcohol (ethyl) (methyl) (without remission) F10.20
    with
      amnestic disorder, persisting F10.26
      anxiety disorder F10.280
      dementia, persisting F10.27
      intoxication F10.229
        with delirium F10.221
        uncomplicated F10.220
      mood disorder F10.24
      psychotic disorder F10.259
        with
          delusions F10.250
          hallucinations F10.251
      remission F10.21
      sexual dysfunction F10.281

☑ **Additional Character Required — Refer to the Tabular List for Character Selection**   ▽ **Subterms under main terms may continue to next column or page**

Index

Dependence — continued
  alcohol — continued
    with — continued
      sleep disorder F10.282
      specified disorder NEC F10.288
      withdrawal F10.239
        with
          delirium F10.231
          perceptual disturbance F10.232
        uncomplicated F10.230
    counseling and surveillance Z71.41
  amobarbital — see Dependence, drug, sedative
  amphetamine(s) (type) — see Dependence, drug, stimulant NEC
  amytal (sodium) — see Dependence, drug, sedative
  analgesic NEC F55.8
  anesthetic (agent) (gas) (general) (local) NEC — see Dependence, drug, psychoactive NEC
  anxiolytic NEC — see Dependence, drug, sedative
  barbital(s) — see Dependence, drug, sedative
  barbiturate(s) (compounds) (drugs classifiable to T42) — see Dependence, drug, sedative
  benzedrine — see Dependence, drug, stimulant NEC
  bhang — see Dependence, drug, cannabis
  bromide(s) NEC — see Dependence, drug, sedative
  caffeine — see Dependence, drug, stimulant NEC
  cannabis (sativa) (indica) (resin) (derivatives) (type) — see Dependence, drug, cannabis
  chloral (betaine) (hydrate) — see Dependence, drug, sedative
  chlordiazepoxide — see Dependence, drug, sedative
  coca (leaf) (derivatives) — see Dependence, drug, cocaine
  cocaine — see Dependence, drug, cocaine
  codeine — see Dependence, drug, opioid
  combinations of drugs F19.20
  dagga — see Dependence, drug, cannabis
  demerol — see Dependence, drug, opioid
  dexamphetamine — see Dependence, drug, stimulant NEC
  dexedrine — see Dependence, drug, stimulant NEC
  dextromethorphan — see Dependence, drug, opioid
  dextromoramide — see Dependence, drug, opioid
  dextro-nor-pseudo-ephedrine — see Dependence, drug, stimulant NEC
  dextrorphan — see Dependence, drug, opioid
  diazepam — see Dependence, drug, sedative
  dilaudid — see Dependence, drug, opioid
  D-lysergic acid diethylamide — see Dependence, drug, hallucinogen
  drug NEC F19.20
    with sleep disorder F19.282
    cannabis F12.20
      with
        anxiety disorder F12.280
        intoxication F12.229
          with
            delirium F12.221
            perceptual disturbance F12.222
          uncomplicated F12.220
        other specified disorder F12.288
        psychosis F12.259
          delusions F12.250
          hallucinations F12.251
        unspecified disorder F12.29
      in remission F12.21
    cocaine F14.20
      with
        anxiety disorder F14.280
        intoxication F14.229
          with
            delirium F14.221
            perceptual disturbance F14.222
          uncomplicated F14.220
        mood disorder F14.24
        other specified disorder F14.288
        psychosis F14.259
          delusions F14.250
          hallucinations F14.251
        sexual dysfunction F14.281
        sleep disorder F14.282
        unspecified disorder F14.29
        withdrawal F14.23
      in remission F14.21
      withdrawal symptoms in newborn P96.1
    counseling and surveillance Z71.51
    hallucinogen F16.20

Dependence — continued
  drug — continued
    hallucinogen — continued
      with
        anxiety disorder F16.280
        flashbacks F16.283
        intoxication F16.229
          with delirium F16.221
          uncomplicated F16.220
        mood disorder F16.24
        other specified disorder F16.288
        perception disorder, persisting F16.283
        psychosis F16.259
          delusions F16.250
          hallucinations F16.251
        unspecified disorder F16.29
      in remission F16.21
    in remission F19.21
    inhalant F18.20
      with
        anxiety disorder F18.280
        dementia, persisting F18.27
        intoxication F18.229
          with delirium F18.221
          uncomplicated F18.220
        mood disorder F18.24
        other specified disorder F18.288
        psychosis F18.259
          delusions F18.250
          hallucinations F18.251
        unspecified disorder F18.29
      in remission F18.21
    nicotine F17.200
      with disorder F17.209
      in remission F17.201
      specified disorder NEC F17.208
      withdrawal F17.203
      chewing tobacco F17.220
        with disorder F17.229
        in remission F17.221
        specified disorder NEC F17.228
        withdrawal F17.223
      cigarettes F17.210
        with disorder F17.219
        in remission F17.211
        specified disorder NEC F17.218
        withdrawal F17.213
      specified product NEC F17.290
        with disorder F17.299
        remission F17.291
        specified disorder NEC F17.298
        withdrawal F17.293
    opioid F11.20
      with
        intoxication F11.229
          with
            delirium F11.221
            perceptual disturbance F11.222
          uncomplicated F11.220
        mood disorder F11.24
        other specified disorder F11.288
        psychosis F11.259
          delusions F11.250
          hallucinations F11.251
        sexual dysfunction F11.281
        sleep disorder F11.282
        unspecified disorder F11.29
        withdrawal F11.23
      in remission F11.21
    psychoactive NEC F19.20
      with
        amnestic disorder F19.26
        anxiety disorder F19.280
        dementia F19.27
        intoxication F19.229
          with
            delirium F19.221
            perceptual disturbance F19.222
          uncomplicated F19.220
        mood disorder F19.24
        other specified disorder F19.288
        psychosis F19.259
          delusions F19.250
          hallucinations F19.251
        sexual dysfunction F19.281
        sleep disorder F19.282
        unspecified disorder F19.29
        withdrawal F19.239

Dependence — continued
  drug — continued
    psychoactive — continued
      with — continued
        withdrawal — continued
          with
            delirium F19.231
            perceptual disturbance F19.232
          uncomplicated F19.230
    sedative, hypnotic or anxiolytic F13.20
      with
        amnestic disorder F13.26
        anxiety disorder F13.280
        dementia, persisting F13.27
        intoxication F13.229
          with delirium F13.221
          uncomplicated F13.220
        mood disorder F13.24
        other specified disorder F13.288
        psychosis F13.259
          delusions F13.250
          hallucinations F13.251
        sexual dysfunction F13.281
        sleep disorder F13.282
        unspecified disorder F13.29
        withdrawal F13.239
          with
            delirium F13.231
            perceptual disturbance F13.232
          uncomplicated F13.230
      in remission F13.21
    stimulant NEC F15.20
      with
        anxiety disorder F15.280
        intoxication F15.229
          with
            delirium F15.221
            perceptual disturbance F15.222
          uncomplicated F15.220
        mood disorder F15.24
        other specified disorder F15.288
        psychosis F15.259
          delusions F15.250
          hallucinations F15.251
        sexual dysfunction F15.281
        sleep disorder F15.282
        unspecified disorder F15.29
        withdrawal F15.23
      in remission F15.21
  ethyl
    alcohol (without remission) F10.20
      with remission F10.21
    bromide — see Dependence, drug, sedative
    carbamate F19.20
    chloride F19.20
    morphine — see Dependence, drug, opioid
  ganja — see Dependence, drug, cannabis
  glue (airplane) (sniffing) — see Dependence, drug, inhalant
  glutethimide — see Dependence, drug, sedative
  hallucinogenics — see Dependence, drug, hallucinogen
  hashish — see Dependence, drug, cannabis
  hemp — see Dependence, drug, cannabis
  heroin (salt) (any) — see Dependence, drug, opioid
  hypnotic NEC — see Dependence, drug, sedative
  Indian hemp — see Dependence, drug, cannabis
  inhalants — see Dependence, drug, inhalant
  khat — see Dependence, drug, stimulant NEC
  laudanum — see Dependence, drug, opioid
  LSD (-25) (derivatives) — see Dependence, drug, hallucinogen
  luminal — see Dependence, drug, sedative
  lysergic acid — see Dependence, drug, hallucinogen
  maconha — see Dependence, drug, cannabis
  marihuana — see Dependence, drug, cannabis
  meprobamate — see Dependence, drug, sedative
  mescaline — see Dependence, drug, hallucinogen
  methadone — see Dependence, drug, opioid
  methamphetamine(s) — see Dependence, drug, stimulant NEC
  methaqualone — see Dependence, drug, sedative
  methyl
    alcohol (without remission) F10.20
      with remission F10.21
    bromide — see Dependence, drug, sedative
    morphine — see Dependence, drug, opioid

Dependence — Dependence

Dependence — continued
methyl — continued
phenidate — see Dependence, drug, stimulant NEC
sulfonal — see Dependence, drug, sedative
morphine (sulfate) (sulfite) (type) — see Dependence, drug, opioid
narcotic (drug) NEC — see Dependence, drug, opioid
nembutal — see Dependence, drug, sedative
neraval — see Dependence, drug, sedative
neravan — see Dependence, drug, sedative
neurobarb — see Dependence, drug, sedative
nicotine — see Dependence, drug, nicotine
nitrous oxide F19.20
nonbarbiturate sedatives and tranquilizers with similar effect — see Dependence, drug, sedative
on
artificial heart (fully implantable) (mechanical) Z95.812
aspirator Z99.0
care provider (because of) Z74.9
impaired mobility Z74.09
need for
assistance with personal care Z74.1
continuous supervision Z74.3
no other household member able to render care Z74.2
specified reason NEC Z74.8
machine Z99.89
enabling NEC Z99.89
specified type NEC Z99.89
renal dialysis (hemodialysis) (peritoneal) Z99.2
respirator Z99.11
ventilator Z99.11
wheelchair Z99.3
opiate — see Dependence, drug, opioid
opioids — see Dependence, drug, opioid
opium (alkaloids) (derivatives) (tincture) — see Dependence, drug, opioid
oxygen (long-term) (supplemental) Z99.81
paraldehyde — see Dependence, drug, sedative
paregoric — see Dependence, drug, opioid
PCP (phencyclidine) (or related substance) — see Dependence, drug, hallucinogen
pentobarbital — see Dependence, drug, sedative
pentobarbitone (sodium) — see Dependence, drug, sedative
pentothal — see Dependence, drug, sedative
peyote — see Dependence, drug, hallucinogen
phencyclidine (PCP) (or related substance) — see Dependence, drug, hallucinogen
phenmetrazine — see Dependence, drug, stimulant NEC
phenobarbital — see Dependence, drug, sedative
polysubstance F19.20
psilocibin, psilocin, psilocyn, psilocyline — see Dependence, drug, hallucinogen
psychostimulant NEC — see Dependence, drug, stimulant NEC
secobarbital — see Dependence, drug, sedative
seconal — see Dependence, drug, sedative
sedative NEC — see Dependence, drug, sedative
specified drug NEC — see Dependence, drug
stimulant NEC — see Dependence, drug, stimulant NEC
substance NEC — see Dependence, drug
supplemental oxygen Z99.81
tobacco — see Dependence, drug, nicotine
counseling and surveillance Z71.6
tranquilizer NEC — see Dependence, drug, sedative
vitamin B6 E53.1
volatile solvents — see Dependence, drug, inhalant

Dependency
care-provider Z74.9
passive F60.7
reactions (persistent) F60.7

Depersonalization (in neurotic state) (neurotic) (syndrome) F48.1

Depletion
extracellular fluid E86.9
plasma E86.1
potassium E87.6
nephropathy N25.89
salt or sodium E87.1
causing heat exhaustion or prostration T67.4 ☑
nephropathy N28.9
volume NOS E86.9

Deployment (current) (military) status Z56.82
in theater or in support of military war, peacekeeping and humanitarian operations Z56.82
personal history of Z91.82
military war, peacekeeping and humanitarian deployment (current or past conflict) Z91.82
returned from Z91.82

Depolarization, premature I49.40
atrial I49.1
junctional I49.2
specified NEC I49.49
ventricular I49.3

Deposit
bone in Boeck's sarcoid D86.89
calcareous, calcium — see Calcification
cholesterol
retina H35.89
vitreous (body) (humor) — see Deposit, crystalline
conjunctiva H11.11- ☑
cornea H18.00- ☑
argentous H18.02- ☑
due to metabolic disorder H18.03- ☑
Kayser-Fleischer ring H18.04- ☑
pigmentation — see Pigmentation, cornea
crystalline, vitreous (body) (humor) H43.2- ☑
hemosiderin in old scars of cornea — see Pigmentation, cornea, stromal
metallic in lens — see Cataract, specified NEC
skin R23.8
tooth, teeth (betel) (black) (green) (materia alba) (orange) (tobacco) K03.6
urate, kidney — see Calculus, kidney

Depraved appetite — see Pica

Depressed
HDL cholesterol E78.6

Depression (acute) (mental) F32.9
agitated (single episode) F32.2
anaclitic — see Disorder, adjustment
anxiety F41.8
persistent F34.1
arches (see also Deformity, limb, flat foot)
atypical (single episode) F32.89
recurrent episode F33.8
basal metabolic rate R94.8
bone marrow D75.89
central nervous system R09.2
cerebral R29.818
newborn P91.4
cerebrovascular I67.9
chest wall M95.4
climacteric (single episode) F32.89
recurrent episode F33.8
endogenous (without psychotic symptoms) F33.2
with psychotic symptoms F33.3
functional activity R68.89
hysterical F44.89
involutional (single episode) F32.89
recurrent episode F33.8
major F32.9
with psychotic symptoms F32.3
recurrent — see Disorder, depressive, recurrent
manic-depressive — see Disorder, depressive, recurrent
masked (single episode) F32.89
medullary G93.89
menopausal (single episode) F32.89
recurrent episode F33.8
metatarsus — see Depression, arches
monopolar F33.9
nervous F34.1
neurotic F34.1
nose M95.0
postnatal F53
postpartum F53
post-psychotic of schizophrenia F32.89
post-schizophrenic F32.89
psychogenic (reactive) (single episode) F32.9
psychoneurotic F34.1
psychotic (single episode) F32.3
recurrent F33.3
reactive (psychogenic) (single episode) F32.9
psychotic (single episode) F32.3
recurrent — see Disorder, depressive, recurrent
respiratory center G93.89
seasonal — see Disorder, depressive, recurrent
senile F03 ☑
severe, single episode F32.2
situational F43.21

Depression — continued
skull Q67.4
specified NEC (single episode) F32.89
sternum M95.4
visual field — see Defect, visual field
vital (recurrent) (without psychotic symptoms) F33.2
with psychotic symptoms F33.3
single episode F32.2

Deprivation
cultural Z60.3
effects NOS T73.9 ☑
specified NEC T73.8 ☑
emotional NEC Z65.8
affecting infant or child — see Maltreatment, child, psychological
food T73.0 ☑
protein — see Malnutrition
sleep Z72.820
social Z60.4
affecting infant or child — see Maltreatment, child, psychological
specified NEC T73.8 ☑
vitamins — see Deficiency, vitamin
water T73.1 ☑

Derangement
ankle (internal) — see Derangement, joint, ankle
cartilage (articular) NEC — see Derangement, joint, articular cartilage, by site
recurrent — see Dislocation, recurrent
cruciate ligament, anterior, current injury — see Sprain, knee, cruciate, anterior
elbow (internal) — see Derangement, joint, elbow
hip (joint) (internal) (old) — see Derangement, joint, hip
joint (internal) M24.9
ankylosis — see Ankylosis
articular cartilage M24.10
ankle M24.17- ☑
elbow M24.12- ☑
foot M24.17- ☑
hand M24.14- ☑
hip M24.15- ☑
knee NEC M23.9- ☑
loose body — see Loose, body
shoulder M24.11- ☑
wrist M24.13- ☑
contracture — see Contraction, joint
current injury (see also Dislocation)
knee, meniscus or cartilage — see Tear, meniscus
dislocation
pathological — see Dislocation, pathological
recurrent — see Dislocation, recurrent
knee — see Derangement, knee
ligament — see Disorder, ligament
loose body — see Loose, body
recurrent — see Dislocation, recurrent
specified type NEC M24.80
ankle M24.87- ☑
elbow M24.82- ☑
foot joint M24.87- ☑
hand joint M24.84- ☑
hip M24.85- ☑
shoulder M24.81- ☑
wrist M24.83- ☑
temporomandibular M26.69
knee (recurrent) M23.9- ☑
ligament disruption, spontaneous M23.60- ☑
anterior cruciate M23.61- ☑
capsular M23.67- ☑
instability, chronic M23.5- ☑
lateral collateral M23.64- ☑
medial collateral M23.63- ☑
posterior cruciate M23.62- ☑
loose body M23.4- ☑
meniscus M23.30- ☑
cystic M23.00- ☑
lateral M23.002
anterior horn M23.04- ☑
posterior horn M23.05- ☑
specified NEC M23.06- ☑
medial M23.005
anterior horn M23.01- ☑
posterior horn M23.02- ☑
specified NEC M23.03- ☑

☑ Additional Character Required — Refer to the Tabular List for Character Selection ⬚ Subterms under main terms may continue to next column or page

Derangement — *continued*
  knee — *continued*
    meniscus — *continued*
      degenerate — *see* Derangement, knee, meniscus, specified NEC
      detached — *see* Derangement, knee, meniscus, specified NEC
      due to old tear or injury M23.20- ☑
        lateral M23.20- ☑
          anterior horn M23.24- ☑
          posterior horn M23.25- ☑
          specified NEC M23.26- ☑
        medial M23.20- ☑
          anterior horn M23.21- ☑
          posterior horn M23.22- ☑
          specified NEC M23.23- ☑
      retained — *see* Derangement, knee, meniscus, specified NEC
      specified NEC M23.30- ☑
        lateral M23.30- ☑
          anterior horn M23.34- ☑
          posterior horn M23.35- ☑
          specified NEC M23.36- ☑
        medial M23.30- ☑
          anterior horn M23.31- ☑
          posterior horn M23.32- ☑
          specified NEC M23.33- ☑
    old M23.8X- ☑
    specified NEC — *see* subcategory M23.8 ☑
  low back NEC — *see* Dorsopathy, specified NEC
  meniscus — *see* Derangement, knee, meniscus
  mental — *see* Psychosis
  patella, specified NEC — *see* Disorder, patella, derangement NEC
  semilunar cartilage (knee) — *see* Derangement, knee, meniscus, specified NEC
  shoulder (internal) — *see* Derangement, joint, shoulder
Dercum's disease E88.2
Derealization (neurotic) F48.1
Dermal — *see* condition
Dermaphytid — *see* Dermatophytosis
Dermatitis (eczematous) L30.9
  ab igne L59.0
  acarine B88.0
  actinic (due to sun) L57.8
    other than from sun L59.8
  allergic — *see* Dermatitis, contact, allergic
  ambustionis, due to burn or scald — *see* Burn
  amebic A06.7
  ammonia L22
  arsenical (ingested) L27.8
  artefacta L98.1
    psychogenic F54
  atopic L20.9
    psychogenic F54
    specified NEC L20.89
  autoimmune progesterone L30.8
  berlock, berloque L56.2
  blastomycotic B40.3
  blister beetle L24.89
  bullous, bullosa L13.9
    mucosynechial, atrophic L12.1
    seasonal L30.8
    specified NEC L13.8
  calorica L59.0
    due to burn or scald — *see* Burn
  caterpillar L24.89
  cercarial B65.3
  combustionis L59.0
    due to burn or scald — *see* Burn
  congelationis T69.1 ☑
  contact (occupational) L25.9
    allergic L23.9
      due to
        adhesives L23.1
        cement L23.5
        chemical products NEC L23.5
        chromium L23.0
        cosmetics L23.2
        dander (cat) (dog) L23.81
        drugs in contact with skin L23.3
        dyes L23.4
        food in contact with skin L23.6
        hair (cat) (dog) L23.81
        insecticide L23.5
        metals L23.0

Dermatitis — *continued*
  contact — *continued*
    allergic — *continued*
      due to — *continued*
        nickel L23.0
        plants, non-food L23.7
        plastic L23.5
        rubber L23.5
        specified agent NEC L23.89
      due to
        cement L25.3
        chemical products NEC L25.3
        cosmetics L25.0
        dander (cat) (dog) L23.81
        drugs in contact with skin L25.1
        dyes L25.2
        food in contact with skin L25.4
        hair (cat) (dog) L23.81
        plants, non-food L25.5
        specified agent NEC L25.8
    irritant L24.9
      due to
        cement L24.5
        chemical products NEC L24.5
        cosmetics L24.3
        detergents L24.0
        drugs in contact with skin L24.4
        food in contact with skin L24.6
        oils and greases L24.1
        plants, non-food L24.7
        solvents L24.2
        specified agent NEC L24.89
  contusiformis L52
  diabetic — *see* E08-E13 with .620
  diaper L22
  diphtheritica A36.3
  dry skin L85.3
  due to
    acetone (contact) (irritant) L24.2
    acids (contact) (irritant) L24.5
    adhesive(s) (allergic) (contact) (plaster) L23.1
      irritant L24.5
    alcohol (irritant) (skin contact) (substances in category T51) L24.2
      taken internally L27.8
    alkalis (contact) (irritant) L24.5
    arsenic (ingested) L27.8
    carbon disulfide (contact) (irritant) L24.2
    caustics (contact) (irritant) L24.5
    cement (contact) L25.3
    cereal (ingested) L27.2
    chemical(s) NEC L25.3
      taken internally L27.8
    chlorocompounds L24.2
    chromium (contact) (irritant) L24.81
    coffee (ingested) L27.2
    cold weather L30.8
    cosmetics (contact) L25.0
      allergic L23.2
      irritant L24.3
    cyclohexanes L24.2
    dander (cat) (dog) L23.81
    Demodex species B88.0
    Dermanyssus gallinae B88.0
    detergents (contact) (irritant) L24.0
    dichromate L24.81
    drugs and medicaments (generalized) (internal use) L27.0
      external — *see* Dermatitis, due to, drugs, in contact with skin
      in contact with skin L25.1
        allergic L23.3
        irritant L24.4
      localized skin eruption L27.1
      specified substance — *see* Table of Drugs and Chemicals
    dyes (contact) L25.2
      allergic L23.4
      irritant L24.89
    epidermophytosis — *see* Dermatophytosis
    esters L24.2
    external irritant NEC L24.9
    fish (ingested) L27.2
    flour (ingested) L27.2
    food (ingested) L27.2
      in contact with skin L25.4
    fruit (ingested) L27.2
    furs (allergic) (contact) L23.81
    glues — *see* Dermatitis, due to, adhesives

Dermatitis — *continued*
  due to — *continued*
    glycols L24.2
    greases NEC (contact) (irritant) L24.1
    hair (cat) (dog) L23.81
    hot
      objects and materials — *see* Burn
      weather or places L59.0
    hydrocarbons L24.2
    infrared rays L59.8
    ingestion, ingested substance L27.9
      chemical NEC L27.8
      drugs and medicaments — *see* Dermatitis, due to, drugs
      food L27.2
      specified NEC L27.8
    insecticide in contact with skin L24.5
    internal agent L27.9
      drugs and medicaments (generalized) — *see* Dermatitis, due to, drugs
      food L27.2
    irradiation — *see* Dermatitis, due to, radioactive substance
    ketones L24.2
    lacquer tree (allergic) (contact) L23.7
    light (sun) NEC L57.8
      acute L56.8
      other L59.8
    Liponyssoides sanguineus B88.0
    low temperature L30.8
    meat (ingested) L27.2
    metals, metal salts (contact) (irritant) L24.81
    milk (ingested) L27.2
    nickel (contact) (irritant) L24.81
    nylon (contact) (irritant) L24.5
    oils NEC (contact) (irritant) L24.1
    paint solvent (contact) (irritant) L24.2
    petroleum products (contact) (irritant) (substances in T52.0) L24.2
    plants NEC (contact) L25.5
      allergic L23.7
      irritant L24.7
    plasters (adhesive) (any) (allergic) (contact) L23.1
      irritant L24.5
    plastic (contact) L25.3
    preservatives (contact) — *see* Dermatitis, due to, chemical, in contact with skin
    primrose (allergic) (contact) L23.7
    primula (allergic) (contact) L23.7
    radiation L59.8
      nonionizing (chronic exposure) L57.8
      sun NEC L57.8
        acute L56.8
    radioactive substance L58.9
      acute L58.0
      chronic L58.1
    radium L58.9
      acute L58.0
      chronic L58.1
    ragweed (allergic) (contact) L23.7
    Rhus (allergic) (contact) (diversiloba) (radicans) (toxicodendron) (venenata) (verniciflua) L23.7
    rubber (contact) L24.5
    Senecio jacobaea (allergic) (contact) L23.7
    solvents (contact) (irritant) (substances in category T52) L24.2
    specified agent NEC (contact) L25.8
      allergic L23.89
      irritant L24.89
    sunshine NEC L57.8
      acute L56.8
    tetrachlorethylene (contact) (irritant) L24.2
    toluene (contact) (irritant) L24.2
    turpentine (contact) L24.2
    ultraviolet rays (sun NEC) (chronic exposure) L57.8
      acute L56.8
    vaccine or vaccination L27.0
      specified substance — *see* Table of Drugs and Chemicals
    varicose veins — *see* Varix, leg, with, inflammation
    X-rays L58.9
      acute L58.0
      chronic L58.1
  dyshydrotic L30.1
  dysmenorrheica N94.6
  escharotica — *see* Burn
  exfoliative, exfoliativa (generalized) L26

◣ Subterms under main terms may continue to next column or page   ☑ Additional Character Required — Refer to the Tabular List for Character Selection   **95**

Derangement — Dermatitis

Dermatitis — *continued*
- exfoliative, exfoliativa — *continued*
  - neonatorum L00
- eyelid (*see also* Dermatosis, eyelid)
  - allergic H01.119
    - left H01.116
      - lower H01.115
      - upper H01.114
    - right H01.113
      - lower H01.112
      - upper H01.111
  - contact — *see* Dermatitis, eyelid, allergic
  - due to
    - Demodex species B88.0
    - herpes (zoster) B02.39
      - simplex B00.59
  - eczematous H01.139
    - left H01.136
      - lower H01.135
      - upper H01.134
    - right H01.133
      - lower H01.132
      - upper H01.131
- facta, factitia, factitial L98.1
  - psychogenic F54
- flexural NEC L20.82
- friction L30.4
- fungus B36.9
  - specified type NEC B36.8
- gangrenosa, gangrenous infantum L08.0
- harvest mite B88.0
- heat L59.0
- herpesviral, vesicular (ear) (lip) B00.1
- herpetiformis (bullous) (erythematous) (pustular) (vesicular) L13.0
  - juvenile L12.2
  - senile L12.0
- hiemalis L30.8
- hypostatic, hypostatica — *see* Varix, leg, with, inflammation
- infectious eczematoid L30.3
- infective L30.3
- irritant — *see* Dermatitis, contact, irritant
- Jacquet's (diaper dermatitis) L22
- Leptus B88.0
- lichenified NEC L28.0
- medicamentosa (generalized) (internal use) — *see* Dermatitis, due to drugs
- mite B88.0
- multiformis L13.0
  - juvenile L12.2
- napkin L22
- neurotica L13.0
- nummular L30.0
- papillaris capillitii L73.0
- pellagrous E52
- perioral L71.0
- photocontact L56.2
- polymorpha dolorosa L13.0
- pruriginosa L13.0
- pruritic NEC L30.8
- psychogenic F54
- purulent L08.0
- pustular
  - contagious B08.02
  - subcorneal L13.1
- pyococcal L08.0
- pyogenica L08.0
- repens L40.2
- Ritter's (exfoliativa) L00
- Schamberg's L81.7
- schistosome B65.3
- seasonal bullous L30.8
- seborrheic L21.9
  - infantile L21.1
  - specified NEC L21.8
- sensitization NOS L23.9
- septic L08.0
- solare L57.8
- specified NEC L30.8
- stasis I87.2
  - with
    - varicose ulcer — *see* Varix, leg, with ulcer, with inflammation
    - varicose veins — *see* Varix, leg, with, inflammation
  - due to postthrombotic syndrome — *see* Syndrome, postthrombotic

Dermatitis — *continued*
- suppurative L08.0
- traumatic NEC L30.4
- trophoneurotica L13.0
- ultraviolet (sun) (chronic exposure) L57.8
  - acute L56.8
- varicose — *see* Varix, leg, with, inflammation
- vegetans L10.1
- verrucosa B43.0
- vesicular, herpesviral B00.1

Dermatoarthritis, lipoid E78.81
Dermatochalasis, eyelid H02.839
- left H02.836
  - lower H02.835
  - upper H02.834
- right H02.833
  - lower H02.832
  - upper H02.831

Dermatofibroma (lenticulare) — *see* Neoplasm, skin, benign
- protuberans — *see* Neoplasm, skin, uncertain behavior

Dermatofibrosarcoma (pigmented) (protuberans) — *see* Neoplasm, skin, malignant
Dermatographia L50.3
Dermatolysis (exfoliativa) (congenital) Q82.8
- acquired L57.4
- eyelids — *see* Blepharochalasis
- palpebrarum — *see* Blepharochalasis
- senile L57.4

Dermatomegaly NEC Q82.8
Dermatomucosomyositis M33.10
- with
  - myopathy M33.12
  - respiratory involvement M33.11
  - specified organ involvement NEC M33.19

Dermatomycosis B36.9
- furfuracea B36.0
- specified type NEC B36.8

Dermatomyositis (acute) (chronic) (*see also* Dermatopolymyositis)
- adult (*see also* Dermatomyositis, specified NEC) M33.10
- in (due to) neoplastic disease (*see also* Neoplasm) D49.9 [M36.0]
- juvenile M33.00
  - with
    - myopathy M33.02
    - respiratory involvement M33.01
    - specified organ involvement NEC M33.09
  - without myopathy M33.03
- specified NEC M33.10
  - with
    - myopathy M33.12
    - respiratory involvement M33.11
    - specified organ involvement NEC M33.19
  - without myopathy M33.13

Dermatoneuritis of children — *see* Poisoning, mercury
Dermatophilosis A48.8
Dermatophytid L30.2
Dermatophytide — *see* Dermatophytosis
Dermatophytosis (epidermophyton) (infection) (Microsporum) (tinea) (Trichophyton) B35.9
- beard B35.0
- body B35.4
- capitis B35.0
- corporis B35.4
- deep-seated B35.8
- disseminated B35.8
- foot B35.3
- granulomatous B35.8
- groin B35.6
- hand B35.2
- nail B35.1
- perianal (area) B35.6
- scalp B35.0
- specified NEC B35.8

Dermatopolymyositis M33.90
- with
  - myopathy M33.92
  - respiratory involvement M33.91
  - specified organ involvement NEC M33.99
- without myopathy M33.93
- in neoplastic disease (*see also* Neoplasm) D49.9 [M36.0]
- juvenile M33.00
  - with
    - myopathy M33.02
    - respiratory involvement M33.01
    - specified organ involvement NEC M33.09

Dermatopolymyositis — *continued*
- specified NEC M33.10
  - myopathy M33.12
  - respiratory involvement M33.11
  - specified organ involvement NEC M33.19

Dermatopolyneuritis — *see* Poisoning, mercury
Dermatorrhexis Q79.6
- acquired L57.4

Dermatosclerosis (*see also* Scleroderma)
- localized L94.0

Dermatosis L98.9
- Andrews' L08.89
- Bowen's — *see* Neoplasm, skin, in situ
- bullous L13.9
  - specified NEC L13.8
- exfoliativa L26
- eyelid (noninfectious)
  - dermatitis — *see* Dermatitis, eyelid
  - discoid lupus erythematosus — *see* Lupus, erythematosus, eyelid
  - xeroderma — *see* Xeroderma, acquired, eyelid
- factitial L98.1
- febrile neutrophilic L98.2
- gonococcal A54.89
- herpetiformis L13.0
  - juvenile L12.2
- linear IgA L13.8
- menstrual NEC L98.8
- neutrophilic, febrile L98.2
- occupational — *see* Dermatitis, contact
- papulosa nigra L82.1
- pigmentary L81.9
  - progressive L81.7
  - Schamberg's L81.7
- psychogenic F54
- purpuric, pigmented L81.7
- pustular, subcorneal L13.1
- transient acantholytic L11.1

Dermographia, dermographism L50.3
Dermoid (cyst) (*see also* Neoplasm, benign, by site)
- with malignant transformation C56- ☑
- due to radiation (nonionizing) L57.8

Dermopathy
- infiltrative with thyrotoxicosis — *see* Thyrotoxicosis
- nephrogenic fibrosing L90.8

Dermophytosis — *see* Dermatophytosis
Descemetocele H18.73- ☑
Descemet's membrane — *see* condition
Descending — *see* condition
Descensus uteri — *see* Prolapse, uterus
Desert
- rheumatism B38.0
- sore — *see* Ulcer, skin

Desertion (newborn) — *see* Maltreatment
Desmoid (extra-abdominal) (tumor) — *see* Neoplasm, connective tissue, uncertain behavior
- abdominal D48.1

Despondency F32.9
Desquamation, skin R23.4
Destruction, destructive (*see also* Damage)
- articular facet (*see also* Derangement, joint, specified type NEC)
  - knee M23.8X- ☑
  - vertebra — *see* Spondylosis
- bone (*see also* Disorder, bone, specified type NEC)
  - syphilitic A52.77
- joint (*see also* Derangement, joint, specified type NEC)
  - sacroiliac M53.3
- rectal sphincter K62.89
- septum (nasal) J34.89
- tuberculous NEC — *see* Tuberculosis
- tympanum, tympanic membrane (nontraumatic) — *see* Disorder, tympanic membrane, specified NEC
- vertebral disc — *see* Degeneration, intervertebral disc

Destructiveness (*see also* Disorder, conduct)
- adjustment reaction — *see* Disorder, adjustment

Desultory labor O62.2
Detachment
- cartilage — *see* Sprain
- cervix, annular N88.8
  - complicating delivery O71.3
- choroid (old) (postinfectional) (simple) (spontaneous) H31.40- ☑
  - hemorrhagic H31.41- ☑
  - serous H31.42- ☑
- ligament — *see* Sprain

Detachment — *continued*
  meniscus (knee) (*see also* Derangement, knee, meniscus, specified NEC)
    current injury — *see* Tear, meniscus
    due to old tear or injury — *see* Derangement, knee, meniscus, due to old tear
  retina (without retinal break) (serous) H33.2- ☑
    with retinal:
      break H33.00- ☑
        giant H33.03- ☑
        multiple H33.02- ☑
        single H33.01- ☑
      dialysis H33.04- ☑
    pigment epithelium — *see* Degeneration, retina, separation of layers, pigment epithelium detachment
    rhegmatogenous — *see* Detachment, retina, with retinal, break
    specified NEC H33.8
    total H33.05- ☑
    traction H33.4- ☑
  vitreous (body) H43.81 ☑
Detergent asthma J69.8
Deterioration
  epileptic F06.8
  general physical R53.81
  heart, cardiac — *see* Degeneration, myocardial
  mental — *see* Psychosis
  myocardial, myocardium — *see* Degeneration, myocardial
  senile (simple) R54
Deuteranomaly (anomalous trichromat) H53.53
Deuteranopia (complete) (incomplete) H53.53
Development
  abnormal, bone Q79.9
  arrested R62.50
    bone — *see* Arrest, development or growth, bone
    child R62.50
    due to malnutrition E45
  defective, congenital (*see also* Anomaly, by site)
    cauda equina Q06.3
    left ventricle Q24.8
      in hypoplastic left heart syndrome Q23.4
    valve Q24.8
      pulmonary Q22.3
  delayed (*see also* Delay, development) R62.50
    arithmetical skills F81.2
    language (skills) (expressive) F80.1
    learning skill F81.9
    mixed skills F88
    motor coordination F82
    reading F81.0
    specified learning skill NEC F81.89
    speech F80.9
    spelling F81.81
    written expression F81.81
  imperfect, congenital (*see also* Anomaly, by site)
    heart Q24.9
    lungs Q33.6
  incomplete
    bronchial tree Q32.4
    organ or site not listed — *see* Hypoplasia, by site
    respiratory system Q34.9
  sexual, precocious NEC E30.1
  tardy, mental (*see also* Disability, intellectual) F79
Developmental — *see* condition
  testing, infant or child — *see* Examination, child
Devergie's disease (pityriasis rubra pilaris) L44.0
Deviation (in)
  conjugate palsy (eye) (spastic) H51.0
  esophagus (acquired) K22.8
  eye, skew H51.8
  midline (jaw) (teeth) (dental arch) M26.29
    specified site NEC — *see* Malposition
  nasal septum J34.2
    congenital Q67.4
  opening and closing of the mandible M26.53
  organ or site, congenital NEC — *see* Malposition, congenital
  septum (nasal) (acquired) J34.2
    congenital Q67.4
  sexual F65.9
    bestiality F65.89
    erotomania F52.8
    exhibitionism F65.2
    fetishism, fetishistic F65.0
      transvestism F65.1
    frotteurism F65.81

Deviation — *continued*
  sexual — *continued*
    masochism F65.51
    multiple F65.89
    necrophilia F65.89
    nymphomania F52.8
    pederosis F65.4
    pedophilia F65.4
    sadism, sadomasochism F65.52
    satyriasis F52.8
    specified type NEC F65.89
    transvestism F64.1
    voyeurism F65.3
  teeth, midline M26.29
  trachea J39.8
  ureter, congenital Q62.61
Device
  cerebral ventricle (communicating) in situ Z98.2
  contraceptive — *see* Contraceptive, device
  drainage, cerebrospinal fluid, in situ Z98.2
Devic's disease G36.0
Devil's
  grip B33.0
  pinches (purpura simplex) D69.2
Devitalized tooth K04.99
Devonshire colic — *see* Poisoning, lead
Dextraposition, aorta Q20.3
  in tetralogy of Fallot Q21.3
Dextrinosis, limit (debrancher enzyme deficiency) E74.03
Dextrocardia (true) Q24.0
  with
    complete transposition of viscera Q89.3
    situs inversus Q89.3
Dextrotransposition, aorta Q20.3
d-glycericacidemia E72.59
Dhat syndrome F48.8
Dhobi itch B35.6
Di George's syndrome D82.1
Di Guglielmo's disease C94.0- ☑
Diabetes, diabetic (mellitus) (sugar) E11.9
  with
    amyotrophy E11.44
    arthropathy NEC E11.618
    autonomic (poly)neuropathy E11.43
    cataract E11.36
    Charcot's joints E11.610
    chronic kidney disease E11.22
    circulatory complication NEC E11.59
    complication E11.8
      specified NEC E11.69
    dermatitis E11.620
    foot ulcer E11.621
    gangrene E11.52
    gastroparalysis E11.43
    gastroparesis E11.43
    glomerulonephrosis, intracapillary E11.21
    glomerulosclerosis, intercapillary E11.21
    hyperglycemia E11.65
    hyperosmolarity E11.00
      with coma E11.01
    hypoglycemia E11.649
      with coma E11.641
    ketoacidosis E11.10
      with coma E11.11
    kidney complications NEC E11.29
    Kimmelstiel-Wilson disease E11.21
    loss of protective sensation (LOPS) — *see* Diabetes, by type, with neuropathy
    mononeuropathy E11.41
    myasthenia E11.44
    necrobiosis lipoidica E11.620
    nephropathy E11.21
    neuralgia E11.42
    neurologic complication NEC E11.49
    neuropathic arthropathy E11.610
    neuropathy E11.40
    ophthalmic complication NEC E11.39
    oral complication NEC E11.638
    osteomyelitis E11.69
    periodontal disease E11.630
    peripheral angiopathy E11.51
      with gangrene E11.52
    polyneuropathy E11.42
    renal complication NEC E11.29
    renal tubular degeneration E11.29
    retinopathy E11.319
      with macular edema E11.311

Diabetes, diabetic — *continued*
  with — *continued*
    retinopathy — *continued*
      with macular edema — *continued*
        resolved following treatment E11.37 ☑
      nonproliferative E11.329 ☑
        with macular edema E11.321 ☑
        mild E11.329 ☑
          with macular edema E11.321 ☑
        moderate E11.339 ☑
          with macular edema E11.331 ☑
        severe E11.349 ☑
          with macular edema E11.341 ☑
      proliferative E11.359 ☑
        with
          combined traction retinal detachment and rhegmatogenous retinal detachment E11.354 ☑
          macular edema E11.351 ☑
          stable proliferative diabetic retinopathy E11.355 ☑
          traction retinal detachment involving the macula E11.352 ☑
          traction retinal detachment not involving the macula E11.353 ☑
    skin complication NEC E11.628
    skin ulcer NEC E11.622
  brittle — *see* Diabetes, type 1
  bronzed E83.110
  complicating pregnancy — *see* Pregnancy, complicated by, diabetes
  dietary counseling and surveillance Z71.3
  due to
    autoimmune process — *see* Diabetes, type 1
    immune mediated pancreatic islet beta-cell destruction — *see* Diabetes, type 1
  due to drug or chemical E09.9
    with
      amyotrophy E09.44
      arthropathy NEC E09.618
      autonomic (poly)neuropathy E09.43
      cataract E09.36
      Charcot's joints E09.610
      chronic kidney disease E09.22
      circulatory complication NEC E09.59
      complication E09.8
        specified NEC E09.69
      dermatitis E09.620
      foot ulcer E09.621
      gangrene E09.52
      gastroparalysis E09.43
      gastroparesis E09.43
      glomerulonephrosis, intracapillary E09.21
      glomerulosclerosis, intercapillary E09.21
      hyperglycemia E09.65
      hyperosmolarity E09.00
        with coma E09.01
      hypoglycemia E09.649
        with coma E09.641
      ketoacidosis E09.10
        with coma E09.11
      kidney complications NEC E09.29
      Kimmelsteil-Wilson disease E09.21
      mononeuropathy E09.41
      myasthenia E09.44
      necrobiosis lipoidica E09.620
      nephropathy E09.21
      neuralgia E09.42
      neurologic complication NEC E09.49
      neuropathic arthropathy E09.610
      neuropathy E09.40
      ophthalmic complication NEC E09.39
      oral complication NEC E09.638
      periodontal disease E09.630
      peripheral angiopathy E09.51
        with gangrene E09.52
      polyneuropathy E09.42
      renal complication NEC E09.29
      renal tubular degeneration E09.29
      retinopathy E09.319
        with macular edema E09.311
        nonproliferative E09.329 ☑
          with macular edema E09.321 ☑
          mild E09.329 ☑
            with macular edema E09.321 ☑
          moderate E09.339 ☑
            with macular edema E09.331 ☑
          severe E09.349 ☑

▼ Subterms under main terms may continue to next column or page   ☑ Additional Character Required — Refer to the Tabular List for Character Selection   97

Detachment — Diabetes, diabetic

Index

Diabetes, diabetic — Diabetes, diabetic

Diabetes, diabetic — *continued*
due to drug or chemical — *continued*
with — *continued*
retinopathy — *continued*
nonproliferative — *continued*
severe — *continued*
with macular edema E09.341 ☑
proliferative E09.359 ☑
with
combined traction retinal detachment and rhegmatogenous
retinal detachment E09.354 ☑
macular edema E09.351 ☑
stable proliferative diabetic
retinopathy E09.355 ☑
traction retinal detachment involving
the macula E09.352 ☑
traction retinal detachment not involving the macula E09.353 ☑
resolved following treatment E09.37 ☑
skin complication NEC E09.628
skin ulcer NEC E09.622
due to underlying condition E08.9
with
amyotrophy E08.44
arthropathy NEC E08.618
autonomic (poly)neuropathy E08.43
cataract E08.36
Charcot's joints E08.610
chronic kidney disease E08.22
circulatory complication NEC E08.59
complication E08.8
specified NEC E08.69
dermatitis E08.620
foot ulcer E08.621
gangrene E08.52
gastroparalysis E08.43
gastroparesis E08.43
glomerulonephrosis, intracapillary E08.21
glomerulosclerosis, intercapillary E08.21
hyperglycemia E08.65
hyperosmolarity E08.00
with coma E08.01
hypoglycemia E08.649
with coma E08.641
ketoacidosis E08.10
with coma E08.11
kidney complications NEC E08.29
Kimmelsteil-WIlson disease E08.21
mononeuropathy E08.41
myasthenia E08.44
necrobiosis lipoidica E08.620
nephropathy E08.21
neuralgia E08.42
neurologic complication NEC E08.49
neuropathic arthropathy E08.610
neuropathy E08.40
ophthalmic complication NEC E08.39
oral complication NEC E08.638
periodontal disease E08.630
peripheral angiopathy E08.51
with gangrene E08.52
polyneuropathy E08.42
renal complication NEC E08.29
renal tubular degeneration E08.29
retinopathy E08.319
with macular edema E08.311
nonproliferative E08.329 ☑
with macular edema E08.321 ☑
mild E08.329 ☑
with macular edema E08.321 ☑
moderate E08.339 ☑
with macular edema E08.331 ☑
severe E08.349 ☑
with macular edema E08.341 ☑
proliferative E08.359 ☑
with
combined traction retinal detachment and rhegmatogenous
retinal detachment E08.354 ☑
macular edema E08.351 ☑
stable proliferative diabetic
retinopathy E08.355 ☑
traction retinal detachment involving
the macula E08.352 ☑
traction retinal detachment not involving the macula E08.353 ☑
resolved following treatment E08.37 ☑

Diabetes, diabetic — *continued*
due to underlying condition — *continued*
with — *continued*
skin complication NEC E08.628
skin ulcer NEC E08.622
gestational (in pregnancy) O24.419
affecting newborn P70.0
diet controlled O24.410
in childbirth O24.429
diet controlled O24.420
insulin (and diet) controlled O24.424
oral drug controlled (antidiabetic) (hypoglycemic) O24.425
insulin (and diet) controlled O24.414
oral drug controlled (antidiabetic) (hypoglycemic)
O24.415
puerperal O24.439
diet controlled O24.430
insulin (and diet) controlled O24.434
oral drug controlled (antidiabetic) (hypoglycemic) O24.435
hepatogenous E13.9
idiopathic — *see* Diabetes, type 1
inadequately controlled — *code to* Diabetes, by type,
with hyperglycemia
insipidus E23.2
nephrogenic N25.1
pituitary E23.2
vasopressin resistant N25.1
insulin dependent — *code to* type of diabetes
juvenile-onset — *see* Diabetes, type 1
ketosis-prone — *see* Diabetes, type 1
latent R73.03
neonatal (transient) P70.2
non-insulin dependent — *code to* type of diabetes
out of control — *code to* Diabetes, by type, with hyperglycemia
phosphate E83.39
poorly controlled — *code to* Diabetes, by type, with
hyperglycemia
postpancreatectomy — *see* Diabetes, specified type
NEC
postprocedural — *see* Diabetes, specified type NEC
secondary diabetes mellitus NEC — *see* Diabetes,
specified type NEC
specified type NEC E13.9
with
amyotrophy E13.44
arthropathy NEC E13.618
autonomic (poly)neuropathy E13.43
cataract E13.36
Charcot's joints E13.610
chronic kidney disease E13.22
circulatory complication NEC E13.59
complication E13.8
specified NEC E13.69
dermatitis E13.620
foot ulcer E13.621
gangrene E13.52
gastroparalysis E13.43
gastroparesis E13.43
glomerulonephrosis, intracapillary E13.21
glomerulosclerosis, intercapillary E13.21
hyperglycemia E13.65
hyperosmolarity E13.00
with coma E13.01
hypoglycemia E13.649
with coma E13.641
ketoacidosis E13.10
with coma E13.11
kidney complications NEC E13.29
Kimmelsteil-Wilson disease E13.21
mononeuropathy E13.41
myasthenia E13.44
necrobiosis lipoidica E13.620
nephropathy E13.21
neuralgia E13.42
neurologic complication NEC E13.49
neuropathic arthropathy E13.610
neuropathy E13.40
ophthalmic complication NEC E13.39
oral complication NEC E13.638
periodontal disease E13.630
peripheral angiopathy E13.51
with gangrene E13.52
polyneuropathy E13.42
renal complication NEC E13.29
renal tubular degeneration E13.29

Diabetes, diabetic — *continued*
specified type — *continued*
with — *continued*
retinopathy E13.319
with macular edema E13.311
nonproliferative E13.329 ☑
with macular edema E13.321 ☑
mild E13.329 ☑
with macular edema E13.321 ☑
moderate E13.339 ☑
with macular edema E13.331 ☑
severe E13.349 ☑
with macular edema E13.341 ☑
proliferative E13.359 ☑
with
combined traction retinal detachment and rhegmatogenous
retinal detachment E13.354 ☑
macular edema E13.351 ☑
stable proliferative diabetic
retinopathy E13.355 ☑
traction retinal detachment involving
the macula E13.352 ☑
traction retinal detachment not involving the macula E13.353 ☑
resolved following treatment E13.37 ☑
skin complication NEC E13.628
skin ulcer NEC E13.622
steroid-induced — *see* Diabetes, due to, drug or
chemical
type 1 E10.9
with
amyotrophy E10.44
arthropathy NEC E10.618
autonomic (poly)neuropathy E10.43
cataract E10.36
Charcot's joints E10.610
chronic kidney disease E10.22
circulatory complication NEC E10.59
complication E10.8
specified NEC E10.69
dermatitis E10.620
foot ulcer E10.621
gangrene E10.52
gastroparalysis E10.43
gastroparesis E10.43
glomerulonephrosis, intracapillary E10.21
glomerulosclerosis, intercapillary E10.21
hyperglycemia E10.65
hypoglycemia E10.649
with coma E10.641
ketoacidosis E10.10
with coma E10.11
kidney complications NEC E10.29
Kimmelsteil-Wilson disease E10.21
mononeuropathy E10.41
myasthenia E10.44
necrobiosis lipoidica E10.620
nephropathy E10.21
neuralgia E10.42
neurologic complication NEC E10.49
neuropathic arthropathy E10.610
neuropathy E10.40
ophthalmic complication NEC E10.39
oral complication NEC E10.638
osteomyelitis E10.69
periodontal disease E10.630
peripheral angiopathy E10.51
with gangrene E10.52
polyneuropathy E10.42
renal complication NEC E10.29
renal tubular degeneration E10.29
retinopathy E10.319
with macular edema E10.311
nonproliferative E10.329 ☑
with macular edema E10.321 ☑
mild E10.329 ☑
with macular edema E10.321 ☑
moderate E10.339 ☑
with macular edema E10.331 ☑
severe E10.349 ☑
with macular edema E10.341 ☑
proliferative E10.359 ☑
with
combined traction retinal detachment and rhegmatogenous
retinal detachment E10.354 ☑
macular edema E10.351 ☑

☑ Additional Character Required — Refer to the Tabular List for Character Selection   ▽ Subterms under main terms may continue to next column or page

Diabetes, diabetic — *continued*
  type 1 — *continued*
    with — *continued*
      retinopathy — *continued*
        proliferative — *continued*
          with — *continued*
            stable proliferative diabetic retinopathy E10.355 ☑
            traction retinal detachment involving the macula E10.352 ☑
            traction retinal detachment not involving the macula E10.353 ☑
        resolved following treatment E10.37 ☑
      skin complication NEC E10.628
      skin ulcer NEC E10.622
  type 2 E11.9
    with
      amyotrophy E11.44
      arthropathy NEC E11.618
      autonomic (poly)neuropathy E11.43
      cataract E11.36
      Charcot's joints E11.610
      chronic kidney disease E11.22
      circulatory complication NEC E11.59
      complication E11.8
        specified NEC E11.69
      dermatitis E11.620
      foot ulcer E11.621
      gangrene E11.52
      gastroparalysis E11.43
      gastroparesis E11.43
      glomerulonephrosis, intracapillary E11.21
      glomerulosclerosis, intercapillary E11.21
      hyperglycemia E11.65
      hyperosmolarity E11.00
        with coma E11.01
      hypoglycemia E11.649
        with coma E11.641
      ketoacidosis E11.10
        with coma E11.11
      kidney complications NEC E11.29
      Kimmelstiel-Wilson disease E11.21
      mononeuropathy E11.41
      myasthenia E11.44
      necrobiosis lipoidica E11.620
      nephropathy E11.21
      neuralgia E11.42
      neurologic complication NEC E11.49
      neuropathic arthropathy E11.610
      neuropathy E11.40
      ophthalmic complication NEC E11.39
      oral complication NEC E11.638
      osteomyelitis E11.69
      periodontal disease E11.630
      peripheral angiopathy E11.51
        with gangrene E11.52
      polyneuropathy E11.42
      renal complication NEC E11.29
      renal tubular degeneration E11.29
      retinopathy E11.319
        with macular edema E11.311
        nonproliferative E11.329 ☑
          with macular edema E11.321 ☑
          mild E11.329 ☑
            with macular edema E11.321 ☑
          moderate E11.339 ☑
            with macular edema E11.331 ☑
          severe E11.349 ☑
            with macular edema E11.341 ☑
        proliferative E11.359 ☑
          with
            combined traction retinal detachment and rhegmatogenous retinal detachment E11.354 ☑
            macular edema E11.351 ☑
            stable proliferative diabetic retinopathy E11.355 ☑
            traction retinal detachment involving the macula E11.352 ☑
            traction retinal detachment not involving the macula E11.353 ☑
        resolved following treatment E11.37 ☑
      skin complication NEC E11.628
      skin ulcer NEC E11.622
  uncontrolled
    meaning
      hyperglycemia — *see* Diabetes, by type, with, hyperglycemia

Diabetes, diabetic — *continued*
  uncontrolled — *continued*
    meaning — *continued*
      hypoglycemia — *see* Diabetes, by type, with, hypoglycemia
Diacyclothrombopathia D69.1
Diagnosis deferred R69
Dialysis (intermittent) (treatment)
  noncompliance (with) Z91.15
  renal (hemodialysis) (peritoneal), status Z99.2
  retina, retinal — *see* Detachment, retina, with retinal, dialysis
Diamond-Blackfan anemia (congenital hypoplastic) D61.01
Diamond-Gardener syndrome (autoerythrocyte sensitization) D69.2
Diaper rash L22
Diaphoresis (excessive) R61
Diaphragm — *see* condition
Diaphragmalgia R07.1
Diaphragmatitis, diaphragmitis J98.6
Diaphysial aclasis Q78.6
Diaphysitis — *see* Osteomyelitis, specified type NEC
Diarrhea, diarrheal (disease) (infantile) (inflammatory) R19.7
  achlorhydric K31.83
  allergic K52.29
    due to
      colitis — *see* Colitis, allergic
      enteritis — *see* Enteritis, allergic
  amebic (*see also* Amebiasis) A06.0
    with abscess — *see* Abscess, amebic
    acute A06.0
    chronic A06.1
    nondysenteric A06.2
  bacillary — *see* Dysentery, bacillary
  balantidial A07.0
  cachectic NEC K52.89
  Chilomastix A07.8
  choleriformis A00.1
  chronic (noninfectious) K52.9
  coccidial A07.3
  Cochin-China K90.1
    strongyloidiasis B78.0
  Dientamoeba A07.8
  dietetic (*see also* Diarrhea, allergic) K52.29
  drug-induced K52.1
  due to
    bacteria A04.9
      specified NEC A04.8
    Campylobacter A04.5
    Capillaria philippinensis B81.1
    Clostridium difficile
      not specified as recurrent A04.72
      recurrent A04.71
    Clostridium perfringens (C) (F) A04.8
    Cryptosporidium A07.2
    drugs K52.1
    Escherichia coli A04.4
      enteroaggregative A04.4
      enterohemorrhagic A04.3
      enteroinvasive A04.2
      enteropathogenic A04.0
      enterotoxigenic A04.1
      specified NEC A04.4
    food hypersensitivity (*see also* Diarrhea, allergic) K52.29
    Necator americanus B76.1
    S. japonicum B65.2
    specified organism NEC A08.8
      bacterial A04.8
      viral A08.39
    Staphylococcus A04.8
    Trichuris trichiuria B79
    virus — *see* Enteritis, viral
    Yersinia enterocolitica A04.6
  dysenteric A09
  endemic A09
  epidemic A09
  flagellate A07.9
  Flexner's (ulcerative) A03.1
  functional K59.1
    following gastrointestinal surgery K91.89
    psychogenic F45.8
  Giardia lamblia A07.1
  giardial A07.1
  hill K90.1
  infectious A09

Diarrhea, diarrheal — *continued*
  malarial — *see* Malaria
  mite B88.0
  mycotic NEC B49
  neonatal (noninfectious) P78.3
  nervous F45.8
  neurogenic K59.1
  noninfectious K52.9
  postgastrectomy K91.1
  postvagotomy K91.1
  protozoal A07.9
    specified NEC A07.8
  psychogenic F45.8
  specified
    bacterium NEC A04.8
    virus NEC A08.39
  strongyloidiasis B78.0
  toxic K52.1
  trichomonal A07.8
  tropical K90.1
  tuberculous A18.32
  viral — *see* Enteritis, viral
Diastasis
  cranial bones M84.88
    congenital NEC Q75.8
  joint (traumatic) — *see* Dislocation
  muscle M62.00
    ankle M62.07- ☑
    congenital Q79.8
    foot M62.07- ☑
    forearm M62.03- ☑
    hand M62.04- ☑
    lower leg M62.06- ☑
    pelvic region M62.05- ☑
    shoulder region M62.01- ☑
    specified site NEC M62.08
    thigh M62.05- ☑
    upper arm M62.02- ☑
  recti (abdomen)
    complicating delivery O71.89
    congenital Q79.59
Diastema, tooth, teeth, fully erupted M26.32
Diastematomyelia Q06.2
Diataxia, cerebral G80.4
Diathesis
  allergic — *see* History, allergy
  bleeding (familial) D69.9
  cystine (familial) E72.00
  gouty — *see* Gout
  hemorrhagic (familial) D69.9
    newborn NEC P53
  spasmophilic R29.0
Diaz's disease or osteochondrosis (juvenile) (talus) — *see* Osteochondrosis, juvenile, tarsus
Dibothriocephalus, dibothriocephaliasis (latus) (infection) (infestation) B70.0
  larval B70.1
Dicephalus, dicephaly Q89.4
Dichotomy, teeth K00.2
Dichromat, dichromatopsia (congenital) — *see* Deficiency, color vision
Dichuchwa A65
Dicroceliasis B66.2
Didelphia, didelphys — *see* Double uterus
Didymytis N45.1
  with orchitis N45.3
Dietary
  inadequacy or deficiency E63.9
  surveillance and counseling Z71.3
Dietl's crisis N13.8
Dieulafoy lesion (hemorrhagic)
  duodenum K31.82
  esophagus K22.8
  intestine (colon) K63.81
  stomach K31.82
Difficult, difficulty (in)
  acculturation Z60.3
  feeding R63.3
    newborn P92.9
      breast P92.5
      specified NEC P92.8
    nonorganic (infant or child) F98.29
  intubation, in anesthesia T88.4 ☑
  mechanical, gastroduodenal stoma K91.89
    causing obstruction (*see also* Obstruction, intestine, postoperative) K91.30
  micturition
    need to immediately re-void R39.191

Difficult, difficulty — *continued*
  micturition — *continued*
    position dependent R39.192
    specified NEC R39.198
  reading (developmental) F81.0
    secondary to emotional disorders F93.9
  spelling (specific) F81.81
    with reading disorder F81.89
    due to inadequate teaching Z55.8
  swallowing — *see* Dysphagia
  walking R26.2
  work
    conditions NEC Z56.5
    schedule Z56.3
Diffuse — *see* condition
Digestive — *see* condition
Dihydropyrimidine dehydrogenase disease (DPD)
    E88.89
Diktyoma — *see* Neoplasm, malignant, by site
Dilaceration, tooth K00.4
Dilatation
  anus K59.8
    venule — *see* Hemorrhoids
  aorta (focal) (general) — *see* Ectasia, aorta
    with aneuysm — *see* Aneurysm, aorta
    congenital Q25.44
  artery — *see* Aneurysm
  bladder (sphincter) N32.89
    congenital Q64.79
  blood vessel I99.8
  bronchial J47.9
    with
      exacerbation (acute) J47.1
      lower respiratory infection J47.0
  calyx (due to obstruction) — *see* Hydronephrosis
  capillaries I78.8
  cardiac (acute) (chronic) (*see also* Hypertrophy, cardiac)
    congenital Q24.8
      valve NEC Q24.8
        pulmonary Q22.3
    valve — *see* Endocarditis
  cavum septi pellucidi Q06.8
  cervix (uteri) (*see also* Incompetency, cervix)
    incomplete, poor, slow complicating delivery O62.0
  colon K59.39
    congenital Q43.1
    psychogenic F45.8
    toxic K59.31
  common duct (acquired) K83.8
    congenital Q44.5
  cystic duct (acquired) K82.8
    congenital Q44.5
  duct, mammary — *see* Ectasia, mammary duct
  duodenum K59.8
  esophagus K22.8
    congenital Q39.5
    due to achalasia K22.0
  eustachian tube, congenital Q17.8
  gallbladder K82.8
  gastric — *see* Dilatation, stomach
  heart (acute) (chronic) (*see also* Hypertrophy, cardiac)
    congenital Q24.8
    valve — *see* Endocarditis
  ileum K59.8
    psychogenic F45.8
  jejunum K59.8
    psychogenic F45.8
  kidney (calyx) (collecting structures) (cystic)
      (parenchyma) (pelvis) (idiopathic) N28.89
  lacrimal passages or duct — *see* Disorder, lacrimal
      system, changes
  lymphatic vessel I89.0
  mammary duct — *see* Ectasia, mammary duct
  Meckel's diverticulum (congenital) Q43.0
    malignant — *see* Table of Neoplasms, small intes-
        tine, malignant
  myocardium (acute) (chronic) — *see* Hypertrophy,
      cardiac
  organ or site, congenital NEC — *see* Distortion
  pancreatic duct K86.89
  pericardium — *see* Pericarditis
  pharynx J39.2
  prostate N42.89
  pulmonary
    artery (idiopathic) I28.8
    valve, congenital Q22.3
  pupil H57.04
  rectum K59.39

Dilatation — *continued*
  saccule, congenital Q16.5
  salivary gland (duct) K11.8
  sphincter ani K62.89
  stomach K31.89
    acute K31.0
    psychogenic F45.8
  submaxillary duct K11.8
  trachea, congenital Q32.1
  ureter (idiopathic) N28.82
    congenital Q62.2
    due to obstruction N13.4
  urethra (acquired) N36.8
  vasomotor I73.9
  vein I86.8
  ventricular, ventricle (acute) (chronic) (*see also* Hyper-
      trophy, cardiac)
    cerebral, congenital Q04.8
  venule NEC I86.8
  vesical orifice N32.89
Dilated, dilation — *see* Dilatation
Diminished, diminution
  hearing (acuity) — *see* Deafness
  sense or sensation (cold) (heat) (tactile) (vibratory)
      R20.8
  vision NEC H54.7
  vital capacity R94.2
Diminuta taenia B71.0
Dimitri-Sturge-Weber disease Q85.8
Dimple
  congenital sacral Q82.6
  parasacral Q82.6
  pilonidal or postanal — *see* Cyst, pilonidal
Dioctophyme renalis (infection) (infestation) B83.8
Dipetalonemiasis B74.4
Diphallus Q55.69
Diphtheria, diphtheritic (gangrenous) (hemorrhagic)
    A36.9
  carrier (suspected) Z22.2
  cutaneous A36.3
  faucial A36.0
  infection of wound A36.3
  laryngeal A36.2
  myocarditis A36.81
  nasal, anterior A36.89
  nasopharyngeal A36.1
  neurological complication A36.89
  pharyngeal A36.0
  specified site NEC A36.89
  tonsillar A36.0
Diphyllobothriasis (intestine) B70.0
  larval B70.1
Diplacusis H93.22- ☑
Diplegia (upper limbs) G83.0
  congenital (cerebral) G80.8
  facial G51.0
  lower limbs G82.20
  spastic G80.1
Diplococcus, diplococcal — *see* condition
Diplopia H53.2
Dipsomania F10.20
  with
    psychosis — *see* Psychosis, alcoholic
    remission F10.21
Dipylidiasis B71.1
DIRA (deficiency of interleukin 1 receptor antagonist)
    M04.8
Direction, teeth, abnormal, fully erupted M26.30
Dirofilariasis B74.8
Dirt-eating child F98.3
Disability, disabilities
  heart — *see* Disease, heart
  intellectual F79
    with
      autistic features F84.9
      mild (I.Q. 50-69) F70
      moderate (I.Q. 35-49) F71
      profound (I.Q. under 20) F73
      severe (I.Q. 20-34) F72
      specified level NEC F78
  knowledge acquisition F81.9
  learning F81.9
  limiting activities Z73.6
  spelling, specific F81.81
Disappearance of family member Z63.4
Disarticulation — *see* Amputation
  meaning traumatic amputation — *see* Amputation,
      traumatic

Discharge (from)
  abnormal finding in — *see* Abnormal, specimen
  breast (female) (male) N64.52
  diencephalic autonomic idiopathic — *see* Epilepsy,
      specified NEC
  ear (*see also* Otorrhea)
    blood — *see* Otorrhagia
  excessive urine R35.8
  nipple N64.52
  penile R36.9
  postnasal R09.82
  prison, anxiety concerning Z65.2
  urethral R36.9
    without blood R36.0
    hematospermia R36.1
  vaginal N89.8
Discitis, diskitis M46.40
  cervical region M46.42
  cervicothoracic region M46.43
  lumbar region M46.46
  lumbosacral region M46.47
  multiple sites M46.49
  occipito-atlanto-axial region M46.41
  pyogenic — *see* Infection, intervertebral disc, pyogenic
  sacrococcygeal region M46.48
  thoracic region M46.44
  thoracolumbar region M46.45
Discoid
  meniscus (congenital) Q68.6
  semilunar cartilage (congenital) — *see* Derangement,
      knee, meniscus, specified NEC
Discoloration
  nails L60.8
  teeth (posteruptive) K03.7
    during formation K00.8
Discomfort
  chest R07.89
  visual H53.14- ☑
Discontinuity, ossicles, ear H74.2- ☑
Discord (with)
  boss Z56.4
  classmates Z55.4
  counselor Z64.4
  employer Z56.4
  family Z63.8
  fellow employees Z56.4
  in-laws Z63.1
  landlord Z59.2
  lodgers Z59.2
  neighbors Z59.2
  probation officer Z64.4
  social worker Z64.4
  teachers Z55.4
  workmates Z56.4
Discordant connection
  atrioventricular (congenital) Q20.5
  ventriculoarterial Q20.3
Discrepancy
  centric occlusion maximum intercuspation M26.55
  leg length (acquired) — *see* Deformity, limb, unequal
      length
    congenital — *see* Defect, reduction, lower limb
  uterine size date O26.84- ☑
Discrimination
  ethnic Z60.5
  political Z60.5
  racial Z60.5
  religious Z60.5
  sex Z60.5
Disease, diseased (*see also* Syndrome)
  absorbent system I87.8
  acid-peptic K30
  Acosta's T70.29 ☑
  Adams-Stokes (-Morgagni) (syncope with heart block)
      I45.9
  Addison's anemia (pernicious) D51.0
  adenoids (and tonsils) J35.9
  adrenal (capsule) (cortex) (gland) (medullary) E27.9
    hyperfunction E27.0
    specified NEC E27.8
  ainhum L94.6
  airway
    obstructive, chronic J44.9
      due to
        cotton dust J66.0
        specific organic dusts NEC J66.8
    reactive — *see* Asthma
  akamushi (scrub typhus) A75.3

☑ **Additional Character Required — Refer to the Tabular List for Character Selection**   ▽ **Subterms under main terms may continue to next column or page**

Disease, diseased — *continued*

Albers-Schönberg (marble bones) Q78.2
Albert's — *see* Tendinitis, Achilles
alimentary canal K63.9
alligator-skin Q80.9
    acquired L85.0
alpha heavy chain C88.3
alpine T70.29 ☑
altitude T70.20 ☑
alveolar ridge
    edentulous K06.9
        specified NEC K06.8
alveoli, teeth K08.9
Alzheimer's G30.9 [F02.80]
    with behavioral disturbance G30.9 [F02.81]
    early onset G30.0 [F02.80]
        with behavioral disturbance G30.0 [F02.81]
    late onset G30.1 [F02.80]
        with behavioral disturbance G30.1 [F02.81]
    specified NEC G30.8 [F02.80]
        with behavioral disturbance G30.8 [F02.81]
amyloid — *see* Amyloidosis
Andersen's (glycogenosis IV) E74.09
Andes T70.29 ☑
Andrews' (bacterid) L08.89
angiospastic I73.9
    cerebral G45.9
    vein I87.8
anterior
    chamber H21.9
    horn cell G12.29
antiglomerular basement membrane (anti- GBM) antibody M31.0
    tubulo-interstitial nephritis N12
antral — *see* Sinusitis, maxillary
anus K62.9
    specified NEC K62.89
aorta (nonsyphilitic) I77.9
    syphilitic NEC A52.02
aortic (heart) (valve) I35.9
    rheumatic I06.9
Apollo B30.3
aponeuroses — *see* Enthesopathy
appendix K38.9
    specified NEC K38.8
aqueous (chamber) H21.9
Arnold-Chiari — *see* Arnold-Chiari disease
arterial I77.9
    occlusive — *see* Occlusion, by site
        due to stricture or stenosis I77.1
arteriocardiorenal — *see* Hypertension, cardiorenal
arteriolar (generalized) (obliterative) I77.9
arteriorenal — *see* Hypertension, kidney
arteriosclerotic (*see also* Arteriosclerosis)
    cardiovascular — *see* Disease, heart, ischemic, atherosclerotic
    coronary (artery) — *see* Disease, heart, ischemic, atherosclerotic
    heart — *see* Disease, heart, ischemic, atherosclerotic
artery I77.9
    cerebral I67.9
    coronary I25.10
        with angina pectoris — *see* Arteriosclerosis, coronary (artery)
arthropod-borne NOS (viral) A94
    specified type NEC A93.8
atticoantral, chronic H66.20
    left H66.22
        with right H66.23
    right H66.21
        with left H66.23
auditory canal — *see* Disorder, ear, external
auricle, ear NEC — *see* Disorder, pinna
Australian X A83.4
autoimmune (systemic) NOS M35.9
    hemolytic (cold type) (warm type) D59.1
        drug-induced D59.0
    thyroid E06.3
aviator's — *see* Effect, adverse, high altitude
Ayerza's (pulmonary artery sclerosis with pulmonary hypertension) I27.0
Babington's (familial hemorrhagic telangiectasia) I78.0
bacterial A49.9
    specified NEC A48.8
    zoonotic A28.9
        specified type NEC A28.8
Baelz's (cheilitis glandularis apostematosa) K13.0

Disease, diseased — *continued*

bagasse J67.1
balloon — *see* Effect, adverse, high altitude
Bang's (brucella abortus) A23.1
Bannister's T78.3 ☑
barometer makers' — *see* Poisoning, mercury
Barraquer (-Simons') (progressive lipodystrophy) E88.1
Barrett's — *see* Barrett's, esophagus
Bartholin's gland N75.9
basal ganglia G25.9
    degenerative G23.9
        specified NEC G23.8
    specified NEC G25.89
Basedow's (exophthalmic goiter) — *see* Hyperthyroidism, with, goiter (diffuse)
Bateman's B08.1
Batten-Steinert G71.11
Battey A31.0
Beard's (neurasthenia) F48.8
Becker
    idiopathic mural endomyocardial I42.3
    myotonia congenita G71.12
Begbie's (exophthalmic goiter) — *see* Hyperthyroidism, with, goiter (diffuse)
behavioral, organic F07.9
Beigel's (white piedra) B36.2
Benson's — *see* Deposit, crystalline
Bernard-Soulier (thrombopathy) D69.1
Bernhardt (-Roth) — *see* Mononeuropathy, lower limb, meralgia paresthetica
Biermer's (pernicious anemia) D51.0
bile duct (common) (hepatic) K83.9
    with calculus, stones — *see* Calculus, bile duct
    specified NEC K83.8
biliary (tract) K83.9
    specified NEC K83.8
Billroth's — *see* Spina bifida
bird fancier's J67.2
black lung J60
bladder N32.9
    in (due to)
        schistosomiasis (bilharziasis) B65.0 [N33]
    specified NEC N32.89
bleeder's D66
blood D75.9
    forming organs D75.9
    vessel I99.9
Bloodgood's — *see* Mastopathy, cystic
Bodechtel-Guttmann (subacute sclerosing panencephalitis) A81.1
bone (*see also* Disorder, bone)
    aluminum M83.4
    fibrocystic NEC
        jaw M27.49
bone-marrow D75.9
Borna A83.9
Bornholm (epidemic pleurodynia) B33.0
Bouchard's (myopathic dilatation of the stomach) K31.0
Bouillaud's (rheumatic heart disease) I01.9
Bourneville (-Brissaud) (tuberous sclerosis) Q85.1
Bouveret (-Hoffmann) (paroxysmal tachycardia) I47.9
bowel K63.9
    functional K59.9
        psychogenic F45.8
brain G93.9
    arterial, artery I67.9
    arteriosclerotic I67.2
    congenital Q04.9
    degenerative — *see* Degeneration, brain
    inflammatory — *see* Encephalitis
    organic G93.9
        arteriosclerotic I67.2
    parasitic NEC B71.9 [G94]
    senile NEC G31.1
    specified NEC G93.89
breast (*see also* Disorder, breast) N64.9
    cystic (chronic) — *see* Mastopathy, cystic
    fibrocystic — *see* Mastopathy, cystic
    Paget's
        female, unspecified side C50.91- ☑
        male, unspecified side C50.92- ☑
    specified NEC N64.89
Breda's — *see* Yaws
Bretonneau's (diphtheritic malignant angina) A36.0
Bright's — *see* Nephritis
    arteriosclerotic — *see* Hypertension, kidney
Brill's (recrudescent typhus) A75.1

Disease, diseased — *continued*

Brill-Zinsser (recrudescent typhus) A75.1
Brion-Kayser — *see* Fever, paratyphoid
broad
    beta E78.2
    ligament (noninflammatory) N83.9
        inflammatory — *see* Disease, pelvis, inflammatory
        specified NEC N83.8
Brocq-Duhring (dermatitis herpetiformis) L13.0
Brocq's
    meaning
        dermatitis herpetiformis L13.0
        prurigo L28.2
bronchopulmonary J98.4
bronchus NEC J98.09
bronze Addison's E27.1
    tuberculous A18.7
budgerigar fancier's J67.2
Buerger's (thromboangiitis obliterans) I73.1
bullous L13.9
    chronic of childhood L12.2
    specified NEC L13.8
Bürger-Grütz (essential familial hyperlipemia) E78.3
bursa — *see* Bursopathy
caisson T70.3 ☑
California — *see* Coccidioidomycosis
capillaries I78.9
    specified NEC I78.8
Carapata A68.0
cardiac — *see* Disease, heart
cardiopulmonary, chronic I27.9
cardiorenal (hepatic) (hypertensive) (vascular) — *see* Hypertension, cardiorenal
cardiovascular (atherosclerotic) I25.10
    with angina pectoris — *see* Arteriosclerosis, coronary (artery),
    congenital Q28.9
    hypertensive — *see* Hypertension, heart
    newborn P29.9
        specified NEC P29.89
    renal (hypertensive) — *see* Hypertension, cardiorenal
    syphilitic (asymptomatic) A52.00
cartilage — *see* Disorder, cartilage
Castellani's A69.8
Castleman (unicentric) (multicentric) D47.Z2
    HHV-8-associated (*see also* Herpesvirus, human, 8) D47.Z2
cat-scratch A28.1
Cavare's (familial periodic paralysis) G72.3
cecum K63.9
celiac (adult) (infantile) (with steatorrhea) K90.0
cellular tissue L98.9
central core G71.2
cerebellar, cerebellum — *see* Disease, brain
cerebral (*see also* Disease, brain)
    degenerative — *see* Degeneration, brain
cerebrospinal G96.9
cerebrovascular I67.9
    acute I67.89
        embolic I63.4- ☑
        thrombotic I63.3- ☑
    arteriosclerotic I67.2
    specified NEC I67.89
cervix (uteri) (noninflammatory) N88.9
    inflammatory — *see* Cervicitis
    specified NEC N88.8
Chabert's A22.9
Chandler's (osteochondritis dissecans, hip) — *see* Osteochondritis, dissecans, hip
Charlouis — *see* Yaws
Chédiak-Steinbrinck (-Higashi) (congenital gigantism of peroxidase granules) E70.330
chest J98.9
Chiari's (hepatic vein thrombosis) I82.0
Chicago B40.9
Chignon B36.8
chigo, chigoe B88.1
childhood granulomatous D71
Chinese liver fluke B66.1
chlamydial A74.9
    specified NEC A74.89
cholecystic K82.9
choroid H31.9
    specified NEC H31.8
Christmas D67
chronic bullous of childhood L12.2

Disease, diseased — *continued*

chylomicron retention E78.3
ciliary body H21.9
  specified NEC H21.89
circulatory (system) NEC I99.8
  newborn P29.9
  syphilitic A52.00
    congenital A50.54
coagulation factor deficiency (congenital) — *see* Defect, coagulation
coccidioidal — *see* Coccidioidomycosis
cold
  agglutinin or hemoglobinuria D59.1
    paroxysmal D59.6
  hemagglutinin (chronic) D59.1
collagen NOS (nonvascular) (vascular) M35.9
  specified NEC M35.8
colon K63.9
  functional K59.9
    congenital Q43.2
  ischemic (*see also* Ischemia, intestine, acute) K55.039
colonic inflammatory bowel, unclassified (IBDU) K52.3
combined system — *see* Degeneration, combined
compressed air T70.3 ✓
Concato's (pericardial polyserositis) A19.9
  nontubercular I31.1
  pleural — *see* Pleurisy, with effusion
conjunctiva H11.9
  chlamydial A74.0
  specified NEC H11.89
  viral B30.9
    specified NEC B30.8
connective tissue, systemic (diffuse) M35.9
  in (due to)
    hypogammaglobulinemia D80.1 [M36.8]
    ochronosis E70.29 [M36.8]
  specified NEC M35.8
Conor and Bruch's (boutonneuse fever) A77.1
Cooper's — *see* Mastopathy, cystic
Cori's (glycogenosis III) E74.03
corkhandler's or corkworker's J67.3
cornea H18.9
  specified NEC H18.89- ✓
coronary (artery) — *see* Disease, heart, ischemic, atherosclerotic
  congenital Q24.5
  ostial, syphilitic (aortic) (mitral) (pulmonary) A52.03
corpus cavernosum N48.9
  specified NEC N48.89
Cotugno's — *see* Sciatica
coxsackie (virus) NEC B34.1
cranial nerve NOS G52.9
Creutzfeldt-Jakob — *see* Creutzfeldt-Jakob disease or syndrome
Crocq's (acrocyanosis) I73.89
Crohn's — *see* Enteritis, regional
Curschmann G71.11
cystic
  breast (chronic) — *see* Mastopathy, cystic
  kidney, congenital Q61.9
  liver, congenital Q44.6
  lung J98.4
    congenital Q33.0
cytomegalic inclusion (generalized) B25.9
  with pneumonia B25.0
  congenital P35.1
cytomegaloviral B25.9
  specified NEC B25.8
Czerny's (periodic hydrarthrosis of the knee) — *see* Effusion, joint, knee
Daae (-Finsen) (epidemic pleurodynia) B33.0
Darling's — *see* Histoplasmosis capsulati
de Quervain's (tendon sheath) M65.4
  thyroid (subacute granulomatous thyroiditis) E06.1
Débove's (splenomegaly) R16.1
deer fly — *see* Tularemia
Degos' I77.89
demyelinating, demyelinizating (nervous system) G37.9
  multiple sclerosis G35
  specified NEC G37.8
dense deposit (*see also* N00-N07 with fourth character .6) N05.6
deposition, hydroxyapatite — *see* Disease, hydroxyapatite deposition
Devergie's (pityriasis rubra pilaris) L44.0
Devic's G36.0

diaphorase deficiency D74.0
diaphragm J98.6
diarrheal, infectious NEC A09
digestive system K92.9
  specified NEC K92.89
disc, degenerative — *see* Degeneration, intervertebral disc
discogenic (*see also* Displacement, intervertebral disc NEC)
  with myelopathy — *see* Disorder, disc, with, myelopathy
diverticular — *see* Diverticula
Dubois (thymus) A50.59 [E35]
Duchenne-Griesinger G71.0
Duchenne's
  muscular dystrophy G71.0
  pseudohypertrophy, muscles G71.0
ductless glands E34.9
Duhring's (dermatitis herpetiformis) L13.0
duodenum K31.9
  specified NEC K31.89
Dupré's (meningism) R29.1
Dupuytren's (muscle contracture) M72.0
Durand-Nicholas-Favre (climatic bubo) A55
Duroziez's (congenital mitral stenosis) Q23.2
ear — *see* Disorder, ear
Eberth's — *see* Fever, typhoid
Ebola (virus) A98.4
Ebstein's heart Q22.5
Echinococcus — *see* Echinococcus
echovirus NEC B34.1
Eddowes' (brittle bones and blue sclera) Q78.0
edentulous (alveolar) ridge K06.9
  specified NEC K06.8
Edsall's T67.2 ✓
Eichstedt's (pityriasis versicolor) B36.0
Eisenmenger's (irreversible) I27.83
Ellis-van Creveld (chondroectodermal dysplasia) Q77.6
end stage renal (ESRD) N18.6
  due to hypertension I12.0
endocrine glands or system NEC E34.9
endomyocardial (eosinophilic) I42.3
English (rickets) E55.0
enteroviral, enterovirus NEC B34.1
  central nervous system NEC A88.8
epidemic B99.9
  specified NEC B99.8
epididymis N50.9
Erb (-Landouzy) G71.0
Erdheim-Chester (ECD) E88.89
esophagus K22.9
  functional K22.4
  psychogenic F45.8
  specified NEC K22.8
Eulenburg's (congenital paramyotonia) G71.19
eustachian tube — *see* Disorder, eustachian tube
external
  auditory canal — *see* Disorder, ear, external
  ear — *see* Disorder, ear, external
extrapyramidal G25.9
  specified NEC G25.89
eye H57.9
  anterior chamber H21.9
  inflammatory NEC H57.8
  muscle (external) — *see* Strabismus
  specified NEC H57.8
  syphilitic — *see* Oculopathy, syphilitic
eyeball H44.9
  specified NEC H44.89
eyelid — *see* Disorder, eyelid
  specified NEC — *see* Disorder, eyelid, specified type NEC
eyeworm of Africa B74.3
facial nerve (seventh) G51.9
  newborn (birth injury) P11.3
Fahr (of brain) G23.8
Fahr Volhard (of kidney) I12.- ✓
fallopian tube (noninflammatory) N83.9
  inflammatory — *see* Salpingo-oophoritis
  specified NEC N83.8
familial periodic paralysis G72.3
Fanconi's (congenital pancytopenia) D61.09
fascia NEC (*see also* Disorder, muscle)
  inflammatory — *see* Myositis
  specified NEC M62.89
Fauchard's (periodontitis) — *see* Periodontitis
Favre-Durand-Nicolas (climatic bubo) A55

Fede's K14.0
Feer's — *see* Poisoning, mercury
female pelvic inflammatory (*see also* Disease, pelvis, inflammatory) N73.9
  syphilitic (secondary) A51.42
  tuberculous A18.17
Fernels' (aortic aneurysm) I71.9
fibrocaseous of lung — *see* Tuberculosis, pulmonary
fibrocystic — *see* Fibrocystic disease
Fiedler's (leptospiral jaundice) A27.0
fifth B08.3
file-cutter's — *see* Poisoning, lead
fish-skin Q80.9
  acquired L85.0
Flajani (-Basedow) (exophthalmic goiter) — *see* Hyperthyroidism, with, goiter (diffuse)
flax-dresser's J66.1
fluke — *see* Infestation, fluke
foot and mouth B08.8
foot process N04.9
Forbes' (glycogenosis III) E74.03
Fordyce-Fox (apocrine miliaria) L75.2
Fordyce's (ectopic sebaceous glands) (mouth) Q38.6
Forestier's (rhizomelic pseudopolyarthritis) M35.3
  meaning ankylosing hyperostosis — *see* Hyperostosis, ankylosing
Fothergill's
  neuralgia — *see* Neuralgia, trigeminal
  scarlatina anginosa A38.9
Fournier (gangrene) N49.3
  female N76.89
fourth B08.8
Fox (-Fordyce) (apocrine miliaria) L75.2
Francis' — *see* Tularemia
Franklin C88.2
Frei's (climatic bubo) A55
Friedreich's
  combined systemic or ataxia G11.1
  myoclonia G25.3
frontal sinus — *see* Sinusitis, frontal
fungus NEC B49
Gaisböck's (polycythemia hypertonica) D75.1
gallbladder K82.9
  calculus — *see* Calculus, gallbladder
  cholecystitis — *see* Cholecystitis
  cholesterolosis K82.4
  fistula — *see* Fistula, gallbladder
  hydrops K82.1
  obstruction — *see* Obstruction, gallbladder
  perforation K82.2
  specified NEC K82.8
gamma heavy chain C88.2
Gamna's (siderotic splenomegaly) D73.2
Gamstorp's (adynamia episodica hereditaria) G72.3
Gandy-Nanta (siderotic splenomegaly) D73.2
ganister J62.8
gastric — *see* Disease, stomach
gastroesophageal reflux (GERD) K21.9
  with esophagitis K21.0
gastrointestinal (tract) K92.9
  amyloid E85.4
  functional K59.9
    psychogenic F45.8
  specified NEC K92.89
Gee (-Herter) (-Heubner) (-Thaysen) (nontropical sprue) K90.0
genital organs
  female N94.9
  male N50.9
Gerhardt's (erythromelalgia) I73.81
Gibert's (pityriasis rosea) L42
Gierke's (glycogenosis I) E74.01
Gilles de la Tourette's (motor-verbal tic) F95.2
gingiva K06.9
  plaque induced K05.00
  specified NEC K06.8
gland (lymph) I89.9
Glanzmann's (hereditary hemorrhagic thrombasthenia) D69.1
glass-blower's (cataract) — *see* Cataract, specified NEC
  salivary gland hypertrophy K11.1
Glisson's — *see* Rickets
globe H44.9
  specified NEC H44.89
glomerular (*see also* Glomerulonephritis)
  with edema — *see* Nephrosis
  acute — *see* Nephritis, acute

✓ **Additional Character Required** — Refer to the Tabular List for Character Selection   ▽ Subterms under main terms may continue to next column or page

Disease, diseased — continued
  glomerular (see also Glomerulonephritis) — contin-
    ued
    chronic — see Nephritis, chronic
    minimal change N05.0
    rapidly progressive N01.9
  glycogen storage E74.00
    Andersen's E74.09
    Cori's E74.03
    Forbes' E74.03
    generalized E74.00
    glucose-6-phosphatase deficiency E74.01
    heart E74.02 [I43]
    hepatorenal E74.09
    Hers' E74.09
    liver and kidney E74.09
    McArdle's E74.04
    muscle phosphofructokinase E74.09
    myocardium E74.02 [I43]
    Pompe's E74.02
    Tauri's E74.09
    type 0 E74.09
    type I E74.01
    type II E74.02
    type III E74.03
    type IV E74.09
    type V E74.04
    type VI-XI E74.09
    Von Gierke's E74.01
  Goldstein's (familial hemorrhagic telangiectasia) I78.0
  gonococcal NOS A54.9
  graft-versus-host (GVH) D89.813
    acute D89.810
    acute on chronic D89.812
    chronic D89.811
  grainhandler's J67.8
  granulomatous (childhood) (chronic) D71
  Graves' (exophthalmic goiter) — see Hyperthyroidism,
    with, goiter (diffuse)
  Griesinger's — see Ancylostomiasis
  Grisel's M43.6
  Gruby's (tinea tonsurans) B35.0
  Guillain-Barré G61.0
  Guinon's (motor-verbal tic) F95.2
  gum K06.9
  gynecological N94.9
  H (Hartnup's) E72.02
  Haff — see Poisoning, mercury
  Hageman (congenital factor XII deficiency) D68.2
  hair (color) (shaft) L67.9
    follicles L73.9
      specified NEC L73.8
  Hamman's (spontaneous mediastinal emphysema)
    J98.2
  hand, foot and mouth B08.4
  Hansen's — see Leprosy
  Hantavirus, with pulmonary manifestations B33.4
    with renal manifestations A98.5
  Harada's H30.81- ☑
  Hartnup (pellagra-cerebellar ataxia-renal
    aminoaciduria) E72.02
  Hart's (pellagra-cerebellar ataxia-renal aminoaciduria)
    E72.02
  Hashimoto's (struma lymphomatosa) E06.3
  Hb — see Disease, hemoglobin
  heart (organic) I51.9
    with
      pulmonary edema (acute) (see also Failure,
        ventricular, left) I50.1
      rheumatic fever (conditions in I00)
        active I01.9
          with chorea I02.0
          specified NEC I01.8
        inactive or quiescent (with chorea) I09.9
          specified NEC I09.89
    amyloid E85.4 [I43]
    aortic (valve) I35.9
    arteriosclerotic or sclerotic (senile) — see Disease,
      heart, ischemic, atherosclerotic
    artery, arterial — see Disease, heart, ischemic,
      atherosclerotic
    beer drinkers' I42.6
    beriberi (wet) E51.12
    black I27.0
    congenital Q24.9
      cyanotic Q24.9
      specified NEC Q24.8
    coronary — see Disease, heart, ischemic

Disease, diseased — continued
  heart — continued
    cryptogenic I51.9
    fibroid — see Myocarditis
    functional I51.89
      psychogenic F45.8
    glycogen storage E74.02 [I43]
    gonococcal A54.83
    hypertensive — see Hypertension, heart
    hyperthyroid (see also Hyperthyroidism)
      E05.90 [I43]
      with thyroid storm E05.91 [I43]
    ischemic (chronic or with a stated duration of over
      4 weeks) I25.9
      atherosclerotic (of) I25.10
        with angina pectoris — see Arteriosclerosis,
          coronary (artery)
        coronary artery bypass graft — see Arte-
          riosclerosis, coronary (artery),
      cardiomyopathy I25.5
      diagnosed on ECG or other special investiga-
        tion, but currently presenting no symp-
        toms I25.6
      silent I25.6
      specified form NEC I25.89
    kyphoscoliotic I27.1
    meningococcal A39.50
      endocarditis A39.51
      myocarditis A39.52
      pericarditis A39.53
    mitral I05.9
      specified NEC I05.8
    muscular — see Degeneration, myocardial
    psychogenic (functional) F45.8
    pulmonary (chronic) I27.9
      in schistosomiasis B65.9 [I52]
      specified NEC I27.89
    rheumatic (chronic) (inactive) (old) (quiescent)
      (with chorea) I09.9
      active or acute I01.9
        with chorea (acute) (rheumatic) (Syden-
          ham's) I02.0
      specified NEC I09.89
    senile — see Myocarditis
    syphilitic A52.06
      aortic A52.03
        aneurysm A52.01
      congenital A50.54 [I52]
    thyrotoxic (see also Thyrotoxicosis) E05.90 [I43]
      with thyroid storm E05.91 [I43]
    valve, valvular (obstructive) (regurgitant) (see also
      Endocarditis)
      congenital NEC Q24.8
        pulmonary Q22.3
    vascular — see Disease, cardiovascular
  heavy chain NEC C88.2
    alpha C88.3
    gamma C88.2
    mu C88.2
  Hebra's
    pityriasis
      maculata et circinata L42
      rubra pilaris L44.0
    prurigo L28.2
  hematopoietic organs D75.9
  hemoglobin or Hb
    abnormal (mixed) NEC D58.2
      with thalassemia D56.9
    AS genotype D57.3
    Bart's D56.0
    C (Hb-C) D58.2
      with other abnormal hemoglobin NEC D58.2
      elliptocytosis D58.1
      Hb-S D57.2- ☑
      sickle-cell D57.2- ☑
      thalassemia D56.8
    Constant Spring D58.2
    D (Hb-D) D58.2
    E (Hb-E) D58.2
    E-beta thalassemia D56.5
    elliptocytosis D58.1
    H (Hb-H) (thalassemia) D56.0
      with other abnormal hemoglobin NEC D56.9
      Constant Spring D56.0
    I thalassemia D56.9
    M D74.0
    S or SS D57.1
    SC D57.2- ☑

Disease, diseased — continued
  hemoglobin or Hb — continued
    SD D57.8- ☑
    SE D57.8- ☑
    spherocytosis D58.0
    unstable, hemolytic D58.2
  hemolytic (newborn) P55.9
    autoimmune (cold type) (warm type) D59.1
    drug-induced D59.0
    due to or with
      incompatibility
        ABO (blood group) P55.1
        blood (group) (Duffy) (K(ell)) (Kidd) (Lewis)
          (M) (S) NEC P55.8
        Rh (blood group) (factor) P55.0
        Rh negative mother P55.0
    specified type NEC P55.8
    unstable hemoglobin D58.2
  hemorrhagic D69.9
    newborn P53
  Henoch (-Schönlein) (purpura nervosa) D69.0
  hepatic — see Disease, liver
  hepatolenticular E83.01
  heredodegenerative NEC
    spinal cord G95.89
  herpesviral, disseminated B00.7
  Hers' (glycogenosis VI) E74.09
  Herter (-Gee) (-Heubner) (nontropical sprue) K90.0
  Heubner-Herter (nontropical sprue) K90.0
  high fetal gene or hemoglobin thalassemia D56.9
  Hildenbrand's — see Typhus
  hip (joint) M25.9
    congenital Q65.89
    suppurative M00.9
    tuberculous A18.02
  His (-Werner) (trench fever) A79.0
  Hodgson's I71.2
    ruptured I71.1
  Holla — see Spherocytosis
  hookworm B76.9
    specified NEC B76.8
  host-versus-graft D89.813
    acute D89.810
    acute on chronic D89.812
    chronic D89.811
  human immunodeficiency virus (HIV) B20
  Huntington's G10
    with dementia G10 [F02.80]
  Hutchinson's (cheiropompholyx) — see Hutchinson's
    disease
  hyaline (diffuse) (generalized)
    membrane (lung) (newborn) P22.0
      adult J80
  hydatid — see Echinococcus
  hydroxyapatite deposition M11.00
    ankle M11.07- ☑
    elbow M11.02- ☑
    foot joint M11.07- ☑
    hand joint M11.04- ☑
    hip M11.05- ☑
    knee M11.06- ☑
    multiple site M11.09
    shoulder M11.01- ☑
    vertebra M11.08
    wrist M11.03- ☑
  hyperkinetic — see Hyperkinesia
  hypertensive — see Hypertension
  hypophysis E23.7
  Iceland G93.3
  I-cell E77.0
  immune D89.9
  immunoproliferative (malignant) C88.9
    small intestinal C88.3
    specified NEC C88.8
  inclusion B25.9
    salivary gland B25.9
  infectious, infective B99.9
    congenital P37.9
      specified NEC P37.8
      viral P35.9
        specified type NEC P35.8
    specified NEC B99.8
  inflammatory
    penis N48.29
      abscess N48.21
      cellulitis N48.22
    prepuce N47.7
      balanoposthitis N47.6

Disease, diseased — *continued*
inflammatory — *continued*
  tubo-ovarian — *see* Salpingo-oophoritis
 intervertebral disc (*see also* Disorder, disc)
  with myelopathy — *see* Disorder, disc, with,
   myelopathy
  cervical, cervicothoracic — *see* Disorder, disc, cervical
   with
    myelopathy — *see* Disorder, disc, cervical,
     with myelopathy
    neuritis, radiculitis or radiculopathy — *see*
     Disorder, disc, cervical, with neuritis
    specified NEC — *see* Disorder, disc, cervical,
     specified type NEC
  lumbar (with)
   myelopathy M51.06
   neuritis, radiculitis, radiculopathy or sciatica
    M51.16
   specified NEC M51.86
  lumbosacral (with)
   neuritis, radiculitis, radiculopathy or sciatica
    M51.17
   specified NEC M51.87
  specified NEC — *see* Disorder, disc, specified NEC
  thoracic (with)
   myelopathy M51.04
   neuritis, radiculitis or radiculopathy M51.14
   specified NEC M51.84
  thoracolumbar (with)
   myelopathy M51.05
   neuritis, radiculitis or radiculopathy M51.15
   specified NEC M51.85
 intestine K63.9
  functional K59.9
   psychogenic F45.8
   specified NEC K59.8
  organic K63.9
  protozoal A07.9
  specified NEC K63.89
 iris H21.9
  specified NEC H21.89
 iron metabolism or storage E83.10
 island (scrub typhus) A75.3
 itai-itai — *see* Poisoning, cadmium
 Jakob-Creutzfeldt — *see* Creutzfeldt-Jakob disease or
  syndrome
 jaw M27.9
  fibrocystic M27.49
  specified NEC M27.8
 jigger B88.1
 joint (*see also* Disorder, joint)
  Charcot's — *see* Arthropathy, neuropathic (Charcot)
  degenerative — *see* Osteoarthritis
   multiple M15.9
   spine — *see* Spondylosis
  hypertrophic — *see* Osteoarthritis
  sacroiliac M53.3
  specified NEC — *see* Disorder, joint, specified type
   NEC
  spine NEC — *see* Dorsopathy
  suppurative — *see* Arthritis, pyogenic or pyemic
 Jourdain's (acute gingivitis) K05.00
  nonplaque induced K05.01
  plaque induced K05.00
 Kaschin-Beck (endemic polyarthritis) M12.10
  ankle M12.17- ☑
  elbow M12.12- ☑
  foot joint M12.17- ☑
  hand joint M12.14- ☑
  hip M12.15- ☑
  knee M12.16- ☑
  multiple site M12.19
  shoulder M12.11- ☑
  vertebra M12.18
  wrist M12.13- ☑
 Katayama B65.2
 Kedani (scrub typhus) A75.3
 Keshan E59
 kidney (functional) (pelvis) N28.9
  chronic N18.9
   hypertensive — *see* Hypertension, kidney
   stage 1 N18.1
   stage 2 (mild) N18.2
   stage 3 (moderate) N18.3
   stage 4 (severe) N18.4
   stage 5 N18.5

Disease, diseased — *continued*
kidney — *continued*
  complicating pregnancy — *see* Pregnancy, complicated by, renal disease
  cystic (congenital) Q61.9
  fibrocystic (congenital) Q61.8
  hypertensive — *see* Hypertension, kidney
  in (due to)
   schistosomiasis (bilharziasis) B65.9 [N29]
  multicystic Q61.4
  polycystic Q61.3
   adult type Q61.2
   childhood type NEC Q61.19
    collecting duct dilatation Q61.11
 Kimmelstiel (-Wilson) (intercapillary polycystic (congenital) glomerulosclerosis) — *see* E08-E13 with
  .21
 Kinnier Wilson's (hepatolenticular degeneration)
  E83.01
 kissing — *see* Mononucleosis, infectious
 Klebs' (*see also* Glomerulonephritis) N05- ☑
 Klippel-Feil (brevicollis) Q76.1
 Köhler-Pellegrini-Stieda (calcification, knee joint) —
  see Bursitis, tibial collateral
 Kok Q89.8
 König's (osteochondritis dissecans) — *see* Osteochon-
  dritis, dissecans
 Korsakoff's (nonalcoholic) F04
  alcoholic F10.96
   with dependence F10.26
 Kostmann's (infantile genetic agranulocytosis) D70.0
 kuru A81.81
 Kyasanur Forest A98.2
 labyrinth, ear — *see* Disorder, ear, inner
 lacrimal system — *see* Disorder, lacrimal system
 Lafora's — *see* Epilepsy, generalized, idiopathic
 Lancereaux-Mathieu (leptospiral jaundice) A27.0
 Landry's G61.0
 Larrey-Weil (leptospiral jaundice) A27.0
 larynx J38.7
 legionnaires' A48.1
  nonpneumonic A48.2
 Lenegre's I44.2
 lens H27.9
  specified NEC H27.8
 Lev's (acquired complete heart block) I44.2
 Lewy body (dementia) G31.83 [F02.80]
  with behavioral disturbance G31.83 [F02.81]
 Lichtheim's (subacute combined sclerosis with pernicious anemia) D51.0
 Lightwood's (renal tubular acidosis) N25.89
 Lignac's (cystinosis) E72.04
 lip K13.0
 lipid-storage E75.6
  specified NEC E75.5
 Lipschütz's N76.6
 liver (chronic) (organic) K76.9
  alcoholic (chronic) K70.9
   acute — *see* Disease, liver, alcoholic, hepatitis
   cirrhosis K70.30
    with ascites K70.31
   failure K70.40
    with coma K70.41
   fatty liver K70.0
   fibrosis K70.2
   hepatitis K70.10
    with ascites K70.11
   sclerosis K70.2
  cystic, congenital Q44.6
  drug-induced (idiosyncratic) (toxic) (predictable)
   (unpredictable) — *see* Disease, liver, toxic
  end stage K72.90
   due to hepatitis — *see* Hepatitis
  fatty, nonalcoholic (NAFLD) K76.0
   alcoholic K70.0
  fibrocystic (congenital) Q44.6
  fluke
   Chinese B66.1
   oriental B66.1
   sheep B66.3
  gestational alloimmune (GALD) P78.84
  glycogen storage E74.09 [K77]
  in (due to)
   schistosomiasis (bilharziasis) B65.9 [K77]
  inflammatory K75.9
   alcoholic K70.1 ☑
   specified NEC K75.89
  polycystic (congenital) Q44.6

Disease, diseased — *continued*
liver — *continued*
  toxic K71.9
   with
    cholestasis K71.0
    cirrhosis (liver) K71.7
    fibrosis (liver) K71.7
    focal nodular hyperplasia K71.8
    hepatic granuloma K71.8
    hepatic necrosis K71.10
     with coma K71.11
    hepatitis NEC K71.6
     acute K71.2
     chronic
      active K71.50
       with ascites K71.51
      lobular K71.4
      persistent K71.3
    lupoid K71.50
     with ascites K71.51
    peliosis hepatis K71.8
    veno-occlusive disease (VOD) of liver K71.8
  veno-occlusive K76.5
 Lobo's (keloid blastomycosis) B48.0
 Lobstein's (brittle bones and blue sclera) Q78.0
 Ludwig's (submaxillary cellulitis) K12.2
 lumbosacral region M53.87
 lung J98.4
  black J60
  congenital Q33.9
  cystic J98.4
   congenital Q33.0
  fibroid (chronic) — *see* Fibrosis, lung
  fluke B66.4
   oriental B66.4
  in
   amyloidosis E85.4 [J99]
   sarcoidosis D86.0
   Sjögren's syndrome M35.02
   systemic
    lupus erythematosus M32.13
    sclerosis M34.81
  interstitial J84.9
   of childhood, specified NEC J84.848
   respiratory bronchiolitis J84.115
   specified NEC J84.89
  obstructive (chronic) J44.9
   with
    acute
     bronchitis J44.0
     exacerbation NEC J44.1
     lower respiratory infection J44.0
    alveolitis, allergic J67.9
    asthma J44.9
    bronchiectasis J47.9
     with
      exacerbation (acute) J47.1
      lower respiratory infection J47.0
    bronchitis J44.9
     with
      exacerbation (acute) J44.1
      lower respiratory infection J44.0
    emphysema J43.9
    hypersensitivity pneumonitis J67.9
   decompensated J44.1
    with
     exacerbation (acute) J44.1
  polycystic J98.4
   congenital Q33.0
  rheumatoid (diffuse) (interstitial) — *see* Rheumatoid, lung
 Lutembacher's (atrial septal defect with mitral stenosis)
  Q21.1
 Lyme A69.20
 lymphatic (gland) (system) (channel) (vessel) I89.9
 lymphoproliferative D47.9
  specified NEC D47.Z9 (*following* D47.4)
  T-gamma D47.Z9 (*following* D47.4)
  X-linked D82.3
 Magitot's M27.2
 malarial — *see* Malaria
 malignant (*see also* Neoplasm, malignant, by site)
 Manson's B65.1
 maple bark J67.6
 maple-syrup-urine E71.0
 Marburg (virus) A98.3
 Marion's (bladder neck obstruction) N32.0
 Marsh's (exophthalmic goiter) — *see* Hyperthyroidism,
  with, goiter (diffuse)

☑ **Additional Character Required — Refer to the Tabular List for Character Selection**

🔄 **Subterms under main terms may continue to next column or page**

Disease, diseased — continued
  mastoid (process) — see Disorder, ear, middle
  Mathieu's (leptospiral jaundice) A27.Ø
  Maxcy's A75.2
  McArdle (-Schmid-Pearson) (glycogenosis V) E74.Ø4
  mediastinum J98.59
  medullary center (idiopathic) (respiratory) G93.89
  Meige's (chronic hereditary edema) Q82.Ø
  meningococcal — see Infection, meningococcal
  mental F99
    organic FØ9
  mesenchymal M35.9
  mesenteric embolic (see also Ischemia, intestine, acute)
      K55.Ø39
  metabolic, metabolism E88.9
    bilirubin E8Ø.7
  metal-polisher's J62.8
  metastatic (see also Neoplasm, secondary, by site)
      C79.9
  microvascular - code to condition
  microvillus
    atrophy Q43.8
    inclusion (MVD) Q43.8
  middle ear — see Disorder, ear, middle
  Mikulicz' (dryness of mouth, absent or decreased
      lacrimation) K11.8
  Milroy's (chronic hereditary edema) Q82.Ø
  Minamata — see Poisoning, mercury
  minicore G71.2
  Minor's G95.19
  Minot's (hemorrhagic disease, newborn) P53
  Minot-von Willebrand-Jürgens (angiohemophilia)
      D68.Ø
  Mitchell's (erythromelalgia) I73.81
  mitral (valve) IØ5.9
    nonrheumatic I34.9
  mixed connective tissue M35.1
  moldy hay J67.Ø
  Monge's T7Ø.29 ☑
  Morgagni-Adams-Stokes (syncope with heart block)
      I45.9
  Morgagni's (syndrome) (hyperostosis frontalis interna)
      M85.2
  Morton's (with metatarsalgia) — see Lesion, nerve,
      plantar
  Morvan's G6Ø.8
  motor neuron (bulbar) (mixed type) (spinal) G12.2Ø
    amyotrophic lateral sclerosis G12.21
    familial G12.24
    progressive bulbar palsy G12.22
    specified NEC G12.29
  moyamoya I67.5
  mu heavy chain disease C88.2
  multicore G71.2
  muscle (see also Disorder, muscle)
    inflammatory — see Myositis
    ocular (external) — see Strabismus
  musculoskeletal system, soft tissue — see also Disor-
      der, soft tissue
    specified NEC — see Disorder, soft tissue, specified
        type NEC
  mushroom workers' J67.5
  mycotic B49
  myelodysplastic, not classified C94.6
  myeloproliferative, not classified C94.6
    chronic D47.1
  myocardium, myocardial (see also Degeneration, my-
      ocardial) I51.5
    primary (idiopathic) I42.9
  myoneural G7Ø.9
  Naegeli's D69.1
  nails L6Ø.9
    specified NEC L6Ø.8
  Nairobi (sheep virus) A93.8
  nasal J34.9
  nemaline body G71.2
  nerve — see Disorder, nerve
  nervous system G98.8
    autonomic G9Ø.9
    central G96.9
      specified NEC G96.8
    congenital QØ7.9
    parasympathetic G9Ø.9
    specified NEC G98.8
    sympathetic G9Ø.9
    vegetative G9Ø.9
  neuromuscular system G7Ø.9
  Newcastle B3Ø.8

Disease, diseased — continued
  Nicolas (-Durand)-Favre (climatic bubo) A55
  nipple N64.9
    Paget's C5Ø.Ø1- ☑
      female C5Ø.Ø1- ☑
      male C5Ø.Ø2- ☑
  Nishimoto (-Takeuchi) I67.5
  nonarthropod-borne NOS (viral) B34.9
    enterovirus NEC B34.1
  nonautoimmune hemolytic D59.4
    drug-induced D59.2
  Nonne-Milroy-Meige (chronic hereditary edema) Q82.Ø
  nose J34.9
  nucleus pulposus — see Disorder, disc
  nutritional E63.9
  oast-house-urine E72.19
    ocular
      herpesviral BØØ.5Ø
      zoster BØ2.3Ø
  obliterative vascular I77.1
  Ohara's — see Tularemia
  Opitz's (congestive splenomegaly) D73.2
  Oppenheim-Urbach (necrobiosis lipoidica diabetico-
      rum) — see EØ8-E13 with .62Ø
  optic nerve NEC — see Disorder, nerve, optic
  orbit — see Disorder, orbit
  Oriental liver fluke B66.1
  Oriental lung fluke B66.4
  Ormond's N13.5
  Oropouche virus A93.Ø
  Osler-Rendu (familial hemorrhagic telangiectasia) I78.Ø
  osteofibrocystic E21.Ø
  Otto's M24.7
  outer ear — see Disorder, ear, external
  ovary (noninflammatory) N83.9
    cystic N83.2Ø- ☑
    inflammatory — see Salpingo-oophoritis
    polycystic E28.2
    specified NEC N83.8
  Owren's (congenital) — see Defect, coagulation
  pancreas K86.9
    cystic K86.2
    fibrocystic E84.9
    specified NEC K86.89
  panvalvular IØ8.9
    specified NEC IØ8.8
  parametrium (noninflammatory) N83.9
  parasitic B89
    cerebral NEC B71.9 [G94]
    intestinal NOS B82.9
    mouth B37.Ø
    skin NOS B88.9
    specified type — see Infestation
    tongue B37.Ø
  parathyroid (gland) E21.5
    specified NEC E21.4
  Parkinson's G2Ø
  parodontal KØ5.6
  Parrot's (syphilitic osteochondritis) A5Ø.Ø2
  Parry's (exophthalmic goiter) — see Hyperthyroidism,
      with, goiter (diffuse)
  Parson's (exophthalmic goiter) — see Hyperthyroidism,
      with, goiter (diffuse)
  Paxton's (white piedra) B36.2
  pearl-worker's — see Osteomyelitis, specified type
      NEC
  Pellegrini-Stieda (calcification, knee joint) — see Bur-
      sitis, tibial collateral
  pelvis, pelvic
    female NOS N94.9
      specified NEC N94.89
    gonococcal (acute) (chronic) A54.24
    inflammatory (female) N73.9
      acute N73.Ø
      chlamydial A56.11
      chronic N73.1
      specified NEC N73.8
      syphilitic (secondary) A51.42
        late A52.76
      tuberculous A18.17
    organ, female N94.9
    peritoneum, female NEC N94.89
  penis N48.9
    inflammatory N48.29
      abscess N48.21
      cellulitis N48.22
    specified NEC N48.89
  periapical tissues NOS KØ4.9Ø

Disease, diseased — continued
  periodontal KØ5.6
    specified NEC KØ5.5
  periosteum — see Disorder, bone, specified type NEC
  peripheral
    arterial I73.9
    autonomic nervous system G9Ø.9
    nerves — see Polyneuropathy
    vascular NOS I73.9
  peritoneum K66.9
    pelvic, female NEC N94.89
    specified NEC K66.8
  persistent mucosal (middle ear) H66.2Ø
    left H66.22
      with right H66.23
    right H66.21
      with left H66.23
  Petit's — see Hernia, abdomen, specified site NEC
  pharynx J39.2
    specified NEC J39.2
  Phocas' — see Mastopathy, cystic
  photochromogenic (acid-fast bacilli) (pulmonary)
      A31.Ø
    nonpulmonary A31.9
  Pick's G31.Ø1 [FØ2.8Ø]
    with behavioral disturbance G31.Ø1 [FØ2.81]
    brain G31.Ø1 [FØ2.8Ø]
      with behavioral disturbance G31.Ø1 [FØ2.81]
    of pericardium (pericardial pseudocirrhosis of liver)
        I31.1
  pigeon fancier's J67.2
  pineal gland E34.8
  pink — see Poisoning, mercury
  Pinkus' (lichen nitidus) L44.1
  pinworm B8Ø
  Piry virus A93.8
  pituitary (gland) E23.7
  pituitary-snuff-taker's J67.8
  pleura (cavity) J94.9
    specified NEC J94.8
  pneumatic drill (hammer) T75.21 ☑
  Pollitzer's (hidradenitis suppurativa) L73.2
  polycystic
    kidney or renal Q61.3
      adult type Q61.2
      childhood type NEC Q61.19
        collecting duct dilatation Q61.11
    liver or hepatic Q44.6
    lung or pulmonary J98.4
      congenital Q33.Ø
    ovary, ovaries E28.2
    spleen Q89.Ø9
  polyethylene T84.Ø5- ☑
  Pompe's (glycogenosis II) E74.Ø2
  Posadas-Wernicke B38.9
  Potain's (pulmonary edema) — see Edema, lung
  prepuce N47.8
    inflammatory N47.7
      balanoposthitis N47.6
  Pringle's (tuberous sclerosis) Q85.1
  prion, central nervous system A81.9
    specified NEC A81.89
  prostate N42.9
    specified NEC N42.89
  protozoal B64
    acanthamebiasis — see Acanthamebiasis
    African trypanosomiasis — see African trypanoso-
        miasis
    babesiosis B6Ø.Ø
    Chagas disease — see Chagas disease
    intestine, intestinal AØ7.9
    leishmaniasis — see Leishmaniasis
    malaria — see Malaria
    naegleriasis B6Ø.2
    pneumocystosis B59
    specified organism NEC B6Ø.8
    toxoplasmosis — see Toxoplasmosis
  pseudo-Hurler's E77.Ø
  psychiatric F99
  psychotic — see Psychosis
  Puente's (simple glandular cheilitis) K13.Ø
  puerperal (see also Puerperal) O9Ø.89
  pulmonary (see also Disease, lung)
    artery I28.9
    chronic obstructive J44.9
      with
        acute bronchitis J44.Ø
        exacerbation (acute) J44.1

Disease, diseased — *continued*
pulmonary (*see also* Disease, lung) — *continued*
  chronic obstructive — *continued*
    with — *continued*
      lower respiratory infection (acute) J44.0
    decompensated J44.1
      with
        exacerbation (acute) J44.1
  heart I27.9
    specified NEC I27.89
  hypertensive (vascular) (*see also* Hypertension, pulmonary) I27.20
    primary (idiopathic) I27.0
    NEC I27.2 ☑
  valve I37.9
    rheumatic I09.89
pulp (dental) NOS K04.90
pulseless M31.4
Putnam's (subacute combined sclerosis with pernicious anemia) D51.0
Pyle (-Cohn) (metaphyseal dysplasia) Q78.5
ragpicker's or ragsorter's A22.1
Raynaud's — *see* Raynaud's disease
reactive airway — *see* Asthma
Reclus' (cystic) — *see* Mastopathy, cystic
rectum K62.9
  specified NEC K62.89
Refsum's (heredopathia atactica polyneuritiformis) G60.1
renal (functional) (pelvis) (*see also* Disease, kidney) N28.9
  with
    edema — *see* Nephrosis
    glomerular lesion — *see* Glomerulonephritis
      with edema — *see* Nephrosis
    interstitial nephritis N12
  acute N28.9
  chronic (*see also* Disease, kidney, chronic) N18.9
  cystic, congenital Q61.9
  diabetic — *see* E08-E13 with .22
  end-stage (failure) N18.6
    due to hypertension I12.0
  fibrocystic (congenital) Q61.8
  hypertensive — *see* Hypertension, kidney
  lupus M32.14
  phosphate-losing (tubular) N25.0
  polycystic (congenital) Q61.3
    adult type Q61.2
    childhood type NEC Q61.19
      collecting duct dilatation Q61.11
  rapidly progressive N01.9
  subacute N01.9
Rendu-Osler-Weber (familial hemorrhagic telangiectasia) I78.0
renovascular (arteriosclerotic) — *see* Hypertension, kidney
respiratory (tract) J98.9
  acute or subacute NOS J06.9
    due to
      chemicals, gases, fumes or vapors (inhalation) J68.3
      external agent J70.9
        specified NEC J70.8
      radiation J70.0
      smoke inhalation J70.5
    noninfectious J39.8
  chronic NOS J98.9
    due to
      chemicals, gases, fumes or vapors J68.4
      external agent J70.9
        specified NEC J70.8
      radiation J70.1
    newborn P27.9
      specified NEC P27.8
  due to
    chemicals, gases, fumes or vapors J68.9
      acute or subacute NEC J68.3
      chronic J68.4
    external agent J70.9
      specified NEC J70.8
    newborn P28.9
      specified type NEC P28.89
  upper J39.9
    acute or subacute J06.9
    noninfectious NEC J39.8
    specified NEC J39.8
    streptococcal J06.9
retina, retinal H35.9

Disease, diseased — *continued*
retina, retinal — *continued*
  Batten's or Batten-Mayou E75.4 [H36]
  specified NEC H35.89
rheumatoid — *see* Arthritis, rheumatoid
rickettsial NOS A79.9
  specified type NEC A79.89
Riga (-Fede) (cachectic aphthae) K14.0
Riggs' (compound periodontitis) — *see* Periodontitis
Ritter's L00
Rivalta's (cervicofacial actinomycosis) A42.2
Robles' (onchocerciasis) B73.01
Roger's (congenital interventricular septal defect) Q21.0
Rosenthal's (factor XI deficiency) D68.1
Ross River B33.1
Rossbach's (hyperchlorhydria) K30
Rotes Quérol — *see* Hyperostosis, ankylosing
Roth (-Bernhardt) — *see* Mononeuropathy, lower limb, meralgia paresthetica
Runeberg's (progressive pernicious anemia) D51.0
sacroiliac NEC M53.3
salivary gland or duct K11.9
  inclusion B25.9
  specified NEC K11.8
  virus B25.9
sandworm B76.9
Schimmelbusch's — *see* Mastopathy, cystic
Schmorl's — *see* Schmorl's disease or nodes
Schönlein (-Henoch) (purpura rheumatica) D69.0
Schottmüller's — *see* Fever, paratyphoid
Schultz's (agranulocytosis) — *see* Agranulocytosis
Schwalbe-Ziehen-Oppenheim G24.1
Schwartz-Jampel G71.13
sclera H15.9
  specified NEC H15.89
scrofulous (tuberculous) A18.2
scrotum N50.9
sebaceous glands L73.9
semilunar cartilage, cystic (*see also* Derangement, knee, meniscus, cystic)
seminal vesicle N50.9
serum NEC (*see also* Reaction, serum) T80.69 ☑
sexually transmitted A64
  anogenital
    herpesviral infection — *see* Herpes, anogenital
    warts A63.0
  chancroid A57
  chlamydial infection — *see* Chlamydia
  gonorrhea — *see* Gonorrhea
  granuloma inguinale A58
  specified organism NEC A63.8
  syphilis — *see* Syphilis
  trichomoniasis — *see* Trichomoniasis
Sézary C84.1- ☑
shimamushi (scrub typhus) A75.3
shipyard B30.0
sickle-cell D57.1
  with crisis (vasoocclusive pain) D57.00
    with
      acute chest syndrome D57.01
      splenic sequestration D57.02
  elliptocytosis D57.8- ☑
  Hb-C D57.20
    with crisis (vasoocclusive pain) D57.219
      with
        acute chest syndrome D57.211
        splenic sequestration D57.212
    without crisis D57.20
  Hb-SD D57.80
    with crisis D57.819
      with
        acute chest syndrome D57.811
        splenic sequestration D57.812
  Hb-SE D57.80
    with crisis D57.819
      with
        acute chest syndrome D57.811
        splenic sequestration D57.812
  specified NEC D57.80
    with crisis D57.819
      with
        acute chest syndrome D57.811
        splenic sequestration D57.812
  spherocytosis D57.80
    with crisis D57.819
      with
        acute chest syndrome D57.811

Disease, diseased — *continued*
sickle-cell — *continued*
  spherocytosis — *continued*
    with crisis — *continued*
      with — *continued*
        splenic sequestration D57.812
  thalassemia D57.40
    with crisis (vasoocclusive pain) D57.419
      with
        acute chest syndrome D57.411
        splenic sequestration D57.412
    without crisis D57.40
silo-filler's J68.8
  bronchitis J68.0
  pneumonitis J68.0
  pulmonary edema J68.1
simian B B00.4
Simons' (progressive lipodystrophy) E88.1
sin nombre virus B33.4
sinus — *see* Sinusitis
Sirkari's B55.0
sixth B08.20
  due to human herpesvirus 6 B08.21
  due to human herpesvirus 7 B08.22
skin L98.9
  due to metabolic disorder NEC E88.9 [L99]
  specified NEC L98.8
slim (HIV) B20
small vessel I73.9
Sneddon-Wilkinson (subcorneal pustular dermatosis) L13.1
South African creeping B88.0
spinal (cord) G95.9
  congenital Q06.9
  specified NEC G95.89
spine (*see also* Spondylopathy)
  joint — *see* Dorsopathy
  tuberculous A18.01
spinocerebellar (hereditary) G11.9
  specified NEC G11.8
spleen D73.9
  amyloid E85.4 [D77]
  organic D73.9
  polycystic Q89.09
  postinfectional D73.89
sponge-diver's — *see* Toxicity, venom, marine animal, sea anemone
Startle Q89.8
Steinert's G71.11
Sticker's (erythema infectiosum) B08.3
Stieda's (calcification, knee joint) — *see* Bursitis, tibial collateral
Stokes' (exophthalmic goiter) — *see* Hyperthyroidism, with, goiter (diffuse)
Stokes-Adams (syncope with heart block) I45.9
stomach K31.9
  functional, psychogenic F45.8
  specified NEC K31.89
stonemason's J62.8
storage
  glycogen — *see* Disease, glycogen storage
  mucopolysaccharide — *see* Mucopolysaccharidosis
striatopallidal system NEC G25.89
Stuart-Prower (congenital factor X deficiency) D68.2
Stuart's (congenital factor X deficiency) D68.2
subcutaneous tissue — *see* Disease, skin
supporting structures of teeth K08.9
  specified NEC K08.89
suprarenal (capsule) (gland) E27.9
  hyperfunction E27.0
  specified NEC E27.8
sweat glands L74.9
  specified NEC L74.8
Sweeley-Klionsky E75.21
Swift (-Feer) — *see* Poisoning, mercury
swimming-pool granuloma A31.1
Sylvest's (epidemic pleurodynia) B33.0
sympathetic nervous system G90.9
synovium — *see* Disorder, synovium
syphilitic — *see* Syphilis
systemic tissue mast cell C96.20
tanapox (virus) B08.71
Tangier E78.6
Tarral-Besnier (pityriasis rubra pilaris) L44.0
Tauri's E74.09
tear duct — *see* Disorder, lacrimal system
tendon, tendinous (*see also* Disorder, tendon)
  nodular — *see* Trigger finger

☑ **Additional Character Required** — Refer to the Tabular List for Character Selection   ▽ Subterms under main terms may continue to next column or page

Disease, diseased — *continued*
  terminal vessel I73.9
  testis N50.9
  thalassemia Hb-S — *see* Disease, sickle-cell, tha-
      lassemia
  Thaysen-Gee (nontropical sprue) K90.0
  Thomsen G71.12
  throat J39.2
    septic J02.0
  thromboembolic — *see* Embolism
  thymus (gland) E32.9
    specified NEC E32.8
  thyroid (gland) E07.9
    heart (*see also* Hyperthyroidism) E05.90 [I43]
      with thyroid storm E05.91 [I43]
    specified NEC E07.89
  Tietze's M94.0
  tongue K14.9
    specified NEC K14.8
  tonsils, tonsillar (and adenoids) J35.9
  tooth, teeth K08.9
    hard tissues K03.9
      specified NEC K03.89
    pulp NEC K04.99
    specified NEC K08.89
  Tourette's F95.2
  trachea NEC J39.8
  tricuspid I07.9
    nonrheumatic I36.9
  triglyceride-storage E75.5
  trophoblastic — *see* Mole, hydatidiform
  tsutsugamushi A75.3
  tube (fallopian) (noninflammatory) N83.9
    inflammatory — *see* Salpingitis
    specified NEC N83.8
  tuberculous NEC — *see* Tuberculosis
  tubo-ovarian (noninflammatory) N83.9
    inflammatory — *see* Salpingo-oophoritis
    specified NEC N83.8
  tubotympanic, chronic — *see* Otitis, media, suppura-
      tive, chronic, tubotympanic
  tubulo-interstitial N15.9
    specified NEC N15.8
  tympanum — *see* Disorder, tympanic membrane
  Uhl's Q24.8
  Underwood's (sclerema neonatorum) P83.0
  Unverricht (-Lundborg) — *see* Epilepsy, generalized,
      idiopathic
  Urbach-Oppenheim (necrobiosis lipoidica diabetico-
      rum) — *see* E08-E13 with .620
  ureter N28.9
    in (due to)
      schistosomiasis (bilharziasis) B65.0 [N29]
  urethra N36.9
    specified NEC N36.8
  urinary (tract) N39.9
    bladder N32.9
      specified NEC N32.89
    specified NEC N39.8
  uterus (noninflammatory) N85.9
    infective — *see* Endometritis
    inflammatory — *see* Endometritis
    specified NEC N85.8
  uveal tract (anterior) H21.9
    posterior H31.9
  vagabond's B85.1
  vagina, vaginal (noninflammatory) N89.9
    inflammatory NEC N76.89
    specified NEC N89.8
  valve, valvular I38
    multiple I08.9
      specified NEC I08.8
  van Creveld-von Gierke (glycogenosis I) E74.01
  vas deferens N50.9
  vascular I99.9
    arteriosclerotic — *see* Arteriosclerosis
    ciliary body NEC — *see* Disorder, iris, vascular
    hypertensive — *see* Hypertension
    iris NEC — *see* Disorder, iris, vascular
    obliterative I77.1
      peripheral I73.9
    occlusive I99.8
    peripheral (occlusive) I73.9
      in diabetes mellitus — *see* E08-E13 with .51
  vasomotor I73.9
  vasospastic I73.9
  vein I87.9
  venereal (*see also* Disease, sexually transmitted) A64

Disease, diseased — *continued*
  venereal (*see also* Disease, sexually transmitted) —
    continued
    chlamydial NEC A56.8
      anus A56.3
      genitourinary NOS A56.2
      pharynx A56.4
      rectum A56.3
    fifth A55
    sixth A55
    specified nature or type NEC A63.8
  vertebra, vertebral (*see also* Spondylopathy)
    disc — *see* Disorder, disc
  vibration — *see* Vibration, adverse effects
  viral, virus (*see also* Disease, by type of virus) B34.9
    arbovirus NOS A94
    arthropod-borne NOS A94
    congenital P35.9
      specified NEC P35.8
    Hanta (with renal manifestations) (Dobrava) (Pu-
      umala) (Seoul) A98.5
      with pulmonary manifestations (Andes) (Bayou)
        (Bermejo) (Black Creek Canal) (Choclo)
        (Juquitiba) (Laguna negra) (Lechiguanas)
        (New York) (Oran) (Sin nombre) B33.4
    Hantaan (Korean hemorrhagic fever) A98.5
    human immunodeficiency (HIV) B20
    Kunjin A83.4
    nonarthropod-borne NOS B34.9
    Powassan A84.8
    Rocio (encephalitis) A83.6
    Sin nombre (Hantavirus) (cardio)-pulmonary syn-
      drome) B33.4
    Tahyna B33.8
    vesicular stomatitis A93.8
  vitreous H43.9
    specified NEC H43.89
  vocal cord J38.3
  Volkmann's, acquired T79.6 ☑
  von Eulenburg's (congenital paramyotonia) G71.19
  von Gierke's (glycogenosis I) E74.01
  von Graefe's — *see* Strabismus, paralytic, ophthalmo-
      plegia, progressive
  von Willebrand (-Jürgens) (angiohemophilia) D68.0
  Vrolik's (osteogenesis imperfecta) Q78.0
  vulva (noninflammatory) N90.9
    inflammatory NEC N76.89
    specified NEC N90.89
  Wallgren's (obstruction of splenic vein with collateral
      circulation) I87.8
  Wassilieff's (leptospiral jaundice) A27.0
  wasting NEC R64
    due to malnutrition E41
  Waterhouse-Friderichsen A39.1
  Wegner's (syphilitic osteochondritis) A50.02
  Weil's (leptospiral jaundice of lung) A27.0
  Weir Mitchell's (erythromelalgia) I73.81
  Werdnig-Hoffmann G12.0
  Wermer's E31.21
  Werner-His (trench fever) A79.0
  Werner-Schultz (neutropenic splenomegaly) D73.81
  Wernicke-Posadas B38.9
  whipworm B79
  white blood cells D72.9
    specified NEC D72.89
  white matter R90.82
  white-spot, meaning lichen sclerosus et atrophicus
      L90.0
    penis N48.0
    vulva N90.4
  Wilkie's K55.1
  Wilkinson-Sneddon (subcorneal pustular dermatosis)
      L13.1
  Willis' — *see* Diabetes
  Wilson's (hepatolenticular degeneration) E83.01
  woolsorter's A22.1
  yaba monkey tumor B08.72
  yaba pox (virus) B08.72
  Zika virus A92.5
  zoonotic, bacterial A28.9
    specified type NEC A28.8
Disfigurement (due to scar) L90.5
Disgerminoma — *see* Dysgerminoma
DISH (diffuse idiopathic skeletal hyperostosis) — *see*
    Hyperostosis, ankylosing
Disinsertion, retina — *see* Detachment, retina
Dislocatable hip, congenital Q65.6

Dislocation (articular)
  with fracture — *see* Fracture
  acromioclavicular (joint) S43.10- ☑
    with displacement
      100%-200% S43.12- ☑
      more than 200% S43.13- ☑
    inferior S43.14- ☑
    posterior S43.15- ☑
  ankle S93.0- ☑
  astragalus — *see* Dislocation, ankle
  atlantoaxial S13.121 ☑
  atlantooccipital S13.111 ☑
  atloidooccipital S13.111 ☑
  breast bone S23.29 ☑
  capsule, joint — *code by* site under Dislocation
  carpal (bone) — *see* Dislocation, wrist
  carpometacarpal (joint) NEC S63.05- ☑
    thumb S63.04- ☑
  cartilage (joint) — *code by* site under Dislocation
  cervical spine (vertebra) — *see* Dislocation, vertebra,
      cervical
  chronic — *see* Dislocation, recurrent
  clavicle — *see* Dislocation, acromioclavicular joint
  coccyx S33.2 ☑
  congenital NEC Q68.8
  coracoid — *see* Dislocation, shoulder
  costal cartilage S23.29 ☑
  costochondral S23.29 ☑
  cricoarytenoid articulation S13.29 ☑
  cricothyroid articulation S13.29 ☑
  dorsal vertebra — *see* Dislocation, vertebra, thoracic
  ear ossicle — *see* Discontinuity, ossicles, ear
  elbow S53.10- ☑
    congenital Q68.8
    pathological — *see* Dislocation, pathological NEC,
      elbow
    radial head alone — *see* Dislocation, radial head
    recurrent — *see* Dislocation, recurrent, elbow
    traumatic S53.10- ☑
      anterior S53.11- ☑
      lateral S53.14- ☑
      medial S53.13- ☑
      posterior S53.12- ☑
      specified type NEC S53.19- ☑
  eye, nontraumatic — *see* Luxation, globe
  eyeball, nontraumatic — *see* Luxation, globe
  femur
    distal end — *see* Dislocation, knee
    proximal end — *see* Dislocation, hip
  fibula
    distal end — *see* Dislocation, ankle
    proximal end — *see* Dislocation, knee
  finger S63.25- ☑
    index S63.25- ☑
    interphalangeal S63.27- ☑
      distal S63.29- ☑
        index S63.29- ☑
        little S63.29- ☑
        middle S63.29- ☑
        ring S63.29- ☑
      index S63.27- ☑
      little S63.27- ☑
      middle S63.27- ☑
      proximal S63.28- ☑
        index S63.28- ☑
        little S63.28- ☑
        middle S63.28- ☑
        ring S63.28- ☑
      ring S63.27- ☑
    little S63.25- ☑
    metacarpophalangeal S63.26- ☑
      index S63.26- ☑
      little S63.26- ☑
      middle S63.26- ☑
      ring S63.26- ☑
    middle S63.25- ☑
    recurrent — *see* Dislocation, recurrent, finger
    ring S63.25- ☑
    thumb — *see* Dislocation, thumb
  foot S93.30- ☑
    recurrent — *see* Dislocation, recurrent, foot
    specified site NEC S93.33- ☑
    tarsal joint S93.31- ☑
    tarsometatarsal joint S93.32- ☑
    toe — *see* Dislocation, toe
  fracture — *see* Fracture

Dislocation — *continued*
glenohumeral (joint) — *see* Dislocation, shoulder
glenoid — *see* Dislocation, shoulder
habitual — *see* Dislocation, recurrent
hip S73.00- ☑
  anterior S73.03- ☑
    obturator S73.02- ☑
  central S73.04- ☑
  congenital (total) Q65.2
    bilateral Q65.1
    partial Q65.5
      bilateral Q65.4
      unilateral Q65.3-
    unilateral Q65.0-
  developmental M24.85- ☑
  pathological — *see* Dislocation, pathological NEC, hip
  posterior S73.01- ☑
  recurrent — *see* Dislocation, recurrent, hip
humerus, proximal end — *see* Dislocation, shoulder
incomplete — *see* Subluxation, by site
incus — *see* Discontinuity, ossicles, ear
infracoracoid — *see* Dislocation, shoulder
innominate (pubic junction) (sacral junction) S33.39 ☑
  acetabulum — *see* Dislocation, hip
interphalangeal (joint(s))
  finger S63.279 ☑
    distal S63.29- ☑
      index S63.29- ☑
      little S63.29- ☑
      middle S63.29- ☑
      ring S63.29- ☑
    index S63.27- ☑
    little S63.27- ☑
    middle S63.27- ☑
    proximal S63.28- ☑
      index S63.28- ☑
      little S63.28- ☑
      middle S63.28- ☑
      ring S63.28- ☑
    ring S63.27- ☑
  foot or toe — *see* Dislocation, toe
  thumb S63.12- ☑
    distal joint S63.14- ☑
    proximal joint S63.13- ☑
jaw (cartilage) (meniscus) S03.0- ☑
joint prosthesis — *see* Complications, joint prosthesis, mechanical, displacement, by site
knee S83.106 ☑
  cap — *see* Dislocation, patella
  congenital Q68.2
  old M23.8X- ☑
  patella — *see* Dislocation, patella
  pathological — *see* Dislocation, pathological NEC, knee
  proximal tibia
    anteriorly S83.11- ☑
    laterally S83.14- ☑
    medially S83.13- ☑
    posteriorly S83.12- ☑
  recurrent (*see also* Derangement, knee, specified NEC)
  specified type NEC S83.19- ☑
lacrimal gland H04.16- ☑
lens (complete) H27.10
  anterior H27.12- ☑
  congenital Q12.1
  ocular implant — *see* Complications, intraocular lens
  partial H27.11- ☑
  posterior H27.13- ☑
  traumatic S05.8X- ☑
ligament — *code by* site under Dislocation
lumbar (vertebra) — *see* Dislocation, vertebra, lumbar
lumbosacral (vertebra) (*see also* Dislocation, vertebra, lumbar)
  congenital Q76.49
mandible S03.0- ☑
meniscus (knee) — *see* Tear, meniscus
  other sites - code by site under Dislocation
metacarpal (bone)
  distal end — *see* Dislocation, finger
  proximal end S63.06- ☑
metacarpophalangeal (joint)
  finger S63.26- ☑
    index S63.26- ☑

Dislocation — *continued*
metacarpophalangeal — *continued*
  finger — *continued*
    little S63.26- ☑
    middle S63.26- ☑
    ring S63.26- ☑
    thumb S63.11- ☑
metatarsal (bone) — *see* Dislocation, foot
metatarsophalangeal (joint(s)) — *see* Dislocation, toe
midcarpal (joint) S63.03- ☑
midtarsal (joint) — *see* Dislocation, foot
neck S13.20 ☑
  specified site NEC S13.29 ☑
  vertebra — *see* Dislocation, vertebra, cervical
nose (septal cartilage) S03.1 ☑
occipitoatloid S13.111 ☑
old — *see* Derangement, joint, specified type NEC
ossicles, ear — *see* Discontinuity, ossicles, ear
partial — *see* Subluxation, by site
patella S83.006 ☑
  congenital Q74.1
  lateral S83.01- ☑
  recurrent (nontraumatic) M22.0- ☑
    incomplete M22.1- ☑
  specified type NEC S83.09- ☑
pathological NEC M24.30
  ankle M24.37- ☑
  elbow M24.32- ☑
  foot joint M24.37- ☑
  hand joint M24.34- ☑
  hip M24.35- ☑
  knee M24.36- ☑
  lumbosacral joint — *see* subcategory M53.2 ☑
  pelvic region — *see* Dislocation, pathological, hip
  sacroiliac — *see* subcategory M53.2 ☑
  shoulder M24.31- ☑
  wrist M24.33- ☑
pelvis NEC S33.30 ☑
  specified NEC S33.39 ☑
phalanx
  finger or hand — *see* Dislocation, finger
  foot or toe — *see* Dislocation, toe
prosthesis, internal — *see* Complications, prosthetic device, by site, mechanical
radial head S53.006 ☑
  anterior S53.01- ☑
  posterior S53.02- ☑
  specified type NEC S53.09- ☑
radiocarpal (joint) S63.02- ☑
radiohumeral (joint) — *see* Dislocation, radial head
radioulnar (joint)
  distal S63.01- ☑
  proximal — *see* Dislocation, elbow
radius
  distal end — *see* Dislocation, wrist
  proximal end — *see* Dislocation, radial head
recurrent M24.40
  ankle M24.47- ☑
  elbow M24.42- ☑
  finger M24.44- ☑
  foot joint M24.47- ☑
  hand joint M24.44- ☑
  hip M24.45- ☑
  knee M24.46- ☑
    patella — *see* Dislocation, patella, recurrent
  patella — *see* Dislocation, patella, recurrent
  sacroiliac — *see* subcategory M53.2 ☑
  shoulder M24.41- ☑
  toe M24.47- ☑
  vertebra (*see also* subcategory) M43.5 ☑
    atlantoaxial M43.4
      with myelopathy M43.3
  wrist M24.43- ☑
rib (cartilage) S23.29 ☑
sacrococcygeal S33.2 ☑
sacroiliac (joint) (ligament) S33.2 ☑
  congenital Q74.2
  recurrent — *see* subcategory M53.2 ☑
sacrum S33.2 ☑
scaphoid (bone) (hand) (wrist) — *see* Dislocation, wrist
  foot — *see* Dislocation, foot
scapula — *see* Dislocation, shoulder, girdle, scapula
semilunar cartilage, knee — *see* Tear, meniscus
septal cartilage (nose) S03.1 ☑
septum (nasal) (old) J34.2

Dislocation — *continued*
sesamoid bone — *code by* site under Dislocation
shoulder (blade) (ligament) (joint) (traumatic) S43.006 ☑
  acromioclavicular — *see* Dislocation, acromioclavicular
  chronic — *see* Dislocation, recurrent, shoulder
  congenital Q68.8
  girdle S43.30- ☑
    scapula S43.31- ☑
    specified site NEC S43.39- ☑
  humerus S43.00- ☑
    anterior S43.01- ☑
    inferior S43.03- ☑
    posterior S43.02- ☑
  pathological — *see* Dislocation, pathological NEC, shoulder
  recurrent — *see* Dislocation, recurrent, shoulder
  specified type NEC S43.08- ☑
spine
  cervical — *see* Dislocation, vertebra, cervical
  congenital Q76.49
  due to birth trauma P11.5
  lumbar — *see* Dislocation, vertebra, lumbar
  thoracic — *see* Dislocation, vertebra, thoracic
spontaneous — *see* Dislocation, pathological
sternoclavicular (joint) S43.206 ☑
  anterior S43.21- ☑
  posterior S43.22- ☑
sternum S23.29 ☑
subglenoid — *see* Dislocation, shoulder
symphysis pubis S33.4 ☑
talus — *see* Dislocation, ankle
tarsal (bone(s)) (joint(s)) — *see* Dislocation, foot
tarsometatarsal (joint(s)) — *see* Dislocation, foot
temporomandibular (joint) S03.0- ☑
thigh, proximal end — *see* Dislocation, hip
thorax S23.20 ☑
  specified site NEC S23.29 ☑
  vertebra — *see* Dislocation, vertebra
thumb S63.10- ☑
  interphalangeal joint — *see* Dislocation, interphalangeal (joint), thumb
  metacarpophalangeal joint — *see* Dislocation, metacarpophalangeal (joint), thumb
thyroid cartilage S13.29 ☑
tibia
  distal end — *see* Dislocation, ankle
  proximal end — *see* Dislocation, knee
tibiofibular (joint)
  distal — *see* Dislocation, ankle
  superior — *see* Dislocation, knee
toe(s) S93.106 ☑
  great S93.10- ☑
    interphalangeal joint S93.11- ☑
    metatarsophalangeal joint S93.12- ☑
  interphalangeal joint S93.119 ☑
  lesser S93.106 ☑
    interphalangeal joint S93.11- ☑
    metatarsophalangeal joint S93.12- ☑
  metatarsophalangeal joint S93.12- ☑
tooth S03.2 ☑
trachea S23.29 ☑
ulna
  distal end S63.07- ☑
  proximal end — *see* Dislocation, elbow
ulnohumeral (joint) — *see* Dislocation, elbow
vertebra (articular process) (body) (traumatic)
  cervical S13.101 ☑
    atlantoaxial joint S13.121 ☑
    atlantooccipital joint S13.111 ☑
    atloidooccipital joint S13.111 ☑
    joint between
      C0 and C1 S13.111 ☑
      C1 and C2 S13.121 ☑
      C2 and C3 S13.131 ☑
      C3 and C4 S13.141 ☑
      C4 and C5 S13.151 ☑
      C5 and C6 S13.161 ☑
      C6 and C7 S13.171 ☑
      C7 and T1 S13.181 ☑
    occipitoatloid joint S13.111 ☑
  congenital Q76.49
  lumbar S33.101 ☑
    joint between
      L1 and L2 S33.111 ☑

☑ **Additional Character Required** — Refer to the Tabular List for Character Selection
◥ᴺᴱᵂ **Subterms under main terms may continue to next column or page**

Dislocation — continued
  vertebra — continued
    lumbar — continued
      joint between — continued
        L2 and L3 S33.121 ☑
        L3 and L4 S33.131 ☑
        L4 and L5 S33.141 ☑
    nontraumatic — see Displacement, intervertebral disc
    partial — see Subluxation, by site
    recurrent NEC — see subcategory M43.5 ☑
    thoracic S23.101 ☑
      joint between
        T1 and T2 S23.111 ☑
        T2 and T3 S23.121 ☑
        T3 and T4 S23.123 ☑
        T4 and T5 S23.131 ☑
        T5 and T6 S23.133 ☑
        T6 and T7 S23.141 ☑
        T7 and T8 S23.143 ☑
        T8 and T9 S23.151 ☑
        T9 and T10 S23.153 ☑
        T10 and T11 S23.161 ☑
        T11 and T12 S23.163 ☑
        T12 and L1 S23.171 ☑
  wrist (carpal bone) S63.006 ☑
    carpometacarpal joint — see Dislocation, carpometacarpal (joint)
    distal radioulnar joint — see Dislocation, radioulnar (joint), distal
    metacarpal bone, proximal — see Dislocation, metacarpal (bone), proximal end
    midcarpal — see Dislocation, midcarpal (joint)
    radiocarpal joint — see Dislocation, radiocarpal (joint)
    recurrent — see Dislocation, recurrent, wrist
    specified site NEC S63.09- ☑
    ulna — see Dislocation, ulna, distal end
  xiphoid cartilage S23.29 ☑
Disorder (of) (see also Disease)
  acantholytic L11.9
    specified NEC L11.8
  acute
    psychotic — see Psychosis, acute
    stress F43.0
  adjustment (grief) F43.20
    with
      anxiety F43.22
        with depressed mood F43.23
      conduct disturbance F43.24
        with emotional disturbance F43.25
      depressed mood F43.21
        with anxiety F43.23
      other specified symptom F43.29
  adrenal (capsule) (gland) (medullary) E27.9
    specified NEC E27.8
  adrenogenital E25.9
    drug-induced E25.8
    iatrogenic E25.8
    idiopathic E25.8
  adult personality (and behavior) F69
    specified NEC F68.8
  affective (mood) — see Disorder, mood
  aggressive, unsocialized F91.1
  alcohol use
    mild F10.10
      with
        alcohol intoxication F10.129
          delirium F10.121
        alcohol-induced
          anxiety disorder F10.180
          bipolar and related disorder F10.14
          depressive disorder F10.14
          psychotic disorder F10.159
          sexual dysfunction F10.181
          sleep disorder F10.182
      in remission (early) (sustained) F10.11
    moderate or severe F10.20
      with
        alcohol intoxication F10.229
          delirium F10.221
        alcohol-induced
          anxiety disorder F10.280
          bipolar and related disorder F10.24
          depressive disorder F10.24
          major neurocognitive disorder, amnestic-confabulatory type F10.26

Disorder — continued
  alcohol use — continued
    moderate or severe — continued
      with — continued
        alcohol-induced — continued
          major neurocognitive disorder, non-amnestic-confabulatory type F10.27
          mild neurocognitive disorder F10.288
          psychotic disorder F10.259
          sexual dysfunction F10.281
          sleep disorder F10.282
      in remission (early) (sustained) F10.21
  alcohol-related F10.99
    with
      amnestic disorder, persisting F10.96
      anxiety disorder F10.980
      dementia, persisting F10.97
      intoxication F10.929
        with delirium F10.921
        uncomplicated F10.920
      mood disorder F10.94
      other specified F10.988
      psychotic disorder F10.959
        with
          delusions F10.950
          hallucinations F10.951
      sexual dysfunction F10.981
      sleep disorder F10.982
  allergic — see Allergy
  alveolar NEC J84.09
  amino-acid
    cystathioninuria E72.19
    cystinosis E72.04
    cystinuria E72.01
    glycinuria E72.09
    homocystinuria E72.11
    metabolism — see Disturbance, metabolism, amino-acid
    specified NEC E72.8
    neonatal, transitory P74.8
    renal transport NEC E72.09
    transport NEC E72.09
  amnesic, amnestic
    alcohol-induced F10.96
      with dependence F10.26
    due to (secondary to) general medical condition F04
    psychoactive NEC-induced F19.96
      with
        abuse F19.16
        dependence F19.26
    sedative, hypnotic or anxiolytic-induced F13.96
      with dependence F13.26
  amphetamine (or other stimulant) use
    mild
      with
        amphetamine, cocaine, or other stimulant intoxication
          with perceptual disturbances F15.122
          without perceptual disturbances F15.129
        amphetamine (or other stimulant) -induced
          anxiety disorder F15.180
          bipolar and related disorder F15.14
          depressive disorder F15.14
          obsessive-compulsive and related disorder F15.188
          psychotic disorder F15.159
          sexual dysfunction F15.181
        intoxication delirium F15.121
    moderate or severe
      with
        amphetamine, cocaine, or other stimulant intoxication
          with perceptual disturbances F15.222
          without perceptual disturbances F15.229
        amphetamine (or other stimulant) -induced
          anxiety disorder F15.280
          bipolar and related disorder F15.24
          depressive disorder F15.24
          obsessive-compulsive and related disorder F15.288
          psychotic disorder F15.259
          sexual dysfunction F15.281
        intoxication delirium F15.221
  amphetamine-type substance use
    mild F15.10
      in remission (early) (sustained) F15.11
    moderate F15.20

Disorder — continued
  amphetamine-type substance use — continued
    moderate — continued
      in remission (early) (sustained) F15.21
    severe F15.20
      in remission (early) (sustained) F15.21
  anaerobic glycolysis with anemia D55.2
  anxiety F41.9
    due to (secondary to)
      alcohol F10.980
        in
          abuse F10.180
          dependence F10.280
      amphetamine F15.980
        in
          abuse F15.180
          dependence F15.280
      anxiolytic F13.980
        in
          abuse F13.180
          dependence F13.280
      caffeine F15.980
        in
          abuse F15.180
          dependence F15.280
      cannabis F12.980
        in
          abuse F12.180
          dependence F12.280
      cocaine F14.980
        in
          abuse F14.180
          dependence F14.180
      general medical condition F06.4
      hallucinogen F16.980
        in
          abuse F16.180
          dependence F16.280
      hypnotic F13.980
        in
          abuse F13.180
          dependence F13.280
      inhalant F18.980
        in
          abuse F18.180
          dependence F18.280
      phencyclidine F16.980
        in
          abuse F16.180
          dependence F16.280
      psychoactive substance NEC F19.980
        in
          abuse F19.180
          dependence F19.280
      sedative F13.980
        in
          abuse F13.180
          dependence F13.280
      volatile solvents F18.980
        in
          abuse F18.180
          dependence F18.280
    generalized F41.1
    illness F45.21
    mixed
      with depression (mild) F41.8
      specified NEC F41.3
    organic F06.4
    phobic F40.9
      of childhood F40.8
    specified NEC F41.8
  aortic valve — see Endocarditis, aortic
  aromatic amino-acid metabolism E70.9
    specified NEC E70.8
  arteriole NEC I77.89
  artery NEC I77.89
  articulation — see Disorder, joint
  attachment (childhood)
    disinhibited F94.2
    reactive F94.1
  attention-deficit hyperactivity (adolescent) (adult) (child) F90.9
    combined
      presentation F90.2
      type F90.2
    hyperactive
      impulsive presentation F90.1
      type F90.1

▧ **Subterms under main terms may continue to next column or page**   ☑ **Additional Character Required — Refer to the Tabular List for Character Selection**   **109**

Dislocation — Disorder

Disorder — *continued*
attention-deficit hyperactivity — *continued*
inattentive
presentation F90.0
type F90.0
specified type NEC F90.8
attention-deficit without hyperactivity (adolescent) (adult) (child) F98.8
auditory processing (central) H93.25
autism spectrum F84.0
autistic F84.0
autoimmune D89.89
autonomic nervous system G90.9
specified NEC G90.8
avoidant
child or adolescent F40.10
restrictive food intake F50.82
balance
acid-base E87.8
mixed E87.4
electrolyte E87.8
fluid NEC E87.8
behavioral (disruptive) — *see* Disorder, conduct
beta-amino-acid metabolism E72.8
bile acid and cholesterol metabolism E78.70
Barth syndrome E78.71
other specified E78.79
Smith-Lemli-Opitz syndrome E78.72
bilirubin excretion E80.6
binge eating F50.81
binocular
movement H51.9
convergence
excess H51.12
insufficiency H51.11
internuclear ophthalmoplegia — *see* Ophthalmoplegia, internuclear
palsy of conjugate gaze H51.0
specified type NEC H51.8
vision NEC — *see* Disorder, vision, binocular
bipolar (I) (type I) F31.9
and related due to a known physiological condition
with
manic features F06.33
manic- or hypomanic-like episodes F06.33
mixed features F06.34
current (or most recent) episode
depressed F31.9
with psychotic features F31.5
without psychotic features F31.30
mild F31.31
moderate F31.32
severe (without psychotic features) F31.4
with psychotic features F31.5
hypomanic F31.0
manic F31.9
with psychotic features F31.2
without psychotic features F31.10
mild F31.11
moderate F31.12
severe (without psychotic features) F31.13
with psychotic features F31.2
mixed F31.60
mild F31.61
moderate F31.62
severe (without psychotic features) F31.63
with psychotic features F31.64
severe depression (without psychotic features) F31.4
with psychotic features F31.5
in remission (currently) F31.70
in full remission
most recent episode
depressed F31.76
hypomanic F31.72
manic F31.74
mixed F31.78
in partial remission
most recent episode
depressed F31.75
hypomanic F31.71
manic F31.73
mixed F31.77
organic F06.30
single manic episode F30.9
mild F30.11
moderate F30.12
severe (without psychotic symptoms) F30.13

Disorder — *continued*
bipolar — *continued*
single manic episode — *continued*
severe — *continued*
with psychotic symptoms F30.2
specified NEC F31.89
bipolar II (type 2) F31.81
bladder N32.9
functional NEC N31.9
in schistosomiasis B65.0 [N33]
specified NEC N32.89
bleeding D68.9
blood D75.9
in congenital early syphilis A50.09 [D77]
body dysmorphic F45.22
bone M89.9
continuity M84.9
specified type NEC M84.80
ankle M84.87- ☑
fibula M84.86- ☑
foot M84.87- ☑
hand M84.84- ☑
humerus M84.82- ☑
neck M84.88
pelvis M84.859
radius M84.83- ☑
rib M84.88
shoulder M84.81- ☑
skull M84.88
thigh M84.85- ☑
tibia M84.86- ☑
ulna M84.83- ☑
vertebra M84.88
density and structure M85.9
cyst (*see also* Cyst, bone, specified type NEC)
aneurysmal — *see* Cyst, bone, aneurysmal
solitary — *see* Cyst, bone, solitary
diffuse idiopathic skeletal hyperostosis — *see* Hyperostosis, ankylosing
fibrous dysplasia (monostotic) — *see* Dysplasia, fibrous, bone
fluorosis — *see* Fluorosis, skeletal
hyperostosis of skull M85.2
osteitis condensans — *see* Osteitis, condensans
specified type NEC M85.8- ☑
ankle M85.87- ☑
foot M85.87- ☑
forearm M85.83- ☑
hand M85.84- ☑
lower leg M85.86- ☑
multiple sites M85.89
neck M85.88
rib M85.88
shoulder M85.81- ☑
skull M85.88
thigh M85.85- ☑
upper arm M85.82- ☑
vertebra M85.88
development and growth NEC M89.20
carpus M89.24- ☑
clavicle M89.21- ☑
femur M89.25- ☑
fibula M89.26- ☑
finger M89.24- ☑
humerus M89.22- ☑
ilium M89.259
ischium M89.259
metacarpus M89.24- ☑
metatarsus M89.27- ☑
multiple sites M89.29
neck M89.28
radius M89.23- ☑
rib M89.28
scapula M89.21- ☑
skull M89.28
tarsus M89.27- ☑
tibia M89.26- ☑
toe M89.27- ☑
ulna M89.23- ☑
vertebra M89.28
specified type NEC M89.8X- ☑
brachial plexus G54.0
branched-chain amino-acid metabolism E71.2
specified NEC E71.19
breast N64.9
agalactia — *see* Agalactia

Disorder — *continued*
breast — *continued*
associated with
lactation O92.70
specified NEC O92.79
pregnancy O92.20
specified NEC O92.29
puerperium O92.20
specified NEC O92.29
cracked nipple — *see* Cracked nipple
galactorrhea — *see* Galactorrhea
hypogalactia O92.4
lactation disorder NEC O92.79
mastitis — *see* Mastitis
nipple infection — *see* Infection, nipple
retracted nipple — *see* Retraction, nipple
specified type NEC N64.89
Briquet's F45.0
bullous, in diseases classified elsewhere L14
caffeine use
mild
with
caffeine-induced
anxiety disorder F15.180
sleep disorder F15.182
moderate or severe
with
caffeine-induced
anxiety disorder F15.280
sleep disorder F15.282
cannabis use
mild F12.10
with
cannabis intoxication delirium F12.121
with perceptual disturbances F12.122
without perceptual disturbances F12.129
cannabis-induced
anxiety disorder F12.180
psychotic disorder F12.159
sleep disorder F12.188
in remission (early) (sustained) F12.11
moderate or severe F12.20
with
cannabis intoxication
with perceptual disturbances F12.222
without perceptual disturbances F12.229
cannabis-induced
anxiety disorder F12.280
psychotic disorder F12.259
sleep disorder F12.288
delirium F12.221
in remission (early) (sustained) F12.21
carbohydrate
absorption, intestinal NEC E74.39
metabolism (congenital) E74.9
specified NEC E74.8
cardiac, functional I51.89
carnitine metabolism E71.40
cartilage M94.9
articular NEC — *see* Derangement, joint, articular cartilage
chondrocalcinosis — *see* Chondrocalcinosis
specified type NEC M94.8X- ☑
articular — *see* Derangement, joint, articular cartilage
multiple sites M94.8X0
catatonia (due to known physiological condition) (with another mental disorder) F06.1
catatonic
due to (secondary to) known physiological condition F06.1
organic F06.1
central auditory processing H93.25
cervical
region NEC M53.82
root (nerve) NEC G54.2
character NOS F60.9
childhood disintegrative NEC F84.3
cholesterol and bile acid metabolism E78.70
Barth syndrome E78.71
other specified E78.79
Smith-Lemli-Opitz syndrome E78.72
choroid H31.9
atrophy — *see* Atrophy, choroid
degeneration — *see* Degeneration, choroid
detachment — *see* Detachment, choroid
dystrophy — *see* Dystrophy, choroid
hemorrhage — *see* Hemorrhage, choroid

☑ **Additional Character Required — Refer to the Tabular List for Character Selection**   ⩗ **Subterms under main terms may continue to next column or page**

Disorder — *continued*
 choroid — *continued*
  rupture — *see* Rupture, choroid
  scar — *see* Scar, chorioretinal
  solar retinopathy — *see* Retinopathy, solar
  specified type NEC H31.8
 ciliary body — *see* Disorder, iris
  degeneration — *see* Degeneration, ciliary body
 coagulation (factor) (*see also* Defect, coagulation) D68.9
  newborn, transient P61.6
 cocaine use
  mild F14.10
   with
    amphetamine, cocaine, or other stimulant intoxication
     with perceptual disturbances F14.122
     without perceptual disturbances F14.129
    cocaine intoxication delirium F14.121
    cocaine-induced
     anxiety disorder F14.180
     bipolar and related disorder F14.14
     depressive disorder F14.14
     obsessive-compulsive and related disorder F14.188
     psychotic disorder F14.159
     sexual dysfunction F14.181
     sleep disorder F14.182
   in remission (early) (sustained) F14.11
  moderate or severe F14.20
   with
    amphetamine, cocaine, or other stimulant intoxication
     with perceptual disturbances F14.222
     without perceptual disturbances F14.229
    cocaine intoxication delirium F14.221
    cocaine-induced
     anxiety disorder F14.280
     bipolar and related disorder F14.24
     depressive disorder F14.24
     obsessive-compulsive and related disorder F14.288
     psychotic disorder F14.259
     sexual dysfunction F14.281
     sleep disorder F14.282
   in remission (early) (sustained) F14.21
 coccyx NEC M53.3
 cognitive F09
  due to (secondary to) general medical condition F09
  persisting R41.89
   due to
    alcohol F10.97
     with dependence F10.27
    anxiolytics F13.97
     with dependence F13.27
    hypnotics F13.97
     with dependence F13.27
    sedatives F13.97
     with dependence F13.27
    specified substance NEC F19.97
     with
      abuse F19.17
      dependence F19.27
 communication F80.9
  social pragmatic F80.82
 conduct (childhood) F91.9
  adjustment reaction — *see* Disorder, adjustment
  adolescent onset type F91.2
  childhood onset type F91.1
  compulsive F63.9
  confined to family context F91.0
  depressive F91.8
  group type F91.2
  hyperkinetic — *see* Disorder, attention-deficit hyperactivity
  oppositional defiance F91.3
  socialized F91.2
  solitary aggressive type F91.1
  specified NEC F91.8
  unsocialized (aggressive) F91.1
 conduction, heart I45.9
 congenital glycosylation (CDG) E74.8
 conjunctiva H11.9
  infection — *see* Conjunctivitis
 connective tissue, localized L94.9
  specified NEC L94.8

Disorder — *continued*
 conversion (functional neurological symptom disorder)
  with
   abnormal movement F44.4
   anesthesia or sensory loss F44.6
   attacks or seizures F44.5
   mixed symptoms F44.7
   special sensory symptoms F44.6
   speech symptoms F44.4
   swallowing symptoms F44.4
   weakness or paralysis F44.4
 convulsive (secondary) — *see* Convulsions
 cornea H18.9
  deformity — *see* Deformity, cornea
  degeneration — *see* Degeneration, cornea
  deposits — *see* Deposit, cornea
  due to contact lens H18.82- ☑
   specified as edema — *see* Edema, cornea
  edema — *see* Edema, cornea
  keratitis — *see* Keratitis
  keratoconjunctivitis — *see* Keratoconjunctivitis
  membrane change — *see* Change, corneal membrane
  neovascularization — *see* Neovascularization, cornea
  scar — *see* Opacity, cornea
  specified type NEC H18.89- ☑
  ulcer — *see* Ulcer, cornea
 corpus cavernosum N48.9
 cranial nerve — *see* Disorder, nerve, cranial
 cyclothymic F34.0
 defiant oppositional F91.3
 delusional (persistent) (systematized) F22
  induced F24
 depersonalization F48.1
 depressive F32.9
  due to known physiological condition
   with
    depressive features F06.31
    major depressive-like episode F06.32
    mixed features F06.34
  major F32.9
   with psychotic symptoms F32.3
   in remission (full) F32.5
    partial F32.4
   recurrent F33.9
    with psychotic features F33.3
   single episode F32.9
    mild F32.0
    moderate F32.1
    severe (without psychotic symptoms) F32.2
     with psychotic symptoms F32.3
  organic F06.31
  persistent F34.1
  recurrent F33.9
   current episode
    mild F33.0
    moderate F33.1
    severe (without psychotic symptoms) F33.2
     with psychotic symptoms F33.3
   in remission F33.40
    full F33.42
    partial F33.41
   specified NEC F33.8
  single episode — *see* Episode, depressive
  specified NEC F32.89
 developmental F89
  arithmetical skills F81.2
  coordination (motor) F82
  expressive writing F81.81
  language F80.9
   expressive F80.1
   mixed receptive and expressive F80.2
   receptive type F80.2
   specified NEC F80.89
  learning F81.9
   arithmetical F81.2
   reading F81.0
  mixed F88
  motor coordination or function F82
  pervasive F84.9
   specified NEC F84.8
  phonological F80.0
  reading F81.0
  scholastic skills (*see also* Disorder, learning)
   mixed F81.89
  specified NEC F88
  speech F80.9

Disorder — *continued*
 developmental — *continued*
  speech — *continued*
   articulation F80.0
   specified NEC F80.89
  written expression F81.81
 diaphragm J98.6
 digestive (system) K92.9
  newborn P78.9
   specified NEC P78.89
  postprocedural — *see* Complication, gastrointestinal
  psychogenic F45.8
 disc (intervertebral) M51.9
  with
   myelopathy
    cervical region M50.00
    cervicothoracic region M50.03
    high cervical region M50.01
    lumbar region M51.06
    mid-cervical region M50.020
    sacrococcygeal region M53.3
    thoracic region M51.04
    thoracolumbar region M51.05
   radiculopathy
    cervical region M50.10
    cervicothoracic region M50.13
    high cervical region M50.11
    lumbar region M51.16
    lumbosacral region M51.17
    mid-cervical region M50.120
    sacrococcygeal region M53.3
    thoracic region M51.14
    thoracolumbar region M51.15
  cervical M50.90
   with
    myelopathy M50.00
     C2-C3 M50.01
     C3-C4 M50.01
     C4-C5 M50.021
     C5-C6 M50.022
     C6-C7 M50.023
     C7-T1 M50.03
     cervicothoracic region M50.03
     high cervical region M50.01
     mid-cervical region M50.020
    neuritis, radiculitis or radiculopathy M50.10
     C2-C3 M50.11
     C3-C4 M50.11
     C4-C5 M50.121
     C5-C6 M50.122
     C6-C7 M50.123
     C7-T1 M50.13
     cervicothoracic region M50.13
     high cervical region M50.11
     mid-cervical region M50.120
   C2-C3 M50.91
   C3-C4 M50.91
   C4-C5 M50.921
   C5-C6 M50.922
   C6-C7 M50.923
   C7-T1 M50.93
   cervicothoracic region M50.93
   degeneration M50.30
    C2-C3 M50.31
    C3-C4 M50.31
    C4-C5 M50.321
    C5-C6 M50.322
    C6-C7 M50.323
    C7-T1 M50.33
    cervicothoracic region M50.33
    high cervical region M50.31
    mid-cervical region M50.320
   displacement M50.20
    C2-C3 M50.21
    C3-C4 M50.21
    C4-C5 M50.221
    C5-C6 M50.222
    C6-C7 M50.223
    C7-T1 M50.23
    cervicothoracic region M50.23
    high cervical region M50.21
    mid-cervical region M50.220
   high cervical region M50.91
   mid-cervical region M50.920
   specified type NEC M50.80
    C2-C3 M50.81
    C3-C4 M50.81
    C4-C5 M50.821

Disorder — *continued*
  disc — *continued*
    cervical — *continued*
      specified type — *continued*
        C5-C6 M50.822
        C6-C7 M50.823
        C7-T1 M50.83
        cervicothoracic region M50.83
        high cervical region M50.81
        mid-cervical region M50.820
      specified NEC
        lumbar region M51.86
        lumbosacral region M51.87
        sacrococcygeal region M53.3
        thoracic region M51.84
        thoracolumbar region M51.85
    disinhibited attachment (childhood) F94.2
    disintegrative, childhood NEC F84.3
    disruptive F91.9
      mood dysregulation F34.81
      specified NEC F91.8
    disruptive behavior — *see* Disorder, conduct
    dissocial personality F60.2
    dissociative F44.9
      affecting
        motor function F44.4
          and sensation F44.7
        sensation F44.6
          and motor function F44.7
      brief reactive F43.0
      due to (secondary to) general medical condition
        F06.8
      mixed F44.7
      organic F06.8
      other specified NEC F44.89
    double heterozygous sickling — *see* Disease, sickle-
      cell
    dream anxiety F51.5
    drug induced hemorrhagic D68.32
    drug related F19.99
      abuse — *see* Abuse, drug
      dependence — *see* Dependence, drug
    dysmorphic body F45.22
    dysthymic F34.1
    ear H93.9- ☑
      bleeding — *see* Otorrhagia
      deafness — *see* Deafness
      degenerative H93.09- ☑
      discharge — *see* Otorrhea
      external H61.9- ☑
        auditory canal stenosis — *see* Stenosis, external
          ear canal
        exostosis — *see* Exostosis, external ear canal
        impacted cerumen — *see* Impaction, cerumen
        otitis — *see* Otitis, externa
        perichondritis — *see* Perichondritis, ear
        pinna — *see* Disorder, pinna
        specified type NEC H61.89- ☑
      inner H83.9- ☑
        vestibular dysfunction — *see* Disorder,
          vestibular function
      middle H74.9- ☑
        adhesive H74.1- ☑
        ossicle — *see* Abnormal, ear ossicles
        polyp — *see* Polyp, ear (middle)
        specified NEC, in diseases classified elsewhere
          H75.8- ☑
      postprocedural — *see* Complications, ear, proce-
        dure
      specified NEC, in diseases classified elsewhere
        H94.8- ☑
    eating (adult) (psychogenic) F50.9
      anorexia — *see* Anorexia
      binge F50.81
      bulimia F50.2
      child F98.29
        pica F98.3
        rumination disorder F98.21
      pica F50.89
        childhood F98.3
    electrolyte (balance) NEC E87.8
      with
        abortion — *see* Abortion by type complicated
          by specified condition NEC
        ectopic pregnancy O08.5
        molar pregnancy O08.5
      acidosis (metabolic) (respiratory) E87.2
      alkalosis (metabolic) (respiratory) E87.3

Disorder — *continued*
  elimination, transepidermal L87.9
    specified NEC L87.8
  emotional (persistent) F34.9
    of childhood F93.9
      specified NEC F93.8
  endocrine E34.9
    postprocedural E89.89
    specified NEC E89.89
  erectile (male) (organic) (*see also* Dysfunction, sexual,
    male, erectile) N52.9
    nonorganic F52.21
  erythematous — *see* Erythema
  esophagus K22.9
    functional K22.4
    psychogenic F45.8
  eustachian tube H69.9- ☑
    infection — *see* Salpingitis, eustachian
    obstruction — *see* Obstruction, eustachian tube
    patulous — *see* Patulous, eustachian tube
    specified NEC H69.8- ☑
  exhibitionistic F65.2
  extrapyramidal G25.9
    in deseases classified elsewhere — *see* category
      G26
    specified type NEC G25.89
  eye H57.9
    postprocedural — *see* Complication, postprocedu-
      ral, eye
  eyelid H02.9
    cyst — *see* Cyst, eyelid
    degenerative H02.70
      chloasma — *see* Chloasma, eyelid
      madarosis — *see* Madarosis
      specified type NEC H02.79
      vitiligo — *see* Vitiligo, eyelid
      xanthelasma — *see* Xanthelasma
    dermatochalasis — *see* Dermatochalasis
    edema — *see* Edema, eyelid
    elephantiasis — *see* Elephantiasis, eyelid
    foreign body, retained — *see* Foreign body, re-
      tained, eyelid
    function H02.59
      abnormal innervation syndrome — *see* Syn-
        drome, abnormal innervation
      blepharochalasis — *see* Blepharochalasis
      blepharoclonus — *see* Blepharoclonus
      blepharophimosis — *see* Blepharophimosis
      blepharoptosis — *see* Blepharoptosis
      lagophthalmos — *see* Lagophthalmos
      lid retraction — *see* Retraction, lid
    hypertrichosis — *see* Hypertrichosis, eyelid
    specified type NEC H02.89
    vascular H02.879
      left H02.876
        lower H02.875
        upper H02.874
      right H02.873
        lower H02.872
        upper H02.871
  factitious F68.10
    with predominantly
      physical symptoms F68.12
        with psychological symptoms F68.13
      psychological symptoms F68.11
        with physical symptoms F68.13
  factor, coagulation — *see* Defect, coagulation
  fatty acid
    metabolism E71.30
      specified NEC E71.39
    oxidation
      LCAD E71.310
      MCAD E71.311
      SCAD E71.312
      specified deficiency NEC E71.318
  feeding (infant or child) (*see also* Disorder, eating)
    R63.3
    or eating disorder F50.9
    specified NEC F50.9
  feigned (with obvious motivation) Z76.5
    without obvious motivation — *see* Disorder, facti-
      tious
  female
    hypoactive sexual desire F52.0
    orgasmic F52.31
    sexual interest/arousal F52.22
  fetishistic F65.0
  fibroblastic M72.9

Disorder — *continued*
  fibroblastic — *continued*
    specified NEC M72.8
  fluency
    adult onset F98.5
    childhood onset F80.81
    following
      cerebral infarction I69.323
      cerebrovascular disease I69.923
        specified disease NEC I69.823
      intracerebral hemorrhage I69.123
      nontraumatic intracranial hemorrhage NEC
        I69.223
      subarachnoid hemorrhage I69.023
    in conditions classified elsewhere R47.82
  fluid balance E87.8
  follicular (skin) L73.9
    specified NEC L73.8
  frotteuristic F65.81
  fructose metabolism E74.10
    essential fructosuria E74.11
    fructokinase deficiency E74.11
    fructose-1, 6-diphosphatase deficiency E74.19
    hereditary fructose intolerance E74.12
    other specified E74.19
  functional polymorphonuclear neutrophils D71
  gallbladder, biliary tract and pancreas in diseases
    classified elsewhere K87
  gambling F63.0
  gamma-glutamyl cycle E72.8
  gastric (functional) K31.9
    motility K30
    psychogenic F45.8
    secretion K30
  gastrointestinal (functional) NOS K92.9
    newborn P78.9
    psychogenic F45.8
  gender-identity or -role F64.9
    childhood F64.2
    effect on relationship F66
    of adolescence or adulthood F64.0
      nontranssexual F64.8
    specified NEC F64.8
    uncertainty F66
  genito-pelvic pain penetration F52.6
  genitourinary system
    female N94.9
    male N50.9
    psychogenic F45.8
  globe H44.9
    degenerated condition H44.50
      absolute glaucoma H44.51- ☑
      atrophy H44.52- ☑
      leucocoria H44.53- ☑
    degenerative H44.30
      chalcosis H44.31- ☑
      myopia (*see also* Myopia, degenerative)
        H44.2- ☑
      siderosis H44.32- ☑
      specified type NEC H44.39- ☑
    endophthalmitis — *see* Endophthalmitis
    foreign body, retained — *see* Foreign body, intraoc-
      ular, old, retained
    hemophthalmos — *see* Hemophthalmos
    hypotony H44.40
      due to
        ocular fistula H44.42- ☑
        specified disorder NEC H44.43- ☑
      flat anterior chamber H44.41- ☑
      primary H44.44- ☑
    luxation — *see* Luxation, globe
    specified type NEC H44.89
  glomerular (in) N05.9
    amyloidosis E85.4 [N08]
    cryoglobulinemia D89.1 [N08]
    disseminated intravascular coagulation D65 [N08]
    Fabry's disease E75.21 [N08]
    familial lecithin cholesterol acyltransferase deficien-
      cy E78.6 [N08]
    Goodpasture's syndrome M31.0
    hemolytic-uremic syndrome D59.3
    Henoch (-Schönlein) purpura D69.0 [N08]
    malariae malaria B52.0
    microscopic polyangiitis M31.7 [N08]
    multiple myeloma C90.0- ☑ [N08]
    mumps B26.83
    schistosomiasis B65.9 [N08]
    sepsis NEC A41.- ☑ [N08]

☑ **Additional Character Required** — **Refer to the Tabular List for Character Selection**   ▽ Subterms under main terms may continue to next column or page

Disorder — *continued*
　glomerular — *continued*
　　sepsis — *continued*
　　　streptococcal A40.- ☑ [N08]
　　sickle-cell disorders D57.- ☑ [N08]
　　strongyloidiasis B78.9 [N08]
　　subacute bacterial endocarditis I33.0 [N08]
　　syphilis A52.75
　　systemic lupus erythematosus M32.14
　　thrombotic thrombocytopenic purpura
　　　M31.1 [N08]
　　Waldenström macroglobulinemia C88.0 [N08]
　　Wegener's granulomatosis M31.31
　gluconeogenesis E74.4
　glucosaminoglycan metabolism — *see* Disorder,
　　metabolism, glucosaminoglycan
　glycine metabolism E72.50
　　d-glycericacidemia E72.59
　　hyperhydroxyprolinemia E72.59
　　hyperoxaluria E72.53
　　hyperprolinemia E72.59
　　non-ketotic hyperglycinemia E72.51
　　oxalosis E72.53
　　oxaluria E72.53
　　sarcosinemia E72.59
　　trimethylaminuria E72.52
　glycoprotein metabolism E77.9
　　specified NEC E77.8
　habit (and impulse) F63.9
　　involving sexual behavior NEC F65.9
　　specified NEC F63.89
　hallucinogen use
　　mild F16.10
　　　with
　　　　hallucinogen intoxication delirium F16.121
　　　　hallucinogen-induced
　　　　　anxiety disorder F16.180
　　　　　bipolar and related disorder F16.14
　　　　　depressive disorder F16.14
　　　　　psychotic disorder F16.159
　　　　other hallucinogen intoxication F16.129
　　　in remission (early) (sustained) F16.11
　　moderate or severe F16.20
　　　with
　　　　hallucinogen intoxication delirium F16.221
　　　　hallucinogen-induced
　　　　　anxiety disorder F16.280
　　　　　bipolar and related disorder F16.24
　　　　　depressive disorder F16.24
　　　　　psychotic disorder F16.259
　　　　other hallucinogen intoxication F16.229
　　　in remission (early) (sustained) F16.21
　heart action I49.9
　hematological D75.9
　　newborn (transient) P61.9
　　specified NEC P61.8
　hematopoietic organs D75.9
　hemorrhagic NEC D69.9
　　drug-induced D68.32
　　due to
　　　extrinsic circulating anticoagulants D68.32
　　　increase in
　　　　anti-IIa D68.32
　　　　anti-Xa D68.32
　　　intrinsic
　　　　circulating anticoagulants D68.318
　　　　increase in
　　　　　anti-IXa D68.318
　　　　　antithrombin D68.318
　　　　　anti-VIIIa D68.318
　　　　　anti-XIa D68.318
　　following childbirth O72.3
　hemostasis — *see* Defect, coagulation
　histidine metabolism E70.40
　　histidinemia E70.41
　　other specified E70.49
　hoarding F42.3
　hyperkinetic — *see* Disorder, attention-deficit hyper-
　　activity
　hyperleucine-isoleucinemia E71.19
　hypervalinemia E71.19
　hypoactive sexual desire F52.0
　hypochondriacal F45.20
　　body dysmorphic F45.22
　　neurosis F45.21
　　other specified F45.29
　identity
　　dissociative F44.81
　　illness anxiety F45.21

Disorder — *continued*
　identity — *continued*
　　of childhood F93.8
　immune mechanism (immunity) D89.9
　　specified type NEC D89.89
　impaired renal tubular function N25.9
　　specified NEC N25.89
　impulse (control) F63.9
　inflammatory
　　pelvic, in diseases classified elsewhere — *see* cate-
　　　gory N74
　　penis N48.29
　　　abscess N48.21
　　　cellulitis N48.22
　inhalant use
　　mild F18.10
　　　with
　　　　inhalant intoxication F18.129
　　　　inhalant intoxication delirium F18.121
　　　　inhalant-induced
　　　　　anxiety disorder F18.180
　　　　　depressive disorder F18.14
　　　　　major neurocognitive disorder F18.17
　　　　　mild neurocognitive disorder F18.188
　　　　　psychotic disorder F18.159
　　　in remission (early) (sustained) F18.11
　　moderate or severe F18.20
　　　with
　　　　inhalant intoxication F18.229
　　　　inhalant intoxication delirium F18.221
　　　　inhalant-induced
　　　　　anxiety disorder F18.280
　　　　　depressive disorder F18.24
　　　　　major neurocognitive disorder F18.27
　　　　　mild neurocognitive disorder F18.288
　　　　　psychotic disorder F18.259
　　　in remission (early) (sustained) F18.21
　integument, newborn P83.9
　　specified NEC P83.88
　intermittent explosive F63.81
　internal secretion pancreas — *see* Increased, secretion,
　　pancreas, endocrine
　intestine, intestinal
　　carbohydrate absorption NEC E74.39
　　　postoperative K91.2
　　functional NEC K59.9
　　　postoperative K91.89
　　psychogenic F45.8
　　vascular K55.9
　　　chronic K55.1
　　　specified NEC K55.8
　intraoperative (intraprocedural) — *see* Complications,
　　intraoperative
　involuntary emotional expression (IEED) F07.89
　iris H21.9
　　adhesions — *see* Adhesions, iris
　　atrophy — *see* Atrophy, iris
　　chamber angle recession — *see* Recession, cham-
　　　ber angle
　　cyst — *see* Cyst, iris
　　degeneration — *see* Degeneration, iris
　　in diseases classified elsewhere H22
　　iridodialysis — *see* Iridodialysis
　　iridoschisis — *see* Iridoschisis
　　miotic pupillary cyst — *see* Cyst, pupillary
　　pupillary
　　　abnormality — *see* Abnormality, pupillary
　　　membrane — *see* Membrane, pupillary
　　specified type NEC H21.89
　　vascular NEC H21.1X- ☑
　iron metabolism E83.10
　　specified NEC E83.19
　isovaleric acidemia E71.110
　jaw, developmental M27.40
　　temporomandibular (*see also* Anomaly, dentofacial,
　　　temporomandibular joint) M26.60- ☑
　joint M25.9
　　derangement — *see* Derangement, joint
　　effusion — *see* Effusion, joint
　　fistula — *see* Fistula, joint
　　hemarthrosis — *see* Hemarthrosis
　　instability — *see* Instability, joint
　　osteophyte — *see* Osteophyte
　　pain — *see* Pain, joint
　　psychogenic F45.8
　　specified type NEC M25.80
　　　ankle M25.87- ☑
　　　elbow M25.82- ☑

Disorder — *continued*
　joint — *continued*
　　specified type — *continued*
　　　foot joint M25.87- ☑
　　　hand joint M25.84- ☑
　　　hip M25.85- ☑
　　　knee M25.86- ☑
　　　shoulder M25.81- ☑
　　　wrist M25.83- ☑
　　stiffness — *see* Stiffness, joint
　ketone metabolism E71.32
　kidney N28.9
　　functional (tubular) N25.9
　　in
　　　schistosomiasis B65.9 [N29]
　　tubular function N25.9
　　　specified NEC N25.89
　lacrimal system H04.9
　　changes H04.69
　　　fistula — *see* Fistula, lacrimal
　　gland H04.19
　　　atrophy — *see* Atrophy, lacrimal gland
　　　cyst — *see* Cyst, lacrimal, gland
　　　dacryops — *see* Dacryops
　　　dislocation — *see* Dislocation, lacrimal gland
　　　dry eye syndrome — *see* Syndrome, dry eye
　　　infection — *see* Dacryoadenitis
　　　granuloma — *see* Granuloma, lacrimal
　　　inflammation — *see* Inflammation, lacrimal
　　　obstruction — *see* Obstruction, lacrimal
　　specified NEC H04.89
　lactation NEC O92.79
　language (developmental) F80.9
　　expressive F80.1
　　mixed receptive and expressive F80.2
　　receptive F80.2
　late luteal phase dysphoric N94.89
　learning (specific) F81.9
　　acalculia R48.8
　　alexia R48.0
　　mathematics F81.2
　　reading F81.0
　　specified
　　　with impairment in
　　　　mathematics F81.2
　　　　reading F81.0
　　　　written expression F81.81
　　specified NEC F81.89
　　spelling F81.81
　　written expression F81.81
　lens H27.9
　　aphakia — *see* Aphakia
　　cataract — *see* Cataract
　　dislocation — *see* Dislocation, lens
　　specified type NEC H27.8
　ligament M24.20
　　ankle M24.27- ☑
　　attachment, spine — *see* Enthesopathy, spinal
　　elbow M24.22- ☑
　　foot joint M24.27- ☑
　　hand joint M24.24- ☑
　　hip M24.25- ☑
　　knee — *see* Derangement, knee, specified NEC
　　shoulder M24.21- ☑
　　vertebra M24.28
　　wrist M24.23- ☑
　ligamentous attachments (*see also* Enthesopathy)
　　spine — *see* Enthesopathy, spinal
　lipid
　　metabolism, congenital E78.9
　　storage E75.6
　　　specified NEC E75.5
　lipoprotein
　　deficiency (familial) E78.6
　　metabolism E78.9
　　　specified NEC E78.89
　liver K76.9
　　malarial B54 [K77]
　low back (*see also* Dorsopathy, specified NEC)
　lumbosacral
　　plexus G54.1
　　root (nerve) NEC G54.4
　lung, interstitial, drug-induced J70.4
　　acute J70.2
　　chronic J70.3
　lymphoproliferative, post-transplant (PTLD) D47.Z1
　　(*following* D47.4)
　lysine and hydroxylysine metabolism E72.3

Disorder — *continued*
  major neurocognitive — *see* Dementia, in (due to)
  male
    erectile (organic) (*see also* Dysfunction, sexual, male, erectile) N52.9
      nonorganic F52.21
    hypoactive sexual desire F52.0
    orgasmic F52.32
  manic F30.9
    organic F06.33
  mast cell activation — *see* Activation, mast cell
  mastoid (*see also* Disorder, ear, middle)
    postprocedural — *see* Complications, ear, procedure
  meniscus — *see* Derangement, knee, meniscus
  menopausal N95.9
    specified NEC N95.8
  menstrual N92.6
    psychogenic F45.8
    specified NEC N92.5
  mental (or behavioral) (nonpsychotic) F99
    due to (secondary to)
      amphetamine
        due to drug abuse — *see* Abuse, drug, stimulant
        due to drug dependence — *see* Dependence, drug, stimulant
      brain disease, damage and dysfunction F09
      caffeine use
        due to drug abuse — *see* Abuse, drug, stimulant
        due to drug dependence — *see* Dependence, drug, stimulant
      cannabis use
        due to drug abuse — *see* Abuse, drug, cannabis
        due to drug dependence — *see* Dependence, drug, cannabis
      general medical condition F09
      sedative or hypnotic use
        due to drug abuse — *see* Abuse, drug, sedative
        due to drug dependence — *see* Dependence, drug, sedative
      tobacco (nicotine) use — *see* Dependence, drug, nicotine
    following organic brain damage F07.9
      frontal lobe syndrome F07.0
      personality change F07.0
      postconcussional syndrome F07.81
      specified NEC F07.89
    infancy, childhood or adolescence F98.9
    neurotic — *see* Neurosis
    organic or symptomatic F09
    presenile, psychotic F03 ☑
    problem NEC
    psychoneurotic — *see* Neurosis
    psychotic — *see* Psychosis
    puerperal F53
    senile, psychotic NEC F03 ☑
  metabolic, amino acid, transitory, newborn P74.8
  metabolism NOS E88.9
    amino-acid E72.9
      aromatic E70.9
        albinism — *see* Albinism
        histidine E70.40
          histidinemia E70.41
          other specified E70.49
        hyperphenylalaninemia E70.1
          classical phenylketonuria E70.0
        other specified E70.8
        tryptophan E70.5
        tyrosine E70.20
          hypertyrosinemia E70.21
          other specified E70.29
      branched chain E71.2
        3-methylglutaconic aciduria E71.111
        hyperleucine-isoleucinemia E71.19
        hypervalinemia E71.19
        isovaleric acidemia E71.110
        maple syrup urine disease E71.0
        methylmalonic acidemia E71.120
        organic aciduria NEC E71.118
        other specified E71.19
        proprionate NEC E71.128
        proprionic acidemia E71.121
      glycine E72.50
        d-glycericacidemia E72.59

Disorder — *continued*
  metabolism — *continued*
    amino-acid — *continued*
      glycine — *continued*
        hyperhydroxyprolinemia E72.59
        hyperoxaluria E72.53
        hyperprolinemia E72.59
        non-ketotic hyperglycinemia E72.51
        other specified E72.59
        sarcosinemia E72.59
        trimethylaminuria E72.52
      hydroxylysine E72.3
      lysine E72.3
      ornithine E72.4
      other specified E72.8
        beta-amino acid E72.8
        gamma-glutamyl cycle E72.8
      straight-chain E72.8
      sulfur-bearing E72.10
        homocystinuria E72.11
        methylenetetrahydrofolate reductase deficiency E72.12
        other specified E72.19
    bile acid and cholesterol metabolism E78.70
    bilirubin E80.7
      specified NEC E80.6
    calcium E83.50
      hypercalcemia E83.52
      hypocalcemia E83.51
      other specified E83.59
    carbohydrate E74.9
      specified NEC E74.8
    cholesterol and bile acid metabolism E78.70
    congenital E88.9
    copper E83.00
      specified type NEC E83.09
      Wilson's disease E83.01
    cystinuria E72.01
    fructose E74.10
    galactose E74.20
    glucosaminoglycan E76.9
      mucopolysaccharidosis — *see* Mucopolysaccharidosis
      specified NEC E76.8
    glutamine E72.8
    glycine E72.50
    glycogen storage (hepatorenal) E74.09
    glycoprotein E77.9
      specified NEC E77.8
    glycosaminoglycan E76.9
      specified NEC E76.8
    in labor and delivery O75.89
    iron E83.10
    isoleucine E71.19
    leucine E71.19
    lipoid E78.9
    lipoprotein E78.9
      specified NEC E78.89
    magnesium E83.40
      hypermagnesemia E83.41
      hypomagnesemia E83.42
      other specified E83.49
    mineral E83.9
      specified NEC E83.89
    mitochondrial E88.40
      MELAS syndrome E88.41
      MERRF syndrome (myoclonic epilepsy associated with ragged-red fibers) E88.42
      other specified E88.49
    ornithine E72.4
    phosphatases E83.30
    phosphorus E83.30
      acid phosphatase deficiency E83.39
      hypophosphatasia E83.39
      hypophosphatemia E83.39
        familial E83.31
      other specified E83.39
      pseudovitamin D deficiency E83.32
    plasma protein NEC E88.09
    porphyrin — *see* Porphyria
    postprocedural E89.89
      specified NEC E89.89
    purine E79.9
      specified NEC E79.8
    pyrimidine E79.9
      specified NEC E79.8
    pyruvate E74.4
    serine E72.8
    sodium E87.8

Disorder — *continued*
  metabolism — *continued*
    specified NEC E88.89
    threonine E72.8
    valine E71.19
    zinc E83.2
  methylmalonic acidemia E71.120
  micturition NEC (*see also* Difficulty, micturition) R39.198
    feeling of incomplete emptying R39.14
    hesitancy R39.11
    poor stream R39.12
    psychogenic F45.8
    split stream R39.13
    straining R39.16
    urgency R39.15
  mild neurocognitive G31.84
  mitochondrial metabolism E88.40
  mitral (valve) — *see* Endocarditis, mitral
  mixed
    anxiety and depressive F41.8
    of scholastic skills (developmental) F81.89
    receptive expressive language F80.2
  mood F39
    bipolar — *see* Disorder, bipolar
    depressive — *see* Disorder, depressive
    due to (secondary to)
      alcohol F10.94
      amphetamine F15.94
        in
          abuse F15.14
          dependence F15.24
      anxiolytic F13.94
        in
          abuse F13.14
          dependence F13.24
      cocaine F14.94
        in
          abuse F14.14
          dependence F14.24
      general medical condition F06.30
      hallucinogen F16.94
        in
          abuse F16.14
          dependence F16.24
      hypnotic F13.94
        in
          abuse F13.14
          dependence F13.24
      inhalant F18.94
        in
          abuse F18.14
          dependence F18.24
      opioid F11.94
        in
          abuse F11.14
          dependence F11.24
      phencyclidine (PCP) F16.94
        in
          abuse F16.14
          dependence F16.24
      physiological condition F06.30
        with
          depressive features F06.31
          major depressive-like episode F06.32
          manic features F06.33
          mixed features F06.34
      psychoactive substance NEC F19.94
        in
          abuse F19.14
          dependence F19.24
      sedative F13.94
        in
          abuse F13.14
          dependence F13.24
      volatile solvents F18.94
        in
          abuse F18.14
          dependence F18.24
    manic episode F30.9
      with psychotic symptoms F30.2
      without psychotic symptoms F30.10
        mild F30.11
        moderate F30.12
        severe F30.13
      in remission (full) F30.4
        partial F30.3
      specified type NEC F30.8
    organic F06.30

☑ **Additional Character Required** — Refer to the Tabular List for Character Selection   ▽ **Subterms under main terms may continue to next column or page**

Index

Disorder — Disorder

Disorder — *continued*
  mood — *continued*
    organic — *continued*
      right hemisphere F07.89
    persistent F34.9
      cyclothymia F34.0
      dysthymia F34.1
      specified type NEC F34.89
    recurrent F39
    right hemisphere organic F07.89
  movement G25.9
    drug-induced G25.70
      akathisia G25.71
      specified NEC G25.79
    hysterical F44.4
    in diseases classified elsewhere — *see* category
      G26
    periodic limb G47.61
      sleep related G47.61
    sleep related NEC G47.69
    specified NEC G25.89
    stereotyped F98.4
    treatment-induced G25.9
  multiple personality F44.81
  muscle M62.9
    attachment, spine — *see* Enthesopathy, spinal
    in trichinellosis — *see* Trichinellosis, with muscle
      disorder
    psychogenic F45.8
    specified type NEC M62.89
    tone, newborn P94.9
      specified NEC P94.8
  muscular
    attachments (*see also* Enthesopathy)
      spine — *see* Enthesopathy, spinal
    urethra N36.44
  musculoskeletal system, soft tissue — *see* Disorder,
    soft tissue
    postprocedural M96.89
    psychogenic F45.8
  myoneural G70.9
    due to lead G70.1
    specified NEC G70.89
    toxic G70.1
  myotonic NEC G71.19
  nail, in diseases classified elsewhere L62
  neck region NEC — *see* Dorsopathy, specified NEC
  neonatal onset multisystemic inflammatory (NOMID)
    M04.2
  nerve G58.9
    abducent NEC — *see* Strabismus, paralytic, sixth
      nerve
    accessory G52.8
    acoustic — *see* subcategory H93.3 ☑
    auditory — *see* subcategory H93.3 ☑
    auriculotemporal G50.8
    axillary G54.0
    cerebral — *see* Disorder, nerve, cranial
    cranial G52.9
      eighth — *see* subcategory H93.3 ☑
      eleventh G52.8
      fifth G50.9
      first G52.0
      fourth NEC — *see* Strabismus, paralytic, fourth
        nerve
      multiple G52.7
      ninth G52.1
      second NEC — *see* Disorder, nerve, optic
      seventh NEC G51.8
      sixth NEC — *see* Strabismus, paralytic, sixth
        nerve
      specified NEC G52.8
      tenth G52.2
      third NEC — *see* Strabismus, paralytic, third
        nerve
      twelfth G52.3
    entrapment — *see* Neuropathy, entrapment
    facial G51.9
      specified NEC G51.8
    femoral — *see* Lesion, nerve, femoral
    glossopharyngeal NEC G52.1
    hypoglossal G52.3
    intercostal G58.0
    lateral
      cutaneous of thigh — *see* Mononeuropathy,
        lower limb, meralgia paresthetica
      popliteal — *see* Lesion, nerve, popliteal
      lower limb — *see* Mononeuropathy, lower limb

Disorder — *continued*
  nerve — *continued*
    medial popliteal — *see* Lesion, nerve, popliteal,
      medial
    median NEC — *see* Lesion, nerve, median
    multiple G58.7
    oculomotor NEC — *see* Strabismus, paralytic, third
      nerve
    olfactory G52.0
    optic NEC H47.09- ☑
      hemorrhage into sheath — *see* Hemorrhage,
        optic nerve
      ischemic H47.01- ☑
    peroneal — *see* Lesion, nerve, popliteal
    phrenic G58.8
    plantar — *see* Lesion, nerve, plantar
    pneumogastric G52.2
    posterior tibial — *see* Syndrome, tarsal tunnel
    radial — *see* Lesion, nerve, radial
    recurrent laryngeal G52.2
    root G54.9
      cervical G54.2
      lumbosacral G54.1
      specified NEC G54.8
      thoracic G54.3
    sciatic NEC — *see* Lesion, nerve, sciatic
    specified NEC G58.8
      lower limb — *see* Mononeuropathy, lower limb,
        specified NEC
      upper limb — *see* Mononeuropathy, upper
        limb, specified NEC
    sympathetic G90.9
    tibial — *see* Lesion, nerve, popliteal, medial
    trigeminal G50.9
      specified NEC G50.8
    trochlear NEC — *see* Strabismus, paralytic, fourth
      nerve
    ulnar — *see* Lesion, nerve, ulnar
    upper limb — *see* Mononeuropathy, upper limb
    vagus G52.2
  nervous system G98.8
    autonomic (peripheral) G90.9
      specified NEC G90.8
    central G96.9
      specified NEC G96.8
    parasympathetic G90.9
    specified NEC G98.8
    sympathetic G90.9
    vegetative G90.9
  neurocognitive R41.9
    major
      with
        aggressive behavior F01.51
        combative behavior F01.51
        violent behavior F01.51
      without behavioral disturbance F01.50
      due to vascular disease, with behavioral distur-
        bance F01.51
      in (due to) (other diseases classified elsewhere)
        (*see also* Dementia, in (due to)) F02.80
        with
          aggressive behavior F02.81
          combative behavior F02.81
          violent behavior F02.81
    mild G31.84
  neurodevelopmental F89
    specified NEC F88
  neurohypophysis NEC E23.3
  neurological NEC R29.818
  neuromuscular G70.9
    hereditary NEC G71.9
    specified NEC G70.89
    toxic G70.1
  neurotic F48.9
    specified NEC F48.8
  neutrophil, polymorphonuclear D71
  nicotine use — *see* Dependence, drug, nicotine
  nightmare F51.5
  non-rapid eye movement sleep arousal
    sleep terror type F51.4
    sleepwalking type F51.3
  nose J34.9
    specified NEC J34.89
  obsessive-compulsive F42.9
    and related disorder due to a known physiological
      condition F06.8
  odontogenesis NOS K00.9

Disorder — *continued*
  opioid use
    with
      opioid-induced psychotic disorder F11.959
        with
          delusions F11.950
          hallucinations F11.951
    due to drug abuse — *see* Abuse, drug, opioid
    due to drug dependence — *see* Dependence, drug,
      opioid
    mild F11.10
      with
        opioid intoxication
          with perceptual disturbances F11.122
          without perceptual disturbances F11.129
          delirium F11.121
        opioid-induced
          anxiety disorder F11.188
          depressive disorder F11.14
          sexual dysfunction F11.181
      in remission (early) (sustained) F11.11
    moderate or severe F11.20
      with
        opioid intoxication
          with perceptual disturbances F11.222
          without perceptual disturbances F11.229
          delirium F11.221
        opioid-induced
          anxiety disorder F11.288
          anxiety disorder F11.988
          depressive disorder F11.24
          depressive disorder F11.94
          sexual dysfunction F11.281
          sexual dysfunction F11.981
      in remission (early) (sustained) F11.21
  oppositional defiant F91.3
  optic
    chiasm H47.49
      due to
        inflammatory disorder H47.41
        neoplasm H47.42
        vascular disorder H47.43
    disc H47.39- ☑
      coloboma — *see* Coloboma, optic disc
      drusen — *see* Drusen, optic disc
      pseudopapilledema — *see* Pseudopapilledema
    radiations — *see* Disorder, visual, pathway
    tracts — *see* Disorder, visual, pathway
  orbit H05.9
    cyst — *see* Cyst, orbit
    deformity — *see* Deformity, orbit
    edema — *see* Edema, orbit
    enophthalmos — *see* Enophthalmos
    exophthalmos — *see* Exophthalmos
    hemorrhage — *see* Hemorrhage, orbit
    inflammation — *see* Inflammation, orbit
    myopathy — *see* Myopathy, extraocular muscles
    retained foreign body — *see* Foreign body, orbit,
      old
    specified type NEC H05.89
  organic
    anxiety F06.4
    catatonic F06.1
    delusional F06.2
    dissociative F06.8
    emotionally labile (asthenic) F06.8
    mood (affective) F06.30
    schizophrenia-like F06.2
  orgasmic (female) F52.31
    male F52.32
  ornithine metabolism E72.4
  overanxious F41.1
    of childhood F93.8
  pain
    with related psychological factors F45.42
    exclusively related to psychological factors F45.41
    genito-pelvic penetration disorder F52.6
  pancreatic internal secretion E16.9
    specified NEC E16.8
  panic F41.0
    with agoraphobia F40.01
  papulosquamous L44.9
    in diseases classified elsewhere L45
    specified NEC L44.8
  paranoid F22
    induced F24
    shared F24
  paraphilic F65.9

Index

Disorder — Disorder

Index

Disorder — Disorder

Disorder — continued
paraphilic — continued
specified NEC F65.89
parathyroid (gland) E21.5
specified NEC E21.4
parietoalveolar NEC J84.09
paroxysmal, mixed R56.9
patella M22.9- ☑
chondromalacia — see Chondromalacia, patella
derangement NEC M22.3X- ☑
recurrent
dislocation — see Dislocation, patella, recurrent
subluxation — see Dislocation, patella, recurrent, incomplete
specified NEC M22.8X- ☑
patellofemoral M22.2X- ☑
pedophilic F65.4
pentose phosphate pathway with anemia D55.1
perception, due to hallucinogens F16.983
in
abuse F16.183
dependence F16.283
peripheral nervous system NEC G64
peroxisomal E71.50
biogenesis
neonatal adrenoleukodystrophy E71.511
specified disorder NEC E71.518
Zellweger syndrome E71.510
rhizomelic chondrodysplasia punctata E71.540
specified form NEC E71.548
group 1 E71.518
group 2 E71.53
group 3 E71.542
X-linked adrenoleukodystrophy E71.529
adolescent E71.521
adrenomyeloneuropathy E71.522
childhood E71.520
specified form NEC E71.528
Zellweger-like syndrome E71.541
persistent
(somatoform) pain F45.41
affective (mood) F34.9
personality (see also Personality) F60.9
affective F34.0
aggressive F60.3
amoral F60.2
anankastic F60.5
antisocial F60.2
anxious F60.6
asocial F60.2
asthenic F60.7
avoidant F60.6
borderline F60.3
change (secondary) due to general medical condition F07.0
compulsive F60.5
cyclothymic F34.0
dependent (passive) F60.7
depressive F34.1
dissocial F60.2
emotional instability F60.3
expansive paranoid F60.0
explosive F60.3
following organic brain damage F07.9
histrionic F60.4
hyperthymic F34.0
hypothymic F34.1
hysterical F60.4
immature F60.89
inadequate F60.7
labile F60.3
mixed (nonspecific) F60.89
moral deficiency F60.2
narcissistic F60.81
negativistic F60.89
obsessional F60.5
obsessive (-compulsive) F60.5
organic F07.9
overconscientious F60.5
paranoid F60.0
passive (-dependent) F60.7
passive-aggressive F60.89
pathological NEC F60.9
pseudosocial F60.2
psychopathic F60.2
schizoid F60.1
schizotypal F21
self-defeating F60.7

Disorder — continued
personality (see also Personality) — continued
specified NEC F60.89
type A F60.5
unstable (emotional) F60.3
pervasive, developmental F84.9
phencyclidine use
mild F16.10
with
phencyclidine intoxication F16.129
phencyclidine intoxication delirium F16.121
phencyclidine-induced
anxiety disorder F16.180
bipolar and related disorder F16.14
depressive disorder F16.14
psychotic disorder F16.159
in remission (early) (sustained) F16.11
moderate or severe F16.20
with
phencyclidine intoxication F16.229
phencyclidine intoxication delirium F16.221
phencyclidine-induced
anxiety disorder F16.280
bipolar and related disorder F16.14
depressive disorder F16.24
psychotic disorder F16.259
in remission (early) (sustained) F16.21
phobic anxiety, childhood F40.8
phosphate-losing tubular N25.0
pigmentation L81.9
choroid, congenital Q14.3
diminished melanin formation L81.6
iron L81.8
specified NEC L81.8
pinna (noninfective) H61.10- ☑
deformity, acquired H61.11- ☑
hematoma H61.12- ☑
perichondritis — see Perichondritis, ear
specified type NEC H61.19- ☑
pituitary gland E23.7
iatrogenic (postprocedural) E89.3
specified NEC E23.6
platelets D69.1
plexus G54.9
specified NEC G54.8
polymorphonuclear neutrophils D71
porphyrin metabolism — see Porphyria
postconcussional F07.81
posthallucinogen perception F16.983
in
abuse F16.183
dependence F16.283
postmenopausal N95.9
specified NEC N95.8
postprocedural (postoperative) — see Complications, postprocedural
post-transplant lymphoproliferative D47.Z1 (following D47.4)
post-traumatic stress (PTSD) F43.10
acute F43.11
chronic F43.12
premenstrual dysphoric (PMDD) F32.81
prepuce N47.8
propionic acidemia E71.121
prostate N42.9
specified NEC N42.89
psychogenic NOS (see also condition) F45.9
anxiety F41.8
appetite F50.9
asthenic F48.8
cardiovascular (system) F45.8
compulsive F42.8
cutaneous F54
depressive F32.9
digestive (system) F45.8
dysmenorrheic F45.8
dyspneic F45.8
endocrine (system) F54
eye NEC F45.8
feeding — see Disorder, eating
functional NEC F45.8
gastric F45.8
gastrointestinal (system) F45.8
genitourinary (system) F45.8
heart (function) (rhythm) F45.8
hyperventilatory F45.8
hypochondriacal — see Disorder, hypochondriacal
intestinal F45.8

Disorder — continued
psychogenic (see also condition) — continued
joint F45.8
learning F81.9
limb F45.8
lymphatic (system) F45.8
menstrual F45.8
micturition F45.8
monoplegic NEC F44.4
motor F44.4
muscle F45.8
musculoskeletal F45.8
neurocirculatory F45.8
obsessive F42.8
occupational F48.8
organ or part of body NEC F45.8
paralytic NEC F44.4
phobic F40.9
physical NEC F45.8
rectal F45.8
respiratory (system) F45.8
rheumatic F45.8
sexual (function) F52.9
skin (allergic) (eczematous) F54
sleep F51.9
specified part of body NEC F45.8
stomach F45.8
psychological F99
associated with
disease classified elsewhere F54
sexual
development F66
relationship F66
uncertainty about gender identity F64.9
psychomotor NEC F44.4
hysterical F44.4
psychoneurotic (see also Neurosis)
mixed NEC F48.8
psychophysiologic — see Disorder, somatoform
psychosexual F65.9
development F66
identity of childhood F64.2
psychosomatic NOS — see Disorder, somatoform
multiple F45.0
undifferentiated F45.1
psychotic — see Psychosis
transient (acute) F23
puberty E30.9
specified NEC E30.8
pulmonary (valve) — see Endocarditis, pulmonary
purine metabolism E79.9
pyrimidine metabolism E79.9
pyruvate metabolism E74.4
reactive attachment (childhood) F94.1
reading R48.0
developmental (specific) F81.0
receptive language F80.2
receptor, hormonal, peripheral (see also Syndrome, androgen insensitivity) E34.50
recurrent brief depressive F33.8
reflex R29.2
refraction H52.7
aniseikonia H52.32
anisometropia H52.31
astigmatism — see Astigmatism
hypermetropia — see Hypermetropia
myopia — see Myopia
presbyopia H52.4
specified NEC H52.6
relationship F68.8
due to sexual orientation F66
REM sleep behavior G47.52
renal function, impaired (tubular) N25.9
resonance R49.9
specified NEC R49.8
respiratory function, impaired (see also Failure, respiration)
postprocedural — see Complication, postoperative, respiratory system
psychogenic F45.8
retina H35.9
angioid streaks H35.33
changes in vascular appearance H35.01- ☑
degeneration — see Degeneration, retina
dystrophy (hereditary) — see Dystrophy, retina
edema H35.81
hemorrhage — see Hemorrhage, retina
ischemia H35.82

☑ Additional Character Required — Refer to the Tabular List for Character Selection   ▽ Subterms under main terms may continue to next column or page

Disorder — *continued*
  retina — *continued*
    macular degeneration — *see* Degeneration, macula
    microaneurysms H35.04- ☑
    microvascular abnormality NEC H35.09
    neovascularization — *see* Neovascularization, retina
    retinopathy — *see* Retinopathy
    separation of layers H35.70
      central serous chorioretinopathy H35.71- ☑
      pigment epithelium detachment (serous) H35.72- ☑
      hemorrhagic H35.73- ☑
    specified type NEC H35.89
    telangiectasis — *see* Telangiectasis, retina
    vasculitis — *see* Vasculitis, retina
  retroperitoneal K68.9
  right hemisphere organic affective F07.89
  rumination (infant or child) F98.21
  sacrum, sacrococcygeal NEC M53.3
  schizoaffective F25.9
    bipolar type F25.0
    depressive type F25.1
    manic type F25.0
    mixed type F25.0
    specified NEC F25.8
  schizoid of childhood F84.5
  schizophrenia spectrum and other psychotic disorder F29
    specified NEC F28
  schizophreniform F20.81
    brief F23
  schizotypal (personality) F21
  secretion, thyrocalcitonin E07.0
  sedative, hypnotic, or anxiolytic use
    mild F13.10
      with
        sedative, hypnotic, or anxiolytic intoxication F13.129
        sedative, hypnotic, or anxiolytic intoxication delirium F13.121
        sedative, hypnotic, or anxiolytic-induced
          anxiety disorder F13.180
          bipolar and related disorder F13.14
          depressive disorder F13.14
          psychotic disorder F13.159
          sexual dysfunction F13.181
      in remission (early) (sustained) F13.11
    moderate or severe F13.20
      with
        sedative, hypnotic, or anxiolytic intoxication F13.229
        sedative, hypnotic, or anxiolytic intoxication delirium F13.221
        sedative, hypnotic, or anxiolytic-induced
          anxiety disorder F13.280
          bipolar and related disorder F13.24
          depressive disorder F13.24
          major neurocognitive disorder F13.27
          mild neurocognitive disorder F13.288
          psychotic disorder F13.259
          sexual dysfunction F13.281
      in remission (early) (sustained) F13.21
  seizure (*see also* Epilepsy) G40.909
    intractable G40.919
      with status epilepticus G40.911
  semantic pragmatic F80.89
    with autism F84.0
  sense of smell R43.1
    psychogenic F45.8
  separation anxiety, of childhood F93.0
  sexual
    aversion F52.1
    function, psychogenic F52.9
    interest/arousal, female F52.22
    masochism F65.51
    maturation F66
    nonorganic F52.9
    preference (*see also* Deviation, sexual) F65.9
      fetishistic transvestism F65.1
    relationship F66
    sadism F65.52
  shyness, of childhood and adolescence F40.10
  sibling rivalry F93.8
  sickle-cell (sickling) (homozygous) — *see* Disease, sickle-cell
    heterozygous D57.3
    specified type NEC D57.8- ☑

Disorder — *continued*
  sickle-cell — *see* Disease, sickle-cell — *continued*
    trait D57.3
  sinus (nasal) J34.9
    specified NEC J34.89
  skin L98.9
    atrophic L90.9
      specified NEC L90.8
    granulomatous L92.9
      specified NEC L92.8
    hypertrophic L91.9
      specified NEC L91.8
    infiltrative NEC L98.6
    newborn P83.9
      specified NEC P83.88
    picking F42.4
    psychogenic (allergic) (eczematous) F54
  sleep G47.9
    breathing-related — *see* Apnea, sleep
    circadian rhythm G47.20
      advance sleep phase type G47.22
      delayed sleep phase type G47.21
      due to
        alcohol
          abuse F10.182
          dependence F10.282
          use F10.982
        amphetamines
          abuse F15.182
          dependence F15.282
          use F15.982
        caffeine
          abuse F15.182
          dependence F15.282
          use F15.982
        cocaine
          abuse F14.182
          dependence F14.282
          use F14.982
        drug NEC
          abuse F19.182
          dependence F19.282
          use F19.982
        opioid
          abuse F11.182
          dependence F11.282
          use F11.982
        psychoactive substance NEC
          abuse F19.182
          dependence F19.282
          use F19.982
        sedative, hypnotic, or anxiolytic
          abuse F13.182
          dependence F13.282
          use F13.982
        stimulant NEC
          abuse F15.182
          dependence F15.282
          use F15.982
      free running type G47.24
      in conditions classified elsewhere G47.27
      irregular sleep wake type G47.23
      jet lag type G47.25
      non-24-hour sleep-wake type G47.24
      shift work type G47.26
      specified NEC G47.29
    due to
      alcohol
        abuse F10.182
        dependence F10.282
        use F10.982
      amphetamine
        abuse F15.182
        dependence F15.282
        use F15.982
      anxiolytic
        abuse F13.182
        dependence F13.282
        use F13.982
      caffeine
        abuse F15.182
        dependence F15.282
        use F15.982
      cocaine
        abuse F14.182
        dependence F14.282
        use F14.982
      drug NEC
        abuse F19.182

Disorder — *continued*
  sleep — *continued*
    due to — *continued*
      drug — *continued*
        dependence F19.282
        use F19.982
      hypnotic
        abuse F13.182
        dependence F13.282
        use F13.982
      opioid
        abuse F11.182
        dependence F11.282
        use F11.982
      psychoactive substance NEC
        abuse F19.182
        dependence F19.282
        use F19.982
      sedative
        abuse F13.182
        dependence F13.282
        use F13.982
      stimulant NEC
        abuse F15.182
        dependence F15.282
        use F15.982
    emotional F51.9
    excessive somnolence — *see* Hypersomnia
    hypersomnia type — *see* Hypersomnia
    initiating or maintaining — *see* Insomnia
    nightmares F51.5
    nonorganic F51.9
      specified NEC F51.8
    parasomnia type G47.50
    specified NEC G47.8
    terrors F51.4
    walking F51.3
  sleep-wake pattern or schedule (*see also* Disorder, sleep, circadian rhythm) G47.9
    specified NEC G47.8
  social
    anxiety (of childhood) F40.10
      generalized F40.11
    functioning in childhood F94.9
      specified NEC F94.8
    pragmatic F80.82
  soft tissue M79.9
    ankle M79.9
    due to use, overuse and pressure M70.90
      ankle M70.97- ☑
      bursitis — *see* Bursitis
      foot M70.97- ☑
      forearm M70.93- ☑
      hand M70.94- ☑
      lower leg M70.96- ☑
      multiple sites M70.99
      pelvic region M70.95- ☑
      shoulder region M70.91- ☑
      specified site NEC M70.98
      specified type NEC M70.80
        ankle M70.87- ☑
        foot M70.87- ☑
        forearm M70.83- ☑
        hand M70.84- ☑
        lower leg M70.86- ☑
        multiple sites M70.89
        pelvic region M70.85- ☑
        shoulder region M70.81- ☑
        specified site NEC M70.88
        thigh M70.85- ☑
        upper arm M70.82- ☑
      thigh M70.95- ☑
      upper arm M70.92- ☑
    foot M79.9
    forearm M79.9
    hand M79.9
    lower leg M79.9
    multiple sites M79.9
    occupational — *see* Disorder, soft tissue, due to use, overuse and pressure
    pelvic region M79.9
    shoulder region M79.9
    specified type NEC M79.89
    thigh M79.9
    upper arm M79.9
  somatic symptom F45.1
  somatization F45.0
  somatoform F45.9

Disorder — continued
somatoform — continued
  pain (persistent) F45.41
  somatization (multiple) (long-lasting) F45.0
  specified NEC F45.8
  undifferentiated F45.1
somnolence, excessive — see Hypersomnia
specific
  arithmetical F81.2
  developmental, of motor F82
  reading F81.0
  speech and language F80.9
  spelling F81.81
  written expression F81.81
speech R47.9
  articulation (functional) (specific) F80.0
  developmental F80.9
  specified NEC R47.89
speech-sound F80.0
spelling (specific) F81.81
spine (see also Dorsopathy)
  ligamentous or muscular attachments, peripheral
    — see Enthesopathy, spinal
  specified NEC — see Dorsopathy, specified NEC
stereotyped, habit or movement F98.4
stimulant use (other) (unspecified)
  mild F15.10
    in remission (early) (sustained) F15.11
  moderate or severe F15.20
    in remission (early) (sustained) F15.21
stomach (functional) — see Disorder, gastric
stress F43.9
  acute F43.0
  post-traumatic F43.10
    acute F43.11
    chronic F43.12
substance use (other) (unknown)
  mild F19.10
    with substance-induced
      anxiety disorder F19.180
      bipolar and related disorder F19.14
      depressive disorder F19.14
      major neurocognitive disorder F19.17
      mild neurocognitive disorder F19.188
      obsessive-compulsive and related disorder
        F19.188
      sexual dysfunction F19.181
    substance intoxication F19.129
    substance intoxication delirium F19.121
  moderate or severe F19.20
    with substance-induced
      anxiety disorder F19.280
      bipolar and related disorder F19.24
      depressive disorder F19.24
      major neurocognitive disorder F19.27
      mild neurocognitive disorder F19.288
      obsessive-compulsive and related disorder
        F19.288
      sexual dysfunction F19.281
    in remission (early) (sustained) F19.21
    substance intoxication F19.229
    substance intoxication delirium F19.221
sulfur-bearing amino-acid metabolism E72.10
sweat gland (eccrine) L74.9
  apocrine L75.9
    specified NEC L75.8
  specified NEC L74.8
synovium M67.90
  acromioclavicular M67.91- ☑
  ankle M67.97- ☑
  elbow M67.92- ☑
  foot M67.97- ☑
  forearm M67.93- ☑
  hand M67.94- ☑
  hip M67.95- ☑
  knee M67.96- ☑
  multiple sites M67.99
  rupture — see Rupture, synovium
  shoulder M67.91- ☑
  specified type NEC M67.80
    acromioclavicular M67.81- ☑
    ankle M67.87- ☑
    elbow M67.82- ☑
    foot M67.87- ☑
    hand M67.84- ☑
    hip M67.85- ☑
    knee M67.86- ☑
    multiple sites M67.89

Disorder — continued
synovium — continued
  specified type — continued
    wrist M67.83- ☑
  synovitis — see Synovitis
  upper arm M67.92- ☑
  wrist M67.93- ☑
temperature regulation, newborn P81.9
  specified NEC P81.8
temporomandibular joint M26.60- ☑
tendon M67.90
  acromioclavicular M67.91- ☑
  ankle M67.97- ☑
  contracture — see Contracture, tendon
  elbow M67.92- ☑
  foot M67.97- ☑
  forearm M67.93- ☑
  hand M67.94- ☑
  hip M67.95- ☑
  knee M67.96- ☑
  multiple sites M67.99
  rupture — see Rupture, tendon
  shoulder M67.91- ☑
  specified type NEC M67.80
    acromioclavicular M67.81- ☑
    ankle M67.87- ☑
    elbow M67.82- ☑
    foot M67.87- ☑
    hand M67.84- ☑
    hip M67.85- ☑
    knee M67.86- ☑
    multiple sites M67.89
    trunk M67.88
    wrist M67.83- ☑
  synovitis — see Synovitis
  tendinitis — see Tendinitis
  tenosynovitis — see Tenosynovitis
  trunk M67.98
  upper arm M67.92- ☑
  wrist M67.93- ☑
thoracic root (nerve) NEC G54.3
thyrocalcitonin hypersecretion E07.0
thyroid (gland) E07.9
  function NEC, neonatal, transitory P72.2
  iodine-deficiency related E01.8
  specified NEC E07.89
tic — see Tic
tobacco use
  chewing tobacco (mild) (moderate) (severe)
    in remission (early) (sustained) F17.221
  cigarettes (mild) (moderate) (severe)
    in remission (early) (sustained) F17.211
  mild Z72.0
    in remission (early) (sustained) F17.201
  moderate F17.200
    in remission (early) (sustained) F17.201
  severe F17.200
    in remission (early) (sustained) F17.201
  specified product NEC (mild) (moderate) (severe)
    in remission (early) (sustained) F17.291
tooth K08.9
  development K00.9
    specified NEC K00.8
  eruption K00.6
Tourette's F95.2
trance and possession F44.89
transvestic F65.1
trauma and stressor-related F43.9
  other specified F43.8
tricuspid (valve) — see Endocarditis, tricuspid
tryptophan metabolism E70.5
tubular, phosphate-losing N25.0
tubulo-interstitial (in)
  brucellosis A23.9 [N16]
  cystinosis E72.04
  diphtheria A36.84
  glycogen storage disease E74.00 [N16]
  leukemia NEC C95.9- ☑ [N16]
  lymphoma NEC C85.9- ☑ [N16]
  mixed cryoglobulinemia D89.1 [N16]
  multiple myeloma C90.0- ☑ [N16]
  Salmonella infection A02.25
  sarcoidosis D86.84
  sepsis A41.9 [N16]
    streptococcal A40.9 [N16]
  systemic lupus erythematosus M32.15
  toxoplasmosis B58.83

Disorder — continued
tubulo-interstitial — continued
  transplant rejection T86.91 [N16]
  Wilson's disease E83.01 [N16]
tubulo-renal function, impaired N25.9
  specified NEC N25.89
tympanic membrane H73.9- ☑
  atrophy — see Atrophy, tympanic membrane
  infection — see Myringitis
  perforation — see Perforation, tympanum
  specified NEC H73.89- ☑
unsocialized aggressive F91.1
urea cycle metabolism E72.20
  argininemia E72.21
  argininosuccinic aciduria E72.22
  citrullinemia E72.23
  ornithine transcarbamylase deficiency E72.4
  other specified E72.29
ureter (in) N28.9
  schistosomiasis B65.0 [N29]
  tuberculosis A18.11
urethra N36.9
  specified NEC N36.8
urinary system N39.9
  specified NEC N39.8
valve, heart
  aortic — see Endocarditis, aortic
  mitral — see Endocarditis, mitral
  pulmonary — see Endocarditis, pulmonary
  rheumatic
    aortic — see Endocarditis, aortic, rheumatic
    mitral — see Endocarditis, mitral
    pulmonary — see Endocarditis, pulmonary,
      rheumatic
    tricuspid — see Endocarditis, tricuspid
  tricuspid — see Endocarditis, tricuspid
vestibular function H81.9- ☑
  specified NEC — see subcategory H81.8 ☑
    in diseases classified elsewhere H82.- ☑
  vertigo — see Vertigo
vision, binocular H53.30
  abnormal retinal correspondence H53.31
  diplopia H53.2
  fusion with defective stereopsis H53.32
  simultaneous perception H53.33
  suppression H53.34
visual
  cortex
    blindness H47.619
      left brain H47.612
      right brain H47.611
    due to
      inflammatory disorder H47.629
        left brain H47.622
        right brain H47.621
      neoplasm H47.639
        left brain H47.632
        right brain H47.631
      vascular disorder H47.649
        left brain H47.642
        right brain H47.641
  pathway H47.9
    due to
      inflammatory disorder H47.51- ☑
      neoplasm H47.52- ☑
      vascular disorder H47.53- ☑
    optic chiasm — see Disorder, optic, chiasm
vitreous body H43.9
  crystalline deposits — see Deposit, crystalline
  degeneration — see Degeneration, vitreous
  hemorrhage — see Hemorrhage, vitreous
  opacities — see Opacity, vitreous
  prolapse — see Prolapse, vitreous
  specified type NEC H43.89
voice R49.9
  specified type NEC R49.8
volatile solvent use
  due to drug abuse — see Abuse, drug, inhalant
  due to drug dependence — see Dependence, drug,
    inhalant
voyeuristic F65.3
white blood cells D72.9
  specified NEC D72.89
withdrawing, child or adolescent F40.10
Disorientation R41.0
Displacement, displaced
  acquired traumatic of bone, cartilage, joint, tendon
    NEC — see Dislocation

☑ Additional Character Required — Refer to the Tabular List for Character Selection
🔻 Subterms under main terms may continue to next column or page

Displacement, displaced — *continued*
  adrenal gland (congenital) Q89.1
  appendix, retrocecal (congenital) Q43.8
  auricle (congenital) Q17.4
  bladder (acquired) N32.89
    congenital Q64.19
  brachial plexus (congenital) Q07.8
  brain stem, caudal (congenital) Q04.8
  canaliculus (lacrimalis), congenital Q10.6
  cardia through esophageal hiatus (congenital) Q40.1
  cerebellum, caudal (congenital) Q04.8
  cervix — *see* Malposition, uterus
  colon (congenital) Q43.3
  device, implant or graft (*see also* Complications, by site and type, mechanical) T85.628 ☑
    arterial graft NEC — *see* Complication, cardiovascular device, mechanical, vascular
    breast (implant) T85.42 ☑
    catheter NEC T85.628 ☑
      dialysis (renal) T82.42 ☑
        intraperitoneal T85.621 ☑
      infusion NEC T82.524 ☑
        spinal (epidural) (subdural) T85.620 ☑
      urinary
        cystostomy T83.020 ☑
        Hopkins T83.028 ☑
        ileostomy T83.028 ☑
        indwelling T83.021 ☑
        nephrostomy T83.022 ☑
        specified NEC T83.028 ☑
        urostomy T83.028 ☑
    electronic (electrode) (pulse generator) (stimulator) — *see* Complication, electronic stimulator
    fixation, internal (orthopedic) NEC — *see* Complication, fixation device, mechanical
    gastrointestinal — *see* Complications, prosthetic device, mechanical, gastrointestinal device
    genital NEC T83.428 ☑
      intrauterine contraceptive device (string) T83.32 ☑
      penile prosthesis (cylinder) (implanted) (pump) (reservoir) T83.420 ☑
      testicular prosthesis T83.421 ☑
    heart NEC — *see* Complication, cardiovascular device, mechanical
    joint prosthesis — *see* Complications, joint prosthesis, mechanical
    ocular — *see* Complications, prosthetic device, mechanical, ocular device
    orthopedic NEC — *see* Complication, orthopedic, device or graft, mechanical
    specified NEC T85.628 ☑
    urinary NEC T83.128 ☑
      graft T83.22 ☑
      sphincter, implanted T83.121 ☑
      stent (ileal conduit) (nephroureteral) T83.123 ☑
      ureteral indwelling T83.122 ☑
    vascular NEC — *see* Complication, cardiovascular device, mechanical
    ventricular intracranial shunt T85.02 ☑
  electronic stimulator
    bone T84.320 ☑
    cardiac — *see* Complications, cardiac device, electronic
    nervous system — *see* Complication, prosthetic device, mechanical, electronic nervous system stimulator
    urinary — *see* Complications, electronic stimulator, urinary
  esophageal mucosa into cardia of stomach, congenital Q39.8
  esophagus (acquired) K22.8
    congenital Q39.8
  eyeball (acquired) (lateral) (old) — *see* Displacement, globe
    congenital Q15.8
    current — *see* Avulsion, eye
  fallopian tube (acquired) N83.4- ☑
    congenital Q50.6
    opening (congenital) Q50.6
  gallbladder (congenital) Q44.1
  gastric mucosa (congenital) Q40.2
  globe (acquired) (old) (lateral) H05.21- ☑
    current — *see* Avulsion, eye
  heart (congenital) Q24.8
    acquired I51.89
  hymen (upward) (congenital) Q52.4

Displacement, displaced — *continued*
  intervertebral disc NEC
    with myelopathy — *see* Disorder, disc, with, myelopathy
    cervical, cervicothoracic (with) M50.20
      myelopathy — *see* Disorder, disc, cervical, with myelopathy
      neuritis, radiculitis or radiculopathy — *see* Disorder, disc, cervical, with neuritis
    due to trauma — *see* Dislocation, vertebra
    lumbar region M51.26
      with
        myelopathy M51.06
        neuritis, radiculitis, radiculopathy or sciatica M51.16
    lumbosacral region M51.27
      with
        neuritis, radiculitis, radiculopathy or sciatica M51.17
    sacrococcygeal region M53.3
    thoracic region M51.24
      with
        myelopathy M51.04
        neuritis, radiculitis, radiculopathy M51.14
    thoracolumbar region M51.25
      with
        myelopathy M51.05
        neuritis, radiculitis, radiculopathy M51.15
  intrauterine device (string) T83.32 ☑
  kidney (acquired) N28.83
    congenital Q63.2
  lachrymal, lacrimal apparatus or duct (congenital) Q10.6
  lens, congenital Q12.1
  macula (congenital) Q14.1
  Meckel's diverticulum Q43.0
    malignant — *see* Table of Neoplasms, small intestine, malignant
  nail (congenital) Q84.6
    acquired L60.8
  opening of Wharton's duct in mouth Q38.4
  organ or site, congenital NEC — *see* Malposition, congenital
  ovary (acquired) N83.4- ☑
    congenital Q50.39
    free in peritoneal cavity (congenital) Q50.39
    into hernial sac N83.4- ☑
  oviduct (acquired) N83.4- ☑
    congenital Q50.6
  parathyroid (gland) E21.4
  parotid gland (congenital) Q38.4
  punctum lacrimale (congenital) Q10.6
  sacro-iliac (joint) (congenital) Q74.2
    current injury S33.2 ☑
    old — *see* subcategory M53.2 ☑
  salivary gland (any) (congenital) Q38.4
  spleen (congenital) Q89.09
  stomach, congenital Q40.2
  sublingual duct Q38.4
  tongue (downward) (congenital) Q38.3
  tooth, teeth, fully erupted M26.30
    horizontal M26.33
    vertical M26.34
  trachea (congenital) Q32.1
  ureter or ureteric opening or orifice (congenital) Q62.62
  uterine opening of oviducts or fallopian tubes Q50.6
  uterus, uterine — *see* Malposition, uterus
  ventricular septum Q21.0
    with rudimentary ventricle Q20.4

Disproportion
  between native and reconstructed breast N65.1
  fiber-type G71.2
Disruptio uteri — *see* Rupture, uterus
Disruption (of)
  ciliary body NEC H21.89
  closure of
    cornea T81.31 ☑
    craniotomy T81.32 ☑
    fascia (muscular) (superficial) T81.32 ☑
    internal organ or tissue T81.32 ☑
    laceration (external) (internal) T81.33 ☑
    ligament T81.32 ☑
    mucosa T81.31 ☑
    muscle or muscle flap T81.32 ☑
    ribs or rib cage T81.32 ☑
    skin and subcutaneous tissue (full-thickness) (superficial) T81.31 ☑

Disruption — *continued*
  closure of — *continued*
    skull T81.32 ☑
    sternum (sternotomy) T81.32 ☑
    tendon T81.32 ☑
    traumatic laceration (external) (internal) T81.33 ☑
  family Z63.8
    due to
      absence of family member due to military deployment Z63.31
      absence of family member NEC Z63.32
      alcoholism and drug addiction in family Z63.72
      bereavement Z63.4
      death (assumed) or disappearance of family member Z63.4
      divorce or separation Z63.5
      drug addiction in family Z63.72
      return of family member from military deployment (current or past conflict) Z63.71
      stressful life events NEC Z63.79
  iris NEC H21.89
  ligament(s) (*see also* Sprain)
    knee
      current injury — *see* Dislocation, knee
      old (chronic) — *see* Derangement, knee, instability
      spontaneous NEC — *see* Derangement, knee, disruption ligament
  ossicular chain — *see* Discontinuity, ossicles, ear
  pelvic ring (stable) S32.810 ☑
    unstable S32.811 ☑
  traumatic injury wound repair T81.33 ☑
  wound T81.30 ☑
    episiotomy O90.1
    operation T81.31 ☑
      cesarean O90.0
      external operation wound (superficial) T81.31 ☑
      internal operation wound (deep) T81.32 ☑
    perineal (obstetric) O90.1
    traumatic injury repair T81.33 ☑
Dissatisfaction with
  employment Z56.9
  school environment Z55.4
Dissecting — *see* condition
Dissection
  aorta I71.00
    abdominal I71.02
    thoracic I71.01
    thoracoabdominal I71.03
  artery I77.70
    basilar (trunk) I77.75
    carotid I77.71
    cerebral (nonruptured) I67.0
      ruptured — *see* Hemorrhage, intracranial, subarachnoid
    coronary I25.42
    extremity
      lower I77.77
      upper I77.76
    iliac I77.72
    precerebral
      congenital (nonruptured) Q28.1
      specified site NEC I77.75
    renal I77.73
    specified NEC I77.79
    vertebral I77.74
  precerebral artery, congenital (nonruptured) Q28.1
  Heartland A93.8
  traumatic — *see* Wound, open, by site
  vascular I99.8
  wound — *see* Wound, open
Disseminated — *see* condition
Dissociation
  auriculoventricular or atrioventricular (AV) (any degree) (isorhythmic) I45.89
    with heart block I44.2
  interference I45.89
Dissociative reaction, state F44.9
Dissolution, vertebra — *see* Osteoporosis
Distension, distention
  abdomen R14.0
  bladder N32.89
  cecum K63.89
  colon K63.89
  gallbladder K82.8
  intestine K63.89
  kidney N28.89

Distension, distention — continued
  liver K76.89
  seminal vesicle N50.89
  stomach K31.89
    acute K31.0
    psychogenic F45.8
  ureter — see Dilatation, ureter
  uterus N85.8
Distoma hepaticum infestation B66.3
Distomiasis B66.9
  bile passages B66.3
  hemic B65.9
  hepatic B66.3
    due to Clonorchis sinensis B66.1
  intestinal B66.5
  liver B66.3
    due to Clonorchis sinensis B66.1
  lung B66.4
  pulmonary B66.4
Distomolar (fourth molar) K00.1
Disto-occlusion (Division I) (Division II) M26.212
Distortion(s) (congenital)
  adrenal (gland) Q89.1
  arm NEC Q68.8
  bile duct or passage Q44.5
  bladder Q64.79
  brain Q04.9
  cervix (uteri) Q51.9
  chest (wall) Q67.8
    bones Q76.8
  clavicle Q74.0
  clitoris Q52.6
  coccyx Q76.49
  common duct Q44.5
  coronary Q24.5
  cystic duct Q44.5
  ear (auricle) (external) Q17.3
    inner Q16.5
    middle Q16.4
      ossicles Q16.3
  endocrine NEC Q89.2
  eustachian tube Q17.8
  eye (adnexa) Q15.8
  face bone(s) NEC Q75.8
  fallopian tube Q50.6
  femur NEC Q68.8
  fibula NEC Q68.8
  finger(s) Q68.1
  foot Q66.9
  genitalia, genital organ(s)
    female Q52.8
      external Q52.79
      internal NEC Q52.8
  gyri Q04.8
  hand bone(s) Q68.1
  heart (auricle) (ventricle) Q24.8
    valve (cusp) Q24.8
  hepatic duct Q44.5
  humerus NEC Q68.8
  hymen Q52.4
  intrafamilial communications Z63.8
  jaw NEC M26.89
  labium (majus) (minus) Q52.79
  leg NEC Q68.8
  lens Q12.8
  liver Q44.7
  lumbar spine Q76.49
    with disproportion O33.8
      causing obstructed labor O65.0
  lumbosacral (joint) (region) Q76.49
    kyphosis — see Kyphosis, congenital
    lordosis — see Lordosis, congenital
  nerve Q07.8
  nose Q30.8
  organ
    of Corti Q16.5
    or site not listed — see Anomaly, by site
  ossicles, ear Q16.3
  oviduct Q50.6
  pancreas Q45.3
  parathyroid (gland) Q89.2
  pituitary (gland) Q89.2
  radius NEC Q68.8
  sacroiliac joint Q74.2
  sacrum Q76.49
  scapula Q74.0
  shoulder girdle Q74.0
  skull bone(s) NEC Q75.8

Distortion(s) — continued
  skull bone(s) — continued
    with
      anencephalus Q00.0
      encephalocele — see Encephalocele
      hydrocephalus Q03.9
        with spina bifida — see Spina bifida, with
          hydrocephalus
      microcephaly Q02
  spinal cord Q06.8
  spine Q76.49
    kyphosis — see Kyphosis, congenital
    lordosis — see Lordosis, congenital
  spleen Q89.09
  sternum NEC Q76.7
  thorax (wall) Q67.8
    bony Q76.8
  thymus (gland) Q89.2
  thyroid (gland) Q89.2
  tibia NEC Q68.8
  toe(s) Q66.9
  tongue Q38.3
  trachea (cartilage) Q32.1
  ulna NEC Q68.8
  ureter Q62.8
  urethra Q64.79
    causing obstruction Q64.39
  uterus Q51.9
  vagina Q52.4
  vertebra Q76.49
    kyphosis — see Kyphosis, congenital
    lordosis — see Lordosis, congenital
  visual (see also Disturbance, vision)
    shape and size H53.15
  vulva Q52.79
  wrist (bones) (joint) Q68.8
Distress
  abdomen — see Pain, abdominal
  acute respiratory R06.03
    syndrome (adult) (child) J80
  epigastric R10.13
  fetal P84
    complicating pregnancy — see Stress, fetal
  gastrointestinal (functional) K30
    psychogenic F45.8
  intestinal (functional) NOS K59.9
    psychogenic F45.8
  maternal, during labor and delivery O75.0
  relationship, with spouse or intimate partner Z63.0
  respiratory (adult) (child) R06.03
    newborn P22.9
      specified NEC P22.8
    orthopnea R06.01
    psychogenic F45.8
    shortness of breath R06.02
    specified type NEC R06.09
Distribution vessel, atypical Q27.9
  coronary artery Q24.5
  precerebral Q28.1
Districhiasis L68.8
Disturbance(s) (see also Disease)
  absorption K90.9
    calcium E58
    carbohydrate K90.49
    fat K90.49
      pancreatic K90.3
    protein K90.49
    starch K90.49
    vitamin — see Deficiency, vitamin
  acid-base equilibrium E87.8
    mixed E87.4
  activity and attention (with hyperkinesis) — see Disorder, attention-deficit hyperactivity
  amino acid transport E72.00
  assimilation, food K90.9
  auditory nerve, except deafness — see subcategory H93.3 ☑
  behavior — see Disorder, conduct
  blood clotting (mechanism) (see also Defect, coagulation) D68.9
  cerebral
    nerve — see Disorder, nerve, cranial
    status, newborn P91.9
      specified NEC P91.88
  circulatory I99.9
  conduct (see also Disorder, conduct) F91.9
    adjustment reaction — see Disorder, adjustment
    compulsive F63.9

Disturbance(s) — continued
  conduct (see also Disorder, conduct) — continued
    disruptive F91.9
    hyperkinetic — see Disorder, attention-deficit hyperactivity
    socialized F91.2
    specified NEC F91.8
    unsocialized F91.1
  coordination R27.8
  cranial nerve — see Disorder, nerve, cranial
  deep sensibility — see Disturbance, sensation
  digestive K30
    psychogenic F45.8
  electrolyte (see also Imbalance, electrolyte)
    newborn, transitory P74.4
      hyperammonemia P74.6
      potassium balance P74.3
      sodium balance P74.2
      specified type NEC P74.4
  emotions specific to childhood and adolescence F93.9
    with
      anxiety and fearfulness NEC F93.8
      elective mutism F94.0
      oppositional disorder F91.3
      sensitivity (withdrawal) F40.10
      shyness F40.10
      social withdrawal F40.10
    involving relationship problems F93.8
    mixed F93.8
    specified NEC F93.8
  endocrine (gland) E34.9
    neonatal, transitory P72.9
      specified NEC P72.8
  equilibrium R42
  fructose metabolism E74.10
  gait — see Gait
    hysterical F44.4
    psychogenic F44.4
  gastrointestinal (functional) K30
    psychogenic F45.8
  habit, child F98.9
  hearing, except deafness and tinnitus — see Abnormal, auditory perception
  heart, functional (conditions in I44-I50)
    due to presence of (cardiac) prosthesis I97.19- ☑
    postoperative I97.89
      cardiac surgery (see also Infarct, myocardium, associated with revascularization procedure) I97.19- ☑
  hormones E34.9
  innervation uterus (parasympathetic) (sympathetic) N85.8
  keratinization NEC
    gingiva K05.10
      nonplaque induced K05.11
      plaque induced K05.10
    lip K13.0
    oral (mucosa) (soft tissue) K13.29
    tongue K13.29
  learning (specific) — see Disorder, learning
  memory — see Amnesia
    mild, following organic brain damage F06.8
  mental F99
    associated with diseases classified elsewhere F54
  metabolism E88.9
    with
      abortion — see Abortion, by type with other specified complication
      ectopic pregnancy O08.5
      molar pregnancy O08.5
    amino-acid E72.9
      aromatic E70.9
      branched-chain E71.2
      straight-chain E72.8
      sulfur-bearing E72.10
    ammonia E72.20
    arginine E72.21
    arginosuccinic acid E72.22
    carbohydrate E74.9
    cholesterol E78.9
    citrulline E72.23
    cystathionine E72.19
    general E88.9
    glutamine E72.8
    histidine E70.40
    homocystine E72.19
    hydroxylysine E72.3
    in labor or delivery O75.89

☑ **Additional Character Required** — Refer to the Tabular List for Character Selection   ▽ **Subterms under main terms may continue to next column or page**

Disturbance(s) — continued
- metabolism — continued
  - iron E83.10
  - lipoid E78.9
  - lysine E72.3
  - methionine E72.19
  - neonatal, transitory P74.9
    - calcium and magnesium P71.9
      - specified type NEC P71.8
    - carbohydrate metabolism P70.9
      - specified type NEC P70.8
    - specified NEC P74.8
  - ornithine E72.4
  - phosphate E83.39
  - sodium NEC E87.8
  - threonine E72.8
  - tryptophan E70.5
  - tyrosine E70.20
  - urea cycle E72.20
- motor R29.2
- nervous, functional R45.0
- neuromuscular mechanism (eye), due to syphilis A52.15
- nutritional E63.9
  - nail L60.3
- ocular motion H51.9
  - psychogenic F45.8
- oculogyric H51.8
  - psychogenic F45.8
- oculomotor H51.9
  - psychogenic F45.8
- olfactory nerve R43.1
- optic nerve NEC — see Disorder, nerve, optic
- oral epithelium, including tongue NEC K13.29
- perceptual due to
  - alcohol withdrawal F10.232
  - amphetamine intoxication F15.922
    - in
      - abuse F15.122
      - dependence F15.222
  - anxiolytic withdrawal F13.232
  - cannabis intoxication (acute) F12.922
    - in
      - abuse F12.122
      - dependence F12.222
  - cocaine intoxication (acute) F14.922
    - in
      - abuse F14.122
      - dependence F14.222
  - hypnotic withdrawal F13.232
  - opioid intoxication (acute) F11.922
    - in
      - abuse F11.122
      - dependence F11.222
  - phencyclidine intoxication (acute) F16.122
  - sedative withdrawal F13.232
- personality (pattern) (trait) (see also Disorder, personality) F60.9
  - following organic brain damage F07.9
- polyglandular E31.9
  - specified NEC E31.8
- potassium balance, newborn P74.3
- psychogenic F45.9
- psychomotor F44.4
- psychophysical visual H53.16
- pupillary — see Anomaly, pupil, function
- reflex R29.2
- rhythm, heart I49.9
- salivary secretion K11.7
- sensation (cold) (heat) (localization) (tactile discrimination) (texture) (vibratory) NEC R20.9
  - hysterical F44.6
  - skin R20.9
    - anesthesia R20.0
    - hyperesthesia R20.3
    - hypoesthesia R20.1
    - paresthesia R20.2
    - specified type NEC R20.8
  - smell R43.9
    - and taste (mixed) R43.8
    - anosmia R43.0
    - parosmia R43.1
    - specified NEC R43.8
  - taste R43.9
    - and smell (mixed) R43.8
    - parageusia R43.2
    - specified NEC R43.8
- sensory — see Disturbance, sensation

Disturbance(s) — continued
- situational (transient) (see also Disorder, adjustment)
  - acute F43.0
- sleep G47.9
  - nonorganic origin F51.9
- smell — see Disturbance, sensation, smell
- sociopathic F60.2
- sodium balance, newborn P74.2
- speech R47.9
  - developmental F80.9
  - specified NEC R47.89
- stomach (functional) K31.9
- sympathetic (nerve) G90.9
- taste — see Disturbance, sensation, taste
- temperature
  - regulation, newborn P81.9
    - specified NEC P81.8
  - sense R20.8
    - hysterical F44.6
- tooth
  - eruption K00.6
  - formation K00.4
  - structure, hereditary NEC K00.5
- touch — see Disturbance, sensation
- vascular I99.9
  - arteriosclerotic — see Arteriosclerosis
- vasomotor I73.9
- vasospastic I73.9
- vision, visual H53.9
  - following
    - cerebral infarction I69.398
    - cerebrovascular disease I69.998
      - specified NEC I69.898
    - intracerebral hemorrhage I69.198
    - nontraumatic intracranial hemorrhage NEC I69.298
    - specified disease NEC I69.898
    - subarachnoid hemorrhage I69.098
  - psychophysical H53.16
  - specified NEC H53.8
  - subjective H53.10
    - day blindness H53.11
    - discomfort H53.14- ☑
    - distortions of shape and size H53.15
    - loss
      - sudden H53.13- ☑
      - transient H53.12- ☑
    - specified type NEC H53.19
- voice R49.9
  - psychogenic F44.4
  - specified NEC R49.8

Diuresis R35.8
Diver's palsy, paralysis or squeeze T70.3 ☑
Diverticulitis (acute) K57.92
- bladder — see Cystitis
- ileum — see Diverticulitis, intestine, small
- intestine K57.92
  - with
    - abscess, perforation or peritonitis K57.80
      - with bleeding K57.81
    - bleeding K57.93
  - congenital Q43.8
  - large K57.32
    - with
      - abscess, perforation or peritonitis K57.20
        - with bleeding K57.21
      - bleeding K57.33
      - small intestine K57.52
        - with
          - abscess, perforation or peritonitis K57.40
            - with bleeding K57.41
          - bleeding K57.53
  - small K57.12
    - with
      - abscess, perforation or peritonitis K57.00
        - with bleeding K57.01
      - bleeding K57.13
      - large intestine K57.52
        - with
          - abscess, perforation or peritonitis K57.40
            - with bleeding K57.41
          - bleeding K57.53
Diverticulosis K57.90
- with bleeding K57.91
- large intestine K57.30

Diverticulosis — continued
- large intestine — continued
  - with
    - bleeding K57.31
    - small intestine K57.50
      - with bleeding K57.51
- small intestine K57.10
  - with
    - bleeding K57.11
    - large intestine K57.50
      - with bleeding K57.51
Diverticulum, diverticula (multiple) K57.90
- appendix (noninflammatory) K38.2
- bladder (sphincter) N32.3
  - congenital Q64.6
- bronchus (congenital) Q32.4
  - acquired J98.09
- calyx, calyceal (kidney) N28.89
- cardia (stomach) K31.4
- cecum — see Diverticulosis, intestine, large
  - congenital Q43.8
- colon — see Diverticulosis, intestine, large
  - congenital Q43.8
- duodenum — see Diverticulosis, intestine, small
  - congenital Q43.8
- epiphrenic (esophagus) K22.5
- esophagus (congenital) Q39.6
  - acquired (epiphrenic) (pulsion) (traction) K22.5
- eustachian tube — see Disorder, eustachian tube, specified NEC
- fallopian tube N83.8
- gastric K31.4
- heart (congenital) Q24.8
- ileum — see Diverticulosis, intestine, small
- jejunum — see Diverticulosis, intestine, small
- kidney (pelvis) (calyces) N28.89
  - with calculus — see Calculus, kidney
- Meckel's (displaced) (hypertrophic) Q43.0
  - malignant — see Table of Neoplasms, small intestine, malignant
- midthoracic K22.5
- organ or site, congenital NEC — see Distortion
- pericardium (congenital) (cyst) Q24.8
  - acquired I31.8
- pharyngoesophageal (congenital) Q39.6
  - acquired K22.5
- pharynx (congenital) Q38.7
- rectosigmoid — see Diverticulosis, intestine, large
  - congenital Q43.8
- rectum — see Diverticulosis, intestine, large
- Rokitansky's K22.5
- seminal vesicle N50.89
- sigmoid — see Diverticulosis, intestine, large
  - congenital Q43.8
- stomach (acquired) K31.4
  - congenital Q40.2
- trachea (acquired) J39.8
- ureter (acquired) N28.89
  - congenital Q62.8
- ureterovesical orifice N28.89
- urethra (acquired) N36.1
  - congenital Q64.79
- ventricle, left (congenital) Q24.8
- vesical N32.3
  - congenital Q64.6
- Zenker's (esophagus) K22.5
Division
- cervix uteri (acquired) N88.8
- glans penis Q55.69
- labia minora (congenital) Q52.79
- ligament (partial or complete) (current) (see also Sprain)
  - with open wound — see Wound, open
- muscle (partial or complete) (current) (see also Injury, muscle)
  - with open wound — see Wound, open
- nerve (traumatic) — see Injury, nerve
- spinal cord — see Injury, spinal cord, by region
- vein I87.8
Divorce, causing family disruption Z63.5
Dix-Hallpike neurolabyrinthitis — see Neuronitis, vestibular
Dizziness R42
- hysterical F44.89
- psychogenic F45.8
DMAC (disseminated mycobacterium avium- intracellulare complex) A31.2
DNR (do not resuscitate) Z66

Doan-Wiseman syndrome (primary splenic neutropenia) — see Agranulocytosis
Doehle-Heller aortitis A52.02
Dog bite — see Bite
Dohle body panmyelopathic syndrome D72.0
Dolichocephaly Q67.2
Dolichocolon Q43.8
Dolichostenomelia — see Syndrome, Marfan's
Donohue's syndrome E34.8
Donor (organ or tissue) Z52.9
　blood (whole) Z52.000
　　autologous Z52.010
　　specified component (lymphocytes) (platelets) NEC Z52.008
　　　autologous Z52.018
　　　specified donor NEC Z52.098
　　specified donor NEC Z52.090
　　stem cells Z52.001
　　　autologous Z52.011
　　　specified donor NEC Z52.091
　bone Z52.20
　　autologous Z52.21
　　marrow Z52.3
　　specified type NEC Z52.29
　cornea Z52.5
　egg (Oocyte) Z52.819
　　age 35 and over Z52.812
　　　anonymous recipient Z52.812
　　　designated recipient Z52.813
　　under age 35 Z52.810
　　　anonymous recipient Z52.810
　　　designated recipient Z52.811
　kidney Z52.4
　liver Z52.6
　lung Z52.89
　lymphocyte — see Donor, blood, specified components NEC
　Oocyte — see Donor, egg
　platelets Z52.008
　potential, examination of Z00.5
　semen Z52.89
　skin Z52.10
　　autologous Z52.11
　　specified type NEC Z52.19
　specified organ or tissue NEC Z52.89
　sperm Z52.89
Donovanosis A58
Dorsalgia M54.9
　psychogenic F45.41
　specified NEC M54.89
Dorsopathy M53.9
　deforming M43.9
　　specified NEC — see subcategory M43.8 ☑
　specified NEC M53.80
　　cervical region M53.82
　　cervicothoracic region M53.83
　　lumbar region M53.86
　　lumbosacral region M53.87
　　occipito-atlanto-axial region M53.81
　　sacrococcygeal region M53.88
　　thoracic region M53.84
　　thoracolumbar region M53.85
Double
　albumin E88.09
　aortic arch Q25.45
　auditory canal Q17.8
　auricle (heart) Q20.8
　bladder Q64.79
　cervix Q51.820
　　with doubling of uterus (and vagina) Q51.10
　　　with obstruction Q51.11
　inlet ventricle Q20.4
　kidney with double pelvis (renal) Q63.0
　meatus urinarius Q64.75
　monster Q89.4
　outlet
　　left ventricle Q20.2
　　right ventricle Q20.1
　pelvis (renal) with double ureter Q62.5
　tongue Q38.3
　ureter (one or both sides) Q62.5
　　with double pelvis (renal) Q62.5
　urethra Q64.74
　urinary meatus Q64.75
　uterus Q51.2
　　with
　　　doubling of cervix (and vagina) Q51.10
　　　　with obstruction Q51.11

Double — continued
　uterus — continued
　　in pregnancy or childbirth O34.59- ☑
　　　causing obstructed labor O65.5
　vagina Q52.10
　　with doubling of uterus (and cervix) Q51.10
　　　with obstruction Q51.11
　vision H53.2
　vulva Q52.79
Douglas' pouch, cul-de-sac — see condition
Down syndrome Q90.9
　meiotic nondisjunction Q90.0
　mitotic nondisjunction Q90.1
　mosaicism Q90.1
　translocation Q90.2
DPD (dihydropyrimidine dehydrogenase deficiency) E88.89
Dracontiasis B72
Dracunculiasis, dracunculosis B72
Dream state, hysterical F44.89
Drepanocytic anemia — see Disease, sickle-cell
Dresbach's syndrome (elliptocytosis) D58.1
Dreschlera (hawaiiensis) (infection) B43.8
Dressler's syndrome I24.1
Drift, ulnar — see Deformity, limb, specified type NEC, forearm
Drinking (alcohol)
　excessive, to excess NEC (without dependence) F10.10
　　habitual (continual) (without remission) F10.20
　　　with remission F10.21
Drip, postnasal (chronic) R09.82
　due to
　　allergic rhinitis — see Rhinitis, allergic
　　common cold J00
　　gastroesophageal reflux — see Reflux, gastroesophageal
　　nasopharyngitis — see Nasopharyngitis
　　other known condition — code to condition
　　sinusitis — see Sinusitis
Droop
　facial R29.810
　　cerebrovascular disease I69.992
　　　cerebral infarction I69.392
　　　intracerebral hemorrhage I69.192
　　　nontraumatic intracranial hemorrhage NEC I69.292
　　　specified disease NEC I69.892
　　　subarachnoid hemorrhage I69.092
Drop (in)
　attack NEC R55
　finger — see Deformity, finger
　foot — see Deformity, limb, foot, drop
　hematocrit (precipitous) R71.0
　hemoglobin R71.0
　toe — see Deformity, toe, specified NEC
　wrist — see Deformity, limb, wrist drop
Dropped heart beats I45.9
Dropsy, dropsical (see also Hydrops)
　abdomen R18.8
　brain — see Hydrocephalus
　cardiac, heart — see Failure, heart, congestive
　gangrenous — see Gangrene
　heart — see Failure, heart, congestive
　kidney — see Nephrosis
　lung — see Edema, lung
　newborn due to isoimmunization P56.0
　pericardium — see Pericarditis
Drowned, drowning (near) T75.1 ☑
Drowsiness R40.0
Drug
　abuse counseling and surveillance Z71.51
　addiction — see Dependence
　dependence — see Dependence
　habit — see Dependence
　harmful use — see Abuse, drug
　induced fever R50.2
　overdose — see Table of Drugs and Chemicals, by drug, poisoning
　poisoning — see Table of Drugs and Chemicals, by drug, poisoning
　resistant organism infection (see also Resistant, organism, to, drug) Z16.30
　therapy
　　long term (current) (prophylactic) — see Therapy, drug long-term (current) (prophylactic)

Drug — continued
　therapy — continued
　　short term — omit code
　wrong substance given or taken in error — see Table of Drugs and Chemicals, by drug, poisoning
Drunkenness (without dependence) F10.129
　acute in alcoholism F10.229
　chronic (without remission) F10.20
　　with remission F10.21
　pathological (without dependence) F10.129
　　with dependence F10.229
　sleep F51.9
Drusen
　macula (degenerative) (retina) — see Degeneration, macula, drusen
　optic disc H47.32- ☑
Dry, dryness (see also condition)
　larynx J38.7
　mouth R68.2
　　due to dehydration E86.0
　nose J34.89
　socket (teeth) M27.3
　throat J39.2
DSAP L56.5
Duane's syndrome H50.81- ☑
Dubin-Johnson disease or syndrome E80.6
Dubois' disease (thymus gland) A50.59 [E35]
Dubowitz' syndrome Q87.1
Duchenne-Aran muscular atrophy G12.21
Duchenne-Griesinger disease G71.0
Duchenne's
　disease or syndrome
　　motor neuron disease G12.22
　　muscular dystrophy G71.0
　locomotor ataxia (syphilitic) A52.11
　paralysis
　　birth injury P14.0
　　due to or associated with
　　　motor neuron disease G12.22
　　　muscular dystrophy G71.0
Ducrey's chancre A57
Duct, ductus — see condition
Duhring's disease (dermatitis herpetiformis) L13.0
Dullness, cardiac (decreased) (increased) R01.2
Dumb ague — see Malaria
Dumbness — see Aphasia
Dumdum fever B55.0
Dumping syndrome (postgastrectomy) K91.1
Duodenitis (nonspecific) (peptic) K29.80
　with bleeding K29.81
Duodenocholangitis — see Cholangitis
Duodenum, duodenal — see condition
Duplay's bursitis or periarthritis — see Tendinitis, calcific, shoulder
Duplication, duplex (see also Accessory)
　alimentary tract Q45.8
　anus Q43.4
　appendix (and cecum) Q43.4
　biliary duct (any) Q44.5
　bladder Q64.79
　cecum (and appendix) Q43.4
　cervix Q51.820
　chromosome NEC
　　with complex rearrangements NEC Q92.5
　　seen only at prometaphase Q92.8
　cystic duct Q44.5
　digestive organs Q45.8
　esophagus Q39.8
　frontonasal process Q75.8
　intestine (large) (small) Q43.4
　kidney Q63.0
　liver Q44.7
　pancreas Q45.3
　penis Q55.69
　respiratory organs NEC Q34.8
　salivary duct Q38.4
　spinal cord (incomplete) Q06.2
　stomach Q40.2
Dupré's disease (meningism) R29.1
Dupuytren's contraction or disease M72.0
Durand-Nicolas-Favre disease A55
Durotomy (inadvertent) (incidental) G97.41
Duroziez's disease (congenital mitral stenosis) Q23.2
Dutton's relapsing fever (West African) A68.1
Dwarfism E34.3
　achondroplastic Q77.4
　congenital E34.3
　constitutional E34.3

Dwarfism — *continued*
  hypochondroplastic Q77.4
  hypophyseal E23.0
  infantile E34.3
  Laron-type E34.3
  Lorain (-Levi) type E23.0
  metatropic Q77.8
  nephrotic-glycosuric (with hypophosphatemic rickets)
      E72.09
  nutritional E45
  pancreatic K86.89
  pituitary E23.0
  renal N25.0
  thanatophoric Q77.1
Dyke-Young anemia (secondary) (symptomatic) D59.1
Dysacusis — *see* Abnormal, auditory perception
Dysadrenocortism E27.9
  hyperfunction E27.0
Dysarthria R47.1
  following
      cerebral infarction I69.322
      cerebrovascular disease I69.922
          specified disease NEC I69.822
      intracerebral hemorrhage I69.122
      nontraumatic intracranial hemorrhage NEC I69.222
      subarachnoid hemorrhage I69.022
Dysautonomia (familial) G90.1
Dysbarism T70.3 ☑
Dysbasia R26.2
  angiosclerotica intermittens I73.9
  hysterical F44.4
  lordotica (progressiva) G24.1
  nonorganic origin F44.4
  psychogenic F44.4
Dysbetalipoproteinemia (familial) E78.2
Dyscalculia R48.8
  developmental F81.2
Dyschezia K59.00
Dyschondroplasia (with hemangiomata) Q78.4
Dyschromia (skin) L81.9
Dyscollagenosis M35.9
Dyscranio-pygo-phalangy Q87.0
Dyscrasia
  blood (with) D75.9
      antepartum hemorrhage — *see* Hemorrhage, an-
          tepartum, with coagulation defect
      intrapartum hemorrhage O67.0
      newborn P61.9
          specified type NEC P61.8
      puerperal, postpartum O72.3
  polyglandular, pluriglandular E31.9
Dysendocrinism E34.9
Dysentery, dysenteric (catarrhal) (diarrhea) (epidemic)
    (hemorrhagic) (infectious) (sporadic) (tropical) A09
  abscess, liver A06.4
  amebic (*see also* Amebiasis) A06.0
      with abscess — *see* Abscess, amebic
      acute A06.0
      chronic A06.1
  arthritis (*see also* category M01) A09
      bacillary (*see also* category M01) A03.9
  bacillary A03.9
      arthritis (*see also* category M01) A03.9
      Boyd A03.2
      Flexner A03.1
      Schmitz (-Stutzer) A03.0
      Shiga (-Kruse) A03.0
      Shigella A03.9
          boydii A03.2
          dysenteriae A03.0
          flexneri A03.1
          group A A03.0
          group B A03.1
          group C A03.2
          group D A03.3
          sonnei A03.3
          specified type NEC A03.8
      Sonne A03.3
      specified type NEC A03.8
  balantidial A07.0
  Balantidium coli A07.0
  Boyd's A03.2
  candidal B37.82
  Chilomastix A07.8
  Chinese A03.9
  coccidial A07.3
  Dientamoeba (fragilis) A07.8
  Embadomonas A07.8

Dysentery, dysenteric — *continued*
  Entamoeba, entamebic — *see* Dysentery, amebic
  Flexner-Boyd A03.2
  Flexner's A03.1
  Giardia lamblia A07.1
  Hiss-Russell A03.1
  Lamblia A07.1
  leishmanial B55.0
  malarial — *see* Malaria
  metazoal B82.0
  monilial B37.82
  protozoal A07.9
  Salmonella A02.0
  schistosomal B65.1
  Schmitz (-Stutzer) A03.0
  Shiga (-Kruse) A03.0
  Shigella NOS — *see* Dysentery, bacillary
  Sonne A03.3
  strongyloidiasis B78.0
  trichomonal A07.8
  viral (*see also* Enteritis, viral) A08.4
Dysequilibrium R42
Dysesthesia R20.8
  hysterical F44.6
Dysfibrinogenemia (congenital) D68.2
Dysfunction
  adrenal E27.9
      hyperfunction E27.0
  autonomic
      due to alcohol G31.2
      somatoform F45.8
  bladder N31.9
      neurogenic NOS — *see* Dysfunction, bladder,
          neuromuscular
      neuromuscular NOS N31.9
          atonic (motor) (sensory) N31.2
          autonomous N31.2
          flaccid N31.2
          nonreflex N31.2
          reflex N31.1
          specified NEC N31.8
          uninhibited N31.0
  bleeding, uterus N93.8
  cerebral G93.89
  colon K59.9
      psychogenic F45.8
  colostomy K94.03
  cystic duct K82.8
  cystostomy (stoma) — *see* Complications, cystostomy
  ejaculatory N53.19
      anejaculatory orgasm N53.13
      painful N53.12
      premature F52.4
      retarded N53.11
  endocrine NOS E34.9
  endometrium N85.8
  enterostomy K94.13
  erectile — *see* Dysfunction, sexual, male, erectile
  gallbladder K82.8
  gastrostomy (stoma) K94.23
  gland, glandular NOS E34.9
  heart I51.89
  hemoglobin D75.89
  hepatic K76.89
  hypophysis E23.7
  hypothalamic NEC E23.3
  ileostomy (stoma) K94.13
  jejunostomy (stoma) K94.13
  kidney — *see* Disease, renal
  labyrinthine — *see* subcategory H83.2 ☑
  left ventricular, following sudden emotional stress
      I51.81
  liver K76.89
  male — *see* Dysfunction, sexual, male
  orgasmic (female) F52.31
      male F52.32
  ovary E28.9
      specified NEC E28.8
  papillary muscle I51.89
  parathyroid E21.4
  physiological NEC R68.89
      psychogenic F59
  pineal gland E34.8
  pituitary (gland) E23.3
  platelets D69.1
  polyglandular E31.9
      specified NEC E31.8
  psychophysiologic F59

Dysfunction — *continued*
  psychosexual F52.9
      with
          dyspareunia F52.6
          premature ejaculation F52.4
          vaginismus F52.5
  pylorus K31.9
  rectum K59.9
      psychogenic F45.8
  reflex (sympathetic) — *see* Syndrome, pain, complex
      regional I
  segmental — *see* Dysfunction, somatic
  senile R54
  sexual (due to) R37
      alcohol F10.981
      amphetamine F15.981
          in
              abuse F15.181
              dependence F15.281
      anxiolytic F13.981
          in
              abuse F13.181
              dependence F13.281
      cocaine F14.981
          in
              abuse F14.181
              dependence F14.281
      excessive sexual drive F52.8
      failure of genital response (male) F52.21
          female F52.22
      female N94.9
          aversion F52.1
          dyspareunia N94.10
              psychogenic F52.6
          frigidity F52.22
          nymphomania F52.8
          orgasmic F52.31
          psychogenic F52.9
              aversion F52.1
              dyspareunia F52.6
              frigidity F52.22
              nymphomania F52.8
              orgasmic F52.31
              vaginismus F52.5
          vaginismus N94.2
              psychogenic F52.5
      hypnotic F13.981
          in
              abuse F13.181
              dependence F13.281
      inhibited orgasm (female) F52.31
          male F52.32
      lack
          of sexual enjoyment F52.1
          or loss of sexual desire F52.0
      male N53.9
          anejaculatory orgasm N53.13
          ejaculatory N53.19
              painful N53.12
              premature F52.4
              retarded N53.11
          erectile N52.9
              drug induced N52.2
              due to
                  disease classified elsewhere N52.1
                  drug N52.2
              postoperative (postprocedural) N52.39
                  following
                      cryotherapy N52.37
                      interstitial seed therapy N52.36
                      prostate ablative therapy N52.37
                      prostatectomy N52.34
                          radical N52.31
                      radiation therapy N52.35
                      radical cystectomy N52.32
                      ultrasound ablative therapy N52.37
                      urethral surgery N52.33
              psychogenic F52.21
              specified cause NEC N52.8
              vasculogenic
                  arterial insufficiency N52.01
                      with corporo-venous occlusive
                          N52.03
                  corporo-venous occlusive N52.02
                      with arterial insufficiency N52.03
          impotence — *see* Dysfunction, sexual, male,
              erectile
          psychogenic F52.9
              aversion F52.1

Dysfunction — continued
  sexual — continued
    male — continued
      psychogenic — continued
        erectile F52.21
        orgasmic F52.32
        premature ejaculation F52.4
        satyriasis F52.8
        specified type NEC F52.8
      specified type NEC N53.8
    nonorganic F52.9
      specified NEC F52.8
    opioid F11.981
      in
        abuse F11.181
        dependence F11.281
    orgasmic dysfunction (female) F52.31
      male F52.32
    premature ejaculation F52.4
    psychoactive substances NEC F19.981
      in
        abuse F19.181
        dependence F19.281
    psychogenic F52.9
    sedative F13.981
      in
        abuse F13.181
        dependence F13.281
    sexual aversion F52.1
    vaginismus (nonorganic) (psychogenic) F52.5
  sinoatrial node I49.5
  somatic M99.09
    abdomen M99.09
    acromioclavicular M99.07
    cervical region M99.01
    cervicothoracic M99.01
    costochondral M99.08
    costovertebral M99.08
    head region M99.00
    hip M99.05
    lower extremity M99.06
    lumbar region M99.03
    lumbosacral M99.03
    occipitocervical M99.00
    pelvic region M99.05
    pubic M99.05
    rib cage M99.08
    sacral region M99.04
    sacrococcygeal M99.04
    sacroiliac M99.04
    specified NEC M99.09
    sternochondral M99.08
    sternoclavicular M99.07
    thoracic region M99.02
    thoracolumbar M99.02
    upper extremity M99.07
  somatoform autonomic F45.8
  stomach K31.89
    psychogenic F45.8
  suprarenal E27.9
    hyperfunction E27.0
  symbolic R48.9
    specified type NEC R48.8
  temporomandibular (joint) M26.69
    joint-pain syndrome M26.62- ☑
  testicular (endocrine) E29.9
    specified NEC E29.8
  thymus E32.9
  thyroid E07.9
  ureterostomy (stoma) — see Complications, stoma, urinary tract
  urethrostomy (stoma) — see Complications, stoma, urinary tract
  uterus, complicating delivery O62.9
    hypertonic O62.4
    hypotonic O62.2
      primary O62.0
      secondary O62.1
  ventricular I51.9
    with congestive heart failure (see also Failure, heart) I50.9
    left, reversible, following sudden emotional stress I51.81
Dysgenesis
  gonadal (due to chromosomal anomaly) Q96.9
    pure Q99.1
  renal Q60.5
    bilateral Q60.4
    unilateral Q60.3

Dysgenesis — continued
  reticular D72.0
  tidal platelet D69.3
Dysgerminoma
  specified site — see Neoplasm, malignant, by site
  unspecified site
    female C56.9
    male C62.90
Dysgeusia R43.2
Dysgraphia R27.8
Dyshidrosis, dysidrosis L30.1
Dyskaryotic cervical smear R87.619
Dyskeratosis L85.8
  cervix — see Dysplasia, cervix
  congenital Q82.8
  uterus NEC N85.8
Dyskinesia G24.9
  biliary (cystic duct or gallbladder) K82.8
  drug induced
    orofacial G24.01
  esophagus K22.4
  hysterical F44.4
  intestinal K59.8
  nonorganic origin F44.4
  orofacial (idiopathic) G24.4
    drug induced G24.01
  psychogenic F44.4
  subacute, drug induced G24.01
  tardive G24.01
    neuroleptic induced G24.01
  trachea J39.8
  tracheobronchial J98.09
Dyslalia (developmental) F80.0
Dyslexia R48.0
  developmental F81.0
Dyslipidemia E78.5
  depressed HDL cholesterol E78.6
  elevated fasting triglycerides E78.1
Dysmaturity (see also Light for dates)
  pulmonary (newborn) (Wilson-Mikity) P27.0
Dysmenorrhea (essential) (exfoliative) N94.6
  congestive (syndrome) N94.6
  primary N94.4
  psychogenic F45.8
  secondary N94.5
Dysmetabolic syndrome X E88.81
Dysmetria R27.8
Dysmorphism (due to)
  alcohol Q86.0
  exogenous cause NEC Q86.8
  hydantoin Q86.1
  warfarin Q86.2
Dysmorphophobia (nondelusional) F45.22
  delusional F22
Dysnomia R47.01
Dysorexia R63.0
  psychogenic F50.89
Dysostosis
  cleidocranial, cleidocranialis Q74.0
  craniofacial Q75.1
  Fairbank's (idiopathic familial generalized osteophytosis) Q78.9
  mandibulofacial (incomplete) Q75.4
  multiplex E76.01
  oculomandibular Q75.5
Dyspareunia (female) N94.10
  deep N94.12
  male N53.12
  nonorganic F52.6
  psychogenic F52.6
  secondary N94.19
  specified NEC N94.19
  superficial (introital) N94.11
Dyspepsia R10.13
  atonic K30
  functional (allergic) (congenital) (gastrointestinal) (occupational) (reflex) K30
  intestinal K59.8
  nervous F45.8
  neurotic F45.8
  psychogenic F45.8
Dysphagia R13.10
  cervical R13.19
  following
    cerebral infarction I69.391
    cerebrovascular disease I69.991
      specified NEC I69.891
    intracerebral hemorrhage I69.191

Dysphagia — continued
  following — continued
    nontraumatic intracranial hemorrhage NEC I69.291
    specified disease NEC I69.891
    subarachnoid hemorrhage I69.091
  functional (hysterical) F45.8
  hysterical F45.8
  nervous (hysterical) F45.8
  neurogenic R13.19
  oral phase R13.11
  oropharyngeal phase R13.12
  pharyngeal phase R13.13
  pharyngoesophageal phase R13.14
  psychogenic F45.8
  sideropenic D50.1
  spastica K22.4
  specified NEC R13.19
Dysphagocytosis, congenital D71
Dysphasia R47.02
  developmental
    expressive type F80.1
    receptive type F80.2
  following
    cerebrovascular disease I69.921
      cerebral infarction I69.321
      intracerebral hemorrhage I69.121
      nontraumatic intracranial hemorrhage NEC I69.221
      specified disease NEC I69.821
      subarachnoid hemorrhage I69.021
Dysphonia R49.0
  functional F44.4
  hysterical F44.4
  psychogenic F44.4
  spastica J38.3
Dysphoria
  gender F64.9
    in
      adolescence and adulthood F64.0
      children F64.2
    specified NEC F64.8
  postpartal O90.6
Dyspituitarism E23.3
Dysplasia (see also Anomaly)
  acetabular, congenital Q65.89
  alveolar capillary, with vein misalignment J84.843
  anus (histologically confirmed) (mild) (moderate) K62.82
    severe D01.3
  arrhythmogenic right ventricular I42.8
  arterial, fibromuscular I77.3
  asphyxiating thoracic (congenital) Q77.2
  brain Q07.9
  bronchopulmonary, perinatal P27.1
  cervix (uteri) N87.9
    mild N87.0
    moderate N87.1
    severe D06.9
  chondroectodermal Q77.6
  colon D12.6
  craniometaphyseal Q78.8
  dentinal K00.5
  diaphyseal, progressive Q78.3
  dystrophic Q77.5
  ectodermal (anhidrotic) (congenital) (hereditary) Q82.4
    hydrotic Q82.8
  epithelial, uterine cervix — see Dysplasia, cervix
  eye (congenital) Q11.2
  fibrous
    bone NEC (monostotic) M85.00
      ankle M85.07- ☑
      foot M85.07- ☑
      forearm M85.03- ☑
      hand M85.04- ☑
      lower leg M85.06- ☑
      multiple site M85.09
      neck M85.08
      rib M85.08
      shoulder M85.01- ☑
      skull M85.08
      specified site NEC M85.08
      thigh M85.05- ☑
      toe M85.07- ☑
      upper arm M85.02- ☑
      vertebra M85.08
    diaphyseal, progressive Q78.3
    jaw M27.8
    polyostotic Q78.1

☑ **Additional Character Required — Refer to the Tabular List for Character Selection**   ▽ Subterms under main terms may continue to next column or page

Dysplasia — *continued*
  florid osseous (*see also* Cyst, calcifying odontogenic)
  high grade, focal D12.6
  hip, congenital Q65.89
  joint, congenital Q74.8
  kidney Q61.4
    multicystic Q61.4
  leg Q74.2
  lung, congenital (not associated with short gestation) Q33.6
  mammary (gland) (benign) N60.9- ☑
    cyst (solitary) — *see* Cyst, breast
    cystic — *see* Mastopathy, cystic
    duct ectasia — *see* Ectasia, mammary duct
    fibroadenosis — *see* Fibroadenosis, breast
    fibrosclerosis — *see* Fibrosclerosis, breast
    specified type NEC N60.8- ☑
  metaphyseal Q78.5
  muscle Q79.8
  oculodentodigital Q87.0
  periapical (cemental) (cemento-osseous) — *see* Cyst, calcifying odontogenic
  periosteum — *see* Disorder, bone, specified type NEC
  polyostotic fibrous Q78.1
  prostate (*see also* Neoplasia, intraepithelial, prostate) N42.30
    severe D07.5
    specified NEC N42.39
  renal Q61.4
    multicystic Q61.4
  retinal, congenital Q14.1
  right ventricular, arrhythmogenic I42.8
  septo-optic Q04.4
  skin L98.8
  spinal cord Q06.1
  spondyloepiphyseal Q77.7
  thymic, with immunodeficiency D82.1
  vagina N89.3
    mild N89.0
    moderate N89.1
    severe NEC D07.2
  vulva N90.3
    mild N90.0
    moderate N90.1
    severe NEC D07.1

Dyspnea (nocturnal) (paroxysmal) R06.00
  asthmatic (bronchial) J45.909
    with
      bronchitis J45.909
        with
          exacerbation (acute) J45.901
          status asthmaticus J45.902
        chronic J44.9
      exacerbation (acute) J45.901
      status asthmaticus J45.902
    cardiac — *see* Failure, ventricular, left
  cardiac — *see* Failure, ventricular, left
  functional F45.8
  hyperventilation R06.4
  hysterical F45.8
  newborn P28.89
  orthopnea R06.01
  psychogenic F45.8
  shortness of breath R06.02
  specified type NEC R06.09

Dyspraxia R27.8
  developmental (syndrome) F82

Dysproteinemia E88.09

Dysreflexia, autonomic G90.4

Dysrhythmia
  cardiac I49.9
    newborn
      bradycardia P29.12
      occurring before birth P03.819
        before onset of labor P03.810
        during labor P03.811
      tachycardia P29.11
    postoperative I97.89
  cerebral or cortical — *see* Epilepsy

Dyssomnia — *see* Disorder, sleep

Dyssynergia
  biliary K83.8
  bladder sphincter N36.44
  cerebellaris myoclonica (Hunt's ataxia) G11.1

Dysthymia F34.1

Dysthyroidism E07.9

Dystocia O66.9
  affecting newborn P03.1

Dystocia — *continued*
  cervical (hypotonic) O62.2
    affecting newborn P03.6
    primary O62.0
    secondary O62.1
  contraction ring O62.4
  fetal O66.9
    abnormality NEC O66.3
    conjoined twins O66.3
    oversize O66.2
  maternal O66.9
  positional O64.9 ☑
  shoulder (girdle) O66.0
    causing obstructed labor O66.0
  uterine NEC O62.4

Dystonia G24.9
  deformans progressiva G24.1
  drug induced NEC G24.09
    acute G24.02
    specified NEC G24.09
  familial G24.1
  idiopathic G24.1
    familial G24.1
    nonfamilial G24.2
    orofacial G24.4
  lenticularis G24.8
  musculorum deformans G24.1
  neuroleptic induced (acute) G24.02
  orofacial (idiopathic) G24.4
  oromandibular G24.4
    due to drug G24.01
  specified NEC G24.8
  torsion (familial) (idiopathic) G24.1
    acquired G24.8
    genetic G24.1
    symptomatic (nonfamilial) G24.2

Dystonic movements R25.8

Dystrophy, dystrophia
  adiposogenital E23.6
  Becker's type G71.0
  cervical sympathetic G90.2
  choroid (hereditary) H31.20
    central areolar H31.22
    choroideremia H31.21
    gyrate atrophy H31.23
    specified type NEC H31.29
  cornea (hereditary) H18.50
    endothelial H18.51
    epithelial H18.52
    granular H18.53
    lattice H18.54
    macular H18.55
    specified type NEC H18.59
  Duchenne's type G71.0
  due to malnutrition E45
  Erb's G71.0
  Fuchs' H18.51
  Gower's muscular G71.0
  hair L67.8
  infantile neuraxonal G31.89
  Landouzy-Déjérine G71.0
  Leyden-Möbius G71.0
  muscular G71.0
    benign (Becker type) G71.0
    congenital (hereditary) (progressive) (with specific morphological abnormalities of the muscle fiber) G71.0
      myotonic G71.11
    distal G71.0
    Duchenne type G71.0
    Emery-Dreifuss G71.0
    Erb type G71.0
    facioscapulohumeral G71.0
    Gower's G71.0
    hereditary (progressive) G71.0
    Landouzy-Déjérine type G71.0
    limb-girdle G71.0
    myotonic G71.11
    progressive (hereditary) G71.0
      Charcot-Marie (-Tooth) type G60.0
    pseudohypertrophic (infantile) G71.0
    severe (Duchenne type) G71.0
  myocardium, myocardial — *see* Degeneration, myocardial
  nail L60.3
    congenital Q84.6
  nutritional E45
  ocular G71.0
  oculocerebrorenal E72.03

Dystrophy, dystrophia — *continued*
  oculopharyngeal G71.0
  ovarian N83.8
  polyglandular E31.8
  reflex (neuromuscular) (sympathetic) — *see* Syndrome, pain, complex regional I
  retinal (hereditary) H35.50
    in
      lipid storage disorders E75.6 [H36]
      systemic lipidoses E75.6 [H36]
    involving
      pigment epithelium H35.54
      sensory area H35.53
    pigmentary H35.52
    vitreoretinal H35.51
  Salzmann's nodular — *see* Degeneration, cornea, nodular
  scapuloperoneal G71.0
  skin NEC L98.8
  sympathetic (reflex) — *see* Syndrome, pain, complex regional I
    cervical G90.2
  tapetoretinal H35.54
  thoracic, asphyxiating Q77.2
  unguium L60.3
    congenital Q84.6
  vitreoretinal H35.51
  vulva N90.4
  yellow (liver) — *see* Failure, hepatic

Dysuria R30.0
  psychogenic F45.8

E

Eales' disease H35.06- ☑

Ear (*see also* condition)
  piercing Z41.3
  tropical NEC B36.9 [H62.40]
    in
      aspergillosis B44.89
      candidiasis B37.84
      moniliasis B37.84
  wax (impacted) H61.20
    left H61.22
      with right H61.23
    right H61.21
      with left H61.23

Earache — *see* subcategory H92.0 ☑

Early satiety R68.81

Eaton-Lambert syndrome — *see* Syndrome, Lambert-Eaton

Eberth's disease (typhoid fever) A01.00

Ebola virus disease A98.4

Ebstein's anomaly or syndrome (heart) Q22.5

Eccentro-osteochondrodysplasia E76.29

Ecchondroma — *see* Neoplasm, bone, benign

Ecchondrosis D48.0

Ecchymosis R58
  conjunctiva — *see* Hemorrhage, conjunctiva
  eye (traumatic) — *see* Contusion, eyeball
  eyelid (traumatic) — *see* Contusion, eyelid
  newborn P54.5
  spontaneous R23.3
  traumatic — *see* Contusion

Echinococciasis — *see* Echinococcus

Echinococcosis — *see* Echinococcus

Echinococcus (infection) B67.90
  granulosus B67.4
    bone B67.2
    liver B67.0
    lung B67.1
    multiple sites B67.32
    specified site NEC B67.39
    thyroid B67.31
  liver NOS B67.8
    granulosus B67.0
    multilocularis B67.5
  lung NEC B67.99
    granulosus B67.1
    multilocularis B67.69
  multilocularis B67.7
    liver B67.5
    multiple sites B67.61
    specified site NEC B67.69
  specified site NEC B67.99
    granulosus B67.39
    multilocularis B67.69
  thyroid NEC B67.99

◢ Subterms under main terms may continue to next column or page   ☑ Additional Character Required — Refer to the Tabular List for Character Selection   **125**

Dysplasia — Echinococcus

Echinococcus — *continued*
  thyroid — *continued*
    granulosus B67.31
    multilocularis B67.69 [E35]
Echinorhynchiasis B83.8
Echinostomiasis B66.8
Echolalia R48.8
Echovirus, as cause of disease classified elsewhere
    B97.12
Eclampsia, eclamptic (coma) (convulsions) (delirium)
    (with hypertension) NEC O15.9
  complicating
    labor and delivery O15.1
    postpartum O15.2
    pregnancy O15.0- ☑
    puerperium O15.2
Economic circumstances affecting care Z59.9
Economo's disease A85.8
Ectasia, ectasis
  annuloaortic I35.8
  aorta I77.819
    with aneurysm — *see* Aneurysm, aorta
    abdominal I77.811
    thoracic I77.810
    thoracoabdominal I77.812
  breast — *see* Ectasia, mammary duct
  capillary I78.8
  cornea H18.71- ☑
  gastric antral vascular (GAVE) K31.819
    with hemorrhage K31.811
    without hemorrhage K31.819
  mammary duct N60.4- ☑
  salivary gland (duct) K11.8
  sclera — *see* Sclerectasia
Ecthyma L08.0
  contagiosum B08.02
  gangrenosum L08.0
  infectiosum B08.02
Ectocardia Q24.8
Ectodermal dysplasia (anhidrotic) Q82.4
Ectodermosis erosiva pluriorificialis L51.1
Ectopic, ectopia (congenital)
  abdominal viscera Q45.8
    due to defect in anterior abdominal wall Q79.59
  ACTH syndrome E24.3
  adrenal gland Q89.1
  anus Q43.5
  atrial beats I49.1
  beats I49.49
    atrial I49.1
    ventricular I49.3
  bladder Q64.10
  bone and cartilage in lung Q33.5
  brain Q04.8
  breast tissue Q83.8
  cardiac Q24.8
  cerebral Q04.8
  cordis Q24.8
  endometrium — *see* Endometriosis
  gastric mucosa Q40.2
  gestation — *see* Pregnancy, by site
  heart Q24.8
  hormone secretion NEC E34.2
  kidney (crossed) (pelvis) Q63.2
  lens, lentis Q12.1
  mole — *see* Pregnancy, by site
  organ or site NEC — *see* Malposition, congenital
  pancreas Q45.3
  pregnancy — *see* Pregnancy, ectopic
  pupil — *see* Abnormality, pupillary
  renal Q63.2
  sebaceous glands of mouth Q38.6
  spleen Q89.09
  testis Q53.00
    bilateral Q53.02
    unilateral Q53.01
  thyroid Q89.2
  tissue in lung Q33.5
  ureter Q62.63
  ventricular beats I49.3
  vesicae Q64.10
Ectromelia Q73.8
  lower limb — *see* Defect, reduction, limb, lower,
    specified type NEC
  upper limb — *see* Defect, reduction, limb, upper,
    specified type NEC
Ectropion H02.109
  cervix N86

Ectropion — *continued*
  cervix — *continued*
    with cervicitis N72
  congenital Q10.1
  eyelid (paralytic) H02.109
    cicatricial H02.119
      left H02.116
        lower H02.115
        upper H02.114
      right H02.113
        lower H02.112
        upper H02.111
    congenital Q10.1
    left H02.106
      lower H02.105
      upper H02.104
    mechanical H02.129
      left H02.126
        lower H02.125
        upper H02.124
      right H02.123
        lower H02.122
        upper H02.121
    right H02.103
      lower H02.102
      upper H02.101
    senile H02.139
      left H02.136
        lower H02.135
        upper H02.134
      right H02.133
        lower H02.132
        upper H02.131
    spastic H02.149
      left H02.146
        lower H02.145
        upper H02.144
      right H02.143
        lower H02.142
        upper H02.141
  iris H21.89
  lip (acquired) K13.0
    congenital Q38.0
  urethra N36.8
  uvea H21.89
Eczema (acute) (chronic) (erythematous) (fissum)
    (rubrum) (squamous) (*see also* Dermatitis) L30.9
  contact — *see* Dermatitis, contact
  dyshydrotic L30.1
  external ear — *see* Otitis, externa, acute, eczematoid
  flexural L20.82
  herpeticum B00.0
  hypertrophicum L28.0
  hypostatic — *see* Varix, leg, with, inflammation
  impetiginous L01.1
  infantile (due to any substance) L20.83
    intertriginous L21.1
    seborrheic L21.1
  intertriginous NEC L30.4
    infantile L21.1
  intrinsic (allergic) L20.84
  lichenified NEC L28.0
  marginatum (hebrae) B35.6
  pustular L30.3
  stasis I87.2
    with varicose veins — *see* Varix, leg, with, inflam-
      mation
  vaccination, vaccinatum T88.1 ☑
  varicose — *see* Varix, leg, with, inflammation
Eczematid L30.2
Eddowes (-Spurway) **syndrome** Q78.0
Edema, edematous (infectious) (pitting) (toxic) R60.9
  with nephritis — *see* Nephrosis
  allergic T78.3 ☑
  amputation stump (surgical) (sequelae) (late effect))
    T87.89
  angioneurotic (allergic) (any site) (with urticaria)
    T78.3 ☑
    hereditary D84.1
  angiospastic I73.9
  Berlin's (traumatic) S05.8X- ☑
  brain (cytotoxic) (vasogenic) G93.6
    due to birth injury P11.0
    newborn (anoxia or hypoxia) P52.4
      birth injury P11.0
    traumatic — *see* Injury, intracranial, cerebral edema
  cardiac — *see* Failure, heart, congestive
  cardiovascular — *see* Failure, heart, congestive

Edema, edematous — *continued*
  cerebral — *see* Edema, brain
  cerebrospinal — *see* Edema, brain
  cervix (uteri) (acute) N88.8
    puerperal, postpartum O90.89
  chronic hereditary Q82.0
  circumscribed, acute T78.3 ☑
    hereditary D84.1
  conjunctiva H11.42- ☑
  cornea H18.2- ☑
    idiopathic H18.22- ☑
    secondary H18.23- ☑
      due to contact lens H18.21- ☑
  due to
    lymphatic obstruction I89.0
    salt retention E87.0
  epiglottis — *see* Edema, glottis
  essential, acute T78.3 ☑
    hereditary D84.1
  extremities, lower — *see* Edema, legs
  eyelid NEC H02.849
    left H02.846
      lower H02.845
      upper H02.844
    right H02.843
      lower H02.842
      upper H02.841
  familial, hereditary Q82.0
  famine — *see* Malnutrition, severe
  generalized R60.1
  glottis, glottic, glottidis (obstructive) (passive) J38.4
    allergic T78.3 ☑
    hereditary D84.1
  heart — *see* Failure, heart, congestive
  heat T67.7 ☑
  hereditary Q82.0
  inanition — *see* Malnutrition, severe
  intracranial G93.6
  iris H21.89
  joint — *see* Effusion, joint
  larynx — *see* Edema, glottis
  legs R60.0
    due to venous obstruction I87.1
    hereditary Q82.0
  localized R60.0
    due to venous obstruction I87.1
  lower limbs — *see* Edema, legs
  lung J81.1
    with heart condition or failure — *see* Failure, ven-
      tricular, left
    acute J81.0
    chemical (acute) J68.1
      chronic J68.1
    chronic J81.1
      due to
        chemicals, gases, fumes or vapors (inhala-
          tion) J68.1
        external agent J70.9
          specified NEC J70.8
        radiation J70.1
    due to
      chemicals, fumes or vapors (inhalation) J68.1
      external agent J70.9
        specified NEC J70.8
      high altitude T70.29 ☑
      near drowning T75.1 ☑
      radiation J70.0
    meaning failure, left ventricle I50.1
  lymphatic I89.0
    due to mastectomy I97.2
  macula H35.81
    cystoid, following cataract surgery — *see* Complica-
      tions, postprocedural, following cataract
      surgery
    diabetic — *see* Diabetes, by type, with, retinopathy,
      with macular edema
  malignant — *see* Gangrene, gas
  Milroy's Q82.0
  nasopharynx J39.2
  newborn P83.30
    hydrops fetalis — *see* Hydrops, fetalis
    specified NEC P83.39
  nutritional (*see also* Malnutrition, severe)
    with dyspigmentation, skin and hair E40
  optic disc or nerve — *see* Papilledema
  orbit H05.22- ☑
  pancreas K86.89
  papilla, optic — *see* Papilledema

☑ Additional Character Required — Refer to the Tabular List for Character Selection   ▽ Subterms under main terms may continue to next column or page

Edema, edematous — *continued*
- penis N48.89
- periodic T78.3 ☑
  - hereditary D84.1
- pharynx J39.2
- pulmonary — *see* Edema, lung
- Quincke's T78.3 ☑
  - hereditary D84.1
- renal — *see* Nephrosis
- retina H35.81
  - diabetic — *see* Diabetes, by type, with, retinopathy, with macular edema
- salt E87.0
- scrotum N50.89
- seminal vesicle N50.89
- spermatic cord N50.89
- spinal (cord) (vascular) (nontraumatic) G95.19
- starvation — *see* Malnutrition, severe
- stasis — *see* Hypertension, venous, (chronic)
- subglottic — *see* Edema, glottis
- supraglottic — *see* Edema, glottis
- testis N44.8
- tunica vaginalis N50.89
- vas deferens N50.89
- vulva (acute) N90.89

Edentulism — *see* Absence, teeth, acquired
Edsall's disease T67.2 ☑
Educational handicap Z55.9
- specified NEC Z55.8
Edward's syndrome — *see* Trisomy, 18
Effect(s) (of) (from) — *see* Effect, adverse NEC
Effect, adverse
- abnormal gravitational (G) forces or states T75.81 ☑
- abuse — *see* Maltreatment
- air pressure T70.9 ☑
  - specified NEC T70.8 ☑
- altitude (high) — *see* Effect, adverse, high altitude
- anesthesia (*see also* Anesthesia) T88.59 ☑
  - in labor and delivery O74.9
  - local, toxic
    - in labor and delivery O74.4
    - in pregnancy NEC O29.3- ☑
    - postpartum, puerperal O89.3
  - postpartum, puerperal O89.9
  - specified NEC T88.59 ☑
    - in labor and delivery O74.8
    - postpartum, puerperal O89.8
  - spinal and epidural T88.59 ☑
    - headache T88.59 ☑
      - in labor and delivery O74.5
      - postpartum, puerperal O89.4
    - specified NEC
      - in labor and delivery O74.6
      - postpartum, puerperal O89.5
- antitoxin — *see* Complications, vaccination
- atmospheric pressure T70.9 ☑
  - due to explosion T70.8 ☑
  - high T70.3 ☑
  - low — *see* Effect, adverse, high altitude
  - specified effect NEC T70.8 ☑
- biological, correct substance properly administered — *see* Effect, adverse, drug
- blood (derivatives) (serum) (transfusion) — *see* Complications, transfusion
- chemical substance — *see* Table of Drugs and Chemicals
- cold (temperature) (weather) T69.9 ☑
  - chilblains T69.1 ☑
  - frostbite — *see* Frostbite
  - specified effect NEC T69.8 ☑
- drugs and medicaments T88.7 ☑
  - specified drug — *see* Table of Drugs and Chemicals, by drug, adverse effect
  - specified effect — *see* *code to* condition
- electric current, electricity (shock) T75.4 ☑
  - burn — *see* Burn
- exertion (excessive) T73.3 ☑
- exposure — *see* Exposure
- external cause NEC T75.89 ☑
- foodstuffs T78.1 ☑
  - allergic reaction — *see* Allergy, food
    - causing anaphylaxis — *see* Shock, anaphylactic, due to food
  - noxious — *see* Poisoning, food, noxious
- gases, fumes, or vapors T59.9- ☑
  - specified agent — *see* Table of Drugs and Chemicals

Effect, adverse — *continued*
- glue (airplane) sniffing
  - due to drug abuse — *see* Abuse, drug, inhalant
  - due to drug dependence — *see* Dependence, drug, inhalant
- heat — *see* Heat
- high altitude NEC T70.29 ☑
  - anoxia T70.29 ☑
  - on
    - ears T70.0 ☑
    - sinuses T70.1 ☑
  - polycythemia D75.1
- high pressure fluids T70.4 ☑
- hot weather — *see* Heat
- hunger T73.0 ☑
- immersion, foot — *see* Immersion
- immunization — *see* Complications, vaccination
- immunological agents — *see* Complications, vaccination
- infrared (radiation) (rays) NOS T66 ☑
  - dermatitis or eczema L59.8
- infusion — *see* Complications, infusion
- lack of care of infants — *see* Maltreatment, child
- lightning — *see* Lightning
- medical care T88.9 ☑
  - specified NEC T88.8 ☑
- medicinal substance, correct, properly administered — *see* Effect, adverse, drug
- motion T75.3 ☑
- noise, on inner ear — *see* subcategory H83.3 ☑
- overheated places — *see* Heat
- psychosocial, of work environment Z56.5
- radiation (diagnostic) (infrared) (natural source) (therapeutic) (ultraviolet) (X-ray) NOS T66 ☑
  - dermatitis or eczema — *see* Dermatitis, due to, radiation
  - fibrosis of lung J70.1
  - pneumonitis J70.0
  - pulmonary manifestations
    - acute J70.0
    - chronic J70.1
  - skin L59.9
- radioactive substance NOS
  - dermatitis or eczema — *see* Radiodermatitis
- reduced temperature T69.9 ☑
  - immersion foot or hand — *see* Immersion
  - specified effect NEC T69.8 ☑
- serum NEC (*see also* Reaction, serum) T80.69 ☑
- specified NEC T78.8 ☑
  - external cause NEC T75.89 ☑
- strangulation — *see* Asphyxia, traumatic
- submersion T75.1 ☑
- thirst T73.1 ☑
- toxic — *see* Toxicity
- transfusion — *see* Complications, transfusion
- ultraviolet (radiation) (rays) NOS T66 ☑
  - burn — *see* Burn
  - dermatitis or eczema — *see* Dermatitis, due to, ultraviolet rays
    - acute L56.8
- vaccine (any) — *see* Complications, vaccination
- vibration — *see* Vibration, adverse effects
- water pressure NEC T70.9 ☑
  - specified NEC T70.8 ☑
- weightlessness T75.82 ☑
- whole blood — *see* Complications, transfusion
- work environment Z56.5
Effects, late — *see* Sequelae
Effluvium
- anagen L65.1
- telogen L65.0
Effort syndrome (psychogenic) F45.8
Effusion
- amniotic fluid — *see* Pregnancy, complicated by, premature rupture of membranes
- brain (serous) G93.6
- bronchial — *see* Bronchitis
- cerebral G93.6
- cerebrospinal (*see also* Meningitis)
  - vessel G93.6
- chest — *see* Effusion, pleura
- chylous, chyliform (pleura) J94.0
- intracranial G93.6
- joint M25.40
  - ankle M25.47- ☑
  - elbow M25.42- ☑
  - foot joint M25.47- ☑

Effusion — *continued*
- joint — *continued*
  - hand joint M25.44- ☑
  - hip M25.45- ☑
  - knee M25.46- ☑
  - shoulder M25.41- ☑
  - specified joint NEC M25.48
  - wrist M25.43- ☑
- malignant pleural J91.0
- meninges — *see* Meningitis
- pericardium, pericardial (noninflammatory) I31.3
  - acute — *see* Pericarditis, acute
- peritoneal (chronic) R18.8
- pleura, pleurisy, pleuritic, pleuropericardial J90
  - chylous, chyliform J94.0
  - due to systemic lupus erythematosis M32.13
  - in conditions classified elsewhere J91.8
  - influenzal — *see* Influenza, with, respiratory manifestations NEC
  - malignant J91.0
  - newborn P28.89
  - tuberculous NEC A15.6
    - primary (progressive) A15.7
- spinal — *see* Meningitis
- thorax, thoracic — *see* Effusion, pleura
Egg shell nails L60.3
- congenital Q84.6
Egyptian splenomegaly B65.1
Ehlers-Danlos syndrome Q79.6
Ehrlichiosis A77.40
- due to
  - E. chafeensis A77.41
  - E. sennetsu A79.81
  - specified organism NEC A77.49
Eichstedt's disease B36.0
Eisenmenger's
- complex or syndrome I27.83
- defect Q21.8
Ejaculation
- delayed F52.32
- painful N53.12
- premature F52.4
- retarded N53.11
- retrograde N53.14
- semen, painful N53.12
  - psychogenic F52.6
Ekbom's syndrome (restless legs) G25.81
Ekman's syndrome (brittle bones and blue sclera) Q78.0
Elastic skin Q82.8
- acquired L57.4
Elastofibroma — *see* Neoplasm, connective tissue, benign
Elastoma (juvenile) Q82.8
- Miescher's L87.2
Elastomyofibrosis I42.4
Elastosis
- actinic, solar L57.8
- atrophicans (senile) L57.4
- perforans serpiginosa L87.2
- senilis L57.4
Elbow — *see* condition
Electric current, electricity, effects (concussion) (fatal) (nonfatal) (shock) T75.4 ☑
- burn — *see* Burn
Electric feet syndrome E53.8
Electrocution T75.4 ☑
- from electroshock gun (taser) T75.4 ☑
Electrolyte imbalance E87.8
- with
  - abortion — *see* Abortion by type, complicated by, electrolyte imbalance
  - ectopic pregnancy O08.5
  - molar pregnancy O08.5
Elephantiasis (nonfilarial) I89.0
- arabicum — *see* Infestation, filarial
- bancroftian B74.0
- congenital (any site) (hereditary) Q82.0
- due to
  - Brugia (malayi) B74.1
    - timori B74.2
  - mastectomy I97.2
  - Wuchereria (bancrofti) B74.0
- eyelid H02.859
  - left H02.856
    - lower H02.855
    - upper H02.854
  - right H02.853
    - lower H02.852

Elephantiasis — *continued*
  eyelid — *continued*
    right — *continued*
      upper H02.851
  filarial, filariensis — *see* Infestation, filarial
  glandular I89.0
  graecorum A30.9
  lymphangiectatic I89.0
  lymphatic vessel I89.0
    due to mastectomy I97.2
  scrotum (nonfilarial) I89.0
  streptococcal I89.0
  surgical I97.89
    postmastectomy I97.2
  telangiectodes I89.0
  vulva (nonfilarial) N90.89
Elevated, elevation
  antibody titer R76.0
  basal metabolic rate R94.8
  blood pressure (*see also* Hypertension)
    reading (incidental) (isolated) (nonspecific), no di-
      agnosis of hypertension R03.0
  blood sugar R73.9
  body temperature (of unknown origin) R50.9
  cancer antigen 125 [CA 125] R97.1
  carcinoembryonic antigen [CEA] R97.0
  cholesterol E78.00
    with high triglycerides E78.2
  conjugate, eye H51.0
  C-reactive protein (CRP) R79.82
  diaphragm, congenital Q79.1
  erythrocyte sedimentation rate R70.0
  fasting glucose R73.01
  fasting triglycerides E78.1
  finding on laboratory examination — *see* Findings,
    abnormal, inconclusive, without diagnosis, by
    type of exam
  GFR (glomerular filtration rate) — *see* Findings, abnor-
    mal, inconclusive, without diagnosis, by type of
    exam
  glucose tolerance (oral) R73.02
  immunoglobulin level R76.8
  indoleacetic acid R82.5
  lactic acid dehydrogenase (LDH) level R74.0
  leukocytes D72.829
  lipoprotein a level E78.8 ☑
  liver function
    study R94.5
    test R79.89
      alkaline phosphatase R74.8
      aminotransferase R74.0
      bilirubin R17
      hepatic enzyme R74.8
      lactate dehydrogenase R74.0
  lymphocytes D72.820
  prostate specific antigen [PSA] R97.20
  Rh titer — *see* Complication(s), transfusion, incompat-
    ibility reaction, Rh (factor)
  scapula, congenital Q74.0
  sedimentation rate R70.0
  SGOT R74.0
  SGPT R74.0
  transaminase level R74.0
  triglycerides E78.1
    with high cholesterol E78.2
  tumor associated antigens [TAA] NEC R97.8
  tumor specific antigens [TSA] NEC R97.8
  urine level of
    17-ketosteroids R82.5
    catecholamine R82.5
    indoleacetic acid R82.5
    steroids R82.5
    vanillylmandelic acid (VMA) R82.5
  venous pressure I87.8
  white blood cell count D72.829
    specified NEC D72.828
Elliptocytosis (congenital) (hereditary) D58.1
  Hb C (disease) D58.1
  hemoglobin disease D58.1
  sickle-cell (disease) D57.8- ☑
    trait D57.3
Ellison-Zollinger syndrome E16.4
Ellis-van Creveld syndrome (chondroectodermal dysplasia) Q77.6
Elongated, elongation (congenital) (*see also* Distortion)
  bone Q79.9
  cervix (uteri) Q51.828
    acquired N88.4

Elongated, elongation — *continued*
  cervix — *continued*
    hypertrophic N88.4
  colon Q43.8
  common bile duct Q44.5
  cystic duct Q44.5
  frenulum, penis Q55.69
  labia minora (acquired) N90.69
  ligamentum patellae Q74.1
  petiolus (epiglottidis) Q31.8
  tooth, teeth K00.2
  uvula Q38.6
Eltor cholera A00.1
Emaciation (due to malnutrition) E41
Embadomoniasis A07.8
Embedded tooth, teeth K01.0
  root only K08.3
Embolic — *see* condition
Embolism (multiple) (paradoxical) I74.9
  air (any site) (traumatic) T79.0 ☑
    following
      abortion — *see* Abortion by type complicated
        by embolism
      ectopic pregnancy O08.2
      infusion, therapeutic injection or transfusion
        T80.0 ☑
      molar pregnancy O08.2
    procedure NEC
      artery T81.719 ☑
        mesenteric T81.710 ☑
        renal T81.711 ☑
        specified NEC T81.718 ☑
      vein T81.72 ☑
    in pregnancy, childbirth or puerperium — *see*
      Embolism, obstetric
  amniotic fluid (pulmonary) (*see also* Embolism, obstet-
    ric)
    following
      abortion — *see* Abortion by type complicated
        by embolism
      ectopic pregnancy O08.2
      molar pregnancy O08.2
  aorta, aortic I74.10
    abdominal I74.09
      saddle I74.01
    bifurcation I74.09
    saddle I74.01
    thoracic I74.11
  artery I74.9
    auditory, internal I65.8
    basilar — *see* Occlusion, artery, basilar
    carotid (common) (internal) — *see* Occlusion,
      artery, carotid
    cerebellar (anterior inferior) (posterior inferior)
      (superior) I66.3
    cerebral — *see* Occlusion, artery, cerebral
    choroidal (anterior) I65.8
    communicating posterior I65.8
    coronary (*see also* Infarct, myocardium)
      not resulting in infarction I24.0
    extremity I74.4
      lower I74.3
      upper I74.2
    hypophyseal I65.8
    iliac I74.5
    limb I74.4
      lower I74.3
      upper I74.2
    mesenteric (with gangrene) (*see also* Ischemia, in-
      testine, acute) K55.059
    ophthalmic — *see* Occlusion, artery, retina
    peripheral I74.4
    pontine I65.8
    precerebral — *see* Occlusion, artery, precerebral
    pulmonary — *see* Embolism, pulmonary
    renal N28.0
    retinal — *see* Occlusion, artery, retina
    septic I76
    specified NEC I74.8
    vertebral — *see* Occlusion, artery, vertebral
  basilar (artery) I65.1
  blood clot
    following
      abortion — *see* Abortion by type complicated
        by embolism
      ectopic or molar pregnancy O08.2
    in pregnancy, childbirth or puerperium — *see*
      Embolism, obstetric

Embolism — *continued*
  brain (*see also* Occlusion, artery, cerebral)
    following
      abortion — *see* Abortion by type complicated
        by embolism
      ectopic or molar pregnancy O08.2
    puerperal, postpartum, childbirth — *see* Embolism,
      obstetric
  capillary I78.8
  cardiac (*see also* Infarct, myocardium)
    not resulting in infarction I51.3
  carotid (artery) (common) (internal) — *see* Occlusion,
    artery, carotid
  cavernous sinus (venous) — *see* Embolism, intracranial
    venous sinus
  cerebral — *see* Occlusion, artery, cerebral
  cholesterol — *see* Atheroembolism
  coronary (artery or vein) (systemic) — *see* Occlusion,
    coronary
  due to device, implant or graft (*see also* Complications,
    by site and type, specified NEC)
    arterial graft NEC T82.818 ☑
    breast (implant) T85.818 ☑
    catheter NEC T85.818 ☑
      dialysis (renal) T82.818 ☑
        intraperitoneal T85.818 ☑
      infusion NEC T82.818 ☑
        spinal (epidural) (subdural) T85.810 ☑
      urinary (indwelling) T83.81 ☑
    electronic (electrode) (pulse generator) (stimulator)
      bone T84.81 ☑
      cardiac T82.817 ☑
      nervous system (brain) (peripheral nerve)
        (spinal) T85.810 ☑
      urinary T83.81 ☑
    fixation, internal (orthopedic) NEC T84.81 ☑
    gastrointestinal (bile duct) (esophagus) T85.818 ☑
    genital NEC T83.81 ☑
    heart (graft) (valve) T82.817 ☑
    joint prosthesis T84.81 ☑
    ocular (corneal graft) (orbital implant) T85.818 ☑
    orthopedic (bone graft) NEC T86.838
    specified NEC T85.818 ☑
    urinary (graft) NEC T83.81 ☑
    vascular NEC T82.818 ☑
    ventricular intracranial shunt T85.810 ☑
  extremities
    lower — *see* Embolism, vein, lower extremity
      arterial I74.3
    upper I74.2
  eye H34.9
  fat (cerebral) (pulmonary) (systemic) T79.1 ☑
    complicating delivery — *see* Embolism, obstetric
    following
      abortion — *see* Abortion by type complicated
        by embolism
      ectopic or molar pregnancy O08.2
  following
    abortion — *see* Abortion by type complicated by
      embolism
    ectopic or molar pregnancy O08.2
    infusion, therapeutic injection or transfusion
      air T80.0 ☑
  heart (fatty) (*see also* Infarct, myocardium)
    not resulting in infarction I51.3
  hepatic (vein) I82.0
  in pregnancy, childbirth or puerperium — *see* Em-
    bolism, obstetric
  intestine (artery) (vein) (with gangrene) (*see also* Is-
    chemia, intestine, acute) K55.039
  intracranial (*see also* Occlusion, artery, cerebral)
    venous sinus (any) G08
      nonpyogenic I67.6
  intraspinal venous sinuses or veins G08
    nonpyogenic G95.19
  kidney (artery) N28.0
  lateral sinus (venous) — *see* Embolism, intracranial,
    venous sinus
  leg — *see* Embolism, vein, lower extremity
    arterial I74.3
  longitudinal sinus (venous) — *see* Embolism, intracra-
    nial, venous sinus
  lung (massive) — *see* Embolism, pulmonary
  meninges I66.8
  mesenteric (artery) (vein) (with gangrene) (*see also*
    Ischemia, intestine, acute) K55.059

☑ **Additional Character Required — Refer to the Tabular List for Character Selection**   ⩔ **Subterms under main terms may continue to next column or page**

Embolism — continued
　obstetric (in) (pulmonary)
　　childbirth O88.22
　　　air O88.02
　　　amniotic fluid O88.12
　　　blood clot O88.22
　　　fat O88.82
　　　pyemic O88.32
　　　septic O88.32
　　　specified type NEC O88.82
　　pregnancy O88.21- ☑
　　　air O88.01- ☑
　　　amniotic fluid O88.11- ☑
　　　blood clot O88.21- ☑
　　　fat O88.81- ☑
　　　pyemic O88.31- ☑
　　　septic O88.31- ☑
　　　specified type NEC O88.81- ☑
　　puerperal O88.23
　　　air O88.03
　　　amniotic fluid O88.13
　　　blood clot O88.23
　　　fat O88.83
　　　pyemic O88.33
　　　septic O88.33
　　　specified type NEC O88.83
　ophthalmic — see Occlusion, artery, retina
　penis N48.81
　peripheral artery NOS I74.4
　pituitary E23.6
　popliteal (artery) I74.3
　portal (vein) I81
　postoperative, postprocedural
　　artery T81.719 ☑
　　　mesenteric T81.710 ☑
　　　renal T81.711 ☑
　　　specified NEC T81.718 ☑
　　vein T81.72 ☑
　precerebral artery — see Occlusion, artery, precerebral
　puerperal — see Embolism, obstetric
　pulmonary (acute) (artery) (vein) I26.99
　　with acute cor pulmonale I26.09
　　chronic I27.82
　　following
　　　abortion — see Abortion by type complicated
　　　　　by embolism
　　　ectopic or molar pregnancy O08.2
　　healed or old Z86.711
　　in pregnancy, childbirth or puerperium — see
　　　　Embolism, obstetric
　　personal history of Z86.711
　　saddle I26.92
　　　with acute cor pulmonale I26.02
　　septic I26.90
　　　with acute cor pulmonale I26.01
　pyemic (multiple) I76
　　following
　　　abortion — see Abortion by type complicated
　　　　　by embolism
　　　ectopic or molar pregnancy O08.2
　　Hemophilus influenzae A41.3
　　pneumococcal A40.3
　　　with pneumonia J13
　　puerperal, postpartum, childbirth (any organism)
　　　　— see Embolism, obstetric
　　specified organism NEC A41.89
　　staphylococcal A41.2
　　streptococcal A40.9
　renal (artery) N28.0
　　vein I82.3
　retina, retinal — see Occlusion, artery, retina
　saddle
　　abdominal aorta I74.01
　　pulmonary artery I26.92
　　　with acute cor pulmonale I26.02
　septic (arterial) I76
　　complicating abortion — see Abortion, by type,
　　　　complicated by, embolism
　sinus — see Embolism, intracranial, venous sinus
　soap complicating abortion — see Abortion, by type,
　　　complicated by, embolism
　spinal cord G95.19
　　pyogenic origin G06.1
　spleen, splenic (artery) I74.8
　upper extremity I74.2
　vein (acute) I82.90
　　antecubital I82.61- ☑
　　　chronic I82.71- ☑

Embolism — continued
　vein — continued
　　axillary I82.A1- ☑ (following I82.7)
　　　chronic I82.A2- ☑ (following I82.7)
　　basilic I82.61- ☑
　　　chronic I82.71- ☑
　　brachial I82.62- ☑
　　　chronic I82.72- ☑
　　brachiocephalic (innominate) I82.290
　　　chronic I82.291
　　cephalic I82.61- ☑
　　　chronic I82.71- ☑
　　chronic I82.91
　　deep (DVT) I82.40- ☑
　　　calf I82.4Z- ☑
　　　　chronic I82.5Z- ☑
　　　lower leg I82.4Z- ☑
　　　　chronic I82.5Z- ☑
　　　thigh I82.4Y- ☑
　　　　chronic I82.5Y- ☑
　　　upper leg I82.4Y ☑
　　　　chronic I82.5Y-
　　femoral I82.41- ☑
　　　chronic I82.51- ☑
　　iliac (iliofemoral) I82.42- ☑
　　　chronic I82.52- ☑
　　innominate I82.290
　　　chronic I82.291
　　internal jugular I82.C1- ☑ (following I82.7)
　　　chronic I82.C2- ☑ (following I82.7)
　　lower extremity
　　　deep I82.40- ☑
　　　　chronic I82.50- ☑
　　　　specified NEC I82.49- ☑
　　　　　chronic NEC I82.59- ☑
　　　distal
　　　　deep I82.4Z- ☑
　　　proximal
　　　　deep I82.4Y- ☑
　　　　　chronic I82.5Y- ☑
　　　superficial I82.81- ☑
　　popliteal I82.43- ☑
　　　chronic I82.53- ☑
　　radial I82.62- ☑
　　　chronic I82.72- ☑
　　renal I82.3
　　saphenous (greater) (lesser) I82.81- ☑
　　specified NEC I82.890
　　　chronic NEC I82.891
　　subclavian I82.B1- ☑ (following I82.7)
　　　chronic I82.B2- ☑ (following I82.7)
　　thoracic NEC I82.290
　　　chronic I82.291
　　tibial I82.44- ☑
　　　chronic I82.54- ☑
　　ulnar I82.62- ☑
　　　chronic I82.72- ☑
　　upper extremity I82.60- ☑
　　　chronic I82.70- ☑
　　　deep I82.62- ☑
　　　　chronic I82.72- ☑
　　　superficial I82.61- ☑
　　　　chronic I82.71- ☑
　　vena cava
　　　inferior (acute) I82.220
　　　　chronic I82.221
　　　superior (acute) I82.210
　　　　chronic I82.211
　　venous sinus G08
　　vessels of brain — see Occlusion, artery, cerebral
Embolus — see Embolism
Embryoma (see also Neoplasm, uncertain behavior, by
　　site)
　benign — see Neoplasm, benign, by site
　kidney C64.- ☑
　liver C22.0
　malignant (see also Neoplasm, malignant, by site)
　　kidney C64.- ☑
　　liver C22.0
　　testis C62.9- ☑
　　　descended (scrotal) C62.1- ☑
　　　undescended C62.0- ☑
　testis C62.9- ☑
　　descended (scrotal) C62.1- ☑
　　undescended C62.0- ☑

Embryonic
　circulation Q28.9
　heart Q28.9
　vas deferens Q55.4
Embryopathia NOS Q89.9
Embryotoxon Q13.4
Emesis — see Vomiting
Emotional lability R45.86
Emotionality, pathological F60.3
Emotogenic disease — see Disorder, psychogenic
Emphysema (atrophic) (bullous) (chronic) (interlobular)
　　(lung) (obstructive) (pulmonary) (senile) (vesicular)
　　J43.9
　cellular tissue (traumatic) T79.7 ☑
　　surgical T81.82 ☑
　centrilobular J43.2
　compensatory J98.3
　congenital (interstitial) P25.0
　conjunctiva H11.89
　connective tissue (traumatic) T79.7 ☑
　　surgical T81.82 ☑
　due to chemicals, gases, fumes or vapors J68.4
　eyelid(s) — see Disorder, eyelid, specified type NEC
　　surgical T81.82 ☑
　　traumatic T79.7 ☑
　interstitial J98.2
　　congenital P25.0
　　perinatal period P25.0
　laminated tissue T79.7 ☑
　　surgical T81.82 ☑
　mediastinal J98.2
　　newborn P25.2
　orbit, orbital — see Disorder, orbit, specified type NEC
　panacinar J43.1
　panlobular J43.1
　specified NEC J43.8
　subcutaneous (traumatic) T79.7 ☑
　　nontraumatic J98.2
　　postprocedural T81.82 ☑
　　surgical T81.82 ☑
　surgical T81.82 ☑
　thymus (gland) (congenital) E32.8
　traumatic (subcutaneous) T79.7 ☑
　unilateral J43.0
Empty nest syndrome Z60.0
Empyema (acute) (chest) (double) (pleura) (supradi-
　　aphragmatic) (thorax) J86.9
　with fistula J86.0
　accessory sinus (chronic) — see Sinusitis
　antrum (chronic) — see Sinusitis, maxillary
　brain (any part) — see Abscess, brain
　ethmoidal (chronic) (sinus) — see Sinusitis, ethmoidal
　extradural — see Abscess, extradural
　frontal (chronic) (sinus) — see Sinusitis, frontal
　gallbladder K81.0
　mastoid (process) (acute) — see Mastoiditis, acute
　maxilla, maxillary M27.2
　　sinus (chronic) — see Sinusitis, maxillary
　nasal sinus (chronic) — see Sinusitis
　sinus (accessory) (chronic) (nasal) — see Sinusitis
　sphenoidal (sinus) (chronic) — see Sinusitis, sphe-
　　　noidal
　subarachnoid — see Abscess, extradural
　subdural — see Abscess, subdural
　tuberculous A15.6
　ureter — see Ureteritis
　ventricular — see Abscess, brain
En coup de sabre lesion L94.1
Enamel pearls K00.2
Enameloma K00.2
Enanthema, viral B09
Encephalitis (chronic) (hemorrhagic) (idiopathic)
　　(nonepidemic) (spurious) (subacute) G04.90
　acute (see also Encephalitis, viral) A86
　　disseminated G04.00
　　　infectious G04.01
　　　noninfectious G04.81
　　　postimmunization (postvaccination) G04.02
　　　postinfectious G04.01
　　inclusion body A85.8
　　necrotizing hemorrhagic G04.30
　　　postimmunization G04.32
　　　postinfectious G04.31
　　　specified NEC G04.39
　arboviral, arbovirus NEC A85.2
　arthropod-borne NEC (viral) A85.2
　Australian A83.4

Encephalitis — continued
- California (virus) A83.5
- Central European (tick-borne) A84.1
- Czechoslovakian A84.1
- Dawson's (inclusion body) A81.1
- diffuse sclerosing A81.1
- disseminated, acute G04.00
- due to
  - cat scratch disease A28.1
  - human immunodeficiency virus (HIV) disease B20 [G05.3]
  - malaria — see Malaria
  - rickettsiosis — see Rickettsiosis
  - smallpox inoculation G04.02
  - typhus — see Typhus
- Eastern equine A83.2
- endemic (viral) A86
- epidemic NEC (viral) A86
- equine (acute) (infectious) (viral) A83.9
  - Eastern A83.2
  - Venezuelan A92.2
  - Western A83.1
- Far Eastern (tick-borne) A84.0
- following vaccination or other immunization procedure G04.02
- herpes zoster B02.0
- herpesviral B00.4
  - due to herpesvirus 6 B10.01
  - due to herpesvirus 7 B10.09
  - specified NEC B10.09
- Ilheus (virus) A83.8
- in (due to)
  - actinomycosis A42.82
  - adenovirus A85.1
  - African trypanosomiasis B56.9 [G05.3]
  - Chagas' disease (chronic) B57.42
  - cytomegalovirus B25.8
  - enterovirus A85.0
  - herpes (simplex) virus B00.4
    - due to herpesvirus 6 B10.01
    - due to herpesvirus 7 B10.09
    - specified NEC B10.09
  - infectious disease NEC B99 ☑ [G05.3]
  - influenza — see Influenza, with, encephalopathy
  - listeriosis A32.12
  - measles B05.0
  - mumps B26.2
  - naegleriasis B60.2
  - parasitic disease NEC B89 [G05.3]
  - poliovirus A80.9 [G05.3]
  - rubella B06.01
  - syphilis
    - congenital A50.42
    - late A52.14
  - systemic lupus erythematosus M32.19
  - toxoplasmosis (acquired) B58.2
    - congenital P37.1
  - tuberculosis A17.82
  - zoster B02.0
- inclusion body A81.1
- infectious (acute) (virus) NEC A86
- Japanese (B type) A83.0
- La Crosse A83.5
- lead — see Poisoning, lead
- lethargica (acute) (infectious) A85.8
- louping ill A84.8
- lupus erythematosus, systemic M32.19
- lymphatica A87.2
- Mengo A85.8
- meningococcal A39.81
- Murray Valley A83.4
- otitic NEC H66.40 [G05.3]
- parasitic NOS B71.9
- periaxial G37.0
- periaxialis (concentrica) (diffuse) G37.5
- postchickenpox B01.11
- postexanthematous NEC B09
- postimmunization G04.02
- postinfectious NEC G04.01
- postmeasles B05.0
- postvaccinal G04.02
- postvaricella B01.11
- postviral NEC A86
- Powassan A84.8
- Rasmussen G04.81
- Rio Bravo A85.8
- Russian
  - autumnal A83.0
  - spring-summer (taiga) A84.0

Encephalitis — continued
- saturnine — see Poisoning, lead
- specified NEC G04.81
- St. Louis A83.3
- subacute sclerosing A81.1
- summer A83.0
- suppurative G04.81
- tick-borne A84.9
- Torula, torular (cryptococcal) B45.1
- toxic NEC G92
- trichinosis B75 [G05.3]
- type
  - B A83.0
  - C A83.3
- van Bogaert's A81.1
- Venezuelan equine A92.2
- Vienna A85.8
- viral, virus A86
  - arthropod-borne NEC A85.2
    - mosquito-borne A83.9
      - Australian X disease A83.4
      - California virus A83.5
      - Eastern equine A83.2
      - Japanese (B type) A83.0
      - Murray Valley A83.4
      - specified NEC A83.8
      - St. Louis A83.3
      - type B A83.0
      - type C A83.3
      - Western equine A83.1
    - tick-borne A84.9
      - biundulant A84.1
      - central European A84.1
      - Czechoslovakian A84.1
      - diphasic meningoencephalitis A84.1
      - Far Eastern A84.0
      - Russian spring-summer (taiga) A84.0
      - specified NEC A84.8
  - specified type NEC A85.8
- Western equine A83.1

Encephalocele Q01.9
- frontal Q01.0
- nasofrontal Q01.1
- occipital Q01.2
- specified NEC Q01.8

Encephalocystocele — see Encephalocele
Encephaloduroarteriomyosynangiosis (EDAMS) I67.5
Encephalomalacia (brain) (cerebellar) (cerebral) — see Softening, brain
Encephalomeningitis — see Meningoencephalitis
Encephalomeningocele — see Encephalocele
Encephalomeningomyelitis — see Meningoencephalitis
Encephalomyelitis (see also Encephalitis) G04.90
- acute disseminated G04.00
  - infectious G04.01
  - noninfectious G04.81
  - postimmunization G04.02
  - postinfectious G04.01
- acute necrotizing hemorrhagic G04.30
  - postimmunization G04.32
  - postinfectious G04.31
  - specified NEC G04.39
- benign myalgic G93.3
- equine A83.9
  - Eastern A83.2
  - Venezuelan A92.2
  - Western A83.1
- in diseases classified elsewhere G05.3
- myalgic, benign G93.3
- postchickenpox B01.11
- postinfectious NEC G04.01
- postmeasles B05.0
- postvaccinal G04.02
- postvaricella B01.11
- rubella B06.01
- specified NEC G04.81
- Venezuelan equine A92.2

Encephalomyelocele — see Encephalocele
Encephalomyelomeningitis — see Meningoencephalitis
Encephalomyelopathy G96.9
Encephalomyeloradiculitis (acute) G61.0
Encephalomyeloradiculoneuritis (acute) (Guillain-Barré) G61.0
Encephalomyeloradiculopathy G96.9
Encephalopathia hyperbilirubinemica, newborn P57.9

Encephalopathia hyperbilirubinemica, newborn — continued
- due to isoimmunization (conditions in P55) P57.0
Encephalopathy (acute) G93.40
- acute necrotizing hemorrhagic G04.30
  - postimmunization G04.32
  - postinfectious G04.31
  - specified NEC G04.39
- alcoholic G31.2
- anoxic — see Damage, brain, anoxic
- arteriosclerotic I67.2
- centrolobar progressive (Schilder) G37.0
- congenital Q07.9
- degenerative, in specified disease NEC G32.89
- demyelinating callosal G37.1
- due to
  - drugs (see also Table of Drugs and Chemicals) G92
  - hepatic — see Failure, hepatic
  - hyperbilirubinemic, newborn P57.9
    - due to isoimmunization (conditions in P55) P57.0
- hypertensive I67.4
- hypoglycemic E16.2
- hypoxic — see Damage, brain, anoxic
- hypoxic ischemic P91.60
  - mild P91.61
  - moderate P91.62
  - severe P91.63
- in (due to) (with)
  - birth injury P11.1
  - hyperinsulinism E16.1 [G94]
  - influenza — see Influenza, with, encephalopathy
  - lack of vitamin (see also Deficiency, vitamin) E56.9 [G32.89]
  - neoplastic disease (see also Neoplasm) D49.9 [G13.1]
  - serum (see also Reaction, serum) T80.69 ☑
  - syphilis A52.17
  - trauma (postconcussional) F07.81
    - current injury — see Injury, intracranial
  - vaccination G04.02
- lead — see Poisoning, lead
- metabolic G93.41
  - drug induced G92
  - toxic G92
- myoclonic, early, symptomatic — see Epilepsy, generalized, specified NEC
- necrotizing, subacute (Leigh) G31.82
- neonatal P91.819
  - in diseases classified elsewhere P91.811
- pellagrous E52 [G32.89]
- portosystemic — see Failure, hepatic
- postcontusional F07.81
  - current injury — see Injury, intracranial, diffuse
- posthypoglycemic (coma) E16.1 [G94]
- postradiation G93.89
- saturnine — see Poisoning, lead
- septic G93.41
- specified NEC G93.49
- spongiform, subacute (viral) A81.09
- toxic G92
  - metabolic G92
- traumatic (postconcussional) F07.81
  - current injury — see Injury, intracranial
- vitamin B deficiency NEC E53.9 [G32.89]
  - vitamin B1 E51.2
- Wernicke's E51.2

Encephalorrhagia — see Hemorrhage, intracranial, intracerebral
Encephalosis, posttraumatic F07.81
Enchondroma (see also Neoplasm, bone, benign)
Enchondromatosis (cartilaginous) (multiple) Q78.4
Encopresis R15.9
- functional F98.1
- nonorganic origin F98.1
- psychogenic F98.1
Encounter (with health service) (for) Z76.89
- adjustment and management (of)
  - breast implant Z45.81 ☑
  - implanted device NEC Z45.89
  - myringotomy device (stent) (tube) Z45.82
- administrative purpose only Z02.9
  - examination for
    - adoption Z02.82
    - armed forces Z02.3
    - disability determination Z02.71
    - driving license Z02.4
    - employment Z02.1
    - insurance Z02.6

Encounter — *continued*
- administrative purpose only — *continued*
  - examination for — *continued*
    - medical certificate NEC Z02.79
    - paternity testing Z02.81
    - residential institution admission Z02.2
    - school admission Z02.0
    - sports Z02.5
    - specified reason NEC Z02.89
- aftercare — *see* Aftercare
- antenatal screening Z36.9
  - cervical length Z36.86
  - chromosomal anomalies Z36.0
  - congenital cardiac abnormalities Z36.83
  - elevated maternal serum alphafetoprotein Z36.1
  - fetal growth retardation Z36.4
  - fetal lung maturity Z36.84
  - fetal macrosomia Z36.88
  - hydrops fetalis Z36.81
  - intrauterine growth restriction (IUGR) /small-for-dates Z36.4
  - isoimmunization Z36.5
  - large-for-dates Z36.88
  - malformations Z36.3
  - non-visualized anatomy on a previous scan Z36.2
  - nuchal translucency Z36.82
  - raised alphafetoprotein level Z36.1
  - risk of pre-term labor Z36.86
  - specified follow-up NEC Z36.2
  - specified genetic defects NEC Z36.8A
  - specified type NEC Z36.89
  - Streptococcus B Z36.85
  - suspected anomaly Z36.3
  - uncertain dates Z36.87
- assisted reproductive fertility procedure cycle Z31.83
- blood typing Z01.83
  - Rh typing Z01.83
- breast augmentation or reduction Z41.1
- breast implant exchange (different material) (different size) Z45.81 ☑
- breast reconstruction following mastectomy Z42.1
- check-up — *see* Examination
- chemotherapy for neoplasm Z51.11
- colonoscopy, screening Z12.11
- counseling — *see* Counseling
- delivery, full-term, uncomplicated O80
  - cesarean, without indication O82
- desensitization to allergens Z51.6
- ear piercing Z41.3
- examination — *see* Examination
- expectant parent(s) (adoptive) pre-birth pediatrician visit Z76.81
- fertility preservation procedure (prior to cancer therapy) (prior to removal of gonads) Z31.84
- fitting (of) — *see* Fitting (and adjustment) (of)
- genetic
  - counseling
    - nonprocreative Z71.83
    - procreative Z31.5
  - testing — *see* Test, genetic
- hearing conservation and treatment Z01.12
- immunotherapy for neoplasm Z51.12
- in vitro fertilization cycle Z31.83
- insulin pump titration Z46.81
- joint prosthesis insertion following prior explantation of joint prosthesis (staged procedure)
  - hip Z47.32
  - knee Z47.33
  - shoulder Z47.31
- laboratory (as part of a general medical examination) Z00.00
  - with abnormal findings Z00.01
- mental health services (for)
  - abuse NEC
    - perpetrator Z69.82
    - victim Z69.81
  - child abuse
    - nonparental
      - perpetrator Z69.021
      - victim Z69.020
    - parental
      - perpetrator Z69.011

Encounter — *continued*
- mental health services — *continued*
  - child abuse — *continued*
    - parental — *continued*
      - victim Z69.010
  - child neglect
    - nonparental
      - perpetrator Z69.021
      - victim Z69.020
    - parental
      - perpetrator Z69.011
      - victim Z69.010
  - child psychological abuse
    - nonparental
      - perpetrator Z69.021
      - victim Z69.020
    - parental
      - perpetrator Z69.011
      - victim Z69.010
  - child sexual abuse
    - nonparental
      - perpetrator Z69.021
      - victim Z69.020
    - parental
      - perpetrator Z69.011
      - victim Z69.010
  - non-spousal adult abuse (perpetrator) (victim) Z69.81
  - spousal or partner
    - abuse
      - perpetrator Z69.12
      - victim Z69.11
    - neglect
      - perpetrator Z69.12
      - victim Z69.11
    - psychological abuse
      - perpetrator Z69.12
      - victim Z69.11
    - violence
      - perpetrator (physical) (sexual) Z69.12
      - victim (physical) Z69.11
        - sexual Z69.81
- observation (for) (ruled out)
  - exposure to (suspected)
    - anthrax Z03.810
    - biological agent NEC Z03.818
- pediatrician visit, by expectant parent(s) (adoptive) Z76.81
- placental sample (taken vaginally) (*see also* Encounter, antenatal screening) Z36.9
- plastic and reconstructive surgery following medical procedure or healed injury NEC Z42.8
- pregnancy
  - supervision of — *see* Pregnancy, supervision of
  - test Z32.00
    - result negative Z32.02
    - result positive Z32.01
- procreative management and counseling for gestational carrier Z31.7
- prophylactic measures Z29.9
  - antivenin Z29.12
  - fluoride administration Z29.3
  - immunotherapy for respiratory syncytial virus (RSV) Z29.11
  - rabies immune globin Z29.14
  - Rho (D) immune globulin Z29.13
  - specified NEC Z29.8
- radiation therapy (antineoplastic) Z51.0
- radiological (as part of a general medical examination) Z00.00
  - with abnormal findings Z00.01
- reconstructive surgery following medical procedure or healed injury NEC Z42.8
- removal (of) (*see also* Removal)
  - artificial
    - arm Z44.00- ☑
      - complete Z44.01- ☑
      - partial Z44.02- ☑
    - eye Z44.2- ☑
    - leg Z44.10- ☑
      - complete Z44.11- ☑
      - partial Z44.12- ☑
    - breast implant Z45.81 ☑
      - tissue expander (without synchronous insertion of permanent implant) Z45.81 ☑
  - device Z46.9
    - specified NEC Z46.89

Encounter — *continued*
- removal (*see also* Removal) — *continued*
  - external
    - fixation device — *code to* fracture with seventh character D
    - prosthesis, prosthetic device Z44.9
      - breast Z44.3- ☑
      - specified NEC Z44.8
  - implanted device NEC Z45.89
  - insulin pump Z46.81
  - internal fixation device Z47.2
  - myringotomy device (stent) (tube) Z45.82
  - nervous system device NEC Z46.2
    - brain neuropacemaker Z46.2
    - visual substitution device Z46.2
      - implanted Z45.31
  - non-vascular catheter Z46.82
  - orthodontic device Z46.4
  - stent
    - ureteral Z46.6
  - urinary device Z46.6
- repeat cervical smear to confirm findings of recent normal smear following initial abnormal smear Z01.42
- respirator [ventilator] use during power failure Z99.12
- Rh typing Z01.83
- screening — *see* Screening
- specified NEC Z76.89
- sterilization Z30.2
- suspected condition, ruled out
  - amniotic cavity and membrane Z03.71
  - cervical shortening Z03.75
  - fetal anomaly Z03.73
  - fetal growth Z03.74
  - maternal and fetal conditions NEC Z03.79
  - oligohydramnios Z03.71
  - placental problem Z03.72
  - polyhydramnios Z03.71
- suspected exposure (to), ruled out
  - anthrax Z03.810
  - biological agents NEC Z03.818
- termination of pregnancy, elective Z33.2
- testing — *see* Test
- therapeutic drug level monitoring Z51.81
- titration, insulin pump Z46.81
- to determine fetal viability of pregnancy O36.80 ☑
- training
  - insulin pump Z46.81
- X-ray of chest (as part of a general medical examination) Z00.00
  - with abnormal findings Z00.01

Encystment — *see* Cyst
Endarteritis (bacterial, subacute) (infective) I77.6
- brain I67.7
- cerebral or cerebrospinal I67.7
- deformans — *see* Arteriosclerosis
- embolic — *see* Embolism
- obliterans (*see also* Arteriosclerosis)
  - pulmonary I28.8
- pulmonary I28.8
- retina — *see* Vasculitis, retina
- senile — *see* Arteriosclerosis
- syphilitic A52.09
  - brain or cerebral A52.04
  - congenital A50.54 [I79.8]
- tuberculous A18.89
Endemic — *see* condition
Endocarditis (chronic) (marantic) (nonbacterial) (thrombotic) (valvular) I38
- with rheumatic fever (conditions in I00)
  - active — *see* Endocarditis, acute, rheumatic
  - inactive or quiescent (with chorea) I09.1
- acute or subacute I33.9
  - infective I33.0
  - rheumatic (aortic) (mitral) (pulmonary) (tricuspid) I01.1
    - with chorea (acute) (rheumatic) (Sydenham's) I02.0
- aortic (heart) (nonrheumatic) (valve) I35.8
  - with
    - mitral disease I08.0
      - with tricuspid (valve) disease I08.3
      - active or acute I01.1
        - with chorea (acute) (rheumatic) (Sydenham's) I02.0
    - rheumatic fever (conditions in I00)
      - active — *see* Endocarditis, acute, rheumatic
      - inactive or quiescent (with chorea) I06.9

Endocarditis — *continued*
aortic — *continued*
  with — *continued*
    tricuspid (valve) disease I08.2
      with mitral (valve) disease I08.3
    acute or subacute I33.9
    arteriosclerotic I35.8
    rheumatic I06.9
      with mitral disease I08.0
        with tricuspid (valve) disease I08.3
          active or acute I01.1
            with chorea (acute) (rheumatic) (Sydenham's) I02.0
        active or acute I01.1
          with chorea (acute) (rheumatic) (Sydenham's) I02.0
      specified NEC I06.8
    specified cause NEC I35.8
    syphilitic A52.03
  arteriosclerotic I38
  atypical verrucous (Libman-Sacks) M32.11
  bacterial (acute) (any valve) (subacute) I33.0
  candidal B37.6
  congenital Q24.8
  constrictive I33.0
  Coxiella burnetii A78 [I39]
  Coxsackie B33.21
  due to
    prosthetic cardiac valve T82.6 ☑
    Q fever A78 [I39]
    Serratia marcescens I33.0
    typhoid (fever) A01.02
  gonococcal A54.83
  infectious or infective (acute) (any valve) (subacute) I33.0
  lenta (acute) (any valve) (subacute) I33.0
  Libman-Sacks M32.11
  listerial A32.82
  Löffler's I42.3
  malignant (acute) (any valve) (subacute) I33.0
  meningococcal A39.51
  mitral (chronic) (double) (fibroid) (heart) (inactive) (valve) (with chorea) I05.9
    with
      aortic (valve) disease I08.0
        with tricuspid (valve) disease I08.3
          active or acute I01.1
            with chorea (acute) (rheumatic) (Sydenham's) I02.0
      rheumatic fever (conditions in I00)
        active — *see* Endocarditis, acute, rheumatic
        inactive or quiescent (with chorea) I05.9
      tricuspid (valve) disease I08.1
        with aortic (valve) disease I08.3
    active or acute I01.1
      with chorea (acute) (rheumatic) (Sydenham's) I02.0
    bacterial I33.0
    arteriosclerotic I34.8
    nonrheumatic I34.8
      acute or subacute I33.9
    specified NEC I05.8
  monilial B37.6
  multiple valves I08.9
    specified disorders I08.8
  mycotic (acute) (any valve) (subacute) I33.0
  pneumococcal (acute) (any valve) (subacute) I33.0
  pulmonary (chronic) (heart) (valve) I37.8
    with rheumatic fever (conditions in I00)
      active — *see* Endocarditis, acute, rheumatic
      inactive or quiescent (with chorea) I09.89
        with aortic, mitral or tricuspid disease I08.8
    acute or subacute I33.9
      rheumatic I01.1
        with chorea (acute) (rheumatic) (Sydenham's) I02.0
    arteriosclerotic I37.8
    congenital Q22.2
    rheumatic (chronic) (inactive) (with chorea) I09.89
      active or acute I01.1
        with chorea (acute) (rheumatic) (Sydenham's) I02.0
    syphilitic A52.03
  purulent (acute) (any valve) (subacute) I33.0
  Q fever A78 [I39]
  rheumatic (chronic) (inactive) (with chorea) I09.1
    active or acute (aortic) (mitral) (pulmonary) (tricuspid) I01.1

Endocarditis — *continued*
rheumatic — *continued*
  active or acute — *continued*
    with chorea (acute) (rheumatic) (Sydenham's) I02.0
  rheumatoid — *see* Rheumatoid, carditis
  septic (acute) (any valve) (subacute) I33.0
  streptococcal (acute) (any valve) (subacute) I33.0
  subacute — *see* Endocarditis, acute
  suppurative (acute) (any valve) (subacute) I33.0
  syphilitic A52.03
  toxic I33.9
  tricuspid (chronic) (heart) (inactive) (rheumatic) (valve) (with chorea) I07.9
    with
      aortic (valve) disease I08.2
        mitral (valve) disease I08.3
      mitral (valve) disease I08.1
        aortic (valve) disease I08.3
      rheumatic fever (conditions in I00)
        active — *see* Endocarditis, acute, rheumatic
        inactive or quiescent (with chorea) I07.8
    active or acute I01.1
      with chorea (acute) (rheumatic) (Sydenham's) I02.0
    arteriosclerotic I36.8
    nonrheumatic I36.8
      acute or subacute I33.9
    specified cause, except rheumatic I36.8
  tuberculous — *see* Tuberculosis, endocarditis
  typhoid A01.02
  ulcerative (acute) (any valve) (subacute) I33.0
  vegetative (acute) (any valve) (subacute) I33.0
  verrucous (atypical) (nonbacterial) (nonrheumatic) M32.11

Endocardium, endocardial (*see also* condition)
  cushion defect Q21.2
Endocervicitis (*see also* Cervicitis)
  due to intrauterine (contraceptive) device T83.69 ☑
  hyperplastic N72
Endocrine — *see* condition
Endocrinopathy, pluriglandular E31.9
Endodontic
  overfill M27.52
  underfill M27.53
Endodontitis K04.01
  irreversible K04.02
  reversible K04.01
Endomastoiditis — *see* Mastoiditis
Endometrioma N80.9
Endometriosis N80.9
  appendix N80.5
  bladder N80.8
  bowel N80.5
  broad ligament N80.3
  cervix N80.0
  colon N80.5
  cul-de-sac (Douglas') N80.3
  exocervix N80.0
  fallopian tube N80.2
  female genital organ NEC N80.8
  gallbladder N80.8
  in scar of skin N80.6
  internal N80.0
  intestine N80.5
  lung N80.8
  myometrium N80.0
  ovary N80.1
  parametrium N80.3
  pelvic peritoneum N80.3
  peritoneal (pelvic) N80.3
  rectovaginal septum N80.4
  rectum N80.5
  round ligament N80.3
  skin (scar) N80.6
  specified site NEC N80.8
  stromal D39.0
  thorax N80.8
  umbilicus N80.8
  uterus (internal) N80.0
  vagina N80.4
  vulva N80.8
Endometritis (decidual) (nonspecific) (purulent) (senile) (atrophic) (suppurative) N71.9
  with ectopic pregnancy O08.0
  acute N71.0
  blenorrhagic (gonococcal) (acute) (chronic) A54.24

Endometritis — *continued*
  cervix, cervical (with erosion or ectropion) (*see also* Cervicitis)
    hyperplastic N72
  chlamydial A56.11
  chronic N71.1
  following
    abortion — *see* Abortion by type complicated by genital infection
    ectopic or molar pregnancy O08.0
  gonococcal, gonorrheal (acute) (chronic) A54.24
  hyperplastic (*see also* Hyperplasia, endometrial) N85.00
    cervix N72
  puerperal, postpartum, childbirth O86.12
  subacute N71.0
  tuberculous A18.17
Endometrium — *see* condition
Endomyocardiopathy, South African I42.3
Endomyocarditis — *see* Endocarditis
Endomyofibrosis I42.3
Endomyometritis — *see* Endometritis
Endopericarditis — *see* Endocarditis
Endoperineuritis — *see* Disorder, nerve
Endophlebitis — *see* Phlebitis
Endophthalmia — *see* Endophthalmitis, purulent
Endophthalmitis (acute) (infective) (metastatic) (subacute) H44.009
  bleb associated (*see also* Bleb, inflamed (infected), postprocedural H59.4 ☑
  gonorrheal A54.39
  in (due to)
    cysticercosis B69.1
    onchocerciasis B73.01
    toxocariasis B83.0
  panuveitis — *see* Panuveitis
  parasitic H44.12- ☑
  purulent H44.00- ☑
    panophthalmitis — *see* Panophthalmitis
    vitreous abscess H44.02- ☑
  specified NEC H44.19
  sympathetic — *see* Uveitis, sympathetic
Endosalpingioma D28.2
Endosalpingiosis N94.89
Endosteitis — *see* Osteomyelitis
Endothelioma, bone — *see* Neoplasm, bone, malignant
Endotheliosis (hemorrhagic infectional) D69.8
Endotoxemia — code to condition
Endotrachelitis — *see* Cervicitis
Engelmann (-Camurati) **syndrome** Q78.3
English disease — *see* Rickets
Engman's disease L30.3
Engorgement
  breast N64.59
    newborn P83.4
    puerperal, postpartum O92.79
  lung (passive) — *see* Edema, lung
  pulmonary (passive) — *see* Edema, lung
  stomach K31.89
  venous, retina — *see* Occlusion, retina, vein, engorgement
Enlargement, enlarged (*see also* Hypertrophy)
  adenoids J35.2
    with tonsils J35.3
  alveolar ridge K08.89
    congenital — *see* Anomaly, alveolar
  apertures of diaphragm (congenital) Q79.1
  gingival K06.1
  heart, cardiac — *see* Hypertrophy, cardiac
  labium majus, childhood asymmetric (CALME) N90.61
  lacrimal gland, chronic H04.03- ☑
  liver — *see* Hypertrophy, liver
  lymph gland or node R59.9
    generalized R59.1
    localized R59.0
  orbit H05.34- ☑
  organ or site, congenital NEC — *see* Anomaly, by site
  parathyroid (gland) E21.0
  pituitary fossa R93.0
  prostate N40.0
    with lower urinary tract symptoms (LUTS) N40.1
    without lower urinary tract symtpoms (LUTS) N40.0
  sella turcica R93.0
  spleen — *see* Splenomegaly
  thymus (gland) (congenital) E32.0
  thyroid (gland) — *see* Goiter
  tongue K14.8
  tonsils J35.1

Enlargement, enlarged — *continued*
  tonsils — *continued*
    with adenoids J35.3
  uterus N85.2
  vestibular aqueduct Q16.5
Enophthalmos H05.40- ☑
  due to
    orbital tissue atrophy H05.41- ☑
    trauma or surgery H05.42- ☑
Enostosis M27.8
Entamebic, entamebiasis — *see* Amebiasis
Entanglement
  umbilical cord(s) O69.82 ☑
    with compression O69.2 ☑
    without compression O69.82 ☑
    around neck (with compression) O69.81 ☑
      with compression O69.1 ☑
      without compression O69.81 ☑
    of twins in monoamniotic sac O69.2 ☑
Enteralgia — *see* Pain, abdominal
Enteric — *see* condition
Enteritis (acute) (diarrheal) (hemorrhagic) (noninfective)
    K52.9
  adenovirus A08.2
  aertrycke infection A02.0
  allergic K52.29
    with
      eosinophilic gastritis or gastroenteritis K52.81
      food protein-induced enterocolitis syndrome
        K52.21
      food protein-induced enteropathy K52.22
  amebic (acute) A06.0
    with abscess — *see* Abscess, amebic
    chronic A06.1
      with abscess — *see* Abscess, amebic
      nondysenteric A06.2
    nondysenteric A06.2
  astrovirus A08.32
  bacillary NOS A03.9
  bacterial A04.9
    specified NEC A04.8
  calicivirus A08.31
  candidal B37.82
  Chilomastix A07.8
  choleriformis A00.1
  chronic (noninfectious) K52.9
    ulcerative — *see* Colitis, ulcerative
  cicatrizing (chronic) — *see* Enteritis, regional, small
    intestine
  Clostridium
    botulinum (food poisoning) A05.1
    difficile
      not specified as recurrent A04.72
      recurrent A04.71
  coccidial A07.3
  coxsackie virus A08.39
  dietetic (*see also* Enteritis, allergic) K52.29
  drug-induced K52.1
  due to
    astrovirus A08.32
    calicivirus A08.31
    coxsackie virus A08.39
    drugs K52.1
    echovirus A08.39
    enterovirus NEC A08.39
    food hypersensitivity (*see also* Enteritis, allergic)
      K52.29
    infectious organism (bacterial) (viral) — *see* Enteri-
      tis, infectious
    torovirus A08.39
    Yersinia enterocolitica A04.6
  echovirus A08.39
  eltor A00.1
  enterovirus NEC A08.39
  eosinophilic K52.81
  epidemic (infectious) A09
  fulminant (*see also* Ischemia, intestine, acute) K55.019
  gangrenous — *see* Enteritis, infectious
  giardial A07.1
  infectious NOS A09
    due to
      adenovirus A08.2
      Aerobacter aerogenes A04.8
      Arizona (bacillus) A02.0
      bacteria NOS A04.9
        specified NEC A04.8
      Campylobacter A04.5

Enteritis — *continued*
  infectious — *continued*
    due to — *continued*
      Clostridium difficile
        not specified as recurrent A04.72
        recurrent A04.71
      Clostridium perfringens A04.8
      Enterobacter aerogenes A04.8
      enterovirus A08.39
      Escherichia coli A04.4
        enteroaggregative A04.4
        enterohemorrhagic A04.3
        enteroinvasive A04.2
        enteropathogenic A04.0
        enterotoxigenic A04.1
        specified NEC A04.4
      specified
        bacteria NEC A04.8
        virus NEC A08.39
      Staphylococcus A04.8
      virus NEC A08.4
        specified type NEC A08.39
      Yersinia enterocolitica A04.6
    specified organism NEC A08.8
  influenzal — *see* Influenza, with, digestive manifesta-
    tions
  ischemic K55.9
    acute (*see also* Ischemia, intestine, acute) K55.019
    chronic K55.1
  microsporidial A07.8
  mucomembranous, myxomembranous — *see* Syn-
    drome, irritable bowel
  mucous — *see* Syndrome, irritable bowel
  necroticans A05.2
  necrotizing of newborn — *see* Enterocolitis, necrotiz-
    ing, in newborn
  neurogenic — *see* Syndrome, irritable bowel
  newborn necrotizing — *see* Enterocolitis, necrotizing,
    in newborn
  noninfectious K52.9
  norovirus A08.11
  parasitic NEC B82.9
  paratyphoid (fever) — *see* Fever, paratyphoid
  protozoal A07.9
    specified NEC A07.8
  radiation K52.0
  regional (of) K50.90
    with
      complication K50.919
        abscess K50.914
        fistula K50.913
        intestinal obstruction K50.912
        rectal bleeding K50.911
        specified complication NEC K50.918
    colon — *see* Enteritis, regional, large intestine
    duodenum — *see* Enteritis, regional, small intestine
    ileum — *see* Enteritis, regional, small intestine
    jejunum — *see* Enteritis, regional, small intestine
    large bowel — *see* Enteritis, regional, large intes-
      tine
    large intestine (colon) (rectum) K50.10
      with
        complication K50.119
          abscess K50.114
          fistula K50.113
          intestinal obstruction K50.112
          rectal bleeding K50.111
          small intestine (duodenum) (ileum) (je-
            junum) involvement K50.80
            with
              complication K50.819
                abscess K50.814
                fistula K50.813
                intestinal obstruction K50.812
                rectal bleeding K50.811
                specified complication NEC
                  K50.818
          specified complication NEC K50.118
    rectum — *see* Enteritis, regional, large intestine
    small intestine (duodenum) (ileum) (jejunum)
      K50.00
      with
        complication K50.019
          abscess K50.014
          fistula K50.013
          intestinal obstruction K50.012
          large intestine (colon) (rectum) involve-
            ment K50.80

Enteritis — *continued*
  regional — *continued*
    small intestine — *continued*
      with — *continued*
        complication — *continued*
          large intestine involvement — *contin-
            ued*
            with
              complication K50.819
                abscess K50.814
                fistula K50.813
                intestinal obstruction K50.812
                rectal bleeding K50.811
                specified complication NEC
                  K50.818
          rectal bleeding K50.011
          specified complication NEC K50.018
  rotaviral A08.0
  Salmonella, salmonellosis (arizonae) (cholerae-suis)
    (enteritidis) (typhimurium) A02.0
  segmental — *see* Enteritis, regional
  septic A09
  Shigella — *see* Infection, Shigella
  small round structured NEC A08.19
  spasmodic, spastic — *see* Syndrome, irritable bowel
  staphylococcal A04.8
    due to food A05.0
  torovirus A08.39
  toxic NEC K52.1
    due to Clostridium difficile
      not specified as recurrent A04.72
      recurrent A04.71
  trichomonal A07.8
  tuberculous A18.32
  typhosa A01.00
  ulcerative (chronic) — *see* Colitis, ulcerative
  viral A08.4
    adenovirus A08.2
    enterovirus A08.39
    Rotavirus A08.0
    small round structured NEC A08.19
    specified NEC A08.39
    virus specified NEC A08.39
Enterobiasis B80
Enterobius vermicularis (infection) (infestation) B80
Enterocele (*see also* Hernia, abdomen)
  pelvic, pelvis (acquired) (congenital) N81.5
  vagina, vaginal (acquired) (congenital) NEC N81.5
Enterocolitis (*see also* Enteritis) K52.9
  due to Clostridium difficile
    not specified as recurrent A04.72
    recurrent A04.71
  fulminant ischemic (*see also* Ischemia, intestine, acute)
    K55.059
  granulomatous — *see* Enteritis, regional
  hemorrhagic (acute) (*see also* Ischemia, intestine,
    acute) K55.059
    chronic K55.1
  infectious NEC A09
  ischemic K55.9
  necrotizing K55.30
    with
      perforation K55.33
      pneumatosis K55.32
        and perforation K55.33
    without pneumatosis or perforation K55.31
    due to Clostridium difficile
      not specified as recurrent A04.72
      recurrent A04.71
    in newborn P77.9
      stage 1 (without pneumatosis, without perfora-
        tion) P77.1
      stage 2 (with pneumatosis, without perforation)
        P77.2
      stage 3 (with pneumatosis, with perforation)
        P77.3
    in non-newborn K55.30
      stage 1 (without pneumatosis, without perfora-
        tion) K55.31
      stage 2 (with pneumatosis, without perforation)
        K55.32
      stage 3 (with pneumatosis, with perforation)
        K55.33
  noninfectious K52.9
    newborn — *see* Enterocolitis, necrotizing, in new-
      born
  pseudomembranous (newborn)
    not specified as recurrent A04.72

⚐ Subterms under main terms may continue to next column or page   ☑ Additional Character Required — Refer to the Tabular List for Character Selection   **133**

Enlargement, enlarged — Enterocolitis

Enterocolitis — *continued*
  pseudomembranous — *continued*
    recurrent A04.71
  radiation K52.0
    newborn — *see* Enterocolitis, necrotizing, in new-
      born
  ulcerative (chronic) — *see* Pancolitis, ulcerative
    (chronic)
Enterogastritis — *see* Enteritis
Enteropathy K63.9
  celiac-gluten-sensitive K90.0
    non-celiac K90.41
  food protein-induced enterocolitis K52.22
  hemorrhagic, terminal (*see also* Ischemia, intestine,
    acute) K55.059
  protein-losing K90.49
Enteroperitonitis — *see* Peritonitis
Enteroptosis K63.4
Enterorrhagia K92.2
Enterospasm (*see also* Syndrome, irritable, bowel)
  psychogenic F45.8
Enterostenosis (*see also* Obstruction, intestine, specified
  NEC) K56.699
Enterostomy
  complication — *see* Complication, enterostomy
  status Z93.4
Enterovirus, as cause of disease classified elsewhere
  B97.10
  coxsackievirus B97.11
  echovirus B97.12
  other specified B97.19
Enthesopathy (peripheral) M77.9
  Achilles tendinitis — *see* Tendinitis, Achilles
  ankle and tarsus M77.9
    specified type NEC — *see* Enthesopathy, foot,
      specified type NEC
  anterior tibial syndrome M76.81- ☑
  calcaneal spur — *see* Spur, bone, calcaneal
  elbow region M77.8
    lateral epicondylitis — *see* Epicondylitis, lateral
    medial epicondylitis — *see* Epicondylitis, medial
  foot NEC M77.9
    metatarsalgia — *see* Metatarsalgia
    specified type NEC M77.5- ☑
  forearm M77.9
  gluteal tendinitis — *see* Tendinitis, gluteal
  hand M77.9
  hip — *see* Enthesopathy, lower limb, specified type
    NEC
  iliac crest spur — *see* Spur, bone, iliac crest
  iliotibial band syndrome — *see* Syndrome, iliotibial
    band
  knee — *see* Enthesopathy, lower limb, lower leg,
    specified type NEC
  lateral epicondylitis — *see* Epicondylitis, lateral
  lower limb (excluding foot) M76.9
    Achilles tendinitis — *see* Tendinitis, Achilles
    anterior tibial syndrome M76.81- ☑
    gluteal tendinitis — *see* Tendinitis, gluteal
    iliac crest spur — *see* Spur, bone, iliac crest
    iliotibial band syndrome — *see* Syndrome, iliotibial
      band
    patellar tendinitis — *see* Tendinitis, patellar
    pelvic region — *see* Enthesopathy, lower limb,
      specified type NEC
    peroneal tendinitis — *see* Tendinitis, peroneal
    posterior tibial syndrome M76.82- ☑
    psoas tendinitis — *see* Tendinitis, psoas
    shoulder M77.9
    specified type NEC M76.89- ☑
    tibial collateral bursitis — *see* Bursitis, tibial collat-
      eral
  medial epicondylitis — *see* Epicondylitis, medial
  metatarsalgia — *see* Metatarsalgia
  multiple sites M77.9
  patellar tendinitis — *see* Tendinitis, patellar
  pelvis M77.9
  periarthritis of wrist — *see* Periarthritis, wrist
  peroneal tendinitis — *see* Tendinitis, peroneal
  posterior tibial syndrome M76.82- ☑
  psoas tendinitis — *see* Tendinitis, psoas
  shoulder region — *see* Lesion, shoulder
  specified site NEC M77.9
  specified type NEC M77.8
  spinal M46.00
    cervical region M46.02
    cervicothoracic region M46.03

Enthesopathy — *continued*
  spinal — *continued*
    lumbar region M46.06
    lumbosacral region M46.07
    multiple sites M46.09
    occipito-atlanto-axial region M46.01
    sacrococcygeal region M46.08
    thoracic region M46.04
    thoracolumbar region M46.05
  tibial collateral bursitis — *see* Bursitis, tibial collateral
  upper arm M77.9
  wrist and carpus NEC M77.8
    calcaneal spur — *see* Spur, bone, calcaneal
    periarthritis of wrist — *see* Periarthritis, wrist
Entomophobia F40.218
Entomophthoromycosis B46.8
Entrance, air into vein — *see* Embolism, air
Entrapment, nerve — *see* Neuropathy, entrapment
Entropion (eyelid) (paralytic) H02.009
  cicatricial H02.019
    left H02.016
      lower H02.015
      upper H02.014
    right H02.013
      lower H02.012
      upper H02.011
  congenital Q10.2
  left H02.006
    lower H02.005
    upper H02.004
  mechanical H02.029
    left H02.026
      lower H02.025
      upper H02.024
    right H02.023
      lower H02.022
      upper H02.021
  right H02.003
    lower H02.002
    upper H02.001
  senile H02.039
    left H02.036
      lower H02.035
      upper H02.034
    right H02.033
      lower H02.032
      upper H02.031
  spastic H02.049
    left H02.046
      lower H02.045
      upper H02.044
    right H02.043
      lower H02.042
      upper H02.041
Enucleated eye (traumatic, current) S05.7- ☑
Enuresis R32
  functional F98.0
  habit disturbance F98.0
  nocturnal N39.44
    psychogenic F98.0
  nonorganic origin F98.0
  psychogenic F98.0
Eosinopenia — *see* Agranulocytosis
Eosinophilia (allergic) (hereditary) (idiopathic) (secondary) D72.1
  with
    angiolymphoid hyperplasia (ALHE) D18.01
  infiltrative J82
  Löffler's J82
  peritoneal — *see* Peritonitis, eosinophilic
  pulmonary NEC J82
  tropical (pulmonary) J82
Eosinophilia-myalgia syndrome M35.8
Ependymitis (acute) (cerebral) (chronic) (granular) —
  see Encephalomyelitis
Ependymoblastoma
  specified site — *see* Neoplasm, malignant, by site
  unspecified site C71.9
Ependymoma (epithelial) (malignant)
  anaplastic
    specified site — *see* Neoplasm, malignant, by site
    unspecified site C71.9
  benign
    specified site — *see* Neoplasm, benign, by site
    unspecified site D33.2
  myxopapillary D43.2
    specified site — *see* Neoplasm, uncertain behavior,
      by site

Ependymoma — *continued*
  myxopapillary — *continued*
    unspecified site D43.2
  papillary D43.2
    specified site — *see* Neoplasm, uncertain behavior,
      by site
    unspecified site D43.2
  specified site — *see* Neoplasm, malignant, by site
  unspecified site C71.9
Ependymopathy G93.89
Ephelis, ephelides L81.2
Epiblepharon (congenital) Q10.3
Epicanthus, epicanthic fold (eyelid) (congenital) Q10.3
Epicondylitis (elbow)
  lateral M77.1- ☑
  medial M77.0- ☑
Epicystitis — *see* Cystitis
Epidemic — *see* condition
Epidermidalization, cervix — *see* Dysplasia, cervix
Epidermis, epidermal — *see* condition
Epidermodysplasia verruciformis B07.8
Epidermolysis
  bullosa (congenital) Q81.9
    acquired L12.30
      drug-induced L12.31
        specified cause NEC L12.35
    dystrophica Q81.2
    letalis Q81.1
    simplex Q81.0
    specified NEC Q81.8
  necroticans combustiformis L51.2
    due to drug — *see* Table of Drugs and Chemicals,
      by drug
Epidermophytid — *see* Dermatophytosis
Epidermophytosis (infected) — *see* Dermatophytosis
Epididymis — *see* condition
Epididymitis (acute) (nonvenereal) (recurrent) (residual)
  N45.1
  with orchitis N45.3
  blennorrhagic (gonococcal) A54.23
  caseous (tuberculous) A18.15
  chlamydial A56.19
  filarial (*see also* Infestation, filarial) B74.9 [N51]
  gonococcal A54.23
  syphilitic A52.76
  tuberculous A18.15
Epididymo-orchitis (*see also* Epididymitis) N45.3
Epidural — *see* condition
Epigastrium, epigastric — *see* condition
Epigastrocele — *see* Hernia, ventral
Epiglottis — *see* condition
Epiglottitis, epiglottiditis (acute) J05.10
  with obstruction J05.11
  chronic J37.0
Epignathus Q89.4
Epilepsia partialis continua (*see also* Kozhevnikof's
  epilepsy) G40.1- ☑
Epilepsy, epileptic, epilepsia (attack) (cerebral) (con-
  vulsion) (fit) (seizure) G40.909

*Note: the following terms are to be considered
equivalent to intractable: pharmacoresistant
(pharmacologically resistant), treatment resistant,
refractory (medically) and poorly controlled*

  with
    complex partial seizures — *see* Epilepsy, localiza-
      tion-related, symptomatic, with complex
      partial seizures
    grand mal seizures on awakening — *see* Epilepsy,
      generalized, specified NEC
    myoclonic absences — *see* Epilepsy, generalized,
      specified NEC
    myoclonic-astatic seizures — *see* Epilepsy, gener-
      alized, specified NEC
    simple partial seizures — *see* Epilepsy, localization-
      related, symptomatic, with simple partial
      seizures
  akinetic — *see* Epilepsy, generalized, specified NEC
  benign childhood with centrotemporal EEG spikes —
    see Epilepsy, localization-related, idiopathic
  benign myoclonic in infancy G40.80- ☑
  Bravais-jacksonian — *see* Epilepsy, localization-related,
    symptomatic, with simple partial seizures
  childhood
    with occipital EEG paroxysms — *see* Epilepsy, local-
      ization-related, idiopathic
    absence G40.A09 (*following* G40.3)

Epilepsy, epileptic, epilepsia — *continued*
  childhood — *continued*
    absence — *continued*
      intractable G40.A19 (*following G40.3*)
        with status epilepticus G40.A11 (*following G40.3*)
        without status epilepticus G40.A19 (*following G40.3*)
      not intractable G40.A09 (*following G40.3*)
        with status epilepticus G40.A01 (*following G40.3*)
        without status epilepticus G40.A09 (*following G40.3*)
  climacteric — *see* Epilepsy, specified NEC
  cysticercosis B69.0
  deterioration (mental) F06.8
  due to syphilis A52.19
  focal — *see* Epilepsy, localization-related, symptomatic, with simple partial seizures
  generalized
    idiopathic G40.309
      intractable G40.319
        with status epilepticus G40.311
        without status epilepticus G40.319
      not intractable G40.309
        with status epilepticus G40.301
        without status epilepticus G40.309
    specified NEC G40.409
      intractable G40.419
        with status epilepticus G40.411
        without status epilepticus G40.419
      not intractable G40.409
        with status epilepticus G40.401
        without status epilepticus G40.409
  impulsive petit mal — *see* Epilepsy, juvenile myoclonic
  intractable G40.919
    with status epilepticus G40.911
    without status epilepticus G40.919
  juvenile absence G40.A09 (*following G40.3*)
    intractable G40.A19 (*following G40.3*)
      with status epilepticus G40.A11 (*following G40.3*)
      without status epilepticus G40.A19 (*following G40.3*)
    not intractable G40.A09 (*following G40.3*)
      with status epilepticus G40.A01 (*following G40.3*)
      without status epilepticus G40.A09 (*following G40.3*)
  juvenile myoclonic G40.B09 (*following G40.3*)
    intractable G40.B19 (*following G40.3*)
      with status epilepticus G40.B11 (*following G40.3*)
      without status epilepticus G40.B19 (*following G40.3*)
    not intractable G40.B09 (*following G40.3*)
      with status epilepticus G40.B01 (*following G40.3*)
      without status epilepticus G40.B09 (*following G40.3*)
  localization-related (focal) (partial)
    idiopathic G40.009
      with seizures of localized onset G40.009
        intractable G40.019
          with status epilepticus G40.011
          without status epilepticus G40.019
        not intractable G40.009
          with status epilepticus G40.001
          without status epilepticus G40.009
    symptomatic
      with complex partial seizures G40.209
        intractable G40.219
          with status epilepticus G40.211
          without status epilepticus G40.219
        not intractable G40.209
          with status epilepticus G40.201
          without status epilepticus G40.209
      with simple partial seizures G40.109
        intractable G40.119
          with status epilepticus G40.111
          without status epilepticus G40.119
        not intractable G40.109
          with status epilepticus G40.101
          without status epilepticus G40.109
  myoclonus, myoclonic — *see* Epilepsy, generalized, specified NEC
    progressive — *see* Epilepsy, generalized, idiopathic
  not intractable G40.909
    with status epilepticus G40.901

Epilepsy, epileptic, epilepsia — *continued*
  not intractable — *continued*
    without status epilepticus G40.909
  on awakening — *see* Epilepsy, generalized, specified NEC
  parasitic NOS B71.9 [G94]
  partialis continua (*see also* Kozhevnikof's epilepsy) G40.1- ☑
  peripheral — *see* Epilepsy, specified NEC
  procursiva — *see* Epilepsy, localization-related, symptomatic, with simple partial seizures
  progressive (familial) myoclonic — *see* Epilepsy, generalized, idiopathic
  reflex — *see* Epilepsy, specified NEC
  related to
    alcohol G40.509
      not intractable G40.509
        with status epilepticus G40.501
        without status epliepticus G40.509
    drugs G40.509
      not intractable G40.509
        with status epilepticus G40.501
        without status epilepticus G40.509
    external causes G40.509
      not intractable G40.509
        with status epilepticus G40.501
        without status epilepticus G40.509
    hormonal changes G40.509
      not intractable G40.509
        with status epilepticus G40.501
        without status epilepticus G40.509
    sleep deprivation G40.509
      not intractable G40.509
        with status epilepticus G40.501
        without status epilepticus G40.509
    stress G40.509
      not intractable G40.509
        with status epilepticus G40.501
        without status epliepticus G40.509
  somatomotor — *see* Epilepsy, localization-related, symptomatic, with simple partial seizures
  somatosensory — *see* Epilepsy, localization-related, symptomatic, with simple partial seizures
  spasms G40.822
    intractable G40.824
      with status epilepticus G40.823
      without status epilepticus G40.824
    not intractable G40.822
      with status epilepticus G40.821
      without status epilepticus G40.822
  specified NEC G40.802
    intractable G40.804
      with status epilepticus G40.803
      without status epilepticus G40.804
    not intractable G40.802
      with status epilepticus G40.801
      without status epilepticus G40.802
  syndromes
    generalized
      idiopathic G40.309
        intractable G40.319
          with status epilepticus G40.311
          without status epilepticus G40.319
        not intractable G40.309
          with status epilepticus G40.301
          without status epilepticus G40.309
      specified NEC G40.409
        intractable G40.419
          with status epilepticus G40.411
          without status epilepticus G40.419
        not intractable G40.409
          with status epilepticus G40.401
          without status epilepticus G40.409
    localization-related (focal) (partial)
      idiopathic G40.009
        with seizures of localized onset G40.009
          intractable G40.019
            with status epilepticus G40.011
            without status epilepticus G40.019
          not intractable G40.009
            with status epilepticus G40.001
            without status epilepticus G40.009
    symptomatic
      with complex partial seizures G40.209
        intractable G40.219
          with status epilepticus G40.211
          without status epilepticus G40.219
        not intractable G40.209

Epilepsy, epileptic, epilepsia — *continued*
  syndromes — *continued*
    localization-related — *continued*
      symptomatic — *continued*
        with complex partial seizures — *continued*
          not intractable — *continued*
            with status epilepticus G40.201
            without status epilepticus G40.209
        with simple partial seizures G40.109
          intractable G40.119
            with status epilepticus G40.111
            without status epilepticus G40.119
          not intractable G40.109
            with status epilepticus G40.101
            without status epilepticus G40.109
      specified NEC G40.802
        intractable G40.804
          with status epilepticus G40.803
          without status epilepticus G40.804
        not intractable G40.802
          with status epilepticus G40.801
          without status epilepticus G40.802
  tonic (-clonic) — *see* Epilepsy, generalized, specified NEC
  twilight F05
  uncinate (gyrus) — *see* Epilepsy, localization-related, symptomatic, with complex partial seizures
  Unverricht (-Lundborg) (familial myoclonic) — *see* Epilepsy, generalized, idiopathic
  visceral — *see* Epilepsy, specified NEC
  visual — *see* Epilepsy, specified NEC
Epiloia Q85.1
Epimenorrhea N92.0
Epipharyngitis — *see* Nasopharyngitis
Epiphora H04.20- ☑
  due to
    excess lacrimation H04.21- ☑
    insufficient drainage H04.22- ☑
Epiphyseal arrest — *see* Arrest, epiphyseal
Epiphyseolysis, epiphysiolysis — *see* Osteochondropathy
Epiphysitis (*see also* Osteochondropathy)
  juvenile M92.9
  syphilitic (congenital) A50.02
Epiplocele — *see* Hernia, abdomen
Epiploitis — *see* Peritonitis
Epiplosarcomphalocele — *see* Hernia, umbilicus
Episcleritis (suppurative) H15.10- ☑
  in (due to)
    syphilis A52.71
    tuberculosis A18.51
  nodular H15.12- ☑
  periodica fugax H15.11- ☑
    angioneurotic — *see* Edema, angioneurotic
  syphilitic (late) A52.71
  tuberculous A18.51
Episode
  affective, mixed F39
  depersonalization (in neurotic state) F48.1
  depressive F32.9
    major F32.9
      mild F32.0
      moderate F32.1
      severe (without psychotic symptoms) F32.2
        with psychotic symptoms F32.3
      recurrent F33.9
        brief F33.8
      specified NEC F32.89
  hypomanic F30.8
  manic F30.9
    with
      psychotic symptoms F30.2
      remission (full) F30.4
        partial F30.3
    without psychotic symptoms F30.10
      mild F30.11
      moderate F30.12
      severe (without psychotic symptoms) F30.13
        with psychotic symptoms F30.2
    other specified F30.8
    recurrent F31.89
  psychotic F23
    organic F06.8
  schizophrenic (acute) NEC, brief F23
Epispadias (female) (male) Q64.0
Episplenitis D73.89
Epistaxis (multiple) R04.0

Epistaxis — *continued*
  hereditary I78.0
  vicarious menstruation N94.89
Epithelioma (malignant) (*see also* Neoplasm, malignant, by site)
  adenoides cysticum — *see* Neoplasm, skin, benign
  basal cell — *see* Neoplasm, skin, malignant
  benign — *see* Neoplasm, benign, by site
  Bowen's — *see* Neoplasm, skin, in situ
  calcifying, of Malherbe — *see* Neoplasm, skin, benign
  external site — *see* Neoplasm, skin, malignant
  intraepidermal, Jadassohn — *see* Neoplasm, skin, benign
  squamous cell — *see* Neoplasm, malignant, by site
Epitheliomatosis pigmented Q82.1
Epitheliopathy, multifocal placoid pigment H30.14- ☑
Epithelium, epithelial — *see* condition
Epituberculosis (with atelectasis) (allergic) A15.7
Eponychia Q84.6
Epstein's
  nephrosis or syndrome — *see* Nephrosis
  pearl K09.8
Epulis (gingiva) (fibrous) (giant cell) K06.8
Equinia A24.0
Equinovarus (congenital) (talipes) Q66.0
  acquired — *see* Deformity, limb, clubfoot
Equivalent
  convulsive (abdominal) — *see* Epilepsy, specified NEC
  epileptic (psychic) — *see* Epilepsy, localization-related, symptomatic, with complex partial seizures
Erb (-Duchenne) **paralysis** (birth injury) (newborn) P14.0
Erb-Goldflam disease or syndrome G70.00
  with exacerbation (acute) G70.01
  in crisis G70.01
Erb's
  disease G71.0
  palsy, paralysis (brachial) (birth) (newborn) P14.0
    spinal (spastic) syphilitic A52.17
  pseudohypertrophic muscular dystrophy G71.0
Erdheim's syndrome (acromegalic macrospondylitis) E22.0
Erection, painful (persistent) — *see* Priapism
Ergosterol deficiency (vitamin D) E55.9
  with
    adult osteomalacia M83.8
    rickets — *see* Rickets
Ergotism (*see also* Poisoning, food, noxious, plant)
  from ergot used as drug (migraine therapy) — *see* Table of Drugs and Chemicals
Erosio interdigitalis blastomycetica B37.2
Erosion
  artery I77.2
    without rupture I77.89
  bone — *see* Disorder, bone, density and structure, specified NEC
  bronchus J98.09
  cartilage (joint) — *see* Disorder, cartilage, specified type NEC
  cervix (uteri) (acquired) (chronic) (congenital) N86
    with cervicitis N72
  cornea (nontraumatic) — *see* Ulcer, cornea
    recurrent H18.83- ☑
    traumatic — *see* Abrasion, cornea
  dental (idiopathic) (occupational) (due to diet, drugs or vomiting) K03.2
  duodenum, postpyloric — *see* Ulcer, duodenum
  esophagus K22.10
    with bleeding K22.11
  gastric — *see* Ulcer, stomach
  gastrojejunal — *see* Ulcer, gastrojejunal
  implanted mesh — *see* Complications, mesh
  intestine K63.3
  lymphatic vessel I89.8
  pylorus, pyloric (ulcer) — *see* Ulcer, stomach
  spine, aneurysmal A52.09
  stomach — *see* Ulcer, stomach
  subcutaneous device pocket
    nervous system prosthetic device, implant, or graft T85.890 ☑
    other internal prosthetic device, implant, or graft T85.898 ☑
  teeth (idiopathic) (occupational) (due to diet, drugs or vomiting) K03.2
  urethra N36.8
  uterus N85.8
Erotomania F52.8

Error
  metabolism, inborn — *see* Disorder, metabolism
  refractive — *see* Disorder, refraction
Eructation R14.2
  nervous or psychogenic F45.8
Eruption
  creeping B76.9
  drug (generalized) (taken internally) L27.0
    fixed L27.1
    in contact with skin — *see* Dermatitis, due to drugs
    localized L27.1
  Hutchinson, summer L56.4
  Kaposi's varicelliform B00.0
  napkin L22
  polymorphous light (sun) L56.4
  recalcitrant pustular L13.8
  ringed R23.8
  skin (nonspecific) R21
    creeping (meaning hookworm) B76.9
    due to inoculation/vaccination (generalized) (*see also* Dermatitis, due to, vaccine) L27.0
      localized L27.1
    erysipeloid A26.0
    feigned L98.1
    Kaposi's varicelliform B00.0
    lichenoid L28.0
    meaning dermatitis — *see* Dermatitis
    toxic NEC L53.0
  tooth, teeth, abnormal (incomplete) (late) (premature) (sequence) K00.6
  vesicular R23.8
Erysipelas (gangrenous) (infantile) (newborn) (phlegmonous) (suppurative) A46
  external ear A46 [H62.40]
  puerperal, postpartum O86.89
Erysipeloid A26.9
  cutaneous (Rosenbach's) A26.0
  disseminated A26.8
  sepsis A26.7
  specified NEC A26.8
Erythema, erythematous (infectional) (inflammation) L53.9
  ab igne L59.0
  annulare (centrifugum) (rheumaticum) L53.1
  arthriticum epidemicum A25.1
  brucellum — *see* Brucellosis
  chronic figurate NEC L53.3
  chronicum migrans (Borrelia burgdorferi) A69.20
  diaper L22
  due to
    chemical NEC L53.0
      in contact with skin L24.5
    drug (internal use) — *see* Dermatitis, due to, drugs
  elevatum diutinum L95.1
  endemic E52
  epidemic, arthritic A25.1
  figuratum perstans L53.3
  gluteal L22
  heat — *code by site under* Burn, first degree
  ichthyosiforme congenitum bullous Q80.3
  in diseases classified elsewhere L54
  induratum (nontuberculous) L52
    tuberculous A18.4
  infectiosum B08.3
  intertrigo L30.4
  iris L51.9
  marginatum L53.2
    in (due to) acute rheumatic fever I00
  medicamentosum — *see* Dermatitis, due to, drugs
  migrans A26.0
    chronicum A69.20
    tongue K14.1
  multiforme (major) (minor) L51.9
    bullous, bullosum L51.1
    conjunctiva L51.1
    nonbullous L51.0
    pemphigoides L12.0
    specified NEC L51.8
  napkin L22
  neonatorum P83.88
    toxic P83.1
  nodosum L52
    tuberculous A18.4
  palmar L53.8
  pernio T69.1 ☑
  rash, newborn P83.88
  scarlatiniform (recurrent) (exfoliative) L53.8
  solare L55.0

Erythema, erythematous — *continued*
  specified NEC L53.8
  toxic, toxicum NEC L53.0
    newborn P83.1
  tuberculous (primary) A18.4
Erythematous, erythematosus — *see* condition
Erythermalgia (primary) I73.81
Erythralgia I73.81
Erythrasma L08.1
Erythredema (polyneuropathy) — *see* Poisoning, mercury
Erythremia (acute) C94.0- ☑
  chronic D45
  secondary D75.1
Erythroblastopenia (*see also* Aplasia, red cell) D60.9
  congenital D61.01
Erythroblastophthisis D61.09
Erythroblastosis (fetalis) (newborn) P55.9
  due to
    ABO (antibodies) (incompatibility) (isoimmunization) P55.1
    Rh (antibodies) (incompatibility) (isoimmunization) P55.0
Erythrocyanosis (crurum) I73.89
Erythrocythemia — *see* Erythremia
Erythrocytosis (megalosplenic) (secondary) D75.1
  familial D75.0
  oval, hereditary — *see* Elliptocytosis
  secondary D75.1
  stress D75.1
Erythroderma (secondary) (*see also* Erythema) L53.9
  bullous ichthyosiform, congenital Q80.3
  desquamativum L21.1
  ichthyosiform, congenital (bullous) Q80.3
  neonatorum P83.88
  psoriaticum L40.8
Erythrodysesthesia, palmar plantar (PPE) L27.1
Erythrogenesis imperfecta D61.09
Erythroleukemia C94.0- ☑
Erythromelalgia I73.81
Erythrophagocytosis D75.89
Erythrophobia F40.298
Erythroplakia, oral epithelium, and tongue K13.29
Erythroplasia (Queyrat) D07.4
  specified site — *see* Neoplasm, skin, in situ
  unspecified site D07.4
Escherichia coli (E. coli), **as cause of disease classified elsewhere** B96.20
  non-O157 Shiga toxin-producing (with known O group) B96.22
  non-Shiga toxin-producing B96.29
  O157 B96.21
  O157 with confirmation of Shiga toxin when H antigen is unknown, or is not H7 B96.21
  O157:H- (nonmotile) with confirmation of Shiga toxin B96.21
  O157:H7 with or without confirmation of Shiga toxin-production B96.21
  Shiga toxin-producing (with unspecified O group) (STEC) B96.23
  specified NEC B96.29
Esophagismus K22.4
Esophagitis (acute) (alkaline) (chemical) (chronic) (infectional) (necrotic) (peptic) (postoperative) K20.9
  candidal B37.81
  due to gastrointestinal reflux disease K21.0
  eosinophilic K20.0
  reflux K21.0
  specified NEC K20.8
  tuberculous A18.83
  ulcerative K22.10
    with bleeding K22.11
Esophagocele K22.5
Esophagomalacia K22.8
Esophagospasm K22.4
Esophagostenosis K22.2
Esophagostomiasis B81.8
Esophagotracheal — *see* condition
Esophagus — *see* condition
Esophoria H50.51
  convergence, excess H51.12
  divergence, insufficiency H51.8
Esotropia — *see* Strabismus, convergent concomitant
Espundia B55.2
Essential — *see* condition
Esthesioneuroblastoma C30.0
Esthesioneurocytoma C30.0

Esthesioneuroepithelioma C30.0
Esthiomene A55
Estivo-autumnal malaria (fever) B50.9
Estrangement (marital) Z63.5
  parent-child NEC Z62.890
Estriasis — *see* Myiasis
Ethanolism — *see* Alcoholism
Etherism — *see* Dependence, drug, inhalant
Ethmoid, ethmoidal — *see* condition
Ethmoiditis (chronic) (nonpurulent) (purulent) (*see also* Sinusitis, ethmoidal)
  influenzal — *see* Influenza, with, respiratory manifestations NEC
  Woakes' J33.1
Ethylism — *see* Alcoholism
Eulenburg's disease (congenital paramyotonia) G71.19
Eumycetoma B47.0
Eunuchoidism E29.1
  hypogonadotropic E23.0
European blastomycosis — *see* Cryptococcosis
Eustachian — *see* condition
Evaluation (for) (of)
  development state
    adolescent Z00.3
    period of
      delayed growth in childhood Z00.70
        with abnormal findings Z00.71
      rapid growth in childhood Z00.2
      puberty Z00.3
  growth and developmental state (period of rapid growth) Z00.2
    delayed growth Z00.70
      with abnormal findings Z00.71
  mental health (status) Z00.8
    requested by authority Z04.6
  period of
    delayed growth in childhood Z00.70
      with abnormal findings Z00.71
    rapid growth in childhood Z00.2
  suspected condition — *see* Observation
Evans syndrome D69.41
Event
  apparent life threatening in newborn and infant (ALTE) R68.13
  brief resolved unexplained event (BRUE) R68.13
Eventration (*see also* Hernia, ventral)
  colon into chest — *see* Hernia, diaphragm
  diaphragm (congenital) Q79.1
Eversion
  bladder N32.89
  cervix (uteri) N86
    with cervicitis N72
  foot NEC (*see also* Deformity, valgus, ankle)
    congenital Q66.6
  punctum lacrimale (postinfectional) (senile) H04.52- ☑
  ureter (meatus) N28.89
  urethra (meatus) N36.8
  uterus N81.4
Evidence
  cytologic
    of malignancy on anal smear R85.614
    of malignancy on cervical smear R87.614
    of malignancy on vaginal smear R87.624
Evisceration
  birth injury P15.8
  traumatic NEC
    eye — *see* Enucleated eye
Evulsion — *see* Avulsion
Ewing's sarcoma or tumor — *see* Neoplasm, bone, malignant
Examination (for) (following) (general) (of) (routine) Z00.00
  with abnormal findings Z00.01
  abuse, physical (alleged), ruled out
    adult Z04.71
    child Z04.72
  adolescent (development state) Z00.3
  alleged rape or sexual assault (victim), ruled out
    adult Z04.41
    child Z04.42
  allergy Z01.82
  annual (adult) (periodic) (physical) Z00.00
    with abnormal findings Z00.01
    gynecological Z01.419
      with abnormal findings Z01.411
  antibody response Z01.84
  blood — *see* Examination, laboratory
  blood pressure Z01.30

Examination — *continued*
  blood pressure — *continued*
    with abnormal findings Z01.31
  cancer staging — *see* Neoplasm, malignant, by site
  cervical Papanicolaou smear Z12.4
    as part of routine gynecological examination Z01.419
    with abnormal findings Z01.411
  child (over 28 days old) Z00.129
    with abnormal findings Z00.121
    under 28 days old — *see* Newborn, examination
  clinical research control or normal comparison (control) (participant) Z00.6
  contraceptive (drug) maintenance (routine) Z30.8
    device (intrauterine) Z30.431
  dental Z01.20
    with abnormal findings Z01.21
  developmental — *see* Examination, child
  donor (potential) Z00.5
  ear Z01.10
    with abnormal findings NEC Z01.118
  eye Z01.00
    with abnormal findings Z01.01
  following
    accident NEC Z04.3
      transport Z04.1
      work Z04.2
    assault, alleged, ruled out
      adult Z04.71
      child Z04.72
    motor vehicle accident Z04.1
    treatment (for) Z09
      combined NEC Z09
        fracture Z09
        malignant neoplasm Z08
      malignant neoplasm Z08
      mental disorder Z09
      specified condition NEC Z09
  follow-up (routine) (following) Z09
    chemotherapy NEC Z09
      malignant neoplasm Z08
    fracture Z09
    malignant neoplasm Z08
    postpartum Z39.2
    psychotherapy Z09
    radiotherapy NEC Z09
      malignant neoplasm Z08
    surgery NEC Z09
      malignant neoplasm Z08
  gynecological Z01.419
    with abnormal findings Z01.411
    for contraceptive maintenance Z30.8
  health — *see* Examination, medical
  hearing Z01.10
    with abnormal findings NEC Z01.118
    following failed hearing screening Z01.110
  immunity status testing Z01.84
  laboratory (as part of a general medical examination) Z00.00
    with abnormal findings Z00.01
    preprocedural Z01.812
  lactating mother Z39.1
  medical (adult) (for) (of) Z00.00
    with abnormal findings Z00.01
    administrative purpose only Z02.9
      specified NEC Z02.89
    admission to
      armed forces Z02.3
      old age home Z02.2
      prison Z02.89
      residential institution Z02.2
      school Z02.0
        following illness or medical treatment Z02.0
      summer camp Z02.89
    adoption Z02.82
    blood alcohol or drug level Z02.83
    camp (summer) Z02.89
    clinical research, normal subject (control) (participant) Z00.6
    control subject in clinical research (normal comparison) (participant) Z00.6
    donor (potential) Z00.5
    driving license Z02.4
    general (adult) Z00.00
      with abnormal findings Z00.01
    immigration Z02.89
    insurance purposes Z02.6
    marriage Z02.89
    medicolegal reasons NEC Z04.8

Examination — *continued*
  medical — *continued*
    naturalization Z02.89
    participation in sport Z02.5
    paternity testing Z02.81
    population survey Z00.8
    pre-employment Z02.1
    pre-operative — *see* Examination, pre-procedural
    pre-procedural
      cardiovascular Z01.810
      respiratory Z01.811
      specified NEC Z01.818
    preschool children
      for admission to school Z02.0
    prisoners
      for entrance into prison Z02.89
    recruitment for armed forces Z02.3
    specified NEC Z00.8
    sport competition Z02.5
  medicolegal reason NEC Z04.8
  newborn — *see* Newborn, examination
  pelvic (annual) (periodic) Z01.419
    with abnormal findings Z01.411
  period of rapid growth in childhood Z00.2
  periodic (adult) (annual) (routine) Z00.00
    with abnormal findings Z00.01
  physical (adult) (*see also* Examination, medical) Z00.00
    sports Z02.5
  postpartum
    immediately after delivery Z39.0
    routine follow-up Z39.2
  pre-chemotherapy (antineoplastic) Z01.818
  prenatal (normal pregnancy) (*see also* Pregnancy, normal) Z34.9- ☑
  pre-procedural (pre-operative)
    cardiovascular Z01.810
    laboratory Z01.812
    respiratory Z01.811
    specified NEC Z01.818
  prior to chemotherapy (antineoplastic) Z01.818
  psychiatric NEC Z00.8
    follow-up not needing further care Z09
    requested by authority Z04.6
  radiological (as part of a general medical examination) Z00.00
    with abnormal findings Z00.01
  repeat cervical smear to confirm findings of recent normal smear following initial abnormal smear Z01.42
  skin (hypersensitivity) Z01.82
  special (*see also* Examination, by type) Z01.89
    specified type NEC Z01.89
  specified type or reason NEC Z04.8
  teeth Z01.20
    with abnormal findings Z01.21
  urine — *see* Examination, laboratory
  vision Z01.00
    with abnormal findings Z01.01
Exanthem, exanthema (*see also* Rash)
  with enteroviral vesicular stomatitis B08.4
  Boston A88.0
  epidemic with meningitis A88.0 [G02]
  subitum B08.20
    due to human herpesvirus 6 B08.21
    due to human herpesvirus 7 B08.22
  viral, virus B09
    specified type NEC B08.8
Excess, excessive, excessively
  alcohol level in blood R78.0
  androgen (ovarian) E28.1
  attrition, tooth, teeth K03.0
  carotene, carotin (dietary) E67.1
  cold, effects of T69.9 ☑
    specified effect NEC T69.8 ☑
  convergence H51.12
  crying
    in child, adolescent, or adult R45.83
    in infant R68.11
  development, breast N62
  divergence H51.8
  drinking (alcohol) NEC (without dependence) F10.10
    habitual (continual) (without remission) F10.20
  eating R63.2
  estrogen E28.0
  fat (*see also* Obesity)
    in heart — *see* Degeneration, myocardial
    localized E65
  foreskin N47.8

Excess, excessive, excessively — *continued*
  gas R14.0
  glucagon E16.3
  heat — *see* Heat
  intermaxillary vertical dimension of fully erupted teeth M26.37
  interocclusal distance of fully erupted teeth M26.37
  kalium E87.5
  large
    colon K59.39
      congenital Q43.8
    infant P08.0
    organ or site, congenital NEC — *see* Anomaly, by site
  long
    organ or site, congenital NEC — *see* Anomaly, by site
  menstruation (with regular cycle) N92.0
    with irregular cycle N92.1
  napping Z72.821
  natrium E87.0
  number of teeth K00.1
  nutrient (dietary) NEC R63.2
  potassium (K) E87.5
  salivation K11.7
  secretion (*see also* Hypersecretion)
    milk O92.6
    sputum R09.3
    sweat R61
  sexual drive F52.8
  short
    organ or site, congenital NEC — *see* Anomaly, by site
    umbilical cord in labor or delivery O69.3 ☑
  skin L98.7
    and subcutaneous tissue L98.7
    eyelid (acquired) — *see* Blepharochalasis
      congenital Q10.3
  sodium (Na) E87.0
  spacing of fully erupted teeth M26.32
  sputum R09.3
  sweating R61
  thirst R63.1
    due to deprivation of water T73.1 ☑
  tuberosity of jaw M26.07
  vitamin
    A (dietary) E67.0
      administered as drug (prolonged intake) — *see* Table of Drugs and Chemicals, vitamins, adverse effect
      overdose or wrong substance given or taken — *see* Table of Drugs and Chemicals, vitamins, poisoning
    D (dietary) E67.3
      administered as drug (prolonged intake) — *see* Table of Drugs and Chemicals, vitamins, adverse effect
      overdose or wrong substance given or taken — *see* Table of Drugs and Chemicals, vitamins, poisoning
  weight
    gain R63.5
    loss R63.4
Excitability, abnormal, under minor stress (personality disorder) F60.3
Excitation
  anomalous atrioventricular I45.6
  psychogenic F30.8
  reactive (from emotional stress, psychological trauma) F30.8
Excitement
  hypomanic F30.8
  manic F30.9
  mental, reactive (from emotional stress, psychological trauma) F30.8
  state, reactive (from emotional stress, psychological trauma) F30.8
Excoriation (traumatic) (*see also* Abrasion)
  neurotic L98.1
  skin picking disorder F42.4
Exfoliation
  due to erythematous conditions according to extent of body surface involved L49.0
    less than 10 percent of body surface L49.0
    10-19 percent of body surface L49.1
    20-29 percent of body surface L49.2
    30-39 percent of body surface L49.3
    40-49 percent of body surface L49.4

Exfoliation — *continued*
  due to erythematous conditions according to extent of body surface involved — *continued*
    50-59 percent of body surface L49.5
    60-69 percent of body surface L49.6
    70-79 percent of body surface L49.7
    80-89 percent of body surface L49.8
    90-99 percent of body surface L49.9
  teeth, due to systemic causes K08.0
Exfoliative — *see* condition
Exhaustion, exhaustive (physical NEC) R53.83
  battle F43.0
  cardiac — *see* Failure, heart
  delirium F43.0
  due to
    cold T69.8 ☑
    excessive exertion T73.3 ☑
    exposure T73.2 ☑
    neurasthenia F48.8
  heart — *see* Failure, heart
  heat (*see also* Heat, exhaustion) T67.5 ☑
    due to
      salt depletion T67.4 ☑
      water depletion T67.3 ☑
  maternal, complicating delivery O75.81
  mental F48.8
  myocardium, myocardial — *see* Failure, heart
  nervous F48.8
  old age R54
  psychogenic F48.8
  psychosis F43.0
  senile R54
  vital NEC Z73.0
Exhibitionism F65.2
Exocervicitis — *see* Cervicitis
Exomphalos Q79.2
  meaning hernia — *see* Hernia, umbilicus
Exophoria H50.52
  convergence, insufficiency H51.11
  divergence, excess H51.8
Exophthalmos H05.2- ☑
  congenital Q15.8
  constant NEC H05.24- ☑
  displacement, globe — *see* Displacement, globe
  due to thyrotoxicosis (hyperthyroidism) — *see* Hyperthyroidism, with, goiter (diffuse)
  dysthyroid — *see* Hyperthyroidism, with, goiter (diffuse)
  goiter — *see* Hyperthyroidism, with, goiter (diffuse)
  intermittent NEC H05.25- ☑
  malignant — *see* Hyperthyroidism, with, goiter (diffuse)
  orbital
    edema — *see* Edema, orbit
    hemorrhage — *see* Hemorrhage, orbit
  pulsating NEC H05.26- ☑
  thyrotoxic, thyrotropic — *see* Hyperthyroidism, with, goiter (diffuse)
Exostosis (*see also* Disorder, bone)
  cartilaginous — *see* Neoplasm, bone, benign
  congenital (multiple) Q78.6
  external ear canal H61.81- ☑
  gonococcal A54.49
  jaw (bone) M27.8
  multiple, congenital Q78.6
  orbit H05.35- ☑
  osteocartilaginous — *see* Neoplasm, bone, benign
  syphilitic A52.77
Exotropia — *see* Strabismus, divergent concomitant
Explanation of
  investigation finding Z71.2
  medication Z71.89
Exposure (to) (*see also* Contact, with) T75.89 ☑
  acariasis Z20.7
  AIDS virus Z20.6
  air pollution Z77.110
  algae and algae toxins Z77.121
  algae bloom Z77.121
  anthrax Z20.810
  aromatic amines Z77.020
  aromatic (hazardous) compounds NEC Z77.028
  aromatic dyes NOS Z77.028
  arsenic Z77.010
  asbestos Z77.090
  bacterial disease NEC Z20.818
  benzene Z77.021
  blue-green algae bloom Z77.121

Exposure — *continued*
  body fluids (potentially hazardous) Z77.21
  brown tide Z77.121
  chemicals (chiefly nonmedicinal) (hazardous) NEC Z77.098
  cholera Z20.09
  chromium compounds Z77.018
  cold, effects of T69.9 ☑
    specified effect NEC T69.8 ☑
  communicable disease Z20.9
    bacterial NEC Z20.818
    specified NEC Z20.89
    viral NEC Z20.828
  cyanobacteria bloom Z77.121
  disaster Z65.5
  discrimination Z60.5
  dyes Z77.098
  effects of T73.9 ☑
  environmental tobacco smoke (acute) (chronic) Z77.22
  Escherichia coli (E. coli) Z20.01
  exhaustion due to T73.2 ☑
  fiberglass — *see* Table of Drugs and Chemicals, fiberglass
  German measles Z20.4
  gonorrhea Z20.2
  hazardous metals NEC Z77.018
  hazardous substances NEC Z77.29
  hazards in the physical environment NEC Z77.128
  hazards to health NEC Z77.9
  human immunodeficiency virus (HIV) Z20.6
  human T-lymphotropic virus type-1 (HTLV-1) Z20.89
  implanted
    mesh — *see* Complications, mesh
    prosthetic materials NEC — *see* Complications, prosthetic materials NEC
  infestation (parasitic) NEC Z20.7
  intestinal infectious disease NEC Z20.09
    Escherichia coli (E. coli) Z20.01
  lead Z77.011
  meningococcus Z20.811
  mold (toxic) Z77.120
  nickel dust Z77.018
  noise Z77.122
  occupational
    air contaminants NEC Z57.39
    dust Z57.2
    environmental tobacco smoke Z57.31
    extreme temperature Z57.6
    noise Z57.0
    radiation Z57.1
    risk factors Z57.9
      specified NEC Z57.8
    toxic agents (gases) (liquids) (solids) (vapors) in agriculture Z57.4
    toxic agents (gases) (liquids) (solids) (vapors) in industry NEC Z57.5
    vibration Z57.7
  parasitic disease NEC Z20.7
  pediculosis Z20.7
  persecution Z60.5
  pfiesteria piscicida Z77.121
  poliomyelitis Z20.89
  pollution
    air Z77.110
    environmental NEC Z77.118
    soil Z77.112
    water Z77.111
  polycyclic aromatic hydrocarbons Z77.028
  prenatal (drugs) (toxic chemicals) — *see* Newborn, affected by, noxious substances transmitted via placenta or breast milk
  rabies Z20.3
  radiation, naturally occurring NEC Z77.123
  radon Z77.123
  red tide (Florida) Z77.121
  rubella Z20.4
  second hand tobacco smoke (acute) (chronic) Z77.22
    in the perinatal period P96.81
  sexually-transmitted disease Z20.2
  smallpox (laboratory) Z20.89
  syphilis Z20.2
  terrorism Z65.4
  torture Z65.4
  tuberculosis Z20.1
  uranium Z77.012
  varicella Z20.820
  venereal disease Z20.2
  viral disease NEC Z20.828

Exposure — *continued*
  war Z65.5
  water pollution Z77.111
Exsanguination — *see* Hemorrhage
Exstrophy
  abdominal contents Q45.8
  bladder Q64.10
    cloacal Q64.12
    specified type NEC Q64.19
    supravesical fissure Q64.11
Extensive — *see* condition
Extra (*see also* Accessory)
  marker chromosomes (normal individual) Q92.61
    in abnormal individual Q92.62
  rib Q76.6
    cervical Q76.5
Extrasystoles (supraventricular) I49.49
  atrial I49.1
  auricular I49.1
  junctional I49.2
  ventricular I49.3
Extrauterine gestation or pregnancy — *see* Pregnancy, by site
Extravasation
  blood R58
  chyle into mesentery I89.8
  pelvicalyceal N13.8
  pyelosinus N13.8
  urine (from ureter) R39.0
  vesicant agent
    antineoplastic chemotherapy T80.810 ☑
    other agent NEC T80.818 ☑
Extremity — *see* condition, limb
Extrophy — *see* Exstrophy
Extroversion
  bladder Q64.19
  uterus N81.4
    complicating delivery O71.2
    postpartal (old) N81.4
Extruded tooth (teeth) M26.34
Extrusion
  breast implant (prosthetic) T85.42 ☑
  eye implant (globe) (ball) T85.328 ☑
  intervertebral disc — *see* Displacement, intervertebral disc
  ocular lens implant (prosthetic) — *see* Complications, intraocular lens
  vitreous — *see* Prolapse, vitreous
Exudate
  pleural — *see* Effusion, pleura
  retina H35.89
Exudative — *see* condition
Eye, eyeball, eyelid — *see* condition
Eyestrain — *see* Disturbance, vision, subjective
Eyeworm disease of Africa B74.3

F

Faber's syndrome (achlorhydric anemia) D50.9
Fabry (-Anderson) **disease** E75.21
Faciocephalalgia, autonomic (*see also* Neuropathy, peripheral, autonomic) G90.09
Factor(s)
  psychic, associated with diseases classified elsewhere F54
  psychological
    affecting physical conditions F54
    or behavioral
      affecting general medical condition F54
      associated with disorders or diseases classified elsewhere F54
Fahr disease (of brain) G23.8
Fahr Volhard disease (of kidney) I12.- ☑
Failure, failed
  abortion — *see* Abortion, attempted
  aortic (valve) I35.8
    rheumatic I06.8
  attempted abortion — *see* Abortion, attempted
  biventricular I50.82
    due to left heart failure I50.814
  bone marrow — *see* Anemia, aplastic
  cardiac — *see* Failure, heart
  cardiorenal (chronic) (*see also* Failure, renal, and Failure, heart) I50.9
    hypertensive I13.2
  cardiorespiratory (*see also* Failure, heart) R09.2
  cardiovascular (chronic) — *see* Failure, heart

Failure, failed — *continued*
  cerebrovascular I67.9
  cervical dilatation in labor O62.0
  circulation, circulatory (peripheral) R57.9
    newborn P29.89
  compensation — *see* Disease, heart
  compliance with medical treatment or regimen — *see* Noncompliance
  congestive — *see* Failure, heart, congestive
  dental implant (endosseous) M27.69
    due to
      failure of dental prosthesis M27.63
      lack of attached gingiva M27.62
      occlusal trauma (poor prosthetic design) M27.62
      parafunctional habits M27.62
      periodontal infection (peri-implantitis) M27.62
      poor oral hygiene M27.62
    osseointegration M27.61
      due to
        complications of systemic disease M27.61
        poor bone quality M27.61
      iatrogenic M27.61
    post-osseointegration
      biological M27.62
      due to complications of systemic disease M27.62
      iatrogenic M27.62
      mechanical M27.63
    pre-integration M27.61
    pre-osseointegration M27.61
    specified NEC M27.69
  descent of head (at term) of pregnancy (mother) O32.4 ☑
  endosseous dental implant — *see* Failure, dental implant
  engagement of head (term of pregnancy) (mother) O32.4 ☑
  erection (penile) (*see also* Dysfunction, sexual, male, erectile) N52.9
    nonorganic F52.21
  examination(s), anxiety concerning Z55.2
  expansion terminal respiratory units (newborn) (primary) P28.0
  forceps NOS (with subsequent cesarean delivery) O66.5
  gain weight (child over 28 days old) R62.51
    adult R62.7
    newborn P92.6
  genital response (male) F52.21
    female F52.22
  heart (acute) (senile) (sudden) I50.9
    with
      acute pulmonary edema — *see* Failure, ventricular, left
      decompensation (*see also* Failure, heart, by type as diastolic or systolic, acute and chronic) I50.9
      dilatation — *see* Disease, heart
      normal ejection fraction — *see* Failure, heart, diastolic
      preserved ejection fraction — *see* Failure, heart, diastolic
      reduced ejection fraction — *see* Failure, heart, systolic
    arteriosclerotic I70.90
    biventricular I50.82
      due to left heart failure I50.814
    combined left-right sided I50.82
      due to left heart failure I50.814
    compensated (*see also* Failure, heart, by type as diastolic or systolic, chronic) I50.9
    complicating
      anesthesia (general) (local) or other sedation in labor and delivery O74.2
        in pregnancy O29.12- ☑
        postpartum, puerperal O89.1
      delivery (cesarean) (instrumental) O75.4
    congestive I50.9
      with rheumatic fever (conditions in I00)
        active I01.8
        inactive or quiescent (with chorea) I09.81
      newborn P29.0
      rheumatic (chronic) (inactive) (with chorea) I09.81
        active or acute I01.8
          with chorea I02.0
    decompensated (*see also* Failure, heart, by type as diastolic or systolic, acute and chronic) I50.9

Failure, failed — *continued*
  heart — *continued*
    degenerative — *see* Degeneration, myocardial
    diastolic (congestive) (left ventricular) I50.30
      acute (congestive) I50.31
        and (on) chronic (congestive) I50.33
      chronic (congestive) I50.32
        and (on) acute (congestive) I50.33
      combined with systolic (congestive) I50.40
        acute (congestive) I50.41
          and (on) chronic (congestive) I50.43
        chronic (congestive) I50.42
          and (on) acute (congestive) I50.43
    due to presence of cardiac prosthesis I97.13- ☑
    end stage (*see also* Failure, heart, type as diastolic or systolic, chronic) I50.84
    following cardiac surgery I97.13- ☑
    high output NOS I50.83
    hypertensive — *see* Hypertension, heart
    left (ventricular) (*see also* Failure, ventricular, left)
      combined diastolic and systolic — *see* Failure, heart, diastolic, combined with systolic
      diastolic — *see* Failure, heart, diastolic
      systolic — *see* Failure, heart, systolic
    low output (syndrome) NOS I50.9
    newborn P29.0
    organic — *see* Disease, heart
    peripartum O90.3
    postprocedural I97.13- ☑
    rheumatic (chronic) (inactive) I09.9
    right (isolated) (ventricular) I50.810
      acute I50.811
        and (on) chronic I50.813
      chronic I50.812
        and acute I50.813
      secondary to left heart failure I50.814
    specified NEC I50.89

> Note: heart failure stages A, B, C, and D are based on the American College of Cardiology and American Heart Association stages of heart failure, which complement and should not be confused with the New York Heart Association Classification of Heart Failure, into Class I, Class II, Class III, and Class IV

    stage A Z91.89
    stage B (*see also* Failure, heart, by type as diastolic or systolic) I50.9
    stage C (*see also* Failure, heart, by type as diastolic or systolic) I50.9
    stage D (*see also* Failure, heart, by type as diastolic or systolic, chronic) I50.84
    systolic (congestive) (left ventricular) I50.20
      acute (congestive) I50.21
        and (on) chronic (congestive) I50.23
      chronic (congestive) I50.22
        and (on) acute (congestive) I50.23
      combined with diastolic (congestive) I50.40
        acute (congestive) I50.41
          and (on) chronic (congestive) I50.43
        chronic (congestive) I50.42
          and (on) acute (congestive) I50.43
    thyrotoxic (*see also* Thyrotoxicosis) E05.90 [I43]
      with
        high output (*see also* Thyrotoxicosis) I50.83
        thyroid storm E05.91 [I43]
          high output (*see also* Thyrotoxicosis) I50.83
    valvular — *see* Endocarditis
  hepatic K72.90
    with coma K72.91
    acute or subacute K72.00
      with coma K72.01
      due to drugs K71.10
        with coma K71.11
    alcoholic (acute) (chronic) (subacute) K70.40
      with coma K70.41
    chronic K72.10
      with coma K72.11
      due to drugs (acute) (subacute) (chronic) K71.10
        with coma K71.11
    due to drugs (acute) (subacute) (chronic) K71.10
      with coma K71.11
    postprocedural K91.82
  hepatorenal K76.7
  induction (of labor) O61.9
    abortion — *see* Abortion, attempted
    by
      oxytocic drugs O61.0

☜ Subterms under main terms may continue to next column or page   ☑ Additional Character Required — Refer to the Tabular List for Character Selection   139

Exposure — Failure, failed

Failure, failed — *continued*
  induction — *continued*
    by — *continued*
      prostaglandins O61.0
    instrumental O61.1
    mechanical O61.1
    medical O61.0
    specified NEC O61.8
    surgical O61.1
  intubation during anesthesia T88.4 ☑
    in pregnancy O29.6- ☑
    labor and delivery O74.7
    postpartum, puerperal O89.6
  involution, thymus (gland) E32.0
  kidney (*see also* Disease, kidney, chronic) N19
    acute (*see also* Failure, renal, acute) N17.9
  lactation (complete) O92.3
    partial O92.4
  Leydig's cell, adult E29.1
  liver — *see* Failure, hepatic
  menstruation at puberty N91.0
  mitral I05.8
  myocardial, myocardium (*see also* Failure, heart) I50.9
    chronic (*see also* Failure, heart, congestive) I50.9
    congestive (*see also* Failure, heart, congestive) I50.9
  orgasm (female) (psychogenic) F52.31
    male F52.32
  ovarian (primary) E28.39
    iatrogenic E89.40
      asymptomatic E89.40
      symptomatic E89.41
    postprocedural (postablative) (postirradiation) (postsurgical) E89.40
      asymptomatic E89.40
      symptomatic E89.41
  ovulation causing infertility N97.0
  polyglandular, autoimmune E31.0
  prosthetic joint implant — *see* Complications, joint prosthesis, mechanical, breakdown, by site
  renal N19
    with
      tubular necrosis (acute) N17.0
    acute N17.9
      with
        cortical necrosis N17.1
        medullary necrosis N17.2
        tubular necrosis N17.0
      specified NEC N17.8
    chronic N18.9
      hypertensive — *see* Hypertension, kidney
    congenital P96.0
    end stage (chronic) N18.6
      due to hypertension I12.0
    following
      abortion — *see* Abortion by type complicated by specified condition NEC
      crushing T79.5 ☑
      ectopic or molar pregnancy O08.4
      labor and delivery (acute) O90.4
    hypertensive — *see* Hypertension, kidney
    postprocedural N99.0
  respiration, respiratory J96.90
    with
      hypercapnia J96.92
      hypercarbia J96.02
      hypoxia J96.91
    acute J96.00
      with
        hypercapnia J96.02
        hypercarbia J96.02
        hypoxia J96.01
    acute and (on) chronic J96.20
      with
        hypercapnia J96.22
        hypercarbia J96.22
        hypoxia J96.21
    center G93.89
    chronic J96.10
      with
        hypercapnia J96.12
        hypercarbia J96.12
        hypoxia J96.11
    newborn P28.5
    postprocedural (acute) J95.821
      acute and chronic J95.822
  rotation
    cecum Q43.3
    colon Q43.3

Failure, failed — *continued*
  rotation — *continued*
    intestine Q43.3
    kidney Q63.2
  sedation (conscious) (moderate) during procedure T88.52 ☑
    history of Z92.83
  segmentation (*see also* Fusion)
    fingers — *see* Syndactylism, complex, fingers
    vertebra Q76.49
      with scoliosis Q76.3
  seminiferous tubule, adult E29.1
  senile (general) R54
  sexual arousal (male) F52.21
    female F52.22
  testicular endocrine function E29.1
  to thrive (child over 28 days old) R62.51
    adult R62.7
    newborn P92.6
  transplant T86.92
    bone T86.831
      marrow T86.02
    cornea T86.841
    heart T86.22
      with lung(s) T86.32
    intestine T86.851
    kidney T86.12
    liver T86.42
    lung(s) T86.811
      with heart T86.32
    pancreas T86.891
    skin (allograft) (autograft) T86.821
    specified organ or tissue NEC T86.891
    stem cell (peripheral blood) (umbilical cord) T86.5
  trial of labor (with subsequent cesarean delivery) O66.40
    following previous cesarean delivery O66.41
  tubal ligation N99.89
  urinary — *see* Disease, kidney, chronic
  vacuum extraction NOS (with subsequent cesarean delivery) O66.5
  vasectomy N99.89
  ventouse NOS (with subsequent cesarean delivery) O66.5
  ventricular (*see also* Failure, heart) I50.9
    left (*see also* Failure, heart, left) I50.1
      with rheumatic fever (conditions in I00)
        active I01.8
          with chorea I02.0
        inactive or quiescent (with chorea) I09.81
        rheumatic (chronic) (inactive) (with chorea) I09.81
          active or acute I01.8
            with chorea I02.0
    right — *see* Failure, heart, right
  vital centers, newborn P91.88
Fainting (fit) R55
Fallen arches — *see* Deformity, limb, flat foot
Falling, falls (repeated) R29.6
  any organ or part — *see* Prolapse
Fallopian
  insufflation Z31.41
  tube — *see* condition
Fallot's
  pentalogy Q21.8
  tetrad or tetralogy Q21.3
  triad or trilogy Q22.3
False (*see also* condition)
  croup J38.5
  joint — *see* Nonunion, fracture
  labor (pains) O47.9
    at or after 37 completed weeks of gestation O47.1
    before 37 completed weeks of gestation O47.0- ☑
  passage, urethra (prostatic) N36.5
  pregnancy F45.8
Family, familial (*see also* condition)
  disruption Z63.8
    involving divorce or separation Z63.5
  Li-Fraumeni (syndrome) Z15.01
  planning advice Z30.09
  problem Z63.9
    specified NEC Z63.8
  retinoblastoma C69.2- ☑
Famine (effects of) T73.0 ☑
  edema — *see* Malnutrition, severe
Fanconi (-de Toni)(-Debré) **syndrome** E72.09
  with cystinosis E72.04
Fanconi's anemia (congenital pancytopenia) D61.09

Farber's disease or syndrome E75.29
Farcy A24.0
Farmer's
  lung J67.0
  skin L57.8
Farsightedness — *see* Hypermetropia
Fascia — *see* condition
Fasciculation R25.3
Fasciitis M72.9
  diffuse (eosinophilic) M35.4
  infective M72.8
    necrotizing M72.6
  necrotizing M72.6
  nodular M72.4
  perirenal (with ureteral obstruction) N13.5
    with infection N13.6
  plantar M72.2
  specified NEC M72.8
  traumatic (old) M72.8
    current — *code by* site under Sprain
Fascioliasis B66.3
Fasciolopsis, fasciolopsiasis (intestinal) B66.5
Fascioscapulohumeral myopathy G71.0
Fast pulse R00.0
Fat
  embolism — *see* Embolism, fat
  excessive (*see also* Obesity)
    in heart — *see* Degeneration, myocardial
  in stool R19.5
  localized (pad) E65
    heart — *see* Degeneration, myocardial
    knee M79.4
    retropatellar M79.4
  necrosis
    breast N64.1
    mesentery K65.4
    omentum K65.4
  pad E65
    knee M79.4
Fatigue R53.83
  auditory deafness — *see* Deafness
  chronic R53.82
  combat F43.0
  general R53.83
    psychogenic F48.8
  heat (transient) T67.6 ☑
  muscle M62.89
  myocardium — *see* Failure, heart
  neoplasm-related R53.0
  nervous, neurosis F48.8
  operational F48.8
  psychogenic (general) F48.8
  senile R54
  voice R49.8
Fatness — *see* Obesity
Fatty (*see also* condition)
  apron E65
  degeneration — *see* Degeneration, fatty
  heart (enlarged) — *see* Degeneration, myocardial
  liver NEC K76.0
    alcoholic K70.0
    nonalcoholic K76.0
  necrosis — *see* Degeneration, fatty
Fauces — *see* condition
Fauchard's disease (periodontitis) — *see* Periodontitis
Faucitis J02.9
Favism (anemia) D55.0
Favus — *see* Dermatophytosis
Fazio-Londe disease or syndrome G12.1
Fear complex or reaction F40.9
Fear of — *see* Phobia
Feared complaint unfounded Z71.1
Febris, febrile (*see also* Fever)
  flava (*see also* Fever, yellow) A95.9
  melitensis A23.0
  pestis — *see* Plague
  recurrens — *see* Fever, relapsing
  rubra A38.9
Fecal
  incontinence R15.9
  smearing R15.1
  soiling R15.1
  urgency R15.2
Fecalith (impaction) K56.41
  appendix K38.1
  congenital P76.8
Fede's disease K14.0

Feeble rapid pulse due to shock following injury
  T79.4 ☑
Feeble-minded F70
Feeding
  difficulties R63.3
  problem R63.3
    newborn P92.9
      specified NEC P92.8
    nonorganic (adult) — see Disorder, eating
Feeling (of)
  foreign body in throat R09.89
Feer's disease — see Poisoning, mercury
Feet — see condition
Feigned illness Z76.5
Feil-Klippel syndrome (brevicollis) Q76.1
Feinmesser's (hidrotic) **ectodermal dysplasia** Q82.4
Felinophobia F40.218
Felon (see also Cellulitis, digit)
  with lymphangitis — see Lymphangitis, acute, digit
Felty's syndrome M05.00
  ankle M05.07- ☑
  elbow M05.02- ☑
  foot joint M05.07- ☑
  hand joint M05.04- ☑
  hip M05.05- ☑
  knee M05.06- ☑
  multiple site M05.09
  shoulder M05.01- ☑
  vertebra — see Spondylitis, ankylosing
  wrist M05.03- ☑
Female genital cutting status — see Female genital
    mutilation status (FGM)
Female genital mutilation status (FGM) N90.810
  specified NEC N90.818
  type I (clitorectomy status) N90.811
  type II (clitorectomy with excision of labia minora sta-
    tus) N90.812
  type III (infibulation status) N90.813
  type IV N90.818
Femur, femoral — see condition
Fenestration, fenestrated (see also Imperfect, closure)
  aortico-pulmonary Q21.4
  cusps, heart valve NEC Q24.8
    pulmonary Q22.3
  pulmonic cusps Q22.3
Fernell's disease (aortic aneurysm) I71.9
Fertile eunuch syndrome E23.0
Fetid
  breath R19.6
  sweat L75.0
Fetishism F65.0
  transvestic F65.1
Fetus, fetal (see also condition)
  alcohol syndrome (dysmorphic) Q86.0
  compressus O31.0- ☑
  hydantoin syndrome Q86.1
  lung tissue P28.0
  papyraceous O31.0- ☑
Fever (inanition) (of unknown origin) (persistent) (with
    chills) (with rigor) R50.9
  abortus A23.1
  Aden (dengue) A90
  African tick-borne A68.1
  American
    mountain (tick) A93.2
    spotted A77.0
  aphthous B08.8
  arbovirus, arboviral A94
    hemorrhagic A94
    specified NEC A93.8
  Argentinian hemorrhagic A96.0
  Assam B55.0
  Australian Q A78
  Bangkok hemorrhagic A91
  Barmah forest A92.8
  Bartonella A44.0
  bilious, hemoglobinuric B50.8
  blackwater B50.8
  blister B00.1
  Bolivian hemorrhagic A96.1
  Bonvale dam T73.3 ☑
  boutonneuse A77.1
  brain — see Encephalitis
  Brazilian purpuric A48.4
  breakbone A90
  Bullis A77.0
  Bunyamwera A92.8

Fever — continued
  Burdwan B55.0
  Bwamba A92.8
  Cameroon — see Malaria
  Canton A75.9
  catarrhal (acute) J00
    chronic J31.0
  cat-scratch A28.1
  Central Asian hemorrhagic A98.0
  cerebral — see Encephalitis
  cerebrospinal meningococcal A39.0
  Chagres B50.9
  Chandipura A92.8
  Changuinola A93.1
  Charcot's (biliary) (hepatic) (intermittent) — see Calcu-
    lus, bile duct
  Chikungunya (viral) (hemorrhagic) A92.0
  Chitral A93.1
  Colombo — see Fever, paratyphoid
  Colorado tick (virus) A93.2
  congestive (remittent) — see Malaria
  Congo virus A98.0
  continued malarial B50.9
  Corsican — see Malaria
  Crimean-Congo hemorrhagic A98.0
  Cyprus — see Brucellosis
  dandy A90
  deer fly — see Tularemia
  dengue (virus) A90
    hemorrhagic A91
    sandfly A93.1
  desert B38.0
  drug induced R50.2
  due to
    conditions classified elsewhere R50.81
    heat T67.0 ☑
  enteric A01.00
  enteroviral exanthematous (Boston exanthem) A88.0
  ephemeral (of unknown origin) R50.9
  epidemic hemorrhagic A98.5
  erysipelatous — see Erysipelas
  estivo-autumnal (malarial) B50.9
  famine A75.0
  five day A79.0
  following delivery O86.4
  Fort Bragg A27.89
  gastroenteric A01.00
  gastromalarial — see Malaria
  Gibraltar — see Brucellosis
  glandular — see Mononucleosis, infectious
  Guama (viral) A92.8
  Haverhill A25.1
  hay (allergic) J30.1
    with asthma (bronchial) J45.909
      with
        exacerbation (acute) J45.901
        status asthmaticus J45.902
    due to
      allergen other than pollen J30.89
      pollen, any plant or tree J30.1
  heat (effects) T67.0 ☑
  hematuric, bilious B50.8
  hemoglobinuric (malarial) (bilious) B50.8
  hemorrhagic (arthropod-borne) NOS A94
    with renal syndrome A98.5
    arenaviral A96.9
      specified NEC A96.8
    Argentinian A96.0
    Bangkok A91
    Bolivian A96.1
    Central Asian A98.0
    Chikungunya A92.0
    Crimean-Congo A98.0
    dengue (virus) A91
    epidemic A98.5
    Junin (virus) A96.0
    Korean A98.5
    Kyasanur forest A98.2
    Machupo (virus) A96.1
    mite-borne A93.8
    mosquito-borne A92.8
    Omsk A98.1
    Philippine A91
    Russian A98.5
    Singapore A91
    Southeast Asia A91
    Thailand A91
    tick-borne NEC A93.8

Fever — continued
  hemorrhagic — continued
    viral A99
      specified NEC A98.8
  hepatic — see Cholecystitis
  herpetic — see Herpes
  icterohemorrhagic A27.0
  Indiana A93.8
  infective B99.9
    specified NEC B99.8
  intermittent (bilious) (see also Malaria)
    of unknown origin R50.9
    pernicious B50.9
  iodide R50.2
  Japanese river A75.3
  jungle (see also Malaria)
    yellow A95.0
  Junin (virus) hemorrhagic A96.0
  Katayama B65.2
  kedani A75.3
  Kenya (tick) A77.1
  Kew Garden A79.1
  Korean hemorrhagic A98.5
  Lassa A96.2
  Lone Star A77.0
  Machupo (virus) hemorrhagic A96.1
  malaria, malarial — see Malaria
  Malta A23.9
  Marseilles A77.1
  marsh — see Malaria
  Mayaro (viral) A92.8
  Mediterranean (see also Brucellosis) A23.9
    familial M04.1
    tick A77.1
  meningeal — see Meningitis
  Meuse A79.0
  Mexican A75.2
  mianeh A68.1
  miasmatic — see Malaria
  mosquito-borne (viral) A92.9
    hemorrhagic A92.8
  mountain (see also Brucellosis)
    meaning Rocky Mountain spotted fever A77.0
    tick (American) (Colorado) (viral) A93.2
  Mucambo (viral) A92.8
  mud A27.9
  Neapolitan — see Brucellosis
  neutropenic D70.9
  newborn P81.9
    environmental P81.0
  Nine-Mile A78
  non-exanthematous tick A93.2
  North Asian tick-borne A77.2
  Omsk hemorrhagic A98.1
  O'nyong-nyong (viral) A92.1
  Oropouche (viral) A93.0
  Oroya A44.0
  paludal — see Malaria
  Panama (malarial) B50.9
  Pappataci A93.1
  paratyphoid A01.4
    A A01.1
    B A01.2
    C A01.3
  parrot A70
  periodic (Mediterranean) M04.1
  persistent (of unknown origin) R50.9
  petechial A39.0
  pharyngoconjunctival B30.2
  Philippine hemorrhagic A91
  phlebotomus A93.1
  Piry (virus) A93.8
  Pixuna (viral) A92.8
  Plasmodium ovale B53.0
  polioviral (nonparalytic) A80.4
  Pontiac A48.2
  postimmunization R50.83
  postoperative R50.82
    due to infection T81.4 ☑
  posttransfusion R50.84
  postvaccination R50.83
  presenting with conditions classified elsewhere R50.81
  pretibial A27.89
  puerperal O86.4
  Q A78
  quadrilateral A78
  quartan (malaria) B52.9
  Queensland (coastal) (tick) A77.3

Fever — *continued*
  quintan A79.0
  rabbit — *see* Tularemia
  rat-bite A25.9
    due to
      Spirillum A25.0
      Streptobacillus moniliformis A25.1
  recurrent — *see* Fever, relapsing
  relapsing (Borrelia) A68.9
    Carter's (Asiatic) A68.1
    Dutton's (West African) A68.1
    Koch's A68.9
    louse-borne A68.0
    Novy's
      louse-borne A68.0
      tick-borne A68.1
    Obermeyer's (European) A68.0
    tick-borne A68.1
  remittent (bilious) (congestive) (gastric) — *see* Malaria
  rheumatic (active) (acute) (chronic) (subacute) I00
    with central nervous system involvement I02.9
    active with heart involvement — *see* category
        I01 ☑
    inactive or quiescent with
      cardiac hypertrophy I09.89
      carditis I09.9
      endocarditis I09.1
        aortic (valve) I06.9
          with mitral (valve) disease I08.0
        mitral (valve) I05.9
          with aortic (valve) disease I08.0
        pulmonary (valve) I09.89
        tricuspid (valve) I07.8
      heart disease NEC I09.89
      heart failure (congestive) (conditions in I50.)
          I09.81
      left ventricular failure (conditions in I50.1-I50.4-)
          I09.81
      myocarditis, myocardial degeneration (condi-
          tions in I51.4) I09.0
      pancarditis I09.9
      pericarditis I09.2
  Rift Valley (viral) A92.4
  Rocky Mountain spotted A77.0
  rose J30.1
  Ross River B33.1
  Russian hemorrhagic A98.5
  San Joaquin (Valley) B38.0
  sandfly A93.1
  Sao Paulo A77.0
  scarlet A38.9
  seven day (leptospirosis) (autumnal) (Japanese) A27.89
    dengue A90
  shin-bone A79.0
  Singapore hemorrhagic A91
  solar A90
  Songo A98.5
  sore B00.1
  South African tick-bite A68.1
  Southeast Asia hemorrhagic A91
  spinal — *see* Meningitis
  spirillary A25.0
  splenic — *see* Anthrax
  spotted A77.9
    American A77.0
    Brazilian A77.0
    cerebrospinal meningitis A39.0
    Colombian A77.0
    due to Rickettsia
      australis A77.3
      conorii A77.1
      rickettsii A77.0
      sibirica A77.2
      specified type NEC A77.8
    Ehrlichiosis A77.40
      due to
        E. chafeensis A77.41
        specified organism NEC A77.49
    Rocky Mountain A77.0
  steroid R50.2
  streptobacillary A25.1
  subtertian B50.9
  Sumatran mite A75.3
  sun A90
  swamp A27.9
  swine A02.8
  sylvatic, yellow A95.0
  Tahyna B33.8

Fever — *continued*
  tertian — *see* Malaria, tertian
  Thailand hemorrhagic A91
  thermic T67.0 ☑
  three-day A93.1
  tick
    American mountain A93.2
    Colorado A93.2
    Kemerovo A93.8
    Mediterranean A77.1
    mountain A93.2
    nonexanthematous A93.2
    Quaranfil A93.8
  tick-bite NEC A93.8
  tick-borne (hemorrhagic) NEC A93.8
  trench A79.0
  tsutsugamushi A75.3
  typhogastric A01.00
  typhoid (abortive) (hemorrhagic) (intermittent) (ma-
      lignant) A01.00
    complicated by
      arthritis A01.04
      heart involvement A01.02
      meningitis A01.01
      osteomyelitis A01.05
      pneumonia A01.03
      specified NEC A01.09
  typhomalarial — *see* Malaria
  typhus — *see* Typhus (fever)
  undulant — *see* Brucellosis
  unknown origin R50.9
  uveoparotid D86.89
  valley B38.0
  Venezuelan equine A92.2
  vesicular stomatitis A93.8
  viral hemorrhagic — *see* Fever, hemorrhagic, by type
      of virus
  Volhynian A79.0
  Wesselsbron (viral) A92.8
  West
    African B50.8
    Nile (viral) A92.30
      with
        complications NEC A92.39
        cranial nerve disorders A92.32
        encephalitis A92.31
        encephalomyelitis A92.31
        neurologic manifestation NEC A92.32
        optic neuritis A92.32
        polyradiculitis A92.32
  Whitmore's — *see* Melioidosis
  Wolhynian A79.0
  worm B83.9
  yellow A95.9
    jungle A95.0
    sylvatic A95.0
    urban A95.1
  Zika virus A92.5
Fibrillation
  atrial or auricular (established) I48.91
    chronic I48.2
    paroxysmal I48.0
    permanent I48.2
    persistent I48.1
  cardiac I49.8
  heart I49.8
  muscular M62.89
  ventricular I49.01
Fibrin
  ball or bodies, pleural (sac) J94.1
  chamber, anterior (eye) (gelatinous exudate) — *see*
      Iridocyclitis, acute
Fibrinogenolysis — *see* Fibrinolysis
Fibrinogenopenia D68.8
  acquired D65
  congenital D68.2
Fibrinolysis (hemorrhagic) (acquired) D65
  antepartum hemorrhage — *see* Hemorrhage, antepar-
      tum, with coagulation defect
  following
    abortion — *see* Abortion by type complicated by
        hemorrhage
    ectopic or molar pregnancy O08.1
  intrapartum O67.0
  newborn, transient P60
  postpartum O72.3
Fibrinopenia (hereditary) D68.2
  acquired D68.4

Fibrinopurulent — *see* condition
Fibrinous — *see* condition
Fibroadenoma
  cellular intracanalicular D24- ☑
  giant D24- ☑
  intracanalicular
    cellular D24- ☑
    giant D24- ☑
    specified site — *see* Neoplasm, benign, by site
    unspecified site D24- ☑
  juvenile D24- ☑
  pericanalicular
    specified site — *see* Neoplasm, benign, by site
    unspecified site D24- ☑
  phyllodes D24- ☑
  prostate D29.1
  specified site NEC — *see* Neoplasm, benign, by site
  unspecified site D24- ☑
Fibroadenosis, breast (chronic) (cystic) (diffuse) (peri-
    odic) (segmental) N60.2- ☑
Fibroangioma (*see also* Neoplasm, benign, by site)
  juvenile
    specified site — *see* Neoplasm, benign, by site
    unspecified site D10.6
Fibrochondrosarcoma — *see* Neoplasm, cartilage,
    malignant
Fibrocystic
  disease (*see also* Fibrosis, cystic)
    breast — *see* Mastopathy, cystic
    jaw M27.49
    kidney (congenital) Q61.8
    liver Q44.6
    pancreas E84.9
  kidney (congenital) Q61.8
Fibrodysplasia ossificans progressiva — *see* Myositis,
    ossificans, progressiva
Fibroelastosis (cordis) (endocardial) (endomyocardial)
    I42.4
Fibroid (tumor) (*see also* Neoplasm, connective tissue,
    benign)
  disease, lung (chronic) — *see* Fibrosis, lung
  heart (disease) — *see* Myocarditis
  in pregnancy or childbirth O34.1- ☑
    causing obstructed labor O65.5
  induration, lung (chronic) — *see* Fibrosis, lung
  lung — *see* Fibrosis, lung
  pneumonia (chronic) — *see* Fibrosis, lung
  uterus (*see also* Leiomyoma, uterus) D25.9
Fibrolipoma — *see* Lipoma
Fibroliposarcoma — *see* Neoplasm, connective tissue,
    malignant
Fibroma (*see also* Neoplasm, connective tissue, benign)
  ameloblastic — *see* Cyst, calcifying odontogenic
  bone (nonossifying) — *see* Disorder, bone, specified
      type NEC
    ossifying — *see* Neoplasm, bone, benign
  cementifying — *see* Neoplasm, bone, benign
  chondromyxoid — *see* Neoplasm, bone, benign
  desmoplastic — *see* Neoplasm, connective tissue,
      uncertain behavior
  durum — *see* Neoplasm, connective tissue, benign
  fascial — *see* Neoplasm, connective tissue, benign
  invasive — *see* Neoplasm, connective tissue, uncertain
      behavior
  molle — *see* Lipoma
  myxoid — *see* Neoplasm, connective tissue, benign
  nasopharynx, nasopharyngeal (juvenile) D10.6
  nonosteogenic (nonossifying) — *see* Dysplasia, fibrous
  odontogenic (central) — *see* Cyst, calcifying odonto-
      genic
  ossifying — *see* Neoplasm, bone, benign
  periosteal — *see* Neoplasm, bone, benign
  soft — *see* Lipoma
Fibromatosis M72.9
  abdominal — *see* Neoplasm, connective tissue, uncer-
      tain behavior
  aggressive — *see* Neoplasm, connective tissue, uncer-
      tain behavior
  congenital generalized — *see* Neoplasm, connective
      tissue, uncertain behavior
  Dupuytren's M72.0
  gingival K06.1
  palmar (fascial) M72.0
  plantar (fascial) M72.2
  pseudosarcomatous (proliferative) (subcutaneous)
      M72.4
  retroperitoneal D48.3

☑ **Additional Character Required — Refer to the Tabular List for Character Selection**   ▼ **Subterms under main terms may continue to next column or page**

Fibromatosis — *continued*
  specified NEC M72.8
Fibromyalgia M79.7
Fibromyoma (*see also* Neoplasm, connective tissue, benign)
  uterus (corpus) (*see also* Leiomyoma, uterus)
    in pregnancy or childbirth — *see* Fibroid, in pregnancy or childbirth
      causing obstructed labor O65.5
Fibromyositis M79.7
Fibromyxolipoma D17.9
Fibromyxoma — *see* Neoplasm, connective tissue, benign
Fibromyxosarcoma — *see* Neoplasm, connective tissue, malignant
Fibro-odontoma, ameloblastic — *see* Cyst, calcifying odontogenic
Fibro-osteoma — *see* Neoplasm, bone, benign
Fibroplasia, retrolental H35.17- ☑
Fibropurulent — *see* condition
Fibrosarcoma (*see also* Neoplasm, connective tissue, malignant)
  ameloblastic C41.1
    upper jaw (bone) C41.0
  congenital — *see* Neoplasm, connective tissue, malignant
  fascial — *see* Neoplasm, connective tissue, malignant
  infantile — *see* Neoplasm, connective tissue, malignant
  odontogenic C41.1
    upper jaw (bone) C41.0
  periosteal — *see* Neoplasm, bone, malignant
Fibrosclerosis
  breast N60.3- ☑
  multifocal M35.5
  penis (corpora cavernosa) N48.6
Fibrosis, fibrotic
  adrenal (gland) E27.8
  amnion O41.8X- ☑
  anal papillae K62.89
  arteriocapillary — *see* Arteriosclerosis
  bladder N32.89
    interstitial — *see* Cystitis, chronic, interstitial
    localized submucosal — *see* Cystitis, chronic, interstitial
    panmural — *see* Cystitis, chronic, interstitial
  breast — *see* Fibrosclerosis, breast
  capillary (*see also* Arteriosclerosis) I70.90
    lung (chronic) — *see* Fibrosis, lung
  cardiac — *see* Myocarditis
  cervix N88.8
  chorion O41.8X- ☑
  corpus cavernosum (sclerosing) N48.6
  cystic (of pancreas) E84.9
    with
      distal intestinal obstruction syndrome E84.19
      fecal impaction E84.19
      intestinal manifestations NEC E84.19
      pulmonary manifestations E84.0
      specified manifestations NEC E84.8
    due to device, implant or graft (*see also* Complications, by site and type, specified NEC) T85.828 ☑
      arterial graft NEC T82.828 ☑
      breast (implant) T85.828 ☑
      catheter NEC T85.828 ☑
        dialysis (renal) T82.828 ☑
          intraperitoneal T85.828 ☑
        infusion NEC T82.828 ☑
          spinal (epidural) (subdural) T85.820 ☑
        urinary (indwelling) T83.82 ☑
      electronic (electrode) (pulse generator) (stimulator)
        bone T84.82 ☑
        cardiac T82.827 ☑
        nervous system (brain) (peripheral nerve) (spinal) T85.820 ☑
        urinary T83.82 ☑
      fixation, internal (orthopedic) NEC T84.82 ☑
      gastrointestinal (bile duct) (esophagus) T85.828 ☑
      genital NEC T83.82 ☑
      heart NEC T82.827 ☑
      joint prosthesis T84.82 ☑
      ocular (corneal graft) (orbital implant) NEC T85.828 ☑
      orthopedic NEC T84.82 ☑
      specified NEC T85.828 ☑
      urinary NEC T83.82 ☑
      vascular NEC T82.828 ☑

Fibrosis, fibrotic — *continued*
  due to device, implant or graft (*see also* Complications, by site and type) — *continued*
    ventricular intracranial shunt T85.820 ☑
  ejaculatory duct N50.89
  endocardium — *see* Endocarditis
  endomyocardial (tropical) I42.3
  epididymis N50.89
  eye muscle — *see* Strabismus, mechanical
  heart — *see* Myocarditis
  hepatic — *see* Fibrosis, liver
  hepatolienal (portal hypertension) K76.6
  hepatosplenic (portal hypertension) K76.6
  infrapatellar fat pad M79.4
  intrascrotal N50.89
  kidney N26.9
  liver K74.0
    with sclerosis K74.2
    alcoholic K70.2
  lung (atrophic) (chronic) (confluent) (massive) (perialveolar) (peribronchial) J84.10
    with
      anthracosilicosis J60
      anthracosis J60
      asbestosis J61
      bagassosis J67.1
      bauxite J63.1
      berylliosis J63.2
      byssinosis J66.0
      calcicosis J62.8
      chalicosis J62.8
      dust reticulation J64
      farmer's lung J67.0
      ganister disease J62.8
      graphite J63.3
      pneumoconiosis NOS J64
      siderosis J63.4
      silicosis J62.8
    capillary J84.10
    congenital P27.8
    diffuse (idiopathic) J84.10
      chemicals, gases, fumes or vapors (inhalation) J68.4
      interstitial J84.10
        acute J84.114
      talc J62.0
    following radiation J70.1
    idiopathic J84.112
    postinflammatory J84.10
    silicotic J62.8
    tuberculous — *see* Tuberculosis, pulmonary
  lymphatic gland I89.8
  median bar — *see* Hyperplasia, prostate
  mediastinum (idiopathic) J98.59
  meninges G96.19
  myocardium, myocardial — *see* Myocarditis
  ovary N83.8
  oviduct N83.8
  pancreas K86.89
  penis NEC N48.6
  pericardium I31.0
  perineum, in pregnancy or childbirth O34.7- ☑
    causing obstructed labor O65.5
  pleura J94.1
  popliteal fat pad M79.4
  prostate (chronic) — *see* Hyperplasia, prostate
  pulmonary (*see also* Fibrosis, lung) J84.10
    congenital P27.8
    idiopathic J84.112
  rectal sphincter K62.89
  retroperitoneal, idiopathic (with ureteral obstruction) N13.5
    with infection N13.6
  sclerosing mesenteric (idiopathic) K65.4
  scrotum N50.89
  seminal vesicle N50.89
  senile R54
  skin L90.5
  spermatic cord N50.89
  spleen D73.89
    in schistosomiasis (bilharziasis) B65.9 [D77]
  subepidermal nodular — *see* Neoplasm, skin, benign
  submucous (oral) (tongue) K13.5
  testis N44.8
    chronic, due to syphilis A52.76
  thymus (gland) E32.8
  tongue, submucous K13.5
  tunica vaginalis N50.89

Fibrosis, fibrotic — *continued*
  uterus (non-neoplastic) N85.8
  vagina N89.8
  valve, heart — *see* Endocarditis
  vas deferens N50.89
  vein I87.8
Fibrositis (periarticular) M79.7
  nodular, chronic (Jaccoud's) (rheumatoid) — *see* Arthropathy, postrheumatic, chronic
Fibrothorax J94.1
Fibrotic — *see* Fibrosis
Fibrous — *see* condition
Fibroxanthoma (*see also* Neoplasm, connective tissue, benign)
  atypical — *see* Neoplasm, connective tissue, uncertain behavior
  malignant — *see* Neoplasm, connective tissue, malignant
Fibroxanthosarcoma — *see* Neoplasm, connective tissue, malignant
Fiedler's
  disease (icterohemorrhagic leptospirosis) A27.0
  myocarditis (acute) I40.1
Fifth disease B08.3
  venereal A55
Filaria, filarial, filariasis — *see* Infestation, filarial
Filatov's disease — *see* Mononucleosis, infectious
File-cutter's disease — *see* Poisoning, lead
Filling defect
  biliary tract R93.2
  bladder R93.41
  duodenum R93.3
  gallbladder R93.2
  gastrointestinal tract R93.3
  intestine R93.3
  kidney R93.42- ☑
  stomach R93.3
  ureter R93.41
  urinary organs, specified NEC R93.49
Fimbrial cyst Q50.4
Financial problem affecting care NOS Z59.9
  bankruptcy Z59.8
  foreclosure on loan Z59.8
Findings, abnormal, inconclusive, without diagnosis
  (*see also* Abnormal)
  17-ketosteroids, elevated R82.5
  acetonuria R82.4
  alcohol in blood R78.0
  anisocytosis R71.8
  antenatal screening of mother O28.9
    biochemical O28.1
    chromosomal O28.5
    cytological O28.2
    genetic O28.5
    hematological O28.0
    radiological O28.4
    specified NEC O28.8
    ultrasonic O28.3
  antibody titer, elevated R76.0
  anticardiolipin antibody R76.0
  antiphosphatidylglycerol antibody R76.0
  antiphosphatidylinositol antibody R76.0
  antiphosphatidylserine antibody R76.0
  antiphospholipid antibody R76.0
  bacteriuria R82.71
  bicarbonate E87.8
  bile in urine R82.2
  blood sugar R73.09
    high R73.9
    low (transient) E16.2
  body fluid or substance, specified NEC R88.8
  casts, urine R82.99
  catecholamines R82.5
  cells, urine R82.99
  chloride E87.8
  cholesterol E78.9
    high E78.00
      with high triglycerides E78.2
  chyluria R82.0
  cloudy
    dialysis effluent R88.0
    urine R82.90
  creatinine clearance R94.4
  crystals, urine R82.99
  culture
    blood R78.81
    positive — *see* Positive, culture
  echocardiogram R93.1

Findings, abnormal, inconclusive, without diagnosis
— *continued*
electrolyte level, urinary R82.99
function study NEC R94.8
  bladder R94.8
  endocrine NEC R94.7
    thyroid R94.6
  kidney R94.4
  liver R94.5
  pancreas R94.8
  placenta R94.8
  pulmonary R94.2
  spleen R94.8
gallbladder, nonvisualization R93.2
glucose (tolerance test) (non-fasting) R73.09
glycosuria R81
heart
  shadow R93.1
  sounds R01.2
hematinuria R82.3
hematocrit drop (precipitous) R71.0
hemoglobinuria R82.3
human papillomavirus (HPV) DNA test positive
  cervix
    high risk R87.810
    low risk R87.820
  vagina
    high risk R87.811
    low risk R87.821
in blood (of substance not normally found in blood) R78.9
  addictive drug NEC R78.4
  alcohol (excessive level) R78.0
  cocaine R78.2
  hallucinogen R78.3
  heavy metals (abnormal level) R78.79
  lead R78.71
  lithium (abnormal level) R78.89
  opiate drug R78.1
  psychotropic drug R78.5
  specified substance NEC R78.89
  steroid agent R78.6
indoleacetic acid, elevated R82.5
ketonuria R82.4
lactic acid dehydrogenase (LDH) R74.0
liver function test R79.89
mammogram NEC R92.8
  calcification (calculus) R92.1
  inconclusive result (due to dense breasts) R92.2
  microcalcification R92.0
mediastinal shift R93.8
melanin, urine R82.99
myoglobinuria R82.1
neonatal screening P09
nonvisualization of gallbladder R93.2
odor of urine NOS R82.90
Papanicolaou cervix R87.619
  non-atypical endometrial cells R87.618
pneumoencephalogram R93.0
poikilocytosis R71.8
potassium (deficiency) E87.6
  excess E87.5
PPD R76.11
radiologic (X-ray) R93.8
  abdomen R93.5
  biliary tract R93.2
  breast R92.8
  gastrointestinal tract R93.3
  genitourinary organs R93.8
  head R93.0
  inconclusive due to excess body fat of patient R93.9
  intrathoracic organs NEC R93.1
  placenta R93.8
  retroperitoneum R93.5
  skin R93.8
  skull R93.0
  subcutaneous tissue R93.8
red blood cell (count) (morphology) (sickling) (volume) R71.8
scan NEC R94.8
  bladder R94.8
  bone R94.8
  kidney R94.4
  liver R93.2
  lung R94.2
  pancreas R94.8
  placental R94.8
  spleen R94.8
  thyroid R94.6

Findings, abnormal, inconclusive, without diagnosis
— *continued*
sedimentation rate, elevated R70.0
SGOT R74.0
SGPT R74.0
sodium (deficiency) E87.1
  excess E87.0
specified body fluid NEC R88.8
stress test R94.39
thyroid (function) (metabolic rate) (scan) (uptake) R94.6
transaminase (level) R74.0
triglycerides E78.9
  high E78.1
  with high cholesterol E78.2
tuberculin skin test (without active tuberculosis) R76.11
urine R82.90
  acetone R82.4
  bacteria R82.71
  bile R82.2
  casts or cells R82.99
  chyle R82.0
  culture positive R82.79
  glucose R81
  hemoglobin R82.3
  ketone R82.4
  sugar R81
vanillylmandelic acid (VMA), elevated R82.5
vectorcardiogram (VCG) R94.39
ventriculogram R93.0
white blood cell (count) (differential) (morphology) D72.9
xerography R92.8
Finger — *see* condition
Fire, Saint Anthony's — *see* Erysipelas
Fire-setting
pathological (compulsive) F63.1
Fish hook stomach K31.89
Fishmeal-worker's lung J67.8
Fissure, fissured
anus, anal K60.2
  acute K60.0
  chronic K60.1
  congenital Q43.8
ear, lobule, congenital Q17.8
epiglottis (congenital) Q31.8
larynx J38.7
  congenital Q31.8
lip K13.0
  congenital — *see* Cleft, lip
nipple N64.0
  associated with
    lactation O92.13
    pregnancy O92.11- ☑
    puerperium O92.12
nose Q30.2
palate (congenital) — *see* Cleft, palate
skin R23.4
spine (congenital) (*see also* Spina bifida)
  with hydrocephalus — *see* Spina bifida, by site, with hydrocephalus
tongue (acquired) K14.5
  congenital Q38.3
Fistula (cutaneous) L98.8
abdomen (wall) K63.2
  bladder N32.2
  intestine NEC K63.2
  ureter N28.89
  uterus N82.5
abdominorectal K63.2
abdominosigmoidal K63.2
abdominothoracic J86.0
abdominouterine N82.5
  congenital Q51.7
abdominovesical N32.2
accessory sinuses — *see* Sinusitis
actinomycotic — *see* Actinomycosis
alveolar antrum — *see* Sinusitis, maxillary
alveolar process K04.6
anorectal K60.5
antrobuccal — *see* Sinusitis, maxillary
antrum — *see* Sinusitis, maxillary
anus, anal (recurrent) (infectional) K60.3
  congenital Q43.6
    with absence, atresia and stenosis Q42.2
  tuberculous A18.32
aorta-duodenal I77.2

Fistula — *continued*
appendix, appendicular K38.3
arteriovenous (acquired) (nonruptured) I77.0
  brain I67.1
    congenital Q28.2
      ruptured I60.8
    ruptured I60.8
  cerebral — *see* Fistula, arteriovenous, brain
  congenital (peripheral) (*see also* Malformation, arteriovenous)
    brain Q28.2
      ruptured I60.8
    coronary Q24.5
    pulmonary Q25.72
  coronary I25.41
    congenital Q24.5
  pulmonary I28.0
    congenital Q25.72
  surgically created (for dialysis) Z99.2
    complication — *see* Complication, arteriovenous, fistula, surgically created
  traumatic — *see* Injury, blood vessel
artery I77.2
aural (mastoid) — *see* Mastoiditis, chronic
auricle (*see also* Disorder, pinna, specified type NEC)
  congenital Q18.1
Bartholin's gland N82.8
bile duct (common) (hepatic) K83.3
  with calculus, stones — *see* Calculus, bile duct
biliary (tract) — *see* Fistula, bile duct
bladder (sphincter) NEC (*see also* Fistula, vesico-) N32.2
  into seminal vesicle N32.2
bone (*see also* Disorder, bone, specified type NEC)
  with osteomyelitis, chronic — *see* Osteomyelitis, chronic, with draining sinus
brain G93.89
  arteriovenous (acquired) I67.1
    congenital Q28.2
branchial (cleft) Q18.0
branchiogenous Q18.0
breast N61.0
  puerperal, postpartum or gestational, due to mastitis (purulent) — *see* Mastitis, obstetric, purulent
bronchial J86.0
bronchocutaneous, bronchomediastinal, bronchopleural, bronchopleuromediastinal (infective) J86.0
  tuberculous NEC A15.5
bronchoesophageal J86.0
  congenital Q39.2
    with atresia of esophagus Q39.1
bronchovisceral J86.0
buccal cavity (infective) K12.2
cecosigmoidal K63.2
cecum K63.2
cerebrospinal (fluid) G96.0
cervical, lateral Q18.1
cervicoaural Q18.1
cervicosigmoidal N82.4
cervicovesical N82.1
cervix N82.8
chest (wall) J86.0
cholecystenteric — *see* Fistula, gallbladder
cholecystocolic — *see* Fistula, gallbladder
cholecystocolonic — *see* Fistula, gallbladder
cholecystoduodenal — *see* Fistula, gallbladder
cholecystogastric — *see* Fistula, gallbladder
cholecystointestinal — *see* Fistula, gallbladder
choledochoduodenal — *see* Fistula, bile duct
cholocolic K82.3
coccyx — *see* Sinus, pilonidal
colon K63.2
colostomy K94.09
common duct — *see* Fistula, bile duct
congenital, site not listed — *see* Anomaly, by site
coronary, arteriovenous I25.41
  congenital Q24.5
costal region J86.0
cul-de-sac, Douglas' N82.8
cystic duct (*see also* Fistula, gallbladder)
  congenital Q44.5
dental K04.6
diaphragm J86.0
duodenum K31.6
ear (external) (canal) — *see* Disorder, ear, external, specified type NEC
enterocolic K63.2
enterocutaneous K63.2

Fistula — *continued*
  enterouterine N82.4
    congenital Q51.7
  enterovaginal N82.4
    congenital Q52.2
    large intestine N82.3
    small intestine N82.2
  enterovesical N32.1
  epididymis N50.89
    tuberculous A18.15
  esophagobronchial J86.0
    congenital Q39.2
      with atresia of esophagus Q39.1
  esophagocutaneous K22.8
  esophagopleural-cutaneous J86.0
  esophagotracheal J86.0
    congenital Q39.2
      with atresia of esophagus Q39.1
  esophagus K22.8
    congenital Q39.2
      with atresia of esophagus Q39.1
  ethmoid — *see* Sinusitis, ethmoidal
  eyeball (cornea) (sclera) — *see* Disorder, globe, hy-
    potony
  eyelid H01.8
  fallopian tube, external N82.5
  fecal K63.2
    congenital Q43.6
  from periapical abscess K04.6
  frontal sinus — *see* Sinusitis, frontal
  gallbladder K82.3
    with calculus, cholelithiasis, stones — *see* Calculus,
      gallbladder
  gastric K31.6
  gastrocolic K31.6
    congenital Q40.2
    tuberculous A18.32
  gastroenterocolic K31.6
  gastroesophageal K31.6
  gastrojejunal K31.6
  gastrojejunocolic K31.6
  genital tract (female) N82.9
    specified NEC N82.8
    to intestine NEC N82.4
    to skin N82.5
  hepatic artery-portal vein, congenital Q26.6
  hepatopleural J86.0
  hepatopulmonary J86.0
  ileorectal or ileosigmoidal K63.2
  ileovaginal N82.2
  ileovesical N32.1
  ileum K63.2
  in ano K60.3
    tuberculous A18.32
  inner ear (labyrinth) — *see* subcategory H83.1 ☑
  intestine NEC K63.2
  intestinocolonic (abdominal) K63.2
  intestinoureteral N28.89
  intestinouterine N82.4
  intestinovaginal N82.4
    large intestine N82.3
    small intestine N82.2
  intestinovesical N32.1
  ischiorectal (fossa) K61.3
  jejunum K63.2
  joint M25.10
    ankle M25.17- ☑
    elbow M25.12- ☑
    foot joint M25.17- ☑
    hand joint M25.14- ☑
    hip M25.15- ☑
    knee M25.16- ☑
    shoulder M25.11- ☑
    specified joint NEC M25.18
    tuberculous — *see* Tuberculosis, joint
    vertebrae M25.18
    wrist M25.13- ☑
  kidney N28.89
  labium (majus) (minus) N82.8
  labyrinth — *see* subcategory H83.1 ☑
  lacrimal (gland) (sac) H04.61- ☑
  lacrimonasal duct — *see* Fistula, lacrimal
  laryngotracheal, congenital Q34.8
  larynx J38.7
  lip K13.0
    congenital Q38.0
  lumbar, tuberculous A18.01
  lung J86.0

Fistula — *continued*
  lymphatic I89.8
  mammary (gland) N61.0
  mastoid (process) (region) — *see* Mastoiditis, chronic
  maxillary J32.0
  medial, face and neck Q18.8
  mediastinal J86.0
  mediastinobronchial J86.0
  mediastinocutaneous J86.0
  middle ear — *see* subcategory H74.8 ☑
  mouth K12.2
  nasal J34.89
    sinus — *see* Sinusitis
  nasopharynx J39.2
  nipple N64.0
  nose J34.89
  oral (cutaneous) K12.2
    maxillary J32.0
    nasal (with cleft palate) — *see* Cleft, palate
  orbit, orbital — *see* Disorder, orbit, specified type NEC
  oroantral J32.0
  oviduct, external N82.5
  palate (hard) M27.8
  pancreatic K86.89
  pancreaticoduodenal K86.89
  parotid (gland) K11.4
    region K12.2
  penis N48.89
  perianal K60.3
  pericardium (pleura) (sac) — *see* Pericarditis
  pericecal K63.2
  perineorectal K60.4
  perineosigmoidal K63.2
  perineum, perineal (with urethral involvement) NEC
    N36.0
    tuberculous A18.13
    ureter N28.89
  perirectal K60.4
    tuberculous A18.32
  peritoneum K65.9
  pharyngoesophageal J39.2
  pharynx J39.2
    branchial cleft (congenital) Q18.0
  pilonidal (infected) (rectum) — *see* Sinus, pilonidal
  pleura, pleural, pleurocutaneous, pleuroperitoneal
    J86.0
    tuberculous NEC A15.6
  pleuropericardial I31.8
  portal vein-hepatic artery, congenital Q26.6
  postauricular H70.81- ☑
  postoperative, persistent T81.83 ☑
    specified site — *see* Fistula, by site
  preauricular (congenital) Q18.1
  prostate N42.89
  pulmonary J86.0
    arteriovenous I28.0
      congenital Q25.72
    tuberculous — *see* Tuberculosis, pulmonary
  pulmonoperitoneal J86.0
  rectolabial N82.4
  rectosigmoid (intercommunicating) K63.2
  rectoureteral N28.89
  rectourethral N36.0
    congenital Q64.73
  rectouterine N82.4
    congenital Q51.7
  rectovaginal N82.3
    congenital Q52.2
    tuberculous A18.18
  rectovesical N32.1
    congenital Q64.79
  rectovesicovaginal N82.3
  rectovulval N82.4
    congenital Q52.79
  rectum (to skin) K60.4
    congenital Q43.6
      with absence, atresia and stenosis Q42.0
    tuberculous A18.32
  renal N28.89
  retroauricular — *see* Fistula, postauricular
  salivary duct or gland (any) K11.4
    congenital Q38.4
  scrotum (urinary) N50.89
    tuberculous A18.15
  semicircular canals — *see* subcategory H83.1 ☑
  sigmoid K63.2
    to bladder N32.1
  sinus — *see* Sinusitis

Fistula — *continued*
  skin L98.8
    to genital tract (female) N82.5
  splenocolic D73.89
  stercoral K63.2
  stomach K31.6
  sublingual gland K11.4
  submandibular gland K11.4
  submaxillary (gland) K11.4
    region K12.2
  thoracic J86.0
    duct I89.8
  thoracoabdominal J86.0
  thoracogastric J86.0
  thoracointestinal J86.0
  thorax J86.0
  thyroglossal duct Q89.2
  thyroid E07.89
  trachea, congenital (external) (internal) Q32.1
  tracheoesophageal J86.0
    congenital Q39.2
      with atresia of esophagus Q39.1
    following tracheostomy J95.04
  traumatic arteriovenous — *see* Injury, blood vessel,
    by site
  tuberculous — *code by* site under Tuberculosis
  typhoid A01.09
  umbilicourinary Q64.8
  urachus, congenital Q64.4
  ureter (persistent) N28.89
  ureteroabdominal N28.89
  ureterorectal N28.89
  ureterosigmoido-abdominal N28.89
  ureterovaginal N82.1
  ureterovesical N32.2
  urethra N36.0
    congenital Q64.79
    tuberculous A18.13
  urethroperineal N36.0
  urethroperineovesical N32.2
  urethrorectal N36.0
    congenital Q64.73
  urethroscrotal N50.89
  urethrovaginal N82.1
  urethrovesical N32.2
  urinary (tract) (persistent) (recurrent) N36.0
  uteroabdominal N82.5
    congenital Q51.7
  uteroenteric, uterointestinal N82.4
    congenital Q51.7
  uterorectal N82.4
    congenital Q51.7
  uteroureteric N82.1
  uterourethral Q51.7
  uterovaginal N82.8
  uterovesical N82.1
    congenital Q51.7
  uterus N82.8
  vagina (postpartal) (wall) N82.8
  vaginocutaneous (postpartal) N82.5
  vaginointestinal NEC N82.4
    large intestine N82.3
    small intestine N82.2
  vaginoperineal N82.5
  vasocutaneous, congenital Q55.7
  vesical NEC N32.2
  vesicoabdominal N32.2
  vesicocervicovaginal N82.1
  vesicocolic N32.1
  vesicocutaneous N32.2
  vesicoenteric N32.1
  vesicointestinal N32.1
  vesicometrorectal N82.4
  vesicoperineal N32.2
  vesicorectal N32.1
    congenital Q64.79
  vesicosigmoidal N32.1
  vesicosigmoidovaginal N82.3
  vesicoureteral N32.2
  vesicoureterovaginal N82.1
  vesicourethral N32.2
  vesicourethrorectal N32.1
  vesicouterine N82.1
    congenital Q51.7
  vesicovaginal N82.0
  vulvorectal N82.4
    congenital Q52.79
Fit R56.9
  epileptic — *see* Epilepsy

Fit — *continued*
  fainting R55
  hysterical F44.5
  newborn P90
Fitting (and adjustment) (of)
  artificial
    arm — *see* Admission, adjustment, artificial, arm
    breast Z44.3 ☑
    eye Z44.2 ☑
    leg — *see* Admission, adjustment, artificial, leg
  automatic implantable cardiac defibrillator (with synchronous cardiac pacemaker) Z45.02
  brain neuropacemaker Z46.2
    implanted Z45.42
  cardiac defibrillator — *see* Fitting (and adjustment) (of), automatic implantable cardiac defibrillator
  catheter, non-vascular Z46.82
  colostomy belt Z46.89
  contact lenses Z46.0
  CRT-D (resynchronization therapy defibrillator) Z45.02
  CRT-P (cardiac resynchronization therapy pacemaker) Z45.018
    pulse generator Z45.010
  cystostomy device Z46.6
  defibrillator, cardiac — *see* Fitting (and adjustment) (of), automatic implantable cardiac defibrillator
  dentures Z46.3
  device NOS Z46.9
    abdominal Z46.89
    gastrointestinal NEC Z46.59
    implanted NEC Z45.89
    nervous system Z46.2
      implanted — *see* Admission, adjustment, device, implanted, nervous system
    orthodontic Z46.4
    orthoptic Z46.0
    orthotic Z46.89
    prosthetic (external) Z44.9
      breast Z44.3 ☑
      dental Z46.3
      eye Z44.2 ☑
      specified NEC Z44.8
    specified NEC Z46.89
    substitution
      auditory Z46.2
        implanted — *see* Admission, adjustment, device, implanted, hearing device
      nervous system Z46.2
        implanted — *see* Admission, adjustment, device, implanted, nervous system
      visual Z46.2
        implanted Z45.31
    urinary Z46.6
  gastric lap band Z46.51
  gastrointestinal appliance NEC Z46.59
  glasses (reading) Z46.0
  hearing aid Z46.1
  ileostomy device Z46.89
  insulin pump Z46.81
  intestinal appliance NEC Z46.89
  myringotomy device (stent) (tube) Z45.82
  neuropacemaker Z46.2
    implanted Z45.42
  non-vascular catheter Z46.82
  orthodontic device Z46.4
  orthopedic device (brace) (cast) (corset) (shoes) Z46.89
  pacemaker (cardiac) (cardiac resynchronization therapy (CRT-P)) Z45.018
    nervous system (brain) (peripheral nerve) (spinal cord) Z46.2
      implanted Z45.42
    pulse generator Z45.010
  portacath (port-a-cath) Z45.2
  prosthesis (external) Z44.9
    arm — *see* Admission, adjustment, artificial, arm
    breast Z44.3 ☑
    dental Z46.3
    eye Z44.2 ☑
    leg — *see* Admission, adjustment, artificial, leg
    specified NEC Z44.8
  spectacles Z46.0
  wheelchair Z46.89
Fitzhugh-Curtis syndrome
  due to
    Chlamydia trachomatis A74.81
    Neisseria gonorrhorea (gonococcal peritonitis) A54.85

Fitz's syndrome (acute hemorrhagic pancreatitis) (*see also* Pancreatitis, acute) K85.80
Fixation
  joint — *see* Ankylosis
  larynx J38.7
  stapes — *see* Ankylosis, ear ossicles
    deafness — *see* Deafness, conductive
  uterus (acquired) — *see* Malposition, uterus
  vocal cord J38.3
Flabby ridge K06.8
Flaccid (*see also* condition)
  palate, congenital Q38.5
Flail
  chest S22.5 ☑
    newborn (birth injury) P13.8
  joint (paralytic) M25.20
    ankle M25.27- ☑
    elbow M25.22- ☑
    foot joint M25.27- ☑
    hand joint M25.24- ☑
    hip M25.25- ☑
    knee M25.26- ☑
    shoulder M25.21- ☑
    specified joint NEC M25.28
    wrist M25.23- ☑
Flajani's disease — *see* Hyperthyroidism, with, goiter (diffuse)
Flap, liver K71.3
Flashbacks (residual to hallucinogen use) F16.283
Flat
  chamber (eye) — *see* Disorder, globe, hypotony, flat anterior chamber
  chest, congenital Q67.8
  foot (acquired) (fixed type) (painful) (postural) (*see also* Deformity, limb, flat foot)
    congenital (rigid) (spastic) (everted) Q66.5- ☑
    rachitic sequelae (late effect) E64.3
  organ or site, congenital NEC — *see* Anomaly, by site
  pelvis M95.5
    with disproportion (fetopelvic) O33.0
      causing obstructed labor O65.0
    congenital Q74.2
Flatau-Schilder disease G37.0
Flatback syndrome M40.30
  lumbar region M40.36
  lumbosacral region M40.37
  thoracolumbar region M40.35
Flattening
  head, femur M89.8X5
  hip — *see* Coxa, plana
  lip (congenital) Q18.8
  nose (congenital) Q67.4
    acquired M95.0
Flatulence R14.3
  psychogenic F45.8
Flatus R14.3
  vaginalis N89.8
Flax-dresser's disease J66.1
Flea bite — *see* Injury, bite, by site, superficial, insect
Flecks, glaucomatous (subcapsular) — *see* Cataract, complicated
Fleischer (-Kayser) **ring** (cornea) H18.04- ☑
Fleshy mole O02.0
Flexibilitas cerea — *see* Catalepsy
Flexion
  amputation stump (surgical) T87.89
  cervix — *see* Malposition, uterus
  contracture, joint — *see* Contraction, joint
  deformity, joint (*see also* Deformity, limb, flexion) M21.20
    hip, congenital Q65.89
  uterus (*see also* Malposition, uterus)
    lateral — *see* Lateroversion, uterus
Flexner-Boyd dysentery A03.2
Flexner's dysentery A03.1
Flexure — *see* Flexion
Flint murmur (aortic insufficiency) I35.1
Floater, vitreous — *see* Opacity, vitreous
Floating
  cartilage (joint) (*see also* Loose, body, joint)
    knee — *see* Derangement, knee, loose body
  gallbladder, congenital Q44.1
  kidney N28.89
    congenital Q63.8
  spleen D73.89
Flooding N92.0
Floor — *see* condition

Floppy
  baby syndrome (nonspecific) P94.2
  iris syndrome (intraoperative) (IFIS) H21.81
  nonrheumatic mitral valve syndrome I34.1
Flu (*see also* Influenza)
  avian (*see also* Influenza, due to, identified novel influenza A virus) J09.X2
  bird (*see also* Influenza, due to, identified novel influenza A virus) J09.X2
  intestinal NEC A08.4
  swine (viruses that normally cause infections in pigs) (*see also* Influenza, due to, identified novel influenza A virus) J09.X2
Fluctuating blood pressure I99.8
Fluid
  abdomen R18.8
  chest J94.8
  heart — *see* Failure, heart, congestive
  joint — *see* Effusion, joint
  loss (acute) E86.9
  lung — *see* Edema, lung
  overload E87.70
    specified NEC E87.79
  peritoneal cavity R18.8
  pleural cavity J94.8
  retention R60.9
Flukes NEC (*see also* Infestation, fluke)
  blood NEC — *see* Schistosomiasis
  liver B66.3
Fluor (vaginalis) N89.8
  trichomonal or due to Trichomonas (vaginalis) A59.00
Fluorosis
  dental K00.3
  skeletal M85.10
    ankle M85.17- ☑
    foot M85.17- ☑
    forearm M85.13- ☑
    hand M85.14- ☑
    lower leg M85.16- ☑
    multiple site M85.19
    neck M85.18
    rib M85.18
    shoulder M85.11- ☑
    skull M85.18
    specified site NEC M85.18
    thigh M85.15- ☑
    toe M85.17- ☑
    upper arm M85.12- ☑
    vertebra M85.18
Flush syndrome E34.0
Flushing R23.2
  menopausal N95.1
Flutter
  atrial or auricular I48.92
    atypical I48.4
    type I I48.3
    type II I48.4
    typical I48.3
  heart I49.8
    atrial or auricular I48.92
      atypical I48.4
      type I I48.3
      type II I48.4
      typical I48.3
    ventricular I49.02
  ventricular I49.02
FNHTR (febrile nonhemolytic transfusion reaction) R50.84
Fochier's abscess — *code by* site under Abscess
Focus, Assmann's — *see* Tuberculosis, pulmonary
Fogo selvagem L10.3
Foix-Alajouanine syndrome G95.19
Fold, folds (anomalous) (*see also* Anomaly, by site)
  Descemet's membrane — *see* Change, corneal membrane, Descemet's, fold
  epicanthic Q10.3
  heart Q24.8
Folie à deux F24
Follicle
  cervix (nabothian) (ruptured) N88.8
  graafian, ruptured, with hemorrhage N83.0- ☑
  nabothian N88.8
Follicular — *see* condition
Folliculitis (superficial) L73.9
  abscedens et suffodiens L66.3
  cyst N83.0- ☑
  decalvans L66.2
  deep — *see* Furuncle, by site

☑ **Additional Character Required — Refer to the Tabular List for Character Selection**   ▽ Subterms under main terms may continue to next column or page

Folliculitis — *continued*
  gonococcal (acute) (chronic) A54.01
  keloid, keloidalis L73.0
  pustular L01.02
  ulerythematosa reticulata L66.4
Folliculome lipidique
  specified site — *see* Neoplasm, benign, by site
  unspecified site
    female D27.9
    male D29.20
Følling's disease E70.0
Follow-up — *see* Examination, follow-up
Fong's syndrome (hereditary osteo-onychodysplasia)
  Q87.2
Food
  allergy L27.2
  asphyxia (from aspiration or inhalation) — *see* Foreign
    body, by site
  choked on — *see* Foreign body, by site
  deprivation T73.0
    specified kind of food NEC E63.8
  intoxication — *see* Poisoning, food
  lack of T73.0 ☑
  poisoning — *see* Poisoning, food
  rejection NEC — *see* Disorder, eating
  strangulation or suffocation — *see* Foreign body, by
    site
  toxemia — *see* Poisoning, food
Foot — *see* condition
Foramen ovale (nonclosure) (patent) (persistent) Q21.1
Forbes' glycogen storage disease E74.03
Fordyce-Fox disease L75.2
Fordyce's disease (mouth) Q38.6
Forearm — *see* condition
Foreign body
  with
    laceration — *see* Laceration, by site, with foreign
      body
    puncture wound — *see* Puncture, by site, with
      foreign body
  accidentally left following a procedure T81.509 ☑
    aspiration T81.506 ☑
      resulting in
        adhesions T81.516 ☑
        obstruction T81.526 ☑
        perforation T81.536 ☑
        specified complication NEC T81.596 ☑
    cardiac catheterization T81.505 ☑
      resulting in
        acute reaction T81.60 ☑
          aseptic peritonitis T81.61 ☑
          specified NEC T81.69 ☑
        adhesions T81.515 ☑
        obstruction T81.525 ☑
        perforation T81.535 ☑
        specified complication NEC T81.595 ☑
    causing
      acute reaction T81.60 ☑
        aseptic peritonitis T81.61 ☑
        specified complication NEC T81.69 ☑
      adhesions T81.519 ☑
      aseptic peritonitis T81.61 ☑
      obstruction T81.529 ☑
      perforation T81.539 ☑
      specified complication NEC T81.599 ☑
    endoscopy T81.504 ☑
      resulting in
        adhesions T81.514 ☑
        obstruction T81.524 ☑
        perforation T81.534 ☑
        specified complication NEC T81.594 ☑
    immunization T81.503 ☑
      resulting in
        adhesions T81.513 ☑
        obstruction T81.523 ☑
        perforation T81.533 ☑
        specified complication NEC T81.593 ☑
    infusion T81.501 ☑
      resulting in
        adhesions T81.511 ☑
        obstruction T81.521 ☑
        perforation T81.531 ☑
        specified complication NEC T81.591 ☑
    injection T81.503 ☑
      resulting in
        adhesions T81.513 ☑

Foreign body — *continued*
  accidentally left following a procedure — *continued*
    injection — *continued*
      resulting in — *continued*
        obstruction T81.523 ☑
        perforation T81.533 ☑
        specified complication NEC T81.593 ☑
    kidney dialysis T81.502 ☑
      resulting in
        adhesions T81.512 ☑
        obstruction T81.522 ☑
        perforation T81.532 ☑
        specified complication NEC T81.592 ☑
    packing removal T81.507 ☑
      resulting in
        acute reaction T81.60 ☑
          aseptic peritonitis T81.61 ☑
          specified NEC T81.69 ☑
        adhesions T81.517 ☑
        obstruction T81.527 ☑
        perforation T81.537 ☑
        specified complication NEC T81.597 ☑
    puncture T81.506 ☑
      resulting in
        adhesions T81.516 ☑
        obstruction T81.526 ☑
        perforation T81.536 ☑
        specified complication NEC T81.596 ☑
    specified procedure NEC T81.508 ☑
      resulting in
        acute reaction T81.60 ☑
          aseptic peritonitis T81.61 ☑
          specified NEC T81.69 ☑
        adhesions T81.518 ☑
        obstruction T81.528 ☑
        perforation T81.538 ☑
        specified complication NEC T81.598 ☑
    surgical operation T81.500 ☑
      resulting in
        acute reaction T81.60 ☑
          aseptic peritonitis T81.61 ☑
          specified NEC T81.69 ☑
        adhesions T81.510 ☑
        obstruction T81.520 ☑
        perforation T81.530 ☑
        specified complication NEC T81.590 ☑
    transfusion T81.501 ☑
      resulting in
        adhesions T81.511 ☑
        obstruction T81.521 ☑
        perforation T81.531 ☑
        specified complication NEC T81.591 ☑
  alimentary tract T18.9 ☑
    anus T18.5 ☑
    colon T18.4 ☑
    esophagus — *see* Foreign body, esophagus
    mouth T18.0 ☑
    multiple sites T18.8 ☑
    rectosigmoid (junction) T18.5 ☑
    rectum T18.5 ☑
    small intestine T18.3 ☑
    specified site NEC T18.8 ☑
    stomach T18.2 ☑
  anterior chamber (eye) S05.5- ☑
  auditory canal — *see* Foreign body, entering through
    orifice, ear
  bronchus T17.508 ☑
    causing
      asphyxiation T17.500 ☑
        food (bone) (seed) T17.520 ☑
        gastric contents (vomitus) T17.510 ☑
        specified type NEC T17.590 ☑
      injury NEC T17.508 ☑
        food (bone) (seed) T17.528 ☑
        gastric contents (vomitus) T17.518 ☑
        specified type NEC T17.598 ☑
  canthus — *see* Foreign body, conjunctival sac
  ciliary body (eye) S05.5- ☑
  conjunctival sac T15.1- ☑
  cornea T15.0- ☑
  entering through orifice
    accessory sinus T17.0 ☑
    alimentary canal T18.9 ☑
      multiple parts T18.8 ☑
      specified part NEC T18.8 ☑

Foreign body — *continued*
  entering through orifice — *continued*
    alveolar process T18.0 ☑
    antrum (Highmore's) T17.0 ☑
    anus T18.5 ☑
    appendix T18.4 ☑
    auditory canal — *see* Foreign body, entering
      through orifice, ear
    auricle — *see* Foreign body, entering through ori-
      fice, ear
    bladder T19.1 ☑
    bronchioles — *see* Foreign body, respiratory tract,
      specified site NEC
    bronchus (main) — *see* Foreign body, bronchus
    buccal cavity T18.0 ☑
    canthus (inner) — *see* Foreign body, conjunctival
      sac
    cecum T18.4 ☑
    cervix (canal) (uteri) T19.3 ☑
    colon T18.4 ☑
    conjunctival sac — *see* Foreign body, conjunctival
      sac
    cornea — *see* Foreign body, cornea
    digestive organ or tract NOS T18.9 ☑
      multiple parts T18.8 ☑
      specified part NEC T18.8 ☑
    duodenum T18.3 ☑
    ear (external) T16.- ☑
    esophagus — *see* Foreign body, esophagus
    eye (external) NOS T15.9- ☑
      conjunctival sac — *see* Foreign body, conjunc-
        tival sac
      cornea — *see* Foreign body, cornea
      specified part NEC T15.8- ☑
    eyeball (*see also* Foreign body, entering through
      orifice, eye, specified part NEC)
      with penetrating wound — *see* Puncture, eye-
        ball
    eyelid (*see also* Foreign body, conjunctival sac)
      with
        laceration — *see* Laceration, eyelid, with
          foreign body
        puncture — *see* Puncture, eyelid, with for-
          eign body
        superficial injury — *see* Foreign body, super-
          ficial, eyelid
    gastrointestinal tract T18.9 ☑
      multiple parts T18.8 ☑
      specified part NEC T18.8 ☑
    genitourinary tract T19.9 ☑
      multiple parts T19.8 ☑
      specified part NEC T19.8 ☑
    globe — *see* Foreign body, entering through ori-
      fice, eyeball
    gum T18.0 ☑
    Highmore's antrum T17.0 ☑
    hypopharynx — *see* Foreign body, pharynx
    ileum T18.3 ☑
    intestine (small) T18.3 ☑
      large T18.4 ☑
    lacrimal apparatus (punctum) — *see* Foreign body,
      entering through orifice, eye, specified part
      NEC
    large intestine T18.4 ☑
    larynx — *see* Foreign body, larynx
    lung — *see* Foreign body, respiratory tract, speci-
      fied site NEC
    maxillary sinus T17.0 ☑
    mouth T18.0 ☑
    nasal sinus T17.0 ☑
    nasopharynx — *see* Foreign body, pharynx
    nose (passage) T17.1 ☑
    nostril T17.1 ☑
    oral cavity T18.0 ☑
    palate T18.0 ☑
    penis T19.4 ☑
    pharynx — *see* Foreign body, pharynx
    piriform sinus — *see* Foreign body, pharynx
    rectosigmoid (junction) T18.5 ☑
    rectum T18.5 ☑
    respiratory tract — *see* Foreign body, respiratory
      tract
    sinus (accessory) (frontal) (maxillary) (nasal)
      T17.0 ☑
      piriform — *see* Foreign body, pharynx
    small intestine T18.3 ☑

☜ **Subterms under main terms may continue to next column or page**   ☑ **Additional Character Required — Refer to the Tabular List for Character Selection**   **147**

Folliculitis — Foreign body

Foreign body — *continued*
  entering through orifice — *continued*
    stomach T18.2 ☑
    suffocation by — *see* Foreign body, by site
    tear ducts or glands — *see* Foreign body, entering through orifice, eye, specified part NEC
    throat — *see* Foreign body, pharynx
    tongue T18.0 ☑
    tonsil, tonsillar (fossa) — *see* Foreign body, pharynx
    trachea — *see* Foreign body, trachea
    ureter T19.8 ☑
    urethra T19.0 ☑
    uterus (any part) T19.3 ☑
    vagina T19.2 ☑
    vulva T19.2 ☑
  esophagus T18.108 ☑
    causing
      injury NEC T18.108 ☑
        food (bone) (seed) T18.128 ☑
        gastric contents (vomitus) T18.118 ☑
        specified type NEC T18.198 ☑
      tracheal compression T18.100 ☑
        food (bone) (seed) T18.120 ☑
        gastric contents (vomitus) T18.110 ☑
        specified type NEC T18.190 ☑
  feeling of, in throat R09.89
  fragment — *see* Retained, foreign body fragments (type of)
  genitourinary tract T19.9 ☑
    bladder T19.1 ☑
    multiple parts T19.8 ☑
    penis T19.4 ☑
    specified site NEC T19.8 ☑
    urethra T19.0 ☑
    uterus T19.3 ☑
      IUD Z97.5
    vagina T19.2 ☑
      contraceptive device Z97.5
    vulva T19.2 ☑
  granuloma (old) (soft tissue) (*see also* Granuloma, foreign body)
    skin L92.3
  in
    laceration — *see* Laceration, by site, with foreign body
    puncture wound — *see* Puncture, by site, with foreign body
    soft tissue (residual) M79.5
  inadvertently left in operation wound — *see* Foreign body, accidentally left during a procedure
  ingestion, ingested NOS T18.9 ☑
  inhalation or inspiration — *see* Foreign body, by site
  internal organ, not entering through a natural orifice — code as specific injury with foreign body
  intraocular S05.5- ☑
    old, retained (nonmagnetic) H44.70- ☑
      anterior chamber H44.71- ☑
      ciliary body H44.72- ☑
      iris H44.72- ☑
      lens H44.73- ☑
      magnetic H44.60- ☑
        anterior chamber H44.61- ☑
        ciliary body H44.62- ☑
        iris H44.62- ☑
        lens H44.63- ☑
        posterior wall H44.64- ☑
        specified site NEC H44.69- ☑
        vitreous body H44.65- ☑
      posterior wall H44.74- ☑
      specified site NEC H44.79- ☑
      vitreous body H44.75- ☑
  iris — *see* Foreign body, intraocular
  lacrimal punctum — *see* Foreign body, entering through orifice, eye, specified part NEC
  larynx T17.308 ☑
    causing
      asphyxiation T17.300 ☑
        food (bone) (seed) T17.320 ☑
        gastric contents (vomitus) T17.310 ☑
        specified type NEC T17.390 ☑
      injury NEC T17.308 ☑
        food (bone) (seed) T17.328 ☑
        gastric contents (vomitus) T17.318 ☑
        specified type NEC T17.398 ☑
  lens — *see* Foreign body, intraocular
  ocular muscle S05.4- ☑

Foreign body — *continued*
  ocular muscle — *continued*
    old, retained — *see* Foreign body, orbit, old
  old or residual
    soft tissue (residual) M79.5
  operation wound, left accidentally — *see* Foreign body, accidentally left during a procedure
  orbit S05.4- ☑
    old, retained H05.5- ☑
  pharynx T17.208 ☑
    causing
      asphyxiation T17.200 ☑
        food (bone) (seed) T17.220 ☑
        gastric contents (vomitus) T17.210 ☑
        specified type NEC T17.290 ☑
      injury NEC T17.208 ☑
        food (bone) (seed) T17.228 ☑
        gastric contents (vomitus) T17.218 ☑
        specified type NEC T17.298 ☑
  respiratory tract T17.908 ☑
    bronchioles — *see* Foreign body, respiratory tract, specified site NEC
    bronchus — *see* Foreign body, bronchus
    causing
      asphyxiation T17.900 ☑
        food (bone) (seed) T17.920 ☑
        gastric contents (vomitus) T17.910 ☑
        specified type NEC T17.990 ☑
      injury NEC T17.908 ☑
        food (bone) (seed) T17.928 ☑
        gastric contents (vomitus) T17.918 ☑
        specified type NEC T17.998 ☑
    larynx — *see* Foreign body, larynx
    lung — *see* Foreign body, respiratory tract, specified site NEC
    multiple parts — *see* Foreign body, respiratory tract, specified site NEC
    nasal sinus T17.0 ☑
    nasopharynx — *see* Foreign body, pharynx
    nose T17.1 ☑
    nostril T17.1 ☑
    pharynx — *see* Foreign body, pharynx
    specified site NEC T17.808 ☑
      causing
        asphyxiation T17.800 ☑
          food (bone) (seed) T17.820 ☑
          gastric contents (vomitus) T17.810 ☑
          specified type NEC T17.890 ☑
        injury NEC T17.808 ☑
          food (bone) (seed) T17.828 ☑
          gastric contents (vomitus) T17.818 ☑
          specified type NEC T17.898 ☑
    throat — *see* Foreign body, pharynx
    trachea — *see* Foreign body, trachea
  retained (old) (nonmagnetic) (in)
    anterior chamber (eye) — *see* Foreign body, intraocular, old, retained, anterior chamber
      magnetic — *see* Foreign body, intraocular, old, retained, magnetic, anterior chamber
    ciliary body — *see* Foreign body, intraocular, old, retained, ciliary body
      magnetic — *see* Foreign body, intraocular, old, retained, magnetic, ciliary body
    eyelid H02.819
      left H02.816
        lower H02.815
        upper H02.814
      right H02.813
        lower H02.812
        upper H02.811
    fragments — *see* Retained, foreign body fragments (type of)
    globe — *see* Foreign body, intraocular, old, retained
      magnetic — *see* Foreign body, intraocular, old, retained, magnetic
    intraocular — *see* Foreign body, intraocular, old, retained
      magnetic — *see* Foreign body, intraocular, old, retained, magnetic
    iris — *see* Foreign body, intraocular, old, retained, iris
      magnetic — *see* Foreign body, intraocular, old, retained, magnetic, iris
    lens — *see* Foreign body, intraocular, old, retained, lens

Foreign body — *continued*
  retained — *continued*
    lens — *see* Foreign body, intraocular, old, retained, lens — *continued*
      magnetic — *see* Foreign body, intraocular, old, retained, magnetic, lens
    muscle — *see* Foreign body, retained, soft tissue
    orbit — *see* Foreign body, orbit, old
    posterior wall of globe — *see* Foreign body, intraocular, old, retained, posterior wall
      magnetic — *see* Foreign body, intraocular, old, retained, magnetic, posterior wall
    retrobulbar — *see* Foreign body, orbit, old, retrobulbar
    soft tissue M79.5
    vitreous — *see* Foreign body, intraocular, old, retained, vitreous body
      magnetic — *see* Foreign body, intraocular, old, retained, magnetic, vitreous body
  retina S05.5- ☑
  superficial, without open wound
    abdomen, abdominal (wall) S30.851 ☑
    alveolar process S00.552 ☑
    ankle S90.55- ☑
    antecubital space — *see* Foreign body, superficial, forearm
    anus S30.857 ☑
    arm (upper) S40.85- ☑
    auditory canal — *see* Foreign body, superficial, ear
    auricle — *see* Foreign body, superficial, ear
    axilla — *see* Foreign body, superficial, arm
    back, lower S30.850 ☑
    breast S20.15- ☑
    brow S00.85 ☑
    buttock S30.850 ☑
    calf — *see* Foreign body, superficial, leg
    canthus — *see* Foreign body, superficial, eyelid
    cheek S00.85 ☑
      internal S00.552 ☑
    chest wall — *see* Foreign body, superficial, thorax
    chin S00.85 ☑
    clitoris S30.854 ☑
    costal region — *see* Foreign body, superficial, thorax
    digit(s)
      foot — *see* Foreign body, superficial, toe
      hand — *see* Foreign body, superficial, finger
    ear S00.45- ☑
    elbow S50.35- ☑
    epididymis S30.853 ☑
    epigastric region S30.851 ☑
    epiglottis S10.15 ☑
    esophagus, cervical S10.15 ☑
    eyebrow — *see* Foreign body, superficial, eyelid
    eyelid S00.25- ☑
    face S00.85 ☑
    finger(s) S60.459 ☑
      index S60.45- ☑
      little S60.45- ☑
      middle S60.45- ☑
      ring S60.45- ☑
    flank S30.851 ☑
    foot (except toe(s) alone) S90.85- ☑
      toe — *see* Foreign body, superficial, toe
    forearm S50.85- ☑
      elbow only — *see* Foreign body, superficial, elbow
    forehead S00.85 ☑
    genital organs, external
      female S30.856 ☑
      male S30.855 ☑
    groin S30.851 ☑
    gum S00.552 ☑
    hand S60.55- ☑
    head S00.95 ☑
      ear — *see* Foreign body, superficial, ear
      eyelid — *see* Foreign body, superficial, eyelid
      lip S00.551 ☑
      nose S00.35 ☑
      oral cavity S00.552 ☑
      scalp S00.05 ☑
      specified site NEC S00.85 ☑
    heel — *see* Foreign body, superficial, foot
    hip S70.25- ☑
    inguinal region S30.851 ☑
    interscapular region S20.459 ☑

☑ Additional Character Required — Refer to the Tabular List for Character Selection   ▽ Subterms under main terms may continue to next column or page

Foreign body — *continued*
  superficial, without open wound — *continued*
    jaw S00.85 ☑
    knee S80.25- ☑
    labium (majus) (minus) S30.854 ☑
    larynx S10.15 ☑
    leg (lower) S80.85- ☑
      knee — *see* Foreign body, superficial, knee
      upper — *see* Foreign body, superficial, thigh
    lip S00.551 ☑
    lower back S30.850 ☑
    lumbar region S30.850 ☑
    malar region S00.85 ☑
    mammary — *see* Foreign body, superficial, breast
    mastoid region S00.85 ☑
    mouth S00.552 ☑
    nail
      finger — *see* Foreign body, superficial, finger
      toe — *see* Foreign body, superficial, toe
    nape S10.85 ☑
    nasal S00.35 ☑
    neck S10.95 ☑
      specified site NEC S10.85 ☑
      throat S10.15 ☑
    nose S00.35 ☑
    occipital region S00.05 ☑
    oral cavity S00.552 ☑
    orbital region — *see* Foreign body, superficial, eyelid
    palate S00.552 ☑
    palm — *see* Foreign body, superficial, hand
    parietal region S00.05 ☑
    pelvis S30.850 ☑
    penis S30.852 ☑
    perineum
      female S30.854 ☑
      male S30.850 ☑
    periocular area — *see* Foreign body, superficial, eyelid
    phalanges
      finger — *see* Foreign body, superficial, finger
      toe — *see* Foreign body, superficial, toe
    pharynx S10.15 ☑
    pinna — *see* Foreign body, superficial, ear
    popliteal space — *see* Foreign body, superficial, knee
    prepuce S30.852 ☑
    pubic region S30.850 ☑
    pudendum
      female S30.856 ☑
      male S30.855 ☑
    sacral region S30.850 ☑
    scalp S00.05 ☑
    scapular region — *see* Foreign body, superficial, shoulder
    scrotum S30.853 ☑
    shin — *see* Foreign body, superficial, leg
    shoulder S40.25- ☑
    sternal region S20.359 ☑
    submaxillary region S00.85 ☑
    submental region S00.85 ☑
    subungual
      finger(s) — *see* Foreign body, superficial, finger
      toe(s) — *see* Foreign body, superficial, toe
    supraclavicular fossa S10.85 ☑
    supraorbital S00.85 ☑
    temple S00.85 ☑
    temporal region S00.85 ☑
    testis S30.853 ☑
    thigh S70.35- ☑
    thorax, thoracic (wall) S20.95 ☑
      back S20.45- ☑
      front S20.35- ☑
    throat S10.15 ☑
    thumb S60.35- ☑
    toe(s) (lesser) S90.456 ☑
      great S90.45- ☑
    tongue S00.552 ☑
    trachea S10.15 ☑
    tunica vaginalis S30.853 ☑
    tympanum, tympanic membrane — *see* Foreign body, superficial, ear
    uvula S00.552 ☑
    vagina S30.854 ☑
    vocal cords S10.15 ☑
    vulva S30.854 ☑

Foreign body — *continued*
  superficial, without open wound — *continued*
    wrist S60.85- ☑
  swallowed T18.9 ☑
  trachea T17.408 ☑
    causing
      asphyxiation T17.400 ☑
        food (bone) (seed) T17.420 ☑
        gastric contents (vomitus) T17.410 ☑
        specified type NEC T17.490 ☑
      injury NEC T17.408 ☑
        food (bone) (seed) T17.428 ☑
        gastric contents (vomitus) T17.418 ☑
        specified type NEC T17.498 ☑
  type of fragment — *see* Retained, foreign body fragments (type of)
  vitreous (humor) S05.5- ☑
Forestier's disease (rhizomelic pseudopolyarthritis) M35.3
  meaning ankylosing hyperostosis — *see* Hyperostosis, ankylosing
Formation
  hyalin in cornea — *see* Degeneration, cornea
  sequestrum in bone (due to infection) — *see* Osteomyelitis, chronic
  valve
    colon, congenital Q43.8
    ureter (congenital) Q62.39
Formication R20.2
Fort Bragg fever A27.89
Fossa (*see also* condition)
  pyriform — *see* condition
Foster-Kennedy syndrome H47.14- ☑
Fothergill's
  disease (trigeminal neuralgia) (*see also* Neuralgia, trigeminal)
  scarlatina anginosa A38.9
Foul breath R19.6
Foundling Z76.1
Fournier disease or gangrene N49.3
  female N76.89
Fourth
  cranial nerve — *see* condition
  molar K00.1
Foville's (peduncular) **disease or syndrome** G46.3
Fox (-Fordyce) disease (apocrine miliaria) L75.2
Fracture, burst — *see* Fracture, traumatic, by site
Fracture, chronic — *see* Fracture, pathological, by site
Fracture, insufficiency — *see* Fracture, pathological, by site
Fracture, nontraumatic, NEC
  atypical
    femur M84.750- ☑
      complete
        oblique M84.759 ☑
          left side M84.758 ☑
          right side M84.757 ☑
        transverse M84.756 ☑
          left side M84.755 ☑
          right side M84.754 ☑
      incomplete M84.753 ☑
        left side M84.752 ☑
        right side M84.751 ☑
Fracture, pathological (pathologic) (*see also* Fracture, traumatic) M84.40 ☑
  ankle M84.47- ☑
  carpus M84.44- ☑
  clavicle M84.41- ☑
  compression (not due to trauma) (*see also* Collapse, vertebra) M48.50- ☑
  dental implant M27.63
  dental restorative material K08.539
    with loss of material K08.531
    without loss of material K08.530
  due to
    neoplastic disease NEC (*see also* Neoplasm) M84.50 ☑
      ankle M84.57- ☑
      carpus M84.54- ☑
      clavicle M84.51- ☑
      femur M84.55- ☑
      fibula M84.56- ☑
      finger M84.54- ☑
      hip M84.559 ☑
      humerus M84.52- ☑
      ilium M84.550 ☑

Fracture, pathological — *continued*
  due to — *continued*
    neoplastic disease (*see also* Neoplasm) — *continued*
      ischium M84.550 ☑
      metacarpus M84.54- ☑
      metatarsus M84.57- ☑
      neck M84.58 ☑
      pelvis M84.550 ☑
      radius M84.53- ☑
      rib M84.58 ☑
      scapula M84.51- ☑
      skull M84.58 ☑
      specified site NEC M84.58 ☑
      tarsus M84.57- ☑
      tibia M84.56- ☑
      toe M84.57- ☑
      ulna M84.53- ☑
      vertebra M84.58 ☑
    osteoporosis M80.00 ☑
      disuse — *see* Osteoporosis, specified type NEC, with pathological fracture
      drug-induced — *see* Osteoporosis, drug-induced, with pathological fracture
      idiopathic — *see* Osteoporosis, specified type NEC, with pathological fracture
      postmenopausal — *see* Osteoporosis, postmenopausal, with pathological fracture
      postoophorectomy — *see* Osteoporosis, postoophorectomy, with pathological fracture
      postsurgical malabsorption — *see* Osteoporosis, specified type NEC, with pathological fracture
      specified cause NEC — *see* Osteoporosis, specified type NEC, with pathological fracture
    specified disease NEC M84.60 ☑
      ankle M84.67- ☑
      carpus M84.64- ☑
      clavicle M84.61- ☑
      femur M84.65- ☑
      fibula M84.66- ☑
      finger M84.64- ☑
      hip M84.65- ☑
      humerus M84.62- ☑
      ilium M84.650 ☑
      ischium M84.650 ☑
      metacarpus M84.64- ☑
      metatarsus M84.67- ☑
      neck M84.68 ☑
      radius M84.63- ☑
      rib M84.68 ☑
      scapula M84.61- ☑
      skull M84.68 ☑
      tarsus M84.67- ☑
      tibia M84.66- ☑
      toe M84.67- ☑
      ulna M84.63- ☑
      vertebra M84.68 ☑
  femur M84.45- ☑
  fibula M84.46- ☑
  finger M84.44- ☑
  hip M84.459 ☑
  humerus M84.42- ☑
  ilium M84.454 ☑
  ischium M84.454 ☑
  joint prosthesis — *see* Complications, joint prosthesis, mechanical, breakdown, by site
    periprosthetic — *see* Fracture, pathological, periprosthetic
  metacarpus M84.44- ☑
  metatarsus M84.47- ☑
  neck M84.48 ☑
  pelvis M84.454 ☑
  periprosthetic M97.9 ☑
    ankle M97.2- ☑
    elbow M97.4- ☑
    finger M97.8 ☑
    hip M97.0- ☑
    knee M97.1- ☑
    other specified joint M97.8 ☑
    shoulder M97.3- ☑
    spinal joint M97.8 ☑
    toe joint M97.8 ☑
    wrist joint M97.8 ☑
  radius M84.43- ☑

Fracture, pathological — *continued*
  restorative material (dental) K08.539
    with loss of material K08.531
    without loss of material K08.530
  rib M84.48 ☑
  scapula M84.41- ☑
  skull M84.48 ☑
  tarsus M84.47- ☑
  tibia M84.46- ☑
  toe M84.47- ☑
  ulna M84.43- ☑
  vertebra M84.48 ☑
Fracture, traumatic (abduction) (adduction) (separation)
    (*see also* Fracture, pathological) T14.8 ☑
  acetabulum S32.40- ☑
    column
      anterior (displaced) (iliopubic) S32.43- ☑
        nondisplaced S32.436 ☑
      posterior (displaced) (ilioischial) S32.443 ☑
        nondisplaced S32.44- ☑
    dome (displaced) S32.48- ☑
      nondisplaced S32.48 ☑
    specified NEC S32.49- ☑
    transverse (displaced) S32.45- ☑
      with associated posterior wall fracture (displaced) S32.46- ☑
        nondisplaced S32.46- ☑
      nondisplaced S32.45- ☑
    wall
      anterior (displaced) S32.41- ☑
        nondisplaced S32.41- ☑
      medial (displaced) S32.47- ☑
        nondisplaced S32.47- ☑
      posterior (displaced) S32.42- ☑
        with associated transverse fracture (displaced) S32.46- ☑
          nondisplaced S32.46- ☑
        nondisplaced S32.42- ☑
  acromion — *see* Fracture, scapula, acromial process
  ankle S82.899 ☑
    bimalleolar (displaced) S82.84- ☑
      nondisplaced S82.84- ☑
    lateral malleolus only (displaced) S82.6- ☑
      nondisplaced S82.6- ☑
    medial malleolus (displaced) S82.5- ☑
      associated with Maisonneuve's fracture — *see* Fracture, Maisonneuve's
      nondisplaced S82.5- ☑
    talus — *see* Fracture, tarsal, talus
    trimalleolar (displaced) S82.85- ☑
      nondisplaced S82.85- ☑
  arm (upper) (*see also* Fracture, humerus, shaft)
    humerus — *see* Fracture, humerus
    radius — *see* Fracture, radius
    ulna — *see* Fracture, ulna
  astragalus — *see* Fracture, tarsal, talus
  atlas — *see* Fracture, neck, cervical vertebra, first
  axis — *see* Fracture, neck, cervical vertebra, second
  back — *see* Fracture, vertebra
  Barton's — *see* Barton's fracture
  base of skull — *see* Fracture, skull, base
  basicervical (basal) (femoral) S72.0 ☑
  Bennett's — *see* Bennett's fracture
  bimalleolar — *see* Fracture, ankle, bimalleolar
  blow-out S02.3- ☑
  bone NEC T14.8 ☑
    birth injury P13.9
    following insertion of orthopedic implant, joint prosthesis or bone plate — *see* Fracture, following insertion of orthopedic implant, joint prosthesis or bone plate
    in (due to) neoplastic disease NEC — *see* Fracture, pathological, due to, neoplastic disease
    pathological (cause unknown) — *see* Fracture, pathological
  breast bone — *see* Fracture, sternum
  bucket handle (semilunar cartilage) — *see* Tear, meniscus
  burst — *see* Fracture, traumatic, by site
  calcaneus — *see* Fracture, tarsal, calcaneus
  carpal bone(s) S62.10- ☑
    capitate (displaced) S62.13- ☑
      nondisplaced S62.13- ☑
    cuneiform — *see* Fracture, carpal bone, triquetrum
    hamate (body) (displaced) S62.143 ☑
      hook process (displaced) S62.15- ☑

Fracture, traumatic — *continued*
  carpal bone(s) — *continued*
    hamate — *continued*
      hook process — *continued*
        nondisplaced S62.15- ☑
      nondisplaced S62.14- ☑
    larger multangular — *see* Fracture, carpal bones, trapezium
    lunate (displaced) S62.12- ☑
      nondisplaced S62.12- ☑
    navicular S62.00- ☑
      distal pole (displaced) S62.01- ☑
        nondisplaced S62.01- ☑
      middle third (displaced) S62.02- ☑
        nondisplaced S62.02- ☑
      proximal third (displaced) S62.03- ☑
        nondisplaced S62.03- ☑
      volar tuberosity — *see* Fracture, carpal bones, navicular, distal pole
    os magnum — *see* Fracture, carpal bones, capitate
    pisiform (displaced) S62.16- ☑
      nondisplaced S62.16- ☑
    semilunar — *see* Fracture, carpal bones, lunate
    smaller multangular — *see* Fracture, carpal bones, trapezoid
    trapezium (displaced) S62.17- ☑
      nondisplaced S62.17- ☑
    trapezoid (displaced) S62.18- ☑
      nondisplaced S62.18- ☑
    triquetrum (displaced) S62.11- ☑
      nondisplaced S62.11- ☑
    unciform — *see* Fracture, carpal bones, hamate
  cervical — *see* Fracture, vertebra, cervical
  clavicle S42.00- ☑
    acromial end (displaced) S42.03- ☑
      nondisplaced S42.03- ☑
    birth injury P13.4
    lateral end — *see* Fracture, clavicle, acromial end
    shaft (displaced) S42.02- ☑
      nondisplaced S42.02- ☑
    sternal end (anterior) (displaced) S42.01- ☑
      nondisplaced S42.01- ☑
      posterior S42.01- ☑
  coccyx S32.2 ☑
  collapsed — *see* Collapse, vertebra
  collar bone — *see* Fracture, clavicle
  Colles' — *see* Colles' fracture
  coronoid process — *see* Fracture, ulna, upper end, coronoid process
  corpus cavernosum penis S39.840 ☑
  costochondral cartilage S23.41 ☑
  costochondral, costosternal junction — *see* Fracture, rib
  cranium — *see* Fracture, skull
  cricoid cartilage S12.8 ☑
  cuboid (ankle) — *see* Fracture, tarsal, cuboid
  cuneiform
    foot — *see* Fracture, tarsal, cuneiform
    wrist — *see* Fracture, carpal, triquetrum
  delayed union — *see* Delay, union, fracture
  dental restorative material K08.539
    with loss of material K08.531
    without loss of material K08.530
  due to
    birth injury — *see* Birth, injury, fracture
    osteoporosis — *see* Osteoporosis, with fracture
  Dupuytren's — *see* Fracture, ankle, lateral malleolus
  elbow S42.40- ☑
  ethmoid (bone) (sinus) — *see* Fracture, skull, base
  face bone S02.92 ☑
  fatigue (*see also* Fracture, stress)
    vertebra M48.40 ☑
      cervical region M48.42 ☑
      cervicothoracic region M48.43 ☑
      lumbar region M48.46 ☑
      lumbosacral region M48.47 ☑
      occipito-atlanto-axial region M48.41 ☑
      sacrococcygeal region M48.48 ☑
      thoracic region M48.44 ☑
      thoracolumbar region M48.45 ☑
  femur, femoral S72.9- ☑
    basicervical (basal) S72.0 ☑
    birth injury P13.2
    capital epiphyseal S79.01- ☑
    condyles, epicondyles — *see* Fracture, femur, lower end

Fracture, traumatic — *continued*
  femur, femoral — *continued*
    distal end — *see* Fracture, femur, lower end
    epiphysis
      head — *see* Fracture, femur, upper end, epiphysis
      lower — *see* Fracture, femur, lower end, epiphysis
      upper — *see* Fracture, femur, upper end, epiphysis
    following insertion of implant, prosthesis or plate M96.66- ☑
    head — *see* Fracture, femur, upper end, head
    intertrochanteric — *see* Fracture, femur, trochanteric
    intratrochanteric — *see* Fracture, femur, trochanteric
    lower end S72.40- ☑
      condyle (displaced) S72.41- ☑
        lateral (displaced) S72.42- ☑
          nondisplaced S72.42- ☑
        medial (displaced) S72.43- ☑
          nondisplaced S72.43- ☑
        nondisplaced S72.41- ☑
      epiphysis (displaced) S72.44- ☑
        nondisplaced S72.44- ☑
      physeal S79.10- ☑
        Salter-Harris
          Type I S79.11- ☑
          Type II S79.12- ☑
          Type III S79.13- ☑
          Type IV S79.14- ☑
          specified NEC S79.19- ☑
      specified NEC S72.49- ☑
      supracondylar (displaced) S72.45- ☑
        with intracondylar extension (displaced) S72.46- ☑
          nondisplaced S72.46- ☑
        nondisplaced S72.45- ☑
      torus S72.47- ☑
    neck — *see* Fracture, femur, upper end, neck
    pertrochanteric — *see* Fracture, femur, trochanteric
    shaft (lower third) (middle third) (upper third) S72.30- ☑
      comminuted (displaced) S72.35- ☑
        nondisplaced S72.35- ☑
      oblique (displaced) S72.33- ☑
        nondisplaced S72.33- ☑
      segmental (displaced) S72.36- ☑
        nondisplaced S72.36- ☑
      specified NEC S72.39- ☑
      spiral (displaced) S72.34- ☑
        nondisplaced S72.34- ☑
      transverse (displaced) S72.32- ☑
        nondisplaced S72.32- ☑
    specified site NEC — *see* subcategory S72.8 ☑
    subcapital (displaced) S72.01- ☑
    subtrochanteric (region) (section) (displaced) S72.2- ☑
      nondisplaced S72.2- ☑
    transcervical — *see* Fracture, femur, upper end, neck
    transtrochanteric — *see* Fracture, femur, trochanteric
    trochanteric S72.10- ☑
      apophyseal (displaced) S72.13- ☑
        nondisplaced S72.13- ☑
      greater trochanter (displaced) S72.11- ☑
        nondisplaced S72.11- ☑
      intertrochanteric (displaced) S72.14- ☑
        nondisplaced S72.14- ☑
      lesser trochanter (displaced) S72.12- ☑
        nondisplaced S72.12- ☑
    upper end S72.00- ☑
      apophyseal (displaced) S72.13- ☑
        nondisplaced S72.13- ☑
      cervicotrochanteric — *see* Fracture, femur, upper end, neck, base
      epiphysis (displaced) S72.02- ☑
        nondisplaced S72.02- ☑
      head S72.05- ☑
        articular (displaced) S72.06- ☑
          nondisplaced S72.06- ☑
        specified NEC S72.09- ☑
      intertrochanteric (displaced) S72.14- ☑

☑ Additional Character Required — Refer to the Tabular List for Character Selection   ▽ Subterms under main terms may continue to next column or page

Fracture, traumatic — *continued*
  femur, femoral — *continued*
    upper end — *continued*
      intertrochanteric — *continued*
        nondisplaced S72.14- ☑
      intracapsular S72.01- ☑
      midcervical (displaced) S72.03- ☑
        nondisplaced S72.03- ☑
      neck S72.00- ☑
        base (displaced) S72.04- ☑
          nondisplaced S72.04- ☑
        specified NEC S72.09- ☑
      pertrochanteric — *see* Fracture, femur, upper
        end, trochanteric
      physeal S79.00- ☑
        Salter-Harris type I S79.01- ☑
        specified NEC S79.09- ☑
      subcapital (displaced) S72.01- ☑
      subtrochanteric (displaced) S72.2- ☑
        nondisplaced S72.2- ☑
      transcervical — *see* Fracture, femur, upper end,
        midcervical
      trochanteric S72.10- ☑
        greater (displaced) S72.11- ☑
          nondisplaced S72.11- ☑
        lesser (displaced) S72.12- ☑
          nondisplaced S72.12- ☑
  fibula (shaft) (styloid) S82.40- ☑
    comminuted (displaced) S82.45- ☑
      nondisplaced S82.45- ☑
    following insertion of implant, prosthesis or plate
      M96.67- ☑
    involving ankle or malleolus — *see* Fracture, fibula,
      lateral malleolus
    lateral malleolus (displaced) S82.6- ☑
      nondisplaced S82.6- ☑
    lower end
      physeal S89.30- ☑
        Salter-Harris
          Type I S89.31- ☑
          Type II S89.32- ☑
        specified NEC S89.39- ☑
      specified NEC S82.83- ☑
      torus S82.82- ☑
    oblique (displaced) S82.43- ☑
      nondisplaced S82.43- ☑
    segmental (displaced) S82.46- ☑
      nondisplaced S82.46- ☑
    specified NEC S82.49- ☑
    spiral (displaced) S82.44- ☑
      nondisplaced S82.44- ☑
    transverse (displaced) S82.42- ☑
      nondisplaced S82.42- ☑
    upper end
      physeal S89.20- ☑
        Salter-Harris
          Type I S89.21- ☑
          Type II S89.22- ☑
        specified NEC S89.29- ☑
      specified NEC S82.83- ☑
      torus S82.81- ☑
  finger (except thumb) S62.60- ☑
    distal phalanx (displaced) S62.63- ☑
      nondisplaced S62.66- ☑
    index S62.60- ☑
      distal phalanx (displaced) S62.63- ☑
        nondisplaced S62.66- ☑
      medial phalanx (displaced) S62.62- ☑
        nondisplaced S62.65- ☑
      proximal phalanx (displaced) S62.61- ☑
        nondisplaced S62.64- ☑
    little S62.60- ☑
      distal phalanx (displaced) S62.63- ☑
        nondisplaced S62.66- ☑
      medial phalanx (displaced) S62.62- ☑
        nondisplaced S62.65- ☑
      proximal phalanx (displaced) S62.61- ☑
        nondisplaced S62.64- ☑
    medial phalanx (displaced) S62.62- ☑
      nondisplaced S62.65- ☑
    middle S62.60- ☑
      distal phalanx (displaced) S62.63- ☑
        nondisplaced S62.66- ☑
      medial phalanx (displaced) S62.62- ☑
        nondisplaced S62.65- ☑
      proximal phalanx (displaced) S62.61- ☑

Fracture, traumatic — *continued*
  finger — *continued*
    middle — *continued*
      proximal phalanx — *continued*
        nondisplaced S62.64- ☑
    proximal phalanx (displaced) S62.61- ☑
      nondisplaced S62.64- ☑
    ring S62.60- ☑
      distal phalanx (displaced) S62.63- ☑
        nondisplaced S62.66- ☑
      medial phalanx (displaced) S62.62- ☑
        nondisplaced S62.65- ☑
      proximal phalanx (displaced) S62.61- ☑
        nondisplaced S62.64- ☑
    thumb — *see* Fracture, thumb
  following insertion (intraoperative) (postoperative) of
    orthopedic implant, joint prosthesis or bone
    plate M96.69
    femur M96.66- ☑
    fibula M96.67- ☑
    humerus M96.62- ☑
    pelvis M96.65
    radius M96.63- ☑
    specified bone NEC M96.69
    tibia M96.67- ☑
    ulna M96.63- ☑
  foot S92.90- ☑
    astragalus — *see* Fracture, tarsal, talus
    calcaneus — *see* Fracture, tarsal, calcaneus
    cuboid — *see* Fracture, tarsal, cuboid
    cuneiform — *see* Fracture, tarsal, cuneiform
    metatarsal — *see* Fracture, metatarsal
    navicular — *see* Fracture, tarsal, navicular
    sesamoid S92.81- ☑
    specified NEC S92.81- ☑
    talus — *see* Fracture, tarsal, talus
    tarsal — *see* Fracture, tarsal
    toe — *see* Fracture, toe
  forearm S52.9- ☑
    radius — *see* Fracture, radius
    ulna — *see* Fracture, ulna
  fossa (anterior) (middle) (posterior) S02.19 ☑
  frontal (bone) (skull) S02.0 ☑
    sinus S02.19 ☑
  glenoid (cavity) (scapula) — *see* Fracture, scapula,
    glenoid cavity
  greenstick — *see* Fracture, by site
  hallux — *see* Fracture, toe, great
  hand S62.9- ☑
    carpal — *see* Fracture, carpal bone
    finger (except thumb) — *see* Fracture, finger
    metacarpal — *see* Fracture, metacarpal
    navicular (scaphoid) (hand) — *see* Fracture, carpal
      bone, navicular
    thumb — *see* Fracture, thumb
  healed or old
    with complications — *code by* Nature of the com-
      plication
  heel bone — *see* Fracture, tarsal, calcaneus
  Hill-Sachs S42.29- ☑
  hip — *see* Fracture, femur, neck
  humerus S42.30- ☑
    anatomical neck — *see* Fracture, humerus, upper
      end
    articular process — *see* Fracture, humerus, lower
      end
    capitellum — *see* Fracture, humerus, lower end,
      condyle, lateral
    distal end — *see* Fracture, humerus, lower end
    epiphysis
      lower — *see* Fracture, humerus, lower end,
        physeal
      upper — *see* Fracture, humerus, upper end,
        physeal
    external condyle — *see* Fracture, humerus, lower
      end, condyle, lateral
    following insertion of implant, prosthesis or plate
      M96.62- ☑
    great tuberosity — *see* Fracture, humerus, upper
      end, greater tuberosity
    intercondylar — *see* Fracture, humerus, lower end
    internal epicondyle — *see* Fracture, humerus,
      lower end, epicondyle, medial
    lesser tuberosity — *see* Fracture, humerus, upper
      end, lesser tuberosity
    lower end S42.40- ☑

Fracture, traumatic — *continued*
  humerus — *continued*
    lower end — *continued*
      condyle
        lateral (displaced) S42.45- ☑
          nondisplaced S42.45- ☑
        medial (displaced) S42.46- ☑
          nondisplaced S42.46- ☑
      epicondyle
        lateral (displaced) S42.43- ☑
          nondisplaced S42.43- ☑
        medial (displaced) S42.44- ☑
          incarcerated S42.44- ☑
          nondisplaced S42.44- ☑
      physeal S49.10- ☑
        Salter-Harris
          Type I S49.11- ☑
          Type II S49.12- ☑
          Type III S49.13- ☑
          Type IV S49.14- ☑
        specified NEC S49.19- ☑
      specified NEC (displaced) S42.49- ☑
        nondisplaced S42.49- ☑
      supracondylar (simple) (displaced) S42.41- ☑
        with intercondylar fracture — *see* Fracture,
          humerus, lower end
        comminuted (displaced) S42.42- ☑
          nondisplaced S42.42- ☑
        nondisplaced S42.41- ☑
      torus S42.48- ☑
      transcondylar (displaced) S42.47- ☑
        nondisplaced S42.47- ☑
    proximal end — *see* Fracture, humerus, upper end
    shaft S42.30- ☑
      comminuted (displaced) S42.35- ☑
        nondisplaced S42.35- ☑
      greenstick S42.31- ☑
      oblique (displaced) S42.33- ☑
        nondisplaced S42.33- ☑
      segmental (displaced) S42.36- ☑
        nondisplaced S42.36- ☑
      specified NEC S42.39- ☑
      spiral (displaced) S42.34- ☑
        nondisplaced S42.34- ☑
      transverse (displaced) S42.32- ☑
        nondisplaced S42.32- ☑
    supracondylar — *see* Fracture, humerus, lower end
    surgical neck — *see* Fracture, humerus, upper end,
      surgical neck
    trochlea — *see* Fracture, humerus, lower end,
      condyle, medial
    tuberosity — *see* Fracture, humerus, upper end
    upper end S42.20- ☑
      anatomical neck — *see* Fracture, humerus, up-
        per end, specified NEC
      articular head — *see* Fracture, humerus, upper
        end, specified NEC
      epiphysis — *see* Fracture, humerus, upper end,
        physeal
      greater tuberosity (displaced) S42.25- ☑
        nondisplaced S42.25- ☑
      lesser tuberosity (displaced) S42.26- ☑
        nondisplaced S42.26- ☑
      physeal S49.00- ☑
        Salter-Harris
          Type I S49.01- ☑
          Type II S49.02- ☑
          Type III S49.03- ☑
          Type IV S49.04- ☑
        specified NEC S49.09- ☑
      specified NEC (displaced) S42.29- ☑
        nondisplaced S42.29- ☑
      surgical neck (displaced) S42.21- ☑
        four-part S42.24- ☑
        nondisplaced S42.21- ☑
        three-part S42.23- ☑
        two-part (displaced) S42.22- ☑
          nondisplaced S42.22- ☑
      torus S42.27- ☑
      transepiphyseal — *see* Fracture, humerus, up-
        per end, physeal
  hyoid bone S12.8 ☑
  ilium S32.30- ☑
    with disruption of pelvic ring — *see* Disruption,
      pelvic ring
    avulsion (displaced) S32.31- ☑

Fracture, traumatic — *continued*
  ilium — *continued*
    avulsion — *continued*
      nondisplaced S32.31- ☑
      specified NEC S32.39- ☑
    impaction, impacted — *code as* Fracture, by site
    innominate bone — *see* Fracture, ilium
    instep — *see* Fracture, foot
    ischium S32.60- ☑
      with disruption of pelvic ring — *see* Disruption, pelvic ring
      avulsion (displaced) S32.61- ☑
        nondisplaced S32.61- ☑
      specified NEC S32.69- ☑
    jaw (bone) (lower) — *see* Fracture, mandible
      upper — *see* Fracture, maxilla
    joint prosthesis — *see* Complications, joint prosthesis, mechanical, breakdown, by site
      periprosthetic — *see* Fracture, traumatic, periprosthetic
    knee cap — *see* Fracture, patella
    larynx S12.8 ☑
    late effects — *see* Sequelae, fracture
    leg (lower) S82.9- ☑
      ankle — *see* Fracture, ankle
      femur — *see* Fracture, femur
      fibula — *see* Fracture, fibula
      malleolus — *see* Fracture, ankle
      patella — *see* Fracture, patella
      specified site NEC S82.89- ☑
      tibia — *see* Fracture, tibia
    lumbar spine — *see* Fracture, vertebra, lumbar
    lumbosacral spine S32.9 ☑
    Maisonneuve's (displaced) S82.86- ☑
      nondisplaced S82.86- ☑
    malar bone (*see also* Fracture, maxilla) S02.400 ☑
      left side S02.40B ☑
      right side S02.40A ☑
    malleolus — *see* Fracture, ankle
    malunion — *see* Fracture, by site
    mandible (lower jaw (bone)) S02.609 ☑
      alveolus S02.67- ☑
      angle (of jaw) S02.65- ☑
      body, unspecified S02.600 ☑
        left side S02.602 ☑
        right side S02.601 ☑
      condylar process S02.61- ☑
      coronoid process S02.63- ☑
      ramus, unspecified S02.64- ☑
      specified site NEC S02.69 ☑
      subcondylar process S02.62- ☑
      symphysis S02.66 ☑
    manubrium (sterni) S22.21 ☑
      dissociation from sternum S22.23 ☑
    march — *see* Fracture, traumatic, stress, by site
    maxilla, maxillary (bone) (sinus) (superior) (upper jaw) S02.401 ☑
      alveolus S02.42 ☑
      inferior — *see* Fracture, mandible
      LeFort I S02.411 ☑
      LeFort II S02.412 ☑
      LeFort III S02.413 ☑
      left side S02.40D ☑
      right side S02.40C ☑
    metacarpal S62.309 ☑
      base (displaced) S62.319 ☑
        nondisplaced S62.349 ☑
      fifth S62.30- ☑
        base (displaced) S62.31- ☑
          nondisplaced S62.34- ☑
        neck (displaced) S62.33- ☑
          nondisplaced S62.36- ☑
        shaft (displaced) S62.32- ☑
          nondisplaced S62.35- ☑
        specified NEC S62.398 ☑
      first S62.20- ☑
        base NEC (displaced) S62.23- ☑
          nondisplaced S62.23- ☑
        Bennett's — *see* Bennett's fracture
        neck (displaced) S62.25- ☑
          nondisplaced S62.25- ☑
        shaft (displaced) S62.24- ☑
          nondisplaced S62.24- ☑
        specified NEC S62.29- ☑
      fourth S62.30- ☑
        base (displaced) S62.31- ☑

Fracture, traumatic — *continued*
  metacarpal — *continued*
    fourth — *continued*
      base — *continued*
        nondisplaced S62.34- ☑
      neck (displaced) S62.33- ☑
        nondisplaced S62.36- ☑
      shaft (displaced) S62.32- ☑
        nondisplaced S62.35- ☑
      specified NEC S62.39- ☑
      neck (displaced) S62.33- ☑
      nondisplaced S62.36- ☑
      Rolando's — *see* Rolando's fracture
      second S62.30- ☑
        base (displaced) S62.31- ☑
          nondisplaced S62.34- ☑
        neck (displaced) S62.33- ☑
          nondisplaced S62.36- ☑
        shaft (displaced) S62.32- ☑
          nondisplaced S62.35- ☑
        specified NEC S62.39- ☑
      shaft (displaced) S62.32- ☑
        nondisplaced S62.35- ☑
      specified NEC S62.399 ☑
      third S62.30- ☑
        base (displaced) S62.31- ☑
          nondisplaced S62.34- ☑
        neck (displaced) S62.33- ☑
          nondisplaced S62.36- ☑
        shaft (displaced) S62.32- ☑
          nondisplaced S62.35- ☑
        specified NEC S62.39- ☑
    metastatic — *see* Fracture, pathological, due to, neoplastic disease (*see also* Neoplasm)
    metatarsal bone S92.30- ☑
      fifth (displaced) S92.35- ☑
        nondisplaced S92.35- ☑
      first (displaced) S92.31- ☑
        nondisplaced S92.31- ☑
      fourth (displaced) S92.34- ☑
        nondisplaced S92.34- ☑
      physeal S99.10- ☑
        Salter-Harris
          Type I S99.11- ☑
          Type II S99.12- ☑
          Type III S99.13- ☑
          Type IV S99.14- ☑
        specified NEC S99.19- ☑
      second (displaced) S92.32- ☑
        nondisplaced S92.32- ☑
      third (displaced) S92.33- ☑
        nondisplaced S92.33- ☑
    Monteggia's — *see* Monteggia's fracture
    multiple
      hand (and wrist) NEC — *see* Fracture, by site
      ribs — *see* Fracture, rib, multiple
    nasal (bone(s)) S02.2 ☑
    navicular (scaphoid) (foot) (*see also* Fracture, tarsal, navicular)
      hand — *see* Fracture, carpal, navicular
    neck S12.9 ☑
      cervical vertebra S12.9 ☑
        fifth (displaced) S12.400 ☑
          nondisplaced S12.401 ☑
          specified type NEC (displaced) S12.490 ☑
            nondisplaced S12.491 ☑
        first (displaced) S12.000 ☑
          burst (stable) S12.01 ☑
            unstable S12.02 ☑
          lateral mass (displaced) S12.040 ☑
            nondisplaced S12.041 ☑
          nondisplaced S12.001 ☑
          posterior arch (displaced) S12.030 ☑
            nondisplaced S12.031 ☑
          specified type NEC (displaced) S12.090 ☑
            nondisplaced S12.091 ☑
        fourth (displaced) S12.300 ☑
          nondisplaced S12.301 ☑
          specified type NEC (displaced) S12.390 ☑
            nondisplaced S12.391 ☑
        second (displaced) S12.100 ☑
          dens (anterior) (displaced) (type II) S12.110 ☑
            nondisplaced S12.112 ☑
            posterior S12.111 ☑

Fracture, traumatic — *continued*
  neck — *continued*
    cervical vertebra — *continued*
      second — *continued*
        dens — *continued*
          specified type NEC (displaced) S12.120 ☑
            nondisplaced S12.121 ☑
        nondisplaced S12.101 ☑
        specified type NEC (displaced) S12.190 ☑
          nondisplaced S12.191 ☑
      seventh (displaced) S12.600 ☑
        nondisplaced S12.601 ☑
        specified type NEC (displaced) S12.690 ☑
          nondisplaced S12.691 ☑
      sixth (displaced) S12.500 ☑
        nondisplaced S12.501 ☑
        specified type NEC (displaced) S12.590 ☑
          nondisplaced S12.591 ☑
      third (displaced) S12.200 ☑
        nondisplaced S12.201 ☑
        specified type NEC (displaced) S12.290 ☑
          nondisplaced S12.291 ☑
    hyoid bone S12.8 ☑
    larynx S12.8 ☑
    specified site NEC S12.8 ☑
    thyroid cartilage S12.8 ☑
    trachea S12.8 ☑
  neoplastic NEC — *see* Fracture, pathological, due to, neoplastic disease
  neural arch — *see* Fracture, vertebra
  newborn — *see* Birth, injury, fracture
  nontraumatic — *see* Fracture, pathological
  nonunion — *see* Nonunion, fracture
  nose, nasal (bone) (septum) S02.2 ☑
  occiput — *see* Fracture, skull, base, occiput
  odontoid process — *see* Fracture, neck, cervical vertebra, second
  olecranon (process) (ulna) — *see* Fracture, ulna, upper end, olecranon process
  orbit, orbital (bone) (region) S02.8- ☑
    floor (blow-out) S02.3- ☑
    roof S02.19 ☑
  os
    calcis — *see* Fracture, tarsal, calcaneus
    magnum — *see* Fracture, carpal, capitate
    pubis — *see* Fracture, pubis
  palate S02.8- ☑
  parietal bone (skull) S02.0 ☑
  patella S82.00- ☑
    comminuted (displaced) S82.04- ☑
      nondisplaced S82.04- ☑
    longitudinal (displaced) S82.02- ☑
      nondisplaced S82.02- ☑
    osteochondral (displaced) S82.01- ☑
      nondisplaced S82.01- ☑
    specified NEC S82.09- ☑
    transverse (displaced) S82.03- ☑
      nondisplaced S82.03- ☑
  pedicle (of vertebral arch) — *see* Fracture, vertebra
  pelvis, pelvic (bone) S32.9 ☑
    acetabulum — *see* Fracture, acetabulum
    circle — *see* Disruption, pelvic ring
    following insertion of implant, prosthesis or plate M96.65
    ilium — *see* Fracture, ilium
    ischium — *see* Fracture, ischium
    multiple
      with disruption of pelvic ring (circle) — *see* Disruption, pelvic ring
      without disruption of pelvic ring (circle) S32.82 ☑
    pubis — *see* Fracture, pubis
    sacrum — *see* Fracture, sacrum
    specified site NEC S32.89 ☑
  periprosthetic, around internal prosthetic joint M97.9 ☑
    ankle M97.2- ☑
    elbow M97.4- ☑
    finger M97.8 ☑
    hip M97.0- ☑
    knee M97.1- ☑
    shoulder M97.3- ☑
    specified joint NEC M97.8 ☑
    spine M97.8 ☑
    toe M97.8 ☑

Fracture, traumatic — *continued*
  periprosthetic, around internal prosthetic joint —
        continued
     wrist M97.8 ☑
  phalanx
     foot — *see* Fracture, toe
     hand — *see* Fracture, finger
  pisiform — *see* Fracture, carpal, pisiform
  pond — *see* Fracture, skull
  prosthetic device, internal — *see* Complications,
        prosthetic device, by site, mechanical
  pubis S32.50- ☑
     with disruption of pelvic ring — *see* Disruption,
           pelvic ring
     specified site NEC S32.59- ☑
     superior rim S32.51- ☑
  radius S52.9- ☑
     distal end — *see* Fracture, radius, lower end
     following insertion of implant, prosthesis or plate
           M96.63- ☑
     head — *see* Fracture, radius, upper end, head
     lower end S52.50- ☑
        Barton's — *see* Barton's fracture
        Colles' — *see* Colles' fracture
        extraarticular NEC S52.55- ☑
        intraarticular NEC S52.57- ☑
        physeal S59.20- ☑
           Salter-Harris
              Type I S59.21- ☑
              Type II S59.22- ☑
              Type III S59.23- ☑
              Type IV S59.24- ☑
              specified NEC S59.29- ☑
        Smith's — *see* Smith's fracture
        specified NEC S52.59- ☑
        styloid process (displaced) S52.51- ☑
           nondisplaced S52.51- ☑
        torus S52.52- ☑
     neck — *see* Fracture, radius, upper end
     proximal end — *see* Fracture, radius, upper end
     shaft S52.30- ☑
        bent bone S52.38- ☑
        comminuted (displaced) S52.35- ☑
           nondisplaced S52.35- ☑
        Galeazzi's — *see* Galeazzi's fracture
        greenstick S52.31- ☑
        oblique (displaced) S52.33- ☑
           nondisplaced S52.33- ☑
        segmental (displaced) S52.36- ☑
           nondisplaced S52.36- ☑
        specified NEC S52.39- ☑
        spiral (displaced) S52.34- ☑
           nondisplaced S52.34- ☑
        transverse (displaced) S52.32- ☑
           nondisplaced S52.32- ☑
     upper end S52.10- ☑
        head (displaced) S52.12- ☑
           nondisplaced S52.12- ☑
        neck (displaced) S52.13- ☑
           nondisplaced S52.13- ☑
        physeal S59.10- ☑
           Salter-Harris
              Type I S59.11- ☑
              Type II S59.12- ☑
              Type III S59.13- ☑
              Type IV S59.14- ☑
              specified NEC S59.19- ☑
        specified NEC S52.18- ☑
        torus S52.11- ☑
  ramus
     inferior or superior, pubis — *see* Fracture, pubis
     mandible — *see* Fracture, mandible
  restorative material (dental) K08.539
        with loss of material K08.531
        without loss of material K08.530
  rib S22.3- ☑
     with flail chest — *see* Flail, chest
     multiple S22.4- ☑
        with flail chest — *see* Flail, chest
  root, tooth — *see* Fracture, tooth
  sacrum S32.10 ☑
     specified NEC S32.19 ☑
     Type
        1 S32.14 ☑
        2 S32.15 ☑
        3 S32.16 ☑

Fracture, traumatic — *continued*
  sacrum — *continued*
     Type — *continued*
        4 S32.17 ☑
     Zone
        I S32.119 ☑
           displaced (minimally) S32.111 ☑
              severely S32.112 ☑
           nondisplaced S32.110 ☑
        II S32.129 ☑
           displaced (minimally) S32.121 ☑
              severely S32.122 ☑
           nondisplaced S32.120 ☑
        III S32.139 ☑
           displaced (minimally) S32.131 ☑
              severely S32.132 ☑
           nondisplaced S32.130 ☑
  scaphoid (hand) (*see also* Fracture, carpal, navicular)
     foot — *see* Fracture, tarsal, navicular
  scapula S42.10- ☑
     acromial process (displaced) S42.12- ☑
        nondisplaced S42.12- ☑
     body (displaced) S42.11- ☑
        nondisplaced S42.11- ☑
     coracoid process (displaced) S42.13- ☑
        nondisplaced S42.13- ☑
     glenoid cavity (displaced) S42.14- ☑
        nondisplaced S42.14- ☑
     neck (displaced) S42.15- ☑
        nondisplaced S42.15- ☑
     specified NEC S42.19- ☑
  semilunar bone, wrist — *see* Fracture, carpal, lunate
  sequelae — *see* Sequelae, fracture
  sesamoid bone
     foot S92.81- ☑
     hand — *see* Fracture, carpal
     other — *see* Fracture, traumatic, by site
  shepherd's — *see* Fracture, tarsal, talus
  shoulder (girdle) S42.9- ☑
     blade — *see* Fracture, scapula
  sinus (ethmoid) (frontal) S02.19 ☑
  skull S02.91 ☑
     base S02.10- ☑
        occiput S02.119 ☑
           condyle S02.113 ☑
              specified NEC S02.118 ☑
                 left side S02.11H ☑
                 right side S02.11G ☑
              type I S02.110 ☑
                 left side S02.11B ☑
                 right side S02.11A ☑
              type II S02.111 ☑
                 left side S02.11D ☑
                 right side S02.11C ☑
              type III S02.112 ☑
                 left side S02.11F ☑
                 right side S02.11E ☑
        specified NEC S02.19 ☑
     birth injury P13.0
     frontal bone S02.0 ☑
     parietal bone S02.0 ☑
     specified site NEC S02.8- ☑
     temporal bone S02.19 ☑
     vault S02.0 ☑
  Smith's — *see* Smith's fracture
  sphenoid (bone) (sinus) S02.19 ☑
  spine — *see* Fracture, vertebra
  spinous process — *see* Fracture, vertebra
  spontaneous (cause unknown) — *see* Fracture,
        pathological
  stave (of thumb) — *see* Fracture, metacarpal, first
  sternum S22.20 ☑
     with flail chest — *see* Flail, chest
     body S22.22 ☑
     manubrium S22.21 ☑
     xiphoid (process) S22.24 ☑
  stress M84.30 ☑
     ankle M84.37- ☑
     carpus M84.34- ☑
     clavicle M84.31- ☑
     femoral neck M84.359 ☑
     femur M84.35- ☑
     fibula M84.36- ☑
     finger M84.34- ☑
     hip M84.359 ☑
     humerus M84.32- ☑

Fracture, traumatic — *continued*
  stress — *continued*
     ilium M84.350 ☑
     ischium M84.350 ☑
     metacarpus M84.34- ☑
     metatarsus M84.37- ☑
     neck — *see* Fracture, fatigue, vertebra
     pelvis M84.350 ☑
     radius M84.33- ☑
     rib M84.38 ☑
     scapula M84.31- ☑
     skull M84.38 ☑
     tarsus M84.37- ☑
     tibia M84.36- ☑
     toe M84.37- ☑
     ulna M84.33- ☑
     vertebra — *see* Fracture, fatigue, vertebra
  supracondylar, elbow — *see* Fracture, humerus, lower
        end, supracondylar
  symphysis pubis — *see* Fracture, pubis
  talus (ankle bone) — *see* Fracture, tarsal, talus
  tarsal bone(s) S92.20- ☑
     astragalus — *see* Fracture, tarsal, talus
     calcaneus S92.00- ☑
        anterior process (displaced) S92.02- ☑
           nondisplaced S92.02- ☑
        body (displaced) S92.01- ☑
           nondisplaced S92.01- ☑
        extraarticular NEC (displaced) S92.05- ☑
           nondisplaced S92.05- ☑
        intraarticular (displaced) S92.06- ☑
           nondisplaced S92.06- ☑
        physeal S99.00- ☑
           Salter-Harris
              Type I S99.01- ☑
              Type II S99.02- ☑
              Type III S99.03- ☑
              Type IV S99.04- ☑
              specified NEC S99.09- ☑
        tuberosity (displaced) S92.04- ☑
           avulsion (displaced) S92.03- ☑
              nondisplaced S92.03- ☑
           nondisplaced S92.04- ☑
     cuboid (displaced) S92.21- ☑
        nondisplaced S92.21- ☑
     cuneiform
        intermediate (displaced) S92.23- ☑
           nondisplaced S92.23- ☑
        lateral (displaced) S92.22- ☑
           nondisplaced S92.22- ☑
        medial (displaced) S92.24- ☑
           nondisplaced S92.24- ☑
     navicular (displaced) S92.25- ☑
        nondisplaced S92.25- ☑
     scaphoid — *see* Fracture, tarsal, navicular
     talus S92.10- ☑
        avulsion (displaced) S92.15- ☑
           nondisplaced S92.15- ☑
        body (displaced) S92.12- ☑
           nondisplaced S92.12- ☑
        dome (displaced) S92.14- ☑
           nondisplaced S92.14- ☑
        head (displaced) S92.12- ☑
           nondisplaced S92.12- ☑
        lateral process (displaced) S92.14- ☑
           nondisplaced S92.14- ☑
        neck (displaced) S92.11- ☑
           nondisplaced S92.11- ☑
        posterior process (displaced) S92.13- ☑
           nondisplaced S92.13- ☑
        specified NEC S92.19- ☑
  temporal bone (styloid) S02.19 ☑
  thorax (bony) S22.9 ☑
     with flail chest — *see* Flail, chest
     rib S22.3- ☑
        multiple S22.4- ☑
           with flail chest — *see* Flail, chest
     sternum S22.20 ☑
        body S22.22 ☑
        manubrium S22.21 ☑
        xiphoid process S22.24 ☑
     vertebra (displaced) S22.009 ☑
        burst (stable) S22.001 ☑
           unstable S22.002 ☑
        eighth S22.069 ☑
           burst (stable) S22.061 ☑

Fracture, traumatic — *continued*
 thorax — *continued*
  vertebra — *continued*
   eighth — *continued*
    burst — *continued*
     unstable S22.062 ☑
    specified type NEC S22.068 ☑
    wedge compression S22.060 ☑
   eleventh S22.089 ☑
    burst (stable) S22.081 ☑
     unstable S22.082 ☑
    specified type NEC S22.088 ☑
    wedge compression S22.080 ☑
   fifth S22.059 ☑
    burst (stable) S22.051 ☑
     unstable S22.052 ☑
    specified type NEC S22.058 ☑
    wedge compression S22.050 ☑
   first S22.019 ☑
    burst (stable) S22.011 ☑
     unstable S22.012 ☑
    specified type NEC S22.018 ☑
    wedge compression S22.010 ☑
   fourth S22.049 ☑
    burst (stable) S22.041 ☑
     unstable S22.042 ☑
    specified type NEC S22.048 ☑
    wedge compression S22.040 ☑
   ninth S22.079 ☑
    burst (stable) S22.071 ☑
     unstable S22.072 ☑
    specified type NEC S22.078 ☑
    wedge compression S22.070 ☑
   nondisplaced S22.001 ☑
   second S22.029 ☑
    burst (stable) S22.021 ☑
     unstable S22.022 ☑
    specified type NEC S22.028 ☑
    wedge compression S22.020 ☑
   seventh S22.069 ☑
    burst (stable) S22.061 ☑
     unstable S22.062 ☑
    specified type NEC S22.068 ☑
    wedge compression S22.060 ☑
   sixth S22.059 ☑
    burst (stable) S22.051 ☑
     unstable S22.052 ☑
    specified type NEC S22.058 ☑
    wedge compression S22.050 ☑
   specified type NEC S22.008 ☑
   tenth S22.079 ☑
    burst (stable) S22.071 ☑
     unstable S22.072 ☑
    specified type NEC S22.078 ☑
    wedge compression S22.070 ☑
   third S22.039 ☑
    burst (stable) S22.031 ☑
     unstable S22.032 ☑
    specified type NEC S22.038 ☑
    wedge compression S22.030 ☑
   twelfth S22.089 ☑
    burst (stable) S22.081 ☑
     unstable S22.082 ☑
    specified type NEC S22.088 ☑
    wedge compression S22.080 ☑
   wedge compression S22.000 ☑
 thumb S62.50- ☑
  distal phalanx (displaced) S62.52- ☑
   nondisplaced S62.52- ☑
  proximal phalanx (displaced) S62.51- ☑
   nondisplaced S62.51- ☑
 thyroid cartilage S12.8 ☑
 tibia (shaft) S82.20- ☑
  comminuted (displaced) S82.25- ☑
   nondisplaced S82.25- ☑
  condyles — *see* Fracture, tibia, upper end
  distal end — *see* Fracture, tibia, lower end
  epiphysis
   lower — *see* Fracture, tibia, lower end
   upper — *see* Fracture, tibia, upper end
  following insertion of implant, prosthesis or plate
   M96.67- ☑
  head (involving knee joint) — *see* Fracture, tibia,
   upper end
  intercondyloid eminence — *see* Fracture, tibia,
   upper end

Fracture, traumatic — *continued*
 tibia — *continued*
  involving ankle or malleolus — *see* Fracture, ankle,
   medial malleolus
  lower end S82.30- ☑
   physeal S89.10- ☑
    Salter-Harris
     Type I S89.11- ☑
     Type II S89.12- ☑
     Type III S89.13- ☑
     Type IV S89.14- ☑
    specified NEC S89.19- ☑
   pilon (displaced) S82.87- ☑
    nondisplaced S82.87- ☑
   specified NEC S82.39- ☑
   torus S82.31- ☑
  malleolus — *see* Fracture, ankle, medial malleolus
  oblique (displaced) S82.23- ☑
   nondisplaced S82.23- ☑
  pilon — *see* Fracture, tibia, lower end, pilon
  proximal end — *see* Fracture, tibia, upper end
  segmental (displaced) S82.26- ☑
   nondisplaced S82.26- ☑
  specified NEC S82.29- ☑
  spine — *see* Fracture, tibia, upper end, spine
  spiral (displaced) S82.24- ☑
   nondisplaced S82.24- ☑
  transverse (displaced) S82.22- ☑
   nondisplaced S82.22- ☑
  tuberosity — *see* Fracture, tibia, upper end,
   tuberosity
  upper end S82.10- ☑
   bicondylar (displaced) S82.14- ☑
    nondisplaced S82.14- ☑
   lateral condyle (displaced) S82.12- ☑
    nondisplaced S82.12- ☑
   medial condyle (displaced) S82.13- ☑
    nondisplaced S82.13- ☑
   physeal S89.00- ☑
    Salter-Harris
     Type I S89.01- ☑
     Type II S89.02- ☑
     Type III S89.03- ☑
     Type IV S89.04- ☑
    specified NEC S89.09- ☑
   plateau — *see* Fracture, tibia, upper end, bi-
    condylar
   specified NEC S82.19- ☑
   spine (displaced) S82.11- ☑
    nondisplaced S82.11- ☑
   torus S82.16- ☑
   tuberosity (displaced) S82.15- ☑
    nondisplaced S82.15- ☑
 toe S92.91- ☑
  great (displaced) S92.40- ☑
   distal phalanx (displaced) S92.42- ☑
    nondisplaced S92.42- ☑
   nondisplaced S92.40- ☑
   proximal phalanx (displaced) S92.41- ☑
    nondisplaced S92.41- ☑
   specified NEC S92.49- ☑
  lesser (displaced) S92.50- ☑
   distal phalanx (displaced) S92.53- ☑
    nondisplaced S92.53- ☑
   medial phalanx (displaced) S92.52- ☑
    nondisplaced S92.52- ☑
   nondisplaced S92.50- ☑
   proximal phalanx (displaced) S92.51- ☑
    nondisplaced S92.51- ☑
   specified NEC S92.59- ☑
  physeal
   phalanx S99.20- ☑
    Salter-Harris
     Type I S99.21- ☑
     Type II S99.22- ☑
     Type III S99.23- ☑
     Type IV S99.24- ☑
    specified NEC S99.29- ☑
 tooth (root) S02.5 ☑
 trachea (cartilage) S12.8 ☑
 transverse process — *see* Fracture, vertebra
 trapezium or trapezoid bone — *see* Fracture, carpal
 trimalleolar — *see* Fracture, ankle, trimalleolar
 triquetrum (cuneiform of carpus) — *see* Fracture,
  carpal, triquetrum
 trochanter — *see* Fracture, femur, trochanteric

Fracture, traumatic — *continued*
 tuberosity (external) — *see* Fracture, traumatic, by site
 ulna (shaft) S52.20- ☑
  bent bone S52.28- ☑
  coronoid process — *see* Fracture, ulna, upper end,
   coronoid process
  distal end — *see* Fracture, ulna, lower end
  following insertion of implant, prosthesis or plate
   M96.63- ☑
  head S52.60- ☑
  lower end S52.60- ☑
   physeal S59.00- ☑
    Salter-Harris
     Type I S59.01- ☑
     Type II S59.02- ☑
     Type III S59.03- ☑
     Type IV S59.04- ☑
    specified NEC S59.09- ☑
   specified NEC S52.69- ☑
   styloid process (displaced) S52.61- ☑
    nondisplaced S52.61- ☑
   torus S52.62- ☑
  proximal end — *see* Fracture, ulna, upper end
  shaft S52.20- ☑
   comminuted (displaced) S52.25- ☑
    nondisplaced S52.25- ☑
   greenstick S52.21- ☑
   Monteggia's — *see* Monteggia's fracture
   oblique (displaced) S52.23- ☑
    nondisplaced S52.23- ☑
   segmental (displaced) S52.26- ☑
    nondisplaced S52.26- ☑
   specified NEC S52.29- ☑
   spiral (displaced) S52.24- ☑
    nondisplaced S52.24- ☑
   transverse (displaced) S52.22- ☑
    nondisplaced S52.22- ☑
  upper end S52.00- ☑
   coronoid process (displaced) S52.04- ☑
    nondisplaced S52.04- ☑
   olecranon process (displaced) S52.02- ☑
    with intraarticular extension S52.03- ☑
    nondisplaced S52.02- ☑
     with intraarticular extension S52.03- ☑
   specified NEC S52.09- ☑
   torus S52.01- ☑
 unciform — *see* Fracture, carpal, hamate
 vault of skull S02.0 ☑
 vertebra, vertebral (arch) (body) (column) (neural arch)
  (pedicle) (spinous process) (transverse process)
  atlas — *see* Fracture, neck, cervical vertebra, first
  axis — *see* Fracture, neck, cervical vertebra, second
  cervical (teardrop) S12.9 ☑
   axis — *see* Fracture, neck, cervical vertebra,
    second
   first (atlas) — *see* Fracture, neck, cervical verte-
    bra, first
   second (axis) — *see* Fracture, neck, cervical
    vertebra, second
  chronic M84.48 ☑
  coccyx S32.2 ☑
  dorsal — *see* Fracture, thorax, vertebra
  lumbar S32.009 ☑
   burst (stable) S32.001 ☑
    unstable S32.002 ☑
   fifth S32.059 ☑
    burst (stable) S32.051 ☑
     unstable S32.052 ☑
    specified type NEC S32.058 ☑
    wedge compression S32.050 ☑
   first S32.019 ☑
    burst (stable) S32.011 ☑
     unstable S32.012 ☑
    specified type NEC S32.018 ☑
    wedge compression S32.010 ☑
   fourth S32.049 ☑
    burst (stable) S32.041 ☑
     unstable S32.042 ☑
    specified type NEC S32.048 ☑
    wedge compression S32.040 ☑
   second S32.029 ☑
    burst (stable) S32.021 ☑
     unstable S32.022 ☑
    specified type NEC S32.028 ☑
    wedge compression S32.020 ☑
   specified type NEC S32.008 ☑

☑ **Additional Character Required — Refer to the Tabular List for Character Selection**   ▽ **Subterms under main terms may continue to next column or page**

Index

Fracture, traumatic — Fracture, traumatic

Fracture, traumatic — *continued*
  vertebra, vertebral — *continued*
    lumbar — *continued*
      third S32.Ø39 ☑
        burst (stable) S32.Ø31 ☑
          unstable S32.Ø32 ☑
        specified type NEC S32.Ø38 ☑
        wedge compression S32.Ø3Ø ☑
        wedge compression S32.ØØØ ☑
    metastatic — *see* Collapse, vertebra, in, specified
        disease NEC (*see also* Neoplasm)
    newborn (birth injury) P11.5
    sacrum S32.1Ø ☑
      specified NEC S32.19 ☑
      Type
        1 S32.14 ☑
        2 S32.15 ☑
        3 S32.16 ☑
        4 S32.17 ☑
      Zone
        I S32.119 ☑
          displaced (minimally) S32.111 ☑
            severely S32.112 ☑
          nondisplaced S32.11Ø ☑
        II S32.129 ☑
          displaced (minimally) S32.121 ☑
            severely S32.122 ☑
          nondisplaced S32.12Ø ☑
        III S32.139 ☑
          displaced (minimally) S32.131 ☑
            severely S32.132 ☑
          nondisplaced S32.13Ø ☑
    thoracic — *see* Fracture, thorax, vertebra
  vertex SØ2.Ø ☑
  vomer (bone) SØ2.2 ☑
  wrist S62.1Ø- ☑
    carpal — *see* Fracture, carpal bone
    navicular (scaphoid) (hand) — *see* Fracture, carpal,
        navicular
  xiphisternum, xiphoid (process) S22.24 ☑
  zygoma SØ2.4Ø2 ☑
    left side SØ2.4ØF ☑
    right side SØ2.4ØE ☑
Fragile, fragility
  autosomal site Q95.5
  bone, congenital (with blue sclera) Q78.Ø
  capillary (hereditary) D69.8
  hair L67.8
  nails L6Ø.3
  non-sex chromosome site Q95.5
  X chromosome Q99.2
Fragilitas
  crinium L67.8
  ossium (with blue sclerae) (hereditary) Q78.Ø
  unguium L6Ø.3
    congenital Q84.6
Fragments, cataract (lens), **following cataract surgery**
      H59.Ø2- ☑
  retained foreign body — *see* Retained, foreign body
      fragments (type of)
Frailty (frail) R54
  mental R41.81
Frambesia, frambesial (tropica) (*see also* Yaws)
  initial lesion or ulcer A66.Ø
  primary A66.Ø
Frambeside
  gummatous A66.4
  of early yaws A66.2
Frambesioma A66.1
Franceschetti-Klein (-Wildervanck) **disease or syn-
      drome** Q75.4
Francis' disease — *see* Tularemia
Franklin disease C88.2
Frank's essential thrombocytopenia D69.3
Fraser's syndrome Q87.Ø
Freckle(s) L81.2
  malignant melanoma in — *see* Melanoma
  melanotic (Hutchinson's) — *see* Melanoma, in situ
  retinal D49.81
Frederickson's hyperlipoproteinemia, type
  I and V E78.3
  IIA E78.ØØ
  IIB and III E78.2
  IV E78.1
Freeman Sheldon syndrome Q87.Ø
Freezing (*see also* Effect, adverse, cold) T69.9 ☑

Freiberg's disease (infraction of metatarsal head or os-
    teochondrosis) — *see* Osteochondrosis, juvenile,
    metatarsus
Frei's disease A55
Fremitus, friction, cardiac RØ1.2
Frenum, frenulum
  external os Q51.828
  tongue (shortening) (congenital) Q38.1
Frequency micturition (nocturnal) R35.Ø
  psychogenic F45.8
Frey's syndrome
  auriculotemporal G5Ø.8
  hyperhidrosis L74.52
Friction
  burn — *see* Burn, by site
  fremitus, cardiac RØ1.2
  precordial RØ1.2
  sounds, chest RØ9.89
Friderichsen-Waterhouse syndrome or disease A39.1
Friedländer's B (bacillus) **NEC** (*see also* condition) A49.8
Friedreich's
  ataxia G11.1
  combined systemic disease G11.1
  facial hemihypertrophy Q67.4
  sclerosis (cerebellum) (spinal cord) G11.1
Frigidity F52.22
Fröhlich's syndrome E23.6
Frontal (*see also* condition)
  lobe syndrome FØ7.Ø
Frostbite (superficial) T33.9Ø ☑
  with
    partial thickness skin loss — *see* Frostbite (superfi-
        cial), by site
    tissue necrosis T34.9Ø ☑
  abdominal wall T33.3 ☑
    with tissue necrosis T34.3 ☑
  ankle T33.81- ☑
    with tissue necrosis T34.81- ☑
  arm T33.4- ☑
    with tissue necrosis T34.4- ☑
    finger(s) — *see* Frostbite, finger
    hand — *see* Frostbite, hand
    wrist — *see* Frostbite, wrist
  ear T33.Ø1- ☑
    with tissue necrosis T34.Ø1- ☑
  face T33.Ø9 ☑
    with tissue necrosis T34.Ø9 ☑
  finger T33.53- ☑
    with tissue necrosis T34.53- ☑
  foot T33.82- ☑
    with tissue necrosis T34.82- ☑
  hand T33.52- ☑
    with tissue necrosis T34.52- ☑
  head T33.Ø9 ☑
    with tissue necrosis T34.Ø9 ☑
    ear — *see* Frostbite, ear
    nose — *see* Frostbite, nose
  hip (and thigh) T33.6- ☑
    with tissue necrosis T34.6- ☑
  knee T33.7- ☑
    with tissue necrosis T34.7- ☑
  leg T33.9- ☑
    with tissue necrosis T34.9- ☑
    ankle — *see* Frostbite, ankle
    foot — *see* Frostbite, foot
    knee — *see* Frostbite, knee
    lower T33.7- ☑
      with tissue necrosis T34.7- ☑
    thigh — *see* Frostbite, hip
    toe — *see* Frostbite, toe
  limb
    lower T33.99 ☑
      with tissue necrosis T34.99 ☑
    upper — *see* Frostbite, arm
  neck T33.1 ☑
    with tissue necrosis T34.1 ☑
  nose T33.Ø2 ☑
    with tissue necrosis T34.Ø2 ☑
  pelvis T33.3 ☑
    with tissue necrosis T34.3 ☑
  specified site NEC T33.99 ☑
    with tissue necrosis T34.99 ☑
  thigh — *see* Frostbite, hip
  thorax T33.2 ☑
    with tissue necrosis T34.2 ☑
  toes T33.83- ☑

Frostbite — *continued*
  toes — *continued*
    with tissue necrosis T34.83- ☑
  trunk T33.99 ☑
    with tissue necrosis T34.99 ☑
  wrist T33.51- ☑
    with tissue necrosis T34.51- ☑
Frotteurism F65.81
Frozen (*see also* Effect, adverse, cold) T69.9 ☑
  pelvis (female) N94.89
    male K66.8
  shoulder — *see* Capsulitis, adhesive
Fructokinase deficiency E74.11
Fructose 1,6 diphosphatase deficiency E74.19
Fructosemia (benign) (essential) E74.12
Fructosuria (benign) (essential) E74.11
Fuchs'
  black spot (myopic) (*see also* Myopia, degenerative)
      H44.2- ☑
  dystrophy (corneal endothelium) H18.51
  heterochromic cyclitis — *see* Cyclitis, Fuchs' hete-
      rochromic
Fucosidosis E77.1
Fugue R68.89
  dissociative F44.1
  hysterical (dissociative) F44.1
  postictal in epilepsy — *see* Epilepsy
  reaction to exceptional stress (transient) F43.Ø
Fulminant, fulminating — *see* condition
Functional (*see also* condition)
  bleeding (uterus) N93.8
Functioning, intellectual, borderline R41.83
Fundus — *see* condition
Fungemia NOS B49
Fungus, fungous
  cerebral G93.89
  disease NOS B49
  infection — *see* Infection, fungus
Funiculitis (acute) (chronic) (endemic) N49.1
  gonococcal (acute) (chronic) A54.23
  tuberculous A18.15
Funnel
  breast (acquired) M95.4
    congenital Q67.6
    sequelae (late effect) of rickets E64.3
  chest (acquired) M95.4
    congenital Q67.6
    sequelae (late effect) of rickets E64.3
  pelvis (acquired) M95.5
    with disproportion (fetopelvic) O33.3 ☑
      causing obstructed labor O65.3
    congenital Q74.2
FUO (fever of unknown origin) R5Ø.9
Furfur L21.Ø
  microsporon B36.Ø
Furrier's lung J67.8
Furrowed K14.5
  nail(s) (transverse) L6Ø.4
    congenital Q84.6
  tongue K14.5
    congenital Q38.3
Furuncle LØ2.92
  abdominal wall LØ2.221
  ankle — *see* Furuncle, lower limb
  antecubital space — *see* Furuncle, upper limb
  anus K61.Ø
  arm — *see* Furuncle, upper limb
  auditory canal, external — *see* Abscess, ear, external
  auricle (ear) — *see* Abscess, ear, external
  axilla (region) LØ2.42- ☑
  back (any part) LØ2.222
  breast N61.1
  buttock LØ2.32
  cheek (external) LØ2.Ø2
  chest wall LØ2.223
  chin LØ2.Ø2
  corpus cavernosum N48.21
  ear, external — *see* Abscess, ear, external
  external auditory canal — *see* Abscess, ear, external
  eyelid — *see* Abscess, eyelid
  face LØ2.Ø2
  femoral (region) — *see* Furuncle, lower limb
  finger — *see* Furuncle, hand
  flank LØ2.221
  foot LØ2.62- ☑
  forehead LØ2.Ø2
  gluteal (region) LØ2.32

Furuncle — *continued*
  groin L02.224
  hand L02.52- ☑
  head L02.821
    face L02.02
  hip — *see* Furuncle, lower limb
  kidney — *see* Abscess, kidney
  knee — *see* Furuncle, lower limb
  labium (majus) (minus) N76.4
  lacrimal
    gland — *see* Dacryoadenitis
    passages (duct) (sac) — *see* Inflammation, lacrimal,
      passages, acute
  leg (any part) — *see* Furuncle, lower limb
  lower limb L02.42- ☑
  malignant A22.0
  mouth K12.2
  navel L02.226
  neck L02.12
  nose J34.0
  orbit, orbital — *see* Abscess, orbit
  palmar (space) — *see* Furuncle, hand
  partes posteriores L02.32
  pectoral region L02.223
  penis N48.21
  perineum L02.225
  pinna — *see* Abscess, ear, external
  popliteal — *see* Furuncle, lower limb
  prepatellar — *see* Furuncle, lower limb
  scalp L02.821
  seminal vesicle N49.0
  shoulder — *see* Furuncle, upper limb
  specified site NEC L02.828
  submandibular K12.2
  temple (region) L02.02
  thumb — *see* Furuncle, hand
  toe — *see* Furuncle, foot
  trunk L02.229
    abdominal wall L02.221
    back L02.222

Furuncle — *continued*
  trunk — *continued*
    chest wall L02.223
    groin L02.224
    perineum L02.225
    umbilicus L02.226
  umbilicus L02.226
  upper limb L02.42- ☑
  vulva N76.4
Furunculosis — *see* Furuncle
Fused — *see* Fusion, fused
Fusion, fused (congenital)
  astragaloscaphoid Q74.2
  atria Q21.1
  auditory canal Q16.1
  auricles, heart Q21.1
  binocular with defective stereopsis H53.32
  bone Q79.8
  cervical spine M43.22
  choanal Q30.0
  commissure, mitral valve Q23.2
  cusps, heart valve NEC Q24.8
    mitral Q23.2
    pulmonary Q22.1
    tricuspid Q22.4
  ear ossicles Q16.3
  fingers Q70.0 ☑
  hymen Q52.3
  joint (acquired) (*see also* Ankylosis)
    congenital Q74.8
  kidneys (incomplete) Q63.1
  labium (majus) (minus) Q52.5
  larynx and trachea Q34.8
  limb, congenital Q74.8
    lower Q74.2
    upper Q74.0
  lobes, lung Q33.8
  lumbosacral (acquired) M43.27
    arthrodesis status Z98.1
    congenital Q76.49

Fusion, fused — *continued*
  lumbosacral — *continued*
    postprocedural status Z98.1
  nares, nose, nasal, nostril(s) Q30.0
  organ or site not listed — *see* Anomaly, by site
  ossicles Q79.9
    auditory Q16.3
  pulmonic cusps Q22.1
  ribs Q76.6
  sacroiliac (joint) (acquired) M43.28
    arthrodesis status Z98.1
    congenital Q74.2
    postprocedural status Z98.1
  spine (acquired) NEC M43.20
    arthrodesis status Z98.1
    cervical region M43.22
    cervicothoracic region M43.23
    congenital Q76.49
    lumbar M43.26
    lumbosacral region M43.27
    occipito-atlanto-axial region M43.21
    postoperative status Z98.1
    sacrococcygeal region M43.28
    thoracic region M43.24
    thoracolumbar region M43.25
  sublingual duct with submaxillary duct at opening in
    mouth Q38.4
  testes Q55.1
  toes Q70.2- ☑
  tooth, teeth K00.2
  trachea and esophagus Q39.8
  twins Q89.4
  vagina Q52.4
  ventricles, heart Q21.0
  vertebra (arch) — *see* Fusion, spine
  vulva Q52.5
Fusospirillosis (mouth) (tongue) (tonsil) A69.1
Fussy baby R68.12

G

Gain in weight (abnormal) (excessive) (*see also* Weight, gain)

Gaisböck's disease (polycythemia hypertonica) D75.1

Gait abnormality R26.9
- ataxic R26.0
- falling R29.6
- hysterical (ataxic) (staggering) F44.4
- paralytic R26.1
- spastic R26.1
- specified type NEC R26.89
- staggering R26.0
- unsteadiness R26.81
- walking difficulty NEC R26.2

Galactocele (breast) N64.89
- puerperal, postpartum O92.79

Galactokinase deficiency E74.29

Galactophoritis N61.0
- gestational, puerperal, postpartum O91.2- ☑

Galactorrhea O92.6
- not associated with childbirth N64.3

Galactosemia (classic) (congenital) E74.21

Galactosuria E74.29

Galacturia R82.0
- schistosomiasis (bilharziasis) B65.0

GALD (gestational alloimmune liver disease) P78.84

Galeazzi's fracture S52.37- ☑

Galen's vein — *see* condition

Galeophobia F40.218

Gall duct — *see* condition

Gallbladder (*see also* condition)
- acute K81.0

Gallop rhythm R00.8

Gallstone (colic) (cystic duct) (gallbladder) (impacted) (multiple) (*see also* Calculus, gallbladder)
- with
  - cholecystitis — *see* Calculus, gallbladder, with cholecystitis
- bile duct (common) (hepatic) — *see* Calculus, bile duct
  - causing intestinal obstruction K56.3
- specified NEC K80.80
  - with obstruction K80.81

Gambling Z72.6
- pathological (compulsive) F63.0

Gammopathy (of undetermined significance [MGUS]) D47.2
- associated with lymphoplasmacytic dyscrasia D47.2
- monoclonal D47.2
- polyclonal D89.0

Gamna's disease (sideriotic splenomegaly) D73.1

Gamophobia F40.298

Gampsodactylia (congenital) Q66.7

Gamstorp's disease (adynamia episodica hereditaria) G72.3

Gandy-Nanta disease (sideriotic splenomegaly) D73.1

Gang
- membership offenses Z72.810

Gangliocytoma D36.10

Ganglioglioma — *see* Neoplasm, uncertain behavior, by site

Ganglion (compound) (diffuse) (joint) (tendon (sheath)) M67.40
- ankle M67.47- ☑
- foot M67.47- ☑
- forearm M67.43- ☑
- hand M67.44- ☑
- lower leg M67.46- ☑
- multiple sites M67.49
- of yaws (early) (late) A66.6
- pelvic region M67.45- ☑
- periosteal — *see* Periostitis
- shoulder region M67.41- ☑
- specified site NEC M67.48
- thigh region M67.45- ☑
- tuberculous A18.09
- upper arm M67.42- ☑
- wrist M67.43- ☑

Ganglioneuroblastoma — *see* Neoplasm, nerve, malignant

Ganglioneuroma D36.10
- malignant — *see* Neoplasm, nerve, malignant

Ganglioneuromatosis D36.10

Ganglionitis
- fifth nerve — *see* Neuralgia, trigeminal
- gasserian (postherpetic) (postzoster) B02.21

Ganglionitis — *continued*
- geniculate G51.1
  - newborn (birth injury) P11.3
  - postherpetic, postzoster B02.21
- herpes zoster B02.21
- postherpetic geniculate B02.21

Gangliosidosis E75.10
- GM1 E75.19
- GM2 E75.00
  - other specified E75.09
  - Sandhoff disease E75.01
  - Tay-Sachs disease E75.02
- GM3 E75.19
- mucolipidosis IV E75.11

Gangosa A66.5

Gangrene, gangrenous (connective tissue) (dropsical) (dry) (moist) (skin) (ulcer) (*see also* Necrosis) I96
- with diabetes (mellitus) — *see* Diabetes, gangrene
- abdomen (wall) I96
- alveolar M27.3
- appendix K35.80
  - with
    - perforation or rupture K35.2
    - peritoneal abscess K35.3
    - peritonitis NEC K35.3
      - generalized (with perforation or rupture) K35.2
      - localized (with perforation or rupture) K35.3
- arteriosclerotic (general) (senile) — *see* Arteriosclerosis, extremities, with, gangrene
- auricle I96
- Bacillus welchii A48.0
- bladder (infectious) — *see* Cystitis, specified type NEC
- bowel, cecum, or colon — *see* Gangrene, intestine
- Clostridium perfringens or welchii A48.0
- cornea H18.89- ☑
- corpora cavernosa N48.29
  - noninfective N48.89
- cutaneous, spreading I96
- decubital — *see* Ulcer, pressure, by site
- diabetic (any site) — *see* Diabetes, gangrene
- emphysematous — *see* Gangrene, gas
- epidemic — *see* Poisoning, food, noxious, plant
- epididymis (infectional) N45.1
- erysipelas — *see* Erysipelas
- extremity (lower) (upper) I96
- Fournier N49.3
  - female N76.89
- fusospirochetal A69.0
- gallbladder — *see* Cholecystitis, acute
- gas (bacillus) A48.0
  - following
    - abortion — *see* Abortion by type complicated by infection
    - ectopic or molar pregnancy O08.0
- glossitis K14.0
- hernia — *see* Hernia, by site, with gangrene
- intestine, intestinal (hemorrhagic) (massive) (*see also* Infarct, intestine) K55.069
  - with
    - mesenteric embolism (*see also* Infarct, intestine) K55.069
    - obstruction — *see* Obstruction, intestine
- laryngitis J04.0
- limb (lower) (upper) I96
- lung J85.0
  - spirochetal A69.8
- lymphangitis I89.1
- Meleney's (synergistic) — *see* Ulcer, skin
- mesentery (*see also* Infarct, intestine) K55.069
  - with
    - embolism (*see also* Infarct, intestine) K55.069
    - intestinal obstruction — *see* Obstruction, intestine
- mouth A69.0
- ovary — *see* Oophoritis
- pancreas — *see* Pancreatitis, acute
- penis N48.29
  - noninfective N48.89
- perineum I96
- pharynx (*see also* Pharyngitis)
  - Vincent's A69.1
- presenile I73.1
- progressive synergistic — *see* Ulcer, skin
- pulmonary J85.0
- pulpal (dental) K04.1
- quinsy J36
- Raynaud's (symmetric gangrene) I73.01

Gangrene, gangrenous — *continued*
- retropharyngeal J39.2
- scrotum N49.3
  - noninfective N50.89
- senile (atherosclerotic) — *see* Arteriosclerosis, extremities, with, gangrene
- spermatic cord N49.1
  - noninfective N50.89
- spine I96
- spirochetal NEC A69.8
- spreading cutaneous I96
- stomatitis A69.0
- symmetrical I73.01
- testis (infectional) N45.2
  - noninfective N44.8
- throat (*see also* Pharyngitis)
  - diphtheritic A36.0
  - Vincent's A69.1
- thyroid (gland) E07.89
- tooth (pulp) K04.1
- tuberculous NEC — *see* Tuberculosis
- tunica vaginalis N49.1
  - noninfective N50.89
- umbilicus I96
- uterus — *see* Endometritis
- uvulitis K12.2
- vas deferens N49.1
  - noninfective N50.89
- vulva N76.89

Ganister disease J62.8

Ganser's syndrome (hysterical) F44.89

Gardner-Diamond syndrome (autoerythrocyte sensitization) D69.2

Gargoylism E76.01

Garré's disease, osteitis (sclerosing), osteomyelitis — *see* Osteomyelitis, specified type NEC

Garrod's pad, knuckle M72.1

Gartner's duct
- cyst Q52.4
- persistent Q50.6

Gas R14.3
- asphyxiation, inhalation, poisoning, suffocation NEC — *see* Table of Drugs and Chemicals
- excessive R14.0
- gangrene A48.0
  - following
    - abortion — *see* Abortion by type complicated by infection
    - ectopic or molar pregnancy O08.0
- on stomach R14.0
- pains R14.1

Gastralgia (*see also* Pain, abdominal)

Gastrectasis K31.0
- psychogenic F45.8

Gastric — *see* condition

Gastrinoma
- malignant
  - pancreas C25.4
  - specified site NEC — *see* Neoplasm, malignant, by site
  - unspecified site C25.4
- specified site — *see* Neoplasm, uncertain behavior
- unspecified site D37.9

Gastritis (simple) K29.70
- with bleeding K29.71
- acute (erosive) K29.00
  - with bleeding K29.01
- alcoholic K29.20
  - with bleeding K29.21
- allergic K29.60
  - with bleeding K29.61
- atrophic (chronic) K29.40
  - with bleeding K29.41
- chronic (antral) (fundal) K29.50
  - with bleeding K29.51
  - atrophic K29.40
    - with bleeding K29.41
  - superficial K29.30
    - with bleeding K29.31
- dietary counseling and surveillance Z71.3
- due to diet deficiency E63.9
- eosinophilic K52.81
- giant hypertrophic K29.60
  - with bleeding K29.61
- granulomatous K29.60
  - with bleeding K29.61
- hypertrophic (mucosa) K29.60
  - with bleeding K29.61

Index

Gastritis — Glaucoma

Gastritis — *continued*
- nervous F54
- spastic K29.60
  - with bleeding K29.61
  - specified NEC K29.60
    - with bleeding K29.61
- superficial chronic K29.30
  - with bleeding K29.31
- tuberculous A18.83
- viral NEC A08.4

Gastrocarcinoma — *see* Neoplasm, malignant, stomach

Gastrocolic — *see* condition

Gastrodisciasis, gastrodiscoidiasis B66.8

Gastroduodenitis K29.90
- with bleeding K29.91
- virus, viral A08.4
  - specified type NEC A08.39

Gastrodynia — *see* Pain, abdominal

Gastroenteritis (acute) (chronic) (noninfectious) (*see also* Enteritis) K52.9
- allergic K52.29
  - with
    - eosinophilic gastritis or gastroenteritis K52.81
    - food protein-induced enterocolitis syndrome K52.21
    - food protein-induced enteropathy K52.22
- dietetic (*see also* Gastroenteritis, allergic) K52.29
- drug-induced K52.1
- due to
  - Cryptosporidium A07.2
  - drugs K52.1
  - food poisoning — *see* Intoxication, foodborne
  - radiation K52.0
- eosinophilic K52.81
- epidemic (infectious) A09
- food hypersensitivity (*see also* Gastroenteritis, allergic) K52.29
- infectious — *see* Enteritis, infectious
- influenzal — *see* Influenza, with gastroenteritis
- noninfectious K52.9
  - specified NEC K52.89
- rotaviral A08.0
- Salmonella A02.0
- toxic K52.1
- viral NEC A08.4
  - acute infectious A08.39
    - type Norwalk A08.11
  - infantile (acute) A08.39
  - Norwalk agent A08.11
  - rotaviral A08.0
  - severe of infants A08.39
  - specified type NEC A08.39

Gastroenteropathy (*see also* Gastroenteritis) K52.9
- acute, due to Norovirus A08.11
- acute, due to Norwalk agent A08.11
- infectious A09

Gastroenteroptosis K63.4

Gastroesophageal laceration- hemorrhage syndrome K22.6

Gastrointestinal — *see* condition

Gastrojejunal — *see* condition

Gastrojejunitis (*see also* Enteritis) K52.9

Gastrojejunocolic — *see* condition

Gastroliths K31.89

Gastromalacia K31.89

Gastroparalysis K31.84
- diabetic — *see* Diabetes, gastroparalysis

Gastroparesis K31.84
- diabetic — *see* Diabetes, by type, with gastroparesis

Gastropathy K31.9
- congestive portal K31.89
- erythematous K29.70
- exudative K90.89
- portal hypertensive K31.89

Gastroptosis K31.89

Gastrorrhagia K92.2
- psychogenic F45.8

Gastroschisis (congenital) Q79.3

Gastrospasm (neurogenic) (reflex) K31.89
- neurotic F45.8
- psychogenic F45.8

Gastrostaxis — *see* Gastritis, with bleeding

Gastrostenosis K31.89

Gastrostomy
- attention to Z43.1
- status Z93.1

Gastrosuccorrhea (continuous) (intermittent) K31.89
- neurotic F45.8

Gastrosuccorrhea — *continued*
- psychogenic F45.8

Gatophobia F40.218

Gaucher's disease or splenomegaly (adult) (infantile) E75.22

Gee (-Herter)(-Thaysen) **disease** (nontropical sprue) K90.0

Gélineau's syndrome G47.419
- with cataplexy G47.411

Gemination, tooth, teeth K00.2

Gemistocytoma
- specified site — *see* Neoplasm, malignant, by site
- unspecified site C71.9

General, generalized — *see* condition

Genetic
- carrier (status)
  - cystic fibrosis Z14.1
  - hemophilia A (asymptomatic) Z14.01
    - symptomatic Z14.02
  - specified NEC Z14.8
- susceptibility to disease NEC Z15.89
  - malignant neoplasm Z15.09
    - breast Z15.01
    - endometrium Z15.04
    - ovary Z15.02
    - prostate Z15.03
    - specified NEC Z15.09
  - multiple endocrine neoplasia Z15.81

Genital — *see* condition

Genito-anorectal syndrome A55

Genitourinary system — *see* condition

Genu
- congenital Q74.1
- extrorsum (acquired) (*see also* Deformity, varus, knee)
  - congenital Q74.1
  - sequelae (late effect) of rickets E64.3
- introrsum (acquired) (*see also* Deformity, valgus, knee)
  - congenital Q74.1
  - sequelae (late effect) of rickets E64.3
- rachitic (old) E64.3
- recurvatum (acquired) (*see also* Deformity, limb, specified type NEC, lower leg)
  - congenital Q68.2
  - sequelae (late effect) of rickets E64.3
- valgum (acquired) (knock-knee) M21.06- ☑
  - congenital Q74.1
  - sequelae (late effect) of rickets E64.3
- varum (acquired) (bowleg) M21.16- ☑
  - congenital Q74.1
  - sequelae (late effect) of rickets E64.3

Geographic tongue K14.1

Geophagia — *see* Pica

Geotrichosis B48.3
- stomatitis B48.3

Gephyrophobia F40.242

Gerbode defect Q21.0

GERD (gastroesophageal reflux disease) K21.9

Gerhardt's
- disease (erythromelalgia) I73.81
- syndrome (vocal cord paralysis) J38.00
  - bilateral J38.02
  - unilateral J38.01

German measles (*see also* Rubella)
- exposure to Z20.4

Germinoblastoma (diffuse) C85.9- ☑
- follicular C82.9- ☑

Germinoma — *see* Neoplasm, malignant, by site

Gerontoxon — *see* Degeneration, cornea, senile

Gerstmann's syndrome R48.8
- developmental F81.2

Gerstmann-Sträussler-Scheinker syndrome (GSS) A81.82

Gestation (period) (*see also* Pregnancy)
- ectopic — *see* Pregnancy, by site
- multiple O30.9- ☑
  - greater than quadruplets — *see* Pregnancy, multiple (gestation), specified NEC
  - specified NEC — *see* Pregnancy, multiple (gestation), specified NEC

Gestational
- mammary abscess O91.11- ☑
- purulent mastitis O91.11- ☑
- subareolar abscess O91.11- ☑

Ghon tubercle, primary infection A15.7

Ghost
- teeth K00.4
- vessels (cornea) H16.41- ☑

Ghoul hand A66.3

Gianotti-Crosti disease L44.4

Giant
- cell
  - epulis K06.8
  - peripheral granuloma K06.8
- esophagus, congenital Q39.5
- kidney, congenital Q63.3
- urticaria T78.3 ☑
  - hereditary D84.1

Giardiasis A07.1

Gibert's disease or pityriasis L42

Giddiness R42
- hysterical F44.89
- psychogenic F45.8

Gierke's disease (glycogenosis I) E74.01

Gigantism (cerebral) (hypophyseal) (pituitary) E22.0
- constitutional E34.4

Gilbert's disease or syndrome E80.4

Gilchrist's disease B40.9

Gilford-Hutchinson disease E34.8

Gilles de la Tourette's disease or syndrome (motor-verbal tic) F95.2

Gingivitis K05.10
- acute (catarrhal) K05.00
  - necrotizing A69.1
  - nonplaque induced K05.01
  - plaque induced K05.00
- chronic (desquamative) (hyperplastic) (simple marginal) (pregnancy associated) (ulcerative) K05.10
  - nonplaque induced K05.11
  - plaque induced K05.10
- expulsiva — *see* Periodontitis
- necrotizing ulcerative (acute) A69.1
- pellagrous E52
  - acute necrotizing A69.1
- Vincent's A69.1

Gingivoglossitis K14.0

Gingivopericementitis — *see* Periodontitis

Gingivosis — *see* Gingivitis, chronic

Gingivostomatitis K05.10
- herpesviral B00.2
- necrotizing ulcerative (acute) A69.1

Gland, glandular — *see* condition

Glanders A24.0

Glanzmann (-Naegeli) **disease or thrombasthenia** D69.1

Glasgow coma scale
- total score
  - 3-8 R40.243 ☑
  - 9-12 R40.242 ☑
  - 13-15 R40.241 ☑

Glass-blower's disease (cataract) — *see* Cataract, specified NEC

Glaucoma H40.9
- with
  - increased episcleral venous pressure H40.81- ☑
  - pseudoexfoliation of lens — *see* Glaucoma, open angle, primary, capsular
- absolute H44.51- ☑
- angle-closure (primary) H40.20- ☑
  - acute (attack) (crisis) H40.21- ☑
  - chronic H40.22- ☑
  - intermittent H40.23- ☑
  - residual stage H40.24- ☑
- borderline H40.00- ☑
- capsular (with pseudoexfoliation of lens) — *see* Glaucoma, open angle, primary, capsular
- childhood Q15.0
- closed angle — *see* Glaucoma, angle-closure
- congenital Q15.0
- corticosteroid-induced — *see* Glaucoma, secondary, drugs
- hypersecretion H40.82- ☑
- in (due to)
  - amyloidosis E85.4 [H42]
  - aniridia Q13.1 [H42]
  - concussion of globe — *see* Glaucoma, secondary, trauma
  - dislocation of lens — *see* Glaucoma, secondary
  - disorder of lens NEC — *see* Glaucoma, secondary
  - drugs — *see* Glaucoma, secondary, drugs
  - endocrine disease NOS E34.9 [H42]
  - eye
    - inflammation — *see* Glaucoma, secondary, inflammation
    - trauma — *see* Glaucoma, secondary, trauma

Glaucoma — *continued*
  in — *continued*
    hypermature cataract — *see* Glaucoma, secondary
    iridocyclitis — *see* Glaucoma, secondary, inflammation
    lens disorder — *see* Glaucoma, secondary
    Lowe's syndrome E72.03 [H42]
    metabolic disease NOS E88.9 [H42]
    ocular disorders NEC — *see* Glaucoma, secondary
    onchocerciasis B73.02
    pupillary block — *see* Glaucoma, secondary
    retinal vein occlusion — *see* Glaucoma, secondary
    Rieger's anomaly Q13.81 [H42]
    rubeosis of iris — *see* Glaucoma, secondary
    tumor of globe — *see* Glaucoma, secondary
  infantile Q15.0
  low tension — *see* Glaucoma, open angle, primary, low-tension
  malignant H40.83- ☑
  narrow angle — *see* Glaucoma, angle-closure
  newborn Q15.0
  noncongestive (chronic) — *see* Glaucoma, open angle
  nonobstructive — *see* Glaucoma, open angle
  obstructive (*see also* Glaucoma, angle-closure)
    due to lens changes — *see* Glaucoma, secondary
  open angle H40.10- ☑
    primary H40.11-
      capsular (with pseudoexfoliation of lens) H40.14- ☑
      low-tension H40.12- ☑
      pigmentary H40.13- ☑
      residual stage H40.15- ☑
  phacolytic — *see* Glaucoma, secondary
  pigmentary — *see* Glaucoma, open angle, primary, pigmentary
  postinfectious — *see* Glaucoma, secondary, inflammation
  secondary (to) H40.5- ☑
    drugs H40.6- ☑
    inflammation H40.4- ☑
    trauma H40.3- ☑
  simple (chronic) H40.11- ☑
  simplex H40.11- ☑
  specified type NEC H40.89
  suspect H40.00- ☑
  syphilitic A52.71
  traumatic (*see also* Glaucoma, secondary, trauma)
    newborn (birth injury) P15.3
  tuberculous A18.59
Glaucomatous flecks (subcapsular) — *see* Cataract, complicated
Glazed tongue K14.4
Gleet (gonococcal) A54.01
Glénard's disease K63.4
Glioblastoma (multiforme)
  with sarcomatous component
    specified site — *see* Neoplasm, malignant, by site
    unspecified site C71.9
  giant cell
    specified site — *see* Neoplasm, malignant, by site
    unspecified site C71.9
  specified site — *see* Neoplasm, malignant, by site
  unspecified site C71.9
Glioma (malignant)
  astrocytic
    specified site — *see* Neoplasm, malignant, by site
    unspecified site C71.9
  mixed
    specified site — *see* Neoplasm, malignant, by site
    unspecified site C71.9
  nose Q30.8
  specified site NEC — *see* Neoplasm, malignant, by site
  subependymal D43.2
    specified site — *see* Neoplasm, uncertain behavior, by site
    unspecified site D43.2
  unspecified site C71.9
Gliomatosis cerebri C71.0
Glioneuroma — *see* Neoplasm, uncertain behavior, by site
Gliosarcoma
  specified site — *see* Neoplasm, malignant, by site
  unspecified site C71.9
Gliosis (cerebral) G93.89
  spinal G95.89
Glisson's disease — *see* Rickets
Globinuria R82.3

Globus (hystericus) F45.8
Glomangioma D18.00
  intra-abdominal D18.03
  intracranial D18.02
  skin D18.01
  specified site NEC D18.09
Glomangiomyoma D18.00
  intra-abdominal D18.03
  intracranial D18.02
  skin D18.01
  specified site NEC D18.09
Glomangiosarcoma — *see* Neoplasm, connective tissue, malignant
Glomerular
  disease in syphilis A52.75
  nephritis — *see* Glomerulonephritis
Glomerulitis — *see* Glomerulonephritis
Glomerulonephritis (*see also* Nephritis) N05.9
  with
    edema — *see* Nephrosis
    minimal change N05.0
    minor glomerular abnormality N05.0
  acute N00.9
  chronic N03.9
  crescentic (diffuse) NEC (*see also* N00-N07 with fourth character .7) N05.7
  dense deposit (*see also* N00-N07 with fourth character .6) N05.6
  diffuse
    crescentic (*see also* N00-N07 with fourth character .7) N05.7
    endocapillary proliferative (*see also* N00-N07 with fourth character .4) N05.4
    membranous (*see also* N00-N07 with fourth character .2) N05.2
    mesangial proliferative (*see also* N00-N07 with fourth character .3) N05.3
    mesangiocapillary (*see also* N00-N07 with fourth character .5) N05.5
    sclerosing N18.9
  endocapillary proliferative (diffuse) NEC (*see also* N00-N07 with fourth character .4) N05.4
  extracapillary NEC (*see also* N00-N07 with fourth character .7) N05.7
  focal (and segmental) (*see also* N00-N07 with fourth character .1) N05.1
  hypocomplementemic — *see* Glomerulonephritis, membranoproliferative
  IgA — *see* Nephropathy, IgA
  immune complex (circulating) NEC N05.8
  in (due to)
    amyloidosis E85.4 [N08]
    bilharziasis B65.9 [N08]
    cryoglobulinemia D89.1 [N08]
    defibrination syndrome D65 [N08]
    diabetes mellitus — *see* Diabetes, glomerulosclerosis
    disseminated intravascular coagulation D65 [N08]
    Fabry (-Anderson) disease E75.21 [N08]
    Goodpasture's syndrome M31.0
    hemolytic-uremic syndrome D59.3
    Henoch (-Schönlein) purpura D69.0 [N08]
    lecithin cholesterol acyltransferase deficiency E78.6 [N08]
    microscopic polyangiitis M31.7 [N08]
    multiple myeloma C90.0- ☑ [N08]
    Plasmodium malariae B52.0
    schistosomiasis B65.9 [N08]
    sepsis A41.9 [N08]
      streptococcal A40- ☑ [N08]
    sickle-cell disorders D57.- ☑ [N08]
    strongyloidiasis B78.9 [N08]
    subacute bacterial endocarditis I33.0 [N08]
    syphilis (late) congenital A50.59 [N08]
    systemic lupus erythematosus M32.14
    thrombotic thrombocytopenic purpura M31.1 [N08]
    typhoid fever A01.09
    Waldenström macroglobulinemia C88.0 [N08]
    Wegener's granulomatosis M31.31
  latent or quiescent N03.9
  lobular, lobulonodular — *see* Glomerulonephritis, membranoproliferative
  membranoproliferative (diffuse)(type 1 or 3) (*see also* N00-N07 with fourth character .5) N05.5
    dense deposit (type 2) NEC (*see also* N00-N07 with fourth character .6) N05.6

Glomerulonephritis — *continued*
  membranous (diffuse) NEC (*see also* N00-N07 with fourth character .2) N05.2
  mesangial
    IgA/IgG — *see* Nephropathy, IgA
    proliferative (diffuse) NEC (*see also* N00-N07 with fourth character .3) N05.3
  mesangiocapillary (diffuse) NEC (*see also* N00-N07 with fourth character .5) N05.5
  necrotic, necrotizing NEC (*see also* N00- N07 with fourth character .8) N05.8
  nodular — *see* Glomerulonephritis, membranoproliferative
  poststreptococcal NEC N05.9
    acute N00.9
    chronic N03.9
    rapidly progressive N01.9
  proliferative NEC (*see also* N00-N07 with fourth character .8) N05.8
    diffuse (lupus) M32.14
  rapidly progressive N01.9
  sclerosing, diffuse N18.9
  specified pathology NEC (*see also* N00- N07 with fourth character .8) N05.8
  subacute N01.9
Glomerulopathy — *see* Glomerulonephritis
Glomerulosclerosis (*see also* Sclerosis, renal)
  intercapillary (nodular) (with diabetes) — *see* Diabetes, glomerulosclerosis
  intracapillary — *see* Diabetes, glomerulosclerosis
Glossagra K14.6
Glossalgia K14.6
Glossitis (chronic superficial) (gangrenous) (Moeller's) K14.0
  areata exfoliativa K14.1
  atrophic K14.4
  benign migratory K14.1
  cortical superficial, sclerotic K14.0
  Hunter's D51.0
  interstitial, sclerous K14.0
  median rhomboid K14.2
  pellagrous E52
  superficial, chronic K14.0
Glossocele K14.8
Glossodynia K14.6
  exfoliativa K14.4
Glossoncus K14.8
Glossopathy K14.9
Glossophytia K14.3
Glossoplegia K14.8
Glossoptosis K14.8
Glossopyrosis K14.6
Glossotrichia K14.3
Glossy skin L90.8
Glottis — *see* condition
Glottitis (*see also* Laryngitis) J04.0
Glucagonoma
  pancreas
    benign D13.7
    malignant C25.4
    uncertain behavior D37.8
  specified site NEC
    benign — *see* Neoplasm, benign, by site
    malignant — *see* Neoplasm, malignant, by site
    uncertain behavior — *see* Neoplasm, uncertain behavior, by site
  unspecified site
    benign D13.7
    malignant C25.4
    uncertain behavior D37.8
Glucoglycinuria E72.51
Glucose-galactose malabsorption E74.39
Glue
  ear — *see* Otitis, media, nonsuppurative, chronic, mucoid
  sniffing (airplane) — *see* Abuse, drug, inhalant
    dependence — *see* Dependence, drug, inhalant
Glutaric aciduria E72.3
Glycinemia E72.51
Glycinuria (renal) (with ketosis) E72.09
Glycogen
  infiltration — *see* Disease, glycogen storage
  storage disease — *see* Disease, glycogen storage
Glycogenosis (diffuse) (generalized) (*see also* Disease, glycogen storage)
  cardiac E74.02 [I43]

Glycogenosis — *continued*
  diabetic, secondary — *see* Diabetes, glycogenosis, secondary
  pulmonary interstitial J84.842
Glycopenia E16.2
Glycosuria R81
  renal E74.8
Gnathostoma spinigerum (infection) (infestation), **gnathostomiasis** (wandering swelling) B83.1
Goiter (plunging) (substernal) E04.9
  with
    hyperthyroidism (recurrent) — *see* Hyperthyroidism, with, goiter
    thyrotoxicosis — *see* Hyperthyroidism, with, goiter
  adenomatous — *see* Goiter, nodular
  cancerous C73
  congenital (nontoxic) E03.0
    diffuse E03.0
    parenchymatous E03.0
    transitory, with normal functioning P72.0
  cystic E04.2
    due to iodine-deficiency E01.1
  due to
    enzyme defect in synthesis of thyroid hormone E07.1
    iodine-deficiency (endemic) E01.2
  dyshormonogenetic (familial) E07.1
  endemic (iodine-deficiency) E01.2
    diffuse E01.0
    multinodular E01.1
  exophthalmic — *see* Hyperthyroidism, with, goiter
  iodine-deficiency (endemic) E01.2
    diffuse E01.0
    multinodular E01.1
    nodular E01.1
  lingual Q89.2
  lymphadenoid E06.3
  malignant C73
  multinodular (cystic) (nontoxic) E04.2
    toxic or with hyperthyroidism E05.20
      with thyroid storm E05.21
  neonatal NEC P72.0
  nodular (nontoxic) (due to) E04.9
    with
      hyperthyroidism E05.20
        with thyroid storm E05.21
      thyrotoxicosis E05.20
        with thyroid storm E05.21
    endemic E01.1
    iodine-deficiency E01.1
    sporadic E04.9
    toxic E05.20
      with thyroid storm E05.21
  nontoxic E04.9
    diffuse (colloid) E04.0
    multinodular E04.2
    simple E04.0
    specified NEC E04.8
    uninodular E04.1
  simple E04.0
  toxic — *see* Hyperthyroidism, with, goiter
  uninodular (nontoxic) E04.1
    toxic or with hyperthyroidism E05.10
      with thyroid storm E05.11
Goiter-deafness syndrome E07.1
Goldberg syndrome Q89.8
Goldberg-Maxwell syndrome E34.51
Goldblatt's hypertension or kidney I70.1
Goldenhar (-Gorlin) **syndrome** Q87.0
Goldflam-Erb disease or syndrome G70.00
  with exacerbation (acute) G70.01
  in crisis G70.01
Goldscheider's disease Q81.8
Goldstein's disease (familial hemorrhagic telangiectasia) I78.0
Golfer's elbow — *see* Epicondylitis, medial
Gonadoblastoma
  specified site — *see* Neoplasm, uncertain behavior, by site
  unspecified site
    female D39.10
    male D40.10
Gonecystitis — *see* Vesiculitis
Gongylonemiasis B83.8
Goniosynechiae — *see* Adhesions, iris, goniosynechiae
Gonococcemia A54.86
Gonococcus, gonococcal (disease) (infection) (*see also* condition) A54.9

Gonococcus, gonococcal — *continued*
  anus A54.6
  bursa, bursitis A54.49
  conjunctiva, conjunctivitis (neonatorum) A54.31
  endocardium A54.83
  eye A54.30
    conjunctivitis A54.31
    iridocyclitis A54.32
    keratitis A54.33
    newborn A54.31
    other specified A54.39
  fallopian tubes (acute) (chronic) A54.24
  genitourinary (organ) (system) (tract) (acute) A54.00
    lower A54.00
      with abscess (accessory gland) (periurethral) A54.1
    upper (*see also* condition) A54.29
  heart A54.83
  iridocyclitis A54.32
  joint A54.42
  lymphatic (gland) (node) A54.89
  meninges, meningitis A54.81
  musculoskeletal A54.40
    arthritis A54.42
    osteomyelitis A54.43
    other specified A54.49
    spondylopathy A54.41
  pelviperitonitis A54.24
  pelvis (acute) (chronic) A54.24
  pharynx A54.5
  proctitis A54.6
  pyosalpinx (acute) (chronic) A54.24
  rectum A54.6
  skin A54.89
  specified site NEC A54.89
  tendon sheath A54.49
  throat A54.5
  urethra (acute) (chronic) A54.01
    with abscess (accessory gland) (periurethral) A54.1
  vulva (acute) (chronic) A54.02
Gonocytoma
  specified site — *see* Neoplasm, uncertain behavior, by site
  unspecified site
    female D39.10
    male D40.10
Gonorrhea (acute) (chronic) A54.9
  Bartholin's gland (acute) (chronic) (purulent) A54.02
    with abscess (accessory gland) (periurethral) A54.1
  bladder A54.01
  cervix A54.03
  conjunctiva, conjunctivitis (neonatorum) A54.31
  contact Z20.2
  Cowper's gland (with abscess) A54.1
  exposure to Z20.2
  fallopian tube (acute) (chronic) A54.24
  kidney (acute) (chronic) A54.21
  lower genitourinary tract A54.00
    with abscess (accessory gland) (periurethral) A54.1
  ovary (acute) (chronic) A54.24
  pelvis (acute) (chronic) A54.24
    female pelvic inflammatory disease A54.24
  penis A54.09
  prostate (acute) (chronic) A54.22
  seminal vesicle (acute) (chronic) A54.23
  specified site not listed (*see also* Gonococcus) A54.89
  spermatic cord (acute) (chronic) A54.23
  urethra A54.01
    with abscess (accessory gland) (periurethral) A54.1
  vagina A54.02
  vas deferens (acute) (chronic) A54.23
  vulva A54.02
Goodall's disease A08.19
Goodpasture's syndrome M31.0
Gopalan's syndrome (burning feet) E53.0
Gorlin-Chaudry-Moss syndrome Q87.0
Gottron's papules L94.4
Gougerot-Blum syndrome (pigmented purpuric lichenoid dermatitis) L81.7
Gougerot-Carteaud disease or syndrome (confluent reticulate papillomatosis) L83
Gougerot's syndrome (trisymptomatic) L81.7
Gouley's syndrome (constrictive pericarditis) I31.1
Goundou A66.6
Gout, chronic (*see also* Gout, gouty) M1A.9 ☑ (*following* M08)
  drug-induced M1A.20 ☑ (*following* M08)
    ankle M1A.27- ☑ (*following* M08)

Gout, chronic — *continued*
  drug-induced — *continued*
    elbow M1A.22- ☑ (*following* M08)
    foot joint M1A.27- ☑ (*following* M08)
    hand joint M1A.24- ☑ (*following* M08)
    hip M1A.25- ☑ (*following* M08)
    knee M1A.26- ☑ (*following* M08)
    multiple site M1A.29- ☑ (*following* M08)
    shoulder M1A.21- ☑ (*following* M08)
    vertebrae M1A.28 ☑ (*following* M08)
    wrist M1A.23- ☑ (*following* M08)
  idiopathic M1A.00 ☑ (*following* M08)
    ankle M1A.07- ☑ (*following* M08)
    elbow M1A.02- ☑ (*following* M08)
    foot joint M1A.07- ☑ (*following* M08)
    hand joint M1A.04- ☑ (*following* M08)
    hip M1A.05- ☑ (*following* M08)
    knee M1A.06- ☑ (*following* M08)
    multiple site M1A.09 ☑ (*following* M08)
    shoulder M1A.01- ☑ (*following* M08)
    vertebrae M1A.08 ☑ (*following* M08)
    wrist M1A.03- ☑ (*following* M08)
  in (due to) renal impairment M1A.30 ☑ (*following* M08)
    ankle M1A.37- ☑ (*following* M08)
    elbow M1A.32- ☑ (*following* M08)
    foot joint M1A.37- ☑ (*following* M08)
    hand joint M1A.34- ☑ (*following* M08)
    hip M1A.35- ☑ (*following* M08)
    knee M1A.36- ☑ (*following* M08)
    multiple site M1A.39 ☑ (*following* M08)
    shoulder M1A.31- ☑ (*following* M08)
    vertebrae M1A.38 ☑ (*following* M08)
    wrist M1A.33- ☑ (*following* M08)
  lead-induced M1A.10 ☑ (*following* M08)
    ankle M1A.17- ☑ (*following* M08)
    elbow M1A.12- ☑ (*following* M08)
    foot joint M1A.17- ☑ (*following* M08)
    hand joint M1A.14- ☑ (*following* M08)
    hip M1A.15- ☑ (*following* M08)
    knee M1A.16- ☑ (*following* M08)
    multiple site M1A.19 ☑ (*following* M08)
    shoulder M1A.11- ☑ (*following* M08)
    vertebrae M1A.18 ☑ (*following* M08)
    wrist M1A.13- ☑ (*following* M08)
  primary — *see* Gout, chronic, idiopathic
  saturnine — *see* Gout, chronic, lead-induced
  secondary NEC M1A.40 ☑ (*following* M08)
    ankle M1A.47- ☑ (*following* M08)
    elbow M1A.42- ☑ (*following* M08)
    foot joint M1A.47- ☑ (*following* M08)
    hand joint M1A.44- ☑ (*following* M08)
    hip M1A.45- ☑ (*following* M08)
    knee M1A.46- ☑ (*following* M08)
    multiple site M1A.49 ☑ (*following* M08)
    shoulder M1A.41- ☑ (*following* M08)
    vertebrae M1A.48 ☑ (*following* M08)
    wrist M1A.43- ☑ (*following* M08)
  syphilitic (*see also* subcategory M14.8-) A52.77
  tophi M1A.9 ☑ (*following* M08)
Gout, gouty (acute) (attack) (flare) (*see also* Gout, chronic) M10.9
  drug-induced M10.20
    ankle M10.27- ☑
    elbow M10.22- ☑
    foot joint M10.27- ☑
    hand joint M10.24- ☑
    hip M10.25- ☑
    knee M10.26- ☑
    multiple site M10.29
    shoulder M10.21- ☑
    vertebrae M10.28
    wrist M10.23- ☑
  idiopathic M10.00
    ankle M10.07- ☑
    elbow M10.02- ☑
    foot joint M10.07- ☑
    hand joint M10.04- ☑
    hip M10.05- ☑
    knee M10.06- ☑
    multiple site M10.09
    shoulder M10.01- ☑
    vertebrae M10.08
    wrist M10.03- ☑
  in (due to) renal impairment M10.30
    ankle M10.37- ☑

Gout, gouty — *continued*
  in renal impairment — *continued*
    elbow M10.32- ☑
    foot joint M10.37- ☑
    hand joint M10.34- ☑
    hip M10.35- ☑
    knee M10.36- ☑
    multiple site M10.39
    shoulder M10.31- ☑
    vertebrae M10.38
    wrist M10.33- ☑
  lead-induced M10.10
    ankle M10.17- ☑
    elbow M10.12- ☑
    foot joint M10.17- ☑
    hand joint M10.14- ☑
    hip M10.15- ☑
    knee M10.16- ☑
    multiple site M10.19
    shoulder M10.11- ☑
    vertebrae M10.18
    wrist M10.13- ☑
  primary — *see* Gout, idiopathic
  saturnine — *see* Gout, lead-induced
  secondary NEC M10.40
    ankle M10.47- ☑
    elbow M10.42- ☑
    foot joint M10.47- ☑
    hand joint M10.44- ☑
    hip M10.45- ☑
    knee M10.46- ☑
    multiple site M10.49
    shoulder M10.41- ☑
    vertebrae M10.48
    wrist M10.43- ☑
  syphilitic (*see also* subcategory M14.8-) A52.77
  tophi — *see* Gout, chronic
Gower's
  muscular dystrophy G71.0
  syndrome (vasovagal attack) R55
Gradenigo's syndrome — *see* Otitis, media, suppurative, acute
Graefe's disease — *see* Strabismus, paralytic, ophthal-moplegia, progressive
Graft-versus-host disease D89.813
  acute D89.810
  acute on chronic D89.812
  chronic D89.811
Grain mite (itch) B88.0
Grainhandler's disease or lung J67.8
Grand mal — *see* Epilepsy, generalized, specified NEC
Grand multipara status only (not pregnant) Z64.1
  pregnant — *see* Pregnancy, complicated by, grand multiparity
Granite worker's lung J62.8
Granular (*see also* condition)
  inflammation, pharynx J31.2
  kidney (contracting) — *see* Sclerosis, renal
  liver K74.69
Granulation tissue (abnormal) (excessive) L92.9
  postmastoidectomy cavity — *see* Complications, postmastoidectomy, granulation
Granulocytopenia (primary) (malignant) — *see* Agran-ulocytosis
Granuloma L92.9
  abdomen K66.8
    from residual foreign body L92.3
    pyogenicum L98.0
  actinic L57.5
  annulare (perforating) L92.0
  apical K04.5
  aural — *see* Otitis, externa, specified NEC
  beryllium (skin) L92.3
  bone
    eosinophilic C96.6
    from residual foreign body — *see* Osteomyelitis, specified type NEC
    lung C96.6
  brain (any site) G06.0
    schistosomiasis B65.9 [G07]
  canaliculus lacrimalis — *see* Granuloma, lacrimal
  candidal (cutaneous) B37.2
  cerebral (any site) G06.0
  coccidioidal (primary) (progressive) B38.7
    lung B38.1
    meninges B38.4
  colon K63.89

Granuloma — *continued*
  conjunctiva H11.22- ☑
  dental K04.5
  ear, middle — *see* Cholesteatoma
  eosinophilic C96.6
    bone C96.6
    lung C96.6
    oral mucosa K13.4
    skin L92.2
  eyelid H01.8
  facial (e) L92.2
  foreign body (in soft tissue) NEC M60.20
    ankle M60.27- ☑
    foot M60.27- ☑
    forearm M60.23- ☑
    hand M60.24- ☑
    in operation wound — *see* Foreign body, acciden-tally left during a procedure
    lower leg M60.26- ☑
    pelvic region M60.25- ☑
    shoulder region M60.21- ☑
    skin L92.3
    specified site NEC M60.28
    subcutaneous tissue L92.3
    thigh M60.25- ☑
    upper arm M60.22- ☑
  gangraenescens M31.2
  genito-inguinale A58
  giant cell (central) (reparative) (jaw) M27.1
    gingiva (peripheral) K06.8
  gland (lymph) I88.8
  hepatic NEC K75.3
    in (due to)
      berylliosis J63.2 [K77]
      sarcoidosis D86.89
  Hodgkin C81.9 ☑
  ileum K63.89
  infectious B99.9
    specified NEC B99.8
  inguinale (Donovan) (venereal) A58
  intestine NEC K63.89
  intracranial (any site) G06.0
  intraspinal (any part) G06.1
  iridocyclitis — *see* Iridocyclitis, chronic
  jaw (bone) (central) M27.1
    reparative giant cell M27.1
  kidney (*see also* Infection, kidney) N15.8
  lacrimal H04.81- ☑
  larynx J38.7
  lethal midline (faciale(e)) M31.2
  liver NEC — *see* Granuloma, hepatic
  lung (infectious) (*see also* Fibrosis, lung)
    coccidioidal B38.1
    eosinophilic C96.6
  Majocchi's B35.8
  malignant (facial(e)) M31.2
  mandible (central) M27.1
  midline (lethal) M31.2
  monilial (cutaneous) B37.2
  nasal sinus — *see* Sinusitis
  operation wound T81.89 ☑
    foreign body — *see* Foreign body, accidentally left during a procedure
    stitch T81.89 ☑
    talc — *see* Foreign body, accidentally left during a procedure
  oral mucosa K13.4
  orbit, orbital H05.11- ☑
  paracoccidioidal B41.8
  penis, venereal A58
  periapical K04.5
  peritoneum K66.8
    due to ova of helminths NOS (*see also* Helminthia-sis) B83.9 [K67]
  postmastoidectomy cavity — *see* Complications, postmastoidectomy, recurrent cholesteatoma
  prostate N42.89
  pudendi (ulcerating) A58
  pulp, internal (tooth) K03.3
  pyogenic, pyogenicum (of) (skin) L98.0
    gingiva K06.8
    maxillary alveolar ridge K04.5
    oral mucosa K13.4
  rectum K62.89
  reticulohistiocytic D76.3
  rubrum nasi L74.8
  Schistosoma — *see* Schistosomiasis
  septic (skin) L98.0

Granuloma — *continued*
  silica (skin) L92.3
  sinus (accessory) (infective) (nasal) — *see* Sinusitis
  skin L92.9
    from residual foreign body L92.3
    pyogenicum L98.0
  spine
    syphilitic (epidural) A52.19
    tuberculous A18.01
  stitch (postoperative) T81.89 ☑
  suppurative (skin) L98.0
  swimming pool A31.1
  talc (*see also* Granuloma, foreign body)
    in operation wound — *see* Foreign body, acciden-tally left during a procedure
  telangiectaticum (skin) L98.0
  tracheostomy J95.09
  trichophyticum B35.8
  tropicum A66.4
  umbilical P83.81
  umbilicus P83.81
  urethra N36.8
  uveitis — *see* Iridocyclitis, chronic
  vagina A58
  venereum A58
  vocal cord J38.3
Granulomatosis L92.9
  lymphoid C83.8- ☑
  miliary (listerial) A32.89
  necrotizing, respiratory M31.30
  progressive septic D71
  specified NEC L92.8
  Wegener's M31.30
    with renal involvement M31.31
Granulomatous tissue (abnormal) (excessive) L92.9
Granulosis rubra nasi L74.8
Graphite fibrosis (of lung) J63.3
Graphospasm F48.8
  organic G25.89
Grating scapula M89.8X1
Gravel (urinary) — *see* Calculus, urinary
Graves' disease — *see* Hyperthyroidism, with, goiter
Gravis — *see* condition
Grawitz tumor C64.- ☑
Gray syndrome (newborn) P93.0
Grayness, hair (premature) L67.1
  congenital Q84.2
Green sickness D50.8
Greenfield's disease
  meaning
    concentric sclerosis (encephalitis periaxialis concen-trica) G37.5
    metachromatic leukodystrophy E75.25
Greenstick fracture — *code as* Fracture, by site
Grey syndrome (newborn) P93.0
Grief F43.21
  prolonged F43.29
  reaction (*see also* Disorder, adjustment) F43.20
Griesinger's disease B76.9
Grinder's lung or pneumoconiosis J62.8
Grinding, teeth
  psychogenic F45.8
  sleep related G47.63
Grip
  Dabney's B33.0
  devil's B33.0
Grippe, grippal (*see also* Influenza)
  Balkan A78
  summer, of Italy A93.1
Grisel's disease M43.6
Groin — *see* condition
Grooved tongue K14.5
Ground itch B76.9
Grover's disease or syndrome L11.1
Growing pains, children R29.898
Growth (fungoid) (neoplastic) (new) (*see also* Neoplasm)
  adenoid (vegetative) J35.8
  benign — *see* Neoplasm, benign, by site
  malignant — *see* Neoplasm, malignant, by site
  rapid, childhood Z00.2
  secondary — *see* Neoplasm, secondary, by site
Gruby's disease B35.0
Gubler-Millard paralysis or syndrome G46.3
Guerin-Stern syndrome Q74.3
Guidance, insufficient anterior (occlusal) M26.54
Guillain-Barré disease or syndrome G61.0
  sequelae G65.0

Guinea worms (infection) (infestation) B72
Guinon's disease (motor-verbal tic) F95.2
Gull's disease E03.4
Gum — see condition
Gumboil K04.7
  with sinus K04.6
Gumma (syphilitic) A52.79
  artery A52.09
    cerebral A52.04
  bone A52.77
    of yaws (late) A66.6
  brain A52.19
  cauda equina A52.19
  central nervous system A52.3
  ciliary body A52.71
  congenital A50.59
  eyelid A52.71
  heart A52.06
  intracranial A52.19
  iris A52.71
  kidney A52.75
  larynx A52.73
  leptomeninges A52.19
  liver A52.74
  meninges A52.19
  myocardium A52.06
  nasopharynx A52.73
  neurosyphilitic A52.3
  nose A52.73
  orbit A52.71
  palate (soft) A52.79
  penis A52.76
  pericardium A52.06
  pharynx A52.73
  pituitary A52.79
  scrofulous (tuberculous) A18.4
  skin A52.79
  specified site NEC A52.79
  spinal cord A52.19
  tongue A52.79
  tonsil A52.73
  trachea A52.73
  tuberculous A18.4
  ulcerative due to yaws A66.4
  ureter A52.75
  yaws A66.4
    bone A66.6
Gunn's syndrome Q07.8
Gunshot wound (see also Wound, open)
  fracture — code as Fracture, by site
  internal organs — see Injury, by site
Gynandrism Q56.0
Gynandroblastoma
  specified site — see Neoplasm, uncertain behavior, by site
  unspecified site
    female D39.10
    male D40.10
Gynecological examination (periodic) (routine) Z01.419
  with abnormal findings Z01.411
Gynecomastia N62
Gynephobia F40.291
Gyrate scalp Q82.8

H

H (Hartnup's) **disease** E72.02
Haas' disease or osteochondrosis (juvenile) (head of humerus) — see Osteochondrosis, juvenile, humerus
Habit, habituation
  bad sleep Z72.821
  chorea F95.8
  disturbance, child F98.9
  drug — see Dependence, drug
  irregular sleep Z72.821
  laxative F55.2
  spasm — see Tic
  tic — see Tic
Haemophilus (H.) **influenzae, as cause of disease classified elsewhere** B96.3
Haff disease — see Poisoning, mercury
Hageman's factor defect, deficiency or disease D68.2
Haglund's disease or osteochondrosis (juvenile) (os tibiale externum) — see Osteochondrosis, juvenile, tarsus
Hailey-Hailey disease Q82.8

Hair (see also condition)
  plucking F63.3
    in stereotyped movement disorder F98.4
  tourniquet syndrome (see also Constriction, external, by site)
    finger S60.44- ☑
    penis S30.842 ☑
    thumb S60.34- ☑
    toe S90.44- ☑
Hairball in stomach T18.2 ☑
Hair-pulling, pathological (compulsive) F63.3
Hairy black tongue K14.3
Half vertebra Q76.49
Halitosis R19.6
Hallerman-Streiff syndrome Q87.0
Hallervorden-Spatz disease G23.0
Hallopeau's acrodermatitis or disease L40.2
Hallucination R44.3
  auditory R44.0
  gustatory R44.2
  olfactory R44.2
  specified NEC R44.2
  tactile R44.2
  visual R44.1
Hallucinosis (chronic) F28
  alcoholic (acute) F10.951
    in
      abuse F10.151
      dependence F10.251
  drug-induced F19.951
    cannabis F12.951
    cocaine F14.951
    hallucinogen F16.151
    in
      abuse F19.151
        cannabis F12.151
        cocaine F14.151
        hallucinogen F16.151
        inhalant F18.151
        opioid F11.151
        sedative, anxiolytic or hypnotic F13.151
        stimulant NEC F15.151
      dependence F19.251
        cannabis F12.251
        cocaine F14.251
        hallucinogen F16.251
        inhalant F18.251
        opioid F11.251
        sedative, anxiolytic or hypnotic F13.251
        stimulant NEC F15.251
    inhalant F18.951
    opioid F11.951
    sedative, anxiolytic or hypnotic F13.951
    stimulant NEC F15.951
  organic F06.0
Hallux
  deformity (acquired) NEC M20.5X- ☑
  limitus M20.5X- ☑
  malleus (acquired) NEC M20.3- ☑
  rigidus (acquired) M20.2- ☑
    congenital Q74.2
    sequelae (late effect) of rickets E64.3
  valgus (acquired) M20.1- ☑
    congenital Q66.6
  varus (acquired) M20.3- ☑
    congenital Q66.3
Halo, visual H53.19
Hamartoma, hamartoblastoma Q85.9
  epithelial (gingival), odontogenic, central or peripheral — see Cyst, calcifying odontogenic
Hamartosis Q85.9
Hamman-Rich syndrome J84.114
Hammer toe (acquired) NEC (see also Deformity, toe, hammer toe)
  congenital Q66.89
  sequelae (late effect) of rickets E64.3
Hand — see condition
Hand-foot syndrome L27.1
Handicap, handicapped
  educational Z55.9
    specified NEC Z55.8
Hand-Schüller-Christian disease or syndrome C96.5
Hanging (asphyxia) (strangulation) (suffocation) — see Asphyxia, traumatic, due to mechanical threat
Hangnail (see also Cellulitis, digit)
  with lymphangitis — see Lymphangitis, acute, digit
Hangover (alcohol) F10.129

Hanhart's syndrome Q87.0
Hanot-Chauffard (-Troisier) **syndrome** E83.19
Hanot's cirrhosis or disease K74.3
Hansen's disease — see Leprosy
Hantaan virus disease (Korean hemorrhagic fever) A98.5
Hantavirus disease (with renal manifestations) (Dobrava) (Puumala) (Seoul) A98.5
  with pulmonary manifestations (Andes) (Bayou) (Bermejo) (Black Creek Canal) (Choclo) (Juquitiba) (Laguna negra) (Lechiguanas) (New York) (Oran) (Sin nombre) B33.4
Happy puppet syndrome Q93.5
Harada's disease or syndrome H30.81- ☑
Hardening
  artery — see Arteriosclerosis
  brain G93.89
Harelip (complete) (incomplete) — see Cleft, lip
Harlequin (newborn) Q80.4
Harley's disease D59.6
Harmful use (of)
  alcohol F10.10
  anxiolytics — see Abuse, drug, sedative
  cannabinoids — see Abuse, drug, cannabis
  cocaine — see Abuse, drug, cocaine
  drug — see Abuse, drug
  hallucinogens — see Abuse, drug, hallucinogen
  hypnotics — see Abuse, drug, sedative
  opioids — see Abuse, drug, opioid
  PCP (phencyclidine) — see Abuse, drug, hallucinogen
  sedatives — see Abuse, drug, sedative
  stimulants NEC — see Abuse, drug, stimulant
Harris' lines — see Arrest, epiphyseal
Hartnup's disease E72.02
Harvester's lung J67.0
Harvesting ovum for in vitro fertilization Z31.83
Hashimoto's disease or thyroiditis E06.3
Hashitoxicosis (transient) E06.3
Hassal-Henle bodies or warts (cornea) H18.49
Haut mal — see Epilepsy, generalized, specified NEC
Haverhill fever A25.1
Hay fever (see also Fever, hay) J30.1
Hayem-Widal syndrome D59.8
Haygarth's nodes M15.8
Haymaker's lung J67.0
Hb (abnormal)
  Bart's disease D56.0
  disease — see Disease, hemoglobin
  trait — see Trait
Head — see condition
Headache R51
  allergic NEC G44.89
  associated with sexual activity G44.82
  chronic daily R51
  cluster G44.009
    chronic G44.029
      intractable G44.021
      not intractable G44.029
    episodic G44.019
      intractable G44.011
      not intractable G44.019
    intractable G44.001
    not intractable G44.009
  cough (primary) G44.83
  daily chronic R51
  drug-induced NEC G44.40
    intractable G44.41
    not intractable G44.40
  exertional (primary) G44.84
  histamine G44.009
    intractable G44.001
    not intractable G44.009
  hypnic G44.81
  lumbar puncture G97.1
  medication overuse G44.40
    intractable G44.41
    not intractable G44.40
  menstrual — see Migraine, menstrual
  migraine (type) (see also Migraine) G43.909
  nasal septum R51
  neuralgiform, short lasting unilateral, with conjunctival injection and tearing (SUNCT) G44.059
    intractable G44.051
    not intractable G44.059
  new daily persistent (NDPH) G44.52
  orgasmic G44.82
  periodic syndromes in adults and children G43.C0
    (following G43.7)

☑ **Additional Character Required** — Refer to the Tabular List for Character Selection   ▽ **Subterms under main terms may continue to next column or page**

Headache — *continued*
  periodic syndromes in adults and children — *contin-ued*
    with refractory migraine G43.C1 (*following* G43.7)
    without refractory migraine G43.C0 (*following* G43.7)
    intractable G43.C1 (*following* G43.7)
    not intractable G43.C0 (*following* G43.7)
  postspinal puncture G97.1
  post-traumatic G44.309
    acute G44.319
      intractable G44.311
      not intractable G44.319
    chronic G44.329
      intractable G44.321
      not intractable G44.329
    intractable G44.301
    not intractable G44.309
  pre-menstrual — *see* Migraine, menstrual
  preorgasmic G44.82
  primary
    cough G44.83
    exertional G44.84
    stabbing G44.85
    thunderclap G44.53
  rebound G44.40
    intractable G44.41
    not intractable G44.40
  short lasting unilateral neuralgiform, with conjunctival injection and tearing (SUNCT) G44.059
    intractable G44.051
    not intractable G44.059
  specified syndrome NEC G44.89
  spinal and epidural anesthesia - induced T88.59 ☑
    in labor and delivery O74.5
    in pregnancy O29.4- ☑
    postpartum, puerperal O89.4
  spinal fluid loss (from puncture) G97.1
  stabbing (primary) G44.85
  tension (-type) G44.209
    chronic G44.229
      intractable G44.221
      not intractable G44.229
    episodic G44.219
      intractable G44.211
      not intractable G44.219
    intractable G44.201
    not intractable G44.209
  thunderclap (primary) G44.53
  vascular NEC G44.1
Healthy
  infant
    accompanying sick mother Z76.3
    receiving care Z76.2
  person accompanying sick person Z76.3
Hearing examination Z01.10
  with abnormal findings NEC Z01.118
  following failed hearing screening Z01.110
  for hearing conservation and treatment Z01.12
Heart — *see* condition
Heart beat
  abnormality R00.9
    specified NEC R00.8
  awareness R00.2
  rapid R00.0
  slow R00.1
Heartburn R12
  psychogenic F45.8
Heartland virus disease A93.8
Heat (effects) T67.9 ☑
  apoplexy T67.0 ☑
  burn (*see also* Burn) L55.9
  collapse T67.1 ☑
  cramps T67.2 ☑
  dermatitis or eczema L59.0
  edema T67.7 ☑
  erythema — *code by site under* Burn, first degree
  excessive T67.9 ☑
    specified effect NEC T67.8 ☑
  exhaustion T67.5 ☑
    anhydrotic T67.3 ☑
    due to
      salt (and water) depletion T67.4 ☑
      water depletion T67.3 ☑
        with salt depletion T67.4 ☑
  fatigue (transient) T67.6 ☑
  fever T67.0 ☑
  hyperpyrexia T67.0 ☑

Heat — *continued*
  prickly L74.0
  prostration — *see* Heat, exhaustion
  pyrexia T67.0 ☑
  rash L74.0
  specified effect NEC T67.8 ☑
  stroke T67.0 ☑
  sunburn — *see* Sunburn
  syncope T67.1 ☑
Heavy-for-dates NEC (infant) (4000g to 4499g) P08.1
  exceptionally (4500g or more) P08.0
Hebephrenia, hebephrenic (schizophrenia) F20.1
Heberden's disease or nodes (with arthropathy) M15.1
Hebra's
  pityriasis L26
  prurigo L28.2
Heel — *see* condition
Heerfordt's disease D86.89
Hegglin's anomaly or syndrome D72.0
Heilmeyer-Schoner disease D45
Heine-Medin disease A80.9
Heinz body anemia, congenital D58.2
Heliophobia F40.228
Heller's disease or syndrome F84.3
HELLP syndrome (hemolysis, elevated liver enzymes and low platelet count) O14.2- ☑
  complicating
    childbirth O14.24
    puerperium O14.25
Helminthiasis (*see also* Infestation, helminth)
  Ancylostoma B76.0
  intestinal B82.0
    mixed types (types classifiable to more than one of the titles B65.0-B81.3 and B81.8) B81.4
    specified type NEC B81.8
  mixed types (intestinal) (types classifiable to more than one of the titles B65.0-B81.3 and B81.8) B81.4
  Necator (americanus) B76.1
  specified type NEC B83.8
Heloma L84
Hemangioblastoma — *see* Neoplasm, connective tissue, uncertain behavior
  malignant — *see* Neoplasm, connective tissue, malignant
Hemangioendothelioma (*see also* Neoplasm, uncertain behavior, by site)
  benign D18.00
    intra-abdominal D18.03
    intracranial D18.02
    skin D18.01
    specified site NEC D18.09
  bone (diffuse) — *see* Neoplasm, bone, malignant
  epithelioid (*see also* Neoplasm, uncertain behavior, by site)
    malignant — *see* Neoplasm, malignant, by site
  malignant — *see* Neoplasm, connective tissue, malignant
Hemangiofibroma — *see* Neoplasm, benign, by site
Hemangiolipoma — *see* Lipoma
Hemangioma D18.00
  arteriovenous D18.00
    intra-abdominal D18.03
    intracranial D18.02
    skin D18.01
    specified site NEC D18.09
  capillary D18.00
    intra-abdominal D18.03
    intracranial D18.02
    skin D18.01
    specified site NEC D18.09
  cavernous D18.00
    intra-abdominal D18.03
    intracranial D18.02
    skin D18.01
    specified site NEC D18.09
  epithelioid D18.00
    intra-abdominal D18.03
    intracranial D18.02
    skin D18.01
    specified site NEC D18.09
  histiocytoid D18.00
    intra-abdominal D18.03
    intracranial D18.02
    skin D18.01
    specified site NEC D18.09
  infantile D18.00
    intra-abdominal D18.03

Hemangioma — *continued*
  infantile — *continued*
    intracranial D18.02
    skin D18.01
    specified site NEC D18.09
  intra-abdominal D18.03
  intracranial D18.02
  intramuscular D18.00
    intra-abdominal D18.03
    intracranial D18.02
    skin D18.01
    specified site NEC D18.09
  intrathoracic structures D18.09
  juvenile D18.00
  malignant — *see* Neoplasm,connective tissue, malignant
  plexiform D18.00
    intra-abdominal D18.03
    intracranial D18.02
    skin D18.01
    specified site NEC D18.09
  racemose D18.00
    intra-abdominal D18.03
    intracranial D18.02
    skin D18.01
    specified site NEC D18.09
  sclerosing — *see* Neoplasm, skin, benign
  simplex D18.00
    intra-abdominal D18.03
    intracranial D18.02
    skin D18.01
    specified site NEC D18.09
  skin D18.01
  specified site NEC D18.09
  venous D18.00
    intra-abdominal D18.03
    intracranial D18.02
    skin D18.01
    specified site NEC D18.09
  verrucous keratotic D18.00
    intra-abdominal D18.03
    intracranial D18.02
    skin D18.01
    specified site NEC D18.09
Hemangiomatosis (systemic) I78.8
  involving single site — *see* Hemangioma
Hemangiopericytoma (*see also* Neoplasm, connective tissue, uncertain behavior)
  benign — *see* Neoplasm, connective tissue, benign
  malignant — *see* Neoplasm, connective tissue, malignant
Hemangiosarcoma — *see* Neoplasm, connective tissue, malignant
Hemarthrosis (nontraumatic) M25.00
  ankle M25.07- ☑
  elbow M25.02- ☑
  foot joint M25.07- ☑
  hand joint M25.04- ☑
  hip M25.05- ☑
  in hemophilic arthropathy — *see* Arthropathy, hemophilic
  knee M25.06- ☑
  shoulder M25.01- ☑
  specified joint NEC M25.08
  traumatic — *see* Sprain, by site
  vertebrae M25.08
  wrist M25.03- ☑
Hematemesis K92.0
  with ulcer — *code by site under* Ulcer, with hemorrhage K27.4
  newborn, neonatal P54.0
    due to swallowed maternal blood P78.2
Hematidrosis L74.8
Hematinuria (*see also* Hemoglobinuria)
  malarial B50.8
Hematobilia K83.8
Hematocele
  female NEC N94.89
    with ectopic pregnancy O00.90
      with intrauterine pregnancy O00.91
    ovary N83.8
  male N50.1
Hematochezia (*see also* Melena) K92.1
Hematochyluria (*see also* Infestation, filarial)
  schistosomiasis (bilharziasis) B65.0
Hematocolpos (with hematometra or hematosalpinx) N89.7
Hematocornea — *see* Pigmentation, cornea, stromal

Hematogenous — *see* condition
Hematoma (traumatic) (skin surface intact) (*see also* Contusion)
  with
    injury of internal organs — *see* Injury, by site
    open wound — *see* Wound, open
  amputation stump (surgical) (late) T87.89
  aorta, dissecting I71.00
    abdominal I71.02
    thoracic I71.01
    thoracoabdominal I71.03
  aortic intramural — *see* Dissection, aorta
  arterial (complicating trauma) — *see* Injury, blood vessel, by site
  auricle — *see* Contusion, ear
    nontraumatic — *see* Disorder, pinna, hematoma
  birth injury NEC P15.8
  brain (traumatic)
    with
      cerebral laceration or contusion (diffuse) — *see* Injury, intracranial, diffuse
        focal — *see* Injury, intracranial, focal
    cerebellar, traumatic S06.37- ✓
    intracerebral, traumatic — *see* Injury, intracranial, intracerebral hemorrhage
    newborn NEC P52.4
      birth injury P10.1
    nontraumatic — *see* Hemorrhage, intracranial
    subarachnoid, arachnoid, traumatic — *see* Injury, intracranial, subarachnoid hemorrhage
    subdural, traumatic — *see* Injury, intracranial, subdural hemorrhage
  breast (nontraumatic) N64.89
  broad ligament (nontraumatic) N83.7
    traumatic S37.892 ✓
  cerebellar, traumatic S06.37- ✓
  cerebral — *see* Hematoma, brain
  cerebrum S06.36- ✓
    left S06.35- ✓
    right S06.34- ✓
  cesarean delivery wound O90.2
  complicating delivery (perineal) (pelvic) (vagina) (vulva) O71.7
  corpus cavernosum (nontraumatic) N48.89
  epididymis (nontraumatic) N50.1
  epidural (traumatic) — *see* Injury, intracranial, epidural hemorrhage
    spinal — *see* Injury, spinal cord, by region
  episiotomy O90.2
  face, birth injury P15.4
  genital organ NEC (nontraumatic)
    female (nonobstetric) N94.89
      traumatic S30.202 ✓
    male N50.1
      traumatic S30.201 ✓
  internal organs — *see* Injury, by site
  intracerebral, traumatic — *see* Injury, intracranial, intracerebral hemorrhage
  intraoperative — *see* Complications, intraoperative, hemorrhage
  labia (nontraumatic) (nonobstetric) N90.89
  liver (subcapsular) (nontraumatic) K76.89
    birth injury P15.0
  mediastinum — *see* Injury, intrathoracic
  mesosalpinx (nontraumatic) N83.7
    traumatic S37.898 ✓
  muscle — code by site under Contusion
  nontraumatic
    muscle M79.81
    soft tissue M79.81
  obstetrical surgical wound O90.2
  orbit, orbital (nontraumatic) (*see also* Hemorrhage, orbit)
    traumatic — *see* Contusion, orbit
  pelvis (female) (nontraumatic) (nonobstetric) N94.89
    obstetric O71.7
    traumatic — *see* Injury, by site
  penis (nontraumatic) N48.89
    birth injury P15.5
  perianal (nontraumatic) K64.5
  perineal S30.23 ✓
    complicating delivery O71.7
  perirenal — *see* Injury, kidney
  pinna — *see* Contusion, ear
    nontraumatic — *see* Disorder, pinna, hematoma
  placenta O43.89- ✓

Hematoma — *continued*
  postoperative (postprocedural) — *see* Complication, postprocedural, hematoma
  retroperitoneal (nontraumatic) K66.1
    traumatic S36.892 ✓
  scrotum, superficial S30.22 ✓
    birth injury P15.5
  seminal vesicle (nontraumatic) N50.1
    traumatic S37.892 ✓
  spermatic cord (traumatic) S37.892 ✓
    nontraumatic N50.1
  spinal (cord) (meninges) (*see also* Injury, spinal cord, by region)
    newborn (birth injury) P11.5
  spleen D73.5
    intraoperative — *see* Complications, intraoperative, hemorrhage, spleen
    postprocedural (postoperative) — *see* Complications, postprocedural, hemorrhage, spleen
  sternocleidomastoid, birth injury P15.2
  sternomastoid, birth injury P15.2
  subarachnoid (traumatic) — *see* Injury, intracranial, subarachnoid hemorrhage
    newborn (nontraumatic) P52.5
      due to birth injury P10.3
    nontraumatic — *see* Hemorrhage, intracranial, subarachnoid
  subdural (traumatic) — *see* Injury, intracranial, subdural hemorrhage
    newborn (localized) P52.8
      birth injury P10.0
    nontraumatic — *see* Hemorrhage, intracranial, subdural
  superficial, newborn P54.5
  testis (nontraumatic) N50.1
    birth injury P15.5
  tunica vaginalis (nontraumatic) N50.1
  umbilical cord, complicating delivery O69.5 ✓
  uterine ligament (broad) (nontraumatic) N83.7
    traumatic S37.892 ✓
  vagina (ruptured) (nontraumatic) N89.8
    complicating delivery O71.7
  vas deferens (nontraumatic) N50.1
    traumatic S37.892 ✓
  vitreous — *see* Hemorrhage, vitreous
  vulva (nontraumatic) (nonobstetric) N90.89
    complicating delivery O71.7
    newborn (birth injury) P15.5
Hematometra N85.7
  with hematocolpos N89.7
Hematomyelia (central) G95.19
  newborn (birth injury) P11.5
  traumatic T14.8 ✓
Hematomyelitis G04.90
Hematoperitoneum — *see* Hemoperitoneum
Hematophobia F40.230
Hematopneumothorax (see Hemothorax)
Hematopoiesis, cyclic D70.4
Hematoporphyria — *see* Porphyria
Hematorachis, hematorrhachis G95.19
  newborn (birth injury) P11.5
Hematosalpinx N83.6
  with
    hematocolpos N89.7
    hematometra N85.7
      with hematocolpos N89.7
  infectional — *see* Salpingitis
Hematospermia R36.1
Hematothorax (see Hemothorax)
Hematuria R31.9
  benign (familial) (of childhood) (*see also* Hematuria, idiopathic)
    essential microscopic R31.1
  due to sulphonamide, sulfonamide — *see* Table of Drugs and Chemicals, by drug
  endemic (*see also* Schistosomiasis) B65.0
  gross R31.0
  idiopathic N02.9
    with glomerular lesion
      crescentic (diffuse) glomerulonephritis N02.7
      dense deposit disease N02.6
      endocapillary proliferative glomerulonephritis N02.4
      focal and segmental hyalinosis or sclerosis N02.1
      membranoproliferative (diffuse) N02.5
      membranous (diffuse) N02.2
      mesangial proliferative (diffuse) N02.3

Hematuria — *continued*
  idiopathic — *continued*
    with glomerular lesion — *continued*
      mesangiocapillary (diffuse) N02.5
      minor abnormality N02.0
      proliferative NEC N02.8
      specified pathology NEC N02.8
  intermittent — *see* Hematuria, idiopathic
  malarial B50.8
  microscopic NEC (with symptoms) R31.29
    asymptomatic R31.21
    benign essential R31.1
  paroxysmal (*see also* Hematuria, idiopathic)
    nocturnal D59.5
  persistent — *see* Hematuria, idiopathic
  recurrent — *see* Hematuria, idiopathic
  tropical (*see also* Schistosomiasis) B65.0
  tuberculous A18.13
Hemeralopia (day blindness) H53.11
  vitamin A deficiency E50.5
Hemi-akinesia R41.4
Hemianalgesia R20.0
Hemianencephaly Q00.0
Hemianesthesia R20.0
Hemianopia, hemianopsia (heteronymous) H53.47
  homonymous H53.46- ✓
  syphilitic A52.71
Hemiathetosis R25.8
Hemiatrophy R68.89
  cerebellar G31.9
  face, facial, progressive (Romberg) G51.8
  tongue K14.8
Hemiballism (us) G25.5
Hemicardia Q24.8
Hemicephalus, hemicephaly Q00.0
Hemichorea G25.5
Hemicolitis, left — *see* Colitis, left sided
Hemicrania
  congenital malformation Q00.0
  continua G44.51
  meaning migraine (*see also* Migraine) G43.909
  paroxysmal G44.039
    chronic G44.049
      intractable G44.041
      not intractable G44.049
    episodic G44.039
      intractable G44.031
      not intractable G44.039
    intractable G44.031
    not intractable G44.039
Hemidystrophy — *see* Hemiatrophy
Hemiectromelia Q73.8
Hemihypalgesia R20.8
Hemihypesthesia R20.1
Hemi-inattention R41.4
Hemimelia Q73.8
  lower limb — *see* Defect, reduction, lower limb, specified type NEC
  upper limb — *see* Defect, reduction, upper limb, specified type NEC
Hemiparalysis — *see* Hemiplegia
Hemiparesis — *see* Hemiplegia
Hemiparesthesia R20.2
Hemiparkinsonism G20
Hemiplegia G81.9- ✓
  alternans facialis G83.89
  ascending NEC G81.90
    spinal G95.89
  congenital (cerebral) G80.8
    spastic G80.2
  embolic (current episode) I63.4- ✓
  flaccid G81.0- ✓
  following
    cerebrovascular disease I69.959
      cerebral infarction I69.35- ✓
      intracerebral hemorrhage I69.15- ✓
      nontraumatic intracranial hemorrhage NEC I69.25- ✓
      specified disease NEC I69.85- ✓
      stroke NOS I69.35- ✓
      subarachnoid hemorrhage I69.05- ✓
  hysterical F44.4
  newborn NEC P91.88
    birth injury P11.9
  spastic G81.1- ✓
    congenital G80.2
  thrombotic (current episode) I63.3- ✓

Hemisection, spinal cord — *see* Injury, spinal cord, by region
Hemispasm (facial) R25.2
Hemisporosis B48.8
Hemitremor R25.1
Hemivertebra Q76.49
  failure of segmentation with scoliosis Q76.3
  fusion with scoliosis Q76.3
Hemochromatosis E83.119
  with refractory anemia D46.1
  due to repeated red blood cell transfusion E83.111
  hereditary (primary) E83.110
  neonatal P78.84
  primary E83.110
  specified NEC E83.118
Hemoglobin (*see also* condition)
  abnormal (disease) — *see* Disease, hemoglobin
  AS genotype D57.3
  Constant Spring D58.2
  E-beta thalassemia D56.5
  fetal, hereditary persistence (HPFH) D56.4
  H Constant Spring D56.0
  low NOS D64.9
  S (Hb S), heterozygous D57.3
Hemoglobinemia D59.9
  due to blood transfusion T80.89 ☑
  paroxysmal D59.6
    nocturnal D59.5
Hemoglobinopathy (mixed) D58.2
  with thalassemia D56.8
  sickle-cell D57.1
    with thalassemia D57.40
      with crisis (vasoocclusive pain) D57.419
        with
          acute chest syndrome D57.411
          splenic sequestration D57.412
      without crisis D57.40
Hemoglobinuria R82.3
  with anemia, hemolytic, acquired (chronic) NEC D59.6
  cold (agglutinin) (paroxysmal) (with Raynaud's syndrome) D59.6
  due to exertion or hemolysis NEC D59.6
  intermittent D59.6
  malarial B50.8
  march D59.6
  nocturnal (paroxysmal) D59.5
  paroxysmal (cold) D59.6
    nocturnal D59.5
Hemolymphangioma D18.1
Hemolysis
  intravascular
    with
      abortion — *see* Abortion, by type, complicated by, hemorrhage
      ectopic or molar pregnancy O08.1
      hemorrhage
        antepartum — *see* Hemorrhage, antepartum, with coagulation defect
        intrapartum (*see also* Hemorrhage, complicating, delivery) O67.0
      postpartum O72.3
  neonatal (excessive) P58.9
    specified NEC P58.8
Hemolytic — *see* condition
Hemopericardium I31.2
  following acute myocardial infarction (current complication) I23.0
  newborn P54.8
  traumatic — *see* Injury, heart, with hemopericardium
Hemoperitoneum K66.1
  infectional K65.9
  traumatic S36.899 ☑
    with open wound — *see* Wound, open, with penetration into peritoneal cavity
Hemophilia (classical) (familial) (hereditary) D66
  A D66
  acquired D68.311
  autoimmune D68.311
  B D67
  C D68.1
  calcipriva (*see also* Defect, coagulation) D68.4
  nonfamilial (*see also* Defect, coagulation) D68.4
  secondary D68.311
  vascular D68.0
Hemophthalmos H44.81- ☑
Hemopneumothorax (*see also* Hemothorax)
  traumatic S27.2 ☑
Hemoptysis R04.2

Hemoptysis — *continued*
  newborn P26.9
  tuberculous — *see* Tuberculosis, pulmonary
Hemorrhage, hemorrhagic (concealed) R58
  abdomen R58
  accidental antepartum — *see* Hemorrhage, antepartum
  acute idiopathic pulmonary, in infants R04.81
  adenoid J35.8
  adrenal (capsule) (gland) E27.49
    medulla E27.8
    newborn P54.4
  after delivery — *see* Hemorrhage, postpartum
  alveolar
    lung, newborn P26.8
    process K08.89
  alveolus K08.89
  amputation stump (surgical) T87.89
  anemia (chronic) D50.0
    acute D62
  antepartum (with) O46.90
    with coagulation defect O46.00- ☑
      afibrinogenemia O46.01- ☑
      disseminated intravascular coagulation O46.02- ☑
      hypofibrinogenemia O46.01- ☑
      specified defect NEC O46.09- ☑
    before 20 weeks gestation O20.9
      specified type NEC O20.8
      threatened abortion O20.0
    due to
      abruptio placenta (*see also* Abruptio placentae) O45.9- ☑
      leiomyoma, uterus — *see* Hemorrhage, antepartum, specified cause NEC
      placenta previa O44.1- ☑
    specified cause NEC — *see* subcategory O46.8X- ☑
  anus (sphincter) K62.5
  apoplexy (stroke) — *see* Hemorrhage, intracranial, intracerebral
  arachnoid — *see* Hemorrhage, intracranial, subarachnoid
  artery R58
    brain — *see* Hemorrhage, intracranial, intracerebral
  basilar (ganglion) I61.0
  bladder N32.89
  bowel K92.2
    newborn P54.3
  brain (miliary) (nontraumatic) — *see* Hemorrhage, intracranial, intracerebral
    due to
      birth injury P10.1
      syphilis A52.05
    epidural or extradural (traumatic) — *see* Injury, intracranial, epidural hemorrhage
    newborn P52.4
      birth injury P10.1
    subarachnoid — *see* Hemorrhage, intracranial, subarachnoid
    subdural — *see* Hemorrhage, intracranial, subdural
  brainstem (nontraumatic) I61.3
    traumatic S06.38- ☑
  breast N64.59
  bronchial tube — *see* Hemorrhage, lung
  bronchopulmonary — *see* Hemorrhage, lung
  bronchus — *see* Hemorrhage, lung
  bulbar I61.5
  capillary I78.8
    primary D69.8
  cecum K92.2
  cerebellar, cerebellum (nontraumatic) I61.4
    newborn P52.6
    traumatic S06.37- ☑
  cerebral, cerebrum (*see also* Hemorrhage, intracranial, intracerebral)
    lobe I61.1
    newborn (anoxic) P52.4
      birth injury P10.1
  cerebromeningeal I61.8
  cerebrospinal — *see* Hemorrhage, intracranial, intracerebral
  cervix (uteri) (stump) NEC N88.8
  chamber, anterior (eye) — *see* Hyphema
  childbirth — *see* Hemorrhage, complicating, delivery
  choroid H31.30- ☑
    expulsive H31.31- ☑
  ciliary body — *see* Hyphema
  cochlea — *see* subcategory H83.8 ☑

Hemorrhage, hemorrhagic — *continued*
  colon K92.2
  complicating
    abortion — *see* Abortion, by type, complicated by, hemorrhage
    delivery O67.9
      associated with coagulation defect (afibrinogenemia) (DIC) (hyperfibrinolysis) O67.0
      specified cause NEC O67.8
    surgical procedure — *see* Hemorrhage, intraoperative
  conjunctiva H11.3- ☑
    newborn P54.8
  cord, newborn (stump) P51.9
  corpus luteum (ruptured) cyst N83.1- ☑
  cortical (brain) I61.1
  cranial — *see* Hemorrhage, intracranial
  cutaneous R23.3
    due to autosensitivity, erythrocyte D69.2
    newborn P54.5
  delayed
    following ectopic or molar pregnancy O08.1
    postpartum O72.2
  diathesis (familial) D69.9
  disease D69.9
    newborn P53
    specified type NEC D69.8
  due to or associated with
    afibrinogenemia or other coagulation defect (conditions in categories D65- D69)
      antepartum — *see* Hemorrhage, antepartum, with coagulation defect
      intrapartum O67.0
    dental implant M27.61
    device, implant or graft (*see also* Complications, by site and type, specified NEC) T85.838 ☑
      arterial graft NEC T82.838 ☑
      breast T85.838 ☑
      catheter NEC T85.838 ☑
        dialysis (renal) T82.838 ☑
          intraperitoneal T85.838 ☑
        infusion NEC T82.838 ☑
          spinal (epidural) (subdural) T85.830 ☑
        urinary (indwelling) T83.83 ☑
      electronic (electrode) (pulse generator) (stimulator)
        bone T84.83 ☑
        cardiac T82.837 ☑
        nervous system (brain) (peripheral nerve) (spinal) T85.830 ☑
        urinary T83.83 ☑
      fixation, internal (orthopedic) NEC T84.83 ☑
      gastrointestinal (bile duct) (esophagus) T85.838 ☑
      genital NEC T83.83 ☑
      heart NEC T82.837 ☑
      joint prosthesis T84.83 ☑
      ocular (corneal graft) (orbital implant) NEC T85.838 ☑
      orthopedic NEC T84.83 ☑
        bone graft T86.838
      specified NEC T85.838 ☑
      urinary NEC T83.83 ☑
      vascular NEC T82.838 ☑
      ventricular intracranial shunt T85.830 ☑
  duodenum, duodenal K92.2
    ulcer — *see* Ulcer, duodenum, with hemorrhage
  dura mater — *see* Hemorrhage, intracranial, subdural
  endotracheal — *see* Hemorrhage, lung
  epicranial subaponeurotic (massive), birth injury P12.2
  epidural (traumatic) (*see also* Injury, intracranial, epidural hemorrhage)
    nontraumatic I62.1
  esophagus K22.8
    varix I85.01
      secondary I85.11
  excessive, following ectopic gestation (subsequent episode) O08.1
  extradural (traumatic) — *see* Injury, intracranial, epidural hemorrhage
    birth injury P10.8
    newborn (anoxic) (nontraumatic) P52.8
    nontraumatic I62.1
  eye NEC H57.8
    fundus — *see* Hemorrhage, retina
    lid — *see* Disorder, eyelid, specified type NEC
  fallopian tube N83.6

Hemorrhage, hemorrhagic — *continued*
fibrinogenolysis — *see* Fibrinolysis
fibrinolytic (acquired) — *see* Fibrinolysis
from
    ear (nontraumatic) — *see* Otorrhagia
    tracheostomy stoma J95.01
fundus, eye — *see* Hemorrhage, retina
funis — *see* Hemorrhage, umbilicus, cord
gastric — *see* Hemorrhage, stomach
gastroenteric K92.2
    newborn P54.3
gastrointestinal (tract) K92.2
    newborn P54.3
genital organ, male N50.1
genitourinary (tract) NOS R31.9
gingiva K06.8
globe (eye) — *see* Hemophthalmos
graafian follicle cyst (ruptured) N83.0- ☑
gum K06.8
heart I51.89
hypopharyngeal (throat) R04.1
intermenstrual (regular) N92.3
    irregular N92.1
internal (organs) NEC R58
    capsule I61.0
    ear — *see* subcategory H83.8 ☑
    newborn P54.8
intestine K92.2
    newborn P54.3
intra-abdominal R58
intra-alveolar (lung), newborn P26.8
intracerebral (nontraumatic) — *see* Hemorrhage, intracranial, intracerebral
intracranial (nontraumatic) I62.9
    birth injury P10.9
    epidural, nontraumatic I62.1
    extradural, nontraumatic I62.1
    intracerebral (nontraumatic) (in) I61.9
        brain stem I61.3
        cerebellum I61.4
        hemisphere I61.2
            cortical (superficial) I61.1
            subcortical (deep) I61.0
        intraoperative
            during a nervous system procedure G97.31
            during other procedure G97.32
        intraventricular I61.5
        multiple localized I61.6
        newborn P52.4
            birth injury P10.1
        postprocedural
            following a nervous system procedure G97.51
            following other procedure G97.52
        specified NEC I61.8
        superficial I61.1
        traumatic (diffuse) — *see* Injury, intracranial, diffuse
            focal — *see* Injury, intracranial, focal
    newborn P52.9
        specified NEC P52.8
    subarachnoid (nontraumatic) (from) I60.9
        intracranial (cerebral) artery I60.7
            anterior communicating I60.2
            basilar I60.4
            carotid siphon and bifurcation I60.0- ☑
            communicating I60.7
                 anterior I60.2
                posterior I60.3- ☑
            middle cerebral I60.1- ☑
            posterior communicating I60.3- ☑
            specified artery NEC I60.6
            vertebral I60.5- ☑
        newborn P52.5
            birth injury P10.3
        specified NEC I60.8
        traumatic S06.6X- ☑
    subdural (nontraumatic) I62.00
        acute I62.01
        birth injury P10.0
        chronic I62.03
        newborn (anoxic) (hypoxic) P52.8
            birth injury P10.0
        spinal G95.19
        subacute I62.02
        traumatic — *see* Injury, intracranial, subdural hemorrhage

Hemorrhage, hemorrhagic — *continued*
intracranial — *continued*
    traumatic — *see* Injury, intracranial, focal brain injury
intramedullary NEC G95.19
intraocular — *see* Hemophthalmos
intraoperative, intraprocedural — *see* Complication, hemorrhage (hematoma), intraoperative (intraprocedural), by site
intrapartum — *see* Hemorrhage, complicating, delivery
intrapelvic
    female N94.89
    male K66.1
intraperitoneal K66.1
intrapontine I61.3
intraprocedural — *see* Complication, hemorrhage (hematoma), intraoperative (intraprocedural), by site
intrauterine N85.7
    complicating delivery (*see also* Hemorrhage, complicating, delivery) O67.9
    postpartum — *see* Hemorrhage, postpartum
intraventricular I61.5
    newborn (nontraumatic) (*see also* Newborn, affected by, hemorrhage) P52.3
        due to birth injury P10.2
        grade
            1 P52.0
            2 P52.1
            3 P52.21
            4 P52.22
intravesical N32.89
iris (postinfectional) (postinflammatory) (toxic) — *see* Hyphema
joint (nontraumatic) — *see* Hemarthrosis
kidney N28.89
knee (joint) (nontraumatic) — *see* Hemarthrosis, knee
labyrinth — *see* subcategory H83.8 ☑
lenticular striate artery I61.0
ligature, vessel — *see* Hemorrhage, postoperative
liver K76.89
lung R04.89
    newborn P26.9
        massive P26.1
        specified NEC P26.8
    tuberculous — *see* Tuberculosis, pulmonary
massive umbilical, newborn P51.0
mediastinum — *see* Hemorrhage, lung
medulla I61.3
membrane (brain) I60.8
    spinal cord — *see* Hemorrhage, spinal cord
meninges, meningeal (brain) (middle) I60.8
    spinal cord — *see* Hemorrhage, spinal cord
mesentery K66.1
metritis — *see* Endometritis
mouth K13.79
mucous membrane NEC R58
    newborn P54.8
muscle M62.89
nail (subungual) L60.8
nasal turbinate R04.0
    newborn P54.8
navel, newborn P51.9
newborn P54.9
    specified NEC P54.8
nipple N64.59
nose R04.0
    newborn P54.8
omentum K66.1
optic nerve (sheath) H47.02- ☑
orbit, orbital H05.23- ☑
ovary NEC N83.8
oviduct N83.6
pancreas K86.89
parathyroid (gland) (spontaneous) E21.4
parturition — *see* Hemorrhage, complicating, delivery
penis N48.89
pericardium, pericarditis I31.2
peritoneum, peritoneal K66.1
peritonsillar tissue J35.8
    due to infection J36
petechial R23.3
    due to autosensitivity, erythrocyte D69.2
pituitary (gland) E23.6
pleura — *see* Hemorrhage, lung
polioencephalitis, superior E51.2
polymyositis — *see* Polymyositis

Hemorrhage, hemorrhagic — *continued*
pons, pontine I61.3
posterior fossa (nontraumatic) I61.8
    newborn P52.6
postmenopausal N95.0
postnasal R04.0
postoperative — *see* Complications, postprocedural, hemorrhage, by site
postpartum NEC (following delivery of placenta) O72.1
    delayed or secondary O72.2
    retained placenta O72.0
    third stage O72.0
pregnancy — *see* Hemorrhage, antepartum
preretinal — *see* Hemorrhage, retina
prostate N42.1
puerperal — *see* Hemorrhage, postpartum
    delayed or secondary O72.2
pulmonary R04.89
    newborn P26.9
        massive P26.1
        specified NEC P26.8
    tuberculous — *see* Tuberculosis, pulmonary
purpura (primary) D69.3
rectum (sphincter) K62.5
    newborn P54.2
recurring, following initial hemorrhage at time of injury T79.2 ☑
renal N28.89
respiratory passage or tract R04.9
    specified NEC R04.89
retina, retinal (vessels) H35.6- ☑
    diabetic — *see* Diabetes, retinal, hemorrhage
retroperitoneal R58
scalp R58
scrotum N50.1
secondary (nontraumatic) R58
    following initial hemorrhage at time of injury T79.2 ☑
seminal vesicle N50.1
skin R23.3
    newborn P54.5
slipped umbilical ligature P51.8
spermatic cord N50.1
spinal (cord) G95.19
    newborn (birth injury) P11.5
spleen D73.5
    intraoperative — *see* Complications, intraoperative, hemorrhage, spleen
    postprocedural — *see* Complications, postprocedural, hemorrhage, spleen
stomach K92.2
    newborn P54.3
    ulcer — *see* Ulcer, stomach, with hemorrhage
subarachnoid (nontraumatic) — *see* Hemorrhage, intracranial, subarachnoid
subconjunctival (*see also* Hemorrhage, conjunctiva)
    birth injury P15.3
subcortical (brain) I61.0
subcutaneous R23.3
subdiaphragmatic R58
subdural (acute) (nontraumatic) — *see* Hemorrhage, intracranial, subdural
subependymal
    newborn P52.0
        with intraventricular extension P52.1
            and intracerebral extension P52.22
subgaleal P12.2
subhyaloid — *see* Hemorrhage, retina
subperiosteal — *see* Disorder, bone, specified type NEC
subretinal — *see* Hemorrhage, retina
subtentorial — *see* Hemorrhage, intracranial, subdural
subungual L60.8
suprarenal (capsule) (gland) E27.49
    newborn P54.4
tentorium (traumatic) NEC — *see* Hemorrhage, brain
    newborn (birth injury) P10.4
testis N50.1
third stage (postpartum) O72.0
thorax — *see* Hemorrhage, lung
throat R04.1
thymus (gland) E32.8
thyroid (cyst) (gland) E07.89
tongue K14.8
tonsil J35.8
trachea — *see* Hemorrhage, lung
tracheobronchial R04.89
    newborn P26.0

☑ **Additional Character Required — Refer to the Tabular List for Character Selection**

▽ **Subterms under main terms may continue to next column or page**

Hemorrhage, hemorrhagic — *continued*
  traumatic — *code to* specific injury
    cerebellar — *see* Hemorrhage, brain
    intracranial — *see* Hemorrhage, brain
    recurring or secondary (following initial hemor-
      rhage at time of injury) T79.2 ☑
  tuberculous NEC (*see also* Tuberculosis, pulmonary)
    A15.0
  tunica vaginalis N50.1
  ulcer — *code by* site under Ulcer, with hemorrhage
    K27.4
  umbilicus, umbilical
    cord
      after birth, newborn P51.9
      complicating delivery O69.5 ☑
    newborn P51.9
      massive P51.0
      slipped ligature P51.8
    stump P51.9
  urethra (idiopathic) N36.8
  uterus, uterine (abnormal) N93.9
    climacteric N92.4
    complicating delivery — *see* Hemorrhage, compli-
      cating, delivery
    dysfunctional or functional N93.8
    intermenstrual (regular) N92.3
      irregular N92.1
    postmenopausal N95.0
    postpartum — *see* Hemorrhage, postpartum
    preclimacteric or premenopausal N92.4
    prepubertal N93.8
    pubertal N92.2
  vagina (abnormal) N93.9
    newborn P54.6
  vas deferens N50.1
  vasa previa O69.4 ☑
  ventricular I61.5
  vesical N32.89
  viscera NEC R58
    newborn P54.8
  vitreous (humor) (intraocular) H43.1- ☑
  vulva N90.89
Hemorrhoids (bleeding) (without mention of degree)
  K64.9
  1st degree (grade/stage I) (without prolapse outside
    of anal canal) K64.0
  2nd degree (grade/stage II) (that prolapse with
    straining but retract spontaneously) K64.1
  3rd degree (grade/stage III) (that prolapse with
    straining and require manual replacement back
    inside anal canal) K64.2
  4th degree (grade/stage IV) (with prolapsed tissue that
    cannot be manually replaced) K64.3
  complicating
    pregnancy O22.4 ☑
    puerperium O87.2
  external K64.4
    with
      thrombosis K64.5
  internal (without mention of degree) K64.8
  prolapsed K64.8
  skin tags
    anus K64.4
    residual K64.4
  specified NEC K64.8
  strangulated (*see also* Hemorrhoids, by degree) K64.8
  thrombosed (*see also* Hemorrhoids, by degree) K64.5
  ulcerated (*see also* Hemorrhoids, by degree) K64.8
Hemosalpinx N83.6
  with
    hematocolpos N89.7
    hematometra N85.7
      with hematocolpos N89.7
Hemosiderosis (dietary) E83.19
  pulmonary, idiopathic E83.1- ☑ [J84.03]
  transfusion T80.89 ☑
Hemothorax (bacterial) (nontuberculous) J94.2
  newborn P54.8
  traumatic S27.1 ☑
    with pneumothorax S27.2 ☑
  tuberculous NEC A15.6
Henoch (-Schönlein) **disease or syndrome** (purpura)
  D69.0
Henpue, henpuye A66.6
Hepar lobatum (syphilitic) A52.74
Hepatalgia K76.89
Hepatitis K75.9
  acute B17.9

Hepatitis — *continued*
  acute — *continued*
    with coma K72.01
    with hepatic failure — *see* Failure, hepatic
    alcoholic — *see* Hepatitis, alcoholic
    infectious B17.9
    non-viral K72.0 ☑
    viral B17.9
  alcoholic (acute) (chronic) K70.10
    with ascites K70.11
  amebic — *see* Abscess, liver, amebic
  anicteric, (viral) — *see* Hepatitis, viral
  antigen-associated (HAA) — *see* Hepatitis, B
  Australia-antigen (positive) — *see* Hepatitis, B
  autoimmune K75.4
  B B19.10
    with hepatic coma B19.11
    acute B16.9
      with
        delta-agent (coinfection) (without hepatic
          coma) B16.1
          with hepatic coma B16.0
        hepatic coma (without delta-agent coinfec-
          tion) B16.2
    chronic B18.1
      with delta-agent B18.0
  bacterial NEC K75.89
  C (viral) B19.20
    with hepatic coma B19.21
    acute B17.10
      with hepatic coma B17.11
    chronic B18.2
  catarrhal (acute) B15.9
    with hepatic coma B15.0
  cholangiolitic K75.89
  cholestatic K75.89
  chronic K73.9
    active NEC K73.2
    lobular NEC K73.1
    persistent NEC K73.0
    specified NEC K73.8
  cytomegaloviral B25.1
  due to ethanol (acute) (chronic) — *see* Hepatitis, alco-
    holic
  epidemic B15.9
    with hepatic coma B15.0
  fulminant NEC (viral) — *see* Hepatitis, viral
  granulomatous NEC K75.3
  herpesviral B00.81
  history of
    B Z86.19
    C Z86.19
  homologous serum — *see* Hepatitis, viral, type B
  in (due to)
    mumps B26.81
    toxoplasmosis (acquired) B58.1
      congenital (active) P37.1 [K77]
  infectious, infective B15.9
    acute (subacute) B17.9
    chronic B18.9
  inoculation — *see* Hepatitis, viral, type B
  interstitial (chronic) K74.69
  lupoid NEC K75.4
  malignant NEC (with hepatic failure) K72.90
    with coma K72.91
  neonatal (idiopathic) (toxic) P59.29
  neonatal giant cell P59.29
  newborn P59.29
  non-viral K72.0 ☑
  postimmunization — *see* Hepatitis, viral, type B
  post-transfusion — *see* Hepatitis, viral, type B
  reactive, nonspecific K75.2
  serum — *see* Hepatitis, viral, type B
  specified type NEC
    with hepatic failure — *see* Failure, hepatic
  syphilitic (late) A52.74
    congenital (early) A50.08 [K77]
      late A50.59 [K77]
    secondary A51.45
  toxic (*see also* Disease, liver, toxic) K71.6
  tuberculous A18.83
  viral, virus B19.9
    with hepatic coma B19.0
    acute B17.9
    chronic B18.9
      specified NEC B18.8
      type
        B B18.1

Hepatitis — *continued*
  viral, virus — *continued*
    chronic — *continued*
      type — *continued*
        B — *continued*
          with delta-agent B18.0
        C B18.2
    congenital P35.3
    coxsackie B33.8 [K77]
    cytomegalic inclusion B25.1
    in remission, any type — *code to* Hepatitis, chronic,
      by type
    non-A, non-B B17.8
    specified type NEC (with or without coma) B17.8
    type
      A B15.9
        with hepatic coma B15.0
      B B19.10
        with hepatic coma B19.11
        acute B16.9
          with
            delta-agent (coinfection) (without
              hepatic coma) B16.1
              with hepatic coma B16.0
            hepatic coma (without delta-agent
              coinfection) B16.2
        chronic B18.1
          with delta-agent B18.0
      C B19.20
        with hepatic coma B19.21
        acute B17.10
          with hepatic coma B17.11
        chronic B18.2
      E B17.2
      non-A, non-B B17.8
Hepatization lung (acute) — *see* Pneumonia, lobar
Hepatoblastoma C22.2
Hepatocarcinoma C22.0
Hepatocholangiocarcinoma C22.0
Hepatocholangioma, benign D13.4
Hepatocholangitis K75.89
Hepatolenticular degeneration E83.01
Hepatoma (malignant) C22.0
  benign D13.4
  embryonal C22.0
Hepatomegaly (*see also* Hypertrophy, liver)
  with splenomegaly R16.2
  congenital Q44.7
  in mononucleosis
    gammaherpesviral B27.09
    infectious specified NEC B27.89
Hepatoptosis K76.89
Hepatorenal syndrome following labor and delivery
  O90.4
Hepatosis K76.89
Hepatosplenomegaly R16.2
  hyperlipemic (Bürger-Grütz type) E78.3 [K77]
Hereditary — *see* condition
Heredodegeneration, macular — *see* Dystrophy, retina
Heredopathia atactica polyneuritiformis G60.1
Heredosyphilis — *see* Syphilis, congenital
Herlitz' syndrome Q81.1
Hermansky-Pudlak syndrome E70.331
Hermaphrodite, hermaphroditism (true) Q56.0
  46,XX with streak gonads Q99.1
  46,XX/46,XY Q99.0
  46,XY with streak gonads Q99.1
  chimera 46,XX/46,XY Q99.0
Hernia, hernial (acquired) (recurrent) K46.9
  with
    gangrene — *see* Hernia, by site, with, gangrene
    incarceration — *see* Hernia, by site, with, obstruc-
      tion
    irreducible — *see* Hernia, by site, with, obstruction
    obstruction — *see* Hernia, by site, with, obstruction
    strangulation — *see* Hernia, by site, with, obstruc-
      tion
  abdomen, abdominal K46.9
    with
      gangrene (and obstruction) K46.1
      obstruction K46.0
    femoral — *see* Hernia, femoral
    incisional — *see* Hernia, incisional
    inguinal — *see* Hernia, inguinal
    specified site NEC K45.8
      with
        gangrene (and obstruction) K45.1
        obstruction K45.0

Hernia, hernial — *continued*
  abdomen, abdominal — *continued*
    umbilical — *see* Hernia, umbilical
    wall — *see* Hernia, ventral
  appendix — *see* Hernia, abdomen
  bladder (mucosa) (sphincter)
    congenital (female) (male) Q79.51
    female — *see* Cystocele
    male N32.89
  brain, congenital — *see* Encephalocele
  cartilage, vertebra — *see* Displacement, intervertebral disc
  cerebral, congenital (*see also* Encephalocele)
    endaural Q01.8
  ciliary body (traumatic) S05.2- ☑
  colon — *see* Hernia, abdomen
  Cooper's — *see* Hernia, abdomen, specified site NEC
  crural — *see* Hernia, femoral
  diaphragm, diaphragmatic K44.9
    with
      gangrene (and obstruction) K44.1
      obstruction K44.0
    congenital Q79.0
  direct (inguinal) — *see* Hernia, inguinal
  diverticulum, intestine — *see* Hernia, abdomen
  double (inguinal) — *see* Hernia, inguinal, bilateral
  due to adhesions (with obstruction) K56.50
  epigastric (*see also* Hernia, ventral) K43.9
  esophageal hiatus — *see* Hernia, hiatal
  external (inguinal) — *see* Hernia, inguinal
  fallopian tube N83.4- ☑
  fascia M62.89
  femoral K41.90
    with
      gangrene (and obstruction) K41.40
        not specified as recurrent K41.40
        recurrent K41.41
      obstruction K41.30
        not specified as recurrent K41.30
        recurrent K41.31
    bilateral K41.20
      with
        gangrene (and obstruction) K41.10
          not specified as recurrent K41.10
          recurrent K41.11
        obstruction K41.00
          not specified as recurrent K41.00
          recurrent K41.01
      not specified as recurrent K41.20
      recurrent K41.21
    not specified as recurrent K41.90
    recurrent K41.91
    unilateral K41.90
      with
        gangrene (and obstruction) K41.40
          not specified as recurrent K41.40
          recurrent K41.41
        obstruction K41.30
          not specified as recurrent K41.30
          recurrent K41.31
      not specified as recurrent K41.90
      recurrent K41.91
  foramen magnum G93.5
    congenital Q01.8
  funicular (umbilical) (*see also* Hernia, umbilicus)
    spermatic (cord) — *see* Hernia, inguinal
  gastrointestinal tract — *see* Hernia, abdomen
  Hesselbach's — *see* Hernia, femoral, specified site NEC
  hiatal (esophageal) (sliding) K44.9
    with
      gangrene (and obstruction) K44.1
      obstruction K44.0
    congenital Q40.1
  hypogastric — *see* Hernia, ventral
  incarcerated (*see also* Hernia, by site, with obstruction)
    with gangrene — *see* Hernia, by site, with gangrene
  incisional K43.2
    with
      gangrene (and obstruction) K43.1
      obstruction K43.0
  indirect (inguinal) — *see* Hernia, inguinal
  inguinal (direct) (external) (funicular) (indirect) (internal) (oblique) (scrotal) (sliding) K40.90
    with
      gangrene (and obstruction) K40.40
        not specified as recurrent K40.40
        recurrent K40.41

Hernia, hernial — *continued*
  inguinal — *continued*
    with — *continued*
      obstruction K40.30
        not specified as recurrent K40.30
        recurrent K40.31
    bilateral K40.20
      with
        gangrene (and obstruction) K40.10
          not specified as recurrent K40.10
          recurrent K40.11
        obstruction K40.00
          not specified as recurrent K40.00
          recurrent K40.01
      not specified as recurrent K40.20
      recurrent K40.21
    not specified as recurrent K40.90
    recurrent K40.91
    unilateral K40.90
      with
        gangrene (and obstruction) K40.40
          not specified as recurrent K40.40
          recurrent K40.41
        obstruction K40.30
          not specified as recurrent K40.30
          recurrent K40.31
      not specified as recurrent K40.90
      recurrent K40.91
  internal (*see also* Hernia, abdomen)
    inguinal — *see* Hernia, inguinal
  interstitial — *see* Hernia, abdomen
  intervertebral cartilage or disc — *see* Displacement, intervertebral disc
  intestine, intestinal — *see* Hernia, by site
  intra-abdominal — *see* Hernia, abdomen
  iris (traumatic) S05.2- ☑
  irreducible (*see also* Hernia, by site, with obstruction)
    with gangrene — *see* Hernia, by site, with gangrene
  ischiatic — *see* Hernia, abdomen, specified site NEC
  ischiorectal — *see* Hernia, abdomen, specified site NEC
  lens (traumatic) S05.2- ☑
  linea (alba) (semilunaris) — *see* Hernia, ventral
  Littre's — *see* Hernia, abdomen
  lumbar — *see* Hernia, abdomen, specified site NEC
  lung (subcutaneous) J98.4
  mediastinum J98.59
  mesenteric (internal) — *see* Hernia, abdomen
  midline — *see* Hernia, ventral
  muscle (sheath) M62.89
  nucleus pulposus — *see* Displacement, intervertebral disc
  oblique (inguinal) — *see* Hernia, inguinal
  obstructive (*see also* Hernia, by site, with obstruction)
    with gangrene — *see* Hernia, by site, with gangrene
  obturator — *see* Hernia, abdomen, specified site NEC
  omental — *see* Hernia, abdomen
  ovary N83.4- ☑
  oviduct N83.4- ☑
  paraesophageal (*see also* Hernia, diaphragm)
    congenital Q40.1
  parastomal K43.5
    with
      gangrene (and obstruction) K43.4
      obstruction K43.3
  paraumbilical — *see* Hernia, umbilicus
  perineal — *see* Hernia, abdomen, specified site NEC
  Petit's — *see* Hernia, abdomen, specified site NEC
  postoperative — *see* Hernia, incisional
  pregnant uterus — *see* Abnormal, uterus in pregnancy or childbirth
  prevesical N32.89
  properitoneal — *see* Hernia, abdomen, specified site NEC
  pudendal — *see* Hernia, abdomen, specified site NEC
  rectovaginal N81.6
  retroperitoneal — *see* Hernia, abdomen, specified site NEC
  Richter's — *see* Hernia, abdomen, with obstruction
  Rieux's, Riex's — *see* Hernia, abdomen, specified site NEC
  sac condition (adhesion) (dropsy) (inflammation) (laceration) (suppuration) — *code by site under* Hernia
  sciatic — *see* Hernia, abdomen, specified site NEC

Hernia, hernial — *continued*
  scrotum, scrotal — *see* Hernia, inguinal
  sliding (inguinal) (*see also* Hernia, inguinal)
    hiatus — *see* Hernia, hiatal
  spigelian — *see* Hernia, ventral
  spinal — *see* Spina bifida
  strangulated (*see also* Hernia, by site, with obstruction)
    with gangrene — *see* Hernia, by site, with gangrene
  subxiphoid — *see* Hernia, ventral
  supra-umbilicus — *see* Hernia, ventral
  tendon — *see* Disorder, tendon, specified type NEC
  Treitz's (fossa) — *see* Hernia, abdomen, specified site NEC
  tunica vaginalis Q55.29
  umbilicus, umbilical K42.9
    with
      gangrene (and obstruction) K42.1
      obstruction K42.0
  ureter N28.89
  urethra, congenital Q64.79
  urinary meatus, congenital Q64.79
  uterus N81.4
    pregnant — *see* Abnormal, uterus in pregnancy or childbirth
  vaginal (anterior) (wall) — *see* Cystocele
  Velpeau's — *see* Hernia, femoral
  ventral K43.9
    with
      gangrene (and obstruction) K43.7
      obstruction K43.6
    incisional K43.2
      with
        gangrene (and obstruction) K43.1
        obstruction K43.0
      recurrent — *see* Hernia, incisional
    specified NEC K43.9
      with
        gangrene (and obstruction) K43.7
        obstruction K43.6
  vesical
    congenital (female) (male) Q79.51
    female — *see* Cystocele
    male N32.89
  vitreous (into wound) S05.2- ☑
    into anterior chamber — *see* Prolapse, vitreous
Herniation (*see also* Hernia)
  brain (stem) G93.5
  cerebral G93.5
  mediastinum J98.59
  nucleus pulposus — *see* Displacement, intervertebral disc
Herpangina B08.5
Herpes, herpesvirus, herpetic B00.9
  anogenital A60.9
    perianal skin A60.1
    rectum A60.1
    urogenital tract A60.00
      cervix A60.03
      male genital organ NEC A60.02
      penis A60.01
      specified site NEC A60.09
      vagina A60.04
      vulva A60.04
  blepharitis (zoster) B02.39
    simplex B00.59
  circinatus B35.4
    bullosus L12.0
  conjunctivitis (simplex) B00.53
    zoster B02.31
  cornea B02.33
  encephalitis B00.4
    due to herpesvirus 6 B10.01
    due to herpesvirus 7 B10.09
    specified NEC B10.09
  eye (zoster) B02.30
    simplex B00.50
  eyelid (zoster) B02.39
    simplex B00.59
  facialis B00.1
  febrilis B00.1
  geniculate ganglionitis B02.21
  genital, genitalis A60.00
    female A60.09
    male A60.02
  gestational, gestationis O26.4- ☑
  gingivostomatitis B00.2
  human B00.9

☑ **Additional Character Required** — Refer to the Tabular List for Character Selection

▽ **Subterms under main terms may continue to next column or page**

Herpes, herpesvirus, herpetic — *continued*
- human — *continued*
  - 1 — *see* Herpes, simplex
  - 2 — *see* Herpes, simplex
  - 3 — *see* Varicella
  - 4 — *see* Mononucleosis, Epstein-Barr (virus)
  - 5 — *see* Disease, cytomegalic inclusion (generalized)
  - 6
    - encephalitis B10.01
    - specified NEC B10.81
  - 7
    - encephalitis B10.09
    - specified NEC B10.82
  - 8 B10.89
- infection NEC B10.89
  - Kaposi's sarcoma associated B10.89
- iridocyclitis (simplex) B00.51
  - zoster B02.32
- iris (vesicular erythema multiforme) L51.9
- iritis (simplex) B00.51
  - Kaposi's sarcoma associated B10.89
- keratitis (simplex) (dendritic) (disciform) (interstitial) B00.52
  - zoster (interstitial) B02.33
- keratoconjunctivitis (simplex) B00.52
  - zoster B02.33
- labialis B00.1
- lip B00.1
- meningitis (simplex) B00.3
  - zoster B02.1
- ophthalmicus (zoster) NEC B02.30
  - simplex B00.50
- penis A60.01
- perianal skin A60.1
- pharyngitis, pharyngotonsillitis B00.2
- rectum A60.1
- scrotum A60.02
- sepsis B00.7
- simplex B00.9
  - complicated NEC B00.89
  - congenital P35.2
  - conjunctivitis B00.53
  - external ear B00.1
  - eyelid B00.59
  - hepatitis B00.81
  - keratitis (interstitial) B00.52
  - myleitis B00.82
  - specified complication NEC B00.89
  - visceral B00.89
- stomatitis B00.2
- tonsurans B35.0
- visceral B00.89
- vulva A60.04
- whitlow B00.89
- zoster (*see also* condition) B02.9
  - auricularis B02.21
  - complicated NEC B02.8
  - conjunctivitis B02.31
  - disseminated B02.7
  - encephalitis B02.0
  - eye (lid) B02.39
  - geniculate ganglionitis B02.21
  - keratitis (interstitial) B02.33
  - meningitis B02.1
  - myelitis B02.24
  - neuritis, neuralgia B02.29
  - ophthalmicus NEC B02.30
  - oticus B02.21
  - polyneuropathy B02.23
  - specified complication NEC B02.8
  - trigeminal neuralgia B02.22

Herpesvirus (human) — *see* Herpes
Herpetophobia F40.218
Herrick's anemia — *see* Disease, sickle-cell
Hers' disease E74.09
Herter-Gee syndrome K90.0
Herxheimer's reaction R68.89
Hesitancy
- of micturition R39.11
- urinary R39.11

Hesselbach's hernia — *see* Hernia, femoral, specified site NEC
Heterochromia (congenital) Q13.2
- cataract — *see* Cataract, complicated
- cyclitis (Fuchs) — *see* Cyclitis, Fuchs' heterochromic
- hair L67.1
- iritis — *see* Cyclitis, Fuchs' heterochromic

Heterochromia — *continued*
- retained metallic foreign body (nonmagnetic) — *see* Foreign body, intraocular, old, retained
  - magnetic — *see* Foreign body, intraocular, old, retained, magnetic
- uveitis — *see* Cyclitis, Fuchs' heterochromic
Heterophoria — *see* Strabismus, heterophoria
Heterophyes, heterophyiasis (small intestine) B66.8
Heterotopia, heterotopic (*see also* Malposition, congenital)
- cerebralis Q04.8
Heterotropia — *see* Strabismus
Heubner-Herter disease K90.0
Hexadactylism Q69.9
HGSIL (cytology finding) (high grade squamous intraepithelial lesion on cytologic smear) (Pap smear finding)
- anus R85.613
- cervix R87.613
  - biopsy (histology) finding — *see* Neoplasia, intraepithelial, cervix, grade II or grade III
- vagina R87.623
  - biopsy (histology) finding — *see* Neoplasia, intraepithelial, cervix, grade II or grade III
Hibernoma — *see* Lipoma
Hiccup, hiccough R06.6
- epidemic B33.0
- psychogenic F45.8
Hidden penis (congenital) Q55.64
- acquired N48.83
Hidradenitis (axillaris) (suppurative) L73.2
Hidradenoma (nodular) (*see also* Neoplasm, skin, benign)
- clear cell — *see* Neoplasm, skin, benign
- papillary — *see* Neoplasm, skin, benign
Hidrocystoma — *see* Neoplasm, skin, benign
High
- altitude effects T70.20 ☑
  - anoxia T70.29 ☑
  - on
    - ears T70.0 ☑
    - sinuses T70.1 ☑
  - polycythemia D75.1
- arch
  - foot Q66.7
  - palate, congenital Q38.5
- arterial tension — *see* Hypertension
- basal metabolic rate R94.8
- blood pressure (*see also* Hypertension)
  - borderline R03.0
  - reading (incidental) (isolated) (nonspecific), without diagnosis of hypertension R03.0
- cholesterol E78.00
  - with high triglycerides E78.2
- diaphragm (congenital) Q79.1
- expressed emotional level within family Z63.8
- head at term O32.4 ☑
- palate, congenital Q38.5
- risk
  - infant NEC Z76.2
  - sexual behavior (heterosexual) Z72.51
    - bisexual Z72.53
    - homosexual Z72.52
- scrotal testis, testes
  - bilateral Q53.23
  - unilateral Q53.13
- temperature (of unknown origin) R50.9
- thoracic rib Q76.6
- triglycerides E78.1
  - with high cholesterol E78.2
Hildenbrand's disease A75.0
Hilum — *see* condition
Hip — *see* condition
Hippel's disease Q85.8
Hippophobia F40.218
Hippus H57.09
Hirschsprung's disease or megacolon Q43.1
Hirsutism, hirsuties L68.0
Hirudiniasis
- external B88.3
- internal B83.4
Hiss-Russell dysentery A03.1
Histidinemia, histidinuria E70.41
Histiocytoma (*see also* Neoplasm, skin, benign)
- fibrous (*see also* Neoplasm, skin, benign)
  - atypical — *see* Neoplasm, connective tissue, uncertain behavior

Histiocytoma — *continued*
- fibrous (*see also* Neoplasm, skin, benign) — *continued*
  - malignant — *see* Neoplasm, connective tissue, malignant
Histiocytosis D76.3
- acute differentiated progressive C96.0
- Langerhans' cell NEC C96.6
  - multifocal X
    - multisystemic (disseminated) C96.0
    - unisystemic C96.5
  - pulmonary, adult (adult PLCH) J84.82
  - unifocal (X) C96.6
- lipid, lipoid D76.3
  - essential E75.29
- malignant C96.A (*following* C96.6)
- mononuclear phagocytes NEC D76.1
  - Langerhans' cells C96.6
- non-Langerhans cell D76.3
- polyostotic sclerosing D76.3
- sinus, with massive lymphadenopathy D76.3
- syndrome NEC D76.3
- X NEC C96.6
  - acute (progressive) C96.0
  - chronic C96.6
  - multifocal C96.5
  - multisystemic C96.0
  - unifocal C96.6
Histoplasmosis B39.9
- with pneumonia NEC B39.2
- African B39.5
- American — *see* Histoplasmosis, capsulati
- capsulati B39.4
  - disseminated B39.3
  - generalized B39.3
  - pulmonary B39.2
    - acute B39.0
    - chronic B39.1
- Darling's B39.4
- duboisii B39.5
- lung NEC B39.2
History
- family (of) (*see also* History, personal (of))
  - alcohol abuse Z81.1
  - allergy NEC Z84.89
  - anemia Z83.2
  - arthritis Z82.61
  - asthma Z82.5
  - blindness Z82.1
  - cardiac death (sudden) Z82.41
  - carrier of genetic disease Z84.81
  - chromosomal anomaly Z82.79
  - chronic
    - disabling disease NEC Z82.8
    - lower respiratory disease Z82.5
  - colonic polyps Z83.71
  - congenital malformations and deformations Z82.79
    - polycystic kidney Z82.71
  - consanguinity Z84.3
  - deafness Z82.2
  - diabetes mellitus Z83.3
  - disability NEC Z82.8
  - disease or disorder (of)
    - allergic NEC Z84.89
    - behavioral NEC Z81.8
    - blood and blood-forming organs Z83.2
    - cardiovascular NEC Z82.49
    - chronic disabling NEC Z82.8
    - digestive Z83.79
    - ear NEC Z83.52
    - endocrine NEC Z83.49
    - eye NEC Z83.518
      - glaucoma Z83.511
    - familial hypercholesterolemia Z83.42
    - genitourinary NEC Z84.2
    - glaucoma Z83.511
    - hematological Z83.2
    - immune mechanism Z83.2
    - infectious NEC Z83.1
    - ischemic heart Z82.49
    - kidney Z84.1
    - mental NEC Z81.8
    - metabolic Z83.49
    - musculoskeletal NEC Z82.69
    - neurological NEC Z82.0
    - nutritional Z83.49
    - parasitic NEC Z83.1
    - psychiatric NEC Z81.8
    - respiratory NEC Z83.6

History — *continued*
  family (*see also* History, personal) — *continued*
    disease or disorder — *continued*
      skin and subcutaneous tissue NEC Z84.0
      specified NEC Z84.89
    drug abuse NEC Z81.3
    epilepsy Z82.0
    familial hypercholesterolemia Z83.42
    genetic disease carrier Z84.81
    glaucoma Z83.511
    hearing loss Z82.2
    human immunodeficiency virus (HIV) infection Z83.0
    Huntington's chorea Z82.0
    intellectual disability Z81.0
    leukemia Z80.6
    malignant neoplasm (of) NOS Z80.9
      bladder Z80.52
      breast Z80.3
      bronchus Z80.1
      digestive organ Z80.0
      gastrointestinal tract Z80.0
      genital organ Z80.49
        ovary Z80.41
        prostate Z80.42
        specified organ NEC Z80.49
        testis Z80.43
      hematopoietic NEC Z80.7
      intrathoracic organ NEC Z80.2
      kidney Z80.51
      lung Z80.1
      lymphatic NEC Z80.7
      ovary Z80.41
      prostate Z80.42
      respiratory organ NEC Z80.2
      specified site NEC Z80.8
      testis Z80.43
      trachea Z80.1
      urinary organ or tract Z80.59
        bladder Z80.52
        kidney Z80.51
    mental
      disorder NEC Z81.8
    multiple endocrine neoplasia (MEN) syndrome Z83.41
    osteoporosis Z82.62
    polycystic kidney Z82.71
    polyps (colon) Z83.71
    psychiatric disorder Z81.8
    psychoactive substance abuse NEC Z81.3
    respiratory condition NEC Z83.6
      asthma and other lower respiratory conditions Z82.5
    self-harmful behavior Z81.8
    SIDS (sudden infant death syndrome) Z84.82
    skin condition Z84.0
    specified condition NEC Z84.89
    stroke (cerebrovascular) Z82.3
    substance abuse NEC Z81.4
      alcohol Z81.1
      drug NEC Z81.3
      psychoactive NEC Z81.3
      tobacco Z81.2
    sudden
      cardiac death Z82.41
      infant death syndrome (SIDS) Z84.82
    tobacco abuse Z81.2
    violence, violent behavior Z81.8
    visual loss Z82.1
  personal (of) (*see also* History, family (of))
    abuse
      adult Z91.419
        physical and sexual Z91.410
        psychological Z91.411
      childhood Z62.819
        physical Z62.810
        psychological Z62.811
        sexual Z62.810
    alcohol dependence F10.21
    allergy (to) Z88.9
      analgesic agent NEC Z88.6
      anesthetic Z88.4
      antibiotic agent NEC Z88.1
      anti-infective agent NEC Z88.3
      contrast media Z91.041
      drugs, medicaments and biological substances Z88.9
        specified NEC Z88.8
      food Z91.018

History — *continued*
  personal (*see also* History, family) — *continued*
    allergy — *continued*
      food — *continued*
        additives Z91.02
        eggs Z91.012
        milk products Z91.011
        peanuts Z91.010
        seafood Z91.013
        specified food NEC Z91.018
      insect Z91.038
        bee Z91.030
      latex Z91.040
      medicinal agents Z88.9
        specified NEC Z88.8
      narcotic agent NEC Z88.5
      nonmedicinal agents Z91.048
      penicillin Z88.0
      serum Z88.7
      specified NEC Z91.09
      sulfonamides Z88.2
      vaccine Z88.7
    anaphylactic shock Z87.892
    anaphylaxis Z87.892
    behavioral disorders Z86.59
    benign carcinoid tumor Z86.012
    benign neoplasm Z86.018
      brain Z86.011
      carcinoid Z86.012
      colonic polyps Z86.010
    brain injury (traumatic) Z87.820
    breast implant removal Z98.86
    calculi, renal Z87.442
    cancer — *see* History, personal (of), malignant neoplasm (of)
    cardiac arrest (death), successfully resuscitated Z86.74
    cerebral infarction without residual deficit Z86.73
    cervical dysplasia Z87.410
    chemotherapy for neoplastic condition Z92.21
    childhood abuse — *see* History, personal (of), abuse
    cleft lip (corrected) Z87.730
    cleft palate (corrected) Z87.730
    collapsed vertebra (healed) Z87.311
      due to osteoporosis Z87.310
    combat and operational stress reaction Z86.51
    congenital malformation (corrected) Z87.798
      circulatory system (corrected) Z87.74
      digestive system (corrected) NEC Z87.738
      ear (corrected) Z87.721
      eye (corrected) Z87.720
      face and neck (corrected) Z87.790
      genitourinary system (corrected) NEC Z87.718
      heart (corrected) Z87.74
      integument (corrected) Z87.76
      limb(s) (corrected) Z87.76
      musculoskeletal system (corrected) Z87.76
      neck (corrected) Z87.790
      nervous system (corrected) NEC Z87.728
      respiratory system (corrected) Z87.75
      sense organs (corrected) NEC Z87.728
      specified NEC Z87.798
    contraception Z92.0
    deployment (military) Z91.82
    diabetic foot ulcer Z86.31
    disease or disorder (of) Z87.898
      anaphylaxis Z87.892
      blood and blood-forming organs Z86.2
      circulatory system Z86.79
        specified condition NEC Z86.79
      connective tissue Z87.39
      digestive system Z87.19
        colonic polyp Z86.010
        peptic ulcer disease Z87.11
        specified condition NEC Z87.19
      ear Z86.69
      endocrine Z86.39
        diabetic foot ulcer Z86.31
        gestational diabetes Z86.32
        specified type NEC Z86.39
      eye Z86.69
      genital (track) system NEC
        female Z87.42
        male Z87.438
      hematological Z86.2
      Hodgkin Z85.71
      immune mechanism Z86.2
      infectious Z86.19

History — *continued*
  personal (*see also* History, family) — *continued*
    disease or disorder — *continued*
      infectious — *continued*
        malaria Z86.13
        Methicillin resistant Staphylococcus aureus (MRSA) Z86.14
        poliomyelitis Z86.12
        specified NEC Z86.19
        tuberculosis Z86.11
      mental NEC Z86.59
      metabolic Z86.39
        diabetic foot ulcer Z86.31
        gestational diabetes Z86.32
        specified type NEC Z86.39
      musculoskeletal NEC Z87.39
      nervous system Z86.69
      nutritional Z86.39
      parasitic Z86.19
      respiratory system NEC Z87.09
      sense organs Z86.69
      skin Z87.2
      specified site or type NEC Z87.898
      subcutaneous tissue Z87.2
      trophoblastic Z87.59
      urinary system NEC Z87.448
    drug dependence — *see* Dependence, drug, by type, in remission
    drug therapy
      antineoplastic chemotherapy Z92.21
      estrogen Z92.23
      immunosupression Z92.25
      inhaled steroids Z92.240
      monoclonal drug Z92.22
      specified NEC Z92.29
      steroid Z92.241
      systemic steroids Z92.241
    dysplasia
      cervical (mild) (moderate) Z87.410
        severe (grade III) Z86.001
      prostatic Z87.430
      vaginal (mild) (moderate) Z87.411
        severe (grade III) Z86.008
      vulvar (mild) (moderate) Z87.412
        severe (grade III) Z86.008
    embolism (venous) Z86.718
      pulmonary Z86.711
    encephalitis Z86.61
    estrogen therapy Z92.23
    extracorporeal membrane oxygenation (ECMO) Z92.81
    failed conscious sedation Z92.83
    failed moderate sedation Z92.83
    fall, falling Z91.81
    fracture (healed)
      fatigue Z87.312
      fragility Z87.310
      osteoporosis Z87.310
      pathological NEC Z87.311
      stress Z87.312
      traumatic Z87.81
    gestational diabetes Z86.32
    hepatitis
      B Z86.19
      C Z86.19
    Hodgkin disease Z85.71
    hyperthermia, malignant Z88.4
    hypospadias (corrected) Z87.710
    hysterectomy Z90.710
    immunosupression therapy Z92.25
    in situ neoplasm
      breast Z86.000
      cervix uteri Z86.001
      specified NEC Z86.008
    in utero procedure during pregnancy Z98.870
    in utero procedure while a fetus Z98.871
    infection NEC Z86.19
      central nervous system Z86.61
      Methicillin resistant Staphylococcus aureus (MRSA) Z86.14
      urinary (recurrent) (tract) Z87.440
    injury NEC Z87.828
    irradiation Z92.3
    kidney stones Z87.442
    leukemia Z85.6
    lymphoma (non-Hodgkin) Z85.72
    malignant melanoma (skin) Z85.820
    malignant neoplasm (of) Z85.9
      accessory sinuses Z85.22

☑ **Additional Character Required — Refer to the Tabular List for Character Selection**   ▽ **Subterms under main terms may continue to next column or page**

History — *continued*
　personal (*see also* History, family) — *continued*
　　malignant neoplasm — *continued*
　　　anus NEC Z85.048
　　　　carcinoid Z85.040
　　　bladder Z85.51
　　　bone Z85.830
　　　brain Z85.841
　　　breast Z85.3
　　　bronchus NEC Z85.118
　　　　carcinoid Z85.110
　　　carcinoid — *see* History, personal (of), malignant neoplasm, by site, carcinoid
　　　cervix Z85.41
　　　colon NEC Z85.038
　　　　carcinoid Z85.030
　　　digestive organ Z85.00
　　　　specified NEC Z85.09
　　　endocrine gland NEC Z85.858
　　　epididymis Z85.48
　　　esophagus Z85.01
　　　eye Z85.840
　　　gastrointestinal tract — *see* History, malignant neoplasm, digestive organ
　　　genital organ
　　　　female Z85.40
　　　　　specified NEC Z85.44
　　　　male Z85.45
　　　　　specified NEC Z85.49
　　　hematopoietic NEC Z85.79
　　　intrathoracic organ Z85.20
　　　kidney NEC Z85.528
　　　　carcinoid Z85.520
　　　large intestine NEC Z85.038
　　　　carcinoid Z85.030
　　　larynx Z85.21
　　　liver Z85.05
　　　lung NEC Z85.118
　　　　carcinoid Z85.110
　　　mediastinum Z85.29
　　　Merkel cell Z85.821
　　　middle ear Z85.22
　　　nasal cavities Z85.22
　　　nervous system NEC Z85.848
　　　oral cavity Z85.819
　　　　specified site NEC Z85.818
　　　ovary Z85.43
　　　pancreas Z85.07
　　　pelvis Z85.53
　　　pharynx Z85.819
　　　　specified site NEC Z85.818
　　　pleura Z85.29
　　　prostate Z85.46
　　　rectosigmoid junction NEC Z85.048
　　　　carcinoid Z85.040
　　　rectum NEC Z85.048
　　　　carcinoid Z85.040
　　　respiratory organ Z85.20
　　　sinuses, accessory Z85.22
　　　skin NEC Z85.828
　　　　melanoma Z85.820
　　　　Merkel cell Z85.821
　　　small intestine NEC Z85.068
　　　　carcinoid Z85.060
　　　soft tissue Z85.831
　　　specified site NEC Z85.89
　　　stomach NEC Z85.028
　　　　carcinoid Z85.020
　　　testis Z85.47
　　　thymus NEC Z85.238
　　　　carcinoid Z85.230
　　　thyroid Z85.850
　　　tongue Z85.810
　　　trachea Z85.12
　　　urinary organ or tract Z85.50
　　　　specified NEC Z85.59
　　　uterus Z85.42
　　maltreatment Z91.89
　　medical treatment NEC Z92.89
　　melanoma (malignant) (skin) Z85.820
　　meningitis Z86.61
　　mental disorder Z86.59
　　Merkel cell carcinoma (skin) Z85.821
　　Methicillin resistant Staphylococcus aureus (MRSA) Z86.14
　　military deployment Z91.82
　　military war, peacekeeping and humanitarian deployment (current or past conflict) Z91.82
　　myocardial infarction (old) I25.2

History — *continued*
　personal (*see also* History, family) — *continued*
　　neglect (in)
　　　adult Z91.412
　　　childhood Z62.812
　　neoplasm
　　　benign Z86.018
　　　　brain Z86.011
　　　　colon polyp Z86.010
　　　in situ
　　　　breast Z86.000
　　　　cervix uteri Z86.001
　　　　specified NEC Z86.008
　　　malignant — *see* History of, malignant neoplasm
　　　uncertain behavior Z86.03
　　nephrotic syndrome Z87.441
　　nicotine dependence Z87.891
　　noncompliance with medical treatment or regimen — *see* Noncompliance
　　nutritional deficiency Z86.39
　　obstetric complications Z87.59
　　　childbirth Z87.59
　　　pregnancy Z87.59
　　　pre-term labor Z87.51
　　　puerperium Z87.59
　　osteoporosis fractures Z87.31 ☑
　　parasuicide (attempt) Z91.5
　　physical trauma NEC Z87.828
　　　self-harm or suicide attempt Z91.5
　　pneumonia (recurrent) Z87.01
　　poisoning Z91.89
　　　self-harm or suicide attempt Z91.5
　　poor personal hygiene Z91.89
　　preterm labor Z87.51
　　procedure during pregnancy Z98.870
　　procedure while a fetus Z98.871
　　prolonged reversible ischemic neurologic deficit (PRIND) Z86.73
　　prostatic dysplasia Z87.430
　　psychological
　　　abuse
　　　　adult Z91.411
　　　　child Z62.811
　　　trauma, specified NEC Z91.49
　　radiation therapy Z92.3
　　removal
　　　implant
　　　　breast Z98.86
　　renal calculi Z87.442
　　respiratory condition NEC Z87.09
　　retained foreign body fully removed Z87.821
　　risk factors NEC Z91.89
　　self-harm Z91.5
　　self-poisoning attempt Z91.5
　　sex reassignment Z87.890
　　sleep-wake cycle problem Z72.821
　　specified NEC Z87.898
　　steroid therapy (systemic) Z92.241
　　　inhaled Z92.240
　　stroke without residual deficits Z86.73
　　substance abuse NEC F10-F19
　　sudden cardiac arrest Z86.74
　　sudden cardiac death successfully resuscitated Z86.74
　　suicide attempt Z91.5
　　surgery NEC Z98.890
　　　with uterine scar Z98.891
　　　sex reassignment Z87.890
　　　transplant — *see* Transplant
　　thrombophlebitis Z86.72
　　thrombosis (venous) Z86.718
　　　pulmonary Z86.711
　　tobacco dependence Z87.891
　　transient ischemic attack (TIA) without residual deficits Z86.73
　　trauma (physical) NEC Z87.828
　　　psychological NEC Z91.49
　　　self-harm Z91.5
　　traumatic brain injury Z87.820
　　unhealthy sleep-wake cycle Z72.821
　　unintended awareness under general anesthesia Z92.84
　　urinary calculi Z87.442
　　urinary (recurrent) (tract) infection(s) Z87.440
　　uterine scar from previous surgery Z98.891
　　vaginal dysplasia Z87.411
　　venous thrombosis or embolism Z86.718
　　　pulmonary Z86.711

History — *continued*
　personal (*see also* History, family) — *continued*
　　vulvar dysplasia Z87.412
His-Werner disease A79.0
HIV (*see also* Human, immunodeficiency virus) B20
　laboratory evidence (nonconclusive) R75
　nonconclusive test (in infants) R75
　positive, seropositive Z21
Hives (bold) — *see* Urticaria
Hoarseness R49.0
Hobo Z59.0
Hodgkin disease — *see* Lymphoma, Hodgkin
Hodgson's disease I71.2
　ruptured I71.1
Hoffa-Kastert disease E88.89
Hoffa's disease E88.89
Hoffmann-Bouveret syndrome I47.9
Hoffmann's syndrome E03.9 [G73.7]
Hole (round)
　macula H35.34- ☑
　retina (without detachment) — *see* Break, retina, round hole
　　with detachment — *see* Detachment, retina, with retinal, break
Holiday relief care Z75.5
Hollenhorst's plaque — *see* Occlusion, artery, retina
Hollow foot (congenital) Q66.7
　acquired — *see* Deformity, limb, foot, specified NEC
Holoprosencephaly Q04.2
Holt-Oram syndrome Q87.2
Homelessness Z59.0
Homesickness — *see* Disorder, adjustment
Homocystinemia, homocystinuria E72.11
Homogentisate 1,2-dioxygenase deficiency E70.29
Homologous serum hepatitis (prophylactic) (therapeutic) — *see* Hepatitis, viral, type B
Honeycomb lung J98.4
　congenital Q33.0
Hooded
　clitoris Q52.6
　penis Q55.69
Hookworm (anemia) (disease) (infection) (infestation) B76.9
　specified NEC B76.8
Hordeolum (eyelid) (externum) (recurrent) H00.019
　internum H00.029
　　left H00.026
　　　lower H00.025
　　　upper H00.024
　　right H00.023
　　　lower H00.022
　　　upper H00.021
　left H00.016
　　lower H00.015
　　upper H00.014
　right H00.013
　　lower H00.012
　　upper H00.011
Horn
　cutaneous L85.8
　nail L60.2
　　congenital Q84.6
Horner (-Claude Bernard) **syndrome** G90.2
　traumatic — *see* Injury, nerve, cervical sympathetic
Horseshoe kidney (congenital) Q63.1
Horton's headache or neuralgia G44.099
　intractable G44.091
　not intractable G44.099
Hospital hopper syndrome — *see* Disorder, factitious
Hospitalism in children — *see* Disorder, adjustment
Hostility R45.5
　towards child Z62.3
Hot flashes
　menopausal N95.1
Hourglass (contracture) (*see also* Contraction, hourglass)
　stomach K31.89
　　congenital Q40.2
　　stricture K31.2
Household, housing circumstance affecting care Z59.9
　specified NEC Z59.8
Housemaid's knee — *see* Bursitis, prepatellar
Hudson (-Stähli) **line** (cornea) — *see* Pigmentation, cornea, anterior
Human
　bite (open wound) (*see also* Bite)
　　intact skin surface — *see* Bite, superficial

Human — continued
  herpesvirus — see Herpes
  immunodeficiency virus (HIV) disease (infection) B20
    asymptomatic status Z21
    contact Z20.6
    counseling Z71.7
    dementia B20 [F02.80]
      with behavioral disturbance B20 [F02.81]
    exposure to Z20.6
    laboratory evidence R75
    type-2 (HIV 2) as cause of disease classified else-
      where B97.35
  papillomavirus (HPV)
    DNA test positive
      high risk
        cervix R87.810
        vagina R87.811
      low risk
        cervix R87.820
        vagina R87.821
    screening for Z11.51
  T-cell lymphotropic virus
    type-1 (HTLV-I) infection B33.3
      as cause of disease classified elsewhere B97.33
      carrier Z22.6
    type-2 (HTLV-II) as cause of disease classified else-
      where B97.34
Humidifier lung or pneumonitis J67.7
Humiliation (experience) **in childhood** Z62.898
Humpback (acquired) — see Kyphosis
Hunchback (acquired) — see Kyphosis
Hunger T73.0- ☑
  air, psychogenic F45.8
Hungry bone syndrome E83.81
Hunner's ulcer — see Cystitis, chronic, interstitial
Hunter's
  glossitis D51.0
  syndrome E76.1
Huntington's disease or chorea G10
  with dementia G10 [F02.80]
    with behavioral disturbance G10 [F02.81]
Hunt's
  disease or syndrome (herpetic geniculate ganglionitis)
    B02.21
  dyssynergia cerebellaris myoclonica G11.1
  neuralgia B02.21
Hurler (-Scheie) **disease or syndrome** E76.02
Hurst's disease G36.1
Hurthle cell
  adenocarcinoma C73
  adenoma D34
  carcinoma C73
  tumor D34
Hutchinson-Boeck disease or syndrome — see Sarcoidosis
Hutchinson-Gilford disease or syndrome E34.8
Hutchinson's
  disease, meaning
    angioma serpiginosum L81.7
    pompholyx (cheiropompholyx) L30.1
    prurigo estivalis L56.4
    summer eruption or summer prurigo L56.4
  melanotic freckle — see Melanoma, in situ
    malignant melanoma in — see Melanoma
  teeth or incisors (congenital syphilis) A50.52
  triad (congenital syphilis) A50.53
Hyalin plaque, sclera, senile H15.89
Hyaline membrane (disease) (lung) (pulmonary) (newborn) P22.0
Hyalinosis
  cutis (et mucosae) E78.89
  focal and segmental (glomerular) (see also N00-N07
    with fourth character .1) N05.1
Hyalitis, hyalosis, asteroid (see also Deposit, crystalline)
  syphilitic (late) A52.71
Hydatid
  cyst or tumor — see Echinococcus
  mole — see Hydatidiform mole
  Morgagni
    female Q50.5
    male (epididymal) Q55.4
      testicular Q55.29
Hydatidiform mole (benign) (complicating pregnancy)
  (delivered) (undelivered) O01.9
  classical O01.0
  complete O01.0
  incomplete O01.1
  invasive D39.2

Hydatidiform mole — continued
  malignant D39.2
  partial O01.1
Hydatidosis — see Echinococcus
Hydradenitis (axillaris) (suppurative) L73.2
Hydradenoma — see Hidradenoma
Hydramnios O40.- ☑
Hydrancephaly, hydranencephaly Q04.3
  with spina bifida — see Spina bifida, with hydro-
    cephalus
Hydrargyrism NEC — see Poisoning, mercury
Hydrarthrosis (see also Effusion, joint)
  gonococcal A54.42
  intermittent M12.40
    ankle M12.47- ☑
    elbow M12.42- ☑
    foot joint M12.47- ☑
    hand joint M12.44- ☑
    hip M12.45- ☑
    knee M12.46- ☑
    multiple site M12.49
    shoulder M12.41- ☑
    specified joint NEC M12.48
    wrist M12.43- ☑
  of yaws (early) (late) (see also subcategory M14.8-)
    A66.6
  syphilitic (late) A52.77
    congenital A50.55 [M12.80]
Hydremia D64.89
Hydrencephalocele (congenital) — see Encephalocele
Hydrencephalomeningocele (congenital) — see Encephalocele
Hydroa R23.8
  aestivale L56.4
  vacciniforme L56.4
Hydroadenitis (axillaris) (suppurative) L73.2
Hydrocalycosis — see Hydronephrosis
Hydrocele (spermatic cord) (testis) (tunica vaginalis)
  N43.3
  canal of Nuck N94.89
  communicating N43.2
    congenital P83.5
  congenital P83.5
  encysted N43.0
  female NEC N94.89
  infected N43.1
  newborn P83.5
  round ligament N94.89
  specified NEC N43.2
  spinalis — see Spina bifida
  vulva N90.89
Hydrocephalus (acquired) (external) (internal) (malignant) (recurrent) G91.9
  aqueduct Sylvius stricture Q03.0
  causing disproportion O33.6 ☑
    with obstructed labor O66.3
  communicating G91.0
  congenital (external) (internal) Q03.9
    with spina bifida Q05.4
      cervical Q05.0
      dorsal Q05.1
      lumbar Q05.2
      lumbosacral Q05.2
      sacral Q05.3
      thoracic Q05.1
      thoracolumbar Q05.1
    specified NEC Q03.8
  due to toxoplasmosis (congenital) P37.1
  foramen Magendie block (acquired) G91.1
    congenital (see also Hydrocephalus, congenital)
      Q03.1
  in (due to)
    infectious disease NEC B89 [G91.4]
    neoplastic disease NEC (see also Neoplasm) G91.4
    parasitic disease B89 [G91.4]
  newborn Q03.9
    with spina bifida — see Spina bifida, with hydro-
      cephalus
  noncommunicating G91.1
  normal pressure G91.2
    secondary G91.0
  obstructive G91.1
  otitic G93.2
  post-traumatic NEC G91.3
  secondary G91.4
    post-traumatic G91.3
  specified NEC G91.8
  syphilitic, congenital A50.49

Hydrocolpos (congenital) N89.8
Hydrocystoma — see Neoplasm, skin, benign
Hydroencephalocele (congenital) — see Encephalocele
Hydroencephalomeningocele (congenital) — see En-
  cephalocele
Hydrohematopneumothorax — see Hemothorax
Hydromeningitis — see Meningitis
Hydromeningocele (spinal) (see also Spina bifida)
  cranial — see Encephalocele
Hydrometra N85.8
Hydrometrocolpos N89.8
Hydromicrocephaly Q02
Hydromphalos (since birth) Q45.8
Hydromyelia Q06.4
Hydromyelocele — see Spina bifida
Hydronephrosis (atrophic) (early) (functionless) (inter-
  mittent) (primary) (secondary) NEC N13.30
  with
    infection N13.6
    obstruction (by) (of)
      renal calculus N13.2
        with infection N13.6
      ureteral NEC N13.1
        with infection N13.6
        calculus N13.2
          with infection N13.6
      ureteropelvic junction (congenital) Q62.11
        acquired N13.0
          with infection N13.6
      ureteral stricture NEC N13.1
        with infection N13.6
  congenital Q62.0
  due to acquired occlusion of ureteropelvic junction
    N13.0
  specified type NEC N13.39
  tuberculous A18.11
Hydropericarditis — see Pericarditis
Hydropericardium — see Pericarditis
Hydroperitoneum R18.8
Hydrophobia — see Rabies
Hydrophthalmos Q15.0
Hydropneumohemothorax — see Hemothorax
Hydropneumopericarditis — see Pericarditis
Hydropneumopericardium — see Pericarditis
Hydropneumothorax J94.8
  traumatic — see Injury, intrathoracic, lung
  tuberculous NEC A15.6
Hydrops R60.9
  abdominis R18.8
  articulorum intermittens — see Hydrarthrosis, inter-
    mittent
  cardiac — see Failure, heart, congestive
  causing obstructed labor (mother) O66.3
  endolymphatic H81.0- ☑
  fetal — see Pregnancy, complicated by, hydrops, fetalis
  fetalis P83.2
    due to
      ABO isoimmunization P56.0
      alpha thalassemia D56.0
      hemolytic disease P56.90
        specified NEC P56.99
      isoimmunization (ABO) (Rh) P56.0
      other specified nonhemolytic disease NEC P83.2
      Rh incompatibility P56.0
    during pregnancy — see Pregnancy, complicated
      by, hydrops, fetalis
  gallbladder K82.1
  joint — see Effusion, joint
  labyrinth H81.0- ☑
  newborn (idiopathic) P83.2
    due to
      ABO isoimmunization P56.0
      alpha thalassemia D56.0
      hemolytic disease P56.90
        specified NEC P56.99
      isoimmunization (ABO) (Rh) P56.0
      Rh incompatibility P56.0
  nutritional — see Malnutrition, severe
  pericardium — see Pericarditis
  pleura — see Hydrothorax
  spermatic cord — see Hydrocele
Hydropyonephrosis N13.6
Hydrorachis Q06.4
Hydrorrhea (nasal) J34.89
  pregnancy — see Rupture, membranes, premature
Hydrosadenitis (axillaris) (suppurative) L73.2
Hydrosalpinx (fallopian tube) (follicularis) N70.11

Hydrothorax (double) (pleura) J94.8
  chylous (nonfilarial) I89.8
    filarial (see also Infestation, filarial) B74.9 [J91.8]
  traumatic — see Injury, intrathoracic
  tuberculous NEC (non primary) A15.6
Hydroureter (see also Hydronephrosis) N13.4
  with infection N13.6
  congenital Q62.39
Hydroureteronephrosis — see Hydronephrosis
Hydrourethra N36.8
Hydroxykynureninuria E70.8
Hydroxylysinemia E72.3
Hydroxyprolinemia E72.59
Hygiene, sleep
  abuse Z72.821
  inadequate Z72.821
  poor Z72.821
Hygroma (congenital) (cystic) D18.1
  praepatellare, prepatellar — see Bursitis, prepatellar
  subdural I62.03
Hymen — see condition
Hymenolepis, hymenolepiasis (diminuta) (infection)
    (infestation) (nana) B71.0
Hypalgesia R20.8
Hyperacidity (gastric) K31.89
  psychogenic F45.8
Hyperactive, hyperactivity F90.9
  basal cell, uterine cervix — see Dysplasia, cervix
  bowel sounds R19.12
  cervix epithelial (basal) — see Dysplasia, cervix
  child F90.9
    attention deficit — see Disorder, attention-deficit
        hyperactivity
  detrusor muscle N32.81
  gastrointestinal K31.89
    psychogenic F45.8
  nasal mucous membrane J34.3
  stomach K31.89
  thyroid (gland) — see Hyperthyroidism
Hyperacusis H93.23- ☑
Hyperadrenalism E27.5
Hyperadrenocorticism E24.9
  congenital E25.0
  iatrogenic E24.2
    correct substance properly administered — see
        Table of Drugs and Chemicals, by drug, ad-
        verse effect
    overdose or wrong substance given or taken —
        see Table of Drugs and Chemicals, by drug,
        poisoning
  not associated with Cushing's syndrome E27.0
  pituitary-dependent E24.0
Hyperaldosteronism E26.9
  familial (type I) E26.02
  glucocorticoid-remediable E26.02
  primary (due to (bilateral) adrenal hyperplasia) E26.09
  primary NEC E26.09
  secondary E26.1
  specified NEC E26.89
Hyperalgesia R20.8
Hyperalimentation R63.2
  carotene, carotin E67.1
  specified NEC E67.8
  vitamin
    A E67.0
    D E67.3
Hyperaminoaciduria
  arginine E72.21
  cystine E72.01
  lysine E72.3
  ornithine E72.4
Hyperammonemia (congenital) E72.20
Hyperazotemia — see Uremia
Hyperbetalipoproteinemia (familial) E78.00
  with prebetalipoproteinemia E78.2
Hyperbilirubinemia
  constitutional E80.6
  familial conjugated E80.6
  neonatal (transient) — see Jaundice, newborn
Hypercalcemia, hypocalciuric, familial E83.52
Hypercalciuria, idiopathic E83.52
Hypercapnia R06.89
  newborn P84
Hypercarotenemia, hypercarotinemia (dietary) E67.1
Hypercementosis K03.4
Hyperchloremia E87.8
Hyperchlorhydria K31.89

Hyperchlorhydria — continued
  neurotic F45.8
  psychogenic F45.8
Hypercholesterinemia — see Hypercholesterolemia
Hypercholesterolemia (essential) (primary) (pure)
    E78.00
  with hyperglyceridemia, endogenous E78.2
  dietary counseling and surveillance Z71.3
  familial E78.01
  hereditary E78.01
Hyperchylia gastrica, psychogenic F45.8
Hyperchylomicronemia (familial) (primary) E78.3
  with hyperbetalipoproteinemia E78.3
Hypercoagulable (state) D68.59
  activated protein C resistance D68.51
  antithrombin (III) deficiency D68.59
  factor V Leiden mutation D68.51
  primary NEC D68.59
  protein C deficiency D68.59
  protein S deficiency D68.59
  prothrombin gene mutation D68.52
  secondary D68.69
  specified NEC D68.69
Hypercoagulation (state) D68.59
Hypercorticalism, pituitary-dependent E24.0
Hypercorticosolism — see Cushing's, syndrome
Hypercorticosteronism E24.2
  correct substance properly administered — see Table
      of Drugs and Chemicals, by drug, adverse effect
  overdose or wrong substance given or taken — see
      Table of Drugs and Chemicals, by drug, poison-
      ing
Hypercortisonism E24.2
  correct substance properly administered — see Table
      of Drugs and Chemicals, by drug, adverse effect
  overdose or wrong substance given or taken — see
      Table of Drugs and Chemicals, by drug, poison-
      ing
Hyperekplexia Q89.8
Hyperelectrolytemia E87.8
Hyperemesis R11.10
  with nausea R11.2
  gravidarum (mild) O21.0
    with
      carbohydrate depletion O21.1
      dehydration O21.1
      electrolyte imbalance O21.1
      metabolic disturbance O21.1
    severe (with metabolic disturbance) O21.1
  projectile R11.12
  psychogenic F45.8
Hyperemia (acute) (passive) R68.89
  anal mucosa K62.89
  bladder N32.89
  cerebral I67.89
  conjunctiva H11.43- ☑
  ear internal, acute — see subcategory H83.0 ☑
  enteric K59.8
  eye — see Hyperemia, conjunctiva
  eyelid (active) (passive) — see Disorder, eyelid, speci-
      fied type NEC
  intestine K59.8
  iris — see Disorder, iris, vascular
  kidney N28.89
  labyrinth — see subcategory H83.0 ☑
  liver (active) K76.89
  lung (passive) — see Edema, lung
  pulmonary (passive) — see Edema, lung
  renal N28.89
  retina H35.89
  stomach K31.89
Hyperesthesia (body surface) R20.3
  larynx (reflex) J38.7
    hysterical F44.89
  pharynx (reflex) J39.2
    hysterical F44.89
Hyperestrogenism (drug-induced) (iatrogenic) E28.0
Hyperexplexia Q89.8
Hyperfibrinolysis — see Fibrinolysis
Hyperfructosemia E74.19
Hyperfunction
  adrenal cortex, not associated with Cushing's syn-
      drome E27.0
  medulla E27.5
    adrenomedullary E27.5
  virilism E25.9
    congenital E25.0
  ovarian E28.8

Hyperfunction — continued
  pancreas K86.89
  parathyroid (gland) E21.3
  pituitary (gland) (anterior) E22.9
    specified NEC E22.8
  polyglandular E31.1
  testicular E29.0
Hypergammaglobulinemia D89.2
  polyclonal D89.0
  Waldenström D89.0
Hypergastrinemia E16.4
Hyperglobulinemia R77.1
Hyperglycemia, hyperglycemic (transient) R73.9
  coma — see Diabetes, by type, with coma
  postpancreatectomy E89.1
Hyperglyceridemia (endogenous) (essential) (familial)
    (hereditary) (pure) E78.1
  mixed E78.3
Hyperglycinemia (non-ketotic) E72.51
Hypergonadism
  ovarian E28.8
  testicular (primary) (infantile) E29.0
Hyperheparinemia D68.32
Hyperhidrosis, hyperidrosis R61
  focal
    primary L74.519
      axilla L74.510
      face L74.511
      palms L74.512
      soles L74.513
    secondary L74.52
  generalized R61
  localized
    primary L74.519
      axilla L74.510
      face L74.511
      palms L74.512
      soles L74.513
    secondary L74.52
  psychogenic F45.8
  secondary R61
    focal L74.52
Hyperhistidinemia E70.41
Hyperhomocysteinemia E72.11
Hyperhydroxyprolinemia E72.59
Hyperinsulinism (functional) E16.1
  with
    coma (hypoglycemic) E15
    encephalopathy E16.1 [G94]
  ectopic E16.1
  therapeutic misadventure (from administration of in-
      sulin) — see subcategory T38.3 ☑
Hyperkalemia E87.5
Hyperkeratosis (see also Keratosis) L85.9
  cervix N88.0
  due to yaws (early) (late) (palmar or plantar) A66.3
  follicularis Q82.8
    penetrans (in cutem) L87.0
  palmoplantaris climacterica L85.1
  pinta A67.1
  senile (with pruritus) L57.0
  universalis congenita Q80.8
  vocal cord J38.3
  vulva N90.4
Hyperkinesia, hyperkinetic (disease) (reaction) (syn-
    drome) (childhood) (adolescence) (see also Disorder,
    attention-deficit hyperactivity)
  heart I51.89
Hyperleucine-isoleucinemia E71.19
Hyperlipemia, hyperlipidemia E78.5
  combined E78.2
    familial E78.4
  group
    A E78.00
    B E78.1
    C E78.2
    D E78.3
  mixed E78.2
  specified NEC E78.4
Hyperlipidosis E75.6
  hereditary NEC E75.5
Hyperlipoproteinemia E78.5
  Fredrickson's type
    I E78.3
    IIa E78.00
    IIb E78.2
    III E78.2
    IV E78.1

Index

Hydrothorax — Hyperlipoproteinemia

Hyperlipoproteinemia — *continued*
  Fredrickson's type — *continued*
    V E78.3
    low-density-lipoprotein-type (LDL) E78.00
    very-low-density-lipoprotein-type (VLDL) E78.1
Hyperlucent lung, unilateral J43.0
Hyperlysinemia E72.3
Hypermagnesemia E83.41
  neonatal P71.8
Hypermenorrhea N92.0
Hypermethioninemia E72.19
Hypermetropia (congenital) H52.0- ☑
Hypermobility, hypermotility
  cecum — *see* Syndrome, irritable bowel
  coccyx — *see* subcategory M53.2 ☑
  colon — *see* Syndrome, irritable bowel
    psychogenic F45.8
  ileum K58.9
  intestine (*see also* Syndrome, irritable bowel) K58.9
    psychogenic F45.8
  meniscus (knee) — *see* Derangement, knee, meniscus
  scapula — *see* Instability, joint, shoulder
  stomach K31.89
    psychogenic F45.8
  syndrome M35.7
  urethra N36.41
    with intrinsic sphincter deficiency N36.43
Hypernasality R49.21
Hypernatremia E87.0
Hypernephroma C64.- ☑
Hyperopia — *see* Hypermetropia
Hyperorexia nervosa F50.2
Hyperornithinemia E72.4
Hyperosmia R43.1
Hyperosmolality E87.0
Hyperostosis (monomelic) (*see also* Disorder, bone, density and structure, specified NEC)
  ankylosing (spine) M48.10
    cervical region M48.12
    cervicothoracic region M48.13
    lumbar region M48.16
    lumbosacral region M48.17
    multiple sites M48.19
    occipito-atlanto-axial region M48.11
    sacrococcygeal region M48.18
    thoracic region M48.14
    thoracolumbar region M48.15
  cortical (skull) M85.2
    infantile M89.8X- ☑
  frontal, internal of skull M85.2
  interna frontalis M85.2
  skeletal, diffuse idiopathic — *see* Hyperostosis, ankylosing
  skull M85.2
    congenital Q75.8
  vertebral, ankylosing — *see* Hyperostosis, ankylosing
Hyperovarism E28.8
Hyperoxaluria (primary) E72.53
Hyperparathyroidism E21.3
  primary E21.0
  secondary (renal) N25.81
    non-renal E21.1
  specified NEC E21.2
  tertiary E21.2
Hyperpathia R20.8
Hyperperistalsis R19.2
  psychogenic F45.8
Hyperpermeability, capillary I78.8
Hyperphagia R63.2
Hyperphenylalaninemia NEC E70.1
Hyperphoria (alternating) H50.53
Hyperphosphatemia E83.39
Hyperpiesis, hyperpiesia — *see* Hypertension
Hyperpigmentation (*see also* Pigmentation)
  melanin NEC L81.4
  postinflammatory L81.0
Hyperpinealism E34.8
Hyperpituitarism E22.9
Hyperplasia, hyperplastic
  adenoids J35.2
  adrenal (capsule) (cortex) (gland) E27.8
    with
      sexual precocity (male) E25.9
        congenital E25.0
      virilism, adrenal E25.9
        congenital E25.0
      virilization (female) E25.9

Hyperplasia, hyperplastic — *continued*
  adrenal — *continued*
    with — *continued*
      virilization — *continued*
        congenital E25.0
    congenital E25.0
    salt-losing E25.0
  adrenomedullary E27.5
  angiolymphoid, eosinophilia (ALHE) D18.01
  appendix (lymphoid) K38.0
  artery, fibromuscular I77.3
  bone (*see also* Hypertrophy, bone)
    marrow D75.89
  breast (*see also* Hypertrophy, breast)
    ductal (atypical) N60.9- ☑
  C-cell, thyroid E07.0
  cementation (tooth) (teeth) K03.4
  cervical gland R59.0
  cervix (uteri) (basal cell) (endometrium) (polypoid) (*see also* Dysplasia, cervix)
    congenital Q51.828
  clitoris, congenital Q52.6
  denture K06.2
  endocervicitis N72
  endometrium, endometrial (adenomatous) (benign) (cystic) (glandular) (glandular-cystic) (polypoid) N85.00
    with atypia N85.02
    cervix — *see* Dysplasia, cervix
    complex (without atypia) N85.01
    simple (without atypia) N85.01
  epithelial L85.9
    focal, oral, including tongue K13.29
    nipple N62
    skin L85.9
    tongue K13.29
    vaginal wall N89.3
  erythroid D75.89
  fibromuscular of artery (carotid) (renal) I77.3
  genital
    female NEC N94.89
    male N50.89
  gingiva K06.1
  glandularis cystica uteri (interstitialis) (*see also* Hyperplasia, endometrial) N85.00
  gum K06.1
  hymen, congenital Q52.4
  irritative, edentulous (alveolar) K06.2
  jaw M26.09
    alveolar M26.79
    lower M26.03
      alveolar M26.72
    upper M26.01
      alveolar M26.71
  kidney (congenital) Q63.3
  labia N90.69
    epithelial N90.3
  liver (congenital) Q44.7
    nodular, focal K76.89
  lymph gland or node R59.9
  mandible, mandibular M26.03
    alveolar M26.72
    unilateral condylar M27.8
  maxilla, maxillary M26.01
    alveolar M26.71
  myometrium, myometrial N85.2
  neuroendocrine cell, of infancy J84.841
  nose
    lymphoid J34.89
    polypoid J33.9
  oral mucosa (irritative) K13.6
  organ or site, congenital NEC — *see* Anomaly, by site
  ovary N83.8
  palate, papillary (irritative) K13.6
  pancreatic islet cells E16.9
    alpha E16.8
      with excess
        gastrin E16.4
        glucagon E16.3
    beta E16.1
  parathyroid (gland) E21.0
  pharynx (lymphoid) J39.2
  prostate (adenofibromatous) (nodular) N40.0
    with lower urinary tract symptoms (LUTS) N40.1
    without lower urinary tract symptpoms (LUTS) N40.0
  renal artery I77.89
  reticulo-endothelial (cell) D75.89
  salivary gland (any) K11.1

Hyperplasia, hyperplastic — *continued*
  Schimmelbusch's — *see* Mastopathy, cystic
  suprarenal capsule (gland) E27.8
  thymus (gland) (persistent) E32.0
  thyroid (gland) — *see* Goiter
  tonsils (faucial) (infective) (lingual) (lymphoid) J35.1
    with adenoids J35.3
  unilateral condylar M27.8
  uterus, uterine N85.2
    endometrium (glandular) (*see also* Hyperplasia, endometrial) N85.00
  vulva N90.69
    epithelial N90.3
Hyperpnea — *see* Hyperventilation
Hyperpotassemia E87.5
Hyperprebetalipoproteinemia (familial) E78.1
Hyperprolactinemia E22.1
Hyperprolinemia (type I) (type II) E72.59
Hyperproteinemia E88.09
Hyperprothrombinemia, causing coagulation factor deficiency D68.4
Hyperpyrexia R50.9
  heat (effects) T67.0 ☑
  malignant, due to anesthetic T88.3 ☑
  rheumatic — *see* Fever, rheumatic
  unknown origin R50.9
Hyper-reflexia R29.2
Hypersalivation K11.7
Hypersecretion
  ACTH (not associated with Cushing's syndrome) E27.0
    pituitary E24.0
  adrenaline E27.5
  adrenomedullary E27.5
  androgen (testicular) E29.0
    ovarian (drug-induced) (iatrogenic) E28.1
  calcitonin E07.0
  catecholamine E27.5
  corticoadrenal E24.9
  cortisol E24.9
  epinephrine E27.5
  estrogen E28.0
  gastric K31.89
    psychogenic F45.8
  gastrin E16.4
  glucagon E16.3
  hormone(s)
    ACTH (not associated with Cushing's syndrome) E27.0
      pituitary E24.0
    antidiuretic E22.2
    growth E22.0
    intestinal NEC E34.1
    ovarian androgen E28.1
    pituitary E22.9
    testicular E29.0
    thyroid stimulating E05.80
      with thyroid storm E05.81
  insulin — *see* Hyperinsulinism
  lacrimal glands — *see* Epiphora
  medulloadrenal E27.5
  milk O92.6
  ovarian androgens E28.1
  salivary gland (any) K11.7
  thyrocalcitonin E07.0
  upper respiratory J39.8
Hypersegmentation, leukocytic, hereditary D72.0
Hypersensitive, hypersensitiveness, hypersensitivity (*see also* Allergy)
  carotid sinus G90.01
  colon — *see* Irritable, colon
  drug T88.7 ☑
  gastrointestinal K52.29
    immediate K52.29
    psychogenic F45.8
  labyrinth — *see* subcategory H83.2 ☑
  pain R20.8
  pneumonitis — *see* Pneumonitis, allergic
  reaction T78.40 ☑
    upper respiratory tract NEC J39.3
Hypersomnia (organic) G47.10
  due to
    alcohol
      abuse F10.182
      dependence F10.282
      use F10.982
    amphetamines
      abuse F15.182
      dependence F15.282

☑ Additional Character Required — Refer to the Tabular List for Character Selection   Subterms under main terms may continue to next column or page

Hypersomnia — *continued*
 due to — *continued*
  amphetamines — *continued*
   use F15.982
  caffeine
   abuse F15.182
   dependence F15.282
   use F15.982
  cocaine
   abuse F14.182
   dependence F14.282
   use F14.982
  drug NEC
   abuse F19.182
   dependence F19.282
   use F19.982
  medical condition G47.14
  mental disorder F51.13
  opioid
   abuse F11.182
   dependence F11.282
   use F11.982
  psychoactive substance NEC
   abuse F19.182
   dependence F19.282
   use F19.982
  sedative, hypnotic, or anxiolytic
   abuse F13.182
   dependence F13.282
   use F13.982
  stimulant NEC
   abuse F15.182
   dependence F15.282
   use F15.982
 idiopathic G47.11
  with long sleep time G47.11
  without long sleep time G47.12
 menstrual related G47.13
 nonorganic origin F51.11
  specified NEC F51.19
 not due to a substance or known physiological condition F51.11
  specified NEC F51.19
 primary F51.11
 recurrent G47.13
 specified NEC G47.19
Hypersplenia, hypersplenism D73.1
Hyperstimulation, ovaries (associated with induced ovulation) N98.1
Hypersusceptibility — *see* Allergy
Hypertelorism (ocular) (orbital) Q75.2
Hypertension, hypertensive (accelerated) (benign) (essential) (idiopathic) (malignant) (systemic) I10
 with
  heart failure (congestive) I11.0
  heart involvement (conditions in I50.-, I51.4- I51.9 due to hypertension) — *see* Hypertension, heart
  kidney involvement — *see* Hypertension, kidney
 benign, intracranial G93.2
 borderline R03.0
 cardiorenal (disease) I13.10
  with heart failure I13.0
   with stage 1 through stage 4 chronic kidney disease I13.0
   with stage 5 or end stage renal disease I13.2
  without heart failure I13.10
   with stage 1 through stage 4 chronic kidney disease I13.10
   with stage 5 or end stage renal disease I13.11
 cardiovascular
  disease (arteriosclerotic) (sclerotic) — *see* Hypertension, heart
  renal (disease) — *see* Hypertension, cardiorenal
 chronic venous — *see* Hypertension, venous (chronic)
 complicating
  childbirth (labor) O16.4
   pre-existing O10.92
    with
     heart disease O10.12
      with renal disease O10.32
     pre-eclampsia O11.4
     renal disease O10.22
      with heart disease O10.32
     essential O10.02
    secondary O10.42
  pregnancy O16.- ☑
   with edema (*see also* Pre-eclampsia) O14.9- ☑

Hypertension, hypertensive — *continued*
 complicating — *continued*
  pregnancy — *continued*
   gestational (pregnancy induced) (without proteinuria) O13.- ☑
    with proteinuria O14.9- ☑
     mild pre-eclampsia O14.0- ☑
     moderate pre-eclampsia O14.0- ☑
     severe pre-eclampsia O14.1- ☑
      with hemolysis, elevated liver enzymes and low platelet count (HELLP) O14.2- ☑
   pre-existing O10.91- ☑
    with
     heart disease O10.11- ☑
      with renal disease O10.31- ☑
     pre-eclampsia — *see* category O11
     renal disease O10.21- ☑
      with heart disease O10.31- ☑
    essential O10.01- ☑
    secondary O10.41- ☑
   transient O13- ☑
  puerperium, pre-existing O16.5
   pre-existing
    with
     heart disease O10.13
      with renal disease O10.33
     pre-eclampsia O11.5
     renal disease O10.23
      with heart disease O10.33
    essential O10.03
   pregnancy-induced O13.9
   secondary O10.43
 crisis I16.9
 due to
  endocrine disorders I15.2
  pheochromocytoma I15.2
  renal disorders NEC I15.1
   arterial I15.0
  renovascular disorders I15.0
  specified disease NEC I15.8
 emergency I16.1
 encephalopathy I67.4
 gestational (without significant proteinuria) (pregnancy-induced) (transient) O13.- ☑
  with significant proteinuria — *see* Pre-eclampsia
  complicating
   delivery O13.4
   puerperium O13.5
 Goldblatt's I70.1
 heart (disease) (conditions in I51.4-I51.9 due to hypertension) I11.9
  with
   heart failure (congestive) I11.0
   kidney disease (chronic) — *see* Hypertension, cardiorenal
 intracranial (benign) G93.2
 kidney I12.9
  with
   heart disease — *see* Hypertension, cardiorenal
   stage 1 through stage 4 chronic kidney disease I12.9
   stage 5 chronic kidney disease (CKD) or end stage renal disease (ESRD) I12.0
 lesser circulation I27.0
 maternal O16- ☑
 newborn P29.2
  pulmonary (persistent) P29.30
 ocular H40.05- ☑
 pancreatic duct — *code to* underlying condition
  with chronic pancreatitis K86.1
 portal (due to chronic liver disease) (idiopathic) K76.6
  gastropathy K31.89
  in (due to) schistosomiasis (bilharziasis) B65.9 [K77]
 postoperative I97.3
 psychogenic F45.8
 pulmonary I27.20
  with
   cor pulmonale (chronic) I27.29
    acute I26.09
   right heart ventricular strain/failure I27.29
    acute I26.09
   right to left shunt related to congenital heart disease I27.83
   unclear multifactorial mechanisms I27.29
  arterial (associated) (drug-induced) (toxin-induced) I27.21
  chronic thromboembolic I27.24

Hypertension, hypertensive — *continued*
 pulmonary — *continued*
  due to
   hematologic disorders I27.29
   left heart disease I27.22
   lung diseases and hypoxia I27.23
   metabolic disorders I27.29
   specified systemic disorders I27.29
  group 1 (associated) (drug-induced) (toxin-induced) I27.21
  group 2 I27.22
  group 3 I27.23
  group 4 I27.24
  group 5 I27.29
  of newborn (persistent) P29.30
  primary (idiopathic) I27.0
  secondary
   arterial I27.21
   specified NEC I27.29
 renal — *see* Hypertension, kidney
 renovascular I15.0
 secondary NEC I15.9
  due to
   endocrine disorders I15.2
   pheochromocytoma I15.2
   renal disorders NEC I15.1
    arterial I15.0
   renovascular disorders I15.0
  specified NEC I15.8
 transient, of pregnancy O13- ☑
 urgency I16.0
 venous (chronic)
  due to
   deep vein thrombosis — *see* Syndrome, postthrombotic
   idiopathic I87.309
    with
     inflammation I87.32- ☑
      with ulcer I87.33- ☑
     specified complication NEC I87.39- ☑
     ulcer I87.31- ☑
      with inflammation I87.33- ☑
    asymptomatic I87.30- ☑
Hypertensive urgency — *see* Hypertension
Hyperthecosis ovary E28.8
Hyperthermia (of unknown origin) (*see also* Hyperpyrexia)
 malignant, due to anesthesia T88.3 ☑
 newborn P81.9
  environmental P81.0
Hyperthyroid (recurrent) — *see* Hyperthyroidism
Hyperthyroidism (latent) (pre-adult) (recurrent) E05.90
 with
  goiter (diffuse) E05.00
   with thyroid storm E05.01
   nodular (multinodular) E05.20
    with thyroid storm E05.21
    uninodular E05.10
     with thyroid storm E05.11
  storm E05.91
 due to ectopic thyroid tissue E05.30
  with thyroid storm E05.31
 neonatal, transitory P72.1
 specified NEC E05.80
  with thyroid storm E05.81
Hypertony, hypertonia, hypertonicity
 bladder N31.8
 congenital P94.1
 stomach K31.89
  psychogenic F45.8
 uterus, uterine (contractions) (complicating delivery) O62.4
Hypertrichosis L68.9
 congenital Q84.2
 eyelid H02.869
  left H02.866
   lower H02.865
   upper H02.864
  right H02.863
   lower H02.862
   upper H02.861
 lanuginosa Q84.2
  acquired L68.1
 localized L68.2
 specified NEC L68.8
Hypertriglyceridemia, essential E78.1

Hypertrophy, hypertrophic

adenofibromatous, prostate — *see* Enlargement, enlarged, prostate
adenoids (infective) J35.2
  with tonsils J35.3
adrenal cortex E27.8
alveolar process or ridge — *see* Anomaly, alveolar
anal papillae K62.89
artery I77.89
  congenital NEC Q27.8
    digestive system Q27.8
    lower limb Q27.8
    specified site NEC Q27.8
    upper limb Q27.8
auricular — *see* Hypertrophy, cardiac
Bartholin's gland N75.8
bile duct (common) (hepatic) K83.8
bladder (sphincter) (trigone) N32.89
bone M89.30
  carpus M89.34- ☑
  clavicle M89.31- ☑
  femur M89.35- ☑
  fibula M89.36- ☑
  finger M89.34- ☑
  humerus M89.32- ☑
  ilium M89.359
  ischium M89.359
  metacarpus M89.34- ☑
  metatarsus M89.37- ☑
  multiple sites M89.39
  neck M89.38
  radius M89.33- ☑
  rib M89.38
  scapula M89.31- ☑
  skull M89.38
  tarsus M89.37- ☑
  tibia M89.36- ☑
  toe M89.37- ☑
  ulna M89.33- ☑
  vertebra M89.38
brain G93.89
breast N62
  cystic — *see* Mastopathy, cystic
  newborn P83.4
  pubertal, massive N62
  puerperal, postpartum — *see* Disorder, breast, specified type NEC
  senile (parenchymatous) N62
cardiac (chronic) (idiopathic) I51.7
  with rheumatic fever (conditions in I00)
    active I01.8
    inactive or quiescent (with chorea) I09.89
  congenital NEC Q24.8
  fatty — *see* Degeneration, myocardial
  hypertensive — *see* Hypertension, heart
  rheumatic (with chorea) I09.89
    active or acute I01.8
      with chorea I02.0
  valve — *see* Endocarditis
cartilage — *see* Disorder, cartilage, specified type NEC
cecum — *see* Megacolon
cervix (uteri) N88.8
  congenital Q51.828
  elongation N88.4
clitoris (cirrhotic) N90.89
  congenital Q52.6
colon (*see also* Megacolon)
  congenital Q43.2
conjunctiva, lymphoid H11.89
corpora cavernosa N48.89
cystic duct K82.8
duodenum K31.89
endometrium (glandular) (*see also* Hyperplasia, endometrial) N85.00
  cervix N88.8
epididymis N50.89
esophageal hiatus (congenital) Q79.1
  with hernia — *see* Hernia, hiatal
eyelid — *see* Disorder, eyelid, specified type NEC
fat pad E65
  knee (infrapatellar) (popliteal) (prepatellar) (retropatellar) M79.4
foot (congenital) Q74.2
frenulum, frenum (tongue) K14.8
  lip K13.0
gallbladder K82.8
gastric mucosa K29.60
  with bleeding K29.61

Hypertrophy, hypertrophic — continued

gland, glandular R59.9
  generalized R59.1
  localized R59.0
gum (mucous membrane) K06.1
heart (idiopathic) (*see also* Hypertrophy, cardiac)
  valve (*see also* Endocarditis) I38
hemifacial Q67.4
hepatic — *see* Hypertrophy, liver
hiatus (esophageal) Q79.1
hilus gland R59.0
hymen, congenital Q52.4
ileum K63.89
intestine NEC K63.89
jejunum K63.89
kidney (compensatory) N28.81
  congenital Q63.3
labium (majus) (minus) N90.60
ligament — *see* Disorder, ligament
lingual tonsil (infective) J35.1
  with adenoids J35.3
lip K13.0
  congenital Q18.6
liver R16.0
  acute K76.89
  cirrhotic — *see* Cirrhosis, liver
  congenital Q44.7
  fatty — *see* Fatty, liver
lymph, lymphatic gland R59.9
  generalized R59.1
  localized R59.0
  tuberculous — *see* Tuberculosis, lymph gland
mammary gland — *see* Hypertrophy, breast
Meckel's diverticulum (congenital) Q43.0
  malignant — *see* Table of Neoplasms, small intestine, malignant
median bar — *see* Hyperplasia, prostate
meibomian gland — *see* Chalazion
meniscus, knee, congenital Q74.1
metatarsal head — *see* Hypertrophy, bone, metatarsus
metatarsus — *see* Hypertrophy, bone, metatarsus
mucous membrane
  alveolar ridge K06.2
  gum K06.1
  nose (turbinate) J34.3
muscle M62.89
muscular coat, artery I77.89
myocardium (*see also* Hypertrophy, cardiac)
  idiopathic I42.2
myometrium N85.2
nail L60.2
  congenital Q84.5
nasal J34.89
  alae J34.89
  bone J34.89
  cartilage J34.89
  mucous membrane (septum) J34.3
  sinus J34.89
  turbinate J34.3
nasopharynx, lymphoid (infectional) (tissue) (wall) J35.2
nipple N62
organ or site, congenital NEC — *see* Anomaly, by site
ovary N83.8
palate (hard) M27.8
  soft K13.79
pancreas, congenital Q45.3
parathyroid (gland) E21.0
parotid gland K11.1
penis N48.89
pharyngeal tonsil J35.2
pharynx J39.2
  lymphoid (infectional) (tissue) (wall) J35.2
pituitary (anterior) (fossa) (gland) E23.6
prepuce (congenital) N47.8
  female N90.89
prostate — *see* Enlargement, enlarged, prostate
  congenital Q55.4
pseudomuscular G71.0
pylorus (adult) (muscle) (sphincter) K31.1
  congenital or infantile Q40.0
rectal, rectum (sphincter) K62.89
rhinitis (turbinate) J31.0
salivary gland (any) K11.1
  congenital Q38.4
scaphoid (tarsal) — *see* Hypertrophy, bone, tarsus
scar L91.0
scrotum N50.89

Hypertrophy, hypertrophic — continued

seminal vesicle N50.89
sigmoid — *see* Megacolon
skin L91.9
  specified NEC L91.8
spermatic cord N50.89
spleen — *see* Splenomegaly
spondylitis — *see* Spondylosis
stomach K31.89
sublingual gland K11.1
submandibular gland K11.1
suprarenal cortex (gland) E27.8
synovial NEC M67.20
  acromioclavicular M67.21- ☑
  ankle M67.27- ☑
  elbow M67.22- ☑
  foot M67.27- ☑
  hand M67.24- ☑
  hip M67.25- ☑
  knee M67.26- ☑
  multiple sites M67.29
  specified site NEC M67.28
  wrist M67.23- ☑
tendon — *see* Disorder, tendon, specified type NEC
testis N44.8
  congenital Q55.29
thymic, thymus (gland) (congenital) E32.0
thyroid (gland) — *see* Goiter
toe (congenital) Q74.2
  acquired (*see also* Deformity, toe, specified NEC)
tongue K14.8
  congenital Q38.2
  papillae (foliate) K14.3
tonsils (faucial) (infective) (lingual) (lymphoid) J35.1
  with adenoids J35.3
tunica vaginalis N50.89
ureter N28.89
urethra N36.8
uterus N85.2
  neck (with elongation) N88.4
  puerperal O90.89
uvula K13.79
vagina N89.8
vas deferens N50.89
vein I87.8
ventricle, ventricular (heart) (*see also* Hypertrophy, cardiac)
  congenital Q24.8
  in tetralogy of Fallot Q21.3
verumontanum N36.8
vocal cord J38.3
vulva N90.60
  stasis (nonfilarial) N90.69

Hypertropia H50.2- ☑
Hypertyrosinemia E70.21
Hyperuricemia (asymptomatic) E79.0
Hypervalinemia E71.19
Hyperventilation (tetany) R06.4
  hysterical F45.8
  psychogenic F45.8
  syndrome F45.8
Hypervitaminosis (dietary) NEC E67.8
  A E67.0
    administered as drug (prolonged intake) — *see* Table of Drugs and Chemicals, vitamins, adverse effect
    overdose or wrong substance given or taken — *see* Table of Drugs and Chemicals, vitamins, poisoning
  B6 E67.2
  D E67.3
    administered as drug (prolonged intake) — *see* Table of Drugs and Chemicals, vitamins, adverse effect
    overdose or wrong substance given or taken — *see* Table of Drugs and Chemicals, vitamins, poisoning
  K E67.8
    administered as drug (prolonged intake) — *see* Table of Drugs and Chemicals, vitamins, adverse effect
    overdose or wrong substance given or taken — *see* Table of Drugs and Chemicals, vitamins, poisoning
Hypervolemia E87.70
  specified NEC E87.79
Hypesthesia R20.1
  cornea — *see* Anesthesia, cornea

☑ **Additional Character Required — Refer to the Tabular List for Character Selection**
▽ **Subterms under main terms may continue to next column or page**

Hyphema H21.0- ☑
  traumatic S05.1- ☑
Hypoacidity, gastric K31.89
  psychogenic F45.8
Hypoadrenalism, hypoadrenia E27.40
  primary E27.1
  tuberculous A18.7
Hypoadrenocorticism E27.40
  pituitary E23.0
  primary E27.1
Hypoalbuminemia E88.09
Hypoaldosteronism E27.40
Hypoalphalipoproteinemia E78.6
Hypobarism T70.29 ☑
Hypobaropathy T70.29 ☑
Hypobetalipoproteinemia (familial) E78.6
Hypocalcemia E83.51
  dietary E58
  neonatal P71.1
    due to cow's milk P71.0
  phosphate-loading (newborn) P71.1
Hypochloremia E87.8
Hypochlorhydria K31.89
  neurotic F45.8
  psychogenic F45.8
Hypochondria, hypochondriac, hypochondriasis
  (reaction) F45.21
  sleep F51.03
Hypochondrogenesis Q77.0
Hypochondroplasia Q77.4
Hypochromasia, blood cells D50.8
Hypodontia — see Anodontia
Hypoeosinophilia D72.89
Hypoesthesia R20.1
Hypofibrinogenemia D68.8
  acquired D65
  congenital (hereditary) D68.2
Hypofunction
  adrenocortical E27.40
    drug-induced E27.3
    postprocedural E89.6
    primary E27.1
  adrenomedullary, postprocedural E89.6
  cerebral R29.818
  corticoadrenal NEC E27.40
  intestinal K59.8
  labyrinth — see subcategory H83.2 ☑
  ovary E28.39
  pituitary (gland) (anterior) E23.0
  testicular E29.1
    postprocedural (postsurgical) (postirradiation) (ia-
      trogenic) E89.5
Hypogalactia O92.4
Hypogammaglobulinemia (see also Agammaglobulinemia) D80.1
  hereditary D80.0
  nonfamilial D80.1
  transient, of infancy D80.7
Hypogenitalism (congenital) — see Hypogonadism
Hypoglossia Q38.3
Hypoglycemia (spontaneous) E16.2
  coma E15
    diabetic — see Diabetes, by type, with hypo-
      glycemia, with coma
  diabetic — see Diabetes, hypoglycemia
  dietary counseling and surveillance Z71.3
  drug-induced E16.0
    with coma (nondiabetic) E15
  due to insulin E16.0
    with coma (nondiabetic) E15
    therapeutic misadventure — see subcategory
      T38.3 ☑
  functional, nonhyperinsulinemic E16.1
  iatrogenic E16.0
    with coma (nondiabetic) E15
  in infant of diabetic mother P70.1
    gestational diabetes P70.0
  infantile E16.1
  leucine-induced E71.19
  neonatal (transitory) P70.4
    iatrogenic P70.3
  reactive (not drug-induced) E16.1
  transitory neonatal P70.4
Hypogonadism
  female E28.39
  hypogonadotropic E23.0
  male E29.1
  ovarian (primary) E28.39

Hypogonadism — continued
  pituitary E23.0
  testicular (primary) E29.1
Hypohidrosis, hypoidrosis L74.4
Hypoinsulinemia, postprocedural E89.1
Hypokalemia E87.6
Hypoleukocytosis — see Agranulocytosis
Hypolipoproteinemia (alpha) (beta) E78.6
Hypomagnesemia E83.42
  neonatal P71.2
Hypomania, hypomanic reaction F30.8
Hypomenorrhea — see Oligomenorrhea
Hypometabolism R63.8
Hypomotility
  gastrointestinal (tract) K31.89
    psychogenic F45.8
  intestine K59.8
    psychogenic F45.8
  stomach K31.89
    psychogenic F45.8
Hyponasality R49.22
Hyponatremia E87.1
Hypo-osmolality E87.1
Hypo-ovarianism, hypo-ovarism E28.39
Hypoparathyroidism E20.9
  familial E20.8
  idiopathic E20.0
  neonatal, transitory P71.4
  postprocedural E89.2
  specified NEC E20.8
Hypoperfusion (in)
  newborn P96.89
Hypopharyngitis — see Laryngopharyngitis
Hypophoria H50.53
Hypophosphatemia, hypophosphatasia (acquired)
  (congenital) (renal) E83.39
  familial E83.31
Hypophyseal, hypophysis (see also condition)
  dwarfism E23.0
  gigantism E22.0
Hypopiesis — see Hypotension
Hypopinealism E34.8
Hypopituitarism (juvenile) E23.0
  drug-induced E23.1
  due to
    hypophysectomy E89.3
    radiotherapy E89.3
  iatrogenic NEC E23.1
  postirradiation E89.3
  postpartum O99.285
  postprocedural E89.3
Hypoplasia, hypoplastic
  adrenal (gland), congenital Q89.1
  alimentary tract, congenital Q45.8
    upper Q40.8
  anus, anal (canal) Q42.3
    with fistula Q42.2
  aorta, aortic Q25.42
    ascending, in hypoplastic left heart syndrome
      Q23.4
    valve Q23.1
      in hypoplastic left heart syndrome Q23.4
  areola, congenital Q83.8
  arm (congenital) — see Defect, reduction, upper limb
  artery (peripheral) Q27.8
    brain (congenital) Q28.3
    coronary Q24.5
    digestive system Q27.8
    lower limb Q27.8
    pulmonary Q25.79
      functional, unilateral J43.0
    retinal (congenital) Q14.1
    specified site NEC Q27.8
    umbilical Q27.0
    upper limb Q27.8
  auditory canal Q17.8
    causing impairment of hearing Q16.9
  biliary duct or passage Q44.5
  bone NOS Q79.9
    face Q75.8
    marrow D61.9
      megakaryocytic D69.49
    skull — see Hypoplasia, skull
  brain Q02
    gyri Q04.3
    part of Q04.3
  breast (areola) N64.82
  bronchus Q32.4

Hypoplasia, hypoplastic — continued
  cardiac Q24.8
  carpus — see Defect, reduction, upper limb, specified
    type NEC
  cartilage hair Q78.8
  cecum Q42.8
  cementum K00.4
  cephalic Q02
  cerebellum Q04.3
  cervix (uteri), congenital Q51.821
  clavicle (congenital) Q74.0
  coccyx Q76.49
  colon Q42.9
    specified NEC Q42.8
  corpus callosum Q04.0
  cricoid cartilage Q31.2
  digestive organ(s) or tract NEC Q45.8
    upper (congenital) Q40.8
  ear (auricle) (lobe) Q17.2
    middle Q16.4
  enamel of teeth (neonatal) (postnatal) (prenatal) K00.4
  endocrine (gland) NEC Q89.2
  endometrium N85.8
  epididymis (congenital) Q55.4
  epiglottis Q31.2
  erythroid, congenital D61.01
  esophagus (congenital) Q39.8
  eustachian tube Q17.8
  eye Q11.2
  eyelid (congenital) Q10.3
  face Q18.8
    bone(s) Q75.8
  femur (congenital) — see Defect, reduction, lower
    limb, specified type NEC
  fibula (congenital) — see Defect, reduction, lower
    limb, specified type NEC
  finger (congenital) — see Defect, reduction, upper
    limb, specified type NEC
  focal dermal Q82.8
  foot — see Defect, reduction, lower limb, specified
    type NEC
  gallbladder Q44.0
  genitalia, genital organ(s)
    female, congenital Q52.8
      external Q52.79
      internal NEC Q52.8
    in adiposogenital dystrophy E23.6
  glottis Q31.2
  hair Q84.2
  hand (congenital) — see Defect, reduction, upper limb,
    specified type NEC
  heart Q24.8
  humerus (congenital) — see Defect, reduction, upper
    limb, specified type NEC
  intestine (small) Q41.9
    large Q42.9
      specified NEC Q42.8
  jaw M26.09
    alveolar M26.79
    lower M26.04
      alveolar M26.74
    upper M26.02
      alveolar M26.73
  kidney(s) Q60.5
    bilateral Q60.4
    unilateral Q60.3
  labium (majus) (minus), congenital Q52.79
  larynx Q31.2
  left heart syndrome Q23.4
  leg (congenital) — see Defect, reduction, lower limb
  limb Q73.8
    lower (congenital) — see Defect, reduction, lower
      limb
    upper (congenital) — see Defect, reduction, upper
      limb
  liver Q44.7
  lung (lobe) (not associated with short gestation) Q33.6
    associated with immaturity, low birth weight, pre-
      maturity, or short gestation P28.0
  mammary (areola), congenital Q83.8
  mandible, mandibular M26.04
    alveolar M26.74
    unilateral condylar M27.8
  maxillary M26.02
    alveolar M26.73
  medullary D61.9
  megakaryocytic D69.49

Hypoplasia, hypoplastic — *continued*
  metacarpus — *see* Defect, reduction, upper limb, specified type NEC
  metatarsus — *see* Defect, reduction, lower limb, specified type NEC
  muscle Q79.8
  nail(s) Q84.6
  nose, nasal Q30.1
  optic nerve H47.03- ☑
  osseous meatus (ear) Q17.8
  ovary, congenital Q50.39
  pancreas Q45.0
  parathyroid (gland) Q89.2
  parotid gland Q38.4
  patella Q74.1
  pelvis, pelvic girdle Q74.2
  penis (congenital) Q55.62
  peripheral vascular system Q27.8
    digestive system Q27.8
    lower limb Q27.8
    specified site NEC Q27.8
    upper limb Q27.8
  pituitary (gland) (congenital) Q89.2
  pulmonary (not associated with short gestation) Q33.6
    artery, functional J43.0
    associated with short gestation P28.0
  radioulnar — *see* Defect, reduction, upper limb, specified type NEC
  radius — *see* Defect, reduction, upper limb
  rectum Q42.1
    with fistula Q42.0
  respiratory system NEC Q34.8
  rib Q76.6
  right heart syndrome Q22.6
  sacrum Q76.49
  scapula Q74.0
  scrotum Q55.1
  shoulder girdle Q74.0
  skin Q82.8
  skull (bone) Q75.8
    with
      anencephaly Q00.0
      encephalocele — *see* Encephalocele
      hydrocephalus Q03.9
        with spina bifida — *see* Spina bifida, by site, with hydrocephalus
      microcephaly Q02
  spinal (cord) (ventral horn cell) Q06.1
  spine Q76.49
  sternum Q76.7
  tarsus — *see* Defect, reduction, lower limb, specified type NEC
  testis Q55.1
  thymic, with immunodeficiency D82.1
  thymus (gland) Q89.2
    with immunodeficiency D82.1
  thyroid (gland) E03.1
    cartilage Q31.2
  tibiofibular (congenital) — *see* Defect, reduction, lower limb, specified type NEC
  toe — *see* Defect, reduction, lower limb, specified type NEC
  tongue Q38.3
  Turner's K00.4
  ulna (congenital) — *see* Defect, reduction, upper limb
  umbilical artery Q27.0
  unilateral condylar M27.8
  ureter Q62.8
  uterus, congenital Q51.811
  vagina Q52.4
  vascular NEC peripheral Q27.8
    brain Q28.3
    digestive system Q27.8
    lower limb Q27.8
    specified site NEC Q27.8
    upper limb Q27.8
  vein(s) (peripheral) Q27.8
    brain Q28.3
    digestive system Q27.8
    great Q26.8
    lower limb Q27.8
    specified site NEC Q27.8
    upper limb Q27.8
  vena cava (inferior) (superior) Q26.8
  vertebra Q76.49
  vulva, congenital Q52.79
  zonule (ciliary) Q12.8
Hypopnea, obstructive sleep apnea G47.33

Hypopotassemia E87.6
Hypoproconvertinemia, congenital (hereditary) D68.2
Hypoproteinemia E77.8
Hypoprothrombinemia (congenital) (hereditary) (idiopathic) D68.2
  acquired D68.4
  newborn, transient P61.6
Hypoptyalism K11.7
Hypopyon (eye) (anterior chamber) — *see* Iridocyclitis, acute, hypopyon
Hypopyrexia R68.0
Hyporeflexia R29.2
Hyposecretion
  ACTH E23.0
  antidiuretic hormone E23.2
  ovary E28.39
  salivary gland (any) K11.7
  vasopressin E23.2
Hyposegmentation, leukocytic, hereditary D72.0
Hyposiderinemia D50.9
Hypospadias Q54.9
  balanic Q54.0
  coronal Q54.0
  glandular Q54.0
  penile Q54.1
  penoscrotal Q54.2
  perineal Q54.3
  specified NEC Q54.8
Hypospermatogenesis — *see* Oligospermia
Hyposplenism D73.0
Hypostasis pulmonary, passive — *see* Edema, lung
Hypostatic — *see* condition
Hyposthenuria N28.89
Hypotension (arterial) (constitutional) I95.9
  chronic I95.89
  drug-induced I95.2
  due to (of) hemodialysis I95.3
  iatrogenic I95.89
  idiopathic (permanent) I95.0
  intracranial, following ventricular shunting (ventriculostomy) G97.2
  intra-dialytic I95.3
  maternal, syndrome (following labor and delivery) O26.5- ☑
  neurogenic, orthostatic G90.3
  orthostatic (chronic) I95.1
    due to drugs I95.2
    neurogenic G90.3
  postoperative I95.81
  postural I95.1
  specified NEC I95.89
Hypothermia (accidental) T68 ☑
  due to anesthesia, anesthetic T88.51 ☑
  low environmental temperature T68 ☑
  neonatal P80.9
    environmental (mild) NEC P80.8
    mild P80.8
    severe (chronic) (cold injury syndrome) P80.0
    specified NEC P80.8
  not associated with low environmental temperature R68.0
Hypothyroidism (acquired) E03.9
  autoimmune — *see* Thyroiditis, autoimmune
  congenital (without goiter) E03.1
    with goiter (diffuse) E03.0
  due to
    exogenous substance NEC E03.2
    iodine-deficiency, acquired E01.8
      subclinical E02
    irradiation therapy E89.0
    medicament NEC E03.2
    P-aminosalicylic acid (PAS) E03.2
    phenylbutazone E03.2
    resorcinol E03.2
    sulfonamide E03.2
    surgery E89.0
    thiourea group drugs E03.2
  iatrogenic NEC E03.2
  iodine-deficiency (acquired) E01.8
    congenital — *see* Syndrome, iodine- deficiency, congenital
    subclinical E02
  neonatal, transitory P72.2
  postinfectious E03.3
  postirradiation E89.0
  postprocedural E89.0
  postsurgical E89.0
  specified NEC E03.8

Hypothyroidism — *continued*
  subclinical, iodine-deficiency related E02
Hypotonia, hypotonicity, hypotony
  bladder N31.2
  congenital (benign) P94.2
  eye — *see* Disorder, globe, hypotony
Hypotrichosis — *see* Alopecia
Hypotropia H50.2- ☑
Hypoventilation R06.89
  congenital central alveolar G47.35
  sleep related
    idiopathic nonobstructive alveolar G47.34
    in conditions classified elsewhere G47.36
Hypovitaminosis — *see* Deficiency, vitamin
Hypovolemia E86.1
  surgical shock T81.19 ☑
  traumatic (shock) T79.4 ☑
Hypoxemia R09.02
  newborn P84
  sleep related, in conditions classified elsewhere G47.36
Hypoxia (*see also* Anoxia) R09.02
  cerebral, during a procedure NEC G97.81
    postprocedural NEC G97.82
  intrauterine P84
  myocardial — *see* Insufficiency, coronary
  newborn P84
  sleep-related G47.34
Hypsarrhythmia — *see* Epilepsy, generalized, specified NEC
Hysteralgia, pregnant uterus O26.89- ☑
Hysteria, hysterical (conversion) (dissociative state) F44.9
  anxiety F41.8
  convulsions F44.5
  psychosis, acute F44.9
Hysteroepilepsy F44.5

IBDU (colonic inflammatory bowel dissease unclassified) K52.3
Ichthyoparasitism due to Vandellia cirrhosa B88.8
Ichthyosis (congenital) Q80.9
  acquired L85.0
  fetalis Q80.4
  hystrix Q80.8
  lamellar Q80.2
  lingual K13.29
  palmaris and plantaris Q82.8
  simplex Q80.0
  vera Q80.8
  vulgaris Q80.0
  X-linked Q80.1
Ichthyotoxism — *see* Poisoning, fish
  bacterial — *see* Intoxication, foodborne
Icteroanemia, hemolytic (acquired) D59.9
  congenital — *see* Spherocytosis
Icterus (*see also* Jaundice)
  conjunctiva R17
  gravis, newborn P55.0
  hematogenous (acquired) D59.9
  hemolytic (acquired) D59.9
    congenital — *see* Spherocytosis
  hemorrhagic (acute) (leptospiral) (spirochetal) A27.0
    newborn P53
  infectious B15.9
    with hepatic coma B15.0
    leptospiral A27.0
    spirochetal A27.0
  neonatorum — *see* Jaundice, newborn
  newborn P59.9
  spirochetal A27.0
Ictus solaris, solis T67.0 ☑
Id reaction (due to bacteria) L30.2
Ideation
  homicidal R45.850
  suicidal R45.851
Identity disorder (child) F64.9
  gender role F64.2
  psychosexual F64.2
Idioglossia F80.0
Idiopathic — *see* condition
Idiot, idiocy (congenital) F73
  amaurotic (Bielschowsky(-Jansky)) (family) (infantile (late)) (juvenile (late)) (Vogt-Spielmeyer) E75.4
  microcephalic Q02
IgE asthma J45.909

☑ **Additional Character Required — Refer to the Tabular List for Character Selection**   ◥ **Subterms under main terms may continue to next column or page**

IIAC (idiopathic infantile arterial calcification) Q28.8
Ileitis (chronic) (noninfectious) (see also Enteritis) K52.9
  backwash — see Pancolitis, ulcerative (chronic)
  infectious A09
  regional (ulcerative) — see Enteritis, regional, small
     intestine
  segmental — see Enteritis, regional
  terminal (ulcerative) — see Enteritis, regional, small
     intestine
Ileocolitis (see also Enteritis) K52.9
  infectious A09
  regional — see Enteritis, regional
  ulcerative K51.0- ☑
Ileostomy
  attention to Z43.2
  malfunctioning K94.13
  status Z93.2
    with complication — see Complications, enteros-
     tomy
Ileotyphus — see Typhoid
Ileum — see condition
Ileus (bowel) (colon) (inhibitory) (intestine) K56.7
  adynamic K56.0
  due to gallstone (in intestine) K56.3
  duodenal (chronic) K31.5
  gallstone K56.3
  mechanical NEC (see also Obstruction, intestine,
    specified NEC) K56.699
  meconium P76.0
    in cystic fibrosis E84.11
    meaning meconium plug (without cystic fibrosis)
     P76.0
  myxedema K59.8
  neurogenic K56.0
    Hirschsprung's disease or megacolon Q43.1
  newborn
    due to meconium P76.0
     in cystic fibrosis E84.11
     meaning meconium plug (without cystic fibro-
      sis) P76.0
    transitory P76.1
  obstructive (see also Obstruction, intestine, specified
    NEC) K56.699
  paralytic K56.0
  postoperative K91.89
Iliac — see condition
Iliotibial band syndrome M76.3- ☑
Illiteracy Z55.0
Illness (see also Disease) R69
  manic-depressive — see Disorder, bipolar
Imbalance R26.89
  autonomic G90.8
  constituents of food intake E63.1
  electrolyte E87.8
    with
     abortion — see Abortion by type, complicated
      by, electrolyte imbalance
     molar pregnancy O08.5
    due to hyperemesis gravidarum O21.1
    following ectopic or molar pregnancy O08.5
    neonatal, transitory NEC P74.4
     potassium P74.3
     sodium P74.2
  endocrine E34.9
  eye muscle NOS H50.9
  hormone E34.9
  hysterical F44.4
  labyrinth — see subcategory H83.2 ☑
  posture R29.3
  protein-energy — see Malnutrition
  sympathetic G90.8
Imbecile, imbecility (I.Q. 35-49) F71
Imbedding, intrauterine device T83.39 ☑
Imbibition, cholesterol (gallbladder) K82.4
Imbrication, teeth,, fully erupted M26.30
Imerslund (-Gräsbeck) **syndrome** D51.1
Immature (see also Immaturity)
  birth (less than 37 completed weeks) — see Preterm,
    newborn
    extremely (less than 28 completed weeks) — see
     Immaturity, extreme
  personality F60.89
Immaturity (less than 37 completed weeks) (see also
  Preterm, newborn)
  extreme of newborn (less than 28 completed weeks
    of gestation) (less than 196 completed days of
    gestation) (unspecified weeks of gestation)
    P07.20

Immaturity — continued
  extreme of newborn — continued
    gestational age
     less than 23 completed weeks P07.21
     23 completed weeks (23 weeks, 0 days through
      23 weeks, 6 days) P07.22
     24 completed weeks (24 weeks, 0 days through
      24 weeks, 6 days) P07.23
     25 completed weeks (25 weeks, 0 days through
      25 weeks, 6 days) P07.24
     26 completed weeks (26 weeks, 0 days through
      26 weeks, 6 days) P07.25
     27 completed weeks (27 weeks, 0 days through
      27 weeks, 6 days) P07.26
  fetus or infant light-for-dates — see Light-for-dates
  lung, newborn P28.0
  organ or site NEC — see Hypoplasia
  pulmonary, newborn P28.0
  reaction F60.89
  sexual (female) (male), after puberty E30.0
Immersion T75.1 ☑
  foot T69.02- ☑
  hand T69.01- ☑
Immobile, immobility
  complete, due to severe physical disability or frailty
    R53.2
  intestine K59.8
  syndrome (paraplegic) M62.3
Immune reconstitution (inflammatory) syndrome [IRIS]
  D89.3
Immunization (see also Vaccination)
  ABO — see Incompatibility, ABO
    in newborn P55.1
  complication — see Complications, vaccination
  encounter for Z23
  not done (not carried out) Z28.9
    because (of)
     acute illness of patient Z28.01
     allergy to vaccine (or component) Z28.04
     caregiver refusal Z28.82
     chronic illness of patient Z28.02
     contraindication NEC Z28.09
     group pressure Z28.1
     guardian refusal Z28.82
     immune compromised state of patient Z28.03
     parent refusal Z28.82
     patient had disease being vaccinated against
      Z28.81
     patient refusal Z28.21
     patient's belief Z28.1
     religious beliefs of patient Z28.1
     specified reason NEC Z28.89
      of patient Z28.29
     unspecified patient reason Z28.20
  Rh factor
    affecting management of pregnancy NEC
     O36.09- ☑
    anti-D antibody O36.01- ☑
    from transfusion — see Complication(s), transfu-
     sion, incompatibility reaction, Rh (factor)
Immunocytoma C83.0- ☑
Immunodeficiency D84.9
  with
    adenosine-deaminase deficiency D81.3
    antibody defects D80.9
     specified type NEC D80.8
    hyperimmunoglobulinemia D80.6
    increased immunoglobulin M (IgM) D80.5
    major defect D82.9
     specified type NEC D82.8
    partial albinism D82.8
    short-limbed stature D82.2
    thrombocytopenia and eczema D82.0
  antibody with
    hyperimmunoglobulinemia D80.6
    near-normal immunoglobulins D80.6
  autosomal recessive, Swiss type D80.0
  combined D81.9
    biotin-dependent carboxylase D81.819
     biotinidase D81.810
     holocarboxylase synthetase D81.818
     specified type NEC D81.818
    severe (SCID) D81.9
     with
      low or normal B-cell numbers D81.2
      low T- and B-cell numbers D81.1
      reticular dysgenesis D81.0
    specified type NEC D81.89

Immunodeficiency — continued
  common variable D83.9
    with
     abnormalities of B-cell numbers and function
      D83.0
     autoantibodies to B- or T-cells D83.2
     immunoregulatory T-cell disorders D83.1
    specified type NEC D83.8
  following hereditary defective response to Epstein-
    Barr virus (EBV) D82.3
  selective, immunoglobulin
    A (IgA) D80.2
    G (IgG) (subclasses) D80.3
    M (IgM) D80.4
  severe combined (SCID) D81.9
  specified type NEC D84.8
  X-linked, with increased IgM D80.5
Immunotherapy (encounter for)
  antineoplastic Z51.12
Impaction, impacted
  bowel, colon, rectum (see also Impaction, fecal) K56.49
    by gallstone K56.3
  calculus — see Calculus
  cerumen (ear) (external) H61.2- ☑
  cuspid — see Impaction, tooth
  dental (same or adjacent tooth) K01.1
  fecal, feces K56.41
  fracture — see Fracture, by site
  gallbladder — see Calculus, gallbladder
  gallstone(s) — see Calculus, gallbladder
    bile duct (common) (hepatic) — see Calculus, bile
     duct
    cystic duct — see Calculus, gallbladder
    in intestine, with obstruction (any part) K56.3
  intestine (calculous) NEC (see also Impaction, fecal)
    K56.49
    gallstone, with ileus K56.3
  intrauterine device (IUD) T83.39 ☑
  molar — see Impaction, tooth
  shoulder, causing obstructed labor O66.0
  tooth, teeth K01.1
  turbinate J34.89
Impaired, impairment (function)
  auditory discrimination — see Abnormal, auditory
    perception
  cognitive, mild, so stated G31.84
  dual sensory Z73.82
  fasting glucose R73.01
  glucose tolerance (oral) R73.02
  hearing — see Deafness
  heart — see Disease, heart
  kidney N28.9
    disorder resulting from N25.9
     specified NEC N25.89
  liver K72.90
    with coma K72.91
  mastication K08.89
  mild cognitive, so stated G31.84
  mobility
    ear ossicles — see Ankylosis, ear ossicles
    requiring care provider Z74.09
  myocardium, myocardial — see Insufficiency, myocar-
    dial
  rectal sphincter R19.8
  renal (acute) (chronic) N28.9
    disorder resulting from N25.9
     specified NEC N25.89
  vision NEC H54.7
    both eyes H54.3
Impediment, speech R47.9
  psychogenic (childhood) F98.8
  slurring R47.81
  specified NEC R47.89
Impending
  coronary syndrome I20.0
  delirium tremens F10.239
  myocardial infarction I20.0
Imperception auditory (acquired) (see also Deafness)
  congenital H93.25
Imperfect
  aeration, lung (newborn) NEC — see Atelectasis
  closure (congenital)
    alimentary tract NEC Q45.8
     lower Q43.8
     upper Q40.8
    atrioventricular ostium Q21.2
    atrium (secundum) Q21.1
    branchial cleft NOS Q18.2

Imperfect — continued
  closure — continued
    branchial cleft — continued
      cyst Q18.Ø
      fistula Q18.Ø
      sinus Q18.Ø
    choroid Q14.3
    cricoid cartilage Q31.8
    cusps, heart valve NEC Q24.8
      pulmonary Q22.3
    ductus
      arteriosus Q25.Ø
      Botalli Q25.Ø
    ear drum (causing impairment of hearing) Q16.4
    esophagus with communication to bronchus or trachea Q39.1
    eyelid Q1Ø.3
    foramen
      botalli Q21.1
      ovale Q21.1
    genitalia, genital organ(s) or system
      female Q52.8
        external Q52.79
        internal NEC Q52.8
      male Q55.8
    glottis Q31.8
    interatrial ostium or septum Q21.1
    interauricular ostium or septum Q21.1
    interventricular ostium or septum Q21.Ø
    larynx Q31.8
    lip — see Cleft, lip
    nasal septum Q3Ø.3
    nose Q3Ø.2
    omphalomesenteric duct Q43.Ø
    optic nerve entry Q14.2
    organ or site not listed — see Anomaly, by site
    ostium
      interatrial Q21.1
      interauricular Q21.1
      interventricular Q21.Ø
    palate — see Cleft, palate
    preauricular sinus Q18.1
    retina Q14.1
    roof of orbit Q75.8
    sclera Q13.5
    septum
      aorticopulmonary Q21.4
      atrial (secundum) Q21.1
      between aorta and pulmonary artery Q21.4
      heart Q21.9
      interatrial (secundum) Q21.1
      interauricular (secundum) Q21.1
      interventricular Q21.Ø
        in tetralogy of Fallot Q21.3
      nasal Q3Ø.3
      ventricular Q21.Ø
        with pulmonary stenosis or atresia, dextra-position of aorta, and hypertrophy of right ventricle Q21.3
        in tetralogy of Fallot Q21.3
    skull Q75.Ø
      with
        anencephaly QØØ.Ø
        encephalocele — see Encephalocele
        hydrocephalus QØ3.9
          with spina bifida — see Spina bifida, by site, with hydrocephalus
        microcephaly QØ2
    spine (with meningocele) — see Spina bifida, by site
    trachea Q32.1
    tympanic membrane (causing impairment of hearing) Q16.4
    uterus Q51.818
    vitelline duct Q43.Ø
  erection — see Dysfunction, sexual, male, erectile
  fusion — see Imperfect, closure
  inflation, lung (newborn) — see Atelectasis
  posture R29.3
  rotation, intestine Q43.3
  septum, ventricular Q21.Ø
Imperfectly descended testis — see Cryptorchid
Imperforate (congenital) (see also Atresia)
  anus Q42.3
    with fistula Q42.2
  cervix (uteri) Q51.828
  esophagus Q39.Ø
    with tracheoesophageal fistula Q39.1
  hymen Q52.3

Imperforate — continued
  jejunum Q41.1
  pharynx Q38.8
  rectum Q42.1
    with fistula Q42.Ø
  urethra Q64.39
  vagina Q52.4
Impervious (congenital) (see also Atresia)
  anus Q42.3
    with fistula Q42.2
  bile duct Q44.2
  esophagus Q39.Ø
    with tracheoesophageal fistula Q39.1
  intestine (small) Q41.9
    large Q42.9
      specified NEC Q42.8
  rectum Q42.1
    with fistula Q42.Ø
  ureter — see Atresia, ureter
  urethra Q64.39
Impetiginization of dermatoses LØ1.1
Impetigo (any organism) (any site) (circinate) (conta-giosa) (simplex) (vulgaris) LØ1.ØØ
  Bockhart's LØ1.Ø2
  bullous, bullosa LØ1.Ø3
  external ear LØ1.ØØ [H62.4Ø]
  follicularis LØ1.Ø2
  furfuracea L3Ø.5
  herpetiformis L4Ø.1
    nonobstetrical L4Ø.1
  neonatorum LØ1.Ø3
  nonbullous LØ1.Ø1
  specified type NEC LØ1.Ø9
  ulcerative LØ1.Ø9
Impingement (on teeth)
  soft tissue
    anterior M26.81
    posterior M26.82
Implant, endometrial N8Ø.9
Implantation
  anomalous — see Anomaly, by site
    ureter Q62.63
  cyst
    external area or site (skin) NEC L72.Ø
    iris — see Cyst, iris, implantation
    vagina N89.8
    vulva N9Ø.7
  dermoid (cyst) — see Implantation, cyst
Impotence (sexual) N52.9
  counseling Z7Ø.1
  organic origin (see also Dysfunction, sexual, male, erectile) N52.9
  psychogenic F52.21
Impression, basilar Q75.8
Imprisonment, anxiety concerning Z65.1
Improper care (child) (newborn) — see Maltreatment
Improperly tied umbilical cord (causing hemorrhage) P51.8
Impulsiveness (impulsive) R45.87
Inability to swallow — see Aphagia
Inaccessible, inaccessibility
  health care NEC Z75.3
    due to
      waiting period Z75.2
        for admission to facility elsewhere Z75.1
    other helping agencies Z75.4
Inactive — see condition
Inadequate, inadequacy
  aesthetics of dental restoration KØ8.56
  biologic, constitutional, functional, or social F6Ø.7
  development
    child R62.5Ø
    genitalia
      after puberty NEC E3Ø.Ø
      congenital
        female Q52.8
          external Q52.79
          internal Q52.8
          male Q55.8
    lungs Q33.6
      associated with short gestation P28.Ø
    organ or site not listed — see Anomaly, by site
  diet (causing nutritional deficiency) E63.9
  eating habits Z72.4
  environment, household Z59.1
  family support Z63.8
  food (supply) NEC Z59.4
    hunger effects T73.Ø ☑

Inadequate, inadequacy — continued
  functional F6Ø.7
  household care, due to
    family member
      handicapped or ill Z74.2
      on vacation Z75.5
      temporarily away from home Z74.2
    technical defects in home Z59.1
    temporary absence from home of person rendering care Z74.2
  housing (heating) (space) Z59.1
  income (financial) Z59.6
  intrafamilial communication Z63.8
  material resources Z59.9
  mental — see Disability, intellectual
  parental supervision or control of child Z62.Ø
  personality F6Ø.7
  pulmonary
    function RØ6.89
      newborn P28.5
    ventilation, newborn P28.5
  sample of cytologic smear
    anus R85.615
    cervix R87.615
    vagina R87.625
  social F6Ø.7
    insurance Z59.7
    skills NEC Z73.4
  supervision of child by parent Z62.Ø
  teaching affecting education Z55.8
  welfare support Z59.7
Inanition R64
  with edema — see Malnutrition, severe
  due to
    deprivation of food T73.Ø ☑
    malnutrition — see Malnutrition
  fever R5Ø.9
Inappropriate
  change in quantitative human chorionic gonadotropin (hCG) in early pregnancy OØ2.81
  diet or eating habits Z72.4
  level of quantitative human chorionic gonadotropin (hCG) for gestational age in early pregnancy OØ2.81
  secretion
    antidiuretic hormone (ADH) (excessive) E22.2
      deficiency E23.2
    pituitary (posterior) E22.2
Inattention at or after birth — see Neglect
Incarceration, incarcerated
  enterocele K46.Ø
    gangrenous K46.1
  epiplocele K46.Ø
    gangrenous K46.1
  exomphalos K42.Ø
    gangrenous K42.1
  hernia (see also Hernia, by site, with obstruction)
    with gangrene — see Hernia, by site, with gan-grene
  iris, in wound — see Injury, eye, laceration, with pro-lapse
  lens, in wound — see Injury, eye, laceration, with prolapse
  omphalocele K42.Ø
  prison, anxiety concerning Z65.1
  rupture — see Hernia, by site
  sarcoepiplocele K46.Ø
    gangrenous K46.1
  sarcoepiplomphalocele K42.Ø
    with gangrene K42.1
  uterus N85.8
    gravid O34.51- ☑
      causing obstructed labor O65.5
Incised wound
  external — see Laceration
  internal organs — see Injury, by site
Incision, incisional
  hernia K43.2
    with
      gangrene (and obstruction) K43.1
      obstruction K43.Ø
  surgical, complication — see Complications, surgical procedure
  traumatic
    external — see Laceration
    internal organs — see Injury, by site
Inclusion
  azurophilic leukocytic D72.Ø

Inclusion — continued
  blennorrhea (neonatal) (newborn) P39.1
  gallbladder in liver (congenital) Q44.1

Incompatibility
  ABO
    affecting management of pregnancy O36.11- ☑
      anti-A sensitization O36.11- ☑
      anti-B sensitization O36.19- ☑
      specified NEC O36.19- ☑
    infusion or transfusion reaction — see Complica-
      tion(s), transfusion, incompatibility reaction,
      ABO
    newborn P55.1
  blood (group) (Duffy) (K(ell)) (Kidd) (Lewis) (M) (S) NEC
    affecting management of pregnancy O36.11- ☑
      anti-A sensitization O36.11- ☑
      anti-B sensitization O36.19- ☑
    infusion or transfusion reaction T80.89 ☑
    newborn P55.8
  divorce or estrangement Z63.5
  Rh (blood group) (factor) Z31.82
    affecting management of pregnancy NEC
      O36.09- ☑
      anti-D antibody O36.01- ☑
    infusion or transfusion reaction — see Complica-
      tion(s), transfusion, incompatibility reaction,
      Rh (factor)
    newborn P55.0
  rhesus — see Incompatibility, Rh

Incompetency, incompetent, incompetence
  annular
    aortic (valve) — see Insufficiency, aortic
    mitral (valve) I34.0
    pulmonary valve (heart) I37.1
  aortic (valve) — see Insufficiency, aortic
  cardiac valve — see Endocarditis
  cervix, cervical (os) N88.3
    in pregnancy O34.3- ☑
  chronotropic I45.89
    with
      autonomic dysfunction G90.8
      ischemic heart disease I25.89
      left ventricular dysfunction I51.89
      sinus node dysfunction I49.8
  esophagogastric (junction) (sphincter) K22.0
  mitral (valve) — see Insufficiency, mitral
  pelvic fundus N81.89
  pubocervical tissue N81.82
  pulmonary valve (heart) I37.1
    congenital Q22.3
  rectovaginal tissue N81.83
  tricuspid (annular) (valve) — see Insufficiency, tricuspid
  valvular — see Endocarditis
    congenital Q24.8
  vein, venous (saphenous) (varicose) — see Varix, leg

Incomplete (see also condition)
  bladder, emptying R33.9
  defecation R15.0
  expansion lungs (newborn) NEC — see Atelectasis
  rotation, intestine Q43.3

Inconclusive
  diagnostic imaging due to excess body fat of patient
    R93.9
  findings on diagnostic imaging of breast NEC R92.8
  mammogram (due to dense breasts) R92.2

Incontinence R32
  anal sphincter R15.9
  coital N39.491
  feces R15.9
    nonorganic origin F98.1
  insensible (urinary) N39.42
  overflow N39.490
  postural (urinary) N39.492
  psychogenic F45.8
  rectal R15.9
  reflex N39.498
  stress (female) (male) N39.3
    and urge N39.46
  urethral sphincter R32
  urge N39.41
    and stress (female) (male) N39.46
  urine (urinary) R32
    continuous N39.45
    due to cognitive impairment, or severe physical
      disability or immobility R39.81
    functional R39.81
    insensible N39.42
    mixed (stress and urge) N39.46

Incontinence — continued
  urine — continued
    nocturnal N39.44
    nonorganic origin F98.0
    overflow N39.490
    post dribbling N39.43
    postural N39.492
    reflex N39.498
    specified NEC N39.498
    stress (female) (male) N39.3
      and urge N39.46
    total N39.498
    unaware N39.42
    urge N39.41
      and stress (female) (male) N39.46

Incontinentia pigmenti Q82.3

Incoordinate, incoordination
  esophageal-pharyngeal (newborn) — see Dysphagia
  muscular R27.8
  uterus (action) (contractions) (complicating delivery)
    O62.4

Increase, increased
  abnormal, in development R63.8
  androgens (ovarian) E28.1
  anticoagulants (antithrombin) (anti-VIIIa) (anti-IXa)
    (anti-Xa) (anti-XIa) — see Circulating anticoagu-
    lants
  cold sense R20.8
  estrogen E28.0
  function
    adrenal
      cortex — see Cushing's, syndrome
      medulla E27.5
    pituitary (gland) (anterior) (lobe) E22.9
      posterior E22.2
  heat sense R20.8
  intracranial pressure (benign) G93.2
  permeability, capillaries I78.8
  pressure, intracranial G93.2
  secretion
    gastrin E16.4
    glucagon E16.3
    pancreas, endocrine E16.9
      growth hormone-releasing hormone E16.8
      pancreatic polypeptide E16.8
      somatostatin E16.8
      vasoactive-intestinal polypeptide E16.8
  sphericity, lens Q12.4
  splenic activity D73.1
  venous pressure I87.8
    portal K76.6

Increta placenta O43.22- ☑

Incrustation, cornea, foreign body (lead)(zinc) — see
  Foreign body, cornea

Incyclophoria H50.54

Incyclotropia — see Cyclotropia

Indeterminate sex Q56.4

India rubber skin Q82.8

Indigestion (acid) (bilious) (functional) K30
  catarrhal K31.89
  due to decomposed food NOS A05.9
  nervous F45.8
  psychogenic F45.8

Indirect — see condition

Induratio penis plastica N48.6

Induration, indurated
  brain G93.89
  breast (fibrous) N64.51
    puerperal, postpartum O92.29
  broad ligament N83.8
  chancre
    anus A51.1
    congenital A50.07
    extragenital NEC A51.2
  corpora cavernosa (penis) (plastic) N48.6
  liver (chronic) K76.89
  lung (black) (chronic) (fibroid) (see also Fibrosis, lung)
    J84.10
    essential brown J84.03
  penile (plastic) N48.6
  phlebitic — see Phlebitis
  skin R23.4

Inebriety (without dependence) — see Alcohol, intoxication

Inefficiency, kidney N28.9

Inelasticity, skin R23.4

Inequality, leg (length) (acquired) (see also Deformity,
  limb, unequal length)
  congenital — see Defect, reduction, lower limb

Inequality, leg — continued
  lower leg — see Deformity, limb, unequal
    length

Inertia
  bladder (neurogenic) N31.2
  stomach K31.89
    psychogenic F45.8
  uterus, uterine during labor O62.2
    during latent phase of labor O62.0
    primary O62.0
    secondary O62.1
  vesical (neurogenic) N31.2

Infancy, infantile, infantilism (see also condition)
  celiac K90.0
  genitalia, genitals (after puberty) E30.0
  Herter's (nontropical sprue) K90.0
  intestinal K90.0
  Lorain E23.0
  pancreatic K86.89
  pelvis M95.5
    with disproportion (fetopelvic) O33.1
      causing obstructed labor O65.1
  pituitary E23.0
  renal N25.0
  uterus — see Infantile, genitalia

Infant(s) (see also Infancy)
  excessive crying R68.11
  irritable child R68.12
  lack of care — see Neglect
  liveborn (singleton) Z38.2
    born in hospital Z38.00
      by cesarean Z38.01
    born outside hospital Z38.1
    multiple NEC Z38.8
      born in hospital Z38.68
        by cesarean Z38.69
      born outside hospital Z38.7
    quadruplet Z38.8
      born in hospital Z38.63
        by cesarean Z38.64
      born outside hospital Z38.7
    quintuplet Z38.8
      born in hospital Z38.65
        by cesarean Z38.66
      born outside hospital Z38.7
    triplet Z38.8
      born in hospital Z38.61
        by cesarean Z38.62
      born outside hospital Z38.7
    twin Z38.5
      born in hospital Z38.30
        by cesarean Z38.31
      born outside hospital Z38.4
  of diabetic mother (syndrome of) P70.1
    gestational diabetes P70.0

Infantile (see also condition)
  genitalia, genitals E30.0
  os, uterine E30.0
  penis E30.0
  testis E29.1
  uterus E30.0

Infantilism — see Infancy

Infarct, infarction
  adrenal (capsule) (gland) E27.49
  appendices epiploicae (see also Infarct, intestine)
    K55.069
  bowel (see also Infarct, intestine) K55.069
  brain (stem) — see Infarct, cerebral
  breast N64.89
  brewer's (kidney) N28.0
  cardiac — see Infarct, myocardium
  cerebellar — see Infarct, cerebral
  cerebral (see also Occlusion, artery cerebral or precere-
    bral, with infarction) I63.9
    aborted I63.9
    cortical I63.9
    due to
      cerebral venous thrombosis, nonpyogenic I63.6
      embolism
        cerebral arteries I63.4- ☑
        precerebral arteries I63.1- ☑
      occlusion NEC
        cerebral arteries I63.5- ☑
        precerebral arteries I63.2- ☑
      stenosis NEC
        cerebral arteries I63.5- ☑
        precerebral arteries I63.2- ☑

Infarct, infarction — *continued*
cerebral (*see also* Occlusion, artery cerebral or precerebral, with infarction) — *continued*
  due to — *continued*
    thrombosis
      cerebral artery I63.3- ☑
      precerebral artery I63.0- ☑
    intraoperative
      during cardiac surgery I97.810
      during other surgery I97.811
    postprocedural
      following cardiac surgery I97.820
      following other surgery I97.821
    specified NEC I63.8
colon (acute) (agnogenic) (embolic) (hemorrhagic) (nonocclusive) (nonthrombotic) (occlusive) (segmental) (thrombotic) (with gangrene) (*see also* Infarct, intestine) K55.049
coronary artery — *see* Infarct, myocardium
embolic — *see* Embolism
fallopian tube N83.8
gallbladder K82.8
heart — *see* Infarct, myocardium
hepatic K76.3
hypophysis (anterior lobe) E23.6
impending (myocardium) I20.0
intestine (acute) (agnogenic) (embolic) (hemorrhagic) (nonocclusive) (nonthrombotic) (occlusive) (thrombotic) (with gangrene) K55.069
  diffuse K55.062
  focal K55.061
  large K55.049
    diffuse K55.042
    focal K55.041
  small K55.029
    diffuse K55.022
    focal K55.021
kidney N28.0
liver K76.3
lung (embolic) (thrombotic) — *see* Embolism, pulmonary
lymph node I89.8
mesentery, mesenteric (embolic) (thrombotic) (with gangrene) (*see also* Infarct, intestine) K55.069
muscle (ischemic) M62.20
  ankle M62.27- ☑
  foot M62.27- ☑
  forearm M62.23- ☑
  hand M62.24- ☑
  lower leg M62.26- ☑
  pelvic region M62.25- ☑
  shoulder region M62.21- ☑
  specified site NEC M62.28
  thigh M62.25- ☑
  upper arm M62.22- ☑
myocardium, myocardial (acute) (with stated duration of 4 weeks or less) I21.9
  associated with revascularization procedure I21.A9
  diagnosed on ECG, but presenting no symptoms I25.2
  due to
    demand ischemia I21.A1
    ischemic imbalance I21.A1
  healed or old I25.2
  intraoperative (*see also* Infarct, myocardium, associated with revascularization procedure)
    during cardiac surgery I97.790
    during other surgery I97.791
  non-Q wave I21.4
  non-ST elevation (NSTEMI) I21.4
    subsequent I22.2
  nontransmural I21.4
  past (diagnosed on ECG or other investigation, but currently presenting no symptoms) I25.2
  postprocedural (*see also* Infarct, myocardium, associated with revascularization procedure)
    following cardiac surgery (*see also* Infarct, myocardium, type 4 or type 5) I97.190
    following other surgery I97.191
  Q wave (see also, Infarct, myocardium, by site) I21.3
  secondary to
    demand ischemia I21.A1
    ischemic imbalance I21.A1
  ST elevation (STEMI) I21.3
    anterior (anteroapical) (anterolateral) (anteroseptal) (Q wave) (wall) I21.09
      subsequent I22.0

Infarct, infarction — *continued*
myocardium, myocardial — *continued*
  ST elevation — *continued*
    inferior (diaphragmatic) (inferolateral) (inferoposterior) (wall) NEC I21.19
      subsequent I22.1
    inferoposterior transmural (Q wave) I21.11
    involving
      coronary artery of anterior wall NEC I21.09
      coronary artery of inferior wall NEC I21.19
      diagonal coronary artery I21.02
      left anterior descending coronary artery I21.02
      left circumflex coronary artery I21.21
      left main coronary artery I21.01
      oblique marginal coronary artery I21.21
      right coronary artery I21.11
    lateral (apical-lateral) (basal-lateral) (high) I21.29
      subsequent I22.8
    posterior (posterobasal) (posterolateral) (posteroseptal) (true) I21.29
      subsequent I22.8
    septal I21.29
      subsequent I22.8
    specified NEC I21.29
      subsequent I22.8
    subsequent I22.9
  subsequent (recurrent) (reinfarction) I22.9
    anterior (anteroapical) (anterolateral) (anteroseptal) (wall) I22.0
    diaphragmatic (wall) I22.1
    inferior (diaphragmatic) (inferolateral) (inferoposterior) (wall) I22.1
    lateral (apical-lateral) (basal-lateral) (high) I22.8
    non-ST elevation (NSTEMI) I22.2
    posterior (posterobasal) (posterolateral) (posteroseptal) (true) I22.8
    septal I22.8
    specified NEC I22.8
    ST elevation I22.9
      anterior (anteroapical) (anterolateral) (anteroseptal) (wall) I22.0
      inferior (diaphragmatic) (inferolateral) (inferoposterior) (wall) I22.1
      specified NEC I22.8
    subendocardial I22.2
    transmural I22.9
      anterior (anteroapical) (anterolateral) (anteroseptal) (wall) I22.0
      diaphragmatic (wall) I22.1
      inferior (diaphragmatic) (inferolateral) (inferoposterior) (wall) I22.1
      lateral (apical-lateral) (basal-lateral) (high) I22.8
      posterior (posterobasal) (posterolateral) (posteroseptal) (true) I22.8
      specified NEC I22.8
    type 1 (*see also* Infarction, myocardial, subsequent, by site, or by ST elevation or non-ST elevation) I22.9
    type 2 I21.A1
    type 3 I21.A9
    type 4 I21.A9
    type 5 I21.A9
  syphilitic A52.06
  transmural I21.9
    anterior (anteroapical) (anterolateral) (anteroseptal) (Q wave) (wall) NEC I21.09
    inferior (diaphragmatic) (inferolateral) (inferoposterior) (Q wave) (wall) NEC I21.19
    inferoposterior (Q wave) I21.11
    lateral (apical-lateral) (basal-lateral) (high) NEC I21.29
    posterior (posterobasal) (posterolateral) (posteroseptal) (true) NEC I21.29
    septal NEC I21.29
    specified NEC I21.29
    type 1 (*see also* Infarction, myocardial, by site, or by ST elevation or non-ST elevation) I21.9
    type 2 I21.A1
    type 3 I21.A9
    type 4 (a) (b) (c) I21.A9
    type 5 I21.A9
  nontransmural I21.4
omentum (*see also* Infarct, intestine) K55.069
ovary N83.8
pancreas K86.89
papillary muscle — *see* Infarct, myocardium

Infarct, infarction — *continued*
parathyroid gland E21.4
pituitary (gland) E23.6
placenta O43.81- ☑
prostate N42.89
pulmonary (artery) (vein) (hemorrhagic) — *see* Embolism, pulmonary
renal (embolic) (thrombotic) N28.0
retina, retinal (artery) — *see* Occlusion, artery, retina
spinal (cord) (acute) (embolic) (nonembolic) G95.11
spleen D73.5
  embolic or thrombotic I74.8
subendocardial (acute) (nontransmural) I21.4
suprarenal (capsule) (gland) E27.49
testis N50.1
thrombotic (*see also* Thrombosis)
  artery, arterial — *see* Embolism
thyroid (gland) E07.89
ventricle (heart) — *see* Infarct, myocardium
Infecting — *see* condition
Infection, infected, infective (opportunistic) B99.9
  with
    drug resistant organism — *see* Resistance (to), drug (*see also* specific organism)
    lymphangitis — *see* Lymphangitis
    organ dysfunction (acute) R65.20
      with septic shock R65.21
  abscess (skin) — *code by* site under Abscess
  Absidia — *see* Mucormycosis
  Acanthamoeba — *see* Acanthamebiasis
  Acanthocheilonema (perstans) (streptocerca) B74.4
  accessory sinus (chronic) — *see* Sinusitis
  achorion — *see* Dermatophytosis
  Acremonium falciforme B47.0
  acromioclavicular M00.9
  Actinobacillus (actinomycetem-comitans) A28.8
    mallei A24.0
    muris A25.1
  Actinomadura B47.1
  Actinomyces (israelii) (*see also* Actinomycosis) A42.9
  Actinomycetales — *see* Actinomycosis
  actinomycotic NOS — *see* Actinomycosis
  adenoid (and tonsil) J03.90
    chronic J35.02
  adenovirus NEC
    as cause of disease classified elsewhere B97.0
    unspecified nature or site B34.0
  aerogenes capsulatus A48.0
  aertrycke — *see* Infection, salmonella
  alimentary canal NOS — *see* Enteritis, infectious
  Allescheria boydii B48.2
  Alternaria B48.8
  alveolus, alveolar (process) K04.7
  Ameba, amebic (histolytica) — *see* Amebiasis
  amniotic fluid, sac or cavity O41.10- ☑
    chorioamnionitis O41.12- ☑
    placentitis O41.14- ☑
  amputation stump (surgical) — *see* Complication, amputation stump, infection
  Ancylostoma (duodenalis) B76.0
  Anisakiasis, Anisakis larvae B81.0
  anthrax — *see* Anthrax
  antrum (chronic) — *see* Sinusitis, maxillary
  anus, anal (papillae) (sphincter) K62.89
  arbovirus (arbor virus) A94
    specified type NEC A93.8
  artificial insemination N98.0
  Ascaris lumbricoides — *see* Ascariasis
  Ascomycetes B47.0
  Aspergillus (flavus) (fumigatus) (terreus) — *see* Aspergillosis
  atypical
    acid-fast (bacilli) — *see* Mycobacterium, atypical
    mycobacteria — *see* Mycobacterium, atypical
    virus A81.9
      specified type NEC A81.89
  auditory meatus (external) — *see* Otitis, externa, infective
  auricle (ear) — *see* Otitis, externa, infective
  axillary gland (lymph) L04.2
  Bacillus A49.9
    abortus A23.1
    anthracis — *see* Anthrax
    Ducrey's (any location) A57
    Flexner's A03.1
    Friedländer's NEC A49.8
    gas (gangrene) A48.0
    mallei A24.0

Infection, infected, infective — *continued*
  Bacillus — *continued*
    melitensis A23.0
    paratyphoid, paratyphosus A01.4
      A A01.1
      B A01.2
      C A01.3
    Shiga (-Kruse) A03.0
    suipestifer — *see* Infection, salmonella
    swimming pool A31.1
    typhosa A01.00
    welchii — *see* Gangrene, gas
  bacterial NOS A49.9
    as cause of disease classified elsewhere B96.89
      Bacteroides fragilis [B. fragilis] B96.6
      Clostridium perfringens [C. perfringens] B96.7
      Enterobacter sakazakii B96.89
      Enterococcus B95.2
      Escherichia coli [E. coli] (*see also* Escherichia
        coli) B96.20
      Helicobacter pylori [H.pylori] B96.81
      Hemophilus influenzae [H. influenzae] B96.3
      Klebsiella pneumoniae [K. pneumoniae] B96.1
      Mycoplasma pneumoniae [M. pneumoniae]
        B96.0
      Proteus (mirabilis) (morganii) B96.4
      Pseudomonas (aeruginosa) (mallei) (pseudoma-
        llei) B96.5
      Staphylococcus B95.8
        aureus (methicillin susceptible) (MSSA)
          B95.61
          methicillin resistant (MRSA) B95.62
        specified NEC B95.7
      Streptococcus B95.5
        group A B95.0
        group B B95.1
        pneumoniae B95.3
        specified NEC B95.4
      Vibrio vulnificus B96.82
    specified NEC A48.8
  Bacterium
    paratyphosum A01.4
      A A01.1
      B A01.2
      C A01.3
    typhosum A01.00
  Bacteroides NEC A49.8
    fragilis, as cause of disease classified elsewhere
      B96.6
  Balantidium coli A07.0
  Bartholin's gland N75.8
  Basidiobolus B46.8
  bile duct (common) (hepatic) — *see* Cholangitis
  bladder — *see* Cystitis
  Blastomyces, blastomycotic (*see also* Blastomycosis)
    brasiliensis — *see* Paracoccidioidomycosis
    dermatitidis — *see* Blastomycosis
    European — *see* Cryptococcosis
    Loboi B48.0
    North American B40.9
    South American — *see* Paracoccidioidomycosis
  bleb, postprocedure — *see* Blebitis
  bone — *see* Osteomyelitis
  Bordetella — *see* Whooping cough
  Borrelia bergdorfi A69.20
  brain (*see also* Encephalitis) G04.90
    membranes — *see* Meningitis
    septic G06.0
      meninges — *see* Meningitis, bacterial
  branchial cyst Q18.0
  breast — *see* Mastitis
  bronchus — *see* Bronchitis
  Brucella A23.9
    abortus A23.1
    canis A23.3
    melitensis A23.0
    mixed A23.8
    specified NEC A23.8
    suis A23.2
  Brugia (malayi) B74.1
    timori B74.2
  bursa — *see* Bursitis, infective
  buttocks (skin) L08.9
  Campylobacter, intestinal A04.5
    as cause of disease classified elsewhere B96.81
  Candida (albicans) (tropicalis) — *see* Candidiasis
  candiru B88.8
  Capillaria (intestinal) B81.1

Infection, infected, infective — *continued*
  Capillaria — *continued*
    hepatica B83.8
    philippinensis B81.1
  cartilage — *see* Disorder, cartilage, specified type NEC
  cat liver fluke B66.0
  catheter-related bloodstream (CRBSI) T80.211 ☑
  cellulitis — *code by* site under Cellulitis
  central line-associated T80.219 ☑
    bloodstream (CLABSI) T80.211 ☑
    specified NEC T80.218 ☑
  Cephalosporium falciforme B47.0
  cerebrospinal — *see* Meningitis
  cervical gland (lymph) L04.0
  cervix — *see* Cervicitis
  cesarean delivery wound (puerperal) O86.0
  cestodes — *see* Infestation, cestodes
  chest J22
  Chilomastix (intestinal) A07.8
  Chlamydia, chlamydial A74.9
    anus A56.3
    genitourinary tract A56.2
      lower A56.00
      specified NEC A56.19
    lymphogranuloma A55
    pharynx A56.4
    psittaci A70
    rectum A56.3
    sexually transmitted NEC A56.8
  cholera — *see* Cholera
  Cladosporium
    bantianum (brain abscess) B43.1
    carrionii B43.0
    castellanii B36.1
    trichoides (brain abscess) B43.1
    werneckii B36.1
  Clonorchis (sinensis) (liver) B66.1
  Clostridium NEC
    bifermentans A48.0
    botulinum (food poisoning) A05.1
      infant A48.51
      wound A48.52
    difficile
      as cause of disease classified elsewhere B96.89
      foodborne (disease)
        not specified as recurrent A04.72
        recurrent A04.71
      gas gangrene A48.0
      necrotizing enterocolitis
        not specified as recurrent A04.72
        recurrent A04.71
      sepsis A41.4
    gas-forming NEC A48.0
    histolyticum A48.0
    novyi, causing gas gangrene A48.0
    oedematiens A48.0
    perfringens
      as cause of disease classified elsewhere B96.7
      due to food A05.2
      foodborne (disease) A05.2
      gas gangrene A48.0
      sepsis A41.4
    septicum, causing gas gangrene A48.0
    sordellii, causing gas gangrene A48.0
    welchii
      as cause of disease classified elsewhere B96.7
      foodborne (disease) A05.2
      gas gangrene A48.0
      necrotizing enteritis A05.2
      sepsis A41.4
  Coccidioides (immitis) — *see* Coccidioidomycosis
  colon — *see* Enteritis, infectious
  colostomy K94.02
  common duct — *see* Cholangitis
  congenital P39.9
    Candida (albicans) P37.5
    cytomegalovirus P35.1
    hepatitis, viral P35.3
    herpes simplex P35.2
    infectious or parasitic disease P37.9
      specified NEC P37.8
    listeriosis (disseminated) P37.2
    malaria NEC P37.4
      falciparum P37.3
    Plasmodium falciparum P37.3
    poliomyelitis P35.8
    rubella P35.0
    skin P39.4

Infection, infected, infective — *continued*
  congenital — *continued*
    toxoplasmosis (acute) (subacute) (chronic) P37.1
    tuberculosis P37.0
    urinary (tract) P39.3
    vaccinia P35.8
    virus P35.9
      specified type NEC P35.8
  Conidiobolus B46.8
  coronavirus NEC B34.2
    as cause of disease classified elsewhere B97.29
    severe acute respiratory syndrome (SARS associat-
      ed) B97.21
  corpus luteum — *see* Salpingo-oophoritis
  Corynebacterium diphtheriae — *see* Diphtheria
  cotia virus B08.8
  Coxiella burnetii A78
  coxsackie — *see* Coxsackie
  Cryptococcus neoformans — *see* Cryptococcosis
  Cryptosporidium A07.2
  Cunninghamella — *see* Mucormycosis
  cyst — *see* Cyst
  cystic duct (*see also* Cholecystitis) K81.9
  Cysticercus cellulosae — *see* Cysticercosis
  cytomegalovirus, cytomegaloviral B25.9
    congenital P35.1
    maternal, maternal care for (suspected) damage
      to fetus O35.3 ☑
    mononucleosis B27.10
      with
        complication NEC B27.19
        meningitis B27.12
        polyneuropathy B27.11
  delta-agent (acute), in hepatitis B carrier B17.0
  dental (pulpal origin) K04.7
  Deuteromycetes B47.0
  Dicrocoelium dendriticum B66.2
  Dipetalonema (perstans) (streptocerca) B74.4
  diphtherial — *see* Diphtheria
  Diphyllobothrium (adult) (latum) (pacificum) B70.0
    larval B70.1
  Diplogonoporus (grandis) B71.8
  Dipylidium caninum B67.4
  Dirofilaria B74.8
  Dracunculus medinensis B72
  Drechslera (hawaiiensis) B43.8
  Ducrey Haemophilus (any location) A57
  due to or resulting from
    artificial insemination N98.0
    central venous catheter T80.219 ☑
      bloodstream T80.211 ☑
      exit or insertion site T80.212 ☑
      localized T80.212 ☑
      port or reservoir T80.212 ☑
      specified NEC T80.218 ☑
      tunnel T80.212 ☑
    device, implant or graft (*see also* Complications,
      by site and type, infection or inflammation)
      T85.79 ☑
      arterial graft NEC T82.7 ☑
      breast (implant) T85.79 ☑
      catheter NEC T85.79 ☑
        dialysis (renal) T82.7 ☑
          intraperitoneal T85.71 ☑
        infusion NEC T82.7 ☑
          cranial T85.735 ☑
          intrathecal T85.735 ☑
          spinal (epidural) (subdural) T85.735 ☑
          subarachnoid T85.735 ☑
        urinary T83.518 ☑
          cystostomy T83.510 ☑
          Hopkins T83.518 ☑
          ileostomy T83.518 ☑
          nephrostomy T83.512 ☑
          specified NEC T83.518 ☑
          urethral indwelling T83.511 ☑
          urostomy T83.518 ☑
      electronic (electrode) (pulse generator) (stimu-
        lator)
        bone T84.7 ☑
        cardiac T82.7 ☑
        nervous system T85.738 ☑
          brain T85.731 ☑
          cranial nerve T85.732 ☑
          gastric nerve T85.732 ☑
          generator pocket T85.734 ☑
          neurostimulator generator T85.734 ☑

Infection, infected, infective — *continued*
  due to or resulting from — *continued*
    device, implant or graft (*see also* Complications, by
      site and type, infection or inflammation) —
      continued
      electronic — *continued*
        nervous system — *continued*
          peripheral nerve T85.732 ☑
          sacral nerve T85.732 ☑
          spinal cord T85.733 ☑
          vagal nerve T85.732 ☑
          urinary (indwelling) T83.51 ☑
      fixation, internal (orthopedic) NEC — *see*
        Complication, fixation device, infection
      gastrointestinal (bile duct) (esophagus)
        T85.79 ☑
        neurostimulator electrode (lead) T85.732 ☑
      genital NEC T83.69 ☑
      heart NEC T82.7 ☑
        valve (prosthesis) T82.6 ☑
          graft T82.7 ☑
      joint prosthesis — *see* Complication, joint
        prosthesis, infection
      ocular (corneal graft) (orbital implant) NEC
        T85.79 ☑
      orthopedic NEC T84.7 ☑
      penile (cylinder) (pump) (resevoir) T83.61 ☑
      specified NEC T85.79 ☑
      testicular T83.62 ☑
      urinary NEC T83.598 ☑
        ileal conduit stent T83.593 ☑
        implanted neurostimulation T83.590 ☑
        implanted sphincter T83.591 ☑
        indwelling ureteral stent T83.592 ☑
        nephroureteral stent T83.593 ☑
        specified stent NEC T83.593 ☑
      vascular NEC T82.7 ☑
      ventricular intracranial (communicating) shunt
        T85.730 ☑
    Hickman catheter T80.219 ☑
      bloodstream T80.211 ☑
      localized T80.212 ☑
      specified NEC T80.218 ☑
    immunization or vaccination T88.0 ☑
    infusion, injection or transfusion NEC T80.29 ☑
    injury NEC — *code by* site under Wound, open
    peripherally inserted central catheter (PICC)
      T80.219 ☑
      bloodstream T80.211 ☑
      localized T80.212 ☑
      specified NEC T80.218 ☑
    portacath (port-a-cath) T80.219 ☑
      bloodstream T80.211 ☑
      localized T80.212 ☑
      specified NEC T80.218 ☑
    pulmonary artery catheter — *see* Infection, due to
      or resulting from, central venous catheter
    surgery T81.4 ☑
    Swan Ganz catheter — *see* Infection, due to or re-
      sulting from, central venous catheter
    triple lumen catheter T80.219 ☑
      bloodstream T80.211 ☑
      localized T80.212 ☑
      specified NEC T80.218 ☑
    umbilical venous catheter T80.219 ☑
      bloodstream T80.211 ☑
      localized T80.212 ☑
      specified NEC T80.218 ☑
  during labor NEC O75.3
  ear (middle) (*see also* Otitis media)
    external — *see* Otitis, externa, infective
    inner — *see* subcategory H83.0 ☑
  Eberthella typhosa A01.00
  Echinococcus — *see* Echinococcus
  echovirus
    as cause of disease classified elsewhere B97.12
    unspecified nature or site B34.1
  endocardium I33.0
  endocervix — *see* Cervicitis
  Entamoeba — *see* Amebiasis
  enteric — *see* Enteritis, infectious
  Enterobacter sakazakii B96.89
  Enterobius vermicularis B80
  enterostomy K94.12
  enterovirus B34.1
    as cause of disease classified elsewhere B97.10

Infection, infected, infective — *continued*
  enterovirus — *continued*
    as cause of disease classified elsewhere — *contin-ued*
      coxsackievirus B97.11
      echovirus B97.12
      specified NEC B97.19
  Entomophthora B46.8
  Epidermophyton — *see* Dermatophytosis
  epididymis — *see* Epididymitis
  episiotomy (puerperal) O86.0
  Erysipelothrix (insidiosa) (rhusiopathiae) — *see*
    Erysipeloid
  erythema infectiosum B08.3
  Escherichia (E.) coli NEC A49.8
    as cause of disease classified elsewhere (*see also*
      Escherichia coli) B96.20
    congenital P39.8
      sepsis P36.4
    generalized A41.51
    intestinal — *see* Enteritis, infectious, due to, Es-
      cherichia coli
  ethmoidal (chronic) (sinus) — *see* Sinusitis, ethmoidal
  eustachian tube (ear) — *see* Salpingitis, eustachian
  external auditory canal (meatus) NEC — *see* Otitis,
    externa, infective
  eye (purulent) — *see* Endophthalmitis, purulent
  eyelid — *see* Inflammation, eyelid
  fallopian tube — *see* Salpingo-oophoritis
  Fasciola (gigantica) (hepatica) (indica) B66.3
  Fasciolopsis (buski) B66.5
  filarial — *see* Infestation, filarial
  finger (skin) L08.9
    nail L03.01- ☑
      fungus B35.1
  fish tapeworm B70.0
    larval B70.1
  flagellate, intestinal A07.9
  fluke — *see* Infestation, fluke
  focal
    teeth (pulpal origin) K04.7
    tonsils J35.01
  Fonsecaea (compactum) (pedrosoi) B43.0
  food — *see* Intoxication, foodborne
  foot (skin) L08.9
    dermatophytic fungus B35.3
  Francisella tularensis — *see* Tularemia
  frontal (sinus) (chronic) — *see* Sinusitis, frontal
  fungus NOS B49
    beard B35.0
    dermatophytic — *see* Dermatophytosis
    foot B35.3
    groin B35.6
    hand B35.2
    nail B35.1
    pathogenic to compromised host only B48.8
    perianal (area) B35.6
    scalp B35.0
    skin B36.9
      foot B35.3
      hand B35.2
      toenails B35.1
  Fusarium B48.8
  gallbladder — *see* Cholecystitis
  gas bacillus — *see* Gangrene, gas
  gastrointestinal — *see* Enteritis, infectious
  generalized NEC — *see* Sepsis
  generator pocket, implanted electronic neurostimula-
    tor T85.734 ☑
  genital organ or tract
    female — *see* Disease, pelvis, inflammatory
    male N49.9
      multiple sites N49.8
      specified NEC N49.8
  Ghon tubercle, primary A15.7
  Giardia lamblia A07.1
  gingiva (chronic) K05.10
    acute K05.00
      nonplaque induced K05.01
      plaque induced K05.00
    nonplaque induced K05.11
    plaque induced K05.10
  glanders A24.0
  glenosporopsis B48.0
  Gnathostoma (spinigerum) B83.1
  Gongylonema B83.8
  gonococcal — *see* Gonococcus
  gram-negative bacilli NOS A49.9

Infection, infected, infective — *continued*
  guinea worm B72
  gum (chronic) K05.10
    acute K05.00
      nonplaque induced K05.01
      plaque induced K05.00
    nonplaque induced K05.11
    plaque induced K05.10
  Haemophilus — *see* Infection, Hemophilus
  heart — *see* Carditis
  Helicobacter pylori A04.8
    as cause of disease classified elsewhere B96.81
  helminths B83.9
    intestinal B82.0
      mixed (types classifiable to more than one of
        the titles B65.0-B81.3 and B81.8) B81.4
      specified type NEC B81.8
    specified type NEC B83.8
  Hemophilus
    aegyptius, systemic A48.4
    ducrey (any location) A57
    generalized A41.3
    influenzae NEC A49.2
      as cause of disease classified elsewhere B96.3
  herpes (simplex) (*see also* Herpes)
    congenital P35.2
    disseminated B00.7
    zoster B02.9
  herpesvirus, herpesviral — *see* Herpes
  Heterophyes (heterophyes) B66.8
  hip (joint) NEC M00.9
    due to internal joint prosthesis
      left T84.52 ☑
      right T84.51 ☑
    skin NEC L08.9
  Histoplasma — *see* Histoplasmosis
    American B39.4
    capsulatum B39.4
  hookworm B76.9
  human
    papilloma virus A63.0
    T-cell lymphotropic virus type-1 (HTLV-1) B33.3
  hydrocele N43.0
  Hymenolepis B71.0
  hypopharynx — *see* Pharyngitis
  inguinal (lymph) glands L04.1
    due to soft chancre A57
  intervertebral disc, pyogenic M46.30
    cervical region M46.32
    cervicothoracic region M46.33
    lumbar region M46.36
    lumbosacral region M46.37
    multiple sites M46.39
    occipito-atlanto-axial region M46.31
    sacrococcygeal region M46.38
    thoracic region M46.34
    thoracolumbar region M46.35
  intestine, intestinal — *see* Enteritis, infectious
    specified NEC A08.8
  intra-amniotic affecting newborn NEC P39.2
  Isospora belli or hominis A07.3
  Japanese B encephalitis A83.0
  jaw (bone) (lower) (upper) M27.2
  joint NEC M00.9
    due to internal joint prosthesis T84.50 ☑
  kidney (cortex) (hematogenous) N15.9
    with calculus N20.0
      with hydronephrosis N13.6
    following ectopic gestation O08.83
    pelvis and ureter (cystic) N28.85
    puerperal (postpartum) O86.21
    specified NEC N15.8
  Klebsiella (K.) pneumoniae NEC A49.8
    as cause of disease classified elsewhere B96.1
  knee (joint) NEC M00.9
    due to internal joint prosthesis
      left T84.54 ☑
      right T84.53 ☑
    joint M00.9
    skin L08.9
  Koch's — *see* Tuberculosis
  labia (majora) (minora) (acute) — *see* Vulvitis
  lacrimal
    gland — *see* Dacryoadenitis
    passages (duct) (sac) — *see* Inflammation, lacrimal,
      passages
  lancet fluke B66.2
  larynx NEC J38.7

☑ **Additional Character Required — Refer to the Tabular List for Character Selection**   ▽ **Subterms under main terms may continue to next column or page**

Infection, infected, infective — *continued*
  leg (skin) NOS L08.9
  Legionella pneumophila A48.1
    nonpneumonic A48.2
  Leishmania (*see also* Leishmaniasis)
    aethiopica B55.1
    braziliensis B55.2
    chagasi B55.0
    donovani B55.0
    infantum B55.0
    major B55.1
    mexicana B55.1
    tropica B55.1
  lentivirus, as cause of disease classified elsewhere
      B97.31
  Leptosphaeria senegalensis B47.0
  Leptospira interrogans A27.9
    autumnalis A27.89
    canicola A27.89
    hebdomadis A27.89
    icterohaemorrhagiae A27.0
    pomona A27.89
    specified type NEC A27.89
  leptospirochetal NEC — *see* Leptospirosis
  Listeria monocytogenes (*see also* Listeriosis)
    congenital P37.2
  Loa loa B74.3
    with conjunctival infestation B74.3
    eyelid B74.3
  Loboa loboi B48.0
  local, skin (staphylococcal) (streptococcal) L08.9
    abscess — *code by* site under Abscess
    cellulitis — *code by* site under Cellulitis
    specified NEC L08.89
    ulcer — *see* Ulcer, skin
  Loefflerella mallei A24.0
  lung (*see also* Pneumonia) J18.9
    atypical Mycobacterium A31.0
    spirochetal A69.8
    tuberculous — *see* Tuberculosis, pulmonary
    virus — *see* Pneumonia, viral
  lymph gland (*see also* Lymphadenitis, acute)
    mesenteric I88.0
  lymphoid tissue, base of tongue or posterior pharynx,
      NEC (chronic) J35.03
  Madurella (grisea) (mycetomii) B47.0
  major
    following ectopic or molar pregnancy O08.0
    puerperal, postpartum, childbirth O85
  Malassezia furfur B36.0
  Malleomyces
    mallei A24.0
    pseudomallei (whitmori) — *see* Melioidosis
  mammary gland N61.0
  Mansonella (ozzardi) (perstans) (streptocerca) B74.4
  mastoid — *see* Mastoiditis
  maxilla, maxillary M27.2
    sinus (chronic) — *see* Sinusitis, maxillary
  mediastinum J98.51
  Medina (worm) B72
  meibomian cyst or gland — *see* Hordeolum
  meninges — *see* Meningitis, bacterial
  meningococcal (*see also* condition) A39.9
    adrenals A39.1
    brain A39.81
    cerebrospinal A39.0
    conjunctiva A39.89
    endocardium A39.51
    heart A39.50
      endocardium A39.51
      myocardium A39.52
      pericardium A39.53
    joint A39.83
    meninges A39.0
    meningococcemia A39.4
      acute A39.2
      chronic A39.3
    myocardium A39.52
    pericardium A39.53
    retrobulbar neuritis A39.82
    specified site NEC A39.89
  mesenteric lymph nodes or glands NEC I88.0
  Metagonimus B66.8
  metatarsophalangeal M00.9
  methicillin
    resistant Staphylococcus aureus (MRSA) A49.02
    susceptible Staphylococcus aureus (MSSA) A49.01
  Microsporum, microsporic — *see* Dermatophytosis

Infection, infected, infective — *continued*
  mixed flora (bacterial) NEC A49.8
  Monilia — *see* Candidiasis
  Monosporium apiospermum B48.2
  mouth, parasitic B37.0
  Mucor — *see* Mucormycosis
  muscle NEC — *see* Myositis, infective
  mycelium NOS B49
  mycetoma B47.9
    actinomycotic NEC B47.1
    mycotic NEC B47.0
  Mycobacterium, mycobacterial — *see* Mycobacterium
  Mycoplasma NEC A49.3
    pneumoniae, as cause of disease classified else-
        where B96.0
  mycotic NOS B49
    pathogenic to compromised host only B48.8
    skin NOS B36.9
  myocardium NEC I40.0
  nail (chronic)
    with lymphangitis — *see* Lymphangitis, acute,
        digit
    finger L03.01- ☑
      fungus B35.1
    ingrowing L60.0
    toe L03.03- ☑
      fungus B35.1
  nasal sinus (chronic) — *see* Sinusitis
  nasopharynx — *see* Nasopharyngitis
  navel L08.82
  Necator americanus B76.1
  Neisseria — *see* Gonococcus
  Neotestudina rosatii B47.0
  newborn P39.9
    intra-amniotic NEC P39.2
    skin P39.4
    specified type NEC P39.8
  nipple N61.0
    associated with
      lactation O91.03
      pregnancy O91.01- ☑
      puerperium O91.02
  Nocardia — *see* Nocardiosis
  obstetrical surgical wound (puerperal) O86.0
  Oesophagostomum (apiostomum) B81.8
  Oestrus ovis — *see* Myiasis
  Oidium albicans B37.9
  Onchocerca (volvulus) — *see* Onchocerciasis
  oncovirus, as cause of disease classified elsewhere
      B97.32
  operation wound T81.4 ☑
  Opisthorchis (felineus) (viverrini) B66.0
  orbit, orbital — *see* Inflammation, orbit
  orthopoxvirus NEC B08.09
  ovary — *see* Salpingo-oophoritis
  Oxyuris vermicularis B80
  pancreas (acute) — *see* Pancreatitis, acute
    abscess — *see* Pancreatitis, acute
    specified NEC (*see also* Pancreatitis, acute) K85.80
  papillomavirus, as cause of disease classified elsewhere
      B97.7
  papovavirus NEC B34.4
  Paracoccidioides brasiliensis — *see* Paracoccidioidomy-
      cosis
  Paragonimus (westermani) B66.4
  parainfluenza virus B34.8
  parameningococcus NOS A39.9
  parapoxvirus B08.60
    specified NEC B08.69
  parasitic B89
  Parastrongylus
    cantonensis B83.2
    costaricensis B81.3
    paratyphoid A01.4
      Type A A01.1
      Type B A01.2
      Type C A01.3
  paraurethral ducts N34.2
  parotid gland — *see* Sialoadenitis
  parvovirus NEC B34.3
    as cause of disease classified elsewhere B97.6
  Pasteurella NEC A28.0
    multocida A28.0
    pestis — *see* Plague
    pseudotuberculosis A28.0
    septica (cat bite) (dog bite) A28.0
    tularensis — *see* Tularemia
  pelvic, female — *see* Disease, pelvis, inflammatory

Infection, infected, infective — *continued*
  Penicillium (marneffei) B48.4
  penis (glans) (retention) NEC N48.29
  periapical K04.5
  peridental, periodontal K05.20
    generalized — *see* Peridontitis, aggressive, gener-
        alized
    localized — *see* Peridontitis, aggressive, localized
  perinatal period P39.9
    specified type NEC P39.8
  perineal repair (puerperal) O86.0
  periorbital — *see* Inflammation, orbit
  perirectal K62.89
  perirenal — *see* Infection, kidney
  peritoneal — *see* Peritonitis
  periureteral N28.89
  Petriellidium boydii B48.2
  pharynx (*see also* Pharyngitis)
    coxsackievirus B08.5
    posterior, lymphoid (chronic) J35.03
  Phialophora
    gougerotii (subcutaneous abscess or cyst) B43.2
    jeanselmei (subcutaneous abscess or cyst) B43.2
    verrucosa (skin) B43.0
  Piedraia hortae B36.3
  pinta A67.9
    intermediate A67.1
    late A67.2
    mixed A67.3
    primary A67.0
  pinworm B80
  pityrosporum furfur B36.0
  pleuro-pneumonia-like organism (PPLO) NEC A49.3
    as cause of disease classified elsewhere B96.0
  pneumococcus, pneumococcal NEC A49.1
    as cause of disease classified elsewhere B95.3
    generalized (purulent) A40.3
      with pneumonia J13
  Pneumocystis carinii (pneumonia) B59
  Pneumocystis jiroveci (pneumonia) B59
  port or reservoir T80.212 ☑
  postoperative T81.4 ☑
  postoperative wound T81.4 ☑
  postprocedural T81.4 ☑
  postvaccinal T88.0 ☑
  prepuce NEC N47.7
    with penile inflammation N47.6
  prion — *see* Disease, prion, central nervous system
  prostate (capsule) — *see* Prostatitis
  Proteus (mirabilis) (morganii) (vulgaris) NEC A49.8
    as cause of disease classified elsewhere B96.4
  protozoal NEC B64
    intestinal A07.9
      specified NEC A07.8
    specified NEC B60.8
  Pseudallescheria boydii B48.2
  Pseudomonas NEC A49.8
    as cause of disease classified elsewhere B96.5
    mallei A24.0
    pneumonia J15.1
    pseudomallei — *see* Melioidosis
  puerperal O86.4
    genitourinary tract NEC O86.89
    major or generalized O85
    minor O86.4
    specified NEC O86.89
  pulmonary — *see* Infection, lung
  purulent — *see* Abscess
  Pyrenochaeta romeroi B47.0
  Q fever A78
  rectum (sphincter) K62.89
  renal (*see also* Infection, kidney)
    pelvis and ureter (cystic) N28.85
  reovirus, as cause of disease classified elsewhere B97.5
  respiratory (tract) NEC J98.8
    acute J22
    chronic J98.8
    influenzal (upper) (acute) — *see* Influenza, with,
        respiratory manifestations NEC
    lower (acute) J22
      chronic — *see* Bronchitis, chronic
    rhinovirus J00
    syncytial virus, as cause of disease classified else-
        where B97.4
    upper (acute) NOS J06.9
      chronic J39.8
      streptococcal J06.9
      viral NOS J06.9

Infection, infected, infective — *continued*
  resulting from
    presence of internal prosthesis, implant, graft —
          see Complications, by site and type, infection
  retortamoniasis A07.8
  retroperitoneal NEC K68.9
  retrovirus B33.3
    as cause of disease classified elsewhere B97.30
      human
        immunodeficiency, type 2 (HIV 2) B97.35
        T-cell lymphotropic
            type I (HTLV-I) B97.33
            type II (HTLV-II) B97.34
      lentivirus B97.31
      oncovirus B97.32
      specified NEC B97.39
  Rhinosporidium (seeberi) B48.1
  rhinovirus
    as cause of disease classified elsewhere B97.89
    unspecified nature or site B34.8
  Rhizopus — *see* Mucormycosis
  rickettsial NOS A79.9
  roundworm (large) NEC B82.0
    Ascariasis (*see also* Ascariasis) B77.9
  rubella — *see* Rubella
  Saccharomyces — *see* Candidiasis
  salivary duct or gland (any) — *see* Sialoadenitis
  Salmonella (aertrycke) (arizonae) (callinarum)
        (cholerae-suis) (enteritidis) (suipestifer) (ty-
        phimurium) A02.9
    with
      (gastro)enteritis A02.0
      sepsis A02.1
      specified manifestation NEC A02.8
    due to food (poisoning) A02.9
    hirschfeldii A01.3
    localized A02.20
      arthritis A02.23
      meningitis A02.21
      osteomyelitis A02.24
      pneumonia A02.22
      pyelonephritis A02.25
      specified NEC A02.29
    paratyphi A01.4
      A A01.1
      B A01.2
      C A01.3
    schottmuelleri A01.2
    typhi, typhosa — *see* Typhoid
  Sarcocystis A07.8
  scabies B86
  Schistosoma — *see* Infestation, Schistosoma
  scrotum (acute) NEC N49.2
  seminal vesicle — *see* Vesiculitis
  septic
    localized, skin — *see* Abscess
  sheep liver fluke B66.3
  Shigella A03.9
    boydii A03.2
    dysenteriae A03.0
    flexneri A03.1
    group
      A A03.0
      B A03.1
      C A03.2
      D A03.3
    Schmitz (-Stutzer) A03.0
    schmitzii A03.0
    shigae A03.0
    sonnei A03.3
    specified NEC A03.8
  shoulder (joint) NEC M00.9
    due to internal joint prosthesis T84.59 ☑
    skin NEC L08.9
  sinus (accessory) (chronic) (nasal) (*see also* Sinusitis)
    pilonidal — *see* Sinus, pilonidal
    skin NEC L08.89
  Skene's duct or gland — *see* Urethritis
  skin (local) (staphylococcal) (streptococcal) L08.9
    abscess — *code by* site under Abscess
    cellulitis — *code by* site under Cellulitis
    due to fungus B36.9
      specified type NEC B36.8
    mycotic B36.9
      specified type NEC B36.8
    newborn P39.4
    ulcer — *see* Ulcer, skin
  slow virus A81.9

Infection, infected, infective — *continued*
  slow virus — *continued*
    specified NEC A81.89
  Sparganum (mansoni) (proliferum) (baxteri) B70.1
  specific (*see also* Syphilis)
    to perinatal period — *see* Infection, congenital
  specified NEC B99.8
  spermatic cord NEC N49.1
  sphenoidal (sinus) — *see* Sinusitis, sphenoidal
  spinal cord NOS (*see also* Myelitis) G04.91
    abscess G06.1
    meninges — *see* Meningitis
    streptococcal G04.89
  Spirillum A25.0
  spirochetal NOS A69.9
    lung A69.8
    specified NEC A69.8
  spleen D73.89
  Sporotrichum, Sporothrix (schenckii) — *see* Sporotri-
        chosis
  staphylococcal, unspecified site
    as cause of disease classified elsewhere B95.8
      aureus (methicillin susceptible) (MSSA) B95.61
        methicillin resistant (MRSA) B95.62
      specified NEC B95.7
    aureus (methicillin susceptible) (MSSA) A49.01
      methicillin resistant (MRSA) A49.02
    food poisoning A05.0
    generalized (purulent) A41.2
    pneumonia — *see* Pneumonia, staphylococcal
  Stellantchasmus falcatus B66.8
  streptobacillus moniliformis A25.1
  streptococcal NEC A49.1
    as cause of disease classified elsewhere B95.5
    B genitourinary complicating
      childbirth O98.82
      pregnancy O98.81- ☑
      puerperium O98.83
    congenital
      sepsis P36.10
        group B P36.0
        specified NEC P36.19
    generalized (purulent) A40.9
  Streptomyces B47.1
  Strongyloides (stercoralis) — *see* Strongyloidiasis
  stump (amputation) (surgical) — *see* Complication,
        amputation stump, infection
  subcutaneous tissue, local L08.9
  suipestifer — *see* Infection, salmonella
  swimming pool bacillus A31.1
  Taenia — *see* Infestation, Taenia
  Taeniarhynchus saginatus B68.1
  tapeworm — *see* Infestation, tapeworm
  tendon (sheath) — *see* Tenosynovitis, infective NEC
  Ternidens diminutus B81.8
  testis — *see* Orchitis
  threadworm B80
  throat — *see* Pharyngitis
  thyroglossal duct K14.8
  toe (skin) L08.9
    cellulitis L03.03- ☑
      fungus B35.1
    nail L03.03- ☑
      fungus B35.1
  tongue NEC K14.0
    parasitic B37.0
  tonsil (and adenoid) (faucial) (lingual) (pharyngeal) —
        see Tonsillitis
  tooth, teeth K04.7
    periapical K04.7
    peridental, periodontal K05.20
      generalized — *see* Peridontitis, aggressive,
          generalized
      localized — *see* Peridontitis, aggressive, local-
          ized
    pulp K04.01
      irreversible K04.02
      reversible K04.01
    socket M27.3
  TORCH — *see* Infection, congenital
    without active infection P00.2
  Torula histolytica — *see* Cryptococcosis
  Toxocara (canis) (cati) (felis) B83.0
  Toxoplasma gondii — *see* Toxoplasma
  trachea, chronic J42
  trematode NEC — *see* Infestation, fluke
  trench fever A79.0

Infection, infected, infective — *continued*
  Treponema pallidum — *see* Syphilis
  Trichinella (spiralis) B75
  Trichomonas A59.9
    cervix A59.09
    intestine A07.8
    prostate A59.02
    specified site NEC A59.8
    urethra A59.03
    urogenitalis A59.00
    vagina A59.01
    vulva A59.01
  Trichophyton, trichophytic — *see* Dermatophytosis
  Trichosporon (beigelii) cutaneum B36.2
  Trichostrongylus B81.2
  Trichuris (trichiura) B79
  Trombicula (irritans) B88.0
  Trypanosoma
    brucei
      gambiense B56.0
      rhodesiense B56.1
    cruzi — *see* Chagas' disease
  tubal — *see* Salpingo-oophoritis
  tuberculous NEC — *see* Tuberculosis
  tubo-ovarian — *see* Salpingo-oophoritis
  tunica vaginalis N49.1
  tunnel T80.212 ☑
  tympanic membrane NEC — *see* Myringitis
  typhoid (abortive) (ambulant) (bacillus) — *see* Typhoid
  typhus A75.9
    flea-borne A75.2
    mite-borne A75.3
    recrudescent A75.1
    tick-borne A77.9
      African A77.1
      North Asian A77.2
  umbilicus L08.82
  ureter N28.86
  urethra — *see* Urethritis
  urinary (tract) N39.0
    bladder — *see* Cystitis
    complicating
      pregnancy O23.4- ☑
        specified type NEC O23.3- ☑
    kidney — *see* Infection, kidney
    newborn P39.3
    puerperal (postpartum) O86.20
    tuberculous A18.13
    urethra — *see* Urethritis
  uterus, uterine — *see* Endometritis
  vaccination T88.0 ☑
  vaccinia not from vaccination B08.011
  vagina (acute) — *see* Vaginitis
  varicella B01.9
  varicose veins — *see* Varix
  vas deferens NEC N49.1
  vesical — *see* Cystitis
  Vibrio
    cholerae A00.0
      El Tor A00.1
    parahaemolyticus (food poisoning) A05.3
    vulnificus
      as cause of disease classified elsewhere B96.82
      foodborne intoxication A05.5
  Vincent's (gum) (mouth) (tonsil) A69.1
  virus, viral NOS B34.9
    adenovirus
      as cause of disease classified elsewhere B97.0
      unspecified nature or site B34.0
    arbovirus, arbovirus arthropod-borne A94
    as cause of disease classified elsewhere B97.89
      adenovirus B97.0
      coronavirus B97.29
        SARS-associated B97.21
      coxsackievirus B97.11
      echovirus B97.12
      enterovirus B97.10
        coxsackievirus B97.11
        echovirus B97.12
        specified NEC B97.19
      human
        immunodeficiency, type 2 (HIV 2) B97.35
        metapneumovirus B97.81
        T-cell lymphotropic,
            type I (HTLV-I) B97.33
            type II (HTLV-II) B97.34
      papillomavirus B97.7
      parvovirus B97.6

Infection, infected, infective — continued
  virus, viral — continued
    as cause of disease classified elsewhere — continued
      reovirus B97.5
      respiratory syncytial B97.4
      retrovirus B97.30
        human
          immunodeficiency, type 2 (HIV 2) B97.35
          T-cell lymphotropic,
            type I (HTLV-I) B97.33
            type II (HTLV-II) B97.34
        lentivirus B97.31
        oncovirus B97.32
        specified NEC B97.39
      specified NEC B97.89
    central nervous system A89
      atypical A81.9
        specified NEC A81.89
      enterovirus NEC A88.8
        meningitis A87.0
      slow virus A81.9
        specified NEC A81.89
      specified NEC A88.8
    chest J98.8
    cotia B08.8
    coxsackie (see also Infection, coxsackie) B34.1
      as cause of disease classified elsewhere B97.11
    ECHO
      as cause of disease classified elsewhere B97.12
      unspecified nature or site B34.1
    encephalitis, tick-borne A84.9
    enterovirus, as cause of disease classified elsewhere
        B97.10
      coxsackievirus B97.11
      echovirus B97.12
      specified NEC B97.19
    exanthem NOS B09
    human metapneumovirus as cause of disease
        classified elsewhere B97.81
    human papilloma as cause of disease classified
        elsewhere B97.7
    intestine — see Enteritis, viral
    respiratory syncytial
      as cause of disease classified elsewhere B97.4
        bronchopneumonia J12.1
        common cold syndrome J00
        nasopharyngitis (acute) J00
    rhinovirus
      as cause of disease classified elsewhere B97.89
      unspecified nature or site B34.8
    slow A81.9
      specified NEC A81.89
    specified type NEC B33.8
      as cause of disease classified elsewhere B97.89
      unspecified nature or site B34.8
    unspecified nature or site B34.9
    West Nile — see Virus, West Nile
  vulva (acute) — see Vulvitis
  West Nile — see Virus, West Nile
  whipworm B79
  worms B83.9
    specified type NEC B83.8
  Wuchereria (bancrofti) B74.0
    malayi B74.1
  yatapoxvirus B08.70
    specified NEC B08.79
  yeast (see also Candidiasis) B37.9
  yellow fever — see Fever, yellow
  Yersinia
    enterocolitica (intestinal) A04.6
    pestis — see Plague
    pseudotuberculosis A28.2
  Zeis' gland — see Hordeolum
  Zika virus A92.5
  zoonotic bacterial NOS A28.9
  Zopfia senegalensis B47.0
Infective, infectious — see condition
Infertility
  female N97.9
    age-related N97.8
    associated with
      anovulation N97.0
      cervical (mucus) disease or anomaly N88.3
      congenital anomaly
        cervix N88.3
        fallopian tube N97.1
        uterus N97.2

Infertility — continued
  female — continued
    associated with — continued
      congenital anomaly — continued
        vagina N97.8
      dysmucorrhea N88.3
      fallopian tube disease or anomaly N97.1
      pituitary-hypothalamic origin E23.0
      specified origin NEC N97.8
      Stein-Leventhal syndrome E28.2
      uterine disease or anomaly N97.2
      vaginal disease or anomaly N97.8
    due to
      cervical anomaly N88.3
      fallopian tube anomaly N97.1
      ovarian failure E28.39
      Stein-Leventhal syndrome E28.2
      uterine anomaly N97.2
      vaginal anomaly N97.8
    nonimplantation N97.2
    origin
      cervical N88.3
      tubal (block) (occlusion) (stenosis) N97.1
      uterine N97.2
      vaginal N97.8
  male N46.9
    azoospermia N46.01
      extratesticular cause N46.029
        drug therapy N46.021
        efferent duct obstruction N46.023
        infection N46.022
        radiation N46.024
        specified cause NEC N46.029
        systemic disease N46.025
    oligospermia N46.11
      extratesticular cause N46.129
        drug therapy N46.121
        efferent duct obstruction N46.123
        infection N46.122
        radiation N46.124
        specified cause NEC N46.129
        systemic disease N46.125
    specified type NEC N46.8
Infestation B88.9
  Acanthocheilonema (perstans) (streptocerca) B74.4
  Acariasis B88.0
    demodex folliculorum B88.0
    sarcoptes scabiei B86
    trombiculae B88.0
  Agamofilaria streptocerca B74.4
  Ancylostoma, ankylostoma (braziliense) (caninum)
      (ceylanicum) (duodenale) B76.0
    americanum B76.1
    new world B76.1
  Anisakis larvae, anisakiasis B81.0
  arthropod NEC B88.2
  Ascaris lumbricoides — see Ascariasis
  Balantidium coli A07.0
  beef tapeworm B68.1
  Bothriocephalus (latus) B70.0
    larval B70.1
  broad tapeworm B70.0
    larval B70.1
  Brugia (malayi) B74.1
    timori B74.2
  candiru B88.8
  Capillaria
    hepatica B83.8
    philippinensis B81.1
  cat liver fluke B66.0
  cestodes B71.9
    diphyllobothrium — see Infestation, diphyllobothrium
    dipylidiasis B71.1
    hymenolepiasis B71.0
    specified type NEC B71.8
  chigger B88.0
  chigo, chigoe B88.1
  Clonorchis (sinensis) (liver) B66.1
  coccidial A07.3
  crab-lice B85.3
  Cysticercus cellulosae — see Cysticercosis
  Demodex (folliculorum) B88.0
  Dermanyssus gallinae B88.0
  Dermatobia (hominis) — see Myiasis
  Dibothriocephalus (latus) B70.0
    larval B70.1
  Dicrocoelium dendriticum B66.2

Infestation — continued
  Diphyllobothrium (adult) (latum) (intestinal) (pacificum) B70.0
    larval B70.1
  Diplogonoporus (grandis) B71.8
  Dipylidium caninum B67.4
  Distoma hepaticum B66.3
  dog tapeworm B67.4
  Dracunculus medinensis B72
  dragon worm B72
  dwarf tapeworm B71.0
  Echinococcus — see Echinococcus
  Echinostomum ilocanum B66.8
  Entamoeba (histolytica) — see Infection, Ameba
  Enterobius vermicularis B80
  eyelid
    in (due to)
      leishmaniasis B55.1
      loiasis B74.3
      onchocerciasis B73.09
      phthiriasis B85.3
    parasitic NOS B89
  eyeworm B74.3
  Fasciola (gigantica) (hepatica) (indica) B66.3
  Fasciolopsis (buski) (intestine) B66.5
  filarial B74.9
    bancroftian B74.0
    conjunctiva B74.9
    due to
      Acanthocheilonema (perstans) (streptocerca)
          B74.4
      Brugia (malayi) B74.1
        timori B74.2
      Dracunculus medinensis B72
      guinea worm B72
      loa loa B74.3
      Mansonella (ozzardi) (perstans) (streptocerca)
          B74.4
      Onchocerca volvulus B73.00
        eye B73.00
        eyelid B73.09
      Wuchereria (bancrofti) B74.0
    Malayan B74.1
    ozzardi B74.4
    specified type NEC B74.8
  fish tapeworm B70.0
    larval B70.1
  fluke B66.9
    blood NOS — see Schistosomiasis
    cat liver B66.0
    intestinal B66.5
    lancet B66.2
    liver (sheep) B66.3
      cat B66.0
      Chinese B66.1
      due to clonorchiasis B66.1
      oriental B66.1
    lung (oriental) B66.4
    sheep liver B66.3
    specified type NEC B66.8
  fly larvae — see Myiasis
  Gasterophilus (intestinalis) — see Myiasis
  Gastrodiscoides hominis B66.8
  Giardia lamblia A07.1
  Gnathostoma (spinigerum) B83.1
  Gongylonema B83.8
  guinea worm B72
  helminth B83.9
    angiostrongyliasis B83.2
      intestinal B81.3
    gnathostomiasis B83.1
    hirudiniasis, internal B83.4
    intestinal B82.0
      angiostrongyliasis B81.3
      anisakiasis B81.0
      ascariasis — see Ascariasis
      capillariasis B81.1
      cysticercosis — see Cysticercosis
      diphyllobothriasis — see Infestation, diphyllobothriasis
      dracunculiasis B72
      echinococcus — see Echinococcosis
      enterobiasis B80
      filariasis — see Infestation, filarial
      fluke — see Infestation, fluke
      hookworm — see Infestation, hookworm
      mixed (types classifiable to more than one of
          the titles B65.0-B81.3 and B81.8) B81.4

Infestation — continued
 helminth — continued
  intestinal — continued
   onchocerciasis — see Onchocerciasis
   schistosomiasis — see Infestation, schistosoma
   specified
    cestode NEC — see Infestation, cestode
    type NEC B81.8
   strongyloidiasis — see Strongyloidiasis
   taenia — see Infestation, taenia
   trichinellosis B75
   trichostrongyliasis B81.2
   trichuriasis B79
  specified type NEC B83.8
  syngamiasis B83.3
  visceral larva migrans B83.0
 Heterophyes (heterophyes) B66.8
 hookworm B76.9
  ancylostomiasis B76.0
  necatoriasis B76.1
  specified type NEC B76.8
 Hymenolepis (diminuta) (nana) B71.0
 intestinal NEC B82.9
 leeches (aquatic) (land) — see Hirudiniasis
 Leishmania — see Leishmaniasis
 lice, louse — see Infestation, Pediculus
 Linguatula B88.8
 Liponyssoides sanguineus B88.0
 Loa loa B74.3
  conjunctival B74.3
  eyelid B74.3
 louse — see Infestation, Pediculus
 maggots — see Myiasis
 Mansonella (ozzardi) (perstans) (streptocerca) B74.4
 Medina (worm) B72
 Metagonimus (yokogawai) B66.8
 microfilaria streptocerca — see Onchocerciasis
  eye B73.00
  eyelid B73.09
 mites B88.9
  scabic B86
 Monilia (albicans) — see Candidiasis
 mouth B37.0
 Necator americanus B76.1
 nematode NEC (intestinal) B82.0
  Ancylostoma B76.0
  conjunctiva NEC B83.9
  Enterobius vermicularis B80
  Gnathostoma spinigerum B83.1
  physaloptera B80
  specified NEC B81.8
  trichostrongylus B81.2
  trichuris (trichuria) B79
 Oesophagostomum (apiostomum) B81.8
 Oestrus ovis (see also Myiasis) B87.9
 Onchocerca (volvulus) — see Onchocerciasis
 orbit, parasitic NOS B89
 Oxyuris vermicularis B80
 Paragonimus (westermani) B66.4
 parasite, parasitic B89
  eyelid B89
  intestinal NOS B82.9
  mouth B37.0
  skin B88.9
  tongue B37.0
 Parastrongylus
  cantonensis B83.2
  costaricensis B81.3
 Pediculus B85.2
  body B85.1
  capitis (humanus) (any site) B85.0
  corporis (humanus) (any site) B85.1
  head B85.0
  mixed (classifiable to more than one of the titles
   B85.0 - B85.3) B85.4
  pubis (any site) B85.3
 Pentastoma B88.8
 Phthirus (pubis) (any site) B85.3
  with any infestation classifiable to B85.0 - B85.2
   B85.4
 pinworm B80
 pork tapeworm (adult) B68.0
 protozoal NEC B64
  intestinal A07.9
   specified NEC A07.8
  specified NEC B60.8
 pubic, louse B85.3

Infestation — continued
 rat tapeworm B71.0
 red bug B88.0
 roundworm (large) NEC B82.0
  Ascariasis (see also Ascariasis) B77.9
 sandflea B88.1
 Sarcoptes scabiei B86
 scabies B86
 Schistosoma B65.9
  bovis B65.8
  cercariae B65.3
  haematobium B65.0
  intercalatum B65.8
  japonicum B65.2
  mansoni B65.1
  mattheei B65.8
  mekongi B65.8
  specified type NEC B65.8
  spindale B65.8
 screw worms — see Myiasis
 skin NOS B88.9
 Sparganum (mansoni) (proliferum) (baxteri) B70.1
  larval B70.1
 specified type NEC B88.8
 Spirometra larvae B70.1
 Stellantchasmus falcatus B66.8
 Strongyloides stercoralis — see Strongyloidiasis
 Taenia B68.9
  diminuta B71.0
  echinococcus — see Echinococcus
  mediocanellata B68.1
  nana B71.0
  saginata B68.1
  solium (intestinal form) B68.0
   larval form — see Cysticercosis
 Taeniarhynchus saginatus B68.1
 tapeworm B71.9
  beef B68.1
  broad B70.0
   larval B70.1
  dog B67.4
  dwarf B71.0
  fish B70.0
   larval B70.1
  pork B68.0
  rat B71.0
 Ternidens diminutus B81.8
 Tetranychus molestissimus B88.0
 threadworm B80
 tongue B37.0
 Toxocara (canis) (cati) (felis) B83.0
 trematode(s) NEC — see Infestation, fluke
 Trichinella (spiralis) B75
 Trichocephalus B79
 Trichomonas — see Trichomoniasis
 Trichostrongylus B81.2
 Trichuris (trichiura) B79
 Trombicula (irritans) B88.0
 Tunga penetrans B88.1
 Uncinaria americana B76.1
 Vandellia cirrhosa B88.8
 whipworm B79
 worms B83.9
  intestinal B82.0
 Wuchereria (bancrofti) B74.0
Infiltrate, infiltration
 amyloid (generalized) (localized) — see Amyloidosis
 calcareous NEC R89.7
  localized — see Degeneration, by site
 calcium salt R89.7
 cardiac
  fatty — see Degeneration, myocardial
  glycogenic E74.02 [I43]
 corneal — see Edema, cornea
 eyelid — see Inflammation, eyelid
 glycogen, glycogenic — see Disease, glycogen storage
 heart, cardiac
  fatty — see Degeneration, myocardial
  glycogenic E74.02 [I43]
 inflammatory in vitreous H43.89
 kidney N28.89
 leukemic — see Leukemia
 liver K76.89
  fatty — see Fatty, liver NEC
  glycogen (see also Disease, glycogen storage)
   E74.03 [K77]
 lung R91.8
  eosinophilic J82

Infiltrate, infiltration — continued
 lymphatic (see also Leukemia, lymphatic) C91.9- ☑
  gland I88.9
 muscle, fatty M62.89
 myocardium, myocardial
  fatty — see Degeneration, myocardial
  glycogenic E74.02 [I43]
 on chest x-ray R91.8
 pulmonary R91.8
  with eosinophilia J82
 skin (lymphocytic) L98.6
 thymus (gland) (fatty) E32.8
 urine R39.0
 vesicant agent
  antineoplastic chemotherapy T80.810 ☑
  other agent NEC T80.818 ☑
 vitreous body H43.89
Infirmity R68.89
 senile R54
Inflammation, inflamed, inflammatory (with exudation)
 abducent (nerve) — see Strabismus, paralytic, sixth
  nerve
 accessory sinus (chronic) — see Sinusitis
 adrenal (gland) E27.8
 alveoli, teeth M27.3
  scorbutic E54
 anal canal, anus K62.89
 antrum (chronic) — see Sinusitis, maxillary
 appendix — see Appendicitis
 arachnoid — see Meningitis
 areola N61.0
  puerperal, postpartum or gestational — see Infection, nipple
 areolar tissue NOS L08.9
 artery — see Arteritis
 auditory meatus (external) — see Otitis, externa
 Bartholin's gland N75.8
 bile duct (common) (hepatic) or passage — see
  Cholangitis
 bladder — see Cystitis
 bone — see Osteomyelitis
 brain (see also Encephalitis)
  membrane — see Meningitis
 breast N61.0
  puerperal, postpartum, gestational — see Mastitis,
   obstetric
 broad ligament — see Disease, pelvis, inflammatory
 bronchi — see Bronchitis
 catarrhal J00
 cecum — see Appendicitis
 cerebral (see also Encephalitis)
  membrane — see Meningitis
 cerebrospinal
  meningococcal A39.0
 cervix (uteri) — see Cervicitis
 chest J98.8
 chorioretinal H30.9- ☑
  cyclitis — see Cyclitis
  disseminated H30.10- ☑
   generalized H30.13- ☑
   peripheral H30.12- ☑
   posterior pole H30.11- ☑
  epitheliopathy — see Epitheliopathy
  focal H30.00- ☑
   juxtapapillary H30.01- ☑
   macular H30.04- ☑
   paramacular — see Inflammation, chorioretinal,
    focal, macular
   peripheral H30.03- ☑
   posterior pole H30.02- ☑
  specified type NEC H30.89- ☑
 choroid — see Inflammation, chorioretinal
 chronic, postmastoidectomy cavity — see Complications, postmastoidectomy, inflammation
 colon — see Enteritis
 connective tissue (diffuse) NEC — see Disorder, soft
  tissue, specified type NEC
 cornea — see Keratitis
 corpora cavernosa N48.29
 cranial nerve — see Disorder, nerve, cranial
 Douglas' cul-de-sac or pouch (chronic) N73.2
 due to device, implant or graft (see also Complications,
  by site and type, infection or inflammation)
  arterial graft T82.7 ☑
  breast (implant) T85.79 ☑
  catheter T85.79 ☑

Inflammation, inflamed, inflammatory —
continued
  due to device, implant or graft (*see also* Complications,
    by site and type, infection or inflammation) —
    continued
    catheter — *continued*
      dialysis (renal) T82.7 ☑
        intraperitoneal T85.71 ☑
      infusion T82.7 ☑
        cranial T85.735 ☑
        intrathecal T85.735 ☑
        spinal (epidural) (subdural) T85.735 ☑
        subarachnoid T85.735 ☑
      urinary T83.518 ☑
        cystostomy T83.510 ☑
        Hopkins T83.518 ☑
        ileostomy T83.518 ☑
        nephrostomy T83.512 ☑
        specified NEC T83.518 ☑
        urethral indwelling T83.511 ☑
        urostomy T83.518 ☑
    electronic (electrode) (pulse generator) (stimulator)
      bone T84.7 ☑
      cardiac T82.7 ☑
      nervous system T85.738 ☑
        brain T85.731 ☑
        cranial nerve T85.732 ☑
        gastric nerve T85.732 ☑
        neurostimulator generator T85.734 ☑
        peripheral nerve T85.732 ☑
        sacral nerve T85.732 ☑
        spinal cord T85.733 ☑
        vagal nerve T85.732 ☑
      urinary T83.590 ☑
    fixation, internal (orthopedic) NEC — *see* Compli-
      cation, fixation device, infection
    gastrointestinal (bile duct) (esophagus) T85.79 ☑
      neurostimulator electrode (lead) T85.732 ☑
    genital NEC T83.69 ☑
    heart NEC T82.7 ☑
      valve (prosthesis) T82.6 ☑
      graft T82.7 ☑
    joint prosthesis — *see* Complication, joint prosthe-
      sis, infection
    ocular (corneal graft) (orbital implant) NEC
      T85.79 ☑
    orthopedic NEC T84.7 ☑
    penile (cylinder) (pump) (resevoir) T83.61 ☑
    specified NEC T85.79 ☑
    testicular T83.62 ☑
    urinary NEC T83.598 ☑
      ileal conduit stent T83.593 ☑
      implanted neurostimulation T83.590 ☑
      implanted sphincter T83.591 ☑
      indwelling ureteral stent T83.592 ☑
      nephroureteral stent T83.593 ☑
      specified stent NEC T83.593 ☑
    vascular NEC T82.7 ☑
    ventricular intracranial (communicating) shunt
      T85.730 ☑
  duodenum K29.80
    with bleeding K29.81
  dura mater — *see* Meningitis
  ear (middle) (*see also* Otitis, media)
    external — *see* Otitis, externa
    inner — *see* subcategory H83.0 ☑
  epididymis — *see* Epididymitis
  esophagus K20.9
  ethmoidal (sinus) (chronic) — *see* Sinusitis, ethmoidal
  eustachian tube (catarrhal) — *see* Salpingitis, eustachi-
    an
  eyelid H01.9
    abscess — *see* Abscess, eyelid
    blepharitis — *see* Blepharitis
    chalazion — *see* Chalazion
    dermatosis (noninfectious) — *see* Dermatosis,
      eyelid
    hordeolum — *see* Hordeolum
    specified NEC H01.8
  fallopian tube — *see* Salpingo-oophoritis
  fascia — *see* Myositis
  follicular, pharynx J31.2
  frontal (sinus) (chronic) — *see* Sinusitis, frontal
  gallbladder — *see* Cholecystitis
  gastric — *see* Gastritis
  gastrointestinal — *see* Enteritis

Inflammation, inflamed, inflammatory —
continued
  genital organ (internal) (diffuse)
    female — *see* Disease, pelvis, inflammatory
    male N49.9
      multiple sites N49.8
      specified NEC N49.8
  gland (lymph) — *see* Lymphadenitis
  glottis — *see* Laryngitis
  granular, pharynx J31.2
  gum K05.10
    nonplaque induced K05.11
    plaque induced K05.10
  heart — *see* Carditis
  hepatic duct — *see* Cholangitis
  ileoanal (internal) pouch K91.850
  ileum (*see also* Enteritis)
    regional or terminal — *see* Enteritis, regional
  intestinal pouch K91.850
  intestine (any part) — *see* Enteritis
  jaw (acute) (bone) (chronic) (lower) (suppurative)
    (upper) M27.2
  joint NEC — *see* Arthritis
    sacroiliac M46.1
  kidney — *see* Nephritis
  knee (joint) M13.169
    tuberculous A18.02
  labium (majus) (minus) — *see* Vulvitis
  lacrimal
    gland — *see* Dacryoadenitis
    passages (duct) (sac) (*see also* Dacryocystitis)
      canaliculitis — *see* Canaliculitis, lacrimal
  larynx — *see* Laryngitis
  leg NOS L08.9
  lip K13.0
  liver (capsule) (*see also* Hepatitis)
    chronic K73.9
    suppurative K75.0
  lung (acute) (*see also* Pneumonia)
    chronic J98.4
  lymph gland or node — *see* Lymphadenitis
  lymphatic vessel — *see* Lymphangitis
  maxilla, maxillary M27.2
    sinus (chronic) — *see* Sinusitis, maxillary
  membranes of brain or spinal cord — *see* Meningitis
  meninges — *see* Meningitis
  mouth K12.1
  muscle — *see* Myositis
  myocardium — *see* Myocarditis
  nasal sinus (chronic) — *see* Sinusitis
  nasopharynx — *see* Nasopharyngitis
  navel L08.82
  nerve NEC — *see* Neuralgia
  nipple N61.0
    puerperal, postpartum or gestational — *see* Infec-
      tion, nipple
  nose — *see* Rhinitis
  oculomotor (nerve) — *see* Strabismus, paralytic, third
    nerve
  optic nerve — *see* Neuritis, optic
  orbit (chronic) H05.10
    acute H05.00
      abscess — *see* Abscess, orbit
      cellulitis — *see* Cellulitis, orbit
      osteomyelitis — *see* Osteomyelitis, orbit
      periostitis — *see* Periostitis, orbital
      tenonitis — *see* Tenonitis, eye
    granuloma — *see* Granuloma, orbit
    myositis — *see* Myositis, orbital
  ovary — *see* Salpingo-oophoritis
  oviduct — *see* Salpingo-oophoritis
  pancreas (acute) — *see* Pancreatitis
  parametrium N73.0
  parotid region L08.9
  pelvis, female — *see* Disease, pelvis, inflammatory
  penis (corpora cavernosa) N48.29
  perianal K62.89
  pericardium — *see* Pericarditis
  perineum (female) (male) L08.9
  perirectal K62.89
  peritoneum — *see* Peritonitis
  periuterine — *see* Disease, pelvis, inflammatory
  perivesical — *see* Cystitis
  petrous bone (acute) (chronic) — *see* Petrositis
  pharynx (acute) — *see* Pharyngitis
  pia mater — *see* Meningitis
  pleura — *see* Pleurisy

Inflammation, inflamed, inflammatory —
continued
  polyp, colon (*see also* Polyp, colon, inflammatory)
    K51.40
  prostate (*see also* Prostatitis)
    specified type NEC N41.8
  rectosigmoid — *see* Rectosigmoiditis
  rectum (*see also* Proctitis) K62.89
  respiratory, upper (*see also* Infection, respiratory, up-
    per) J06.9
    acute, due to radiation J70.0
    chronic, due to external agent — *see* condition,
      respiratory, chronic, due to
    due to
      chemicals, gases, fumes or vapors (inhalation)
        J68.2
      radiation J70.1
  retina — *see* Chorioretinitis
  retrocecal — *see* Appendicitis
  retroperitoneal — *see* Peritonitis
  salivary duct or gland (any) (suppurative) — *see*
    Sialoadenitis
  scorbutic, alveoli, teeth E54
  scrotum N49.2
  seminal vesicle — *see* Vesiculitis
  sigmoid — *see* Enteritis
  sinus — *see* Sinusitis
  Skene's duct or gland — *see* Urethritis
  skin L08.9
  spermatic cord N49.1
  sphenoidal (sinus) — *see* Sinusitis, sphenoidal
  spinal
    cord — *see* Encephalitis
    membrane — *see* Meningitis
    nerve — *see* Disorder, nerve
  spine — *see* Spondylopathy, inflammatory
  spleen (capsule) D73.89
  stomach — *see* Gastritis
  subcutaneous tissue L08.9
  suprarenal (gland) E27.8
  synovial — *see* Tenosynovitis
  tendon (sheath) NEC — *see* Tenosynovitis
  testis — *see* Orchitis
  throat (acute) — *see* Pharyngitis
  thymus (gland) E32.8
  thyroid (gland) — *see* Thyroiditis
  tongue K14.0
  tonsil — *see* Tonsillitis
  trachea — *see* Tracheitis
  trochlear (nerve) — *see* Strabismus, paralytic, fourth
    nerve
  tubal — *see* Salpingo-oophoritis
  tuberculous NEC — *see* Tuberculosis
  tubo-ovarian — *see* Salpingo-oophoritis
  tunica vaginalis N49.1
  tympanic membrane — *see* Tympanitis
  umbilicus, umbilical L08.82
  uterine ligament — *see* Disease, pelvis, inflammatory
  uterus (catarrhal) — *see* Endometritis
  uveal tract (anterior) NOS (*see also* Iridocyclitis)
    posterior — *see* Chorioretinitis
  vagina — *see* Vaginitis
  vas deferens N49.1
  vein (*see also* Phlebitis)
    intracranial or intraspinal (septic) G08
    thrombotic I80.9
      leg — *see* Phlebitis, leg
      lower extremity — *see* Phlebitis, leg
  vocal cord J38.3
  vulva — *see* Vulvitis
  Wharton's duct (suppurative) — *see* Sialoadenitis
Inflation, lung, imperfect (newborn) — *see* Atelectasis
Influenza (bronchial) (epidemic) (respiratory (upper))
  (unidentified influenza virus) J11.1
  with
    digestive manifestations J11.2
    encephalopathy J11.81
    enteritis J11.2
    gastroenteritis J11.2
    gastrointestinal manifestations J11.2
    laryngitis J11.1
    myocarditis J11.82
    otitis media J11.83
    pharyngitis J11.1
    pneumonia J11.00
      specified type J11.08
    respiratory manifestations NEC J11.1

Index

Influenza — Injury

Influenza — *continued*
with — *continued*
specified manifestation NEC J11.89
A/H5N1 (*see also* Influenza, due to, identified novel influenza A virus) J09.X2
avian (*see also* Influenza, due to, identified novel influenza A virus) J09.X2
bird (*see also* Influenza, due to, identified novel influenza A virus) J09.X2
due to
avian (*see also* Influenza, due to, identified novel influenza A virus) J09.X2
identified influenza virus NEC J10.1
with
digestive manifestations J10.2
encephalopathy J10.81
enteritis J10.2
gastroenteritis J10.2
gastrointestinal manifestations J10.2
laryngitis J10.1
myocarditis J10.82
otitis media J10.83
pharyngitis J10.1
pneumonia (unspecified type) J10.00
with same identified influenza virus J10.01
specified type NEC J10.08
respiratory manifestations NEC J10.1
specified manifestation NEC J10.89
identified novel influenza A virus J09.X2
with
digestive manifestations J09.X3
encephalopathy J09.X9
enteritis J09.X3
gastroenteritis J09.X3
gastrointestinal manifestations J09.X3
laryngitis J09.X2
myocarditis J09.X9
otitis media J09.X9
pharyngitis J09.X2
pneumonia J09.X1
respiratory manifestations NEC J09.X2
specified manifestation NEC J09.X9
upper respiratory symptoms J09.X2
novel (2009) H1N1 influenza (*see also* Influenza, due to, identified influenza virus NEC) J10.1
novel influenza A/H1N1 (*see also* Influenza, due to, identified influenza virus NEC) J10.1
of other animal origin, not bird or swine (*see also* Influenza, due to, identified novel influenza A virus) J09.X2
swine (viruses that normally cause infections in pigs) (*see also* Influenza, due to, identified novel influenza A virus) J09.X2
Influenzal — *see* Influenza
Influenza-like disease — *see* Influenza
Infraction, Freiberg's (metatarsal head) — *see* Osteochondrosis, juvenile, metatarsus
Infraeruption of tooth (teeth) M26.34
Infusion complication, misadventure, or reaction — *see* Complications, infusion
Ingestion
chemical — *see* Table of Drugs and Chemicals, by substance, poisoning
drug or medicament
correct substance properly administered — *see* Table of Drugs and Chemicals, by drug, adverse effect
overdose or wrong substance given or taken — *see* Table of Drugs and Chemicals, by drug, poisoning
foreign body — *see* Foreign body, alimentary tract
tularemia A21.3
Ingrowing
hair (beard) L73.1
nail (finger) (toe) L60.0
Inguinal (*see also* condition)
testicle Q53.9
bilateral Q53.212
unilateral Q53.112
Inhalant-induced
anxiety disorder F18.980
depressive disorder F18.94
major neurocognitive disorder F18.97
mild neurocognitive disorder F18.988
psychotic disorder F18.959
Inhalation
anthrax A22.1

Inhalation — *continued*
flame T27.3 ☑
food or foreign body — *see* Foreign body, by site
gases, fumes, or vapors NEC T59.9- ☑
specified agent — *see* Table of Drugs and Chemicals, by substance
liquid or vomitus — *see* Asphyxia
meconium (newborn) P24.00
with
with respiratory symptoms P24.01
pneumonia (pneumonitis) P24.01
mucus — *see* Asphyxia, mucus
oil or gasoline (causing suffocation) — *see* Foreign body, by site
smoke J70.5
due to chemicals, gases, fumes and vapors J68.9
steam — *see* Toxicity, vapors
stomach contents or secretions — *see* Foreign body, by site
due to anesthesia (general) (local) or other sedation T88.59 ☑
in labor and delivery O74.0
in pregnancy O29.01- ☑
postpartum, puerperal O89.01
Inhibition, orgasm
female F52.31
male F52.32
Inhibitor, systemic lupus erythematosus (presence of) D68.62
Iniencephalus, iniencephaly Q00.2
Injection, traumatic jet (air) (industrial) (water) (paint or dye) T70.4 ☑
Injury (*see also* specified injury type) T14.90 ☑
abdomen, abdominal S39.91 ☑
blood vessel — *see* Injury, blood vessel, abdomen
cavity — *see* Injury, intra-abdominal
contusion S30.1 ☑
internal — *see* Injury, intra-abdominal
intra-abdominal organ — *see* Injury, intra-abdominal
nerve — *see* Injury, nerve, abdomen
open — *see* Wound, open, abdomen
specified NEC S39.81 ☑
superficial — *see* Injury, superficial, abdomen
Achilles tendon S86.00- ☑
laceration S86.02- ☑
specified type NEC S86.09- ☑
strain S86.01- ☑
acoustic, resulting in deafness — *see* Injury, nerve, acoustic
adrenal (gland) S37.819 ☑
contusion S37.812 ☑
laceration S37.813 ☑
specified type NEC S37.818 ☑
alveolar (process) S09.93 ☑
ankle S99.91- ☑
contusion — *see* Contusion, ankle
dislocation — *see* Dislocation, ankle
fracture — *see* Fracture, ankle
nerve — *see* Injury, nerve, ankle
open — *see* Wound, open, ankle
specified type NEC S99.81- ☑
sprain — *see* Sprain, ankle
superficial — *see* Injury, superficial, ankle
anterior chamber, eye — *see* Injury, eye, specified site NEC
anus — *see* Injury, abdomen
aorta (thoracic) S25.00 ☑
abdominal S35.00 ☑
laceration (minor) (superficial) S35.01 ☑
major S35.02 ☑
specified type NEC S35.09 ☑
laceration (minor) (superficial) S25.01 ☑
major S25.02 ☑
specified type NEC S25.09 ☑
arm (upper) S49.9- ☑
blood vessel — *see* Injury, blood vessel, arm
contusion — *see* Contusion, arm, upper
fracture — *see* Fracture, humerus
lower — *see* Injury, forearm
muscle — *see* Injury, muscle, shoulder
nerve — *see* Injury, nerve, arm
open — *see* Wound, open, arm
specified type NEC S49.8- ☑
superficial — *see* Injury, superficial, arm

Injury — *continued*
artery (complicating trauma) (*see also* Injury, blood vessel, by site)
cerebral or meningeal — *see* Injury, intracranial
auditory canal (external) (meatus) S09.91 ☑
auricle, auris, ear S09.91 ☑
axilla — *see* Injury, shoulder
back — *see* Injury, back, lower
bile duct S36.13 ☑
birth (*see also* Birth, injury) P15.9
bladder (sphincter) S37.20 ☑
at delivery O71.5
contusion S37.22 ☑
laceration S37.23 ☑
obstetrical trauma O71.5
specified type NEC S37.29 ☑
blast (air) (hydraulic) (immersion) (underwater) NEC T14.8 ☑
acoustic nerve trauma — *see* Injury, nerve, acoustic
bladder — *see* Injury, bladder
brain — *see* Concussion
colon — *see* Injury, intestine, large
ear (primary) S09.31- ☑
secondary S09.39- ☑
generalized T70.8 ☑
lung — *see* Injury, intrathoracic, lung
multiple body organs T70.8 ☑
peritoneum S36.81 ☑
rectum S36.61 ☑
retroperitoneum S36.898 ☑
small intestine S36.419 ☑
duodenum S36.410 ☑
specified site NEC S36.418 ☑
specified
intra-abdominal organ NEC S36.898 ☑
pelvic organ NEC S37.899 ☑
blood vessel NEC T14.8 ☑
abdomen S35.9 ☑
aorta — *see* Injury, aorta, abdominal
celiac artery — *see* Injury, blood vessel, celiac artery
iliac vessel — *see* Injury, blood vessel, iliac
laceration S35.91 ☑
mesenteric vessel — *see* Injury, mesenteric
portal vein — *see* Injury, blood vessel, portal vein
renal vessel — *see* Injury, blood vessel, renal
specified vessel NEC S35.8X- ☑
splenic vessel — *see* Injury, blood vessel, splenic
vena cava — *see* Injury, vena cava, inferior
ankle — *see* Injury, blood vessel, foot
aorta (abdominal) (thoracic) — *see* Injury, aorta
arm (upper) NEC S45.90- ☑
forearm — *see* Injury, blood vessel, forearm
laceration S45.91- ☑
specified
site NEC S45.80- ☑
laceration S45.81- ☑
specified type NEC S45.89- ☑
type NEC S45.99- ☑
superficial vein S45.30- ☑
laceration S45.31- ☑
specified type NEC S45.39- ☑
axillary
artery S45.00- ☑
laceration S45.01- ☑
specified type NEC S45.09- ☑
vein S45.20- ☑
laceration S45.21- ☑
specified type NEC S45.29- ☑
azygos vein — *see* Injury, blood vessel, thoracic, specified site NEC
brachial
artery S45.10- ☑
laceration S45.11- ☑
specified type NEC S45.19- ☑
vein S45.20- ☑
laceration S45.219 ☑
specified type NEC S45.29- ☑
carotid artery (common) (external) (internal, extracranial) S15.00- ☑
internal, intracranial S06.8- ☑
laceration (minor) (superficial) S15.01- ☑
major S15.02- ☑
specified type NEC S15.09- ☑

190
☑ Additional Character Required — Refer to the Tabular List for Character Selection
🔻 Subterms under main terms may continue to next column or page

Injury — *continued*
  blood vessel — *continued*
    celiac artery S35.219 ✓
      branch S35.299 ✓
        laceration (minor) (superficial) S35.291 ✓
          major S35.292 ✓
        specified NEC S35.298 ✓
      laceration (minor) (superficial) S35.211 ✓
        major S35.212 ✓
      specified type NEC S35.218 ✓
    cerebral — *see* Injury, intracranial
    deep plantar — *see* Injury, blood vessel, plantar artery
    digital (hand) — *see* Injury, blood vessel, finger
    dorsal
      artery (foot) S95.00- ✓
        laceration S95.01- ✓
        specified type NEC S95.09- ✓
      vein (foot) S95.20- ✓
        laceration S95.21- ✓
        specified type NEC S95.29- ✓
    due to accidental laceration during procedure — *see* Laceration, accidental complicating surgery
    extremity — *see* Injury, blood vessel, limb
    femoral
      artery (common) (superficial) S75.00- ✓
        laceration (minor) (superficial) S75.01- ✓
          major S75.02- ✓
        specified type NEC S75.09- ✓
      vein (hip level) (thigh level) S75.10- ✓
        laceration (minor) (superficial) S75.11- ✓
          major S75.12- ✓
        specified type NEC S75.19- ✓
    finger S65.50- ✓
      index S65.50- ✓
        laceration S65.51- ✓
        specified type NEC S65.59- ✓
      laceration S65.51- ✓
      little S65.50- ✓
        laceration S65.51- ✓
        specified type NEC S65.59- ✓
      middle S65.50- ✓
        laceration S65.51- ✓
        specified type NEC S65.59- ✓
      specified type NEC S65.59- ✓
      thumb — *see* Injury, blood vessel, thumb
    foot S95.90- ✓
      dorsal
        artery — *see* Injury, blood vessel, dorsal, artery
        vein — *see* Injury, blood vessel, dorsal, vein
      laceration S95.91- ✓
      plantar artery — *see* Injury, blood vessel, plantar artery
      specified
        site NEC S95.80- ✓
          laceration S95.81- ✓
          specified type NEC S95.89- ✓
        specified type NEC S95.99- ✓
    forearm S55.90- ✓
      laceration S55.91- ✓
      radial artery — *see* Injury, blood vessel, radial artery
      specified
        site NEC S55.80- ✓
          laceration S55.81- ✓
          specified type NEC S55.89- ✓
        type NEC S55.99- ✓
      ulnar artery — *see* Injury, blood vessel, ulnar artery
      vein S55.20- ✓
        laceration S55.21- ✓
        specified type NEC S55.29- ✓
    gastric
      artery — *see* Injury, mesenteric, artery, branch
      vein — *see* Injury, blood vessel, abdomen
    gastroduodenal artery — *see* Injury, mesenteric, artery, branch
    greater saphenous vein (lower leg level) S85.30- ✓
      hip (and thigh) level S75.20- ✓
        laceration (minor) (superficial) S75.21- ✓
          major S75.22- ✓
        specified type NEC S75.29- ✓
      laceration S85.31- ✓
      specified type NEC S85.39- ✓

Injury — *continued*
  blood vessel — *continued*
    hand (level) S65.90- ✓
      finger — *see* Injury, blood vessel, finger
      laceration S65.91- ✓
      palmar arch — *see* Injury, blood vessel, palmar arch
      radial artery — *see* Injury, blood vessel, radial artery, hand
      specified
        site NEC S65.80- ✓
          laceration S65.81- ✓
          specified type NEC S65.89- ✓
        type NEC S65.99- ✓
      thumb — *see* Injury, blood vessel, thumb
      ulnar artery — *see* Injury, blood vessel, ulnar artery, hand
    head S09.0 ✓
      intracranial — *see* Injury, intracranial
      multiple S09.0 ✓
    hepatic
      artery — *see* Injury, mesenteric, artery
      vein — *see* Injury, vena cava, inferior
    hip S75.90- ✓
      femoral artery — *see* Injury, blood vessel, femoral, artery
      femoral vein — *see* Injury, blood vessel, femoral, vein
      greater saphenous vein — *see* Injury, blood vessel, greater saphenous, hip level
      laceration S75.91- ✓
      specified
        site NEC S75.80- ✓
          laceration S75.81- ✓
          specified type NEC S75.89- ✓
        type NEC S75.99- ✓
    hypogastric (artery) (vein) — *see* Injury, blood vessel, iliac
    iliac S35.5- ✓
      artery S35.51- ✓
      specified vessel NEC S35.5- ✓
      uterine vessel — *see* Injury, blood vessel, uterine
      vein S35.51- ✓
    innominate — *see* Injury, blood vessel, thoracic, innominate
    intercostal (artery) (vein) — *see* Injury, blood vessel, thoracic, intercostal
    jugular vein (external) S15.20- ✓
      internal S15.30- ✓
        laceration (minor) (superficial) S15.31- ✓
          major S15.32- ✓
        specified type NEC S15.39- ✓
      laceration (minor) (superficial) S15.21- ✓
        major S15.22- ✓
      specified type NEC S15.29- ✓
    leg (level) (lower) S85.90- ✓
      greater saphenous — *see* Injury, blood vessel, greater saphenous
      laceration S85.91- ✓
      lesser saphenous — *see* Injury, blood vessel, lesser saphenous
      peroneal artery — *see* Injury, blood vessel, peroneal artery
      popliteal
        artery — *see* Injury, blood vessel, popliteal, artery
        vein — *see* Injury, blood vessel, popliteal, vein
      specified
        site NEC S85.80- ✓
          laceration S85.81- ✓
          specified type NEC S85.89- ✓
        type NEC S85.99- ✓
      thigh — *see* Injury, blood vessel, hip
      tibial artery — *see* Injury, blood vessel, tibial artery
    lesser saphenous vein (lower leg level) S85.40- ✓
      laceration S85.41- ✓
      specified type NEC S85.49- ✓
    limb
      lower — *see* Injury, blood vessel, leg
      upper — *see* Injury, blood vessel, arm
    lower back — *see* Injury, blood vessel, abdomen
      specified NEC — *see* Injury, blood vessel, abdomen, specified, site NEC

Injury — *continued*
  blood vessel — *continued*
    mammary (artery) (vein) — *see* Injury, blood vessel, thoracic, specified site NEC
    mesenteric (inferior) (superior)
      artery — *see* Injury, mesenteric, artery
      vein — *see* Injury, blood vessel, mesenteric, vein
    neck S15.9 ✓
      specified site NEC S15.8 ✓
    ovarian (artery) (vein) — *see* subcategory S35.8 ✓
    palmar arch (superficial) S65.20- ✓
      deep S65.30- ✓
        laceration S65.31- ✓
        specified type NEC S65.39- ✓
      laceration S65.21- ✓
      specified type NEC S65.29- ✓
    pelvis — *see* Injury, blood vessel, abdomen
      specified NEC — *see* Injury, blood vessel, abdomen, specified, site NEC
    peroneal artery S85.20- ✓
      laceration S85.21- ✓
      specified type NEC S85.29- ✓
    plantar artery (deep) (foot) S95.10- ✓
      laceration S95.11- ✓
      specified type NEC S95.19- ✓
    popliteal
      artery S85.00- ✓
        laceration S85.01- ✓
        specified type NEC S85.09- ✓
      vein S85.50- ✓
        laceration S85.51- ✓
        specified type NEC S85.59- ✓
    portal vein S35.319 ✓
      laceration S35.311 ✓
      specified type NEC S35.318 ✓
    precerebral — *see* Injury, blood vessel, neck
    pulmonary (artery) (vein) — *see* Injury, blood vessel, thoracic, pulmonary
    radial artery (forearm level) S55.10- ✓
      hand and wrist (level) S65.10- ✓
        laceration S65.11- ✓
        specified type NEC S65.19- ✓
      laceration S55.11- ✓
      specified type NEC S55.19- ✓
    renal
      artery S35.40- ✓
        laceration S35.41- ✓
        specified NEC S35.49- ✓
      vein S35.40- ✓
        laceration S35.41- ✓
        specified NEC S35.49- ✓
    saphenous vein (greater) (lower leg level) — *see* Injury, blood vessel, greater saphenous
      hip and thigh level — *see* Injury, blood vessel, greater saphenous, hip level
      lesser — *see* Injury, blood vessel, lesser saphenous
    shoulder
      specified NEC — *see* Injury, blood vessel, arm, specified site NEC
      superficial vein — *see* Injury, blood vessel, arm, superficial vein
    specified NEC T14.8 ✓
    splenic
      artery — *see* Injury, blood vessel, celiac artery, branch
      vein S35.329 ✓
        laceration S35.321 ✓
        specified NEC S35.328 ✓
    subclavian — *see* Injury, blood vessel, thoracic, innominate
    thigh — *see* Injury, blood vessel, hip
    thoracic S25.90 ✓
      aorta S25.00 ✓
        laceration (minor) (superficial) S25.01 ✓
          major S25.02 ✓
        specified type NEC S25.09 ✓
      azygos vein — *see* Injury, blood vessel, thoracic, specified, site NEC
      innominate
        artery S25.10- ✓
          laceration (minor) (superficial) S25.11- ✓
            major S25.12- ✓
          specified type NEC S25.19- ✓

Injury — continued
  blood vessel — continued
    thoracic — continued
      innominate — continued
        vein S25.30- ☑
          laceration (minor) (superficial)
            S25.31- ☑
          major S25.32- ☑
          specified type NEC S25.39- ☑
      intercostal S25.50- ☑
        laceration S25.51- ☑
        specified type NEC S25.59- ☑
      laceration S25.91 ☑
      mammary vessel — see Injury, blood vessel,
        thoracic, specified, site NEC
      pulmonary S25.40- ☑
        laceration (minor) (superficial) S25.41- ☑
        major S25.42- ☑
        specified type NEC S25.49- ☑
      specified
        site NEC S25.80- ☑
          laceration S25.81 ☑
          specified type NEC S25.89 ☑
        type NEC S25.99 ☑
      subclavian — see Injury, blood vessel, thoracic,
        innominate
      vena cava (superior) S25.20 ☑
        laceration (minor) (superficial) S25.21 ☑
        major S25.22 ☑
        specified type NEC S25.29 ☑
    thumb S65.40- ☑
      laceration S65.41- ☑
      specified type NEC S65.49- ☑
    tibial artery S85.10- ☑
      anterior S85.13- ☑
        laceration S85.14- ☑
        specified injury NEC S85.15- ☑
      laceration S85.11- ☑
      posterior S85.16- ☑
        laceration S85.17- ☑
        specified injury NEC S85.18- ☑
      specified injury NEC S85.12- ☑
    ulnar artery (forearm level) S55.00- ☑
      hand and wrist (level) S65.00- ☑
        laceration S65.01- ☑
        specified type NEC S65.09- ☑
      laceration S55.01- ☑
      specified type NEC S55.09- ☑
    upper arm (level) — see Injury, blood vessel, arm
      superficial vein — see Injury, blood vessel, arm,
        superficial vein
    uterine S35.5- ☑
      artery S35.53- ☑
      vein S35.53- ☑
    vena cava — see Injury, vena cava
    vertebral artery S15.10- ☑
      laceration (minor) (superficial) S15.11- ☑
        major S15.12- ☑
      specified type NEC S15.19- ☑
    wrist (level) — see Injury, blood vessel, hand
  brachial plexus S14.3 ☑
    newborn P14.3
  brain (traumatic) S06.9- ☑
    diffuse (axonal) S06.2X- ☑
    focal S06.30- ☑
  brainstem S06.38- ☑
  breast NOS S29.9
  broad ligament — see Injury, pelvic organ, specified
    site NEC
  bronchus, bronchi — see Injury, intrathoracic,
    bronchus
  brow S09.90 ☑
  buttock S39.92 ☑
  canthus, eye S05.90 ☑
  cardiac plexus — see Injury, nerve, thorax, sympathetic
  cauda equina S34.3 ☑
  cavernous sinus — see Injury, intracranial
  cecum — see Injury, colon
  celiac ganglion or plexus — see Injury, nerve, lum-
    bosacral, sympathetic
  cerebellum — see Injury, intracranial
  cerebral — see Injury, intracranial
  cervix (uteri) — see Injury, uterus
  cheek (wall) S09.93 ☑
  chest — see Injury, thorax

Injury — continued
  childbirth (newborn) (see also Birth, injury)
    maternal NEC O71.9
  chin S09.93 ☑
  choroid (eye) — see Injury, eye, specified site NEC
  clitoris S39.94 ☑
  coccyx (see also Injury, back, lower)
    complicating delivery O71.6
  colon — see Injury, intestine, large
  common bile duct — see Injury, liver
  conjunctiva (superficial) — see Injury, eye, conjunctiva
  conus medullaris — see Injury, spinal, sacral
  cord
    spermatic (pelvic region) S37.898 ☑
      scrotal region S39.848 ☑
    spinal — see Injury, spinal cord, by region
  cornea — see Injury, eye, specified site NEC
    abrasion — see Injury, eye, cornea, abrasion
  cortex (cerebral) (see also Injury, intracranial)
    visual — see Injury, nerve, optic
  costal region NEC S29.9
  costochondral NEC S29.9
  cranial
    cavity — see Injury, intracranial
    nerve — see Injury, nerve, cranial
  crushing — see Crush
  cutaneous sensory nerve
  cystic duct — see Injury, liver
  deep tissue — see Contusion, by site
    meaning pressure ulcer — see Ulcer, pressure, un-
      stageable, by site
  delivery (newborn) P15.9
    maternal NEC O71.9
  Descemet's membrane — see Injury, eyeball, penetrat-
    ing
  diaphragm — see Injury, intrathoracic, diaphragm
  duodenum — see Injury, intestine, small, duodenum
  ear (auricle) (external) (canal) S09.91 ☑
    abrasion — see Abrasion, ear
    bite — see Bite, ear
    blister — see Blister, ear
    bruise — see Contusion, ear
    contusion — see Contusion, ear
    external constriction — see Constriction, external,
      ear
    hematoma — see Hematoma, ear
    inner — see Injury, ear, middle
    laceration — see Laceration, ear
    middle S09.30- ☑
      blast — see Injury, blast, ear
      specified NEC S09.39- ☑
    puncture — see Puncture, ear
    superficial — see Injury, superficial, ear
  eighth cranial nerve (acoustic or auditory) — see Injury,
    nerve, acoustic
  elbow S59.90- ☑
    contusion — see Contusion, elbow
    dislocation — see Dislocation, elbow
    fracture — see Fracture, ulna, upper end
    open — see Wound, open, elbow
    specified NEC S59.80- ☑
    sprain — see Sprain, elbow
    superficial — see Injury, superficial, elbow
  eleventh cranial nerve (accessory) — see Injury, nerve,
    accessory
  epididymis S39.94 ☑
  epigastric region S39.91 ☑
  epiglottis NEC S19.89 ☑
  esophageal plexus — see Injury, nerve, thorax, sympa-
    thetic
  esophagus (thoracic part) (see also Injury, intrathoracic,
    esophagus)
    cervical NEC S19.85 ☑
  eustachian tube S09.30 ☑
  eye S05.9- ☑
    avulsion S05.7- ☑
    ball — see Injury, eyeball
    conjunctiva S05.0- ☑
    cornea
      abrasion S05.0- ☑
      laceration S05.3- ☑
        with prolapse S05.2- ☑
    lacrimal apparatus S05.8X- ☑
    orbit penetration S05.4- ☑
    specified site NEC S05.8X- ☑
  eyeball S05.8X- ☑

Injury — continued
  eyeball — continued
    contusion S05.1- ☑
    penetrating S05.6- ☑
      with
        foreign body S05.5- ☑
        prolapse or loss of intraocular tissue
          S05.2- ☑
        without prolapse or loss of intraocular tissue
          S05.3- ☑
    specified type NEC S05.8- ☑
  eyebrow S09.93 ☑
  eyelid S09.93 ☑
    abrasion — see Abrasion, eyelid
    contusion — see Contusion, eyelid
    open — see Wound, open, eyelid
  face S09.93 ☑
  fallopian tube S37.509 ☑
    bilateral S37.502 ☑
      blast injury S37.512 ☑
      contusion S37.522 ☑
      laceration S37.532 ☑
      specified type NEC S37.592 ☑
    blast injury (primary) S37.519 ☑
      bilateral S37.512 ☑
      secondary — see Injury, fallopian tube, speci-
        fied type NEC
      unilateral S37.511 ☑
    contusion S37.529 ☑
      bilateral S37.522 ☑
      unilateral S37.521 ☑
    laceration S37.539 ☑
      bilateral S37.532 ☑
      unilateral S37.531 ☑
    specified type NEC S37.599 ☑
      bilateral S37.592 ☑
      unilateral S37.591 ☑
    unilateral S37.501 ☑
      blast injury S37.511 ☑
      contusion S37.521 ☑
      laceration S37.531 ☑
      specified type NEC S37.591 ☑
  fascia — see Injury, muscle
  fifth cranial nerve (trigeminal) — see Injury, nerve,
    trigeminal
  finger (nail) S69.9- ☑
    blood vessel — see Injury, blood vessel, finger
    contusion — see Contusion, finger
    dislocation — see Dislocation, finger
    fracture — see Fracture, finger
    muscle — see Injury, muscle, finger
    nerve — see Injury, nerve, digital, finger
    open — see Wound, open, finger
    specified NEC S69.8- ☑
    sprain — see Sprain, finger
    superficial — see Injury, superficial, finger
  first cranial nerve (olfactory) — see Injury, nerve, olfac-
    tory
  flank — see Injury, abdomen
  foot S99.92- ☑
    blood vessel — see Injury, blood vessel, foot
    contusion — see Contusion, foot
    dislocation — see Dislocation, foot
    fracture — see Fracture, foot
    muscle — see Injury, muscle, foot
    open — see Wound, open, foot
    specified type NEC S99.82- ☑
    sprain — see Sprain, foot
    superficial — see Injury, superficial, foot
  forceps NOS P15.9
  forearm S59.91- ☑
    blood vessel — see Injury, blood vessel, forearm
    contusion — see Contusion, forearm
    fracture — see Fracture, forearm
    muscle — see Injury, muscle, forearm
    nerve — see Injury, nerve, forearm
    open — see Wound, open, forearm
    specified NEC S59.81- ☑
    superficial — see Injury, superficial, forearm
  forehead S09.90 ☑
  fourth cranial nerve (trochlear) — see Injury, nerve,
    trochlear
  gallbladder S36.129 ☑
    contusion S36.122 ☑
    laceration S36.123 ☑
    specified NEC S36.128 ☑

Injury — *continued*
  ganglion
    celiac, coeliac — *see* Injury, nerve, lumbosacral, sympathetic
    gasserian — *see* Injury, nerve, trigeminal
    stellate — *see* Injury, nerve, thorax, sympathetic
    thoracic sympathetic — *see* Injury, nerve, thorax, sympathetic
  gasserian ganglion — *see* Injury, nerve, trigeminal
  gastric artery — *see* Injury, blood vessel, celiac artery, branch
  gastroduodenal artery — *see* Injury, blood vessel, celiac artery, branch
  gastrointestinal tract — *see* Injury, intra-abdominal
    with open wound into abdominal cavity — *see* Wound, open, with penetration into peritoneal cavity
    colon — *see* Injury, intestine, large
    rectum — *see* Injury, intestine, large, rectum
      with open wound into abdominal cavity S36.61 ☑
    small intestine — *see* Injury, intestine, small
    specified site NEC — *see* Injury, intra-abdominal, specified, site NEC
    stomach — *see* Injury, stomach
  genital organ(s)
    external S39.94 ☑
      specified NEC S39.848 ☑
    internal S37.90 ☑
      fallopian tube — *see* Injury, fallopian tube
      ovary — *see* Injury, ovary
      prostate — *see* Injury, prostate
      seminal vesicle — *see* Injury, pelvis, organ, specified site NEC
      uterus — *see* Injury, uterus
      vas deferens — *see* Injury, pelvis, organ, specified site NEC
    obstetrical trauma O71.9
  gland
    lacrimal laceration — *see* Injury, eye, specified site NEC
    salivary S09.93 ☑
    thyroid NEC S19.84 ☑
  globe (eye) S05.90 ☑
    specified NEC S05.8X- ☑
  groin — *see* Injury, abdomen
  gum S09.90 ☑
  hand S69.9- ☑
    blood vessel — *see* Injury, blood vessel, hand
    contusion — *see* Contusion, hand
    fracture — *see* Fracture, hand
    muscle — *see* Injury, muscle, hand
    nerve — *see* Injury, nerve, hand
    open — *see* Wound, open, hand
    specified NEC S69.8- ☑
    sprain — *see* Sprain, hand
    superficial — *see* Injury, superficial, hand
  head S09.90 ☑
    with loss of consciousness S06.9- ☑
    specified NEC S09.8 ☑
  heart S26.90 ☑
    with hemopericardium S26.00 ☑
      contusion S26.01 ☑
      laceration (mild) S26.020 ☑
        major S26.022 ☑
        moderate S26.021 ☑
      specified type NEC S26.09 ☑
    without hemopericardium S26.10 ☑
      contusion S26.11 ☑
      laceration S26.12 ☑
      specified type NEC S26.19 ☑
    contusion S26.91 ☑
    laceration S26.92 ☑
    specified type NEC S26.99 ☑
  heel — *see* Injury, foot
  hepatic
    artery — *see* Injury, blood vessel, celiac artery, branch
    duct — *see* Injury, liver
    vein — *see* Injury, vena cava, inferior
  hip S79.91- ☑
    blood vessel — *see* Injury, blood vessel, hip
    contusion — *see* Contusion, hip
    dislocation — *see* Dislocation, hip
    fracture — *see* Fracture, femur, neck
    muscle — *see* Injury, muscle, hip

Injury — *continued*
  hip — *continued*
    nerve — *see* Injury, nerve, hip
    open — *see* Wound, open, hip
    specified NEC S79.81- ☑
    sprain — *see* Sprain, hip
    superficial — *see* Injury, superficial, hip
  hymen S39.94 ☑
  hypogastric
    blood vessel — *see* Injury, blood vessel, iliac
    plexus — *see* Injury, nerve, lumbosacral, sympathetic
  ileum — *see* Injury, intestine, small
  iliac region S39.91 ☑
  instrumental (during surgery) — *see* Laceration, accidental complicating surgery
    birth injury — *see* Birth, injury
    nonsurgical — *see* Injury, by site
    obstetrical O71.9
      bladder O71.5
      cervix O71.3
      high vaginal O71.4
      perineal NOS O70.9
      urethra O71.5
      uterus O71.5
        with rupture or perforation O71.1
  internal T14.8 ☑
    aorta — *see* Injury, aorta
    bladder (sphincter) — *see* Injury, bladder
      with
        ectopic or molar pregnancy O08.6
        following ectopic or molar pregnancy O08.6
        obstetrical trauma O71.5
    bronchus, bronchi — *see* Injury, intrathoracic, bronchus
    cecum — *see* Injury, intestine, large
    cervix (uteri) (*see also* Injury, uterus)
      with ectopic or molar pregnancy O08.6
      following ectopic or molar pregnancy O08.6
      obstetrical trauma O71.3
    chest — *see* Injury, intrathoracic
    gastrointestinal tract — *see* Injury, intra-abdominal
    heart — *see* Injury, heart
    intestine NEC — *see* Injury, intestine
    intrauterine — *see* Injury, uterus
    mesentery — *see* Injury, intra-abdominal, specified, site NEC
    pelvis, pelvic (organ) S37.90 ☑
      following ectopic or molar pregnancy (subsequent episode) O08.6
      obstetrical trauma NEC O71.5
        rupture or perforation O71.1
      specified NEC S39.83 ☑
    rectum — *see* Injury, intestine, large, rectum
    stomach — *see* Injury, stomach
    ureter — *see* Injury, ureter
    urethra (sphincter) following ectopic or molar pregnancy O08.6
    uterus — *see* Injury, uterus
  interscapular area — *see* Injury, thorax
  intestine
    large S36.509 ☑
      ascending (right) S36.500 ☑
        blast injury (primary) S36.510 ☑
          secondary S36.590 ☑
        contusion S36.520 ☑
        laceration S36.530 ☑
        specified type NEC S36.590 ☑
      blast injury (primary) S36.519 ☑
        ascending (right) S36.510 ☑
        descending (left) S36.512 ☑
        rectum S36.61 ☑
        sigmoid S36.513 ☑
        specified site NEC S36.518 ☑
        transverse S36.511 ☑
      contusion S36.529 ☑
        ascending (right) S36.520 ☑
        descending (left) S36.522 ☑
        rectum S36.62 ☑
        sigmoid S36.523 ☑
        specified site NEC S36.528 ☑
        transverse S36.521 ☑
      descending (left) S36.502 ☑
        blast injury (primary) S36.512 ☑
          secondary S36.592 ☑
        contusion S36.522 ☑
        laceration S36.532 ☑

Injury — *continued*
  intestine — *continued*
    large — *continued*
      descending — *continued*
        specified type NEC S36.592 ☑
      laceration S36.539 ☑
        ascending (right) S36.530 ☑
        descending (left) S36.532 ☑
        rectum S36.63 ☑
        sigmoid S36.533 ☑
        specified site NEC S36.538 ☑
        transverse S36.531 ☑
      rectum S36.60 ☑
        blast injury (primary) S36.61 ☑
          secondary S36.69 ☑
        contusion S36.62 ☑
        laceration S36.63 ☑
        specified type NEC S36.69 ☑
      sigmoid S36.503 ☑
        blast injury (primary) S36.513 ☑
          secondary S36.593 ☑
        contusion S36.523 ☑
        laceration S36.533 ☑
        specified type NEC S36.593 ☑
      specified
        site NEC S36.508 ☑
          blast injury (primary) S36.518 ☑
            secondary S36.598 ☑
          contusion S36.528 ☑
          laceration S36.538 ☑
          specified type NEC S36.598 ☑
        type NEC S36.599 ☑
          ascending (right) S36.590 ☑
          descending (left) S36.592 ☑
          rectum S36.69 ☑
          sigmoid S36.593 ☑
          specified site NEC S36.598 ☑
          transverse S36.591 ☑
      transverse S36.501 ☑
        blast injury (primary) S36.511 ☑
          secondary S36.591 ☑
        contusion S36.521 ☑
        laceration S36.531 ☑
        specified type NEC S36.591 ☑
    small S36.409 ☑
      blast injury (primary) S36.419 ☑
        duodenum S36.410 ☑
        secondary S36.499 ☑
          duodenum S36.490 ☑
          specified site NEC S36.498 ☑
        specified site NEC S36.418 ☑
      contusion S36.429 ☑
        duodenum S36.420 ☑
        specified site NEC S36.428 ☑
      duodenum S36.400 ☑
        blast injury (primary) S36.410 ☑
          secondary S36.490 ☑
        contusion S36.420 ☑
        laceration S36.430 ☑
        specified NEC S36.490 ☑
      laceration S36.439 ☑
        duodenum S36.430 ☑
        specified site NEC S36.438 ☑
      specified
        site NEC S36.408 ☑
        type NEC S36.499 ☑
          duodenum S36.490 ☑
          specified site NEC S36.498 ☑
  intra-abdominal S36.90 ☑
    adrenal gland — *see* Injury, adrenal gland
    bladder — *see* Injury, bladder
    colon — *see* Injury, intestine, large
    contusion S36.92 ☑
    fallopian tube — *see* Injury, fallopian tube
    gallbladder — *see* Injury, gallbladder
    intestine — *see* Injury, intestine
    kidney — *see* Injury, kidney
    laceration S36.93 ☑
    liver — *see* Injury, liver
    ovary — *see* Injury, ovary
    pancreas — *see* Injury, pancreas
    pelvic NOS S37.90 ☑
    peritoneum — *see* Injury, intra-abdominal, specified, site NEC
    prostate — *see* Injury, prostate
    rectum — *see* Injury, intestine, large, rectum

Injury — *continued*
  intra-abdominal — *continued*
    retroperitoneum — *see* Injury, intra-abdominal, specified, site NEC
    seminal vesicle — *see* Injury, pelvis, organ, specified site NEC
    small intestine — *see* Injury, intestine, small
    specified
      pelvic S37.90 ☑
        specified
          site NEC S37.899 ☑
            specified type NEC S37.898 ☑
          type NEC S37.99 ☑
      site NEC S36.899 ☑
        contusion S36.892 ☑
        laceration S36.893 ☑
        specified type NEC S36.898 ☑
        type NEC S36.99 ☑
    spleen — *see* Injury, spleen
    stomach — *see* Injury, stomach
    ureter — *see* Injury, ureter
    urethra — *see* Injury, urethra
    uterus — *see* Injury, uterus
    vas deferens — *see* Injury, pelvis, organ, specified site NEC
  intracranial (traumatic) S06.9- ☑
    cerebellar hemorrhage, traumatic — *see* Injury, intracranial, focal
    cerebral edema, traumatic S06.1X- ☑
      diffuse S06.1X- ☑
      focal S06.1X- ☑
    diffuse (axonal) S06.2X- ☑
    epidural hemorrhage (traumatic) S06.4X- ☑
    focal brain injury S06.30- ☑
      contusion — *see* Contusion, cerebral
      laceration — *see* Laceration, cerebral
    intracerebral hemorrhage, traumatic S06.36- ☑
      left side S06.35- ☑
      right side S06.34- ☑
    subarachnoid hemorrhage, traumatic S06.6X- ☑
    subdural hemorrhage, traumatic S06.5X- ☑
  intraocular — *see* Injury, eyeball, penetrating
  intrathoracic S27.9 ☑
    bronchus S27.409 ☑
      bilateral S27.402 ☑
      blast injury (primary) S27.419 ☑
        bilateral S27.412 ☑
        secondary — *see* Injury, intrathoracic, bronchus, specified type NEC
        unilateral S27.411 ☑
      contusion S27.429 ☑
        bilateral S27.422 ☑
        unilateral S27.421 ☑
      laceration S27.439 ☑
        bilateral S27.432 ☑
        unilateral S27.431 ☑
      specified type NEC S27.499 ☑
        bilateral S27.492 ☑
        unilateral S27.491 ☑
      unilateral S27.401 ☑
    diaphragm S27.809 ☑
      contusion S27.802 ☑
      laceration S27.803 ☑
      specified type NEC S27.808 ☑
    esophagus (thoracic) S27.819 ☑
      contusion S27.812 ☑
      laceration S27.813 ☑
      specified type NEC S27.818 ☑
    heart — *see* Injury, heart
    hemopneumothorax S27.2 ☑
    hemothorax S27.1 ☑
    lung S27.309 ☑
      aspiration J69.0
      bilateral S27.302 ☑
      blast injury (primary) S27.319 ☑
        bilateral S27.312 ☑
        secondary — *see* Injury, intrathoracic, lung, specified type NEC
        unilateral S27.311 ☑
      contusion S27.329 ☑
        bilateral S27.322 ☑
        unilateral S27.321 ☑
      laceration S27.339 ☑
        bilateral S27.332 ☑
        unilateral S27.331 ☑
      specified type NEC S27.399 ☑

Injury — *continued*
  intrathoracic — *continued*
    lung — *continued*
      specified type — *continued*
        bilateral S27.392 ☑
        unilateral S27.391 ☑
      unilateral S27.301 ☑
    pleura S27.60 ☑
      laceration S27.63 ☑
      specified type NEC S27.69 ☑
    pneumothorax S27.0 ☑
    specified organ NEC S27.899 ☑
      contusion S27.892 ☑
      laceration S27.893 ☑
      specified type NEC S27.898 ☑
    thoracic duct — *see* Injury, intrathoracic, specified organ NEC
    thymus gland — *see* Injury, intrathoracic, specified organ NEC
    trachea, thoracic S27.50 ☑
      blast (primary) S27.51 ☑
      contusion S27.52 ☑
      laceration S27.53 ☑
      specified type NEC S27.59 ☑
  iris — *see* Injury, eye, specified site NEC
    penetrating — *see* Injury, eyeball, penetrating
  jaw S09.93 ☑
  jejunum — *see* Injury, intestine, small
  joint NOS T14.8 ☑
    old or residual — *see* Disorder, joint, specified type NEC
  kidney S37.00- ☑
    acute (nontraumatic) N17.9
    contusion — *see* Contusion, kidney
    laceration — *see* Laceration, kidney
    specified NEC S37.09- ☑
  knee S89.9- ☑
    contusion — *see* Contusion, knee
    dislocation — *see* Dislocation, knee
    meniscus (lateral) (medial) — *see* Sprain, knee, specified site NEC
      old injury or tear — *see* Derangement, knee, meniscus, due to old injury
    open — *see* Wound, open, knee
    specified NEC S89.8- ☑
    sprain — *see* Sprain, knee
    superficial — *see* Injury, superficial, knee
  labium (majus) (minus) S39.94 ☑
  labyrinth, ear S09.30- ☑
  lacrimal apparatus, duct, gland, or sac — *see* Injury, eye, specified site NEC
  larynx NEC S19.81 ☑
  leg (lower) S89.9- ☑
    blood vessel — *see* Injury, blood vessel, leg
    contusion — *see* Contusion, leg
    fracture — *see* Fracture, leg
    muscle — *see* Injury, muscle, leg
    nerve — *see* Injury, nerve, leg
    open — *see* Wound, open, leg
    specified NEC S89.8- ☑
    superficial — *see* Injury, superficial, leg
  lens, eye — *see* Injury, eye, specified site NEC
    penetrating — *see* Injury, eyeball, penetrating
  limb NEC T14.8 ☑
  lip S09.93 ☑
  liver S36.119 ☑
    contusion S36.112 ☑
    laceration S36.113 ☑
      major (stellate) S36.116 ☑
      minor S36.114 ☑
      moderate S36.115 ☑
    specified NEC S36.118 ☑
  lower back S39.92 ☑
    specified NEC S39.82 ☑
  lumbar, lumbosacral (region) S39.92 ☑
    plexus — *see* Injury, lumbosacral plexus
  lumbosacral plexus S34.4 ☑
  lung (*see also* Injury, intrathoracic, lung)
    aspiration J69.0
    transfusion-related (TRALI) J95.84
  lymphatic thoracic duct — *see* Injury, intrathoracic, specified organ NEC
  malar region S09.93 ☑
  mastoid region S09.90 ☑
  maxilla S09.93 ☑

Injury — *continued*
  mediastinum — *see* Injury, intrathoracic, specified organ NEC
  membrane, brain — *see* Injury, intracranial
  meningeal artery — *see* Injury, intracranial, subdural hemorrhage
  meninges (cerebral) — *see* Injury, intracranial
  mesenteric
    artery
      branch S35.299 ☑
        laceration (minor) (superficial) S35.291 ☑
          major S35.292 ☑
        specified NEC S35.298 ☑
      inferior S35.239 ☑
        laceration (minor) (superficial) S35.231 ☑
          major S35.232 ☑
        specified NEC S35.238 ☑
      superior S35.229 ☑
        laceration (minor) (superficial) S35.221 ☑
          major S35.222 ☑
        specified NEC S35.228 ☑
    plexus (inferior) (superior) — *see* Injury, nerve, lumbosacral, sympathetic
    vein
      inferior S35.349 ☑
        laceration S35.341 ☑
        specified NEC S35.348 ☑
      superior S35.339 ☑
        laceration S35.331 ☑
        specified NEC S35.338 ☑
  mesentery — *see* Injury, intra-abdominal, specified site NEC
  mesosalpinx — *see* Injury, pelvic organ, specified site NEC
  middle ear S09.30- ☑
  midthoracic region NOS S29.9 ☑
  mouth S09.93 ☑
  multiple NOS T07 ☑
  muscle (and fascia) (and tendon)
    abdomen S39.001 ☑
      laceration S39.021 ☑
      specified type NEC S39.091 ☑
      strain S39.011 ☑
    abductor
      thumb, forearm level — *see* Injury, muscle, thumb, abductor
    adductor
      thigh S76.20- ☑
        laceration S76.22- ☑
        specified type NEC S76.29- ☑
        strain S76.21- ☑
    ankle — *see* Injury, muscle, foot
    anterior muscle group, at leg level (lower) S86.20- ☑
      laceration S86.22- ☑
      specified type NEC S86.29- ☑
      strain S86.21- ☑
    arm (upper) — *see* Injury, muscle, shoulder
    biceps (parts NEC) S46.20- ☑
      laceration S46.22- ☑
      long head S46.10- ☑
        laceration S46.12- ☑
        specified type NEC S46.19- ☑
        strain S46.11- ☑
      specified type NEC S46.29- ☑
      strain S46.21- ☑
    extensor
      finger(s) (other than thumb) — *see* Injury, muscle, finger by site, extensor
      forearm level, specified NEC — *see* Injury, muscle, forearm, extensor
      thumb — *see* Injury, muscle, thumb, extensor
      toe (large) (ankle level) (foot level) — *see* Injury, muscle, toe, extensor
    finger
      extensor (forearm level) S56.40- ☑
        hand level S66.309 ☑
          laceration S66.329 ☑
          specified type NEC S66.399 ☑
          strain S66.319 ☑
        laceration S56.429 ☑
        specified type NEC S56.499 ☑
        strain S56.419 ☑
      flexor (forearm level) S56.10- ☑
        hand level S66.109 ☑
          laceration S66.129 ☑

☑ Additional Character Required — Refer to the Tabular List for Character Selection   🔽 Subterms under main terms may continue to next column or page

Injury — *continued*
  muscle — *continued*
    finger — *continued*
      flexor — *continued*
        hand level — *continued*
          specified type NEC S66.199 ☑
          strain S66.119 ☑
        laceration S56.129 ☑
        specified type NEC S56.199 ☑
        strain S56.119 ☑
      index
        extensor (forearm level)
          hand level S66.308 ☑
            laceration S66.32- ☑
            specified type NEC S66.39- ☑
            strain S66.31- ☑
          specified type NEC S56.492- ☑
        flexor (forearm level)
          hand level S66.108 ☑
            laceration S66.12- ☑
            specified type NEC S66.19- ☑
            strain S66.11- ☑
          specified type NEC S56.19- ☑
          strain S56.11- ☑
        intrinsic S66.50- ☑
          laceration S66.52- ☑
          specified type NEC S66.59- ☑
          strain S66.51- ☑
      intrinsic S66.509 ☑
        laceration S66.529 ☑
        specified type NEC S66.599 ☑
        strain S66.519 ☑
      little
        extensor (forearm level)
          hand level S66.30- ☑
            laceration S66.32- ☑
            specified type NEC S66.39- ☑
            strain S66.31- ☑
          laceration S56.42- ☑
          specified type NEC S56.49- ☑
          strain S56.41- ☑
        flexor (forearm level)
          hand level S66.10- ☑
            laceration S66.12- ☑
            specified type NEC S66.19- ☑
            strain S66.11- ☑
          laceration S56.12- ☑
          specified type NEC S56.19- ☑
          strain S56.11- ☑
        intrinsic S66.50- ☑
          laceration S66.52- ☑
          specified type NEC S66.59- ☑
          strain S66.51- ☑
      middle
        extensor (forearm level)
          hand level S66.30- ☑
            laceration S66.32- ☑
            specified type NEC S66.39- ☑
            strain S66.31- ☑
          laceration S56.42- ☑
          specified type NEC S56.49- ☑
          strain S56.41- ☑
        flexor (forearm level)
          hand level S66.10- ☑
            laceration S66.12- ☑
            specified type NEC S66.19- ☑
            strain S66.11- ☑
          laceration S56.12- ☑
          specified type NEC S56.19- ☑
          strain S56.11- ☑
        intrinsic S66.50- ☑
          laceration S66.52- ☑
          specified type NEC S66.59- ☑
          strain S66.51- ☑
      ring
        extensor (forearm level)
          hand level S66.30- ☑
            laceration S66.32- ☑
            specified type NEC S66.39- ☑
            strain S66.31- ☑
          laceration S56.42- ☑
          specified type NEC S56.49- ☑
          strain S56.41- ☑
        flexor (forearm level)
          hand level S66.10- ☑
            laceration S66.12- ☑

Injury — *continued*
  muscle — *continued*
    finger — *continued*
      ring — *continued*
        flexor — *continued*
          hand level — *continued*
            specified type NEC S66.19- ☑
            strain S66.11- ☑
          laceration S56.12- ☑
          specified type NEC S56.19- ☑
          strain S56.11- ☑
        intrinsic S66.50- ☑
          laceration S66.52- ☑
          specified type NEC S66.59- ☑
          strain S66.51- ☑
    flexor
      finger(s) (other than thumb) — *see* Injury,
        muscle, finger
      forearm level, specified NEC — *see* Injury,
        muscle, forearm, flexor
      thumb — *see* Injury, muscle, thumb, flexor
      toe (long) (ankle level) (foot level) — *see* Injury,
        muscle, toe, flexor
    foot S96.90- ☑
      intrinsic S96.20- ☑
        laceration S96.22- ☑
        specified type NEC S96.29- ☑
        strain S96.21- ☑
      laceration S96.92- ☑
      long extensor, toe — *see* Injury, muscle, toe,
        extensor
      long flexor, toe — *see* Injury, muscle, toe, flexor
      specified
        site NEC S96.80- ☑
          laceration S96.82- ☑
          specified type NEC S96.89- ☑
          strain S96.81- ☑
        type S96.99- ☑
      strain S96.91- ☑
    forearm (level) S56.90- ☑
      extensor S56.50- ☑
        laceration S56.52- ☑
        specified type NEC S56.59- ☑
        strain S56.51- ☑
      flexor S56.20- ☑
        laceration S56.22- ☑
        specified type NEC S56.29- ☑
        strain S56.21- ☑
      laceration S56.92- ☑
      specified S56.99- ☑
        site NEC S56.80- ☑
          laceration S56.82- ☑
          strain S56.81- ☑
          type NEC S56.89- ☑
      strain S56.91- ☑
    hand (level) S66.90- ☑
      laceration S66.92- ☑
      specified
        site NEC S66.80- ☑
          laceration S66.82- ☑
          specified type NEC S66.89- ☑
          strain S66.81- ☑
        type NEC S66.99- ☑
      strain S66.91- ☑
    head S09.10 ☑
      laceration S09.12 ☑
      specified type NEC S09.19 ☑
      strain S09.11 ☑
    hip NEC S76.00- ☑
      laceration S76.02- ☑
      specified type NEC S76.09- ☑
      strain S76.01- ☑
    intrinsic
      ankle and foot level — *see* Injury, muscle, foot,
        intrinsic
      finger (other than thumb) — *see* Injury, muscle,
        finger by site, intrinsic
      foot (level) — *see* Injury, muscle, foot, intrinsic
      thumb — *see* Injury, muscle, thumb, intrinsic
    leg (level) (lower) S86.90- ☑
      Achilles tendon — *see* Injury, Achilles tendon
      anterior muscle group — *see* Injury, muscle,
        anterior muscle group
      laceration S86.92- ☑
      peroneal muscle group — *see* Injury, muscle,
        peroneal muscle group

Injury — *continued*
  muscle — *continued*
    leg — *continued*
      posterior muscle group — *see* Injury, muscle,
        posterior muscle group, leg level
      specified
        site NEC S86.80- ☑
          laceration S86.82- ☑
          specified type NEC S86.89- ☑
          strain S86.81- ☑
        type NEC S86.99- ☑
      strain S86.91- ☑
    long
      extensor toe, at ankle and foot level — *see* In-
        jury, muscle, toe, extensor
      flexor, toe, at ankle and foot level — *see* Injury,
        muscle, toe, flexor
      head, biceps — *see* Injury, muscle, biceps, long
        head
    lower back S39.002 ☑
      laceration S39.022 ☑
      specified type NEC S39.092 ☑
      strain S39.012 ☑
    neck (level) S16.9 ☑
      laceration S16.2 ☑
      specified type NEC S16.8 ☑
      strain S16.1 ☑
    pelvis S39.003 ☑
      laceration S39.023 ☑
      specified type NEC S39.093 ☑
      strain S39.013 ☑
    peroneal muscle group, at leg level (lower)
      S86.30- ☑
      laceration S86.32- ☑
      specified type NEC S86.39- ☑
      strain S86.31- ☑
    posterior muscle (group)
      leg level (lower) S86.10- ☑
        laceration S86.12- ☑
        specified type NEC S86.19- ☑
        strain S86.11- ☑
      thigh level S76.30- ☑
        laceration S76.32- ☑
        specified type NEC S76.39- ☑
        strain S76.31- ☑
    quadriceps (thigh) S76.10- ☑
      laceration S76.12- ☑
      specified type NEC S76.19- ☑
      strain S76.11- ☑
    shoulder S46.90- ☑
      laceration S46.92- ☑
      rotator cuff — *see* Injury, rotator cuff
      specified site NEC S46.80- ☑
        laceration S46.82- ☑
        specified type NEC S46.89- ☑
        strain S46.81- ☑
      specified type NEC S46.99- ☑
      strain S46.91- ☑
    thigh NEC (level) S76.90- ☑
      adductor — *see* Injury, muscle, adductor, thigh
      laceration S76.92- ☑
      posterior muscle (group) — *see* Injury, muscle,
        posterior muscle, thigh level
      quadriceps — *see* Injury, muscle, quadriceps
      specified
        site NEC S76.80- ☑
          laceration S76.82- ☑
          specified type NEC S76.89- ☑
          strain S76.81- ☑
        type NEC S76.99- ☑
      strain S76.91- ☑
    thorax (level) S29.009 ☑
      back wall S29.002 ☑
      front wall S29.001 ☑
      laceration S29.029 ☑
        back wall S29.022 ☑
        front wall S29.021 ☑
      specified type NEC S29.099 ☑
        back wall S29.092 ☑
        front wall S29.091 ☑
      strain S29.019 ☑
        back wall S29.012 ☑
        front wall S29.011 ☑
    thumb
      abductor (forearm level) S56.30- ☑
        laceration S56.32- ☑

Injury — *continued*
- muscle — *continued*
  - thumb — *continued*
    - abductor — *continued*
      - specified type NEC S56.39- ☑
      - strain S56.31- ☑
    - extensor (forearm level) S56.30- ☑
      - hand level S66.20- ☑
        - laceration S66.22- ☑
        - specified type NEC S66.29- ☑
        - strain S66.21- ☑
      - laceration S56.32- ☑
      - specified type NEC S56.39- ☑
      - strain S56.31- ☑
    - flexor (forearm level) S56.00- ☑
      - hand level S66.00- ☑
        - laceration S66.02- ☑
        - specified type NEC S66.09- ☑
        - strain S66.01- ☑
      - laceration S56.02- ☑
      - specified type NEC S56.09- ☑
      - strain S56.01- ☑
      - wrist level — *see* Injury, muscle, thumb, flexor, hand level
    - intrinsic S66.40- ☑
      - laceration S66.42- ☑
      - specified type NEC S66.49- ☑
      - strain S66.41- ☑
  - toe (*see also* Injury, muscle, foot)
    - extensor, long S96.10- ☑
      - laceration S96.12- ☑
      - specified type NEC S96.19- ☑
      - strain S96.11- ☑
    - flexor, long S96.00- ☑
      - laceration S96.02- ☑
      - specified type NEC S96.09- ☑
      - strain S96.01- ☑
  - triceps S46.30- ☑
    - laceration S46.32- ☑
    - specified type NEC S46.39- ☑
    - strain S46.31- ☑
  - wrist (and hand) level — *see* Injury, muscle, hand
- musculocutaneous nerve — *see* Injury, nerve, musculocutaneous
- myocardium — *see* Injury, heart
- nape — *see* Injury, neck
- nasal (septum) (sinus) S09.92 ☑
- nasopharynx S09.92 ☑
- neck S19.9 ☑
  - specified NEC S19.80 ☑
    - specified site NEC S19.89 ☑
- nerve NEC T14.8 ☑
  - abdomen S34.9 ☑
    - peripheral S34.6 ☑
    - specified site NEC S34.8 ☑
  - abducens S04.4- ☑
    - contusion S04.4- ☑
    - laceration S04.4- ☑
    - specified type NEC S04.4- ☑
  - abducent — *see* Injury, nerve, abducens
  - accessory S04.7- ☑
    - contusion S04.7- ☑
    - laceration S04.7- ☑
    - specified type NEC S04.7- ☑
  - acoustic S04.6- ☑
    - contusion S04.6- ☑
    - laceration S04.6- ☑
    - specified type NEC S04.6- ☑
  - ankle S94.9- ☑
    - cutaneous sensory S94.3- ☑
    - specified site NEC — *see* subcategory S94.8 ☑
  - anterior crural, femoral — *see* Injury, nerve, femoral
  - arm (upper) S44.9- ☑
    - axillary — *see* Injury, nerve, axillary
    - cutaneous — *see* Injury, nerve, cutaneous, arm
    - median — *see* Injury, nerve, median, upper arm
    - musculocutaneous — *see* Injury, nerve, musculocutaneous
    - radial — *see* Injury, nerve, radial, upper arm
    - specified site NEC — *see* subcategory S44.8 ☑
    - ulnar — *see* Injury, nerve, ulnar, arm
  - auditory — *see* Injury, nerve, acoustic
  - axillary S44.3- ☑
  - brachial plexus — *see* Injury, brachial plexus
  - cervical sympathetic S14.5 ☑
  - cranial S04.9 ☑

Injury — *continued*
- nerve — *continued*
  - cranial — *continued*
    - contusion S04.9 ☑
    - eighth (acoustic or auditory) — *see* Injury, nerve, acoustic
    - eleventh (accessory) — *see* Injury, nerve, accessory
    - fifth (trigeminal) — *see* Injury, nerve, trigeminal
    - first (olfactory) — *see* Injury, nerve, olfactory
    - fourth (trochlear) — *see* Injury, nerve, trochlear
    - laceration S04.9 ☑
    - ninth (glossopharyngeal) — *see* Injury, nerve, glossopharyngeal
    - second (optic) — *see* Injury, nerve, optic
    - seventh (facial) — *see* Injury, nerve, facial
    - sixth (abducent) — *see* Injury, nerve, abducens
    - specified
      - nerve NEC S04.89- ☑
        - contusion S04.89- ☑
        - laceration S04.89- ☑
        - specified type NEC S04.89- ☑
      - type NEC S04.9 ☑
    - tenth (pneumogastric or vagus) — *see* Injury, nerve, vagus
    - third (oculomotor) — *see* Injury, nerve, oculomotor
    - twelfth (hypoglossal) — *see* Injury, nerve, hypoglossal
  - cutaneous sensory
    - ankle (level) S94.3- ☑
    - arm (upper) (level) S44.5- ☑
    - foot (level) — *see* Injury, nerve, cutaneous sensory, ankle
    - forearm (level) S54.3- ☑
    - hip (level) S74.2- ☑
    - leg (lower level) S84.2- ☑
    - shoulder (level) — *see* Injury, nerve, cutaneous sensory, arm
    - thigh (level) — *see* Injury, nerve, cutaneous sensory, hip
  - deep peroneal — *see* Injury, nerve, peroneal, foot
  - digital
    - finger S64.4- ☑
      - index S64.49- ☑
      - little S64.49- ☑
      - middle S64.49- ☑
      - ring S64.49- ☑
    - thumb S64.3- ☑
    - toe — *see* Injury, nerve, ankle, specified site NEC
  - eighth cranial (acoustic or auditory) — *see* Injury, nerve, acoustic
  - eleventh cranial (accessory) — *see* Injury, nerve, accessory
  - facial S04.5- ☑
    - contusion S04.5- ☑
    - laceration S04.5- ☑
    - newborn P11.3
    - specified type NEC S04.5- ☑
  - femoral (hip level) (thigh level) S74.1- ☑
  - fifth cranial (trigeminal) — *see* Injury, nerve, trigeminal
  - finger (digital) — *see* Injury, nerve, digital, finger
  - first cranial (olfactory) — *see* Injury, nerve, olfactory
  - foot S94.9- ☑
    - cutaneous sensory S94.3- ☑
    - deep peroneal S94.2- ☑
    - lateral plantar S94.0- ☑
    - medial plantar S94.1- ☑
    - specified site NEC — *see* subcategory S94.8 ☑
  - forearm (level) S54.9- ☑
    - cutaneous sensory — *see* Injury, nerve, cutaneous sensory, forearm
    - median — *see* Injury, nerve, median
    - radial — *see* Injury, nerve, radial
    - specified site NEC — *see* subcategory S54.8 ☑
    - ulnar — *see* Injury, nerve, ulnar
  - fourth cranial (trochlear) — *see* Injury, nerve, trochlear
  - glossopharyngeal S04.89- ☑
    - specified type NEC S04.89- ☑
  - hand S64.9- ☑
    - median — *see* Injury, nerve, median, hand
    - radial — *see* Injury, nerve, radial, hand
    - specified NEC — *see* subcategory S64.8 ☑

Injury — *continued*
- nerve — *continued*
  - hand — *continued*
    - ulnar — *see* Injury, nerve, ulnar, hand
  - hip (level) S74.9- ☑
    - cutaneous sensory — *see* Injury, nerve, cutaneous sensory, hip
    - femoral — *see* Injury, nerve, femoral
    - sciatic — *see* Injury, nerve, sciatic
    - specified site NEC — *see* subcategory S74.8 ☑
  - hypoglossal S04.89- ☑
    - specified type NEC S04.89- ☑
  - lateral plantar S94.0- ☑
  - leg (lower) S84.9- ☑
    - cutaneous sensory — *see* Injury, nerve, cutaneous sensory, leg
    - peroneal — *see* Injury, nerve, peroneal
    - specified site NEC — *see* subcategory S84.8 ☑
    - tibial — *see* Injury, nerve, tibial
    - upper — *see* Injury, nerve, thigh
  - lower
    - back — *see* Injury, nerve, abdomen, specified site NEC
      - peripheral — *see* Injury, nerve, abdomen, peripheral
    - limb — *see* Injury, nerve, leg
  - lumbar plexus — *see* Injury, nerve, lumbosacral, sympathetic
  - lumbar spinal — *see* Injury, nerve, spinal, lumbar
  - lumbosacral
    - plexus — *see* Injury, nerve, lumbosacral, sympathetic
    - sympathetic S34.5 ☑
  - medial plantar S94.1- ☑
  - median (forearm level) S54.1- ☑
    - hand (level) S64.1- ☑
    - upper arm (level) S44.1- ☑
    - wrist (level) — *see* Injury, nerve, median, hand
  - musculocutaneous S44.4- ☑
  - musculospiral (upper arm level) — *see* Injury, nerve, radial, upper arm
  - neck S14.9 ☑
    - peripheral S14.4 ☑
    - specified site NEC S14.8 ☑
    - sympathetic S14.5 ☑
  - ninth cranial (glossopharyngeal) — *see* Injury, nerve, glossopharyngeal
  - oculomotor S04.1- ☑
    - contusion S04.1- ☑
    - laceration S04.1- ☑
    - specified type NEC S04.1- ☑
  - olfactory S04.81- ☑
    - specified type NEC S04.81- ☑
  - optic S04.01- ☑
    - contusion S04.01- ☑
    - laceration S04.01- ☑
    - specified type NEC S04.01- ☑
  - pelvic girdle — *see* Injury, nerve, hip
  - pelvis — *see* Injury, nerve, abdomen, specified site NEC
    - peripheral — *see* Injury, nerve, abdomen, peripheral
  - peripheral NEC T14.8 ☑
    - abdomen — *see* Injury, nerve, abdomen, peripheral
    - lower back — *see* Injury, nerve, abdomen, peripheral
    - neck — *see* Injury, nerve, neck, peripheral
    - pelvis — *see* Injury, nerve, abdomen, peripheral
    - specified NEC T14.8 ☑
  - peroneal (lower leg level) S84.1- ☑
    - foot S94.2- ☑
  - plexus
    - brachial — *see* Injury, brachial plexus
    - celiac, coeliac — *see* Injury, nerve, lumbosacral, sympathetic
    - mesenteric, inferior — *see* Injury, nerve, lumbosacral, sympathetic
    - sacral — *see* Injury, lumbosacral plexus
    - spinal
      - brachial — *see* Injury, brachial plexus
      - lumbosacral — *see* Injury, lumbosacral plexus
  - pneumogastric — *see* Injury, nerve, vagus
  - radial (forearm level) S54.2- ☑
    - hand (level) S64.2- ☑

Injury — continued
  nerve — continued
    radial — continued
      upper arm (level) S44.2- ☑
      wrist (level) — see Injury, nerve, radial, hand
    root — see Injury, nerve, spinal, root
    sacral plexus — see Injury, lumbosacral plexus
    sacral spinal — see Injury, nerve, spinal, sacral
    sciatic (hip level) (thigh level) S74.0- ☑
    second cranial (optic) — see Injury, nerve, optic
    seventh cranial (facial) — see Injury, nerve, facial
    shoulder — see Injury, nerve, arm
    sixth cranial (abducent) — see Injury, nerve, abducens
    spinal
      plexus — see Injury, nerve, plexus, spinal
      root
        cervical S14.2 ☑
        dorsal S24.2 ☑
        lumbar S34.21 ☑
        sacral S34.22 ☑
        thoracic — see Injury, nerve, spinal, root, dorsal
    splanchnic — see Injury, nerve, lumbosacral, sympathetic
    sympathetic NEC — see Injury, nerve, lumbosacral, sympathetic
      cervical — see Injury, nerve, cervical sympathetic
    tenth cranial (pneumogastric or vagus) — see Injury, nerve, vagus
    thigh (level) — see Injury, nerve, hip
      cutaneous sensory — see Injury, nerve, cutaneous sensory, hip
      femoral — see Injury, nerve, femoral
      sciatic — see Injury, nerve, sciatic
      specified NEC — see Injury, nerve, hip
    third cranial (oculomotor) — see Injury, nerve, oculomotor
    thorax S24.9 ☑
      peripheral S24.3 ☑
      specified site NEC S24.8 ☑
      sympathetic S24.4 ☑
    thumb, digital — see Injury, nerve, digital, thumb
    tibial (lower leg level) (posterior) S84.0- ☑
    toe — see Injury, nerve, ankle
    trigeminal S04.3- ☑
      contusion S04.3- ☑
      laceration S04.3- ☑
      specified type NEC S04.3- ☑
    trochlear S04.2- ☑
      contusion S04.2- ☑
      laceration S04.2- ☑
      specified type NEC S04.2- ☑
    twelfth cranial (hypoglossal) — see Injury, nerve, hypoglossal
    ulnar (forearm level) S54.0- ☑
      arm (upper) (level) S44.0- ☑
      hand (level) S64.0- ☑
      wrist (level) — see Injury, nerve, ulnar, hand
    vagus S04.89- ☑
      specified type NEC S04.89- ☑
    wrist (level) — see Injury, nerve, hand
  ninth cranial nerve (glossopharyngeal) — see Injury, nerve, glossopharyngeal
  nose (septum) S09.92 ☑
  obstetrical O71.9
    specified NEC O71.89
  occipital (region) (scalp) S09.90 ☑
    lobe — see Injury, intracranial
  optic chiasm S04.02 ☑
  optic radiation S04.03- ☑
  optic tract and pathways S04.03- ☑
  orbit, orbital (region) — see Injury, eye
    penetrating (with foreign body) — see Injury, eye, orbit, penetrating
    specified NEC — see Injury, eye, specified site NEC
  ovary, ovarian S37.409 ☑
    bilateral S37.402 ☑
      contusion S37.422 ☑
      laceration S37.432 ☑
      specified type NEC S37.492 ☑
    blood vessel — see Injury, blood vessel, ovarian
    contusion S37.429 ☑
      bilateral S37.422 ☑
      unilateral S37.421 ☑

Injury — continued
  ovary, ovarian — continued
    laceration S37.439 ☑
      bilateral S37.432 ☑
      unilateral S37.431 ☑
    specified type NEC S37.499 ☑
      bilateral S37.492 ☑
      unilateral S37.491 ☑
    unilateral S37.401 ☑
      contusion S37.421 ☑
      laceration S37.431 ☑
      specified type NEC S37.491 ☑
  palate (hard) (soft) S09.93 ☑
  pancreas S36.209 ☑
    body S36.201 ☑
      contusion S36.221 ☑
      laceration S36.231 ☑
        major S36.261 ☑
        minor S36.241 ☑
        moderate S36.251 ☑
      specified type NEC S36.291 ☑
    contusion S36.229 ☑
    head S36.200 ☑
      contusion S36.220 ☑
      laceration S36.230 ☑
        major S36.260 ☑
        minor S36.240 ☑
        moderate S36.250 ☑
      specified type NEC S36.290 ☑
    laceration S36.239 ☑
      major S36.269 ☑
      minor S36.249 ☑
      moderate S36.259 ☑
    specified type NEC S36.299 ☑
    tail S36.202 ☑
      contusion S36.222 ☑
      laceration S36.232 ☑
        major S36.262 ☑
        minor S36.242 ☑
        moderate S36.252 ☑
      specified type NEC S36.292 ☑
  parietal (region) (scalp) S09.90 ☑
    lobe — see Injury, intracranial
  patellar ligament (tendon) S76.10- ☑
    laceration S76.12- ☑
    specified NEC S76.19- ☑
    strain S76.11- ☑
  pelvis, pelvic (floor) S39.93 ☑
    complicating delivery O70.1
    joint or ligament, complicating delivery O71.6
    organ S37.90 ☑
      with ectopic or molar pregnancy O08.6
      complication of abortion — see Abortion
      contusion S37.92 ☑
      following ectopic or molar pregnancy O08.6
      laceration S37.93 ☑
      obstetrical trauma NEC O71.5
      specified
        site NEC S37.899 ☑
          contusion S37.892 ☑
          laceration S37.893 ☑
          specified type NEC S37.898 ☑
        type NEC S37.99 ☑
    specified NEC S39.83 ☑
  penis S39.94 ☑
  perineum S39.94 ☑
  peritoneum S36.81 ☑
    laceration S36.893 ☑
  periurethral tissue — see Injury, urethra
    complicating delivery O71.82
  phalanges
    foot — see Injury, foot
    hand — see Injury, hand
  pharynx NEC S19.85 ☑
  pleura — see Injury, intrathoracic, pleura
  plexus
    brachial — see Injury, brachial plexus
    cardiac — see Injury, nerve, thorax, sympathetic
    celiac, coeliac — see Injury, nerve, lumbosacral, sympathetic
    esophageal — see Injury, nerve, thorax, sympathetic
    hypogastric — see Injury, nerve, lumbosacral, sympathetic
    lumbar, lumbosacral — see Injury, lumbosacral plexus

Injury — continued
  plexus — continued
    mesenteric — see Injury, nerve, lumbosacral, sympathetic
    pulmonary — see Injury, nerve, thorax, sympathetic
  postcardiac surgery (syndrome) I97.0
  prepuce S39.94 ☑
  prostate S37.829 ☑
    contusion S37.822 ☑
    laceration S37.823 ☑
    specified type NEC S37.828 ☑
  pubic region S39.94 ☑
  pudendum S39.94 ☑
  pulmonary plexus — see Injury, nerve, thorax, sympathetic
  rectovaginal septum NEC S39.83 ☑
  rectum — see Injury, intestine, large, rectum
  retina — see Injury, eye, specified site NEC
    penetrating — see Injury, eyeball, penetrating
  retroperitoneal — see Injury, intra-abdominal, specified site NEC
  rotator cuff (muscle(s)) (tendon(s)) S46.00- ☑
    laceration S46.02- ☑
    specified type NEC S46.09- ☑
    strain S46.01- ☑
  round ligament — see Injury, pelvic organ, specified site NEC
  sacral plexus — see Injury, lumbosacral plexus
  salivary duct or gland S09.93 ☑
  scalp S09.90 ☑
    newborn (birth injury) P12.9
      due to monitoring (electrode) (sampling incision) P12.4
      specified NEC P12.89
        caput succedaneum P12.81
  scapular region — see Injury, shoulder
  sclera — see Injury, eye, specified site NEC
    penetrating — see Injury, eyeball, penetrating
  scrotum S39.94 ☑
  second cranial nerve (optic) — see Injury, nerve, optic
  seminal vesicle — see Injury, pelvic organ, specified site NEC
  seventh cranial nerve (facial) — see Injury, nerve, facial
  shoulder S49.9- ☑
    blood vessel — see Injury, blood vessel, arm
    contusion — see Contusion, shoulder
    dislocation — see Dislocation, shoulder
    fracture — see Fracture, shoulder
    muscle — see Injury, muscle, shoulder
    nerve — see Injury, nerve, shoulder
    open — see Wound, open, shoulder
    specified type NEC S49.8- ☑
    sprain — see Sprain, shoulder girdle
    superficial — see Injury, superficial, shoulder
  sinus
    cavernous — see Injury, intracranial
    nasal S09.92 ☑
  sixth cranial nerve (abducent) — see Injury, nerve, abducens
  skeleton, birth injury P13.9
    specified part NEC P13.8
  skin NEC T14.8 ☑
    surface intact — see Injury, superficial
  skull NEC S09.90 ☑
  specified NEC T14.8 ☑
  spermatic cord (pelvic region) S37.898 ☑
    scrotal region S39.848 ☑
  spinal (cord)
    cervical (neck) S14.109 ☑
      anterior cord syndrome S14.139 ☑
        C1 level S14.131 ☑
        C2 level S14.132 ☑
        C3 level S14.133 ☑
        C4 level S14.134 ☑
        C5 level S14.135 ☑
        C6 level S14.136 ☑
        C7 level S14.137 ☑
        C8 level S14.138 ☑
      Brown-Séquard syndrome S14.149 ☑
        C1 level S14.141 ☑
        C2 level S14.142 ☑
        C3 level S14.143 ☑
        C4 level S14.144 ☑
        C5 level S14.145 ☑
        C6 level S14.146 ☑

▽ Subterms under main terms may continue to next column or page   ☑ Additional Character Required — Refer to the Tabular List for Character Selection   **197**

Injury — Injury

Injury — *continued*
 spinal — *continued*
  cervical — *continued*
   Brown-Séquard syndrome — *continued*
    C7 level S14.147 ☑
    C8 level S14.148 ☑
   C1 level S14.101 ☑
   C2 level S14.102 ☑
   C3 level S14.103 ☑
   C4 level S14.104 ☑
   C5 level S14.105 ☑
   C6 level S14.106 ☑
   C7 level S14.107 ☑
   C8 level S14.108 ☑
   central cord syndrome S14.129 ☑
    C1 level S14.121 ☑
    C2 level S14.122 ☑
    C3 level S14.123 ☑
    C4 level S14.124 ☑
    C5 level S14.125 ☑
    C6 level S14.126 ☑
    C7 level S14.127 ☑
    C8 level S14.128 ☑
   complete lesion S14.119 ☑
    C1 level S14.111 ☑
    C2 level S14.112 ☑
    C3 level S14.113 ☑
    C4 level S14.114 ☑
    C5 level S14.115 ☑
    C6 level S14.116 ☑
    C7 level S14.117 ☑
    C8 level S14.118 ☑
   concussion S14.0 ☑
   edema S14.0 ☑
   incomplete lesion specified NEC S14.159 ☑
    C1 level S14.151 ☑
    C2 level S14.152 ☑
    C3 level S14.153 ☑
    C4 level S14.154 ☑
    C5 level S14.155 ☑
    C6 level S14.156 ☑
    C7 level S14.157 ☑
    C8 level S14.158 ☑
   posterior cord syndrome S14.159 ☑
    C1 level S14.151 ☑
    C2 level S14.152 ☑
    C3 level S14.153 ☑
    C4 level S14.154 ☑
    C5 level S14.155 ☑
    C6 level S14.156 ☑
    C7 level S14.157 ☑
    C8 level S14.158 ☑
  dorsal — *see* Injury, spinal, thoracic
  lumbar S34.109 ☑
   complete lesion S34.119 ☑
    L1 level S34.111 ☑
    L2 level S34.112 ☑
    L3 level S34.113 ☑
    L4 level S34.114 ☑
    L5 level S34.115 ☑
   concussion S34.01 ☑
   edema S34.01 ☑
   incomplete lesion S34.129 ☑
    L1 level S34.121 ☑
    L2 level S34.122 ☑
    L3 level S34.123 ☑
    L4 level S34.124 ☑
    L5 level S34.125 ☑
   L1 level S34.101 ☑
   L2 level S34.102 ☑
   L3 level S34.103 ☑
   L4 level S34.104 ☑
   L5 level S34.105 ☑
  nerve root NEC
   cervical — *see* Injury, nerve, spinal, root, cervical
   dorsal — *see* Injury, nerve, spinal, root, dorsal
   lumbar S34.21 ☑
   sacral S34.22 ☑
   thoracic — *see* Injury, nerve, spinal, root, dorsal
  plexus
   brachial — *see* Injury, brachial plexus
   lumbosacral — *see* Injury, lumbosacral plexus
  sacral S34.139 ☑
   complete lesion S34.131 ☑
   incomplete lesion S34.132 ☑

Injury — *continued*
 spinal — *continued*
  thoracic S24.109 ☑
   anterior cord syndrome S24.139 ☑
    T1 level S24.131 ☑
    T2-T6 level S24.132 ☑
    T7-T10 level S24.133 ☑
    T11-T12 level S24.134 ☑
   Brown-Séquard syndrome S24.149 ☑
    T1 level S24.141 ☑
    T2-T6 level S24.142 ☑
    T7-T10 level S24.143 ☑
    T11-T12 level S24.144 ☑
   complete lesion S24.119 ☑
    T1 level S24.111 ☑
    T2-T6 level S24.112 ☑
    T7-T10 level S24.113 ☑
    T11-T12 level S24.114 ☑
   concussion S24.0 ☑
   edema S24.0 ☑
   incomplete lesion specified NEC S24.159 ☑
    T1 level S24.151 ☑
    T2-T6 level S24.152 ☑
    T7-T10 level S24.153 ☑
    T11-T12 level S24.154 ☑
   posterior cord syndrome S24.159 ☑
    T1 level S24.151 ☑
    T2-T6 level S24.152 ☑
    T7-T10 level S24.153 ☑
    T11-T12 level S24.154 ☑
   T1 level S24.101 ☑
   T2-T6 level S24.102 ☑
   T7-T10 level S24.103 ☑
   T11-T12 level S24.104 ☑
 splanchnic nerve — *see* Injury, nerve, lumbosacral, sympathetic
 spleen S36.00 ☑
  contusion S36.029 ☑
   major S36.021 ☑
   minor S36.020 ☑
  laceration S36.039 ☑
   major (massive) (stellate) S36.032 ☑
   moderate S36.031 ☑
   superficial (capsular) (minor) S36.030 ☑
  specified type NEC S36.09 ☑
 splenic artery — *see* Injury, blood vessel, celiac artery, branch
 stellate ganglion — *see* Injury, nerve, thorax, sympathetic
 sternal region S29.9 ☑
 stomach S36.30 ☑
  contusion S36.32 ☑
  laceration S36.33 ☑
  specified type NEC S36.39 ☑
 subconjunctival — *see* Injury, eye, conjunctiva
 subcutaneous NEC T14.8 ☑
 submaxillary region S09.93 ☑
 submental region S09.93 ☑
 subungual
  fingers — *see* Injury, hand
  toes — *see* Injury, foot
 superficial NEC T14.8 ☑
  abdomen, abdominal (wall) S30.92 ☑
   abrasion S30.811 ☑
   bite S30.871 ☑
    insect S30.861 ☑
   contusion S30.1 ☑
   external constriction S30.841 ☑
   foreign body S30.851 ☑
  abrasion — *see* Abrasion, by site
  adnexa, eye NEC — *see* Injury, eye, specified site NEC
  alveolar process — *see* Injury, superficial, oral cavity
  ankle S90.91- ☑
   abrasion — *see* Abrasion, ankle
   bite — *see* Bite, ankle
   blister — *see* Blister, ankle
   contusion — *see* Contusion, ankle
   external constriction — *see* Constriction, external, ankle
   foreign body — *see* Foreign body, superficial, ankle
  anus S30.98 ☑
  arm (upper) S40.92- ☑
   abrasion — *see* Abrasion, arm

Injury — *continued*
 superficial — *continued*
  arm — *continued*
   bite — *see* Bite, superficial, arm
   blister — *see* Blister, arm (upper)
   contusion — *see* Contusion, arm
   external constriction — *see* Constriction, external, arm
   foreign body — *see* Foreign body, superficial, arm
  auditory canal (external) (meatus) — *see* Injury, superficial, ear
  auricle — *see* Injury, superficial, ear
  axilla — *see* Injury, superficial, arm
  back (see also Injury, superficial, thorax, back)
   lower S30.91 ☑
    abrasion S30.810 ☑
    contusion S30.0 ☑
    external constriction S30.840 ☑
    superficial
     bite NEC S30.870 ☑
      insect S30.860 ☑
     foreign body S30.850 ☑
  bite NEC — *see* Bite, superficial NEC, by site
  blister — *see* Blister, by site
  breast S20.10- ☑
   abrasion — *see* Abrasion, breast
   bite — *see* Bite, superficial, breast
   contusion — *see* Contusion, breast
   external constriction — *see* Constriction, external, breast
   foreign body — *see* Foreign body, superficial, breast
  brow — *see* Injury, superficial, head, specified NEC
  buttock S30.91 ☑
  calf — *see* Injury, superficial, leg
  canthus, eye — *see* Injury, superficial, periocular area
  cheek (external) — *see* Injury, superficial, head, specified NEC
   internal — *see* Injury, superficial, oral cavity
  chest wall — *see* Injury, superficial, thorax
  chin — *see* Injury, superficial, head NEC
  clitoris S30.95 ☑
  conjunctiva — *see* Injury, eye, conjunctiva
   with foreign body (in conjunctival sac) — *see* Foreign body, conjunctival sac
  contusion — *see* Contusion, by site
  costal region — *see* Injury, superficial, thorax
  digit(s)
   hand — *see* Injury, superficial, finger
  ear (auricle) (canal) (external) S00.40- ☑
   abrasion — *see* Abrasion, ear
   bite — *see* Bite, superficial, ear
   contusion — *see* Contusion, ear
   external constriction — *see* Constriction, external, ear
   foreign body — *see* Foreign body, superficial, ear
  elbow S50.90- ☑
   abrasion — *see* Abrasion, elbow
   bite — *see* Bite, superficial, elbow
   blister — *see* Blister, elbow
   contusion — *see* Contusion, elbow
   external constriction — *see* Constriction, external, elbow
   foreign body — *see* Foreign body, superficial, elbow
  epididymis S30.94 ☑
  epigastric region S30.92 ☑
  epiglottis — *see* Injury, superficial, throat
  esophagus
   cervical — *see* Injury, superficial, throat
  external constriction — *see* Constriction, external, by site
  extremity NEC T14.8 ☑
  eyeball NEC — *see* Injury, eye, specified site NEC
  eyebrow — *see* Injury, superficial, periocular area
  eyelid S00.20- ☑
   abrasion — *see* Abrasion, eyelid
   bite — *see* Bite, superficial, eyelid
   contusion — *see* Contusion, eyelid
   external constriction — *see* Constriction, external, eyelid
   foreign body — *see* Foreign body, superficial, eyelid

☑ **Additional Character Required — Refer to the Tabular List for Character Selection**   ▽ **Subterms under main terms may continue to next column or page**

Injury — continued
  superficial — continued
    face NEC — see Injury, superficial, head, specified NEC
    finger(s) S60.949 ☑
      abrasion — see Abrasion, finger
      bite — see Bite, superficial, finger
      blister — see Blister, finger
      contusion — see Contusion, finger
      external constriction — see Constriction, external, finger
      foreign body — see Foreign body, superficial, finger
      index S60.94- ☑
      insect bite — see Bite, by site, superficial, insect
      little S60.94- ☑
      middle S60.94- ☑
      ring S60.94- ☑
    flank S30.92 ☑
    foot S90.92- ☑
      abrasion — see Abrasion, foot
      bite — see Bite, foot
      blister — see Blister, foot
      contusion — see Contusion, foot
      external constriction — see Constriction, external, foot
      foreign body — see Foreign body, superficial, foot
    forearm S50.91- ☑
      abrasion — see Abrasion, forearm
      bite — see Bite, forearm, superficial
      blister — see Blister, forearm
      contusion — see Contusion, forearm
      elbow only — see Injury, superficial, elbow
      external constriction — see Constriction, external, forearm
      foreign body — see Foreign body, superficial, forearm
    forehead — see Injury, superficial, head NEC
    foreign body — see Foreign body, superficial
    genital organs, external
      female S30.97 ☑
      male S30.96 ☑
    globe (eye) — see Injury, eye, specified site NEC
    groin S30.92 ☑
    gum — see Injury, superficial, oral cavity
    hand S60.92- ☑
      abrasion — see Abrasion, hand
      bite — see Bite, superficial, hand
      contusion — see Contusion, hand
      external constriction — see Constriction, external, hand
      foreign body — see Foreign body, superficial, hand
    head S00.90 ☑
      ear — see Injury, superficial, ear
      eyelid — see Injury, superficial, eyelid
      nose S00.30 ☑
      oral cavity S00.502 ☑
      scalp S00.00 ☑
      specified site NEC S00.80 ☑
    heel — see Injury, superficial, foot
    hip S70.91- ☑
      abrasion — see Abrasion, hip
      bite — see Bite, superficial, hip
      blister — see Blister, hip
      contusion — see Contusion, hip
      external constriction — see Constriction, external, hip
      foreign body — see Foreign body, superficial, hip
    iliac region — see Injury, superficial, abdomen
    inguinal region — see Injury, superficial, abdomen
    insect bite — see Bite, by site, superficial, insect
    interscapular region — see Injury, superficial, thorax, back
    jaw — see Injury, superficial, head, specified NEC
    knee S80.91- ☑
      abrasion — see Abrasion, knee
      bite — see Bite, superficial, knee
      blister — see Blister, knee
      contusion — see Contusion, knee
      external constriction — see Constriction, external, knee
      foreign body — see Foreign body, superficial, knee

Injury — continued
  superficial — continued
    labium (majus) (minus) S30.95 ☑
    lacrimal (apparatus) (gland) (sac) — see Injury, eye, specified site NEC
    larynx — see Injury, superficial, throat
    leg (lower) S80.92- ☑
      abrasion — see Abrasion, leg
      bite — see Bite, superficial, leg
      contusion — see Contusion, leg
      external constriction — see Constriction, external, leg
      foreign body — see Foreign body, superficial, leg
      knee — see Injury, superficial, knee
    limb NEC T14.8 ☑
    lip S00.501 ☑
    lower back S30.91 ☑
    lumbar region S30.91 ☑
    malar region — see Injury, superficial, head, specified NEC
    mammary — see Injury, superficial, breast
    mastoid region — see Injury, superficial, head, specified NEC
    mouth — see Injury, superficial, oral cavity
    muscle NEC T14.8 ☑
    nail NEC T14.8 ☑
      finger — see Injury, superficial, finger
      toe — see Injury, superficial, toe
    nasal (septum) — see Injury, superficial, nose
    neck S10.90 ☑
      specified site NEC S10.80 ☑
    nose (septum) S00.30 ☑
    occipital region — see Injury, superficial, scalp
    oral cavity S00.502 ☑
    orbital region — see Injury, superficial, periocular area
    palate — see Injury, superficial, oral cavity
    palm — see Injury, superficial, hand
    parietal region — see Injury, superficial, scalp
    pelvis S30.91 ☑
      girdle — see Injury, superficial, hip
    penis S30.93 ☑
    perineum
      female S30.95 ☑
      male S30.91 ☑
    periocular area S00.20- ☑
      abrasion — see Abrasion, eyelid
      bite — see Bite, superficial, eyelid
      contusion — see Contusion, eyelid
      external constriction — see Constriction, external, eyelid
      foreign body — see Foreign body, superficial, eyelid
    phalanges
      finger — see Injury, superficial, finger
      toe — see Injury, superficial, toe
    pharynx — see Injury, superficial, throat
    pinna — see Injury, superficial, ear
    popliteal space — see Injury, superficial, knee
    prepuce S30.93 ☑
    pubic region S30.91 ☑
    pudendum
      female S30.97 ☑
      male S30.96 ☑
    sacral region S30.91 ☑
    scalp S00.00 ☑
    scapular region — see Injury, superficial, shoulder
    sclera — see Injury, eye, specified site NEC
    scrotum S30.94 ☑
    shin — see Injury, superficial, leg
    shoulder S40.91- ☑
      abrasion — see Abrasion, shoulder
      bite — see Bite, superficial, shoulder
      blister — see Blister, shoulder
      contusion — see Contusion, shoulder
      external constriction — see Constriction, external, shoulder
      foreign body — see Foreign body, superficial, shoulder
    skin NEC T14.8 ☑
    sternal region — see Injury, superficial, thorax, front
    subconjunctival — see Injury, eye, specified site NEC
    subcutaneous NEC T14.8 ☑

Injury — continued
  superficial — continued
    submaxillary region — see Injury, superficial, head, specified NEC
    submental region — see Injury, superficial, head, specified NEC
    subungual
      finger(s) — see Injury, superficial, finger
      toe(s) — see Injury, superficial, toe
    supraclavicular fossa — see Injury, superficial, neck
    supraorbital — see Injury, superficial, head, specified NEC
    temple — see Injury, superficial, head, specified NEC
    temporal region — see Injury, superficial, head, specified NEC
    testis S30.94 ☑
    thigh S70.92- ☑
      abrasion — see Abrasion, thigh
      bite — see Bite, superficial, thigh
      blister — see Blister, thigh
      contusion — see Contusion, thigh
      external constriction — see Constriction, external, thigh
      foreign body — see Foreign body, superficial, thigh
    thorax, thoracic (wall) S20.90 ☑
      abrasion — see Abrasion, thorax
      back S20.40- ☑
      bite — see Bite, thorax, superficial
      blister — see Blister, thorax
      contusion — see Contusion, thorax
      external constriction — see Constriction, external, thorax
      foreign body — see Foreign body, superficial, thorax
      front S20.30- ☑
    throat S10.10 ☑
      abrasion S10.11 ☑
      bite S10.17 ☑
        insect S10.16 ☑
      blister S10.12 ☑
      contusion S10.0 ☑
      external constriction S10.14 ☑
      foreign body S10.15 ☑
    thumb S60.93- ☑
      abrasion — see Abrasion, thumb
      bite — see Bite, superficial, thumb
      blister — see Blister, thumb
      contusion — see Contusion, thumb
      external constriction — see Constriction, external, thumb
      foreign body — see Foreign body, superficial, thumb
      insect bite — see Bite, by site, superficial, insect
      specified type NEC S60.39 ☑
    toe(s) S90.93- ☑
      abrasion — see Abrasion, toe
      bite — see Bite, toe
      blister — see Blister, toe
      contusion — see Contusion, toe
      external constriction — see Constriction, external, toe
      foreign body — see Foreign body, superficial, toe
      great S90.93- ☑
    tongue — see Injury, superficial, oral cavity
    tooth, teeth — see Injury, superficial, oral cavity
    trachea S10.10 ☑
    tunica vaginalis S30.94 ☑
    tympanum, tympanic membrane — see Injury, superficial, ear
    uvula — see Injury, superficial, oral cavity
    vagina S30.95 ☑
    vocal cords — see Injury, superficial, throat
    vulva S30.95 ☑
    wrist S60.91- ☑
  supraclavicular region — see Injury, neck
  supraorbital S09.93 ☑
  suprarenal gland (multiple) — see Injury, adrenal
  surgical complication (external or internal site) — see Laceration, accidental complicating surgery
  temple S09.90 ☑
  temporal region S09.90 ☑
  tendon (see also Injury, muscle, by site)
    abdomen — see Injury, muscle, abdomen

Injury — *continued*
  tendon (*see also* Injury, muscle, by site) — *continued*
    Achilles — *see* Injury, Achilles tendon
    lower back — *see* Injury, muscle, lower back
    pelvic organs — *see* Injury, muscle, pelvis
  tenth cranial nerve (pneumogastric or vagus) — *see* Injury, nerve, vagus
  testis S39.94 ☑
  thigh S79.92- ☑
    blood vessel — *see* Injury, blood vessel, hip
    contusion — *see* Contusion, thigh
    fracture — *see* Fracture, femur
    muscle — *see* Injury, muscle, thigh
    nerve — *see* Injury, nerve, thigh
    open — *see* Wound, open, thigh
    specified NEC S79.82- ☑
    superficial — *see* Injury, superficial, thigh
  third cranial nerve (oculomotor) — *see* Injury, nerve, oculomotor
  thorax, thoracic S29.9 ☑
    blood vessel — *see* Injury, blood vessel, thorax
    cavity — *see* Injury, intrathoracic
    dislocation — *see* Dislocation, thorax
    external (wall) S29.9 ☑
      contusion — *see* Contusion, thorax
      nerve — *see* Injury, nerve, thorax
      open — *see* Wound, open, thorax
      specified NEC S29.8 ☑
      sprain — *see* Sprain, thorax
      superficial — *see* Injury, superficial, thorax
    fracture — *see* Fracture, thorax
    internal — *see* Injury, intrathoracic
    intrathoracic organ — *see* Injury, intrathoracic
    sympathetic ganglion — *see* Injury, nerve, thorax, sympathetic
  throat (*see also* Injury, neck) S19.9 ☑
  thumb S69.9- ☑
    blood vessel — *see* Injury, blood vessel, thumb
    contusion — *see* Contusion, thumb
    dislocation — *see* Dislocation, thumb
    fracture — *see* Fracture, thumb
    muscle — *see* Injury, muscle, thumb
    nerve — *see* Injury, nerve, digital, thumb
    open — *see* Wound, open, thumb
    specified NEC S69.8- ☑
    sprain — *see* Sprain, thumb
    superficial — *see* Injury, superficial, thumb
  thymus (gland) — *see* Injury, intrathoracic, specified organ NEC
  thyroid (gland) NEC S19.84 ☑
  toe S99.92- ☑
    contusion — *see* Contusion, toe
    dislocation — *see* Dislocation, toe
    fracture — *see* Fracture, toe
    muscle — *see* Injury, muscle, toe
    open — *see* Wound, open, toe
    specified type NEC S99.82- ☑
    sprain — *see* Sprain, toe
    superficial — *see* Injury, superficial, toe
  tongue S09.93 ☑
  tonsil S09.93 ☑
  tooth S09.93 ☑
  trachea (cervical) NEC S19.82 ☑
    thoracic — *see* Injury, intrathoracic, trachea, thoracic
  transfusion-related acute lung (TRALI) J95.84
  tunica vaginalis S39.94 ☑
  twelfth cranial nerve (hypoglossal) — *see* Injury, nerve, hypoglossal
  ureter S37.10 ☑
    contusion S37.12 ☑
    laceration S37.13 ☑
    specified type NEC S37.19 ☑
  urethra (sphincter) S37.30 ☑
    at delivery O71.5
    contusion S37.32 ☑
    laceration S37.33 ☑
    specified type NEC S37.39 ☑
  urinary organ S37.90 ☑
    contusion S37.92 ☑
    laceration S37.93 ☑
    specified
      site NEC S37.899 ☑
        contusion S37.892 ☑
        laceration S37.893 ☑

Injury — *continued*
  urinary organ — *continued*
    specified — *continued*
      site — *continued*
        specified type NEC S37.898 ☑
      type NEC S37.99 ☑
  uterus, uterine S37.60 ☑
    with ectopic or molar pregnancy O08.6
    blood vessel — *see* Injury, blood vessel, iliac
    contusion S37.62 ☑
    laceration S37.63 ☑
      cervix at delivery O71.3
    rupture associated with obstetrics — *see* Rupture, uterus
    specified type NEC S37.69 ☑
  uvula S09.93 ☑
  vagina S39.93 ☑
    abrasion S30.814 ☑
    bite S31.45 ☑
      insect S30.864 ☑
      superficial NEC S30.874 ☑
    contusion S30.23 ☑
    crush S38.03 ☑
    during delivery — *see* Laceration, vagina, during delivery
    external constriction S30.844 ☑
    insect bite S30.864 ☑
    laceration S31.41 ☑
      with foreign body S31.42 ☑
    open wound S31.40 ☑
    puncture S31.43 ☑
      with foreign body S31.44 ☑
    superficial S30.95 ☑
      foreign body S30.854 ☑
  vas deferens — *see* Injury, pelvic organ, specified site NEC
  vascular NEC T14.8 ☑
  vein — *see* Injury, blood vessel
  vena cava (superior) S25.20 ☑
    inferior S35.10 ☑
      laceration (minor) (superficial) S35.11 ☑
        major S35.12 ☑
      specified type NEC S35.19 ☑
    laceration (minor) (superficial) S25.21 ☑
      major S25.22 ☑
    specified type NEC S25.29 ☑
  vesical (sphincter) — *see* Injury, bladder
  visual cortex S04.04- ☑
  vitreous (humor) S05.90 ☑
    specified NEC S05.8X- ☑
  vocal cord NEC S19.83 ☑
  vulva S39.94 ☑
    abrasion S30.814 ☑
    bite S31.45 ☑
      insect S30.864 ☑
      superficial NEC S30.874 ☑
    contusion S30.23 ☑
    crush S38.03 ☑
    during delivery — *see* Laceration, perineum, female, during delivery
    external constriction S30.844 ☑
    insect bite S30.864 ☑
    laceration S31.41 ☑
      with foreign body S31.42 ☑
    open wound S31.40 ☑
    puncture S31.43 ☑
      with foreign body S31.44 ☑
    superficial S30.95 ☑
      foreign body S30.854 ☑
  whiplash (cervical spine) S13.4 ☑
  wrist S69.9- ☑
    blood vessel — *see* Injury, blood vessel, hand
    contusion — *see* Contusion, wrist
    dislocation — *see* Dislocation, wrist
    fracture — *see* Fracture, wrist
    muscle — *see* Injury, muscle, hand
    nerve — *see* Injury, nerve, hand
    open — *see* Wound, open, wrist
    specified NEC S69.8- ☑
    sprain — *see* Sprain, wrist
    superficial — *see* Injury, superficial, wrist
Inoculation (*see also* Vaccination)
  complication or reaction — *see* Complications, vaccination
Insanity, insane (*see also* Psychosis)
  adolescent — *see* Schizophrenia

Insanity, insane — *continued*
  confusional F28
    acute or subacute F05
  delusional F22
  senile F03 ☑
Insect
  bite — *see* Bite, by site, superficial, insect
  venomous, poisoning NEC (by) — *see* Venom, arthropod
Insensitivity
  adrenocorticotropin hormone (ACTH) E27.49
  androgen E34.50
    complete E34.51
    partial E34.52
Insertion
  cord (umbilical) lateral or velamentous O43.12- ☑
  intrauterine contraceptive device (encounter for) — *see* Intrauterine contraceptive device
Insolation (sunstroke) T67.0 ☑
Insomnia (organic) G47.00
  without objective findings F51.02
  adjustment F51.02
  adjustment disorder F51.02
  behavioral, of childhood Z73.819
    combined type Z73.812
    limit setting type Z73.811
    sleep-onset association type Z73.810
  childhood Z73.819
  chronic F51.04
    somatized tension F51.04
  conditioned F51.04
  due to
    alcohol
      abuse F10.182
      dependence F10.282
      use F10.982
    amphetamines
      abuse F15.182
      dependence F15.282
      use F15.982
    anxiety disorder F51.05
    caffeine
      abuse F15.182
      dependence F15.282
      use F15.982
    cocaine
      abuse F14.182
      dependence F14.282
      use F14.982
    depression F51.05
    drug NEC
      abuse F19.182
      dependence F19.282
      use F19.982
    medical condition G47.01
    mental disorder NEC F51.05
    opioid
      abuse F11.182
      dependence F11.282
      use F11.982
    psychoactive substance NEC
      abuse F19.182
      dependence F19.182
      use F19.982
    sedative, hypnotic, or anxiolytic
      abuse F13.182
      dependence F13.282
      use F13.982
    stimulant NEC
      abuse F15.182
      dependence F15.282
      use F15.982
  fatal familial (FFI) A81.83
  idiopathic F51.01
  learned F51.3
  nonorganic origin F51.01
  not due to a substance or known physiological condition F51.01
    specified NEC F51.09
  paradoxical F51.03
  primary F51.01
  psychiatric F51.05
  psychophysiologic F51.04
  related to psychopathology F51.05
  short-term F51.02
  specified NEC G47.09
  stress-related F51.02
  transient F51.02

☑ **Additional Character Required** — Refer to the Tabular List for Character Selection   ▽ **Subterms under main terms may continue to next column or page**

Inspiration
　food or foreign body — *see* Foreign body, by site
　mucus — *see* Asphyxia, mucus
Inspissated bile syndrome (newborn) P59.1
Instability
　emotional (excessive) F60.3
　joint (post-traumatic) M25.30
　　ankle M25.37- ☑
　　due to old ligament injury — *see* Disorder, ligament
　　elbow M25.32- ☑
　　flail — *see* Flail, joint
　　foot M25.37- ☑
　　hand M25.34- ☑
　　hip M25.35- ☑
　　knee M25.36- ☑
　　lumbosacral — *see* subcategory M53.2 ☑
　　prosthesis — *see* Complications, joint prosthesis, mechanical, displacement, by site
　　sacroiliac — *see* subcategory M53.2 ☑
　　secondary to
　　　old ligament injury — *see* Disorder, ligament
　　　removal of joint prosthesis M96.89
　　shoulder (region) M25.31- ☑
　　spine — *see* subcategory M53.2 ☑
　　wrist M25.33- ☑
　knee (chronic) M23.5- ☑
　lumbosacral — *see* subcategory M53.2 ☑
　nervous F48.8
　personality (emotional) F60.3
　spine — *see* Instability, joint, spine
　vasomotor R55
Institutional syndrome (childhood) F94.2
Institutionalization, affecting child Z62.22
　disinhibited attachment F94.2
Insufficiency, insufficient
　accommodation, old age H52.4
　adrenal (gland) E27.40
　　primary E27.1
　adrenocortical E27.40
　　drug-induced E27.3
　　iatrogenic E27.3
　　primary E27.1
　anatomic crown height K08.89
　anterior (occlusal) guidance M26.54
　anus K62.89
　aortic (valve) I35.1
　　with
　　　mitral (valve) disease I08.0
　　　　with tricuspid (valve) disease I08.3
　　　stenosis I35.2
　　　tricuspid (valve) disease I08.2
　　　　with mitral (valve) disease I08.3
　　congenital Q23.1
　　rheumatic I06.1
　　　with
　　　　mitral (valve) disease I08.0
　　　　　with tricuspid (valve) disease I08.3
　　　　stenosis I06.2
　　　　　with mitral (valve) disease I08.0
　　　　　　with tricuspid (valve) disease I08.3
　　　　tricuspid (valve) disease I08.2
　　　　　with mitral (valve) disease I08.3
　　specified cause NEC I35.1
　　syphilitic A52.03
　arterial I77.1
　　basilar G45.0
　　carotid (hemispheric) G45.1
　　cerebral I67.81
　　coronary (acute or subacute) I24.8
　　mesenteric K55.1
　　peripheral I73.9
　　precerebral (multiple) (bilateral) G45.2
　　vertebral G45.0
　arteriovenous I99.8
　biliary K83.8
　cardiac (*see also* Insufficiency, myocardial)
　　due to presence of (cardiac) prosthesis I97.11- ☑
　　postprocedural I97.11- ☑
　cardiorenal, hypertensive I13.2
　cardiovascular — *see* Disease, cardiovascular
　cerebrovascular (acute) I67.81
　　with transient focal neurological signs and symptoms G45.8
　circulatory NEC I99.8
　　newborn P29.89
　clinical crown length K08.89
　convergence H51.11

Insufficiency, insufficient — *continued*
　coronary (acute or subacute) I24.8
　　chronic or with a stated duration of over 4 weeks I25.89
　corticoadrenal E27.40
　　primary E27.1
　dietary E63.9
　divergence H51.8
　food T73.0 ☑
　gastroesophageal K22.8
　gonadal
　　ovary E28.39
　　testis E29.1
　heart (*see also* Insufficiency, myocardial)
　　newborn P29.0
　　valve — *see* Endocarditis
　hepatic — *see* Failure, hepatic
　idiopathic autonomic G90.09
　interocclusal distance of fully erupted teeth (ridge) M26.36
　kidney N28.9
　　acute N28.9
　　chronic N18.9
　lacrimal (secretion) H04.12- ☑
　　passages — *see* Stenosis, lacrimal
　liver — *see* Failure, hepatic
　lung — *see* Insufficiency, pulmonary
　mental (congenital) — *see* Disability, intellectual
　mesenteric K55.1
　mitral (valve) I34.0
　　with
　　　aortic valve disease I08.0
　　　　with tricuspid (valve) disease I08.3
　　　obstruction or stenosis I05.2
　　　　with aortic valve disease I08.0
　　　tricuspid (valve) disease I08.1
　　　　with aortic (valve) disease I08.3
　　congenital Q23.3
　　rheumatic I05.1
　　　with
　　　　aortic valve disease I08.0
　　　　　with tricuspid (valve) disease I08.3
　　　　obstruction or stenosis I05.2
　　　　　with aortic valve disease I08.0
　　　　　　with tricuspid (valve) disease I08.3
　　　　tricuspid (valve) disease I08.1
　　　　　with aortic (valve) disease I08.3
　　　active or acute I01.1
　　　　with chorea, rheumatic (Sydenham's) I02.0
　　specified cause, except rheumatic I34.0
　muscle (*see also* Disease, muscle)
　　heart — *see* Insufficiency, myocardial
　　ocular NEC H50.9
　myocardial, myocardium (with arteriosclerosis) (*see also* Failure, heart) I50.9
　　with
　　　rheumatic fever (conditions in I00) I09.0
　　　　active, acute or subacute I01.2
　　　　　with chorea I02.0
　　　　inactive or quiescent (with chorea) I09.0
　　congenital Q24.8
　　hypertensive — *see* Hypertension, heart
　　newborn P29.0
　　rheumatic I09.0
　　　active, acute, or subacute I01.2
　　syphilitic A52.06
　nourishment T73.0 ☑
　pancreatic K86.89
　　exocrine K86.81
　parathyroid (gland) E20.9
　peripheral vascular (arterial) I73.9
　pituitary E23.0
　placental (mother) O36.51- ☑
　platelets D69.6
　prenatal care affecting management of pregnancy O09.3- ☑
　progressive pluriglandular E31.0
　pulmonary J98.4
　　acute, following surgery (nonthoracic) J95.2
　　　thoracic J95.1
　　chronic, following surgery J95.3
　　following
　　　shock J98.4
　　　trauma J98.4
　　newborn P28.5
　　valve I37.1
　　　with stenosis I37.2
　　　congenital Q22.2

Insufficiency, insufficient — *continued*
　pulmonary — *continued*
　　valve — *continued*
　　　rheumatic I09.89
　　　　with aortic, mitral or tricuspid (valve) disease I08.8
　pyloric K31.89
　renal (acute) N28.9
　　chronic N18.9
　respiratory R06.89
　　newborn P28.5
　rotation — *see* Malrotation
　sleep syndrome F51.12
　social insurance Z59.7
　suprarenal E27.40
　　primary E27.1
　tarso-orbital fascia, congenital Q10.3
　testis E29.1
　thyroid (gland) (acquired) E03.9
　　congenital E03.1
　tricuspid (valve) (rheumatic) I07.1
　　with
　　　aortic (valve) disease I08.2
　　　　with mitral (valve) disease I08.3
　　　mitral (valve) disease I08.1
　　　　with aortic (valve) disease I08.3
　　　obstruction or stenosis I07.2
　　　　with aortic (valve) disease I08.2
　　　　　with mitral (valve) disease I08.3
　　congenital Q22.8
　　nonrheumatic I36.1
　　　with stenosis I36.2
　urethral sphincter R32
　valve, valvular (heart) I38
　　aortic — *see* Insufficiency, aortic (valve)
　　congenital Q24.8
　　mitral — *see* Insufficiency, mitral (valve)
　　pulmonary — *see* Insufficiency, pulmonary, valve
　　tricuspid — *see* Insufficiency, tricuspid (valve)
　vascular I99.8
　　intestine K55.9
　　　acute (*see also* Ischemia, intestine, acute) K55.059
　　mesenteric K55.1
　　peripheral I73.9
　　renal — *see* Hypertension, kidney
　velopharyngeal
　　acquired K13.79
　　congenital Q38.8
　venous (chronic) (peripheral) I87.2
　ventricular — *see* Insufficiency, myocardial
　welfare support Z59.7
Insufflation, fallopian Z31.41
Insular — *see* condition
Insulinoma
　pancreas
　　benign D13.7
　　malignant C25.4
　　uncertain behavior D37.8
　specified site
　　benign — *see* Neoplasm, by site, benign
　　malignant — *see* Neoplasm, by site, malignant
　　uncertain behavior — *see* Neoplasm, by site, uncertain behavior
　unspecified site
　　benign D13.7
　　malignant C25.4
　　uncertain behavior D37.8
Insuloma — *see* Insulinoma
Interference
　balancing side M26.56
　non-working side M26.56
Intermenstrual — *see* condition
Intermittent — *see* condition
Internal — *see* condition
Interrogation
　cardiac defibrillator (automatic) (implantable) Z45.02
　cardiac pacemaker Z45.018
　cardiac (event) (loop) recorder Z45.09
　infusion pump (implanted) (intrathecal) Z45.1
　neurostimulator Z46.2
Interruption
　aortic arch Q25.21
　bundle of His I44.30
　phase-shift, sleep cycle — *see* Disorder, sleep, circadian rhythm
　sleep phase-shift, or 24 hour sleep-wake cycle — *see* Disorder, sleep, circadian rhythm

---

Interstitial — see condition
Intertrigo L30.4
  labialis K13.0
Intervertebral disc — see condition
Intestine, intestinal — see condition
Intolerance
  carbohydrate K90.49
  disaccharide, hereditary E73.0
  fat NEC K90.49
    pancreatic K90.3
  food K90.49
    dietary counseling and surveillance Z71.3
  fructose E74.10
    hereditary E74.12
  glucose (-galactose) E74.39
  gluten K90.41
  lactose E73.9
    specified NEC E73.8
  lysine E72.3
  milk NEC K90.49
    lactose E73.9
  protein K90.49
  starch NEC K90.49
  sucrose (-isomaltose) E74.31
Intoxicated NEC (without dependence) — see Alcohol,
    intoxication
Intoxication
  acid E87.2
  alcoholic (acute) (without dependence) — see Alcohol,
    intoxication
  alimentary canal K52.1
  amphetamine (without dependence) — see Abuse,
    drug, stimulant, with intoxication
    with dependence — see Dependence, drug, stim-
      ulant, with intoxication
  anxiolytic (acute) (without dependence) — see Abuse,
    drug, sedative, with intoxication
    with dependence — see Dependence, drug, seda-
      tive, with intoxication
  caffeine F15.929
    with dependence — see Dependence, drug, stim-
      ulant, with intoxication
  cannabinoids (acute) (without dependence) — see
    Use, cannabis, with intoxication
    with
      abuse — see Abuse, drug, cannabis, with intox-
        ication
      dependence — see Dependence, drug,
        cannabis, with intoxication
  chemical — see Table of Drugs and Chemicals
    via placenta or breast milk — see - Absorption,
      chemical, through placenta
  cocaine (acute) (without dependence) — see Abuse,
    drug, cocaine, with intoxication
    with dependence — see Dependence, drug, co-
      caine, with intoxication
  drug
    acute (without dependence) — see Abuse, drug,
      by type with intoxication
      with dependence — see Dependence, drug, by
        type with intoxication
    addictive
      via placenta or breast milk — see Absorption,
        drug, addictive, through placenta
    newborn P93.8
      gray baby syndrome P93.0
    overdose or wrong substance given or taken —
      see Table of Drugs and Chemicals, by drug,
      poisoning
  enteric K52.1
  foodborne A05.9
    bacterial A05.9
    classical (Clostridium botulinum) A05.1
    due to
      Bacillus cereus A05.4
      bacterium A05.9
        specified NEC A05.8
      Clostridium
        botulinum A05.1
        perfringens A05.2
        welchii A05.2
      Salmonella A02.9
        with
          (gastro)enteritis A02.0
          localized infection(s) A02.20
            arthritis A02.23
            meningitis A02.21
            osteomyelitis A02.24

Intoxication — continued
  foodborne — continued
    due to — continued
      Salmonella — continued
        with — continued
          localized infection(s) — continued
            pneumonia A02.22
            pyelonephritis A02.25
            specified NEC A02.29
          sepsis A02.1
          specified manifestation NEC A02.8
      Staphylococcus A05.0
      Vibrio
        parahaemolyticus A05.3
        vulnificus A05.5
    enterotoxin, staphylococcal A05.0
    noxious — see Poisoning, food, noxious
  gastrointestinal K52.1
  hallucinogenic (without dependence) — see Abuse,
    drug, hallucinogen, with intoxication
    with dependence — see Dependence, drug, hallu-
      cinogen, with intoxication
  hypnotic (acute) (without dependence) — see Abuse,
    drug, sedative, with intoxication
    with dependence — see Dependence, drug, seda-
      tive, with intoxication
  inhalant (acute) (without dependence) — see Abuse,
    drug, inhalant, with intoxication
    with dependence — see Dependence, drug, in-
      halant, with intoxication
  meaning
    inebriation — see category F10 ✓
    poisoning — see Table of Drugs and Chemicals
  methyl alcohol (acute) (without dependence) — see
    Alcohol, intoxication
  opioid (acute) (without dependence) — see Abuse,
    drug, opioid, with intoxication
    with dependence — see Dependence, drug, opioid,
      with intoxication
  pathologic NEC (without dependence) — see Alcohol,
    intoxication
  phencyclidine (without dependence) — see Abuse,
    drug, hallucinogen, with intoxication
    with dependence — see Dependence, drug, hallu-
      cinogen, with intoxication
  potassium (K) E87.5
  psychoactive substance NEC (without dependence)
    — see Abuse, drug, psychoactive NEC, with in-
      toxication
    with dependence — see Dependence, drug, psy-
      choactive NEC, with intoxication
  sedative (acute) (without dependence) — see Abuse,
    drug, sedative, with intoxication
    with dependence — see Dependence, drug, seda-
      tive, with intoxication
  serum (see also Reaction, serum) T80.69 ✓
  uremic — see Uremia
  volatile solvents (acute) (without dependence) — see
    Abuse, drug, inhalant, with intoxication
    with dependence — see Dependence, drug, in-
      halant, with intoxication
  water E87.79
Intraabdominal testis, testes
  bilateral Q53.211
  unilateral Q53.111
Intracranial — see condition
Intrahepatic gallbladder Q44.1
Intraligamentous — see condition
Intrathoracic (see also condition)
  kidney Q63.2
Intrauterine contraceptive device
  checking Z30.431
  in situ Z97.5
  insertion Z30.430
    immediately following removal Z30.433
  management Z30.431
  reinsertion Z30.433
  removal Z30.432
  replacement Z30.433
  retention in pregnancy O26.3- ✓
Intraventricular — see condition
Intrinsic deformity — see Deformity
Intubation, difficult or failed T88.4 ✓
Intumescence, lens (eye) (cataract) — see Cataract
Intussusception (bowel) (colon) (enteric) (ileocecal)
    (ileocolic) (intestine) (rectum) K56.1
  appendix K38.8
  congenital Q43.8

Intussusception — continued
  ureter (with obstruction) N13.5
Invagination (bowel, colon, intestine or rectum) K56.1
Inversion
  albumin-globulin (A-G) ratio E88.09
  bladder N32.89
  cecum — see Intussusception
  cervix N88.8
  chromosome in normal individual Q95.1
  circadian rhythm — see Disorder, sleep, circadian
    rhythm
  nipple N64.59
    congenital Q83.8
    gestational — see Retraction, nipple
    puerperal, postpartum — see Retraction, nipple
  nyctohemeral rhythm — see Disorder, sleep, circadian
    rhythm
  optic papilla Q14.2
  organ or site, congenital NEC — see Anomaly, by site
  sleep rhythm — see Disorder, sleep, circadian rhythm
  testis (congenital) Q55.29
  uterus (chronic) (postinfectional) (postpartal, old)
    N85.5
    postpartum O71.2
  vagina (posthysterectomy) N99.3
  ventricular Q20.5
Investigation (see also Examination) Z04.9
  clinical research subject (control) (normal comparison)
    (participant) Z00.6
Involuntary movement, abnormal R25.9
Involution, involutional (see also condition)
  breast, cystic — see Dysplasia, mammary, specified
    type NEC
  depression (single episode) F32.89
    recurrent episode F33.9
  melancholia (single episode) F32.89
    recurrent episode F33.8
  ovary, senile — see Atrophy, ovary
  thymus failure E32.8
I.Q.
  under 20 F73
  20-34 F72
  35-49 F71
  50-69 F70
IRDS (type I) P22.0
  type II P22.1
Irideremia Q13.1
Iridis rubeosis — see Disorder, iris, vascular
Iridochoroiditis (panuveitis) — see Panuveitis
Iridocyclitis H20.9
  acute H20.0- ✓
    hypopyon H20.05- ✓
    primary H20.01- ✓
    recurrent H20.02- ✓
    secondary (noninfectious) H20.04- ✓
      infectious H20.03- ✓
  chronic H20.1- ✓
  due to allergy — see Iridocyclitis, acute, secondary
  endogenous — see Iridocyclitis, acute, primary
  Fuchs' — see Cyclitis, Fuchs' heterochromic
  gonococcal A54.32
  granulomatous — see Iridocyclitis, chronic
  herpes, herpetic (simplex) B00.51
    zoster B02.32
  hypopyon — see Iridocyclitis, acute, hypopyon
  in (due to)
    ankylosing spondylitis M45.9
    gonococcal infection A54.32
    herpes (simplex) virus B00.51
      zoster B02.32
    infectious disease NOS B99 ✓
    parasitic disease NOS B89 [H22]
    sarcoidosis D86.83
    syphilis A51.43
    tuberculosis A18.54
    zoster B02.32
  lens-induced H20.2- ✓
  nongranulomatous — see Iridocyclitis, acute
  recurrent — see Iridocyclitis, acute, recurrent
  rheumatic — see Iridocyclitis, chronic
  subacute — see Iridocyclitis, acute
  sympathetic — see Uveitis, sympathetic
  syphilitic (secondary) A51.43
  tuberculous (chronic) A18.54
  Vogt-Koyanagi H20.82- ✓
Iridocyclochoroiditis (panuveitis) — see Panuveitis
Iridodialysis H21.53- ✓

✓ Additional Character Required — Refer to the Tabular List for Character Selection   ▽ Subterms under main terms may continue to next column or page

Iridodonesis H21.89
Iridoplegia (complete) (partial) (reflex) H57.09
Iridoschisis H21.25- ☑
Iris (*see also* condition)
 bombé — *see* Membrane, pupillary
Iritis (*see also* Iridocyclitis)
 chronic — *see* Iridocyclitis, chronic
 diabetic — *see* E08-E13 with .39
 due to
  herpes simplex B00.51
  leprosy A30.9 [H22]
 gonococcal A54.32
 gouty (*see also* Gout, by type) M10.9 [H22]
 granulomatous — *see* Iridocyclitis, chronic
 lens induced — *see* Iridocyclitis, lens-induced
 papulosa (syphilitic) A52.71
 rheumatic — *see* Iridocyclitis, chronic
 syphilitic (secondary) A51.43
  congenital (early) A50.01
  late A52.71
 tuberculous A18.54
Iron — *see* condition
Iron-miner's lung J63.4
Irradiated enamel (tooth, teeth) K03.89
Irradiation effects, adverse T66 ☑
Irreducible, irreducibility — *see* condition
Irregular, irregularity
 action, heart I49.9
 alveolar process K08.89
 bleeding N92.6
 breathing R06.89
 contour of cornea (acquired) — *see* Deformity, cornea
  congenital Q13.4
 contour, reconstructed breast N65.0
 dentin (in pulp) K04.3
 eye movements H55.89
  nystagmus — *see* Nystagmus
  saccadic H55.81
 labor O62.2
 menstruation (cause unknown) N92.6
 periods N92.6
 prostate N42.9
 pupil — *see* Abnormality, pupillary
 reconstructed breast N65.0
 respiratory R06.89
 septum (nasal) J34.2
 shape, organ or site, congenital NEC — *see* Distortion
 sleep-wake pattern (rhythm) G47.23
Irritable, irritability R45.4
 bladder N32.89
 bowel (syndrome) K58.9
  with
   constipation K58.1
   diarrhea K58.0
  mixed K58.2
  psychogenic F45.8
  specified NEC K58.8
 bronchial — *see* Bronchitis
 cerebral, in newborn P91.3
 colon (*see also* Irritable, bowel) K58.9
  with diarrhea K58.0
  psychogenic F45.8
 duodenum K59.8
 heart (psychogenic) F45.8
 hip — *see* Derangement, joint, specified type NEC, hip
 ileum K59.8
 infant R68.12
 jejunum K59.8
 rectum K59.8
 stomach K31.89
  psychogenic F45.8
 sympathetic G90.8
 urethra N36.8
Irritation
 anus K62.89
 axillary nerve G54.0
 bladder N32.89
 brachial plexus G54.0
 bronchial — *see* Bronchitis
 cervical plexus G54.2
 cervix — *see* Cervicitis
 choroid, sympathetic — *see* Endophthalmitis
 cranial nerve — *see* Disorder, nerve, cranial
 gastric K31.89
  psychogenic F45.8
 globe, sympathetic — *see* Uveitis, sympathetic
 labyrinth — *see* subcategory H83.2 ☑
 lumbosacral plexus G54.1

Irritation — *continued*
 meninges (traumatic) — *see* Injury, intracranial
  nontraumatic — *see* Meningismus
 nerve — *see* Disorder, nerve
 nervous R45.0
 penis N48.89
 perineum NEC L29.3
 peripheral autonomic nervous system G90.8
 peritoneum — *see* Peritonitis
 pharynx J39.2
 plantar nerve — *see* Lesion, nerve, plantar
 spinal (cord) (traumatic) (*see also* Injury, spinal cord, by region)
  nerve G58.9
   root NEC — *see* Radiculopathy
  nontraumatic — *see* Myelopathy
 stomach K31.89
  psychogenic F45.8
 sympathetic nerve NEC G90.8
 ulnar nerve — *see* Lesion, nerve, ulnar
 vagina N89.8
Ischemia, ischemic I99.8
 bowel (transient)
  acute (*see also* Ischemia, intestine, acute) K55.059
  chronic K55.1
  due to mesenteric artery insufficiency K55.1
 brain — *see* Ischemia, cerebral
 cardiac (see Disease, heart, ischemic)
 cardiomyopathy I25.5
 cerebral (chronic) (generalized) I67.82
  arteriosclerotic I67.2
  intermittent G45.9
  newborn P91.0
  recurrent focal G45.8
  transient G45.9
 colon chronic (due to mesenteric artery insufficiency) K55.1
 coronary — *see* Disease, heart, ischemic
 demand (coronary) (*see also* Angina) I24.8
  with myocardial infarction I21.A1
  resulting in myocardial infarction I21.A1
 heart (chronic or with a stated duration of over 4 weeks) I25.9
  acute or with a stated duration of 4 weeks or less I24.9
  subacute I24.9
 infarction, muscle — *see* Infarct, muscle
 intestine (large) (small) (transient) K55.9
  acute K55.059
   diffuse K55.052
   focal K55.051
   large K55.039
    diffuse K55.032
    focal K55.031
   small K55.019
    diffuse K55.012
    focal K55.011
  chronic K55.1
  due to mesenteric artery insufficiency K55.1
 kidney N28.0
 mesenteric, acute (*see also* Ischemia, intestine, acute) K55.059
 muscle, traumatic T79.6 ☑
 myocardium, myocardial (chronic or with a stated duration of over 4 weeks) I25.9
  acute, without myocardial infarction I51.3
  silent (asymptomatic) I25.6
  transient of newborn P29.4
 renal N28.0
 retina, retinal — *see* Occlusion, artery, retina
 small bowel
  acute K55.019
   diffuse K55.012
   focal K55.011
  chronic K55.1
  due to mesenteric artery insufficiency K55.1
 spinal cord G95.11
 subendocardial — *see* Insufficiency, coronary
 supply (coronary) (*see also* Angina) I25.9
  due to vasospasm I20.1
Ischial spine — *see* condition
Ischialgia — *see* Sciatica
Ischiopagus Q89.4
Ischium, ischial — *see* condition
Ischuria R34
Iselin's disease or osteochondrosis — *see* Osteochondrosis, juvenile, metatarsus

Islands of
 parotid tissue in
  lymph nodes Q38.6
  neck structures Q38.6
 submaxillary glands in
  fascia Q38.6
  lymph nodes Q38.6
  neck muscles Q38.6
Islet cell tumor, pancreas D13.7
Isoimmunization NEC (*see also* Incompatibility)
 affecting management of pregnancy (ABO) (with hydrops fetalis) O36.11- ☑
  anti-A sensitization O36.11- ☑
  anti-B sensitization O36.19- ☑
  anti-c sensitization O36.09- ☑
  anti-C sensitization O36.09- ☑
  anti-e sensitization O36.09- ☑
  anti-E sensitization O36.09- ☑
  Rh NEC O36.09- ☑
   anti-D antibody O36.01- ☑
  specified NEC O36.19- ☑
 newborn P55.9
  with
   hydrops fetalis P56.0
   kernicterus P57.0
  ABO (blood groups) P55.1
  Rhesus (Rh) factor P55.0
  specified type NEC P55.8
Isolation, isolated
 dwelling Z59.8
 family Z63.79
 social Z60.4
Isoleucinosis E71.19
Isomerism atrial appendages (with asplenia or polysplenia) Q20.6
Isosporiasis, isosporosis A07.3
Isovaleric acidemia E71.110
Issue of
 medical certificate Z02.79
  for disability determination Z02.71
 repeat prescription (appliance) (glasses) (medicinal substance, medicament, medicine) Z76.0
  contraception — *see* Contraception
Itch, itching (*see also* Pruritus)
 baker's L23.6
 barber's B35.0
 bricklayer's L24.5
 cheese B88.0
 clam digger's B65.3
 coolie B76.9
 copra B88.0
 dew B76.9
 dhobi B35.6
 filarial — *see* Infestation, filarial
 grain B88.0
 grocer's B88.0
 ground B76.9
 harvest B88.0
 jock B35.6
 Malabar B35.5
  beard B35.0
  foot B35.3
  scalp B35.0
 meaning scabies B86
 Norwegian B86
 perianal L29.0
 poultrymen's B88.0
 sarcoptic B86
 scabies B86
 scrub B88.0
 straw B88.0
 swimmer's B65.3
 water B76.9
 winter L29.8
Ivemark's syndrome (asplenia with congenital heart disease) Q89.01
Ivory bones Q78.2
Ixodiasis NEC B88.8

J

Jaccoud's syndrome — *see* Arthropathy, postrheumatic, chronic
Jackson's
 membrane Q43.3
 paralysis or syndrome G83.89
 veil Q43.3
Jacquet's dermatitis (diaper dermatitis) L22

⬇ Subterms under main terms may continue to next column or page   ☑ Additional Character Required — Refer to the Tabular List for Character Selection   **203**

Iridodonesis — Jacquet's dermatitis

Jadassohn-Pellizari's disease or anetoderma L90.2
Jadassohn's
 blue nevus — *see* Nevus
 intraepidermal epithelioma — *see* Neoplasm, skin,
  benign
Jaffe-Lichtenstein (-Uehlinger) **syndrome** — *see* Dys-
 plasia, fibrous, bone NEC
Jakob-Creutzfeldt disease or syndrome — *see*
 Creutzfeldt-Jakob disease or syndrome
Jaksch-Luzet disease D64.89
Jamaican
 neuropathy G92
 paraplegic tropical ataxic-spastic syndrome G92
Janet's disease F48.8
Janiceps Q89.4
Jansky-Bielschowsky amaurotic idiocy E75.4
Japanese
 B-type encephalitis A83.0
 river fever A75.3
Jaundice (yellow) R17
 acholuric (familial) (splenomegalic) (*see also* Spherocytosis)
  acquired D59.8
 breast-milk (inhibitor) P59.3
 catarrhal (acute) B15.9
  with hepatic coma B15.0
 cholestatic (benign) R17
 due to or associated with
  delayed conjugation P59.8
   associated with (due to) preterm delivery P59.0
  preterm delivery P59.0
 epidemic (catarrhal) B15.9
  with hepatic coma B15.0
  leptospiral A27.0
  spirochetal A27.0
 familial nonhemolytic (congenital) (Gilbert) E80.4
  Crigler-Najjar E80.5
 febrile (acute) B15.9
  with hepatic coma B15.0
  leptospiral A27.0
  spirochetal A27.0
 hematogenous D59.9
 hemolytic (acquired) D59.9
  congenital — *see* Spherocytosis
 hemorrhagic (acute) (leptospiral) (spirochetal) A27.0
 infectious (acute) (subacute) B15.9
  with hepatic coma B15.0
  leptospiral A27.0
  spirochetal A27.0
 leptospiral (hemorrhagic) A27.0
 malignant (without coma) K72.90
  with coma K72.91
 neonatal — *see* Jaundice, newborn
 newborn P59.9
  due to or associated with
   ABO
    antibodies P55.1
    incompatibility, maternal/fetal P55.1
    isoimmunization P55.1
   absence or deficiency of enzyme system for
    bilirubin conjugation (congenital) P59.8
   bleeding P58.1
   breast milk inhibitors to conjugation P59.3
    associated with preterm delivery P59.0
   bruising P58.0
   Crigler-Najjar syndrome E80.5
   delayed conjugation P59.8
    associated with preterm delivery P59.0
   drugs or toxins
    given to newborn P58.42
    transmitted from mother P58.41
   excessive hemolysis P58.9
    due to
     bleeding P58.1
     bruising P58.0
     drugs or toxins
      given to newborn P58.42
      transmitted from mother P58.41
     infection P58.2
     polycythemia P58.3
     swallowed maternal blood P58.5
    specified type NEC P58.8
   galactosemia E74.21
   Gilbert syndrome E80.4
   hemolytic disease P55.9
    ABO isoimmunization P55.1
    Rh isoimmunization P55.0
    specified NEC P55.8

Jaundice — *continued*
 newborn — *continued*
  due to or associated with — *continued*
   hepatocellular damage P59.20
    specified NEC P59.29
   hereditary hemolytic anemia P58.8
   hypothyroidism, congenital E03.1
   incompatibility, maternal/fetal NOS P55.9
   infection P58.2
   inspissated bile syndrome P59.1
   isoimmunization NOS P55.9
   mucoviscidosis E84.9
   polycythemia P58.3
   preterm delivery P59.0
   Rh
    antibodies P55.0
    incompatibility, maternal/fetal P55.0
    isoimmunization P55.0
   specified cause NEC P59.8
   swallowed maternal blood P58.5
   spherocytosis (congenital) D58.0
  nonhemolytic congenital familial (Gilbert) E80.4
  nuclear, newborn (*see also* Kernicterus of newborn)
   P57.9
 obstructive (*see also* Obstruction, bile duct) K83.1
 post-immunization — *see* Hepatitis, viral, type, B
 post-transfusion — *see* Hepatitis, viral, type, B
 regurgitation (*see also* Obstruction, bile duct) K83.1
 serum (homologous) (prophylactic) (therapeutic) —
  see Hepatitis, viral, type, B
 spirochetal (hemorrhagic) A27.0
 symptomatic R17
  newborn P59.9
Jaw — *see* condition
Jaw-winking phenomenon or syndrome Q07.8
Jealousy
 alcoholic F10.988
 childhood F93.8
 sibling F93.8
Jejunitis — *see* Enteritis
Jejunostomy status Z93.4
Jejunum, jejunal — *see* condition
Jensen's disease — *see* Inflammation, chorioretinal, fo-
 cal, juxtapapillary
Jerks, myoclonic G25.3
Jervell-Lange-Nielsen syndrome I45.81
Jeune's disease Q77.2
Jigger disease B88.1
Job's syndrome (chronic granulomatous disease) D71
Joint (*see also* condition)
 mice — *see* Loose, body, joint
 knee M23.4- ☑
Jordan's anomaly or syndrome D72.0
Joseph-Diamond-Blackfan anemia (congenital hy-
 poplastic) D61.01
Jungle yellow fever A95.0
Jüngling's disease — *see* Sarcoidosis
Juvenile — *see* condition

K

Kahler's disease C90.0- ☑
Kakke E51.11
Kala-azar B55.0
Kallmann's syndrome E23.0
Kanner's syndrome (autism) — *see* Psychosis, childhood
Kaposi's
 dermatosis (xeroderma pigmentosum) Q82.1
 lichen ruber L44.0
  acuminatus L44.0
 sarcoma
  colon C46.4
  connective tissue C46.1
  gastrointestinal organ C46.4
  lung C46.5- ☑
  lymph node (multiple) C46.3
  palate (hard) (soft) C46.2
  rectum C46.4
  skin (multiple sites) C46.0
  specified site NEC C46.7
  stomach C46.4
  unspecified site C46.9
 varicelliform eruption B00.0
  vaccinia T88.1 ☑
Kartagener's syndrome or triad (sinusitis, bronchiectasis, situs inversus) Q89.3

Karyotype
 with abnormality except iso (Xq) Q96.2
 45,X Q96.0
 46,X
  iso (Xq) Q96.1
 46,XX Q98.3
  with streak gonads Q50.32
  hermaphrodite (true) Q99.1
  male Q98.3
 46,XY
  with streak gonads Q56.1
  female Q97.3
  hermaphrodite (true) Q99.1
 47,XXX Q97.0
 47,XXY Q98.0
 47,XYY Q98.5
Kaschin-Beck disease — *see* Disease, Kaschin-Beck
Katayama's disease or fever B65.2
Kawasaki's syndrome M30.3
Kayser-Fleischer ring (cornea) (pseudosclerosis)
 H18.04- ☑
Kaznelson's syndrome (congenital hypoplastic anemia)
 D61.01
Kearns-Sayre syndrome H49.81- ☑
Kedani fever A75.3
Kelis L91.0
Kelly (-Patterson) **syndrome** (sideropenic dysphagia)
 D50.1
Keloid, cheloid L91.0
 acne L73.0
 Addison's L94.0
 cornea — *see* Opacity, cornea
 Hawkin's L91.0
 scar L91.0
Keloma L91.0
Kenya fever A77.1
Keratectasia (*see also* Ectasia, cornea)
 congenital Q13.4
Keratinization of alveolar ridge mucosa
 excessive K13.23
 minimal K13.22
Keratinized residual ridge mucosa
 excessive K13.23
 minimal K13.22
Keratitis (nodular) (nonulcerative) (simple) (zonular)
 H16.9
 with ulceration (central) (marginal) (perforated) (ring)
  — *see* Ulcer, cornea
 actinic — *see* Photokeratitis
 arborescens (herpes simplex) B00.52
 areolar H16.11- ☑
 bullosa H16.8
 deep H16.309
  specified type NEC H16.399
 dendritic (a) (herpes simplex) B00.52
 disciform (is) (herpes simplex) B00.52
  varicella B01.81
 filamentary H16.12- ☑
 gonococcal (congenital or prenatal) A54.33
 herpes, herpetic (simplex) B00.52
  zoster B02.33
 in (due to)
  acanthamebiasis B60.13
  adenovirus B30.0
  exanthema (*see also* Exanthem) B09
  herpes (simplex) virus B00.52
  measles B05.81
  syphilis A50.31
  tuberculosis A18.52
  zoster B02.33
 interstitial (nonsyphilitic) H16.30- ☑
  diffuse H16.32- ☑
  herpes, herpetic (simplex) B00.52
   zoster B02.33
  sclerosing H16.33- ☑
  specified type NEC H16.39- ☑
  syphilitic (congenital) (late) A50.31
  tuberculous A18.52
 macular H16.11- ☑
 nummular H16.11- ☑
 oyster shuckers' H16.8
 parenchymatous — *see* Keratitis, interstitial
 petrificans H16.8
 postmeasles B05.81
 punctata
  leprosa A30.9 [H16.14-] ☑
  syphilitic (profunda) A50.31
 punctate H16.14- ☑

☑ **Additional Character Required** — Refer to the Tabular List for Character Selection

▽ **Subterms under main terms may continue to next column or page**

Keratitis — *continued*
  purulent H16.8
  rosacea L71.8
  sclerosing H16.33- ☑
  specified type NEC H16.8
  stellate H16.11- ☑
  striate H16.11- ☑
  superficial H16.10- ☑
    with conjunctivitis — *see* Keratoconjunctivitis
    due to light — *see* Photokeratitis
  suppurative H16.8
  syphilitic (congenital) (prenatal) A50.31
  trachomatous A71.1
    sequelae B94.0
  tuberculous A18.52
  vesicular H16.8
  xerotic (*see also* Keratomalacia) H16.8
    vitamin A deficiency E50.4
Keratoacanthoma L85.8
Keratocele — *see* Descemetocele
Keratoconjunctivitis H16.20- ☑
  Acanthamoeba B60.13
  adenoviral B30.0
  epidemic B30.0
  exposure H16.21- ☑
  herpes, herpetic (simplex) B00.52
    zoster B02.33
  in exanthema (*see also* Exanthem) B09
  infectious B30.0
  lagophthalmic — *see* Keratoconjunctivitis, specified
    type NEC
  neurotrophic H16.23- ☑
  phlyctenular H16.25- ☑
  postmeasles B05.81
  shipyard B30.0
  sicca (Sjogren's) M35.0- ☑
    not Sjogren's H16.22- ☑
  specified type NEC H16.29- ☑
  tuberculous (phlyctenular) A18.52
  vernal H16.26- ☑
Keratoconus H18.60- ☑
  congenital Q13.4
  stable H18.61- ☑
  unstable H18.62- ☑
Keratocyst (dental) (odontogenic) — *see* Cyst, calcifying
  odontogenic
Keratoderma, keratodermia (congenital) (palmaris et
  plantaris) (symmetrical) Q82.8
  acquired L85.1
    in diseases classified elsewhere L86
  climactericum L85.1
  gonococcal A54.89
  gonorrheal A54.89
  punctata L85.2
  Reiter's — *see* Reiter's disease
Keratodermatocele — *see* Descemetocele
Keratoglobus H18.79 ☑
  congenital Q15.8
    with glaucoma Q15.0
Keratohemia — *see* Pigmentation, cornea, stromal
Keratoiritis (*see also* Iridocyclitis)
  syphilitic A50.39
  tuberculous A18.54
Keratoma L57.0
  palmaris and plantaris hereditarium Q82.8
  senile L57.0
Keratomalacia H18.44- ☑
  vitamin A deficiency E50.4
Keratomegaly Q13.4
Keratomycosis B49
  nigrans, nigricans (palmaris) B36.1
Keratopathy H18.9
  band H18.42- ☑
  bullous (aphakic), following cataract surgery
    H59.01- ☑
  bullous H18.1- ☑
Keratoscleritis, tuberculous A18.52
Keratosis L57.0
  actinic L57.0
  arsenical L85.8
  congenital, specified NEC Q80.8
  female genital NEC N94.89
  follicularis Q82.8
    acquired L11.0
    congenita Q82.8
    et parafollicularis in cutem penetrans L87.0
    spinulosa (decalvans) Q82.8

Keratosis — *continued*
  follicularis — *continued*
    vitamin A deficiency E50.8
  gonococcal A54.89
  male genital (external) N50.89
  nigricans L83
  obturans, external ear (canal) — *see* Cholesteatoma,
    external ear
  palmaris et plantaris (inherited) (symmetrical) Q82.8
    acquired L85.1
  penile N48.89
  pharynx J39.2
  pilaris, acquired L85.8
  punctata (palmaris et plantaris) L85.2
  scrotal N50.89
  seborrheic L82.1
    inflamed L82.0
  senile L57.0
  solar L57.0
  tonsillaris J35.8
  vagina N89.4
  vegetans Q82.8
  vitamin A deficiency E50.8
  vocal cord J38.3
Kerato-uveitis — *see* Iridocyclitis
Kerion (celsi) B35.0
Kernicterus of newborn (not due to isoimmunization)
  P57.9
  due to isoimmunization (conditions in P55.0-P55.9)
    P57.0
  specified type NEC P57.8
Kerunoparalysis T75.09 ☑
Keshan disease E59
Ketoacidosis E87.2
  diabetic — *see* Diabetes, by type, with ketoacidosis
Ketonuria R82.4
Ketosis NEC E88.89
  diabetic — *see* Diabetes, by type, with with ketoacido-
    sis
Kew Garden fever A79.1
Kidney — *see* condition
Kienböck's disease (*see also* Osteochondrosis, juvenile,
  hand, carpal lunate)
  adult M93.1
Kimmelstiel (-Wilson) **disease** — *see* Diabetes, Kimmelstiel (-Wilson) disease
Kink, kinking
  artery I77.1
  hair (acquired) L67.8
  ileum or intestine — *see* Obstruction, intestine
  Lane's — *see* Obstruction, intestine
  organ or site, congenital NEC — *see* Anomaly, by site
  ureter (pelvic junction) N13.5
    with
      hydronephrosis N13.1
        with infection N13.6
      pyelonephritis (chronic) N11.1
    congenital Q62.39
  vein(s) I87.8
    caval I87.1
    peripheral I87.1
Kinnier Wilson's disease (hepatolenticular degeneration) E83.01
Kissing spine M48.20
  cervical region M48.22
  cervicothoracic region M48.23
  lumbar region M48.26
  lumbosacral region M48.27
  occipito-atlanto-axial region M48.21
  thoracic region M48.24
  thoracolumbar region M48.25
Klatskin's tumor C22.1
Klauder's disease A26.8
Klebs' disease (*see also* Glomerulonephritis) N05- ☑
Klebsiella (K.) **pneumoniae, as cause of disease**
  classified elsewhere B96.1
Klein (e)-**Levin syndrome** G47.13
Kleptomania F63.2
Klinefelter's syndrome Q98.4
  karyotype 47,XXY Q98.0
  male with more than two X chromosomes Q98.1
Klippel-Feil deficiency, disease, or syndrome (brevi-
  collis) Q76.1
Klippel's disease I67.2
Klippel-Trenaunay (-Weber) **syndrome** Q87.2
Klumpke (-Déjerine) **palsy, paralysis** (birth) (newborn)
  P14.1
Knee — *see* condition

Knock knee (acquired) M21.06- ☑
  congenital Q74.1
Knot(s)
  intestinal, syndrome (volvulus) K56.2
  surfer S89.8- ☑
  umbilical cord (true) O69.2 ☑
Knotting (of)
  hair L67.8
  intestine K56.2
Knuckle pad (Garrod's) M72.1
Koch's
  infection — *see* Tuberculosis
  relapsing fever A68.9
Koch-Weeks' conjunctivitis — *see* Conjunctivitis, acute,
  mucopurulent
Köebner's syndrome Q81.8
Köenig's disease (osteochondritis dissecans) — *see* Osteochondritis, dissecans
Köhler-Pellegrini-Steida disease or syndrome (calcification, knee joint) — *see* Bursitis, tibial collateral
Köhler's disease
  patellar — *see* Osteochondrosis, juvenile, patella
  tarsal navicular — *see* Osteochondrosis, juvenile, tarsus
Koilonychia L60.3
  congenital Q84.6
Kojevnikov's, epilepsy — *see* Kozhevnikof's epilepsy
Koplik's spots B05.9
Kopp's asthma E32.8
Korsakoff's (Wernicke) **disease, psychosis or syn-**
  drome (alcoholic) F10.96
  with dependence F10.26
  drug-induced
    due to drug abuse — *see* Abuse, drug, by type,
      with amnestic disorder
    due to drug dependence — *see* Dependence, drug,
      by type, with amnestic disorder
  nonalcoholic F04
Korsakov's disease, psychosis or syndrome — *see*
  Korsakoff's disease
Korsakow's disease, psychosis or syndrome — *see*
  Korsakoff's disease
Kostmann's disease or syndrome (infantile genetic
  agranulocytosis) — *see* Agranulocytosis
Kozhevnikof's epilepsy G40.109
  intractable G40.119
    with status epilepticus G40.111
    without status epilepticus G40.119
  not intractable G40.109
    with status epilepticus G40.101
    without status epilepticus G40.109
Krabbe's
  disease E75.23
  syndrome, congenital muscle hypoplasia Q79.8
Kraepelin-Morel disease — *see* Schizophrenia
Kraft-Weber-Dimitri disease Q85.8
Kraurosis
  ani K62.89
  penis N48.0
  vagina N89.8
  vulva N90.4
Kreotoxism A05.9
Krukenberg's
  spindle — *see* Pigmentation, cornea, posterior
  tumor C79.6- ☑
Kufs' disease E75.4
Kugelberg-Welander disease G12.1
Kuhnt-Junius degeneration (*see also* Degeneration,
  macula) H35.32- ☑
Kümmell's disease or spondylitis — *see* Spondylopa-
  thy, traumatic
Kupffer cell sarcoma C22.3
Kuru A81.81
Kussmaul's
  disease M30.0
  respiration E87.2
    in diabetic acidosis — *see* Diabetes, by type, with
      ketoacidosis
Kwashiorkor E40
  marasmic, marasmus type E42
Kyasanur Forest disease A98.2
Kyphoscoliosis, kyphoscoliotic (acquired) (*see also*
  Scoliosis) M41.9
  congenital Q67.5
  heart (disease) I27.1
  sequelae of rickets E64.3
  tuberculous A18.01
Kyphosis, kyphotic (acquired) M40.209

Kyphosis, kyphotic — *continued*
  cervical region M40.202
  cervicothoracic region M40.203
  congenital Q76.419
    cervical region Q76.412
    cervicothoracic region Q76.413
    occipito-atlanto-axial region Q76.411
    thoracic region Q76.414
    thoracolumbar region Q76.415
  Morquio-Brailsford type (spinal) (*see also* subcategory M49.8) E76.219
  postlaminectomy M96.3
  postradiation therapy M96.2
  postural (adolescent) M40.00
    cervicothoracic region M40.03
    thoracic region M40.04
    thoracolumbar region M40.05
  secondary NEC M40.10
    cervical region M40.12
    cervicothoracic region M40.13
    thoracic region M40.14
    thoracolumbar region M40.15
  sequelae of rickets E64.3
  specified type NEC M40.299
    cervical region M40.292
    cervicothoracic region M40.293
    thoracic region M40.294
    thoracolumbar region M40.295
  syphilitic, congenital A50.56
  thoracic region M40.204
  thoracolumbar region M40.205
  tuberculous A18.01
Kyrle disease L87.0

L

Labia, labium — *see* condition
Labile
  blood pressure R09.89
  vasomotor system I73.9
Labioglossal paralysis G12.29
Labium leporinum — *see* Cleft, lip
Labor — *see* Delivery
Labored breathing — *see* Hyperventilation
Labyrinthitis (circumscribed) (destructive) (diffuse) (inner ear) (latent) (purulent) (suppurative) (*see also* subcategory) H83.0 ☑
  syphilitic A52.79
Laceration
  with abortion — *see* Abortion, by type, complicated by laceration of pelvic organs
  abdomen, abdominal
    wall S31.119 ☑
      with
        foreign body S31.129 ☑
        penetration into peritoneal cavity S31.619 ☑
          with foreign body S31.629 ☑
      epigastric region S31.112 ☑
        with
          foreign body S31.122 ☑
          penetration into peritoneal cavity S31.612 ☑
            with foreign body S31.622 ☑
      left
        lower quadrant S31.114 ☑
          with
            foreign body S31.124 ☑
            penetration into peritoneal cavity S31.614 ☑
              with foreign body S31.624 ☑
        upper quadrant S31.111 ☑
          with
            foreign body S31.121 ☑
            penetration into peritoneal cavity S31.611 ☑
              with foreign body S31.621 ☑
      periumbilic region S31.115 ☑
        with
          foreign body S31.125 ☑
          penetration into peritoneal cavity S31.615 ☑
            with foreign body S31.625 ☑
      right
        lower quadrant S31.113 ☑
          with
            foreign body S31.123 ☑

Laceration — *continued*
  abdomen, abdominal — *continued*
    wall — *continued*
      right — *continued*
        lower quadrant — *continued*
          with — *continued*
            penetration into peritoneal cavity S31.613 ☑
              with foreign body S31.623 ☑
        upper quadrant S31.110 ☑
          with
            foreign body S31.120 ☑
            penetration into peritoneal cavity S31.610 ☑
              with foreign body S31.620 ☑
  accidental, complicating surgery — *see* Complications, surgical, accidental puncture or laceration
  Achilles tendon S86.02- ☑
  adrenal gland S37.813 ☑
  alveolar (process) — *see* Laceration, oral cavity
  ankle S91.01- ☑
    with
      foreign body S91.02- ☑
  antecubital space — *see* Laceration, elbow
  anus (sphincter) S31.831 ☑
    with
      ectopic or molar pregnancy O08.6
      foreign body S31.832 ☑
    complicating delivery — *see* Delivery, complicated, by, laceration, anus (sphincter)
    following ectopic or molar pregnancy O08.6
    nontraumatic, nonpuerperal — *see* Fissure, anus
  arm (upper) S41.11- ☑
    with foreign body S41.12- ☑
    lower — *see* Laceration, forearm
  auditory canal (external) (meatus) — *see* Laceration, ear
  auricle, ear — *see* Laceration, ear
  axilla — *see* Laceration, arm
  back (*see also* Laceration, thorax, back)
    lower S31.010 ☑
      with
        foreign body S31.020 ☑
          with penetration into retroperitoneal space S31.021 ☑
        penetration into retroperitoneal space S31.011 ☑
  bile duct S36.13 ☑
  bladder S37.23 ☑
    with ectopic or molar pregnancy O08.6
    following ectopic or molar pregnancy O08.6
    obstetrical trauma O71.5
  blood vessel — *see* Injury, blood vessel
  bowel (*see also* Laceration, intestine)
    with ectopic or molar pregnancy O08.6
    complicating abortion — *see* Abortion, by type, complicated by, specified condition NEC
    following ectopic or molar pregnancy O08.6
    obstetrical trauma O71.5
  brain (any part) (cortex) (diffuse) (membrane) (*see also* Injury, intracranial, diffuse)
    during birth P10.8
      with hemorrhage P10.1
    focal — *see* Injury, intracranial, focal brain injury
  brainstem S06.38- ☑
  breast S21.01- ☑
    with foreign body S21.02- ☑
  broad ligament S37.893 ☑
    with ectopic or molar pregnancy O08.6
    following ectopic or molar pregnancy O08.6
    laceration syndrome N83.8
    obstetrical trauma O71.6
    syndrome (laceration) N83.8
  buttock S31.801 ☑
    with foreign body S31.802 ☑
    left S31.821 ☑
      with foreign body S31.822 ☑
    right S31.811 ☑
      with foreign body S31.812 ☑
  calf — *see* Laceration, leg
  canaliculus lacrimalis — *see* Laceration, eyelid
  canthus, eye — *see* Laceration, eyelid
  capsule, joint — *see* Sprain
  causing eversion of cervix uteri (old) N86
  central (perineal), complicating delivery O70.9
  cerebellum, traumatic S06.37- ☑
  cerebral S06.33- ☑

Laceration — *continued*
  cerebral — *continued*
    during birth P10.8
      with hemorrhage P10.1
    left side S06.32- ☑
    right side S06.31- ☑
  cervix (uteri)
    with ectopic or molar pregnancy O08.6
    following ectopic or molar pregnancy O08.6
    nonpuerperal, nontraumatic N88.1
    obstetrical trauma (current) O71.3
    old (postpartal) N88.1
    traumatic S37.63
  cheek (external) S01.41- ☑
    with foreign body S01.42- ☑
    internal — *see* Laceration, oral cavity
  chest wall — *see* Laceration, thorax
  chin — *see* Laceration, head, specified site NEC
  chordae tendinae NEC I51.1
    concurrent with acute myocardial infarction — *see* Infarct, myocardium
    following acute myocardial infarction (current complication) I23.4
  clitoris — *see* Laceration, vulva
  colon — *see* Laceration, intestine, large, colon
  common bile duct S36.13 ☑
  cortex (cerebral) — *see* Injury, intracranial, diffuse
  costal region — *see* Laceration, thorax
  cystic duct S36.13 ☑
  diaphragm S27.803 ☑
  digit(s)
    foot — *see* Laceration, toe
    hand — *see* Laceration, finger
  duodenum S36.430 ☑
  ear (canal) (external) S01.31- ☑
    with foreign body S01.32- ☑
    drum S09.2- ☑
  elbow S51.01- ☑
    with
      foreign body S51.02- ☑
  epididymis — *see* Laceration, testis
  epigastric region — *see* Laceration, abdomen, wall, epigastric region
  esophagus K22.8
    traumatic
      cervical S11.21 ☑
        with foreign body S11.22 ☑
      thoracic S27.813 ☑
  eye (ball) S05.3- ☑
    with prolapse or loss of intraocular tissue S05.2- ☑
    penetrating S05.6- ☑
  eyebrow — *see* Laceration, eyelid
  eyelid S01.11- ☑
    with foreign body S01.12- ☑
  face NEC — *see* Laceration, head, specified site NEC
  fallopian tube S37.539 ☑
    bilateral S37.532 ☑
    unilateral S37.531 ☑
  finger(s) S61.219 ☑
    with
      damage to nail S61.319 ☑
        with
          foreign body S61.329 ☑
      foreign body S61.229 ☑
    index S61.218 ☑
      with
        damage to nail S61.318 ☑
          with
            foreign body S61.328 ☑
        foreign body S61.228 ☑
      left S61.211 ☑
        with
          damage to nail S61.311 ☑
            with
              foreign body S61.321 ☑
          foreign body S61.221 ☑
        right S61.210 ☑
          with
            damage to nail S61.310 ☑
              with
                foreign body S61.320 ☑
            foreign body S61.220 ☑
    little S61.218 ☑
      with
        damage to nail S61.318 ☑
          with
            foreign body S61.328 ☑

☑ **Additional Character Required — Refer to the Tabular List for Character Selection**   ⛛ **Subterms under main terms may continue to next column or page**

Laceration — *continued*
  finger(s) — *continued*
    little — *continued*
      with — *continued*
        foreign body S61.228 ☑
      left S61.217 ☑
        with
          damage to nail S61.317 ☑
            with
              foreign body S61.327 ☑
          foreign body S61.227 ☑
      right S61.216 ☑
        with
          damage to nail S61.316 ☑
            with
              foreign body S61.326 ☑
          foreign body S61.226 ☑
    middle S61.218 ☑
      with
        damage to nail S61.318 ☑
          with
            foreign body S61.328 ☑
        foreign body S61.228 ☑
      left S61.213 ☑
        with
          damage to nail S61.313 ☑
            with
              foreign body S61.323 ☑
          foreign body S61.223 ☑
      right S61.212 ☑
        with
          damage to nail S61.312 ☑
            with
              foreign body S61.322 ☑
          foreign body S61.222 ☑
    ring S61.218 ☑
      with
        damage to nail S61.318 ☑
          with
            foreign body S61.328 ☑
        foreign body S61.228 ☑
      left S61.215 ☑
        with
          damage to nail S61.315 ☑
            with
              foreign body S61.325 ☑
          foreign body S61.225 ☑
      right S61.214 ☑
        with
          damage to nail S61.314 ☑
            with
              foreign body S61.324 ☑
          foreign body S61.224 ☑
  flank S31.119 ☑
    with foreign body S31.129 ☑
  foot (except toe(s) alone) S91.319 ☑
    with foreign body S91.329 ☑
    left S91.312 ☑
      with foreign body S91.322 ☑
    right S91.311 ☑
      with foreign body S91.321 ☑
    toe — *see* Laceration, toe
  forearm S51.819 ☑
    with
      foreign body S51.829 ☑
    elbow only — *see* Laceration, elbow
    left S51.812 ☑
      with
        foreign body S51.822 ☑
    right S51.811 ☑
      with
        foreign body S51.821 ☑
  forehead S01.81 ☑
    with foreign body S01.82 ☑
  fourchette O70.0
    with ectopic or molar pregnancy O08.6
    complicating delivery O70.0
    following ectopic or molar pregnancy O08.6
  gallbladder S36.123 ☑
  genital organs, external
    female S31.512 ☑
      with foreign body S31.522 ☑
      vagina — *see* Laceration, vagina
      vulva — *see* Laceration, vulva
    male S31.511 ☑
      with foreign body S31.521 ☑

Laceration — *continued*
  genital organs, external — *continued*
    male — *continued*
      penis — *see* Laceration, penis
      scrotum — *see* Laceration, scrotum
      testis — *see* Laceration, testis
  groin — *see* Laceration, abdomen, wall
  gum — *see* Laceration, oral cavity
  hand S61.419 ☑
    with
      foreign body S61.429 ☑
    finger — *see* Laceration, finger
    left S61.412 ☑
      with
        foreign body S61.422 ☑
    right S61.411 ☑
      with
        foreign body S61.421 ☑
    thumb — *see* Laceration, thumb
  head S01.91 ☑
    with foreign body S01.92 ☑
    cheek — *see* Laceration, cheek
    ear — *see* Laceration, ear
    eyelid — *see* Laceration, eyelid
    lip — *see* Laceration, lip
    nose — *see* Laceration, nose
    oral cavity — *see* Laceration, oral cavity
    scalp S01.01 ☑
      with foreign body S01.02 ☑
    specified site NEC S01.81 ☑
      with foreign body S01.82 ☑
    temporomandibular area — *see* Laceration, cheek
  heart — *see* Injury, heart, laceration
  heel — *see* Laceration, foot
  hepatic duct S36.13 ☑
  hip S71.019 ☑
    with foreign body S71.029 ☑
    left S71.012 ☑
      with foreign body S71.022 ☑
    right S71.011 ☑
      with foreign body S71.021 ☑
  hymen — *see* Laceration, vagina
  hypochondrium — *see* Laceration, abdomen, wall
  hypogastric region — *see* Laceration, abdomen, wall
  ileum S36.438 ☑
  inguinal region — *see* Laceration, abdomen, wall
  instep — *see* Laceration, foot
  internal organ — *see* Injury, by site
  interscapular region — *see* Laceration, thorax, back
  intestine
    large
      colon S36.539 ☑
        ascending S36.530 ☑
        descending S36.532 ☑
        sigmoid S36.533 ☑
        specified site NEC S36.538 ☑
      rectum S36.63 ☑
        transverse S36.531 ☑
    small S36.439 ☑
      duodenum S36.430 ☑
      specified site NEC S36.438 ☑
  intra-abdominal organ S36.93 ☑
    intestine — *see* Laceration, intestine
    liver — *see* Laceration, liver
    pancreas — *see* Laceration, pancreas
    peritoneum S36.81 ☑
    specified site NEC S36.893 ☑
    spleen — *see* Laceration, spleen
    stomach — *see* Laceration, stomach
  intracranial NEC (*see also* Injury, intracranial, diffuse)
    birth injury P10.9
  jaw — *see* Laceration, head, specified site NEC
  jejunum S36.438 ☑
  joint capsule — *see* Sprain, by site
  kidney S37.03- ☑
    major (greater than 3 cm) (massive) (stellate) S37.06- ☑
    minor (less than 1 cm) S37.04- ☑
    moderate (1 to 3 cm) S37.05- ☑
    multiple S37.06- ☑
  knee S81.01- ☑
    with foreign body S81.02- ☑
  labium (majus) (minus) — *see* Laceration, vulva
  lacrimal duct — *see* Laceration, eyelid
  large intestine — *see* Laceration, intestine, large
  larynx S11.011 ☑

Laceration — *continued*
  larynx — *continued*
    with foreign body S11.012 ☑
  leg (lower) S81.819 ☑
    with foreign body S81.829 ☑
    foot — *see* Laceration, foot
    knee — *see* Laceration, knee
    left S81.812 ☑
      with foreign body S81.822 ☑
    right S81.811 ☑
      with foreign body S81.821 ☑
    upper — *see* Laceration, thigh
  ligament — *see* Sprain
  lip S01.511 ☑
    with foreign body S01.521 ☑
  liver S36.113 ☑
    major (stellate) S36.116 ☑
    minor S36.114 ☑
    moderate S36.115 ☑
  loin — *see* Laceration, abdomen, wall
  lower back — *see* Laceration, back, lower
  lumbar region — *see* Laceration, back, lower
  lung S27.339 ☑
    bilateral S27.332 ☑
    unilateral S27.331 ☑
  malar region — *see* Laceration, head, specified site NEC
  mammary — *see* Laceration, breast
  mastoid region — *see* Laceration, head, specified site NEC
  meninges — *see* Injury, intracranial, diffuse
  meniscus — *see* Tear, meniscus
  mesentery S36.893 ☑
  mesosalpinx S37.893 ☑
  mouth — *see* Laceration, oral cavity
  muscle — *see* Injury, muscle, by site, laceration
  nail
    finger — *see* Laceration, finger, with damage to nail
    toe — *see* Laceration, toe, with damage to nail
  nasal (septum) (sinus) — *see* Laceration, nose
  nasopharynx — *see* Laceration, head, specified site NEC
  neck S11.91 ☑
    with foreign body S11.92 ☑
    involving
      cervical esophagus S11.21 ☑
        with foreign body S11.22 ☑
      larynx — *see* Laceration, larynx
      pharynx — *see* Laceration, pharynx
      thyroid gland — *see* Laceration, thyroid gland
      trachea — *see* Laceration, trachea
    specified site NEC S11.81 ☑
      with foreign body S11.82 ☑
  nerve — *see* Injury, nerve
  nose (septum) (sinus) S01.21 ☑
    with foreign body S01.22 ☑
  ocular NOS S05.3- ☑
    adnexa NOS S01.11- ☑
  oral cavity S01.512 ☑
    with foreign body S01.522 ☑
  orbit (eye) — *see* Wound, open, ocular, orbit
  ovary S37.439 ☑
    bilateral S37.432 ☑
    unilateral S37.431 ☑
  palate — *see* Laceration, oral cavity
  palm — *see* Laceration, hand
  pancreas S36.239 ☑
  pelvic S31.010 ☑
    with
      foreign body S31.020 ☑
        penetration into retroperitoneal cavity S31.021 ☑
      penetration into retroperitoneal cavity S31.011 ☑
    floor (*see also* Laceration, back, lower)
      with ectopic or molar pregnancy O08.6
      complicating delivery O70.1
      following ectopic or molar pregnancy O08.6
      old (postpartal) N81.89
    organ S37.93 ☑
  penis S31.21 ☑
    with foreign body S31.22 ☑
  perineum
    female S31.41 ☑

Laceration — *continued*
  perineum — *continued*
    female — *continued*
      with
        ectopic or molar pregnancy O08.6
        foreign body S31.42 ☑
      during delivery O70.9
        first degree O70.0
        fourth degree O70.3
        second degree O70.1
        third degree (*see also* Delivery, complicated,
          by, laceration, perineum, third de-
          gree) O70.20
      old (postpartal) N81.89
      postpartal N81.89
      secondary (postpartal) O90.1
    male S31.119 ☑
      with foreign body S31.129 ☑
  periocular area (with or without lacrimal passages) —
    see Laceration, eyelid
  peritoneum S36.893 ☑
  periumbilic region — *see* Laceration, abdomen, wall,
    periumbilic
  periurethral tissue — *see* Laceration, urethra
  phalanges
    finger — *see* Laceration, finger
    toe — *see* Laceration, toe
  pharynx S11.21 ☑
    with foreign body S11.22 ☑
  pinna — *see* Laceration, ear
  popliteal space — *see* Laceration, knee
  prepuce — *see* Laceration, penis
  prostate S37.823 ☑
  pubic region S31.119 ☑
    with foreign body S31.129 ☑
  pudendum — *see* Laceration, genital organs, external
  rectovaginal septum — *see* Laceration, vagina
  rectum S36.63 ☑
  retroperitoneum S36.893 ☑
  round ligament S37.893 ☑
  sacral region — *see* Laceration, back, lower
  sacroiliac region — *see* Laceration, back, lower
  salivary gland — *see* Laceration, oral cavity
  scalp S01.01 ☑
    with foreign body S01.02 ☑
  scapular region — *see* Laceration, shoulder
  scrotum S31.31 ☑
    with foreign body S31.32 ☑
  seminal vesicle S37.893 ☑
  shin — *see* Laceration, leg
  shoulder S41.019 ☑
    with foreign body S41.029 ☑
    left S41.012 ☑
      with foreign body S41.022 ☑
    right S41.011 ☑
      with foreign body S41.021 ☑
  small intestine — *see* Laceration, intestine, small
  spermatic cord — *see* Laceration, testis
  spinal cord (meninges) (*see also* Injury, spinal cord, by
    region)
    due to injury at birth P11.5
    newborn (birth injury) P11.5
  spleen S36.039 ☑
    major (massive) (stellate) S36.032 ☑
    moderate S36.031 ☑
    superficial (minor) S36.030 ☑
  sternal region — *see* Laceration, thorax, front
  stomach S36.33 ☑
  submaxillary region — *see* Laceration, head, specified
    site NEC
  submental region — *see* Laceration, head, specified
    site NEC
  subungual
    finger(s) — *see* Laceration, finger, with damage to
      nail
    toe(s) — *see* Laceration, toe, with damage to nail
  suprarenal gland — *see* Laceration, adrenal gland
  temple, temporal region — *see* Laceration, head,
    specified site NEC
  temporomandibular area — *see* Laceration, cheek
  tendon — *see* Injury, muscle, by site, laceration
    Achilles S86.02- ☑
  tentorium cerebelli — *see* Injury, intracranial, diffuse
  testis S31.31 ☑
    with foreign body S31.32 ☑
  thigh S71.11- ☑
    with foreign body S71.12- ☑

Laceration — *continued*
  thorax, thoracic (wall) S21.91 ☑
    with foreign body S21.92 ☑
    back S21.22- ☑
      with penetration into thoracic cavity
        S21.42- ☑
    front S21.12- ☑
      with penetration into thoracic cavity
        S21.32- ☑
    back S21.21- ☑
      with
        foreign body S21.22- ☑
          with penetration into thoracic cavity
            S21.42- ☑
        penetration into thoracic cavity S21.41- ☑
    breast — *see* Laceration, breast
    front S21.11- ☑
      with
        foreign body S21.12- ☑
          with penetration into thoracic cavity
            S21.32- ☑
        penetration into thoracic cavity S21.31- ☑
  thumb S61.019 ☑
    with
      damage to nail S61.119 ☑
        with
          foreign body S61.129 ☑
      foreign body S61.029 ☑
    left S61.012 ☑
      with
        damage to nail S61.112 ☑
          with
            foreign body S61.122 ☑
        foreign body S61.022 ☑
    right S61.011 ☑
      with
        damage to nail S61.111 ☑
          with
            foreign body S61.121 ☑
        foreign body S61.021 ☑
  thyroid gland S11.11 ☑
    with foreign body S11.12 ☑
  toe(s) S91.119 ☑
    with
      damage to nail S91.219 ☑
        with
          foreign body S91.229 ☑
      foreign body S91.129 ☑
    great S91.113 ☑
      with
        damage to nail S91.213 ☑
          with
            foreign body S91.223 ☑
        foreign body S91.123 ☑
      left S91.112 ☑
        with
          damage to nail S91.212 ☑
            with
              foreign body S91.222 ☑
          foreign body S91.122 ☑
      right S91.111 ☑
        with
          damage to nail S91.211 ☑
            with
              foreign body S91.221 ☑
          foreign body S91.121 ☑
    lesser S91.116 ☑
      with
        damage to nail S91.216 ☑
          with
            foreign body S91.226 ☑
        foreign body S91.126 ☑
      left S91.115 ☑
        with
          damage to nail S91.215 ☑
            with
              foreign body S91.225 ☑
          foreign body S91.125 ☑
      right S91.114 ☑
        with
          damage to nail S91.214 ☑
            with
              foreign body S91.224 ☑
          foreign body S91.124 ☑
  tongue — *see* Laceration, oral cavity
  trachea S11.021 ☑

Laceration — *continued*
  trachea — *continued*
    with foreign body S11.022 ☑
  tunica vaginalis — *see* Laceration, testis
  tympanum, tympanic membrane — *see* Laceration,
    ear, drum
  umbilical region S31.115 ☑
    with foreign body S31.125 ☑
  ureter S37.13 ☑
  urethra S37.33 ☑
    with or following ectopic or molar pregnancy O08.6
    obstetrical trauma O71.5
  urinary organ NEC S37.893 ☑
  uterus S37.63 ☑
    with ectopic or molar pregnancy O08.6
    following ectopic or molar pregnancy O08.6
    nonpuerperal, nontraumatic N85.8
    obstetrical trauma NEC O71.81
    old (postpartal) N85.8
  uvula — *see* Laceration, oral cavity
  vagina S31.41 ☑
    with
      ectopic or molar pregnancy O08.6
      foreign body S31.42 ☑
    during delivery O71.4
      with perineal laceration — *see* Laceration, per-
        ineum, female, during delivery
    following ectopic or molar pregnancy O08.6
    nonpuerperal, nontraumatic N89.8
    old (postpartal) N89.8
  vas deferens S37.893 ☑
  vesical — *see* Laceration, bladder
  vocal cords S11.031 ☑
    with foreign body S11.032 ☑
  vulva S31.41 ☑
    with
      ectopic or molar pregnancy O08.6
      foreign body S31.42 ☑
    complicating delivery O70.0
    following ectopic or molar pregnancy O08.6
    nonpuerperal, nontraumatic N90.89
    old (postpartal) N90.89
  wrist S61.519 ☑
    with
      foreign body S61.529 ☑
    left S61.512 ☑
      with
        foreign body S61.522 ☑
    right S61.511 ☑
      with
        foreign body S61.521 ☑

Lack of
  achievement in school Z55.3
  adequate
    food Z59.4
    intermaxillary vertical dimension of fully erupted
      teeth M26.36
    sleep Z72.820
  appetite (see Anorexia) R63.0
  awareness R41.9
  care
    in home Z74.2
    of infant (at or after birth) T76.02 ☑
      confirmed T74.02 ☑
  cognitive functions R41.9
  coordination R27.9
    ataxia R27.0
    specified type NEC R27.8
  development (physiological) R62.50
    failure to thrive (child over 28 days old) R62.51
      adult R62.7
      newborn P92.6
    short stature R62.52
    specified type NEC R62.59
  energy R53.83
  financial resources Z59.6
  food T73.0 ☑
  growth R62.52
  heating Z59.1
  housing (permanent) (temporary) Z59.0
    adequate Z59.1
  learning experiences in childhood Z62.898
  leisure time (affecting life-style) Z73.2
  material resources Z59.9
  memory (*see also* Amnesia)
    mild, following organic brain damage F06.8
  ovulation N97.0
  parental supervision or control of child Z62.0

Lack of — *continued*
  person able to render necessary care Z74.2
  physical exercise Z72.3
  play experience in childhood Z62.898
  posterior occlusal support M26.57
  relaxation (affecting life-style) Z73.2
  sexual
    desire F52.0
    enjoyment F52.1
  shelter Z59.0
  sleep (adequate) Z72.820
  supervision of child by parent Z62.0
  support, posterior occlusal M26.57
  water T73.1 ☑
Lacrimal — *see* condition
Lacrimation, abnormal — *see* Epiphora
Lacrimonasal duct — *see* condition
Lactation, lactating (breast) (puerperal, postpartum)
  associated
    cracked nipple O92.13
    retracted nipple O92.03
  defective O92.4
  disorder NEC O92.79
  excessive O92.6
  failed (complete) O92.3
    partial O92.4
  mastitis NEC — *see* Mastitis, obstetric
  mother (care and/or examination) Z39.1
  nonpuerperal N64.3
Lacticemia, excessive E87.2
Lacunar skull Q75.8
Laennec's cirrhosis K70.30
  with ascites K70.31
  nonalcoholic K74.69
Lafora's disease — *see* Epilepsy, generalized, idiopathic
Lag, lid (nervous) — *see* Retraction, lid
Lagophthalmos (eyelid) (nervous) H02.209
  cicatricial H02.219
    left H02.216
      lower H02.215
      upper H02.214
    right H02.213
      lower H02.212
      upper H02.211
  keratoconjunctivitis — *see* Keratoconjunctivitis
  left H02.206
    lower H02.205
    upper H02.204
  mechanical H02.229
    left H02.226
      lower H02.225
      upper H02.224
    right H02.223
      lower H02.222
      upper H02.221
  paralytic H02.239
    left H02.236
      lower H02.235
      upper H02.234
    right H02.233
      lower H02.232
      upper H02.231
  right H02.203
    lower H02.202
    upper H02.201
Laki-Lorand factor deficiency — *see* Defect, coagulation, specified type NEC
Lalling F80.0
Lambert-Eaton syndrome — *see* Syndrome, Lambert-Eaton
Lambliasis, lambliosis A07.1
Landau-Kleffner syndrome — *see* Epilepsy, specified NEC
Landouzy-Déjérine dystrophy or facioscapulohumeral atrophy G71.0
Landouzy's disease (icterohemorrhagic leptospirosis) A27.0
Landry-Guillain-Barré, syndrome or paralysis G61.0
Landry's disease or paralysis G61.0
Lane's
  band Q43.3
  kink — *see* Obstruction, intestine
  syndrome K90.2
Langdon Down syndrome — *see* Trisomy, 21
Lapsed immunization schedule status Z28.3
Large
  baby (regardless of gestational age) (4000g to 4499g) P08.1

Large — *continued*
  ear, congenital Q17.1
  physiological cup Q14.2
  stature R68.89
Large-for-dates NEC (infant) (4000g to 4499g) P08.1
  affecting management of pregnancy O36.6- ☑
  exceptionally (4500g or more) P08.0
Larsen-Johansson disease orosteochondrosis — *see* Osteochondrosis, juvenile, patella
Larsen's syndrome (flattened facies and multiple congenital dislocations) Q74.8
Larva migrans
  cutaneous B76.9
    Ancylostoma B76.0
  visceral B83.0
Laryngeal — *see* condition
Laryngismus (stridulus) J38.5
  congenital P28.89
  diphtheritic A36.2
Laryngitis (acute) (edematous) (fibrinous) (infective) (infiltrative) (malignant) (membranous) (phlegmonous) (pneumococcal) (pseudomembranous) (septic) (subglottic) (suppurative) (ulcerative) J04.0
  with
    influenza, flu, or grippe — *see* Influenza, with, laryngitis
    tracheitis (acute) — *see* Laryngotracheitis
  atrophic J37.0
  catarrhal J37.0
  chronic J37.0
    with tracheitis (chronic) J37.1
  diphtheritic A36.2
  due to external agent — *see* Inflammation, respiratory, upper, due to
  H. influenzae J04.0
  Hemophilus influenzae J04.0
  hypertrophic J37.0
  influenzal — *see* Influenza, with, respiratory manifestations NEC
  obstructive J05.0
  sicca J37.0
  spasmodic J05.0
    acute J04.0
  streptococcal J04.0
  stridulous J05.0
  syphilitic (late) A52.73
    congenital A50.59 [J99]
    early A50.03 [J99]
  tuberculous A15.5
  Vincent's A69.1
Laryngocele (congenital) (ventricular) Q31.3
Laryngofissure J38.7
  congenital Q31.8
Laryngomalacia (congenital) Q31.5
Laryngopharyngitis (acute) J06.0
  chronic J37.0
  due to external agent — *see* Inflammation, respiratory, upper, due to
Laryngoplegia J38.00
  bilateral J38.02
  unilateral J38.01
Laryngoptosis J38.7
Laryngospasm J38.5
Laryngostenosis J38.6
Laryngotracheitis (acute) (Infectional) (infective) (viral) J04.2
  atrophic J37.1
  catarrhal J37.1
  chronic J37.1
  diphtheritic A36.2
  due to external agent — *see* Inflammation, respiratory, upper, due to
  Hemophilus influenzae J04.2
  hypertrophic J37.1
  influenzal — *see* Influenza, with, respiratory manifestations NEC
  pachydermic J38.7
  sicca J37.1
  spasmodic J38.5
    acute J05.0
  streptococcal J04.2
  stridulous J38.5
  syphilitic (late) A52.73
    congenital A50.59 [J99]
    early A50.03 [J99]
  tuberculous A15.5
  Vincent's A69.1
Laryngotracheobronchitis — *see* Bronchitis

Larynx, laryngeal — *see* condition
Lassa fever A96.2
Lassitude — *see* Weakness
Late
  talker R62.0
  walker R62.0
Late effect(s) — *see* Sequelae
Latent — *see* condition
Laterocession — *see* Lateroversion
Lateroflexion — *see* Lateroversion
Lateroversion
  cervix — *see* Lateroversion, uterus
  uterus, uterine (cervix) (postinfectional) (postpartal, old) N85.4
    congenital Q51.818
    in pregnancy or childbirth O34.59- ☑
Lathyrism — *see* Poisoning, food, noxious, plant
Launois' syndrome (pituitary gigantism) E22.0
Launois-Bensaude adenolipomatosis E88.89
Laurence-Moon (-Bardet)-**Biedl syndrome** Q87.89
Lax, laxity (*see also* Relaxation)
  ligament (ous) (*see also* Disorder, ligament)
    familial M35.7
    knee — *see* Derangement, knee
  skin (acquired) L57.4
    congenital Q82.8
Laxative habit F55.2
Lazy leukocyte syndrome D70.8
Lead miner's lung J63.6
Leak, leakage
  air NEC J93.82
    postprocedural J95.812
  amniotic fluid — *see* Rupture, membranes, premature
  blood (microscopic), fetal, into maternal circulation affecting management of pregnancy — *see* Pregnancy, complicated by
  cerebrospinal fluid G96.0
    from spinal (lumbar) puncture G97.0
  device, implant or graft (*see also* Complications, by site and type, mechanical)
    arterial graft NEC — *see* Complication, cardiovascular device, mechanical, vascular
    breast (implant) T85.43 ☑
    catheter NEC T85.638 ☑
      dialysis (renal) T82.43 ☑
        intraperitoneal T85.631 ☑
      infusion NEC T82.534 ☑
        spinal (epidural) (subdural) T85.630 ☑
      urinary T83.038 ☑
        cystostomy T83.030 ☑
        Hopkins T83.038 ☑
        ileostomy T83.038 ☑
        indwelling T83.031 ☑
        nephrostomy T83.032 ☑
        specified T83.038 ☑
        urostomy T83.038 ☑
    gastrointestinal — *see* Complications, prosthetic device, mechanical, gastrointestinal device
    genital NEC T83.498 ☑
      penile prosthesis (cylinder) (implanted) (pump) (reservoir) T83.490 ☑
      testicular prosthesis T83.491 ☑
    heart NEC — *see* Complication, cardiovascular device, mechanical
    joint prosthesis — *see* Complications, joint prosthesis, mechanical, specified NEC, by site
    ocular NEC — *see* Complications, prosthetic device, mechanical, ocular device
    orthopedic NEC — *see* Complication, orthopedic, device, mechanical
    persistent air J93.82
    specified NEC T85.638 ☑
    urinary NEC (*see also* Complication, genitourinary, device, urinary, mechanical)
      graft T83.23 ☑
    vascular NEC — *see* Complication, cardiovascular device, mechanical
    ventricular intracranial shunt T85.03 ☑
  urine — *see* Incontinence
Leaky heart — *see* Endocarditis
Learning defect (specific) F81.9
Leather bottle stomach C16.9
Leber's
  congenital amaurosis H35.50
  optic atrophy (hereditary) H47.22
Lederer's anemia D59.1
Leeches (external) — *see* Hirudiniasis

Leg — see condition
Legg (-Calvé)-**Perthes disease, syndrome or osteo-**
chondrosis M91.1- ☑
Legionellosis A48.1
    nonpneumonic A48.2
Legionnaires'
    disease A48.1
        nonpneumonic A48.2
        pneumonia A48.1
Leigh's disease G31.82
Leiner's disease L21.1
Leiofibromyoma — see Leiomyoma
Leiomyoblastoma — see Neoplasm, connective tissue,
    benign
Leiomyofibroma (see also Neoplasm, connective tissue,
    benign)
    uterus (cervix) (corpus) D25.9
Leiomyoma (see also Neoplasm, connective tissue, be-
    nign)
    bizarre — see Neoplasm, connective tissue, benign
    cellular — see Neoplasm, connective tissue, benign
    epithelioid — see Neoplasm, connective tissue, benign
    uterus (cervix) (corpus) D25.9
        intramural D25.1
        submucous D25.0
        subserosal D25.2
    vascular — see Neoplasm, connective tissue, benign
Leiomyoma, leiomyomatosis (intravascular) — see
    Neoplasm, connective tissue, uncertain behavior
Leiomyosarcoma (see also Neoplasm, connective tissue,
    malignant)
    epithelioid — see Neoplasm, connective tissue, malig-
        nant
    myxoid — see Neoplasm, connective tissue, malignant
Leishmaniasis B55.9
    American (mucocutaneous) B55.2
        cutaneous B55.1
    Asian Desert B55.1
    Brazilian B55.2
    cutaneous (any type) B55.1
    dermal (see also Leishmaniasis, cutaneous)
        post-kala-azar B55.0
    eyelid B55.1
    infantile B55.0
    Mediterranean B55.0
    mucocutaneous (American) (New World) B55.2
    naso-oral B55.2
    nasopharyngeal B55.2
    old world B55.1
    tegumentaria diffusa B55.1
    visceral B55.0
Leishmanoid, dermal (see also Leishmaniasis, cuta-
    neous)
    post-kala-azar B55.0
Lenegre's disease I44.2
Lengthening, leg — see Deformity, limb, unequal length
Lennert's lymphoma — see Lymphoma, Lennert's
Lennox-Gastaut syndrome G40.812
    intractable G40.814
        with status epilepticus G40.813
        without status epilepticus G40.814
    not intractable G40.812
        with status epilepticus G40.811
        without status epilepticus G40.812
Lens — see condition
Lenticonus (anterior) (posterior) (congenital) Q12.8
Lenticular degeneration, progressive E83.01
Lentiglobus (posterior) (congenital) Q12.8
Lentigo (congenital) L81.4
    maligna (see also Melanoma, in situ)
        melanoma — see Melanoma
Lentivirus, as cause of disease classified elsewhere
    B97.31
Leontiasis
    ossium M85.2
    syphilitic (late) A52.78
        congenital A50.59
Lepothrix A48.8
Lepra — see Leprosy
Leprechaunism E34.8
Leprosy A30.- ☑
    with muscle disorder A30.9 [M63.80]
        ankle A30.9 [M63.87-] ☑
        foot A30.9 [M63.87-] ☑
        forearm A30.9 [M63.83-] ☑
        hand A30.9 [M63.84-] ☑
        lower leg A30.9 [M63.86-] ☑

Leprosy — continued
    with muscle disorder — continued
        multiple sites A30.9 [M63.89]
        pelvic region A30.9 [M63.85-] ☑
        shoulder region A30.9 [M63.81-] ☑
        specified site NEC A30.9 [M63.88]
        thigh A30.9 [M63.85-] ☑
        upper arm A30.9 [M63.82-] ☑
    anesthetic A30.9
    BB A30.3
    BL A30.4
    borderline (infiltrated) (neuritic) A30.3
        lepromatous A30.4
        tuberculoid A30.2
    BT A30.2
    dimorphous (infiltrated) (neuritic) A30.3
    I A30.0
    indeterminate (macular) (neuritic) A30.0
    lepromatous (diffuse) (infiltrated) (macular) (neuritic)
        (nodular) A30.5
    LL A30.5
    macular (early) (neuritic) (simple) A30.9
    maculoanesthetic A30.9
    mixed A30.3
    neural A30.9
    nodular A30.5
    primary neuritic A30.3
    specified type NEC A30.8
    TT A30.1
    tuberculoid (major) (minor) A30.1
Leptocytosis, hereditary D56.9
Leptomeningitis (chronic) (circumscribed) (hemorrhagic)
    (nonsuppurative) — see Meningitis
Leptomeningopathy G96.19
Leptospiral — see condition
Leptospirochetal — see condition
Leptospirosis A27.9
    canicola A27.89
    due to Leptospira interrogans serovar icterohaemor-
        rhagiae A27.0
    icterohemorrhagica A27.0
    pomona A27.89
    Weil's disease A27.0
Leptus dermatitis B88.0
Leriche's syndrome (aortic bifurcation occlusion) I74.09
Leri's pleonosteosis Q78.8
Leri-Weill syndrome Q77.8
Lermoyez' syndrome — see Vertigo, peripheral NEC
Lesch-Nyhan syndrome E79.1
Leser-Trélat disease L82.1
    inflamed L82.0
Lesion(s) (nontraumatic)
    abducens nerve — see Strabismus, paralytic, sixth
        nerve
    alveolar process K08.9
    angiocentric immunoproliferative D47.Z9 (following
        D47.4)
    anorectal K62.9
    aortic (valve) I35.9
    auditory nerve — see subcategory H93.3 ☑
    basal ganglion G25.9
    bile duct — see Disease, bile duct
    biomechanical M99.9
        specified type NEC M99.89
            abdomen M99.89
            acromioclavicular M99.87
            cervical region M99.81
            cervicothoracic M99.81
            costochondral M99.88
            costovertebral M99.88
            head region M99.80
            hip M99.85
            lower extremity M99.86
            lumbar region M99.83
            lumbosacral M99.83
            occipitocervical M99.80
            pelvic region M99.85
            pubic M99.85
            rib cage M99.88
            sacral region M99.84
            sacrococcygeal M99.84
            sacroiliac M99.84
            specified NEC M99.89
            sternochondral M99.88
            sternoclavicular M99.87
            thoracic region M99.82
            thoracolumbar M99.82
            upper extremity M99.87

Lesion(s) — continued
    bladder N32.9
    bone — see Disorder, bone
    brachial plexus G54.0
    brain G93.9
        congenital Q04.9
        vascular I67.9
            degenerative I67.9
            hypertensive I67.4
    buccal cavity K13.79
    calcified — see Calcification
    canthus — see Disorder, eyelid
    carate — see Pinta, lesions
    cardia K31.9
    cardiac (see also Disease, heart) I51.9
        congenital Q24.9
        valvular — see Endocarditis
    cauda equina G83.4
    cecum K63.9
    cerebral — see Lesion, brain
    cerebrovascular I67.9
        degenerative I67.9
        hypertensive I67.4
    cervical (nerve) root NEC G54.2
    chiasmal — see Disorder, optic, chiasm
    chorda tympani G51.8
    coin, lung R91.1
    colon K63.9
    combined periodontic - endodontic K05.5
    congenital — see Anomaly, by site
    conjunctiva H11.9
    conus medullaris — see Injury, conus medullaris
    coronary artery — see Ischemia, heart
    cranial nerve G52.9
        eighth — see Disorder, ear
        eleventh G52.9
        fifth G50.9
        first G52.0
        fourth — see Strabismus, paralytic, fourth nerve
        seventh G51.9
        sixth — see Strabismus, paralytic, sixth nerve
        tenth G52.2
        twelfth G52.3
    cystic — see Cyst
    degenerative — see Degeneration
    duodenum K31.9
    edentulous (alveolar) ridge, associated with trauma,
        due to traumatic occlusion K06.2
    en coup de sabre L94.1
    eyelid — see Disorder, eyelid
    gasserian ganglion G50.8
    gastric K31.9
    gastroduodenal K31.9
    gastrointestinal K63.9
    gingiva, associated with trauma K06.2
    glomerular
        focal and segmental (see also N00-N07 with fourth
            character .1) N05.1
        minimal change (see also N00-N07 with fourth
            character .0) N05.0
    heart (organic) — see Disease, heart
    hyperchromic, due to pinta (carate) A67.1
    hyperkeratotic — see Hyperkeratosis
    hypothalamic E23.7
    ileocecal K63.9
    ileum K63.9
    iliohypogastric nerve G57.8- ☑
    inflammatory — see Inflammation
    intestine K63.9
    intracerebral — see Lesion, brain
    intrachiasmal (optic) — see Disorder, optic, chiasm
    intracranial, space-occupying R90.0
    joint — see Disorder, joint
        sacroiliac (old) M53.3
    keratotic — see Keratosis
    kidney — see Disease, renal
    laryngeal nerve (recurrent) G52.2
    lip K13.0
    liver K76.9
    lumbosacral
        plexus G54.1
        root (nerve) NEC G54.4
    lung (coin) R91.1
    maxillary sinus J32.0
    mitral I05.9
    Morel-Lavallée — see Hematoma, by site
    motor cortex NEC G93.89
    mouth K13.79

Lesion(s) — *continued*
  nerve G58.9
    femoral G57.2- ☑
    median G56.1- ☑
      carpal tunnel syndrome — *see* Syndrome, carpal tunnel
    plantar G57.6- ☑
    popliteal (lateral) G57.3- ☑
      medial G57.4- ☑
    radial G56.3- ☑
    sciatic G57.0- ☑
    spinal — *see* Injury, nerve, spinal
    ulnar G56.2- ☑
  nervous system, congenital Q07.9
  nonallopathic — *see* Lesion, biomechanical
  nose (internal) J34.89
  obstructive — *see* Obstruction
  obturator nerve G57.8- ☑
  oral mucosa K13.70
  organ or site NEC — *see* Disease, by site
  osteolytic — *see* Osteolysis
  peptic K27.9
  periodontal, due to traumatic occlusion K05.5
  pharynx J39.2
  pigment, pigmented (skin) L81.9
  pinta — *see* Pinta, lesions
  polypoid — *see* Polyp
  prechiasmal (optic) — *see* Disorder, optic, chiasm
  primary (*see also* Syphilis, primary) A51.0
    carate A67.0
    pinta A67.0
    yaws A66.0
  pulmonary J98.4
    valve I37.9
  pylorus K31.9
  rectosigmoid K63.9
  retina, retinal H35.9
  sacroiliac (joint) (old) M53.3
  salivary gland K11.9
    benign lymphoepithelial K11.8
  saphenous nerve G57.8- ☑
  sciatic nerve G57.0- ☑
  secondary — *see* Syphilis, secondary
  shoulder (region) M75.9- ☑
    specified NEC M75.8- ☑
  sigmoid K63.9
  sinus (accessory) (nasal) J34.89
  skin L98.9
    suppurative L08.0
  SLAP S43.43- ☑
  spinal cord G95.9
    congenital Q06.9
  spleen D73.89
  stomach K31.9
  superior glenoid labrum S43.43- ☑
  syphilitic — *see* Syphilis
  tertiary — *see* Syphilis, tertiary
  thoracic root (nerve) NEC G54.3
  tonsillar fossa J35.9
  tooth, teeth K08.9
    white spot
      chewing surface K02.51
      pit and fissure surface K02.51
      smooth surface K02.61
  traumatic — *see* specific type of injury by site
  tricuspid (valve) I07.9
    nonrheumatic I36.9
  trigeminal nerve G50.9
  ulcerated or ulcerative — *see* Ulcer, skin
  uterus N85.9
  vagus nerve G52.2
  valvular — *see* Endocarditis
  vascular I99.9
    affecting central nervous system I67.9
    following trauma NEC T14.8 ☑
    umbilical cord, complicating delivery O69.5 ☑
  warty — *see* Verruca
  white spot (tooth)
    chewing surface K02.51
    pit and fissure surface K02.51
    smooth surface K02.61
Lethargic — *see* condition
Lethargy R53.83
Letterer-Siwe's disease C96.0
Leukemia, leukemic C95.9- ☑
  acute basophilic C94.8- ☑
  acute bilineal C95.0- ☑

Leukemia, leukemic — *continued*
  acute erythroid C94.0- ☑
  acute lymphoblastic C91.0- ☑
  acute megakaryoblastic C94.2- ☑
  acute megakaryocytic C94.2- ☑
  acute mixed lineage C95.0- ☑
  acute monoblastic (monoblastic/monocytic) C93.0- ☑
  acute monocytic (monoblastic/monocytic) C93.0- ☑
  acute myeloblastic (minimal differentiation) (with maturation) C92.0- ☑
  acute myeloid
    with
      11q23-abnormality C92.6- ☑
      dysplasia of remaining hematopoesis and/or myelodysplastic disease in its history C92.A- ☑ (*following* C92.6)
      multilineage dysplasia C92.A- ☑ (*following* C92.6)
      variation of MLL-gene C92.6- ☑
    M6 (a)(b) C94.0- ☑
    M7 C94.2- ☑
  acute myelomonocytic C92.5- ☑
  acute promyelocytic C92.4- ☑
  adult T-cell (HTLV-1-associated) (acute variant) (chronic variant) (lymphomatoid variant) (smouldering variant) C91.5- ☑
  aggressive NK-cell C94.8- ☑
  AML (1/ETO) (M0) (M1) (M2) (without a FAB classification) C92.0- ☑
  AML M3 C92.4- ☑
  AML M4 (Eo with inv(16) or t(16;16)) C92.5- ☑
  AML M5 C93.0- ☑
  AML M5a C93.0- ☑
  AML M5b C93.0- ☑
  AML Me with t (15;17) and variants C92.4- ☑
  atypical chronic myeloid, BCR/ABL-negative C92.2- ☑
  biphenotypic acute C95.0- ☑
  blast cell C95.0- ☑
  Burkitt-type, mature B-cell C91.A- ☑ (*following* C91.6)
  chronic lymphocytic, of B-cell type C91.1- ☑
  chronic monocytic C93.1- ☑
  chronic myelogenous (Philadelphia chromosome (Ph1) positive) (t(9;22)) (q34;q11) (with crisis of blast cells) C92.1- ☑
  chronic myeloid, BCR/ABL-positive C92.1- ☑
    atypical, BCR/ABL-negative C92.2- ☑
  chronic myelomonocytic C93.1- ☑
  chronic neutrophilic D47.1
  CMML (-1) (-2) (with eosinophilia) C93.1- ☑
  granulocytic (*see also* Category C92) C92.9- ☑
  hairy cell C91.4- ☑
  juvenile myelomonocytic C93.3- ☑
  lymphoid C91.9- ☑
    specified NEC C91.Z- ☑ (*following* C91.6)
  mast cell C94.3- ☑
  mature B-cell, Burkitt-type C91.A- ☑ (*following* C91.6)
  monocytic (subacute) C93.9- ☑
    specified NEC C93.Z- ☑ (*following* C93.3)
  myelogenous (*see also* Category C92) C92.9- ☑
  myeloid C92.9- ☑
    specified NEC C92.Z- ☑ (*following* C92.6)
  plasma cell C90.1- ☑
  plasmacytic C90.1- ☑
  prolymphocytic
    of B-cell type C91.3- ☑
    of T-cell type C91.6- ☑
  specified NEC C94.8- ☑
  stem cell, of unclear lineage C95.0- ☑
  subacute lymphocytic C91.9- ☑
  T-cell large granular lymphocytic C91.Z- ☑ (*following* C91.6)
  unspecified cell type C95.9- ☑
    acute C95.0- ☑
    chronic C95.1- ☑
Leukemoid reaction (*see also* Reaction, leukemoid) D72.823
Leukoaraiosis (hypertensive) I67.81
Leukoariosis — *see* Leukoaraiosis
Leukocoria — *see* Disorder, globe, degenerated condition, leucocoria
Leukocytopenia D72.819
Leukocytosis D72.829
  eosinophilic D72.1
Leukoderma, leukodermia NEC L81.5
  syphilitic A51.39
    late A52.79

Leukodystrophy E75.29
Leukoedema, oral epithelium K13.29
Leukoencephalitis G04.81
  acute (subacute) hemorrhagic G36.1
    postimmunization or postvaccinal G04.02
  postinfectious G04.01
  subacute sclerosing A81.1
  van Bogaert's (sclerosing) A81.1
Leukoencephalopathy (*see also* Encephalopathy) G93.49
  Binswanger's I67.3
  heroin vapor G92
  metachromatic E75.25
  multifocal (progressive) A81.2
  postimmunization and postvaccinal G04.02
  progressive multifocal A81.2
  reversible, posterior G93.6
  van Bogaert's (sclerosing) A81.1
  vascular, progressive I67.3
Leukoerythroblastosis D75.9
Leukokeratosis (*see also* Leukoplakia)
  mouth K13.21
  nicotina palati K13.24
  oral mucosa K13.21
  tongue K13.21
  vocal cord J38.3
Leukokraurosis vulva (e) N90.4
Leukoma (cornea) (*see also* Opacity, cornea)
  adherent H17.0- ☑
  interfering with central vision — *see* Opacity, cornea, central
Leukomalacia, cerebral, newborn P91.2
  periventricular P91.2
Leukomelanopathy, hereditary D72.0
Leukonychia (punctata) (striata) L60.8
  congenital Q84.4
Leukopathia unguium L60.8
  congenital Q84.4
Leukopenia D72.819
  basophilic D72.818
  chemotherapy (cancer) induced D70.1
  congenital D70.0
  cyclic D70.0
  drug induced NEC D70.2
    due to cytoreductive cancer chemotherapy D70.1
  eosinophilic D72.818
  familial D70.0
  infantile genetic D70.0
  malignant D70.9
  periodic D70.0
  transitory neonatal P61.5
Leukopenic — *see* condition
Leukoplakia
  anus K62.89
  bladder (postinfectional) N32.89
  buccal K13.21
  cervix (uteri) N88.0
  esophagus K22.8
  gingiva K13.21
  hairy (oral mucosa) (tongue) K13.3
  kidney (pelvis) N28.89
  larynx J38.7
  lip K13.21
  mouth K13.21
  oral epithelium, including tongue (mucosa) K13.21
  palate K13.21
  pelvis (kidney) N28.89
  penis (infectional) N48.0
  rectum K62.89
  syphilitic (late) A52.79
  tongue K13.21
  ureter (postinfectional) N28.89
  urethra (postinfectional) N36.8
  uterus N85.8
  vagina N89.4
  vocal cord J38.3
  vulva N90.4
Leukorrhea N89.8
  due to Trichomonas (vaginalis) A59.00
  trichomonal A59.00
Leukosarcoma C85.9- ☑
Levocardia (isolated) Q24.1
  with situs inversus Q89.3
Levotransposition Q20.5
Lev's disease or syndrome (acquired complete heart block) I44.2
Levulosuria — *see* Fructosuria
Levurid L30.2

Lewy body (ies) (dementia) (disease) G31.83
Leyden-Moebius dystrophy G71.0
Leydig cell
  carcinoma
    specified site — *see* Neoplasm, malignant, by site
    unspecified site
      female C56.9
      male C62.9- ☑
  tumor
    benign
      specified site — *see* Neoplasm, benign, by site
      unspecified site
        female D27.- ☑
        male D29.2- ☑
    malignant
      specified site — *see* Neoplasm, malignant, by
        site
      unspecified site
        female C56.- ☑
        male C62.9- ☑
    specified site — *see* Neoplasm, uncertain behavior,
      by site
    unspecified site
      female D39.1- ☑
      male D40.1- ☑
Leydig-Sertoli cell tumor
  specified site — *see* Neoplasm, benign, by site
  unspecified site
    female D27.- ☑
    male D29.2- ☑
LGSIL (Low grade squamous intraepithelial lesion on cytologic smear of)
  anus R85.612
  cervix R87.612
  vagina R87.622
Liar, pathologic F60.2
Libido
  decreased R68.82
Libman-Sacks disease M32.11
Lice (infestation) B85.2
  body (Pediculus corporis) B85.1
  crab B85.3
  head (Pediculus capitis) B85.0
  mixed (classifiable to more than one of the titles B85.0-B85.3) B85.4
  pubic (Phthirus pubis) B85.3
Lichen L28.0
  albus L90.0
    penis N48.0
    vulva N90.4
  amyloidosis E85.4 [L99]
  atrophicus L90.0
    penis N48.0
    vulva N90.4
  congenital Q82.8
  myxedematosus L98.5
  nitidus L44.1
  pilaris Q82.8
    acquired L85.8
  planopilaris L66.1
  planus (chronicus) L43.9
    annularis L43.8
    bullous L43.1
    follicular L66.1
    hypertrophic L43.0
    moniliformis L44.3
    of Wilson L43.9
    specified NEC L43.8
    subacute (active) L43.3
    tropicus L43.3
  ruber
    acuminatus L44.0
    moniliformis L44.3
    planus L43.9
  sclerosus (et atrophicus) L90.0
    penis N48.0
    vulva N90.4
  scrofulosus (primary) (tuberculous) A18.4
  simplex (chronicus) (circumscriptus) L28.0
  striatus L44.2
  urticatus L28.2
Lichenification L28.0
Lichenoides tuberculosis (primary) A18.4
Lichtheim's disease or syndrome — *see* Degeneration, combined
Lien migrans D73.89
Ligament — *see* condition

Light
  for gestational age — *see* Light for dates
  headedness R42
Light-for-dates (infant) P05.00
  with weight of
    1000-1249 grams P05.04
    1250-1499 grams P05.05
    1500-1749 grams P05.06
    1750-1999 grams P05.07
    2000-2499 grams P05.08
    2500 grams and over P05.09
    499 grams or less P05.01
    500-749 grams P05.02
    750-999 grams P05.03
  affecting management of pregnancy O36.59- ☑
  and small-for-dates — *see* Small for dates
  specified NEC P05.09
Lightning (effects) (stroke) (struck by) T75.00 ☑
  burn — *see* Burn
  foot E53.8
  shock T75.01 ☑
  specified effect NEC T75.09 ☑
Lightwood-Albright syndrome N25.89
Lightwood's disease or syndrome (renal tubular acidosis) N25.89
Lignac (-de Toni) (-Fanconi) (-Debré) **disease or syndrome** E72.09
  with cystinosis E72.04
Ligneous thyroiditis E06.5
Likoff's syndrome I20.8
Limb — *see* condition
Limbic epilepsy personality syndrome F07.0
Limitation, limited
  activities due to disability Z73.6
  cardiac reserve — *see* Disease, heart
  eye muscle duction, traumatic — *see* Strabismus, mechanical
  mandibular range of motion M26.52
Lindau (-von Hippel) **disease** Q85.8
Line(s)
  Beau's L60.4
  Harris' — *see* Arrest, epiphyseal
  Hudson's (cornea) — *see* Pigmentation, cornea, anterior
  Stähli's (cornea) — *see* Pigmentation, cornea, anterior
Linea corneae senilis — *see* Change, cornea, senile
Lingua
  geographica K14.1
  nigra (villosa) K14.3
  plicata K14.5
  tylosis K13.29
Lingual — *see* condition
Linguatulosis B88.8
Linitis (gastric) **plastica** C16.9
Lip — *see* condition
Lipedema — *see* Edema
Lipemia (*see also* Hyperlipidemia)
  retina, retinalis E78.3
Lipidosis E75.6
  cerebral (infantile) (juvenile) (late) E75.4
  cerebroretinal E75.4
  cerebroside E75.22
  cholesterol (cerebral) E75.5
  glycolipid E75.21
  hepatosplenomegalic E78.3
  sphingomyelin — *see* Niemann-Pick disease or syndrome
  sulfatide E75.29
Lipoadenoma — *see* Neoplasm, benign, by site
Lipoblastoma — *see* Lipoma
Lipoblastomatosis — *see* Lipoma
Lipochondrodystrophy E76.01
Lipochrome histiocytosis (familial) D71
Lipodermatosclerosis — *see* Varix, leg, with, inflammation
  ulcerated — *see* Varix, leg, with, ulcer, with inflammation by site
Lipodystrophia progressiva E88.1
Lipodystrophy (progressive) E88.1
  insulin E88.1
  intestinal K90.81
  mesenteric K65.4
Lipofibroma — *see* Lipoma
Lipofuscinosis, neuronal (with ceroidosis) E75.4
Lipogranuloma, sclerosing L92.8
Lipogranulomatosis E78.89
Lipoid (*see also* condition)

Lipoid — *continued*
  histiocytosis D76.3
    essential E75.29
  nephrosis N04.9
  proteinosis of Urbach E78.89
Lipoidemia — *see* Hyperlipidemia
Lipoidosis — *see* Lipidosis
Lipoma D17.9
  fetal D17.9
    fat cell D17.9
  infiltrating D17.9
  intramuscular D17.9
  pleomorphic D17.9
  site classification
    arms (skin) (subcutaneous) D17.2- ☑
    connective tissue D17.30
      intra-abdominal D17.5
      intrathoracic D17.4
      peritoneum D17.79
      retroperitoneum D17.79
      specified site NEC D17.39
      spermatic cord D17.6
    face (skin) (subcutaneous) D17.0
    genitourinary organ NEC D17.72
    head (skin) (subcutaneous) D17.0
    intra-abdominal D17.5
    intrathoracic D17.4
    kidney D17.71
    legs (skin) (subcutaneous) D17.2- ☑
    neck (skin) (subcutaneous) D17.0
    peritoneum D17.79
    retroperitoneum D17.79
    skin D17.30
      specified site NEC D17.39
    specified site NEC D17.79
    spermatic cord D17.6
    subcutaneous D17.30
      specified site NEC D17.39
    trunk (skin) (subcutaneous) D17.1
    unspecified D17.9
  spindle cell D17.9
Lipomatosis E88.2
  dolorosa (Dercum) E88.2
  fetal — *see* Lipoma
  Launois-Bensaude E88.89
Lipomyoma — *see* Lipoma
Lipomyxoma — *see* Lipoma
Lipomyxosarcoma — *see* Neoplasm, connective tissue, malignant
Lipoprotein metabolism disorder E78.9
Lipoproteinemia E78.5
  broad-beta E78.2
  floating-beta E78.2
  hyper-pre-beta E78.1
Liposarcoma (*see also* Neoplasm, connective tissue, malignant)
  dedifferentiated — *see* Neoplasm, connective tissue, malignant
  differentiated type — *see* Neoplasm, connective tissue, malignant
  embryonal — *see* Neoplasm, connective tissue, malignant
  mixed type — *see* Neoplasm, connective tissue, malignant
  myxoid — *see* Neoplasm, connective tissue, malignant
  pleomorphic — *see* Neoplasm, connective tissue, malignant
  round cell — *see* Neoplasm, connective tissue, malignant
  well differentiated type — *see* Neoplasm, connective tissue, malignant
Liposynovitis prepatellaris E88.89
Lipping, cervix N86
Lipschütz disease or ulcer N76.6
Lipuria R82.0
  schistosomiasis (bilharziasis) B65.0
Lisping F80.0
Lissauer's paralysis A52.17
Lissencephalia, lissencephaly Q04.3
Listeriosis, listerellosis A32.9
  congenital (disseminated) P37.2
  cutaneous A32.0
  neonatal, newborn (disseminated) P37.2
  oculoglandular A32.81
  specified NEC A32.89
Lithemia E79.0
Lithiasis — *see* Calculus
Lithosis J62.8

☑ **Additional Character Required — Refer to the Tabular List for Character Selection**　　　🔻 **Subterms under main terms may continue to next column or page**

Lithuria R82.99
Litigation, anxiety concerning Z65.3
Little leaguer's elbow — *see* Epicondylitis, medial
Little's disease G80.9
Littre's
   gland — *see* condition
   hernia — *see* Hernia, abdomen
Littritis — *see* Urethritis
Livedo (annularis) (racemosa) (reticularis) R23.1
Liver — *see* condition
Living alone (problems with) Z60.2
   with handicapped person Z74.2
Lloyd's syndrome — *see* Adenomatosis, endocrine
Loa loa, loaiasis, loasis B74.3
Lobar — *see* condition
Lobomycosis B48.0
Lobo's disease B48.0
Lobotomy syndrome F07.0
Lobstein (-Ekman) **disease or syndrome** Q78.0
Lobster-claw hand Q71.6- ☑
Lobulation (congenital) (*see also* Anomaly, by site)
   kidney, Q63.1
   liver, abnormal Q44.7
   spleen Q89.09
Lobule, lobular — *see* condition
Local, localized — *see* condition
Locked twins causing obstructed labor O66.1
Locked-in state G83.5
Locking
   joint — *see* Derangement, joint, specified type NEC
      knee — *see* Derangement, knee
Lockjaw — *see* Tetanus
Löffler's
   endocarditis I42.3
   eosinophilia J82
   pneumonia J82
   syndrome (eosinophilic pneumonitis) J82
Loiasis (with conjunctival infestation) (eyelid) B74.3
Lone Star fever A77.0
Long
   labor O63.9
      first stage O63.0
      second stage O63.1
   QT syndrome I45.81
Longitudinal stripes or grooves, nails L60.8
   congenital Q84.6
Long-term (current) (prophylactic) **drug therapy** (use of)
   agents affecting estrogen receptors and estrogen levels NEC Z79.818
   anastrozole (Arimidex) Z79.811
   antibiotics Z79.2
      short-term use — *omit code*
   anticoagulants Z79.01
   anti-inflammatory, non-steroidal (NSAID) Z79.1
   antiplatelet Z79.02
   antithrombotics Z79.02
   aromatase inhibitors Z79.811
   aspirin Z79.82
   birth control pill or patch Z79.3
   bisphosphonates Z79.83
   contraceptive, oral Z79.3
   drug, specified NEC Z79.899
   estrogen receptor downregulators Z79.818
   Evista Z79.810
   exemestane (Aromasin) Z79.811
   Fareston Z79.810
   fulvestrant (Faslodex) Z79.818
   gonadotropin-releasing hormone (GnRH) agonist Z79.818
   goserelin acetate (Zoladex) Z79.818
   hormone replacement Z79.890
   insulin Z79.4
   letrozole (Femara) Z79.811
   leuprolide acetate (leuprorelin) (Lupron) Z79.818
   megestrol acetate (Megace) Z79.818
   methadone for pain management Z79.891
   Nolvadex Z79.810
   non-steroidal anti-inflammatories (NSAID) Z79.1
   opiate analgesic Z79.891
   oral
      antidiabetic Z79.84
      contraceptive Z79.3
      hypoglycemic Z79.84
   raloxifene (Evista) Z79.810
   selective estrogen receptor modulators (SERMs) Z79.810

Long-term (current) (prophylactic) **drug therapy** — *continued*
   steroids
      inhaled Z79.51
      systemic Z79.52
   tamoxifen (Nolvadex) Z79.810
   toremifene (Fareston) Z79.810
Loop
   intestine — *see* Volvulus
   vascular on papilla (optic) Q14.2
Loose (*see also* condition)
   body
      joint M24.00
         ankle M24.07- ☑
         elbow M24.02- ☑
         hand M24.04- ☑
         hip M24.05- ☑
         knee M23.4- ☑
         shoulder (region) M24.01- ☑
         specified site NEC M24.08
         toe M24.07- ☑
         vertebra M24.08
         wrist M24.03- ☑
      knee M23.4- ☑
      sheath, tendon — *see* Disorder, tendon, specified type NEC
   cartilage — *see* Loose, body, joint
   skin and subcutaneous tissue (following bariatric surgery weight loss) (following dietary weight loss) L98.7
   tooth, teeth K08.89
Loosening
   aseptic
      joint prosthesis — *see* Complications, joint prosthesis, mechanical, loosening, by site
   epiphysis — *see* Osteochondropathy
   mechanical
      joint prosthesis — *see* Complications, joint prosthesis, mechanical, loosening, by site
Looser-Milkman (-Debray) **syndrome** M83.8
Lop ear (deformity) Q17.3
Lorain (-Levi) **short stature syndrome** E23.0
Lordosis M40.50
   acquired — *see* Lordosis, specified type NEC
   congenital Q76.429
      lumbar region Q76.426
      lumbosacral region Q76.427
      sacral region Q76.428
      sacrococcygeal region Q76.428
      thoracolumbar region Q76.425
   lumbar region M40.56
   lumbosacral region M40.57
   postsurgical M96.4
   postural — *see* Lordosis, specified type NEC
   rachitic (late effect) (sequelae) E64.3
   sequelae of rickets E64.3
   specified type NEC M40.40
      lumbar region M40.46
      lumbosacral region M40.47
      thoracolumbar region M40.45
   thoracolumbar region M40.55
   tuberculous A18.01
Loss (of)
   appetite (*see also* Anorexia) R63.0
      hysterical F50.89
      nonorganic origin F50.89
      psychogenic F50.89
   blood — *see* Hemorrhage
   bone —*see* Loss, substance of, bone
   consciousness, transient R55
      traumatic — *see* Injury, intracranial
   control, sphincter, rectum R15.9
      nonorganic origin F98.1
   elasticity, skin R23.4
   family (member) in childhood Z62.898
   fluid (acute) E86.9
   function of labyrinth — *see* subcategory H83.2 ☑
   hair, nonscarring — *see* Alopecia
   hearing (*see also* Deafness)
      central NOS H90.5
      conductive H90.2
         bilateral H90.0
         unilateral
            with
               restricted hearing on the contralateral side H90.A1- ☑
               unrestricted hearing on the contralateral side H90.1- ☑

Loss — *continued*
   hearing (*see also* Deafness) — *continued*
      mixed conductive and sensorineural hearing loss H90.8
         bilateral H90.6
         unilateral
            with
               restricted hearing on the contralateral side H90.A3- ☑
               unrestricted hearing on the contralateral side H90.7- ☑
      neural NOS H90.5
      perceptive NOS H90.5
      sensorineural NOS H90.5
         bilateral H90.3
         unilateral
            with
               restricted hearing onthe contralateral side H90.A2- ☑
               unrestricted hearing on the contralateral side H90.4- ☑
      sensory NOS H90.5
   height R29.890
   limb or member, traumatic, current — *see* Amputation, traumatic
   love relationship in childhood Z62.898
   memory (*see also* Amnesia)
      mild, following organic brain damage F06.8
   mind — *see* Psychosis
   occlusal vertical dimension of fully erupted teeth M26.37
   organ or part — *see* Absence, by site, acquired
   ossicles, ear (partial) H74.32- ☑
   parent in childhood Z63.4
   pregnancy, recurrent N96
      without current pregnancy N96
      care in current pregnancy O26.2- ☑
   recurrent pregnancy — *see* Loss, pregnancy, recurrent
   self-esteem, in childhood Z62.898
   sense of
      smell — *see* Disturbance, sensation, smell
      taste — *see* Disturbance, sensation, taste
      touch R20.8
   sensory R44.9
      dissociative F44.6
   sexual desire F52.0
   sight (acquired) (complete) (congenital) — *see* Blindness
   substance of
      bone — *see* Disorder, bone, density and structure, specified NEC
         horizontal alveolar K06.3
      cartilage — *see* Disorder, cartilage, specified type NEC
         auricle (ear) — *see* Disorder, pinna, specified type NEC
      vitreous (humor) H15.89
   tooth, teeth — *see* Absence, teeth, acquired
   vision, visual H54.7
      both eyes H54.3
      one eye H54.60
         left (normal vision on right) H54.62
         right (normal vision on left) H54.61
      specified as blindness — *see* Blindness
      subjective
         sudden H53.13- ☑
         transient H53.12- ☑
   vitreous — *see* Prolapse, vitreous
   voice — *see* Aphonia
   weight (abnormal) (cause unknown) R63.4
Louis-Bar syndrome (ataxia-telangiectasia) G11.3
Louping ill (encephalitis) A84.8
Louse, lousiness — *see* Lice
Low
   achiever, school Z55.3
   back syndrome M54.5
   basal metabolic rate R94.8
   birthweight (2499 grams or less) P07.10
      with weight of
         1000-1249 grams P07.14
         1250-1499 grams P07.15
         1500-1749 grams P07.16
         1750-1999 grams P07.17
         2000-2499 grams P07.18
      extreme (999 grams or less) P07.00
        with weight of
         499 grams or less P07.01
         500-749 grams P07.02

Low — *continued*
 birthweight — *continued*
  extreme — *continued*
   with weight of — *continued*
    750-999 grams P07.03
  for gestational age — *see* Light for dates
 blood pressure (*see also* Hypotension)
  reading (incidental) (isolated) (nonspecific) R03.1
 cardiac reserve — *see* Disease, heart
 function (*see also* Hypofunction)
  kidney N28.9
 hematocrit D64.9
 hemoglobin D64.9
 income Z59.6
 level of literacy Z55.0
 lying
  kidney N28.89
  organ or site, congenital — *see* Malposition, congenital
 output syndrome (cardiac) — *see* Failure, heart
 platelets (blood) — *see* Thrombocytopenia
 reserve, kidney N28.89
 salt syndrome E87.1
 self esteem R45.81
 set ears Q17.4
 vision H54.2X- ☑
  one eye (other eye normal) H54.50
   left (normal vision on right) H54.52A- ☑
   other eye blind — *see* Blindness
   right (normal vision on left) H54.511- ☑
Low-density-lipoprotein-type (LDL) **hyperlipoproteinemia** E78.00
Lowe's syndrome E72.03
Lown-Ganong-Levine syndrome I45.6
LSD reaction (acute) (without dependence) F16.90
 with dependence F16.20
L-shaped kidney Q63.8
Ludwig's angina or disease K12.2
Lues (venerea), **luetic** — *see* Syphilis
Luetscher's syndrome (dehydration) E86.0
Lumbago, lumbalgia M54.5
 with sciatica M54.4- ☑
  due to intervertebral disc disorder M51.17
 due to displacement, intervertebral disc M51.27
  with sciatica M51.17
Lumbar — *see* condition
Lumbarization, vertebra, congenital Q76.49
Lumbermen's itch B88.0
Lump (*see also* Mass)
 breast N63.0
  axillary tail
   left N63.32
   right N63.31
  left
   lower inner quadrant N63.24
   lower outer quadrant N63.23
   unspecified quadrant N63.20
   upper inner quadrant N63.22
   upper outer quadrant N63.21
  right
   lower inner quadrant N63.14
   lower outer quadrant N63.13
   unspecified quadrant N63.10
   upper inner quadrant N63.12
   upper outer quadrant N63.11
  subareolar
   left N63.42
   right N63.41
Lunacy — *see* Psychosis
Lung — *see* condition
Lupoid (miliary) **of Boeck** D86.3
Lupus
 anticoagulant D68.62
  with
   hemorrhagic disorder D68.312
   hypercoagulable state D68.62
  finding without diagnosis R76.0
 discoid (local) L93.0
 erythematosus (discoid) (local) L93.0
  disseminated — *see* Lupus, erythematosus, systemic
  eyelid H01.129
   left H01.126
    lower H01.125
    upper H01.124
   right H01.123
    lower H01.122
    upper H01.121

Lupus — *continued*
 erythematosus — *continued*
  profundus L93.2
  specified NEC L93.2
  subacute cutaneous L93.1
  systemic M32.9
   with organ or system involvement M32.10
    endocarditis M32.11
    lung M32.13
    pericarditis M32.12
    renal (glomerular) M32.14
     tubulo-interstitial M32.15
    specified organ or system NEC M32.19
   drug-induced M32.0
   inhibitor (presence of) D68.62
    with
     hemorrhagic disorder D68.312
     hypercoagulable state D68.62
    finding without diagnosis R76.0
   specified NEC M32.8
 exedens A18.4
 hydralazine M32.0
  correct substance properly administered — *see* Table of Drugs and Chemicals, by drug, adverse effect
  overdose or wrong substance given or taken — *see* Table of Drugs and Chemicals, by drug, poisoning
 nephritis (chronic) M32.14
 nontuberculous, not disseminated L93.0
 panniculitis L93.2
 pernio (Besnier) D86.3
 systemic — *see* Lupus, erythematosus, systemic
 tuberculous A18.4
  eyelid A18.4
 vulgaris A18.4
  eyelid A18.4
Luteinoma D27.- ☑
Lutembacher's disease or syndrome (atrial septal defect with mitral stenosis) Q21.1
Luteoma D27.- ☑
Lutz (-Splendore-de Almeida) **disease** — *see* Paracoccidioidomycosis
Luxation (*see also* Dislocation)
 eyeball (nontraumatic) — *see* Luxation, globe
  birth injury P15.3
 globe, nontraumatic H44.82- ☑
 lacrimal gland — *see* Dislocation, lacrimal gland
 lens (old) (partial) (spontaneous)
  congenital Q12.1
  syphilitic A50.39
Lycanthropy F22
Lyell's syndrome L51.2
 due to drug L51.2
  correct substance properly administered — *see* Table of Drugs and Chemicals, by drug, adverse effect
  overdose or wrong substance given or taken — *see* Table of Drugs and Chemicals, by drug, poisoning
Lyme disease A69.20
Lymph
 gland or node — *see* condition
 scrotum — *see* Infestation, filarial
Lymphadenitis I88.9
 with ectopic or molar pregnancy O08.0
 acute L04.9
  axilla L04.2
  face L04.0
  head L04.0
  hip L04.3
  limb
   lower L04.3
   upper L04.2
  neck L04.0
  shoulder L04.2
  specified site NEC L04.8
  trunk L04.1
 anthracosis (occupational) J60
 any site, except mesenteric I88.9
  chronic I88.1
  subacute I88.1
 breast
  gestational — *see* Mastitis, obstetric
  puerperal, postpartum (nonpurulent) O91.22
 chancroidal (congenital) A57
 chronic I88.1
  mesenteric I88.0

Lymphadenitis — *continued*
 due to
  Brugia (malayi) B74.1
   timori B74.2
  chlamydial lymphogranuloma A55
  diphtheria (toxin) A36.89
  lymphogranuloma venereum A55
  Wuchereria bancrofti B74.0
 following ectopic or molar pregnancy O08.0
 gonorrheal A54.89
 infective — *see* Lymphadenitis, acute
 mesenteric (acute) (chronic) (nonspecific) (subacute) I88.0
  due to Salmonella typhi A01.09
  tuberculous A18.39
 mycobacterial A31.8
 purulent — *see* Lymphadenitis, acute
 pyogenic — *see* Lymphadenitis, acute
 regional, nonbacterial I88.8
 septic — *see* Lymphadenitis, acute
 subacute, unspecified site I88.1
 suppurative — *see* Lymphadenitis, acute
 syphilitic (early) (secondary) A51.49
  late A52.79
 tuberculous — *see* Tuberculosis, lymph gland
 venereal (chlamydial) A55
Lymphadenoid goiter E06.3
Lymphadenopathy (generalized) R59.1
 angioimmunoblastic, with dysproteinemia (AILD) C86.5
 due to toxoplasmosis (acquired) B58.89
  congenital (acute) (subacute) (chronic) P37.1
 localized R59.0
 syphilitic (early) (secondary) A51.49
Lymphadenosis R59.1
Lymphangiectasis I89.0
 conjunctiva H11.89
 postinfectional I89.0
 scrotum I89.0
Lymphangiectatic elephantiasis, nonfilarial I89.0
Lymphangioendothelioma D18.1
 malignant — *see* Neoplasm, connective tissue, malignant
Lymphangioleiomyomatosis J84.81
Lymphangioma D18.1
 capillary D18.1
 cavernous D18.1
 cystic D18.1
 malignant — *see* Neoplasm, connective tissue, malignant
Lymphangiomyoma D18.1
Lymphangiomyomatosis J84.81
Lymphangiosarcoma — *see* Neoplasm, connective tissue, malignant
Lymphangitis I89.1
 with
  abscess — *code by* site under Abscess
  cellulitis — *code by* site under Cellulitis
  ectopic or molar pregnancy O08.0
 acute L03.91
  abdominal wall L03.321
  ankle — *see* Lymphangitis, acute, lower limb
  arm — *see* Lymphangitis, acute, upper limb
  auricle (ear) — *see* Lymphangitis, acute, ear
  axilla L03.12- ☑
  back (any part) L03.322
  buttock L03.327
  cervical (meaning neck) L03.222
  cheek (external) L03.212
  chest wall L03.323
  digit
   finger — *see* Lymphangitis, acute, finger
   toe — *see* Lymphangitis, acute, toe
  ear (external) H60.1- ☑
  external auditory canal — *see* Lymphangitis, acute, ear
  eyelid — *see* Abscess, eyelid
  face NEC L03.212
  finger (intrathecal) (periosteal) (subcutaneous) (subcuticular) L03.02- ☑
  foot — *see* Lymphangitis, acute, lower limb
  gluteal (region) L03.327
  groin L03.324
  hand — *see* Lymphangitis, acute, upper limb
  head NEC L03.891
   face (any part, except ear, eye and nose) L03.212
  heel — *see* Lymphangitis, acute, lower limb

☑ **Additional Character Required** — **Refer to the Tabular List for Character Selection**   ▽ **Subterms under main terms may continue to next column or page**

Lymphangitis — *continued*
  acute — *continued*
    hip — *see* Lymphangitis, acute, lower limb
    jaw (region) L03.212
    knee — *see* Lymphangitis, acute, lower limb
    leg — *see* Lymphangitis, acute, lower limb
    lower limb L03.12- ☑
      toe — *see* Lymphangitis, acute, toe
    navel L03.326
    neck (region) L03.222
    orbit, orbital — *see* Cellulitis, orbit
    pectoral (region) L03.323
    perineal, perineum L03.325
    scalp (any part) L03.891
    shoulder — *see* Lymphangitis, acute, upper limb
    specified site NEC L03.898
    thigh — *see* Lymphangitis, acute, lower limb
    thumb (intrathecal) (periosteal) (subcutaneous) (subcuticular) — *see* Lymphangitis, acute, finger
    toe (intrathecal) (periosteal) (subcutaneous) (subcuticular) L03.04- ☑
    trunk L03.329
      abdominal wall L03.321
      back (any part) L03.322
      buttock L03.327
      chest wall L03.323
      groin L03.324
      perineal, perineum L03.325
      umbilicus L03.326
    umbilicus L03.326
    upper limb L03.12- ☑
      axilla — *see* Lymphangitis, acute, axilla
      finger — *see* Lymphangitis, acute, finger
      thumb — *see* Lymphangitis, acute, finger
    wrist — *see* Lymphangitis, acute, upper limb
  breast
    gestational — *see* Mastitis, obstetric
  chancroidal A57
  chronic (any site) I89.1
  due to
    Brugia (malayi) B74.1
      timori B74.2
    Wuchereria bancrofti B74.0
  following ectopic or molar pregnancy O08.89
  penis
    acute N48.29
    gonococcal (acute) (chronic) A54.09
  puerperal, postpartum, childbirth O86.89
  strumous, tuberculous A18.2
  subacute (any site) I89.1
  tuberculous — *see* Tuberculosis, lymph gland
Lymphatic (vessel) — *see* condition
Lymphatism E32.8
Lymphectasia I89.0
Lymphedema (acquired) (*see also* Elephantiasis)
  congenital Q82.0
  hereditary (chronic) (idiopathic) Q82.0
  postmastectomy I97.2
  praecox I89.0
  secondary I89.0
  surgical NEC I97.89
    postmastectomy (syndrome) I97.2
Lymphoblastic — *see* condition
Lymphoblastoma (diffuse) — *see* Lymphoma, lymphoblastic (diffuse)
  giant follicular — *see* Lymphoma, lymphoblastic (diffuse)
  macrofollicular — *see* Lymphoma, lymphoblastic (diffuse)
Lymphocele I89.8
Lymphocytic
  chorioencephalitis (acute) (serous) A87.2
  choriomeningitis (acute) (serous) A87.2
  meningoencephalitis A87.2
Lymphocytoma, benign cutis L98.8
Lymphocytopenia D72.810
Lymphocytosis (symptomatic) D72.820
  infectious (acute) B33.8
Lymphoepithelioma — *see* Neoplasm, malignant, by site
Lymphogranuloma (malignant) (*see also* Lymphoma, Hodgkin)
  chlamydial A55
  inguinale A55
  venereum (any site) (chlamydial) (with stricture of rectum) A55

Lymphogranulomatosis (malignant) (*see also* Lymphoma, Hodgkin)
  benign (Boeck's sarcoid) (Schaumann's) D86.1
Lymphohistiocytosis, hemophagocytic (familial) D76.1
Lymphoid — *see* condition
Lymphoma (of) (malignant) C85.90
  adult T-cell (HTLV-1-associated) (acute variant) (chronic variant) (lymphomatoid variant) (smouldering variant) C91.5- ☑
  anaplastic large cell
    ALK-negative C84.7- ☑
    ALK-positive C84.6- ☑
    CD30-positive C84.6- ☑
    primary cutaneous C86.6
  angioimmunoblastic T-cell C86.5
  BALT C88.4
  B-cell C85.1- ☑
  blastic NK-cell C86.4
  blastic plasmacytoid dendritic cell neoplasm (BPDCN) C86.4
  B-precursor C83.5- ☑
  bronchial-associated lymphoid tissue [BALT-lymphoma] C88.4
  Burkitt (atypical) C83.7- ☑
  Burkitt-like C83.7- ☑
  centrocytic C83.1- ☑
  cutaneous follicle center C82.6- ☑
  cutaneous T-cell C84.A- ☑ (*following* C84.7)
  diffuse follicle center C82.5- ☑
  diffuse large cell C83.3- ☑
    anaplastic C83.3- ☑
    B-cell C83.3- ☑
    CD30-positive C83.3- ☑
    centroblastic C83.3- ☑
    immunoblastic C83.3- ☑
    plasmablastic C83.3- ☑
    subtype not specified C83.3- ☑
    T-cell rich C83.3- ☑
  enteropathy-type (associated) (intestinal) T-cell C86.2
  extranodal marginal zone B-cell lymphoma of mucosa-associated lymphoid tissue [MALT-lymphoma] C88.4
  extranodal NK/T-cell, nasal type C86.0
  follicular C82.9- ☑
    grade
      I C82.0- ☑
      II C82.1- ☑
      III C82.2- ☑
      IIIa C82.3- ☑
      IIIb C82.4- ☑
    specified NEC C82.8- ☑
  hepatosplenic T-cell (alpha-beta) (gamma-delta) C86.1
  histiocytic C85.9- ☑
    true C96.A (*following* C96.6)
  Hodgkin C81.9 ☑
    lymphocyte depleted (classical) C81.3- ☑
    lymphocyte-rich (classical) C81.4- ☑
    mixed cellularity (classical) C81.2- ☑
    nodular
      lymphocyte predominant C81.0- ☑
      sclerosis (classical) C81.1- ☑
    nodular sclerosis (classical) C81.1- ☑
    specified NEC (classical) C81.7- ☑
  intravascular large B-cell C83.8- ☑
  Lennert's C84.4- ☑
  lymphoblastic (diffuse) C83.5- ☑
  lymphoblastic B-cell C83.5- ☑
  lymphoblastic T-cell C83.5- ☑
  lymphoepithelioid C84.4- ☑
  lymphoplasmacytic C83.0- ☑
    with IgM-production C88.0
  MALT C88.4
  mantle cell C83.1- ☑
  mature T-cell NEC C84.4- ☑
  mature T/NK-cell C84.9- ☑
    specified NEC C84.Z- ☑ (*following* C84.7)
  mediastinal (thymic) large B-cell C85.2- ☑
  Mediterranean C88.3
  mucosa-associated lymphoid tissue [MALT-lymphoma] C88.4
  NK/T cell C84.9- ☑
  nodal marginal zone C83.0- ☑
  non-follicular (diffuse) C83.9- ☑
    specified NEC C83.8- ☑
  non-Hodgkin (*see also* Lymphoma, by type) C85.9- ☑
    specified NEC C85.8- ☑

Lymphoma — *continued*
  non-leukemic variant of B-CLL C83.0- ☑
  peripheral T-cell, not classified C84.4- ☑
  primary cutaneous
    anaplastic large cell C86.6
    CD30-positive large T-cell C86.6
  primary effusion B-cell C83.8- ☑
  SALT C88.4
  skin-associated lymphoid tissue [SALT-lymphoma] C88.4
  small cell B-cell C83.0- ☑
  splenic marginal zone C83.0- ☑
  subcutaneous panniculitis-like T-cell C86.3
  T-precursor C83.5- ☑
  true histiocytic C96.A (*following* C96.6)
Lymphomatosis — *see* Lymphoma
Lymphopathia venereum, veneris A55
Lymphopenia D72.810
Lymphoplasmacytic leukemia — *see* Leukemia, chronic lymphocytic, B-cell type
Lymphoproliferation, X-linked disease D82.3
Lymphoreticulosis, benign (of inoculation) A28.1
Lymphorrhea I89.8
Lymphosarcoma (diffuse) (*see also* Lymphoma) C85.9- ☑
Lymphostasis I89.8
Lypemania — *see* Melancholia
Lysine and hydroxylysine metabolism disorder E72.3
Lyssa — *see* Rabies

M

Macacus ear Q17.3
Maceration, wet feet, tropical (syndrome) T69.02- ☑
MacLeod's syndrome J43.0
Macrocephalia, macrocephaly Q75.3
Macrocheilia, macrochilia (congenital) Q18.6
Macrocolon (*see also* Megacolon) Q43.1
Macrocornea Q15.8
  with glaucoma Q15.0
Macrocytic — *see* condition
Macrocytosis D75.89
Macrodactylia, macrodactylism (fingers) (thumbs) Q74.0
  toes Q74.2
Macrodontia K00.2
Macrogenia M26.05
Macrogenitosomia (adrenal) (male) (praecox) E25.9
  congenital E25.0
Macroglobulinemia (idiopathic) (primary) C88.0
  monoclonal (essential) D47.2
  Waldenström C88.0
Macroglossia (congenital) Q38.2
  acquired K14.8
Macrognathia, macrognathism (congenital) (mandibular) (maxillary) M26.09
Macrogyria (congenital) Q04.8
Macrohydrocephalus — *see* Hydrocephalus
Macromastia — *see* Hypertrophy, breast
Macrophthalmos Q11.3
  in congenital glaucoma Q15.0
Macropsia H53.15
Macrosigmoid K59.39
  congenital Q43.2
Macrospondylitis , acromegalic E22.0
Macrostomia (congenital) Q18.4
Macrotia (external ear) (congenital) Q17.1
Macula
  cornea, corneal — *see* Opacity, cornea
  degeneration (atrophic) (exudative) (senile) (*see also* Degeneration, macula)
    hereditary — *see* Dystrophy, retina
Maculae ceruleae B85.1
Maculopathy, toxic — *see* Degeneration, macula, toxic
Madarosis (eyelid) H02.729
  left H02.726
    lower H02.725
    upper H02.724
  right H02.723
    lower H02.722
    upper H02.721
Madelung's
  deformity (radius) Q74.0
  disease
    radial deformity Q74.0
    symmetrical lipomas, neck E88.89
Madness — *see* Psychosis

Madura
  foot B47.9
    actinomycotic B47.1
    mycotic B47.0
Maduromycosis B47.0
Maffucci's syndrome Q78.4
Magnesium metabolism disorder — *see* Disorder,
    metabolism, magnesium
Main en griffe (acquired) (*see also* Deformity, limb,
    clawhand)
  congenital Q74.0
Maintenance (encounter for)
  antineoplastic chemotherapy Z51.11
  antineoplastic radiation therapy Z51.0
  methadone F11.20
Majocchi's
  disease L81.7
  granuloma B35.8
Major — *see* condition
Mal de los pintos — *see* Pinta
Mal de mer T75.3 ☑
Malabar itch (any site) B35.5
Malabsorption K90.9
  calcium K90.89
  carbohydrate K90.49
  disaccharide E73.9
  fat K90.49
  galactose E74.20
  glucose (-galactose) E74.39
  intestinal K90.9
    specified NEC K90.89
  isomaltose E74.31
  lactose E73.9
  methionine E72.19
  monosaccharide E74.39
  postgastrectomy K91.2
  postsurgical K91.2
  protein K90.49
  starch K90.49
  sucrose E74.39
  syndrome K90.9
    postsurgical K91.2
Malacia, bone (adult) M83.9
  juvenile — *see* Rickets
Malacoplakia
  bladder N32.89
  pelvis (kidney) N28.89
  ureter N28.89
  urethra N36.8
Malacosteon, juvenile — *see* Rickets
Maladaptation — *see* Maladjustment
Maladie de Roger Q21.0
Maladjustment
  conjugal Z63.0
    involving divorce or estrangement Z63.5
  educational Z55.4
  family Z63.9
  marital Z63.0
    involving divorce or estrangement Z63.5
  occupational NEC Z56.89
  simple, adult — *see* Disorder, adjustment
  situational — *see* Disorder, adjustment
  social Z60.9
    due to
      acculturation difficulty Z60.3
      discrimination and persecution (perceived)
        Z60.5
      exclusion and isolation Z60.4
      life-cycle (phase of life) transition Z60.0
      rejection Z60.4
      specified reason NEC Z60.8
Malaise R53.81
Malakoplakia — *see* Malacoplakia
Malaria, malarial (fever) B54
  with
    blackwater fever B50.8
      hemoglobinuric (bilious) B50.8
    hemoglobinuria B50.8
  accidentally induced (therapeutically) — *code by* type
    under Malaria
  algid B50.9
  cerebral B50.0 [G94]
  clinically diagnosed (without parasitological confirma-
    tion) B54
  congenital NEC P37.4
    falciparum P37.3
  congestion, congestive B54
  continued (fever) B50.9

Malaria, malarial — *continued*
  estivo-autumnal B50.9
  falciparum B50.9
    with complications NEC B50.8
      cerebral B50.0 [G94]
      severe B50.8
  hemorrhagic B54
  malariae B52.9
    with
      complications NEC B52.8
      glomerular disorder B52.0
  malignant (tertian) — *see* Malaria, falciparum
  mixed infections — *code to* first listed type in B50-B53
  ovale B53.0
  parasitologically confirmed NEC B53.8
  pernicious, acute — *see* Malaria, falciparum
  Plasmodium (P.)
    falciparum NEC — *see* Malaria, falciparum
    malariae NEC B52.9
      with Plasmodium
        falciparum (and or vivax) — *see* Malaria,
          falciparum
        vivax (*see also* Malaria, vivax)
          and falciparum — *see* Malaria, falci-
            parum
    ovale B53.0
      with Plasmodium malariae (*see also* Malaria,
        malariae)
        and vivax (*see also* Malaria, vivax)
          and falciparum — *see* Malaria, falci-
            parum
    simian B53.1
      with Plasmodium malariae (*see also* Malaria,
        malariae)
        and vivax (*see also* Malaria, vivax)
          and falciparum — *see* Malaria, falci-
            parum
    vivax NEC B51.9
      with Plasmodium falciparum — *see* Malaria,
        falciparum
  quartan — *see* Malaria, malariae
  quotidian — *see* Malaria, falciparum
  recurrent B54
  remittent B54
  specified type NEC (parasitologically confirmed) B53.8
  spleen B54
  subtertian (fever) — *see* Malaria, falciparum
  tertian (benign) (*see also* Malaria, vivax)
    malignant B50.9
  tropical B50.9
  typhoid B54
  vivax B51.9
    with
      complications NEC B51.8
      ruptured spleen B51.0
Malassez's disease (cystic) N50.89
Malassimilation K90.9
Maldescent, testis Q53.9
  bilateral Q53.20
    abdominal Q53.211
    perineal Q53.22
  unilateral Q53.10
    abdominal Q53.111
    perineal Q53.12
Maldevelopment (*see also* Anomaly)
  brain Q07.9
  colon Q43.9
  hip Q74.2
    congenital dislocation Q65.2
      bilateral Q65.1
      unilateral Q65.0- ☑
  mastoid process Q75.8
  middle ear Q16.4
    except ossicles Q16.4
    ossicles Q16.3
  ossicles Q16.3
  spine Q76.49
  toe Q74.2
Male type pelvis Q74.2
  with disproportion (fetopelvic) O33.3 ☑
    causing obstructed labor O65.3
Malformation (congenital) (*see also* Anomaly)
  adrenal gland Q89.1
  affecting multiple systems with skeletal changes NEC
    Q87.5
  alimentary tract Q45.9
    specified type NEC Q45.8
    upper Q40.9

Malformation — *continued*
  alimentary tract — *continued*
    upper — *continued*
      specified type NEC Q40.8
  aorta Q25.40
    absence Q25.41
    aneurysm, congenital Q25.43
    aplasia Q25.41
    atresia Q25.29
      aortic arch Q25.21
    coarctation (preductal) (postductal) Q25.1
    dilatation, congenital Q25.44
    hypoplasia Q25.42
    patent ductus arteriosus Q25.0
    specified type NEC Q25.49
    stenosis Q25.1
      supravalvular Q25.3
  aortic valve Q23.9
    specified NEC Q23.8
  arteriovenous, aneurysmatic (congenital) Q27.30
    brain Q28.2
    cerebral Q28.2
    peripheral Q27.30
      digestive system Q27.33
      lower limb Q27.32
      other specified site Q27.39
      renal vessel Q27.34
      upper limb Q27.31
    precerebral vessels (nonruptured) Q28.0
  auricle
    ear (congenital) Q17.3
      acquired H61.119
        left H61.112
          with right H61.113
        right H61.111
          with left H61.113
  bile duct Q44.5
  bladder Q64.79
    aplasia Q64.5
    diverticulum Q64.6
    exstrophy — *see* Exstrophy, bladder
    neck obstruction Q64.31
  bone Q79.9
    face Q75.9
      specified type NEC Q75.8
    skull Q75.9
      specified type NEC Q75.8
  brain (multiple) Q04.9
    arteriovenous Q28.2
    specified type NEC Q04.8
  branchial cleft Q18.2
  breast Q83.9
    specified type NEC Q83.8
  broad ligament Q50.6
  bronchus Q32.4
  bursa Q79.9
  cardiac
    chambers Q20.9
      specified type NEC Q20.8
    septum Q21.9
      specified type NEC Q21.8
  cerebral Q04.9
    vessels Q28.3
  cervix uteri Q51.9
    specified type NEC Q51.828
  Chiari
    Type I G93.5
    Type II Q07.01
  choroid (congenital) Q14.3
    plexus Q07.8
  circulatory system Q28.9
  cochlea Q16.5
  cornea Q13.4
  coronary vessels Q24.5
  corpus callosum (congenital) Q04.0
  diaphragm Q79.1
  digestive system NEC, specified type NEC Q45.8
  dura Q07.9
    brain Q04.9
    spinal Q06.9
  ear Q17.9
    causing impairment of hearing Q16.9
    external Q17.9
      accessory auricle Q17.0
      causing impairment of hearing Q16.9
        absence of
          auditory canal Q16.1
          auricle Q16.0
        macrotia Q17.1

☑ **Additional Character Required** — Refer to the Tabular List for Character Selection   ▽ **Subterms under main terms may continue to next column or page**

Malformation — *continued*
  ear — *continued*
    external — *continued*
      microtia Q17.2
      misplacement Q17.4
      misshapen NEC Q17.3
      prominence Q17.5
      specified type NEC Q17.8
    inner Q16.5
    middle Q16.4
      absence of eustachian tube Q16.2
      ossicles (fusion) Q16.3
    ossicles Q16.3
    specified type NEC Q17.8
  epididymis Q55.4
  esophagus Q39.9
    specified type NEC Q39.8
  eye Q15.9
    lid Q10.3
    specified NEC Q15.8
  fallopian tube Q50.6
  genital organ — *see* Anomaly, genitalia
  great
    artery Q25.9
      aorta — *see* Malformation, aorta
      pulmonary artery — *see* Malformation, pul-
        monary, artery
      specified type NEC Q25.8
    vein Q26.9
      anomalous
        portal venous connection Q26.5
        pulmonary venous connection Q26.4
          partial Q26.3
          total Q26.2
      persistent left superior vena cava Q26.1
      portal vein-hepatic artery fistula Q26.6
      specified type NEC Q26.8
      vena cava stenosis, congenital Q26.0
  gum Q38.6
  hair Q84.2
  heart Q24.9
    specified type NEC Q24.8
  integument Q84.9
    specified type NEC Q84.8
  internal ear Q16.5
  intestine Q43.9
    specified type NEC Q43.8
  iris Q13.2
  joint Q74.9
    ankle Q74.2
    lumbosacral Q76.49
    sacroiliac Q74.2
    specified type NEC Q74.8
  kidney Q63.9
    accessory Q63.0
    giant Q63.3
    horseshoe Q63.1
    hydronephrosis Q62.0
    malposition Q63.2
    specified type NEC Q63.8
  lacrimal apparatus Q10.6
  lingual Q38.3
  lip Q38.0
  liver Q44.7
  lung Q33.9
  meninges or membrane (congenital) Q07.9
    cerebral Q04.8
    spinal (cord) Q06.9
  middle ear Q16.4
    ossicles Q16.3
  mitral valve Q23.9
    specified NEC Q23.8
  Mondini's (congenital) (malformation, cochlea) Q16.5
  mouth (congenital) Q38.6
  multiple types NEC Q89.7
  musculoskeletal system Q79.9
  myocardium Q24.8
  nail Q84.6
  nervous system (central) Q07.9
  nose Q30.9
    specified type NEC Q30.8
  optic disc Q14.2
  orbit Q10.7
  ovary Q50.39
  palate Q38.5
  parathyroid gland Q89.2
  pelvic organs or tissues NEC
    in pregnancy or childbirth O34.8- ☑
      causing obstructed labor O65.5

Malformation — *continued*
  penis Q55.69
    aplasia Q55.5
    curvature (lateral) Q55.61
    hypoplasia Q55.62
  pericardium Q24.8
  peripheral vascular system Q27.9
    specified type NEC Q27.8
  pharynx Q38.8
  precerebral vessels Q28.1
  prostate Q55.4
  pulmonary
    arteriovenous Q25.72
    artery Q25.9
      atresia Q25.5
      specified type NEC Q25.79
      stenosis Q25.6
    valve Q22.3
  renal artery Q27.2
  respiratory system Q34.9
  retina Q14.1
  scrotum — *see* Malformation, testis and scrotum
  seminal vesicles Q55.4
  sense organs NEC Q07.9
  skin Q82.9
  specified NEC Q89.8
  spinal
    cord Q06.9
    nerve root Q07.8
  spine Q76.49
    kyphosis — *see* Kyphosis, congenital
    lordosis — *see* Lordosis, congenital
  spleen Q89.09
  stomach Q40.3
    specified type NEC Q40.2
  teeth, tooth K00.9
  tendon Q79.9
  testis and scrotum Q55.20
    aplasia Q55.0
    hypoplasia Q55.1
    polyorchism Q55.21
    retractile testis Q55.22
    scrotal transposition Q55.23
    specified NEC Q55.29
  thorax, bony Q76.9
  throat Q38.8
  thyroid gland Q89.2
  tongue (congenital) Q38.3
    hypertrophy Q38.2
    tie Q38.1
  trachea Q32.1
  tricuspid valve Q22.9
    specified type NEC Q22.8
  umbilical cord NEC (complicating delivery) O69.89 ☑
  umbilicus Q89.9
  ureter Q62.8
    agenesis Q62.4
    duplication Q62.5
    malposition — *see* Malposition, congenital, ureter
    obstructive defect — *see* Defect, obstructive, ureter
    vesico-ureteric-renal reflux Q62.7
  urethra Q64.79
    aplasia Q64.5
    duplication Q64.74
    posterior valves Q64.2
    prolapse Q64.71
    stricture Q64.32
  urinary system Q64.9
  uterus Q51.9
    specified type NEC Q51.818
  vagina Q52.4
  vas deferens Q55.4
    atresia Q55.3
  vascular system, peripheral Q27.9
  venous — *see* Anomaly, vein(s)
  vulva Q52.70
Malfunction (*see also* Dysfunction)
  cardiac electronic device T82.119 ☑
    electrode T82.110 ☑
    pulse generator T82.111 ☑
    specified type NEC T82.118 ☑
  catheter device NEC T85.618 ☑
    cystostomy T83.010 ☑
    dialysis (renal) (vascular) T82.41 ☑
      intraperitoneal T85.611 ☑
    infusion NEC T82.514 ☑
      cranial T85.610 ☑
      epidural T85.610 ☑

Malfunction — *continued*
  catheter device — *continued*
    infusion — *continued*
      intrathecal T85.610 ☑
      spinal T85.610 ☑
      subarachnoid T85.610 ☑
      subdural T85.610 ☑
    urinary (*see also* Breakdown, device, catheter)
      T83.018 ☑
    colostomy K94.03
    valve K94.03
    cystostomy (stoma) N99.512
    catheter T83.010 ☑
    enteric stoma K94.13
    enterostomy K94.13
    esophagostomy K94.33
    gastroenteric K31.89
    gastrostomy K94.23
    ileostomy K94.13
    valve K94.13
    intrathecal infusion pump T85.615 ☑
    jejunostomy K94.13
    nervous system device, implant or graft, specified NEC
      T85.615 ☑
    pacemaker — *see* Malfunction, cardiac electronic de-
      vice
    prosthetic device, internal — *see* Complications,
      prosthetic device, by site, mechanical
    tracheostomy J95.03
    urinary device NEC — *see* Complication, genitourinary,
      device, urinary, mechanical
    valve
      colostomy K94.03
      heart T82.09 ☑
      ileostomy K94.13
    vascular graft or shunt NEC — *see* Complication, car-
      diovascular device, mechanical, vascular
    ventricular (communicating shunt) T85.01 ☑
Malherbe's tumor — *see* Neoplasm, skin, benign
Malibu disease L98.8
Malignancy (*see also* Neoplasm, malignant, by site)
  unspecified site (primary) C80.1
Malignant — *see* condition
Malingerer, malingering Z76.5
Mallet finger (acquired) — *see* Deformity, finger, mallet
  finger
  congenital Q74.0
  sequelae of rickets E64.3
Malleus A24.0
Mallory's bodies R89.7
Mallory-Weiss syndrome K22.6
Malnutrition E46
  degree
    first E44.1
    mild (protein) E44.1
    moderate (protein) E44.0
    second E44.0
    severe (protein-energy) E43
      intermediate form E42
        with
          kwashiorkor (and marasmus) E42
          marasmus E41
    third E43
  following gastrointestinal surgery K91.2
  intrauterine
    light-for-dates — *see* Light for dates
    small-for-dates — *see* Small for dates
  lack of care, or neglect (child) (infant) T76.02 ☑
    confirmed T74.02 ☑
  malignant E40
  protein E46
    calorie E46
      mild E44.1
      moderate E44.0
      severe E43
        intermediate form E42
          with
            kwashiorkor (and marasmus) E42
            marasmus E41
    energy E46
      mild E44.1
      moderate E44.0
      severe E43
        intermediate form E42
          with
            kwashiorkor (and marasmus) E42
            marasmus E41
  severe (protein-energy) E43

Index

Malnutrition — continued
  severe — continued
    with
      kwashiorkor (and marasmus) E42
      marasmus E41
Malocclusion (teeth) M26.4
  Angle's M26.219
    class I M26.211
    class II M26.212
    class III M26.213
  due to
    abnormal swallowing M26.59
    mouth breathing M26.59
    tongue, lip or finger habits M26.59
  temporomandibular (joint) M26.69
Malposition
  cervix — see Malposition, uterus
  congenital
    adrenal (gland) Q89.1
    alimentary tract Q45.8
      lower Q43.8
      upper Q40.8
    aorta Q25.49
    appendix Q43.8
    arterial trunk Q20.0
    artery (peripheral) Q27.8
      coronary Q24.5
      digestive system Q27.8
      lower limb Q27.8
      pulmonary Q25.79
      specified site NEC Q27.8
      upper limb Q27.8
    auditory canal Q17.8
      causing impairment of hearing Q16.9
    auricle (ear) Q17.4
      causing impairment of hearing Q16.9
      cervical Q18.2
    biliary duct or passage Q44.5
    bladder (mucosa) — see Exstrophy, bladder
    brachial plexus Q07.8
    brain tissue Q04.8
    breast Q83.8
    bronchus Q32.4
    cecum Q43.8
    clavicle Q74.0
    colon Q43.8
    digestive organ or tract NEC Q45.8
      lower Q43.8
      upper Q40.8
    ear (auricle) (external) Q17.4
      ossicles Q16.3
    endocrine (gland) NEC Q89.2
    epiglottis Q31.8
    eustachian tube Q17.8
    eye Q15.8
    facial features Q18.8
    fallopian tube Q50.6
    finger(s) Q68.1
      supernumerary Q69.0
    foot Q66.9
    gallbladder Q44.1
    gastrointestinal tract Q45.8
    genitalia, genital organ(s) or tract
      female Q52.8
        external Q52.79
        internal NEC Q52.8
      male Q55.8
    glottis Q31.8
    hand Q68.1
    heart Q24.8
      dextrocardia Q24.0
        with complete transposition of viscera Q89.3
    hepatic duct Q44.5
    hip (joint) Q65.89
    intestine (large) (small) Q43.8
      with anomalous adhesions, fixation or malrotation Q43.3
    joint NEC Q68.8
    kidney Q63.2
    larynx Q31.8
    limb Q68.8
      lower Q68.8
      upper Q68.8
    liver Q44.7
    lung (lobe) Q33.8
    nail(s) Q84.6
    nerve Q07.8
    nervous system NEC Q07.8
    nose, nasal (septum) Q30.8

Malposition — continued
  congenital — continued
    organ or site not listed — see Anomaly, by site
    ovary Q50.39
    pancreas Q45.3
    parathyroid (gland) Q89.2
    patella Q74.1
    peripheral vascular system Q27.8
    pituitary (gland) Q89.2
    respiratory organ or system NEC Q34.8
    rib (cage) Q76.6
      supernumerary in cervical region Q76.5
    scapula Q74.0
    shoulder Q74.0
    spinal cord Q06.8
    spleen Q89.09
    sternum NEC Q76.7
    stomach Q40.2
    symphysis pubis Q74.2
    thymus (gland) Q89.2
    thyroid (gland) (tissue) Q89.2
      cartilage Q31.8
    toe(s) Q66.9
      supernumerary Q69.2
    tongue Q38.3
    trachea Q32.1
    ureter Q62.60
      deviation Q62.61
      displacement Q62.62
      ectopia Q62.63
      specified type NEC Q62.69
    uterus Q51.818
    vein(s) (peripheral) Q27.8
      great Q26.8
    vena cava (inferior) (superior) Q26.8
  device, implant or graft (see also Complications, by site and type, mechanical) T85.628 ☑
    arterial graft NEC — see Complication, cardiovascular device, mechanical, vascular
    breast (implant) T85.42 ☑
    catheter NEC T85.628 ☑
      cystostomy T83.020 ☑
      dialysis (renal) T82.42 ☑
        intraperitoneal T85.621 ☑
      infusion NEC T82.524 ☑
        spinal (epidural) (subdural) T85.620 ☑
      urinary (see also Displacement, device, catheter, urinary) T83.028 ☑
    electronic (electrode) (pulse generator) (stimulator)
      bone T84.320 ☑
      cardiac T82.129 ☑
        electrode T82.120 ☑
        pulse generator T82.121 ☑
        specified type NEC T82.128 ☑
      nervous system — see Complication, prosthetic device, mechanical, electronic nervous system stimulator
      urinary — see Complication, genitourinary, device, urinary, mechanical
    fixation, internal (orthopedic) NEC — see Complication, fixation device, mechanical
    gastrointestinal — see Complications, prosthetic device, mechanical, gastrointestinal device
    genital NEC T83.428 ☑
      intrauterine contraceptive device (string) T83.32 ☑
      penile prosthesis (cylinder) (implanted) (pump) (reservoir) T83.420 ☑
      testicular prosthesis T83.421 ☑
    heart NEC — see Complication, cardiovascular device, mechanical
    joint prosthesis — see Complication, joint prosthesis, mechanical
    ocular NEC — see Complications, prosthetic device, mechanical, ocular device
    orthopedic NEC — see Complication, orthopedic, device, mechanical
    specified NEC T85.628 ☑
    urinary NEC (see also Complication, genitourinary, device, urinary, mechanical)
      graft T83.22 ☑
    vascular NEC — see Complication, cardiovascular device, mechanical
    ventricular intracranial shunt T85.02 ☑
  fetus — see Pregnancy, complicated by (management affected by), presentation, fetal
  gallbladder K82.8

Malposition — continued
  gastrointestinal tract, congenital Q45.8
  heart, congenital NEC Q24.8
  joint prosthesis — see Complications, joint prosthesis, mechanical, displacement, by site
  stomach K31.89
    congenital Q40.2
  tooth, teeth, fully erupted M26.30
  uterus (acute) (acquired) (adherent) (asymptomatic) (postinfectional) (postpartal, old) N85.4
    anteflexion or anteversion N85.4
      congenital Q51.818
    flexion N85.4
      lateral — see Lateroversion, uterus
    inversion N85.5
    lateral (flexion) (version) — see Lateroversion, uterus
      in pregnancy or childbirth — see subcategory O34.5 ☑
    retroflexion or retroversion — see Retroversion, uterus
Malposture R29.3
Malrotation
  cecum Q43.3
  colon Q43.3
  intestine Q43.3
  kidney Q63.2
Malta fever — see Brucellosis
Maltreatment
  adult
    abandonment
      confirmed T74.01 ☑
      suspected T76.01 ☑
    confirmed T74.91 ☑
    history of Z91.419
    neglect
      confirmed T74.01 ☑
      suspected T76.01 ☑
    physical abuse
      confirmed T74.11 ☑
      suspected T76.11 ☑
    psychological abuse
      confirmed T74.31 ☑
      history of Z91.411
      suspected T76.31 ☑
    sexual abuse
      confirmed T74.21 ☑
      suspected T76.21 ☑
    suspected T76.91 ☑
  child
    abandonment
      confirmed T74.02 ☑
      suspected T76.02 ☑
    confirmed T74.92 ☑
    history of — see History, personal (of), abuse
    neglect
      confirmed T74.02 ☑
      history of — see History, personal (of), abuse
      suspected T76.02 ☑
    physical abuse
      confirmed T74.12 ☑
      history of — see History, personal (of), abuse
      suspected T76.12 ☑
    psychological abuse
      confirmed T74.32 ☑
      history of — see History, personal (of), abuse
      suspected T76.32 ☑
    sexual abuse
      confirmed T74.22 ☑
      history of — see History, personal (of), abuse
      suspected T76.22 ☑
    suspected T76.92 ☑
  personal history of Z91.89
Maltworker's lung J67.4
Malunion, fracture — see Fracture, by site
Mammillitis N61.0
  puerperal, postpartum O91.02
Mammitis — see Mastitis
Mammogram (examination) Z12.39
  routine Z12.31
Mammoplasia N62
Management (of)
  bone conduction hearing device (implanted) Z45.320
  cardiac pacemaker NEC Z45.018
  cerebrospinal fluid drainage device Z45.41
  cochlear device (implanted) Z45.321
  contraceptive Z30.9

☑ **Additional Character Required** — Refer to the Tabular List for Character Selection   ▽ **Subterms under main terms may continue to next column or page**

Malnutrition — Management

Management — *continued*
  contraceptive — *continued*
    specified NEC Z30.8
    implanted device Z45.9
      specified NEC Z45.89
    infusion pump Z45.1
    procreative Z31.9
      male factor infertility in female Z31.81
      specified NEC Z31.89
    prosthesis (external) (*see also* Fitting) Z44.9
      implanted Z45.9
        specified NEC Z45.89
    renal dialysis catheter Z49.01
    vascular access device Z45.2
Mangled — *see* specified injury by site
Mania (monopolar) (*see also* Disorder, mood, manic
    episode)
  with psychotic symptoms F30.2
  without psychotic symptoms F30.10
    mild F30.11
    moderate F30.12
    severe F30.13
  Bell's F30.8
  chronic (recurrent) F31.89
  hysterical F44.89
  puerperal F30.8
  recurrent F31.89
Manic depression F31.9
Manic-depressive insanity, psychosis, or syndrome
    — *see* Disorder, bipolar
Mannosidosis E77.1
Mansonelliasis, mansonellosis B74.4
Manson's
  disease B65.1
  schistosomiasis B65.1
Manual — *see* condition
Maple-bark-stripper's lung (disease) J67.6
Maple-syrup-urine disease E71.0
Marable's syndrome (celiac artery compression) I77.4
Marasmus E41
  due to malnutrition E41
  intestinal E41
  nutritional E41
  senile R54
  tuberculous NEC — *see* Tuberculosis
Marble
  bones Q78.2
  skin R23.8
Marburg virus disease A98.3
March
  fracture — *see* Fracture, traumatic, stress, by site
  hemoglobinuria D59.6
Marchesani (-Weill) **syndrome** Q87.0
Marchiafava (-Bignami) **syndrome or disease** G37.1
Marchiafava-Micheli syndrome D59.5
Marcus Gunn's syndrome Q07.8
Marfan's syndrome — *see* Syndrome, Marfan's
Marie-Bamberger disease — *see* Osteoarthropathy,
    hypertrophic, specified NEC
Marie-Charcot-Tooth neuropathic muscular atrophy
    G60.0
Marie's
  cerebellar ataxia (late-onset) G11.2
  disease or syndrome (acromegaly) E22.0
Marie-Strümpell arthritis, disease or spondylitis —
    see Spondylitis, ankylosing
Marion's disease (bladder neck obstruction) N32.0
Marital conflict Z63.0
Mark
  port wine Q82.5
  raspberry Q82.5
  strawberry Q82.5
  stretch L90.6
  tattoo L81.8
Marker heterochromatin — *see* Extra, marker chromo-
    somes
Maroteaux-Lamy syndrome (mild) (severe) E76.29
Marrow (bone)
  arrest D61.9
  poor function D75.89
Marseilles fever A77.1
Marsh fever — *see* Malaria
Marshall's (hidrotic) **ectodermal dysplasia** Q82.4
Marsh's disease (exophthalmic goiter) E05.00
  with storm E05.01
Masculinization (female) **with adrenal hyperplasia**
    E25.9

Masculinization (female) **with adrenal hyperplasia**
    — *continued*
  congenital E25.0
Masculinovoblastoma D27.- ☑
Masochism (sexual) F65.51
Mason's lung J62.8
Mass
  abdominal R19.00
    epigastric R19.06
    generalized R19.07
    left lower quadrant R19.04
    left upper quadrant R19.02
    periumbilic R19.05
    right lower quadrant R19.03
    right upper quadrant R19.01
    specified site NEC R19.09
  breast (*see also* Lump, breast) N63.0
  chest R22.2
  cystic — *see* Cyst
  ear H93.8- ☑
  head R22.0
  intra-abdominal (diffuse) (generalized) — *see* Mass,
    abdominal
  kidney N28.89
  liver R16.0
  localized (skin) R22.9
    chest R22.2
    head R22.0
    limb
      lower R22.4- ☑
      upper R22.3- ☑
    neck R22.1
    trunk R22.2
  lung R91.8
  malignant — *see* Neoplasm, malignant, by site
  neck R22.1
  pelvic (diffuse) (generalized) — *see* Mass, abdominal
  specified organ NEC — *see* Disease, by site
  splenic R16.1
  substernal thyroid — *see* Goiter
  superficial (localized) R22.9
  umbilical (diffuse) (generalized) R19.09
Massive — *see* condition
Mast cell
  disease, systemic tissue D47.02
  leukemia C94.3- ☑
  neoplasm
    malignant C96.20
      specified type NEC C96.29
    of uncertain behavior NEC D47.09
  sarcoma C96.22
  tumor D47.09
Mastalgia N64.4
Masters-Allen syndrome N83.8
Mastitis (acute) (diffuse) (nonpuerperal) (subacute) N61.0
  with abscess N61.1
  without abscess N61.0
  chronic (cystic) — *see* Mastopathy, cystic
  cystic (Schimmelbusch's type) — *see* Mastopathy,
    cystic
  fibrocystic — *see* Mastopathy, cystic
  infective N61.0
    newborn P39.0
  interstitial, gestational or puerperal — *see* Mastitis,
    obstetric
  neonatal (noninfective) P83.4
    infective P39.0
  obstetric (interstitial) (nonpurulent)
    associated with
      lactation O91.23
      pregnancy O91.21- ☑
      puerperium O91.22
    purulent
      associated with
        lactation O91.13
        pregnancy O91.11- ☑
        puerperium O91.12
  periductal — *see* Ectasia, mammary duct
  phlegmonous — *see* Mastopathy, cystic
  plasma cell — *see* Ectasia, mammary duct
Mastocytoma (extracutaneous) D47.09
  malignant C96.29
  solitary D47.01
Mastocytosis D47.09
  aggressive systemic C96.21
  cutaneous (diffuse) (maculopapular) D47.01
    congenital Q82.2
    of neonatal onset Q82.2

Mastocytosis — *continued*
  cutaneous — *continued*
    of newborn onset Q82.2
  indolent systemic D47.02
  isolated bone marrow D47.02
  malignant C96.29
  systemic (indolent) (smoldering)
    with an associated hematological non-mast cell
      lineage disease (SM-AHNMD) D47.02
Mastodynia N64.4
Mastoid — *see* condition
Mastoidalgia — *see* subcategory H92.0 ☑
Mastoiditis (coalescent) (hemorrhagic) (suppurative)
    H70.9- ☑
  acute, subacute H70.00- ☑
    complicated NEC H70.09- ☑
    subperiosteal H70.01- ☑
  chronic (necrotic) (recurrent) H70.1- ☑
  in (due to)
    infectious disease NEC B99 [H75.0-] ☑
    parasitic disease NEC B89 [H75.0-] ☑
    tuberculosis A18.03
  petrositis — *see* Petrositis
  postauricular fistula — *see* Fistula, postauricular
  specified NEC H70.89- ☑
  tuberculous A18.03
Mastopathy, mastopathia N64.9
  chronica cystica — *see* Mastopathy, cystic
  cystic (chronic) (diffuse) N60.1- ☑
    with epithelial proliferation N60.3- ☑
  diffuse cystic — *see* Mastopathy, cystic
  estrogenic, oestrogenica N64.89
  ovarian origin N64.89
Mastoplasia, mastoplastia N62
Masturbation (excessive) F98.8
Maternal care (for) — *see* Pregnancy (complicated by)
    (management affected by)
Matheiu's disease (leptospiral jaundice) A27.0
Mauclaire's disease or osteochondrosis — *see* Osteo-
    chondrosis, juvenile, hand, metacarpal
Maxcy's disease A75.2
Maxilla, maxillary — *see* condition
May (-Hegglin) **anomaly or syndrome** D72.0
McArdle (-Schmid)(-Pearson) **disease** (glycogen storage)
    E74.04
McCune-Albright syndrome Q78.1
McQuarrie's syndrome (idiopathic familial hypo-
    glycemia) E16.2
Meadow's syndrome Q86.1
Measles (black) (hemorrhagic) (suppressed) B05.9
  with
    complications NEC B05.89
    encephalitis B05.0
    intestinal complications B05.4
    keratitis (keratoconjunctivitis) B05.81
    meningitis B05.1
    otitis media B05.3
    pneumonia B05.2
  French — *see* Rubella
  German — *see* Rubella
  Liberty — *see* Rubella
Meatitis, urethral — *see* Urethritis
Meatus, meatal — *see* condition
Meat-wrappers' asthma J68.9
Meckel-Gruber syndrome Q61.9
Meckel's diverticulitis, diverticulum (displaced) (hy-
    pertrophic) Q43.0
  malignant — *see* Table of Neoplasms, small intestine,
    malignant
Meconium
  ileus, newborn P76.0
    in cystic fibrosis E84.11
    meaning meconium plug (without cystic fibrosis)
      P76.0
  obstruction, newborn P76.0
    due to fecaliths P76.0
    in mucoviscidosis E84.11
  peritonitis P78.0
  plug syndrome (newborn) NEC P76.0
Median (*see also* condition)
  arcuate ligament syndrome I77.4
  bar (prostate) (vesical orifice) — *see* Hyperplasia,
    prostate
  rhomboid glossitis K14.2
Mediastinal shift R93.8
Mediastinitis (acute) (chronic) J98.51
  syphilitic A52.73

▽ **Subterms under main terms may continue to next column or page**   ☑ **Additional Character Required — Refer to the Tabular List for Character Selection**   **219**

Management — Mediastinitis

Mediastinitis — *continued*
tuberculous A15.8
Mediastinopericarditis (*see also* Pericarditis)
acute I30.9
adhesive I31.0
chronic I31.8
rheumatic I09.2
Mediastinum, mediastinal — *see* condition
Medicine poisoning — *see* Table of Drugs and Chemicals, by drug, poisoning
Mediterranean
fever — *see* Brucellosis
familial M04.1
tick A77.1
kala-azar B55.0
leishmaniasis B55.0
tick fever A77.1
Medulla — *see* condition
Medullary cystic kidney Q61.5
Medullated fibers
optic (nerve) Q14.8
retina Q14.1
Medulloblastoma
desmoplastic C71.6
specified site — *see* Neoplasm, malignant, by site
unspecified site C71.6
Medulloepithelioma (*see also* Neoplasm, malignant, by site)
teratoid — *see* Neoplasm, malignant, by site
Medullomyoblastoma
specified site — *see* Neoplasm, malignant, by site
unspecified site C71.6
Meekeren-Ehlers-Danlos syndrome Q79.6
Megacolon (acquired) (functional) (not Hirschsprung's disease) (in) K59.39
Chagas' disease B57.32
congenital, congenitum (aganglionic) Q43.1
Hirschsprung's (disease) Q43.1
toxic NEC K59.31
due to Clostridium difficile
not specified as recurrent A04.72
recurrent A04.71
Megaesophagus (functional) K22.0
congenital Q39.5
in (due to) Chagas' disease B57.31
Megalencephaly Q04.5
Megalerythema (epidemic) B08.3
Megaloappendix Q43.8
Megalocephalus, megalocephaly NEC Q75.3
Megalocornea Q15.8
with glaucoma Q15.0
Megalocytic anemia D53.1
Megalodactylia (fingers) (thumbs) (congenital) Q74.0
toes Q74.2
Megaloduodenum Q43.8
Megaloesophagus (functional) K22.0
congenital Q39.5
Megalogastria (acquired) K31.89
congenital Q40.2
Megalophthalmos Q11.3
Megalopsia H53.15
Megalosplenia — *see* Splenomegaly
Megaloureter N28.82
congenital Q62.2
Megarectum K62.89
Megasigmoid K59.39
congenital Q43.2
Megaureter N28.82
congenital Q62.2
Megavitamin-B6 syndrome E67.2
Megrim — *see* Migraine
Meibomian
cyst, infected — *see* Hordeolum
gland — *see* condition
sty, stye — *see* Hordeolum
Meibomitis — *see* Hordeolum
Meige-Milroy disease (chronic hereditary edema) Q82.0
Meige's syndrome Q82.0
Melalgia, nutritional E53.8
Melancholia F32.9
climacteric (single episode) F32.89
recurrent episode F33.8
hypochondriac F45.29
intermittent (single episode) F32.89
recurrent episode F33.8
involutional (single episode) F32.89
recurrent episode F33.8

Melancholia — *continued*
menopausal (single episode) F32.89
recurrent episode F33.8
puerperal F32.89
reactive (emotional stress or trauma) F32.3
recurrent F33.9
senile F03 ☑
stuporous (single episode) F32.89
recurrent episode F33.8
Melanemia R79.89
Melanoameloblastoma — *see* Neoplasm, bone, benign
Melanoblastoma — *see* Melanoma
Melanocarcinoma — *see* Melanoma
Melanocytoma, eyeball D31.9- ☑
Melanocytosis, neurocutaneous Q82.8
Melanoderma, melanodermia L81.4
Melanodontia, infantile K03.89
Melanodontoclasia K03.89
Melanoepithelioma — *see* Melanoma
Melanoma (malignant) C43.9
acral lentiginous, malignant — *see* Melanoma, skin, by site
amelanotic — *see* Melanoma, skin, by site
balloon cell — *see* Melanoma, skin, by site
benign — *see* Nevus
desmoplastic, malignant — *see* Melanoma, skin, by site
epithelioid cell — *see* Melanoma, skin, by site
with spindle cell, mixed — *see* Melanoma, skin, by site
in
giant pigmented nevus — *see* Melanoma, skin, by site
Hutchinson's melanotic freckle — *see* Melanoma, skin, by site
junctional nevus — *see* Melanoma, skin, by site
precancerous melanosis — *see* Melanoma, skin, by site
in situ D03.9
abdominal wall D03.59
ala nasi D03.39
ankle D03.7- ☑
anus, anal (margin) (skin) D03.51
arm D03.6- ☑
auditory canal D03.2- ☑
auricle (ear) D03.2- ☑
auricular canal (external) D03.2- ☑
axilla, axillary fold D03.59
back D03.59
breast D03.52
brow D03.39
buttock D03.59
canthus (eye) D03.1- ☑
cheek (external) D03.39
chest wall D03.59
chin D03.39
choroid D03.8
conjunctiva D03.8
ear (external) D03.2- ☑
external meatus (ear) D03.2- ☑
eye D03.8
eyebrow D03.39
eyelid (lower) (upper) D03.1- ☑
face D03.30
specified NEC D03.39
female genital organ (external) NEC D03.8
finger D03.6- ☑
flank D03.59
foot D03.7- ☑
forearm D03.6- ☑
forehead D03.39
foreskin D03.8
gluteal region D03.59
groin D03.59
hand D03.6- ☑
heel D03.7- ☑
helix D03.2- ☑
hip D03.7- ☑
interscapular region D03.59
iris D03.8
jaw D03.39
knee D03.7- ☑
labium (majus) (minus) D03.8
lacrimal gland D03.8
leg D03.7- ☑
lip (lower) (upper) D03.0
lower limb NEC D03.7- ☑

Melanoma — *continued*
in situ — *continued*
male genital organ (external) NEC D03.8
nail D03.9
finger D03.6- ☑
toe D03.7- ☑
neck D03.4
nose (external) D03.39
orbit D03.8
penis D03.8
perianal skin D03.51
perineum D03.51
pinna D03.2- ☑
popliteal fossa or space D03.7- ☑
prepuce D03.8
pudendum D03.8
retina D03.8
retrobulbar D03.8
scalp D03.4
scrotum D03.8
shoulder D03.6- ☑
specified site NEC D03.8
submammary fold D03.52
temple D03.39
thigh D03.7- ☑
toe D03.7- ☑
trunk NEC D03.59
umbilicus D03.59
upper limb NEC D03.6- ☑
vulva D03.8
juvenile — *see* Nevus
malignant, of soft parts except skin — *see* Neoplasm, connective tissue, malignant
metastatic
breast C79.81
genital organ C79.82
specified site NEC C79.89
neurotropic, malignant — *see* Melanoma, skin, by site
nodular — *see* Melanoma, skin, by site
regressing, malignant — *see* Melanoma, skin, by site
skin C43.9
abdominal wall C43.59
ala nasi C43.31
ankle C43.7- ☑
anus, anal (skin) C43.51
arm C43.6- ☑
auditory canal (external) C43.2- ☑
auricle (ear) C43.2- ☑
auricular canal (external) C43.2- ☑
axilla, axillary fold C43.59
back C43.59
breast (female) (male) C43.52
brow C43.39
buttock C43.59
canthus (eye) C43.1- ☑
cheek (external) C43.39
chest wall C43.59
chin C43.39
ear (external) C43.2- ☑
elbow C43.6- ☑
external meatus (ear) C43.2- ☑
eyebrow C43.39
eyelid (lower) (upper) C43.1- ☑
face C43.30
specified NEC C43.39
female genital organ (external) NEC C51.9
finger C43.6- ☑
flank C43.59
foot C43.7- ☑
forearm C43.6- ☑
forehead C43.39
foreskin C60.0
glabella C43.39
gluteal region C43.59
groin C43.59
hand C43.6- ☑
heel C43.7- ☑
helix C43.2- ☑
hip C43.7- ☑
interscapular region C43.59
jaw (external) C43.39
knee C43.7- ☑
labium C51.9
majus C51.0
minus C51.1
leg C43.7- ☑
lip (lower) (upper) C43.0

Melanoma — *continued*
  skin — *continued*
    lower limb NEC C43.7- ☑
    male genital organ (external) NEC C63.9
    nail
      finger C43.6- ☑
      toe C43.7- ☑
    nasolabial groove C43.39
    nates C43.59
    neck C43.4
    nose (external) C43.31
    overlapping site C43.8
    palpebra C43.1- ☑
    penis C60.9
    perianal skin C43.51
    perineum C43.51
    pinna C43.2- ☑
    popliteal fossa or space C43.7- ☑
    prepuce C60.0
    pudendum C51.9
    scalp C43.4
    scrotum C63.2
    shoulder C43.6- ☑
    skin NEC C43.9
    submammary fold C43.52
    temple C43.39
    thigh C43.7- ☑
    toe C43.7- ☑
    trunk NEC C43.59
    umbilicus C43.59
    upper limb NEC C43.6- ☑
    vulva C51.9
      overlapping sites C51.8
  spindle cell
    with epithelioid, mixed — *see* Melanoma, skin, by
      site
    type A C69.4- ☑
    type B C69.4- ☑
  superficial spreading — *see* Melanoma, skin, by site
Melanosarcoma (*see also* Melanoma)
  epithelioid cell — *see* Melanoma
Melanosis L81.4
  addisonian E27.1
    tuberculous A18.7
  adrenal E27.1
  colon K63.89
  conjunctiva — *see* Pigmentation, conjunctiva
    congenital Q13.89
  cornea (presenile) (senile) (*see also* Pigmentation,
    cornea)
    congenital Q13.4
  eye NEC H57.8
    congenital Q15.8
  lenticularis progressiva Q82.1
  liver K76.89
  precancerous (*see also* Melanoma, in situ)
    malignant melanoma in — *see* Melanoma
  Riehl's L81.4
  sclera H15.89
    congenital Q13.89
  suprarenal E27.1
  tar L81.4
  toxic L81.4
Melanuria R82.99
MELAS syndrome E88.41
Melasma L81.1
  adrenal (gland) E27.1
  suprarenal (gland) E27.1
Melena K92.1
  with ulcer — *code by* site under Ulcer, with hemor-
    rhage K27.4
  due to swallowed maternal blood P78.2
  newborn, neonatal P54.1
    due to swallowed maternal blood P78.2
Meleney's
  gangrene (cutaneous) — *see* Ulcer, skin
  ulcer (chronic undermining) — *see* Ulcer, skin
Melioidosis A24.9
  acute A24.1
  chronic A24.2
  fulminating A24.1
  pneumonia A24.1
  pulmonary (chronic) A24.2
    acute A24.1
    subacute A24.2
  sepsis A24.1
  specified NEC A24.3
  subacute A24.2

Melitensis, febris A23.0
Melkersson (-Rosenthal) **syndrome** G51.2
Mellitus, diabetes — *see* Diabetes
Melorheostosis (bone) — *see* Disorder, bone, density
  and structure, specified NEC
Meloschisis Q18.4
Melotia Q17.4
Membrana
  capsularis lentis posterior Q13.89
  epipapillaris Q14.2
Membranacea placenta O43.19- ☑
Membranaceous uterus N85.8
Membrane(s), membranous (*see also* condition)
  cyclitic — *see* Membrane, pupillary
  folds, congenital — *see* Web
  Jackson's Q43.3
  over face of newborn P28.9
  premature rupture — *see* Rupture, membranes, pre-
    mature
  pupillary H21.4- ☑
    persistent Q13.89
  retained (with hemorrhage) (complicating delivery)
    O72.2
    without hemorrhage O73.1
  secondary cataract — *see* Cataract, secondary
  unruptured (causing asphyxia) — *see* Asphyxia, new-
    born
  vitreous — *see* Opacity, vitreous, membranes and
    strands
Membranitis — *see* Chorioamnionitis
Memory disturbance, lack or loss (*see also* Amnesia)
  mild, following organic brain damage F06.8
Menadione deficiency E56.1
Menarche
  delayed E30.0
  precocious E30.1
Mendacity, pathologic F60.2
Mendelson's syndrome (due to anesthesia) J95.4
  in labor and delivery O74.0
  in pregnancy O29.01- ☑
  obstetric O74.0
  postpartum, puerperal O89.01
Ménétrier's disease or syndrome K29.60
  with bleeding K29.61
Ménière's disease, syndrome or vertigo H81.0- ☑
Meninges, meningeal — *see* condition
Meningioma (*see also* Neoplasm, meninges, benign)
  angioblastic — *see* Neoplasm, meninges, benign
  angiomatous — *see* Neoplasm, meninges, benign
  endotheliomatous — *see* Neoplasm, meninges, benign
  fibroblastic — *see* Neoplasm, meninges, benign
  fibrous — *see* Neoplasm, meninges, benign
  hemangioblastic — *see* Neoplasm, meninges, benign
  hemangiopericytic — *see* Neoplasm, meninges, be-
    nign
  malignant — *see* Neoplasm, meninges, malignant
  meningiothelial — *see* Neoplasm, meninges, benign
  meningotheliomatous — *see* Neoplasm, meninges,
    benign
  mixed — *see* Neoplasm, meninges, benign
  multiple — *see* Neoplasm, meninges, uncertain behav-
    ior
  papillary — *see* Neoplasm, meninges, uncertain behav-
    ior
  psammomatous — *see* Neoplasm, meninges, benign
  syncytial — *see* Neoplasm, meninges, benign
  transitional — *see* Neoplasm, meninges, benign
Meningiomatosis (diffuse) — *see* Neoplasm, meninges,
  uncertain behavior
Meningism — *see* Meningismus
Meningismus (infectional) (pneumococcal) R29.1
  due to serum or vaccine R29.1
  influenzal — *see* Influenza, with, manifestations NEC
Meningitis (basal) (basic) (brain) (cerebral) (cervical)
  (congestive) (diffuse) (hemorrhagic) (infantile)
  (membranous) (metastatic) (nonspecific) (pontine)
  (progressive) (simple) (spinal) (subacute) (sympathetic) (toxic) G03.9
  abacterial G03.0
  actinomycotic A42.81
  adenoviral A87.1
  arbovirus A87.8
  aseptic (acute) G03.0
  bacterial G00.9
    Escherichia coli (E. coli) G00.8
    Friedländer (bacillus) G00.8
    gram-negative G00.9

Meningitis — *continued*
  bacterial — *continued*
    H. influenzae G00.0
    Klebsiella G00.8
    pneumococcal G00.1
    specified organism NEC G00.8
    staphylococcal G00.3
    streptococcal (acute) G00.2
  benign recurrent (Mollaret) G03.2
  candidal B37.5
  caseous (tuberculous) A17.0
  cerebrospinal A39.0
  chronic NEC G03.1
  clear cerebrospinal fluid NEC G03.0
  coxsackievirus A87.0
  cryptococcal B45.1
  diplococcal (gram positive) A39.0
  echovirus A87.0
  enteroviral A87.0
  eosinophilic B83.2
  epidemic NEC A39.0
  Escherichia coli (E. coli) G00.8
  fibrinopurulent G00.9
    specified organism NEC G00.8
  Friedländer (bacillus) G00.8
  gonococcal A54.81
  gram-negative cocci G00.9
  gram-positive cocci G00.9
  H. influenzae G00.0
  Haemophilus (influenzae) G00.0
  in (due to)
    adenovirus A87.1
    African trypanosomiasis B56.9 [G02]
    anthrax A22.8
    bacterial disease NEC A48.8 [G01]
    Chagas' disease (chronic) B57.41
    chickenpox B01.0
    coccidioidomycosis B38.4
    Diplococcus pneumoniae G00.1
    enterovirus A87.0
    herpes (simplex) virus B00.3
      zoster B02.1
    infectious mononucleosis B27.92
    leptospirosis A27.81
    Listeria monocytogenes A32.11
    Lyme disease A69.21
    measles B05.1
    mumps (virus) B26.1
    neurosyphilis (late) A52.13
    parasitic disease NEC B89 [G02]
    poliovirus A80.9 [G02]
    preventive immunization, inoculation or vaccina-
      tion G03.8
    rubella B06.02
    Salmonella infection A02.21
    specified cause NEC G03.8
    Streptococcal pneumoniae G00.1
    typhoid fever A01.01
    varicella B01.0
    viral disease NEC A87.8
    whooping cough A37.90
    zoster B02.1
  infectious G00.9
  influenzal (H. influenzae) G00.0
  Klebsiella G00.8
  leptospiral (aseptic) A27.81
  lymphocytic (acute) (benign) (serous) A87.2
  meningococcal A39.0
  Mima polymorpha G00.8
  Mollaret (benign recurrent) G03.2
  monilial B37.5
  mycotic NEC B49 [G02]
  Neisseria A39.0
  nonbacterial G03.0
  nonpyogenic NEC G03.0
  ossificans G96.19
  pneumococcal streptococcus pneumoniae G00.1
  poliovirus A80.9 [G02]
  postmeasles B05.1
  purulent G00.9
    specified organism NEC G00.8
  pyogenic G00.9
    specified organism NEC G00.8
  Salmonella (arizonae) (Cholerae-Suis) (enteritidis) (ty-
    phimurium) A02.21
  septic G00.9
    specified organism NEC G00.8
  serosa circumscripta NEC G03.0
  serous NEC G93.2

Meningitis — *continued*
  specified organism NEC G00.8
  sporotrichosis B42.81
  staphylococcal G00.3
  sterile G03.0
  Streptococcal (acute) G00.2
    pneumoniae G00.1
  suppurative G00.9
    specified organism NEC G00.8
  syphilitic (late) (tertiary) A52.13
    acute A51.41
    congenital A50.41
    secondary A51.41
  Torula histolytica (cryptococcal) B45.1
  traumatic (complication of injury) T79.8 ☑
  tuberculous A17.0
  typhoid A01.01
  viral NEC A87.9
  Yersinia pestis A20.3
Meningocele (spinal) (*see also* Spina bifida)
  with hydrocephalus — *see* Spina bifida, by site, with
    hydrocephalus
  acquired (traumatic) G96.19
  cerebral — *see* Encephalocele
Meningocerebritis — *see* Meningoencephalitis
Meningococcemia A39.4
  acute A39.2
  chronic A39.3
Meningococcus, meningococcal (*see also* condition)
    A39.9
  adrenalitis, hemorrhagic A39.1
  carrier (suspected) of Z22.31
  meningitis (cerebrospinal) A39.0
Meningoencephalitis (*see also* Encephalitis) G04.90
  acute NEC (*see also* Encephalitis, viral) A86
  bacterial NEC G04.2
  California A83.5
  diphasic A84.1
  eosinophilic B83.2
  epidemic A39.81
  herpesviral, herpetic B00.4
    due to herpesvirus 6 B10.01
    due to herpesvirus 7 B10.09
    specified NEC B10.09
  in (due to)
    blastomycosis NEC B40.81
    diseases classified elsewhere G05.3
    free-living amebae B60.2
    H. influenzae G00.0
    Hemophilus influenzae (H .influenzae) G00.0
    herpes B00.4
      due to herpesvirus 6 B10.01
      due to herpesvirus 7 B10.09
      specified NEC B10.09
    Lyme disease A69.22
    mercury — *see* subcategory T56.1 ☑
    mumps B26.2
    Naegleria (amebae) (organisms) (fowleri) B60.2
    Parastrongylus cantonensis B83.2
    toxoplasmosis (acquired) B58.2
      congenital P37.1
  infectious (acute) (viral) A86
  influenzal (H. influenzae) G00.0
  Listeria monocytogenes A32.12
  lymphocytic (serous) A87.2
  mumps B26.2
  parasitic NEC B89 [G05.3]
  pneumococcal G04.2
  primary amebic B60.2
  specific (syphilitic) A52.14
  specified organism NEC G04.81
  staphylococcal G04.2
  streptococcal G04.2
  syphilitic A52.14
  toxic NEC G92
    due to mercury — *see* subcategory T56.1 ☑
  tuberculous A17.82
  virus NEC A86
Meningoencephalocele (*see also* Encephalocele)
  syphilitic A52.19
    congenital A50.49
Meningoencephalomyelitis (*see also* Meningoen-
    cephalitis)
  acute NEC (viral) A86
    disseminated G04.00
      postimmunization or postvaccination G04.02
      postinfectious G04.01

Meningoencephalomyelitis — *continued*
  due to
    actinomycosis A42.82
    Torula B45.1
    Toxoplasma or toxoplasmosis (acquired) B58.2
      congenital P37.1
  postimmunization or postvaccination G04.02
Meningoencephalomyelopathy G96.9
Meningoencephalopathy G96.9
Meningomyelitis (*see also* Meningoencephalitis)
  bacterial NEC G04.2
  blastomycotic NEC B40.81
  cryptococcal B45.1
  in diseases classified elsewhere G05.4
  meningococcal A39.81
  syphilitic A52.14
  tuberculous A17.82
Meningomyelocele (*see also* Spina bifida)
  syphilitic A52.19
Meningomyeloneuritis — *see* Meningoencephalitis
Meningoradiculitis — *see* Meningitis
Meningovascular — *see* condition
Menkes' disease or syndrome E83.09
  meaning maple-syrup-urine disease E71.0
Menometrorrhagia N92.1
Menopause, menopausal (asymptomatic) (state) Z78.0
  arthritis (any site) NEC — *see* Arthritis, specified form
    NEC
  bleeding N92.4
  depression (single episode) F32.89
    agitated (single episode) F32.2
      recurrent episode F33.9
    psychotic (single episode) F32.89
      recurrent episode F33.9
    recurrent episode F33.8
  melancholia (single episode) F32.89
    recurrent episode F33.8
  paranoid state F22
  premature E28.319
    asymptomatic E28.319
      postirradiation E89.40
      postsurgical E89.40
    symptomatic E28.310
      postirradiation E89.41
      postsurgical E89.41
  psychosis NEC F28
  symptomatic N95.1
  toxic polyarthritis NEC — *see* Arthritis, specified form
    NEC
Menorrhagia (primary) N92.0
  climacteric N92.4
    menopausal N92.4
  menopausal N92.4
  postclimacteric N95.0
  postmenopausal N95.0
  preclimacteric or premenopausal N92.4
  pubertal (menses retained) N92.2
Menostaxis N92.0
Menses, retention N94.89
Menstrual — *see* Menstruation
Menstruation
  absent — *see* Amenorrhea
  anovulatory N97.0
  cycle, irregular N92.6
  delayed N91.0
  disorder N93.9
    psychogenic F45.8
  during pregnancy O20.8
  excessive (with regular cycle) N92.0
    with irregular cycle N92.1
    at puberty N92.2
  frequent N92.0
  infrequent — *see* Oligomenorrhea
  irregular N92.6
    specified NEC N92.5
  latent N92.5
  membranous N92.5
  painful (*see also* Dysmenorrhea) N94.6
    primary N94.4
    psychogenic F45.8
    secondary N94.5
  passage of clots N92.0
  precocious E30.1
  protracted N92.5
  rare — *see* Oligomenorrhea
  retained N94.89
  retrograde N92.5
  scanty — *see* Oligomenorrhea

Menstruation — *continued*
  suppression N94.89
  vicarious (nasal) N94.89
Mental (*see also* condition)
  deficiency — *see* Disability, intellectual
  deterioration — *see* Psychosis
  disorder — *see* Disorder, mental
  exhaustion F48.8
  insufficiency (congenital) — *see* Disability, intellectual
  observation without need for further medical care
    Z03.89
  retardation — *see* Disability, intellectual
  subnormality — *see* Disability, intellectuall
  upset — *see* Disorder, mental
Meralgia paresthetica G57.1- ☑
Mercurial — *see* condition
Mercurialism — *see* subcategory T56.1 ☑
Merkel cell tumor — *see* Carcinoma, Merkel cell
Merocele — *see* Hernia, femoral
Meromelia
  lower limb — *see* Defect, reduction, lower limb
    intercalary
      femur — *see* Defect, reduction, lower limb,
        specified type NEC
        tibiofibular (complete) (incomplete) — *see*
          Defect, reduction, lower limb
  upper limb — *see* Defect, reduction, upper limb
    intercalary, humeral, radioulnar — *see* Agenesis,
      arm, with hand present
MERRF syndrome (myoclonic epilepsy associated with
    ragged-red fiber) E88.42
Merzbacher-Pelizaeus disease E75.29
Mesaortitis — *see* Aortitis
Mesarteritis — *see* Arteritis
Mesencephalitis — *see* Encephalitis
Mesenchymoma (*see also* Neoplasm, connective tissue,
    uncertain behavior)
  benign — *see* Neoplasm, connective tissue, benign
  malignant — *see* Neoplasm, connective tissue, malig-
    nant
Mesenteritis K65.4
  retractile K65.4
  sclerosing K65.4
Mesentery, mesenteric — *see* condition
Mesiodens, mesiodentes K00.1
Mesio-occlusion M26.213
Mesocolon — *see* condition
Mesonephroma (malignant) — *see* Neoplasm, malig-
    nant, by site
  benign — *see* Neoplasm, benign, by site
Mesophlebitis — *see* Phlebitis
Mesostromal dysgenesia Q13.89
Mesothelioma (malignant) C45.9
  benign
    mesentery D19.1
    mesocolon D19.1
    omentum D19.1
    peritoneum D19.1
    pleura D19.0
    specified site NEC D19.7
    unspecified site D19.9
  biphasic C45.9
    benign
      mesentery D19.1
      mesocolon D19.1
      omentum D19.1
      peritoneum D19.1
      pleura D19.0
      specified site NEC D19.7
      unspecified site D19.9
  cystic D48.4
  epithelioid C45.9
    benign
      mesentery D19.1
      mesocolon D19.1
      omentum D19.1
      peritoneum D19.1
      pleura D19.0
      specified site NEC D19.7
      unspecified site D19.9
  fibrous C45.9
    benign
      mesentery D19.1
      mesocolon D19.1
      omentum D19.1
      peritoneum D19.1
      pleura D19.0
      specified site NEC D19.7

Mesothelioma — *continued*
  fibrous — *continued*
    benign — *continued*
      unspecified site D19.9
    site classification
      liver C45.7
      lung C45.7
      mediastinum C45.7
      mesentery C45.1
      mesocolon C45.1
      omentum C45.1
      pericardium C45.2
      peritoneum C45.1
      pleura C45.0
        parietal C45.0
      retroperitoneum C45.7
      specified site NEC C45.7
      unspecified C45.9
Metabolic syndrome E88.81
Metagonimiasis B66.8
Metagonimus infestation (intestine) B66.8
Metal
  pigmentation L81.8
  polisher's disease J62.8
Metamorphopsia H53.15
Metaplasia
  apocrine (breast) — *see* Dysplasia, mammary, specified
    type NEC
  cervix (squamous) — *see* Dysplasia, cervix
  endometrium (squamous) (uterus) N85.8
  esophagus K22.7- ☑
  kidney (pelvis) (squamous) N28.89
  myelogenous D73.1
  myeloid (agnogenic) (megakaryocytic) D73.1
  spleen D73.1
  squamous cell, bladder N32.89
Metastasis, metastatic
  abscess — *see* Abscess
  calcification E83.59
  cancer
    from specified site — *see* Neoplasm, malignant,
      by site
    to specified site — *see* Neoplasm, secondary, by
      site
  deposits (in) — *see* Neoplasm, secondary, by site
  disease (*see also* Neoplasm, secondary, by site) C79.9
  spread (to) — *see* Neoplasm, secondary, by site
Metastrongyliasis B83.8
Metatarsalgia M77.4- ☑
  anterior G57.6- ☑
  Morton's G57.6- ☑
Metatarsus, metatarsal (*see also* condition)
  adductus, congenital Q66.22
  valgus (abductus), congenital Q66.6
  varus (congenital) Q66.22
    primus Q66.21
Methadone use — *see* Use, opioid
Methemoglobinemia D74.9
  acquired (with sulfhemoglobinemia) D74.8
  congenital D74.0
  enzymatic (congenital) D74.0
  Hb M disease D74.0
  hereditary D74.0
  toxic D74.8
Methemoglobinuria — *see* Hemoglobinuria
Methioninemia E72.19
Methylmalonic acidemia E71.120
Metritis (catarrhal) (hemorrhagic) (septic) (suppurative)
  (*see also* Endometritis)
  cervical — *see* Cervicitis
Metropathia hemorrhagica N93.8
Metroperitonitis — *see* Peritonitis, pelvic, female
Metrorrhagia N92.1
  climacteric N92.4
  menopausal N92.4
  postpartum NEC (atonic) (following delivery of placen-
    ta) O72.1
    delayed or secondary O72.2
  preclimacteric or premenopausal N92.4
  psychogenic F45.8
Metrorrhexis — *see* Rupture, uterus
Metrosalpingitis N70.91
Metrostaxis N93.8
Metrovaginitis — *see* Endometritis
Meyer-Schwickerath and Weyers syndrome Q87.0
Meynert's amentia (nonalcoholic) F04
  alcoholic F10.96

Meynert's amentia — *continued*
  alcoholic — *continued*
    with dependence F10.26
Mibelli's disease (porokeratosis) Q82.8
Mice, joint — *see* Loose, body, joint
  knee M23.4- ☑
Micrencephalon, micrencephaly Q02
Microalbuminuria R80.9
Microaneurysm, retinal (*see also* Disorder, retina, mi-
  croaneurysms)
  diabetic — *see* E08-E13 with .31
Microangiopathy (peripheral) I73.9
  thrombotic M31.1
Microcalcifications, breast R92.0
Microcephalus, microcephalic, microcephaly Q02
  due to toxoplasmosis (congenital) P37.1
Microcheilia Q18.7
Microcolon (congenital) Q43.8
Microcornea (congenital) Q13.4
Microcytic — *see* condition
Microdeletions NEC Q93.88
Microdontia K00.2
Microdrepanocytosis D57.40
  with crisis (vasoocclusive pain) D57.419
    with
      acute chest syndrome D57.411
      splenic sequestration D57.412
Microembolism
  atherothrombotic — *see* Atheroembolism
  retinal — *see* Occlusion, artery, retina
Microencephalon Q02
Microfilaria streptocerca infestation — *see* Onchocer-
  ciasis
Microgastria (congenital) Q40.2
Microgenia M26.06
Microgenitalia, congenital
  female Q52.8
  male Q55.8
Microglioma — *see* Lymphoma, non-Hodgkin, specified
  NEC
Microglossia (congenital) Q38.3
Micrognathia, micrognathism (congenital)
  (mandibular) (maxillary) M26.09
Microgyria (congenital) Q04.3
Microinfarct of heart — *see* Insufficiency, coronary
Microlentia (congenital) Q12.8
Microlithiasis, alveolar, pulmonary J84.02
Micromastia N64.82
Micromyelia (congenital) Q06.8
Micropenis Q55.62
Microphakia (congenital) Q12.8
Microphthalmos, microphthalmia (congenital) Q11.2
  due to toxoplasmosis P37.1
Micropsia H53.15
Microscopic polyangiitis (polyarteritis) M31.7
Microsporidiosis B60.8
  intestinal A07.8
Microsporon furfur infestation B36.0
Microsporosis (*see also* Dermatophytosis)
  nigra B36.1
Microstomia (congenital) Q18.5
Microtia (congenital) (external ear) Q17.2
Microtropia H50.40
Microvillus inclusion disease (MVD) (MVID) Q43.8
Micturition
  disorder NEC (*see also* Difficulty, micturition) R39.198
    psychogenic F45.8
  frequency R35.0
    psychogenic F45.8
  hesitancy R39.11
  incomplete emptying R39.14
  nocturnal R35.1
  painful R30.9
    dysuria R30.0
    psychogenic F45.8
    tenesmus R30.1
  poor stream R39.12
  position dependent R39.192
  split stream R39.13
  straining R39.16
  urgency R39.15
Mid plane — *see* condition
Middle
  ear — *see* condition
  lobe (right) syndrome J98.19
Miescher's elastoma L87.2
Mietens' syndrome Q87.2

Migraine (idiopathic) G43.909
  with aura (acute-onset) (prolonged) (typical) (without
    headache) G43.109
    with refractory migraine G43.119
      with status migrainosus G43.111
      without status migrainosus G43.119
    without mention of refractory migraine G43.109
      with status migrainosus G43.101
      without status migrainosus G43.109
    intractable G43.119
      with status migrainosus G43.111
      without status migrainosus G43.119
    not intractable G43.109
      with status migrainosus G43.101
      without status migrainosus G43.109
    persistent G43.509
      with cerebral infarction G43.609
        with refractory migraine G43.619
          with status migrainosus G43.611
          without status migrainosus G43.619
        without refractory migraine G43.609
          with status migrainosus G43.601
          without status migrainosus G43.609
        intractable G43.619
          with status migrainosus G43.611
          without status migrainosus G43.619
        not intractable G43.609
          with status migrainosus G43.601
          without status migrainosus G43.609
      without cerebral infarction G43.509
        with refractory migraine G43.519
          with status migrainosus G43.511
          without status migrainosus G43.519
        without refractory migraine G43.509
          with status migrainosus G43.501
          without status migrainosus G43.509
        intractable G43.519
          with status migrainosus G43.511
          without status migrainosus G43.519
        not intractable G43.509
          with status migrainosus G43.501
          without status migrainosus G43.509
  with refractory migraine G43.919
    with status migrainosus G43.911
    without status migrainosus G43.919
  without aura G43.009
    with refractory migraine G43.019
      with status migrainosus G43.011
      without status migrainosus G43.019
    without mention of refractory migraine G43.009
      with status migrainosus G43.001
      without status migrainosus G43.009
    chronic G43.709
      with refractory migraine G43.719
        with status migrainosus G43.711
        without status migrainosus G43.719
      without refractory migraine G43.709
        with status migrainosus G43.701
        without status migrainosus G43.709
      intractable
        with status migrainosus G43.711
        without status migrainosus G43.719
      not intractable
        with status migrainosus G43.701
        without status migrainosus G43.709
    intractable
      with status migrainosus G43.011
      without status migrainosus G43.019
    not intractable
      with status migrainosus G43.001
      without status migrainosus G43.009
  without refractory migraine G43.909
    with status migrainosus G43.901
    without status migrainosus G43.919
  abdominal G43.D0 (*following* G43.7)
    with refractory migraine G43.D1 (*following* G43.7)
    without refractory migraine G43.D0 (*following*
      G43.7)
    intractable G43.D1 (*following* G43.7)
    not intractable G43.D0 (*following* G43.7)
  basilar — *see* Migraine, with aura
  classical — *see* Migraine, with aura
  common — *see* Migraine, without aura
  complicated G43.109
  equivalents — *see* Migraine, with aura
  familiar — *see* Migraine, hemiplegic
  hemiplegic G43.409
    with refractory migraine G43.419
      with status migrainosus G43.411

Migraine — continued
  hemiplegic — continued
    with refractory migraine — continued
      without status migrainosus G43.419
    without refractory migraine G43.409
      with status migrainosus G43.401
      without status migrainosus G43.409
    intractable G43.419
      with status migrainosus G43.411
      without status migrainosus G43.419
    not intractable G43.409
      with status migrainosus G43.401
      without status migrainosus G43.409
    intractable G43.919
      with status migrainosus G43.911
      without status migrainosus G43.919
  menstrual G43.829
    with refractory migraine G43.839
      with status migrainosus G43.831
      without status migrainosus G43.839
    without refractory migraine G43.829
      with status migrainosus G43.821
      without status migrainosus G43.829
    intractable G43.839
      with status migrainosus G43.831
      without status migrainosus G43.839
    not intractable 4G43.829
      with status migrainosus G43.821
      without status migrainosus G43.829
  menstrually related — see Migraine, menstrual
  not intractable G43.909
    with status migrainosus G43.901
    without status migrainosus G43.919
  ophthalmoplegic G43.B0 (following G43.7)
    with refractory migraine G43.B1 (following G43.7)
    without refractory migraine G43.B0 (following G43.7)
    intractable G43.B1 (following G43.7)
    not intractable G43.B0 (following G43.7)
  persistent aura (with, without) cerebral infarction — see Migraine, with aura, persistent
  preceded or accompanied by transient focal neurological phenomena — see Migraine, with aura
  pre-menstrual — see Migraine, menstrual
  pure menstrual — see Migraine, menstrual
  retinal — see Migraine, with aura
  specified NEC G43.809
    intractable G43.819
      with status migrainosus G43.811
      without status migrainosus G43.819
    not intractable G43.809
      with status migrainosus G43.801
      without status migrainosus G43.809
  sporadic — see Migraine, hemiplegic
  transformed — see Migraine, without aura, chronic
  triggered seizures — see Migraine, with aura
Migrant, social Z59.0
Migration, anxiety concerning Z60.3
Migratory, migrating (see also condition)
  person Z59.0
  testis Q55.29
Mikity-Wilson disease or syndrome P27.0
Mikulicz' disease or syndrome K11.8
Miliaria L74.3
  alba L74.1
  apocrine L75.2
  crystallina L74.1
  profunda L74.2
  rubra L74.0
  tropicalis L74.2
Miliary — see condition
Milium L72.0
  colloid L57.8
Milk
  crust L21.0
  excessive secretion O92.6
  poisoning — see Poisoning, food, noxious
  retention O92.79
  sickness — see Poisoning, food, noxious
  spots I31.0
Milk-alkali disease or syndrome E83.52
Milk-leg (deep vessels) (nonpuerperal) — see Embolism, vein, lower extremity
  complicating pregnancy O22.3- ☑
  puerperal, postpartum, childbirth O87.1
Milkman's disease or syndrome M83.8
Milky urine — see Chyluria
Millard-Gubler (-Foville) **paralysis or syndrome** G46.3

Millar's asthma J38.5
Miller Fisher syndrome G61.0
Mills' disease — see Hemiplegia
Millstone maker's pneumoconiosis J62.8
Milroy's disease (chronic hereditary edema) Q82.0
Minamata disease T56.1 ☑
Miners' asthma or lung J60
Minkowski-Chauffard syndrome — see Spherocytosis
Minor — see condition
Minor's disease (hematomyelia) G95.19
Minot's disease (hemorrhagic disease), newborn P53
Minot-von Willebrand-Jurgens disease or syndrome (angiohemophilia) D68.0
Minus (and plus) **hand** (intrinsic) — see Deformity, limb, specified type NEC, forearm
Miosis (pupil) H57.03
Mirizzi's syndrome (hepatic duct stenosis) K83.1
Mirror writing F81.0
Misadventure (of) (prophylactic) (therapeutic) (see also Complications) T88.9 ☑
  administration of insulin (by accident) — see subcategory T38.3 ☑
  infusion — see Complications, infusion
  local applications (of fomentations, plasters, etc.) T88.9 ☑
    burn or scald — see Burn
    specified NEC T88.8 ☑
  medical care (early) (late) T88.9 ☑
    adverse effect of drugs or chemicals — see Table of Drugs and Chemicals
    burn or scald — see Burn
    specified NEC T88.8 ☑
  specified NEC T88.8 ☑
  surgical procedure (early) (late) — see Complications, surgical procedure
  transfusion — see Complications, transfusion
  vaccination or other immunological procedure — see Complications, vaccination
Miscarriage O03.9
Misdirection, aqueous H40.83- ☑
Misperception, sleep state F51.02
Misplaced, misplacement
  ear Q17.4
  kidney (acquired) N28.89
    congenital Q63.2
  organ or site, congenital NEC — see Malposition, congenital
Missed
  abortion O02.1
  delivery O36.4 ☑
Missing (see also Absence)
  string of intrauterine contraceptive device T83.32- ☑
Misuse of drugs F19.99
Mitchell's disease (erythromelalgia) I73.81
Mite(s) (infestation) B88.9
  diarrhea B88.0
  grain (itch) B88.0
  hair follicle (itch) B88.0
  in sputum B88.0
Mitral — see condition
Mittelschmerz N94.0
Mixed — see condition
MMN (multifocal motor neuropathy) G61.82
MNGIE (Mitochondrial Neurogastrointestinal Encephalopathy) **syndrome** E88.49
Mobile, mobility
  cecum Q43.3
  excessive — see Hypermobility
  gallbladder, congenital Q44.1
  kidney N28.89
  organ or site, congenital NEC — see Malposition, congenital
Mobitz heart block (atrioventricular) I44.1
Moebius, Möbius
  disease (ophthalmoplegic migraine) — see Migraine, ophthalmoplegic
  syndrome Q87.0
    congenital oculofacial paralysis (with other anomalies) Q87.0
    ophthalmoplegic migraine — see Migraine, ophthalmoplegic
Moeller's glossitis K14.0
Mohr's syndrome (Types I and II) Q87.0
Mola destruens D39.2
Molar pregnancy O02.0
Molarization of premolars K00.2

Molding, head (during birth) — omit code
Mole (pigmented) (see also Nevus)
  blood O02.0
  Breus' O02.0
  cancerous — see Melanoma
  carneous O02.0
  destructive D39.2
  fleshy O02.0
  hydatid, hydatidiform (benign) (complicating pregnancy) (delivered) (undelivered) O01.9
    classical O01.0
    complete O01.0
    incomplete O01.1
    invasive D39.2
    malignant D39.2
    partial O01.1
  intrauterine O02.0
  invasive (hydatidiform) D39.2
  malignant
    meaning
      malignant hydatidiform mole D39.2
      melanoma — see Melanoma
  nonhydatidiform O02.0
  nonpigmented — see Nevus
  pregnancy NEC O02.0
  skin — see Nevus
  tubal O00.10- ☑
    with intrauterine pregnancy O00.11- ☑
  vesicular — see Mole, hydatidiform
Molimen, molimina (menstrual) N94.3
Molluscum contagiosum (epitheliale) B08.1
Mönckeberg's arteriosclerosis, disease, or sclerosis — see Arteriosclerosis, extremities
Mondini's malformation (cochlea) Q16.5
Mondor's disease I80.8
Monge's disease T70.29 ☑
Monilethrix (congenital) Q84.1
Moniliasis (see also Candidiasis) B37.9
  neonatal P37.5
Monitoring (encounter for)
  therapeutic drug level Z51.81
Monkey malaria B53.1
Monkeypox B04
Monoarthritis M13.10
  ankle M13.17- ☑
  elbow M13.12- ☑
  foot joint M13.17- ☑
  hand joint M13.14- ☑
  hip M13.15- ☑
  knee M13.16- ☑
  shoulder M13.11- ☑
  wrist M13.13- ☑
Monoblastic — see condition
Monochromat (ism), monochromatopsia (acquired) (congenital) H53.51
Monocytic — see condition
Monocytopenia D72.818
Monocytosis (symptomatic) D72.821
Monomania — see Psychosis
Mononeuritis G58.9
  cranial nerve — see Disorder, nerve, cranial
  femoral nerve G57.2- ☑
  lateral
    cutaneous nerve of thigh G57.1- ☑
    popliteal nerve G57.3- ☑
  lower limb G57.9- ☑
    specified nerve NEC G57.8- ☑
  medial popliteal nerve G57.4- ☑
  median nerve G56.1- ☑
  multiplex G58.7
  plantar nerve G57.6- ☑
  posterior tibial nerve G57.5- ☑
  radial nerve G56.3- ☑
  sciatic nerve G57.0- ☑
  specified NEC G58.8
  tibial nerve G57.4- ☑
  ulnar nerve G56.2- ☑
  upper limb G56.9- ☑
    specified nerve NEC G56.8- ☑
  vestibular — see subcategory H93.3 ☑
Mononeuropathy G58.9
  carpal tunnel syndrome — see Syndrome, carpal tunnel
  diabetic NEC — see E08-E13 with .41
  femoral nerve — see Lesion, nerve, femoral
  ilioinguinal nerve G57.8- ☑
  in diseases classified elsewhere — see category G59

Mononeuropathy — *continued*
  intercostal G58.0
  lower limb G57.9- ☑
    causalgia — *see* Causalgia, lower limb
    femoral nerve — *see* Lesion, nerve, femoral
    meralgia paresthetica G57.1- ☑
    plantar nerve — *see* Lesion, nerve, plantar
    popliteal nerve — *see* Lesion, nerve, popliteal
    sciatic nerve — *see* Lesion, nerve, sciatic
    specified NEC G57.8- ☑
    tarsal tunnel syndrome — *see* Syndrome, tarsal
        tunnel
  median nerve — *see* Lesion, nerve, median
  multiplex G58.7
  obturator nerve G57.8- ☑
  popliteal nerve — *see* Lesion, nerve, popliteal
  radial nerve — *see* Lesion, nerve, radial
  saphenous nerve G57.8- ☑
  specified NEC G58.8
  tarsal tunnel syndrome — *see* Syndrome, tarsal tunnel
  tuberculous A17.83
  ulnar nerve — *see* Lesion, nerve, ulnar
  upper limb G56.9- ☑
    carpal tunnel syndrome — *see* Syndrome, carpal
        tunnel
    causalgia — *see* Causalgia
    median nerve — *see* Lesion, nerve, median
    radial nerve — *see* Lesion, nerve, radial
    specified site NEC G56.8- ☑
    ulnar nerve — *see* Lesion, nerve, ulnar
Mononucleosis, infectious B27.90
  with
    complication NEC B27.99
    meningitis B27.92
    polyneuropathy B27.91
  cytomegaloviral B27.10
    with
      complication NEC B27.19
      meningitis B27.12
      polyneuropathy B27.11
  Epstein-Barr (virus) B27.00
    with
      complication NEC B27.09
      meningitis B27.02
      polyneuropathy B27.01
  gammaherpesviral B27.00
    with
      complication NEC B27.09
      meningitis B27.02
      polyneuropathy B27.01
  specified NEC B27.80
    with
      complication NEC B27.89
      meningitis B27.82
      polyneuropathy B27.81
Monoplegia G83.3- ☑
  congenital (cerebral) G80.8
    spastic G80.1
  embolic (current episode) I63.4- ☑
  following
    cerebrovascular disease
      cerebral infarction
        lower limb I69.34- ☑
        upper limb I69.33- ☑
      intracerebral hemorrhage
        lower limb I69.14- ☑
        upper limb I69.13- ☑
      lower limb I69.94- ☑
      nontraumatic intracranial hemorrhage NEC
        lower limb I69.24- ☑
        upper limb I69.23- ☑
      specified disease NEC
        lower limb I69.84- ☑
        upper limb I69.83- ☑
      stroke NOS
        lower limb I69.34- ☑
        upper limb I69.33- ☑
      subarachnoid hemorrhage
        lower limb I69.04- ☑
        upper limb I69.03- ☑
      upper limb I69.93- ☑
  hysterical (transient) F44.4
  lower limb G83.1- ☑
  psychogenic (conversion reaction) F44.4
  thrombotic (current episode) I63.3- ☑
  transient R29.818
  upper limb G83.2- ☑

Monorchism, monorchidism Q55.0
Monosomy (*see also* Deletion, chromosome) Q93.9
  specified NEC Q93.89
  whole chromosome
    meiotic nondisjunction Q93.0
    mitotic nondisjunction Q93.1
    mosaicism Q93.1
  X Q96.9
Monster, monstrosity (single) Q89.7
  acephalic Q00.0
  twin Q89.4
Monteggia's fracture (-dislocation) S52.27- ☑
Mooren's ulcer (cornea) — *see* Ulcer, cornea, Mooren's
Moore's syndrome — *see* Epilepsy, specified NEC
Mooser-Neill reaction A75.2
Mooser's bodies A75.2
Morbidity not stated or unknown R69
Morbilli — *see* Measles
Morbus (*see also* Disease)
  angelicus, anglorum E55.0
  Beigel B36.2
  caducus — *see* Epilepsy
  celiacus K90.0
  comitialis — *see* Epilepsy
  cordis (*see also* Disease, heart) I51.9
    valvulorum — *see* Endocarditis
  coxae senilis M16.9
    tuberculous A18.02
  hemorrhagicus neonatorum P53
  maculosus neonatorum P54.5
Morel (-Stewart)(-Morgagni) **syndrome** M85.2
Morel-Kraepelin disease — *see* Schizophrenia
Morel-Moore syndrome M85.2
Morgagni's
  cyst, organ, hydatid, or appendage
    female Q50.5
    male (epididymal) Q55.4
      testicular Q55.29
  syndrome M85.2
Morgagni-Stewart-Morel syndrome M85.2
Morgagni-Stokes-Adams syndrome I45.9
Morgagni-Turner (-Albright) **syndrome** Q96.9
Moria F07.0
Moron (I.Q. 50-69) F70
Morphea L94.0
Morphinism (without remission) F11.20
  with remission F11.21
Morphinomania (without remission) F11.20
  with remission F11.21
Morquio (-Ullrich)(-Brailsford) **disease or syndrome** —
  see Mucopolysaccharidosis
Mortification (dry) (moist) — *see* Gangrene
Morton's metatarsalgia (neuralgia)(neuroma) (syn-
  drome) G57.6- ☑
Morvan's disease or syndrome G60.8
Mosaicism, mosaic (autosomal) (chromosomal)
  45,X/46,XX Q96.3
  45,X/other cell lines NEC with abnormal sex chromo-
      some Q96.4
  sex chromosome
    female Q97.8
    lines with various numbers of X chromosomes
        Q97.2
    male Q98.7
  XY Q96.3
Moschowitz' disease M31.1
Mother yaw A66.0
Motion sickness (from travel, any vehicle) (from round-
  abouts or swings) T75.3 ☑
Mottled, mottling, teeth (enamel) (endemic) (nonen-
  demic) K00.3
Mounier-Kuhn syndrome Q32.4
  with bronchiectasis J47.9
    exacerbation (acute) J47.1
    lower respiratory infection J47.0
  acquired J98.09
    with bronchiectasis J47.9
      with
        exacerbation (acute) J47.1
        lower respiratory infection J47.0
Mountain
  sickness T70.29 ☑
    with polycythemia , acquired (acute) D75.1
  tick fever A93.2
Mouse, joint — *see* Loose, body, joint
  knee M23.4- ☑
Mouth — *see* condition

Movable
  coccyx — *see* subcategory M53.2 ☑
  kidney N28.89
    congenital Q63.8
  spleen D73.89
Movements, dystonic R25.8
Moyamoya disease I67.5
MRSA (Methicillin resistant Staphylococcus aureus)
  infection A49.02
    as the cause of diseases classified elsewhere B95.62
  sepsis A41.02
MSSA (Methicillin susceptible Staphylococcus aureus)
  infection A49.01
    as the cause of diseases classified elsewhere B95.61
  sepsis A41.01
Mucha-Habermann disease L41.0
Mucinosis (cutaneous) (focal) (papular) (skin) L98.5
  oral K13.79
Mucocele
  appendix K38.8
  buccal cavity K13.79
  gallbladder K82.1
  lacrimal sac, chronic H04.43- ☑
  nasal sinus J34.1
  nose J34.1
  salivary gland (any) K11.6
  sinus (accessory) (nasal) J34.1
  turbinate (bone) (middle) (nasal) J34.1
  uterus N85.8
Mucolipidosis
  I E77.1
  II, III E77.0
  IV E75.11
Mucopolysaccharidosis E76.3
  beta-gluduronidase deficiency E76.29
  cardiopathy E76.3 [I52]
  Hunter's syndrome E76.1
  Hurler's syndrome E76.01
  Hurler-Scheie syndrome E76.02
  Maroteaux-Lamy syndrome E76.29
  Morquio syndrome E76.219
    A E76.210
    B E76.211
    classic E76.210
  Sanfilippo syndrome E76.22
  Scheie's syndrome E76.03
  specified NEC E76.29
  type
    I
      Hurler's syndrome E76.01
      Hurler-Scheie syndrome E76.02
      Scheie's syndrome E76.03
    II E76.1
    III E76.22
    IV E76.219
    IVA E76.210
    IVB E76.211
    VI E76.29
    VII E76.29
Mucormycosis B46.5
  cutaneous B46.3
  disseminated B46.4
  gastrointestinal B46.2
  generalized B46.4
  pulmonary B46.0
  rhinocerebral B46.1
  skin B46.3
  subcutaneous B46.3
Mucositis (ulcerative) K12.30
  due to drugs NEC K12.32
  gastrointestinal K92.81
  mouth (oral) (oropharyngeal) K12.30
    due to antineoplastic therapy K12.31
    due to drugs NEC K12.32
    due to radiation K12.33
    specified NEC K12.39
    viral K12.39
  nasal J34.81
  oral cavity — *see* Mucositis, mouth
  oral soft tissues — *see* Mucositis, mouth
  vagina and vulva N76.81
Mucositis necroticans agranulocytica — *see* Agranulocytosis
Mucous (*see also* condition)
  patches (syphilitic) A51.39
    congenital A50.07
Mucoviscidosis E84.9
  with meconium obstruction E84.11

Mucus
asphyxia or suffocation — *see* Asphyxia, mucus
in stool R19.5
plug — *see* Asphyxia, mucus
Muguet B37.0
Mulberry molars (congenital syphilis) A50.52
Müllerian mixed tumor
specified site — *see* Neoplasm, malignant, by site
unspecified site C54.9
Multicystic kidney (development) Q61.4
Multiparity (grand) Z64.1
affecting management of pregnancy, labor and delivery (supervision only) O09.4- ☑
requiring contraceptive management — *see* Contraception
Multipartita placenta O43.19- ☑
Multiple, multiplex (*see also* condition)
digits (congenital) Q69.9
endocrine neoplasia — *see* Neoplasia, endocrine, multiple (MEN)
personality F44.81
Mumps B26.9
arthritis B26.85
complication NEC B26.89
encephalitis B26.2
hepatitis B26.81
meningitis (aseptic) B26.1
meningoencephalitis B26.2
myocarditis B26.82
oophoritis B26.89
orchitis B26.0
pancreatitis B26.3
polyneuropathy B26.84
Mumu (*see also* Infestation, filarial) B74.9 [N51]
Münchhausen's syndrome — *see* Disorder, factitious
Münchmeyer's syndrome — *see* Myositis, ossificans, progressiva
Mural — *see* condition
Murmur (cardiac) (heart) (organic) R01.1
abdominal R19.15
aortic (valve) — *see* Endocarditis, aortic
benign R01.0
diastolic — *see* Endocarditis
Flint I35.1
functional R01.0
Graham Steell I37.1
innocent R01.0
mitral (valve) — *see* Insufficiency, mitral
nonorganic R01.0
presystolic, mitral — *see* Insufficiency, mitral
pulmonic (valve) I37.8
systolic R01.1
tricuspid (valve) I07.9
valvular — *see* Endocarditis
Murri's disease (intermittent hemoglobinuria) D59.6
Muscle, muscular (*see also* condition)
carnitine (palmityltransferase) deficiency E71.314
Musculoneuralgia — *see* Neuralgia
Mushrooming hip — *see* Derangement, joint, specified NEC, hip
Mushroom-workers' (pickers') **disease or lung** J67.5
Mutation(s)
factor V Leiden D68.51
prothrombin gene D68.52
surfactant, of lung J84.83
Mutism (*see also* Aphasia)
deaf (acquired) (congenital) NEC H91.3
elective (adjustment reaction) (childhood) F94.0
hysterical F44.4
selective (childhood) F94.0
MVD (microvillus inclusion disease) Q43.8
MVID (microvillus inclusion disease) Q43.8
Myalgia M79.1
epidemic (cervical) B33.0
traumatic NEC T14.8 ☑
Myasthenia G70.9
congenital G70.2
cordis — *see* Failure, heart
developmental G70.2
gravis G70.00
with exacerbation (acute) G70.01
in crisis G70.01
neonatal, transient P94.0
pseudoparalytica G70.00
with exacerbation (acute) G70.01
in crisis G70.01
stomach, psychogenic F45.8

Myasthenia — *continued*
syndrome
in
diabetes mellitus — *see* E08-E13 with .44
neoplastic disease (*see also* Neoplasm) D49.9 [G73.3]
pernicious anemia D51.0 [G73.3]
thyrotoxicosis E05.90 [G73.3]
with thyroid storm E05.91 [G73.3]
Myasthenic M62.81
Mycelium infection B49
Mycetismus — *see* Poisoning, food, noxious, mushroom
Mycetoma B47.9
actinomycotic B47.1
bone (mycotic) B47.9 [M90.80]
eumycotic B47.0
foot B47.9
actinomycotic B47.1
mycotic B47.0
madurae NEC B47.9
mycotic B47.0
maduromycotic B47.0
mycotic B47.0
nocardial B47.1
Mycobacteriosis — *see* Mycobacterium
Mycobacterium, mycobacterial (infection) A31.9
anonymous A31.9
atypical A31.9
cutaneous A31.1
pulmonary A31.0
tuberculous — *see* Tuberculosis, pulmonary
specified site NEC A31.8
avium (intracellulare complex) A31.0
balnei A31.1
Battey A31.0
chelonei A31.8
cutaneous A31.1
extrapulmonary systemic A31.8
fortuitum A31.8
intracellulare (Battey bacillus) A31.0
kakaferifu A31.8
kansasii (yellow bacillus) A31.0
kasongo A31.8
leprae (*see also* Leprosy) A30.9
luciflavum A31.1
marinum (M. balnei) A31.1
nonspecific — *see* Mycobacterium, atypical
pulmonary (atypical) A31.0
tuberculous — *see* Tuberculosis, pulmonary
scrofulaceum A31.8
simiae A31.8
systemic, extrapulmonary A31.8
szulgai A31.8
terrae A31.8
triviale A31.8
tuberculosis (human, bovine) — *see* Tuberculosis
ulcerans A31.1
xenopi A31.8
Mycoplasma (M.) **pneumoniae, as cause of disease classified elsewhere** B96.0
Mycosis, mycotic B49
cutaneous NEC B36.9
ear B36.9
in
aspergillosis B44.89
candidiasis B37.84
moniliasis B37.84
fungoides (extranodal) (solid organ) C84.0- ☑
mouth B37.0
nails B35.1
opportunistic B48.8
skin NEC B36.9
specified NEC B48.8
stomatitis B37.0
vagina, vaginitis (candidal) B37.3
Mydriasis (pupil) H57.04
Myelatelia Q06.1
Myelinolysis, pontine, central G37.2
Myelitis (acute) (ascending) (childhood) (chronic) (descending) (diffuse) (disseminated) (idiopathic) (pressure) (progressive) (spinal cord) (subacute) (*see also* Encephalitis) G04.91
herpes simplex B00.82
herpes zoster B02.24
in diseases classified elsewhere G05.4
necrotizing, subacute G37.4
optic neuritis in G36.0
postchickenpox B01.12

Myelitis — *continued*
postherpetic B02.24
postimmunization G04.02
postinfectious NEC G04.89
postvaccinal G04.02
specified NEC G04.89
syphilitic (transverse) A52.14
toxic G92
transverse (in demyelinating diseases of central nervous system) G37.3
tuberculous A17.82
varicella B01.12
Myeloblastic — *see* condition
Myeloblastoma
granular cell (*see also* Neoplasm, connective tissue)
malignant — *see* Neoplasm, connective tissue, malignant
tongue D10.1
Myelocele — *see* Spina bifida
Myelocystocele — *see* Spina bifida
Myelocytic — *see* condition
Myelodysplasia D46.9
specified NEC D46.Z (*following* D46.4)
spinal cord (congenital) Q06.1
Myelodysplastic syndrome D46.9
with
5q deletion D46.C (*following* D46.2)
isolated del (5q) chromosomal abnormality D46.C (*following* D46.2)
specified NEC D46.Z (*following* D46.4)
Myeloencephalitis — *see* Encephalitis
Myelofibrosis D75.81
with myeloid metaplasia D47.4
acute C94.4- ☑
idiopathic (chronic) D47.4
primary D47.1
secondary D75.81
in myeloproliferative disease D47.4
Myelogenous — *see* condition
Myeloid — *see* condition
Myelokathexis D70.9
Myeloleukodystrophy E75.29
Myelolipoma — *see* Lipoma
Myeloma (multiple) C90.0- ☑
monostotic C90.3 ☑
plasma cell C90.0- ☑
plasma cell C90.0- ☑
solitary (*see also* Plasmacytoma, solitary) C90.3- ☑
Myelomalacia G95.89
Myelomatosis C90.0- ☑
Myelomeningitis — *see* Meningoencephalitis
Myelomeningocele (spinal cord) — *see* Spina bifida
Myelo-osteo-musculodysplasia hereditaria Q79.8
Myelopathic
anemia D64.89
muscle atrophy — *see* Atrophy, muscle, spinal
pain syndrome G89.0
Myelopathy (spinal cord) G95.9
drug-induced G95.89
in (due to)
degeneration or displacement, intervertebral disc NEC — *see* Disorder, disc, with, myelopathy
infection — *see* Encephalitis
intervertebral disc disorder (*see also* Disorder, disc, with, myelopathy)
mercury — *see* subcategory T56.1 ☑
neoplastic disease (*see also* Neoplasm) D49.9 [G99.2]
pernicious anemia D51.0 [G99.2]
spondylosis — *see* Spondylosis, with myelopathy NEC
necrotic (subacute) (vascular) G95.19
radiation-induced G95.89
spondylogenic NEC — *see* Spondylosis, with myelopathy NEC
toxic G95.89
transverse, acute G37.3
vascular G95.19
vitamin B12 E53.8 [G32.0]
Myelophthisis D61.82
Myeloradiculitis G04.91
Myeloradiculodysplasia (spinal) Q06.1
Myelosarcoma C92.3- ☑
Myelosclerosis D75.89
with myeloid metaplasia D47.4
disseminated, of nervous system G35
megakaryocytic D47.4

☑ **Additional Character Required — Refer to the Tabular List for Character Selection**   ⬇ **Subterms under main terms may continue to next column or page**

Myelosclerosis — *continued*
  megakaryocytic — *continued*
    with myeloid metaplasia D47.4
Myelosis
  acute C92.0- ☑
  aleukemic C92.9- ☑
  chronic D47.1
  erythremic (acute) C94.0- ☑
  megakaryocytic C94.2- ☑
  nonleukemic D72.828
  subacute C92.9- ☑
Myiasis (cavernous) B87.9
  aural B87.4
  creeping B87.0
  cutaneous B87.0
  dermal B87.0
  ear (external) (middle) B87.4
  eye B87.2
  genitourinary B87.81
  intestinal B87.82
  laryngeal B87.3
  nasopharyngeal B87.3
  ocular B87.2
  orbit B87.2
  skin B87.0
  specified site NEC B87.89
  traumatic B87.1
  wound B87.1
Myoadenoma, prostate — *see* Hyperplasia, prostate
Myoblastoma
  granular cell (*see also* Neoplasm, connective tissue, benign)
    malignant — *see* Neoplasm, connective tissue, malignant
  tongue D10.1
Myocardial — *see* condition
Myocardiopathy (congestive) (constrictive) (familial) (hypertrophic nonobstructive) (idiopathic) (infiltrative) (obstructive) (primary) (restrictive) (sporadic) (*see also* Cardiomyopathy) I42.9
  alcoholic I42.6
  cobalt-beer I42.6
  glycogen storage E74.02 [I43]
  hypertrophic obstructive I42.1
  in (due to)
    beriberi E51.12
    cardiac glycogenosis E74.02 [I43]
    Friedreich's ataxia G11.1 [I43]
    myotonia atrophica G71.11 [I43]
    progressive muscular dystrophy G71.0 [I43]
  obscure (African) I42.8
  secondary I42.9
  thyrotoxic E05.90 [I43]
    with storm E05.91 [I43]
  toxic NEC I42.7
Myocarditis (with arteriosclerosis)(chronic)(fibroid) (interstitial) (old) (progressive) (senile) I51.4
  with
    rheumatic fever (conditions in I00) I09.0
      active — *see* Myocarditis, acute, rheumatic
      inactive or quiescent (with chorea) I09.0
  active I40.9
    rheumatic I01.2
      with chorea (acute) (rheumatic) (Sydenham's) I02.0
  acute or subacute (interstitial) I40.9
    due to
      streptococcus (beta-hemolytic) I01.2
    idiopathic I40.1
    rheumatic I01.2
      with chorea (acute) (rheumatic) (Sydenham's) I02.0
    specified NEC I40.8
  aseptic of newborn B33.22
  bacterial (acute) I40.0
  Coxsackie (virus) B33.22
  diphtheritic A36.81
  eosinophilic I40.1
  epidemic of newborn (Coxsackie) B33.22
  Fiedler's (acute) (isolated) I40.1
  giant cell (acute) (subacute) I40.1
  gonococcal A54.83
  granulomatous (idiopathic) (isolated) (nonspecific) I40.1
  hypertensive — *see* Hypertension, heart
  idiopathic (granulomatous) I40.1
  in (due to)
    diphtheria A36.81

Myocarditis — *continued*
  in — *continued*
    epidemic louse-borne typhus A75.0 [I41]
    Lyme disease A69.29
    sarcoidosis D86.85
    scarlet fever A38.1
    toxoplasmosis (acquired) B58.81
    typhoid A01.02
    typhus NEC A75.9 [I41]
  infective I40.0
  influenzal — *see* Influenza, with, myocarditis
  isolated (acute) I40.1
  meningococcal A39.52
  mumps B26.82
  nonrheumatic, active I40.9
  parenchymatous I40.9
  pneumococcal I40.0
  rheumatic (chronic) (inactive) (with chorea) I09.0
    active or acute I01.2
      with chorea (acute) (rheumatic) (Sydenham's) I02.0
  rheumatoid — *see* Rheumatoid, carditis
  septic I40.0
  staphylococcal I40.0
  suppurative I40.0
  syphilitic (chronic) A52.06
  toxic I40.8
    rheumatic — *see* Myocarditis, acute, rheumatic
  tuberculous A18.84
  typhoid A01.02
  valvular — *see* Endocarditis
  virus, viral I40.0
    of newborn (Coxsackie) B33.22
Myocardium, myocardial — *see* condition
Myocardosis — *see* Cardiomyopathy
Myoclonus, myoclonic, myoclonia (familial) (essential) (multifocal) (simplex) G25.3
  drug-induced G25.3
  epilepsy (*see also* Epilepsy, generalized, specified NEC) G40.4- ☑
    familial (progressive) G25.3
  epileptica G40.409
    with status epilepticus G40.401
  facial G51.3
  familial progressive G25.3
  Friedreich's G25.3
  jerks G25.3
  massive G25.3
  palatal G25.3
  pharyngeal G25.3
Myocytolysis I51.5
Myodiastasis — *see* Diastasis, muscle
Myoendocarditis — *see* Endocarditis
Myoepithelioma — *see* Neoplasm, benign, by site
Myofasciitis (acute) — *see* Myositis
Myofibroma (*see also* Neoplasm, connective tissue, benign)
  uterus (cervix) (corpus) — *see* Leiomyoma
Myofibromatosis D48.1
  infantile Q89.8
Myofibrosis M62.89
  heart — *see* Myocarditis
  scapulohumeral — *see* Lesion, shoulder, specified NEC
Myofibrositis M79.7
  scapulohumeral — *see* Lesion, shoulder, specified NEC
Myoglobulinuria, myoglobinuria (primary) R82.1
Myokymia, facial G51.4
Myolipoma — *see* Lipoma
Myoma (*see also* Neoplasm, connective tissue, benign)
  malignant — *see* Neoplasm, connective tissue, malignant
  prostate D29.1
  uterus (cervix) (corpus) — *see* Leiomyoma
Myomalacia M62.89
Myometritis — *see* Endometritis
Myometrium — *see* condition
Myonecrosis, clostridial A48.0
Myopathy G72.9
  acute
    necrotizing G72.81
    quadriplegic G72.81
  alcoholic G72.1
  benign congenital G71.2
  central core G71.2
  centronuclear G71.2
  congenital (benign) G71.2
  critical illness G72.81
  distal G71.0

Myopathy — *continued*
  drug-induced G72.0
  endocrine NEC E34.9 [G73.7]
  extraocular muscles H05.82- ☑
  facioscapulohumeral G71.0
  hereditary G71.9
    specified NEC G71.8
  immune NEC G72.49
  in (due to)
    Addison's disease E27.1 [G73.7]
    alcohol G72.1
    amyloidosis E85.0 [G73.7]
    cretinism E00.9 [G73.7]
    Cushing's syndrome E24.9 [G73.7]
    drugs G72.0
    endocrine disease NEC E34.9 [G73.7]
    giant cell arteritis M31.6 [G73.7]
    glycogen storage disease E74.00 [G73.7]
    hyperadrenocorticism E24.9 [G73.7]
    hyperparathyroidism NEC E21.3 [G73.7]
    hypoparathyroidism E20.9 [G73.7]
    hypopituitarism E23.0 [G73.7]
    hypothyroidism E03.9 [G73.7]
    infectious disease NEC B99 ☑ [G73.7]
    lipid storage disease E75.6 [G73.7]
    metabolic disease NEC E88.9 [G73.7]
    myxedema E03.9 [G73.7]
    parasitic disease NEC B89 [G73.7]
    polyarteritis nodosa M30.0 [G73.7]
    rheumatoid arthritis — *see* Rheumatoid, myopathy
    sarcoidosis D86.87
    scleroderma M34.82
    sicca syndrome M35.03
    Sjögren's syndrome M35.03
    systemic lupus erythematosus M32.19
    thyrotoxicosis (hyperthyroidism) E05.90 [G73.7]
      with thyroid storm E05.91 [G73.7]
    toxic agent NEC G72.2
  inflammatory NEC G72.49
  intensive care (ICU) G72.81
  limb-girdle G71.0
  mitochondrial NEC G71.3
  myotubular G71.2
  mytonic, proximal (PROMM) G71.11
  nemaline G71.2
  ocular G71.0
  oculopharyngeal G71.0
  of critical illness G72.81
  primary G71.9
    specified NEC G71.8
  progressive NEC G72.89
  proximal myotonic (PROMM) G71.11
  rod G71.2
  scapulohumeral G71.0
  specified NEC G72.89
  toxic G72.2
Myopericarditis (*see also* Pericarditis)
  chronic rheumatic I09.2
Myopia (axial) (congenital) H52.1- ☑
  degenerative (malignant) H44.20
    with
      choroidal neovascularization H44.2A- ☑
      foveoschisis H44.2D- ☑
      macular hole H44.2B- ☑
      retinal detachment H44.2C- ☑
      specified maculopathy NEC H44.2E- ☑
    bilateral H44.23
    left eye H44.22
    right eye H44.21
  malignant (*see also* Myopia, degenerative) H44.2- ☑
  pernicious (*see also* Myopia, degenerative) H44.2- ☑
  progressive high (degenerative) (*see also* Myopia, degenerative) H44.2- ☑
Myosarcoma — *see* Neoplasm, connective tissue, malignant
Myosis (pupil) H57.03
  stromal (endolymphatic) D39.0
Myositis M60.9
  clostridial A48.0
  due to posture — *see* Myositis, specified type NEC
  epidemic B33.0
  fibrosa or fibrous (chronic), Volkmann's T79.6 ☑
  foreign body granuloma — *see* Granuloma, foreign body
  in (due to)
    bilharziasis B65.9 [M63.8-] ☑
    cysticercosis B69.81
    leprosy A30.9 [M63.8-] ☑

Myositis — *continued*
in — *continued*
mycosis B49 [M63.8-] ☑
sarcoidosis D86.87
schistosomiasis B65.9 [M63.8-] ☑
syphilis
late A52.78
secondary A51.49
toxoplasmosis (acquired) B58.82
trichinellosis B75 [M63.8-] ☑
tuberculosis A18.09
inclusion body [IBM] G72.41
infective M60.009
arm M60.002
left M60.001
right M60.000
leg M60.005
left M60.004
right M60.003
lower limb M60.005
ankle M60.07- ☑
foot M60.07- ☑
lower leg M60.06- ☑
thigh M60.05- ☑
toe M60.07- ☑
multiple sites M60.09
specified site NEC M60.08
upper limb M60.002
finger M60.04- ☑
forearm M60.03- ☑
hand M60.04- ☑
shoulder region M60.01- ☑
upper arm M60.02- ☑
interstitial M60.10
ankle M60.17- ☑
foot M60.17- ☑
forearm M60.13- ☑
hand M60.14- ☑
lower leg M60.16- ☑
multiple sites M60.19
shoulder region M60.11- ☑
specified site NEC M60.18
thigh M60.15- ☑
upper arm M60.12- ☑
mycotic B49 [M63.8-] ☑
orbital, chronic H05.12- ☑
ossificans or ossifying (circumscripta) (*see also* Ossification, muscle, specified NEC)
in (due to)
burns M61.30
ankle M61.37- ☑
foot M61.37- ☑
forearm M61.33- ☑
hand M61.34- ☑
lower leg M61.36- ☑
multiple sites M61.39
pelvic region M61.35- ☑

Myositis — *continued*
ossificans or ossifying (*see also* Ossification, muscle, specified) — *continued*
in — *continued*
burns — *continued*
shoulder region M61.31- ☑
specified site NEC M61.38
thigh M61.35- ☑
upper arm M61.32- ☑
quadriplegia or paraplegia M61.20
ankle M61.27- ☑
foot M61.27- ☑
forearm M61.23- ☑
hand M61.24- ☑
lower leg M61.26- ☑
multiple sites M61.29
pelvic region M61.25- ☑
shoulder region M61.21- ☑
specified site NEC M61.28
thigh M61.25- ☑
upper arm M61.22- ☑
progressiva M61.10
ankle M61.17- ☑
finger M61.14- ☑
foot M61.17- ☑
forearm M61.13- ☑
hand M61.14- ☑
lower leg M61.16- ☑
multiple sites M61.19
pelvic region M61.15- ☑
shoulder region M61.11- ☑
specified site NEC M61.18
thigh M61.15- ☑
toe M61.17- ☑
upper arm M61.12- ☑
traumatica M61.00
ankle M61.07- ☑
foot M61.07- ☑
forearm M61.03- ☑
hand M61.04- ☑
lower leg M61.06- ☑
multiple sites M61.09
pelvic region M61.05- ☑
shoulder region M61.01- ☑
specified site NEC M61.08
thigh M61.05- ☑
upper arm M61.02- ☑
purulent — *see* Myositis, infective
specified type NEC M60.80
ankle M60.87- ☑
foot M60.87- ☑
forearm M60.83- ☑
hand M60.84- ☑
lower leg M60.86- ☑
multiple sites M60.89
pelvic region M60.85- ☑
shoulder region M60.81- ☑

Myositis — *continued*
specified type — *continued*
specified site NEC M60.88
thigh M60.85- ☑
upper arm M60.82- ☑
suppurative — *see* Myositis, infective
traumatic (old) — *see* Myositis, specified type NEC
Myospasia impulsiva F95.2
Myotonia (acquisita) (intermittens) M62.89
atrophica G71.11
chondrodystrophic G71.13
congenita (acetazolamide responsive) (dominant) (recessive) G71.12
drug-induced G71.14
dystrophica G71.11
fluctuans G71.19
levior G71.12
permanens G71.19
symptomatic G71.19
Myotonic pupil — *see* Anomaly, pupil, function, tonic pupil
Myriapodiasis B88.2
Myringitis H73.2- ☑
with otitis media — *see* Otitis, media
acute H73.00- ☑
bullous H73.01- ☑
specified NEC H73.09- ☑
bullous — *see* Myringitis, acute, bullous
chronic H73.1- ☑
Mysophobia F40.228
Mytilotoxism — *see* Poisoning, fish
Myxadenitis labialis K13.0
Myxedema (adult) (idiocy) (infantile) (juvenile) (*see also* Hypothyroidism) E03.9
circumscribed E05.90
with storm E05.91
coma E03.5
congenital E00.1
cutis L98.5
localized (pretibial) E05.90
with storm E05.91
papular L98.5
Myxochondrosarcoma — *see* Neoplasm, cartilage, malignant
Myxofibroma — *see* Neoplasm, connective tissue, benign
odontogenic — *see* Cyst, calcifying odontogenic
Myxofibrosarcoma — *see* Neoplasm, connective tissue, malignant
Myxolipoma D17.9
Myxoliposarcoma — *see* Neoplasm, connective tissue, malignant
Myxoma (*see also* Neoplasm, connective tissue, benign)
nerve sheath — *see* Neoplasm, nerve, benign
odontogenic — *see* Cyst, calcifying odontogenic
Myxosarcoma — *see* Neoplasm, connective tissue, malignant

N

Naegeli's
  disease Q82.8
  leukemia, monocytic C93.1- ☑
Naegleriasis (with meningoencephalitis) B60.2
Naffziger's syndrome G54.0
Naga sore — *see* Ulcer, skin
Nägele's pelvis M95.5
  with disproportion (fetopelvic) O33.0
    causing obstructed labor O65.0
Nail (*see also* condition)
  biting F98.8
  patella syndrome Q87.2
Nanism, nanosomia — *see* Dwarfism
Nanophyetiasis B66.8
Nanukayami A27.89
Napkin rash L22
Narcolepsy G47.419
  with cataplexy G47.411
  in conditions classified elsewhere G47.429
    with cataplexy G47.421
Narcosis R06.89
Narcotism — *see* Dependence
NARP (Neuropathy, Ataxia and Retinitis pigmentosa) syndrome E88.49
Narrow
  anterior chamber angle H40.03- ☑
  gingival width (of periodontal soft tissue) K05.5
  pelvis — *see* Contraction, pelvis
Narrowing (*see also* Stenosis)
  artery I77.1
    auditory, internal I65.8
    basilar — *see* Occlusion, artery, basilar
    carotid — *see* Occlusion, artery, carotid
    cerebellar — *see* Occlusion, artery, cerebellar
    cerebral — *see* Occlusion artery, cerebral
    choroidal — *see* Occlusion, artery, cerebral, specified NEC
    communicating posterior — *see* Occlusion, artery, cerebral, specified NEC
    coronary (*see also* Disease, heart, ischemic, atherosclerotic)
      congenital Q24.5
      syphilitic A50.54 [I52]
      due to syphilis NEC A52.06
    hypophyseal — *see* Occlusion, artery, cerebral, specified NEC
    pontine — *see* Occlusion, artery, cerebral, specified NEC
    precerebral — *see* Occlusion, artery, precerebral
    vertebral — *see* Occlusion, artery, vertebral
  auditory canal (external) — *see* Stenosis, external ear canal
  eustachian tube — *see* Obstruction, eustachian tube
  eyelid — *see* Disorder, eyelid function
  larynx J38.6
  mesenteric artery (*see also* Ischemia, intestine, acute) K55.059
  palate M26.89
  palpebral fissure — *see* Disorder, eyelid function
  ureter N13.5
    with infection N13.6
  urethra — *see* Stricture, urethra
Narrowness, abnormal, eyelid Q10.3
Nasal — *see* condition
Nasolachrymal, nasolacrimal — *see* condition
Nasopharyngeal (*see also* condition)
  pituitary gland Q89.2
  torticollis M43.6
Nasopharyngitis (acute) (infective) (streptococcal) (subacute) J00
  chronic (suppurative) (ulcerative) J31.1
Nasopharynx, nasopharyngeal — *see* condition
Natal tooth, teeth K00.6
Nausea (without vomiting) R11.0
  with vomiting R11.2
  gravidarum — *see* Hyperemesis, gravidarum
  marina T75.3 ☑
  navalis T75.3 ☑
Navel — *see* condition
Neapolitan fever — *see* Brucellosis
Near drowning T75.1 ☑
Nearsightedness — *see* Myopia
Near-syncope R55
Nebula, cornea — *see* Opacity, cornea

Necator americanus infestation B76.1
Necatoriasis B76.1
Neck — *see* condition
Necrobiosis R68.89
  lipoidica NEC L92.1
    with diabetes — *see* E08-E13 with .620
Necrolysis, toxic epidermal L51.2
  due to drug
    correct substance properly administered — *see* Table of Drugs and Chemicals, by drug, adverse effect
    overdose or wrong substance given or taken — *see* Table of Drugs and Chemicals, by drug, poisoning
Necrophilia F65.89
Necrosis, necrotic (ischemic) (*see also* Gangrene)
  adrenal (capsule) (gland) E27.49
  amputation stump (surgical) (late) T87.50
    arm T87.5- ☑
    leg T87.5- ☑
  antrum J32.0
  aorta (hyaline) (*see also* Aneurysm, aorta)
    cystic medial — *see* Dissection, aorta
  artery I77.5
  bladder (aseptic) (sphincter) N32.89
  bone (*see also* Osteonecrosis) M87.9
    aseptic or avascular — *see* Osteonecrosis
      idiopathic M87.00
    ethmoid J32.2
    jaw M27.2
    tuberculous — *see* Tuberculosis, bone
  brain I67.89
  breast (aseptic) (fat) (segmental) N64.1
  bronchus J98.09
  central nervous system NEC I67.89
  cerebellar I67.89
  cerebral I67.89
  colon (*see also* Infarct, intestine) K55.049
  cornea H18.89- ☑
  cortical (acute) (renal) N17.1
  cystic medial (aorta) — *see* Dissection, aorta
  dental pulp K04.1
  esophagus K22.8
  ethmoid (bone) J32.2
  eyelid — *see* Disorder, eyelid, degenerative
  fat, fatty (generalized) (*see also* Disorder, soft tissue, specified type NEC)
    abdominal wall K65.4
    breast (aseptic) (segmental) N64.1
    localized — *see* Degeneration, by site, fatty
    mesentery K65.4
    omentum K65.4
    pancreas K86.89
    peritoneum K65.4
    skin (subcutaneous), newborn P83.0
    subcutaneous, due to birth injury P15.6
  gallbladder — *see* Cholecystitis, acute
  heart — *see* Infarct, myocardium
  hip, aseptic or avascular — *see* Osteonecrosis, by type, femur
  intestine (acute) (hemorrhagic) (massive) (*see also* Infarct, intestine) K55.069
  jaw M27.2
  kidney (bilateral) N28.0
    acute N17.9
    cortical (acute) (bilateral) N17.1
      with ectopic or molar pregnancy O08.4
    medullary (bilateral) (in acute renal failure) (papillary) N17.2
    papillary (bilateral) (in acute renal failure) N17.2
    tubular N17.0
      with ectopic or molar pregnancy O08.4
      complicating
        abortion — *see* Abortion, by type, complicated by, tubular necrosis
        ectopic or molar pregnancy O08.4
        pregnancy — *see* Pregnancy, complicated by, diseases of, specified type or system NEC
      following ectopic or molar pregnancy O08.4
      traumatic T79.5 ☑
  larynx J38.7
  liver (with hepatic failure) (cell) — *see* Failure, hepatic
    hemorrhagic, central K76.2
  lung J85.0
  lymphatic gland — *see* Lymphadenitis, acute
  mammary gland (fat) (segmental) N64.1
  mastoid (chronic) — *see* Mastoiditis, chronic

Necrosis, necrotic — *continued*
  medullary (acute) (renal) N17.2
  mesentery (*see also* Infarct, intestine) K55.069
    fat K65.4
  mitral valve — *see* Insufficiency, mitral
  myocardium, myocardial — *see* Infarct, myocardium
  nose J34.0
  omentum (with mesenteric infarction) (*see also* Infarct, intestine) K55.069
    fat K65.4
  orbit, orbital — *see* Osteomyelitis, orbit
  ossicles, ear — *see* Abnormal, ear ossicles
  ovary N70.92
  pancreas (aseptic) (duct) (fat) K86.89
    acute (infective) — *see* Pancreatitis, acute
    infective — *see* Pancreatitis, acute
  papillary (acute) (renal) N17.2
  perineum N90.89
  peritoneum (with mesenteric infarction) (*see also* Infarct, intestine) K55.069
    fat K65.4
  pharynx J02.9
    in granulocytopenia — *see* Neutropenia
    Vincent's A69.1
  phosphorus — *see* subcategory T54.2 ☑
  pituitary (gland) E23.0
    postpartum O99.285
    Sheehan O99.285
  pressure — *see* Ulcer, pressure, by site
  pulmonary J85.0
  pulp (dental) K04.1
  radiation — *see* Necrosis, by site
  radium — *see* Necrosis, by site
  renal — *see* Necrosis, kidney
  sclera H15.89
  scrotum N50.89
  skin or subcutaneous tissue NEC I96
  spine, spinal (column) (*see also* Osteonecrosis, by type, vertebra)
    cord G95.19
  spleen D73.5
  stomach K31.89
  stomatitis (ulcerative) A69.0
  subcutaneous fat, newborn P83.88
  subendocardial (acute) I21.4
    chronic I25.89
  suprarenal (capsule) (gland) E27.49
  testis N50.89
  thymus (gland) E32.8
  tonsil J35.8
  trachea J39.8
  tuberculous NEC — *see* Tuberculosis
  tubular (acute) (anoxic) (renal) (toxic) N17.0
    postprocedural N99.0
  vagina N89.8
  vertebra (*see also* Osteonecrosis, by type, vertebra)
    tuberculous A18.01
  vulva N90.89
  X-ray — *see* Necrosis, by site
Necrospermia — *see* Infertility, male
Need (for)
  care provider because (of)
    assistance with personal care Z74.1
    continuous supervision required Z74.3
    impaired mobility Z74.09
    no other household member able to render care Z74.2
    specified reason NEC Z74.8
  immunization — *see* Vaccination
  vaccination — *see* Vaccination
Neglect
  adult
    confirmed T74.01 ☑
    history of Z91.412
    suspected T76.01 ☑
  child (childhood)
    confirmed T74.02 ☑
    history of Z62.812
    suspected T76.02 ☑
  emotional, in childhood Z62.898
  hemispatial R41.4
  left-sided R41.4
  sensory R41.4
  visuospatial R41.4
Neisserian infection NEC — *see* Gonococcus
Nelaton's syndrome G60.8
Nelson's syndrome E24.1
Nematodiasis (intestinal) B82.0

▽ Subterms under main terms may continue to next column or page   ☑ Additional Character Required — Refer to the Tabular List for Character Selection   229

Naegeli's — Nematodiasis

Nematodiasis — *continued*
  Ancylostoma B76.0
Neonatal (*see also* Newborn)
  acne L70.4
  bradycardia P29.12
  screening, abnormal findings on P09
  tachycardia P29.11
  tooth, teeth K00.6
Neonatorum — *see* condition
Neoplasia
  endocrine, multiple (MEN) E31.20
    type I E31.21
    type IIA E31.22
    type IIB E31.23
  intraepithelial (histologically confirmed)
    anal (AIN) (histologically confirmed) K62.82
      grade I K62.82
      grade II K62.82
      severe D01.3
    cervical glandular (histologically confirmed) D06.9
    cervix (uteri) (CIN) (histologically confirmed) N87.9
      glandular D06.9
      grade I N87.0
      grade II N87.1
      grade III (severe dysplasia) (*see also* Carcinoma,
        cervix uteri, in situ) D06.9
    prostate (histologically confirmed) (PIN) N42.31
      grade I N42.31
      grade II N42.31
      grade III (severe dysplasia) D07.5
    vagina (histologically confirmed) (VAIN) N89.3
      grade I N89.0
      grade II N89.1
      grade III (severe dysplasia) D07.2
    vulva (histologically confirmed) (VIN) N90.3
      grade I N90.0
      grade II N90.1
      grade III (severe dysplasia) D07.1
Neoplasm, neoplastic (*see also* Table of Neoplasms)
  lipomatous, benign — *see* Lipoma
  malignant mast cell C96.20
    specified type NEC C96.29
  mast cell, of uncertain behavior NEC D47.09
Neovascularization
  ciliary body — *see* Disorder, iris, vascular
  cornea H16.40- ☑
    deep H16.44- ☑
    ghost vessels — *see* Ghost, vessels
    localized H16.43- ☑
    pannus — *see* Pannus
  iris — *see* Disorder, iris, vascular
  retina H35.05- ☑
Nephralgia N23
Nephritis, nephritic (albuminuric) (azotemic) (congenital) (disseminated) (epithelial) (familial) (focal) (granulomatous) (hemorrhagic) (infantile) (nonsuppurative, excretory) (uremic) N05.9
  with
    dense deposit disease N05.6
    diffuse
      crescentic glomerulonephritis N05.7
      endocapillary proliferative glomerulonephritis N05.4
      membranous glomerulonephritis N05.2
      mesangial proliferative glomerulonephritis N05.3
      mesangiocapillary glomerulonephritis N05.5
    edema — *see* Nephrosis
    focal and segmental glomerular lesions N05.1
    foot process disease N04.9
    glomerular lesion
      diffuse sclerosing N05.8
      hypocomplementemic — *see* Nephritis, membranoproliferative
      IgA — *see* Nephropathy, IgA
      lobular, lobulonodular — *see* Nephritis, membranoproliferative
      nodular — *see* Nephritis, membranoproliferative
    lesion of
      glomerulonephritis, proliferative N05.8
      renal necrosis N05.9
    minor glomerular abnormality N05.0
    specified morphological changes NEC N05.8
  acute N00.9
    with
      dense deposit disease N00.6

Nephritis, nephritic — *continued*
  acute — *continued*
    with — *continued*
      diffuse
        crescentic glomerulonephritis N00.7
        endocapillary proliferative glomerulonephritis N00.4
        membranous glomerulonephritis N00.2
        mesangial proliferative glomerulonephritis N00.3
        mesangiocapillary glomerulonephritis N00.5
      focal and segmental glomerular lesions N00.1
      minor glomerular abnormality N00.0
      specified morphological changes NEC N00.8
  amyloid E85.4 [N08]
  antiglomerular basement membrane (anti-GBM) antibody NEC
    in Goodpasture's syndrome M31.0
  antitubular basement membrane (tubulo-interstitial) NEC N12
    toxic — *see* Nephropathy, toxic
  arteriolar — *see* Hypertension, kidney
  arteriosclerotic — *see* Hypertension, kidney
  ascending — *see* Nephritis, tubulo-interstitial
  atrophic N03.9
  Balkan (endemic) N15.0
  calculous, calculus — *see* Calculus, kidney
  cardiac — *see* Hypertension, kidney
  cardiovascular — *see* Hypertension, kidney
  chronic N03.9
    with
      dense deposit disease N03.6
      diffuse
        crescentic glomerulonephritis N03.7
        endocapillary proliferative glomerulonephritis N03.4
        membranous glomerulonephritis N03.2
        mesangial proliferative glomerulonephritis N03.3
        mesangiocapillary glomerulonephritis N03.5
      focal and segmental glomerular lesions N03.1
      minor glomerular abnormality N03.0
      specified morphological changes NEC N03.8
    arteriosclerotic — *see* Hypertension, kidney
  cirrhotic N26.9
  complicating pregnancy O26.83- ☑
  croupous N00.9
  degenerative — *see* Nephrosis
  diffuse sclerosing N05.8
  due to
    diabetes mellitus — *see* E08-E13 with .21
    subacute bacterial endocarditis I33.0
    systemic lupus erythematosus (chronic) M32.14
    typhoid fever A01.09
  gonococcal (acute) (chronic) A54.21
  hypocomplementemic — *see* Nephritis, membranoproliferative
  IgA — *see* Nephropathy, IgA
  immune complex (circulating) NEC N05.8
  infective — *see* Nephritis, tubulo-interstitial
  interstitial — *see* Nephritis, tubulo-interstitial
  lead N14.3
  membranoproliferative (diffuse) (type 1 or 3) (*see also* N00-N07 with fourth character .5) N05.5
    type 2 (*see also* N00-N07 with fourth character .6) N05.6
  minimal change N05.0
  necrotic, necrotizing NEC (*see also* N00-N07 with fourth character .8) N05.8
  nephrotic — *see* Nephrosis
  nodular — *see* Nephritis, membranoproliferative
  polycystic Q61.3
    adult type Q61.2
    autosomal
      dominant Q61.2
      recessive NEC Q61.19
    childhood type NEC Q61.19
    infantile type NEC Q61.19
  poststreptococcal N05.9
    acute N00.9
    chronic N03.9
    rapidly progressive N01.9
  proliferative NEC (*see also* N00-N07 with fourth character .8) N05.8
  purulent — *see* Nephritis, tubulo-interstitial
  rapidly progressive N01.9
    with
      dense deposit disease N01.6

Nephritis, nephritic — *continued*
  rapidly progressive — *continued*
    with — *continued*
      diffuse
        crescentic glomerulonephritis N01.7
        endocapillary proliferative glomerulonephritis N01.4
        membranous glomerulonephritis N01.2
        mesangial proliferative glomerulonephritis N01.3
        mesangiocapillary glomerulonephritis N01.5
      focal and segmental glomerular lesions N01.1
      minor glomerular abnormality N01.0
      specified morphological changes NEC N01.8
  salt losing or wasting NEC N28.89
  saturnine N14.3
  sclerosing, diffuse N05.8
  septic — *see* Nephritis, tubulo-interstitial
  specified pathology NEC (*see also* N00-N07 with fourth character .8) N05.8
  subacute N01.9
  suppurative — *see* Nephritis, tubulo-interstitial
  syphilitic (late) A52.75
    congenital A50.59 [N08]
    early (secondary) A51.44
  toxic — *see* Nephropathy, toxic
  tubal, tubular — *see* Nephritis, tubulo-interstitial
  tuberculous A18.11
  tubulo-interstitial (in) N12
    acute (infectious) N10
    chronic (infectious) N11.9
      nonobstructive N11.8
        reflux-associated N11.0
      obstructive N11.1
      specified NEC N11.8
    due to
      brucellosis A23.9 [N16]
      cryoglobulinemia D89.1 [N16]
      glycogen storage disease E74.00 [N16]
    Sjögren's syndrome M35.04
  vascular — *see* Hypertension, kidney
  war N00.9
Nephroblastoma (epithelial) (mesenchymal) C64- ☑
Nephrocalcinosis E83.59 [N29]
Nephrocystitis, pustular — *see* Nephritis, tubulo-interstitial
Nephrolithiasis (congenital) (pelvis) (recurrent) (*see also* Calculus, kidney)
Nephroma C64- ☑
  mesoblastic D41.0- ☑
Nephronephritis — *see* Nephrosis
Nephronophthisis Q61.5
Nephropathia epidemica A98.5
Nephropathy (*see also* Nephritis) N28.9
  with
    edema — *see* Nephrosis
    glomerular lesion — *see* Glomerulonephritis
  amyloid, hereditary E85.0
  analgesic N14.0
    with medullary necrosis, acute N17.2
  Balkan (endemic) N15.0
  chemical — *see* Nephropathy, toxic
  diabetic — *see* E08-E13 with .21
  drug-induced N14.2
    specified NEC N14.1
  focal and segmental hyalinosis or sclerosis N02.1
  heavy metal-induced N14.3
  hereditary NEC N07.9
    with
      dense deposit disease N07.6
      diffuse
        crescentic glomerulonephritis N07.7
        endocapillary proliferative glomerulonephritis N07.4
        membranous glomerulonephritis N07.2
        mesangial proliferative glomerulonephritis N07.3
        mesangiocapillary glomerulonephritis N07.5
      focal and segmental glomerular lesions N07.1
      minor glomerular abnormality N07.0
      specified morphological changes NEC N07.8
  hypercalcemic N25.89
  hypertensive — *see* Hypertension, kidney
  hypokalemic (vacuolar) N25.89
  IgA N02.8
    with glomerular lesion N02.9
      focal and segmental hyalinosis or sclerosis N02.1

Nephropathy — *continued*
  IgA — *continued*
    with glomerular lesion — *continued*
      membranoproliferative (diffuse) N02.5
      membranous (diffuse) N02.2
      mesangial proliferative (diffuse) N02.3
      mesangiocapillary (diffuse) N02.5
      proliferative NEC N02.8
      specified pathology NEC N02.8
  lead N14.3
  membranoproliferative (diffuse) N02.5
  membranous (diffuse) N02.2
  mesangial (IgA/IgG) — *see* Nephropathy, IgA
    proliferative (diffuse) N02.3
  mesangiocapillary (diffuse) N02.5
  obstructive N13.8
  phenacetin N17.2
  phosphate-losing N25.0
  potassium depletion N25.89
  pregnancy-related O26.83- ☑
  proliferative NEC (*see also* N00-N07 with fourth character .8) N05.8
  protein-losing N25.89
  saturnine N14.3
  sickle-cell D57.- ☑ [N08]
  toxic NEC N14.4
    due to
      drugs N14.2
        analgesic N14.0
        specified NEC N14.1
      heavy metals N14.3
  vasomotor N17.0
  water-losing N25.89
Nephroptosis N28.83
Nephropyosis — *see* Abscess, kidney
Nephrorrhagia N28.89
Nephrosclerosis (arteriolar)(arteriosclerotic) (chronic) (hyaline) (*see also* Hypertension, kidney)
  hyperplastic — *see* Hypertension, kidney
  senile N26.9
Nephrosis, nephrotic (Epstein's) (syndrome) (congenital) N04.9
  with
    foot process disease N04.9
    glomerular lesion N04.1
    hypocomplementemic N04.5
  acute N04.9
  anoxic — *see* Nephrosis, tubular
  chemical — *see* Nephrosis, tubular
  cholemic K76.7
  diabetic — *see* E08-E13 with .21
  Finnish type (congenital) Q89.8
  hemoglobin N10
  hemoglobinuric — *see* Nephrosis, tubular
  in
    amyloidosis E85.4 [N08]
    diabetes mellitus — *see* E08-E13 with .21
    epidemic hemorrhagic fever A98.5
    malaria (malariae) B52.0
  ischemic — *see* Nephrosis, tubular
  lipoid N04.9
  lower nephron — *see* Nephrosis, tubular
  malarial (malariae) B52.0
  minimal change N04.0
  myoglobin N10
  necrotizing — *see* Nephrosis, tubular
  osmotic (sucrose) N25.89
  radiation N04.9
  syphilitic (late) A52.75
  toxic — *see* Nephrosis, tubular
  tubular (acute) N17.0
    postprocedural N99.0
    radiation N04.9
Nephrosonephritis, hemorrhagic (endemic) A98.5
Nephrostomy
  attention to Z43.6
  status Z93.6
Nerve (*see also* condition)
  injury — *see* Injury, nerve, by body site
Nerves R45.0
Nervous (*see also* condition) R45.0
  heart F45.8
  stomach F45.8
  tension R45.0
Nervousness R45.0
Nesidioblastoma
  pancreas D13.7
  specified site NEC — *see* Neoplasm, benign, by site

Nesidioblastoma — *continued*
  unspecified site D13.7
Nettleship's syndrome — *see* Urticaria pigmentosa
Neumann's disease or syndrome L10.1
Neuralgia, neuralgic (acute) M79.2
  accessory (nerve) G52.8
  acoustic (nerve) — *see* subcategory H93.3 ☑
  auditory (nerve) — *see* subcategory H93.3 ☑
  ciliary G44.009
    intractable G44.001
    not intractable G44.009
  cranial
    nerve (*see also* Disorder, nerve, cranial)
      fifth or trigeminal — *see* Neuralgia, trigeminal
      postherpetic, postzoster B02.29
  ear — *see* subcategory H92.0 ☑
  facialis vera G51.1
  Fothergill's — *see* Neuralgia, trigeminal
  glossopharyngeal (nerve) G52.1
  Horton's G44.009
    intractable G44.091
    not intractable G44.099
  Hunt's B02.21
  hypoglossal (nerve) G52.3
  infraorbital — *see* Neuralgia, trigeminal
  malarial — *see* Malaria
  migrainous G44.009
    intractable G44.001
    not intractable G44.009
  Morton's G57.6- ☑
  nerve, cranial — *see* Disorder, nerve, cranial
  nose G52.0
  occipital M54.81
  olfactory G52.0
  penis N48.9
  perineum R10.2
  postherpetic NEC B02.29
    trigeminal B02.22
  pubic region R10.2
  scrotum R10.2
  Sluder's G44.89
  specified nerve NEC G58.8
  spermatic cord R10.2
  sphenopalatine (ganglion) G90.09
  trifacial — *see* Neuralgia, trigeminal
  trigeminal G50.0
    postherpetic, postzoster B02.22
  vagus (nerve) G52.2
  writer's F48.8
    organic G25.89
Neurapraxia — *see* Injury, nerve
Neurasthenia F48.8
  cardiac F45.8
  gastric F45.8
  heart F45.8
Neurilemmoma (*see also* Neoplasm, nerve, benign)
  acoustic (nerve) D33.3
  malignant (*see also* Neoplasm, nerve, malignant)
    acoustic (nerve) C72.4- ☑
Neurilemmosarcoma — *see* Neoplasm, nerve, malignant
Neurinoma — *see* Neoplasm, nerve, benign
Neurinomatosis — *see* Neoplasm, nerve, uncertain behavior
Neuritis (rheumatoid) M79.2
  abducens (nerve) — *see* Strabismus, paralytic, sixth nerve
  accessory (nerve) G52.8
  acoustic (nerve) (*see also* subcategory) H93.3 ☑
    in (due to)
      infectious disease NEC B99 ☑ [H94.0-] ☑
      parasitic disease NEC B89 [H94.0-] ☑
    syphilitic A52.15
  alcoholic G62.1
    with psychosis — *see* Psychosis, alcoholic
  amyloid, any site E85.4 [G63]
  auditory (nerve) — *see* subcategory H93.3 ☑
  brachial — *see* Radiculopathy
    due to displacement, intervertebral disc — *see* Disorder, disc, cervical, with neuritis
  cranial nerve
    due to Lyme disease A69.22
    eighth or acoustic or auditory — *see* subcategory H93.3 ☑
    eleventh or accessory G52.8
    fifth or trigeminal G51.0
    first or olfactory G52.0

Neuritis — *continued*
  cranial nerve — *continued*
    fourth or trochlear — *see* Strabismus, paralytic, fourth nerve
    second or optic — *see* Neuritis, optic
    seventh or facial G51.8
      newborn (birth injury) P11.3
    sixth or abducent — *see* Strabismus, paralytic, sixth nerve
    tenth or vagus G52.2
    third or oculomotor — *see* Strabismus, paralytic, third nerve
    twelfth or hypoglossal G52.3
  Déjérine-Sottas G60.0
  diabetic (mononeuropathy) — *see* E08-E13 with .41
    polyneuropathy — *see* E08-E13 with .42
  due to
    beriberi E51.11
    displacement, prolapse or rupture, intervertebral disc — *see* Disorder, disc, with, radiculopathy
    herniation, nucleus pulposus M51.9 [G55]
  endemic E51.11
  facial G51.8
    newborn (birth injury) P11.3
  general — *see* Polyneuropathy
  geniculate ganglion G51.1
    due to herpes (zoster) B02.21
  gouty (*see also* Gout, by type) M10.9 [G63]
  hypoglossal (nerve) G52.3
  ilioinguinal (nerve) G57.9- ☑
  infectious (multiple) NEC G61.0
  interstitial hypertrophic progressive G60.0
  lumbar M54.16
  lumbosacral M54.17
  multiple (*see also* Polyneuropathy)
    endemic E51.11
    infective, acute G61.0
  multiplex endemica E51.11
  nerve root — *see* Radiculopathy
  oculomotor (nerve) — *see* Strabismus, paralytic, third nerve
  olfactory nerve G52.0
  optic (nerve) (hereditary) (sympathetic) H46.9
    with demyelination G36.0
    in myelitis G36.0
    nutritional H46.2
    papillitis — *see* Papillitis, optic
    retrobulbar H46.1- ☑
    specified type NEC H46.8
    toxic H46.3
  peripheral (nerve) G62.9
    multiple — *see* Polyneuropathy
    single — *see* Mononeuritis
  pneumogastric (nerve) G52.2
  postherpetic, postzoster B02.29
  progressive hypertrophic interstitial G60.0
  retrobulbar (*see also* Neuritis, optic, retrobulbar)
    in (due to)
      late syphilis A52.15
      meningococcal infection A39.82
    meningococcal A39.82
    syphilitic A52.15
  sciatic (nerve) (*see also* Sciatica)
    due to displacement of intervertebral disc — *see* Disorder, disc, with, radiculopathy
  serum (*see also* Reaction, serum) T80.69 ☑
  shoulder-girdle G54.5
  specified nerve NEC G58.8
  spinal (nerve) root — *see* Radiculopathy
  syphilitic A52.15
  thenar (median) G56.1- ☑
  thoracic M54.14
  toxic NEC G62.2
  trochlear (nerve) — *see* Strabismus, paralytic, fourth nerve
  vagus (nerve) G52.2
Neuroastrocytoma — *see* Neoplasm, uncertain behavior, by site
Neuroavitaminosis E56.9 [G99.8]
Neuroblastoma
  olfactory C30.0
  specified site — *see* Neoplasm, malignant, by site
  unspecified site C74.90
Neurochorioretinitis — *see* Chorioretinitis
Neurocirculatory asthenia F45.8
Neurocysticercosis B69.0
Neurocytoma — *see* Neoplasm, benign, by site

Neurodermatitis (circumscribed) (circumscripta) (local) L28.0
 atopic L20.81
 diffuse (Brocq) L20.81
 disseminated L20.81
Neuroencephalomyelopathy, optic G36.0
Neuroepithelioma (see also Neoplasm, malignant, by site)
 olfactory C30.0
Neurofibroma (see also Neoplasm, nerve, benign)
 melanotic — see Neoplasm, nerve, benign
 multiple — see Neurofibromatosis
 plexiform — see Neoplasm, nerve, benign
Neurofibromatosis (multiple) (nonmalignant) Q85.00
 acoustic Q85.02
 malignant — see Neoplasm, nerve, malignant
 specified NEC Q85.09
 type 1 (von Recklinghausen) Q85.01
 type 2 Q85.02
Neurofibrosarcoma — see Neoplasm, nerve, malignant
Neurogenic (see also condition)
 bladder (see also Dysfunction, bladder, neuromuscular) N31.9
  cauda equina syndrome G83.4
 bowel NEC K59.2
 heart F45.8
Neuroglioma — see Neoplasm, uncertain behavior, by site
Neurolabyrinthitis (of Dix and Hallpike) — see Neuronitis, vestibular
Neurolathyrism — see Poisoning, food, noxious, plant
Neuroleprosy A30.9
Neuroma (see also Neoplasm, nerve, benign)
 acoustic (nerve) D33.3
 amputation (stump) (traumatic) (surgical complication) (late) T87.3- ☑
  arm T87.3- ☑
  leg T87.3- ☑
 digital (toe) G57.6- ☑
 interdigital G58.8
  lower limb (toe) G57.8- ☑
  upper limb G56.8- ☑
 intermetatarsal G57.8- ☑
 Morton's G57.6- ☑
 nonneoplastic
  arm G56.9- ☑
  leg G57.9- ☑
  lower extremity G57.9- ☑
  upper extremity G56.9- ☑
 optic (nerve) D33.3
 plantar G57.6- ☑
 plexiform — see Neoplasm, nerve, benign
 surgical (nonneoplastic)
  arm G56.9- ☑
  leg G57.9- ☑
  lower extremity G57.9- ☑
  upper extremity G56.9- ☑
Neuromyalgia — see Neuralgia
Neuromyasthenia (epidemic) (postinfectious) G93.3
Neuromyelitis G36.9
 ascending G61.0
 optica G36.0
Neuromyopathy G70.9
 paraneoplastic D49.9 [G13.0]
Neuromyotonia (Isaacs) G71.19
Neuronevus — see Nevus
Neuronitis G58.9
 ascending (acute) G57.2- ☑
 vestibular H81.2- ☑
Neuroparalytic — see condition
Neuropathy, neuropathic G62.9
 acute motor G62.81
 alcoholic G62.1
  with psychosis — see Psychosis, alcoholic
 arm G56.9- ☑
 autonomic, peripheral — see Neuropathy, peripheral, autonomic
 axillary G56.9- ☑
 bladder N31.9
  atonic (motor) (sensory) N31.2
  autonomous N31.2
  flaccid N31.2
  nonreflex N31.2
  reflex N31.1
  uninhibited N31.0
 brachial plexus G54.0
 cervical plexus G54.2

Neuropathy, neuropathic — continued
 chronic
  progressive segmentally demyelinating G62.89
  relapsing demyelinating G62.89
 Déjérine-Sottas G60.0
 diabetic — see E08-E13 with .40
  mononeuropathy — see E08-E13 with .41
  polyneuropathy — see E08-E13 with .42
 entrapment G58.9
  iliohypogastric nerve G57.8- ☑
  ilioinguinal nerve G57.8- ☑
  lateral cutaneous nerve of thigh G57.1- ☑
  median nerve G56.0- ☑
  obturator nerve G57.8- ☑
  peroneal nerve G57.3- ☑
  posterior tibial nerve G57.5- ☑
  saphenous nerve G57.8- ☑
  ulnar nerve G56.2- ☑
 facial nerve G51.9
 hereditary G60.9
  motor and sensory (types I-IV) G60.0
  sensory G60.8
  specified NEC G60.8
 hypertrophic G60.0
  Charcot-Marie-Tooth G60.0
  Déjérine-Sottas G60.0
  interstitial progressive G60.0
  of infancy G60.0
  Refsum G60.1
 idiopathic G60.9
  progressive G60.3
  specified NEC G60.8
 in association with hereditary ataxia G60.2
 intercostal G58.0
 ischemic — see Disorder, nerve
 Jamaica (ginger) G62.2
 leg NEC G57.9- ☑
 lower extremity G57.9- ☑
 lumbar plexus G54.1
 median nerve G56.1- ☑
 motor and sensory (see also Polyneuropathy)
  hereditary (types I-IV) G60.0
 multifocal motor (MMN) G61.82
 multiple (acute) (chronic) — see Polyneuropathy
 optic (nerve) (see also Neuritis, optic)
  ischemic H47.01- ☑
 paraneoplastic (sensorial) (Denny Brown) D49.9 [G13.0]
 peripheral (nerve) (see also Polyneuropathy) G62.9
  autonomic G90.9
   idiopathic G90.09
   in (due to)
    amyloidosis E85.4 [G99.0]
    diabetes mellitus — see E08-E13 with .43
    endocrine disease NEC E34.9 [G99.0]
    gout M10.00 [G99.0]
    hyperthyroidism E05.90 [G99.0]
     with thyroid storm E05.91 [G99.0]
    metabolic disease NEC E88.9 [G99.0]
  idiopathic G60.9
   progressive G60.3
  in (due to)
   antitetanus serum G62.0
   arsenic G62.2
   drugs NEC G62.0
   lead G62.2
   organophosphate compounds G62.2
   toxic agent NEC G62.2
 plantar nerves G57.6- ☑
 progressive
  hypertrophic interstitial G60.0
  inflammatory G62.81
 radicular NEC — see Radiculopathy
 sacral plexus G54.1
 sciatic G57.0- ☑
 serum G61.1
 toxic NEC G62.2
 trigeminal sensory G50.8
 ulnar nerve G56.2- ☑
 uremic N18.9 [G63]
 vitamin B12 E53.8 [G63]
  with anemia (pernicious) D51.0 [G63]
   due to dietary deficiency D51.3 [G63]
Neurophthisis (see also Disorder, nerve)
 peripheral, diabetic — see E08-E13 with .42
Neuroretinitis — see Chorioretinitis
Neuroretinopathy, hereditary optic H47.22
Neurosarcoma — see Neoplasm, nerve, malignant
Neurosclerosis — see Disorder, nerve

Neurosis, neurotic F48.9
 anankastic F42.8
 anxiety (state) F41.1
  panic type F41.0
 asthenic F48.8
 bladder F45.8
 cardiac (reflex) F45.8
 cardiovascular F45.8
 character F60.9
 colon F45.8
 compensation F68.1 ☑
 compulsive, compulsion F42.8
 conversion F44.9
 craft F48.8
 cutaneous F45.8
 depersonalization F48.1
 depressive (reaction) (type) F34.1
 environmental F48.8
 excoriation L98.1
 fatigue F48.8
 functional — see Disorder, somatoform
 gastric F45.8
 gastrointestinal F45.8
 heart F45.8
 hypochondriacal F45.21
 hysterical F44.9
 incoordination F45.8
  larynx F45.8
  vocal cord F45.8
 intestine F45.8
 larynx (sensory) F45.8
  hysterical F44.4
 mixed NEC F48.8
 musculoskeletal F45.8
 obsessional F42.8
 obsessive-compulsive F42.8
 occupational F48.8
 ocular NEC F45.8
 organ — see Disorder, somatoform
 pharynx F45.8
 phobic F40.9
 posttraumatic (situational) F43.10
  acute F43.11
  chronic F43.12
 psychasthenic (type) F48.8
 railroad F48.8
 rectum F45.8
 respiratory F45.8
 rumination F45.8
 sexual F65.9
 situational F48.8
 social F40.10
  generalized F40.11
 specified type NEC F48.8
 state F48.9
  with depersonalization episode F48.1
 stomach F45.8
 traumatic F43.10
  acute F43.11
  chronic F43.12
 vasomotor F45.8
 visceral F45.8
 war F48.8
Neurospongioblastosis diffusa Q85.1
Neurosyphilis (arrested) (early) (gumma) (late) (latent) (recurrent) (relapse) A52.3
 with ataxia (cerebellar) (locomotor) (spastic) (spinal) A52.19
 aneurysm (cerebral) A52.05
 arachnoid (adhesive) A52.13
 arteritis (any artery) (cerebral) A52.04
 asymptomatic A52.2
 congenital A50.40
 dura (mater) A52.13
 general paresis A52.17
 hemorrhagic A52.05
 juvenile (asymptomatic) (meningeal) A50.40
 leptomeninges (aseptic) A52.13
 meningeal, meninges (adhesive) A52.13
 meningitis A52.13
 meningovascular (diffuse) A52.13
 optic atrophy A52.15
 parenchymatous (degenerative) A52.19
 paresis, paretic A52.17
  juvenile A50.45
 remission in (sustained) A52.3
 serological (without symptoms) A52.2
 specified nature or site NEC A52.19
 tabes, tabetic (dorsalis) A52.11

☑ **Additional Character Required** — Refer to the Tabular List for Character Selection

▽ Subterms under main terms may continue to next column or page

Neurosyphilis — *continued*
  tabes, tabetic — *continued*
    juvenile A50.45
  taboparesis A52.17
    juvenile A50.45
  thrombosis (cerebral) A52.05
  vascular (cerebral) NEC A52.05
Neurothekeoma — *see* Neoplasm, nerve, benign
Neurotic — *see* Neurosis
Neurotoxemia — *see* Toxemia
Neutroclusion M26.211
Neutropenia, neutropenic (chronic) (genetic) (idiopathic) (immune) (infantile) (malignant) (pernicious) (splenic) D70.9
  congenital (primary) D70.0
  cyclic D70.4
  cytoreductive cancer chemotherapy sequela D70.1
  drug-induced D70.2
    due to cytoreductive cancer chemotherapy D70.1
  due to infection D70.3
  fever D70.9
  neonatal, transitory (isoimmune) (maternal transfer) P61.5
  periodic D70.4
  secondary (cyclic) (periodic) (splenic) D70.4
    drug-induced D70.2
      due to cytoreductive cancer chemotherapy D70.1
  toxic D70.8
Neutrophilia, hereditary giant D72.0
Nevocarcinoma — *see* Melanoma
Nevus D22.9
  achromic — *see* Neoplasm, skin, benign
  amelanotic — *see* Neoplasm, skin, benign
  angiomatous D18.00
    intra-abdominal D18.03
    intracranial D18.02
    skin D18.01
    specified site NEC D18.09
  araneus I78.1
  balloon cell — *see* Neoplasm, skin, benign
  bathing trunk D48.5
  blue — *see* Neoplasm, skin, benign
    cellular — *see* Neoplasm, skin, benign
    giant — *see* Neoplasm, skin, benign
    Jadassohn's — *see* Neoplasm, skin, benign
    malignant — *see* Melanoma
  capillary D18.00
    intra-abdominal D18.03
    intracranial D18.02
    skin D18.01
    specified site NEC D18.09
  cavernous D18.00
    intra-abdominal D18.03
    intracranial D18.02
    skin D18.01
    specified site NEC D18.09
  cellular — *see* Neoplasm, skin, benign
    blue — *see* Neoplasm, skin, benign
  choroid D31.3- ☑
  comedonicus Q82.5
  conjunctiva D31.0- ☑
  dermal — *see* Neoplasm, skin, benign
    with epidermal nevus — *see* Neoplasm, skin, benign
  dysplastic — *see* Neoplasm, skin, benign
  eye D31.9- ☑
  flammeus Q82.5
  hemangiomatous D18.00
    intra-abdominal D18.03
    intracranial D18.02
    skin D18.01
    specified site NEC D18.09
  iris D31.4- ☑
  lacrimal gland D31.5- ☑
  lymphatic D18.1
  magnocellular
    specified site — *see* Neoplasm, benign, by site
    unspecified site D31.40
  malignant — *see* Melanoma
  meaning hemangioma D18.00
    intra-abdominal D18.03
    intracranial D18.02
    skin D18.01
    specified site NEC D18.09
  mouth (mucosa) D10.30
    specified site NEC D10.39
    white sponge Q38.6

Nevus — *continued*
  multiplex Q85.1
  non-neoplastic I78.1
  oral mucosa D10.30
    specified site NEC D10.39
    white sponge Q38.6
  orbit D31.6- ☑
  pigmented
    giant (*see also* Neoplasm, skin, uncertain behavior) D48.5
      malignant melanoma in — *see* Melanoma
  portwine Q82.5
  retina D31.2- ☑
  retrobulbar D31.6- ☑
  sanguineous Q82.5
  senile I78.1
  skin D22.9
    abdominal wall D22.5
    ala nasi D22.39
    ankle D22.7- ☑
    anus, anal D22.5
    arm D22.6- ☑
    auditory canal (external) D22.2- ☑
    auricle (ear) D22.2- ☑
    auricular canal (external) D22.2- ☑
    axilla, axillary fold D22.5
    back D22.5
    breast D22.5
    brow D22.39
    buttock D22.5
    canthus (eye) D22.1- ☑
    cheek (external) D22.39
    chest wall D22.5
    chin D22.39
    ear (external) D22.2- ☑
    external meatus (ear) D22.2- ☑
    eyebrow D22.39
    eyelid (lower) (upper) D22.1- ☑
    face D22.30
      specified NEC D22.39
    female genital organ (external) NEC D28.0
    finger D22.6- ☑
    flank D22.5
    foot D22.7- ☑
    forearm D22.6- ☑
    forehead D22.39
    foreskin D29.0
    genital organ (external) NEC
      female D28.0
      male D29.9
    gluteal region D22.5
    groin D22.5
    hand D22.6- ☑
    heel D22.7- ☑
    helix D22.2- ☑
    hip D22.7- ☑
    interscapular region D22.5
    jaw D22.39
    knee D22.7- ☑
    labium (majus) (minus) D28.0
    leg D22.7- ☑
    lip (lower) (upper) D22.0
    lower limb D22.7- ☑
    male genital organ (external) D29.9
    nail D22.9
      finger D22.6- ☑
      toe D22.7- ☑
    nasolabial groove D22.39
    nates D22.5
    neck D22.4
    nose (external) D22.39
    palpebra D22.1- ☑
    penis D29.0
    perianal skin D22.5
    perineum D22.5
    pinna D22.2- ☑
    popliteal fossa or space D22.7- ☑
    prepuce D29.0
    pudendum D28.0
    scalp D22.4
    scrotum D29.4
    shoulder D22.6- ☑
    submammary fold D22.5
    temple D22.39
    thigh D22.7- ☑
    toe D22.7- ☑
    trunk NEC D22.5

Nevus — *continued*
  skin — *continued*
    umbilicus D22.5
    upper limb D22.6- ☑
    vulva D28.0
    specified site NEC — *see* Neoplasm, by site, benign
  spider I78.1
  stellar I78.1
  strawberry Q82.5
  Sutton's benign D22.9
  unius lateris Q82.5
  Unna's Q82.5
  vascular Q82.5
  verrucous Q82.5
Newborn (infant) (liveborn) (singleton) Z38.2
  abstinence syndrome P96.1
  acne L70.4
  affected by
    abnormalities of membranes P02.9
      specified NEC P02.8
    abruptio placenta P02.1
    amino-acid metabolic disorder, transitory P74.8
    amniocentesis (while in utero) P00.6
    amnionitis P02.7
    apparent life threatening event (ALTE) R68.13
    bleeding (into)
      cerebral cortex P52.22
      germinal matrix P52.0
      ventricles P52.1
    breech delivery P03.0
    cardiac arrest P29.81
    cardiomyopathy I42.8
      congenital I42.4
    cerebral ischemia P91.0
    Cesarean delivery P03.4
    chemotherapy agents P04.1
    chorioamnionitis P02.7
    cocaine (crack) P04.41
    complications of labor and delivery P03.9
      specified NEC P03.89
    compression of umbilical cord NEC P02.5
    contracted pelvis P03.1
    delivery P03.9
      Cesarean P03.4
      forceps P03.2
      vacuum extractor P03.3
    entanglement (knot) in umbilical cord P02.5
    environmental chemicals P04.6
    fetal (intrauterine)
      growth retardation P05.9
      malnutrition not light or small for gestational age P05.2
    forceps delivery P03.2
    heart rate abnormalities
      bradycardia P29.12
      intrauterine P03.819
        before onset of labor P03.810
        during labor P03.811
      tachycardia P29.11
    hemorrhage (antepartum) P02.1
      cerebellar (nontraumatic) P52.6
      intracerebral (nontraumatic) P52.4
      intracranial (nontraumatic) P52.9
        specified NEC P52.8
      intraventricular (nontraumatic) P52.3
        grade 1 P52.0
        grade 2 P52.1
        grade 3 P52.21
        grade 4 P52.22
      posterior fossa (nontraumatic) P52.6
      subarachnoid (nontraumatic) P52.5
      subependymal P52.0
        with intracerebral extension P52.22
        with intraventricular extension P52.1
          with enlargment of ventricles P52.21
          without intraventricular extension P52.0
    hypoxic ischemic encephalopathy [HIE] P91.60
      mild P91.61
      moderate P91.62
      severe P91.63
    induction of labor P03.89
    intestinal perforation P78.0
    intrauterine (fetal) blood loss P50.9
      due to (from)
        cut end of co-twin cord P50.5
        hemorrhage into
          co-twin P50.3
          maternal circulation P50.4
          placenta P50.2

Newborn — continued
  affected by — continued
    intrauterine blood loss — continued
      due to — continued
        ruptured cord blood P50.1
        vasa previa P50.0
      specified NEC P50.8
    intrauterine (fetal) hemorrhage P50.9
    intrauterine (in utero) procedure P96.5
    malpresentation (malposition) NEC P03.1
    maternal (complication of) (use of)
      alcohol P04.3
      analgesia (maternal) P04.0
      anesthesia (maternal) P04.0
      blood loss P02.1
      circulatory disease P00.3
      condition P00.9
        specified NEC P00.89
      delivery P03.9
        Cesarean P03.4
        forceps P03.2
        vacuum extractor P03.3
      diabetes mellitus (pre-existing) P70.1
      disorder P00.9
        specified NEC P00.89
      drugs (addictive) (illegal) NEC P04.49
      ectopic pregnancy P01.4
      gestational diabetes P70.0
      hemorrhage P02.1
      hypertensive disorder P00.0
      incompetent cervix P01.0
      infectious disease P00.2
      injury P00.5
      labor and delivery P03.9
      malpresentation before labor P01.7
      maternal death P01.6
      medical procedure P00.7
      medication P04.1
      multiple pregnancy P01.5
      nutritional disorder P00.4
      oligohydramnios P01.2
      parasitic disease P00.2
      periodontal disease P00.81
      placenta previa P02.0
      polyhydramnios P01.3
      precipitate delivery P03.5
      pregnancy P01.9
        specified P01.8
      premature rupture of membranes P01.1
      renal disease P00.1
      respiratory disease P00.3
      surgical procedure P00.6
      urinary tract disease P00.1
      uterine contraction (abnormal) P03.6
    meconium peritonitis P78.0
    medication (legal) (maternal use) (prescribed) P04.1
    membrane abnormalities P02.9
      specified NEC P02.8
    membranitis P02.7
    methamphetamine(s) P04.49
    mixed metabolic and respiratory acidosis P84
    neonatal abstinence syndrome P96.1
    noxious substances transmitted via placenta or
      breast milk P04.9
      specified NEC P04.8
    nutritional supplements P04.5
    placenta previa P02.0
    placental
      abnormality (functional) (morphological)
        P02.20
        specified NEC P02.29
      dysfunction P02.29
      infarction P02.29
      insufficiency P02.29
      separation NEC P02.1
      transfusion syndromes P02.3
    placentitis P02.7
    precipitate delivery P03.5
    prolapsed cord P02.4
    respiratory arrest P28.81
    slow intrauterine growth P05.9
    tobacco P04.2
    twin to twin transplacental transfusion P02.3
    umbilical cord (tightly) around neck P02.5
    umbilical cord condition P02.60
      short cord P02.69
      specified NEC P02.69
    uterine contractions (abnormal) P03.6
    vasa previa P02.69

Newborn — continued
  affected by — continued
    vasa previa — continued
      from intrauterine blood loss P50.0
    apnea P28.4
      obstructive P28.4
      primary P28.3
      sleep (central) (obstructive) (primary) P28.3
    born in hospital Z38.00
      by cesarean Z38.01
    born outside hospital Z38.1
    breast buds P96.89
    breast engorgement P83.4
    check-up — see Newborn, examination
    convulsion P90
    dehydration P74.1
    examination
      8 to 28 days old Z00.111
      under 8 days old Z00.110
    fever P81.9
      environmentally-induced P81.0
    hyperbilirubinemia P59.9
      of prematurity P59.0
    hypernatremia P74.2
    hyponatremia P74.2
    infection P39.9
      candidal P37.5
      specified NEC P39.8
      urinary tract P39.3
    jaundice P59.9
      due to
        breast milk inhibitor P59.3
        hepatocellular damage P59.20
          specified NEC P59.29
        preterm delivery P59.0
      of prematurity P59.0
      specified NEC P59.8
    late metabolic acidosis P74.0
    mastitis P39.0
      infective P39.0
      noninfective P83.4
    multiple born NEC Z38.8
      born in hospital Z38.68
        by cesarean Z38.69
      born outside hospital Z38.7
    omphalitis P38.9
      with mild hemorrhage P38.1
      without hemorrhage P38.9
    post-term P08.21
    prolonged gestation (over 42 completed weeks)
      P08.22
    quadruplet Z38.8
      born in hospital Z38.63
        by cesarean Z38.64
      born outside hospital Z38.7
    quintuplet Z38.8
      born in hospital Z38.65
        by cesarean Z38.66
      born outside hospital Z38.7
    seizure P90
    sepsis (congenital) P36.9
      due to
        anaerobes NEC P36.5
        Escherichia coli P36.4
        Staphylococcus P36.30
          aureus P36.2
          specified NEC P36.39
        Streptococcus P36.10
          group B P36.0
          specified NEC P36.19
      specified NEC P36.8
    triplet Z38.8
      born in hospital Z38.61
        by cesarean Z38.62
      born outside hospital Z38.7
    twin Z38.5
      born in hospital Z38.30
        by cesarean Z38.31
      born outside hospital Z38.4
    vomiting P92.09
      bilious P92.01
    weight check Z00.111
Newcastle conjunctivitis or disease B30.8
Nezelof's syndrome (pure alymphocytosis) D81.4
Niacin (amide) **deficiency** E52
Nicolas (-Durand)-**Favre disease** A55
Nicotine — see Tobacco
Nicotinic acid deficiency E52

Niemann-Pick disease or syndrome E75.249
  specified NEC E75.248
  type
    A E75.240
    B E75.241
    C E75.242
    D E75.243
Night
  blindness — see Blindness, night
  sweats R61
  terrors (child) F51.4
Nightmares (REM sleep type) F51.5
NIHSS (National Institutes of Health Stroke Scale) **score**
  R29.7- ☑
Nipple — see condition
Nisbet's chancre A57
Nishimoto (-Takeuchi) **disease** I67.5
Nitritoid crisis or reaction — see Crisis, nitritoid
Nitrosohemoglobinemia D74.8
Njovera A65
Nocardiosis, nocardiasis A43.9
  cutaneous A43.1
  lung A43.0
  pneumonia A43.0
  pulmonary A43.0
  specified site NEC A43.8
Nocturia R35.1
  psychogenic F45.8
Nocturnal — see condition
Nodal rhythm I49.8
Node(s) (see also Nodule)
  Bouchard's (with arthropathy) M15.2
  Haygarth's M15.8
  Heberden's (with arthropathy) M15.1
  larynx J38.7
  lymph — see condition
  milker's B08.03
  Osler's I33.0
  Schmorl's — see Schmorl's disease
  singer's J38.2
  teacher's J38.2
  tuberculous — see Tuberculosis, lymph gland
  vocal cord J38.2
Nodule(s), nodular
  actinomycotic — see Actinomycosis
  breast NEC (see also Lump, breast) N63.0
  colloid (cystic), thyroid E04.1
  cutaneous — see Swelling, localized
  endometrial (stromal) D26.1
  Haygarth's M15.8
  inflammatory — see Inflammation
  juxta-articular
    syphilitic A52.77
    yaws A66.7
  larynx J38.7
  lung, solitary (subsegmental branch of the bronchial
    tree) R91.1
    multiple R91.8
  milker's B08.03
  prostate N40.2
    with lower urinary tract symptoms (LUTS) N40.3
    without lower urinary tract symptoms (LUTS) N40.2
  pulmonary, solitary (subsegmental branch of the
    bronchial tree) R91.1
  retrocardiac R09.89
  rheumatoid M06.30
    ankle M06.37- ☑
    elbow M06.32- ☑
    foot joint M06.37- ☑
    hand joint M06.34- ☑
    hip M06.35- ☑
    knee M06.36- ☑
    multiple site M06.39
    shoulder M06.31- ☑
    vertebra M06.38
    wrist M06.33- ☑
  scrotum (inflammatory) N49.2
  singer's J38.2
  solitary, lung (subsegmental branch of the bronchial
    tree) R91.1
    multiple R91.8
  subcutaneous — see Swelling, localized
  teacher's J38.2
  thyroid (cold) (gland) (nontoxic) E04.1
    with thyrotoxicosis E05.20
      with thyroid storm E05.21
    toxic or with hyperthyroidism E05.20
      with thyroid storm E05.21

☑ **Additional Character Required** — Refer to the Tabular List for Character Selection   ▽ Subterms under main terms may continue to next column or page

Nodule(s), nodular — *continued*
   vocal cord J38.2
Noma (gangrenous) (hospital) (infective) A69.0
   auricle I96
   mouth A69.0
   pudendi N76.89
   vulvae N76.89
Nomad, nomadism Z59.0
NOMID (neonatal onset multisystemic inflammatory disorder) M04.2
Nonadherence to medical treatment Z91.19
Nonautoimmune hemolytic anemia D59.4
   drug-induced D59.2
Nonclosure (*see also* Imperfect, closure)
   ductus arteriosus (Botallo's) Q25.0
   foramen
      botalli Q21.1
      ovale Q21.1
Noncompliance Z91.19
   with
      dialysis Z91.15
      dietary regimen Z91.11
      medical treatment Z91.19
      medication regimen NEC Z91.14
         underdosing (*see also* Table of Drugs and Chemicals, categories T36-T50, with final character 6) Z91.14
            intentional NEC Z91.128
               due to financial hardship of patient Z91.120
            unintentional NEC Z91.138
               due to patient's age related debility Z91.130
      renal dialysis Z91.15
Nondescent (congenital) (*see also* Malposition, congenital)
   cecum Q43.3
   colon Q43.3
   testicle Q53.9
      bilateral Q53.20
         abdominal Q53.211
         perineal Q53.22
      unilateral Q53.10
         abdominal Q53.111
         perineal Q53.12
Nondevelopment
   brain Q02
      part of Q04.3
   heart Q24.8
   organ or site, congenital NEC — *see* Hypoplasia
Nonengagement
   head NEC O32.4 ☑
      in labor, causing obstructed labor O64.8 ☑
Nonexanthematous tick fever A93.2
Nonexpansion, lung (newborn) P28.0
Nonfunctioning
   cystic duct (*see also* Disease, gallbladder) K82.8
   gallbladder (*see also* Disease, gallbladder) K82.8
   kidney N28.9
   labyrinth — *see* subcategory H83.2 ☑
Non-Hodgkin lymphoma NEC — *see* Lymphoma, non-Hodgkin
Nonimplantation, ovum N97.2
Noninsufflation, fallopian tube N97.1
Non-ketotic hyperglycinemia E72.51
Nonne-Milroy syndrome Q82.0
Nonovulation N97.0
Non-palpable testicle(s)
   bilateral R39.84
   unilateral R39.83
Nonpatent fallopian tube N97.1
Nonpneumatization, lung NEC P28.0
Nonrotation — *see* Malrotation
Nonsecretion, urine — *see* Anuria
Nonunion
   fracture — *see* Fracture, by site
   joint, following fusion or arthrodesis M96.0
   organ or site, congenital NEC — *see* Imperfect, closure
   symphysis pubis, congenital Q74.2
Nonvisualization, gallbladder R93.2
Nonvital, nonvitalized tooth K04.99
Non-working side interference M26.56
Noonan's syndrome Q87.1
Normocytic anemia (infectional) due to blood loss (chronic) D50.0
   acute D62
Norrie's disease (congenital) Q15.8

North American blastomycosis B40.9
Norwegian itch B86
Nose, nasal — *see* condition
Nosebleed R04.0
Nose-picking F98.8
Nosomania F45.21
Nosophobia F45.22
Nostalgia F43.20
Notch of iris Q13.2
Notching nose, congenital (tip) Q30.2
Nothnagel's
   syndrome — *see* Strabismus, paralytic, third nerve
   vasomotor acroparesthesia I73.89
Novy's relapsing fever A68.9
   louse-borne A68.0
   tick-borne A68.1
Noxious
   foodstuffs, poisoning by — *see* Poisoning, food, noxious, plant
   substances transmitted through placenta or breast milk P04.9
Nucleus pulposus — *see* condition
Numbness R20.0
Nuns' knee — *see* Bursitis, prepatellar
Nursemaid's elbow S53.03- ☑
Nutcracker esophagus K22.4
Nutmeg liver K76.1
Nutrient element deficiency E61.9
   specified NEC E61.8
Nutrition deficient or insufficient (*see also* Malnutrition) E46
   due to
      insufficient food T73.0 ☑
      lack of
         care (child) T76.02 ☑
            adult T76.01 ☑
         food T73.0 ☑
Nutritional stunting E45
Nyctalopia (night blindness) — *see* Blindness, night
Nycturia R35.1
   psychogenic F45.8
Nymphomania F52.8
Nystagmus H55.00
   benign paroxysmal — *see* Vertigo, benign paroxysmal
   central positional H81.4- ☑
   congenital H55.01
   dissociated H55.04
   latent H55.02
   miners' H55.09
   positional
      benign paroxysmal H81.4- ☑
      central H81.4- ☑
   specified form NEC H55.09
   visual deprivation H55.03

O

Obermeyer's relapsing fever (European) A68.0
Obesity E66.9
   with alveolar hypoventilation E66.2
   adrenal E27.8
   complicating
      childbirth O99.214
      pregnancy O99.21- ☑
      puerperium O99.215
   constitutional E66.8
   dietary counseling and surveillance Z71.3
   drug-induced E66.1
   due to
      drug E66.1
      excess calories E66.09
         morbid E66.01
         severe E66.01
   endocrine E66.8
   endogenous E66.8
   exogenous E66.09
   familial E66.8
   glandular E66.8
   hypothyroid — *see* Hypothyroidism
   hypoventilation syndrome (OHS) E66.2
   morbid E66.01
      with
         alveolar hypoventilation E66.2
         obesity hypoventilation syndrome (OHS) E66.2
      due to excess calories E66.01
   nutritional E66.09
   pituitary E23.6

Obesity — *continued*
   severe E66.01
   specified type NEC E66.8
Oblique — *see* condition
Obliteration
   appendix (lumen) K38.8
   artery I77.1
   bile duct (noncalculous) K83.1
   common duct (noncalculous) K83.1
   cystic duct — *see* Obstruction, gallbladder
   disease, arteriolar I77.1
   endometrium N85.8
   eye, anterior chamber — *see* Disorder, globe, hypotony
   fallopian tube N97.1
   lymphatic vessel I89.0
      due to mastectomy I97.2
   organ or site, congenital NEC — *see* Atresia, by site
   ureter N13.5
      with infection N13.6
   urethra — *see* Stricture, urethra
   vein I87.8
   vestibule (oral) K08.89
Observation (following) (for) (without need for further medical care) Z04.9
   accident NEC Z04.3
      at work Z04.2
      transport Z04.1
   adverse effect of drug Z03.6
   alleged rape or sexual assault (victim), ruled out
      adult Z04.41
      child Z04.42
   criminal assault Z04.8
   development state
      adolescent Z00.3
      period of rapid growth in childhood Z00.2
      puberty Z00.3
   disease, specified NEC Z03.89
   following work accident Z04.2
   growth and development state — *see* Observation, development state
   injuries (accidental) NEC (*see also* Observation, accident)
   newborn (for)
      suspected condition, related to exposure from the mother or birth process — *see* Newborn, affected by, maternal
         ruled out Z05.9
            cardiac Z05.0
            connective tissue Z05.73
            gastrointestinal Z05.5
            genetic Z05.41
            genitourinary Z05.6
            immunologic Z05.43
            infectious Z05.1
            metabolic Z05.42
            musculoskeletal Z05.72
            neurological Z05.2
            respiratory Z05.3
            skin and subcutaneous tissue Z05.71
            specified condition NEC Z05.8
   postpartum
      immediately after delivery Z39.0
      routine follow-up Z39.2
   pregnancy (normal) (without complication) Z34.9- ☑
      high risk O09.9- ☑
   suicide attempt, alleged NEC Z03.89
      self-poisoning Z03.6
   suspected, ruled out (*see also* Suspected condition, ruled out)
      abuse, physical
         adult Z04.71
         child Z04.72
      accident at work Z04.2
      adult battering victim Z04.71
      child battering victim Z04.72
      condition NEC Z03.89
         newborn (*see also* Observation, newborn (for), suspected condition, ruled out) Z05.9
      drug poisoning or adverse effect Z03.6
      exposure (to)
         anthrax Z03.810
         biological agent NEC Z03.818
      inflicted injury NEC Z04.8
      suicide attempt, alleged Z03.89
         self-poisoning Z03.6
      toxic effects from ingested substance (drug) (poison) Z03.6

Index

Observation — *continued*
toxic effects from ingested substance (drug) (poison) Z03.6
Obsession, obsessional state F42.8
mixed thoughts and acts F42.2
Obsessive-compulsive neurosis or reaction F42.8
Obstetric embolism, septic — *see* Embolism, obstetric, septic
Obstetrical trauma (complicating delivery) O71.9
with or following ectopic or molar pregnancy O08.6
specified type NEC O71.89
Obstipation — *see* Constipation
Obstruction, obstructed, obstructive
airway J98.8
with
allergic alveolitis J67.9
asthma J45.909
with
exacerbation (acute) J45.901
status asthmaticus J45.902
bronchiectasis J47.9
with
exacerbation (acute) J47.1
lower respiratory infection J47.0
bronchitis (chronic) J44.9
emphysema J43.9
chronic J44.9
with
allergic alveolitis — *see* Pneumonitis, hypersensitivity
bronchiectasis J47.9
with
exacerbation (acute) J47.1
lower respiratory infection J47.0
due to
foreign body — *see* Foreign body, by site, causing asphyxia
inhalation of fumes or vapors J68.9
laryngospasm J38.5
ampulla of Vater K83.1
aortic (heart) (valve) — *see* Stenosis, aortic
aortoiliac I74.09
aqueduct of Sylvius G91.1
congenital Q03.0
with spina bifida — *see* Spina bifida, by site, with hydrocephalus
Arnold-Chiari — *see* Arnold-Chiari disease
artery (*see also* Atherosclerosis, artery) I70.9 ☑
basilar (complete) (partial) — *see* Occlusion, artery, basilar
carotid (complete) (partial) — *see* Occlusion, artery, carotid
cerebellar — *see* Occlusion, artery, cerebellar
cerebral (anterior) (middle) (posterior) — *see* Occlusion, artery, cerebral
precerebral — *see* Occlusion, artery, precerebral
renal N28.0
retinal NEC — *see* Occlusion, artery, retina
stent — *see* Restenosis, stent
vertebral (complete) (partial) — *see* Occlusion, artery, vertebral
band (intestinal) (*see also* Obstruction, intestine, specified NEC) K56.699
bile duct or passage (common) (hepatic) (noncalculous) K83.1
with calculus K80.51
congenital (causing jaundice) Q44.3
biliary (duct) (tract) K83.1
gallbladder K82.0
bladder-neck (acquired) N32.0
congenital Q64.31
due to hyperplasia (hypertrophy) of prostate — *see* Hyperplasia, prostate
bowel — *see* Obstruction, intestine
bronchus J98.09
canal, ear — *see* Stenosis, external ear canal
cardia K22.2
caval veins (inferior) (superior) I87.1
cecum — *see* Obstruction, intestine
circulatory I99.8
colon — *see* Obstruction, intestine
common duct (noncalculous) K83.1
coronary (artery) — *see* Occlusion, coronary
cystic duct (*see also* Obstruction, gallbladder)
with calculus K80.21
device, implant or graft (*see also* Complications, by site and type, mechanical) T85.698 ☑

Obstruction, obstructed, obstructive — *continued*
device, implant or graft (*see also* Complications, by site and type, mechanical) — *continued*
arterial graft NEC — *see* Complication, cardiovascular device, mechanical, vascular
catheter NEC T85.628 ☑
cystostomy T83.090 ☑
dialysis (renal) T82.49 ☑
intraperitoneal T85.691 ☑
Hopkins T83.098 ☑
ileostomy T83.098 ☑
infusion NEC T82.594 ☑
spinal (epidural) (subdural) T85.690 ☑
nephrostomy T83.092 ☑
urethral indwelling T83.091 ☑
urinary T83.098 ☑
urostomy T83.098 ☑
due to infection T85.79 ☑
gastrointestinal — *see* Complications, prosthetic device, mechanical, gastrointestinal device
genital NEC T83.498 ☑
intrauterine contraceptive device T83.39 ☑
penile prosthesis (cylinder) (implanted) (pump) (resevoir) T83.490 ☑
testicular prosthesis T83.491 ☑
heart NEC — *see* Complication, cardiovascular device, mechanical
joint prosthesis — *see* Complications, joint prosthesis, mechanical, specified NEC, by site
orthopedic NEC — *see* Complication, orthopedic, device, mechanical
specified NEC T85.628 ☑
urinary NEC (*see also* Complication, genitourinary, device, urinary, mechanical)
graft T83.29 ☑
vascular NEC — *see* Complication, cardiovascular device, mechanical
ventricular intracranial shunt T85.09 ☑
due to foreign body accidentally left in operative wound T81.529 ☑
duodenum K31.5
ejaculatory duct N50.89
esophagus K22.2
eustachian tube (complete) (partial) H68.10- ☑
cartilagenous (extrinsic) H68.13- ☑
intrinsic H68.12- ☑
osseous H68.11- ☑
fallopian tube (bilateral) N97.1
fecal K56.41
with hernia — *see* Hernia, by site, with obstruction
foramen of Monro (congenital) Q03.8
with spina bifida — *see* Spina bifida, by site, with hydrocephalus
foreign body — *see* Foreign body
gallbladder K82.0
with calculus, stones K80.21
congenital Q44.1
gastric outlet K31.1
gastrointestinal — *see* Obstruction, intestine
hepatic K76.89
duct (noncalculous) K83.1
ileum — *see* Obstruction, intestine
iliofemoral (artery) I74.5
intestine K56.609
with
adhesions (intestinal) (peritoneal) K56.50
complete K56.52
incomplete K56.51
partial K56.51
adynamic K56.0
by gallstone K56.3
complete K56.601
congenital (small) Q41.9
large Q42.9
specified part NEC Q42.8
incomplete K56.600
neurogenic K56.0
Hirschsprung's disease or megacolon Q43.1
newborn P76.9
due to
fecaliths P76.8
inspissated milk P76.2
meconium (plug) P76.0
in mucoviscidosis E84.11
specified NEC P76.8
partial K56.600
postoperative K91.30

Obstruction, obstructed, obstructive — *continued*
intestine — *continued*
postoperative — *continued*
complete K91.32
incomplete K91.31
partial K91.31
reflex K56.0
specified NEC K56.699
complete K56.691
incomplete K56.690
partial K56.690
volvulus K56.2
intracardiac ball valve prosthesis T82.09 ☑
jejunum — *see* Obstruction, intestine
joint prosthesis — *see* Complications, joint prosthesis, mechanical, specified NEC, by site
kidney (calices) N28.89
labor — *see* Delivery
lacrimal (passages) (duct)
by
dacryolith — *see* Dacryolith
stenosis — *see* Stenosis, lacrimal
congenital Q10.5
neonatal H04.53- ☑
lacrimonasal duct — *see* Obstruction, lacrimal
lacteal, with steatorrhea K90.2
laryngitis — *see* Laryngitis
larynx NEC J38.6
congenital Q31.8
lung J98.4
disease, chronic J44.9
lymphatic I89.0
meconium (plug)
newborn P76.0
due to fecaliths P76.0
in mucoviscidosis E84.11
mitral — *see* Stenosis, mitral
nasal J34.89
nasolacrimal duct (*see also* Obstruction, lacrimal)
congenital Q10.5
nasopharynx J39.2
nose J34.89
organ or site, congenital NEC — *see* Atresia, by site
pancreatic duct K86.89
parotid duct or gland K11.8
pelviureteral junction N13.5
with hydronephrosis N13.0
congenital Q62.39
pharynx J39.2
portal (circulation) (vein) I81
prostate (*see also* Hyperplasia, prostate)
valve (urinary) N32.0
pulmonary valve (heart) I37.0
pyelonephritis (chronic) N11.1
pylorus
adult K31.1
congenital or infantile Q40.0
rectosigmoid — *see* Obstruction, intestine
rectum K62.4
renal N28.89
outflow N13.8
pelvis, congenital Q62.39
respiratory J98.8
chronic J44.9
retinal (vessels) H34.9
salivary duct (any) K11.8
with calculus K11.5
sigmoid — *see* Obstruction, intestine
sinus (accessory) (nasal) J34.89
Stensen's duct K11.8
stomach NEC K31.89
acute K31.0
congenital Q40.2
due to pylorospasm K31.3
submandibular duct K11.8
submaxillary gland K11.8
with calculus K11.5
thoracic duct I89.0
thrombotic — *see* Thrombosis
trachea J39.8
tracheostomy airway J95.03
tricuspid (valve) — *see* Stenosis, tricuspid
upper respiratory, congenital Q34.8
ureter (functional) (pelvic junction) NEC N13.5
with
hydronephrosis N13.1
with infection N13.6
pyelonephritis (chronic) N11.1

☑ **Additional Character Required — Refer to the Tabular List for Character Selection**   ⩗ **Subterms under main terms may continue to next column or page**

Observation — Obstruction, obstructed, obstructive

Obstruction, obstructed, obstructive — *continued*
  ureter — *continued*
    congenital Q62.39
    due to calculus — *see* Calculus, ureter
  urethra NEC N36.8
    congenital Q64.39
  urinary (moderate) N13.9
    due to hyperplasia (hypertrophy) of prostate —
      see Hyperplasia, prostate
    organ or tract (lower) N13.9
    prostatic valve N32.0
    specified NEC N13.8
  uropathy N13.9
  uterus N85.8
  vagina N89.5
  valvular — *see* Endocarditis
  vein, venous I87.1
    caval (inferior) (superior) I87.1
    thrombotic — *see* Thrombosis
  vena cava (inferior) (superior) I87.1
  vesical NEC N32.0
  vesicourethral orifice N32.0
    congenital Q64.31
  vessel NEC I99.8
    stent — *see* Restenosis, stent
Obturator — *see* condition
Occlusal wear, teeth K03.0
Occlusio pupillae — *see* Membrane, pupillary
Occlusion, occluded
  anus K62.4
    congenital Q42.3
      with fistula Q42.2
  aortoiliac (chronic) I74.09
  aqueduct of Sylvius G91.1
    congenital Q03.0
      with spina bifida — *see* Spina bifida, by site,
        with hydrocephalus
  artery (*see also* Atherosclerosis, artery) I70.9 ☑
    auditory, internal I65.8
    basilar I65.1
      with
        infarction I63.22
          due to
            embolism I63.12
            thrombosis I63.02
    brain or cerebral I66.9
      with infarction (due to) I63.5- ☑
        embolism I63.4- ☑
        thrombosis I63.3- ☑
    carotid I65.2- ☑
      with
        infarction I63.23- ☑
          due to
            embolism I63.13- ☑
            thrombosis I63.03- ☑
    cerebellar (anterior inferior) (posterior inferior)
      (superior) I66.3
      with infarction I63.54- ☑
        due to
          embolism I63.44- ☑
          thrombosis I63.34- ☑
    cerebral I66.9
      with infarction I63.50
        due to
          embolism I63.40
            specified NEC I63.49
          thrombosis I63.30
            specified NEC I63.39
      anterior I66.1- ☑
        with infarction I63.52- ☑
          due to
            embolism I63.42- ☑
            thrombosis I63.32- ☑
      middle I66.0- ☑
        with infarction I63.51- ☑
          due to
            embolism I63.41- ☑
            thrombosis I63.31- ☑
      posterior I66.2- ☑
        with infarction I63.53- ☑
          due to
            embolism I63.43- ☑
            thrombosis I63.33- ☑
      specified NEC I66.8
        with infarction I63.59
          due to
            embolism I63.4- ☑

Occlusion, occluded — *continued*
  artery (*see also* Atherosclerosis, artery) — *continued*
    cerebral — *continued*
      specified — *continued*
        with infarction — *continued*
          due to — *continued*
            thrombosis I63.3- ☑
    choroidal (anterior) — *see* Occlusion, artery, pre-
      cerebral, specified NEC
    communicating posterior — *see* Occlusion, artery,
      precerebral, specified NEC
    complete
      coronary I25.82
      extremities I70.92
    coronary (acute) (thrombotic) (without myocardial
      infarction) I24.0
      with myocardial infarction — *see* Infarction,
        myocardium
      chronic total I25.82
      complete I25.82
      healed or old I25.2
      total (chronic) I25.82
    hypophyseal — *see* Occlusion, artery, precerebral,
      specified NEC
    iliac I74.5
    lower extremities due to stenosis or stricture I77.1
    mesenteric (embolic) (thrombotic) (*see also* Infarct,
      intestine) K55.069
    perforating — *see* Occlusion, artery, cerebral,
      specified NEC
    peripheral I77.9
      thrombotic or embolic I74.4
    pontine — *see* Occlusion, artery, precerebral,
      specified NEC
    precerebral I65.9
      with infarction I63.20
        due to
          embolism I63.10
            specified NEC I63.19
          thrombosis I63.00
            specified NEC I63.09
        specified NEC I63.29
      basilar — *see* Occlusion, artery, basilar
      carotid — *see* Occlusion, artery, carotid
      puerperal O88.23
      specified NEC I65.8
        with infarction I63.29
          due to
            embolism I63.19
            thrombosis I63.09
      vertebral — *see* Occlusion, artery, vertebral
    renal N28.0
    retinal
      branch H34.23- ☑
      central H34.1- ☑
      partial H34.21- ☑
      transient H34.0- ☑
    spinal — *see* Occlusion, artery, precerebral, verte-
      bral
    total (chronic)
      coronary I25.82
      extremities I70.92
    vertebral I65.0- ☑
      with
        infarction I63.21- ☑
          due to
            embolism I63.11- ☑
            thrombosis I63.01- ☑
  basilar artery — *see* Occlusion, artery, basilar
  bile duct (common) (hepatic) (noncalculous) K83.1
  bowel — *see* Obstruction, intestine
  carotid (artery) (common) (internal) — *see* Occlusion,
    artery, carotid
  centric (of teeth) M26.59
    maximum intercuspation discrepancy M26.55
  cerebellar (artery) — *see* Occlusion, artery, cerebellar
  cerebral (artery) — *see* Occlusion, artery, cerebral
  cerebrovascular (*see also* Occlusion, artery, cerebral)
    with infarction I63.5- ☑
  cervical canal — *see* Stricture, cervix
  cervix (uteri) — *see* Stricture, cervix
  choanal Q30.0
  choroidal (artery) — *see* Occlusion, artery, precerebral,
    specified NEC
  colon — *see* Obstruction, intestine
  communicating posterior artery — *see* Occlusion,
    artery, precerebral, specified NEC

Occlusion, occluded — *continued*
  coronary (artery) (vein) (thrombotic) (*see also* Infarct,
    myocardium)
    chronic total I25.82
    healed or old I25.2
    not resulting in infarction I24.0
    total (chronic) I25.82
  cystic duct — *see* Obstruction, gallbladder
  embolic — *see* Embolism
  fallopian tube N97.1
    congenital Q50.6
  gallbladder (*see also* Obstruction, gallbladder)
    congenital (causing jaundice) Q44.1
  gingiva, traumatic K06.2
  hymen N89.6
    congenital Q52.3
  hypophyseal (artery) — *see* Occlusion, artery, precere-
    bral, specified NEC
  iliac artery I74.5
  intestine — *see* Obstruction, intestine
  lacrimal passages — *see* Obstruction, lacrimal
  lung J98.4
  lymph or lymphatic channel I89.0
  mammary duct N64.89
  mesenteric artery (embolic) (thrombotic) (*see also* In-
    farct, intestine) K55.069
  nose J34.89
    congenital Q30.0
  organ or site, congenital NEC — *see* Atresia, by site
  oviduct N97.1
    congenital Q50.6
  peripheral arteries
    due to stricture or stenosis I77.1
    upper extremity I74.2
  pontine (artery) — *see* Occlusion, artery, precerebral,
    specified NEC
  posterior lingual, of mandibular teeth M26.29
  precerebral artery — *see* Occlusion, artery, precerebral
  punctum lacrimale — *see* Obstruction, lacrimal
  pupil — *see* Membrane, pupillary
  pylorus, adult (*see also* Stricture, pylorus) K31.1
  renal artery N28.0
  retina, retinal
    artery — *see* Occlusion, artery, retinal
    vein (central) H34.81- ☑
      engorgement H34.82- ☑
      tributary H34.83- ☑
    vessels H34.9
  spinal artery — *see* Occlusion, artery, precerebral,
    vertebral
  teeth (mandibular) (posterior lingual) M26.29
  thoracic duct I89.0
  thrombotic — *see* Thrombosis, artery
  traumatic
    edentulous (alveolar) ridge K06.2
    gingiva K06.2
    periodontal K05.5
  tubal N97.1
  ureter (complete) (partial) N13.5
    congenital Q62.10
  ureteropelvic junction N13.5
    congenital Q62.11
  ureterovesical orifice N13.5
    congenital Q62.12
  urethra — *see* Stricture, urethra
  uterus N85.8
  vagina N89.5
  vascular NEC I99.8
  vein — *see* Thrombosis
    retinal — *see* Occlusion, retinal, vein
  vena cava (inferior) (superior) — *see* Embolism, vena
    cava
  ventricle (brain) NEC G91.1
  vertebral (artery) — *see* Occlusion, artery, vertebral
  vessel (blood) I99.8
  vulva N90.5
Occult
  blood in feces (stools) R19.5
Occupational
  problems NEC Z56.89
Ochlophobia — *see* Agoraphobia
Ochronosis (endogenous) E70.29
Ocular muscle — *see* condition
Oculogyric crisis or disturbance H51.8
  psychogenic F45.8
Oculomotor syndrome H51.9
Oculopathy
  syphilitic NEC A52.71

Oculopathy — *continued*
  syphilitic — *continued*
    congenital
      early A50.01
      late A50.30
    early (secondary) A51.43
    late A52.71
Oddi's sphincter spasm K83.4
Odontalgia K08.89
Odontoameloblastoma — *see* Cyst, calcifying odontogenic
Odontoclasia K03.89
Odontodysplasia, regional K00.4
Odontogenesis imperfecta K00.5
Odontoma (ameloblastic) (complex) (compound) (fibroameloblastic) — *see* Cyst, calcifying odontogenic
Odontomyelitis (closed) (open) K04.01
  irreversible K04.02
  reversible K04.01
Odontorrhagia K08.89
Odontosarcoma, ameloblastic C41.1
  upper jaw (bone) C41.0
Oestriasis — *see* Myiasis
Oguchi's disease H53.63
Ohara's disease — *see* Tularemia
OHS (obesity hypoventilation syndrome) E66.2
Oidiomycosis — *see* Candidiasis
Oidium albicans infection — *see* Candidiasis
Old age (without mention of debility) R54
  dementia F03 ☑
Old (previous) **myocardial infarction** I25.2
Olfactory — *see* condition
Oligemia — *see* Anemia
Oligoastrocytoma
  specified site — *see* Neoplasm, malignant, by site
  unspecified site C71.9
Oligocythemia D64.9
Oligodendroblastoma
  specified site — *see* Neoplasm, malignant
  unspecified site C71.9
Oligodendroglioma
  anaplastic type
    specified site — *see* Neoplasm, malignant, by site
    unspecified site C71.9
  specified site — *see* Neoplasm, malignant, by site
  unspecified site C71.9
Oligodontia — *see* Anodontia
Oligoencephalon Q02
Oligohidrosis L74.4
Oligohydramnios O41.0- ☑
Oligohydrosis L74.4
Oligomenorrhea N91.5
  primary N91.3
  secondary N91.4
Oligophrenia (*see also* Disability, intellectual)
  phenylpyruvic E70.0
Oligospermia N46.11
  due to
    drug therapy N46.121
    efferent duct obstruction N46.123
    infection N46.122
    radiation N46.124
    specified cause NEC N46.129
    systemic disease N46.125
Oligotrichia — *see* Alopecia
Oliguria R34
  postprocedural N99.0
  with, complicating or following ectopic or molar pregnancy O08.4
Ollier's disease Q78.4
Omenotocele — *see* Hernia, abdomen, specified site NEC
Omentitis — *see* Peritonitis
Omentum, omental — *see* condition
Omphalitis (congenital) (newborn) P38.9
  with mild hemorrhage P38.1
  without hemorrhage P38.9
  not of newborn L08.82
  tetanus A33
Omphalocele Q79.2
Omphalomesenteric duct, persistent Q43.0
Omphalorrhagia, newborn P51.9
Omsk hemorrhagic fever A98.1
Onanism (excessive) F98.8
Onchocerciasis, onchocercosis B73.1
  with
    eye disease B73.00

Onchocerciasis, onchocercosis — *continued*
  with — *continued*
    eye disease — *continued*
      endophthalmitis B73.01
      eyelid B73.09
      glaucoma B73.02
      specified NEC B73.09
  eyelid B73.09
  eye NEC B73.09
Oncocytoma — *see* Neoplasm, benign, by site
Oncovirus, as cause of disease classified elsewhere B97.32
Ondine's curse — *see* Apnea, sleep
Oneirophrenia F23
Onychauxis L60.2
  congenital Q84.5
Onychia (*see also* Cellulitis, digit)
  with lymphangitis — *see* Lymphangitis, acute, digit
  candidal B37.2
  dermatophytic B35.1
Onychitis (*see also* Cellulitis, digit)
  with lymphangitis — *see* Lymphangitis, acute, digit
Onychocryptosis L60.0
Onychodystrophy L60.3
  congenital Q84.6
Onychogryphosis, onychogryposis L60.2
Onycholysis L60.1
Onychomadesis L60.8
Onychomalacia L60.3
Onychomycosis (finger) (toe) B35.1
Onycho-osteodysplasia Q87.2
Onychophagia F98.8
Onychophosis L60.8
Onychoptosis L60.8
Onychorrhexis L60.3
  congenital Q84.6
Onychoschizia L60.3
Onyxis (finger) (toe) L60.0
Onyxitis (*see also* Cellulitis, digit)
  with lymphangitis — *see* Lymphangitis, acute, digit
Oophoritis (cystic) (infectional) (interstitial) N70.92
  with salpingitis N70.93
  acute N70.02
    with salpingitis N70.03
  chronic N70.12
    with salpingitis N70.13
  complicating abortion — *see* Abortion, by type, complicated by, oophoritis
Oophorocele N83.4- ☑
Opacity, opacities
  cornea H17.- ☑
    central H17.1- ☑
    congenital Q13.3
    degenerative — *see* Degeneration, cornea
    hereditary — *see* Dystrophy, cornea
    inflammatory — *see* Keratitis
    minor H17.81- ☑
    peripheral H17.82- ☑
    sequelae of trachoma (healed) B94.0
    specified NEC H17.89
  enamel (teeth) (fluoride) (nonfluoride) K00.3
  lens — *see* Cataract
  snowball — *see* Deposit, crystalline
  vitreous (humor) NEC H43.39- ☑
    congenital Q14.0
    membranes and strands H43.31- ☑
Opalescent dentin (hereditary) K00.5
Open, opening
  abnormal, organ or site, congenital — *see* Imperfect, closure
  angle with
    borderline
      findings
        high risk H40.02- ☑
        low risk H40.01- ☑
      intraocular pressure H40.00- ☑
    cupping of discs H40.01- ☑
    glaucoma (primary) — *see* Glaucoma, open angle
  bite
    anterior M26.220
    posterior M26.221
  false — *see* Imperfect, closure
  margin on tooth restoration K08.51
  restoration margins of tooth K08.51
  wound — *see* Wound, open
Operational fatigue F48.8
Operative — *see* condition

Operculitis — *see* Periodontitis
Operculum — *see* Break, retina
Ophiasis L63.2
Ophthalmia (*see also* Conjunctivitis) H10.9
  actinic rays — *see* Photokeratitis
  allergic (acute) — *see* Conjunctivitis, acute, atopic
  blennorrhagic (gonococcal) (neonatorum) A54.31
  diphtheritic A36.86
  Egyptian A71.1
  electrica — *see* Photokeratitis
  gonococcal (neonatorum) A54.31
  metastatic — *see* Endophthalmitis, purulent
  migraine — *see* Migraine, ophthalmoplegic
  neonatorum, newborn P39.1
    gonococcal A54.31
  nodosa H16.24- ☑
  purulent — *see* Conjunctivitis, acute, mucopurulent
  spring — *see* Conjunctivitis, acute, atopic
  sympathetic — *see* Uveitis, sympathetic
Ophthalmitis — *see* Ophthalmia
Ophthalmocele (congenital) Q15.8
Ophthalmoneuromyelitis G36.0
Ophthalmoplegia (*see also* Strabismus, paralytic)
  anterior internuclear — *see* Ophthalmoplegia, internuclear
  ataxia-areflexia G61.0
  diabetic — *see* E08-E13 with .39
  exophthalmic E05.00
    with thyroid storm E05.01
  external H49.88- ☑
    progressive H49.4- ☑
      with pigmentary retinopathy — *see* Kearns-Sayre syndrome
    total H49.3- ☑
  internal (complete) (total) H52.51- ☑
  internuclear H51.2- ☑
  migraine — *see* Migraine, ophthalmoplegic
  Parinaud's H49.88- ☑
  progressive external — *see* Ophthalmoplegia, external, progressive
  supranuclear, progressive G23.1
  total (external) — *see* Ophthalmoplegia, external, total
Opioid(s)
  abuse — *see* Abuse, drug, opioids
  dependence — *see* Dependence, drug, opioids
  induced, without use disorder
    anxiety disorder F11.988
    delirium F11.921
    depressive disorder F11.94
    sexual dysfunction F11.981
    sleep disorder F11.982
Opisthognathism M26.09
Opisthorchiasis (felineus) (viverrini) B66.0
Opitz' disease D73.2
Opiumism — *see* Dependence, drug, opioid
Oppenheim's disease G70.2
Oppenheim-Urbach disease (necrobiosis lipoidica diabeticorum) — *see* E08-E13 with .620
Optic nerve — *see* condition
Orbit — *see* condition
Orchioblastoma C62.9- ☑
Orchitis (gangrenous) (nonspecific) (septic) (suppurative) N45.2
  blennorrhagic (gonococcal) (acute) (chronic) A54.23
  chlamydial A56.19
  filarial (*see also* Infestation, filarial) B74.9 [N51]
  gonococcal (acute) (chronic) A54.23
  mumps B26.0
  syphilitic A52.76
  tuberculous A18.15
Orf (virus disease) B08.02
Organic (*see also* condition)
  brain syndrome F09
  heart — *see* Disease, heart
  mental disorder F09
  psychosis F09
Orgasm
  anejaculatory N53.13
Oriental
  bilharziasis B65.2
  schistosomiasis B65.2
Orifice — *see* condition
Origin of both great vessels from right ventricle Q20.1
Ormond's disease (with ureteral obstruction) N13.5
  with infection N13.6
Ornithine metabolism disorder E72.4

Ornithinemia (Type I) (Type II) E72.4
Ornithosis A70
Orotaciduria, oroticaciduria (congenital) (hereditary) (pyrimidine deficiency) E79.8
  anemia D53.0
Orthodontics
  adjustment Z46.4
  fitting Z46.4
Orthopnea R06.01
Orthopoxvirus B08.09
  specified NEC B08.09
Os, uterus — see condition
Osgood-Schlatter disease or osteochondrosis — see Osteochondrosis, juvenile, tibia
Osler (-Weber)-**Rendu disease** I78.0
Osler's nodes I33.0
Osmidrosis L75.0
Osseous — see condition
Ossification
  artery — see Arteriosclerosis
  auricle (ear) — see Disorder, pinna, specified type NEC
  bronchial J98.09
  cardiac — see Degeneration, myocardial
  cartilage (senile) — see Disorder, cartilage, specified type NEC
  coronary (artery) — see Disease, heart, ischemic, atherosclerotic
  diaphragm J98.6
  ear, middle — see Otosclerosis
  falx cerebri G96.19
  fontanel, premature Q75.0
  heart (see also Degeneration, myocardial)
    valve — see Endocarditis
  larynx J38.7
  ligament — see Disorder, tendon, specified type NEC
    posterior longitudinal — see Spondylopathy, specified NEC
  meninges (cerebral) (spinal) G96.19
  multiple, eccentric centers — see Disorder, bone, development or growth
  muscle (see also Calcification, muscle)
    due to burns — see Myositis, ossificans, in, burns
    paralytic — see Myositis, ossificans, in, quadriplegia
    progressive — see Myositis, ossificans, progressiva
    specified NEC M61.50
      ankle M61.57- ☑
      foot M61.57- ☑
      forearm M61.53- ☑
      hand M61.54- ☑
      lower leg M61.56- ☑
      multiple sites M61.59
      pelvic region M61.55- ☑
      shoulder region M61.51- ☑
      specified site NEC M61.58
      thigh M61.55- ☑
      upper arm M61.52- ☑
    traumatic — see Myositis, ossificans, traumatica
  myocardium, myocardial — see Degeneration, myocardial
  penis N48.89
  periarticular — see Disorder, joint, specified type NEC
  pinna — see Disorder, pinna, specified type NEC
  rider's bone — see Ossification, muscle, specified NEC
  sclera H15.89
  subperiosteal, post-traumatic M89.8X- ☑
  tendon — see Disorder, tendon, specified type NEC
  trachea J39.8
  tympanic membrane — see Disorder, tympanic membrane, specified NEC
  vitreous (humor) — see Deposit, crystalline
Osteitis (see also Osteomyelitis)
  alveolar M27.3
  condensans M85.30
    ankle M85.37- ☑
    foot M85.37- ☑
    forearm M85.33- ☑
    hand M85.34- ☑
    lower leg M85.36- ☑
    multiple site M85.39
    neck M85.38
    rib M85.38
    shoulder M85.31- ☑
    skull M85.38
    specified site NEC M85.38
    thigh M85.35- ☑
    toe M85.37- ☑
    upper arm M85.32- ☑

Osteitis — continued
  condensans — continued
    vertebra M85.38
  deformans M88.9
    in (due to)
      malignant neoplasm of bone C41.9 [M90.60]
      neoplastic disease (see also Neoplasm) D49.9 [M90.60]
        carpus D49.9 [M90.64-] ☑
        clavicle D49.9 [M90.61-] ☑
        femur D49.9 [M90.65-] ☑
        fibula D49.9 [M90.66-] ☑
        finger D49.9 [M90.64-] ☑
        humerus D49.9 [M90.62-] ☑
        ilium D49.9 [M90.65-] ☑
        ischium D49.9 [M90.65-] ☑
        metacarpus D49.9 [M90.64-] ☑
        metatarsus D49.9 [M90.67-] ☑
        multiple sites D49.9 [M90.69]
        neck D49.9 [M90.68]
        radius D49.9 [M90.63-] ☑
        rib D49.9 [M90.68]
        scapula D49.9 [M90.61-] ☑
        skull D49.9 [M90.68]
        tarsus D49.9 [M90.67-] ☑
        tibia D49.9 [M90.66-] ☑
        toe D49.9 [M90.67-] ☑
        ulna D49.9 [M90.63-] ☑
        vertebra D49.9 [M90.68]
    skull M88.0
    specified NEC — see Paget's disease, bone, by site
    vertebra M88.1
  due to yaws A66.6
  fibrosa NEC — see Cyst, bone, by site
    circumscripta — see Dysplasia, fibrous, bone NEC
    cystica (generalisata) E21.0
    disseminata Q78.1
    osteoplastica E21.0
  fragilitans Q78.0
  Garr's (sclerosing) — see Osteomyelitis, specified type NEC
  jaw (acute) (chronic) (lower) (suppurative) (upper) M27.2
  parathyroid E21.0
  petrous bone (acute) (chronic) — see Petrositis
  sclerotic, nonsuppurative — see Osteomyelitis, specified type NEC
  tuberculosa A18.09
    cystica D86.89
    multiplex cystoides D86.89
Osteoarthritis M19.90
  ankle M19.07- ☑
  elbow M19.02- ☑
  foot joint M19.07- ☑
  generalized M15.9
    erosive M15.4
    primary M15.0
    specified NEC M15.8
  hand joint M19.04- ☑
    first carpometacarpal joint M18.9
  hip M16.1- ☑
    bilateral M16.0
    due to hip dysplasia (unilateral) M16.3- ☑
      bilateral M16.2
  interphalangeal
    distal (Heberden) M15.1
    proximal (Bouchard) M15.2
  knee M17.1- ☑
    bilateral M17.0
  post-traumatic NEC M19.92
    ankle M19.17- ☑
    elbow M19.12- ☑
    foot joint M19.17- ☑
    hand joint M19.14- ☑
      first carpometacarpal joint M18.3- ☑
        bilateral M18.2
    hip M16.5- ☑
      bilateral M16.4
    knee M17.3- ☑
      bilateral M17.2
    shoulder M19.11- ☑
    wrist M19.13- ☑
  primary M19.91
    ankle M19.07- ☑
    elbow M19.02- ☑
    foot joint M19.07- ☑
    hand joint M19.04- ☑

Osteoarthritis — continued
  primary — continued
    hand joint — continued
      first carpometacarpal joint M18.1- ☑
        bilateral M18.0
    hip M16.1- ☑
      bilateral M16.0
    knee M17.1- ☑
      bilateral M17.0
    shoulder M19.01- ☑
    spine — see Spondylosis
    wrist M19.03- ☑
  secondary M19.93
    ankle M19.27- ☑
    elbow M19.22- ☑
    foot joint M19.27- ☑
    hand joint M19.24- ☑
      first carpometacarpal joint M18.5- ☑
        bilateral M18.4
    hip M16.7
      bilateral M16.6
    knee M17.5
      bilateral M17.4
    multiple M15.3
    shoulder M19.21- ☑
    spine — see Spondylosis
    wrist M19.23- ☑
  shoulder M19.01- ☑
  spine — see Spondylosis
  wrist M19.03- ☑
Osteoarthropathy (hypertrophic) M19.90
  ankle — see Osteoarthritis, primary, ankle
  elbow — see Osteoarthritis, primary, elbow
  foot joint — see Osteoarthritis, primary, foot
  hand joint — see Osteoarthritis, primary, hand joint
  knee joint — see Osteoarthritis, primary, knee
  multiple site — see Osteoarthritis, primary, multiple joint
  pulmonary (see also Osteoarthropathy, specified type NEC)
    hypertrophic — see Osteoarthropathy, hypertrophic, specified type NEC
  secondary — see Osteoarthropathy, specified type NEC
  secondary hypertrophic — see Osteoarthropathy, specified type NEC
  shoulder — see Osteoarthritis, primary, shoulder
  specified joint NEC — see Osteoarthritis, primary, specified joint NEC
  specified type NEC M89.40
    carpus M89.44- ☑
    clavicle M89.41- ☑
    femur M89.45- ☑
    fibula M89.46- ☑
    finger M89.44- ☑
    humerus M89.42- ☑
    ilium M89.459
    ischium M89.459
    metacarpus M89.44- ☑
    metatarsus M89.47- ☑
    multiple sites M89.49
    neck M89.48
    radius M89.43- ☑
    rib M89.48
    scapula M89.41- ☑
    skull M89.48
    tarsus M89.47- ☑
    tibia M89.46- ☑
    toe M89.47- ☑
    ulna M89.43- ☑
    vertebra M89.48
  spine — see Spondylosis
  wrist — see Osteoarthritis, primary, wrist
Osteoarthrosis (degenerative) (hypertrophic) (joint) (see also Osteoarthritis)
  deformans alkaptonurica E70.29 [M36.8]
  erosive M15.4
  generalized M15.9
    primary M15.0
  polyarticular M15.9
  spine — see Spondylosis
Osteoblastoma — see Neoplasm, bone, benign
  aggressive — see Neoplasm, bone, uncertain behavior
Osteochondritis (see also Osteochondropathy, by site)
  Brailsford's — see Osteochondrosis, juvenile, radius
  dissecans M93.20
    ankle M93.27- ☑

Osteochondritis — *continued*
dissecans — *continued*
elbow M93.22- ☑
foot M93.27- ☑
hand M93.24- ☑
hip M93.25- ☑
knee M93.26- ☑
multiple sites M93.29
shoulder joint M93.21- ☑
specified site NEC M93.28
wrist M93.23- ☑
juvenile M92.9
patellar — *see* Osteochondrosis, juvenile, patella
syphilitic (congenital) (early) A50.02 [M90.80]
ankle A50.02 [M90.87-] ☑
elbow A50.02 [M90.82-] ☑
foot A50.02 [M90.87-] ☑
forearm A50.02 [M90.83-] ☑
hand A50.02 [M90.84-] ☑
hip A50.02 [M90.85-] ☑
knee A50.02 [M90.86-] ☑
multiple sites A50.02 [M90.89]
shoulder joint A50.02 [M90.81-] ☑
specified site NEC A50.02 [M90.88]
Osteochondroarthrosis deformans endemica — *see* Disease, Kaschin-Beck
Osteochondrodysplasia Q78.9
with defects of growth of tubular bones and spine Q77.9
specified NEC Q77.8
specified NEC Q78.8
Osteochondrodystrophy E78.9
Osteochondrolysis — *see* Osteochondritis, dissecans
Osteochondroma — *see* Neoplasm, bone, benign
Osteochondromatosis D48.0
syndrome Q78.4
Osteochondromyxosarcoma — *see* Neoplasm, bone, malignant
Osteochondropathy M93.90
ankle M93.97- ☑
elbow M93.92- ☑
foot M93.97- ☑
hand M93.94- ☑
hip M93.95- ☑
Kienböck's disease of adults M93.1
knee M93.96- ☑
multiple joints M93.99
osteochondritis dissecans — *see* Osteochondritis, dissecans
osteochondrosis — *see* Osteochondrosis
shoulder region M93.91- ☑
slipped upper femoral epiphysis — *see* Slipped, epiphysis, upper femoral
specified joint NEC M93.98
specified type NEC M93.80
ankle M93.87- ☑
elbow M93.82- ☑
foot M93.87- ☑
hand M93.84- ☑
hip M93.85- ☑
knee M93.86- ☑
multiple joints M93.89
shoulder region M93.81- ☑
specified joint NEC M93.88
wrist M93.83- ☑
syphilitic, congenital
early A50.02 [M90.80]
late A50.56 [M90.80]
wrist M93.93- ☑
Osteochondrosarcoma — *see* Neoplasm, bone, malignant
Osteochondrosis (*see also* Osteochondropathy, by site)
acetabulum (juvenile) M91.0
adult — *see* Osteochondropathy, specified type NEC, by site
astragalus (juvenile) — *see* Osteochondrosis, juvenile, tarsus
Blount's — *see* Osteochondrosis, juvenile, tibia
Buchanan's M91.0
Burns' — *see* Osteochondrosis, juvenile, ulna
calcaneus (juvenile) — *see* Osteochondrosis, juvenile, tarsus
capitular epiphysis (femur) (juvenile) — *see* Legg-Calvé-Perthes disease
carpal (juvenile) (lunate) (scaphoid) — *see* Osteochondrosis, juvenile, hand, carpal lunate
adult M93.1

Osteochondrosis — *continued*
coxae juvenilis — *see* Legg-Calvé-Perthes disease
deformans juvenilis, coxae — *see* Legg-Calvé-Perthes disease
Diaz's — *see* Osteochondrosis, juvenile, tarsus
dissecans (knee) (shoulder) — *see* Osteochondritis, dissecans
femoral capital epiphysis (juvenile) — *see* Legg-Calvé-Perthes disease
femur (head), juvenile — *see* Legg-Calvé-Perthes disease
fibula (juvenile) — *see* Osteochondrosis, juvenile, fibula
foot NEC (juvenile) M92.8
Freiberg's — *see* Osteochondrosis, juvenile, metatarsus
Haas' (juvenile) — *see* Osteochondrosis, juvenile, humerus
Haglund's — *see* Osteochondrosis, juvenile, tarsus
hip (juvenile) — *see* Legg-Calvé-Perthes disease
humerus (capitulum) (head) (juvenile) — *see* Osteochondrosis, juvenile, humerus
ilium, iliac crest (juvenile) M91.0
ischiopubic synchondrosis M91.0
Iselin's — *see* Osteochondrosis, juvenile, metatarsus
juvenile, juvenilis M92.9
after congenital dislocation of hip reduction — *see* Osteochondrosis, juvenile, hip, specified NEC
arm — *see* Osteochondrosis, juvenile, upper limb NEC
capitular epiphysis (femur) — *see* Legg-Calvé-Perthes disease
clavicle, sternal epiphysis — *see* Osteochondrosis, juvenile, upper limb NEC
coxae — *see* Legg-Calvé-Perthes disease
deformans M92.9
fibula M92.5- ☑
foot NEC M92.8
hand M92.20- ☑
carpal lunate M92.21- ☑
metacarpal head M92.22- ☑
specified site NEC M92.29- ☑
head of femur — *see* Legg-Calvé-Perthes disease
hip and pelvis M91.9- ☑
coxa plana — *see* Coxa, plana
femoral head — *see* Legg-Calvé-Perthes disease
pelvis M91.0
pseudocoxalgia — *see* Pseudocoxalgia
specified NEC M91.8- ☑
humerus M92.0- ☑
limb
lower NEC M92.8
upper NEC — *see* Osteochondrosis, juvenile, upper limb NEC
medial cuneiform bone — *see* Osteochondrosis, juvenile, tarsus
metatarsus M92.7- ☑
patella M92.4- ☑
radius M92.1- ☑
specified site NEC M92.8
spine M42.00
cervical region M42.02
cervicothoracic region M42.03
lumbar region M42.06
lumbosacral region M42.07
multiple sites M42.09
occipito-atlanto-axial region M42.01
sacrococcygeal region M42.08
thoracic region M42.04
thoracolumbar region M42.05
tarsus M92.6- ☑
tibia M92.5- ☑
ulna M92.1- ☑
upper limb NEC M92.3- ☑
vertebra (body) (epiphyseal plates) (Calvé's) (Scheuermann's) — *see* Osteochondrosis, juvenile, spine
Kienböck's — *see* Osteochondrosis, juvenile, hand, carpal lunate
adult M93.1
Köhler's
patellar — *see* Osteochondrosis, juvenile, patella
tarsal navicular — *see* Osteochondrosis, juvenile, tarsus
Legg-Perthes (-Calvé)(-Waldenström) — *see* Legg-Calvé-Perthes disease
limb
lower NEC (juvenile) M92.8

Osteochondrosis — *continued*
limb — *continued*
upper NEC (juvenile) — *see* Osteochondrosis, juvenile, upper limb NEC
lunate bone (carpal) (juvenile) (*see also* Osteochondrosis, juvenile, hand, carpal lunate)
adult M93.1
Mauclaire's — *see* Osteochondrosis, juvenile, hand, metacarpal
metacarpal (head) (juvenile) — *see* Osteochondrosis, juvenile, hand, metacarpal
metatarsus (fifth) (head) (juvenile) (second) — *see* Osteochondrosis, juvenile, metatarsus
navicular (juvenile) — *see* Osteochondrosis, juvenile, tarsus
os
calcis (juvenile) — *see* Osteochondrosis, juvenile, tarsus
tibiale externum (juvenile) — *see* Osteochondrosis, juvenile, tarsus
Osgood-Schlatter — *see* Osteochondrosis, juvenile, tibia
Panner's — *see* Osteochondrosis, juvenile, humerus
patellar center (juvenile) (primary) (secondary) — *see* Osteochondrosis, juvenile, patella
pelvis (juvenile) M91.0
Pierson's M91.0
radius (head) (juvenile) — *see* Osteochondrosis, juvenile, radius
Scheuermann's — *see* Osteochondrosis, juvenile, spine
Sever's — *see* Osteochondrosis, juvenile, tarsus
Sinding-Larsen — *see* Osteochondrosis, juvenile, patella
spine M42.9
adult M42.10
cervical region M42.12
cervicothoracic region M42.13
lumbar region M42.16
lumbosacral region M42.17
multiple sites M42.19
occipito-atlanto-axial region M42.11
sacrococcygeal region M42.18
thoracic region M42.14
thoracolumbar region M42.15
juvenile — *see* Osteochondrosis, juvenile, spine
symphysis pubis (juvenile) M91.0
syphilitic (congenital) A50.02
talus (juvenile) — *see* Osteochondrosis, juvenile, tarsus
tarsus (navicular) (juvenile) — *see* Osteochondrosis, juvenile, tarsus
tibia (proximal) (tubercle) (juvenile) — *see* Osteochondrosis, juvenile, tibia
tuberculous — *see* Tuberculosis, bone
ulna (lower) (juvenile) — *see* Osteochondrosis, juvenile, ulna
van Neck's M91.0
vertebral — *see* Osteochondrosis, spine
Osteoclastoma D48.0
malignant — *see* Neoplasm, bone, malignant
Osteodynia — *see* Disorder, bone, specified type NEC
Osteodystrophy Q78.9
azotemic N25.0
congenital Q78.9
parathyroid, secondary E21.1
renal N25.0
Osteofibroma — *see* Neoplasm, bone, benign
Osteofibrosarcoma — *see* Neoplasm, bone, malignant
Osteogenesis imperfecta Q78.0
Osteogenic — *see* condition
Osteolysis M89.50
carpus M89.54- ☑
clavicle M89.51- ☑
femur M89.55- ☑
fibula M89.56- ☑
finger M89.54- ☑
humerus M89.52- ☑
ilium M89.559
ischium M89.559
joint prosthesis (periprosthetic) — *see* Complications, joint prosthesis, mechanical, periprosthetic, osteolysis, by site
metacarpus M89.54- ☑
metatarsus M89.57- ☑
multiple sites M89.59
neck M89.58
periprosthetic — *see* Complications, joint prosthesis, mechanical, periprosthetic, osteolysis, by site

☑ **Additional Character Required — Refer to the Tabular List for Character Selection**   ▽ Subterms under main terms may continue to next column or page

Osteolysis — continued
  radius M89.53- ☑
  rib M89.58
  scapula M89.51- ☑
  skull M89.58
  tarsus M89.57- ☑
  tibia M89.56- ☑
  toe M89.57- ☑
  ulna M89.53- ☑
  vertebra M89.58
Osteoma (see also Neoplasm, bone, benign)
  osteoid (see also Neoplasm, bone, benign)
    giant — see Neoplasm, bone, benign
Osteomalacia M83.9
  adult M83.9
    drug-induced NEC M83.5
    due to
      malabsorption (postsurgical) M83.2
      malnutrition M83.3
    specified NEC M83.8
  aluminium-induced M83.4
  infantile — see Rickets
  juvenile — see Rickets
  oncogenic E83.89
  pelvis M83.8
  puerperal M83.0
  senile M83.1
  vitamin-D-resistant in adults E83.31 [M90.8-] ☑
    carpus E83.31 [M90.84-] ☑
    clavicle E83.31 [M90.81-] ☑
    femur E83.31 [M90.85-] ☑
    fibula E83.31 [M90.86-] ☑
    finger E83.31 [M90.84-] ☑
    humerus E83.31 [M90.82-] ☑
    ilium E83.31 [M90.859]
    ischium E83.31 [M90.859]
    metacarpus E83.31 [M90.84-] ☑
    metatarsus E83.31 [M90.87-] ☑
    multiple sites E83.31 [M90.89]
    neck E83.31 [M90.88]
    radius E83.31 [M90.83-] ☑
    rib E83.31 [M90.88]
    scapula E83.31 [M90.819]
    skull E83.31 [M90.88]
    tarsus E83.31 [M90.879]
    tibia E83.31 [M90.869]
    toe E83.31 [M90.879]
    ulna E83.31 [M90.839]
    vertebra E83.31 [M90.88]
Osteomyelitis (general) (infective) (localized) (neonatal) (purulent) (septic) (staphylococcal) (streptococcal) (suppurative) (with periostitis) M86.9
  acute M86.10
    carpus M86.14- ☑
    clavicle M86.11- ☑
    femur M86.15- ☑
    fibula M86.16- ☑
    finger M86.14- ☑
    hematogenous M86.00
      carpus M86.04- ☑
      clavicle M86.01- ☑
      femur M86.05- ☑
      fibula M86.06- ☑
      finger M86.04- ☑
      humerus M86.02- ☑
      ilium M86.059
      ischium M86.059
      mandible M27.2
      metacarpus M86.04- ☑
      metatarsus M86.07- ☑
      multiple sites M86.09
      neck M86.08
      orbit H05.02- ☑
      petrous bone — see Petrositis
      radius M86.03- ☑
      rib M86.08
      scapula M86.01- ☑
      skull M86.08
      tarsus M86.07- ☑
      tibia M86.06- ☑
      toe M86.07- ☑
      ulna M86.03- ☑
      vertebra — see Osteomyelitis, vertebra
    humerus M86.12- ☑
    ilium M86.159
    ischium M86.159
    mandible M27.2

Osteomyelitis — continued
  acute — continued
    metacarpus M86.14- ☑
    metatarsus M86.17- ☑
    multiple sites M86.19
    neck M86.18
    orbit H05.02- ☑
    petrous bone — see Petrositis
    radius M86.13- ☑
    rib M86.18
    scapula M86.11- ☑
    skull M86.18
    tarsus M86.17- ☑
    tibia M86.16- ☑
    toe M86.17- ☑
    ulna M86.13- ☑
    vertebra — see Osteomyelitis, vertebra
  chronic (or old) M86.60
    with draining sinus M86.40
      carpus M86.44- ☑
      clavicle M86.41- ☑
      femur M86.45- ☑
      fibula M86.46- ☑
      finger M86.44- ☑
      humerus M86.42- ☑
      ilium M86.459
      ischium M86.459
      mandible M27.2
      metacarpus M86.44- ☑
      metatarsus M86.47- ☑
      multiple sites M86.49
      neck M86.48
      orbit H05.02- ☑
      petrous bone — see Petrositis
      radius M86.43- ☑
      rib M86.48
      scapula M86.41- ☑
      skull M86.48
      tarsus M86.47- ☑
      tibia M86.46- ☑
      toe M86.47- ☑
      ulna M86.43- ☑
      vertebra — see Osteomyelitis, vertebra
    carpus M86.64- ☑
    clavicle M86.61- ☑
    femur M86.65- ☑
    fibula M86.66- ☑
    finger M86.64- ☑
    hematogenous NEC M86.50
      carpus M86.54- ☑
      clavicle M86.51- ☑
      femur M86.55- ☑
      fibula M86.56- ☑
      finger M86.54- ☑
      humerus M86.52- ☑
      ilium M86.559
      ischium M86.559
      mandible M27.2
      metacarpus M86.54- ☑
      metatarsus M86.57- ☑
      multifocal M86.30
        carpus M86.34- ☑
        clavicle M86.31- ☑
        femur M86.35- ☑
        fibula M86.36- ☑
        finger M86.34- ☑
        humerus M86.32- ☑
        ilium M86.359
        ischium M86.359
        metacarpus M86.34- ☑
        metatarsus M86.37- ☑
        multiple sites M86.39
        neck M86.38
        radius M86.33- ☑
        rib M86.38
        scapula M86.31- ☑
        skull M86.38
        tarsus M86.37- ☑
        tibia M86.36- ☑
        toe M86.37- ☑
        ulna M86.33- ☑
        vertebra — see Osteomyelitis, vertebra
      multiple sites M86.59
      neck M86.58
      orbit H05.02- ☑
      petrous bone — see Petrositis

Osteomyelitis — continued
  chronic — continued
    hematogenous — continued
      radius M86.53- ☑
      rib M86.58
      scapula M86.51- ☑
      skull M86.58
      tarsus M86.57- ☑
      tibia M86.56- ☑
      toe M86.57- ☑
      ulna M86.53- ☑
      vertebra — see Osteomyelitis, vertebra
    humerus M86.62- ☑
    ilium M86.659
    ischium M86.659
    mandible M27.2
    metacarpus M86.64- ☑
    metatarsus M86.67- ☑
    multifocal — see Osteomyelitis, chronic, hematogenous, multifocal
    multiple sites M86.69
    neck M86.68
    orbit H05.02- ☑
    petrous bone — see Petrositis
    radius M86.63- ☑
    rib M86.68
    scapula M86.61- ☑
    skull M86.68
    tarsus M86.67- ☑
    tibia M86.66- ☑
    toe M86.67- ☑
    ulna M86.63- ☑
    vertebra — see Osteomyelitis, vertebra
  echinococcal B67.2
  Garr's — see Osteomyelitis, specified type NEC
  in diabetes mellitus — see E08-E13 with .69
  jaw (acute) (chronic) (lower) (neonatal) (suppurative) (upper) M27.2
  nonsuppurating — see Osteomyelitis, specified type NEC
  orbit H05.02- ☑
  petrous bone — see Petrositis
  Salmonella (arizonae) (cholerae-suis) (enteritidis) (ty-phimurium) A02.24
  sclerosing, nonsuppurative — see Osteomyelitis, specified type NEC
  specified type NEC (see also subcategory) M86.8X- ☑
    mandible M27.2
    orbit H05.02- ☑
    petrous bone — see Petrositis
    vertebra — see Osteomyelitis, vertebra
  subacute M86.20
    carpus M86.24- ☑
    clavicle M86.21- ☑
    femur M86.25- ☑
    fibula M86.26- ☑
    finger M86.24- ☑
    humerus M86.22- ☑
    mandible M27.2
    metacarpus M86.24- ☑
    metatarsus M86.27- ☑
    multiple sites M86.29
    neck M86.28
    orbit H05.02- ☑
    petrous bone — see Petrositis
    radius M86.23- ☑
    rib M86.28
    scapula M86.21- ☑
    skull M86.28
    tarsus M86.27- ☑
    tibia M86.26- ☑
    toe M86.27- ☑
    ulna M86.23- ☑
    vertebra — see Osteomyelitis, vertebra
  syphilitic A52.77
    congenital (early) A50.02 [M90.80]
  tuberculous — see Tuberculosis, bone
  typhoid A01.05
  vertebra M46.20
    cervical region M46.22
    cervicothoracic region M46.23
    lumbar region M46.26
    lumbosacral region M46.27
    occipito-atlanto-axial region M46.21
    sacrococcygeal region M46.28
    thoracic region M46.24
    thoracolumbar region M46.25

Osteomyelofibrosis D47.4
Osteomyelosclerosis D75.89
Osteonecrosis M87.9
  due to
    drugs — *see* Osteonecrosis, secondary, due to,
      drugs
    trauma — *see* Osteonecrosis, secondary, due to,
      trauma
  idiopathic aseptic M87.00
    ankle M87.07- ☑
    carpus M87.03- ☑
    clavicle M87.01- ☑
    femur M87.05- ☑
    fibula M87.06- ☑
    finger M87.04- ☑
    humerus M87.02- ☑
    ilium M87.050
    ischium M87.050
    metacarpus M87.04- ☑
    metatarsus M87.07- ☑
    multiple sites M87.09
    neck M87.08
    pelvis M87.050
    radius M87.03- ☑
    rib M87.08
    scapula M87.01- ☑
    skull M87.08
    tarsus M87.07- ☑
    tibia M87.06- ☑
    toe M87.07- ☑
    ulna M87.03- ☑
    vertebra M87.08
  secondary NEC M87.30
    carpus M87.33- ☑
    clavicle M87.31- ☑
    due to
      drugs M87.10
        carpus M87.13- ☑
        clavicle M87.11- ☑
        femur M87.15- ☑
        fibula M87.16- ☑
        finger M87.14- ☑
        humerus M87.12- ☑
        ilium M87.159
        ischium M87.159
        jaw M87.180
        metacarpus M87.14- ☑
        metatarsus M87.17- ☑
        multiple sites M87.19
        neck M87.18 ☑
        radius M87.13- ☑
        rib M87.18 ☑
        scapula M87.11- ☑
        skull M87.18 ☑
        tarsus M87.17- ☑
        tibia M87.16- ☑
        toe M87.17- ☑
        ulna M87.13- ☑
        vertebra M87.18 ☑
      hemoglobinopathy NEC D58.2 [M90.50]
        carpus D58.2 [M90.54-] ☑
        clavicle D58.2 [M90.51-] ☑
        femur D58.2 [M90.55-] ☑
        fibula D58.2 [M90.56-] ☑
        finger D58.2 [M90.54-] ☑
        humerus D58.2 [M90.52-] ☑
        ilium D58.2 [M90.55-] ☑
        ischium D58.2 [M90.55-] ☑
        metacarpus D58.2 [M90.54-] ☑
        metatarsus D58.2 [M90.57-] ☑
        multiple sites D58.2 [M90.58]
        neck D58.2 [M90.58]
        radius D58.2 [M90.53-] ☑
        rib D58.2 [M90.58]
        scapula D58.2 [M90.51-] ☑
        skull D58.2 [M90.58]
        tarsus D58.2 [M90.57-] ☑
        tibia D58.2 [M90.56-] ☑
        toe D58.2 [M90.57-] ☑
        ulna D58.2 [M90.53-] ☑
        vertebra D58.2 [M90.58]
      trauma (previous) M87.20
        carpus M87.23- ☑
        clavicle M87.21- ☑
        femur M87.25- ☑
        fibula M87.26- ☑

Osteonecrosis — *continued*
  secondary — *continued*
    due to — *continued*
      trauma — *continued*
        finger M87.24- ☑
        humerus M87.22- ☑
        ilium M87.25- ☑
        ischium M87.25- ☑
        metacarpus M87.24- ☑
        metatarsus M87.27- ☑
        multiple sites M87.29
        neck M87.28
        radius M87.23- ☑
        rib M87.28
        scapula M87.21- ☑
        skull M87.28
        tarsus M87.27- ☑
        tibia M87.26- ☑
        toe M87.27- ☑
        ulna M87.23- ☑
        vertebra M87.28
    femur M87.35- ☑
    fibula M87.36- ☑
    finger M87.34- ☑
    humerus M87.32- ☑
    ilium M87.350
    in
      caisson disease T70.3 ☑ [M90.50]
        carpus T70.3 ☑ [M90.54-] ☑
        clavicle T70.3 ☑ [M90.51-] ☑
        femur T70.3 ☑ [M90.55-] ☑
        fibula T70.3 ☑ [M90.56-] ☑
        finger T70.3 ☑ [M90.54-] ☑
        humerus T70.3 ☑ [M90.52-] ☑
        ilium T70.3 ☑ [M90.55-] ☑
        ischium T70.3 ☑ [M90.55-] ☑
        metacarpus T70.3 ☑ [M90.54-] ☑
        metatarsus T70.3 ☑ [M90.57-] ☑
        multiple sites T70.3 ☑ [M90.59]
        neck T70.3 ☑ [M90.58]
        radius T70.3 ☑ [M90.53-] ☑
        rib T70.3 ☑ [M90.58]
        scapula T70.3 ☑ [M90.51-] ☑
        skull T70.3 ☑ [M90.58]
        tarsus T70.3 ☑ [M90.57-] ☑
        tibia T70.3 ☑ [M90.56-] ☑
        toe T70.3 ☑ [M90.57-] ☑
        ulna T70.3 ☑ [M90.53-] ☑
        vertebra T70.3 ☑ [M90.58]
    ischium M87.350
    metacarpus M87.34- ☑
    metatarsus M87.37- ☑
    multiple site M87.39
    neck M87.38
    radius M87.33- ☑
    rib M87.38
    scapula M87.319
    skull M87.38
    tarsus M87.379
    tibia M87.366
    toe M87.379
    ulna M87.33- ☑
    vertebra M87.38
  specified type NEC M87.80
    carpus M87.83- ☑
    clavicle M87.81- ☑
    femur M87.85- ☑
    fibula M87.86- ☑
    finger M87.84- ☑
    humerus M87.82- ☑
    ilium M87.85- ☑
    ischium M87.85- ☑
    metacarpus M87.84- ☑
    metatarsus M87.87- ☑
    multiple sites M87.89
    neck M87.88
    radius M87.83- ☑
    rib M87.88
    scapula M87.81- ☑
    skull M87.88
    tarsus M87.87- ☑
    tibia M87.86- ☑
    toe M87.87- ☑
    ulna M87.83- ☑
    vertebra M87.88
Osteo-onycho-arthro-dysplasia Q87.2

Osteo-onychodysplasia, hereditary Q87.2
Osteopathia condensans disseminata Q78.8
Osteopathy (*see also* Osteomyelitis, Osteonecrosis, Osteoporosis)
  after poliomyelitis M89.60
    carpus M89.64- ☑
    clavicle M89.61- ☑
    femur M89.65- ☑
    fibula M89.66- ☑
    finger M89.64- ☑
    humerus M89.62- ☑
    ilium M89.659
    ischium M89.659
    metacarpus M89.64- ☑
    metatarsus M89.67- ☑
    multiple sites M89.69
    neck M89.68
    radius M89.63- ☑
    rib M89.68
    scapula M89.61- ☑
    skull M89.68
    tarsus M89.67- ☑
    tibia M89.66- ☑
    toe M89.67- ☑
    ulna M89.63- ☑
    vertebra M89.68
  in (due to)
    renal osteodystrophy N25.0
    specified diseases classified elsewhere — *see* sub-
      category M90.8 ☑
Osteopenia M85.8- ☑
  borderline M85.8- ☑
Osteoperiostitis — *see* Osteomyelitis, specified type
  NEC
Osteopetrosis (familial) Q78.2
Osteophyte M25.70
  ankle M25.77- ☑
  elbow M25.72- ☑
  foot joint M25.77- ☑
  hand joint M25.74- ☑
  hip M25.75- ☑
  knee M25.76- ☑
  shoulder M25.71- ☑
  spine M25.78
  vertebrae M25.78
  wrist M25.73- ☑
Osteopoikilosis Q78.8
Osteoporosis (female) (male) M81.0
  with current pathological fracture M80.00 ☑
  age-related M81.0
    with current pathologic fracture M80.00 ☑
      carpus M80.04- ☑
      clavicle M80.01- ☑
      fibula M80.06- ☑
      finger M80.04- ☑
      humerus M80.02- ☑
      ilium M80.05- ☑
      ischium M80.05- ☑
      metacarpus M80.04- ☑
      metatarsus M80.07- ☑
      pelvis M80.05- ☑
      radius M80.03- ☑
      scapula M80.01- ☑
      tarsus M80.07- ☑
      tibia M80.06- ☑
      toe M80.07- ☑
      ulna M80.03- ☑
      vertebra M80.08 ☑
  disuse M81.8
    with current pathological fracture M80.80 ☑
      carpus M80.84- ☑
      clavicle M80.81- ☑
      fibula M80.86- ☑
      finger M80.84- ☑
      humerus M80.82- ☑
      ilium M80.85- ☑
      ischium M80.85- ☑
      metacarpus M80.84- ☑
      metatarsus M80.87- ☑
      pelvis M80.85- ☑
      radius M80.83- ☑
      scapula M80.81- ☑
      tarsus M80.87- ☑
      tibia M80.86- ☑
      toe M80.87- ☑
      ulna M80.83- ☑

☑ **Additional Character Required — Refer to the Tabular List for Character Selection**   ▽ Subterms under main terms may continue to next column or page

Osteoporosis — *continued*
  disuse — *continued*
    with current pathological fracture — *continued*
      vertebra M80.88 ☑
  drug-induced — *see* Osteoporosis, specified type NEC
  idiopathic — *see* Osteoporosis, specified type NEC
  involutional — *see* Osteoporosis, age-related
  Lequesne M81.6
  localized M81.6
  postmenopausal M81.0
    with pathological fracture M80.00 ☑
      carpus M80.04- ☑
      clavicle M80.01- ☑
      fibula M80.06- ☑
      finger M80.04- ☑
      humerus M80.02- ☑
      ilium M80.05- ☑
      ischium M80.05- ☑
      metacarpus M80.04- ☑
      metatarsus M80.07- ☑
      pelvis M80.05- ☑
      radius M80.03- ☑
      scapula M80.01- ☑
      tarsus M80.07- ☑
      tibia M80.06- ☑
      toe M80.07- ☑
      ulna M80.03- ☑
      vertebra M80.08 ☑
  postoophorectomy — *see* Osteoporosis, specified type NEC
  postsurgical malabsorption — *see* Osteoporosis, specified type NEC
  post-traumatic — *see* Osteoporosis, specified type NEC
  senile — *see* Osteoporosis, age-related
  specified type NEC M81.8
    with pathological fracture M80.80 ☑
      carpus M80.84- ☑
      clavicle M80.81- ☑
      fibula M80.86- ☑
      finger M80.84- ☑
      humerus M80.82- ☑
      ilium M80.85- ☑
      ischium M80.85- ☑
      metacarpus M80.84- ☑
      metatarsus M80.87- ☑
      pelvis M80.85- ☑
      radius M80.83- ☑
      scapula M80.81- ☑
      tarsus M80.87- ☑
      tibia M80.86- ☑
      toe M80.87- ☑
      ulna M80.83- ☑
      vertebra M80.88 ☑
Osteopsathyrosis (idiopathica) Q78.0
Osteoradionecrosis, jaw (acute) (chronic) (lower) (suppurative) (upper) M27.2
Osteosarcoma (any form) — *see* Neoplasm, bone, malignant
Osteosclerosis Q78.2
  acquired M85.8- ☑
  congenita Q77.4
  fragilitas (generalisata) Q78.2
  myelofibrosis D75.81
Osteosclerotic anemia D64.89
Osteosis
  cutis L94.2
  renal fibrocystic N25.0
Österreicher-Turner syndrome Q87.2
Ostium
  atrioventriculare commune Q21.2
  primum (arteriosum) (defect) (persistent) Q21.2
  secundum (arteriosum) (defect) (patent) (persistent) Q21.1
Ostrum-Furst syndrome Q75.8
Otalgia H92.0 ☑
Otitis (acute) H66.90
  with effusion (*see also* Otitis, media, nonsuppurative)
    purulent — *see* Otitis, media, suppurative
  adhesive — *see* subcategory H74.1 ☑
  chronic (*see also* Otitis, media, chronic)
    with effusion (*see also* Otitis, media, nonsuppurative, chronic)
  externa H60.9- ☑
    abscess — *see* Abscess, ear, external
    acute (noninfective) H60.50- ☑

Otitis — *continued*
  externa — *continued*
    acute — *continued*
      actinic H60.51- ☑
      chemical H60.52- ☑
      contact H60.53- ☑
      eczematoid H60.54- ☑
      infective — *see* Otitis, externa, infective
      reactive H60.55- ☑
      specified NEC H60.59- ☑
    cellulitis — *see* Cellulitis, ear
    chronic H60.6- ☑
    diffuse — *see* Otitis, externa, infective, diffuse
    hemorrhagic — *see* Otitis, externa, infective, hemorrhagic
    in (due to)
      aspergillosis B44.89
      candidiasis B37.84
      erysipelas A46 [H62.40]
      herpes (simplex) virus infection B00.1
        zoster B02.8
      impetigo L01.00 [H62.40]
      infectious disease NEC B99 ☑ [H62.4-] ☑
      mycosis NEC B36.9 [H62.40]
      parasitic disease NEC B89 [H62.40]
      viral disease NEC B34.9 [H62.40]
      zoster B02.8
    infective NEC H60.39- ☑
      abscess — *see* Abscess, ear, external
      cellulitis — *see* Cellulitis, ear
      diffuse H60.31- ☑
      hemorrhagic H60.32- ☑
      swimmer's ear — *see* Swimmer's, ear
    malignant H60.2- ☑
    mycotic NEC B36.9 [H62.40]
      in
        aspergillosis B44.89
        candidiasis B37.84
        moniliasis B37.84
    necrotizing — *see* Otitis, externa, malignant
    Pseudomonas aeruginosa — *see* Otitis, externa, malignant
    reactive — *see* Otitis, externa, acute, reactive
    specified NEC — *see* subcategory H60.8 ☑
    tropical NEC B36.9 [H62.40]
      in
        aspergillosis B44.89
        candidiasis B37.84
        moniliasis B37.84
  insidiosa — *see* Otosclerosis
  interna H83.0 ☑
  media (hemorrhagic) (staphylococcal) (streptococcal) H66.9- ☑
    with effusion (nonpurulent) — *see* Otitis, media, nonsuppurative
    acute, subacute H66.90
      allergic — *see* Otitis, media, nonsuppurative, acute, allergic
      exudative — *see* Otitis, media, suppurative, acute
      mucoid — *see* Otitis, media, nonsuppurative, acute
      necrotizing (*see also* Otitis, media, suppurative, acute)
        in
          measles B05.3
          scarlet fever A38.0
      nonsuppurative NEC — *see* Otitis, media, nonsuppurative, acute
      purulent — *see* Otitis, media, suppurative, acute
      sanguinous — *see* Otitis, media, nonsuppurative, acute
      secretory — *see* Otitis, media, nonsuppurative, acute, serous
      seromucinous — *see* Otitis, media, nonsuppurative, acute
      serous — *see* Otitis, media, nonsuppurative, acute, serous
      suppurative — *see* Otitis, media, suppurative, acute
    allergic — *see* Otitis, media, nonsuppurative
    catarrhal — *see* Otitis, media, nonsuppurative
    chronic H66.90
      with effusion (nonpurulent) — *see* Otitis, media, nonsuppurative, chronic

Otitis — *continued*
  media — *continued*
    chronic — *continued*
      allergic — *see* Otitis, media, nonsuppurative, chronic, allergic
      benign suppurative — *see* Otitis, media, suppurative, chronic, tubotympanic
      catarrhal — *see* Otitis, media, nonsuppurative, chronic, serous
      exudative — *see* Otitis, media, nonsuppurative, chronic
      mucinous — *see* Otitis, media, nonsuppurative, chronic, mucoid
      mucoid — *see* Otitis, media, nonsuppurative, chronic, mucoid
      nonsuppurative NEC — *see* Otitis, media, nonsuppurative, chronic
      purulent — *see* Otitis, media, suppurative, chronic
      secretory — *see* Otitis, media, nonsuppurative, chronic, mucoid
      seromucinous — *see* Otitis, media, nonsuppurative, chronic
      serous — *see* Otitis, media, nonsuppurative, chronic, serous
      suppurative — *see* Otitis, media, suppurative, chronic
      transudative — *see* Otitis, media, nonsuppurative, chronic, mucoid
    exudative — *see* Otitis, media, suppurative
    in (due to) (with)
      influenza — *see* Influenza, with, otitis media
      measles B05.3
      scarlet fever A38.0
      tuberculosis A18.6
      viral disease NEC B34.- ☑ [H67.-] ☑
    mucoid — *see* Otitis, media, nonsuppurative
    nonsuppurative H65.9- ☑
      acute or subacute NEC H65.19- ☑
        allergic H65.11- ☑
          recurrent H65.11- ☑
        recurrent H65.19- ☑
        secretory — *see* Otitis, media, nonsuppurative, serous
        serous H65.0- ☑
          recurrent H65.0- ☑
      chronic H65.49- ☑
        allergic H65.41- ☑
        mucoid H65.3- ☑
        serous H65.2- ☑
    postmeasles B05.3
    purulent — *see* Otitis, media, suppurative
    secretory — *see* Otitis, media, nonsuppurative
    seromucinous — *see* Otitis, media, nonsuppurative
    serous — *see* Otitis, media, nonsuppurative
    suppurative H66.4- ☑
      acute H66.00- ☑
        with rupture of ear drum H66.01- ☑
        recurrent H66.00- ☑
          with rupture of ear drum H66.01- ☑
      chronic (*see also* subcategory) H66.3 ☑
        atticoantral H66.2- ☑
        benign — *see* Otitis, media, suppurative, chronic, tubotympanic
        tubotympanic H66.1- ☑
    transudative — *see* Otitis, media, nonsuppurative
    tuberculous A18.6
Otocephaly Q18.2
Otolith syndrome — *see* subcategory H81.8 ☑
Otomycosis (diffuse) **NEC** B36.9 [H62.40]
  in
    aspergillosis B44.89
    candidiasis B37.84
    moniliasis B37.84
Otoporosis — *see* Otosclerosis
Otorrhagia (nontraumatic) H92.2- ☑
  traumatic — *code by* Type of injury
Otorrhea H92.1- ☑
  cerebrospinal G96.0
Otosclerosis (general) H80.9- ☑
  cochlear (endosteal) H80.2- ☑
  involving
    otic capsule — *see* Otosclerosis, cochlear
    oval window
      nonobliterative H80.0- ☑
      obliterative H80.1- ☑
    round window — *see* Otosclerosis, cochlear

▽ **Subterms under main terms may continue to next column or page**   ☑ **Additional Character Required — Refer to the Tabular List for Character Selection**   **243**

Osteoporosis — Otosclerosis

Otosclerosis — *continued*
  nonobliterative — *see* Otosclerosis, involving, oval
    window, nonobliterative
  obliterative — *see* Otosclerosis, involving, oval win-
    dow, obliterative
  specified NEC H80.8- ☑
Otospongiosis — *see* Otosclerosis
Otto's disease or pelvis M24.7
Outcome of delivery Z37.9
  multiple births Z37.9
    all liveborn Z37.50
      quadruplets Z37.52
      quintuplets Z37.53
      sextuplets Z37.54
      specified number NEC Z37.59
      triplets Z37.51
    all stillborn Z37.7
    some liveborn Z37.60
      quadruplets Z37.62
      quintuplets Z37.63
      sextuplets Z37.64
      specified number NEC Z37.69
      triplets Z37.61
  single NEC Z37.9
    liveborn Z37.0
    stillborn Z37.1
  twins NEC Z37.9
    both liveborn Z37.2
    both stillborn Z37.4
    one liveborn, one stillborn Z37.3
Outlet — *see* condition
Ovalocytosis (congenital) (hereditary) — *see* Elliptocytosis
Ovarian — *see* Condition
Ovariocele N83.4- ☑
Ovaritis (cystic) — *see* Oophoritis
Ovary, ovarian (*see also* condition)
  resistant syndrome E28.39
  vein syndrome N13.8
Overactive (*see also* Hyperfunction)
  adrenal cortex NEC E27.0
  bladder N32.81
  hypothalamus E23.3
  thyroid — *see* Hyperthyroidism
Overactivity R46.3
  child — *see* Disorder, attention-deficit hyperactivity
Overbite (deep) (excessive) (horizontal) (vertical) M26.29
Overbreathing — *see* Hyperventilation
Overconscientious personality F60.5
Overdevelopment — *see* Hypertrophy
Overdistension — *see* Distension
Overdose, overdosage (drug) — *see* Table of Drugs and
  Chemicals, by drug, poisoning
Overeating R63.2
  nonorganic origin F50.89
  psychogenic F50.89
Overexertion (effects) (exhaustion) T73.3 ☑
Overexposure (effects) T73.9 ☑
  exhaustion T73.2 ☑
Overfeeding — *see* Overeating
  newborn P92.4
Overfill, endodontic M27.52
Overgrowth, bone — *see* Hypertrophy, bone
Overhanging of dental restorative material (unre-
  pairable) K08.52
Overheated (places) (effects) — *see* Heat
Overjet (excessive horizontal) M26.23
Overlaid, overlying (suffocation) — *see* Asphyxia,
  traumatic, due to mechanical threat
Overlap, excessive horizontal (teeth) M26.23
Overlapping toe (acquired) (*see also* Deformity, toe,
  specified NEC)
  congenital (fifth toe) Q66.89
Overload
  circulatory, due to transfusion (blood) (blood compo-
    nents) (TACO) E87.71
  fluid E87.70
    due to transfusion (blood) (blood components)
      E87.71
    specified NEC E87.79
  iron, due to repeated red blood cell transfusions
    E83.111
  potassium (K) E87.5
  sodium (Na) E87.0
Overnutrition — *see* Hyperalimentation
Overproduction (*see also* Hypersecretion)
  ACTH E27.0

Overproduction — *continued*
  catecholamine E27.5
  growth hormone E22.0
Overprotection, child by parent Z62.1
Overriding
  aorta Q25.49
  finger (acquired) — *see* Deformity, finger
    congenital Q68.1
  toe (acquired) (*see also* Deformity, toe, specified NEC)
    congenital Q66.89
Overstrained R53.83
  heart — *see* Hypertrophy, cardiac
Overuse, muscle NEC M70.8- ☑
Overweight E66.3
Overworked R53.83
Oviduct — *see* condition
Ovotestis Q56.0
Ovulation (cycle)
  failure or lack of N97.0
  pain N94.0
Ovum — *see* condition
Owren's disease or syndrome (parahemophilia) D68.2
Ox heart — *see* Hypertrophy, cardiac
Oxalosis E72.53
Oxaluria E72.53
Oxycephaly, oxycephalic Q75.0
  syphilitic, congenital A50.02
Oxyuriasis B80
Oxyuris vermicularis (infestation) B80
Ozena J31.0

P

Pachyderma, pachydermia L85.9
  larynx (verrucosa) J38.7
Pachydermatocele (congenital) Q82.8
Pachydermoperiostosis (*see also* Osteoarthropathy,
  hypertrophic, specified type NEC)
  clubbed nail M89.40 [L62]
Pachygyria Q04.3
Pachymeningitis (adhesive) (basal) (brain) (cervical)
  (chronic)(circumscribed) (external) (fibrous) (hemorrhagic) (hypertrophic) (internal) (purulent) (spinal)
  (suppurative) — *see* Meningitis
Pachyonychia (congenital) Q84.5
Pacinian tumor — *see* Neoplasm, skin, benign
Pad, knuckle or Garrod's M72.1
Paget's disease
  with infiltrating duct carcinoma — *see* Neoplasm,
    breast, malignant
  bone M88.9
    carpus M88.84- ☑
    clavicle M88.81- ☑
    femur M88.85- ☑
    fibula M88.86- ☑
    finger M88.84- ☑
    humerus M88.82- ☑
    ilium M88.85- ☑
    in neoplastic disease — *see* Osteitis, deformans, in
      neoplastic disease
    ischium M88.85- ☑
    metacarpus M88.84- ☑
    metatarsus M88.87- ☑
    multiple sites M88.89
    neck M88.88
    radius M88.83- ☑
    rib M88.88
    scapula M88.81- ☑
    skull M88.0
    tarsus M88.87- ☑
    tibia M88.86- ☑
    toe M88.87- ☑
    ulna M88.83- ☑
    vertebra M88.88
  breast (female) C50.01- ☑
    male C50.02- ☑
  extramammary (*see also* Neoplasm, skin, malignant)
    anus C21.0
      margin C44.590
      skin C44.590
  intraductal carcinoma — *see* Neoplasm, breast, malig-
    nant
  malignant — *see* Neoplasm, skin, malignant
    breast (female) C50.01- ☑
      male C50.02- ☑
    unspecified site (female) C50.01- ☑
      male C50.02- ☑

Paget's disease — *continued*
  mammary — *see* Paget's disease, breast
  nipple — *see* Paget's disease, breast
  osteitis deformans — *see* Paget's disease, bone
Paget-Schroetter syndrome I82.890
Pain(s) (*see also* Painful) R52
  abdominal R10.9
    colic R10.83
    generalized R10.84
      with acute abdomen R10.0
    lower R10.30
      left quadrant R10.32
      pelvic or perineal R10.2
      periumbilical R10.33
      right quadrant R10.31
    rebound — *see* Tenderness, abdominal, rebound
    severe with abdominal rigidity R10.0
    tenderness — *see* Tenderness, abdominal
    upper R10.10
      epigastric R10.13
      left quadrant R10.12
      right quadrant R10.11
  acute R52
    due to trauma G89.11
    neoplasm related G89.3
    postprocedural NEC G89.18
    post-thoracotomy G89.12
    specified by site — *code to* Pain, by site
  adnexa (uteri) R10.2
  anginoid — *see* Pain, precordial
  anus K62.89
  arm — *see* Pain, limb, upper
  axillary (axilla) M79.62- ☑
  back (postural) M54.9
  bladder R39.89
    associated with micturition — *see* Micturition,
      painful
    chronic R39.82
  bone — *see* Disorder, bone, specified type NEC
  breast N64.4
  broad ligament R10.2
  cancer associated (acute) (chronic) G89.3
  cecum — *see* Pain, abdominal
  cervicobrachial M53.1
  chest (central) R07.9
    anterior wall R07.89
    atypical R07.89
    ischemic I20.9
    musculoskeletal R07.89
    non-cardiac R07.89
    on breathing R07.1
    pleurodynia R07.81
    precordial R07.2
    wall (anterior) R07.89
  chronic G89.29
    associated with significant psychosocial dysfunc-
      tion G89.4
    due to trauma G89.21
    neoplasm related G89.3
    postoperative NEC G89.28
    postprocedural NEC G89.28
    post-thoracotomy G89.22
    specified NEC G89.29
  coccyx M53.3
  colon — *see* Pain, abdominal
  coronary — *see* Angina
  costochondral R07.1
  diaphragm R07.1
  due to cancer G89.3
  due to device, implant or graft (*see also* Complications,
    by site and type, specified NEC) T85.848 ☑
    arterial graft NEC T82.848 ☑
    breast (implant) T85.848 ☑
    catheter NEC T85.848 ☑
      dialysis (renal) T82.848 ☑
        intraperitoneal T85.848 ☑
      infusion NEC T82.848 ☑
        spinal (epidural) (subdural) T85.840 ☑
      urinary (indwelling) T83.84 ☑
    electronic (electrode) (pulse generator) (stimulator)
      bone T85.840 ☑
      cardiac T82.847 ☑
      nervous system (brain) (peripheral nerve)
        (spinal) T85.84 ☑
      urinary T83.84 ☑
    fixation, internal (orthopedic) NEC T84.84 ☑
    gastrointestinal (bile duct) (esophagus) T85.848 ☑
    genital NEC T83.84 ☑

☑ **Additional Character Required** — Refer to the Tabular List for Character Selection   ▽ Subterms under main terms may continue to next column or page

Pain(s) — *continued*
  due to device, implant or graft (*see also* Complications, by site and type, specified) — *continued*
    heart NEC T82.847 ☑
    infusion NEC T85.848 ☑
    joint prosthesis T84.84 ☑
    ocular (corneal graft) (orbital implant) NEC T85.848 ☑
    orthopedic NEC T84.84 ☑
    specified NEC T85.848 ☑
    urinary NEC T83.84 ☑
    vascular NEC T82.848 ☑
    ventricular intracranial shunt T85.840 ☑
  due to malignancy (primary) (secondary) G89.3
  ear — *see* subcategory H92.0 ☑
  epigastric, epigastrium R10.13
  eye — *see* Pain, ocular
  face, facial R51
    atypical G50.1
  female genital organs NEC N94.89
  finger — *see* Pain, limb, upper
  flank — *see* Pain, abdominal
  foot — *see* Pain, limb, lower
  gallbladder K82.9
  gas (intestinal) R14.1
  gastric — *see* Pain, abdominal
  generalized NOS R52
  genital organ
    female N94.89
    male N50.89
  groin — *see* Pain, abdominal, lower
  hand — *see* Pain, limb, upper
  head — *see* Headache
  heart — *see* Pain, precordial
  infra-orbital — *see* Neuralgia, trigeminal
  intercostal R07.82
  intermenstrual N94.0
  jaw R68.84
  joint M25.50
    ankle M25.57- ☑
    elbow M25.52- ☑
    finger M25.54- ☑
    foot M25.57- ☑
    hand M25.54- ☑
    hip M25.55- ☑
    knee M25.56- ☑
    shoulder M25.51- ☑
    toe M25.57- ☑
    wrist M25.53- ☑
  kidney N23
  laryngeal R07.0
  leg — *see* Pain, limb, lower
  limb M79.609
    lower M79.60- ☑
      foot M79.67- ☑
      lower leg M79.66- ☑
      thigh M79.65- ☑
      toe M79.67- ☑
    upper M79.60- ☑
      axilla M79.62- ☑
      finger M79.64- ☑
      forearm M79.63- ☑
      hand M79.64- ☑
      upper arm M79.62- ☑
  loin M54.5
  low back M54.5
  lumbar region M54.5
  mandibular R68.84
  mastoid — *see* subcategory H92.0 ☑
  maxilla R68.84
  menstrual (*see also* Dysmenorrhea) N94.6
  metacarpophalangeal (joint) — *see* Pain, joint, hand
  metatarsophalangeal (joint) — *see* Pain, joint, foot
  mouth K13.79
  muscle — *see* Myalgia
  musculoskeletal (*see also* Pain, by site) M79.1
  myofascial M79.1
  nasal J34.89
  nasopharynx J39.2
  neck NEC M54.2
  nerve NEC — *see* Neuralgia
  neuromuscular — *see* Neuralgia
  nose J34.89
  ocular H57.1- ☑
  ophthalmic — *see* Pain, ocular
  orbital region — *see* Pain, ocular
  ovary N94.89

Pain(s) — *continued*
  over heart — *see* Pain, precordial
  ovulation N94.0
  pelvic (female) R10.2
  penis N48.89
  pericardial — *see* Pain, precordial
  perineal, perineum R10.2
  pharynx J39.2
  pleura, pleural, pleuritic R07.81
  postoperative NOS G89.18
  postprocedural NOS G89.18
  post-thoracotomy G89.12
  precordial (region) R07.2
  premenstrual N94.3
  psychogenic (persistent) (any site) F45.41
  radicular (spinal) — *see* Radiculopathy
  rectum K62.89
  respiration R07.1
  retrosternal R07.2
  rheumatoid, muscular — *see* Myalgia
  rib R07.81
  root (spinal) — *see* Radiculopathy
  round ligament (stretch) R10.2
  sacroiliac M53.3
  sciatic — *see* Sciatica
  scrotum N50.82
  seminal vesicle N50.89
  shoulder M25.51- ☑
  spermatic cord N50.89
  spinal root — *see* Radiculopathy
  spine M54.9
    cervical M54.2
    low back M54.5
      with sciatica M54.4- ☑
    thoracic M54.6
  stomach — *see* Pain, abdominal
  substernal R07.2
  temporomandibular (joint) M26.62- ☑
  testis N50.81- ☑
  thoracic spine M54.6
    with radicular and visceral pain M54.14
  throat R07.0
  tibia — *see* Pain, limb, lower
  toe — *see* Pain, limb, lower
  tongue K14.6
  tooth K08.89
  trigeminal — *see* Neuralgia, trigeminal
  tumor associated G89.3
  ureter N23
  urinary (organ) (system) N23
  uterus NEC N94.89
  vagina R10.2
  vertebrogenic (syndrome) M54.89
  vesical R39.89
    associated with micturition — *see* Micturition, painful
  vulva R10.2
Painful (*see also* Pain)
  coitus
    female N94.10
    male N53.12
    psychogenic F52.6
  ejaculation (semen) N53.12
    psychogenic F52.6
  erection — *see* Priapism
  feet syndrome E53.8
  joint replacement (hip) (knee) T84.84 ☑
  menstruation — *see* Dysmenorrhea
    psychogenic F45.8
  micturition — *see* Micturition, painful
  respiration R07.1
  scar NEC L90.5
  wire sutures T81.89 ☑
Painter's colic — *see* subcategory T56.0 ☑
Palate — *see* condition
Palatoplegia K13.79
Palatoschisis — *see* Cleft, palate
Palilalia R48.8
Palliative care Z51.5
Pallor R23.1
  optic disc, temporal — *see* Atrophy, optic
Palmar (*see also* condition)
  fascia — *see* condition
Palpable
  cecum K63.89
  kidney N28.89
  ovary N83.8
  prostate N42.9

Palpable — *continued*
  spleen — *see* Splenomegaly
Palpitations (heart) R00.2
  psychogenic F45.8
Palsy (*see also* Paralysis) G83.9
  atrophic diffuse (progressive) G12.22
  Bell's (*see also* Palsy, facial)
    newborn P11.3
  brachial plexus NEC G54.0
    newborn (birth injury) P14.3
  brain — *see* Palsy, cerebral
  bulbar (progressive) (chronic) G12.22
    of childhood (Fazio-Londe) G12.1
    pseudo NEC G12.29
    supranuclear (progressive) G23.1
  cerebral (congenital) G80.9
    ataxic G80.4
    athetoid G80.3
    choreathetoid G80.3
    diplegic G80.8
      spastic G80.1
    dyskinetic G80.3
      athetoid G80.3
      choreathetoid G80.3
      distonic G80.3
    dystonic G80.3
    hemiplegic G80.8
      spastic G80.2
    mixed G80.8
    monoplegic G80.8
      spastic G80.1
    paraplegic G80.8
      spastic G80.1
    quadriplegic G80.8
      spastic G80.0
    spastic G80.1
      diplegic G80.1
      hemiplegic G80.2
      monoplegic G80.1
      quadriplegic G80.0
      specified NEC G80.1
      tetrapelgic G80.0
    specified NEC G80.8
    syphilitic A52.12
      congenital A50.49
    tetraplegic G80.8
      spastic G80.0
  cranial nerve (*see also* Disorder, nerve, cranial)
    multiple G52.7
      in
        infectious disease B99 ☑ [G53]
        neoplastic disease (*see also* Neoplasm) D49.9 [G53]
        parasitic disease B89 [G53]
        sarcoidosis D86.82
  creeping G12.22
  diver's T70.3 ☑
  Erb's P14.0
  facial G51.0
    newborn (birth injury) P11.3
  glossopharyngeal G52.1
  Klumpke (-Déjérine) P14.1
  lead — *see* subcategory T56.0 ☑
  median nerve (tardy) G56.1- ☑
  nerve G58.9
    specified NEC G58.8
  peroneal nerve (acute) (tardy) G57.3- ☑
  progressive supranuclear G23.1
  pseudobulbar NEC G12.29
  radial nerve (acute) G56.3- ☑
  seventh nerve (*see also* Palsy, facial)
    newborn P11.3
  shaking — *see* Parkinsonism
  spastic (cerebral) (spinal) G80.1
  ulnar nerve (tardy) G56.2- ☑
  wasting G12.29
Paludism — *see* Malaria
Panangiitis M30.0
Panaris, panaritium (*see also* Cellulitis, digit)
  with lymphangitis — *see* Lymphangitis, acute, digit
Panarteritis nodosa M30.0
  brain or cerebral I67.7
Pancake heart R93.1
  with cor pulmonale (chronic) I27.81
Pancarditis (acute) (chronic) I51.89
  rheumatic I09.89
    active or acute I01.8
Pancoast's syndrome or tumor C34.1- ☑

Pancolitis, ulcerative (chronic) K51.00
  with
    abscess K51.014
    complication K51.019
    fistula K51.013
    obstruction K51.012
    rectal bleeding K51.011
    specified complication NEC K51.018
Pancreas, pancreatic — *see* condition
Pancreatitis (annular) (apoplectic) (calcareous) (edematous) (hemorrhagic) (malignant) (recurrent) (subacute) (suppurative) K85.90
  with necrosis (uninfected) K85.91
    infected K85.92
  acute (without necrosis or infection) K85.90
    with necrosis (uninfected) K85.91
      infected K85.92
    alcohol induced (without necrosis or infection) K85.20
      with necrosis (uninfected) K85.21
        infected K85.22
    biliary (without necrosis or infection) K85.10
      with necrosis (uninfected) K85.11
        infected K85.12
    drug induced (without necrosis or infection) K85.30
      with necrosis (uninfected) K85.31
        infected K85.32
    gallstone (without necrosis or infection) K85.10
      with necrosis (uninfected) K85.11
        infected K85.12
    idiopathic (without necrosis or infection) K85.00
      with necrosis (uninfected) K85.01
        infected K85.02
    specified NEC (without necrosis or infection) K85.80
      with necrosis (uninfected) K85.81
        infected K85.82
  chronic (infectious) K86.1
    alcohol-induced K86.0
    recurrent K86.1
    relapsing K86.1
  cystic (chronic) K86.1
  cytomegaloviral B25.2
  fibrous (chronic) K86.1
  gallstone (without necrosis or infection) K85.10
    with necrosis (uninfected) K85.11
      infected K85.12
  gangrenous — *see* Pancreatitis, acute
  interstitial (chronic) K86.1
    acute (*see also* Pancreatitis, acute) K85.80
  mumps B26.3
  recurrent (chronic) K86.1
  relapsing, chronic K86.1
  syphilitic A52.74
Pancreatoblastoma — *see* Neoplasm, pancreas, malignant
Pancreolithiasis K86.89
Pancytolysis D75.89
Pancytopenia (acquired) D61.818
  with
    malformations D61.09
    myelodysplastic syndrome — *see* Syndrome, myelodysplastic
  antineoplastic chemotherapy induced D61.810
  congenital D61.09
  drug-induced NEC D61.811
PANDAS (pediatric autoimmune neuropsychiatric disorders associated with streptococcal infections syndrome) D89.89
Panencephalitis, subacute, sclerosing A81.1
Panhematopenia D61.9
  congenital D61.09
  constitutional D61.09
  splenic, primary D73.1
Panhemocytopenia D61.9
  congenital D61.09
  constitutional D61.09
Panhypogonadism E29.1
Panhypopituitarism E23.0
  prepubertal E23.0
Panic (attack) (state) F41.0
  reaction to exceptional stress (transient) F43.0
Panmyelopathy, familial, constitutional D61.09
Panmyelophthisis D61.82
  congenital D61.09
Panmyelosis (acute) (with myelofibrosis) C94.4- ☑
Panner's disease — *see* Osteochondrosis, juvenile, humerus
Panneuritis endemica E51.11

Panniculitis (nodular) (nonsuppurative) M79.3
  back M54.00
    cervical region M54.02
    cervicothoracic region M54.03
    lumbar region M54.06
    lumbosacral region M54.07
    multiple sites M54.09
    occipito-atlanto-axial region M54.01
    sacrococcygeal region M54.08
    thoracic region M54.04
    thoracolumbar region M54.05
  lupus L93.2
  mesenteric K65.4
  neck M54.02
    cervicothoracic region M54.03
    occipito-atlanto-axial region M54.01
  relapsing M35.6
Panniculus adiposus (abdominal) E65
Pannus (allergic) (cornea) (degenerativus) (keratic) H16.42- ☑
  abdominal (symptomatic) E65
  trachomatosus, trachomatous (active) A71.1
Panophthalmitis H44.01- ☑
Pansinusitis (chronic) (hyperplastic) (nonpurulent) (purulent) J32.4
  acute J01.40
    recurrent J01.41
  tuberculous A15.8
Panuveitis (sympathetic) H44.11- ☑
Panvalvular disease I08.9
  specified NEC I08.8
PAPA (pyogenic arthritis, pyoderma gangrenosum, and acne syndrome) M04.8
Papanicolaou smear, cervix Z12.4
  as part of routine gynecological examination Z01.419
    with abnormal findings Z01.411
  for suspected neoplasm Z12.4
  nonspecific abnormal finding R87.619
  routine Z01.419
    with abnormal findings Z01.411
Papilledema (choked disc) H47.10
  associated with
    decreased ocular pressure H47.12
    increased intracranial pressure H47.11
    retinal disorder H47.13
  Foster-Kennedy syndrome H47.14- ☑
Papillitis H46.00
  anus K62.89
  chronic lingual K14.4
  necrotizing, kidney N17.2
  optic H46.0- ☑
  rectum K62.89
  renal, necrotizing N17.2
  tongue K14.0
Papilloma (*see also* Neoplasm, benign, by site)
  acuminatum (female) (male) (anogenital) A63.0
  basal cell L82.1
    inflamed L82.0
  benign pinta (primary) A67.0
  bladder (urinary) (transitional cell) D41.4
  choroid plexus (lateral ventricle) (third ventricle) D33.0
    anaplastic C71.5
    fourth ventricle D33.1
    malignant C71.5
  renal pelvis (transitional cell) D41.1- ☑
    benign D30.1- ☑
  Schneiderian
    specified site — *see* Neoplasm, benign, by site
    unspecified site D14.0
  serous surface
    borderline malignancy
      specified site — *see* Neoplasm, uncertain behavior, by site
      unspecified site D39.10
    specified site — *see* Neoplasm, benign, by site
    unspecified site D27.9
  transitional (cell)
    bladder (urinary) D41.4
    inverted type — *see* Neoplasm, uncertain behavior, by site
    renal pelvis D41.1- ☑
    ureter D41.2- ☑
  ureter (transitional cell) D41.2- ☑
    benign D30.2- ☑
  urothelial — *see* Neoplasm, uncertain behavior, by site
  villous — *see* Neoplasm, uncertain behavior, by site

Papilloma — *continued*
  villous — *see* Neoplasm, uncertain behavior, by site — *continued*
    adenocarcinoma in — *see* Neoplasm, malignant, by site
    in situ — *see* Neoplasm, in situ
  yaws, plantar or palmar A66.1
Papillomata, multiple, of yaws A66.1
Papillomatosis (*see also* Neoplasm, benign, by site)
  confluent and reticulated L83
  cystic, breast — *see* Mastopathy, cystic
  ductal, breast — *see* Mastopathy, cystic
  intraductal (diffuse) — *see* Neoplasm, benign, by site
  subareolar duct D24- ☑
Papillomavirus, as cause of disease classified elsewhere B97.7
Papillon-Léage and Psaume syndrome Q87.0
Papule(s) R23.8
  carate (primary) A67.0
  fibrous, of nose D22.39
  Gottron's L94.4
  pinta (primary) A67.0
Papulosis
  lymphomatoid C86.6
  malignant I77.89
Papyraceous fetus O31.0- ☑
Para-albuminemia E88.09
Paracephalus Q89.7
Parachute mitral valve Q23.2
Paracoccidioidomycosis B41.9
  disseminated B41.7
  generalized B41.7
  mucocutaneous-lymphangitic B41.8
  pulmonary B41.0
  specified NEC B41.8
  visceral B41.8
Paradentosis K05.4
Paraffinoma T88.8 ☑
Paraganglioma D44.7
  adrenal D35.0- ☑
    malignant C74.1- ☑
  aortic body D44.7
    malignant C75.5
  carotid body D44.6
    malignant C75.4
  chromaffin (*see also* Neoplasm, benign, by site)
    malignant — *see* Neoplasm, malignant, by site
  extra-adrenal D44.7
    malignant C75.5
      specified site — *see* Neoplasm, malignant, by site
      unspecified site C75.5
    specified site — *see* Neoplasm, uncertain behavior, by site
    unspecified site D44.7
  gangliocytic D13.2
    specified site — *see* Neoplasm, benign, by site
    unspecified site D13.2
  glomus jugulare D44.7
    malignant C75.5
  jugular D44.7
  malignant C75.5
    specified site — *see* Neoplasm, malignant, by site
    unspecified site C75.5
  nonchromaffin D44.7
    malignant C75.5
      specified site — *see* Neoplasm, malignant, by site
      unspecified site C75.5
    specified site — *see* Neoplasm, uncertain behavior, by site
    unspecified site D44.7
  parasympathetic D44.7
    specified site — *see* Neoplasm, uncertain behavior, by site
    unspecified site D44.7
  specified site — *see* Neoplasm, uncertain behavior, by site
  sympathetic D44.7
    specified site — *see* Neoplasm, uncertain behavior, by site
    unspecified site D44.7
  unspecified site D44.7
Parageusia R43.2
  psychogenic F45.8
Paragonimiasis B66.4

Paragranuloma, Hodgkin — *see* Lymphoma, Hodgkin,
   specified NEC
Parahemophilia (*see also* Defect, coagulation) D68.2
Parakeratosis R23.4
   variegata L41.0
Paralysis, paralytic (complete) (incomplete) G83.9
   with
      syphilis A52.17
   abducens, abducent (nerve) — *see* Strabismus, para-
      lytic, sixth nerve
   abductor, lower extremity G57.9- ☑
   accessory nerve G52.8
   accommodation (*see also* Paresis, of accommodation)
      hysterical F44.89
   acoustic nerve (except Deafness) H93.3 ☑
   agitans (*see also* Parkinsonism) G20
      arteriosclerotic G21.4
   alternating (oculomotor) G83.89
   amyotrophic G12.21
   ankle G57.9- ☑
   anus (sphincter) K62.89
   arm — *see* Monoplegia, upper limb
   ascending (spinal), acute G61.0
   association G12.29
   asthenic bulbar G70.00
      with exacerbation (acute) G70.01
      in crisis G70.01
   ataxic (hereditary) G11.9
      general (syphilitic) A52.17
   atrophic G58.9
      infantile, acute — *see* Poliomyelitis, paralytic
      progressive G12.22
      spinal (acute) — *see* Poliomyelitis, paralytic
   axillary G54.0
   Babinski-Nageotte's G83.89
   Bell's G51.0
      newborn P11.3
   Benedikt's G46.3
   birth injury P14.9
      spinal cord P11.5
   bladder (neurogenic) (sphincter) N31.2
   bowel, colon or intestine K56.0
   brachial plexus G54.0
      birth injury P14.3
      newborn (birth injury) P14.3
   brain G83.9
      diplegia G83.0
      triplegia G83.89
   bronchial J98.09
   Brown-Séquard G83.81
   bulbar (chronic) (progressive) G12.22
      infantile — *see* Poliomyelitis, paralytic
      poliomyelitic — *see* Poliomyelitis, paralytic
      pseudo G12.29
   bulbospinal G70.00
      with exacerbation (acute) G70.01
      in crisis G70.01
   cardiac (*see also* Failure, heart) I50.9
   cerebrocerebellar, diplegic G80.1
   cervical
      plexus G54.2
      sympathetic G90.09
   Céstan-Chenais G46.3
   Charcot-Marie-Tooth type G60.0
   Clark's G80.9
   colon K56.0
   compressed air T70.3 ☑
   compression
      arm G56.9- ☑
      leg G57.9- ☑
      lower extremity G57.9- ☑
      upper extremity G56.9- ☑
   congenital (cerebral) — *see* Palsy, cerebral
   conjugate movement (gaze) (of eye) H51.0
      cortical (nuclear) (supranuclear) H51.0
   cordis — *see* Failure, heart
   cranial or cerebral nerve G52.9
   creeping G12.22
   crossed leg G83.89
   crutch — *see* Injury, brachial plexus
   deglutition R13.0
      hysterical F44.4
   dementia A52.17
   descending (spinal) NEC G12.29
   diaphragm (flaccid) J98.6
      due to accidental dissection of phrenic nerve dur-
         ing procedure — *see* Puncture, accidental
         complicating surgery

Paralysis, paralytic — *continued*
   digestive organs NEC K59.8
   diplegic — *see* Diplegia
   divergence (nuclear) H51.8
   diver's T70.3 ☑
   Duchenne's
      birth injury P14.0
      due to or associated with
         motor neuron disease G12.22
         muscular dystrophy G71.0
   due to intracranial or spinal birth injury — *see* Palsy,
      cerebral
   embolic (current episode) I63.4- ☑
   Erb (-Duchenne) (birth) (newborn) P14.0
   Erb's syphilitic spastic spinal A52.17
   esophagus K22.8
   eye muscle (extrinsic) H49.9
      intrinsic (*see also* Paresis, of accommodation)
   facial (nerve) G51.0
      birth injury P11.3
      congenital P11.3
      following operation NEC — *see* Puncture, acciden-
         tal complicating surgery
      newborn (birth injury) P11.3
   familial (recurrent) (periodic) G72.3
      spastic G11.4
   fauces J39.2
   finger G56.9- ☑
   gait R26.1
   gastric nerve (nondiabetic) G52.2
   gaze, conjugate H51.0
   general (progressive) (syphilitic) A52.17
      juvenile A50.45
   glottis J38.00
      bilateral J38.02
      unilateral J38.01
   gluteal G54.1
   Gubler (-Millard) G46.3
   hand — *see* Monoplegia, upper limb
   heart — *see* Arrest, cardiac
   hemiplegic — *see* Hemiplegia
   hyperkalemic periodic (familial) G72.3
   hypoglossal (nerve) G52.3
   hypokalemic periodic G72.3
   hysterical F44.4
   ileus K56.0
   infantile (*see also* Poliomyelitis, paralytic) A80.30
      bulbar — *see* Poliomyelitis, paralytic
      cerebral — *see* Palsy, cerebral
      spastic — *see* Palsy, cerebral, spastic
   infective — *see* Poliomyelitis, paralytic
   inferior nuclear G83.9
   internuclear — *see* Ophthalmoplegia, internuclear
   intestine K56.0
   iris H57.09
      due to diphtheria (toxin) A36.89
   ischemic, Volkmann's (complicating trauma) T79.6 ☑
   Jackson's G83.89
   jake — *see* Poisoning, food, noxious, plant
   Jamaica ginger (jake) G62.2
   juvenile general A50.45
   Klumpke (-Déjérine) (birth) (newborn) P14.1
   labioglossal (laryngeal) (pharyngeal) G12.29
   Landry's G61.0
   laryngeal nerve (recurrent) (superior) (unilateral) J38.00
      bilateral J38.02
      unilateral J38.01
   larynx J38.00
      bilateral J38.02
      due to diphtheria (toxin) A36.2
      unilateral J38.01
   lateral G12.23
   lead T56.0 ☑
   left side — *see* Hemiplegia
   leg G83.1- ☑
      both — *see* Paraplegia
      crossed G83.89
      hysterical F44.4
      psychogenic F44.4
      transient or transitory R29.818
         traumatic NEC — *see* Injury, nerve, leg
   levator palpebrae superioris — *see* Blepharoptosis,
      paralytic
   limb — *see* Monoplegia
   lip K13.0
   Lissauer's A52.17
   lower limb — *see* Monoplegia, lower limb
      both — *see* Paraplegia

Paralysis, paralytic — *continued*
   lung J98.4
   median nerve G56.1- ☑
   medullary (tegmental) G83.89
   mesencephalic NEC G83.89
      tegmental G83.89
   middle alternating G83.89
   Millard-Gubler-Foville G46.3
   monoplegic — *see* Monoplegia
   motor G83.9
   muscle, muscular NEC G72.89
      due to nerve lesion G58.9
      eye (extrinsic) H49.9
         intrinsic — *see* Paresis, of accommodation
         oblique — *see* Strabismus, paralytic, fourth
            nerve
      iris sphincter H21.9
      ischemic (Volkmann's) (complicating trauma)
         T79.6 ☑
      progressive G12.21
      pseudohypertrophic G71.0
   musculocutaneous nerve G56.9- ☑
   musculospiral G56.9- ☑
   nerve (*see also* Disorder, nerve)
      abducent — *see* Strabismus, paralytic, sixth nerve
      accessory G52.8
      auditory (except Deafness) H93.3 ☑
      birth injury P14.9
      cranial or cerebral G52.9
      facial G51.0
         birth injury P11.3
         congenital P11.3
         newborn (birth injury) P11.3
      fourth or trochlear — *see* Strabismus, paralytic,
         fourth nerve
      newborn (birth injury) P14.9
      oculomotor — *see* Strabismus, paralytic, third
         nerve
      phrenic (birth injury) P14.2
      radial G56.3- ☑
      seventh or facial G51.0
         newborn (birth injury) P11.3
      sixth or abducent — *see* Strabismus, paralytic, sixth
         nerve
      syphilitic A52.15
      third or oculomotor — *see* Strabismus, paralytic,
         third nerve
      trigeminal G50.9
      trochlear — *see* Strabismus, paralytic, fourth nerve
      ulnar G56.2- ☑
   normokalemic periodic G72.3
   ocular H49.9
      alternating G83.89
   oculofacial, congenital (Moebius) Q87.0
   oculomotor (external bilateral) (nerve) — *see* Strabis-
      mus, paralytic, third nerve
   palate (soft) K13.79
   paratrigeminal G50.9
   periodic (familial) (hyperkalemic) (hypokalemic) (my-
      otonic) (normokalemic) (potassium sensitive)
      (secondary) G72.3
   peripheral autonomic nervous system — *see* Neuropa-
      thy, peripheral, autonomic
   peroneal (nerve) G57.3- ☑
   pharynx J39.2
   phrenic nerve G56.8- ☑
   plantar nerve(s) G57.6- ☑
   pneumogastric nerve G52.2
   poliomyelitis (current) — *see* Poliomyelitis, paralytic
   popliteal nerve G57.3- ☑
   postepileptic transitory G83.84
   progressive (atrophic) (bulbar) (spinal) G12.22
      general A52.17
      infantile acute — *see* Poliomyelitis, paralytic
      supranuclear G23.1
   pseudobulbar G12.29
   pseudohypertrophic (muscle) G71.0
   psychogenic F44.4
   quadriceps G57.9- ☑
   quadriplegic — *see* Tetraplegia
   radial nerve G56.3- ☑
   rectus muscle (eye) H49.9
   recurrent isolated sleep G47.53
   respiratory (muscle) (system) (tract) R06.81
      center NEC G93.89
      congenital P28.89
      newborn P28.89
   right side — *see* Hemiplegia

Paralysis, paralytic — continued
　saturnine T56.0 ☑
　sciatic nerve G57.0- ☑
　senile G83.9
　shaking — see Parkinsonism
　shoulder G56.9- ☑
　sleep, recurrent isolated G47.53
　spastic G83.9
　　cerebral — see Palsy, cerebral, spastic
　　congenital (cerebral) — see Palsy, cerebral, spastic
　　familial G11.4
　　hereditary G11.4
　　quadriplegic G80.0
　　syphilitic (spinal) A52.17
　sphincter, bladder — see Paralysis, bladder
　spinal (cord) G83.9
　　accessory nerve G52.8
　　acute — see Poliomyelitis, paralytic
　　ascending acute G61.0
　　atrophic (acute) (see also Poliomyelitis, paralytic)
　　　spastic, syphilitic A52.17
　　congenital NEC — see Palsy, cerebral
　　hereditary G95.89
　　infantile — see Poliomyelitis, paralytic
　　progressive G12.21
　　sequelae NEC G83.89
　sternomastoid G52.8
　stomach K31.84
　　diabetic — see Diabetes, by type, with gastroparesis
　　nerve G52.2
　　　diabetic — see Diabetes, by type, with gastroparesis
　stroke — see Infarct, brain
　subcapsularis G56.8- ☑
　supranuclear (progressive) G23.1
　sympathetic G90.8
　　cervical G90.09
　　nervous system — see Neuropathy, peripheral, autonomic
　syndrome G83.9
　　specified NEC G83.89
　syphilitic spastic spinal (Erb's) A52.17
　thigh G57.9- ☑
　throat J39.2
　　diphtheritic A36.0
　　muscle J39.2
　thrombotic (current episode) I63.3- ☑
　thumb G56.9- ☑
　tick — see Toxicity, venom, arthropod, specified NEC
　Todd's (postepileptic transitory paralysis) G83.84
　toe G57.6- ☑
　tongue K14.8
　transient R29.5
　　arm or leg NEC R29.818
　　traumatic NEC — see Injury, nerve
　trapezius G52.8
　traumatic, transient NEC — see Injury, nerve
　trembling — see Parkinsonism
　triceps brachii G56.9- ☑
　trigeminal nerve G50.9
　trochlear (nerve) — see Strabismus, paralytic, fourth nerve
　ulnar nerve G56.2- ☑
　upper limb — see Monoplegia, upper limb
　uremic N18.9 [G99.8]
　uveoparotitic D86.89
　uvula K13.79
　　postdiphtheritic A36.0
　vagus nerve G52.2
　vasomotor NEC G90.8
　velum palati K13.79
　vesical — see Paralysis, bladder
　vestibular nerve (except Vertigo) H93.3 ☑
　vocal cords J38.00
　　bilateral J38.02
　　unilateral J38.01
　Volkmann's (complicating trauma) T79.6 ☑
　wasting G12.29
　Weber's G46.3
　wrist G56.9- ☑
Paramedial urethrovesical orifice Q64.79
Paramenia N92.6
Parametritis (see also Disease, pelvis, inflammatory) N73.2
　acute N73.0

Parametritis — continued
　complicating abortion — see Abortion, by type, complicated by, parametritis
Parametrium, parametric — see condition
Paramnesia — see Amnesia
Paramolar K00.1
Paramyloidosis E85.89
Paramyoclonus multiplex G25.3
Paramyotonia (congenita) G71.19
Parangi — see Yaws
Paranoia (querulans) F22
　senile F03 ☑
Paranoid
　dementia (senile) F03 ☑
　　praecox — see Schizophrenia
　personality F60.0
　psychosis (climacteric) (involutional) (menopausal) F22
　　psychogenic (acute) F23
　　senile F03 ☑
　reaction (acute) F23
　　chronic F22
　schizophrenia F20.0
　state (climacteric) (involutional) (menopausal) (simple) F22
　　senile F03 ☑
　tendencies F60.0
　traits F60.0
　trends F60.0
　type, psychopathic personality F60.0
Paraparesis — see Paraplegia
Paraphasia R47.02
Paraphilia F65.9
Paraphimosis (congenital) N47.2
　chancroidal A57
Paraphrenia, paraphrenic (late) F22
　schizophrenia F20.0
Paraplegia (lower) G82.20
　ataxic — see Degeneration, combined, spinal cord
　complete G82.21
　congenital (cerebral) G80.8
　　spastic G80.1
　familial spastic G11.4
　functional (hysterical) F44.4
　hereditary, spastic G11.4
　hysterical F44.4
　incomplete G82.22
　Pott's A18.01
　psychogenic F44.4
　spastic
　　Erb's spinal, syphilitic A52.17
　　hereditary G11.4
　　tropical G04.1
　syphilitic (spastic) A52.17
　tropical spastic G04.1
Parapoxvirus B08.60
　specified NEC B08.69
Paraproteinemia D89.2
　benign (familial) D89.2
　monoclonal D47.2
　secondary to malignant disease D47.2
Parapsoriasis L41.9
　en plaques L41.4
　guttata L41.1
　large plaque L41.4
　retiform, retiformis L41.5
　small plaque L41.3
　specified NEC L41.8
　varioliformis (acuta) L41.0
Parasitic (see also condition)
　disease NEC B89
　stomatitis B37.0
　sycosis (beard) (scalp) B35.0
　twin Q89.4
Parasitism B89
　intestinal B82.9
　skin B88.9
　specified — see Infestation
Parasitophobia F40.218
Parasomnia G47.50
　due to
　　alcohol
　　　abuse F10.182
　　　dependence F10.282
　　　use F10.982
　　amphetamines
　　　abuse F15.182
　　　dependence F15.282

Parasomnia — continued
　due to — continued
　　amphetamines — continued
　　　use F15.982
　　caffeine
　　　abuse F15.182
　　　dependence F15.282
　　　use F15.982
　　cocaine
　　　abuse F14.182
　　　dependence F14.282
　　　use F14.982
　　drug NEC
　　　abuse F19.182
　　　dependence F19.282
　　　use F19.982
　　opioid
　　　abuse F11.182
　　　dependence F11.282
　　　use F11.982
　　psychoactive substance NEC
　　　abuse F19.182
　　　dependence F19.282
　　　use F19.982
　　sedative, hypnotic, or anxiolytic
　　　abuse F13.182
　　　dependence F13.282
　　　use F13.982
　　stimulant NEC
　　　abuse F15.182
　　　dependence F15.282
　　　use F15.982
　　in conditions classified elsewhere G47.54
　　nonorganic origin F51.8
　　organic G47.50
　　specified NEC G47.59
Paraspadias Q54.9
Paraspasmus facialis G51.8
Parasuicide (attempt)
　history of (personal) Z91.5
　　in family Z81.8
Parathyroid gland — see condition
Parathyroid tetany E20.9
Paratrachoma A74.0
Paratyphilitis — see Appendicitis
Paratyphoid (fever) — see Fever, paratyphoid
Paratyphus — see Fever, paratyphoid
Paraurethral duct Q64.79
　nonorganic origin F51.5
Paraurethritis (see also Urethritis)
　gonococcal (acute) (chronic) (with abscess) A54.1
Paravaccinia NEC B08.04
Paravaginitis — see Vaginitis
Parencephalitis (see also Encephalitis)
　sequelae G09
Parent-child conflict — see Conflict, parent-child
　estrangement NEC Z62.890
Paresis (see also Paralysis)
　accommodation — see Paresis, of accommodation
　Bernhardt's G57.1- ☑
　bladder (sphincter) (see also Paralysis, bladder)
　　tabetic A52.17
　bowel, colon or intestine K56.0
　extrinsic muscle, eye H49.9
　general (progressive) (syphilitic) A52.17
　　juvenile A50.45
　heart — see Failure, heart
　insane (syphilitic) A52.17
　juvenile (general) A50.45
　of accommodation H52.52- ☑
　peripheral progressive (idiopathic) G60.3
　pseudohypertrophic G71.0
　senile G83.9
　syphilitic (general) A52.17
　　congenital A50.45
　vesical NEC N31.2
Paresthesia (see also Disturbance, sensation, skin) R20.2
　Bernhardt G57.1- ☑
Paretic — see condition
Parinaud's
　conjunctivitis H10.89
　oculoglandular syndrome H10.89
　ophthalmoplegia H49.88- ☑
Parkinsonism (idiopathic) (primary) G20
　with neurogenic orthostatic hypotension (symptomatic) G90.3
　arteriosclerotic G21.4
　dementia G31.83 [F02.80]

Parkinsonism — *continued*
  dementia — *continued*
    with behavioral disturbance G31.83 [F02.81]
  due to
    drugs NEC G21.19
      neuroleptic G21.11
    medication-induced NEC G21.19
  neuroleptic induced G21.11
  postencephalitic G21.3
  secondary G21.9
    due to
      arteriosclerosis G21.4
      drugs NEC G21.19
        neuroleptic G21.11
      encephalitis G21.3
      external agents NEC G21.2
      syphilis A52.19
    specified NEC G21.8
  syphilitic A52.19
  treatment-induced NEC G21.19
  vascular G21.4
Parkinson's disease, syndrome or tremor — *see* Parkinsonism
Parodontitis — *see* Periodontitis
Parodontosis K05.4
Paronychia (*see also* Cellulitis, digit)
  with lymphangitis — *see* Lymphangitis, acute, digit
  candidal (chronic) B37.2
  tuberculous (primary) A18.4
Parorexia (psychogenic) F50.89
Parosmia R43.1
  psychogenic F45.8
Parotid gland — *see* condition
Parotitis, parotiditis (allergic)(nonspecific toxic) (purulent) (septic) (suppurative) (*see also* Sialoadenitis)
  epidemic — *see* Mumps
  infectious — *see* Mumps
  postoperative K91.89
  surgical K91.89
Parrot fever A70
Parrot's disease (early congenital syphilitic pseudoparalysis) A50.02
Parry-Romberg syndrome G51.8
Parry's disease or syndrome E05.00
  with thyroid storm E05.01
Pars planitis — *see* Cyclitis
Parsonage (-Aldren)-**Turner syndrome** G54.5
Parson's disease (exophthalmic goiter) E05.00
  with thyroid storm E05.01
Particolored infant Q82.8
Parturition — *see* Delivery
Parulis K04.7
  with sinus K04.6
Parvovirus, as cause of disease classified elsewhere B97.6
Pasini and Pierini's atrophoderma L90.3
Passage
  false, urethra N36.5
  meconium (newborn) during delivery P03.82
  of sounds or bougies — *see* Attention to, artificial, opening
Passive — *see* condition
  smoking Z77.22
Pasteurella septica A28.0
Pasteurellosis — *see* Infection, Pasteurella
PAT (paroxysmal atrial tachycardia) I47.1
Patau's syndrome — *see* Trisomy, 13
Patches
  mucous (syphilitic) A51.39
    congenital A50.07
  smokers' (mouth) K13.24
Patellar — *see* condition
Patent (*see also* Imperfect, closure)
  canal of Nuck Q52.4
  cervix N88.3
  ductus arteriosus or Botallo's Q25.0
  foramen
    botalli Q21.1
    ovale Q21.1
  interauricular septum Q21.1
  interventricular septum Q21.0
  omphalomesenteric duct Q43.0
  os (uteri) — *see* Patent, cervix
  ostium secundum Q21.1
  urachus Q64.4
  vitelline duct Q43.0
Paterson (-Brown)(-Kelly) **syndrome or web** D50.1

Pathologic, pathological (*see also* condition)
  asphyxia R09.01
  fire-setting F63.1
  gambling F63.0
  ovum O02.0
  resorption, tooth K03.3
  stealing F63.2
Pathology (of) — *see* Disease
  periradicular, associated with previous endodontic treatment NEC M27.59
Pattern, sleep-wake, irregular G47.23
Patulous (*see also* Imperfect, closure (congenital))
  alimentary tract Q45.8
    lower Q43.8
    upper Q40.8
  eustachian tube H69.0- ☑
Pause, sinoatrial I49.5
Paxton's disease B36.2
Pearl(s)
  enamel K00.2
  Epstein's K09.8
Pearl-worker's disease — *see* Osteomyelitis, specified type NEC
Pectenosis K62.4
Pectoral — *see* condition
Pectus
  carinatum (congenital) Q67.7
    acquired M95.4
    rachitic sequelae (late effect) E64.3
  excavatum (congenital) Q67.6
    acquired M95.4
    rachitic sequelae (late effect) E64.3
  recurvatum (congenital) Q67.6
Pedatrophia E41
Pederosis F65.4
Pediculosis (infestation) B85.2
  capitis (head-louse) (any site) B85.0
  corporis (body-louse) (any site) B85.1
  eyelid B85.0
  mixed (classifiable to more than one of the titles B85.0-B85.3) B85.4
  pubis (pubic louse) (any site) B85.3
  vestimenti B85.1
  vulvae B85.3
Pediculus (infestation) — *see* Pediculosis
Pedophilia F65.4
Peg-shaped teeth K00.2
Pelade — *see* Alopecia, areata
Pelger-Huët anomaly or syndrome D72.0
Peliosis (rheumatica) D69.0
  hepatis K76.4
    with toxic liver disease K71.8
Pelizaeus-Merzbacher disease E75.29
Pellagra (alcoholic) (with polyneuropathy) E52
Pellagra-cerebellar-ataxia-renal aminoaciduria syndrome E72.02
Pellegrini (-Stieda) **disease or syndrome** — *see* Bursitis, tibial collateral
Pellizzi's syndrome E34.8
Pelvic (*see also* condition)
  examination (periodic) (routine) Z01.419
    with abnormal findings Z01.411
  kidney, congenital Q63.2
Pelviolithiasis — *see* Calculus, kidney
Pelviperitonitis (*see also* Peritonitis, pelvic)
  gonococcal A54.24
  puerperal O85
Pelvis — *see* condition or type
Pemphigoid L12.9
  benign, mucous membrane L12.1
  bullous L12.0
  cicatricial L12.1
  juvenile L12.2
  ocular L12.1
  specified NEC L12.8
Pemphigus L10.9
  benign familial (chronic) Q82.8
  Brazilian L10.3
  circinatus L13.0
  conjunctival L12.1
  drug-induced L10.5
  erythematosus L10.4
  foliaceus L10.2
  gangrenous — *see* Gangrene
  neonatorum L01.03
  ocular L12.1
  paraneoplastic L10.81

Pemphigus — *continued*
  specified NEC L10.89
  syphilitic (congenital) A50.06
  vegetans L10.1
  vulgaris L10.0
  wildfire L10.3
Pendred's syndrome E07.1
Pendulous
  abdomen, in pregnancy — *see* Pregnancy, complicated by, abnormal, pelvic organs or tissues NEC
  breast N64.89
Penetrating wound (*see also* Puncture)
  with internal injury — *see* Injury, by site
  eyeball — *see* Puncture, eyeball
  orbit (with or without foreign body) — *see* Puncture, orbit
  uterus by instrument with or following ectopic or molar pregnancy O08.6
Penicillosis B48.4
Penis — *see* condition
Penitis N48.29
Pentalogy of Fallot Q21.8
Pentasomy X syndrome Q97.1
Pentosuria (essential) E74.8
Percreta placenta - O43.23 ☑
Peregrinating patient — *see* Disorder, factitious
Perforation, perforated (nontraumatic) (of)
  accidental during procedure (blood vessel) (nerve) (organ) — *see* Complication, accidental puncture or laceration
  antrum — *see* Sinusitis, maxillary
  appendix K35.2
    with localized peritonitis K35.3
  atrial septum, multiple Q21.1
  attic, ear — *see* Perforation, tympanum, attic
  bile duct (common) (hepatic) K83.2
    cystic K82.2
  bladder (urinary)
    with or following ectopic or molar pregnancy O08.6
    obstetrical trauma O71.5
    traumatic S37.29 ☑
      at delivery O71.5
  bowel K63.1
    with or following ectopic or molar pregnancy O08.6
    newborn P78.0
    obstetrical trauma O71.5
    traumatic — *see* Laceration, intestine
  broad ligament N83.8
    with or following ectopic or molar pregnancy O08.6
    obstetrical trauma O71.6
  by
    device, implant or graft (*see also* Complications, by site and type, mechanical) T85.628 ☑
      arterial graft NEC — *see* Complication, cardiovascular device, mechanical, vascular
      breast (implant) T85.49 ☑
      catheter NEC T85.698 ☑
        cystostomy T83.090 ☑
        dialysis (renal) T82.49 ☑
          intraperitoneal T85.691 ☑
        infusion NEC T82.594 ☑
          spinal (epidural) (subdural) T85.690 ☑
        urinary (*see also* Complications, catheter, urinary T83.098 ☑
      electronic (electrode) (pulse generator) (stimulator)
        bone T84.390 ☑
        cardiac T82.199 ☑
          electrode T82.190 ☑
          pulse generator T82.191 ☑
          specified type NEC T82.198 ☑
        nervous system — *see* Complication, prosthetic device, mechanical, electronic nervous system stimulator
        urinary — *see* Complication, genitourinary, device, urinary, mechanical
      fixation, internal (orthopedic) NEC — *see* Complication, fixation device, mechanical
      gastrointestinal — *see* Complications, prosthetic device, mechanical, gastrointestinal device
      genital NEC T83.498 ☑
        intrauterine contraceptive device T83.39 ☑
        penile prosthesis T83.490 ☑
      heart NEC — *see* Complication, cardiovascular device, mechanical

---

Perforation, perforated — *continued*
  by — *continued*
    device, implant or graft (*see also* Complications, by
      site and type, mechanical) — *continued*
      joint prosthesis — *see* Complications, joint
        prosthesis, mechanical, specified NEC, by
        site
      ocular NEC — *see* Complications, prosthetic
        device, mechanical, ocular device
      orthopedic NEC — *see* Complication, orthope-
        dic, device, mechanical
        specified NEC T85.628 ☑
      urinary NEC (*see also* Complication, genitouri-
        nary, device, urinary, mechanical)
        graft T83.29 ☑
      vascular NEC — *see* Complication, cardiovascu-
        lar device, mechanical
      ventricular intracranial shunt T85.09 ☑
    foreign body left accidentally in operative wound
      T81.539 ☑
    instrument (any) during a procedure, accidental
      — *see* Puncture, accidental complicating
      surgery
  cecum K35.2
    with localized peritonitis K35.3
  cervix (uteri) N88.8
    with or following ectopic or molar pregnancy O08.6
    obstetrical trauma O71.3
  colon K63.1
    newborn P78.0
    obstetrical trauma O71.5
    traumatic — *see* Laceration, intestine, large
  common duct (bile) K83.2
  cornea (due to ulceration) — *see* Ulcer, cornea, perfo-
    rated
  cystic duct K82.2
  diverticulum (intestine) K57.80
    with bleeding K57.81
    large intestine K57.20
      with
        bleeding K57.21
        small intestine K57.40
          with bleeding K57.41
      small intestine K57.00
      with
        bleeding K57.01
        large intestine K57.40
          with bleeding K57.41
  ear drum — *see* Perforation, tympanum
  esophagus K22.3
  ethmoidal sinus — *see* Sinusitis, ethmoidal
  frontal sinus — *see* Sinusitis, frontal
  gallbladder K82.2
  heart valve — *see* Endocarditis
  ileum K63.1
    newborn P78.0
    obstetrical trauma O71.5
    traumatic — *see* Laceration, intestine, small
  instrumental, surgical (accidental) (blood vessel)
    (nerve) (organ) — *see* Puncture, accidental
    complicating surgery
  intestine NEC K63.1
    with ectopic or molar pregnancy O08.6
    newborn P78.0
    obstetrical trauma O71.5
    traumatic — *see* Laceration, intestine
    ulcerative NEC K63.1
      newborn P78.0
  jejunum, jejunal K63.1
    obstetrical trauma O71.5
    traumatic — *see* Laceration, intestine, small
    ulcer — *see* Ulcer, gastrojejunal, with perforation
  joint prosthesis — *see* Complications, joint prosthesis,
    mechanical, specified NEC, by site
  mastoid (antrum) (cell) — *see* Disorder, mastoid,
    specified NEC
  maxillary sinus — *see* Sinusitis, maxillary
  membrana tympani — *see* Perforation, tympanum
  nasal
    septum J34.89
      congenital Q30.3
      syphilitic A52.73
    sinus J34.89
      congenital Q30.8
      due to sinusitis — *see* Sinusitis
  palate (*see also* Cleft, palate) Q35.9
    syphilitic A52.79
  palatine vault (*see also* Cleft, palate, hard) Q35.1

Perforation, perforated — *continued*
  palatine vault (*see also* Cleft, palate, hard) — *contin-*
    ued
    syphilitic A52.79
      congenital A50.59
  pars flaccida (ear drum) — *see* Perforation, tympanum,
    attic
  pelvic
    floor S31.030 ☑
      with
        ectopic or molar pregnancy O08.6
        penetration into retroperitoneal space
          S31.031 ☑
        retained foreign body S31.040 ☑
          with penetration into retroperitoneal
            space S31.041 ☑
      following ectopic or molar pregnancy O08.6
      obstetrical trauma O70.1
    organ S37.99
      adrenal gland S37.818 ☑
      bladder — *see* Perforation, bladder
      fallopian tube S37.599 ☑
        bilateral S37.592 ☑
        unilateral S37.591 ☑
      kidney S37.09- ☑
      obstetrical trauma O71.5
      ovary S37.499 ☑
        bilateral S37.492 ☑
        unilateral S37.491 ☑
      prostate S37.828 ☑
      specified organ NEC S37.898 ☑
      ureter — *see* Perforation, ureter
      urethra — *see* Perforation, urethra
      uterus — *see* Perforation, uterus
  perineum — *see* Laceration, perineum
  pharynx J39.2
  rectum K63.1
    newborn P78.0
    obstetrical trauma O71.5
    traumatic S36.63 ☑
  root canal space due to endodontic treatment M27.51
  sigmoid K63.1
    newborn P78.0
    obstetrical trauma O71.5
    traumatic S36.533 ☑
  sinus (accessory) (chronic) (nasal) J34.89
  sphenoidal sinus — *see* Sinusitis, sphenoidal
  surgical (accidental) (by instrument) (blood vessel)
    (nerve) (organ) — *see* Puncture, accidental
    complicating surgery
  traumatic
    external — *see* Puncture
    eye — *see* Puncture, eyeball
    internal organ — *see* Injury, by site
  tympanum, tympanic (membrane) (persistent post-
    traumatic) (postinflammatory) H72.9- ☑
    attic H72.1- ☑
      multiple — *see* Perforation, tympanum, multi-
        ple
      total — *see* Perforation, tympanum, total
    central H72.0- ☑
      multiple — *see* Perforation, tympanum, multi-
        ple
      total — *see* Perforation, tympanum, total
    marginal NEC — *see* subcategory H72.2 ☑
    multiple H72.81- ☑
    pars flaccida — *see* Perforation, tympanum, attic
    total H72.82- ☑
    traumatic, current episode S09.2- ☑
  typhoid, gastrointestinal — *see* Typhoid
  ulcer — *see* Ulcer, by site, with perforation
  ureter N28.89
    traumatic S37.19 ☑
  urethra N36.8
    with ectopic or molar pregnancy O08.6
    following ectopic or molar pregnancy O08.6
    obstetrical trauma O71.5
    traumatic S37.39 ☑
      at delivery O71.5
  uterus
    with ectopic or molar pregnancy O08.6
    by intrauterine contraceptive device T83.39 ☑
    following ectopic or molar pregnancy O08.6
    obstetrical trauma O71.1
    traumatic S37.69 ☑
      obstetric O71.1
  uvula K13.79

Perforation, perforated — *continued*
  uvula — *continued*
    syphilitic A52.79
  vagina O71.4
    obstetrical trauma O71.4
    other trauma — *see* Puncture, vagina
Periadenitis mucosa necrotica recurrens K12.0
Periappendicitis (acute) — *see* Appendicitis
Periarteritis nodosa (disseminated) (infectious)
  (necrotizing) M30.0
Periarthritis (joint) (*see also* Enthesopathy)
  Duplay's M75.0- ☑
  gonococcal A54.42
  humeroscapularis — *see* Capsulitis, adhesive
  scapulohumeral — *see* Capsulitis, adhesive
  shoulder — *see* Capsulitis, adhesive
  wrist M77.2- ☑
Periarthrosis (angioneural) — *see* Enthesopathy
Pericapsulitis, adhesive (shoulder) — *see* Capsulitis,
  adhesive
Pericarditis (with decompensation) (with effusion) I31.9
  with rheumatic fever (conditions in I00)
    active — *see* Pericarditis, rheumatic
    inactive or quiescent I09.2
  acute (hemorrhagic) (nonrheumatic) (Sicca) I30.9
    with chorea (acute) (rheumatic) (Sydenham's) I02.0
    benign I30.8
    nonspecific I30.0
    rheumatic I01.0
      with chorea (acute) (Sydenham's) I02.0
  adhesive or adherent (chronic) (external) (internal)
    I31.0
    acute — *see* Pericarditis, acute
    rheumatic I09.2
  bacterial (acute) (subacute) (with serous or seropuru-
    lent effusion) I30.1
  calcareous I31.1
  cholesterol (chronic) I31.8
    acute I30.9
  chronic (nonrheumatic) I31.9
    rheumatic I09.2
  constrictive (chronic) I31.1
  coxsackie B33.23
  fibrinocaseous (tuberculous) A18.84
  fibrinopurulent I30.1
  fibrinous I30.8
  fibrous I31.0
  gonococcal A54.83
  idiopathic I30.0
  in systemic lupus erythematosus M32.12
  infective I30.1
  meningococcal A39.53
  neoplastic (chronic) I31.8
    acute I30.9
  obliterans, obliterating I31.0
  plastic I31.0
  pneumococcal I30.1
  postinfarction I24.1
  purulent I30.1
  rheumatic (active) (acute) (with effusion) (with pneu-
    monia) I01.0
    with chorea (acute) (rheumatic) (Sydenham's) I02.0
    chronic or inactive (with chorea) I09.2
  rheumatoid — *see* Rheumatoid, carditis
  septic I30.1
  serofibrinous I30.8
  staphylococcal I30.1
  streptococcal I30.1
  suppurative I30.1
  syphilitic A52.06
  tuberculous A18.84
  uremic N18.9 [I32]
  viral I30.1
Pericardium, pericardial — *see* condition
Pericellulitis — *see* Cellulitis
Pericementitis (chronic) (suppurative) (*see also* Periodontitis)
  acute K05.20
    generalized — *see* Peridontitis, aggressive, gener-
      alized
    localized — *see* Peridontitis, aggressive, localized
Perichondritis
  auricle — *see* Perichondritis, ear
  bronchus J98.09
  ear (external) H61.00- ☑
    acute H61.01- ☑
    chronic H61.02- ☑
  external auditory canal — *see* Perichondritis, ear

☑ **Additional Character Required — Refer to the Tabular List for Character Selection** ▽ Subterms under main terms may continue to next column or page

Perichondritis — *continued*
 larynx J38.7
  syphilitic A52.73
  typhoid A01.09
 nose J34.89
 pinna — *see* Perichondritis, ear
 trachea J39.8
Periclasia K05.4
Pericoronitis — *see* Periodontitis
Pericystitis N30.90
 with hematuria N30.91
Peridiverticulitis (intestine) K57.92
 cecum — *see* Diverticulitis, intestine, large
 colon — *see* Diverticulitis, intestine, large
 duodenum — *see* Diverticulitis, intestine, small
 intestine — *see* Diverticulitis, intestine
 jejunum — *see* Diverticulitis, intestine, small
 rectosigmoid — *see* Diverticulitis, intestine, large
 rectum — *see* Diverticulitis, intestine, large
 sigmoid — *see* Diverticulitis, intestine, large
Periendocarditis — *see* Endocarditis
Periepididymitis N45.1
Perifolliculitis L01.02
 abscedens, caput, scalp L66.3
 capitis, abscedens (et suffodiens) L66.3
 superficial pustular L01.02
Perihepatitis K65.8
Perilabyrinthitis (acute) — *see* subcategory H83.0 ☑
Perimeningitis — *see* Meningitis
Perimetritis — *see* Endometritis
Perimetrosalpingitis — *see* Salpingo-oophoritis
Perineocele N81.81
Perinephric, perinephritic — *see* condition
Perinephritis (*see also* Infection, kidney)
 purulent — *see* Abscess, kidney
Perineum, perineal — *see* condition
Perineuritis NEC — *see* Neuralgia
Periodic — *see* condition
Periodontitis (chronic) (complex) (compound) (local)
  (simplex) K05.30
 acute K05.20
  generalized K05.229
   moderate K05.222
   severe K05.223
   slight K05.221
  localized K05.219
   moderate K05.212
   severe K05.213
   slight K05.211
 apical K04.5
  acute (pulpal origin) K04.4
 generalized K05.329
  moderate K05.322
  severe K05.323
  slight K05.321
 localized K05.319
  moderate K05.312
  severe K05.313
  slight K05.311
Periodontoclasia K05.4
Periodontosis (juvenile) K05.4
Periods (*see also* Menstruation)
 heavy N92.0
 irregular N92.6
 shortened intervals (irregular) N92.1
Perionychia (*see also* Cellulitis, digit)
 with lymphangitis — *see* Lymphangitis, acute, digit
Perioophoritis — *see* Salpingo-oophoritis
Periorchitis N45.2
Periosteum, periosteal — *see* condition
Periostitis (albuminosa) (circumscribed) (diffuse) (infective) (monomelic) (*see also* Osteomyelitis)
 alveolar M27.3
 alveolodental M27.3
 dental M27.3
 gonorrheal A54.43
 jaw (lower) (upper) M27.2
 orbit H05.03- ☑
 syphilitic A52.77
  congenital (early) A50.02 [M90.80]
  secondary A51.46
 tuberculous — *see* Tuberculosis, bone
 yaws (hypertrophic) (early) (late) A66.6 [M90.80]
Periostosis (hyperplastic) (*see also* Disorder, bone,
  specified type NEC)
 with osteomyelitis — *see* Osteomyelitis, specified type
  NEC

Peripartum
 cardiomyopathy O90.3
Periphlebitis — *see* Phlebitis
Periproctitis K62.89
Periprostatitis — *see* Prostatitis
Perirectal — *see* condition
Perirenal — *see* condition
Perisalpingitis — *see* Salpingo-oophoritis
Perisplenitis (infectional) D73.89
Peristalsis, visible or reversed R19.2
Peritendinitis — *see* Enthesopathy
Peritoneum, peritoneal — *see* condition
Peritonitis (adhesive) (bacterial) (fibrinous) (hemorrhagic) (idiopathic) (localized) (perforative) (primary)
  (with adhesions) (with effusion) K65.9
 with or following
  abscess K65.1
  appendicitis K35.3
   with perforation or rupture K35.2
   generalized K35.2
   localized K35.3
  diverticular disease (intestine) K57.80
   with bleeding K57.81
   ectopic or molar pregnancy O08.0
   large intestine K57.20
    with
     bleeding K57.21
     small intestine K57.40
      with bleeding K57.41
   small intestine K57.00
    with
     bleeding K57.01
     large intestine K57.40
      with bleeding K57.41
 acute (generalized) K65.0
 aseptic T81.61 ☑
 bile, biliary K65.3
 chemical T81.61 ☑
 chlamydial A74.81
 chronic proliferative K65.8
 complicating abortion — *see* Abortion, by type, complicated by, pelvic peritonitis
 congenital P78.1
 diaphragmatic K65.0
 diffuse K65.0
 diphtheritic A36.89
 disseminated K65.0
 due to
  bile K65.3
  foreign
   body or object accidentally left during a proce-
    dure (instrument) (sponge) (swab)
    T81.599 ☑
   substance accidentally left during a procedure
    (chemical) (powder) (talc) T81.61 ☑
  talc T81.61 ☑
  urine K65.8
 eosinophilic K65.8
  acute K65.0
 fibrocaseous (tuberculous) A18.31
 fibropurulent K65.0
 following ectopic or molar pregnancy O08.0
 general (ized) K65.0
 gonococcal A54.85
 meconium (newborn) P78.0
 neonatal P78.1
  meconium P78.0
 pancreatic K65.0
 paroxysmal, familial E85.0
  benign E85.0
 pelvic
  female N73.5
   acute N73.3
   chronic N73.4
    with adhesions N73.6
  male K65.0
 periodic, familial E85.0
 proliferative, chronic K65.8
 puerperal, postpartum, childbirth O85
 purulent K65.0
 septic K65.0
 specified NEC K65.8
 spontaneous bacterial K65.2
 subdiaphragmatic K65.0
 subphrenic K65.0
 suppurative K65.0
 syphilitic A52.74
  congenital (early) A50.08 [K67]

Peritonitis — *continued*
 talc T81.61 ☑
 tuberculous A18.31
 urine K65.8
Peritonsillar — *see* condition
Peritonsillitis J36
Perityphlitis K37
Periureteritis N28.89
Periurethral — *see* condition
Periurethritis (gangrenous) — *see* Urethritis
Periuterine — *see* condition
Perivaginitis — *see* Vaginitis
Perivasculitis, retinal H35.06- ☑
Perivasitis (chronic) N49.1
Perivesiculitis (seminal) — *see* Vesiculitis
Perlèche NEC K13.0
 due to
  candidiasis B37.83
  moniliasis B37.83
  riboflavin deficiency E53.0
  vitamin B2 (riboflavin) deficiency E53.0
Pernicious — *see* condition
Pernio, perniosis T69.1 ☑
Perpetrator (of abuse) — *see* Index to External Causes
  of Injury, Perpetrator
Persecution
 delusion F22
 social Z60.5
Perseveration (tonic) R48.8
Persistence, persistent (congenital)
 anal membrane Q42.3
  with fistula Q42.2
 arteria stapedia Q16.3
 atrioventricular canal Q21.2
 branchial cleft NOS Q18.2
  cyst Q18.0
  fistula Q18.0
  sinus Q18.0
 bulbus cordis in left ventricle Q21.8
 canal of Cloquet Q14.0
 capsule (opaque) Q12.8
 cilioretinal artery or vein Q14.8
 cloaca Q43.7
 communication — *see* Fistula, congenital
 convolutions
  aortic arch Q25.46
  fallopian tube Q50.6
  oviduct Q50.6
  uterine tube Q50.6
 double aortic arch Q25.45
 ductus arteriosus (Botalli) Q25.0
 fetal
  circulation P29.38
  form of cervix (uteri) Q51.828
  hemoglobin, hereditary (HPFH) D56.4
 foramen
  Botalli Q21.1
  ovale Q21.1
 Gartner's duct Q52.4
 hemoglobin, fetal (hereditary) (HPFH) D56.4
 hyaloid
  artery (generally incomplete) Q14.0
  system Q14.8
 hymen, in pregnancy or childbirth — *see* Pregnancy,
  complicated by, abnormal, vulva
 lanugo Q84.2
 left
  posterior cardinal vein Q26.8
  root with right arch of aorta Q25.49
  superior vena cava Q26.1
 Meckel's diverticulum Q43.0
  malignant — *see* Table of Neoplasms, small intestine, malignant
 mucosal disease (middle ear) — *see* Otitis, media,
   suppurative, chronic, tubotympanic
 nail(s), anomalous Q84.6
 omphalomesenteric duct Q43.0
 organ or site not listed — *see* Anomaly, by site
 ostium
  atrioventriculare commune Q21.2
  primum Q21.2
  secundum Q21.1
 ovarian rests in fallopian tube Q50.6
 pancreatic tissue in intestinal tract Q43.8
 primary (deciduous)
  teeth K00.6
  vitreous hyperplasia Q14.0
 pupillary membrane Q13.89

Persistence, persistent — *continued*
rhesus (Rh) titer — *see* Complication(s), transfusion, incompatibility reaction, Rh (factor)
right aortic arch Q25.47
sinus
urogenitalis
female Q52.8
male Q55.8
venosus with imperfect incorporation in right auricle Q26.8
thymus (gland) (hyperplasia) E32.0
thyroglossal duct Q89.2
thyrolingual duct Q89.2
truncus arteriosus or communis Q20.0
tunica vasculosa lentis Q12.2
umbilical sinus Q64.4
urachus Q64.4
vitelline duct Q43.0
Person (with)
admitted for clinical research, as a control subject (normal comparison) (participant) Z00.6
awaiting admission to adequate facility elsewhere Z75.1
concern (normal) about sick person in family Z63.6
consulting on behalf of another Z71.0
feigning illness Z76.5
living (in)
without
adequate housing (heating) (space) Z59.1
housing (permanent) (temporary) Z59.0
person able to render necessary care Z74.2
shelter Z59.0
alone Z60.2
boarding school Z59.3
residential institution Z59.3
on waiting list Z75.1
sick or handicapped in family Z63.6
Personality (disorder) F60.9
accentuation of traits (type A pattern) Z73.1
affective F34.0
aggressive F60.3
amoral F60.2
anacastic, anankastic F60.5
antisocial F60.2
anxious F60.6
asocial F60.2
asthenic F60.7
avoidant F60.6
borderline F60.3
change due to organic condition (enduring) F07.0
compulsive F60.5
cycloid F34.0
cyclothymic F34.0
dependent F60.7
depressive F34.1
dissocial F60.2
dual F44.81
eccentric F60.89
emotionally unstable F60.3
expansive paranoid F60.0
explosive F60.3
fanatic F60.0
haltose type F60.89
histrionic F60.4
hyperthymic F34.0
hypothymic F34.1
hysterical F60.4
immature F60.89
inadequate F60.7
labile (emotional) F60.3
mixed (nonspecific) F60.89
morally defective F60.2
multiple F44.81
narcissistic F60.81
obsessional F60.5
obsessive (-compulsive) F60.5
organic F07.0
overconscientious F60.5
paranoid F60.0
passive (-dependent) F60.7
passive-aggressive F60.89
pathologic F60.9
pattern defect or disturbance F60.9
pseudopsychopathic (organic) F07.0
pseudoretarded (organic) F07.0
psychoinfantile F60.4
psychoneurotic NEC F60.89
psychopathic F60.2
querulant F60.0

Personality — *continued*
sadistic F60.89
schizoid F60.1
self-defeating F60.7
sensitive paranoid F60.0
sociopathic (amoral) (antisocial) (asocial) (dissocial) F60.2
specified NEC F60.89
type A Z73.1
unstable (emotional) F60.3
Perthes' disease — *see* Legg-Calvé-Perthes disease
Pertussis (*see also* Whooping cough) A37.90
Perversion, perverted
appetite F50.89
psychogenic F50.89
function
pituitary gland E23.2
posterior lobe E22.2
sense of smell and taste R43.8
psychogenic F45.8
sexual — *see* Deviation, sexual
Pervious, congenital (*see also* Imperfect, closure)
ductus arteriosus Q25.0
Pes (congenital) (*see also* Talipes)
acquired (*see also* Deformity, limb, foot, specified NEC)
planus — *see* Deformity, limb, flat foot
adductus Q66.89
cavus Q66.7
deformity NEC, acquired — *see* Deformity, limb, foot, specified NEC
planus (acquired) (any degree) (*see also* Deformity, limb, flat foot)
rachitic sequelae (late effect) E64.3
valgus Q66.6
Pest, pestis — *see* Plague
Petechia, petechiae R23.3
newborn P54.5
Petechial typhus A75.9
Peter's anomaly Q13.4
Petit mal seizure — *see* Epilepsy, generalized, specified NEC
Petit's hernia — *see* Hernia, abdomen, specified site NEC
Petrellidosis B48.2
Petrositis H70.20- ☑
acute H70.21- ☑
chronic H70.22- ☑
Peutz-Jeghers disease or syndrome Q85.8
Peyronie's disease N48.6
PFAPA (periodic fever, aphthous stomatitis, pharyngitis, and adenopathy syndrome) M04.8
Pfeiffer's disease — *see* Mononucleosis, infectious
Phagedena (dry) (moist) (sloughing) (*see also* Gangrene)
geometric L88
penis N48.29
tropical — *see* Ulcer, skin
vulva N76.6
Phagedenic — *see* condition
Phakoma H35.89
Phakomatosis (*see also* specific eponymous syndromes) Q85.9
Bourneville's Q85.1
specified NEC Q85.8
Phantom limb syndrome (without pain) G54.7
with pain G54.6
Pharyngeal pouch syndrome D82.1
Pharyngitis (acute) (catarrhal) (gangrenous) (infective) (malignant) (membranous) (phlegmonous) (pseudomembranous) (simple) (subacute) (suppurative) (ulcerative) (viral) J02.9
with influenza, flu, or grippe — *see* Influenza, with, pharyngitis
aphthous B08.5
atrophic J31.2
chlamydial A56.4
chronic (atrophic) (granular) (hypertrophic) J31.2
coxsackievirus B08.5
diphtheritic A36.0
enteroviral vesicular B08.5
follicular (chronic) J31.2
fusospirochetal A69.1
gonococcal A54.5
granular (chronic) J31.2
herpesviral B00.2
hypertrophic J31.2
infectional, chronic J31.2
influenzal — *see* Influenza, with, respiratory manifestations NEC

Pharyngitis — *continued*
lymphonodular, acute (enteroviral) B08.8
pneumococcal J02.8
purulent J02.9
putrid J02.9
septic J02.0
sicca J31.2
specified organism NEC J02.8
staphylococcal J02.8
streptococcal J02.0
syphilitic, congenital (early) A50.03
tuberculous A15.8
vesicular, enteroviral B08.5
viral NEC J02.8
Pharyngoconjunctivitis, viral B30.2
Pharyngolaryngitis (acute) J06.0
chronic J37.0
Pharyngoplegia J39.2
Pharyngotonsillitis, herpesviral B00.2
Pharyngotracheitis, chronic J42
Pharynx, pharyngeal — *see* condition
Phencyclidine-induced
anxiety disorder F16.980
bipolar and related disorder F16.94
depressive disorder F16.94
psychotic disorder F16.959
Phenomenon
Arthus' — *see* Arthus' phenomenon
jaw-winking Q07.8
lupus erythematosus (LE) cell M32.9
Raynaud's (secondary) I73.00
with gangrene I73.01
vasomotor R55
vasospastic I73.9
vasovagal R55
Wenckebach's I44.1
Phenylketonuria E70.1
classical E70.0
maternal E70.1
Pheochromoblastoma
specified site — *see* Neoplasm, malignant, by site
unspecified site C74.10
Pheochromocytoma
malignant
specified site — *see* Neoplasm, malignant, by site
unspecified site C74.10
specified site — *see* Neoplasm, benign, by site
unspecified site D35.00
Pheohyphomycosis — *see* Chromomycosis
Pheomycosis — *see* Chromomycosis
Phimosis (congenital) (due to infection) N47.1
chancroidal A57
Phlebectasia (*see also* Varix)
congenital Q27.4
Phlebitis (infective) (pyemic) (septic) (suppurative) I80.9
antepartum — *see* Thrombophlebitis, antepartum
blue — *see* Phlebitis, leg, deep
breast, superficial I80.8
cavernous (venous) sinus — *see* Phlebitis, intracranial (venous) sinus
cerebral (venous) sinus — *see* Phlebitis, intracranial (venous) sinus
chest wall, superficial I80.8
cranial (venous) sinus — *see* Phlebitis, intracranial (venous) sinus
deep (vessels) — *see* Phlebitis, leg, deep
due to implanted device — *see* Complications, by site and type, specified NEC
during or resulting from a procedure T81.72 ☑
femoral vein (superficial) I80.1- ☑
femoropopliteal vein I80.0- ☑
gestational — *see* Phlebopathy, gestational
hepatic veins I80.8
iliofemoral — *see* Phlebitis, femoral vein
intracranial (venous) sinus (any) G08
nonpyogenic I67.6
intraspinal venous sinuses and veins G08
nonpyogenic G95.19
lateral (venous) sinus — *see* Phlebitis, intracranial (venous) sinus
leg I80.3
antepartum — *see* Thrombophlebitis, antepartum
deep (vessels) NEC I80.20- ☑
iliac I80.21- ☑
popliteal vein I80.22- ☑
specified vessel NEC I80.29- ☑
tibial vein I80.23- ☑

Phlebitis — *continued*
　leg — *continued*
　　femoral vein (superficial) I80.1- ☑
　　superficial (vessels) I80.0- ☑
　longitudinal sinus — *see* Phlebitis, intracranial (venous) sinus
　lower limb — *see* Phlebitis, leg
　migrans, migrating (superficial) I82.1
　pelvic
　　with ectopic or molar pregnancy O08.0
　　following ectopic or molar pregnancy O08.0
　　puerperal, postpartum O87.1
　popliteal vein — *see* Phlebitis, leg, deep, popliteal
　portal (vein) K75.1
　postoperative T81.72 ☑
　pregnancy — *see* Thrombophlebitis, antepartum
　puerperal, postpartum, childbirth O87.0
　　deep O87.1
　　pelvic O87.1
　　superficial O87.0
　retina — *see* Vasculitis, retina
　saphenous (accessory) (great) (long) (small) — *see* Phlebitis, leg, superficial
　sinus (meninges) — *see* Phlebitis, intracranial (venous) sinus
　specified site NEC I80.8
　syphilitic A52.09
　tibial vein — *see* Phlebitis, leg, deep, tibial
　ulcerative I80.9
　　leg — *see* Phlebitis, leg
　umbilicus I80.8
　uterus (septic) — *see* Endometritis
　varicose (leg) (lower limb) — *see* Varix, leg, with, inflammation
Phlebofibrosis I87.8
Phleboliths I87.8
Phlebopathy,
　gestational O22.9- ☑
　puerperal O87.9
Phlebosclerosis I87.8
Phlebothrombosis (*see also* Thrombosis)
　antepartum — *see* Thrombophlebitis, antepartum
　pregnancy — *see* Thrombophlebitis, antepartum
　puerperal — *see* Thrombophlebitis, puerperal
Phlebotomus fever A93.1
Phlegmasia
　alba dolens O87.1
　　nonpuerperal — *see* Phlebitis, femoral vein
　cerulea dolens — *see* Phlebitis, leg, deep
Phlegmon — *see* Abscess
Phlegmonous — *see* condition
Phlyctenulosis (allergic) (keratoconjunctivitis) (nontuberculous) (*see also* Keratoconjunctivitis)
　cornea — *see* Keratoconjunctivitis
　tuberculous A18.52
Phobia, phobic F40.9
　animal F40.218
　　spiders F40.210
　examination F40.298
　reaction F40.9
　simple F40.298
　social F40.10
　　generalized F40.11
　specific (isolated) F40.298
　　animal F40.218
　　　spiders F40.210
　　blood F40.230
　　injection F40.231
　　injury F40.233
　　men F40.290
　　natural environment F40.228
　　　thunderstorms F40.220
　　situational F40.248
　　　bridges F40.242
　　　closed in spaces F40.240
　　　flying F40.243
　　　heights F40.241
　　specified focus NEC F40.298
　　transfusion F40.231
　　women F40.291
　specified NEC F40.8
　　medical care NEC F40.232
　state F40.9
Phocas' disease — *see* Mastopathy, cystic
Phocomelia Q73.1
　lower limb — *see* Agenesis, leg, with foot present
　upper limb — *see* Agenesis, arm, with hand present

Phoria H50.50
Phosphate-losing tubular disorder N25.0
Phosphatemia E83.39
Phosphaturia E83.39
Photodermatitis (sun) L56.8
　chronic L57.8
　due to drug L56.8
　light other than sun L59.8
Photokeratitis H16.13- ☑
Photophobia H53.14- ☑
Photophthalmia — *see* Photokeratitis
Photopsia H53.19
Photoretinitis — *see* Retinopathy, solar
Photosensitivity, photosensitization (sun) skin L56.8
　light other than sun L59.8
Phrenitis — *see* Encephalitis
Phrynoderma (vitamin A deficiency) E50.8
Phthiriasis (pubis) B85.3
　with any infestation classifiable to B85.0-B85.2 B85.4
Phthirus infestation — *see* Phthiriasis
Phthisis (*see also* Tuberculosis)
　bulbi (infectional) — *see* Disorder, globe, degenerated condition, atrophy
　eyeball (due to infection) — *see* Disorder, globe, degenerated condition, atrophy
Phycomycosis — *see* Zygomycosis
Physalopteriasis B81.8
Physical restraint status Z78.1
Phytobezoar T18.9 ☑
　intestine T18.3 ☑
　stomach T18.2 ☑
Pian — *see* Yaws
Pianoma A66.1
Pica F50.89
　in adults F50.89
　infant or child F98.3
Picking, nose F98.8
Pick-Niemann disease — *see* Niemann-Pick disease or syndrome
Pick's
　cerebral atrophy G31.01 [F02.80]
　　with behavioral disturbance G31.01 [F02.81]
　disease or syndrome (brain) G31.01 [F02.80]
　　with behavioral disturbance G31.01 [F02.81]
　　brain G31.01 [F02.80]
　　　with behavioral disturbance G31.01 [F02.81]
　　pericardium (pericardial pseudocirrhosis of liver) I31.1
　syndrome
　　brain G31.01 [F02.80]
　　　with behavioral disturbance G31.01 [F02.81]
　　of heart (pericardial pseudocirrhosis of liver) I31.1
Pickwickian syndrome E66.2
Piebaldism E70.39
Piedra (beard) (scalp) B36.8
　black B36.3
　white B36.2
Pierre Robin deformity or syndrome Q87.0
Pierson's disease or osteochondrosis M91.0
Pig-bel A05.2
Pigeon
　breast or chest (acquired) M95.4
　　congenital Q67.7
　　rachitic sequelae (late effect) E64.3
　breeder's disease or lung J67.2
　fancier's disease or lung J67.2
　toe — *see* Deformity, toe, specified NEC
Pigmentation (abnormal) (anomaly) L81.9
　conjunctiva H11.13- ☑
　cornea (anterior) H18.01- ☑
　　posterior H18.05- ☑
　　stromal H18.06- ☑
　diminished melanin formation NEC L81.6
　iron L81.8
　lids, congenital Q82.8
　limbus corneae — *see* Pigmentation, cornea
　metals L81.8
　optic papilla, congenital Q14.2
　retina, congenital (grouped) (nevoid) Q14.1
　scrotum, congenital Q82.8
　tattoo L81.8
Piles (*see also* Hemorrhoids) K64.9
Pili
　annulati or torti (congenital) Q84.1
　incarnati L73.1
Pill roller hand (intrinsic) — *see* Parkinsonism
Pilomatrixoma — *see* Neoplasm, skin, benign

Pilomatrixoma — *continued*
　malignant — *see* Neoplasm, skin, malignant
Pilonidal — *see* condition
Pimple R23.8
PIN — *see* Neoplasia, intraepithelial, prostate
Pinched nerve — *see* Neuropathy, entrapment
Pindborg tumor — *see* Cyst, calcifying odontogenic
Pineal body or gland — *see* condition
Pinealoblastoma C75.3
Pinealoma D44.5
　malignant C75.3
Pineoblastoma C75.3
Pineocytoma D44.5
Pinguecula H11.15- ☑
Pingueculitis H10.81- ☑
Pinhole meatus (*see also* Stricture, urethra) N35.9
Pink
　disease — *see* subcategory T56.1 ☑
　eye — *see* Conjunctivitis, acute, mucopurulent
Pinkus' disease (lichen nitidus) L44.1
Pinpoint
　meatus — *see* Stricture, urethra
　os (uteri) — *see* Stricture, cervix
Pins and needles R20.2
Pinta A67.9
　cardiovascular lesions A67.2
　chancre (primary) A67.0
　erythematous plaques A67.1
　hyperchromic lesions A67.1
　hyperkeratosis A67.1
　lesions A67.9
　　cardiovascular A67.2
　　hyperchromic A67.1
　　intermediate A67.1
　　late A67.2
　　mixed A67.3
　　primary A67.0
　　skin (achromic) (cicatricial) (dyschromic) A67.2
　　　hyperchromic A67.1
　　　mixed (achromic and hyperchromic) A67.3
　papule (primary) A67.0
　skin lesions (achromic) (cicatricial) (dyschromic) A67.2
　　hyperchromic A67.1
　　mixed (achromic and hyperchromic) A67.3
　vitiligo A67.2
Pintids A67.1
Pinworm (disease) (infection) (infestation) B80
Piroplasmosis B60.0
Pistol wound — *see* Gunshot wound
Pitchers' elbow — *see* Derangement, joint, specified type NEC, elbow
Pithecoid pelvis Q74.2
　with disproportion (fetopelvic) O33.0
　　causing obstructed labor O65.0
Pithiatism F48.8
Pitted — *see* Pitting
Pitting (*see also* Edema) R60.9
　lip R60.0
　nail L60.8
　teeth K00.4
Pituitary gland — *see* condition
Pituitary-snuff-taker's disease J67.8
Pityriasis (capitis) L21.0
　alba L30.5
　circinata (et maculata) L42
　furfuracea L21.0
　Hebra's L26
　lichenoides L41.0
　　chronica L41.1
　　et varioliformis (acuta) L41.0
　maculata (et circinata) L30.5
　nigra B36.1
　pilaris, Hebra's L44.0
　rosea L42
　rotunda L44.8
　rubra (Hebra) pilaris L44.0
　simplex L30.5
　specified type NEC L30.5
　streptogenes L30.5
　versicolor (scrotal) B36.0
Placenta, placental — *see* Pregnancy, complicated by (care of) (management affected by), specified condition
Placentitis O41.14- ☑
Plagiocephaly Q67.3
Plague A20.9
　abortive A20.8

Plague — Pneumonia

Index

Plague — *continued*
  ambulatory A20.8
  asymptomatic A20.8
  bubonic A20.0
  cellulocutaneous A20.1
  cutaneobubonic A20.1
  lymphatic gland A20.0
  meningitis A20.3
  pharyngeal A20.8
  pneumonic (primary) (secondary) A20.2
  pulmonary, pulmonic A20.2
  septicemic A20.7
  tonsillar A20.8
    septicemic A20.7
Planning, family
  contraception Z30.9
  procreation Z31.69
Plaque(s)
  artery, arterial — *see* Arteriosclerosis
  calcareous — *see* Calcification
  coronary, lipid rich I25.83
  epicardial I31.8
  erythematous, of pinta A67.1
  Hollenhorst's — *see* Occlusion, artery, retina
  lipid rich, coronary I25.83
  pleural (without asbestos) J92.9
    with asbestos J92.0
  tongue K13.29
Plasmacytoma C90.3- ☑
  extramedullary C90.2- ☑
  medullary C90.0- ☑
  solitary C90.3- ☑
Plasmacytopenia D72.818
Plasmacytosis D72.822
Plaster ulcer — *see* Ulcer, pressure, by site
Plateau iris syndrome (post-iridectomy) (postprocedural) (without glaucoma) H21.82
  with glaucoma H40.22- ☑
Platybasia Q75.8
Platyonychia (congenital) Q84.6
  acquired L60.8
Platypelloid pelvis M95.5
  with disproportion (fetopelvic) O33.0
    causing obstructed labor O65.0
  congenital Q74.2
Platyspondylisis Q76.49
Plaut (-Vincent) **disease** (*see also* Vincent's) A69.1
Plethora R23.2
  newborn P61.1
Pleura, pleural — *see* condition
Pleuralgia R07.81
Pleurisy (acute) (adhesive) (chronic) (costal) (diaphragmatic) (double) (dry) (fibrinous) (fibrous) (interlobar) (latent) (plastic) (primary) (residual) (sicca) (sterile) (subacute) (unresolved) R09.1
  with
    adherent pleura J86.0
    effusion J90
      chylous, chyliform J94.0
      tuberculous (non primary) A15.6
        primary (progressive) A15.7
    tuberculosis — *see* Pleurisy, tuberculous (non primary)
  encysted — *see* Pleurisy, with effusion
  exudative — *see* Pleurisy, with effusion
  fibrinopurulent, fibropurulent — *see* Pyothorax
  hemorrhagic — *see* Hemothorax
  pneumococcal J90
  purulent — *see* Pyothorax
  septic — *see* Pyothorax
  serofibrinous — *see* Pleurisy, with effusion
  seropurulent — *see* Pyothorax
  serous — *see* Pleurisy, with effusion
  staphylococcal J86.9
  streptococcal J90
  suppurative — *see* Pyothorax
  traumatic (post) (current) — *see* Injury, intrathoracic, pleura
  tuberculous (with effusion) (non primary) A15.6
    primary (progressive) A15.7
Pleuritis sicca — *see* Pleurisy
Pleurobronchopneumonia — *see* Pneumonia, broncho-
Pleurodynia R07.81
  epidemic B33.0
  viral B33.0
Pleuropericarditis (*see also* Pericarditis)
  acute I30.9

Pleuropneumonia (acute) (bilateral) (double) (septic) (*see also* Pneumonia) J18.8
  chronic — *see* Fibrosis, lung
Pleuro-pneumonia-like-organism (PPLO), as cause of disease classified elsewhere B96.0
Pleurorrhea — *see* Pleurisy, with effusion
Plexitis, brachial G54.0
Plica
  polonica B85.0
  syndrome, knee M67.5- ☑
  tonsil J35.8
Plicated tongue K14.5
Plug
  bronchus NEC J98.09
  meconium (newborn) NEC syndrome P76.0
  mucus — *see* Asphyxia, mucus
Plumbism — *see* subcategory T56.0 ☑
Plummer's disease E05.20
  with thyroid storm E05.21
Plummer-Vinson syndrome D50.1
Pluricarential syndrome of infancy E40
Plus (and minus) **hand** (intrinsic) — *see* Deformity, limb, specified type NEC, forearm
Pneumathemia — *see* Air, embolism
Pneumatic hammer (drill) **syndrome** T75.21 ☑
Pneumatocele (lung) J98.4
  intracranial G93.89
  tension J44.9
Pneumatosis
  cystoides intestinalis K63.89
  intestinalis K63.89
  peritonei K66.8
Pneumaturia R39.89
Pneumoblastoma — *see* Neoplasm, lung, malignant
Pneumocephalus G93.89
Pneumococcemia A40.3
Pneumococcus, pneumococcal — *see* condition
Pneumoconiosis (due to) (inhalation of) J64
  with tuberculosis (any type in A15) J65
  aluminum J63.0
  asbestos J61
  bagasse, bagassosis J67.1
  bauxite J63.1
  beryllium J63.2
  coal miners' (simple) J60
  coalworkers' (simple) J60
  collier's J60
  cotton dust J66.0
  diatomite (diatomaceous earth) J62.8
  dust
    inorganic NEC J63.6
    lime J62.8
    marble J62.8
    organic NEC J66.8
  fumes or vapors (from silo) J68.9
  graphite J63.3
  grinder's J62.8
  kaolin J62.8
  mica J62.8
  millstone maker's J62.8
  mineral fibers NEC J61
  miner's J60
  moldy hay J67.0
  potter's J62.8
  rheumatoid — *see* Rheumatoid, lung
  sandblaster's J62.8
  silica, silicate NEC J62.8
    with carbon J60
  stonemason's J62.8
  talc (dust) J62.0
Pneumocystis carinii pneumonia B59
Pneumocystis jiroveci (pneumonia) B59
Pneumocystosis (with pneumonia) B59
Pneumohemopericardium I31.2
Pneumohemothorax J94.2
  traumatic S27.2 ☑
Pneumohydropericardium — *see* Pericarditis
Pneumohydrothorax — *see* Hydrothorax
Pneumomediastinum J98.2
  congenital or perinatal P25.2
Pneumomycosis B49 [J99]
Pneumonia (acute) (double) (migratory) (purulent) (septic) (unresolved) J18.9
  with
    influenza — *see* Influenza, with, pneumonia
    lung abscess J85.1

Pneumonia — *continued*
  with — *continued*
    lung abscess — *continued*
      due to specified organism — *see* Pneumonia, in (due to)
  adenoviral J12.0
  adynamic J18.2
  alba A50.04
  allergic (eosinophilic) J82
  alveolar — *see* Pneumonia, lobar
  anaerobes J15.8
  anthrax A22.1
  apex, apical — *see* Pneumonia, lobar
  Ascaris B77.81
  aspiration J69.0
    due to
      aspiration of microorganisms
        bacterial J15.9
        viral J12.9
      food (regurgitated) J69.0
      gastric secretions J69.0
      milk (regurgitated) J69.0
      oils, essences J69.1
      solids, liquids NEC J69.8
      vomitus J69.0
    newborn P24.81
      amniotic fluid (clear) P24.11
      blood P24.21
      food (regurgitated) P24.31
      liquor (amnii) P24.11
      meconium P24.01
      milk P24.31
      mucus P24.11
      specified NEC P24.81
      stomach contents P24.31
    postprocedural J95.4
  atypical NEC J18.9
  bacillus J15.9
    specified NEC J15.8
  bacterial J15.9
    specified NEC J15.8
  Bacteroides (fragilis) (oralis) (melaninogenicus) J15.8
  basal, basic, basilar — *see* Pneumonia, by type
  bronchiolitis obliterans organized (BOOP) J84.89
  broncho-, bronchial (confluent) (croupous) (diffuse) (disseminated) (hemorrhagic) (involving lobes) (lobar) (terminal) J18.0
    allergic (eosinophilic) J82
    aspiration — *see* Pneumonia, aspiration
    bacterial J15.9
      specified NEC J15.8
    chronic — *see* Fibrosis, lung
    diplococcal J13
    Eaton's agent J15.7
    Escherichia coli (E. coli) J15.5
    Friedländer's bacillus J15.0
    Hemophilus influenzae J14
    hypostatic J18.2
    inhalation (*see also* Pneumonia, aspiration)
      due to fumes or vapors (chemical) J68.0
      of oils or essences J69.1
    Klebsiella (pneumoniae) J15.0
    lipid, lipoid J69.1
      endogenous J84.89
    Mycoplasma (pneumoniae) J15.7
    pleuro-pneumonia-like-organisms (PPLO) J15.7
    pneumococcal J13
    Proteus J15.6
    Pseudomonas J15.1
    Serratia marcescens J15.6
    specified organism NEC J16.8
    staphylococcal — *see* Pneumonia, staphylococcal
    streptococcal NEC J15.4
      group B J15.3
      pneumoniae J13
    viral, virus — *see* Pneumonia, viral
  Butyrivibrio (fibriosolvens) J15.8
  Candida B37.1
  caseous — *see* Tuberculosis, pulmonary
  catarrhal — *see* Pneumonia, broncho
  chlamydial J16.0
    congenital P23.1
  cholesterol J84.89
  cirrhotic (chronic) — *see* Fibrosis, lung
  Clostridium (haemolyticum) (novyi) J15.8
  confluent — *see* Pneumonia, broncho
  congenital (infective) P23.9

☑ **Additional Character Required — Refer to the Tabular List for Character Selection**   ☑ **Subterms under main terms may continue to next column or page**

Pneumonia — *continued*
  congenital — *continued*
    due to
      bacterium NEC P23.6
      Chlamydia P23.1
      Escherichia coli P23.4
      Haemophilus influenzae P23.6
      infective organism NEC P23.8
      Klebsiella pneumoniae P23.6
      Mycoplasma P23.6
      Pseudomonas P23.5
      Staphylococcus P23.2
      Streptococcus (except group B) P23.6
        group B P23.3
      viral agent P23.0
    specified NEC P23.8
  croupous — *see* Pneumonia, lobar
  cryptogenic organizing J84.116
  cytomegalic inclusion B25.0
  cytomegaloviral B25.0
  deglutition — *see* Pneumonia, aspiration
  desquamative interstitial J84.117
  diffuse — *see* Pneumonia, broncho
  diplococcal, diplococcus (broncho-) (lobar) J13
  disseminated (focal) — *see* Pneumonia, broncho
  Eaton's agent J15.7
  embolic, embolism — *see* Embolism, pulmonary
  Enterobacter J15.6
  eosinophilic J82
  Escherichia coli (E. coli) J15.5
  Eubacterium J15.8
  fibrinous — *see* Pneumonia, lobar
  fibroid, fibrous (chronic) — *see* Fibrosis, lung
  Friedländer's bacillus J15.0
  Fusobacterium (nucleatum) J15.8
  gangrenous J85.0
  giant cell (measles) B05.2
  gonococcal A54.84
  gram-negative bacteria NEC J15.6
    anaerobic J15.8
  Hemophilus influenzae (broncho) (lobar) J14
  human metapneumovirus J12.3
  hypostatic (broncho) (lobar) J18.2
  in (due to)
    actinomycosis A42.0
    adenovirus J12.0
    anthrax A22.1
    ascariasis B77.81
    aspergillosis B44.9
    Bacillus anthracis A22.1
    Bacterium anitratum J15.6
    candidiasis B37.1
    chickenpox B01.2
    Chlamydia J16.0
      neonatal P23.1
    coccidioidomycosis B38.2
      acute B38.0
      chronic B38.1
    cytomegalovirus disease B25.0
    Diplococcus (pneumoniae) J13
    Eaton's agent J15.7
    Enterobacter J15.6
    Escherichia coli (E. coli) J15.5
    Friedländer's bacillus J15.0
    fumes and vapors (chemical) (inhalation) J68.0
    gonorrhea A54.84
    Hemophilus influenzae (H. influenzae) J14
    Herellea J15.6
    histoplasmosis B39.2
      acute B39.0
      chronic B39.1
    human metapneumovirus J12.3
    Klebsiella (pneumoniae) J15.0
    measles B05.2
    Mycoplasma (pneumoniae) J15.7
    nocardiosis, nocardiasis A43.0
    ornithosis A70
    parainfluenza virus J12.2
    pleuro-pneumonia-like-organism (PPLO) J15.7
    pneumococcus J13
    pneumocystosis (Pneumocystis carinii) (Pneumocystis jiroveci) B59
    Proteus J15.6
    Pseudomonas NEC J15.1
      pseudomallei A24.1
    psittacosis A70
    Q fever A78
    respiratory syncytial virus J12.1

Pneumonia — *continued*
  in — *continued*
    rheumatic fever I00 [J17]
    rubella B06.81
    Salmonella (infection) A02.22
      typhi A01.03
    schistosomiasis B65.9 [J17]
    Serratia marcescens J15.6
    specified
      bacterium NEC J15.8
      organism NEC J16.8
    spirochetal NEC A69.8
    Staphylococcus J15.20
      aureus (methicillin susceptible) (MSSA) J15.211
        methicillin resistant (MRSA) J15.212
      specified NEC J15.29
    Streptococcus J15.4
      group B J15.3
      pneumoniae J13
      specified NEC J15.4
    toxoplasmosis B58.3
    tularemia A21.2
    typhoid (fever) A01.03
    varicella B01.2
    virus — *see* Pneumonia, viral
    whooping cough A37.91
      due to
        Bordetella parapertussis A37.11
        Bordetella pertussis A37.01
        specified NEC A37.81
    Yersinia pestis A20.2
  inhalation of food or vomit — *see* Pneumonia, aspiration
  interstitial J84.9
    chronic J84.111
    desquamative J84.117
    due to
      collagen vascular disease J84.17
      known underlying cause J84.17
    idiopathic NOS J84.111
    in disease classified elsewhere J84.17
    lymphocytic (due to collagen vascular disease) (in diseases classified elsewhere) J84.17
    lymphoid J84.2
    non-specific J84.89
      due to
        collagen vascular disease J84.17
        known underlying cause J84.17
      idiopathic J84.113
      in diseases classified elsewhere J84.17
    plasma cell B59
    pseudomonas J15.1
    usual J84.112
      due to collagen vascular disease J84.17
      idiopathic J84.112
      in diseases classified elsewhere J84.17
  Klebsiella (pneumoniae) J15.0
  lipid, lipoid (exogenous) J69.1
    endogenous J84.89
  lobar (disseminated) (double) (interstitial) J18.1
    bacterial J15.9
      specified NEC J15.8
    chronic — *see* Fibrosis, lung
    Escherichia coli (E. coli) J15.5
    Friedländer's bacillus J15.0
    Hemophilus influenzae J14
    hypostatic J18.2
    Klebsiella (pneumoniae) J15.0
    pneumococcal J13
    Proteus J15.6
    Pseudomonas J15.1
    specified organism NEC J16.8
    staphylococcal — *see* Pneumonia, staphylococcal
    streptococcal NEC J15.4
    Streptococcus pneumoniae J13
    viral, virus — *see* Pneumonia, viral
  lobular — *see* Pneumonia, broncho
  Löffler's J82
  lymphoid interstitial J84.2
  massive — *see* Pneumonia, lobar
  meconium P24.01
  MRSA (methicillin resistant Staphylococcus aureus) J15.212
  MSSA (methicillin susceptible Staphylococcus aureus) J15.211
  multilobar — *see* Pneumonia, by type
  Mycoplasma (pneumoniae) J15.7
  necrotic J85.0

Pneumonia — *continued*
  neonatal P23.9
    aspiration — *see* Aspiration, by substance, with pneumonia
  nitrogen dioxide J68.0
  organizing J84.89
    due to
      collagen vascular disease J84.17
      known underlying cause J84.17
    in diseases classified elsewhere J84.17
  orthostatic J18.2
  parainfluenza virus J12.2
  parenchymatous — *see* Fibrosis, lung
  passive J18.2
  patchy — *see* Pneumonia, broncho
  Peptococcus J15.8
  Peptostreptococcus J15.8
  plasma cell (of infants) B59
  pleurolobar — *see* Pneumonia, lobar
  pleuro-pneumonia-like organism (PPLO) J15.7
  pneumococcal (broncho) (lobar) J13
  Pneumocystis (carinii) (jiroveci) B59
  postinfectional NEC B99 ☑ [J17]
  postmeasles B05.2
  Proteus J15.6
  Pseudomonas J15.1
  psittacosis A70
  radiation J70.0
  respiratory syncytial virus J12.1
  resulting from a procedure J95.89
  rheumatic I00 [J17]
  Salmonella (arizonae) (cholerae-suis) (enteritidis) (typhimurium) A02.22
    typhi A01.03
    typhoid fever A01.03
  SARS-associated coronavirus J12.81
  segmented, segmental — *see* Pneumonia, broncho-
  Serratia marcescens J15.6
  specified NEC J18.8
    bacterium NEC J15.8
    organism NEC J16.8
    virus NEC J12.89
  spirochetal NEC A69.8
  staphylococcal (broncho) (lobar) J15.20
    aureus (methicillin susceptible) (MSSA) J15.211
      methicillin resistant (MRSA) J15.212
    specified NEC J15.29
  static, stasis J18.2
  streptococcal NEC (broncho) (lobar) J15.4
    group
      A J15.4
      B J15.3
      specified NEC J15.4
  Streptococcus pneumoniae J13
  syphilitic, congenital (early) A50.04
  traumatic (complication) (early) (secondary) T79.8 ☑
  tuberculous (any) — *see* Tuberculosis, pulmonary
  tularemic A21.2
  varicella B01.2
  Veillonella J15.8
  ventilator associated J95.851
  viral, virus (broncho) (interstitial) (lobar) J12.9
    adenoviral J12.0
    congenital P23.0
    human metapneumovirus J12.3
    parainfluenza J12.2
    respiratory syncytial J12.1
    SARS-associated coronavirus J12.81
    specified NEC J12.89
  white (congenital) A50.04
Pneumonic — *see* condition
Pneumonitis (acute) (primary) (*see also* Pneumonia)
  air-conditioner J67.7
  allergic (due to) J67.9
    organic dust NEC J67.8
    red cedar dust J67.8
    sequoiosis J67.8
    wood dust J67.8
  aspiration J69.0
    due to
      anesthesia J95.4
        during
          labor and delivery O74.0
          pregnancy O29.01- ☑
          puerperium O89.01
      fumes or gases J68.0
      obstetric O74.0

Pneumonitis — *continued*
  chemical (due to gases, fumes or vapors) (inhalation) J68.0
    due to anesthesia J95.4
  cholesterol J84.89
  chronic — *see* Fibrosis, lung
  congenital rubella P35.0
  crack (cocaine) J68.0
  due to
    beryllium J68.0
    cadmium J68.0
    crack (cocaine) J68.0
    detergent J69.8
    fluorocarbon-polymer J68.0
    food, vomit (aspiration) J69.0
    fumes or vapors J68.0
    gases, fumes or vapors (inhalation) J68.0
    inhalation
      blood J69.8
      essences J69.1
      food (regurgitated), milk, vomit J69.0
      oils, essences J69.1
      saliva J69.0
      solids, liquids NEC J69.8
    manganese J68.0
    nitrogen dioxide J68.0
    oils, essences J69.1
    solids, liquids NEC J69.8
    toxoplasmosis (acquired) B58.3
      congenital P37.1
    vanadium J68.0
    ventilator J95.851
  eosinophilic J82
  hypersensitivity J67.9
    air conditioner lung J67.7
    bagassosis J67.1
    bird fancier's lung J67.2
    farmer's lung J67.0
    maltworker's lung J67.4
    maple bark-stripper's lung J67.6
    mushroom worker's lung J67.5
    specified organic dust NEC J67.8
    suberosis J67.3
  interstitial (chronic) J84.89
    acute J84.114
    lymphoid J84.2
    non-specific J84.89
      idiopathic J84.113
  lymphoid, interstitial J84.2
  meconium P24.01
  postanesthetic J95.4
    correct substance properly administered — *see* Table of Drugs and Chemicals, by drug, adverse effect
    in labor and delivery O74.0
    in pregnancy O29.01- ☑
    obstetric O74.0
    overdose or wrong substance given or taken (by accident) — *see* Table of Drugs and Chemicals, by drug, poisoning
    postpartum, puerperal O89.01
  postoperative J95.4
    obstetric O74.0
  radiation J70.0
  rubella, congenital P35.0
  ventilation (air-conditioning) J67.7
  ventilator associated J95.851
  wood-dust J67.8
Pneumonoconiosis — *see* Pneumoconiosis
Pneumoparotid K11.8
Pneumopathy NEC J98.4
  alveolar J84.09
  due to organic dust NEC J66.8
  parietoalveolar J84.09
Pneumopericarditis (*see also* Pericarditis)
  acute I30.9
Pneumopericardium (*see also* Pericarditis)
  congenital P25.3
  newborn P25.3
  traumatic (post) — *see* Injury, heart
Pneumophagia (psychogenic) F45.8
Pneumopleurisy, pneumopleuritis (*see also* Pneumonia) J18.8
Pneumopyopericardium I30.1
Pneumopyothorax — *see* Pyopneumothorax
  with fistula J86.0
Pneumorrhagia (*see also* Hemorrhage, lung)
  tuberculous — *see* Tuberculosis, pulmonary

Pneumothorax NOS J93.9
  acute J93.83
  chronic J93.81
  congenital P25.1
  perinatal period P25.1
  postprocedural J95.811
  specified NEC J93.83
  spontaneous NOS J93.83
    newborn P25.1
    primary J93.11
    secondary J93.12
    tension J93.0
  tense valvular, infectional J93.0
  tension (spontaneous) J93.0
  traumatic S27.0 ☑
    with hemothorax S27.2 ☑
  tuberculous — *see* Tuberculosis, pulmonary
Podagra (*see also* Gout) M10.9
Podencephalus Q01.9
Poikilocytosis R71.8
Poikiloderma L81.6
  Civatte's L57.3
  congenital Q82.8
  vasculare atrophicans L94.5
Poikilodermatomyositis M33.10
  with
    myopathy M33.12
    respiratory involvement M33.11
    specified organ involvement NEC M33.19
Pointed ear (congenital) Q17.3
Poison ivy, oak, sumac or other plant dermatitis (allergic) (contact) L23.7
Poisoning (acute) (*see also* Table of Drugs and Chemicals)
  algae and toxins T65.82- ☑
  Bacillus B (aertrycke) (cholerae (suis)) (paratyphosus) (suipestifer) A02.9
    botulinus A05.1
  bacterial toxins A05.9
  berries, noxious — *see* Poisoning, food, noxious, berries
  botulism A05.1
  ciguatera fish T61.0- ☑
  Clostridium botulinum A05.1
  death-cap (Amanita phalloides) (Amanita verna) — *see* Poisoning, food, noxious, mushrooms
  drug — *see* Table of Drugs and Chemicals, by drug, poisoning
  epidemic, fish (noxious) — *see* Poisoning, seafood
    bacterial A05.9
  fava bean D55.0
  fish (noxious) T61.9- ☑
    bacterial — *see* Intoxication, foodborne, by agent
    ciguatera fish — *see* Poisoning, ciguatera fish
    scombroid fish — *see* Poisoning, scombroid fish
    specified type NEC T61.77- ☑
  food (acute) (diseased) (infected) (noxious) NEC T62.9- ☑
    bacterial — *see* Intoxication, foodborne, by agent
    due to
      Bacillus (aertrycke) (choleraesuis) (paratyphosus) (suipestifer) A02.9
        botulinus A05.1
      Clostridium (perfringens) (Welchii) A05.2
      salmonella (aertrycke) (callinarum) (choleraesuis) (enteritidis) (paratyphi) (suipestifer) A02.9
        with
          gastroenteritis A02.0
          sepsis A02.1
      staphylococcus A05.0
      Vibrio
        parahaemolyticus A05.3
        vulnificus A05.5
    noxious or naturally toxic T62.9- ☑
      berries — *see* subcategory T62.1 ☑
      fish — *see* Poisoning, seafood
      mushrooms — *see* subcategory T62.0X ☑
      plants NEC — *see* subcategory T62.2X ☑
      seafood — *see* Poisoning, seafood
      specified NEC — *see* subcategory T62.8X ☑
  ichthyotoxism — *see* Poisoning, seafood
  kreotoxism, food A05.9
  latex T65.81- ☑
  lead T56.0- ☑
  mushroom — *see* Poisoning, food, noxious, mushroom
  mussels (*see also* Poisoning, shellfish)
    bacterial — *see* Intoxication, foodborne, by agent

Poisoning — *continued*
  nicotine (tobacco) T65.2- ☑
  noxious foodstuffs — *see* Poisoning, food, noxious
  plants, noxious — *see* Poisoning, food, noxious, plants NEC
  ptomaine — *see* Poisoning, food
  radiation J70.0
  Salmonella (arizonae) (cholerae-suis) (enteritidis) (typhimurium) A02.9
  scombroid fish T61.1- ☑
  seafood (noxious) T61.9- ☑
    bacterial — *see* Intoxication, foodborne, by agent
    fish — *see* Poisoning, fish
    shellfish — *see* Poisoning, shellfish
    specified NEC — *see* subcategory T61.8X ☑
  shellfish (amnesic) (azaspiracid) (diarrheic) (neurotoxic) (noxious) (paralytic) T61.78- ☑
    bacterial — *see* Intoxication, foodborne, by agent
    ciguatera mollusk — *see* Poisoning, ciguatera fish
  specified substance NEC T65.891 ☑
  Staphylococcus, food A05.0
  tobacco (nicotine) T65.2- ☑
  water E87.79
Poker spine — *see* Spondylitis, ankylosing
Poland syndrome Q79.8
Polioencephalitis (acute) (bulbar) A80.9
  inferior G12.22
  influenzal — *see* Influenza, with, encephalopathy
  superior hemorrhagic (acute) (Wernicke's) E51.2
  Wernicke's E51.2
Polioencephalomyelitis (acute) (anterior) A80.9
  with beriberi E51.2
Polioencephalopathy, superior hemorrhagic E51.2
  with
    beriberi E51.11
    pellagra E52
Poliomeningoencephalitis — *see* Meningoencephalitis
Poliomyelitis (acute) (anterior) (epidemic) A80.9
  with paralysis (bulbar) — *see* Poliomyelitis, paralytic
  abortive A80.4
  ascending (progressive) — *see* Poliomyelitis, paralytic
  bulbar (paralytic) — *see* Poliomyelitis, paralytic
  congenital P35.8
  nonepidemic A80.9
  nonparalytic A80.4
  paralytic A80.30
    specified NEC A80.39
    vaccine-associated A80.0
    wild virus
      imported A80.1
      indigenous A80.2
  spinal, acute A80.9
Poliosis (eyebrow) (eyelashes) L67.1
  circumscripta, acquired L67.1
Pollakiuria R35.0
  psychogenic F45.8
Pollinosis J30.1
Pollitzer's disease L73.2
Polyadenitis (*see also* Lymphadenitis)
  malignant A20.0
Polyalgia M79.89
Polyangiitis M30.0
  microscopic M31.7
  overlap syndrome M30.8
Polyarteritis
  microscopic M31.7
  nodosa M30.0
    with lung involvement M30.1
    juvenile M30.2
    related condition NEC M30.8
Polyarthralgia — *see* Pain, joint
Polyarthritis, polyarthropathy (*see also* Arthritis) M13.0
  due to or associated with other specified conditions — *see* Arthritis
  epidemic (Australian) (with exanthema) B33.1
  infective — *see* Arthritis, pyogenic or pyemic
  inflammatory M06.4
  juvenile (chronic) (seronegative) M08.3
  migratory — *see* Fever, rheumatic
  rheumatic, acute — *see* Fever, rheumatic
Polyarthrosis M15.9
  post-traumatic M15.3
  primary M15.0
  specified NEC M15.8
Polycarential syndrome of infancy E40
Polychondritis (atrophic) (chronic) (*see also* Disorder, cartilage, specified type NEC)
  relapsing M94.1

Polycoria Q13.2
Polycystic (disease)
  degeneration, kidney Q61.3
    autosomal dominant (adult type) Q61.2
    autosomal recessive (infantile type)
      NEC Q61.19
  kidney Q61.3
    autosomal
      dominant Q61.2
      recessive NEC Q61.19
    autosomal dominant (adult type) Q61.2
    autosomal recessive (childhood type) NEC Q61.19
    infantile type NEC Q61.19
  liver Q44.6
  lung J98.4
    congenital Q33.0
  ovary, ovaries E28.2
  spleen Q89.09
Polycythemia (secondary) D75.1
  acquired D75.1
  benign (familial) D75.0
  due to
    donor twin P61.1
    erythropoietin D75.1
    fall in plasma volume D75.1
    high altitude D75.1
    maternal-fetal transfusion P61.1
    stress D75.1
  emotional D75.1
  erythropoietin D75.1
  familial (benign) D75.0
  Gaisböck's (hypertonica) D75.1
  high altitude D75.1
  hypertonica D75.1
  hypoxemic D75.1
  neonatorum P61.1
  nephrogenous D75.1
  relative D75.1
  secondary D75.1
  spurious D75.1
  stress D75.1
  vera D45
Polycytosis cryptogenica D75.1
Polydactylism, polydactyly Q69.9
  toes Q69.2
Polydipsia R63.1
Polydystrophy, pseudo-Hurler E77.0
Polyembryoma — see Neoplasm, malignant, by site
Polyglandular
  deficiency E31.0
  dyscrasia E31.9
  dysfunction E31.9
  syndrome E31.8
Polyhydramnios O40.- ☑
Polymastia Q83.1
Polymenorrhea N92.0
Polymyalgia M35.3
  arteritica, giant cell M31.5
  rheumatica M35.3
    with giant cell arteritis M31.5
Polymyositis (acute) (chronic) (hemorrhagic) M33.20
  with
    myopathy M33.22
    respiratory involvement M33.21
    skin involvement — see Dermatopolymyositis
    specified organ involvement NEC M33.29
  ossificans (generalisata) (progressiva) — see Myositis, ossificans, progressiva
Polyneuritis, polyneuritic (see also Polyneuropathy)
  acute (post-)infective G61.0
  alcoholic G62.1
  cranialis G52.7
  demyelinating, chronic inflammatory (CIDP) G61.81
  diabetic — see Diabetes, polyneuropathy
  diphtheritic A36.83
  due to lack of vitamin NEC E56.9 [G63]
  endemic E51.11
  erythredema — see subcategory T56.1 ☑
  febrile, acute G61.0
  hereditary ataxic G60.1
  idiopathic, acute G61.0
  infective (acute) G61.0
  inflammatory, chronic demyelinating (CIDP) G61.81
  nutritional E63.9 [G63]
  postinfective (acute) G61.0
  specified NEC G62.89
Polyneuropathy (peripheral) G62.9

Polyneuropathy — continued
  alcoholic G62.1
  amyloid (Portuguese) E85.1 [G63]
    transthyretin-related (ATTR) familial E85.1
  arsenical G62.2
  critical illness G62.81
  demyelinating, chronic inflammatory (CIDP) G61.81
  diabetic — see Diabetes, polyneuropathy
  drug-induced G62.0
  hereditary G60.9
    specified NEC G60.8
  idiopathic G60.9
    progressive G60.3
  in (due to)
    alcohol G62.1
      sequelae G65.2
    amyloidosis, familial (Portuguese) E85.1 [G63]
    antitetanus serum G61.1
    arsenic G62.2
      sequelae G65.2
    avitaminosis NEC E56.9 [G63]
    beriberi E51.11
    collagen vascular disease NEC M35.9 [G63]
    deficiency (of)
      B (-complex) vitamins E53.9 [G63]
      vitamin B6 E53.1 [G63]
    diabetes — see Diabetes, polyneuropathy
    diphtheria A36.83
    drug or medicament G62.0
      correct substance properly administered — see Table of Drugs and Chemicals, by drug, adverse effect
      overdose or wrong substance given or taken — see Table of Drugs and Chemicals, by drug, poisoning
    endocrine disease NEC E34.9 [G63]
    herpes zoster B02.23
    hypoglycemia E16.2 [G63]
    infectious
      disease NEC B99 ☑ [G63]
      mononucleosis B27.91
    lack of vitamin NEC E56.9 [G63]
    lead G62.2
      sequelae G65.2
    leprosy A30.9 [G63]
    Lyme disease A69.22
    metabolic disease NEC E88.9 [G63]
    microscopic polyangiitis M31.7 [G63]
    mumps B26.84
    neoplastic disease (see also Neoplasm) D49.9 [G63]
    nutritional deficiency NEC E63.9 [G63]
    organophosphate compounds G62.2
      sequelae G65.2
    parasitic disease NEC B89 [G63]
    pellagra E52 [G63]
    polyarteritis nodosa M30.0
    porphyria E80.20 [G63]
    radiation G62.82
    rheumatoid arthritis — see Rheumatoid, polyneuropathy
    sarcoidosis D86.89
    serum G61.1
    syphilis (late) A52.15
      congenital A50.43
    systemic
      connective tissue disorder M35.9 [G63]
      lupus erythematosus M32.19
    toxic agent NEC G62.2
      sequelae G65.2
  inflammatory G61.9
    chronic demyelinating (CIDP) G61.81
    sequelae G65.1
    specified NEC G61.89
  lead G62.2
    sequelae G65.2
  nutritional NEC E63.9 [G63]
  postherpetic (zoster) B02.23
  progressive G60.3
  radiation-induced G62.82
  sensory (hereditary) (idiopathic) G60.8
  specified NEC G62.89
  syphilitic (late) A52.15
    congenital A50.43
  transthyretin-related (ATTR) familial amyloid E85.1
    triorthocresyl phosphate G62.2
      sequelae G65.2
    tuberculosis A17.89
    uremia N18.9 [G63]

Polyneuropathy — continued
  transthyretin-related familial amyloid — continued
    vitamin B12 deficiency E53.8 [G63]
      with anemia (pernicious) D51.0 [G63]
        due to dietary deficiency D51.3 [G63]
    zoster B02.23
Polyopia H53.8
Polyorchism, polyorchidism Q55.21
Polyosteoarthritis (see also Osteoarthritis, generalized) M15.9
  post-traumatic M15.3
  specified NEC M15.8
Polyostotic fibrous dysplasia Q78.1
Polyotia Q17.0
Polyp, polypus J33.8
  accessory sinus J33.8
  adenocarcinoma in — see Neoplasm, malignant, by site
  adenocarcinoma in situ in — see Neoplasm, in situ, by site
  adenoid tissue J33.0
  adenomatous (see also Neoplasm, benign, by site)
    adenocarcinoma in — see Neoplasm, malignant, by site
    adenocarcinoma in situ in — see Neoplasm, in situ, by site
    carcinoma in — see Neoplasm, malignant, by site
    carcinoma in situ in — see Neoplasm, in situ, by site
    multiple — see Neoplasm, benign
      adenocarcinoma in — see Neoplasm, malignant, by site
      adenocarcinoma in situ in — see Neoplasm, in situ, by site
  antrum J33.8
  anus, anal (canal) K62.0
  Bartholin's gland N84.3
  bladder D41.4
  carcinoma in — see Neoplasm, malignant, by site
  carcinoma in situ in — see Neoplasm, in situ, by site
  cecum D12.0
  cervix (uteri) N84.1
    in pregnancy or childbirth — see Pregnancy, complicated by, abnormal, cervix
    mucous N84.1
    nonneoplastic N84.1
  choanal J33.0
  cholesterol K82.4
  clitoris N84.3
  colon K63.5
    adenomatous D12.6
    ascending D12.2
    cecum D12.0
    descending D12.4
    inflammatory K51.40
      with
        abscess K51.414
        complication K51.419
          specified NEC K51.418
        fistula K51.413
        intestinal obstruction K51.412
        rectal bleeding K51.411
    sigmoid D12.5
    transverse D12.3
  corpus uteri N84.0
  dental K04.01
    irreversible K04.02
    reversible K04.01
  duodenum K31.7
  ear (middle) H74.4- ☑
  endometrium N84.0
  ethmoidal (sinus) J33.8
  fallopian tube N84.8
  female genital tract N84.9
    specified NEC N84.8
  frontal (sinus) J33.8
  gallbladder K82.4
  gingiva, gum K06.8
  labia, labium (majus) (minus) N84.3
  larynx (mucous) J38.1
    adenomatous D14.1
  malignant — see Neoplasm, malignant, by site
  maxillary (sinus) J33.8
  middle ear — see Polyp, ear (middle)
  myometrium N84.0
  nares
    anterior J33.9
    posterior J33.0

Polyp, polypus — *continued*
  nasal (mucous) J33.9
    cavity J33.0
      septum J33.0
  nasopharyngeal J33.0
  nose (mucous) J33.9
  oviduct N84.8
  pharynx J39.2
  placenta O90.89
  prostate — *see* Enlargement, enlarged, prostate
  pudenda, pudendum N84.3
  pulpal (dental) K04.01
    irreversible K04.02
    reversible K04.01
  rectum (nonadenomatous) K62.1
    adenomatous — *see* Polyp, adenomatous
  septum (nasal) J33.0
  sinus (accessory) (ethmoidal) (frontal) (maxillary)
    (sphenoidal) J33.8
  sphenoidal (sinus) J33.8
  stomach K31.7
    adenomatous D13.1
  tube, fallopian N84.8
  turbinate, mucous membrane J33.8
  umbilical, newborn P83.6
  ureter N28.89
  urethra N36.2
  uterus (body) (corpus) (mucous) N84.0
    cervix N84.1
    in pregnancy or childbirth — *see* Pregnancy,
      complicated by, tumor, uterus
  vagina N84.2
  vocal cord (mucous) J38.1
  vulva N84.3
Polyphagia R63.2
Polyploidy Q92.7
Polypoid — *see* condition
Polyposis (*see also* Polyp)
  coli (adenomatous) D12.6
    adenocarcinoma in C18.9
    adenocarcinoma in situ in — *see* Neoplasm, in situ,
      by site
    carcinoma in C18.9
  colon (adenomatous) D12.6
  familial D12.6
    adenocarcinoma in situ in — *see* Neoplasm, in situ,
      by site
  intestinal (adenomatous) D12.6
  malignant lymphomatous C83.1- ☑
  multiple, adenomatous (*see also* Neoplasm, benign)
    D36.9
Polyradiculitis — *see* Polyneuropathy
Polyradiculoneuropathy (acute) (postinfective) (segmentally demyelinating) G61.0
Polyserositis
  due to pericarditis I31.1
  pericardial I31.1
  periodic, familial E85.0
  tuberculous A19.9
    acute A19.1
    chronic A19.8
Polysplenia syndrome Q89.09
Polysyndactyly (*see also* Syndactylism, syndactyly) Q70.4
Polytrichia L68.3
Polyunguia Q84.6
Polyuria R35.8
  nocturnal R35.1
  psychogenic F45.8
Pompe's disease (glycogen storage) E74.02
Pompholyx L30.1
Poncet's disease (tuberculous rheumatism) A18.09
Pond fracture — *see* Fracture, skull
Ponos B55.0
Pons, pontine — *see* condition
Poor
  aesthetic of existing restoration of tooth K08.56
  contractions, labor O62.2
  gingival margin to tooth restoration K08.51
  personal hygiene R46.0
  prenatal care, affecting management of pregnancy
    — *see* Pregnancy, complicated by, insufficient,
    prenatal care
  sucking reflex (newborn) R29.2
  urinary stream R39.12
  vision NEC H54.7
Poradenitis, nostras inguinalis or venerea A55
Porencephaly (congenital) (developmental) (true) Q04.6
  acquired G93.0

Porencephaly — *continued*
  nondevelopmental G93.0
  traumatic (post) F07.89
Porocephaliasis B88.8
Porokeratosis Q82.8
Poroma, eccrine — *see* Neoplasm, skin, benign
Porphyria (South African) E80.20
  acquired E80.20
  acute intermittent (hepatic) (Swedish) E80.21
  cutanea tarda (hereditary) (symptomatic) E80.1
  due to drugs E80.20
    correct substance properly administered — *see*
      Table of Drugs and Chemicals, by drug, ad-
      verse effect
    overdose or wrong substance given or taken —
      see Table of Drugs and Chemicals, by drug,
      poisoning
  erythropoietic (congenital) (hereditary) E80.0
  hepatocutaneous type E80.1
  secondary E80.20
  toxic NEC E80.20
  variegata E80.20
Porphyrinuria — *see* Porphyria
Porphyruria — *see* Porphyria
Port wine nevus, mark, or stain Q82.5
Portal — *see* condition
Posadas-Wernicke disease B38.9
Positive
  culture (nonspecific)
    blood R78.81
    bronchial washings R84.5
    cerebrospinal fluid R83.5
    cervix uteri R87.5
    nasal secretions R84.5
    nipple discharge R89.5
    nose R84.5
      staphylococcus (Methicillin susceptible) Z22.321
        Methicillin resistant Z22.322
    peritoneal fluid R85.5
    pleural fluid R84.5
    prostatic secretions R86.5
    saliva R85.5
    seminal fluid R86.5
    sputum R84.5
    synovial fluid R89.5
    throat scrapings R84.5
    urine R82.79
    vagina R87.5
    vulva R87.5
    wound secretions R89.5
  PPD (skin test) R76.11
  serology for syphilis A53.0
    with signs or symptoms — *code as* Syphilis, by site
      and stage
    false R76.8
  skin test, tuberculin (without active tuberculosis)
    R76.11
  test, human immunodeficiency virus (HIV) R75
  VDRL A53.0
    with signs or symptoms — *code by* site and stage
      under Syphilis A53.9
  Wassermann reaction A53.0
Postcardiotomy syndrome I97.0
Postcaval ureter Q62.62
Postcholecystectomy syndrome K91.5
Postclimacteric bleeding N95.0
Postcommissurotomy syndrome I97.0
Postconcussional syndrome F07.81
Postcontusional syndrome F07.81
Postcricoid region — *see* condition
Post-dates (40-42 weeks) (pregnancy) (mother) O48.0
  more than 42 weeks gestation O48.1
Postencephalitic syndrome F07.89
Posterior — *see* condition
Posterolateral sclerosis (spinal cord) — *see* Degenera-
  tion, combined
Postexanthematous — *see* condition
Postfebrile — *see* condition
Postgastrectomy dumping syndrome K91.1
Posthemiplegic chorea — *see* Monoplegia
Posthemorrhagic anemia (chronic) D50.0
  acute D62
  newborn P61.3
Postherpetic neuralgia (zoster) B02.29
  trigeminal B02.22
Posthitis N47.7
Postimmunization complication or reaction — *see*
  Complications, vaccination

Postinfectious — *see* condition
Postlaminectomy syndrome NEC M96.1
Postleukotomy syndrome F07.0
Postmastectomy lymphedema (syndrome) I97.2
Postmaturity, postmature (over 42 weeks)
  maternal (over 42 weeks gestation) O48.1
  newborn P08.22
Postmeasles complication NEC (*see also* condition)
  B05.89
Postmenopausal
  endometrium (atrophic) N95.8
    suppurative (*see also* Endometritis) N71.9
  osteoporosis — *see* Osteoporosis, postmenopausal
Postnasal drip R09.82
  due to
    allergic rhinitis — *see* Rhinitis, allergic
    common cold J00
    gastroesophageal reflux — *see* Reflux, gastroe-
      sophageal
    nasopharyngitis — *see* Nasopharyngitis
    other known condition — *code to* condition
    sinusitis — *see* Sinusitis
Postnatal — *see* condition
Postoperative (postprocedural) — *see* Complication,
  postoperative
  pneumothorax, therapeutic Z98.3
  state NEC Z98.890
Postpancreatectomy hyperglycemia E89.1
Postpartum — *see* Puerperal
Postphlebitic syndrome — *see* Syndrome, postthrom-
  botic
Postpolio (myelitic) **syndrome** G14
Postpoliomyelitic (*see also* condition)
  osteopathy — *see* Osteopathy, after poliomyelitis
Postprocedural (*see also* Postoperative)
  hypoinsulinemia E89.1
Postschizophrenic depression F32.89
Postsurgery status (*see also* Status (post))
  pneumothorax, therapeutic Z98.3
Post-term (40-42 weeks) (pregnancy) (mother) O48.0
  infant P08.21
  more than 42 weeks gestation (mother) O48.1
Post-traumatic brain syndrome, nonpsychotic F07.81
Post-typhoid abscess A01.09
Postures, hysterical F44.2
Postvaccinal reaction or complication — *see* Complications, vaccination
Postvalvulotomy syndrome I97.0
Potain's
  disease (pulmonary edema) — *see* Edema, lung
  syndrome (gastrectasis with dyspepsia) K31.0
Potter's
  asthma J62.8
  facies Q60.6
  lung J62.8
  syndrome (with renal agenesis) Q60.6
Pott's
  curvature (spinal) A18.01
  disease or paraplegia A18.01
  spinal curvature A18.01
  tumor, puffy — *see* Osteomyelitis, specified type NEC
Pouch
  bronchus Q32.4
  Douglas' — *see* condition
  esophagus, esophageal, congenital Q39.6
    acquired K22.5
  gastric K31.4
  Hartmann's K82.8
  pharynx, pharyngeal (congenital) Q38.7
Pouchitis K91.850
Poultrymen's itch B88.0
Poverty NEC Z59.6
  extreme Z59.5
Poxvirus NEC B08.8
Prader-Willi syndrome Q87.1
Preauricular appendage or tag Q17.0
Prebetalipoproteinemia (acquired) (essential) (familial)
  (hereditary) (primary) (secondary) E78.1
  with chylomicronemia E78.3
Precipitate labor or delivery O62.3
Preclimacteric bleeding (menorrhagia) N92.4
Precocious
  adrenarche E30.1
  menarche E30.1
  menstruation E30.1
  pubarche E30.1
  puberty E30.1

Precocious — *continued*
  puberty — *continued*
    central E22.8
    sexual development NEC E30.1
    thelarche E30.8
Precocity, sexual (constitutional) (cryptogenic) (female) (idiopathic) (male) E30.1
  with adrenal hyperplasia E25.9
    congenital E25.0
Precordial pain R07.2
Predeciduous teeth K00.2
Prediabetes, prediabetic R73.03
  complicating
    pregnancy — *see* Pregnancy, complicated by, diseases of, specified type or system NEC
    puerperium O99.89
Predislocation status of hip at birth Q65.6
Pre-eclampsia O14.9- ☑
  with pre-existing hypertension — *see* Hypertension, complicating pregnancy, pre-existing, with, pre-eclampsia
  complicating
    childbirth O14.94
    puerperium O14.95
  mild O14.0- ☑
    complicating
      childbirth O14.04
      puerperium O14.05
  moderate O14.0- ☑
    complicating
      childbirth O14.04
      puerperium O14.05
  severe O14.1- ☑
    with hemolysis, elevated liver enzymes and low platelet count (HELLP) O14.2- ☑
      complicating
        childbirth O14.24
        puerperium O14.25
    complicating
      childbirth O14.14
      puerperium O14.15
Pre-eruptive color change, teeth, tooth K00.8
Pre-excitation atrioventricular conduction I45.6
Preglaucoma H40.00- ☑
Pregnancy (single) (uterine) (*see also* Delivery and Puerperal)

> Note: The Tabular must be reviewed for assignment of appropriate seventh character for multiple gestation codes in Chapter 15

> Note: The Tabular must be reviewed for assignment of the appropriate character indicating the trimester of the pregnancy

  abdominal (ectopic) O00.00
    with intrauterine pregnancy O00.01
      with viable fetus O36.7- ☑
  ampullar O00.10- ☑
    with intrauterine pregnancy O00.11- ☑
  biochemical O02.81
  broad ligament O00.80
    with intrauterine pregnancy O00.81
  cervical O00.8
    with intrauterine pregnancy O00.81
  chemical O02.81
  complicated by (care of) (management affected by)
    abnormal, abnormality
      cervix O34.4-
        causing obstructed labor O65.5
      cord (umbilical) O69.9 ☑
      fetal heart rate or rhythm O36.83- ☑
      findings on antenatal screening of mother O28.9
        biochemical O28.1
        chromosomal O28.5
        cytological O28.2
        genetic O28.5
        hematological O28.0
        radiological O28.4
        specified NEC O28.8
        ultrasonic O28.3
      glucose (tolerance) NEC O99.810
      pelvic organs O34.9- ☑
        specified NEC O34.8- ☑
          causing obstructed labor O65.5
      pelvis (bony) (major) NEC O33.0
      perineum O34.7- ☑

Pregnancy — *continued*
  complicated by — *continued*
    abnormal, abnormality — *continued*
      position
        placenta O44.0- ☑
          with hemorrhage O44.1- ☑
        uterus O34.59- ☑
      uterus O34.59- ☑
        causing obstructed labor O65.5
        congenital O34.0- ☑
      vagina O34.6-
        causing obstructed labor O65.5
      vulva O34.7-
        causing obstructed labor O65.5
    abruptio placentae — *see* Abruptio placentae
    abscess or cellulitis
      bladder O23.1- ☑
      breast O91.11- ☑
      genital organ or tract O23.9- ☑
    abuse
      physical O9A.31 ☑ (*following* O99)
      psychological O9A.51 ☑ (*following* O99)
      sexual O9A.41 ☑ (*following* O99)
    adverse effect anesthesia O29.9- ☑
      aspiration pneumonitis O29.01- ☑
      cardiac arrest O29.11- ☑
      cardiac complication NEC O29.19- ☑
      cardiac failure O29.12- ☑
      central nervous system complication NEC O29.29- ☑
      cerebral anoxia O29.21- ☑
      failed or difficult intubation O29.6- ☑
      inhalation of stomach contents or secretions NOS O29.01- ☑
      local, toxic reaction O29.3X ☑
      Mendelson's syndrome O29.01- ☑
      pressure collapse of lung O29.02- ☑
      pulmonary complications NEC O29.09- ☑
      specified NEC O29.8X- ☑
      spinal and epidural type NEC O29.5X ☑
        induced headache O29.4- ☑
    albuminuria (*see also* Proteinuria, gestational) O12.1- ☑
    alcohol use O99.31- ☑
    amnionitis O41.12- ☑
    anaphylactoid syndrome of pregnancy O88.01- ☑
    anemia (conditions in D50-D64) (pre-existing) O99.01- ☑
      complicating the puerperium O99.03
    antepartum hemorrhage O46.9- ☑
      with coagulation defect — *see* Hemorrhage, antepartum, with coagulation defect
      specified NEC O46.8X- ☑
    appendicitis O99.61- ☑
    atrophy (yellow) (acute) liver (subacute) O26.61- ☑
    bariatric surgery status O99.84- ☑
    bicornis or bicornuate uterus O34.0- ☑
    biliary tract problems O26.61- ☑
    breech presentation O32.1 ☑
    cardiovascular diseases (conditions in I00-I09, I20-I52, I70-I99) O99.41- ☑
    cerebrovascular disorders (conditions in I60-I69) O99.41- ☑
    cervical shortening O26.87- ☑
    cervicitis O23.51- ☑
    chloasma (gravidarum) O26.89- ☑
    cholecystitis O99.61- ☑
    cholestasis (intrahepatic) O26.61- ☑
    chorioamnionitis O41.12- ☑
    circulatory system disorder (conditions in I00-I09, I20-I99, O99.41-)
    compound presentation O32.6 ☑
    conjoined twins O30.02- ☑
    connective system disorders (conditions in M00-M99) O99.89
    contracted pelvis (general) O33.1
      inlet O33.2
      outlet O33.3 ☑
    convulsions (eclamptic) (uremic) (*see also* Eclampsia) O15.9
    cracked nipple O92.11- ☑
    cystitis O23.1- ☑
    cystocele O34.8- ☑
    death of fetus (near term) O36.4 ☑
      early pregnancy O02.1

Pregnancy — *continued*
  complicated by — *continued*
    death of fetus — *continued*
      of one fetus or more in multiple gestation O31.2- ☑
    deciduitis O41.14- ☑
    decreased fetal movement O36.81- ☑
    dental problems O99.61- ☑
    diabetes (mellitus) O24.91- ☑
      gestational (pregnancy induced) — *see* Diabetes, gestational
      pre-existing O24.31- ☑
        specified NEC O24.81- ☑
        type 1 O24.01- ☑
        type 2 O24.11- ☑
    digestive system disorders (conditions in K00-K93) O99.61- ☑
    diseases of — *see* Pregnancy, complicated by, specified body system disease
      biliary tract O26.61- ☑
      blood NEC (conditions in D65-D77) O99.11- ☑
      liver O26.61- ☑
      specified NEC O99.89
    disorders of — *see* Pregnancy, complicated by, specified body system disorder
      amniotic fluid and membranes O41.9- ☑
        specified NEC O41.8X- ☑
      biliary tract O26.61- ☑
      ear and mastoid process (conditions in H60-H95) O99.89
      eye and adnexa (conditions in H00-H59) O99.89
      liver O26.61- ☑
      skin (conditions in L00-L99) O99.71- ☑
      specified NEC O99.89
    displacement, uterus NEC O34.59- ☑
      causing obstructed labor O65.5
    disproportion (due to) O33.9
      fetal (ascites) (hydrops) (meningomyelocele) (sacral teratoma) (tumor) deformities NEC O33.7 ☑
      generally contracted pelvis O33.1
      hydrocephalic fetus O33.6 ☑
      inlet contraction of pelvis O33.2
      mixed maternal and fetal origin O33.4 ☑
      specified NEC O33.8
    double uterus O34.0- ☑
      causing obstructed labor O65.5
    drug use (conditions in F11-F19) O99.32- ☑
    eclampsia, eclamptic (coma) (convulsions) (delirium) (nephritis) (uremia) (*see also* Eclampsia) O15.- ☑
    ectopic pregnancy — *see* Pregnancy, ectopic
    edema O12.0- ☑
      with
        gestational hypertension, mild (*see also* Pre-eclampsia) O14.0- ☑
        proteinuria O12.2- ☑
    effusion, amniotic fluid — *see* Pregnancy, complicated by, premature rupture of membranes
    elderly
      multigravida O09.52- ☑
      primigravida O09.51- ☑
    embolism (*see also* Embolism, obstetric, pregnancy) O88.- ☑
    endocrine diseases NEC O99.28- ☑
    endometritis O86.12
    excessive weight gain O26.0- ☑
    exhaustion O26.81- ☑
      during labor and delivery O75.81
    face presentation O32.3 ☑
    failed induction of labor O61.9
      instrumental O61.1
      mechanical O61.1
      medical O61.0
      specified NEC O61.8
      surgical O61.1
    failed or difficult intubation for anesthesia O29.6- ☑
    false labor (pains) O47.9
      at or after 37 completed weeks of pregnancy O47.1
      before 37 completed weeks of pregnancy O47.0- ☑
    fatigue O26.81- ☑
      during labor and delivery O75.81
    fatty metamorphosis of liver O26.61- ☑
    female genital mutilation O34.8- ☑ [N90.81-] ☑

☟ Subterms under main terms may continue to next column or page   ☑ Additional Character Required — Refer to the Tabular List for Character Selection   259

Precocious — Pregnancy

Pregnancy — *continued*
  complicated by — *continued*
    fetal (maternal care for)
      abnormality or damage O35.9 ☑
        acid-base balance O68
        specified type NEC O35.8 ☑
      acidemia O68
      acidosis O68
      alkalosis O68
      anemia and thrombocytopenia O36.82- ☑
      anencephaly O35.0 ☑
      chromosomal abnormality (conditions in Q90-Q99) O35.1 ☑
      conjoined twins O30.02- ☑
      damage from
        amniocentesis O35.7 ☑
        biopsy procedures O35.7 ☑
        drug addiction O35.5 ☑
        hematological investigation O35.7 ☑
        intrauterine contraceptive device O35.7 ☑
        maternal
          alcohol addiction O35.4 ☑
          cytomegalovirus infection O35.3 ☑
          disease NEC O35.8 ☑
          drug addiction O35.5 ☑
          listeriosis O35.8 ☑
          rubella O35.3 ☑
          toxoplasmosis O35.8 ☑
          viral infection O35.3 ☑
        medical procedure NEC O35.7 ☑
        radiation O35.6 ☑
      death (near term) O36.4 ☑
        early pregnancy O02.1
      decreased movement O36.81- ☑
      disproportion due to deformity (fetal) O33.7 ☑
      excessive growth (large for dates) O36.6- ☑
      growth retardation O36.59- ☑
        light for dates O36.59- ☑
        small for dates O36.59- ☑
      heart rate irregularity (bradycardia) (decelerations) (tachycardia) O76
      hereditary disease O35.2 ☑
      hydrocephalus O35.0 ☑
      intrauterine death O36.4 ☑
      poor growth O36.59- ☑
        light for dates O36.59- ☑
        small for dates O36.59- ☑
      problem O36.9- ☑
        specified NEC O36.89- ☑
      reduction (elective) O31.3- ☑
      selective termination O31.3- ☑
      spina bifida O35.0 ☑
      thrombocytopenia O36.82- ☑
    fibroid (tumor) (uterus) O34.1- ☑
    fissure of nipple O92.11- ☑
    gallstones O99.61- ☑
    gastric banding status O99.84- ☑
    gastric bypass status O99.84- ☑
    genital herpes (asymptomatic) (history of) (inactive) O98.3- ☑
    genital tract infection O23.9- ☑
    glomerular diseases (conditions in N00-N07) O26.83- ☑
      with hypertension, pre-existing — *see* Hypertension, complicating, pregnancy, pre-existing, with, renal disease
    gonorrhea O98.21- ☑
    grand multiparity O09.4 ☑
    habitual aborter — *see* Pregnancy, complicated by, recurrent pregnancy loss
    HELLP syndrome (hemolysis, elevated liver enzymes and low platelet count) O14.2- ☑
    hemorrhage
      antepartum — *see* Hemorrhage, antepartum
      before 20 completed weeks gestation O20.9
        specified NEC O20.8
      due to premature separation, placenta (see also Abruptio placentae) O45.9- ☑
      early O20.9
        specified NEC O20.8
        threatened abortion O20.0
    hemorrhoids O22.4- ☑
    hepatitis (viral) O98.41- ☑
    herniation of uterus O34.59- ☑
    high
      head at term O32.4 ☑

Pregnancy — *continued*
  complicated by — *continued*
    high — *continued*
      risk — *see* Supervision (of) (for), high-risk
    history of in utero procedure during previous pregnancy O09.82- ☑
    HIV O98.71- ☑
    human immunodeficiency virus (HIV) disease O98.71- ☑
    hydatidiform mole (*see also* Mole, hydatidiform) O01.9
    hydramnios O40.- ☑
    hydrocephalic fetus (disproportion) O33.6 ☑
    hydrops
      amnii O40.- ☑
      fetalis O36.2- ☑
        associated with isoimmunization (*see also* Pregnancy, complicated by, isoimmunization) O36.11- ☑
    hydrorrhea O42.90
    hyperemesis (gravidarum) (mild) (*see also* Hyperemesis, gravidarum) O21.0
    hypertension — *see* Hypertension, complicating pregnancy
    hypertensive
      heart and renal disease, pre-existing — *see* Hypertension, complicating, pregnancy, pre-existing, with, heart disease, with renal disease
      heart disease, pre-existing — *see* Hypertension, complicating, pregnancy, pre-existing, with, heart disease
      renal disease, pre-existing — *see* Hypertension, complicating, pregnancy, pre-existing, with, renal disease
    hypotension O26.5- ☑
    immune disorders NEC (conditions in D80-D89) O99.11- ☑
    incarceration, uterus O34.51- ☑
    incompetent cervix O34.3- ☑
    inconclusive fetal viability O36.80 ☑
    infection(s) O98.91- ☑
      amniotic fluid or sac O41.10- ☑
      bladder O23.1- ☑
      carrier state NEC O99.830
        streptococcus B O99.820
      genital organ or tract O23.9- ☑
        specified NEC O23.59- ☑
      genitourinary tract O23.9- ☑
      gonorrhea O98.21- ☑
      hepatitis (viral) O98.41- ☑
      HIV O98.71- ☑
      human immunodeficiency virus (HIV) O98.71- ☑
      kidney O23.0- ☑
      nipple O91.01- ☑
      parasitic disease O98.91- ☑
        specified NEC O98.81- ☑
      protozoal disease O98.61- ☑
      sexually transmitted NEC O98.31- ☑
      specified type NEC O98.81- ☑
      syphilis O98.11- ☑
      tuberculosis O98.01- ☑
      urethra O23.2- ☑
      urinary (tract) O23.4- ☑
        specified NEC O23.3- ☑
      viral disease O98.51- ☑
    injury or poisoning (conditions in S00-T88) O9A.21- ☑ (*following* O99)
      due to abuse
        physical O9A.31- ☑ (*following* O99)
        psychological O9A.51- ☑ (*following* O99)
        sexual O9A.41- ☑ (*following* O99)
    insufficient
      prenatal care O09.3- ☑
      weight gain O26.1- ☑
    insulin resistance O26.89 ☑
    intrauterine fetal death (near term) O36.4 ☑
      early pregnancy O02.1
      multiple gestation (one fetus or more) O31.2- ☑
    isoimmunization O36.11- ☑
      anti-A sensitization O36.11- ☑
      anti-B sensitization O36.19- ☑
      Rh O36.09- ☑
        anti-D antibody O36.01- ☑

Pregnancy — *continued*
  complicated by — *continued*
    isoimmunization — *continued*
      specified NEC O36.19- ☑
    laceration of uterus NEC O71.81
    malformation
      placenta, placental (vessel) O43.10- ☑
        specified NEC O43.19- ☑
      uterus (congenital) O34.0- ☑
    malnutrition (conditions in E40-E46) O25.1- ☑
    maternal hypotension syndrome O26.5- ☑
    mental disorders (conditions in F01-F09, F20-F99) O99.34- ☑
      alcohol use O99.31- ☑
      drug use O99.32- ☑
      smoking O99.33- ☑
    mentum presentation O32.3 ☑
    metabolic disorders O99.28- ☑
    missed
      abortion O02.1
      delivery O36.4 ☑
    multiple gestations O30.9- ☑
      conjoined twins O30.02- ☑
      quadruplet — *see* Pregnancy, quadruplet
      specified complication NEC O31.8X- ☑
      specified number of multiples NEC — *see* Pregnancy, multiple (gestation), specified NEC
      triplet — *see* Pregnancy, triplet
      twin — *see* Pregnancy, twin
    musculoskeletal condition (conditions is M00-M99) O99.89
    necrosis, liver (conditions in K72) O26.61- ☑
    neoplasm
      benign
        cervix O34.4- ☑
        corpus uteri O34.1- ☑
        uterus O34.1- ☑
      malignant O9A.11- ☑ (*following* O99)
    nephropathy NEC O26.83- ☑
    nervous system condition (conditions in G00-G99) O99.35- ☑
    nutritional diseases NEC O99.28- ☑
    obesity (pre-existing) O99.21- ☑
    obesity surgery status O99.84- ☑
    oblique lie or presentation O32.2 ☑
    older mother — *see* Pregnancy, complicated by, elderly
    oligohydramnios O41.0- ☑
      with premature rupture of membranes (*see also* Pregnancy, complicated by, premature rupture of membranes) O42.- ☑
    onset (spontaneous) of labor after 37 completed weeks of gestation but before 39 completed weeks gestation, with delivery by (planned) cesarean section O75.82
    oophoritis O23.52- ☑
    overdose, drug (*see also* Table of Drugs and Chemicals, by drug, poisoning) O9A.21- ☑ (*following* O99)
    oversize fetus O33.5 ☑
    papyraceous fetus O31.0- ☑
    pelvic inflammatory disease O99.89
    periodontal disease O99.61- ☑
    peripheral neuritis O26.82- ☑
    peritoneal (pelvic) adhesions O99.89
    phlebitis O22.9- ☑
    phlebopathy O22.9- ☑
    phlebothrombosis (superficial) O22.2- ☑
      deep O22.3- ☑
    placenta accreta O43.21- ☑
    placenta increta O43.22- ☑
    placenta percreta O43.23- ☑
    placenta previa O44.0- ☑
      complete O44.0- ☑
        with hemorrhage O44.1- ☑
      marginal O44.2- ☑
        with hemorrhage O44.3- ☑
      partial O44.2- ☑
        with hemorrhage O44.3- ☑
    placental disorder O43.9- ☑
      specified NEC O43.89- ☑
    placental dysfunction O43.89- ☑
    placental infarction O43.81- ☑
    placental insufficiency O36.51- ☑

☑ **Additional Character Required — Refer to the Tabular List for Character Selection**
    ▽ Subterms under main terms may continue to next column or page

Pregnancy — *continued*
　complicated by — *continued*
　　placental transfusion syndromes
　　　fetomaternal O43.01- ☑
　　　fetus to fetus O43.02- ☑
　　　maternofetal O43.01- ☑
　　placentitis O41.14- ☑
　　pneumonia O99.51- ☑
　　poisoning (*see also* Table of Drugs and Chemicals)
　　　O9A.21 ☑ (*following* O99)
　　polyhydramnios O40- ☑
　　polymorphic eruption of pregnancy O26.86
　　poor obstetric history NEC O09.29- ☑
　　postmaturity (post-term) (40 to 42 weeks) O48.0
　　　more than 42 completed weeks gestation
　　　　(prolonged) O48.1
　　pre-eclampsia O14.9- ☑
　　　mild O14.0- ☑
　　　moderate O14.0- ☑
　　　severe O14.1- ☑
　　　　with hemolysis, elevated liver enzymes and
　　　　　low platelet count (HELLP) O14.2- ☑
　　premature labor — *see* Pregnancy, complicated
　　　by, preterm labor
　　premature rupture of membranes O42.90
　　　with onset of labor
　　　　after 24 hours O42.10
　　　　　at or after 37 weeks gestation, onset of
　　　　　　labor more than 24 hours follow-
　　　　　　ing rupture O42.12
　　　　　pre-term (before 37 completed weeks
　　　　　　of gestation) O42.11- ☑
　　　　within 24 hours O42.00
　　　　　at or after 37 weeks gestation, onset of
　　　　　　labor within 24 hours of rupture
　　　　　　O42.02
　　　　　pre-term (before 37 completed weeks
　　　　　　of gestation) O42.01- ☑
　　　at or after 37 weeks gestation, unspecified as
　　　　to length of time between rupture and
　　　　onset of labor O42.92
　　　full-term, unspecified as to length of time be-
　　　　tween rupture and onset of labor O42.92
　　　pre-term (before 37 completed weeks of gesta-
　　　　tion) O42.91- ☑
　　premature separation of placenta (*see also* Abrup-
　　　tio placentae) O45.9- ☑
　　presentation, fetal — *see* Delivery, complicated
　　　by, malposition
　　preterm delivery O60.10 ☑
　　preterm labor
　　　with delivery O60.10 ☑
　　　　preterm O60.10 ☑
　　　　term O60.20 ☑
　　　without delivery O60.00
　　　　second trimester O60.02
　　　　third trimester O60.03
　　　second trimester
　　　　with preterm delivery
　　　　　second trimester O60.12 ☑
　　　　　third trimester O60.13 ☑
　　　　with term delivery O60.22 ☑
　　　　without delivery O60.02
　　　third trimester
　　　　with term delivery O60.23 ☑
　　　　with third trimester preterm delivery
　　　　　O60.14 ☑
　　　　without delivery O60.03
　　previous history of — *see* Pregnancy, supervision
　　　of, high-risk
　　prolapse, uterus O34.52- ☑
　　proteinuria (gestational) (*see also* Proteinuria,
　　　gestational) O12.1- ☑
　　　with edema O12.2- ☑
　　pruritic urticarial papules and plaques of pregnancy
　　　(PUPPP) O26.86
　　pruritus (neurogenic) O26.89- ☑
　　psychosis or psychoneurosis (puerperal) F53
　　ptyalism O26.89- ☑
　　PUPPP (pruritic urticarial papules and plaques of
　　　pregnancy) O26.86
　　pyelitis O23.0- ☑
　　recurrent pregnancy loss O26.2- ☑
　　renal disease or failure NEC O26.83- ☑
　　　with secondary hypertension, pre-existing —
　　　　see Hypertension, complicating, pregnan-
　　　　cy, pre-existing, secondary

Pregnancy — *continued*
　complicated by — *continued*
　　renal disease or failure — *continued*
　　　hypertensive, pre-existing — *see* Hypertension,
　　　　complicating, pregnancy, pre-existing,
　　　　with, renal disease
　　respiratory condition (conditions in J00-J99)
　　　O99.51- ☑
　　retained, retention
　　　dead ovum O02.0
　　　intrauterine contraceptive device O26.3- ☑
　　retroversion, uterus O34.53- ☑
　　Rh immunization, incompatibility or sensitization
　　　NEC O36.09- ☑
　　　anti-D antibody O36.01- ☑
　　rupture
　　　amnion (premature) (*see also* Pregnancy, com-
　　　　plicated by, premature rupture of mem-
　　　　branes) O42- ☑
　　　membranes (premature) (*see also* Pregnancy,
　　　　complicated by, premature rupture of
　　　　membranes) O42- ☑
　　　uterus (during labor) O71.1
　　　　before onset of labor O71.0- ☑
　　salivation (excessive) O26.89- ☑
　　salpingitis O23.52- ☑
　　salpingo-oophoritis O23.52- ☑
　　sepsis (conditions in A40, A41) O98.81- ☑
　　size date discrepancy (uterine) O26.84- ☑
　　skin condition (conditions in L00-L99) O99.71- ☑
　　smoking (tobacco) O99.33- ☑
　　social problem O09.7- ☑
　　specified condition NEC O26.89- ☑
　　spotting O26.85- ☑
　　streptococcus group B (GBS) carrier state O99.820
　　subluxation of symphysis (pubis) O26.71- ☑
　　syphilis (conditions in A50-A53) O98.11- ☑
　　threatened
　　　abortion O20.0
　　　labor O47.9
　　　　at or after 37 completed weeks of gestation
　　　　　O47.1
　　　　before 37 completed weeks of gestation
　　　　　O47.0- ☑
　　thrombophlebitis (superficial) O22.2- ☑
　　thrombosis O22.9- ☑
　　　cerebral venous O22.5- ☑
　　　cerebrovenous sinus O22.5- ☑
　　　deep O22.3- ☑
　　tobacco use disorder (smoking) O99.33- ☑
　　torsion of uterus O34.59- ☑
　　toxemia O14.9- ☑
　　transverse lie or presentation O32.2 ☑
　　tuberculosis (conditions in A15-A19) O98.01- ☑
　　tumor (benign)
　　　cervix O34.4- ☑
　　　malignant O9A.11- ☑ (*following* O99)
　　　uterus O34.1- ☑
　　unstable lie O32.0 ☑
　　upper respiratory infection O99.51- ☑
　　urethritis O23.2- ☑
　　uterine size date discrepancy O26.84- ☑
　　vaginitis or vulvitis O23.59- ☑
　　varicose veins (lower extremities) O22.0- ☑
　　　genitals O22.1- ☑
　　　legs O22.0- ☑
　　　perineal O22.1- ☑
　　　vaginal or vulval O22.1- ☑
　　venereal disease NEC (conditions in A63.8)
　　　O98.31- ☑
　　venous disorders O22.9- ☑
　　　specified NEC O22.8X- ☑
　　very young mother — *see* Pregnancy, complicated
　　　by, young mother
　　viral diseases (conditions in A80-B09, B25-B34)
　　　O98.51- ☑
　　vomiting O21.9
　　　due to diseases classified elsewhere O21.8
　　　hyperemesis gravidarum (mild) (*see also* Hyper-
　　　　emesis, gravidarum) O21.0
　　　late (occurring after 20 weeks of gestation)
　　　　O21.2
　　young mother
　　　multigravida O09.62- ☑
　　　primigravida O09.61- ☑
　complicated NOS O26.9- ☑
　concealed O09.3- ☑

Pregnancy — *continued*
　continuing following
　　elective fetal reduction of one or more fetus
　　　O31.3- ☑
　　intrauterine death of one or more fetus O31.2- ☑
　　spontaneous abortion of one or more fetus
　　　O31.1- ☑
　cornual O00.80
　　with intrauterine pregnancy O00.81
　ectopic (ruptured) O00.90
　　with intrauterine pregnancy O00.91
　　abdominal O00.00
　　　with
　　　　intrauterine pregnancy O00.01
　　　　　viable fetus O36.7- ☑
　　cervical O00.80
　　　with intrauterine pregnancy O00.81
　　complicated (by) O08.9
　　　afibrinogenemia O08.1
　　　cardiac arrest O08.81
　　　chemical damage of pelvic organ(s) O08.6
　　　circulatory collapse O08.3
　　　defibrination syndrome O08.1
　　　electrolyte imbalance O08.5
　　　embolism (amniotic fluid) (blood clot) (pul-
　　　　monary) (septic) O08.2
　　　endometritis O08.0
　　　genital tract and pelvic infection O08.0
　　　hemorrhage (delayed) (excessive) O08.1
　　　infection
　　　　genital tract or pelvic O08.0
　　　　kidney O08.83
　　　　urinary tract O08.3
　　　intravascular coagulation O08.1
　　　laceration of pelvic organ(s) O08.6
　　　metabolic disorder O08.5
　　　oliguria O08.4
　　　oophoritis O08.0
　　　parametritis O08.0
　　　pelvic peritonitis O08.0
　　　perforation of pelvic organ(s) O08.6
　　　renal failure or shutdown O08.4
　　　salpingitis or salpingo-oophoritis O08.0
　　　sepsis O08.82
　　　shock O08.83
　　　　septic O08.82
　　　specified condition NEC O08.89
　　　tubular necrosis (renal) O08.4
　　　uremia O08.4
　　　urinary infection O08.83
　　　venous complication NEC O08.7
　　　　embolism O08.2
　　cornual O00.80
　　　with intrauterine pregnancy O00.81
　　intraligamentous O00.80
　　　with intrauterine pregnancy O00.81
　　mural O00.80
　　　with intrauterine pregnancy O00.81
　　ovarian O00.20- ☑
　　　with intrauterine pregnancy O00.21- ☑
　　specified site NEC O00.80
　　　with intrauterine pregnancy O00.81
　　tubal (ruptured) O00.10- ☑
　　　with intrauterine pregnancy O00.11- ☑
　examination (normal) Z34.9- ☑
　　first Z34.0- ☑
　　high-risk — *see* Pregnancy, supervision of, high-
　　　risk
　　specified Z34.8- ☑
　extrauterine — *see* Pregnancy, ectopic
　fallopian O00.10- ☑
　　with intrauterine pregnancy O00.11- ☑
　false F45.8
　gestational carrier Z33.3
　hidden O09.3- ☑
　high-risk — *see* Pregnancy, supervision of, high-risk
　incidental finding Z33.1
　interstitial O00.80
　　with intrauterine pregnancy O00.81
　intraligamentous O00.80
　　with intrauterine pregnancy O00.81
　intramural O00.80
　　with intrauterine pregnancy O00.81
　intraperitoneal O00.00
　　with intrauterine pregnancy O00.01
　isthmian O00.10- ☑
　　with intrauterine pregnancy O00.11- ☑
　mesometric (mural) O00.80

Pregnancy — *continued*
  mesometric — *continued*
    with intrauterine pregnancy O00.81
  molar NEC O02.0
    complicated (by) O08.9
      afibrinogenemia O08.1
      cardiac arrest O08.81
      chemical damage of pelvic organ(s) O08.6
      circulatory collapse O08.3
      defibrination syndrome O08.1
      electrolyte imbalance O08.5
      embolism (amniotic fluid) (blood clot) (pulmonary) (septic) O08.2
      endometritis O08.0
      genital tract and pelvic infection O08.0
      hemorrhage (delayed) (excessive) O08.1
      infection
        genital tract or pelvic O08.0
        kidney O08.83
        urinary tract O08.83
      intravascular coagulation O08.1
      laceration of pelvic organ(s) O08.6
      metabolic disorder O08.5
      oliguria O08.4
      oophoritis O08.0
      parametritis O08.0
      pelvic peritonitis O08.0
      perforation of pelvic organ(s) O08.6
      renal failure or shutdown O08.4
      salpingitis or salpingo-oophoritis O08.0
      sepsis O08.82
      shock O08.3
        septic O08.82
      specified condition NEC O08.89
      tubular necrosis (renal) O08.4
      uremia O08.4
      urinary infection O08.83
      venous complication NEC O08.7
        embolism O08.2
  hydatidiform (*see also* Mole, hydatidiform) O01.9
  multiple (gestation) O30.9- ☑
    greater than quadruplets — *see* Pregnancy, multiple (gestation), specified NEC
    specified NEC O30.80- ☑
      with
        two or more monoamniotic fetuses O30.82-
        two or more monochorionic fetuses O30.81-
      two or more monoamniotic fetuses O30.82- ☑
      two or more monochorionic fetuses O30.81- ☑
      unable to determine number of placenta and number of amniotic sacs O30.89- ☑
      unspecified number of placenta and unspecified number of amniotic sacs O30.80- ☑
  mural O00.80
    with intrauterine pregnancy O00.81
  normal (supervision of) Z34.9- ☑
    first Z34.0- ☑
    high-risk — *see* Pregnancy, supervision of, high-risk
    specified Z34.8- ☑
  ovarian O00.20- ☑
    with intrauterine pregnancy O00.21- ☑
  postmature (40 to 42 weeks) O48.0
    more than 42 weeks gestation O48.1
  post-term (40 to 42 weeks) O48.0
  prenatal care only Z34.9- ☑
    first Z34.0- ☑
    high-risk — *see* Pregnancy, supervision of, high-risk
    specified Z34.8- ☑
  prolonged (more than 42 weeks gestation) O48.1
  quadruplet O30.20- ☑
    with
      two or more monoamniotic fetuses O30.22- ☑
      two or more monochorionic fetuses O30.21- ☑
    two or more monoamniotic fetuses O30.22- ☑
    two or more monochorionic fetuses O30.21- ☑
    unable to determine number of placenta and number of amniotic sacs O30.29- ☑
    unspecified number of placenta and unspecified number of amniotic sacs O30.20- ☑
  quintuplet — *see* Pregnancy, multiple (gestation), specified NEC
  sextuplet — *see* Pregnancy, multiple (gestation), specified NEC

Pregnancy — *continued*
  supervision of
    concealed pregnancy O09.3- ☑
    elderly mother
      multigravida O09.52- ☑
      primigravida O09.51- ☑
    hidden pregnancy O09.3- ☑
    high-risk O09.9- ☑
      due to (history of)
        ectopic pregnancy O09.1- ☑
        elderly — *see* Pregnancy, supervision, elderly mother
        grand multiparity O09.4 ☑
        in utero procedure during previous pregnancy O09.82- ☑
        in vitro fertilization O09.81- ☑
        infertility O09.0- ☑
        insufficient prenatal care O09.3- ☑
        molar pregnancy O09.A- ☑
        multiple previous pregnancies O09.4- ☑
        older mother — *see* Pregnancy, supervision of, elderly mother
        poor reproductive or obstetric history NEC O09.29- ☑
        pre-term labor O09.21- ☑
        previous
          neonatal death O09.29- ☑
        social problems O09.7- ☑
        specified NEC O09.89- ☑
        very young mother — *see* Pregnancy, supervision, young mother
      resulting from in vitro fertilization O09.81- ☑
    normal Z34.9- ☑
      first Z34.0- ☑
      specified NEC Z34.8- ☑
    young mother
      multigravida O09.62- ☑
      primigravida O09.61- ☑
  triplet O30.10- ☑
    with
      two or more monoamniotic fetuses O30.12- ☑
      two or more monochorionic fetuses O30.11- ☑
    two or more monoamniotic fetuses O30.12- ☑
    two or more monochorionic fetuses O30.11- ☑
    unable to determine number of placenta and number of amniotic sacs O30.19- ☑
    unspecified number of placenta and unspecified number of amniotic sacs O30.10- ☑
  tubal (with abortion) (with rupture) O00.10- ☑
    with intrauterine pregnancy O00.11- ☑
  twin O30.00- ☑
    conjoined O30.02- ☑
    dichorionic/diamniotic (two placenta, two amniotic sacs) O30.04- ☑
    monochorionic/diamniotic (one placenta, two amniotic sacs) O30.03- ☑
    monochorionic/monoamniotic (one placenta, one amniotic sac) O30.01- ☑
    unable to determine number of placenta and number of amniotic sacs O30.09- ☑
    unspecified number of placenta and unspecified number of amniotic sacs O30.00- ☑
  unwanted Z64.0
  weeks of gestation
    less than 8 weeks Z3A.01 (*following* Z36)
    8 weeks Z3A.08 (*following* Z36)
    9 weeks Z3A.09 (*following* Z36)
    10 weeks Z3A.10 (*following* Z36)
    11 weeks Z3A.11 (*following* Z36)
    12 weeks Z3A.12 (*following* Z36)
    13 weeks Z3A.13 (*following* Z36)
    14 weeks Z3A.14 (*following* Z36)
    15 weeks Z3A.15 (*following* Z36)
    16 weeks Z3A.16 (*following* Z36)
    17 weeks Z3A.17 (*following* Z36)
    18 weeks Z3A.18 (*following* Z36)
    19 weeks Z3A.19 (*following* Z36)
    20 weeks Z3A.20 (*following* Z36)
    21 weeks Z3A.21 (*following* Z36)
    22 weeks Z3A.22 (*following* Z36)
    23 weeks Z3A.23 (*following* Z36)
    24 weeks Z3A.24 (*following* Z36)
    25 weeks Z3A.25 (*following* Z36)
    26 weeks Z3A.26 (*following* Z36)
    27 weeks Z3A.27 (*following* Z36)
    28 weeks Z3A.28 (*following* Z36)
    29 weeks Z3A.29 (*following* Z36)

Pregnancy — *continued*
  weeks of gestation — *continued*
    30 weeks Z3A.30 (*following* Z36)
    31 weeks Z3A.31 (*following* Z36)
    32 weeks Z3A.32 (*following* Z36)
    33 weeks Z3A.33 (*following* Z36)
    34 weeks Z3A.34 (*following* Z36)
    35 weeks Z3A.35 (*following* Z36)
    36 weeks Z3A.36 (*following* Z36)
    37 weeks Z3A.37 (*following* Z36)
    38 weeks Z3A.38 (*following* Z36)
    39 weeks Z3A.39 (*following* Z36)
    40 weeks Z3A.40 (*following* Z36)
    41 weeks Z3A.41 (*following* Z36)
    42 weeks Z3A.42 (*following* Z36)
    greater than 42 weeks Z3A.49 (*following* Z36)
    not specified Z3A.00 (*following* Z36)
Preiser's disease — *see* Osteonecrosis, secondary, due to, trauma, metacarpus
Pre-kwashiorkor — *see* Malnutrition, severe
Preleukemia (syndrome) D46.9
Preluxation, hip, congenital Q65.6
Premature (*see also* condition)
  adrenarche E27.0
  aging E34.8
  beats I49.40
    atrial I49.1
    auricular I49.1
    supraventricular I49.1
  birth NEC — *see* Preterm, newborn
  closure, foramen ovale Q21.8
  contraction
    atrial I49.1
    atrioventricular I49.2
    auricular I49.1
    auriculoventricular I49.49
    heart (extrasystole) I49.49
    junctional I49.2
    ventricular I49.3
  delivery (*see also* Pregnancy, complicated by, preterm labor) O60.10 ☑
  ejaculation F52.4
  infant NEC — *see* Preterm, newborn
    light-for-dates — *see* Light for dates
  labor — *see* Pregnancy, complicated by, preterm labor
  lungs P28.0
  menopause E28.319
    asymptomatic E28.319
    symptomatic E28.310
  newborn
    less than 37 completed weeks — *see* Preterm, newborn
    extreme (less than 28 completed weeks) — *see* Immaturity, extreme
  puberty E30.1
  rupture membranes or amnion — *see* Pregnancy, complicated by, premature rupture of membranes
  senility E34.8
  thelarche E30.8
  ventricular systole I49.3
Prematurity NEC (less than 37 completed weeks) — *see* Preterm, newborn
  extreme (less than 28 completed weeks) — *see* Immaturity, extreme
Premenstrual
  dysphoric disorder (PMDD) F32.81
  tension (syndrome) N94.3
Premolarization, cuspids K00.2
Prenatal
  care, normal pregnancy — *see* Pregnancy, normal
  screening of mother (*see also* Encounter, antenatal screening) Z36.9
  teeth K00.6
Preparatory care for subsequent treatment NEC
  for dialysis Z49.01
    peritoneal Z49.02
Prepartum — *see* condition
Preponderance, left or right ventricular I51.7
Prepuce — *see* condition
PRES (posterior reversible encephalopathy syndrome) I67.83
Presbycardia R54
Presbycusis, presbyacusia H91.1- ☑
Presbyesophagus K22.8
Presbyophrenia F03 ☑
Presbyopia H52.4
Prescription of contraceptives (initial) Z30.019

262
☑ Additional Character Required — Refer to the Tabular List for Character Selection
▽ Subterms under main terms may continue to next column or page

Prescription of contraceptives — *continued*
- barrier Z30.018
- diaphragm Z30.018
- emergency (postcoital) Z30.012
- implantable subdermal Z30.017
- injectable Z30.013
- intrauterine contraceptive device Z30.014
- pills Z30.011
- postcoital (emergency) Z30.012
- repeat Z30.40
  - barrier Z30.49
  - diaphragm Z30.49
  - implantable subdermal Z30.46
  - injectable Z30.42
  - pills Z30.41
  - specified type NEC Z30.49
  - transdermal patch hormonal Z30.45
  - vaginal ring hormonal Z30.44
- specified type NEC Z30.018
  - transdermal patch hormonal Z30.016
  - vaginal ring hormonal Z30.015

Presence (of)
- ankle-joint implant (functional) (prosthesis) Z96.66- ☑
- aortocoronary (bypass) graft Z95.1
- arterial-venous shunt (dialysis) Z99.2
- artificial
  - eye (globe) Z97.0
  - heart (fully implantable) (mechanical) Z95.812
    - valve Z95.2
  - larynx Z96.3
  - lens (intraocular) Z96.1
  - limb (complete) (partial) Z97.1- ☑
    - arm Z97.1- ☑
      - bilateral Z97.15
    - leg Z97.1- ☑
      - bilateral Z97.16
- audiological implant (functional) Z96.29
- bladder implant (functional) Z96.0
- bone
  - conduction hearing device Z96.29
  - implant (functional) NEC Z96.7
  - joint (prosthesis) — *see* Presence, joint implant
- cardiac
  - defibrillator (functional) (with synchronous cardiac pacemaker) Z95.810
  - implant or graft Z95.9
    - specified type NEC Z95.818
  - pacemaker Z95.0
  - resynchronization therapy
    - defibrillator Z95.810
    - pacemaker Z95.0
- cardioverter-defibrillator (ICD) Z95.810
- cerebrospinal fluid drainage device Z98.2
- cochlear implant (functional) Z96.21
- contact lens (es) Z97.3
- coronary artery graft or prosthesis Z95.5
- CRT-D (cardiac resynchronization therapy defibrillator) Z95.810
- CRT-P (cardiac resynchronization therapy pacemaker) Z95.0
- CSF shunt Z98.2
- dental prosthesis device Z97.2
- dentures Z97.2
- device (external) NEC Z97.8
  - cardiac NEC Z95.818
    - heart assist Z95.811
    - implanted (functional) Z96.9
      - specified NEC Z96.89
    - prosthetic Z97.8
- ear implant Z96.20
  - cochlear implant Z96.21
  - myringotomy tube Z96.22
  - specified type NEC Z96.29
- elbow-joint implant (functional) (prosthesis) Z96.62- ☑
- endocrine implant (functional) NEC Z96.49
- eustachian tube stent or device (functional) Z96.29
- external hearing-aid or device Z97.4
- finger-joint implant (functional) (prosthetic) Z96.69- ☑
- functional implant Z96.9
  - specified NEC Z96.89
- graft
  - cardiac NEC Z95.818
  - vascular NEC Z95.828
- hearing-aid or device (external) Z97.4
  - implant (bone) (cochlear) (functional) Z96.21
- heart assist device Z95.811
- heart valve implant (functional) Z95.2

Presence — *continued*
- heart valve implant — *continued*
  - prosthetic Z95.2
  - specified type NEC Z95.4
  - xenogenic Z95.3
- hip-joint implant (functional) (prosthesis) Z96.64- ☑
- ICD (cardioverter-defibrillator) Z95.810
- implanted device (artificial) (functional) (prosthetic) Z96.9
  - automatic cardiac defibrillator (with synchronous cardiac pacemaker) Z95.810
  - cardiac pacemaker Z95.0
  - cochlear Z96.21
  - dental Z96.5
  - heart Z95.812
  - heart valve Z95.2
    - prosthetic Z95.2
    - specified NEC Z95.4
    - xenogenic Z95.3
  - insulin pump Z96.41
  - intraocular lens Z96.1
  - joint Z96.60
    - ankle Z96.66- ☑
    - elbow Z96.62- ☑
    - finger Z96.69- ☑
    - hip Z96.64- ☑
    - knee Z96.65- ☑
    - shoulder Z96.61- ☑
    - specified NEC Z96.698
    - wrist Z96.63- ☑
  - larynx Z96.3
  - myringotomy tube Z96.22
  - otological Z96.20
    - cochlear Z96.21
    - eustachian stent Z96.29
    - myringotomy Z96.22
    - specified NEC Z96.29
    - stapes Z96.29
  - skin Z96.81
  - skull plate Z96.7
  - specified NEC Z96.89
  - urogenital Z96.0
- insulin pump (functional) Z96.41
- intestinal bypass or anastomosis Z98.0
- intraocular lens (functional) Z96.1
- intrauterine contraceptive device (IUD) Z97.5
- intravascular implant (functional) (prosthetic) NEC Z95.9
  - coronary artery Z95.5
  - defibrillator (with synchronous cardiac pacemaker) Z95.810
  - peripheral vessel (with angioplasty) Z95.820
- joint implant (prosthetic) (any) Z96.6
  - ankle — *see* Presence, ankle joint implant
  - elbow — *see* Presence, elbow joint implant
  - finger — *see* Presence, finger joint implant
  - hip — *see* Presence, hip joint implant
  - knee — *see* Presence, knee joint implant
  - shoulder — *see* Presence, shoulder joint implant
  - specified joint NEC Z96.698
  - wrist — *see* Presence, wrist joint implant
- knee-joint implant (functional) (prosthesis) Z96.65- ☑
- laryngeal implant (functional) Z96.3
- mandibular implant (dental) Z96.5
- myringotomy tube(s) Z96.22
- orthopedic-joint implant (prosthetic) (any) — *see* Presence, joint implant
- otological implant (functional) Z96.29
- shoulder-joint implant (functional) (prosthesis) Z96.61- ☑
- skull-plate implant Z96.7
- spectacles Z97.3
- stapes implant (functional) Z96.29
- systemic lupus erythematosus [SLE] inhibitor D68.62
- tendon implant (functional) (graft) Z96.7
- tooth root(s) implant Z96.5
- ureteral stent Z96.0
- urethral stent Z96.0
- urogenital implant (functional) Z96.0
- vascular implant or device Z95.9
  - access port device Z95.828
  - specified type NEC Z95.828
- wrist-joint implant (functional) (prosthesis) Z96.63- ☑

Presenile (*see also* condition)
- dementia F03 ☑
- premature aging E34.8

Presentation, fetal — *see* Delivery, complicated by, malposition

Prespondylolisthesis (congenital) Q76.2
Pressure
- area, skin — *see* Ulcer, pressure, by site
- brachial plexus G54.0
- brain G93.5
  - injury at birth NEC P11.1
- cerebral — *see* Pressure, brain
- chest R07.89
- cone, tentorial G93.5
- hyposystolic (*see also* Hypotension)
  - incidental reading, without diagnosis of hypotension R03.1
- increased
  - intracranial (benign) G93.2
    - injury at birth P11.0
  - intraocular H40.05- ☑
- lumbosacral plexus G54.1
- mediastinum J98.59
- necrosis (chronic) — *see* Ulcer, pressure, by site
- parental, inappropriate (excessive) Z62.6
- sore (chronic) — *see* Ulcer, pressure, by site
- spinal cord G95.20
- ulcer (chronic) — *see* Ulcer, pressure, by site
- venous, increased I87.8

Pre-syncope R55
Preterm
- delivery (*see also* Pregnancy, complicated by, preterm labor) O60.10 ☑
- labor — *see* Pregnancy, complicated by, preterm labor
- newborn (infant) P07.30
  - gestational age
    - 28 completed weeks (28 weeks, 0 days through 28 weeks, 6 days) P07.31
    - 29 completed weeks (29 weeks, 0 days through 29 weeks, 6 days) P07.32
    - 30 completed weeks (30 weeks, 0 days through 30 weeks, 6 days) P07.33
    - 31 completed weeks (31 weeks, 0 days through 31 weeks, 6 days) P07.34
    - 32 completed weeks (32 weeks, 0 days through 32 weeks, 6 days) P07.35
    - 33 completed weeks (33 weeks, 0 days through 33 weeks, 6 days) P07.36
    - 34 completed weeks (34 weeks, 0 days through 34 weeks, 6 days) P07.37
    - 35 completed weeks (35 weeks, 0 days through 35 weeks, 6 days) P07.38
    - 36 completed weeks (36 weeks, 0 days through 36 weeks, 6 days) P07.39

Previa
- placenta (total) (without hemorrhage) O44.0- ☑
  - with hemorrhage O44.1- ☑
  - complete O44.0- ☑
    - with hemorrhage O44.1- ☑
  - low (*see also* Delivery, complicated, by, placenta, low) O44.4- ☑
    - with hemorrhage O44.5- ☑
  - marginal O44.2- ☑
    - with hemorrhage O44.3- ☑
  - partial O44.2- ☑
    - with hemorrhage O44.3- ☑
- vasa O69.4 ☑

Priapism N48.30
- due to
  - disease classified elsewhere N48.32
  - drug N48.33
  - specified cause NEC N48.39
  - trauma N48.31

Prickling sensation (skin) R20.2
Prickly heat L74.0
Primary — *see* condition
Primigravida
- elderly, affecting management of pregnancy, labor and delivery (supervision only) — *see* Pregnancy, complicated by, elderly, primigravida
- older, affecting management of pregnancy, labor and delivery (supervision only) — *see* Pregnancy, complicated by, elderly, primigravida
- very young, affecting management of pregnancy, labor and delivery (supervision only) — *see* Pregnancy, complicated by, young mother, primigravida

Primipara
- elderly, affecting management of pregnancy, labor and delivery (supervision only) — *see* Pregnancy, complicated by, elderly, primigravida

Primipara — *continued*
older, affecting management of pregnancy, labor and delivery (supervision only) — *see* Pregnancy, complicated by, elderly, primigravida
very young, affecting management of pregnancy, labor and delivery (supervision only) — *see* Pregnancy, complicated by, young mother, primigravida
Primus varus (bilateral) Q66.2 ☑
PRIND (Prolonged reversible ischemic neurologic deficit) I63.9
Pringle's disease (tuberous sclerosis) Q85.1
Prinzmetal angina I20.1
Prizefighter ear — *see* Cauliflower ear
Problem (with) (related to)
academic Z55.8
acculturation Z60.3
adjustment (to)
change of job Z56.1
life-cycle transition Z60.0
pension Z60.0
retirement Z60.0
adopted child Z62.821
alcoholism in family Z63.72
atypical parenting situation Z62.9
bankruptcy Z59.8
behavioral (adult) F69
drug seeking Z76.5
birth of sibling affecting child Z62.898
care (of)
provider dependency Z74.9
specified NEC Z74.8
sick or handicapped person in family or household Z63.6
child
abuse (affecting the child) — *see* Maltreatment, child
custody or support proceedings Z65.3
in care of non-parental family member Z62.21
in foster care Z62.21
in welfare custody Z62.21
living in orphanage or group home Z62.22
child-rearing Z62.9
specified NEC Z62.898
communication (developmental) F80.9
conflict or discord (with)
boss Z56.4
classmates Z55.4
counselor Z64.4
employer Z56.4
family Z63.9
specified NEC Z63.8
probation officer Z64.4
social worker Z64.4
teachers Z55.4
workmates Z56.4
conviction in legal proceedings Z65.0
with imprisonment Z65.1
counselor Z64.4
creditors Z59.8
digestive K92.9
drug addict in family Z63.72
ear — *see* Disorder, ear
economic Z59.9
affecting care Z59.9
specified NEC Z59.8
education Z55.9
specified NEC Z55.8
employment Z56.9
change of job Z56.1
discord Z56.4
environment Z56.5
sexual harassment Z56.81
specified NEC Z56.89
stressful schedule Z56.3
stress NEC Z56.6
threat of job loss Z56.2
unemployment Z56.0
enuresis, child F98.0
eye H57.9
failed examinations (school) Z55.2
falling Z91.81
family (*see also* Disruption, family) Z63.9
specified NEC Z63.8
feeding (elderly) (infant) R63.3
newborn P92.9
breast P92.5
overfeeding P92.4
slow P92.2

Problem — *continued*
feeding — *continued*
newborn — *continued*
specified NEC P92.8
underfeeding P92.3
nonorganic F50.89
finance Z59.9
specified NEC Z59.8
foreclosure on loan Z59.8
foster child Z62.822
frightening experience(s) in childhood Z62.898
genital NEC
female N94.9
male N50.9
health care Z75.9
specified NEC Z75.8
hearing — *see* Deafness
homelessness Z59.0
housing Z59.9
inadequate Z59.1
isolated Z59.8
specified NEC Z59.8
identity (of childhood) F93.8
illegitimate pregnancy (unwanted) Z64.0
illiteracy Z55.0
impaired mobility Z74.09
imprisonment or incarceration Z65.1
inadequate teaching affecting education Z55.8
inappropriate (excessive) parental pressure Z62.6
influencing health status NEC Z78.9
in-law Z63.1
institutionalization, affecting child Z62.22
intrafamilial communication Z63.8
jealousy, child F93.8
landlord Z59.2
language (developmental) F80.9
learning (developmental) F81.9
legal Z65.3
conviction without imprisonment Z65.0
imprisonment Z65.1
release from prison Z65.2
life-management Z73.9
specified NEC Z73.89
life-style Z72.9
gambling Z72.6
high-risk sexual behavior (heterosexual) Z72.51
bisexual Z72.53
homosexual Z72.52
inappropriate eating habits Z72.4
self-damaging behavior NEC Z72.89
specified NEC Z72.89
tobacco use Z72.0
literacy Z55.9
low level Z55.0
specified NEC Z55.8
living alone Z60.2
lodgers Z59.2
loss of love relationship in childhood Z62.898
marital Z63.0
involving
divorce Z63.5
estrangement Z63.5
gender identity F66
mastication K08.89
medical
care, within family Z63.6
facilities Z75.9
specified NEC Z75.8
mental F48.9
multiparity Z64.1
negative life events in childhood Z62.9
altered pattern of family relationships Z62.898
frightening experience Z62.898
loss of
love relationship Z62.898
self-esteem Z62.898
physical abuse (alleged) — *see* Maltreatment, child
removal from home Z62.29
specified event NEC Z62.898
neighbor Z59.2
neurological NEC R29.818
new step-parent affecting child Z62.898
none (feared complaint unfounded) Z71.1
occupational NEC Z56.89
parent-child — *see* Conflict, parent-child
personal hygiene Z91.89
personality F69
phase-of-life transition, adjustment Z60.0

Problem — *continued*
presence of sick or disabled person in family or household Z63.79
needing care Z63.6
primary support group (family) Z63.9
specified NEC Z63.8
probation officer Z64.4
psychiatric F99
psychosexual (development) F66
psychosocial Z65.9
religious or spiritual Z65.8
specified NEC Z65.8
relationship Z63.9
childhood F93.8
release from prison Z65.2
religious or spiritual Z65.8
removal from home affecting child Z62.29
seeking and accepting known hazardous and harmful
behavioral or psychological interventions Z65.8
chemical, nutritional or physical interventions Z65.8
sexual function (nonorganic) F52.9
sight H54.7
sleep disorder, child F51.9
smell — *see* Disturbance, sensation, smell
social
environment Z60.9
specified NEC Z60.8
exclusion and rejection Z60.4
worker Z64.4
speech R47.9
developmental F80.9
specified NEC R47.89
swallowing — *see* Dysphagia
taste — *see* Disturbance, sensation, taste
tic, child F95.0
underachievement in school Z55.3
unemployment Z56.0
threatened Z56.2
unwanted pregnancy Z64.0
upbringing Z62.9
specified NEC Z62.898
urinary N39.9
voice production R47.89
work schedule (stressful) Z56.3
Procedure (surgical)
converted
arthroscopic to open Z53.33
laparoscopic to open Z53.31
specified procedure NEC to open Z53.39
thoracoscopic to open Z53.32
for purpose other than remedying health state Z41.9
specified NEC Z41.8
not done Z53.9
because of
administrative reasons Z53.8
contraindication Z53.09
smoking Z53.01
patient's decision Z53.20
for reasons of belief or group pressure Z53.1
left against medical advice (AMA) Z53.21
specified reason NEC Z53.29
specified reason NEC Z53.8
Procidentia (uteri) N81.3
Proctalgia K62.89
fugax K59.4
spasmodic K59.4
Proctitis K62.89
amebic (acute) A06.0
chlamydial A56.3
gonococcal A54.6
granulomatous — *see* Enteritis, regional, large intestine
herpetic A60.1
radiation K62.7
tuberculous A18.32
ulcerative (chronic) K51.20
with
complication K51.219
abscess K51.214
fistula K51.213
obstruction K51.212
rectal bleeding K51.211
specified NEC K51.218
Proctocele
female (without uterine prolapse) N81.6
with uterine prolapse N81.2
complete N81.3
male K62.3

☑ **Additional Character Required** — Refer to the Tabular List for Character Selection   ▽ **Subterms under main terms may continue to next column or page**

Proctocolitis
  food protein-induced K52.82
  food-induced eosinophilic K52.82
  milk protein-induced K52.82
  mucosal — *see* Rectosigmoiditis, ulcerative
Proctoptosis K62.3
Proctorrhagia K62.5
Proctosigmoiditis K63.89
  ulcerative (chronic) — *see* Rectosigmoiditis, ulcerative
Proctospasm K59.4
  psychogenic F45.8
Profichet's disease — *see* Disorder, soft tissue, specified
    type NEC
Progeria E34.8
Prognathism (mandibular) (maxillary) M26.19
Progonoma (melanotic) — *see* Neoplasm, benign, by
  site
Progressive — *see* condition
Prolactinoma
  specified site — *see* Neoplasm, benign, by site
  unspecified site D35.2
Prolapse, prolapsed
  anus, anal (canal) (sphincter) K62.2
  arm or hand O32.2 ☑
    causing obstructed labor O64.4 ☑
  bladder (mucosa) (sphincter) (acquired)
    congenital Q79.4
    female — *see* Cystocele
    male N32.89
  breast implant (prosthetic) T85.49 ☑
  cecostomy K94.09
  cecum K63.4
  cervix, cervical (hypertrophied) N81.2
    anterior lip, obstructing labor O65.5
    congenital Q51.828
    postpartal, old N81.2
    stump N81.85
  ciliary body (traumatic) — *see* Laceration, eye(ball),
    with prolapse or loss of interocular tissue
  colon (pedunculated) K63.4
  colostomy K94.09
  disc (intervertebral) — *see* Displacement, interverte-
    bral disc
  eye implant (orbital) T85.398 ☑
    lens (ocular) — *see* Complications, intraocular lens
  fallopian tube N83.4-
  gastric (mucosa) K31.89
  genital, female N81.9
    specified NEC N81.89
  globe, nontraumatic — *see* Luxation, globe
  ileostomy bud K94.19
  intervertebral disc — *see* Displacement, intervertebral
    disc
  intestine (small) K63.4
  iris (traumatic) — *see* Laceration, eye(ball), with pro-
    lapse or loss of interocular tissue
    nontraumatic H21.89
  kidney N28.83
    congenital Q63.2
  laryngeal muscles or ventricle J38.7
  liver K76.89
  meatus urinarius N36.8
  mitral (valve) I34.1
  ocular lens implant — *see* Complications, intraocular
    lens
  organ or site, congenital NEC — *see* Malposition,
    congenital
  ovary N83.4- ☑
  pelvic floor, female N81.89
  perineum, female N81.89
  rectum (mucosa) (sphincter) K62.3
    due to trichuris trichuria B79
  spleen D73.89
  stomach K31.89
  umbilical cord
    complicating delivery O69.0 ☑
  urachus, congenital Q64.4
  ureter N28.89
    with obstruction N13.5
      with infection N13.6
  ureterovesical orifice N28.89
  urethra (acquired) (infected) (mucosa) N36.8
    congenital Q64.71
  urinary meatus N36.8
    congenital Q64.72
  uterovaginal N81.4
    complete N81.3
    incomplete N81.2

Prolapse, prolapsed — *continued*
  uterus (with prolapse of vagina) N81.4
    complete N81.3
    congenital Q51.818
    first degree N81.2
    in pregnancy or childbirth — *see* Pregnancy,
      complicated by, abnormal, uterus
    incomplete N81.2
    postpartal (old) N81.4
    second degree N81.2
    third degree N81.3
  uveal (traumatic) — *see* Laceration, eye(ball), with
    prolapse or loss of interocular tissue
  vagina (anterior) (wall) — *see* Cystocele
    with prolapse of uterus N81.4
      complete N81.3
      incomplete N81.2
    posterior wall N81.6
    posthysterectomy N99.3
  vitreous (humor) H43.0- ☑
    in wound — *see* Laceration, eye(ball), with pro-
      lapse or loss of interocular tissue
  womb — *see* Prolapse, uterus
Prolapsus, female N81.9
  specified NEC N81.89
Proliferation(s)
  primary cutaneous CD30-positive large T-cell C86.6
  prostate, atypical small acinar N42.32
Proliferative — *see* condition
Prolonged, prolongation (of)
  bleeding (time) (idiopathic) R79.1
  coagulation (time) R79.1
  gestation (over 42 completed weeks)
    mother O48.1
    newborn P08.22
  interval I44.0
  labor O63.9
    first stage O63.0
    second stage O63.1
  partial thromboplastin time (PTT) R79.1
  pregnancy (more than 42 weeks gestation) O48.1
  prothrombin time R79.1
  QT interval I45.81
  uterine contractions in labor O62.4
Prominence, prominent
  auricle (congenital) (ear) Q17.5
  ischial spine or sacral promontory
    with disproportion (fetopelvic) O33.0
      causing obstructed labor O65.0
  nose (congenital) acquired M95.0
Promiscuity — *see* High, risk, sexual behavior
Pronation
  ankle — *see* Deformity, limb, foot, specified NEC
  foot (*see also* Deformity, limb, foot, specified NEC)
    congenital Q74.2
Prophylactic
  administration of
    antibiotics, long-term Z79.2
      short-term use — *omit code*
    drug (*see also* Long-term (current) drug therapy
      (use of)) Z79.899
  medication Z79.899
  organ removal (for neoplasia management) Z40.00
    breast Z40.01
    fallopian tube(s) Z40.03
      with ovary(s) Z40.02
    ovary(s) Z40.02
    specified site NEC Z40.09
  surgery Z40.9
    for risk factors related to malignant neoplasm —
      see Prophylactic, organ removal
    specified NEC Z40.8
  vaccination Z23
Propionic acidemia E71.121
Proptosis (ocular) (*see also* Exophthalmos)
  thyroid — *see* Hyperthyroidism, with goiter
Prosecution, anxiety concerning Z65.3
Prosopagnosia R48.3
Prostadynia N42.81
Prostate, prostatic — *see* condition
Prostatism — *see* Hyperplasia, prostate
Prostatitis (congestive) (suppurative) (with cystitis) N41.9
  acute N41.0
  cavitary N41.8
  chronic N41.1
  diverticular N41.8
  due to Trichomonas (vaginalis) A59.02
  fibrous N41.1

Prostatitis — *continued*
  gonococcal (acute) (chronic) A54.22
  granulomatous N41.4
  hypertrophic N41.1
  subacute N41.1
  trichomonal A59.02
  tuberculous A18.14
Prostatocystitis N41.3
Prostatorrhea N42.89
Prostatosis N42.82
Prostration R53.83
  heat (*see also* Heat, exhaustion)
    anhydrotic T67.3 ☑
    due to
      salt (and water) depletion T67.4 ☑
      water depletion T67.3 ☑
  nervous F48.8
  senile R54
Protanomaly (anomalous trichromat) H53.54
Protanopia (complete) (incomplete) H53.54
Protection (against) (from) — *see* Prophylactic
Protein
  deficiency NEC — *see* Malnutrition
  malnutrition — *see* Malnutrition
  sickness (*see also* Reaction, serum) T80.69 ☑
Proteinemia R77.9
Proteinosis
  alveolar (pulmonary) J84.01
  lipid or lipoid (of Urbach) E78.89
Proteinuria R80.9
  Bence Jones R80.3
  complicating pregnancy — *see* Proteinuria, gestational
  gestational
    complicating
      childbirth O12.14
      pregnancy O12.1- ☑
        with edema O12.2- ☑
      puerperium O12.15
  idiopathic R80.0
  isolated R80.0
    with glomerular lesion N06.9
      dense deposit disease N06.6
      diffuse
        crescentic glomerulonephritis N06.7
        endocapillary proliferative glomerulonephri-
          tis N06.4
        mesangiocapillary glomerulonephritis N06.5
      focal and segmental hyalinosis or sclerosis
        N06.1
      membranous (diffuse) N06.2
      mesangial proliferative (diffuse) N06.3
      minimal change N06.0
      specified pathology NEC N06.8
  orthostatic R80.2
    with glomerular lesion — *see* Proteinuria, isolated,
      with glomerular lesion
  persistent R80.1
    with glomerular lesion — *see* Proteinuria, isolated,
      with glomerular lesion
  postural R80.2
    with glomerular lesion — *see* Proteinuria, isolated,
      with glomerular lesion
  pre-eclamptic — *see* Pre-eclampsia
  puerperal O12.15
  specified type NEC R80.8
Proteolysis, pathologic D65
Proteus (mirabilis) (morganii), **as cause of disease**
  classified elsewhere B96.4
Prothrombin gene mutation D68.52
Protoporphyria, erythropoietic E80.0
Protozoal (*see also* condition)
  disease B64
    specified NEC B60.8
Protrusion, protrusio
  acetabuli M24.7
  acetabulum (into pelvis) M24.7
  device, implant or graft (*see also* Complications, by
    site and type, mechanical) T85.698 ☑
    arterial graft NEC — *see* Complication, cardiovas-
      cular device, mechanical, vascular
    breast (implant) T85.49 ☑
    catheter NEC T85.698 ☑
      cystostomy T83.090 ☑
      dialysis (renal) T82.49 ☑
        intraperitoneal T85.691 ☑
      infusion NEC T82.594 ☑
        spinal (epidural) (subdural) T85.690 ☑

Protrusion, protrusio — continued
  device, implant or graft (see also Complications, by site and type, mechanical) — continued
    catheter — continued
      urinary (see also Complications, catheter, urinary) T83.098 ☑
      electronic (electrode) (pulse generator) (stimulator)
        bone T84.390 ☑
        nervous system — see Complication, prosthetic device, mechanical, electronic nervous system stimulator
    fixation, internal (orthopedic) NEC — see Complication, fixation device, mechanical
    gastrointestinal — see Complications, prosthetic device, mechanical, gastrointestinal device
    genital NEC T83.498 ☑
      intrauterine contraceptive device T83.39 ☑
      penile prosthesis (cylinder) (implanted) (pump) (resevoir) T83.490 ☑
      testicular prosthesis T83.491 ☑
    heart NEC — see Complication, cardiovascular device, mechanical
    joint prosthesis — see Complications, joint prosthesis, mechanical, specified NEC, by site
    ocular NEC — see Complication, prosthetic device, mechanical, ocular device
    orthopedic NEC — see Complication, orthopedic, device, mechanical
    specified NEC T85.628 ☑
    urinary NEC (see also Complication, genitourinary, device, urinary, mechanical)
      graft T83.29 ☑
    vascular NEC — see Complication, cardiovascular device, mechanical
    ventricular intracranial shunt T85.09 ☑
  intervertebral disc — see Displacement, intervertebral disc
  joint prosthesis — see Complications, joint prosthesis, mechanical, specified NEC, by site
  nucleus pulposus — see Displacement, intervertebral disc
Prune belly (syndrome) Q79.4
Prurigo (ferox) (gravis) (Hebrae) (Hebra's) (mitis) (simplex) L28.2
  Besnier's L20.0
  estivalis L56.4
  nodularis L28.1
  psychogenic F45.8
Pruritus, pruritic (essential) L29.9
  ani, anus L29.0
    psychogenic F45.8
  anogenital L29.3
    psychogenic F45.8
  due to onchocerca volvulus B73.1
  gravidarum — see Pregnancy, complicated by, specified pregnancy-related condition NEC
  hiemalis L29.8
  neurogenic (any site) F45.8
  perianal L29.0
  psychogenic (any site) F45.8
  scroti, scrotum L29.1
    psychogenic F45.8
  senile, senilis L29.8
  specified NEC L29.8
    psychogenic F45.8
  Trichomonas A59.9
  vulva, vulvae L29.2
    psychogenic F45.8
Pseudarthrosis, pseudoarthrosis (bone) — see Nonunion, fracture
  clavicle, congenital Q74.0
  joint, following fusion or arthrodesis M96.0
Pseudoaneurysm — see Aneurysm
Pseudoangina (pectoris) — see Angina
Pseudoangioma I81
Pseudoarteriosus Q28.8
Pseudoarthrosis — see Pseudarthrosis
Pseudobulbar affect (PBA) F48.2
Pseudochromhidrosis L67.8
Pseudocirrhosis, liver, pericardial I31.1
Pseudocowpox B08.03
Pseudocoxalgia M91.3- ☑
Pseudocroup J38.5
Pseudo-Cushing's syndrome, alcohol-induced E24.4
Pseudocyesis F45.8
Pseudocyst
  lung J98.4

Pseudocyst — continued
  pancreas K86.3
  retina — see Cyst, retina
Pseudoelephantiasis neuroarthritica Q82.0
Pseudoexfoliation, capsule (lens) — see Cataract, specified NEC
Pseudofolliculitis barbae L73.1
Pseudoglioma H44.89
Pseudohemophilia (Bernuth's) (hereditary) (type B) D68.0
  Type A D69.8
  vascular D69.8
Pseudohermaphroditism Q56.3
  adrenal E25.8
  female Q56.2
    with adrenocortical disorder E25.8
    without adrenocortical disorder Q56.2
    adrenal (congenital) E25.0
    unspecified E25.9
  male Q56.1
    with
      5-alpha-reductase deficiency E29.1
      adrenocortical disorder E25.8
      androgen resistance E34.51
      cleft scrotum Q56.1
      feminizing testis E34.51
    without gonadal disorder Q56.1
    adrenal E25.8
    unspecified E25.9
Pseudo-Hurler's polydystrophy E77.0
Pseudohydrocephalus G93.2
Pseudohypertrophic muscular dystrophy (Erb's) G71.0
Pseudohypertrophy, muscle G71.0
Pseudohypoparathyroidism E20.1
Pseudoinsomnia F51.03
Pseudoleukemia, infantile D64.89
Pseudomembranous — see condition
Pseudomeningocele (cerebral) (infective) (post-traumatic) G96.19
  postprocedural (spinal) G97.82
Pseudomenses (newborn) P54.6
Pseudomenstruation (newborn) P54.6
Pseudomonas
  aeruginosa, as cause of disease classified elsewhere B96.5
  mallei infection A24.0
    as cause of disease classified elsewhere B96.5
  pseudomallei, as cause of disease classified elsewhere B96.5
Pseudomyotonia G71.19
Pseudomyxoma peritonei C78.6
Pseudoneuritis, optic (nerve) (disc) (papilla), **congenital** Q14.2
Pseudo-obstruction intestine (acute) (chronic) (idiopathic) (intermittent secondary) (primary) K59.8
Pseudopapilledema H47.33- ☑
  congenital Q14.2
Pseudoparalysis
  arm or leg R29.818
  atonic, congenital P94.2
Pseudopelade L66.0
Pseudophakia Z96.1
Pseudopolyarthritis, rhizomelic M35.3
Pseudopolycythemia D75.1
Pseudopseudohypoparathyroidism E20.1
Pseudopterygium H11.81- ☑
Pseudoptosis (eyelid) — see Blepharochalasis
Pseudopuberty, precocious
  female heterosexual E25.8
  male isosexual E25.8
Pseudorickets (renal) N25.0
Pseudorubella B08.20
Pseudosclerema, newborn P83.88
Pseudosclerosis (brain)
  Jakob's — see Creutzfeldt-Jakob disease or syndrome
  of Westphal (Strümpell) E83.01
  spastic — see Creutzfeldt-Jakob disease or syndrome
Pseudotetanus — see Convulsions
Pseudotetany R29.0
  hysterical F44.5
Pseudotruncus arteriosus Q25.49
Pseudotuberculosis A28.2
  enterocolitis A04.8
  pasteurella (infection) A28.0
Pseudotumor
  cerebri G93.2
  orbital H05.11 ☑

Pseudoxanthoma elasticum Q82.8
Psilosis (sprue) (tropical) K90.1
  nontropical K90.0
Psittacosis A70
Psoitis M60.88
Psoriasis L40.9
  arthropathic L40.50
    arthritis mutilans L40.52
    distal interphalangeal L40.51
    juvenile L40.54
    other specified L40.59
    spondylitis L40.53
  buccal K13.29
  flexural L40.8 ✍
  guttate L40.4
  mouth K13.29
  nummular L40.0
  plaque L40.0
  psychogenic F54
  pustular (generalized) L40.1
    palmaris et plantaris L40.3
  specified NEC L40.8
  vulgaris L40.0
Psychasthenia F48.8
Psychiatric disorder or problem F99
Psychogenic (see also condition)
  factors associated with physical conditions F54
Psychological and behavioral factors affecting medical condition F59
Psychoneurosis, psychoneurotic (see also Neurosis)
  anxiety (state) F41.1
  depersonalization F48.1
  hypochondriacal F45.21
  hysteria F44.9
  neurasthenic F48.8
  personality NEC F60.89
Psychopathy, psychopathic
  affectionless F94.2
  autistic F84.5
  constitution, post-traumatic F07.81
  personality — see Disorder, personality
  sexual — see Deviation, sexual
  state F60.2
Psychosexual identity disorder of childhood F64.2
Psychosis, psychotic F29
  acute (transient) F23
    hysterical F44.9
  affective — see Disorder, mood
  alcoholic F10.959
    with
      abuse F10.159
      anxiety disorder F10.980
        with
          abuse F10.180
          dependence F10.280
      delirium tremens F10.231
      delusions F10.950
        with
          abuse F10.150
          dependence F10.250
      dementia F10.97
        with dependence F10.27
      dependence F10.259
      hallucinosis F10.951
        with
          abuse F10.151
          dependence F10.251
      mood disorder F10.94
        with
          abuse F10.14
          dependence F10.24
      paranoia F10.950
        with
          abuse F10.150
          dependence F10.250
      persisting amnesia F10.96
        with dependence F10.26
    amnestic confabulatory F10.96
      with dependence F10.26
    delirium tremens F10.231
    Korsakoff's, Korsakov's, Korsakow's F10.26
    paranoid type F10.950
      with
        abuse F10.150
        dependence F10.250
  anergastic — see Psychosis, organic
  arteriosclerotic (simple type) (uncomplicated) F01.50
    with behavioral disturbance F01.51

Psychosis, psychotic — *continued*
- childhood F84.0
  - atypical F84.8
- climacteric — *see* Psychosis, involutional
- confusional F29
  - acute or subacute F05
  - reactive F23
- cycloid F23
- depressive — *see* Disorder, depressive
- disintegrative (childhood) F84.3
- drug-induced — *see* F11-F19 with .X59
  - paranoid and hallucinatory states — *see* F11-F19 with .X50 or .X51
- due to or associated with
  - addiction, drug — *see* F11-F19 with .X59
  - dependence
    - alcohol F10.259
    - drug — *see* F11-F19 with .X59
  - epilepsy F06.8
  - Huntington's chorea F06.8
  - ischemia, cerebrovascular (generalized) F06.8
  - multiple sclerosis F06.8
  - physical disease F06.8
  - presenile dementia F03 ☑
  - senile dementia F03 ☑
  - vascular disease (arteriosclerotic) (cerebral) F01.50
    - with behavioral disturbance F01.51
- epileptic F06.8
- episode F23
  - due to or associated with physical condition F06.8
- exhaustive F43.0
- hallucinatory, chronic F28
- hypomanic F30.8
- hysterical (acute) F44.9
- induced F24
- infantile F84.0
  - atypical F84.8
- infective (acute) (subacute) F05
- involutional F28
  - depressive — *see* Disorder, depressive
  - melancholic — *see* Disorder, depressive
  - paranoid (state) F22
- Korsakoff's, Korsakov's, Korsakow's (nonalcoholic) F04
  - alcoholic F10.96
    - in dependence F10.26
  - induced by other psychoactive substance — *see* categories F11-F19 with .X5X
- mania, manic (single episode) F30.2
  - recurrent type F31.89
- manic-depressive — *see* Disorder, bipolar
- menopausal — *see* Psychosis, involutional
- mixed schizophrenic and affective F25.8
- multi-infarct (cerebrovascular) F01.50
  - with behavioral disturbance F01.51
- nonorganic F29
  - specified NEC F28
- organic F09
  - due to or associated with
    - arteriosclerosis (cerebral) — *see* Psychosis, arteriosclerotic
    - cerebrovascular disease, arteriosclerotic — *see* Psychosis, arteriosclerotic
    - childbirth — *see* Psychosis, puerperal
    - Creutzfeldt-Jakob disease or syndrome — *see* Creutzfeldt-Jakob disease or syndrome
    - dependence, alcohol F10.259
    - disease
      - alcoholic liver F10.259
      - brain, arteriosclerotic — *see* Psychosis, arteriosclerotic
      - cerebrovascular F01.50
        - with behavioral disturbance F01.51
      - Creutzfeldt-Jakob — *see* Creutzfeldt-Jakob disease or syndrome
      - endocrine or metabolic F06.8
        - acute or subacute F05
      - liver, alcoholic F10.259
    - epilepsy transient (acute) F05
    - infection
      - brain (intracranial) F06.8
        - acute or subacute F05
    - intoxication
      - alcoholic (acute) F10.259
      - drug F11-F19 with .X59
    - ischemia, cerebrovascular (generalized) — *see* Psychosis, arteriosclerotic
    - puerperium — *see* Psychosis, puerperal

Psychosis, psychotic — *continued*
- organic — *continued*
  - due to or associated with — *continued*
    - trauma, brain (birth) (from electric current) (surgical) F06.8
      - acute or subacute F05
  - infective F06.8
    - acute or subacute F05
  - post-traumatic F06.8
    - acute or subacute F05
- paranoiac F22
- paranoid (climacteric) (involutional) (menopausal) F22
  - psychogenic (acute) F23
  - schizophrenic F20.0
  - senile F03 ☑
- postpartum F53
- presbyophrenic (type) F03 ☑
- presenile F03 ☑
- psychogenic (paranoid) F23
  - depressive F32.3
- puerperal F53
  - specified type — *see* Psychosis, by type
- reactive (brief) (transient) (emotional stress) (psychological trauma) F23
  - depressive F32.3
    - recurrent F33.3
  - excitative type F30.8
- schizoaffective F25.9
  - depressive type F25.1
  - manic type F25.0
- schizophrenia, schizophrenic — *see* Schizophrenia
- schizophrenia-like, in epilepsy F06.2
- schizophreniform F20.81
  - affective type F25.9
  - brief F23
  - confusional type F23
  - mixed type F25.0
- senile NEC F03 ☑
  - depressed or paranoid type F03 ☑
  - simple deterioration F03 ☑
  - specified type — *code to* condition
- shared F24
- situational (reactive) F23
- symbiotic (childhood) F84.3
- symptomatic F09

Psychosomatic — *see* Disorder, psychosomatic
Psychosyndrome, organic F07.9
Psychotic episode due to or associated with physical condition F06.8
Pterygium (eye) H11.00- ☑
- amyloid H11.01- ☑
- central H11.02- ☑
- colli Q18.3
- double H11.03- ☑
- peripheral
  - progressive H11.05- ☑
  - stationary H11.04- ☑
- recurrent H11.06- ☑
Ptilosis (eyelid) — *see* Madarosis
Ptomaine (poisoning) — *see* Poisoning, food
Ptosis (*see also* Blepharoptosis)
- adiposa (false) — *see* Blepharoptosis
- breast N64.81
- cecum K63.4
- colon K63.4
- congenital (eyelid) Q10.0
  - specified site NEC — *see* Anomaly, by site
- eyelid — *see* Blepharoptosis
  - congenital Q10.0
- gastric K31.89
- intestine K63.4
- kidney N28.83
- liver K76.89
- renal N28.83
- splanchnic K63.4
- spleen D73.89
- stomach K31.89
- viscera K63.4
PTP D69.51
Ptyalism (periodic) K11.7
- hysterical F45.8
- pregnancy — *see* Pregnancy, complicated by, specified pregnancy-related condition NEC
- psychogenic F45.8
Ptyalolithiasis K11.5
Pubarche, precocious E30.1
Pubertas praecox E30.1
Puberty (development state) Z00.3

Puberty — *continued*
- bleeding (excessive) N92.2
- delayed E30.0
- precocious (constitutional) (cryptogenic) (idiopathic) E30.1
  - central E22.8
  - due to
    - ovarian hyperfunction E28.1
      - estrogen E28.0
    - testicular hyperfunction E29.0
- premature E30.1
  - due to
    - adrenal cortical hyperfunction E25.8
    - pineal tumor E34.8
    - pituitary (anterior) hyperfunction E22.8
Puckering, macula — *see* Degeneration, macula, puckering
Pudenda, pudendum — *see* condition
Puente's disease (simple glandular cheilitis) K13.0
Puerperal, puerperium (complicated by, complications)
- abnormal glucose (tolerance test) O99.815
- abscess
  - areola O91.02
    - associated with lactation O91.03
  - Bartholin's gland O86.19
  - breast O91.12
    - associated with lactation O91.13
  - cervix (uteri) O86.11
  - genital organ NEC O86.19
  - kidney O86.21
  - mammary O91.12
    - associated with lactation O91.13
  - nipple O91.02
    - associated with lactation O91.03
  - peritoneum O85
  - subareolar O91.12
    - associated with lactation O91.13
  - urinary tract — *see* Puerperal, infection, urinary
  - uterus O86.12
  - vagina (wall) O86.13
  - vaginorectal O86.13
  - vulvovaginal gland O86.13
- adnexitis O86.19
- afibrinogenemia, or other coagulation defect O72.3
- albuminuria (acute) (subacute) — *see* Proteinuria, gestational
- alcohol use O99.315
- anemia O90.81
  - pre-existing (pre-pregnancy) O99.03
- anesthetic death O89.8
- apoplexy O99.43
- bariatric surgery status O99.845
- blood disorder NEC O99.13
- blood dyscrasia O72.3
- cardiomyopathy O90.3
- cerebrovascular disorder (conditions in I60-I69) O99.43
- cervicitis O86.11
- circulatory system disorder O99.43
- coagulopathy (any) O99.13
  - with hemorrhage O72.3
- complications O90.9
  - specified NEC O90.89
- convulsions — *see* Eclampsia
- cystitis O86.22
- cystopyelitis O86.29
- delirium NEC F05
- diabetes O24.93
  - gestational — *see* Puerperal, gestational diabetes
  - pre-existing O24.33
    - specified NEC O24.83
    - type 1 O24.03
    - type 2 O24.13
- digestive system disorder O99.63
- disease O90.9
  - breast NEC O92.29
  - cerebrovascular (acute) O99.43
  - nonobstetric NEC O99.89
  - tubo-ovarian O86.19
  - Valsuani's O99.03
- disorder O90.9
  - biliary tract O26.63
  - lactation O92.70
  - liver O26.63
  - nonobstetric NEC O99.89
- disruption
  - cesarean wound O90.0
  - episiotomy wound O90.1
  - perineal laceration wound O90.1

Puerperal, puerperium — *continued*
- drug use O99.325
- eclampsia (with pre-existing hypertension) O15.2
- embolism (pulmonary) (blood clot) — *see* Embolism, obstetric, puerperal
- endocrine, nutritional or metabolic disease NEC O99.285
- endophlebitis — *see* Puerperal, phlebitis
- endotrachelitis O86.11
- failure
  - lactation (complete) O92.3
    - partial O92.4
  - renal, acute O90.4
- fever (of unknown origin) O86.4
  - septic O85
- fissure, nipple O92.12
  - associated with lactation O92.13
- fistula
  - breast (due to mastitis) O91.12
    - associated with lactation O91.13
  - nipple O91.02
    - associated with lactation O91.03
- galactophoritis O91.22
  - associated with lactation O91.23
- galactorrhea O92.6
- gastric banding status O99.845
- gastric bypass status O99.845
- gastrointestinal disease NEC O99.63
- gestational
  - diabetes O24.439
    - diet controlled O24.430
    - insulin (and diet) controlled O24.434
    - oral drug controlled (antidiabetic) (hypo-glycemic) O24.435
  - edema O12.05
    - with proteinuria O12.25
  - proteinuria O12.15
- gonorrhea O98.23
- hematoma, subdural O99.43
- hemiplegia, cerebral O99.355
  - due to cerbrovascular disorder O99.43
- hemorrhage O72.1
  - brain O99.43
  - bulbar O99.43
  - cerebellar O99.43
  - cerebral O99.43
  - cortical O99.43
  - delayed or secondary O72.2
  - extradural O99.43
  - internal capsule O99.43
  - intracranial O99.43
  - intrapontine O99.43
  - meningeal O99.43
  - pontine O99.43
  - retained placenta O72.0
  - subarachnoid O99.43
  - subcortical O99.43
  - subdural O99.43
  - third stage O72.0
  - uterine, delayed O72.2
  - ventricular O99.43
- hemorrhoids O87.2
- hepatorenal syndrome O90.4
- hypertension — *see* Hypertension, complicating, puerperium
- hypertrophy, breast O92.29
- induration breast (fibrous) O92.29
- infection O86.4
  - cervix O86.11
  - generalized O85
  - genital tract NEC O86.19
    - obstetric surgical wound O86.0
  - kidney (bacillus coli) O86.21
  - maternal O98.93
    - carrier state NEC O99.835
    - gonorrhea O98.23
    - human immunodeficiency virus (HIV) O98.73
    - protozoal O98.63
    - sexually transmitted NEC O98.33
    - specified NEC O98.83
    - streptococcus group B (GBS) carrier state O99.825
    - syphilis O98.13
    - tuberculosis O98.03
    - viral hepatitis O98.43
    - viral NEC O98.53
  - nipple O91.02
    - associated with lactation O91.03
  - peritoneum O85

Puerperal, puerperium — *continued*
- infection — *continued*
  - renal O86.21
  - specified NEC O86.89
  - urinary (asymptomatic) (tract) NEC O86.20
    - bladder O86.22
    - kidney O86.21
    - specified site NEC O86.29
    - urethra O86.22
  - vagina O86.13
  - vein — *see* Puerperal, phlebitis
- ischemia, cerebral O99.43
- lymphangitis O86.89
  - breast O91.22
    - associated with lactation O91.23
- malignancy O9A.13 (*following* O99)
- malnutrition O25.3
- mammillitis O91.02
  - associated with lactation O91.03
- mammitis O91.22
  - associated with lactation O91.23
- mania F30.8
- mastitis O91.22
  - associated with lactation O91.23
  - purulent O91.12
    - associated with lactation O91.13
- melancholia — *see* Disorder, depressive
- mental disorder NEC O99.345
- metroperitonitis O85
- metrorrhagia — *see* Hemorrhage, postpartum
- metrosalpingitis O86.19
- metrovaginitis O86.13
- milk leg O87.1
- monoplegia, cerebral O99.43
- mood disturbance O90.6
- necrosis, liver (acute) (subacute) (conditions in subcategory K72.0) O26.63
  - with renal failure O90.4
- nervous system disorder O99.355
- obesity (pre-existing prior to pregnancy) O99.215
- obesity surgery status O99.845
- occlusion, precerebral artery O99.43
- paralysis
  - bladder (sphincter) O90.89
  - cerebral O99.43
- paralytic stroke O99.43
- parametritis O85
- paravaginitis O86.13
- pelviperitonitis O85
- perimetritis O86.12
- perimetrosalpingitis O86.19
- perinephritis O86.21
- periphlebitis — *see* Puerperal phlebitis
- peritoneal infection O85
- peritonitis (pelvic) O85
- perivaginitis O86.13
- phlebitis O87.0
  - deep O87.1
  - pelvic O87.1
  - superficial O87.0
- phlebothrombosis, deep O87.1
- phlegmasia alba dolens O87.1
- placental polyp O90.89
- pneumonia, embolic — *see* Embolism, obstetric, puerperal
- pre-eclampsia — *see* Pre-eclampsia
- psychosis F53
- pyelitis O86.21
- pyelocystitis O86.29
- pyelonephritis O86.21
- pyelonephrosis O86.21
- pyemia O85
- pyocystitis O86.29
- pyohemia O85
- pyometra O86.12
- pyonephritis O86.21
- pyosalpingitis O86.19
- pyrexia (of unknown origin) O86.4
- renal
  - disease NEC O90.89
  - failure O90.4
- respiratory disease NEC O99.53
- retention
  - decidua — *see* Retention, decidua
  - placenta O72.0
  - secundines — *see* Retention, secundines
- retrated nipple O92.02
- salpingo-ovaritis O86.19

Puerperal, puerperium — *continued*
- salpingoperitonitis O85
- secondary perineal tear O90.1
- sepsis (pelvic) O85
- sepsis O85
- septic thrombophlebitis O86.81
- skin disorder NEC O99.73
- specified condition NEC O99.89
- stroke O99.43
- subinvolution (uterus) O90.89
- subluxation of symphysis (pubis) O26.73
- suppuration — *see* Puerperal, abscess
- tetanus A34
- thelitis O91.02
  - associated with lactation O91.03
- thrombocytopenia O72.3
- thrombophlebitis (superficial) O87.0
  - deep O87.1
  - pelvic O87.1
  - septic O86.81
- thrombosis (venous) — *see* Thrombosis, puerperal
- thyroiditis O90.5
- toxemia (eclamptic) (pre-eclamptic) (with convulsions) O15.2
- trauma, non-obstetric O9A.23 (*following* O99)
  - caused by abuse (physical) (suspected) O9A.33 (*following* O99)
    - confirmed O9A.33 (*following* O99)
    - psychological (suspected) O9A.53 (*following* O99)
      - confirmed O9A.53 (*following* O99)
    - sexual (suspected) O9A.43 (*following* O99)
      - confirmed O9A.43 (*following* O99)
- uremia (due to renal failure) O90.4
- urethritis O86.22
- vaginitis O86.13
- varicose veins (legs) O87.4
  - vulva or perineum O87.8
- venous O87.9
- vulvitis O86.19
- vulvovaginitis O86.13
- white leg O87.1

Puerperium — *see* Puerperal

Pulmolithiasis J98.4

Pulmonary — *see* condition

Pulpitis (acute) (anachoretic) (chronic) (hyperplastic) (putrescent) (suppurative) (ulcerative) K04.01
- irreversible K04.02
- reversible K04.01

Pulpless tooth K04.99

Pulse
- alternating R00.8
- bigeminal R00.8
- fast R00.0
- feeble, rapid due to shock following injury T79.4 ☑
- rapid R00.0
- weak R09.89

Pulsus alternans or trigeminus R00.8

Punch drunk F07.81

Punctum lacrimale occlusion — *see* Obstruction, lacrimal

Puncture
- abdomen, abdominal
  - wall S31.139 ☑
    - with
      - foreign body S31.149 ☑
      - penetration into peritoneal cavity S31.639 ☑
        - with foreign body S31.649 ☑
  - epigastric region S31.132 ☑
    - with
      - foreign body S31.142 ☑
      - penetration into peritoneal cavity S31.632 ☑
        - with foreign body S31.642 ☑
  - left
    - lower quadrant S31.134 ☑
      - with
        - foreign body S31.144 ☑
        - penetration into peritoneal cavity S31.634 ☑
          - with foreign body S31.644 ☑
    - upper quadrant S31.131 ☑
      - with
        - foreign body S31.141 ☑
        - penetration into peritoneal cavity S31.631 ☑
          - with foreign body S31.641 ☑

☑ Additional Character Required — Refer to the Tabular List for Character Selection ▽ Subterms under main terms may continue to next column or page

Puncture — *continued*
  abdomen, abdominal — *continued*
    wall — *continued*
      periumbilic region S31.135 ☑
        with
          foreign body S31.145 ☑
          penetration into peritoneal cavity
            S31.635 ☑
            with foreign body S31.645 ☑
      right
        lower quadrant S31.133 ☑
          with
            foreign body S31.143 ☑
            penetration into peritoneal cavity
              S31.633 ☑
              with foreign body S31.643 ☑
        upper quadrant S31.130 ☑
          with
            foreign body S31.140 ☑
            penetration into peritoneal cavity
              S31.630 ☑
              with foreign body S31.640 ☑
  accidental, complicating surgery — *see* Complication,
    accidental puncture or laceration
  alveolar (process) — *see* Puncture, oral cavity
  ankle S91.039 ☑
    with
      foreign body S91.049 ☑
    left S91.032 ☑
      with
        foreign body S91.042 ☑
    right S91.031 ☑
      with
        foreign body S91.041 ☑
  anus S31.833 ☑
    with foreign body S31.834 ☑
  arm (upper) S41.139 ☑
    with foreign body S41.149 ☑
    left S41.132 ☑
      with foreign body S41.142 ☑
    lower — *see* Puncture, forearm
    right S41.131 ☑
      with foreign body S41.141 ☑
  auditory canal (external) (meatus) — *see* Puncture,
    ear
  auricle, ear — *see* Puncture, ear
  axilla — *see* Puncture, arm
  back (*see also* Puncture, thorax, back)
    lower S31.030 ☑
      with
        foreign body S31.040 ☑
          with penetration into retroperitoneal
            space S31.041 ☑
        penetration into retroperitoneal space
          S31.031 ☑
  bladder (traumatic) S37.29 ☑
    nontraumatic N32.89
  breast S21.039 ☑
    with foreign body S21.049 ☑
    left S21.032 ☑
      with foreign body S21.042 ☑
    right S21.031 ☑
      with foreign body S21.041 ☑
  buttock S31.803 ☑
    with foreign body S31.804 ☑
    left S31.823 ☑
      with foreign body S31.824 ☑
    right S31.813 ☑
      with foreign body S31.814 ☑
  by
    device, implant or graft — *see* Complications, by
      site and type, mechanical
    foreign body left accidentally in operative wound
      T81.539 ☑
    instrument (any) during a procedure, accidental
      — *see* Puncture, accidental complicating
      surgery
  calf — *see* Puncture, leg
  canaliculus lacrimalis — *see* Puncture, eyelid
  canthus, eye — *see* Puncture, eyelid
  cervical esophagus S11.23 ☑
    with foreign body S11.24 ☑
  cheek (external) S01.439 ☑
    with foreign body S01.449 ☑
    internal — *see* Puncture, oral cavity
    left S01.432 ☑

Puncture — *continued*
  cheek — *continued*
    left — *continued*
      with foreign body S01.442 ☑
    right S01.431 ☑
      with foreign body S01.441 ☑
  chest wall — *see* Puncture, thorax
  chin — *see* Puncture, head, specified site NEC
  clitoris — *see* Puncture, vulva
  costal region — *see* Puncture, thorax
  digit(s)
    foot — *see* Puncture, toe
    hand — *see* Puncture, finger
  ear (canal) (external) S01.339 ☑
    with foreign body S01.349 ☑
    drum S09.2- ☑
    left S01.332 ☑
      with foreign body S01.342 ☑
    right S01.331 ☑
      with foreign body S01.341 ☑
  elbow S51.039 ☑
    with
      foreign body S51.049 ☑
    left S51.032 ☑
      with
        foreign body S51.042 ☑
    right S51.031 ☑
      with
        foreign body S51.041 ☑
  epididymis — *see* Puncture, testis
  epigastric region — *see* Puncture, abdomen, wall,
    epigastric
  epiglottis S11.83 ☑
    with foreign body S11.84 ☑
  esophagus
    cervical S11.23 ☑
      with foreign body S11.24 ☑
    thoracic S27.818 ☑
  eyeball S05.6- ☑
    with foreign body S05.5- ☑
  eyebrow — *see* Puncture, eyelid
  eyelid S01.13- ☑
    with foreign body S01.14- ☑
    left S01.132 ☑
      with foreign body S01.142 ☑
    right S01.131 ☑
      with foreign body S01.141 ☑
  face NEC — *see* Puncture, head, specified site NEC
  finger(s) S61.239 ☑
    with
      damage to nail S61.339 ☑
        with
          foreign body S61.349 ☑
      foreign body S61.249 ☑
    index S61.238 ☑
      with
        damage to nail S61.338 ☑
          with
            foreign body S61.348 ☑
        foreign body S61.248 ☑
      left S61.231 ☑
        with
          damage to nail S61.331 ☑
            with
              foreign body S61.341 ☑
          foreign body S61.241 ☑
      right S61.230 ☑
        with
          damage to nail S61.330 ☑
            with
              foreign body S61.340 ☑
          foreign body S61.240 ☑
    little S61.238 ☑
      with
        damage to nail S61.338 ☑
          with
            foreign body S61.348 ☑
        foreign body S61.248 ☑
      left S61.237 ☑
        with
          damage to nail S61.337 ☑
            with
              foreign body S61.347 ☑
          foreign body S61.247 ☑
      right S61.236 ☑

Puncture — *continued*
  finger(s) — *continued*
    little — *continued*
      right — *continued*
        with
          damage to nail S61.336 ☑
            with
              foreign body S61.346 ☑
          foreign body S61.246 ☑
    middle S61.238 ☑
      with
        damage to nail S61.338 ☑
          with
            foreign body S61.348 ☑
        foreign body S61.248 ☑
      left S61.233 ☑
        with
          damage to nail S61.333 ☑
            with
              foreign body S61.343 ☑
          foreign body S61.243 ☑
      right S61.232 ☑
        with
          damage to nail S61.332 ☑
            with
              foreign body S61.342 ☑
          foreign body S61.242 ☑
    ring S61.238 ☑
      with
        damage to nail S61.338 ☑
          with
            foreign body S61.348 ☑
        foreign body S61.248 ☑
      left S61.235 ☑
        with
          damage to nail S61.335 ☑
            with
              foreign body S61.345 ☑
          foreign body S61.245 ☑
      right S61.234 ☑
        with
          damage to nail S61.334 ☑
            with
              foreign body S61.344 ☑
          foreign body S61.244 ☑
  flank S31.139 ☑
    with foreign body S31.149 ☑
  foot (except toe(s) alone) S91.339 ☑
    with foreign body S91.349 ☑
    left S91.332 ☑
      with foreign body S91.342 ☑
    right S91.331 ☑
      with foreign body S91.341 ☑
    toe — *see* Puncture, toe
  forearm S51.839 ☑
    with
      foreign body S51.849 ☑
    elbow only — *see* Puncture, elbow
    left S51.832 ☑
      with
        foreign body S51.842 ☑
    right S51.831 ☑
      with
        foreign body S51.841 ☑
  forehead — *see* Puncture, head, specified site NEC
  genital organs, external
    female S31.532 ☑
      with foreign body S31.542 ☑
      vagina — *see* Puncture, vagina
      vulva — *see* Puncture, vulva
    male S31.531 ☑
      with foreign body S31.541 ☑
      penis — *see* Puncture, penis
      scrotum — *see* Puncture, scrotum
      testis — *see* Puncture, testis
  groin — *see* Puncture, abdomen, wall
  gum — *see* Puncture, oral cavity
  hand S61.439 ☑
    with
      foreign body S61.449 ☑
    finger — *see* Puncture, finger
    left S61.432 ☑
      with
        foreign body S61.442 ☑
    right S61.431 ☑

Puncture — *continued*
  hand — *continued*
    right — *continued*
      with
        foreign body S61.441 ☑
      thumb — *see* Puncture, thumb
  head S01.93 ☑
    with foreign body S01.94 ☑
    cheek — *see* Puncture, cheek
    ear — *see* Puncture, ear
    eyelid — *see* Puncture, eyelid
    lip — *see* Puncture, oral cavity
    nose — *see* Puncture, nose
    oral cavity — *see* Puncture, oral cavity
    scalp S01.03 ☑
      with foreign body S01.04 ☑
    specified site NEC S01.83 ☑
      with foreign body S01.84 ☑
    temporomandibular area — *see* Puncture, cheek
  heart S26.99 ☑
    with hemopericardium S26.09 ☑
    without hemopericardium S26.19 ☑
  heel — *see* Puncture, foot
  hip S71.039 ☑
    with foreign body S71.049 ☑
    left S71.032 ☑
      with foreign body S71.042 ☑
    right S71.031 ☑
      with foreign body S71.041 ☑
  hymen — *see* Puncture, vagina
  hypochondrium — *see* Puncture, abdomen, wall
  hypogastric region — *see* Puncture, abdomen, wall
  inguinal region — *see* Puncture, abdomen, wall
  instep — *see* Puncture, foot
  internal organs — *see* Injury, by site
  interscapular region — *see* Puncture, thorax, back
  intestine
    large
      colon S36.599 ☑
        ascending S36.590 ☑
        descending S36.592 ☑
        sigmoid S36.593 ☑
        specified site NEC S36.598 ☑
        transverse S36.591 ☑
      rectum S36.69 ☑
    small S36.499 ☑
      duodenum S36.490 ☑
      specified site NEC S36.498 ☑
  intra-abdominal organ S36.99 ☑
    gallbladder S36.128 ☑
    intestine — *see* Puncture, intestine
    liver S36.118 ☑
    pancreas — *see* Puncture, pancreas
    peritoneum S36.81 ☑
    specified site NEC S36.898 ☑
    spleen S36.09 ☑
    stomach S36.39 ☑
  jaw — *see* Puncture, head, specified site NEC
  knee S81.039 ☑
    with foreign body S81.049 ☑
    left S81.032 ☑
      with foreign body S81.042 ☑
    right S81.031 ☑
      with foreign body S81.041 ☑
  labium (majus) (minus) — *see* Puncture, vulva
  lacrimal duct — *see* Puncture, eyelid
  larynx S11.013 ☑
    with foreign body S11.014 ☑
  leg (lower) S81.839 ☑
    with foreign body S81.849 ☑
    foot — *see* Puncture, foot
    knee — *see* Puncture, knee
    left S81.832 ☑
      with foreign body S81.842 ☑
    right S81.831 ☑
      with foreign body S81.841 ☑
    upper — *see* Puncture, thigh
  lip S01.531 ☑
    with foreign body S01.541 ☑
  loin — *see* Puncture, abdomen, wall
  lower back — *see* Puncture, back, lower
  lumbar region — *see* Puncture, back, lower
  malar region — *see* Puncture, head, specified site NEC
  mammary — *see* Puncture, breast
  mastoid region — *see* Puncture, head, specified site NEC

Puncture — *continued*
  mouth — *see* Puncture, oral cavity
  nail
    finger — *see* Puncture, finger, with damage to nail
    toe — *see* Puncture, toe, with damage to nail
  nasal (septum) (sinus) — *see* Puncture, nose
  nasopharynx — *see* Puncture, head, specified site NEC
  neck S11.93 ☑
    with foreign body S11.94 ☑
    involving
      cervical esophagus — *see* Puncture, cervical esophagus
      larynx — *see* Puncture, larynx
      pharynx — *see* Puncture, pharynx
      thyroid gland — *see* Puncture, thyroid gland
      trachea — *see* Puncture, trachea
    specified site NEC S11.83 ☑
      with foreign body S11.84 ☑
  nose (septum) (sinus) S01.23 ☑
    with foreign body S01.24 ☑
  ocular — *see* Puncture, eyeball
  oral cavity S01.532 ☑
    with foreign body S01.542 ☑
  orbit S05.4- ☑
  palate — *see* Puncture, oral cavity
  palm — *see* Puncture, hand
  pancreas S36.299 ☑
    body S36.291 ☑
    head S36.290 ☑
    tail S36.292 ☑
  pelvis — *see* Puncture, back, lower
  penis S31.23 ☑
    with foreign body S31.24 ☑
  perineum
    female S31.43 ☑
      with foreign body S31.44 ☑
    male S31.139 ☑
      with foreign body S31.149 ☑
  periocular area (with or without lacrimal passages) — *see* Puncture, eyelid
  phalanges
    finger — *see* Puncture, finger
    toe — *see* Puncture, toe
  pharynx S11.23 ☑
    with foreign body S11.24 ☑
  pinna — *see* Puncture, ear
  popliteal space — *see* Puncture, knee
  prepuce — *see* Puncture, penis
  pubic region S31.139 ☑
    with foreign body S31.149 ☑
  pudendum — *see* Puncture, genital organs, external
  rectovaginal septum — *see* Puncture, vagina
  sacral region — *see* Puncture, back, lower
  sacroiliac region — *see* Puncture, back, lower
  salivary gland — *see* Puncture, oral cavity
  scalp S01.03 ☑
    with foreign body S01.04 ☑
  scapular region — *see* Puncture, shoulder
  scrotum S31.33 ☑
    with foreign body S31.34 ☑
  shin — *see* Puncture, leg
  shoulder S41.039 ☑
    with foreign body S41.049 ☑
    left S41.032 ☑
      with foreign body S41.042 ☑
    right S41.031 ☑
      with foreign body S41.041 ☑
  spermatic cord — *see* Puncture, testis
  sternal region — *see* Puncture, thorax, front
  submaxillary region — *see* Puncture, head, specified site NEC
  submental region — *see* Puncture, head, specified site NEC
  subungual
    finger(s) — *see* Puncture, finger, with damage to nail
    toe — *see* Puncture, toe, with damage to nail
  supraclavicular fossa — *see* Puncture, neck, specified site NEC
  temple, temporal region — *see* Puncture, head, specified site NEC
  temporomandibular area — *see* Puncture, cheek
  testis S31.33 ☑
    with foreign body S31.34 ☑
  thigh S71.139 ☑
    with foreign body S71.149 ☑

Puncture — *continued*
  thigh — *continued*
    left S71.132 ☑
      with foreign body S71.142 ☑
    right S71.131 ☑
      with foreign body S71.141 ☑
  thorax, thoracic (wall) S21.93 ☑
    with foreign body S21.94 ☑
    back S21.23- ☑
      with
        foreign body S21.24- ☑
          with penetration S21.44 ☑
        penetration S21.43 ☑
    breast — *see* Puncture, breast
    front S21.13- ☑
      with
        foreign body S21.14- ☑
          with penetration S21.34 ☑
        penetration S21.33 ☑
  throat — *see* Puncture, neck
  thumb S61.039 ☑
    with
      damage to nail S61.139 ☑
        with
          foreign body S61.149 ☑
      foreign body S61.049 ☑
    left S61.032 ☑
      with
        damage to nail S61.132 ☑
          with
            foreign body S61.142 ☑
        foreign body S61.042 ☑
    right S61.031 ☑
      with
        damage to nail S61.131 ☑
          with
            foreign body S61.141 ☑
        foreign body S61.041 ☑
  thyroid gland S11.13 ☑
    with foreign body S11.14 ☑
  toe(s) S91.139 ☑
    with
      damage to nail S91.239 ☑
        with
          foreign body S91.249 ☑
      foreign body S91.149 ☑
    great S91.133 ☑
      with
        damage to nail S91.233 ☑
          with
            foreign body S91.243 ☑
        foreign body S91.143 ☑
      left S91.132 ☑
        with
          damage to nail S91.232 ☑
            with
              foreign body S91.242 ☑
          foreign body S91.142 ☑
      right S91.131 ☑
        with
          damage to nail S91.231 ☑
            with
              foreign body S91.241 ☑
          foreign body S91.141 ☑
    lesser S91.136 ☑
      with
        damage to nail S91.236 ☑
          with
            foreign body S91.246 ☑
        foreign body S91.146 ☑
      left S91.135 ☑
        with
          damage to nail S91.235 ☑
            with
              foreign body S91.245 ☑
          foreign body S91.145 ☑
      right S91.134 ☑
        with
          damage to nail S91.234 ☑
            with
              foreign body S91.244 ☑
          foreign body S91.144 ☑
  tongue — *see* Puncture, oral cavity
  trachea S11.023 ☑
    with foreign body S11.024 ☑
  tunica vaginalis — *see* Puncture, testis

☑ **Additional Character Required — Refer to the Tabular List for Character Selection**   ▽ **Subterms under main terms may continue to next column or page**

Puncture — *continued*
  tympanum, tympanic membrane S09.2- ☑
  umbilical region S31.135 ☑
    with foreign body S31.145 ☑
  uvula — *see* Puncture, oral cavity
  vagina S31.43 ☑
    with foreign body S31.44 ☑
  vocal cords S11.033 ☑
    with foreign body S11.034 ☑
  vulva S31.43 ☑
    with foreign body S31.44 ☑
  wrist S61.539 ☑
    with
      foreign body S61.549 ☑
    left S61.532 ☑
      with
        foreign body S61.542 ☑
    right S61.531 ☑
      with
        foreign body S61.541 ☑
PUO (pyrexia of unknown origin) R50.9
Pupillary membrane (persistent) Q13.89
Pupillotonia — *see* Anomaly, pupil, function, tonic pupil
Purpura D69.2
  abdominal D69.0
  allergic D69.0
  anaphylactoid D69.0
  annularis telangiectodes L81.7
  arthritic D69.0
  autoerythrocyte sensitization D69.2
  autoimmune D69.0
  bacterial D69.0
  Bateman's (senile) D69.2
  capillary fragility (hereditary) (idiopathic) D69.8
  cryoglobulinemic D89.1
  Devil's pinches D69.2
  fibrinolytic — *see* Fibrinolysis
  fulminans, fulminous D65
  gangrenous D65
  hemorrhagic, hemorrhagica D69.3
    not due to thrombocytopenia D69.0
  Henoch (-Schönlein) (allergic) D69.0
  hypergammaglobulinemic (benign) (Waldenström) D89.0
  idiopathic (thrombocytopenic) D69.3
    nonthrombocytopenic D69.0
  immune thrombocytopenic D69.3
  infectious D69.0
  malignant D69.0
  neonatorum P54.5
  nervosa D69.0
  newborn P54.5
  nonthrombocytopenic D69.2
    hemorrhagic D69.0
    idiopathic D69.0
  nonthrombopenic D69.2
  peliosis rheumatica D69.0
  posttransfusion (post-transfusion) (from (fresh) whole blood or blood products) D69.51
  primary D69.49
  red cell membrane sensitivity D69.2
  rheumatica D69.0
  Schönlein (-Henoch) (allergic) D69.0
  scorbutic E54 [D77]
  senile D69.2
  simplex D69.2
  symptomatica D69.0
  telangiectasia annularis L81.7
  thrombocytopenic D69.49
    congenital D69.42
    hemorrhagic D69.3
    hereditary D69.42
    idiopathic D69.3
    immune D69.3
    neonatal, transitory P61.0
    thrombotic M31.1
  thrombohemolytic — *see* Fibrinolysis
  thrombolytic — *see* Fibrinolysis
  thrombopenic D69.49
  thrombotic, thrombocytopenic M31.1
  toxic D69.0
  vascular D69.0
  visceral symptoms D69.0
Purpuric spots R23.3
Purulent — *see* condition
Pus
  in
    stool R19.5

Pus — *continued*
  in — *continued*
    urine N39.0
  tube (rupture) — *see* Salpingo-oophoritis
Pustular rash L08.0
Pustule (nonmalignant) L08.9
  malignant A22.0
Pustulosis palmaris et plantaris L40.3
Putnam (-Dana) **disease or syndrome** — *see* Degeneration, combined
Putrescent pulp (dental) K04.1
Pyarthritis, pyarthrosis — *see* Arthritis, pyogenic or pyemic
  tuberculous — *see* Tuberculosis, joint
Pyelectasis — *see* Hydronephrosis
Pyelitis (congenital) (uremic) (*see also* Pyelonephritis)
  with
    calculus — *see* category N20 ☑
      with hydronephrosis N13.2
    contracted kidney N11.9
  acute N10
  chronic N11.9
    with calculus — *see* category N20 ☑
      with hydronephrosis N13.2
  cystica N28.84
  puerperal (postpartum) O86.21
  tuberculous A18.11
Pyelocystitis — *see* Pyelonephritis
Pyelonephritis (*see also* Nephritis, tubulo-interstitial)
  with
    calculus — *see* category N20 ☑
      with hydronephrosis N13.2
    contracted kidney N11.9
  acute N10
  calculous — *see* category N20 ☑
    with hydronephrosis N13.2
  chronic N11.9
    with calculus — *see* category N20 ☑
      with hydronephrosis N13.2
    associated with ureteral obstruction or stricture N11.1
    nonobstructive N11.8
      with reflux (vesicoureteral) N11.0
    obstructive N11.1
    specified NEC N11.8
  in (due to)
    brucellosis A23.9 [N16]
    cryoglobulinemia (mixed) D89.1 [N16]
    cystinosis E72.04
    diphtheria A36.84
    glycogen storage disease E74.09 [N16]
    leukemia NEC C95.9- ☑ [N16]
    lymphoma NEC C85.90 [N16]
    multiple myeloma C90.0- ☑ [N16]
    obstruction N11.1
    Salmonella infection A02.25
    sarcoidosis D86.84
    sepsis A41.9 [N16]
    Sjögren's disease M35.04
    toxoplasmosis B58.83
    transplant rejection T86.91 [N16]
    Wilson's disease E83.01 [N16]
  nonobstructive N12
    with reflux (vesicoureteral) N11.0
    chronic N11.8
  syphilitic A52.75
Pyelonephrosis (obstructive) N11.1
  chronic N11.9
Pyelophlebitis I80.8
Pyeloureteritis cystica N28.85
Pyemia, pyemic (fever) (infection) (purulent) (*see also* Sepsis)
  joint — *see* Arthritis, pyogenic or pyemic
  liver K75.1
  pneumococcal A40.3
  portal K75.1
  postvaccinal T88.0 ☑
  puerperal, postpartum, childbirth O85
  specified organism NEC A41.89
  tuberculous — *see* Tuberculosis, miliary
Pygopagus Q89.4
Pyknoepilepsy (idiopathic) — *see* Pyknolepsy
Pyknolepsy G40.A09 (*following* G40.3)
  intractable G40.A19 (*following* G40.3)
    with status epilepticus G40.A11 (*following* G40.3)
    without status epilepticus G40.A19 (*following* G40.3)
  not intractable G40.A09 (*following* G40.3)

Pyknolepsy — *continued*
  not intractable — *continued*
    with status epilepticus G40.A01 (*following* G40.3)
    without status epilepticus G40.A09 (*following* G40.3)
Pylephlebitis K75.1
Pyle's syndrome Q78.5
Pylethrombophlebitis K75.1
Pylethrombosis K75.1
Pyloritis K29.90
  with bleeding K29.91
Pylorospasm (reflex) **NEC** K31.3
  congenital or infantile Q40.0
  neurotic F45.8
  newborn Q40.0
  psychogenic F45.8
Pylorus, pyloric — *see* condition
Pyoarthrosis — *see* Arthritis, pyogenic or pyemic
Pyocele
  mastoid — *see* Mastoiditis, acute
  sinus (accessory) — *see* Sinusitis
  turbinate (bone) J32.9
  urethra (*see also* Urethritis) N34.0
Pyocolpos — *see* Vaginitis
Pyocystitis N30.80
  with hematuria N30.81
Pyoderma, pyodermia L08.0
  gangrenosum L88
  newborn P39.4
  phagedenic L88
  vegetans L08.81
Pyodermatitis L08.0
  vegetans L08.81
Pyogenic — *see* condition
Pyohydronephrosis N13.6
Pyometra, pyometrium, pyometritis — *see* Endometritis
Pyomyositis (tropical) — *see* Myositis, infective
Pyonephritis N12
Pyonephrosis N13.6
  tuberculous A18.11
Pyo-oophoritis — *see* Salpingo-oophoritis
Pyo-ovarium — *see* Salpingo-oophoritis
Pyopericarditis, pyopericardium I30.1
Pyophlebitis — *see* Phlebitis
Pyopneumopericardium I30.1
Pyopneumothorax (infective) J86.9
  with fistula J86.0
  tuberculous NEC A15.6
Pyosalpinx, pyosalpingitis (*see also* Salpingo-oophoritis)
Pyothorax J86.9
  with fistula J86.0
  tuberculous NEC A15.6
Pyoureter N28.89
  tuberculous A18.11
Pyramidopallidonigral syndrome G20
Pyrexia (of unknown origin) R50.9
  atmospheric T67.0 ☑
  during labor NEC O75.2
  heat T67.0 ☑
  newborn P81.9
    environmentally-induced P81.0
  persistent R50.9
  puerperal O86.4
Pyroglobulinemia NEC E88.09
Pyromania F63.1
Pyrosis R12
Pyuria (bacterial) N39.0

Q

Q fever A78
  with pneumonia A78
Quadricuspid aortic valve Q23.8
Quadrilateral fever A78
Quadriparesis — *see* Quadriplegia
  meaning muscle weakness M62.81
Quadriplegia G82.50
  complete
    C1-C4 level G82.51
    C5-C7 level G82.53
  congenital (cerebral) (spinal) G80.8
    spastic G80.0
  embolic (current episode) I63.4- ☑
  functional R53.2

Quadriplegia — *continued*
  incomplete
    C1-C4 level G82.52
    C5-C7 level G82.54
  thrombotic (current episode) I63.3- ☑
  traumatic — *code to* injury with seventh character S
    current episode — *see* Injury, spinal (cord), cervical
Quadruplet, pregnancy — *see* Pregnancy, quadruplet
Quarrelsomeness F60.3
Queensland fever A77.3
Quervain's disease M65.4
  thyroid E06.1
Queyrat's erythroplasia D07.4
  penis D07.4
  specified site — *see* Neoplasm, skin, in situ
  unspecified site D07.4
Quincke's disease or edema T78.3 ☑
  hereditary D84.1
Quinsy (gangrenous) J36
Quintan fever A79.0
Quintuplet, pregnancy — *see* Pregnancy, quintuplet

R

Rabbit fever — *see* Tularemia
Rabies A82.9
  contact Z20.3
  exposure to Z20.3
  inoculation reaction — *see* Complications, vaccination
  sylvatic A82.0
  urban A82.1
Rachischisis — *see* Spina bifida
Rachitic (*see also* condition)
  deformities of spine (late effect) (sequelae) E64.3
  pelvis (late effect) (sequelae) E64.3
    with disproportion (fetopelvic) O33.0
      causing obstructed labor O65.0
Rachitis, rachitism (acute) (tarda) (*see also* Rickets)
  renalis N25.0
  sequelae E64.3
Radial nerve — *see* condition
Radiation
  burn — *see* Burn
  effects NOS T66 ☑
  sickness NOS T66 ☑
  therapy, encounter for Z51.0
Radiculitis (pressure) (vertebrogenic) — *see* Radiculopathy
Radiculomyelitis (*see also* Encephalitis)
  toxic, due to
    Clostridium tetani A35
    Corynebacterium diphtheriae A36.82
Radiculopathy M54.10
  cervical region M54.12
  cervicothoracic region M54.13
  due to
    disc disorder
      C3 M50.11
      C4 M50.11
      C5 M50.121
      C6 M50.122
      C7 M50.123
    displacement of intervertebral disc — *see* Disorder, disc, with, radiculopathy
  leg M54.1- ☑
  lumbar region M54.16
  lumbosacral region M54.17
  occipito-atlanto-axial region M54.11
  postherpetic B02.29
  sacrococcygeal region M54.18
  syphilitic A52.11
  thoracic region (with visceral pain) M54.14
  thoracolumbar region M54.15
Radiodermal burns (acute, chronic, or occupational) — *see* Burn
Radiodermatitis L58.9
  acute L58.0
  chronic L58.1
Radiotherapy session Z51.0
RAEB (refractory anemia with excess blasts) D46.2- ☑
Rage, meaning rabies — *see* Rabies
Ragpicker's disease A22.1
Ragsorter's disease A22.1
Raillietiniasis B71.8
Railroad neurosis F48.8
Railway spine F48.8

Raised (*see also* Elevated)
  antibody titer R76.0
Rake teeth, tooth M26.39
Rales R09.89
Ramifying renal pelvis Q63.8
Ramsay-Hunt disease or syndrome (*see also* Hunt's disease) B02.21
  meaning dyssynergia cerebellaris myoclonica G11.1
Ranula K11.6
  congenital Q38.4
Rape
  adult
    confirmed T74.21 ☑
    suspected T76.21 ☑
  alleged, observation or examination, ruled out
    adult Z04.41
    child Z04.42
  child
    confirmed T74.22 ☑
    suspected T76.22 ☑
Rapid
  feeble pulse, due to shock, following injury T79.4 ☑
  heart (beat) R00.0
    psychogenic F45.8
  second stage (delivery) O62.3
  time-zone change syndrome — *see* Disorder, sleep, circadian rhythm, psychogenic
Rarefaction, bone — *see* Disorder, bone, density and structure, specified NEC
Rash (toxic) R21
  canker A38.9
  diaper L22
  drug (internal use) L27.0
    contact (*see also* Dermatitis, due to, drugs, external) L25.1
  following immunization T88.1 ☑
  food — *see* Dermatitis, due to, food
  heat L74.0
  napkin (psoriasiform) L22
  nettle — *see* Urticaria
  pustular L08.0
  rose R21
    epidemic B06.9
  scarlet A38.9
  serum (*see also* Reaction, serum) T80.69 ☑
  wandering tongue K14.1
Rasmussen aneurysm — *see* Tuberculosis, pulmonary
Rasmussen encephalitis G04.81
Rat-bite fever A25.9
  due to Streptobacillus moniliformis A25.1
  spirochetal (morsus muris) A25.0
Rathke's pouch tumor D44.3
Raymond (-Céstan) **syndrome** I65.8
Raynaud's disease, phenomenon or syndrome (secondary) I73.00
  with gangrene (symmetric) I73.01
RDS (newborn) (type I) P22.0
  type II P22.1
Reaction (*see also* Disorder)
  adaptation — *see* Disorder, adjustment
  adjustment (anxiety) (conduct disorder) (depressiveness) (distress) — *see* Disorder, adjustment
    with
      mutism, elective (child) (adolescent) F94.0
  adverse
    food (any) (ingested) NEC T78.1 ☑
      anaphylactic — *see* Shock, anaphylactic, due to food
  affective — *see* Disorder, mood
  allergic — *see* Allergy
  anaphylactic — *see* Shock, anaphylactic
  anaphylactoid — *see* Shock, anaphylactic
  anesthesia — *see* Anesthesia, complication
  antitoxin (prophylactic) (therapeutic) — *see* Complications, vaccination
  anxiety F41.1
  Arthus — *see* Arthus' phenomenon
  asthenic F48.8
  combat and operational stress F43.0
  compulsive F42.8
  conversion F44.9
  crisis, acute F43.0
  deoxyribonuclease (DNA) (DNase) hypersensitivity D69.2
  depressive (single episode) F32.9
    affective (single episode) F31.4
      recurrent episode F33.9

Reaction — *continued*
  depressive — *continued*
    neurotic F34.1
    psychoneurotic F34.1
    psychotic F32.3
    recurrent — *see* Disorder, depressive, recurrent
  dissociative F44.9
  drug NEC T88.7 ☑
    addictive — *see* Dependence, drug
      transmitted via placenta or breast milk — *see* Absorption, drug, addictive, through placenta
    allergic — *see* Allergy, drug
    lichenoid L43.2
    newborn P93.8
      gray baby syndrome P93.0
    overdose or poisoning (by accident) — *see* Table of Drugs and Chemicals, by drug, poisoning
    photoallergic L56.1
    phototoxic L56.0
    withdrawal — *see* Dependence, by drug, with, withdrawal
      infant of dependent mother P96.1
      newborn P96.1
    wrong substance given or taken (by accident) — *see* Table of Drugs and Chemicals, by drug, poisoning
  fear F40.9
    child (abnormal) F93.8
  febrile nonhemolytic transfusion (FNHTR) R50.84
  fluid loss, cerebrospinal G97.1
  foreign
    body NEC — *see* Granuloma, foreign body
      in operative wound (inadvertently left) — *see* Foreign body, accidentally left during a procedure
    substance accidentally left during a procedure (chemical) (powder) (talc) T81.60 ☑
      aseptic peritonitis T81.61 ☑
      body or object (instrument) (sponge) (swab) — *see* Foreign body, accidentally left during a procedure
      specified reaction NEC T81.69 ☑
  grief — *see* Disorder, adjustment
  Herxheimer's R68.89
  hyperkinetic — *see* Hyperkinesia
  hypochondriacal F45.20
  hypoglycemic, due to insulin E16.0
    with coma (diabetic) — *see* Diabetes, coma
      nondiabetic E15
    therapeutic misadventure — *see* subcategory T38.3 ☑
  hypomanic F30.8
  hysterical F44.9
  immunization — *see* Complications, vaccination
  incompatibility
    ABO blood group (infusion) (transfusion) — *see* Complication(s), transfusion, incompatibility reaction, ABO
    delayed serologic T80.39 ☑
    minor blood group (Duffy) (E) (K(ell)) (Kidd) (Lewis) (M) (N) (P) (S) T80.89 ☑
    Rh (factor) (infusion) (transfusion) — *see* Complication(s), transfusion, incompatibility reaction, Rh (factor)
  inflammatory — *see* Infection
  infusion — *see* Complications, infusion
  inoculation (immune serum) — *see* Complications, vaccination
  insulin T38.3- ☑
  involutional psychotic — *see* Disorder, depressive
  leukemoid D72.823
    basophilic D72.823
    lymphocytic D72.823
    monocytic D72.823
    myelocytic D72.823
    neutrophilic D72.823
  LSD (acute)
    due to drug abuse — *see* Abuse, drug, hallucinogen
    due to drug dependence — *see* Dependence, drug, hallucinogen
  lumbar puncture G97.1
  manic-depressive — *see* Disorder, bipolar
  neurasthenic F48.8
  neurogenic — *see* Neurosis
  neurotic F48.9
  neurotic-depressive F34.1

Reaction — *continued*
- nitritoid — *see* Crisis, nitritoid
- nonspecific
  - to
    - cell mediated immunity measurement of gamma interferon antigen response without active tuberculosis R76.12
    - QuantiFERON-TB test (QFT) without active tuberculosis R76.12
    - tuberculin test (*see also* Reaction, tuberculin skin test) R76.11
- obsessive-compulsive F42.8
- organic, acute or subacute — *see* Delirium
- paranoid (acute) F23
  - chronic F22
  - senile F03 ☑
- passive dependency F60.7
- phobic F40.9
- post-traumatic stress, uncomplicated Z73.3
- psychogenic F99
- psychoneurotic (*see also* Neurosis)
  - compulsive F42.8
  - depersonalization F48.1
  - depressive F34.1
  - hypochondriacal F45.20
  - neurasthenic F48.8
  - obsessive F42.8
- psychophysiologic — *see* Disorder, somatoform
- psychosomatic — *see* Disorder, somatoform
- psychotic — *see* Psychosis
- scarlet fever toxin — *see* Complications, vaccination
- schizophrenic F23
  - acute (brief) (undifferentiated) F23
  - latent F21
  - undifferentiated (acute) (brief) F23
- serological for syphilis — *see* Serology for syphilis
- serum T80.69 ☑
  - anaphylactic (immediate) (*see also* Shock, anaphylactic) T80.59 ☑
  - specified reaction NEC
    - due to
      - administration of blood and blood products T80.61 ☑
      - immunization T80.62 ☑
      - serum specified NEC T80.69 ☑
      - vaccination T80.62 ☑
- situational — *see* Disorder, adjustment
- somatization — *see* Disorder, somatoform
- spinal puncture G97.1
- stress (severe) F43.9
  - acute (agitation) ("daze") (disorientation) (disturbance of consciousness) (flight reaction) (fugue) F43.0
  - specified NEC F43.8
- surgical procedure — *see* Complications, surgical procedure
- tetanus antitoxin — *see* Complications, vaccination
- toxic, to local anesthesia T88.59 ☑
  - in labor and delivery O74.4
  - in pregnancy O29.3X- ☑
  - postpartum, puerperal O89.3
- toxin-antitoxin — *see* Complications, vaccination
- transfusion (blood) (bone marrow) (lymphocytes) (allergic) — *see* Complications, transfusion
- tuberculin skin test, abnormal R76.11
- vaccination (any) — *see* Complications, vaccination
- withdrawing, child or adolescent F93.8

Reactive airway disease — *see* Asthma
Reactive depression — *see* Reaction, depressive
Rearrangement
- chromosomal
  - balanced (in) Q95.9
    - abnormal individual (autosomal) Q95.2
      - non-sex (autosomal) chromosomes Q95.2
      - sex/non-sex chromosomes Q95.3
    - specified NEC Q95.8

Recalcitrant patient — *see* Noncompliance
Recanalization, thrombus — *see* Thrombosis
Recession, receding
- chamber angle (eye) H21.55- ☑
- chin M26.09
- gingival (postinfective) (postoperative)
  - generalized K06.020
    - minimal K06.021
    - moderate K06.022
    - severe K06.023
  - localized K06.010
    - minimal K06.011

Recession, receding — *continued*
- gingival — *continued*
  - localized — *continued*
    - moderate K06.012
    - severe K06.013
Recklinghausen disease Q85.01
- bones E21.0
Reclus' disease (cystic) — *see* Mastopathy, cystic
Recrudescent typhus (fever) A75.1
Recruitment, auditory H93.21- ☑
Rectalgia K62.89
Rectitis K62.89
Rectocele
- female (without uterine prolapse) N81.6
  - with uterine prolapse N81.4
    - incomplete N81.2
- in pregnancy — *see* Pregnancy, complicated by, abnormal, pelvic organs or tissues NEC
- male K62.3
Rectosigmoid junction — *see* condition
Rectosigmoiditis K63.89
- ulcerative (chronic) K51.30
  - with
    - complication K51.319
      - abscess K51.314
      - fistula K51.313
      - obstruction K51.312
      - rectal bleeding K51.311
      - specified NEC K51.318
Rectourethral — *see* condition
Rectovaginal — *see* condition
Rectovesical — *see* condition
Rectum, rectal — *see* condition
Recurrent — *see* condition
- pregnancy loss — *see* Loss (of), pregnancy, recurrent
Red bugs B88.0
Red tide (*see also* Table of Drugs and Chemicals) T65.82- ☑
Red-cedar lung or pneumonitis J67.8
Reduced
- mobility Z74.09
- ventilatory or vital capacity R94.2
Redundant, redundancy
- anus (congenital) Q43.8
- clitoris N90.89
- colon (congenital) Q43.8
- foreskin (congenital) N47.8
- intestine (congenital) Q43.8
- labia N90.69
- organ or site, congenital NEC — *see* Accessory
- panniculus (abdominal) E65
- prepuce (congenital) N47.8
- pylorus K31.89
- rectum (congenital) Q43.8
- scrotum N50.89
- sigmoid (congenital) Q43.8
- skin L98.7
  - and subcutaneous tissue L98.7
  - of face L57.4
    - eyelids — *see* Blepharochalasis
- stomach K31.89
Reduplication — *see* Duplication
Reflex R29.2
- hyperactive gag J39.2
- pupillary, abnormal — *see* Anomaly, pupil, function
- vasoconstriction I73.9
- vasovagal R55
Reflux K21.9
- acid K21.9
- esophageal K21.9
  - with esophagitis K21.0
  - newborn P78.83
- gastroesophageal K21.9
  - with esophagitis K21.0
- mitral — *see* Insufficiency, mitral
- ureteral — *see* Reflux, vesicoureteral
- vesicoureteral (with scarring) N13.70
  - with
    - nephropathy N13.729
      - with hydroureter N13.739
        - bilateral N13.732
        - unilateral N13.731
      - without hydroureter N13.729
        - bilateral N13.722
        - unilateral N13.721
      - bilateral N13.722
      - unilateral N13.721
    - pyelonephritis (chronic) N11.0

Reflux — *continued*
- vesicoureteral — *continued*
  - without nephropathy N13.71
  - congenital Q62.7
Reforming, artificial openings — *see* Attention to, artificial, opening
Refractive error — *see* Disorder, refraction
Refsum's disease or syndrome G60.1
Refusal of
- food, psychogenic F50.89
- treatment (because of) Z53.20
  - left against medical advice (AMA) Z53.21
  - patient's decision NEC Z53.29
  - reasons of belief or group pressure Z53.1
Regional — *see* condition
Regurgitation R11.10
- aortic (valve) — *see* Insufficiency, aortic
- food (*see also* Vomiting)
  - with reswallowing — *see* Rumination
  - newborn P92.1
- gastric contents — *see* Vomiting
- heart — *see* Endocarditis
- mitral (valve) — *see* Insufficiency, mitral
  - congenital Q23.3
- myocardial — *see* Endocarditis
- pulmonary (valve) (heart) I37.1
  - congenital Q22.2
  - syphilitic A52.03
- tricuspid — *see* Insufficiency, tricuspid
- valve, valvular — *see* Endocarditis
  - congenital Q24.8
- vesicoureteral — *see* Reflux, vesicoureteral
Reichmann's disease or syndrome K31.89
Reifenstein syndrome E34.52
Reinsertion
- implantable subdermal contraceptive Z30.46
- intrauterine contraceptive device Z30.433
Reiter's disease, syndrome, or urethritis M02.30
- ankle M02.37- ☑
- elbow M02.32- ☑
- foot joint M02.37- ☑
- hand joint M02.34- ☑
- hip M02.35- ☑
- knee M02.36- ☑
- multiple site M02.39
- shoulder M02.31- ☑
- vertebra M02.38
- wrist M02.33- ☑
Rejection
- food, psychogenic F50.89
- transplant T86.91
  - bone T86.830
    - marrow T86.01
  - cornea T86.840
  - heart T86.21
    - with lung(s) T86.31
  - intestine T86.850
  - kidney T86.11
  - liver T86.41
  - lung(s) T86.810
    - with heart T86.31
  - organ (immune or nonimmune cause) T86.91
  - pancreas T86.890
  - skin (allograft) (autograft) T86.820
  - specified NEC T86.890
  - stem cell (peripheral blood) (umbilical cord) T86.5
Relapsing fever A68.9
- Carter's (Asiatic) A68.1
- Dutton's (West African) A68.1
- Koch's A68.9
- louse-borne (epidemic) A68.0
- Novy's (American) A68.1
- Obermeyers' (European) A68.0
- Spirillum A68.9
- tick-borne (endemic) A68.1
Relationship
- occlusal
  - open anterior M26.220
  - open posterior M26.221
Relaxation
- anus (sphincter) K62.89
  - psychogenic F45.8
- arch (foot) (*see also* Deformity, limb, flat foot)
- back ligaments — *see* Instability, joint, spine
- bladder (sphincter) N31.2
- cardioesophageal K21.9
- cervix — *see* Incompetency, cervix
- diaphragm J98.6

Relaxation — *continued*
  joint (capsule) (ligament) (paralytic) — *see* Flail, joint
    congenital NEC Q74.8
  lumbosacral (joint) — *see* subcategory M53.2 ☑
  pelvic floor N81.89
  perineum N81.89
  posture R29.3
  rectum (sphincter) K62.89
  sacroiliac (joint) — *see* subcategory M53.2 ☑
  scrotum N50.89
  urethra (sphincter) N36.44
  vesical N31.2
Release from prison, anxiety concerning Z65.2
Remains
  canal of Cloquet Q14.0
  capsule (opaque) Q14.8
Remittent fever (malarial) B54
Remnant
  canal of Cloquet Q14.0
  capsule (opaque) Q14.8
  cervix, cervical stump (acquired) (postoperative) N88.8
  cystic duct, postcholecystectomy K91.5
  fingernail L60.8
    congenital Q84.6
  meniscus, knee — *see* Derangement, knee, meniscus, specified NEC
  thyroglossal duct Q89.2
  tonsil J35.8
    infected (chronic) J35.01
  urachus Q64.4
Removal (from) (of)
  artificial
    arm Z44.00- ☑
      complete Z44.01- ☑
      partial Z44.02- ☑
    eye Z44.2- ☑
    leg Z44.10- ☑
      complete Z44.11- ☑
      partial Z44.12- ☑
  breast implant Z45.81 ☑
  cardiac pulse generator (battery) (end-of-life) Z45.010
  catheter (urinary) (indwelling) Z46.6
    from artificial opening — *see* Attention to, artificial, opening
    non-vascular Z46.82
    vascular NEC Z45.2
  device Z46.9
    contraceptive Z30.432
      implantable subdermal Z30.46
    implanted NEC Z45.89
    specified NEC Z46.89
  drains Z48.03
  dressing (nonsurgical) Z48.00
    surgical Z48.01
  external
    fixation device — *code to* fracture with seventh character D
    prosthesis, prosthetic device Z44.9
      breast Z44.3- ☑
      specified NEC Z44.8
  home in childhood (to foster home or institution) Z62.29
  ileostomy Z43.2
  insulin pump Z46.81
  myringotomy device (stent) (tube) Z45.82
  nervous system device NEC Z46.2
    brain neuropacemaker Z46.2
    visual substitution device Z46.2
      implanted Z45.31
  non-vascular catheter Z46.82
  organ, prophylactic (for neoplasia management) — *see* Prophylactic, organ removal
  orthodontic device Z46.4
  staples Z48.02
  stent
    ureteral Z46.6
  suture Z48.02
  urinary device Z46.6
  vascular access device or catheter Z45.2
Ren
  arcuatus Q63.1
  mobile, mobilis N28.89
    congenital Q63.8
  unguliformis Q63.1
Renal — *see* condition
Rendu-Osler-Weber disease or syndrome I78.0
Reninoma D41.0- ☑
Renon-Delille syndrome E23.3

Reovirus, as cause of disease classified elsewhere B97.5
Repeated falls NEC R29.6
Replaced chromosome by dicentric ring Q93.2
Replacement by artificial or mechanical device or prosthesis of
  bladder Z96.0
  blood vessel NEC Z95.828
  bone NEC Z96.7
  cochlea Z96.21
  coronary artery Z95.5
  eustachian tube Z96.29
  eye globe Z97.0
  heart Z95.812
    valve Z95.2
      prosthetic Z95.2
      specified NEC Z95.4
      xenogenic Z95.3
  intestine Z96.89
  joint Z96.60
    hip — *see* Presence, hip joint implant
    knee — *see* Presence, knee joint implant
    specified site NEC Z96.698
  larynx Z96.3
  lens Z96.1
  limb(s) — *see* Presence, artificial, limb
  mandible NEC (for tooth root implant(s)) Z96.5
  organ NEC Z96.89
  peripheral vessel NEC Z95.828
  stapes Z96.29
  teeth Z97.2
  tendon Z96.7
  tissue NEC Z96.89
  tooth root(s) Z96.5
  vessel NEC Z95.828
    coronary (artery) Z95.5
Request for expert evidence Z04.8
Reserve, decreased or low
  cardiac — *see* Disease, heart
  kidney N28.89
Residual (*see also* condition)
  ovary syndrome N99.83
  state, schizophrenic F20.5
  urine R39.198
Resistance, resistant (to)
  activated protein C D68.51
  complicating pregnancy O26.89 ☑
  insulin E88.81
  organism(s)
    to
      drug Z16.30
        aminoglycosides Z16.29
        amoxicillin Z16.11
        ampicillin Z16.11
        antibiotic(s) Z16.20
          multiple Z16.24
          specified NEC Z16.29
        antifungal Z16.32
        antimicrobial (single) Z16.30
          multiple Z16.35
          specified NEC Z16.39
        antimycobacterial (single) Z16.341
          multiple Z16.342
        antiparasitic Z16.31
        antiviral Z16.33
        beta lactam antibiotics Z16.10
          specified NEC Z16.19
        cephalosporins Z16.19
        extended beta lactamase (ESBL) Z16.12
        fluoroquinolones Z16.23
        macrolides Z16.29
        methicillin — *see* MRSA
        multiple drugs (MDRO)
          antibiotics Z16.24
          antimicrobial Z16.35
          antimycobacterials Z16.342
        penicillins Z16.11
        quinine (and related compounds) Z16.31
        quinolones Z16.23
        sulfonamides Z16.29
        tetracyclines Z16.29
        tuberculostatics (single) Z16.341
          multiple Z16.342
        vancomycin Z16.21
          related antibiotics Z16.22
  thyroid hormone E07.89
Resorption
  dental (roots) K03.3

Resorption — *continued*
  dental — *continued*
    alveoli M26.79
  teeth (external) (internal) (pathological) (roots) K03.3
Respiration
  Cheyne-Stokes R06.3
  decreased due to shock, following injury T79.4 ☑
  disorder of, psychogenic F45.8
  insufficient, or poor R06.89
    newborn P28.5
  painful R07.1
  sighing, psychogenic F45.8
Respiratory (*see also* condition)
  distress syndrome (newborn) (type I) P22.0
    type II P22.1
  syncytial virus, as cause of disease classified elsewhere B97.4
Respite care Z75.5
Response (drug)
  photoallergic L56.1
  phototoxic L56.0
Restenosis
  stent
    vascular
      end stent
        adjacent to stent — *see* Arteriosclerosis
        within the stent
          coronary T82.855 ☑
          peripheral T82.856 ☑
      in stent
        coronary vessel T82.855 ☑
        peripheral vessel T82.856 ☑
Restless legs (syndrome) G25.81
Restlessness R45.1
Restoration (of)
  dental
    aesthetically inadequate or displeasing K08.56
    defective K08.50
      specified NEC K08.59
    failure of marginal integrity K08.51
    failure of periodontal anatomical intergrity K08.54
  organ continuity from previous sterilization (tuboplasty) (vasoplasty) Z31.0
    aftercare Z31.42
  tooth (existing)
    contours biologically incompatible with oral health K08.54
    open margins K08.51
    overhanging K08.52
    poor aesthetic K08.56
    poor gingival margins K08.51
  unsatisfactory, of tooth K08.50
    specified NEC K08.59
Restorative material (dental)
  allergy to K08.55
  fractured K08.539
    with loss of material K08.531
    without loss of material K08.530
  unrepairable overhanging of K08.52
Restriction of housing space Z59.1
Rests, ovarian, in fallopian tube Q50.6
Restzustand (schizophrenic) F20.5
Retained (*see also* Retention)
  cholelithiasis following cholecystectomy K91.86
  foreign body fragments (type of) Z18.9
    acrylics Z18.2
    animal quill(s) or spines Z18.31
    cement Z18.83
    concrete Z18.83
    crystalline Z18.83
    depleted isotope Z18.09
    depleted uranium Z18.01
    diethylhexylphthalates Z18.2
    glass Z18.81
    isocyanate Z18.2
    magnetic metal Z18.11
    metal Z18.10
    nonmagnectic metal Z18.12
    nontherapeutic radioactive Z18.09
    organic NEC Z18.39
    plastic Z18.2
    quill(s) (animal) Z18.31
    radioactive (nontherapeutic) NEC Z18.09
    specified NEC Z18.89
    spine(s) (animal) Z18.31
    stone Z18.83
    tooth (teeth) Z18.32
    wood Z18.33

Retained — *continued*
　fragments (type of) Z18.9
　　acrylics Z18.2
　　animal quill(s) or spines Z18.31
　　cement Z18.83
　　concrete Z18.83
　　crystalline Z18.83
　　depleted isotope Z18.09
　　depleted uranium Z18.01
　　diethylhexylphthalates Z18.2
　　glass Z18.81
　　isocyanate Z18.2
　　magnetic metal Z18.11
　　metal Z18.10
　　nonmagnectic metal Z18.12
　　nontherapeutic radioactive Z18.09
　　organic NEC Z18.39
　　plastic Z18.2
　　quill(s) (animal) Z18.31
　　radioactive (nontherapeutic) NEC Z18.09
　　specified NEC Z18.89
　　spine(s) (animal) Z18.31
　　stone Z18.83
　　tooth (teeth) Z18.32
　　wood Z18.33
　gallstones, following cholecystectomy K91.86
Retardation
　development, developmental, specific — *see* Disorder, developmental
　endochondral bone growth — *see* Disorder, bone, development or growth
　growth R62.50
　　due to malnutrition E45
　mental — *see* Disability, intellectual
　motor function, specific F82
　physical (child) R62.52
　　due to malnutrition E45
　reading (specific) F81.0
　spelling (specific) (without reading disorder) F81.81
Retching — *see* Vomiting
Retention (*see also* Retained)
　bladder — *see* Retention, urine
　carbon dioxide E87.2
　cholelithiasis following cholecystectomy K91.86
　cyst — *see* Cyst
　dead
　　fetus (at or near term) (mother) O36.4 ☑
　　　early fetal death O02.1
　　ovum O02.0
　decidua (fragments) (following delivery) (with hemorrhage) O72.2
　　without hemorrhage O73.1
　deciduous tooth K00.6
　dental root K08.3
　fecal — *see* Constipation
　fetus
　　dead O36.4 ☑
　　　early O02.1
　fluid R60.9
　foreign body (*see also* Foreign body, retained)
　　current trauma — *code as* Foreign body, by site or type
　gallstones, following cholecystectomy K91.86
　gastric K31.89
　intrauterine contraceptive device, in pregnancy — *see* Pregnancy, complicated by, retention, intrauterine device
　membranes (complicating delivery) (with hemorrhage) O72.2
　　with abortion — *see* Abortion, by type
　　without hemorrhage O73.1
　meniscus — *see* Derangement, meniscus
　menses N94.89
　milk (puerperal, postpartum) O92.79
　nitrogen, extrarenal R39.2
　ovary syndrome N99.83
　placenta (total) (with hemorrhage) O72.0
　　without hemorrhage O73.0
　　portions or fragments (with hemorrhage) O72.2
　　　without hemorrhage O73.1
　products of conception
　　early pregnancy (dead fetus) O02.1
　　following
　　　delivery (with hemorrhage) O72.2
　　　　without hemorrhage O73.1
　secundines (following delivery) (with hemorrhage) O72.0
　　without hemorrhage O73.0

Retention — *continued*
　secundines — *continued*
　　complicating puerperium (delayed hemorrhage) O72.2
　　partial O72.2
　　　without hemorrhage O73.1
　smegma, clitoris N90.89
　urine R33.9
　　drug-induced R33.0
　　due to hyperplasia (hypertrophy) of prostate — *see* Hyperplasia, prostate
　　organic R33.8
　　　drug-induced R33.0
　　psychogenic F45.8
　　specified NEC R33.8
　water (in tissues) — *see* Edema
Reticulation, dust — *see* Pneumoconiosis
Reticulocytosis R70.1
Reticuloendotheliosis
　acute infantile C96.0
　leukemic C91.4- ☑
　nonlipid C96.0
Reticulohistiocytoma (giant-cell) D76.3
Reticuloid, actinic L57.1
Reticulosis (skin)
　acute of infancy C96.0
　hemophagocytic, familial D76.1
　histiocytic medullary C96.A (*following* C96.6)
　lipomelanotic I89.8
　malignant (midline) C86.0
　polymorphic C83.8- ☑
　Sézary — *see* Sézary disease
Retina, retinal (*see also* condition)
　dark area D49.81
Retinitis (*see also* Inflammation, chorioretinal)
　albuminurica N18.9 [H32]
　diabetic — *see* Diabetes, retinitis
　disciformis — *see* Degeneration, macula
　focal — *see* Inflammation, chorioretinal, focal
　gravidarum — *see* Pregnancy, complicated by, specified pregnancy-related condition NEC
　juxtapapillaris — *see* Inflammation, chorioretinal, focal, juxtapapillary
　luetic — *see* Retinitis, syphilitic
　pigmentosa H35.52
　proliferans — *see* Disorder, globe, degenerative, specified type NEC
　proliferating — *see* Disorder, globe, degenerative, specified type NEC
　renal N18.9 [H32]
　syphilitic (early) (secondary) A51.43
　　central, recurrent A52.71
　　congenital (early) A50.01 [H32]
　　late A52.71
　tuberculous A18.53
Retinoblastoma C69.2- ☑
　differentiated C69.2- ☑
　undifferentiated C69.2- ☑
Retinochoroiditis (*see also* Inflammation, chorioretinal)
　disseminated — *see* Inflammation, chorioretinal, disseminated
　　syphilitic A52.71
　focal — *see* Inflammation, chorioretinal
　juxtapapillaris — *see* Inflammation, chorioretinal, focal, juxtapapillary
Retinopathy (background) H35.00
　arteriosclerotic I70.8 [H35.0-] ☑
　atherosclerotic I70.8 [H35.0-] ☑
　central serous — *see* Chorioretinopathy, central serous
　Coats H35.02- ☑
　diabetic — *see* Diabetes, retinopathy
　exudative H35.02- ☑
　hypertensive H35.03- ☑
　in (due to)
　　diabetes — *see* Diabetes, retinopathy
　　sickle-cell disorders D57.- ☑ [H36]
　of prematurity H35.10- ☑
　　stage 0 H35.11- ☑
　　stage 1 H35.12- ☑
　　stage 2 H35.13- ☑
　　stage 3 H35.14- ☑
　　stage 4 H35.15- ☑
　　stage 5 H35.16- ☑
　pigmentary, congenital — *see* Dystrophy, retina
　proliferative NEC H35.2- ☑
　　diabetic — *see* Diabetes, retinopathy, proliferative
　　sickle-cell D57.- ☑ [H36]

Retinopathy — *continued*
　solar H31.02- ☑
Retinoschisis H33.10- ☑
　congenital Q14.1
　specified type NEC H33.19- ☑
Retortamoniasis A07.8
Retractile testis Q55.22
Retraction
　cervix — *see* Retroversion, uterus
　drum (membrane) — *see* Disorder, tympanic membrane, specified NEC
　finger — *see* Deformity, finger
　lid H02.539
　　left H02.536
　　　lower H02.535
　　　upper H02.534
　　right H02.533
　　　lower H02.532
　　　upper H02.531
　lung J98.4
　mediastinum J98.59
　nipple N64.53
　　associated with
　　　lactation O92.03
　　　pregnancy O92.01- ☑
　　　puerperium O92.02
　　congenital Q83.8
　palmar fascia M72.0
　pleura — *see* Pleurisy
　ring, uterus (Bandl's) (pathological) O62.4
　sternum (congenital) Q76.7
　　acquired M95.4
　uterus — *see* Retroversion, uterus
　valve (heart) — *see* Endocarditis
Retrobulbar — *see* condition
Retrocecal — *see* condition
Retrocession — *see* Retroversion
Retrodisplacement — *see* Retroversion
Retroflection, retroflexion — *see* Retroversion
Retrognathia, retrognathism (mandibular) (maxillary) M26.19
Retrograde menstruation N92.5
Retroperineal — *see* condition
Retroperitoneal — *see* condition
Retroperitonitis K68.9
Retropharyngeal — *see* condition
Retroplacental — *see* condition
Retroposition — *see* Retroversion
Retroprosthetic membrane T85.398 ☑
Retrosternal thyroid (congenital) Q89.2
Retroversion, retroverted
　cervix — *see* Retroversion, uterus
　female NEC — *see* Retroversion, uterus
　iris H21.89
　testis (congenital) Q55.29
　uterus (acquired) (acute) (any degree) (asymptomatic) (cervix) (postinfectional) (postpartal, old) N85.4
　　congenital Q51.818
　　in pregnancy O34.53- ☑
Retrovirus, as cause of disease classified elsewhere B97.30
　human
　　immunodeficiency, type 2 (HIV 2) B97.35
　　T-cell lymphotropic
　　　type I (HTLV-I) B97.33
　　　type II (HTLV-II) B97.34
　lentivirus B97.31
　oncovirus B97.32
　specified NEC B97.39
Retrusion, premaxilla (developmental) M26.09
Rett's disease or syndrome F84.2
Reverse peristalsis R19.2
Reye's syndrome G93.7
Rh (factor)
　hemolytic disease (newborn) P55.0
　incompatibility, immunization or sensitization
　　affecting management of pregnancy NEC O36.09- ☑
　　　anti-D antibody O36.01- ☑
　　newborn P55.0
　　transfusion reaction — *see* Complication(s), transfusion, incompatibility reaction, Rh (factor)
　negative mother affecting newborn P55.0
　titer elevated — *see* Complication(s), transfusion, incompatibility reaction, Rh (factor)
　transfusion reaction — *see* Complication(s), transfusion, incompatibility reaction, Rh (factor)

Rhabdomyolysis (idiopathic) NEC M62.82
traumatic T79.6 ☑
Rhabdomyoma (see also Neoplasm, connective tissue, benign)
adult — see Neoplasm, connective tissue, benign
fetal — see Neoplasm, connective tissue, benign
glycogenic — see Neoplasm, connective tissue, benign
Rhabdomyosarcoma (any type) — see Neoplasm, connective tissue, malignant
Rhabdosarcoma — see Rhabdomyosarcoma
Rhesus (factor) **incompatibility** — see Rh, incompatibility
Rheumatic (acute) (subacute) (chronic)
adherent pericardium I09.2
coronary arteritis I01.9
degeneration, myocardium I09.0
fever (acute) — see Fever, rheumatic
heart — see Disease, heart, rheumatic
myocardial degeneration — see Degeneration, myocardium
myocarditis (chronic) (inactive) (with chorea) I09.0
with chorea (acute) (rheumatic) (Sydenham's) I02.0
active or acute I01.2
pancarditis, acute I01.8
with chorea (acute) (rheumatic) Sydenham's) I02.0
pericarditis (active) (acute) (with effusion) (with pneumonia) I01.0
with chorea (acute) (rheumatic) (Sydenham's) I02.0
chronic or inactive I09.2
pneumonia I00 [J17]
torticollis M43.6
typhoid fever A01.09
Rheumatism (articular) (neuralgic) (nonarticular) M79.0
gout — see Arthritis, rheumatoid
intercostal, meaning Tietze's disease M94.0
palindromic (any site) M12.30
ankle M12.37- ☑
elbow M12.32- ☑
foot joint M12.37- ☑
hand joint M12.34- ☑
hip M12.35- ☑
knee M12.36- ☑
multiple site M12.39
shoulder M12.31- ☑
specified joint NEC M12.38
vertebrae M12.38
wrist M12.33- ☑
sciatic M54.4- ☑
Rheumatoid (see also condition)
arthritis (see also Arthritis, rheumatoid)
with involvement of organs NEC M05.60
ankle M05.67- ☑
elbow M05.62- ☑
foot joint M05.67- ☑
hand joint M05.64- ☑
hip M05.65- ☑
knee M05.66- ☑
multiple site M05.69
shoulder M05.61- ☑
vertebra — see Spondylitis, ankylosing
wrist M05.63- ☑
seronegative — see Arthritis, rheumatoid, seronegative
seropositive — see Arthritis, rheumatoid, seropositive
carditis M05.30
ankle M05.37- ☑
elbow M05.32- ☑
foot joint M05.37- ☑
hand joint M05.34- ☑
hip M05.35- ☑
knee M05.36- ☑
multiple site M05.39
shoulder M05.31- ☑
vertebra — see Spondylitis, ankylosing
wrist M05.33- ☑
endocarditis — see Rheumatoid, carditis
lung (disease) M05.10
ankle M05.17- ☑
elbow M05.12- ☑
foot joint M05.17- ☑
hand joint M05.14- ☑
hip M05.15- ☑
knee M05.16- ☑
multiple site M05.19
shoulder M05.11- ☑
vertebra — see Spondylitis, ankylosing

Rheumatoid — continued
lung — continued
wrist M05.13- ☑
myocarditis — see Rheumatoid, carditis
myopathy M05.40
ankle M05.47- ☑
elbow M05.42- ☑
foot joint M05.47- ☑
hand joint M05.44- ☑
hip M05.45- ☑
knee M05.46- ☑
multiple site M05.49
shoulder M05.41- ☑
vertebra — see Spondylitis, ankylosing
wrist M05.43- ☑
pericarditis — see Rheumatoid, carditis
polyarthritis — see Arthritis, rheumatoid
polyneuropathy M05.50
ankle M05.57- ☑
elbow M05.52- ☑
foot joint M05.57- ☑
hand joint M05.54- ☑
hip M05.55- ☑
knee M05.56- ☑
multiple site M05.59
shoulder M05.51- ☑
vertebra — see Spondylitis, ankylosing
wrist M05.53- ☑
vasculitis M05.20
ankle M05.27- ☑
elbow M05.22- ☑
foot joint M05.27- ☑
hand joint M05.24- ☑
hip M05.25- ☑
knee M05.26- ☑
multiple site M05.29
shoulder M05.21- ☑
vertebra — see Spondylitis, ankylosing
wrist M05.23- ☑
Rhinitis (atrophic) (catarrhal) (chronic) (croupous) (fibrinous) (granulomatous) (hyperplastic) (hypertrophic) (membranous) (obstructive) (purulent) (suppurative) (ulcerative) J31.0
with
sore throat — see Nasopharyngitis
acute J00
allergic J30.9
with asthma J45.909
with
exacerbation (acute) J45.901
status asthmaticus J45.902
due to
food J30.5
pollen J30.1
nonseasonal J30.89
perennial J30.89
seasonal NEC J30.2
specified NEC J30.89
infective J00
pneumococcal J00
syphilitic A52.73
congenital A50.05 [J99]
tuberculous A15.8
vasomotor J30.0
Rhinoantritis (chronic) — see Sinusitis, maxillary
Rhinodacryolith — see Dacryolith
Rhinolith (nasal sinus) J34.89
Rhinomegaly J34.89
Rhinopharyngitis (acute) (subacute) (see also Nasopharyngitis)
chronic J31.1
destructive ulcerating A66.5
mutilans A66.5
Rhinophyma L71.1
Rhinorrhea J34.89
cerebrospinal (fluid) G96.0
paroxysmal — see Rhinitis, allergic
spasmodic — see Rhinitis, allergic
Rhinosalpingitis — see Salpingitis, eustachian
Rhinoscleroma A48.8
Rhinosporidiosis B48.1
Rhinovirus infection NEC B34.8
Rhizomelic chondrodysplasia punctata E71.540
Rhythm
atrioventricular nodal I49.8
disorder I49.9
coronary sinus I49.8

Rhythm — continued
disorder — continued
ectopic I49.8
nodal I49.8
escape I49.9
heart, abnormal I49.9
idioventricular I44.2
nodal I49.8
sleep, inversion G47.2- ☑
nonorganic origin — see Disorder, sleep, circadian rhythm, psychogenic
Rhytidosis facialis L98.8
Rib (see also condition)
cervical Q76.5
Riboflavin deficiency E53.0
Rice bodies (see also Loose, body, joint)
knee M23.4- ☑
Richter syndrome — see Leukemia, chronic lymphocytic, B-cell type
Richter's hernia — see Hernia, abdomen, with obstruction
Ricinism — see Poisoning, food, noxious, plant
Rickets (active) (acute) (adolescent) (chest wall) (congenital) (current) (infantile) (intestinal) E55.0
adult — see Osteomalacia
celiac K90.0
hypophosphatemic with nephrotic-glycosuric dwarfism E72.09
inactive E64.3
kidney N25.0
renal N25.0
sequelae, any E64.3
vitamin-D-resistant E83.31 [M90.80]
Rickettsial disease A79.9
specified type NEC A79.89
Rickettsialpox (Rickettsia akari) A79.1
Rickettsiosis A79.9
due to
Ehrlichia sennetsu A79.81
Rickettsia akari (rickettsialpox) A79.1
specified type NEC A79.89
tick-borne A77.9
vesicular A79.1
Rider's bone — see Ossification, muscle, specified NEC
Ridge, alveolus (see also condition)
flabby K06.8
Ridged ear, congenital Q17.3
Riedel's
lobe, liver Q44.7
struma, thyroiditis or disease E06.5
Rieger's anomaly or syndrome Q13.81
Riehl's melanosis L81.4
Rietti-Greppi-Micheli anemia D56.9
Rieux's hernia — see Hernia, abdomen, specified site NEC
Riga (-Fede) **disease** K14.0
Riggs' disease — see Periodontitis
Right aortic arch Q25.47
Right middle lobe syndrome J98.11
Rigid, rigidity (see also condition)
abdominal R19.30
with severe abdominal pain R10.0
epigastric R19.36
generalized R19.37
left lower quadrant R19.34
left upper quadrant R19.32
periumbilic R19.35
right lower quadrant R19.33
right upper quadrant R19.31
articular, multiple, congenital Q68.8
cervix (uteri) in pregnancy — see Pregnancy, complicated by, abnormal, cervix
hymen (acquired) (congenital) N89.6
nuchal R29.1
pelvic floor in pregnancy — see Pregnancy, complicated by, abnormal, pelvic organs or tissues NEC
perineum or vulva in pregnancy — see Pregnancy, complicated by, abnormal, vulva
spine — see Dorsopathy, specified NEC
vagina in pregnancy — see Pregnancy, complicated by, abnormal, vagina
Rigors R68.89
with fever R50.9
Riley-Day syndrome G90.1
RIND (reversible ischemic neurologic deficit) I63.9
Ring(s)
aorta (vascular) Q25.45
Bandl's O62.4

Ring(s) — *continued*
contraction, complicating delivery O62.4
esophageal, lower (muscular) K22.2
Fleischer's (cornea) H18.04- ☑
hymenal, tight (acquired) (congenital) N89.6
Kayser-Fleischer (cornea) H18.04- ☑
retraction, uterus, pathological O62.4
Schatzki's (esophagus) (lower) K22.2
congenital Q39.3
Soemmerring's — *see* Cataract, secondary
vascular (congenital) Q25.8
aorta Q25.45
Ringed hair (congenital) Q84.1
Ringworm B35.9
beard B35.0
black dot B35.0
body B35.4
Burmese B35.5
corporeal B35.4
foot B35.3
groin B35.6
hand B35.2
honeycomb B35.0
nails B35.1
perianal (area) B35.6
scalp B35.0
specified NEC B35.8
Tokelau B35.5
Rise, venous pressure I87.8
Rising, PSA following treatment for malignant neoplasm of prostate R97.21
Risk
for
dental caries Z91.849
high Z91.843
low Z91.841
moderate Z91.842
suicidal
meaning personal history of attempted suicide Z91.5
meaning suicidal ideation — *see* Ideation, suicidal
Ritter's disease L00
Rivalry, sibling Z62.891
Rivalta's disease A42.2
River blindness B73.01
Robert's pelvis Q74.2
with disproportion (fetopelvic) O33.0
causing obstructed labor O65.0
Robin (-Pierre) **syndrome** Q87.0
Robinow-Silvermann-Smith syndrome Q87.1
Robinson's (hidrotic) **ectodermal dysplasia or syndrome** Q82.4
Robles' disease B73.01
Rocky Mountain (spotted) **fever** A77.0
Roetheln — *see* Rubella
Roger's disease Q21.0
Rokitansky-Aschoff sinuses (gallbladder) K82.8
Rolando's fracture (displaced) S62.22- ☑
nondisplaced S62.22- ☑
Romano-Ward (prolonged QT interval) **syndrome** I45.81
Romberg's disease or syndrome G51.8
Roof, mouth — *see* condition
Rosacea L71.9
acne L71.9
keratitis L71.8
specified NEC L71.8
Rosary, rachitic E55.0
Rose
cold J30.1
fever J30.1
rash R21
epidemic B06.9
Rosenbach's erysipeloid A26.0
Rosenthal's disease or syndrome D68.1
Roseola B09
infantum B08.20
due to human herpesvirus 6 B08.21
due to human herpesvirus 7 B08.22
Ross River disease or fever B33.1
Rossbach's disease K31.89
psychogenic F45.8
Rostan's asthma (cardiac) — *see* Failure, ventricular, left
Rotation
anomalous, incomplete or insufficient, intestine Q43.3
cecum (congenital) Q43.3
colon (congenital) Q43.3

Rotation — *continued*
spine, incomplete or insufficient — *see* Dorsopathy, deforming, specified NEC
tooth, teeth, fully erupted M26.35
vertebra, incomplete or insufficient — *see* Dorsopathy, deforming, specified NEC
Rotes Quérol disease or syndrome — *see* Hyperostosis, ankylosing
Roth (-Bernhardt) **disease or syndrome** — *see* Meralgia paraesthetica
Rothmund (-Thomson) **syndrome** Q82.8
Rotor's disease or syndrome E80.6
Round
back (with wedging of vertebrae) — *see* Kyphosis
sequelae (late effect) of rickets E64.3
worms (large) (infestation) NEC B82.0
Ascariasis (*see also* Ascariasis) B77.9
Roussy-Lévy syndrome G60.0
Rubella (German measles) B06.9
complication NEC B06.09
neurological B06.00
congenital P35.0
contact Z20.4
exposure to Z20.4
maternal
care for (suspected) damage to fetus O35.3 ☑
manifest rubella in infant P35.0
suspected damage to fetus affecting management of pregnancy O35.3 ☑
specified complications NEC B06.89
Rubeola (meaning measles) — *see* Measles
meaning rubella — *see* Rubella
Rubeosis, iris — *see* Disorder, iris, vascular
Rubinstein-Taybi syndrome Q87.2
Rudimentary (congenital) (*see also* Agenesis)
arm — *see* Defect, reduction, upper limb
bone Q79.9
cervix uteri Q51.828
eye Q11.2
lobule of ear Q17.3
patella Q74.1
respiratory organs in thoracopagus Q89.4
tracheal bronchus Q32.4
uterus Q51.818
in male Q56.1
vagina Q52.0
Ruled out condition — *see* Observation, suspected
Rumination R11.10
with nausea R11.2
disorder of infancy F98.21
neurotic F42.8
newborn P92.1
obsessional F42.8
psychogenic F42.8
Runeberg's disease D51.0
Runny nose R09.89
Rupia (syphilitic) A51.39
congenital A50.06
tertiary A52.79
Rupture, ruptured
abscess (spontaneous) — *code by* site under Abscess
aneurysm — *see* Aneurysm
anus (sphincter) — *see* Laceration, anus
aorta, aortic I71.8
abdominal I71.3
arch I71.1
ascending I71.1
descending I71.8
abdominal I71.3
thoracic I71.1
syphilitic A52.01
thoracoabdominal I71.5
thorax, thoracic I71.1
transverse I71.1
traumatic — *see* Injury, aorta, laceration, major
valve or cusp (*see also* Endocarditis, aortic) I35.8
appendix (with peritonitis) K35.2
with localized peritonitis K35.3
arteriovenous fistula, brain I60.8
artery I77.2
brain — *see* Hemorrhage, intracranial, intracerebral
coronary — *see* Infarct, myocardium
heart — *see* Infarct, myocardium
pulmonary I28.8
traumatic (complication) — *see* Injury, blood vessel
bile duct (common) (hepatic) K83.2
cystic K82.2

Rupture, ruptured — *continued*
bladder (sphincter) (nontraumatic) (spontaneous) N32.89
following ectopic or molar pregnancy O08.6
obstetrical trauma O71.5
traumatic S37.29 ☑
blood vessel (*see also* Hemorrhage)
brain — *see* Hemorrhage, intracranial, intracerebral
heart — *see* Infarct, myocardium
traumatic (complication) — *see* Injury, blood vessel, laceration, major, by site
bone — *see* Fracture
bowel (nontraumatic) K63.1
brain
aneurysm (congenital) (*see also* Hemorrhage, intracranial, subarachnoid)
syphilitic A52.05
hemorrhagic — *see* Hemorrhage, intracranial, intracerebral
capillaries I78.8
cardiac (auricle) (ventricle) (wall) I23.3
with hemopericardium I23.0
infectional I40.9
traumatic — *see* Injury, heart
cartilage (articular) (current) (*see also* Sprain)
knee S83.3- ☑
semilunar — *see* Tear, meniscus
cecum (with peritonitis) K65.0
with peritoneal abscess K35.3
traumatic S36.598 ☑
celiac artery, traumatic — *see* Injury, blood vessel, celiac artery, laceration, major
cerebral aneurysm (congenital) (*see* Hemorrhage, intracranial, subarachnoid)
cervix (uteri)
with ectopic or molar pregnancy O08.6
following ectopic or molar pregnancy O08.6
obstetrical trauma O71.3
traumatic S37.69 ☑
chordae tendineae NEC I51.1
concurrent with acute myocardial infarction — *see* Infarct, myocardium
following acute myocardial infarction (current complication) I23.4
choroid (direct) (indirect) (traumatic) H31.32- ☑
circle of Willis I60.6
colon (nontraumatic) K63.1
traumatic — *see* Injury, intestine, large
cornea (traumatic) — *see* Injury, eye, laceration
coronary (artery) (thrombotic) — *see* Infarct, myocardium
corpus luteum (infected) (ovary) N83.1- ☑
cyst — *see* Cyst
cystic duct K82.2
Descemet's membrane — *see* Change, corneal membrane, Descemet's, rupture
traumatic — *see* Injury, eye, laceration
diaphragm, traumatic — *see* Injury, intrathoracic, diaphragm
disc — *see* Rupture, intervertebral disc
diverticulum (intestine) K57.80
with bleeding K57.81
bladder N32.3
large intestine K57.20
with
bleeding K57.21
small intestine K57.40
with bleeding K57.41
small intestine K57.00
with
bleeding K57.01
large intestine K57.40
with bleeding K57.41
duodenal stump K31.89
ear drum (nontraumatic) (*see also* Perforation, tympanum)
traumatic S09.2- ☑
due to blast injury — *see* Injury, blast, ear
esophagus K22.3
eye (without prolapse or loss of intraocular tissue) — *see* Injury, eye, laceration
fallopian tube NEC (nonobstetric) (nontraumatic) N83.8
due to pregnancy O00.10- ☑
with intrauterine pregnancy O00.11- ☑
fontanel P13.1
gallbladder K82.2
traumatic S36.128 ☑

Rupture, ruptured — *continued*
gastric (*see also* Rupture, stomach)
  vessel K92.2
globe (eye) (traumatic) — *see* Injury, eye, laceration
graafian follicle (hematoma) N83.0- ☑
heart — *see* Rupture, cardiac
hymen (nontraumatic) (nonintentional) N89.8
internal organ, traumatic — *see* Injury, by site
intervertebral disc — *see* Displacement, intervertebral
  disc
  traumatic — *see* Rupture, traumatic, intervertebral
    disc
intestine NEC (nontraumatic) K63.1
  traumatic — *see* Injury, intestine
iris (*see also* Abnormality, pupillary)
  traumatic — *see* Injury, eye, laceration
joint capsule, traumatic — *see* Sprain
kidney (traumatic) S37.06- ☑
  birth injury P15.8
  nontraumatic N28.89
lacrimal duct (traumatic) — *see* Injury, eye, specified
  site NEC
lens (cataract) (traumatic) — *see* Cataract, traumatic
ligament, traumatic — *see* Rupture, traumatic, ligament, by site
liver S36.116 ☑
  birth injury P15.0
lymphatic vessel I89.8
marginal sinus (placental) (with hemorrhage) — *see*
  Hemorrhage, antepartum, specified cause NEC
membrana tympani (nontraumatic) — *see* Perforation,
  tympanum
membranes (spontaneous)
  artificial
    delayed delivery following O75.5
  delayed delivery following — *see* Pregnancy,
    complicated by, premature rupture of
    membranes
meningeal artery I60.8
meniscus (knee) (*see also* Tear, meniscus)
  old — *see* Derangement, meniscus
  site other than knee — *code as* Sprain
mesenteric artery, traumatic — *see* Injury, mesenteric,
  artery, laceration, major
mesentery (nontraumatic) K66.8
  traumatic — *see* Injury, intra-abdominal, specified,
    site NEC
mitral (valve) I34.8
muscle (traumatic) (*see also* Strain)
  diastasis — *see* Diastasis, muscle
  nontraumatic M62.10
    ankle M62.17- ☑
    foot M62.17- ☑
    forearm M62.13- ☑
    hand M62.14- ☑
    lower leg M62.16- ☑
    pelvic region M62.15- ☑
    shoulder region M62.11- ☑
    specified site NEC M62.18
    thigh M62.15- ☑
    upper arm M62.12- ☑
  traumatic — *see* Strain, by site
musculotendinous junction NEC, nontraumatic — *see*
  Rupture, tendon, spontaneous
mycotic aneurysm causing cerebral hemorrhage —
  see Hemorrhage, intracranial, subarachnoid
myocardium, myocardial — *see* Rupture, cardiac
  traumatic — *see* Injury, heart
nontraumatic, meaning hernia — *see* Hernia
obstructed — *see* Hernia, by site, obstructed
operation wound — *see* Disruption, wound, operation
ovary, ovarian N83.8
  corpus luteum cyst N83.1- ☑
  follicle (graafian) N83.0- ☑
oviduct (nonobstetric) (nontraumatic) N83.8
  due to pregnancy O00.10- ☑
    with intrauterine pregnancy O00.11- ☑
pancreas (nontraumatic) K86.89
  traumatic S36.299 ☑
papillary muscle NEC I51.2
  following acute myocardial infarction (current
    complication) I23.5
pelvic
  floor, complicating delivery O70.1
  organ NEC, obstetrical trauma O71.5
perineum (nonobstetric) (nontraumatic) N90.89

Rupture, ruptured — *continued*
perineum — *continued*
  complicating delivery — *see* Delivery, complicated,
    by, laceration, anus (sphincter)
postoperative wound — *see* Disruption, wound, operation
prostate (traumatic) S37.828 ☑
pulmonary
  artery I28.8
  valve (heart) I37.8
  vein I28.8
  vessel I28.8
pus tube — *see* Salpingitis
pyosalpinx — *see* Salpingitis
rectum (nontraumatic) K63.1
  traumatic S36.69 ☑
retina, retinal (traumatic) (without detachment) (*see
  also* Break, retina)
  with detachment — *see* Detachment, retina, with
    retinal, break
rotator cuff (nontraumatic) M75.10- ☑
  complete M75.12- ☑
  incomplete M75.11- ☑
sclera — *see* Injury, eye, laceration
sigmoid (nontraumatic) K63.1
  traumatic S36.593 ☑
spinal cord (*see also* Injury, spinal cord, by region)
  due to injury at birth P11.5
  newborn (birth injury) P11.5
spleen (traumatic) S36.09 ☑
  birth injury P15.1
  congenital (birth injury) P15.1
  due to P. vivax malaria B51.0
  nontraumatic D73.5
  spontaneous D73.5
splenic vein R58
  traumatic — *see* Injury, blood vessel, splenic vein
stomach (nontraumatic) (spontaneous) K31.89
  traumatic S36.39 ☑
supraspinatus (complete) (incomplete) (nontraumatic)
  — *see* Tear, rotator cuff
symphysis pubis
  obstetric O71.6
  traumatic S33.4 ☑
synovium (cyst) M66.10
  ankle M66.17- ☑
  elbow M66.12- ☑
  finger M66.14- ☑
  foot M66.17- ☑
  forearm M66.13- ☑
  hand M66.14- ☑
  pelvic region M66.15- ☑
  shoulder region M66.11- ☑
  specified site NEC M66.18
  thigh M66.15- ☑
  toe M66.17- ☑
  upper arm M66.12- ☑
  wrist M66.13- ☑
tendon (traumatic) — *see* Strain
  nontraumatic (spontaneous) M66.9
    ankle M66.87- ☑
    extensor M66.20
      ankle M66.27- ☑
      foot M66.27- ☑
      forearm M66.23- ☑
      hand M66.24- ☑
      lower leg M66.26- ☑
      multiple sites M66.29
      pelvic region M66.25- ☑
      shoulder region M66.21- ☑
      specified site NEC M66.28
      thigh M66.25- ☑
      upper arm M66.22- ☑
    flexor M66.30
      ankle M66.37- ☑
      foot M66.37- ☑
      forearm M66.33- ☑
      hand M66.34- ☑
      lower leg M66.36- ☑
      multiple sites M66.39
      pelvic region M66.35- ☑
      shoulder region M66.31- ☑
      specified site NEC M66.38
      thigh M66.35- ☑
      upper arm M66.32- ☑
    foot M66.87- ☑
    forearm M66.83- ☑

Rupture, ruptured — *continued*
tendon — *see* Strain — *continued*
  nontraumatic — *continued*
    hand M66.84- ☑
    lower leg M66.86- ☑
    multiple sites M66.89
    pelvic region M66.85- ☑
    shoulder region M66.81- ☑
    specified
      site NEC M66.88
      tendon M66.80
    thigh M66.85- ☑
    upper arm M66.82- ☑
thoracic duct I89.8
tonsil J35.8
traumatic
  aorta — *see* Injury, aorta, laceration, major
  diaphragm — *see* Injury, intrathoracic, diaphragm
  external site — *see* Wound, open, by site
  eye — *see* Injury, eye, laceration
  internal organ — *see* Injury, by site
  intervertebral disc
    cervical S13.0 ☑
    lumbar S33.0 ☑
    thoracic S23.0 ☑
  kidney S37.06- ☑
  ligament (*see also* Sprain)
    ankle — *see* Sprain, ankle
    carpus — *see* Rupture, traumatic, ligament,
      wrist
    collateral (hand) — *see* Rupture, traumatic,
      ligament, finger, collateral
    finger (metacarpophalangeal) (interphalangeal)
      S63.40- ☑
      collateral S63.41- ☑
        index S63.41- ☑
        little S63.41- ☑
        middle S63.41- ☑
        ring S63.41- ☑
      index S63.40- ☑
      little S63.40- ☑
      middle S63.40- ☑
      palmar S63.42- ☑
        index S63.42- ☑
        little S63.42- ☑
        middle S63.42- ☑
        ring S63.42- ☑
      ring S63.40- ☑
      specified site NEC S63.499 ☑
        index S63.49- ☑
        little S63.49- ☑
        middle S63.49- ☑
        ring S63.49- ☑
      volar plate S63.43- ☑
        index S63.43- ☑
        little S63.43- ☑
        middle S63.43- ☑
        ring S63.43- ☑
    foot — *see* Sprain, foot
    radial collateral S53.2- ☑
    radiocarpal — *see* Rupture, traumatic, ligament,
      wrist, radiocarpal
    ulnar collateral S53.3- ☑
    ulnocarpal — *see* Rupture, traumatic, ligament,
      wrist, ulnocarpal
    wrist S63.30- ☑
      collateral S63.31- ☑
      radiocarpal S63.32- ☑
      specified site NEC S63.39- ☑
      ulnocarpal (palmar) S63.33- ☑
  liver S36.116 ☑
  membrana tympani — *see* Rupture, ear drum,
    traumatic
  muscle or tendon — *see* Strain
  myocardium — *see* Injury, heart
  pancreas S36.299 ☑
  rectum S36.69 ☑
  sigmoid S36.593 ☑
  spleen S36.09 ☑
  stomach S36.39 ☑
  symphysis pubis S33.4 ☑
  tympanum, tympanic (membrane) — *see* Rupture,
    ear drum, traumatic
  ureter S37.19 ☑
  uterus S37.69 ☑
  vagina — *see* Injury, vagina

Rupture, ruptured — *continued*
  traumatic — *continued*
    vena cava — *see* Injury, vena cava, laceration, major
    tricuspid (heart) (valve) I07.8
    tube, tubal (nonobstetric) (nontraumatic) N83.8
      abscess — *see* Salpingitis
      due to pregnancy O00.10- ☑
        with intrauterine pregnancy O00.11- ☑
      tympanum, tympanic (membrane) (nontraumatic)
        (*see also* Perforation, tympanic membrane)
        H72.9- ☑
        traumatic — *see* Rupture, ear drum, traumatic
    umbilical cord, complicating delivery O69.89 ☑
    ureter (traumatic) S37.19 ☑
      nontraumatic N28.89
    urethra (nontraumatic) N36.8
      with ectopic or molar pregnancy O08.6
      following ectopic or molar pregnancy O08.6
      obstetrical trauma O71.5
      traumatic S37.39 ☑
    uterosacral ligament (nonobstetric) (nontraumatic)
      N83.8
    uterus (traumatic) S37.69 ☑
      before labor O71.0- ☑
      during or after labor O71.1
      nonpuerperal, nontraumatic N85.8
      pregnant (during labor) O71.1
        before labor O71.0- ☑
    vagina — *see* Injury, vagina
    valve, valvular (heart) — *see* Endocarditis
    varicose vein — *see* Varix
    varix — *see* Varix
    vena cava R58
      traumatic — *see* Injury, vena cava, laceration, major
    vesical (urinary) N32.89
    vessel (blood) R58
      pulmonary I28.8
      traumatic — *see* Injury, blood vessel
    viscus R19.8
    vulva complicating delivery O70.0
Russell-Silver syndrome Q87.1
Russian spring-summer type encephalitis A84.0
Rust's disease (tuberculous cervical spondylitis) A18.01
Ruvalcaba-Myhre-Smith syndrome E71.440
Rytand-Lipsitch syndrome I44.2

S

Saber, sabre shin or tibia (syphilitic) A50.56 [M90.8-] ☑
Sac lacrimal — *see* condition
Saccharomyces infection B37.9
Saccharopinuria E72.3
Saccular — *see* condition
Sacculation
  aorta (nonsyphilitic) — *see* Aneurysm, aorta
  bladder N32.3
  intralaryngeal (congenital) (ventricular) Q31.3
  larynx (congenital) (ventricular) Q31.3
  organ or site, congenital — *see* Distortion
  pregnant uterus — *see* Pregnancy, complicated by,
    abnormal, uterus
  ureter N28.89
  urethra N36.1
  vesical N32.3
Sachs' amaurotic familial idiocy or disease E75.02
Sachs-Tay disease E75.02
Sacks-Libman disease M32.11
Sacralgia M53.3
Sacralization Q76.49
Sacropinuria E72.3
Sacrodynia M53.3
Sacroiliac joint — *see* condition
Sacroiliitis NEC M46.1
Sacrum — *see* condition
Saddle
  back — *see* Lordosis
  embolus
    abdominal aorta I74.01
    pulmonary artery I26.92
      with acute cor pulmonale I26.02
  injury — *code to* condition
  nose M95.0
    due to syphilis A50.57
Sadism (sexual) F65.52
Sadness, postpartal O90.6
Sadomasochism F65.50
Saemisch's ulcer (cornea) — *see* Ulcer, cornea, central

Sagging
  skin and subcutaneous tissue (following bariatric
    surgery weight loss) (following dietary weight
    loss) L98.7
Sahib disease B55.0
Sailors' skin L57.8
Saint
  Anthony's fire — *see* Erysipelas
  triad — *see* Hernia, diaphragm
  Vitus' dance — *see* Chorea, Sydenham's
Salaam
  attack(s) — *see* Epilepsy, spasms
  tic R25.8
Salicylism
  abuse F55.8
  overdose or wrong substance given — *see* Table of
    Drugs and Chemicals, by drug, poisoning
Salivary duct or gland — *see* condition
Salivation, excessive K11.7
Salmonella — *see* Infection, Salmonella
Salmonellosis A02.0
Salpingitis (catarrhal) (fallopian tube) (nodular) (pseud-
    ofollicular) (purulent) (septic) N70.91
  with oophoritis N70.93
  acute N70.01
    with oophoritis N70.03
  chlamydial A56.11
  chronic N70.11
    with oophoritis N70.13
  complicating abortion — *see* Abortion, by type, com-
    plicated by, salpingitis
  ear — *see* Salpingitis, eustachian
  eustachian (tube) H68.00- ☑
    acute H68.01- ☑
    chronic H68.02- ☑
  follicularis N70.11
    with oophoritis N70.13
  gonococcal (acute) (chronic) A54.24
  interstitial, chronic N70.11
    with oophoritis N70.13
  isthmica nodosa N70.11
    with oophoritis N70.13
  specific (gonococcal) (acute) (chronic) A54.24
  tuberculous (acute) (chronic) A18.17
  venereal (gonococcal) (acute) (chronic) A54.24
Salpingocele N83.4- ☑
Salpingo-oophoritis (catarrhal) (purulent) (ruptured)
    (septic) (suppurative) N70.93
  acute N70.03
    with ectopic or molar pregnancy O08.0
    following ectopic or molar pregnancy O08.0
    gonococcal A54.24
  chronic N70.13
  following ectopic or molar pregnancy O08.0
  gonococcal (acute) (chronic) A54.24
  puerperal O86.19
  specific (gonococcal) (acute) (chronic) A54.24
  subacute N70.03
  tuberculous (acute) (chronic) A18.17
  venereal (gonococcal) (acute) (chronic) A54.24
Salpingo-ovaritis — *see* Salpingo-oophoritis
Salpingoperitonitis — *see* Salpingo-oophoritis
Salzmann's nodular dystrophy — *see* Degeneration,
    cornea, nodular
Sampson's cyst or tumor N80.1
San Joaquin (Valley) **fever** B38.0
Sandblaster's asthma, lung or pneumoconiosis J62.8
Sander's disease (paranoia) F22
Sandfly fever A93.1
Sandhoff's disease E75.01
Sanfilippo (Type B) (Type C) (Type D) **syndrome** E76.22
Sanger-Brown ataxia G11.2
Sao Paulo fever or typhus A77.0
Saponification, mesenteric K65.8
Sarcocele (benign)
  syphilitic A52.76
    congenital A50.59
Sarcocystosis A07.8
Sarcoepiplocele — *see* Hernia
Sarcoepiplomphalocele Q79.2
Sarcoid (*see also* Sarcoidosis)
  arthropathy D86.86
  Boeck's D86.9
  Darier-Roussy D86.3
  iridocyclitis D86.83
  meningitis D86.81
  myocarditis D86.85

Sarcoid — *continued*
  myositis D86.87
  pyelonephritis D86.84
  Spiegler-Fendt L08.89
Sarcoidosis D86.9
  with
    cranial nerve palsies D86.82
    hepatic granuloma D86.89
    polyarthritis D86.86
    tubulo-interstitial nephropathy D86.84
  combined sites NEC D86.89
  lung D86.0
    and lymph nodes D86.2
  lymph nodes D86.1
    and lung D86.2
  meninges D86.81
  skin D86.3
  specified type NEC D86.89
Sarcoma (of) (*see also* Neoplasm, connective tissue, ma-
    lignant)
  alveolar soft part — *see* Neoplasm, connective tissue,
    malignant
  ameloblastic C41.1
    upper jaw (bone) C41.0
  botryoid — *see* Neoplasm, connective tissue, malig-
    nant
  botryoides — *see* Neoplasm, connective tissue, malig-
    nant
  cerebellar C71.6
    circumscribed (arachnoidal) C71.6
  circumscribed (arachnoidal) cerebellar C71.6
  clear cell (*see also* Neoplasm, connective tissue, malig-
    nant)
    kidney C64.- ☑
  dendritic cells (accessory cells) C96.4
  embryonal — *see* Neoplasm, connective tissue, malig-
    nant
  endometrial (stromal) C54.1
    isthmus C54.0
  epithelioid (cell) — *see* Neoplasm, connective tissue,
    malignant
  Ewing's — *see* Neoplasm, bone, malignant
  follicular dendritic cell C96.4
  germinoblastic (diffuse) — *see* Lymphoma, diffuse
    large cell
    follicular — *see* Lymphoma, follicular, specified
      NEC
  giant cell (except of bone) (*see also* Neoplasm, connec-
    tive tissue, malignant)
    bone — *see* Neoplasm, bone, malignant
  glomoid — *see* Neoplasm, connective tissue, malig-
    nant
  granulocytic C92.3- ☑
  hemangioendothelial — *see* Neoplasm, connective
    tissue, malignant
  hemorrhagic, multiple — *see* Sarcoma, Kaposi's
  histiocytic C96.A (*following* C96.6)
  Hodgkin — *see* Lymphoma, Hodgkin
  immunoblastic (diffuse) — *see* Lymphoma, diffuse
    large cell
  interdigitating dendritic cell C96.4
  Kaposi's
    colon C46.4
    connective tissue C46.1
    gastrointestinal organ C46.4
    lung C46.5- ☑
    lymph node(s) C46.3
    palate (hard) (soft) C46.2
    rectum C46.4
    skin C46.0
    specified site NEC C46.7
    stomach C46.4
    unspecified site C46.9
  Kupffer cell C22.3
  Langerhans cell C96.4
  leptomeningeal — *see* Neoplasm, meninges, malig-
    nant
  liver NEC C22.4
  lymphangioendothelial — *see* Neoplasm, connective
    tissue, malignant
  lymphoblastic — *see* Lymphoma, lymphoblastic (dif-
    fuse)
  lymphocytic — *see* Lymphoma, small cell B-cell
  mast cell C96.22
  melanotic — *see* Melanoma
  meningeal — *see* Neoplasm, meninges, malignant
  meningothelial — *see* Neoplasm, meninges, malignant

Sarcoma — *continued*
  mesenchymal (*see also* Neoplasm, connective tissue, malignant)
    mixed — *see* Neoplasm, connective tissue, malignant
  mesothelial — *see* Mesothelioma
  monstrocellular
    specified site — *see* Neoplasm, malignant, by site
    unspecified site C71.9
  myeloid C92.3- ☑
  neurogenic — *see* Neoplasm, nerve, malignant
  odontogenic C41.1
    upper jaw (bone) C41.0
  osteoblastic — *see* Neoplasm, bone, malignant
  osteogenic (*see also* Neoplasm, bone, malignant)
    juxtacortical — *see* Neoplasm, bone, malignant
    periosteal — *see* Neoplasm, bone, malignant
  periosteal (*see also* Neoplasm, bone, malignant)
    osteogenic — *see* Neoplasm, bone, malignant
  pleomorphic cell — *see* Neoplasm, connective tissue, malignant
  reticulum cell (diffuse) — *see* Lymphoma, diffuse large cell
    nodular — *see* Lymphoma, follicular
    pleomorphic cell type — *see* Lymphoma, diffuse large cell
  rhabdoid — *see* Neoplasm, malignant, by site
  round cell — *see* Neoplasm, connective tissue, malignant
  small cell — *see* Neoplasm, connective tissue, malignant
  soft tissue — *see* Neoplasm, connective tissue, malignant
  spindle cell — *see* Neoplasm, connective tissue, malignant
  stromal (endometrial) C54.1
    isthmus C54.0
  synovial (*see also* Neoplasm, connective tissue, malignant)
    biphasic — *see* Neoplasm, connective tissue, malignant
    epithelioid cell — *see* Neoplasm, connective tissue, malignant
    spindle cell — *see* Neoplasm, connective tissue, malignant
Sarcomatosis
  meningeal — *see* Neoplasm, meninges, malignant
  specified site NEC — *see* Neoplasm, connective tissue, malignant
  unspecified site C80.1
Sarcopenia (age-related) M62.84
Sarcosinemia E72.59
Sarcosporidiosis (intestinal) A07.8
Satiety, early R68.81
Saturnine — *see* condition
Saturnism
  overdose or wrong substance given or taken — *see* Table of Drugs and Chemicals, by drug, poisoning
Satyriasis F52.8
Sauriasis — *see* Ichthyosis
SBE (subacute bacterial endocarditis) I33.0
Scabies (any site) B86
Scabs R23.4
Scaglietti-Dagnini syndrome E22.0
Scald — *see* Burn
Scalenus anticus (anterior) **syndrome** G54.0
Scales R23.4
Scaling, skin R23.4
Scalp — *see* condition
Scapegoating affecting child Z62.3
Scaphocephaly Q75.0
Scapulalgia M89.8X1
Scapulohumeral myopathy G71.0
Scar, scarring (*see also* Cicatrix) L90.5
  adherent L90.5
  atrophic L90.5
  cervix
    in pregnancy or childbirth — *see* Pregnancy, complicated by, abnormal cervix
  cheloid L91.0
  chorioretinal H31.00- ☑
    posterior pole macula H31.01- ☑
    postsurgical H59.81- ☑
    solar retinopathy H31.02- ☑
    specified type NEC H31.09- ☑
  choroid — *see* Scar, chorioretinal

Scar, scarring — *continued*
  conjunctiva H11.24- ☑
  cornea H17.9
    xerophthalmic (*see also* Opacity, cornea)
      vitamin A deficiency E50.6
  duodenum, obstructive K31.5
  hypertrophic L91.0
  keloid L91.0
  labia N90.89
  lung (base) J98.4
  macula — *see* Scar, chorioretinal, posterior pole
  muscle M62.89
  myocardium, myocardial I25.2
  painful L90.5
  posterior pole (eye) — *see* Scar, chorioretinal, posterior pole
  retina — *see* Scar, chorioretinal
  trachea J39.8
  transmural uterine, in pregnancy O34.29
  uterus N85.8
    in pregnancy O34.29
  vagina N89.8
    postoperative N99.2
  vulva N90.89
Scarabiasis B88.2
Scarlatina (anginosa) (maligna) A38.9
  myocarditis (acute) A38.1
    old — *see* Myocarditis
  otitis media A38.0
  ulcerosa A38.8
Scarlet fever (albuminuria) (angina) A38.9
Schamberg's disease (progressive pigmentary dermatosis) L81.7
Schatzki's ring (acquired) (esophagus) (lower) K22.2
  congenital Q39.3
Schaufenster krankheit I20.8
Schaumann's
  benign lymphogranulomatosis D86.1
  disease or syndrome — *see* Sarcoidosis
Scheie's syndrome E76.03
Schenck's disease B42.1
Scheuermann's disease or osteochondrosis — *see* Osteochondrosis, juvenile, spine
Schilder (-Flatau) **disease** G37.0
Schilling-type monocytic leukemia C93.0- ☑
Schimmelbusch's disease, cystic mastitis, or hyperplasia — *see* Mastopathy, cystic
Schistosoma infestation — *see* Infestation, Schistosoma
Schistosomiasis B65.9
  with muscle disorder B65.9 [M63.80]
    ankle B65.9 [M63.87-] ☑
    foot B65.9 [M63.87-] ☑
    forearm B65.9 [M63.83-] ☑
    hand B65.9 [M63.84-] ☑
    lower leg B65.9 [M63.86-] ☑
    multiple sites B65.9 [M63.89]
    pelvic region B65.9 [M63.85-] ☑
    shoulder region B65.9 [M63.81-] ☑
    specified site NEC B65.9 [M63.88]
    thigh B65.9 [M63.85-] ☑
    upper arm B65.9 [M63.82-] ☑
  Asiatic B65.2
  bladder B65.0
  chestermani B65.8
  colon B65.1
  cutaneous B65.3
  due to
    S. haematobium B65.0
    S. japonicum B65.2
    S. mansoni B65.1
    S. mattheii B65.8
  Eastern B65.2
  genitourinary tract B65.0
  intestinal B65.1
  lung NEC B65.9 [J99]
    pneumonia B65.9 [J17]
  Manson's (intestinal) B65.1
  oriental B65.2
  pulmonary NEC B65.9 [J99]
    pneumonia B65.9
  Schistosoma
    haematobium B65.0
    japonicum B65.2
    mansoni B65.1
  specified type NEC B65.8
  urinary B65.0
  vesical B65.0
Schizencephaly Q04.6

Schizoaffective psychosis F25.9
Schizodontia K00.2
Schizoid personality F60.1
Schizophrenia, schizophrenic F20.9
  acute (brief) (undifferentiated) F23
  atypical (form) F20.3
  borderline F21
  catalepsy F20.2
  catatonic (type) (excited) (withdrawn) F20.2
  cenesthopathic, cenesthesiopathic F20.89
  childhood type F84.5
  chronic undifferentiated F20.5
  cyclic F25.0
  disorganized (type) F20.1
  flexibilitas cerea F20.2
  hebephrenic (type) F20.1
  incipient F21
  latent F21
  negative type F20.5
  paranoid (type) F20.0
  paraphrenic F20.0
  post-psychotic depression F32.89
  prepsychotic F21
  prodromal F21
  pseudoneurotic F21
  pseudopsychopathic F21
  reaction F23
  residual (state) (type) F20.5
  restzustand F20.5
  schizoaffective (type) — *see* Psychosis, schizoaffective
  simple (type) F20.89
  simplex F20.89
  specified type NEC F20.89
  spectrum and other psychotic disorder F29
    specified NEC F28
  stupor F20.2
  syndrome of childhood F84.5
  undifferentiated (type) F20.3
    chronic F20.5
Schizothymia (persistent) F60.1
Schlatter-Osgood disease or osteochondrosis — *see* Osteochondrosis, juvenile, tibia
Schlatter's tibia — *see* Osteochondrosis, juvenile, tibia
Schmidt's syndrome (polyglandular, autoimmune) E31.0
Schmincke's carcinoma or tumor — *see* Neoplasm, nasopharynx, malignant
Schmitz (-Stutzer) **dysentery** A03.0
Schmorl's disease or nodes
  lumbar region M51.46
  lumbosacral region M51.47
  sacrococcygeal region M53.3
  thoracic region M51.44
  thoracolumbar region M51.45
Schneiderian
  papilloma — *see* Neoplasm, nasopharynx, benign
    specified site — *see* Neoplasm, benign, by site
    unspecified site D14.0
  specified site — *see* Neoplasm, malignant, by site
    unspecified site C30.0
Scholte's syndrome (malignant carcinoid) E34.0
Scholz (-Bielchowsky-Henneberg) **disease or syndrome** E75.25
Schönlein (-Henoch) disease or purpura (primary) (rheumatic) D69.0
Schottmuller's disease A01.4
Schroeder's syndrome (endocrine hypertensive) E27.0
Schüller-Christian disease or syndrome C96.5
Schultze's type acroparesthesia, simple I73.89
Schultz's disease or syndrome — *see* Agranulocytosis
Schwalbe-Ziehen-Oppenheim disease G24.1
Schwannoma (*see also* Neoplasm, nerve, benign)
  malignant (*see also* Neoplasm, nerve, malignant)
    with rhabdomyoblastic differentiation — *see* Neoplasm, nerve, malignant
  melanocytic — *see* Neoplasm, nerve, benign
  pigmented — *see* Neoplasm, nerve, benign
Schwannomatosis Q85.03
Schwartz (-Jampel) **syndrome** G71.13
Schwartz-Bartter syndrome E22.2
Schweniger-Buzzi anetoderma L90.1
Sciatic — *see* condition
Sciatica (infective)
  with lumbago M54.4- ☑
    due to intervertebral disc disorder — *see* Disorder, disc, with, radiculopathy
  due to displacement of intervertebral disc (with lumbago) — *see* Disorder, disc, with, radiculopathy

☑ **Additional Character Required** — Refer to the Tabular List for Character Selection   ▽ **Subterms under main terms may continue to next column or page**

Sciatica — *continued*
  wallet M54.3- ☑

Scimitar syndrome Q26.8

Sclera — *see* condition

Sclerectasia H15.84- ☑

Scleredema
  adultorum — *see* Sclerosis, systemic
  Buschke's — *see* Sclerosis, systemic
  newborn P83.0

Sclerema (adiposum) (edematosum) (neonatorum) (newborn) P83.0
  adultorum — *see* Sclerosis, systemic

Scleriasis — *see* Scleroderma

Scleritis H15.00- ☑
  with corneal involvement H15.04- ☑
  anterior H15.01- ☑
  brawny H15.02- ☑
  in (due to) zoster B02.34
  posterior H15.03- ☑
  specified type NEC H15.09- ☑
  syphilitic A52.71
  tuberculous (nodular) A18.51

Sclerochoroiditis H31.8

Scleroconjunctivitis — *see* Scleritis

Sclerocystic ovary syndrome E28.2

Sclerodactyly, sclerodactylia L94.3

Scleroderma, sclerodermia (acrosclerotic) (diffuse) (generalized) (progressive) (pulmonary) (*see also* Sclerosis, systemic) M34.9
  circumscribed L94.0
  linear L94.1
  localized L94.0
  newborn P83.88
  systemic M34.9

Sclerokeratitis H16.8
  tuberculous A18.52

Scleroma nasi A48.8

Scleromalacia (perforans) H15.05- ☑

Scleromyxedema L98.5

Sclérose en plaques G35

Sclerosis, sclerotic
  adrenal (gland) E27.8
  Alzheimer's — *see* Disease, Alzheimer's
  amyotrophic (lateral) G12.21
  aorta, aortic I70.0
    valve — *see* Endocarditis, aortic
  artery, arterial, arteriolar, arteriovascular — *see* Arteriosclerosis
  ascending multiple G35
  brain (generalized) (lobular) G37.9
    artery, arterial I67.2
    diffuse G37.0
    disseminated G35
    insular G35
    Krabbe's E75.23
    miliary G35
    multiple G35
    presenile (Alzheimer's) — *see* Disease, Alzheimer's, early onset
    senile (arteriosclerotic) I67.2
    stem, multiple G35
    tuberous Q85.1
  bulbar, multiple G35
  bundle of His I44.39
  cardiac — *see* Disease, heart, ischemic, atherosclerotic
  cardiorenal — *see* Hypertension, cardiorenal
  cardiovascular (*see also* Disease, cardiovascular)
    renal — *see* Hypertension, cardiorenal
  cerebellar — *see* Sclerosis, brain
  cerebral — *see* Sclerosis, brain
  cerebrospinal (disseminated) (multiple) G35
  cerebrovascular I67.2
  choroid — *see* Degeneration, choroid
  combined (spinal cord) (*see also* Degeneration, combined)
    multiple G35
  concentric (Balo) G37.5
  cornea — *see* Opacity, cornea
  coronary (artery) I25.10
    with angina pectoris — *see* Arteriosclerosis, coronary (artery),
  corpus cavernosum
    female N90.89
    male N48.6
  diffuse (brain) (spinal cord) G37.0
  disseminated G35
  dorsal G35

Sclerosis, sclerotic — *continued*
  dorsolateral (spinal cord) — *see* Degeneration, combined
  endometrium N85.5
  extrapyramidal G25.9
  eye, nuclear (senile) — *see* Cataract, senile, nuclear
  focal and segmental (glomerular) (*see also* N00-N07 with fourth character .1) N05.1
  Friedreich's (spinal cord) G11.1
  funicular (spermatic cord) N50.89
  general (vascular) — *see* Arteriosclerosis
  gland (lymphatic) I89.8
  hepatic K74.1
    alcoholic K70.2
  hereditary
    cerebellar G11.9
    spinal (Friedreich's ataxia) G11.1
  hippocampal G93.81
  insular G35
  kidney — *see* Sclerosis, renal
  larynx J38.7
  lateral (amyotrophic) (descending) (spinal) G12.21
    primary G12.23
  lens, senile nuclear — *see* Cataract, senile, nuclear
  liver K74.1
    with fibrosis K74.2
      alcoholic K70.2
    alcoholic K70.2
    cardiac K76.1
  lung — *see* Fibrosis, lung
  mastoid — *see* Mastoiditis, chronic
  mesial temporal G93.81
  mitral I05.8
  Mönckeberg's (medial) — *see* Arteriosclerosis, extremities
  multiple (brain stem) (cerebral) (generalized) (spinal cord) G35
  myocardium, myocardial — *see* Disease, heart, ischemic, atherosclerotic
  nuclear (senile), eye — *see* Cataract, senile, nuclear
  ovary N83.8
  pancreas K86.89
  penis N48.6
  peripheral arteries — *see* Arteriosclerosis, extremities
  plaques G35
  pluriglandular E31.8
  polyglandular E31.8
  posterolateral (spinal cord) — *see* Degeneration, combined
  presenile (Alzheimer's) — *see* Disease, Alzheimer's, early onset
  primary, lateral G12.23
  progressive, systemic M34.0
  pulmonary — *see* Fibrosis, lung
    artery I27.0
    valve (heart) — *see* Endocarditis, pulmonary
  renal N26.9
    with
      cystine storage disease E72.09
      hypertensive heart disease (conditions in I11) — *see* Hypertension, cardiorenal
      arteriolar (hyaline) (hyperplastic) — *see* Hypertension, kidney
  retina (senile) (vascular) H35.00
  senile (vascular) — *see* Arteriosclerosis
  spinal (cord) (progressive) G95.89
    ascending G61.0
    combined (*see also* Degeneration, combined)
      multiple G35
      syphilitic A52.11
    disseminated G35
    dorsolateral — *see* Degeneration, combined
    hereditary (Friedreich's) (mixed form) G11.1
    lateral (amyotrophic) G12.23
    multiple G35
    posterior (syphilitic) A52.11
  stomach K31.89
  subendocardial, congenital I42.4
  systemic M34.9
    with
      lung involvement M34.81
      myopathy M34.82
      polyneuropathy M34.83
    drug-induced M34.2
    due to chemicals NEC M34.2
    progressive M34.0
    specified NEC M34.89
  temporal (mesial) G93.81

Sclerosis, sclerotic — *continued*
  tricuspid (heart) (valve) I07.8
  tuberous (brain) Q85.1
  tympanic membrane — *see* Disorder, tympanic membrane, specified NEC
  valve, valvular (heart) — *see* Endocarditis
  vascular — *see* Arteriosclerosis
  vein I87.8

Scoliosis (acquired) (postural) M41.9
  adolescent (idiopathic) — *see* Scoliosis, idiopathic, adolescent
  congenital Q67.5
    due to bony malformation Q76.3
    failure of segmentation (hemivertebra) Q76.3
    hemivertebra fusion Q76.3
    postural Q67.5
  idiopathic M41.20
    adolescent M41.129
      cervical region M41.122
      cervicothoracic region M41.123
      lumbar region M41.126
      lumbosacral region M41.127
      thoracic region M41.124
      thoracolumbar region M41.125
    cervical region M41.22
    cervicothoracic region M41.23
    infantile M41.00
      cervical region M41.02
      cervicothoracic region M41.03
      lumbar region M41.06
      lumbosacral region M41.07
      sacrococcygeal region M41.08
      thoracic region M41.04
      thoracolumbar region M41.05
    juvenile M41.119
      cervical region M41.112
      cervicothoracic region M41.113
      lumbar region M41.116
      lumbosacral region M41.117
      thoracic region M41.114
      thoracolumbar region M41.115
    lumbar region M41.26
    lumbosacral region M41.27
    thoracic region M41.24
    thoracolumbar region M41.25
  infantile — *see* Scoliosis, idiopathic, infantile
  neuromuscular M41.40
    cervical region M41.42
    cervicothoracic region M41.43
    lumbar region M41.46
    lumbosacral region M41.47
    occipito-atlanto-axial region M41.41
    thoracic region M41.44
    thoracolumbar region M41.45
  paralytic — *see* Scoliosis, neuromuscular
  postradiation therapy M96.5
  rachitic (late effect or sequelae) E64.3 [M49.80]
    cervical region E64.3 [M49.82]
    cervicothoracic region E64.3 [M49.83]
    lumbar region E64.3 [M49.86]
    lumbosacral region E64.3 [M49.87]
    multiple sites E64.3 [M49.89]
    occipito-atlanto-axial region E64.3 [M49.81]
    sacrococcygeal region E64.3 [M49.88]
    thoracic region E64.3 [M49.84]
    thoracolumbar region E64.3 [M49.85]
  sciatic M54.4- ☑
  secondary (to) NEC M41.50
    cerebral palsy, Friedreich's ataxia, poliomyelitis, neuromuscular disorders — *see* Scoliosis, neuromuscular
    cervical region M41.52
    cervicothoracic region M41.53
    lumbar region M41.56
    lumbosacral region M41.57
    thoracic region M41.54
    thoracolumbar region M41.55
  specified form NEC M41.80
    cervical region M41.82
    cervicothoracic region M41.83
    lumbar region M41.86
    lumbosacral region M41.87
    thoracic region M41.84
    thoracolumbar region M41.85
  thoracogenic M41.30
    thoracic region M41.34
    thoracolumbar region M41.35
  tuberculous A18.01

Index

Sciatica — Scoliosis

Scoliotic pelvis
with disproportion (fetopelvic) O33.Ø
causing obstructed labor O65.Ø
Scorbutus, scorbutic (*see also* Scurvy)
anemia D53.2
Score, NIHSS (National Institutes of Health Stroke Scale)
R29.7- ☑
Scotoma (arcuate) (Bjerrum) (central) (ring) (*see also*
Defect, visual field, localized, scotoma)
scintillating H53.19
Scratch — *see* Abrasion
Scratchy throat R09.89
Screening (for) Z13.9
alcoholism Z13.89
anemia Z13.Ø
anomaly, congenital Z13.89
antenatal, of mother (*see also* Encounter, antenatal
screening) Z36.9
arterial hypertension Z13.6
arthropod-borne viral disease NEC Z11.59
bacteriuria, asymptomatic Z13.89
behavioral disorder Z13.89
brain injury, traumatic Z13.85Ø
bronchitis, chronic Z13.83
brucellosis Z11.2
cardiovascular disorder Z13.6
cataract Z13.5
chlamydial diseases Z11.8
cholera Z11.Ø
chromosomal abnormalities (nonprocreative) NEC
Z13.79
colonoscopy Z12.11
congenital
dislocation of hip Z13.89
eye disorder Z13.5
malformation or deformation Z13.89
contamination NEC Z13.88
cystic fibrosis Z13.228
dengue fever Z11.59
dental disorder Z13.84
depression Z13.89
developmental handicap Z13.4
in early childhood Z13.4
infant Z13.4
diabetes mellitus Z13.1
diphtheria Z11.2
disability, intellectual Z13.4
infant Z13.4
disease or disorder Z13.9
bacterial NEC Z11.2
intestinal infectious Z11.Ø
respiratory tuberculosis Z11.1
blood or blood-forming organ Z13.Ø
cardiovascular Z13.6
Chagas' Z11.6
chlamydial Z11.8
dental Z13.89
developmental Z13.4
in child Z13.4
infant Z13.4
digestive tract NEC Z13.818
lower GI Z13.811
upper GI Z13.81Ø
ear Z13.5
endocrine Z13.29
eye Z13.5
genitourinary Z13.89
heart Z13.6
human immunodeficiency virus (HIV) infection
Z11.4
immunity Z13.Ø
infection
intestinal Z11.Ø
specified NEC Z11.6
infectious Z11.9
mental Z13.89
metabolic Z13.228
neurological Z13.89
nutritional Z13.21
metabolic Z13.228
lipoid disorders Z13.22Ø
protozoal Z11.6
intestinal Z11.Ø
respiratory Z13.83
rheumatic Z13.828
rickettsial Z11.8
sexually-transmitted NEC Z11.3
human immunodeficiency virus (HIV) Z11.4

Screening — *continued*
disease or disorder — *continued*
sickle-cell (trait) Z13.Ø
skin Z13.89
specified NEC Z13.89
spirochetal Z11.8
thyroid Z13.29
vascular Z13.6
venereal Z11.3
viral NEC Z11.59
human immunodeficiency virus (HIV) Z11.4
intestinal Z11.Ø
elevated titer Z13.89
emphysema Z13.83
encephalitis, viral (mosquito- or tick-borne) Z11.59
exposure to contaminants (toxic) Z13.88
fever
dengue Z11.59
hemorrhagic Z11.59
yellow Z11.59
filariasis Z11.6
galactosemia Z13.228
gastrointestinal condition Z13.818
genetic (nonprocreative) - for procreative management — *see* Testing, genetic, for procreative
management
disease carrier status (nonprocreative) Z13.71
specified NEC (nonprocreative) Z13.79
genitourinary condition Z13.89
glaucoma Z13.5
gonorrhea Z11.3
gout Z13.89
helminthiasis (intestinal) Z11.6
hematopoietic malignancy Z12.89
hemoglobinopathies NEC Z13.Ø
hemorrhagic fever Z11.59
Hodgkin disease Z12.89
human immunodeficiency virus (HIV) Z11.4
human papillomavirus Z11.51
hypertension Z13.6
immunity disorders Z13.Ø
infection
mycotic Z11.8
parasitic Z11.8
ingestion of radioactive substance Z13.88
intellectual disability Z13.4
infant Z13.4
intestinal
helminthiasis Z11.6
infectious disease Z11.Ø
leishmaniasis Z11.6
leprosy Z11.2
leptospirosis Z11.8
leukemia Z12.89
lymphoma Z12.89
malaria Z11.6
malnutrition Z13.29
metabolic Z13.228
nutritional Z13.21
measles Z11.59
mental disorder Z13.89
metabolic errors, inborn Z13.228
multiphasic Z13.89
musculoskeletal disorder Z13.828
osteoporosis Z13.82Ø
mycoses Z11.8
myocardial infarction (acute) Z13.6
neoplasm (malignant) (of) Z12.9
bladder Z12.6
blood Z12.89
breast Z12.39
routine mammogram Z12.31
cervix Z12.4
colon Z12.11
genitourinary organs NEC Z12.79
bladder Z12.6
cervix Z12.4
ovary Z12.73
prostate Z12.5
testis Z12.71
vagina Z12.72
hematopoietic system Z12.89
intestinal tract Z12.1Ø
colon Z12.11
rectum Z12.12
small intestine Z12.13
lung Z12.2
lymph (glands) Z12.89
nervous system Z12.82

Screening — *continued*
neoplasm — *continued*
oral cavity Z12.81
prostate Z12.5
rectum Z12.12
respiratory organs Z12.2
skin Z12.83
small intestine Z12.13
specified site NEC Z12.89
stomach Z12.Ø
nephropathy Z13.89
nervous system disorders NEC Z13.858
neurological condition Z13.89
osteoporosis Z13.82Ø
parasitic infestation Z11.9
specified NEC Z11.8
phenylketonuria Z13.228
plague Z11.2
poisoning (chemical) (heavy metal) Z13.88
poliomyelitis Z11.59
postnatal, chromosomal abnormalities Z13.89
prenatal, of mother (*see also* Encounter, antenatal
screening) Z36.9
protozoal disease Z11.6
intestinal Z11.Ø
pulmonary tuberculosis Z11.1
radiation exposure Z13.88
respiratory condition Z13.83
respiratory tuberculosis Z11.1
rheumatoid arthritis Z13.828
rubella Z11.59
schistosomiasis Z11.6
sexually-transmitted disease NEC Z11.3
human immunodeficiency virus (HIV) Z11.4
sickle-cell disease or trait Z13.Ø
skin condition Z13.89
sleeping sickness Z11.6
special Z13.9
specified NEC Z13.89
syphilis Z11.3
tetanus Z11.2
trachoma Z11.8
traumatic brain injury Z13.85Ø
trypanosomiasis Z11.6
tuberculosis, respiratory Z11.1
venereal disease Z11.3
viral encephalitis (mosquito- or tick-borne) Z11.59
whooping cough Z11.2
worms, intestinal Z11.6
yaws Z11.8
yellow fever Z11.59
Scrofula, scrofulosis (tuberculosis of cervical lymph
glands) A18.2
Scrofulide (primary) (tuberculous) A18.4
Scrofuloderma, scrofulodermia (any site) (primary)
A18.4
Scrofulosus lichen (primary) (tuberculous) A18.4
Scrofulous — *see* condition
Scrotal tongue K14.5
Scrotum — *see* condition
Scurvy, scorbutic E54
anemia D53.2
gum E54
infantile E54
rickets E55.Ø [M90.8Ø]
Sealpox B08.62
Seasickness T75.3 ☑
Seatworm (infection) (infestation) B8Ø
Sebaceous (*see also* condition)
cyst — *see* Cyst, sebaceous
Seborrhea, seborrheic L21.9
capillitii R23.8
capitis L21.Ø
dermatitis L21.9
infantile L21.1
eczema L21.9
infantile L21.1
sicca L21.Ø
Seckel's syndrome Q87.1
Seclusion, pupil — *see* Membrane, pupillary
Second hand tobacco smoke exposure (acute)
(chronic) Z77.22
in the perinatal period P96.81
Secondary
dentin (in pulp) KØ4.3
neoplasm, secondaries — *see* Table of Neoplasms,
secondary

Secretion
- antidiuretic hormone, inappropriate E22.2
- catecholamine, by pheochromocytoma E27.5
- hormone
  - antidiuretic, inappropriate (syndrome) E22.2
    - by
      - carcinoid tumor E34.0
      - pheochromocytoma E27.5
    - ectopic NEC E34.2
- urinary
  - excessive R35.8
  - suppression R34

Section
- nerve, traumatic — *see* Injury, nerve

Sedative, hypnotic, or anxiolytic-induced
- anxiety disorder F13.980
- bipolar and related disorder F13.94
- delirium F13.921
- depressive disorder F13.94
- major neurocognitive disorder F13.97
- mild neurocognitive disorder F13.988
- psychotic disorder F13.959
- sexual dysfunction F13.981
- sleep disorder F13.982

Segmentation, incomplete (congenital) (*see also* Fusion)
- bone NEC Q78.8
- lumbosacral (joint) (vertebra) Q76.49

Seitelberger's syndrome (infantile neuraxonal dystrophy) G31.89

Seizure(s) (*see also* Convulsions) R56.9
- akinetic — *see* Epilepsy, generalized, specified NEC
- atonic — *see* Epilepsy, generalized, specified NEC
- autonomic (hysterical) F44.5
- convulsive — *see* Convulsions
- cortical (focal) (motor) — *see* Epilepsy, localization-related, symptomatic, with simple partial seizures
- disorder (*see also* Epilepsy) G40.909
- due to stroke — *see* Sequelae (of), disease, cerebrovascular, by type, specified NEC
- epileptic — *see* Epilepsy
- febrile (simple) R56.00
  - with status epilepticus G40.901
  - complex (atypical) (complicated) R56.01
    - with status epilepticus G40.901
- grand mal G40.409
  - intractable G40.419
    - with status epilepticus G40.411
    - without status epilepticus G40.419
  - not intractable G40.409
    - with status epilepticus G40.401
    - without status epilepticus G40.409
- heart — *see* Disease, heart
- hysterical F44.5
- intractable G40.919
  - with status epilepticus G40.911
- Jacksonian (focal) (motor type) (sensory type) — *see* Epilepsy, localization-related, symptomatic, with simple partial seizures
- newborn P90
- nonspecific epileptic
  - atonic — *see* Epilepsy, generalized, specified NEC
  - clonic — *see* Epilepsy, generalized, specified NEC
  - myoclonic — *see* Epilepsy, generalized, specified NEC
  - tonic — *see* Epilepsy, generalized, specified NEC
  - tonic-clonic — *see* Epilepsy, generalized, specified NEC
- partial, developing into secondarily generalized seizures
  - complex — *see* Epilepsy, localization-related, symptomatic, with complex partial seizures
  - simple — *see* Epilepsy, localization-related, symptomatic, with simple partial seizures
- petit mal G40.409
  - intractable G40.419
    - with status epilepticus G40.411
    - without status epilepticus G40.419
  - not intractable G40.409
    - with status epilepticus G40.401
    - without status epilepticus G40.409
- post traumatic R56.1
- recurrent G40.909
- specified NEC G40.89
- uncinate — *see* Epilepsy, localization-related, symptomatic, with complex partial seizures

Selenium deficiency, dietary E59

Self-damaging behavior (life-style) Z72.89
Self-harm (attempted)
- history (personal) Z91.5
  - in family Z81.8

Self-mutilation (attempted)
- history (personal) Z91.5
  - in family Z81.8

Self-poisoning
- history (personal) Z91.5
  - in family Z81.8
- observation following (alleged) attempt Z03.6

Semicoma R40.1
Seminal vesiculitis N49.0
Seminoma C62.9- ☑
- specified site — *see* Neoplasm, malignant, by site

Senear-Usher disease or syndrome L10.4
Senectus R54
Senescence (without mention of psychosis) R54
Senile, senility (*see also* condition) R41.81
- with
  - acute confusional state F05
  - mental changes NOS F03 ☑
  - psychosis NEC — *see* Psychosis, senile
- asthenia R54
- cervix (atrophic) N88.8
- debility R54
- endometrium (atrophic) N85.8
- fallopian tube (atrophic) — *see* Atrophy, fallopian tube
- heart (failure) R54
- ovary (atrophic) — *see* Atrophy, ovary
- premature E34.8
- vagina, vaginitis (atrophic) N95.2
- wart L82.1

Sensation
- burning (skin) R20.8
  - tongue K14.6
- loss of R20.8
- prickling (skin) R20.2
- tingling (skin) R20.2

Sense loss
- smell — *see* Disturbance, sensation, smell
- taste — *see* Disturbance, sensation, taste
- touch R20.8

Sensibility disturbance (cortical) (deep) (vibratory) R20.9
Sensitive, sensitivity (*see also* Allergy)
- carotid sinus G90.01
- child (excessive) F93.8
- cold, autoimmune D59.1
- dentin K03.89
- gluten (non-celiac) K90.41
- latex Z91.040
- methemoglobin D74.8
- tuberculin, without clinical or radiological symptoms R76.11
- visual
  - glare H53.71
  - impaired contrast H53.72

Sensitiver Beziehungswahn F22
Sensitization, auto-erythrocytic D69.2
Separation
- anxiety, abnormal (of childhood) F93.0
- apophysis, traumatic — *code as* Fracture, by site
- choroid — *see* Detachment, choroid
- epiphysis, epiphyseal
  - nontraumatic (*see also* Osteochondropathy, specified type NEC)
    - upper femoral — *see* Slipped, epiphysis, upper femoral
  - traumatic — *code as* Fracture, by site
- fracture — *see* Fracture
- infundibulum cardiac from right ventricle by a partition Q24.3
- joint (traumatic) (current) — *code by* site under Dislocation
- pubic bone, obstetrical trauma O71.6
- retina, retinal — *see* Detachment, retina
- symphysis pubis, obstetrical trauma O71.6
- tracheal ring, incomplete, congenital Q32.1

Sepsis (generalized) (unspecified organism) A41.9
- with
  - organ dysfunction (acute) (multiple) R65.20
    - with septic shock R65.21
- actinomycotic A42.7
- adrenal hemorrhage syndrome (meningococcal) A39.1
- anaerobic A41.4
- Bacillus anthracis A22.7
- Brucella (*see also* Brucellosis) A23.9

Sepsis — *continued*
- candidal B37.7
- cryptogenic A41.9
- due to device, implant or graft T85.79 ☑
  - arterial graft NEC T82.7 ☑
  - breast (implant) T85.79 ☑
  - catheter NEC T85.79 ☑
    - dialysis (renal) T82.7 ☑
      - intraperitoneal T85.71 ☑
    - infusion NEC T82.7 ☑
      - spinal (cranial) (epidural) (intrathecal) (spinal) (subarachnoid) (subdural) T85.735 ☑
    - urethral indwelling T83.511 ☑
    - urinary T83.518 ☑
  - ectopic or molar pregnancy O08.82
  - electronic (electrode) (pulse generator) (stimulator)
    - bone T84.7 ☑
    - cardiac T82.7 ☑
    - nervous system T85.738 ☑
      - brain T85.731 ☑
      - neurostimulator generator T85.734 ☑
      - peripheral nerve T85.732 ☑
      - spinal cord T85.733 ☑
    - urinary T83.590 ☑
  - fixation, internal (orthopedic) — *see* Complication, fixation device, infection
  - gastrointestinal (bile duct) (esophagus) T85.79 ☑
    - neurostimulator electrode (lead) T85.732 ☑
  - genital T83.69 ☑
  - heart NEC T82.7 ☑
    - valve (prosthesis) T82.6 ☑
      - graft T82.7 ☑
  - joint prosthesis — *see* Complication, joint prosthesis, infection
  - ocular (corneal graft) (orbital implant) T85.79 ☑
  - orthopedic NEC T84.7 ☑
    - fixation device, internal — *see* Complication, fixation device, infection
  - specified NEC T85.79 ☑
  - vascular T82.7 ☑
  - ventricular intracranial (communicating) shunt T85.730 ☑
- during labor O75.3
- Enterococcus A41.81
- Erysipelothrix (rhusiopathiae) (erysipeloid) A26.7
- Escherichia coli (E. coli) A41.5 ☑
- extraintestinal yersiniosis A28.2
- following
  - abortion (subsequent episode) O08.0
    - current episode — *see* Abortion
  - ectopic or molar pregnancy O08.82
  - immunization T88.0 ☑
  - infusion, therapeutic injection or transfusion NEC T80.29 ☑
- gangrenous A41.9
- gonococcal A54.86
- Gram-negative (organism) A41.5 ☑
  - anaerobic A41.4
- Haemophilus influenzae A41.3
- herpesviral B00.7
- intra-abdominal K65.1
- intraocular — *see* Endophthalmitis, purulent
- Listeria monocytogenes A32.7
- localized — *code to* specific localized infection
  - in operation wound T81.4 ☑
  - skin — *see* Abscess
- malleus A24.0
- melioidosis A24.1
- meningeal — *see* Meningitis
- meningococcal A39.4
  - acute A39.2
  - chronic A39.3
- MSSA (Methicillin susceptible Staphylococcus aureus) A41.01
- newborn P36.9
  - due to
    - anaerobes NEC P36.5
    - Escherichia coli P36.4
    - Staphylococcus P36.30
      - aureus P36.2
      - specified NEC P36.39
    - Streptococcus P36.10
      - group B P36.0
      - specified NEC P36.19
  - specified NEC P36.8
- Pasteurella multocida A28.0

▽ Subterms under main terms may continue to next column or page   ☑ Additional Character Required — Refer to the Tabular List for Character Selection   283

Secretion — Sepsis

Sepsis — *continued*
  pelvic, puerperal, postpartum, childbirth O85
  pneumococcal A40.3
  postprocedural T81.4 ☑
  puerperal, postpartum, childbirth (pelvic) O85
  Salmonella (arizonae) (cholerae-suis) (enteritidis) (typhimurium) A02.1
  severe R65.20
    with septic shock R65.21
  Shigella (*see also* Dysentery, bacillary) A03.9
  skin, localized — *see* Abscess
  specified organism NEC A41.89
  Staphylococcus, staphylococcal A41.2
    aureus (methicillin susceptible) (MSSA) A41.01
      methicillin resistant (MRSA) A41.02
    coagulase-negative A41.1
    specified NEC A41.1
  Streptococcus, streptococcal A40.9
    agalactiae A40.1
    group
      A A40.0
      B A40.1
      D A41.81
    neonatal P36.10
      group B P36.0
      specified NEC P36.19
    pneumoniae A40.3
    pyogenes A40.0
    specified NEC A40.8
  tracheostomy stoma J95.02
  tularemic A21.7
  umbilical, umbilical cord (newborn) — *see* Sepsis, newborn
  Yersinia pestis A20.7
Septate — *see* Septum
Septic — *see* condition
  arm — *see* Cellulitis, upper limb
    with lymphangitis — *see* Lymphangitis, acute, upper limb
  embolus — *see* Embolism
  finger — *see* Cellulitis, digit
    with lymphangitis — *see* Lymphangitis, acute, digit
  foot — *see* Cellulitis, lower limb
    with lymphangitis — *see* Lymphangitis, acute, lower limb
  gallbladder (acute) K81.0
  hand — *see* Cellulitis, upper limb
    with lymphangitis — *see* Lymphangitis, acute, upper limb
  joint — *see* Arthritis, pyogenic or pyemic
  leg — *see* Cellulitis, lower limb
    with lymphangitis — *see* Lymphangitis, acute, lower limb
  nail (*see also* Cellulitis, digit)
    with lymphangitis — *see* Lymphangitis, acute, digit
  sore (*see also* Abscess)
    throat J02.0
      streptococcal J02.0
  spleen (acute) D73.89
  teeth, tooth (pulpal origin) K04.4
  throat — *see* Pharyngitis
  thrombus — *see* Thrombosis
  toe — *see* Cellulitis, digit
    with lymphangitis — *see* Lymphangitis, acute, digit
  tonsils, chronic J35.01
    with adenoiditis J35.03
  uterus — *see* Endometritis
Septicemia A41.9
  meaning sepsis — *see* Sepsis
Septum, septate (congenital) (*see also* Anomaly, by site)
  anal Q42.3
    with fistula Q42.2
  aqueduct of Sylvius Q03.0
    with spina bifida — *see* Spina bifida, by site, with hydrocephalus
  uterus (complete) (partial) Q51.2
  vagina Q52.10
    in pregnancy — *see* Pregnancy, complicated by, abnormal vagina
      causing obstructed labor O65.5
    longitudinal Q52.129
      microperforate
        left side Q52.124
        right side Q52.123
      nonobstruction Q52.120

Septum, septate — *continued*
  vagina — *continued*
    longitudinal — *continued*
      obstructing Q52.129
        left side Q52.122
        right side Q52.121
    transverse Q52.11
Sequelae (of) (*see also* condition)
  abscess, intracranial or intraspinal (conditions in G06) G09
  amputation — *code to* injury with seventh character S
  burn and corrosion — *code to* injury with seventh character S
  calcium deficiency E64.8
  cerebrovascular disease — *see* Sequelae, disease, cerebrovascular
  childbirth O94
  contusion — *code to* injury with seventh character S
  corrosion — *see* Sequelae, burn and corrosion
  crushing injury — *code to* injury with seventh character S
  disease
    cerebrovascular I69.90
      alteration of sensation I69.998
      aphasia I69.920
      apraxia I69.990
      ataxia I69.993
      cognitive deficits I69.91 ☑
      disturbance of vision I69.998
      dysarthria I69.922
      dysphagia I69.991
      dysphasia I69.921
      facial droop I69.992
      facial weakness I69.992
      fluency disorder I69.923
      hemiplegia I69.95- ☑
      hemorrhage
        intracerebral — *see* Sequelae, hemorrhage, intracerebral
        intracranial, nontraumatic NEC — *see* Sequelae, hemorrhage, intracranial, nontraumatic
        subarachnoid — *see* Sequelae, hemorrhage, subarachnoid
      language deficit I69.928
      monoplegia
        lower limb I69.94- ☑
        upper limb I69.93- ☑
      paralytic syndrome I69.96- ☑
      specified effect NEC I69.998
      specified type NEC I69.80
        alteration of sensation I69.898
        aphasia I69.820
        apraxia I69.890
        ataxia I69.893
        cognitive deficits I69.81 ☑
        disturbance of vision I69.898
        dysarthria I69.822
        dysphagia I69.891
        dysphasia I69.821
        facial droop I69.892
        facial weakness I69.892
        fluency disorder I69.823
        hemiplegia I69.85- ☑
        language deficit I69.828
        monoplegia
          lower limb I69.84- ☑
          upper limb I69.83- ☑
        paralytic syndrome I69.86- ☑
        specified effect NEC I69.898
      speech deficit I69.928
        speech deficit I69.828
      stroke NOS — *see* Sequelae, stroke NOS
  dislocation — *code to* injury with seventh character S
  encephalitis or encephalomyelitis (conditions in G04) G09
    in infectious disease NEC B94.8
    viral B94.1
  external cause — *code to* injury with seventh character S
  foreign body entering natural orifice — *code to* injury with seventh character S
  fracture — *code to* injury with seventh character S
  frostbite — *code to* injury with seventh character S
  Hansen's disease B92
  hemorrhage
    intracerebral I69.10

Sequelae — *continued*
  hemorrhage — *continued*
    intracerebral — *continued*
      alteration of sensation I69.198
      aphasia I69.120
      apraxia I69.190
      ataxia I69.193
      cognitive deficits I69.11 ☑
      disturbance of vision I69.198
      dysarthria I69.122
      dysphagia I69.191
      dysphasia I69.121
      facial droop I69.192
      facial weakness I69.192
      fluency disorder I69.123
      hemiplegia I69.15- ☑
      language deficit NEC I69.128
      monoplegia
        lower limb I69.14- ☑
        upper limb I69.13- ☑
      paralytic syndrome I69.16- ☑
      specified effect NEC I69.198
      speech deficit NEC I69.128
    intracranial, nontraumatic NEC I69.20
      alteration of sensation I69.298
      aphasia I69.220
      apraxia I69.290
      ataxia I69.293
      cognitive deficits I69.21 ☑
      disturbance of vision I69.298
      dysarthria I69.222
      dysphagia I69.291
      dysphasia I69.221
      facial droop I69.292
      facial weakness I69.292
      fluency disorder I69.223
      hemiplegia I69.25- ☑
      language deficit NEC I69.228
      monoplegia
        lower limb I69.24- ☑
        upper limb I69.23- ☑
      paralytic syndrome I69.26- ☑
      specified effect NEC I69.298
      speech deficit NEC I69.228
    subarachnoid I69.00
      alteration of sensation I69.098
      aphasia I69.020
      apraxia I69.090
      ataxia I69.093
      cognitive deficits — *see* subcategory I69.01- ☑
      disturbance of vision I69.098
      dysarthria I69.022
      dysphagia I69.091
      dysphasia I69.021
      facial droop I69.092
      facial weakness I69.092
      fluency disorder I69.023
      hemiplegia I69.05- ☑
      language deficit NEC I69.028
      monoplegia
        lower limb I69.04- ☑
        upper limb I69.03- ☑
      paralytic syndrome I69.06- ☑
      specified effect NEC I69.098
      speech deficit NEC I69.028
  hepatitis, viral B94.2
  hyperalimentation E68
  infarction
    cerebral I69.30
      alteration of sensation I69.398
      aphasia I69.320
      apraxia I69.390
      ataxia I69.393
      cognitive deficits I69.31 ☑
      disturbance of vision I69.398
      dysarthria I69.322
      dysphagia I69.391
      dysphasia I69.321
      facial droop I69.392
      facial weakness I69.392
      fluency disorder I69.323
      hemiplegia I69.35- ☑
      language deficit NEC I69.328
      monoplegia
        lower limb I69.34- ☑
        upper limb I69.33- ☑
      paralytic syndrome I69.36- ☑
      specified effect NEC I69.398

Sequelae — *continued*
  infarction — *continued*
    cerebral — *continued*
      speech deficit NEC I69.328
    infection, pyogenic, intracranial or intraspinal G09
    infectious disease B94.9
      specified NEC B94.8
    injury — *code to* injury with seventh character S
    leprosy B92
    meningitis
      bacterial (conditions in G00) G09
      other or unspecified cause (conditions in G03) G09
    muscle (and tendon) injury — *code to* injury with seventh character S
    myelitis — *see* Sequelae, encephalitis
    niacin deficiency E64.8
    nutritional deficiency E64.9
      specified NEC E64.8
    obstetrical condition O94
    parasitic disease B94.9
    phlebitis or thrombophlebitis of intracranial or in-traspinal venous sinuses and veins (conditions in G08) G09
    poisoning — *code to* poisoning with seventh character S
      nonmedicinal substance — *see* Sequelae, toxic effect, nonmedicinal substance
    poliomyelitis (acute) B91
    pregnancy O94
    protein-energy malnutrition E64.0
    puerperium O94
    rickets E64.3
    selenium deficiency E64.8
    sprain and strain — *code to* injury with seventh character S
    stroke NOS I69.30
      alteration in sensation I69.398
      aphasia I69.320
      apraxia I69.390
      ataxia I69.393
      cognitive deficits I69.31 ☑
      disturbance of vision I69.398
      dysarthria I69.322
      dysphagia I69.391
      dysphasia I69.321
      facial droop I69.392
      facial weakness I69.392
      hemiplegia I69.35- ☑
      language deficit NEC I69.328
      monoplegia
        lower limb I69.34- ☑
        upper limb I69.33- ☑
      paralytic syndrome I69.36- ☑
      specified effect NEC I69.398
      speech deficit NEC I69.328
    tendon and muscle injury — *code to* injury with seventh character S
    thiamine deficiency E64.8
    trachoma B94.0
    tuberculosis B90.9
      bones and joints B90.2
      central nervous system B90.0
      genitourinary B90.1
      pulmonary (respiratory) B90.9
      specified organs NEC B90.8
    viral
      encephalitis B94.1
      hepatitis B94.2
    vitamin deficiency NEC E64.8
      A E64.1
      B E64.8
      C E64.2
    wound, open — *code to* injury with seventh character S
Sequestration (*see also* Sequestrum)
  disk — *see* Displacement, intervertebral disk
  lung, congenital Q33.2
Sequestrum
  bone — *see* Osteomyelitis, chronic
  dental M27.2
  jaw bone M27.2
  orbit — *see* Osteomyelitis, orbit
  sinus (accessory) (nasal) — *see* Sinusitis
Sequoiosis lung or pneumonitis J67.8

Serology for syphilis
  doubtful
    with signs or symptoms — *code by* site and stage under Syphilis
    follow-up of latent syphilis — *see* Syphilis, latent
  negative, with signs or symptoms — *code by* site and stage under Syphilis
  positive A53.0
    with signs or symptoms — *code by* site and stage under Syphilis
  reactivated A53.0
Seroma (*see also* Hematoma)
  postprocedural — *see* Complication, postprocedural, seroma
  traumatic, secondary and recurrent T79.2 ☑
Seropurulent — *see* condition
Serositis, multiple K65.8
  pericardial I31.1
  peritoneal K65.8
Serous — *see* condition
Sertoli cell
  adenoma
    specified site — *see* Neoplasm, benign, by site
    unspecified site
      female D27.9
      male D29.20
  carcinoma
    specified site — *see* Neoplasm, malignant, by site
    unspecified site (male) C62.9- ☑
      female C56.9
  tumor
    with lipid storage
      specified site — *see* Neoplasm, benign, by site
      unspecified site
        female D27.9
        male D29.20
    specified site — *see* Neoplasm, benign, by site
    unspecified site
      female D27.9
      male D29.20
Sertoli-Leydig cell tumor — *see* Neoplasm, benign, by site
  specified site — *see* Neoplasm, benign, by site
  unspecified site
    female D27.9
    male D29.20
Serum
  allergy, allergic reaction (*see also* Reaction, serum) T80.69 ☑
    shock (*see also* Shock, anaphylactic) T80.59 ☑
  arthritis (*see also* Reaction, serum) T80.69 ☑
  complication or reaction NEC (*see also* Reaction, serum) T80.69 ☑
  disease NEC (*see also* Reaction, serum) T80.69 ☑
  hepatitis (*see also* Hepatitis, viral, type B)
    carrier (suspected) of B18.1
  intoxication (*see also* Reaction, serum) T80.69 ☑
  neuritis (*see also* Reaction, serum) T80.69 ☑
  neuropathy G61.1
  poisoning NEC (*see also* Reaction, serum) T80.69 ☑
  rash NEC (*see also* Reaction, serum) T80.69 ☑
  reaction NEC (*see also* Reaction, serum) T80.69 ☑
  sickness NEC (*see also* Reaction, serum) T80.69 ☑
  urticaria (*see also* Reaction, serum) T80.69 ☑
Sesamoiditis M25.8- ☑
Severe sepsis R65.20
  with septic shock R65.21
Sever's disease or osteochondrosis — *see* Osteochondrosis, juvenile, tarsus
Sex
  chromosome mosaics Q97.8
    lines with various numbers of X chromosomes Q97.2
  education Z70.8
  reassignment surgery status Z87.890
Sextuplet pregnancy — *see* Pregnancy, sextuplet
Sexual
  function, disorder of (psychogenic) F52.9
  immaturity (female) (male) E30.0
  impotence (psychogenic) organic origin NEC — *see* Dysfunction, sexual, male
  precocity (constitutional) (cryptogenic) (female) (idio-pathic) (male) E30.1
Sexuality, pathologic — *see* Deviation, sexual
Sézary disease C84.1- ☑
Shadow, lung R91.8
Shaking palsy or paralysis — *see* Parkinsonism

Shallowness, acetabulum — *see* Derangement, joint, specified type NEC, hip
Shaver's disease J63.1
Sheath (tendon) — *see* condition
Sheathing, retinal vessels H35.01- ☑
Shedding
  nail L60.8
  premature, primary (deciduous) teeth K00.6
Sheehan's disease or syndrome E23.0
Shelf, rectal K62.89
Shell teeth K00.5
Shellshock (current) F43.0
  lasting state — *see* Disorder, post-traumatic stress
Shield kidney Q63.1
Shift
  auditory threshold (temporary) H93.24- ☑
  mediastinal R93.8
Shifting sleep-work schedule (affecting sleep) G47.26
Shiga (-Kruse) **dysentery** A03.0
Shiga's bacillus A03.0
Shigella (dysentery) — *see* Dysentery, bacillary
Shigellosis A03.9
  Group A A03.0
  Group B A03.1
  Group C A03.2
  Group D A03.3
Shin splints S86.89- ☑
Shingles — *see* Herpes, zoster
Shipyard disease or eye B30.0
Shirodkar suture, in pregnancy — *see* Pregnancy, complicated by, incompetent cervix
Shock R57.9
  with ectopic or molar pregnancy O08.3
  adrenal (cortical) (Addisonian) E27.2
  adverse food reaction (anaphylactic) — *see* Shock, anaphylactic, due to food
  allergic — *see* Shock, anaphylactic
  anaphylactic T78.2 ☑
    chemical — *see* Table of Drugs and Chemicals
    due to drug or medicinal substance
      correct substance properly administered T88.6 ☑
      overdose or wrong substance given or taken (by accident) — *see* Table of Drugs and Chemicals, by drug, poisoning
    due to food (nonpoisonous) T78.00 ☑
      additives T78.06 ☑
      dairy products T78.07 ☑
      eggs T78.08 ☑
      fish T78.03 ☑
        shellfish T78.02 ☑
      fruit T78.04 ☑
      milk T78.07 ☑
      nuts T78.05 ☑
        multiple types T78.05 ☑
        peanuts T78.01 ☑
      peanuts T78.01 ☑
      seeds T78.05 ☑
      specified type NEC T78.09 ☑
      vegetable T78.04 ☑
    following sting(s) — *see* Venom
    immunization T80.52 ☑
    serum T80.59 ☑
      blood and blood products T80.51 ☑
      immunization T80.52 ☑
      specified NEC T80.59 ☑
      vaccination T80.52 ☑
  anaphylactoid — *see* Shock, anaphylactic
  anesthetic
    correct substance properly administered T88.2 ☑
    overdose or wrong substance given or taken — *see* Table of Drugs and Chemicals, by drug, poisoning
    specified anesthetic — *see* Table of Drugs and Chemicals, by drug, poisoning
  cardiogenic R57.0
  chemical substance — *see* Table of Drugs and Chemicals
  complicating ectopic or molar pregnancy O08.3
  culture — *see* Disorder, adjustment
  drug
    due to correct substance properly administered T88.6 ☑
    overdose or wrong substance given or taken (by accident) — *see* Table of Drugs and Chemicals, by drug, poisoning
  during or after labor and delivery O75.1

▼ **Subterms under main terms may continue to next column or page**   ☑ **Additional Character Required — Refer to the Tabular List for Character Selection**   **285**

Sequelae — Shock

Shock — *continued*
- electric T75.4 ☑
  - (taser) T75.4 ☑
- endotoxic R65.21
  - postprocedural (resulting from a procedure, not elsewhere classified) T81.12 ☑
- following
  - ectopic or molar pregnancy O08.3
  - injury (immediate) (delayed) T79.4 ☑
  - labor and delivery O75.1
- food (anaphylactic) — *see* Shock, anaphylactic, due to food
- from electroshock gun (taser) T75.4 ☑
- gram-negative R65.21
  - postprocedural (resulting from a procedure, not elsewhere classified) T81.12 ☑
- hematologic R57.8
- hemorrhagic R57.8
  - surgery (intraoperative) (postoperative) T81.19 ☑
  - trauma T79.4 ☑
- hypovolemic R57.1
  - surgical T81.19 ☑
  - traumatic T79.4 ☑
- insulin E15
  - therapeutic misadventure — *see* subcategory T38.3 ☑
- kidney N17.0
  - traumatic (following crushing) T79.5 ☑
- lightning T75.01 ☑
- liver K72.00
- lung J80
- obstetric O75.1
  - with ectopic or molar pregnancy O08.3
  - following ectopic or molar pregnancy O08.3
- pleural (surgical) T81.19 ☑
  - due to trauma T79.4 ☑
- postprocedural (postoperative) T81.10 ☑
  - with ectopic or molar pregnancy O08.3
  - cardiogenic T81.11 ☑
  - endotoxic T81.12 ☑
  - following ectopic or molar pregnancy O08.3
  - gram-negative T81.12 ☑
  - hypovolemic T81.19 ☑
  - septic T81.12 ☑
  - specified type NEC T81.19 ☑
- psychic F43.0
- septic (due to severe sepsis) R65.21
- specified NEC R57.8
- surgical T81.10 ☑
- taser gun (taser) T75.4 ☑
- therapeutic misadventure NEC T81.10 ☑
- thyroxin
  - overdose or wrong substance given or taken — *see* Table of Drugs and Chemicals, by drug, poisoning
- toxic, syndrome A48.3
- transfusion — *see* Complications, transfusion
- traumatic (immediate) (delayed) T79.4 ☑

Shoemaker's chest M95.4
Short, shortening, shortness
- arm (acquired) (*see also* Deformity, limb, unequal length)
  - congenital Q71.81- ☑
  - forearm — *see* Deformity, limb, unequal length
- bowel syndrome K91.2
- breath R06.02
- cervical (complicating pregnancy) O26.87- ☑
  - non-gravid uterus N88.3
- common bile duct, congenital Q44.5
- cord (umbilical), complicating delivery O69.3 ☑
- cystic duct, congenital Q44.5
- esophagus (congenital) Q39.8
- femur (acquired) — *see* Deformity, limb, unequal length, femur
  - congenital — *see* Defect, reduction, lower limb, longitudinal, femur
- frenum, frenulum, linguae (congenital) Q38.1
- hip (acquired) (*see also* Deformity, limb, unequal length)
  - congenital Q65.89
- leg (acquired) (*see also* Deformity, limb, unequal length)
  - congenital Q72.81- ☑
  - lower leg (*see also* Deformity, limb, unequal length)
- limbed stature, with immunodeficiency D82.2
- lower limb (acquired) (*see also* Deformity, limb, unequal length)

Short, shortening, shortness — *continued*
- lower limb (*see also* Deformity, limb, unequal length) — *continued*
  - congenital Q72.81- ☑
- organ or site, congenital NEC — *see* Distortion
- palate, congenital Q38.5
- radius (acquired) (*see also* Deformity, limb, unequal length)
  - congenital — *see* Defect, reduction, upper limb, longitudinal, radius
- rib syndrome Q77.2
- stature (child) (hereditary) (idiopathic) NEC R62.52
  - constitutional E34.3
  - due to endocrine disorder E34.3
  - Laron-type E34.3
- tendon (*see also* Contraction, tendon)
  - with contracture of joint — *see* Contraction, joint
  - Achilles (acquired) M67.0- ☑
    - congenital Q66.89
  - congenital Q79.8
- thigh (acquired) (*see also* Deformity, limb, unequal length, femur)
  - congenital — *see* Defect, reduction, lower limb, longitudinal, femur
- tibialis anterior (tendon) — *see* Contraction, tendon
- umbilical cord
  - complicating delivery O69.3 ☑
- upper limb, congenital — *see* Defect, reduction, upper limb, specified type NEC
- urethra N36.8
- uvula, congenital Q38.5
- vagina (congenital) Q52.4

Shortsightedness — *see* Myopia
Shoshin (acute fulminating beriberi) E51.11
Shoulder — *see* condition
Shovel-shaped incisors K00.2
Shower, thromboembolic — *see* Embolism
Shunt
- arterial-venous (dialysis) Z99.2
- arteriovenous, pulmonary (acquired) I28.0
  - congenital Q25.72
- cerebral ventricle (communicating) in situ Z98.2
- surgical, prosthetic, with complications — *see* Complications, cardiovascular, device or implant

Shutdown, renal N28.9
Shy-Drager syndrome G90.3
Sialadenitis, sialadenosis (any gland) (chronic) (periodic) (suppurative) — *see* Sialoadenitis
Sialectasia K11.8
Sialidosis E77.1
Sialitis, silitis (any gland) (chronic) (suppurative) — *see* Sialoadenitis
Sialoadenitis (any gland) (periodic) (suppurative) K11.20
- acute K11.21
  - recurrent K11.22
- chronic K11.23
Sialoadenopathy K11.9
Sialoangitis — *see* Sialoadenitis
Sialodochitis (fibrinosa) — *see* Sialoadenitis
Sialodocholithiasis K11.5
Sialolithiasis K11.5
Sialometaplasia, necrotizing K11.8
Sialorrhea (*see also* Ptyalism)
- periodic — *see* Sialoadenitis
Sialosis K11.7
Siamese twin Q89.4
Sibling rivalry Z62.891
Sicard's syndrome G52.7
Sicca syndrome M35.00
- with
  - keratoconjunctivitis M35.01
  - lung involvement M35.02
  - myopathy M35.03
  - renal tubulo-interstitial disorders M35.04
- specified organ involvement NEC M35.09
Sick R69
- or handicapped person in family Z63.79
  - needing care at home Z63.6
- sinus (syndrome) I49.5
Sick-euthyroid syndrome E07.81
Sickle-cell
- anemia — *see* Disease, sickle-cell
- trait D57.3
Sicklemia (*see also* Disease, sickle-cell)
- trait D57.3
Sickness
- air (travel) T75.3 ☑

Sickness — *continued*
- airplane T75.3 ☑
- alpine T70.29 ☑
- altitude T70.20 ☑
- Andes T70.29 ☑
- aviator's T70.29 ☑
- balloon T70.29 ☑
- car T75.3 ☑
- compressed air T70.3 ☑
- decompression T70.3 ☑
- green D50.8
- milk — *see* Poisoning, food, noxious
- motion T75.3 ☑
- mountain T70.29 ☑
  - acute D75.1
- protein (*see also* Reaction, serum) T80.69 ☑
- radiation T66 ☑
- roundabout (motion) T75.3 ☑
- sea T75.3 ☑
- serum NEC (*see also* Reaction, serum) T80.69 ☑
- sleeping (African) B56.9
  - by Trypanosoma B56.9
    - brucei
      - gambiense B56.0
      - rhodesiense B56.1
  - East African B56.1
  - Gambian B56.0
  - Rhodesian B56.1
  - West African B56.0
- swing (motion) T75.3 ☑
- train (railway) (travel) T75.3 ☑
- travel (any vehicle) T75.3 ☑
Sideropenia — *see* Anemia, iron deficiency
Siderosilicosis J62.8
Siderosis (lung) J63.4
- eye (globe) — *see* Disorder, globe, degenerative, siderosis
Siemens' syndrome (ectodermal dysplasia) Q82.8
Sighing R06.89
- psychogenic F45.8
Sigmoid (*see also* condition)
- flexure — *see* condition
- kidney Q63.1
Sigmoiditis (*see also* Enteritis) K52.9
- infectious A09
- noninfectious K52.9
Silfversköld's syndrome Q78.9
Silicosiderosis J62.8
Silicosis, silicotic (simple) (complicated) J62.8
- with tuberculosis J65
Silicotuberculosis J65
Silo-fillers' disease J68.8
- bronchitis J68.0
- pneumonitis J68.0
- pulmonary edema J68.1
Silver's syndrome Q87.1
Simian malaria B53.1
Simmonds' cachexia or disease E23.0
Simons' disease or syndrome (progressive lipodystrophy) E88.1
Simple, simplex — *see* condition
Simulation, conscious (of illness) Z76.5
Simultanagnosia (asimultagnosia) R48.3
Sin Nombre virus disease (Hantavirus) (cardio)-pulmonary syndrome) B33.4
Sinding-Larsen disease or osteochondrosis — *see* Osteochondrosis, juvenile, patella
Singapore hemorrhagic fever A91
Singer's node or nodule J38.2
Single
- atrium Q21.2
- coronary artery Q24.5
- umbilical artery Q27.0
- ventricle Q20.4
Singultus R06.6
- epidemicus B33.0
Sinus (*see also* Fistula)
- abdominal K63.89
- arrest I45.5
- arrhythmia I49.8
- bradycardia R00.1
- branchial cleft (internal) (external) Q18.0
- coccygeal — *see* Sinus, pilonidal
- dental K04.6
- dermal (congenital) Q06.8
  - with abscess Q06.8
  - coccygeal, pilonidal — *see* Sinus, coccygeal

Sinus — *continued*
  infected, skin NEC L08.89
  marginal, ruptured or bleeding — *see* Hemorrhage, antepartum, specified cause NEC
  medial, face and neck Q18.8
  pause I45.5
  pericranii Q01.9
  pilonidal (infected) (rectum) L05.92
    with abscess L05.02
  preauricular Q18.1
  rectovaginal N82.3
  Rokitansky-Aschoff (gallbladder) K82.8
  sacrococcygeal (dermoid) (infected) — *see* Sinus, pilonidal
  tachycardia R00.0
    paroxysmal I47.1
  tarsi syndrome M25.57- ☑
  testis N50.89
  tract (postinfective) — *see* Fistula
  urachus Q64.4
Sinusitis (accessory) (chronic) (hyperplastic) (nasal) (nonpurulent) (purulent) J32.9
  acute J01.90
    ethmoidal J01.20
      recurrent J01.21
    frontal J01.10
      recurrent J01.11
    involving more than one sinus, other than pansinusitis J01.80
      recurrent J01.81
    maxillary J01.00
      recurrent J01.01
    pansinusitis J01.40
      recurrent J01.41
    recurrent J01.91
    specified NEC J01.80
      recurrent J01.81
    sphenoidal J01.30
      recurrent J01.31
  allergic — *see* Rhinitis, allergic
  due to high altitude T70.1 ☑
  ethmoidal J32.2
    acute J01.20
      recurrent J01.21
  frontal J32.1
    acute J01.10
      recurrent J01.11
  influenzal — *see* Influenza, with, respiratory manifestations NEC
  involving more than one sinus but not pansinusitis J32.8
    acute J01.80
      recurrent J01.81
  maxillary J32.0
    acute J01.00
      recurrent J01.01
  sphenoidal J32.3
    acute J01.30
      recurrent J01.31
  tuberculous, any sinus A15.8
Sinusitis-bronchiectasis-situs inversus (syndrome) (triad) Q89.3
Sipple's syndrome E31.22
Sirenomelia (syndrome) Q87.2
Siriasis T67.0 ☑
Sirkari's disease B55.0
Siti A65
Situation, psychiatric F99
Situational
  disturbance (transient) — *see* Disorder, adjustment
    acute F43.0
  maladjustment — *see* Disorder, adjustment
  reaction — *see* Disorder, adjustment
    acute F43.0
Situs inversus or transversus (abdominalis) (thoracis) Q89.3
Sixth disease B08.20
  due to human herpesvirus 6 B08.21
  due to human herpesvirus 7 B08.22
Sjögren-Larsson syndrome Q87.1
Sjögren's syndrome or disease — *see* Sicca syndrome
Skeletal — *see* condition
Skene's gland — *see* condition
Skenitis — *see* Urethritis
Skerljevo A65
Skevas-Zerfus disease — *see* Toxicity, venom, marine animal, sea anemone
Skin (*see also* condition)

Skin — *continued*
  clammy R23.1
  donor — *see* Donor, skin
  hidebound M35.9
Slate-dressers' or slate-miners' lung J62.8
Sleep
  apnea — *see* Apnea, sleep
  deprivation Z72.820
  disorder or disturbance G47.9
    child F51.9
    nonorganic origin F51.9
    specified NEC G47.8
  disturbance G47.9
    nonorganic origin F51.9
  drunkenness F51.9
  rhythm inversion G47.2- ☑
  terrors F51.4
  walking F51.3
    hysterical F44.89
Sleep hygiene
  abuse Z72.821
  inadequate Z72.821
  poor Z72.821
Sleeping sickness — *see* Sickness, sleeping
Sleeplessness — *see* Insomnia
  menopausal N95.1
Sleep-wake schedule disorder G47.20
Slim disease (in HIV infection) B20
Slipped, slipping
  epiphysis (traumatic) (*see also* Osteochondropathy, specified type NEC)
    capital femoral (traumatic)
      acute (on chronic) S79.01- ☑
    current traumatic — *code as* Fracture, by site
    upper femoral (nontraumatic) M93.00- ☑
      acute M93.01- ☑
        on chronic M93.03- ☑
      chronic M93.02- ☑
  intervertebral disc — *see* Displacement, intervertebral disc
  ligature, umbilical P51.8
  patella — *see* Disorder, patella, derangement NEC
  rib M89.8X8
  sacroiliac joint — *see* subcategory M53.2 ☑
  tendon — *see* Disorder, tendon
  ulnar nerve, nontraumatic — *see* Lesion, nerve, ulnar
  vertebra NEC — *see* Spondylolisthesis
Slocumb's syndrome E27.0
Sloughing (multiple) (phagedena) (skin) (*see also* Gangrene)
  abscess — *see* Abscess
  appendix K38.8
  fascia — *see* Disorder, soft tissue, specified type NEC
  scrotum N50.89
  tendon — *see* Disorder, tendon
  transplanted organ — *see* Rejection, transplant
  ulcer — *see* Ulcer, skin
Slow
  feeding, newborn P92.2
  flow syndrome, coronary I20.8
  heart (beat) R00.1
Slowing, urinary stream R39.198
Sluder's neuralgia (syndrome) G44.89
Slurred, slurring speech R47.81
Small (ness)
  for gestational age — *see* Small for dates
  introitus, vagina N89.6
  kidney (unknown cause) N27.9
    bilateral N27.1
    unilateral N27.0
  ovary (congenital) Q50.39
  pelvis
    with disproportion (fetopelvic) O33.1
      causing obstructed labor O65.1
  uterus N85.8
  white kidney N03.9
Small-and-light-for-dates — *see* Small for dates
Small-for-dates (infant) P05.10
  with weight of
    499 grams or less P05.11
    500-749 grams P05.12
    750-999 grams P05.13
    1000-1249 grams P05.14
    1250-1499 grams P05.15
    1500-1749 grams P05.16
    1750-1999 grams P05.17
    2000-2499 grams P05.18

Small-for-dates — *continued*
  with weight of — *continued*
    2500 grams and over P05.19
  specified NEC P05.19
Smallpox B03
Smearing, fecal R15.1
Smith-Lemli-Opitz syndrome E78.72
Smith's fracture S52.54- ☑
Smoker — *see* Dependence, drug, nicotine
Smoker's
  bronchitis J41.0
  cough J41.0
  palate K13.24
  throat J31.2
  tongue K13.24
Smoking
  passive Z77.22
Smothering spells R06.81
Snaggle teeth, tooth M26.39
Snapping
  finger — *see* Trigger finger
  hip — *see* Derangement, joint, specified type NEC, hip
    involving the iliotiblial band M76.3- ☑
  knee — *see* Derangement, knee
    involving the iliotiblial band M76.3- ☑
Sneddon-Wilkinson disease or syndrome (sub-corneal pustular dermatosis) L13.1
Sneezing (intractable) R06.7
Sniffing
  cocaine
    abuse — *see* Abuse, drug, cocaine
    dependence — *see* Dependence, drug, cocaine
  gasoline
    abuse — *see* Abuse, drug, inhalant
    dependence — *see* Dependence, drug, inhalant
  glue (airplane)
    abuse — *see* Abuse, drug, inhalant
    drug dependence — *see* Dependence, drug, inhalant
Sniffles
  newborn P28.89
Snoring R06.83
Snow blindness — *see* Photokeratitis
Snuffles (non-syphilitic) R06.5
  newborn P28.89
  syphilitic (infant) A50.05 [J99]
Social
  exclusion Z60.4
    due to discrimination or persecution (perceived) Z60.5
  migrant Z59.0
    acculturation difficulty Z60.3
  rejection Z60.4
    due to discrimination or persecution Z60.5
  role conflict NEC Z73.5
  skills inadequacy NEC Z73.4
  transplantation Z60.3
Sodoku A25.0
Soemmering's ring — *see* Cataract, secondary
Soft (*see also* condition)
  nails L60.3
Softening
  bone — *see* Osteomalacia
  brain (necrotic) (progressive) G93.89
    congenital Q04.8
    embolic I63.4- ☑
    hemorrhagic — *see* Hemorrhage, intracranial, intracerebral
    occlusive I63.5- ☑
    thrombotic I63.3- ☑
  cartilage M94.2- ☑
    patella M22.4- ☑
  cerebellar — *see* Softening, brain
  cerebral — *see* Softening, brain
  cerebrospinal — *see* Softening, brain
  myocardial, heart — *see* Degeneration, myocardial
  spinal cord G95.89
  stomach K31.89
Soldier's
  heart F45.8
  patches I31.0
Solitary
  cyst, kidney N28.1
  kidney, congenital Q60.0
Solvent abuse — *see* Abuse, drug, inhalant
  dependence — *see* Dependence, drug, inhalant

☟ Subterms under main terms may continue to next column or page   ☑ Additional Character Required — Refer to the Tabular List for Character Selection   **287**

Sinus — Solvent abuse

Somatization reaction, somatic reaction — *see* Disorder, somatoform
Somnambulism F51.3
  hysterical F44.89
Somnolence R40.0
  nonorganic origin F51.11
Sonne dysentery A03.3
Soor B37.0
Sore
  bed — *see* Ulcer, pressure, by site
  chiclero B55.1
  Delhi B55.1
  desert — *see* Ulcer, skin
  eye H57.1- ☑
  Lahore B55.1
  mouth K13.79
    canker K12.0
  muscle M79.1
  Naga — *see* Ulcer, skin
  of skin — *see* Ulcer, skin
  oriental B55.1
  pressure — *see* Ulcer, pressure, by site
  skin L98.9
  soft A57
  throat (acute) (*see also* Pharyngitis)
    with influenza, flu, or grippe — *see* Influenza, with, respiratory manifestations NEC
    chronic J31.2
    coxsackie (virus) B08.5
    diphtheritic A36.0
    herpesviral B00.2
    influenzal — *see* Influenza, with, respiratory manifestations NEC
    septic J02.0
    streptococcal (ulcerative) J02.0
    viral NEC J02.8
      coxsackie B08.5
  tropical — *see* Ulcer, skin
  veldt — *see* Ulcer, skin
Soto's syndrome (cerebral gigantism) Q87.3
South African cardiomyopathy syndrome I42.8
Southeast Asian hemorrhagic fever A91
Spacing
  abnormal, tooth, teeth, fully erupted M26.30
  excessive, tooth, fully erupted M26.32
Spade-like hand (congenital) Q68.1
Spading nail L60.8
  congenital Q84.6
Spanish collar N47.1
Sparganosis B70.1
Spasm(s), **spastic, spasticity** (*see also* condition) R25.2
  accommodation — *see* Spasm, of accommodation
  ampulla of Vater K83.4
  anus, ani (sphincter) (reflex) K59.4
    psychogenic F45.8
  artery I73.9
    cerebral G45.9
  Bell's G51.3
  bladder (sphincter, external or internal) N32.89
    psychogenic F45.8
  bronchus, bronchiole J98.01
  cardia K22.0
  cardiac I20.1
  carpopedal — *see* Tetany
  cerebral (arteries) (vascular) G45.9
  cervix, complicating delivery O62.4
  ciliary body (of accommodation) — *see* Spasm, of accommodation
  colon (*see also* Irritable, bowel) K58.9
    with diarrhea K58.0
    psychogenic F45.8
  common duct K83.8
  compulsive — *see* Tic
  conjugate H51.8
  coronary (artery) I20.1
  diaphragm (reflex) R06.6
    epidemic B33.0
    psychogenic F45.8
  duodenum K59.8
  epidemic diaphragmatic (transient) B33.0
  esophagus (diffuse) K22.4
    psychogenic F45.8
  facial G51.3
  fallopian tube N83.8
  gastrointestinal (tract) K31.89
    psychogenic F45.8
  glottis J38.5
    hysterical F44.4

Spasm(s), **spastic, spasticity** — *continued*
  glottis — *continued*
    psychogenic F45.8
      conversion reaction F44.4
    reflex through recurrent laryngeal nerve J38.5
  habit — *see* Tic
  heart I20.1
  hemifacial (clonic) G51.3
  hourglass — *see* Contraction, hourglass
  hysterical F44.4
  infantile — *see* Epilepsy, spasms
  inferior oblique, eye H51.8
  intestinal (*see also* Syndrome, irritable bowel) K58.9
    psychogenic F45.8
  larynx, laryngeal J38.5
    hysterical F44.4
    psychogenic F45.8
      conversion reaction F44.4
  levator palpebrae superioris — *see* Disorder, eyelid function
  muscle NEC M62.838
    back M62.830
  nerve, trigeminal G51.0
  nervous F45.8
  nodding F98.4
  occupational F48.8
  oculogyric H51.8
    psychogenic F45.8
  of accommodation H52.53- ☑
  ophthalmic artery — *see* Occlusion, artery, retina
  perineal, female N94.89
  peroneo-extensor (*see also* Deformity, limb, flat foot)
  pharynx (reflex) J39.2
    hysterical F45.8
    psychogenic F45.8
  psychogenic F45.8
  pylorus NEC K31.3
    adult hypertrophic K31.89
    congenital or infantile Q40.0
    psychogenic F45.8
  rectum (sphincter) K59.4
    psychogenic F45.8
  retinal (artery) — *see* Occlusion, artery, retina
  sigmoid (*see also* Syndrome, irritable bowel) K58.9
    psychogenic F45.8
  sphincter of Oddi K83.4
  stomach K31.89
    neurotic F45.8
  throat J39.2
    hysterical F45.8
    psychogenic F45.8
  tic F95.9
    chronic F95.1
    transient of childhood F95.0
  tongue K14.8
  torsion (progressive) G24.1
  trigeminal nerve — *see* Neuralgia, trigeminal
  ureter N13.5
  urethra (sphincter) N35.9
  uterus N85.8
    complicating labor O62.4
  vagina N94.2
    psychogenic F52.5
  vascular I73.9
  vasomotor I73.9
  vein NEC I87.8
  viscera — *see* Pain, abdominal
Spasmodic — *see* condition
Spasmophilia — *see* Tetany
Spasmus nutans F98.4
Spastic, spasticity (*see also* Spasm)
  child (cerebral) (congenital) (paralysis) G80.1
Speaker's throat R49.8
Specific, specified — *see* condition
Speech
  defect, disorder, disturbance, impediment R47.9
    psychogenic, in childhood and adolescence F98.8
    slurring R47.81
    specified NEC R47.89
Spencer's disease A08.19
Spens' syndrome (syncope with heart block) I45.9
Sperm counts (fertility testing) Z31.41
  postvasectomy Z30.8
  reversal Z31.42
Spermatic cord — *see* condition
Spermatocele N43.40
  congenital Q55.4
  multiple N43.42

Spermatocele — *continued*
  single N43.41
Spermatocystitis N49.0
Spermatocytoma C62.9- ☑
  specified site — *see* Neoplasm, malignant, by site
Spermatorrhea N50.89
Sphacelus — *see* Gangrene
Sphenoidal — *see* condition
Sphenoiditis (chronic) — *see* Sinusitis, sphenoidal
Sphenopalatine ganglion neuralgia G90.09
Sphericity, increased, lens (congenital) Q12.4
Spherocytosis (congenital) (familial) (hereditary) D58.0
  hemoglobin disease D58.0
  sickle-cell (disease) D57.8- ☑
Spherophakia Q12.4
Sphincter — *see* condition
Sphincteritis, sphincter of Oddi — *see* Cholangitis
Sphingolipidosis E75.3
  specified NEC E75.29
Sphingomyelinosis E75.3
Spicule tooth K00.2
Spider
  bite — *see* Toxicity, venom, spider
  fingers — *see* Syndrome, Marfan's
  nevus I78.1
  toes — *see* Syndrome, Marfan's
  vascular I78.1
Spiegler-Fendt
  benign lymphocytoma L98.8
  sarcoid L08.89
Spielmeyer-Vogt disease E75.4
Spina bifida (aperta) Q05.9
  with hydrocephalus NEC Q05.4
  cervical Q05.5
    with hydrocephalus Q05.0
  dorsal Q05.6
    with hydrocephalus Q05.1
  lumbar Q05.7
    with hydrocephalus Q05.2
  lumbosacral Q05.7
    with hydrocephalus Q05.2
  occulta Q76.0
  sacral Q05.8
    with hydrocephalus Q05.3
  thoracic Q05.6
    with hydrocephalus Q05.1
  thoracolumbar Q05.6
    with hydrocephalus Q05.1
Spindle, Krukenberg's — *see* Pigmentation, cornea, posterior
Spine, spinal — *see* condition
Spiradenoma (eccrine) — *see* Neoplasm, skin, benign
Spirillosis A25.0
Spirillum
  minus A25.0
  obermeieri infection A68.0
Spirochetal — *see* condition
Spirochetosis A69.9
  arthritic, arthritica A69.9
  bronchopulmonary A69.8
  icterohemorrhagic A27.0
  lung A69.8
Spirometrosis B70.1
Spitting blood — *see* Hemoptysis
Splanchnoptosis K63.4
Spleen, splenic — *see* condition
Splenectasis — *see* Splenomegaly
Splenitis (interstitial) (malignant) (nonspecific) D73.89
  malarial (*see also* Malaria) B54 [D77]
  tuberculous A18.85
Splenocele D73.89
Splenomegaly, splenomegalia (Bengal) (cryptogenic) (idiopathic) (tropical) R16.1
  with hepatomegaly R16.2
  cirrhotic D73.2
  congenital Q89.09
  congestive, chronic D73.2
  Egyptian B65.1
  Gaucher's E75.22
  malarial (*see also* Malaria) B54 [D77]
  neutropenic D73.81
  Niemann-Pick — *see* Niemann-Pick disease or syndrome
  siderotic D73.2
  syphilitic A52.79
    congenital (early) A50.08 [D77]
Splenopathy D73.9

☑ **Additional Character Required — Refer to the Tabular List for Character Selection**   ⍗ **Subterms under main terms may continue to next column or page**

Splenoptosis D73.89
Splenosis D73.89
Splinter — *see* Foreign body, superficial, by site
Split, splitting
    foot Q72.7- ☑
    hand Q71.6 ☑
    heart sounds R01.2
    lip, congenital — *see* Cleft, lip
    nails L60.3
    urinary stream R39.13
Spondylarthrosis — *see* Spondylosis
Spondylitis (chronic) (*see also* Spondylopathy, inflammatory)
    ankylopoietica — *see* Spondylitis, ankylosing
    ankylosing (chronic) M45.9
        with lung involvement M45.9 [J99]
        cervical region M45.2
        cervicothoracic region M45.3
        juvenile M08.1
        lumbar region M45.6
        lumbosacral region M45.7
        multiple sites M45.0
        occipito-atlanto-axial region M45.1
        sacrococcygeal region M45.8
        thoracic region M45.4
        thoracolumbar region M45.5
    atrophic (ligamentous) — *see* Spondylitis, ankylosing
    deformans (chronic) — *see* Spondylosis
    gonococcal A54.41
    gouty (*see also* Gout, by type, vertebrae) M10.08
    in (due to)
        brucellosis A23.9 [M49.80]
            cervical region A23.9 [M49.82]
            cervicothoracic region A23.9 [M49.83]
            lumbar region A23.9 [M49.86]
            lumbosacral region A23.9 [M49.87]
            multiple sites A23.9 [M49.89]
            occipito-atlanto-axial region A23.9 [M49.81]
            sacrococcygeal region A23.9 [M49.88]
            thoracic region A23.9 [M49.84]
            thoracolumbar region A23.9 [M49.85]
        enterobacteria (*see also* subcategory M49.8) A04.9
        tuberculosis A18.01
    infectious NEC — *see* Spondylopathy, infective
    juvenile ankylosing (chronic) M08.1
    Kümmell's — *see* Spondylopathy, traumatic
    Marie-Strümpell — *see* Spondylitis, ankylosing
    muscularis — *see* Spondylopathy, specified NEC
    psoriatic L40.53
    rheumatoid — *see* Spondylitis, ankylosing
    rhizomelica — *see* Spondylitis, ankylosing
    sacroiliac NEC M46.1
    senescent, senile — *see* Spondylosis
    traumatic (chronic) or post-traumatic — *see* Spondylopathy, traumatic
    tuberculous A18.01
    typhosa A01.05
Spondylolisthesis (acquired) (degenerative) M43.10
    with disproportion (fetopelvic) O33.0
        causing obstructed labor O65.0
    cervical region M43.12
    cervicothoracic region M43.13
    congenital Q76.2
    lumbar region M43.16
    lumbosacral region M43.17
    multiple sites M43.19
    occipito-atlanto-axial region M43.11
    sacrococcygeal region M43.18
    thoracic region M43.14
    thoracolumbar region M43.15
    traumatic (old) M43.10
        acute
            fifth cervical (displaced) S12.430 ☑
                nondisplaced S12.431 ☑
                specified type NEC (displaced) S12.450 ☑
                    nondisplaced S12.451 ☑
                type III S12.44 ☑
            fourth cervical (displaced) S12.330 ☑
                nondisplaced S12.331 ☑
                specified type NEC (displaced) S12.350 ☑
                    nondisplaced S12.351 ☑
                type III S12.34 ☑
            second cervical (displaced) S12.130 ☑
                nondisplaced S12.131 ☑
                specified type NEC (displaced) S12.150 ☑
                    nondisplaced S12.151 ☑
                type III S12.14 ☑

Spondylolisthesis — *continued*
    traumatic — *continued*
        acute — *continued*
            seventh cervical (displaced) S12.630 ☑
                nondisplaced S12.631 ☑
                specified type NEC (displaced) S12.650 ☑
                    nondisplaced S12.651 ☑
                type III S12.64 ☑
            sixth cervical (displaced) S12.530 ☑
                nondisplaced S12.531 ☑
                specified type NEC (displaced) S12.550 ☑
                    nondisplaced S12.551 ☑
                type III S12.54 ☑
            third cervical (displaced) S12.230 ☑
                nondisplaced S12.231 ☑
                specified type NEC (displaced) S12.250 ☑
                    nondisplaced S12.251 ☑
                type III S12.24 ☑
Spondylolysis (acquired) M43.00
    cervical region M43.02
    cervicothoracic region M43.03
    congenital Q76.2
    lumbar region M43.06
    lumbosacral region M43.07
        with disproportion (fetopelvic) O33.0
            causing obstructed labor O65.8
    multiple sites M43.09
    occipito-atlanto-axial region M43.01
    sacrococcygeal region M43.08
    thoracic region M43.04
    thoracolumbar region M43.05
Spondylopathy M48.9
    infective NEC M46.50
        cervical region M46.52
        cervicothoracic region M46.53
        lumbar region M46.56
        lumbosacral region M46.57
        multiple sites M46.59
        occipito-atlanto-axial region M46.51
        sacrococcygeal region M46.58
        thoracic region M46.54
        thoracolumbar region M46.55
    inflammatory M46.90
        cervical region M46.92
        cervicothoracic region M46.93
        lumbar region M46.96
        lumbosacral region M46.97
        multiple sites M46.99
        occipito-atlanto-axial region M46.91
        sacrococcygeal region M46.98
        specified type NEC M46.80
            cervical region M46.82
            cervicothoracic region M46.83
            lumbar region M46.86
            lumbosacral region M46.87
            multiple sites M46.89
            occipito-atlanto-axial region M46.81
            sacrococcygeal region M46.88
            thoracic region M46.84
            thoracolumbar region M46.85
        thoracic region M46.94
        thoracolumbar region M46.95
    neuropathic, in
        syringomyelia and syringobulbia G95.0
        tabes dorsalis A52.11
    specified NEC — *see* subcategory M48.8 ☑
    traumatic M48.30
        cervical region M48.32
        cervicothoracic region M48.33
        lumbar region M48.36
        lumbosacral region M48.37
        occipito-atlanto-axial region M48.31
        sacrococcygeal region M48.38
        thoracic region M48.34
        thoracolumbar region M48.35
Spondylosis M47.9
    with
        disproportion (fetopelvic) O33.0
            causing obstructed labor O65.0
        myelopathy NEC M47.10
            cervical region M47.12
            cervicothoracic region M47.13
            lumbar region M47.16
            occipito-atlanto-axial region M47.11
            thoracic region M47.14
            thoracolumbar region M47.15
        radiculopathy M47.20
            cervical region M47.22

Spondylosis — *continued*
    with — *continued*
        radiculopathy — *continued*
            cervicothoracic region M47.23
            lumbar region M47.26
            lumbosacral region M47.27
            occipito-atlanto-axial region M47.21
            sacrococcygeal region M47.28
            thoracic region M47.24
            thoracolumbar region M47.25
    without myelopathy or radiculopathy M47.819
        cervical region M47.812
        cervicothoracic region M47.813
        lumbar region M47.816
        lumbosacral region M47.817
        occipito-atlanto-axial region M47.811
        sacrococcygeal region M47.818
        thoracic region M47.814
        thoracolumbar region M47.815
    specified NEC M47.899
        cervical region M47.892
        cervicothoracic region M47.893
        lumbar region M47.896
        lumbosacral region M47.897
        occipito-atlanto-axial region M47.891
        sacrococcygeal region M47.898
        thoracic region M47.894
        thoracolumbar region M47.895
    traumatic — *see* Spondylopathy, traumatic
Sponge
    inadvertently left in operation wound — *see* Foreign body, accidentally left during a procedure
    kidney (medullary) Q61.5
Sponge-diver's disease — *see* Toxicity, venom, marine animal, sea anemone
Spongioblastoma (any type) — *see* Neoplasm, malignant, by site
    specified site — *see* Neoplasm, malignant, by site
    unspecified site C71.9
Spongioneuroblastoma — *see* Neoplasm, malignant, by site
Spontaneous (*see also* condition)
    fracture (cause unknown) — *see* Fracture, pathological
Spoon nail L60.3
    congenital Q84.6
Sporadic — *see* condition
Sporothrix schenckii infection — *see* Sporotrichosis
Sporotrichosis B42.9
    arthritis B42.82
    disseminated B42.7
    generalized B42.7
    lymphocutaneous (fixed) (progressive) B42.1
    pulmonary B42.0
    specified NEC B42.89
Spots, spotting (in) (of)
    Bitot's (*see also* Pigmentation, conjunctiva)
        in the young child E50.1
        vitamin A deficiency E50.1
    café, au lait L81.3
    Cayenne pepper I78.1
    cotton wool, retina — *see* Occlusion, artery, retina
    de Morgan's (senile angiomas) I78.1
    Fuchs' black (myopic) (*see also* Myopia, degenerative) H44.2- ☑
    intermenstrual (regular) N92.0
        irregular N92.1
    Koplik's B05.9
    liver L81.4
    pregnancy O26.85- ☑
    purpuric R23.3
    ruby I78.1
Spotted fever — *see* Fever, spotted N92.3
Sprain (joint) (ligament)
    acromioclavicular joint or ligament S43.5- ☑
    ankle S93.40- ☑
        calcaneofibular ligament S93.41- ☑
        deltoid ligament S93.42- ☑
        internal collateral ligament — *see* Sprain, ankle, specified ligament NEC
        specified ligament NEC S93.49- ☑
        talofibular ligament — *see* Sprain, ankle, specified ligament NEC
        tibiofibular ligament S93.43- ☑
    anterior longitudinal, cervical S13.4 ☑
    atlas, atlanto-axial, atlanto-occipital S13.4 ☑
    breast bone — *see* Sprain, sternum
    calcaneofibular — *see* Sprain, ankle
    carpal — *see* Sprain, wrist

Sprain — *continued*
carpometacarpal — *see* Sprain, hand, specified site NEC
cartilage
costal S23.41 ☑
semilunar (knee) — *see* Sprain, knee, specified site NEC
with current tear — *see* Tear, meniscus
thyroid region S13.5 ☑
xiphoid — *see* Sprain, sternum
cervical, cervicodorsal, cervicothoracic S13.4 ☑
chondrosternal S23.421 ☑
coracoclavicular S43.8- ☑
coracohumeral S43.41- ☑
coronary, knee — *see* Sprain, knee, specified site NEC
costal cartilage S23.41 ☑
cricoarytenoid articulation or ligament S13.5 ☑
cricothyroid articulation S13.5 ☑
cruciate, knee — *see* Sprain, knee, cruciate
deltoid, ankle — *see* Sprain, ankle
dorsal (spine) S23.3 ☑
elbow S53.40- ☑
radial collateral ligament S53.43- ☑
radiohumeral S53.41- ☑
rupture
radial collateral ligament — *see* Rupture, traumatic, ligament, radial collateral
ulnar collateral ligament — *see* Rupture, traumatic, ligament, ulnar collateral
specified type NEC S53.49- ☑
ulnar collateral ligament S53.44- ☑
ulnohumeral S53.42- ☑
femur, head — *see* Sprain, hip
fibular collateral, knee — *see* Sprain, knee, collateral
fibulocalcaneal — *see* Sprain, ankle
finger(s) S63.61- ☑
index S63.61- ☑
interphalangeal (joint) S63.63- ☑
index S63.63- ☑
little S63.63- ☑
middle S63.63- ☑
ring S63.63- ☑
little S63.61- ☑
metacarpophalangeal (joint) S63.65- ☑
middle S63.61- ☑
ring S63.61- ☑
specified site NEC S63.69- ☑
index S63.69- ☑
little S63.69- ☑
middle S63.69- ☑
ring S63.69- ☑
foot S93.60- ☑
specified ligament NEC S93.69- ☑
tarsal ligament S93.61- ☑
tarsometatarsal ligament S93.62- ☑
toe — *see* Sprain, toe
hand S63.9- ☑
finger — *see* Sprain, finger
specified site NEC — *see* subcategory S63.8 ☑
thumb — *see* Sprain, thumb
head S03.9 ☑
hip S73.10- ☑
iliofemoral ligament S73.11- ☑
ischiocapsular (ligament) S73.12- ☑
specified NEC S73.19- ☑
iliofemoral — *see* Sprain, hip
innominate
acetabulum — *see* Sprain, hip
sacral junction S33.6 ☑
internal
collateral, ankle — *see* Sprain, ankle
semilunar cartilage — *see* Sprain, knee, specified site NEC
interphalangeal
finger — *see* Sprain, finger, interphalangeal (joint)
toe — *see* Sprain, toe, interphalangeal joint
ischiocapsular — *see* Sprain, hip
ischiofemoral — *see* Sprain, hip
jaw (articular disc) (cartilage) (meniscus) S03.4- ☑
old M26.69
knee S83.9- ☑
collateral ligament S83.40- ☑
lateral (fibular) S83.42- ☑
medial (tibial) S83.41- ☑
cruciate ligament S83.50- ☑
anterior S83.51- ☑

Sprain — *continued*
knee — *continued*
cruciate ligament — *continued*
posterior S83.52- ☑
lateral (fibular) collateral ligament S83.42- ☑
medial (tibial) collateral ligament S83.41- ☑
patellar ligament S76.11- ☑
specified site NEC S83.8X- ☑
superior tibiofibular joint (ligament) S83.6- ☑
lateral collateral — *see* Sprain, knee, collateral
lumbar (spine) S33.5 ☑
lumbosacral S33.9 ☑
mandible (articular disc) S03.4- ☑
old M26.69
medial collateral, knee — *see* Sprain, knee, collateral
meniscus
jaw S03.4- ☑
old M26.69
knee — *see* Sprain, knee, specified site NEC
with current tear — *see* Tear, meniscus
old — *see* Derangement, knee, meniscus, due to old tear
mandible S03.4- ☑
old M26.69
metacarpal (distal) (proximal) — *see* Sprain, hand, specified site NEC
metacarpophalangeal — *see* Sprain, finger, metacarpophalangeal (joint)
metatarsophalangeal — *see* Sprain, toe, metatarsophalangeal joint
midcarpal — *see* Sprain, hand, specified site NEC
midtarsal — *see* Sprain, foot, specified site NEC
neck S13.9 ☑
anterior longitudinal cervical ligament S13.4 ☑
atlanto-axial joint S13.4 ☑
atlanto-occipital joint S13.4 ☑
cervical spine S13.4 ☑
cricoarytenoid ligament S13.5 ☑
cricothyroid ligament S13.5 ☑
specified site NEC S13.8 ☑
thyroid region (cartilage) S13.5 ☑
nose S03.8 ☑
orbicular, hip — *see* Sprain, hip
patella — *see* Sprain, knee, specified site NEC
patellar ligament S76.11- ☑
pelvis NEC S33.8 ☑
phalanx
finger — *see* Sprain, finger
toe — *see* Sprain, toe
pubofemoral — *see* Sprain, hip
radiocarpal — *see* Sprain, wrist
radiohumeral — *see* Sprain, elbow
radius, collateral — *see* Rupture, traumatic, ligament, radial collateral
rib (cage) S23.41 ☑
rotator cuff (capsule) S43.42- ☑
sacroiliac (region)
chronic or old — *see* subcategory M53.2 ☑
joint S33.6 ☑
scaphoid (hand) — *see* Sprain, hand, specified site NEC
scapula (r) — *see* Sprain, shoulder girdle, specified site NEC
semilunar cartilage (knee) — *see* Sprain, knee, specified site NEC
with current tear — *see* Tear, meniscus
old — *see* Derangement, knee, meniscus, due to old tear
shoulder joint S43.40- ☑
acromioclavicular joint (ligament) — *see* Sprain, acromioclavicular joint
blade — *see* Sprain, shoulder, girdle, specified site NEC
coracoclavicular joint (ligament) — *see* Sprain, coracoclavicular joint
coracohumeral ligament — *see* Sprain, coracohumeral joint
girdle S43.9- ☑
specified site NEC S43.8- ☑
rotator cuff — *see* Sprain, rotator cuff
specified site NEC S43.49- ☑
sternoclavicular joint (ligament) — *see* Sprain, sternoclavicular joint
spine
cervical S13.4 ☑
lumbar S33.5 ☑

Sprain — *continued*
spine — *continued*
thoracic S23.3 ☑
sternoclavicular joint S43.6- ☑
sternum S23.429 ☑
chondrosternal joint S23.421 ☑
specified site NEC S23.428 ☑
sternoclavicular (joint) (ligament) S23.420 ☑
symphysis
jaw S03.4- ☑
old M26.69
mandibular S03.4- ☑
old M26.69
talofibular — *see* Sprain, ankle
tarsal — *see* Sprain, foot, specified site NEC
tarsometatarsal — *see* Sprain, foot, specified site NEC
temporomandibular S03.4- ☑
old M26.69
thorax S23.9 ☑
ribs S23.41 ☑
specified site NEC S23.8 ☑
spine S23.3 ☑
sternum — *see* Sprain, sternum
thumb S63.60- ☑
interphalangeal (joint) S63.62- ☑
metacarpophalangeal (joint) S63.64- ☑
specified site NEC S63.68- ☑
thyroid cartilage or region S13.5 ☑
tibia (proximal end) — *see* Sprain, knee, specified site NEC
tibial collateral, knee — *see* Sprain, knee, collateral
tibiofibular
distal — *see* Sprain, ankle
superior — *see* Sprain, knee, specified site NEC
toe(s) S93.50- ☑
great S93.50- ☑
interphalangeal joint S93.51- ☑
great S93.51- ☑
lesser S93.51- ☑
lesser S93.50- ☑
metatarsophalangeal joint S93.52- ☑
great S93.52- ☑
lesser S93.52- ☑
ulna, collateral — *see* Rupture, traumatic, ligament, ulnar collateral
ulnohumeral — *see* Sprain, elbow
wrist S63.50- ☑
carpal S63.51- ☑
radiocarpal S63.52- ☑
specified site NEC S63.59- ☑
xiphoid cartilage — *see* Sprain, sternum
Sprengel's deformity (congenital) Q74.0
Sprue (tropical) K90.1
celiac K90.0
idiopathic K90.49
meaning thrush B37.0
nontropical K90.0
Spur, bone (*see also* Enthesopathy)
calcaneal M77.3- ☑
iliac crest M76.2- ☑
nose (septum) J34.89
Spurway's syndrome Q78.0
Sputum
abnormal (amount) (color) (odor) (purulent) R09.3
blood-stained R04.2
excessive (cause unknown) R09.3
Squamous (*see also* condition)
epithelium in
cervical canal (congenital) Q51.828
uterine mucosa (congenital) Q51.818
Squashed nose M95.0
congenital Q67.4
Squeeze, diver's T70.3 ☑
Squint (*see also* Strabismus)
accommodative — *see* Strabismus, convergent concomitant
St. Hubert's disease A82.9
Stab (*see also* Laceration)
internal organs — *see* Injury, by site
Stafne's cyst or cavity M27.0
Staggering gait R26.0
hysterical F44.4
Staghorn calculus — *see* Calculus, kidney
Stähli's line (cornea) (pigment) — *see* Pigmentation, cornea, anterior

☑ **Additional Character Required — Refer to the Tabular List for Character Selection** ▽ **Subterms under main terms may continue to next column or page**

Stain, staining
  meconium (newborn) P96.83
  port wine Q82.5
  tooth, teeth (hard tissues) (extrinsic) K03.6
    due to
      accretions K03.6
      deposits (betel) (black) (green) (materia alba)
          (orange) (soft) (tobacco) K03.6
      metals (copper) (silver) K03.7
      nicotine K03.6
      pulpal bleeding K03.7
      tobacco K03.6
    intrinsic K00.8
Stammering (see also Disorder, fluency) F80.81
Standstill
  auricular I45.5
  cardiac — see Arrest, cardiac
  sinoatrial I45.5
  ventricular — see Arrest, cardiac
Stannosis J63.5
Stanton's disease — see Melioidosis
Staphylitis (acute) (catarrhal) (chronic) (gangrenous)
    (membranous) (suppurative) (ulcerative) K12.2
Staphylococcal scalded skin syndrome L00
Staphylococcemia A41.2
Staphylococcus, staphylococcal (see also condition)
  as cause of disease classified elsewhere B95.8
    aureus (methicillin susceptible) (MSSA) B95.61
      methicillin resistant (MRSA) B95.62
  specified NEC, as cause of disease classified elsewhere
    B95.7
Staphyloma (sclera)
  cornea H18.72- ☑
  equatorial H15.81- ☑
  localized (anterior) H15.82- ☑
  posticum H15.83- ☑
  ring H15.85- ☑
Stargardt's disease — see Dystrophy, retina
Starvation (inanition) (due to lack of food) T73.0 ☑
  edema — see Malnutrition, severe
Stasis
  bile (noncalculous) K83.1
  bronchus J98.09
    with infection — see Bronchitis
  cardiac — see Failure, heart, congestive
  cecum K59.8
  colon K59.8
  dermatitis I87.2
    with
      varicose ulcer — see Varix, leg, with ulcer, with
        inflammation
      varicose veins — see Varix, leg, with, inflamma-
        tion
    due to postthrombotic syndrome — see Syndrome,
        postthrombotic
  duodenal K31.5
  eczema — see Varix, leg, with, inflammation
  edema — see Hypertension, venous (chronic), idiopath-
    ic
  foot T69.0- ☑
  ileocecal coil K59.8
  ileum K59.8
  intestinal K59.8
  jejunum K59.8
  kidney N19
  liver (cirrhotic) K76.1
  lymphatic I89.8
  pneumonia J18.2
  pulmonary — see Edema, lung
  rectal K59.8
  renal N19
    tubular N17.0
  ulcer — see Varix, leg, with, ulcer
    without varicose veins I87.2
  urine — see Retention, urine
  venous I87.8
State (of)
  affective and paranoid, mixed, organic psychotic F06.8
  agitated R45.1
    acute reaction to stress F43.0
  anxiety (neurotic) F41.1
  apprehension F41.1
  burn-out Z73.0
  climacteric, female Z78.0
    symptomatic N95.1
  compulsive F42.8
    mixed with obsessional thoughts F42.2
  confusional (psychogenic) F44.89

State — continued
  confusional — continued
    acute (see also Delirium)
      with
        arteriosclerotic dementia F01.50
          with behavioral disturbance F01.51
        senility or dementia F05
      alcoholic F10.231
    epileptic F05
    reactive (from emotional stress, psychological
        trauma) F44.89
    subacute — see Delirium
  convulsive — see Convulsions
  crisis F43.0
  depressive F32.9
    neurotic F34.1
  dissociative F44.9
  emotional shock (stress) R45.7
  hypercoagulation — see Hypercoagulable
  locked-in G83.5
  menopausal Z78.0
    symptomatic N95.1
  neurotic F48.9
    with depersonalization F48.1
  obsessional F42.8
  oneiroid (schizophrenia-like) F23
  organic
    hallucinatory (nonalcoholic) F06.0
    paranoid (-hallucinatory) F06.2
  panic F41.0
  paranoid F22
    climacteric F22
    involutional F22
    menopausal F22
    organic F06.2
    senile F03 ☑
    simple F22
  persistent vegetative R40.3
  phobic F40.9
  postleukotomy F07.0
  pregnant
    gestational carrier Z33.3
    incidental Z33.1
  psychogenic, twilight F44.89
  psychopathic (constitutional) F60.2
  psychotic, organic (see also Psychosis, organic)
    mixed paranoid and affective F06.8
    senile or presenile F03 ☑
    transient NEC F06.8
      with
        depression F06.31
        hallucinations F06.0
  residual schizophrenic F20.5
  restlessness R45.1
  stress (emotional) R45.7
  tension (mental) F48.9
    specified NEC F48.8
  transient organic psychotic NEC F06.8
    depressive type F06.31
    hallucinatory type F06.0
  twilight
    epileptic F05
    psychogenic F44.89
  vegetative, persistent R40.3
  vital exhaustion Z73.0
  withdrawal, — see Withdrawal, state
Status (post) (see also Presence (of))
  absence, epileptic — see Epilepsy, by type, with status
    epilepticus
  administration of tPA (rtPA) in a different facility
      within the last 24 hours prior to admission to
      current facility Z92.82
  adrenalectomy (unilateral) (bilateral) E89.6
  anastomosis Z98.0
  anginosus I20.9
  angioplasty (peripheral) Z98.62
    with implant Z95.820
    coronary artery Z98.61
      with implant Z95.5
  aortocoronary bypass Z95.1
  arthrodesis Z98.1
  artificial opening (of) Z93.9
    gastrointestinal tract Z93.4
    specified NEC Z93.8
    urinary tract Z93.6
    vagina Z93.8
  asthmaticus — see Asthma, by type, with status asth-
    maticus

Status — continued
  awaiting organ transplant Z76.82
  bariatric surgery Z98.84
  bed confinement Z74.01
  bleb, filtering (vitreous), after glaucoma surgery Z98.83
  breast implant Z98.82
    removal Z98.86
  cataract extraction Z98.4- ☑
  cholecystectomy Z90.49
  clitorectomy N90.811
    with excision of labia minora N90.812
  colectomy (complete) (partial) Z90.49
  colonization — see Carrier (suspected) of
  colostomy Z93.3
  convulsivus idiopathicus — see Epilepsy, by type, with
    status epilepticus
  coronary artery angioplasty — see Status, angioplasty,
    coronary artery
  coronary artery bypass graft Z95.1
  cystectomy (urinary bladder) Z90.6
  cystostomy Z93.50
    appendico-vesicostomy Z93.52
    cutaneous Z93.51
    specified NEC Z93.59
  delinquent immunization Z28.3
  dental Z98.818
    crown Z98.811
    fillings Z98.811
    restoration Z98.811
    sealant Z98.810
    specified NEC Z98.818
  deployment (current) (military) Z56.82
  dialysis (hemodialysis) (peritoneal) Z99.2
  do not resuscitate (DNR) Z66
  donor — see Donor
  embedded fragments — see Retained, foreign body
    fragments (type of)
  embedded splinter — see Retained, foreign body
    fragments (type of)
  enterostomy Z93.4
  epileptic, epilepticus (see also Epilepsy, by type, with
    status epilepticus) G40.901
  estrogen receptor
    negative Z17.1
    positive Z17.0
  female genital cutting — see Female genital mutilation
    status
  female genital mutilation — see Female genital muti-
    lation status
  filtering (vitreous) bleb after glaucoma surgery Z98.83
  gastrectomy (complete) (partial) Z90.3
  gastric banding Z98.84
  gastric bypass for obesity Z98.84
  gastrostomy Z93.1
  human immunodeficiency virus (HIV) infection,
    asymptomatic Z21
  hysterectomy (complete) (total) Z90.710
    partial (with remaining cervial stump) Z90.711
  ileostomy Z93.2
  implant
    breast Z98.82
  infibulation N90.813
  intestinal bypass Z98.0
  jejunostomy Z93.4
  lapsed immunization schedule Z28.3
  laryngectomy Z90.02
  lymphaticus E32.8
  malignancy
    castrate resistant prostate Z19.2
    hormone resistant Z19.2
    hormone sensitive Z19.1
  marmoratus G80.3
  mastectomy (unilateral) (bilateral) Z90.1- ☑
  military deployment status (current) Z56.82
    in theater or in support of military war, peacekeep-
        ing and humanitarian operations Z56.82
  nephrectomy (unilateral) (bilateral) Z90.5
  nephrostomy Z93.6
  obesity surgery Z98.84
  oophorectomy
    bilateral Z90.722
    unilateral Z90.721
  organ replacement
    by artificial or mechanical device or prosthesis of
        artery Z95.828
        bladder Z96.0
        blood vessel Z95.828
        breast Z97.8

Status — *continued*
 organ replacement — *continued*
  by artificial or mechanical device or prosthesis of
   — *continued*
   eye globe Z97.0
   heart Z95.812
    valve Z95.2
   intestine Z97.8
   joint Z96.60
    hip — *see* Presence, hip joint implant
    knee — *see* Presence, knee joint implant
    specified site NEC Z96.698
   kidney Z97.8
   larynx Z96.3
   lens Z96.1
   limbs — *see* Presence, artificial, limb
   liver Z97.8
   lung Z97.8
   pancreas Z97.8
  by organ transplant (heterologous)(homologous)
   — *see* Transplant
 pacemaker
  brain Z96.89
  cardiac Z95.0
  specified NEC Z96.89
 pancreatectomy Z90.410
  complete Z90.410
  partial Z90.411
  total Z90.410
 physical restraint Z78.1
 pneumonectomy (complete) (partial) Z90.2
 pneumothorax, therapeutic Z98.3
 postcommotio cerebri F07.81
 postoperative (postprocedural) NEC Z98.890
  breast implant Z98.82
  dental Z98.818
   crown Z98.811
   fillings Z98.811
   restoration Z98.811
   sealant Z98.810
   specified NEC Z98.818
  pneumothorax, therapeutic Z98.3
  uterine scar Z98.891
 postpartum (routine follow-up) Z39.2
  care immediately after delivery Z39.0
 postsurgical (postprocedural) NEC Z98.890
  pneumothorax, therapeutic Z98.3
 pregnancy, incidental Z33.1
 prosthesis coronary angioplasty Z95.5
 pseudophakia Z96.1
 renal dialysis (hemodialysis) (peritoneal) Z99.2
 retained foreign body — *see* Retained, foreign body
  fragments (type of)
 reversed jejunal transposition (for bypass) Z98.0
 salpingo-oophorectomy
  bilateral Z90.722
  unilateral Z90.721
 sex reassignment surgery status Z87.890
 shunt
  arteriovenous (for dialysis) Z99.2
  cerebrospinal fluid Z98.2
  ventricular (communicating) (for drainage) Z98.2
 splenectomy Z90.81
 thymicolymphaticus E32.8
 thymicus E32.8
 thymolymphaticus E32.8
 thyroidectomy (hypothyroidism) E89.0
 tooth (teeth) extraction (*see also* Absence, teeth, acquired) K08.409
 tPA (rtPA) administration in a different facility within the last 24 hours prior to admission to current facility Z92.82
 tracheostomy Z93.0
 transplant — *see* Transplant
  organ removed Z98.85
 tubal ligation Z98.51
 underimmunization Z28.3
 ureterostomy Z93.6
 urethrostomy Z93.6
 vagina, artificial Z93.8
 vasectomy Z98.52
 wheelchair confinement Z99.3
Stealing
 child problem F91.8
  in company with others Z72.810
 pathological (compulsive) F63.2
Steam burn — *see* Burn
Steatocystoma multiplex L72.2

Steatohepatitis (nonalcoholic) (NASH) K75.81
Steatoma L72.3
 eyelid (cystic) — *see* Dermatosis, eyelid
 infected — *see* Hordeolum
Steatorrhea (chronic) K90.9
 with lacteal obstruction K90.2
 idiopathic (adult) (infantile) K90.9
 pancreatic K90.3
 primary K90.0
 tropical NEC K90.1
Steatosis E88.89
 heart — *see* Degeneration, myocardial
 kidney N28.89
 liver NEC K76.0
Steele-Richardson-Olszewski disease or syndrome G23.1
Steinbrocker's syndrome G90.8
Steinert's disease G71.11
Stein-Leventhal syndrome E28.2
Stein's syndrome E28.2
STEMI (*see also* Infarct, myocardium, ST elevation) I21.3
Stenocardia I20.8
Stenocephaly Q75.8
Stenosis, stenotic (cicatricial) (*see also* Stricture)
 ampulla of Vater K83.1
 anus, anal (canal) (sphincter) K62.4
  and rectum K62.4
  congenital Q42.3
   with fistula Q42.2
 aorta (ascending) (supraventricular) (congenital) Q25.1
  arteriosclerotic I70.0
  calcified I70.0
  supravalvular Q25.3
 aortic (valve) I35.0
  with insufficiency I35.2
  congenital Q23.0
  rheumatic I06.0
   with
    incompetency, insufficiency or regurgitation I06.2
     with mitral (valve) disease I08.0
      with tricuspid (valve) disease I08.3
    mitral (valve) disease I08.0
     with tricuspid (valve) disease I08.3
    tricuspid (valve) disease I08.2
     with mitral (valve) disease I08.3
  specified cause NEC I35.0
  syphilitic A52.03
 aqueduct of Sylvius (congenital) Q03.0
  with spina bifida — *see* Spina bifida, by site, with hydrocephalus
  acquired G91.1
 artery NEC (*see also* Arteriosclerosis) I77.1
  celiac I77.4
  cerebral — *see* Occlusion, artery, cerebral
  extremities — *see* Arteriosclerosis, extremities
  precerebral — *see* Occlusion, artery, precerebral
  pulmonary (congenital) Q25.6
   acquired I28.8
  renal I70.1
  stent
   coronary T82.855 ☑
   peripheral T82.856 ☑
 bile duct (common) (hepatic) K83.1
  congenital Q44.3
 bladder-neck (acquired) N32.0
  congenital Q64.31
 brain G93.89
 bronchus J98.09
  congenital Q32.3
  syphilitic A52.72
 cardia (stomach) K22.2
  congenital Q39.3
 cardiovascular — *see* Disease, cardiovascular
 caudal M48.08
 cervix, cervical (canal) N88.2
  congenital Q51.828
  in pregnancy or childbirth — *see* Pregnancy, complicated by, abnormal cervix
 colon (*see also* Obstruction, intestine)
  congenital Q42.9
   specified NEC Q42.8
 colostomy K94.03
 common (bile) duct K83.1
  congenital Q44.3
 coronary (artery) — *see* Disease, heart, ischemic, atherosclerotic
 cystic duct — *see* Obstruction, gallbladder

Stenosis, stenotic — *continued*
 due to presence of device, implant or graft (*see also* Complications, by site and type, specified NEC) T85.858 ☑
  arterial graft NEC T82.858 ☑
  breast (implant) T85.858 ☑
  catheter T85.858 ☑
   dialysis (renal) T82.858 ☑
    intraperitoneal T85.858 ☑
   infusion NEC T82.858 ☑
    spinal (epidural) (subdural) T85.850 ☑
   urinary (indwelling) T83.85 ☑
  fixation, internal (orthopedic) NEC T84.85 ☑
  gastrointestinal (bile duct) (esophagus) T85.858 ☑
  genital NEC T83.85 ☑
  heart NEC T82.857 ☑
  joint prosthesis T84.85 ☑
  ocular (corneal graft) (orbital implant) NEC T85.858 ☑
  orthopedic NEC T84.85 ☑
  specified NEC T85.858 ☑
  urinary NEC T83.85 ☑
  vascular NEC T82.858 ☑
  ventricular intracranial shunt T85.850 ☑
 duodenum K31.5
  congenital Q41.0
 ejaculatory duct NEC N50.89
  stent
   vascular
    end stent
     adjacent to stent — *see* Arteriosclerosis
     within the stent
      coronary T82.855 ☑
      peripheral T82.856 ☑
    in stent
     coronary vessel T82.855 ☑
     peripheral vessel T82.856 ☑
 endocervical os — *see* Stenosis, cervix
 enterostomy K94.13
 esophagus K22.2
  congenital Q39.3
  syphilitic A52.79
   congenital A50.59 [K23]
 eustachian tube — *see* Obstruction, eustachian tube
 external ear canal (acquired) H61.30- ☑
  congenital Q16.1
  due to
   inflammation H61.32- ☑
   trauma H61.31- ☑
  postprocedural H95.81- ☑
  specified cause NEC H61.39- ☑
 gallbladder — *see* Obstruction, gallbladder
 glottis J38.6
 heart valve (congenital) Q24.8
  aortic Q23.0
  mitral Q23.2
  pulmonary Q22.1
  tricuspid Q22.4
 hepatic duct K83.1
 hymen N89.6
 hypertrophic subaortic (idiopathic) I42.1
 ileum (*see also* Obstruction, intestine, specified NEC) K56.699
  congenital Q41.2
 infundibulum cardia Q24.3
 intervertebral foramina (*see also* Lesion, biomechanical, specified NEC)
  connective tissue M99.79
   abdomen M99.79
   cervical region M99.71
   cervicothoracic M99.71
   head region M99.70
   lumbar region M99.73
   lumbosacral M99.73
   occipitocervical M99.70
   sacral region M99.74
   sacrococcygeal M99.74
   sacroiliac M99.74
   specified NEC M99.79
   thoracic region M99.72
   thoracolumbar M99.72
  disc M99.79
   abdomen M99.79
   cervical region M99.71
   cervicothoracic M99.71
   head region M99.70
   lower extremity M99.76

☑ **Additional Character Required — Refer to the Tabular List for Character Selection** ▽ **Subterms under main terms may continue to next column or page**

Stenosis, stenotic — *continued*
- intervertebral foramina (*see also* Lesion, biomechanical, specified) — *continued*
  - disc — *continued*
    - lumbar region M99.73
    - lumbosacral M99.73
    - occipitocervical M99.70
    - pelvic M99.75
    - rib cage M99.78
    - sacral region M99.74
    - sacrococcygeal M99.74
    - sacroiliac M99.74
    - specified NEC M99.79
    - thoracic region M99.72
    - thoracolumbar M99.72
    - upper extremity M99.77
  - osseous M99.69
    - abdomen M99.69
    - cervical region M99.61
    - cervicothoracic M99.61
    - head region M99.60
    - lower extremity M99.66
    - lumbar region M99.63
    - lumbosacral M99.63
    - occipitocervical M99.60
    - pelvic M99.65
    - rib cage M99.68
    - sacral region M99.64
    - sacrococcygeal M99.64
    - sacroiliac M99.64
    - specified NEC M99.69
    - thoracic region M99.62
    - thoracolumbar M99.62
    - upper extremity M99.67
  - subluxation — *see* Stenosis, intervertebral foramina, osseous
- intestine (*see also* Obstruction, intestine)
  - congenital (small) Q41.9
    - large Q42.9
      - specified NEC Q42.8
    - specified NEC Q41.8
- jejunum (*see also* Obstruction, intestine, specified NEC) K56.699
  - congenital Q41.1
- lacrimal (passage)
  - canaliculi H04.54- ☑
  - congenital Q10.5
  - duct H04.55- ☑
  - punctum H04.56- ☑
  - sac H04.57- ☑
- lacrimonasal duct — *see* Stenosis, lacrimal, duct
  - congenital Q10.5
- larynx J38.6
  - congenital NEC Q31.8
    - subglottic Q31.1
  - syphilitic A52.73
    - congenital A50.59 [J99]
- mitral (chronic) (inactive) (valve) I05.0
  - with
    - aortic valve disease I08.0
    - incompetency, insufficiency or regurgitation I05.2
  - active or acute I01.1
    - with rheumatic or Sydenham's chorea I02.0
  - congenital Q23.2
  - specified cause, except rheumatic I34.2
  - syphilitic A52.03
- myocardium, myocardial (*see also* Degeneration, myocardial)
  - hypertrophic subaortic (idiopathic) I42.1
- nares (anterior) (posterior) J34.89
  - congenital Q30.0
- nasal duct (*see also* Stenosis, lacrimal, duct)
  - congenital Q10.5
- nasolacrimal duct (*see also* Stenosis, lacrimal, duct)
  - congenital Q10.5
- neural canal (*see also* Lesion, biomechanical, specified NEC)
  - connective tissue M99.49
    - abdomen M99.49
    - cervical region M99.41
    - cervicothoracic M99.41
    - head region M99.40
    - lower extremity M99.46
    - lumbar region M99.43
    - lumbosacral M99.43
    - occipitocervical M99.40
    - pelvic M99.45

Stenosis, stenotic — *continued*
- neural canal (*see also* Lesion, biomechanical, specified) — *continued*
  - connective tissue — *continued*
    - rib cage M99.48
    - sacral region M99.44
    - sacrococcygeal M99.44
    - sacroiliac M99.44
    - specified NEC M99.49
    - thoracic region M99.42
    - thoracolumbar M99.42
    - upper extremity M99.47
  - intervertebral disc M99.59
    - abdomen M99.59
    - cervical region M99.51
    - cervicothoracic M99.51
    - head region M99.50
    - lower extremity M99.56
    - lumbar region M99.53
    - lumbosacral M99.53
    - occipitocervical M99.50
    - pelvic M99.55
    - rib cage M99.58
    - sacral region M99.54
    - sacrococcygeal M99.54
    - sacroiliac M99.54
    - specified NEC M99.59
    - thoracic region M99.52
    - thoracolumbar M99.52
    - upper extremity M99.57
  - osseous M99.39
    - abdomen M99.39
    - cervical region M99.31
    - cervicothoracic M99.31
    - head region M99.30
    - lower extremity M99.36
    - lumbar region M99.33
    - lumbosacral M99.33
    - occipitocervical M99.30
    - pelvic M99.35
    - rib cage M99.38
    - sacral region M99.34
    - sacrococcygeal M99.34
    - sacroiliac M99.34
    - specified NEC M99.39
    - thoracic region M99.32
    - thoracolumbar M99.32
    - upper extremity M99.37
  - subluxation M99.29
    - cervical region M99.21
    - cervicothoracic M99.21
    - head region M99.20
    - lower extremity M99.26
    - lumbar region M99.23
    - lumbosacral M99.23
    - occipitocervical M99.20
    - pelvic M99.25
    - rib cage M99.28
    - sacral region M99.24
    - sacrococcygeal M99.24
    - sacroiliac M99.24
    - specified NEC M99.29
    - thoracic region M99.22
    - thoracolumbar M99.22
    - upper extremity M99.27
- organ or site, congenital NEC — *see* Atresia, by site
- papilla of Vater K83.1
- pulmonary (artery) (congenital) Q25.6
  - with ventricular septal defect, transposition of aorta, and hypertrophy of right ventricle Q21.3
  - acquired I28.8
  - in tetralogy of Fallot Q21.3
  - infundibular Q24.3
  - subvalvular Q24.3
  - supravalvular Q25.6
  - valve I37.0
    - with insufficiency I37.2
    - congenital Q22.1
    - rheumatic I09.89
      - with aortic, mitral or tricuspid (valve) disease I08.8
  - vein, acquired I28.8
  - vessel NEC I28.8
- pulmonic (congenital) Q22.1
  - infundibular Q24.3
  - subvalvular Q24.3
- pylorus (hypertrophic) (acquired) K31.1
  - adult K31.1

Stenosis, stenotic — *continued*
- pylorus — *continued*
  - congenital Q40.0
  - infantile Q40.0
- rectum (sphincter) — *see* Stricture, rectum
- renal artery I70.1
  - congenital Q27.1
- salivary duct (any) K11.8
- sphincter of Oddi K83.1
- spinal M48.00
  - cervical region M48.02
  - cervicothoracic region M48.03
  - lumbar region (NOS) (without neurogenic claudication) M48.061
    - with neurogenic claudication M48.062
  - lumbosacral region M48.07
  - occipito-atlanto-axial region M48.01
  - sacrococcygeal region M48.08
  - thoracic region M48.04
  - thoracolumbar region M48.05
- stomach, hourglass K31.2
- subaortic (congenital) Q24.4
  - hypertrophic (idiopathic) I42.1
- subglottic J38.6
  - congenital Q31.1
  - postprocedural J95.5
- trachea J39.8
  - congenital Q32.1
  - syphilitic A52.73
  - tuberculous NEC A15.5
- tracheostomy J95.03
- tricuspid (valve) I07.0
  - with
    - aortic (valve) disease I08.2
    - incompetence, insufficiency or regurgitation I07.2
      - with aortic (valve) disease I08.2
        - with mitral (valve) disease I08.3
    - mitral (valve) disease I08.1
      - with aortic (valve) disease I08.3
  - congenital Q22.4
  - nonrheumatic I36.0
    - with insufficiency I36.2
- tubal N97.1
- ureter — *see* Atresia, ureter
- ureteropelvic junction, congenital Q62.11
- ureterovesical orifice, congenital Q62.12
- urethra (valve) (*see also* Stricture, urethra)
  - congenital Q64.32
- urinary meatus, congenital Q64.33
- vagina N89.5
  - congenital Q52.4
  - in pregnancy — *see* Pregnancy, complicated by, abnormal vagina
    - causing obstructed labor O65.5
- valve (cardiac) (heart) (*see also* Endocarditis) I38
  - congenital Q24.8
    - aortic Q23.0
    - mitral Q23.2
    - pulmonary Q22.1
    - tricuspid Q22.4
- vena cava (inferior) (superior) I87.1
  - congenital Q26.0
- vesicourethral orifice Q64.31
- vulva N90.5

Stent jail T82.897 ☑
Stercolith (impaction) K56.41
- appendix K38.1
Stercoraceous, stercoral ulcer K63.3
- anus or rectum K62.6
Stereotypies NEC F98.4
Sterility — *see* Infertility
Sterilization — *see* Encounter (for), sterilization
Sternalgia — *see* Angina
Sternopagus Q89.4
Sternum bifidum Q76.7
Steroid
- effects (adverse) (adrenocortical) (iatrogenic)
  - cushingoid E24.2
    - correct substance properly administered — *see* Table of Drugs and Chemicals, by drug, adverse effect
    - overdose or wrong substance given or taken — *see* Table of Drugs and Chemicals, by drug, poisoning
  - diabetes — *see* subcategory E09 ☑

Steroid — *continued*
  effects — *continued*
    diabetes — *see* subcategory — *continued*
      correct substance properly administered — *see* Table of Drugs and Chemicals, by drug, adverse effect
      overdose or wrong substance given or taken — *see* Table of Drugs and Chemicals, by drug, poisoning
    fever R50.2
    insufficiency E27.3
      correct substance properly administered — *see* Table of Drugs and Chemicals, by drug, adverse effect
      overdose or wrong substance given or taken — *see* Table of Drugs and Chemicals, by drug, poisoning
  responder H40.04- ☑
Stevens-Johnson disease or syndrome L51.1
  toxic epidermal necrolysis overlap L51.3
Stewart-Morel syndrome M85.2
Sticker's disease B08.3
Sticky eye — *see* Conjunctivitis, acute, mucopurulent
Stieda's disease — *see* Bursitis, tibial collateral
Stiff neck — *see* Torticollis
Stiff-man syndrome G25.82
Stiffness, joint NEC M25.60
  ankle M25.67- ☑
  ankylosis — *see* Ankylosis, joint
  contracture — *see* Contraction, joint
  elbow M25.62- ☑
  foot M25.67- ☑
  hand M25.64- ☑
  hip M25.65- ☑
  knee M25.66- ☑
  shoulder M25.61- ☑
  wrist M25.63- ☑
Stigmata congenital syphilis A50.59
Stillbirth P95
Still-Felty syndrome — *see* Felty's syndrome
Still's disease or syndrome (juvenile) M08.20
  adult-onset M06.1
  ankle M08.27- ☑
  elbow M08.22- ☑
  foot joint M08.27- ☑
  hand joint M08.24- ☑
  hip M08.25- ☑
  knee M08.26- ☑
  multiple site M08.29
  shoulder M08.21- ☑
  vertebra M08.28
  wrist M08.23- ☑
Stimulation, ovary E28.1
Sting (venomous) (with allergic or anaphylactic shock) — *see* Table of Drugs and Chemicals, by animal or substance, poisoning
Stippled epiphyses Q78.8
Stitch
  abscess T81.4 ☑
  burst (in operation wound) — *see* Disruption, wound, operation
Stokes' disease E05.00
  with thyroid storm E05.01
Stokes-Adams disease or syndrome I45.9
Stokvis (-Talma) **disease** D74.8
Stoma malfunction
  colostomy K94.03
  enterostomy K94.13
  gastrostomy K94.23
  ileostomy K94.13
  tracheostomy J95.03
Stomach — *see* condition
Stomatitis (denture) (ulcerative) K12.1
  angular K13.0
    due to dietary or vitamin deficiency E53.0
  aphthous K12.0
  bovine B08.61
  candidal B37.0
  catarrhal K12.1
  diphtheritic A36.89
  due to
    dietary deficiency E53.0
    thrush B37.0
    vitamin deficiency
      B group NEC E53.9
      B2 (riboflavin) E53.0
  epidemic B08.8

Stomatitis — *continued*
  epizootic B08.8
  follicular K12.1
  gangrenous A69.0
  Geotrichum B48.3
  herpesviral, herpetic B00.2
  herpetiformis K12.0
  malignant K12.1
  membranous acute K12.1
  monilial B37.0
  mycotic B37.0
  necrotizing ulcerative A69.0
  parasitic B37.0
  septic K12.1
  spirochetal A69.1
  suppurative (acute) K12.2
  ulceromembranous A69.1
  vesicular K12.1
    with exanthem (enteroviral) B08.4
    virus disease A93.8
  Vincent's A69.1
Stomatocytosis D58.8
Stomatomycosis B37.0
Stomatorrhagia K13.79
Stone(s) (*see also* Calculus)
  bladder (diverticulum) N21.0
  cystine E72.09
  heart syndrome I50.1
  kidney N20.0
  prostate N42.0
  pulpal (dental) K04.2
  renal N20.0
  salivary gland or duct (any) K11.5
  urethra (impacted) N21.1
  urinary (duct) (impacted) (passage) N20.9
    bladder (diverticulum) N21.0
    lower tract N21.9
    specified NEC N21.8
  xanthine E79.8 [N22]
Stonecutter's lung J62.8
Stonemason's asthma, disease, lung or pneumoco-niosis J62.8
Stoppage
  heart — *see* Arrest, cardiac
  urine — *see* Retention, urine
Storm, thyroid — *see* Thyrotoxicosis
Strabismus (congenital) (nonparalytic) H50.9
  concomitant H50.40
    convergent — *see* Strabismus, convergent concomitant
    divergent — *see* Strabismus, divergent concomitant
  convergent concomitant H50.00
    accommodative component H50.43
    alternating H50.05
      with
        A pattern H50.06
        specified nonconcomitances NEC H50.08
        V pattern H50.07
    monocular H50.01- ☑
      with
        A pattern H50.02- ☑
        specified nonconcomitances NEC H50.04- ☑
        V pattern H50.03- ☑
      intermittent H50.31- ☑
        alternating H50.32
  cyclotropia H50.41 ☑
  divergent concomitant H50.10
    alternating H50.15
      with
        A pattern H50.16
        specified nonconcomitances NEC H50.18
        V pattern H50.17
    monocular H50.11- ☑
      with
        A pattern H50.12- ☑
        specified nonconcomitances NEC H50.14- ☑
        V pattern H50.13- ☑
      intermittent H50.33 ☑
        alternating H50.34
  Duane's syndrome H50.81- ☑
  due to adhesions, scars H50.69
  heterophoria H50.50
    alternating H50.55
    cyclophoria H50.54
    esophoria H50.51
    exophoria H50.52
    vertical H50.53

Strabismus — *continued*
  heterotropia H50.40
    intermittent H50.30
  hypertropia H50.2- ☑
  hypotropia — *see* Hypertropia
  latent H50.50
  mechanical H50.60
    Brown's sheath syndrome H50.61- ☑
    specified type NEC H50.69
  monofixation syndrome H50.42
  paralytic H49.9
    abducens nerve H49.2- ☑
    fourth nerve H49.1- ☑
    Kearns-Sayre syndrome H49.81- ☑
    ophthalmoplegia (external)
      progressive H49.4- ☑
        with pigmentary retinopathy H49.81- ☑
      total H49.3- ☑
    sixth nerve H49.2- ☑
    specified type NEC H49.88- ☑
    third nerve H49.0- ☑
    trochlear nerve H49.1- ☑
  specified type NEC H50.89
  vertical H50.2- ☑
Strain
  back S39.012 ☑
  cervical S16.1 ☑
  eye NEC — *see* Disturbance, vision, subjective
  heart — *see* Disease, heart
  low back S39.012 ☑
  mental NOS Z73.3
    work-related Z56.6
  muscle (tendon) — *see* Injury, muscle, by site, strain
  neck S16.1 ☑
  physical NOS Z73.3
    work-related Z56.6
  postural (*see also* Disorder, soft tissue, due to use)
  psychological NEC Z73.3
  tendon — *see* Injury, muscle, by site, strain
Straining, on urination R39.16
Strand, vitreous — *see* Opacity, vitreous, membranes and strands
Strangulation, strangulated (*see also* Asphyxia, traumatic)
  appendix K38.8
  bladder-neck N32.0
  bowel or colon K56.2
  food or foreign body — *see* Foreign body, by site
  hemorrhoids — *see* Hemorrhoids, with complication
  hernia (*see also* Hernia, by site, with obstruction)
    with gangrene — *see* Hernia, by site, with gangrene
  intestine (large) (small) K56.2
    with hernia (*see also* Hernia, by site, with obstruction)
      with gangrene — *see* Hernia, by site, with gangrene
  mesentery K56.2
  mucus — *see* Asphyxia, mucus
  omentum K56.2
  organ or site, congenital NEC — *see* Atresia, by site
  ovary — *see* Torsion, ovary
  penis N48.89
    foreign body T19.4 ☑
  rupture — *see* Hernia, by site, with obstruction
  stomach due to hernia (*see also* Hernia, by site, with obstruction)
    with gangrene — *see* Hernia, by site, with gangrene
  vesicourethral orifice N32.0
Strangury R30.0
Straw itch B88.0
Strawberry
  gallbladder K82.4
  mark Q82.5
  tongue (red) (white) K14.3
Streak(s)
  macula, angioid H35.33
  ovarian Q50.32
Strephosymbolia F81.0
  secondary to organic lesion R48.8
Streptobacillary fever A25.1
Streptobacillosis A25.1
Streptobacillus moniliformis A25.1
Streptococcus, streptococcal (*see also* condition)
  as cause of disease classified elsewhere B95.5

Streptococcus, streptococcal — *continued*
  group
    A, as cause of disease classified elsewhere B95.Ø
    B, as cause of disease classified elsewhere B95.1
    D, as cause of disease classified elsewhere B95.2
  pneumoniae, as cause of disease classified elsewhere
      B95.3
  specified NEC, as cause of disease classified elsewhere
      B95.4
Streptomycosis B47.1
Streptotrichosis A48.8
Stress F43.9
  family — *see* Disruption, family
  fetal P84
    complicating pregnancy O77.9
      due to drug administration O77.1
  mental NEC Z73.3
    work-related Z56.6
  physical NEC Z73.3
    work-related Z56.6
  polycythemia D75.1
  reaction (*see also* Reaction, stress) F43.9
  work schedule Z56.3
Stretching, nerve — *see* Injury, nerve
Striae albicantes, atrophicae or distensae (cutis) L90.6
Stricture (*see also* Stenosis)
  ampulla of Vater K83.1
  anus (sphincter) K62.4
    congenital Q42.3
      with fistula Q42.2
    infantile Q42.3
      with fistula Q42.2
  aorta (ascending) (congenital) Q25.1
    arteriosclerotic I70.Ø
    calcified I70.Ø
    supravalvular, congenital Q25.3
  aortic (valve) — *see* Stenosis, aortic
  aqueduct of Sylvius (congenital) Q03.Ø
    with spina bifida — *see* Spina bifida, by site, with
        hydrocephalus
    acquired G91.1
  artery I77.1
    basilar — *see* Occlusion, artery, basilar
    carotid — *see* Occlusion, artery, carotid
    celiac I77.4
    congenital (peripheral) Q27.8
      cerebral Q28.3
      coronary Q24.5
      digestive system Q27.8
      lower limb Q27.8
      retinal Q14.1
      specified site NEC Q27.8
      umbilical Q27.Ø
      upper limb Q27.8
    coronary — *see* Disease, heart, ischemic,
        atherosclerotic
      congenital Q24.5
    precerebral — *see* Occlusion, artery, precerebral
    pulmonary (congenital) Q25.6
      acquired I28.8
    renal I70.1
    vertebral — *see* Occlusion, artery, vertebral
  auditory canal (external) (congenital)
    acquired — *see* Stenosis, external ear canal
  bile duct (common) (hepatic) K83.1
    congenital Q44.3
    postoperative K91.89
  bladder N32.89
    neck N32.Ø
  bowel — *see* Obstruction, intestine
  brain G93.89
  bronchus J98.Ø9
    congenital Q32.3
    syphilitic A52.72
  cardia (stomach) K22.2
    congenital Q39.3
  cardiac (*see also* Disease, heart)
    orifice (stomach) K22.2
  cecum — *see* Obstruction, intestine
  cervix, cervical (canal) N88.2
    congenital Q51.828
    in pregnancy — *see* Pregnancy, complicated by,
        abnormal cervix
      causing obstructed labor O65.5
  colon (*see also* Obstruction, intestine)
    congenital Q42.9
      specified NEC Q42.8
  colostomy K94.Ø3

Stricture — *continued*
  common (bile) duct K83.1
  coronary (artery) — *see* Disease, heart, ischemic,
      atherosclerotic
  cystic duct — *see* Obstruction, gallbladder
  digestive organs NEC, congenital Q45.8
  duodenum K31.5
    congenital Q41.Ø
  ear canal (external) (congenital) Q16.1
    acquired — *see* Stricture, auditory canal, acquired
  ejaculatory duct N50.89
  enterostomy K94.13
  esophagus K22.2
    congenital Q39.3
    syphilitic A52.79
      congenital A50.59 [K23]
  eustachian tube (*see also* Obstruction, eustachian tube)
    congenital Q17.8
  fallopian tube N97.1
    gonococcal A54.24
    tuberculous A18.17
  gallbladder — *see* Obstruction, gallbladder
  glottis J38.6
  heart (*see also* Disease, heart)
    valve (*see also* Endocarditis) I38
      aortic Q23.Ø
      mitral Q23.2
      pulmonary Q22.1
      tricuspid Q22.4
  hepatic duct K83.1
  hourglass, of stomach K31.2
  hymen N89.6
  hypopharynx J39.2
  ileum (*see also* Obstruction, intestine, specified NEC)
      K56.699
    congenital Q41.2
  intestine (*see also* Obstruction, intestine)
    congenital (small) Q41.9
      large Q42.9
        specified NEC Q42.8
      specified NEC Q41.8
    ischemic K55.1
  jejunum (*see also* Obstruction, intestine, specified NEC)
      K56.699
    congenital Q41.1
  lacrimal passages (*see also* Stenosis, lacrimal)
    congenital Q10.5
  larynx J38.6
    congenital NEC Q31.8
      subglottic Q31.1
    syphilitic A52.73
      congenital A50.59 [J99]
  meatus
    ear (congenital) Q16.1
      acquired — *see* Stricture, auditory canal, ac-
          quired
    osseous (ear) (congenital) Q16.1
      acquired — *see* Stricture, auditory canal, ac-
          quired
    urinarius (*see also* Stricture, urethra)
      congenital Q64.33
  mitral (valve) — *see* Stenosis, mitral
  myocardium, myocardial I51.5
    hypertrophic subaortic (idiopathic) I42.1
  nares (anterior) (posterior) J34.89
    congenital Q30.Ø
  nasal duct (*see also* Stenosis, lacrimal, duct)
    congenital Q10.5
  nasolacrimal duct (*see also* Stenosis, lacrimal, duct)
    congenital Q10.5
  nasopharynx J39.2
    syphilitic A52.73
  nose J34.89
    congenital Q30.Ø
  nostril (anterior) (posterior) J34.89
    congenital Q30.Ø
    syphilitic A52.73
      congenital A50.59 [J99]
  organ or site, congenital NEC — *see* Atresia, by site
  os uteri — *see* Stricture, cervix
  osseous meatus (ear) (congenital) Q16.1
    acquired — *see* Stricture, auditory canal, acquired
  oviduct — *see* Stricture, fallopian tube
  pelviureteric junction (congenital) Q62.11
    acquired, with hydronephrosis N13.Ø
  penis, by foreign body T19.4 ☑
  pharynx J39.2
  prostate N42.89

Stricture — *continued*
  pulmonary, pulmonic
    artery (congenital) Q25.6
      acquired I28.8
      noncongenital I28.8
    infundibulum (congenital) Q24.3
    valve I37.Ø
      congenital Q22.1
    vein, acquired I28.8
    vessel NEC I28.8
  punctum lacrimale (*see also* Stenosis, lacrimal, punc-
      tum)
    congenital Q10.5
  pylorus (hypertrophic) K31.1
    adult K31.1
    congenital Q40.Ø
    infantile Q40.Ø
  rectosigmoid (*see also* Obstruction, intestine, specified
      NEC) K56.699
  rectum (sphincter) K62.4
    congenital Q42.1
      with fistula Q42.Ø
    due to
      chlamydial lymphogranuloma A55
      irradiation K91.89
      lymphogranuloma venereum A55
    gonococcal A54.6
    inflammatory (chlamydial) A55
    syphilitic A52.74
    tuberculous A18.32
  renal artery I70.1
    congenital Q27.1
  salivary duct or gland (any) K11.8
  sigmoid (flexure) — *see* Obstruction, intestine
  spermatic cord N50.89
  stoma (following) (of)
    colostomy K94.Ø3
    enterostomy K94.13
    gastrostomy K94.23
    ileostomy K94.13
    tracheostomy J95.Ø3
  stomach K31.89
    congenital Q40.2
    hourglass K31.2
  subaortic Q24.4
    hypertrophic (acquired) (idiopathic) I42.1
  subglottic J38.6
  syphilitic NEC A52.79
  trachea J39.8
    congenital Q32.1
    syphilitic A52.73
    tuberculous NEC A15.5
  tracheostomy J95.Ø3
  tricuspid (valve) — *see* Stenosis, tricuspid
  tunica vaginalis N50.89
  ureter (postoperative) N13.5
    with
      hydronephrosis N13.1
        with infection N13.6
        pyelonephritis (chronic) N11.1
    congenital — *see* Atresia, ureter
    tuberculous A18.11
  ureteropelvic junction (congenital) Q62.11
    acquired, with hydronephrosis N13.Ø
  ureterovesical orifice N13.5
    with infection N13.6
  urethra (organic) (spasmodic) N35.9
    associated with schistosomiasis B65.Ø [N37]
    congenital Q64.39
      valvular (posterior) Q64.2
    due to
      infection — *see* Stricture, urethra, postinfective
      trauma — *see* Stricture, urethra, post-traumatic
    gonococcal, gonorrheal A54.Ø1
    infective NEC — *see* Stricture, urethra, postinfective
    late effect (sequelae) of injury — *see* Stricture,
        urethra, post-traumatic
    postcatheterization — *see* Stricture, urethra, post-
        procedural
    postinfective NEC
      female N35.12
      male N35.119
        anterior urethra N35.114
        bulbous urethra N35.112
        meatal N35.111
        membranous urethra N35.113
    postobstetric N35.Ø21

Stricture — *continued*
  urethra — *continued*
    postoperative — *see* Stricture, urethra, postproce-
      dural
    postprocedural
      female N99.12
      male N99.114
        anterior bulbous urethra N99.113
        bulbous urethra N99.111
        fossa navicularis N99.115
        meatal N99.110
        membranous urethra N99.112
    post-traumatic
      female N35.028
        due to childbirth N35.021
      male N35.014
        anterior urethra N35.013
        bulbous urethra N35.011
        meatal N35.010
        membranous urethra N35.012
    sequela (late effect) of
      childbirth N35.021
      injury — *see* Stricture, urethra, post-traumatic
    specified cause NEC N35.8
    syphilitic A52.76
    traumatic — *see* Stricture, urethra, post-traumatic
    valvular (posterior), congenital Q64.2
  urinary meatus — *see* Stricture, urethra
  uterus, uterine (synechiae) N85.6
    os (external) (internal) — *see* Stricture, cervix
  vagina (outlet) — *see* Stenosis, vagina
  valve (cardiac) (heart) (*see also* Endocarditis)
    congenital
      aortic Q23.0
      mitral Q23.2
      pulmonary Q22.1
      tricuspid Q22.4
  vas deferens N50.89
    congenital Q55.4
  vein I87.1
  vena cava (inferior) (superior) NEC I87.1
    congenital Q26.0
  vesicourethral orifice N32.0
    congenital Q64.31
  vulva (acquired) N90.5
Stridor R06.1
  congenital (larynx) P28.89
Stridulous — *see* condition
Stroke (apoplectic) (brain) (embolic) (ischemic) (paralytic)
  (thrombotic) I63.9
  cryptogenic (*see also* infarction, cerebral) I63.9
  epileptic — *see* Epilepsy
  heat T67.0 ☑
  in evolution I63.9
  intraoperative
    during cardiac surgery I97.810
    during other surgery I97.811
  lightning — *see* Lightning
  meaning
    cerebral hemorrhage — *code to* Hemorrhage, in-
      tracranial
    cerebral infarction — *code to* Infarction, cerebral
  postprocedural
    following cardiac surgery I97.820
    following other surgery I97.821
  unspecified (NOS) I63.9
Stromatosis, endometrial D39.0
Strongyloidiasis, strongyloidosis B78.9
  cutaneous B78.1
  disseminated B78.7
  intestinal B78.0
Strophulus pruriginosus L28.2
Struck by lightning — *see* Lightning
Struma (*see also* Goiter)
  Hashimoto E06.3
  lymphomatosa E06.3
  nodosa (simplex) E04.9
    endemic E01.2
      multinodular E01.1
    multinodular E04.2
      iodine-deficiency related E01.1
    toxic or with hyperthyroidism E05.20
      with thyroid storm E05.21
      multinodular E05.20
        with thyroid storm E05.21
      uninodular E05.10
        with thyroid storm E05.11
    toxicosa E05.20

Struma — *continued*
  nodosa — *continued*
    toxicosa — *continued*
      with thyroid storm E05.21
      multinodular E05.20
        with thyroid storm E05.21
      uninodular E05.10
        with thyroid storm E05.11
      uninodular E04.1
  ovarii D27.- ☑
  Riedel's E06.5
Strumipriva cachexia E03.4
Strümpell-Marie spine — *see* Spondylitis, ankylosing
Strümpell-Westphal pseudosclerosis E83.01
Stuart deficiency disease (factor X) D68.2
Stuart-Prower factor deficiency (factor X) D68.2
Student's elbow — *see* Bursitis, elbow, olecranon
Stump — *see* Amputation
Stunting, nutritional E45
Stupor (catatonic) R40.1
  depressive (single episode) F32.89
    recurrent episode F33.8
  dissociative F44.2
  manic F30.2
  manic-depressive F31.89
  psychogenic (anergic) F44.2
  reaction to exceptional stress (transient) F43.0
Sturge (-Weber) (-Dimitri) (-Kalischer) **disease or syn-**
  drome Q85.8
Stuttering F80.81
  adult onset F98.5
  childhood onset F80.81
  following cerebrovascular disease — *see* Disorder,
    fluency. following cerebrovascular disease
  in conditions classified elsewhere R47.82
Sty, stye (external) (internal) (meibomian) (zeisian) —
  see Hordeolum
Subacidity, gastric K31.89
  psychogenic F45.8
Subacute — *see* condition
Subarachnoid — *see* condition
Subcortical — *see* condition
Subcostal syndrome, nerve compression — *see*
  Mononeuropathy, upper limb, specified site NEC
Subcutaneous, subcuticular — *see* condition
Subdural — *see* condition
Subendocardium — *see* condition
Subependymoma
  specified site — *see* Neoplasm, uncertain behavior,
    by site
  unspecified site D43.2
Suberosis J67.3
Subglossitis — *see* Glossitis
Subhemophilia D66
Subinvolution
  breast (postlactational) (postpuerperal) N64.89
  puerperal O90.89
  uterus (chronic) (nonpuerperal) N85.3
    puerperal O90.89
Sublingual — *see* condition
Sublinguitis — *see* Sialoadenitis
Subluxatable hip Q65.6
Subluxation (*see also* Dislocation)
  acromioclavicular S43.11- ☑
  ankle S93.0- ☑
  atlantoaxial, recurrent M43.4
    with myelopathy M43.3
  carpometacarpal (joint) NEC S63.05- ☑
    thumb S63.04- ☑
  complex, vertebral — *see* Complex, subluxation
  congenital (*see also* Malposition, congenital)
    hip — *see* Dislocation, hip, congenital, partial
    joint (excluding hip)
      lower limb Q68.8
      shoulder Q68.8
      upper limb Q68.8
  elbow (traumatic) S53.10- ☑
    anterior S53.11- ☑
    lateral S53.14- ☑
    medial S53.13- ☑
    posterior S53.12- ☑
    specified type NEC S53.19- ☑
  finger S63.20- ☑
    index S63.20- ☑
    interphalangeal S63.22- ☑
      distal S63.24- ☑
        index S63.24- ☑

Subluxation — *continued*
  finger — *continued*
    interphalangeal — *continued*
      distal — *continued*
        little S63.24- ☑
        middle S63.24- ☑
        ring S63.24- ☑
      index S63.22- ☑
      little S63.22- ☑
      middle S63.22- ☑
      proximal S63.23- ☑
        index S63.23- ☑
        little S63.23- ☑
        middle S63.23- ☑
        ring S63.23- ☑
      ring S63.22- ☑
    little S63.20- ☑
    metacarpophalangeal S63.21- ☑
      index S63.21- ☑
      little S63.21- ☑
      middle S63.21- ☑
      ring S63.21- ☑
    middle S63.20- ☑
    ring S63.20- ☑
  foot S93.30- ☑
    specified site NEC S93.33- ☑
    tarsal joint S93.31- ☑
    tarsometatarsal joint S93.32- ☑
    toe — *see* Subluxation, toe
  hip S73.00- ☑
    anterior S73.03- ☑
      obturator S73.02- ☑
    central S73.04- ☑
    posterior S73.01- ☑
  interphalangeal (joint)
    finger S63.22- ☑
      distal joint S63.24- ☑
        index S63.24- ☑
        little S63.24- ☑
        middle S63.24- ☑
        ring S63.24- ☑
      index S63.22- ☑
      little S63.22- ☑
      middle S63.22- ☑
      proximal joint S63.23- ☑
        index S63.23- ☑
        little S63.23- ☑
        middle S63.23- ☑
        ring S63.23- ☑
      ring S63.22- ☑
    thumb S63.12- ☑
      distal joint S63.14- ☑
      proximal joint S63.13- ☑
    toe S93.13- ☑
      great S93.13- ☑
      lesser S93.13- ☑
  joint prosthesis — *see* Complications, joint prosthesis,
    mechanical, displacement, by site
  knee S83.10- ☑
    cap — *see* Subluxation, patella
    patella — *see* Subluxation, patella
    proximal tibia
      anteriorly S83.11- ☑
      laterally S83.14- ☑
      medially S83.13- ☑
      posteriorly S83.12- ☑
    specified type NEC S83.19- ☑
  lens — *see* Dislocation, lens, partial
  ligament, traumatic — *see* Sprain, by site
  metacarpal (bone)
    proximal end S63.06- ☑
  metacarpophalangeal (joint)
    finger S63.21- ☑
      index S63.21- ☑
      little S63.21- ☑
      middle S63.21- ☑
      ring S63.21- ☑
    thumb S63.11- ☑
  metatarsophalangeal joint S93.14- ☑
    great toe S93.14- ☑
    lesser toe S93.14- ☑
  midcarpal (joint) S63.03- ☑
  patella S83.00- ☑
    lateral S83.01- ☑
    recurrent (nontraumatic) — *see* Dislocation,
      patella, recurrent, incomplete

☑ **Additional Character Required** — Refer to the Tabular List for Character Selection   ▽ Subterms under main terms may continue to next column or page

Subluxation — continued
- patella — continued
  - specified type NEC S83.09- ☑
- pathological — see Dislocation, pathological
- radial head S53.00- ☑
  - anterior S53.01- ☑
  - nursemaid's elbow S53.03- ☑
  - posterior S53.02- ☑
  - specified type NEC S53.09- ☑
- radiocarpal (joint) S63.02- ☑
- radioulnar (joint)
  - distal S63.01- ☑
  - proximal — see Subluxation, elbow
- shoulder
  - congenital Q68.8
  - girdle S43.30- ☑
    - scapula S43.31- ☑
    - specified site NEC S43.39- ☑
  - traumatic S43.00- ☑
    - anterior S43.01- ☑
    - inferior S43.03- ☑
    - posterior S43.02- ☑
    - specified type NEC S43.08- ☑
- sternoclavicular (joint) S43.20- ☑
  - anterior S43.21- ☑
  - posterior S43.22- ☑
- symphysis (pubis)
- thumb S63.103 ☑
  - interphalangeal joint — see Subluxation, interphalangeal (joint), thumb
  - metacarpophalangeal joint — see Subluxation, metacarpophalangeal (joint), thumb
- toe(s) S93.10- ☑
  - great S93.10- ☑
    - interphalangeal joint S93.13- ☑
    - metatarsophalangeal joint S93.14- ☑
  - interphalangeal joint S93.13- ☑
  - lesser S93.10- ☑
    - interphalangeal joint S93.13- ☑
    - metatarsophalangeal joint S93.14- ☑
  - metatarsophalangeal joint S93.149 ☑
- ulna
  - distal end S63.07- ☑
  - proximal end — see Subluxation, elbow
- ulnohumeral joint — see Subluxation, elbow
- vertebral
  - recurrent NEC — see subcategory M43.5 ☑
  - traumatic
    - cervical S13.100 ☑
      - atlantoaxial joint S13.120 ☑
      - atlantooccipital joint S13.110 ☑
      - atloidooccipital joint S13.110 ☑
      - joint between
        - C0 and C1 S13.110 ☑
        - C1 and C2 S13.120 ☑
        - C2 and C3 S13.130 ☑
        - C3 and C4 S13.140 ☑
        - C4 and C5 S13.150 ☑
        - C5 and C6 S13.160 ☑
        - C6 and C7 S13.170 ☑
        - C7 and T1 S13.180 ☑
      - occipitoatloid joint S13.110 ☑
    - lumbar S33.100 ☑
      - joint between
        - L1 and L2 S33.110 ☑
        - L2 and L3 S33.120 ☑
        - L3 and L4 S33.130 ☑
        - L4 and L5 S33.140 ☑
    - thoracic S23.100 ☑
      - joint between
        - T1 and T2 S23.110 ☑
        - T2 and T3 S23.120 ☑
        - T3 and T4 S23.122 ☑
        - T4 and T5 S23.130 ☑
        - T5 and T6 S23.132 ☑
        - T6 and T7 S23.140 ☑
        - T7 and T8 S23.142 ☑
        - T8 and T9 S23.150 ☑
        - T9 and T10 S23.152 ☑
        - T10 and T11 S23.160 ☑
        - T11 and T12 S23.162 ☑
        - T12 and L1 S23.170 ☑
- wrist (carpal bone) S63.00- ☑
  - carpometacarpal joint — see Subluxation, carpometacarpal (joint)

Subluxation — continued
- wrist — continued
  - distal radioulnar joint — see Subluxation, radioulnar (joint), distal
  - metacarpal bone, proximal — see Subluxation, metacarpal (bone), proximal end
  - midcarpal — see Subluxation, midcarpal (joint)
  - radiocarpal joint — see Subluxation, radiocarpal (joint)
  - recurrent — see Dislocation, recurrent, wrist
  - specified site NEC S63.09- ☑
  - ulna — see Subluxation, ulna, distal end
Submaxillary — see condition
Submersion (fatal) (nonfatal) T75.1 ☑
Submucous — see condition
Subnormal, subnormality
- accommodation (old age) H52.4
- mental — see Disability, intellectual
- temperature (accidental) T68 ☑
Subphrenic — see condition
Subscapular nerve — see condition
Subseptus uterus Q51.2
Subsiding appendicitis K36
Substance (other psychoactive) **-induced**
- anxiety disorder F19.980
- bipolar and related disorder F19.94
- delirium F19.921
- depressive disorder F19.94
- major neurocognitive disorder F19.97
- mild neurocognitive disorder F19.988
- obsessive-compulsive and related disorder F19.988
- psychotic disorder F19.959
- sexual dysfunction F19.981
- sleep disorder F19.982
Substernal thyroid E04.9
- congenital Q89.2
Substitution disorder F44.9
Subtentorial — see condition
Subthyroidism (acquired) (see also Hypothyroidism)
- congenital E03.1
Succenturiate placenta O43.19- ☑
Sucking thumb, child (excessive) F98.8
Sudamen, sudamina L74.1
Sudanese kala-azar B55.0
Sudden
- hearing loss — see Deafness, sudden
- heart failure — see Failure, heart
Sudeck's atrophy, disease, or syndrome — see Algoneurodystrophy
Suffocation — see Asphyxia, traumatic
Sugar
- blood
  - high (transient) R73.9
  - low (transient) E16.2
- in urine R81
Suicide, suicidal (attempted) T14.91 ☑
- by poisoning — see Table of Drugs and Chemicals
- history of (personal) Z91.5
  - in family Z81.8
- ideation — see Ideation, suicidal
- risk
  - meaning personal history of attempted suicide Z91.5
  - meaning suicidal ideation — see Ideation, suicidal
- tendencies
  - meaning personal history of attempted suicide Z91.5
  - meaning suicidal ideation — see Ideation, suicidal
- trauma — see nature of injury by site
Suipestifer infection — see Infection, salmonella
Sulfhemoglobinemia, sulphemoglobinemia (acquired) (with methemoglobinemia) D74.8
Sumatran mite fever A75.3
Summer — see condition
Sunburn L55.9
- due to
  - tanning bed (acute) L56.8
    - chronic L57.8
  - ultraviolet radiation (acute) L56.8
    - chronic L57.8
- first degree L55.0
- second degree L55.1
- third degree L55.2
SUNCT (short lasting unilateral neuralgiform headache with conjunctival injection and tearing) G44.059
- intractable G44.051
- not intractable G44.059

Sundowning F05
Sunken acetabulum — see Derangement, joint, specified type NEC, hip
Sunstroke T67.0 ☑
Superfecundation — see Pregnancy, multiple
Superfetation — see Pregnancy, multiple
Superinvolution (uterus) N85.8
Supernumerary (congenital)
- aortic cusps Q23.8
- auditory ossicles Q16.3
- bone Q79.8
- breast Q83.1
- carpal bones Q74.0
- cusps, heart valve NEC Q24.8
  - aortic Q23.8
  - mitral Q23.2
  - pulmonary Q22.3
- digit(s) Q69.9
- ear (lobule) Q17.0
- fallopian tube Q50.6
- finger Q69.0
- hymen Q52.4
- kidney Q63.0
- lacrimonasal duct Q10.6
- lobule (ear) Q17.0
- mitral cusps Q23.2
- muscle Q79.8
- nipple(s) Q83.3
- organ or site not listed — see Accessory
- ossicles, auditory Q16.3
- ovary Q50.31
- oviduct Q50.6
- pulmonary, pulmonic cusps Q22.3
- rib Q76.6
  - cervical or first (syndrome) Q76.5
- roots (of teeth) K00.2
- spleen Q89.09
- tarsal bones Q74.2
- teeth K00.1
- testis Q55.29
- thumb Q69.1
- toe Q69.2
- uterus Q51.2
- vagina Q52.1 ☑
- vertebra Q76.49
Supervision (of)
- contraceptive — see Prescription, contraceptives
- dietary (for) Z71.3
  - allergy (food) Z71.3
  - colitis Z71.3
  - diabetes mellitus Z71.3
  - food allergy or intolerance Z71.3
  - gastritis Z71.3
  - hypercholesterolemia Z71.3
  - hypoglycemia Z71.3
  - intolerance (food) Z71.3
  - obesity Z71.3
  - specified NEC Z71.3
- healthy infant or child Z76.2
  - foundling Z76.1
- high-risk pregnancy — see Pregnancy, complicated by, high, risk
- lactation Z39.1
- pregnancy — see Pregnancy, supervision of
Supplemental teeth K00.1
Suppression
- binocular vision H53.34
- lactation O92.5
- menstruation N94.89
- ovarian secretion E28.39
- renal N28.9
- urine, urinary secretion R34
Suppuration, suppurative (see also condition)
- accessory sinus (chronic) — see Sinusitis
- adrenal gland
- antrum (chronic) — see Sinusitis, maxillary
- bladder — see Cystitis
- brain G06.0
  - sequelae G09
- breast N61.1
  - puerperal, postpartum or gestational — see Mastitis, obstetric, purulent
- dental periosteum M27.3
- ear (middle) (see also Otitis, media)
  - external NEC — see Otitis, externa, infective
  - internal — see subcategory H83.0 ☑
- ethmoidal (chronic) (sinus) — see Sinusitis, ethmoidal
- fallopian tube — see Salpingo-oophoritis

Suppuration, suppurative — *continued*
  frontal (chronic) (sinus) — *see* Sinusitis, frontal
  gallbladder (acute) K81.0
  gum K05.20
    generalized — *see* Peridontitis, aggressive, generalized
    localized — *see* Peridontitis, aggressive, localized
  intracranial G06.0
  joint — *see* Arthritis, pyogenic or pyemic
  labyrinthine — *see* subcategory H83.0 ☑
  lung — *see* Abscess, lung
  mammary gland N61.1
    puerperal, postpartum O91.12
      associated with lactation O91.13
  maxilla, maxillary M27.2
    sinus (chronic) — *see* Sinusitis, maxillary
  muscle — *see* Myositis, infective
  nasal sinus (chronic) — *see* Sinusitis
  pancreas, acute (*see also* Pancreatitis, acute) K85.80
  parotid gland — *see* Sialoadenitis
  pelvis, pelvic
    female — *see* Disease, pelvis, inflammatory
    male K65.0
  pericranial — *see* Osteomyelitis
  salivary duct or gland (any) — *see* Sialoadenitis
  sinus (accessory) (chronic) (nasal) — *see* Sinusitis
  sphenoidal sinus (chronic) — *see* Sinusitis, sphenoidal
  thymus (gland) E32.1
  thyroid (gland) E06.0
  tonsil — *see* Tonsillitis
  uterus — *see* Endometritis
Supraeruption of tooth (teeth) M26.34
Supraglottitis J04.30
  with obstruction J04.31
Suprarenal (gland) — *see* condition
Suprascapular nerve — *see* condition
Suprasellar — *see* condition
Surfer's knots or nodules S89.8- ☑
Surgical
  emphysema T81.82 ☑
  procedures, complication or misadventure — *see* Complications, surgical procedures
  shock T81.10 ☑
Surveillance (of) (for) (*see also* Observation)
  alcohol abuse Z71.41
  contraceptive — *see* Prescription, contraceptives
  dietary Z71.3
  drug abuse Z71.51
Susceptibility to disease, genetic Z15.89
  malignant neoplasm Z15.09
    breast Z15.01
    endometrium Z15.04
    ovary Z15.02
    prostate Z15.03
    specified NEC Z15.09
  multiple endocrine neoplasia Z15.81
Suspected condition, ruled out (*see also* Observation, suspected)
  amniotic cavity and membrane Z03.71
  cervical shortening Z03.75
  fetal anomaly Z03.73
  fetal growth Z03.74
  maternal and fetal conditions NEC Z03.79
  newborn (*see also* Observation, newborn, suspected condition ruled out) Z05.9
  oligohydramnios Z03.71
  placental problem Z03.72
  polyhydramnios Z03.71
Suspended uterus
  in pregnancy or childbirth — *see* Pregnancy, complicated by, abnormal uterus
Sutton's nevus D22.9
Suture
  burst (in operation wound) T81.31 ☑
    external operation wound T81.31 ☑
    internal operation wound T81.32 ☑
  inadvertently left in operation wound — *see* Foreign body, accidentally left during a procedure
  removal Z48.02
Swab inadvertently left in operation wound — *see* Foreign body, accidentally left during a procedure
Swallowed, swallowing
  difficulty — *see* Dysphagia
  foreign body — *see* Foreign body, alimentary tract
Swan-neck deformity (finger) — *see* Deformity, finger, swan-neck
Swearing, compulsive F42.8

Swearing, compulsive — *continued*
  in Gilles de la Tourette's syndrome F95.2
Sweat, sweats
  fetid L75.0
  night R61
Sweating, excessive R61
Sweeley-Klionsky disease E75.21
Sweet's disease or dermatosis L98.2
Swelling (of) R60.9
  abdomen, abdominal (not referable to any particular organ) — *see* Mass, abdominal
  ankle — *see* Effusion, joint, ankle
  arm M79.89
    forearm M79.89
  breast (*see also* Lump, breast) N63.0
  Calabar B74.3
  cervical gland R59.0
  chest, localized R22.2
  ear H93.8- ☑
  extremity (lower) (upper) — *see* Disorder, soft tissue, specified type NEC
  finger M79.89
  foot M79.89
  glands R59.9
    generalized R59.1
    localized R59.0
  hand M79.89
  head (localized) R22.0
  inflammatory — *see* Inflammation
  intra-abdominal — *see* Mass, abdominal
  joint — *see* Effusion, joint
  leg M79.89
    lower M79.89
  limb — *see* Disorder, soft tissue, specified type NEC
  localized (skin) R22.9
    chest R22.2
    head R22.0
    limb
      lower — *see* Mass, localized, limb, lower
      upper — *see* Mass, localized, limb, upper
    neck R22.1
    trunk R22.2
  neck (localized) R22.1
  pelvic — *see* Mass, abdominal
  scrotum N50.89
  splenic — *see* Splenomegaly
  testis N50.89
  toe M79.89
  umbilical R19.09
  wandering, due to Gnathostoma (spinigerum) B83.1
  white — *see* Tuberculosis, arthritis
Swift (-Feer) **disease**
  overdose or wrong substance given or taken — *see* Table of Drugs and Chemicals, by drug, poisoning
Swimmer's
  cramp T75.1 ☑
  ear H60.33- ☑
  itch B65.3
Swimming in the head R42
Swollen — *see* Swelling
Swyer syndrome Q99.1
Sycosis L73.8
  barbae (not parasitic) L73.8
  contagiosa (mycotic) B35.0
  lupoides L73.8
  mycotic B35.0
  parasitic B35.0
  vulgaris L73.8
Sydenham's chorea — *see* Chorea, Sydenham's
Sylvatic yellow fever A95.0
Sylvest's disease B33.0
Symblepharon H11.23- ☑
  congenital Q10.3
Symond's syndrome G93.2
Sympathetic — *see* condition
Sympatheticotonia G90.8
Sympathicoblastoma
  specified site — *see* Neoplasm, malignant, by site
  unspecified site C74.90
Sympathogonioma — *see* Sympathicoblastoma
Symphalangy (fingers) (toes) Q70.9
Symptoms NEC R68.89
  breast NEC N64.59
  cold J00
  development NEC R63.8
  factitious, self-induced — *see* Disorder, factitious

Symptoms — *continued*
  genital organs, female R10.2
  involving
    abdomen NEC R19.8
    appearance NEC R46.89
    awareness R41.9
      altered mental status R41.82
      amnesia — *see* Amnesia
      borderline intellectual functioning R41.83
      coma — *see* Coma
      disorientation R41.0
      neurologic neglect syndrome R41.4
      senile cognitive decline R41.81
      specified symptom NEC R41.89
    behavior NEC R46.89
    cardiovascular system NEC R09.89
    chest NEC R09.89
    circulatory system NEC R09.89
    cognitive functions R41.9
      altered mental status R41.82
      amnesia — *see* Amnesia
      borderline intellectual functioning R41.83
      coma — *see* Coma
      disorientation R41.0
      neurologic neglect syndrome R41.4
      senile cognitive decline R41.81
      specified symptom NEC R41.89
    development NEC R62.50
    digestive system NEC R19.8
    emotional state NEC R45.89
      emotional lability R45.86
    food and fluid intake R63.8
    general perceptions and sensations R44.9
      specified NEC R44.8
    musculoskeletal system R29.91
      specified NEC R29.898
    nervous system R29.90
      specified NEC R29.818
    pelvis NEC R19.8
    respiratory system NEC R09.89
    skin and integument R23.9
    urinary system R39.9
  menopausal N95.1
  metabolism NEC R63.8
  neurotic F48.8
  of infancy R68.19
  pelvis NEC, female R10.2
  skin and integument NEC R23.9
  subcutaneous tissue NEC R23.9
  viral cold J00
Sympus Q74.2
Syncephalus Q89.4
Synchondrosis
  abnormal (congenital) Q78.8
  ischiopubic M91.0
Synchysis (scintillans) (senile) (vitreous body) H43.89
Syncope (near) (pre-) R55
  anginosa I20.8
  bradycardia R00.1
  cardiac R55
  carotid sinus G90.01
  due to spinal (lumbar) puncture G97.1
  heart R55
  heat T67.1 ☑
  laryngeal R05
  psychogenic F48.8
  tussive R05
  vasoconstriction R55
  vasodepressor R55
  vasomotor R55
  vasovagal R55
Syndactylism, syndactyly Q70.9
  complex (with synostosis)
    fingers Q70.0- ☑
    toes Q70.2- ☑
  simple (without synostosis)
    fingers Q70.1- ☑
    toes Q70.3- ☑
Syndrome (*see also* Disease)
  48,XXXX Q97.1
  49,XXXXX Q97.1
  5q minus NOS D46.C (*following* D46.2)
  abdominal
    acute R10.0
    muscle deficiency Q79.4
  abnormal innervation H02.519
    left H02.516
      lower H02.515

☑ **Additional Character Required — Refer to the Tabular List for Character Selection**   ⬇ Subterms under main terms may continue to next column or page

Syndrome — *continued*
  abnormal innervation — *continued*
    left — *continued*
      upper H02.514
    right H02.513
      lower H02.512
      upper H02.511
  abstinence, neonatal P96.1
  acid pulmonary aspiration, obstetric O74.0
  acquired immunodeficiency — *see* Human, immunod-
    eficiency virus (HIV) disease
  acute abdominal R10.0
  acute respiratory distress (adult) (child) J80
    idiopathic J84.114
  Adair-Dighton Q78.0
  Adams-Stokes (-Morgagni) I45.9
  adiposogenital E23.6
  adrenal
    hemorrhage (meningococcal) A39.1
    meningococcic A39.1
  adrenocortical — *see* Cushing's, syndrome
  adrenogenital E25.9
    congenital, associated with enzyme deficiency
      E25.0
  afferent loop NEC K91.89
  Alagille's Q44.7
  alcohol withdrawal (without convulsions) — *see* De-
    pendence, alcohol, with, withdrawal
  Alder's D72.0
  Aldrich (-Wiskott) D82.0
  alien hand R41.4
  Alport Q87.81
  alveolar hypoventilation E66.2
  alveolocapillary block J84.10
  amnesic, amnestic (confabulatory) (due to) — *see*
    Disorder, amnesic
  amyostatic (Wilson's disease) E83.01
  androgen insensitivity E34.50
    complete E34.51
    partial E34.52
  androgen resistance (*see also* Syndrome, androgen
    insensitivity) E34.50
  Angelman Q93.5
  anginal — *see* Angina
  ankyloglossia superior Q38.1
  anterior
    chest wall R07.89
    cord G83.82
    spinal artery G95.19
      compression M47.019
        cervical region M47.012
        cervicothoracic region M47.013
        lumbar region M47.016
        occipito-atlanto-axial region M47.011
        thoracic region M47.014
        thoracolumbar region M47.015
    tibial M76.81- ☑
  antibody deficiency D80.9
    agammaglobulinemic D80.1
      hereditary D80.0
    congenital D80.1
    hypogammaglobulinemic D80.1
      hereditary D80.0
  anticardiolipin (-antibody) D68.61
  antidepressant discontinuation T43.205 ☑
  antiphospholipid (-antibody) D68.61
  aortic
    arch M31.4
    bifurcation I74.09
  aortomesenteric duodenum occlusion K31.5
  apical ballooning (transient left ventricular) I51.81
  arcuate ligament I77.4
  argentaffin, argintaffinoma E34.0
  Arnold-Chiari — *see* Arnold-Chiari disease
  Arrillaga-Ayerza I27.0
  arterial tortuosity Q87.82
  arteriovenous steal T82.898- ☑
  Asherman's N85.6
  aspiration, of newborn — *see* Aspiration, by substance,
    with pneumonia
    meconium P24.01
  ataxia-telangiectasia G11.3
  auriculotemporal G50.8
  autoerythrocyte sensitization (Gardner-Diamond)
    D69.2
  autoimmune lymphoproliferative [ALPS] D89.82
  autoimmune polyglandular E31.0
  autoinflammatory M04.9

Syndrome — *continued*
  autoinflammatory — *continued*
    specified type NEC M04.8
  autosomal — *see* Abnormal, autosomes
  Avellis' G46.8
  Ayerza (-Arrillaga) I27.0
  Babinski-Nageotte G83.89
  Bakwin-Krida Q78.5
  bare lymphocyte D81.6
  Barré-Guillain G61.0
  Barré-Liéou M53.0
  Barrett's — *see* Barrett's, esophagus
  Barsony-Polgar K22.4
  Bársony-Teschendorf K22.4
  Barth E78.71
  Bartter's E26.81
  basal cell nevus Q87.89
  Basedow's E05.00
    with thyroid storm E05.01
  basilar artery G45.0
  Batten-Steinert G71.11
  battered
    baby or child — *see* Maltreatment, child, physical
      abuse
    spouse — *see* Maltreatment, adult, physical abuse
  Beals Q87.40
  Beau's I51.5
  Beck's I65.8
  Benedikt's G46.3
  Béquez César (-Steinbrinck-Chédiak-Higashi) E70.330
  Bernhardt-Roth — *see* Meralgia paresthetica
  Bernheim's — *see* Failure, heart, right
  big spleen D73.1
  bilateral polycystic ovarian E28.2
  Bing-Horton's — *see* Horton's headache
  Birt-Hogg-Dube syndrome Q87.89
  Björck (-Thorsen) E34.0
  black
    lung J60
    widow spider bite — *see* Toxicity, venom, spider,
      black widow
  Blackfan-Diamond D61.01
  Blau M04.8
  blind loop K90.2
    congenital Q43.8
    postsurgical K91.2
  blue sclera Q78.0 ☑
  blue toe I75.02- ☑
  Boder-Sedgewick G11.3
  Boerhaave's K22.3
  Borjeson Forssman Lehmann Q89.8
  Bouillaud's I01.9
  Bourneville (-Pringle) Q85.1
  Bouveret (-Hoffman) I47.9
  brachial plexus G54.0
  bradycardia-tachycardia I49.5
  brain (nonpsychotic) F09
    with psychosis, psychotic reaction F09
      acute or subacute — *see* Delirium
    congenital — *see* Disability, intellectual
    organic F09
      post-traumatic (nonpsychotic) F07.81
        psychotic F09
      personality change F07.0
    postcontusional F07.81
    post-traumatic, nonpsychotic F07.81
    psycho-organic F09
    psychotic F06.8
  brain stem stroke G46.3
  Brandt's (acrodermatitis enteropathica) E83.2
  broad ligament laceration N83.8
  Brock's J98.11
  bronze baby P83.88
  Brown-Sequard G83.81
  Brugada I49.8
  bubbly lung P27.0
  Buchem's M85.2
  Budd-Chiari I82.0
  bulbar (progressive) G12.22
  Bürger-Grütz E78.3
  Burke's K86.89
  Burnett's (milk-alkali) E83.52
  burning feet E53.9
  Bywaters' T79.5 ☑
  Call-Fleming I67.841
  carbohydrate-deficient glycoprotein (CDGS) E77.8
  carcinogenic thrombophlebitis I82.1
  carcinoid E34.0

Syndrome — *continued*
  cardiac asthma I50.1
  cardiacos negros I27.0
  cardiofaciocutaneous Q87.89
  cardiopulmonary-obesity E66.2
  cardiorenal — *see* Hypertension, cardiorenal
  cardiorespiratory distress (idiopathic), newborn P22.0
  cardiovascular renal — *see* Hypertension, cardiorenal
  carotid
    artery (hemispheric) (internal) G45.1
    body G90.01
    sinus G90.01
  carpal tunnel G56.0- ☑
  Cassidy (-Scholte) E34.0
  cat cry Q93.4
  cat eye Q92.8
  cauda equina G83.4
  causalgia — *see* Causalgia
  celiac K90.0
    artery compression I77.4
    axis I77.4
  central pain G89.0
  cerebellar
    hereditary G11.9
    stroke G46.4
  cerebellomedullary malformation — *see* Spina bifida
  cerebral
    artery
      anterior G46.1
      middle G46.0
      posterior G46.2
    gigantism E22.0
  cervical (root) M53.1
    disc — *see* Disorder, disc, cervical, with neuritis
    fusion Q76.1
    posterior, sympathicus M53.0
    rib Q76.5
    sympathetic paralysis G90.2
  cervicobrachial (diffuse) M53.1
  cervicocranial M53.0
  cervicodorsal outlet G54.2
  cervicothoracic outlet G54.0
  Céstan (-Raymond) I65.8
  Charcot's (angina cruris) (intermittent claudication)
    I73.9
  Charcot-Weiss-Baker G90.09
  CHARGE Q89.8
  Chédiak-Higashi (-Steinbrinck) E70.330
  chest wall R07.1
  Chiari's (hepatic vein thrombosis) I82.0
  Chilaiditi's Q43.3
  child maltreatment — *see* Maltreatment, child
  chondrocostal junction M94.0
  chondroectodermal dysplasia Q77.6
  chromosome 4 short arm deletion Q93.3
  chromosome 5 short arm deletion Q93.4
  chronic
    infantile neurological, cutaneous and articular
      (CINCA) M04.2
    pain G89.4
    personality F68.8
  Clarke-Hadfield K86.89
  Clerambault's automatism G93.89
  Clouston's (hidrotic ectodermal dysplasia) Q82.4
  clumsiness, clumsy child F82
  cluster headache G44.009
    intractable G44.001
    not intractable G44.009
  Coffin-Lowry Q89.8
  cold injury (newborn) P80.0
  combined immunity deficiency D81.9
  compartment (deep) (posterior) (traumatic) T79.A0 ☑
    (*following* T79.7)
    abdomen T79.A3 ☑ (*following* T79.7)
    lower extremity (hip, buttock, thigh, leg, foot, toes)
      T79.A2 ☑ (*following* T79.7)
    nontraumatic
      abdomen M79.A3 (*following* M79.7)
      lower extremity (hip, buttock, thigh, leg, foot,
        toes) M79.A2- ☑ (*following* M79.7)
      specified site NEC M79.A9 (*following* M79.7)
      upper extremity (shoulder, arm, forearm, wrist,
        hand, fingers) M79.A1- ☑ (*following*
        M79.7)
    postprocedural — *see* Syndrome, compartment,
      nontraumatic
    specified site NEC T79.A9 ☑ (*following* T79.7)

Syndrome — *continued*
  compartment — *continued*
    upper extremity (shoulder, arm, forearm, wrist, hand, fingers) T79.A1 ☑ (*following* T79.7)
  complex regional pain — *see* Syndrome, pain, complex regional
  compression T79.5 ☑
    anterior spinal — *see* Syndrome, anterior, spinal artery, compression
    cauda equina G83.4
    celiac artery I77.4
    vertebral artery M47.029
      cervical region M47.022
      occipito-atlanto-axial region M47.021
  concussion F07.81
  congenital
    affecting multiple systems NEC Q87.89
    central alveolar hypoventilation G47.35
    facial diplegia Q87.0
    muscular hypertrophy-cerebral Q87.89
    oculo-auriculovertebral Q87.0
    oculofacial diplegia (Moebius) Q87.0
    rubella (manifest) P35.0
  congestion-fibrosis (pelvic), female N94.89
  congestive dysmenorrhea N94.6
  connective tissue M35.9
    overlap NEC M35.1
  Conn's E26.01
  conus medullaris G95.81
  cord
    anterior G83.82
    posterior G83.83
  coronary
    acute NEC I24.9
    insufficiency or intermediate I20.0
    slow flow I20.8
  Costen's (complex) M26.69
  costochondral junction M94.0
  costoclavicular G54.0
  costovertebral E22.0
  Cowden Q85.8
  craniovertebral M53.0
  Creutzfeldt-Jakob — *see* Creutzfeldt-Jakob disease or syndrome
  crib death R99
  cricopharyngeal — *see* Dysphagia
  cri-du-chat Q93.4
  croup J05.0
  CRPS I — *see* Syndrome, pain, complex regional I
  crush T79.5 ☑
  cryopyrin-associated perodic M04.2
  cryptophthalmos Q87.0
  cubital tunnel — *see* Lesion, nerve, ulnar
  Curschmann (-Batten) (-Steinert) G71.11
  Cushing's E24.9
    alcohol-induced E24.4
    drug-induced E24.2
    due to
      alcohol
      drugs E24.2
      ectopic ACTH E24.3
      overproduction of pituitary ACTH E24.0
      overdose or wrong substance given or taken — *see* Table of Drugs and Chemicals, by drug, poisoning
    pituitary-dependent E24.0
    specified type NEC E24.8
  cystic duct stump K91.5
  Dana-Putnam D51.0
  Danbolt (-Cross) (acrodermatitis enteropathica) E83.2
  Dandy-Walker Q03.1
    with spina bifida Q07.01
  Danlos' Q79.6
  De Quervain E34.51
  de Toni-Fanconi (-Debré) E72.09
    with cystinosis E72.04
  defibrination (*see also* Fibrinolysis)
    with
      antepartum hemorrhage — *see* Hemorrhage, antepartum, with coagulation defect
      intrapartum hemorrhage — *see* Hemorrhage, complicating, delivery
    newborn P60
    postpartum O72.3
  Degos' I77.89
  Déjérine-Roussy G89.0
  delayed sleep phase G47.21
  demyelinating G37.9

Syndrome — *continued*
  dependence — *see* F10-F19 with fourth character .2
  depersonalization (-derealization) F48.1
  di George's D82.1
  diabetes mellitus in newborn infant P70.2
  diabetes mellitus-hypertension-nephrosis — *see* Diabetes, nephrosis
  diabetes-nephrosis — *see* Diabetes, nephrosis
  diabetic amyotrophy — *see* Diabetes, amyotrophy
  dialysis associated steal T82.898- ☑
  Diamond-Blackfan D61.01
  Diamond-Gardener D69.2
  DIC (diffuse or disseminated intravascular coagulopathy) D65
  Dighton's Q78.0
  disequilibrium E87.8
  Döhle body-panmyelopathic D72.0
  dorsolateral medullary G46.4
  double athetosis G80.3
  Down (*see also* Down syndrome) Q90.9
  Dresbach's (elliptocytosis) D58.1
  Dressler's (postmyocardial infarction) I24.1
    postcardiotomy I97.0
  drug withdrawal, infant of dependent mother P96.1
  dry eye H04.12- ☑
  due to abnormality
    chromosomal Q99.9
      sex
        female phenotype Q97.9
        male phenotype Q98.9
        specified NEC Q99.8
  dumping (postgastrectomy) K91.1
    nonsurgical K31.89
  Dupré's (meningism) R29.1
  dysmetabolic X E88.81
  dyspraxia, developmental F82
  Eagle-Barrett Q79.4
  Eaton-Lambert — *see* Syndrome, Lambert-Eaton
  Ebstein's Q22.5
  ectopic ACTH E24.3
  eczema-thrombocytopenia D82.0
  Eddowes' Q78.0
  effort (psychogenic) F45.8
  Ehlers-Danlos Q79.6
  Eisenmenger's I27.83
  Ekman's Q78.0
  electric feet E53.8
  Ellis-van Creveld Q77.6
  empty nest Z60.0
  endocrine-hypertensive E27.0
  entrapment — *see* Neuropathy, entrapment
  eosinophilia-myalgia M35.8
  epileptic (*see also* Epilepsy, by type)
    absence G40.A09 (*following* G40.3)
      intractable G40.A19 (*following* G40.3)
        with status epilepticus G40.A11 (*following* G40.3)
        without status epilepticus G40.A19 (*following* G40.3)
      not intractable G40.A09 (*following* G40.3)
        with status epilepticus G40.A01 (*following* G40.3)
        without status epilepticus G40.A09 (*following* G40.3)
  Erdheim-Chester (ECD) E88.89
  Erdheim's E22.0
  erythrocyte fragmentation D59.4
  Evans D69.41
  exhaustion F48.8
  extrapyramidal G25.9
    specified NEC G25.89
  eye retraction — *see* Strabismus
  eyelid-malar-mandible Q87.0
  Faber's D50.9
  facial pain, paroxysmal G50.0
  Fallot's Q21.3
  familial cold autoinflammatory M04.2
  familial eczema-thrombocytopenia (Wiskott-Aldrich) D82.0
  Fanconi (-de Toni) (-Debré) E72.09
    with cystinosis E72.04
  Fanconi's (anemia) (congenital pancytopenia) D61.09
  fatigue
    chronic R53.82
    psychogenic F48.8
  faulty bowel habit K59.39
  Feil-Klippel (brevicollis) Q76.1
  Felty's — *see* Felty's syndrome

Syndrome — *continued*
  fertile eunuch E23.0
  fetal
    alcohol (dysmorphic) Q86.0
    hydantoin Q86.1
  Fiedler's I40.1
  first arch Q87.0
  fish odor E72.8
  Fisher's G61.0
  Fitzhugh-Curtis
    due to
      Chlamydia trachomatis A74.81
      Neisseria gonorrhorea (gonococcal peritonitis) A54.85
  Fitz's (*see also* Pancreatitis, acute) K85.80
  Flajani (-Basedow) E05.00
    with thyroid storm E05.01
  flatback — *see* Flatback syndrome
  floppy
    baby P94.2
    iris (intraoeprative) (IFIS) H21.81
    mitral valve I34.1
  flush E34.0
  Foix-Alajouanine G95.19
  Fong's Q87.2
  food protein-induced enterocolitis K52.21
  foramen magnum G93.5
  Foster-Kennedy H47.14- ☑
  Foville's (peduncular) G46.3
  fragile X Q99.2
  Franceschetti Q75.4
  Frey's
    auriculotemporal G50.8
    hyperhidrosis L74.52
  Friderichsen-Waterhouse A39.1
  Froin's G95.89
  frontal lobe F07.0
  Fukuhara E88.49
  functional
    bowel K59.9
    prepubertal castrate E29.1
  Gaisböck's D75.1
  ganglion (basal ganglia brain) G25.9
    geniculi G51.1
  Gardner-Diamond D69.2
  gastroesophageal
    junction K22.0
    laceration-hemorrhage K22.6
  gastrojejunal loop obstruction K91.89
  Gee-Herter-Heubner K90.0
  Gelineau's G47.419
    with cataplexy G47.411
  genito-anorectal A55
  Gerstmann-Sträussler-Scheinker (GSS) A81.82
  Gianotti-Crosti L44.4
  giant platelet (Bernard-Soulier) D69.1
  Gilles de la Tourette's F95.2
  goiter-deafness E07.1
  Goldberg Q89.8
  Goldberg-Maxwell E34.51
  Good's D83.8
  Gopalan' (burning feet) E53.8
  Gorlin's Q87.89
  Gougerot-Blum L81.7
  Gouley's I31.1
  Gower's R55
  gray or grey (newborn) P93.0
    platelet D69.1
  Gubler-Millard G46.3
  Guillain-Barré (-Strohl) G61.0
  gustatory sweating G50.8
  Hadfield-Clarke K86.89
  hair tourniquet — *see* Constriction, external, by site
  Hamman's J98.19
  hand-foot L27.1
  hand-shoulder G90.8
  hantavirus (cardio)-pulmonary (HPS) (HCPS) B33.4
  happy puppet Q93.5
  Harada's H30.81- ☑
  Hayem-Faber D50.9
  headache NEC G44.89
    complicated NEC G44.59
  Heberden's I20.8
  Hedinger's E34.0
  Hegglin's D72.0
  HELLP (hemolysis, elevated liver enzymes and low platelet count) O14.2- ☑
    complicating
      childbirth O14.24

Syndrome — continued
　HELLP — continued
　　complicating — continued
　　　puerperium O14.25
　hemolytic-uremic D59.3
　hemophagocytic, infection-associated D76.2
　Henoch-Schönlein D69.0
　hepatic flexure K59.8
　hepatopulmonary K76.81
　hepatorenal K76.7
　　following delivery O90.4
　　postoperative or postprocedural K91.83
　　postpartum, puerperal O90.4
　hepatourologic K76.7
　Herter (-Gee) (nontropical sprue) K90.0
　Heubner-Herter K90.0
　Heyd's K76.7
　Hilger's G90.09
　histamine-like (fish poisoning) — see Poisoning, fish
　histiocytic D76.3
　histiocytosis NEC D76.3
　HIV infection, acute B20
　Hoffmann-Werdnig G12.0
　Hollander-Simons E88.1
　Hoppe-Goldflam G70.00
　　with exacerbation (acute) G70.01
　　in crisis G70.01
　Horner's G90.2
　hungry bone E83.81
　hunterian glossitis D51.0
　Hutchinson's triad A50.53
　hyperabduction G54.0
　hyperammonemia-hyperornithinemia-homocitrulline-
　　mia E72.4
　hypereosinophilic (idiopathic) D72.1
　hyperimmunoglobulin D M04.1
　hyperimmunoglobulin E (IgE) D82.4
　hyperkalemic E87.5
　hyperkinetic — see Hyperkinesia
　hypermobility M35.7
　hypernatremia E87.0
　hyperosmolarity E87.0
　hyperperfusion G97.82
　hypersplenic D73.1
　hypertransfusion, newborn P61.1
　hyperventilation F45.8
　hyperviscosity (of serum)
　　polycythemic D75.1
　　sclerothymic D58.8
　hypoglycemic (familial) (neonatal) E16.2
　hypokalemic E87.6
　hyponatremic E87.1
　hypopituitarism E23.0
　hypoplastic left-heart Q23.4
　hypopotassemia E87.6
　hyposmolality E87.1
　hypotension, maternal O26.5- ☑
　hypothenar hammer I73.89
　hypoventilation, obesity (OHS) E66.2
　ICF (intravascular coagulation-fibrinolysis) D65
　idiopathic
　　cardiorespiratory distress, newborn P22.0
　　nephrotic (infantile) N04.9
　iliotibial band M76.3- ☑
　immobility, immobilization (paraplegic) M62.3
　immune reconstitution D89.3
　immune reconstitution inflammatory [IRIS] D89.3
　immunity deficiency, combined D81.9
　immunodeficiency
　　acquired — see Human, immunodeficiency virus
　　　(HIV) disease
　　combined D81.9
　impending coronary I20.0
　impingement, shoulder M75.4- ☑
　inappropriate secretion of antidiuretic hormone E22.2
　infant
　　gestational diabetes P70.0
　　of diabetic mother P70.1
　infantilism (pituitary) E23.0
　inferior vena cava I87.1
　inspissated bile (newborn) P59.1
　institutional (childhood) F94.2
　insufficient sleep F51.12
　intermediate coronary (artery) I20.0
　interspinous ligament — see Spondylopathy, specified
　　NEC
　intestinal
　　carcinoid E34.0

Syndrome — continued
　intestinal — continued
　　knot K56.2
　intravascular coagulation-fibrinolysis (ICF) D65
　iodine-deficiency, congenital E00.9
　　type
　　　mixed E00.2
　　　myxedematous E00.1
　　　neurological E00.0
　IRDS (idiopathic respiratory distress, newborn) P22.0
　irritable
　　bowel K58.9
　　　with
　　　　constipation K58.1
　　　　diarrhea K58.0
　　　mixed K58.2
　　　psychogenic F45.8
　　　specified NEC K58.8
　　heart (psychogenic) F45.8
　　weakness F48.8
　ischemic
　　bowel (transient) K55.9
　　　chronic K55.1
　　　due to mesenteric artery insufficiency K55.1
　　steal T82.898 ☑
　IVC (intravascular coagulopathy) D65
　Ivemark's Q89.01
　Jaccoud's — see Arthropathy, postrheumatic, chronic
　Jackson's G83.89
　Jakob-Creutzfeldt — see Creutzfeldt-Jakob disease or
　　syndrome
　jaw-winking Q07.8
　Jervell-Lange-Nielsen I45.81
　jet lag G47.25
　Job's D71
　Joseph-Diamond-Blackfan D61.01
　jugular foramen G52.7
　Kabuki Q89.8
　Kanner's (autism) F84.0
　Kartagener's Q89.3
　Kelly's D50.1
　Kimmelstiel-Wilson — see Diabetes, specified type,
　　with Kimmelstiel-Wilson disease
　Klein (e)-Levine G47.13
　Klippel-Feil (brevicollis) Q76.1
　Köhler-Pellegrini-Steida — see Bursitis, tibial collateral
　König's K59.8
　Korsakoff (-Wernicke) (nonalcoholic) F04
　　alcoholic F10.26
　Kostmann's D70.0
　Krabbe's congenital muscle hypoplasia Q79.8
　labyrinthine — see subcategory H83.2 ☑
　lacunar NEC G46.7
　Lambert-Eaton G70.80
　　in
　　　neoplastic disease G73.1
　　　specified disease NEC G70.81
　Landau-Kleffner — see Epilepsy, specified NEC
　Larsen's Q74.8
　lateral
　　cutaneous nerve of thigh G57.1- ☑
　　medullary G46.4
　Launois' E22.0
　lazy
　　leukocyte D70.8
　　posture M62.3
　Lemiere I80.8
　Lennox-Gastaut G40.812
　　intractable G40.814
　　　with status epilepticus G40.813
　　　without status epilepticus G40.814
　　not intractable G40.812
　　　with status epilepticus G40.811
　　　without status epilepticus G40.812
　lenticular, progressive E83.01
　Leopold-Levi's E05.90
　Lev's I44.2
　Lichtheim's D51.0
　Li-Fraumeni Z15.01
　Lightwood's N25.89
　Lignac (de Toni) (-Fanconi) (-Debré) E72.09
　　with cystinosis E72.04
　Likoff's I20.8
　limbic epilepsy personality F07.0
　liver-kidney K76.7
　lobotomy F07.0
　Loffler's J82
　long arm 18 or 21 deletion Q93.89

Syndrome — continued
　long QT I45.81
　Louis-Barré G11.3
　low
　　atmospheric pressure T70.29 ☑
　　back M54.5
　　output (cardiac) I50.9
　lower radicular, newborn (birth injury) P14.8
　Luetscher's (dehydration) E86.0
　Lupus anticoagulant D68.62
　Lutembacher's Q21.1
　macrophage activation D76.1
　　due to infection D76.2
　magnesium-deficiency R29.0
　Majeed M04.8
　Mal de Debarquement R42
　malabsorption K90.9
　　postsurgical K91.2
　malformation, congenital, due to
　　alcohol Q86.0
　　exogenous cause NEC Q86.8
　　hydantoin Q86.1
　　warfarin Q86.2
　malignant
　　carcinoid E34.0
　　neuroleptic G21.0
　Mallory-Weiss K22.6
　mandibulofacial dysostosis Q75.4
　manic-depressive — see Disorder, bipolar
　maple-syrup-urine E71.0
　Marable's I77.4
　Marfan's Q87.40
　　with
　　　cardiovascular manifestations Q87.418
　　　　aortic dilation Q87.410
　　　ocular manifestations Q87.42
　　　skeletal manifestations Q87.43
　Marie's (acromegaly) E22.0
　mast cell activation — see Activation, mast cell
　maternal hypotension — see Syndrome, hypotension,
　　maternal
　May (-Hegglin) D72.0
　McArdle (-Schmidt) (-Pearson) E74.04
　McQuarrie's E16.2
　meconium plug (newborn) P76.0
　median arcuate ligament I77.4
　Meekeren-Ehlers-Danlos Q79.6
　megavitamin-B6 E67.2
　Meige G24.4
　MELAS E88.41
　Mendelson's O74.0
　MERRF (myoclonic epilepsy associated with ragged-
　　red fibers) E88.42
　mesenteric
　　artery (superior) K55.1
　　vascular insufficiency K55.1
　metabolic E88.81
　metastatic carcinoid E34.0
　micrognathia-glossoptosis Q87.0
　midbrain NEC G93.89
　middle lobe (lung) J98.19
　middle radicular G54.0
　migraine (see also Migraine) G43.909
　Mikulicz' K11.8
　milk-alkali E83.52
　Millard-Gubler G46.3
　Miller-Dieker Q93.88
　Miller-Fisher G61.0
　Minkowski-Chauffard D58.0
　Mirizzi's K83.1
　MNGIE (Mitochondrial Neurogastrointestinal En-
　　cephalopathy) E88.49
　Möbius, ophthalmoplegic migraine — see Migraine,
　　ophthalmoplegic
　monofixation H50.42
　Morel-Moore M85.2
　Morel-Morgagni M85.2
　Morgagni (-Morel) (-Stewart) M85.2
　Morgagni-Adams-Stokes I45.9
　Mounier-Kuhn Q32.4
　　with bronchiectasis J47.9
　　　with
　　　　exacerbation (acute) J47.1
　　　　lower respiratory infection J47.0
　　acquired J98.09
　　　with bronchiectasis J47.9
　　　　with
　　　　　exacerbation (acute) J47.1
　　　　　lower respiratory infection J47.0

Syndrome — *continued*
Muckle-Wells M04.2
mucocutaneous lymph node (acute febrile) (MCLS) M30.3
multiple endocrine neoplasia (MEN) — *see* Neoplasia, endocrine, multiple (MEN)
multiple operations — *see* Disorder, factitious
myasthenic G70.9
  in
    diabetes mellitus — *see* Diabetes, amyotrophy
    endocrine disease NEC E34.9 [G73.3]
    neoplastic disease (*see also* Neoplasm) D49.9 [G73.3]
    thyrotoxicosis (hyperthyroidism) E05.90 [G73.3]
      with thyroid storm E05.91 [G73.3]
myelodysplastic D46.9
  with
    5q deletion D46.C (*following* D46.2)
    isolated del (5q) chromosomal abnormality D46.C (*following* D46.2)
  lesions, low grade D46.20
  specified NEC D46.Z (*following* D46.4)
myelopathic pain G89.0
myeloproliferative (chronic) D47.1
myofascial pain M79.1
Naffziger's G54.0
nail patella Q87.2
NARP (Neuropathy, Ataxia and Retinitis pigmentosa) E88.49
neonatal abstinence P96.1
nephritic (*see also* Nephritis)
  with edema — *see* Nephrosis
  acute N00.9
  chronic N03.9
  rapidly progressive N01.9
nephrotic (congenital) (*see also* Nephrosis) N04.9
  with
    dense deposit disease N04.6
    diffuse
      crescentic glomerulonephritis N04.7
      endocapillary proliferative glomerulonephritis N04.4
      membranous glomerulonephritis N04.2
      mesangial proliferative glomerulonephritis N04.3
      mesangiocapillary glomerulonephritis N04.5
    focal and segmental glomerular lesions N04.1
    minor glomerular abnormality N04.0
    specified morphological changes NEC N04.8
  diabetic — *see* Diabetes, nephrosis
neurologic neglect R41.4
Nezelof's D81.4
Nonne-Milroy-Meige Q82.0
Nothnagel's vasomotor acroparesthesia I73.89
obesity hypoventilation (OHS) E66.2
oculomotor H51.9
ophthalmoplegia-cerebellar ataxia — *see* Strabismus, paralytic, third nerve
oral allergy T78.1 ☑
oral-facial-digital Q87.0
organic
  affective F06.30
  amnesic (not alcohol- or drug-induced) F04
  brain F09
  depressive F06.31
  hallucinosis F06.0
  personality F07.0
Ormond's N13.5
oro-facial-digital Q87.0
os trigonum Q68.8
Osler-Weber-Rendu I78.0
osteoporosis-osteomalacia M83.8
Österreicher-Turner Q87.2
otolith — *see* subcategory H81.8 ☑
oto-palatal-digital Q87.0
outlet (thoracic) G54.0
ovary
  polycystic E28.2
  resistant E28.39
  sclerocystic E28.2
Owren's D68.2
Paget-Schroetter I82.890
pain (*see also* Pain)
  complex regional I G90.50
    lower limb G90.52- ☑
    specified site NEC G90.59
    upper limb G90.51- ☑
  complex regional II — *see* Causalgia

Syndrome — *continued*
painful
  bruising D69.2
  feet E53.8
  prostate N42.81
paralysis agitans — *see* Parkinsonism
paralytic G83.9
  specified NEC G83.89
Parinaud's H51.0
parkinsonian — *see* Parkinsonism
Parkinson's — *see* Parkinsonism
paroxysmal facial pain G50.0
Parry's E05.00
  with thyroid storm E05.01
Parsonage (-Aldren)-Turner G54.5
patella clunk M25.86- ☑
Paterson (-Brown) (-Kelly) D50.1
pectoral girdle I77.89
pectoralis minor I77.89
pediatric autoimmune neuropsychiatric disorders associated with streptococcal infections (PANDAS) D89.89
Pelger-Huet D72.0
pellagra-cerebellar ataxia-renal aminoaciduria E72.02
pellagroid E52
Pellegrini-Stieda — *see* Bursitis, tibial collateral
pelvic congestion-fibrosis, female N94.89
penta X Q97.1
peptic ulcer — *see* Ulcer, peptic
perabduction I77.89
periodic fever M04.1
periodic fever, aphthous stomatitis, pharyngitis, and adenopathy [PFAPA] M04.8
periodic headache, in adults and children — *see* Headache, periodic syndromes in adults and children
periurethral fibrosis N13.5
phantom limb (without pain) G54.7
  with pain G54.6
pharyngeal pouch D82.1
Pick's — *see* Disease, Pick's
Pickwickian E66.2
PIE (pulmonary infiltration with eosinophilia) J82
pigmentary pallidal degeneration (progressive) G23.0
pineal E34.8
pituitary E22.0
placental transfusion — *see* Pregnancy, complicated by, placental transfusion syndromes
plantar fascia M72.2
plateau iris (post-iridectomy) (postprocedural) H21.82
Plummer-Vinson D50.1
pluricarential of infancy E40
pluricarential of infancy E40
pluriglandular (compensatory) E31.8
  autoimmune E31.0
pneumatic hammer T75.21 ☑
polyangiitis overlap M30.8
polycarential of infancy E40
polyglandular E31.8
  autoimmune E31.0
polysplenia Q89.09
pontine NEC G93.89
popliteal
  artery entrapment I77.89
  web Q87.89
post chemoembolization — *code to* associated conditions
postcardiac injury
  postcardiotomy I97.0
  postmyocardial infarction I24.1
postcardiotomy I97.0
postcholecystectomy K91.5
postcommissurotomy I97.0
postconcussional F07.81
postcontusional F07.81
postencephalitic F07.89
posterior
  cervical sympathetic M53.0
  cord G83.83
  fossa compression G93.5
  reversible encephalopathy (PRES) I67.83
postgastrectomy (dumping) K91.1
postgastric surgery K91.1
postinfarction I24.1
postlaminectomy NEC M96.1
postleukotomy F07.0
postmastectomy lymphedema I97.2
postmyocardial infarction I24.1

Syndrome — *continued*
postoperative NEC T81.9 ☑
  blind loop K90.2
postpartum panhypopituitary (Sheehan) E23.0
postpolio (myelitic) G14
postthrombotic I87.009
  with
    inflammation I87.02- ☑
      with ulcer I87.03- ☑
    specified complication NEC I87.09- ☑
    ulcer I87.01- ☑
      with inflammation I87.03- ☑
  asymptomatic I87.00- ☑
postvagotomy K91.1
postvalvulotomy I97.0
postviral NEC G93.3
  fatigue G93.3
Potain's K31.0
potassium intoxication E87.5
precerebral artery (multiple) (bilateral) G45.2
preinfarction I20.0
preleukemic D46.9
premature senility E34.8
premenstrual dysphoric F32.89
premenstrual tension N94.3
Prinzmetal-Massumi R07.1
prune belly Q79.4
pseudo -Turner's Q87.1
pseudocarpal tunnel (sublimis) — *see* Syndrome, carpal tunnel
pseudoparalytica G70.00
  with exacerbation (acute) G70.01
  in crisis G70.01
psycho-organic (nonpsychotic severity) F07.9
  acute or subacute F05
  depressive type F06.31
  hallucinatory type F06.0
  nonpsychotic severity F07.0
  specified NEC F07.89
pulmonary
  arteriosclerosis I27.0
  dysmaturity (Wilson-Mikity) P27.0
  hypoperfusion (idiopathic) P22.0
  renal (hemorrhagic) (Goodpasture's) M31.0
pure
  motor lacunar G46.5
  sensory lacunar G46.6
Putnam-Dana D51.0
pyogenic arthritis, pyoderma gangrenosum, and acne [PAPA] M04.8
pyramidopallidonigral G20
pyriformis — *see* Lesion, nerve, sciatic
QT interval prolongation I45.81
radicular NEC — *see* Radiculopathy
  upper limbs, newborn (birth injury) P14.3
rapid time-zone change G47.25
Rasmussen G04.81
Raymond (-Céstan) I65.8
Raynaud's I73.00
  with gangrene I73.01
RDS (respiratory distress syndrome, newborn) P22.0
reactive airways dysfunction J68.3
Refsum's G60.1
Reifenstein E34.52
renal glomerulohyalinosis-diabetic — *see* Diabetes, nephrosis
Rendu-Osler-Weber I78.0
residual ovary N99.83
resistant ovary E28.39
respiratory
  distress
    acute J80
      adult J80
      child J80
    idiopathic J84.114
    newborn (idiopathic) (type I) P22.0
      type II P22.1
restless legs G25.81
retinoblastoma (familial) C69.2 ☑
retroperitoneal fibrosis N13.5
retroviral seroconversion (acute) Z21
Reye's G93.7
Richter — *see* Leukemia, chronic lymphocytic, B-cell type
Ridley's I50.1
right
  heart, hypoplastic Q22.6

☑ Additional Character Required — Refer to the Tabular List for Character Selection   🔺 Subterms under main terms may continue to next column or page

Syndrome — *continued*
  right — *continued*
    ventricular obstruction — *see* Failure, heart, congestive
  Romano-Ward (prolonged QT interval) I45.81
  rotator cuff, shoulder (*see also* Tear, rotator cuff) M75.10- ☑
  Rotes Quérol — *see* Hyperostosis, ankylosing
  Roth — *see* Meralgia paresthetica
  rubella (congenital) P35.0
  Ruvalcaba-Myhre-Smith E71.440
  Rytand-Lipsitch I44.2
  salt
    depletion E87.1
      due to heat NEC T67.8 ☑
        causing heat exhaustion or prostration T67.4 ☑
    low E87.1
  salt-losing N28.89
  Scaglietti-Dagnini E22.0
  scalenus anticus (anterior) G54.0
  scapulocostal — *see* Mononeuropathy, upper limb, specified site NEC
  scapuloperoneal G71.0
  schizophrenic, of childhood NEC F84.5
  Schnitzler D47.2
  Scholte's E34.0
  Schroeder's E27.0
  Schüller-Christian C96.5
  Schwachman's — *see* Syndrome, Shwachman's
  Schwartz (-Jampel) G71.13
  Schwartz-Bartter E22.2
  scimitar Q26.8
  sclerocystic ovary E28.2
  Seitelberger's G31.89
  septicemic adrenal hemorrhage A39.1
  seroconversion, retroviral (acute) Z21
  serous meningitis G93.2
  severe acute respiratory (SARS) J12.81
  shaken infant T74.4 ☑
  shock (traumatic) T79.4 ☑
    kidney N17.0
      following crush injury T79.5 ☑
    toxic A48.3
  shock-lung J80
  Shone's — *code to* specific anomalies
  short
    bowel K91.2
    rib Q77.2
  shoulder-hand — *see* Algoneurodystrophy
  Shwachman's D70.4
  sicca — *see* Sicca syndrome
  sick
    cell E87.1
    sinus I49.5
  sick-euthyroid E07.81
  sideropenic D50.1
  Siemens' ectodermal dysplasia Q82.4
  Silfversköld's Q78.9
  Simons' E88.1
  sinus tarsi M25.57- ☑
  sinusitis-bronchiectasis-situs inversus Q89.3
  Sipple's E31.22
  sirenomelia Q87.2
  Slocumb's E27.0
  slow flow, coronary I20.8
  Sluder's G44.89
  Smith-Magenis Q93.88
  Sneddon-Wilkinson L13.1
  Sotos' Q87.3
  South African cardiomyopathy I42.8
  spasmodic
    upward movement, eyes H51.8
    winking F95.8
  Spen's I45.9
  splenic
    agenesis Q89.01
    flexure K59.8
    neutropenia D73.81
  Spurway's Q78.0
  staphylococcal scalded skin L00
  steal
    arteriovenous T82.898- ☑
    ischemic T82.898- ☑
    subclavian G45.8
  Stein-Leventhal E28.2
  Stein's E28.2
  Stevens-Johnson syndrome L51.1

Syndrome — *continued*
  Stevens-Johnson syndrome — *continued*
    toxic epidermal necrolysis overlap L51.3
  Stewart-Morel M85.2
  Stickler Q89.8
  stiff baby Q89.8
  stiff man G25.82
  Still-Felty — *see* Felty's syndrome
  Stokes (-Adams) I45.9
  stone heart I50.1
  straight back, congenital Q76.49
  subclavian steal G45.8
  subcoracoid-pectoralis minor G54.0
  subcostal nerve compression I77.89
  subphrenic interposition Q43.3
  superior
    cerebellar artery I63.8
    mesenteric artery K55.1
    semi-circular canal dehiscence H83.8X- ☑
    vena cava I87.1
  supine hypotensive (maternal) — *see* Syndrome, hypotension, maternal
  suprarenal cortical E27.0
  supraspinatus (*see also* Tear, rotator cuff) M75.10- ☑
  Susac G93.49
  swallowed blood P78.2
  sweat retention L74.0
  Swyer Q99.1
  Symond's G93.2
  sympathetic
    cervical paralysis G90.2
    pelvic, female N94.89
  systemic inflammatory response (SIRS), of non-infectious origin (without organ dysfunction) R65.10
    with acute organ dysfunction R65.11
  tachycardia-bradycardia I49.5
  takotsubo I51.81
  TAR (thrombocytopenia with absent radius) Q87.2
  tarsal tunnel G57.5- ☑
  teething K00.7
  tegmental G93.89
  telangiectasic-pigmentation-cataract Q82.8
  temporal pyramidal apex — *see* Otitis, media, suppurative, acute
  temporomandibular joint-pain-dysfunction M26.62- ☑
  Terry's (*see also* Myopia, degenerative) H44.2- ☑
  testicular feminization (*see also* Syndrome, androgen insensitivity) E34.51
  thalamic pain (hyperesthetic) G89.0
  thoracic outlet (compression) G54.0
  Thorson-Björck E34.0
  thrombocytopenia with absent radius (TAR) Q87.2
  thyroid-adrenocortical insufficiency E31.0
  tibial
    anterior M76.81- ☑
    posterior M76.82- ☑
  Tietze's M94.0
  time-zone (rapid) G47.25
  Toni-Fanconi E72.09
    with cystinosis E72.04
  Touraine's Q79.8
  tourniquet — *see* Constriction, external, by site
  toxic shock A48.3
  transient left ventricular apical balloning I51.81
  traumatic vasospastic T75.22 ☑
  Treacher Collins Q75.4
  triple X, female Q97.0
  trisomy Q92.9
    13 Q91.7
      meiotic nondisjunction Q91.4
      mitotic nondisjunction Q91.5
      mosaicism Q91.5
      translocation Q91.6
    18 Q91.3
      meiotic nondisjunction Q91.0
      mitotic nondisjunction Q91.1
      mosaicism Q91.1
      translocation Q91.2
    20 (q)(p) Q92.8
    21 Q90.9
      meiotic nondisjunction Q90.0
      mitotic nondisjunction Q90.1
      mosaicism Q90.1
      translocation Q90.2
    22 Q92.8
  tropical wet feet T69.0- ☑
  Trousseau's I82.1

Syndrome — *continued*
  tumor lysis (following antineoplastic chemotherapy) (spontaneous) NEC E88.3
  tumor necrosis factor receptor associated periodic (TRAPS) M04.1
  Twiddler's (due to)
    automatic implantable defibrillator T82.198 ☑
    cardiac pacemaker T82.198 ☑
  Unverricht (-Lundborg) — *see* Epilepsy, generalized, idiopathic
  upward gaze H51.8
  uremia, chronic (*see also* Disease, kidney, chronic) N18.9
  urethral N34.3
  urethro-oculo-articular — *see* Reiter's disease
  urohepatic K76.7
  vago-hypoglossal G52.7
  van Buchem's M85.2
  van der Hoeve's Q78.0
  vascular NEC in cerebrovascular disease G46.8
  vasoconstriction, reversible cerebrovascular I67.841
  vasomotor I73.9
  vasospastic (traumatic) T75.22 ☑
  vasovagal R55
  VATER Q87.2
  velo-cardio-facial Q93.81
  vena cava (inferior) (superior) (obstruction) I87.1
  vertebral
    artery G45.0
      compression — *see* Syndrome, anterior, spinal artery, compression
    steal G45.0
  vertebro-basilar artery G45.0
  vertebrogenic (pain) M54.89
  vertiginous — *see* Disorder, vestibular function
  Vinson-Plummer D50.1
  virus B34.9
  visceral larva migrans B83.0
  visual disorientation H53.8
  vitamin B6 deficiency E53.1
  vitreal corneal H59.01- ☑
  vitreous (touch) H59.01- ☑
  Vogt-Koyanagi H20.82- ☑
  Volkmann's T79.6 ☑
  von Schroetter's I82.890
  von Willebrand (-Jürgen) D68.0
  Waldenström-Kjellberg D50.1
  Wallenberg's G46.3
  water retention E87.79
  Waterhouse (-Friderichsen) A39.1
  Weber-Gubler G46.3
  Weber-Leyden G46.3
  Weber's G46.3
  Wegener's M31.30
    with
      kidney involvement M31.31
      lung involvement M31.30
        with kidney involvement M31.31
  Weingarten's (tropical eosinophilia) J82
  Weiss-Baker G90.09
  Werdnig-Hoffman G12.0
  Wermer's E31.21
  Werner's E34.8
  Wernicke-Korsakoff (nonalcoholic) F04
    alcoholic F10.26
  Westphal-Strümpell E83.01
  West's — *see* Epilepsy, spasms
  wet
    feet (maceration) (tropical) T69.0- ☑
    lung, newborn P22.1
  whiplash S13.4 ☑
  whistling face Q87.0
  Wilkie's K55.1
  Wilkinson-Sneddon L13.1
  Willebrand (-Jürgens) D68.0
  Wilson's (hepatolenticular degeneration) E83.01
  Wiskott-Aldrich D82.0
  withdrawal — *see* Withdrawal, state
    drug
      infant of dependent mother P96.1
      therapeutic use, newborn P96.2
  Woakes' (ethmoiditis) J33.1
  Wright's (hyperabduction) G54.0
  X I20.9
  XXXX Q97.1
  XXXXX Q97.1
  XXXXY Q98.1
  XXY Q98.0

⬙ Subterms under main terms may continue to next column or page   ☑ Additional Character Required — Refer to the Tabular List for Character Selection   303

Syndrome — Syndrome

Syndrome — continued
- yellow nail L60.5
- Zahorsky's B08.5
- Zellweger syndrome E71.510
- Zellweger-like syndrome E71.541

Synechia (anterior) (iris) (posterior) (pupil) (see also Adhesions, iris)
- intra-uterine (traumatic) N85.6

Synesthesia R20.8

Syngamiasis, syngamosis B83.3

Synodontia K00.2

Synorchidism, synorchism Q55.1

Synostosis (congenital) Q78.8
- astragalo-scaphoid Q74.2
- radioulnar Q74.0

Synovial sarcoma — see Neoplasm, connective tissue, malignant

Synovioma (malignant) (see also Neoplasm, connective tissue, malignant)
- benign — see Neoplasm, connective tissue, benign

Synoviosarcoma — see Neoplasm, connective tissue, malignant

Synovitis (see also Tenosynovitis) M65.9
- crepitant
  - hand M70.0- ☑
  - wrist M70.03- ☑
- gonococcal A54.49
- gouty — see Gout
- in (due to)
  - crystals M65.8- ☑
  - gonorrhea A54.49
  - syphilis (late) A52.78
  - use, overuse, pressure — see Disorder, soft tissue, due to use
- infective NEC — see Tenosynovitis, infective NEC
- specified NEC — see Tenosynovitis, specified type NEC
- syphilitic A52.78
  - congenital (early) A50.02
- toxic — see Synovitis, transient
- transient M67.3- ☑
  - ankle M67.37- ☑
  - elbow M67.32- ☑
  - foot joint M67.37- ☑
  - hand joint M67.34- ☑
  - hip M67.35- ☑
  - knee M67.36- ☑
  - multiple site M67.39
  - pelvic region M67.35- ☑
  - shoulder M67.31- ☑
  - specified joint NEC M67.38
  - wrist M67.33- ☑
- traumatic, current — see Sprain
- tuberculous — see Tuberculosis, synovitis
- villonodular (pigmented) M12.2- ☑
  - ankle M12.27- ☑
  - elbow M12.22- ☑
  - foot joint M12.27- ☑
  - hand joint M12.24- ☑
  - hip M12.25- ☑
  - knee M12.26- ☑
  - multiple site M12.29
  - pelvic region M12.25- ☑
  - shoulder M12.21- ☑
  - specified joint NEC M12.28
  - vertebrae M12.28
  - wrist M12.23- ☑

Syphilid A51.39
- congenital A50.06
- newborn A50.06
- tubercular (late) A52.79

Syphilis, syphilitic (acquired) A53.9
- abdomen (late) A52.79
- acoustic nerve A52.15
- adenopathy (secondary) A51.49
- adrenal (gland) (with cortical hypofunction) A52.79
- age under 2 years NOS (see also Syphilis, congenital, early)
  - acquired A51.9
- alopecia (secondary) A51.32
- anemia (late) A52.79 [D63.8]
- aneurysm (aorta) (ruptured) A52.01
  - central nervous system A52.05
  - congenital A50.54 [I79.0]
- anus (late) A52.74
  - primary A51.1
  - secondary A51.39
- aorta (arch) (abdominal) (thoracic) A52.02

Syphilis, syphilitic — continued
- aorta — continued
  - aneurysm A52.01
- aortic (insufficiency) (regurgitation) (stenosis) A52.03
  - aneurysm A52.01
- arachnoid (adhesive) (cerebral) (spinal) A52.13
- asymptomatic — see Syphilis, latent
- ataxia (locomotor) A52.11
- atrophoderma maculatum A51.39
- auricular fibrillation A52.06
- bladder (late) A52.76
- bone A52.77
  - secondary A51.46
- brain A52.17
- breast (late) A52.79
- bronchus (late) A52.72
- bubo (primary) A51.0
- bulbar palsy A52.19
- bursa (late) A52.78
- cardiac decompensation A52.06
- cardiovascular A52.00
- central nervous system (late) (recurrent) (relapse) (tertiary) A52.3
  - with
    - ataxia A52.11
    - general paralysis A52.17
      - juvenile A50.45
    - paresis (general) A52.17
      - juvenile A50.45
    - tabes (dorsalis) A52.11
      - juvenile A50.45
    - taboparesis A52.17
      - juvenile A50.45
  - aneurysm A52.05
  - congenital A50.40
  - juvenile A50.40
  - remission in (sustained) A52.3
  - serology doubtful, negative, or positive A52.3
  - specified nature or site NEC A52.19
  - vascular A52.05
- cerebral A52.17
  - meningovascular A52.13
  - nerves (multiple palsies) A52.15
  - sclerosis A52.17
  - thrombosis A52.05
- cerebrospinal (tabetic type) A52.12
- cerebrovascular A52.05
- cervix (late) A52.76
- chancre (multiple) A51.0
  - extragenital A51.2
  - Rollet's A51.0
- Charcot's joint A52.16
- chorioretinitis A51.43
  - congenital A50.01
  - late A52.71
  - prenatal A50.01
- choroiditis — see Syphilitic chorioretinitis
- choroidoretinitis — see Syphilitic chorioretinitis
- ciliary body (secondary) A51.43
  - late A52.71
- colon (late) A52.74
- combined spinal sclerosis A52.11
- condyloma (latum) A51.31
- congenital A50.9
  - with
    - paresis (general) A50.45
    - tabes (dorsalis) A50.45
    - taboparesis A50.45
  - early, or less than 2 years after birth NEC A50.2
    - with manifestations — see Syphilis, congenital, early, symptomatic
    - latent (without manifestations) A50.1
      - negative spinal fluid test A50.1
      - serology positive A50.1
    - symptomatic A50.09
      - cutaneous A50.06
      - mucocutaneous A50.07
      - oculopathy A50.01
      - osteochondropathy A50.02
      - pharyngitis A50.03
      - pneumonia A50.04
      - rhinitis A50.05
      - visceral A50.08
  - chorioretinitis, choroiditis A50.01 [H32]
  - interstitial keratitis A50.31
  - juvenile neurosyphilis A50.45
  - late, or 2 years or more after birth NEC A50.7
    - chorioretinitis, choroiditis A50.32
    - interstitial keratitis A50.31

Syphilis, syphilitic — continued
- congenital — continued
  - late, or 2 years or more after birth — continued
    - juvenile neurosyphilis A50.45
    - latent (without manifestations) A50.6
      - negative spinal fluid test A50.6
      - serology positive A50.6
    - symptomatic or with manifestations NEC A50.59
      - arthropathy A50.55
      - cardiovascular A50.54
      - Clutton's joints A50.51
      - Hutchinson's teeth A50.52
      - Hutchinson's triad A50.53
      - osteochondropathy A50.56
      - saddle nose A50.57
- conjugal A53.9
  - tabes A52.11
- conjunctiva (late) A52.71
- contact Z20.2
- cord bladder A52.19
- cornea, late A52.71
- coronary (artery) (sclerosis) A52.06
- coryza, congenital A50.05
- cranial nerve A52.15
  - multiple palsies A52.15
- cutaneous — see Syphilis, skin
- dacryocystitis (late) A52.71
- degeneration, spinal cord A52.12
- dementia paralytica A52.17
  - juvenilis A50.45
- destruction of bone A52.77
- dilatation, aorta A52.01
- due to blood transfusion A53.9
- dura mater A52.13
- ear A52.79
  - inner A52.79
    - nerve (eighth) A52.15
    - neurorecurrence A52.15
- early A51.9
  - cardiovascular A52.00
  - central nervous system A52.3
  - latent (without manifestations) (less than 2 years after infection) A51.5
    - negative spinal fluid test A51.5
    - serological relapse after treatment A51.5
    - serology positive A51.5
  - relapse (treated, untreated) A51.9
  - skin A51.39
  - symptomatic A51.9
    - extragenital chancre A51.2
    - primary, except extragenital chancre A51.0
    - secondary (see also Syphilis, secondary) A51.39
      - relapse (treated, untreated) A51.49
    - ulcer A51.39
- eighth nerve (neuritis) A52.15
- endemic A65
- endocarditis A52.03
  - aortic A52.03
  - pulmonary A52.03
- epididymis (late) A52.76
- epiglottis (late) A52.73
- epiphysitis (congenital) (early) A50.02
- episcleritis (late) A52.71
- esophagus A52.79
- eustachian tube A52.73
- exposure to Z20.2
- eye A52.71
  - eyelid (late) (with gumma) A52.71
- fallopian tube (late) A52.76
- fracture A52.77
- gallbladder (late) A52.74
- gastric (polyposis) (late) A52.74
- general A53.9
  - paralysis A52.17
    - juvenile A50.45
- genital (primary) A51.0
- glaucoma A52.71
- gumma NEC A52.79
  - cardiovascular system A52.00
  - central nervous system A52.3
  - congenital A50.59
- heart (block) (decompensation) (disease) (failure) A52.06 [I52]
  - valve NEC A52.03
- hemianesthesia A52.19
- hemianopsia A52.71
- hemiparesis A52.17
- hemiplegia A52.17

☑ **Additional Character Required — Refer to the Tabular List for Character Selection**   ▽ **Subterms under main terms may continue to next column or page**

Syphilis, syphilitic — *continued*
  hepatic artery A52.09
  hepatis A52.74
  hepatomegaly, congenital A50.08
  hereditaria tarda — *see* Syphilis, congenital, late
  hereditary — *see* Syphilis, congenital
  Hutchinson's teeth A50.52
  hyalitis A52.71
  inactive — *see* Syphilis, latent
  infantum — *see* Syphilis, congenital
  inherited — *see* Syphilis, congenital
  internal ear A52.79
  intestine (late) A52.74
  iris, iritis (secondary) A51.43
    late A52.71
  joint (late) A52.77
  keratitis (congenital) (interstitial) (late) A50.31
  kidney (late) A52.75
  lacrimal passages (late) A52.71
  larynx (late) A52.73
  late A52.9
    cardiovascular A52.00
    central nervous system A52.3
    kidney A52.75
    latent or 2 years or more after infection (without
      manifestations) A52.8
      negative spinal fluid test A52.8
      serology positive A52.8
    paresis A52.17
    specified site NEC A52.79
    symptomatic or with manifestations A52.79
    tabes A52.11
  latent A53.0
    with signs or symptoms — *code by* site and stage
      under Syphilis
    early, or less than 2 years after infection A51.5
    central nervous system A52.2
    date of infection unspecified A53.0
    follow-up of latent syphilis A53.0
      date of infection unspecified A53.0
      late, or 2 years or more after infection A52.8
    late, or 2 years or more after infection A52.8
    positive serology (only finding) A53.0
      early, or less than 2 years after infection A51.5
      date of infection unspecified A53.0
      late, or 2 years or more after infection A52.8
  lens (late) A52.71
  leukoderma A51.39
    late A52.79
  lienitis A52.79
  lip A51.39
    chancre (primary) A51.2
    late A52.79
  Lissauer's paralysis A52.17
  liver A52.74
  locomotor ataxia A52.11
  lung A52.72
  lymph gland (early) (secondary) A51.49
    late A52.79
  lymphadenitis (secondary) A51.49
  macular atrophy of skin A51.39
    striated A52.79
  mediastinum (late) A52.73
  meninges (adhesive) (brain) (spinal cord) A52.13
  meningitis A52.13
    acute (secondary) A51.41
    congenital A50.41
  meningoencephalitis A52.14
  meningovascular A52.13
    congenital A50.41
  mesarteritis A52.09
    brain A52.04
  middle ear A52.77
  mitral stenosis A52.03
  monoplegia A52.17
  mouth (secondary) A51.39
    late A52.79
  mucocutaneous (secondary) A51.39
    late A52.79
  mucous
    membrane (secondary) A51.39
      late A52.79
    patches A51.39
      congenital A50.07
  mulberry molars A50.52
  muscle A52.78
  myocardium A52.06
  nasal sinus (late) A52.73

Syphilis, syphilitic — *continued*
  neonatorum — *see* Syphilis, congenital
  nephrotic syndrome (secondary) A51.44
  nerve palsy (any cranial nerve) A52.15
    multiple A52.15
  nervous system, central A52.3
  neuritis A52.15
    acoustic A52.15
  neurorecidive of retina A52.19
  neuroretinitis A52.19
  newborn — *see* Syphilis, congenital
  nodular superficial (late) A52.79
  nonvenereal A65
  nose (late) A52.73
    saddle back deformity A50.57
  occlusive arterial disease A52.09
  oculopathy A52.71
  ophthalmic (late) A52.71
  optic nerve (atrophy) (neuritis) (papilla) A52.15
  orbit (late) A52.71
  organic A53.9
  osseous (late) A52.77
  osteochondritis (congenital) (early) A50.02 [M90.80]
  osteoporosis A52.77
  ovary (late) A52.76
  oviduct (late) A52.76
  palate (late) A52.79
  pancreas (late) A52.74
  paralysis A52.17
    general A52.17
      juvenile A50.45
  paresis (general) A52.17
    juvenile A50.45
  paresthesia A52.19
  Parkinson's disease or syndrome A52.19
  paroxysmal tachycardia A52.06
  pemphigus (congenital) A50.06
  penis (chancre) A51.0
    late A52.76
  pericardium A52.06
  perichondritis, larynx (late) A52.73
  periosteum (late) A52.77
    congenital (early) A50.02 [M90.80]
    early (secondary) A51.46
  peripheral nerve A52.79
  petrous bone (late) A52.77
  pharynx (late) A52.73
    secondary A51.39
  pituitary (gland) A52.79
  pleura (late) A52.73
  pneumonia, white A50.04
  pontine lesion A52.17
  portal vein A52.09
  primary A51.0
    anal A51.1
    and secondary — *see* Syphilis, secondary
    central nervous system A52.3
    extragenital chancre NEC A51.2
    fingers A51.2
    genital A51.0
    lip A51.2
    specified site NEC A51.2
    tonsils A51.2
  prostate (late) A52.76
  ptosis (eyelid) A52.71
  pulmonary (late) A52.72
    artery A52.09
  pyelonephritis (late) A52.75
  recently acquired, symptomatic A51.9
  rectum (late) A52.74
  respiratory tract (late) A52.73
  retina, late A52.71
  retrobulbar neuritis A52.15
  salpingitis A52.76
  sclera (late) A52.71
  sclerosis
    cerebral A52.17
    coronary A52.06
    multiple A52.11
  scotoma (central) A52.71
  scrotum (late) A52.76
  secondary (and primary) A51.49
    adenopathy A51.49
    anus A51.39
    bone A51.46
    chorioretinitis, choroiditis A51.43
    hepatitis A51.45
    liver A51.45
    lymphadenitis A51.49

Syphilis, syphilitic — *continued*
  secondary — *continued*
    meningitis (acute) A51.41
    mouth A51.39
    mucous membranes A51.39
    periosteum, periostitis A51.46
    pharynx A51.39
    relapse (treated, untreated) A51.49
    skin A51.39
    specified form NEC A51.49
    tonsil A51.39
    ulcer A51.39
    viscera NEC A51.49
    vulva A51.39
  seminal vesicle (late) A52.76
  seronegative with signs or symptoms — *code by* site
    and stage under Syphilis
  seropositive
    with signs or symptoms — *code by* site and stage
      under Syphilis
    follow-up of latent syphilis — *see* Syphilis, latent
    only finding — *see* Syphilis, latent
  seventh nerve (paralysis) A52.15
  sinus, sinusitis (late) A52.73
  skeletal system A52.77
  skin (with ulceration) (early) (secondary) A51.39
    late or tertiary A52.79
  small intestine A52.74
  spastic spinal paralysis A52.17
  spermatic cord (late) A52.76
  spinal (cord) A52.12
  spleen A52.79
  splenomegaly A52.79
  spondylitis A52.77
  staphyloma A52.71
  stigmata (congenital) A50.59
  stomach A52.74
  synovium A52.78
  tabes dorsalis (late) A52.11
    juvenile A50.45
  tabetic type A52.11
    juvenile A50.45
  taboparesis A52.17
    juvenile A50.45
  tachycardia A52.06
  tendon (late) A52.78
  tertiary A52.9
    with symptoms NEC A52.79
    cardiovascular A52.00
    central nervous system A52.3
    multiple NEC A52.79
    specified site NEC A52.79
  testis A52.76
  thorax A52.73
  throat A52.73
  thymus (gland) (late) A52.79
  thyroid (late) A52.79
  tongue (late) A52.79
  tonsil (lingual) (late) A52.73
    primary A51.2
    secondary A51.39
  trachea (late) A52.73
  tunica vaginalis (late) A52.76
  ulcer (any site) (early) (secondary) A51.39
    late A52.79
    perforating A52.79
      foot A52.11
  urethra (late) A52.76
  urogenital (late) A52.76
  uterus (late) A52.76
  uveal tract (secondary) A51.43
    late A52.71
  uveitis (secondary) A51.43
    late A52.71
  uvula (late) (perforated) A52.79
  vagina A51.0
    late A52.76
  valvulitis NEC A52.03
  vascular A52.00
    brain (cerebral) A52.05
  ventriculi A52.74
  vesicae urinariae (late) A52.76
  viscera (abdominal) (late) A52.74
    secondary A51.49
  vitreous (opacities) (late) A52.71
    hemorrhage A52.71
  vulva A51.0
    late A52.76
    secondary A51.39

Subterms under main terms may continue to next column or page   ☑ Additional Character Required — Refer to the Tabular List for Character Selection   305

Index

Syphilis, syphilitic — Syphilis, syphilitic

Syphiloma A52.79
  cardiovascular system A52.00
  central nervous system A52.3
  circulatory system A52.00
  congenital A50.59
Syphilophobia F45.29
Syringadenoma (*see also* Neoplasm, skin, benign)
  papillary — *see* Neoplasm, skin, benign

Syringobulbia G95.0
Syringocystadenoma — *see* Neoplasm, skin, benign
  papillary — *see* Neoplasm, skin, benign
Syringoma (*see also* Neoplasm, skin, benign)
  chondroid — *see* Neoplasm, skin, benign
Syringomyelia G95.0
Syringomyelitis — *see* Encephalitis
Syringomyelocele — *see* Spina bifida

Syringopontia G95.0
System, systemic (*see also* condition)
  disease, combined — *see* Degeneration, combined
  inflammatory response syndrome (SIRS) of non-infectious origin (without organ dysfunction) R65.10
    with acute organ dysfunction R65.11
  lupus erythematosus M32.9
    inhibitor present D68.62

T

Tabacism, tabacosis, tabagism (*see also* Poisoning, tobacco)
  meaning dependence (without remission) F17.200
    with
      disorder F17.299
        in remission F17.211
        specified disorder NEC F17.298
        withdrawal F17.203
Tabardillo A75.9
  flea-borne A75.2
  louse-borne A75.0
Tabes, tabetic A52.10
  with
    central nervous system syphilis A52.10
    Charcot's joint A52.16
    cord bladder A52.19
    crisis, viscera (any) A52.19
    paralysis, general A52.17
    paresis (general) A52.17
    perforating ulcer (foot) A52.19
  arthropathy (Charcot) A52.16
  bladder A52.19
  bone A52.11
  cerebrospinal A52.12
  congenital A50.45
  conjugal A52.10
  dorsalis A52.11
    juvenile A50.49
  juvenile A50.49
  latent A52.19
  mesenterica A18.39
  paralysis, insane, general A52.17
  spasmodic A52.17
  syphilis (cerebrospinal) A52.12
Taboparalysis A52.17
Taboparesis (remission) A52.17
  juvenile A50.45
TAC (trigeminal autonomic cephalgia) **NEC** G44.099
  intractable G44.091
  not intractable G44.099
Tache noir S60.22- ☑
Tachyalimentation K91.2
Tachyarrhythmia, tachyrhythmia — *see* Tachycardia
Tachycardia R00.0
  atrial (paroxysmal) I47.1
  auricular I47.1
  AV nodal re-entry (re-entrant) I47.1
  junctional (paroxysmal) I47.1
  newborn P29.11
  nodal (paroxysmal) I47.1
  non-paroxysmal AV nodal I45.89
  paroxysmal (sustained) (nonsustained) I47.9
    with sinus bradycardia I49.5
    atrial (PAT) I47.1
    atrioventricular (AV) (re-entrant) I47.1
      psychogenic F54
    junctional I47.1
      ectopic I47.1
    nodal I47.1
    psychogenic (atrial) (supraventricular) (ventricular) F54
    supraventricular (sustained) I47.1
      psychogenic F54
    ventricular I47.2
      psychogenic F54
  psychogenic F45.8
  sick sinus I49.5
  sinoauricular NOS R00.0
    paroxysmal I47.1
  sinus [sinusal] NOS R00.0
    paroxysmal I47.1
  supraventricular I47.1
  ventricular (paroxysmal) (sustained) I47.2
    psychogenic F54
Tachygastria K31.89
Tachypnea R06.82
  hysterical F45.8
  newborn (idiopathic) (transitory) P22.1
  psychogenic F45.8
  transitory, of newborn P22.1
TACO (transfusion associated circulatory overload) E87.71
Taenia (infection) (infestation) B68.9
  diminuta B71.0
  echinococcal infestation B67.90
  mediocanellata B68.1

Taenia — *continued*
  nana B71.0
  saginata B68.1
  solium (intestinal form) B68.0
    larval form — *see* Cysticercosis
Taeniasis (intestine) — *see* Taenia
Tag (hypertrophied skin) (infected) L91.8
  adenoid J35.8
  anus K64.4
  hemorrhoidal K64.4
  hymen N89.8
  perineal N90.89
  preauricular Q17.0
  sentinel K64.4
  skin L91.8
    accessory (congenital) Q82.8
    anus K64.4
    congenital Q82.8
    preauricular Q17.0
  tonsil J35.8
  urethra, urethral N36.8
  vulva N90.89
Tahyna fever B33.8
Takahara's disease E80.3
Takayasu's disease or syndrome M31.4
Talcosis (pulmonary) J62.0
Talipes (congenital) Q66.89
  acquired, planus — *see* Deformity, limb, flat foot
  asymmetric Q66.89
  calcaneovalgus Q66.4
  calcaneovarus Q66.1
  calcaneus Q66.89
  cavus Q66.7
  equinovalgus Q66.6
  equinovarus Q66.0
  equinus Q66.89
  percavus Q66.7
  planovalgus Q66.6
  planus (acquired) (any degree) (*see also* Deformity, limb, flat foot)
    congenital Q66.5- ☑
    due to rickets (sequelae) E64.3
  valgus Q66.6
  varus Q66.3
Tall stature, constitutional E34.4
Talma's disease M62.89
Talon noir S90.3- ☑
  hand S60.22- ☑
  heel S90.3- ☑
  toe S90.1- ☑
Tamponade, heart I31.4
Tanapox (virus disease) B08.71
Tangier disease E78.6
Tantrum, child problem F91.8
Tapeworm (infection) (infestation) — *see* Infestation, tapeworm
Tapia's syndrome G52.7
TAR (thrombocytopenia with absent radius) **syndrome** Q87.2
Tarral-Besnier disease L44.0
Tarsal tunnel syndrome — *see* Syndrome, tarsal tunnel
Tarsalgia — *see* Pain, limb, lower
Tarsitis (eyelid) H01.8
  syphilitic A52.71
  tuberculous A18.4
Tartar (teeth) (dental calculus) K03.6
Tattoo (mark) L81.8
Tauri's disease E74.09
Taurodontism K00.2
Taussig-Bing syndrome Q20.1
Taybi's syndrome Q87.2
Tay-Sachs amaurotic familial idiocy or disease E75.02
TBI (traumatic brain injury) S06.9 ☑
Teacher's node or nodule J38.2
Tear, torn (traumatic) (*see also* Laceration)
  with abortion — *see* Abortion
  annular fibrosis M51.35
  anus, anal (sphincter) S31.831 ☑
    complicating delivery
      with third degree perineal laceration (*see also* Delivery, complicated, by, laceration, perineum, third degree) O70.20
        with mucosa O70.3
      without third degree perineal laceration O70.4
    nontraumatic (healed) (old) K62.81
  articular cartilage, old — *see* Derangement, joint, articular cartilage, by site

Tear, torn — *continued*
  bladder
    with ectopic or molar pregnancy O08.6
    following ectopic or molar pregnancy O08.6
    obstetrical O71.5
    traumatic — *see* Injury, bladder
  bowel
    with ectopic or molar pregnancy O08.6
    following ectopic or molar pregnancy O08.6
    obstetrical trauma O71.5
  broad ligament
    with ectopic or molar pregnancy O08.6
    following ectopic or molar pregnancy O08.6
    obstetrical trauma O71.6
  bucket handle (knee) (meniscus) — *see* Tear, meniscus
  capsule, joint — *see* Sprain
  cartilage (*see also* Sprain)
    articular, old — *see* Derangement, joint, articular cartilage, by site
  cervix
    with ectopic or molar pregnancy O08.6
    following ectopic or molar pregnancy O08.6
    obstetrical trauma (current) O71.3
    old N88.1
    traumatic — *see* Injury, uterus
  dural G97.41
    nontraumatic G96.11
  internal organ — *see* Injury, by site
  knee cartilage
    articular (current) S83.3- ☑
    old — *see* Derangement, knee, meniscus, due to old tear
  ligament — *see* Sprain
  meniscus (knee) (current injury) S83.209 ☑
    bucket-handle S83.20- ☑
    lateral
      bucket-handle S83.25- ☑
      complex S83.27- ☑
      peripheral S83.26- ☑
      specified type NEC S83.28- ☑
    medial
      bucket-handle S83.21- ☑
      complex S83.23- ☑
      peripheral S83.22- ☑
      specified type NEC S83.24- ☑
    old — *see* Derangement, knee, meniscus, due to old tear
    site other than knee — *code as* Sprain
    specified type NEC S83.20- ☑
  muscle — *see* Strain
  pelvic
    floor, complicating delivery O70.1
    organ NEC, obstetrical trauma O71.5
      with ectopic or molar pregnancy O08.6
      following ectopic or molar pregnancy O08.6
  perineal, secondary O90.1
  periurethral tissue, obstetrical trauma O71.82
    with ectopic or molar pregnancy O08.6
    following ectopic or molar pregnancy O08.6
  rectovaginal septum — *see* Laceration, vagina
  retina, retinal (without detachment) (horseshoe) (*see also* Break, retina, horseshoe)
    with detachment — *see* Detachment, retina, with retinal, break
  rotator cuff (nontraumatic) M75.10- ☑
    complete M75.12- ☑
    incomplete M75.11- ☑
    traumatic S46.01- ☑
      capsule S43.42- ☑
  semilunar cartilage, knee — *see* Tear, meniscus
  supraspinatus (complete) (incomplete) (nontraumatic) (*see also* Tear, rotator cuff) M75.10- ☑
  tendon — *see* Strain
  tentorial, at birth P10.4
  umbilical cord
    complicating delivery O69.89 ☑
  urethra
    with ectopic or molar pregnancy O08.6
    following ectopic or molar pregnancy O08.6
    obstetrical trauma O71.5
  uterus — *see* Injury, uterus
  vagina — *see* Laceration, vagina
  vessel, from catheter — *see* Puncture, accidental complicating surgery
  vulva, complicating delivery O70.0
Tear-stone — *see* Dacryolith

Teeth (see also condition)
grinding
psychogenic F45.8
sleep related G47.63
Teething (syndrome) K00.7
Telangiectasia, telangiectasis (verrucous) I78.1
ataxic (cerebellar) (Louis-Bar) G11.3
familial I78.0
hemorrhagic, hereditary (congenital) (senile) I78.0
hereditary, hemorrhagic (congenital) (senile) I78.0
juxtafoveal H35.07- ☑
macular H35.07- ☑
macularis eruptiva perstans D47.01
parafoveal H35.07- ☑
retinal (idiopathic) (juxtafoveal) (macular) (parafoveal) H35.07- ☑
spider I78.1
Telephone scatologia F65.89
Telescoped bowel or intestine K56.1
congenital Q43.8
Temperature
body, high (of unknown origin) R50.9
cold, trauma from T69.9 ☑
newborn P80.0
specified effect NEC T69.8 ☑
Temple — see condition
Temporal — see condition
Temporomandibular joint pain-dysfunction syndrome M26.62- ☑
Temporosphenoidal — see condition
Tendency
bleeding — see Defect, coagulation
suicide
meaning personal history of attempted suicide Z91.5
meaning suicidal ideation — see Ideation, suicidal
to fall R29.6
Tenderness, abdominal R10.819
epigastric R10.816
generalized R10.817
left lower quadrant R10.814
left upper quadrant R10.812
periumbilic R10.815
rebound R10.829
epigastric R10.826
generalized R10.827
left lower quadrant R10.824
left upper quadrant R10.822
periumbilic R10.825
right lower quadrant R10.823
right upper quadrant R10.821
right lower quadrant R10.813
right upper quadrant R10.811
Tendinitis, tendonitis (see also Enthesopathy)
Achilles M76.6- ☑
adhesive — see Tenosynovitis, specified type NEC
shoulder — see Capsulitis, adhesive
bicipital M75.2- ☑
calcific M65.2- ☑
ankle M65.27- ☑
foot M65.27- ☑
forearm M65.23- ☑
hand M65.24- ☑
lower leg M65.26- ☑
multiple sites M65.29
pelvic region M65.25- ☑
shoulder M75.3- ☑
specified site NEC M65.28
thigh M65.25- ☑
upper arm M65.22- ☑
due to use, overuse, pressure (see also Disorder, soft tissue, due to use)
specified NEC — see Disorder, soft tissue, due to use, specified NEC
gluteal M76.0- ☑
patellar M76.5- ☑
peroneal M76.7- ☑
psoas M76.1- ☑
tibial (posterior) M76.82- ☑
anterior M76.81- ☑
trochanteric — see Bursitis, hip, trochanteric
Tendon — see condition
Tendosynovitis — see Tenosynovitis
Tenesmus (rectal) R19.8
vesical R30.1
Tennis elbow — see Epicondylitis, lateral

Tenonitis (see also Tenosynovitis)
eye (capsule) H05.04- ☑
Tenontosynovitis — see Tenosynovitis
Tenontothecitis — see Tenosynovitis
Tenophyte — see Disorder, synovium, specified type NEC
Tenosynovitis (see also Synovitis) M65.9
adhesive — see Tenosynovitis, specified type NEC
shoulder — see Capsulitis, adhesive
bicipital (calcifying) — see Tendinitis, bicipital
gonococcal A54.49
in (due to)
crystals M65.8- ☑
gonorrhea A54.49
syphilis (late) A52.78
use, overuse, pressure (see also Disorder, soft tissue, due to use)
specified NEC — see Disorder, soft tissue, due to use, specified NEC
infective NEC M65.1- ☑
ankle M65.17- ☑
foot M65.17- ☑
forearm M65.13- ☑
hand M65.14- ☑
lower leg M65.16- ☑
multiple sites M65.19
pelvic region M65.15- ☑
shoulder region M65.11- ☑
specified site NEC M65.18
thigh M65.15- ☑
upper arm M65.12- ☑
radial styloid M65.4
shoulder region M65.81- ☑
adhesive — see Capsulitis, adhesive
specified type NEC M65.88
ankle M65.87- ☑
foot M65.87- ☑
forearm M65.83- ☑
hand M65.84- ☑
lower leg M65.86- ☑
multiple sites M65.89
pelvic region M65.85- ☑
shoulder region M65.81- ☑
specified site NEC M65.88
thigh M65.85- ☑
upper arm M65.82- ☑
tuberculous — see Tuberculosis, tenosynovitis
Tenovaginitis — see Tenosynovitis
Tension
arterial, high (see also Hypertension)
without diagnosis of hypertension R03.0
headache G44.209
intractable G44.201
not intractable G44.209
nervous R45.0
pneumothorax J93.0
premenstrual N94.3
state (mental) F48.9
Tentorium — see condition
Teratencephalus Q89.8
Teratism Q89.7
Teratoblastoma (malignant) — see Neoplasm, malignant, by site
Teratocarcinoma (see also Neoplasm, malignant, by site)
liver C22.7
Teratoma (solid) (see also Neoplasm, uncertain behavior, by site)
with embryonal carcinoma, mixed — see Neoplasm, malignant, by site
with malignant transformation — see Neoplasm, malignant, by site
adult (cystic) — see Neoplasm, benign, by site
benign — see Neoplasm, benign, by site
combined with choriocarcinoma — see Neoplasm, malignant, by site
cystic (adult) — see Neoplasm, benign, by site
differentiated — see Neoplasm, benign, by site
embryonal (see also Neoplasm, malignant, by site)
liver C22.7
immature — see Neoplasm, malignant, by site
liver C22.7
adult, benign, cystic, differentiated type or mature D13.4
malignant (see also Neoplasm, malignant, by site)
anaplastic — see Neoplasm, malignant, by site
intermediate — see Neoplasm, malignant, by site

Teratoma — continued
malignant (see also Neoplasm, malignant, by site) — continued
intermediate — see Neoplasm, malignant, by site — continued
specified site — see Neoplasm, malignant, by site
unspecified site C62.90
undifferentiated — see Neoplasm, malignant, by site
mature — see Neoplasm, uncertain behavior, by site
malignant — see Neoplasm, by site, malignant, by site
ovary D27.- ☑
embryonal, immature or malignant C56- ☑
solid — see Neoplasm, uncertain behavior, by site
testis C62.9- ☑
adult, benign, cystic, differentiated type or mature D29.2- ☑
scrotal C62.1- ☑
undescended C62.0- ☑
Termination
anomalous (see also Malposition, congenital)
right pulmonary vein Q26.3
pregnancy, elective Z33.2
Ternidens diminutus infestation B81.8
Ternidensiasis B81.8
Terror(s) night (child) F51.4
Terrorism, victim of Z65.4
Terry's syndrome (see also Myopia, degenerative) H44.2- ☑
Tertiary — see condition
Test, tests, testing (for)
adequacy (for dialysis)
hemodialysis Z49.31
peritoneal Z49.32
blood pressure Z01.30
abnormal reading — see Blood, pressure
blood typing Z01.83
Rh typing Z01.83
blood-alcohol Z04.8
positive — see Findings, abnormal, in blood
blood-drug Z04.8
positive — see Findings, abnormal, in blood
cardiac pulse generator (battery) Z45.010
fertility Z31.41
genetic
disease carrier status for procreative management
female Z31.430
male Z31.440
male partner of patient with recurrent pregnancy loss Z31.441
procreative management NEC
female Z31.438
male Z31.448
hearing Z01.10
with abnormal findings NEC Z01.118
HIV (human immunodeficiency virus)
nonconclusive (in infants) R75
positive Z21
seropositive Z21
immunity status Z01.84
intelligence NEC Z01.89
laboratory (as part of a general medical examination) Z00.00
with abnormal finding Z00.01
for medicolegal reason NEC Z04.8
male partner of patient with recurrent pregnancy loss Z31.441
Mantoux (for tuberculosis) Z11.1
abnormal result R76.11
pregnancy, positive first pregnancy — see Pregnancy, normal, first
procreative Z31.49
fertility Z31.41
skin, diagnostic
allergy Z01.82
special screening examination — see Screening, by name of disease
Mantoux Z11.1
tuberculin Z11.1
specified NEC Z01.89
tuberculin Z11.1
abnormal result R76.11
vision Z01.00
with abnormal findings Z01.01
Wassermann Z11.3
positive — see Serology for syphilis, positive

☑ **Additional Character Required — Refer to the Tabular List for Character Selection**   ▽ **Subterms under main terms may continue to next column or page**

Testicle, testicular, testis (*see also* condition)
  feminization syndrome (*see also* Syndrome, androgen insensitivity) E34.51
  migrans Q55.29
Tetanus, tetanic (cephalic) (convulsions) A35
  with
    abortion A34
    ectopic or molar pregnancy O08.0
  following ectopic or molar pregnancy O08.0
  inoculation reaction (due to serum) — *see* Complications, vaccination
  neonatorum A33
  obstetrical A34
  puerperal, postpartum, childbirth A34
Tetany (due to) R29.0
  alkalosis E87.3
  associated with rickets E55.0
  convulsions R29.0
    hysterical F44.5
  functional (hysterical) F44.5
  hyperkinetic R29.0
    hysterical F44.5
  hyperpnea R06.4
    hysterical F44.5
    psychogenic F45.8
  hyperventilation (*see also* Hyperventilation) R06.4
    hysterical F44.5
  neonatal (without calcium or magnesium deficiency) P71.3
  parathyroid (gland) E20.9
  parathyroprival E89.2
  post- (para)thyroidectomy E89.2
  postoperative E89.2
  pseudotetany R29.0
  psychogenic (conversion reaction) F44.5
Tetralogy of Fallot Q21.3
Tetraplegia (chronic) (*see also* Quadriplegia) G82.50
Thailand hemorrhagic fever A91
Thalassanemia — *see* Thalassemia
Thalassemia (anemia) (disease) D56.9
  with other hemoglobinopathy D56.8
  alpha (major) (severe) (triple gene defect) D56.0
    minor D56.3
    silent carrier D56.3
    trait D56.3
  beta (severe) D56.1
    homozygous D56.1
    major D56.1
    minor D56.3
    trait D56.3
  delta-beta (homozygous) D56.2
    minor D56.3
    trait D56.3
  dominant D56.8
  hemoglobin
    C D56.8
    E-beta D56.5
  intermedia D56.1
  major D56.1
  minor D56.3
  mixed D56.8
  sickle-cell — *see* Disease, sickle-cell, thalassemia
  specified type NEC D56.8
  trait D56.3
  variants D56.8
Thanatophoric dwarfism or short stature Q77.1
Thaysen-Gee disease (nontropical sprue) K90.0
Thaysen's disease K90.0
Thecoma D27- ☑
  luteinized D27- ☑
  malignant C56- ☑
Thelarche, premature E30.8
Thelaziasis B83.8
Thelitis N61.0
  puerperal, postpartum or gestational — *see* Infection, nipple
Therapeutic — *see* condition
Therapy
  drug, long-term (current) (prophylactic)
    agents affecting estrogen receptors and estrogen levels NEC Z79.818
    anastrozole (Arimidex) Z79.811
    antibiotics Z79.2
      short-term use — *omit code*
    anticoagulants Z79.01
    anti-inflammatory Z79.1
    antiplatelet Z79.02
    antithrombotics Z79.02

Therapy — *continued*
  drug, long-term — *continued*
    aromatase inhibitors Z79.811
    aspirin Z79.82
    birth control pill or patch Z79.3
    bisphosphonates Z79.83
    contraceptive, oral Z79.3
    drug, specified NEC Z79.899
    estrogen receptor downregulators Z79.818
    Evista Z79.810
    exemestane (Aromasin) Z79.811
    Fareston Z79.810
    fulvestrant (Faslodex) Z79.818
    gonadotropin-releasing hormone (GnRH) agonist Z79.818
    goserelin acetate (Zoladex) Z79.818
    hormone replacement Z79.890
    insulin Z79.4
    letrozole (Femara) Z79.811
    leuprolide acetate (leuprorelin) (Lupron) Z79.818
    megestrol acetate (Megace) Z79.818
    methadone
      for pain management Z79.891
      maintenance therapy F11.20
    Nolvadex Z79.810
    opiate analgesic Z79.891
    oral contraceptive Z79.3
    raloxifene (Evista) Z79.810
    selective estrogen receptor modulators (SERMs) Z79.810
    short term — *omit code*
    steroids
      inhaled Z79.51
      systemic Z79.52
    tamoxifen (Nolvadex) Z79.810
    toremifene (Fareston) Z79.810
Thermic — *see* condition
Thermography (abnormal) (*see also* Abnormal, diagnostic imaging) R93.8
  breast R92.8
Thermoplegia T67.0 ☑
Thesaurismosis, glycogen — *see* Disease, glycogen storage
Thiamin deficiency E51.9
  specified NEC E51.8
Thiaminic deficiency with beriberi E51.11
Thibierge-Weissenbach syndrome — *see* Sclerosis, systemic
Thickening
  bone — *see* Hypertrophy, bone
  breast N64.59
  endometrium R93.8
  epidermal L85.9
    specified NEC L85.8
  hymen N89.6
  larynx J38.7
  nail L60.2
    congenital Q84.5
  periosteal — *see* Hypertrophy, bone
  pleura J92.9
    with asbestos J92.0
  skin R23.4
  subepiglottic J38.7
  tongue K14.8
  valve, heart — *see* Endocarditis
Thigh — *see* condition
Thinning vertebra — *see* Spondylopathy, specified NEC
Thirst, excessive R63.1
  due to deprivation of water T73.1 ☑
Thomsen disease G71.12
Thoracic (*see also* condition)
  kidney Q63.2
  outlet syndrome G54.0
Thoracogastroschisis (congenital) Q79.8
Thoracopagus Q89.4
Thorax — *see* condition
Thorn's syndrome N28.89
Thorson-Björck syndrome E34.0
Threadworm (infection) (infestation) B80
Threatened
  abortion O20.0
    with subsequent abortion O03.9
  job loss, anxiety concerning Z56.2
  labor (without delivery) O47.9
    at or after 37 completed weeks of gestation O47.1
    before 37 completed weeks of gestation O47.0- ☑
  loss of job, anxiety concerning Z56.2
  miscarriage O20.0

Threatened — *continued*
  unemployment, anxiety concerning Z56.2
Three-day fever A93.1
Threshers' lung J67.0
Thrix annulata (congenital) Q84.1
Throat — *see* condition
Thrombasthenia (Glanzmann) (hemorrhagic) (hereditary) D69.1
Thromboangiitis I73.1
  obliterans (general) I73.1
    cerebral I67.89
    vessels
      brain I67.89
      spinal cord I67.89
Thromboarteritis — *see* Arteritis
Thromboasthenia (Glanzmann) (hemorrhagic) (hereditary) D69.1
Thrombocytasthenia (Glanzmann) D69.1
Thrombocythemia (essential) (hemorrhagic) (idiopathic) (primary) D47.3
Thrombocytopathy (dystrophic) (granulopenic) D69.1
Thrombocytopenia, thrombocytopenic D69.6
  with absent radius (TAR) Q87.2
  congenital D69.42
  dilutional D69.59
  due to
    (massive) blood transfusion D69.59
    drugs D69.59
    extracorporeal circulation of blood D69.59
    platelet alloimmunization D69.59
  essential D69.3
  heparin induced (HIT) D75.82
  hereditary D69.42
  idiopathic D69.3
  neonatal, transitory P61.0
    due to
      exchange transfusion P61.0
      idiopathic maternal thrombocytopenia P61.0
      isoimmunization P61.0
  primary NEC D69.49
    idiopathic D69.3
  puerperal, postpartum O72.3
  secondary D69.59
  transient neonatal P61.0
Thrombocytosis, essential D47.3
  primary D47.3
Thromboembolism — *see* Embolism
Thrombopathy (Bernard-Soulier) D69.1
  constitutional D68.0
  Willebrand-Jurgens D68.0
Thrombopenia — *see* Thrombocytopenia
Thrombophilia D68.59
  primary NEC D68.59
  secondary NEC D68.69
  specified NEC D68.69
Thrombophlebitis I80.9
  antepartum O22.2- ☑
    deep O22.3- ☑
    superficial O22.2- ☑
  cavernous (venous) sinus G08
    complicating pregnancy O22.5- ☑
    nonpyogenic I67.6
  cerebral (sinus) (vein) G08
    nonpyogenic I67.6
    sequelae G09
  due to implanted device — *see* Complications, by site and type, specified NEC
  during or resulting from a procedure NEC T81.72 ☑
  femoral vein (superficial) I80.1- ☑
  femoropopliteal vein I80.0- ☑
  hepatic (vein) I80.8
  idiopathic, recurrent I82.1
  iliofemoral I80.1- ☑
  intracranial venous sinus (any) G08
    nonpyogenic I67.6
    sequelae G09
  intraspinal venous sinuses and veins G08
    nonpyogenic G95.19
  lateral (venous) sinus G08
    nonpyogenic I67.6
  leg I80.3
    superficial I80.0- ☑
  longitudinal (venous) sinus G08
    nonpyogenic I67.6
  lower extremity I80.299
  migrans, migrating I82.1
  pelvic
    with ectopic or molar pregnancy O08.0

Thrombophlebitis — *continued*
pelvic — *continued*
following ectopic or molar pregnancy O08.0
puerperal O87.1
popliteal vein — *see* Phlebitis, leg, deep, popliteal
portal (vein) K75.1
postoperative T81.72 ☑
pregnancy — *see* Thrombophlebitis, antepartum
puerperal, postpartum, childbirth O87.0
deep O87.1
pelvic O87.1
septic O86.81
superficial O87.0
saphenous (greater) (lesser) I80.0- ☑
sinus (intracranial) G08
nonpyogenic I67.6
specified site NEC I80.8
tibial vein I80.23- ☑
Thrombosis, thrombotic (bland) (multiple) (progressive)
(silent) (vessel) I82.90
anal K64.5
antepartum — *see* Thrombophlebitis, antepartum
aorta, aortic I74.10
abdominal I74.09
saddle I74.01
bifurcation I74.09
saddle I74.01
specified site NEC I74.19
terminal I74.09
thoracic I74.11
valve — *see* Endocarditis, aortic
apoplexy I63.3- ☑
artery, arteries (postinfectional) I74.9
auditory, internal — *see* Occlusion, artery, precerebral, specified NEC
basilar — *see* Occlusion, artery, basilar
carotid (common) (internal) — *see* Occlusion, artery, carotid
cerebellar (anterior inferior) (posterior inferior) (superior) — *see* Occlusion, artery, cerebellar
cerebral — *see* Occlusion, artery, cerebral
choroidal (anterior) — *see* Occlusion, artery, precerebral, specified NEC
communicating, posterior — *see* Occlusion, artery, precerebral, specified NEC
coronary (*see also* Infarct, myocardium)
not resulting in infarction I24.0
hepatic I74.8
hypophyseal — *see* Occlusion, artery, precerebral, specified NEC
iliac I74.5
limb I74.4
lower I74.3
upper I74.2
meningeal, anterior or posterior — *see* Occlusion, artery, cerebral, specified NEC
mesenteric (with gangrene) (*see also* Infarct, intestine) K55.069
ophthalmic — *see* Occlusion, artery, retina
pontine — *see* Occlusion, artery, precerebral, specified NEC
precerebral — *see* Occlusion, artery, precerebral
pulmonary (iatrogenic) — *see* Embolism, pulmonary
renal N28.0
retinal — *see* Occlusion, artery, retina
spinal, anterior or posterior G95.11
traumatic NEC T14.8 ☑
vertebral — *see* Occlusion, artery, vertebral
atrium, auricular (*see also* Infarct, myocardium)
following acute myocardial infarction (current complication) I23.6
not resulting in infarction I51.3
old I51.3
basilar (artery) — *see* Occlusion, artery, basilar
brain (artery) (stem) (*see also* Occlusion, artery, cerebral)
due to syphilis A52.05
puerperal O99.43
sinus — *see* Thrombosis, intracranial venous sinus
capillary I78.8
cardiac (*see also* Infarct, myocardium)
not resulting in infarction I51.3
old I51.3
valve — *see* Endocarditis
carotid (artery) (common) (internal) — *see* Occlusion, artery, carotid

Thrombosis, thrombotic — *continued*
cavernous (venous) sinus — *see* Thrombosis, intracranial venous sinus
cerebellar artery (anterior inferior) (posterior inferior) (superior) I66.3
cerebral (artery) — *see* Occlusion, artery, cerebral
cerebrovenous sinus (*see also* Thrombosis, intracranial venous sinus)
puerperium O87.3
chronic I82.91
coronary (artery) (vein) (*see also* Infarct, myocardium)
not resulting in infarction I24.0
corpus cavernosum N48.89
cortical I66.9
deep — *see* Embolism, vein, lower extremity
due to device, implant or graft (*see also* Complications, by site and type, specified NEC) T85.868 ☑
arterial graft NEC T82.868 ☑
breast (implant) T85.868 ☑
catheter NEC T85.868 ☑
dialysis (renal) T82.868 ☑
intraperitoneal T85.868 ☑
infusion NEC T82.868 ☑
spinal (epidural) (subdural) T85.860 ☑
urinary (indwelling) T83.86 ☑
electronic (electrode) (pulse generator) (stimulator)
bone T84.86 ☑
cardiac T82.867 ☑
nervous system (brain) (peripheral nerve) (spinal) T85.860 ☑
urinary T83.86 ☑
fixation, internal (orthopedic) NEC T84.86 ☑
gastrointestinal (bile duct) (esophagus) T85.868 ☑
genital NEC T83.86 ☑
heart T82.867 ☑
joint prosthesis T84.86 ☑
ocular (corneal graft) (orbital implant) NEC T85.868 ☑
orthopedic NEC T84.86 ☑
specified NEC T85.868 ☑
urinary NEC T83.86 ☑
vascular NEC T82.868 ☑
ventricular intracranial shunt T85.860 ☑
during the puerperium — *see* Thrombosis, puerperal
endocardial (*see also* Infarct, myocardium)
not resulting in infarction I51.3
eye — *see* Occlusion, retina
genital organ
female NEC N94.89
pregnancy — *see* Thrombophlebitis, antepartum
male N50.1
gestational — *see* Phlebopathy, gestational
heart (chamber) (*see also* Infarct, myocardium)
not resulting in infarction I51.3
old I51.3
hepatic (vein) I82.0
artery I74.8
history (of) Z86.718
intestine (with gangrene) (*see also* Infarct, intestine) K55.069
intracardiac NEC (apical) (atrial) (auricular) (ventricular) (old) I51.3
intracranial (arterial) I66.9
venous sinus (any) G08
nonpyogenic origin I67.6
puerperium O87.3
intramural (*see also* Infarct, myocardium)
not resulting in infarction I51.3
old I51.3
intraspinal venous sinuses and veins G08
nonpyogenic G95.19
kidney (artery) N28.0
lateral (venous) sinus — *see* Thrombosis, intracranial venous sinus
leg — *see* Thrombosis, vein, lower extremity
arterial I74.3
liver (venous) I82.0
artery I74.8
portal vein I81
longitudinal (venous) sinus — *see* Thrombosis, intracranial venous sinus
lower limb — *see* Thrombosis, vein, lower extremity
lung (iatrogenic) (postoperative) — *see* Embolism, pulmonary
meninges (brain) (arterial) I66.8

Thrombosis, thrombotic — *continued*
mesenteric (artery) (with gangrene) (*see also* Infarct, intestine) K55.069
vein (inferior) (superior) I81
mitral I34.8
mural (*see also* Infarct, myocardium)
due to syphilis A52.06
not resulting in infarction I51.3
old I51.3
omentum (with gangrene) (*see also* Infarct, intestine) K55.069
ophthalmic — *see* Occlusion, retina
pampiniform plexus (male) N50.1
parietal (*see also* Infarct, myocardium)
not resulting in infarction I24.0
penis, superficial vein N48.81
perianal venous K64.5
peripheral arteries I74.4
upper I74.2
personal history (of) Z86.718
portal I81
due to syphilis A52.09
precerebral artery — *see* Occlusion, artery, precerebral
puerperal, postpartum O87.0
brain (artery) O99.43
venous (sinus) O87.3
cardiac O99.43
cerebral (artery) O99.43
venous (sinus) O87.3
superficial O87.0
pulmonary (artery) (iatrogenic) (postoperative) (vein) — *see* Embolism, pulmonary
renal (artery) N28.0
vein I82.3
resulting from presence of device, implant or graft — *see* Complications, by site and type, specified NEC
retina, retinal — *see* Occlusion, retina
scrotum N50.1
seminal vesicle N50.1
sigmoid (venous) sinus — *see* Thrombosis, intracranial venous sinus
sinus, intracranial (any) — *see* Thrombosis, intracranial venous sinus
specified site NEC I82.890
chronic I82.891
spermatic cord N50.1
spinal cord (arterial) G95.11
due to syphilis A52.09
pyogenic origin G06.1
spleen, splenic D73.5
artery I74.8
testis N50.1
traumatic NEC T14.8 ☑
tricuspid I07.8
tumor — *see* Neoplasm, unspecified behavior, by site
tunica vaginalis N50.1
umbilical cord (vessels), complicating delivery O69.5 ☑
vas deferens N50.1
vein (acute) I82.90
antecubital I82.61- ☑
chronic I82.71- ☑
axillary I82.A1- ☑ (*following* I82.7)
chronic I82.A2- ☑ (*following* I82.7)
basilic I82.61- ☑
chronic I82.71- ☑
brachial I82.62- ☑
chronic I82.72- ☑
brachiocephalic (innominate) I82.290
chronic I82.291
cephalic I82.61- ☑
chronic I82.71- ☑
cerebral, nonpyogenic I67.6
chronic I82.91
deep (DVT) I82.40- ☑
calf I82.4Z- ☑
chronic I82.5Z- ☑
lower leg I82.4Z- ☑
chronic I82.5Z- ☑
thigh I82.4Y- ☑
chronic I82.5Y- ☑
upper leg I82.4Y ☑
chronic I82.5Y- ☑
femoral I82.41- ☑
chronic I82.51- ☑
iliac (iliofemoral) I82.42- ☑
chronic I82.52- ☑

☑ **Additional Character Required — Refer to the Tabular List for Character Selection**   🔄 **Subterms under main terms may continue to next column or page**

Thrombosis, thrombotic — *continued*
  vein — *continued*
    innominate I82.290
      chronic I82.291
    internal jugular I82.C1- ☑ (*following* I82.7)
      chronic I82.C2- ☑ (*following* I82.7)
    lower extremity
      deep I82.40- ☑
        chronic I82.50- ☑
          specified NEC I82.49- ☑
            chronic NEC I82.59- ☑
      distal
        deep I82.4Z- ☑
      proximal
        deep I82.4Y- ☑
          chronic I82.5Y- ☑
      superficial I82.81- ☑
    perianal K64.5
    popliteal I82.43- ☑
      chronic I82.53- ☑
    radial I82.62- ☑
      chronic I82.72- ☑
    renal I82.3
    saphenous (greater) (lesser) I82.81- ☑
    specified NEC I82.890
      chronic NEC I82.891
    subclavian I82.B1- ☑ (*following* I82.7)
      chronic I82.B2- ☑ (*following* I82.7)
    thoracic NEC I82.290
      chronic I82.291
    tibial I82.44- ☑
      chronic I82.54- ☑
    ulnar I82.62- ☑
      chronic I82.72- ☑
    upper extremity I82.60- ☑
      chronic I82.70- ☑
      deep I82.62- ☑
        chronic I82.72- ☑
      superficial I82.61- ☑
        chronic I82.71- ☑
  vena cava
    inferior I82.220
      chronic I82.221
    superior I82.210
      chronic I82.211
  venous, perianal K64.5
  ventricle (*see also* Infarct, myocardium)
    following acute myocardial infarction (current complication) I23.6
    not resulting in infarction I24.0
    old I51.3
Thrombus — *see* Thrombosis
Thrush (*see also* Candidiasis)
  newborn P37.5
  oral B37.0
  vaginal B37.3
Thumb (*see also* condition)
  sucking (child problem) F98.8
Thymitis E32.8
Thymoma (benign) D15.0
  malignant C37
Thymus, thymic (gland) — *see* condition
Thyrocele — *see* Goiter
Thyroglossal (*see also* condition)
  cyst Q89.2
  duct, persistent Q89.2
Thyroid (gland) (body) (*see also* condition)
  hormone resistance E07.89
  lingual Q89.2
  nodule (cystic) (nontoxic) (single) E04.1
Thyroiditis E06.9
  acute (nonsuppurative) (pyogenic) (suppurative) E06.0
  autoimmune E06.3
  chronic (nonspecific) (sclerosing) E06.5
    with thyrotoxicosis, transient E06.2
    fibrous E06.5
    lymphadenoid E06.3
    lymphocytic E06.3
    lymphoid E06.3
  de Quervain's E06.1
  drug-induced E06.4
  fibrous (chronic) E06.5
  giant-cell (follicular) E06.1
  granulomatous (de Quervain) (subacute) E06.1
  Hashimoto's (struma lymphomatosa) E06.3
  iatrogenic E06.4
  ligneous E06.5

Thyroiditis — *continued*
  lymphocytic (chronic) E06.3
  lymphoid E06.3
  lymphomatous E06.3
  nonsuppurative E06.1
  postpartum, puerperal O90.5
  pseudotuberculous E06.1
  pyogenic E06.0
  radiation E06.4
  Riedel's E06.5
  subacute (granulomatous) E06.1
  suppurative E06.0
  tuberculous A18.81
  viral E06.1
  woody E06.5
Thyrolingual duct, persistent Q89.2
Thyromegaly E01.0
Thyrotoxic
  crisis — *see* Thyrotoxicosis
  heart disease or failure (*see also* Thyrotoxicosis) E05.90 [I43]
    with thyroid storm E05.91 [I43]
  storm — *see* Thyrotoxicosis
Thyrotoxicosis (recurrent) E05.90
  with
    goiter (diffuse) E05.00
      with thyroid storm E05.01
      adenomatous uninodular E05.10
        with thyroid storm E05.11
      multinodular E05.20
        with thyroid storm E05.21
      nodular E05.20
        with thyroid storm E05.21
      uninodular E05.10
        with thyroid storm E05.11
    infiltrative
      dermopathy E05.00
        with thyroid storm E05.01
      ophthalmopathy E05.00
        with thyroid storm E05.01
    single thyroid nodule E05.10
      with thyroid storm E05.11
    thyroid storm E05.91
  due to
    ectopic thyroid nodule or tissue E05.30
      with thyroid storm E05.31
    ingestion of (excessive) thyroid material E05.40
      with thyroid storm E05.41
    overproduction of thyroid-stimulating hormone E05.80
      with thyroid storm E05.81
    specified cause NEC E05.80
      with thyroid storm E05.81
  factitia E05.40
    with thyroid storm E05.41
  heart (*see also* Failure, heart, high-output) E05.90 [I43]
    with thyroid storm (*see also* Failure, heart, high-output) E05.91 [I43]
    failure (*see also* Failure, heart, high-output) E05.90 [I43]
  neonatal (transient) P72.1
  transient with chronic thyroiditis E06.2
Tibia vara — *see* Osteochondrosis, juvenile, tibia
Tic (disorder) F95.9
  breathing F95.8
  child problem F95.0
  compulsive F95.1
  de la Tourette F95.2
  degenerative (generalized) (localized) G25.69
    facial G25.69
  disorder
    chronic
      motor F95.1
      vocal F95.1
    combined vocal and multiple motor F95.2
    transient F95.0
  douloureux G50.0
    atypical G50.1
    postherpetic, postzoster B02.22
  drug-induced G25.61
  eyelid F95.8
  habit F95.9
    chronic F95.1
    transient of childhood F95.0
  lid, transient of childhood F95.0
  motor-verbal F95.2
  occupational F48.8
  orbicularis F95.8

Tic — *continued*
  orbicularis — *continued*
    transient of childhood F95.0
  organic origin G25.69
  postchoreic G25.69
  provisional F95.0
  psychogenic, compulsive F95.1
  salaam R25.8
  spasm (motor or vocal) F95.9
    chronic F95.1
    transient of childhood F95.0
  specified NEC F95.8
Tick-borne — *see* condition
Tietze's disease or syndrome M94.0
Tight, tightness
  anus K62.89
  chest R07.89
  fascia (lata) M62.89
  foreskin (congenital) N47.1
  hymen, hymenal ring N89.6
  introitus (acquired) (congenital) N89.6
  rectal sphincter K62.89
  tendon — *see* Short, tendon
  urethral sphincter N35.9
Tilting vertebra — *see* Dorsopathy, deforming, specified NEC
Timidity, child F93.8
Tinea (intersecta) (tarsi) B35.9
  amiantacea L44.8
  asbestina B35.0
  barbae B35.0
  beard B35.0
  black dot B35.0
  blanca B36.2
  capitis B35.0
  corporis B35.4
  cruris B35.6
  flava B36.0
  foot B35.3
  furfuracea B36.0
  imbricata (Tokelau) B35.5
  kerion B35.0
  manuum B35.2
  microsporic — *see* Dermatophytosis
  nigra B36.1
  nodosa — *see* Piedra
  pedis B35.3
  scalp B35.0
  specified NEC B35.8
  sycosis B35.0
  tonsurans B35.0
  trichophytic — *see* Dermatophytosis
  unguium B35.1
  versicolor B36.0
Tingling sensation (skin) R20.2
Tin-miner's lung J63.5
Tinnitus NOS H93.1- ☑
  audible H93.1- ☑
  aurium H93.1- ☑
  pulsatile H93.A- ☑
  subjective H93.1- ☑
Tipped tooth (teeth) M26.33
Tipping
  pelvis M95.5
    with disproportion (fetopelvic) O33.0
      causing obstructed labor O65.0
  tooth (teeth), fully erupted M26.33
Tiredness R53.83
Tissue — *see* condition
Tobacco (nicotine)
  abuse — *see* Tobacco, use
  dependence — *see* Dependence, drug, nicotine
  harmful use Z72.0
  heart — *see* Tobacco, toxic effect
  maternal use, affecting newborn P04.2
  toxic effect — *see* Table of Drugs and Chemicals, by substance, poisoning
    chewing tobacco — *see* Table of Drugs and Chemicals, by substance, poisoning
    cigarettes — *see* Table of Drugs and Chemicals, by substance, poisoning
  use Z72.0
    complicating
      childbirth O99.334
      pregnancy O99.33- ☑
      puerperium O99.335
    counseling and surveillance Z71.6
    history Z87.891

Tobacco — *continued*
  withdrawal state (*see also* Dependence, drug, nicotine) F17.203
Tocopherol deficiency E56.0
Todd's
  cirrhosis K74.3
  paralysis (postepileptic) (transitory) G83.84
Toe — *see* condition
Toilet, artificial opening — *see* Attention to, artificial, opening
Tokelau (ringworm) B35.5
Tollwut — *see* Rabies
Tommaselli's disease R31.9
  correct substance properly administered — *see* Table of Drugs and Chemicals, by drug, adverse effect
  overdose or wrong substance given or taken — *see* Table of Drugs and Chemicals, by drug, poisoning
Tongue (*see also* condition)
  tie Q38.1
Tonic pupil — *see* Anomaly, pupil, function, tonic pupil
Toni-Fanconi syndrome (cystinosis) E72.09
  with cystinosis E72.04
Tonsil — *see* condition
Tonsillitis (acute) (catarrhal) (croupous) (follicular) (gangrenous) (infective) (lacunar) (lingual) (malignant) (membranous) (parenchymatous) (phlegmonous) (pseudomembranous) (purulent) (septic) (subacute) (suppurative) (toxic) (ulcerative) (vesicular) (viral) J03.90
  chronic J35.01
    with adenoiditis J35.03
  diphtheritic A36.0
  hypertrophic J35.01
    with adenoiditis J35.03
  recurrent J03.91
  specified organism NEC J03.80
    recurrent J03.81
  staphylococcal J03.80
    recurrent J03.81
  streptococcal J03.00
    recurrent J03.01
  tuberculous A15.8
  Vincent's A69.1
Tooth, teeth — *see* condition
Toothache K08.89
Topagnosis R20.8
Tophi — *see* Gout, chronic
TORCH infection — *see* Infection, congenital
  without active infection P00.2
Torn — *see* Tear
Tornwaldt's cyst or disease J39.2
Torsion
  accessory tube — *see* Torsion, fallopian tube
  adnexa (female) — *see* Torsion, fallopian tube
  aorta, acquired I77.1
  appendix epididymis N44.04
  appendix testis N44.03
  bile duct (common) (hepatic) K83.8
    congenital Q44.5
  bowel, colon or intestine K56.2
  cervix — *see* Malposition, uterus
  cystic duct K82.8
  dystonia — *see* Dystonia, torsion
  epididymis (appendix) N44.04
  fallopian tube N83.52- ☑
    with ovary N83.53
  gallbladder K82.8
    congenital Q44.1
  hydatid of Morgagni
    female N83.52- ☑
    male N44.03
  kidney (pedicle) (leading to infarction) N28.0
  Meckel's diverticulum (congenital) Q43.0
    malignant — *see* Table of Neoplasms, small intestine, malignant
  mesentery K56.2
  omentum K56.2
  organ or site, congenital NEC — *see* Anomaly, by site
  ovary (pedicle) N83.51- ☑
    with fallopian tube N83.53
    congenital Q50.2
  oviduct — *see* Torsion, fallopian tube
  penis (acquired) N48.82
    congenital Q55.63
  spasm — *see* Dystonia, torsion
  spermatic cord N44.02
    extravaginal N44.01

Torsion — *continued*
  spermatic cord — *continued*
    intravaginal N44.02
  spleen D73.5
  testis, testicle N44.00
    appendix N44.03
  tibia — *see* Deformity, limb, specified type NEC, lower leg
  uterus — *see* Malposition, uterus
Torticollis (intermittent) (spastic) M43.6
  congenital (sternomastoid) Q68.0
  due to birth injury P15.8
  hysterical F44.4
  ocular R29.891
  psychogenic F45.8
    conversion reaction F44.4
  rheumatic M43.6
  rheumatoid M06.88
  spasmodic G24.3
  traumatic, current S13.4 ☑
Tortipelvis G24.1
Tortuous
  aortic arch Q25.46
  artery I77.1
  organ or site, congenital NEC — *see* Distortion
  retinal vessel, congenital Q14.1
  ureter N13.8
  urethra N36.8
  vein — *see* Varix
Torture, victim of Z65.4
Torula, torular (histolytica) (infection) — *see* Cryptococcosis
Torulosis — *see* Cryptococcosis
Torus (mandibularis) (palatinus) M27.0
  fracture — *see* Fracture, by site, torus
Touraine's syndrome Q79.8
Tourette's syndrome F95.2
Tourniquet syndrome — *see* Constriction, external, by site
Tower skull Q75.0
  with exophthalmos Q87.0
Toxemia R68.89
  bacterial — *see* Sepsis
  burn — *see* Burn
  eclamptic (with pre-existing hypertension) — *see* Eclampsia
  erysipelatous — *see* Erysipelas
  fatigue R68.89
  food — *see* Poisoning, food
  gastrointestinal K52.1
  intestinal K52.1
  kidney — *see* Uremia
  malarial — *see* Malaria
  myocardial — *see* Myocarditis, toxic
  of pregnancy — *see* Pre-eclampsia
  pre-eclamptic — *see* Pre-eclampsia
  small intestine K52.1
  staphylococcal, due to food A05.0
  stasis R68.89
  uremic — *see* Uremia
  urinary — *see* Uremia
Toxemica cerebropathia psychica (nonalcoholic) F04
  alcoholic — *see* Alcohol, amnestic disorder
Toxic (poisoning) (*see also* condition) T65.91 ☑
  effect — *see* Table of Drugs and Chemicals, by substance, poisoning
  shock syndrome A48.3
  thyroid (gland) — *see* Thyrotoxicosis
Toxicemia — *see* Toxemia
Toxicity — *see* Table of Drugs and Chemicals, by substance, poisoning
  fava bean D55.0
  food, noxious — *see* Poisoning, food
  from drug or nonmedicinal substance — *see* Table of Drugs and Chemicals, by drug
Toxicosis (*see also* Toxemia)
  capillary, hemorrhagic D69.0
Toxinfection, gastrointestinal K52.1
Toxocariasis B83.0
Toxoplasma, toxoplasmosis (acquired) B58.9
  with
    hepatitis B58.1
    meningoencephalitis B58.2
    ocular involvement B58.00
    other organ involvement B58.89
    pneumonia, pneumonitis B58.3
  congenital (acute) (subacute) (chronic) P37.1

Toxoplasma, toxoplasmosis — *continued*
  maternal, manifest toxoplasmosis in infant (acute) (subacute) (chronic) P37.1
tPA (rtPA) administation in a different facility within the last 24 hours prior to admission to current facility Z92.82
Trabeculation, bladder N32.89
Trachea — *see* condition
Tracheitis (catarrhal) (infantile) (membranous) (plastic) (septal) (suppurative) (viral) J04.10
  with
    bronchitis (15 years of age and above) J40
      acute or subacute — *see* Bronchitis, acute
      chronic J42
      tuberculous NEC A15.5
      under 15 years of age J20.9
    laryngitis (acute) J04.2
      chronic J37.1
      tuberculous NEC A15.5
  acute J04.10
    with obstruction J04.11
  chronic J42
    with
      bronchitis (chronic) J42
      laryngitis (chronic) J37.1
  diphtheritic (membranous) A36.89
  due to external agent — *see* Inflammation, respiratory, upper, due to
  syphilitic A52.73
  tuberculous A15.5
Trachelitis (nonvenereal) — *see* Cervicitis
Tracheobronchial — *see* condition
Tracheobronchitis (15 years of age and above) (*see also* Bronchitis)
  due to
    Bordetella bronchiseptica A37.80
      with pneumonia A37.81
    Francisella tularensis A21.8
Tracheobronchomegaly Q32.4
  with bronchiectasis J47.9
    with
      exacerbation (acute) J47.1
      lower respiratory infection J47.0
  acquired J98.09
    with bronchiectasis J47.9
      with
        exacerbation (acute) J47.1
        lower respiratory infection J47.0
Tracheobronchopneumonitis — *see* Pneumonia, broncho-
Tracheocele (external) (internal) J39.8
  congenital Q32.1
Tracheomalacia J39.8
  congenital Q32.0
Tracheopharyngitis (acute) J06.9
  chronic J42
  due to external agent — *see* Inflammation, respiratory, upper, due to
Tracheostenosis J39.8
Tracheostomy
  complication — *see* Complication, tracheostomy
  status Z93.0
    attention to Z43.0
    malfunctioning J95.03
Trachoma, trachomatous A71.9
  active (stage) A71.1
  contraction of conjunctiva A71.1
  dubium A71.0
  healed or sequelae B94.0
  initial (stage) A71.0
  pannus A71.1
  Türck's J37.0
Traction, vitreomacular H43.82- ☑
Train sickness T75.3 ☑
Trait(s)
  Hb-S D57.3
  hemoglobin
    abnormal NEC D58.2
      with thalassemia D56.3
    C — *see* Disease, hemoglobin C
    S (Hb-S) D57.3
  Lepore D56.3
  personality, accentuated Z73.1
  sickle-cell D57.3
    with elliptocytosis or spherocytosis D57.3
  type A personality Z73.1
Tramp Z59.0
Trance R41.89

Trance — *continued*
  hysterical F44.89
Transaminasemia R74.0
Transection
  abdomen (partial) S38.3 ☑
  aorta (incomplete) (*see also* Injury, aorta)
    complete — *see* Injury, aorta, laceration, major
  carotid artery (incomplete) (*see also* Injury, blood
      vessel, carotid, laceration)
    complete — *see* Injury, blood vessel, carotid, lacer-
        ation, major
  celiac artery (incomplete) S35.211 ☑
    branch (incomplete) S35.291 ☑
      complete S35.292 ☑
    complete S35.212 ☑
  innominate
    artery (incomplete) (*see also* Injury, blood vessel,
        thoracic, innominate, artery, laceration)
      complete — *see* Injury, blood vessel, thoracic,
          innominate, artery, laceration, major
    vein (incomplete) (*see also* Injury, blood vessel,
        thoracic, innominate, vein, laceration)
      complete — *see* Injury, blood vessel, thoracic,
          innominate, vein, laceration, major
  jugular vein (external) (incomplete) (*see also* Injury,
      blood vessel, jugular vein, laceration)
    complete — *see* Injury, blood vessel, jugular vein,
        laceration, major
    internal (incomplete) (*see also* Injury, blood vessel,
        jugular vein, internal, laceration)
      complete — *see* Injury, blood vessel, jugular
          vein, internal, laceration, major
  mesenteric artery (incomplete) (*see also* Injury,
      mesenteric, artery, laceration)
    complete — *see* Injury, mesenteric artery, lacera-
        tion, major
  pulmonary vessel (incomplete) (*see also* Injury, blood
      vessel, thoracic, pulmonary, laceration)
    complete — *see* Injury, blood vessel, thoracic,
        pulmonary, laceration, major
  subclavian — *see* Transection, innominate
  vena cava (incomplete) (*see also* Injury, vena cava)
    complete — *see* Injury, vena cava, laceration, major
  vertebral artery (incomplete) (*see also* Injury, blood
      vessel, vertebral, laceration)
    complete — *see* Injury, blood vessel, vertebral,
        laceration, major
Transfusion
  associated (red blood cell) hemochromatosis E83.111
  blood
    ABO incompatible — *see* Complication(s), transfu-
        sion, incompatibility reaction, ABO
    minor blood group (Duffy) (E) (K(ell)) (Kidd) (Lewis)
        (M) (N) (P) (S) T80.89 ☑
    reaction or complication — *see* Complications,
        transfusion
  fetomaternal (mother) — *see* Pregnancy, complicated
      by, placenta, transfusion syndrome
  maternofetal (mother) — *see* Pregnancy, complicated
      by, placenta, transfusion syndrome
  placental (syndrome) (mother) — *see* Pregnancy,
      complicated by, placenta, transfusion syndrome
  reaction (adverse) — *see* Complications, transfusion
  related acute lung injury (TRALI) J95.84
  twin-to-twin — *see* Pregnancy, complicated by, pla-
      centa, transfusion syndrome, fetus to fetus
Transient (meaning homeless) (*see also* condition) Z59.0
Translocation
  balanced autosomal Q95.9
    in normal individual Q95.0
  chromosomes NEC Q99.8
    balanced and insertion in normal individual Q95.0
  Down syndrome Q90.2
  trisomy
    13 Q91.6
    18 Q91.2
    21 Q90.2
Translucency, iris — *see* Degeneration, iris
**Transmission of chemical substances through the
  placenta** — *see* Absorption, chemical, through
    placenta
Transparency, lung, unilateral J43.0
Transplant (ed) (status) Z94.9
  awaiting organ Z76.82
  bone Z94.6
    marrow Z94.81
  candidate Z76.82

Transplant — *continued*
  complication — *see* Complication, transplant
  cornea Z94.7
  heart Z94.1
    and lung(s) Z94.3
    valve Z95.2
      prosthetic Z95.2
      specified NEC Z95.4
      xenogenic Z95.3
  intestine Z94.82
  kidney Z94.0
  liver Z94.4
  lung(s) Z94.2
    and heart Z94.3
  organ (failure) (infection) (rejection) Z94.9
    removal status Z98.85
  pancreas Z94.83
  skin Z94.5
  social Z60.3
  specified organ or tissue NEC Z94.89
  stem cells Z94.84
  tissue Z94.9
Transplants, ovarian, endometrial N80.1
Transposed — *see* Transposition
Transposition (congenital) (*see also* Malposition, con-
    genital)
  abdominal viscera Q89.3
  aorta (dextra) Q20.3
  appendix Q43.8
  colon Q43.8
  corrected Q20.5
  great vessels (complete) (partial) Q20.3
  heart Q24.0
    with complete transposition of viscera Q89.3
  intestine (large) (small) Q43.8
  reversed jejunal (for bypass) (status) Z98.0
  scrotum Q55.23
  stomach Q40.2
    with general transposition of viscera Q89.3
  tooth, teeth, fully erupted M26.30
  vessels, great (complete) (partial) Q20.3
  viscera (abdominal) (thoracic) Q89.3
Transsexualism F64.0
Transverse (*see also* condition)
  arrest (deep), in labor O64.0 ☑
  lie (mother) O32.2 ☑
    causing obstructed labor O64.8 ☑
Transvestism, transvestitism (dual-role) F64.1
  fetishistic F65.1
Trapped placenta (with hemorrhage) O72.0
  without hemorrhage O73.0
TRAPS (tumor necrosis factor receptor associated periodic
    syndrome) M04.1
Trauma, traumatism (*see also* Injury)
  acoustic — *see* subcategory H83.3 ☑
  birth — *see* Birth, injury
  complicating ectopic or molar pregnancy O08.6
  during delivery O71.9
  following ectopic or molar pregnancy O08.6
  obstetric O71.9
    specified NEC O71.89
  occusal
    primary K08.81
    secondary K08.82
Traumatic (*see also* condition)
  brain injury S06.9 ☑
Treacher Collins syndrome Q75.4
Treitz's hernia — *see* Hernia, abdomen, specified site
    NEC
Trematode infestation — *see* Infestation, fluke
Trematodiasis — *see* Infestation, fluke
Trembling paralysis — *see* Parkinsonism
Tremor(s) R25.1
  drug induced G25.1
  essential (benign) G25.0
  familial G25.0
  hereditary G25.0
  hysterical F44.4
  intention G25.2
  medication induced postural G25.1
  mercurial — *see* subcategory T56.1 ☑
  Parkinson's — *see* Parkinsonism
  psychogenic (conversion reaction) F44.4
  senilis R54
  specified type NEC G25.2
Trench
  fever A79.0
  foot — *see* Immersion, foot

Trench — *continued*
  mouth A69.1
Treponema pallidum infection — *see* Syphilis
Treponematosis
  due to
    T. pallidum — *see* Syphilis
    T. pertenue — *see* Yaws
Triad
  Hutchinson's (congenital syphilis) A50.53
  Kartagener's Q89.3
  Saint's — *see* Hernia, diaphragm
Trichiasis (eyelid) H02.059
  with entropion — *see* Entropion
  left H02.056
    lower H02.055
    upper H02.054
  right H02.053
    lower H02.052
    upper H02.051
Trichinella spiralis (infection) (infestation) B75
Trichinellosis, trichiniasis, trichinelliasis, trichinosis
    B75
  with muscle disorder B75 [M63.80]
    ankle B75 [M63.87-] ☑
    foot B75 [M63.87-] ☑
    forearm B75 [M63.83-] ☑
    hand B75 [M63.84-] ☑
    lower leg B75 [M63.86-] ☑
    multiple sites B75 [M63.89]
    pelvic region B75 [M63.85-] ☑
    shoulder region B75 [M63.81-] ☑
    specified site NEC B75 [M63.88]
    thigh B75 [M63.85-] ☑
    upper arm B75 [M63.82-] ☑
Trichobezoar T18.9 ☑
  intestine T18.3 ☑
  stomach T18.2 ☑
Trichocephaliasis, trichocephalosis B79
Trichocephalus infestation B79
Trichoclasis L67.8
Trichoepithelioma (*see also* Neoplasm, skin, benign)
  malignant — *see* Neoplasm, skin, malignant
Trichofolliculoma — *see* Neoplasm, skin, benign
Tricholemmoma — *see* Neoplasm, skin, benign
Trichomoniasis A59.9
  bladder A59.03
  cervix A59.09
  intestinal A07.8
  prostate A59.02
  seminal vesicles A59.09
  specified site NEC A59.8
  urethra A59.03
  urogenitalis A59.00
  vagina A59.01
  vulva A59.01
Trichomycosis
  axillaris A48.8
  nodosa, nodularis B36.8
Trichonodosis L67.8
Trichophytid, trichophyton infection — *see* Dermato-
    phytosis
Trichophytobezoar T18.9 ☑
  intestine T18.3 ☑
  stomach T18.2 ☑
Trichophytosis — *see* Dermatophytosis
Trichoptilosis L67.8
Trichorrhexis (nodosa) (invaginata) L67.0
Trichosis axillaris A48.8
Trichosporosis nodosa B36.2
Trichostasis spinulosa (congenital) Q84.1
Trichostrongyliasis, trichostrongylosis (small intes-
    tine) B81.2
Trichostrongylus infection B81.2
Trichotillomania F63.3
Trichromat, trichromatopsia, anomalous (congenital)
    H53.55
Trichuriasis B79
Trichuris trichiura (infection) (infestation) (any site) B79
Tricuspid (valve) — *see* condition
Trifid (*see also* Accessory)
  kidney (pelvis) Q63.8
  tongue Q38.3
Trigeminal neuralgia — *see* Neuralgia, trigeminal
Trigeminy R00.8
Trigger finger (acquired) M65.30
  congenital Q74.0
  index finger M65.32- ☑

Index

Trance — Trigger finger

Trigger finger — *continued*
little finger M65.35- ☑
middle finger M65.33- ☑
ring finger M65.34- ☑
thumb M65.31- ☑
Trigonitis (bladder) (chronic) (pseudomembranous) N30.30
with hematuria N30.31
Trigonocephaly Q75.0
Trilocular heart — *see* Cor triloculare
Trimethylaminuria E72.52
Tripartite placenta O43.19- ☑
Triphalangeal thumb Q74.0
Triple (*see also* Accessory)
kidneys Q63.0
uteri Q51.818
X, female Q97.0
Triplegia G83.89
congenital G80.8
Triplet (newborn) (*see also* Newborn, triplet)
complicating pregnancy — *see* Pregnancy, triplet
Triplication — *see* Accessory
Triploidy Q92.7
Trismus R25.2
neonatorum A33
newborn A33
Trisomy (syndrome) Q92.9
13 (partial) Q91.7
meiotic nondisjunction Q91.4
mitotic nondisjunction Q91.5
mosaicism Q91.5
translocation Q91.6
18 (partial) Q91.3
meiotic nondisjunction Q91.0
mitotic nondisjunction Q91.1
mosaicism Q91.1
translocation Q91.2
20 Q92.8
21 (partial) Q90.9
meiotic nondisjunction Q90.0
mitotic nondisjunction Q90.1
mosaicism Q90.1
translocation Q90.2
22 Q92.8
autosomes Q92.9
chromosome specified NEC Q92.8
partial Q92.2
due to unbalanced translocation Q92.5
specified NEC Q92.8
whole (nonsex chromosome)
meiotic nondisjunction Q92.0
mitotic nondisjunction Q92.1
mosaicism Q92.1
due to
dicentrics — *see* Extra, marker chromosomes
extra rings — *see* Extra, marker chromosomes
isochromosomes — *see* Extra, marker chromosomes
specified NEC Q92.8
whole chromosome Q92.9
meiotic nondisjunction Q92.0
mitotic nondisjunction Q92.1
mosaicism Q92.1
partial Q92.9
specified NEC Q92.8
Tritanomaly, tritanopia H53.55
Trombiculosis, trombiculiasis, trombidiosis B88.0
Trophedema (congenital) (hereditary) Q82.0
Trophoblastic disease (*see also* Mole, hydatidiform) O01.9
Tropholymphedema Q82.0
Trophoneurosis NEC G96.8
disseminated M34.9
Tropical — *see* condition
Trouble (*see also* Disease)
heart — *see* Disease, heart
kidney — *see* Disease, renal
nervous R45.0
sinus — *see* Sinusitis
Trousseau's syndrome (thrombophlebitis migrans) I82.1
Truancy, childhood
from school Z72.810
Truncus
arteriosus (persistent) Q20.0
communis Q20.0
Trunk — *see* condition

Trypanosomiasis
African B56.9
by Trypanosoma brucei
gambiense B56.0
rhodesiense B56.1
American — *see* Chagas' disease
Brazilian — *see* Chagas' disease
by Trypanosoma
brucei gambiense B56.0
brucei rhodesiense B56.1
cruzi — *see* Chagas' disease
gambiensis, Gambian B56.0
rhodesiensis, Rhodesian B56.1
South American — *see* Chagas' disease
where
African trypanosomiasis is prevalent B56.9
Chagas' disease is prevalent B57.2
T-shaped incisors K00.2
Tsutsugamushi (disease) (fever) A75.3
Tube, tubal, tubular — *see* condition
Tubercle (*see also* Tuberculosis)
brain, solitary A17.81
Darwin's Q17.8
Ghon, primary infection A15.7
Tuberculid, tuberculide (indurating, subcutaneous) (lichenoid) (miliary) (papulonecrotic) (primary) (skin) A18.4
Tuberculoma (*see also* Tuberculosis)
brain A17.81
meninges (cerebral) (spinal) A17.1
spinal cord A17.81
Tuberculosis, tubercular, tuberculous (calcification) (calcified) (caseous) (chromogenic acid-fast bacilli) (degeneration) (fibrocaseous) (fistula) (interstitial) (isolated circumscribed lesions) (necrosis) (parenchymatous) (ulcerative) A15.9
with pneumoconiosis (any condition in J60-J64) J65
abdomen (lymph gland) A18.39
abscess (respiratory) A15.9
bone A18.03
hip A18.02
knee A18.02
sacrum A18.01
specified site NEC A18.03
spinal A18.01
vertebra A18.01
brain A17.81
breast A18.89
Cowper's gland A18.15
dura (mater) (cerebral) (spinal) A17.81
epidural (cerebral) (spinal) A17.81
female pelvis A18.17
frontal sinus A15.8
genital organs NEC A18.10
genitourinary A18.10
gland (lymphatic) — *see* Tuberculosis, lymph gland
hip A18.02
intestine A18.32
ischiorectal A18.32
joint NEC A18.02
hip A18.02
knee A18.02
specified NEC A18.02
vertebral A18.01
kidney A18.11
knee A18.02
latent R76.11
lumbar (spine) A18.01
lung — *see* Tuberculosis, pulmonary
meninges (cerebral) (spinal) A17.0
muscle A18.09
perianal (fistula) A18.32
perinephritic A18.11
perirectal A18.32
rectum A18.32
retropharyngeal A15.8
sacrum A18.01
scrofulous A18.2
scrotum A18.15
skin (primary) A18.4
spinal cord A17.81
spine or vertebra (column) A18.01
subdiaphragmatic A18.31
testis A18.15
urinary A18.13
uterus A18.17
accessory sinus — *see* Tuberculosis, sinus
Addison's disease A18.7

Tuberculosis, tubercular, tuberculous — *continued*
adenitis — *see* Tuberculosis, lymph gland
adenoids A15.8
adenopathy — *see* Tuberculosis, lymph gland
adherent pericardium A18.84
adnexa (uteri) A18.17
adrenal (capsule) (gland) A18.7
alimentary canal A18.32
anemia A18.89
ankle (joint) (bone) A18.02
anus A18.32
apex, apical — *see* Tuberculosis, pulmonary
appendicitis, appendix A18.32
arachnoid A17.0
artery, arteritis A18.89
cerebral A18.89
arthritis (chronic) (synovial) A18.02
spine or vertebra (column) A18.01
articular — *see* Tuberculosis, joint
ascites A18.31
asthma — *see* Tuberculosis, pulmonary
axilla, axillary (gland) A18.2
bladder A18.12
bone A18.03
hip A18.02
knee A18.02
limb NEC A18.03
sacrum A18.01
spine or vertebral column A18.01
bowel (miliary) A18.32
brain A17.81
breast A18.89
broad ligament A18.17
bronchi, bronchial, bronchus A15.5
ectasia, ectasis (bronchiectasis) — *see* Tuberculosis, pulmonary
fistula A15.5
primary (progressive) A15.7
gland or node A15.4
primary (progressive) A15.7
lymph gland or node A15.4
primary (progressive) A15.7
bronchiectasis — *see* Tuberculosis, pulmonary
bronchitis A15.5
bronchopleural A15.6
bronchopneumonia, bronchopneumonic — *see* Tuberculosis, pulmonary
bronchorrhagia A15.5
bronchotracheal A15.5
bronze disease A18.7
buccal cavity A18.83
bulbourethral gland A18.15
bursa A18.09
cachexia A15.9
cardiomyopathy A18.84
caries — *see* Tuberculosis, bone
cartilage A18.02
intervertebral A18.01
catarrhal — *see* Tuberculosis, respiratory
cecum A18.32
cellulitis (primary) A18.4
cerebellum A17.81
cerebral, cerebrum A17.81
cerebrospinal A17.81
meninges A17.0
cervical (lymph gland or node) A18.2
cervicitis, cervix (uteri) A18.16
chest — *see* Tuberculosis, respiratory
chorioretinitis A18.53
choroid, choroiditis A18.53
ciliary body A18.54
colitis A18.32
collier's J65
colliquativa (primary) A18.4
colon A18.32
complex, primary A15.7
congenital P37.0
conjunctiva A18.59
connective tissue (systemic) A18.89
contact Z20.1
cornea (ulcer) A18.52
Cowper's gland A18.15
coxae A18.02
coxalgia A18.02
cul-de-sac of Douglas A18.17
curvature, spine A18.01
cutis (colliquativa) (primary) A18.4
cyst, ovary A18.18

Tuberculosis, tubercular, tuberculous — continued
cystitis A18.12
dactylitis A18.03
diarrhea A18.32
diffuse — see Tuberculosis, miliary
digestive tract A18.32
disseminated — see Tuberculosis, miliary
duodenum A18.32
dura (mater) (cerebral) (spinal) A17.0
    abscess (cerebral) (spinal) A17.81
dysentery A18.32
ear (inner) (middle) A18.6
    bone A18.03
    external (primary) A18.4
    skin (primary) A18.4
elbow A18.02
emphysema — see Tuberculosis, pulmonary
empyema A15.6
encephalitis A17.82
endarteritis A18.89
endocarditis A18.84
    aortic A18.84
    mitral A18.84
    pulmonary A18.84
    tricuspid A18.84
endocrine glands NEC A18.82
endometrium A18.17
enteric, enterica, enteritis A18.32
enterocolitis A18.32
epididymis, epididymitis A18.15
epidural abscess (cerebral) (spinal) A17.81
epiglottis A15.5
episcleritis A18.51
erythema (induratum) (nodosum) (primary) A18.4
esophagus A18.83
eustachian tube A18.6
exposure (to) Z20.1
exudative — see Tuberculosis, pulmonary
eye A18.50
eyelid (primary) (lupus) A18.4
fallopian tube (acute) (chronic) A18.17
fascia A18.09
fauces A15.8
female pelvic inflammatory disease A18.17
finger A18.03
first infection A15.7
gallbladder A18.83
ganglion A18.09
gastritis A18.83
gastrocolic fistula A18.32
gastroenteritis A18.32
gastrointestinal tract A18.32
general, generalized — see Tuberculosis, miliary
genital organs A18.10
genitourinary A18.10
genu A18.02
glandula suprarenalis A18.7
glandular, general A18.2
glottis A15.5
grinder's J65
gum A18.83
hand A18.03
heart A18.84
hematogenous — see Tuberculosis, miliary
hemoptysis — see Tuberculosis, pulmonary
hemorrhage NEC — see Tuberculosis, pulmonary
hemothorax A15.6
hepatitis A18.83
hilar lymph nodes A15.4
    primary (progressive) A15.7
hip (joint) (disease) (bone) A18.02
hydropneumothorax A15.6
hydrothorax A15.6
hypoadrenalism A18.7
hypopharynx A15.8
ileocecal (hyperplastic) A18.32
ileocolitis A18.32
ileum A18.32
iliac spine (superior) A18.03
immunological findings only A15.7
indurativa (primary) A18.4
infantile A15.7
infection A15.9
    without clinical manifestations A15.7
infraclavicular gland A18.2
inguinal gland A18.2
inguinalis A18.2
intestine (any part) A18.32

Tuberculosis, tubercular, tuberculous — continued
iridocyclitis A18.54
iris, iritis A18.54
ischiorectal A18.32
jaw A18.03
jejunum A18.32
joint A18.02
    vertebral A18.01
keratitis (interstitial) A18.52
keratoconjunctivitis A18.52
kidney A18.11
knee (joint) A18.02
kyphosis, kyphoscoliosis A18.01
laryngitis A15.5
larynx A15.5
latent R76.11
leptomeninges, leptomeningitis (cerebral) (spinal) A17.0
lichenoides (primary) A18.4
linguae A18.83
lip A18.83
liver A18.83
lordosis A18.01
lung — see Tuberculosis, pulmonary
lupus vulgaris A18.4
lymph gland or node (peripheral) A18.2
    abdomen A18.39
    bronchial A15.4
        primary (progressive) A15.7
    cervical A18.2
    hilar A15.4
        primary (progressive) A15.7
    intrathoracic A15.4
        primary (progressive) A15.7
    mediastinal A15.4
        primary (progressive) A15.7
    mesenteric A18.39
    retroperitoneal A18.39
    tracheobronchial A15.4
        primary (progressive) A15.7
lymphadenitis — see Tuberculosis, lymph gland
lymphangitis — see Tuberculosis, lymph gland
lymphatic (gland) (vessel) — see Tuberculosis, lymph gland
mammary gland A18.89
marasmus A15.9
mastoiditis A18.03
mediastinal lymph gland or node A15.4
    primary (progressive) A15.7
mediastinitis A15.8
    primary (progressive) A15.7
mediastinum A15.8
    primary (progressive) A15.7
medulla A17.81
melanosis, Addisonian A18.7
meninges, meningitis (basilar) (cerebral) (cerebrospinal) (spinal) A17.0
meningoencephalitis A17.82
mesentery, mesenteric (gland or node) A18.39
miliary A19.9
    acute A19.2
        multiple sites A19.1
        single specified site A19.0
    chronic A19.8
    specified NEC A19.8
millstone makers' J65
miner's J65
molder's J65
mouth A18.83
multiple A19.9
    acute A19.1
    chronic A19.8
muscle A18.09
myelitis A17.82
myocardium, myocarditis A18.84
nasal (passage) (sinus) A15.8
nasopharynx A15.8
neck gland A18.2
nephritis A18.11
nerve (mononeuropathy) A17.83
nervous system A17.9
nose (septum) A15.8
ocular A18.50
omentum A18.31
oophoritis (acute) (chronic) A18.17
optic (nerve trunk) (papilla) A18.59
orbit A18.59
orchitis A18.15
organ, specified NEC A18.89

Tuberculosis, tubercular, tuberculous — continued
osseous — see Tuberculosis, bone
osteitis — see Tuberculosis, bone
osteomyelitis — see Tuberculosis, bone
otitis media A18.6
ovary, ovaritis (acute) (chronic) A18.17
oviduct (acute) (chronic) A18.17
pachymeningitis A17.0
palate (soft) A18.83
pancreas A18.83
papulonecrotic (a) (primary) A18.4
parathyroid glands A18.82
paronychia (primary) A18.4
parotid gland or region A18.83
pelvis (bony) A18.03
penis A18.15
peribronchitis A15.5
pericardium, pericarditis A18.84
perichondritis, larynx A15.5
periostitis — see Tuberculosis, bone
perirectal fistula A18.32
peritoneum NEC A18.31
peritonitis A18.31
pharynx, pharyngitis A15.8
phlyctenulosis (keratoconjunctivitis) A18.52
phthisis NEC — see Tuberculosis, pulmonary
pituitary gland A18.82
pleura, pleural, pleurisy, pleuritis (fibrinous) (obliterative) (purulent) (simple plastic) (with effusion) A15.6
    primary (progressive) A15.7
pneumonia, pneumonic — see Tuberculosis, pulmonary
pneumothorax (spontaneous) (tense valvular) — see Tuberculosis, pulmonary
polyneuropathy A17.89
polyserositis A19.9
    acute A19.1
    chronic A19.8
potter's J65
prepuce A18.15
primary (complex) A15.7
proctitis A18.32
prostate, prostatitis A18.14
pulmonalis — see Tuberculosis, pulmonary
pulmonary (cavitated) (fibrotic) (infiltrative) (nodular) A15.0
    childhood type or first infection A15.7
    primary (complex) A15.7
pyelitis A18.11
pyelonephritis A18.11
pyemia — see Tuberculosis, miliary
pyonephrosis A18.11
pyopneumothorax A15.6
pyothorax A15.6
rectum (fistula) (with abscess) A18.32
reinfection stage — see Tuberculosis, pulmonary
renal A18.11
renis A18.11
respiratory A15.9
    primary A15.7
    specified site NEC A15.8
retina, retinitis A18.53
retroperitoneal (lymph gland or node) A18.39
rheumatism NEC A18.09
rhinitis A15.8
sacroiliac (joint) A18.01
sacrum A18.01
salivary gland A18.83
salpingitis (acute) (chronic) A18.17
sandblaster's J65
sclera A18.51
scoliosis A18.01
scrofulous A18.2
scrotum A18.15
seminal tract or vesicle A18.15
senile A15.9
septic — see Tuberculosis, miliary
shoulder (joint) A18.02
    blade A18.03
sigmoid A18.32
sinus (any nasal) A15.8
    bone A18.03
    epididymis A18.15
skeletal NEC A18.03
skin (any site) (primary) A18.4
small intestine A18.32
soft palate A18.83

Index

Tuberculosis, tubercular, tuberculous — Tumor

Tuberculosis, tubercular, tuberculous — *continued*
spermatic cord A18.15
spine, spinal (column) A18.01
cord A17.81
medulla A17.81
membrane A17.0
meninges A17.0
spleen, splenitis A18.85
spondylitis A18.01
sternoclavicular joint A18.02
stomach A18.83
stonemason's J65
subcutaneous tissue (cellular) (primary) A18.4
subcutis (primary) A18.4
subdeltoid bursa A18.83
submaxillary (region) A18.83
supraclavicular gland A18.2
suprarenal (capsule) (gland) A18.7
swelling, joint (see also category M01) (see also Tuberculosis, joint) A18.02
symphysis pubis A18.02
synovitis A18.09
articular A18.02
spine or vertebra A18.01
systemic — see Tuberculosis, miliary
tarsitis A18.4
tendon (sheath) — see Tuberculosis, tenosynovitis
tenosynovitis A18.09
spine or vertebra A18.01
testis A18.15
throat A15.8
thymus gland A18.82
thyroid gland A18.81
tongue A18.83
tonsil, tonsillitis A15.8
trachea, tracheal A15.5
lymph gland or node A15.4
primary (progressive) A15.7
tracheobronchial A15.5
lymph gland or node A15.4
primary (progressive) A15.7
tubal (acute) (chronic) A18.17
tunica vaginalis A18.15
ulcer (skin) (primary) A18.4
bowel or intestine A18.32
specified NEC — see Tuberculosis, by site
unspecified site A15.9
ureter A18.11
urethra, urethral (gland) A18.13
urinary organ or tract A18.13
uterus A18.17
uveal tract A18.54
uvula A18.83
vagina A18.18
vas deferens A18.15
verruca, verrucosa (cutis) (primary) A18.4
vertebra (column) A18.01
vesiculitis A18.15
vulva A18.18
wrist (joint) A18.02
Tuberculum
Carabelli — see Excludes Note at K00.2
occlusal — see Excludes Note at K00.2
paramolare K00.2
Tuberosity, enitre maxillary M26.07
Tuberous sclerosis (brain) Q85.1
Tubo-ovarian — see condition
Tuboplasty, after previous sterilization Z31.0
aftercare Z31.42
Tubotympanitis, catarrhal (chronic) — see Otitis, media, nonsuppurative, chronic, serous
Tularemia A21.9
with
conjunctivitis A21.1
pneumonia A21.2
abdominal A21.3
bronchopneumonic A21.2
conjunctivitis A21.1
cryptogenic A21.3
enteric A21.3
gastrointestinal A21.3
generalized A21.7
ingestion A21.3
intestinal A21.3
oculoglandular A21.1
ophthalmic A21.1
pneumonia (any), pneumonic A21.2
pulmonary A21.2

Tularemia — *continued*
sepsis A21.7
specified NEC A21.8
typhoidal A21.7
ulceroglandular A21.0
Tularensis conjunctivitis A21.1
Tumefaction (see also Swelling)
liver — see Hypertrophy, liver
Tumor (see also Neoplasm, unspecified behavior, by site)
acinar cell — see Neoplasm, uncertain behavior, by
site
acinic cell — see Neoplasm, uncertain behavior, by
site
adenocarcinoid — see Neoplasm, malignant, by site
adenomatoid (see also Neoplasm, benign, by site)
odontogenic — see Cyst, calcifying odontogenic
adnexal (skin) — see Neoplasm, skin, benign, by site
adrenal
cortical (benign) D35.0- ☑
malignant C74.0- ☑
rest — see Neoplasm, benign, by site
alpha-cell
malignant
pancreas C25.4
specified site NEC — see Neoplasm, malignant,
by site
unspecified site C25.4
pancreas D13.7
specified site NEC — see Neoplasm, benign, by site
unspecified site D13.7
aneurysmal — see Aneurysm
aortic body D44.7
malignant C75.5
Askin's — see Neoplasm, connective tissue, malignant
basal cell (see also Neoplasm, skin, uncertain behavior)
D48.5
Bednar — see Neoplasm, skin, malignant
benign (unclassified) — see Neoplasm, benign, by site
beta-cell
malignant
pancreas C25.4
specified site NEC — see Neoplasm, malignant,
by site
unspecified site C25.4
pancreas D13.7
specified site NEC — see Neoplasm, benign, by site
unspecified site D13.7
Brenner D27.9
borderline malignancy D39.1- ☑
malignant C56- ☑
proliferating D39.1- ☑
bronchial alveolar, intravascular D38.1
Brooke's — see Neoplasm, skin, benign
brown fat — see Lipoma
Burkitt — see Lymphoma, Burkitt
calcifying epithelial odontogenic — see Cyst, calcifying
odontogenic
carcinoid
benign D3A.00 (following D36)
appendix D3A.020 (following D36)
ascending colon D3A.022 (following D36)
bronchus (lung) D3A.090 (following D36)
cecum D3A.021 (following D36)
colon D3A.029 (following D36)
descending colon D3A.024 (following D36)
duodenum D3A.010 (following D36)
foregut NOS D3A.094 (following D36)
hindgut NOS D3A.096 (following D36)
ileum D3A.012 (following D36)
jejunum D3A.011 (following D36)
kidney D3A.093 (following D36)
large intestine D3A.029 (following D36)
lung (bronchus) D3A.090 (following D36)
midgut NOS D3A.095 (following D36)
rectum D3A.026 (following D36)
sigmoid colon D3A.025 (following D36)
small intestine D3A.019 (following D36)
specified NEC D3A.098 (following D36)
stomach D3A.092 (following D36)
thymus D3A.091 (following D36)
transverse colon D3A.023 (following D36)
malignant C7A.00 (following C75)
appendix C7A.020 (following C75)
ascending colon C7A.022 (following C75)
bronchus (lung) C7A.090 (following C75)
cecum C7A.021 (following C75)
colon C7A.029 (following C75)
descending colon C7A.024 (following C75)

Tumor — *continued*
carcinoid — *continued*
malignant — *continued*
duodenum C7A.010 (following C75)
foregut NOS C7A.094 (following C75)
hindgut NOS C7A.096 (following C75)
ileum C7A.012 (following C75)
jejunum C7A.011 (following C75)
kidney C7A.093 (following C75)
large intestine C7A.029 (following C75)
lung (bronchus) C7A.090 (following C75)
midgut NOS C7A.095 (following C75)
rectum C7A.026 (following C75)
sigmoid colon C7A.025 (following C75)
small intestine C7A.019 (following C75)
specified NEC C7A.098 (following C75)
stomach C7A.092 (following C75)
thymus C7A.091 (following C75)
transverse colon C7A.023 (following C75)
mesentery metastasis C7B.04 (following C75)
secondary C7B.00 (following C75)
bone C7B.03 (following C75)
distant lymph nodes C7B.01 (following C75)
liver C7B.02 (following C75)
peritoneum C7B.04 (following C75)
specified NEC C7B.09 (following C75)
carotid body D44.6
malignant C75.4
cells (see also Neoplasm, unspecified behavior, by site)
benign — see Neoplasm, benign, by site
malignant — see Neoplasm, malignant, by site
uncertain whether benign or malignant — see
Neoplasm, uncertain behavior, by site
cervix, in pregnancy or childbirth — see Pregnancy,
complicated by, tumor, cervix
chondromatous giant cell — see Neoplasm, bone,
benign
chromaffin (see also Neoplasm, benign, by site)
malignant — see Neoplasm, malignant, by site
Cock's peculiar L72.3
Codman's — see Neoplasm, bone, benign
dentigerous, mixed — see Cyst, calcifying odontogenic
dermoid — see Neoplasm, benign, by site
with malignant transformation C56- ☑
desmoid (extra-abdominal) (see also Neoplasm, connective tissue, uncertain behavior)
abdominal — see Neoplasm, connective tissue,
uncertain behavior
embolus — see Neoplasm, secondary, by site
embryonal (mixed) (see also Neoplasm, uncertain behavior, by site)
liver C22.7
endodermal sinus
specified site — see Neoplasm, malignant, by site
unspecified site
female C56.- ☑
male C62.90
epithelial
benign — see Neoplasm, benign, by site
malignant — see Neoplasm, malignant, by site
Ewing's — see Neoplasm, bone, malignant
fatty — see Lipoma
fibroid — see Leiomyoma
G cell
malignant
pancreas C25.4
specified site NEC — see Neoplasm, malignant,
by site
unspecified site C25.4
specified site — see Neoplasm, uncertain behavior,
by site
unspecified site D37.8
germ cell (see also Neoplasm, malignant, by site)
mixed — see Neoplasm, malignant, by site
ghost cell, odontogenic — see Cyst, calcifying odontogenic
giant cell (see also Neoplasm, uncertain behavior, by
site)
bone D48.0
malignant — see Neoplasm, bone, malignant
chondromatous — see Neoplasm, bone, benign
malignant — see Neoplasm, malignant, by site
soft parts — see Neoplasm, connective tissue, uncertain behavior
malignant — see Neoplasm, connective tissue,
malignant
glomus D18.00
intra-abdominal D18.03

☑ **Additional Character Required — Refer to the Tabular List for Character Selection**   ⦾ **Subterms under main terms may continue to next column or page**

Tumor — *continued*
  glomus — *continued*
    intracranial D18.02
    jugulare D44.7
      malignant C75.5
    skin D18.01
    specified site NEC D18.09
  gonadal stromal — *see* Neoplasm, uncertain behavior, by site
  granular cell (*see also* Neoplasm, connective tissue, benign)
    malignant — *see* Neoplasm, connective tissue, malignant
  granulosa cell D39.1- ☑
    juvenile D39.1- ☑
    malignant C56- ☑
  granulosa cell-theca cell D39.1- ☑
    malignant C56- ☑
  Grawitz's C64- ☑
  hemorrhoidal — *see* Hemorrhoids
  hilar cell D27- ☑
  hilus cell D27- ☑
  Hurthle cell (benign) D34
    malignant C73
  hydatid — *see* Echinococcus
  hypernephroid (*see also* Neoplasm, uncertain behavior, by site)
  interstitial cell (*see also* Neoplasm, uncertain behavior, by site)
    benign — *see* Neoplasm, benign, by site
    malignant — *see* Neoplasm, malignant, by site
  intravascular bronchial alveolar D38.1
  islet cell — *see* Neoplasm, benign, by site
    malignant — *see* Neoplasm, malignant, by site
      pancreas C25.4
      specified site NEC — *see* Neoplasm, malignant, by site
      unspecified site C25.4
    pancreas D13.7
    specified site NEC — *see* Neoplasm, benign, by site
    unspecified site D13.7
  juxtaglomerular D41.0- ☑
  Klatskin's C22.1
  Krukenberg's C79.6- ☑
  Leydig cell — *see* Neoplasm, uncertain behavior, by site
    benign — *see* Neoplasm, benign, by site
      specified site — *see* Neoplasm, benign, by site
      unspecified site
        female D27.9
        male D29.20
    malignant — *see* Neoplasm, malignant, by site
      specified site — *see* Neoplasm, malignant, by site
      unspecified site
        female C56.9
        male C62.90
    specified site — *see* Neoplasm, uncertain behavior, by site
    unspecified site
      female D39.10
      male D40.10
  lipid cell, ovary D27- ☑
  lipoid cell, ovary D27- ☑
  malignant (*see also* Neoplasm, malignant, by site) C80.1
    fusiform cell (type) C80.1
    giant cell (type) C80.1
    localized, plasma cell — *see* Plasmacytoma, solitary
    mixed NEC C80.1
    small cell (type) C80.1
    spindle cell (type) C80.1
    unclassified C80.1
  mast cell D47.09
  melanotic, neuroectodermal — *see* Neoplasm, benign, by site
  Merkel cell — *see* Carcinoma, Merkel cell
  mesenchymal
    malignant — *see* Neoplasm, connective tissue, malignant
    mixed — *see* Neoplasm, connective tissue, uncertain behavior
  mesodermal, mixed (*see also* Neoplasm, malignant, by site)
    liver C22.4

Tumor — *continued*
  mesonephric (*see also* Neoplasm, uncertain behavior, by site)
    malignant — *see* Neoplasm, malignant, by site
  metastatic
    from specified site — *see* Neoplasm, malignant, by site
    of specified site — *see* Neoplasm, malignant, by site
    to specified site — *see* Neoplasm, secondary, by site
  mixed NEC (*see also* Neoplasm, benign, by site)
    malignant — *see* Neoplasm, malignant, by site
  mucinous of low malignant potential
    specified site — *see* Neoplasm, malignant, by site
    unspecified site C56.9
  mucocarcinoid
    specified site — *see* Neoplasm, malignant, by site
    unspecified site C18.1
  mucoepidermoid — *see* Neoplasm, uncertain behavior, by site
  Müllerian, mixed
    specified site — *see* Neoplasm, malignant, by site
    unspecified site C54.9
  myoepithelial — *see* Neoplasm, benign, by site
  neuroectodermal (peripheral) — *see* Neoplasm, malignant, by site
    primitive
      specified site — *see* Neoplasm, malignant, by site
      unspecified site C71.9
  neuroendocrine D3A.8 (*following* D36)
    malignant poorly differentiated C7A.1 (*following* C75)
    secondary NEC C7B.8 (*following* C75)
    specified NEC C7A.8 (*following* C75)
  neurogenic olfactory C30.0
  nonencapsulated sclerosing C73
  odontogenic (adenomatoid) (benign) (calcifying epithelial) (keratocystic) (squamous) — *see* Cyst, calcifying odontogenic
    malignant C41.1
      upper jaw (bone) C41.0
  ovarian stromal D39.1- ☑
  ovary, in pregnancy — *see* Pregnancy, complicated by
  pacinian — *see* Neoplasm, skin, benign
  Pancoast's — *see* Pancoast's syndrome
  papillary (*see also* Papilloma)
    cystic D37.9
    mucinous of low malignant potential C56- ☑
      specified site — *see* Neoplasm, malignant, by site
      unspecified site C56.9
    serous of low malignant potential
      specified site — *see* Neoplasm, malignant, by site
      unspecified site C56.9
  pelvic, in pregnancy or childbirth — *see* Pregnancy, complicated by
  phantom F45.8
  phyllodes D48.6- ☑
    benign D24- ☑
    malignant — *see* Neoplasm, breast, malignant
  Pindborg — *see* Cyst, calcifying odontogenic
  placental site trophoblastic D39.2
  plasma cell (malignant) (localized) — *see* Plasmacytoma, solitary
  polyvesicular vitelline
    specified site — *see* Neoplasm, malignant, by site
    unspecified site
      female C56.9
      male C62.90
  Pott's puffy — *see* Osteomyelitis, specified NEC
  Rathke's pouch D44.3
  retinal anlage — *see* Neoplasm, benign, by site
  salivary gland type, mixed — *see* Neoplasm, salivary gland, benign
    malignant — *see* Neoplasm, salivary gland, malignant
  Sampson's N80.1
  Schmincke's — *see* Neoplasm, nasopharynx, malignant
  sclerosing stromal D27- ☑
  sebaceous — *see* Cyst, sebaceous
  secondary — *see* Neoplasm, secondary, by site
    carcinoid C7B.00 (*following* C75)
      bone C7B.03 (*following* C75)
      distant lymph nodes C7B.01 (*following* C75)

Tumor — *continued*
  secondary — *see* Neoplasm, secondary, by site — *continued*
    carcinoid — *continued*
      liver C7B.02 (*following* C75)
      peritoneum C7B.04 (*following* C75)
      specified NEC C7B.09 (*following* C75)
    neuroendocrine NEC C7B.8 (*following* C75)
  serous of low malignant potential
    specified site — *see* Neoplasm, malignant, by site
    unspecified site C56.9
  Sertoli cell — *see* Neoplasm, benign, by site
    with lipid storage
      specified site — *see* Neoplasm, benign, by site
      unspecified site
        female D27.9
        male D29.20
    specified site — *see* Neoplasm, benign, by site
    unspecified site
      female D27.9
      male D29.20
  Sertoli-Leydig cell — *see* Neoplasm, benign, by site
    specified site — *see* Neoplasm, benign, by site
    unspecified site
      female D27.9
      male D29.20
  sex cord (-stromal) — *see* Neoplasm, uncertain behavior, by site
    with annular tubules D39.1- ☑
  skin appendage — *see* Neoplasm, skin, benign
  smooth muscle — *see* Neoplasm, connective tissue, uncertain behavior
  soft tissue
    benign — *see* Neoplasm, connective tissue, benign
    malignant — *see* Neoplasm, connective tissue, malignant
  sternomastoid (congenital) Q68.0
  stromal
    endometrial D39.0
    gastric D48.1
      benign D21.4
      malignant C16.9
      uncertain behavior D48.1
    gastrointestinal C49.A- ☑
      benign D21.4
      esophagus C49.A1
      malignant C49.A0
        colon C49.A4
        duodenum C49.A3
        esophagus C49.A1
        ileum C49.A3
        jejunum C49.A3
        large intestine C49.A4
        Meckel diverticulum C49.A3
        omentum C49.A9
        peritoneum C49.A9
        rectum C49.A5
        small intestine C49.A3
        specified site NEC C49.A9
        stomach C49.A2
      rectum C49.A5
      small intestine C49.A3
      specified site NEC C49.A9
      stomach C49.A2
      uncertain behavior D48.1
    intestine
      benign D21.4
      malignant
        large C49.A4
        small C49.A3
      uncertain behavior D48.1
    ovarian D39.1- ☑
    stomach C49.A2
      benign D21.4
      malignant C49.A2
      uncertain behavior D48.1
  sweat gland (*see also* Neoplasm, skin, uncertain behavior)
    benign — *see* Neoplasm, skin, benign
    malignant — *see* Neoplasm, skin, malignant
  syphilitic, brain A52.17
  testicular D40.10
  testicular stromal D40.1- ☑
  theca cell D27.- ☑
  theca cell-granulosa cell D39.1- ☑
  Triton, malignant — *see* Neoplasm, nerve, malignant
  trophoblastic, placental site D39.2
  turban D23.4

Tumor — *continued*
  uterus (body), in pregnancy or childbirth — *see* Pregnancy, complicated by, tumor, uterus
  vagina, in pregnancy or childbirth — *see* Pregnancy, complicated by
  varicose — *see* Varix
  von Recklinghausen's — *see* Neurofibromatosis
  vulva or perineum, in pregnancy or childbirth — *see* Pregnancy, complicated by
    causing obstructed labor O65.5
  Warthin's — *see* Neoplasm, salivary gland, benign
  Wilms' C64- ☑
  yolk sac — *see* Neoplasm, malignant, by site
    specified site — *see* Neoplasm, malignant, by site
    unspecified site
      female C56.9
      male C62.90
Tumor lysis syndrome (following antineoplastic chemotherapy) (spontaneous) NEC E88.3
Tumorlet — *see* Neoplasm, uncertain behavior, by site
Tungiasis B88.1
Tunica vasculosa lentis Q12.2
Turban tumor D23.4
Türck's trachoma J37.0
Turner-Kieser syndrome Q87.2
Turner-like syndrome Q87.1
Turner's
  hypoplasia (tooth) K00.4
  syndrome Q96.9
    specified NEC Q96.8
  tooth K00.4
Turner-Ullrich syndrome Q96.9
Tussis convulsiva — *see* Whooping cough
Twiddler's syndrome (due to)
  automatic implantable defibrillatorT82.198
  cardiac pacemaker T82.198 ☑
Twilight state
  epileptic F05
  psychogenic F44.89
Twin (newborn) (*see also* Newborn, twin)
  conjoined Q89.4
  pregnancy — *see* Pregnancy, twin
Twinning, teeth K00.2
Twist, twisted
  bowel, colon or intestine K56.2
  hair (congenital) Q84.1
  mesentery K56.2
  omentum K56.2
  organ or site, congenital NEC — *see* Anomaly, by site
  ovarian pedicle — *see* Torsion, ovary
Twitching R25.3
Tylosis (acquired) L84
  buccalis K13.29
  linguae K13.29
  palmaris et plantaris (congenital) (inherited) Q82.8
    acquired L85.1
Tympanism R14.0
Tympanites (abdominal) (intestinal) R14.0
Tympanitis — *see* Myringitis
Tympanosclerosis H74.0 ☑
Tympanum — *see* condition
Tympany
  abdomen R14.0
  chest R09.89
Type A behavior pattern Z73.1
Typhlitis — *see* Appendicitis
Typhoenteritis — *see* Typhoid
Typhoid (abortive) (ambulant) (any site) (clinical) (fever) (hemorrhagic) (infection) (intermittent) (malignant) (rheumatic) (Widal negative) A01.00
  with pneumonia A01.03
  abdominal A01.09
  arthritis A01.04
  carrier (suspected) of Z22.0
  cholecystitis (current) A01.09
  endocarditis A01.02
  heart involvement A01.02
  inoculation reaction — *see* Complications, vaccination
  meningitis A01.01
  mesenteric lymph nodes A01.09
  myocarditis A01.02
  osteomyelitis A01.05
  perichondritis, larynx A01.09
  pneumonia A01.03
  specified NEC A01.09
  spine A01.05
  ulcer (perforating) A01.09

Typhomalaria (fever) — *see* Malaria
Typhomania A01.00
Typhoperitonitis A01.09
Typhus (fever) A75.9
  abdominal, abdominalis — *see* Typhoid
  African tick A77.1
  amarillic A95.9
  brain A75.9 [G94]
  cerebral A75.9 [G94]
  classical A75.0
  due to Rickettsia
    prowazekii A75.0
      recrudescent A75.1
    tsutsugamushi A75.3
    typhi A75.2
  endemic (flea-borne) A75.2
  epidemic (louse-borne) A75.0
  exanthematicus SAI A75.0
    brillii SAI A75.1
    mexicanus SAI A75.2
    typhus murinus A75.2
  exanthematic NEC A75.0
  flea-borne A75.2
  India tick A77.1
  Kenya (tick) A77.1
  louse-borne A75.0
  Mexican A75.2
  mite-borne A75.3
  murine A75.2
  North Asian tick-borne A77.2
  petechial A75.9
  Queensland tick A77.3
  rat A75.2
  recrudescent A75.1
  recurrens — *see* Fever, relapsing
  Sao Paulo A77.0
  scrub (China) (India) (Malaysia) (New Guinea) A75.3
  shop (of Malaysia) A75.2
  Siberian tick A77.2
  tick-borne A77.9
  tropical (mite-borne) A75.3
Tyrosinemia E70.21
  newborn, transitory P74.5
Tyrosinosis E70.21
Tyrosinuria E70.29

U

Uhl's anomaly or disease Q24.8
Ulcer, ulcerated, ulcerating, ulceration, ulcerative
  alveolar process M27.3
  amebic (intestine) A06.1
    skin A06.7
  anastomotic — *see* Ulcer, gastrojejunal
  anorectal K62.6
  antral — *see* Ulcer, stomach
  anus (sphincter) (solitary) K62.6
  aorta — *see* Aneurysm
  aphthous (oral) (recurrent) K12.0
    genital organ(s)
      female N76.6
      male N50.89
  artery I77.2
  atrophic — *see* Ulcer, skin
    decubitus — *see* Ulcer, pressure, by site
  back L98.429
    with
      bone involvement without evidence of necrosis L98.426
      bone necrosis L98.424
      exposed fat layer L98.422
      muscle involvement without evidence of necrosis L98.425
      muscle necrosis L98.423
      skin breakdown only L98.421
      specified severity NEC L98.428
  Barrett's (esophagus) K22.10
    with bleeding K22.11
  bile duct (common) (hepatic) K83.8
  bladder (solitary) (sphincter) NEC N32.89
    bilharzial B65.9 [N33]
    in schistosomiasis (bilharzial) B65.9 [N33]
    submucosal — *see* Cystitis, interstitial
    tuberculous A18.12
  bleeding K27.4
  bone — *see* Osteomyelitis, specified type NEC
  bowel — *see* Ulcer, intestine
  breast N61.1

Ulcer, ulcerated, ulcerating, ulceration, ulcerative — *continued*
  bronchus J98.09
  buccal (cavity) (traumatic) K12.1
  Buruli A31.1
  buttock L98.419
    with
      bone involvement without evidence of necrosis L98.416
      bone necrosis L98.414
      exposed fat layer L98.412
      muscle involvement without evidence of necrosis L98.415
      muscle necrosis L98.413
      skin breakdown only L98.411
      specified severity NEC L98.418
  cancerous — *see* Neoplasm, malignant, by site
  cardia K22.10
    with bleeding K22.11
  cardioesophageal (peptic) K22.10
    with bleeding K22.11
  cecum — *see* Ulcer, intestine
  cervix (uteri) (decubitus) (trophic) N86
    with cervicitis N72
  chancroidal A57
  chiclero B55.1
  chronic (cause unknown) — *see* Ulcer, skin
  Cochin-China B55.1
  colon — *see* Ulcer, intestine
  conjunctiva H10.89
  cornea H16.00- ☑
    with hypopyon H16.03- ☑
    central H16.01- ☑
    dendritic (herpes simplex) B00.52
    marginal H16.04- ☑
    Mooren's H16.05- ☑
    mycotic H16.06- ☑
    perforated H16.07- ☑
    ring H16.02- ☑
    tuberculous (phlyctenular) A18.52
  corpus cavernosum (chronic) N48.5
  crural — *see* Ulcer, lower limb
  Curling's — *see* Ulcer, peptic, acute
  Cushing's — *see* Ulcer, peptic, acute
  cystic duct K82.8
  cystitis (interstitial) — *see* Cystitis, interstitial
  decubitus — *see* Ulcer, pressure, by site
  dendritic, cornea (herpes simplex) B00.52
  diabetes, diabetic — *see* Diabetes, ulcer
  Dieulafoy's K25.0
  due to
    infection NEC — *see* Ulcer, skin
    radiation NEC L59.8
    trophic disturbance (any region) — *see* Ulcer, skin
    X-ray L58.1
  duodenum, duodenal (eroded) (peptic) K26.9
    with
      hemorrhage K26.4
        and perforation K26.6
      perforation K26.5
    acute K26.3
      with
        hemorrhage K26.0
          and perforation K26.2
        perforation K26.1
    chronic K26.7
      with
        hemorrhage K26.4
          and perforation K26.6
        perforation K26.5
  dysenteric A09
  elusive — *see* Cystitis, interstitial
  endocarditis (acute) (chronic) (subacute) I28.8
  epiglottis J38.7
  esophagus (peptic) K22.10
    with bleeding K22.11
    due to
      aspirin K22.10
        with bleeding K22.11
      gastrointestinal reflux disease K21.0
      ingestion of chemical or medicament K22.10
        with bleeding K22.11
    fungal K22.10
      with bleeding K22.11
    infective K22.10
      with bleeding K22.11
    varicose — *see* Varix, esophagus
  eyelid (region) H01.8

☑ **Additional Character Required** — Refer to the Tabular List for Character Selection   ▽ **Subterms under main terms may continue to next column or page**

Ulcer, ulcerated, ulcerating, ulceration, ulcerative
— *continued*
- fauces J39.2
- Fenwick (-Hunner) (solitary) — *see* Cystitis, interstitial
- fistulous — *see* Ulcer, skin
- foot (indolent) (trophic) — *see* Ulcer, lower limb
- frambesial, initial A66.0
- frenum (tongue) K14.0
- gallbladder or duct K82.8
- gangrenous — *see* Gangrene
- gastric — *see* Ulcer, stomach
- gastrocolic — *see* Ulcer, gastrojejunal
- gastroduodenal — *see* Ulcer, peptic
- gastroesophageal — *see* Ulcer, stomach
- gastrointestinal — *see* Ulcer, gastrojejunal
- gastrojejunal (peptic) K28.9
  - with
    - hemorrhage K28.4
      - and perforation K28.6
    - perforation K28.5
  - acute K28.3
    - with
      - hemorrhage K28.0
        - and perforation K28.2
      - perforation K28.1
  - chronic K28.7
    - with
      - hemorrhage K28.4
        - and perforation K28.6
      - perforation K28.5
- gastrojejunocolic — *see* Ulcer, gastrojejunal
- gingiva K06.8
- gingivitis K05.10
  - nonplaque induced K05.11
  - plaque induced K05.10
- glottis J38.7
- granuloma of pudenda A58
- gum K06.8
- gumma, due to yaws A66.4
- heel — *see* Ulcer, lower limb
- hemorrhoid (*see also* Hemorrhoids, by degree) K64.8
- Hunner's — *see* Cystitis, interstitial
- hypopharynx J39.2
- hypopyon (chronic) (subacute) — *see* Ulcer, cornea, with hypopyon
- hypostaticum — *see* Ulcer, varicose
- ileum — *see* Ulcer, intestine
- intestine, intestinal K63.3
  - with perforation K63.1
  - amebic A06.1
  - duodenal — *see* Ulcer, duodenum
  - granulocytopenic (with hemorrhage) — *see* Neutropenia
  - marginal — *see* Ulcer, gastrojejunal
  - perforating K63.1
    - newborn P78.0
  - primary, small intestine K63.3
  - rectum K62.6
  - stercoraceous, stercoral K63.3
  - tuberculous A18.32
  - typhoid (fever) — *see* Typhoid
  - varicose I86.8
- jejunum, jejunal — *see* Ulcer, gastrojejunal
- keratitis — *see* Ulcer, cornea
- knee — *see* Ulcer, lower limb
- labium (majus) (minus) N76.6
- laryngitis — *see* Laryngitis
- larynx (aphthous) (contact) J38.7
  - diphtheritic A36.2
- leg — *see* Ulcer, lower limb
- lip K13.0
- Lipschütz's N76.6
- lower limb (atrophic) (chronic) (neurogenic) (perforating) (pyogenic) (trophic) (tropical) L97.909
  - with
    - bone involvement without evidence of necrosis L97.906
    - bone necrosis L97.904
    - exposed fat layer L97.902
    - muscle involvement without evidence of necrosis L97.905
    - muscle necrosis L97.903
    - skin breakdown only L97.901
    - specified severity NEC L97.908
  - ankle L97.309
    - with
      - bone involvement without evidence of necrosis L97.306

Ulcer, ulcerated, ulcerating, ulceration, ulcerative
— *continued*
- lower limb — *continued*
  - ankle — *continued*
    - with — *continued*
      - bone necrosis L97.304
      - exposed fat layer L97.302
      - muscle involvement without evidence of necrosis L97.305
      - muscle necrosis L97.303
      - skin breakdown only L97.301
      - specified severity NEC L97.308
    - left L97.329
      - with
        - bone involvement without evidence of necrosis L97.326
        - bone necrosis L97.324
        - exposed fat layer L97.322
        - muscle involvement without evidence of necrosis L97.325
        - muscle necrosis L97.323
        - skin breakdown only L97.321
        - specified severity NEC L97.328
    - right L97.319
      - with
        - bone involvement without evidence of necrosis L97.316
        - bone necrosis L97.314
        - exposed fat layer L97.312
        - muscle involvement without evidence of necrosis L97.315
        - muscle necrosis L97.313
        - skin breakdown only L97.311
        - specified severity NEC L97.318
  - calf L97.209
    - with
      - bone involvement without evidence of necrosis L97.206
      - bone necrosis L97.204
      - exposed fat layer L97.202
      - muscle involvement without evidence of necrosis L97.205
      - muscle necrosis L97.203
      - skin breakdown only L97.201
      - specified severity NEC L97.208
    - left L97.229
      - with
        - bone involvement without evidence of necrosis L97.226
        - bone necrosis L97.224
        - exposed fat layer L97.222
        - muscle involvement without evidence of necrosis L97.225
        - muscle necrosis L97.223
        - skin breakdown only L97.221
        - specified severity NEC L97.228
    - right L97.219
      - with
        - bone involvement without evidence of necrosis L97.216
        - bone necrosis L97.214
        - exposed fat layer L97.212
        - muscle involvement without evidence of necrosis L97.215
        - muscle necrosis L97.213
        - skin breakdown only L97.211
        - specified severity NEC L97.218
  - decubitus — *see* Ulcer, pressure, by site
  - foot specified NEC L97.509
    - with
      - bone involvement without evidence of necrosis L97.506
      - bone necrosis L97.504
      - exposed fat layer L97.502
      - muscle involvement without evidence of necrosis L97.505
      - muscle necrosis L97.503
      - skin breakdown only L97.501
      - specified severity NEC L97.508
    - left L97.529
      - with
        - bone involvement without evidence of necrosis L97.526
        - bone necrosis L97.524
        - exposed fat layer L97.522
        - muscle involvement without evidence of necrosis L97.525
        - muscle necrosis L97.523
        - skin breakdown only L97.521

Ulcer, ulcerated, ulcerating, ulceration, ulcerative
— *continued*
- lower limb — *continued*
  - foot specified — *continued*
    - left — *continued*
      - with — *continued*
        - specified severity NEC L97.528
    - right L97.519
      - with
        - bone involvement without evidence of necrosis L97.516
        - bone necrosis L97.514
        - exposed fat layer L97.512
        - muscle involvement without evidence of necrosis L97.515
        - muscle necrosis L97.513
        - skin breakdown only L97.511
        - specified severity NEC L97.518
  - heel L97.409
    - with
      - bone involvement without evidence of necrosis L97.406
      - bone necrosis L97.404
      - exposed fat layer L97.402
      - muscle involvement without evidence of necrosis L97.405
      - muscle necrosis L97.403
      - skin breakdown only L97.401
      - specified severity NEC L97.408
    - left L97.429
      - with
        - bone involvement without evidence of necrosis L97.426
        - bone necrosis L97.424
        - exposed fat layer L97.422
        - muscle involvement without evidence of necrosis L97.425
        - muscle necrosis L97.423
        - skin breakdown only L97.421
        - specified severity NEC L97.428
    - right L97.419
      - with
        - bone involvement without evidence of necrosis L97.416
        - bone necrosis L97.414
        - exposed fat layer L97.412
        - muscle involvement without evidence of necrosis L97.415
        - muscle necrosis L97.413
        - skin breakdown only L97.411
        - specified severity NEC L97.418
  - left L97.929
    - with
      - bone involvement without evidence of necrosis L97.926
      - bone necrosis L97.924
      - exposed fat layer L97.922
      - muscle involvement without evidence of necrosis L97.925
      - muscle necrosis L97.923
      - skin breakdown only L97.921
      - specified severity NEC L97.928
  - leprous A30.1
  - lower leg NOS L97.909
    - with
      - bone involvement without evidence of necrosis L97.906
      - bone necrosis L97.904
      - exposed fat layer L97.902
      - muscle involvement without evidence of necrosis L97.905
      - muscle necrosis L97.903
      - skin breakdown only L97.901
      - specified severity NEC L97.908
    - left L97.929
      - with
        - bone involvement without evidence of necrosis L97.926
        - bone necrosis L97.924
        - exposed fat layer L97.922
        - muscle involvement without evidence of necrosis L97.925
        - muscle necrosis L97.923
        - skin breakdown only L97.921
        - specified severity NEC L97.928
    - right L97.919
      - with
        - bone involvement without evidence of necrosis L97.916

Ulcer, ulcerated, ulcerating, ulceration, ulcerative	Ulcer, ulcerated, ulcerating, ulceration, ulcerative	Ulcer, ulcerated, ulcerating, ulceration, ulcerative
— continued	— continued	— continued

lower limb — *continued*
  lower leg — *continued*
    right — *continued*
      with — *continued*
        bone necrosis L97.914
        exposed fat layer L97.912
        muscle involvement without evidence
          of necrosis L97.915
        muscle necrosis L97.913
        skin breakdown only L97.911
        specified severity NEC L97.918
  specified site NEC L97.809
    with
      bone involvement without evidence of
        necrosis L97.806
      bone necrosis L97.804
      exposed fat layer L97.802
      muscle involvement without evidence
        of necrosis L97.805
      muscle necrosis L97.803
      skin breakdown only L97.801
      specified severity NEC L97.808
    left L97.829
      with
        bone involvement without evidence
          of necrosis L97.826
        bone necrosis L97.824
        exposed fat layer L97.822
        muscle involvement without evi-
          dence of necrosis L97.825
        muscle necrosis L97.823
        skin breakdown only L97.821
        specified severity NEC L97.828
    right L97.819
      with
        bone involvement without evidence
          of necrosis L97.816
        bone necrosis L97.814
        exposed fat layer L97.812
        muscle involvement without evi-
          dence of necrosis L97.815
        muscle necrosis L97.813
        skin breakdown only L97.811
        specified severity NEC L97.818
  midfoot L97.409
    with
      bone involvement without evidence of
        necrosis L97.406
      bone necrosis L97.404
      exposed fat layer L97.402
      muscle involvement without evidence of
        necrosis L97.405
      muscle necrosis L97.403
      skin breakdown only L97.401
      specified severity NEC L97.408
    left L97.429
      with
        bone involvement without evidence of
          necrosis L97.426
        bone necrosis L97.424
        exposed fat layer L97.422
        muscle involvement without evidence of
          necrosis L97.425
        muscle necrosis L97.423
        skin breakdown only L97.421
        specified severity NEC L97.428
    right L97.419
      with
        bone involvement without evidence of
          necrosis L97.416
        bone necrosis L97.414
        exposed fat layer L97.412
        muscle involvement without evidence
          of necrosis L97.415
        muscle necrosis L97.413
        skin breakdown only L97.411
        specified severity NEC L97.418
  right L97.919
    with
      bone involvement without evidence of
        necrosis L97.916
      bone necrosis L97.914
      exposed fat layer L97.912
      muscle involvement without evidence of
        necrosis L97.915
      muscle necrosis L97.913
      skin breakdown only L97.911

lower limb — *continued*
  right — *continued*
    with — *continued*
      specified severity NEC L97.918
  syphilitic A52.19
  thigh L97.109
    with
      bone involvement without evidence of
        necrosis L97.106
      bone necrosis L97.104
      exposed fat layer L97.102
      muscle involvement without evidence of
        necrosis L97.105
      muscle necrosis L97.103
      skin breakdown only L97.101
      specified severity NEC L97.108
    left L97.129
      with
        bone involvement without evidence of
          necrosis L97.126
        bone necrosis L97.124
        exposed fat layer L97.122
        muscle involvement without evidence
          of necrosis L97.125
        muscle necrosis L97.123
        skin breakdown only L97.121
        specified severity NEC L97.128
    right L97.119
      with
        bone involvement without evidence of
          necrosis L97.116
        bone necrosis L97.114
        exposed fat layer L97.112
        muscle involvement without evidence
          of necrosis L97.115
        muscle necrosis L97.113
        skin breakdown only L97.111
        specified severity NEC L97.118
  toe L97.509
    with
      bone involvement without evidence of
        necrosis L97.506
      bone necrosis L97.504
      exposed fat layer L97.502
      muscle involvement without evidence of
        necrosis L97.505
      muscle necrosis L97.503
      skin breakdown only L97.501
      specified severity NEC L97.508
    left L97.529
      with
        bone involvement without evidence of
          necrosis L97.526
        bone necrosis L97.524
        exposed fat layer L97.522
        muscle involvement without evidence
          of necrosis L97.525
        muscle necrosis L97.523
        skin breakdown only L97.521
        specified severity NEC L97.528
    right L97.519
      with
        bone involvement without evidence of
          necrosis L97.516
        bone necrosis L97.514
        exposed fat layer L97.512
        muscle involvement without evidence
          of necrosis L97.515
        muscle necrosis L97.513
        skin breakdown only L97.511
        specified severity NEC L97.518
  varicose — *see* Varix, leg, with, ulcer
luetic — *see* Ulcer, syphilitic
lung J98.4
  tuberculous — *see* Tuberculosis, pulmonary
malignant — *see* Neoplasm, malignant, by site
marginal NEC — *see* Ulcer, gastrojejunal
meatus (urinarius) N34.2
Meckel's diverticulum Q43.0
  malignant — *see* Table of Neoplasms, small intes-
    tine, malignant
Meleney's (chronic undermining) — *see* Ulcer, skin
Mooren's (cornea) — *see* Ulcer, cornea, Mooren's
mycobacterial (skin) A31.1
nasopharynx J39.2
neck, uterus N86

neurogenic NEC — *see* Ulcer, skin
nose, nasal (passage) (infective) (septum) J34.0
  skin — *see* Ulcer, skin
  spirochetal A69.8
  varicose (bleeding) I86.8
oral mucosa (traumatic) K12.1
palate (soft) K12.1
penis (chronic) N48.5
peptic (site unspecified) K27.9
  with
    hemorrhage K27.4
      and perforation K27.6
    perforation K27.5
  acute K27.3
    with
      hemorrhage K27.0
        and perforation K27.2
      perforation K27.1
  chronic K27.7
    with
      hemorrhage K27.4
        and perforation K27.6
      perforation K27.5
  esophagus K22.10
    with bleeding K22.11
  newborn P78.82
perforating K27.5
  skin — *see* Ulcer, skin
peritonsillar J35.8
phagedenic (tropical) — *see* Ulcer, skin
pharynx J39.2
phlebitis — *see* Phlebitis
plaster — *see* Ulcer, pressure, by site
popliteal space — *see* Ulcer, lower limb
postpyloric — *see* Ulcer, duodenum
prepuce N47.7
prepyloric — *see* Ulcer, stomach
pressure (pressure area) L89.9- ☑
  ankle L89.5- ☑
  back L89.1- ☑
  buttock L89.3- ☑
  coccyx L89.15- ☑
  contiguous site of back, buttock, hip L89.4- ☑
  elbow L89.0- ☑
  face L89.81- ☑
  head L89.81- ☑
  heel L89.6- ☑
  hip L89.2- ☑
  sacral region (tailbone) L89.15- ☑
  specified site NEC L89.89- ☑
  stage 1 (healing) (pre-ulcer skin changes limited
      to persistent focal edema)
    ankle L89.5- ☑
    back L89.1- ☑
    buttock L89.3- ☑
    coccyx L89.15- ☑
    contiguous site of back, buttock, hip L89.4- ☑
    elbow L89.0- ☑
    face L89.81- ☑
    head L89.81- ☑
    heel L89.6- ☑
    hip L89.2- ☑
    sacral region (tailbone) L89.15- ☑
    specified site NEC L89.89- ☑
  stage 2 (healing) (abrasion, blister, partial thickness
      skin loss involving epidermis and/or dermis)
    ankle L89.5- ☑
    back L89.1- ☑
    buttock L89.3- ☑
    coccyx L89.15- ☑
    contiguous site of back, buttock, hip L89.4- ☑
    elbow L89.0- ☑
    face L89.81- ☑
    head L89.81- ☑
    heel L89.6- ☑
    hip L89.2- ☑
    sacral region (tailbone) L89.15- ☑
    specified site NEC L89.89- ☑
  stage 3 (healing) (full thickness skin loss involving
      damage or necrosis of subcutaneous tissue)
    ankle L89.5- ☑
    back L89.1- ☑
    buttock L89.3- ☑
    coccyx L89.15- ☑
    contiguous site of back, buttock, hip L89.4- ☑

Ulcer, ulcerated, ulcerating, ulceration, ulcerative
— *continued*
pressure — *continued*
 stage 3 — *continued*
  elbow L89.0- ☑
  face L89.81- ☑
  head L89.81- ☑
  heel L89.6- ☑
  hip L89.2- ☑
  sacral region (tailbone) L89.15- ☑
  specified site NEC L89.89- ☑
 stage 4 (healing) (necrosis of soft tissues through
   to underlying muscle, tendon, or bone)
  ankle L89.5- ☑
  back L89.1- ☑
  buttock L89.3- ☑
  coccyx L89.15- ☑
  contiguous site of back, buttock, hip L89.4- ☑
  elbow L89.0- ☑
  face L89.81- ☑
  head L89.81- ☑
  heel L89.6- ☑
  hip L89.2- ☑
  sacral region (tailbone) L89.15- ☑
  specified site NEC L89.89- ☑
 unspecified stage
  ankle L89.5- ☑
  back L89.1- ☑
  buttock L89.3- ☑
  coccyx L89.15- ☑
  contiguous site of back, buttock, hip L89.4- ☑
  elbow L89.0- ☑
  face L89.81- ☑
  head L89.81- ☑
  heel L89.6- ☑
  hip L89.2- ☑
  sacral region (tailbone) L89.15- ☑
  specified site NEC L89.89- ☑
 unstageable
  ankle L89.5- ☑
  back L89.1- ☑
  buttock L89.3- ☑
  coccyx L89.15- ☑
  contiguous site of back, buttock, hip L89.4- ☑
  elbow L89.0- ☑
  face L89.81- ☑
  head L89.81- ☑
  heel L89.6- ☑
  hip L89.2- ☑
  sacral region (tailbone) L89.15- ☑
  specified site NEC L89.89- ☑
primary of intestine K63.3
 with perforation K63.1
prostate N41.9
pyloric — *see* Ulcer, stomach
rectosigmoid K63.3
 with perforation K63.1
rectum (sphincter) (solitary) K62.6
 stercoraceous, stercoral K62.6
retina — *see* Inflammation, chorioretinal
rodent (*see also* Neoplasm, skin, malignant)
sclera — *see* Scleritis
scrofulous (tuberculous) A18.2
scrotum N50.89
 tuberculous A18.15
 varicose I86.1
seminal vesicle N50.89
sigmoid — *see* Ulcer, intestine
skin (atrophic) (chronic) (neurogenic) (non-healing)
  (perforating) (pyogenic) (trophic) (tropical)
  L98.499
 with gangrene — *see* Gangrene
 amebic A06.7
 back — *see* Ulcer, back
 buttock — *see* Ulcer, buttock
 decubitus — *see* Ulcer, pressure
 lower limb — *see* Ulcer, lower limb
 mycobacterial A31.1
 specified site NEC L98.499
  with
   bone involvement without evidence of
    necrosis L98.496
   bone necrosis L98.494
   exposed fat layer L98.492
   muscle involvement without evidence of
    necrosis L98.495
   muscle necrosis L98.493

Ulcer, ulcerated, ulcerating, ulceration, ulcerative
skin — *continued*
 specified site — *continued*
  with — *continued*
   skin breakdown only L98.491
   specified severity NEC L98.498
 tuberculous (primary) A18.4
 varicose — *see* Ulcer, varicose
sloughing — *see* Ulcer, skin
solitary, anus or rectum (sphincter) K62.6
sore throat J02.9
 streptococcal J02.0
spermatic cord N50.89
spine (tuberculous) A18.01
stasis (venous) — *see* Varix, leg, with, ulcer
 without varicose veins I87.2
stercoraceous, stercoral K63.3
 with perforation K63.1
 anus or rectum K62.6
stoma, stomal — *see* Ulcer, gastrojejunal
stomach (eroded) (peptic) (round) K25.9
 with
  hemorrhage K25.4
   and perforation K25.6
  perforation K25.5
 acute K25.3
  with
   hemorrhage K25.0
    and perforation K25.2
   perforation K25.1
 chronic K25.7
  with
   hemorrhage K25.4
    and perforation K25.6
   perforation K25.5
stomal — *see* Ulcer, gastrojejunal
stomatitis K12.1
stress — *see* Ulcer, peptic
strumous (tuberculous) A18.2
submucosal, bladder — *see* Cystitis, interstitial
syphilitic (any site) (early) (secondary) A51.39
 late A52.79
 perforating A52.79
  foot A52.11
testis N50.89
thigh — *see* Ulcer, lower limb
throat J39.2
 diphtheritic A36.0
toe — *see* Ulcer, lower limb
tongue (traumatic) K14.0
tonsil J35.8
 diphtheritic A36.0
trachea J39.8
trophic — *see* Ulcer, skin
tropical — *see* Ulcer, skin
tuberculous — *see* Tuberculosis, ulcer
tunica vaginalis N50.89
turbinate J34.89
typhoid (perforating) — *see* Typhoid
unspecified site — *see* Ulcer, skin
urethra (meatus) — *see* Urethritis
uterus N85.8
 cervix N86
  with cervicitis N72
 neck N86
  with cervicitis N72
vagina N76.5
 in Behçet's disease M35.2 [N77.0]
 pessary N89.8
valve, heart I33.0
varicose (lower limb, any part) (*see also* Varix, leg, with,
  ulcer)
 broad ligament I86.2
 esophagus — *see* Varix, esophagus
 inflamed or infected — *see* Varix, leg, with ulcer,
   with inflammation
 nasal septum I86.8
 perineum I86.3
 scrotum I86.1
 specified site NEC I86.8
 sublingual I86.0
 vulva I86.3
vas deferens N50.89
vulva (acute) (infectional) N76.6
 in (due to)
  Behçet's disease M35.2 [N77.0]
  herpesviral (herpes simplex) infection A60.04

Ulcer, ulcerated, ulcerating, ulceration, ulcerative
— *continued*
vulva — *continued*
 in — *continued*
  tuberculosis A18.18
vulvobuccal, recurring N76.6
X-ray L58.1
yaws A66.4
Ulcerosa scarlatina A38.8
Ulcus (*see also* Ulcer)
 cutis tuberculosum A18.4
 duodeni — *see* Ulcer, duodenum
 durum (syphilitic) A51.0
  extragenital A51.2
 gastrojejunale — *see* Ulcer, gastrojejunal
 hypostaticum — *see* Ulcer, varicose
 molle (cutis) (skin) A57
 serpens corneae — *see* Ulcer, cornea, central
 ventriculi — *see* Ulcer, stomach
Ulegyria Q04.8
Ulerythema
 ophryogenes, congenital Q84.2
 sycosiforme L73.8
Ullrich (-Bonnevie)(-Turner) **syndrome** (*see also* Turner's
  syndrome) Q87.1
Ullrich-Feichtiger syndrome Q87.0
Ulnar — *see* condition
Ulorrhagia, ulorrhea K06.8
Umbilicus, umbilical — *see* condition
Unacceptable
 contours of tooth K08.54
 morphology of tooth K08.54
Unavailability (of)
 bed at medical facility Z75.1
 health service-related agencies Z75.4
 medical facilities (at) Z75.3
  due to
   investigation by social service agency Z75.2
   lack of services at home Z75.0
   remoteness from facility Z75.3
   waiting list Z75.1
  home Z75.0
  outpatient clinic Z75.3
 schooling Z55.1
 social service agencies Z75.4
Uncinaria americana infestation B76.1
Uncinariasis B76.9
Uncongenial work Z56.5
Unconscious (ness) — *see* Coma
Under observation — *see* Observation
Underachievement in school Z55.3
Underdevelopment (*see also* Undeveloped)
 nose Q30.1
 sexual E30.0
Underdosing (*see also* Table of Drugs and Chemicals,
  categories T36-T50, with final character 6) Z91.14
 intentional NEC Z91.128
  due to financial hardship of patient Z91.120
 unintentional NEC Z91.138
  due to patient's age related debility Z91.130
Underfeeding, newborn P92.3
Underfill, endodontic M27.53
Underimmunization status Z28.3
Undernourishment — *see* Malnutrition
Undernutrition — *see* Malnutrition
Underweight R63.6
 for gestational age — *see* Light for dates
Underwood's disease P83.0
Undescended (*see also* Malposition, congenital)
 cecum Q43.3
 colon Q43.3
 testicle — *see* Cryptorchid
Undeveloped, undevelopment (*see also* Hypoplasia)
 brain (congenital) Q02
 cerebral (congenital) Q02
 heart Q24.8
 lung Q33.6
 testis E29.1
 uterus E30.0
Undiagnosed (disease) R69
Undulant fever — *see* Brucellosis
Unemployment, anxiety concerning Z56.0
 threatened Z56.2
Unequal length (acquired) (limb) (*see also* Deformity,
  limb, unequal length)
 leg (*see also* Deformity, limb, unequal length)
  congenital Q72.9- ☑

Index

Unextracted dental root K08.3
Unguis incarnatus L60.0
Unhappiness R45.2
Unicornate uterus Q51.4
  in pregnancy or childbirth O34.00
Unilateral (*see also* condition)
  development, breast N64.89
  organ or site, congenital NEC — *see* Agenesis, by site
Unilocular heart Q20.8
Union, abnormal (*see also* Fusion)
  larynx and trachea Q34.8
Universal mesentery Q43.3
Unrepairable overhanging of dental restorative
    materials K08.52
Unsatisfactory
  restoration of tooth K08.50
    specified NEC K08.59
  sample of cytologic smear
    anus R85.615
    cervix R87.615
    vagina R87.625
  surroundings Z59.1
    work Z56.5
Unsoundness of mind — *see* Psychosis
Unstable
  back NEC — *see* Instability, joint, spine
  hip (congenital) Q65.6
    acquired — *see* Derangement, joint, specified type
      NEC, hip
  joint — *see* Instability, joint
    secondary to removal of joint prosthesis M96.89
  lie (mother) O32.0 ☑
  lumbosacral joint (congenital)
    acquired — *see* subcategory M53.2 ☑
  sacroiliac — *see* subcategory M53.2 ☑
  spine NEC — *see* Instability, joint, spine
Unsteadiness on feet R26.81
Untruthfulness, child problem F91.8
Unverricht (-Lundborg) **disease or epilepsy** — *see*
    Epilepsy, generalized, idiopathic
Unwanted pregnancy Z64.0
Upbringing, institutional Z62.22
  away from parents NEC Z62.29
  in care of non-parental family member Z62.21
  in foster care Z62.21
  in orphanage or group home Z62.22
  in welfare custody Z62.21
Upper respiratory — *see* condition
Upset
  gastric K30
  gastrointestinal K30
    psychogenic F45.8
  intestinal (large) (small) K59.9
    psychogenic F45.8
  menstruation N93.9
  mental F48.9
  stomach K30
    psychogenic F45.8
Urachus (*see also* condition)
  patent or persistent Q64.4
Urbach-Oppenheim disease (necrobiosis lipoidica dia-
    beticorum) — *see* E08-E13 with .620
Urbach's lipoid proteinosis E78.89
Urbach-Wiethe disease E78.89
Urban yellow fever A95.1
Urea
  blood, high — *see* Uremia
  cycle metabolism disorder — *see* Disorder, urea cycle
    metabolism
Uremia, uremic N19
  with
    ectopic or molar pregnancy O08.4
    polyneuropathy N18.9 [G63]
  chronic NOS (*see also* Disease, kidney, chronic) N18.9
    due to hypertension — *see* Hypertensive, kidney
  complicating
    ectopic or molar pregnancy O08.4
  congenital P96.0
  extrarenal R39.2
  following ectopic or molar pregnancy O08.4
  newborn P96.0
  prerenal R39.2
Ureter, ureteral — *see* condition
Ureteralgia N23
Ureterectasis — *see* Hydroureter
Ureteritis N28.89
  cystica N28.86

Ureteritis — *continued*
  due to calculus N20.1
    with calculus, kidney N20.2
      with hydronephrosis N13.2
  gonococcal (acute) (chronic) A54.21
  nonspecific N28.89
Ureterocele N28.89
  congenital (orthotopic) Q62.31
  ectopic Q62.32
Ureterolith, ureterolithiasis — *see* Calculus, ureter
Ureterostomy
  attention to Z43.6
  status Z93.6
Urethra, urethral — *see* condition
Urethralgia R39.89
Urethritis (anterior) (posterior) N34.2
  calculous N21.1
  candidal B37.41
  chlamydial A56.01
  diplococcal (gonococcal) A54.01
    with abscess (accessory gland) (periurethral) A54.1
  gonococcal A54.01
    with abscess (accessory gland) (periurethral) A54.1
  nongonococcal N34.1
    Reiter's — *see* Reiter's disease
  nonspecific N34.1
  nonvenereal N34.1
  postmenopausal N34.2
  puerperal O86.22
  Reiter's — *see* Reiter's disease
  specified NEC N34.2
  trichomonal or due to Trichomonas (vaginalis) A59.03
Urethrocele N81.0
  with
    cystocele — *see* Cystocele
    prolapse of uterus — *see* Prolapse, uterus
Urethrolithiasis (with colic or infection) N21.1
Urethrorectal — *see* condition
Urethrorrhagia N36.8
Urethrorrhea R36.9
Urethrostomy
  attention to Z43.6
  status Z93.6
Urethrotrigonitis — *see* Trigonitis
Urethrovaginal — *see* condition
Urgency
  fecal R15.2
  hypertensive — *see* Hypertension
  urinary R39.15
Urhidrosis, uridrosis L74.8
Uric acid in blood (increased) E79.0
Uricacidemia (asymptomatic) E79.0
Uricemia (asymptomatic) E79.0
Uricosuria R82.99
Urinary — *see* condition
Urination
  frequent R35.0
  painful R30.9
Urine
  blood in — *see* Hematuria
  discharge, excessive R35.8
  enuresis, nonorganic origin F98.0
  extravasation R39.0
  frequency R35.0
  incontinence R32
    nonorganic origin F98.0
  intermittent stream R39.198
  pus in N39.0
  retention or stasis R33.9
    organic R33.8
      drug-induced R33.0
    psychogenic F45.8
  secretion
    deficient R34
    excessive R35.8
    frequency R35.0
  stream
    intermittent R39.198
    slowing R39.198
    splitting R39.13
    weak R39.12
Urinemia — *see* Uremia
Urinoma, urethra N36.8
Uroarthritis, infectious (Reiter's) — *see* Reiter's disease
Urodialysis R34
Urolithiasis — *see* Calculus, urinary
Uronephrosis — *see* Hydronephrosis
Uropathy N39.9

Uropathy — *continued*
  obstructive N13.9
    specified NEC N13.8
  reflux N13.9
    specified NEC N13.8
  vesicoureteral reflux-associated — *see* Reflux, vesi-
    coureteral
Urosepsis — *code to* condition
Urticaria L50.9
  with angioneurotic edema T78.3 ☑
    hereditary D84.1
  allergic L50.0
  cholinergic L50.5
  chronic L50.8
  cold, familial L50.2
  contact L50.6
  dermatographic L50.3
  due to
    cold or heat L50.2
    drugs L50.0
    food L50.0
    inhalants L50.0
    plants L50.6
    serum (*see also* Reaction, serum) T80.69 ☑
  factitial L50.3
  familial cold M04.2
  giant T78.3 ☑
    hereditary D84.1
  gigantea T78.3 ☑
  idiopathic L50.1
  larynx T78.3 ☑
    hereditary D84.1
  neonatorum P83.88
  nonallergic L50.1
  papulosa (Hebra) L28.2
  pigmentosa D47.01
    congenital Q82.2
    of neonatal onset Q82.2
    of newborn onset Q82.2
  recurrent periodic L50.8
  serum (*see also* Reaction, serum) T80.69 ☑
  solar L56.3
  specified type NEC L50.8
  thermal (cold) (heat) L50.2
  vibratory L50.4
  xanthelasmoidea — *see* Urticaria pigmentosa
Use (of)
  alcohol Z72.89
    with
      intoxication F10.929
      sleep disorder F10.982
    harmful — *see* Abuse, alcohol
  amphetamines — *see* Use, stimulant NEC
  caffeine — *see* Use, stimulant NEC
  cannabis F12.90
    with
      anxiety disorder F12.980
      intoxication F12.929
        with
          delirium F12.921
          perceptual disturbance F12.922
        uncomplicated F12.920
      other specified disorder F12.988
      psychosis F12.959
        delusions F12.950
        hallucinations F12.951
      unspecified disorder F12.99
  cocaine F14.90
    with
      anxiety disorder F14.980
      intoxication F14.929
        with
          delirium F14.921
          perceptual disturbance F14.922
        uncomplicated F14.920
      other specified disorder F14.988
      psychosis F14.959
        delusions F14.950
        hallucinations F14.951
      sexual dysfunction F14.981
      sleep disorder F14.982
      unspecified disorder F14.99
    harmful — *see* Abuse, drug, cocaine
  drug(s) NEC F19.90
    with sleep disorder F19.982
    harmful — *see* Abuse, drug, by type
  hallucinogen NEC F16.90

Unextracted dental root — Use

☑ **Additional Character Required** — **Refer to the Tabular List for Character Selection**   🖝 **Subterms under main terms may continue to next column or page**

Use — *continued*
 hallucinogen — *continued*
  with
   anxiety disorder F16.980
   intoxication F16.929
    with
     delirium F16.921
    uncomplicated F16.920
   mood disorder F16.94
   other specified disorder F16.988
   perception disorder (flashbacks) F16.983
   psychosis F16.959
    delusions F16.950
    hallucinations F16.951
   unspecified disorder F16.99
  harmful — *see* Abuse, drug, hallucinogen NEC
 inhalants F18.90
  with
   anxiety disorder F18.980
   intoxication F18.929
    with delirium F18.921
    uncomplicated F18.920
   mood disorder F18.94
   other specified disorder F18.988
   persisting dementia F18.97
   psychosis F18.959
    delusions F18.950
    hallucinations F18.951
   unspecified disorder F18.99
  harmful — *see* Abuse, drug, inhalant
 methadone — *see* Use, opioid
 nonprescribed drugs F19.90
  harmful — *see* Abuse, non-psychoactive substance
 opioid F11.90
  with
   disorder F11.99
    mood F11.94
    sleep F11.982
    specified type NEC F11.988
   intoxication F11.929
    with
     delirium F11.921
     perceptual disturbance F11.922
    uncomplicated F11.920
   withdrawal F11.93
  harmful — *see* Abuse, drug, opioid
 patent medicines F19.90
  harmful — *see* Abuse, non-psychoactive substance
 psychoactive drug NEC F19.90
  with
   anxiety disorder F19.980
   intoxication F19.929
    with
     delirium F19.921
     perceptual disturbance F19.922
    uncomplicated F19.920
   mood disorder F19.94
   other specified disorder F19.988
   persisting
    amnestic disorder F19.96
    dementia F19.97
   psychosis F19.959
    delusions F19.950
    hallucinations F19.951
   sexual dysfunction F19.981
   sleep disorder F19.982
   unspecified disorder F19.99
   withdrawal F19.939
    with
     delirium F19.931
     perceptual disturbance F19.932
    uncomplicated F19.930
  harmful — *see* Abuse, drug NEC, psychoactive NEC
 sedative, hypnotic, or anxiolytic F13.90
  with
   anxiety disorder F13.980
   intoxication F13.929
    with
     delirium F13.921
    uncomplicated F13.920
   other specified disorder F13.988
   persisting
    amnestic disorder F13.96
    dementia F13.97
   psychosis F13.959
    delusions F13.950
    hallucinations F13.951
   sexual dysfunction F13.981

Use — *continued*
 sedative, hypnotic, or anxiolytic — *continued*
  with — *continued*
   sleep disorder F13.982
   unspecified disorder F13.99
  harmful — *see* Abuse, drug, sedative, hypnotic, or anxiolytic
 stimulant NEC F15.90
  with
   anxiety disorder F15.980
   intoxication F15.929
    with
     delirium F15.921
     perceptual disturbance F15.922
    uncomplicated F15.920
   mood disorder F15.94
   other specified disorder F15.988
   psychosis F15.959
    delusions F15.950
    hallucinations F15.951
   sexual dysfunction F15.981
   sleep disorder F15.982
   unspecified disorder F15.99
   withdrawal F15.93
  harmful — *see* Abuse, drug, stimulant NEC
 tobacco Z72.0
  with dependence — *see* Dependence, drug, nicotine
 volatile solvents (*see also* Use, inhalant) F18.90
  harmful — *see* Abuse, drug, inhalant
Usher-Senear disease or syndrome L10.4
Uta B55.1
Uteromegaly N85.2
Uterovaginal — *see* condition
Uterovesical — *see* condition
Uveal — *see* condition
Uveitis (anterior) (*see also* Iridocyclitis)
 acute — *see* Iridocyclitis, acute
 chronic — *see* Iridocyclitis, chronic
 due to toxoplasmosis (acquired) B58.09
  congenital P37.1
 granulomatous — *see* Iridocyclitis, chronic
 heterochromic — *see* Cyclitis, Fuchs' heterochromic
 lens-induced — *see* Iridocyclitis, lens-induced
 posterior — *see* Chorioretinitis
 sympathetic H44.13- ☑
 syphilitic (secondary) A51.43
  congenital (early) A50.01
  late A52.71
 tuberculous A18.54
Uveoencephalitis — *see* Inflammation, chorioretinal
Uveokeratitis — *see* Iridocyclitis
Uveoparotitis D86.89
Uvula — *see* condition
Uvulitis (acute) (catarrhal) (chronic) (membranous) (suppurative) (ulcerative) K12.2

V

Vaccination (prophylactic)
 complication or reaction — *see* Complications, vaccination
 delayed Z28.9
 encounter for Z23
 not done — *see* Immunization, not done, because of)
Vaccinia (generalized) (localized) T88.1 ☑
 without vaccination B08.011
 congenital P35.8
Vacuum, in sinus (accessory) (nasal) J34.89
Vagabond, vagabondage Z59.0
Vagabond's disease B85.1
Vagina, vaginal — *see* condition
Vaginalitis (tunica) (testis) N49.1
Vaginismus (reflex) N94.2
 functional F52.5
 nonorganic F52.5
 psychogenic F52.5
 secondary N94.2
Vaginitis (acute) (circumscribed) (diffuse) (emphysematous) (nonvenereal) (ulcerative) N76.0
 with ectopic or molar pregnancy O08.0
 amebic A06.82
 atrophic, postmenopausal N95.2
 bacterial N76.0
 blennorrhagic (gonococcal) A54.02
 candidal B37.3
 chlamydial A56.02

Vaginitis — *continued*
 chronic N76.1
 due to Trichomonas (vaginalis) A59.01
 following ectopic or molar pregnancy O08.0
 gonococcal A54.02
  with abscess (accessory gland) (periurethral) A54.1
 granuloma A58
 in (due to)
  candidiasis B37.3
  herpesviral (herpes simplex) infection A60.04
  pinworm infection B80 [N77.1]
 monilial B37.3
 mycotic (candidal) B37.3
 postmenopausal atrophic N95.2
 puerperal (postpartum) O86.13
 senile (atrophic) N95.2
 subacute or chronic N76.1
 syphilitic (early) A51.0
  late A52.76
 trichomonal A59.01
 tuberculous A18.18
Vaginosis — *see* Vaginitis
Vagotonia G52.2
Vagrancy Z59.0
VAIN — *see* Neoplasia, intraepithelial, vagina
Vallecula — *see* condition
Valley fever B38.0
Valsuani's disease — *see* Anemia, obstetric
Valve, valvular (formation) (*see also* condition)
 cerebral ventricle (communicating) in situ Z98.2
 cervix, internal os Q51.828
 congenital NEC — *see* Atresia, by site
 ureter (pelvic junction) (vesical orifice) Q62.39
 urethra (congenital) (posterior) Q64.2
Valvulitis (chronic) — *see* Endocarditis
Valvulopathy — *see* Endocarditis
Van Bogaert's leukoencephalopathy (sclerosing) (subacute) A81.1
Van Bogaert-Scherer-Epstein disease or syndrome E75.5
Van Buchem's syndrome M85.2
Van Creveld-von Gierke disease E74.01
Van der Hoeve (-de Kleyn) **syndrome** Q78.0
Van der Woude's syndrome Q38.0
Van Neck's disease or osteochondrosis M91.0
Vanishing lung J44.9
Vapor asphyxia or suffocation T59.9 ☑
 specified agent — *see* Table of Drugs and Chemicals
Variance, lethal ball, prosthetic heart valve T82.09 ☑
Variants, thalassemic D56.8
Variations in hair color L67.1
Varicella B01.9
 with
  complications NEC B01.89
  encephalitis B01.11
  encephalomyelitis B01.11
  meningitis B01.0
  myelitis B01.12
  pneumonia B01.2
 congenital P35.8
Varices — *see* Varix
Varicocele (scrotum) (thrombosed) I86.1
 ovary I86.2
 perineum I86.3
 spermatic cord (ulcerated) I86.1
Varicose
 aneurysm (ruptured) I77.0
 dermatitis — *see* Varix, leg, with, inflammation
 eczema — *see* Varix, leg, with, inflammation
 phlebitis — *see* Varix, with, inflammation
 tumor — *see* Varix
 ulcer (lower limb, any part) (*see also* Varix, leg, with, ulcer)
  anus (*see also* Hemorrhoids) K64.8
  esophagus — *see* Varix, esophagus
  inflamed or infected — *see* Varix, leg, with ulcer, with inflammation
  nasal septum I86.8
  perineum I86.3
  scrotum I86.1
  specified site NEC I86.8
 vein — *see* Varix
 vessel — *see* Varix, leg
Varicosis, varicosities, varicosity — *see* Varix
Variola (major) (minor) B03
Varioloid B03
Varix (lower limb) (ruptured) I83.90

Use — Varix

Varix — continued
with
  edema I83.899
  inflammation I83.10
    with ulcer (venous) I83.209
  pain I83.819
  specified complication NEC I83.899
  stasis dermatitis I83.10
    with ulcer (venous) I83.209
  swelling I83.899
  ulcer I83.009
    with inflammation I83.209
aneurysmal I77.0
asymptomatic I83.9- ☑
bladder I86.2
broad ligament I86.2
complicating
  childbirth (lower extremity) O87.4
    anus or rectum O87.2
    genital (vagina, vulva or perineum) O87.8
  pregnancy (lower extremity) O22.0- ☑
    anus or rectum O22.4- ☑
    genital (vagina, vulva or perineum) O22.1- ☑
  puerperium (lower extremity) O87.4
    anus or rectum O87.2
    genital (vagina, vulva, perineum) O87.8
congenital (any site) Q27.8
esophagus (idiopathic) (primary) (ulcerated) I85.00
  bleeding I85.01
  congenital Q27.8
  in (due to)
    alcoholic liver disease I85.10
      bleeding I85.11
    cirrhosis of liver I85.10
      bleeding I85.11
    portal hypertension I85.10
      bleeding I85.11
    schistosomiasis I85.10
      bleeding I85.11
    toxic liver disease I85.10
      bleeding I85.11
  secondary I85.10
    bleeding I85.11
gastric I86.4
inflamed or infected I83.10
  ulcerated I83.209
labia (majora) I86.3
leg (asymptomatic) I83.90
  with
    edema I83.899
    inflammation I83.10
      with ulcer — see Varix, leg, with, ulcer, with inflammation by site
    pain I83.819
    specified complication NEC I83.899
    swelling I83.899
    ulcer I83.009
      with inflammation I83.209
      ankle I83.003
        with inflammation I83.203
      calf I83.002
        with inflammation I83.202
      foot NEC I83.005
        with inflammation I83.205
      heel I83.004
        with inflammation I83.204
      lower leg NEC I83.008
        with inflammation I83.208
      midfoot I83.004
        with inflammation I83.204
      thigh I83.001
        with inflammation I83.201
  bilateral (asymptomatic) I83.93
    with
      edema I83.893
      pain I83.813
      specified complication NEC I83.893
      swelling I83.893
      ulcer I83.0- ☑
        with inflammation I83.209
  left (asymptomatic) I83.92
    with
      edema I83.892
      inflammation I83.12
        with ulcer — see Varix, leg, with, ulcer, with inflammation by site
      pain I83.812
      specified complication NEC I83.892

Varix — continued
leg — continued
  left — continued
    with — continued
      swelling I83.892
      ulcer I83.029
        with inflammation I83.229
        ankle I83.023
          with inflammation I83.223
        calf I83.022
          with inflammation I83.222
        foot NEC I83.025
          with inflammation I83.225
        heel I83.024
          with inflammation I83.224
        lower leg NEC I83.028
          with inflammation I83.228
        midfoot I83.024
          with inflammation I83.224
        thigh I83.021
          with inflammation I83.221
  right (asymptomatic) I83.91
    with
      edema I83.891
      inflammation I83.11
        with ulcer — see Varix, leg, with, ulcer, with inflammation by site
      pain I83.811
      specified complication NEC I83.891
      swelling I83.891
      ulcer I83.019
        with inflammation I83.219
        ankle I83.013
          with inflammation I83.213
        calf I83.012
          with inflammation I83.212
        foot NEC I83.015
          with inflammation I83.215
        heel I83.014
          with inflammation I83.214
        lower leg NEC I83.018
          with inflammation I83.218
        midfoot I83.014
          with inflammation I83.214
        thigh I83.011
          with inflammation I83.211
nasal septum I86.8
orbit I86.8
  congenital Q27.8
ovary I86.2
papillary I78.1
pelvis I86.2
perineum I86.3
pharynx I86.8
placenta O43.89- ☑
renal papilla I86.8
retina H35.09
scrotum (ulcerated) I86.1
sigmoid colon I86.8
specified site NEC I86.8
spinal (cord) (vessels) I86.8
spleen, splenic (vein) (with phlebolith) I86.8
stomach I86.4
sublingual I86.0
ulcerated I83.009
  inflamed or infected I83.209
uterine ligament I86.2
vagina I86.8
vocal cord I86.8
vulva I86.3
Vas deferens — see condition
Vas deferentitis N49.1
Vasa previa O69.4 ☑
  hemorrhage from, affecting newborn P50.0
Vascular (see also condition)
  loop on optic papilla Q14.2
  spasm I73.9
  spider I78.1
Vascularization, cornea — see Neovascularization, cornea
Vasculitis I77.6
  allergic D69.0
  cryoglobulinemic D89.1
  disseminated I77.6
  hypocomplementemic M31.8
  kidney I77.89
  livedoid L95.0
  nodular L95.8

Vasculitis — continued
  retina H35.06- ☑
  rheumatic — see Fever, rheumatic
  rheumatoid — see Rheumatoid, vasculitis
  skin (limited to) L95.9
    specified NEC L95.8
  systemic M31.8
Vasculopathy, necrotizing M31.9
  cardiac allograft T86.290
  specified NEC M31.8
Vasitis (nodosa) N49.1
  tuberculous A18.15
Vasodilation I73.9
Vasomotor — see condition
Vasoplasty, after previous sterilization Z31.0
  aftercare Z31.42
Vasospasm (vasoconstriction) I73.9
  cerebral (cerebrovascular) (artery) I67.848
    reversible I67.841
  coronary I20.1
  nerve
    arm — see Mononeuropathy, upper limb
    brachial plexus G54.0
    cervical plexus G54.2
    leg — see Mononeuropathy, lower limb
  peripheral NOS I73.9
  retina (artery) — see Occlusion, artery, retina
Vasospastic — see condition
Vasovagal attack (paroxysmal) R55
  psychogenic F45.8
VATER syndrome Q87.2
Vater's ampulla — see condition
Vegetation, vegetative
  adenoid (nasal fossa) J35.8
  endocarditis (acute) (any valve) (subacute) I33.0
  heart (mycotic) (valve) I33.0
Veil
  Jackson's Q43.3
Vein, venous — see condition
Veldt sore — see Ulcer, skin
Velpeau's hernia — see Hernia, femoral
Venereal
  bubo A55
  disease A64
  granuloma inguinale A58
  lymphogranuloma (Durand-Nicolas-Favre) A55
Venofibrosis I87.8
Venom, venomous — see Table of Drugs and Chemicals, by animal or substance, poisoning
Venous — see condition
Ventilator lung, newborn P27.8
Ventral — see condition
Ventricle, ventricular (see also condition)
  escape I49.3
  inversion Q20.5
Ventriculitis (cerebral) (see also Encephalitis) G04.90
Ventriculostomy status Z98.2
Vernet's syndrome G52.7
Verneuil's disease (syphilitic bursitis) A52.78
Verruca (due to HPV) (filiformis) (simplex) (viral) (vulgaris) B07.9
  acuminata A63.0
  necrogenica (primary) (tuberculosa) A18.4
  plana B07.8
  plantaris B07.0
  seborrheica L82.1
    inflamed L82.0
  senile (seborrheic) L82.1
    inflamed L82.0
  tuberculosa (primary) A18.4
  venereal A63.0
Verrucosities — see Verruca
Verruga peruana, peruviana A44.1
Version
  with extraction
  cervix — see Malposition, uterus
  uterus (postinfectional) (postpartal, old) — see Malposition, uterus
Vertebra, vertebral — see condition
Vertical talus (congenital) Q66.80
  left foot Q66.82
  right foot Q66.81
Vertigo R42
  auditory — see Vertigo, aural
  aural H81.31- ☑
  benign paroxysmal (positional) H81.1- ☑
  central (origin) H81.4- ☑

Vertigo — *continued*
cerebral H81.4- ☑
Dix and Hallpike (epidemic) — *see* Neuronitis, vestibular
due to infrasound T75.23 ☑
epidemic
Dix and Hallpike — *see* Neuronitis, vestibular
Pedersen's — *see* Neuronitis, vestibular
vestibular neuronitis — *see* Neuronitis, vestibular
hysterical F44.89
infrasound T75.23 ☑
labyrinthine — *see* subcategory H81.Ø ☑
laryngeal RØ5
malignant positional H81.4- ☑
Ménière's — *see* subcategory H81.Ø ☑
menopausal N95.1
otogenic — *see* Vertigo, aural
paroxysmal positional, benign — *see* Vertigo, benign paroxysmal
Pedersen's (epidemic) — *see* Neuronitis, vestibular
peripheral NEC H81.39- ☑
positional
benign paroxysmal — *see* Vertigo, benign paroxysmal
malignant H81.4- ☑
Very-low-density-lipoprotein-type (VLDL) **hyper-lipoproteinemia** E78.1
Vesania — *see* Psychosis
Vesical — *see* condition
Vesicle
cutaneous R23.8
seminal — *see* condition
skin R23.8
Vesicocolic — *see* condition
Vesicoperineal — *see* condition
Vesicorectal — *see* condition
Vesicourethrorectal — *see* condition
Vesicovaginal — *see* condition
Vesicular — *see* condition
Vesiculitis (seminal) N49.Ø
amebic AØ6.82
gonorrheal (acute) (chronic) A54.23
trichomonal A59.Ø9
tuberculous A18.15
Vestibulitis (ear) (*see also* subcategory) H83.Ø ☑
nose (external) J34.89
vulvar N94.81Ø
Vestibulopathy , acute peripheral (recurrent) — *see* Neuronitis, vestibular
Vestige, vestigial (*see also* Persistence)
branchial Q18.Ø
structures in vitreous Q14.Ø
Vibration
adverse effects T75.2Ø ☑
pneumatic hammer syndrome T75.21 ☑
specified effect NEC T75.29 ☑
vasospastic syndrome T75.22 ☑
vertigo from infrasound T75.23 ☑
exposure (occupational) Z57.7
vertigo T75.23 ☑
Vibriosis A28.9
Victim (of)
crime Z65.4
disaster Z65.5
terrorism Z65.4
torture Z65.4
war Z65.5
Vidal's disease L28.Ø
Villaret's syndrome G52.7
Villous — *see* condition
VIN — *see* Neoplasia, intraepithelial, vulva
Vincent's infection (angina) (gingivitis) A69.1
stomatitis NEC A69.1
Vinson-Plummer syndrome D5Ø.1
Violence, physical R45.6
Viosterol deficiency — *see* Deficiency, calciferol
Vipoma — *see* Neoplasm, malignant, by site
Viremia B34.9
Virilism (adrenal) E25.9
congenital E25.Ø
Virilization (female) (suprarenal) E25.9
congenital E25.Ø
isosexual E28.2
Virulent bubo A57
Virus, viral (*see also* condition)
as cause of disease classified elsewhere B97.89
cytomegalovirus B25.9

Virus, viral — *continued*
human immunodeficiency (HIV) — *see* Human, immunodeficiency virus (HIV) disease
infection — *see* Infection, virus
specified NEC B34.8
swine influenza (viruses that normally cause infections in pigs) (*see also* Influenza, due to, identified novel influenza A virus) JØ9.X2
West Nile (fever) A92.3Ø
with
complications NEC A92.39
cranial nerve disorders A92.32
encephalitis A92.31
encephalomyelitis A92.31
neurologic manifestation NEC A92.32
optic neuritis A92.32
polyradiculitis A92.32
Viscera, visceral — *see* condition
Visceroptosis K63.4
Visible peristalsis R19.2
Vision, visual
binocular, suppression H53.34
blurred, blurring H53.8
hysterical F44.6
defect, defective NEC H54.7
disorientation (syndrome) H53.8
disturbance H53.9
hysterical F44.6
double H53.2
examination ZØ1.ØØ
with abnormal findings ZØ1.Ø1
field, limitation (defect) — *see* Defect, visual field
hallucinations R44.1
halos H53.19
loss — *see* Loss, vision
sudden — *see* Disturbance, vision, subjective, loss, sudden
low (both eyes) — *see* Low, vision
perception, simultaneous without fusion H53.33
Vitality, lack or want of R53.83
newborn P96.89
Vitamin deficiency — *see* Deficiency, vitamin
Vitelline duct, persistent Q43.Ø
Vitiligo L8Ø
eyelid HØ2.739
left HØ2.736
lower HØ2.735
upper HØ2.734
right HØ2.733
lower HØ2.732
upper HØ2.731
pinta A67.2
vulva N9Ø.89
Vitreal corneal syndrome H59.Ø1- ☑
Vitreoretinopathy, proliferative (*see also* Retinopathy, proliferative)
with retinal detachment — *see* Detachment, retina, traction
Vitreous (*see also* condition)
touch syndrome — *see* Complication, postprocedural, following cataract surgery
Vocal cord — *see* condition
Vogt-Koyanagi syndrome H2Ø.82- ☑
Vogt's disease or syndrome G8Ø.3
Vogt-Spielmeyer amaurotic idiocy or disease E75.4
Voice
change R49.9
specified NEC R49.8
loss — *see* Aphonia
Volhynian fever A79.Ø
Volkmann's ischemic contracture or paralysis (complicating trauma) T79.6 ☑
Volvulus (bowel) (colon) (intestine) K56.2
with perforation K56.2
congenital Q43.8
duodenum K31.5
fallopian tube — *see* Torsion, fallopian tube
oviduct — *see* Torsion, fallopian tube
stomach (due to absence of gastrocolic ligament) K31.89
Vomiting R11.1Ø
with nausea R11.2
without nausea R11.11
asphyxia — *see* Foreign body, by site, causing asphyxia, gastric contents
bilious (cause unknown) R11.14
following gastro-intestinal surgery K91.Ø
in newborn P92.Ø1

Vomiting — *continued*
blood — *see* Hematemesis
causing asphyxia, choking, or suffocation — *see* Foreign body, by site
cyclical G43.AØ (*following* G43.7)
with refractory migraine G43.A1 (*following* G43.7)
without refractory migraine G43.AØ (*following* G43.7)
intractable G43.A1 (*following* G43.7)
not intractable G43.AØ (*following* G43.7)
psychogenic F5Ø.89
fecal mater R11.13
following gastrointestinal surgery K91.Ø
psychogenic F5Ø.89
functional K31.89
hysterical F5Ø.89
nervous F5Ø.89
neurotic F5Ø.89
newborn NEC P92.Ø9
bilious P92.Ø1
periodic R11.1Ø
psychogenic F5Ø.89
projectile R11.12
psychogenic F5Ø.89
uremic — *see* Uremia
Vomito negro — *see* Fever, yellow
Von Bezold's abscess — *see* Mastoiditis, acute
Von Economo-Cruchet disease A85.8
Von Eulenburg's disease G71.19
Von Gierke's disease E74.Ø1
Von Hippel (-Lindau) **disease or syndrome** Q85.8
Von Jaksch's anemia or disease D64.89
Von Recklinghausen
disease (neurofibromatosis) Q85.Ø1
bones E21.Ø
Von Schroetter's syndrome I82.89Ø
Von Willebrand (-Jurgens)(-Minot) **disease or syndrome** D68.Ø
Von Zumbusch's disease L4Ø.1
Voyeurism F65.3
Vrolik's disease Q78.Ø
Vulva — *see* condition
Vulvismus N94.2
Vulvitis (acute) (allergic) (atrophic) (hypertrophic) (intertriginous) (senile) N76.2
with ectopic or molar pregnancy OØ8.Ø
adhesive, congenital Q52.79
blennorrhagic (gonococcal) A54.Ø2
candidal B37.3
chlamydial A56.Ø2
due to Haemophilus ducreyi A57
following ectopic or molar pregnancy OØ8.Ø
gonococcal A54.Ø2
with abscess (accessory gland) (periurethral) A54.1
herpesviral A6Ø.Ø4
leukoplakic N9Ø.4
monilial B37.3
puerperal (postpartum) O86.19
subacute or chronic N76.3
syphilitic (early) A51.Ø
late A52.76
trichomonal A59.Ø1
tuberculous A18.18
Vulvodynia N94.819
specified NEC N94.818
Vulvorectal — *see* condition
Vulvovaginitis (acute) — *see* Vaginitis

W

Waiting list, person on Z75.1
for organ transplant Z76.82
undergoing social agency investigation Z75.2
Waldenström
hypergammaglobulinemia D89.Ø
syndrome or macroglobulinemia C88.Ø
Waldenström-Kjellberg syndrome D5Ø.1
Walking
difficulty R26.2
psychogenic F44.4
sleep F51.3
hysterical F44.89
Wall, abdominal — *see* condition
Wallenberg's disease or syndrome G46.3
Wallgren's disease I87.8
Wandering
gallbladder, congenital Q44.1
in diseases classified elsewhere Z91.83

☞ **Subterms under main terms may continue to next column or page**   ☑ **Additional Character Required — Refer to the Tabular List for Character Selection**   **325**

Vertigo — Wandering

Wandering — *continued*
  kidney, congenital Q63.8
  organ or site, congenital NEC — *see* Malposition, congenital, by site
  pacemaker (heart) I49.8
  spleen D73.89
War neurosis F48.8
Wart (due to HPV) (filiform) (infectious) (viral) B07.9
  anogenital region (venereal) A63.0
  common B07.8
  external genital organs (venereal) A63.0
  flat B07.8
  Hassal-Henle's (of cornea) H18.49
  Peruvian A44.1
  plantar B07.0
  prosector (tuberculous) A18.4
  seborrheic L82.1
    inflamed L82.0
  senile (seborrheic) L82.1
    inflamed L82.0
  tuberculous A18.4
  venereal A63.0
Warthin's tumor — *see* Neoplasm, salivary gland, benign
Wassilieff's disease A27.0
Wasting
  disease R64
    due to malnutrition E41
  extreme (due to malnutrition) E41
  muscle NEC — *see* Atrophy, muscle
Water
  clefts (senile cataract) — *see* Cataract, senile, incipient
  deprivation of T73.1 ☑
  intoxication E87.79
  itch B76.9
  lack of T73.1 ☑
  loading E87.70
  on
    brain — *see* Hydrocephalus
    chest J94.8
  poisoning E87.79
Waterbrash R12
Waterhouse (-Friderichsen) **syndrome or disease** (meningococcal) A39.1
Water-losing nephritis N25.89
Watermelon stomach K31.819
  with hemorrhage K31.811
  without hemorrhage K31.819
Watsoniasis B66.8
Wax in ear — *see* Impaction, cerumen
Weak, weakening, weakness (generalized) R53.1
  arches (acquired) (*see also* Deformity, limb, flat foot)
  bladder (sphincter) R32
  facial R29.810
    following
      cerebrovascular disease I69.992
        cerebral infarction I69.392
        intracerebral hemorrhage I69.192
        nontraumatic intracranial hemorrhage NEC I69.292
        specified disease NEC I69.892
        stroke I69.392
        subarachnoid hemorrhage I69.092
  foot (double) — *see* Weak, arches
  heart, cardiac — *see* Failure, heart
  mind F70
  muscle M62.81
  myocardium — *see* Failure, heart
  newborn P96.89
  pelvic fundus N81.89
  pubocervical tissue N81.82
  rectovaginal tissue N81.83
  senile R54
  urinary stream R39.12
  valvular — *see* Endocarditis
Wear, worn (with normal or routine use)
  articular bearing surface of internal joint prosthesis — *see* Complications, joint prosthesis, mechanical, wear of articular bearing surfaces, by site
  device, implant or graft — *see* Complications, by site, mechanical complication
  tooth, teeth (approximal) (hard tissues) (interproximal) (occlusal) K03.0
Weather, weathered
  effects of
    cold T69.9 ☑
      specified effect NEC T69.8 ☑
    hot — *see* Heat
  skin L57.8

Weaver's syndrome Q87.3
Web, webbed (congenital)
  duodenal Q43.8
  esophagus Q39.4
  fingers Q70.1- ☑
  larynx (glottic) (subglottic) Q31.0
  neck (pterygium colli) Q18.3
  Paterson-Kelly D50.1
  popliteal syndrome Q87.89
  toes Q70.3- ☑
Weber-Christian disease M35.6
Weber-Cockayne syndrome (epidermolysis bullosa) Q81.8
Weber-Gubler syndrome G46.3
Weber-Leyden syndrome G46.3
Weber-Osler syndrome I78.0
Weber's paralysis or syndrome G46.3
Wedge-shaped or wedging vertebra — *see* Collapse, vertebra NEC
Wegener's granulomatosis or syndrome M31.30
  with
    kidney involvement M31.31
    lung involvement M31.30
      with kidney involvement M31.31
Wegner's disease A50.02
Weight
  1000-2499 grams at birth (low) — *see* Low, birth-weight
  999 grams or less at birth (extremely low) — *see* Low, birthweight, extreme
  and length below 10th percentile for gestational age P05.1- ☑
  below but length above 10th percentile for gestational age P05.0- ☑
  gain (abnormal) (excessive) R63.5
    in pregnancy — *see* Pregnancy, complicated by, excessive weight gain
    low — *see* Pregnancy, complicated by, insufficient, weight gain
  loss (abnormal) (cause unknown) R63.4
Weightlessness (effect of) T75.82 ☑
Weil (I)-**Marchesani syndrome** Q87.1
Weil's disease A27.0
Weingarten's syndrome J82
Weir Mitchell's disease I73.81
Weiss-Baker syndrome G90.09
Wells' disease L98.3
Wen — *see* Cyst, sebaceous
Wenckebach's block or phenomenon I44.1
Werdnig-Hoffmann syndrome (muscular atrophy) G12.0
Werlhof's disease D69.3
Wermer's disease or syndrome E31.21
Werner-His disease A79.0
Werner's disease or syndrome E34.8
Wernicke-Korsakoff's syndrome or psychosis (alcoholic) F10.96
  with dependence F10.26
  drug-induced
    due to drug abuse — *see* Abuse, drug, by type, with amnestic disorder
    due to drug dependence — *see* Dependence, drug, by type, with amnestic disorder
  nonalcoholic F04
Wernicke-Posadas disease B38.9
Wernicke's
  developmental aphasia F80.2
  disease or syndrome E51.2
  encephalopathy E51.2
  polioencephalitis, superior E51.2
West African fever B50.8
Westphal-Strümpell syndrome E83.01
West's syndrome — *see* Epilepsy, spasms
Wet
  feet, tropical (maceration) (syndrome) — *see* Immersion, foot
  lung (syndrome), newborn P22.1
Wharton's duct — *see* condition
Wheal — *see* Urticaria
Wheezing R06.2
Whiplash injury S13.4 ☑
Whipple's disease (*see also* subcategory M14.8-) K90.81
Whipworm (disease) (infection) (infestation) B79
Whistling face Q87.0
White (*see also* condition)
  kidney, small N03.9
  leg, puerperal, postpartum, childbirth O87.1

White — *continued*
  mouth B37.0
  patches of mouth K13.29
  spot lesions, teeth
    chewing surface K02.51
    pit and fissure surface K02.51
    smooth surface K02.61
Whitehead L70.0
Whitlow (*see also* Cellulitis, digit)
  with lymphangitis — *see* Lymphangitis, acute, digit
  herpesviral B00.89
Whitmore's disease or fever — *see* Melioidosis
Whooping cough A37.90
  with pneumonia A37.91
    due to Bordetella
      bronchiseptica A37.81
      parapertussis A37.11
      pertussis A37.01
    specified organism NEC A37.81
  due to
    Bordetella
      bronchiseptica A37.80
        with pneumonia A37.81
      parapertussis A37.10
        with pneumonia A37.11
      pertussis A37.00
        with pneumonia A37.01
    specified NEC A37.80
      with pneumonia A37.81
Wichman's asthma J38.5
Wide cranial sutures, newborn P96.3
Widening aorta — *see* Ectasia, aorta
  with aneurysm — *see* Aneurysm, aorta
Wilkie's disease or syndrome K55.1
Wilkinson-Sneddon disease or syndrome L13.1
Willebrand (-Jürgens) **thrombopathy** D68.0
Willige-Hunt disease or syndrome G23.1
Wilms' tumor C64- ☑
Wilson-Mikity syndrome P27.0
Wilson's
  disease or syndrome E83.01
  hepatolenticular degeneration E83.01
  lichen ruber L43.9
Window (*see also* Imperfect, closure)
  aorticopulmonary Q21.4
Winter — *see* condition
Wiskott-Aldrich syndrome D82.0
Withdrawal state (*see also* Dependence, drug by type, with withdrawal)
  alcohol
    with perceptual disturbances F10.232
    without perceptual disturbances F10.239
  caffeine F15.93
  cannabis F12.288
  newborn
    correct therapeutic substance properly administered P96.2
    infant of dependent mother P96.1
  therapeutic substance, neonatal P96.2
Witts' anemia D50.8
Witzelsucht F07.0
Woakes' ethmoiditis or syndrome J33.1
Wolff-Hirschorn syndrome Q93.3
Wolff-Parkinson-White syndrome I45.6
Wolhynian fever A79.0
Wolman's disease E75.5
Wood lung or pneumonitis J67.8
Woolly, wooly hair (congenital) (nevus) Q84.1
Woolsorter's disease A22.1
Word
  blindness (congenital) (developmental) F81.0
  deafness (congenital) (developmental) H93.25
Worm(s) (infection) (infestation) (*see also* Infestation, helminth)
  guinea B72
  in intestine NEC B82.0
Worm-eaten soles A66.3
Worn out — *see* Exhaustion
  cardiac
    defibrillator (with synchronous cardiace pacemaker) Z45.02
    pacemaker
      battery Z45.010
      lead Z45.018
  device, implant or graft — *see* Complications, by site, mechanical
Worried well Z71.1
Worries R45.82

☑ **Additional Character Required — Refer to the Tabular List for Character Selection**   ⬇ **Subterms under main terms may continue to next column or page**

Wound check Z48.0- ☑
    due to injury — *code to* Injury, by site, using appropri-
        ate seventh character for subsequent encounter
Wound, open T14.8- ☑
    abdomen, abdominal
        wall S31.109 ☑
            with penetration into peritoneal cavity
                S31.609 ☑
            bite — *see* Bite, abdomen, wall
            epigastric region S31.102 ☑
                with penetration into peritoneal cavity
                    S31.602 ☑
                bite — *see* Bite, abdomen, wall, epigastric
                    region
                laceration — *see* Laceration, abdomen, wall,
                    epigastric region
                puncture — *see* Puncture, abdomen, wall,
                    epigastric region
            laceration — *see* Laceration, abdomen, wall
            left
                lower quadrant S31.104 ☑
                    with penetration into peritoneal cavity
                        S31.604 ☑
                    bite — *see* Bite, abdomen, wall, left,
                        lower quadrant
                    laceration — *see* Laceration, abdomen,
                        wall, left, lower quadrant
                    puncture — *see* Puncture, abdomen,
                        wall, left, lower quadrant
                upper quadrant S31.101 ☑
                    with penetration into peritoneal cavity
                        S31.601 ☑
                    bite — *see* Bite, abdomen, wall, left, up-
                        per quadrant
                    laceration — *see* Laceration, abdomen,
                        wall, left, upper quadrant
                    puncture — *see* Puncture, abdomen,
                        wall, left, upper quadrant
            periumbilic region S31.105 ☑
                with penetration into peritoneal cavity
                    S31.605 ☑
                bite — *see* Bite, abdomen, wall, periumbilic
                    region
                laceration — *see* Laceration, abdomen, wall,
                    periumbilic region
                puncture — *see* Puncture, abdomen, wall,
                    periumbilic region
            puncture — *see* Puncture, abdomen, wall
            right
                lower quadrant S31.103 ☑
                    with penetration into peritoneal cavity
                        S31.603 ☑
                    bite — *see* Bite, abdomen, wall, right,
                        lower quadrant
                    laceration — *see* Laceration, abdomen,
                        wall, right, lower quadrant
                    puncture — *see* Puncture, abdomen,
                        wall, right, lower quadrant
                upper quadrant S31.100 ☑
                    with penetration into peritoneal cavity
                        S31.600 ☑
                    bite — *see* Bite, abdomen, wall, right,
                        upper quadrant
                    laceration — *see* Laceration, abdomen,
                        wall, right, upper quadrant
                    puncture — *see* Puncture, abdomen,
                        wall, right, upper quadrant
    alveolar (process) — *see* Wound, open, oral cavity
    ankle S91.00- ☑
        bite — *see* Bite, ankle
        laceration — *see* Laceration, ankle
        puncture — *see* Puncture, ankle
    antecubital space — *see* Wound, open, elbow
    anterior chamber, eye — *see* Wound, open, ocular
    anus S31.839 ☑
        bite S31.835 ☑
        laceration — *see* Laceration, anus
        puncture — *see* Puncture, anus
    arm (upper) S41.10- ☑
        with amputation — *see* Amputation, traumatic,
            arm
        bite — *see* Bite, arm
        forearm — *see* Wound, open, forearm
        laceration — *see* Laceration, arm
        puncture — *see* Puncture, arm
    auditory canal (external) (meatus) — *see* Wound, open,
        ear

Wound, open — *continued*
    auricle, ear — *see* Wound, open, ear
    axilla — *see* Wound, open, arm
    back (*see also* Wound, open, thorax, back)
        lower S31.000 ☑
            with penetration into retroperitoneal space
                S31.001 ☑
            bite — *see* Bite, back, lower
            laceration — *see* Laceration, back, lower
            puncture — *see* Puncture, back, lower
    bite — *see* Bite
    blood vessel — *see* Injury, blood vessel
    breast S21.00- ☑
        with amputation — *see* Amputation, traumatic,
            breast
        bite — *see* Bite, breast
        laceration — *see* Laceration, breast
        puncture — *see* Puncture, breast
    buttock S31.809 ☑
        bite — *see* Bite, buttock
        laceration — *see* Laceration, buttock
        left S31.829 ☑
        puncture — *see* Puncture, buttock
        right S31.819 ☑
    calf — *see* Wound, open, leg
    canaliculus lacrimalis — *see* Wound, open, eyelid
    canthus, eye — *see* Wound, open, eyelid
    cervical esophagus S11.20 ☑
        bite S11.25 ☑
        laceration — *see* Laceration, esophagus, traumatic,
            cervical
        puncture — *see* Puncture, cervical esophagus
    cheek (external) S01.40- ☑
        bite — *see* Bite, cheek
        internal — *see* Wound, open, oral cavity
        laceration — *see* Laceration, cheek
        puncture — *see* Puncture, cheek
    chest wall — *see* Wound, open, thorax
    chin — *see* Wound, open, head, specified site NEC
    choroid — *see* Wound, open, ocular
    ciliary body (eye) — *see* Wound, open, ocular
    clitoris S31.40 ☑
        with amputation — *see* Amputation, traumatic,
            clitoris
        bite S31.45 ☑
        laceration — *see* Laceration, vulva
        puncture — *see* Puncture, vulva
    conjunctiva — *see* Wound, open, ocular
    cornea — *see* Wound, open, ocular
    costal region — *see* Wound, open, thorax
    Descemet's membrane — *see* Wound, open, ocular
    digit(s)
        foot — *see* Wound, open, toe
        hand — *see* Wound, open, finger
    ear (canal) (external) S01.30- ☑
        with amputation — *see* Amputation, traumatic,
            ear
        bite — *see* Bite, ear
        drum S09.2- ☑
        laceration — *see* Laceration, ear
        puncture — *see* Puncture, ear
    elbow S51.00- ☑
        bite — *see* Bite, elbow
        laceration — *see* Laceration, elbow
        puncture — *see* Puncture, elbow
    epididymis — *see* Wound, open, testis
    epigastric region S31.102 ☑
        with penetration into peritoneal cavity S31.602 ☑
        bite — *see* Bite, abdomen, wall, epigastric region
        laceration — *see* Laceration, abdomen, wall, epi-
            gastric region
        puncture — *see* Puncture, abdomen, wall, epigas-
            tric region
    epiglottis — *see* Wound, open, neck, specified site
        NEC
    esophagus (thoracic) S27.819 ☑
        cervical — *see* Wound, open, cervical esophagus
        laceration S27.813 ☑
        specified type NEC S27.818 ☑
    eye — *see* Wound, open, ocular
    eyeball — *see* Wound, open, ocular
    eyebrow — *see* Wound, open, eyelid
    eyelid S01.10- ☑
        bite — *see* Bite, eyelid
        laceration — *see* Laceration, eyelid
        puncture — *see* Puncture, eyelid

Wound, open — *continued*
    face NEC — *see* Wound, open, head, specified site NEC
    finger(s) S61.209 ☑
        with
            amputation — *see* Amputation, traumatic, fin-
                ger
            damage to nail S61.309 ☑
        bite — *see* Bite, finger
        index S61.208 ☑
            with
                damage to nail S61.308 ☑
            left S61.201 ☑
                with
                    damage to nail S61.301 ☑
            right S61.200 ☑
                with
                    damage to nail S61.300 ☑
        laceration — *see* Laceration, finger
        little S61.208 ☑
            with
                damage to nail S61.308 ☑
            left S61.207 ☑
                with damage to nail S61.307 ☑
            right S61.206 ☑
                with damage to nail S61.306 ☑
        middle S61.208 ☑
            with
                damage to nail S61.308 ☑
            left S61.203 ☑
                with damage to nail S61.303 ☑
            right S61.202 ☑
                with damage to nail S61.302 ☑
        puncture — *see* Puncture, finger
        ring S61.208 ☑
            with
                damage to nail S61.308 ☑
            left S61.205 ☑
                with damage to nail S61.305 ☑
            right S61.204 ☑
                with damage to nail S61.304 ☑
    flank — *see* Wound, open, abdomen, wall
    foot (except toe(s) alone) S91.30- ☑
        with amputation — *see* Amputation, traumatic,
            foot
        bite — *see* Bite, foot
        laceration — *see* Laceration, foot
        puncture — *see* Puncture, foot
        toe — *see* Wound, open, toe
    forearm S51.80- ☑
        with
            amputation — *see* Amputation, traumatic,
                forearm
        bite — *see* Bite, forearm
        elbow only — *see* Wound, open, elbow
        laceration — *see* Laceration, forearm
        puncture — *see* Puncture, forearm
    forehead — *see* Wound, open, head, specified site NEC
    genital organs, external
        with amputation — *see* Amputation, traumatic,
            genital organs
        bite — *see* Bite, genital organ
        female S31.502 ☑
            vagina S31.40 ☑
            vulva S31.40 ☑
        laceration — *see* Laceration, genital organ
        male S31.501 ☑
            penis S31.20 ☑
            scrotum S31.30 ☑
            testes S31.30 ☑
        puncture — *see* Puncture, genital organ
    globe (eye) — *see* Wound, open, ocular
    groin — *see* Wound, open, abdomen, wall
    gum — *see* Wound, open, oral cavity
    hand S61.40- ☑
        with
            amputation — *see* Amputation, traumatic,
                hand
        bite — *see* Bite, hand
        finger(s) — *see* Wound, open, finger
        laceration — *see* Laceration, hand
        puncture — *see* Puncture, hand
        thumb — *see* Wound, open, thumb
    head S01.90 ☑
        bite — *see* Bite, head
        cheek — *see* Wound, open, cheek
        ear — *see* Wound, open, ear

Wound, open — *continued*
   head — *continued*
      eyelid — *see* Wound, open, eyelid
      laceration — *see* Laceration, head
      lip — *see* Wound, open, lip
      nose S01.20 ✓
      oral cavity — *see* Wound, open, oral cavity
      puncture — *see* Puncture, head
      scalp — *see* Wound, open, scalp
      specified site NEC S01.80 ✓
      temporomandibular area — *see* Wound, open,
         cheek
   heel — *see* Wound, open, foot
   hip S71.00- ✓
      with amputation — *see* Amputation, traumatic,
         hip
      bite — *see* Bite, hip
      laceration — *see* Laceration, hip
      puncture — *see* Puncture, hip
   hymen S31.40 ✓
      bite — *see* Bite, vulva
      laceration — *see* Laceration, vagina
      puncture — *see* Puncture, vagina
   hypochondrium S31.109 ✓
      bite — *see* Bite, hypochondrium
      laceration — *see* Laceration, hypochondrium
      puncture — *see* Puncture, hypochondrium
   hypogastric region S31.109 ✓
      bite — *see* Bite, hypogastric region
      laceration — *see* Laceration, hypogastric region
      puncture — *see* Puncture, hypogastric region
   iliac (region) — *see* Wound, open, inguinal region
   inguinal region S31.109 ✓
      bite — *see* Bite, abdomen, wall, lower quadrant
      laceration — *see* Laceration, inguinal region
      puncture — *see* Puncture, inguinal region
   instep — *see* Wound, open, foot
   interscapular region — *see* Wound, open, thorax, back
   intraocular — *see* Wound, open, ocular
   iris — *see* Wound, open, ocular
   jaw — *see* Wound, open, head, specified site NEC
   knee S81.00- ✓
      bite — *see* Bite, knee
      laceration — *see* Laceration, knee
      puncture — *see* Puncture, knee
   labium (majus) (minus) — *see* Wound, open, vulva
   laceration — *see* Laceration, by site
   lacrimal duct — *see* Wound, open, eyelid
   larynx S11.019 ✓
      bite — *see* Bite, larynx
      laceration — *see* Laceration, larynx
      puncture — *see* Puncture, larynx
   left
      lower quadrant S31.104 ✓
         with penetration into peritoneal cavity
            S31.604 ✓
         bite — *see* Bite, abdomen, wall, left, lower
            quadrant
         laceration — *see* Laceration, abdomen, wall,
            left, lower quadrant
         puncture — *see* Puncture, abdomen, wall, left,
            lower quadrant
      upper quadrant S31.101 ✓
         with penetration into peritoneal cavity
            S31.601 ✓
         bite — *see* Bite, abdomen, wall, left, upper
            quadrant
         laceration — *see* Laceration, abdomen, wall,
            left, upper quadrant
         puncture — *see* Puncture, abdomen, wall, left,
            upper quadrant
   leg (lower) S81.80- ✓
      with amputation — *see* Amputation, traumatic,
         leg
      ankle — *see* Wound, open, ankle
      bite — *see* Bite, leg
      foot — *see* Wound, open, foot
      knee — *see* Wound, open, knee
      laceration — *see* Laceration, leg
      puncture — *see* Puncture, leg
      toe — *see* Wound, open, toe
      upper — *see* Wound, open, thigh
   lip S01.501 ✓
      bite — *see* Bite, lip
      laceration — *see* Laceration, lip
      puncture — *see* Puncture, lip

Wound, open — *continued*
   loin S31.109 ✓
      bite — *see* Bite, abdomen, wall
      laceration — *see* Laceration, loin
      puncture — *see* Puncture, loin
   lower back — *see* Wound, open, back, lower
   lumbar region — *see* Wound, open, back, lower
   malar region — *see* Wound, open, head, specified site
      NEC
   mammary — *see* Wound, open, breast
   mastoid region — *see* Wound, open, head, specified
      site NEC
   mouth — *see* Wound, open, oral cavity
   nail
      finger — *see* Wound, open, finger, with damage
         to nail
      toe — *see* Wound, open, toe, with damage to nail
   nape (neck) — *see* Wound, open, neck
   nasal (septum) (sinus) — *see* Wound, open, nose
   nasopharynx — *see* Wound, open, head, specified site
      NEC
   neck S11.90 ✓
      bite — *see* Bite, neck
      involving
         cervical esophagus S11.20 ✓
         larynx — *see* Wound, open, larynx
         pharynx S11.20 ✓
         thyroid S11.10 ✓
         trachea (cervical) S11.029 ✓
            bite — *see* Bite, trachea
            laceration S11.021 ✓
               with foreign body S11.022 ✓
            puncture S11.023 ✓
               with foreign body S11.024 ✓
      laceration — *see* Laceration, neck
      puncture — *see* Puncture, neck
      specified site NEC S11.80 ✓
      specified type NEC S11.89 ✓
   nose (septum) (sinus) S01.20 ✓
      with amputation — *see* Amputation, traumatic,
         nose
      bite — *see* Bite, nose
      laceration — *see* Laceration, nose
      puncture — *see* Puncture, nose
   ocular S05.90 ✓
      avulsion (traumatic enucleation) S05.7- ✓
      eyeball S05.6- ✓
         with foreign body S05.5- ✓
      eyelid — *see* Wound, open, eyelid
      laceration and rupture S05.3- ✓
         with prolapse or loss of intraocular tissue
            S05.2- ✓
      orbit (penetrating) (with or without foreign body)
         S05.4- ✓
      periocular area — *see* Wound, open, eyelid
      specified NEC S05.8X- ✓
   oral cavity S01.502 ✓
      bite S01.552 ✓
      laceration — *see* Laceration, oral cavity
      puncture — *see* Puncture, oral cavity
   orbit — *see* Wound, open, ocular, orbit
   palate — *see* Wound, open, oral cavity
   palm — *see* Wound, open, hand
   pelvis, pelvic (see also Wound, open, back, lower)
      girdle — *see* Wound, open, hip
   penetrating — *see* Puncture, by site
   penis S31.20 ✓
      with amputation — *see* Amputation, traumatic,
         penis
      bite S31.25 ✓
      laceration — *see* Laceration, penis
      puncture — *see* Puncture, penis
   perineum
      bite — *see* Bite, perineum
      female S31.502 ✓
      laceration — *see* Laceration, perineum
      male S31.501 ✓
      puncture — *see* Puncture, perineum
   periocular area (with or without lacrimal passages) —
      see Wound, open, eyelid
   periumbilic region S31.105 ✓
      with penetration into peritoneal cavity S31.605 ✓
      bite — *see* Bite, abdomen, wall, periumbilic region
      laceration — *see* Laceration, abdomen, wall, peri-
         umbilic region

Wound, open — *continued*
   periumbilic region — *continued*
      puncture — *see* Puncture, abdomen, wall, perium-
         bilic region
   phalanges
      finger — *see* Wound, open, finger
      toe — *see* Wound, open, toe
   pharynx S11.20 ✓
   pinna — *see* Wound, open, ear
   popliteal space — *see* Wound, open, knee
   prepuce — *see* Wound, open, penis
   pubic region — *see* Wound, open, back, lower
   pudendum — *see* Wound, open, genital organs, exter-
      nal
   puncture wound — *see* Puncture
   rectovaginal septum — *see* Wound, open, vagina
   right
      lower quadrant S31.103 ✓
         with penetration into peritoneal cavity
            S31.603 ✓
         bite — *see* Bite, abdomen, wall, right, lower
            quadrant
         laceration — *see* Laceration, abdomen, wall,
            right, lower quadrant
         puncture — *see* Puncture, abdomen, wall, right,
            lower quadrant
      upper quadrant S31.100 ✓
         with penetration into peritoneal cavity
            S31.600 ✓
         bite — *see* Bite, abdomen, wall, right, upper
            quadrant
         laceration — *see* Laceration, abdomen, wall,
            right, upper quadrant
         puncture — *see* Puncture, abdomen, wall, right,
            upper quadrant
   sacral region — *see* Wound, open, back, lower
   sacroiliac region — *see* Wound, open, back, lower
   salivary gland — *see* Wound, open, oral cavity
   scalp S01.00 ✓
      bite S01.05 ✓
      laceration — *see* Laceration, scalp
      puncture — *see* Puncture, scalp
   scalpel, newborn (birth injury) P15.8
   scapular region — *see* Wound, open, shoulder
   sclera — *see* Wound, open, ocular
   scrotum S31.30 ✓
      with amputation — *see* Amputation, traumatic,
         scrotum
      bite S31.35 ✓
      laceration — *see* Laceration, scrotum
      puncture — *see* Puncture, scrotum
   shin — *see* Wound, open, leg
   shoulder S41.00- ✓
      with amputation — *see* Amputation, traumatic,
         arm
      bite — *see* Bite, shoulder
      laceration — *see* Laceration, shoulder
      puncture — *see* Puncture, shoulder
   skin NOS T14.8 ✓
   spermatic cord — *see* Wound, open, testis
   sternal region — *see* Wound, open, thorax, front wall
   submaxillary region — *see* Wound, open, head, speci-
      fied site NEC
   submental region — *see* Wound, open, head, specified
      site NEC
   subungual
      finger(s) — *see* Wound, open, finger
      toe(s) — *see* Wound, open, toe
   supraclavicular region — *see* Wound, open, neck,
      specified site NEC
   temple, temporal region — *see* Wound, open, head,
      specified site NEC
   temporomandibular area — *see* Wound, open, cheek
   testis S31.30 ✓
      with amputation — *see* Amputation, traumatic,
         testes
      bite S31.35 ✓
      laceration — *see* Laceration, testis
      puncture — *see* Puncture, testis
   thigh S71.10- ✓
      with amputation — *see* Amputation, traumatic,
         hip
      bite — *see* Bite, thigh
      laceration — *see* Laceration, thigh
      puncture — *see* Puncture, thigh
   thorax, thoracic (wall) S21.90 ✓
      back S21.20- ✓

Wound, open — *continued*
  thorax, thoracic — *continued*
    back — *continued*
      with penetration S21.40 ☑
    bite — *see* Bite, thorax
    breast — *see* Wound, open, breast
    front S21.10-
      with penetration S21.30 ☑
    laceration — *see* Laceration, thorax
    puncture — *see* Puncture, thorax
  throat — *see* Wound, open, neck
  thumb S61.009 ☑
    with
      amputation — *see* Amputation, traumatic, thumb
      damage to nail S61.109 ☑
    bite — *see* Bite, thumb
    laceration — *see* Laceration, thumb
    left S61.002 ☑
      with
        damage to nail S61.102 ☑
    puncture — *see* Puncture, thumb
    right S61.001 ☑
      with
        damage to nail S61.101 ☑
  thyroid (gland) — *see* Wound, open, neck, thyroid
  toe(s) S91.109 ☑
    with
      amputation — *see* Amputation, traumatic, toe
      damage to nail S91.209 ☑
    bite — *see* Bite, toe
    great S91.103 ☑
      with
        damage to nail S91.203 ☑
      left S91.102 ☑
        with
          damage to nail S91.202 ☑
      right S91.101 ☑
        with
          damage to nail S91.201 ☑
    laceration — *see* Laceration, toe
    lesser S91.106 ☑
      with
        damage to nail S91.206 ☑
      left S91.105 ☑
        with
          damage to nail S91.205 ☑
      right S91.104 ☑
        with
          damage to nail S91.204 ☑
    puncture — *see* Puncture, toe
  tongue — *see* Wound, open, oral cavity
  trachea (cervical region) — *see* Wound, open, neck, trachea
  tunica vaginalis — *see* Wound, open, testis
  tympanum, tympanic membrane S09.2- ☑
    laceration — *see* Laceration, ear, drum
    puncture — *see* Puncture, tympanum
  umbilical region — *see* Wound, open, abdomen, wall, periumbilic region
  uvula — *see* Wound, open, oral cavity
  vagina S31.40 ☑
    bite S31.45 ☑
    laceration — *see* Laceration, vagina
    puncture — *see* Puncture, vagina
  vitreous (humor) — *see* Wound, open, ocular
  vocal cord S11.039 ☑
    bite — *see* Bite, vocal cord
    laceration S11.031 ☑
      with foreign body S11.032 ☑
    puncture S11.033 ☑
      with foreign body S11.034 ☑
  vulva S31.40 ☑
    with amputation — *see* Amputation, traumatic, vulva
    bite S31.45 ☑
    laceration — *see* Laceration, vulva
    puncture — *see* Puncture, vulva
  wrist S61.50- ☑
    bite — *see* Bite, wrist
    laceration — *see* Laceration, wrist
    puncture — *see* Puncture, wrist
Wound, superficial — *see* Injury (*see also* specified injury type)

Wright's syndrome G54.0
Wrist — *see* condition
Wrong drug (by accident) (given in error) — *see* Table of Drugs and Chemicals, by drug, poisoning
Wry neck — *see* Torticollis
Wuchereria (bancrofti) **infestation** B74.0
Wuchereriasis B74.0
Wuchernde Struma Langhans C73

X

Xanthelasma (eyelid) (palpebrarum) H02.60
  left H02.66
    lower H02.65
    upper H02.64
  right H02.63
    lower H02.62
    upper H02.61
Xanthelasmatosis (essential) E78.2
Xanthinuria, hereditary E79.8
Xanthoastrocytoma
  specified site — *see* Neoplasm, malignant, by site
  unspecified site C71.9
Xanthofibroma — *see* Neoplasm, connective tissue, benign
Xanthogranuloma D76.3
Xanthoma(s), xanthomatosis (primary) (familial) (hereditary) E75.5
  with
    hyperlipoproteinemia
      Type I E78.3
      Type III E78.2
      Type IV E78.1
      Type V E78.3
  bone (generalisata) C96.5
  cerebrotendinous E75.5
  cutaneotendinous E75.5
  disseminatum (skin) E78.2
  eruptive E78.2
  hypercholesterinemic E78.00
  hypercholesterolemic E78.00
  hyperlipidemic E78.5
  joint E75.5
  multiple (skin) E78.2
  tendon (sheath) E75.5
  tuberosum E78.2
  tuberous E78.2
  tubo-eruptive E78.2
  verrucous, oral mucosa K13.4
Xanthosis R23.8
Xenophobia F40.10
Xeroderma (*see also* Ichthyosis)
  acquired L85.0
  eyelid H01.149
    left H01.146
      lower H01.145
      upper H01.144
    right H01.143
      lower H01.142
      upper H01.141
  pigmentosum Q82.1
  vitamin A deficiency E50.8
Xerophthalmia (vitamin A deficiency) E50.7
  unrelated to vitamin A deficiency — *see* Keratoconjunctivitis
Xerosis
  conjunctiva H11.14- ☑
    with Bitot's spots (*see also* Pigmentation, conjunctiva)
      vitamin A deficiency E50.1
    vitamin A deficiency E50.0
  cornea H18.89- ☑
    with ulceration — *see* Ulcer, cornea
      vitamin A deficiency E50.3
    vitamin A deficiency E50.2
  cutis L85.3
  skin L85.3
Xerostomia K11.7
Xiphopagus Q89.4
XO syndrome Q96.9
X-ray (of)
  abnormal findings — *see* Abnormal, diagnostic imaging
  breast (mammogram) (routine) Z12.31

X-ray — *continued*
  chest
    routine (as part of a general medical examination) Z00.00
      with abnormal findings Z00.01
  routine (as part of a general medical examination) Z00.00
    with abnormal findings Z00.01
XXXXY syndrome Q98.1
XXY syndrome Q98.0

Y

Yaba pox (virus disease) B08.72
Yatapoxvirus B08.70
  specified NEC B08.79
Yawning R06.89
  psychogenic F45.8
Yaws A66.9
  cutaneous, less than five years after infection A66.2
  bone lesions A66.6
  butter A66.1
  chancre A66.0
  early (cutaneous) (macular) (maculopapular) (micropapular) (papular) A66.2
    frambeside A66.2
    skin lesions NEC A66.2
  eyelid A66.2
  ganglion A66.6
  gangosis, gangosa A66.5
  gumma, gummata A66.4
    bone A66.6
  gummatous
    frambeside A66.4
    osteitis A66.6
    periostitis A66.6
  hydrarthrosis (*see also* subcategory M14.8-) A66.6
  hyperkeratosis (early) (late) A66.3
  initial lesions A66.0
  joint lesions (*see also* subcategory M14.8-) A66.6
  juxta-articular nodules A66.7
  late nodular (ulcerated) A66.4
  latent (without clinical manifestations) (with positive serology) A66.8
  mother A66.0
  mucosal A66.7
  multiple papillomata A66.1
  nodular, late (ulcerated) A66.4
  osteitis A66.6
  papilloma, plantar or palmar A66.1
  periostitis (hypertrophic) A66.6
  specified NEC A66.7
  ulcers A66.4
  wet crab A66.1
Yeast infection (*see also* Candidiasis) B37.9
Yellow
  atrophy (liver) — *see* Failure, hepatic
  fever — *see* Fever, yellow
  jack — *see* Fever, yellow
  jaundice — *see* Jaundice
  nail syndrome L60.5
Yersiniosis (*see also* Infection, Yersinia)
  extraintestinal A28.2
  intestinal A04.6

Z

Zahorsky's syndrome (herpangina) B08.5
Zellweger's syndrome Q87.89
Zenker's diverticulum (esophagus) K22.5
Ziehen-Oppenheim disease G24.1
Zieve's syndrome K70.0
Zika NOS A92.5
Zinc
  deficiency, dietary E60
  metabolism disorder E83.2
Zollinger-Ellison syndrome E16.4
Zona — *see* Herpes, zoster
Zoophobia F40.218
Zoster (herpes) — *see* Herpes, zoster
Zygomycosis B46.9
  specified NEC B46.8
Zymotic — *see* condition

Index

Wound, open — Zymotic

	Malignant Primary	Malignant Secondary	Ca in situ	Benign	Uncertain	Unspecified Behavior

Note: The list below gives the code number for neoplasms by anatomical site. For each site there are six possible code numbers according to whether the neoplasm in question is malignant, benign, in situ, of uncertain behavior, or of unspecified nature. The description of the neoplasm will often indicate which of the six columns is appropriate; e.g., malignant melanoma of skin, benign fibroadenoma of breast, carcinoma in situ of cervix uteri. Where such descriptors are not present, the remainder of the Index should be consulted where guidance is given to the appropriate column for each morphological (histological) variety listed; e.g., Mesonephroma – see Neoplasm, malignant; Embryoma (see also Neoplasm, uncertain behavior); Disease, Bowen's – see Neoplasm, skin, in situ. However, the guidance in the Index can be overridden if one of the descriptors mentioned above is present; e.g., malignant adenoma of colon is coded to C18.9 and not to D12.6 as the adjective "malignant" overrides the Index entry "Adenoma (see also Neoplasm, benign, by site)." Codes listed with a dash -, following the code have a required additional character for laterality. The tabular list must be reviewed for the complete code.

	Malignant Primary	Malignant Secondary	Ca in situ	Benign	Uncertain	Unspecified Behavior
Neoplasm, neoplastic	C80.1	C79.9	D09.9	D36.9	D48.9	D49.9
abdomen, abdominal	C76.2	C79.8-☑	D09.8	D36.7	D48.7	D49.89
cavity	C76.2	C79.8-☑	D09.8	D36.7	D48.7	D49.89
organ	C76.2	C79.8-☑	D09.8	D36.7	D48.7	D49.89
viscera	C76.2	C79.8-☑	D09.8	D36.7	D48.7	D49.89
wall — *see also* Neoplasm, abdomen, wall, skin	C44.509	C79.2	D04.5	D23.5	D48.5	D49.2
connective tissue	C49.4	C79.8-☑	—	D21.4	D48.1	D49.2
skin	C44.509	—	—	—	—	—
basal cell carcinoma	C44.519	—	—	—	—	—
specified type NEC	C44.599	—	—	—	—	—
squamous cell carcinoma	C44.529	—	—	—	—	—
abdominopelvic	C76.8	C79.8-☑	—	D36.7	D48.7	D49.89
accessory sinus — *see* Neoplasm, sinus						
acoustic nerve	C72.4-☑	C79.49		D33.3	D43.3	D49.7
adenoid (pharynx) (tissue)	C11.1	C79.89	D00.08	D10.6	D37.05	D49.0
adipose tissue — *see also* Neoplasm, connective tissue	C49.4	C79.89	—	D21.9	D48.1	D49.2
adnexa (uterine)	C57.4	C79.89	D07.39	D28.7	D39.8	D49.59
adrenal	C74.9-☑	C79.7-☑	D09.3	D35.0-☑	D44.1-☑	D49.7
capsule	C74.9-☑	C79.7-☑	D09.3	D35.0-☑	D44.1-☑	D49.7
cortex	C74.0-☑	C79.7-☑	D09.3	D35.0-☑	D44.1-☑	D49.7
gland	C74.9-☑	C79.7-☑	D09.3	D35.0-☑	D44.1-☑	D49.7
medulla	C74.1-☑	C79.7-☑	D09.3	D35.0-☑	D44.1-☑	D49.7
ala nasi (external) — *see also* Neoplasm, skin, nose	C44.301	C79.2	D04.39	D23.39	D48.5	D49.2
alimentary canal or tract NEC	C26.9	C78.80	D01.9	D13.9	D37.9	D49.0
alveolar	C03.9	C79.89	D00.03	D10.39	D37.09	D49.0
mucosa	C03.9	C79.89	D00.03	D10.39	D37.09	D49.0
lower	C03.1	C79.89	D00.03	D10.39	D37.09	D49.0
upper	C03.0	C79.89	D00.03	D10.39	D37.09	D49.0
ridge or process	C41.1	C79.51	—	D16.5	D48.0	D49.2
carcinoma	C03.9	C79.8-☑	—	—	—	—
lower	C03.1	C79.8-☑	—	—	—	—
upper	C03.0	C79.8-☑	—	—	—	—
lower	C41.1	C79.51	—	D16.5	D48.0	D49.2
mucosa	C03.9	C79.89	D00.03	D10.39	D37.09	D49.0
lower	C03.1	C79.89	D00.03	D10.39	D37.09	D49.0
upper	C03.0	C79.89	D00.03	D10.39	D37.09	D49.0
upper	C41.0	C79.51	—	D16.4	D48.0	D49.2
sulcus	C06.1	C79.89	D00.02	D10.39	D37.09	D49.0
alveolus	C03.9	C79.89	D00.03	D10.39	D37.09	D49.0
lower	C03.1	C79.89	D00.03	D10.39	D37.09	D49.0
upper	C03.0	C79.89	D00.03	D10.39	D37.09	D49.0
ampulla of Vater	C24.1	C78.89	D01.5	D13.5	D37.6	D49.0
ankle NEC	C76.5-☑	C79.89	D04.7-☑	D36.7	D48.7	D49.89
anorectum, anorectal (junction)	C21.8	C78.5	D01.3	D12.9	D37.8	D49.0
antecubital fossa or space	C76.4-☑	C79.89	D04.6-☑	D36.7	D48.7	D49.89

	Malignant Primary	Malignant Secondary	Ca in situ	Benign	Uncertain	Unspecified Behavior
Neoplasm, neoplastic — *continued*						
antrum (Highmore) (maxillary)	C31.0	C78.39	D02.3	D14.0	D38.5	D49.1
pyloric	C16.3	C78.89	D00.2	D13.1	D37.1	D49.0
tympanicum	C30.1	C78.39	D02.3	D14.0	D38.5	D49.1
anus, anal	C21.0	C78.5	D01.3	D12.9	D37.8	D49.0
canal	C21.1	C78.5	D01.3	D12.9	D37.8	D49.0
cloacogenic zone	C21.2	C78.5	D01.3	D12.9	D37.8	D49.0
margin — *see also* Neoplasm, anus, skin	C44.500	C79.2	D04.5	D23.5	D48.5	D49.2
overlapping lesion with rectosigmoid junction or rectum	C21.8	—	—	—	—	—
skin	C44.500	C79.2	D04.5	D23.5	D48.5	D49.2
basal cell carcinoma	C44.510	—	—	—	—	—
specified type NEC	C44.590	—	—	—	—	—
squamous cell carcinoma	C44.520	—	—	—	—	—
sphincter	C21.1	C78.5	D01.3	D12.9	D37.8	D49.0
aorta (thoracic)	C49.3	C79.89	—	D21.3	D48.1	D49.2
abdominal	C49.4	C79.89	—	D21.4	D48.1	D49.2
aortic body	C75.5	C79.89	—	D35.6	D44.7	D49.7
aponeurosis	C49.9	C79.89	—	D21.9	D48.1	D49.2
palmar	C49.1-☑	C79.89	—	D21.1-☑	D48.1	D49.2
plantar	C49.2-☑	C79.89	—	D21.2-☑	D48.1	D49.2
appendix	C18.1	C78.5	D01.0	D12.1	D37.3	D49.0
arachnoid	C70.9	C79.49	—	D32.9	D42.9	D49.7
cerebral	C70.0	C79.32	—	D32.0	D42.0	D49.7
spinal	C70.1	C79.49	—	D32.1	D42.1	D49.7
areola	C50.0-☑	C79.81	D05-☑	D24-☑	D48.6-☑	D49.3
arm NEC	C76.4-☑	C79.89	D04.6-☑	D36.7	D48.7	D49.89
artery — *see* Neoplasm, connective tissue						
aryepiglottic fold	C13.1	C79.89	D00.08	D10.7	D37.05	D49.0
hypopharyngeal aspect	C13.1	C79.89	D00.08	D10.7	D37.05	D49.0
laryngeal aspect	C32.1	C78.39	D02.0	D14.1	D38.0	D49.1
marginal zone	C13.1	C79.89	D00.08	D10.7	D37.05	D49.0
arytenoid (cartilage)	C32.3	C78.39	D02.0	D14.1	D38.0	D49.1
fold — *see* Neoplasm, aryepiglottic						
associated with transplanted organ	C80.2	—	—	—	—	—
atlas	C41.2	C79.51	—	D16.6	D48.0	D49.2
atrium, cardiac	C38.0	C79.89	—	D15.1	D48.7	D49.89
auditory						
canal (external) (skin)	C44.20-☑	C79.2	D04.2-☑	D23.2-☑	D48.5	D49.2
internal	C30.1	C78.39	D02.3	D14.0	D38.5	D49.1
nerve	C72.4-☑	C79.49	—	D33.3	D43.3	D49.7
tube	C30.1	C78.39	D02.3	D14.0	D38.5	D49.1
opening	C11.2	C79.89	D00.08	D10.6	D37.05	D49.0
auricle, ear — *see also* Neoplasm, skin, ear	C44.20-☑	C79.2	D04.2-☑	D23.2-☑	D48.5	D49.2
auricular canal (external) — *see also* Neoplasm, skin, ear	C44.20-☑	C79.2	D04.2-☑	D23.2-☑	D48.5	D49.2
internal	C30.1	C78.39	D02.3	D14.0	D38.5	D49.2
autonomic nerve or nervous system NEC (see Neoplasm, nerve, peripheral)						
axilla, axillary	C76.1	C79.89	D09.8	D36.7	D48.7	D49.89
fold — *see also* Neoplasm, skin, trunk	C44.509	C79.2	D04.5	D23.5	D48.5	D49.2
back NEC	C76.8	C79.89	D04.5	D36.7	D48.7	D49.89
Bartholin's gland	C51.0	C79.82	D07.1	D28.0	D39.8	D49.59
basal ganglia	C71.0	C79.31	—	D33.0	D43.0	D49.6
basis pedunculi	C71.7	C79.31	—	D33.1	D43.1	D49.6
bile or biliary (tract)	C24.9	C78.89	D01.5	D13.5	D37.6	D49.0
canaliculi (biliferi) (intrahepatic)	C22.1	C78.7	D01.5	D13.4	D37.6	D49.0
canals, interlobular	C22.1	C78.89	D01.5	D13.4	D37.6	D49.0

Neoplasm, neoplastic — continued

	Malignant Primary	Malignant Secondary	Ca in situ	Benign	Uncertain	Unspecified Behavior
bile or biliary — *continued*						
duct or passage (common) (cystic) (extrahepatic)	C24.0	C78.89	D01.5	D13.5	D37.6	D49.0
interlobular	C22.1	C78.89	D01.5	D13.4	D37.6	D49.0
intrahepatic	C22.1	C78.7	D01.5	D13.4	D37.6	D49.0
and extrahepatic	C24.8	C78.89	D01.5	D13.5	D37.6	D49.0
bladder (urinary)	C67.9	C79.11	D09.0	D30.3	D41.4	D49.4
dome	C67.1	C79.11	D09.0	D30.3	D41.4	D49.4
neck	C67.5	C79.11	D09.0	D30.3	D41.4	D49.4
orifice	C67.9	C79.11	D09.0	D30.3	D41.4	D49.4
ureteric	C67.6	C79.11	D09.0	D30.3	D41.4	D49.4
urethral	C67.5	C79.11	D09.0	D30.3	D41.4	D49.4
overlapping lesion	C67.8	—	—	—	—	—
sphincter	C67.8	C79.11	D09.0	D30.3	D41.4	D49.4
trigone	C67.0	C79.11	D09.0	D30.3	D41.4	D49.4
urachus	C67.7	C79.11	D09.0	D30.3	D41.4	D49.4
wall	C67.9	C79.11	D09.0	D30.3	D41.4	D49.4
anterior	C67.3	C79.11	D09.0	D30.3	D41.4	D49.4
lateral	C67.2	C79.11	D09.0	D30.3	D41.4	D49.4
posterior	C67.4	C79.11	D09.0	D30.3	D41.4	D49.4
blood vessel — *see* Neoplasm, connective tissue						
bone (periosteum)	C41.9	C79.51	—	D16.9	D48.0	D49.2
acetabulum	C41.4	C79.51	—	D16.8	D48.0	D49.2
ankle	C40.3-✓	C79.51	—	D16.3-✓	—	—
arm NEC	C40.0-✓	C79.51	—	D16.0-✓	—	—
astragalus	C40.3-✓	C79.51	—	D16.3-✓	—	—
atlas	C41.2	C79.51	—	D16.6	D48.0	D49.2
axis	C41.2	C79.51	—	D16.6	D48.0	D49.2
back NEC	C41.2	C79.51	—	D16.6	D48.0	D49.2
calcaneus	C40.3-✓	C79.51	—	D16.3-✓	—	—
calvarium	C41.0	C79.51	—	D16.4	D48.0	D49.2
carpus (any)	C40.1-✓	C79.51	—	D16.1-✓	—	—
cartilage NEC	C41.9	C79.51	—	D16.9	D48.0	D49.2
clavicle	C41.3	C79.51	—	D16.7	D48.0	D49.2
clivus	C41.0	C79.51	—	D16.4	D48.0	D49.2
coccygeal vertebra	C41.4	C79.51	—	D16.8	D48.0	D49.2
coccyx	C41.4	C79.51	—	D16.8	D48.0	D49.2
costal cartilage	C41.3	C79.51	—	D16.7	D48.0	D49.2
costovertebral joint	C41.3	C79.51	—	D16.7	D48.0	D49.2
cranial	C41.0	C79.51	—	D16.4	D48.0	D49.2
cuboid	C40.3-✓	C79.51	—	D16.3-✓	—	—
cuneiform	C41.9	C79.51	—	D16.9	D48.0	D49.2
elbow	C40.0-✓	C79.51	—	D16.0-✓	—	—
ethmoid (labyrinth)	C41.0	C79.51	—	D16.4	D48.0	D49.2
face	C41.0	C79.51	—	D16.4	D48.0	D49.2
femur (any part)	C40.2-✓	C79.51	—	D16.2-✓	—	—
fibula (any part)	C40.2-✓	C79.51	—	D16.2-✓	—	—
finger (any)	C40.1-✓	C79.51	—	D16.1-✓	—	—
foot	C40.3-✓	C79.51	—	D16.3-✓	—	—
forearm	C40.0-✓	C79.51	—	D16.0-✓	—	—
frontal	C41.0	C79.51	—	D16.4	D48.0	D49.2
hand	C40.1-✓	C79.51	—	D16.1-✓	—	—
heel	C40.3-✓	C79.51	—	D16.3-✓	—	—
hip	C41.4	C79.51	—	D16.8	D48.0	D49.2
humerus (any part)	C40.0-✓	C79.51	—	D16.0-✓	—	—
hyoid	C41.0	C79.51	—	D16.4	D48.0	D49.2
ilium	C41.4	C79.51	—	D16.8	D48.0	D49.2
innominate	C41.4	C79.51	—	D16.8	D48.0	D49.2
intervertebral cartilage or disc	C41.2	C79.51	—	D16.6	D48.0	D49.2
ischium	C41.4	C79.51	—	D16.8	D48.0	D49.2
jaw (lower)	C41.1	C79.51	—	D16.5	D48.0	D49.2
knee	C40.2-✓	C79.51	—	D16.2-✓	—	—
leg NEC	C40.2-✓	C79.51	—	D16.2-✓	—	—
limb NEC	C40.9-✓	C79.51	—	D16.9	—	—
lower (long bones)	C40.2-✓	C79.51	—	D16.2-✓	—	—
short bones	C40.3-✓	C79.51	—	D16.3-✓	—	—
upper (long bones)	C40.0-✓	C79.51	—	D16.0-✓	—	—
short bones	C40.1-✓	C79.51	—	D16.1-✓	—	—
malar	C41.0	C79.51	—	D16.4	D48.0	D49.2

Neoplasm, neoplastic — continued

	Malignant Primary	Malignant Secondary	Ca in situ	Benign	Uncertain	Unspecified Behavior
bone — *continued*						
mandible	C41.1	C79.51	—	D16.5	D48.0	D49.2
marrow NEC (any bone)	C96.9	C79.52	—	—	D47.9	D49.89
mastoid	C41.0	C79.51	—	D16.4	D48.0	D49.2
maxilla, maxillary (superior)	C41.0	C79.51	—	D16.4	D48.0	D49.2
inferior	C41.1	C79.51	—	D16.5	D48.0	D49.2
metacarpus (any)	C40.1-✓	C79.51	—	D16.1-✓	—	—
metatarsus (any)	C40.3-✓	C79.51	—	D16.3-✓	—	—
navicular						
ankle	C40.3-✓	C79.51	—	—	—	—
hand	C40.1-✓	C79.51	—	—	—	—
nose, nasal	C41.0	C79.51	—	D16.4	D48.0	D49.2
occipital	C41.0	C79.51	—	D16.4	D48.0	D49.2
orbit	C41.0	C79.51	—	D16.4	D48.0	D49.2
overlapping sites	C40.8-✓	—	—	—	—	—
parietal	C41.0	C79.51	—	D16.4	D48.0	D49.2
patella	C40.2-✓	C79.51	—	—	—	—
pelvic	C41.4	C79.51	—	D16.8	D48.0	D49.2
phalanges						
foot	C40.3-✓	C79.51	—	—	—	—
hand	C40.1-✓	C79.51	—	—	—	—
pubic	C41.4	C79.51	—	D16.8	D48.0	D49.2
radius (any part)	C40.0-✓	C79.51	—	D16.0-✓	—	—
rib	C41.3	C79.51	—	D16.7	D48.0	D49.2
sacral vertebra	C41.4	C79.51	—	D16.8	D48.0	D49.2
sacrum	C41.4	C79.51	—	D16.8	D48.0	D49.2
scaphoid						
of ankle	C40.3-✓	C79.51	—	—	—	—
of hand	C40.1-✓	C79.51	—	—	—	—
scapula (any part)	C40.0-✓	C79.51	—	D16.0-✓	—	—
sella turcica	C41.0	C79.51	—	D16.4	D48.0	D49.2
shoulder	C40.0-✓	C79.51	—	D16.0-✓	—	—
skull	C41.0	C79.51	—	D16.4	D48.0	D49.2
sphenoid	C41.0	C79.51	—	D16.4	D48.0	D49.2
spine, spinal (column)	C41.2	C79.51	—	D16.6	D48.0	D49.2
coccyx	C41.4	C79.51	—	D16.8	D48.0	D49.2
sacrum	C41.4	C79.51	—	D16.8	D48.0	D49.2
sternum	C41.3	C79.51	—	D16.7	D48.0	D49.2
tarsus (any)	C40.3-✓	C79.51	—	—	—	—
temporal	C41.0	C79.51	—	D16.4	D48.0	D49.2
thumb	C40.1-✓	C79.51	—	—	—	—
tibia (any part)	C40.2-✓	C79.51	—	—	—	—
toe (any)	C40.3-✓	C79.51	—	—	—	—
trapezium	C40.1-✓	C79.51	—	—	—	—
trapezoid	C40.1-✓	C79.51	—	—	—	—
turbinate	C41.0	C79.51	—	D16.4	D48.0	D49.2
ulna (any part)	C40.0-✓	C79.51	—	D16.0-✓	—	—
unciform	C40.1-✓	C79.51	—	—	—	—
vertebra (column)	C41.2	C79.51	—	D16.6	D48.0	D49.2
coccyx	C41.4	C79.51	—	D16.8	D48.0	D49.2
sacrum	C41.4	C79.51	—	D16.8	D48.0	D49.2
vomer	C41.0	C79.51	—	D16.4	D48.0	D49.2
wrist	C40.1-✓	C79.51	—	—	—	—
xiphoid process	C41.3	C79.51	—	D16.7	D48.0	D49.2
zygomatic	C41.0	C79.51	—	D16.4	D48.0	D49.2
book-leaf (mouth) — *ventral surface of tongue and floor of mouth*	C06.89	C79.89	D00.00	D10.39	D37.09	D49.0
bowel — *see* Neoplasm, intestine						
brachial plexus	C47.1-✓	C79.89	—	D36.12	D48.2	D49.2
brain NEC	C71.9	C79.31	—	D33.2	D43.2	D49.6
basal ganglia	C71.0	C79.31	—	D33.0	D43.0	D49.6
cerebellopontine angle	C71.6	C79.31	—	D33.1	D43.1	D49.6
cerebellum NOS	C71.6	C79.31	—	D33.1	D43.1	D49.6
cerebrum	C71.0	C79.31	—	D33.0	D43.0	D49.6
choroid plexus	C71.7	C79.31	—	D33.1	D43.1	D49.6
corpus callosum	C71.8	C79.31	—	D33.2	D43.2	D49.6
corpus striatum	C71.0	C79.31	—	D33.0	D43.0	D49.6
cortex (cerebral)	C71.0	C79.31	—	D33.0	D43.0	D49.6
frontal lobe	C71.1	C79.31	—	D33.0	D43.0	D49.6
globus pallidus	C71.0	C79.31	—	D33.0	D43.0	D49.6
hippocampus	C71.2	C79.31	—	D33.0	D43.0	D49.6
hypothalamus	C71.0	C79.31	—	D33.0	D43.0	D49.6
internal capsule	C71.0	C79.31	—	D33.0	D43.0	D49.6

Neoplasm, neoplastic — continued

	Malignant Primary	Malignant Secondary	Ca in situ	Benign	Uncertain	Unspecified Behavior
brain — continued						
medulla						
oblongata	C71.7	C79.31	—	D33.1	D43.1	D49.6
meninges	C70.0	C79.32	—	D32.0	D42.0	D49.7
midbrain	C71.7	C79.31	—	D33.1	D43.1	D49.6
occipital lobe	C71.4	C79.31	—	D33.0	D43.0	D49.6
overlapping lesion	C71.8	C79.31	—	—	—	—
parietal lobe	C71.3	C79.31	—	D33.0	D43.0	D49.6
peduncle	C71.7	C79.31	—	D33.1	D43.1	D49.6
pons	C71.7	C79.31	—	D33.1	D43.1	D49.6
stem	C71.7	C79.31	—	D33.1	D43.1	D49.6
tapetum	C71.8	C79.31	—	D33.2	D43.2	D49.6
temporal lobe	C71.2	C79.31	—	D33.0	D43.0	D49.6
thalamus	C71.0	C79.31	—	D33.0	D43.0	D49.6
uncus	C71.2	C79.31	—	D33.0	D43.0	D49.6
ventricle (floor)	C71.5	C79.31	—	D33.0	D43.0	D49.6
fourth	C71.7	C79.31	—	D33.1	D43.1	D49.6
branchial (cleft) (cyst) (vestiges)	C10.4	C79.89	D00.08	D10.5	D37.05	D49.0
breast (connective tissue) (glandular tissue) (soft parts)	C50.9-✓	C79.81	D05.-✓	D24.-✓	D48.6-✓	D49.3
areola	C50.0-✓	C79.81	D05.-✓	D24.-✓	D48.6-✓	D49.3
axillary tail	C50.6-✓	C79.81	D05.-✓	D24.-✓	D48.6-✓	D49.3
central portion	C50.1-✓	C79.81	D05.-✓	D24.-✓	D48.6-✓	D49.3
inner	C50.8-✓	C79.81	D05.-✓	D24.-✓	D48.6-✓	D49.3
lower	C50.8-✓	C79.81	D05.-✓	D24.-✓	D48.6-✓	D49.3
lower-inner quadrant	C50.3-✓	C79.81	D05.-✓	D24.-✓	D48.6-✓	D49.3
lower-outer quadrant	C50.5-✓	C79.81	D05.-✓	D24.-✓	D48.6-✓	D49.3
mastectomy site (skin) — see also Neoplasm, breast, skin	C44.501	C79.2	—	—	—	—
specified as breast tissue	C50.8-✓	C79.81	—	—	—	—
midline	C50.8-✓	C79.81	D05.-✓	D24.-✓	D48.6-✓	D49.3
nipple	C50.0-✓	C79.81	D05.-✓	D24.-✓	D48.6-✓	D49.3
outer	C50.8-✓	C79.81	D05.-✓	D24.-✓	D48.6-✓	D49.3
overlapping lesion	C50.8-✓	—	—	—	—	—
skin	C44.501	C79.2	D04.5	D23.5	D48.5	D49.2
basal cell carcinoma	C44.511	—	—	—	—	—
specified type NEC	C44.591	—	—	—	—	—
squamous cell carcinoma	C44.521	—	—	—	—	—
tail (axillary)	C50.6-✓	C79.81	D05.-✓	D24.-✓	D48.6-✓	D49.3
upper	C50.8-✓	C79.81	D05.-✓	D24.-✓	D48.6-✓	D49.3
upper-inner quadrant	C50.2-✓	C79.81	D05.-✓	D24.-✓	D48.6-✓	D49.3
upper-outer quadrant	C50.4-✓	C79.81	D05.-✓	D24.-✓	D48.6-✓	D49.3
broad ligament	C57.1-✓	C79.82	D07.39	D28.2	D39.8	D49.59
bronchiogenic, bronchogenic (lung)	C34.9-✓	C78.0-✓	D02.2-✓	D14.3-✓	D38.1	D49.1
bronchiole	C34.9-✓	C78.0-✓	D02.2-✓	D14.3-✓	D38.1	D49.1
bronchus	C34.9-✓	C78.0-✓	D02.2-✓	D14.3-✓	D38.1	D49.1
carina	C34.0-✓	C78.0-✓	D02.2-✓	D14.3-✓	D38.1	D49.1
lower lobe of lung	C34.3-✓	C78.0-✓	D02.2-✓	D14.3-✓	D38.1	D49.1
main	C34.0-✓	C78.0-✓	D02.2-✓	D14.3-✓	D38.1	D49.1
middle lobe of lung	C34.2	C78.0-✓	D02.21	D14.31	D38.1	D49.1
overlapping lesion	C34.8-✓	—	—	—	—	—
upper lobe of lung	C34.1-✓	C78.0-✓	D02.2-✓	D14.3-✓	D38.1	D49.1
brow	C44.309	C79.2	D04.39	D23.39	D48.5	D49.2
basal cell carcinoma	C44.319	—	—	—	—	—
specified type NEC	C44.399	—	—	—	—	—
squamous cell carcinoma	C44.329	—	—	—	—	—
buccal (cavity)	C06.9	C79.89	D00.00	D10.39	D37.09	D49.0
commissure	C06.0	C79.89	D00.02	D10.39	D37.09	D49.0
groove (lower) (upper)	C06.1	C79.89	D00.02	D10.39	D37.09	D49.0
mucosa	C06.0	C79.89	D00.02	D10.39	D37.09	D49.0
sulcus (lower) (upper)	C06.1	C79.89	D00.02	D10.39	D37.09	D49.0

Neoplasm, neoplastic — continued

	Malignant Primary	Malignant Secondary	Ca in situ	Benign	Uncertain	Unspecified Behavior
bulbourethral gland	C68.0	C79.19	D09.19	D30.4	D41.3	D49.59
bursa — see Neoplasm, connective tissue						
buttock NEC	C76.3	C79.89	D04.5	D36.7	D48.7	D49.89
calf	C76.5-✓	C79.89	D04.7-✓	D36.7	D48.7	D49.89
calvarium	C41.0	C79.51	—	D16.4	D48.0	D49.2
calyx, renal	C65.-✓	C79.0-✓	D09.19	D30.1-✓	D41.1-✓	D49.51-✓
canal						
anal	C21.1	C78.5	D01.3	D12.9	D37.8	D49.0
auditory (external) — see also Neoplasm, skin, ear	C44.20-✓	C79.2	D04.2-✓	D23.2-✓	D48.5	D49.2
auricular (external) — see also Neoplasm, skin, ear	C44.20-✓	C79.2	D04.2-✓	D23.2-✓	D48.5	D49.2
canaliculi, biliary (biliferi) (intrahepatic)	C22.1	C78.7	D01.5	D13.4	D37.6	D49.0
canthus (eye) (inner) (outer)	C44.10-✓	C79.2	D04.1-✓	D23.1-✓	D48.5	D49.2
basal cell carcinoma	C44.11-✓	—	—	—	—	—
specified type NEC	C44.19-✓	—	—	—	—	—
squamous cell carcinoma	C44.12-✓	—	—	—	—	—
capillary — see Neoplasm, connective tissue						
caput coli	C18.0	C78.5	D01.0	D12.0	D37.4	D49.0
carcinoid — see Tumor, carcinoid						
cardia (gastric)	C16.0	C78.89	D00.2	D13.1	D37.1	D49.0
cardiac orifice (stomach)	C16.0	C78.89	D00.2	D13.1	D37.1	D49.0
cardio-esophageal junction	C16.0	C78.89	D00.2	D13.1	D37.1	D49.0
cardio-esophagus	C16.0	C78.89	D00.2	D13.1	D37.1	D49.0
carina (bronchus)	C34.0-✓	C78.0-✓	D02.2-✓	D14.3-✓	D38.1	D49.1
carotid (artery)	C49.0	C79.89	—	D21.0	D48.1	D49.2
body	C75.4	C79.89	—	D35.5	D44.6	D49.7
carpus (any bone)	C40.1-✓	C79.51	—	D16.1-✓	—	D49.2
cartilage (articular) (joint) NEC — see also Neoplasm, bone	C41.9	C79.51	—	D16.9	D48.0	D49.2
arytenoid	C32.3	C78.39	D02.0	D14.1	D38.0	D49.1
auricular	C49.0	C79.89	—	D21.0	D48.1	D49.2
bronchi	C34.0-✓	C78.39	—	D14.3-✓	D38.1	D49.1
costal	C41.3	C79.51	—	D16.7	D48.0	D49.2
cricoid	C32.3	C78.39	D02.0	D14.1	D38.0	D49.1
cuneiform	C32.3	C78.39	D02.0	D14.1	D38.0	D49.1
ear (external)	C49.0	C79.89	—	D21.0	D48.1	D49.2
ensiform	C41.3	C79.51	—	D16.7	D48.0	D49.2
epiglottis	C32.1	C78.39	D02.0	D14.1	D38.0	D49.1
anterior surface	C10.1	C79.89	D00.08	D10.5	D37.05	D49.0
eyelid	C49.0	C79.89	—	D21.0	D48.1	D49.2
intervertebral	C41.2	C79.51	—	D16.6	D48.0	D49.2
larynx, laryngeal	C32.3	C78.39	D02.0	D14.1	D38.0	D49.1
nose, nasal	C30.0	C78.39	D02.3	D14.0	D38.5	D49.1
pinna	C49.0	C79.89	—	D21.0	D48.1	D49.2
rib	C41.3	C79.51	—	D16.7	D48.0	D49.2
semilunar (knee)	C40.2-✓	C79.51	—	D16.2-✓	D48.0	D49.2
thyroid	C32.3	C78.39	D02.0	D14.1	D38.0	D49.1
trachea	C33	C78.39	D02.1	D14.2	D38.1	D49.1
cauda equina	C72.1	C79.49	—	D33.4	D43.4	D49.7
cavity						
buccal	C06.9	C79.89	D00.00	D10.30	D37.09	D49.0
nasal	C30.0	C78.39	D02.3	D14.0	D38.5	D49.1
oral	C06.9	C79.89	D00.00	D10.30	D37.09	D49.0
peritoneal	C48.2	C78.6	—	D20.1	D48.4	D49.0
tympanic	C30.1	C78.39	D02.3	D14.0	D38.5	D49.1
cecum	C18.0	C78.5	D01.0	D12.0	D37.4	D49.0
central nervous system	C72.9	C79.40	—	—	—	—
cerebellopontine (angle)	C71.6	C79.31	—	D33.1	D43.1	D49.6
cerebellum, cerebellar	C71.6	C79.31	—	D33.1	D43.1	D49.6
cerebrum, cerebral (cortex) (hemisphere) (white matter)	C71.0	C79.31	—	D33.0	D43.0	D49.6
meninges	C70.0	C79.32	—	D32.0	D42.0	D49.7
peduncle	C71.7	C79.31	—	D33.1	D43.1	D49.6

Neoplasm, neoplastic — continued	Malignant Primary	Malignant Secondary	Ca in situ	Benign	Uncertain	Unspecified Behavior
cerebrum, cerebral — continued						
ventricle	C71.5	C79.31	—	D33.0	D43.0	D49.6
fourth	C71.7	C79.31	—	D33.1	D43.1	D49.6
cervical region	C76.0	C79.89	D09.8	D36.7	D48.7	D49.89
cervix (cervical) (uteri) (uterus)	C53.9	C79.82	D06.9	D26.0	D39.0	D49.59
canal	C53.0	C79.82	D06.0	D26.0	D39.0	D49.59
endocervix (canal) (gland)	C53.0	C79.82	D06.0	D26.0	D39.0	D49.59
exocervix	C53.1	C79.82	D06.1	D26.0	D39.0	D49.59
external os	C53.1	C79.82	D06.1	D26.0	D39.0	D49.59
internal os	C53.0	C79.82	D06.0	D26.0	D39.0	D49.59
nabothian gland	C53.0	C79.82	D06.0	D26.0	D39.0	D49.59
overlapping lesion	C53.8	—	—	—	—	—
squamocolumnar junction	C53.8	C79.82	D06.7	D26.0	D39.0	D49.59
stump	C53.8	C79.82	D06.7	D26.0	D39.0	D49.59
cheek	C76.0	C79.89	D09.8	D36.7	D48.7	D49.89
external	C44.309	C79.2	D04.39	D23.39	D48.5	D49.2
basal cell carcinoma	C44.319	—	—	—	—	—
specified type NEC	C44.399	—	—	—	—	—
squamous cell carcinoma	C44.329	—	—	—	—	—
inner aspect	C06.0	C79.89	D00.02	D10.39	D37.09	D49.0
internal	C06.0	C79.89	D00.02	D10.39	D37.09	D49.0
mucosa	C06.0	C79.89	D00.02	D10.39	D37.09	D49.0
chest (wall) NEC	C76.1	C79.89	D09.8	D36.7	D48.7	D49.89
chiasma opticum	C72.3-✔	C79.49	—	D33.3	D43.3	D49.7
chin	C44.309	C79.2	D04.39	D23.39	D48.5	D49.2
basal cell carcinoma	C44.319	—	—	—	—	—
specified type NEC	C44.399	—	—	—	—	—
squamous cell carcinoma	C44.329	—	—	—	—	—
choana	C11.3	C79.89	D00.08	D10.6	D37.05	D49.0
cholangiole	C22.1	C78.89	D01.5	D13.4	D37.6	D49.0
choledochal duct	C24.0	C78.89	D01.5	D13.5	D37.6	D49.0
choroid	C69.3-✔	C79.49	D09.2-✔	D31.3-✔	D48.7	D49.81
plexus	C71.5	C79.31	—	D33.0	D43.0	D49.6
ciliary body	C69.4-✔	C79.49	D09.2-✔	D31.4-✔	D48.7	D49.89
clavicle	C41.3	C79.51	—	D16.7	D48.0	D49.2
clitoris	C51.2	C79.82	D07.1	D28.0	D39.8	D49.59
clivus	C41.0	C79.51	—	D16.4	D48.0	D49.2
cloacogenic zone	C21.2	C78.5	D01.3	D12.9	D37.8	D49.0
coccygeal						
body or glomus	C49.5	C79.89	—	D21.5	D48.1	D49.2
vertebra	C41.4	C79.51	—	D16.8	D48.0	D49.2
coccyx	C41.4	C79.51	—	D16.8	D48.0	D49.2
colon — see also Neoplasm, intestine, large	C18.9	C78.5	—	—	—	—
with rectum	C19	C78.5	D01.1	D12.7	D37.5	D49.0
columnella — see also Neoplasm, skin, face	C44.390	C79.2	D04.39	D23.39	D48.5	D49.2
column, spinal — see Neoplasm, spine						
commissure						
labial, lip	C00.6	C79.89	D00.01	D10.39	D37.01	D49.0
laryngeal	C32.0	C78.39	D02.0	D14.1	D38.0	D49.1
common (bile) duct	C24.0	C78.89	D01.5	D13.5	D37.6	D49.0
concha — see also Neoplasm, skin, ear	C44.20-✔	C79.2	D04.2-✔	D23.2-✔	D48.5	D49.2
nose	C30.0	C78.39	D02.3	D14.0	D38.5	D49.1
conjunctiva	C69.0-✔	C79.49	D09.2-✔	D31.0-✔	D48.7	D49.89

Neoplasm, neoplastic — continued	Malignant Primary	Malignant Secondary	Ca in situ	Benign	Uncertain	Unspecified Behavior
connective tissue NEC	C49.9	C79.89	—	D21.9	D48.1	D49.2

Note: For neoplasms of connective tissue (blood vessel, bursa, fascia, ligament, muscle, peripheral nerves, sympathetic and parasympathetic nerves and ganglia, synovia, tendon, etc.) or of morphological types that indicate connective tissue, code according to the list under "Neoplasm, connective tissue". For sites that do not appear in this list, code to neoplasm of that site; e.g., fibrosarcoma, pancreas (C25.9)

Note: Morphological types that indicate connective tissue appear in their proper place in the alphabetic index with the instruction "see Neoplasm, connective tissue ...."

	Malignant Primary	Malignant Secondary	Ca in situ	Benign	Uncertain	Unspecified Behavior
abdomen	C49.4	C79.89	—	D21.4	D48.1	D49.2
abdominal wall	C49.4	C79.89	—	D21.4	D48.1	D49.2
ankle	C49.2-✔	C79.89	—	D21.2-✔	D48.1	D49.2
antecubital fossa or space	C49.1-✔	C79.89	—	D21.1-✔	D48.1	D49.2
arm	C49.1-✔	C79.89	—	D21.1-✔	D48.1	D49.2
auricle (ear)	C49.0	C79.89	—	D21.0	D48.1	D49.2
axilla	C49.3	C79.89	—	D21.3	D48.1	D49.2
back	C49.6	C79.89	—	D21.6	D48.1	D49.2
breast — see Neoplasm, breast						
buttock	C49.5	C79.89	—	D21.5	D48.1	D49.2
calf	C49.2-✔	C79.89	—	D21.2-✔	D48.1	D49.2
cervical region	C49.0	C79.89	—	D21.0	D48.1	D49.2
cheek	C49.0	C79.89	—	D21.0	D48.1	D49.2
chest (wall)	C49.3	C79.89	—	D21.3	D48.1	D49.2
chin	C49.0	C79.89	—	D21.0	D48.1	D49.2
diaphragm	C49.3	C79.89	—	D21.3	D48.1	D49.2
ear (external)	C49.0	C79.89	—	D21.0	D48.1	D49.2
elbow	C49.1-✔	C79.89	—	D21.1-✔	D48.1	D49.2
extrarectal	C49.5	C79.89	—	D21.5	D48.1	D49.2
extremity	C49.9	C79.89	—	D21.9	D48.1	D49.2
lower	C49.2-✔	C79.89	—	D21.2-✔	D48.1	D49.2
upper	C49.1-✔	C79.89	—	D21.1-✔	D48.1	D49.2
eyelid	C49.0	C79.89	—	D21.0	D48.1	D49.2
face	C49.0	C79.89	—	D21.0	D48.1	D49.2
finger	C49.1-✔	C79.89	—	D21.1-✔	D48.1	D49.2
flank	C49.6	C79.89	—	D21.6	D48.1	D49.2
foot	C49.2-✔	C79.89	—	D21.2-✔	D48.1	D49.2
forearm	C49.1-✔	C79.89	—	D21.1-✔	D48.1	D49.2
forehead	C49.0	C79.89	—	D21.0	D48.1	D49.2
gastric	C49.4	C79.89	—	D21.4	D48.1	D49.2
gastrointestinal	C49.4	C79.89	—	D21.4	D48.1	D49.2
gluteal region	C49.5	C79.89	—	D21.5	D48.1	D49.2
great vessels NEC	C49.3	C79.89	—	D21.3	D48.1	D49.2
groin	C49.5	C79.89	—	D21.5	D48.1	D49.2
hand	C49.1-✔	C79.89	—	D21.1-✔	D48.1	D49.2
head	C49.0	C79.89	—	D21.0	D48.1	D49.2
heel	C49.2-✔	C79.89	—	D21.2-✔	D48.1	D49.2
hip	C49.2-✔	C79.89	—	D21.2-✔	D48.1	D49.2
hypochondrium	C49.4	C79.89	—	D21.4	D48.1	D49.2
iliopsoas muscle	C49.5	C79.89	—	D21.5	D48.1	D49.2
infraclavicular region	C49.3	C79.89	—	D21.3	D48.1	D49.2
inguinal (canal) (region)	C49.5	C79.89	—	D21.5	D48.1	D49.2
intestinal	C49.4	C79.89	—	D21.4	D48.1	D49.2
intrathoracic	C49.3	C79.89	—	D21.3	D48.1	D49.2
ischiorectal fossa	C49.5	C79.89	—	D21.5	D48.1	D49.2
jaw	C03.9	C79.89	D00.03	D10.39	D48.1	D49.0
knee	C49.2-✔	C79.89	—	D21.2-✔	D48.1	D49.2
leg	C49.2-✔	C79.89	—	D21.2-✔	D48.1	D49.2
limb NEC	C49.9	C79.89	—	D21.9	D48.1	D49.2
lower	C49.2-✔	C79.89	—	D21.2-✔	D48.1	D49.2
upper	C49.1-✔	C79.89	—	D21.1-✔	D48.1	D49.2
nates	C49.5	C79.89	—	D21.5	D48.1	D49.2
neck	C49.0	C79.89	—	D21.0	D48.1	D49.2
orbit	C69.6-✔	C79.49	D09.2-✔	D31.6-✔	D48.1	D49.89
overlapping lesion	C49.8	—	—	—	—	—
pararectal	C49.5	C79.89	—	D21.5	D48.1	D49.2
para-urethral	C49.5	C79.89	—	D21.5	D48.1	D49.2
paravaginal	C49.5	C79.89	—	D21.5	D48.1	D49.2
pelvis (floor)	C49.5	C79.89	—	D21.5	D48.1	D49.2
pelvo-abdominal	C49.8	C79.89	—	D21.6	D48.1	D49.2
perineum	C49.5	C79.89	—	D21.5	D48.1	D49.2
perirectal (tissue)	C49.5	C79.89	—	D21.5	D48.1	D49.2

✔ Additional Character Required — Refer to the Tabular List for Character Selection   Subterms under main terms may continue to next column or page

	Malignant Primary	Malignant Secondary	Ca in situ	Benign	Uncertain	Unspecified Behavior
Neoplasm, neoplastic — *continued*						
connective tissue — *continued*						
periurethral (tissue)	C49.5	C79.89	—	D21.5	D48.1	D49.2
popliteal fossa or space	C49.2-✓	C79.89	—	D21.2-✓	D48.1	D49.2
presacral	C49.5	C79.89	—	D21.5	D48.1	D49.2
psoas muscle	C49.4	C79.89	—	D21.4	D48.1	D49.2
pterygoid fossa	C49.0	C79.89	—	D21.0	D48.1	D49.2
rectovaginal septum or wall	C49.5	C79.89	—	D21.5	D48.1	D49.2
rectovesical	C49.5	C79.89	—	D21.5	D48.1	D49.2
retroperitoneum	C48.0	C78.6	—	D20.0	D48.3	D49.0
sacrococcygeal region	C49.5	C79.89	—	D21.5	D48.1	D49.2
scalp	C49.0	C79.89	—	D21.0	D48.1	D49.2
scapular region	C49.3	C79.89	—	D21.3	D48.1	D49.2
shoulder	C49.1-✓	C79.89	—	D21.1-✓	D48.1	D49.2
skin (dermis) NEC — *see also* Neoplasm, skin, by site	C44.90	C79.2	D04.9	D23.9	D48.5	D49.2
stomach	C49.4	C79.89	—	D21.4	D48.1	D49.2
submental	C49.0	C79.89	—	D21.0	D48.1	D49.2
supraclavicular region	C49.0	C79.89	—	D21.0	D48.1	D49.2
temple	C49.0	C79.89	—	D21.0	D48.1	D49.2
temporal region	C49.0	C79.89	—	D21.0	D48.1	D49.2
thigh	C49.2-✓	C79.89	—	D21.2-✓	D48.1	D49.2
thoracic (duct) (wall)	C49.3	C79.89	—	D21.3	D48.1	D49.2
thorax	C49.3	C79.89	—	D21.3	D48.1	D49.2
thumb	C49.1-✓	C79.89	—	D21.1-✓	D48.1	D49.2
toe	C49.2-✓	C79.89	—	D21.2-✓	D48.1	D49.2
trunk	C49.6	C79.89	—	D21.6	D48.1	D49.2
umbilicus	C49.4	C79.89	—	D21.4	D48.1	D49.2
vesicorectal	C49.5	C79.89	—	D21.5	D48.1	D49.2
wrist	C49.1-✓	C79.89	—	D21.1-✓	D48.1	D49.2
conus medullaris	C72.0	C79.49	—	D33.4	D43.4	D49.7
cord (true) (vocal)	C32.0	C78.39	D02.0	D14.1	D38.0	D49.1
false	C32.1	C78.39	D02.0	D14.1	D38.0	D49.1
spermatic	C63.1-✓	C79.82	D07.69	D29.8	D40.8	D49.59
spinal (cervical) (lumbar) (thoracic)	C72.0	C79.49	—	D33.4	D43.4	D49.7
cornea (limbus)	C69.1-✓	C79.49	D09.2-✓	D31.1-✓	D48.7	D49.89
corpus						
albicans	C56.-✓	C79.6-✓	D07.39	D27.-✓	D39.1-✓	D49.59
callosum, brain	C71.0	C79.31	—	D33.2	D43.2	D49.6
cavernosum	C60.2	C79.82	D07.4	D29.0	D40.8	D49.59
gastric	C16.2	C78.89	D00.2	D13.1	D37.1	D49.0
overlapping sites	C54.8	—	—	—	—	—
penis	C60.2	C79.82	D07.4	D29.0	D40.8	D49.59
striatum, cerebrum	C71.0	C79.31	—	D33.0	D43.0	D49.6
uteri	C54.9	C79.82	D07.0	D26.1	D39.0	D49.59
isthmus	C54.0	C79.82	D07.0	D26.1	D39.0	D49.59
cortex						
adrenal	C74.0-✓	C79.7-✓	D09.3	D35.0-✓	D44.1-✓	D49.7
cerebral	C71.0	C79.31	—	D33.0	D43.0	D49.6
costal cartilage	C41.3	C79.51	—	D16.7	D48.0	D49.2
costovertebral joint	C41.3	C79.51	—	D16.7	D48.0	D49.2
Cowper's gland	C68.0	C79.19	D09.19	D30.4	D41.3	D49.59
cranial (fossa, any)	C71.9	C79.31	—	D33.2	D43.2	D49.6
meninges	C70.0	C79.32	—	D32.0	D42.0	D49.7
nerve	C72.50	C79.49	—	D33.3	D43.3	D49.7
specified NEC	C72.59	C79.49	—	D33.3	D43.3	D49.7
craniobuccal pouch	C75.2	C79.89	D09.3	D35.2	D44.3	D49.7
craniopharyngeal (duct) (pouch)	C75.2	C79.89	D09.3	D35.3	D44.4	D49.7
cricoid	C13.0	C79.89	D00.08	D10.7	D37.05	D49.0
cartilage	C32.3	C78.39	D02.0	D14.1	D38.0	D49.1
cricopharynx	C13.0	C79.89	D00.08	D10.7	D37.05	D49.0
crypt of Morgagni	C21.8	C78.5	D01.3	D12.9	D37.8	D49.0
crystalline lens	C69.4-✓	C79.49	D09.2-✓	D31.4-✓	D48.7	D49.89
cul-de-sac (Douglas')	C48.1	C78.6	—	D20.1	D48.4	D49.0
cuneiform cartilage	C32.3	C78.39	D02.0	D14.1	D38.0	D49.1
cutaneous — *see* Neoplasm, skin						
cutis — *see* Neoplasm, skin						

	Malignant Primary	Malignant Secondary	Ca in situ	Benign	Uncertain	Unspecified Behavior
Neoplasm, neoplastic — *continued*						
cystic (bile) duct (common)	C24.0	C78.89	D01.5	D13.5	D37.6	D49.0
dermis — *see* Neoplasm, skin						
diaphragm	C49.3	C79.89	—	D21.3	D48.1	D49.2
digestive organs, system, tube, or tract NEC	C26.9	C78.89	D01.9	D13.9	D37.9	D49.0
disc, intervertebral	C41.2	C79.51	—	D16.6	D48.0	D49.2
disease, generalized	C80.0	—	—	—	—	—
disseminated	C80.0	—	—	—	—	—
Douglas' cul-de-sac or pouch	C48.1	C78.6	—	D20.1	D48.4	D49.0
duodenojejunal junction	C17.8	C78.4	D01.49	D13.39	D37.2	D49.0
duodenum	C17.0	C78.4	D01.49	D13.2	D37.2	D49.0
dura (cranial) (mater)	C70.9	C79.49	—	D32.9	D42.9	D49.7
cerebral	C70.0	C79.32	—	D32.0	D42.0	D49.7
spinal	C70.1	C79.49	—	D32.1	D42.1	D49.7
ear (external) — *see also* Neoplasm, skin, ear	C44.20-✓	C79.2	D04.2-✓	D23.2-✓	D48.5	D49.2
auricle or auris — *see also* Neoplasm, skin, ear	C44.20-✓	C79.2	D04.2-✓	D23.2-✓	D48.5	D49.2
canal, external — *see also* Neoplasm, skin, ear	C44.20-✓	C79.2	D04.2-✓	D23.2-✓	D48.5	D49.2
cartilage	C49.0	C79.89	—	D21.0	D48.1	D49.2
external meatus — *see also* Neoplasm, skin, ear	C44.20-✓	C79.2	D04.2-✓	D23.2-✓	D48.5	D49.2
inner	C30.1	C78.39	D02.3	D14.0	D38.5	D49.1
lobule — *see also* Neoplasm, skin, ear	C44.20-✓	C79.2	D04.2-✓	D23.2-✓	D48.5	D49.2
middle	C30.1	C78.39	D02.3	D14.0	D38.5	D49.1
overlapping lesion with accessory sinuses	C31.8	—	—	—	—	—
skin	C44.20-✓	C79.2	D04.2-✓	D23.2-✓	D48.5	D49.2
basal cell carcinoma	C44.21-✓	—	—	—	—	—
specified type NEC	C44.29-✓	—	—	—	—	—
squamous cell carcinoma	C44.22-✓	—	—	—	—	—
earlobe	C44.20-✓	C79.2	D04.2-✓	D23.2-✓	D48.5	D49.2
basal cell carcinoma	C44.21-✓	—	—	—	—	—
specified type NEC	C44.29-✓	—	—	—	—	—
squamous cell carcinoma	C44.22-✓	—	—	—	—	—
ejaculatory duct	C63.7	C79.82	D07.69	D29.8	D40.8	D49.59
elbow NEC	C76.4-✓	C79.89	D04.6-✓	D36.7	D48.7	D49.89
endocardium	C38.0	C79.89	—	D15.1	D48.7	D49.89
endocervix (canal) (gland)	C53.0	C79.82	D06.0	D26.0	D39.0	D49.59
endocrine gland NEC	C75.9	C79.89	D09.3	D35.9	D44.9	D49.7
pluriglandular	C75.8	C79.89	D09.3	D35.7	D44.9	D49.7
endometrium (gland) (stroma)	C54.1	C79.82	D07.0	D26.1	D39.0	D49.59
ensiform cartilage	C41.3	C79.51	—	D16.7	D48.0	D49.2
enteric — *see* Neoplasm, intestine						
ependyma (brain)	C71.5	C79.31	—	D33.0	D43.0	D49.6
fourth ventricle	C71.7	C79.31	—	D33.1	D43.1	D49.6
epicardium	C38.0	C79.89	—	D15.1	D48.7	D49.89
epididymis	C63.0-✓	C79.82	D07.69	D29.3-✓	D40.8	D49.59
epidural	C72.9	C79.49	—	D33.9	D43.9	D49.7
epiglottis	C32.1	C78.39	D02.0	D14.1	D38.0	D49.1
anterior aspect or surface	C10.1	C79.89	D00.08	D10.5	D37.05	D49.0
cartilage	C32.3	C78.39	D02.0	D14.1	D38.0	D49.1
free border (margin)	C10.1	C79.89	D00.08	D10.5	D37.05	D49.0
junctional region	C10.8	C79.89	D00.08	D10.5	D37.05	D49.0
posterior (laryngeal) surface	C32.1	C78.39	D02.0	D14.1	D38.0	D49.1

	Malignant Primary	Malignant Secondary	Ca in situ	Benign	Uncertain	Unspecified Behavior
Neoplasm, neoplastic — *continued*						
epiglottis — *continued*						
suprahyoid						
portion	C32.1	C78.39	D02.0	D14.1	D38.0	D49.1
esophagogastric						
junction	C16.0	C78.89	D00.2	D13.1	D37.1	D49.0
esophagus	C15.9	C78.89	D00.1	D13.0	D37.8	D49.0
abdominal	C15.5	C78.89	D00.1	D13.0	D37.8	D49.0
cervical	C15.3	C78.89	D00.1	D13.0	D37.8	D49.0
distal (third)	C15.5	C78.89	D00.1	D13.0	D37.8	D49.0
lower (third)	C15.5	C78.89	D00.1	D13.0	D37.8	D49.0
middle (third)	C15.4	C78.89	D00.1	D13.0	D37.8	D49.0
overlapping lesion	C15.8	—	—	—	—	—
proximal (third)	C15.3	C78.89	D00.1	D13.0	D37.8	D49.0
thoracic	C15.4	C78.89	D00.1	D13.0	D37.8	D49.0
upper (third)	C15.3	C78.89	D00.1	D13.0	D37.8	D49.0
ethmoid (sinus)	C31.1	C78.39	D02.3	D14.0	D38.5	D49.1
bone or labyrinth	C41.0	C79.51	—	D16.4	D48.0	D49.2
eustachian tube	C30.1	C78.39	D02.3	D14.0	D38.5	D49.1
exocervix	C53.1	C79.82	D06.1	D26.0	D39.0	D49.59
external						
meatus (ear) — *see also*						
Neoplasm, skin,						
ear	C44.20-☑	C79.2	D04.2-☑	D23.2-☑	D48.5	D49.2
os, cervix uteri	C53.1	C79.82	D06.1	D26.0	D39.0	D49.59
extradural	C72.9	C79.49	—	D33.9	D43.9	D49.7
extrahepatic (bile)						
duct	C24.0	C78.89	D01.5	D13.5	D37.6	D49.0
overlapping lesion with						
gallbladder	C24.8	—	—	—	—	—
extraocular muscle	C69.6-☑	C79.49	D09.2-☑	D31.6-☑	D48.7	D49.89
extrarectal	C76.3	C79.89	D09.8	D36.7	D48.7	D49.89
extremity	C76.8	C79.89	D04.8	D36.7	D48.7	D49.89
lower	C76.5-☑	C79.89	D04.7-☑	D36.7	D48.7	D49.89
upper	C76.4-☑	C79.89	D04.6-☑	D36.7	D48.7	D49.89
eyeball	C69.9-☑	C79.49	D09.2-☑	D31.9-☑	D48.7	D49.89
eyebrow	C44.309	C79.2	D04.39	D23.39	D48.5	D49.2
basal cell						
carcinoma	C44.319	—	—	—	—	—
specified type NEC	C44.399	—	—	—	—	—
squamous cell						
carcinoma	C44.329	—	—	—	—	—
eyelid (lower) (skin)						
(upper)	C44.10-☑	—	—	—	—	—
basal cell						
carcinoma	C44.11-☑	—	—	—	—	—
cartilage	C49.0	C79.89	—	D21.0	D48.1	D49.2
specified type NEC	C44.19-☑	—	—	—	—	—
squamous cell						
carcinoma	C44.12-☑	—	—	—	—	—
eye NEC	C69.9-☑	C79.49	D09.2-☑	D31.9-☑	D48.7	D49.89
overlapping sites	C69.8-☑	—	—	—	—	—
face NEC	C76.0	C79.89	D04.39	D36.7	D48.7	D49.89
fallopian tube						
(accessory)	C57.0-☑	C79.82	D07.39	D28.2	D39.8	D49.59
falx (cerebella)						
(cerebri)	C70.0	C79.32	—	D32.0	D42.0	D49.7
fascia — *see also*						
Neoplasm, connective						
tissue						
palmar	C49.1-☑	C79.89	—	D21.1-☑	D48.1	D49.2
plantar	C49.2-☑	C79.89	—	D21.2-☑	D48.1	D49.2
fatty tissue — *see*						
Neoplasm, connective						
tissue						
fauces, faucial NEC	C10.9	C79.89	D00.08	D10.5	D37.05	D49.0
pillars	C09.1	C79.89	D00.08	D10.5	D37.05	D49.0
tonsil	C09.9	C79.89	D00.08	D10.4	D37.05	D49.0
femur (any part)	C40.2-☑	—	—	D16.2-☑	—	—
fetal membrane	C58	C79.82	D07.0	D26.7	D39.2	D49.59
fibrous tissue — *see*						
Neoplasm, connective						
tissue						
fibula (any part)	C40.2-☑	C79.51	—	D16.2-☑	—	—
filum terminale	C72.0	C79.49	—	D33.4	D43.4	D49.7
finger NEC	C76.4-☑	C79.89	D04.6-☑	D36.7	D48.7	D49.89
flank NEC	C76.8	C79.89	D04.5	D36.7	D48.7	D49.89
follicle, nabothian	C53.0	C79.82	D06.0	D26.0	D39.0	D49.59
foot NEC	C76.5-☑	C79.89	D04.7-☑	D36.7	D48.7	D49.89
forearm NEC	C76.4-☑	C79.89	D04.6-☑	D36.7	D48.7	D49.89
forehead (skin)	C44.309	C79.2	D04.39	D23.39	D48.5	D49.2

	Malignant Primary	Malignant Secondary	Ca in situ	Benign	Uncertain	Unspecified Behavior
Neoplasm, neoplastic — *continued*						
forehead — *continued*						
basal cell						
carcinoma	C44.319	—	—	—	—	—
specified type NEC	C44.399	—	—			
squamous cell						
carcinoma	C44.329	—	—	—	—	—
foreskin	C60.0	C79.82	D07.4	D29.0	D40.8	D49.59
fornix						
pharyngeal	C11.3	C79.89	D00.08	D10.6	D37.05	D49.0
vagina	C52	C79.82	D07.2	D28.1	D39.8	D49.59
fossa (of)						
anterior (cranial)	C71.9	C79.31	—	D33.2	D43.2	D49.6
cranial	C71.9	C79.31	—	D33.2	D43.2	D49.6
ischiorectal	C76.3	C79.89	D09.8	D36.7	D48.7	D49.89
middle (cranial)	C71.9	C79.31	—	D33.2	D43.2	D49.6
piriform	C12	C79.89	D00.08	D10.7	D37.05	D49.0
pituitary	C75.1	C79.89	D09.3	D35.2	D44.3	D49.7
posterior (cranial)	C71.9	C79.31	—	D33.2	D43.2	D49.6
pterygoid	C49.0	C79.89	—	D21.0	D48.1	D49.2
pyriform	C12	C79.89	D00.08	D10.7	D37.05	D49.0
Rosenmuller	C11.2	C79.89	D00.08	D10.6	D37.05	D49.0
tonsillar	C09.0	C79.89	D00.08	D10.5	D37.05	D49.0
fourchette	C51.9	C79.82	D07.1	D28.0	D39.8	D49.59
frenulum						
labii — *see* Neoplasm,						
lip, internal						
linguae	C02.2	C79.89	D00.07	D10.1	D37.02	D49.0
frontal						
bone	C41.0	C79.51	—	D16.4	D48.0	D49.2
lobe, brain	C71.1	C79.31	—	D33.0	D43.0	D49.6
pole	C71.1	C79.31	—	D33.0	D43.0	D49.6
sinus	C31.2	C78.39	D02.3	D14.0	D38.5	D49.1
fundus						
stomach	C16.1	C78.89	D00.2	D13.1	D37.1	D49.0
uterus	C54.3	C79.82	D07.0	D26.1	D39.0	D49.59
gallbladder	C23	C78.89	D01.5	D13.5	D37.6	D49.0
overlapping lesion with						
extrahepatic bile						
ducts	C24.8	—	—	—	—	—
gall duct						
(extrahepatic)	C24.0	C78.89	D01.5	D13.5	D37.6	D49.0
intrahepatic	C22.1	C78.7	D01.5	D13.4	D37.6	D49.0
ganglia — *see also*						
Neoplasm, nerve,						
peripheral	C47.9	C79.89	—	D36.10	D48.2	D49.2
basal	C71.0	C79.31	—	D33.0	D43.0	D49.6
cranial nerve	C72.50	C79.49	—	D33.3	D43.3	D49.7
Gartner's duct	C52	C79.82	D07.2	D28.1	D39.8	D49.59
gastric — *see* Neoplasm,						
stomach						
gastrocolic	C26.9	C78.89	D01.9	D13.9	D37.9	D49.0
gastroesophageal						
junction	C16.0	C78.89	D00.2	D13.1	D37.1	D49.0
gastrointestinal (tract)						
NEC	C26.9	C78.89	D01.9	D13.9	D37.9	D49.0
generalized	C80.0	—	—	—	—	—
genital organ or tract						
female NEC	C57.9	C79.82	D07.30	D28.9	D39.9	D49.59
overlapping						
lesion	C57.8	—	—	—	—	—
specified site						
NEC	C57.7	C79.82	D07.39	D28.7	D39.8	D49.59
male NEC	C63.9	C79.82	D07.60	D29.9	D40.9	D49.59
overlapping						
lesion	C63.8	—	—	—	—	—
specified site						
NEC	C63.7	C79.82	D07.69	D29.8	D40.8	D49.59
genitourinary tract						
female	C57.9	C79.82	D07.30	D28.9	D39.9	D49.59
male	C63.9	C79.82	D07.60	D29.9	D40.9	D49.59
gingiva (alveolar)						
(marginal)	C03.9	C79.89	D00.03	D10.39	D37.09	D49.0
lower	C03.1	C79.89	D00.03	D10.39	D37.09	D49.0
mandibular	C03.1	C79.89	D00.03	D10.39	D37.09	D49.0
maxillary	C03.0	C79.89	D00.03	D10.39	D37.09	D49.0
upper	C03.0	C79.89	D00.03	D10.39	D37.09	D49.0
gland, glandular						
(lymphatic) (system)						
— *see also* Neoplasm,						
lymph gland						
endocrine NEC	C75.9	C79.89	D09.3	D35.9	D44.9	D49.7

Neoplasm, neoplastic — continued	Malignant Primary	Malignant Secondary	Ca in situ	Benign	Uncertain	Unspecified Behavior
gland, glandular — *see also* Neoplasm, lymph gland — *continued*						
salivary — *see* Neoplasm, salivary gland						
glans penis	C60.1	C79.82	D07.4	D29.0	D40.8	D49.59
globus pallidus	C71.0	C79.31	—	D33.0	D43.0	D49.6
glomus						
coccygeal	C49.5	C79.89	—	D21.5	D48.1	D49.2
jugularis	C75.5	C79.89	—	D35.6	D44.7	D49.7
glosso-epiglottic fold(s)	C10.1	C79.89	D00.08	D10.5	D37.05	D49.0
glossopalatine fold	C09.1	C79.89	D00.08	D10.5	D37.05	D49.0
glossopharyngeal sulcus	C09.0	C79.89	D00.08	D10.5	D37.05	D49.0
glottis	C32.0	C78.39	D02.0	D14.1	D38.0	D49.1
gluteal region	C76.3	C79.89	D04.5	D36.7	D48.7	D49.89
great vessels NEC	C49.3	C79.89	—	D21.3	D48.1	D49.2
groin NEC	C76.3	C79.89	D04.5	D36.7	D48.7	D49.89
gum	C03.9	C79.89	D00.03	D10.39	D37.09	D49.0
lower	C03.1	C79.89	D00.03	D10.39	D37.09	D49.0
upper	C03.0	C79.89	D00.03	D10.39	D37.09	D49.0
hand NEC	C76.4-✓	C79.89	D04.6-✓	D36.7	D48.7	D49.89
head NEC	C76.0	C79.89	D04.4	D36.7	D48.7	D49.89
heart	C38.0	C79.89	—	D15.1	D48.7	D49.89
heel NEC	C76.5-✓	C79.89	D04.7-✓	D36.7	D48.7	D49.89
helix — *see also* Neoplasm, skin, ear	C44.20-✓	C79.2	D04.2-✓	D23.2-✓	D48.5	D49.2
hematopoietic, hemopoietic tissue NEC	C96.9	—	—	—	—	—
specified NEC	C96.Z	—	—	—	—	—
hemisphere, cerebral	C71.0	C79.31	—	D33.0	D43.0	D49.6
hemorrhoidal zone	C21.1	C78.5	D01.3	D12.9	D37.8	D49.0
hepatic — *see also* Index to disease, by histology	C22.9	C78.7	D01.5	D13.4	D37.6	D49.0
duct (bile)	C24.0	C78.89	D01.5	D13.5	D37.6	D49.0
flexure (colon)	C18.3	C78.5	D01.0	D12.3	D37.4	D49.0
primary	C22.8	C78.7	D01.5	D13.4	D37.6	D49.0
hepatobiliary	C24.9	C78.89	D01.5	D13.5	D37.6	D49.0
hepatoblastoma	C22.2	C78.7	D01.5	D13.4	D37.6	D49.0
hepatoma	C22.0	C78.7	D01.5	D13.4	D37.6	D49.0
hilus of lung	C34.0-✓	C78.0-✓	D02.2-✓	D14.3-✓	D38.1	D49.1
hippocampus, brain	C71.2	C79.31	—	D33.0	D43.0	D49.6
hip NEC	C76.5-✓	C79.89	D04.7-✓	D36.7	D48.7	D49.89
humerus (any part)	C40.0-✓	C79.51	—	D16.0-✓	—	—
hymen	C52	C79.82	D07.2	D28.1	D39.8	D49.59
hypopharynx, hypopharyngeal NEC	C13.9	C79.89	D00.08	D10.7	D37.05	D49.0
overlapping lesion	C13.8	—	—	—	—	—
postcricoid region	C13.0	C79.89	D00.08	D10.7	D37.05	D49.0
posterior wall	C13.2	C79.89	D00.08	D10.7	D37.05	D49.0
pyriform fossa (sinus)	C12	C79.89	D00.08	D10.7	D37.05	D49.0
hypophysis	C75.1	C79.89	D09.3	D35.2	D44.3	D49.7
hypothalamus	C71.0	C79.31	—	D33.0	D43.0	D49.6
ileocecum, ileocecal (coil) (junction) (valve)	C18.0	C78.5	D01.0	D12.0	D37.4	D49.0
ileum	C17.2	C78.4	D01.49	D13.39	D37.2	D49.0
ilium	C41.4	C79.51	—	D16.8	D48.0	D49.2
immunoproliferative NEC	C88.9	—	—	—	—	—
infraclavicular (region)	C76.1	C79.89	D04.5	D36.7	D48.7	D49.89
inguinal (region)	C76.3	C79.89	D04.5	D36.7	D48.7	D49.89
insula	C71.0	C79.31	—	D33.0	D43.0	D49.6
insular tissue (pancreas)	C25.4	C78.89	D01.7	D13.7	D37.8	D49.0
brain	C71.0	C79.31	—	D33.0	D43.0	D49.6
interarytenoid fold	C13.1	C78.39	D00.08	D10.7	D37.05	D49.0
hypopharyngeal aspect	C13.1	C79.89	D00.08	D10.7	D37.05	D49.0
laryngeal aspect	C32.1	C79.89	D02.0	D14.1	D38.0	D49.1
marginal zone	C13.1	C79.89	D00.08	D10.7	D37.05	D49.0
interdental papillae	C03.9	C79.89	D00.03	D10.39	D37.09	D49.0
Neoplasm, neoplastic — continued						
interdental papillae — *continued*						
lower	C03.1	C79.89	D00.03	D10.39	D37.09	D49.0
upper	C03.0	C79.89	D00.03	D10.39	D37.09	D49.0
internal						
capsule	C71.0	C79.31	—	D33.0	D43.0	D49.6
os (cervix)	C53.0	C79.82	D06.0	D26.0	D39.0	D49.59
intervertebral cartilage or disc	C41.2	C79.51	—	D16.6	D48.0	D49.2
intestine, intestinal	C26.0	C78.80	D01.40	D13.9	D37.8	D49.0
large	C18.9	C78.5	D01.0	D12.6	D37.4	D49.0
appendix	C18.1	C78.5	D01.0	D12.1	D37.3	D49.0
caput coli	C18.0	C78.5	D01.0	D12.0	D37.4	D49.0
cecum	C18.0	C78.5	D01.0	D12.0	D37.4	D49.0
colon	C18.9	C78.5	D01.0	D12.6	D37.4	D49.0
and rectum	C19	C78.5	D01.1	D12.7	D37.5	D49.0
ascending	C18.2	C78.5	D01.0	D12.2	D37.4	D49.0
caput	C18.0	C78.5	D01.0	D12.0	D37.4	D49.0
descending	C18.6	C78.5	D01.0	D12.4	D37.4	D49.0
distal	C18.6	C78.5	D01.0	D12.4	D37.4	D49.0
left	C18.6	C78.5	D01.0	D12.4	D37.4	D49.0
overlapping lesion	C18.8	—	—	—	—	—
pelvic	C18.7	C78.5	D01.0	D12.5	D37.4	D49.0
right	C18.2	C78.5	D01.0	D12.2	D37.4	D49.0
sigmoid (flexure)	C18.7	C78.5	D01.0	D12.5	D37.4	D49.0
transverse	C18.4	C78.5	D01.0	D12.3	D37.4	D49.0
hepatic flexure	C18.3	C78.5	D01.0	D12.3	D37.4	D49.0
ileocecum, ileocecal (coil) (valve)	C18.0	C78.5	D01.0	D12.0	D37.4	D49.0
overlapping lesion	C18.8	—	—	—	—	—
sigmoid flexure (lower) (upper)	C18.7	C78.5	D01.0	D12.5	D37.4	D49.0
splenic flexure	C18.5	C78.5	D01.0	D12.3	D37.4	D49.0
small	C17.9	C78.4	D01.40	D13.30	D37.2	D49.0
duodenum	C17.0	C78.4	D01.49	D13.2	D37.2	D49.0
ileum	C17.2	C78.4	D01.49	D13.39	D37.2	D49.0
jejunum	C17.1	C78.4	D01.49	D13.39	D37.2	D49.0
overlapping lesion	C17.8	—	—	—	—	—
tract NEC	C26.0	C78.89	D01.40	D13.9	D37.8	D49.0
intra-abdominal	C76.2	C79.89	D09.8	D36.7	D48.7	D49.89
intracranial NEC	C71.9	C79.31	—	D33.2	D43.2	D49.6
intrahepatic (bile) duct	C22.1	C78.7	D01.5	D13.4	D37.6	D49.0
intraocular	C69.9-✓	C79.49	D09.2-✓	D31.9-✓	D48.7	D49.89
intraorbital	C69.6-✓	C79.49	D09.2-✓	D31.6-✓	D48.7	D49.89
intrasellar	C75.1	C79.89	D09.3	D35.2	D44.3	D49.7
intrathoracic (cavity) (organs)	C76.1	C79.89	D09.8	D15.9	D48.7	D49.89
specified NEC	C76.1	C79.89	D09.8	D15.7	—	—
iris	C69.4-✓	C79.49	D09.2-✓	D31.4-✓	D48.7	D49.89
ischiorectal (fossa)	C76.3	C79.89	D09.8	D36.7	D48.7	D49.89
ischium	C41.4	C79.51	—	D16.8	D48.0	D49.2
island of Reil	C71.0	C79.31	—	D33.0	D43.0	D49.6
islands or islets of Langerhans	C25.4	C78.89	D01.7	D13.7	D37.8	D49.0
isthmus uteri	C54.0	C79.82	D07.0	D26.1	D39.0	D49.59
jaw	C76.0	C79.89	D09.8	D36.7	D48.7	D49.89
bone	C41.1	C79.51	—	D16.5	D48.0	D49.2
lower	C41.1	C79.51	—	D16.5	—	—
upper	C41.0	C79.51	—	D16.4	—	—
carcinoma (any type) (lower) (upper)	C76.0	C79.89	—	—	—	—
skin — *see also* Neoplasm, skin, face	C44.309	C79.2	D04.39	D23.39	D48.5	D49.2
soft tissues	C03.9	C79.89	D00.03	D10.39	D37.09	D49.0
lower	C03.1	C79.89	D00.03	D10.39	D37.09	D49.0
upper	C03.0	C79.89	D00.03	D10.39	D37.09	D49.0
jejunum	C17.1	C78.4	D01.49	D13.39	D37.2	D49.0
joint NEC — *see also* Neoplasm, bone	C41.9	C79.51	—	D16.9	D48.0	D49.2
acromioclavicular	C40.0-✓	C79.51	—	D16.0-✓		

Neoplasm, neoplastic — continued

	Malignant Primary	Malignant Secondary	Ca in situ	Benign	Uncertain	Unspecified Behavior
joint — *see also* Neoplasm, bone — *continued*						
bursa or synovial membrane — *see* Neoplasm, connective tissue						
costovertebral	C41.3	C79.51	—	D16.7	D48.0	D49.2
sternocostal	C41.3	C79.51	—	D16.7	D48.0	D49.2
temporomandibular	C41.1	C79.51	—	D16.5	D48.0	D49.2
junction						
anorectal	C21.8	C78.5	D01.3	D12.9	D37.8	D49.0
cardioesophageal	C16.0	C78.89	D00.2	D13.1	D37.1	D49.0
esophagogastric	C16.0	C78.89	D00.2	D13.1	D37.1	D49.0
gastroesophageal	C16.0	C78.89	D00.2	D13.1	D37.1	D49.0
hard and soft palate	C05.9	C79.89	D00.00	D10.39	D37.09	D49.0
ileocecal	C18.0	C78.5	D01.0	D12.0	D37.4	D49.0
pelvirectal	C19	C78.5	D01.1	D12.7	D37.5	D49.0
pelviureteric	C65.-☑	C79.0-☑	D09.19	D30.1-☑	D41.1-☑	D49.59
rectosigmoid	C19	C78.5	D01.1	D12.7	D37.5	D49.0
squamocolumnar, of cervix	C53.8	C79.82	D06.7	D26.0	D39.0	D49.59
Kaposi's sarcoma — *see* Kaposi's, sarcoma						
kidney						
(parenchymal)	C64.-☑	C79.0-☑	D09.19	D30.0-☑	D41.0-☑	D49.51-☑
calyx	C65.-☑	C79.0-☑	D09.19	D30.1-☑	D41.1-☑	D49.51-☑
hilus	C65.-☑	C79.0-☑	D09.19	D30.1-☑	D41.1-☑	D49.51-☑
pelvis	C65.-☑	C79.0-☑	D09.19	D30.1-☑	D41.1-☑	D49.51-☑
knee NEC	C76.5-☑	C79.89	D04.7-☑	D36.7	D48.7	D49.89
labia (skin)	C51.9	C79.82	D07.1	D28.0	D39.8	D49.59
majora	C51.0	C79.82	D07.1	D28.0	D39.8	D49.59
minora	C51.1	C79.82	D07.1	D28.0	D39.8	D49.59
labial — *see also* Neoplasm, lip	C00.9	C79.89	D00.01	D10.0	D37.01	D49.0
sulcus (lower) (upper)	C06.1	C79.89	D00.02	D10.39	D37.09	D49.0
labium (skin)	C51.9	C79.82	D07.1	D28.0	D39.8	D49.59
majus	C51.0	C79.82	D07.1	D28.0	D39.8	D49.59
minus	C51.1	C79.82	D07.1	D28.0	D39.8	D49.59
lacrimal						
canaliculi	C69.5-☑	C79.49	D09.2-☑	D31.5-☑	D48.7	D49.89
duct (nasal)	C69.5-☑	C79.49	D09.2-☑	D31.5-☑	D48.7	D49.89
gland	C69.5-☑	C79.49	D09.2-☑	D31.5-☑	D48.7	D49.89
punctum	C69.5-☑	C79.49	D09.2-☑	D31.5-☑	D48.7	D49.89
sac	C69.5-☑	C79.49	D09.2-☑	D31.5-☑	D48.7	D49.89
Langerhans, islands or islets	C25.4	C78.89	D01.7	D13.7	D37.8	D49.0
laryngopharynx	C13.9	C79.89	D00.08	D10.7	D37.05	D49.0
larynx, laryngeal NEC	C32.9	C78.39	D02.0	D14.1	D38.0	D49.1
aryepiglottic fold	C32.1	C78.39	D02.0	D14.1	D38.0	D49.1
cartilage (arytenoid) (cricoid) (cuneiform) (thyroid)	C32.3	C78.39	D02.0	D14.1	D38.0	D49.1
commissure (anterior) (posterior)	C32.0	C78.39	D02.0	D14.1	D38.0	D49.1
extrinsic NEC	C32.1	C78.39	D02.0	D14.1	D38.0	D49.1
meaning hypopharynx	C13.9	C79.89	D00.08	D10.7	D37.05	D49.0
interarytenoid fold	C32.1	C78.39	D02.0	D14.1	D38.0	D49.1
intrinsic	C32.0	C78.39	D02.0	D14.1	D38.0	D49.1
overlapping lesion	C32.8	—	—	—	—	—
ventricular band	C32.1	C78.39	D02.0	D14.1	D38.0	D49.1
leg NEC	C76.5-☑	C79.89	D04.7-☑	D36.7	D48.7	D49.89
lens, crystalline	C69.4-☑	C79.49	D09.2-☑	D31.4-☑	D48.7	D49.89
lid (lower) (upper)	C44.10-☑	C79.2	D04.1-☑	D23.1-☑	D48.5	D49.2
basal cell carcinoma	C44.11-☑	—	—	—	—	—
specified type NEC	C44.19-☑	—	—	—	—	—
squamous cell carcinoma	C44.12-☑	—	—	—	—	—

Neoplasm, neoplastic — continued

	Malignant Primary	Malignant Secondary	Ca in situ	Benign	Uncertain	Unspecified Behavior
ligament — *see also* Neoplasm, connective tissue						
broad	C57.1-☑	C79.82	D07.39	D28.2	D39.8	D49.59
Mackenrodt's	C57.7	C79.82	D07.39	D28.7	D39.8	D49.59
non-uterine — *see* Neoplasm, connective tissue						
round	C57.2-☑	C79.82	—	D28.2	D39.8	D49.59
sacro-uterine	C57.3	C79.82	—	D28.2	D39.8	D49.59
uterine	C57.3	C79.82	—	D28.2	D39.8	D49.59
utero-ovarian	C57.7	C79.82	D07.39	D28.2	D39.8	D49.59
uterosacral	C57.3	C79.82	—	D28.2	D39.8	D49.59
limb	C76.8	C79.89	D04.8	D36.7	D48.7	D49.89
lower	C76.5-☑	C79.89	D04.7-☑	D36.7	D48.7	D49.89
upper	C76.4-☑	C79.89	D04.6-☑	D36.7	D48.7	D49.89
limbus of cornea	C69.1-☑	C79.49	D09.2-☑	D31.1-☑	D48.7	D49.89
lingual NEC — *see also* Neoplasm, tongue	C02.9	C79.89	D00.07	D10.1	D37.02	D49.0
lingula, lung	C34.1-☑	C78.0-☑	D02.2-☑	D14.3-☑	D38.1	D49.1
lip	C00.9	C79.89	D00.01	D10.0	D37.01	D49.0
buccal aspect — *see* Neoplasm, lip, internal						
commissure	C00.6	C79.89	D00.01	D10.0	D37.01	D49.0
external	C00.2	C79.89	D00.01	D10.0	D37.01	D49.0
lower	C00.1	C79.89	D00.01	D10.0	D37.01	D49.0
upper	C00.0	C79.89	D00.01	D10.0	D37.01	D49.0
frenulum — *see* Neoplasm, lip, internal						
inner aspect — *see* Neoplasm, lip, internal						
internal	C00.5	C79.89	D00.01	D10.0	D37.01	D49.0
lower	C00.4	C79.89	D00.01	D10.0	D37.01	D49.0
upper	C00.3	C79.89	D00.01	D10.0	D37.01	D49.0
lipstick area	C00.2	C79.89	D00.01	D10.0	D37.01	D49.0
lower	C00.1	C79.89	D00.01	D10.0	D37.01	D49.0
upper	C00.0	C79.89	D00.01	D10.0	D37.01	D49.0
lower	C00.1	C79.89	D00.01	D10.0	D37.01	D49.0
internal	C00.4	C79.89	D00.01	D10.0	D37.01	D49.0
mucosa — *see* Neoplasm, lip, internal						
oral aspect — *see* Neoplasm, lip, internal						
overlapping lesion	C00.8	—	—	—	—	—
with oral cavity or pharynx	C14.8	—	—	—	—	—
skin (commissure) (lower) (upper)	C44.00	C79.2	D04.0	D23.0	D48.5	D49.2
basal cell carcinoma	C44.01	—	—	—	—	—
specified type NEC	C44.09	—	—	—	—	—
squamous cell carcinoma	C44.02	—	—	—	—	—
upper	C00.0	C79.89	D00.01	D10.0	D37.01	D49.0
internal	C00.3	C79.89	D00.01	D10.0	D37.01	D49.0
vermilion border	C00.2	C79.89	D00.01	D10.0	D37.01	D49.0
lower	C00.1	C79.89	D00.01	D10.0	D37.01	D49.0
upper	C00.0	C79.89	D00.01	D10.0	D37.01	D49.0
lipomatous — *see* Lipoma, by site						
liver — *see also* Index to disease, by						
histology	C22.9	C78.7	D01.5	D13.4	D37.6	D49.0
primary	C22.8	C78.7	D01.5	D13.4	D37.6	D49.0
lumbosacral plexus	C47.5	C79.89	—	D36.16	D48.2	D49.2
lung	C34.9-☑	C78.0-☑	D02.2-☑	D14.3-☑	D38.1	D49.1
azygos lobe	C34.1-☑	C78.0-☑	D02.2-☑	D14.3-☑	D38.1	D49.1
carina	C34.0-☑	C78.0-☑	D02.2-☑	D14.3-☑	D38.1	D49.1
hilus	C34.0-☑	C78.0-☑	D02.2-☑	D14.3-☑	D38.1	D49.1
lingula	C34.1-☑	C78.0-☑	D02.2-☑	D14.3-☑	D38.1	D49.1
lobe NEC	C34.9-☑	C78.0-☑	D02.2-☑	D14.3-☑	D38.1	D49.1
lower lobe	C34.3-☑	C78.0-☑	D02.2-☑	D14.3-☑	D38.1	D49.1

☑ Additional Character Required — Refer to the Tabular List for Character Selection   ▽ Subterms under main terms may continue to next column or page

Neoplasm, neoplastic — continued

	Malignant Primary	Malignant Secondary	Ca in situ	Benign	Uncertain	Unspecified Behavior
lung — continued						
main bronchus	C34.0-☑	C78.0-☑	D02.2-☑	D14.3-☑	D38.1	D49.1
mesothelioma — see Mesothelioma						
middle lobe	C34.2	C78.0-☑	D02.21	D14.31	D38.1	D49.1
overlapping lesion	C34.8-☑	—	—	—	—	—
upper lobe	C34.1-☑	C78.0-☑	D02.2-☑	D14.3-☑	D38.1	D49.1
lymph, lymphatic channel						
NEC	C49.9	C79.89	—	D21.9	D48.1	D49.2
gland (secondary)	—	C77.9	—	D36.0	D48.7	D49.89
abdominal	—	C77.2	—	D36.0	D48.7	D49.89
aortic	—	C77.2	—	D36.0	D48.7	D49.89
arm	—	C77.3	—	D36.0	D48.7	D49.89
auricular (anterior) (posterior)	—	C77.0	—	D36.0	D48.7	D49.89
axilla, axillary	—	C77.3	—	D36.0	D48.7	D49.89
brachial	—	C77.3	—	D36.0	D48.7	D49.89
bronchial	—	C77.1	—	D36.0	D48.7	D49.89
bronchopulmonary	—	C77.1	—	D36.0	D48.7	D49.89
celiac	—	C77.2	—	D36.0	D48.7	D49.89
cervical	—	C77.0	—	D36.0	D48.7	D49.89
cervicofacial	—	C77.0	—	D36.0	D48.7	D49.89
Cloquet	—	C77.4	—	D36.0	D48.7	D49.89
colic	—	C77.2	—	D36.0	D48.7	D49.89
common duct	—	C77.2	—	D36.0	D48.7	D49.89
cubital	—	C77.3	—	D36.0	D48.7	D49.89
diaphragmatic	—	C77.1	—	D36.0	D48.7	D49.89
epigastric, inferior	—	C77.2	—	D36.0	D48.7	D49.89
epitrochlear	—	C77.3	—	D36.0	D48.7	D49.89
esophageal	—	C77.1	—	D36.0	D48.7	D49.89
face	—	C77.0	—	D36.0	D48.7	D49.89
femoral	—	C77.4	—	D36.0	D48.7	D49.89
gastric	—	C77.2	—	D36.0	D48.7	D49.89
groin	—	C77.4	—	D36.0	D48.7	D49.89
head	—	C77.0	—	D36.0	D48.7	D49.89
hepatic	—	C77.2	—	D36.0	D48.7	D49.89
hilar (pulmonary)	—	C77.1	—	D36.0	D48.7	D49.89
splenic	—	C77.2	—	D36.0	D48.7	D49.89
hypogastric	—	C77.5	—	D36.0	D48.7	D49.89
ileocolic	—	C77.2	—	D36.0	D48.7	D49.89
iliac	—	C77.5	—	D36.0	D48.7	D49.89
infraclavicular	—	C77.3	—	D36.0	D48.7	D49.89
inguina, inguinal	—	C77.4	—	D36.0	D48.7	D49.89
innominate	—	C77.1	—	D36.0	D48.7	D49.89
intercostal	—	C77.1	—	D36.0	D48.7	D49.89
intestinal	—	C77.2	—	D36.0	D48.7	D49.89
intrabdominal	—	C77.2	—	D36.0	D48.7	D49.89
intrapelvic	—	C77.5	—	D36.0	D48.7	D49.89
intrathoracic	—	C77.1	—	D36.0	D48.7	D49.89
jugular	—	C77.0	—	D36.0	D48.7	D49.89
leg	—	C77.4	—	D36.0	D48.7	D49.89
limb						
lower	—	C77.4	—	D36.0	D48.7	D49.89
upper	—	C77.3	—	D36.0	D48.7	D49.89
lower limb	—	C77.4	—	D36.0	D48.7	D49.89
lumbar	—	C77.2	—	D36.0	D48.7	D49.89
mandibular	—	C77.0	—	D36.0	D48.7	D49.89
mediastinal	—	C77.1	—	D36.0	D48.7	D49.89
mesenteric (inferior) (superior)	—	C77.2	—	D36.0	D48.7	D49.89
midcolic	—	C77.2	—	D36.0	D48.7	D49.89
multiple sites in categories C77.0-C77.5	—	C77.8	—	D36.0	D48.7	D49.89
neck	—	C77.0	—	D36.0	D48.7	D49.89
obturator	—	C77.5	—	D36.0	D48.7	D49.89
occipital	—	C77.0	—	D36.0	D48.7	D49.89
pancreatic	—	C77.2	—	D36.0	D48.7	D49.89
para-aortic	—	C77.2	—	D36.0	D48.7	D49.89
paracervical	—	C77.5	—	D36.0	D48.7	D49.89
parametrial	—	C77.5	—	D36.0	D48.7	D49.89
parasternal	—	C77.1	—	D36.0	D48.7	D49.89
parotid	—	C77.0	—	D36.0	D48.7	D49.89
pectoral	—	C77.3	—	D36.0	D48.7	D49.89
pelvic	—	C77.5	—	D36.0	D48.7	D49.89
peri-aortic	—	C77.2	—	D36.0	D48.7	D49.89
peripancreatic	—	C77.2	—	D36.0	D48.7	D49.89
popliteal	—	C77.4	—	D36.0	D48.7	D49.89
porta hepatis	—	C77.2	—	D36.0	D48.7	D49.89

Neoplasm, neoplastic — continued

	Malignant Primary	Malignant Secondary	Ca in situ	Benign	Uncertain	Unspecified Behavior
lymph, lymphatic channel — continued						
gland — continued						
portal	—	C77.2	—	D36.0	D48.7	D49.89
preauricular	—	C77.0	—	D36.0	D48.7	D49.89
prelaryngeal	—	C77.0	—	D36.0	D48.7	D49.89
presymphysial	—	C77.5	—	D36.0	D48.7	D49.89
pretracheal	—	C77.0	—	D36.0	D48.7	D49.89
primary (any site) NEC	C96.9	—	—	—	—	—
pulmonary (hiler)	—	C77.1	—	D36.0	D48.7	D49.89
pyloric	—	C77.2	—	D36.0	D48.7	D49.89
retroperitoneal	—	C77.2	—	D36.0	D48.7	D49.89
retropharyngeal	—	C77.0	—	D36.0	D48.7	D49.89
Rosenmuller's	—	C77.4	—	D36.0	D48.7	D49.89
sacral	—	C77.5	—	D36.0	D48.7	D49.89
scalene	—	C77.0	—	D36.0	D48.7	D49.89
site NEC	—	C77.9	—	D36.0	D48.7	D49.89
splenic (hilar)	—	C77.2	—	D36.0	D48.7	D49.89
subclavicular	—	C77.3	—	D36.0	D48.7	D49.89
subinguinal	—	C77.4	—	D36.0	D48.7	D49.89
sublingual	—	C77.0	—	D36.0	D48.7	D49.89
submandibular	—	C77.0	—	D36.0	D48.7	D49.89
submaxillary	—	C77.0	—	D36.0	D48.7	D49.89
submental	—	C77.0	—	D36.0	D48.7	D49.89
subscapular	—	C77.3	—	D36.0	D48.7	D49.89
supraclavicular	—	C77.0	—	D36.0	D48.7	D49.89
thoracic	—	C77.1	—	D36.0	D48.7	D49.89
tibial	—	C77.4	—	D36.0	D48.7	D49.89
tracheal	—	C77.1	—	D36.0	D48.7	D49.89
tracheobronchial	—	C77.1	—	D36.0	D48.7	D49.89
upper limb	—	C77.3	—	D36.0	D48.7	D49.89
Virchow's	—	C77.0	—	D36.0	D48.7	D49.89
node — see also Neoplasm, lymph gland						
primary NEC	C96.9	—	—	—	—	—
vessel — see also Neoplasm, connective tissue	C49.9	C79.89	—	D21.9	D48.1	D49.2
Mackenrodt's ligament	C57.7	C79.82	D07.39	D28.7	D39.8	D49.59
malar	C41.0	C79.51	—	D16.4	D48.0	D49.2
region — see Neoplasm, cheek						
mammary gland — see Neoplasm, breast						
mandible	C41.1	C79.51	—	D16.5	D48.0	D49.2
alveolar						
mucosa (carcinoma)	C03.1	C79.89	D00.03	D10.39	D37.09	D49.0
ridge or process	C41.1	C79.51	—	D16.5	D48.0	D49.2
marrow (bone) NEC	C96.9	C79.52	—	—	D47.9	D49.89
mastectomy site (skin) — see also Neoplasm, breast, skin	C44.501	C79.2	—	—	—	—
specified as breast tissue	C50.8-☑	C79.81	—	—	—	—
mastoid (air cells) (antrum) (cavity)	C30.1	C78.39	D02.3	D14.0	D38.5	D49.1
bone or process	C41.0	C79.51	—	D16.4	D48.0	D49.2
maxilla, maxillary (superior)	C41.0	C79.51	—	D16.4	D48.0	D49.2
alveolar						
mucosa	C03.0	C79.89	D00.03	D10.39	D37.09	D49.0
ridge or process (carcinoma)	C41.0	C79.51	—	D16.4	D48.0	D49.2
antrum	C31.0	C78.39	D02.3	D14.0	D38.5	D49.1
carcinoma	C03.0	C79.51	—	—	—	—
inferior — see Neoplasm, mandible						
sinus	C31.0	C78.39	D02.3	D14.0	D38.5	D49.1
meatus external (ear) — see also Neoplasm, skin, ear	C44.20-☑	C79.2	D04.2-☑	D23.2-☑	D48.5	D49.2
Meckel diverticulum, malignant	C17.3	C78.4	D01.49	D13.39	D37.2	D49.0
mediastinum, mediastinal	C38.3	C78.1	—	D15.2	D38.3	D49.89

Neoplasm, neoplastic — continued	Malignant Primary	Malignant Secondary	Ca in situ	Benign	Uncertain	Unspecified Behavior
mediastinum, mediastinal — continued						
anterior	C38.1	C78.1	—	D15.2	D38.3	D49.89
posterior	C38.2	C78.1	—	D15.2	D38.3	D49.89
medulla						
adrenal	C74.1-✓	C79.7-✓	D09.3	D35.0-✓	D44.1-✓	D49.7
oblongata	C71.7	C79.31	—	D33.1	D43.1	D49.6
meibomian gland	C44.10-✓	C79.2	D04.1-✓	D23.1-✓	D48.5	D49.2
basal cell carcinoma	C44.11-✓	—	—	—	—	—
specified type NEC	C44.19-✓	—	—	—	—	—
squamous cell carcinoma	C44.12-✓	—	—	—	—	—
melanoma — *see* Melanoma						
meninges	C70.9	C79.49	—	D32.9	D42.9	D49.7
brain	C70.0	C79.32	—	D32.0	D42.0	D49.7
cerebral	C70.0	C79.32	—	D32.0	D42.0	D49.7
crainial	C70.0	C79.32	—	D32.0	D42.0	D49.7
intracranial	C70.0	C79.32	—	D32.0	D42.0	D49.7
spinal (cord)	C70.1	C79.49	—	D32.1	D42.1	D49.7
meniscus, knee joint (lateral) (medial)	C40.2-✓	C79.51	—	D16.2-✓	D48.0	D49.2
Merkel cell — *see* Carcinoma, Merkel cell						
mesentery, mesenteric	C48.1	C78.6	—	D20.1	D48.4	D49.0
mesoappendix	C48.1	C78.6	—	D20.1	D48.4	D49.0
mesocolon	C48.1	C78.6	—	D20.1	D48.4	D49.0
mesopharynx — *see* Neoplasm, oropharynx						
mesosalpinx	C57.1-✓	C79.82	D07.39	D28.2	D39.8	D49.59
mesothelial tissue — *see* Mesothelioma						
mesothelioma — *see* Mesothelioma						
mesovarium	C57.1-✓	C79.82	D07.39	D28.2	D39.8	D49.59
metacarpus (any bone)	C40.1-✓	C79.51	—	D16.1-✓	—	—
metastatic NEC — *see also* Neoplasm, by site, secondary	—	C79.9	—	—	—	—
metatarsus (any bone)	C40.3-✓	C79.51	—	D16.3-✓	—	—
midbrain	C71.7	C79.31	—	D33.1	D43.1	D49.6
milk duct — *see* Neoplasm, breast						
mons						
pubis	C51.9	C79.82	D07.1	D28.0	D39.8	D49.59
veneris	C51.9	C79.82	D07.1	D28.0	D39.8	D49.59
motor tract	C72.9	C79.49	—	D33.9	D43.9	D49.7
brain	C71.9	C79.31	—	D33.2	D43.2	D49.6
cauda equina	C72.1	C79.49	—	D33.4	D43.4	D49.7
spinal	C72.0	C79.49	—	D33.4	D43.4	D49.7
mouth	C06.9	C79.89	D00.00	D10.30	D37.09	D49.0
book-leaf	C06.89	C79.89	—	—	—	—
floor	C04.9	C79.89	D00.06	D10.2	D37.09	D49.0
anterior portion	C04.0	C79.89	D00.06	D10.2	D37.09	D49.0
lateral portion	C04.1	C79.89	D00.06	D10.2	D37.09	D49.0
overlapping lesion	C04.8	—	—	—	—	—
overlapping NEC	C06.80	—	—	—	—	—
roof	C05.9	C79.89	D00.00	D10.39	D37.09	D49.0
specified part NEC	C06.89	C79.89	D00.00	D10.39	D37.09	D49.0
vestibule	C06.1	C79.89	D00.00	D10.39	D37.09	D49.0
mucosa						
alveolar (ridge or process)	C03.9	C79.89	D00.03	D10.39	D37.09	D49.0
lower	C03.1	C79.89	D00.03	D10.39	D37.09	D49.0
upper	C03.0	C79.89	D00.03	D10.39	D37.09	D49.0
buccal	C06.0	C79.89	D00.02	D10.39	D37.09	D49.0
cheek	C06.0	C79.89	D00.02	D10.39	D37.09	D49.0
lip — *see* Neoplasm, lip, internal						
nasal	C30.0	C78.39	D02.3	D14.0	D38.5	D49.1
oral	C06.0	C79.89	D00.02	D10.39	D37.09	D49.0
Mullerian duct						
female	C57.7	C79.82	D07.39	D28.7	D39.8	D49.59
male	C63.7	C79.82	D07.69	D29.8	D40.8	D49.59

Neoplasm, neoplastic — continued	Malignant Primary	Malignant Secondary	Ca in situ	Benign	Uncertain	Unspecified Behavior
muscle — *see also* Neoplasm, connective tissue						
extraocular	C69.6-✓	C79.49	D09.2-✓	D31.6-✓	D48.7	D49.89
myocardium	C38.0	C79.89	—	D15.1	D48.7	D49.89
myometrium	C54.2	C79.82	D07.0	D26.1	D39.0	D49.59
myopericardium	C38.0	C79.89	—	D15.1	D48.7	D49.89
nabothian gland (follicle)	C53.0	C79.82	D06.0	D26.0	D39.0	D49.59
nail — *see also* Neoplasm, skin, limb	C44.90	C79.2	D04.9	D23.9	D48.5	D49.2
finger — *see also* Neoplasm, skin, limb, upper	C44.60-✓	C79.2	D04.6-✓	D23.6-✓	D48.5	D49.2
toe — *see also* Neoplasm, skin, limb, lower	C44.70-✓	C79.2	D04.7-✓	D23.7-✓	D48.5	D49.2
nares, naris (anterior) (posterior)	C30.0	C78.39	D02.3	D14.0	D38.5	D49.1
nasal — *see* Neoplasm, nose						
nasolabial groove — *see also* Neoplasm, skin, face	C44.309	C79.2	D04.39	D23.39	D48.5	D49.2
nasolacrimal duct	C69.5-✓	C79.49	D09.2-✓	D31.5-✓	D48.7	D49.89
nasopharynx, nasopharyngeal	C11.9	C79.89	D00.08	D10.6	D37.05	D49.0
floor	C11.3	C79.89	D00.08	D10.6	D37.05	D49.0
overlapping lesion	C11.8	—	—	—	—	—
roof	C11.0	C79.89	D00.08	D10.6	D37.05	D49.0
wall	C11.9	C79.89	D00.08	D10.6	D37.05	D49.0
anterior	C11.3	C79.89	D00.08	D10.6	D37.05	D49.0
lateral	C11.2	C79.89	D00.08	D10.6	D37.05	D49.0
posterior	C11.1	C79.89	D00.08	D10.6	D37.05	D49.0
superior	C11.0	C79.89	D00.08	D10.6	D37.05	D49.0
nates — *see also* Neoplasm, skin, trunk	C44.509	C79.2	D04.5	D23.5	D48.5	D49.2
neck NEC	C76.0	C79.89	D09.8	D36.7	D48.7	D49.89
skin	C44.40	—	—	—	—	—
basal cell carcinoma	C44.41	—	—	—	—	—
specified type NEC	C44.49	—	—	—	—	—
squamous cell carcinoma	C44.42	—	—	—	—	—
nerve (ganglion)	C47.9	C79.89	—	D36.10	D48.2	D49.2
abducens	C72.59	C79.49	—	D33.3	D43.3	D49.7
accessory (spinal)	C72.59	C79.49	—	D33.3	D43.3	D49.7
acoustic	C72.4-✓	C79.49	—	D33.3	D43.3	D49.7
auditory	C72.4-✓	C79.49	—	D33.3	D43.3	D49.7
autonomic NEC — *see also* Neoplasm, nerve, peripheral	C47.9	C79.89	—	D36.10	D48.2	D49.2
brachial	C47.1-✓	C79.89	—	D36.12	D48.2	D49.2
cranial	C72.50	C79.49	—	D33.3	D43.3	D49.7
specified NEC	C72.59	C79.49	—	D33.3	D43.3	D49.7
facial	C72.59	C79.49	—	D33.3	D43.3	D49.7
femoral	C47.2-✓	C79.89	—	D36.13	D48.2	D49.2
ganglion NEC — *see also* Neoplasm, nerve, peripheral	C47.9	C79.89	—	D36.10	D48.2	D49.2
glossopharyngeal	C72.59	C79.49	—	D33.3	D43.3	D49.7
hypoglossal	C72.59	C79.49	—	D33.3	D43.3	D49.7
intercostal	C47.3	C79.89	—	D36.14	D48.2	D49.2
lumbar	C47.6	C79.89	—	D36.17	D48.2	D49.2
median	C47.1-✓	C79.89	—	D36.12	D48.2	D49.2
obturator	C47.2-✓	C79.89	—	D36.13	D48.2	D49.2
oculomotor	C72.59	C79.49	—	D33.3	D43.3	D49.7
olfactory	C72.2-✓	C79.49	—	D33.3	D43.3	D49.7
optic	C72.3-✓	C79.49	—	D33.3	D43.3	D49.7
parasympathetic NEC	C47.9	C79.89	—	D36.10	D48.2	D49.2
peripheral NEC	C47.9	C79.89	—	D36.10	D48.2	D49.2
abdomen	C47.4	C79.89	—	D36.15	D48.2	D49.2
abdominal wall	C47.4	C79.89	—	D36.15	D48.2	D49.2
ankle	C47.2-✓	C79.89	—	D36.13	D48.2	D49.2
antecubital fossa or space	C47.1-✓	C79.89	—	D36.12	D48.2	D49.2

✓ Additional Character Required — Refer to the Tabular List for Character Selection   ▽ Subterms under main terms may continue to next column or page

Neoplasm, neoplastic — continued

	Malignant Primary	Malignant Secondary	Ca in situ	Benign	Uncertain	Unspecified Behavior
nerve — continued						
peripheral — continued						
arm	C47.1-☑	C79.89	—	D36.12	D48.2	D49.2
auricle (ear)	C47.0	C79.89	—	D36.11	D48.2	D49.2
axilla	C47.3	C79.89	—	D36.12	D48.2	D49.2
back	C47.6	C79.89	—	D36.17	D48.2	D49.2
buttock	C47.5	C79.89	—	D36.16	D48.2	D49.2
calf	C47.2-☑	C79.89	—	D36.13	D48.2	D49.2
cervical region	C47.0	C79.89	—	D36.11	D48.2	D49.2
cheek	C47.0	C79.89	—	D36.11	D48.2	D49.2
chest (wall)	C47.3	C79.89	—	D36.14	D48.2	D49.2
chin	C47.0	C79.89	—	D36.11	D48.2	D49.2
ear (external)	C47.0	C79.89	—	D36.11	D48.2	D49.2
elbow	C47.1-☑	C79.89	—	D36.12	D48.2	D49.2
extrarectal	C47.5	C79.89	—	D36.16	D48.2	D49.2
extremity	C47.9	C79.89	—	D36.10	D48.2	D49.2
lower	C47.2-☑	C79.89	—	D36.13	D48.2	D49.2
upper	C47.1-☑	C79.89	—	D36.12	D48.2	D49.2
eyelid	C47.0	C79.89	—	D36.11	D48.2	D49.2
face	C47.0	C79.89	—	D36.11	D48.2	D49.2
finger	C47.1-☑	C79.89	—	D36.12	D48.2	D49.2
flank	C47.6	C79.89	—	D36.17	D48.2	D49.2
foot	C47.2-☑	C79.89	—	D36.13	D48.2	D49.2
forearm	C47.1-☑	C79.89	—	D36.12	D48.2	D49.2
forehead	C47.0	C79.89	—	D36.11	D48.2	D49.2
gluteal region	C47.5	C79.89	—	D36.16	D48.2	D49.2
groin	C47.5	C79.89	—	D36.16	D48.2	D49.2
hand	C47.1-☑	C79.89	—	D36.12	D48.2	D49.2
head	C47.0	C79.89	—	D36.11	D48.2	D49.2
heel	C47.2-☑	C79.89	—	D36.13	D48.2	D49.2
hip	C47.2-☑	C79.89	—	D36.13	D48.2	D49.2
infraclavicular region	C47.3	C79.89	—	D36.14	D48.2	D49.2
inguinal (canal) (region)	C47.5	C79.89	—	D36.16	D48.2	D49.2
intrathoracic	C47.3	C79.89	—	D36.14	D48.2	D49.2
ischiorectal fossa	C47.5	C79.89	—	D36.16	D48.2	D49.2
knee	C47.2-☑	C79.89	—	D36.13	D48.2	D49.2
leg	C47.2-☑	C79.89	—	D36.13	D48.2	D49.2
limb NEC	C47.9	C79.89	—	D36.10	D48.2	D49.2
lower	C47.2-☑	C79.89	—	D36.13	D48.2	D49.2
upper	C47.1-☑	C79.89	—	D36.12	D48.2	D49.2
nates	C47.5	C79.89	—	D36.16	D48.2	D49.2
neck	C47.0	C79.89	—	D36.11	D48.2	D49.2
orbit	C69.6-☑	C79.49	—	D31.6-☑	D48.7	D49.2
pararectal	C47.5	C79.89	—	D36.16	D48.2	D49.2
paraurethral	C47.5	C79.89	—	D36.16	D48.2	D49.2
paravaginal	C47.5	C79.89	—	D36.16	D48.2	D49.2
pelvis (floor)	C47.5	C79.89	—	D36.16	D48.2	D49.2
pelvoabdominal	C47.8	C79.89	—	D36.17	D48.2	D49.2
perineum	C47.5	C79.89	—	D36.16	D48.2	D49.2
perirectal (tissue)	C47.5	C79.89	—	D36.16	D48.2	D49.2
periurethral (tissue)	C47.5	C79.89	—	D36.16	D48.2	D49.2
popliteal fossa or space	C47.2-☑	C79.89	—	D36.13	D48.2	D49.2
presacral	C47.5	C79.89	—	D36.16	D48.2	D49.2
pterygoid fossa	C47.0	C79.89	—	D36.11	D48.2	D49.2
rectovaginal septum or wall	C47.5	C79.89	—	D36.16	D48.2	D49.2
rectovesical	C47.5	C79.89	—	D36.16	D48.2	D49.2
sacrococcygeal region	C47.5	C79.89	—	D36.16	D48.2	D49.2
scalp	C47.0	C79.89	—	D36.11	D48.2	D49.2
scapular region	C47.3	C79.89	—	D36.14	D48.2	D49.2
shoulder	C47.1-☑	C79.89	—	D36.12	D48.2	D49.2
submental	C47.0	C79.89	—	D36.11	D48.2	D49.2
supraclavicular region	C47.0	C79.89	—	D36.11	D48.2	D49.2
temple	C47.0	C79.89	—	D36.11	D48.2	D49.2
temporal region	C47.0	C79.89	—	D36.11	D48.2	D49.2
thigh	C47.2-☑	C79.89	—	D36.13	D48.2	D49.2
thoracic (duct) (wall)	C47.3	C79.89	—	D36.14	D48.2	D49.2
thorax	C47.3	C79.89	—	D36.14	D48.2	D49.2
thumb	C47.1-☑	C79.89	—	D36.12	D48.2	D49.2
toe	C47.2-☑	C79.89	—	D36.13	D48.2	D49.2
trunk	C47.6	C79.89	—	D36.17	D48.2	D49.2

Neoplasm, neoplastic — continued

	Malignant Primary	Malignant Secondary	Ca in situ	Benign	Uncertain	Unspecified Behavior
nerve — continued						
peripheral — continued						
umbilicus	C47.4	C79.89	—	D36.15	D48.2	D49.2
vesicorectal	C47.5	C79.89	—	D36.16	D48.2	D49.2
wrist	C47.1-☑	C79.89	—	D36.12	D48.2	D49.2
radial	C47.1-☑	C79.89	—	D36.12	D48.2	D49.2
sacral	C47.5	C79.89	—	D36.16	D48.2	D49.2
sciatic	C47.2-☑	C79.89	—	D36.13	D48.2	D49.2
spinal NEC	C47.9	C79.89	—	D36.10	D48.2	D49.2
accessory	C72.59	C79.49	—	D33.3	D43.3	D49.7
sympathetic NEC — see also Neoplasm, nerve, peripheral	C47.9	C79.89	—	D36.10	D48.2	D49.2
trigeminal	C72.59	C79.49	—	D33.3	D43.3	D49.7
trochlear	C72.59	C79.49	—	D33.3	D43.3	D49.7
ulnar	C47.1-☑	C79.89	—	D36.12	D48.2	D49.2
vagus	C72.59	C79.49	—	D33.3	D43.3	D49.7
nervous system (central)	C72.9	C79.40	—	D33.9	D43.9	D49.7
autonomic — see Neoplasm, nerve, peripheral						
parasympathetic — see Neoplasm, nerve, peripheral						
specified site NEC	—	C79.49	—	D33.7	D43.8	—
sympathetic — see Neoplasm, nerve, peripheral						
nevus — see Nevus						
nipple	C50.0-☑	C79.81	D05.-☑	D24.-☑	—	—
nose, nasal	C76.0	C79.89	D09.8	D36.7	D48.7	D49.89
ala (external) (nasi) — see also Neoplasm, nose, skin	C44.301	C79.2	D04.39	D23.39	D48.5	D49.2
bone	C41.0	C79.51	—	D16.4	D48.0	D49.2
cartilage	C30.0	C78.39	D02.3	D14.0	D38.5	D49.1
cavity	C30.0	C78.39	D02.3	D14.0	D38.5	D49.1
choana	C11.3	C79.89	D00.08	D10.6	D37.05	D49.0
external (skin) — see also Neoplasm, nose, skin	C44.301	C79.2	D04.39	D23.39	D48.5	D49.2
fossa	C30.0	C78.39	D02.3	D14.0	D38.5	D49.1
internal	C30.0	C78.39	D02.3	D14.0	D38.5	D49.1
mucosa	C30.0	C78.39	D02.3	D14.0	D38.5	D49.1
septum	C30.0	C78.39	D02.3	D14.0	D38.5	D49.1
posterior margin	C11.3	C79.89	D00.08	D10.6	D37.05	D49.0
sinus — see Neoplasm, sinus						
skin	C44.301	C79.2	D04.39	D23.39	D48.5	D49.2
basal cell carcinoma	C44.311	—	—	—	—	—
specified type NEC	C44.391	—	—	—	—	—
squamous cell carcinoma	C44.321	—	—	—	—	—
turbinate (mucosa)	C30.0	C78.39	D02.3	D14.0	D38.5	D49.1
bone	C41.0	C79.51	—	D16.4	D48.0	D49.2
vestibule	C30.0	C78.39	D02.3	D14.0	D38.5	D49.1
nostril	C30.0	C78.39	D02.3	D14.0	D38.5	D49.1
nucleus pulposus	C41.2	C79.51	—	D16.6	D48.0	D49.2
occipital						
bone	C41.0	C79.51	—	D16.4	D48.0	D49.2
lobe or pole, brain	C71.4	C79.31	—	D33.0	D43.0	D49.6
odontogenic — see Neoplasm, jaw bone						
olfactory nerve or bulb	C72.2-☑	C79.49	—	D33.3	D43.3	D49.7
olive (brain)	C71.7	C79.31	—	D33.1	D43.1	D49.6
omentum	C48.1	C78.6	—	D20.1	D48.4	D49.0
operculum (brain)	C71.0	C79.31	—	D33.0	D43.0	D49.6
optic nerve, chiasm, or tract	C72.3-☑	C79.49	—	D33.3	D43.3	D49.7
oral (cavity)	C06.9	C79.89	D00.00	D10.30	D37.09	D49.0
ill-defined	C14.8	C79.89	D00.00	D10.30	D37.09	D49.0
mucosa	C06.0	C79.89	D00.02	D10.39	D37.09	D49.0
orbit	C69.6-☑	C79.49	D09.2-☑	D31.6-☑	D48.7	D49.89
autonomic nerve	C69.6-☑	C79.49	—	D31.6-☑	D48.7	D49.2
bone	C41.0	C79.51	—	D16.4	D48.0	D49.2

Neoplasm, neoplastic — continued

	Malignant Primary	Malignant Secondary	Ca in situ	Benign	Uncertain	Unspecified Behavior
orbit — *continued*						
eye	C69.6-☑	C79.49	D09.2-☑	D31.6-☑	D48.7	D49.89
peripheral nerves	C69.6-☑	C79.49	—	D31.6-☑	D48.7	D49.2
soft parts	C69.6-☑	C79.49	D09.2-☑	D31.6-☑	D48.7	D49.89
organ of Zuckerkandl	C75.5	C79.89	—	D35.6	D44.7	D49.7
oropharynx	C10.9	C79.89	D00.08	D10.5	D37.05	D49.0
branchial cleft (vestige)	C10.4	C79.89	D00.08	D10.5	D37.05	D49.0
junctional region	C10.8	C79.89	D00.08	D10.5	D37.05	D49.0
lateral wall	C10.2	C79.89	D00.08	D10.5	D37.05	D49.0
overlapping lesion	C10.8	—	—	—	—	—
pillars or fauces	C09.1	C79.89	D00.08	D10.5	D37.05	D49.0
posterior wall	C10.3	C79.89	D00.08	D10.5	D37.05	D49.0
vallecula	C10.0	C79.89	D00.08	D10.5	D37.05	D49.0
os						
external	C53.1	C79.82	D06.1	D26.0	D39.0	D49.59
internal	C53.0	C79.82	D06.0	D26.0	D39.0	D49.59
ovary	C56.-☑	C79.6-☑	D07.39	D27.-☑	D39.1-☑	D49.59
oviduct	C57.0-☑	C79.82	D07.39	D28.2	D39.8	D49.59
palate	C05.9	C79.89	D00.00	D10.39	D37.09	D49.0
hard	C05.0	C79.89	D00.05	D10.39	D37.09	D49.0
junction of hard and soft palate	C05.9	C79.89	D00.00	D10.39	D37.09	D49.0
overlapping lesions	C05.8	—	—	—	—	—
soft	C05.1	C79.89	D00.04	D10.39	D37.09	D49.0
nasopharyngeal surface	C11.3	C79.89	D00.08	D10.6	D37.05	D49.0
posterior surface	C11.3	C79.89	D00.08	D10.6	D37.05	D49.0
superior surface	C11.3	C79.89	D00.08	D10.6	D37.05	D49.0
palatoglossal arch	C09.1	C79.89	D00.00	D10.5	D37.09	D49.0
palatopharyngeal arch	C09.1	C79.89	D00.00	D10.5	D37.09	D49.0
pallium	C71.0	C79.31	—	D33.0	D43.0	D49.6
palpebra	C44.10-☑	C79.2	D04.1-☑	D23.1-☑	D48.5	D49.2
basal cell carcinoma	C44.11-☑	—	—	—	—	—
specified type NEC	C44.19-☑	—	—	—	—	—
squamous cell carcinoma	C44.12-☑	—	—	—	—	—
pancreas	C25.9	C78.89	D01.7	D13.6	D37.8	D49.0
body	C25.1	C78.89	D01.7	D13.6	D37.8	D49.0
duct (of Santorini) (of Wirsung)	C25.3	C78.89	D01.7	D13.6	D37.8	D49.0
ectopic tissue	C25.7	C78.89	—	D13.6	D37.8	D49.0
head	C25.0	C78.89	D01.7	D13.6	D37.8	D49.0
islet cells	C25.4	C78.89	D01.7	D13.7	D37.8	D49.0
neck	C25.7	C78.89	D01.7	D13.6	D37.8	D49.0
overlapping lesion	C25.8	—	—	—	—	—
tail	C25.2	C78.89	D01.7	D13.6	D37.8	D49.0
para-aortic body	C75.5	C79.89	—	D35.6	D44.7	D49.7
paraganglion NEC	C75.5	C79.89	—	D35.6	D44.7	D49.7
parametrium	C57.3	C79.82	—	D28.2	D39.8	D49.59
paranephric	C48.0	C78.6	—	D20.0	D48.3	D49.0
pararectal	C76.3	C79.89	—	D36.7	D48.7	D49.89
parasagittal (region)	C76.0	C79.89	D09.8	D36.7	D48.7	D49.89
parasellar	C72.9	C79.49	—	D33.9	D43.8	D49.7
parathyroid (gland)	C75.0	C79.89	D09.3	D35.1	D44.2	D49.7
paraurethral	C76.3	C79.89	—	D36.7	D48.7	D49.89
gland	C68.1	C79.19	D09.19	D30.8	D41.8	D49.59
paravaginal	C76.3	C79.89	—	D36.7	D48.7	D49.89
parenchyma, kidney	C64.-☑	C79.0-☑	D09.19	D30.0-☑	D41.0-☑	D49.51-☑
parietal						
bone	C41.0	C79.51	—	D16.4	D48.0	D49.2
lobe, brain	C71.3	C79.31	—	D33.0	D43.0	D49.6
paroophoron	C57.1-☑	C79.82	D07.39	D28.2	D39.8	D49.59
parotid (duct) (gland)	C07	C79.89	D00.00	D11.0	D37.030	D49.0
parovarium	C57.1-☑	C79.82	D07.39	D28.2	D39.8	D49.59
patella	C40.20	C79.51	—	—	—	—
peduncle, cerebral	C71.7	C79.31	—	D33.1	D43.1	D49.6
pelvirectal junction	C19	C78.5	D01.1	D12.7	D37.5	D49.0
pelvis, pelvic	C76.3	C79.89	D09.8	D36.7	D48.7	D49.89
bone	C41.4	C79.51	—	D16.8	D48.0	D49.2
floor	C76.3	C79.89	D09.8	D36.7	D48.7	D49.89
renal	C65.-☑	C79.0-☑	D09.19	D30.1-☑	D41.1-☑	D49.51-☑
viscera	C76.3	C79.89	D09.8	D36.7	D48.7	D49.89
wall	C76.3	C79.89	D09.8	D36.7	D48.7	D49.89
pelvo-abdominal	C76.8	C79.89	D09.8	D36.7	D48.7	D49.89
penis	C60.9	C79.82	D07.4	D29.0	D40.8	D49.59

Neoplasm, neoplastic — continued

	Malignant Primary	Malignant Secondary	Ca in situ	Benign	Uncertain	Unspecified Behavior
penis — *continued*						
body	C60.2	C79.82	D07.4	D29.0	D40.8	D49.59
corpus (cavernosum)	C60.2	C79.82	D07.4	D29.0	D40.8	D49.59
glans	C60.1	C79.82	D07.4	D29.0	D40.8	D49.59
overlapping sites	C60.8	—	—	—	—	—
skin NEC	C60.9	C79.82	D07.4	D29.0	D40.8	D49.59
periadrenal (tissue)	C48.0	C78.6	—	D20.0	D48.3	D49.0
perianal (skin) — *see also* Neoplasm, anus, skin	C44.500	C79.2	D04.5	D23.5	D48.5	D49.2
pericardium	C38.0	C79.89	—	D15.1	D48.7	D49.89
perinephric	C48.0	C78.6	—	D20.0	D48.3	D49.0
perineum	C76.3	C79.89	D09.8	D36.7	D48.7	D49.89
periodontal tissue NEC	C03.9	C79.89	D00.03	D10.39	D37.09	D49.0
periosteum — *see* Neoplasm, bone						
peripancreatic	C48.0	C78.6	—	D20.0	D48.3	D49.0
peripheral nerve NEC	C47.9	C79.89	—	D36.10	D48.2	D49.2
perirectal (tissue)	C76.3	C79.89	—	D36.7	D48.7	D49.89
perirenal (tissue)	C48.0	C78.6	—	D20.0	D48.3	D49.0
peritoneum, peritoneal (cavity)	C48.2	C78.6	—	D20.1	D48.4	D49.0
benign mesothelial tissue — *see* Mesothelioma, benign						
overlapping lesion with digestive organs	C48.8	—	—	—	—	—
	C26.9	—	—	—	—	—
parietal	C48.1	C78.6	—	D20.1	D48.4	D49.0
pelvic	C48.1	C78.6	—	D20.1	D48.4	D49.0
specified part NEC	C48.1	C78.6	—	D20.1	D48.4	D49.0
peritonsillar (tissue)	C76.0	C79.89	D09.8	D36.7	D48.7	D49.89
periurethral tissue	C76.3	C79.89	—	D36.7	D48.7	D49.89
phalanges						
foot	C40.3-☑	C79.51	—	D16.3-☑	—	—
hand	C40.1-☑	C79.51	—	D16.1-☑	—	—
pharynx, pharyngeal	C14.0	C79.89	D00.08	D10.9	D37.05	D49.0
bursa	C11.1	C79.89	D00.08	D10.6	D37.05	D49.0
fornix	C11.3	C79.89	D00.08	D10.6	D37.05	D49.0
recess	C11.2	C79.89	D00.08	D10.6	D37.05	D49.0
region	C14.0	C79.89	D00.08	D10.9	D37.05	D49.0
tonsil	C11.1	C79.89	D00.08	D10.6	D37.05	D49.0
wall (lateral) (posterior)	C14.0	C79.89	D00.08	D10.9	D37.05	D49.0
pia mater	C70.9	C79.40	—	D32.9	D42.9	D49.7
cerebral	C70.0	C79.32	—	D32.0	D42.0	D49.7
cranial	C70.0	C79.32	—	D32.0	D42.0	D49.7
spinal	C70.1	C79.49	—	D32.1	D42.1	D49.7
pillars of fauces	C09.1	C79.89	D00.08	D10.5	D37.05	D49.0
pineal (body) (gland)	C75.3	C79.89	D09.3	D35.4	D44.5	D49.7
pinna (ear) NEC — *see also* Neoplasm, skin, ear	C44.20-☑	C79.2	D04.2-☑	D23.2-☑	D48.5	D49.2
piriform fossa or sinus	C12	C79.89	D00.08	D10.7	D37.05	D49.0
pituitary (body) (fossa) (gland) (lobe)	C75.1	C79.89	D09.3	D35.2	D44.3	D49.7
placenta	C58	C79.82	D07.0	D26.7	D39.2	D49.59
pleura, pleural (cavity)	C38.4	C78.2	—	D19.0	D38.2	D49.1
overlapping lesion with heart or mediastinum	C38.8	—	—	—	—	—
parietal	C38.4	C78.2	—	D19.0	D38.2	D49.1
visceral	C38.4	C78.2	—	D19.0	D38.2	D49.1
plexus						
brachial	C47.1-☑	C79.89	—	D36.12	D48.2	D49.2
cervical	C47.0	C79.89	—	D36.11	D48.2	D49.2
choroid	C71.5	C79.31	—	D33.0	D43.0	D49.6
lumbosacral	C47.5	C79.89	—	D36.16	D48.2	D49.2
sacral	C47.5	C79.89	—	D36.16	D48.2	D49.2
pluriendocrine	C75.8	C79.89	D09.3	D35.7	D44.9	D49.7
pole						
frontal	C71.1	C79.31	—	D33.0	D43.0	D49.6
occipital	C71.4	C79.31	—	D33.0	D43.0	D49.6
pons (varolii)	C71.7	C79.31	—	D33.1	D43.1	D49.6

☑ Additional Character Required — Refer to the Tabular List for Character Selection   ▽ Subterms under main terms may continue to next column or page

Neoplasm, neoplastic — continued	Malignant Primary	Malignant Secondary	Ca in situ	Benign	Uncertain	Unspecified Behavior
popliteal fossa or space	C76.5-☑	C79.89	D04.7-☑	D36.7	D48.7	D49.89
postcricoid (region)	C13.0	C79.89	D00.08	D10.7	D37.05	D49.0
posterior fossa (cranial)	C71.9	C79.31	—	D33.2	D43.2	D49.6
postnasal space	C11.9	C79.89	D00.08	D10.6	D37.05	D49.0
prepuce	C60.0	C79.82	D07.4	D29.0	D40.8	D49.59
prepylorus	C16.4	C78.89	D00.2	D13.1	D37.1	D49.0
presacral (region)	C76.3	C79.89	—	D36.7	D48.7	D49.89
prostate (gland)	C61	C79.82	D07.5	D29.1	D40.0	D49.59
utricle	C68.0	C79.19	D09.19	D30.4	D41.3	D49.59
pterygoid fossa	C49.0	C79.89	—	D21.0	D48.1	D49.2
pubic bone	C41.4	C79.51	—	D16.8	D48.0	D49.2
pudenda, pudendum (female)	C51.9	C79.82	D07.1	D28.0	D39.8	D49.59
pulmonary — see also Neoplasm, lung	C34.9-☑	C78.0-☑	D02.2-☑	D14.3-☑	D38.1	D49.1
putamen	C71.0	C79.31	—	D33.0	D43.0	D49.6
pyloric						
antrum	C16.3	C78.89	D00.2	D13.1	D37.1	D49.0
canal	C16.4	C78.89	D00.2	D13.1	D37.1	D49.0
pylorus	C16.4	C78.89	D00.2	D13.1	D37.1	D49.0
pyramid (brain)	C71.7	C79.31	—	D33.1	D43.1	D49.6
pyriform fossa or sinus	C12	C79.89	D00.08	D10.7	D37.05	D49.0
radius (any part)	C40.0-☑	C79.51	—	D16.0-☑	—	—
Rathke's pouch	C75.1	C79.89	D09.3	D35.2	D44.3	D49.7
rectosigmoid (junction)	C19	C78.5	D01.1	D12.7	D37.5	D49.0
overlapping lesion with anus or rectum	C21.8	—	—	—	—	—
rectouterine pouch	C48.1	C78.6	—	D20.1	D48.4	D49.0
rectovaginal septum or wall	C76.3	C79.89	D09.8	D36.7	D48.7	D49.89
rectovesical septum	C76.3	C79.89	D09.8	D36.7	D48.7	D49.89
rectum (ampulla)	C20	C78.5	D01.2	D12.8	D37.5	D49.0
and colon	C19	C78.5	D01.1	D12.7	D37.5	D49.0
overlapping lesion with anus or rectosigmoid junction	C21.8	—	—	—	—	—
renal	C64.-☑	C79.0-☑	D09.19	D30.0-☑	D41.0-☑	D49.51-☑
calyx	C65.-☑	C79.0-☑	D09.19	D30.1-☑	D41.1-☑	D49.51-☑
hilus	C65.-☑	C79.0-☑	D09.19	D30.1-☑	D41.1-☑	D49.51-☑
parenchyma	C64.-☑	C79.0-☑	D09.19	D30.0-☑	D41.0-☑	D49.51-☑
pelvis	C65.-☑	C79.0-☑	D09.19	D30.1-☑	D41.1-☑	D49.51-☑
respiratory						
organs or system NEC	C39.9	C78.30	D02.4	D14.4	D38.6	D49.1
tract NEC	C39.9	C78.30	D02.4	D14.4	D38.5	D49.1
upper	C39.0	C78.30	D02.4	D14.4	D38.5	D49.1
retina	C69.2-☑	C79.49	D09.2-☑	D31.2-☑	D48.7	D49.81
retrobulbar	C69.6-☑	C79.49	—	D31.6-☑	D48.7	D49.89
retrocecal	C48.0	C78.6	—	D20.0	D48.3	D49.0
retromolar (area) (triangle) (trigone)	C06.2	C79.89	D00.00	D10.39	D37.09	D49.0
retro-orbital	C76.0	C79.89	D09.8	D36.7	D48.7	D49.89
retroperitoneal (space) (tissue)	C48.0	C78.6	—	D20.0	D48.3	D49.0
retroperitoneum	C48.0	C78.6	—	D20.0	D48.3	D49.0
retropharyngeal	C14.0	C79.89	D00.08	D10.9	D37.05	D49.0
retrovesical (septum)	C76.3	C79.89	D09.8	D36.7	D48.7	D49.89
rhinencephalon	C71.0	C79.31	—	D33.0	D43.0	D49.6
rib	C41.3	C79.51	—	D16.7	D48.0	D49.2
Rosenmuller's fossa	C11.2	C79.89	D00.08	D10.6	D37.05	D49.0
round ligament	C57.2-☑	C79.82	—	D28.2	D39.8	D49.59
sacrococcyx, sacrococcygeal region	C41.4	C79.51	—	D16.8	D48.0	D49.2
	C76.3	C79.89	D09.8	D36.7	D48.7	D49.89
sacrouterine ligament	C57.3	C79.82	—	D28.2	D39.8	D49.59
sacrum, sacral (vertebra)	C41.4	C79.51	—	D16.8	D48.0	D49.2
salivary gland or duct (major)	C08.9	C79.89	D00.00	D11.9	D37.039	D49.0
minor NEC	C06.9	C79.89	D00.00	D10.39	D37.04	D49.0
overlapping lesion	C08.9	—	—	—	—	—
parotid	C07	C79.89	D00.00	D11.0	D37.030	D49.0

Neoplasm, neoplastic — continued	Malignant Primary	Malignant Secondary	Ca in situ	Benign	Uncertain	Unspecified Behavior
salivary gland or duct — continued						
pluriglandular	C08.9	C79.89	D00.00	D11.9	D37.039	D49.0
sublingual	C08.1	C79.89	D00.00	D11.7	D37.031	D49.0
submandibular	C08.0	C79.89	D00.00	D11.7	D37.032	D49.0
submaxillary	C08.0	C79.89	D00.00	D11.7	D37.032	D49.0
salpinx (uterine)	C57.0-☑	C79.82	D07.39	D28.2	D39.8	D49.59
Santorini's duct	C25.3	C78.89	D01.7	D13.6	D37.8	D49.0
scalp	C44.40	C79.2	D04.4	D23.4	D48.5	D49.2
basal cell carcinoma	C44.41	—	—	—	—	—
specified type NEC	C44.49	—	—	—	—	—
squamous cell carcinoma	C44.42	—	—	—	—	—
scapula (any part)	C40.0-☑	C79.51	—	D16.0-☑	—	—
scapular region	C76.1	C79.89	D09.8	D36.7	D48.7	D49.89
scar NEC — see also Neoplasm, skin, by site	C44.90	C79.2	D04.9	D23.9	D48.5	D49.2
sciatic nerve	C47.2-☑	C79.89	—	D36.13	D48.2	D49.2
sclera	C69.4-☑	C79.49	D09.2-☑	D31.4-☑	D48.7	D49.89
scrotum (skin)	C63.2	C79.82	D07.61	D29.4	D40.8	D49.59
sebaceous gland — see Neoplasm, skin						
sella turcica	C75.1	C79.89	D09.3	D35.2	D44.3	D49.7
bone	C41.0	C79.51	—	D16.4	D48.0	D49.2
semilunar cartilage (knee)	C40.2-☑	C79.51	—	D16.2-☑	D48.0	D49.2
seminal vesicle	C63.7	C79.82	D07.69	D29.8	D40.8	D49.59
septum						
nasal	C30.0	C78.39	D02.3	D14.0	D38.5	D49.1
posterior margin	C11.3	C79.89	D00.08	D10.6	D37.05	D49.0
rectovaginal	C76.3	C79.89	D09.8	D36.7	D48.7	D49.89
rectovesical	C76.3	C79.89	D09.8	D36.7	D48.7	D49.89
urethrovaginal	C57.9	C79.82	D07.30	D28.9	D39.9	D49.59
vesicovaginal	C57.9	C79.82	D07.30	D28.9	D39.9	D49.59
shoulder NEC	C76.4-☑	C79.89	D04.6-☑	D36.7	D48.7	D49.89
sigmoid flexure (lower) (upper)	C18.7	C78.5	D01.0	D12.5	D37.4	D49.0
sinus (accessory)	C31.9	C78.39	D02.3	D14.0	D38.5	D49.1
bone (any)	C41.0	C79.51	—	D16.4	D48.0	D49.2
ethmoidal	C31.1	C78.39	D02.3	D14.0	D38.5	D49.1
frontal	C31.2	C78.39	D02.3	D14.0	D38.5	D49.1
maxillary	C31.0	C78.39	D02.3	D14.0	D38.5	D49.1
nasal, paranasal NEC	C31.9	C78.39	D02.3	D14.0	D38.5	D49.1
overlapping lesion	C31.8	—	—	—	—	—
pyriform	C12	C79.89	D00.08	D10.7	D37.05	D49.0
sphenoid	C31.3	C78.39	D02.3	D14.0	D38.5	D49.1
skeleton, skeletal NEC	C41.9	C79.51	—	D16.9	D48.0	D49.2
Skene's gland	C68.1	C79.19	D09.19	D30.8	D41.8	D49.59
skin NOS	C44.90	C79.2	D04.9	D23.9	D48.5	D49.2
abdominal wall	C44.509	C79.2	D04.5	D23.5	D48.5	D49.2
basal cell carcinoma	C44.519	—	—	—	—	—
specified type NEC	C44.599	—	—	—	—	—
squamous cell carcinoma	C44.529	—	—	—	—	—
ala nasi — see also Neoplasm, nose, skin	C44.301	C79.2	D04.39	D23.39	D48.5	D49.2
ankle — see also Neoplasm, skin, limb, lower	C44.70-☑	C79.2	D04.7-☑	D23.7-☑	D48.5	D49.2
antecubital space — see also Neoplasm, skin, limb, upper	C44.60-☑	C79.2	D04.6-☑	D23.6-☑	D48.5	D49.2
anus	C44.500	C79.2	D04.5	D23.5	D48.5	D49.2
basal cell carcinoma	C44.510	—	—	—	—	—
specified type NEC	C44.590	—	—	—	—	—
squamous cell carcinoma	C44.520	—	—	—	—	—
arm — see also Neoplasm, skin, limb, upper	C44.60-☑	C79.2	D04.6-☑	D23.6-☑	D48.5	D49.2

Neoplasm, neoplastic — continued	Malignant Primary	Malignant Secondary	Ca in situ	Benign	Uncertain	Unspecified Behavior
skin — continued						
auditory canal (external) — see also Neoplasm, skin, ear	C44.20-☑	C79.2	D04.2-☑	D23.2-☑	D48.5	D49.2
auricle (ear) — see also Neoplasm, skin, ear	C44.20-☑	C79.2	D04.2-☑	D23.2-☑	D48.5	D49.2
auricular canal (external) — see also Neoplasm, skin, ear	C44.20-☑	C79.2	D04.2-☑	D23.2-☑	D48.5	D49.2
axilla, axillary fold — see also Neoplasm, skin, trunk	C44.509	C79.2	D04.5	D23.5	D48.5	D49.2
back — see also Neoplasm, skin, trunk	C44.509	C79.2	D04.5	D23.5	D48.5	D49.2
basal cell carcinoma	C44.91	—	—	—	—	—
breast	C44.501	C79.2	D04.5	D23.5	D48.5	D49.2
basal cell carcinoma	C44.511	—	—	—	—	—
specified type NEC	C44.591	—	—	—	—	—
squamous cell carcinoma	C44.521	—	—	—	—	—
brow — see also Neoplasm, skin, face	C44.309	C79.2	D04.39	D23.39	D48.5	D49.2
buttock — see also Neoplasm, skin, trunk	C44.509	C79.2	D04.5	D23.5	D48.5	D49.2
calf — see also Neoplasm, skin, limb, lower	C44.70-☑	C79.2	D04.7-☑	D23.7-☑	D48.5	D49.2
canthus (eye) (inner) (outer)	C44.10-☑	C79.2	D04.1-☑	D23.1-☑	D48.5	D49.2
basal cell carcinoma	C44.11-☑	—	—	—	—	—
specified type NEC	C44.19-☑	—	—	—	—	—
squamous cell carcinoma	C44.12-☑	—	—	—	—	—
cervical region — see also Neoplasm, skin, neck	C44.40	C79.2	D04.4	D23.4	D48.5	D49.2
cheek (external) — see also Neoplasm, skin, face	C44.309	C79.2	D04.39	D23.39	D48.5	D49.2
chest (wall) — see also Neoplasm, skin, trunk	C44.509	C79.2	D04.5	D23.5	D48.5	D49.2
chin — see also Neoplasm, skin, face	C44.309	C79.2	D04.39	D23.39	D48.5	D49.2
clavicular area — see also Neoplasm, skin, trunk	C44.509	C79.2	D04.5	D23.5	D48.5	D49.2
clitoris	C51.2	C79.82	D07.1	D28.0	D39.8	D49.59
columnella — see also Neoplasm, skin, face	C44.309	C79.2	D04.39	D23.39	D48.5	D49.2
concha — see also Neoplasm, skin, ear	C44.20-☑	C79.2	D04.2-☑	D23.2-☑	D48.5	D49.2
ear (external)	C44.20-☑	C79.2	D04.2-☑	D23.2-☑	D48.5	D49.2
basal cell carcinoma	C44.21-☑	—	—	—	—	—
specified type NEC	C44.29-☑	—	—	—	—	—
squamous cell carcinoma	C44.22-☑	—	—	—	—	—
elbow — see also Neoplasm, skin, limb, upper	C44.60-☑	C79.2	D04.6-☑	D23.6-☑	D48.5	D49.2
eyebrow — see also Neoplasm, skin, face	C44.309	C79.2	D04.39	D23.39	D48.5	D49.2
eyelid	C44.10-☑	C79.2	D04.1-☑	D23.1-☑	D48.5	D49.2

Neoplasm, neoplastic — continued	Malignant Primary	Malignant Secondary	Ca in situ	Benign	Uncertain	Unspecified Behavior
skin — continued						
eyelid — continued						
basal cell carcinoma	C44.11-☑	—	—	—	—	—
specified type NEC	C44.19-☑	—	—	—	—	—
squamous cell carcinoma	C44.12-☑	—	—	—	—	—
face NOS	C44.300	C79.2	D04.30	D23.30	D48.5	D49.2
basal cell carcinoma	C44.310					
specified type NEC	C44.390					
squamous cell carcinoma	C44.320					
female genital organs (external)	C51.9	C79.82	D07.1	D28.0	D39.8	D49.59
clitoris	C51.2	C79.82	D07.1	D28.0	D39.8	D49.59
labium NEC	C51.9	C79.82	D07.1	D28.0	D39.8	D49.59
majus	C51.0	C79.82	D07.1	D28.0	D39.8	D49.59
minus	C51.1	C79.82	D07.1	D28.0	D39.8	D49.59
pudendum	C51.9	C79.82	D07.1	D28.0	D39.8	D49.59
vulva	C51.9	C79.82	D07.1	D28.0	D39.8	D49.59
finger — see also Neoplasm, skin, limb, upper	C44.60-☑	C79.2	D04.6-☑	D23.6-☑	D48.5	D49.2
flank — see also Neoplasm, skin, trunk	C44.509	C79.2	D04.5	D23.5	D48.5	D49.2
foot — see also Neoplasm, skin, limb, lower	C44.70-☑	C79.2	D04.7-☑	D23.7-☑	D48.5	D49.2
forearm — see also Neoplasm, skin, limb, upper	C44.60-☑	C79.2	D04.6-☑	D23.6-☑	D48.5	D49.2
forehead — see also Neoplasm, skin, face	C44.309	C79.2	D04.39	D23.39	D48.5	D49.2
glabella — see also Neoplasm, skin, face	C44.309	C79.2	D04.39	D23.39	D48.5	D49.2
gluteal region — see also Neoplasm, skin, trunk	C44.509	C79.2	D04.5	D23.5	D48.5	D49.2
groin — see also Neoplasm, skin, trunk	C44.509	C79.2	D04.5	D23.5	D48.5	D49.2
hand — see also Neoplasm, skin, limb, upper	C44.60-☑	C79.2	D04.6-☑	D23.6-☑	D48.5	D49.2
head NEC — see also Neoplasm, skin, scalp	C44.40	C79.2	D04.4	D23.4	D48.5	D49.2
heel — see also Neoplasm, skin, limb, lower	C44.70-☑	C79.2	D04.7-☑	D23.7-☑	D48.5	D49.2
helix — see also Neoplasm, skin, ear	C44.20-☑	C79.2	D04.2-☑	D23.2-☑	D48.5	D49.2
hip — see also Neoplasm, skin, limb, lower	C44.70-☑	C79.2	D04.7-☑	D23.7-☑	D48.5	D49.2
infraclavicular region — see also Neoplasm, skin, trunk	C44.509	C79.2	D04.5	D23.5	D48.5	D49.2
inguinal region — see also Neoplasm, skin, trunk	C44.509	C79.2	D04.5	D23.5	D48.5	D49.2
jaw — see also Neoplasm, skin, face	C44.309	C79.2	D04.39	D23.39	D48.5	D49.2
Kaposi's sarcoma — see Kaposi's, sarcoma, skin						
knee — see also Neoplasm, skin, limb, lower	C44.70-☑	C79.2	D04.7-☑	D23.7-☑	D48.5	D49.2
labia						
majora	C51.0	C79.82	D07.1	D28.0	D39.8	D49.59
minora	C51.1	C79.82	D07.1	D28.0	D39.8	D49.59

☑ Additional Character Required — Refer to the Tabular List for Character Selection　　　▽ Subterms under main terms may continue to next column or page

Neoplasm, neoplastic — continued
skin — continued

	Malignant Primary	Malignant Secondary	Ca in situ	Benign	Uncertain	Unspecified Behavior
leg — see also Neoplasm, skin, limb, lower	C44.70-☑	C79.2	D04.7-☑	D23.7-☑	D48.5	D49.2
lid (lower) (upper)	C44.10-☑	C79.2	D04.1-☑	D23.1-☑	D48.5	D49.2
basal cell carcinoma	C44.11-☑	—	—	—	—	—
specified type NEC	C44.19-☑	—	—	—	—	—
squamous cell carcinoma	C44.12-☑	—	—	—	—	—
limb NEC	C44.90	C79.2	D04.9	D23.9	D48.5	D49.2
basal cell carcinoma	C44.91	—	—	—	—	—
lower	C44.70-☑	C79.2	D04.7-☑	D23.7-☑	D48.5	D49.2
basal cell carcinoma	C44.71-☑	—	—	—	—	—
specified type NEC	C44.79-☑	—	—	—	—	—
squamous cell carcinoma	C44.72-☑	—	—	—	—	—
upper	C44.60-☑	C79.2	D04.6-☑	D23.6-☑	D48.5	D49.2
basal cell carcinoma	C44.61-☑	—	—	—	—	—
specified type NEC	C44.69-☑	—	—	—	—	—
squamous cell carcinoma	C44.62-☑	—	—	—	—	—
lip (lower) (upper)	C44.00	C79.2	D04.0	D23.0	D48.5	D49.2
basal cell carcinoma	C44.01	—	—	—	—	—
specified type NEC	C44.09	—	—	—	—	—
squamous cell carcinoma	C44.02	—	—	—	—	—
male genital organs	C63.9	C79.82	D07.60	D29.9	D40.8	D49.59
penis	C60.9	C79.82	D07.4	D29.0	D40.8	D49.59
prepuce	C60.0	C79.82	D07.4	D29.0	D40.8	D49.59
scrotum	C63.2	C79.82	D07.61	D29.4	D40.8	D49.59
mastectomy site (skin) — see also Neoplasm, skin, breast	C44.501	C79.2				
specified as breast tissue	C50.8-☑	C79.81				
meatus, acoustic (external) — see also Neoplasm, skin, ear	C44.20-☑	C79.2	D04.2-☑	D23.2-☑	D48.5	D49.2
melanotic — see Melanoma						
Merkel cell — see Carcinoma, Merkel cell						
nates — see also Neoplasm, skin, trunk	C44.509	C79.2	D04.5	D23.5	D48.5	D49.2
neck	C44.40	C79.2	D04.4	D23.4	D48.5	D49.2
basal cell carcinoma	C44.41	—	—	—	—	—
specified type NEC	C44.49	—	—	—	—	—
squamous cell carcinoma	C44.42	—	—	—	—	—
nevus — see Nevus, skin						
nose (external) — see also Neoplasm, nose, skin	C44.301	C79.2	D04.39	D23.39	D48.5	D49.2
overlapping lesion	C44.80	—	—	—	—	—
basal cell carcinoma	C44.81	—	—	—	—	—
specified type NEC	C44.89	—	—	—	—	—
squamous cell carcinoma	C44.82	—	—	—	—	—
palm — see also Neoplasm, skin, limb, upper	C44.60-☑	C79.2	D04.6-☑	D23.6-☑	D48.5	D49.2
palpebra	C44.10-☑	C79.2	D04.1-☑	D23.1-☑	D48.5	D49.2
palpebra — continued						
basal cell carcinoma	C44.11-☑	—	—	—	—	—
specified type NEC	C44.19-☑	—	—	—	—	—
squamous cell carcinoma	C44.12-☑	—	—	—	—	—
penis NEC	C60.9	C79.82	D07.4	D29.0	D40.8	D49.59
perianal — see also Neoplasm, skin, anus	C44.500	C79.2	D04.5	D23.5	D48.5	D49.2
perineum — see also Neoplasm, skin, anus	C44.500	C79.2	D04.5	D23.5	D48.5	D49.2
pinna — see also Neoplasm, skin, ear	C44.20-☑	C79.2	D04.2-☑	D23.2-☑	D48.5	D49.2
plantar — see also Neoplasm, skin, limb, lower	C44.70-☑	C79.2	D04.7-☑	D23.7-☑	D48.5	D49.2
popliteal fossa or space — see also Neoplasm, skin, limb, lower	C44.70-☑	C79.2	D04.7-☑	D23.7-☑	D48.5	D49.2
prepuce	C60.0	C79.82	D07.4	D29.0	D40.8	D49.59
pubes — see also Neoplasm, skin, trunk	C44.509	C79.2	D04.5	D23.5	D48.5	D49.2
sacrococcygeal region — see also Neoplasm, skin, trunk	C44.509	C79.2	D04.5	D23.5	D48.5	D49.2
scalp	C44.40	C79.2	D04.4	D23.4	D48.5	D49.2
basal cell carcinoma	C44.41	—	—	—	—	—
specified type NEC	C44.49	—	—	—	—	—
squamous cell carcinoma	C44.42	—	—	—	—	—
scapular region — see also Neoplasm, skin, trunk	C44.509	C79.2	D04.5	D23.5	D48.5	D49.2
scrotum	C63.2	C79.82	D07.61	D29.4	D40.8	D49.59
shoulder — see also Neoplasm, skin, limb, upper	C44.60-☑	C79.2	D04.6-☑	D23.6-☑	D48.5	D49.2
sole (foot) — see also Neoplasm, skin, limb, lower	C44.70-☑	C79.2	D04.7-☑	D23.7-☑	D48.5	D49.2
specified sites NEC	C44.80	C79.2	D04.8	D23.9	D48.5	D49.2
basal cell carcinoma	C44.81	—	—	—	—	—
specified type NEC	C44.89	—	—	—	—	—
squamous cell carcinoma	C44.82	—	—	—	—	—
specified type NEC	C44.99	—	—	—	—	—
squamous cell carcinoma	C44.92	—	—	—	—	—
submammary fold — see also Neoplasm, skin, trunk	C44.509	C79.2	D04.5	D23.5	D48.5	D49.2
supraclavicular region — see also Neoplasm, skin, neck	C44.40	C79.2	D04.4	D23.4	D48.5	D49.2
temple — see also Neoplasm, skin, face	C44.309	C79.2	D04.39	D23.39	D48.5	D49.2
thigh — see also Neoplasm, skin, limb, lower	C44.70-☑	C79.2	D04.7-☑	D23.7-☑	D48.5	D49.2
thoracic wall — see also Neoplasm, skin, trunk	C44.509	C79.2	D04.5	D23.5	D48.5	D49.2
thumb — see also Neoplasm, skin, limb, upper	C44.60-☑	C79.2	D04.6-☑	D23.6-☑	D48.5	D49.2
toe — see also Neoplasm, skin, limb, lower	C44.70-☑	C79.2	D04.7-☑	D23.7-☑	D48.5	D49.2

Neoplasm, neoplastic — continued

	Malignant Primary	Malignant Secondary	Ca in situ	Benign	Uncertain	Unspecified Behavior
skin — continued						
tragus — see also Neoplasm, skin, ear	C44.20-☑	C79.2	D04.2-☑	D23.2-☑	D48.5	D49.2
trunk	C44.509	C79.2	D04.5	D23.5	D48.5	D49.2
basal cell carcinoma	C44.519	—	—	—	—	—
specified type NEC	C44.599	—	—	—	—	—
squamous cell carcinoma	C44.529	—	—	—	—	—
umbilicus — see also Neoplasm, skin, trunk	C44.509	C79.2	D04.5	D23.5	D48.5	D49.2
vulva	C51.9	C79.82	D07.1	D28.0	D39.8	D49.59
overlapping lesion	C51.8	—	—	—	—	—
wrist — see also Neoplasm, skin, limb, upper	C44.60-☑	C79.2	D04.6-☑	D23.6-☑	D48.5	D49.2
skull	C41.0	C79.51		D16.4	D48.0	D49.2
soft parts or tissues — see Neoplasm, connective tissue						
specified site NEC	C76.8	C79.89	D09.8	D36.7	D48.7	D49.89
spermatic cord	C63.1-☑	C79.82	D07.69	D29.8	D40.8	D49.59
sphenoid	C31.3	C78.39	D02.3	D14.0	D38.5	D49.1
bone	C41.0	C79.51		D16.4	D48.0	D49.2
sinus	C31.3	C78.39	D02.3	D14.0	D38.5	D49.1
sphincter						
anal	C21.1	C78.5	D01.3	D12.9	D37.8	D49.0
of Oddi	C24.0	C78.89	D01.5	D13.5	D37.6	D49.0
spine, spinal (column)	C41.2	C79.51		D16.6	D48.0	D49.2
bulb	C71.7	C79.31		D33.1	D43.1	D49.6
coccyx	C41.4	C79.51		D16.8	D48.0	D49.2
cord (cervical) (lumbar) (sacral) (thoracic)	C72.0	C79.49		D33.4	D43.4	D49.7
dura mater	C70.1	C79.49		D32.1	D42.1	D49.7
lumbosacral	C41.2	C79.51		D16.6	D48.0	D49.2
marrow NEC	C96.9	C79.52		—	D47.9	D49.89
membrane	C70.1	C79.49		D32.1	D42.1	D49.7
meninges	C70.1	C79.49		D32.1	D42.1	D49.7
nerve (root)	C47.9	C79.89		D36.10	D48.2	D49.2
pia mater	C70.1	C79.49		D32.1	D42.1	D49.7
root	C47.9	C79.89		D36.10	D48.2	D49.2
sacrum	C41.4	C79.51		D16.8	D48.0	D49.2
spleen, splenic NEC	C26.1	C78.89	D01.7	D13.9	D37.8	D49.0
flexure (colon)	C18.5	C78.5	D01.0	D12.3	D37.4	D49.0
stem, brain	C71.7	C79.31		D33.1	D43.1	D49.6
Stensen's duct	C07	C79.89	D00.00	D11.0	D37.030	D49.0
sternum	C41.3	C79.51		D16.7	D48.0	D49.2
stomach	C16.9	C78.89	D00.2	D13.1	D37.1	D49.0
antrum (pyloric)	C16.3	C78.89	D00.2	D13.1	D37.1	D49.0
body	C16.2	C78.89	D00.2	D13.1	D37.1	D49.0
cardia	C16.0	C78.89	D00.2	D13.1	D37.1	D49.0
cardiac orifice	C16.0	C78.89	D00.2	D13.1	D37.1	D49.0
corpus	C16.2	C78.89	D00.2	D13.1	D37.1	D49.0
fundus	C16.1	C78.89	D00.2	D13.1	D37.1	D49.0
greater curvature NEC	C16.6	C78.89	D00.2	D13.1	D37.1	D49.0
lesser curvature NEC	C16.5	C78.89	D00.2	D13.1	D37.1	D49.0
overlapping lesion	C16.8	—	—	—	—	—
prepylorus	C16.4	C78.89	D00.2	D13.1	D37.1	D49.0
pylorus	C16.4	C78.89	D00.2	D13.1	D37.1	D49.0
wall NEC	C16.9	C78.89	D00.2	D13.1	D37.1	D49.0
anterior NEC	C16.8	C78.89	D00.2	D13.1	D37.1	D49.0
posterior NEC	C16.8	C78.89	D00.2	D13.1	D37.1	D49.0
stroma, endometrial	C54.1	C79.82	D07.0	D26.1	D39.0	D49.59
stump, cervical	C53.8	C79.82	D06.7	D26.0	D39.0	D49.59
subcutaneous (nodule) (tissue) NEC — see Neoplasm, connective tissue						
subdural	C70.9	C79.32		D32.9	D42.9	D49.7
subglottis, subglottic	C32.2	C78.39	D02.0	D14.1	D38.0	D49.1
sublingual	C04.9	C79.89	D00.06	D10.2	D37.09	D49.0
gland or duct	C08.1	C79.89	D00.00	D11.7	D37.031	D49.0

Neoplasm, neoplastic — continued

	Malignant Primary	Malignant Secondary	Ca in situ	Benign	Uncertain	Unspecified Behavior
submandibular gland	C08.0	C79.89	D00.00	D11.7	D37.032	D49.0
submaxillary gland or duct	C08.0	C79.89	D00.00	D11.7	D37.032	D49.0
submental	C76.0	C79.89	D09.8	D36.7	D48.7	D49.89
subpleural	C34.9-☑	C78.0-☑	D02.2-☑	D14.3-☑	D38.1	D49.1
substernal	C38.1	C78.1	—	D15.2	D38.3	D49.89
sudoriferous, sudoriparous gland, site unspecified	C44.90	C79.2	D04.9	D23.9	D48.5	D49.2
specified site — see Neoplasm, skin						
supraclavicular region	C76.0	C79.89	D09.8	D36.7	D48.7	D49.89
supraglottis	C32.1	C78.39	D02.0	D14.1	D38.0	D49.1
suprarenal	C74.9-☑	C79.7-☑	D09.3	D35.0-☑	D44.1-☑	D49.7
capsule	C74.9-☑	C79.7-☑	D09.3	D35.0-☑	D44.1-☑	D49.7
cortex	C74.0-☑	C79.7-☑	D09.3	D35.0-☑	D44.1-☑	D49.7
gland	C74.9-☑	C79.7-☑	D09.3	D35.0-☑	D44.1-☑	D49.7
medulla	C74.1-☑	C79.7-☑	D09.3	D35.0-☑	D44.1-☑	D49.7
suprasellar (region)	C71.9	C79.31	—	D33.2	D43.2	D49.6
supratentorial (brain) NEC	C71.0	C79.31	—	D33.0	D43.0	D49.6
sweat gland (apocrine) (eccrine), site unspecified	C44.90	C79.2	D04.9	D23.9	D48.5	D49.2
specified site — see Neoplasm, skin						
sympathetic nerve or nervous system NEC	C47.9	C79.89	—	D36.10	D48.2	D49.2
symphysis pubis	C41.4	C79.51	—	D16.8	D48.0	D49.2
synovial membrane — see Neoplasm, connective tissue						
tapetum, brain	C71.8	C79.31	—	D33.2	D43.2	D49.6
tarsus (any bone)	C40.3-☑	C79.51	—	D16.3-☑	—	—
temple (skin) — see also Neoplasm, skin, face	C44.309	C79.2	D04.39	D23.39	D48.5	D49.2
temporal						
bone	C41.0	C79.51	—	D16.4	D48.0	D49.2
lobe or pole	C71.2	C79.31	—	D33.0	D43.0	D49.6
region	C76.0	C79.89	D09.8	D36.7	D48.7	D49.89
skin — see also Neoplasm, skin, face	C44.309	C79.2	D04.39	D23.39	D48.5	D49.2
tendon (sheath) — see Neoplasm, connective tissue						
tentorium (cerebelli)	C70.0	C79.32	—	D32.0	D42.0	D49.7
testis, testes	C62.9-☑	C79.82	D07.69	D29.2-☑	D40.1-☑	D49.59
descended	C62.1-☑	C79.82	D07.69	D29.2-☑	D40.1-☑	D49.59
ectopic	C62.0-☑	C79.82	D07.69	D29.2-☑	D40.1-☑	D49.59
retained	C62.0-☑	C79.82	D07.69	D29.2-☑	D40.1-☑	D49.59
scrotal	C62.1-☑	C79.82	D07.69	D29.2-☑	D40.1-☑	D49.59
undescended	C62.0-☑	C79.82	D07.69	D29.2-☑	D40.1-☑	D49.59
unspecified whether descended or undescended	C62.9-☑	C79.82	D07.69	D29.2-☑	D40.1-☑	D49.59
thalamus	C71.0	C79.31	—	D33.0	D43.0	D49.6
thigh NEC	C76.5-☑	C79.89	D04.7-☑	D36.7	D48.7	D49.89
thorax, thoracic (cavity) (organs NEC)	C76.1	C79.89	D09.8	D36.7	D48.7	D49.89
duct	C49.3	C79.89	—	D21.3	D48.1	D49.2
wall NEC	C76.1	C79.89	D09.8	D36.7	D48.7	D49.89
throat	C14.0	C79.89	D00.08	D10.9	D37.05	D49.0
thumb NEC	C76.4-☑	C79.89	D04.6-☑	D36.7	D48.7	D49.89
thymus (gland)	C37	C79.89	D09.3	D15.0	D38.4	D49.89
thyroglossal duct	C73	C79.89	D09.3	D34	D44.0	D49.7
thyroid (gland)	C73	C79.89	D09.3	D34	D44.0	D49.7
cartilage	C32.3	C78.39	D02.0	D14.1	D38.0	D49.1
tibia (any part)	C40.2-☑	C79.51	—	D16.2-☑	—	—
toe NEC	C76.5-☑	C79.89	D04.7-☑	D36.7	D48.7	D49.89
tongue	C02.9	C79.89	D00.07	D10.1	D37.02	D49.0
anterior (two-thirds) NEC	C02.3	C79.89	D00.07	D10.1	D37.02	D49.0
dorsal surface	C02.0	C79.89	D00.07	D10.1	D37.02	D49.0
ventral surface	C02.2	C79.89	D00.07	D10.1	D37.02	D49.0

Neoplasm, neoplastic — continued	Malignant Primary	Malignant Secondary	Ca in situ	Benign	Uncertain	Unspecified Behavior
tongue — continued						
base (dorsal surface)	C01	C79.89	D00.07	D10.1	D37.02	D49.0
border (lateral)	C02.1	C79.89	D00.07	D10.1	D37.02	D49.0
dorsal surface NEC	C02.0	C79.89	D00.07	D10.1	D37.02	D49.0
fixed part NEC	C01	C79.89	D00.07	D10.1	D37.02	D49.0
foreamen cecum	C02.0	C79.89	D00.07	D10.1	D37.02	D49.0
frenulum linguae	C02.2	C79.89	D00.07	D10.1	D37.02	D49.0
junctional zone	C02.8	C79.89	D00.07	D10.1	D37.02	D49.0
margin (lateral)	C02.1	C79.89	D00.07	D10.1	D37.02	D49.0
midline NEC	C02.1	C79.89	D00.07	D10.1	D37.02	D49.0
mobile part NEC	C02.3	C79.89	D00.07	D10.1	D37.02	D49.0
overlapping lesion	C02.8	—	—	—	—	—
posterior (third)	C01	C79.89	D00.07	D10.1	D37.02	D49.0
root	C01	C79.89	D00.07	D10.1	D37.02	D49.0
surface (dorsal)	C02.0	C79.89	D00.07	D10.1	D37.02	D49.0
base	C01	C79.89	D00.07	D10.1	D37.02	D49.0
ventral	C02.2	C79.89	D00.07	D10.1	D37.02	D49.0
tip	C02.1	C79.89	D00.07	D10.1	D37.02	D49.0
tonsil	C02.4	C79.89	D00.07	D10.1	D37.02	D49.0
tonsil	C09.9	C79.89	D00.08	D10.4	D37.05	D49.0
fauces, faucial	C09.9	C79.89	D00.08	D10.4	D37.05	D49.0
lingual	C02.4	C79.89	D00.07	D10.1	D37.02	D49.0
overlapping sites	C09.8	—	—	—	—	—
palatine	C09.9	C79.89	D00.08	D10.4	D37.05	D49.0
pharyngeal	C11.1	C79.89	D00.08	D10.6	D37.05	D49.0
pillar (anterior) (posterior)	C09.1	C79.89	D00.08	D10.5	D37.05	D49.0
tonsillar fossa	C09.0	C79.89	D00.08	D10.5	D37.05	D49.0
tooth socket NEC	C03.9	C79.89	D00.03	D10.39	D37.09	D49.0
trachea (cartilage) (mucosa)	C33	C78.39	D02.1	D14.2	D38.1	D49.1
overlapping lesion with bronchus or lung	C34.8-☑	—	—	—	—	—
tracheobronchial	C34.8-☑	C78.39	D02.1	D14.2	D38.1	D49.1
overlapping lesion with lung	C34.8-☑	—	—	—	—	—
tragus — see also Neoplasm, skin, ear	C44.20-☑	C79.2	D04.2-☑	D23.2-☑	D48.5	D49.2
trunk NEC	C76.8	C79.89	D04.5	D36.7	D48.7	D49.89
tubo-ovarian	C57.8	C79.82	D07.39	D28.7	D39.8	D49.59
tunica vaginalis	C63.7	C79.82	D07.69	D29.8	D40.8	D49.59
turbinate (bone)	C41.0	C79.51	—	D16.4	D48.0	D49.2
nasal	C30.0	C78.39	D02.3	D14.0	D38.5	D49.1
tympanic cavity	C30.1	C78.39	D02.3	D14.0	D38.5	D49.1
ulna (any part)	C40.0-☑	C79.51	—	D16.0-☑	—	—
umbilicus, umbilical — see also Neoplasm, skin, trunk	C44.509	C79.2	D04.5	D23.5	D48.5	D49.2
uncus, brain	C71.2	C79.31	—	D33.0	D43.0	D49.6
unknown site or unspecified	C80.1	C79.9	D09.9	D36.9	D48.9	D49.9
urachus	C67.7	C79.11	D09.0	D30.3	D41.4	D49.4
ureter-bladder (junction)	C67.6	C79.11	D09.0	D30.3	D41.4	D49.4
ureter, ureteral	C66.-☑	C79.19	D09.19	D30.2-☑	D41.2-☑	D49.59
orifice (bladder)	C67.6	C79.11	D09.0	D30.3	D41.4	D49.4
urethra, urethral (gland)	C68.0	C79.19	D09.19	D30.4	D41.3	D49.59
orifice, internal	C67.5	C79.11	D09.0	D30.3	D41.4	D49.4
urethrovaginal (septum)	C57.9	C79.82	D07.30	D28.9	D39.8	D49.59
urinary organ or system	C68.9	C79.10	D09.10	D30.9	D41.9	D49.59
bladder — see Neoplasm, bladder						
overlapping lesion	C68.8	—	—	—	—	—
specified sites NEC	C68.8	C79.19	D09.19	D30.8	D41.8	D49.59
utero-ovarian	C57.8	C79.82	D07.39	D28.7	D39.8	D49.59
ligament	C57.1-☑	C79.82	D07.39	D28.2	D39.8	D49.59
uterosacral ligament	C57.3	C79.82	—	D28.2	D39.8	D49.59
uterus, uteri, uterine	C55	C79.82	D07.0	D26.9	D39.0	D49.59
adnexa NEC	C57.4	C79.82	D07.39	D28.7	D39.8	D49.59
body	C54.9	C79.82	D07.0	D26.1	D39.0	D49.59
cervix	C53.9	C79.82	D06.9	D26.0	D39.0	D49.59
cornu	C54.9	C79.82	D07.0	D26.1	D39.0	D49.59
corpus	C54.9	C79.82	D07.0	D26.1	D39.0	D49.59
endocervix (canal) (gland)	C53.0	C79.82	D06.0	D26.0	D39.0	D49.59

Neoplasm, neoplastic — continued	Malignant Primary	Malignant Secondary	Ca in situ	Benign	Uncertain	Unspecified Behavior
uterus, uteri, uterine — continued						
endometrium	C54.1	C79.82	D07.0	D26.1	D39.0	D49.59
exocervix	C53.1	C79.82	D06.1	D26.0	D39.0	D49.59
external os	C53.1	C79.82	D06.1	D26.0	D39.0	D49.59
fundus	C54.3	C79.82	D07.0	D26.1	D39.0	D49.59
internal os	C53.0	C79.82	D06.0	D26.0	D39.0	D49.59
isthmus	C54.0	C79.82	D07.0	D26.1	D39.0	D49.59
ligament	C57.3	C79.82	—	D28.2	D39.8	D49.59
broad	C57.1-☑	C79.82	D07.39	D28.2	D39.8	D49.59
round	C57.2-☑	C79.82	—	D28.2	D39.8	D49.59
lower segment	C54.0	C79.82	D07.0	D26.1	D39.0	D49.59
myometrium	C54.2	C79.82	D07.0	D26.1	D39.0	D49.59
overlapping sites	C54.8	—	—	—	—	—
squamocolumnar junction	C53.8	C79.82	D06.7	D26.0	D39.0	D49.59
tube	C57.0-☑	C79.82	D07.39	D28.2	D39.8	D49.59
utricle, prostatic	C68.0	C79.19	D09.19	D30.4	D41.3	D49.59
uveal tract	C69.4-☑	C79.49	D09.2-☑	D31.4-☑	D48.7	D49.89
uvula	C05.2	C79.89	D00.04	D10.39	D37.09	D49.0
vagina, vaginal (fornix) (vault) (wall)	C52	C79.82	D07.2	D28.1	D39.8	D49.59
vaginovesical	C57.9	C79.82	D07.30	D28.9	D39.9	D49.59
septum	C57.9	C79.82	D07.30	D28.9	D39.9	D49.59
vallecula (epiglottis)	C10.0	C79.89	D00.08	D10.5	D37.05	D49.0
vascular — see Neoplasm, connective tissue						
vas deferens	C63.1-☑	C79.82	D07.69	D29.8	D40.8	D49.59
Vater's ampulla	C24.1	C78.89	D01.5	D13.5	D37.6	D49.0
vein, venous — see Neoplasm, connective tissue						
vena cava (abdominal) (inferior)	C49.4	C79.89	—	D21.4	D48.1	D49.2
superior	C49.3	C79.89	—	D21.3	D48.1	D49.2
ventricle (cerebral) (floor) (lateral) (third)	C71.5	C79.31	—	D33.0	D43.0	D49.6
cardiac (left) (right)	C38.0	C79.89	—	D15.1	D48.7	D49.89
fourth	C71.7	C79.31	—	D33.1	D43.1	D49.6
ventricular band of larynx	C32.1	C78.39	D02.0	D14.1	D38.0	D49.1
ventriculus — see Neoplasm, stomach						
vermillion border — see Neoplasm, lip						
vermis, cerebellum	C71.6	C79.31	—	D33.1	D43.1	D49.6
vertebra (column)	C41.2	C79.51	—	D16.6	D48.0	D49.2
coccyx	C41.4	C79.51	—	D16.8	D48.0	D49.2
marrow NEC	C96.9	C79.52	—	—	D47.9	D49.89
sacrum	C41.4	C79.51	—	D16.8	D48.0	D49.2
vesical — see Neoplasm, bladder						
vesicle, seminal	C63.7	C79.82	D07.69	D29.8	D40.8	D49.59
vesicocervical tissue	C57.9	C79.82	D07.30	D28.9	D39.9	D49.59
vesicorectal	C76.3	C79.82	D09.8	D36.7	D48.7	D49.89
vesicovaginal	C57.9	C79.82	D07.30	D28.9	D39.9	D49.59
septum	C57.9	C79.82	D07.30	D28.9	D39.8	D49.59
vessel (blood) — see Neoplasm, connective tissue						
vestibular gland, greater	C51.0	C79.82	D07.1	D28.0	D39.8	D49.59
vestibule						
mouth	C06.1	C79.89	D00.00	D10.39	D37.09	D49.0
nose	C30.0	C78.39	D02.3	D14.0	D38.5	D49.1
Virchow's gland	C77.0	C77.0	—	D36.0	D48.7	D49.89
viscera NEC	C76.8	C79.89	D09.8	D36.7	D48.7	D49.89
vocal cords (true)	C32.0	C78.39	D02.0	D14.1	D38.0	D49.1
false	C32.1	C78.39	D02.0	D14.1	D38.0	D49.1
vomer	C41.0	C79.51	—	D16.4	D48.0	D49.2
vulva	C51.9	C79.82	D07.1	D28.0	D39.8	D49.59
vulvovaginal gland	C51.0	C79.82	D07.1	D28.0	D39.8	D49.59
Waldeyer's ring	C14.2	C79.89	D00.08	D10.9	D37.05	D49.0
Wharton's duct	C08.0	C79.89	D00.00	D11.7	D37.032	D49.0
white matter (central) (cerebral)	C71.0	C79.31	—	D33.0	D43.0	D49.6
windpipe	C33	C78.39	D02.1	D14.2	D38.1	D49.1
Wirsung's duct	C25.3	C78.89	D01.7	D13.6	D37.8	D49.0
wolffian (body) (duct) female	C57.7	C79.82	D07.39	D28.7	D39.8	D49.59

	Malignant Primary	Malignant Secondary	Ca in situ	Benign	Uncertain	Unspecified Behavior
Neoplasm, neoplastic — *continued*						
wolffian — *continued*						
male	C63.7	C79.82	D07.69	D29.8	D40.8	D49.59
womb — *see* Neoplasm, uterus						
wrist NEC	C76.4-☑	C79.89	D04.6-☑	D36.7	D48.7	D49.89
xiphoid process	C41.3	C79.51	—	D16.7	D48.0	D49.2
Zuckerkandl organ	C75.5	C79.89	—	D35.6	D44.7	D49.7

☑ Additional Character Required — Refer to the Tabular List for Character Selection   ▽ Subterms under main terms may continue to next column or page

Table of Drugs and Chemicals

Substance	Poisoning, Accidental (unintentional)	Poisoning, Intentional Self-harm	Poisoning, Assault	Poisoning, Undetermined	Adverse Effect	Under-dosing
14-Hydroxydihydromorphinone	T40.2X1	T40.2X2	T40.2X3	T40.2X4	T40.2X5	T40.2X6
1-Propanol	T51.3X1	T51.3X2	T51.3X3	T51.3X4	—	—
2,3,7,8-Tetrachlorodibenzo-p-dioxin	T53.7X1	T53.7X2	T53.7X3	T53.7X4	—	—
2,4,5-T (trichlorophenoxyacetic acid)	T60.1X1	T60.1X2	T60.1X3	T60.1X4	—	—
2,4,5-Trichlorophenoxyacetic acid	T60.3X1	T60.3X2	T60.3X3	T60.3X4	—	—
2,4-D (dichlorophenoxyacetic acid)	T60.3X1	T60.3X2	T60.3X3	T60.3X4	—	—
2,4-Toluene diisocyanate	T65.0X1	T65.0X2	T65.0X3	T65.0X4	—	—
2-Deoxy-5-fluorouridine	T45.1X1	T45.1X2	T45.1X3	T45.1X4	T45.1X5	T45.1X6
2-Ethoxyethanol	T52.3X1	T52.3X2	T52.3X3	T52.3X4	—	—
2-Methoxyethanol	T52.3X1	T52.3X2	T52.3X3	T52.3X4	—	—
2-Propanol	T51.2X1	T51.2X2	T51.2X3	T51.2X4	—	—
4-Aminobutyric acid	T43.8X1	T43.8X2	T43.8X3	T43.8X4	T43.8X5	T43.8X6
4-Aminophenol derivatives	T39.1X1	T39.1X2	T39.1X3	T39.1X4	T39.1X5	T39.1X6
5-Deoxy-5-fluorouridine	T45.1X1	T45.1X2	T45.1X3	T45.1X4	T45.1X5	T45.1X6
5-Methoxypsoralen (5-MOP)	T50.991	T50.992	T50.993	T50.994	T50.995	T50.996
8-Aminoquinoline drugs	T37.2X1	T37.2X2	T37.2X3	T37.2X4	T37.2X5	T37.2X6
8-Methoxypsoralen (8-MOP)	T50.991	T50.992	T50.993	T50.994	T50.995	T50.996
ABOB	T37.5X1	T37.5X2	T37.5X3	T37.5X4	T37.5X5	T37.5X6
Abrine	T62.2X1	T62.2X2	T62.2X3	T62.2X4	—	—
Abrus (seed)	T62.2X1	T62.2X2	T62.2X3	T62.2X4	—	—
Absinthe	T51.0X1	T51.0X2	T51.0X3	T51.0X4	—	—
beverage	T51.0X1	T51.0X2	T51.0X3	T51.0X4	—	—
Acaricide	T60.8X1	T60.8X2	T60.8X3	T60.8X4	—	—
Acebutolol	T44.7X1	T44.7X2	T44.7X3	T44.7X4	T44.7X5	T44.7X6
Acecarbromal	T42.6X1	T42.6X2	T42.6X3	T42.6X4	T42.6X5	T42.6X6
Aceclidine	T44.1X1	T44.1X2	T44.1X3	T44.1X4	T44.1X5	T44.1X6
Acedapsone	T37.0X1	T37.0X2	T37.0X3	T37.0X4	T37.0X5	T37.0X6
Acefylline piperazine	T48.6X1	T48.6X2	T48.6X3	T48.6X4	T48.6X5	T48.6X6
Acemorphan	T40.2X1	T40.2X2	T40.2X3	T40.2X4	T40.2X5	T40.2X6
Acenocoumarin	T45.511	T45.512	T45.513	T45.514	T45.515	T45.516
Acenocoumarol	T45.511	T45.512	T45.513	T45.514	T45.515	T45.516
Acepifylline	T48.6X1	T48.6X2	T48.6X3	T48.6X4	T48.6X5	T48.6X6
Acepromazine	T43.3X1	T43.3X2	T43.3X3	T43.3X4	T43.3X5	T43.3X6
Acesulfamethoxypyridazine	T37.0X1	T37.0X2	T37.0X3	T37.0X4	T37.0X5	T37.0X6
Acetal	T52.8X1	T52.8X2	T52.8X3	T52.8X4	—	—
Acetaldehyde (vapor)	T52.8X1	T52.8X2	T52.8X3	T52.8X4	—	—
liquid	T65.891	T65.892	T65.893	T65.894	—	—
Acetaminophen	T39.1X1	T39.1X2	T39.1X3	T39.1X4	T39.1X5	T39.1X6
Acetaminosalol	T39.1X1	T39.1X2	T39.1X3	T39.1X4	T39.1X5	T39.1X6
Acetanilide	T39.1X1	T39.1X2	T39.1X3	T39.1X4	T39.1X5	T39.1X6
Acetarsol	T37.3X1	T37.3X2	T37.3X3	T37.3X4	T37.3X5	T37.3X6
Acetazolamide	T50.2X1	T50.2X2	T50.2X3	T50.2X4	T50.2X5	T50.2X6
Acetiamine	T45.2X1	T45.2X2	T45.2X3	T45.2X4	T45.2X5	T45.2X6
Acetic						
acid	T54.2X1	T54.2X2	T54.2X3	T54.2X4	—	—
with sodium acetate (ointment)	T49.3X1	T49.3X2	T49.3X3	T49.3X4	T49.3X5	T49.3X6
ester (solvent)(vapor)	T52.8X1	T52.8X2	T52.8X3	T52.8X4	—	—
irrigating solution	T50.3X1	T50.3X2	T50.3X3	T50.3X4	T50.3X5	T50.3X6
medicinal (lotion)	T49.2X1	T49.2X2	T49.2X3	T49.2X4	T49.2X5	T49.2X6
anhydride	T65.891	T65.892	T65.893	T65.894	—	—
ether (vapor)	T52.8X1	T52.8X2	T52.8X3	T52.8X4	—	—
Acetohexamide	T38.3X1	T38.3X2	T38.3X3	T38.3X4	T38.3X5	T38.3X6
Acetohydroxamic acid	T50.991	T50.992	T50.993	T50.994	T50.995	T50.996
Acetomenaphthone	T45.7X1	T45.7X2	T45.7X3	T45.7X4	T45.7X5	T45.7X6
Acetomorphine	T40.1X1	T40.1X2	T40.1X3	T40.1X4	—	—
Acetone (oils)	T52.4X1	T52.4X2	T52.4X3	T52.4X4	—	—
chlorinated	T52.4X1	T52.4X2	T52.4X3	T52.4X4	—	—
vapor	T52.4X1	T52.4X2	T52.4X3	T52.4X4	—	—
Acetonitrile	T52.8X1	T52.8X2	T52.8X3	T52.8X4	—	—
Acetophenazine	T43.3X1	T43.3X2	T43.3X3	T43.3X4	T43.3X5	T43.3X6
Acetophenetedin	T39.1X1	T39.1X2	T39.1X3	T39.1X4	T39.1X5	T39.1X6
Acetophenone	T52.4X1	T52.4X2	T52.4X3	T52.4X4	—	—
Acetorphine	T40.2X1	T40.2X2	T40.2X3	T40.2X4	—	—
Acetosulfone (sodium)	T37.1X1	T37.1X2	T37.1X3	T37.1X4	T37.1X5	T37.1X6
Acetrizoate (sodium)	T50.8X1	T50.8X2	T50.8X3	T50.8X4	T50.8X5	T50.8X6
Acetrizoic acid	T50.8X1	T50.8X2	T50.8X3	T50.8X4	T50.8X5	T50.8X6
Acetyl						
bromide	T53.6X1	T53.6X2	T53.6X3	T53.6X4	—	—
chloride	T53.6X1	T53.6X2	T53.6X3	T53.6X4	—	—
Acetylcarbromal	T42.6X1	T42.6X2	T42.6X3	T42.6X4	T42.6X5	T42.6X6
Acetylcholine						
chloride	T44.1X1	T44.1X2	T44.1X3	T44.1X4	T44.1X5	T44.1X6
derivative	T44.1X1	T44.1X2	T44.1X3	T44.1X4	T44.1X5	T44.1X6
Acetylcysteine	T48.4X1	T48.4X2	T48.4X3	T48.4X4	T48.4X5	T48.4X6
Acetyldigitoxin	T46.0X1	T46.0X2	T46.0X3	T46.0X4	T46.0X5	T46.0X6
Acetyldigoxin	T46.0X1	T46.0X2	T46.0X3	T46.0X4	T46.0X5	T46.0X6
Acetyldihydrocodeine	T40.2X1	T40.2X2	T40.2X3	T40.2X4	—	—
Acetyldihydrocodeinone	T40.2X1	T40.2X2	T40.2X3	T40.2X4	—	—
Acetylene (gas)	T59.891	T59.892	T59.893	T59.894	—	—
dichloride	T53.6X1	T53.6X2	T53.6X3	T53.6X4	—	—
incomplete combustion of	T58.11	T58.12	T58.13	T58.14		
industrial	T59.891	T59.892	T59.893	T59.894	—	—
tetrachloride	T53.6X1	T53.6X2	T53.6X3	T53.6X4	—	—
vapor	T53.6X1	T53.6X2	T53.6X3	T53.6X4	—	—
Acetylpheneturide	T42.6X1	T42.6X2	T42.6X3	T42.6X4	T42.6X5	T42.6X6
Acetylphenylhydrazine	T39.8X1	T39.8X2	T39.8X3	T39.8X4	T39.8X5	T39.8X6
Acetylsalicylic acid (salts)	T39.011	T39.012	T39.013	T39.014	T39.015	T39.016
enteric coated	T39.011	T39.012	T39.013	T39.014	T39.015	T39.016
Acetylsulfamethoxypyridazine	T37.0X1	T37.0X2	T37.0X3	T37.0X4	T37.0X5	T37.0X6
Achromycin	T36.4X1	T36.4X2	T36.4X3	T36.4X4	T36.4X5	T36.4X6
ophthalmic preparation	T49.5X1	T49.5X2	T49.5X3	T49.5X4	T49.5X5	T49.5X6
topical NEC	T49.0X1	T49.0X2	T49.0X3	T49.0X4	T49.0X5	T49.0X6
Aciclovir	T37.5X1	T37.5X2	T37.5X3	T37.5X4	T37.5X5	T37.5X6
Acidifying agent NEC	T50.901	T50.902	T50.903	T50.904	T50.905	T50.906
Acid (corrosive) NEC	T54.2X1	T54.2X2	T54.2X3	T54.2X4	—	—
Acipimox	T46.6X1	T46.6X2	T46.6X3	T46.6X4	T46.6X5	T46.6X6
Acitretin	T50.991	T50.992	T50.993	T50.994	T50.995	T50.996
Aclarubicin	T45.1X1	T45.1X2	T45.1X3	T45.1X4	T45.1X5	T45.1X6
Aclatonium napadisilate	T48.1X1	T48.1X2	T48.1X3	T48.1X4	T48.1X5	T48.1X6
Aconite (wild)	T46.991	T46.992	T46.993	T46.994	T46.995	T46.996
Aconitine	T46.991	T46.992	T46.993	T46.994	T46.995	T46.996
Aconitum ferox	T46.991	T46.992	T46.993	T46.994	T46.995	T46.996
Acridine	T65.6X1	T65.6X2	T65.6X3	T65.6X4	—	—
vapor	T59.891	T59.892	T59.893	T59.894	—	—
Acriflavine	T37.91	T37.92	T37.93	T37.94	T37.95	T37.96
Acriflavinium chloride	T49.0X1	T49.0X2	T49.0X3	T49.0X4	T49.0X5	T49.0X6
Acrinol	T49.0X1	T49.0X2	T49.0X3	T49.0X4	T49.0X5	T49.0X6
Acrisorcin	T49.0X1	T49.0X2	T49.0X3	T49.0X4	T49.0X5	T49.0X6
Acrivastine	T45.0X1	T45.0X2	T45.0X3	T45.0X4	T45.0X5	T45.0X6
Acrolein (gas)	T59.891	T59.892	T59.893	T59.894	—	—
liquid	T54.1X1	T54.1X2	T54.1X3	T54.1X4	—	—
Acrylamide	T65.891	T65.892	T65.893	T65.894	—	—
Acrylic resin	T49.3X1	T49.3X2	T49.3X3	T49.3X4	T49.3X5	T49.3X6
Acrylonitrile	T65.891	T65.892	T65.893	T65.894	—	—
Actaea spicata	T62.2X1	T62.2X2	T62.2X3	T62.2X4	—	—
berry	T62.1X1	T62.1X2	T62.1X3	T62.1X4	—	—
Acterol	T37.3X1	T37.3X2	T37.3X3	T37.3X4	T37.3X5	T37.3X6
ACTH	T38.811	T38.812	T38.813	T38.814	T38.815	T38.816
Actinomycin C	T45.1X1	T45.1X2	T45.1X3	T45.1X4	T45.1X5	T45.1X6
Actinomycin D	T45.1X1	T45.1X2	T45.1X3	T45.1X4	T45.1X5	T45.1X6
Activated charcoal — see also Charcoal, medicinal	T47.6X1	T47.6X2	T47.6X3	T47.6X4	T47.6X5	T47.6X6
Acyclovir	T37.5X1	T37.5X2	T37.5X3	T37.5X4	T37.5X5	T37.5X6
Adenine	T45.2X1	T45.2X2	T45.2X3	T45.2X4	T45.2X5	T45.2X6
arabinoside	T37.5X1	T37.5X2	T37.5X3	T37.5X4	T37.5X5	T37.5X6
Adenosine (phosphate)	T46.2X1	T46.2X2	T46.2X3	T46.2X4	T46.2X5	T46.2X6
ADH	T38.891	T38.892	T38.893	T38.894	T38.895	T38.896
Adhesive NEC	T65.891	T65.892	T65.893	T65.894	—	—
Adicillin	T36.0X1	T36.0X2	T36.0X3	T36.0X4	T36.0X5	T36.0X6
Adiphenine	T44.3X1	T44.3X2	T44.3X3	T44.3X4	T44.3X5	T44.3X6
Adipiodone	T50.8X1	T50.8X2	T50.8X3	T50.8X4	T50.8X5	T50.8X6
Adjunct, pharmaceutical	T50.901	T50.902	T50.903	T50.904	T50.905	T50.906
Adrenal (extract, cortex or medulla) (glucocorticoids) (hormones) (mineralocorticoids)	T38.0X1	T38.0X2	T38.0X3	T38.0X4	T38.0X5	T38.0X6
ENT agent	T49.6X1	T49.6X2	T49.6X3	T49.6X4	T49.6X5	T49.6X6
ophthalmic preparation	T49.5X1	T49.5X2	T49.5X3	T49.5X4	T49.5X5	T49.5X6
topical NEC	T49.0X1	T49.0X2	T49.0X3	T49.0X4	T49.0X5	T49.0X6
Adrenalin — see Adrenaline						
Adrenaline	T44.5X1	T44.5X2	T44.5X3	T44.5X4	T44.5X5	T44.5X6
Adrenergic NEC	T44.901	T44.902	T44.903	T44.904	T44.905	T44.906
blocking agent NEC	T44.8X1	T44.8X2	T44.8X3	T44.8X4	T44.8X5	T44.8X6
beta, heart	T44.7X1	T44.7X2	T44.7X3	T44.7X4	T44.7X5	T44.7X6
specified NEC	T44.991	T44.992	T44.993	T44.994	T44.995	T44.996
Adrenochrome						
derivative	T46.991	T46.992	T46.993	T46.994	T46.995	T46.996
(mono) semicarbazone	T46.991	T46.992	T46.993	T46.994	T46.995	T46.996
Adrenocorticotrophic hormone	T38.811	T38.812	T38.813	T38.814	T38.815	T38.816
Adrenocorticotrophin	T38.811	T38.812	T38.813	T38.814	T38.815	T38.816
Adriamycin	T45.1X1	T45.1X2	T45.1X3	T45.1X4	T45.1X5	T45.1X6
Aerosol spray NEC	T65.91	T65.92	T65.93	T65.94	—	—
Aerosporin	T36.8X1	T36.8X2	T36.8X3	T36.8X4	T36.8X5	T36.8X6
ENT agent	T49.6X1	T49.6X2	T49.6X3	T49.6X4	T49.6X5	T49.6X6
ophthalmic preparation	T49.5X1	T49.5X2	T49.5X3	T49.5X4	T49.5X5	T49.5X6
topical NEC	T49.0X1	T49.0X2	T49.0X3	T49.0X4	T49.0X5	T49.0X6
Aethusa cynapium	T62.2X1	T62.2X2	T62.2X3	T62.2X4	—	—
Afghanistan black	T40.7X1	T40.7X2	T40.7X3	T40.7X4	T40.7X5	T40.7X6

14-Hydroxydihydromorphinone — Afghanistan black

Table of Drugs and Chemicals

Aflatoxin — Amanita phalloides

Substance	Poisoning, Accidental (unintentional)	Poisoning, Intentional Self-harm	Poisoning, Assault	Poisoning, Undetermined	Adverse Effect	Underdosing
Aflatoxin	T64.01	T64.02	T64.03	T64.04	—	—
Afloqualone	T42.8X1	T42.8X2	T42.8X3	T42.8X4	T42.8X5	T42.8X6
African boxwood	T62.2X1	T62.2X2	T62.2X3	T62.2X4		
Agar	T47.4X1	T47.4X2	T47.4X3	T47.4X4	T47.4X5	T47.4X6
Agonist						
predominantly						
alpha-adrenoreceptor	T44.4X1	T44.4X2	T44.4X3	T44.4X4	T44.4X5	T44.4X6
beta-adrenoreceptor	T44.5X1	T44.5X2	T44.5X3	T44.5X4	T44.5X5	T44.5X6
Agricultural agent NEC	T65.91	T65.92	T65.93	T65.94	—	—
Agrypnal	T42.3X1	T42.3X2	T42.3X3	T42.3X4	T42.3X5	T42.3X6
AHLG	T50.Z11	T50.Z12	T50.Z13	T50.Z14	T50.Z15	T50.Z16
Air contaminant(s), source/type NOS	T65.91	T65.92	T65.93	T65.94	—	—
Ajmaline	T46.2X1	T46.2X2	T46.2X3	T46.2X4	T46.2X5	T46.2X6
Akee	T62.1X1	T62.1X2	T62.1X3	T62.1X4		
Akrinol	T49.0X1	T49.0X2	T49.0X3	T49.0X4	T49.0X5	T49.0X6
Akritoin	T37.8X1	T37.8X2	T37.8X3	T37.8X4	T37.8X5	T37.8X6
Alacepril	T46.4X1	T46.4X2	T46.4X3	T46.4X4	T46.4X5	T46.4X6
Alantolactone	T37.4X1	T37.4X2	T37.4X3	T37.4X4	T37.4X5	T37.4X6
Albamycin	T36.8X1	T36.8X2	T36.8X3	T36.8X4	T36.8X5	T36.8X6
Albendazole	T37.4X1	T37.4X2	T37.4X3	T37.4X4	T37.4X5	T37.4X6
Albumin						
bovine	T45.8X1	T45.8X2	T45.8X3	T45.8X4	T45.8X5	T45.8X6
human serum	T45.8X1	T45.8X2	T45.8X3	T45.8X4	T45.8X5	T45.8X6
salt-poor	T45.8X1	T45.8X2	T45.8X3	T45.8X4	T45.8X5	T45.8X6
normal human serum	T45.8X1	T45.8X2	T45.8X3	T45.8X4	T45.8X5	T45.8X6
Albuterol	T48.6X1	T48.6X2	T48.6X3	T48.6X4	T48.6X5	T48.6X6
Albutoin	T42.0X1	T42.0X2	T42.0X3	T42.0X4	T42.0X5	T42.0X6
Alclometasone	T49.0X1	T49.0X2	T49.0X3	T49.0X4	T49.0X5	T49.0X6
Alcohol	T51.91	T51.92	T51.93	T51.94	—	—
absolute	T51.0X1	T51.0X2	T51.0X3	T51.0X4	—	—
beverage	T51.0X1	T51.0X2	T51.0X3	T51.0X4	—	—
allyl	T51.8X1	T51.8X2	T51.8X3	T51.8X4	—	—
amyl	T51.3X1	T51.3X2	T51.3X3	T51.3X4	—	—
antifreeze	T51.1X1	T51.1X2	T51.1X3	T51.1X4	—	—
beverage	T51.0X1	T51.0X2	T51.0X3	T51.0X4	—	—
butyl	T51.3X1	T51.3X2	T51.3X3	T51.3X4	—	—
dehydrated	T51.0X1	T51.0X2	T51.0X3	T51.0X4	—	—
beverage	T51.0X1	T51.0X2	T51.0X3	T51.0X4	—	—
denatured	T51.0X1	T51.0X2	T51.0X3	T51.0X4	—	—
deterrent NEC	T50.6X1	T50.6X2	T50.6X3	T50.6X4	T50.6X5	T50.6X6
diagnostic (gastric function)	T50.8X1	T50.8X2	T50.8X3	T50.8X4	T50.8X5	T50.8X6
ethyl	T51.0X1	T51.0X2	T51.0X3	T51.0X4	—	—
beverage	T51.0X1	T51.0X2	T51.0X3	T51.0X4	—	—
grain	T51.0X1	T51.0X2	T51.0X3	T51.0X4	—	—
beverage	T51.0X1	T51.0X2	T51.0X3	T51.0X4	—	—
industrial	T51.0X1	T51.0X2	T51.0X3	T51.0X4	—	—
isopropyl	T51.2X1	T51.2X2	T51.2X3	T51.2X4	—	—
methyl	T51.1X1	T51.1X2	T51.1X3	T51.1X4	—	—
preparation for consumption	T51.0X1	T51.0X2	T51.0X3	T51.0X4	—	—
propyl	T51.3X1	T51.3X2	T51.3X3	T51.3X4	—	—
secondary	T51.2X1	T51.2X2	T51.2X3	T51.2X4	—	—
radiator	T51.1X1	T51.1X2	T51.1X3	T51.1X4	—	—
rubbing	T51.2X1	T51.2X2	T51.2X3	T51.2X4	—	—
specified type NEC	T51.8X1	T51.8X2	T51.8X3	T51.8X4	—	—
surgical	T51.0X1	T51.0X2	T51.0X3	T51.0X4	—	—
vapor (from any type of Alcohol)	T59.891	T59.892	T59.893	T59.894	—	—
wood	T51.1X1	T51.1X2	T51.1X3	T51.1X4	—	—
Alcuronium (chloride)	T48.1X1	T48.1X2	T48.1X3	T48.1X4	T48.1X5	T48.1X6
Aldactone	T50.0X1	T50.0X2	T50.0X3	T50.0X4	T50.0X5	T50.0X6
Aldesulfone sodium	T37.1X1	T37.1X2	T37.1X3	T37.1X4	T37.1X5	T37.1X6
Aldicarb	T60.0X1	T60.0X2	T60.0X3	T60.0X4	—	—
Aldomet	T46.5X1	T46.5X2	T46.5X3	T46.5X4	T46.5X5	T46.5X6
Aldosterone	T50.0X1	T50.0X2	T50.0X3	T50.0X4	T50.0X5	T50.0X6
Aldrin (dust)	T60.1X1	T60.1X2	T60.1X3	T60.1X4	—	—
Aleve — see Naproxen						
Alexitol sodium	T47.1X1	T47.1X2	T47.1X3	T47.1X4	T47.1X5	T47.1X6
Alfacalcidol	T45.2X1	T45.2X2	T45.2X3	T45.2X4	T45.2X5	T45.2X6
Alfadolone	T41.1X1	T41.1X2	T41.1X3	T41.1X4	T41.1X5	T41.1X6
Alfaxalone	T41.1X1	T41.1X2	T41.1X3	T41.1X4	T41.1X5	T41.1X6
Alfentanil	T40.4X1	T40.4X2	T40.4X3	T40.4X4	T40.4X5	T40.4X6
Alfuzosin (hydrochloride)	T44.8X1	T44.8X2	T44.8X3	T44.8X4	T44.8X5	T44.8X6
Algae (harmful) (toxin)	T65.821	T65.822	T65.823	T65.824	—	—
Algeldrate	T47.1X1	T47.1X2	T47.1X3	T47.1X4	T47.1X5	T47.1X6
Algin	T47.8X1	T47.8X2	T47.8X3	T47.8X4	T47.8X5	T47.8X6
Alglucerase	T45.3X1	T45.3X2	T45.3X3	T45.3X4	T45.3X5	T45.3X6
Alidase	T45.3X1	T45.3X2	T45.3X3	T45.3X4	T45.3X5	T45.3X6
Alimemazine	T43.3X1	T43.3X2	T43.3X3	T43.3X4	T43.3X5	T43.3X6
Aliphatic thiocyanates	T65.0X1	T65.0X2	T65.0X3	T65.0X4	—	—
Alizapride	T45.0X1	T45.0X2	T45.0X3	T45.0X4	T45.0X5	T45.0X6

Substance	Poisoning, Accidental (unintentional)	Poisoning, Intentional Self-harm	Poisoning, Assault	Poisoning, Undetermined	Adverse Effect	Underdosing
Alkali (caustic)	T54.3X1	T54.3X2	T54.3X3	T54.3X4	—	—
Alkaline antiseptic solution (aromatic)	T49.6X1	T49.6X2	T49.6X3	T49.6X4	T49.6X5	T49.6X6
Alkalinizing agents (medicinal)	T50.901	T50.902	T50.903	T50.904	T50.905	T50.906
Alkalizing agent NEC	T50.901	T50.902	T50.903	T50.904	T50.905	T50.906
Alka-seltzer	T39.011	T39.012	T39.013	T39.014	T39.015	T39.016
Alkavervir	T46.5X1	T46.5X2	T46.5X3	T46.5X4	T46.5X5	T46.5X6
Alkonium (bromide)	T49.0X1	T49.0X2	T49.0X3	T49.0X4	T49.0X5	T49.0X6
Alkylating drug NEC	T45.1X1	T45.1X2	T45.1X3	T45.1X4	T45.1X5	T45.1X6
antimyeloproliferative	T45.1X1	T45.1X2	T45.1X3	T45.1X4	T45.1X5	T45.1X6
lymphatic	T45.1X1	T45.1X2	T45.1X3	T45.1X4	T45.1X5	T45.1X6
Alkylisocyanate	T65.0X1	T65.0X2	T65.0X3	T65.0X4	—	—
Allantoin	T49.4X1	T49.4X2	T49.4X3	T49.4X4	T49.4X5	T49.4X6
Allegron	T43.011	T43.012	T43.013	T43.014	T43.015	T43.016
Allethrin	T49.0X1	T49.0X2	T49.0X3	T49.0X4	T49.0X5	T49.0X6
Allobarbital	T42.3X1	T42.3X2	T42.3X3	T42.3X4	T42.3X5	T42.3X6
Allopurinol	T50.4X1	T50.4X2	T50.4X3	T50.4X4	T50.4X5	T50.4X6
Allyl						
alcohol	T51.8X1	T51.8X2	T51.8X3	T51.8X4	—	—
disulfide	T46.6X1	T46.6X2	T46.6X3	T46.6X4	T46.6X5	T46.6X6
Allylestrenol	T38.5X1	T38.5X2	T38.5X3	T38.5X4	T38.5X5	T38.5X6
Allylisopropylacetylurea	T42.6X1	T42.6X2	T42.6X3	T42.6X4	T42.6X5	T42.6X6
Allylisopropylmalonylurea	T42.3X1	T42.3X2	T42.3X3	T42.3X4	T42.3X5	T42.3X6
Allylthiourea	T49.3X1	T49.3X2	T49.3X3	T49.3X4	T49.3X5	T49.3X6
Allyltribromide	T42.6X1	T42.6X2	T42.6X3	T42.6X4	T42.6X5	T42.6X6
Allylpropymal	T42.3X1	T42.3X2	T42.3X3	T42.3X4	T42.3X5	T42.3X6
Almagate	T47.1X1	T47.1X2	T47.1X3	T47.1X4	T47.1X5	T47.1X6
Almasilate	T47.1X1	T47.1X2	T47.1X3	T47.1X4	T47.1X5	T47.1X6
Almitrine	T50.7X1	T50.7X2	T50.7X3	T50.7X4	T50.7X5	T50.7X6
Aloes	T47.2X1	T47.2X2	T47.2X3	T47.2X4	T47.2X5	T47.2X6
Aloglutamol	T47.1X1	T47.1X2	T47.1X3	T47.1X4	T47.1X5	T47.1X6
Aloin	T47.2X1	T47.2X2	T47.2X3	T47.2X4	T47.2X5	T47.2X6
Aloxidone	T42.2X1	T42.2X2	T42.2X3	T42.2X4	T42.2X5	T42.2X6
Alpha						
acetyldigoxin	T46.0X1	T46.0X2	T46.0X3	T46.0X4	T46.0X5	T46.0X6
adrenergic blocking drug	T44.6X1	T44.6X2	T44.6X3	T44.6X4	T44.6X5	T44.6X6
amylase	T45.3X1	T45.3X2	T45.3X3	T45.3X4	T45.3X5	T45.3X6
tocoferol (acetate)	T45.2X1	T45.2X2	T45.2X3	T45.2X4	T45.2X5	T45.2X6
tocopherol	T45.2X1	T45.2X2	T45.2X3	T45.2X4	T45.2X5	T45.2X6
Alphadolone	T41.1X1	T41.1X2	T41.1X3	T41.1X4	T41.1X5	T41.1X6
Alphaprodine	T40.4X1	T40.4X2	T40.4X3	T40.4X4	T40.4X5	T40.4X6
Alphaxalone	T41.1X1	T41.1X2	T41.1X3	T41.1X4	T41.1X5	T41.1X6
Alprazolam	T42.4X1	T42.4X2	T42.4X3	T42.4X4	T42.4X5	T42.4X6
Alprenolol	T44.7X1	T44.7X2	T44.7X3	T44.7X4	T44.7X5	T44.7X6
Alprostadil	T46.7X1	T46.7X2	T46.7X3	T46.7X4	T46.7X5	T46.7X6
Alsactide	T38.811	T38.812	T38.813	T38.814	T38.815	T38.816
Alseroxylon	T46.5X1	T46.5X2	T46.5X3	T46.5X4	T46.5X5	T46.5X6
Alteplase	T45.611	T45.612	T45.613	T45.614	T45.615	T45.616
Altizide	T50.2X1	T50.2X2	T50.2X3	T50.2X4	T50.2X5	T50.2X6
Altretamine	T45.1X1	T45.1X2	T45.1X3	T45.1X4	T45.1X5	T45.1X6
Alum (medicinal)	T49.4X1	T49.4X2	T49.4X3	T49.4X4	T49.4X5	T49.4X6
nonmedicinal (ammonium) (potassium)	T56.891	T56.892	T56.893	T56.894	—	—
Aluminium, aluminum						
acetate	T49.2X1	T49.2X2	T49.2X3	T49.2X4	T49.2X5	T49.2X6
solution	T49.0X1	T49.0X2	T49.0X3	T49.0X4	T49.0X5	T49.0X6
aspirin	T39.011	T39.012	T39.013	T39.014	T39.015	T39.016
bis (acetylsalicylate)	T39.011	T39.012	T39.013	T39.014	T39.015	T39.016
carbonate (gel, basic)	T47.1X1	T47.1X2	T47.1X3	T47.1X4	T47.1X5	T47.1X6
chlorhydroxide-complex	T47.1X1	T47.1X2	T47.1X3	T47.1X4	T47.1X5	T47.1X6
chloride	T49.2X1	T49.2X2	T49.2X3	T49.2X4	T49.2X5	T49.2X6
clofibrate	T46.6X1	T46.6X2	T46.6X3	T46.6X4	T46.6X5	T46.6X6
diacetate	T49.2X1	T49.2X2	T49.2X3	T49.2X4	T49.2X5	T49.2X6
glycinate	T47.1X1	T47.1X2	T47.1X3	T47.1X4	T47.1X5	T47.1X6
hydroxide (gel)	T47.1X1	T47.1X2	T47.1X3	T47.1X4	T47.1X5	T47.1X6
hydroxide-magnesium carb. gel	T47.1X1	T47.1X2	T47.1X3	T47.1X4	T47.1X5	T47.1X6
magnesium silicate	T47.1X1	T47.1X2	T47.1X3	T47.1X4	T47.1X5	T47.1X6
nicotinate	T46.7X1	T46.7X2	T46.7X3	T46.7X4	T46.7X5	T46.7X6
ointment (surgical) (topical)	T49.3X1	T49.3X2	T49.3X3	T49.3X4	T49.3X5	T49.3X6
phosphate	T47.1X1	T47.1X2	T47.1X3	T47.1X4	T47.1X5	T47.1X6
salicylate	T39.091	T39.092	T39.093	T39.094	T39.095	T39.096
silicate	T47.1X1	T47.1X2	T47.1X3	T47.1X4	T47.1X5	T47.1X6
sodium silicate	T47.1X1	T47.1X2	T47.1X3	T47.1X4	T47.1X5	T47.1X6
subacetate	T49.2X1	T49.2X2	T49.2X3	T49.2X4	T49.2X5	T49.2X6
sulfate	T49.0X1	T49.0X2	T49.0X3	T49.0X4	T49.0X5	T49.0X6
tannate	T47.6X1	T47.6X2	T47.6X3	T47.6X4	T47.6X5	T47.6X6
topical NEC	T49.3X1	T49.3X2	T49.3X3	T49.3X4	T49.3X5	T49.3X6
Alurate	T42.3X1	T42.3X2	T42.3X3	T42.3X4	T42.3X5	T42.3X6
Alverine	T44.3X1	T44.3X2	T44.3X3	T44.3X4	T44.3X5	T44.3X6
Alvodine	T40.2X1	T40.2X2	T40.2X3	T40.2X4	T40.2X5	T40.2X6
Amanita phalloides	T62.0X1	T62.0X2	T62.0X3	T62.0X4	—	—

Additional Character May Be Required — Refer to the Tabular List for Character Selection ▽ Subterms under main terms may continue to next column or page

Substance	Poisoning, Accidental (unintentional)	Poisoning, Intentional Self-harm	Poisoning, Assault	Poisoning, Undetermined	Adverse Effect	Under-dosing
Amanitine	T62.0X1	T62.0X2	T62.0X3	T62.0X4	—	—
Amantadine	T42.8X1	T42.8X2	T42.8X3	T42.8X4	T42.8X5	T42.8X6
Ambazone	T49.6X1	T49.6X2	T49.6X3	T49.6X4	T49.6X5	T49.6X6
Ambenonium (chloride)	T44.0X1	T44.0X2	T44.0X3	T44.0X4	T44.0X5	T44.0X6
Ambroxol	T48.4X1	T48.4X2	T48.4X3	T48.4X4	T48.4X5	T48.4X6
Ambuphylline	T48.6X1	T48.6X2	T48.6X3	T48.6X4	T48.6X5	T48.6X6
Ambutonium bromide	T44.3X1	T44.3X2	T44.3X3	T44.3X4	T44.3X5	T44.3X6
Amcinonide	T49.0X1	T49.0X2	T49.0X3	T49.0X4	T49.0X5	T49.0X6
Amdinocilline	T36.0X1	T36.0X2	T36.0X3	T36.0X4	T36.0X5	T36.0X6
Ametazole	T50.8X1	T50.8X2	T50.8X3	T50.8X4	T50.8X5	T50.8X6
Amethocaine	T41.3X1	T41.3X2	T41.3X3	T41.3X4	T41.3X5	T41.3X6
regional	T41.3X1	T41.3X2	T41.3X3	T41.3X4	T41.3X5	T41.3X6
spinal	T41.3X1	T41.3X2	T41.3X3	T41.3X4	T41.3X5	T41.3X6
Amethopterin	T45.1X1	T45.1X2	T45.1X3	T45.1X4	T45.1X5	T45.1X6
Amezinium metilsulfate	T44.991	T44.992	T44.993	T44.994	T44.995	T44.996
Amfebutamone	T43.291	T43.292	T43.293	T43.294	T43.295	T43.296
Amfepramone	T50.5X1	T50.5X2	T50.5X3	T50.5X4	T50.5X5	T50.5X6
Amfetamine	T43.621	T43.622	T43.623	T43.624	T43.625	T43.626
Amfetaminil	T43.621	T43.622	T43.623	T43.624	T43.625	T43.626
Amfomycin	T36.8X1	T36.8X2	T36.8X3	T36.8X4	T36.8X5	T36.8X6
Amidefrine mesilate	T48.5X1	T48.5X2	T48.5X3	T48.5X4	T48.5X5	T48.5X6
Amidone	T40.3X1	T40.3X2	T40.3X3	T40.3X4	T40.3X5	T40.3X6
Amidopyrine	T39.2X1	T39.2X2	T39.2X3	T39.2X4	T39.2X5	T39.2X6
Amidotrizoate	T50.8X1	T50.8X2	T50.8X3	T50.8X4	T50.8X5	T50.8X6
Amiflamine	T43.1X1	T43.1X2	T43.1X3	T43.1X4	T43.1X5	T43.1X6
Amikacin	T36.5X1	T36.5X2	T36.5X3	T36.5X4	T36.5X5	T36.5X6
Amikhelline	T46.3X1	T46.3X2	T46.3X3	T46.3X4	T46.3X5	T46.3X6
Amiloride	T50.2X1	T50.2X2	T50.2X3	T50.2X4	T50.2X5	T50.2X6
Aminacrine	T49.0X1	T49.0X2	T49.0X3	T49.0X4	T49.0X5	T49.0X6
Amineptine	T43.011	T43.012	T43.013	T43.014	T43.015	T43.016
Aminitrozole	T37.3X1	T37.3X2	T37.3X3	T37.3X4	T37.3X5	T37.3X6
Aminoacetic acid (derivatives)	T50.3X1	T50.3X2	T50.3X3	T50.3X4	T50.3X5	T50.3X6
Amino acids	T50.3X1	T50.3X2	T50.3X3	T50.3X4	T50.3X5	T50.3X6
Aminoacridine	T49.0X1	T49.0X2	T49.0X3	T49.0X4	T49.0X5	T49.0X6
Aminobenzoic acid (-p)	T49.3X1	T49.3X2	T49.3X3	T49.3X4	T49.3X5	T49.3X6
Aminocaproic acid	T45.621	T45.622	T45.623	T45.624	T45.625	T45.626
Aminoethylisothiourium	T45.8X1	T45.8X2	T45.8X3	T45.8X4	T45.8X5	T45.8X6
Aminofenazone	T39.2X1	T39.2X2	T39.2X3	T39.2X4	T39.2X5	T39.2X6
Aminoglutethimide	T45.1X1	T45.1X2	T45.1X3	T45.1X4	T45.1X5	T45.1X6
Aminohippuric acid	T50.8X1	T50.8X2	T50.8X3	T50.8X4	T50.8X5	T50.8X6
Aminomethylbenzoic acid	T45.691	T45.692	T45.693	T45.694	T45.695	T45.696
Aminometradine	T50.2X1	T50.2X2	T50.2X3	T50.2X4	T50.2X5	T50.2X6
Aminopentamide	T44.3X1	T44.3X2	T44.3X3	T44.3X4	T44.3X5	T44.3X6
Aminophenazone	T39.2X1	T39.2X2	T39.2X3	T39.2X4	T39.2X5	T39.2X6
Aminophenol	T54.0X1	T54.0X2	T54.0X3	T54.0X4	—	—
Aminophenylpyridone	T43.591	T43.592	T43.593	T43.594	T43.595	T43.596
Aminophylline	T48.6X1	T48.6X2	T48.6X3	T48.6X4	T48.6X5	T48.6X6
Aminopterin sodium	T45.1X1	T45.1X2	T45.1X3	T45.1X4	T45.1X5	T45.1X6
Aminopyrine	T39.2X1	T39.2X2	T39.2X3	T39.2X4	T39.2X5	T39.2X6
Aminorex	T50.5X1	T50.5X2	T50.5X3	T50.5X4	T50.5X5	T50.5X6
Aminosalicylic acid	T37.1X1	T37.1X2	T37.1X3	T37.1X4	T37.1X5	T37.1X6
Aminosalylum	T37.1X1	T37.1X2	T37.1X3	T37.1X4	T37.1X5	T37.1X6
Amiodarone	T46.2X1	T46.2X2	T46.2X3	T46.2X4	T46.2X5	T46.2X6
Amiphenazole	T50.7X1	T50.7X2	T50.7X3	T50.7X4	T50.7X5	T50.7X6
Amiquinsin	T46.5X1	T46.5X2	T46.5X3	T46.5X4	T46.5X5	T46.5X6
Amisometradine	T50.2X1	T50.2X2	T50.2X3	T50.2X4	T50.2X5	T50.2X6
Amisulpride	T43.591	T43.592	T43.593	T43.594	T43.595	T43.596
Amitriptyline	T43.011	T43.012	T43.013	T43.014	T43.015	T43.016
Amitriptylinoxide	T43.011	T43.012	T43.013	T43.014	T43.015	T43.016
Amlexanox	T48.6X1	T48.6X2	T48.6X3	T48.6X4	T48.6X5	T48.6X6
Ammonia (fumes) (gas) (vapor)	T59.891	T59.892	T59.893	T59.894	—	—
aromatic spirit	T48.991	T48.992	T48.993	T48.994	T48.995	T48.996
liquid (household)	T54.3X1	T54.3X2	T54.3X3	T54.3X4	—	—
Ammoniated mercury	T49.0X1	T49.0X2	T49.0X3	T49.0X4	T49.0X5	T49.0X6
Ammonium						
acid tartrate	T49.5X1	T49.5X2	T49.5X3	T49.5X4	T49.5X5	T49.5X6
bromide	T42.6X1	T42.6X2	T42.6X3	T42.6X4	T42.6X5	T42.6X6
carbonate	T54.3X1	T54.3X2	T54.3X3	T54.3X4	—	—
chloride	T50.991	T50.992	T50.993	T50.994	T50.995	T50.996
expectorant	T48.4X1	T48.4X2	T48.4X3	T48.4X4	T48.4X5	T48.4X6
compounds (household) NEC	T54.3X1	T54.3X2	T54.3X3	T54.3X4	—	—
fumes (any usage)	T59.891	T59.892	T59.893	T59.894	—	—
industrial	T54.3X1	T54.3X2	T54.3X3	T54.3X4	—	—
ichthyosulronate	T49.4X1	T49.4X2	T49.4X3	T49.4X4	T49.4X5	T49.4X6
mandelate	T37.91	T37.92	T37.93	T37.94	T37.95	T37.96
sulfamate	T60.3X1	T60.3X2	T60.3X3	T60.3X4	—	—
sulfonate resin	T47.8X1	T47.8X2	T47.8X3	T47.8X4	T47.8X5	T47.8X6
Amobarbital (sodium)	T42.3X1	T42.3X2	T42.3X3	T42.3X4	T42.3X5	T42.3X6
Amodiaquine	T37.2X1	T37.2X2	T37.2X3	T37.2X4	T37.2X5	T37.2X6
Amopyroquin (e)	T37.2X1	T37.2X2	T37.2X3	T37.2X4	T37.2X5	T37.2X6

Substance	Poisoning, Accidental (unintentional)	Poisoning, Intentional Self-harm	Poisoning, Assault	Poisoning, Undetermined	Adverse Effect	Under-dosing
Amoxapine	T43.011	T43.012	T43.013	T43.014	T43.015	T43.016
Amoxicillin	T36.0X1	T36.0X2	T36.0X3	T36.0X4	T36.0X5	T36.0X6
Amperozide	T43.591	T43.592	T43.593	T43.594	T43.595	T43.596
Amphenidone	T43.591	T43.592	T43.593	T43.594	T43.595	T43.596
Amphetamine NEC	T43.621	T43.622	T43.623	T43.624	T43.625	T43.626
Amphomycin	T36.8X1	T36.8X2	T36.8X3	T36.8X4	T36.8X5	T36.8X6
Amphotalide	T37.4X1	T37.4X2	T37.4X3	T37.4X4	T37.4X5	T37.4X6
Amphotericin B	T36.7X1	T36.7X2	T36.7X3	T36.7X4	T36.7X5	T36.7X6
topical	T49.0X1	T49.0X2	T49.0X3	T49.0X4	T49.0X5	T49.0X6
Ampicillin	T36.0X1	T36.0X2	T36.0X3	T36.0X4	T36.0X5	T36.0X6
Amprotropine	T44.3X1	T44.3X2	T44.3X3	T44.3X4	T44.3X5	T44.3X6
Amsacrine	T45.1X1	T45.1X2	T45.1X3	T45.1X4	T45.1X5	T45.1X6
Amygdaline	T62.2X1	T62.2X2	T62.2X3	T62.2X4	—	—
Amyl						
acetate	T52.8X1	T52.8X2	T52.8X3	T52.8X4		
vapor	T59.891	T59.892	T59.893	T59.894		
alcohol	T51.3X1	T51.3X2	T51.3X3	T51.3X4	—	—
chloride	T53.6X1	T53.6X2	T53.6X3	T53.6X4		
formate	T52.8X1	T52.8X2	T52.8X3	T52.8X4		
nitrite	T46.3X1	T46.3X2	T46.3X3	T46.3X4	T46.3X5	T46.3X6
propionate	T65.891	T65.892	T65.893	T65.894		
Amylase	T47.5X1	T47.5X2	T47.5X3	T47.5X4	T47.5X5	T47.5X6
Amyleine, regional	T41.3X1	T41.3X2	T41.3X3	T41.3X4	T41.3X5	T41.3X6
Amylene						
dichloride	T53.6X1	T53.6X2	T53.6X3	T53.6X4	—	—
hydrate	T51.3X1	T51.3X2	T51.3X3	T51.3X4	—	—
Amylmetacresol	T49.6X1	T49.6X2	T49.6X3	T49.6X4	T49.6X5	T49.6X6
Amylobarbitone	T42.3X1	T42.3X2	T42.3X3	T42.3X4	T42.3X5	T42.3X6
Amylocaine, regional	T41.3X1	T41.3X2	T41.3X3	T41.3X4	T41.3X5	T41.3X6
infiltration (subcutaneous)	T41.3X1	T41.3X2	T41.3X3	T41.3X4	T41.3X5	T41.3X6
nerve block (peripheral) (plexus)	T41.3X1	T41.3X2	T41.3X3	T41.3X4	T41.3X5	T41.3X6
spinal	T41.3X1	T41.3X2	T41.3X3	T41.3X4	T41.3X5	T41.3X6
topical (surface)	T41.3X1	T41.3X2	T41.3X3	T41.3X4	T41.3X5	T41.3X6
Amylopectin	T47.6X1	T47.6X2	T47.6X3	T47.6X4	T47.6X5	T47.6X6
Amytal (sodium)	T42.3X1	T42.3X2	T42.3X3	T42.3X4	T42.3X5	T42.3X6
Anabolic steroid	T38.7X1	T38.7X2	T38.7X3	T38.7X4	T38.7X5	T38.7X6
Analeptic NEC	T50.7X1	T50.7X2	T50.7X3	T50.7X4	T50.7X5	T50.7X6
Analgesic	T39.91	T39.92	T39.93	T39.94	T39.95	T39.96
anti-inflammatory NEC	T39.91	T39.92	T39.93	T39.94	T39.95	T39.96
propionic acid derivative	T39.311	T39.312	T39.313	T39.314	T39.315	T39.316
antirheumatic NEC	T39.4X1	T39.4X2	T39.4X3	T39.4X4	T39.4X5	T39.4X6
aromatic NEC	T39.1X1	T39.1X2	T39.1X3	T39.1X4	T39.1X5	T39.1X6
narcotic NEC	T40.601	T40.602	T40.603	T40.604	T40.605	T40.606
combination	T40.601	T40.602	T40.603	T40.604	T40.605	T40.606
obstetric	T40.601	T40.602	T40.603	T40.604	T40.605	T40.606
non-narcotic NEC	T39.91	T39.92	T39.93	T39.94	T39.95	T39.96
combination	T39.91	T39.92	T39.93	T39.94	T39.95	T39.96
pyrazole	T39.2X1	T39.2X2	T39.2X3	T39.2X4	T39.2X5	T39.2X6
specified NEC	T39.8X1	T39.8X2	T39.8X3	T39.8X4	T39.8X5	T39.8X6
Analgin	T39.2X1	T39.2X2	T39.2X3	T39.2X4	T39.2X5	T39.2X6
Anamirta cocculus	T62.1X1	T62.1X2	T62.1X3	T62.1X4	—	—
Ancillin	T36.0X1	T36.0X2	T36.0X3	T36.0X4	T36.0X5	T36.0X6
Ancrod	T45.691	T45.692	T45.693	T45.694	T45.695	T45.696
Androgen	T38.7X1	T38.7X2	T38.7X3	T38.7X4	T38.7X5	T38.7X6
Androgen-estrogen mixture	T38.7X1	T38.7X2	T38.7X3	T38.7X4	T38.7X5	T38.7X6
Androstalone	T38.7X1	T38.7X2	T38.7X3	T38.7X4	T38.7X5	T38.7X6
Androstanolone	T38.7X1	T38.7X2	T38.7X3	T38.7X4	T38.7X5	T38.7X6
Androsterone	T38.7X1	T38.7X2	T38.7X3	T38.7X4	T38.7X5	T38.7X6
Anemone pulsatilla	T62.2X1	T62.2X2	T62.2X3	T62.2X4	—	—
Anesthesia						
caudal	T41.3X1	T41.3X2	T41.3X3	T41.3X4	T41.3X5	T41.3X6
endotracheal	T41.0X1	T41.0X2	T41.0X3	T41.0X4	T41.0X5	T41.0X6
epidural	T41.3X1	T41.3X2	T41.3X3	T41.3X4	T41.3X5	T41.3X6
inhalation	T41.0X1	T41.0X2	T41.0X3	T41.0X4	T41.0X5	T41.0X6
local	T41.3X1	T41.3X2	T41.3X3	T41.3X4	T41.3X5	T41.3X6
mucosal	T41.3X1	T41.3X2	T41.3X3	T41.3X4	T41.3X5	T41.3X6
muscle relaxation	T48.1X1	T48.1X2	T48.1X3	T48.1X4	T48.1X5	T48.1X6
nerve blocking	T41.3X1	T41.3X2	T41.3X3	T41.3X4	T41.3X5	T41.3X6
plexus blocking	T41.3X1	T41.3X2	T41.3X3	T41.3X4	T41.3X5	T41.3X6
potentiated	T41.201	T41.202	T41.203	T41.204	T41.205	T41.206
rectal	T41.201	T41.202	T41.203	T41.204	T41.205	T41.206
general	T41.201	T41.202	T41.203	T41.204	T41.205	T41.206
local	T41.3X1	T41.3X2	T41.3X3	T41.3X4	T41.3X5	T41.3X6
regional	T41.3X1	T41.3X2	T41.3X3	T41.3X4	T41.3X5	T41.3X6
surface	T41.3X1	T41.3X2	T41.3X3	T41.3X4	T41.3X5	T41.3X6
Anesthetic NEC — *see also* Anesthesia	T41.41	T41.42	T41.43	T41.44	T41.45	T41.46
with muscle relaxant	T41.201	T41.202	T41.203	T41.204	T41.205	T41.206
general	T41.201	T41.202	T41.203	T41.204	T41.205	T41.206
local	T41.3X1	T41.3X2	T41.3X3	T41.3X4	T41.3X5	T41.3X6
gaseous NEC	T41.0X1	T41.0X2	T41.0X3	T41.0X4	T41.0X5	T41.0X6

Substance	Poisoning, Accidental (unintentional)	Poisoning, Intentional Self-harm	Poisoning, Assault	Poisoning, Undetermined	Adverse Effect	Under-dosing
Anesthetic — *see also* Anesthesia — *continued*						
general NEC	T41.201	T41.202	T41.203	T41.204	T41.205	T41.206
halogenated hydrocarbon derivatives NEC	T41.0X1	T41.0X2	T41.0X3	T41.0X4	T41.0X5	T41.0X6
infiltration NEC	T41.3X1	T41.3X2	T41.3X3	T41.3X4	T41.3X5	T41.3X6
intravenous NEC	T41.1X1	T41.1X2	T41.1X3	T41.1X4	T41.1X5	T41.1X6
local NEC	T41.3X1	T41.3X2	T41.3X3	T41.3X4	T41.3X5	T41.3X6
rectal	T41.201	T41.202	T41.203	T41.204	T41.205	T41.206
general	T41.201	T41.202	T41.203	T41.204	T41.205	T41.206
local	T41.3X1	T41.3X2	T41.3X3	T41.3X4	T41.3X5	T41.3X6
regional NEC	T41.3X1	T41.3X2	T41.3X3	T41.3X4	T41.3X5	T41.3X6
spinal NEC	T41.3X1	T41.3X2	T41.3X3	T41.3X4	T41.3X5	T41.3X6
thiobarbiturate	T41.1X1	T41.1X2	T41.1X3	T41.1X4	T41.1X5	T41.1X6
topical	T41.3X1	T41.3X2	T41.3X3	T41.3X4	T41.3X5	T41.3X6
Aneurine	T45.2X1	T45.2X2	T45.2X3	T45.2X4	T45.2X5	T45.2X6
Angio-Conray	T50.8X1	T50.8X2	T50.8X3	T50.8X4	T50.8X5	T50.8X6
Angiotensin	T44.5X1	T44.5X2	T44.5X3	T44.5X4	T44.5X5	T44.5X6
Angiotensinamide	T44.991	T44.992	T44.993	T44.994	T44.995	T44.996
Anhydrohydroxy-progesterone	T38.5X1	T38.5X2	T38.5X3	T38.5X4	T38.5X5	T38.5X6
Anhydron	T50.2X1	T50.2X2	T50.2X3	T50.2X4	T50.2X5	T50.2X6
Anileridine	T40.4X1	T40.4X2	T40.4X3	T40.4X4	T40.4X5	T40.4X6
Aniline (dye) (liquid)	T65.3X1	T65.3X2	T65.3X3	T65.3X4	—	—
analgesic	T39.1X1	T39.1X2	T39.1X3	T39.1X4	T39.1X5	T39.1X6
derivatives, therapeutic NEC	T39.1X1	T39.1X2	T39.1X3	T39.1X4	T39.1X5	T39.1X6
vapor	T65.3X1	T65.3X2	T65.3X3	T65.3X4	—	—
Aniscoropine	T44.3X1	T44.3X2	T44.3X3	T44.3X4	T44.3X5	T44.3X6
Anise oil	T47.5X1	T47.5X2	T47.5X3	T47.5X4	T47.5X5	T47.5X6
Anisidine	T65.3X1	T65.3X2	T65.3X3	T65.3X4	—	—
Anisindione	T45.511	T45.512	T45.513	T45.514	T45.515	T45.516
Anisotropine methyl-bromide	T44.3X1	T44.3X2	T44.3X3	T44.3X4	T44.3X5	T44.3X6
Anistreplase	T45.611	T45.612	T45.613	T45.614	T45.615	T45.616
Anorexiant (central)	T50.5X1	T50.5X2	T50.5X3	T50.5X4	T50.5X5	T50.5X6
Anorexic agents	T50.5X1	T50.5X2	T50.5X3	T50.5X4	T50.5X5	T50.5X6
Ansamycin	T36.6X1	T36.6X2	T36.6X3	T36.6X4	T36.6X5	T36.6X6
Ant (bite) (sting)	T63.421	T63.422	T63.423	T63.424	—	—
Antabuse	T50.6X1	T50.6X2	T50.6X3	T50.6X4	T50.6X5	T50.6X6
Antacid NEC	T47.1X1	T47.1X2	T47.1X3	T47.1X4	T47.1X5	T47.1X6
Antagonist						
Aldosterone	T50.0X1	T50.0X2	T50.0X3	T50.0X4	T50.0X5	T50.0X6
alpha-adrenoreceptor	T44.6X1	T44.6X2	T44.6X3	T44.6X4	T44.6X5	T44.6X6
anticoagulant	T45.7X1	T45.7X2	T45.7X3	T45.7X4	T45.7X5	T45.7X6
beta-adrenoreceptor	T44.7X1	T44.7X2	T44.7X3	T44.7X4	T44.7X5	T44.7X6
extrapyramidal NEC	T44.3X1	T44.3X2	T44.3X3	T44.3X4	T44.3X5	T44.3X6
folic acid	T45.1X1	T45.1X2	T45.1X3	T45.1X4	T45.1X5	T45.1X6
H2 receptor	T47.0X1	T47.0X2	T47.0X3	T47.0X4	T47.0X5	T47.0X6
heavy metal	T45.8X1	T45.8X2	T45.8X3	T45.8X4	T45.8X5	T45.8X6
narcotic analgesic	T50.7X1	T50.7X2	T50.7X3	T50.7X4	T50.7X5	T50.7X6
opiate	T50.7X1	T50.7X2	T50.7X3	T50.7X4	T50.7X5	T50.7X6
pyrimidine	T45.1X1	T45.1X2	T45.1X3	T45.1X4	T45.1X5	T45.1X6
serotonin	T46.5X1	T46.5X2	T46.5X3	T46.5X4	T46.5X5	T46.5X6
Antazolin(e)	T45.0X1	T45.0X2	T45.0X3	T45.0X4	T45.0X5	T45.0X6
Anterior pituitary hormone NEC	T38.811	T38.812	T38.813	T38.814	T38.815	T38.816
Anthelmintic NEC	T37.4X1	T37.4X2	T37.4X3	T37.4X4	T37.4X5	T37.4X6
Anthiolimine	T37.4X1	T37.4X2	T37.4X3	T37.4X4	T37.4X5	T37.4X6
Anthralin	T49.4X1	T49.4X2	T49.4X3	T49.4X4	T49.4X5	T49.4X6
Anthramycin	T45.1X1	T45.1X2	T45.1X3	T45.1X4	T45.1X5	T45.1X6
Antiadrenergic NEC	T44.8X1	T44.8X2	T44.8X3	T44.8X4	T44.8X5	T44.8X6
Antiallergic NEC	T45.0X1	T45.0X2	T45.0X3	T45.0X4	T45.0X5	T45.0X6
Antiandrogen NEC	T38.6X1	T38.6X2	T38.6X3	T38.6X4	T38.6X5	T38.6X6
Anti-anemic (drug) (preparation)	T45.8X1	T45.8X2	T45.8X3	T45.8X4	T45.8X5	T45.8X6
Antianxiety drug NEC	T43.501	T43.502	T43.503	T43.504	T43.505	T43.506
Antiaris toxicaria	T65.891	T65.892	T65.893	T65.894	—	—
Antiarteriosclerotic drug	T46.6X1	T46.6X2	T46.6X3	T46.6X4	T46.6X5	T46.6X6
Antiasthmatic drug NEC	T48.6X1	T48.6X2	T48.6X3	T48.6X4	T48.6X5	T48.6X6
Antibiotic NEC	T36.91	T36.92	T36.93	T36.94	T36.95	T36.96
aminoglycoside	T36.5X1	T36.5X2	T36.5X3	T36.5X4	T36.5X5	T36.5X6
anticancer	T45.1X1	T45.1X2	T45.1X3	T45.1X4	T45.1X5	T45.1X6
antifungal	T36.7X1	T36.7X2	T36.7X3	T36.7X4	T36.7X5	T36.7X6
antimycobacterial	T36.5X1	T36.5X2	T36.5X3	T36.5X4	T36.5X5	T36.5X6
antineoplastic	T45.1X1	T45.1X2	T45.1X3	T45.1X4	T45.1X5	T45.1X6
b-lactam NEC	T36.1X1	T36.1X2	T36.1X3	T36.1X4	T36.1X5	T36.1X6
cephalosporin (group)	T36.1X1	T36.1X2	T36.1X3	T36.1X4	T36.1X5	T36.1X6
chloramphenicol (group)	T36.2X1	T36.2X2	T36.2X3	T36.2X4	T36.2X5	T36.2X6
ENT	T49.6X1	T49.6X2	T49.6X3	T49.6X4	T49.6X5	T49.6X6
eye	T49.5X1	T49.5X2	T49.5X3	T49.5X4	T49.5X5	T49.5X6
fungicidal (local)	T49.0X1	T49.0X2	T49.0X3	T49.0X4	T49.0X5	T49.0X6
intestinal	T36.8X1	T36.8X2	T36.8X3	T36.8X4	T36.8X5	T36.8X6
local	T49.0X1	T49.0X2	T49.0X3	T49.0X4	T49.0X5	T49.0X6

Substance	Poisoning, Accidental (unintentional)	Poisoning, Intentional Self-harm	Poisoning, Assault	Poisoning, Undetermined	Adverse Effect	Under-dosing
Antibiotic — *continued*						
macrolides	T36.3X1	T36.3X2	T36.3X3	T36.3X4	T36.3X5	T36.3X6
polypeptide	T36.8X1	T36.8X2	T36.8X3	T36.8X4	T36.8X5	T36.8X6
specified NEC	T36.8X1	T36.8X2	T36.8X3	T36.8X4	T36.8X5	T36.8X6
tetracycline (group)	T36.4X1	T36.4X2	T36.4X3	T36.4X4	T36.4X5	T36.4X6
throat	T49.6X1	T49.6X2	T49.6X3	T49.6X4	T49.6X5	T49.6X6
Anticancer agents NEC	T45.1X1	T45.1X2	T45.1X3	T45.1X4	T45.1X5	T45.1X6
Anticholesterolemic drug NEC	T46.6X1	T46.6X2	T46.6X3	T46.6X4	T46.6X5	T46.6X6
Anticholinergic NEC	T44.3X1	T44.3X2	T44.3X3	T44.3X4	T44.3X5	T44.3X6
Anticholinesterase	T44.0X1	T44.0X2	T44.0X3	T44.0X4	T44.0X5	T44.0X6
organophosphorus	T44.0X1	T44.0X2	T44.0X3	T44.0X4	T44.0X5	T44.0X6
insecticide	T60.0X1	T60.0X2	T60.0X3	T60.0X4	—	—
nerve gas	T59.891	T59.892	T59.893	T59.894	—	—
reversible	T44.0X1	T44.0X2	T44.0X3	T44.0X4	T44.0X5	T44.0X6
ophthalmological	T49.5X1	T49.5X2	T49.5X3	T49.5X4	T49.5X5	T49.5X6
Anticoagulant NEC	T45.511	T45.512	T45.513	T45.514	T45.515	T45.516
Antagonist	T45.7X1	T45.7X2	T45.7X3	T45.7X4	T45.7X5	T45.7X6
Anti-common-cold drug NEC	T48.5X1	T48.5X2	T48.5X3	T48.5X4	T48.5X5	T48.5X6
Anticonvulsant	T42.71	T42.72	T42.73	T42.74	T42.75	T42.76
barbiturate	T42.3X1	T42.3X2	T42.3X3	T42.3X4	T42.3X5	T42.3X6
combination (with barbiturate)	T42.3X1	T42.3X2	T42.3X3	T42.3X4	T42.3X5	T42.3X6
hydantoin	T42.0X1	T42.0X2	T42.0X3	T42.0X4	T42.0X5	T42.0X6
hypnotic NEC	T42.6X1	T42.6X2	T42.6X3	T42.6X4	T42.6X5	T42.6X6
oxazolidinedione	T42.2X1	T42.2X2	T42.2X3	T42.2X4	T42.2X5	T42.2X6
pyrimidinedione	T42.6X1	T42.6X2	T42.6X3	T42.6X4	T42.6X5	T42.6X6
specified NEC	T42.6X1	T42.6X2	T42.6X3	T42.6X4	T42.6X5	T42.6X6
succinimide	T42.2X1	T42.2X2	T42.2X3	T42.2X4	T42.2X5	T42.2X6
Antidepressant	T43.201	T43.202	T43.203	T43.204	T43.205	T43.206
monoamine oxidase inhibitor	T43.1X1	T43.1X2	T43.1X3	T43.1X4	T43.1X5	T43.1X6
selective serotonin norepinephrine reuptake inhibitor	T43.211	T43.212	T43.213	T43.214	T43.215	T43.216
selective serotonin reuptake inhibitor	T43.221	T43.222	T43.223	T43.224	T43.225	T43.226
specified NEC	T43.291	T43.292	T43.293	T43.294	T43.295	T43.296
tetracyclic	T43.021	T43.022	T43.023	T43.024	T43.025	T43.026
triazolopyridine	T43.211	T43.212	T43.213	T43.214	T43.215	T43.216
tricyclic	T43.011	T43.012	T43.013	T43.014	T43.015	T43.016
Antidiabetic NEC	T38.3X1	T38.3X2	T38.3X3	T38.3X4	T38.3X5	T38.3X6
biguanide	T38.3X1	T38.3X2	T38.3X3	T38.3X4	T38.3X5	T38.3X6
and sulfonyl combined	T38.3X1	T38.3X2	T38.3X3	T38.3X4	T38.3X5	T38.3X6
combined	T38.3X1	T38.3X2	T38.3X3	T38.3X4	T38.3X5	T38.3X6
sulfonylurea	T38.3X1	T38.3X2	T38.3X3	T38.3X4	T38.3X5	T38.3X6
Antidiarrheal drug NEC	T47.6X1	T47.6X2	T47.6X3	T47.6X4	T47.6X5	T47.6X6
absorbent	T47.6X1	T47.6X2	T47.6X3	T47.6X4	T47.6X5	T47.6X6
Anti-D immunoglobulin (human)	T50.Z11	T50.Z12	T50.Z13	T50.Z14	T50.Z15	T50.Z16
Antidiphtheria serum	T50.Z11	T50.Z12	T50.Z13	T50.Z14	T50.Z15	T50.Z16
Antidiuretic hormone	T38.891	T38.892	T38.893	T38.894	T38.895	T38.896
Antidote NEC	T50.6X1	T50.6X2	T50.6X3	T50.6X4	T50.6X5	T50.6X6
heavy metal	T45.8X1	T45.8X2	T45.8X3	T45.8X4	T45.8X5	T45.8X6
Antidysrhythmic NEC	T46.2X1	T46.2X2	T46.2X3	T46.2X4	T46.2X5	T46.2X6
Antiemetic drug	T45.0X1	T45.0X2	T45.0X3	T45.0X4	T45.0X5	T45.0X6
Antiepilepsy agent	T42.71	T42.72	T42.73	T42.74	T42.75	T42.76
combination	T42.5X1	T42.5X2	T42.5X3	T42.5X4	T42.5X5	T42.5X6
mixed	T42.5X1	T42.5X2	T42.5X3	T42.5X4	T42.5X5	T42.5X6
specified, NEC	T42.6X1	T42.6X2	T42.6X3	T42.6X4	T42.6X5	T42.6X6
Antiestrogen NEC	T38.6X1	T38.6X2	T38.6X3	T38.6X4	T38.6X5	T38.6X6
Antifertility pill	T38.4X1	T38.4X2	T38.4X3	T38.4X4	T38.4X5	T38.4X6
Antifibrinolytic drug	T45.621	T45.622	T45.623	T45.624	T45.625	T45.626
Antifilarial drug	T37.4X1	T37.4X2	T37.4X3	T37.4X4	T37.4X5	T37.4X6
Antiflatulent	T47.5X1	T47.5X2	T47.5X3	T47.5X4	T47.5X5	T47.5X6
Antifreeze	T65.91	T65.92	T65.93	T65.94	—	—
alcohol	T51.1X1	T51.1X2	T51.1X3	T51.1X4	—	—
ethylene glycol	T51.8X1	T51.8X2	T51.8X3	T51.8X4	—	—
Antifungal						
antibiotic (systemic)	T36.7X1	T36.7X2	T36.7X3	T36.7X4	T36.7X5	T36.7X6
anti-infective NEC	T37.91	T37.92	T37.93	T37.94	T37.95	T37.96
disinfectant, local	T49.0X1	T49.0X2	T49.0X3	T49.0X4	T49.0X5	T49.0X6
nonmedicinal (spray)	T60.3X1	T60.3X2	T60.3X3	T60.3X4	—	—
topical	T49.0X1	T49.0X2	T49.0X3	T49.0X4	T49.0X5	T49.0X6
Anti-gastric-secretion drug NEC	T47.1X1	T47.1X2	T47.1X3	T47.1X4	T47.1X5	T47.1X6
Antigonadotrophin NEC	T38.6X1	T38.6X2	T38.6X3	T38.6X4	T38.6X5	T38.6X6
Antihallucinogen	T43.501	T43.502	T43.503	T43.504	T43.505	T43.506
Antihelmintics	T37.4X1	T37.4X2	T37.4X3	T37.4X4	T37.4X5	T37.4X6
Antihemophilic						
factor	T45.8X1	T45.8X2	T45.8X3	T45.8X4	T45.8X5	T45.8X6
fraction	T45.8X1	T45.8X2	T45.8X3	T45.8X4	T45.8X5	T45.8X6

352

Additional Character May Be Required — Refer to the Tabular List for Character Selection ▽ Subterms under main terms may continue to next column or page

Substance	Poisoning, Accidental (unintentional)	Poisoning, Intentional Self-harm	Poisoning, Assault	Poisoning, Undetermined	Adverse Effect	Under-dosing
Antihemophilic — *continued*						
globulin concentrate	T45.7X1	T45.7X2	T45.7X3	T45.7X4	T45.7X5	T45.7X6
human plasma	T45.8X1	T45.8X2	T45.8X3	T45.8X4	T45.8X5	T45.8X6
plasma, dried	T45.7X1	T45.7X2	T45.7X3	T45.7X4	T45.7X5	T45.7X6
Antihemorrhoidal preparation	T49.2X1	T49.2X2	T49.2X3	T49.2X4	T49.2X5	T49.2X6
Antiheparin drug	T45.7X1	T45.7X2	T45.7X3	T45.7X4	T45.7X5	T45.7X6
Antihistamine	T45.0X1	T45.0X2	T45.0X3	T45.0X4	T45.0X5	T45.0X6
Antihookworm drug	T37.4X1	T37.4X2	T37.4X3	T37.4X4	T37.4X5	T37.4X6
Anti-human lymphocytic globulin	T50.Z11	T50.Z12	T50.Z13	T50.Z14	T50.Z15	T50.Z16
Antihyperlipidemic drug	T46.6X1	T46.6X2	T46.6X3	T46.6X4	T46.6X5	T46.6X6
Antihypertensive drug NEC	T46.5X1	T46.5X2	T46.5X3	T46.5X4	T46.5X5	T46.5X6
Anti-infective NEC	T37.91	T37.92	T37.93	T37.94	T37.95	T37.96
anthelmintic	T37.4X1	T37.4X2	T37.4X3	T37.4X4	T37.4X5	T37.4X6
antibiotics	T36.91	T36.92	T36.93	T36.94	T36.95	T36.96
specified NEC	T36.8X1	T36.8X2	T36.8X3	T36.8X4	T36.8X5	T36.8X6
antimalarial	T37.2X1	T37.2X2	T37.2X3	T37.2X4	T37.2X5	T37.2X6
antimycobacterial NEC	T37.1X1	T37.1X2	T37.1X3	T37.1X4	T37.1X5	T37.1X6
antibiotics	T36.5X1	T36.5X2	T36.5X3	T36.5X4	T36.5X5	T36.5X6
antiprotozoal NEC	T37.3X1	T37.3X2	T37.3X3	T37.3X4	T37.3X5	T37.3X6
blood	T37.2X1	T37.2X2	T37.2X3	T37.2X4	T37.2X5	T37.2X6
antiviral	T37.5X1	T37.5X2	T37.5X3	T37.5X4	T37.5X5	T37.5X6
arsenical	T37.8X1	T37.8X2	T37.8X3	T37.8X4	T37.8X5	T37.8X6
bismuth, local	T49.0X1	T49.0X2	T49.0X3	T49.0X4	T49.0X5	T49.0X6
ENT	T49.6X1	T49.6X2	T49.6X3	T49.6X4	T49.6X5	T49.6X6
eye NEC	T49.5X1	T49.5X2	T49.5X3	T49.5X4	T49.5X5	T49.5X6
heavy metals NEC	T37.8X1	T37.8X2	T37.8X3	T37.8X4	T37.8X5	T37.8X6
local NEC	T49.0X1	T49.0X2	T49.0X3	T49.0X4	T49.0X5	T49.0X6
specified NEC	T49.0X1	T49.0X2	T49.0X3	T49.0X4	T49.0X5	T49.0X6
mixed	T37.91	T37.92	T37.93	T37.94	T37.95	T37.96
ophthalmic preparation	T49.5X1	T49.5X2	T49.5X3	T49.5X4	T49.5X5	T49.5X6
topical NEC	T49.0X1	T49.0X2	T49.0X3	T49.0X4	T49.0X5	T49.0X6
Anti-inflammatory drug NEC	T39.391	T39.392	T39.393	T39.394	T39.395	T39.396
local	T49.0X1	T49.0X2	T49.0X3	T49.0X4	T49.0X5	T49.0X6
nonsteroidal NEC	T39.391	T39.392	T39.393	T39.394	T39.395	T39.396
propionic acid derivative	T39.311	T39.312	T39.313	T39.314	T39.315	T39.316
specified NEC	T39.391	T39.392	T39.393	T39.394	T39.395	T39.396
Antikaluretic	T50.3X1	T50.3X2	T50.3X3	T50.3X4	T50.3X5	T50.3X6
Antiknock (tetraethyl lead)	T56.0X1	T56.0X2	T56.0X3	T56.0X4	—	—
Antilipemic drug NEC	T46.6X1	T46.6X2	T46.6X3	T46.6X4	T46.6X5	T46.6X6
Antimalarial	T37.2X1	T37.2X2	T37.2X3	T37.2X4	T37.2X5	T37.2X6
prophylactic NEC	T37.2X1	T37.2X2	T37.2X3	T37.2X4	T37.2X5	T37.2X6
pyrimidine derivative	T37.2X1	T37.2X2	T37.2X3	T37.2X4	T37.2X5	T37.2X6
Antimetabolite	T45.1X1	T45.1X2	T45.1X3	T45.1X4	T45.1X5	T45.1X6
Antimitotic agent	T45.1X1	T45.1X2	T45.1X3	T45.1X4	T45.1X5	T45.1X6
Antimony (compounds) (vapor) **NEC**	T56.891	T56.892	T56.893	T56.894	—	—
anti-infectives	T37.8X1	T37.8X2	T37.8X3	T37.8X4	T37.8X5	T37.8X6
dimercaptosuccinate	T37.3X1	T37.3X2	T37.3X3	T37.3X4	T37.3X5	T37.3X6
hydride	T56.891	T56.892	T56.893	T56.894	—	—
pesticide (vapor)	T60.8X1	T60.8X2	T60.8X3	T60.8X4	—	—
potassium (sodium) tartrate	T37.8X1	T37.8X2	T37.8X3	T37.8X4	T37.8X5	T37.8X6
sodium dimercaptosuccinate	T37.3X1	T37.3X2	T37.3X3	T37.3X4	T37.3X5	T37.3X6
tartrated	T37.8X1	T37.8X2	T37.8X3	T37.8X4	T37.8X5	T37.8X6
Antimuscarinic NEC	T44.3X1	T44.3X2	T44.3X3	T44.3X4	T44.3X5	T44.3X6
Antimycobacterial drug NEC	T37.1X1	T37.1X2	T37.1X3	T37.1X4	T37.1X5	T37.1X6
antibiotics	T36.5X1	T36.5X2	T36.5X3	T36.5X4	T36.5X5	T36.5X6
combination	T37.1X1	T37.1X2	T37.1X3	T37.1X4	T37.1X5	T37.1X6
Antinausea drug	T45.0X1	T45.0X2	T45.0X3	T45.0X4	T45.0X5	T45.0X6
Antinematode drug	T37.4X1	T37.4X2	T37.4X3	T37.4X4	T37.4X5	T37.4X6
Antineoplastic NEC	T45.1X1	T45.1X2	T45.1X3	T45.1X4	T45.1X5	T45.1X6
alkaloidal	T45.1X1	T45.1X2	T45.1X3	T45.1X4	T45.1X5	T45.1X6
antibiotics	T45.1X1	T45.1X2	T45.1X3	T45.1X4	T45.1X5	T45.1X6
combination	T45.1X1	T45.1X2	T45.1X3	T45.1X4	T45.1X5	T45.1X6
estrogen	T38.5X1	T38.5X2	T38.5X3	T38.5X4	T38.5X5	T38.5X6
steroid	T38.7X1	T38.7X2	T38.7X3	T38.7X4	T38.7X5	T38.7X6
Antiparasitic drug (systemic)	T37.91	T37.92	T37.93	T37.94	T37.95	T37.96
local	T49.0X1	T49.0X2	T49.0X3	T49.0X4	T49.0X5	T49.0X6
specified NEC	T37.8X1	T37.8X2	T37.8X3	T37.8X4	T37.8X5	T37.8X6
Antiparkinsonism drug NEC	T42.8X1	T42.8X2	T42.8X3	T42.8X4	T42.8X5	T42.8X6
Antiperspirant NEC	T49.2X1	T49.2X2	T49.2X3	T49.2X4	T49.2X5	T49.2X6
Antiphlogistic NEC	T39.4X1	T39.4X2	T39.4X3	T39.4X4	T39.4X5	T39.4X6
Antiplatyhelmintic drug	T37.4X1	T37.4X2	T37.4X3	T37.4X4	T37.4X5	T37.4X6
Antiprotozoal drug NEC	T37.3X1	T37.3X2	T37.3X3	T37.3X4	T37.3X5	T37.3X6
blood	T37.2X1	T37.2X2	T37.2X3	T37.2X4	T37.2X5	T37.2X6
local	T49.0X1	T49.0X2	T49.0X3	T49.0X4	T49.0X5	T49.0X6

Substance	Poisoning, Accidental (unintentional)	Poisoning, Intentional Self-harm	Poisoning, Assault	Poisoning, Undetermined	Adverse Effect	Under-dosing
Antipruritic drug NEC	T49.1X1	T49.1X2	T49.1X3	T49.1X4	T49.1X5	T49.1X6
Antipsychotic drug	T43.501	T43.502	T43.503	T43.504	T43.505	T43.506
specified NEC	T43.591	T43.592	T43.593	T43.594	T43.595	T43.596
Antipyretic	T39.91	T39.92	T39.93	T39.94	T39.95	T39.96
specified NEC	T39.8X1	T39.8X2	T39.8X3	T39.8X4	T39.8X5	T39.8X6
Antipyrine	T39.2X1	T39.2X2	T39.2X3	T39.2X4	T39.2X5	T39.2X6
Antirabies hyperimmune serum	T50.Z11	T50.Z12	T50.Z13	T50.Z14	T50.Z15	T50.Z16
Antirheumatic NEC	T39.4X1	T39.4X2	T39.4X3	T39.4X4	T39.4X5	T39.4X6
Antirigidity drug NEC	T42.8X1	T42.8X2	T42.8X3	T42.8X4	T42.8X5	T42.8X6
Antischistosomal drug	T37.4X1	T37.4X2	T37.4X3	T37.4X4	T37.4X5	T37.4X6
Antiscorpion sera	T50.Z11	T50.Z12	T50.Z13	T50.Z14	T50.Z15	T50.Z16
Antiseborrheics	T49.4X1	T49.4X2	T49.4X3	T49.4X4	T49.4X5	T49.4X6
Antiseptics (external) (medicinal)	T49.0X1	T49.0X2	T49.0X3	T49.0X4	T49.0X5	T49.0X6
Antistine	T45.0X1	T45.0X2	T45.0X3	T45.0X4	T45.0X5	T45.0X6
Antitapeworm drug	T37.4X1	T37.4X2	T37.4X3	T37.4X4	T37.4X5	T37.4X6
Antitetanus immunoglobulin	T50.Z11	T50.Z12	T50.Z13	T50.Z14	T50.Z15	T50.Z16
Antithrombotic	T45.521	T45.522	T45.523	T45.524	T45.525	T45.526
Antithyroid drug NEC	T38.2X1	T38.2X2	T38.2X3	T38.2X4	T38.2X5	T38.2X6
Antitoxin	T50.Z11	T50.Z12	T50.Z13	T50.Z14	T50.Z15	T50.Z16
diphtheria	T50.Z11	T50.Z12	T50.Z13	T50.Z14	T50.Z15	T50.Z16
gas gangrene	T50.Z11	T50.Z12	T50.Z13	T50.Z14	T50.Z15	T50.Z16
tetanus	T50.Z11	T50.Z12	T50.Z13	T50.Z14	T50.Z15	T50.Z16
Antitrichomonal drug	T37.3X1	T37.3X2	T37.3X3	T37.3X4	T37.3X5	T37.3X6
Antituberculars	T37.1X1	T37.1X2	T37.1X3	T37.1X4	T37.1X5	T37.1X6
antibiotics	T36.5X1	T36.5X2	T36.5X3	T36.5X4	T36.5X5	T36.5X6
Antitussive NEC	T48.3X1	T48.3X2	T48.3X3	T48.3X4	T48.3X5	T48.3X6
codeine mixture	T40.2X1	T40.2X2	T40.2X3	T40.2X4	T40.2X5	T40.2X6
opiate	T40.2X1	T40.2X2	T40.2X3	T40.2X4	T40.2X5	T40.2X6
Antivaricose drug	T46.8X1	T46.8X2	T46.8X3	T46.8X4	T46.8X5	T46.8X6
Antivenin, antivenom (sera)	T50.Z11	T50.Z12	T50.Z13	T50.Z14	T50.Z15	T50.Z16
crotaline	T50.Z11	T50.Z12	T50.Z13	T50.Z14	T50.Z15	T50.Z16
spider bite	T50.Z11	T50.Z12	T50.Z13	T50.Z14	T50.Z15	T50.Z16
Antivertigo drug	T45.0X1	T45.0X2	T45.0X3	T45.0X4	T45.0X5	T45.0X6
Antiviral drug NEC	T37.5X1	T37.5X2	T37.5X3	T37.5X4	T37.5X5	T37.5X6
eye	T49.5X1	T49.5X2	T49.5X3	T49.5X4	T49.5X5	T49.5X6
Antiwhipworm drug	T37.4X1	T37.4X2	T37.4X3	T37.4X4	T37.4X5	T37.4X6
Ant poison — *see* Insecticide						
Antrol — *see also* by specific chemical substance	T60.91	T60.92	T60.93	T60.94		
fungicide	T60.91	T60.92	T60.93	T60.94	—	—
ANTU (alpha naphthylthiourea)	T60.4X1	T60.4X2	T60.4X3	T60.4X4	—	—
Apalcillin	T36.0X1	T36.0X2	T36.0X3	T36.0X4	T36.0X5	T36.0X6
APC	T48.5X1	T48.5X2	T48.5X3	T48.5X4	T48.5X5	T48.5X6
Aplonidine	T44.4X1	T44.4X2	T44.4X3	T44.4X4	T44.4X5	T44.4X6
Apomorphine	T47.7X1	T47.7X2	T47.7X3	T47.7X4	T47.7X5	T47.7X6
Appetite depressants, central	T50.5X1	T50.5X2	T50.5X3	T50.5X4	T50.5X5	T50.5X6
Apraclonidine (hydrochloride)	T44.4X1	T44.4X2	T44.4X3	T44.4X4	T44.4X5	T44.4X6
Apresoline	T46.5X1	T46.5X2	T46.5X3	T46.5X4	T46.5X5	T46.5X6
Aprindine	T46.2X1	T46.2X2	T46.2X3	T46.2X4	T46.2X5	T46.2X6
Aprobarbital	T42.3X1	T42.3X2	T42.3X3	T42.3X4	T42.3X5	T42.3X6
Apronalide	T42.6X1	T42.6X2	T42.6X3	T42.6X4	T42.6X5	T42.6X6
Aprotinin	T45.621	T45.622	T45.623	T45.624	T45.625	T45.626
Aptocaine	T41.3X1	T41.3X2	T41.3X3	T41.3X4	T41.3X5	T41.3X6
Aqua fortis	T54.2X1	T54.2X2	T54.2X3	T54.2X4	—	—
Ara-A	T37.5X1	T37.5X2	T37.5X3	T37.5X4	T37.5X5	T37.5X6
Ara-C	T45.1X1	T45.1X2	T45.1X3	T45.1X4	T45.1X5	T45.1X6
Arachis oil	T49.3X1	T49.3X2	T49.3X3	T49.3X4	T49.3X5	T49.3X6
cathartic	T47.4X1	T47.4X2	T47.4X3	T47.4X4	T47.4X5	T47.4X6
Aralen	T37.2X1	T37.2X2	T37.2X3	T37.2X4	T37.2X5	T37.2X6
Arecoline	T44.1X1	T44.1X2	T44.1X3	T44.1X4	T44.1X5	T44.1X6
Arginine	T50.991	T50.992	T50.993	T50.994	T50.995	T50.996
glutamate	T50.991	T50.992	T50.993	T50.994	T50.995	T50.996
Argyrol	T49.0X1	T49.0X2	T49.0X3	T49.0X4	T49.0X5	T49.0X6
ENT agent	T49.6X1	T49.6X2	T49.6X3	T49.6X4	T49.6X5	T49.6X6
ophthalmic preparation	T49.5X1	T49.5X2	T49.5X3	T49.5X4	T49.5X5	T49.5X6
Aristocort	T38.0X1	T38.0X2	T38.0X3	T38.0X4	T38.0X5	T38.0X6
ENT agent	T49.6X1	T49.6X2	T49.6X3	T49.6X4	T49.6X5	T49.6X6
ophthalmic preparation	T49.5X1	T49.5X2	T49.5X3	T49.5X4	T49.5X5	T49.5X6
topical NEC	T49.0X1	T49.0X2	T49.0X3	T49.0X4	T49.0X5	T49.0X6
Aromatics, corrosive	T54.1X1	T54.1X2	T54.1X3	T54.1X4	—	—
disinfectants	T54.1X1	T54.1X2	T54.1X3	T54.1X4	—	—
Arsenate of lead	T57.0X1	T57.0X2	T57.0X3	T57.0X4	—	—
herbicide	T57.0X1	T57.0X2	T57.0X3	T57.0X4	—	—
Arsenic, arsenicals (compounds) (dust) (vapor) **NEC**	T57.0X1	T57.0X2	T57.0X3	T57.0X4	—	—
anti-infectives	T37.8X1	T37.8X2	T37.8X3	T37.8X4	T37.8X5	T37.8X6
pesticide (dust) (fumes)	T57.0X1	T57.0X2	T57.0X3	T57.0X4	—	—

Substance	Poisoning, Accidental (unintentional)	Poisoning, Intentional Self-harm	Poisoning, Assault	Poisoning, Undetermined	Adverse Effect	Under-dosing
Arsine (gas)	T57.0X1	T57.0X2	T57.0X3	T57.0X4	—	—
Arsphenamine (silver)	T37.8X1	T37.8X2	T37.8X3	T37.8X4	T37.8X5	T37.8X6
Arsthinol	T37.3X1	T37.3X2	T37.3X3	T37.3X4	T37.3X5	T37.3X6
Artane	T44.3X1	T44.3X2	T44.3X3	T44.3X4	T44.3X5	T44.3X6
Arthropod (venomous) **NEC**	T63.481	T63.482	T63.483	T63.484	—	—
Articaine	T41.3X1	T41.3X2	T41.3X3	T41.3X4	T41.3X5	T41.3X6
Asbestos	T57.8X1	T57.8X2	T57.8X3	T57.8X4	—	—
Ascaridole	T37.4X1	T37.4X2	T37.4X3	T37.4X4	T37.4X5	T37.4X6
Ascorbic acid	T45.2X1	T45.2X2	T45.2X3	T45.2X4	T45.2X5	T45.2X6
Asiaticoside	T49.0X1	T49.0X2	T49.0X3	T49.0X4	T49.0X5	T49.0X6
Asparaginase	T45.1X1	T45.1X2	T45.1X3	T45.1X4	T45.1X5	T45.1X6
Aspidium (oleoresin)	T37.4X1	T37.4X2	T37.4X3	T37.4X4	T37.4X5	T37.4X6
Aspirin (aluminum) (soluble)	T39.011	T39.012	T39.013	T39.014	T39.015	T39.016
Aspoxicillin	T36.0X1	T36.0X2	T36.0X3	T36.0X4	T36.0X5	T36.0X6
Astemizole	T45.0X1	T45.0X2	T45.0X3	T45.0X4	T45.0X5	T45.0X6
Astringent (local)	T49.2X1	T49.2X2	T49.2X3	T49.2X4	T49.2X5	T49.2X6
specified NEC	T49.2X1	T49.2X2	T49.2X3	T49.2X4	T49.2X5	T49.2X6
Astromicin	T36.5X1	T36.5X2	T36.5X3	T36.5X4	T36.5X5	T36.5X6
Ataractic drug NEC	T43.501	T43.502	T43.503	T43.504	T43.505	T43.506
Atenolol	T44.7X1	T44.7X2	T44.7X3	T44.7X4	T44.7X5	T44.7X6
Atonia drug, intestinal	T47.4X1	T47.4X2	T47.4X3	T47.4X4	T47.4X5	T47.4X6
Atophan	T50.4X1	T50.4X2	T50.4X3	T50.4X4	T50.4X5	T50.4X6
Atracurium besilate	T48.1X1	T48.1X2	T48.1X3	T48.1X4	T48.1X5	T48.1X6
Atropine	T44.3X1	T44.3X2	T44.3X3	T44.3X4	T44.3X5	T44.3X6
derivative	T44.3X1	T44.3X2	T44.3X3	T44.3X4	T44.3X5	T44.3X6
methonitrate	T44.3X1	T44.3X2	T44.3X3	T44.3X4	T44.3X5	T44.3X6
Attapulgite	T47.6X1	T47.6X2	T47.6X3	T47.6X4	T47.6X5	T47.6X6
Auramine	T65.891	T65.892	T65.893	T65.894	—	—
dye	T65.6X1	T65.6X2	T65.6X3	T65.6X4	—	—
fungicide	T60.3X1	T60.3X2	T60.3X3	T60.3X4	—	—
Auranofin	T39.4X1	T39.4X2	T39.4X3	T39.4X4	T39.4X5	T39.4X6
Aurantiin	T46.991	T46.992	T46.993	T46.994	T46.995	T46.996
Aureomycin	T36.4X1	T36.4X2	T36.4X3	T36.4X4	T36.4X5	T36.4X6
ophthalmic preparation	T49.5X1	T49.5X2	T49.5X3	T49.5X4	T49.5X5	T49.5X6
topical NEC	T49.0X1	T49.0X2	T49.0X3	T49.0X4	T49.0X5	T49.0X6
Aurothioglucose	T39.4X1	T39.4X2	T39.4X3	T39.4X4	T39.4X5	T39.4X6
Aurothioglycanide	T39.4X1	T39.4X2	T39.4X3	T39.4X4	T39.4X5	T39.4X6
Aurothiomalate sodium	T39.4X1	T39.4X2	T39.4X3	T39.4X4	T39.4X5	T39.4X6
Aurotioprol	T39.4X1	T39.4X2	T39.4X3	T39.4X4	T39.4X5	T39.4X6
Automobile fuel	T52.0X1	T52.0X2	T52.0X3	T52.0X4	—	—
Autonomic nervous system agent NEC	T44.901	T44.902	T44.903	T44.904	T44.905	T44.906
Avlosulfon	T37.1X1	T37.1X2	T37.1X3	T37.1X4	T37.1X5	T37.1X6
Avomine	T42.6X1	T42.6X2	T42.6X3	T42.6X4	T42.6X5	T42.6X6
Axerophthol	T45.2X1	T45.2X2	T45.2X3	T45.2X4	T45.2X5	T45.2X6
Azacitidine	T45.1X1	T45.1X2	T45.1X3	T45.1X4	T45.1X5	T45.1X6
Azacyclonol	T43.591	T43.592	T43.593	T43.594	T43.595	T43.596
Azadirachta	T60.2X1	T60.2X2	T60.2X3	T60.2X4	—	—
Azanidazole	T37.3X1	T37.3X2	T37.3X3	T37.3X4	T37.3X5	T37.3X6
Azapetine	T46.7X1	T46.7X2	T46.7X3	T46.7X4	T46.7X5	T46.7X6
Azapropazone	T39.2X1	T39.2X2	T39.2X3	T39.2X4	T39.2X5	T39.2X6
Azaribine	T45.1X1	T45.1X2	T45.1X3	T45.1X4	T45.1X5	T45.1X6
Azaserine	T45.1X1	T45.1X2	T45.1X3	T45.1X4	T45.1X5	T45.1X6
Azatadine	T45.0X1	T45.0X2	T45.0X3	T45.0X4	T45.0X5	T45.0X6
Azatepa	T45.1X1	T45.1X2	T45.1X3	T45.1X4	T45.1X5	T45.1X6
Azathioprine	T45.1X1	T45.1X2	T45.1X3	T45.1X4	T45.1X5	T45.1X6
Azelaic acid	T49.0X1	T49.0X2	T49.0X3	T49.0X4	T49.0X5	T49.0X6
Azelastine	T45.0X1	T45.0X2	T45.0X3	T45.0X4	T45.0X5	T45.0X6
Azidocillin	T36.0X1	T36.0X2	T36.0X3	T36.0X4	T36.0X5	T36.0X6
Azidothymidine	T37.5X1	T37.5X2	T37.5X3	T37.5X4	T37.5X5	T37.5X6
Azinphos (ethyl) (methyl)	T60.0X1	T60.0X2	T60.0X3	T60.0X4	—	—
Aziridine (chelating)	T54.1X1	T54.1X2	T54.1X3	T54.1X4	—	—
Azithromycin	T36.3X1	T36.3X2	T36.3X3	T36.3X4	T36.3X5	T36.3X6
Azlocillin	T36.0X1	T36.0X2	T36.0X3	T36.0X4	T36.0X5	T36.0X6
Azobenzene smoke	T65.3X1	T65.3X2	T65.3X3	T65.3X4	—	—
acaricide	T60.8X1	T60.8X2	T60.8X3	T60.8X4	—	—
Azosulfamide	T37.0X1	T37.0X2	T37.0X3	T37.0X4	T37.0X5	T37.0X6
AZT	T37.5X1	T37.5X2	T37.5X3	T37.5X4	T37.5X5	T37.5X6
Aztreonam	T36.1X1	T36.1X2	T36.1X3	T36.1X4	T36.1X5	T36.1X6
Azulfidine	T37.0X1	T37.0X2	T37.0X3	T37.0X4	T37.0X5	T37.0X6
Azuresin	T50.8X1	T50.8X2	T50.8X3	T50.8X4	T50.8X5	T50.8X6
b-acetyldigoxin	T46.0X1	T46.0X2	T46.0X3	T46.0X4	T46.0X5	T46.0X6
P-Acetamidophenol	T39.1X1	T39.1X2	T39.1X3	T39.1X4	T39.1X5	T39.1X6
Bacampicillin	T36.0X1	T36.0X2	T36.0X3	T36.0X4	T36.0X5	T36.0X6
Bacillus						
lactobacillus	T47.8X1	T47.8X2	T47.8X3	T47.8X4	T47.8X5	T47.8X6
subtilis	T47.6X1	T47.6X2	T47.6X3	T47.6X4	T47.6X5	T47.6X6
Bacimycin	T49.0X1	T49.0X2	T49.0X3	T49.0X4	T49.0X5	T49.0X6
ophthalmic preparation	T49.5X1	T49.5X2	T49.5X3	T49.5X4	T49.5X5	T49.5X6
Bacitracin zinc	T49.0X1	T49.0X2	T49.0X3	T49.0X4	T49.0X5	T49.0X6
with neomycin	T49.0X1	T49.0X2	T49.0X3	T49.0X4	T49.0X5	T49.0X6
ENT agent	T49.6X1	T49.6X2	T49.6X3	T49.6X4	T49.6X5	T49.6X6
ophthalmic preparation	T49.5X1	T49.5X2	T49.5X3	T49.5X4	T49.5X5	T49.5X6

Substance	Poisoning, Accidental (unintentional)	Poisoning, Intentional Self-harm	Poisoning, Assault	Poisoning, Undetermined	Adverse Effect	Under-dosing
Bacitracin zinc — *continued*						
topical NEC	T49.0X1	T49.0X2	T49.0X3	T49.0X4	T49.0X5	T49.0X6
Baclofen	T42.8X1	T42.8X2	T42.8X3	T42.8X4	T42.8X5	T42.8X6
Baking soda	T50.991	T50.992	T50.993	T50.994	T50.995	T50.996
BAL	T45.8X1	T45.8X2	T45.8X3	T45.8X4	T45.8X5	T45.8X6
Bambuterol	T48.6X1	T48.6X2	T48.6X3	T48.6X4	T48.6X5	T48.6X6
Bamethan (sulfate)	T46.7X1	T46.7X2	T46.7X3	T46.7X4	T46.7X5	T46.7X6
Bamifylline	T48.6X1	T48.6X2	T48.6X3	T48.6X4	T48.6X5	T48.6X6
Bamipine	T45.0X1	T45.0X2	T45.0X3	T45.0X4	T45.0X5	T45.0X6
Baneberry — *see* Actaea spicata						
Banewort — *see* Belladonna						
Barbenyl	T42.3X1	T42.3X2	T42.3X3	T42.3X4	T42.3X5	T42.3X6
Barbexaclone	T42.6X1	T42.6X2	T42.6X3	T42.6X4	T42.6X5	T42.6X6
Barbital	T42.3X1	T42.3X2	T42.3X3	T42.3X4	T42.3X5	T42.3X6
sodium	T42.3X1	T42.3X2	T42.3X3	T42.3X4	T42.3X5	T42.3X6
Barbitone	T42.3X1	T42.3X2	T42.3X3	T42.3X4	T42.3X5	T42.3X6
Barbiturate NEC	T42.3X1	T42.3X2	T42.3X3	T42.3X4	T42.3X5	T42.3X6
with tranquilizer	T42.3X1	T42.3X2	T42.3X3	T42.3X4	T42.3X5	T42.3X6
anesthetic (intravenous)	T41.1X1	T41.1X2	T41.1X3	T41.1X4	T41.1X5	T41.1X6
Barium (carbonate) (chloride) (sulfite)	T57.8X1	T57.8X2	T57.8X3	T57.8X4	—	—
diagnostic agent	T50.8X1	T50.8X2	T50.8X3	T50.8X4	T50.8X5	T50.8X6
pesticide	T60.4X1	T60.4X2	T60.4X3	T60.4X4	—	—
rodenticide	T60.4X1	T60.4X2	T60.4X3	T60.4X4	—	—
sulfate (medicinal)	T50.8X1	T50.8X2	T50.8X3	T50.8X4	T50.8X5	T50.8X6
Barrier cream	T49.3X1	T49.3X2	T49.3X3	T49.3X4	T49.3X5	T49.3X6
Basic fuchsin	T49.0X1	T49.0X2	T49.0X3	T49.0X4	T49.0X5	T49.0X6
Battery acid or fluid	T54.2X1	T54.2X2	T54.2X3	T54.2X4	—	—
Bay rum	T51.8X1	T51.8X2	T51.8X3	T51.8X4	—	—
b-benzalbutyramide	T46.6X1	T46.6X2	T46.6X3	T46.6X4	T46.6X5	T46.6X6
BCG (vaccine)	T50.A91	T50.A92	T50.A93	T50.A94	T50.A95	T50.A96
BCNU	T45.1X1	T45.1X2	T45.1X3	T45.1X4	T45.1X5	T45.1X6
Bearsfoot	T62.2X1	T62.2X2	T62.2X3	T62.2X4	—	—
Beclamide	T42.6X1	T42.6X2	T42.6X3	T42.6X4	T42.6X5	T42.6X6
Beclomethasone	T44.5X1	T44.5X2	T44.5X3	T44.5X4	T44.5X5	T44.5X6
Bee (sting) (venom)	T63.441	T63.442	T63.443	T63.444	—	—
Befunolol	T49.5X1	T49.5X2	T49.5X3	T49.5X4	T49.5X5	T49.5X6
Bekanamycin	T36.5X1	T36.5X2	T36.5X3	T36.5X4	T36.5X5	T36.5X6
Belladonna — *see also* Nightshade						
alkaloids	T44.3X1	T44.3X2	T44.3X3	T44.3X4	T44.3X5	T44.3X6
extract	T44.3X1	T44.3X2	T44.3X3	T44.3X4	T44.3X5	T44.3X6
herb	T44.3X1	T44.3X2	T44.3X3	T44.3X4	T44.3X5	T44.3X6
Bemegride	T50.7X1	T50.7X2	T50.7X3	T50.7X4	T50.7X5	T50.7X6
Benactyzine	T44.3X1	T44.3X2	T44.3X3	T44.3X4	T44.3X5	T44.3X6
Benadryl	T45.0X1	T45.0X2	T45.0X3	T45.0X4	T45.0X5	T45.0X6
Benaprizine	T44.3X1	T44.3X2	T44.3X3	T44.3X4	T44.3X5	T44.3X6
Benazepril	T46.4X1	T46.4X2	T46.4X3	T46.4X4	T46.4X5	T46.4X6
Bencyclane	T46.7X1	T46.7X2	T46.7X3	T46.7X4	T46.7X5	T46.7X6
Bendazol	T46.3X1	T46.3X2	T46.3X3	T46.3X4	T46.3X5	T46.3X6
Bendrofluazide	T50.2X1	T50.2X2	T50.2X3	T50.2X4	T50.2X5	T50.2X6
Bendroflumethiazide	T50.2X1	T50.2X2	T50.2X3	T50.2X4	T50.2X5	T50.2X6
Benemid	T50.4X1	T50.4X2	T50.4X3	T50.4X4	T50.4X5	T50.4X6
Benethamine penicillin	T36.0X1	T36.0X2	T36.0X3	T36.0X4	T36.0X5	T36.0X6
Benexate	T47.1X1	T47.1X2	T47.1X3	T47.1X4	T47.1X5	T47.1X6
Benfluorex	T46.6X1	T46.6X2	T46.6X3	T46.6X4	T46.6X5	T46.6X6
Benfotiamine	T45.2X1	T45.2X2	T45.2X3	T45.2X4	T45.2X5	T45.2X6
Benisone	T49.0X1	T49.0X2	T49.0X3	T49.0X4	T49.0X5	T49.0X6
Benomyl	T60.0X1	T60.0X2	T60.0X3	T60.0X4	—	—
Benoquin	T49.8X1	T49.8X2	T49.8X3	T49.8X4	T49.8X5	T49.8X6
Benoxinate	T41.3X1	T41.3X2	T41.3X3	T41.3X4	T41.3X5	T41.3X6
Benperidol	T43.4X1	T43.4X2	T43.4X3	T43.4X4	T43.4X5	T43.4X6
Benproperine	T48.3X1	T48.3X2	T48.3X3	T48.3X4	T48.3X5	T48.3X6
Benserazide	T42.8X1	T42.8X2	T42.8X3	T42.8X4	T42.8X5	T42.8X6
Bentazepam	T42.4X1	T42.4X2	T42.4X3	T42.4X4	T42.4X5	T42.4X6
Bentiromide	T50.8X1	T50.8X2	T50.8X3	T50.8X4	T50.8X5	T50.8X6
Bentonite	T49.3X1	T49.3X2	T49.3X3	T49.3X4	T49.3X5	T49.3X6
Benzalbutyramide	T46.6X1	T46.6X2	T46.6X3	T46.6X4	T46.6X5	T46.6X6
Benzalkonium (chloride)	T49.0X1	T49.0X2	T49.0X3	T49.0X4	T49.0X5	T49.0X6
ophthalmic preparation	T49.5X1	T49.5X2	T49.5X3	T49.5X4	T49.5X5	T49.5X6
Benzamidosalicylate (calcium)	T37.1X1	T37.1X2	T37.1X3	T37.1X4	T37.1X5	T37.1X6
Benzamine	T41.3X1	T41.3X2	T41.3X3	T41.3X4	T41.3X5	T41.3X6
lactate	T49.1X1	T49.1X2	T49.1X3	T49.1X4	T49.1X5	T49.1X6
Benzamphetamine	T50.5X1	T50.5X2	T50.5X3	T50.5X4	T50.5X5	T50.5X6
Benzapril hydrochloride	T46.5X1	T46.5X2	T46.5X3	T46.5X4	T46.5X5	T46.5X6
Benzathine benzylpenicillin	T36.0X1	T36.0X2	T36.0X3	T36.0X4	T36.0X5	T36.0X6
Benzathine penicillin	T36.0X1	T36.0X2	T36.0X3	T36.0X4	T36.0X5	T36.0X6
Benzatropine	T42.8X1	T42.8X2	T42.8X3	T42.8X4	T42.8X5	T42.8X6
Benzbromarone	T50.4X1	T50.4X2	T50.4X3	T50.4X4	T50.4X5	T50.4X6
Benzcarbimine	T45.1X1	T45.1X2	T45.1X3	T45.1X4	T45.1X5	T45.1X6
Benzedrex	T44.991	T44.992	T44.993	T44.994	T44.995	T44.996

Substance	Poisoning, Accidental (unintentional)	Poisoning, Intentional Self-harm	Poisoning, Assault	Poisoning, Undetermined	Adverse Effect	Under-dosing
Benzedrine (amphetamine)	T43.621	T43.622	T43.623	T43.624	T43.625	T43.626
Benzenamine	T65.3X1	T65.3X2	T65.3X3	T65.3X4	—	—
Benzene	T52.1X1	T52.1X2	T52.1X3	T52.1X4	—	—
homologues (acetyl) (dimethyl) (methyl) (solvent)	T52.2X1	T52.2X2	T52.2X3	T52.2X4	—	—
Benzethonium (chloride)	T49.0X1	T49.0X2	T49.0X3	T49.0X4	T49.0X5	T49.0X6
Benzfetamine	T50.5X1	T50.5X2	T50.5X3	T50.5X4	T50.5X5	T50.5X6
Benzhexol	T44.3X1	T44.3X2	T44.3X3	T44.3X4	T44.3X5	T44.3X6
Benzhydramine (chloride)	T45.0X1	T45.0X2	T45.0X3	T45.0X4	T45.0X5	T45.0X6
Benzidine	T65.891	T65.892	T65.893	T65.894	—	—
Benzilonium bromide	T44.3X1	T44.3X2	T44.3X3	T44.3X4	T44.3X5	T44.3X6
Benzimidazole	T60.3X1	T60.3X2	T60.3X3	T60.3X4	—	—
Benzin (e) — see Ligroin						
Benziodarone	T46.3X1	T46.3X2	T46.3X3	T46.3X4	T46.3X5	T46.3X6
Benznidazole	T37.3X1	T37.3X2	T37.3X3	T37.3X4	T37.3X5	T37.3X6
Benzocaine	T41.3X1	T41.3X2	T41.3X3	T41.3X4	T41.3X5	T41.3X6
Benzodiapin	T42.4X1	T42.4X2	T42.4X3	T42.4X4	T42.4X5	T42.4X6
Benzodiazepine NEC	T42.4X1	T42.4X2	T42.4X3	T42.4X4	T42.4X5	T42.4X6
Benzoic acid	T49.0X1	T49.0X2	T49.0X3	T49.0X4	T49.0X5	T49.0X6
with salicylic acid	T49.0X1	T49.0X2	T49.0X3	T49.0X4	T49.0X5	T49.0X6
Benzoin (tincture)	T48.5X1	T48.5X2	T48.5X3	T48.5X4	T48.5X5	T48.5X6
Benzol (benzene)	T52.1X1	T52.1X2	T52.1X3	T52.1X4	—	—
vapor	T52.0X1	T52.0X2	T52.0X3	T52.0X4	—	—
Benzomorphan	T40.2X1	T40.2X2	T40.2X3	T40.2X4	T40.2X5	T40.2X6
Benzonatate	T48.3X1	T48.3X2	T48.3X3	T48.3X4	T48.3X5	T48.3X6
Benzophenones	T49.3X1	T49.3X2	T49.3X3	T49.3X4	T49.3X5	T49.3X6
Benzopyrone	T46.991	T46.992	T46.993	T46.994	T46.995	T46.996
Benzothiadiazides	T50.2X1	T50.2X2	T50.2X3	T50.2X4	T50.2X5	T50.2X6
Benzoxonium chloride	T49.0X1	T49.0X2	T49.0X3	T49.0X4	T49.0X5	T49.0X6
Benzoylpas calcium	T37.1X1	T37.1X2	T37.1X3	T37.1X4	T37.1X5	T37.1X6
Benzoyl peroxide	T49.0X1	T49.0X2	T49.0X3	T49.0X4	T49.0X5	T49.0X6
Benzperidin	T43.591	T43.592	T43.593	T43.594	T43.595	T43.596
Benzperidol	T43.591	T43.592	T43.593	T43.594	T43.595	T43.596
Benzphetamine	T50.5X1	T50.5X2	T50.5X3	T50.5X4	T50.5X5	T50.5X6
Benzpyrinium bromide	T44.1X1	T44.1X2	T44.1X3	T44.1X4	T44.1X5	T44.1X6
Benzquinamide	T45.0X1	T45.0X2	T45.0X3	T45.0X4	T45.0X5	T45.0X6
Benzthiazide	T50.2X1	T50.2X2	T50.2X3	T50.2X4	T50.2X5	T50.2X6
Benztropine						
anticholinergic	T44.3X1	T44.3X2	T44.3X3	T44.3X4	T44.3X5	T44.3X6
antiparkinson	T42.8X1	T42.8X2	T42.8X3	T42.8X4	T42.8X5	T42.8X6
Benzydamine	T49.0X1	T49.0X2	T49.0X3	T49.0X4	T49.0X5	T49.0X6
Benzyl						
acetate	T52.8X1	T52.8X2	T52.8X3	T52.8X4	—	—
alcohol	T49.0X1	T49.0X2	T49.0X3	T49.0X4	T49.0X5	T49.0X6
benzoate	T49.0X1	T49.0X2	T49.0X3	T49.0X4	T49.0X5	T49.0X6
Benzoic acid	T49.0X1	T49.0X2	T49.0X3	T49.0X4	T49.0X5	T49.0X6
morphine	T40.2X1	T40.2X2	T40.2X3	T40.2X4	—	—
nicotinate	T46.6X1	T46.6X2	T46.6X3	T46.6X4	T46.6X5	T46.6X6
penicillin	T36.0X1	T36.0X2	T36.0X3	T36.0X4	T36.0X5	T36.0X6
Benzylhydrochlorthiazide	T50.2X1	T50.2X2	T50.2X3	T50.2X4	T50.2X5	T50.2X6
Benzylpenicillin	T36.0X1	T36.0X2	T36.0X3	T36.0X4	T36.0X5	T36.0X6
Benzylthiouracil	T38.2X1	T38.2X2	T38.2X3	T38.2X4	T38.2X5	T38.2X6
Bephenium	T37.4X1	T37.4X2	T37.4X3	T37.4X4	T37.4X5	T37.4X6
hydroxynaphthoate						
Bepridil	T46.1X1	T46.1X2	T46.1X3	T46.1X4	T46.1X5	T46.1X6
Bergamot oil	T65.891	T65.892	T65.893	T65.894	—	—
Bergapten	T50.991	T50.992	T50.993	T50.994	T50.995	T50.996
Berries, poisonous	T62.1X1	T62.1X2	T62.1X3	T62.1X4	—	—
Beryllium (compounds)	T56.7X1	T56.7X2	T56.7X3	T56.7X4	—	—
beta adrenergic blocking agent, heart	T44.7X1	T44.7X2	T44.7X3	T44.7X4	T44.7X5	T44.7X6
Betacarotene	T45.2X1	T45.2X2	T45.2X3	T45.2X4	T45.2X5	T45.2X6
Beta-Chlor	T42.6X1	T42.6X2	T42.6X3	T42.6X4	T42.6X5	T42.6X6
Betahistine	T46.7X1	T46.7X2	T46.7X3	T46.7X4	T46.7X5	T46.7X6
Betaine	T47.5X1	T47.5X2	T47.5X3	T47.5X4	T47.5X5	T47.5X6
Betamethasone	T49.0X1	T49.0X2	T49.0X3	T49.0X4	T49.0X5	T49.0X6
topical	T49.0X1	T49.0X2	T49.0X3	T49.0X4	T49.0X5	T49.0X6
Betamicin	T36.8X1	T36.8X2	T36.8X3	T36.8X4	T36.8X5	T36.8X6
Betanidine	T46.5X1	T46.5X2	T46.5X3	T46.5X4	T46.5X5	T46.5X6
Betaxolol	T44.7X1	T44.7X2	T44.7X3	T44.7X4	T44.7X5	T44.7X6
Betazole	T50.8X1	T50.8X2	T50.8X3	T50.8X4	T50.8X5	T50.8X6
Bethanechol	T44.1X1	T44.1X2	T44.1X3	T44.1X4	T44.1X5	T44.1X6
chloride	T44.1X1	T44.1X2	T44.1X3	T44.1X4	T44.1X5	T44.1X6
Bethanidine	T46.5X1	T46.5X2	T46.5X3	T46.5X4	T46.5X5	T46.5X6
Betoxycaine	T41.3X1	T41.3X2	T41.3X3	T41.3X4	T41.3X5	T41.3X6
Betula oil	T49.3X1	T49.3X2	T49.3X3	T49.3X4	T49.3X5	T49.3X6
Bevantolol	T44.7X1	T44.7X2	T44.7X3	T44.7X4	T44.7X5	T44.7X6
Bevonium metilsulfate	T44.3X1	T44.3X2	T44.3X3	T44.3X4	T44.3X5	T44.3X6
Bezafibrate	T46.6X1	T46.6X2	T46.6X3	T46.6X4	T46.6X5	T46.6X6
Bezitramide	T40.4X1	T40.4X2	T40.4X3	T40.4X4	T40.4X5	T40.4X6
BHA	T50.991	T50.992	T50.993	T50.994	T50.995	T50.996
Bhang	T40.7X1	T40.7X2	T40.7X3	T40.7X4	T40.7X5	T40.7X6
BHC (medicinal)	T49.0X1	T49.0X2	T49.0X3	T49.0X4	T49.0X5	T49.0X6

Substance	Poisoning, Accidental (unintentional)	Poisoning, Intentional Self-harm	Poisoning, Assault	Poisoning, Undetermined	Adverse Effect	Under-dosing
BHC — continued						
nonmedicinal (vapor)	T53.6X1	T53.6X2	T53.6X3	T53.6X4	—	—
Bialamicol	T37.3X1	T37.3X2	T37.3X3	T37.3X4	T37.3X5	T37.3X6
Bibenzonium bromide	T48.3X1	T48.3X2	T48.3X3	T48.3X4	T48.3X5	T48.3X6
Bibrocathol	T49.5X1	T49.5X2	T49.5X3	T49.5X4	T49.5X5	T49.5X6
Bichloride of mercury — see Mercury, chloride						
Bichromates (calcium) (potassium)(sodium) (crystals)	T57.8X1	T57.8X2	T57.8X3	T57.8X4		
fumes	T56.2X1	T56.2X2	T56.2X3	T56.2X4	—	—
Biclotymol	T49.6X1	T49.6X2	T49.6X3	T49.6X4	T49.6X5	T49.6X6
Bicucculine	T50.7X1	T50.7X2	T50.7X3	T50.7X4	T50.7X5	T50.7X6
Bifemelane	T43.291	T43.292	T43.293	T43.294	T43.295	T43.296
Biguanide derivatives, oral	T38.3X1	T38.3X2	T38.3X3	T38.3X4	T38.3X5	T38.3X6
Bile salts	T47.5X1	T47.5X2	T47.5X3	T47.5X4	T47.5X5	T47.5X6
Biligrafin	T50.8X1	T50.8X2	T50.8X3	T50.8X4	T50.8X5	T50.8X6
Bilopaque	T50.8X1	T50.8X2	T50.8X3	T50.8X4	T50.8X5	T50.8X6
Binifibrate	T46.6X1	T46.6X2	T46.6X3	T46.6X4	T46.6X5	T46.6X6
Binitrobenzol	T65.3X1	T65.3X2	T65.3X3	T65.3X4	—	—
Bioflavonoid(s)	T46.991	T46.992	T46.993	T46.994	T46.995	T46.996
Biological substance NEC	T50.901	T50.902	T50.903	T50.904	T50.905	T50.906
Biotin	T45.2X1	T45.2X2	T45.2X3	T45.2X4	T45.2X5	T45.2X6
Biperiden	T44.3X1	T44.3X2	T44.3X3	T44.3X4	T44.3X5	T44.3X6
Bisacodyl	T47.2X1	T47.2X2	T47.2X3	T47.2X4	T47.2X5	T47.2X6
Bisbentiamine	T45.2X1	T45.2X2	T45.2X3	T45.2X4	T45.2X5	T45.2X6
Bisbutiamine	T45.2X1	T45.2X2	T45.2X3	T45.2X4	T45.2X5	T45.2X6
Bisdequalinium (salts) (diacetate)	T49.6X1	T49.6X2	T49.6X3	T49.6X4	T49.6X5	T49.6X6
Bishydroxycoumarin	T45.511	T45.512	T45.513	T45.514	T45.515	T45.516
Bismarsen	T37.8X1	T37.8X2	T37.8X3	T37.8X4	T37.8X5	T37.8X6
Bismuth salts	T47.6X1	T47.6X2	T47.6X3	T47.6X4	T47.6X5	T47.6X6
aluminate	T47.1X1	T47.1X2	T47.1X3	T47.1X4	T47.1X5	T47.1X6
anti-infectives	T37.8X1	T37.8X2	T37.8X3	T37.8X4	T37.8X5	T37.8X6
formic iodide	T49.0X1	T49.0X2	T49.0X3	T49.0X4	T49.0X5	T49.0X6
glycolylarsenate	T49.0X1	T49.0X2	T49.0X3	T49.0X4	T49.0X5	T49.0X6
nonmedicinal (compounds) NEC	T65.91	T65.92	T65.93	T65.94	—	—
subcarbonate	T47.6X1	T47.6X2	T47.6X3	T47.6X4	T47.6X5	T47.6X6
subsalicylate	T37.8X1	T37.8X2	T37.8X3	T37.8X4	T37.8X5	T37.8X6
sulfarsphenamine	T37.8X1	T37.8X2	T37.8X3	T37.8X4	T37.8X5	T37.8X6
Bisoprolol	T44.7X1	T44.7X2	T44.7X3	T44.7X4	T44.7X5	T44.7X6
Bisoxatin	T47.2X1	T47.2X2	T47.2X3	T47.2X4	T47.2X5	T47.2X6
Bisulepin (hydrochloride)	T45.0X1	T45.0X2	T45.0X3	T45.0X4	T45.0X5	T45.0X6
Bithionol	T37.8X1	T37.8X2	T37.8X3	T37.8X4	T37.8X5	T37.8X6
anthelminthic	T37.4X1	T37.4X2	T37.4X3	T37.4X4	T37.4X5	T37.4X6
Bitolterol	T48.6X1	T48.6X2	T48.6X3	T48.6X4	T48.6X5	T48.6X6
Bitoscanate	T37.4X1	T37.4X2	T37.4X3	T37.4X4	T37.4X5	T37.4X6
Bitter almond oil	T62.8X1	T62.8X2	T62.8X3	T62.8X4	—	—
Bittersweet	T62.2X1	T62.2X2	T62.2X3	T62.2X4	—	—
Black						
flag	T60.91	T60.92	T60.93	T60.94	—	—
henbane	T62.2X1	T62.2X2	T62.2X3	T62.2X4	—	—
leaf (40)	T60.91	T60.92	T60.93	T60.94	—	—
widow spider (bite)	T63.311	T63.312	T63.313	T63.314	—	—
antivenin	T50.Z11	T50.Z12	T50.Z13	T50.Z14	T50.Z15	T50.Z16
Blast furnace gas (carbon monoxide from)	T58.8X1	T58.8X2	T58.8X3	T58.8X4	—	—
Bleach	T54.91	T54.92	T54.93	T54.94	—	—
Bleaching agent (medicinal)	T49.4X1	T49.4X2	T49.4X3	T49.4X4	T49.4X5	T49.4X6
Bleomycin	T45.1X1	T45.1X2	T45.1X3	T45.1X4	T45.1X5	T45.1X6
Blockain	T41.3X1	T41.3X2	T41.3X3	T41.3X4	T41.3X5	T41.3X6
infiltration (subcutaneous)	T41.3X1	T41.3X2	T41.3X3	T41.3X4	T41.3X5	T41.3X6
nerve block (peripheral) (plexus)	T41.3X1	T41.3X2	T41.3X3	T41.3X4	T41.3X5	T41.3X6
topical (surface)	T41.3X1	T41.3X2	T41.3X3	T41.3X4	T41.3X5	T41.3X6
Blockers, calcium channel	T46.1X1	T46.1X2	T46.1X3	T46.1X4	T46.1X5	T46.1X6
Blood (derivatives) (natural) (plasma) (whole)	T45.8X1	T45.8X2	T45.8X3	T45.8X4	T45.8X5	T45.8X6
dried	T45.8X1	T45.8X2	T45.8X3	T45.8X4	T45.8X5	T45.8X6
drug affecting NEC	T45.91	T45.92	T45.93	T45.94	T45.95	T45.96
expander NEC	T45.8X1	T45.8X2	T45.8X3	T45.8X4	T45.8X5	T45.8X6
fraction NEC	T45.8X1	T45.8X2	T45.8X3	T45.8X4	T45.8X5	T45.8X6
substitute (macromolecular)	T45.8X1	T45.8X2	T45.8X3	T45.8X4	T45.8X5	T45.8X6
Blue velvet	T40.2X1	T40.2X2	T40.2X3	T40.2X4	—	—
Bone meal	T62.8X1	T62.8X2	T62.8X3	T62.8X4	—	—
Bonine	T45.0X1	T45.0X2	T45.0X3	T45.0X4	T45.0X5	T45.0X6
Bopindolol	T44.7X1	T44.7X2	T44.7X3	T44.7X4	T44.7X5	T44.7X6
Boracic acid	T49.0X1	T49.0X2	T49.0X3	T49.0X4	T49.0X5	T49.0X6
ENT agent	T49.6X1	T49.6X2	T49.6X3	T49.6X4	T49.6X5	T49.6X6
ophthalmic preparation	T49.5X1	T49.5X2	T49.5X3	T49.5X4	T49.5X5	T49.5X6
Borane complex	T57.8X1	T57.8X2	T57.8X3	T57.8X4	—	—

Substance	Poisoning, Accidental (unintentional)	Poisoning, Intentional Self-harm	Poisoning, Assault	Poisoning, Undetermined	Adverse Effect	Under-dosing
Borate(s)	T57.8X1	T57.8X2	T57.8X3	T57.8X4	—	—
buffer	T50.991	T50.992	T50.993	T50.994	T50.995	T50.996
cleanser	T54.91	T54.92	T54.93	T54.94	—	—
sodium	T57.8X1	T57.8X2	T57.8X3	T57.8X4	—	—
Borax (cleanser)	T54.91	T54.92	T54.93	T54.94	—	—
Bordeaux mixture	T60.3X1	T60.3X2	T60.3X3	T60.3X4	—	—
Boric acid	T49.0X1	T49.0X2	T49.0X3	T49.0X4	T49.0X5	T49.0X6
ENT agent	T49.6X1	T49.6X2	T49.6X3	T49.6X4	T49.6X5	T49.6X6
ophthalmic preparation	T49.5X1	T49.5X2	T49.5X3	T49.5X4	T49.5X5	T49.5X6
Bornaprine	T44.3X1	T44.3X2	T44.3X3	T44.3X4	T44.3X5	T44.3X6
Boron	T57.8X1	T57.8X2	T57.8X3	T57.8X4	—	—
hydride NEC	T57.8X1	T57.8X2	T57.8X3	T57.8X4	—	—
fumes or gas	T57.8X1	T57.8X2	T57.8X3	T57.8X4	—	—
trifluoride	T59.891	T59.892	T59.893	T59.894	—	—
Botox	T48.291	T48.292	T48.293	T48.294	T48.295	T48.296
Botulinus anti-toxin (type A, B)	T50.Z11	T50.Z12	T50.Z13	T50.Z14	T50.Z15	T50.Z16
Brake fluid vapor	T59.891	T59.892	T59.893	T59.894	—	—
Brallobarbital	T42.3X1	T42.3X2	T42.3X3	T42.3X4	T42.3X5	T42.3X6
Bran (wheat)	T47.4X1	T47.4X2	T47.4X3	T47.4X4	T47.4X5	T47.4X6
Brass (fumes)	T56.891	T56.892	T56.893	T56.894	—	—
Brasso	T52.0X1	T52.0X2	T52.0X3	T52.0X4	—	—
Bretylium tosilate	T46.2X1	T46.2X2	T46.2X3	T46.2X4	T46.2X5	T46.2X6
Brevital (sodium)	T41.1X1	T41.1X2	T41.1X3	T41.1X4	T41.1X5	T41.1X6
Brinase	T45.3X1	T45.3X2	T45.3X3	T45.3X4	T45.3X5	T45.3X6
British antilewisite	T45.8X1	T45.8X2	T45.8X3	T45.8X4	T45.8X5	T45.8X6
Brodifacoum	T60.4X1	T60.4X2	T60.4X3	T60.4X4	—	—
Bromal (hydrate)	T42.6X1	T42.6X2	T42.6X3	T42.6X4	T42.6X5	T42.6X6
Bromazepam	T42.4X1	T42.4X2	T42.4X3	T42.4X4	T42.4X5	T42.4X6
Bromazine	T45.0X1	T45.0X2	T45.0X3	T45.0X4	T45.0X5	T45.0X6
Brombenzylcyanide	T59.3X1	T59.3X2	T59.3X3	T59.3X4	—	—
Bromelains	T45.3X1	T45.3X2	T45.3X3	T45.3X4	T45.3X5	T45.3X6
Bromethalin	T60.4X1	T60.4X2	T60.4X3	T60.4X4	—	—
Bromhexine	T48.4X1	T48.4X2	T48.4X3	T48.4X4	T48.4X5	T48.4X6
Bromide salts	T42.6X1	T42.6X2	T42.6X3	T42.6X4	T42.6X5	T42.6X6
Bromindione	T45.511	T45.512	T45.513	T45.514	T45.515	T45.516
Bromine						
compounds (medicinal)	T42.6X1	T42.6X2	T42.6X3	T42.6X4	T42.6X5	T42.6X6
sedative	T42.6X1	T42.6X2	T42.6X3	T42.6X4	T42.6X5	T42.6X6
vapor	T59.891	T59.892	T59.893	T59.894	—	—
Bromisoval	T42.6X1	T42.6X2	T42.6X3	T42.6X4	T42.6X5	T42.6X6
Bromisovalum	T42.6X1	T42.6X2	T42.6X3	T42.6X4	T42.6X5	T42.6X6
Bromobenzylcyanide	T59.3X1	T59.3X2	T59.3X3	T59.3X4	—	—
Bromochlorosalicylani-lide	T49.0X1	T49.0X2	T49.0X3	T49.0X4	T49.0X5	T49.0X6
Bromocriptine	T42.8X1	T42.8X2	T42.8X3	T42.8X4	T42.8X5	T42.8X6
Bromodiphenhydramine	T45.0X1	T45.0X2	T45.0X3	T45.0X4	T45.0X5	T45.0X6
Bromoform	T42.6X1	T42.6X2	T42.6X3	T42.6X4	T42.6X5	T42.6X6
Bromophenol blue reagent	T50.991	T50.992	T50.993	T50.994	T50.995	T50.996
Bromopride	T47.8X1	T47.8X2	T47.8X3	T47.8X4	T47.8X5	T47.8X6
Bromosalicylchloranitide	T49.0X1	T49.0X2	T49.0X3	T49.0X4	T49.0X5	T49.0X6
Bromosalicylhydroxamic acid	T37.1X1	T37.1X2	T37.1X3	T37.1X4	T37.1X5	T37.1X6
Bromo-seltzer	T39.1X1	T39.1X2	T39.1X3	T39.1X4	T39.1X5	T39.1X6
Bromoxynil	T60.3X1	T60.3X2	T60.3X3	T60.3X4	—	—
Bromperidol	T43.4X1	T43.4X2	T43.4X3	T43.4X4	T43.4X5	T43.4X6
Brompheniramine	T45.0X1	T45.0X2	T45.0X3	T45.0X4	T45.0X5	T45.0X6
Bromsulfophthalein	T50.8X1	T50.8X2	T50.8X3	T50.8X4	T50.8X5	T50.8X6
Bromural	T42.6X1	T42.6X2	T42.6X3	T42.6X4	T42.6X5	T42.6X6
Bromvaletone	T42.6X1	T42.6X2	T42.6X3	T42.6X4	T42.6X5	T42.6X6
Bronchodilator NEC	T48.6X1	T48.6X2	T48.6X3	T48.6X4	T48.6X5	T48.6X6
Brotizolam	T42.4X1	T42.4X2	T42.4X3	T42.4X4	T42.4X5	T42.4X6
Brovincamine	T46.7X1	T46.7X2	T46.7X3	T46.7X4	T46.7X5	T46.7X6
Brown recluse spider (bite) (venom)	T63.331	T63.332	T63.333	T63.334	—	—
Brown spider (bite) (venom)	T63.391	T63.392	T63.393	T63.394	—	—
Broxaterol	T48.6X1	T48.6X2	T48.6X3	T48.6X4	T48.6X5	T48.6X6
Broxuridine	T45.1X1	T45.1X2	T45.1X3	T45.1X4	T45.1X5	T45.1X6
Broxyquinoline	T37.8X1	T37.8X2	T37.8X3	T37.8X4	T37.8X5	T37.8X6
Bruceine	T48.291	T48.292	T48.293	T48.294	T48.295	T48.296
Brucia	T62.2X1	T62.2X2	T62.2X3	T62.2X4	—	—
Brucine	T65.1X1	T65.1X2	T65.1X3	T65.1X4	—	—
Brunswick green — see Copper						
Bruten — see Ibuprofen						
Bryonia	T47.2X1	T47.2X2	T47.2X3	T47.2X4	T47.2X5	T47.2X6
Buclizine	T45.0X1	T45.0X2	T45.0X3	T45.0X4	T45.0X5	T45.0X6
Buclosamide	T49.0X1	T49.0X2	T49.0X3	T49.0X4	T49.0X5	T49.0X6
Budesonide	T44.5X1	T44.5X2	T44.5X3	T44.5X4	T44.5X5	T44.5X6
Budralazine	T46.5X1	T46.5X2	T46.5X3	T46.5X4	T46.5X5	T46.5X6
Bufferin	T39.011	T39.012	T39.013	T39.014	T39.015	T39.016
Buflomedil	T46.7X1	T46.7X2	T46.7X3	T46.7X4	T46.7X5	T46.7X6
Buformin	T38.3X1	T38.3X2	T38.3X3	T38.3X4	T38.3X5	T38.3X6
Bufotenine	T40.991	T40.992	T40.993	T40.994		
Bufrolin	T48.6X1	T48.6X2	T48.6X3	T48.6X4	T48.6X5	T48.6X6
Bufylline	T48.6X1	T48.6X2	T48.6X3	T48.6X4	T48.6X5	T48.6X6
Bulk filler	T50.5X1	T50.5X2	T50.5X3	T50.5X4	T50.5X5	T50.5X6
cathartic	T47.4X1	T47.4X2	T47.4X3	T47.4X4	T47.4X5	T47.4X6
Bumetanide	T50.1X1	T50.1X2	T50.1X3	T50.1X4	T50.1X5	T50.1X6
Bunaftine	T46.2X1	T46.2X2	T46.2X3	T46.2X4	T46.2X5	T46.2X6
Bunamiodyl	T50.8X1	T50.8X2	T50.8X3	T50.8X4	T50.8X5	T50.8X6
Bunazosin	T44.6X1	T44.6X2	T44.6X3	T44.6X4	T44.6X5	T44.6X6
Bunitrolol	T44.7X1	T44.7X2	T44.7X3	T44.7X4	T44.7X5	T44.7X6
Buphenine	T46.7X1	T46.7X2	T46.7X3	T46.7X4	T46.7X5	T46.7X6
Bupivacaine	T41.3X1	T41.3X2	T41.3X3	T41.3X4	T41.3X5	T41.3X6
infiltration (subcutaneous)	T41.3X1	T41.3X2	T41.3X3	T41.3X4	T41.3X5	T41.3X6
nerve block (peripheral) (plexus)	T41.3X1	T41.3X2	T41.3X3	T41.3X4	T41.3X5	T41.3X6
spinal	T41.3X1	T41.3X2	T41.3X3	T41.3X4	T41.3X5	T41.3X6
Bupranolol	T44.7X1	T44.7X2	T44.7X3	T44.7X4	T44.7X5	T44.7X6
Buprenorphine	T40.4X1	T40.4X2	T40.4X3	T40.4X4	T40.4X5	T40.4X6
Bupropion	T43.291	T43.292	T43.293	T43.294	T43.295	T43.296
Burimamide	T47.1X1	T47.1X2	T47.1X3	T47.1X4	T47.1X5	T47.1X6
Buserelin	T38.891	T38.892	T38.893	T38.894	T38.895	T38.896
Buspirone	T43.591	T43.592	T43.593	T43.594	T43.595	T43.596
Busulfan, busulphan	T45.1X1	T45.1X2	T45.1X3	T45.1X4	T45.1X5	T45.1X6
Butabarbital (sodium)	T42.3X1	T42.3X2	T42.3X3	T42.3X4	T42.3X5	T42.3X6
Butabarbitone	T42.3X1	T42.3X2	T42.3X3	T42.3X4	T42.3X5	T42.3X6
Butabarpal	T42.3X1	T42.3X2	T42.3X3	T42.3X4	T42.3X5	T42.3X6
Butacaine	T41.3X1	T41.3X2	T41.3X3	T41.3X4	T41.3X5	T41.3X6
Butalamine	T46.7X1	T46.7X2	T46.7X3	T46.7X4	T46.7X5	T46.7X6
Butalbital	T42.3X1	T42.3X2	T42.3X3	T42.3X4	T42.3X5	T42.3X6
Butallylonal	T42.3X1	T42.3X2	T42.3X3	T42.3X4	T42.3X5	T42.3X6
Butamben	T41.3X1	T41.3X2	T41.3X3	T41.3X4	T41.3X5	T41.3X6
Butamirate	T48.3X1	T48.3X2	T48.3X3	T48.3X4	T48.3X5	T48.3X6
Butane (distributed in mobile container)	T59.891	T59.892	T59.893	T59.894	—	—
distributed through pipes	T59.891	T59.892	T59.893	T59.894	—	—
incomplete combustion	T58.11	T58.12	T58.13	T58.14	—	—
Butanilicaine	T41.3X1	T41.3X2	T41.3X3	T41.3X4	T41.3X5	T41.3X6
Butanol	T51.3X1	T51.3X2	T51.3X3	T51.3X4	—	—
Butanone, 2-butanone	T52.4X1	T52.4X2	T52.4X3	T52.4X4	—	—
Butantrone	T49.4X1	T49.4X2	T49.4X3	T49.4X4	T49.4X5	T49.4X6
Butaperazine	T43.3X1	T43.3X2	T43.3X3	T43.3X4	T43.3X5	T43.3X6
Butazolidin	T39.2X1	T39.2X2	T39.2X3	T39.2X4	T39.2X5	T39.2X6
Butetamate	T48.6X1	T48.6X2	T48.6X3	T48.6X4	T48.6X5	T48.6X6
Butethal	T42.3X1	T42.3X2	T42.3X3	T42.3X4	T42.3X5	T42.3X6
Butethamate	T44.3X1	T44.3X2	T44.3X3	T44.3X4	T44.3X5	T44.3X6
Buthalitone (sodium)	T41.1X1	T41.1X2	T41.1X3	T41.1X4	T41.1X5	T41.1X6
Butisol (sodium)	T42.3X1	T42.3X2	T42.3X3	T42.3X4	T42.3X5	T42.3X6
Butizide	T50.2X1	T50.2X2	T50.2X3	T50.2X4	T50.2X5	T50.2X6
Butobarbital	T42.3X1	T42.3X2	T42.3X3	T42.3X4	T42.3X5	T42.3X6
sodium	T42.3X1	T42.3X2	T42.3X3	T42.3X4	T42.3X5	T42.3X6
Butobarbitone	T42.3X1	T42.3X2	T42.3X3	T42.3X4	T42.3X5	T42.3X6
Butoconazole (nitrate)	T49.0X1	T49.0X2	T49.0X3	T49.0X4	T49.0X5	T49.0X6
Butorphanol	T40.4X1	T40.4X2	T40.4X3	T40.4X4	T40.4X5	T40.4X6
Butriptyline	T43.011	T43.012	T43.013	T43.014	T43.015	T43.016
Butropium bromide	T44.3X1	T44.3X2	T44.3X3	T44.3X4	T44.3X5	T44.3X6
Buttercups	T62.2X1	T62.2X2	T62.2X3	T62.2X4	—	—
Butter of antimony — see Antimony						
Butyl						
acetate (secondary)	T52.8X1	T52.8X2	T52.8X3	T52.8X4	—	—
alcohol	T51.3X1	T51.3X2	T51.3X3	T51.3X4	—	—
aminobenzoate	T41.3X1	T41.3X2	T41.3X3	T41.3X4	T41.3X5	T41.3X6
butyrate	T52.8X1	T52.8X2	T52.8X3	T52.8X4	—	—
carbinol	T51.3X1	T51.3X2	T51.3X3	T51.3X4	—	—
carbitol	T52.3X1	T52.3X2	T52.3X3	T52.3X4	—	—
cellosolve	T52.3X1	T52.3X2	T52.3X3	T52.3X4	—	—
chloral (hydrate)	T42.6X1	T42.6X2	T42.6X3	T42.6X4	T42.6X5	T42.6X6
formate	T52.8X1	T52.8X2	T52.8X3	T52.8X4	—	—
lactate	T52.8X1	T52.8X2	T52.8X3	T52.8X4	—	—
propionate	T52.8X1	T52.8X2	T52.8X3	T52.8X4	—	—
scopolamine bromide	T44.3X1	T44.3X2	T44.3X3	T44.3X4	T44.3X5	T44.3X6
thiobarbital sodium	T41.1X1	T41.1X2	T41.1X3	T41.1X4	T41.1X5	T41.1X6
Butylated hydroxyanisole	T50.991	T50.992	T50.993	T50.994	T50.995	T50.996
Butylchloral hydrate	T42.6X1	T42.6X2	T42.6X3	T42.6X4	T42.6X5	T42.6X6
Butyltoluene	T52.2X1	T52.2X2	T52.2X3	T52.2X4	—	—
Butyn	T41.3X1	T41.3X2	T41.3X3	T41.3X4	T41.3X5	T41.3X6
Butyrophenone (-based tranquilizers)	T43.4X1	T43.4X2	T43.4X3	T43.4X4	T43.4X5	T43.4X6
Caberpoline	T42.8X1	T42.8X2	T42.8X3	T42.8X4	T42.8X5	T42.8X6
Cacodyl, cacodylic acid	T57.0X1	T57.0X2	T57.0X3	T57.0X4	—	—
Cactinomycin	T45.1X1	T45.1X2	T45.1X3	T45.1X4	T45.1X5	T45.1X6
Cade oil	T49.4X1	T49.4X2	T49.4X3	T49.4X4	T49.4X5	T49.4X6
Cadexomer iodine	T49.0X1	T49.0X2	T49.0X3	T49.0X4	T49.0X5	T49.0X6
Cadmium (chloride) (fumes) (oxide)	T56.3X1	T56.3X2	T56.3X3	T56.3X4	—	—

356

Additional Character May Be Required — Refer to the Tabular List for Character Selection   ▼ Subterms under main terms may continue to next column or page

Substance	Poisoning, Accidental (unintentional)	Poisoning, Intentional Self-harm	Poisoning, Assault	Poisoning, Undetermined	Adverse Effect	Under-dosing
Cadmium — continued						
sulfide (medicinal) NEC	T49.4X1	T49.4X2	T49.4X3	T49.4X4	T49.4X5	T49.4X6
Cadralazine	T46.5X1	T46.5X2	T46.5X3	T46.5X4	T46.5X5	T46.5X6
Caffeine	T43.611	T43.612	T43.613	T43.614	T43.615	T43.616
Calabar bean	T62.2X1	T62.2X2	T62.2X3	T62.2X4	—	—
Caladium seguinum	T62.2X1	T62.2X2	T62.2X3	T62.2X4	—	—
Calamine (lotion)	T49.3X1	T49.3X2	T49.3X3	T49.3X4	T49.3X5	T49.3X6
Calcifediol	T45.2X1	T45.2X2	T45.2X3	T45.2X4	T45.2X5	T45.2X6
Calciferol	T45.2X1	T45.2X2	T45.2X3	T45.2X4	T45.2X5	T45.2X6
Calcitonin	T50.991	T50.992	T50.993	T50.994	T50.995	T50.996
Calcitriol	T45.2X1	T45.2X2	T45.2X3	T45.2X4	T45.2X5	T45.2X6
Calcium	T50.3X1	T50.3X2	T50.3X3	T50.3X4	T50.3X5	T50.3X6
actylsalicylate	T39.011	T39.012	T39.013	T39.014	T39.015	T39.016
benzamidosalicylate	T37.1X1	T37.1X2	T37.1X3	T37.1X4	T37.1X5	T37.1X6
bromide	T42.6X1	T42.6X2	T42.6X3	T42.6X4	T42.6X5	T42.6X6
bromolactobionate	T42.6X1	T42.6X2	T42.6X3	T42.6X4	T42.6X5	T42.6X6
carbaspirin	T39.011	T39.012	T39.013	T39.014	T39.015	T39.016
carbimide	T50.6X1	T50.6X2	T50.6X3	T50.6X4	T50.6X5	T50.6X6
carbonate	T47.1X1	T47.1X2	T47.1X3	T47.1X4	T47.1X5	T47.1X6
chloride	T50.991	T50.992	T50.993	T50.994	T50.995	T50.996
anhydrous	T50.991	T50.992	T50.993	T50.994	T50.995	T50.996
cyanide	T57.8X1	T57.8X2	T57.8X3	T57.8X4	—	—
dioctyl sulfosuccinate	T47.4X1	T47.4X2	T47.4X3	T47.4X4	T47.4X5	T47.4X6
disodium edathamil	T45.8X1	T45.8X2	T45.8X3	T45.8X4	T45.8X5	T45.8X6
disodium edetate	T45.8X1	T45.8X2	T45.8X3	T45.8X4	T45.8X5	T45.8X6
dobesilate	T46.991	T46.992	T46.993	T46.994	T46.995	T46.996
EDTA	T45.8X1	T45.8X2	T45.8X3	T45.8X4	T45.8X5	T45.8X6
ferrous citrate	T45.4X1	T45.4X2	T45.4X3	T45.4X4	T45.4X5	T45.4X6
folinate	T45.8X1	T45.8X2	T45.8X3	T45.8X4	T45.8X5	T45.8X6
glubionate	T50.3X1	T50.3X2	T50.3X3	T50.3X4	T50.3X5	T50.3X6
gluconate	T50.3X1	T50.3X2	T50.3X3	T50.3X4	T50.3X5	T50.3X6
gluconogalactogluconate	T50.3X1	T50.3X2	T50.3X3	T50.3X4	T50.3X5	T50.3X6
hydrate, hydroxide	T54.3X1	T54.3X2	T54.3X3	T54.3X4	—	—
hypochlorite	T54.3X1	T54.3X2	T54.3X3	T54.3X4	—	—
iodide	T48.4X1	T48.4X2	T48.4X3	T48.4X4	T48.4X5	T48.4X6
ipodate	T50.8X1	T50.8X2	T50.8X3	T50.8X4	T50.8X5	T50.8X6
lactate	T50.3X1	T50.3X2	T50.3X3	T50.3X4	T50.3X5	T50.3X6
leucovorin	T45.8X1	T45.8X2	T45.8X3	T45.8X4	T45.8X5	T45.8X6
mandelate	T37.91	T37.92	T37.93	T37.94	T37.95	T37.96
oxide	T54.3X1	T54.3X2	T54.3X3	T54.3X4	—	—
pantothenate	T45.2X1	T45.2X2	T45.2X3	T45.2X4	T45.2X5	T45.2X6
phosphate	T50.3X1	T50.3X2	T50.3X3	T50.3X4	T50.3X5	T50.3X6
salicylate	T39.091	T39.092	T39.093	T39.094	T39.095	T39.096
salts	T50.3X1	T50.3X2	T50.3X3	T50.3X4	T50.3X5	T50.3X6
Calculus-dissolving drug	T50.991	T50.992	T50.993	T50.994	T50.995	T50.996
Calomel	T49.0X1	T49.0X2	T49.0X3	T49.0X4	T49.0X5	T49.0X6
Caloric agent	T50.3X1	T50.3X2	T50.3X3	T50.3X4	T50.3X5	T50.3X6
Calusterone	T38.7X1	T38.7X2	T38.7X3	T38.7X4	T38.7X5	T38.7X6
Camazepam	T42.4X1	T42.4X2	T42.4X3	T42.4X4	T42.4X5	T42.4X6
Camomile	T49.0X1	T49.0X2	T49.0X3	T49.0X4	T49.0X5	T49.0X6
Camoquin	T37.2X1	T37.2X2	T37.2X3	T37.2X4	T37.2X5	T37.2X6
Camphor						
insecticide	T60.2X1	T60.2X2	T60.2X3	T60.2X4	—	—
medicinal	T49.8X1	T49.8X2	T49.8X3	T49.8X4	T49.8X5	T49.8X6
Camylofin	T44.3X1	T44.3X2	T44.3X3	T44.3X4	T44.3X5	T44.3X6
Cancer chemotherapy drug regimen	T45.1X1	T45.1X2	T45.1X3	T45.1X4	T45.1X5	T45.1X6
Candeptin	T49.0X1	T49.0X2	T49.0X3	T49.0X4	T49.0X5	T49.0X6
Candicidin	T49.0X1	T49.0X2	T49.0X3	T49.0X4	T49.0X5	T49.0X6
Cannabinol	T40.7X1	T40.7X2	T40.7X3	T40.7X4	T40.7X5	T40.7X6
Cannabis (derivatives)	T40.7X1	T40.7X2	T40.7X3	T40.7X4	T40.7X5	T40.7X6
Canned heat	T51.1X1	T51.1X2	T51.1X3	T51.1X4	—	—
Canrenoic acid	T50.0X1	T50.0X2	T50.0X3	T50.0X4	T50.0X5	T50.0X6
Canrenone	T50.0X1	T50.0X2	T50.0X3	T50.0X4	T50.0X5	T50.0X6
Cantharides, cantharidin, cantharis	T49.8X1	T49.8X2	T49.8X3	T49.8X4	T49.8X5	T49.8X6
Canthaxanthin	T50.991	T50.992	T50.993	T50.994	T50.995	T50.996
Capillary-active drug NEC	T46.901	T46.902	T46.903	T46.904	T46.905	T46.906
Capreomycin	T36.8X1	T36.8X2	T36.8X3	T36.8X4	T36.8X5	T36.8X6
Capsicum	T49.4X1	T49.4X2	T49.4X3	T49.4X4	T49.4X5	T49.4X6
Captafol	T60.3X1	T60.3X2	T60.3X3	T60.3X4	—	—
Captan	T60.3X1	T60.3X2	T60.3X3	T60.3X4	—	—
Captodiame, captodiamine	T43.591	T43.592	T43.593	T43.594	T43.595	T43.596
Captopril	T46.4X1	T46.4X2	T46.4X3	T46.4X4	T46.4X5	T46.4X6
Caramiphen	T44.3X1	T44.3X2	T44.3X3	T44.3X4	T44.3X5	T44.3X6
Carazolol	T44.7X1	T44.7X2	T44.7X3	T44.7X4	T44.7X5	T44.7X6
Carbachol	T44.1X1	T44.1X2	T44.1X3	T44.1X4	T44.1X5	T44.1X6
Carbacrylamine (resin)	T50.3X1	T50.3X2	T50.3X3	T50.3X4	T50.3X5	T50.3X6
Carbamate (insecticide)	T60.0X1	T60.0X2	T60.0X3	T60.0X4	—	—
Carbamate (sedative)	T42.6X1	T42.6X2	T42.6X3	T42.6X4	T42.6X5	T42.6X6
herbicide	T60.0X1	T60.0X2	T60.0X3	T60.0X4	—	—
insecticide	T60.0X1	T60.0X2	T60.0X3	T60.0X4	—	—
Carbamazepine	T42.1X1	T42.1X2	T42.1X3	T42.1X4	T42.1X5	T42.1X6

Substance	Poisoning, Accidental (unintentional)	Poisoning, Intentional Self-harm	Poisoning, Assault	Poisoning, Undetermined	Adverse Effect	Under-dosing
Carbamide	T47.3X1	T47.3X2	T47.3X3	T47.3X4	T47.3X5	T47.3X6
peroxide	T49.0X1	T49.0X2	T49.0X3	T49.0X4	T49.0X5	T49.0X6
topical	T49.8X1	T49.8X2	T49.8X3	T49.8X4	T49.8X5	T49.8X6
Carbamylcholine chloride	T44.1X1	T44.1X2	T44.1X3	T44.1X4	T44.1X5	T44.1X6
Carbaril	T60.0X1	T60.0X2	T60.0X3	T60.0X4	—	—
Carbarsone	T37.3X1	T37.3X2	T37.3X3	T37.3X4	T37.3X5	T37.3X6
Carbaryl	T60.0X1	T60.0X2	T60.0X3	T60.0X4	—	—
Carbaspirin	T39.011	T39.012	T39.013	T39.014	T39.015	T39.016
Carbazochrome (salicylate) (sodium sulfonate)	T49.4X1	T49.4X2	T49.4X3	T49.4X4	T49.4X5	T49.4X6
Carbenicillin	T36.0X1	T36.0X2	T36.0X3	T36.0X4	T36.0X5	T36.0X6
Carbenoxolone	T47.1X1	T47.1X2	T47.1X3	T47.1X4	T47.1X5	T47.1X6
Carbetapentane	T48.3X1	T48.3X2	T48.3X3	T48.3X4	T48.3X5	T48.3X6
Carbethyl salicylate	T39.091	T39.092	T39.093	T39.094	T39.095	T39.096
Carbidopa (with levodopa)	T42.8X1	T42.8X2	T42.8X3	T42.8X4	T42.8X5	T42.8X6
Carbimazole	T38.2X1	T38.2X2	T38.2X3	T38.2X4	T38.2X5	T38.2X6
Carbinol	T51.1X1	T51.1X2	T51.1X3	T51.1X4	—	—
Carbinoxamine	T45.0X1	T45.0X2	T45.0X3	T45.0X4	T45.0X5	T45.0X6
Carbiphene	T39.8X1	T39.8X2	T39.8X3	T39.8X4	T39.8X5	T39.8X6
Carbitol	T52.3X1	T52.3X2	T52.3X3	T52.3X4	—	—
Carbocaine	T41.3X1	T41.3X2	T41.3X3	T41.3X4	T41.3X5	T41.3X6
infiltration (subcutaneous)	T41.3X1	T41.3X2	T41.3X3	T41.3X4	T41.3X5	T41.3X6
nerve block (peripheral) (plexus)	T41.3X1	T41.3X2	T41.3X3	T41.3X4	T41.3X5	T41.3X6
topical (surface)	T41.3X1	T41.3X2	T41.3X3	T41.3X4	T41.3X5	T41.3X6
Carbocisteine	T48.4X1	T48.4X2	T48.4X3	T48.4X4	T48.4X5	T48.4X6
Carbocromen	T46.3X1	T46.3X2	T46.3X3	T46.3X4	T46.3X5	T46.3X6
Carbol fuchsin	T49.0X1	T49.0X2	T49.0X3	T49.0X4	T49.0X5	T49.0X6
Carbolic acid — see also Phenol	T54.0X1	T54.0X2	T54.0X3	T54.0X4	—	—
Carbolonium (bromide)	T48.1X1	T48.1X2	T48.1X3	T48.1X4	T48.1X5	T48.1X6
Carbo medicinalis	T47.6X1	T47.6X2	T47.6X3	T47.6X4	T47.6X5	T47.6X6
Carbomycin	T36.8X1	T36.8X2	T36.8X3	T36.8X4	T36.8X5	T36.8X6
Carbon						
bisulfide (liquid)	T65.4X1	T65.4X2	T65.4X3	T65.4X4	—	—
vapor	T65.4X1	T65.4X2	T65.4X3	T65.4X4	—	—
dioxide (gas)	T59.7X1	T59.7X2	T59.7X3	T59.7X4	—	—
medicinal	T41.5X1	T41.5X2	T41.5X3	T41.5X4	T41.5X5	T41.5X6
nonmedicinal	T59.7X1	T59.7X2	T59.7X3	T59.7X4	—	—
snow	T49.4X1	T49.4X2	T49.4X3	T49.4X4	T49.4X5	T49.4X6
disulfide (liquid)	T65.4X1	T65.4X2	T65.4X3	T65.4X4	—	—
vapor	T65.4X1	T65.4X2	T65.4X3	T65.4X4	—	—
monoxide (from incomplete combustion)	T58.91	T58.92	T58.93	T58.94	—	—
blast furnace gas	T58.8X1	T58.8X2	T58.8X3	T58.8X4	—	—
butane (distributed in mobile container)	T58.11	T58.12	T58.13	T58.14	—	—
distributed through pipes	T58.11	T58.12	T58.13	T58.14	—	—
charcoal fumes	T58.2X1	T58.2X2	T58.2X3	T58.2X4	—	—
coal	T58.2X1	T58.2X2	T58.2X3	T58.2X4	—	—
coke (in domestic stoves, fireplaces)	T58.2X1	T58.2X2	T58.2X3	T58.2X4	—	—
exhaust gas (motor) not in transit	T58.01	T58.02	T58.03	T58.04	—	—
combustion engine, any not in watercraft	T58.01	T58.02	T58.03	T58.04	—	—
farm tractor, not in transit	T58.01	T58.02	T58.03	T58.04	—	—
gas engine	T58.01	T58.02	T58.03	T58.04	—	—
motor pump	T58.01	T58.02	T58.03	T58.04	—	—
motor vehicle, not in transit	T58.01	T58.02	T58.03	T58.04	—	—
fuel (in domestic use)	T58.2X1	T58.2X2	T58.2X3	T58.2X4	—	—
gas (piped)	T58.11	T58.12	T58.13	T58.14	—	—
in mobile container	T58.11	T58.12	T58.13	T58.14	—	—
piped (natural)	T58.11	T58.12	T58.13	T58.14	—	—
utility	T58.11	T58.12	T58.13	T58.14	—	—
in mobile container	T58.11	T58.12	T58.13	T58.14	—	—
gas (piped)	T58.11	T58.12	T58.13	T58.14	—	—
illuminating gas	T58.11	T58.12	T58.13	T58.14	—	—
industrial fuels or gases, any	T58.8X1	T58.8X2	T58.8X3	T58.8X4	—	—
kerosene (in domestic stoves, fireplaces)	T58.2X1	T58.2X2	T58.2X3	T58.2X4	—	—
kiln gas or vapor	T58.8X1	T58.8X2	T58.8X3	T58.8X4	—	—
motor exhaust gas, not in transit	T58.01	T58.02	T58.03	T58.04	—	—
piped gas (manufactured) (natural)	T58.11	T58.12	T58.13	T58.14	—	—
producer gas	T58.8X1	T58.8X2	T58.8X3	T58.8X4	—	—
propane (distributed in mobile container)	T58.11	T58.12	T58.13	T58.14	—	—

Table of Drugs and Chemicals

Carbon — Central nervous system

Substance	Poisoning, Accidental (unintentional)	Poisoning, Intentional Self-harm	Poisoning, Assault	Poisoning, Undetermined	Adverse Effect	Under-dosing
Carbon — continued						
monoxide — continued						
propane — continued						
distributed through pipes	T58.11	T58.12	T58.13	T58.14	—	—
solid (in domestic stoves, fireplaces)	T58.2X1	T58.2X2	T58.2X3	T58.2X4	—	—
specified source NEC	T58.8X1	T58.8X2	T58.8X3	T58.8X4	—	—
stove gas	T58.11	T58.12	T58.13	T58.14	—	—
piped	T58.11	T58.12	T58.13	T58.14	—	—
utility gas	T58.11	T58.12	T58.13	T58.14	—	—
piped	T58.11	T58.12	T58.13	T58.14	—	—
water gas	T58.11	T58.12	T58.13	T58.14	—	—
wood (in domestic stoves, fireplaces)	T58.2X1	T58.2X2	T58.2X3	T58.2X4	—	—
tetrachloride (vapor) NEC	T53.0X1	T53.0X2	T53.0X3	T53.0X4	—	—
liquid (cleansing agent) NEC	T53.0X1	T53.0X2	T53.0X3	T53.0X4	—	—
solvent	T53.0X1	T53.0X2	T53.0X3	T53.0X4	—	—
Carbonic acid gas	T59.7X1	T59.7X2	T59.7X3	T59.7X4	—	—
anhydrase inhibitor NEC	T50.2X1	T50.2X2	T50.2X3	T50.2X4	T50.2X5	T50.2X6
Carbophenothion	T60.0X1	T60.0X2	T60.0X3	T60.0X4	—	—
Carboplatin	T45.1X1	T45.1X2	T45.1X3	T45.1X4	T45.1X5	T45.1X6
Carboprost	T48.0X1	T48.0X2	T48.0X3	T48.0X4	T48.0X5	T48.0X6
Carboquone	T45.1X1	T45.1X2	T45.1X3	T45.1X4	T45.1X5	T45.1X6
Carbowax	T49.3X1	T49.3X2	T49.3X3	T49.3X4	T49.3X5	T49.3X6
Carboxymethylcellulose	T47.4X1	T47.4X2	T47.4X3	T47.4X4	T47.4X5	T47.4X6
Carbrital	T42.3X1	T42.3X2	T42.3X3	T42.3X4	T42.3X5	T42.3X6
Carbromal	T42.6X1	T42.6X2	T42.6X3	T42.6X4	T42.6X5	T42.6X6
Carbutamide	T38.3X1	T38.3X2	T38.3X3	T38.3X4	T38.3X5	T38.3X6
Carbuterol	T48.6X1	T48.6X2	T48.6X3	T48.6X4	T48.6X5	T48.6X6
Cardiac						
depressants	T46.2X1	T46.2X2	T46.2X3	T46.2X4	T46.2X5	T46.2X6
rhythm regulator	T46.2X1	T46.2X2	T46.2X3	T46.2X4	T46.2X5	T46.2X6
specified NEC	T46.2X1	T46.2X2	T46.2X3	T46.2X4	T46.2X5	T46.2X6
Cardiografin	T50.8X1	T50.8X2	T50.8X3	T50.8X4	T50.8X5	T50.8X6
Cardiogreen	T50.8X1	T50.8X2	T50.8X3	T50.8X4	T50.8X5	T50.8X6
Cardiotonic (glycoside) NEC	T46.0X1	T46.0X2	T46.0X3	T46.0X4	T46.0X5	T46.0X6
Cardiovascular drug NEC	T46.901	T46.902	T46.903	T46.904	T46.905	T46.906
Cardrase	T50.2X1	T50.2X2	T50.2X3	T50.2X4	T50.2X5	T50.2X6
Carfecillin	T36.0X1	T36.0X2	T36.0X3	T36.0X4	T36.0X5	T36.0X6
Carfenazine	T43.3X1	T43.3X2	T43.3X3	T43.3X4	T43.3X5	T43.3X6
Carfusin	T49.0X1	T49.0X2	T49.0X3	T49.0X4	T49.0X5	T49.0X6
Carindacillin	T36.0X1	T36.0X2	T36.0X3	T36.0X4	T36.0X5	T36.0X6
Carisoprodol	T42.8X1	T42.8X2	T42.8X3	T42.8X4	T42.8X5	T42.8X6
Carmellose	T47.4X1	T47.4X2	T47.4X3	T47.4X4	T47.4X5	T47.4X6
Carminative	T47.5X1	T47.5X2	T47.5X3	T47.5X4	T47.5X5	T47.5X6
Carmofur	T45.1X1	T45.1X2	T45.1X3	T45.1X4	T45.1X5	T45.1X6
Carmustine	T45.1X1	T45.1X2	T45.1X3	T45.1X4	T45.1X5	T45.1X6
Carotene	T45.2X1	T45.2X2	T45.2X3	T45.2X4	T45.2X5	T45.2X6
Carphenazine	T43.3X1	T43.3X2	T43.3X3	T43.3X4	T43.3X5	T43.3X6
Carpipramine	T42.4X1	T42.4X2	T42.4X3	T42.4X4	T42.4X5	T42.4X6
Carprofen	T39.311	T39.312	T39.313	T39.314	T39.315	T39.316
Carpronium chloride	T44.3X1	T44.3X2	T44.3X3	T44.3X4	T44.3X5	T44.3X6
Carrageenan	T47.8X1	T47.8X2	T47.8X3	T47.8X4	T47.8X5	T47.8X6
Carteolol	T44.7X1	T44.7X2	T44.7X3	T44.7X4	T44.7X5	T44.7X6
Carter's Little Pills	T47.2X1	T47.2X2	T47.2X3	T47.2X4	T47.2X5	T47.2X6
Cascara (sagrada)	T47.2X1	T47.2X2	T47.2X3	T47.2X4	T47.2X5	T47.2X6
Cassava	T62.2X1	T62.2X2	T62.2X3	T62.2X4	—	—
Castellani's paint	T49.0X1	T49.0X2	T49.0X3	T49.0X4	T49.0X5	T49.0X6
Castor						
bean	T62.2X1	T62.2X2	T62.2X3	T62.2X4	—	—
oil	T47.2X1	T47.2X2	T47.2X3	T47.2X4	T47.2X5	T47.2X6
Catalase	T45.3X1	T45.3X2	T45.3X3	T45.3X4	T45.3X5	T45.3X6
Caterpillar (sting)	T63.431	T63.432	T63.433	T63.434	—	—
Catha (edulis) (tea)	T43.691	T43.692	T43.693	T43.694	—	—
Cathartic NEC	T47.4X1	T47.4X2	T47.4X3	T47.4X4	T47.4X5	T47.4X6
anthacene derivative	T47.2X1	T47.2X2	T47.2X3	T47.2X4	T47.2X5	T47.2X6
bulk	T47.4X1	T47.4X2	T47.4X3	T47.4X4	T47.4X5	T47.4X6
contact	T47.2X1	T47.2X2	T47.2X3	T47.2X4	T47.2X5	T47.2X6
emollient NEC	T47.4X1	T47.4X2	T47.4X3	T47.4X4	T47.4X5	T47.4X6
irritant NEC	T47.2X1	T47.2X2	T47.2X3	T47.2X4	T47.2X5	T47.2X6
mucilage	T47.4X1	T47.4X2	T47.4X3	T47.4X4	T47.4X5	T47.4X6
saline	T47.3X1	T47.3X2	T47.3X3	T47.3X4	T47.3X5	T47.3X6
vegetable	T47.2X1	T47.2X2	T47.2X3	T47.2X4	T47.2X5	T47.2X6
Cathine	T50.5X1	T50.5X2	T50.5X3	T50.5X4	T50.5X5	T50.5X6
Cathomycin	T36.8X1	T36.8X2	T36.8X3	T36.8X4	T36.8X5	T36.8X6
Cation exchange resin	T50.3X1	T50.3X2	T50.3X3	T50.3X4	T50.3X5	T50.3X6
Caustic(s) NEC	T54.91	T54.92	T54.93	T54.94	—	—
alkali	T54.3X1	T54.3X2	T54.3X3	T54.3X4	—	—
hydroxide	T54.3X1	T54.3X2	T54.3X3	T54.3X4	—	—
potash	T54.3X1	T54.3X2	T54.3X3	T54.3X4	—	—
soda	T54.3X1	T54.3X2	T54.3X3	T54.3X4	—	—

Substance	Poisoning, Accidental (unintentional)	Poisoning, Intentional Self-harm	Poisoning, Assault	Poisoning, Undetermined	Adverse Effect	Under-dosing
Caustic(s) NEC — continued						
specified NEC	T54.91	T54.92	T54.93	T54.94	—	—
Ceepryn	T49.0X1	T49.0X2	T49.0X3	T49.0X4	T49.0X5	T49.0X6
ENT agent	T49.6X1	T49.6X2	T49.6X3	T49.6X4	T49.6X5	T49.6X6
lozenges	T49.6X1	T49.6X2	T49.6X3	T49.6X4	T49.6X5	T49.6X6
Cefacetrile	T36.1X1	T36.1X2	T36.1X3	T36.1X4	T36.1X5	T36.1X6
Cefaclor	T36.1X1	T36.1X2	T36.1X3	T36.1X4	T36.1X5	T36.1X6
Cefadroxil	T36.1X1	T36.1X2	T36.1X3	T36.1X4	T36.1X5	T36.1X6
Cefalexin	T36.1X1	T36.1X2	T36.1X3	T36.1X4	T36.1X5	T36.1X6
Cefaloglycin	T36.1X1	T36.1X2	T36.1X3	T36.1X4	T36.1X5	T36.1X6
Cefaloridine	T36.1X1	T36.1X2	T36.1X3	T36.1X4	T36.1X5	T36.1X6
Cefalosporins	T36.1X1	T36.1X2	T36.1X3	T36.1X4	T36.1X5	T36.1X6
Cefalotin	T36.1X1	T36.1X2	T36.1X3	T36.1X4	T36.1X5	T36.1X6
Cefamandole	T36.1X1	T36.1X2	T36.1X3	T36.1X4	T36.1X5	T36.1X6
Cefamycin antibiotic	T36.1X1	T36.1X2	T36.1X3	T36.1X4	T36.1X5	T36.1X6
Cefapirin	T36.1X1	T36.1X2	T36.1X3	T36.1X4	T36.1X5	T36.1X6
Cefatrizine	T36.1X1	T36.1X2	T36.1X3	T36.1X4	T36.1X5	T36.1X6
Cefazedone	T36.1X1	T36.1X2	T36.1X3	T36.1X4	T36.1X5	T36.1X6
Cefazolin	T36.1X1	T36.1X2	T36.1X3	T36.1X4	T36.1X5	T36.1X6
Cefbuperazone	T36.1X1	T36.1X2	T36.1X3	T36.1X4	T36.1X5	T36.1X6
Cefetamet	T36.1X1	T36.1X2	T36.1X3	T36.1X4	T36.1X5	T36.1X6
Cefixime	T36.1X1	T36.1X2	T36.1X3	T36.1X4	T36.1X5	T36.1X6
Cefmenoxime	T36.1X1	T36.1X2	T36.1X3	T36.1X4	T36.1X5	T36.1X6
Cefmetazole	T36.1X1	T36.1X2	T36.1X3	T36.1X4	T36.1X5	T36.1X6
Cefminox	T36.1X1	T36.1X2	T36.1X3	T36.1X4	T36.1X5	T36.1X6
Cefonicid	T36.1X1	T36.1X2	T36.1X3	T36.1X4	T36.1X5	T36.1X6
Cefoperazone	T36.1X1	T36.1X2	T36.1X3	T36.1X4	T36.1X5	T36.1X6
Ceforanide	T36.1X1	T36.1X2	T36.1X3	T36.1X4	T36.1X5	T36.1X6
Cefotaxime	T36.1X1	T36.1X2	T36.1X3	T36.1X4	T36.1X5	T36.1X6
Cefotetan	T36.1X1	T36.1X2	T36.1X3	T36.1X4	T36.1X5	T36.1X6
Cefotiam	T36.1X1	T36.1X2	T36.1X3	T36.1X4	T36.1X5	T36.1X6
Cefoxitin	T36.1X1	T36.1X2	T36.1X3	T36.1X4	T36.1X5	T36.1X6
Cefpimizole	T36.1X1	T36.1X2	T36.1X3	T36.1X4	T36.1X5	T36.1X6
Cefpiramide	T36.1X1	T36.1X2	T36.1X3	T36.1X4	T36.1X5	T36.1X6
Cefradine	T36.1X1	T36.1X2	T36.1X3	T36.1X4	T36.1X5	T36.1X6
Cefroxadine	T36.1X1	T36.1X2	T36.1X3	T36.1X4	T36.1X5	T36.1X6
Cefsulodin	T36.1X1	T36.1X2	T36.1X3	T36.1X4	T36.1X5	T36.1X6
Ceftazidime	T36.1X1	T36.1X2	T36.1X3	T36.1X4	T36.1X5	T36.1X6
Cefteram	T36.1X1	T36.1X2	T36.1X3	T36.1X4	T36.1X5	T36.1X6
Ceftezole	T36.1X1	T36.1X2	T36.1X3	T36.1X4	T36.1X5	T36.1X6
Ceftizoxime	T36.1X1	T36.1X2	T36.1X3	T36.1X4	T36.1X5	T36.1X6
Ceftriaxone	T36.1X1	T36.1X2	T36.1X3	T36.1X4	T36.1X5	T36.1X6
Cefuroxime	T36.1X1	T36.1X2	T36.1X3	T36.1X4	T36.1X5	T36.1X6
Cefuzonam	T36.1X1	T36.1X2	T36.1X3	T36.1X4	T36.1X5	T36.1X6
Celestone	T38.0X1	T38.0X2	T38.0X3	T38.0X4	T38.0X5	T38.0X6
topical	T49.0X1	T49.0X2	T49.0X3	T49.0X4	T49.0X5	T49.0X6
Celiprolol	T44.7X1	T44.7X2	T44.7X3	T44.7X4	T44.7X5	T44.7X6
Cellosolve	T52.91	T52.92	T52.93	T52.94	—	—
Cell stimulants and proliferants	T49.8X1	T49.8X2	T49.8X3	T49.8X4	T49.8X5	T49.8X6
Cellulose						
cathartic	T47.4X1	T47.4X2	T47.4X3	T47.4X4	T47.4X5	T47.4X6
hydroxyethyl	T47.4X1	T47.4X2	T47.4X3	T47.4X4	T47.4X5	T47.4X6
nitrates (topical)	T49.3X1	T49.3X2	T49.3X3	T49.3X4	T49.3X5	T49.3X6
oxidized	T49.4X1	T49.4X2	T49.4X3	T49.4X4	T49.4X5	T49.4X6
Centipede (bite)	T63.411	T63.412	T63.413	T63.414	—	—
Central nervous system						
depressants	T42.71	T42.72	T42.73	T42.74	T42.75	T42.76
anesthetic (general) NEC	T41.201	T41.202	T41.203	T41.204	T41.205	T41.206
gases NEC	T41.0X1	T41.0X2	T41.0X3	T41.0X4	T41.0X5	T41.0X6
intravenous	T41.1X1	T41.1X2	T41.1X3	T41.1X4	T41.1X5	T41.1X6
barbiturates	T42.3X1	T42.3X2	T42.3X3	T42.3X4	T42.3X5	T42.3X6
benzodiazepines	T42.4X1	T42.4X2	T42.4X3	T42.4X4	T42.4X5	T42.4X6
bromides	T42.6X1	T42.6X2	T42.6X3	T42.6X4	T42.6X5	T42.6X6
cannabis sativa	T40.7X1	T40.7X2	T40.7X3	T40.7X4	T40.7X5	T40.7X6
chloral hydrate	T42.6X1	T42.6X2	T42.6X3	T42.6X4	T42.6X5	T42.6X6
ethanol	T51.0X1	T51.0X2	T51.0X3	T51.0X4	—	—
hallucinogenics	T40.901	T40.902	T40.903	T40.904	T40.905	T40.906
hypnotics	T42.71	T42.72	T42.73	T42.74	T42.75	T42.76
specified NEC	T42.6X1	T42.6X2	T42.6X3	T42.6X4	T42.6X5	T42.6X6
muscle relaxants	T42.8X1	T42.8X2	T42.8X3	T42.8X4	T42.8X5	T42.8X6
paraldehyde	T42.6X1	T42.6X2	T42.6X3	T42.6X4	T42.6X5	T42.6X6
sedatives; sedative-hypnotics	T42.71	T42.72	T42.73	T42.74	T42.75	T42.76
mixed NEC	T42.6X1	T42.6X2	T42.6X3	T42.6X4	T42.6X5	T42.6X6
specified NEC	T42.6X1	T42.6X2	T42.6X3	T42.6X4	T42.6X5	T42.6X6
muscle-tone depressants	T42.8X1	T42.8X2	T42.8X3	T42.8X4	T42.8X5	T42.8X6
stimulants	T43.601	T43.602	T43.603	T43.604	T43.605	T43.606
amphetamines	T43.621	T43.622	T43.623	T43.624	T43.625	T43.626
analeptics	T50.7X1	T50.7X2	T50.7X3	T50.7X4	T50.7X5	T50.7X6
antidepressants	T43.201	T43.202	T43.203	T43.204	T43.205	T43.206
opiate antagonists	T50.7X1	T50.7X2	T50.7X3	T50.7X4	T50.7X5	T50.7X6
specified NEC	T43.691	T43.692	T43.693	T43.694	T43.695	T43.696

Substance	Poisoning, Accidental (unintentional)	Poisoning, Intentional Self-harm	Poisoning, Assault	Poisoning, Undetermined	Adverse Effect	Under-dosing
Cephalexin	T36.1X1	T36.1X2	T36.1X3	T36.1X4	T36.1X5	T36.1X6
Cephaloglycin	T36.1X1	T36.1X2	T36.1X3	T36.1X4	T36.1X5	T36.1X6
Cephaloridine	T36.1X1	T36.1X2	T36.1X3	T36.1X4	T36.1X5	T36.1X6
Cephalosporins	T36.1X1	T36.1X2	T36.1X3	T36.1X4	T36.1X5	T36.1X6
N (adicillin)	T36.0X1	T36.0X2	T36.0X3	T36.0X4	T36.0X5	T36.0X6
Cephalothin	T36.1X1	T36.1X2	T36.1X3	T36.1X4	T36.1X5	T36.1X6
Cephalotin	T36.1X1	T36.1X2	T36.1X3	T36.1X4	T36.1X5	T36.1X6
Cephradine	T36.1X1	T36.1X2	T36.1X3	T36.1X4	T36.1X5	T36.1X6
Cerbera (odallam)	T62.2X1	T62.2X2	T62.2X3	T62.2X4	—	—
Cerberin	T46.0X1	T46.0X2	T46.0X3	T46.0X4	T46.0X5	T46.0X6
Cerebral stimulants	T43.601	T43.602	T43.603	T43.604	T43.605	T43.606
psychotherapeutic	T43.601	T43.602	T43.603	T43.604	T43.605	T43.606
specified NEC	T43.691	T43.692	T43.693	T43.694	T43.695	T43.696
Cerium oxalate	T45.0X1	T45.0X2	T45.0X3	T45.0X4	T45.0X5	T45.0X6
Cerous oxalate	T45.0X1	T45.0X2	T45.0X3	T45.0X4	T45.0X5	T45.0X6
Ceruletide	T50.8X1	T50.8X2	T50.8X3	T50.8X4	T50.8X5	T50.8X6
Cetalkonium (chloride)	T49.0X1	T49.0X2	T49.0X3	T49.0X4	T49.0X5	T49.0X6
Cethexonium chloride	T49.0X1	T49.0X2	T49.0X3	T49.0X4	T49.0X5	T49.0X6
Cetiedil	T46.7X1	T46.7X2	T46.7X3	T46.7X4	T46.7X5	T46.7X6
Cetirizine	T45.0X1	T45.0X2	T45.0X3	T45.0X4	T45.0X5	T45.0X6
Cetomacrogol	T50.991	T50.992	T50.993	T50.994	T50.995	T50.996
Cetotiamine	T45.2X1	T45.2X2	T45.2X3	T45.2X4	T45.2X5	T45.2X6
Cetoxime	T45.0X1	T45.0X2	T45.0X3	T45.0X4	T45.0X5	T45.0X6
Cetraxate	T47.1X1	T47.1X2	T47.1X3	T47.1X4	T47.1X5	T47.1X6
Cetrimide	T49.0X1	T49.0X2	T49.0X3	T49.0X4	T49.0X5	T49.0X6
Cetrimonium (bromide)	T49.0X1	T49.0X2	T49.0X3	T49.0X4	T49.0X5	T49.0X6
Cetylpyridinium chloride	T49.0X1	T49.0X2	T49.0X3	T49.0X4	T49.0X5	T49.0X6
ENT agent	T49.6X1	T49.6X2	T49.6X3	T49.6X4	T49.6X5	T49.6X6
lozenges	T49.6X1	T49.6X2	T49.6X3	T49.6X4	T49.6X5	T49.6X6
Cevadilla — see Sabadilla						
Cevitamic acid	T45.2X1	T45.2X2	T45.2X3	T45.2X4	T45.2X5	T45.2X6
Chalk, precipitated	T47.1X1	T47.1X2	T47.1X3	T47.1X4	T47.1X5	T47.1X6
Chamomile	T49.0X1	T49.0X2	T49.0X3	T49.0X4	T49.0X5	T49.0X6
Ch'an su	T46.0X1	T46.0X2	T46.0X3	T46.0X4	T46.0X5	T46.0X6
Charcoal	T47.6X1	T47.6X2	T47.6X3	T47.6X4	T47.6X5	T47.6X6
activated — see also Charcoal, medicinal	T47.6X1	T47.6X2	T47.6X3	T47.6X4	T47.6X5	T47.6X6
fumes (Carbon monoxide)	T58.2X1	T58.2X2	T58.2X3	T58.2X4	—	—
industrial	T58.8X1	T58.8X2	T58.8X3	T58.8X4	—	—
medicinal (activated)	T47.6X1	T47.6X2	T47.6X3	T47.6X4	T47.6X5	T47.6X6
antidiarrheal	T47.6X1	T47.6X2	T47.6X3	T47.6X4	T47.6X5	T47.6X6
poison control	T47.8X1	T47.8X2	T47.8X3	T47.8X4	T47.8X5	T47.8X6
specified use other than for diarrhea	T47.8X1	T47.8X2	T47.8X3	T47.8X4	T47.8X5	T47.8X6
topical	T49.8X1	T49.8X2	T49.8X3	T49.8X4	T49.8X5	T49.8X6
Chaulmosulfone	T37.1X1	T37.1X2	T37.1X3	T37.1X4	T37.1X5	T37.1X6
Chelating agent NEC	T50.6X1	T50.6X2	T50.6X3	T50.6X4	T50.6X5	T50.6X6
Chelidonium majus	T62.2X1	T62.2X2	T62.2X3	T62.2X4	—	—
Chemical substance NEC	T65.91	T65.92	T65.93	T65.94	—	—
Chenodeoxycholic acid	T47.5X1	T47.5X2	T47.5X3	T47.5X4	T47.5X5	T47.5X6
Chenodiol	T47.5X1	T47.5X2	T47.5X3	T47.5X4	T47.5X5	T47.5X6
Chenopodium	T37.4X1	T37.4X2	T37.4X3	T37.4X4	T37.4X5	T37.4X6
Cherry laurel	T62.2X1	T62.2X2	T62.2X3	T62.2X4	—	—
Chinidin (e)	T46.2X1	T46.2X2	T46.2X3	T46.2X4	T46.2X5	T46.2X6
Chiniofon	T37.8X1	T37.8X2	T37.8X3	T37.8X4	T37.8X5	T37.8X6
Chlophedianol	T48.3X1	T48.3X2	T48.3X3	T48.3X4	T48.3X5	T48.3X6
Chloral	T42.6X1	T42.6X2	T42.6X3	T42.6X4	T42.6X5	T42.6X6
derivative	T42.6X1	T42.6X2	T42.6X3	T42.6X4	T42.6X5	T42.6X6
hydrate	T42.6X1	T42.6X2	T42.6X3	T42.6X4	T42.6X5	T42.6X6
Chloralamide	T42.6X1	T42.6X2	T42.6X3	T42.6X4	T42.6X5	T42.6X6
Chloralodol	T42.6X1	T42.6X2	T42.6X3	T42.6X4	T42.6X5	T42.6X6
Chloralose	T60.4X1	T60.4X2	T60.4X3	T60.4X4	—	—
Chlorambucil	T45.1X1	T45.1X2	T45.1X3	T45.1X4	T45.1X5	T45.1X6
Chloramine	T57.8X1	T57.8X2	T57.8X3	T57.8X4	—	—
T	T49.0X1	T49.0X2	T49.0X3	T49.0X4	T49.0X5	T49.0X6
topical	T49.0X1	T49.0X2	T49.0X3	T49.0X4	T49.0X5	T49.0X6
Chloramphenicol	T36.2X1	T36.2X2	T36.2X3	T36.2X4	T36.2X5	T36.2X6
ENT agent	T49.6X1	T49.6X2	T49.6X3	T49.6X4	T49.6X5	T49.6X6
ophthalmic preparation	T49.5X1	T49.5X2	T49.5X3	T49.5X4	T49.5X5	T49.5X6
topical NEC	T49.0X1	T49.0X2	T49.0X3	T49.0X4	T49.0X5	T49.0X6
Chlorate (potassium) (sodium) NEC	T60.3X1	T60.3X2	T60.3X3	T60.3X4	—	—
herbicide	T60.3X1	T60.3X2	T60.3X3	T60.3X4	—	—
Chlorazanil	T50.2X1	T50.2X2	T50.2X3	T50.2X4	T50.2X5	T50.2X6
Chlorbenzene, chlorbenzol	T53.7X1	T53.7X2	T53.7X3	T53.7X4	—	—
Chlorbenzoxamine	T44.3X1	T44.3X2	T44.3X3	T44.3X4	T44.3X5	T44.3X6
Chlorbutol	T42.6X1	T42.6X2	T42.6X3	T42.6X4	T42.6X5	T42.6X6
Chlorcyclizine	T45.0X1	T45.0X2	T45.0X3	T45.0X4	T45.0X5	T45.0X6
Chlordan (e) (dust)	T60.1X1	T60.1X2	T60.1X3	T60.1X4	—	—
Chlordantoin	T49.0X1	T49.0X2	T49.0X3	T49.0X4	T49.0X5	T49.0X6
Chlordiazepoxide	T42.4X1	T42.4X2	T42.4X3	T42.4X4	T42.4X5	T42.4X6
Chlordiethyl benzamide	T49.3X1	T49.3X2	T49.3X3	T49.3X4	T49.3X5	T49.3X6
Chloresium	T49.8X1	T49.8X2	T49.8X3	T49.8X4	T49.8X5	T49.8X6
Chlorethiazol	T42.6X1	T42.6X2	T42.6X3	T42.6X4	T42.6X5	T42.6X6
Chlorethyl — see Ethyl chloride						
Chloretone	T42.6X1	T42.6X2	T42.6X3	T42.6X4	T42.6X5	T42.6X6
Chlorex	T53.6X1	T53.6X2	T53.6X3	T53.6X4	—	—
insecticide	T60.1X1	T60.1X2	T60.1X3	T60.1X4	—	—
Chlorfenvinphos	T60.0X1	T60.0X2	T60.0X3	T60.0X4	—	—
Chlorhexadol	T42.6X1	T42.6X2	T42.6X3	T42.6X4	T42.6X5	T42.6X6
Chlorhexamide	T45.1X1	T45.1X2	T45.1X3	T45.1X4	T45.1X5	T45.1X6
Chlorhexidine	T49.0X1	T49.0X2	T49.0X3	T49.0X4	T49.0X5	T49.0X6
Chlorhydroxyquinolin	T49.0X1	T49.0X2	T49.0X3	T49.0X4	T49.0X5	T49.0X6
Chloride of lime (bleach)	T54.3X1	T54.3X2	T54.3X3	T54.3X4	—	—
Chlorimipramine	T43.011	T43.012	T43.013	T43.014	T43.015	T43.016
Chlorinated						
camphene	T53.6X1	T53.6X2	T53.6X3	T53.6X4	—	—
diphenyl	T53.7X1	T53.7X2	T53.7X3	T53.7X4	—	—
hydrocarbons NEC	T53.91	T53.92	T53.93	T53.94	—	—
solvents	T53.91	T53.92	T53.93	T53.94	—	—
lime (bleach)	T54.3X1	T54.3X2	T54.3X3	T54.3X4	—	—
and boric acid solution	T49.0X1	T49.0X2	T49.0X3	T49.0X4	T49.0X5	T49.0X6
naphthalene (insecticide)	T60.1X1	T60.1X2	T60.1X3	T60.1X4	—	—
industrial (non-pesticide)	T53.7X1	T53.7X2	T53.7X3	T53.7X4	—	—
pesticide NEC	T60.8X1	T60.8X2	T60.8X3	T60.8X4	—	—
soda — see also sodium hypochlorite						
solution	T49.0X1	T49.0X2	T49.0X3	T49.0X4	T49.0X5	T49.0X6
Chlorine (fumes) (gas)	T59.4X1	T59.4X2	T59.4X3	T59.4X4	—	—
bleach	T54.3X1	T54.3X2	T54.3X3	T54.3X4	—	—
compound gas NEC	T59.4X1	T59.4X2	T59.4X3	T59.4X4	—	—
disinfectant	T59.4X1	T59.4X2	T59.4X3	T59.4X4	—	—
releasing agents NEC	T59.4X1	T59.4X2	T59.4X3	T59.4X4	—	—
Chlorisondamine chloride	T46.991	T46.992	T46.993	T46.994	T46.995	T46.996
Chlormadinone	T38.5X1	T38.5X2	T38.5X3	T38.5X4	T38.5X5	T38.5X6
Chlormephos	T60.0X1	T60.0X2	T60.0X3	T60.0X4	—	—
Chlormerodrin	T50.2X1	T50.2X2	T50.2X3	T50.2X4	T50.2X5	T50.2X6
Chlormethiazole	T42.6X1	T42.6X2	T42.6X3	T42.6X4	T42.6X5	T42.6X6
Chlormethine	T45.1X1	T45.1X2	T45.1X3	T45.1X4	T45.1X5	T45.1X6
Chlormethylenecycline	T36.4X1	T36.4X2	T36.4X3	T36.4X4	T36.4X5	T36.4X6
Chlormezanone	T42.6X1	T42.6X2	T42.6X3	T42.6X4	T42.6X5	T42.6X6
Chloroacetic acid	T60.3X1	T60.3X2	T60.3X3	T60.3X4	—	—
Chloroacetone	T59.3X1	T59.3X2	T59.3X3	T59.3X4	—	—
Chloroacetophenone	T59.3X1	T59.3X2	T59.3X3	T59.3X4	—	—
Chloroaniline	T53.7X1	T53.7X2	T53.7X3	T53.7X4	—	—
Chlorobenzene, chlorobenzol	T53.7X1	T53.7X2	T53.7X3	T53.7X4	—	—
Chlorobromomethane (fire extinguisher)	T53.6X1	T53.6X2	T53.6X3	T53.6X4	—	—
Chlorobutanol	T49.0X1	T49.0X2	T49.0X3	T49.0X4	T49.0X5	T49.0X6
Chlorocresol	T49.0X1	T49.0X2	T49.0X3	T49.0X4	T49.0X5	T49.0X6
Chlorodehydromethyltestosterone	T38.7X1	T38.7X2	T38.7X3	T38.7X4	T38.7X5	T38.7X6
Chlorodinitrobenzene	T53.7X1	T53.7X2	T53.7X3	T53.7X4	—	—
dust or vapor	T53.7X1	T53.7X2	T53.7X3	T53.7X4	—	—
Chlorodiphenyl	T53.7X1	T53.7X2	T53.7X3	T53.7X4	—	—
Chloroethane — see Ethyl chloride						
Chloroethylene	T53.6X1	T53.6X2	T53.6X3	T53.6X4	—	—
Chlorofluorocarbons	T53.5X1	T53.5X2	T53.5X3	T53.5X4	—	—
Chloroform (fumes) (vapor)	T53.1X1	T53.1X2	T53.1X3	T53.1X4	—	—
anesthetic	T41.0X1	T41.0X2	T41.0X3	T41.0X4	—	—
solvent	T53.1X1	T53.1X2	T53.1X3	T53.1X4	—	—
water, concentrated	T41.0X1	T41.0X2	T41.0X3	T41.0X4	T41.0X5	T41.0X6
Chloroguanide	T37.2X1	T37.2X2	T37.2X3	T37.2X4	T37.2X5	T37.2X6
Chloromycetin	T36.2X1	T36.2X2	T36.2X3	T36.2X4	T36.2X5	T36.2X6
ENT agent	T49.6X1	T49.6X2	T49.6X3	T49.6X4	T49.6X5	T49.6X6
ophthalmic preparation	T49.5X1	T49.5X2	T49.5X3	T49.5X4	T49.5X5	T49.5X6
otic solution	T49.6X1	T49.6X2	T49.6X3	T49.6X4	T49.6X5	T49.6X6
topical NEC	T49.0X1	T49.0X2	T49.0X3	T49.0X4	T49.0X5	T49.0X6
Chloronitrobenzene	T53.7X1	T53.7X2	T53.7X3	T53.7X4	—	—
dust or vapor	T53.7X1	T53.7X2	T53.7X3	T53.7X4	—	—
Chlorophacinone	T60.4X1	T60.4X2	T60.4X3	T60.4X4	—	—
Chlorophenol	T53.7X1	T53.7X2	T53.7X3	T53.7X4	—	—
Chlorophenothane	T60.1X1	T60.1X2	T60.1X3	T60.1X4	—	—
Chlorophyll	T50.991	T50.992	T50.993	T50.994	T50.995	T50.996
Chloropicrin (fumes)	T53.6X1	T53.6X2	T53.6X3	T53.6X4	—	—
fumigant	T60.8X1	T60.8X2	T60.8X3	T60.8X4	—	—
fungicide	T60.3X1	T60.3X2	T60.3X3	T60.3X4	—	—
pesticide	T60.8X1	T60.8X2	T60.8X3	T60.8X4	—	—
Chloroprocaine	T41.3X1	T41.3X2	T41.3X3	T41.3X4	T41.3X5	T41.3X6
infiltration (subcutaneous)	T41.3X1	T41.3X2	T41.3X3	T41.3X4	T41.3X5	T41.3X6
nerve block (peripheral) (plexus)	T41.3X1	T41.3X2	T41.3X3	T41.3X4	T41.3X5	T41.3X6
spinal	T41.3X1	T41.3X2	T41.3X3	T41.3X4	T41.3X5	T41.3X6
Chloroptic	T49.5X1	T49.5X2	T49.5X3	T49.5X4	T49.5X5	T49.5X6
Chloropurine	T45.1X1	T45.1X2	T45.1X3	T45.1X4	T45.1X5	T45.1X6

Substance	Poisoning, Accidental (unintentional)	Poisoning, Intentional Self-harm	Poisoning, Assault	Poisoning, Undetermined	Adverse Effect	Under-dosing
Chloropyramine	T45.0X1	T45.0X2	T45.0X3	T45.0X4	T45.0X5	T45.0X6
Chloropyrifos	T60.0X1	T60.0X2	T60.0X3	T60.0X4	—	—
Chloropyrilene	T45.0X1	T45.0X2	T45.0X3	T45.0X4	T45.0X5	T45.0X6
Chloroquine	T37.2X1	T37.2X2	T37.2X3	T37.2X4	T37.2X5	T37.2X6
Chlorothalonil	T60.3X1	T60.3X2	T60.3X3	T60.3X4	—	—
Chlorothen	T45.0X1	T45.0X2	T45.0X3	T45.0X4	T45.0X5	T45.0X6
Chlorothiazide	T50.2X1	T50.2X2	T50.2X3	T50.2X4	T50.2X5	T50.2X6
Chlorothymol	T49.4X1	T49.4X2	T49.4X3	T49.4X4	T49.4X5	T49.4X6
Chlorotrianisene	T38.5X1	T38.5X2	T38.5X3	T38.5X4	T38.5X5	T38.5X6
Chlorovinyldichloroarsine, not in war	T57.0X1	T57.0X2	T57.0X3	T57.0X4	—	—
Chloroxine	T49.4X1	T49.4X2	T49.4X3	T49.4X4	T49.4X5	T49.4X6
Chloroxylenol	T49.0X1	T49.0X2	T49.0X3	T49.0X4	T49.0X5	T49.0X6
Chlorphenamine	T45.0X1	T45.0X2	T45.0X3	T45.0X4	T45.0X5	T45.0X6
Chlorphenesin	T42.8X1	T42.8X2	T42.8X3	T42.8X4	T42.8X5	T42.8X6
topical (antifungal)	T49.0X1	T49.0X2	T49.0X3	T49.0X4	T49.0X5	T49.0X6
Chlorpheniramine	T45.0X1	T45.0X2	T45.0X3	T45.0X4	T45.0X5	T45.0X6
Chlorphenoxamine	T45.0X1	T45.0X2	T45.0X3	T45.0X4	T45.0X5	T45.0X6
Chlorphentermine	T50.5X1	T50.5X2	T50.5X3	T50.5X4	T50.5X5	T50.5X6
Chlorprocaine — see Chloroprocaine						
Chlorproguanil	T37.2X1	T37.2X2	T37.2X3	T37.2X4	T37.2X5	T37.2X6
Chlorpromazine	T43.3X1	T43.3X2	T43.3X3	T43.3X4	T43.3X5	T43.3X6
Chlorpropamide	T38.3X1	T38.3X2	T38.3X3	T38.3X4	T38.3X5	T38.3X6
Chlorprothixene	T43.4X1	T43.4X2	T43.4X3	T43.4X4	T43.4X5	T43.4X6
Chlorquinaldol	T49.0X1	T49.0X2	T49.0X3	T49.0X4	T49.0X5	T49.0X6
Chlorquinol	T49.0X1	T49.0X2	T49.0X3	T49.0X4	T49.0X5	T49.0X6
Chlortalidone	T50.2X1	T50.2X2	T50.2X3	T50.2X4	T50.2X5	T50.2X6
Chlortetracycline	T36.4X1	T36.4X2	T36.4X3	T36.4X4	T36.4X5	T36.4X6
Chlorthalidone	T50.2X1	T50.2X2	T50.2X3	T50.2X4	T50.2X5	T50.2X6
Chlorthion	T60.0X1	T60.0X2	T60.0X3	T60.0X4	—	—
Chlorthiophos	T60.0X1	T60.0X2	T60.0X3	T60.0X4	—	—
Chlortrianisene	T38.5X1	T38.5X2	T38.5X3	T38.5X4	T38.5X5	T38.5X6
Chlor-Trimeton	T45.0X1	T45.0X2	T45.0X3	T45.0X4	T45.0X5	T45.0X6
Chlorzoxazone	T42.8X1	T42.8X2	T42.8X3	T42.8X4	T42.8X5	T42.8X6
Choke damp	T59.7X1	T59.7X2	T59.7X3	T59.7X4	—	—
Cholagogues	T47.5X1	T47.5X2	T47.5X3	T47.5X4	T47.5X5	T47.5X6
Cholebrine	T50.8X1	T50.8X2	T50.8X3	T50.8X4	T50.8X5	T50.8X6
Cholecalciferol	T45.2X1	T45.2X2	T45.2X3	T45.2X4	T45.2X5	T45.2X6
Cholecystokinin	T50.8X1	T50.8X2	T50.8X3	T50.8X4	T50.8X5	T50.8X6
Cholera vaccine	T50.A91	T50.A92	T50.A93	T50.A94	T50.A95	T50.A96
Choleretic	T47.5X1	T47.5X2	T47.5X3	T47.5X4	T47.5X5	T47.5X6
Cholesterol-lowering agents	T46.6X1	T46.6X2	T46.6X3	T46.6X4	T46.6X5	T46.6X6
Cholestyramine (resin)	T46.6X1	T46.6X2	T46.6X3	T46.6X4	T46.6X5	T46.6X6
Cholic acid	T47.5X1	T47.5X2	T47.5X3	T47.5X4	T47.5X5	T47.5X6
Choline	T48.6X1	T48.6X2	T48.6X3	T48.6X4	T48.6X5	T48.6X6
chloride	T50.991	T50.992	T50.993	T50.994	T50.995	T50.996
dihydrogen citrate	T50.991	T50.992	T50.993	T50.994	T50.995	T50.996
salicylate	T39.091	T39.092	T39.093	T39.094	T39.095	T39.096
theophyllinate	T48.6X1	T48.6X2	T48.6X3	T48.6X4	T48.6X5	T48.6X6
Cholinergic (drug) NEC	T44.1X1	T44.1X2	T44.1X3	T44.1X4	T44.1X5	T44.1X6
muscle tone enhancer	T44.1X1	T44.1X2	T44.1X3	T44.1X4	T44.1X5	T44.1X6
organophosphorus	T44.0X1	T44.0X2	T44.0X3	T44.0X4	T44.0X5	T44.0X6
insecticide	T60.0X1	T60.0X2	T60.0X3	T60.0X4	—	—
nerve gas	T59.891	T59.892	T59.893	T59.894	—	—
trimethyl ammonium propanediol	T44.1X1	T44.1X2	T44.1X3	T44.1X4	T44.1X5	T44.1X6
Cholinesterase reactivator	T50.6X1	T50.6X2	T50.6X3	T50.6X4	T50.6X5	T50.6X6
Cholografin	T50.8X1	T50.8X2	T50.8X3	T50.8X4	T50.8X5	T50.8X6
Chorionic gonadotropin	T38.891	T38.892	T38.893	T38.894	T38.895	T38.896
Chromate	T56.2X1	T56.2X2	T56.2X3	T56.2X4	—	—
dust or mist	T56.2X1	T56.2X2	T56.2X3	T56.2X4	—	—
lead — see also lead	T56.0X1	T56.0X2	T56.0X3	T56.0X4	—	—
paint	T56.0X1	T56.0X2	T56.0X3	T56.0X4	—	—
Chromic						
acid	T56.2X1	T56.2X2	T56.2X3	T56.2X4	—	—
dust or mist	T56.2X1	T56.2X2	T56.2X3	T56.2X4	—	—
phosphate 32P	T45.1X1	T45.1X2	T45.1X3	T45.1X4	T45.1X5	T45.1X6
Chromium	T56.2X1	T56.2X2	T56.2X3	T56.2X4	—	—
compounds — see Chromate						
sesquioxide	T50.8X1	T50.8X2	T50.8X3	T50.8X4	T50.8X5	T50.8X6
Chromomycin A3	T45.1X1	T45.1X2	T45.1X3	T45.1X4	T45.1X5	T45.1X6
Chromonar	T46.3X1	T46.3X2	T46.3X3	T46.3X4	T46.3X5	T46.3X6
Chromyl chloride	T56.2X1	T56.2X2	T56.2X3	T56.2X4	—	—
Chrysarobin	T49.4X1	T49.4X2	T49.4X3	T49.4X4	T49.4X5	T49.4X6
Chrysazin	T47.2X1	T47.2X2	T47.2X3	T47.2X4	T47.2X5	T47.2X6
Chymar	T45.3X1	T45.3X2	T45.3X3	T45.3X4	T45.3X5	T45.3X6
ophthalmic preparation	T49.5X1	T49.5X2	T49.5X3	T49.5X4	T49.5X5	T49.5X6
Chymopapain	T45.3X1	T45.3X2	T45.3X3	T45.3X4	T45.3X5	T45.3X6
Chymotrypsin	T45.3X1	T45.3X2	T45.3X3	T45.3X4	T45.3X5	T45.3X6
ophthalmic preparation	T49.5X1	T49.5X2	T49.5X3	T49.5X4	T49.5X5	T49.5X6
Cianidanol	T50.991	T50.992	T50.993	T50.994	T50.995	T50.996

Substance	Poisoning, Accidental (unintentional)	Poisoning, Intentional Self-harm	Poisoning, Assault	Poisoning, Undetermined	Adverse Effect	Under-dosing
Cianopramine	T43.011	T43.012	T43.013	T43.014	T43.015	T43.016
Cibenzoline	T46.2X1	T46.2X2	T46.2X3	T46.2X4	T46.2X5	T46.2X6
Ciclacillin	T36.0X1	T36.0X2	T36.0X3	T36.0X4	T36.0X5	T36.0X6
Ciclobarbital — see Hexobarbital						
Ciclonicate	T46.7X1	T46.7X2	T46.7X3	T46.7X4	T46.7X5	T46.7X6
Ciclopirox (olamine)	T49.0X1	T49.0X2	T49.0X3	T49.0X4	T49.0X5	T49.0X6
Ciclosporin	T45.1X1	T45.1X2	T45.1X3	T45.1X4	T45.1X5	T45.1X6
Cicuta maculata or virosa	T62.2X1	T62.2X2	T62.2X3	T62.2X4	—	—
Cicutoxin	T62.2X1	T62.2X2	T62.2X3	T62.2X4	—	—
Cigarette lighter fluid	T52.0X1	T52.0X2	T52.0X3	T52.0X4	—	—
Cigarettes (tobacco)	T65.221	T65.222	T65.223	T65.224	—	—
Ciguatoxin	T61.01	T61.02	T61.03	T61.04	—	—
Cilazapril	T46.4X1	T46.4X2	T46.4X3	T46.4X4	T46.4X5	T46.4X6
Cimetidine	T47.0X1	T47.0X2	T47.0X3	T47.0X4	T47.0X5	T47.0X6
Cimetropium bromide	T44.3X1	T44.3X2	T44.3X3	T44.3X4	T44.3X5	T44.3X6
Cinchocaine	T41.3X1	T41.3X2	T41.3X3	T41.3X4	T41.3X5	T41.3X6
topical (surface)	T41.3X1	T41.3X2	T41.3X3	T41.3X4	T41.3X5	T41.3X6
Cinchona	T37.2X1	T37.2X2	T37.2X3	T37.2X4	T37.2X5	T37.2X6
Cinchonine alkaloids	T37.2X1	T37.2X2	T37.2X3	T37.2X4	T37.2X5	T37.2X6
Cinchophen	T50.4X1	T50.4X2	T50.4X3	T50.4X4	T50.4X5	T50.4X6
Cinepazide	T46.7X1	T46.7X2	T46.7X3	T46.7X4	T46.7X5	T46.7X6
Cinnamedrine	T48.5X1	T48.5X2	T48.5X3	T48.5X4	T48.5X5	T48.5X6
Cinnarizine	T45.0X1	T45.0X2	T45.0X3	T45.0X4	T45.0X5	T45.0X6
Cinoxacin	T37.8X1	T37.8X2	T37.8X3	T37.8X4	T37.8X5	T37.8X6
Ciprofibrate	T46.6X1	T46.6X2	T46.6X3	T46.6X4	T46.6X5	T46.6X6
Ciprofloxacin	T36.8X1	T36.8X2	T36.8X3	T36.8X4	T36.8X5	T36.8X6
Cisapride	T47.8X1	T47.8X2	T47.8X3	T47.8X4	T47.8X5	T47.8X6
Cisplatin	T45.1X1	T45.1X2	T45.1X3	T45.1X4	T45.1X5	T45.1X6
Citalopram	T43.221	T43.222	T43.223	T43.224	T43.225	T43.226
Citanest	T41.3X1	T41.3X2	T41.3X3	T41.3X4	T41.3X5	T41.3X6
infiltration (subcutaneous)	T41.3X1	T41.3X2	T41.3X3	T41.3X4	T41.3X5	T41.3X6
nerve block (peripheral) (plexus)	T41.3X1	T41.3X2	T41.3X3	T41.3X4	T41.3X5	T41.3X6
Citric acid	T47.5X1	T47.5X2	T47.5X3	T47.5X4	T47.5X5	T47.5X6
Citrovorum (factor)	T45.8X1	T45.8X2	T45.8X3	T45.8X4	T45.8X5	T45.8X6
Claviceps purpurea	T62.2X1	T62.2X2	T62.2X3	T62.2X4	—	—
Clavulanic acid	T36.1X1	T36.1X2	T36.1X3	T36.1X4	T36.1X5	T36.1X6
Cleaner, cleansing agent, type not specified	T65.891	T65.892	T65.893	T65.894	—	—
of paint or varnish	T52.91	T52.92	T52.93	T52.94	—	—
specified type NEC	T65.891	T65.892	T65.893	T65.894	—	—
Clebopride	T47.8X1	T47.8X2	T47.8X3	T47.8X4	T47.8X5	T47.8X6
Clefamide	T37.3X1	T37.3X2	T37.3X3	T37.3X4	T37.3X5	T37.3X6
Clemastine	T45.0X1	T45.0X2	T45.0X3	T45.0X4	T45.0X5	T45.0X6
Clematis vitalba	T62.2X1	T62.2X2	T62.2X3	T62.2X4	—	—
Clemizole	T45.0X1	T45.0X2	T45.0X3	T45.0X4	T45.0X5	T45.0X6
penicillin	T36.0X1	T36.0X2	T36.0X3	T36.0X4	T36.0X5	T36.0X6
Clenbuterol	T48.6X1	T48.6X2	T48.6X3	T48.6X4	T48.6X5	T48.6X6
Clidinium bromide	T44.3X1	T44.3X2	T44.3X3	T44.3X4	T44.3X5	T44.3X6
Clindamycin	T36.8X1	T36.8X2	T36.8X3	T36.8X4	T36.8X5	T36.8X6
Clinofibrate	T46.6X1	T46.6X2	T46.6X3	T46.6X4	T46.6X5	T46.6X6
Clioquinol	T37.8X1	T37.8X2	T37.8X3	T37.8X4	T37.8X5	T37.8X6
Cliradon	T40.2X1	T40.2X2	T40.2X3	T40.2X4	—	—
Clobazam	T42.4X1	T42.4X2	T42.4X3	T42.4X4	T42.4X5	T42.4X6
Clobenzorex	T50.5X1	T50.5X2	T50.5X3	T50.5X4	T50.5X5	T50.5X6
Clobetasol	T49.0X1	T49.0X2	T49.0X3	T49.0X4	T49.0X5	T49.0X6
Clobetasone	T49.0X1	T49.0X2	T49.0X3	T49.0X4	T49.0X5	T49.0X6
Clobutinol	T48.3X1	T48.3X2	T48.3X3	T48.3X4	T48.3X5	T48.3X6
Clocortolone	T38.0X1	T38.0X2	T38.0X3	T38.0X4	T38.0X5	T38.0X6
Clodantoin	T49.0X1	T49.0X2	T49.0X3	T49.0X4	T49.0X5	T49.0X6
Clodronic acid	T50.991	T50.992	T50.993	T50.994	T50.995	T50.996
Clofazimine	T37.1X1	T37.1X2	T37.1X3	T37.1X4	T37.1X5	T37.1X6
Clofedanol	T48.3X1	T48.3X2	T48.3X3	T48.3X4	T48.3X5	T48.3X6
Clofenamide	T50.2X1	T50.2X2	T50.2X3	T50.2X4	T50.2X5	T50.2X6
Clofenotane	T49.0X1	T49.0X2	T49.0X3	T49.0X4	T49.0X5	T49.0X6
Clofezone	T39.2X1	T39.2X2	T39.2X3	T39.2X4	T39.2X5	T39.2X6
Clofibrate	T46.6X1	T46.6X2	T46.6X3	T46.6X4	T46.6X5	T46.6X6
Clofibride	T46.6X1	T46.6X2	T46.6X3	T46.6X4	T46.6X5	T46.6X6
Cloforex	T50.5X1	T50.5X2	T50.5X3	T50.5X4	T50.5X5	T50.5X6
Clomethiazole	T42.6X1	T42.6X2	T42.6X3	T42.6X4	T42.6X5	T42.6X6
Clometocillin	T36.0X1	T36.0X2	T36.0X3	T36.0X4	T36.0X5	T36.0X6
Clomifene	T38.5X1	T38.5X2	T38.5X3	T38.5X4	T38.5X5	T38.5X6
Clomiphene	T38.5X1	T38.5X2	T38.5X3	T38.5X4	T38.5X5	T38.5X6
Clomipramine	T43.011	T43.012	T43.013	T43.014	T43.015	T43.016
Clomocycline	T36.4X1	T36.4X2	T36.4X3	T36.4X4	T36.4X5	T36.4X6
Clonazepam	T42.4X1	T42.4X2	T42.4X3	T42.4X4	T42.4X5	T42.4X6
Clonidine	T46.5X1	T46.5X2	T46.5X3	T46.5X4	T46.5X5	T46.5X6
Clonixin	T39.8X1	T39.8X2	T39.8X3	T39.8X4	T39.8X5	T39.8X6
Clopamide	T50.2X1	T50.2X2	T50.2X3	T50.2X4	T50.2X5	T50.2X6
Clopenthixol	T43.4X1	T43.4X2	T43.4X3	T43.4X4	T43.4X5	T43.4X6
Cloperastine	T48.3X1	T48.3X2	T48.3X3	T48.3X4	T48.3X5	T48.3X6
Clophedianol	T48.3X1	T48.3X2	T48.3X3	T48.3X4	T48.3X5	T48.3X6
Cloponone	T36.2X1	T36.2X2	T36.2X3	T36.2X4	T36.2X5	T36.2X6

Additional Character May Be Required — Refer to the Tabular List for Character Selection ▽ **Subterms under main terms may continue to next column or page**

Substance	Poisoning, Accidental (unintentional)	Poisoning, Intentional Self-harm	Poisoning, Assault	Poisoning, Undetermined	Adverse Effect	Under-dosing
Cloprednol	T38.0X1	T38.0X2	T38.0X3	T38.0X4	T38.0X5	T38.0X6
Cloral betaine	T42.6X1	T42.6X2	T42.6X3	T42.6X4	T42.6X5	T42.6X6
Cloramfenicol	T36.2X1	T36.2X2	T36.2X3	T36.2X4	T36.2X5	T36.2X6
Clorazepate (dipotassium)	T42.4X1	T42.4X2	T42.4X3	T42.4X4	T42.4X5	T42.4X6
Clorexolone	T50.2X1	T50.2X2	T50.2X3	T50.2X4	T50.2X5	T50.2X6
Clorfenamine	T45.0X1	T45.0X2	T45.0X3	T45.0X4	T45.0X5	T45.0X6
Clorgiline	T43.1X1	T43.1X2	T43.1X3	T43.1X4	T43.1X5	T43.1X6
Clorotepine	T44.3X1	T44.3X2	T44.3X3	T44.3X4	T44.3X5	T44.3X6
Clorox (bleach)	T54.91	T54.92	T54.93	T54.94	—	—
Clorprenaline	T48.6X1	T48.6X2	T48.6X3	T48.6X4	T48.6X5	T48.6X6
Clortermine	T50.5X1	T50.5X2	T50.5X3	T50.5X4	T50.5X5	T50.5X6
Clotiapine	T43.591	T43.592	T43.593	T43.594	T43.595	T43.596
Clotiazepam	T42.4X1	T42.4X2	T42.4X3	T42.4X4	T42.4X5	T42.4X6
Clotibric acid	T46.6X1	T46.6X2	T46.6X3	T46.6X4	T46.6X5	T46.6X6
Clotrimazole	T49.0X1	T49.0X2	T49.0X3	T49.0X4	T49.0X5	T49.0X6
Cloxacillin	T36.0X1	T36.0X2	T36.0X3	T36.0X4	T36.0X5	T36.0X6
Cloxazolam	T42.4X1	T42.4X2	T42.4X3	T42.4X4	T42.4X5	T42.4X6
Cloxiquine	T49.0X1	T49.0X2	T49.0X3	T49.0X4	T49.0X5	T49.0X6
Clozapine	T42.4X1	T42.4X2	T42.4X3	T42.4X4	T42.4X5	T42.4X6
Coagulant NEC	T45.7X1	T45.7X2	T45.7X3	T45.7X4	T45.7X5	T45.7X6
Coal (carbon monoxide from) — see also Carbon, monoxide, coal	T58.2X1	T58.2X2	T58.2X3	T58.2X4	—	—
oil — see Kerosene						
tar	T49.1X1	T49.1X2	T49.1X3	T49.1X4	T49.1X5	T49.1X6
fumes	T59.891	T59.892	T59.893	T59.894	—	—
medicinal (ointment)	T49.4X1	T49.4X2	T49.4X3	T49.4X4	T49.4X5	T49.4X6
analgesics NEC	T39.2X1	T39.2X2	T39.2X3	T39.2X4	T39.2X5	T39.2X6
naphtha (solvent)	T52.0X1	T52.0X2	T52.0X3	T52.0X4	—	—
Cobalamine	T45.2X1	T45.2X2	T45.2X3	T45.2X4	T45.2X5	T45.2X6
Cobalt (nonmedicinal) (fumes) (industrial)	T56.891	T56.892	T56.893	T56.894	—	—
medicinal (trace) (chloride)	T45.8X1	T45.8X2	T45.8X3	T45.8X4	T45.8X5	T45.8X6
Cobra (venom)	T63.041	T63.042	T63.043	T63.044	—	—
Coca (leaf)	T40.5X1	T40.5X2	T40.5X3	T40.5X4	T40.5X5	T40.5X6
Cocaine	T40.5X1	T40.5X2	T40.5X3	T40.5X4	T40.5X5	T40.5X6
topical anesthetic	T41.3X1	T41.3X2	T41.3X3	T41.3X4	T41.3X5	T41.3X6
Cocarboxylase	T45.3X1	T45.3X2	T45.3X3	T45.3X4	T45.3X5	T45.3X6
Coccidioidin	T50.8X1	T50.8X2	T50.8X3	T50.8X4	T50.8X5	T50.8X6
Cocculus indicus	T62.1X1	T62.1X2	T62.1X3	T62.1X4	—	—
Cochineal	T65.6X1	T65.6X2	T65.6X3	T65.6X4	—	—
medicinal products	T50.991	T50.992	T50.993	T50.994	T50.995	T50.996
Codeine	T40.2X1	T40.2X2	T40.2X3	T40.2X4	T40.2X5	T40.2X6
Cod-liver oil	T45.2X1	T45.2X2	T45.2X3	T45.2X4	T45.2X5	T45.2X6
Coenzyme A	T50.991	T50.992	T50.993	T50.994	T50.995	T50.996
Coffee	T62.8X1	T62.8X2	T62.8X3	T62.8X4	—	—
Cogalactoisomerase	T50.991	T50.992	T50.993	T50.994	T50.995	T50.996
Cogentin	T44.3X1	T44.3X2	T44.3X3	T44.3X4	T44.3X5	T44.3X6
Coke fumes or gas (carbon monoxide)	T58.2X1	T58.2X2	T58.2X3	T58.2X4	—	—
industrial use	T58.8X1	T58.8X2	T58.8X3	T58.8X4	—	—
Colace	T47.4X1	T47.4X2	T47.4X3	T47.4X4	T47.4X5	T47.4X6
Colaspase	T45.1X1	T45.1X2	T45.1X3	T45.1X4	T45.1X5	T45.1X6
Colchicine	T50.4X1	T50.4X2	T50.4X3	T50.4X4	T50.4X5	T50.4X6
Colchicum	T62.2X1	T62.2X2	T62.2X3	T62.2X4	—	—
Cold cream	T49.3X1	T49.3X2	T49.3X3	T49.3X4	T49.3X5	T49.3X6
Colecalciferol	T45.2X1	T45.2X2	T45.2X3	T45.2X4	T45.2X5	T45.2X6
Colestipol	T46.6X1	T46.6X2	T46.6X3	T46.6X4	T46.6X5	T46.6X6
Colestyramine	T46.6X1	T46.6X2	T46.6X3	T46.6X4	T46.6X5	T46.6X6
Colimycin	T36.8X1	T36.8X2	T36.8X3	T36.8X4	T36.8X5	T36.8X6
Colistimethate	T36.8X1	T36.8X2	T36.8X3	T36.8X4	T36.8X5	T36.8X6
Colistin	T36.8X1	T36.8X2	T36.8X3	T36.8X4	T36.8X5	T36.8X6
sulfate (eye preparation)	T49.5X1	T49.5X2	T49.5X3	T49.5X4	T49.5X5	T49.5X6
Collagen	T50.991	T50.992	T50.993	T50.994	T50.995	T50.996
Collagenase	T49.4X1	T49.4X2	T49.4X3	T49.4X4	T49.4X5	T49.4X6
Collodion	T49.3X1	T49.3X2	T49.3X3	T49.3X4	T49.3X5	T49.3X6
Colocynth	T47.2X1	T47.2X2	T47.2X3	T47.2X4	T47.2X5	T47.2X6
Colophony adhesive	T49.3X1	T49.3X2	T49.3X3	T49.3X4	T49.3X5	T49.3X6
Colorant — see also Dye	T50.991	T50.992	T50.993	T50.994	T50.995	T50.996
Coloring matter — see Dye(s)						
Combustion gas (after combustion) — see Carbon, monoxide						
prior to combustion	T59.891	T59.892	T59.893	T59.894	—	—
Compazine	T43.3X1	T43.3X2	T43.3X3	T43.3X4	T43.3X5	T43.3X6
Compound						
42 (warfarin)	T60.4X1	T60.4X2	T60.4X3	T60.4X4	—	—
269 (endrin)	T60.1X1	T60.1X2	T60.1X3	T60.1X4	—	—
497 (dieldrin)	T60.1X1	T60.1X2	T60.1X3	T60.1X4	—	—
1080 (sodium fluoroacetate)	T60.4X1	T60.4X2	T60.4X3	T60.4X4	—	—
3422 (parathion)	T60.0X1	T60.0X2	T60.0X3	T60.0X4	—	—
3911 (phorate)	T60.0X1	T60.0X2	T60.0X3	T60.0X4	—	—
Compound — continued						
3956 (toxaphene)	T60.1X1	T60.1X2	T60.1X3	T60.1X4	—	—
4049 (malathion)	T60.0X1	T60.0X2	T60.0X3	T60.0X4	—	—
4069 (malathion)	T60.0X1	T60.0X2	T60.0X3	T60.0X4	—	—
4124 (dicapthon)	T60.0X1	T60.0X2	T60.0X3	T60.0X4	—	—
E (cortisone)	T38.0X1	T38.0X2	T38.0X3	T38.0X4	T38.0X5	T38.0X6
F (hydrocortisone)	T38.0X1	T38.0X2	T38.0X3	T38.0X4	T38.0X5	T38.0X6
Congener, anabolic	T38.7X1	T38.7X2	T38.7X3	T38.7X4	T38.7X5	T38.7X6
Congo red	T50.8X1	T50.8X2	T50.8X3	T50.8X4	T50.8X5	T50.8X6
Coniine, conine	T62.2X1	T62.2X2	T62.2X3	T62.2X4	—	—
Conium (maculatum)	T62.2X1	T62.2X2	T62.2X3	T62.2X4	—	—
Conjugated estrogenic substances	T38.5X1	T38.5X2	T38.5X3	T38.5X4	T38.5X5	T38.5X6
Contac	T48.5X1	T48.5X2	T48.5X3	T48.5X4	T48.5X5	T48.5X6
Contact lens solution	T49.5X1	T49.5X2	T49.5X3	T49.5X4	T49.5X5	T49.5X6
Contraceptive (oral)	T38.4X1	T38.4X2	T38.4X3	T38.4X4	T38.4X5	T38.4X6
vaginal	T49.8X1	T49.8X2	T49.8X3	T49.8X4	T49.8X5	T49.8X6
Contrast medium, radiography	T50.8X1	T50.8X2	T50.8X3	T50.8X4	T50.8X5	T50.8X6
Convallaria glycosides	T46.0X1	T46.0X2	T46.0X3	T46.0X4	T46.0X5	T46.0X6
Convallaria majalis	T62.2X1	T62.2X2	T62.2X3	T62.2X4	—	—
berry	T62.1X1	T62.1X2	T62.1X3	T62.1X4	—	—
Copperhead snake (bite) (venom)	T63.061	T63.062	T63.063	T63.064	—	—
Copper (dust) (fumes) (nonmedicinal) NEC	T56.4X1	T56.4X2	T56.4X3	T56.4X4	—	—
arsenate, arsenite	T57.0X1	T57.0X2	T57.0X3	T57.0X4	—	—
insecticide	T60.2X1	T60.2X2	T60.2X3	T60.2X4	—	—
emetic	T47.7X1	T47.7X2	T47.7X3	T47.7X4	T47.7X5	T47.7X6
fungicide	T60.3X1	T60.3X2	T60.3X3	T60.3X4	—	—
gluconate	T49.0X1	T49.0X2	T49.0X3	T49.0X4	T49.0X5	T49.0X6
insecticide	T60.2X1	T60.2X2	T60.2X3	T60.2X4	—	—
medicinal (trace)	T45.8X1	T45.8X2	T45.8X3	T45.8X4	T45.8X5	T45.8X6
oleate	T49.0X1	T49.0X2	T49.0X3	T49.0X4	T49.0X5	T49.0X6
sulfate	T56.4X1	T56.4X2	T56.4X3	T56.4X4	—	—
cupric	T56.4X1	T56.4X2	T56.4X3	T56.4X4	—	—
fungicide	T60.3X1	T60.3X2	T60.3X3	T60.3X4	—	—
medicinal						
ear	T49.6X1	T49.6X2	T49.6X3	T49.6X4	T49.6X5	T49.6X6
emetic	T47.7X1	T47.7X2	T47.7X3	T47.7X4	T47.7X5	T47.7X6
eye	T49.5X1	T49.5X2	T49.5X3	T49.5X4	T49.5X5	T49.5X6
cuprous	T56.4X1	T56.4X2	T56.4X3	T56.4X4	—	—
fungicide	T60.3X1	T60.3X2	T60.3X3	T60.3X4	—	—
medicinal						
ear	T49.6X1	T49.6X2	T49.6X3	T49.6X4	T49.6X5	T49.6X6
emetic	T47.7X1	T47.7X2	T47.7X3	T47.7X4	T47.7X5	T47.7X6
eye	T49.5X1	T49.5X2	T49.5X3	T49.5X4	T49.5X5	T49.5X6
Coral (sting)	T63.691	T63.692	T63.693	T63.694	—	—
snake (bite) (venom)	T63.021	T63.022	T63.023	T63.024	—	—
Corbadrine	T49.6X1	T49.6X2	T49.6X3	T49.6X4	T49.6X5	T49.6X6
Cordite	T65.891	T65.892	T65.893	T65.894	—	—
vapor	T59.891	T59.892	T59.893	T59.894	—	—
Cordran	T49.0X1	T49.0X2	T49.0X3	T49.0X4	T49.0X5	T49.0X6
Corn cures	T49.4X1	T49.4X2	T49.4X3	T49.4X4	T49.4X5	T49.4X6
Cornhusker's lotion	T49.3X1	T49.3X2	T49.3X3	T49.3X4	T49.3X5	T49.3X6
Corn starch	T49.3X1	T49.3X2	T49.3X3	T49.3X4	T49.3X5	T49.3X6
Coronary vasodilator NEC	T46.3X1	T46.3X2	T46.3X3	T46.3X4	T46.3X5	T46.3X6
Corrosive NEC	T54.91	T54.92	T54.93	T54.94	—	—
acid NEC	T54.2X1	T54.2X2	T54.2X3	T54.2X4	—	—
aromatics	T54.1X1	T54.1X2	T54.1X3	T54.1X4	—	—
disinfectant	T54.1X1	T54.1X2	T54.1X3	T54.1X4	—	—
fumes NEC	T54.91	T54.92	T54.93	T54.94	—	—
specified NEC	T54.91	T54.92	T54.93	T54.94	—	—
sublimate	T56.1X1	T56.1X2	T56.1X3	T56.1X4	—	—
Cortate	T38.0X1	T38.0X2	T38.0X3	T38.0X4	T38.0X5	T38.0X6
Cort-Dome	T38.0X1	T38.0X2	T38.0X3	T38.0X4	T38.0X5	T38.0X6
ENT agent	T49.6X1	T49.6X2	T49.6X3	T49.6X4	T49.6X5	T49.6X6
ophthalmic preparation	T49.5X1	T49.5X2	T49.5X3	T49.5X4	T49.5X5	T49.5X6
topical NEC	T49.0X1	T49.0X2	T49.0X3	T49.0X4	T49.0X5	T49.0X6
Cortef	T38.0X1	T38.0X2	T38.0X3	T38.0X4	T38.0X5	T38.0X6
ENT agent	T49.6X1	T49.6X2	T49.6X3	T49.6X4	T49.6X5	T49.6X6
ophthalmic preparation	T49.5X1	T49.5X2	T49.5X3	T49.5X4	T49.5X5	T49.5X6
topical NEC	T49.0X1	T49.0X2	T49.0X3	T49.0X4	T49.0X5	T49.0X6
Corticosteroid	T38.0X1	T38.0X2	T38.0X3	T38.0X4	T38.0X5	T38.0X6
ENT agent	T49.6X1	T49.6X2	T49.6X3	T49.6X4	T49.6X5	T49.6X6
mineral	T50.0X1	T50.0X2	T50.0X3	T50.0X4	T50.0X5	T50.0X6
ophthalmic	T49.5X1	T49.5X2	T49.5X3	T49.5X4	T49.5X5	T49.5X6
topical NEC	T49.0X1	T49.0X2	T49.0X3	T49.0X4	T49.0X5	T49.0X6
Corticotropin	T38.811	T38.812	T38.813	T38.814	T38.815	T38.816
Cortisol	T38.0X1	T38.0X2	T38.0X3	T38.0X4	T38.0X5	T38.0X6
ENT agent	T49.6X1	T49.6X2	T49.6X3	T49.6X4	T49.6X5	T49.6X6
ophthalmic preparation	T49.5X1	T49.5X2	T49.5X3	T49.5X4	T49.5X5	T49.5X6
topical NEC	T49.0X1	T49.0X2	T49.0X3	T49.0X4	T49.0X5	T49.0X6

Substance	Poisoning, Accidental (unintentional)	Poisoning, Intentional Self-harm	Poisoning, Assault	Poisoning, Undetermined	Adverse Effect	Under-dosing
Cortisone (acetate)	T38.0X1	T38.0X2	T38.0X3	T38.0X4	T38.0X5	T38.0X6
ENT agent	T49.6X1	T49.6X2	T49.6X3	T49.6X4	T49.6X5	T49.6X6
ophthalmic preparation	T49.5X1	T49.5X2	T49.5X3	T49.5X4	T49.5X5	T49.5X6
topical NEC	T49.0X1	T49.0X2	T49.0X3	T49.0X4	T49.0X5	T49.0X6
Cortivazol	T38.0X1	T38.0X2	T38.0X3	T38.0X4	T38.0X5	T38.0X6
Cortogen	T38.0X1	T38.0X2	T38.0X3	T38.0X4	T38.0X5	T38.0X6
ENT agent	T49.6X1	T49.6X2	T49.6X3	T49.6X4	T49.6X5	T49.6X6
ophthalmic preparation	T49.5X1	T49.5X2	T49.5X3	T49.5X4	T49.5X5	T49.5X6
Cortone	T38.0X1	T38.0X2	T38.0X3	T38.0X4	T38.0X5	T38.0X6
ENT agent	T49.6X1	T49.6X2	T49.6X3	T49.6X4	T49.6X5	T49.6X6
ophthalmic preparation	T49.5X1	T49.5X2	T49.5X3	T49.5X4	T49.5X5	T49.5X6
Cortril	T38.0X1	T38.0X2	T38.0X3	T38.0X4	T38.0X5	T38.0X6
ENT agent	T49.6X1	T49.6X2	T49.6X3	T49.6X4	T49.6X5	T49.6X6
ophthalmic preparation	T49.5X1	T49.5X2	T49.5X3	T49.5X4	T49.5X5	T49.5X6
topical NEC	T49.0X1	T49.0X2	T49.0X3	T49.0X4	T49.0X5	T49.0X6
Corynebacterium parvum	T45.1X1	T45.1X2	T45.1X3	T45.1X4	T45.1X5	T45.1X6
Cosmetic preparation	T49.8X1	T49.8X2	T49.8X3	T49.8X4	T49.8X5	T49.8X6
Cosmetics	T49.8X1	T49.8X2	T49.8X3	T49.8X4	T49.8X5	T49.8X6
Cosyntropin	T38.811	T38.812	T38.813	T38.814	T38.815	T38.816
Cotarnine	T45.7X1	T45.7X2	T45.7X3	T45.7X4	T45.7X5	T45.7X6
Co-trimoxazole	T36.8X1	T36.8X2	T36.8X3	T36.8X4	T36.8X5	T36.8X6
Cottonseed oil	T49.3X1	T49.3X2	T49.3X3	T49.3X4	T49.3X5	T49.3X6
Cough mixture (syrup)	T48.4X1	T48.4X2	T48.4X3	T48.4X4	T48.4X5	T48.4X6
containing opiates	T40.2X1	T40.2X2	T40.2X3	T40.2X4	T40.2X5	T40.2X6
expectorants	T48.4X1	T48.4X2	T48.4X3	T48.4X4	T48.4X5	T48.4X6
Coumadin	T45.511	T45.512	T45.513	T45.514	T45.515	T45.516
rodenticide	T60.4X1	T60.4X2	T60.4X3	T60.4X4	—	—
Coumaphos	T60.0X1	T60.0X2	T60.0X3	T60.0X4	—	—
Coumarin	T45.511	T45.512	T45.513	T45.514	T45.515	T45.516
Coumetarol	T45.511	T45.512	T45.513	T45.514	T45.515	T45.516
Cowbane	T62.2X1	T62.2X2	T62.2X3	T62.2X4	—	—
Cozyme	T45.2X1	T45.2X2	T45.2X3	T45.2X4	T45.2X5	T45.2X6
Crack	T40.5X1	T40.5X2	T40.5X3	T40.5X4	—	—
Crataegus extract	T46.0X1	T46.0X2	T46.0X3	T46.0X4	T46.0X5	T46.0X6
Creolin	T54.1X1	T54.1X2	T54.1X3	T54.1X4	—	—
disinfectant	T54.1X1	T54.1X2	T54.1X3	T54.1X4	—	—
Creosol (compound)	T49.0X1	T49.0X2	T49.0X3	T49.0X4	T49.0X5	T49.0X6
Creosote (coal tar)	T49.0X1	T49.0X2	T49.0X3	T49.0X4	T49.0X5	T49.0X6
(beechwood)						
medicinal (expectorant)	T48.4X1	T48.4X2	T48.4X3	T48.4X4	T48.4X5	T48.4X6
syrup	T48.4X1	T48.4X2	T48.4X3	T48.4X4	T48.4X5	T48.4X6
Cresol(s)	T49.0X1	T49.0X2	T49.0X3	T49.0X4	T49.0X5	T49.0X6
and soap solution	T49.0X1	T49.0X2	T49.0X3	T49.0X4	T49.0X5	T49.0X6
Cresyl acetate	T49.0X1	T49.0X2	T49.0X3	T49.0X4	T49.0X5	T49.0X6
Cresylic acid	T49.0X1	T49.0X2	T49.0X3	T49.0X4	T49.0X5	T49.0X6
Crimidine	T60.4X1	T60.4X2	T60.4X3	T60.4X4	—	—
Croconazole	T37.8X1	T37.8X2	T37.8X3	T37.8X4	T37.8X5	T37.8X6
Cromoglicic acid	T48.6X1	T48.6X2	T48.6X3	T48.6X4	T48.6X5	T48.6X6
Cromolyn	T48.6X1	T48.6X2	T48.6X3	T48.6X4	T48.6X5	T48.6X6
Cromonar	T46.3X1	T46.3X2	T46.3X3	T46.3X4	T46.3X5	T46.3X6
Cropropamide	T39.8X1	T39.8X2	T39.8X3	T39.8X4	T39.8X5	T39.8X6
with crotethamide	T50.7X1	T50.7X2	T50.7X3	T50.7X4	T50.7X5	T50.7X6
Crotamiton	T49.0X1	T49.0X2	T49.0X3	T49.0X4	T49.0X5	T49.0X6
Crotethamide	T39.8X1	T39.8X2	T39.8X3	T39.8X4	T39.8X5	T39.8X6
with cropropamide	T50.7X1	T50.7X2	T50.7X3	T50.7X4	T50.7X5	T50.7X6
Croton (oil)	T47.2X1	T47.2X2	T47.2X3	T47.2X4	T47.2X5	T47.2X6
chloral	T42.6X1	T42.6X2	T42.6X3	T42.6X4	T42.6X5	T42.6X6
Crude oil	T52.0X1	T52.0X2	T52.0X3	T52.0X4	—	—
Cryogenine	T39.8X1	T39.8X2	T39.8X3	T39.8X4	T39.8X5	T39.8X6
Cryolite (vapor)	T60.1X1	T60.1X2	T60.1X3	T60.1X4	—	—
insecticide	T60.1X1	T60.1X2	T60.1X3	T60.1X4	—	—
Cryptenamine (tannates)	T46.5X1	T46.5X2	T46.5X3	T46.5X4	T46.5X5	T46.5X6
Crystal violet	T49.0X1	T49.0X2	T49.0X3	T49.0X4	T49.0X5	T49.0X6
Cuckoopint	T62.2X1	T62.2X2	T62.2X3	T62.2X4	—	—
Cumetharol	T45.511	T45.512	T45.513	T45.514	T45.515	T45.516
Cupric						
acetate	T60.3X1	T60.3X2	T60.3X3	T60.3X4	—	—
acetoarsenite	T57.0X1	T57.0X2	T57.0X3	T57.0X4	—	—
arsenate	T57.0X1	T57.0X2	T57.0X3	T57.0X4	—	—
gluconate	T49.0X1	T49.0X2	T49.0X3	T49.0X4	T49.0X5	T49.0X6
oleate	T49.0X1	T49.0X2	T49.0X3	T49.0X4	T49.0X5	T49.0X6
sulfate	T56.4X1	T56.4X2	T56.4X3	T56.4X4	—	—
Cuprous sulfate — see also	T56.4X1	T56.4X2	T56.4X3	T56.4X4	—	—
Copper sulfate						
Curare, curarine	T48.1X1	T48.1X2	T48.1X3	T48.1X4	T48.1X5	T48.1X6
Cyamemazine	T43.3X1	T43.3X2	T43.3X3	T43.3X4	T43.3X5	T43.3X6
Cyamopsis tetragonoloba	T46.6X1	T46.6X2	T46.6X3	T46.6X4	T46.6X5	T46.6X6
Cyanacetyl hydrazide	T37.1X1	T37.1X2	T37.1X3	T37.1X4	T37.1X5	T37.1X6
Cyanic acid (gas)	T59.891	T59.892	T59.893	T59.894	—	—
Cyanide(s) (compounds) (potassium) (sodium)	T65.0X1	T65.0X2	T65.0X3	T65.0X4	—	—
NEC						
dust or gas (inhalation) NEC	T57.3X1	T57.3X2	T57.3X3	T57.3X4	—	—
Cyanide(s) (compounds) (potassium) (sodium) NEC — continued						
fumigant	T65.0X1	T65.0X2	T65.0X3	T65.0X4	—	—
hydrogen	T57.3X1	T57.3X2	T57.3X3	T57.3X4	—	—
mercuric — see Mercury						
pesticide (dust) (fumes)	T65.0X1	T65.0X2	T65.0X3	T65.0X4	—	—
Cyanoacrylate adhesive	T49.3X1	T49.3X2	T49.3X3	T49.3X4	T49.3X5	T49.3X6
Cyanocobalamin	T45.8X1	T45.8X2	T45.8X3	T45.8X4	T45.8X5	T45.8X6
Cyanogen (chloride) (gas) NEC	T59.891	T59.892	T59.893	T59.894		
Cyclacillin	T36.0X1	T36.0X2	T36.0X3	T36.0X4	T36.0X5	T36.0X6
Cyclaine	T41.3X1	T41.3X2	T41.3X3	T41.3X4	T41.3X5	T41.3X6
Cyclamate	T50.991	T50.992	T50.993	T50.994	T50.995	T50.996
Cyclamen europaeum	T62.2X1	T62.2X2	T62.2X3	T62.2X4	—	—
Cyclandelate	T46.7X1	T46.7X2	T46.7X3	T46.7X4	T46.7X5	T46.7X6
Cyclazocine	T50.7X1	T50.7X2	T50.7X3	T50.7X4	T50.7X5	T50.7X6
Cyclizine	T45.0X1	T45.0X2	T45.0X3	T45.0X4	T45.0X5	T45.0X6
Cyclobarbital	T42.3X1	T42.3X2	T42.3X3	T42.3X4	T42.3X5	T42.3X6
Cyclobarbitone	T42.3X1	T42.3X2	T42.3X3	T42.3X4	T42.3X5	T42.3X6
Cyclobenzaprine	T48.1X1	T48.1X2	T48.1X3	T48.1X4	T48.1X5	T48.1X6
Cyclodrine	T44.3X1	T44.3X2	T44.3X3	T44.3X4	T44.3X5	T44.3X6
Cycloguanil embonate	T37.2X1	T37.2X2	T37.2X3	T37.2X4	T37.2X5	T37.2X6
Cyclohexane	T52.8X1	T52.8X2	T52.8X3	T52.8X4	—	—
Cyclohexanol	T51.8X1	T51.8X2	T51.8X3	T51.8X4	—	—
Cyclohexanone	T52.4X1	T52.4X2	T52.4X3	T52.4X4	—	—
Cycloheximide	T60.3X1	T60.3X2	T60.3X3	T60.3X4	—	—
Cyclohexyl acetate	T52.8X1	T52.8X2	T52.8X3	T52.8X4	—	—
Cycloleucin	T45.1X1	T45.1X2	T45.1X3	T45.1X4	T45.1X5	T45.1X6
Cyclomethycaine	T41.3X1	T41.3X2	T41.3X3	T41.3X4	T41.3X5	T41.3X6
Cyclopentamine	T44.4X1	T44.4X2	T44.4X3	T44.4X4	T44.4X5	T44.4X6
Cyclopenthiazide	T50.2X1	T50.2X2	T50.2X3	T50.2X4	T50.2X5	T50.2X6
Cyclopentolate	T44.3X1	T44.3X2	T44.3X3	T44.3X4	T44.3X5	T44.3X6
Cyclophosphamide	T45.1X1	T45.1X2	T45.1X3	T45.1X4	T45.1X5	T45.1X6
Cycloplegic drug	T49.5X1	T49.5X2	T49.5X3	T49.5X4	T49.5X5	T49.5X6
Cyclopropane	T41.291	T41.292	T41.293	T41.294	T41.295	T41.296
Cyclopyrabital	T39.8X1	T39.8X2	T39.8X3	T39.8X4	T39.8X5	T39.8X6
Cycloserine	T37.1X1	T37.1X2	T37.1X3	T37.1X4	T37.1X5	T37.1X6
Cyclosporin	T45.1X1	T45.1X2	T45.1X3	T45.1X4	T45.1X5	T45.1X6
Cyclothiazide	T50.2X1	T50.2X2	T50.2X3	T50.2X4	T50.2X5	T50.2X6
Cycrimine	T44.3X1	T44.3X2	T44.3X3	T44.3X4	T44.3X5	T44.3X6
Cyhalothrin	T60.1X1	T60.1X2	T60.1X3	T60.1X4	—	—
Cymarin	T46.0X1	T46.0X2	T46.0X3	T46.0X4	T46.0X5	T46.0X6
Cypermethrin	T60.1X1	T60.1X2	T60.1X3	T60.1X4	—	—
Cyphenothrin	T60.2X1	T60.2X2	T60.2X3	T60.2X4	—	—
Cyproheptadine	T45.0X1	T45.0X2	T45.0X3	T45.0X4	T45.0X5	T45.0X6
Cyproterone	T38.6X1	T38.6X2	T38.6X3	T38.6X4	T38.6X5	T38.6X6
Cysteamine	T50.6X1	T50.6X2	T50.6X3	T50.6X4	T50.6X5	T50.6X6
Cytarabine	T45.1X1	T45.1X2	T45.1X3	T45.1X4	T45.1X5	T45.1X6
Cytisus						
laburnum	T62.2X1	T62.2X2	T62.2X3	T62.2X4	—	—
scoparius	T62.2X1	T62.2X2	T62.2X3	T62.2X4	—	—
Cytochrome C	T47.5X1	T47.5X2	T47.5X3	T47.5X4	T47.5X5	T47.5X6
Cytomel	T38.1X1	T38.1X2	T38.1X3	T38.1X4	T38.1X5	T38.1X6
Cytosine arabinoside	T45.1X1	T45.1X2	T45.1X3	T45.1X4	T45.1X5	T45.1X6
Cytoxan	T45.1X1	T45.1X2	T45.1X3	T45.1X4	T45.1X5	T45.1X6
Cytozyme	T45.7X1	T45.7X2	T45.7X3	T45.7X4	T45.7X5	T45.7X6
S-Carboxymethylcysteine	T48.4X1	T48.4X2	T48.4X3	T48.4X4	T48.4X5	T48.4X6
Dacarbazine	T45.1X1	T45.1X2	T45.1X3	T45.1X4	T45.1X5	T45.1X6
Dactinomycin	T45.1X1	T45.1X2	T45.1X3	T45.1X4	T45.1X5	T45.1X6
DADPS	T37.1X1	T37.1X2	T37.1X3	T37.1X4	T37.1X5	T37.1X6
Dakin's solution	T49.0X1	T49.0X2	T49.0X3	T49.0X4	T49.0X5	T49.0X6
Dalapon (sodium)	T60.3X1	T60.3X2	T60.3X3	T60.3X4	—	—
Dalmane	T42.4X1	T42.4X2	T42.4X3	T42.4X4	T42.4X5	T42.4X6
Danazol	T38.6X1	T38.6X2	T38.6X3	T38.6X4	T38.6X5	T38.6X6
Danilone	T45.511	T45.512	T45.513	T45.514	T45.515	T45.516
Danthron	T47.2X1	T47.2X2	T47.2X3	T47.2X4	T47.2X5	T47.2X6
Dantrolene	T42.8X1	T42.8X2	T42.8X3	T42.8X4	T42.8X5	T42.8X6
Dantron	T47.2X1	T47.2X2	T47.2X3	T47.2X4	T47.2X5	T47.2X6
Daphne (gnidium) (mezereum)	T62.2X1	T62.2X2	T62.2X3	T62.2X4	—	—
berry	T62.1X1	T62.1X2	T62.1X3	T62.1X4	—	—
Dapsone	T37.1X1	T37.1X2	T37.1X3	T37.1X4	T37.1X5	T37.1X6
Daraprim	T37.2X1	T37.2X2	T37.2X3	T37.2X4	T37.2X5	T37.2X6
Darnel	T62.2X1	T62.2X2	T62.2X3	T62.2X4	—	—
Darvon	T39.8X1	T39.8X2	T39.8X3	T39.8X4	T39.8X5	T39.8X6
Daunomycin	T45.1X1	T45.1X2	T45.1X3	T45.1X4	T45.1X5	T45.1X6
Daunorubicin	T45.1X1	T45.1X2	T45.1X3	T45.1X4	T45.1X5	T45.1X6
DBI	T38.3X1	T38.3X2	T38.3X3	T38.3X4	T38.3X5	T38.3X6
D-Con	T60.91	T60.92	T60.93	T60.94	—	—
insecticide	T60.2X1	T60.2X2	T60.2X3	T60.2X4	—	—
rodenticide	T60.4X1	T60.4X2	T60.4X3	T60.4X4	—	—
DDAVP	T38.891	T38.892	T38.893	T38.894	T38.895	T38.896

Additional Character May Be Required — Refer to the Tabular List for Character Selection ▽ Subterms under main terms may continue to next column or page

Substance	Poisoning, Accidental (unintentional)	Poisoning, Intentional Self-harm	Poisoning, Assault	Poisoning, Undetermined	Adverse Effect	Under-dosing
DDE (bis(chlorophenyl)-dichloroethylene)	T60.2X1	T60.2X2	T60.2X3	T60.2X4	—	—
DDS	T37.1X1	T37.1X2	T37.1X3	T37.1X4	T37.1X5	T37.1X6
DDT (dust)	T60.1X1	T60.1X2	T60.1X3	T60.1X4	—	—
Deadly nightshade — see also Belladonna	T62.2X1	T62.2X2	T62.2X3	T62.2X4	—	—
berry	T62.1X1	T62.1X2	T62.1X3	T62.1X4	—	—
Deamino-D-arginine vasopressin	T38.891	T38.892	T38.893	T38.894	T38.895	T38.896
Deanol (aceglumate)	T50.991	T50.992	T50.993	T50.994	T50.995	T50.996
Debrisoquine	T46.5X1	T46.5X2	T46.5X3	T46.5X4	T46.5X5	T46.5X6
Decaborane	T57.8X1	T57.8X2	T57.8X3	T57.8X4	—	—
fumes	T59.891	T59.892	T59.893	T59.894	—	—
Decadron	T38.0X1	T38.0X2	T38.0X3	T38.0X4	T38.0X5	T38.0X6
ENT agent	T49.6X1	T49.6X2	T49.6X3	T49.6X4	T49.6X5	T49.6X6
ophthalmic preparation	T49.5X1	T49.5X2	T49.5X3	T49.5X4	T49.5X5	T49.5X6
topical NEC	T49.0X1	T49.0X2	T49.0X3	T49.0X4	T49.0X5	T49.0X6
Decahydronaphthalene	T52.8X1	T52.8X2	T52.8X3	T52.8X4	—	—
Decalin	T52.8X1	T52.8X2	T52.8X3	T52.8X4	—	—
Decamethonium (bromide)	T48.1X1	T48.1X2	T48.1X3	T48.1X4	T48.1X5	T48.1X6
Decholin	T47.5X1	T47.5X2	T47.5X3	T47.5X4	T47.5X5	T47.5X6
Declomycin	T36.4X1	T36.4X2	T36.4X3	T36.4X4	T36.4X5	T36.4X6
Decongestant, nasal (mucosa)	T48.5X1	T48.5X2	T48.5X3	T48.5X4	T48.5X5	T48.5X6
combination	T48.5X1	T48.5X2	T48.5X3	T48.5X4	T48.5X5	T48.5X6
Deet	T60.8X1	T60.8X2	T60.8X3	T60.8X4	—	—
Deferoxamine	T45.8X1	T45.8X2	T45.8X3	T45.8X4	T45.8X5	T45.8X6
Deflazacort	T38.0X1	T38.0X2	T38.0X3	T38.0X4	T38.0X5	T38.0X6
Deglycyrrhizinized extract of licorice	T48.4X1	T48.4X2	T48.4X3	T48.4X4	T48.4X5	T48.4X6
Dehydrocholic acid	T47.5X1	T47.5X2	T47.5X3	T47.5X4	T47.5X5	T47.5X6
Dehydroemetine	T37.3X1	T37.3X2	T37.3X3	T37.3X4	T37.3X5	T37.3X6
Dekalin	T52.8X1	T52.8X2	T52.8X3	T52.8X4	—	—
Delalutin	T38.5X1	T38.5X2	T38.5X3	T38.5X4	T38.5X5	T38.5X6
Delorazepam	T42.4X1	T42.4X2	T42.4X3	T42.4X4	T42.4X5	T42.4X6
Delphinium	T62.2X1	T62.2X2	T62.2X3	T62.2X4	—	—
Deltamethrin	T60.1X1	T60.1X2	T60.1X3	T60.1X4	—	—
Deltasone	T38.0X1	T38.0X2	T38.0X3	T38.0X4	T38.0X5	T38.0X6
Deltra	T38.0X1	T38.0X2	T38.0X3	T38.0X4	T38.0X5	T38.0X6
Delvinal	T42.3X1	T42.3X2	T42.3X3	T42.3X4	T42.3X5	T42.3X6
Demecarium (bromide)	T49.5X1	T49.5X2	T49.5X3	T49.5X4	T49.5X5	T49.5X6
Demeclocycline	T36.4X1	T36.4X2	T36.4X3	T36.4X4	T36.4X5	T36.4X6
Demecolcine	T45.1X1	T45.1X2	T45.1X3	T45.1X4	T45.1X5	T45.1X6
Demegestone	T38.5X1	T38.5X2	T38.5X3	T38.5X4	T38.5X5	T38.5X6
Demelanizing agents	T49.8X1	T49.8X2	T49.8X3	T49.8X4	T49.8X5	T49.8X6
Demephion -O and -S	T60.0X1	T60.0X2	T60.0X3	T60.0X4	—	—
Demerol	T40.2X1	T40.2X2	T40.2X3	T40.2X4	T40.2X5	T40.2X6
Demethylchlortetracycline	T36.4X1	T36.4X2	T36.4X3	T36.4X4	T36.4X5	T36.4X6
Demethyltetracycline	T36.4X1	T36.4X2	T36.4X3	T36.4X4	T36.4X5	T36.4X6
Demeton -O and -S	T60.0X1	T60.0X2	T60.0X3	T60.0X4	—	—
Demulcent (external)	T49.3X1	T49.3X2	T49.3X3	T49.3X4	T49.3X5	T49.3X6
specified NEC	T49.3X1	T49.3X2	T49.3X3	T49.3X4	T49.3X5	T49.3X6
Demulen	T38.4X1	T38.4X2	T38.4X3	T38.4X4	T38.4X5	T38.4X6
Denatured alcohol	T51.0X1	T51.0X2	T51.0X3	T51.0X4	—	—
Dendrid	T49.5X1	T49.5X2	T49.5X3	T49.5X4	T49.5X5	T49.5X6
Dental drug, topical application NEC	T49.7X1	T49.7X2	T49.7X3	T49.7X4	T49.7X5	T49.7X6
Dentifrice	T49.7X1	T49.7X2	T49.7X3	T49.7X4	T49.7X5	T49.7X6
Deodorant spray (feminine hygiene)	T49.8X1	T49.8X2	T49.8X3	T49.8X4	T49.8X5	T49.8X6
Deoxycortone	T50.0X1	T50.0X2	T50.0X3	T50.0X4	T50.0X5	T50.0X6
Deoxyribonuclease (pancreatic)	T45.3X1	T45.3X2	T45.3X3	T45.3X4	T45.3X5	T45.3X6
Depilatory	T49.4X1	T49.4X2	T49.4X3	T49.4X4	T49.4X5	T49.4X6
Deprenalin	T42.8X1	T42.8X2	T42.8X3	T42.8X4	T42.8X5	T42.8X6
Deprenyl	T42.8X1	T42.8X2	T42.8X3	T42.8X4	T42.8X5	T42.8X6
Depressant						
appetite (central)	T50.5X1	T50.5X2	T50.5X3	T50.5X4	T50.5X5	T50.5X6
cardiac	T46.2X1	T46.2X2	T46.2X3	T46.2X4	T46.2X5	T46.2X6
central nervous system (anesthetic) — see also Central nervous system, depressants	T42.71	T42.72	T42.73	T42.74	T42.75	T42.76
general anesthetic	T41.201	T41.202	T41.203	T41.204	T41.205	T41.206
muscle tone	T42.8X1	T42.8X2	T42.8X3	T42.8X4	T42.8X5	T42.8X6
muscle tone, central	T42.8X1	T42.8X2	T42.8X3	T42.8X4	T42.8X5	T42.8X6
psychotherapeutic	T43.501	T43.502	T43.503	T43.504	T43.505	T43.506
Depressant, appetite	T50.5X1	T50.5X2	T50.5X3	T50.5X4	T50.5X5	T50.5X6
Deptropine	T45.0X1	T45.0X2	T45.0X3	T45.0X4	T45.0X5	T45.0X6
Dequalinium (chloride)	T49.0X1	T49.0X2	T49.0X3	T49.0X4	T49.0X5	T49.0X6
Derris root	T60.2X1	T60.2X2	T60.2X3	T60.2X4	—	—
Deserpidine	T46.5X1	T46.5X2	T46.5X3	T46.5X4	T46.5X5	T46.5X6
Desferrioxamine	T45.8X1	T45.8X2	T45.8X3	T45.8X4	T45.8X5	T45.8X6
Desipramine	T43.011	T43.012	T43.013	T43.014	T43.015	T43.016
Deslanoside	T46.0X1	T46.0X2	T46.0X3	T46.0X4	T46.0X5	T46.0X6
Desloughing agent	T49.4X1	T49.4X2	T49.4X3	T49.4X4	T49.4X5	T49.4X6
Desmethylimipramine	T43.011	T43.012	T43.013	T43.014	T43.015	T43.016
Desmopressin	T38.891	T38.892	T38.893	T38.894	T38.895	T38.896
Desocodeine	T40.2X1	T40.2X2	T40.2X3	T40.2X4	T40.2X5	T40.2X6
Desogestrel	T38.5X1	T38.5X2	T38.5X3	T38.5X4	T38.5X5	T38.5X6
Desomorphine	T40.2X1	T40.2X2	T40.2X3	T40.2X4	—	—
Desonide	T49.0X1	T49.0X2	T49.0X3	T49.0X4	T49.0X5	T49.0X6
Desoximetasone	T49.0X1	T49.0X2	T49.0X3	T49.0X4	T49.0X5	T49.0X6
Desoxycorticosteroid	T50.0X1	T50.0X2	T50.0X3	T50.0X4	T50.0X5	T50.0X6
Desoxycortone	T50.0X1	T50.0X2	T50.0X3	T50.0X4	T50.0X5	T50.0X6
Desoxyephedrine	T43.621	T43.622	T43.623	T43.624	T43.625	T43.626
Detaxtran	T46.6X1	T46.6X2	T46.6X3	T46.6X4	T46.6X5	T46.6X6
Detergent						
external medication	T49.2X1	T49.2X2	T49.2X3	T49.2X4	T49.2X5	T49.2X6
local	T49.2X1	T49.2X2	T49.2X3	T49.2X4	T49.2X5	T49.2X6
medicinal	T49.2X1	T49.2X2	T49.2X3	T49.2X4	T49.2X5	T49.2X6
nonmedicinal	T55.1X1	T55.1X2	T55.1X3	T55.1X4	—	—
specified NEC	T55.1X1	T55.1X2	T55.1X3	T55.1X4	—	—
Deterrent, alcohol	T50.6X1	T50.6X2	T50.6X3	T50.6X4	T50.6X5	T50.6X6
Detoxifying agent	T50.6X1	T50.6X2	T50.6X3	T50.6X4	T50.6X5	T50.6X6
Detrothyronine	T38.1X1	T38.1X2	T38.1X3	T38.1X4	T38.1X5	T38.1X6
Dettol (external medication)	T49.0X1	T49.0X2	T49.0X3	T49.0X4	T49.0X5	T49.0X6
Dexamethasone	T38.0X1	T38.0X2	T38.0X3	T38.0X4	T38.0X5	T38.0X6
ENT agent	T49.6X1	T49.6X2	T49.6X3	T49.6X4	T49.6X5	T49.6X6
ophthalmic preparation	T49.5X1	T49.5X2	T49.5X3	T49.5X4	T49.5X5	T49.5X6
topical NEC	T49.0X1	T49.0X2	T49.0X3	T49.0X4	T49.0X5	T49.0X6
Dexamfetamine	T43.621	T43.622	T43.623	T43.624	T43.625	T43.626
Dexamphetamine	T43.621	T43.622	T43.623	T43.624	T43.625	T43.626
Dexbrompheniramine	T45.0X1	T45.0X2	T45.0X3	T45.0X4	T45.0X5	T45.0X6
Dexchlorpheniramine	T45.0X1	T45.0X2	T45.0X3	T45.0X4	T45.0X5	T45.0X6
Dexedrine	T43.621	T43.622	T43.623	T43.624	T43.625	T43.626
Dexetimide	T44.3X1	T44.3X2	T44.3X3	T44.3X4	T44.3X5	T44.3X6
Dexfenfluramine	T50.5X1	T50.5X2	T50.5X3	T50.5X4	T50.5X5	T50.5X6
Dexpanthenol	T45.2X1	T45.2X2	T45.2X3	T45.2X4	T45.2X5	T45.2X6
Dextran (40) (70) (150)	T45.8X1	T45.8X2	T45.8X3	T45.8X4	T45.8X5	T45.8X6
Dextriferron	T45.4X1	T45.4X2	T45.4X3	T45.4X4	T45.4X5	T45.4X6
Dextroamphetamine	T43.621	T43.622	T43.623	T43.624	T43.625	T43.626
Dextro calcium pantothenate	T45.2X1	T45.2X2	T45.2X3	T45.2X4	T45.2X5	T45.2X6
Dextromethorphan	T48.3X1	T48.3X2	T48.3X3	T48.3X4	T48.3X5	T48.3X6
Dextromoramide	T40.4X1	T40.4X2	T40.4X3	T40.4X4	—	—
topical	T49.8X1	T49.8X2	T49.8X3	T49.8X4	T49.8X5	T49.8X6
Dextro pantothenyl alcohol	T45.2X1	T45.2X2	T45.2X3	T45.2X4	T45.2X5	T45.2X6
Dextropropoxyphene	T40.4X1	T40.4X2	T40.4X3	T40.4X4	T40.4X5	T40.4X6
Dextrorphan	T40.2X1	T40.2X2	T40.2X3	T40.2X4	T40.2X5	T40.2X6
Dextrose	T50.3X1	T50.3X2	T50.3X3	T50.3X4	T50.3X5	T50.3X6
concentrated solution, intravenous	T46.8X1	T46.8X2	T46.8X3	T46.8X4	T46.8X5	T46.8X6
Dextrothyroxin	T38.1X1	T38.1X2	T38.1X3	T38.1X4	T38.1X5	T38.1X6
Dextrothyroxine sodium	T38.1X1	T38.1X2	T38.1X3	T38.1X4	T38.1X5	T38.1X6
DFP	T44.0X1	T44.0X2	T44.0X3	T44.0X4	T44.0X5	T44.0X6
DHE	T37.3X1	T37.3X2	T37.3X3	T37.3X4	T37.3X5	T37.3X6
45	T46.5X1	T46.5X2	T46.5X3	T46.5X4	T46.5X5	T46.5X6
Diabinese	T38.3X1	T38.3X2	T38.3X3	T38.3X4	T38.3X5	T38.3X6
Diacetone alcohol	T52.4X1	T52.4X2	T52.4X3	T52.4X4	—	—
Diacetyl monoxime	T50.991	T50.992	T50.993	T50.994	—	—
Diacetylmorphine	T40.1X1	T40.1X2	T40.1X3	T40.1X4	—	—
Diachylon plaster	T49.4X1	T49.4X2	T49.4X3	T49.4X4	T49.4X5	T49.4X6
Diaethylstilboestrolum	T38.5X1	T38.5X2	T38.5X3	T38.5X4	T38.5X5	T38.5X6
Diagnostic agent NEC	T50.8X1	T50.8X2	T50.8X3	T50.8X4	T50.8X5	T50.8X6
Dial (soap)	T49.2X1	T49.2X2	T49.2X3	T49.2X4	T49.2X5	T49.2X6
sedative	T42.3X1	T42.3X2	T42.3X3	T42.3X4	T42.3X5	T42.3X6
Dialkyl carbonate	T52.91	T52.92	T52.93	T52.94	—	—
Diallylbarbituric acid	T42.3X1	T42.3X2	T42.3X3	T42.3X4	T42.3X5	T42.3X6
Diallymal	T42.3X1	T42.3X2	T42.3X3	T42.3X4	T42.3X5	T42.3X6
Dialysis solution (intraperitoneal)	T50.3X1	T50.3X2	T50.3X3	T50.3X4	T50.3X5	T50.3X6
Diaminodiphenylsulfone	T37.1X1	T37.1X2	T37.1X3	T37.1X4	T37.1X5	T37.1X6
Diamorphine	T40.1X1	T40.1X2	T40.1X3	T40.1X4	—	—
Diamox	T50.2X1	T50.2X2	T50.2X3	T50.2X4	T50.2X5	T50.2X6
Diamthazole	T49.0X1	T49.0X2	T49.0X3	T49.0X4	T49.0X5	T49.0X6
Dianthone	T47.2X1	T47.2X2	T47.2X3	T47.2X4	T47.2X5	T47.2X6
Diaphenylsulfone	T37.0X1	T37.0X2	T37.0X3	T37.0X4	T37.0X5	T37.0X6
Diasone (sodium)	T37.1X1	T37.1X2	T37.1X3	T37.1X4	T37.1X5	T37.1X6
Diastase	T47.5X1	T47.5X2	T47.5X3	T47.5X4	T47.5X5	T47.5X6
Diatrizoate	T50.8X1	T50.8X2	T50.8X3	T50.8X4	T50.8X5	T50.8X6
Diazepam	T42.4X1	T42.4X2	T42.4X3	T42.4X4	T42.4X5	T42.4X6
Diazinon	T60.0X1	T60.0X2	T60.0X3	T60.0X4	—	—
Diazomethane (gas)	T59.891	T59.892	T59.893	T59.894	—	—
Diazoxide	T46.5X1	T46.5X2	T46.5X3	T46.5X4	T46.5X5	T46.5X6
Dibekacin	T36.5X1	T36.5X2	T36.5X3	T36.5X4	T36.5X5	T36.5X6

Substance	Poisoning, Accidental (unintentional)	Poisoning, Intentional Self-harm	Poisoning, Assault	Poisoning, Undetermined	Adverse Effect	Under-dosing
Dibenamine	T44.6X1	T44.6X2	T44.6X3	T44.6X4	T44.6X5	T44.6X6
Dibenzepin	T43.011	T43.012	T43.013	T43.014	T43.015	T43.016
Dibenzheptropine	T45.0X1	T45.0X2	T45.0X3	T45.0X4	T45.0X5	T45.0X6
Dibenzyline	T44.6X1	T44.6X2	T44.6X3	T44.6X4	T44.6X5	T44.6X6
Diborane (gas)	T59.891	T59.892	T59.893	T59.894	—	—
Dibromochloropropane	T60.8X1	T60.8X2	T60.8X3	T60.8X4	—	—
Dibromodulcitol	T45.1X1	T45.1X2	T45.1X3	T45.1X4	T45.1X5	T45.1X6
Dibromoethane	T53.6X1	T53.6X2	T53.6X3	T53.6X4	—	—
Dibromomannitol	T45.1X1	T45.1X2	T45.1X3	T45.1X4	T45.1X5	T45.1X6
Dibromopropamidine isethionate	T49.0X1	T49.0X2	T49.0X3	T49.0X4	T49.0X5	T49.0X6
Dibrompropamidine	T49.0X1	T49.0X2	T49.0X3	T49.0X4	T49.0X5	T49.0X6
Dibucaine	T41.3X1	T41.3X2	T41.3X3	T41.3X4	T41.3X5	T41.3X6
topical (surface)	T41.3X1	T41.3X2	T41.3X3	T41.3X4	T41.3X5	T41.3X6
Dibunate sodium	T48.3X1	T48.3X2	T48.3X3	T48.3X4	T48.3X5	T48.3X6
Dibutoline sulfate	T44.3X1	T44.3X2	T44.3X3	T44.3X4	T44.3X5	T44.3X6
Dicamba	T60.3X1	T60.3X2	T60.3X3	T60.3X4	—	—
Dicapthon	T60.0X1	T60.0X2	T60.0X3	T60.0X4	—	—
Dichlobenil	T60.3X1	T60.3X2	T60.3X3	T60.3X4	—	—
Dichlone	T60.3X1	T60.3X2	T60.3X3	T60.3X4	—	—
Dichloralphenozone	T42.6X1	T42.6X2	T42.6X3	T42.6X4	T42.6X5	T42.6X6
Dichlorbenzidine	T65.3X1	T65.3X2	T65.3X3	T65.3X4	—	—
Dichlorhydrin	T52.8X1	T52.8X2	T52.8X3	T52.8X4	—	—
Dichlorhydroxyquinoline	T37.8X1	T37.8X2	T37.8X3	T37.8X4	T37.8X5	T37.8X6
Dichlorobenzene	T53.7X1	T53.7X2	T53.7X3	T53.7X4	—	—
Dichlorobenzyl alcohol	T49.6X1	T49.6X2	T49.6X3	T49.6X4	T49.6X5	T49.6X6
Dichlorodifluoromethane	T53.5X1	T53.5X2	T53.5X3	T53.5X4	—	—
Dichloroethane	T52.8X1	T52.8X2	T52.8X3	T52.8X4	—	—
Dichloroethylene	T53.6X1	T53.6X2	T53.6X3	T53.6X4	—	—
Dichloroethyl sulfide, not in war	T59.891	T59.892	T59.893	T59.894	—	—
Dichloroformoxine, not in war	T59.891	T59.892	T59.893	T59.894	—	—
Dichlorohydrin, alpha-dichlorohydrin	T52.8X1	T52.8X2	T52.8X3	T52.8X4	—	—
Dichloromethane (solvent)	T53.4X1	T53.4X2	T53.4X3	T53.4X4	—	—
vapor	T53.4X1	T53.4X2	T53.4X3	T53.4X4	—	—
Dichloronaphthoquinone	T60.3X1	T60.3X2	T60.3X3	T60.3X4	—	—
Dichlorophen	T37.4X1	T37.4X2	T37.4X3	T37.4X4	T37.4X5	T37.4X6
Dichloropropene	T60.3X1	T60.3X2	T60.3X3	T60.3X4	—	—
Dichloropropionic acid	T60.3X1	T60.3X2	T60.3X3	T60.3X4	—	—
Dichlorphenamide	T50.2X1	T50.2X2	T50.2X3	T50.2X4	T50.2X5	T50.2X6
Dichlorvos	T60.0X1	T60.0X2	T60.0X3	T60.0X4	—	—
Diclofenac	T39.391	T39.392	T39.393	T39.394	T39.395	T39.396
Diclofenamide	T50.2X1	T50.2X2	T50.2X3	T50.2X4	T50.2X5	T50.2X6
Diclofensine	T43.291	T43.292	T43.293	T43.294	T43.295	T43.296
Diclonixine	T39.8X1	T39.8X2	T39.8X3	T39.8X4	T39.8X5	T39.8X6
Dicloxacillin	T36.0X1	T36.0X2	T36.0X3	T36.0X4	T36.0X5	T36.0X6
Dicophane	T49.0X1	T49.0X2	T49.0X3	T49.0X4	T49.0X5	T49.0X6
Dicoumarol, dicoumarin, dicumarol	T45.511	T45.512	T45.513	T45.514	T45.515	T45.516
Dicrotophos	T60.0X1	T60.0X2	T60.0X3	T60.0X4	—	—
Dicyanogen (gas)	T65.0X1	T65.0X2	T65.0X3	T65.0X4	—	—
Dicyclomine	T44.3X1	T44.3X2	T44.3X3	T44.3X4	T44.3X5	T44.3X6
Dicycloverine	T44.3X1	T44.3X2	T44.3X3	T44.3X4	T44.3X5	T44.3X6
Dideoxycytidine	T37.5X1	T37.5X2	T37.5X3	T37.5X4	T37.5X5	T37.5X6
Dideoxyinosine	T37.5X1	T37.5X2	T37.5X3	T37.5X4	T37.5X5	T37.5X6
Dieldrin (vapor)	T60.1X1	T60.1X2	T60.1X3	T60.1X4	—	—
Diemal	T42.3X1	T42.3X2	T42.3X3	T42.3X4	T42.3X5	T42.3X6
Dienestrol	T38.5X1	T38.5X2	T38.5X3	T38.5X4	T38.5X5	T38.5X6
Dienoestrol	T38.5X1	T38.5X2	T38.5X3	T38.5X4	T38.5X5	T38.5X6
Dietetic drug NEC	T50.901	T50.902	T50.903	T50.904	T50.905	T50.906
Diethazine	T42.8X1	T42.8X2	T42.8X3	T42.8X4	T42.8X5	T42.8X6
Diethyl						
barbituric acid	T42.3X1	T42.3X2	T42.3X3	T42.3X4	T42.3X5	T42.3X6
carbamazine	T37.4X1	T37.4X2	T37.4X3	T37.4X4	T37.4X5	T37.4X6
carbinol	T51.3X1	T51.3X2	T51.3X3	T51.3X4	—	—
carbonate	T52.8X1	T52.8X2	T52.8X3	T52.8X4	—	—
ether (vapor) — see also ether	T41.0X1	T41.0X2	T41.0X3	T41.0X4	T41.0X5	T41.0X6
oxide	T52.8X1	T52.8X2	T52.8X3	T52.8X4	—	—
propion	T50.5X1	T50.5X2	T50.5X3	T50.5X4	T50.5X5	T50.5X6
stilbestrol	T38.5X1	T38.5X2	T38.5X3	T38.5X4	T38.5X5	T38.5X6
toluamide (nonmedicinal)	T60.8X1	T60.8X2	T60.8X3	T60.8X4	—	—
medicinal	T49.3X1	T49.3X2	T49.3X3	T49.3X4	T49.3X5	T49.3X6
Diethylcarbamazine	T37.4X1	T37.4X2	T37.4X3	T37.4X4	T37.4X5	T37.4X6
Diethylene						
dioxide	T52.8X1	T52.8X2	T52.8X3	T52.8X4	—	—
glycol (monoacetate) (monobutyl ether) (monoethyl ether)	T52.3X1	T52.3X2	T52.3X3	T52.3X4	—	—
Diethylhexylphthalate	T65.891	T65.892	T65.893	T65.894	—	—
Diethylpropion	T50.5X1	T50.5X2	T50.5X3	T50.5X4	T50.5X5	T50.5X6
Diethylstilbestrol	T38.5X1	T38.5X2	T38.5X3	T38.5X4	T38.5X5	T38.5X6
Diethylstilboestrol	T38.5X1	T38.5X2	T38.5X3	T38.5X4	T38.5X5	T38.5X6
Diethylsulfone-diethylmethane	T42.6X1	T42.6X2	T42.6X3	T42.6X4	T42.6X5	T42.6X6
Diethyltoluamide	T49.0X1	T49.0X2	T49.0X3	T49.0X4	T49.0X5	T49.0X6
Diethyltryptamine (DET)	T40.991	T40.992	T40.993	T40.994	—	—
Difebarbamate	T42.3X1	T42.3X2	T42.3X3	T42.3X4	T42.3X5	T42.3X6
Difencloxazine	T40.2X1	T40.2X2	T40.2X3	T40.2X4	T40.2X5	T40.2X6
Difenidol	T45.0X1	T45.0X2	T45.0X3	T45.0X4	T45.0X5	T45.0X6
Difenoxin	T47.6X1	T47.6X2	T47.6X3	T47.6X4	T47.6X5	T47.6X6
Difetarsone	T37.3X1	T37.3X2	T37.3X3	T37.3X4	T37.3X5	T37.3X6
Diffusin	T45.3X1	T45.3X2	T45.3X3	T45.3X4	T45.3X5	T45.3X6
Diflorasone	T49.0X1	T49.0X2	T49.0X3	T49.0X4	T49.0X5	T49.0X6
Diflos	T44.0X1	T44.0X2	T44.0X3	T44.0X4	T44.0X5	T44.0X6
Diflubenzuron	T60.1X1	T60.1X2	T60.1X3	T60.1X4	—	—
Diflucortolone	T49.0X1	T49.0X2	T49.0X3	T49.0X4	T49.0X5	T49.0X6
Diflunisal	T39.091	T39.092	T39.093	T39.094	T39.095	T39.096
Difluoromethyldopa	T42.8X1	T42.8X2	T42.8X3	T42.8X4	T42.8X5	T42.8X6
Difluorophate	T44.0X1	T44.0X2	T44.0X3	T44.0X4	T44.0X5	T44.0X6
Digestant NEC	T47.5X1	T47.5X2	T47.5X3	T47.5X4	T47.5X5	T47.5X6
Digitalin (e)	T46.0X1	T46.0X2	T46.0X3	T46.0X4	T46.0X5	T46.0X6
Digitalis (leaf)(glycoside)	T46.0X1	T46.0X2	T46.0X3	T46.0X4	T46.0X5	T46.0X6
lanata	T46.0X1	T46.0X2	T46.0X3	T46.0X4	T46.0X5	T46.0X6
purpurea	T46.0X1	T46.0X2	T46.0X3	T46.0X4	T46.0X5	T46.0X6
Digitoxin	T46.0X1	T46.0X2	T46.0X3	T46.0X4	T46.0X5	T46.0X6
Digitoxose	T46.0X1	T46.0X2	T46.0X3	T46.0X4	T46.0X5	T46.0X6
Digoxin	T46.0X1	T46.0X2	T46.0X3	T46.0X4	T46.0X5	T46.0X6
Digoxine	T46.0X1	T46.0X2	T46.0X3	T46.0X4	T46.0X5	T46.0X6
Dihydralazine	T46.5X1	T46.5X2	T46.5X3	T46.5X4	T46.5X5	T46.5X6
Dihydrazine	T46.5X1	T46.5X2	T46.5X3	T46.5X4	T46.5X5	T46.5X6
Dihydrocodeine	T40.2X1	T40.2X2	T40.2X3	T40.2X4	T40.2X5	T40.2X6
Dihydrocodeinone	T40.2X1	T40.2X2	T40.2X3	T40.2X4	T40.2X5	T40.2X6
Dihydroergocornine	T46.7X1	T46.7X2	T46.7X3	T46.7X4	T46.7X5	T46.7X6
Dihydroergocristine (mesilate)	T46.7X1	T46.7X2	T46.7X3	T46.7X4	T46.7X5	T46.7X6
Dihydroergokryptine	T46.7X1	T46.7X2	T46.7X3	T46.7X4	T46.7X5	T46.7X6
Dihydroergotamine	T46.5X1	T46.5X2	T46.5X3	T46.5X4	T46.5X5	T46.5X6
Dihydroergotoxine	T46.7X1	T46.7X2	T46.7X3	T46.7X4	T46.7X5	T46.7X6
mesilate	T46.7X1	T46.7X2	T46.7X3	T46.7X4	T46.7X5	T46.7X6
Dihydrohydroxycodeinone	T40.2X1	T40.2X2	T40.2X3	T40.2X4	T40.2X5	T40.2X6
Dihydrohydroxymorphinone	T40.2X1	T40.2X2	T40.2X3	T40.2X4	T40.2X5	T40.2X6
Dihydroisocodeine	T40.2X1	T40.2X2	T40.2X3	T40.2X4	T40.2X5	T40.2X6
Dihydromorphine	T40.2X1	T40.2X2	T40.2X3	T40.2X4	—	—
Dihydromorphinone	T40.2X1	T40.2X2	T40.2X3	T40.2X4	T40.2X5	T40.2X6
Dihydrostreptomycin	T36.5X1	T36.5X2	T36.5X3	T36.5X4	T36.5X5	T36.5X6
Dihydrotachysterol	T45.2X1	T45.2X2	T45.2X3	T45.2X4	T45.2X5	T45.2X6
Dihydroxyaluminum aminoacetate	T47.1X1	T47.1X2	T47.1X3	T47.1X4	T47.1X5	T47.1X6
Dihydroxyaluminum sodium carbonate	T47.1X1	T47.1X2	T47.1X3	T47.1X4	T47.1X5	T47.1X6
Dihydroxyanthraquinone	T47.2X1	T47.2X2	T47.2X3	T47.2X4	T47.2X5	T47.2X6
Dihydroxycodeinone	T40.2X1	T40.2X2	T40.2X3	T40.2X4	T40.2X5	T40.2X6
Dihydroxypropyl theophylline	T50.2X1	T50.2X2	T50.2X3	T50.2X4	T50.2X5	T50.2X6
Diiodohydroxyquin	T37.8X1	T37.8X2	T37.8X3	T37.8X4	T37.8X5	T37.8X6
topical	T49.0X1	T49.0X2	T49.0X3	T49.0X4	T49.0X5	T49.0X6
Diiodohydroxyquinoline	T37.8X1	T37.8X2	T37.8X3	T37.8X4	T37.8X5	T37.8X6
Diiodotyrosine	T38.2X1	T38.2X2	T38.2X3	T38.2X4	T38.2X5	T38.2X6
Diisopromine	T44.3X1	T44.3X2	T44.3X3	T44.3X4	T44.3X5	T44.3X6
Diisopropylamine	T46.3X1	T46.3X2	T46.3X3	T46.3X4	T46.3X5	T46.3X6
Diisopropylfluorophosphonate	T44.0X1	T44.0X2	T44.0X3	T44.0X4	T44.0X5	T44.0X6
Dilantin	T42.0X1	T42.0X2	T42.0X3	T42.0X4	T42.0X5	T42.0X6
Dilaudid	T40.2X1	T40.2X2	T40.2X3	T40.2X4	T40.2X5	T40.2X6
Dilazep	T46.3X1	T46.3X2	T46.3X3	T46.3X4	T46.3X5	T46.3X6
Dill	T47.5X1	T47.5X2	T47.5X3	T47.5X4	T47.5X5	T47.5X6
Diloxanide	T37.3X1	T37.3X2	T37.3X3	T37.3X4	T37.3X5	T37.3X6
Diltiazem	T46.1X1	T46.1X2	T46.1X3	T46.1X4	T46.1X5	T46.1X6
Dimazole	T49.0X1	T49.0X2	T49.0X3	T49.0X4	T49.0X5	T49.0X6
Dimefline	T50.7X1	T50.7X2	T50.7X3	T50.7X4	T50.7X5	T50.7X6
Dimefox	T60.0X1	T60.0X2	T60.0X3	T60.0X4	—	—
Dimemorfan	T48.3X1	T48.3X2	T48.3X3	T48.3X4	T48.3X5	T48.3X6
Dimenhydrinate	T45.0X1	T45.0X2	T45.0X3	T45.0X4	T45.0X5	T45.0X6
Dimercaprol (British anti-lewisite)	T45.8X1	T45.8X2	T45.8X3	T45.8X4	T45.8X5	T45.8X6
Dimercaptopropanol	T45.8X1	T45.8X2	T45.8X3	T45.8X4	T45.8X5	T45.8X6
Dimestrol	T38.5X1	T38.5X2	T38.5X3	T38.5X4	T38.5X5	T38.5X6
Dimetane	T45.0X1	T45.0X2	T45.0X3	T45.0X4	T45.0X5	T45.0X6
Dimethicone	T47.1X1	T47.1X2	T47.1X3	T47.1X4	T47.1X5	T47.1X6
Dimethindene	T45.0X1	T45.0X2	T45.0X3	T45.0X4	T45.0X5	T45.0X6
Dimethisoquin	T49.1X1	T49.1X2	T49.1X3	T49.1X4	T49.1X5	T49.1X6
Dimethisterone	T38.5X1	T38.5X2	T38.5X3	T38.5X4	T38.5X5	T38.5X6
Dimethoate	T60.0X1	T60.0X2	T60.0X3	T60.0X4	—	—
Dimethocaine	T41.3X1	T41.3X2	T41.3X3	T41.3X4	T41.3X5	T41.3X6
Dimethoxanate	T48.3X1	T48.3X2	T48.3X3	T48.3X4	T48.3X5	T48.3X6

Additional Character May Be Required — Refer to the Tabular List for Character Selection

▽ Subterms under main terms may continue to next column or page

Substance	Poisoning, Accidental (unintentional)	Poisoning, Intentional Self-harm	Poisoning, Assault	Poisoning, Undetermined	Adverse Effect	Under-dosing
Dimethyl						
arsine, arsinic acid	T57.0X1	T57.0X2	T57.0X3	T57.0X4	—	—
carbinol	T51.2X1	T51.2X2	T51.2X3	T51.2X4	—	—
carbonate	T52.8X1	T52.8X2	T52.8X3	T52.8X4	—	—
diguanide	T38.3X1	T38.3X2	T38.3X3	T38.3X4	T38.3X5	T38.3X6
ketone	T52.4X1	T52.4X2	T52.4X3	T52.4X4	—	—
vapor	T52.4X1	T52.4X2	T52.4X3	T52.4X4	—	—
meperidine	T40.2X1	T40.2X2	T40.2X3	T40.2X4	T40.2X5	T40.2X6
parathion	T60.0X1	T60.0X2	T60.0X3	T60.0X4	—	—
phthlate	T49.3X1	T49.3X2	T49.3X3	T49.3X4	T49.3X5	T49.3X6
polysiloxane	T47.8X1	T47.8X2	T47.8X3	T47.8X4	T47.8X5	T47.8X6
sulfate (fumes)	T59.891	T59.892	T59.893	T59.894	—	—
liquid	T65.891	T65.892	T65.893	T65.894	—	—
sulfoxide (nonmedicinal)	T52.8X1	T52.8X2	T52.8X3	T52.8X4	—	—
medicinal	T49.4X1	T49.4X2	T49.4X3	T49.4X4	T49.4X5	T49.4X6
tryptamine	T40.991	T40.992	T40.993	T40.994	—	—
tubocurarine	T48.1X1	T48.1X2	T48.1X3	T48.1X4	T48.1X5	T48.1X6
Dimethylamine sulfate	T49.4X1	T49.4X2	T49.4X3	T49.4X4	T49.4X5	T49.4X6
Dimethylformamide	T52.8X1	T52.8X2	T52.8X3	T52.8X4	—	—
Dimethyltubocurarinium chloride	T48.1X1	T48.1X2	T48.1X3	T48.1X4	T48.1X5	T48.1X6
Dimeticone	T47.1X1	T47.1X2	T47.1X3	T47.1X4	T47.1X5	T47.1X6
Dimetilan	T60.0X1	T60.0X2	T60.0X3	T60.0X4	—	—
Dimetindene	T45.0X1	T45.0X2	T45.0X3	T45.0X4	T45.0X5	T45.0X6
Dimetotiazine	T43.3X1	T43.3X2	T43.3X3	T43.3X4	T43.3X5	T43.3X6
Dimorpholamine	T50.7X1	T50.7X2	T50.7X3	T50.7X4	T50.7X5	T50.7X6
Dimoxyline	T46.3X1	T46.3X2	T46.3X3	T46.3X4	T46.3X5	T46.3X6
Dinitrobenzene	T65.3X1	T65.3X2	T65.3X3	T65.3X4	—	—
vapor	T59.891	T59.892	T59.893	T59.894	—	—
Dinitrobenzol	T65.3X1	T65.3X2	T65.3X3	T65.3X4	—	—
vapor	T59.891	T59.892	T59.893	T59.894	—	—
Dinitrobutylphenol	T65.3X1	T65.3X2	T65.3X3	T65.3X4	—	—
Dinitro (-ortho-)cresol (pesticide) (spray)	T65.3X1	T65.3X2	T65.3X3	T65.3X4	—	—
Dinitrocyclohexylphenol	T65.3X1	T65.3X2	T65.3X3	T65.3X4	—	—
Dinitrophenol	T65.3X1	T65.3X2	T65.3X3	T65.3X4	—	—
Dinoprost	T48.0X1	T48.0X2	T48.0X3	T48.0X4	T48.0X5	T48.0X6
Dinoprostone	T48.0X1	T48.0X2	T48.0X3	T48.0X4	T48.0X5	T48.0X6
Dinoseb	T60.3X1	T60.3X2	T60.3X3	T60.3X4	—	—
Dioctyl sulfosuccinate (calcium) (sodium)	T47.4X1	T47.4X2	T47.4X3	T47.4X4	T47.4X5	T47.4X6
Diodone	T50.8X1	T50.8X2	T50.8X3	T50.8X4	T50.8X5	T50.8X6
Diodoquin	T37.8X1	T37.8X2	T37.8X3	T37.8X4	T37.8X5	T37.8X6
Dionin	T40.2X1	T40.2X2	T40.2X3	T40.2X4	T40.2X5	T40.2X6
Diosmin	T46.991	T46.992	T46.993	T46.994	T46.995	T46.996
Dioxane	T52.8X1	T52.8X2	T52.8X3	T52.8X4	—	—
Dioxathion	T60.0X1	T60.0X2	T60.0X3	T60.0X4	—	—
Dioxin	T53.7X1	T53.7X2	T53.7X3	T53.7X4	—	—
Dioxopromethazine	T43.3X1	T43.3X2	T43.3X3	T43.3X4	T43.3X5	T43.3X6
Dioxyline	T46.3X1	T46.3X2	T46.3X3	T46.3X4	T46.3X5	T46.3X6
Dipentene	T52.8X1	T52.8X2	T52.8X3	T52.8X4	—	—
Diperodon	T41.3X1	T41.3X2	T41.3X3	T41.3X4	T41.3X5	T41.3X6
Diphacinone	T60.4X1	T60.4X2	T60.4X3	T60.4X4	—	—
Diphemanil	T44.3X1	T44.3X2	T44.3X3	T44.3X4	T44.3X5	T44.3X6
metilsulfate	T44.3X1	T44.3X2	T44.3X3	T44.3X4	T44.3X5	T44.3X6
Diphenadione	T45.511	T45.512	T45.513	T45.514	T45.515	T45.516
rodenticide	T60.4X1	T60.4X2	T60.4X3	T60.4X4	—	—
Diphenhydramine	T45.0X1	T45.0X2	T45.0X3	T45.0X4	T45.0X5	T45.0X6
Diphenidol	T45.0X1	T45.0X2	T45.0X3	T45.0X4	T45.0X5	T45.0X6
Diphenoxylate	T47.6X1	T47.6X2	T47.6X3	T47.6X4	T47.6X5	T47.6X6
Diphenylamine	T65.3X1	T65.3X2	T65.3X3	T65.3X4	—	—
Diphenylbutazone	T39.2X1	T39.2X2	T39.2X3	T39.2X4	T39.2X5	T39.2X6
Diphenylchloroarsine, not in war	T57.0X1	T57.0X2	T57.0X3	T57.0X4	—	—
Diphenylhydantoin	T42.0X1	T42.0X2	T42.0X3	T42.0X4	T42.0X5	T42.0X6
Diphenylmethane dye	T52.1X1	T52.1X2	T52.1X3	T52.1X4	—	—
Diphenylpyraline	T45.0X1	T45.0X2	T45.0X3	T45.0X4	T45.0X5	T45.0X6
Diphtheria						
antitoxin	T50.Z11	T50.Z12	T50.Z13	T50.Z14	T50.Z15	T50.Z16
toxoid	T50.A91	T50.A92	T50.A93	T50.A94	T50.A95	T50.A96
with tetanus toxoid	T50.A21	T50.A22	T50.A23	T50.A24	T50.A25	T50.A26
with pertussis component	T50.A11	T50.A12	T50.A13	T50.A14	T50.A15	T50.A16
vaccine	T50.A91	T50.A92	T50.A93	T50.A94	T50.A95	T50.A96
combination						
without pertussis	T50.A21	T50.A22	T50.A23	T50.A24	T50.A25	T50.A26
including pertussis	T50.A11	T50.A12	T50.A13	T50.A14	T50.A15	T50.A16
Diphylline	T50.2X1	T50.2X2	T50.2X3	T50.2X4	T50.2X5	T50.2X6
Dipipanone	T40.4X1	T40.4X2	T40.4X3	T40.4X4	—	—
Dipivefrine	T49.5X1	T49.5X2	T49.5X3	T49.5X4	T49.5X5	T49.5X6
Diplovax	T50.B91	T50.B92	T50.B93	T50.B94	T50.B95	T50.B96
Diprophylline	T50.2X1	T50.2X2	T50.2X3	T50.2X4	T50.2X5	T50.2X6
Dipropyline	T48.291	T48.292	T48.293	T48.294	T48.295	T48.296
Dipyridamole	T46.3X1	T46.3X2	T46.3X3	T46.3X4	T46.3X5	T46.3X6
Dipyrone	T39.2X1	T39.2X2	T39.2X3	T39.2X4	T39.2X5	T39.2X6
Diquat (dibromide)	T60.3X1	T60.3X2	T60.3X3	T60.3X4	—	—
Disinfectant	T65.891	T65.892	T65.893	T65.894	—	—
alkaline	T54.3X1	T54.3X2	T54.3X3	T54.3X4	—	—
aromatic	T54.1X1	T54.1X2	T54.1X3	T54.1X4	—	—
intestinal	T37.8X1	T37.8X2	T37.8X3	T37.8X4	T37.8X5	T37.8X6
Disipal	T42.8X1	T42.8X2	T42.8X3	T42.8X4	T42.8X5	T42.8X6
Disodium edetate	T50.6X1	T50.6X2	T50.6X3	T50.6X4	T50.6X5	T50.6X6
Disoprofol	T41.291	T41.292	T41.293	T41.294	T41.295	T41.296
Disopyramide	T46.2X1	T46.2X2	T46.2X3	T46.2X4	T46.2X5	T46.2X6
Distigmine (bromide)	T44.0X1	T44.0X2	T44.0X3	T44.0X4	T44.0X5	T44.0X6
Disulfamide	T50.2X1	T50.2X2	T50.2X3	T50.2X4	T50.2X5	T50.2X6
Disulfanilamide	T37.0X1	T37.0X2	T37.0X3	T37.0X4	T37.0X5	T37.0X6
Disulfiram	T50.6X1	T50.6X2	T50.6X3	T50.6X4	T50.6X5	T50.6X6
Disulfoton	T60.0X1	T60.0X2	T60.0X3	T60.0X4	—	—
Dithiazanine iodide	T37.4X1	T37.4X2	T37.4X3	T37.4X4	T37.4X5	T37.4X6
Dithiocarbamate	T60.0X1	T60.0X2	T60.0X3	T60.0X4	—	—
Dithranol	T49.4X1	T49.4X2	T49.4X3	T49.4X4	T49.4X5	T49.4X6
Diucardin	T50.2X1	T50.2X2	T50.2X3	T50.2X4	T50.2X5	T50.2X6
Diupres	T50.2X1	T50.2X2	T50.2X3	T50.2X4	T50.2X5	T50.2X6
Diuretic NEC	T50.2X1	T50.2X2	T50.2X3	T50.2X4	T50.2X5	T50.2X6
benzothiadiazine	T50.2X1	T50.2X2	T50.2X3	T50.2X4	T50.2X5	T50.2X6
carbonic acid anhydrase inhibitors	T50.2X1	T50.2X2	T50.2X3	T50.2X4	T50.2X5	T50.2X6
furfuryl NEC	T50.2X1	T50.2X2	T50.2X3	T50.2X4	T50.2X5	T50.2X6
loop (high-ceiling)	T50.1X1	T50.1X2	T50.1X3	T50.1X4	T50.1X5	T50.1X6
mercurial NEC	T50.2X1	T50.2X2	T50.2X3	T50.2X4	T50.2X5	T50.2X6
osmotic	T50.2X1	T50.2X2	T50.2X3	T50.2X4	T50.2X5	T50.2X6
purine NEC	T50.2X1	T50.2X2	T50.2X3	T50.2X4	T50.2X5	T50.2X6
saluretic NEC	T50.2X1	T50.2X2	T50.2X3	T50.2X4	T50.2X5	T50.2X6
sulfonamide	T50.2X1	T50.2X2	T50.2X3	T50.2X4	T50.2X5	T50.2X6
thiazide NEC	T50.2X1	T50.2X2	T50.2X3	T50.2X4	T50.2X5	T50.2X6
xanthine	T50.2X1	T50.2X2	T50.2X3	T50.2X4	T50.2X5	T50.2X6
Diurgin	T50.2X1	T50.2X2	T50.2X3	T50.2X4	T50.2X5	T50.2X6
Diuril	T50.2X1	T50.2X2	T50.2X3	T50.2X4	T50.2X5	T50.2X6
Diuron	T60.3X1	T60.3X2	T60.3X3	T60.3X4	—	—
Divalproex	T42.6X1	T42.6X2	T42.6X3	T42.6X4	T42.6X5	T42.6X6
Divinyl ether	T41.0X1	T41.0X2	T41.0X3	T41.0X4	T41.0X5	T41.0X6
Dixanthogen	T49.0X1	T49.0X2	T49.0X3	T49.0X4	T49.0X5	T49.0X6
Dixyrazine	T43.3X1	T43.3X2	T43.3X3	T43.3X4	T43.3X5	T43.3X6
D-lysergic acid diethylamide	T40.8X1	T40.8X2	T40.8X3	T40.8X4	—	—
DMCT	T36.4X1	T36.4X2	T36.4X3	T36.4X4	T36.4X5	T36.4X6
DMSO — see Dimethyl sulfoxide						
DNBP	T60.3X1	T60.3X2	T60.3X3	T60.3X4	—	—
DNOC	T65.3X1	T65.3X2	T65.3X3	T65.3X4	—	—
Dobutamine	T44.5X1	T44.5X2	T44.5X3	T44.5X4	T44.5X5	T44.5X6
DOCA	T38.0X1	T38.0X2	T38.0X3	T38.0X4	T38.0X5	T38.0X6
Docusate sodium	T47.4X1	T47.4X2	T47.4X3	T47.4X4	T47.4X5	T47.4X6
Dodicin	T49.0X1	T49.0X2	T49.0X3	T49.0X4	T49.0X5	T49.0X6
Dofamium chloride	T49.0X1	T49.0X2	T49.0X3	T49.0X4	T49.0X5	T49.0X6
Dolophine	T40.3X1	T40.3X2	T40.3X3	T40.3X4	T40.3X5	T40.3X6
Doloxene	T39.8X1	T39.8X2	T39.8X3	T39.8X4	—	—
Domestic gas (after combustion) — see Gas, utility						
prior to combustion	T59.891	T59.892	T59.893	T59.894	—	—
Domiodol	T48.4X1	T48.4X2	T48.4X3	T48.4X4	T48.4X5	T48.4X6
Domiphen (bromide)	T49.0X1	T49.0X2	T49.0X3	T49.0X4	T49.0X5	T49.0X6
Domperidone	T45.0X1	T45.0X2	T45.0X3	T45.0X4	T45.0X5	T45.0X6
Dopa	T42.8X1	T42.8X2	T42.8X3	T42.8X4	T42.8X5	T42.8X6
Dopamine	T44.991	T44.992	T44.993	T44.994	T44.995	T44.996
Doriden	T42.6X1	T42.6X2	T42.6X3	T42.6X4	T42.6X5	T42.6X6
Dormiral	T42.3X1	T42.3X2	T42.3X3	T42.3X4	T42.3X5	T42.3X6
Dormison	T42.6X1	T42.6X2	T42.6X3	T42.6X4	T42.6X5	T42.6X6
Dornase	T48.4X1	T48.4X2	T48.4X3	T48.4X4	T48.4X5	T48.4X6
Dorsacaine	T41.3X1	T41.3X2	T41.3X3	T41.3X4	T41.3X5	T41.3X6
Dosulepin	T43.011	T43.012	T43.013	T43.014	T43.015	T43.016
Dothiepin	T43.011	T43.012	T43.013	T43.014	T43.015	T43.016
Doxantrazole	T48.6X1	T48.6X2	T48.6X3	T48.6X4	T48.6X5	T48.6X6
Doxapram	T50.7X1	T50.7X2	T50.7X3	T50.7X4	T50.7X5	T50.7X6
Doxazosin	T44.6X1	T44.6X2	T44.6X3	T44.6X4	T44.6X5	T44.6X6
Doxepin	T43.011	T43.012	T43.013	T43.014	T43.015	T43.016
Doxifluridine	T45.1X1	T45.1X2	T45.1X3	T45.1X4	T45.1X5	T45.1X6
Doxorubicin	T45.1X1	T45.1X2	T45.1X3	T45.1X4	T45.1X5	T45.1X6
Doxycycline	T36.4X1	T36.4X2	T36.4X3	T36.4X4	T36.4X5	T36.4X6
Doxylamine	T45.0X1	T45.0X2	T45.0X3	T45.0X4	T45.0X5	T45.0X6
Dramamine	T45.0X1	T45.0X2	T45.0X3	T45.0X4	T45.0X5	T45.0X6
Drano (drain cleaner)	T54.3X1	T54.3X2	T54.3X3	T54.3X4	—	—
Dressing, live pulp	T49.7X1	T49.7X2	T49.7X3	T49.7X4	T49.7X5	T49.7X6
Drocode	T40.2X1	T40.2X2	T40.2X3	T40.2X4	T40.2X5	T40.2X6
Dromoran	T40.2X1	T40.2X2	T40.2X3	T40.2X4	T40.2X5	T40.2X6
Dromostanolone	T38.7X1	T38.7X2	T38.7X3	T38.7X4	T38.7X5	T38.7X6

Substance	Poisoning, Accidental (unintentional)	Poisoning, Intentional Self-harm	Poisoning, Assault	Poisoning, Undetermined	Adverse Effect	Under-dosing
Dronabinol	T40.7X1	T40.7X2	T40.7X3	T40.7X4	T40.7X5	T40.7X6
Droperidol	T43.591	T43.592	T43.593	T43.594	T43.595	T43.596
Dropropizine	T48.3X1	T48.3X2	T48.3X3	T48.3X4	T48.3X5	T48.3X6
Drostanolone	T38.7X1	T38.7X2	T38.7X3	T38.7X4	T38.7X5	T38.7X6
Drotaverine	T44.3X1	T44.3X2	T44.3X3	T44.3X4	T44.3X5	T44.3X6
Drotrecogin alfa	T45.511	T45.512	T45.513	T45.514	T45.515	T45.516
Drug NEC	T50.901	T50.902	T50.903	T50.904	T50.905	T50.906
specified NEC	T50.991	T50.992	T50.993	T50.994	T50.995	T50.996
DTIC	T45.1X1	T45.1X2	T45.1X3	T45.1X4	T45.1X5	T45.1X6
Duboisine	T44.3X1	T44.3X2	T44.3X3	T44.3X4	T44.3X5	T44.3X6
Dulcolax	T47.2X1	T47.2X2	T47.2X3	T47.2X4	T47.2X5	T47.2X6
Duponol (C) (EP)	T49.2X1	T49.2X2	T49.2X3	T49.2X4	T49.2X5	T49.2X6
Durabolin	T38.7X1	T38.7X2	T38.7X3	T38.7X4	T38.7X5	T38.7X6
Dyclone	T41.3X1	T41.3X2	T41.3X3	T41.3X4	T41.3X5	T41.3X6
Dyclonine	T41.3X1	T41.3X2	T41.3X3	T41.3X4	T41.3X5	T41.3X6
Dydrogesterone	T38.5X1	T38.5X2	T38.5X3	T38.5X4	T38.5X5	T38.5X6
Dye NEC	T65.6X1	T65.6X2	T65.6X3	T65.6X4	—	—
antiseptic	T49.0X1	T49.0X2	T49.0X3	T49.0X4	T49.0X5	T49.0X6
diagnostic agents	T50.8X1	T50.8X2	T50.8X3	T50.8X4	T50.8X5	T50.8X6
pharmaceutical NEC	T50.901	T50.902	T50.903	T50.904	T50.905	T50.906
Dyflos	T44.0X1	T44.0X2	T44.0X3	T44.0X4	T44.0X5	T44.0X6
Dymelor	T38.3X1	T38.3X2	T38.3X3	T38.3X4	T38.3X5	T38.3X6
Dynamite	T65.3X1	T65.3X2	T65.3X3	T65.3X4	—	—
fumes	T59.891	T59.892	T59.893	T59.894	—	—
Dyphylline	T44.3X1	T44.3X2	T44.3X3	T44.3X4	T44.3X5	T44.3X6
b-eucaine	T49.1X1	T49.1X2	T49.1X3	T49.1X4	T49.1X5	T49.1X6
Ear drug NEC	T49.6X1	T49.6X2	T49.6X3	T49.6X4	T49.6X5	T49.6X6
Ear preparations	T49.6X1	T49.6X2	T49.6X3	T49.6X4	T49.6X5	T49.6X6
Echothiophate, echothiopate, ecothiopate	T49.5X1	T49.5X2	T49.5X3	T49.5X4	T49.5X5	T49.5X6
Econazole	T49.0X1	T49.0X2	T49.0X3	T49.0X4	T49.0X5	T49.0X6
Ecothiopate iodide	T49.5X1	T49.5X2	T49.5X3	T49.5X4	T49.5X5	T49.5X6
Ecstasy	T43.621	T43.622	T43.623	T43.624	T43.625	T43.626
Ectylurea	T42.6X1	T42.6X2	T42.6X3	T42.6X4	T42.6X5	T42.6X6
Edathamil disodium	T45.8X1	T45.8X2	T45.8X3	T45.8X4	T45.8X5	T45.8X6
Edecrin	T50.1X1	T50.1X2	T50.1X3	T50.1X4	T50.1X5	T50.1X6
Edetate, disodium (calcium)	T45.8X1	T45.8X2	T45.8X3	T45.8X4	T45.8X5	T45.8X6
Edoxudine	T49.5X1	T49.5X2	T49.5X3	T49.5X4	T49.5X5	T49.5X6
Edrophonium	T44.0X1	T44.0X2	T44.0X3	T44.0X4	T44.0X5	T44.0X6
chloride	T44.0X1	T44.0X2	T44.0X3	T44.0X4	T44.0X5	T44.0X6
EDTA	T50.6X1	T50.6X2	T50.6X3	T50.6X4	T50.6X5	T50.6X6
Eflornithine	T37.2X1	T37.2X2	T37.2X3	T37.2X4	T37.2X5	T37.2X6
Efloxate	T46.3X1	T46.3X2	T46.3X3	T46.3X4	T46.3X5	T46.3X6
Elase	T49.8X1	T49.8X2	T49.8X3	T49.8X4	T49.8X5	T49.8X6
Elastase	T45.7X1	T45.7X2	T45.7X3	T45.7X4	T45.7X5	T45.7X6
Elaterium	T47.2X1	T47.2X2	T47.2X3	T47.2X4	T47.2X5	T47.2X6
Elcatonin	T50.991	T50.992	T50.993	T50.994	T50.995	T50.996
Elder	T62.2X1	T62.2X2	T62.2X3	T62.2X4	—	—
berry, (unripe)	T62.1X1	T62.1X2	T62.1X3	T62.1X4	—	—
Electrolyte balance drug	T50.3X1	T50.3X2	T50.3X3	T50.3X4	T50.3X5	T50.3X6
Electrolytes NEC	T50.3X1	T50.3X2	T50.3X3	T50.3X4	T50.3X5	T50.3X6
Electrolytic agent NEC	T50.3X1	T50.3X2	T50.3X3	T50.3X4	T50.3X5	T50.3X6
Elemental diet	T50.901	T50.902	T50.903	T50.904	T50.905	T50.906
Elliptinium acetate	T45.1X1	T45.1X2	T45.1X3	T45.1X4	T45.1X5	T45.1X6
Embramine	T45.0X1	T45.0X2	T45.0X3	T45.0X4	T45.0X5	T45.0X6
Emepronium (salts)	T44.3X1	T44.3X2	T44.3X3	T44.3X4	T44.3X5	T44.3X6
bromide	T44.3X1	T44.3X2	T44.3X3	T44.3X4	T44.3X5	T44.3X6
Emetic NEC	T47.7X1	T47.7X2	T47.7X3	T47.7X4	T47.7X5	T47.7X6
Emetine	T37.3X1	T37.3X2	T37.3X3	T37.3X4	T37.3X5	T37.3X6
Emollient NEC	T49.3X1	T49.3X2	T49.3X3	T49.3X4	T49.3X5	T49.3X6
Emorfazone	T39.8X1	T39.8X2	T39.8X3	T39.8X4	T39.8X5	T39.8X6
Emylcamate	T43.591	T43.592	T43.593	T43.594	T43.595	T43.596
Enalapril	T46.4X1	T46.4X2	T46.4X3	T46.4X4	T46.4X5	T46.4X6
Enalaprilat	T46.4X1	T46.4X2	T46.4X3	T46.4X4	T46.4X5	T46.4X6
Encainide	T46.2X1	T46.2X2	T46.2X3	T46.2X4	T46.2X5	T46.2X6
Endocaine	T41.3X1	T41.3X2	T41.3X3	T41.3X4	T41.3X5	T41.3X6
Endosulfan	T60.2X1	T60.2X2	T60.2X3	T60.2X4	—	—
Endothall	T60.3X1	T60.3X2	T60.3X3	T60.3X4	—	—
Endralazine	T46.5X1	T46.5X2	T46.5X3	T46.5X4	T46.5X5	T46.5X6
Endrin	T60.1X1	T60.1X2	T60.1X3	T60.1X4	—	—
Enflurane	T41.0X1	T41.0X2	T41.0X3	T41.0X4	T41.0X5	T41.0X6
Enhexymal	T42.3X1	T42.3X2	T42.3X3	T42.3X4	T42.3X5	T42.3X6
Enocitabine	T45.1X1	T45.1X2	T45.1X3	T45.1X4	T45.1X5	T45.1X6
Enovid	T38.4X1	T38.4X2	T38.4X3	T38.4X4	T38.4X5	T38.4X6
Enoxacin	T36.8X1	T36.8X2	T36.8X3	T36.8X4	T36.8X5	T36.8X6
Enoxaparin (sodium)	T45.511	T45.512	T45.513	T45.514	T45.515	T45.516
Enpiprazole	T43.591	T43.592	T43.593	T43.594	T43.595	T43.596
Enprofylline	T48.6X1	T48.6X2	T48.6X3	T48.6X4	T48.6X5	T48.6X6
Enprostil	T47.1X1	T47.1X2	T47.1X3	T47.1X4	T47.1X5	T47.1X6
Enterogastrone	T38.891	T38.892	T38.893	T38.894	T38.895	T38.896
ENT preparations (anti-infectives)	T49.6X1	T49.6X2	T49.6X3	T49.6X4	T49.6X5	T49.6X6
Enviomycin	T36.8X1	T36.8X2	T36.8X3	T36.8X4	T36.8X5	T36.8X6
Enzodase	T45.3X1	T45.3X2	T45.3X3	T45.3X4	T45.3X5	T45.3X6
Enzyme NEC	T45.3X1	T45.3X2	T45.3X3	T45.3X4	T45.3X5	T45.3X6
depolymerizing	T49.8X1	T49.8X2	T49.8X3	T49.8X4	T49.8X5	T49.8X6
fibrolytic	T45.3X1	T45.3X2	T45.3X3	T45.3X4	T45.3X5	T45.3X6
gastric	T47.5X1	T47.5X2	T47.5X3	T47.5X4	T47.5X5	T47.5X6
intestinal	T47.5X1	T47.5X2	T47.5X3	T47.5X4	T47.5X5	T47.5X6
local action	T49.4X1	T49.4X2	T49.4X3	T49.4X4	T49.4X5	T49.4X6
proteolytic	T45.3X1	T45.3X2	T45.3X3	T45.3X4	T45.3X5	T45.3X6
thrombolytic	T45.3X1	T45.3X2	T45.3X3	T45.3X4	T45.3X5	T45.3X6
EPAB	T41.3X1	T41.3X2	T41.3X3	T41.3X4	T41.3X5	T41.3X6
Epanutin	T42.0X1	T42.0X2	T42.0X3	T42.0X4	T42.0X5	T42.0X6
Ephedra	T44.991	T44.992	T44.993	T44.994	T44.995	T44.996
Ephedrine	T44.991	T44.992	T44.993	T44.994	T44.995	T44.996
Epichlorhydrin, epichlorohydrin	T52.8X1	T52.8X2	T52.8X3	T52.8X4	—	—
Epicillin	T36.0X1	T36.0X2	T36.0X3	T36.0X4	T36.0X5	T36.0X6
Epiestriol	T38.5X1	T38.5X2	T38.5X3	T38.5X4	T38.5X5	T38.5X6
Epilim — see Sodium valproate						
Epimestrol	T38.5X1	T38.5X2	T38.5X3	T38.5X4	T38.5X5	T38.5X6
Epinephrine	T44.5X1	T44.5X2	T44.5X3	T44.5X4	T44.5X5	T44.5X6
Epirubicin	T45.1X1	T45.1X2	T45.1X3	T45.1X4	T45.1X5	T45.1X6
Epitiostanol	T38.7X1	T38.7X2	T38.7X3	T38.7X4	T38.7X5	T38.7X6
Epitizide	T50.2X1	T50.2X2	T50.2X3	T50.2X4	T50.2X5	T50.2X6
EPN	T60.0X1	T60.0X2	T60.0X3	T60.0X4	—	—
EPO	T45.8X1	T45.8X2	T45.8X3	T45.8X4	T45.8X5	T45.8X6
Epoetin alpha	T45.8X1	T45.8X2	T45.8X3	T45.8X4	T45.8X5	T45.8X6
Epomediol	T50.991	T50.992	T50.993	T50.994	T50.995	T50.996
Epoprostenol	T45.521	T45.522	T45.523	T45.524	T45.525	T45.526
Epoxy resin	T65.891	T65.892	T65.893	T65.894	—	—
Eprazinone	T48.4X1	T48.4X2	T48.4X3	T48.4X4	T48.4X5	T48.4X6
Epsilon aminocaproic acid	T45.621	T45.622	T45.623	T45.624	T45.625	T45.626
Epsom salt	T47.3X1	T47.3X2	T47.3X3	T47.3X4	T47.3X5	T47.3X6
Eptazocine	T40.4X1	T40.4X2	T40.4X3	T40.4X4	T40.4X5	T40.4X6
Equanil	T43.591	T43.592	T43.593	T43.594	T43.595	T43.596
Equisetum	T62.2X1	T62.2X2	T62.2X3	T62.2X4	—	—
diuretic	T50.2X1	T50.2X2	T50.2X3	T50.2X4	T50.2X5	T50.2X6
Ergobasine	T48.0X1	T48.0X2	T48.0X3	T48.0X4	T48.0X5	T48.0X6
Ergocalciferol	T45.2X1	T45.2X2	T45.2X3	T45.2X4	T45.2X5	T45.2X6
Ergoloid mesylates	T46.7X1	T46.7X2	T46.7X3	T46.7X4	T46.7X5	T46.7X6
Ergometrine	T48.0X1	T48.0X2	T48.0X3	T48.0X4	T48.0X5	T48.0X6
Ergonovine	T48.0X1	T48.0X2	T48.0X3	T48.0X4	T48.0X5	T48.0X6
Ergotamine	T46.5X1	T46.5X2	T46.5X3	T46.5X4	T46.5X5	T46.5X6
Ergotocine	T48.0X1	T48.0X2	T48.0X3	T48.0X4	T48.0X5	T48.0X6
Ergotrate	T48.0X1	T48.0X2	T48.0X3	T48.0X4	T48.0X5	T48.0X6
Ergot NEC	T64.81	T64.82	T64.83	T64.84	—	—
derivative	T48.0X1	T48.0X2	T48.0X3	T48.0X4	T48.0X5	T48.0X6
medicinal (alkaloids)	T48.0X1	T48.0X2	T48.0X3	T48.0X4	T48.0X5	T48.0X6
prepared	T48.0X1	T48.0X2	T48.0X3	T48.0X4	T48.0X5	T48.0X6
Eritrityl tetranitrate	T46.3X1	T46.3X2	T46.3X3	T46.3X4	T46.3X5	T46.3X6
Erythrityl tetranitrate	T46.3X1	T46.3X2	T46.3X3	T46.3X4	T46.3X5	T46.3X6
Erythrol tetranitrate	T46.3X1	T46.3X2	T46.3X3	T46.3X4	T46.3X5	T46.3X6
Erythromycin (salts)	T36.3X1	T36.3X2	T36.3X3	T36.3X4	T36.3X5	T36.3X6
ophthalmic preparation	T49.5X1	T49.5X2	T49.5X3	T49.5X4	T49.5X5	T49.5X6
topical NEC	T49.0X1	T49.0X2	T49.0X3	T49.0X4	T49.0X5	T49.0X6
Erythropoietin	T45.8X1	T45.8X2	T45.8X3	T45.8X4	T45.8X5	T45.8X6
human	T45.8X1	T45.8X2	T45.8X3	T45.8X4	T45.8X5	T45.8X6
Escin	T46.991	T46.992	T46.993	T46.994	T46.995	T46.996
Esculin	T45.2X1	T45.2X2	T45.2X3	T45.2X4	T45.2X5	T45.2X6
Esculoside	T45.2X1	T45.2X2	T45.2X3	T45.2X4	T45.2X5	T45.2X6
ESDT (ether-soluble tar distillate)	T49.1X1	T49.1X2	T49.1X3	T49.1X4	T49.1X5	T49.1X6
Eserine	T49.5X1	T49.5X2	T49.5X3	T49.5X4	T49.5X5	T49.5X6
Esflurbiprofen	T39.311	T39.312	T39.313	T39.314	T39.315	T39.316
Eskabarb	T42.3X1	T42.3X2	T42.3X3	T42.3X4	T42.3X5	T42.3X6
Eskalith	T43.8X1	T43.8X2	T43.8X3	T43.8X4	T43.8X5	T43.8X6
Esmolol	T44.7X1	T44.7X2	T44.7X3	T44.7X4	T44.7X5	T44.7X6
Estanozolol	T38.7X1	T38.7X2	T38.7X3	T38.7X4	T38.7X5	T38.7X6
Estazolam	T42.4X1	T42.4X2	T42.4X3	T42.4X4	T42.4X5	T42.4X6
Estradiol	T38.5X1	T38.5X2	T38.5X3	T38.5X4	T38.5X5	T38.5X6
with testosterone	T38.7X1	T38.7X2	T38.7X3	T38.7X4	T38.7X5	T38.7X6
benzoate	T38.5X1	T38.5X2	T38.5X3	T38.5X4	T38.5X5	T38.5X6
Estramustine	T45.1X1	T45.1X2	T45.1X3	T45.1X4	T45.1X5	T45.1X6
Estriol	T38.5X1	T38.5X2	T38.5X3	T38.5X4	T38.5X5	T38.5X6
Estrogen	T38.5X1	T38.5X2	T38.5X3	T38.5X4	T38.5X5	T38.5X6
with progesterone	T38.5X1	T38.5X2	T38.5X3	T38.5X4	T38.5X5	T38.5X6
conjugated	T38.5X1	T38.5X2	T38.5X3	T38.5X4	T38.5X5	T38.5X6
Estrone	T38.5X1	T38.5X2	T38.5X3	T38.5X4	T38.5X5	T38.5X6
Estropipate	T38.5X1	T38.5X2	T38.5X3	T38.5X4	T38.5X5	T38.5X6
Etacrynate sodium	T50.1X1	T50.1X2	T50.1X3	T50.1X4	T50.1X5	T50.1X6
Etacrynic acid	T50.1X1	T50.1X2	T50.1X3	T50.1X4	T50.1X5	T50.1X6
Etafedrine	T48.6X1	T48.6X2	T48.6X3	T48.6X4	T48.6X5	T48.6X6
Etafenone	T46.3X1	T46.3X2	T46.3X3	T46.3X4	T46.3X5	T46.3X6
Etambutol	T37.1X1	T37.1X2	T37.1X3	T37.1X4	T37.1X5	T37.1X6

366

Additional Character May Be Required — Refer to the Tabular List for Character Selection   ▽ Subterms under main terms may continue to next column or page

Substance	Poisoning, Accidental (unintentional)	Poisoning, Intentional Self-harm	Poisoning, Assault	Poisoning, Undetermined	Adverse Effect	Under-dosing
Etamiphyllin	T48.6X1	T48.6X2	T48.6X3	T48.6X4	T48.6X5	T48.6X6
Etamivan	T50.7X1	T50.7X2	T50.7X3	T50.7X4	T50.7X5	T50.7X6
Etamsylate	T45.7X1	T45.7X2	T45.7X3	T45.7X4	T45.7X5	T45.7X6
Etebenecid	T50.4X1	T50.4X2	T50.4X3	T50.4X4	T50.4X5	T50.4X6
Ethacridine	T49.0X1	T49.0X2	T49.0X3	T49.0X4	T49.0X5	T49.0X6
Ethacrynic acid	T50.1X1	T50.1X2	T50.1X3	T50.1X4	T50.1X5	T50.1X6
Ethadione	T42.2X1	T42.2X2	T42.2X3	T42.2X4	T42.2X5	T42.2X6
Ethambutol	T37.1X1	T37.1X2	T37.1X3	T37.1X4	T37.1X5	T37.1X6
Ethamide	T50.2X1	T50.2X2	T50.2X3	T50.2X4	T50.2X5	T50.2X6
Ethamivan	T50.7X1	T50.7X2	T50.7X3	T50.7X4	T50.7X5	T50.7X6
Ethamsylate	T45.7X1	T45.7X2	T45.7X3	T45.7X4	T45.7X5	T45.7X6
Ethanol	T51.0X1	T51.0X2	T51.0X3	T51.0X4	—	—
beverage	T51.0X1	T51.0X2	T51.0X3	T51.0X4	—	—
Ethanolamine oleate	T46.8X1	T46.8X2	T46.8X3	T46.8X4	T46.8X5	T46.8X6
Ethaverine	T44.3X1	T44.3X2	T44.3X3	T44.3X4	T44.3X5	T44.3X6
Ethchlorvynol	T42.6X1	T42.6X2	T42.6X3	T42.6X4	T42.6X5	T42.6X6
Ethebenecid	T50.4X1	T50.4X2	T50.4X3	T50.4X4	T50.4X5	T50.4X6
Ether (vapor)	T41.0X1	T41.0X2	T41.0X3	T41.0X4	T41.0X5	T41.0X6
anesthetic	T41.0X1	T41.0X2	T41.0X3	T41.0X4	T41.0X5	T41.0X6
divinyl	T41.0X1	T41.0X2	T41.0X3	T41.0X4	T41.0X5	T41.0X6
ethyl (medicinal)	T41.0X1	T41.0X2	T41.0X3	T41.0X4	T41.0X5	T41.0X6
nonmedicinal	T52.8X1	T52.8X2	T52.8X3	T52.8X4	—	—
petroleum — see Ligroin						
solvent	T52.8X1	T52.8X2	T52.8X3	T52.8X4	—	—
Ethiazide	T50.2X1	T50.2X2	T50.2X3	T50.2X4	T50.2X5	T50.2X6
Ethidium chloride (vapor)	T59.891	T59.892	T59.893	T59.894		
Ethinamate	T42.6X1	T42.6X2	T42.6X3	T42.6X4	T42.6X5	T42.6X6
Ethinylestradiol, ethinyloestradiol	T38.5X1	T38.5X2	T38.5X3	T38.5X4	T38.5X5	T38.5X6
with						
levonorgestrel	T38.4X1	T38.4X2	T38.4X3	T38.4X4	T38.4X5	T38.4X6
norethisterone	T38.4X1	T38.4X2	T38.4X3	T38.4X4	T38.4X5	T38.4X6
Ethiodized oil (131 I)	T50.8X1	T50.8X2	T50.8X3	T50.8X4	T50.8X5	T50.8X6
Ethion	T60.0X1	T60.0X2	T60.0X3	T60.0X4	—	—
Ethionamide	T37.1X1	T37.1X2	T37.1X3	T37.1X4	T37.1X5	T37.1X6
Ethioniamide	T37.1X1	T37.1X2	T37.1X3	T37.1X4	T37.1X5	T37.1X6
Ethisterone	T38.5X1	T38.5X2	T38.5X3	T38.5X4	T38.5X5	T38.5X6
Ethobral	T42.3X1	T42.3X2	T42.3X3	T42.3X4	T42.3X5	T42.3X6
Ethocaine (infiltration) (topical)	T41.3X1	T41.3X2	T41.3X3	T41.3X4	T41.3X5	T41.3X6
nerve block (peripheral) (plexus)	T41.3X1	T41.3X2	T41.3X3	T41.3X4	T41.3X5	T41.3X6
spinal	T41.3X1	T41.3X2	T41.3X3	T41.3X4	T41.3X5	T41.3X6
Ethoheptazine	T40.4X1	T40.4X2	T40.4X3	T40.4X4	T40.4X5	T40.4X6
Ethopropazine	T44.3X1	T44.3X2	T44.3X3	T44.3X4	T44.3X5	T44.3X6
Ethosuximide	T42.2X1	T42.2X2	T42.2X3	T42.2X4	T42.2X5	T42.2X6
Ethotoin	T42.0X1	T42.0X2	T42.0X3	T42.0X4	T42.0X5	T42.0X6
Ethoxazene	T37.91	T37.92	T37.93	T37.94	T37.95	T37.96
Ethoxazorutoside	T46.991	T46.992	T46.993	T46.994	T46.995	T46.996
Ethoxzolamide	T50.2X1	T50.2X2	T50.2X3	T50.2X4	T50.2X5	T50.2X6
Ethyl						
acetate	T52.8X1	T52.8X2	T52.8X3	T52.8X4	—	—
alcohol	T51.0X1	T51.0X2	T51.0X3	T51.0X4	—	—
beverage	T51.0X1	T51.0X2	T51.0X3	T51.0X4	—	—
aldehyde (vapor)	T59.891	T59.892	T59.893	T59.894	—	—
liquid	T52.8X1	T52.8X2	T52.8X3	T52.8X4	—	—
aminobenzoate	T41.3X1	T41.3X2	T41.3X3	T41.3X4	T41.3X5	T41.3X6
aminophenothiazine	T43.3X1	T43.3X2	T43.3X3	T43.3X4	T43.3X5	T43.3X6
benzoate	T52.8X1	T52.8X2	T52.8X3	T52.8X4	—	—
biscoumacetate	T45.511	T45.512	T45.513	T45.514	T45.515	T45.516
bromide (anesthetic)	T41.0X1	T41.0X2	T41.0X3	T41.0X4	T41.0X5	T41.0X6
carbamate	T45.1X1	T45.1X2	T45.1X3	T45.1X4	T45.1X5	T45.1X6
carbinol	T51.3X1	T51.3X2	T51.3X3	T51.3X4	—	—
carbonate	T52.8X1	T52.8X2	T52.8X3	T52.8X4	—	—
chaulmoograte	T37.1X1	T37.1X2	T37.1X3	T37.1X4	T37.1X5	T37.1X6
chloride (anesthetic)	T41.0X1	T41.0X2	T41.0X3	T41.0X4	T41.0X5	T41.0X6
anesthetic (local)	T41.3X1	T41.3X2	T41.3X3	T41.3X4	T41.3X5	T41.3X6
inhaled	T41.0X1	T41.0X2	T41.0X3	T41.0X4	T41.0X5	T41.0X6
local	T49.4X1	T49.4X2	T49.4X3	T49.4X4	T49.4X5	T49.4X6
solvent	T53.6X1	T53.6X2	T53.6X3	T53.6X4	—	—
dibunate	T48.3X1	T48.3X2	T48.3X3	T48.3X4	T48.3X5	T48.3X6
dichloroarsine (vapor)	T57.0X1	T57.0X2	T57.0X3	T57.0X4	—	—
estranol	T38.7X1	T38.7X2	T38.7X3	T38.7X4	T38.7X5	T38.7X6
ether — see also ether	T52.8X1	T52.8X2	T52.8X3	T52.8X4	—	—
formate NEC (solvent)	T52.0X1	T52.0X2	T52.0X3	T52.0X4	—	—
fumarate	T49.4X1	T49.4X2	T49.4X3	T49.4X4	T49.4X5	T49.4X6
hydroxyisobutyrate NEC (solvent)	T52.8X1	T52.8X2	T52.8X3	T52.8X4	—	—
iodoacetate	T59.3X1	T59.3X2	T59.3X3	T59.3X4	—	—
lactate NEC (solvent)	T52.8X1	T52.8X2	T52.8X3	T52.8X4	—	—
loflazepate	T42.4X1	T42.4X2	T42.4X3	T42.4X4	T42.4X5	T42.4X6
mercuric chloride	T56.1X1	T56.1X2	T56.1X3	T56.1X4	—	—
methylcarbinol	T51.8X1	T51.8X2	T51.8X3	T51.8X4	—	—
Ethyl — continued						
morphine	T40.2X1	T40.2X2	T40.2X3	T40.2X4	T40.2X5	T40.2X6
noradrenaline	T48.6X1	T48.6X2	T48.6X3	T48.6X4	T48.6X5	T48.6X6
oxybutyrate NEC (solvent)	T52.8X1	T52.8X2	T52.8X3	T52.8X4	—	—
Ethylene (gas)	T59.891	T59.892	T59.893	T59.894		
anesthetic (general)	T41.0X1	T41.0X2	T41.0X3	T41.0X4	T41.0X5	T41.0X6
chlorohydrin	T52.8X1	T52.8X2	T52.8X3	T52.8X4	—	—
vapor	T53.6X1	T53.6X2	T53.6X3	T53.6X4	—	—
dichloride	T52.8X1	T52.8X2	T52.8X3	T52.8X4	—	—
vapor	T53.6X1	T53.6X2	T53.6X3	T53.6X4	—	—
dinitrate	T52.3X1	T52.3X2	T52.3X3	T52.3X4	—	—
glycol(s)	T52.8X1	T52.8X2	T52.8X3	T52.8X4	—	—
dinitrate	T52.3X1	T52.3X2	T52.3X3	T52.3X4	—	—
monobutyl ether	T52.3X1	T52.3X2	T52.3X3	T52.3X4	—	—
imine	T54.1X1	T54.1X2	T54.1X3	T54.1X4	—	—
oxide (fumigant) (nonmedicinal)	T59.891	T59.892	T59.893	T59.894	—	—
medicinal	T49.0X1	T49.0X2	T49.0X3	T49.0X4	T49.0X5	T49.0X6
Ethylenediaminetetra-acetic acid	T50.6X1	T50.6X2	T50.6X3	T50.6X4	T50.6X5	T50.6X6
Ethylenediamine theophylline	T48.6X1	T48.6X2	T48.6X3	T48.6X4	T48.6X5	T48.6X6
Ethylenedinitrilotetra-acetate	T50.6X1	T50.6X2	T50.6X3	T50.6X4	T50.6X5	T50.6X6
Ethylestrenol	T38.7X1	T38.7X2	T38.7X3	T38.7X4	T38.7X5	T38.7X6
Ethylhydroxycellulose	T47.4X1	T47.4X2	T47.4X3	T47.4X4	T47.4X5	T47.4X6
Ethylidene						
chloride NEC	T53.6X1	T53.6X2	T53.6X3	T53.6X4	—	—
diacetate	T60.3X1	T60.3X2	T60.3X3	T60.3X4	—	—
dicoumarin	T45.511	T45.512	T45.513	T45.514	T45.515	T45.516
dicoumarol	T45.511	T45.512	T45.513	T45.514	T45.515	T45.516
diethyl ether	T52.0X1	T52.0X2	T52.0X3	T52.0X4	—	—
Ethylmorphine	T40.2X1	T40.2X2	T40.2X3	T40.2X4	T40.2X5	T40.2X6
Ethylnorepinephrine	T48.6X1	T48.6X2	T48.6X3	T48.6X4	T48.6X5	T48.6X6
Ethylparachlorophen-oxyisobutyrate	T46.6X1	T46.6X2	T46.6X3	T46.6X4	T46.6X5	T46.6X6
Ethynodiol	T38.4X1	T38.4X2	T38.4X3	T38.4X4	T38.4X5	T38.4X6
with mestranol diacetate	T38.4X1	T38.4X2	T38.4X3	T38.4X4	T38.4X5	T38.4X6
Etidocaine	T41.3X1	T41.3X2	T41.3X3	T41.3X4	T41.3X5	T41.3X6
infiltration (subcutaneous)	T41.3X1	T41.3X2	T41.3X3	T41.3X4	T41.3X5	T41.3X6
nerve (peripheral) (plexus)	T41.3X1	T41.3X2	T41.3X3	T41.3X4	T41.3X5	T41.3X6
Etidronate	T50.991	T50.992	T50.993	T50.994	T50.995	T50.996
Etidronic acid (disodium salt)	T50.991	T50.992	T50.993	T50.994	T50.995	T50.996
Etifoxine	T42.6X1	T42.6X2	T42.6X3	T42.6X4	T42.6X5	T42.6X6
Etilefrine	T44.4X1	T44.4X2	T44.4X3	T44.4X4	T44.4X5	T44.4X6
Etilfen	T42.3X1	T42.3X2	T42.3X3	T42.3X4	T42.3X5	T42.3X6
Etinodiol	T38.4X1	T38.4X2	T38.4X3	T38.4X4	T38.4X5	T38.4X6
Etiroxate	T46.6X1	T46.6X2	T46.6X3	T46.6X4	T46.6X5	T46.6X6
Etizolam	T42.4X1	T42.4X2	T42.4X3	T42.4X4	T42.4X5	T42.4X6
Etodolac	T39.391	T39.392	T39.393	T39.394	T39.395	T39.396
Etofamide	T37.3X1	T37.3X2	T37.3X3	T37.3X4	T37.3X5	T37.3X6
Etofibrate	T46.6X1	T46.6X2	T46.6X3	T46.6X4	T46.6X5	T46.6X6
Etofylline	T46.7X1	T46.7X2	T46.7X3	T46.7X4	T46.7X5	T46.7X6
clofibrate	T46.6X1	T46.6X2	T46.6X3	T46.6X4	T46.6X5	T46.6X6
Etoglucid	T45.1X1	T45.1X2	T45.1X3	T45.1X4	T45.1X5	T45.1X6
Etomidate	T41.1X1	T41.1X2	T41.1X3	T41.1X4	T41.1X5	T41.1X6
Etomide	T39.8X1	T39.8X2	T39.8X3	T39.8X4	T39.8X5	T39.8X6
Etomidoline	T44.3X1	T44.3X2	T44.3X3	T44.3X4	T44.3X5	T44.3X6
Etoposide	T45.1X1	T45.1X2	T45.1X3	T45.1X4	T45.1X5	T45.1X6
Etorphine	T40.2X1	T40.2X2	T40.2X3	T40.2X4	T40.2X5	T40.2X6
Etoval	T42.3X1	T42.3X2	T42.3X3	T42.3X4	T42.3X5	T42.3X6
Etozolin	T50.1X1	T50.1X2	T50.1X3	T50.1X4	T50.1X5	T50.1X6
Etretinate	T50.991	T50.992	T50.993	T50.994	T50.995	T50.996
Etryptamine	T43.691	T43.692	T43.693	T43.694	T43.695	T43.696
Etybenzatropine	T44.3X1	T44.3X2	T44.3X3	T44.3X4	T44.3X5	T44.3X6
Etynodiol	T38.4X1	T38.4X2	T38.4X3	T38.4X4	T38.4X5	T38.4X6
Eucaine	T41.3X1	T41.3X2	T41.3X3	T41.3X4	T41.3X5	T41.3X6
Eucalyptus oil	T49.7X1	T49.7X2	T49.7X3	T49.7X4	T49.7X5	T49.7X6
Eucatropine	T49.5X1	T49.5X2	T49.5X3	T49.5X4	T49.5X5	T49.5X6
Eucodal	T40.2X1	T40.2X2	T40.2X3	T40.2X4	T40.2X5	T40.2X6
Euneryl	T42.3X1	T42.3X2	T42.3X3	T42.3X4	T42.3X5	T42.3X6
Euphthalmine	T44.3X1	T44.3X2	T44.3X3	T44.3X4	T44.3X5	T44.3X6
Eurax	T49.0X1	T49.0X2	T49.0X3	T49.0X4	T49.0X5	T49.0X6
Euresol	T49.4X1	T49.4X2	T49.4X3	T49.4X4	T49.4X5	T49.4X6
Euthroid	T38.1X1	T38.1X2	T38.1X3	T38.1X4	T38.1X5	T38.1X6
Evans blue	T50.8X1	T50.8X2	T50.8X3	T50.8X4	T50.8X5	T50.8X6
Evipal	T42.3X1	T42.3X2	T42.3X3	T42.3X4	T42.3X5	T42.3X6
sodium	T41.1X1	T41.1X2	T41.1X3	T41.1X4	T41.1X5	T41.1X6
Evipan	T42.3X1	T42.3X2	T42.3X3	T42.3X4	T42.3X5	T42.3X6
sodium	T41.1X1	T41.1X2	T41.1X3	T41.1X4	T41.1X5	T41.1X6
Exalamide	T49.0X1	T49.0X2	T49.0X3	T49.0X4	T49.0X5	T49.0X6
Exalgin	T39.1X1	T39.1X2	T39.1X3	T39.1X4	T39.1X5	T39.1X6
Excipients, pharmaceutical	T50.901	T50.902	T50.903	T50.904	T50.905	T50.906

Table of Drugs and Chemicals

Exhaust gas — Fluorinated corticosteroids

Substance	Poisoning, Accidental (unintentional)	Poisoning, Intentional Self-harm	Poisoning, Assault	Poisoning, Undetermined	Adverse Effect	Under-dosing
Exhaust gas (engine) (motor vehicle)	T58.01	T58.02	T58.03	T58.04	—	—
Ex-Lax (phenolphthalein)	T47.2X1	T47.2X2	T47.2X3	T47.2X4	T47.2X5	T47.2X6
Expectorant NEC	T48.4X1	T48.4X2	T48.4X3	T48.4X4	T48.4X5	T48.4X6
Extended insulin zinc suspension	T38.3X1	T38.3X2	T38.3X3	T38.3X4	T38.3X5	T38.3X6
External medications (skin) (mucous membrane)	T49.91	T49.92	T49.93	T49.94	T49.95	T49.96
dental agent	T49.7X1	T49.7X2	T49.7X3	T49.7X4	T49.7X5	T49.7X6
ENT agent	T49.6X1	T49.6X2	T49.6X3	T49.6X4	T49.6X5	T49.6X6
ophthalmic preparation	T49.5X1	T49.5X2	T49.5X3	T49.5X4	T49.5X5	T49.5X6
specified NEC	T49.8X1	T49.8X2	T49.8X3	T49.8X4	T49.8X5	T49.8X6
Extrapyramidal antagonist NEC	T44.3X1	T44.3X2	T44.3X3	T44.3X4	T44.3X5	T44.3X6
Eye agents (anti-infective)	T49.5X1	T49.5X2	T49.5X3	T49.5X4	T49.5X5	T49.5X6
Eye drug NEC	T49.5X1	T49.5X2	T49.5X3	T49.5X4	T49.5X5	T49.5X6
FAC (fluorouracil + doxorubicin + cyclophosphamide)	T45.1X1	T45.1X2	T45.1X3	T45.1X4	T45.1X5	T45.1X6
Factor						
I (fibrinogen)	T45.8X1	T45.8X2	T45.8X3	T45.8X4	T45.8X5	T45.8X6
III (thromboplastin)	T45.8X1	T45.8X2	T45.8X3	T45.8X4	T45.8X5	T45.8X6
VIII (antihemophilic Factor) (concentrate)	T45.8X1	T45.8X2	T45.8X3	T45.8X4	T45.8X5	T45.8X6
IX complex	T45.7X1	T45.7X2	T45.7X3	T45.7X4	T45.7X5	T45.7X6
human	T45.8X1	T45.8X2	T45.8X3	T45.8X4	T45.8X5	T45.8X6
Famotidine	T47.0X1	T47.0X2	T47.0X3	T47.0X4	T47.0X5	T47.0X6
Fat suspension, intravenous	T50.991	T50.992	T50.993	T50.994	T50.995	T50.996
Fazadinium bromide	T48.1X1	T48.1X2	T48.1X3	T48.1X4	T48.1X5	T48.1X6
Febarbamate	T42.3X1	T42.3X2	T42.3X3	T42.3X4	T42.3X5	T42.3X6
Fecal softener	T47.4X1	T47.4X2	T47.4X3	T47.4X4	T47.4X5	T47.4X6
Fedrilate	T48.3X1	T48.3X2	T48.3X3	T48.3X4	T48.3X5	T48.3X6
Felodipine	T46.1X1	T46.1X2	T46.1X3	T46.1X4	T46.1X5	T46.1X6
Felypressin	T38.891	T38.892	T38.893	T38.894	T38.895	T38.896
Femoxetine	T43.221	T43.222	T43.223	T43.224	T43.225	T43.226
Fenalcomine	T46.3X1	T46.3X2	T46.3X3	T46.3X4	T46.3X5	T46.3X6
Fenamisal	T37.1X1	T37.1X2	T37.1X3	T37.1X4	T37.1X5	T37.1X6
Fenazone	T39.2X1	T39.2X2	T39.2X3	T39.2X4	T39.2X5	T39.2X6
Fenbendazole	T37.4X1	T37.4X2	T37.4X3	T37.4X4	T37.4X5	T37.4X6
Fenbutrazate	T50.5X1	T50.5X2	T50.5X3	T50.5X4	T50.5X5	T50.5X6
Fencamfamine	T43.691	T43.692	T43.693	T43.694	T43.695	T43.696
Fendiline	T46.1X1	T46.1X2	T46.1X3	T46.1X4	T46.1X5	T46.1X6
Fenetylline	T43.691	T43.692	T43.693	T43.694	T43.695	T43.696
Fenflumizole	T39.391	T39.392	T39.393	T39.394	T39.395	T39.396
Fenfluramine	T50.5X1	T50.5X2	T50.5X3	T50.5X4	T50.5X5	T50.5X6
Fenobarbital	T42.3X1	T42.3X2	T42.3X3	T42.3X4	T42.3X5	T42.3X6
Fenofibrate	T46.6X1	T46.6X2	T46.6X3	T46.6X4	T46.6X5	T46.6X6
Fenoprofen	T39.311	T39.312	T39.313	T39.314	T39.315	T39.316
Fenoterol	T48.6X1	T48.6X2	T48.6X3	T48.6X4	T48.6X5	T48.6X6
Fenoverine	T44.3X1	T44.3X2	T44.3X3	T44.3X4	T44.3X5	T44.3X6
Fenoxazoline	T48.5X1	T48.5X2	T48.5X3	T48.5X4	T48.5X5	T48.5X6
Fenproporex	T50.5X1	T50.5X2	T50.5X3	T50.5X4	T50.5X5	T50.5X6
Fenquizone	T50.2X1	T50.2X2	T50.2X3	T50.2X4	T50.2X5	T50.2X6
Fentanyl	T40.4X1	T40.4X2	T40.4X3	T40.4X4	T40.4X5	T40.4X6
Fentazin	T43.3X1	T43.3X2	T43.3X3	T43.3X4	T43.3X5	T43.3X6
Fenthion	T60.0X1	T60.0X2	T60.0X3	T60.0X4	—	—
Fenticlor	T49.0X1	T49.0X2	T49.0X3	T49.0X4	T49.0X5	T49.0X6
Fenylbutazone	T39.2X1	T39.2X2	T39.2X3	T39.2X4	T39.2X5	T39.2X6
Feprazone	T39.2X1	T39.2X2	T39.2X3	T39.2X4	T39.2X5	T39.2X6
Fer de lance (bite) (venom)	T63.061	T63.062	T63.063	T63.064	—	—
Ferric — see also Iron						
chloride	T45.4X1	T45.4X2	T45.4X3	T45.4X4	T45.4X5	T45.4X6
citrate	T45.4X1	T45.4X2	T45.4X3	T45.4X4	T45.4X5	T45.4X6
hydroxide						
colloidal	T45.4X1	T45.4X2	T45.4X3	T45.4X4	T45.4X5	T45.4X6
polymaltose	T45.4X1	T45.4X2	T45.4X3	T45.4X4	T45.4X5	T45.4X6
pyrophosphate	T45.4X1	T45.4X2	T45.4X3	T45.4X4	T45.4X5	T45.4X6
Ferritin	T45.4X1	T45.4X2	T45.4X3	T45.4X4	T45.4X5	T45.4X6
Ferrocholinate	T45.4X1	T45.4X2	T45.4X3	T45.4X4	T45.4X5	T45.4X6
Ferrodextrane	T45.4X1	T45.4X2	T45.4X3	T45.4X4	T45.4X5	T45.4X6
Ferropolimaler	T45.4X1	T45.4X2	T45.4X3	T45.4X4	T45.4X5	T45.4X6
Ferrous — see also Iron						
phosphate	T45.4X1	T45.4X2	T45.4X3	T45.4X4	T45.4X5	T45.4X6
salt	T45.4X1	T45.4X2	T45.4X3	T45.4X4	T45.4X5	T45.4X6
with folic acid	T45.4X1	T45.4X2	T45.4X3	T45.4X4	T45.4X5	T45.4X6
Ferrous fumerate, gluconate, lactate, salt NEC, sulfate (medicinal)	T45.4X1	T45.4X2	T45.4X3	T45.4X4	T45.4X5	T45.4X6
Ferrovanadium (fumes)	T59.891	T59.892	T59.893	T59.894	—	—
Ferrum — see Iron						
Fertilizers NEC	T65.891	T65.892	T65.893	T65.894	—	—
with herbicide mixture	T60.3X1	T60.3X2	T60.3X3	T60.3X4	—	—
Fetoxilate	T47.6X1	T47.6X2	T47.6X3	T47.6X4	T47.6X5	T47.6X6
Fiber, dietary	T47.4X1	T47.4X2	T47.4X3	T47.4X4	T47.4X5	T47.4X6
Fiberglass	T65.831	T65.832	T65.833	T65.834	—	—
Fibrinogen (human)	T45.8X1	T45.8X2	T45.8X3	T45.8X4	T45.8X5	T45.8X6
Fibrinolysin (human)	T45.691	T45.692	T45.693	T45.694	T45.695	T45.696
Fibrinolysis						
affecting drug	T45.601	T45.602	T45.603	T45.604	T45.605	T45.606
inhibitor NEC	T45.621	T45.622	T45.623	T45.624	T45.625	T45.626
Fibrinolytic drug	T45.611	T45.612	T45.613	T45.614	T45.615	T45.616
Filix mas	T37.4X1	T37.4X2	T37.4X3	T37.4X4	T37.4X5	T37.4X6
Filtering cream	T49.3X1	T49.3X2	T49.3X3	T49.3X4	T49.3X5	T49.3X6
Fiorinal	T39.011	T39.012	T39.013	T39.014	T39.015	T39.016
Firedamp	T59.891	T59.892	T59.893	T59.894		
Fish, noxious, nonbacterial	T61.91	T61.92	T61.93	T61.94	—	—
ciguatera	T61.01	T61.02	T61.03	T61.04	—	—
scombroid	T61.11	T61.12	T61.13	T61.14	—	—
shell	T61.781	T61.782	T61.783	T61.784	—	—
specified NEC	T61.771	T61.772	T61.773	T61.774	—	—
Flagyl	T37.3X1	T37.3X2	T37.3X3	T37.3X4	T37.3X5	T37.3X6
Flavine adenine dinucleotide	T45.2X1	T45.2X2	T45.2X3	T45.2X4	T45.2X5	T45.2X6
Flavodic acid	T46.991	T46.992	T46.993	T46.994	T46.995	T46.996
Flavoxate	T44.3X1	T44.3X2	T44.3X3	T44.3X4	T44.3X5	T44.3X6
Flaxedil	T48.1X1	T48.1X2	T48.1X3	T48.1X4	T48.1X5	T48.1X6
Flaxseed (medicinal)	T49.3X1	T49.3X2	T49.3X3	T49.3X4	T49.3X5	T49.3X6
Flecainide	T46.2X1	T46.2X2	T46.2X3	T46.2X4	T46.2X5	T46.2X6
Fleroxacin	T36.8X1	T36.8X2	T36.8X3	T36.8X4	T36.8X5	T36.8X6
Floctafenine	T39.8X1	T39.8X2	T39.8X3	T39.8X4	T39.8X5	T39.8X6
Flomax	T44.6X1	T44.6X2	T44.6X3	T44.6X4	T44.6X5	T44.6X6
Flomoxef	T36.1X1	T36.1X2	T36.1X3	T36.1X4	T36.1X5	T36.1X6
Flopropione	T44.3X1	T44.3X2	T44.3X3	T44.3X4	T44.3X5	T44.3X6
Florantyrone	T47.5X1	T47.5X2	T47.5X3	T47.5X4	T47.5X5	T47.5X6
Floraquin	T37.8X1	T37.8X2	T37.8X3	T37.8X4	T37.8X5	T37.8X6
Florinef	T38.0X1	T38.0X2	T38.0X3	T38.0X4	T38.0X5	T38.0X6
ENT agent	T49.6X1	T49.6X2	T49.6X3	T49.6X4	T49.6X5	T49.6X6
ophthalmic preparation	T49.5X1	T49.5X2	T49.5X3	T49.5X4	T49.5X5	T49.5X6
topical NEC	T49.0X1	T49.0X2	T49.0X3	T49.0X4	T49.0X5	T49.0X6
Flowers of sulfur	T49.4X1	T49.4X2	T49.4X3	T49.4X4	T49.4X5	T49.4X6
Floxuridine	T45.1X1	T45.1X2	T45.1X3	T45.1X4	T45.1X5	T45.1X6
Fluanisone	T43.4X1	T43.4X2	T43.4X3	T43.4X4	T43.4X5	T43.4X6
Flubendazole	T37.4X1	T37.4X2	T37.4X3	T37.4X4	T37.4X5	T37.4X6
Fluclorolone acetonide	T49.0X1	T49.0X2	T49.0X3	T49.0X4	T49.0X5	T49.0X6
Flucloxacillin	T36.0X1	T36.0X2	T36.0X3	T36.0X4	T36.0X5	T36.0X6
Fluconazole	T37.8X1	T37.8X2	T37.8X3	T37.8X4	T37.8X5	T37.8X6
Flucytosine	T37.8X1	T37.8X2	T37.8X3	T37.8X4	T37.8X5	T37.8X6
Fludeoxyglucose (18F)	T50.8X1	T50.8X2	T50.8X3	T50.8X4	T50.8X5	T50.8X6
Fludiazepam	T42.4X1	T42.4X2	T42.4X3	T42.4X4	T42.4X5	T42.4X6
Fludrocortisone	T50.0X1	T50.0X2	T50.0X3	T50.0X4	T50.0X5	T50.0X6
ENT agent	T49.6X1	T49.6X2	T49.6X3	T49.6X4	T49.6X5	T49.6X6
ophthalmic preparation	T49.5X1	T49.5X2	T49.5X3	T49.5X4	T49.5X5	T49.5X6
topical NEC	T49.0X1	T49.0X2	T49.0X3	T49.0X4	T49.0X5	T49.0X6
Fludroxycortide	T49.0X1	T49.0X2	T49.0X3	T49.0X4	T49.0X5	T49.0X6
Flufenamic acid	T39.391	T39.392	T39.393	T39.394	T39.395	T39.396
Fluindione	T45.511	T45.512	T45.513	T45.514	T45.515	T45.516
Flumequine	T37.8X1	T37.8X2	T37.8X3	T37.8X4	T37.8X5	T37.8X6
Flumethasone	T49.0X1	T49.0X2	T49.0X3	T49.0X4	T49.0X5	T49.0X6
Flumethiazide	T50.2X1	T50.2X2	T50.2X3	T50.2X4	T50.2X5	T50.2X6
Flumidin	T37.5X1	T37.5X2	T37.5X3	T37.5X4	T37.5X5	T37.5X6
Flunarizine	T46.7X1	T46.7X2	T46.7X3	T46.7X4	T46.7X5	T46.7X6
Flunidazole	T37.8X1	T37.8X2	T37.8X3	T37.8X4	T37.8X5	T37.8X6
Flunisolide	T48.6X1	T48.6X2	T48.6X3	T48.6X4	T48.6X5	T48.6X6
Flunitrazepam	T42.4X1	T42.4X2	T42.4X3	T42.4X4	T42.4X5	T42.4X6
Fluocinolone (acetonide)	T49.0X1	T49.0X2	T49.0X3	T49.0X4	T49.0X5	T49.0X6
Fluocinonide	T49.0X1	T49.0X2	T49.0X3	T49.0X4	T49.0X5	T49.0X6
Fluocortin (butyl)	T49.0X1	T49.0X2	T49.0X3	T49.0X4	T49.0X5	T49.0X6
Fluocortolone	T49.0X1	T49.0X2	T49.0X3	T49.0X4	T49.0X5	T49.0X6
Fluohydrocortisone	T38.0X1	T38.0X2	T38.0X3	T38.0X4	T38.0X5	T38.0X6
ENT agent	T49.6X1	T49.6X2	T49.6X3	T49.6X4	T49.6X5	T49.6X6
ophthalmic preparation	T49.5X1	T49.5X2	T49.5X3	T49.5X4	T49.5X5	T49.5X6
topical NEC	T49.0X1	T49.0X2	T49.0X3	T49.0X4	T49.0X5	T49.0X6
Fluonid	T49.0X1	T49.0X2	T49.0X3	T49.0X4	T49.0X5	T49.0X6
Fluopromazine	T43.3X1	T43.3X2	T43.3X3	T43.3X4	T43.3X5	T43.3X6
Fluoracetate	T60.8X1	T60.8X2	T60.8X3	T60.8X4	—	—
Fluorescein	T50.8X1	T50.8X2	T50.8X3	T50.8X4	T50.8X5	T50.8X6
Fluorhydrocortisone	T50.0X1	T50.0X2	T50.0X3	T50.0X4	T50.0X5	T50.0X6
Fluoride (nonmedicinal) (pesticide) (sodium) NEC	T60.8X1	T60.8X2	T60.8X3	T60.8X4	—	—
hydrogen — see Hydrofluoric acid						
medicinal NEC	T50.991	T50.992	T50.993	T50.994	T50.995	T50.996
dental use	T49.7X1	T49.7X2	T49.7X3	T49.7X4	T49.7X5	T49.7X6
not pesticide NEC	T54.91	T54.92	T54.93	T54.94	—	—
stannous	T49.7X1	T49.7X2	T49.7X3	T49.7X4	T49.7X5	T49.7X6
Fluorinated corticosteroids	T38.0X1	T38.0X2	T38.0X3	T38.0X4	T38.0X5	T38.0X6

Additional Character May Be Required — Refer to the Tabular List for Character Selection   ▽ Subterms under main terms may continue to next column or page

Substance	Poisoning, Accidental (unintentional)	Poisoning, Intentional Self-harm	Poisoning, Assault	Poisoning, Undetermined	Adverse Effect	Under-dosing
Fluorine (gas)	T59.5X1	T59.5X2	T59.5X3	T59.5X4	—	—
salt — see Fluoride(s)						
Fluoristan	T49.7X1	T49.7X2	T49.7X3	T49.7X4	T49.7X5	T49.7X6
Fluormetholone	T49.0X1	T49.0X2	T49.0X3	T49.0X4	T49.0X5	T49.0X6
Fluoroacetate	T60.8X1	T60.8X2	T60.8X3	T60.8X4	—	—
Fluorocarbon monomer	T53.6X1	T53.6X2	T53.6X3	T53.6X4	—	—
Fluorocytosine	T37.8X1	T37.8X2	T37.8X3	T37.8X4	T37.8X5	T37.8X6
Fluorodeoxyuridine	T45.1X1	T45.1X2	T45.1X3	T45.1X4	T45.1X5	T45.1X6
Fluorometholone	T49.0X1	T49.0X2	T49.0X3	T49.0X4	T49.0X5	T49.0X6
ophthalmic preparation	T49.5X1	T49.5X2	T49.5X3	T49.5X4	T49.5X5	T49.5X6
Fluorophosphate insecticide	T60.0X1	T60.0X2	T60.0X3	T60.0X4	—	—
Fluorosol	T46.3X1	T46.3X2	T46.3X3	T46.3X4	T46.3X5	T46.3X6
Fluorouracil	T45.1X1	T45.1X2	T45.1X3	T45.1X4	T45.1X5	T45.1X6
Fluorphenylalanine	T49.5X1	T49.5X2	T49.5X3	T49.5X4	T49.5X5	T49.5X6
Fluothane	T41.0X1	T41.0X2	T41.0X3	T41.0X4	T41.0X5	T41.0X6
Fluoxetine	T43.221	T43.222	T43.223	T43.224	T43.225	T43.226
Fluoxymesterone	T38.7X1	T38.7X2	T38.7X3	T38.7X4	T38.7X5	T38.7X6
Flupenthixol	T43.4X1	T43.4X2	T43.4X3	T43.4X4	T43.4X5	T43.4X6
Flupentixol	T43.4X1	T43.4X2	T43.4X3	T43.4X4	T43.4X5	T43.4X6
Fluphenazine	T43.3X1	T43.3X2	T43.3X3	T43.3X4	T43.3X5	T43.3X6
Fluprednidene	T49.0X1	T49.0X2	T49.0X3	T49.0X4	T49.0X5	T49.0X6
Fluprednisolone	T38.0X1	T38.0X2	T38.0X3	T38.0X4	T38.0X5	T38.0X6
Fluradoline	T39.8X1	T39.8X2	T39.8X3	T39.8X4	T39.8X5	T39.8X6
Flurandrenolide	T49.0X1	T49.0X2	T49.0X3	T49.0X4	T49.0X5	T49.0X6
Flurandrenolone	T49.0X1	T49.0X2	T49.0X3	T49.0X4	T49.0X5	T49.0X6
Flurazepam	T42.4X1	T42.4X2	T42.4X3	T42.4X4	T42.4X5	T42.4X6
Flurbiprofen	T39.311	T39.312	T39.313	T39.314	T39.315	T39.316
Flurobate	T49.0X1	T49.0X2	T49.0X3	T49.0X4	T49.0X5	T49.0X6
Fluroxene	T41.0X1	T41.0X2	T41.0X3	T41.0X4	T41.0X5	T41.0X6
Fluspirilene	T43.591	T43.592	T43.593	T43.594	T43.595	T43.596
Flutamide	T38.6X1	T38.6X2	T38.6X3	T38.6X4	T38.6X5	T38.6X6
Flutazolam	T38.0X1	T38.0X2	T38.0X3	T38.0X4	T38.0X5	T38.0X6
Fluticasone propionate	T38.0X1	T38.0X2	T38.0X3	T38.0X4	T38.0X5	T38.0X6
Flutoprazepam	T42.4X1	T42.4X2	T42.4X3	T42.4X4	T42.4X5	T42.4X6
Flutropium bromide	T48.6X1	T48.6X2	T48.6X3	T48.6X4	T48.6X5	T48.6X6
Fluvoxamine	T43.221	T43.222	T43.223	T43.224	T43.225	T43.226
Folacin	T45.8X1	T45.8X2	T45.8X3	T45.8X4	T45.8X5	T45.8X6
Folic acid	T45.8X1	T45.8X2	T45.8X3	T45.8X4	T45.8X5	T45.8X6
with ferrous salt	T45.2X1	T45.2X2	T45.2X3	T45.2X4	T45.2X5	T45.2X6
antagonist	T45.1X1	T45.1X2	T45.1X3	T45.1X4	T45.1X5	T45.1X6
Folinic acid	T45.8X1	T45.8X2	T45.8X3	T45.8X4	T45.8X5	T45.8X6
Folium stramoniae	T48.6X1	T48.6X2	T48.6X3	T48.6X4	T48.6X5	T48.6X6
Follicle-stimulating hormone, human	T38.811	T38.812	T38.813	T38.814	T38.815	T38.816
Folpet	T60.3X1	T60.3X2	T60.3X3	T60.3X4	—	—
Fominoben	T48.3X1	T48.3X2	T48.3X3	T48.3X4	T48.3X5	T48.3X6
Food, foodstuffs, noxious, nonbacterial, NEC	T62.91	T62.92	T62.93	T62.94	—	—
berries	T62.1X1	T62.1X2	T62.1X3	T62.1X4	—	—
fish — see also Fish	T61.91	T61.92	T61.93	T61.94	—	—
mushrooms	T62.0X1	T62.0X2	T62.0X3	T62.0X4	—	—
plants	T62.2X1	T62.2X2	T62.2X3	T62.2X4	—	—
seafood	T61.91	T61.92	T61.93	T61.94	—	—
specified NEC	T61.8X1	T61.8X2	T61.8X3	T61.8X4	—	—
seeds	T62.2X1	T62.2X2	T62.2X3	T62.2X4	—	—
shellfish	T61.781	T61.782	T61.783	T61.784	—	—
specified NEC	T62.8X1	T62.8X2	T62.8X3	T62.8X4	—	—
Fool's parsley	T62.2X1	T62.2X2	T62.2X3	T62.2X4	—	—
Formaldehyde (solution), gas or vapor	T59.2X1	T59.2X2	T59.2X3	T59.2X4	—	—
fungicide	T60.3X1	T60.3X2	T60.3X3	T60.3X4	—	—
Formalin	T59.2X1	T59.2X2	T59.2X3	T59.2X4	—	—
fungicide	T60.3X1	T60.3X2	T60.3X3	T60.3X4	—	—
vapor	T59.2X1	T59.2X2	T59.2X3	T59.2X4	—	—
Formic acid	T54.2X1	T54.2X2	T54.2X3	T54.2X4	—	—
vapor	T59.891	T59.892	T59.893	T59.894	—	—
Foscarnet sodium	T37.5X1	T37.5X2	T37.5X3	T37.5X4	T37.5X5	T37.5X6
Fosfestrol	T38.5X1	T38.5X2	T38.5X3	T38.5X4	T38.5X5	T38.5X6
Fosfomycin	T36.8X1	T36.8X2	T36.8X3	T36.8X4	T36.8X5	T36.8X6
Fosfonet sodium	T37.5X1	T37.5X2	T37.5X3	T37.5X4	T37.5X5	T37.5X6
Fosinopril	T46.4X1	T46.4X2	T46.4X3	T46.4X4	T46.4X5	T46.4X6
sodium	T46.4X1	T46.4X2	T46.4X3	T46.4X4	T46.4X5	T46.4X6
Fowler's solution	T57.0X1	T57.0X2	T57.0X3	T57.0X4	—	—
Foxglove	T62.2X1	T62.2X2	T62.2X3	T62.2X4	—	—
Framycetin	T36.5X1	T36.5X2	T36.5X3	T36.5X4	T36.5X5	T36.5X6
Frangula	T47.2X1	T47.2X2	T47.2X3	T47.2X4	T47.2X5	T47.2X6
extract	T47.2X1	T47.2X2	T47.2X3	T47.2X4	T47.2X5	T47.2X6
Frei antigen	T50.8X1	T50.8X2	T50.8X3	T50.8X4	T50.8X5	T50.8X6
Freon	T53.5X1	T53.5X2	T53.5X3	T53.5X4	—	—
Fructose	T50.3X1	T50.3X2	T50.3X3	T50.3X4	T50.3X5	T50.3X6
Frusemide	T50.1X1	T50.1X2	T50.1X3	T50.1X4	T50.1X5	T50.1X6
FSH	T38.811	T38.812	T38.813	T38.814	T38.815	T38.816

Substance	Poisoning, Accidental (unintentional)	Poisoning, Intentional Self-harm	Poisoning, Assault	Poisoning, Undetermined	Adverse Effect	Under-dosing
Ftorafur	T45.1X1	T45.1X2	T45.1X3	T45.1X4	T45.1X5	T45.1X6
Fuel						
automobile	T52.0X1	T52.0X2	T52.0X3	T52.0X4	—	—
exhaust gas, not in transit	T58.01	T58.02	T58.03	T58.04	—	—
vapor NEC	T52.0X1	T52.0X2	T52.0X3	T52.0X4	—	—
gas (domestic use) — see also Carbon, monoxide, fuel, utility	T59.891	T59.892	T59.893	T59.894	—	—
utility	T59.891	T59.892	T59.893	T59.894	—	—
incomplete combustion of — see Carbon, monoxide, fuel, utility						
in mobile container	T59.891	T59.892	T59.893	T59.894	—	—
piped (natural)	T59.891	T59.892	T59.893	T59.894	—	—
industrial, incomplete combustion	T58.8X1	T58.8X2	T58.8X3	T58.8X4	—	—
Fugillin	T36.8X1	T36.8X2	T36.8X3	T36.8X4	T36.8X5	T36.8X6
Fulminate of mercury	T56.1X1	T56.1X2	T56.1X3	T56.1X4	—	—
Fulvicin	T36.7X1	T36.7X2	T36.7X3	T36.7X4	T36.7X5	T36.7X6
Fumadil	T36.8X1	T36.8X2	T36.8X3	T36.8X4	T36.8X5	T36.8X6
Fumagillin	T36.8X1	T36.8X2	T36.8X3	T36.8X4	T36.8X5	T36.8X6
Fumaric acid	T49.4X1	T49.4X2	T49.4X3	T49.4X4	T49.4X5	T49.4X6
Fumes (from)	T59.91	T59.92	T59.93	T59.94	—	—
carbon monoxide — see Carbon, monoxide						
charcoal (domestic use) — see Charcoal, fumes						
chloroform — see Chloroform						
coke (in domestic stoves, fireplaces) — see Coke fumes						
corrosive NEC	T54.91	T54.92	T54.93	T54.94	—	—
ether — see ether						
freons	T53.5X1	T53.5X2	T53.5X3	T53.5X4	—	—
hydrocarbons	T59.891	T59.892	T59.893	T59.894	—	—
petroleum (liquefied)	T59.891	T59.892	T59.893	T59.894	—	—
distributed through pipes (pure or mixed with air)	T59.891	T59.892	T59.893	T59.894	—	—
lead — see lead						
metal — see Metals, or the specified metal						
nitrogen dioxide	T59.0X1	T59.0X2	T59.0X3	T59.0X4	—	—
pesticides — see Pesticides						
petroleum (liquefied)	T59.891	T59.892	T59.893	T59.894	—	—
distributed through pipes (pure or mixed with air)	T59.891	T59.892	T59.893	T59.894	—	—
polyester	T59.891	T59.892	T59.893	T59.894	—	—
specified source NEC — see also substance specified	T59.891	T59.892	T59.893	T59.894	—	—
sulfur dioxide	T59.1X1	T59.1X2	T59.1X3	T59.1X4	—	—
Fumigant NEC	T60.91	T60.92	T60.93	T60.94	—	—
Fungicide NEC (nonmedicinal)	T60.3X1	T60.3X2	T60.3X3	T60.3X4	—	—
Fungi, noxious, used as food	T62.0X1	T62.0X2	T62.0X3	T62.0X4	—	—
Fungizone	T36.7X1	T36.7X2	T36.7X3	T36.7X4	T36.7X5	T36.7X6
topical	T49.0X1	T49.0X2	T49.0X3	T49.0X4	T49.0X5	T49.0X6
Furacin	T49.0X1	T49.0X2	T49.0X3	T49.0X4	T49.0X5	T49.0X6
Furadantin	T37.91	T37.92	T37.93	T37.94	T37.95	T37.96
Furazolidone	T37.8X1	T37.8X2	T37.8X3	T37.8X4	T37.8X5	T37.8X6
Furazolium chloride	T49.0X1	T49.0X2	T49.0X3	T49.0X4	T49.0X5	T49.0X6
Furfural	T52.8X1	T52.8X2	T52.8X3	T52.8X4	—	—
Furnace (coal burning) (domestic), gas from	T58.2X1	T58.2X2	T58.2X3	T58.2X4	—	—
industrial	T58.8X1	T58.8X2	T58.8X3	T58.8X4	—	—
Furniture polish	T65.891	T65.892	T65.893	T65.894	—	—
Furosemide	T50.1X1	T50.1X2	T50.1X3	T50.1X4	T50.1X5	T50.1X6
Furoxone	T37.91	T37.92	T37.93	T37.94	T37.95	T37.96
Fursultiamine	T45.2X1	T45.2X2	T45.2X3	T45.2X4	T45.2X5	T45.2X6
Fusafungine	T36.8X1	T36.8X2	T36.8X3	T36.8X4	T36.8X5	T36.8X6
Fusel oil (any) (amyl) (butyl) (propyl), vapor	T51.3X1	T51.3X2	T51.3X3	T51.3X4	—	—
Fusidate (ethanolamine) (sodium)	T36.8X1	T36.8X2	T36.8X3	T36.8X4	T36.8X5	T36.8X6
Fusidic acid	T36.8X1	T36.8X2	T36.8X3	T36.8X4	T36.8X5	T36.8X6
Fytic acid, nonasodium	T50.6X1	T50.6X2	T50.6X3	T50.6X4	T50.6X5	T50.6X6
b-Galactosidase	T47.5X1	T47.5X2	T47.5X3	T47.5X4	T47.5X5	T47.5X6
GABA	T43.8X1	T43.8X2	T43.8X3	T43.8X4	T43.8X5	T43.8X6
Gadopentetic acid	T50.8X1	T50.8X2	T50.8X3	T50.8X4	T50.8X5	T50.8X6
Galactose	T50.3X1	T50.3X2	T50.3X3	T50.3X4	T50.3X5	T50.3X6
Galantamine	T44.0X1	T44.0X2	T44.0X3	T44.0X4	T44.0X5	T44.0X6

Table of Drugs and Chemicals

Substance	Poisoning, Accidental (unintentional)	Poisoning, Intentional Self-harm	Poisoning, Assault	Poisoning, Undetermined	Adverse Effect	Under-dosing
Gallamine (triethiodide)	T48.1X1	T48.1X2	T48.1X3	T48.1X4	T48.1X5	T48.1X6
Gallium citrate	T50.991	T50.992	T50.993	T50.994	T50.995	T50.996
Gallopamil	T46.1X1	T46.1X2	T46.1X3	T46.1X4	T46.1X5	T46.1X6
Gamboge	T47.2X1	T47.2X2	T47.2X3	T47.2X4	T47.2X5	T47.2X6
Gamimune	T50.Z11	T50.Z12	T50.Z13	T50.Z14	T50.Z15	T50.Z16
Gamma-aminobutyric acid	T43.8X1	T43.8X2	T43.8X3	T43.8X4	T43.8X5	T43.8X6
Gamma-benzene hexachloride (medicinal)	T49.0X1	T49.0X2	T49.0X3	T49.0X4	T49.0X5	T49.0X6
nonmedicinal, vapor	T53.6X1	T53.6X2	T53.6X3	T53.6X4	—	—
Gamma-BHC (medicinal) — *see also* Gamma-benzene hexachloride	T49.0X1	T49.0X2	T49.0X3	T49.0X4	T49.0X5	T49.0X6
Gamma globulin	T50.Z11	T50.Z12	T50.Z13	T50.Z14	T50.Z15	T50.Z16
Gamulin	T50.Z11	T50.Z12	T50.Z13	T50.Z14	T50.Z15	T50.Z16
Ganciclovir (sodium)	T37.5X1	T37.5X2	T37.5X3	T37.5X4	T37.5X5	T37.5X6
Ganglionic blocking drug NEC	T44.2X1	T44.2X2	T44.2X3	T44.2X4	T44.2X5	T44.2X6
specified NEC	T44.2X1	T44.2X2	T44.2X3	T44.2X4	T44.2X5	T44.2X6
Ganja	T40.7X1	T40.7X2	T40.7X3	T40.7X4	T40.7X5	T40.7X6
Garamycin	T36.5X1	T36.5X2	T36.5X3	T36.5X4	T36.5X5	T36.5X6
ophthalmic preparation	T49.5X1	T49.5X2	T49.5X3	T49.5X4	T49.5X5	T49.5X6
topical NEC	T49.0X1	T49.0X2	T49.0X3	T49.0X4	T49.0X5	T49.0X6
Gardenal	T42.3X1	T42.3X2	T42.3X3	T42.3X4	T42.3X5	T42.3X6
Gardepanyl	T42.3X1	T42.3X2	T42.3X3	T42.3X4	T42.3X5	T42.3X6
Gaseous substance — *see* Gas						
Gasoline	T52.0X1	T52.0X2	T52.0X3	T52.0X4	—	—
vapor	T52.0X1	T52.0X2	T52.0X3	T52.0X4	—	—
Gastric enzymes	T47.5X1	T47.5X2	T47.5X3	T47.5X4	T47.5X5	T47.5X6
Gastrografin	T50.8X1	T50.8X2	T50.8X3	T50.8X4	T50.8X5	T50.8X6
Gastrointestinal drug	T47.91	T47.92	T47.93	T47.94	T47.95	T47.96
biological	T47.8X1	T47.8X2	T47.8X3	T47.8X4	T47.8X5	T47.8X6
specified NEC	T47.8X1	T47.8X2	T47.8X3	T47.8X4	T47.8X5	T47.8X6
Gas NEC	T59.91	T59.92	T59.93	T59.94	—	—
acetylene	T59.891	T59.892	T59.893	T59.894	—	—
incomplete combustion of	T58.11	T58.12	T58.13	T58.14	—	—
air contaminants, source or type not specified	T59.91	T59.92	T59.93	T59.94	—	—
anesthetic	T41.0X1	T41.0X2	T41.0X3	T41.0X4	T41.0X5	T41.0X6
blast furnace	T58.8X1	T58.8X2	T58.8X3	T58.8X4	—	—
butane — *see* butane						
carbon monoxide — *see* Carbon, monoxide						
chlorine	T59.4X1	T59.4X2	T59.4X3	T59.4X4	—	—
coal	T58.2X1	T58.2X2	T58.2X3	T58.2X4	—	—
cyanide	T57.3X1	T57.3X2	T57.3X3	T57.3X4	—	—
dicyanogen	T65.0X1	T65.0X2	T65.0X3	T65.0X4	—	—
domestic — *see* Domestic gas						
exhaust	T58.01	T58.02	T58.03	T58.04	—	—
from utility (for cooking, heating, or lighting) (after combustion) — *see* Carbon, monoxide, fuel, utility						
prior to combustion	T59.891	T59.892	T59.893	T59.894	—	—
from wood- or coal-burning stove or fireplace	T58.2X1	T58.2X2	T58.2X3	T58.2X4	—	—
fuel (domestic use) (after combustion) — *see also* Carbon, monoxide, fuel						
industrial use	T58.8X1	T58.8X2	T58.8X3	T58.8X4	—	—
prior to combustion	T59.891	T59.892	T59.893	T59.894	—	—
utility	T59.891	T59.892	T59.893	T59.894	—	—
incomplete combustion of — *see* Carbon, monoxide, fuel, utility						
in mobile container	T59.891	T59.892	T59.893	T59.894	—	—
piped (natural)	T59.891	T59.892	T59.893	T59.894	—	—
garage	T58.01	T58.02	T58.03	T58.04	—	—
hydrocarbon NEC	T59.891	T59.892	T59.893	T59.894	—	—
incomplete combustion of — *see* Carbon, monoxide, fuel, utility						
liquefied — *see* butane						
piped	T59.891	T59.892	T59.893	T59.894	—	—
hydrocyanic acid	T65.0X1	T65.0X2	T65.0X3	T65.0X4	—	—
illuminating (after combustion)	T58.11	T58.12	T58.13	T58.14	—	—
prior to combustion	T59.891	T59.892	T59.893	T59.894	—	—
incomplete combustion, any — *see* Carbon, monoxide						
kiln	T58.8X1	T58.8X2	T58.8X3	T58.8X4	—	—
lacrimogenic	T59.3X1	T59.3X2	T59.3X3	T59.3X4	—	—

Substance	Poisoning, Accidental (unintentional)	Poisoning, Intentional Self-harm	Poisoning, Assault	Poisoning, Undetermined	Adverse Effect	Under-dosing
Gas — *continued*						
liquefied petroleum — *see* butane						
marsh	T59.891	T59.892	T59.893	T59.894	—	—
motor exhaust, not in transit	T58.01	T58.02	T58.03	T58.04	—	—
mustard, not in war	T59.891	T59.892	T59.893	T59.894	—	—
natural	T59.891	T59.892	T59.893	T59.894	—	—
nerve, not in war	T59.91	T59.92	T59.93	T59.94	—	—
oil	T52.0X1	T52.0X2	T52.0X3	T52.0X4	—	—
petroleum (liquefied) (distributed in mobile containers)	T59.891	T59.892	T59.893	T59.894	—	—
piped (pure or mixed with air)	T59.891	T59.892	T59.893	T59.894	—	—
piped (manufactured) (natural) NEC	T59.891	T59.892	T59.893	T59.894	—	—
producer	T58.8X1	T58.8X2	T58.8X3	T58.8X4	—	—
propane — *see* propane						
refrigerant (chlorofluoro-carbon)	T53.5X1	T53.5X2	T53.5X3	T53.5X4	—	—
not chlorofluoro-carbon	T59.891	T59.892	T59.893	T59.894	—	—
sewer	T59.91	T59.92	T59.93	T59.94	—	—
specified source NEC	T59.91	T59.92	T59.93	T59.94	—	—
stove (after combustion)	T58.11	T58.12	T58.13	T58.14	—	—
prior to combustion	T59.891	T59.892	T59.893	T59.894	—	—
tear	T59.3X1	T59.3X2	T59.3X3	T59.3X4	—	—
therapeutic	T41.5X1	T41.5X2	T41.5X3	T41.5X4	T41.5X5	T41.5X6
utility (for cooking, heating, or lighting) (piped) NEC	T59.891	T59.892	T59.893	T59.894	—	—
incomplete combustion of — *see* Carbon, monoxide, fuel, utility						
in mobile container	T59.891	T59.892	T59.893	T59.894	—	—
piped (natural)	T59.891	T59.892	T59.893	T59.894	—	—
water	T58.11	T58.12	T58.13	T58.14	—	—
incomplete combustion of — *see* Carbon, monoxide, fuel, utility						
Gaultheria procumbens	T62.2X1	T62.2X2	T62.2X3	T62.2X4	—	—
Gefarnate	T44.3X1	T44.3X2	T44.3X3	T44.3X4	T44.3X5	T44.3X6
Gelatin (intravenous)	T45.8X1	T45.8X2	T45.8X3	T45.8X4	T45.8X5	T45.8X6
absorbable (sponge)	T45.7X1	T45.7X2	T45.7X3	T45.7X4	T45.7X5	T45.7X6
Gelfilm	T49.8X1	T49.8X2	T49.8X3	T49.8X4	T49.8X5	T49.8X6
Gelfoam	T45.7X1	T45.7X2	T45.7X3	T45.7X4	T45.7X5	T45.7X6
Gelsemine	T50.991	T50.992	T50.993	T50.994	T50.995	T50.996
Gelsemium (sempervirens)	T62.2X1	T62.2X2	T62.2X3	T62.2X4	—	—
Gemeprost	T48.0X1	T48.0X2	T48.0X3	T48.0X4	T48.0X5	T48.0X6
Gemfibrozil	T46.6X1	T46.6X2	T46.6X3	T46.6X4	T46.6X5	T46.6X6
Gemonil	T42.3X1	T42.3X2	T42.3X3	T42.3X4	T42.3X5	T42.3X6
Gentamicin	T36.5X1	T36.5X2	T36.5X3	T36.5X4	T36.5X5	T36.5X6
ophthalmic preparation	T49.5X1	T49.5X2	T49.5X3	T49.5X4	T49.5X5	T49.5X6
topical NEC	T49.0X1	T49.0X2	T49.0X3	T49.0X4	T49.0X5	T49.0X6
Gentian	T47.5X1	T47.5X2	T47.5X3	T47.5X4	T47.5X5	T47.5X6
violet	T49.0X1	T49.0X2	T49.0X3	T49.0X4	T49.0X5	T49.0X6
Gepefrine	T44.4X1	T44.4X2	T44.4X3	T44.4X4	T44.4X5	T44.4X6
Gestonorone caproate	T38.5X1	T38.5X2	T38.5X3	T38.5X4	T38.5X5	T38.5X6
Gexane	T49.0X1	T49.0X2	T49.0X3	T49.0X4	T49.0X5	T49.0X6
Gila monster (venom)	T63.111	T63.112	T63.113	T63.114	—	—
Ginger	T47.5X1	T47.5X2	T47.5X3	T47.5X4	T47.5X5	T47.5X6
Jamaica — *see* Jamaica, ginger						
Gitalin	T46.0X1	T46.0X2	T46.0X3	T46.0X4	T46.0X5	T46.0X6
amorphous	T46.0X1	T46.0X2	T46.0X3	T46.0X4	T46.0X5	T46.0X6
Gitaloxin	T46.0X1	T46.0X2	T46.0X3	T46.0X4	T46.0X5	T46.0X6
Gitoxin	T46.0X1	T46.0X2	T46.0X3	T46.0X4	T46.0X5	T46.0X6
Glafenine	T39.8X1	T39.8X2	T39.8X3	T39.8X4	T39.8X5	T39.8X6
Glandular extract (medicinal) NEC	T50.Z91	T50.Z92	T50.Z93	T50.Z94	T50.Z95	T50.Z96
Glaucarubin	T37.3X1	T37.3X2	T37.3X3	T37.3X4	T37.3X5	T37.3X6
Glibenclamide	T38.3X1	T38.3X2	T38.3X3	T38.3X4	T38.3X5	T38.3X6
Glibornuride	T38.3X1	T38.3X2	T38.3X3	T38.3X4	T38.3X5	T38.3X6
Gliclazide	T38.3X1	T38.3X2	T38.3X3	T38.3X4	T38.3X5	T38.3X6
Glimidine	T38.3X1	T38.3X2	T38.3X3	T38.3X4	T38.3X5	T38.3X6
Glipizide	T38.3X1	T38.3X2	T38.3X3	T38.3X4	T38.3X5	T38.3X6
Gliquidone	T38.3X1	T38.3X2	T38.3X3	T38.3X4	T38.3X5	T38.3X6
Glisolamide	T38.3X1	T38.3X2	T38.3X3	T38.3X4	T38.3X5	T38.3X6
Glisoxepide	T38.3X1	T38.3X2	T38.3X3	T38.3X4	T38.3X5	T38.3X6
Globin zinc insulin	T38.3X1	T38.3X2	T38.3X3	T38.3X4	T38.3X5	T38.3X6
Globulin						
antilymphocytic	T50.Z11	T50.Z12	T50.Z13	T50.Z14	T50.Z15	T50.Z16
antirhesus	T50.Z11	T50.Z12	T50.Z13	T50.Z14	T50.Z15	T50.Z16
antivenin	T50.Z11	T50.Z12	T50.Z13	T50.Z14	T50.Z15	T50.Z16
antiviral	T50.Z11	T50.Z12	T50.Z13	T50.Z14	T50.Z15	T50.Z16

Gallamine — Globulin

Additional Character May Be Required — Refer to the Tabular List for Character Selection

▽ Subterms under main terms may continue to next column or page

Table of Drugs and Chemicals

Substance	Poisoning, Accidental (unintentional)	Poisoning, Intentional Self-harm	Poisoning, Assault	Poisoning, Undetermined	Adverse Effect	Under-dosing
Glucagon	T38.3X1	T38.3X2	T38.3X3	T38.3X4	T38.3X5	T38.3X6
Glucocorticoids	T38.0X1	T38.0X2	T38.0X3	T38.0X4	T38.0X5	T38.0X6
Glucocorticosteroid	T38.0X1	T38.0X2	T38.0X3	T38.0X4	T38.0X5	T38.0X6
Gluconic acid	T50.991	T50.992	T50.993	T50.994	T50.995	T50.996
Glucosamine sulfate	T39.4X1	T39.4X2	T39.4X3	T39.4X4	T39.4X5	T39.4X6
Glucose	T50.3X1	T50.3X2	T50.3X3	T50.3X4	T50.3X5	T50.3X6
with sodium chloride	T50.3X1	T50.3X2	T50.3X3	T50.3X4	T50.3X5	T50.3X6
Glucosulfone sodium	T37.1X1	T37.1X2	T37.1X3	T37.1X4	T37.1X5	T37.1X6
Glucurolactone	T47.8X1	T47.8X2	T47.8X3	T47.8X4	T47.8X5	T47.8X6
Glue NEC	T52.8X1	T52.8X2	T52.8X3	T52.8X4	—	—
Glutamic acid	T47.5X1	T47.5X2	T47.5X3	T47.5X4	T47.5X5	T47.5X6
Glutaral (medicinal)	T49.0X1	T49.0X2	T49.0X3	T49.0X4	T49.0X5	T49.0X6
nonmedicinal	T65.891	T65.892	T65.893	T65.894	—	—
Glutaraldehyde (nonmedicinal)	T65.891	T65.892	T65.893	T65.894	—	—
medicinal	T49.0X1	T49.0X2	T49.0X3	T49.0X4	T49.0X5	T49.0X6
Glutathione	T50.6X1	T50.6X2	T50.6X3	T50.6X4	T50.6X5	T50.6X6
Glutethimide	T42.6X1	T42.6X2	T42.6X3	T42.6X4	T42.6X5	T42.6X6
Glyburide	T38.3X1	T38.3X2	T38.3X3	T38.3X4	T38.3X5	T38.3X6
Glycerin	T47.4X1	T47.4X2	T47.4X3	T47.4X4	T47.4X5	T47.4X6
Glycerol	T47.4X1	T47.4X2	T47.4X3	T47.4X4	T47.4X5	T47.4X6
borax	T49.6X1	T49.6X2	T49.6X3	T49.6X4	T49.6X5	T49.6X6
intravenous	T50.3X1	T50.3X2	T50.3X3	T50.3X4	T50.3X5	T50.3X6
iodinated	T48.4X1	T48.4X2	T48.4X3	T48.4X4	T48.4X5	T48.4X6
Glycerophosphate	T50.991	T50.992	T50.993	T50.994	T50.995	T50.996
Glyceryl						
gualacolate	T48.4X1	T48.4X2	T48.4X3	T48.4X4	T48.4X5	T48.4X6
nitrate	T46.3X1	T46.3X2	T46.3X3	T46.3X4	T46.3X5	T46.3X6
triacetate (topical)	T49.0X1	T49.0X2	T49.0X3	T49.0X4	T49.0X5	T49.0X6
trinitrate	T46.3X1	T46.3X2	T46.3X3	T46.3X4	T46.3X5	T46.3X6
Glycine	T50.3X1	T50.3X2	T50.3X3	T50.3X4	T50.3X5	T50.3X6
Glyclopyramide	T38.3X1	T38.3X2	T38.3X3	T38.3X4	T38.3X5	T38.3X6
Glycobiarsol	T37.3X1	T37.3X2	T37.3X3	T37.3X4	T37.3X5	T37.3X6
Glycols (ether)	T52.3X1	T52.3X2	T52.3X3	T52.3X4	—	—
Glyconiazide	T37.1X1	T37.1X2	T37.1X3	T37.1X4	T37.1X5	T37.1X6
Glycopyrrolate	T44.3X1	T44.3X2	T44.3X3	T44.3X4	T44.3X5	T44.3X6
Glycopyrronium	T44.3X1	T44.3X2	T44.3X3	T44.3X4	T44.3X5	T44.3X6
bromide	T44.3X1	T44.3X2	T44.3X3	T44.3X4	T44.3X5	T44.3X6
Glycoside, cardiac (stimulant)	T46.0X1	T46.0X2	T46.0X3	T46.0X4	T46.0X5	T46.0X6
Glycyclamide	T38.3X1	T38.3X2	T38.3X3	T38.3X4	T38.3X5	T38.3X6
Glycyrrhiza extract	T48.4X1	T48.4X2	T48.4X3	T48.4X4	T48.4X5	T48.4X6
Glycyrrhizic acid	T48.4X1	T48.4X2	T48.4X3	T48.4X4	T48.4X5	T48.4X6
Glycyrrhizinate potassium	T48.4X1	T48.4X2	T48.4X3	T48.4X4	T48.4X5	T48.4X6
Glymidine sodium	T38.3X1	T38.3X2	T38.3X3	T38.3X4	T38.3X5	T38.3X6
Glyphosate	T60.3X1	T60.3X2	T60.3X3	T60.3X4	—	—
Glyphylline	T48.6X1	T48.6X2	T48.6X3	T48.6X4	T48.6X5	T48.6X6
Gold						
colloidal (I98Au)	T45.1X1	T45.1X2	T45.1X3	T45.1X4	T45.1X5	T45.1X6
salts	T39.4X1	T39.4X2	T39.4X3	T39.4X4	T39.4X5	T39.4X6
Golden sulfide of antimony	T56.891	T56.892	T56.893	T56.894	—	—
Goldylocks	T62.2X1	T62.2X2	T62.2X3	T62.2X4	—	—
Gonadal tissue extract	T38.901	T38.902	T38.903	T38.904	T38.905	T38.906
female	T38.5X1	T38.5X2	T38.5X3	T38.5X4	T38.5X5	T38.5X6
male	T38.7X1	T38.7X2	T38.7X3	T38.7X4	T38.7X5	T38.7X6
Gonadorelin	T38.891	T38.892	T38.893	T38.894	T38.895	T38.896
Gonadotropin	T38.891	T38.892	T38.893	T38.894	T38.895	T38.896
chorionic	T38.891	T38.892	T38.893	T38.894	T38.895	T38.896
pituitary	T38.811	T38.812	T38.813	T38.814	T38.815	T38.816
Goserelin	T45.1X1	T45.1X2	T45.1X3	T45.1X4	T45.1X5	T45.1X6
Grain alcohol	T51.0X1	T51.0X2	T51.0X3	T51.0X4	—	—
Gramicidin	T49.0X1	T49.0X2	T49.0X3	T49.0X4	T49.0X5	T49.0X6
Granisetron	T45.0X1	T45.0X2	T45.0X3	T45.0X4	T45.0X5	T45.0X6
Gratiola officinalis	T62.2X1	T62.2X2	T62.2X3	T62.2X4	—	—
Grease	T65.891	T65.892	T65.893	T65.894	—	—
Green hellebore	T62.2X1	T62.2X2	T62.2X3	T62.2X4	—	—
Green soap	T49.2X1	T49.2X2	T49.2X3	T49.2X4	T49.2X5	T49.2X6
Grifulvin	T36.7X1	T36.7X2	T36.7X3	T36.7X4	T36.7X5	T36.7X6
Griseofulvin	T36.7X1	T36.7X2	T36.7X3	T36.7X4	T36.7X5	T36.7X6
Growth hormone	T38.811	T38.812	T38.813	T38.814	T38.815	T38.816
Guaiacol derivatives	T48.4X1	T48.4X2	T48.4X3	T48.4X4	T48.4X5	T48.4X6
Guaiac reagent	T50.991	T50.992	T50.993	T50.994	T50.995	T50.996
Guaifenesin	T48.4X1	T48.4X2	T48.4X3	T48.4X4	T48.4X5	T48.4X6
Guaimesal	T48.4X1	T48.4X2	T48.4X3	T48.4X4	T48.4X5	T48.4X6
Guaiphenesin	T48.4X1	T48.4X2	T48.4X3	T48.4X4	T48.4X5	T48.4X6
Guamecycline	T36.4X1	T36.4X2	T36.4X3	T36.4X4	T36.4X5	T36.4X6
Guanabenz	T46.5X1	T46.5X2	T46.5X3	T46.5X4	T46.5X5	T46.5X6
Guanacline	T46.5X1	T46.5X2	T46.5X3	T46.5X4	T46.5X5	T46.5X6
Guanadrel	T46.5X1	T46.5X2	T46.5X3	T46.5X4	T46.5X5	T46.5X6
Guanatol	T37.2X1	T37.2X2	T37.2X3	T37.2X4	T37.2X5	T37.2X6
Guanethidine	T46.5X1	T46.5X2	T46.5X3	T46.5X4	T46.5X5	T46.5X6
Guanfacine	T46.5X1	T46.5X2	T46.5X3	T46.5X4	T46.5X5	T46.5X6
Guano	T65.891	T65.892	T65.893	T65.894	—	—
Guanochlor	T46.5X1	T46.5X2	T46.5X3	T46.5X4	T46.5X5	T46.5X6
Guanoclor	T46.5X1	T46.5X2	T46.5X3	T46.5X4	T46.5X5	T46.5X6
Guanoctine	T46.5X1	T46.5X2	T46.5X3	T46.5X4	T46.5X5	T46.5X6
Guanoxabenz	T46.5X1	T46.5X2	T46.5X3	T46.5X4	T46.5X5	T46.5X6
Guanoxan	T46.5X1	T46.5X2	T46.5X3	T46.5X4	T46.5X5	T46.5X6
Guar gum (medicinal)	T46.6X1	T46.6X2	T46.6X3	T46.6X4	T46.6X5	T46.6X6
Hachimycin	T36.7X1	T36.7X2	T36.7X3	T36.7X4	T36.7X5	T36.7X6
Hair						
dye	T49.4X1	T49.4X2	T49.4X3	T49.4X4	T49.4X5	T49.4X6
preparation NEC	T49.4X1	T49.4X2	T49.4X3	T49.4X4	T49.4X5	T49.4X6
Halazepam	T42.4X1	T42.4X2	T42.4X3	T42.4X4	T42.4X5	T42.4X6
Halcinolone	T49.0X1	T49.0X2	T49.0X3	T49.0X4	T49.0X5	T49.0X6
Halcinonide	T49.0X1	T49.0X2	T49.0X3	T49.0X4	T49.0X5	T49.0X6
Halethazole	T49.0X1	T49.0X2	T49.0X3	T49.0X4	T49.0X5	T49.0X6
Hallucinogen NEC	T40.901	T40.902	T40.903	T40.904	T40.905	T40.906
Halofantrine	T37.2X1	T37.2X2	T37.2X3	T37.2X4	T37.2X5	T37.2X6
Halofenate	T46.6X1	T46.6X2	T46.6X3	T46.6X4	T46.6X5	T46.6X6
Halometasone	T49.0X1	T49.0X2	T49.0X3	T49.0X4	T49.0X5	T49.0X6
Haloperidol	T43.4X1	T43.4X2	T43.4X3	T43.4X4	T43.4X5	T43.4X6
Haloprogin	T49.0X1	T49.0X2	T49.0X3	T49.0X4	T49.0X5	T49.0X6
Halotex	T49.0X1	T49.0X2	T49.0X3	T49.0X4	T49.0X5	T49.0X6
Halothane	T41.0X1	T41.0X2	T41.0X3	T41.0X4	T41.0X5	T41.0X6
Haloxazolam	T42.4X1	T42.4X2	T42.4X3	T42.4X4	T42.4X5	T42.4X6
Halquinols	T49.0X1	T49.0X2	T49.0X3	T49.0X4	T49.0X5	T49.0X6
Hamamelis	T49.2X1	T49.2X2	T49.2X3	T49.2X4	T49.2X5	T49.2X6
Haptendextran	T45.8X1	T45.8X2	T45.8X3	T45.8X4	T45.8X5	T45.8X6
Harmonyl	T46.5X1	T46.5X2	T46.5X3	T46.5X4	T46.5X5	T46.5X6
Hartmann's solution	T50.3X1	T50.3X2	T50.3X3	T50.3X4	T50.3X5	T50.3X6
Hashish	T40.7X1	T40.7X2	T40.7X3	T40.7X4	T40.7X5	T40.7X6
Hawaiian Woodrose seeds	T40.991	T40.992	T40.993	T40.994	—	—
HCB	T60.3X1	T60.3X2	T60.3X3	T60.3X4	—	—
HCH	T53.6X1	T53.6X2	T53.6X3	T53.6X4	—	—
medicinal	T49.0X1	T49.0X2	T49.0X3	T49.0X4	T49.0X5	T49.0X6
HCN	T57.3X1	T57.3X2	T57.3X3	T57.3X4	—	—
Headache cures, drugs, powders NEC	T50.901	T50.902	T50.903	T50.904	T50.905	T50.906
Heavenly Blue (morning glory)	T40.991	T40.992	T40.993	T40.994	—	—
Heavy metal antidote	T45.8X1	T45.8X2	T45.8X3	T45.8X4	T45.8X5	T45.8X6
Hedaquinium	T49.0X1	T49.0X2	T49.0X3	T49.0X4	T49.0X5	T49.0X6
Hedge hyssop	T62.2X1	T62.2X2	T62.2X3	T62.2X4	—	—
Heet	T49.8X1	T49.8X2	T49.8X3	T49.8X4	T49.8X5	T49.8X6
Helenin	T37.4X1	T37.4X2	T37.4X3	T37.4X4	T37.4X5	T37.4X6
Helium (nonmedicinal) NEC	T59.891	T59.892	T59.893	T59.894	—	—
medicinal	T48.991	T48.992	T48.993	T48.994	T48.995	T48.996
Hellebore (black) (green) (white)	T62.2X1	T62.2X2	T62.2X3	T62.2X4	—	—
Hematin	T45.8X1	T45.8X2	T45.8X3	T45.8X4	T45.8X5	T45.8X6
Hematinic preparation	T45.8X1	T45.8X2	T45.8X3	T45.8X4	T45.8X5	T45.8X6
Hematological agent	T45.91	T45.92	T45.93	T45.94	T45.95	T45.96
specified NEC	T45.8X1	T45.8X2	T45.8X3	T45.8X4	T45.8X5	T45.8X6
Hemlock	T62.2X1	T62.2X2	T62.2X3	T62.2X4	—	—
Hemostatic	T45.621	T45.622	T45.623	T45.624	T45.625	T45.626
drug, systemic	T45.621	T45.622	T45.623	T45.624	T45.625	T45.626
Hemostyptic	T49.4X1	T49.4X2	T49.4X3	T49.4X4	T49.4X5	T49.4X6
Henbane	T62.2X1	T62.2X2	T62.2X3	T62.2X4	—	—
Heparin (sodium)	T45.511	T45.512	T45.513	T45.514	T45.515	T45.516
action reverser	T45.7X1	T45.7X2	T45.7X3	T45.7X4	T45.7X5	T45.7X6
Heparin-fraction	T45.511	T45.512	T45.513	T45.514	T45.515	T45.516
Heparinoid (systemic)	T45.511	T45.512	T45.513	T45.514	T45.515	T45.516
Hepatic secretion stimulant	T47.8X1	T47.8X2	T47.8X3	T47.8X4	T47.8X5	T47.8X6
Hepatitis B						
immune globulin	T50.Z11	T50.Z12	T50.Z13	T50.Z14	T50.Z15	T50.Z16
vaccine	T50.B91	T50.B92	T50.B93	T50.B94	T50.B95	T50.B96
Hepronicate	T46.7X1	T46.7X2	T46.7X3	T46.7X4	T46.7X5	T46.7X6
Heptabarb	T42.3X1	T42.3X2	T42.3X3	T42.3X4	T42.3X5	T42.3X6
Heptabarbital	T42.3X1	T42.3X2	T42.3X3	T42.3X4	T42.3X5	T42.3X6
Heptabarbitone	T42.3X1	T42.3X2	T42.3X3	T42.3X4	T42.3X5	T42.3X6
Heptachlor	T60.1X1	T60.1X2	T60.1X3	T60.1X4	—	—
Heptalgin	T40.2X1	T40.2X2	T40.2X3	T40.2X4	T40.2X5	T40.2X6
Heptaminol	T46.3X1	T46.3X2	T46.3X3	T46.3X4	T46.3X5	T46.3X6
Herbicide NEC	T60.3X1	T60.3X2	T60.3X3	T60.3X4	—	—
Heroin	T40.1X1	T40.1X2	T40.1X3	T40.1X4	—	—
Herplex	T49.5X1	T49.5X2	T49.5X3	T49.5X4	T49.5X5	T49.5X6
HES	T45.8X1	T45.8X2	T45.8X3	T45.8X4	T45.8X5	T45.8X6
Hesperidin	T46.991	T46.992	T46.993	T46.994	T46.995	T46.996
Hetacillin	T36.0X1	T36.0X2	T36.0X3	T36.0X4	T36.0X5	T36.0X6
Hetastarch	T45.8X1	T45.8X2	T45.8X3	T45.8X4	T45.8X5	T45.8X6
HETP	T60.0X1	T60.0X2	T60.0X3	T60.0X4	—	—
Hexachlorobenzene (vapor)	T60.3X1	T60.3X2	T60.3X3	T60.3X4	—	—
Hexachlorocyclohexane	T53.6X1	T53.6X2	T53.6X3	T53.6X4	—	—
Hexachlorophene	T49.0X1	T49.0X2	T49.0X3	T49.0X4	T49.0X5	T49.0X6

Glucagon — Hexachlorophene

Table of Drugs and Chemicals

Substance	Poisoning, Accidental (unintentional)	Poisoning, Intentional Self-harm	Poisoning, Assault	Poisoning, Undetermined	Adverse Effect	Under-dosing
Hexadiline	T46.3X1	T46.3X2	T46.3X3	T46.3X4	T46.3X5	T46.3X6
Hexadimethrine (bromide)	T45.7X1	T45.7X2	T45.7X3	T45.7X4	T45.7X5	T45.7X6
Hexadylamine	T46.3X1	T46.3X2	T46.3X3	T46.3X4	T46.3X5	T46.3X6
Hexaethyl tetraphosphate	T60.0X1	T60.0X2	T60.0X3	T60.0X4	—	—
Hexafluorenium bromide	T48.1X1	T48.1X2	T48.1X3	T48.1X4	T48.1X5	T48.1X6
Hexafluronium (bromide)	T48.1X1	T48.1X2	T48.1X3	T48.1X4	T48.1X5	T48.1X6
Hexa-germ	T49.2X1	T49.2X2	T49.2X3	T49.2X4	T49.2X5	T49.2X6
Hexahydrobenzol	T52.8X1	T52.8X2	T52.8X3	T52.8X4	—	—
Hexahydrocresol(s)	T51.8X1	T51.8X2	T51.8X3	T51.8X4	—	—
arsenide	T57.0X1	T57.0X2	T57.0X3	T57.0X4	—	—
arseniurated	T57.0X1	T57.0X2	T57.0X3	T57.0X4	—	—
cyanide	T57.3X1	T57.3X2	T57.3X3	T57.3X4	—	—
gas	T59.891	T59.892	T59.893	T59.894	—	—
Fluoride (liquid)	T57.8X1	T57.8X2	T57.8X3	T57.8X4	—	—
vapor	T59.891	T59.892	T59.893	T59.894	—	—
phophorated	T60.0X1	T60.0X2	T60.0X3	T60.0X4	—	—
sulfate	T57.8X1	T57.8X2	T57.8X3	T57.8X4	—	—
sulfide (gas)	T59.6X1	T59.6X2	T59.6X3	T59.6X4	—	—
arseniurated	T57.0X1	T57.0X2	T57.0X3	T57.0X4	—	—
sulfurated	T57.8X1	T57.8X2	T57.8X3	T57.8X4	—	—
Hexahydrophenol	T51.8X1	T51.8X2	T51.8X3	T51.8X4	—	—
Hexalen	T51.8X1	T51.8X2	T51.8X3	T51.8X4	—	—
Hexamethonium bromide	T44.2X1	T44.2X2	T44.2X3	T44.2X4	T44.2X5	T44.2X6
Hexamethylene	T52.8X1	T52.8X2	T52.8X3	T52.8X4	—	—
Hexamethylmelamine	T45.1X1	T45.1X2	T45.1X3	T45.1X4	T45.1X5	T45.1X6
Hexamidine	T49.0X1	T49.0X2	T49.0X3	T49.0X4	T49.0X5	T49.0X6
Hexamine (mandelate)	T37.8X1	T37.8X2	T37.8X3	T37.8X4	T37.8X5	T37.8X6
Hexanone, 2-hexanone	T52.4X1	T52.4X2	T52.4X3	T52.4X4	—	—
Hexanuorenium	T48.1X1	T48.1X2	T48.1X3	T48.1X4	T48.1X5	T48.1X6
Hexapropymate	T42.6X1	T42.6X2	T42.6X3	T42.6X4	T42.6X5	T42.6X6
Hexasonium iodide	T44.3X1	T44.3X2	T44.3X3	T44.3X4	T44.3X5	T44.3X6
Hexcarbacholine bromide	T48.1X1	T48.1X2	T48.1X3	T48.1X4	T48.1X5	T48.1X6
Hexemal	T42.3X1	T42.3X2	T42.3X3	T42.3X4	T42.3X5	T42.3X6
Hexestrol	T38.5X1	T38.5X2	T38.5X3	T38.5X4	T38.5X5	T38.5X6
Hexethal (sodium)	T42.3X1	T42.3X2	T42.3X3	T42.3X4	T42.3X5	T42.3X6
Hexetidine	T37.8X1	T37.8X2	T37.8X3	T37.8X4	T37.8X5	T37.8X6
Hexobarbital	T42.3X1	T42.3X2	T42.3X3	T42.3X4	T42.3X5	T42.3X6
rectal	T41.291	T41.292	T41.293	T41.294	T41.295	T41.296
sodium	T41.1X1	T41.1X2	T41.1X3	T41.1X4	T41.1X5	T41.1X6
Hexobendine	T46.3X1	T46.3X2	T46.3X3	T46.3X4	T46.3X5	T46.3X6
Hexocyclium	T44.3X1	T44.3X2	T44.3X3	T44.3X4	T44.3X5	T44.3X6
metilsulfate	T44.3X1	T44.3X2	T44.3X3	T44.3X4	T44.3X5	T44.3X6
Hexoestrol	T38.5X1	T38.5X2	T38.5X3	T38.5X4	T38.5X5	T38.5X6
Hexone	T52.4X1	T52.4X2	T52.4X3	T52.4X4	—	—
Hexoprenaline	T48.6X1	T48.6X2	T48.6X3	T48.6X4	T48.6X5	T48.6X6
Hexylcaine	T41.3X1	T41.3X2	T41.3X3	T41.3X4	T41.3X5	T41.3X6
Hexylresorcinol	T52.2X1	T52.2X2	T52.2X3	T52.2X4	—	—
HGH (human growth hormone)	T38.811	T38.812	T38.813	T38.814	T38.815	T38.816
Hinkle's pills	T47.2X1	T47.2X2	T47.2X3	T47.2X4	T47.2X5	T47.2X6
Histalog	T50.8X1	T50.8X2	T50.8X3	T50.8X4	T50.8X5	T50.8X6
Histamine (phosphate)	T50.8X1	T50.8X2	T50.8X3	T50.8X4	T50.8X5	T50.8X6
Histoplasmin	T50.8X1	T50.8X2	T50.8X3	T50.8X4	T50.8X5	T50.8X6
Holly berries	T62.2X1	T62.2X2	T62.2X3	T62.2X4	—	—
Homatropine	T44.3X1	T44.3X2	T44.3X3	T44.3X4	T44.3X5	T44.3X6
methylbromide	T44.3X1	T44.3X2	T44.3X3	T44.3X4	T44.3X5	T44.3X6
Homochlorcyclizine	T45.0X1	T45.0X2	T45.0X3	T45.0X4	T45.0X5	T45.0X6
Homosalate	T49.3X1	T49.3X2	T49.3X3	T49.3X4	T49.3X5	T49.3X6
Homo-tet	T50.Z11	T50.Z12	T50.Z13	T50.Z14	T50.Z15	T50.Z16
Hormone	T38.801	T38.802	T38.803	T38.804	T38.805	T38.806
adrenal cortical steroids	T38.0X1	T38.0X2	T38.0X3	T38.0X4	T38.0X5	T38.0X6
androgenic	T38.7X1	T38.7X2	T38.7X3	T38.7X4	T38.7X5	T38.7X6
anterior pituitary NEC	T38.811	T38.812	T38.813	T38.814	T38.815	T38.816
antidiabetic agents	T38.3X1	T38.3X2	T38.3X3	T38.3X4	T38.3X5	T38.3X6
antidiuretic	T38.891	T38.892	T38.893	T38.894	T38.895	T38.896
cancer therapy	T45.1X1	T45.1X2	T45.1X3	T45.1X4	T45.1X5	T45.1X6
follicle stimulating	T38.811	T38.812	T38.813	T38.814	T38.815	T38.816
gonadotropic	T38.891	T38.892	T38.893	T38.894	T38.895	T38.896
pituitary	T38.811	T38.812	T38.813	T38.814	T38.815	T38.816
growth	T38.811	T38.812	T38.813	T38.814	T38.815	T38.816
luteinizing	T38.811	T38.812	T38.813	T38.814	T38.815	T38.816
ovarian	T38.5X1	T38.5X2	T38.5X3	T38.5X4	T38.5X5	T38.5X6
oxytocic	T48.0X1	T48.0X2	T48.0X3	T48.0X4	T48.0X5	T48.0X6
parathyroid (derivatives)	T50.991	T50.992	T50.993	T50.994	T50.995	T50.996
pituitary (posterior) NEC	T38.891	T38.892	T38.893	T38.894	T38.895	T38.896
anterior	T38.811	T38.812	T38.813	T38.814	T38.815	T38.816
specified, NEC	T38.891	T38.892	T38.893	T38.894	T38.895	T38.896
thyroid	T38.1X1	T38.1X2	T38.1X3	T38.1X4	T38.1X5	T38.1X6
Hornet (sting)	T63.451	T63.452	T63.453	T63.454	—	—
Horse anti-human lymphocytic serum	T50.Z11	T50.Z12	T50.Z13	T50.Z14	T50.Z15	T50.Z16
Horticulture agent NEC	T65.91	T65.92	T65.93	T65.94	—	—
with pesticide	T60.91	T60.92	T60.93	T60.94	—	—
Human						
albumin	T45.8X1	T45.8X2	T45.8X3	T45.8X4	T45.8X5	T45.8X6
growth hormone (HGH)	T38.811	T38.812	T38.813	T38.814	T38.815	T38.816
immune serum	T50.Z11	T50.Z12	T50.Z13	T50.Z14	T50.Z15	T50.Z16
Hyaluronidase	T45.3X1	T45.3X2	T45.3X3	T45.3X4	T45.3X5	T45.3X6
Hyazyme	T45.3X1	T45.3X2	T45.3X3	T45.3X4	T45.3X5	T45.3X6
Hycodan	T40.2X1	T40.2X2	T40.2X3	T40.2X4	T40.2X5	T40.2X6
Hydantoin derivative NEC	T42.0X1	T42.0X2	T42.0X3	T42.0X4	T42.0X5	T42.0X6
Hydeltra	T38.0X1	T38.0X2	T38.0X3	T38.0X4	T38.0X5	T38.0X6
Hydergine	T44.6X1	T44.6X2	T44.6X3	T44.6X4	T44.6X5	T44.6X6
Hydrabamine penicillin	T36.0X1	T36.0X2	T36.0X3	T36.0X4	T36.0X5	T36.0X6
Hydralazine	T46.5X1	T46.5X2	T46.5X3	T46.5X4	T46.5X5	T46.5X6
Hydrargaphen	T49.0X1	T49.0X2	T49.0X3	T49.0X4	T49.0X5	T49.0X6
Hydrargyri aminochloridum	T49.0X1	T49.0X2	T49.0X3	T49.0X4	T49.0X5	T49.0X6
Hydrastine	T48.291	T48.292	T48.293	T48.294	T48.295	T48.296
Hydrazine	T54.1X1	T54.1X2	T54.1X3	T54.1X4	—	—
monoamine oxidase inhibitors	T43.1X1	T43.1X2	T43.1X3	T43.1X4	T43.1X5	T43.1X6
Hydrazoic acid, azides	T54.2X1	T54.2X2	T54.2X3	T54.2X4	—	—
Hydriodic acid	T48.4X1	T48.4X2	T48.4X3	T48.4X4	T48.4X5	T48.4X6
Hydrocarbon gas	T59.891	T59.892	T59.893	T59.894	—	—
incomplete combustion of — see Carbon, monoxide, fuel, utility						
liquefied (mobile container)	T59.891	T59.892	T59.893	T59.894	—	—
piped (natural)	T59.891	T59.892	T59.893	T59.894	—	—
Hydrochloric acid (liquid)	T54.2X1	T54.2X2	T54.2X3	T54.2X4	—	—
medicinal (digestant)	T47.5X1	T47.5X2	T47.5X3	T47.5X4	T47.5X5	T47.5X6
vapor	T59.891	T59.892	T59.893	T59.894	—	—
Hydrochlorothiazide	T50.2X1	T50.2X2	T50.2X3	T50.2X4	T50.2X5	T50.2X6
Hydrocodone	T40.2X1	T40.2X2	T40.2X3	T40.2X4	T40.2X5	T40.2X6
Hydrocortisone (derivatives)	T38.0X1	T38.0X2	T38.0X3	T38.0X4	T38.0X5	T38.0X6
aceponate	T49.0X1	T49.0X2	T49.0X3	T49.0X4	T49.0X5	T49.0X6
ENT agent	T49.6X1	T49.6X2	T49.6X3	T49.6X4	T49.6X5	T49.6X6
ophthalmic preparation	T49.5X1	T49.5X2	T49.5X3	T49.5X4	T49.5X5	T49.5X6
topical NEC	T49.0X1	T49.0X2	T49.0X3	T49.0X4	T49.0X5	T49.0X6
Hydrocortone	T38.0X1	T38.0X2	T38.0X3	T38.0X4	T38.0X5	T38.0X6
ENT agent	T49.6X1	T49.6X2	T49.6X3	T49.6X4	T49.6X5	T49.6X6
ophthalmic preparation	T49.5X1	T49.5X2	T49.5X3	T49.5X4	T49.5X5	T49.5X6
topical NEC	T49.0X1	T49.0X2	T49.0X3	T49.0X4	T49.0X5	T49.0X6
Hydrocyanic acid (liquid)	T57.3X1	T57.3X2	T57.3X3	T57.3X4	—	—
gas	T65.0X1	T65.0X2	T65.0X3	T65.0X4	—	—
Hydroflumethiazide	T50.2X1	T50.2X2	T50.2X3	T50.2X4	T50.2X5	T50.2X6
Hydrofluoric acid (liquid)	T54.2X1	T54.2X2	T54.2X3	T54.2X4	—	—
vapor	T59.891	T59.892	T59.893	T59.894	—	—
Hydrogen	T59.891	T59.892	T59.893	T59.894	—	—
arsenide	T57.0X1	T57.0X2	T57.0X3	T57.0X4	—	—
arseniureted	T57.0X1	T57.0X2	T57.0X3	T57.0X4	—	—
chloride	T57.8X1	T57.8X2	T57.8X3	T57.8X4	—	—
cyanide (salts)	T57.3X1	T57.3X2	T57.3X3	T57.3X4	—	—
gas	T57.3X1	T57.3X2	T57.3X3	T57.3X4	—	—
Fluoride	T59.5X1	T59.5X2	T59.5X3	T59.5X4	—	—
vapor	T59.5X1	T59.5X2	T59.5X3	T59.5X4	—	—
peroxide	T49.0X1	T49.0X2	T49.0X3	T49.0X4	T49.0X5	T49.0X6
phosphureted	T57.1X1	T57.1X2	T57.1X3	T57.1X4	—	—
sulfide	T59.6X1	T59.6X2	T59.6X3	T59.6X4	—	—
arseniureted	T57.0X1	T57.0X2	T57.0X3	T57.0X4	—	—
sulfureted	T59.6X1	T59.6X2	T59.6X3	T59.6X4	—	—
Hydromethylpyridine	T46.7X1	T46.7X2	T46.7X3	T46.7X4	T46.7X5	T46.7X6
Hydromorphinol	T40.2X1	T40.2X2	T40.2X3	T40.2X4	—	—
Hydromorphinone	T40.2X1	T40.2X2	T40.2X3	T40.2X4	T40.2X5	T40.2X6
Hydromorphone	T40.2X1	T40.2X2	T40.2X3	T40.2X4	T40.2X5	T40.2X6
Hydromox	T50.2X1	T50.2X2	T50.2X3	T50.2X4	T50.2X5	T50.2X6
Hydrophilic lotion	T49.3X1	T49.3X2	T49.3X3	T49.3X4	T49.3X5	T49.3X6
Hydroquinidine	T46.2X1	T46.2X2	T46.2X3	T46.2X4	T46.2X5	T46.2X6
Hydroquinone	T52.2X1	T52.2X2	T52.2X3	T52.2X4	—	—
vapor	T59.891	T59.892	T59.893	T59.894	—	—
Hydrosulfuric acid (gas)	T59.6X1	T59.6X2	T59.6X3	T59.6X4	—	—
Hydrotalcite	T47.1X1	T47.1X2	T47.1X3	T47.1X4	—	T47.1X6
Hydrous wool fat	T49.3X1	T49.3X2	T49.3X3	T49.3X4	T49.3X5	T49.3X6
Hydroxide, caustic	T54.3X1	T54.3X2	T54.3X3	T54.3X4	—	—
Hydroxocobalamin	T45.8X1	T45.8X2	T45.8X3	T45.8X4	T45.8X5	T45.8X6
Hydroxyamphetamine	T49.5X1	T49.5X2	T49.5X3	T49.5X4	T49.5X5	T49.5X6
Hydroxycarbamide	T45.1X1	T45.1X2	T45.1X3	T45.1X4	T45.1X5	T45.1X6
Hydroxychloroquine	T37.8X1	T37.8X2	T37.8X3	T37.8X4	T37.8X5	T37.8X6
Hydroxydihydrocodeinone	T40.2X1	T40.2X2	T40.2X3	T40.2X4	T40.2X5	T40.2X6
Hydroxyestrone	T38.5X1	T38.5X2	T38.5X3	T38.5X4	T38.5X5	T38.5X6
Hydroxyethyl starch	T45.8X1	T45.8X2	T45.8X3	T45.8X4	T45.8X5	T45.8X6
Hydroxymethylpentanone	T52.4X1	T52.4X2	T52.4X3	T52.4X4	—	—
Hydroxyphenamate	T43.591	T43.592	T43.593	T43.594	T43.595	T43.596
Hydroxyphenylbutazone	T39.2X1	T39.2X2	T39.2X3	T39.2X4	T39.2X5	T39.2X6
Hydroxyprogesterone	T38.5X1	T38.5X2	T38.5X3	T38.5X4	T38.5X5	T38.5X6

Additional Character May Be Required — Refer to the Tabular List for Character Selection ▽ Subterms under main terms may continue to next column or page

Hexadiline — Hydroxyprogesterone

Substance	Poisoning, Accidental (unintentional)	Poisoning, Intentional Self-harm	Poisoning, Assault	Poisoning, Undetermined	Adverse Effect	Under-dosing
Hydroxyprogesterone — *continued*						
caproate	T38.5X1	T38.5X2	T38.5X3	T38.5X4	T38.5X5	T38.5X6
Hydroxyquinoline (derivatives) **NEC**	T37.8X1	T37.8X2	T37.8X3	T37.8X4	T37.8X5	T37.8X6
Hydroxystilbamidine	T37.3X1	T37.3X2	T37.3X3	T37.3X4	T37.3X5	T37.3X6
Hydroxytoluene (nonmedicinal)	T54.0X1	T54.0X2	T54.0X3	T54.0X4	—	—
medicinal	T49.0X1	T49.0X2	T49.0X3	T49.0X4	T49.0X5	T49.0X6
Hydroxyurea	T45.1X1	T45.1X2	T45.1X3	T45.1X4	T45.1X5	T45.1X6
Hydroxyzine	T43.591	T43.592	T43.593	T43.594	T43.595	T43.596
Hyoscine	T44.3X1	T44.3X2	T44.3X3	T44.3X4	T44.3X5	T44.3X6
Hyoscyamine	T44.3X1	T44.3X2	T44.3X3	T44.3X4	T44.3X5	T44.3X6
Hyoscyamus	T44.3X1	T44.3X2	T44.3X3	T44.3X4	T44.3X5	T44.3X6
dry extract	T44.3X1	T44.3X2	T44.3X3	T44.3X4	T44.3X5	T44.3X6
Hypaque	T50.8X1	T50.8X2	T50.8X3	T50.8X4	T50.8X5	T50.8X6
Hypertussis	T50.Z11	T50.Z12	T50.Z13	T50.Z14	T50.Z15	T50.Z16
Hypnotic	T42.71	T42.72	T42.73	T42.74	T42.75	T42.76
anticonvulsant	T42.71	T42.72	T42.73	T42.74	T42.75	T42.76
specified NEC	T42.6X1	T42.6X2	T42.6X3	T42.6X4	T42.6X5	T42.6X6
Hypochlorite	T49.0X1	T49.0X2	T49.0X3	T49.0X4	T49.0X5	T49.0X6
Hypophysis, posterior	T38.891	T38.892	T38.893	T38.894	T38.895	T38.896
Hypotensive NEC	T46.5X1	T46.5X2	T46.5X3	T46.5X4	T46.5X5	T46.5X6
Hypromellose	T49.5X1	T49.5X2	T49.5X3	T49.5X4	T49.5X5	T49.5X6
Ibacitabine	T37.5X1	T37.5X2	T37.5X3	T37.5X4	T37.5X5	T37.5X6
Ibopamine	T44.991	T44.992	T44.993	T44.994	T44.995	T44.996
Ibufenac	T39.311	T39.312	T39.313	T39.314	T39.315	T39.316
Ibuprofen	T39.311	T39.312	T39.313	T39.314	T39.315	T39.316
Ibuproxam	T39.311	T39.312	T39.313	T39.314	T39.315	T39.316
Ibuterol	T48.6X1	T48.6X2	T48.6X3	T48.6X4	T48.6X5	T48.6X6
Ichthammol	T49.0X1	T49.0X2	T49.0X3	T49.0X4	T49.0X5	T49.0X6
Ichthyol	T49.4X1	T49.4X2	T49.4X3	T49.4X4	T49.4X5	T49.4X6
Idarubicin	T45.1X1	T45.1X2	T45.1X3	T45.1X4	T45.1X5	T45.1X6
Idrocilamide	T42.8X1	T42.8X2	T42.8X3	T42.8X4	T42.8X5	T42.8X6
Ifenprodil	T46.7X1	T46.7X2	T46.7X3	T46.7X4	T46.7X5	T46.7X6
Ifosfamide	T45.1X1	T45.1X2	T45.1X3	T45.1X4	T45.1X5	T45.1X6
Iletin	T38.3X1	T38.3X2	T38.3X3	T38.3X4	T38.3X5	T38.3X6
Ilex	T62.2X1	T62.2X2	T62.2X3	T62.2X4	—	—
Illuminating gas (after combustion)	T58.11	T58.12	T58.13	T58.14	—	—
prior to combustion	T59.891	T59.892	T59.893	T59.894	—	—
Ilopan	T45.2X1	T45.2X2	T45.2X3	T45.2X4	T45.2X5	T45.2X6
Iloprost	T46.7X1	T46.7X2	T46.7X3	T46.7X4	T46.7X5	T46.7X6
Ilotycin	T36.3X1	T36.3X2	T36.3X3	T36.3X4	T36.3X5	T36.3X6
ophthalmic preparation	T49.5X1	T49.5X2	T49.5X3	T49.5X4	T49.5X5	T49.5X6
topical NEC	T49.0X1	T49.0X2	T49.0X3	T49.0X4	T49.0X5	T49.0X6
Imidazole-4-carboxamide	T45.1X1	T45.1X2	T45.1X3	T45.1X4	T45.1X5	T45.1X6
Iminostilbene	T42.1X1	T42.1X2	T42.1X3	T42.1X4	T42.1X5	T42.1X6
Imipenem	T36.0X1	T36.0X2	T36.0X3	T36.0X4	T36.0X5	T36.0X6
Imipramine	T43.011	T43.012	T43.013	T43.014	T43.015	T43.016
Immu-G	T50.Z11	T50.Z12	T50.Z13	T50.Z14	T50.Z15	T50.Z16
Immuglobin	T50.Z11	T50.Z12	T50.Z13	T50.Z14	T50.Z15	T50.Z16
Immune						
globulin	T50.Z11	T50.Z12	T50.Z13	T50.Z14	T50.Z15	T50.Z16
serum globulin	T50.Z11	T50.Z12	T50.Z13	T50.Z14	T50.Z15	T50.Z16
Immunoglobin human (intravenous) (normal)	T50.Z11	T50.Z12	T50.Z13	T50.Z14	T50.Z15	T50.Z16
unmodified	T50.Z11	T50.Z12	T50.Z13	T50.Z14	T50.Z15	T50.Z16
Immunosuppressive drug	T45.1X1	T45.1X2	T45.1X3	T45.1X4	T45.1X5	T45.1X6
Immu-tetanus	T50.Z11	T50.Z12	T50.Z13	T50.Z14	T50.Z15	T50.Z16
Indalpine	T43.221	T43.222	T43.223	T43.224	T43.225	T43.226
Indanazoline	T48.5X1	T48.5X2	T48.5X3	T48.5X4	T48.5X5	T48.5X6
Indandione (derivatives)	T45.511	T45.512	T45.513	T45.514	T45.515	T45.516
Indapamide	T46.5X1	T46.5X2	T46.5X3	T46.5X4	T46.5X5	T46.5X6
Indendione (derivatives)	T45.511	T45.512	T45.513	T45.514	T45.515	T45.516
Indenolol	T44.7X1	T44.7X2	T44.7X3	T44.7X4	T44.7X5	T44.7X6
Inderal	T44.7X1	T44.7X2	T44.7X3	T44.7X4	T44.7X5	T44.7X6
Indian						
hemp	T40.7X1	T40.7X2	T40.7X3	T40.7X4	T40.7X5	T40.7X6
tobacco	T62.2X1	T62.2X2	T62.2X3	T62.2X4	—	—
Indigo carmine	T50.8X1	T50.8X2	T50.8X3	T50.8X4	T50.8X5	T50.8X6
Indobufen	T45.521	T45.522	T45.523	T45.524	T45.525	T45.526
Indocin	T39.2X1	T39.2X2	T39.2X3	T39.2X4	T39.2X5	T39.2X6
Indocyanine green	T50.8X1	T50.8X2	T50.8X3	T50.8X4	T50.8X5	T50.8X6
Indometacin	T39.391	T39.392	T39.393	T39.394	T39.395	T39.396
Indomethacin	T39.391	T39.392	T39.393	T39.394	T39.395	T39.396
farnesil	T39.4X1	T39.4X2	T39.4X3	T39.4X4	T39.4X5	T39.4X6
Indoramin	T44.6X1	T44.6X2	T44.6X3	T44.6X4	T44.6X5	T44.6X6
Industrial						
alcohol	T51.0X1	T51.0X2	T51.0X3	T51.0X4	—	—
fumes	T59.891	T59.892	T59.893	T59.894	—	—
solvents (fumes) (vapors)	T52.91	T52.92	T52.93	T52.94	—	—
Influenza vaccine	T50.B91	T50.B92	T50.B93	T50.B94	T50.B95	T50.B96
Ingested substance NEC	T65.91	T65.92	T65.93	T65.94	—	—
INH	T37.1X1	T37.1X2	T37.1X3	T37.1X4	T37.1X5	T37.1X6
Inhalation, gas (noxious) — *see* Gas						
Inhibitor						
angiotensin-converting enzyme	T46.4X1	T46.4X2	T46.4X3	T46.4X4	T46.4X5	T46.4X6
carbonic anhydrase	T50.2X1	T50.2X2	T50.2X3	T50.2X4	T50.2X5	T50.2X6
fibrinolysis	T45.621	T45.622	T45.623	T45.624	T45.625	T45.626
monoamine oxidase NEC	T43.1X1	T43.1X2	T43.1X3	T43.1X4	T43.1X5	T43.1X6
hydrazine	T43.1X1	T43.1X2	T43.1X3	T43.1X4	T43.1X5	T43.1X6
postsynaptic	T43.8X1	T43.8X2	T43.8X3	T43.8X4	T43.8X5	T43.8X6
prothrombin synthesis	T45.511	T45.512	T45.513	T45.514	T45.515	T45.516
Ink	T65.891	T65.892	T65.893	T65.894	—	—
Inorganic substance NEC	T57.91	T57.92	T57.93	T57.94	—	—
Inosine pranobex	T37.5X1	T37.5X2	T37.5X3	T37.5X4	T37.5X5	T37.5X6
Inositol	T50.991	T50.992	T50.993	T50.994	T50.995	T50.996
nicotinate	T46.7X1	T46.7X2	T46.7X3	T46.7X4	T46.7X5	T46.7X6
Inproquone	T45.1X1	T45.1X2	T45.1X3	T45.1X4	T45.1X5	T45.1X6
Insecticide NEC	T60.91	T60.92	T60.93	T60.94	—	—
carbamate	T60.0X1	T60.0X2	T60.0X3	T60.0X4	—	—
chlorinated	T60.1X1	T60.1X2	T60.1X3	T60.1X4	—	—
mixed	T60.91	T60.92	T60.93	T60.94	—	—
organochlorine	T60.1X1	T60.1X2	T60.1X3	T60.1X4	—	—
organophosphorus	T60.0X1	T60.0X2	T60.0X3	T60.0X4	—	—
Insect (sting), venomous	T63.481	T63.482	T63.483	T63.484	—	—
ant	T63.421	T63.422	T63.423	T63.424	—	—
bee	T63.441	T63.442	T63.443	T63.444	—	—
caterpillar	T63.431	T63.432	T63.433	T63.434	—	—
hornet	T63.451	T63.452	T63.453	T63.454	—	—
wasp	T63.461	T63.462	T63.463	T63.464	—	—
Insular tissue extract	T38.3X1	T38.3X2	T38.3X3	T38.3X4	T38.3X5	T38.3X6
Insulin (amorphous) (globin) (isophane) (Lente) (NPH) (Semilente) (Ultralente)	T38.3X1	T38.3X2	T38.3X3	T38.3X4	T38.3X5	T38.3X6
defalan	T38.3X1	T38.3X2	T38.3X3	T38.3X4	T38.3X5	T38.3X6
human	T38.3X1	T38.3X2	T38.3X3	T38.3X4	T38.3X5	T38.3X6
injection, soluble	T38.3X1	T38.3X2	T38.3X3	T38.3X4	T38.3X5	T38.3X6
biphasic	T38.3X1	T38.3X2	T38.3X3	T38.3X4	T38.3X5	T38.3X6
intermediate acting	T38.3X1	T38.3X2	T38.3X3	T38.3X4	T38.3X5	T38.3X6
protamine zinc	T38.3X1	T38.3X2	T38.3X3	T38.3X4	T38.3X5	T38.3X6
slow acting	T38.3X1	T38.3X2	T38.3X3	T38.3X4	T38.3X5	T38.3X6
zinc						
protamine injection	T38.3X1	T38.3X2	T38.3X3	T38.3X4	T38.3X5	T38.3X6
suspension (amorphous) (crystalline)	T38.3X1	T38.3X2	T38.3X3	T38.3X4	T38.3X5	T38.3X6
Interferon (alpha) (beta) (gamma)	T37.5X1	T37.5X2	T37.5X3	T37.5X4	T37.5X5	T37.5X6
Intestinal motility control drug	T47.6X1	T47.6X2	T47.6X3	T47.6X4	T47.6X5	T47.6X6
biological	T47.8X1	T47.8X2	T47.8X3	T47.8X4	T47.8X5	T47.8X6
Intranarcon	T41.1X1	T41.1X2	T41.1X3	T41.1X4	T41.1X5	T41.1X6
Intravenous						
amino acids	T50.991	T50.992	T50.993	T50.994	T50.995	T50.996
fat suspension	T50.991	T50.992	T50.993	T50.994	T50.995	T50.996
Inulin	T50.8X1	T50.8X2	T50.8X3	T50.8X4	T50.8X5	T50.8X6
Invert sugar	T50.3X1	T50.3X2	T50.3X3	T50.3X4	T50.3X5	T50.3X6
Inza — *see* Naproxen						
Iobenzamic acid	T50.8X1	T50.8X2	T50.8X3	T50.8X4	T50.8X5	T50.8X6
Iocarmic acid	T50.8X1	T50.8X2	T50.8X3	T50.8X4	T50.8X5	T50.8X6
Iocetamic acid	T50.8X1	T50.8X2	T50.8X3	T50.8X4	T50.8X5	T50.8X6
Iodamide	T50.8X1	T50.8X2	T50.8X3	T50.8X4	T50.8X5	T50.8X6
Iodide NEC — *see also* Iodine	T49.0X1	T49.0X2	T49.0X3	T49.0X4	T49.0X5	T49.0X6
mercury (ointment)	T49.0X1	T49.0X2	T49.0X3	T49.0X4	T49.0X5	T49.0X6
methylate	T49.0X1	T49.0X2	T49.0X3	T49.0X4	T49.0X5	T49.0X6
potassium (expectorant) NEC	T48.4X1	T48.4X2	T48.4X3	T48.4X4	T48.4X5	T48.4X6
Iodinated						
contrast medium	T50.8X1	T50.8X2	T50.8X3	T50.8X4	T50.8X5	T50.8X6
glycerol	T48.4X1	T48.4X2	T48.4X3	T48.4X4	T48.4X5	T48.4X6
human serum albumin (131I)	T50.8X1	T50.8X2	T50.8X3	T50.8X4	T50.8X5	T50.8X6
Iodine (antiseptic, external) (tincture) **NEC**	T49.0X1	T49.0X2	T49.0X3	T49.0X4	T49.0X5	T49.0X6
125 — *see also* Radiation sickness, and Exposure to radioactivce isotopes	T50.8X1	T50.8X2	T50.8X3	T50.8X4	T50.8X5	T50.8X6
therapeutic	T50.991	T50.992	T50.993	T50.994	T50.995	T50.996
131 — *see also* Radiation sickness, and Exposure to radioactivce isotopes	T50.8X1	T50.8X2	T50.8X3	T50.8X4	T50.8X5	T50.8X6
therapeutic	T38.2X1	T38.2X2	T38.2X3	T38.2X4	T38.2X5	T38.2X6
diagnostic	T50.8X1	T50.8X2	T50.8X3	T50.8X4	T50.8X5	T50.8X6

Substance	Poisoning, Accidental (unintentional)	Poisoning, Intentional Self-harm	Poisoning, Assault	Poisoning, Undetermined	Adverse Effect	Under-dosing
Iodine (antiseptic, external)						
(tincture) **NEC** — continued						
for thyroid conditions	T38.2X1	T38.2X2	T38.2X3	T38.2X4	T38.2X5	T38.2X6
(antithyroid)						
solution	T49.0X1	T49.0X2	T49.0X3	T49.0X4	T49.0X5	T49.0X6
vapor	T59.891	T59.892	T59.893	T59.894	—	—
Iodipamide	T50.8X1	T50.8X2	T50.8X3	T50.8X4	T50.8X5	T50.8X6
Iodized (poppy seed) oil	T50.8X1	T50.8X2	T50.8X3	T50.8X4	T50.8X5	T50.8X6
Iodobismitol	T37.8X1	T37.8X2	T37.8X3	T37.8X4	T37.8X5	T37.8X6
Iodochlorhydroxyquin	T37.8X1	T37.8X2	T37.8X3	T37.8X4	T37.8X5	T37.8X6
topical	T49.0X1	T49.0X2	T49.0X3	T49.0X4	T49.0X5	T49.0X6
Iodochlorhydroxyquinoline	T37.8X1	T37.8X2	T37.8X3	T37.8X4	T37.8X5	T37.8X6
Iodocholesterol (131I)	T50.8X1	T50.8X2	T50.8X3	T50.8X4	T50.8X5	T50.8X6
Iodoform	T49.0X1	T49.0X2	T49.0X3	T49.0X4	T49.0X5	T49.0X6
Iodohippuric acid	T50.8X1	T50.8X2	T50.8X3	T50.8X4	T50.8X5	T50.8X6
Iodopanoic acid	T50.8X1	T50.8X2	T50.8X3	T50.8X4	T50.8X5	T50.8X6
Iodophthalein (sodium)	T50.8X1	T50.8X2	T50.8X3	T50.8X4	T50.8X5	T50.8X6
Iodopyracet	T50.8X1	T50.8X2	T50.8X3	T50.8X4	T50.8X5	T50.8X6
Iodoquinol	T37.8X1	T37.8X2	T37.8X3	T37.8X4	T37.8X5	T37.8X6
Iodoxamic acid	T50.8X1	T50.8X2	T50.8X3	T50.8X4	T50.8X5	T50.8X6
Iofendylate	T50.8X1	T50.8X2	T50.8X3	T50.8X4	T50.8X5	T50.8X6
Ioglycamic acid	T50.8X1	T50.8X2	T50.8X3	T50.8X4	T50.8X5	T50.8X6
Iohexol	T50.8X1	T50.8X2	T50.8X3	T50.8X4	T50.8X5	T50.8X6
Ion exchange resin						
anion	T47.8X1	T47.8X2	T47.8X3	T47.8X4	T47.8X5	T47.8X6
cation	T50.3X1	T50.3X2	T50.3X3	T50.3X4	T50.3X5	T50.3X6
cholestyramine	T46.6X1	T46.6X2	T46.6X3	T46.6X4	T46.6X5	T46.6X6
intestinal	T47.8X1	T47.8X2	T47.8X3	T47.8X4	T47.8X5	T47.8X6
Iopamidol	T50.8X1	T50.8X2	T50.8X3	T50.8X4	T50.8X5	T50.8X6
Iopanoic acid	T50.8X1	T50.8X2	T50.8X3	T50.8X4	T50.8X5	T50.8X6
Iophenoic acid	T50.8X1	T50.8X2	T50.8X3	T50.8X4	T50.8X5	T50.8X6
Iopodate, sodium	T50.8X1	T50.8X2	T50.8X3	T50.8X4	T50.8X5	T50.8X6
Iopodic acid	T50.8X1	T50.8X2	T50.8X3	T50.8X4	T50.8X5	T50.8X6
Iopromide	T50.8X1	T50.8X2	T50.8X3	T50.8X4	T50.8X5	T50.8X6
Iopydol	T50.8X1	T50.8X2	T50.8X3	T50.8X4	T50.8X5	T50.8X6
Iotalamic acid	T50.8X1	T50.8X2	T50.8X3	T50.8X4	T50.8X5	T50.8X6
Iothalamate	T50.8X1	T50.8X2	T50.8X3	T50.8X4	T50.8X5	T50.8X6
Iothiouracil	T38.2X1	T38.2X2	T38.2X3	T38.2X4	T38.2X5	T38.2X6
Iotrol	T50.8X1	T50.8X2	T50.8X3	T50.8X4	T50.8X5	T50.8X6
Iotrolan	T50.8X1	T50.8X2	T50.8X3	T50.8X4	T50.8X5	T50.8X6
Iotroxate	T50.8X1	T50.8X2	T50.8X3	T50.8X4	T50.8X5	T50.8X6
Iotroxic acid	T50.8X1	T50.8X2	T50.8X3	T50.8X4	T50.8X5	T50.8X6
Ioversol	T50.8X1	T50.8X2	T50.8X3	T50.8X4	T50.8X5	T50.8X6
Ioxaglate	T50.8X1	T50.8X2	T50.8X3	T50.8X4	T50.8X5	T50.8X6
Ioxaglic acid	T50.8X1	T50.8X2	T50.8X3	T50.8X4	T50.8X5	T50.8X6
Ioxitalamic acid	T50.8X1	T50.8X2	T50.8X3	T50.8X4	T50.8X5	T50.8X6
Ipecac	T47.7X1	T47.7X2	T47.7X3	T47.7X4	T47.7X5	T47.7X6
Ipecacuanha	T48.4X1	T48.4X2	T48.4X3	T48.4X4	T48.4X5	T48.4X6
Ipodate, calcium	T50.8X1	T50.8X2	T50.8X3	T50.8X4	T50.8X5	T50.8X6
Ipral	T42.3X1	T42.3X2	T42.3X3	T42.3X4	T42.3X5	T42.3X6
Ipratropium (bromide)	T48.6X1	T48.6X2	T48.6X3	T48.6X4	T48.6X5	T48.6X6
Ipriflavone	T46.3X1	T46.3X2	T46.3X3	T46.3X4	T46.3X5	T46.3X6
Iprindole	T43.011	T43.012	T43.013	T43.014	T43.015	T43.016
Iproclozide	T43.1X1	T43.1X2	T43.1X3	T43.1X4	T43.1X5	T43.1X6
Iprofenin	T50.8X1	T50.8X2	T50.8X3	T50.8X4	T50.8X5	T50.8X6
Iproheptine	T49.2X1	T49.2X2	T49.2X3	T49.2X4	T49.2X5	T49.2X6
Iproniazid	T43.1X1	T43.1X2	T43.1X3	T43.1X4	T43.1X5	T43.1X6
Iproplatin	T45.1X1	T45.1X2	T45.1X3	T45.1X4	T45.1X5	T45.1X6
Iproveratril	T46.1X1	T46.1X2	T46.1X3	T46.1X4	T46.1X5	T46.1X6
Iron (compounds) (medicinal)	T45.4X1	T45.4X2	T45.4X3	T45.4X4	T45.4X5	T45.4X6
NEC						
ammonium	T45.4X1	T45.4X2	T45.4X3	T45.4X4	T45.4X5	T45.4X6
dextran injection	T45.4X1	T45.4X2	T45.4X3	T45.4X4	T45.4X5	T45.4X6
nonmedicinal	T56.891	T56.892	T56.893	T56.894	—	—
salts	T45.4X1	T45.4X2	T45.4X3	T45.4X4	T45.4X5	T45.4X6
sorbitex	T45.4X1	T45.4X2	T45.4X3	T45.4X4	T45.4X5	T45.4X6
sorbitol citric acid complex	T45.4X1	T45.4X2	T45.4X3	T45.4X4	T45.4X5	T45.4X6
Irrigating fluid (vaginal)	T49.8X1	T49.8X2	T49.8X3	T49.8X4	T49.8X5	T49.8X6
eye	T49.5X1	T49.5X2	T49.5X3	T49.5X4	T49.5X5	T49.5X6
Isepamicin	T36.5X1	T36.5X2	T36.5X3	T36.5X4	T36.5X5	T36.5X6
Isoaminile (citrate)	T48.3X1	T48.3X2	T48.3X3	T48.3X4	T48.3X5	T48.3X6
Isoamyl nitrite	T46.3X1	T46.3X2	T46.3X3	T46.3X4	T46.3X5	T46.3X6
Isobenzan	T60.1X1	T60.1X2	T60.1X3	T60.1X4	—	—
Isobutyl acetate	T52.8X1	T52.8X2	T52.8X3	T52.8X4	—	—
Isocarboxazid	T43.1X1	T43.1X2	T43.1X3	T43.1X4	T43.1X5	T43.1X6
Isoconazole	T49.0X1	T49.0X2	T49.0X3	T49.0X4	T49.0X5	T49.0X6
Isocyanate	T65.0X1	T65.0X2	T65.0X3	T65.0X4	—	—
Isoephedrine	T44.991	T44.992	T44.993	T44.994	T44.995	T44.996
Isoetarine	T48.6X1	T48.6X2	T48.6X3	T48.6X4	T48.6X5	T48.6X6
Isoethadione	T42.2X1	T42.2X2	T42.2X3	T42.2X4	T42.2X5	T42.2X6
Isoetharine	T44.5X1	T44.5X2	T44.5X3	T44.5X4	T44.5X5	T44.5X6
Isoflurane	T41.0X1	T41.0X2	T41.0X3	T41.0X4	T41.0X5	T41.0X6
Isoflurophate	T44.0X1	T44.0X2	T44.0X3	T44.0X4	T44.0X5	T44.0X6

Substance	Poisoning, Accidental (unintentional)	Poisoning, Intentional Self-harm	Poisoning, Assault	Poisoning, Undetermined	Adverse Effect	Under-dosing
Isomaltose, ferric complex	T45.4X1	T45.4X2	T45.4X3	T45.4X4	T45.4X5	T45.4X6
Isometheptene	T44.3X1	T44.3X2	T44.3X3	T44.3X4	T44.3X5	T44.3X6
Isoniazid	T37.1X1	T37.1X2	T37.1X3	T37.1X4	T37.1X5	T37.1X6
with						
rifampicin	T36.6X1	T36.6X2	T36.6X3	T36.6X4	T36.6X5	T36.6X6
thioacetazone	T37.1X1	T37.1X2	T37.1X3	T37.1X4	T37.1X5	T37.1X6
Isonicotinic acid hydrazide	T37.1X1	T37.1X2	T37.1X3	T37.1X4	T37.1X5	T37.1X6
Isonipecaine	T40.4X1	T40.4X2	T40.4X3	T40.4X4	T40.4X5	T40.4X6
Isopentaquine	T37.2X1	T37.2X2	T37.2X3	T37.2X4	T37.2X5	T37.2X6
Isophane insulin	T38.3X1	T38.3X2	T38.3X3	T38.3X4	T38.3X5	T38.3X6
Isophorone	T65.891	T65.892	T65.893	T65.894		
Isophosphamide	T45.1X1	T45.1X2	T45.1X3	T45.1X4	T45.1X5	T45.1X6
Isopregnenone	T38.5X1	T38.5X2	T38.5X3	T38.5X4	T38.5X5	T38.5X6
Isoprenaline	T48.6X1	T48.6X2	T48.6X3	T48.6X4	T48.6X5	T48.6X6
Isopromethazine	T43.3X1	T43.3X2	T43.3X3	T43.3X4	T43.3X5	T43.3X6
Isopropamide	T44.3X1	T44.3X2	T44.3X3	T44.3X4	T44.3X5	T44.3X6
iodide	T44.3X1	T44.3X2	T44.3X3	T44.3X4	T44.3X5	T44.3X6
Isopropanol	T51.2X1	T51.2X2	T51.2X3	T51.2X4	—	—
Isopropyl						
acetate	T52.8X1	T52.8X2	T52.8X3	T52.8X4	—	—
alcohol	T51.2X1	T51.2X2	T51.2X3	T51.2X4	—	—
medicinal	T49.4X1	T49.4X2	T49.4X3	T49.4X4	T49.4X5	T49.4X6
ether	T52.8X1	T52.8X2	T52.8X3	T52.8X4	—	—
Isopropylaminophenazone	T39.2X1	T39.2X2	T39.2X3	T39.2X4	T39.2X5	T39.2X6
Isoproterenol	T48.6X1	T48.6X2	T48.6X3	T48.6X4	T48.6X5	T48.6X6
Isosorbide dinitrate	T46.3X1	T46.3X2	T46.3X3	T46.3X4	T46.3X5	T46.3X6
Isothipendyl	T45.0X1	T45.0X2	T45.0X3	T45.0X4	T45.0X5	T45.0X6
Isotretinoin	T50.991	T50.992	T50.993	T50.994	T50.995	T50.996
Isoxazolyl penicillin	T36.0X1	T36.0X2	T36.0X3	T36.0X4	T36.0X5	T36.0X6
Isoxicam	T39.391	T39.392	T39.393	T39.394	T39.395	T39.396
Isoxsuprine	T46.7X1	T46.7X2	T46.7X3	T46.7X4	T46.7X5	T46.7X6
Ispagula	T47.4X1	T47.4X2	T47.4X3	T47.4X4	T47.4X5	T47.4X6
husk	T47.4X1	T47.4X2	T47.4X3	T47.4X4	T47.4X5	T47.4X6
Isradipine	T46.1X1	T46.1X2	T46.1X3	T46.1X4	T46.1X5	T46.1X6
I-thyroxine sodium	T38.1X1	T38.1X2	T38.1X3	T38.1X4	T38.1X5	T38.1X6
Itraconazole	T37.8X1	T37.8X2	T37.8X3	T37.8X4	T37.8X5	T37.8X6
Itramin tosilate	T46.3X1	T46.3X2	T46.3X3	T46.3X4	T46.3X5	T46.3X6
Ivermectin	T37.4X1	T37.4X2	T37.4X3	T37.4X4	T37.4X5	T37.4X6
Izoniazid	T37.1X1	T37.1X2	T37.1X3	T37.1X4	T37.1X5	T37.1X6
with thioacetazone	T37.1X1	T37.1X2	T37.1X3	T37.1X4	T37.1X5	T37.1X6
Jalap	T47.2X1	T47.2X2	T47.2X3	T47.2X4	T47.2X5	T47.2X6
Jamaica						
dogwood (bark)	T39.8X1	T39.8X2	T39.8X3	T39.8X4	T39.8X5	T39.8X6
ginger	T65.891	T65.892	T65.893	T65.894	—	—
root	T62.2X1	T62.2X2	T62.2X3	T62.2X4	—	—
Jatropha	T62.2X1	T62.2X2	T62.2X3	T62.2X4	—	—
curcas	T62.2X1	T62.2X2	T62.2X3	T62.2X4	—	—
Jectofer	T45.4X1	T45.4X2	T45.4X3	T45.4X4	T45.4X5	T45.4X6
Jellyfish (sting)	T63.621	T63.622	T63.623	T63.624	—	—
Jequirity (bean)	T62.2X1	T62.2X2	T62.2X3	T62.2X4	—	—
Jimson weed (stramonium)	T62.2X1	T62.2X2	T62.2X3	T62.2X4	—	—
seeds	T62.2X1	T62.2X2	T62.2X3	T62.2X4	—	—
Josamycin	T36.3X1	T36.3X2	T36.3X3	T36.3X4	T36.3X5	T36.3X6
Juniper tar	T49.1X1	T49.1X2	T49.1X3	T49.1X4	T49.1X5	T49.1X6
Kallidinogenase	T46.7X1	T46.7X2	T46.7X3	T46.7X4	T46.7X5	T46.7X6
Kallikrein	T46.7X1	T46.7X2	T46.7X3	T46.7X4	T46.7X5	T46.7X6
Kanamycin	T36.5X1	T36.5X2	T36.5X3	T36.5X4	T36.5X5	T36.5X6
Kantrex	T36.5X1	T36.5X2	T36.5X3	T36.5X4	T36.5X5	T36.5X6
Kaolin	T47.6X1	T47.6X2	T47.6X3	T47.6X4	T47.6X5	T47.6X6
light	T47.6X1	T47.6X2	T47.6X3	T47.6X4	T47.6X5	T47.6X6
Karaya (gum)	T47.4X1	T47.4X2	T47.4X3	T47.4X4	T47.4X5	T47.4X6
Kebuzone	T39.2X1	T39.2X2	T39.2X3	T39.2X4	T39.2X5	T39.2X6
Kelevan	T60.1X1	T60.1X2	T60.1X3	T60.1X4	—	—
Kemithal	T41.1X1	T41.1X2	T41.1X3	T41.1X4	T41.1X5	T41.1X6
Kenacort	T38.0X1	T38.0X2	T38.0X3	T38.0X4	T38.0X5	T38.0X6
Keratolytic drug NEC	T49.4X1	T49.4X2	T49.4X3	T49.4X4	T49.4X5	T49.4X6
anthracene	T49.4X1	T49.4X2	T49.4X3	T49.4X4	T49.4X5	T49.4X6
Keratoplastic NEC	T49.4X1	T49.4X2	T49.4X3	T49.4X4	T49.4X5	T49.4X6
Kerosene, kerosine (fuel)	T52.0X1	T52.0X2	T52.0X3	T52.0X4	—	—
(solvent) **NEC**						
insecticide	T52.0X1	T52.0X2	T52.0X3	T52.0X4	—	—
vapor	T52.0X1	T52.0X2	T52.0X3	T52.0X4	—	—
Ketamine	T41.291	T41.292	T41.293	T41.294	T41.295	T41.296
Ketazolam	T42.4X1	T42.4X2	T42.4X3	T42.4X4	T42.4X5	T42.4X6
Ketazon	T39.2X1	T39.2X2	T39.2X3	T39.2X4	T39.2X5	T39.2X6
Ketobemidone	T40.4X1	T40.4X2	T40.4X3	T40.4X4	—	—
Ketoconazole	T49.0X1	T49.0X2	T49.0X3	T49.0X4	T49.0X5	T49.0X6
Ketols	T52.4X1	T52.4X2	T52.4X3	T52.4X4	—	—
Ketone oils	T52.4X1	T52.4X2	T52.4X3	T52.4X4	—	—
Ketoprofen	T39.311	T39.312	T39.313	T39.314	T39.315	T39.316
Ketorolac	T39.8X1	T39.8X2	T39.8X3	T39.8X4	T39.8X5	T39.8X6
Ketotifen	T45.0X1	T45.0X2	T45.0X3	T45.0X4	T45.0X5	T45.0X6
Khat	T43.691	T43.692	T43.693	T43.694	—	—

Substance	Poisoning, Accidental (unintentional)	Poisoning, Intentional Self-harm	Poisoning, Assault	Poisoning, Undetermined	Adverse Effect	Under-dosing
Khellin	T46.3X1	T46.3X2	T46.3X3	T46.3X4	T46.3X5	T46.3X6
Khelloside	T46.3X1	T46.3X2	T46.3X3	T46.3X4	T46.3X5	T46.3X6
Kiln gas or vapor (carbon monoxide)	T58.8X1	T58.8X2	T58.8X3	T58.8X4	—	—
Kitasamycin	T36.3X1	T36.3X2	T36.3X3	T36.3X4	T36.3X5	T36.3X6
Konsyl	T47.4X1	T47.4X2	T47.4X3	T47.4X4	T47.4X5	T47.4X6
Kosam seed	T62.2X1	T62.2X2	T62.2X3	T62.2X4		
Krait (venom)	T63.091	T63.092	T63.093	T63.094		
Kwell (insecticide)	T60.1X1	T60.1X2	T60.1X3	T60.1X4	—	—
anti-infective (topical)	T49.0X1	T49.0X2	T49.0X3	T49.0X4	T49.0X5	T49.0X6
Labetalol	T44.8X1	T44.8X2	T44.8X3	T44.8X4	T44.8X5	T44.8X6
Laburnum (seeds)	T62.2X1	T62.2X2	T62.2X3	T62.2X4	—	—
leaves	T62.2X1	T62.2X2	T62.2X3	T62.2X4	—	—
Lachesine	T49.5X1	T49.5X2	T49.5X3	T49.5X4	T49.5X5	T49.5X6
Lacidipine	T46.5X1	T46.5X2	T46.5X3	T46.5X4	T46.5X5	T46.5X6
Lacquer	T65.6X1	T65.6X2	T65.6X3	T65.6X4	—	—
Lacrimogenic gas	T59.3X1	T59.3X2	T59.3X3	T59.3X4	—	—
Lactated potassic saline	T50.3X1	T50.3X2	T50.3X3	T50.3X4	T50.3X5	T50.3X6
Lactic acid	T49.8X1	T49.8X2	T49.8X3	T49.8X4	T49.8X5	T49.8X6
Lactobacillus						
acidophilus	T47.6X1	T47.6X2	T47.6X3	T47.6X4	T47.6X5	T47.6X6
compound	T47.6X1	T47.6X2	T47.6X3	T47.6X4	T47.6X5	T47.6X6
bifidus, lyophilized	T47.6X1	T47.6X2	T47.6X3	T47.6X4	T47.6X5	T47.6X6
bulgaricus	T47.6X1	T47.6X2	T47.6X3	T47.6X4	T47.6X5	T47.6X6
sporogenes	T47.6X1	T47.6X2	T47.6X3	T47.6X4	T47.6X5	T47.6X6
Lactoflavin	T45.2X1	T45.2X2	T45.2X3	T45.2X4	T45.2X5	T45.2X6
Lactose (as excipient)	T50.901	T50.902	T50.903	T50.904	T50.905	T50.906
Lactuca (virosa) (extract)	T42.6X1	T42.6X2	T42.6X3	T42.6X4	T42.6X5	T42.6X6
Lactucarium	T42.6X1	T42.6X2	T42.6X3	T42.6X4	T42.6X5	T42.6X6
Lactulose	T47.3X1	T47.3X2	T47.3X3	T47.3X4	T47.3X5	T47.3X6
Laevo — see Levo-						
Lanatosides	T46.0X1	T46.0X2	T46.0X3	T46.0X4	T46.0X5	T46.0X6
Lanolin	T49.3X1	T49.3X2	T49.3X3	T49.3X4	T49.3X5	T49.3X6
Largactil	T43.3X1	T43.3X2	T43.3X3	T43.3X4	T43.3X5	T43.3X6
Larkspur	T62.2X1	T62.2X2	T62.2X3	T62.2X4	—	—
Laroxyl	T43.011	T43.012	T43.013	T43.014	T43.015	T43.016
Lasix	T50.1X1	T50.1X2	T50.1X3	T50.1X4	T50.1X5	T50.1X6
Lassar's paste	T49.4X1	T49.4X2	T49.4X3	T49.4X4	T49.4X5	T49.4X6
Latamoxef	T36.1X1	T36.1X2	T36.1X3	T36.1X4	T36.1X5	T36.1X6
Latex	T65.811	T65.812	T65.813	T65.814	—	—
Lathyrus (seed)	T62.2X1	T62.2X2	T62.2X3	T62.2X4	—	—
Laudanum	T40.0X1	T40.0X2	T40.0X3	T40.0X4	T40.0X5	T40.0X6
Laudexium	T48.1X1	T48.1X2	T48.1X3	T48.1X4	T48.1X5	T48.1X6
Laughing gas	T41.0X1	T41.0X2	T41.0X3	T41.0X4	T41.0X5	T41.0X6
Laurel, black or cherry	T62.2X1	T62.2X2	T62.2X3	T62.2X4	—	—
Laurolinium	T49.0X1	T49.0X2	T49.0X3	T49.0X4	T49.0X5	T49.0X6
Lauryl sulfoacetate	T49.2X1	T49.2X2	T49.2X3	T49.2X4	T49.2X5	T49.2X6
Laxative NEC	T47.4X1	T47.4X2	T47.4X3	T47.4X4	T47.4X5	T47.4X6
osmotic	T47.3X1	T47.3X2	T47.3X3	T47.3X4	T47.3X5	T47.3X6
saline	T47.3X1	T47.3X2	T47.3X3	T47.3X4	T47.3X5	T47.3X6
stimulant	T47.2X1	T47.2X2	T47.2X3	T47.2X4	T47.2X5	T47.2X6
L-dopa	T42.8X1	T42.8X2	T42.8X3	T42.8X4	T42.8X5	T42.8X6
Lead (dust) (fumes) (vapor)	T56.0X1	T56.0X2	T56.0X3	T56.0X4	—	—
NEC						
acetate	T49.2X1	T49.2X2	T49.2X3	T49.2X4	T49.2X5	T49.2X6
alkyl (fuel additive)	T56.0X1	T56.0X2	T56.0X3	T56.0X4	—	—
anti-infectives	T37.8X1	T37.8X2	T37.8X3	T37.8X4	T37.8X5	T37.8X6
antiknock compound (tetraethyl)	T56.0X1	T56.0X2	T56.0X3	T56.0X4	—	—
arsenate, arsenite (dust)(herbicide) (insecticide) (vapor)	T57.0X1	T57.0X2	T57.0X3	T57.0X4	—	—
carbonate	T56.0X1	T56.0X2	T56.0X3	T56.0X4	—	—
paint	T56.0X1	T56.0X2	T56.0X3	T56.0X4	—	—
chromate	T56.0X1	T56.0X2	T56.0X3	T56.0X4	—	—
paint	T56.0X1	T56.0X2	T56.0X3	T56.0X4	—	—
dioxide	T56.0X1	T56.0X2	T56.0X3	T56.0X4	—	—
inorganic	T56.0X1	T56.0X2	T56.0X3	T56.0X4	—	—
iodide	T56.0X1	T56.0X2	T56.0X3	T56.0X4	—	—
pigment (paint)	T56.0X1	T56.0X2	T56.0X3	T56.0X4	—	—
monoxide (dust)	T56.0X1	T56.0X2	T56.0X3	T56.0X4	—	—
paint	T56.0X1	T56.0X2	T56.0X3	T56.0X4	—	—
organic	T56.0X1	T56.0X2	T56.0X3	T56.0X4	—	—
oxide	T56.0X1	T56.0X2	T56.0X3	T56.0X4	—	—
paint	T56.0X1	T56.0X2	T56.0X3	T56.0X4	—	—
paint	T56.0X1	T56.0X2	T56.0X3	T56.0X4	—	—
salts	T56.0X1	T56.0X2	T56.0X3	T56.0X4	—	—
specified compound NEC	T56.0X1	T56.0X2	T56.0X3	T56.0X4	—	—
tetra-ethyl	T56.0X1	T56.0X2	T56.0X3	T56.0X4	—	—
Lebanese red	T40.7X1	T40.7X2	T40.7X3	T40.7X4	T40.7X5	T40.7X6
Lefetamine	T39.8X1	T39.8X2	T39.8X3	T39.8X4	T39.8X5	T39.8X6
Lenperone	T43.4X1	T43.4X2	T43.4X3	T43.4X4	T43.4X5	T43.4X6
Lente Iletin (insulin)	T38.3X1	T38.3X2	T38.3X3	T38.3X4	T38.3X5	T38.3X6

Substance	Poisoning, Accidental (unintentional)	Poisoning, Intentional Self-harm	Poisoning, Assault	Poisoning, Undetermined	Adverse Effect	Under-dosing
Leptazol	T50.7X1	T50.7X2	T50.7X3	T50.7X4	T50.7X5	T50.7X6
Leptophos	T60.0X1	T60.0X2	T60.0X3	T60.0X4	—	—
Leritine	T40.2X1	T40.2X2	T40.2X3	T40.2X4	T40.2X5	T40.2X6
Letosteine	T48.4X1	T48.4X2	T48.4X3	T48.4X4	T48.4X5	T48.4X6
Letter	T38.1X1	T38.1X2	T38.1X3	T38.1X4	T38.1X5	T38.1X6
Lettuce opium	T42.6X1	T42.6X2	T42.6X3	T42.6X4	T42.6X5	T42.6X6
Leucinocaine	T41.3X1	T41.3X2	T41.3X3	T41.3X4	T41.3X5	T41.3X6
Leucocianidol	T46.991	T46.992	T46.993	T46.994	T46.995	T46.996
Leucovorin (factor)	T45.8X1	T45.8X2	T45.8X3	T45.8X4	T45.8X5	T45.8X6
Leukeran	T45.1X1	T45.1X2	T45.1X3	T45.1X4	T45.1X5	T45.1X6
Leuprolide	T38.891	T38.892	T38.893	T38.894	T38.895	T38.896
Levalbuterol	T48.6X1	T48.6X2	T48.6X3	T48.6X4	T48.6X5	T48.6X6
Levallorphan	T50.7X1	T50.7X2	T50.7X3	T50.7X4	T50.7X5	T50.7X6
Levamisole	T37.4X1	T37.4X2	T37.4X3	T37.4X4	T37.4X5	T37.4X6
Levanil	T42.6X1	T42.6X2	T42.6X3	T42.6X4	T42.6X5	T42.6X6
Levarterenol	T44.4X1	T44.4X2	T44.4X3	T44.4X4	T44.4X5	T44.4X6
Levdropropizine	T48.3X1	T48.3X2	T48.3X3	T48.3X4	T48.3X5	T48.3X6
Levobunolol	T49.5X1	T49.5X2	T49.5X3	T49.5X4	T49.5X5	T49.5X6
Levocabastine (hydrochloride)	T45.0X1	T45.0X2	T45.0X3	T45.0X4	T45.0X5	T45.0X6
Levocarnitine	T50.991	T50.992	T50.993	T50.994	T50.995	T50.996
Levodopa	T42.8X1	T42.8X2	T42.8X3	T42.8X4	T42.8X5	T42.8X6
with carbidopa	T42.8X1	T42.8X2	T42.8X3	T42.8X4	T42.8X5	T42.8X6
Levo-dromoran	T40.2X1	T40.2X2	T40.2X3	T40.2X4	T40.2X5	T40.2X6
Levoglutamide	T50.991	T50.992	T50.993	T50.994	T50.995	T50.996
Levoid	T38.1X1	T38.1X2	T38.1X3	T38.1X4	T38.1X5	T38.1X6
Levo-isomethadone	T40.3X1	T40.3X2	T40.3X3	T40.3X4	T40.3X5	T40.3X6
Levomepromazine	T43.3X1	T43.3X2	T43.3X3	T43.3X4	T43.3X5	T43.3X6
Levonordefrin	T49.6X1	T49.6X2	T49.6X3	T49.6X4	T49.6X5	T49.6X6
Levonorgestrel	T38.4X1	T38.4X2	T38.4X3	T38.4X4	T38.4X5	T38.4X6
with ethinylestradiol	T38.5X1	T38.5X2	T38.5X3	T38.5X4	T38.5X5	T38.5X6
Levopromazine	T43.3X1	T43.3X2	T43.3X3	T43.3X4	T43.3X5	T43.3X6
Levoprome	T42.6X1	T42.6X2	T42.6X3	T42.6X4	T42.6X5	T42.6X6
Levopropoxyphene	T40.4X1	T40.4X2	T40.4X3	T40.4X4	T40.4X5	T40.4X6
Levopropylhexedrine	T50.5X1	T50.5X2	T50.5X3	T50.5X4	T50.5X5	T50.5X6
Levoproxyphylline	T48.6X1	T48.6X2	T48.6X3	T48.6X4	T48.6X5	T48.6X6
Levorphanol	T40.4X1	T40.4X2	T40.4X3	T40.4X4	T40.4X5	T40.4X6
Levothyroxine	T38.1X1	T38.1X2	T38.1X3	T38.1X4	T38.1X5	T38.1X6
sodium	T38.1X1	T38.1X2	T38.1X3	T38.1X4	T38.1X5	T38.1X6
Levsin	T44.3X1	T44.3X2	T44.3X3	T44.3X4	T44.3X5	T44.3X6
Levulose	T50.3X1	T50.3X2	T50.3X3	T50.3X4	T50.3X5	T50.3X6
Lewisite (gas), not in war	T57.0X1	T57.0X2	T57.0X3	T57.0X4	—	—
Librium	T42.4X1	T42.4X2	T42.4X3	T42.4X4	T42.4X5	T42.4X6
Lidex	T49.0X1	T49.0X2	T49.0X3	T49.0X4	T49.0X5	T49.0X6
Lidocaine	T41.3X1	T41.3X2	T41.3X3	T41.3X4	T41.3X5	T41.3X6
regional	T41.3X1	T41.3X2	T41.3X3	T41.3X4	T41.3X5	T41.3X6
spinal	T41.3X1	T41.3X2	T41.3X3	T41.3X4	T41.3X5	T41.3X6
Lidofenin	T50.8X1	T50.8X2	T50.8X3	T50.8X4	T50.8X5	T50.8X6
Lidoflazine	T46.1X1	T46.1X2	T46.1X3	T46.1X4	T46.1X5	T46.1X6
Lighter fluid	T52.0X1	T52.0X2	T52.0X3	T52.0X4	—	—
Lignin hemicellulose	T47.6X1	T47.6X2	T47.6X3	T47.6X4	T47.6X5	T47.6X6
Lignocaine	T41.3X1	T41.3X2	T41.3X3	T41.3X4	T41.3X5	T41.3X6
regional	T41.3X1	T41.3X2	T41.3X3	T41.3X4	T41.3X5	T41.3X6
spinal	T41.3X1	T41.3X2	T41.3X3	T41.3X4	T41.3X5	T41.3X6
Ligroin (e) (solvent)	T52.0X1	T52.0X2	T52.0X3	T52.0X4	—	—
vapor	T59.891	T59.892	T59.893	T59.894	—	—
Ligustrum vulgare	T62.2X1	T62.2X2	T62.2X3	T62.2X4	—	—
Lily of the valley	T62.2X1	T62.2X2	T62.2X3	T62.2X4	—	—
Lime (chloride)	T54.3X1	T54.3X2	T54.3X3	T54.3X4	—	—
Limonene	T52.8X1	T52.8X2	T52.8X3	T52.8X4	—	—
Lincomycin	T36.8X1	T36.8X2	T36.8X3	T36.8X4	T36.8X5	T36.8X6
Lindane (insecticide) (nonmedicinal) (vapor)	T53.6X1	T53.6X2	T53.6X3	T53.6X4	—	—
medicinal	T49.0X1	T49.0X2	T49.0X3	T49.0X4	T49.0X5	T49.0X6
Liniments NEC	T49.91	T49.92	T49.93	T49.94	T49.95	T49.96
Linoleic acid	T46.6X1	T46.6X2	T46.6X3	T46.6X4	T46.6X5	T46.6X6
Linolenic acid	T46.6X1	T46.6X2	T46.6X3	T46.6X4	T46.6X5	T46.6X6
Linseed	T47.4X1	T47.4X2	T47.4X3	T47.4X4	T47.4X5	T47.4X6
Liothyronine	T38.1X1	T38.1X2	T38.1X3	T38.1X4	T38.1X5	T38.1X6
Liotrix	T38.1X1	T38.1X2	T38.1X3	T38.1X4	T38.1X5	T38.1X6
Lipancreatin	T47.5X1	T47.5X2	T47.5X3	T47.5X4	T47.5X5	T47.5X6
Lipo-alprostadil	T46.7X1	T46.7X2	T46.7X3	T46.7X4	T46.7X5	T46.7X6
Lipo-Lutin	T38.5X1	T38.5X2	T38.5X3	T38.5X4	T38.5X5	T38.5X6
Lipotropic drug NEC	T50.901	T50.902	T50.903	T50.904	T50.905	T50.906
Liquefied petroleum gases	T59.891	T59.892	T59.893	T59.894	—	—
piped (pure or mixed with air)	T59.891	T59.892	T59.893	T59.894	—	—
Liquid						
paraffin	T47.4X1	T47.4X2	T47.4X3	T47.4X4	T47.4X5	T47.4X6
petrolatum	T47.4X1	T47.4X2	T47.4X3	T47.4X4	T47.4X5	T47.4X6
topical	T49.3X1	T49.3X2	T49.3X3	T49.3X4	T49.3X5	T49.3X6
specified NEC	T65.891	T65.892	T65.893	T65.894	—	—
substance	T65.91	T65.92	T65.93	T65.94	—	—

Table of Drugs and Chemicals

Liquor creosolis compositus — Meladrazine

Substance	Poisoning, Accidental (unintentional)	Poisoning, Intentional Self-harm	Poisoning, Assault	Poisoning, Undetermined	Adverse Effect	Under-dosing
Liquor creosolis compositus	T65.891	T65.892	T65.893	T65.894	—	—
Liquorice	T48.4X1	T48.4X2	T48.4X3	T48.4X4	T48.4X5	T48.4X6
extract	T47.8X1	T47.8X2	T47.8X3	T47.8X4	T47.8X5	T47.8X6
Lisinopril	T46.4X1	T46.4X2	T46.4X3	T46.4X4	T46.4X5	T46.4X6
Lisuride	T42.8X1	T42.8X2	T42.8X3	T42.8X4	T42.8X5	T42.8X6
Lithane	T43.8X1	T43.8X2	T43.8X3	T43.8X4	T43.8X5	T43.8X6
Lithium	T56.891	T56.892	T56.893	T56.894		
gluconate	T43.591	T43.592	T43.593	T43.594	T43.595	T43.596
salts (carbonate)	T43.591	T43.592	T43.593	T43.594	T43.595	T43.596
Lithonate	T43.8X1	T43.8X2	T43.8X3	T43.8X4	T43.8X5	T43.8X6
Liver						
extract	T45.8X1	T45.8X2	T45.8X3	T45.8X4	T45.8X5	T45.8X6
for parenteral use	T45.8X1	T45.8X2	T45.8X3	T45.8X4	T45.8X5	T45.8X6
fraction 1	T45.8X1	T45.8X2	T45.8X3	T45.8X4	T45.8X5	T45.8X6
hydrolysate	T45.8X1	T45.8X2	T45.8X3	T45.8X4	T45.8X5	T45.8X6
Lizard (bite) (venom)	T63.121	T63.122	T63.123	T63.124	—	—
LMD	T45.8X1	T45.8X2	T45.8X3	T45.8X4	T45.8X5	T45.8X6
Lobelia	T62.2X1	T62.2X2	T62.2X3	T62.2X4		
Lobeline	T50.7X1	T50.7X2	T50.7X3	T50.7X4	T50.7X5	T50.7X6
Local action drug NEC	T49.8X1	T49.8X2	T49.8X3	T49.8X4	T49.8X5	T49.8X6
Locorten	T49.0X1	T49.0X2	T49.0X3	T49.0X4	T49.0X5	T49.0X6
Lofepramine	T43.011	T43.012	T43.013	T43.014	T43.015	T43.016
Lolium temulentum	T62.2X1	T62.2X2	T62.2X3	T62.2X4	—	—
Lomotil	T47.6X1	T47.6X2	T47.6X3	T47.6X4	T47.6X5	T47.6X6
Lomustine	T45.1X1	T45.1X2	T45.1X3	T45.1X4	T45.1X5	T45.1X6
Lonidamine	T45.1X1	T45.1X2	T45.1X3	T45.1X4	T45.1X5	T45.1X6
Loperamide	T47.6X1	T47.6X2	T47.6X3	T47.6X4	T47.6X5	T47.6X6
Loprazolam	T42.4X1	T42.4X2	T42.4X3	T42.4X4	T42.4X5	T42.4X6
Lorajmine	T46.2X1	T46.2X2	T46.2X3	T46.2X4	T46.2X5	T46.2X6
Loratidine	T45.0X1	T45.0X2	T45.0X3	T45.0X4	T45.0X5	T45.0X6
Lorazepam	T42.4X1	T42.4X2	T42.4X3	T42.4X4	T42.4X5	T42.4X6
Lorcainide	T46.2X1	T46.2X2	T46.2X3	T46.2X4	T46.2X5	T46.2X6
Lormetazepam	T42.4X1	T42.4X2	T42.4X3	T42.4X4	T42.4X5	T42.4X6
Lotions NEC	T49.91	T49.92	T49.93	T49.94	T49.95	T49.96
Lotusate	T42.3X1	T42.3X2	T42.3X3	T42.3X4	T42.3X5	T42.3X6
Lovastatin	T46.6X1	T46.6X2	T46.6X3	T46.6X4	T46.6X5	T46.6X6
Lowila	T49.2X1	T49.2X2	T49.2X3	T49.2X4	T49.2X5	T49.2X6
Loxapine	T43.591	T43.592	T43.593	T43.594	T43.595	T43.596
Lozenges (throat)	T49.6X1	T49.6X2	T49.6X3	T49.6X4	T49.6X5	T49.6X6
LSD	T40.8X1	T40.8X2	T40.8X3	T40.8X4	—	—
L-Tryptophan — see amino acid						
Lubricant, eye	T49.5X1	T49.5X2	T49.5X3	T49.5X4	T49.5X5	T49.5X6
Lubricating oil NEC	T52.0X1	T52.0X2	T52.0X3	T52.0X4	—	—
Lucanthone	T37.4X1	T37.4X2	T37.4X3	T37.4X4	T37.4X5	T37.4X6
Luminal	T42.3X1	T42.3X2	T42.3X3	T42.3X4	T42.3X5	T42.3X6
Lung irritant (gas) NEC	T59.91	T59.92	T59.93	T59.94	—	—
Luteinizing hormone	T38.811	T38.812	T38.813	T38.814	T38.815	T38.816
Lutocylol	T38.5X1	T38.5X2	T38.5X3	T38.5X4	T38.5X5	T38.5X6
Lutromone	T38.5X1	T38.5X2	T38.5X3	T38.5X4	T38.5X5	T38.5X6
Lututrin	T48.291	T48.292	T48.293	T48.294	T48.295	T48.296
Lye (concentrated)	T54.3X1	T54.3X2	T54.3X3	T54.3X4	—	—
Lygranum (skin test)	T50.8X1	T50.8X2	T50.8X3	T50.8X4	T50.8X5	T50.8X6
Lymecycline	T36.4X1	T36.4X2	T36.4X3	T36.4X4	T36.4X5	T36.4X6
Lymphogranuloma venereum antigen	T50.8X1	T50.8X2	T50.8X3	T50.8X4	T50.8X5	T50.8X6
Lynestrenol	T38.4X1	T38.4X2	T38.4X3	T38.4X4	T38.4X5	T38.4X6
Lyovac Sodium Edecrin	T50.1X1	T50.1X2	T50.1X3	T50.1X4	T50.1X5	T50.1X6
Lypressin	T38.891	T38.892	T38.893	T38.894	T38.895	T38.896
Lysergic acid diethylamide	T40.8X1	T40.8X2	T40.8X3	T40.8X4	—	—
Lysergide	T40.8X1	T40.8X2	T40.8X3	T40.8X4	—	—
Lysine vasopressin	T38.891	T38.892	T38.893	T38.894	T38.895	T38.896
Lysol	T54.1X1	T54.1X2	T54.1X3	T54.1X4	—	—
Lysozyme	T49.0X1	T49.0X2	T49.0X3	T49.0X4	T49.0X5	T49.0X6
Lytta (vitatta)	T49.8X1	T49.8X2	T49.8X3	T49.8X4	T49.8X5	T49.8X6
Mace	T59.3X1	T59.3X2	T59.3X3	T59.3X4		
Macrogol	T50.991	T50.992	T50.993	T50.994	T50.995	T50.996
Macrolide						
anabolic drug	T38.7X1	T38.7X2	T38.7X3	T38.7X4	T38.7X5	T38.7X6
antibiotic	T36.3X1	T36.3X2	T36.3X3	T36.3X4	T36.3X5	T36.3X6
Mafenide	T49.0X1	T49.0X2	T49.0X3	T49.0X4	T49.0X5	T49.0X6
Magaldrate	T47.1X1	T47.1X2	T47.1X3	T47.1X4	T47.1X5	T47.1X6
Magic mushroom	T40.991	T40.992	T40.993	T40.994	—	—
Magnamycin	T36.8X1	T36.8X2	T36.8X3	T36.8X4	T36.8X5	T36.8X6
Magnesia magma	T47.1X1	T47.1X2	T47.1X3	T47.1X4	T47.1X5	T47.1X6
Magnesium NEC	T56.891	T56.892	T56.893	T56.894	—	—
carbonate	T47.1X1	T47.1X2	T47.1X3	T47.1X4	T47.1X5	T47.1X6
citrate	T47.4X1	T47.4X2	T47.4X3	T47.4X4	T47.4X5	T47.4X6
hydroxide	T47.1X1	T47.1X2	T47.1X3	T47.1X4	T47.1X5	T47.1X6
oxide	T47.1X1	T47.1X2	T47.1X3	T47.1X4	T47.1X5	T47.1X6
peroxide	T49.0X1	T49.0X2	T49.0X3	T49.0X4	T49.0X5	T49.0X6
salicylate	T39.091	T39.092	T39.093	T39.094	T39.095	T39.096
silicofluoride	T50.3X1	T50.3X2	T50.3X3	T50.3X4	T50.3X5	T50.3X6
Magnesium — continued						
sulfate	T47.4X1	T47.4X2	T47.4X3	T47.4X4	T47.4X5	T47.4X6
thiosulfate	T45.0X1	T45.0X2	T45.0X3	T45.0X4	T45.0X5	T45.0X6
trisilicate	T47.1X1	T47.1X2	T47.1X3	T47.1X4	T47.1X5	T47.1X6
Malathion (medicinal)	T49.0X1	T49.0X2	T49.0X3	T49.0X4	T49.0X5	T49.0X6
insecticide	T60.0X1	T60.0X2	T60.0X3	T60.0X4		
Male fern extract	T37.4X1	T37.4X2	T37.4X3	T37.4X4	T37.4X5	T37.4X6
M-AMSA	T45.1X1	T45.1X2	T45.1X3	T45.1X4	T45.1X5	T45.1X6
Mandelic acid	T37.8X1	T37.8X2	T37.8X3	T37.8X4	T37.8X5	T37.8X6
Manganese (dioxide) (salts)	T57.2X1	T57.2X2	T57.2X3	T57.2X4	—	—
medicinal	T50.991	T50.992	T50.993	T50.994	T50.995	T50.996
Mannitol	T47.3X1	T47.3X2	T47.3X3	T47.3X4	T47.3X5	T47.3X6
hexanitrate	T46.3X1	T46.3X2	T46.3X3	T46.3X4	T46.3X5	T46.3X6
Mannomustine	T45.1X1	T45.1X2	T45.1X3	T45.1X4	T45.1X5	T45.1X6
MAO inhibitors	T43.1X1	T43.1X2	T43.1X3	T43.1X4	T43.1X5	T43.1X6
Mapharsen	T37.8X1	T37.8X2	T37.8X3	T37.8X4	T37.8X5	T37.8X6
Maphenide	T49.0X1	T49.0X2	T49.0X3	T49.0X4	T49.0X5	T49.0X6
Maprotiline	T43.021	T43.022	T43.023	T43.024	T43.025	T43.026
Marcaine	T41.3X1	T41.3X2	T41.3X3	T41.3X4	T41.3X5	T41.3X6
infiltration (subcutaneous)	T41.3X1	T41.3X2	T41.3X3	T41.3X4	T41.3X5	T41.3X6
nerve block (peripheral) (plexus)	T41.3X1	T41.3X2	T41.3X3	T41.3X4	T41.3X5	T41.3X6
Marezine	T45.0X1	T45.0X2	T45.0X3	T45.0X4	T45.0X5	T45.0X6
Marihuana	T40.7X1	T40.7X2	T40.7X3	T40.7X4	T40.7X5	T40.7X6
Marijuana	T40.7X1	T40.7X2	T40.7X3	T40.7X4	T40.7X5	T40.7X6
Marine (sting)	T63.691	T63.692	T63.693	T63.694	—	—
animals (sting)	T63.691	T63.692	T63.693	T63.694	—	—
plants (sting)	T63.711	T63.712	T63.713	T63.714	—	—
Marplan	T43.1X1	T43.1X2	T43.1X3	T43.1X4	T43.1X5	T43.1X6
Marsh gas	T59.891	T59.892	T59.893	T59.894		
Marsilid	T43.1X1	T43.1X2	T43.1X3	T43.1X4	T43.1X5	T43.1X6
Matulane	T45.1X1	T45.1X2	T45.1X3	T45.1X4	T45.1X5	T45.1X6
Mazindol	T50.5X1	T50.5X2	T50.5X3	T50.5X4	T50.5X5	T50.5X6
MCPA	T60.3X1	T60.3X2	T60.3X3	T60.3X4	—	—
MDMA	T43.621	T43.622	T43.623	T43.624	T43.625	T43.626
Meadow saffron	T62.2X1	T62.2X2	T62.2X3	T62.2X4	—	—
Measles virus vaccine (attenuated)	T50.B91	T50.B92	T50.B93	T50.B94	T50.B95	T50.B96
Meat, noxious	T62.8X1	T62.8X2	T62.8X3	T62.8X4	—	—
Meballymal	T42.3X1	T42.3X2	T42.3X3	T42.3X4	T42.3X5	T42.3X6
Mebanazine	T43.1X1	T43.1X2	T43.1X3	T43.1X4	T43.1X5	T43.1X6
Mebaral	T42.3X1	T42.3X2	T42.3X3	T42.3X4	T42.3X5	T42.3X6
Mebendazole	T37.4X1	T37.4X2	T37.4X3	T37.4X4	T37.4X5	T37.4X6
Mebeverine	T44.3X1	T44.3X2	T44.3X3	T44.3X4	T44.3X5	T44.3X6
Mebhydrolin	T45.0X1	T45.0X2	T45.0X3	T45.0X4	T45.0X5	T45.0X6
Mebumal	T42.3X1	T42.3X2	T42.3X3	T42.3X4	T42.3X5	T42.3X6
Mebutamate	T43.591	T43.592	T43.593	T43.594	T43.595	T43.596
Mecamylamine	T44.2X1	T44.2X2	T44.2X3	T44.2X4	T44.2X5	T44.2X6
Mechlorethamine	T45.1X1	T45.1X2	T45.1X3	T45.1X4	T45.1X5	T45.1X6
Mecillinam	T36.0X1	T36.0X2	T36.0X3	T36.0X4	T36.0X5	T36.0X6
Meclizine (hydrochloride)	T45.0X1	T45.0X2	T45.0X3	T45.0X4	T45.0X5	T45.0X6
Meclocycline	T36.4X1	T36.4X2	T36.4X3	T36.4X4	T36.4X5	T36.4X6
Meclofenamate	T39.391	T39.392	T39.393	T39.394	T39.395	T39.396
Meclofenamic acid	T39.391	T39.392	T39.393	T39.394	T39.395	T39.396
Meclofenoxate	T43.691	T43.692	T43.693	T43.694	T43.695	T43.696
Meclozine	T45.0X1	T45.0X2	T45.0X3	T45.0X4	T45.0X5	T45.0X6
Mecobalamin	T45.8X1	T45.8X2	T45.8X3	T45.8X4	T45.8X5	T45.8X6
Mecoprop	T60.3X1	T60.3X2	T60.3X3	T60.3X4	—	—
Mecrilate	T49.3X1	T49.3X2	T49.3X3	T49.3X4	T49.3X5	T49.3X6
Mecysteine	T48.4X1	T48.4X2	T48.4X3	T48.4X4	T48.4X5	T48.4X6
Medazepam	T42.4X1	T42.4X2	T42.4X3	T42.4X4	T42.4X5	T42.4X6
Medicament NEC	T50.901	T50.902	T50.903	T50.904	T50.905	T50.906
Medinal	T42.3X1	T42.3X2	T42.3X3	T42.3X4	T42.3X5	T42.3X6
Medomin	T42.3X1	T42.3X2	T42.3X3	T42.3X4	T42.3X5	T42.3X6
Medrogestone	T38.5X1	T38.5X2	T38.5X3	T38.5X4	T38.5X5	T38.5X6
Medroxalol	T44.8X1	T44.8X2	T44.8X3	T44.8X4	T44.8X5	T44.8X6
Medroxyprogesterone acetate (depot)	T38.5X1	T38.5X2	T38.5X3	T38.5X4	T38.5X5	T38.5X6
Medrysone	T49.0X1	T49.0X2	T49.0X3	T49.0X4	T49.0X5	T49.0X6
Mefenamic acid	T39.391	T39.392	T39.393	T39.394	T39.395	T39.396
Mefenorex	T50.5X1	T50.5X2	T50.5X3	T50.5X4	T50.5X5	T50.5X6
Mefloquine	T37.2X1	T37.2X2	T37.2X3	T37.2X4	T37.2X5	T37.2X6
Mefruside	T50.2X1	T50.2X2	T50.2X3	T50.2X4	T50.2X5	T50.2X6
Megahallucinogen	T40.901	T40.902	T40.903	T40.904	T40.905	T40.906
Megestrol	T38.5X1	T38.5X2	T38.5X3	T38.5X4	T38.5X5	T38.5X6
Meglumine						
antimoniate	T37.8X1	T37.8X2	T37.8X3	T37.8X4	T37.8X5	T37.8X6
diatrizoate	T50.8X1	T50.8X2	T50.8X3	T50.8X4	T50.8X5	T50.8X6
iodipamide	T50.8X1	T50.8X2	T50.8X3	T50.8X4	T50.8X5	T50.8X6
iotroxate	T50.8X1	T50.8X2	T50.8X3	T50.8X4	T50.8X5	T50.8X6
MEK (methyl ethyl ketone)	T52.4X1	T52.4X2	T52.4X3	T52.4X4	—	—
Meladinin	T49.3X1	T49.3X2	T49.3X3	T49.3X4	T49.3X5	T49.3X6
Meladrazine	T44.3X1	T44.3X2	T44.3X3	T44.3X4	T44.3X5	T44.3X6

Additional Character May Be Required — Refer to the Tabular List for Character Selection   ▽ Subterms under main terms may continue to next column or page

Substance	Poisoning, Accidental (unintentional)	Poisoning, Intentional Self-harm	Poisoning, Assault	Poisoning, Undetermined	Adverse Effect	Under-dosing
Melaleuca alternifolia oil	T49.0X1	T49.0X2	T49.0X3	T49.0X4	T49.0X5	T49.0X6
Melanizing agents	T49.3X1	T49.3X2	T49.3X3	T49.3X4	T49.3X5	T49.3X6
Melanocyte-stimulating hormone	T38.891	T38.892	T38.893	T38.894	T38.895	T38.896
Melarsonyl potassium	T37.3X1	T37.3X2	T37.3X3	T37.3X4	T37.3X5	T37.3X6
Melarsoprol	T37.3X1	T37.3X2	T37.3X3	T37.3X4	T37.3X5	T37.3X6
Melia azedarach	T62.2X1	T62.2X2	T62.2X3	T62.2X4	—	—
Melitracen	T43.011	T43.012	T43.013	T43.014	T43.015	T43.016
Mellaril	T43.3X1	T43.3X2	T43.3X3	T43.3X4	T43.3X5	T43.3X6
Meloxine	T49.3X1	T49.3X2	T49.3X3	T49.3X4	T49.3X5	T49.3X6
Melperone	T43.4X1	T43.4X2	T43.4X3	T43.4X4	T43.4X5	T43.4X6
Melphalan	T45.1X1	T45.1X2	T45.1X3	T45.1X4	T45.1X5	T45.1X6
Memantine	T43.8X1	T43.8X2	T43.8X3	T43.8X4	T43.8X5	T43.8X6
Menadiol	T45.7X1	T45.7X2	T45.7X3	T45.7X4	T45.7X5	T45.7X6
sodium sulfate	T45.7X1	T45.7X2	T45.7X3	T45.7X4	T45.7X5	T45.7X6
Menadione	T45.7X1	T45.7X2	T45.7X3	T45.7X4	T45.7X5	T45.7X6
sodium bisulfite	T45.7X1	T45.7X2	T45.7X3	T45.7X4	T45.7X5	T45.7X6
Menaphthone	T45.7X1	T45.7X2	T45.7X3	T45.7X4	T45.7X5	T45.7X6
Menaquinone	T45.7X1	T45.7X2	T45.7X3	T45.7X4	T45.7X5	T45.7X6
Menatetrenone	T45.7X1	T45.7X2	T45.7X3	T45.7X4	T45.7X5	T45.7X6
Meningococcal vaccine	T50.A91	T50.A92	T50.A93	T50.A94	T50.A95	T50.A96
Menningovax (-AC) (-C)	T50.A91	T50.A92	T50.A93	T50.A94	T50.A95	T50.A96
Menotropins	T38.811	T38.812	T38.813	T38.814	T38.815	T38.816
Menthol	T48.5X1	T48.5X2	T48.5X3	T48.5X4	T48.5X5	T48.5X6
Mepacrine	T37.2X1	T37.2X2	T37.2X3	T37.2X4	T37.2X5	T37.2X6
Meparfynol	T42.6X1	T42.6X2	T42.6X3	T42.6X4	T42.6X5	T42.6X6
Mepartricin	T36.7X1	T36.7X2	T36.7X3	T36.7X4	T36.7X5	T36.7X6
Mepazine	T43.3X1	T43.3X2	T43.3X3	T43.3X4	T43.3X5	T43.3X6
Mepenzolate	T44.3X1	T44.3X2	T44.3X3	T44.3X4	T44.3X5	T44.3X6
bromide	T44.3X1	T44.3X2	T44.3X3	T44.3X4	T44.3X5	T44.3X6
Meperidine	T40.4X1	T40.4X2	T40.4X3	T40.4X4	T40.4X5	T40.4X6
Mephebarbital	T42.3X1	T42.3X2	T42.3X3	T42.3X4	T42.3X5	T42.3X6
Mephenamin (e)	T42.8X1	T42.8X2	T42.8X3	T42.8X4	T42.8X5	T42.8X6
Mephenesin	T42.8X1	T42.8X2	T42.8X3	T42.8X4	T42.8X5	T42.8X6
Mephenhydramine	T45.0X1	T45.0X2	T45.0X3	T45.0X4	T45.0X5	T45.0X6
Mephenoxalone	T42.8X1	T42.8X2	T42.8X3	T42.8X4	T42.8X5	T42.8X6
Mephentermine	T44.991	T44.992	T44.993	T44.994	T44.995	T44.996
Mephenytoin	T42.0X1	T42.0X2	T42.0X3	T42.0X4	T42.0X5	T42.0X6
with phenobarbital	T42.3X1	T42.3X2	T42.3X3	T42.3X4	T42.3X5	T42.3X6
Mephobarbital	T42.3X1	T42.3X2	T42.3X3	T42.3X4	T42.3X5	T42.3X6
Mephosfolan	T60.0X1	T60.0X2	T60.0X3	T60.0X4	—	—
Mepindolol	T44.7X1	T44.7X2	T44.7X3	T44.7X4	T44.7X5	T44.7X6
Mepiperphenidol	T44.3X1	T44.3X2	T44.3X3	T44.3X4	T44.3X5	T44.3X6
Mepitiostane	T38.7X1	T38.7X2	T38.7X3	T38.7X4	T38.7X5	T38.7X6
Mepivacaine	T41.3X1	T41.3X2	T41.3X3	T41.3X4	T41.3X5	T41.3X6
epidural	T41.3X1	T41.3X2	T41.3X3	T41.3X4	T41.3X5	T41.3X6
Meprednisone	T38.0X1	T38.0X2	T38.0X3	T38.0X4	T38.0X5	T38.0X6
Meprobam	T43.591	T43.592	T43.593	T43.594	T43.595	T43.596
Meprobamate	T43.591	T43.592	T43.593	T43.594	T43.595	T43.596
Meproscillarin	T46.0X1	T46.0X2	T46.0X3	T46.0X4	T46.0X5	T46.0X6
Meprylcaine	T41.3X1	T41.3X2	T41.3X3	T41.3X4	T41.3X5	T41.3X6
Meptazinol	T39.8X1	T39.8X2	T39.8X3	T39.8X4	T39.8X5	T39.8X6
Mepyramine	T45.0X1	T45.0X2	T45.0X3	T45.0X4	T45.0X5	T45.0X6
Mequitazine	T43.3X1	T43.3X2	T43.3X3	T43.3X4	T43.3X5	T43.3X6
Meralluride	T50.2X1	T50.2X2	T50.2X3	T50.2X4	T50.2X5	T50.2X6
Merbaphen	T50.2X1	T50.2X2	T50.2X3	T50.2X4	T50.2X5	T50.2X6
Merbromin	T49.0X1	T49.0X2	T49.0X3	T49.0X4	T49.0X5	T49.0X6
Mercaptobenzothiazole salts	T49.0X1	T49.0X2	T49.0X3	T49.0X4	T49.0X5	T49.0X6
Mercaptomerin	T50.2X1	T50.2X2	T50.2X3	T50.2X4	T50.2X5	T50.2X6
Mercaptopurine	T45.1X1	T45.1X2	T45.1X3	T45.1X4	T45.1X5	T45.1X6
Mercumatilin	T50.2X1	T50.2X2	T50.2X3	T50.2X4	T50.2X5	T50.2X6
Mercuramide	T50.2X1	T50.2X2	T50.2X3	T50.2X4	T50.2X5	T50.2X6
Mercurochrome	T49.0X1	T49.0X2	T49.0X3	T49.0X4	T49.0X5	T49.0X6
Mercurophylline	T50.2X1	T50.2X2	T50.2X3	T50.2X4	T50.2X5	T50.2X6
Mercury, mercurial, mercuric, mercurous (compounds) (cyanide) (fumes) (nonmedicinal) (vapor) NEC	T56.1X1	T56.1X2	T56.1X3	T56.1X4	—	—
ammoniated	T49.0X1	T49.0X2	T49.0X3	T49.0X4	T49.0X5	T49.0X6
anti-infective						
local	T49.0X1	T49.0X2	T49.0X3	T49.0X4	T49.0X5	T49.0X6
systemic	T37.8X1	T37.8X2	T37.8X3	T37.8X4	T37.8X5	T37.8X6
topical	T49.0X1	T49.0X2	T49.0X3	T49.0X4	T49.0X5	T49.0X6
chloride (ammoniated)	T49.0X1	T49.0X2	T49.0X3	T49.0X4	T49.0X5	T49.0X6
fungicide	T56.1X1	T56.1X2	T56.1X3	T56.1X4	—	—
diuretic NEC	T50.2X1	T50.2X2	T50.2X3	T50.2X4	T50.2X5	T50.2X6
fungicide	T56.1X1	T56.1X2	T56.1X3	T56.1X4	—	—
organic (fungicide)	T56.1X1	T56.1X2	T56.1X3	T56.1X4	—	—
oxide, yellow	T49.0X1	T49.0X2	T49.0X3	T49.0X4	T49.0X5	T49.0X6
Mersalyl	T50.2X1	T50.2X2	T50.2X3	T50.2X4	T50.2X5	T50.2X6
Merthiolate	T49.0X1	T49.0X2	T49.0X3	T49.0X4	T49.0X5	T49.0X6

Substance	Poisoning, Accidental (unintentional)	Poisoning, Intentional Self-harm	Poisoning, Assault	Poisoning, Undetermined	Adverse Effect	Under-dosing
Merthiolate — *continued*						
ophthalmic preparation	T49.5X1	T49.5X2	T49.5X3	T49.5X4	T49.5X5	T49.5X6
Meruvax	T50.B91	T50.B92	T50.B93	T50.B94	T50.B95	T50.B96
Mesalazine	T47.8X1	T47.8X2	T47.8X3	T47.8X4	T47.8X5	T47.8X6
Mescal buttons	T40.991	T40.992	T40.993	T40.994	—	—
Mescaline	T40.991	T40.992	T40.993	T40.994	—	—
Mesna	T48.4X1	T48.4X2	T48.4X3	T48.4X4	T48.4X5	T48.4X6
Mesoglycan	T46.6X1	T46.6X2	T46.6X3	T46.6X4	T46.6X5	T46.6X6
Mesoridazine	T43.3X1	T43.3X2	T43.3X3	T43.3X4	T43.3X5	T43.3X6
Mestanolone	T38.7X1	T38.7X2	T38.7X3	T38.7X4	T38.7X5	T38.7X6
Mesterolone	T38.7X1	T38.7X2	T38.7X3	T38.7X4	T38.7X5	T38.7X6
Mestranol	T38.5X1	T38.5X2	T38.5X3	T38.5X4	T38.5X5	T38.5X6
Mesulergine	T42.8X1	T42.8X2	T42.8X3	T42.8X4	T42.8X5	T42.8X6
Mesulfen	T49.0X1	T49.0X2	T49.0X3	T49.0X4	T49.0X5	T49.0X6
Mesuximide	T42.2X1	T42.2X2	T42.2X3	T42.2X4	T42.2X5	T42.2X6
Metabutethamine	T41.3X1	T41.3X2	T41.3X3	T41.3X4	T41.3X5	T41.3X6
Metactesylacetate	T49.0X1	T49.0X2	T49.0X3	T49.0X4	T49.0X5	T49.0X6
Metacycline	T36.4X1	T36.4X2	T36.4X3	T36.4X4	T36.4X5	T36.4X6
Metaldehyde (snail killer) NEC	T60.8X1	T60.8X2	T60.8X3	T60.8X4	—	—
Metals (heavy) (nonmedicinal)	T56.91	T56.92	T56.93	T56.94	—	—
dust, fumes, or vapor NEC	T56.91	T56.92	T56.93	T56.94	—	—
light NEC	T56.91	T56.92	T56.93	T56.94	—	—
dust, fumes, or vapor NEC	T56.91	T56.92	T56.93	T56.94	—	—
specified NEC	T56.891	T56.892	T56.893	T56.894	—	—
thallium	T56.811	T56.812	T56.813	T56.814	—	—
Metamfetamine	T43.621	T43.622	T43.623	T43.624	T43.625	T43.626
Metamizole sodium	T39.2X1	T39.2X2	T39.2X3	T39.2X4	T39.2X5	T39.2X6
Metampicillin	T36.0X1	T36.0X2	T36.0X3	T36.0X4	T36.0X5	T36.0X6
Metamucil	T47.4X1	T47.4X2	T47.4X3	T47.4X4	T47.4X5	T47.4X6
Metandienone	T38.7X1	T38.7X2	T38.7X3	T38.7X4	T38.7X5	T38.7X6
Metandrostenolone	T38.7X1	T38.7X2	T38.7X3	T38.7X4	T38.7X5	T38.7X6
Metaphen	T49.0X1	T49.0X2	T49.0X3	T49.0X4	T49.0X5	T49.0X6
Metaphos	T60.0X1	T60.0X2	T60.0X3	T60.0X4	—	—
Metapramine	T43.011	T43.012	T43.013	T43.014	T43.015	T43.016
Metaproterenol	T48.291	T48.292	T48.293	T48.294	T48.295	T48.296
Metaraminol	T44.4X1	T44.4X2	T44.4X3	T44.4X4	T44.4X5	T44.4X6
Metaxalone	T42.8X1	T42.8X2	T42.8X3	T42.8X4	T42.8X5	T42.8X6
Metenolone	T38.7X1	T38.7X2	T38.7X3	T38.7X4	T38.7X5	T38.7X6
Metergoline	T42.8X1	T42.8X2	T42.8X3	T42.8X4	T42.8X5	T42.8X6
Metescufylline	T46.991	T46.992	T46.993	T46.994	T46.995	T46.996
Metetoin	T42.0X1	T42.0X2	T42.0X3	T42.0X4	T42.0X5	T42.0X6
Metformin	T38.3X1	T38.3X2	T38.3X3	T38.3X4	T38.3X5	T38.3X6
Methacholine	T44.1X1	T44.1X2	T44.1X3	T44.1X4	T44.1X5	T44.1X6
Methacycline	T36.4X1	T36.4X2	T36.4X3	T36.4X4	T36.4X5	T36.4X6
Methadone	T40.3X1	T40.3X2	T40.3X3	T40.3X4	T40.3X5	T40.3X6
Methallenestril	T38.5X1	T38.5X2	T38.5X3	T38.5X4	T38.5X5	T38.5X6
Methallenoestril	T38.5X1	T38.5X2	T38.5X3	T38.5X4	T38.5X5	T38.5X6
Methamphetamine	T43.621	T43.622	T43.623	T43.624	T43.625	T43.626
Methampyrone	T39.2X1	T39.2X2	T39.2X3	T39.2X4	T39.2X5	T39.2X6
Methandienone	T38.7X1	T38.7X2	T38.7X3	T38.7X4	T38.7X5	T38.7X6
Methandriol	T38.7X1	T38.7X2	T38.7X3	T38.7X4	T38.7X5	T38.7X6
Methandrostenolone	T38.7X1	T38.7X2	T38.7X3	T38.7X4	T38.7X5	T38.7X6
Methane	T59.891	T59.892	T59.893	T59.894	—	—
Methanethiol	T59.891	T59.892	T59.893	T59.894	—	—
Methaniazide	T37.1X1	T37.1X2	T37.1X3	T37.1X4	T37.1X5	T37.1X6
Methanol (vapor)	T51.1X1	T51.1X2	T51.1X3	T51.1X4	—	—
Methantheline	T44.3X1	T44.3X2	T44.3X3	T44.3X4	T44.3X5	T44.3X6
Methanthelinium bromide	T44.3X1	T44.3X2	T44.3X3	T44.3X4	T44.3X5	T44.3X6
Methaphenilene	T45.0X1	T45.0X2	T45.0X3	T45.0X4	T45.0X5	T45.0X6
Methapyrilene	T45.0X1	T45.0X2	T45.0X3	T45.0X4	T45.0X5	T45.0X6
Methaqualone (compound)	T42.6X1	T42.6X2	T42.6X3	T42.6X4	T42.6X5	T42.6X6
Metharbital	T42.3X1	T42.3X2	T42.3X3	T42.3X4	T42.3X5	T42.3X6
Methazolamide	T50.2X1	T50.2X2	T50.2X3	T50.2X4	T50.2X5	T50.2X6
Methdilazine	T43.3X1	T43.3X2	T43.3X3	T43.3X4	T43.3X5	T43.3X6
Methedrine	T43.621	T43.622	T43.623	T43.624	T43.625	T43.626
Methenamine (mandelate)	T37.8X1	T37.8X2	T37.8X3	T37.8X4	T37.8X5	T37.8X6
Methenolone	T38.7X1	T38.7X2	T38.7X3	T38.7X4	T38.7X5	T38.7X6
Methergine	T48.0X1	T48.0X2	T48.0X3	T48.0X4	T48.0X5	T48.0X6
Methetoin	T42.0X1	T42.0X2	T42.0X3	T42.0X4	T42.0X5	T42.0X6
Methiacil	T38.2X1	T38.2X2	T38.2X3	T38.2X4	T38.2X5	T38.2X6
Methicillin	T36.0X1	T36.0X2	T36.0X3	T36.0X4	T36.0X5	T36.0X6
Methimazole	T38.2X1	T38.2X2	T38.2X3	T38.2X4	T38.2X5	T38.2X6
Methiodal sodium	T50.8X1	T50.8X2	T50.8X3	T50.8X4	T50.8X5	T50.8X6
Methionine	T50.991	T50.992	T50.993	T50.994	T50.995	T50.996
Methisazone	T37.5X1	T37.5X2	T37.5X3	T37.5X4	T37.5X5	T37.5X6
Methisoprinol	T37.5X1	T37.5X2	T37.5X3	T37.5X4	T37.5X5	T37.5X6
Methitural	T42.3X1	T42.3X2	T42.3X3	T42.3X4	T42.3X5	T42.3X6
Methixene	T44.3X1	T44.3X2	T44.3X3	T44.3X4	T44.3X5	T44.3X6
Methobarbital, methobarbitone	T42.3X1	T42.3X2	T42.3X3	T42.3X4	T42.3X5	T42.3X6
Methocarbamol	T42.8X1	T42.8X2	T42.8X3	T42.8X4	T42.8X5	T42.8X6

Substance	Poisoning, Accidental (unintentional)	Poisoning, Intentional Self-harm	Poisoning, Assault	Poisoning, Undetermined	Adverse Effect	Under-dosing
Methocarbamol — *continued*						
skeletal muscle relaxant	T48.1X1	T48.1X2	T48.1X3	T48.1X4	T48.1X5	T48.1X6
Methohexital	T41.1X1	T41.1X2	T41.1X3	T41.1X4	T41.1X5	T41.1X6
Methohexitone	T41.1X1	T41.1X2	T41.1X3	T41.1X4	T41.1X5	T41.1X6
Methoin	T42.0X1	T42.0X2	T42.0X3	T42.0X4	T42.0X5	T42.0X6
Methopholine	T39.8X1	T39.8X2	T39.8X3	T39.8X4	T39.8X5	T39.8X6
Methopromazine	T43.3X1	T43.3X2	T43.3X3	T43.3X4	T43.3X5	T43.3X6
Methorate	T48.3X1	T48.3X2	T48.3X3	T48.3X4	T48.3X5	T48.3X6
Methoserpidine	T46.5X1	T46.5X2	T46.5X3	T46.5X4	T46.5X5	T46.5X6
Methotrexate	T45.1X1	T45.1X2	T45.1X3	T45.1X4	T45.1X5	T45.1X6
Methotrimeprazine	T43.3X1	T43.3X2	T43.3X3	T43.3X4	T43.3X5	T43.3X6
Methoxa-Dome	T49.3X1	T49.3X2	T49.3X3	T49.3X4	T49.3X5	T49.3X6
Methoxamine	T44.4X1	T44.4X2	T44.4X3	T44.4X4	T44.4X5	T44.4X6
Methoxsalen	T50.991	T50.992	T50.993	T50.994	T50.995	T50.996
Methoxyaniline	T65.3X1	T65.3X2	T65.3X3	T65.3X4	—	—
Methoxybenzyl penicillin	T36.0X1	T36.0X2	T36.0X3	T36.0X4	T36.0X5	T36.0X6
Methoxychlor	T53.7X1	T53.7X2	T53.7X3	T53.7X4	—	—
Methoxy-DDT	T53.7X1	T53.7X2	T53.7X3	T53.7X4	—	—
Methoxyflurane	T41.0X1	T41.0X2	T41.0X3	T41.0X4	T41.0X5	T41.0X6
Methoxyphenamine	T48.6X1	T48.6X2	T48.6X3	T48.6X4	T48.6X5	T48.6X6
Methoxypromazine	T43.3X1	T43.3X2	T43.3X3	T43.3X4	T43.3X5	T43.3X6
Methscopolamine bromide	T44.3X1	T44.3X2	T44.3X3	T44.3X4	T44.3X5	T44.3X6
Methsuximide	T42.2X1	T42.2X2	T42.2X3	T42.2X4	T42.2X5	T42.2X6
Methyclothiazide	T50.2X1	T50.2X2	T50.2X3	T50.2X4	T50.2X5	T50.2X6
Methyl						
acetate	T52.4X1	T52.4X2	T52.4X3	T52.4X4	—	—
acetone	T52.4X1	T52.4X2	T52.4X3	T52.4X4	—	—
acrylate	T65.891	T65.892	T65.893	T65.894	—	—
alcohol	T51.1X1	T51.1X2	T51.1X3	T51.1X4	—	—
aminophenol	T65.3X1	T65.3X2	T65.3X3	T65.3X4	—	—
amphetamine	T43.621	T43.622	T43.623	T43.624	T43.625	T43.626
androstanolone	T38.7X1	T38.7X2	T38.7X3	T38.7X4	T38.7X5	T38.7X6
atropine	T44.3X1	T44.3X2	T44.3X3	T44.3X4	T44.3X5	T44.3X6
benzene	T52.2X1	T52.2X2	T52.2X3	T52.2X4	—	—
benzoate	T52.8X1	T52.8X2	T52.8X3	T52.8X4	—	—
benzol	T52.2X1	T52.2X2	T52.2X3	T52.2X4	—	—
bromide (gas)	T59.891	T59.892	T59.893	T59.894	—	—
fumigant	T60.8X1	T60.8X2	T60.8X3	T60.8X4	—	—
butanol	T51.3X1	T51.3X2	T51.3X3	T51.3X4	—	—
carbinol	T51.1X1	T51.1X2	T51.1X3	T51.1X4	—	—
carbonate	T52.8X1	T52.8X2	T52.8X3	T52.8X4	—	—
CCNU	T45.1X1	T45.1X2	T45.1X3	T45.1X4	T45.1X5	T45.1X6
cellosolve	T52.91	T52.92	T52.93	T52.94	—	—
cellulose	T47.4X1	T47.4X2	T47.4X3	T47.4X4	T47.4X5	T47.4X6
chloride (gas)	T59.891	T59.892	T59.893	T59.894	—	—
chloroformate	T59.3X1	T59.3X2	T59.3X3	T59.3X4	—	—
cyclohexane	T52.8X1	T52.8X2	T52.8X3	T52.8X4	—	—
cyclohexanol	T51.8X1	T51.8X2	T51.8X3	T51.8X4	—	—
cyclohexanone	T52.8X1	T52.8X2	T52.8X3	T52.8X4	—	—
cyclohexyl acetate	T52.8X1	T52.8X2	T52.8X3	T52.8X4	—	—
demeton	T60.0X1	T60.0X2	T60.0X3	T60.0X4	—	—
dihydromorphinone	T40.2X1	T40.2X2	T40.2X3	T40.2X4	T40.2X5	T40.2X6
ergometrine	T48.0X1	T48.0X2	T48.0X3	T48.0X4	T48.0X5	T48.0X6
ergonovine	T48.0X1	T48.0X2	T48.0X3	T48.0X4	T48.0X5	T48.0X6
ethyl ketone	T52.4X1	T52.4X2	T52.4X3	T52.4X4	—	—
glucamine antimonate	T37.8X1	T37.8X2	T37.8X3	T37.8X4	T37.8X5	T37.8X6
hydrazine	T65.891	T65.892	T65.893	T65.894	—	—
iodide	T65.3X1	T65.3X2	T65.3X3	T65.3X4	—	—
isobutyl ketone	T52.4X1	T52.4X2	T52.4X3	T52.4X4	—	—
isothiocyanate	T60.3X1	T60.3X2	T60.3X3	T60.3X4	—	—
mercaptan	T59.891	T59.892	T59.893	T59.894	—	—
morphine NEC	T40.2X1	T40.2X2	T40.2X3	T40.2X4	T40.2X5	T40.2X6
nicotinate	T49.4X1	T49.4X2	T49.4X3	T49.4X4	T49.4X5	T49.4X6
paraben	T49.0X1	T49.0X2	T49.0X3	T49.0X4	T49.0X5	T49.0X6
parafynol	T42.6X1	T42.6X2	T42.6X3	T42.6X4	T42.6X5	T42.6X6
parathion	T60.0X1	T60.0X2	T60.0X3	T60.0X4	—	—
peridol	T43.4X1	T43.4X2	T43.4X3	T43.4X4	T43.4X5	T43.4X6
phenidate	T43.631	T43.632	T43.633	T43.634	T43.635	T43.636
prednisolone	T38.0X1	T38.0X2	T38.0X3	T38.0X4	T38.0X5	T38.0X6
ENT agent	T49.6X1	T49.6X2	T49.6X3	T49.6X4	T49.6X5	T49.6X6
ophthalmic preparation	T49.5X1	T49.5X2	T49.5X3	T49.5X4	T49.5X5	T49.5X6
topical NEC	T49.0X1	T49.0X2	T49.0X3	T49.0X4	T49.0X5	T49.0X6
propylcarbinol	T51.3X1	T51.3X2	T51.3X3	T51.3X4	—	—
rosaniline NEC	T49.0X1	T49.0X2	T49.0X3	T49.0X4	T49.0X5	T49.0X6
salicylate	T49.2X1	T49.2X2	T49.2X3	T49.2X4	T49.2X5	T49.2X6
sulfate (fumes)	T59.891	T59.892	T59.893	T59.894	—	—
liquid	T52.8X1	T52.8X2	T52.8X3	T52.8X4	—	—
sulfonal	T42.6X1	T42.6X2	T42.6X3	T42.6X4	T42.6X5	T42.6X6
testosterone	T38.7X1	T38.7X2	T38.7X3	T38.7X4	T38.7X5	T38.7X6
thiouracil	T38.2X1	T38.2X2	T38.2X3	T38.2X4	T38.2X5	T38.2X6
Methylamphetamine	T43.621	T43.622	T43.623	T43.624	T43.625	T43.626
Methylated spirit	T51.1X1	T51.1X2	T51.1X3	T51.1X4	—	—
Methylatropine nitrate	T44.3X1	T44.3X2	T44.3X3	T44.3X4	T44.3X5	T44.3X6
Methylbenactyzium bromide	T44.3X1	T44.3X2	T44.3X3	T44.3X4	T44.3X5	T44.3X6
Methylbenzethonium chloride	T49.0X1	T49.0X2	T49.0X3	T49.0X4	T49.0X5	T49.0X6
Methylcellulose	T47.4X1	T47.4X2	T47.4X3	T47.4X4	T47.4X5	T47.4X6
laxative	T47.4X1	T47.4X2	T47.4X3	T47.4X4	T47.4X5	T47.4X6
Methylchlorophenoxyacetic acid	T60.3X1	T60.3X2	T60.3X3	T60.3X4	—	—
Methyldopa	T46.5X1	T46.5X2	T46.5X3	T46.5X4	T46.5X5	T46.5X6
Methyldopate	T46.5X1	T46.5X2	T46.5X3	T46.5X4	T46.5X5	T46.5X6
Methylene						
blue	T50.6X1	T50.6X2	T50.6X3	T50.6X4	T50.6X5	T50.6X6
chloride or dichloride (solvent) NEC	T53.4X1	T53.4X2	T53.4X3	T53.4X4	—	—
Methylenedioxyamphetamine	T43.621	T43.622	T43.623	T43.624	T43.625	T43.626
Methylenedioxymethamphetamine	T43.621	T43.622	T43.623	T43.624	T43.625	T43.626
Methylergometrine	T48.0X1	T48.0X2	T48.0X3	T48.0X4	T48.0X5	T48.0X6
Methylergonovine	T48.0X1	T48.0X2	T48.0X3	T48.0X4	T48.0X5	T48.0X6
Methylestrenolone	T38.5X1	T38.5X2	T38.5X3	T38.5X4	T38.5X5	T38.5X6
Methylethyl cellulose	T50.991	T50.992	T50.993	T50.994	T50.995	T50.996
Methylhexabital	T42.3X1	T42.3X2	T42.3X3	T42.3X4	T42.3X5	T42.3X6
Methylmorphine	T40.2X1	T40.2X2	T40.2X3	T40.2X4	T40.2X5	T40.2X6
Methylparaben (ophthalmic)	T49.5X1	T49.5X2	T49.5X3	T49.5X4	T49.5X5	T49.5X6
Methylparafynol	T42.6X1	T42.6X2	T42.6X3	T42.6X4	T42.6X5	T42.6X6
Methylpentynol, methylpenthynol	T42.6X1	T42.6X2	T42.6X3	T42.6X4	T42.6X5	T42.6X6
Methylphenidate	T43.631	T43.632	T43.633	T43.634	T43.635	T43.636
Methylphenobarbital	T42.3X1	T42.3X2	T42.3X3	T42.3X4	T42.3X5	T42.3X6
Methylpolysiloxane	T47.1X1	T47.1X2	T47.1X3	T47.1X4	T47.1X5	T47.1X6
Methylprednisolone — *see* Methyl, prednisolone						
Methylrosaniline	T49.0X1	T49.0X2	T49.0X3	T49.0X4	T49.0X5	T49.0X6
Methylrosanilinium chloride	T49.0X1	T49.0X2	T49.0X3	T49.0X4	T49.0X5	T49.0X6
Methyltestosterone	T38.7X1	T38.7X2	T38.7X3	T38.7X4	T38.7X5	T38.7X6
Methylthionine chloride	T50.6X1	T50.6X2	T50.6X3	T50.6X4	T50.6X5	T50.6X6
Methylthioninium chloride	T50.6X1	T50.6X2	T50.6X3	T50.6X4	T50.6X5	T50.6X6
Methylthiouracil	T38.2X1	T38.2X2	T38.2X3	T38.2X4	T38.2X5	T38.2X6
Methyprylon	T42.6X1	T42.6X2	T42.6X3	T42.6X4	T42.6X5	T42.6X6
Methysergide	T46.5X1	T46.5X2	T46.5X3	T46.5X4	T46.5X5	T46.5X6
Metiamide	T47.1X1	T47.1X2	T47.1X3	T47.1X4	T47.1X5	T47.1X6
Meticillin	T36.0X1	T36.0X2	T36.0X3	T36.0X4	T36.0X5	T36.0X6
Meticrane	T50.2X1	T50.2X2	T50.2X3	T50.2X4	T50.2X5	T50.2X6
Metildigoxin	T46.0X1	T46.0X2	T46.0X3	T46.0X4	T46.0X5	T46.0X6
Metipranolol	T49.5X1	T49.5X2	T49.5X3	T49.5X4	T49.5X5	T49.5X6
Metirosine	T46.5X1	T46.5X2	T46.5X3	T46.5X4	T46.5X5	T46.5X6
Metisazone	T37.5X1	T37.5X2	T37.5X3	T37.5X4	T37.5X5	T37.5X6
Metixene	T44.3X1	T44.3X2	T44.3X3	T44.3X4	T44.3X5	T44.3X6
Metizoline	T48.5X1	T48.5X2	T48.5X3	T48.5X4	T48.5X5	T48.5X6
Metoclopramide	T45.0X1	T45.0X2	T45.0X3	T45.0X4	T45.0X5	T45.0X6
Metofenazate	T43.3X1	T43.3X2	T43.3X3	T43.3X4	T43.3X5	T43.3X6
Metofoline	T39.8X1	T39.8X2	T39.8X3	T39.8X4	T39.8X5	T39.8X6
Metolazone	T50.2X1	T50.2X2	T50.2X3	T50.2X4	T50.2X5	T50.2X6
Metopon	T40.2X1	T40.2X2	T40.2X3	T40.2X4	T40.2X5	T40.2X6
Metoprine	T45.1X1	T45.1X2	T45.1X3	T45.1X4	T45.1X5	T45.1X6
Metoprolol	T44.7X1	T44.7X2	T44.7X3	T44.7X4	T44.7X5	T44.7X6
Metrifonate	T60.0X1	T60.0X2	T60.0X3	T60.0X4	—	—
Metrizamide	T50.8X1	T50.8X2	T50.8X3	T50.8X4	T50.8X5	T50.8X6
Metrizoic acid	T50.8X1	T50.8X2	T50.8X3	T50.8X4	T50.8X5	T50.8X6
Metronidazole	T37.8X1	T37.8X2	T37.8X3	T37.8X4	T37.8X5	T37.8X6
Metycaine	T41.3X1	T41.3X2	T41.3X3	T41.3X4	T41.3X5	T41.3X6
infiltration (subcutaneous)	T41.3X1	T41.3X2	T41.3X3	T41.3X4	T41.3X5	T41.3X6
nerve block (peripheral) (plexus)	T41.3X1	T41.3X2	T41.3X3	T41.3X4	T41.3X5	T41.3X6
topical (surface)	T41.3X1	T41.3X2	T41.3X3	T41.3X4	T41.3X5	T41.3X6
Metyrapone	T50.8X1	T50.8X2	T50.8X3	T50.8X4	T50.8X5	T50.8X6
Mevinphos	T60.0X1	T60.0X2	T60.0X3	T60.0X4	—	—
Mexazolam	T42.4X1	T42.4X2	T42.4X3	T42.4X4	T42.4X5	T42.4X6
Mexenone	T49.3X1	T49.3X2	T49.3X3	T49.3X4	T49.3X5	T49.3X6
Mexiletine	T46.2X1	T46.2X2	T46.2X3	T46.2X4	T46.2X5	T46.2X6
Mezereon	T62.2X1	T62.2X2	T62.2X3	T62.2X4	—	—
berries	T62.1X1	T62.1X2	T62.1X3	T62.1X4	—	—
Mezlocillin	T36.0X1	T36.0X2	T36.0X3	T36.0X4	T36.0X5	T36.0X6
Mianserin	T43.021	T43.022	T43.023	T43.024	T43.025	T43.026
Micatin	T49.0X1	T49.0X2	T49.0X3	T49.0X4	T49.0X5	T49.0X6
Miconazole	T49.0X1	T49.0X2	T49.0X3	T49.0X4	T49.0X5	T49.0X6
Micronomicin	T36.5X1	T36.5X2	T36.5X3	T36.5X4	T36.5X5	T36.5X6
Midazolam	T42.4X1	T42.4X2	T42.4X3	T42.4X4	T42.4X5	T42.4X6
Midecamycin	T36.3X1	T36.3X2	T36.3X3	T36.3X4	T36.3X5	T36.3X6
Mifepristone	T38.6X1	T38.6X2	T38.6X3	T38.6X4	T38.6X5	T38.6X6
Milk of magnesia	T47.1X1	T47.1X2	T47.1X3	T47.1X4	T47.1X5	T47.1X6

Substance	Poisoning, Accidental (unintentional)	Poisoning, Intentional Self-harm	Poisoning, Assault	Poisoning, Undetermined	Adverse Effect	Under-dosing
Millipede (tropical)	T63.411	T63.412	T63.413	T63.414	—	—
(venomous)						
Miltown	T43.591	T43.592	T43.593	T43.594	T43.595	T43.596
Milverine	T44.3X1	T44.3X2	T44.3X3	T44.3X4	T44.3X5	T44.3X6
Minaprine	T43.291	T43.292	T43.293	T43.294	T43.295	T43.296
Minaxolone	T41.291	T41.292	T41.293	T41.294	T41.295	T41.296
Mineral						
acids	T54.2X1	T54.2X2	T54.2X3	T54.2X4	—	—
oil (laxative)(medicinal)	T47.4X1	T47.4X2	T47.4X3	T47.4X4	T47.4X5	T47.4X6
emulsion	T47.2X1	T47.2X2	T47.2X3	T47.2X4	T47.2X5	T47.2X6
nonmedicinal	T52.0X1	T52.0X2	T52.0X3	T52.0X4	—	—
topical	T49.3X1	T49.3X2	T49.3X3	T49.3X4	T49.3X5	T49.3X6
salt NEC	T50.3X1	T50.3X2	T50.3X3	T50.3X4	T50.3X5	T50.3X6
spirits	T52.0X1	T52.0X2	T52.0X3	T52.0X4	—	—
Mineralocorticosteroid	T50.0X1	T50.0X2	T50.0X3	T50.0X4	T50.0X5	T50.0X6
Minocycline	T36.4X1	T36.4X2	T36.4X3	T36.4X4	T36.4X5	T36.4X6
Minoxidil	T46.7X1	T46.7X2	T46.7X3	T46.7X4	T46.7X5	T46.7X6
Miokamycin	T36.3X1	T36.3X2	T36.3X3	T36.3X4	T36.3X5	T36.3X6
Miotic drug	T49.5X1	T49.5X2	T49.5X3	T49.5X4	T49.5X5	T49.5X6
Mipafox	T60.0X1	T60.0X2	T60.0X3	T60.0X4	—	—
Mirex	T60.1X1	T60.1X2	T60.1X3	T60.1X4	—	—
Mirtazapine	T43.021	T43.022	T43.023	T43.024	T43.025	T43.026
Misonidazole	T37.3X1	T37.3X2	T37.3X3	T37.3X4	T37.3X5	T37.3X6
Misoprostol	T47.1X1	T47.1X2	T47.1X3	T47.1X4	T47.1X5	T47.1X6
Mithramycin	T45.1X1	T45.1X2	T45.1X3	T45.1X4	T45.1X5	T45.1X6
Mitobronitol	T45.1X1	T45.1X2	T45.1X3	T45.1X4	T45.1X5	T45.1X6
Mitoguazone	T45.1X1	T45.1X2	T45.1X3	T45.1X4	T45.1X5	T45.1X6
Mitolactol	T45.1X1	T45.1X2	T45.1X3	T45.1X4	T45.1X5	T45.1X6
Mitomycin	T45.1X1	T45.1X2	T45.1X3	T45.1X4	T45.1X5	T45.1X6
Mitopodozide	T45.1X1	T45.1X2	T45.1X3	T45.1X4	T45.1X5	T45.1X6
Mitotane	T45.1X1	T45.1X2	T45.1X3	T45.1X4	T45.1X5	T45.1X6
Mitoxantrone	T45.1X1	T45.1X2	T45.1X3	T45.1X4	T45.1X5	T45.1X6
Mivacurium chloride	T48.1X1	T48.1X2	T48.1X3	T48.1X4	T48.1X5	T48.1X6
Miyari bacteria	T47.6X1	T47.6X2	T47.6X3	T47.6X4	T47.6X5	T47.6X6
Moclobemide	T43.1X1	T43.1X2	T43.1X3	T43.1X4	T43.1X5	T43.1X6
Moderil	T46.5X1	T46.5X2	T46.5X3	T46.5X4	T46.5X5	T46.5X6
Mofebutazone	T39.2X1	T39.2X2	T39.2X3	T39.2X4	T39.2X5	T39.2X6
Mogadon — *see* Nitrazepam						
Molindone	T43.591	T43.592	T43.593	T43.594	T43.595	T43.596
Molsidomine	T46.3X1	T46.3X2	T46.3X3	T46.3X4	T46.3X5	T46.3X6
Mometasone	T49.0X1	T49.0X2	T49.0X3	T49.0X4	T49.0X5	T49.0X6
Monistat	T49.0X1	T49.0X2	T49.0X3	T49.0X4	T49.0X5	T49.0X6
Monkshood	T62.2X1	T62.2X2	T62.2X3	T62.2X4	—	—
Monoamine oxidase inhibitor NEC	T43.1X1	T43.1X2	T43.1X3	T43.1X4	T43.1X5	T43.1X6
hydrazine	T43.1X1	T43.1X2	T43.1X3	T43.1X4	T43.1X5	T43.1X6
Monobenzone	T49.4X1	T49.4X2	T49.4X3	T49.4X4	T49.4X5	T49.4X6
Monochloroacetic acid	T60.3X1	T60.3X2	T60.3X3	T60.3X4	—	—
Monochlorobenzene	T53.7X1	T53.7X2	T53.7X3	T53.7X4	—	—
Monoethanolamine	T46.8X1	T46.8X2	T46.8X3	T46.8X4	T46.8X5	T46.8X6
oleate	T46.8X1	T46.8X2	T46.8X3	T46.8X4	T46.8X5	T46.8X6
Monooctanoin	T50.991	T50.992	T50.993	T50.994	T50.995	T50.996
Monophenylbutazone	T39.2X1	T39.2X2	T39.2X3	T39.2X4	T39.2X5	T39.2X6
Monosodium glutamate	T65.891	T65.892	T65.893	T65.894	—	—
Monosulfiram	T49.0X1	T49.0X2	T49.0X3	T49.0X4	T49.0X5	T49.0X6
Monoxide, carbon — *see* Carbon, monoxide						
Monoxidine hydrochloride	T46.1X1	T46.1X2	T46.1X3	T46.1X4	T46.1X5	T46.1X6
Monuron	T60.3X1	T60.3X2	T60.3X3	T60.3X4	—	—
Moperone	T43.4X1	T43.4X2	T43.4X3	T43.4X4	T43.4X5	T43.4X6
Mopidamol	T45.1X1	T45.1X2	T45.1X3	T45.1X4	T45.1X5	T45.1X6
MOPP (mechloreth-amine + vincristine + prednisone + procarba-zine)	T45.1X1	T45.1X2	T45.1X3	T45.1X4	T45.1X5	T45.1X6
Morfin	T40.2X1	T40.2X2	T40.2X3	T40.2X4	T40.2X5	T40.2X6
Morinamide	T37.1X1	T37.1X2	T37.1X3	T37.1X4	T37.1X5	T37.1X6
Morning glory seeds	T40.991	T40.992	T40.993	T40.994		
Moroxydine	T37.5X1	T37.5X2	T37.5X3	T37.5X4	T37.5X5	T37.5X6
Morphazinamide	T37.1X1	T37.1X2	T37.1X3	T37.1X4	T37.1X5	T37.1X6
Morphine	T40.2X1	T40.2X2	T40.2X3	T40.2X4	T40.2X5	T40.2X6
antagonist	T50.7X1	T50.7X2	T50.7X3	T50.7X4	T50.7X5	T50.7X6
Morpholinylethylmorphine	T40.2X1	T40.2X2	T40.2X3	T40.2X4	—	—
Morsuximide	T42.2X1	T42.2X2	T42.2X3	T42.2X4	T42.2X5	T42.2X6
Mosapramine	T43.591	T43.592	T43.593	T43.594	T43.595	T43.596
Moth balls — *see also* Pesticides	T60.2X1	T60.2X2	T60.2X3	T60.2X4	—	—
naphthalene	T60.2X1	T60.2X2	T60.2X3	T60.2X4	—	—
paradichlorobenzene	T60.1X1	T60.1X2	T60.1X3	T60.1X4	—	—
Motor exhaust gas	T58.01	T58.02	T58.03	T58.04		
Mouthwash (antiseptic) (zinc chloride)	T49.6X1	T49.6X2	T49.6X3	T49.6X4	T49.6X5	T49.6X6
Moxastine	T45.0X1	T45.0X2	T45.0X3	T45.0X4	T45.0X5	T45.0X6
Moxaverine	T44.3X1	T44.3X2	T44.3X3	T44.3X4	T44.3X5	T44.3X6
Moxisylyte	T46.7X1	T46.7X2	T46.7X3	T46.7X4	T46.7X5	T46.7X6
Mucilage, plant	T47.4X1	T47.4X2	T47.4X3	T47.4X4	T47.4X5	T47.4X6
Mucolytic drug	T48.4X1	T48.4X2	T48.4X3	T48.4X4	T48.4X5	T48.4X6
Mucomyst	T48.4X1	T48.4X2	T48.4X3	T48.4X4	T48.4X5	T48.4X6
Mucous membrane agents (external)	T49.91	T49.92	T49.93	T49.94	T49.95	T49.96
specified NEC	T49.8X1	T49.8X2	T49.8X3	T49.8X4	T49.8X5	T49.8X6
Mumps						
immune globulin (human)	T50.Z11	T50.Z12	T50.Z13	T50.Z14	T50.Z15	T50.Z16
skin test antigen	T50.8X1	T50.8X2	T50.8X3	T50.8X4	T50.8X5	T50.8X6
vaccine	T50.B91	T50.B92	T50.B93	T50.B94	T50.B95	T50.B96
Mumpsvax	T50.B91	T50.B92	T50.B93	T50.B94	T50.B95	T50.B96
Mupirocin	T49.0X1	T49.0X2	T49.0X3	T49.0X4	T49.0X5	T49.0X6
Muriatic acid — *see* Hydrochloric acid						
Muromonab-CD3	T45.1X1	T45.1X2	T45.1X3	T45.1X4	T45.1X5	T45.1X6
Muscle-action drug NEC	T48.201	T48.202	T48.203	T48.204	T48.205	T48.206
Muscle affecting agents NEC	T48.201	T48.202	T48.203	T48.204	T48.205	T48.206
oxytocic	T48.0X1	T48.0X2	T48.0X3	T48.0X4	T48.0X5	T48.0X6
relaxants	T48.201	T48.202	T48.203	T48.204	T48.205	T48.206
central nervous system	T42.8X1	T42.8X2	T42.8X3	T42.8X4	T42.8X5	T42.8X6
skeletal	T48.1X1	T48.1X2	T48.1X3	T48.1X4	T48.1X5	T48.1X6
smooth	T44.3X1	T44.3X2	T44.3X3	T44.3X4	T44.3X5	T44.3X6
Muscle relaxant — *see* Relaxant, muscle						
Muscle-tone depressant, central NEC	T42.8X1	T42.8X2	T42.8X3	T42.8X4	T42.8X5	T42.8X6
specified NEC	T42.8X1	T42.8X2	T42.8X3	T42.8X4	T42.8X5	T42.8X6
Mushroom, noxious	T62.0X1	T62.0X2	T62.0X3	T62.0X4	—	—
Mussel, noxious	T61.781	T61.782	T61.783	T61.784	—	—
Mustard (emetic)	T47.7X1	T47.7X2	T47.7X3	T47.7X4	T47.7X5	T47.7X6
black	T47.7X1	T47.7X2	T47.7X3	T47.7X4	T47.7X5	T47.7X6
gas, not in war	T59.91	T59.92	T59.93	T59.94		
nitrogen	T45.1X1	T45.1X2	T45.1X3	T45.1X4	T45.1X5	T45.1X6
Mustine	T45.1X1	T45.1X2	T45.1X3	T45.1X4	T45.1X5	T45.1X6
M-vac	T45.1X1	T45.1X2	T45.1X3	T45.1X4	T45.1X5	T45.1X6
Mycifradin	T36.5X1	T36.5X2	T36.5X3	T36.5X4	T36.5X5	T36.5X6
topical	T49.0X1	T49.0X2	T49.0X3	T49.0X4	T49.0X5	T49.0X6
Mycitracin	T36.8X1	T36.8X2	T36.8X3	T36.8X4	T36.8X5	T36.8X6
ophthalmic preparation	T49.5X1	T49.5X2	T49.5X3	T49.5X4	T49.5X5	T49.5X6
Mycostatin	T36.7X1	T36.7X2	T36.7X3	T36.7X4	T36.7X5	T36.7X6
topical	T49.0X1	T49.0X2	T49.0X3	T49.0X4	T49.0X5	T49.0X6
Mycotoxins	T64.81	T64.82	T64.83	T64.84	—	—
aflatoxin	T64.01	T64.02	T64.03	T64.04	—	—
specified NEC	T64.81	T64.82	T64.83	T64.84	—	—
Mydriacyl	T44.3X1	T44.3X2	T44.3X3	T44.3X4	T44.3X5	T44.3X6
Mydriatic drug	T49.5X1	T49.5X2	T49.5X3	T49.5X4	T49.5X5	T49.5X6
Myelobromal	T45.1X1	T45.1X2	T45.1X3	T45.1X4	T45.1X5	T45.1X6
Myleran	T45.1X1	T45.1X2	T45.1X3	T45.1X4	T45.1X5	T45.1X6
Myochrysin (e)	T39.2X1	T39.2X2	T39.2X3	T39.2X4	T39.2X5	T39.2X6
Myoneural blocking agents	T48.1X1	T48.1X2	T48.1X3	T48.1X4	T48.1X5	T48.1X6
Myralact	T49.0X1	T49.0X2	T49.0X3	T49.0X4	T49.0X5	T49.0X6
Myristica fragrans	T62.2X1	T62.2X2	T62.2X3	T62.2X4	—	—
Myristicin	T65.891	T65.892	T65.893	T65.894	—	—
Mysoline	T42.3X1	T42.3X2	T42.3X3	T42.3X4	T42.3X5	T42.3X6
Nabilone	T40.7X1	T40.7X2	T40.7X3	T40.7X4	T40.7X5	T40.7X6
Nabumetone	T39.391	T39.392	T39.393	T39.394	T39.395	T39.396
Nadolol	T44.7X1	T44.7X2	T44.7X3	T44.7X4	T44.7X5	T44.7X6
Nafcillin	T36.0X1	T36.0X2	T36.0X3	T36.0X4	T36.0X5	T36.0X6
Nafoxidine	T38.6X1	T38.6X2	T38.6X3	T38.6X4	T38.6X5	T38.6X6
Naftazone	T46.991	T46.992	T46.993	T46.994	T46.995	T46.996
Naftidrofuryl (oxalate)	T46.7X1	T46.7X2	T46.7X3	T46.7X4	T46.7X5	T46.7X6
Naftifine	T49.0X1	T49.0X2	T49.0X3	T49.0X4	T49.0X5	T49.0X6
Nail polish remover	T52.91	T52.92	T52.93	T52.94	—	—
Nalbuphine	T40.4X1	T40.4X2	T40.4X3	T40.4X4	T40.4X5	T40.4X6
Naled	T60.0X1	T60.0X2	T60.0X3	T60.0X4	—	—
Nalidixic acid	T37.8X1	T37.8X2	T37.8X3	T37.8X4	T37.8X5	T37.8X6
Nalorphine	T50.7X1	T50.7X2	T50.7X3	T50.7X4	T50.7X5	T50.7X6
Naloxone	T50.7X1	T50.7X2	T50.7X3	T50.7X4	T50.7X5	T50.7X6
Naltrexone	T50.7X1	T50.7X2	T50.7X3	T50.7X4	T50.7X5	T50.7X6
Namenda	T43.8X1	T43.8X2	T43.8X3	T43.8X4	T43.8X5	T43.8X6
Nandrolone	T38.7X1	T38.7X2	T38.7X3	T38.7X4	T38.7X5	T38.7X6
Naphazoline	T48.5X1	T48.5X2	T48.5X3	T48.5X4	T48.5X5	T48.5X6
Naphtha (painters') (petroleum)	T52.0X1	T52.0X2	T52.0X3	T52.0X4	—	—
solvent	T52.0X1	T52.0X2	T52.0X3	T52.0X4	—	—
vapor	T52.0X1	T52.0X2	T52.0X3	T52.0X4	—	—
Naphthalene (non-chlorinated)	T60.2X1	T60.2X2	T60.2X3	T60.2X4	—	—
chlorinated	T60.1X1	T60.1X2	T60.1X3	T60.1X4	—	—
vapor	T60.1X1	T60.1X2	T60.1X3	T60.1X4	—	—

Substance	Poisoning, Accidental (unintentional)	Poisoning, Intentional Self-harm	Poisoning, Assault	Poisoning, Undetermined	Adverse Effect	Under-dosing
Naphthalene — continued						
insecticide or moth repellent	T60.2X1	T60.2X2	T60.2X3	T60.2X4	—	—
chlorinated	T60.1X1	T60.1X2	T60.1X3	T60.1X4	—	—
vapor	T60.2X1	T60.2X2	T60.2X3	T60.2X4	—	—
chlorinated	T60.1X1	T60.1X2	T60.1X3	T60.1X4	—	—
Naphthol	T65.891	T65.892	T65.893	T65.894	—	—
Naphthylamine	T65.891	T65.892	T65.893	T65.894	—	—
Naphthylthiourea (ANTU)	T60.4X1	T60.4X2	T60.4X3	T60.4X4	—	—
Naprosyn — see Naproxen						
Naproxen	T39.311	T39.312	T39.313	T39.314	T39.315	T39.316
Narcotic (drug)	T40.601	T40.602	T40.603	T40.604	T40.605	T40.606
analgesic NEC	T40.601	T40.602	T40.603	T40.604	T40.605	T40.606
antagonist	T50.7X1	T50.7X2	T50.7X3	T50.7X4	T50.7X5	T50.7X6
specified NEC	T40.691	T40.692	T40.693	T40.694	T40.695	T40.696
synthetic	T40.4X1	T40.4X2	T40.4X3	T40.4X4	T40.4X5	T40.4X6
Narcotine	T48.3X1	T48.3X2	T48.3X3	T48.3X4	T48.3X5	T48.3X6
Nardil	T43.1X1	T43.1X2	T43.1X3	T43.1X4	T43.1X5	T43.1X6
Nasal drug NEC	T49.6X1	T49.6X2	T49.6X3	T49.6X4	T49.6X5	T49.6X6
Natamycin	T49.0X1	T49.0X2	T49.0X3	T49.0X4	T49.0X5	T49.0X6
Natrium cyanide — see Cyanide(s)						
Natural						
blood (product)	T45.8X1	T45.8X2	T45.8X3	T45.8X4	T45.8X5	T45.8X6
gas (piped)	T59.891	T59.892	T59.893	T59.894	—	—
incomplete combustion	T58.11	T58.12	T58.13	T58.14	—	—
Nealbarbital	T42.3X1	T42.3X2	T42.3X3	T42.3X4	T42.3X5	T42.3X6
Nectadon	T48.3X1	T48.3X2	T48.3X3	T48.3X4	T48.3X5	T48.3X6
Nedocromil	T48.6X1	T48.6X2	T48.6X3	T48.6X4	T48.6X5	T48.6X6
Nefopam	T39.8X1	T39.8X2	T39.8X3	T39.8X4	T39.8X5	T39.8X6
Nematocyst (sting)	T63.691	T63.692	T63.693	T63.694	—	—
Nembutal	T42.3X1	T42.3X2	T42.3X3	T42.3X4	T42.3X5	T42.3X6
Nemonapride	T43.591	T43.592	T43.593	T43.594	T43.595	T43.596
Neoarsphenamine	T37.8X1	T37.8X2	T37.8X3	T37.8X4	T37.8X5	T37.8X6
Neocinchophen	T50.4X1	T50.4X2	T50.4X3	T50.4X4	T50.4X5	T50.4X6
Neomycin (derivatives)	T36.5X1	T36.5X2	T36.5X3	T36.5X4	T36.5X5	T36.5X6
with						
bacitracin	T49.0X1	T49.0X2	T49.0X3	T49.0X4	T49.0X5	T49.0X6
neostigmine	T44.0X1	T44.0X2	T44.0X3	T44.0X4	T44.0X5	T44.0X6
ENT agent	T49.6X1	T49.6X2	T49.6X3	T49.6X4	T49.6X5	T49.6X6
ophthalmic preparation	T49.5X1	T49.5X2	T49.5X3	T49.5X4	T49.5X5	T49.5X6
topical NEC	T49.0X1	T49.0X2	T49.0X3	T49.0X4	T49.0X5	T49.0X6
Neonal	T42.3X1	T42.3X2	T42.3X3	T42.3X4	T42.3X5	T42.3X6
Neoprontosil	T37.0X1	T37.0X2	T37.0X3	T37.0X4	T37.0X5	T37.0X6
Neosalvarsan	T37.8X1	T37.8X2	T37.8X3	T37.8X4	T37.8X5	T37.8X6
Neosilversalvarsan	T37.8X1	T37.8X2	T37.8X3	T37.8X4	T37.8X5	T37.8X6
Neosporin	T36.8X1	T36.8X2	T36.8X3	T36.8X4	T36.8X5	T36.8X6
ENT agent	T49.6X1	T49.6X2	T49.6X3	T49.6X4	T49.6X5	T49.6X6
opthalmic preparation	T49.5X1	T49.5X2	T49.5X3	T49.5X4	T49.5X5	T49.5X6
topical NEC	T49.0X1	T49.0X2	T49.0X3	T49.0X4	T49.0X5	T49.0X6
Neostigmine bromide	T44.0X1	T44.0X2	T44.0X3	T44.0X4	T44.0X5	T44.0X6
Neraval	T42.3X1	T42.3X2	T42.3X3	T42.3X4	T42.3X5	T42.3X6
Neravan	T42.3X1	T42.3X2	T42.3X3	T42.3X4	T42.3X5	T42.3X6
Nerium oleander	T62.2X1	T62.2X2	T62.2X3	T62.2X4	—	—
Nerve gas, not in war	T59.91	T59.92	T59.93	T59.94	—	—
Nesacaine	T41.3X1	T41.3X2	T41.3X3	T41.3X4	T41.3X5	T41.3X6
infiltration (subcutaneous)	T41.3X1	T41.3X2	T41.3X3	T41.3X4	T41.3X5	T41.3X6
nerve block (peripheral) (plexus)	T41.3X1	T41.3X2	T41.3X3	T41.3X4	T41.3X5	T41.3X6
Netilmicin	T36.5X1	T36.5X2	T36.5X3	T36.5X4	T36.5X5	T36.5X6
Neurobarb	T42.3X1	T42.3X2	T42.3X3	T42.3X4	T42.3X5	T42.3X6
Neuroleptic drug NEC	T43.501	T43.502	T43.503	T43.504	T43.505	T43.506
Neuromuscular blocking drug	T48.1X1	T48.1X2	T48.1X3	T48.1X4	T48.1X5	T48.1X6
Neutral insulin injection	T38.3X1	T38.3X2	T38.3X3	T38.3X4	T38.3X5	T38.3X6
Neutral spirits	T51.0X1	T51.0X2	T51.0X3	T51.0X4	—	—
beverage	T51.0X1	T51.0X2	T51.0X3	T51.0X4	—	—
Niacin	T46.7X1	T46.7X2	T46.7X3	T46.7X4	T46.7X5	T46.7X6
Niacinamide	T45.2X1	T45.2X2	T45.2X3	T45.2X4	T45.2X5	T45.2X6
Nialamide	T43.1X1	T43.1X2	T43.1X3	T43.1X4	T43.1X5	T43.1X6
Niaprazine	T42.6X1	T42.6X2	T42.6X3	T42.6X4	T42.6X5	T42.6X6
Nicametate	T46.7X1	T46.7X2	T46.7X3	T46.7X4	T46.7X5	T46.7X6
Nicardipine	T46.1X1	T46.1X2	T46.1X3	T46.1X4	T46.1X5	T46.1X6
Nicergoline	T46.7X1	T46.7X2	T46.7X3	T46.7X4	T46.7X5	T46.7X6
Nickel (carbonyl) (tetra-carbonyl) (fumes) (vapor)	T56.891	T56.892	T56.893	T56.894	—	—
Nickelocene	T56.891	T56.892	T56.893	T56.894	—	—
Niclosamide	T37.4X1	T37.4X2	T37.4X3	T37.4X4	T37.4X5	T37.4X6
Nicofuranose	T46.7X1	T46.7X2	T46.7X3	T46.7X4	T46.7X5	T46.7X6
Nicomorphine	T40.2X1	T40.2X2	T40.2X3	T40.2X4	—	—
Nicorandil	T46.3X1	T46.3X2	T46.3X3	T46.3X4	T46.3X5	T46.3X6
Nicotiana (plant)	T62.2X1	T62.2X2	T62.2X3	T62.2X4	—	—
Nicotinamide	T45.2X1	T45.2X2	T45.2X3	T45.2X4	T45.2X5	T45.2X6

Substance	Poisoning, Accidental (unintentional)	Poisoning, Intentional Self-harm	Poisoning, Assault	Poisoning, Undetermined	Adverse Effect	Under-dosing
Nicotine (insecticide) (spray) (sulfate) **NEC**	T60.2X1	T60.2X2	T60.2X3	T60.2X4	—	—
from tobacco	T65.291	T65.292	T65.293	T65.294	—	—
cigarettes	T65.221	T65.222	T65.223	T65.224	—	—
not insecticide	T65.291	T65.292	T65.293	T65.294	—	—
Nicotinic acid	T46.7X1	T46.7X2	T46.7X3	T46.7X4	T46.7X5	T46.7X6
Nicotinyl alcohol	T46.7X1	T46.7X2	T46.7X3	T46.7X4	T46.7X5	T46.7X6
Nicoumalone	T45.511	T45.512	T45.513	T45.514	T45.515	T45.516
Nifedipine	T46.1X1	T46.1X2	T46.1X3	T46.1X4	T46.1X5	T46.1X6
Nifenazone	T39.2X1	T39.2X2	T39.2X3	T39.2X4	T39.2X5	T39.2X6
Nifuraldezone	T37.91	T37.92	T37.93	T37.94	T37.95	T37.96
Nifuratel	T37.8X1	T37.8X2	T37.8X3	T37.8X4	T37.8X5	T37.8X6
Nifurtimox	T37.3X1	T37.3X2	T37.3X3	T37.3X4	T37.3X5	T37.3X6
Nifurtoinol	T37.8X1	T37.8X2	T37.8X3	T37.8X4	T37.8X5	T37.8X6
Nightshade, deadly (solanum) — see also Belladonna	T62.2X1	T62.2X2	T62.2X3	T62.2X4	—	—
berry	T62.1X1	T62.1X2	T62.1X3	T62.1X4	—	—
Nikethamide	T50.7X1	T50.7X2	T50.7X3	T50.7X4	T50.7X5	T50.7X6
Nilstat	T36.7X1	T36.7X2	T36.7X3	T36.7X4	T36.7X5	T36.7X6
topical	T49.0X1	T49.0X2	T49.0X3	T49.0X4	T49.0X5	T49.0X6
Nilutamide	T38.6X1	T38.6X2	T38.6X3	T38.6X4	T38.6X5	T38.6X6
Nimesulide	T39.391	T39.392	T39.393	T39.394	T39.395	T39.396
Nimetazepam	T42.4X1	T42.4X2	T42.4X3	T42.4X4	T42.4X5	T42.4X6
Nimodipine	T46.1X1	T46.1X2	T46.1X3	T46.1X4	T46.1X5	T46.1X6
Nimorazole	T37.3X1	T37.3X2	T37.3X3	T37.3X4	T37.3X5	T37.3X6
Nimustine	T45.1X1	T45.1X2	T45.1X3	T45.1X4	T45.1X5	T45.1X6
Niridazole	T37.4X1	T37.4X2	T37.4X3	T37.4X4	T37.4X5	T37.4X6
Nisentil	T40.2X1	T40.2X2	T40.2X3	T40.2X4	T40.2X5	T40.2X6
Nisoldipine	T46.1X1	T46.1X2	T46.1X3	T46.1X4	T46.1X5	T46.1X6
Nitramine	T65.3X1	T65.3X2	T65.3X3	T65.3X4	—	—
Nitrate, organic	T46.3X1	T46.3X2	T46.3X3	T46.3X4	T46.3X5	T46.3X6
Nitrazepam	T42.4X1	T42.4X2	T42.4X3	T42.4X4	T42.4X5	T42.4X6
Nitrefazole	T50.6X1	T50.6X2	T50.6X3	T50.6X4	T50.6X5	T50.6X6
Nitrendipine	T46.1X1	T46.1X2	T46.1X3	T46.1X4	T46.1X5	T46.1X6
Nitric						
acid (liquid)	T54.2X1	T54.2X2	T54.2X3	T54.2X4	—	—
vapor	T59.891	T59.892	T59.893	T59.894	—	—
oxide (gas)	T59.0X1	T59.0X2	T59.0X3	T59.0X4	—	—
Nitrimidazine	T37.3X1	T37.3X2	T37.3X3	T37.3X4	T37.3X5	T37.3X6
Nitrite, amyl (medicinal) (vapor)	T46.3X1	T46.3X2	T46.3X3	T46.3X4	T46.3X5	T46.3X6
Nitroaniline	T65.3X1	T65.3X2	T65.3X3	T65.3X4	—	—
vapor	T59.891	T59.892	T59.893	T59.894	—	—
Nitrobenzene, nitrobenzol	T65.3X1	T65.3X2	T65.3X3	T65.3X4	—	—
vapor	T65.3X1	T65.3X2	T65.3X3	T65.3X4	—	—
Nitrocellulose	T65.891	T65.892	T65.893	T65.894	—	—
lacquer	T65.891	T65.892	T65.893	T65.894	—	—
Nitrodiphenyl	T65.3X1	T65.3X2	T65.3X3	T65.3X4	—	—
Nitrofural	T49.0X1	T49.0X2	T49.0X3	T49.0X4	T49.0X5	T49.0X6
Nitrofurantoin	T37.8X1	T37.8X2	T37.8X3	T37.8X4	T37.8X5	T37.8X6
Nitrofurazone	T49.0X1	T49.0X2	T49.0X3	T49.0X4	T49.0X5	T49.0X6
Nitrogen	T59.0X1	T59.0X2	T59.0X3	T59.0X4	—	—
mustard	T45.1X1	T45.1X2	T45.1X3	T45.1X4	T45.1X5	T45.1X6
Nitroglycerin, nitroglycerol (medicinal)	T46.3X1	T46.3X2	T46.3X3	T46.3X4	T46.3X5	T46.3X6
nonmedicinal	T65.5X1	T65.5X2	T65.5X3	T65.5X4	—	—
fumes	T65.5X1	T65.5X2	T65.5X3	T65.5X4	—	—
Nitroglycol	T52.3X1	T52.3X2	T52.3X3	T52.3X4	—	—
Nitrohydrochloric acid	T54.2X1	T54.2X2	T54.2X3	T54.2X4	—	—
Nitromersol	T49.0X1	T49.0X2	T49.0X3	T49.0X4	T49.0X5	T49.0X6
Nitronaphthalene	T65.891	T65.892	T65.893	T65.894	—	—
Nitrophenol	T54.0X1	T54.0X2	T54.0X3	T54.0X4	—	—
Nitropropane	T52.8X1	T52.8X2	T52.8X3	T52.8X4	—	—
Nitroprusside	T46.5X1	T46.5X2	T46.5X3	T46.5X4	T46.5X5	T46.5X6
Nitrosodimethylamine	T65.3X1	T65.3X2	T65.3X3	T65.3X4	—	—
Nitrothiazol	T37.4X1	T37.4X2	T37.4X3	T37.4X4	T37.4X5	T37.4X6
Nitrotoluene, nitrotoluol	T65.3X1	T65.3X2	T65.3X3	T65.3X4	—	—
vapor	T65.3X1	T65.3X2	T65.3X3	T65.3X4	—	—
Nitrous						
acid (liquid)	T54.2X1	T54.2X2	T54.2X3	T54.2X4	—	—
fumes	T59.891	T59.892	T59.893	T59.894	—	—
ether spirit	T46.3X1	T46.3X2	T46.3X3	T46.3X4	T46.3X5	T46.3X6
oxide	T41.0X1	T41.0X2	T41.0X3	T41.0X4	T41.0X5	T41.0X6
Nitroxoline	T37.8X1	T37.8X2	T37.8X3	T37.8X4	T37.8X5	T37.8X6
Nitrozone	T49.0X1	T49.0X2	T49.0X3	T49.0X4	T49.0X5	T49.0X6
Nizatidine	T47.0X1	T47.0X2	T47.0X3	T47.0X4	T47.0X5	T47.0X6
Nizofenone	T43.8X1	T43.8X2	T43.8X3	T43.8X4	T43.8X5	T43.8X6
Noctec	T42.6X1	T42.6X2	T42.6X3	T42.6X4	T42.6X5	T42.6X6
Noludar	T42.6X1	T42.6X2	T42.6X3	T42.6X4	T42.6X5	T42.6X6
Nomegestrol	T38.5X1	T38.5X2	T38.5X3	T38.5X4	T38.5X5	T38.5X6
Nomifensine	T43.291	T43.292	T43.293	T43.294	T43.295	T43.296
Nonoxinol	T49.8X1	T49.8X2	T49.8X3	T49.8X4	T49.8X5	T49.8X6

Substance	Poisoning, Accidental (unintentional)	Poisoning, Intentional Self-harm	Poisoning, Assault	Poisoning, Undetermined	Adverse Effect	Under-dosing
Nonylphenoxy	T49.8X1	T49.8X2	T49.8X3	T49.8X4	T49.8X5	T49.8X6
(polyethoxyethanol)						
Noptil	T42.3X1	T42.3X2	T42.3X3	T42.3X4	T42.3X5	T42.3X6
Noradrenaline	T44.4X1	T44.4X2	T44.4X3	T44.4X4	T44.4X5	T44.4X6
Noramidopyrine	T39.2X1	T39.2X2	T39.2X3	T39.2X4	T39.2X5	T39.2X6
methanesulfonate sodium	T39.2X1	T39.2X2	T39.2X3	T39.2X4	T39.2X5	T39.2X6
Norbormide	T60.4X1	T60.4X2	T60.4X3	T60.4X4	—	—
Nordazepam	T42.4X1	T42.4X2	T42.4X3	T42.4X4	T42.4X5	T42.4X6
Norepinephrine	T44.4X1	T44.4X2	T44.4X3	T44.4X4	T44.4X5	T44.4X6
Norethandrolone	T38.7X1	T38.7X2	T38.7X3	T38.7X4	T38.7X5	T38.7X6
Norethindrone	T38.4X1	T38.4X2	T38.4X3	T38.4X4	T38.4X5	T38.4X6
Norethisterone (acetate)	T38.4X1	T38.4X2	T38.4X3	T38.4X4	T38.4X5	T38.4X6
(enantate)						
with ethinylestradiol	T38.5X1	T38.5X2	T38.5X3	T38.5X4	T38.5X5	T38.5X6
Noretynodrel	T38.5X1	T38.5X2	T38.5X3	T38.5X4	T38.5X5	T38.5X6
Norfenefrine	T44.4X1	T44.4X2	T44.4X3	T44.4X4	T44.4X5	T44.4X6
Norfloxacin	T36.8X1	T36.8X2	T36.8X3	T36.8X4	T36.8X5	T36.8X6
Norgestrel	T38.4X1	T38.4X2	T38.4X3	T38.4X4	T38.4X5	T38.4X6
Norgestrienone	T38.4X1	T38.4X2	T38.4X3	T38.4X4	T38.4X5	T38.4X6
Norlestrin	T38.4X1	T38.4X2	T38.4X3	T38.4X4	T38.4X5	T38.4X6
Norlutin	T38.4X1	T38.4X2	T38.4X3	T38.4X4	T38.4X5	T38.4X6
Normal serum albumin (human),	T45.8X1	T45.8X2	T45.8X3	T45.8X4	T45.8X5	T45.8X6
salt-poor						
Normethandrone	T38.5X1	T38.5X2	T38.5X3	T38.5X4	T38.5X5	T38.5X6
Normison — *see*						
Benzodiazepines						
Normorphine	T40.2X1	T40.2X2	T40.2X3	T40.2X4	—	—
Norpseudoephedrine	T50.5X1	T50.5X2	T50.5X3	T50.5X4	T50.5X5	T50.5X6
Nortestosterone	T38.7X1	T38.7X2	T38.7X3	T38.7X4	T38.7X5	T38.7X6
(furanpropionate)						
Nortriptyline	T43.011	T43.012	T43.013	T43.014	T43.015	T43.016
Noscapine	T48.3X1	T48.3X2	T48.3X3	T48.3X4	T48.3X5	T48.3X6
Nose preparations	T49.6X1	T49.6X2	T49.6X3	T49.6X4	T49.6X5	T49.6X6
Novobiocin	T36.5X1	T36.5X2	T36.5X3	T36.5X4	T36.5X5	T36.5X6
Novocain (infiltration)	T41.3X1	T41.3X2	T41.3X3	T41.3X4	T41.3X5	T41.3X6
(topical)						
nerve block (peripheral)	T41.3X1	T41.3X2	T41.3X3	T41.3X4	T41.3X5	T41.3X6
(plexus)						
spinal	T41.3X1	T41.3X2	T41.3X3	T41.3X4	T41.3X5	T41.3X6
Noxious foodstuff	T62.91	T62.92	T62.93	T62.94	—	—
specified NEC	T62.8X1	T62.8X2	T62.8X3	T62.8X4	—	—
Noxiptiline	T43.011	T43.012	T43.013	T43.014	T43.015	T43.016
Noxytiolin	T49.0X1	T49.0X2	T49.0X3	T49.0X4	T49.0X5	T49.0X6
NPH Iletin (insulin)	T38.3X1	T38.3X2	T38.3X3	T38.3X4	T38.3X5	T38.3X6
Numorphan	T40.2X1	T40.2X2	T40.2X3	T40.2X4	T40.2X5	T40.2X6
Nunol	T42.3X1	T42.3X2	T42.3X3	T42.3X4	T42.3X5	T42.3X6
Nupercaine (spinal	T41.3X1	T41.3X2	T41.3X3	T41.3X4	T41.3X5	T41.3X6
anesthetic)						
topical (surface)	T41.3X1	T41.3X2	T41.3X3	T41.3X4	T41.3X5	T41.3X6
Nutmeg oil (liniment)	T49.3X1	T49.3X2	T49.3X3	T49.3X4	T49.3X5	T49.3X6
Nutritional supplement	T50.901	T50.902	T50.903	T50.904	T50.905	T50.906
Nux vomica	T65.1X1	T65.1X2	T65.1X3	T65.1X4	—	—
Nydrazid	T37.1X1	T37.1X2	T37.1X3	T37.1X4	T37.1X5	T37.1X6
Nylidrin	T46.7X1	T46.7X2	T46.7X3	T46.7X4	T46.7X5	T46.7X6
Nystatin	T36.7X1	T36.7X2	T36.7X3	T36.7X4	T36.7X5	T36.7X6
topical	T49.0X1	T49.0X2	T49.0X3	T49.0X4	T49.0X5	T49.0X6
Nytol	T45.0X1	T45.0X2	T45.0X3	T45.0X4	T45.0X5	T45.0X6
Obidoxime chloride	T50.6X1	T50.6X2	T50.6X3	T50.6X4	T50.6X5	T50.6X6
Octafonium (chloride)	T49.3X1	T49.3X2	T49.3X3	T49.3X4	T49.3X5	T49.3X6
Octamethyl	T60.0X1	T60.0X2	T60.0X3	T60.0X4	—	—
pyrophosphoramide						
Octanoin	T50.991	T50.992	T50.993	T50.994	T50.995	T50.996
Octatropine	T44.3X1	T44.3X2	T44.3X3	T44.3X4	T44.3X5	T44.3X6
methylbromide						
Octotiamine	T45.2X1	T45.2X2	T45.2X3	T45.2X4	T45.2X5	T45.2X6
Octoxinol (9)	T49.8X1	T49.8X2	T49.8X3	T49.8X4	T49.8X5	T49.8X6
Octreotide	T38.991	T38.992	T38.993	T38.994	T38.995	T38.996
Octyl nitrite	T46.3X1	T46.3X2	T46.3X3	T46.3X4	T46.3X5	T46.3X6
Oestradiol	T38.5X1	T38.5X2	T38.5X3	T38.5X4	T38.5X5	T38.5X6
Oestriol	T38.5X1	T38.5X2	T38.5X3	T38.5X4	T38.5X5	T38.5X6
Oestrogen	T38.5X1	T38.5X2	T38.5X3	T38.5X4	T38.5X5	T38.5X6
Oestrone	T38.5X1	T38.5X2	T38.5X3	T38.5X4	T38.5X5	T38.5X6
Ofloxacin	T36.8X1	T36.8X2	T36.8X3	T36.8X4	T36.8X5	T36.8X6
Oil (of)	T65.891	T65.892	T65.893	T65.894	—	—
bitter almond	T62.8X1	T62.8X2	T62.8X3	T62.8X4	—	—
cloves	T49.7X1	T49.7X2	T49.7X3	T49.7X4	T49.7X5	T49.7X6
colors	T65.6X1	T65.6X2	T65.6X3	T65.6X4	—	—
fumes	T59.891	T59.892	T59.893	T59.894	—	—
lubricating	T52.0X1	T52.0X2	T52.0X3	T52.0X4	—	—
Niobe	T52.8X1	T52.8X2	T52.8X3	T52.8X4	—	—
vitriol (liquid)	T54.2X1	T54.2X2	T54.2X3	T54.2X4	—	—
fumes	T54.2X1	T54.2X2	T54.2X3	T54.2X4	—	—
wintergreen (bitter) NEC	T49.3X1	T49.3X2	T49.3X3	T49.3X4	T49.3X5	T49.3X6
Oily preparation (for skin)	T49.3X1	T49.3X2	T49.3X3	T49.3X4	T49.3X5	T49.3X6
Ointment NEC	T49.3X1	T49.3X2	T49.3X3	T49.3X4	T49.3X5	T49.3X6
Olanzapine	T43.591	T43.592	T43.593	T43.594	T43.595	T43.596
Oleander	T62.2X1	T62.2X2	T62.2X3	T62.2X4	—	—
Oleandomycin	T36.3X1	T36.3X2	T36.3X3	T36.3X4	T36.3X5	T36.3X6
Oleandrin	T46.0X1	T46.0X2	T46.0X3	T46.0X4	T46.0X5	T46.0X6
Oleic acid	T46.6X1	T46.6X2	T46.6X3	T46.6X4	T46.6X5	T46.6X6
Oleovitamin A	T45.2X1	T45.2X2	T45.2X3	T45.2X4	T45.2X5	T45.2X6
Oleum ricini	T47.2X1	T47.2X2	T47.2X3	T47.2X4	T47.2X5	T47.2X6
Olive oil (medicinal) NEC	T47.4X1	T47.4X2	T47.4X3	T47.4X4	T47.4X5	T47.4X6
Olivomycin	T45.1X1	T45.1X2	T45.1X3	T45.1X4	T45.1X5	T45.1X6
Olsalazine	T47.8X1	T47.8X2	T47.8X3	T47.8X4	T47.8X5	T47.8X6
Omeprazole	T47.1X1	T47.1X2	T47.1X3	T47.1X4	T47.1X5	T47.1X6
OMPA	T60.0X1	T60.0X2	T60.0X3	T60.0X4	—	—
Oncovin	T45.1X1	T45.1X2	T45.1X3	T45.1X4	T45.1X5	T45.1X6
Ondansetron	T45.0X1	T45.0X2	T45.0X3	T45.0X4	T45.0X5	T45.0X6
Ophthaine	T41.3X1	T41.3X2	T41.3X3	T41.3X4	T41.3X5	T41.3X6
Ophthetic	T41.3X1	T41.3X2	T41.3X3	T41.3X4	T41.3X5	T41.3X6
Opiate NEC	T40.601	T40.602	T40.603	T40.604	T40.605	T40.606
antagonists	T50.7X1	T50.7X2	T50.7X3	T50.7X4	T50.7X5	T50.7X6
Opioid NEC	T40.2X1	T40.2X2	T40.2X3	T40.2X4	T40.2X5	T40.2X6
Opipramol	T43.011	T43.012	T43.013	T43.014	T43.015	T43.016
Opium alkaloids (total)	T40.0X1	T40.0X2	T40.0X3	T40.0X4	T40.0X5	T40.0X6
standardized powdered	T40.0X1	T40.0X2	T40.0X3	T40.0X4	T40.0X5	T40.0X6
tincture (camphorated)	T40.0X1	T40.0X2	T40.0X3	T40.0X4	T40.0X5	T40.0X6
Oracon	T38.4X1	T38.4X2	T38.4X3	T38.4X4	T38.4X5	T38.4X6
Oragrafin	T50.8X1	T50.8X2	T50.8X3	T50.8X4	T50.8X5	T50.8X6
Oral contraceptives	T38.4X1	T38.4X2	T38.4X3	T38.4X4	T38.4X5	T38.4X6
Oral rehydration salts	T50.3X1	T50.3X2	T50.3X3	T50.3X4	T50.3X5	T50.3X6
Orazamide	T50.991	T50.992	T50.993	T50.994	T50.995	T50.996
Orciprenaline	T48.291	T48.292	T48.293	T48.294	T48.295	T48.296
Organidin	T48.4X1	T48.4X2	T48.4X3	T48.4X4	T48.4X5	T48.4X6
Organonitrate NEC	T46.3X1	T46.3X2	T46.3X3	T46.3X4	T46.3X5	T46.3X6
Organophosphates	T60.0X1	T60.0X2	T60.0X3	T60.0X4	—	—
Orimune	T50.B91	T50.B92	T50.B93	T50.B94	T50.B95	T50.B96
Orinase	T38.3X1	T38.3X2	T38.3X3	T38.3X4	T38.3X5	T38.3X6
Ormeloxifene	T38.6X1	T38.6X2	T38.6X3	T38.6X4	T38.6X5	T38.6X6
Ornidazole	T37.3X1	T37.3X2	T37.3X3	T37.3X4	T37.3X5	T37.3X6
Ornithine aspartate	T50.991	T50.992	T50.993	T50.994	T50.995	T50.996
Ornoprostil	T47.1X1	T47.1X2	T47.1X3	T47.1X4	T47.1X5	T47.1X6
Orphenadrine	T42.8X1	T42.8X2	T42.8X3	T42.8X4	T42.8X5	T42.8X6
(hydrochloride)						
Ortal (sodium)	T42.3X1	T42.3X2	T42.3X3	T42.3X4	T42.3X5	T42.3X6
Orthoboric acid	T49.0X1	T49.0X2	T49.0X3	T49.0X4	T49.0X5	T49.0X6
ENT agent	T49.6X1	T49.6X2	T49.6X3	T49.6X4	T49.6X5	T49.6X6
ophthalmic preparation	T49.5X1	T49.5X2	T49.5X3	T49.5X4	T49.5X5	T49.5X6
Orthocaine	T41.3X1	T41.3X2	T41.3X3	T41.3X4	T41.3X5	T41.3X6
Orthodichlorobenzene	T53.7X1	T53.7X2	T53.7X3	T53.7X4	—	—
Ortho-Novum	T38.4X1	T38.4X2	T38.4X3	T38.4X4	T38.4X5	T38.4X6
Orthotolidine (reagent)	T54.2X1	T54.2X2	T54.2X3	T54.2X4	—	—
Osmic acid (liquid)	T54.2X1	T54.2X2	T54.2X3	T54.2X4	—	—
fumes	T54.2X1	T54.2X2	T54.2X3	T54.2X4	—	—
Osmotic diuretics	T50.2X1	T50.2X2	T50.2X3	T50.2X4	T50.2X5	T50.2X6
Otilonium bromide	T44.3X1	T44.3X2	T44.3X3	T44.3X4	T44.3X5	T44.3X6
Otorhinolaryngological drug NEC	T49.6X1	T49.6X2	T49.6X3	T49.6X4	T49.6X5	T49.6X6
Ouabain (e)	T46.0X1	T46.0X2	T46.0X3	T46.0X4	T46.0X5	T46.0X6
Ovarian						
hormone	T38.5X1	T38.5X2	T38.5X3	T38.5X4	T38.5X5	T38.5X6
stimulant	T38.5X1	T38.5X2	T38.5X3	T38.5X4	T38.5X5	T38.5X6
Ovral	T38.4X1	T38.4X2	T38.4X3	T38.4X4	T38.4X5	T38.4X6
Ovulen	T38.4X1	T38.4X2	T38.4X3	T38.4X4	T38.4X5	T38.4X6
Oxacillin	T36.0X1	T36.0X2	T36.0X3	T36.0X4	T36.0X5	T36.0X6
Oxalic acid	T54.2X1	T54.2X2	T54.2X3	T54.2X4	—	—
ammonium salt	T50.991	T50.992	T50.993	T50.994	T50.995	T50.996
Oxamniquine	T37.4X1	T37.4X2	T37.4X3	T37.4X4	T37.4X5	T37.4X6
Oxanamide	T43.591	T43.592	T43.593	T43.594	T43.595	T43.596
Oxandrolone	T38.7X1	T38.7X2	T38.7X3	T38.7X4	T38.7X5	T38.7X6
Oxantel	T37.4X1	T37.4X2	T37.4X3	T37.4X4	T37.4X5	T37.4X6
Oxapium iodide	T44.3X1	T44.3X2	T44.3X3	T44.3X4	T44.3X5	T44.3X6
Oxaprotiline	T43.021	T43.022	T43.023	T43.024	T43.025	T43.026
Oxaprozin	T39.311	T39.312	T39.313	T39.314	T39.315	T39.316
Oxatomide	T45.0X1	T45.0X2	T45.0X3	T45.0X4	T45.0X5	T45.0X6
Oxazepam	T42.4X1	T42.4X2	T42.4X3	T42.4X4	T42.4X5	T42.4X6
Oxazimedrine	T50.5X1	T50.5X2	T50.5X3	T50.5X4	T50.5X5	T50.5X6
Oxazolam	T42.4X1	T42.4X2	T42.4X3	T42.4X4	T42.4X5	T42.4X6
Oxazolidine derivatives	T42.2X1	T42.2X2	T42.2X3	T42.2X4	T42.2X5	T42.2X6
Oxazolidinedione	T42.2X1	T42.2X2	T42.2X3	T42.2X4	T42.2X5	T42.2X6
(derivative)						
Ox bile extract	T47.5X1	T47.5X2	T47.5X3	T47.5X4	T47.5X5	T47.5X6
Oxcarbazepine	T42.1X1	T42.1X2	T42.1X3	T42.1X4	T42.1X5	T42.1X6
Oxedrine	T44.4X1	T44.4X2	T44.4X3	T44.4X4	T44.4X5	T44.4X6
Oxeladin (citrate)	T48.3X1	T48.3X2	T48.3X3	T48.3X4	T48.3X5	T48.3X6

Substance	Poisoning, Accidental (unintentional)	Poisoning, Intentional Self-harm	Poisoning, Assault	Poisoning, Undetermined	Adverse Effect	Under-dosing
Oxendolone	T38.5X1	T38.5X2	T38.5X3	T38.5X4	T38.5X5	T38.5X6
Oxetacaine	T41.3X1	T41.3X2	T41.3X3	T41.3X4	T41.3X5	T41.3X6
Oxethazine	T41.3X1	T41.3X2	T41.3X3	T41.3X4	T41.3X5	T41.3X6
Oxetorone	T39.8X1	T39.8X2	T39.8X3	T39.8X4	T39.8X5	T39.8X6
Oxiconazole	T49.0X1	T49.0X2	T49.0X3	T49.0X4	T49.0X5	T49.0X6
Oxidizing agent NEC	T54.91	T54.92	T54.93	T54.94	—	—
Oxipurinol	T50.4X1	T50.4X2	T50.4X3	T50.4X4	T50.4X5	T50.4X6
Oxitriptan	T43.291	T43.292	T43.293	T43.294	T43.295	T43.296
Oxitropium bromide	T48.6X1	T48.6X2	T48.6X3	T48.6X4	T48.6X5	T48.6X6
Oxodipine	T46.1X1	T46.1X2	T46.1X3	T46.1X4	T46.1X5	T46.1X6
Oxolamine	T48.3X1	T48.3X2	T48.3X3	T48.3X4	T48.3X5	T48.3X6
Oxolinic acid	T37.8X1	T37.8X2	T37.8X3	T37.8X4	T37.8X5	T37.8X6
Oxomemazine	T43.3X1	T43.3X2	T43.3X3	T43.3X4	T43.3X5	T43.3X6
Oxophenarsine	T37.3X1	T37.3X2	T37.3X3	T37.3X4	T37.3X5	T37.3X6
Oxprenolol	T44.7X1	T44.7X2	T44.7X3	T44.7X4	T44.7X5	T44.7X6
Oxsoralen	T49.3X1	T49.3X2	T49.3X3	T49.3X4	T49.3X5	T49.3X6
Oxtriphylline	T48.6X1	T48.6X2	T48.6X3	T48.6X4	T48.6X5	T48.6X6
Oxybate sodium	T41.291	T41.292	T41.293	T41.294	T41.295	T41.296
Oxybuprocaine	T41.3X1	T41.3X2	T41.3X3	T41.3X4	T41.3X5	T41.3X6
Oxybutynin	T44.3X1	T44.3X2	T44.3X3	T44.3X4	T44.3X5	T44.3X6
Oxychlorosene	T49.0X1	T49.0X2	T49.0X3	T49.0X4	T49.0X5	T49.0X6
Oxycodone	T40.2X1	T40.2X2	T40.2X3	T40.2X4	T40.2X5	T40.2X6
Oxyfedrine	T46.3X1	T46.3X2	T46.3X3	T46.3X4	T46.3X5	T46.3X6
Oxygen	T41.5X1	T41.5X2	T41.5X3	T41.5X4	T41.5X5	T41.5X6
Oxylone	T49.0X1	T49.0X2	T49.0X3	T49.0X4	T49.0X5	T49.0X6
ophthalmic preparation	T49.5X1	T49.5X2	T49.5X3	T49.5X4	T49.5X5	T49.5X6
Oxymesterone	T38.7X1	T38.7X2	T38.7X3	T38.7X4	T38.7X5	T38.7X6
Oxymetazoline	T48.5X1	T48.5X2	T48.5X3	T48.5X4	T48.5X5	T48.5X6
Oxymetholone	T38.7X1	T38.7X2	T38.7X3	T38.7X4	T38.7X5	T38.7X6
Oxymorphone	T40.2X1	T40.2X2	T40.2X3	T40.2X4	T40.2X5	T40.2X6
Oxypertine	T43.591	T43.592	T43.593	T43.594	T43.595	T43.596
Oxyphenbutazone	T39.2X1	T39.2X2	T39.2X3	T39.2X4	T39.2X5	T39.2X6
Oxyphencyclimine	T44.3X1	T44.3X2	T44.3X3	T44.3X4	T44.3X5	T44.3X6
Oxyphenisatine	T47.2X1	T47.2X2	T47.2X3	T47.2X4	T47.2X5	T47.2X6
Oxyphenonium bromide	T44.3X1	T44.3X2	T44.3X3	T44.3X4	T44.3X5	T44.3X6
Oxypolygelatin	T45.8X1	T45.8X2	T45.8X3	T45.8X4	T45.8X5	T45.8X6
Oxyquinoline (derivatives)	T37.8X1	T37.8X2	T37.8X3	T37.8X4	T37.8X5	T37.8X6
Oxytetracycline	T36.4X1	T36.4X2	T36.4X3	T36.4X4	T36.4X5	T36.4X6
Oxytocic drug NEC	T48.0X1	T48.0X2	T48.0X3	T48.0X4	T48.0X5	T48.0X6
Oxytocin (synthetic)	T48.0X1	T48.0X2	T48.0X3	T48.0X4	T48.0X5	T48.0X6
Ozone	T59.891	T59.892	T59.893	T59.894		
PABA	T49.3X1	T49.3X2	T49.3X3	T49.3X4	T49.3X5	T49.3X6
Packed red cells	T45.8X1	T45.8X2	T45.8X3	T45.8X4	T45.8X5	T45.8X6
Padimate	T49.3X1	T49.3X2	T49.3X3	T49.3X4	T49.3X5	T49.3X6
Paint NEC	T65.6X1	T65.6X2	T65.6X3	T65.6X4	—	—
cleaner	T52.91	T52.92	T52.93	T52.94	—	—
fumes NEC	T59.891	T59.892	T59.893	T59.894	—	—
lead (fumes)	T56.0X1	T56.0X2	T56.0X3	T56.0X4	—	—
solvent NEC	T52.8X1	T52.8X2	T52.8X3	T52.8X4	—	—
stripper	T52.8X1	T52.8X2	T52.8X3	T52.8X4	—	—
Palfium	T40.2X1	T40.2X2	T40.2X3	T40.2X4	—	—
Palm kernel oil	T50.991	T50.992	T50.993	T50.994	T50.995	T50.996
Paludrine	T37.2X1	T37.2X2	T37.2X3	T37.2X4	T37.2X5	T37.2X6
PAM (pralidoxime)	T50.6X1	T50.6X2	T50.6X3	T50.6X4	T50.6X5	T50.6X6
Pamaquine (naphthoute)	T37.2X1	T37.2X2	T37.2X3	T37.2X4	T37.2X5	T37.2X6
Panadol	T39.1X1	T39.1X2	T39.1X3	T39.1X4	T39.1X5	T39.1X6
Pancreatic						
digestive secretion stimulant	T47.8X1	T47.8X2	T47.8X3	T47.8X4	T47.8X5	T47.8X6
dornase	T45.3X1	T45.3X2	T45.3X3	T45.3X4	T45.3X5	T45.3X6
Pancreatin	T47.5X1	T47.5X2	T47.5X3	T47.5X4	T47.5X5	T47.5X6
Pancrelipase	T47.5X1	T47.5X2	T47.5X3	T47.5X4	T47.5X5	T47.5X6
Pancuronium (bromide)	T48.1X1	T48.1X2	T48.1X3	T48.1X4	T48.1X5	T48.1X6
Pangamic acid	T45.2X1	T45.2X2	T45.2X3	T45.2X4	T45.2X5	T45.2X6
Panthenol	T45.2X1	T45.2X2	T45.2X3	T45.2X4	T45.2X5	T45.2X6
topical	T49.8X1	T49.8X2	T49.8X3	T49.8X4	T49.8X5	T49.8X6
Pantopon	T40.0X1	T40.0X2	T40.0X3	T40.0X4	T40.0X5	T40.0X6
Pantothenic acid	T45.2X1	T45.2X2	T45.2X3	T45.2X4	T45.2X5	T45.2X6
Panwarfin	T45.511	T45.512	T45.513	T45.514	T45.515	T45.516
Papain	T47.5X1	T47.5X2	T47.5X3	T47.5X4	T47.5X5	T47.5X6
digestant	T47.5X1	T47.5X2	T47.5X3	T47.5X4	T47.5X5	T47.5X6
Papaveretum	T40.0X1	T40.0X2	T40.0X3	T40.0X4	T40.0X5	T40.0X6
Papaverine	T44.3X1	T44.3X2	T44.3X3	T44.3X4	T44.3X5	T44.3X6
Para-acetamidophenol	T39.1X1	T39.1X2	T39.1X3	T39.1X4	T39.1X5	T39.1X6
Para-aminobenzoic acid	T49.3X1	T49.3X2	T49.3X3	T49.3X4	T49.3X5	T49.3X6
Para-aminophenol derivatives	T39.1X1	T39.1X2	T39.1X3	T39.1X4	T39.1X5	T39.1X6
Para-aminosalicylic acid	T37.1X1	T37.1X2	T37.1X3	T37.1X4	T37.1X5	T37.1X6
Paracetaldehyde	T42.6X1	T42.6X2	T42.6X3	T42.6X4	T42.6X5	T42.6X6
Paracetamol	T39.1X1	T39.1X2	T39.1X3	T39.1X4	T39.1X5	T39.1X6
Parachlorophenol (camphorated)	T49.0X1	T49.0X2	T49.0X3	T49.0X4	T49.0X5	T49.0X6
Paracodin	T40.2X1	T40.2X2	T40.2X3	T40.2X4	T40.2X5	T40.2X6

Substance	Poisoning, Accidental (unintentional)	Poisoning, Intentional Self-harm	Poisoning, Assault	Poisoning, Undetermined	Adverse Effect	Under-dosing
Paradione	T42.2X1	T42.2X2	T42.2X3	T42.2X4	T42.2X5	T42.2X6
Paraffin(s) (wax)	T52.0X1	T52.0X2	T52.0X3	T52.0X4	—	—
liquid (medicinal)	T47.4X1	T47.4X2	T47.4X3	T47.4X4	T47.4X5	T47.4X6
nonmedicinal	T52.0X1	T52.0X2	T52.0X3	T52.0X4	—	—
Paraformaldehyde	T60.3X1	T60.3X2	T60.3X3	T60.3X4	—	—
Paraldehyde	T42.6X1	T42.6X2	T42.6X3	T42.6X4	T42.6X5	T42.6X6
Paramethadione	T42.2X1	T42.2X2	T42.2X3	T42.2X4	T42.2X5	T42.2X6
Paramethasone	T38.0X1	T38.0X2	T38.0X3	T38.0X4	T38.0X5	T38.0X6
acetate	T49.0X1	T49.0X2	T49.0X3	T49.0X4	T49.0X5	T49.0X6
Paraoxon	T60.0X1	T60.0X2	T60.0X3	T60.0X4	—	—
Paraquat	T60.3X1	T60.3X2	T60.3X3	T60.3X4	—	—
Parasympatholytic NEC	T44.3X1	T44.3X2	T44.3X3	T44.3X4	T44.3X5	T44.3X6
Parasympathomimetic drug NEC	T44.1X1	T44.1X2	T44.1X3	T44.1X4	T44.1X5	T44.1X6
Parathion	T60.0X1	T60.0X2	T60.0X3	T60.0X4	—	—
Parathormone	T50.991	T50.992	T50.993	T50.994	T50.995	T50.996
Parathyroid extract	T50.991	T50.992	T50.993	T50.994	T50.995	T50.996
Paratyphoid vaccine	T50.A91	T50.A92	T50.A93	T50.A94	T50.A95	T50.A96
Paredrine	T44.4X1	T44.4X2	T44.4X3	T44.4X4	T44.4X5	T44.4X6
Paregoric	T40.0X1	T40.0X2	T40.0X3	T40.0X4	T40.0X5	T40.0X6
Pargyline	T46.5X1	T46.5X2	T46.5X3	T46.5X4	T46.5X5	T46.5X6
Paris green	T57.0X1	T57.0X2	T57.0X3	T57.0X4	—	—
insecticide	T57.0X1	T57.0X2	T57.0X3	T57.0X4	—	—
Parnate	T43.1X1	T43.1X2	T43.1X3	T43.1X4	T43.1X5	T43.1X6
Paromomycin	T36.5X1	T36.5X2	T36.5X3	T36.5X4	T36.5X5	T36.5X6
Paroxypropione	T45.1X1	T45.1X2	T45.1X3	T45.1X4	T45.1X5	T45.1X6
Parzone	T40.2X1	T40.2X2	T40.2X3	T40.2X4	T40.2X5	T40.2X6
PAS	T37.1X1	T37.1X2	T37.1X3	T37.1X4	T37.1X5	T37.1X6
Pasiniazid	T37.1X1	T37.1X2	T37.1X3	T37.1X4	T37.1X5	T37.1X6
PBB (polybrominated biphenyls)	T65.891	T65.892	T65.893	T65.894	—	—
PCB	T65.891	T65.892	T65.893	T65.894	—	—
PCP						
meaning pentachlorophenol	T60.1X1	T60.1X2	T60.1X3	T60.1X4	—	—
fungicide	T60.3X1	T60.3X2	T60.3X3	T60.3X4	—	—
herbicide	T60.3X1	T60.3X2	T60.3X3	T60.3X4	—	—
insecticide	T60.1X1	T60.1X2	T60.1X3	T60.1X4	—	—
meaning phencyclidine	T40.991	T40.992	T40.993	T40.994	—	—
Peach kernel oil (emulsion)	T47.4X1	T47.4X2	T47.4X3	T47.4X4	T47.4X5	T47.4X6
Peanut oil (emulsion) NEC	T47.4X1	T47.4X2	T47.4X3	T47.4X4	T47.4X5	T47.4X6
topical	T49.3X1	T49.3X2	T49.3X3	T49.3X4	T49.3X5	T49.3X6
Pearly Gates (morning glory seeds)	T40.991	T40.992	T40.993	T40.994	—	—
Pecazine	T43.3X1	T43.3X2	T43.3X3	T43.3X4	T43.3X5	T43.3X6
Pectin	T47.6X1	T47.6X2	T47.6X3	T47.6X4	T47.6X5	T47.6X6
Pefloxacin	T37.8X1	T37.8X2	T37.8X3	T37.8X4	T37.8X5	T37.8X6
Pegademase, bovine	T50.Z91	T50.Z92	T50.Z93	T50.Z94	T50.Z95	T50.Z96
Pelletierine tannate	T37.4X1	T37.4X2	T37.4X3	T37.4X4	T37.4X5	T37.4X6
Pemirolast (potassium)	T48.6X1	T48.6X2	T48.6X3	T48.6X4	T48.6X5	T48.6X6
Pemoline	T50.7X1	T50.7X2	T50.7X3	T50.7X4	T50.7X5	T50.7X6
Pempidine	T44.2X1	T44.2X2	T44.2X3	T44.2X4	T44.2X5	T44.2X6
Penamecillin	T36.0X1	T36.0X2	T36.0X3	T36.0X4	T36.0X5	T36.0X6
Penbutolol	T44.7X1	T44.7X2	T44.7X3	T44.7X4	T44.7X5	T44.7X6
Penethamate	T36.0X1	T36.0X2	T36.0X3	T36.0X4	T36.0X5	T36.0X6
Penfluridol	T43.591	T43.592	T43.593	T43.594	T43.595	T43.596
Penflutizide	T50.2X1	T50.2X2	T50.2X3	T50.2X4	T50.2X5	T50.2X6
Pengitoxin	T46.0X1	T46.0X2	T46.0X3	T46.0X4	T46.0X5	T46.0X6
Penicillamine	T50.6X1	T50.6X2	T50.6X3	T50.6X4	T50.6X5	T50.6X6
Penicillin (any)	T36.0X1	T36.0X2	T36.0X3	T36.0X4	T36.0X5	T36.0X6
Penicillinase	T45.3X1	T45.3X2	T45.3X3	T45.3X4	T45.3X5	T45.3X6
Penicilloyl polylysine	T50.8X1	T50.8X2	T50.8X3	T50.8X4	T50.8X5	T50.8X6
Penimepicycline	T36.4X1	T36.4X2	T36.4X3	T36.4X4	T36.4X5	T36.4X6
Pentachloroethane	T53.6X1	T53.6X2	T53.6X3	T53.6X4	—	—
Pentachloronaphthalene	T53.7X1	T53.7X2	T53.7X3	T53.7X4	—	—
Pentachlorophenol (pesticide)	T60.1X1	T60.1X2	T60.1X3	T60.1X4	—	—
fungicide	T60.3X1	T60.3X2	T60.3X3	T60.3X4	—	—
herbicide	T60.3X1	T60.3X2	T60.3X3	T60.3X4	—	—
insecticide	T60.1X1	T60.1X2	T60.1X3	T60.1X4	—	—
Pentaerythritol	T46.3X1	T46.3X2	T46.3X3	T46.3X4	T46.3X5	T46.3X6
chloral	T42.6X1	T42.6X2	T42.6X3	T42.6X4	T42.6X5	T42.6X6
tetranitrate NEC	T46.3X1	T46.3X2	T46.3X3	T46.3X4	T46.3X5	T46.3X6
Pentaerythrityl tetranitrate	T46.3X1	T46.3X2	T46.3X3	T46.3X4	T46.3X5	T46.3X6
Pentagastrin	T50.8X1	T50.8X2	T50.8X3	T50.8X4	T50.8X5	T50.8X6
Pentalin	T53.6X1	T53.6X2	T53.6X3	T53.6X4	—	—
Pentamethonium bromide	T44.2X1	T44.2X2	T44.2X3	T44.2X4	T44.2X5	T44.2X6
Pentamidine	T37.3X1	T37.3X2	T37.3X3	T37.3X4	T37.3X5	T37.3X6
Pentanol	T51.3X1	T51.3X2	T51.3X3	T51.3X4	—	—
Pentapyrrolinium (bitartrate)	T44.2X1	T44.2X2	T44.2X3	T44.2X4	T44.2X5	T44.2X6
Pentaquine	T37.2X1	T37.2X2	T37.2X3	T37.2X4	T37.2X5	T37.2X6

Substance	Poisoning, Accidental (unintentional)	Poisoning, Intentional Self-harm	Poisoning, Assault	Poisoning, Undetermined	Adverse Effect	Under-dosing
Pentazocine	T40.4X1	T40.4X2	T40.4X3	T40.4X4	T40.4X5	T40.4X6
Pentetrazole	T50.7X1	T50.7X2	T50.7X3	T50.7X4	T50.7X5	T50.7X6
Penthienate bromide	T44.3X1	T44.3X2	T44.3X3	T44.3X4	T44.3X5	T44.3X6
Pentifylline	T46.7X1	T46.7X2	T46.7X3	T46.7X4	T46.7X5	T46.7X6
Pentobarbital	T42.3X1	T42.3X2	T42.3X3	T42.3X4	T42.3X5	T42.3X6
sodium	T42.3X1	T42.3X2	T42.3X3	T42.3X4	T42.3X5	T42.3X6
Pentobarbitone	T42.3X1	T42.3X2	T42.3X3	T42.3X4	T42.3X5	T42.3X6
Pentolonium tartrate	T44.2X1	T44.2X2	T44.2X3	T44.2X4	T44.2X5	T44.2X6
Pentosan polysulfate	T39.8X1	T39.8X2	T39.8X3	T39.8X4	T39.8X5	T39.8X6
(sodium)						
Pentostatin	T45.1X1	T45.1X2	T45.1X3	T45.1X4	T45.1X5	T45.1X6
Pentothal	T41.1X1	T41.1X2	T41.1X3	T41.1X4	T41.1X5	T41.1X6
Pentoxifylline	T46.7X1	T46.7X2	T46.7X3	T46.7X4	T46.7X5	T46.7X6
Pentoxyverine	T48.3X1	T48.3X2	T48.3X3	T48.3X4	T48.3X5	T48.3X6
Pentrinat	T46.3X1	T46.3X2	T46.3X3	T46.3X4	T46.3X5	T46.3X6
Pentylenetetrazole	T50.7X1	T50.7X2	T50.7X3	T50.7X4	T50.7X5	T50.7X6
Pentylsalicylamide	T37.1X1	T37.1X2	T37.1X3	T37.1X4	T37.1X5	T37.1X6
Pentymal	T42.3X1	T42.3X2	T42.3X3	T42.3X4	T42.3X5	T42.3X6
Peplomycin	T45.1X1	T45.1X2	T45.1X3	T45.1X4	T45.1X5	T45.1X6
Peppermint (oil)	T47.5X1	T47.5X2	T47.5X3	T47.5X4	T47.5X5	T47.5X6
Pepsin	T47.5X1	T47.5X2	T47.5X3	T47.5X4	T47.5X5	T47.5X6
digestant	T47.5X1	T47.5X2	T47.5X3	T47.5X4	T47.5X5	T47.5X6
Pepstatin	T47.1X1	T47.1X2	T47.1X3	T47.1X4	T47.1X5	T47.1X6
Peptavlon	T50.8X1	T50.8X2	T50.8X3	T50.8X4	T50.8X5	T50.8X6
Perazine	T43.3X1	T43.3X2	T43.3X3	T43.3X4	T43.3X5	T43.3X6
Percaine (spinal)	T41.3X1	T41.3X2	T41.3X3	T41.3X4	T41.3X5	T41.3X6
topical (surface)	T41.3X1	T41.3X2	T41.3X3	T41.3X4	T41.3X5	T41.3X6
Perchloroethylene	T53.3X1	T53.3X2	T53.3X3	T53.3X4	—	—
medicinal	T37.4X1	T37.4X2	T37.4X3	T37.4X4	T37.4X5	T37.4X6
vapor	T53.3X1	T53.3X2	T53.3X3	T53.3X4		
Percodan	T40.2X1	T40.2X2	T40.2X3	T40.2X4	T40.2X5	T40.2X6
Percogesic — see also	T45.0X1	T45.0X2	T45.0X3	T45.0X4	T45.0X5	T45.0X6
acetaminophen						
Percorten	T38.0X1	T38.0X2	T38.0X3	T38.0X4	T38.0X5	T38.0X6
Pergolide	T42.8X1	T42.8X2	T42.8X3	T42.8X4	T42.8X5	T42.8X6
Pergonal	T38.811	T38.812	T38.813	T38.814	T38.815	T38.816
Perhexilene	T46.3X1	T46.3X2	T46.3X3	T46.3X4	T46.3X5	T46.3X6
Perhexiline (maleate)	T46.3X1	T46.3X2	T46.3X3	T46.3X4	T46.3X5	T46.3X6
Periactin	T45.0X1	T45.0X2	T45.0X3	T45.0X4	T45.0X5	T45.0X6
Periciazine	T43.3X1	T43.3X2	T43.3X3	T43.3X4	T43.3X5	T43.3X6
Periclor	T42.6X1	T42.6X2	T42.6X3	T42.6X4	T42.6X5	T42.6X6
Perindopril	T46.4X1	T46.4X2	T46.4X3	T46.4X4	T46.4X5	T46.4X6
Perisoxal	T39.8X1	T39.8X2	T39.8X3	T39.8X4	T39.8X5	T39.8X6
Peritoneal dialysis solution	T50.3X1	T50.3X2	T50.3X3	T50.3X4	T50.3X5	T50.3X6
Peritrate	T46.3X1	T46.3X2	T46.3X3	T46.3X4	T46.3X5	T46.3X6
Perlapine	T42.4X1	T42.4X2	T42.4X3	T42.4X4	T42.4X5	T42.4X6
Permanganate	T65.891	T65.892	T65.893	T65.894	—	—
Permethrin	T60.1X1	T60.1X2	T60.1X3	T60.1X4	—	—
Pernocton	T42.3X1	T42.3X2	T42.3X3	T42.3X4	T42.3X5	T42.3X6
Pernoston	T42.3X1	T42.3X2	T42.3X3	T42.3X4	T42.3X5	T42.3X6
Peronine	T40.2X1	T40.2X2	T40.2X3	T40.2X4	—	—
Perphenazine	T43.3X1	T43.3X2	T43.3X3	T43.3X4	T43.3X5	T43.3X6
Pertofrane	T43.011	T43.012	T43.013	T43.014	T43.015	T43.016
Pertussis						
immune serum (human)	T50.Z11	T50.Z12	T50.Z13	T50.Z14	T50.Z15	T50.Z16
vaccine (with diphtheria toxoid)	T50.A11	T50.A12	T50.A13	T50.A14	T50.A15	T50.A16
(with tetanus toxoid)						
Peruvian balsam	T49.0X1	T49.0X2	T49.0X3	T49.0X4	T49.0X5	T49.0X6
Peruvoside	T46.0X1	T46.0X2	T46.0X3	T46.0X4	T46.0X5	T46.0X6
Pesticide (dust) (fumes) (vapor)	T60.91	T60.92	T60.93	T60.94	—	—
NEC						
arsenic	T57.0X1	T57.0X2	T57.0X3	T57.0X4	—	—
chlorinated	T60.1X1	T60.1X2	T60.1X3	T60.1X4	—	—
cyanide	T65.0X1	T65.0X2	T65.0X3	T65.0X4	—	—
kerosene	T52.0X1	T52.0X2	T52.0X3	T52.0X4	—	—
mixture (of compounds)	T60.91	T60.92	T60.93	T60.94	—	—
naphthalene	T60.2X1	T60.2X2	T60.2X3	T60.2X4	—	—
organochlorine	T60.1X1	T60.1X2	T60.1X3	T60.1X4	—	—
(compounds)						
petroleum (distillate) (products) NEC	T60.8X1	T60.8X2		T60.8X4	—	—
specified ingredient NEC	T60.8X1	T60.8X2	T60.8X3	T60.8X4	—	—
strychnine	T65.1X1	T65.1X2	T65.1X3	T65.1X4	—	—
thallium	T60.4X1	T60.4X2	T60.4X3	T60.4X4	—	—
Pethidine	T40.4X1	T40.4X2	T40.4X3	T40.4X4	T40.4X5	T40.4X6
Petrichloral	T42.6X1	T42.6X2	T42.6X3	T42.6X4	T42.6X5	T42.6X6
Petrol	T52.0X1	T52.0X2	T52.0X3	T52.0X4	—	—
vapor	T52.0X1	T52.0X2	T52.0X3	T52.0X4	—	—
Petrolatum	T49.3X1	T49.3X2	T49.3X3	T49.3X4	T49.3X5	T49.3X6
hydrophilic	T49.3X1	T49.3X2	T49.3X3	T49.3X4	T49.3X5	T49.3X6
liquid	T47.4X1	T47.4X2	T47.4X3	T47.4X4	T47.4X5	T47.4X6
topical	T49.3X1	T49.3X2	T49.3X3	T49.3X4	T49.3X5	T49.3X6
nonmedicinal	T52.0X1	T52.0X2	T52.0X3	T52.0X4	—	—

Substance	Poisoning, Accidental (unintentional)	Poisoning, Intentional Self-harm	Poisoning, Assault	Poisoning, Undetermined	Adverse Effect	Under-dosing
Petrolatum — continued						
red veterinary	T49.3X1	T49.3X2	T49.3X3	T49.3X4	T49.3X5	T49.3X6
white	T49.3X1	T49.3X2	T49.3X3	T49.3X4	T49.3X5	T49.3X6
Petroleum (products) NEC	T52.0X1	T52.0X2	T52.0X3	T52.0X4	—	—
benzine(s) — see Ligroin						
ether — see Ligroin						
jelly — see Petrolatum						
naphtha — see Ligroin						
pesticide	T60.8X1	T60.8X2	T60.8X3	T60.8X4	—	—
solids	T52.0X1	T52.0X2	T52.0X3	T52.0X4	—	—
solvents	T52.0X1	T52.0X2	T52.0X3	T52.0X4	—	—
vapor	T52.0X1	T52.0X2	T52.0X3	T52.0X4	—	—
Peyote	T40.991	T40.992	T40.993	T40.994	—	—
Phanodorm, phanodorn	T42.3X1	T42.3X2	T42.3X3	T42.3X4	T42.3X5	T42.3X6
Phanquinone	T37.3X1	T37.3X2	T37.3X3	T37.3X4	T37.3X5	T37.3X6
Phanquone	T37.3X1	T37.3X2	T37.3X3	T37.3X4	T37.3X5	T37.3X6
Pharmaceutical						
adjunct NEC	T50.901	T50.902	T50.903	T50.904	T50.905	T50.906
excipient NEC	T50.901	T50.902	T50.903	T50.904	T50.905	T50.906
sweetener	T50.901	T50.902	T50.903	T50.904	T50.905	T50.906
viscous agent	T50.901	T50.902	T50.903	T50.904	T50.905	T50.906
Phemitone	T42.3X1	T42.3X2	T42.3X3	T42.3X4	T42.3X5	T42.3X6
Phenacaine	T41.3X1	T41.3X2	T41.3X3	T41.3X4	T41.3X5	T41.3X6
Phenacemide	T42.6X1	T42.6X2	T42.6X3	T42.6X4	T42.6X5	T42.6X6
Phenacetin	T39.1X1	T39.1X2	T39.1X3	T39.1X4	T39.1X5	T39.1X6
Phenadoxone	T40.2X1	T40.2X2	T40.2X3	T40.2X4		
Phenaglycodol	T43.591	T43.592	T43.593	T43.594	T43.595	T43.596
Phenantoin	T42.0X1	T42.0X2	T42.0X3	T42.0X4	T42.0X5	T42.0X6
Phenaphthazine reagent	T50.991	T50.992	T50.993	T50.994	T50.995	T50.996
Phenazocine	T40.4X1	T40.4X2	T40.4X3	T40.4X4	T40.4X5	T40.4X6
Phenazone	T39.2X1	T39.2X2	T39.2X3	T39.2X4	T39.2X5	T39.2X6
Phenazopyridine	T39.8X1	T39.8X2	T39.8X3	T39.8X4	T39.8X5	T39.8X6
Phenbenicillin	T36.0X1	T36.0X2	T36.0X3	T36.0X4	T36.0X5	T36.0X6
Phenbutrazate	T50.5X1	T50.5X2	T50.5X3	T50.5X4	T50.5X5	T50.5X6
Phencyclidine	T40.991	T40.992	T40.993	T40.994	T40.995	T40.996
Phendimetrazine	T50.5X1	T50.5X2	T50.5X3	T50.5X4	T50.5X5	T50.5X6
Phenelzine	T43.1X1	T43.1X2	T43.1X3	T43.1X4	T43.1X5	T43.1X6
Phenemal	T42.3X1	T42.3X2	T42.3X3	T42.3X4	T42.3X5	T42.3X6
Phenergan	T42.6X1	T42.6X2	T42.6X3	T42.6X4	T42.6X5	T42.6X6
Pheneticillin	T36.0X1	T36.0X2	T36.0X3	T36.0X4	T36.0X5	T36.0X6
Pheneturide	T42.6X1	T42.6X2	T42.6X3	T42.6X4	T42.6X5	T42.6X6
Phenformin	T38.3X1	T38.3X2	T38.3X3	T38.3X4	T38.3X5	T38.3X6
Phenglutarimide	T44.3X1	T44.3X2	T44.3X3	T44.3X4	T44.3X5	T44.3X6
Phenicarbazide	T39.8X1	T39.8X2	T39.8X3	T39.8X4	T39.8X5	T39.8X6
Phenindamine	T45.0X1	T45.0X2	T45.0X3	T45.0X4	T45.0X5	T45.0X6
Phenindione	T45.511	T45.512	T45.513	T45.514	T45.515	T45.516
Pheniprazine	T43.1X1	T43.1X2	T43.1X3	T43.1X4	T43.1X5	T43.1X6
Pheniramine	T45.0X1	T45.0X2	T45.0X3	T45.0X4	T45.0X5	T45.0X6
Phenisatin	T47.2X1	T47.2X2	T47.2X3	T47.2X4	T47.2X5	T47.2X6
Phenmetrazine	T50.5X1	T50.5X2	T50.5X3	T50.5X4	T50.5X5	T50.5X6
Phenobal	T42.3X1	T42.3X2	T42.3X3	T42.3X4	T42.3X5	T42.3X6
Phenobarbital	T42.3X1	T42.3X2	T42.3X3	T42.3X4	T42.3X5	T42.3X6
with						
mephenytoin	T42.3X1	T42.3X2	T42.3X3	T42.3X4	T42.3X5	T42.3X6
phenytoin	T42.3X1	T42.3X2	T42.3X3	T42.3X4	T42.3X5	T42.3X6
sodium	T42.3X1	T42.3X2	T42.3X3	T42.3X4	T42.3X5	T42.3X6
Phenobarbitone	T42.3X1	T42.3X2	T42.3X3	T42.3X4	T42.3X5	T42.3X6
Phenobutiodil	T50.8X1	T50.8X2	T50.8X3	T50.8X4	T50.8X5	T50.8X6
Phenoctide	T49.0X1	T49.0X2	T49.0X3	T49.0X4	T49.0X5	T49.0X6
Phenol	T49.0X1	T49.0X2	T49.0X3	T49.0X4	T49.0X5	T49.0X6
disinfectant	T54.0X1	T54.0X2	T54.0X3	T54.0X4		
in oil injection	T46.8X1	T46.8X2	T46.8X3	T46.8X4	T46.8X5	T46.8X6
medicinal	T49.1X1	T49.1X2	T49.1X3	T49.1X4	T49.1X5	T49.1X6
nonmedicinal NEC	T54.0X1	T54.0X2	T54.0X3	T54.0X4		
pesticide	T60.8X1	T60.8X2	T60.8X3	T60.8X4		
red	T50.8X1	T50.8X2	T50.8X3	T50.8X4	T50.8X5	T50.8X6
Phenolic preparation	T49.1X1	T49.1X2	T49.1X3	T49.1X4	T49.1X5	T49.1X6
Phenolphthalein	T47.2X1	T47.2X2	T47.2X3	T47.2X4	T47.2X5	T47.2X6
Phenolsulfonphthalein	T50.8X1	T50.8X2	T50.8X3	T50.8X4	T50.8X5	T50.8X6
Phenomorphan	T40.2X1	T40.2X2	T40.2X3	T40.2X4	—	—
Phenonyl	T42.3X1	T42.3X2	T42.3X3	T42.3X4	T42.3X5	T42.3X6
Phenoperidine	T40.4X1	T40.4X2	T40.4X3	T40.4X4	—	—
Phenopyrazone	T46.991	T46.992	T46.993	T46.994	T46.995	T46.996
Phenoquin	T50.4X1	T50.4X2	T50.4X3	T50.4X4	T50.4X5	T50.4X6
Phenothiazine (psychotropic)	T43.3X1	T43.3X2	T43.3X3	T43.3X4	T43.3X5	T43.3X6
NEC						
insecticide	T60.2X1	T60.2X2	T60.2X3	T60.2X4	—	—
Phenothrin	T49.0X1	T49.0X2	T49.0X3	T49.0X4	T49.0X5	T49.0X6
Phenoxybenzamine	T46.7X1	T46.7X2	T46.7X3	T46.7X4	T46.7X5	T46.7X6
Phenoxyethanol	T49.0X1	T49.0X2	T49.0X3	T49.0X4	T49.0X5	T49.0X6
Phenoxymethyl penicillin	T36.0X1	T36.0X2	T36.0X3	T36.0X4	T36.0X5	T36.0X6
Phenprobamate	T42.8X1	T42.8X2	T42.8X3	T42.8X4	T42.8X5	T42.8X6
Phenprocoumon	T45.511	T45.512	T45.513	T45.514	T45.515	T45.516

Table of Drugs and Chemicals

Substance	Poisoning, Accidental (unintentional)	Poisoning, Intentional Self-harm	Poisoning, Assault	Poisoning, Undetermined	Adverse Effect	Under-dosing
Phensuximide	T42.2X1	T42.2X2	T42.2X3	T42.2X4	T42.2X5	T42.2X6
Phentermine	T50.5X1	T50.5X2	T50.5X3	T50.5X4	T50.5X5	T50.5X6
Phenthicillin	T36.0X1	T36.0X2	T36.0X3	T36.0X4	T36.0X5	T36.0X6
Phentolamine	T46.7X1	T46.7X2	T46.7X3	T46.7X4	T46.7X5	T46.7X6
Phenyl						
butazone	T39.2X1	T39.2X2	T39.2X3	T39.2X4	T39.2X5	T39.2X6
enediamine	T65.3X1	T65.3X2	T65.3X3	T65.3X4	—	—
hydrazine	T65.3X1	T65.3X2	T65.3X3	T65.3X4	—	—
antineoplastic	T45.1X1	T45.1X2	T45.1X3	T45.1X4	T45.1X5	T45.1X6
mercuric compounds — see						
Mercury						
salicylate	T49.3X1	T49.3X2	T49.3X3	T49.3X4	T49.3X5	T49.3X6
Phenylalanine mustard	T45.1X1	T45.1X2	T45.1X3	T45.1X4	T45.1X5	T45.1X6
Phenylbutazone	T39.2X1	T39.2X2	T39.2X3	T39.2X4	T39.2X5	T39.2X6
Phenylenediamine	T65.3X1	T65.3X2	T65.3X3	T65.3X4	—	—
Phenylephrine	T44.4X1	T44.4X2	T44.4X3	T44.4X4	T44.4X5	T44.4X6
Phenylethylbiguanide	T38.3X1	T38.3X2	T38.3X3	T38.3X4	T38.3X5	T38.3X6
Phenylmercuric						
acetate	T49.0X1	T49.0X2	T49.0X3	T49.0X4	T49.0X5	T49.0X6
borate	T49.0X1	T49.0X2	T49.0X3	T49.0X4	T49.0X5	T49.0X6
nitrate	T49.0X1	T49.0X2	T49.0X3	T49.0X4	T49.0X5	T49.0X6
Phenylmethylbarbitone	T42.3X1	T42.3X2	T42.3X3	T42.3X4	T42.3X5	T42.3X6
Phenylpropanol	T47.5X1	T47.5X2	T47.5X3	T47.5X4	T47.5X5	T47.5X6
Phenylpropanolamine	T44.991	T44.992	T44.993	T44.994	T44.995	T44.996
Phenylsulfthion	T60.0X1	T60.0X2	T60.0X3	T60.0X4	—	—
Phenyltoloxamine	T45.0X1	T45.0X2	T45.0X3	T45.0X4	T45.0X5	T45.0X6
Phenyramidol, phenyramidon	T39.8X1	T39.8X2	T39.8X3	T39.8X4	T39.8X5	T39.8X6
Phenytoin	T42.0X1	T42.0X2	T42.0X3	T42.0X4	T42.0X5	T42.0X6
with Phenobarbital	T42.3X1	T42.3X2	T42.3X3	T42.3X4	T42.3X5	T42.3X6
pHisoHex	T49.2X1	T49.2X2	T49.2X3	T49.2X4	T49.2X5	T49.2X6
Pholcodine	T48.3X1	T48.3X2	T48.3X3	T48.3X4	T48.3X5	T48.3X6
Pholedrine	T46.991	T46.992	T46.993	T46.994	T46.995	T46.996
Phorate	T60.0X1	T60.0X2	T60.0X3	T60.0X4	—	—
Phosdrin	T60.0X1	T60.0X2	T60.0X3	T60.0X4	—	—
Phosfolan	T60.0X1	T60.0X2	T60.0X3	T60.0X4	—	—
Phosgene (gas)	T59.891	T59.892	T59.893	T59.894	—	—
Phosphamidon	T60.0X1	T60.0X2	T60.0X3	T60.0X4	—	—
Phosphate	T65.891	T65.892	T65.893	T65.894	—	—
laxative	T47.4X1	T47.4X2	T47.4X3	T47.4X4	T47.4X5	T47.4X6
organic	T60.0X1	T60.0X2	T60.0X3	T60.0X4	—	—
solvent	T52.91	T52.92	T52.93	T52.94	—	—
tricresyl	T65.891	T65.892	T65.893	T65.894	—	—
Phosphine	T57.1X1	T57.1X2	T57.1X3	T57.1X4	—	—
fumigant	T57.1X1	T57.1X2	T57.1X3	T57.1X4	—	—
Phospholine	T49.5X1	T49.5X2	T49.5X3	T49.5X4	T49.5X5	T49.5X6
Phosphoric acid	T54.2X1	T54.2X2	T54.2X3	T54.2X4	—	—
Phosphorus (compound) NEC	T57.1X1	T57.1X2	T57.1X3	T57.1X4	—	—
pesticide	T60.0X1	T60.0X2	T60.0X3	T60.0X4	—	—
Phthalates	T65.891	T65.892	T65.893	T65.894	—	—
Phthalic anhydride	T65.891	T65.892	T65.893	T65.894	—	—
Phthalimidoglutarimide	T42.6X1	T42.6X2	T42.6X3	T42.6X4	T42.6X5	T42.6X6
Phthalylsulfathiazole	T37.0X1	T37.0X2	T37.0X3	T37.0X4	T37.0X5	T37.0X6
Phylloquinone	T45.7X1	T45.7X2	T45.7X3	T45.7X4	T45.7X5	T45.7X6
Physeptone	T40.3X1	T40.3X2	T40.3X3	T40.3X4	T40.3X5	T40.3X6
Physostigma venenosum	T62.2X1	T62.2X2	T62.2X3	T62.2X4	—	—
Physostigmine	T49.5X1	T49.5X2	T49.5X3	T49.5X4	T49.5X5	T49.5X6
Phytolacca decandra	T62.2X1	T62.2X2	T62.2X3	T62.2X4	—	—
berries	T62.1X1	T62.1X2	T62.1X3	T62.1X4	—	—
Phytomenadione	T45.7X1	T45.7X2	T45.7X3	T45.7X4	T45.7X5	T45.7X6
Phytonadione	T45.7X1	T45.7X2	T45.7X3	T45.7X4	T45.7X5	T45.7X6
Picoperine	T48.3X1	T48.3X2	T48.3X3	T48.3X4	T48.3X5	T48.3X6
Picosulfate (sodium)	T47.2X1	T47.2X2	T47.2X3	T47.2X4	T47.2X5	T47.2X6
Picric (acid)	T54.2X1	T54.2X2	T54.2X3	T54.2X4	—	—
Picrotoxin	T50.7X1	T50.7X2	T50.7X3	T50.7X4	T50.7X5	T50.7X6
Piketoprofen	T49.0X1	T49.0X2	T49.0X3	T49.0X4	T49.0X5	T49.0X6
Pilocarpine	T44.1X1	T44.1X2	T44.1X3	T44.1X4	T44.1X5	T44.1X6
Pilocarpus (jaborandi) extract	T44.1X1	T44.1X2	T44.1X3	T44.1X4	T44.1X5	T44.1X6
Pilsicainide (hydrochloride)	T46.2X1	T46.2X2	T46.2X3	T46.2X4	T46.2X5	T46.2X6
Pimaricin	T36.7X1	T36.7X2	T36.7X3	T36.7X4	T36.7X5	T36.7X6
Pimeclone	T50.7X1	T50.7X2	T50.7X3	T50.7X4	T50.7X5	T50.7X6
Pimelic ketone	T52.8X1	T52.8X2	T52.8X3	T52.8X4	—	—
Pimethixene	T45.0X1	T45.0X2	T45.0X3	T45.0X4	T45.0X5	T45.0X6
Piminodine	T40.2X1	T40.2X2	T40.2X3	T40.2X4	T40.2X5	T40.2X6
Pimozide	T43.591	T43.592	T43.593	T43.594	T43.595	T43.596
Pinacidil	T46.5X1	T46.5X2	T46.5X3	T46.5X4	T46.5X5	T46.5X6
Pinaverium bromide	T44.3X1	T44.3X2	T44.3X3	T44.3X4	T44.3X5	T44.3X6
Pinazepam	T42.4X1	T42.4X2	T42.4X3	T42.4X4	T42.4X5	T42.4X6
Pindolol	T44.7X1	T44.7X2	T44.7X3	T44.7X4	T44.7X5	T44.7X6
Pindone	T60.4X1	T60.4X2	T60.4X3	T60.4X4	—	—
Pine oil (disinfectant)	T65.891	T65.892	T65.893	T65.894	—	—
Pinkroot	T37.4X1	T37.4X2	T37.4X3	T37.4X4	T37.4X5	T37.4X6
Pipadone	T40.2X1	T40.2X2	T40.2X3	T40.2X4	—	—
Pipamazine	T45.0X1	T45.0X2	T45.0X3	T45.0X4	T45.0X5	T45.0X6
Pipamperone	T43.4X1	T43.4X2	T43.4X3	T43.4X4	T43.4X5	T43.4X6
Pipazetate	T48.3X1	T48.3X2	T48.3X3	T48.3X4	T48.3X5	T48.3X6
Pipemidic acid	T37.8X1	T37.8X2	T37.8X3	T37.8X4	T37.8X5	T37.8X6
Pipenzolate bromide	T44.3X1	T44.3X2	T44.3X3	T44.3X4	T44.3X5	T44.3X6
Piperacetazine	T43.3X1	T43.3X2	T43.3X3	T43.3X4	T43.3X5	T43.3X6
Piperacillin	T36.0X1	T36.0X2	T36.0X3	T36.0X4	T36.0X5	T36.0X6
Piperazine	T37.4X1	T37.4X2	T37.4X3	T37.4X4	T37.4X5	T37.4X6
estrone sulfate	T38.5X1	T38.5X2	T38.5X3	T38.5X4	T38.5X5	T38.5X6
Piper cubeba	T62.2X1	T62.2X2	T62.2X3	T62.2X4		
Piperidione	T48.3X1	T48.3X2	T48.3X3	T48.3X4	T48.3X5	T48.3X6
Piperidolate	T44.3X1	T44.3X2	T44.3X3	T44.3X4	T44.3X5	T44.3X6
Piperocaine	T41.3X1	T41.3X2	T41.3X3	T41.3X4	T41.3X5	T41.3X6
infiltration (subcutaneous)	T41.3X1	T41.3X2	T41.3X3	T41.3X4	T41.3X5	T41.3X6
nerve block (peripheral) (plexus)	T41.3X1	T41.3X2	T41.3X3	T41.3X4	T41.3X5	T41.3X6
topical (surface)	T41.3X1	T41.3X2	T41.3X3	T41.3X4	T41.3X5	T41.3X6
Piperonyl butoxide	T60.8X1	T60.8X2	T60.8X3	T60.8X4	—	—
Pipethanate	T44.3X1	T44.3X2	T44.3X3	T44.3X4	T44.3X5	T44.3X6
Pipobroman	T45.1X1	T45.1X2	T45.1X3	T45.1X4	T45.1X5	T45.1X6
Pipotiazine	T43.3X1	T43.3X2	T43.3X3	T43.3X4	T43.3X5	T43.3X6
Pipoxizine	T45.0X1	T45.0X2	T45.0X3	T45.0X4	T45.0X5	T45.0X6
Pipradrol	T43.691	T43.692	T43.693	T43.694	T43.695	T43.696
Piprinhydrinate	T45.0X1	T45.0X2	T45.0X3	T45.0X4	T45.0X5	T45.0X6
Pirarubicin	T45.1X1	T45.1X2	T45.1X3	T45.1X4	T45.1X5	T45.1X6
Pirazinamide	T37.1X1	T37.1X2	T37.1X3	T37.1X4	T37.1X5	T37.1X6
Pirbuterol	T48.6X1	T48.6X2	T48.6X3	T48.6X4	T48.6X5	T48.6X6
Pirenzepine	T47.1X1	T47.1X2	T47.1X3	T47.1X4	T47.1X5	T47.1X6
Piretanide	T50.1X1	T50.1X2	T50.1X3	T50.1X4	T50.1X5	T50.1X6
Piribedil	T42.8X1	T42.8X2	T42.8X3	T42.8X4	T42.8X5	T42.8X6
Piridoxilate	T46.3X1	T46.3X2	T46.3X3	T46.3X4	T46.3X5	T46.3X6
Piritramide	T40.4X1	T40.4X2	T40.4X3	T40.4X4	—	—
Piromidic acid	T37.8X1	T37.8X2	T37.8X3	T37.8X4	T37.8X5	T37.8X6
Piroxicam	T39.391	T39.392	T39.393	T39.394	T39.395	T39.396
beta-cyclodextrin complex	T39.8X1	T39.8X2	T39.8X3	T39.8X4	T39.8X5	T39.8X6
Pirozadil	T46.6X1	T46.6X2	T46.6X3	T46.6X4	T46.6X5	T46.6X6
Piscidia (bark) (erythrina)	T39.8X1	T39.8X2	T39.8X3	T39.8X4	T39.8X5	T39.8X6
Pitch	T65.891	T65.892	T65.893	T65.894		
Pitkin's solution	T41.3X1	T41.3X2	T41.3X3	T41.3X4	T41.3X5	T41.3X6
Pitocin	T48.0X1	T48.0X2	T48.0X3	T48.0X4	T48.0X5	T48.0X6
Pitressin (tannate)	T38.891	T38.892	T38.893	T38.894	T38.895	T38.896
Pituitary extracts (posterior)	T38.891	T38.892	T38.893	T38.894	T38.895	T38.896
anterior	T38.811	T38.812	T38.813	T38.814	T38.815	T38.816
Pituitrin	T38.891	T38.892	T38.893	T38.894	T38.895	T38.896
Pivampicillin	T36.0X1	T36.0X2	T36.0X3	T36.0X4	T36.0X5	T36.0X6
Pivmecillinam	T36.0X1	T36.0X2	T36.0X3	T36.0X4	T36.0X5	T36.0X6
Placental hormone	T38.891	T38.892	T38.893	T38.894	T38.895	T38.896
Placidyl	T42.6X1	T42.6X2	T42.6X3	T42.6X4	T42.6X5	T42.6X6
Plague vaccine	T50.A91	T50.A92	T50.A93	T50.A94	T50.A95	T50.A96
Plant						
food or fertilizer NEC	T65.891	T65.892	T65.893	T65.894	—	—
containing herbicide	T60.3X1	T60.3X2	T60.3X3	T60.3X4	—	—
noxious, used as food	T62.2X1	T62.2X2	T62.2X3	T62.2X4	—	—
berries	T62.1X1	T62.1X2	T62.1X3	T62.1X4	—	—
seeds	T62.2X1	T62.2X2	T62.2X3	T62.2X4	—	—
specified type NEC	T62.2X1	T62.2X2	T62.2X3	T62.2X4	—	—
Plasma	T45.8X1	T45.8X2	T45.8X3	T45.8X4	T45.8X5	T45.8X6
expander NEC	T45.8X1	T45.8X2	T45.8X3	T45.8X4	T45.8X5	T45.8X6
protein fraction (human)	T45.8X1	T45.8X2	T45.8X3	T45.8X4	T45.8X5	T45.8X6
Plasmanate	T45.8X1	T45.8X2	T45.8X3	T45.8X4	T45.8X5	T45.8X6
Plasminogen (tissue) activator	T45.611	T45.612	T45.613	T45.614	T45.615	T45.616
Plaster dressing	T49.3X1	T49.3X2	T49.3X3	T49.3X4	T49.3X5	T49.3X6
Plastic dressing	T49.3X1	T49.3X2	T49.3X3	T49.3X4	T49.3X5	T49.3X6
Plegicil	T43.3X1	T43.3X2	T43.3X3	T43.3X4	T43.3X5	T43.3X6
Plicamycin	T45.1X1	T45.1X2	T45.1X3	T45.1X4	T45.1X5	T45.1X6
Podophyllotoxin	T49.8X1	T49.8X2	T49.8X3	T49.8X4	T49.8X5	T49.8X6
Podophyllum (resin)	T49.4X1	T49.4X2	T49.4X3	T49.4X4	T49.4X5	T49.4X6
Poisonous berries	T62.1X1	T62.1X2	T62.1X3	T62.1X4	—	—
Poison NEC	T65.91	T65.92	T65.93	T65.94	—	—
Pokeweed (any part)	T62.2X1	T62.2X2	T62.2X3	T62.2X4	—	—
Poldine metilsulfate	T44.3X1	T44.3X2	T44.3X3	T44.3X4	T44.3X5	T44.3X6
Polidexide (sulfate)	T46.6X1	T46.6X2	T46.6X3	T46.6X4	T46.6X5	T46.6X6
Polidocanol	T46.8X1	T46.8X2	T46.8X3	T46.8X4	T46.8X5	T46.8X6
Poliomyelitis vaccine	T50.B91	T50.B92	T50.B93	T50.B94	T50.B95	T50.B96
Polish (car) (floor) (furniture) (metal) (porcelain) (silver)	T65.891	T65.892	T65.893	T65.894	—	—
abrasive	T65.891	T65.892	T65.893	T65.894	—	—
porcelain	T65.891	T65.892	T65.893	T65.894	—	—
Poloxalkol	T47.4X1	T47.4X2	T47.4X3	T47.4X4	T47.4X5	T47.4X6
Poloxamer	T47.4X1	T47.4X2	T47.4X3	T47.4X4	T47.4X5	T47.4X6

Phensuximide — Poloxamer

Substance	Poisoning, Accidental (unintentional)	Poisoning, Intentional Self-harm	Poisoning, Assault	Poisoning, Undetermined	Adverse Effect	Under-dosing
Polyaminostyrene resins	T50.3X1	T50.3X2	T50.3X3	T50.3X4	T50.3X5	T50.3X6
Polycarbophil	T47.4X1	T47.4X2	T47.4X3	T47.4X4	T47.4X5	T47.4X6
Polychlorinated biphenyl	T65.891	T65.892	T65.893	T65.894	—	—
Polycycline	T36.4X1	T36.4X2	T36.4X3	T36.4X4	T36.4X5	T36.4X6
Polyester fumes	T59.891	T59.892	T59.893	T59.894	—	—
Polyester resin hardener	T52.91	T52.92	T52.93	T52.94	—	—
fumes	T59.891	T59.892	T59.893	T59.894	—	—
Polyestradiol phosphate	T38.5X1	T38.5X2	T38.5X3	T38.5X4	T38.5X5	T38.5X6
Polyethanolamine alkyl sulfate	T49.2X1	T49.2X2	T49.2X3	T49.2X4	T49.2X5	T49.2X6
Polyethylene adhesive	T49.3X1	T49.3X2	T49.3X3	T49.3X4	T49.3X5	T49.3X6
Polyferose	T45.4X1	T45.4X2	T45.4X3	T45.4X4	T45.4X5	T45.4X6
Polygeline	T45.8X1	T45.8X2	T45.8X3	T45.8X4	T45.8X5	T45.8X6
Polymyxin	T36.8X1	T36.8X2	T36.8X3	T36.8X4	T36.8X5	T36.8X6
B	T36.8X1	T36.891	T36.8X2	T36.8X4	T36.8X5	T36.8X6
ENT agent	T49.6X1	T49.6X2	T49.6X3	T49.6X4	T49.6X5	T49.6X6
ophthalmic preparation	T49.5X1	T49.5X2	T49.5X3	T49.5X4	T49.5X5	T49.5X6
topical NEC	T49.0X1	T49.0X2	T49.0X3	T49.0X4	T49.0X5	T49.0X6
E sulfate (eye preparation)	T49.5X1	T49.5X2	T49.5X3	T49.5X4	T49.5X5	T49.5X6
Polynoxylin	T49.0X1	T49.0X2	T49.0X3	T49.0X4	T49.0X5	T49.0X6
Polyoestradiol phosphate	T38.5X1	T38.5X2	T38.5X3	T38.5X4	T38.5X5	T38.5X6
Polyoxymethyleneurea	T49.0X1	T49.0X2	T49.0X3	T49.0X4	T49.0X5	T49.0X6
Polysilane	T47.8X1	T47.8X2	T47.8X3	T47.8X4	T47.8X5	T47.8X6
Polytetrafluoroethylene (inhaled)	T59.891	T59.892	T59.893	T59.894	—	—
Polythiazide	T50.2X1	T50.2X2	T50.2X3	T50.2X4	T50.2X5	T50.2X6
Polyvidone	T45.8X1	T45.8X2	T45.8X3	T45.8X4	T45.8X5	T45.8X6
Polyvinylpyrrolidone	T45.8X1	T45.8X2	T45.8X3	T45.8X4	T45.8X5	T45.8X6
Pontocaine (hydrochloride) (infiltration) (topical)	T41.3X1	T41.3X2	T41.3X3	T41.3X4	T41.3X5	T41.3X6
nerve block (peripheral) (plexus)	T41.3X1	T41.3X2	T41.3X3	T41.3X4	T41.3X5	T41.3X6
spinal	T41.3X1	T41.3X2	T41.3X3	T41.3X4	T41.3X5	T41.3X6
Porfiromycin	T45.1X1	T45.1X2	T45.1X3	T45.1X4	T45.1X5	T45.1X6
Posterior pituitary hormone NEC	T38.891	T38.892	T38.893	T38.894	T38.895	T38.896
Pot	T40.7X1	T40.7X2	T40.7X3	T40.7X4	T40.7X5	T40.7X6
Potash (caustic)	T54.3X1	T54.3X2	T54.3X3	T54.3X4	—	—
Potassic saline injection (lactated)	T50.3X1	T50.3X2	T50.3X3	T50.3X4	T50.3X5	T50.3X6
Potassium-removing resin	T50.3X1	T50.3X2	T50.3X3	T50.3X4	T50.3X5	T50.3X6
Potassium-retaining drug	T50.3X1	T50.3X2	T50.3X3	T50.3X4	T50.3X5	T50.3X6
Potassium (salts) NEC	T50.3X1	T50.3X2	T50.3X3	T50.3X4	T50.3X5	T50.3X6
aminobenzoate	T45.8X1	T45.8X2	T45.8X3	T45.8X4	T45.8X5	T45.8X6
aminosalicylate	T37.1X1	T37.1X2	T37.1X3	T37.1X4	T37.1X5	T37.1X6
antimony ' tartrate'	T37.8X1	T37.8X2	T37.8X3	T37.8X4	T37.8X5	T37.8X6
arsenite (solution)	T57.0X1	T57.0X2	T57.0X3	T57.0X4	—	—
bichromate	T56.2X1	T56.2X2	T56.2X3	T56.2X4	—	—
bisulfate	T47.3X1	T47.3X2	T47.3X3	T47.3X4	T47.3X5	T47.3X6
bromide	T42.6X1	T42.6X2	T42.6X3	T42.6X4	T42.6X5	T42.6X6
canrenoate	T50.0X1	T50.0X2	T50.0X3	T50.0X4	T50.0X5	T50.0X6
carbonate	T54.3X1	T54.3X2	T54.3X3	T54.3X4	—	—
chlorate NEC	T65.891	T65.892	T65.893	T65.894	—	—
chloride	T50.3X1	T50.3X2	T50.3X3	T50.3X4	T50.3X5	T50.3X6
citrate	T50.991	T50.992	T50.993	T50.994	T50.995	T50.996
cyanide	T65.0X1	T65.0X2	T65.0X3	T65.0X4	—	—
ferric hexacyanoferrate (medicinal)	T50.6X1	T50.6X2	T50.6X3	T50.6X4	T50.6X5	T50.6X6
nonmedicinal	T65.891	T65.892	T65.893	T65.894	—	—
Fluoride	T57.8X1	T57.8X2	T57.8X3	T57.8X4	—	—
glucaldrate	T47.1X1	T47.1X2	T47.1X3	T47.1X4	T47.1X5	T47.1X6
hydroxide	T54.3X1	T54.3X2	T54.3X3	T54.3X4	—	—
iodate	T49.0X1	T49.0X2	T49.0X3	T49.0X4	T49.0X5	T49.0X6
iodide	T48.4X1	T48.4X2	T48.4X3	T48.4X4	T48.4X5	T48.4X6
nitrate	T57.8X1	T57.8X2	T57.8X3	T57.8X4	—	—
oxalate	T65.891	T65.892	T65.893	T65.894	—	—
perchlorate (nonmedicinal) NEC	T65.891	T65.892	T65.893	T65.894	—	—
antithyroid	T38.2X1	T38.2X2	T38.2X3	T38.2X4	T38.2X5	T38.2X6
medicinal	T38.2X1	T38.2X2	T38.2X3	T38.2X4	T38.2X5	T38.2X6
Permanganate (nonmedicinal)	T65.891	T65.892	T65.893	T65.894	—	—
medicinal	T49.0X1	T49.0X2	T49.0X3	T49.0X4	T49.0X5	T49.0X6
sulfate	T47.2X1	T47.2X2	T47.2X3	T47.2X4	T47.2X5	T47.2X6
Povidone	T45.8X1	T45.8X2	T45.8X3	T45.8X4	T45.8X5	T45.8X6
iodine	T49.0X1	T49.0X2	T49.0X3	T49.0X4	T49.0X5	T49.0X6
Practolol	T44.7X1	T44.7X2	T44.7X3	T44.7X4	T44.7X5	T44.7X6
Prajmalium bitartrate	T46.2X1	T46.2X2	T46.2X3	T46.2X4	T46.2X5	T46.2X6
Pralidoxime (iodide)	T50.6X1	T50.6X2	T50.6X3	T50.6X4	T50.6X5	T50.6X6
chloride	T50.6X1	T50.6X2	T50.6X3	T50.6X4	T50.6X5	T50.6X6
Pramiverine	T44.3X1	T44.3X2	T44.3X3	T44.3X4	T44.3X5	T44.3X6
Pramocaine	T49.1X1	T49.1X2	T49.1X3	T49.1X4	T49.1X5	T49.1X6
Pramoxine	T49.1X1	T49.1X2	T49.1X3	T49.1X4	T49.1X5	T49.1X6
Prasterone	T38.7X1	T38.7X2	T38.7X3	T38.7X4	T38.7X5	T38.7X6
Pravastatin	T46.6X1	T46.6X2	T46.6X3	T46.6X4	T46.6X5	T46.6X6
Prazepam	T42.4X1	T42.4X2	T42.4X3	T42.4X4	T42.4X5	T42.4X6
Praziquantel	T37.4X1	T37.4X2	T37.4X3	T37.4X4	T37.4X5	T37.4X6
Prazitone	T43.291	T43.292	T43.293	T43.294	T43.295	T43.296
Prazosin	T44.6X1	T44.6X2	T44.6X3	T44.6X4	T44.6X5	T44.6X6
Prednicarbate	T49.0X1	T49.0X2	T49.0X3	T49.0X4	T49.0X5	T49.0X6
Prednimustine	T45.1X1	T45.1X2	T45.1X3	T45.1X4	T45.1X5	T45.1X6
Prednisolone	T38.0X1	T38.0X2	T38.0X3	T38.0X4	T38.0X5	T38.0X6
ENT agent	T49.6X1	T49.6X2	T49.6X3	T49.6X4	T49.6X5	T49.6X6
ophthalmic preparation	T49.5X1	T49.5X2	T49.5X3	T49.5X4	T49.5X5	T49.5X6
steaglate	T49.0X1	T49.0X2	T49.0X3	T49.0X4	T49.0X5	T49.0X6
topical NEC	T49.0X1	T49.0X2	T49.0X3	T49.0X4	T49.0X5	T49.0X6
Prednisone	T38.0X1	T38.0X2	T38.0X3	T38.0X4	T38.0X5	T38.0X6
Prednylidene	T38.0X1	T38.0X2	T38.0X3	T38.0X4	T38.0X5	T38.0X6
Pregnandiol	T38.5X1	T38.5X2	T38.5X3	T38.5X4	T38.5X5	T38.5X6
Pregneninolone	T38.5X1	T38.5X2	T38.5X3	T38.5X4	T38.5X5	T38.5X6
Preludin	T43.691	T43.692	T43.693	T43.694	T43.695	T43.696
Premarin	T38.5X1	T38.5X2	T38.5X3	T38.5X4	T38.5X5	T38.5X6
Premedication anesthetic	T41.201	T41.202	T41.203	T41.204	T41.205	T41.206
Prenalterol	T44.5X1	T44.5X2	T44.5X3	T44.5X4	T44.5X5	T44.5X6
Prenoxdiazine	T48.3X1	T48.3X2	T48.3X3	T48.3X4	T48.3X5	T48.3X6
Prenylamine	T46.3X1	T46.3X2	T46.3X3	T46.3X4	T46.3X5	T46.3X6
Preparation H	T49.8X1	T49.8X2	T49.8X3	T49.8X4	T49.8X5	T49.8X6
Preparation, local	T49.4X1	T49.4X2	T49.4X3	T49.4X4	T49.4X5	T49.4X6
Preservative (nonmedicinal)	T65.891	T65.892	T65.893	T65.894	—	—
medicinal	T50.901	T50.902	T50.903	T50.904	T50.905	T50.906
wood	T60.91	T60.92	T60.93	T60.94	—	—
Prethcamide	T50.7X1	T50.7X2	T50.7X3	T50.7X4	T50.7X5	T50.7X6
Pride of China	T62.2X1	T62.2X2	T62.2X3	T62.2X4	—	—
Pridinol	T44.3X1	T44.3X2	T44.3X3	T44.3X4	T44.3X5	T44.3X6
Prifinium bromide	T44.3X1	T44.3X2	T44.3X3	T44.3X4	T44.3X5	T44.3X6
Prilocaine	T41.3X1	T41.3X2	T41.3X3	T41.3X4	T41.3X5	T41.3X6
infiltration (subcutaneous)	T41.3X1	T41.3X2	T41.3X3	T41.3X4	T41.3X5	T41.3X6
nerve block (peripheral) (plexus)	T41.3X1	T41.3X2	T41.3X3	T41.3X4	T41.3X5	T41.3X6
regional	T41.3X1	T41.3X2	T41.3X3	T41.3X4	T41.3X5	T41.3X6
Primaquine	T37.2X1	T37.2X2	T37.2X3	T37.2X4	T37.2X5	T37.2X6
Primidone	T42.6X1	T42.6X2	T42.6X3	T42.6X4	T42.6X5	T42.6X6
Primula (veris)	T62.2X1	T62.2X2	T62.2X3	T62.2X4	—	—
Prinadol	T40.2X1	T40.2X2	T40.2X3	T40.2X4	T40.2X5	T40.2X6
Priscol, Priscoline	T44.6X1	T44.6X2	T44.6X3	T44.6X4	T44.6X5	T44.6X6
Pristinamycin	T36.3X1	T36.3X2	T36.3X3	T36.3X4	T36.3X5	T36.3X6
Privet	T62.2X1	T62.2X2	T62.2X3	T62.2X4	—	—
berries	T62.1X1	T62.1X2	T62.1X3	T62.1X4	—	—
Privine	T44.4X1	T44.4X2	T44.4X3	T44.4X4	T44.4X5	T44.4X6
Pro-Banthine	T44.3X1	T44.3X2	T44.3X3	T44.3X4	T44.3X5	T44.3X6
Probarbital	T42.3X1	T42.3X2	T42.3X3	T42.3X4	T42.3X5	T42.3X6
Probenecid	T50.4X1	T50.4X2	T50.4X3	T50.4X4	T50.4X5	T50.4X6
Probucol	T46.6X1	T46.6X2	T46.6X3	T46.6X4	T46.6X5	T46.6X6
Procainamide	T46.2X1	T46.2X2	T46.2X3	T46.2X4	T46.2X5	T46.2X6
Procaine	T41.3X1	T41.3X2	T41.3X3	T41.3X4	T41.3X5	T41.3X6
benzylpenicillin	T36.0X1	T36.0X2	T36.0X3	T36.0X4	T36.0X5	T36.0X6
nerve block (periphreal) (plexus)	T41.3X1	T41.3X2	T41.3X3	T41.3X4	T41.3X5	T41.3X6
penicillin G	T36.0X1	T36.0X2	T36.0X3	T36.0X4	T36.0X5	T36.0X6
regional	T41.3X1	T41.3X2	T41.3X3	T41.3X4	T41.3X5	T41.3X6
spinal	T41.3X1	T41.3X2	T41.3X3	T41.3X4	T41.3X5	T41.3X6
Procalmidol	T43.591	T43.592	T43.593	T43.594	T43.595	T43.596
Procarbazine	T45.1X1	T45.1X2	T45.1X3	T45.1X4	T45.1X5	T45.1X6
Procaterol	T44.5X1	T44.5X2	T44.5X3	T44.5X4	T44.5X5	T44.5X6
Prochlorperazine	T43.3X1	T43.3X2	T43.3X3	T43.3X4	T43.3X5	T43.3X6
Procyclidine	T44.3X1	T44.3X2	T44.3X3	T44.3X4	T44.3X5	T44.3X6
Producer gas	T58.8X1	T58.8X2	T58.8X3	T58.8X4	—	—
Profadol	T40.4X1	T40.4X2	T40.4X3	T40.4X4	T40.4X5	T40.4X6
Profenamine	T44.3X1	T44.3X2	T44.3X3	T44.3X4	T44.3X5	T44.3X6
Profenil	T44.3X1	T44.3X2	T44.3X3	T44.3X4	T44.3X5	T44.3X6
Proflavine	T49.0X1	T49.0X2	T49.0X3	T49.0X4	T49.0X5	T49.0X6
Progabide	T42.6X1	T42.6X2	T42.6X3	T42.6X4	T42.6X5	T42.6X6
Progesterone	T38.5X1	T38.5X2	T38.5X3	T38.5X4	T38.5X5	T38.5X6
Progestin	T38.5X1	T38.5X2	T38.5X3	T38.5X4	T38.5X5	T38.5X6
oral contraceptive	T38.4X1	T38.4X2	T38.4X3	T38.4X4	T38.4X5	T38.4X6
Progestogen NEC	T38.5X1	T38.5X2	T38.5X3	T38.5X4	T38.5X5	T38.5X6
Progestone	T38.5X1	T38.5X2	T38.5X3	T38.5X4	T38.5X5	T38.5X6
Proglumide	T47.1X1	T47.1X2	T47.1X3	T47.1X4	T47.1X5	T47.1X6
Proguanil	T37.2X1	T37.2X2	T37.2X3	T37.2X4	T37.2X5	T37.2X6
Prolactin	T38.811	T38.812	T38.813	T38.814	T38.815	T38.816
Prolintane	T43.691	T43.692	T43.693	T43.694	T43.695	T43.696
Proloid	T38.1X1	T38.1X2	T38.1X3	T38.1X4	T38.1X5	T38.1X6
Proluton	T38.5X1	T38.5X2	T38.5X3	T38.5X4	T38.5X5	T38.5X6
Promacetin	T37.1X1	T37.1X2	T37.1X3	T37.1X4	T37.1X5	T37.1X6
Promazine	T43.3X1	T43.3X2	T43.3X3	T43.3X4	T43.3X5	T43.3X6
Promedol	T40.2X1	T40.2X2	T40.2X3	T40.2X4	—	—

Substance	Poisoning, Accidental (unintentional)	Poisoning, Intentional Self-harm	Poisoning, Assault	Poisoning, Undetermined	Adverse Effect	Under-dosing
Promegestone	T38.5X1	T38.5X2	T38.5X3	T38.5X4	T38.5X5	T38.5X6
Promethazine (teoclate)	T43.3X1	T43.3X2	T43.3X3	T43.3X4	T43.3X5	T43.3X6
Promin	T37.1X1	T37.1X2	T37.1X3	T37.1X4	T37.1X5	T37.1X6
Pronase	T45.3X1	T45.3X2	T45.3X3	T45.3X4	T45.3X5	T45.3X6
Pronestyl (hydrochloride)	T46.2X1	T46.2X2	T46.2X3	T46.2X4	T46.2X5	T46.2X6
Pronetalol	T44.7X1	T44.7X2	T44.7X3	T44.7X4	T44.7X5	T44.7X6
Prontosil	T37.0X1	T37.0X2	T37.0X3	T37.0X4	T37.0X5	T37.0X6
Propachlor	T60.3X1	T60.3X2	T60.3X3	T60.3X4	—	—
Propafenone	T46.2X1	T46.2X2	T46.2X3	T46.2X4	T46.2X5	T46.2X6
Propallylonal	T42.3X1	T42.3X2	T42.3X3	T42.3X4	T42.3X5	T42.3X6
Propamidine	T49.0X1	T49.0X2	T49.0X3	T49.0X4	T49.0X5	T49.0X6
Propane (distributed in mobile container)	T59.891	T59.892	T59.893	T59.894	—	—
distributed through pipes	T59.891	T59.892	T59.893	T59.894	—	—
incomplete combustion	T58.11	T58.12	T58.13	T58.14	—	—
Propanidid	T41.291	T41.292	T41.293	T41.294	T41.295	T41.296
Propanil	T60.3X1	T60.3X2	T60.3X3	T60.3X4	—	—
Propantheline	T44.3X1	T44.3X2	T44.3X3	T44.3X4	T44.3X5	T44.3X6
bromide	T44.3X1	T44.3X2	T44.3X3	T44.3X4	T44.3X5	T44.3X6
Proparacaine	T41.3X1	T41.3X2	T41.3X3	T41.3X4	T41.3X5	T41.3X6
Propatylnitrate	T46.3X1	T46.3X2	T46.3X3	T46.3X4	T46.3X5	T46.3X6
Propicillin	T36.0X1	T36.0X2	T36.0X3	T36.0X4	T36.0X5	T36.0X6
Propiolactone	T49.0X1	T49.0X2	T49.0X3	T49.0X4	T49.0X5	T49.0X6
Propiomazine	T45.0X1	T45.0X2	T45.0X3	T45.0X4	T45.0X5	T45.0X6
Propionaldehyde (medicinal)	T42.6X1	T42.6X2	T42.6X3	T42.6X4	T42.6X5	T42.6X6
Propionate (calcium) (sodium)	T49.0X1	T49.0X2	T49.0X3	T49.0X4	T49.0X5	T49.0X6
Propion gel	T49.0X1	T49.0X2	T49.0X3	T49.0X4	T49.0X5	T49.0X6
Propitocaine	T41.3X1	T41.3X2	T41.3X3	T41.3X4	T41.3X5	T41.3X6
infiltration (subcutaneous)	T41.3X1	T41.3X2	T41.3X3	T41.3X4	T41.3X5	T41.3X6
nerve block (peripheral) (plexus)	T41.3X1	T41.3X2	T41.3X3	T41.3X4	T41.3X5	T41.3X6
Propofol	T41.291	T41.292	T41.293	T41.294	T41.295	T41.296
Propoxur	T60.0X1	T60.0X2	T60.0X3	T60.0X4	—	—
Propoxycaine	T41.3X1	T41.3X2	T41.3X3	T41.3X4	T41.3X5	T41.3X6
infiltration (subcutaneous)	T41.3X1	T41.3X2	T41.3X3	T41.3X4	T41.3X5	T41.3X6
nerve block (peripheral) (plexus)	T41.3X1	T41.3X2	T41.3X3	T41.3X4	T41.3X5	T41.3X6
topical (surface)	T41.3X1	T41.3X2	T41.3X3	T41.3X4	T41.3X5	T41.3X6
Propoxyphene	T40.4X1	T40.4X2	T40.4X3	T40.4X4	T40.4X5	T40.4X6
Propranolol	T44.7X1	T44.7X2	T44.7X3	T44.7X4	T44.7X5	T44.7X6
Propyl						
alcohol	T51.3X1	T51.3X2	T51.3X3	T51.3X4	—	—
carbinol	T51.3X1	T51.3X2	T51.3X3	T51.3X4	—	—
hexadrine	T44.4X1	T44.4X2	T44.4X3	T44.4X4	T44.4X5	T44.4X6
iodone	T50.8X1	T50.8X2	T50.8X3	T50.8X4	T50.8X5	T50.8X6
thiouracil	T38.2X1	T38.2X2	T38.2X3	T38.2X4	T38.2X5	T38.2X6
Propylaminophenothiazine	T43.3X1	T43.3X2	T43.3X3	T43.3X4	T43.3X5	T43.3X6
Propylene	T59.891	T59.892	T59.893	T59.894	—	—
Propylhexedrine	T48.5X1	T48.5X2	T48.5X3	T48.5X4	T48.5X5	T48.5X6
Propyliodone	T50.8X1	T50.8X2	T50.8X3	T50.8X4	T50.8X5	T50.8X6
Propylparaben (ophthalmic)	T49.5X1	T49.5X2	T49.5X3	T49.5X4	T49.5X5	T49.5X6
Propylthiouracil	T38.2X1	T38.2X2	T38.2X3	T38.2X4	T38.2X5	T38.2X6
Propyphenazone	T39.2X1	T39.2X2	T39.2X3	T39.2X4	T39.2X5	T39.2X6
Proquazone	T39.391	T39.392	T39.393	T39.394	T39.395	T39.396
Proscillaridin	T46.0X1	T46.0X2	T46.0X3	T46.0X4	T46.0X5	T46.0X6
Prostacyclin	T45.521	T45.522	T45.523	T45.524	T45.525	T45.526
Prostaglandin (I2)	T45.521	T45.522	T45.523	T45.524	T45.525	T45.526
E1	T46.7X1	T46.7X2	T46.7X3	T46.7X4	T46.7X5	T46.7X6
E2	T48.0X1	T48.0X2	T48.0X3	T48.0X4	T48.0X5	T48.0X6
F2 alpha	T48.0X1	T48.0X2	T48.0X3	T48.0X4	T48.0X5	T48.0X6
Prostigmin	T44.0X1	T44.0X2	T44.0X3	T44.0X4	T44.0X5	T44.0X6
Prosultiamine	T45.2X1	T45.2X2	T45.2X3	T45.2X4	T45.2X5	T45.2X6
Protamine sulfate	T45.7X1	T45.7X2	T45.7X3	T45.7X4	T45.7X5	T45.7X6
zinc insulin	T38.3X1	T38.3X2	T38.3X3	T38.3X4	T38.3X5	T38.3X6
Protease	T47.5X1	T47.5X2	T47.5X3	T47.5X4	T47.5X5	T47.5X6
Protectant, skin NEC	T49.3X1	T49.3X2	T49.3X3	T49.3X4	T49.3X5	T49.3X6
Protein hydrolysate	T50.991	T50.992	T50.993	T50.994	T50.995	T50.996
Prothiaden — see Dothiepin hydrochloride						
Prothionamide	T37.1X1	T37.1X2	T37.1X3	T37.1X4	T37.1X5	T37.1X6
Prothipendyl	T43.591	T43.592	T43.593	T43.594	T43.595	T43.596
Prothoate	T60.0X1	T60.0X2	T60.0X3	T60.0X4	—	—
Prothrombin						
activator	T45.7X1	T45.7X2	T45.7X3	T45.7X4	T45.7X5	T45.7X6
synthesis inhibitor	T45.511	T45.512	T45.513	T45.514	T45.515	T45.516
Protionamide	T37.1X1	T37.1X2	T37.1X3	T37.1X4	T37.1X5	T37.1X6
Protirelin	T38.891	T38.892	T38.893	T38.894	T38.895	T38.896
Protokylol	T48.6X1	T48.6X2	T48.6X3	T48.6X4	T48.6X5	T48.6X6
Protopam	T50.6X1	T50.6X2	T50.6X3	T50.6X4	T50.6X5	T50.6X6
Protoveratrine(s) (A) (B)	T46.5X1	T46.5X2	T46.5X3	T46.5X4	T46.5X5	T46.5X6
Protriptyline	T43.011	T43.012	T43.013	T43.014	T43.015	T43.016

Substance	Poisoning, Accidental (unintentional)	Poisoning, Intentional Self-harm	Poisoning, Assault	Poisoning, Undetermined	Adverse Effect	Under-dosing
Provera	T38.5X1	T38.5X2	T38.5X3	T38.5X4	T38.5X5	T38.5X6
Provitamin A	T45.2X1	T45.2X2	T45.2X3	T45.2X4	T45.2X5	T45.2X6
Proxibarbal	T42.3X1	T42.3X2	T42.3X3	T42.3X4	T42.3X5	T42.3X6
Proxymetacaine	T41.3X1	T41.3X2	T41.3X3	T41.3X4	T41.3X5	T41.3X6
Proxyphylline	T48.6X1	T48.6X2	T48.6X3	T48.6X4	T48.6X5	T48.6X6
Prozac — see Fluoxetine hydrochloride						
Prunus						
laurocerasus	T62.2X1	T62.2X2	T62.2X3	T62.2X4	—	—
virginiana	T62.2X1	T62.2X2	T62.2X3	T62.2X4	—	—
Prussian blue						
commercial	T65.891	T65.892	T65.893	T65.894	—	—
therapeutic	T50.6X1	T50.6X2	T50.6X3	T50.6X4	T50.6X5	T50.6X6
Prussic acid	T65.0X1	T65.0X2	T65.0X3	T65.0X4	—	—
vapor	T57.3X1	T57.3X2	T57.3X3	T57.3X4	—	—
Pseudoephedrine	T44.991	T44.992	T44.993	T44.994	T44.995	T44.996
Psilocin	T40.991	T40.992	T40.993	T40.994	—	—
Psilocybin	T40.991	T40.992	T40.993	T40.994	—	—
Psilocybine	T40.991	T40.992	T40.993	T40.994	—	—
Psoralene (nonmedicinal)	T65.891	T65.892	T65.893	T65.894	—	—
Psoralens (medicinal)	T50.991	T50.992	T50.993	T50.994	T50.995	T50.996
PSP (phenolsulfonphthalein)	T50.8X1	T50.8X2	T50.8X3	T50.8X4	T50.8X5	T50.8X6
Psychodysleptic drug NEC	T40.901	T40.902	T40.903	T40.904	T40.905	T40.906
Psychostimulant	T43.601	T43.602	T43.603	T43.604	T43.605	T43.606
amphetamine	T43.621	T43.622	T43.623	T43.624	T43.625	T43.626
caffeine	T43.611	T43.612	T43.613	T43.614	T43.615	T43.616
methylphenidate	T43.631	T43.632	T43.633	T43.634	T43.635	T43.636
specified NEC	T43.691	T43.692	T43.693	T43.694	T43.695	T43.696
Psychotherapeutic drug NEC	T43.91	T43.92	T43.93	T43.94	T43.95	T43.96
antidepressants — see also Antidepressant	T43.201	T43.202	T43.203	T43.204	T43.205	T43.206
specified NEC	T43.8X1	T43.8X2	T43.8X3	T43.8X4	T43.8X5	T43.8X6
tranquilizers NEC	T43.501	T43.502	T43.503	T43.504	T43.505	T43.506
Psychotomimetic agents	T40.901	T40.902	T40.903	T40.904	T40.905	T40.906
Psychotropic drug NEC	T43.91	T43.92	T43.93	T43.94	T43.95	T43.96
specified NEC	T43.8X1	T43.8X2	T43.8X3	T43.8X4	T43.8X5	T43.8X6
Psyllium hydrophilic mucilloid	T47.4X1	T47.4X2	T47.4X3	T47.4X4	T47.4X5	T47.4X6
Pteroylglutamic acid	T45.8X1	T45.8X2	T45.8X3	T45.8X4	T45.8X5	T45.8X6
Pteroyltriglutamate	T45.1X1	T45.1X2	T45.1X3	T45.1X4	T45.1X5	T45.1X6
PTFE — see Polytetrafluoroethylene						
Pulp						
devitalizing paste	T49.7X1	T49.7X2	T49.7X3	T49.7X4	T49.7X5	T49.7X6
dressing	T49.7X1	T49.7X2	T49.7X3	T49.7X4	T49.7X5	T49.7X6
Pulsatilla	T62.2X1	T62.2X2	T62.2X3	T62.2X4	—	—
Pumpkin seed extract	T37.4X1	T37.4X2	T37.4X3	T37.4X4	T37.4X5	T37.4X6
Purex (bleach)	T54.91	T54.92	T54.93	T54.94	—	—
Purgative NEC — see also Cathartic	T47.4X1	T47.4X2	T47.4X3	T47.4X4	T47.4X5	T47.4X6
Purine analogue (antineoplastic)	T45.1X1	T45.1X2	T45.1X3	T45.1X4	T45.1X5	T45.1X6
Purine diuretics	T50.2X1	T50.2X2	T50.2X3	T50.2X4	T50.2X5	T50.2X6
Purinethol	T45.1X1	T45.1X2	T45.1X3	T45.1X4	T45.1X5	T45.1X6
PVP	T45.8X1	T45.8X2	T45.8X3	T45.8X4	T45.8X5	T45.8X6
Pyrabital	T39.8X1	T39.8X2	T39.8X3	T39.8X4	T39.8X5	T39.8X6
Pyramidon	T39.2X1	T39.2X2	T39.2X3	T39.2X4	T39.2X5	T39.2X6
Pyrantel	T37.4X1	T37.4X2	T37.4X3	T37.4X4	T37.4X5	T37.4X6
Pyrathiazine	T45.0X1	T45.0X2	T45.0X3	T45.0X4	T45.0X5	T45.0X6
Pyrazinamide	T37.1X1	T37.1X2	T37.1X3	T37.1X4	T37.1X5	T37.1X6
Pyrazinoic acid (amide)	T37.1X1	T37.1X2	T37.1X3	T37.1X4	T37.1X5	T37.1X6
Pyrazole (derivatives)	T39.2X1	T39.2X2	T39.2X3	T39.2X4	T39.2X5	T39.2X6
Pyrazolone analgesic NEC	T39.2X1	T39.2X2	T39.2X3	T39.2X4	T39.2X5	T39.2X6
Pyrethrin, pyrethrum (nonmedicinal)	T60.2X1	T60.2X2	T60.2X3	T60.2X4	—	—
Pyrethrum extract	T49.0X1	T49.0X2	T49.0X3	T49.0X4	T49.0X5	T49.0X6
Pyribenzamine	T45.0X1	T45.0X2	T45.0X3	T45.0X4	T45.0X5	T45.0X6
Pyridine	T52.8X1	T52.8X2	T52.8X3	T52.8X4	—	—
aldoxime methiodide	T50.6X1	T50.6X2	T50.6X3	T50.6X4	T50.6X5	T50.6X6
aldoxime methyl chloride	T50.6X1	T50.6X2	T50.6X3	T50.6X4	T50.6X5	T50.6X6
vapor	T59.891	T59.892	T59.893	T59.894	—	—
Pyridium	T39.8X1	T39.8X2	T39.8X3	T39.8X4	T39.8X5	T39.8X6
Pyridostigmine bromide	T44.0X1	T44.0X2	T44.0X3	T44.0X4	T44.0X5	T44.0X6
Pyridoxal phosphate	T45.2X1	T45.2X2	T45.2X3	T45.2X4	T45.2X5	T45.2X6
Pyridoxine	T45.2X1	T45.2X2	T45.2X3	T45.2X4	T45.2X5	T45.2X6
Pyrilamine	T45.0X1	T45.0X2	T45.0X3	T45.0X4	T45.0X5	T45.0X6
Pyrimethamine	T37.2X1	T37.2X2	T37.2X3	T37.2X4	T37.2X5	T37.2X6
with sulfadoxine	T37.2X1	T37.2X2	T37.2X3	T37.2X4	T37.2X5	T37.2X6
Pyrimidine antagonist	T45.1X1	T45.1X2	T45.1X3	T45.1X4	T45.1X5	T45.1X6
Pyriminil	T60.4X1	T60.4X2	T60.4X3	T60.4X4	—	—
Pyrithione zinc	T49.4X1	T49.4X2	T49.4X3	T49.4X4	T49.4X5	T49.4X6
Pyrithyldione	T42.6X1	T42.6X2	T42.6X3	T42.6X4	T42.6X5	T42.6X6

Additional Character May Be Required — Refer to the Tabular List for Character Selection ▽ Subterms under main terms may continue to next column or page

Substance	Poisoning, Accidental (unintentional)	Poisoning, Intentional Self-harm	Poisoning, Assault	Poisoning, Undetermined	Adverse Effect	Under-dosing
Pyrogallic acid	T49.0X1	T49.0X2	T49.0X3	T49.0X4	T49.0X5	T49.0X6
Pyrogallol	T49.0X1	T49.0X2	T49.0X3	T49.0X4	T49.0X5	T49.0X6
Pyroxylin	T49.3X1	T49.3X2	T49.3X3	T49.3X4	T49.3X5	T49.3X6
Pyrrobutamine	T45.0X1	T45.0X2	T45.0X3	T45.0X4	T45.0X5	T45.0X6
Pyrrolizidine alkaloids	T62.8X1	T62.8X2	T62.8X3	T62.8X4	—	—
Pyrvinium chloride	T37.4X1	T37.4X2	T37.4X3	T37.4X4	T37.4X5	T37.4X6
PZI	T38.3X1	T38.3X2	T38.3X3	T38.3X4	T38.3X5	T38.3X6
Quaalude	T42.6X1	T42.6X2	T42.6X3	T42.6X4	T42.6X5	T42.6X6
Quarternary ammonium						
anti-infective	T49.0X1	T49.0X2	T49.0X3	T49.0X4	T49.0X5	T49.0X6
ganglion blocking	T44.2X1	T44.2X2	T44.2X3	T44.2X4	T44.2X5	T44.2X6
parasympatholytic	T44.3X1	T44.3X2	T44.3X3	T44.3X4	T44.3X5	T44.3X6
Quazepam	T42.4X1	T42.4X2	T42.4X3	T42.4X4	T42.4X5	T42.4X6
Quicklime	T54.3X1	T54.3X2	T54.3X3	T54.3X4	—	—
Quillaja extract	T48.4X1	T48.4X2	T48.4X3	T48.4X4	T48.4X5	T48.4X6
Quinacrine	T37.2X1	T37.2X2	T37.2X3	T37.2X4	T37.2X5	T37.2X6
Quinaglute	T46.2X1	T46.2X2	T46.2X3	T46.2X4	T46.2X5	T46.2X6
Quinalbarbital	T42.3X1	T42.3X2	T42.3X3	T42.3X4	T42.3X5	T42.3X6
Quinalbarbitone sodium	T42.3X1	T42.3X2	T42.3X3	T42.3X4	T42.3X5	T42.3X6
Quinalphos	T60.0X1	T60.0X2	T60.0X3	T60.0X4	—	—
Quinapril	T46.4X1	T46.4X2	T46.4X3	T46.4X4	T46.4X5	T46.4X6
Quinestradiol	T38.5X1	T38.5X2	T38.5X3	T38.5X4	T38.5X5	T38.5X6
Quinestradol	T38.5X1	T38.5X2	T38.5X3	T38.5X4	T38.5X5	T38.5X6
Quinestrol	T38.5X1	T38.5X2	T38.5X3	T38.5X4	T38.5X5	T38.5X6
Quinethazone	T50.2X1	T50.2X2	T50.2X3	T50.2X4	T50.2X5	T50.2X6
Quingestanol	T38.4X1	T38.4X2	T38.4X3	T38.4X4	T38.4X5	T38.4X6
Quinidine	T46.2X1	T46.2X2	T46.2X3	T46.2X4	T46.2X5	T46.2X6
Quinine	T37.2X1	T37.2X2	T37.2X3	T37.2X4	T37.2X5	T37.2X6
Quiniobine	T37.8X1	T37.8X2	T37.8X3	T37.8X4	T37.8X5	T37.8X6
Quinisocaine	T49.1X1	T49.1X2	T49.1X3	T49.1X4	T49.1X5	T49.1X6
Quinocide	T37.2X1	T37.2X2	T37.2X3	T37.2X4	T37.2X5	T37.2X6
Quinoline (derivatives) NEC	T37.8X1	T37.8X2	T37.8X3	T37.8X4	T37.8X5	T37.8X6
Quinupramine	T43.011	T43.012	T43.013	T43.014	T43.015	T43.016
Quotane	T41.3X1	T41.3X2	T41.3X3	T41.3X4	T41.3X5	T41.3X6
Rabies						
immune globulin (human)	T50.Z11	T50.Z12	T50.Z13	T50.Z14	T50.Z15	T50.Z16
vaccine	T50.B91	T50.B92	T50.B93	T50.B94	T50.B95	T50.B96
Racemoramide	T40.2X1	T40.2X2	T40.2X3	T40.2X4	—	—
Racemorphan	T40.2X1	T40.2X2	T40.2X3	T40.2X4	T40.2X5	T40.2X6
Racepinefrin	T44.5X1	T44.5X2	T44.5X3	T44.5X4	T44.5X5	T44.5X6
Raclopride	T43.591	T43.592	T43.593	T43.594	T43.595	T43.596
Radiator alcohol	T51.1X1	T51.1X2	T51.1X3	T51.1X4	—	—
Radioactive drug NEC	T50.8X1	T50.8X2	T50.8X3	T50.8X4	T50.8X5	T50.8X6
Radio-opaque (drugs) (materials)	T50.8X1	T50.8X2	T50.8X3	T50.8X4	T50.8X5	T50.8X6
Ramifenazone	T39.2X1	T39.2X2	T39.2X3	T39.2X4	T39.2X5	T39.2X6
Ramipril	T46.4X1	T46.4X2	T46.4X3	T46.4X4	T46.4X5	T46.4X6
Ranitidine	T47.0X1	T47.0X2	T47.0X3	T47.0X4	T47.0X5	T47.0X6
Ranunculus	T62.2X1	T62.2X2	T62.2X3	T62.2X4	—	—
Rat poison NEC	T60.4X1	T60.4X2	T60.4X3	T60.4X4	—	—
Rattlesnake (venom)	T63.011	T63.012	T63.013	T63.014	—	—
Raubasine	T46.7X1	T46.7X2	T46.7X3	T46.7X4	T46.7X5	T46.7X6
Raudixin	T46.5X1	T46.5X2	T46.5X3	T46.5X4	T46.5X5	T46.5X6
Rautensin	T46.5X1	T46.5X2	T46.5X3	T46.5X4	T46.5X5	T46.5X6
Rautina	T46.5X1	T46.5X2	T46.5X3	T46.5X4	T46.5X5	T46.5X6
Rautotal	T46.5X1	T46.5X2	T46.5X3	T46.5X4	T46.5X5	T46.5X6
Rauwiloid	T46.5X1	T46.5X2	T46.5X3	T46.5X4	T46.5X5	T46.5X6
Rauwoldin	T46.5X1	T46.5X2	T46.5X3	T46.5X4	T46.5X5	T46.5X6
Rauwolfia (alkaloids)	T46.5X1	T46.5X2	T46.5X3	T46.5X4	T46.5X5	T46.5X6
Razoxane	T45.1X1	T45.1X2	T45.1X3	T45.1X4	T45.1X5	T45.1X6
Realgar	T57.0X1	T57.0X2	T57.0X3	T57.0X4	—	—
Recombinant (R) — see specific protein						
Red blood cells, packed	T45.8X1	T45.8X2		T45.8X4	T45.8X5	T45.8X6
Red squill (scilliroside)	T60.4X1	T60.4X2	T60.4X3	T60.4X4	—	—
Reducing agent, industrial NEC	T65.891	T65.892	T65.893	T65.894	—	—
Refrigerant gas (chlorofluorocarbon)	T53.5X1	T53.5X2	T53.5X3	T53.5X4	—	—
not chlorofluorocarbon	T59.891	T59.892	T59.893	T59.894	—	—
Regroton	T50.2X1	T50.2X2	T50.2X3	T50.2X4	T50.2X5	T50.2X6
Rehydration salts (oral)	T50.3X1	T50.3X2	T50.3X3	T50.3X4	T50.3X5	T50.3X6
Rela	T42.8X1	T42.8X2	T42.8X3	T42.8X4	T42.8X5	T42.8X6
Relaxant, muscle						
anesthetic	T48.1X1	T48.1X2	T48.1X3	T48.1X4	T48.1X5	T48.1X6
central nervous system	T42.8X1	T42.8X2	T42.8X3	T42.8X4	T42.8X5	T42.8X6
skeletal NEC	T48.1X1	T48.1X2	T48.1X3	T48.1X4	T48.1X5	T48.1X6
smooth NEC	T44.3X1	T44.3X2	T44.3X3	T44.3X4	T44.3X5	T44.3X6
Remoxipride	T43.591	T43.592	T43.593	T43.594	T43.595	T43.596
Renese	T50.2X1	T50.2X2	T50.2X3	T50.2X4	T50.2X5	T50.2X6
Renografin	T50.8X1	T50.8X2	T50.8X3	T50.8X4	T50.8X5	T50.8X6
Replacement solution	T50.3X1	T50.3X2	T50.3X3	T50.3X4	T50.3X5	T50.3X6
Reproterol	T48.6X1	T48.6X2	T48.6X3	T48.6X4	T48.6X5	T48.6X6
Rescinnamine	T46.5X1	T46.5X2	T46.5X3	T46.5X4	T46.5X5	T46.5X6
Reserpin (e)	T46.5X1	T46.5X2	T46.5X3	T46.5X4	T46.5X5	T46.5X6
Resorcin, resorcinol (nonmedicinal)	T65.891	T65.892	T65.893	T65.894		
medicinal	T49.4X1	T49.4X2	T49.4X3	T49.4X4	T49.4X5	T49.4X6
Respaire	T48.4X1	T48.4X2	T48.4X3	T48.4X4	T48.4X5	T48.4X6
Respiratory drug NEC	T48.901	T48.902	T48.903	T48.904	T48.905	T48.906
antiasthmatic NEC	T48.6X1	T48.6X2	T48.6X3	T48.6X4	T48.6X5	T48.6X6
anti-common-cold NEC	T48.5X1	T48.5X2	T48.5X3	T48.5X4	T48.5X5	T48.5X6
expectorant NEC	T48.4X1	T48.4X2	T48.4X3	T48.4X4	T48.4X5	T48.4X6
stimulant	T48.901	T48.902	T48.903	T48.904	T48.905	T48.906
Retinoic acid	T49.0X1	T49.0X2	T49.0X3	T49.0X4	T49.0X5	T49.0X6
Retinol	T45.2X1	T45.2X2	T45.2X3	T45.2X4	T45.2X5	T45.2X6
Rh (D) immune globulin (human)	T50.Z11	T50.Z12	T50.Z13	T50.Z14	T50.Z15	T50.Z16
Rhodine	T39.011	T39.012	T39.013	T39.014	T39.015	T39.016
RhoGAM	T50.Z11	T50.Z12	T50.Z13	T50.Z14	T50.Z15	T50.Z16
Rhubarb						
dry extract	T47.2X1	T47.2X2	T47.2X3	T47.2X4	T47.2X5	T47.2X6
tincture, compound	T47.2X1	T47.2X2	T47.2X3	T47.2X4	T47.2X5	T47.2X6
Ribavirin	T37.5X1	T37.5X2	T37.5X3	T37.5X4	T37.5X5	T37.5X6
Riboflavin	T45.2X1	T45.2X2	T45.2X3	T45.2X4	T45.2X5	T45.2X6
Ribostamycin	T36.5X1	T36.5X2	T36.5X3	T36.5X4	T36.5X5	T36.5X6
Ricin	T62.2X1	T62.2X2	T62.2X3	T62.2X4	—	—
Ricinus communis	T62.2X1	T62.2X2	T62.2X3	T62.2X4	—	—
Rickettsial vaccine NEC	T50.A91	T50.A92	T50.A93	T50.A94	T50.A95	T50.A96
Rifabutin	T36.6X1	T36.6X2	T36.6X3	T36.6X4	T36.6X5	T36.6X6
Rifamide	T36.6X1	T36.6X2	T36.6X3	T36.6X4	T36.6X5	T36.6X6
Rifampicin	T36.6X1	T36.6X2	T36.6X3	T36.6X4	T36.6X5	T36.6X6
with isoniazid	T37.1X1	T37.1X2	T37.1X3	T37.1X4	T37.1X5	T37.1X6
Rifampin	T36.6X1	T36.6X2	T36.6X3	T36.6X4	T36.6X5	T36.6X6
Rifamycin	T36.6X1	T36.6X2	T36.6X3	T36.6X4	T36.6X5	T36.6X6
Rifaximin	T36.6X1	T36.6X2	T36.6X3	T36.6X4	T36.6X5	T36.6X6
Rimantadine	T37.5X1	T37.5X2	T37.5X3	T37.5X4	T37.5X5	T37.5X6
Rimazolium metilsulfate	T39.8X1	T39.8X2	T39.8X3	T39.8X4	T39.8X5	T39.8X6
Rimifon	T37.1X1	T37.1X2	T37.1X3	T37.1X4	T37.1X5	T37.1X6
Rimiterol	T48.6X1	T48.6X2	T48.6X3	T48.6X4	T48.6X5	T48.6X6
Ringer (lactate) solution	T50.3X1	T50.3X2	T50.3X3	T50.3X4	T50.3X5	T50.3X6
Ristocetin	T36.8X1	T36.8X2	T36.8X3	T36.8X4	T36.8X5	T36.8X6
Ritalin	T43.631	T43.632	T43.633	T43.634	T43.635	T43.636
Ritodrine	T44.5X1	T44.5X2	T44.5X3	T44.5X4	T44.5X5	T44.5X6
Roach killer — see Insecticide						
Rociverine	T44.3X1	T44.3X2	T44.3X3	T44.3X4	T44.3X5	T44.3X6
Rocky Mountain spotted fever vaccine	T50.A91	T50.A92	T50.A93	T50.A94	T50.A95	T50.A96
Rodenticide NEC	T60.4X1	T60.4X2	T60.4X3	T60.4X4	—	—
Rohypnol	T42.4X1	T42.4X2	T42.4X3	T42.4X4	T42.4X5	T42.4X6
Rokitamycin	T36.3X1	T36.3X2	T36.3X3	T36.3X4	T36.3X5	T36.3X6
Rolaids	T47.1X1	T47.1X2	T47.1X3	T47.1X4	T47.1X5	T47.1X6
Rolitetracycline	T36.4X1	T36.4X2	T36.4X3	T36.4X4	T36.4X5	T36.4X6
Romilar	T48.3X1	T48.3X2	T48.3X3	T48.3X4	T48.3X5	T48.3X6
Ronifibrate	T46.6X1	T46.6X2	T46.6X3	T46.6X4	T46.6X5	T46.6X6
Rosaprostol	T47.1X1	T47.1X2	T47.1X3	T47.1X4	T47.1X5	T47.1X6
Rose bengal sodium (131I)	T50.8X1	T50.8X2	T50.8X3	T50.8X4	T50.8X5	T50.8X6
Rose water ointment	T49.3X1	T49.3X2	T49.3X3	T49.3X4	T49.3X5	T49.3X6
Rosoxacin	T37.8X1	T37.8X2	T37.8X3	T37.8X4	T37.8X5	T37.8X6
Rotenone	T60.2X1	T60.2X2	T60.2X3	T60.2X4	—	—
Rotoxamine	T45.0X1	T45.0X2	T45.0X3	T45.0X4	T45.0X5	T45.0X6
Rough-on-rats	T60.4X1	T60.4X2	T60.4X3	T60.4X4	—	—
Roxatidine	T47.0X1	T47.0X2	T47.0X3	T47.0X4	T47.0X5	T47.0X6
Roxithromycin	T36.3X1	T36.3X2	T36.3X3	T36.3X4	T36.3X5	T36.3X6
Rt-PA	T45.611	T45.612	T45.613	T45.614	T45.615	T45.616
Rubbing alcohol	T51.2X1	T51.2X2	T51.2X3	T51.2X4	—	—
Rubefacient	T49.4X1	T49.4X2	T49.4X3	T49.4X4	T49.4X5	T49.4X6
Rubella vaccine	T50.B91	T50.B92	T50.B93	T50.B94	T50.B95	T50.B96
Rubeola vaccine	T50.B91	T50.B92	T50.B93	T50.B94	T50.B95	T50.B96
Rubidium chloride Rb82	T50.8X1	T50.8X2	T50.8X3	T50.8X4	T50.8X5	T50.8X6
Rubidomycin	T45.1X1	T45.1X2	T45.1X3	T45.1X4	T45.1X5	T45.1X6
Rue	T62.2X1	T62.2X2	T62.2X3	T62.2X4	—	—
Rufocromomycin	T45.1X1	T45.1X2	T45.1X3	T45.1X4	T45.1X5	T45.1X6
Russel's viper venin	T45.7X1	T45.7X2	T45.7X3	T45.7X4	T45.7X5	T45.7X6
Ruta (graveolens)	T62.2X1	T62.2X2	T62.2X3	T62.2X4	—	—
Rutinum	T46.991	T46.992	T46.993	T46.994	T46.995	T46.996
Rutoside	T46.991	T46.992	T46.993	T46.994	T46.995	T46.996
b-sitosterol(s)	T46.6X1	T46.6X2	T46.6X3	T46.6X4	T46.6X5	T46.6X6
Sabadilla (plant)	T62.2X1	T62.2X2	T62.2X3	T62.2X4	—	—
pesticide	T60.2X1	T60.2X2	T60.2X3	T60.2X4	—	—
Saccharated iron oxide	T45.8X1	T45.8X2		T45.8X4	T45.8X5	T45.8X6
Saccharin	T50.901	T50.902	T50.903	T50.904	T50.905	T50.906
Saccharomyces boulardii	T47.6X1	T47.6X2	T47.6X3	T47.6X4	T47.6X5	T47.6X6
Safflower oil	T46.6X1	T46.6X2	T46.6X3	T46.6X4	T46.6X5	T46.6X6
Safrazine	T43.1X1	T43.1X2	T43.1X3	T43.1X4	T43.1X5	T43.1X6
Salazosulfapyridine	T37.0X1	T37.0X2	T37.0X3	T37.0X4	T37.0X5	T37.0X6

Substance	Poisoning, Accidental (unintentional)	Poisoning, Intentional Self-harm	Poisoning, Assault	Poisoning, Undetermined	Adverse Effect	Under-dosing
Salbutamol	T48.6X1	T48.6X2	T48.6X3	T48.6X4	T48.6X5	T48.6X6
Salicylamide	T39.091	T39.092	T39.093	T39.094	T39.095	T39.096
Salicylate NEC	T39.091	T39.092	T39.093	T39.094	T39.095	T39.096
methyl	T49.3X1	T49.3X2	T49.3X3	T49.3X4	T49.3X5	T49.3X6
theobromine calcium	T50.2X1	T50.2X2	T50.2X3	T50.2X4	T50.2X5	T50.2X6
Salicylazosulfapyridine	T37.0X1	T37.0X2	T37.0X3	T37.0X4	T37.0X5	T37.0X6
Salicylhydroxamic acid	T49.0X1	T49.0X2	T49.0X3	T49.0X4	T49.0X5	T49.0X6
Salicylic acid	T49.4X1	T49.4X2	T49.4X3	T49.4X4	T49.4X5	T49.4X6
with benzoic acid	T49.4X1	T49.4X2	T49.4X3	T49.4X4	T49.4X5	T49.4X6
congeners	T39.091	T39.092	T39.093	T39.094	T39.095	T39.096
derivative	T39.091	T39.092	T39.093	T39.094	T39.095	T39.096
salts	T39.091	T39.092	T39.093	T39.094	T39.095	T39.096
Salinazid	T37.1X1	T37.1X2	T37.1X3	T37.1X4	T37.1X5	T37.1X6
Salmeterol	T48.6X1	T48.6X2	T48.6X3	T48.6X4	T48.6X5	T48.6X6
Salol	T49.3X1	T49.3X2	T49.3X3	T49.3X4	T49.3X5	T49.3X6
Salsalate	T39.091	T39.092	T39.093	T39.094	T39.095	T39.096
Salt-replacing drug	T50.901	T50.902	T50.903	T50.904	T50.905	T50.906
Salt-retaining mineralocorticoid	T50.0X1	T50.0X2	T50.0X3	T50.0X4	T50.0X5	T50.0X6
Salt substitute	T50.901	T50.902	T50.903	T50.904	T50.905	T50.906
Saluretic NEC	T50.2X1	T50.2X2	T50.2X3	T50.2X4	T50.2X5	T50.2X6
Saluron	T50.2X1	T50.2X2	T50.2X3	T50.2X4	T50.2X5	T50.2X6
Salvarsan 606 (neosilver) (silver)	T37.8X1	T37.8X2	T37.8X3	T37.8X4	T37.8X5	T37.8X6
Sambucus canadensis	T62.2X1	T62.2X2	T62.2X3	T62.2X4	—	—
berry	T62.1X1	T62.1X2	T62.1X3	T62.1X4	—	—
Sandril	T46.5X1	T46.5X2	T46.5X3	T46.5X4	T46.5X5	T46.5X6
Sanguinaria canadensis	T62.2X1	T62.2X2	T62.2X3	T62.2X4	—	—
Saniflush (cleaner)	T54.2X1	T54.2X2	T54.2X3	T54.2X4	—	—
Santonin	T37.4X1	T37.4X2	T37.4X3	T37.4X4	T37.4X5	T37.4X6
Santyl	T49.8X1	T49.8X2	T49.8X3	T49.8X4	T49.8X5	T49.8X6
Saralasin	T46.5X1	T46.5X2	T46.5X3	T46.5X4	T46.5X5	T46.5X6
Sarcolysin	T45.1X1	T45.1X2	T45.1X3	T45.1X4	T45.1X5	T45.1X6
Sarkomycin	T45.1X1	T45.1X2	T45.1X3	T45.1X4	T45.1X5	T45.1X6
Saroten	T43.011	T43.012	T43.013	T43.014	T43.015	T43.016
Saturnine — *see* Lead						
Savin (oil)	T49.4X1	T49.4X2	T49.4X3	T49.4X4	T49.4X5	T49.4X6
Scammony	T47.2X1	T47.2X2	T47.2X3	T47.2X4	T47.2X5	T47.2X6
Scarlet red	T49.8X1	T49.8X2	T49.8X3	T49.8X4	T49.8X5	T49.8X6
Scheele's green	T57.0X1	T57.0X2	T57.0X3	T57.0X4	—	—
insecticide	T57.0X1	T57.0X2	T57.0X3	T57.0X4	—	—
Schizontozide (blood)	T37.2X1	T37.2X2	T37.2X3	T37.2X4	T37.2X5	T37.2X6
(tissue)	T37.2X1	T37.2X2	T37.2X3	T37.2X4	T37.2X5	T37.2X6
Schradan	T60.0X1	T60.0X2	T60.0X3	T60.0X4	—	—
Schweinfurth green	T57.0X1	T57.0X2	T57.0X3	T57.0X4	—	—
insecticide	T57.0X1	T57.0X2	T57.0X3	T57.0X4	—	—
Scilla, rat poison	T60.4X1	T60.4X2	T60.4X3	T60.4X4	—	—
Scillaren	T60.4X1	T60.4X2	T60.4X3	T60.4X4	—	—
Sclerosing agent	T46.8X1	T46.8X2	T46.8X3	T46.8X4	T46.8X5	T46.8X6
Scombrotoxin	T61.11	T61.12	T61.13	T61.14	—	—
Scopolamine	T44.3X1	T44.3X2	T44.3X3	T44.3X4	T44.3X5	T44.3X6
Scopolia extract	T44.3X1	T44.3X2	T44.3X3	T44.3X4	T44.3X5	T44.3X6
Scouring powder	T65.891	T65.892	T65.893	T65.894	—	—
Sea						
anemone (sting)	T63.631	T63.632	T63.633	T63.634	—	—
cucumber (sting)	T63.691	T63.692	T63.693	T63.694	—	—
snake (bite) (venom)	T63.091	T63.092	T63.093	T63.094	—	—
urchin spine (puncture)	T63.691	T63.692	T63.693	T63.694	—	—
Seafood	T61.91	T61.92	T61.93	T61.94	—	—
specified NEC	T61.8X1	T61.8X2	T61.8X3	T61.8X4	—	—
Secbutabarbital	T42.3X1	T42.3X2	T42.3X3	T42.3X4	T42.3X5	T42.3X6
Secbutabarbitone	T42.3X1	T42.3X2	T42.3X3	T42.3X4	T42.3X5	T42.3X6
Secnidazole	T37.3X1	T37.3X2	T37.3X3	T37.3X4	T37.3X5	T37.3X6
Secobarbital	T42.3X1	T42.3X2	T42.3X3	T42.3X4	T42.3X5	T42.3X6
Seconal	T42.3X1	T42.3X2	T42.3X3	T42.3X4	T42.3X5	T42.3X6
Secretin	T50.8X1	T50.8X2	T50.8X3	T50.8X4	T50.8X5	T50.8X6
Sedative NEC	T42.71	T42.72	T42.73	T42.74	T42.75	T42.76
mixed NEC	T42.6X1	T42.6X2	T42.6X3	T42.6X4	T42.6X5	T42.6X6
Sedormid	T42.6X1	T42.6X2	T42.6X3	T42.6X4	T42.6X5	T42.6X6
Seed disinfectant or dressing	T60.8X1	T60.8X2	T60.8X3	T60.8X4	—	—
Seeds (poisonous)	T62.2X1	T62.2X2	T62.2X3	T62.2X4	—	—
Selegiline	T42.8X1	T42.8X2	T42.8X3	T42.8X4	T42.8X5	T42.8X6
Selenium NEC	T56.891	T56.892	T56.893	T56.894	—	—
disulfide or sulfide	T49.4X1	T49.4X2	T49.4X3	T49.4X4	T49.4X5	T49.4X6
fumes	T59.891	T59.892	T59.893	T59.894	—	—
sulfide	T49.4X1	T49.4X2	T49.4X3	T49.4X4	T49.4X5	T49.4X6
Selenomethionine (75Se)	T50.8X1	T50.8X2	T50.8X3	T50.8X4	T50.8X5	T50.8X6
Selsun	T49.4X1	T49.4X2	T49.4X3	T49.4X4	T49.4X5	T49.4X6
Semustine	T45.1X1	T45.1X2	T45.1X3	T45.1X4	T45.1X5	T45.1X6
Senega syrup	T48.4X1	T48.4X2	T48.4X3	T48.4X4	T48.4X5	T48.4X6
Senna	T47.2X1	T47.2X2	T47.2X3	T47.2X4	T47.2X5	T47.2X6
Sennoside A+B	T47.2X1	T47.2X2	T47.2X3	T47.2X4	T47.2X5	T47.2X6

Substance	Poisoning, Accidental (unintentional)	Poisoning, Intentional Self-harm	Poisoning, Assault	Poisoning, Undetermined	Adverse Effect	Under-dosing
Septisol	T49.2X1	T49.2X2	T49.2X3	T49.2X4	T49.2X5	T49.2X6
Seractide	T38.811	T38.812	T38.813	T38.814	T38.815	T38.816
Serax	T42.4X1	T42.4X2	T42.4X3	T42.4X4	T42.4X5	T42.4X6
Serenesil	T42.6X1	T42.6X2	T42.6X3	T42.6X4	T42.6X5	T42.6X6
Serenium (hydrochloride)	T37.91	T37.92	T37.93	T37.94	T37.95	T37.96
Serepax — *see* Oxazepam						
Sermorelin	T38.891	T38.892	T38.893	T38.894	T38.895	T38.896
Sernyl	T41.1X1	T41.1X2	T41.1X3	T41.1X4	T41.1X5	T41.1X6
Serotonin	T50.991	T50.992	T50.993	T50.994	T50.995	T50.996
Serpasil	T46.5X1	T46.5X2	T46.5X3	T46.5X4	T46.5X5	T46.5X6
Serrapeptase	T45.3X1	T45.3X2	T45.3X3	T45.3X4	T45.3X5	T45.3X6
Serum						
antibotulinus	T50.Z11	T50.Z12	T50.Z13	T50.Z14	T50.Z15	T50.Z16
anticytotoxic	T50.Z11	T50.Z12	T50.Z13	T50.Z14	T50.Z15	T50.Z16
antidiphtheria	T50.Z11	T50.Z12	T50.Z13	T50.Z14	T50.Z15	T50.Z16
antimeningococcus	T50.Z11	T50.Z12	T50.Z13	T50.Z14	T50.Z15	T50.Z16
anti-Rh	T50.Z11	T50.Z12	T50.Z13	T50.Z14	T50.Z15	T50.Z16
anti-snake-bite	T50.Z11	T50.Z12	T50.Z13	T50.Z14	T50.Z15	T50.Z16
antitetanic	T50.Z11	T50.Z12	T50.Z13	T50.Z14	T50.Z15	T50.Z16
antitoxic	T50.Z11	T50.Z12	T50.Z13	T50.Z14	T50.Z15	T50.Z16
complement (inhibitor)	T45.8X1	T45.8X2	T45.8X3	T45.8X4	T45.8X5	T45.8X6
convalescent	T50.Z11	T50.Z12	T50.Z13	T50.Z14	T50.Z15	T50.Z16
hemolytic complement	T45.8X1	T45.8X2	T45.8X3	T45.8X4	T45.8X5	T45.8X6
immune (human)	T50.Z11	T50.Z12	T50.Z13	T50.Z14	T50.Z15	T50.Z16
protective NEC	T50.Z11	T50.Z12	T50.Z13	T50.Z14	T50.Z15	T50.Z16
Setastine	T45.0X1	T45.0X2	T45.0X3	T45.0X4	T45.0X5	T45.0X6
Setoperone	T43.591	T43.592	T43.593	T43.594	T43.595	T43.596
Sewer gas	T59.91	T59.92	T59.93	T59.94	—	—
Shampoo	T55.0X1	T55.0X2	T55.0X3	T55.0X4	—	—
Shellfish, noxious, nonbacterial	T61.781	T61.782	T61.783	T61.784	—	—
Sildenafil	T46.7X1	T46.7X2	T46.7X3	T46.7X4	T46.7X5	T46.7X6
Silibinin	T50.991	T50.992	T50.993	T50.994	T50.995	T50.996
Silicone NEC	T65.891	T65.892	T65.893	T65.894	—	—
medicinal	T49.3X1	T49.3X2	T49.3X3	T49.3X4	T49.3X5	T49.3X6
Silvadene	T49.0X1	T49.0X2	T49.0X3	T49.0X4	T49.0X5	T49.0X6
Silver	T49.0X1	T49.0X2	T49.0X3	T49.0X4	T49.0X5	T49.0X6
anti-infectives	T49.0X1	T49.0X2	T49.0X3	T49.0X4	T49.0X5	T49.0X6
arsphenamine	T37.8X1	T37.8X2	T37.8X3	T37.8X4	T37.8X5	T37.8X6
colloidal	T49.0X1	T49.0X2	T49.0X3	T49.0X4	T49.0X5	T49.0X6
nitrate	T49.0X1	T49.0X2	T49.0X3	T49.0X4	T49.0X5	T49.0X6
ophthalmic preparation	T49.5X1	T49.5X2	T49.5X3	T49.5X4	T49.5X5	T49.5X6
toughened (keratolytic)	T49.4X1	T49.4X2	T49.4X3	T49.4X4	T49.4X5	T49.4X6
nonmedicinal (dust)	T56.891	T56.892	T56.893	T56.894	—	—
protein	T49.5X1	T49.5X2	T49.5X3	T49.5X4	T49.5X5	T49.5X6
salvarsan	T37.8X1	T37.8X2	T37.8X3	T37.8X4	T37.8X5	T37.8X6
sulfadiazine	T49.4X1	T49.4X2	T49.4X3	T49.4X4	T49.4X5	T49.4X6
Silymarin	T50.991	T50.992	T50.993	T50.994	T50.995	T50.996
Simaldrate	T47.1X1	T47.1X2	T47.1X3	T47.1X4	T47.1X5	T47.1X6
Simazine	T60.3X1	T60.3X2	T60.3X3	T60.3X4	—	—
Simethicone	T47.1X1	T47.1X2	T47.1X3	T47.1X4	T47.1X5	T47.1X6
Simfibrate	T46.6X1	T46.6X2	T46.6X3	T46.6X4	T46.6X5	T46.6X6
Simvastatin	T46.6X1	T46.6X2	T46.6X3	T46.6X4	T46.6X5	T46.6X6
Sincalide	T50.8X1	T50.8X2	T50.8X3	T50.8X4	T50.8X5	T50.8X6
Sinequan	T43.011	T43.012	T43.013	T43.014	T43.015	T43.016
Singoserp	T46.5X1	T46.5X2	T46.5X3	T46.5X4	T46.5X5	T46.5X6
Sintrom	T45.511	T45.512	T45.513	T45.514	T45.515	T45.516
Sisomicin	T36.5X1	T36.5X2	T36.5X3	T36.5X4	T36.5X5	T36.5X6
Sitosterols	T46.6X1	T46.6X2	T46.6X3	T46.6X4	T46.6X5	T46.6X6
Skeletal muscle relaxants	T48.1X1	T48.1X2	T48.1X3	T48.1X4	T48.1X5	T48.1X6
Skin						
agents (external)	T49.91	T49.92	T49.93	T49.94	T49.95	T49.96
specified NEC	T49.8X1	T49.8X2	T49.8X3	T49.8X4	T49.8X5	T49.8X6
test antigen	T50.8X1	T50.8X2	T50.8X3	T50.8X4	T50.8X5	T50.8X6
Sleep-eze	T45.0X1	T45.0X2	T45.0X3	T45.0X4	T45.0X5	T45.0X6
Sleeping draught, pill	T42.71	T42.72	T42.73	T42.74	T42.75	T42.76
Smallpox vaccine	T50.B11	T50.B12	T50.B13	T50.B14	T50.B15	T50.B16
Smelter fumes NEC	T56.91	T56.92	T56.93	T56.94	—	—
Smog	T59.1X1	T59.1X2	T59.1X3	T59.1X4	—	—
Smoke NEC	T59.811	T59.812	T59.813	T59.814	—	—
Smooth muscle relaxant	T44.3X1	T44.3X2	T44.3X3	T44.3X4	T44.3X5	T44.3X6
Snail killer NEC	T60.8X1	T60.8X2	T60.8X3	T60.8X4	—	—
Snake venom or bite	T63.001	T63.002	T63.003	T63.004	—	—
hemocoagulase	T45.7X1	T45.7X2	T45.7X3	T45.7X4	T45.7X5	T45.7X6
Snuff	T65.211	T65.212	T65.213	T65.214	—	—
Soap (powder) (product)	T55.0X1	T55.0X2	T55.0X3	T55.0X4	—	—
enema	T47.4X1	T47.4X2	T47.4X3	T47.4X4	T47.4X5	T47.4X6
medicinal, soft	T49.2X1	T49.2X2	T49.2X3	T49.2X4	T49.2X5	T49.2X6
superfatted	T49.2X1	T49.2X2	T49.2X3	T49.2X4	T49.2X5	T49.2X6
Sobrerol	T48.4X1	T48.4X2	T48.4X3	T48.4X4	T48.4X5	T48.4X6
Soda (caustic)	T54.3X1	T54.3X2	T54.3X3	T54.3X4	—	—
bicarb	T47.1X1	T47.1X2	T47.1X3	T47.1X4	T47.1X5	T47.1X6

Substance	Poisoning, Accidental (unintentional)	Poisoning, Intentional Self-harm	Poisoning, Assault	Poisoning, Undetermined	Adverse Effect	Under-dosing
Soda — *continued*						
chlorinated — *see* Sodium, hypochlorite						
Sodium						
acetosulfone	T37.1X1	T37.1X2	T37.1X3	T37.1X4	T37.1X5	T37.1X6
acetrizoate	T50.8X1	T50.8X2	T50.8X3	T50.8X4	T50.8X5	T50.8X6
acid phosphate	T50.3X1	T50.3X2	T50.3X3	T50.3X4	T50.3X5	T50.3X6
alginate	T47.8X1	T47.8X2	T47.8X3	T47.8X4	T47.8X5	T47.8X6
amidotrizoate	T50.8X1	T50.8X2	T50.8X3	T50.8X4	T50.8X5	T50.8X6
aminopterin	T45.1X1	T45.1X2	T45.1X3	T45.1X4	T45.1X5	T45.1X6
amylosulfate	T47.8X1	T47.8X2	T47.8X3	T47.8X4	T47.8X5	T47.8X6
amytal	T42.3X1	T42.3X2	T42.3X3	T42.3X4	T42.3X5	T42.3X6
antimony gluconate	T37.3X1	T37.3X2	T37.3X3	T37.3X4	T37.3X5	T37.3X6
arsenate	T57.0X1	T57.0X2	T57.0X3	T57.0X4	—	—
aurothiomalate	T39.4X1	T39.4X2	T39.4X3	T39.4X4	T39.4X5	T39.4X6
aurothiosulfate	T39.4X1	T39.4X2	T39.4X3	T39.4X4	T39.4X5	T39.4X6
barbiturate	T42.3X1	T42.3X2	T42.3X3	T42.3X4	T42.3X5	T42.3X6
basic phosphate	T47.4X1	T47.4X2	T47.4X3	T47.4X4	T47.4X5	T47.4X6
bicarbonate	T47.1X1	T47.1X2	T47.1X3	T47.1X4	T47.1X5	T47.1X6
bichromate	T57.8X1	T57.8X2	T57.8X3	T57.8X4	—	—
biphosphate	T50.3X1	T50.3X2	T50.3X3	T50.3X4	T50.3X5	T50.3X6
bisulfate	T65.891	T65.892	T65.893	T65.894	—	—
borate						
cleanser	T57.8X1	T57.8X2	T57.8X3	T57.8X4	—	—
eye	T49.5X1	T49.5X2	T49.5X3	T49.5X4	T49.5X5	T49.5X6
therapeutic	T49.8X1	T49.8X2	T49.8X3	T49.8X4	T49.8X5	T49.8X6
bromide	T42.6X1	T42.6X2	T42.6X3	T42.6X4	T42.6X5	T42.6X6
cacodylate (nonmedicinal) NEC	T50.8X1	T50.8X2	T50.8X3	T50.8X4	T50.8X5	T50.8X6
anti-infective	T37.8X1	T37.8X2	T37.8X3	T37.8X4	T37.8X5	T37.8X6
herbicide	T60.3X1	T60.3X2	T60.3X3	T60.3X4	—	—
calcium edetate	T45.8X1	T45.8X2	T45.8X3	T45.8X4	T45.8X5	T45.8X6
carbonate NEC	T54.3X1	T54.3X2	T54.3X3	T54.3X4	—	—
chlorate NEC	T65.891	T65.892	T65.893	T65.894	—	—
herbicide	T54.91	T54.92	T54.93	T54.94	—	—
chloride	T50.3X1	T50.3X2	T50.3X3	T50.3X4	T50.3X5	T50.3X6
with glucose	T50.3X1	T50.3X2	T50.3X3	T50.3X4	T50.3X5	T50.3X6
chromate	T65.891	T65.892	T65.893	T65.894	—	—
citrate	T50.991	T50.992	T50.993	T50.994	T50.995	T50.996
cromoglicate	T48.6X1	T48.6X2	T48.6X3	T48.6X4	T48.6X5	T48.6X6
cyanide	T65.0X1	T65.0X2	T65.0X3	T65.0X4	—	—
cyclamate	T50.3X1	T50.3X2	T50.3X3	T50.3X4	T50.3X5	T50.3X6
dehydrocholate	T45.8X1	T45.8X2	T45.8X3	T45.8X4	T45.8X5	T45.8X6
diatrizoate	T50.8X1	T50.8X2	T50.8X3	T50.8X4	T50.8X5	T50.8X6
dibunate	T48.4X1	T48.4X2	T48.4X3	T48.4X4	T48.4X5	T48.4X6
dioctyl sulfosuccinate	T47.4X1	T47.4X2	T47.4X3	T47.4X4	T47.4X5	T47.4X6
dipantoyl ferrate	T45.8X1	T45.8X2	T45.8X3	T45.8X4	T45.8X5	T45.8X6
edetate	T45.8X1	T45.8X2	T45.8X3	T45.8X4	T45.8X5	T45.8X6
ethacrynate	T50.1X1	T50.1X2	T50.1X3	T50.1X4	T50.1X5	T50.1X6
feredetate	T45.8X1	T45.8X2	T45.8X3	T45.8X4	T45.8X5	T45.8X6
Fluoride — *see* Fluoride						
fluoroacetate (dust) (pesticide)	T60.4X1	T60.4X2	T60.4X3	T60.4X4	—	—
free salt	T50.3X1	T50.3X2	T50.3X3	T50.3X4	T50.3X5	T50.3X6
fusidate	T36.8X1	T36.8X2	T36.8X3	T36.8X4	T36.8X5	T36.8X6
glucaldrate	T47.1X1	T47.1X2	T47.1X3	T47.1X4	T47.1X5	T47.1X6
glucosulfone	T37.1X1	T37.1X2	T37.1X3	T37.1X4	T37.1X5	T37.1X6
glutamate	T45.8X1	T45.8X2	T45.8X3	T45.8X4	T45.8X5	T45.8X6
hydrogen carbonate	T50.3X1	T50.3X2	T50.3X3	T50.3X4	T50.3X5	T50.3X6
hydroxide	T54.3X1	T54.3X2	T54.3X3	T54.3X4	—	—
hypochlorite (bleach) NEC	T54.3X1	T54.3X2	T54.3X3	T54.3X4	—	—
disinfectant	T54.3X1	T54.3X2	T54.3X3	T54.3X4	—	—
medicinal (anti-infective) (external)	T49.0X1	T49.0X2	T49.0X3	T49.0X4	T49.0X5	T49.0X6
vapor	T54.3X1	T54.3X2	T54.3X3	T54.3X4	—	—
hyposulfite	T49.0X1	T49.0X2	T49.0X3	T49.0X4	T49.0X5	T49.0X6
indigotin disulfonate	T50.8X1	T50.8X2	T50.8X3	T50.8X4	T50.8X5	T50.8X6
iodide	T50.991	T50.992	T50.993	T50.994	T50.995	T50.996
I-131	T50.8X1	T50.8X2	T50.8X3	T50.8X4	T50.8X5	T50.8X6
therapeutic	T38.2X1	T38.2X2	T38.2X3	T38.2X4	T38.2X5	T38.2X6
iodohippurate (131I)	T50.8X1	T50.8X2	T50.8X3	T50.8X4	T50.8X5	T50.8X6
iopodate	T50.8X1	T50.8X2	T50.8X3	T50.8X4	T50.8X5	T50.8X6
iothalamate	T50.8X1	T50.8X2	T50.8X3	T50.8X4	T50.8X5	T50.8X6
iron edetate	T45.4X1	T45.4X2	T45.4X3	T45.4X4	T45.4X5	T45.4X6
lactate (compound solution)	T45.8X1	T45.8X2	T45.8X3	T45.8X4	T45.8X5	T45.8X6
lauryl (sulfate)	T49.2X1	T49.2X2	T49.2X3	T49.2X4	T49.2X5	T49.2X6
L-triiodothyronine	T38.1X1	T38.1X2	T38.1X3	T38.1X4	T38.1X5	T38.1X6
magnesium citrate	T50.991	T50.992	T50.993	T50.994	T50.995	T50.996
mersalate	T50.2X1	T50.2X2	T50.2X3	T50.2X4	T50.2X5	T50.2X6
metasilicate	T65.891	T65.892	T65.893	T65.894	—	—
metrizoate	T50.8X1	T50.8X2	T50.8X3	T50.8X4	T50.8X5	T50.8X6
Sodium — *continued*						
monofluoroacetate (pesticide)	T60.1X1	T60.1X2	T60.1X3	T60.1X4	—	—
morrhuate	T46.8X1	T46.8X2	T46.8X3	T46.8X4	T46.8X5	T46.8X6
nafcillin	T36.0X1	T36.0X2	T36.0X3	T36.0X4	T36.0X5	T36.0X6
nitrate (oxidizing agent)	T65.891	T65.892	T65.893	T65.894	—	—
nitrite	T50.6X1	T50.6X2	T50.6X3	T50.6X4	T50.6X5	T50.6X6
nitroferricyanide	T46.5X1	T46.5X2	T46.5X3	T46.5X4	T46.5X5	T46.5X6
nitroprusside	T46.5X1	T46.5X2	T46.5X3	T46.5X4	T46.5X5	T46.5X6
oxalate	T65.891	T65.892	T65.893	T65.894	—	—
oxide/peroxide	T65.891	T65.892	T65.893	T65.894	—	—
oxybate	T41.291	T41.292	T41.293	T41.294	T41.295	T41.296
para-aminohippurate	T50.8X1	T50.8X2	T50.8X3	T50.8X4	T50.8X5	T50.8X6
perborate (nonmedicinal) NEC	T65.891	T65.892	T65.893	T65.894	—	—
medicinal	T49.0X1	T49.0X2	T49.0X3	T49.0X4	T49.0X5	T49.0X6
soap	T55.0X1	T55.0X2	T55.0X3	T55.0X4	—	—
percarbonate — *see* Sodium, perborate						
pertechnetate Tc99m	T50.8X1	T50.8X2	T50.8X3	T50.8X4	T50.8X5	T50.8X6
phosphate						
cellulose	T45.8X1	T45.8X2	T45.8X3	T45.8X4	T45.8X5	T45.8X6
dibasic	T47.2X1	T47.2X2	T47.2X3	T47.2X4	T47.2X5	T47.2X6
monobasic	T47.2X1	T47.2X2	T47.2X3	T47.2X4	T47.2X5	T47.2X6
phytate	T50.6X1	T50.6X2	T50.6X3	T50.6X4	T50.6X5	T50.6X6
picosulfate	T47.2X1	T47.2X2	T47.2X3	T47.2X4	T47.2X5	T47.2X6
polyhydroxyaluminium monocarbonate	T47.1X1	T47.1X2	T47.1X3	T47.1X4	T47.1X5	T47.1X6
polystyrene sulfonate	T50.3X1	T50.3X2	T50.3X3	T50.3X4	T50.3X5	T50.3X6
propionate	T49.0X1	T49.0X2	T49.0X3	T49.0X4	T49.0X5	T49.0X6
propyl hydroxybenzoate	T50.991	T50.992	T50.993	T50.994	T50.995	T50.996
psylliate	T46.8X1	T46.8X2	T46.8X3	T46.8X4	T46.8X5	T46.8X6
removing resins	T50.3X1	T50.3X2	T50.3X3	T50.3X4	T50.3X5	T50.3X6
salicylate	T39.091	T39.092	T39.093	T39.094	T39.095	T39.096
salt NEC	T50.3X1	T50.3X2	T50.3X3	T50.3X4	T50.3X5	T50.3X6
selenate	T60.2X1	T60.2X2	T60.2X3	T60.2X4	—	—
stibogluconate	T37.3X1	T37.3X2	T37.3X3	T37.3X4	T37.3X5	T37.3X6
sulfate	T47.4X1	T47.4X2	T47.4X3	T47.4X4	T47.4X5	T47.4X6
sulfoxone	T37.1X1	T37.1X2	T37.1X3	T37.1X4	T37.1X5	T37.1X6
tetradecyl sulfate	T46.8X1	T46.8X2	T46.8X3	T46.8X4	T46.8X5	T46.8X6
thiopental	T41.1X1	T41.1X2	T41.1X3	T41.1X4	T41.1X5	T41.1X6
thiosalicylate	T39.091	T39.092	T39.093	T39.094	T39.095	T39.096
thiosulfate	T50.6X1	T50.6X2	T50.6X3	T50.6X4	T50.6X5	T50.6X6
tolbutamide	T38.3X1	T38.3X2	T38.3X3	T38.3X4	T38.3X5	T38.3X6
(L)-triiodothyronine	T38.1X1	T38.1X2	T38.1X3	T38.1X4	T38.1X5	T38.1X6
tyropanoate	T50.8X1	T50.8X2	T50.8X3	T50.8X4	T50.8X5	T50.8X6
valproate	T42.6X1	T42.6X2	T42.6X3	T42.6X4	T42.6X5	T42.6X6
versenate	T50.6X1	T50.6X2	T50.6X3	T50.6X4	T50.6X5	T50.6X6
Sodium-free salt	T50.901	T50.902	T50.903	T50.904	T50.905	T50.906
Sodium-removing resin	T50.3X1	T50.3X2	T50.3X3	T50.3X4	T50.3X5	T50.3X6
Soft soap	T55.0X1	T55.0X2	T55.0X3	T55.0X4	—	—
Solanine	T62.2X1	T62.2X2	T62.2X3	T62.2X4	—	—
berries	T62.1X1	T62.1X2	T62.1X3	T62.1X4	—	—
Solanum dulcamara	T62.2X1	T62.2X2	T62.2X3	T62.2X4	—	—
berries	T62.1X1	T62.1X2	T62.1X3	T62.1X4	—	—
Solapsone	T37.1X1	T37.1X2	T37.1X3	T37.1X4	T37.1X5	T37.1X6
Solar lotion	T49.3X1	T49.3X2	T49.3X3	T49.3X4	T49.3X5	T49.3X6
Solasulfone	T37.1X1	T37.1X2	T37.1X3	T37.1X4	T37.1X5	T37.1X6
Soldering fluid	T65.891	T65.892	T65.893	T65.894	—	—
Solid substance	T65.91	T65.92	T65.93	T65.94	—	—
specified NEC	T65.891	T65.892	T65.893	T65.894	—	—
Solvent, industrial NEC	T52.91	T52.92	T52.93	T52.94	—	—
naphtha	T52.0X1	T52.0X2	T52.0X3	T52.0X4	—	—
petroleum	T52.0X1	T52.0X2	T52.0X3	T52.0X4	—	—
specified NEC	T52.8X1	T52.8X2	T52.8X3	T52.8X4	—	—
Soma	T42.8X1	T42.8X2	T42.8X3	T42.8X4	T42.8X5	T42.8X6
Somatorelin	T38.891	T38.892	T38.893	T38.894	T38.895	T38.896
Somatostatin	T38.991	T38.992	T38.993	T38.994	T38.995	T38.996
Somatotropin	T38.811	T38.812	T38.813	T38.814	T38.815	T38.816
Somatrem	T38.811	T38.812	T38.813	T38.814	T38.815	T38.816
Somatropin	T38.811	T38.812	T38.813	T38.814	T38.815	T38.816
Sominex	T45.0X1	T45.0X2	T45.0X3	T45.0X4	T45.0X5	T45.0X6
Somnos	T42.6X1	T42.6X2	T42.6X3	T42.6X4	T42.6X5	T42.6X6
Somonal	T42.3X1	T42.3X2	T42.3X3	T42.3X4	T42.3X5	T42.3X6
Soneryl	T42.3X1	T42.3X2	T42.3X3	T42.3X4	T42.3X5	T42.3X6
Soothing syrup	T50.901	T50.902	T50.903	T50.904	T50.905	T50.906
Sopor	T42.6X1	T42.6X2	T42.6X3	T42.6X4	T42.6X5	T42.6X6
Soporific	T42.71	T42.72	T42.73	T42.74	T42.75	T42.76
Soporific drug	T42.71	T42.72	T42.73	T42.74	T42.75	T42.76
specified type NEC	T42.6X1	T42.6X2	T42.6X3	T42.6X4	T42.6X5	T42.6X6
Sorbide nitrate	T46.3X1	T46.3X2	T46.3X3	T46.3X4	T46.3X5	T46.3X6
Sorbitol	T47.4X1	T47.4X2	T47.4X3	T47.4X4	T47.4X5	T47.4X6
Sotalol	T44.7X1	T44.7X2	T44.7X3	T44.7X4	T44.7X5	T44.7X6

Subterms under main terms may continue to next column or page — Additional Character May Be Required — Refer to the Tabular List for Character Selection — 389

Soda — Sotalol

Table of Drugs and Chemicals

Sotradecol — Sulfanilylguanidine

Substance	Poisoning, Accidental (unintentional)	Poisoning, Intentional Self-harm	Poisoning, Assault	Poisoning, Undetermined	Adverse Effect	Under-dosing
Sotradecol	T46.8X1	T46.8X2	T46.8X3	T46.8X4	T46.8X5	T46.8X6
Soysterol	T46.6X1	T46.6X2	T46.6X3	T46.6X4	T46.6X5	T46.6X6
Spacoline	T44.3X1	T44.3X2	T44.3X3	T44.3X4	T44.3X5	T44.3X6
Spanish fly	T49.8X1	T49.8X2	T49.8X3	T49.8X4	T49.8X5	T49.8X6
Sparine	T43.3X1	T43.3X2	T43.3X3	T43.3X4	T43.3X5	T43.3X6
Sparteine	T48.0X1	T48.0X2	T48.0X3	T48.0X4	T48.0X5	T48.0X6
Spasmolytic						
anticholinergics	T44.3X1	T44.3X2	T44.3X3	T44.3X4	T44.3X5	T44.3X6
autonomic	T44.3X1	T44.3X2	T44.3X3	T44.3X4	T44.3X5	T44.3X6
bronchial NEC	T48.6X1	T48.6X2	T48.6X3	T48.6X4	T48.6X5	T48.6X6
quaternary ammonium	T44.3X1	T44.3X2	T44.3X3	T44.3X4	T44.3X5	T44.3X6
skeletal muscle NEC	T48.1X1	T48.1X2	T48.1X3	T48.1X4	T48.1X5	T48.1X6
Spectinomycin	T36.5X1	T36.5X2	T36.5X3	T36.5X4	T36.5X5	T36.5X6
Speed	T43.621	T43.622	T43.623	T43.624	T43.625	T43.626
Spermicide	T49.8X1	T49.8X2	T49.8X3	T49.8X4	T49.8X5	T49.8X6
Spider (bite) (venom)	T63.391	T63.392	T63.393	T63.394		
antivenin	T50.Z11	T50.Z12	T50.Z13	T50.Z14	T50.Z15	T50.Z16
Spigelia (root)	T37.4X1	T37.4X2	T37.4X3	T37.4X4	T37.4X5	T37.4X6
Spindle inactivator	T50.4X1	T50.4X2	T50.4X3	T50.4X4	T50.4X5	T50.4X6
Spiperone	T43.4X1	T43.4X2	T43.4X3	T43.4X4	T43.4X5	T43.4X6
Spiramycin	T36.3X1	T36.3X2	T36.3X3	T36.3X4	T36.3X5	T36.3X6
Spirapril	T46.4X1	T46.4X2	T46.4X3	T46.4X4	T46.4X5	T46.4X6
Spirilene	T43.591	T43.592	T43.593	T43.594	T43.595	T43.596
Spirit(s) (neutral) **NEC**	T51.0X1	T51.0X2	T51.0X3	T51.0X4	—	—
beverage	T51.0X1	T51.0X2	T51.0X3	T51.0X4	—	—
industrial	T51.0X1	T51.0X2	T51.0X3	T51.0X4	—	—
mineral	T52.0X1	T52.0X2	T52.0X3	T52.0X4	—	—
of salt — see Hydrochloric acid						
surgical	T51.0X1	T51.0X2	T51.0X3	T51.0X4	—	—
Spironolactone	T50.0X1	T50.0X2	T50.0X3	T50.0X4	T50.0X5	T50.0X6
Spiroperidol	T43.4X1	T43.4X2	T43.4X3	T43.4X4	T43.4X5	T43.4X6
Sponge, absorbable (gelatin)	T45.7X1	T45.7X2	T45.7X3	T45.7X4	T45.7X5	T45.7X6
Sporostacin	T49.0X1	T49.0X2	T49.0X3	T49.0X4	T49.0X5	T49.0X6
Spray (aerosol)	T65.91	T65.92	T65.93	T65.94	—	—
cosmetic	T65.891	T65.892	T65.893	T65.894	—	—
medicinal NEC	T50.901	T50.902	T50.903	T50.904	T50.905	T50.906
pesticides — see Pesticides						
specified content — see specific substance						
Spurge flax	T62.2X1	T62.2X2	T62.2X3	T62.2X4	—	—
Spurges	T62.2X1	T62.2X2	T62.2X3	T62.2X4	—	—
Sputum viscosity-lowering drug	T48.4X1	T48.4X2	T48.4X3	T48.4X4	T48.4X5	T48.4X6
Squill	T46.0X1	T46.0X2	T46.0X3	T46.0X4	T46.0X5	T46.0X6
rat poison	T60.4X1	T60.4X2	T60.4X3	T60.4X4	—	—
Squirting cucumber (cathartic)	T47.2X1	T47.2X2	T47.2X3	T47.2X4	T47.2X5	T47.2X6
Stains	T65.6X1	T65.6X2	T65.6X3	T65.6X4	—	—
Stannous fluoride	T49.7X1	T49.7X2	T49.7X3	T49.7X4	T49.7X5	T49.7X6
Stanolone	T38.7X1	T38.7X2	T38.7X3	T38.7X4	T38.7X5	T38.7X6
Stanozolol	T38.7X1	T38.7X2	T38.7X3	T38.7X4	T38.7X5	T38.7X6
Staphisagria or stavesacre (pediculicide)	T49.0X1	T49.0X2	T49.0X3	T49.0X4	T49.0X5	T49.0X6
Starch	T50.901	T50.902	T50.903	T50.904	T50.905	T50.906
Stelazine	T43.3X1	T43.3X2	T43.3X3	T43.3X4	T43.3X5	T43.3X6
Stemetil	T43.3X1	T43.3X2	T43.3X3	T43.3X4	T43.3X5	T43.3X6
Stepronin	T48.4X1	T48.4X2	T48.4X3	T48.4X4	T48.4X5	T48.4X6
Sterculia	T47.4X1	T47.4X2	T47.4X3	T47.4X4	T47.4X5	T47.4X6
Sternutator gas	T59.891	T59.892	T59.893	T59.894	—	—
Steroid	T38.0X1	T38.0X2	T38.0X3	T38.0X4	T38.0X5	T38.0X6
anabolic	T38.7X1	T38.7X2	T38.7X3	T38.7X4	T38.7X5	T38.7X6
androgenic	T38.7X1	T38.7X2	T38.7X3	T38.7X4	T38.7X5	T38.7X6
antineoplastic, hormone	T38.7X1	T38.7X2	T38.7X3	T38.7X4	T38.7X5	T38.7X6
estrogen	T38.5X1	T38.5X2	T38.5X3	T38.5X4	T38.5X5	T38.5X6
ENT agent	T49.6X1	T49.6X2	T49.6X3	T49.6X4	T49.6X5	T49.6X6
ophthalmic preparation	T49.5X1	T49.5X2	T49.5X3	T49.5X4	T49.5X5	T49.5X6
topical NEC	T49.0X1	T49.0X2	T49.0X3	T49.0X4	T49.0X5	T49.0X6
Stibine	T56.891	T56.892	T56.893	T56.894	—	—
Stibogluconate	T37.3X1	T37.3X2	T37.3X3	T37.3X4	T37.3X5	T37.3X6
Stibophen	T37.4X1	T37.4X2	T37.4X3	T37.4X4	T37.4X5	T37.4X6
Stilbamidine (isetionate)	T37.3X1	T37.3X2	T37.3X3	T37.3X4	T37.3X5	T37.3X6
Stilbestrol	T38.5X1	T38.5X2	T38.5X3	T38.5X4	T38.5X5	T38.5X6
Stilboestrol	T38.5X1	T38.5X2	T38.5X3	T38.5X4	T38.5X5	T38.5X6
Stimulant						
central nervous system — see also Psychostimulant	T43.601	T43.602	T43.603	T43.604	T43.605	T43.606
analeptics	T50.7X1	T50.7X2	T50.7X3	T50.7X4	T50.7X5	T50.7X6
opiate antagonist	T50.7X1	T50.7X2	T50.7X3	T50.7X4	T50.7X5	T50.7X6
psychotherapeutic NEC — see also Psychotherapeutic drug	T43.601	T43.602	T43.603	T43.604	T43.605	T43.606
specified NEC	T43.691	T43.692	T43.693	T43.694	T43.695	T43.696
Stimulant — continued						
respiratory	T48.901	T48.902	T48.903	T48.904	T48.905	T48.906
Stone-dissolving drug	T50.901	T50.902	T50.903	T50.904	T50.905	T50.906
Storage battery (cells) (acid)	T54.2X1	T54.2X2	T54.2X3	T54.2X4	—	—
Stovaine	T41.3X1	T41.3X2	T41.3X3	T41.3X4	T41.3X5	T41.3X6
infiltration (subcutaneous)	T41.3X1	T41.3X2	T41.3X3	T41.3X4	T41.3X5	T41.3X6
nerve block (peripheral) (plexus)	T41.3X1	T41.3X2	T41.3X3	T41.3X4	T41.3X5	T41.3X6
spinal	T41.3X1	T41.3X2	T41.3X3	T41.3X4	T41.3X5	T41.3X6
topical (surface)	T41.3X1	T41.3X2	T41.3X3	T41.3X4	T41.3X5	T41.3X6
Stovarsal	T37.8X1	T37.8X2	T37.8X3	T37.8X4	T37.8X5	T37.8X6
Stove gas — see Gas, stove						
Stoxil	T49.5X1	T49.5X2	T49.5X3	T49.5X4	T49.5X5	T49.5X6
Stramonium	T48.6X1	T48.6X2	T48.6X3	T48.6X4	T48.6X5	T48.6X6
natural state	T62.2X1	T62.2X2	T62.2X3	T62.2X4	—	—
Streptodornase	T45.3X1	T45.3X2	T45.3X3	T45.3X4	T45.3X5	T45.3X6
Streptoduocin	T36.5X1	T36.5X2	T36.5X3	T36.5X4	T36.5X5	T36.5X6
Streptokinase	T45.611	T45.612	T45.613	T45.614	T45.615	T45.616
Streptomycin (derivative)	T36.5X1	T36.5X2	T36.5X3	T36.5X4	T36.5X5	T36.5X6
Streptonivicin	T36.5X1	T36.5X2	T36.5X3	T36.5X4	T36.5X5	T36.5X6
Streptovarycin	T36.5X1	T36.5X2	T36.5X3	T36.5X4	T36.5X5	T36.5X6
Streptozocin	T45.1X1	T45.1X2	T45.1X3	T45.1X4	T45.1X5	T45.1X6
Streptozotocin	T45.1X1	T45.1X2	T45.1X3	T45.1X4	T45.1X5	T45.1X6
Stripper (paint) (solvent)	T52.8X1	T52.8X2	T52.8X3	T52.8X4	—	—
Strobane	T60.1X1	T60.1X2	T60.1X3	T60.1X4	—	—
Strofantina	T46.0X1	T46.0X2	T46.0X3	T46.0X4	T46.0X5	T46.0X6
Strophanthin (g) (k)	T46.0X1	T46.0X2	T46.0X3	T46.0X4	T46.0X5	T46.0X6
Strophanthus	T46.0X1	T46.0X2	T46.0X3	T46.0X4	T46.0X5	T46.0X6
Strophantin	T46.0X1	T46.0X2	T46.0X3	T46.0X4	T46.0X5	T46.0X6
Strophantin-g	T46.0X1	T46.0X2	T46.0X3	T46.0X4	T46.0X5	T46.0X6
Strychnine (nonmedicinal) (pesticide) (salts)	T65.1X1	T65.1X2	T65.1X3	T65.1X4	—	—
medicinal	T48.291	T48.292	T48.293	T48.294	T48.295	T48.296
Strychnos (ignatii) — see Strychnine						
Styramate	T42.8X1	T42.8X2	T42.8X3	T42.8X4	T42.8X5	T42.8X6
Styrene	T65.891	T65.892	T65.893	T65.894		
Succinimide, antiepileptic or anticonvulsant	T42.2X1	T42.2X2	T42.2X3	T42.2X4	T42.2X5	T42.2X6
mercuric — see Mercury						
Succinylcholine	T48.1X1	T48.1X2	T48.1X3	T48.1X4	T48.1X5	T48.1X6
Succinylsulfathiazole	T37.0X1	T37.0X2	T37.0X3	T37.0X4	T37.0X5	T37.0X6
Sucralfate	T47.1X1	T47.1X2	T47.1X3	T47.1X4	T47.1X5	T47.1X6
Sucrose	T50.3X1	T50.3X2	T50.3X3	T50.3X4	T50.3X5	T50.3X6
Sufentanil	T40.4X1	T40.4X2	T40.4X3	T40.4X4	T40.4X5	T40.4X6
Sulbactam	T36.0X1	T36.0X2	T36.0X3	T36.0X4	T36.0X5	T36.0X6
Sulbenicillin	T36.0X1	T36.0X2	T36.0X3	T36.0X4	T36.0X5	T36.0X6
Sulbentine	T49.0X1	T49.0X2	T49.0X3	T49.0X4	T49.0X5	T49.0X6
Sulfacetamide	T49.0X1	T49.0X2	T49.0X3	T49.0X4	T49.0X5	T49.0X6
ophthalmic preparation	T49.5X1	T49.5X2	T49.5X3	T49.5X4	T49.5X5	T49.5X6
Sulfachlorpyridazine	T37.0X1	T37.0X2	T37.0X3	T37.0X4	T37.0X5	T37.0X6
Sulfacitine	T37.0X1	T37.0X2	T37.0X3	T37.0X4	T37.0X5	T37.0X6
Sulfadiasulfone sodium	T37.0X1	T37.0X2	T37.0X3	T37.0X4	T37.0X5	T37.0X6
Sulfadiazine	T37.0X1	T37.0X2	T37.0X3	T37.0X4	T37.0X5	T37.0X6
silver (topical)	T49.0X1	T49.0X2	T49.0X3	T49.0X4	T49.0X5	T49.0X6
Sulfadimethoxine	T37.0X1	T37.0X2	T37.0X3	T37.0X4	T37.0X5	T37.0X6
Sulfadimidine	T37.0X1	T37.0X2	T37.0X3	T37.0X4	T37.0X5	T37.0X6
Sulfadoxine	T37.0X1	T37.0X2	T37.0X3	T37.0X4	T37.0X5	T37.0X6
with pyrimethamine	T37.2X1	T37.2X2	T37.2X3	T37.2X4	T37.2X5	T37.2X6
Sulfaethidole	T37.0X1	T37.0X2	T37.0X3	T37.0X4	T37.0X5	T37.0X6
Sulfafurazole	T37.0X1	T37.0X2	T37.0X3	T37.0X4	T37.0X5	T37.0X6
Sulfaguanidine	T37.0X1	T37.0X2	T37.0X3	T37.0X4	T37.0X5	T37.0X6
Sulfalene	T37.0X1	T37.0X2	T37.0X3	T37.0X4	T37.0X5	T37.0X6
Sulfaloxate	T37.0X1	T37.0X2	T37.0X3	T37.0X4	T37.0X5	T37.0X6
Sulfaloxic acid	T37.0X1	T37.0X2	T37.0X3	T37.0X4	T37.0X5	T37.0X6
Sulfamazone	T39.2X1	T39.2X2	T39.2X3	T39.2X4	T39.2X5	T39.2X6
Sulfamerazine	T37.0X1	T37.0X2	T37.0X3	T37.0X4	T37.0X5	T37.0X6
Sulfameter	T37.0X1	T37.0X2	T37.0X3	T37.0X4	T37.0X5	T37.0X6
Sulfamethazine	T37.0X1	T37.0X2	T37.0X3	T37.0X4	T37.0X5	T37.0X6
Sulfamethizole	T37.0X1	T37.0X2	T37.0X3	T37.0X4	T37.0X5	T37.0X6
Sulfamethoxazole	T37.0X1	T37.0X2	T37.0X3	T37.0X4	T37.0X5	T37.0X6
with trimethoprim	T36.8X1	T36.8X2	T36.8X3	T36.8X4	T36.8X5	T36.8X6
Sulfamethoxydiazine	T37.0X1	T37.0X2	T37.0X3	T37.0X4	T37.0X5	T37.0X6
Sulfamethoxypyridazine	T37.0X1	T37.0X2	T37.0X3	T37.0X4	T37.0X5	T37.0X6
Sulfamethylthiazole	T37.0X1	T37.0X2	T37.0X3	T37.0X4	T37.0X5	T37.0X6
Sulfametoxydiazine	T37.0X1	T37.0X2	T37.0X3	T37.0X4	T37.0X5	T37.0X6
Sulfamidopyrine	T39.2X1	T39.2X2	T39.2X3	T39.2X4	T39.2X5	T39.2X6
Sulfamonomethoxine	T37.0X1	T37.0X2	T37.0X3	T37.0X4	T37.0X5	T37.0X6
Sulfamoxole	T37.0X1	T37.0X2	T37.0X3	T37.0X4	T37.0X5	T37.0X6
Sulfamylon	T49.0X1	T49.0X2	T49.0X3	T49.0X4	T49.0X5	T49.0X6
Sulfan blue (diagnostic dye)	T50.8X1	T50.8X2	T50.8X3	T50.8X4	T50.8X5	T50.8X6
Sulfanilamide	T37.0X1	T37.0X2	T37.0X3	T37.0X4	T37.0X5	T37.0X6
Sulfanilylguanidine	T37.0X1	T37.0X2	T37.0X3	T37.0X4	T37.0X5	T37.0X6

Additional Character May Be Required — Refer to the Tabular List for Character Selection   ▽ Subterms under main terms may continue to next column or page

Substance	Poisoning, Accidental (unintentional)	Poisoning, Intentional Self-harm	Poisoning, Assault	Poisoning, Undetermined	Adverse Effect	Under-dosing
Sulfaperin	T37.0X1	T37.0X2	T37.0X3	T37.0X4	T37.0X5	T37.0X6
Sulfaphenazole	T37.0X1	T37.0X2	T37.0X3	T37.0X4	T37.0X5	T37.0X6
Sulfaphenylthiazole	T37.0X1	T37.0X2	T37.0X3	T37.0X4	T37.0X5	T37.0X6
Sulfaproxyline	T37.0X1	T37.0X2	T37.0X3	T37.0X4	T37.0X5	T37.0X6
Sulfapyridine	T37.0X1	T37.0X2	T37.0X3	T37.0X4	T37.0X5	T37.0X6
Sulfapyrimidine	T37.0X1	T37.0X2	T37.0X3	T37.0X4	T37.0X5	T37.0X6
Sulfarsphenamine	T37.8X1	T37.8X2	T37.8X3	T37.8X4	T37.8X5	T37.8X6
Sulfasalazine	T37.0X1	T37.0X2	T37.0X3	T37.0X4	T37.0X5	T37.0X6
Sulfasuxidine	T37.0X1	T37.0X2	T37.0X3	T37.0X4	T37.0X5	T37.0X6
Sulfasymazine	T37.0X1	T37.0X2	T37.0X3	T37.0X4	T37.0X5	T37.0X6
Sulfated amylopectin	T47.8X1	T47.8X2	T47.8X3	T47.8X4	T47.8X5	T47.8X6
Sulfathiazole	T37.0X1	T37.0X2	T37.0X3	T37.0X4	T37.0X5	T37.0X6
Sulfatostearate	T49.2X1	T49.2X2	T49.2X3	T49.2X4	T49.2X5	T49.2X6
Sulfinpyrazone	T50.4X1	T50.4X2	T50.4X3	T50.4X4	T50.4X5	T50.4X6
Sulfiram	T49.0X1	T49.0X2	T49.0X3	T49.0X4	T49.0X5	T49.0X6
Sulfisomidine	T37.0X1	T37.0X2	T37.0X3	T37.0X4	T37.0X5	T37.0X6
Sulfisoxazole	T37.0X1	T37.0X2	T37.0X3	T37.0X4	T37.0X5	T37.0X6
ophthalmic preparation	T49.5X1	T49.5X2	T49.5X3	T49.5X4	T49.5X5	T49.5X6
Sulfobromophthalein (sodium)	T50.8X1	T50.8X2	T50.8X3	T50.8X4	T50.8X5	T50.8X6
Sulfobromphthalein	T50.8X1	T50.8X2	T50.8X3	T50.8X4	T50.8X5	T50.8X6
Sulfogaiacol	T48.4X1	T48.4X2	T48.4X3	T48.4X4	T48.4X5	T48.4X6
Sulfomyxin	T36.8X1	T36.8X2	T36.8X3	T36.8X4	T36.8X5	T36.8X6
Sulfonal	T42.6X1	T42.6X2	T42.6X3	T42.6X4	T42.6X5	T42.6X6
Sulfonamide NEC	T37.0X1	T37.0X2	T37.0X3	T37.0X4	T37.0X5	T37.0X6
eye	T49.5X1	T49.5X2	T49.5X3	T49.5X4	T49.5X5	T49.5X6
Sulfonazide	T37.1X1	T37.1X2	T37.1X3	T37.1X4	T37.1X5	T37.1X6
Sulfones	T37.1X1	T37.1X2	T37.1X3	T37.1X4	T37.1X5	T37.1X6
Sulfonethylmethane	T42.6X1	T42.6X2	T42.6X3	T42.6X4	T42.6X5	T42.6X6
Sulfonmethane	T42.6X1	T42.6X2	T42.6X3	T42.6X4	T42.6X5	T42.6X6
Sulfonphthal, sulfonphthol	T50.8X1	T50.8X2	T50.8X3	T50.8X4	T50.8X5	T50.8X6
Sulfonylurea derivatives, oral	T38.3X1	T38.3X2	T38.3X3	T38.3X4	T38.3X5	T38.3X6
Sulforidazine	T43.3X1	T43.3X2	T43.3X3	T43.3X4	T43.3X5	T43.3X6
Sulfoxone	T37.1X1	T37.1X2	T37.1X3	T37.1X4	T37.1X5	T37.1X6
Sulfuric acid	T54.2X1	T54.2X2	T54.2X3	T54.2X4	—	—
Sulfur, sulfurated, sulfuric, sulfurous, sulfuryl (compounds NEC) (medicinal)	T49.4X1	T49.4X2	T49.4X3	T49.4X4	T49.4X5	T49.4X6
acid	T54.2X1	T54.2X2	T54.2X3	T54.2X4	—	—
dioxide (gas)	T59.1X1	T59.1X2	T59.1X3	T59.1X4	—	—
ether — see Ether(s)						
hydrogen	T59.6X1	T59.6X2	T59.6X3	T59.6X4	—	—
medicinal (keratolytic) (ointment) NEC	T49.4X1	T49.4X2	T49.4X3	T49.4X4	T49.4X5	T49.4X6
ointment	T49.0X1	T49.0X2	T49.0X3	T49.0X4	T49.0X5	T49.0X6
pesticide (vapor)	T60.91	T60.92	T60.93	T60.94	—	—
vapor NEC	T59.891	T59.892	T59.893	T59.894	—	—
Sulglicotide	T47.1X1	T47.1X2	T47.1X3	T47.1X4	T47.1X5	T47.1X6
Sulindac	T39.391	T39.392	T39.393	T39.394	T39.395	T39.396
Sulisatin	T47.2X1	T47.2X2	T47.2X3	T47.2X4	T47.2X5	T47.2X6
Sulisobenzone	T49.3X1	T49.3X2	T49.3X3	T49.3X4	T49.3X5	T49.3X6
Sulkowitch's reagent	T50.8X1	T50.8X2	T50.8X3	T50.8X4	T50.8X5	T50.8X6
Sulmetozine	T44.3X1	T44.3X2	T44.3X3	T44.3X4	T44.3X5	T44.3X6
Suloctidil	T46.7X1	T46.7X2	T46.7X3	T46.7X4	T46.7X5	T46.7X6
Sulph- — see also Sulf-						
Sulphadiazine	T37.0X1	T37.0X2	T37.0X3	T37.0X4	T37.0X5	T37.0X6
Sulphadimethoxine	T37.0X1	T37.0X2	T37.0X3	T37.0X4	T37.0X5	T37.0X6
Sulphadimidine	T37.0X1	T37.0X2	T37.0X3	T37.0X4	T37.0X5	T37.0X6
Sulphadione	T37.1X1	T37.1X2	T37.1X3	T37.1X4	T37.1X5	T37.1X6
Sulphafurazole	T37.0X1	T37.0X2	T37.0X3	T37.0X4	T37.0X5	T37.0X6
Sulphamethizole	T37.0X1	T37.0X2	T37.0X3	T37.0X4	T37.0X5	T37.0X6
Sulphamethoxazole	T37.0X1	T37.0X2	T37.0X3	T37.0X4	T37.0X5	T37.0X6
Sulphan blue	T50.8X1	T50.8X2	T50.8X3	T50.8X4	T50.8X5	T50.8X6
Sulphaphenazole	T37.0X1	T37.0X2	T37.0X3	T37.0X4	T37.0X5	T37.0X6
Sulphapyridine	T37.0X1	T37.0X2	T37.0X3	T37.0X4	T37.0X5	T37.0X6
Sulphasalazine	T37.0X1	T37.0X2	T37.0X3	T37.0X4	T37.0X5	T37.0X6
Sulphinpyrazone	T50.4X1	T50.4X2	T50.4X3	T50.4X4	T50.4X5	T50.4X6
Sulpiride	T43.591	T43.592	T43.593	T43.594	T43.595	T43.596
Sulprostone	T48.0X1	T48.0X2	T48.0X3	T48.0X4	T48.0X5	T48.0X6
Sulpyrine	T39.2X1	T39.2X2	T39.2X3	T39.2X4	T39.2X5	T39.2X6
Sultamicillin	T36.0X1	T36.0X2	T36.0X3	T36.0X4	T36.0X5	T36.0X6
Sulthiame	T42.6X1	T42.6X2	T42.6X3	T42.6X4	T42.6X5	T42.6X6
Sultiame	T42.6X1	T42.6X2	T42.6X3	T42.6X4	T42.6X5	T42.6X6
Sultopride	T43.591	T43.592	T43.593	T43.594	T43.595	T43.596
Sumatriptan	T39.8X1	T39.8X2	T39.8X3	T39.8X4	T39.8X5	T39.8X6
Sunflower seed oil	T46.6X1	T46.6X2	T46.6X3	T46.6X4	T46.6X5	T46.6X6
Superinone	T48.4X1	T48.4X2	T48.4X3	T48.4X4	T48.4X5	T48.4X6
Suprofen	T39.311	T39.312	T39.313	T39.314	T39.315	T39.316
Suramin (sodium)	T37.4X1	T37.4X2	T37.4X3	T37.4X4	T37.4X5	T37.4X6
Surfacaine	T41.3X1	T41.3X2	T41.3X3	T41.3X4	T41.3X5	T41.3X6
Surital	T41.1X1	T41.1X2	T41.1X3	T41.1X4	T41.1X5	T41.1X6
Sutilains	T45.3X1	T45.3X2	T45.3X3	T45.3X4	T45.3X5	T45.3X6
Suxamethonium (chloride)	T48.1X1	T48.1X2	T48.1X3	T48.1X4	T48.1X5	T48.1X6
Suxethonium (chloride)	T48.1X1	T48.1X2	T48.1X3	T48.1X4	T48.1X5	T48.1X6
Suxibuzone	T39.2X1	T39.2X2	T39.2X3	T39.2X4	T39.2X5	T39.2X6
Sweetener	T50.901	T50.902	T50.903	T50.904	T50.905	T50.906
Sweet niter spirit	T46.3X1	T46.3X2	T46.3X3	T46.3X4	T46.3X5	T46.3X6
Sweet oil (birch)	T49.3X1	T49.3X2	T49.3X3	T49.3X4	T49.3X5	T49.3X6
Sym-dichloroethyl ether	T53.6X1	T53.6X2	T53.6X3	T53.6X4	—	—
Sympatholytic NEC	T44.8X1	T44.8X2	T44.8X3	T44.8X4	T44.8X5	T44.8X6
haloalkylamine	T44.8X1	T44.8X2	T44.8X3	T44.8X4	T44.8X5	T44.8X6
Sympathomimetic NEC	T44.901	T44.902	T44.903	T44.904	T44.905	T44.906
anti-common-cold	T48.5X1	T48.5X2	T48.5X3	T48.5X4	T48.5X5	T48.5X6
bronchodilator	T48.6X1	T48.6X2	T48.6X3	T48.6X4	T48.6X5	T48.6X6
specified NEC	T44.991	T44.992	T44.993	T44.994	T44.995	T44.996
Synagis	T50.B91	T50.B92	T50.B93	T50.B94	T50.B95	T50.B96
Synalar	T49.0X1	T49.0X2	T49.0X3	T49.0X4	T49.0X5	T49.0X6
Synthroid	T38.1X1	T38.1X2	T38.1X3	T38.1X4	T38.1X5	T38.1X6
Syntocinon	T48.0X1	T48.0X2	T48.0X3	T48.0X4	T48.0X5	T48.0X6
Syrosingopine	T46.5X1	T46.5X2	T46.5X3	T46.5X4	T46.5X5	T46.5X6
Systemic drug	T45.91	T45.92	T45.93	T45.94	T45.95	T45.96
specified NEC	T45.8X1	T45.8X2	T45.8X3	T45.8X4	T45.8X5	T45.8X6
Tablets — see also specified substance	T50.901	T50.902	T50.903	T50.904	T50.905	T50.906
Tace	T38.5X1	T38.5X2	T38.5X3	T38.5X4	T38.5X5	T38.5X6
Tacrine	T44.0X1	T44.0X2	T44.0X3	T44.0X4	T44.0X5	T44.0X6
Tadalafil	T46.7X1	T46.7X2	T46.7X3	T46.7X4	T46.7X5	T46.7X6
Talampicillin	T36.0X1	T36.0X2	T36.0X3	T36.0X4	T36.0X5	T36.0X6
Talbutal	T42.3X1	T42.3X2	T42.3X3	T42.3X4	T42.3X5	T42.3X6
Talc powder	T49.3X1	T49.3X2	T49.3X3	T49.3X4	T49.3X5	T49.3X6
Talcum	T49.3X1	T49.3X2	T49.3X3	T49.3X4	T49.3X5	T49.3X6
Taleranol	T38.6X1	T38.6X2	T38.6X3	T38.6X4	T38.6X5	T38.6X6
Tamoxifen	T38.6X1	T38.6X2	T38.6X3	T38.6X4	T38.6X5	T38.6X6
Tamsulosin	T44.6X1	T44.6X2	T44.6X3	T44.6X4	T44.6X5	T44.6X6
Tandearil, tanderil	T39.2X1	T39.2X2	T39.2X3	T39.2X4	T39.2X5	T39.2X6
Tannic acid	T49.2X1	T49.2X2	T49.2X3	T49.2X4	T49.2X5	T49.2X6
medicinal (astringent)	T49.2X1	T49.2X2	T49.2X3	T49.2X4	T49.2X5	T49.2X6
Tannin — see Tannic acid						
Tansy	T62.2X1	T62.2X2	T62.2X3	T62.2X4	—	—
TAO	T36.3X1	T36.3X2	T36.3X3	T36.3X4	T36.3X5	T36.3X6
Tapazole	T38.2X1	T38.2X2	T38.2X3	T38.2X4	T38.2X5	T38.2X6
Taractan	T43.591	T43.592	T43.593	T43.594	T43.595	T43.596
Tarantula (venomous)	T63.321	T63.322	T63.323	T63.324		
Tartar emetic	T37.8X1	T37.8X2	T37.8X3	T37.8X4	T37.8X5	T37.8X6
Tartaric acid	T65.891	T65.892	T65.893	T65.894	—	—
Tartrated antimony (anti-infective)	T37.8X1	T37.8X2	T37.8X3	T37.8X4	T37.8X5	T37.8X6
Tartrate, laxative	T47.4X1	T47.4X2	T47.4X3	T47.4X4	T47.4X5	T47.4X6
Tar NEC	T52.0X1	T52.0X2	T52.0X3	T52.0X4	—	—
camphor	T60.1X1	T60.1X2	T60.1X3	T60.1X4	—	—
distillate	T49.1X1	T49.1X2	T49.1X3	T49.1X4	T49.1X5	T49.1X6
fumes	T59.891	T59.892	T59.893	T59.894	—	—
medicinal	T49.1X1	T49.1X2	T49.1X3	T49.1X4	T49.1X5	T49.1X6
ointment	T49.1X1	T49.1X2	T49.1X3	T49.1X4	T49.1X5	T49.1X6
Tauromustine	T45.1X1	T45.1X2	T45.1X3	T45.1X4	T45.1X5	T45.1X6
TCA — see Trichloroacetic acid						
TCDD	T53.7X1	T53.7X2	T53.7X3	T53.7X4	—	—
TDI (vapor)	T65.0X1	T65.0X2	T65.0X3	T65.0X4	—	—
Tear						
gas	T59.3X1	T59.3X2	T59.3X3	T59.3X4	—	—
solution	T49.5X1	T49.5X2	T49.5X3	T49.5X4	T49.5X5	T49.5X6
Teclothiazide	T50.2X1	T50.2X2	T50.2X3	T50.2X4	T50.2X5	T50.2X6
Teclozan	T37.3X1	T37.3X2	T37.3X3	T37.3X4	T37.3X5	T37.3X6
Tegafur	T45.1X1	T45.1X2	T45.1X3	T45.1X4	T45.1X5	T45.1X6
Tegretol	T42.1X1	T42.1X2	T42.1X3	T42.1X4	T42.1X5	T42.1X6
Teicoplanin	T36.8X1	T36.8X2	T36.8X3	T36.8X4	T36.8X5	T36.8X6
Telepaque	T50.8X1	T50.8X2	T50.8X3	T50.8X4	T50.8X5	T50.8X6
Tellurium	T56.891	T56.892	T56.893	T56.894	—	—
fumes	T56.891	T56.892	T56.893	T56.894	—	—
TEM	T45.1X1	T45.1X2	T45.1X3	T45.1X4	T45.1X5	T45.1X6
Temazepam	T42.4X1	T42.4X2	T42.4X3	T42.4X4	T42.4X5	T42.4X6
Temocillin	T36.0X1	T36.0X2	T36.0X3	T36.0X4	T36.0X5	T36.0X6
Tenamfetamine	T43.621	T43.622	T43.623	T43.624	T43.625	T43.626
Teniposide	T45.1X1	T45.1X2	T45.1X3	T45.1X4	T45.1X5	T45.1X6
Tenitramine	T46.3X1	T46.3X2	T46.3X3	T46.3X4	T46.3X5	T46.3X6
Tenoglicin	T48.4X1	T48.4X2	T48.4X3	T48.4X4	T48.4X5	T48.4X6
Tenonitrozole	T37.3X1	T37.3X2	T37.3X3	T37.3X4	T37.3X5	T37.3X6
Tenoxicam	T39.391	T39.392	T39.393	T39.394	T39.395	T39.396
TEPA	T45.1X1	T45.1X2	T45.1X3	T45.1X4	T45.1X5	T45.1X6
TEPP	T60.0X1	T60.0X2	T60.0X3	T60.0X4	—	—
Teprotide	T46.5X1	T46.5X2	T46.5X3	T46.5X4	T46.5X5	T46.5X6
Terazosin	T44.6X1	T44.6X2	T44.6X3	T44.6X4	T44.6X5	T44.6X6
Terbufos	T60.0X1	T60.0X2	T60.0X3	T60.0X4	—	—
Terbutaline	T48.6X1	T48.6X2	T48.6X3	T48.6X4	T48.6X5	T48.6X6

Terconazole

ICD-10-CM 2018

Table of Drugs and Chemicals

Terconazole — Ticlatone

392   Additional Character May Be Required — Refer to the Tabular List for Character Selection   ▽ Subterms under main terms may continue to next column or page

Substance	Poisoning, Accidental (unintentional)	Poisoning, Intentional Self-harm	Poisoning, Assault	Poisoning, Undetermined	Adverse Effect	Under-dosing
Terconazole	T49.0X1	T49.0X2	T49.0X3	T49.0X4	T49.0X5	T49.0X6
Terfenadine	T45.0X1	T45.0X2	T45.0X3	T45.0X4	T45.0X5	T45.0X6
Teriparatide (acetate)	T50.991	T50.992	T50.993	T50.994	T50.995	T50.996
Terizidone	T37.1X1	T37.1X2	T37.1X3	T37.1X4	T37.1X5	T37.1X6
Terlipressin	T38.891	T38.892	T38.893	T38.894	T38.895	T38.896
Terodiline	T46.3X1	T46.3X2	T46.3X3	T46.3X4	T46.3X5	T46.3X6
Teroxalene	T37.4X1	T37.4X2	T37.4X3	T37.4X4	T37.4X5	T37.4X6
Terpin (cis) **hydrate**	T48.4X1	T48.4X2	T48.4X3	T48.4X4	T48.4X5	T48.4X6
Terramycin	T36.4X1	T36.4X2	T36.4X3	T36.4X4	T36.4X5	T36.4X6
Tertatolol	T44.7X1	T44.7X2	T44.7X3	T44.7X4	T44.7X5	T44.7X6
Tessalon	T48.3X1	T48.3X2	T48.3X3	T48.3X4	T48.3X5	T48.3X6
Testolactone	T38.7X1	T38.7X2	T38.7X3	T38.7X4	T38.7X5	T38.7X6
Testosterone	T38.7X1	T38.7X2	T38.7X3	T38.7X4	T38.7X5	T38.7X6
Tetanus toxoid or vaccine	T50.A91	T50.A92	T50.A93	T50.A94	T50.A95	T50.A96
antitoxin	T50.Z11	T50.Z12	T50.Z13	T50.Z14	T50.Z15	T50.Z16
immune globulin (human)	T50.Z11	T50.Z12	T50.Z13	T50.Z14	T50.Z15	T50.Z16
toxoid	T50.A91	T50.A92	T50.A93	T50.A94	T50.A95	T50.A96
with diphtheria toxoid	T50.A21	T50.A22	T50.A23	T50.A24	T50.A25	T50.A26
with pertussis	T50.A11	T50.A12	T50.A13	T50.A14	T50.A15	T50.A16
Tetrabenazine	T43.591	T43.592	T43.593	T43.594	T43.595	T43.596
Tetracaine	T41.3X1	T41.3X2	T41.3X3	T41.3X4	T41.3X5	T41.3X6
nerve block (peripheral) (plexus)	T41.3X1	T41.3X2	T41.3X3	T41.3X4	T41.3X5	T41.3X6
regional	T41.3X1	T41.3X2	T41.3X3	T41.3X4	T41.3X5	T41.3X6
spinal	T41.3X1	T41.3X2	T41.3X3	T41.3X4	T41.3X5	T41.3X6
Tetrachlorethylene — see Tetrachloroethylene						
Tetrachlormethiazide	T50.2X1	T50.2X2	T50.2X3	T50.2X4	T50.2X5	T50.2X6
Tetrachloroethane	T53.6X1	T53.6X2	T53.6X3	T53.6X4	—	—
vapor	T53.6X1	T53.6X2	T53.6X3	T53.6X4	—	—
paint or varnish	T53.6X1	T53.6X2	T53.6X3	T53.6X4	—	—
Tetrachloroethylene (liquid)	T53.3X1	T53.3X2	T53.3X3	T53.3X4	—	—
medicinal	T37.4X1	T37.4X2	T37.4X3	T37.4X4	T37.4X5	T37.4X6
vapor	T53.3X1	T53.3X2	T53.3X3	T53.3X4	—	—
Tetrachloromethane — see Carbon tetrachloride						
Tetracosactide	T38.811	T38.812	T38.813	T38.814	T38.815	T38.816
Tetracosactrin	T38.811	T38.812	T38.813	T38.814	T38.815	T38.816
Tetracycline	T36.4X1	T36.4X2	T36.4X3	T36.4X4	T36.4X5	T36.4X6
ophthalmic preparation	T49.5X1	T49.5X2	T49.5X3	T49.5X4	T49.5X5	T49.5X6
topical NEC	T49.0X1	T49.0X2	T49.0X3	T49.0X4	T49.0X5	T49.0X6
Tetradifon	T60.8X1	T60.8X2	T60.8X3	T60.8X4	—	—
Tetradotoxin	T61.771	T61.772	T61.773	T61.774	—	—
Tetraethyl						
lead	T56.0X1	T56.0X2	T56.0X3	T56.0X4	—	—
pyrophosphate	T60.0X1	T60.0X2	T60.0X3	T60.0X4	—	—
Tetraethylammonium chloride	T44.2X1	T44.2X2	T44.2X3	T44.2X4	T44.2X5	T44.2X6
Tetraethylthiuram disulfide	T50.6X1	T50.6X2	T50.6X3	T50.6X4	T50.6X5	T50.6X6
Tetrahydroaminoacridine	T44.0X1	T44.0X2	T44.0X3	T44.0X4	T44.0X5	T44.0X6
Tetrahydrocannabinol	T40.7X1	T40.7X2	T40.7X3	T40.7X4	T40.7X5	T40.7X6
Tetrahydrofuran	T52.8X1	T52.8X2	T52.8X3	T52.8X4	—	—
Tetrahydronaphthalene	T52.8X1	T52.8X2	T52.8X3	T52.8X4	—	—
Tetrahydrozoline	T49.5X1	T49.5X2	T49.5X3	T49.5X4	T49.5X5	T49.5X6
Tetralin	T52.8X1	T52.8X2	T52.8X3	T52.8X4	—	—
Tetramethrin	T60.2X1	T60.2X2	T60.2X3	T60.2X4	—	—
Tetramethylthiuram (disulfide) **NEC**	T60.3X1	T60.3X2	T60.3X3	T60.3X4	—	—
medicinal	T49.0X1	T49.0X2	T49.0X3	T49.0X4	T49.0X5	T49.0X6
Tetramisole	T37.4X1	T37.4X2	T37.4X3	T37.4X4	T37.4X5	T37.4X6
Tetranicotinoyl fructose	T46.7X1	T46.7X2	T46.7X3	T46.7X4	T46.7X5	T46.7X6
Tetrazepam	T42.4X1	T42.4X2	T42.4X3	T42.4X4	T42.4X5	T42.4X6
Tetronal	T42.6X1	T42.6X2	T42.6X3	T42.6X4	T42.6X5	T42.6X6
Tetryl	T65.3X1	T65.3X2	T65.3X3	T65.3X4	—	—
Tetrylammonium chloride	T44.2X1	T44.2X2	T44.2X3	T44.2X4	T44.2X5	T44.2X6
Tetryzoline	T49.5X1	T49.5X2	T49.5X3	T49.5X4	T49.5X5	T49.5X6
Thalidomide	T45.1X1	T45.1X2	T45.1X3	T45.1X4	T45.1X5	T45.1X6
Thallium (compounds) (dust) **NEC**	T56.811	T56.812	T56.813	T56.814	—	—
pesticide	T60.4X1	T60.4X2	T60.4X3	T60.4X4	—	—
THC	T40.7X1	T40.7X2	T40.7X3	T40.7X4	T40.7X5	T40.7X6
Thebacon	T48.3X1	T48.3X2	T48.3X3	T48.3X4	T48.3X5	T48.3X6
Thebaine	T40.2X1	T40.2X2	T40.2X3	T40.2X4	T40.2X5	T40.2X6
Thenoic acid	T49.6X1	T49.6X2	T49.6X3	T49.6X4	T49.6X5	T49.6X6
Thenyldiamine	T45.0X1	T45.0X2	T45.0X3	T45.0X4	T45.0X5	T45.0X6
Theobromine (calcium salicylate)	T48.6X1	T48.6X2	T48.6X3	T48.6X4	T48.6X5	T48.6X6
sodium salicylate	T48.6X1	T48.6X2	T48.6X3	T48.6X4	T48.6X5	T48.6X6
Theophyllamine	T48.6X1	T48.6X2	T48.6X3	T48.6X4	T48.6X5	T48.6X6
Theophylline	T48.6X1	T48.6X2	T48.6X3	T48.6X4	T48.6X5	T48.6X6
aminobenzoic acid	T48.6X1	T48.6X2	T48.6X3	T48.6X4	T48.6X5	T48.6X6

Substance	Poisoning, Accidental (unintentional)	Poisoning, Intentional Self-harm	Poisoning, Assault	Poisoning, Undetermined	Adverse Effect	Under-dosing
Theophylline — *continued*						
ethylenediamine	T48.6X1	T48.6X2	T48.6X3	T48.6X4	T48.6X5	T48.6X6
piperazine	T48.6X1	T48.6X2	T48.6X3	T48.6X4	T48.6X5	T48.6X6
p-amino-benzoate						
Thiabendazole	T37.4X1	T37.4X2	T37.4X3	T37.4X4	T37.4X5	T37.4X6
Thialbarbital	T41.1X1	T41.1X2	T41.1X3	T41.1X4	T41.1X5	T41.1X6
Thiamazole	T38.2X1	T38.2X2	T38.2X3	T38.2X4	T38.2X5	T38.2X6
Thiambutosine	T37.1X1	T37.1X2	T37.1X3	T37.1X4	T37.1X5	T37.1X6
Thiamine	T45.2X1	T45.2X2	T45.2X3	T45.2X4	T45.2X5	T45.2X6
Thiamphenicol	T36.2X1	T36.2X2	T36.2X3	T36.2X4	T36.2X5	T36.2X6
Thiamylal	T41.1X1	T41.1X2	T41.1X3	T41.1X4	T41.1X5	T41.1X6
sodium	T41.1X1	T41.1X2	T41.1X3	T41.1X4	T41.1X5	T41.1X6
Thiazesim	T43.291	T43.292	T43.293	T43.294	T43.295	T43.296
Thiazides (diuretics)	T50.2X1	T50.2X2	T50.2X3	T50.2X4	T50.2X5	T50.2X6
Thiazinamium metilsulfate	T43.3X1	T43.3X2	T43.3X3	T43.3X4	T43.3X5	T43.3X6
Thiethylperazine	T43.3X1	T43.3X2	T43.3X3	T43.3X4	T43.3X5	T43.3X6
Thimerosal	T49.0X1	T49.0X2	T49.0X3	T49.0X4	T49.0X5	T49.0X6
ophthalmic preparation	T49.5X1	T49.5X2	T49.5X3	T49.5X4	T49.5X5	T49.5X6
Thioacetazone	T37.1X1	T37.1X2	T37.1X3	T37.1X4	T37.1X5	T37.1X6
with isoniazid	T37.1X1	T37.1X2	T37.1X3	T37.1X4	T37.1X5	T37.1X6
Thiobarbital sodium	T41.1X1	T41.1X2	T41.1X3	T41.1X4	T41.1X5	T41.1X6
Thiobarbiturate anesthetic	T41.1X1	T41.1X2	T41.1X3	T41.1X4	T41.1X5	T41.1X6
Thiobismol	T37.8X1	T37.8X2	T37.8X3	T37.8X4	T37.8X5	T37.8X6
Thiobutabarbital sodium	T41.1X1	T41.1X2	T41.1X3	T41.1X4	T41.1X5	T41.1X6
Thiocarbamate (insecticide)	T60.0X1	T60.0X2	T60.0X3	T60.0X4	—	—
Thiocarbamide	T38.2X1	T38.2X2	T38.2X3	T38.2X4	T38.2X5	T38.2X6
Thiocarbarsone	T37.8X1	T37.8X2	T37.8X3	T37.8X4	T37.8X5	T37.8X6
Thiocarlide	T37.1X1	T37.1X2	T37.1X3	T37.1X4	T37.1X5	T37.1X6
Thioctamide	T50.991	T50.992	T50.993	T50.994	T50.995	T50.996
Thioctic acid	T50.991	T50.992	T50.993	T50.994	T50.995	T50.996
Thiofos	T60.0X1	T60.0X2	T60.0X3	T60.0X4	—	—
Thioglycolate	T49.4X1	T49.4X2	T49.4X3	T49.4X4	T49.4X5	T49.4X6
Thioglycolic acid	T65.891	T65.892	T65.893	T65.894		
Thioguanine	T45.1X1	T45.1X2	T45.1X3	T45.1X4	T45.1X5	T45.1X6
Thiomercaptomerin	T50.2X1	T50.2X2	T50.2X3	T50.2X4	T50.2X5	T50.2X6
Thiomerin	T50.2X1	T50.2X2	T50.2X3	T50.2X4	T50.2X5	T50.2X6
Thiomersal	T49.0X1	T49.0X2	T49.0X3	T49.0X4	T49.0X5	T49.0X6
Thionazin	T60.0X1	T60.0X2	T60.0X3	T60.0X4	—	—
Thiopental (sodium)	T41.1X1	T41.1X2	T41.1X3	T41.1X4	T41.1X5	T41.1X6
Thiopentone (sodium)	T41.1X1	T41.1X2	T41.1X3	T41.1X4	T41.1X5	T41.1X6
Thiopropazate	T43.3X1	T43.3X2	T43.3X3	T43.3X4	T43.3X5	T43.3X6
Thioproperazine	T43.3X1	T43.3X2	T43.3X3	T43.3X4	T43.3X5	T43.3X6
Thioridazine	T43.3X1	T43.3X2	T43.3X3	T43.3X4	T43.3X5	T43.3X6
Thiosinamine	T49.3X1	T49.3X2	T49.3X3	T49.3X4	T49.3X5	T49.3X6
Thiotepa	T45.1X1	T45.1X2	T45.1X3	T45.1X4	T45.1X5	T45.1X6
Thiothixene	T43.4X1	T43.4X2	T43.4X3	T43.4X4	T43.4X5	T43.4X6
Thiouracil (benzyl) (methyl) (propyl)	T38.2X1	T38.2X2	T38.2X3	T38.2X4	T38.2X5	T38.2X6
Thiourea	T38.2X1	T38.2X2	T38.2X3	T38.2X4	T38.2X5	T38.2X6
Thiphenamil	T44.3X1	T44.3X2	T44.3X3	T44.3X4	T44.3X5	T44.3X6
Thiram	T60.3X1	T60.3X2	T60.3X3	T60.3X4	—	—
medicinal	T49.2X1	T49.2X2	T49.2X3	T49.2X4	T49.2X5	T49.2X6
Thonzylamine (systemic)	T45.0X1	T45.0X2	T45.0X3	T45.0X4	T45.0X5	T45.0X6
mucosal decongestant	T48.5X1	T48.5X2	T48.5X3	T48.5X4	T48.5X5	T48.5X6
Thorazine	T43.3X1	T43.3X2	T43.3X3	T43.3X4	T43.3X5	T43.3X6
Thorium dioxide suspension	T50.8X1	T50.8X2	T50.8X3	T50.8X4	T50.8X5	T50.8X6
Thornapple	T62.2X1	T62.2X2	T62.2X3	T62.2X4	—	—
Throat drug NEC	T49.6X1	T49.6X2	T49.6X3	T49.6X4	T49.6X5	T49.6X6
Thrombin	T45.7X1	T45.7X2	T45.7X3	T45.7X4	T45.7X5	T45.7X6
Thrombolysin	T45.611	T45.612	T45.613	T45.614	T45.615	T45.616
Thromboplastin	T45.7X1	T45.7X2	T45.7X3	T45.7X4	T45.7X5	T45.7X6
Thurfyl nicotinate	T46.7X1	T46.7X2	T46.7X3	T46.7X4	T46.7X5	T46.7X6
Thymol	T49.0X1	T49.0X2	T49.0X3	T49.0X4	T49.0X5	T49.0X6
Thymopentin	T37.5X1	T37.5X2	T37.5X3	T37.5X4	T37.5X5	T37.5X6
Thymoxamine	T46.7X1	T46.7X2	T46.7X3	T46.7X4	T46.7X5	T46.7X6
Thymus extract	T38.891	T38.892	T38.893	T38.894	T38.895	T38.896
Thyreotrophic hormone	T38.811	T38.812	T38.813	T38.814	T38.815	T38.816
Thyroglobulin	T38.1X1	T38.1X2	T38.1X3	T38.1X4	T38.1X5	T38.1X6
Thyroid (hormone)	T38.1X1	T38.1X2	T38.1X3	T38.1X4	T38.1X5	T38.1X6
Thyrolar	T38.1X1	T38.1X2	T38.1X3	T38.1X4	T38.1X5	T38.1X6
Thyrotrophin	T38.811	T38.812	T38.813	T38.814	T38.815	T38.816
Thyrotropic hormone	T38.811	T38.812	T38.813	T38.814	T38.815	T38.816
Thyroxine	T38.1X1	T38.1X2	T38.1X3	T38.1X4	T38.1X5	T38.1X6
Tiabendazole	T37.4X1	T37.4X2	T37.4X3	T37.4X4	T37.4X5	T37.4X6
Tiamizide	T50.2X1	T50.2X2	T50.2X3	T50.2X4	T50.2X5	T50.2X6
Tianeptine	T43.291	T43.292	T43.293	T43.294	T43.295	T43.296
Tiapamil	T46.1X1	T46.1X2	T46.1X3	T46.1X4	T46.1X5	T46.1X6
Tiapride	T43.591	T43.592	T43.593	T43.594	T43.595	T43.596
Tiaprofenic acid	T39.311	T39.312	T39.313	T39.314	T39.315	T39.316
Tiaramide	T39.8X1	T39.8X2	T39.8X3	T39.8X4	T39.8X5	T39.8X6
Ticarcillin	T36.0X1	T36.0X2	T36.0X3	T36.0X4	T36.0X5	T36.0X6
Ticlatone	T49.0X1	T49.0X2	T49.0X3	T49.0X4	T49.0X5	T49.0X6

Substance	Poisoning, Accidental (unintentional)	Poisoning, Intentional Self-harm	Poisoning, Assault	Poisoning, Undetermined	Adverse Effect	Under-dosing
Ticlopidine	T45.521	T45.522	T45.523	T45.524	T45.525	T45.526
Ticrynafen	T50.1X1	T50.1X2	T50.1X3	T50.1X4	T50.1X5	T50.1X6
Tidiacic	T50.991	T50.992	T50.993	T50.994	T50.995	T50.996
Tiemonium	T44.3X1	T44.3X2	T44.3X3	T44.3X4	T44.3X5	T44.3X6
iodide	T44.3X1	T44.3X2	T44.3X3	T44.3X4	T44.3X5	T44.3X6
Tienilic acid	T50.1X1	T50.1X2	T50.1X3	T50.1X4	T50.1X5	T50.1X6
Tifenamil	T44.3X1	T44.3X2	T44.3X3	T44.3X4	T44.3X5	T44.3X6
Tigan	T45.0X1	T45.0X2	T45.0X3	T45.0X4	T45.0X5	T45.0X6
Tigloidine	T44.3X1	T44.3X2	T44.3X3	T44.3X4	T44.3X5	T44.3X6
Tilactase	T47.5X1	T47.5X2	T47.5X3	T47.5X4	T47.5X5	T47.5X6
Tiletamine	T41.291	T41.292	T41.293	T41.294	T41.295	T41.296
Tilidine	T40.4X1	T40.4X2	T40.4X3	T40.4X4	—	—
Timepidium bromide	T44.3X1	T44.3X2	T44.3X3	T44.3X4	T44.3X5	T44.3X6
Timiperone	T43.4X1	T43.4X2	T43.4X3	T43.4X4	T43.4X5	T43.4X6
Timolol	T44.7X1	T44.7X2	T44.7X3	T44.7X4	T44.7X5	T44.7X6
Tincture, iodine — *see* Iodine						
Tindal	T43.3X1	T43.3X2	T43.3X3	T43.3X4	T43.3X5	T43.3X6
Tinidazole	T37.3X1	T37.3X2	T37.3X3	T37.3X4	T37.3X5	T37.3X6
Tinoridine	T39.8X1	T39.8X2	T39.8X3	T39.8X4	T39.8X5	T39.8X6
Tin (chloride) (dust) (oxide)	T56.6X1	T56.6X2	T56.6X3	T56.6X4	—	—
NEC						
anti-infectives	T37.8X1	T37.8X2	T37.8X3	T37.8X4	T37.8X5	T37.8X6
Tiocarlide	T37.1X1	T37.1X2	T37.1X3	T37.1X4	T37.1X5	T37.1X6
Tioclomarol	T45.511	T45.512	T45.513	T45.514	T45.515	T45.516
Tioconazole	T49.0X1	T49.0X2	T49.0X3	T49.0X4	T49.0X5	T49.0X6
Tioguanine	T45.1X1	T45.1X2	T45.1X3	T45.1X4	T45.1X5	T45.1X6
Tiopronin	T50.991	T50.992	T50.993	T50.994	T50.995	T50.996
Tiotixene	T43.4X1	T43.4X2	T43.4X3	T43.4X4	T43.4X5	T43.4X6
Tioxolone	T49.4X1	T49.4X2	T49.4X3	T49.4X4	T49.4X5	T49.4X6
Tipepidine	T48.3X1	T48.3X2	T48.3X3	T48.3X4	T48.3X5	T48.3X6
Tiquizium bromide	T44.3X1	T44.3X2	T44.3X3	T44.3X4	T44.3X5	T44.3X6
Tiratricol	T38.1X1	T38.1X2	T38.1X3	T38.1X4	T38.1X5	T38.1X6
Tisopurine	T50.4X1	T50.4X2	T50.4X3	T50.4X4	T50.4X5	T50.4X6
Titanium (compounds)	T56.891	T56.892	T56.893	T56.894	—	—
(vapor)						
dioxide	T49.3X1	T49.3X2	T49.3X3	T49.3X4	T49.3X5	T49.3X6
ointment	T49.3X1	T49.3X2	T49.3X3	T49.3X4	T49.3X5	T49.3X6
oxide	T49.3X1	T49.3X2	T49.3X3	T49.3X4	T49.3X5	T49.3X6
tetrachloride	T56.891	T56.892	T56.893	T56.894	—	—
Titanocene	T56.891	T56.892	T56.893	T56.894	—	—
Titroid	T38.1X1	T38.1X2	T38.1X3	T38.1X4	T38.1X5	T38.1X6
Tizanidine	T42.8X1	T42.8X2	T42.8X3	T42.8X4	T42.8X5	T42.8X6
TMTD	T60.3X1	T60.3X2	T60.3X3	T60.3X4	—	—
TNT (fumes)	T65.3X1	T65.3X2	T65.3X3	T65.3X4	—	—
Toadstool	T62.0X1	T62.0X2	T62.0X3	T62.0X4	—	—
Tobacco NEC	T65.291	T65.292	T65.293	T65.294	—	—
cigarettes	T65.221	T65.222	T65.223	T65.224	—	—
Indian	T62.2X1	T62.2X2	T62.2X3	T62.2X4	—	—
smoke, second-hand	T65.221	T65.222	T65.223	T65.224	—	—
Tobramycin	T36.5X1	T36.5X2	T36.5X3	T36.5X4	T36.5X5	T36.5X6
Tocainide	T46.2X1	T46.2X2	T46.2X3	T46.2X4	T46.2X5	T46.2X6
Tocoferol	T45.2X1	T45.2X2	T45.2X3	T45.2X4	T45.2X5	T45.2X6
Tocopherol	T45.2X1	T45.2X2	T45.2X3	T45.2X4	T45.2X5	T45.2X6
acetate	T45.2X1	T45.2X2	T45.2X3	T45.2X4	T45.2X5	T45.2X6
Tocosamine	T48.0X1	T48.0X2	T48.0X3	T48.0X4	T48.0X5	T48.0X6
Todralazine	T46.5X1	T46.5X2	T46.5X3	T46.5X4	T46.5X5	T46.5X6
Tofisopam	T42.4X1	T42.4X2	T42.4X3	T42.4X4	T42.4X5	T42.4X6
Tofranil	T43.011	T43.012	T43.013	T43.014	T43.015	T43.016
Toilet deodorizer	T65.891	T65.892	T65.893	T65.894	—	—
Tolamolol	T44.7X1	T44.7X2	T44.7X3	T44.7X4	T44.7X5	T44.7X6
Tolazamide	T38.3X1	T38.3X2	T38.3X3	T38.3X4	T38.3X5	T38.3X6
Tolazoline	T46.7X1	T46.7X2	T46.7X3	T46.7X4	T46.7X5	T46.7X6
Tolbutamide (sodium)	T38.3X1	T38.3X2	T38.3X3	T38.3X4	T38.3X5	T38.3X6
Tolciclate	T49.0X1	T49.0X2	T49.0X3	T49.0X4	T49.0X5	T49.0X6
Tolmetin	T39.391	T39.392	T39.393	T39.394	T39.395	T39.396
Tolnaftate	T49.0X1	T49.0X2	T49.0X3	T49.0X4	T49.0X5	T49.0X6
Tolonidine	T46.5X1	T46.5X2	T46.5X3	T46.5X4	T46.5X5	T46.5X6
Toloxatone	T42.6X1	T42.6X2	T42.6X3	T42.6X4	T42.6X5	T42.6X6
Tolperisone	T44.3X1	T44.3X2	T44.3X3	T44.3X4	T44.3X5	T44.3X6
Tolserol	T42.8X1	T42.8X2	T42.8X3	T42.8X4	T42.8X5	T42.8X6
Toluene (liquid)	T52.2X1	T52.2X2	T52.2X3	T52.2X4	—	—
diisocyanate	T65.0X1	T65.0X2	T65.0X3	T65.0X4	—	—
Toluidine	T65.891	T65.892	T65.893	T65.894	—	—
vapor	T59.891	T59.892	T59.893	T59.894	—	—
Toluol (liquid)	T52.2X1	T52.2X2	T52.2X3	T52.2X4	—	—
vapor	T52.2X1	T52.2X2	T52.2X3	T52.2X4	—	—
Toluylenediamine	T65.3X1	T65.3X2	T65.3X3	T65.3X4	—	—
Tolylene-2,4-diisocyanate	T65.0X1	T65.0X2	T65.0X3	T65.0X4	—	—
Tonic NEC	T50.901	T50.902	T50.903	T50.904	T50.905	T50.906
Topical action drug NEC	T49.91	T49.92	T49.93	T49.94	T49.95	T49.96
ear, nose or throat	T49.6X1	T49.6X2	T49.6X3	T49.6X4	T49.6X5	T49.6X6
eye	T49.5X1	T49.5X2	T49.5X3	T49.5X4	T49.5X5	T49.5X6
skin	T49.91	T49.92	T49.93	T49.94	T49.95	T49.96
Topical action drug — *continued*						
specified NEC	T49.8X1	T49.8X2	T49.8X3	T49.8X4	T49.8X5	T49.8X6
Toquizine	T44.3X1	T44.3X2	T44.3X3	T44.3X4	T44.3X5	T44.3X6
Toremifene	T38.6X1	T38.6X2	T38.6X3	T38.6X4	T38.6X5	T38.6X6
Tosylchloramide sodium	T49.8X1	T49.8X2	T49.8X3	T49.8X4	T49.8X5	T49.8X6
Toxaphene (dust) (spray)	T60.1X1	T60.1X2	T60.1X3	T60.1X4	—	—
Toxin, diphtheria (Schick Test)	T50.8X1	T50.8X2	T50.8X3	T50.8X4	T50.8X5	T50.8X6
Toxoid						
combined	T50.A21	T50.A22	T50.A23	T50.A24	T50.A25	T50.A26
diphtheria	T50.A91	T50.A92	T50.A93	T50.A94	T50.A95	T50.A96
tetanus	T50.A91	T50.A92	T50.A93	T50.A94	T50.A95	T50.A96
Trace element NEC	T45.8X1	T45.8X2	T45.8X3	T45.8X4	T45.8X5	T45.8X6
Tractor fuel NEC	T52.0X1	T52.0X2	T52.0X3	T52.0X4	—	—
Tragacanth	T50.991	T50.992	T50.993	T50.994	T50.995	T50.996
Tramadol	T40.4X1	T40.4X2	T40.4X3	T40.4X4	T40.4X5	T40.4X6
Tramazoline	T48.5X1	T48.5X2	T48.5X3	T48.5X4	T48.5X5	T48.5X6
Tranexamic acid	T45.621	T45.622	T45.623	T45.624	T45.625	T45.626
Tranilast	T45.0X1	T45.0X2	T45.0X3	T45.0X4	T45.0X5	T45.0X6
Tranquilizer NEC	T43.501	T43.502	T43.503	T43.504	T43.505	T43.506
with hypnotic or sedative	T42.6X1	T42.6X2	T42.6X3	T42.6X4	T42.6X5	T42.6X6
benzodiazepine NEC	T42.4X1	T42.4X2	T42.4X3	T42.4X4	T42.4X5	T42.4X6
butyrophenone NEC	T43.591	T43.592	T43.593	T43.594	T43.595	T43.596
carbamate	T43.591	T43.592	T43.593	T43.594	T43.595	T43.596
dimethylamine	T43.3X1	T43.3X2	T43.3X3	T43.3X4	T43.3X5	T43.3X6
ethylamine	T43.3X1	T43.3X2	T43.3X3	T43.3X4	T43.3X5	T43.3X6
hydroxyzine	T43.591	T43.592	T43.593	T43.594	T43.595	T43.596
major NEC	T43.501	T43.502	T43.503	T43.504	T43.505	T43.506
penothiazine NEC	T43.3X1	T43.3X2	T43.3X3	T43.3X4	T43.3X5	T43.3X6
phenothiazine-based	T43.3X1	T43.3X2	T43.3X3	T43.3X4	T43.3X5	T43.3X6
piperazine NEC	T43.3X1	T43.3X2	T43.3X3	T43.3X4	T43.3X5	T43.3X6
piperidine	T43.3X1	T43.3X2	T43.3X3	T43.3X4	T43.3X5	T43.3X6
propylamine	T43.3X1	T43.3X2	T43.3X3	T43.3X4	T43.3X5	T43.3X6
specified NEC	T43.591	T43.592	T43.593	T43.594	T43.595	T43.596
thioxanthene NEC	T43.591	T43.592	T43.593	T43.594	T43.595	T43.596
Tranxene	T42.4X1	T42.4X2	T42.4X3	T42.4X4	T42.4X5	T42.4X6
Tranylcypromine	T43.1X1	T43.1X2	T43.1X3	T43.1X4	T43.1X5	T43.1X6
Trapidil	T46.3X1	T46.3X2	T46.3X3	T46.3X4	T46.3X5	T46.3X6
Trasentine	T44.3X1	T44.3X2	T44.3X3	T44.3X4	T44.3X5	T44.3X6
Travert	T50.3X1	T50.3X2	T50.3X3	T50.3X4	T50.3X5	T50.3X6
Trazodone	T43.211	T43.212	T43.213	T43.214	T43.215	T43.216
Trecator	T37.1X1	T37.1X2	T37.1X3	T37.1X4	T37.1X5	T37.1X6
Treosulfan	T45.1X1	T45.1X2	T45.1X3	T45.1X4	T45.1X5	T45.1X6
Tretamine	T45.1X1	T45.1X2	T45.1X3	T45.1X4	T45.1X5	T45.1X6
Tretinoin	T49.0X1	T49.0X2	T49.0X3	T49.0X4	T49.0X5	T49.0X6
Tretoquinol	T48.6X1	T48.6X2	T48.6X3	T48.6X4	T48.6X5	T48.6X6
Triacetin	T49.0X1	T49.0X2	T49.0X3	T49.0X4	T49.0X5	T49.0X6
Triacetoxyanthracene	T49.4X1	T49.4X2	T49.4X3	T49.4X4	T49.4X5	T49.4X6
Triacetyloleandomycin	T36.3X1	T36.3X2	T36.3X3	T36.3X4	T36.3X5	T36.3X6
Triamcinolone	T38.0X1	T38.0X2	T38.0X3	T38.0X4	T38.0X5	T38.0X6
ENT agent	T49.6X1	T49.6X2	T49.6X3	T49.6X4	T49.6X5	T49.6X6
hexacetonide	T49.0X1	T49.0X2	T49.0X3	T49.0X4	T49.0X5	T49.0X6
ophthalmic preparation	T49.5X1	T49.5X2	T49.5X3	T49.5X4	T49.5X5	T49.5X6
topical NEC	T49.0X1	T49.0X2	T49.0X3	T49.0X4	T49.0X5	T49.0X6
Triampyzine	T44.3X1	T44.3X2	T44.3X3	T44.3X4	T44.3X5	T44.3X6
Triamterene	T50.2X1	T50.2X2	T50.2X3	T50.2X4	T50.2X5	T50.2X6
Triazine (herbicide)	T60.3X1	T60.3X2	T60.3X3	T60.3X4	—	—
Triaziquone	T45.1X1	T45.1X2	T45.1X3	T45.1X4	T45.1X5	T45.1X6
Triazolam	T42.4X1	T42.4X2	T42.4X3	T42.4X4	T42.4X5	T42.4X6
Triazole (herbicide)	T60.3X1	T60.3X2	T60.3X3	T60.3X4	—	—
Tribenoside	T46.991	T46.992	T46.993	T46.994	T46.995	T46.996
Tribromacetaldehyde	T42.6X1	T42.6X2	T42.6X3	T42.6X4	T42.6X5	T42.6X6
Tribromoethanol, rectal	T41.291	T41.292	T41.293	T41.294	T41.295	T41.296
Tribromomethane	T42.6X1	T42.6X2	T42.6X3	T42.6X4	T42.6X5	T42.6X6
Trichlorethane	T53.2X1	T53.2X2	T53.2X3	T53.2X4	—	—
Trichlorethylene	T53.2X1	T53.2X2	T53.2X3	T53.2X4	—	—
Trichlorfon	T60.0X1	T60.0X2	T60.0X3	T60.0X4	—	—
Trichlormethiazide	T50.2X1	T50.2X2	T50.2X3	T50.2X4	T50.2X5	T50.2X6
Trichlormethine	T45.1X1	T45.1X2	T45.1X3	T45.1X4	T45.1X5	T45.1X6
Trichloroacetic acid, Trichloracetic acid	T54.2X1	T54.2X2	T54.2X3	T54.2X4	—	—
medicinal	T49.4X1	T49.4X2	T49.4X3	T49.4X4	T49.4X5	T49.4X6
Trichloroethane	T53.2X1	T53.2X2	T53.2X3	T53.2X4	—	—
Trichloroethanol	T42.6X1	T42.6X2	T42.6X3	T42.6X4	T42.6X5	T42.6X6
Trichloroethylene (liquid)	T53.2X1	T53.2X2	T53.2X3	T53.2X4	—	—
(vapor)						
anesthetic (gas)	T41.0X1	T41.0X2	T41.0X3	T41.0X4	T41.0X5	T41.0X6
vapor NEC	T53.2X1	T53.2X2	T53.2X3	T53.2X4	—	—
Trichloroethyl phosphate	T42.6X1	T42.6X2	T42.6X3	T42.6X4	T42.6X5	T42.6X6
Trichlorofluoromethane NEC	T53.5X1	T53.5X2	T53.5X3	T53.5X4	—	—
Trichloronate	T60.0X1	T60.0X2	T60.0X3	T60.0X4	—	—
Trichloropropane	T53.6X1	T53.6X2	T53.6X3	T53.6X4	—	—

Table of Drugs and Chemicals

Substance	Poisoning, Accidental (unintentional)	Poisoning, Intentional Self-harm	Poisoning, Assault	Poisoning, Undetermined	Adverse Effect	Under-dosing
Trichlorotriethylamine	T45.1X1	T45.1X2	T45.1X3	T45.1X4	T45.1X5	T45.1X6
Trichomonacides NEC	T37.3X1	T37.3X2	T37.3X3	T37.3X4	T37.3X5	T37.3X6
Trichomycin	T36.7X1	T36.7X2	T36.7X3	T36.7X4	T36.7X5	T36.7X6
Triclobisonium chloride	T49.0X1	T49.0X2	T49.0X3	T49.0X4	T49.0X5	T49.0X6
Triclocarban	T49.0X1	T49.0X2	T49.0X3	T49.0X4	T49.0X5	T49.0X6
Triclofos	T42.6X1	T42.6X2	T42.6X3	T42.6X4	T42.6X5	T42.6X6
Triclosan	T49.0X1	T49.0X2	T49.0X3	T49.0X4	T49.0X5	T49.0X6
Tricresyl phosphate	T65.891	T65.892	T65.893	T65.894	—	—
solvent	T52.91	T52.92	T52.93	T52.94	—	—
Tricyclamol chloride	T44.3X1	T44.3X2	T44.3X3	T44.3X4	T44.3X5	T44.3X6
Tridesilon	T49.0X1	T49.0X2	T49.0X3	T49.0X4	T49.0X5	T49.0X6
Tridihexethyl iodide	T44.3X1	T44.3X2	T44.3X3	T44.3X4	T44.3X5	T44.3X6
Tridione	T42.2X1	T42.2X2	T42.2X3	T42.2X4	T42.2X5	T42.2X6
Trientine	T45.8X1	T45.8X2	T45.8X3	T45.8X4	T45.8X5	T45.8X6
Triethanolamine NEC	T54.3X1	T54.3X2	T54.3X3	T54.3X4	—	—
detergent	T54.3X1	T54.3X2	T54.3X3	T54.3X4	—	—
trinitrate (biphosphate)	T46.3X1	T46.3X2	T46.3X3	T46.3X4	T46.3X5	T46.3X6
Triethanomelamine	T45.1X1	T45.1X2	T45.1X3	T45.1X4	T45.1X5	T45.1X6
Triethylenemelamine	T45.1X1	T45.1X2	T45.1X3	T45.1X4	T45.1X5	T45.1X6
Triethylenephosphoramide	T45.1X1	T45.1X2	T45.1X3	T45.1X4	T45.1X5	T45.1X6
Triethylenethiophosphoramide	T45.1X1	T45.1X2	T45.1X3	T45.1X4	T45.1X5	T45.1X6
Trifluoperazine	T43.3X1	T43.3X2	T43.3X3	T43.3X4	T43.3X5	T43.3X6
Trifluoroethyl vinyl ether	T41.0X1	T41.0X2	T41.0X3	T41.0X4	T41.0X5	T41.0X6
Trifluperidol	T43.4X1	T43.4X2	T43.4X3	T43.4X4	T43.4X5	T43.4X6
Triflupromazine	T43.3X1	T43.3X2	T43.3X3	T43.3X4	T43.3X5	T43.3X6
Trifluridine	T37.5X1	T37.5X2	T37.5X3	T37.5X4	T37.5X5	T37.5X6
Triflusal	T45.521	T45.522	T45.523	T45.524	T45.525	T45.526
Trihexyphenidyl	T44.3X1	T44.3X2	T44.3X3	T44.3X4	T44.3X5	T44.3X6
Triiodothyronine	T38.1X1	T38.1X2	T38.1X3	T38.1X4	T38.1X5	T38.1X6
Trilene	T41.0X1	T41.0X2	T41.0X3	T41.0X4	T41.0X5	T41.0X6
Trilostane	T38.991	T38.992	T38.993	T38.994	T38.995	T38.996
Trimebutine	T44.3X1	T44.3X2	T44.3X3	T44.3X4	T44.3X5	T44.3X6
Trimecaine	T41.3X1	T41.3X2	T41.3X3	T41.3X4	T41.3X5	T41.3X6
Trimeprazine (tartrate)	T44.3X1	T44.3X2	T44.3X3	T44.3X4	T44.3X5	T44.3X6
Trimetaphan camsilate	T44.2X1	T44.2X2	T44.2X3	T44.2X4	T44.2X5	T44.2X6
Trimetazidine	T46.7X1	T46.7X2	T46.7X3	T46.7X4	T46.7X5	T46.7X6
Trimethadione	T42.2X1	T42.2X2	T42.2X3	T42.2X4	T42.2X5	T42.2X6
Trimethaphan	T44.2X1	T44.2X2	T44.2X3	T44.2X4	T44.2X5	T44.2X6
Trimethidinium	T44.2X1	T44.2X2	T44.2X3	T44.2X4	T44.2X5	T44.2X6
Trimethobenzamide	T45.0X1	T45.0X2	T45.0X3	T45.0X4	T45.0X5	T45.0X6
Trimethoprim	T37.8X1	T37.8X2	T37.8X3	T37.8X4	T37.8X5	T37.8X6
with sulfamethoxazole	T36.8X1	T36.8X2	T36.8X3	T36.8X4	T36.8X5	T36.8X6
Trimethylcarbinol	T51.3X1	T51.3X2	T51.3X3	T51.3X4	—	—
Trimethylpsoralen	T49.3X1	T49.3X2	T49.3X3	T49.3X4	T49.3X5	T49.3X6
Trimeton	T45.0X1	T45.0X2	T45.0X3	T45.0X4	T45.0X5	T45.0X6
Trimetrexate	T45.1X1	T45.1X2	T45.1X3	T45.1X4	T45.1X5	T45.1X6
Trimipramine	T43.011	T43.012	T43.013	T43.014	T43.015	T43.016
Trimustine	T45.1X1	T45.1X2	T45.1X3	T45.1X4	T45.1X5	T45.1X6
Trinitrine	T46.3X1	T46.3X2	T46.3X3	T46.3X4	T46.3X5	T46.3X6
Trinitrobenzol	T65.3X1	T65.3X2	T65.3X3	T65.3X4	—	—
Trinitrophenol	T65.3X1	T65.3X2	T65.3X3	T65.3X4	—	—
Trinitrotoluene (fumes)	T65.3X1	T65.3X2	T65.3X3	T65.3X4	—	—
Trional	T42.6X1	T42.6X2	T42.6X3	T42.6X4	T42.6X5	T42.6X6
Triorthocresyl phosphate	T65.891	T65.892	T65.893	T65.894	—	—
Trioxide of arsenic	T57.0X1	T57.0X2	T57.0X3	T57.0X4	—	—
Trioxysalen	T49.4X1	T49.4X2	T49.4X3	T49.4X4	T49.4X5	T49.4X6
Tripamide	T50.2X1	T50.2X2	T50.2X3	T50.2X4	T50.2X5	T50.2X6
Triparanol	T46.6X1	T46.6X2	T46.6X3	T46.6X4	T46.6X5	T46.6X6
Tripelennamine	T45.0X1	T45.0X2	T45.0X3	T45.0X4	T45.0X5	T45.0X6
Triperiden	T44.3X1	T44.3X2	T44.3X3	T44.3X4	T44.3X5	T44.3X6
Triperidol	T43.4X1	T43.4X2	T43.4X3	T43.4X4	T43.4X5	T43.4X6
Triphenylphosphate	T65.891	T65.892	T65.893	T65.894	—	—
Triple						
bromides	T42.6X1	T42.6X2	T42.6X3	T42.6X4	T42.6X5	T42.6X6
carbonate	T47.1X1	T47.1X2	T47.1X3	T47.1X4	T47.1X5	T47.1X6
vaccine						
DPT	T50.A11	T50.A12	T50.A13	T50.A14	T50.A15	T50.A16
including pertussis	T50.A11	T50.A12	T50.A13	T50.A14	T50.A15	T50.A16
MMR	T50.B91	T50.B92	T50.B93	T50.B94	T50.B95	T50.B96
Triprolidine	T45.0X1	T45.0X2	T45.0X3	T45.0X4	T45.0X5	T45.0X6
Trisodium hydrogen edetate	T50.6X1	T50.6X2	T50.6X3	T50.6X4	T50.6X5	T50.6X6
Trisoralen	T49.3X1	T49.3X2	T49.3X3	T49.3X4	T49.3X5	T49.3X6
Trisulfapyrimidines	T37.0X1	T37.0X2	T37.0X3	T37.0X4	T37.0X5	T37.0X6
Trithiozine	T44.3X1	T44.3X2	T44.3X3	T44.3X4	T44.3X5	T44.3X6
Tritiozine	T44.3X1	T44.3X2	T44.3X3	T44.3X4	T44.3X5	T44.3X6
Tritoqualine	T45.0X1	T45.0X2	T45.0X3	T45.0X4	T45.0X5	T45.0X6
Trofosfamide	T45.1X1	T45.1X2	T45.1X3	T45.1X4	T45.1X5	T45.1X6
Troleandomycin	T36.3X1	T36.3X2	T36.3X3	T36.3X4	T36.3X5	T36.3X6
Trolnitrate (phosphate)	T46.3X1	T46.3X2	T46.3X3	T46.3X4	T46.3X5	T46.3X6
Tromantadine	T37.5X1	T37.5X2	T37.5X3	T37.5X4	T37.5X5	T37.5X6
Trometamol	T50.2X1	T50.2X2	T50.2X3	T50.2X4	T50.2X5	T50.2X6
Tromethamine	T50.2X1	T50.2X2	T50.2X3	T50.2X4	T50.2X5	T50.2X6

Substance	Poisoning, Accidental (unintentional)	Poisoning, Intentional Self-harm	Poisoning, Assault	Poisoning, Undetermined	Adverse Effect	Under-dosing
Tronothane	T41.3X1	T41.3X2	T41.3X3	T41.3X4	T41.3X5	T41.3X6
Tropacine	T44.3X1	T44.3X2	T44.3X3	T44.3X4	T44.3X5	T44.3X6
Tropatepine	T44.3X1	T44.3X2	T44.3X3	T44.3X4	T44.3X5	T44.3X6
Tropicamide	T44.3X1	T44.3X2	T44.3X3	T44.3X4	T44.3X5	T44.3X6
Trospium chloride	T44.3X1	T44.3X2	T44.3X3	T44.3X4	T44.3X5	T44.3X6
Troxerutin	T46.991	T46.992	T46.993	T46.994	T46.995	T46.996
Troxidone	T42.2X1	T42.2X2	T42.2X3	T42.2X4	T42.2X5	T42.2X6
Tryparsamide	T37.3X1	T37.3X2	T37.3X3	T37.3X4	T37.3X5	T37.3X6
Trypsin	T45.3X1	T45.3X2	T45.3X3	T45.3X4	T45.3X5	T45.3X6
Tryptizol	T43.011	T43.012	T43.013	T43.014	T43.015	T43.016
TSH	T38.811	T38.812	T38.813	T38.814	T38.815	T38.816
Tuaminoheptane	T48.5X1	T48.5X2	T48.5X3	T48.5X4	T48.5X5	T48.5X6
Tuberculin, purified protein derivative (PPD)	T50.8X1	T50.8X2	T50.8X3	T50.8X4	T50.8X5	T50.8X6
Tubocurare	T48.1X1	T48.1X2	T48.1X3	T48.1X4	T48.1X5	T48.1X6
Tubocurarine (chloride)	T48.1X1	T48.1X2	T48.1X3	T48.1X4	T48.1X5	T48.1X6
Tulobuterol	T48.6X1	T48.6X2	T48.6X3	T48.6X4	T48.6X5	T48.6X6
Turpentine (spirits of)	T52.8X1	T52.8X2	T52.8X3	T52.8X4	—	—
vapor	T52.8X1	T52.8X2	T52.8X3	T52.8X4	—	—
Tybamate	T43.591	T43.592	T43.593	T43.594	T43.595	T43.596
Tyloxapol	T48.4X1	T48.4X2	T48.4X3	T48.4X4	T48.4X5	T48.4X6
Tymazoline	T48.5X1	T48.5X2	T48.5X3	T48.5X4	T48.5X5	T48.5X6
Typhoid-paratyphoid vaccine	T50.A91	T50.A92	T50.A93	T50.A94	T50.A95	T50.A96
Typhus vaccine	T50.A91	T50.A92	T50.A93	T50.A94	T50.A95	T50.A96
Tyropanoate	T50.8X1	T50.8X2	T50.8X3	T50.8X4	T50.8X5	T50.8X6
Tyrothricin	T49.6X1	T49.6X2	T49.6X3	T49.6X4	T49.6X5	T49.6X6
ENT agent	T49.6X1	T49.6X2	T49.6X3	T49.6X4	T49.6X5	T49.6X6
ophthalmic preparation	T49.5X1	T49.5X2	T49.5X3	T49.5X4	T49.5X5	T49.5X6
Ufenamate	T39.391	T39.392	T39.393	T39.394	T39.395	T39.396
Ultraviolet light protectant	T49.3X1	T49.3X2	T49.3X3	T49.3X4	T49.3X5	T49.3X6
Undecenoic acid	T49.0X1	T49.0X2	T49.0X3	T49.0X4	T49.0X5	T49.0X6
Undecoylium	T49.0X1	T49.0X2	T49.0X3	T49.0X4	T49.0X5	T49.0X6
Undecylenic acid (derivatives)	T49.0X1	T49.0X2	T49.0X3	T49.0X4	T49.0X5	T49.0X6
Unna's boot	T49.3X1	T49.3X2	T49.3X3	T49.3X4	T49.3X5	T49.3X6
Unsaturated fatty acid	T46.6X1	T46.6X2	T46.6X3	T46.6X4	T46.6X5	T46.6X6
Uracil mustard	T45.1X1	T45.1X2	T45.1X3	T45.1X4	T45.1X5	T45.1X6
Uramustine	T45.1X1	T45.1X2	T45.1X3	T45.1X4	T45.1X5	T45.1X6
Urapidil	T46.5X1	T46.5X2	T46.5X3	T46.5X4	T46.5X5	T46.5X6
Urari	T48.1X1	T48.1X2	T48.1X3	T48.1X4	T48.1X5	T48.1X6
Urate oxidase	T50.4X1	T50.4X2	T50.4X3	T50.4X4	T50.4X5	T50.4X6
Urea	T47.3X1	T47.3X2	T47.3X3	T47.3X4	T47.3X5	T47.3X6
peroxide	T49.0X1	T49.0X2	T49.0X3	T49.0X4	T49.0X5	T49.0X6
stibamine	T37.4X1	T37.4X2	T37.4X3	T37.4X4	T37.4X5	T37.4X6
topical	T49.8X1	T49.8X2	T49.8X3	T49.8X4	T49.8X5	T49.8X6
Urethane	T45.1X1	T45.1X2	T45.1X3	T45.1X4	T45.1X5	T45.1X6
Urginea (maritima) (scilla) — *see* Squill						
Uric acid metabolism drug NEC	T50.4X1	T50.4X2	T50.4X3	T50.4X4	T50.4X5	T50.4X6
Uricosuric agent	T50.4X1	T50.4X2	T50.4X3	T50.4X4	T50.4X5	T50.4X6
Urinary anti-infective	T37.8X1	T37.8X2	T37.8X3	T37.8X4	T37.8X5	T37.8X6
Urofollitropin	T38.811	T38.812	T38.813	T38.814	T38.815	T38.816
Urokinase	T45.611	T45.612	T45.613	T45.614	T45.615	T45.616
Urokon	T50.8X1	T50.8X2	T50.8X3	T50.8X4	T50.8X5	T50.8X6
Ursodeoxycholic acid	T50.991	T50.992	T50.993	T50.994	T50.995	T50.996
Ursodiol	T50.991	T50.992	T50.993	T50.994	T50.995	T50.996
Urtica	T62.2X1	T62.2X2	T62.2X3	T62.2X4	—	—
Utility gas — *see* Gas, utility						
Vaccine NEC	T50.Z91	T50.Z92	T50.Z93	T50.Z94	T50.Z95	T50.Z96
antineoplastic	T50.Z91	T50.Z92	T50.Z93	T50.Z94	T50.Z95	T50.Z96
bacterial NEC	T50.A91	T50.A92	T50.A93	T50.A94	T50.A95	T50.A96
with						
other bacterial component	T50.A21	T50.A22	T50.A23	T50.A24	T50.A25	T50.A26
pertussis component	T50.A11	T50.A12	T50.A13	T50.A14	T50.A15	T50.A16
viral-rickettsial component	T50.A21	T50.A22	T50.A23	T50.A24	T50.A25	T50.A26
mixed NEC	T50.A21	T50.A22	T50.A23	T50.A24	T50.A25	T50.A26
BCG	T50.A91	T50.A92	T50.A93	T50.A94	T50.A95	T50.A96
cholera	T50.A91	T50.A92	T50.A93	T50.A94	T50.A95	T50.A96
diphtheria	T50.A91	T50.A92	T50.A93	T50.A94	T50.A95	T50.A96
with tetanus	T50.A21	T50.A22	T50.A23	T50.A24	T50.A25	T50.A26
and pertussis	T50.A11	T50.A12	T50.A13	T50.A14	T50.A15	T50.A16
influenza	T50.B91	T50.B92	T50.B93	T50.B94	T50.B95	T50.B96
measles	T50.B91	T50.B92	T50.B93	T50.B94	T50.B95	T50.B96
with mumps and rubella	T50.B91	T50.B92	T50.B93	T50.B94	T50.B95	T50.B96
meningococcal	T50.A91	T50.A92	T50.A93	T50.A94	T50.A95	T50.A96
mumps	T50.B91	T50.B92	T50.B93	T50.B94	IC50.B95	T50.B96
paratyphoid	T50.A91	T50.A92	T50.A93	T50.A94	T50.A95	T50.A96
pertussis	T50.A11	T50.A12	T50.A13	T50.A14	T50.A15	T50.A16
with diphtheria	T50.A11	T50.A12	T50.A13	T50.A14	T50.A15	T50.A16

Additional Character May Be Required — Refer to the Tabular List for Character Selection

▽ Subterms under main terms may continue to next column or page

Trichlorotriethylamine — Vaccine NEC

Substance	Poisoning, Accidental (unintentional)	Poisoning, Intentional Self-harm	Poisoning, Assault	Poisoning, Undetermined	Adverse Effect	Under-dosing
Vaccine — *continued*						
pertussis — *continued*						
with diphtheria — *continued*						
and tetanus	T50.A11	T50.A12	T50.A13	T50.A14	T50.A15	T50.A16
with other component	T50.A11	T50.A12	T50.A13	T50.A14	T50.A15	T50.A16
plague	T50.A91	T50.A92	T50.A93	T50.A94	T50.A95	T50.A96
poliomyelitis	T50.B91	T50.B92	T50.B93	T50.B94	T50.B95	T50.B96
poliovirus	T50.B91	T50.B92	T50.B93	T50.B94	T50.B95	T50.B96
rabies	T50.B91	T50.B92	T50.B93	T50.B94	T50.B95	T50.B96
respiratory syncytial virus	T50.B91	T50.B92	T50.B93	T50.B94	T50.B95	T50.B96
rickettsial NEC	T50.A91	T50.A92	T50.A93	T50.A94	T50.A95	T50.A96
with						
bacterial component	T50.A21	T50.A22	T50.A23	T50.A24	T50.A25	T50.A26
Rocky Mountain spotted fever	T50.A91	T50.A92	T50.A93	T50.A94	T50.A95	T50.A96
rubella	T50.B91	T50.B92	T50.B93	T50.B94	T50.B95	T50.B96
sabin oral	T50.B91	T50.B92	T50.B93	T50.B94	T50.B95	T50.B96
smallpox	T50.B11	T50.B12	T50.B13	T50.B14	T50.B15	T50.B16
TAB	T50.A91	T50.A92	T50.A93	T50.A94	T50.A95	T50.A96
tetanus	T50.A91	T50.A92	T50.A93	T50.A94	T50.A95	T50.A96
typhoid	T50.A91	T50.A92	T50.A93	T50.A94	T50.A95	T50.A96
typhus	T50.A91	T50.A92	T50.A93	T50.A94	T50.A95	T50.A96
viral NEC	T50.B91	T50.B92	T50.B93	T50.B94	T50.B95	T50.B96
yellow fever	T50.B91	T50.B92	T50.B93	T50.B94	T50.B95	T50.B96
Vaccinia immune globulin	T50.Z11	T50.Z12	T50.Z13	T50.Z14	T50.Z15	T50.Z16
Vaginal contraceptives	T49.8X1	T49.8X2	T49.8X3	T49.8X4	T49.8X5	T49.8X6
Valerian						
root	T42.6X1	T42.6X2	T42.6X3	T42.6X4	T42.6X5	T42.6X6
tincture	T42.6X1	T42.6X2	T42.6X3	T42.6X4	T42.6X5	T42.6X6
Valethamate bromide	T44.3X1	T44.3X2	T44.3X3	T44.3X4	T44.3X5	T44.3X6
Valisone	T49.0X1	T49.0X2	T49.0X3	T49.0X4	T49.0X5	T49.0X6
Valium	T42.4X1	T42.4X2	T42.4X3	T42.4X4	T42.4X5	T42.4X6
Valmid	T42.6X1	T42.6X2	T42.6X3	T42.6X4	T42.6X5	T42.6X6
Valnoctamide	T42.6X1	T42.6X2	T42.6X3	T42.6X4	T42.6X5	T42.6X6
Valproate (sodium)	T42.6X1	T42.6X2	T42.6X3	T42.6X4	T42.6X5	T42.6X6
Valproic acid	T42.6X1	T42.6X2	T42.6X3	T42.6X4	T42.6X5	T42.6X6
Valpromide	T42.6X1	T42.6X2	T42.6X3	T42.6X4	T42.6X5	T42.6X6
Vanadium	T56.891	T56.892	T56.893	T56.894	—	—
Vancomycin	T36.8X1	T36.8X2	T36.8X3	T36.8X4	T36.8X5	T36.8X6
Vapor — *see also* Gas	T59.91	T59.92	T59.93	T59.94	—	—
kiln (carbon monoxide)	T58.8X1	T58.8X2	T58.8X3	T58.8X4	—	—
lead — *see* lead						
specified source NEC	T59.891	T59.892	T59.893	T59.894	—	—
Vardenafil	T46.7X1	T46.7X2	T46.7X3	T46.7X4	T46.7X5	T46.7X6
Varicose reduction drug	T46.8X1	T46.8X2	T46.8X3	T46.8X4	T46.8X5	T46.8X6
Varnish	T65.4X1	T65.4X2	T65.4X3	T65.4X4	—	—
cleaner	T52.91	T52.92	T52.93	T52.94	—	—
Vaseline	T49.3X1	T49.3X2	T49.3X3	T49.3X4	T49.3X5	T49.3X6
Vasodilan	T46.7X1	T46.7X2	T46.7X3	T46.7X4	T46.7X5	T46.7X6
Vasodilator						
coronary NEC	T46.3X1	T46.3X2	T46.3X3	T46.3X4	T46.3X5	T46.3X6
peripheral NEC	T46.7X1	T46.7X2	T46.7X3	T46.7X4	T46.7X5	T46.7X6
Vasopressin	T38.891	T38.892	T38.893	T38.894	T38.895	T38.896
Vasopressor drugs	T38.891	T38.892	T38.893	T38.894	T38.895	T38.896
Vecuronium bromide	T48.1X1	T48.1X2	T48.1X3	T48.1X4	T48.1X5	T48.1X6
Vegetable extract, astringent	T49.2X1	T49.2X2	T49.2X3	T49.2X4	T49.2X5	T49.2X6
Venlafaxine	T43.211	T43.212	T43.213	T43.214	T43.215	T43.216
Venom, venomous (bite) (sting)	T63.91	T63.92	T63.93	T63.94	—	—
amphibian NEC	T63.831	T63.832	T63.833	T63.834	—	—
animal NEC	T63.891	T63.892	T63.893	T63.894	—	—
ant	T63.421	T63.422	T63.423	T63.424	—	—
arthropod NEC	T63.481	T63.482	T63.483	T63.484	—	—
bee	T63.441	T63.442	T63.443	T63.444	—	—
centipede	T63.411	T63.412	T63.413	T63.414	—	—
fish	T63.591	T63.592	T63.593	T63.594	—	—
frog	T63.811	T63.812	T63.813	T63.814	—	—
hornet	T63.451	T63.452	T63.453	T63.454	—	—
insect NEC	T63.481	T63.482	T63.483	T63.484	—	—
lizard	T63.121	T63.122	T63.123	T63.124	—	—
marine						
animals						
bluebottle	T63.611	T63.612	T63.613	T63.614	—	—
jellyfish NEC	T63.621	T63.622	T63.623	T63.624	—	—
Portugese Man-o-war	T63.611	T63.612	T63.613	T63.614	—	—
sea anemone	T63.631	T63.632	T63.633	T63.634	—	—
specified NEC	T63.691	T63.692	T63.693	T63.694	—	—
fish	T63.591	T63.592	T63.593	T63.594	—	—
plants	T63.711	T63.712	T63.713	T63.714	—	—
sting ray	T63.511	T63.512	T63.513	T63.514	—	—
millipede (tropical)	T63.411	T63.412	T63.413	T63.414	—	—
plant NEC	T63.791	T63.792	T63.793	T63.794	—	—

Substance	Poisoning, Accidental (unintentional)	Poisoning, Intentional Self-harm	Poisoning, Assault	Poisoning, Undetermined	Adverse Effect	Under-dosing
Venom, venomous — *continued*						
plant — *continued*						
marine	T63.711	T63.712	T63.713	T63.714	—	—
reptile	T63.191	T63.192	T63.193	T63.194	—	—
gila monster	T63.111	T63.112	T63.113	T63.114	—	—
lizard NEC	T63.121	T63.122	T63.123	T63.124	—	—
scorpion	T63.2X1	T63.2X2	T63.2X3	T63.2X4	—	—
snake	T63.001	T63.002	T63.003	T63.004	—	—
African NEC	T63.081	T63.082	T63.083	T63.084	—	—
American (North) (South) NEC	T63.061	T63.062	T63.063	T63.064	—	—
Asian	T63.081	T63.082	T63.083	T63.084	—	—
Australian	T63.071	T63.072	T63.073	T63.074	—	—
cobra	T63.041	T63.042	T63.043	T63.044	—	—
coral snake	T63.021	T63.022	T63.023	T63.024	—	—
rattlesnake	T63.011	T63.012	T63.013	T63.014	—	—
specified NEC	T63.091	T63.092	T63.093	T63.094	—	—
taipan	T63.031	T63.032	T63.033	T63.034	—	—
specified NEC	T63.891	T63.892	T63.893	T63.894	—	—
spider	T63.301	T63.302	T63.303	T63.304	—	—
black widow	T63.311	T63.312	T63.313	T63.314	—	—
brown recluse	T63.331	T63.332	T63.333	T63.334	—	—
specified NEC	T63.391	T63.392	T63.393	T63.394	—	—
tarantula	T63.321	T63.322	T63.323	T63.324	—	—
sting ray	T63.511	T63.512	T63.513	T63.514	—	—
toad	T63.821	T63.822	T63.823	T63.824	—	—
wasp	T63.461	T63.462	T63.463	T63.464	—	—
Venous sclerosing drug NEC	T46.8X1	T46.8X2	T46.8X3	T46.8X4	T46.8X5	T46.8X6
Ventolin — *see* Albuterol						
Veramon	T42.3X1	T42.3X2	T42.3X3	T42.3X4	T42.3X5	T42.3X6
Verapamil	T46.1X1	T46.1X2	T46.1X3	T46.1X4	T46.1X5	T46.1X6
Veratrine	T46.5X1	T46.5X2	T46.5X3	T46.5X4	T46.5X5	T46.5X6
Veratrum						
album	T62.2X1	T62.2X2	T62.2X3	T62.2X4	—	—
alkaloids	T46.5X1	T46.5X2	T46.5X3	T46.5X4	T46.5X5	T46.5X6
viride	T62.2X1	T62.2X2	T62.2X3	T62.2X4	—	—
Verdigris	T60.3X1	T60.3X2	T60.3X3	T60.3X4	—	—
Veronal	T42.3X1	T42.3X2	T42.3X3	T42.3X4	T42.3X5	T42.3X6
Veroxil	T37.4X1	T37.4X2	T37.4X3	T37.4X4	T37.4X5	T37.4X6
Versenate	T50.6X1	T50.6X2	T50.6X3	T50.6X4	T50.6X5	T50.6X6
Versidyne	T39.8X1	T39.8X2	T39.8X3	T39.8X4	T39.8X5	T39.8X6
Vetrabutine	T48.0X1	T48.0X2	T48.0X3	T48.0X4	T48.0X5	T48.0X6
Vidarabine	T37.5X1	T37.5X2	T37.5X3	T37.5X4	T37.5X5	T37.5X6
Vienna						
green	T57.0X1	T57.0X2	T57.0X3	T57.0X4	—	—
insecticide	T60.2X1	T60.2X2	T60.2X3	T60.2X4	—	—
red	T57.0X1	T57.0X2	T57.0X3	T57.0X4	—	—
pharmaceutical dye	T50.991	T50.992	T50.993	T50.994	T50.995	T50.996
Vigabatrin	T42.6X1	T42.6X2	T42.6X3	T42.6X4	T42.6X5	T42.6X6
Viloxazine	T43.291	T43.292	T43.293	T43.294	T43.295	T43.296
Viminol	T39.8X1	T39.8X2	T39.8X3	T39.8X4	T39.8X5	T39.8X6
Vinbarbital, vinbarbitone	T42.3X1	T42.3X2	T42.3X3	T42.3X4	T42.3X5	T42.3X6
Vinblastine	T45.1X1	T45.1X2	T45.1X3	T45.1X4	T45.1X5	T45.1X6
Vinburnine	T46.7X1	T46.7X2	T46.7X3	T46.7X4	T46.7X5	T46.7X6
Vincamine	T45.1X1	T45.1X2	T45.1X3	T45.1X4	T45.1X5	T45.1X6
Vincristine	T45.1X1	T45.1X2	T45.1X3	T45.1X4	T45.1X5	T45.1X6
Vindesine	T45.1X1	T45.1X2	T45.1X3	T45.1X4	T45.1X5	T45.1X6
Vinesthene, vinethene	T41.0X1	T41.0X2	T41.0X3	T41.0X4	T41.0X5	T41.0X6
Vinorelbine tartrate	T45.1X1	T45.1X2	T45.1X3	T45.1X4	T45.1X5	T45.1X6
Vinpocetine	T46.7X1	T46.7X2	T46.7X3	T46.7X4	T46.7X5	T46.7X6
Vinyl						
acetate	T65.891	T65.892	T65.893	T65.894	—	—
bital	T42.3X1	T42.3X2	T42.3X3	T42.3X4	T42.3X5	T42.3X6
bromide	T65.891	T65.892	T65.893	T65.894	—	—
chloride	T59.891	T59.892	T59.893	T59.894	—	—
ether	T41.0X1	T41.0X2	T41.0X3	T41.0X4	T41.0X5	T41.0X6
Vinylbital	T42.3X1	T42.3X2	T42.3X3	T42.3X4	T42.3X5	T42.3X6
Vinylidene chloride	T65.891	T65.892	T65.893	T65.894	—	—
Vioform	T37.8X1	T37.8X2	T37.8X3	T37.8X4	T37.8X5	T37.8X6
topical	T49.0X1	T49.0X2	T49.0X3	T49.0X4	T49.0X5	T49.0X6
Viomycin	T36.8X1	T36.8X2	T36.8X3	T36.8X4	T36.8X5	T36.8X6
Viosterol	T45.2X1	T45.2X2	T45.2X3	T45.2X4	T45.2X5	T45.2X6
Viper (venom)	T63.091	T63.092	T63.093	T63.094	—	—
Viprynium	T37.4X1	T37.4X2	T37.4X3	T37.4X4	T37.4X5	T37.4X6
Viquidil	T46.7X1	T46.7X2	T46.7X3	T46.7X4	T46.7X5	T46.7X6
Viral vaccine NEC	T50.B91	T50.B92	T50.B93	T50.B94	T50.B95	T50.B96
Virginiamycin	T36.8X1	T36.8X2	T36.8X3	T36.8X4	T36.8X5	T36.8X6
Virugon	T37.5X1	T37.5X2	T37.5X3	T37.5X4	T37.5X5	T37.5X6
Viscous agent	T50.901	T50.902	T50.903	T50.904	T50.905	T50.906
Visine	T49.5X1	T49.5X2	T49.5X3	T49.5X4	T49.5X5	T49.5X6
Visnadine	T46.3X1	T46.3X2	T46.3X3	T46.3X4	T46.3X5	T46.3X6
Vitamin NEC	T45.2X1	T45.2X2	T45.2X3	T45.2X4	T45.2X5	T45.2X6

▼ Subterms under main terms may continue to next column or page　　　　Additional Character May Be Required — Refer to the Tabular List for Character Selection

Table of Drugs and Chemicals

Substance	Poisoning, Accidental (unintentional)	Poisoning, Intentional Self-harm	Poisoning, Assault	Poisoning, Undetermined	Adverse Effect	Under-dosing
Vitamin — continued						
A	T45.2X1	T45.2X2	T45.2X3	T45.2X4	T45.2X5	T45.2X6
B1	T45.2X1	T45.2X2	T45.2X3	T45.2X4	T45.2X5	T45.2X6
B2	T45.2X1	T45.2X2	T45.2X3	T45.2X4	T45.2X5	T45.2X6
B6	T45.2X1	T45.2X2	T45.2X3	T45.2X4	T45.2X5	T45.2X6
B12	T45.2X1	T45.2X2	T45.2X3	T45.2X4	T45.2X5	T45.2X6
B15	T45.2X1	T45.2X2	T45.2X3	T45.2X4	T45.2X5	T45.2X6
B NEC	T45.2X1	T45.2X2	T45.2X3	T45.2X4	T45.2X5	T45.2X6
nicotinic acid	T46.7X1	T46.7X2	T46.7X3	T46.7X4	T46.7X5	T46.7X6
C	T45.2X1	T45.2X2	T45.2X3	T45.2X4	T45.2X5	T45.2X6
D	T45.2X1	T45.2X2	T45.2X3	T45.2X4	T45.2X5	T45.2X6
D2	T45.2X1	T45.2X2	T45.2X3	T45.2X4	T45.2X5	T45.2X6
D3	T45.2X1	T45.2X2	T45.2X3	T45.2X4	T45.2X5	T45.2X6
E	T45.2X1	T45.2X2	T45.2X3	T45.2X4	T45.2X5	T45.2X6
E acetate	T45.2X1	T45.2X2	T45.2X3	T45.2X4	T45.2X5	T45.2X6
hematopoietic	T45.8X1	T45.8X2	T45.8X3	T45.8X4	T45.8X5	T45.8X6
K1	T45.7X1	T45.7X2	T45.7X3	T45.7X4	T45.7X5	T45.7X6
K2	T45.7X1	T45.7X2	T45.7X3	T45.7X4	T45.7X5	T45.7X6
K NEC	T45.7X1	T45.7X2	T45.7X3	T45.7X4	T45.7X5	T45.7X6
PP	T45.2X1	T45.2X2	T45.2X3	T45.2X4	T45.2X5	T45.2X6
ulceroprotectant	T47.1X1	T47.1X2	T47.1X3	T47.1X4	T47.1X5	T47.1X6
Vleminckx's solution	T49.4X1	T49.4X2	T49.4X3	T49.4X4	T49.4X5	T49.4X6
Voltaren — see Diclofenac						
sodium						
Warfarin	T45.511	T45.512	T45.513	T45.514	T45.515	T45.516
rodenticide	T45.511	T45.512	T45.513	T45.514	T45.515	T45.516
sodium	T45.511	T45.512	T45.513	T45.514	T45.515	T45.516
Wasp (sting)	T63.461	T63.462	T63.463	T63.464	—	—
Water						
balance drug	T50.3X1	T50.3X2	T50.3X3	T50.3X4	T50.3X5	T50.3X6
distilled	T50.3X1	T50.3X2	T50.3X3	T50.3X4	T50.3X5	T50.3X6
gas — see Gas, water						
incomplete combustion of —						
see Carbon, monoxide,						
fuel, utility						
hemlock	T62.2X1	T62.2X2	T62.2X3	T62.2X4	—	—
moccasin (venom)	T63.061	T63.062	T63.063	T63.064	—	—
purified	T50.3X1	T50.3X2	T50.3X3	T50.3X4	T50.3X5	T50.3X6
Wax (paraffin) (petroleum)	T52.0X1	T52.0X2	T52.0X3	T52.0X4	—	—
automobile	T65.891	T65.892	T65.893	T65.894	—	—
floor	T52.0X1	T52.0X2	T52.0X3	T52.0X4	—	—
Weed killers NEC	T60.3X1	T60.3X2	T60.3X3	T60.3X4	—	—
Welldorm	T42.6X1	T42.6X2	T42.6X3	T42.6X4	T42.6X5	T42.6X6
White						
arsenic	T57.0X1	T57.0X2	T57.0X3	T57.0X4	—	—
hellebore	T62.2X1	T62.2X2	T62.2X3	T62.2X4	—	—
lotion (keratolytic)	T49.4X1	T49.4X2	T49.4X3	T49.4X4	T49.4X5	T49.4X6
spirit	T52.0X1	T52.0X2	T52.0X3	T52.0X4	—	—
Whitewash	T65.891	T65.892	T65.893	T65.894	—	—
Whole blood (human)	T45.8X1	T45.8X2	T45.8X3	T45.8X4	T45.8X5	T45.8X6
Wild						
black cherry	T62.2X1	T62.2X2	T62.2X3	T62.2X4	—	—
poisonous plants NEC	T62.2X1	T62.2X2	T62.2X3	T62.2X4	—	—
Window cleaning fluid	T65.891	T65.892	T65.893	T65.894	—	—
Wintergreen (oil)	T49.3X1	T49.3X2	T49.3X3	T49.3X4	T49.3X5	T49.3X6
Wisterine	T62.2X1	T62.2X2	T62.2X3	T62.2X4	—	—
Witch hazel	T49.2X1	T49.2X2	T49.2X3	T49.2X4	T49.2X5	T49.2X6
Wood alcohol or spirit	T51.1X1	T51.1X2	T51.1X3	T51.1X4	—	—
Wool fat (hydrous)	T49.3X1	T49.3X2	T49.3X3	T49.3X4	T49.3X5	T49.3X6
Woorali	T48.1X1	T48.1X2	T48.1X3	T48.1X4	T48.1X5	T48.1X6
Wormseed, American	T37.4X1	T37.4X2	T37.4X3	T37.4X4	T37.4X5	T37.4X6
Xamoterol	T44.5X1	T44.5X2	T44.5X3	T44.5X4	T44.5X5	T44.5X6
Xanthine diuretics	T50.2X1	T50.2X2	T50.2X3	T50.2X4	T50.2X5	T50.2X6
Xanthinol nicotinate	T46.7X1	T46.7X2	T46.7X3	T46.7X4	T46.7X5	T46.7X6
Xanthotoxin	T49.3X1	T49.3X2	T49.3X3	T49.3X4	T49.3X5	T49.3X6
Xantinol nicotinate	T46.7X1	T46.7X2	T46.7X3	T46.7X4	T46.7X5	T46.7X6
Xantocillin	T36.0X1	T36.0X2	T36.0X3	T36.0X4	T36.0X5	T36.0X6
Xenon (127Xe) (133Xe)	T50.8X1	T50.8X2	T50.8X3	T50.8X4	T50.8X5	T50.8X6
Xenysalate	T49.4X1	T49.4X2	T49.4X3	T49.4X4	T49.4X5	T49.4X6
Xibornol	T37.8X1	T37.8X2	T37.8X3	T37.8X4	T37.8X5	T37.8X6
Xigris	T45.511	T45.512	T45.513	T45.514	T45.515	T45.516
Xipamide	T50.2X1	T50.2X2	T50.2X3	T50.2X4	T50.2X5	T50.2X6
Xylene (vapor)	T52.2X1	T52.2X2	T52.2X3	T52.2X4	—	—
Xylocaine (infiltration) (topical)	T41.3X1	T41.3X2	T41.3X3	T41.3X4	T41.3X5	T41.3X6
nerve block (peripheral) (plexus)	T41.3X1	T41.3X2	T41.3X3	T41.3X4	T41.3X5	T41.3X6
spinal	T41.3X1	T41.3X2	T41.3X3	T41.3X4	T41.3X5	T41.3X6
Xylol (vapor)	T52.2X1	T52.2X2	T52.2X3	T52.2X4	—	—
Xylometazoline	T48.5X1	T48.5X2	T48.5X3	T48.5X4	T48.5X5	T48.5X6
Yeast	T45.2X1	T45.2X2	T45.2X3	T45.2X4	T45.2X5	T45.2X6
dried	T45.2X1	T45.2X2	T45.2X3	T45.2X4	T45.2X5	T45.2X6

Substance	Poisoning, Accidental (unintentional)	Poisoning, Intentional Self-harm	Poisoning, Assault	Poisoning, Undetermined	Adverse Effect	Under-dosing
Yellow						
fever vaccine	T50.B91	T50.B92	T50.B93	T50.B94	T50.B95	T50.B96
jasmine	T62.2X1	T62.2X2	T62.2X3	T62.2X4	—	—
phenolphthalein	T47.2X1	T47.2X2	T47.2X3	T47.2X4	T47.2X5	T47.2X6
Yew	T62.2X1	T62.2X2	T62.2X3	T62.2X4	—	—
Yohimbic acid	T40.991	T40.992	T40.993	T40.994	T40.995	T40.996
Zactane	T39.8X1	T39.8X2	T39.8X3	T39.8X4	T39.8X5	T39.8X6
Zalcitabine	T37.5X1	T37.5X2	T37.5X3	T37.5X4	T37.5X5	T37.5X6
Zaroxolyn	T50.2X1	T50.2X2	T50.2X3	T50.2X4	T50.2X5	T50.2X6
Zephiran (topical)	T49.0X1	T49.0X2	T49.0X3	T49.0X4	T49.0X5	T49.0X6
ophthalmic preparation	T49.5X1	T49.5X2	T49.5X3	T49.5X4	T49.5X5	T49.5X6
Zeranol	T38.7X1	T38.7X2	T38.7X3	T38.7X4	T38.7X5	T38.7X6
Zerone	T51.1X1	T51.1X2	T51.1X3	T51.1X4	—	—
Zidovudine	T37.5X1	T37.5X2	T37.5X3	T37.5X4	T37.5X5	T37.5X6
Zimeldine	T43.221	T43.222	T43.223	T43.224	T43.225	T43.226
Zinc (compounds) (fumes) (vapor)	T56.5X1	T56.5X2	T56.5X3	T56.5X4	—	—
NEC						
anti-infectives	T49.0X1	T49.0X2	T49.0X3	T49.0X4	T49.0X5	T49.0X6
antivaricose	T46.8X1	T46.8X2	T46.8X3	T46.8X4	T46.8X5	T46.8X6
bacitracin	T49.0X1	T49.0X2	T49.0X3	T49.0X4	T49.0X5	T49.0X6
chloride (mouthwash)	T49.6X1	T49.6X2	T49.6X3	T49.6X4	T49.6X5	T49.6X6
chromate	T56.5X1	T56.5X2	T56.5X3	T56.5X4	—	—
gelatin	T49.3X1	T49.3X2	T49.3X3	T49.3X4	T49.3X5	T49.3X6
oxide	T49.3X1	T49.3X2	T49.3X3	T49.3X4	T49.3X5	T49.3X6
plaster	T49.3X1	T49.3X2	T49.3X3	T49.3X4	T49.3X5	T49.3X6
peroxide	T49.0X1	T49.0X2	T49.0X3	T49.0X4	T49.0X5	T49.0X6
pesticides	T56.5X1	T56.5X2	T56.5X3	T56.5X4	—	—
phosphide	T60.4X1	T60.4X2	T60.4X3	T60.4X4	—	—
pyrithionate	T49.4X1	T49.4X2	T49.4X3	T49.4X4	T49.4X5	T49.4X6
stearate	T49.3X1	T49.3X2	T49.3X3	T49.3X4	T49.3X5	T49.3X6
sulfate	T49.5X1	T49.5X2	T49.5X3	T49.5X4	T49.5X5	T49.5X6
ENT agent	T49.6X1	T49.6X2	T49.6X3	T49.6X4	T49.6X5	T49.6X6
ophthalmic solution	T49.5X1	T49.5X2	T49.5X3	T49.5X4	T49.5X5	T49.5X6
topical NEC	T49.0X1	T49.0X2	T49.0X3	T49.0X4	T49.0X5	T49.0X6
undecylenate	T49.0X1	T49.0X2	T49.0X3	T49.0X4	T49.0X5	T49.0X6
Zineb	T60.0X1	T60.0X2	T60.0X3	T60.0X4	—	—
Zinostatin	T45.1X1	T45.1X2	T45.1X3	T45.1X4	T45.1X5	T45.1X6
Zipeprol	T48.3X1	T48.3X2	T48.3X3	T48.3X4	T48.3X5	T48.3X6
Zofenopril	T46.4X1	T46.4X2	T46.4X3	T46.4X4	T46.4X5	T46.4X6
Zolpidem	T42.6X1	T42.6X2	T42.6X3	T42.6X4	T42.6X5	T42.6X6
Zomepirac	T39.391	T39.392	T39.393	T39.394	T39.395	T39.396
Zopiclone	T42.6X1	T42.6X2	T42.6X3	T42.6X4	T42.6X5	T42.6X6
Zorubicin	T45.1X1	T45.1X2	T45.1X3	T45.1X4	T45.1X5	T45.1X6
Zotepine	T43.591	T43.592	T43.593	T43.594	T43.595	T43.596
Zovant	T45.511	T45.512	T45.513	T45.514	T45.515	T45.516
Zoxazolamine	T42.8X1	T42.8X2	T42.8X3	T42.8X4	T42.8X5	T42.8X6
Zuclopenthixol	T43.4X1	T43.4X2	T43.4X3	T43.4X4	T43.4X5	T43.4X6
Zygadenus (venenosus)	T62.2X1	T62.2X2	T62.2X3	T62.2X4	—	—
Zyprexa	T43.591	T43.592	T43.593	T43.594	T43.595	T43.596

396

Additional Character May Be Required — Refer to the Tabular List for Character Selection   ▽ Subterms under main terms may continue to next column or page

Vitamin NEC — Zyprexa

A

Abandonment (causing exposure to weather conditions) (with intent to injure or kill) NEC X58 ☑
Abuse (adult) (child) (mental) (physical) (sexual) X58 ☑
Accident (to) X58 ☑
  aircraft (in transit) (powered) (*see also* Accident, transport, aircraft)
    due to, caused by cataclysm — *see* Forces of nature, by type
  animal-drawn vehicle — *see* Accident, transport, animal-drawn vehicle occupant
  animal-rider — *see* Accident, transport, animal-rider
  automobile — *see* Accident, transport, car occupant
  bare foot water skier V94.4 ☑
  boat, boating (*see also* Accident, watercraft)
    striking swimmer
      powered V94.11 ☑
      unpowered V94.12 ☑
  bus — *see* Accident, transport, bus occupant
  cable car, not on rails V98.0 ☑
    on rails — *see* Accident, transport, streetcar occupant
  car — *see* Accident, transport, car occupant
  caused by, due to
    animal NEC W64 ☑
    chain hoist W24.0 ☑
    cold (excessive) — *see* Exposure, cold
    corrosive liquid, substance — *see* Table of Drugs and Chemicals
    cutting or piercing instrument — *see* Contact, with, by type of instrument
    drive belt W24.0 ☑
    electric
      current — *see* Exposure, electric current
      motor (*see also* Contact, with, by type of machine) W31.3 ☑
        current (of) W86.8 ☑
    environmental factor NEC X58 ☑
    explosive material — *see* Explosion
    fire, flames — *see* Exposure, fire
    firearm missile — *see* Discharge, firearm by type
    heat (excessive) — *see* Heat
    hot — *see* Contact, with, hot
    ignition — *see* Ignition
    lifting device W24.0 ☑
    lightning — *see* subcategory T75.0 ☑
      causing fire — *see* Exposure, fire
    machine, machinery — *see* Contact, with, by type of machine
    natural factor NEC X58 ☑
    pulley (block) W24.0 ☑
    radiation — *see* Radiation
    steam X13.1 ☑
      inhalation X13.0 ☑
      pipe X16 ☑
    thunderbolt — *see* subcategory T75.0 ☑
      causing fire — *see* Exposure, fire
    transmission device W24.1 ☑
  coach — *see* Accident, transport, bus occupant
  coal car — *see* Accident, transport, industrial vehicle occupant
  diving (*see also* Fall, into, water)
    with
      drowning or submersion — *see* Drowning
  forklift — *see* Accident, transport, industrial vehicle occupant
  heavy transport vehicle NOS — *see* Accident, transport, truck occupant
  ice yacht V98.2 ☑
  in
    medical, surgical procedure
      as, or due to misadventure — *see* Misadventure
      causing an abnormal reaction or later complication without mention of misadventure (*see also* Complication of or following, by type of procedure) Y84.9
  land yacht V98.1 ☑
  late effect of — *see* W00-X58 with 7th character S
  logging car — *see* Accident, transport, industrial vehicle occupant
  machine, machinery (*see also* Contact, with, by type of machine)
    on board watercraft V93.69 ☑
      explosion — *see* Explosion, in, watercraft

Accident — *continued*
  machine, machinery (*see also* Contact, with, by type of machine) — *continued*
    on board watercraft — *continued*
      fire — *see* Burn, on board watercraft
      powered craft V93.63 ☑
        ferry boat V93.61 ☑
        fishing boat V93.62 ☑
        jetskis V93.63 ☑
        liner V93.61 ☑
        merchant ship V93.60 ☑
        passenger ship V93.61 ☑
        sailboat V93.64 ☑
  mine tram — *see* Accident, transport, industrial vehicle occupant
  mobility scooter (motorized) — *see* Accident, transport, pedestrian, conveyance, specified type NEC
  motor scooter — *see* Accident, transport, motorcyclist
  motor vehicle NOS (traffic) (*see also* Accident, transport) V89.2 ☑
    nontraffic V89.0 ☑
    three-wheeled NOS — *see* Accident, transport, three-wheeled motor vehicle occupant
  motorcycle NOS — *see* Accident, transport, motorcyclist
  nonmotor vehicle NOS (nontraffic) (*see also* Accident, transport) V89.1 ☑
    traffic NOS V89.3 ☑
  nontraffic (victim's mode of transport NOS) V88.9 ☑
    collision (between) V88.7 ☑
      bus and truck V88.5 ☑
      car and:
        bus V88.3 ☑
        pickup V88.2 ☑
        three-wheeled motor vehicle V88.0 ☑
        train V88.6 ☑
        truck V88.4 ☑
        two-wheeled motor vehicle V88.0 ☑
        van V88.2 ☑
      specified vehicle NEC and:
        three-wheeled motor vehicle V88.1 ☑
        two-wheeled motor vehicle V88.1 ☑
    known mode of transport — *see* Accident, transport, by type of vehicle
    noncollision V88.8 ☑
  on board watercraft V93.89 ☑
    powered craft V93.83 ☑
      ferry boat V93.81 ☑
      fishing boat V93.82 ☑
      jetskis V93.83 ☑
      liner V93.81 ☑
      merchant ship V93.80 ☑
      passenger ship V93.81 ☑
    unpowered craft V93.88 ☑
      canoe V93.85 ☑
      inflatable V93.86 ☑
        in tow
          recreational V94.31 ☑
          specified NEC V94.32 ☑
      kayak V93.85 ☑
      sailboat V93.84 ☑
      surf-board V93.88 ☑
      water skis V93.87 ☑
      windsurfer V93.88 ☑
  parachutist V97.29 ☑
    entangled in object V97.21 ☑
    injured on landing V97.22 ☑
  pedal cycle — *see* Accident, transport, pedal cyclist
  pedestrian (on foot)
    with
      another pedestrian W51 ☑
        with fall W03 ☑
          due to ice or snow W00.0 ☑
      on pedestrian conveyance NEC V00.09 ☑
      roller skater (in-line) V00.01 ☑
      skate boarder V00.02 ☑
      transport vehicle — *see* Accident, transport
    on pedestrian conveyance — *see* Accident, transport, pedestrian, conveyance
  pick-up truck or van — *see* Accident, transport, pickup truck occupant
  quarry truck — *see* Accident, transport, industrial vehicle occupant
  railway vehicle (any) (in motion) — *see* Accident, transport, railway vehicle occupant
    due to cataclysm — *see* Forces of nature, by type

Accident — *continued*
  scooter (non-motorized) — *see* Accident, transport, pedestrian, conveyance, scooter
  sequelae of — *see* categories W00-X58 with 7th character S
  skateboard — *see* Accident, transport, pedestrian, conveyance, skateboard
  ski(ing) — *see* Accident, transport, pedestrian, conveyance
    lift V98.3 ☑
  specified cause NEC X58 ☑
  streetcar — *see* Accident, transport, streetcar occupant
  traffic (victim's mode of transport NOS) V87.9 ☑
    collision (between) V87.7 ☑
      bus and truck V87.5 ☑
      car and:
        bus V87.3 ☑
        pickup V87.2 ☑
        three-wheeled motor vehicle V87.0 ☑
        train V87.6 ☑
        truck V87.4 ☑
        two-wheeled motor vehicle V87.0 ☑
        van V87.2 ☑
      specified vehicle NEC and:
        three-wheeled motor vehicle V87.1 ☑
        two-wheeled motor vehicle V87.1 ☑
    known mode of transport — *see* Accident, transport, by type of vehicle
    noncollision V87.8 ☑
  transport (involving injury to) V99 ☑
    18 wheeler — *see* Accident, transport, truck occupant
    agricultural vehicle occupant (nontraffic) V84.9 ☑
      driver V84.5 ☑
      hanger-on V84.7 ☑
      passenger V84.6 ☑
      traffic V84.3 ☑
        driver V84.0 ☑
        hanger-on V84.2 ☑
        passenger V84.1 ☑
      while boarding or alighting V84.4 ☑
    aircraft NEC V97.89 ☑
      military NEC V97.818 ☑
        with civlian aircraft V97.810 ☑
        civilian injured by V97.811 ☑
      occupant injured (in)
        nonpowered craft accident V96.9 ☑
          balloon V96.00 ☑
            collision V96.03 ☑
            crash V96.01 ☑
            explosion V96.05 ☑
            fire V96.04 ☑
            forced landing V96.02 ☑
            specified type NEC V96.09 ☑
          glider V96.20 ☑
            collision V96.23 ☑
            crash V96.21 ☑
            explosion V96.25 ☑
            fire V96.24 ☑
            forced landing V96.22 ☑
            specified type NEC V96.29 ☑
          hang glider V96.10 ☑
            collision V96.13 ☑
            crash V96.11 ☑
            explosion V96.15 ☑
            fire V96.14 ☑
            forced landing V96.12 ☑
            specified type NEC V96.19 ☑
          specified craft NEC V96.8 ☑
        powered craft accident V95.9 ☑
          fixed wing NEC
            commercial V95.30 ☑
              collision V95.33 ☑
              crash V95.31 ☑
              explosion V95.35 ☑
              fire V95.34 ☑
              forced landing V95.32 ☑
              specified type NEC V95.39 ☑
            private V95.20 ☑
              collision V95.23 ☑
              crash V95.21 ☑
              explosion V95.25 ☑
              fire V95.24 ☑
              forced landing V95.22 ☑
              specified type NEC V95.29 ☑
          glider V95.10 ☑

Accident — *continued*
  transport — *continued*
    aircraft — *continued*
      occupant injured — *continued*
        powered craft accident — *continued*
          glider — *continued*
            collision V95.13 ✓
            crash V95.11 ✓
            explosion V95.15 ✓
            fire V95.14 ✓
            forced landing V95.12 ✓
            specified type NEC V95.19 ✓
          helicopter V95.00 ✓
            collision V95.03 ✓
            crash V95.01 ✓
            explosion V95.05 ✓
            fire V95.04 ✓
            forced landing V95.02 ✓
            specified type NEC V95.09 ✓
          spacecraft V95.40 ✓
            collision V95.43 ✓
            crash V95.41 ✓
            explosion V95.45 ✓
            fire V95.44 ✓
            forced landing V95.42 ✓
            specified type NEC V95.49 ✓
          specified craft NEC V95.8 ✓
          ultralight V95.10 ✓
            collision V95.13 ✓
            crash V95.11 ✓
            explosion V95.15 ✓
            fire V95.14 ✓
            forced landing V95.12 ✓
            specified type NEC V95.19 ✓
        specified accident NEC V97.0 ✓
        while boarding or alighting V97.1 ✓
      person (injured by)
        falling from, in or on aircraft V97.0 ✓
        machinery on aircraft V97.89 ✓
        on ground with aircraft involvement V97.39 ✓
        rotating propeller V97.32 ✓
        struck by object falling from aircraft V97.31 ✓
        sucked into aircraft jet V97.33 ✓
        while boarding or alighting aircraft V97.1 ✓
    airport (battery-powered) passenger vehicle — *see* Accident, transport, industrial vehicle occupant
    all-terrain vehicle occupant (nontraffic) V86.95 ✓
      driver V86.55 ✓
      dune buggy — *see* Accident, transport, dune buggy occupant
      hanger-on V86.75 ✓
      passenger V86.65 ✓
      snowmobile — *see* Accident, transport, snowmobile occupant
      specified type NEC V86.99 ✓
      traffic V86.35 ✓
        driver V86.05 ✓
        hanger-on V86.25 ✓
        passenger V86.15 ✓
      while boarding or alighting V86.45 ✓
    ambulance occupant (traffic) V86.31 ✓
      driver V86.01 ✓
      hanger-on V86.21 ✓
      nontraffic V86.91 ✓
        driver V86.51 ✓
        hanger-on V86.71 ✓
        passenger V86.61 ✓
      passenger V86.11 ✓
      while boarding or alighting V86.41 ✓
    animal-drawn vehicle occupant (in) V80.929 ✓
      collision (with)
        animal V80.12 ✓
          being ridden V80.711 ✓
        animal-drawn vehicle V80.721 ✓
        bus V80.42 ✓
        car V80.42 ✓
        fixed or stationary object V80.82 ✓
        military vehicle V80.920 ✓
        nonmotor vehicle V80.791 ✓
        pedal cycle V80.22 ✓
        pedestrian V80.12 ✓
        pickup V80.42 ✓
        railway train or vehicle V80.62 ✓

Accident — *continued*
  transport — *continued*
    animal-drawn vehicle occupant — *continued*
      collision — *continued*
        specified motor vehicle NEC V80.52 ✓
        streetcar V80.731 ✓
        truck V80.42 ✓
        two- or three-wheeled motor vehicle V80.32 ✓
        van V80.42 ✓
      noncollision V80.02 ✓
      specified circumstance NEC V80.928 ✓
    animal-rider V80.919 ✓
      collision (with)
        animal V80.11 ✓
          being ridden V80.710 ✓
        animal-drawn vehicle V80.720 ✓
        bus V80.41 ✓
        car V80.41 ✓
        fixed or stationary object V80.81 ✓
        military vehicle V80.910 ✓
        nonmotor vehicle V80.790 ✓
        pedal cycle V80.21 ✓
        pedestrian V80.11 ✓
        pickup V80.41 ✓
        railway train or vehicle V80.61 ✓
        specified motor vehicle NEC V80.51 ✓
        streetcar V80.730 ✓
        truck V80.41 ✓
        two- or three-wheeled motor vehicle V80.31 ✓
        van V80.41 ✓
      noncollision V80.018 ✓
        specified as horse rider V80.010 ✓
      specified circumstance NEC V80.918 ✓
    armored car — *see* Accident, transport, truck occupant
    battery-powered truck (baggage) (mail) — *see* Accident, transport, industrial vehicle occupant
    bus occupant V79.9 ✓
      collision (with)
        animal (traffic) V70.9 ✓
          being ridden (traffic) V76.9 ✓
            nontraffic V76.3 ✓
            while boarding or alighting V76.4 ✓
          nontraffic V70.3 ✓
          while boarding or alighting V70.4 ✓
        animal-drawn vehicle (traffic) V76.9 ✓
          nontraffic V76.3 ✓
          while boarding or alighting V76.4 ✓
        bus (traffic) V74.9 ✓
          nontraffic V74.3 ✓
          while boarding or alighting V74.4 ✓
        car (traffic) V73.9 ✓
          nontraffic V73.3 ✓
          while boarding or alighting V73.4 ✓
        motor vehicle NOS (traffic) V79.60 ✓
          nontraffic V79.20 ✓
          specified type NEC (traffic) V79.69 ✓
            nontraffic V79.29 ✓
        pedal cycle (traffic) V71.9 ✓
          nontraffic V71.3 ✓
          while boarding or alighting V71.4 ✓
        pickup truck (traffic) V73.9 ✓
          nontraffic V73.3 ✓
          while boarding or alighting V73.4 ✓
        railway vehicle (traffic) V75.9 ✓
          nontraffic V75.3 ✓
          while boarding or alighting V75.4 ✓
        specified vehicle NEC (traffic) V76.9 ✓
          nontraffic V76.3 ✓
          while boarding or alighting V76.4 ✓
        stationary object (traffic) V77.9 ✓
          nontraffic V77.3 ✓
          while boarding or alighting V77.4 ✓
        streetcar (traffic) V76.9 ✓
          nontraffic V76.3 ✓
          while boarding or alighting V76.4 ✓
        three wheeled motor vehicle (traffic) V72.9 ✓
          nontraffic V72.3 ✓
          while boarding or alighting V72.4 ✓
        truck (traffic) V74.9 ✓
          nontraffic V74.3 ✓
          while boarding or alighting V74.4 ✓

Accident — *continued*
  transport — *continued*
    bus occupant — *continued*
      collision — *continued*
        two wheeled motor vehicle (traffic) V72.9 ✓
          nontraffic V72.3 ✓
          while boarding or alighting V72.4 ✓
        van (traffic) V73.9 ✓
          nontraffic V73.3 ✓
          while boarding or alighting V73.4 ✓
      driver
        collision (with)
          animal (traffic) V70.5 ✓
            being ridden (traffic) V76.5 ✓
              nontraffic V76.0 ✓
            nontraffic V70.0 ✓
          animal-drawn vehicle (traffic) V76.5 ✓
            nontraffic V76.0 ✓
          bus (traffic) V74.5 ✓
            nontraffic V74.0 ✓
          car (traffic) V73.5 ✓
            nontraffic V73.0 ✓
          motor vehicle NOS (traffic) V79.40 ✓
            nontraffic V79.00 ✓
            specified type NEC (traffic) V79.49 ✓
              nontraffic V79.09 ✓
          pedal cycle (traffic) V71.5 ✓
            nontraffic V71.0 ✓
          pickup truck (traffic) V73.5 ✓
            nontraffic V73.0 ✓
          railway vehicle (traffic) V75.5 ✓
            nontraffic V75.0 ✓
          specified vehicle NEC (traffic) V76.5 ✓
            nontraffic V76.0 ✓
          stationary object (traffic) V77.5 ✓
            nontraffic V77.0 ✓
          streetcar (traffic) V76.5 ✓
            nontraffic V76.0 ✓
          three wheeled motor vehicle (traffic) V72.5 ✓
            nontraffic V72.0 ✓
          truck (traffic) V74.5 ✓
            nontraffic V74.0 ✓
          two wheeled motor vehicle (traffic) V72.5 ✓
            nontraffic V72.0 ✓
          van (traffic) V73.5 ✓
            nontraffic V73.0 ✓
        noncollision accident (traffic) V78.5 ✓
          nontraffic V78.0 ✓
      hanger-on
        collision (with)
          animal (traffic) V70.7 ✓
            being ridden (traffic) V76.7 ✓
              nontraffic V76.2 ✓
            nontraffic V70.2 ✓
          animal-drawn vehicle (traffic) V76.7 ✓
            nontraffic V76.2 ✓
          bus (traffic) V74.7 ✓
            nontraffic V74.2 ✓
          car (traffic) V73.7 ✓
            nontraffic V73.2 ✓
          pedal cycle (traffic) V71.7 ✓
            nontraffic V71.2 ✓
          pickup truck (traffic) V73.7 ✓
            nontraffic V73.2 ✓
          railway vehicle (traffic) V75.7 ✓
            nontraffic V75.2 ✓
          specified vehicle NEC (traffic) V76.7 ✓
            nontraffic V76.2 ✓
          stationary object (traffic) V77.7 ✓
            nontraffic V77.2 ✓
          streetcar (traffic) V76.7 ✓
            nontraffic V76.2 ✓
          three wheeled motor vehicle (traffic) V72.7 ✓
            nontraffic V72.2 ✓
          truck (traffic) V74.7 ✓
            nontraffic V74.2 ✓
          two wheeled motor vehicle (traffic) V72.7 ✓
            nontraffic V72.2 ✓
          van (traffic) V73.7 ✓
            nontraffic V73.2 ✓
        noncollision accident (traffic) V78.7 ✓
          nontraffic V78.2 ✓

Accident — *continued*
  transport — *continued*
    bus occupant — *continued*
      noncollision accident (traffic) V78.9 ☑
        nontraffic V78.3 ☑
        while boarding or alighting V78.4 ☑
      nontraffic V79.3 ☑
      passenger
        collision (with)
          animal (traffic) V70.6 ☑
            being ridden (traffic) V76.6 ☑
              nontraffic V76.1 ☑
            nontraffic V70.1 ☑
          animal-drawn vehicle (traffic) V76.6 ☑
            nontraffic V76.1 ☑
          bus (traffic) V74.6 ☑
            nontraffic V74.1 ☑
          car (traffic) V73.6 ☑
            nontraffic V73.1 ☑
          motor vehicle NOS (traffic) V79.50 ☑
            nontraffic V79.10 ☑
            specified type NEC (traffic) V79.59 ☑
              nontraffic V79.19 ☑
          pedal cycle (traffic) V71.6 ☑
            nontraffic V71.1 ☑
          pickup truck (traffic) V73.6 ☑
            nontraffic V73.1 ☑
          railway vehicle (traffic) V75.6 ☑
            nontraffic V75.1 ☑
          specified vehicle NEC (traffic) V76.6 ☑
            nontraffic V76.1 ☑
          stationary object (traffic) V77.6 ☑
            nontraffic V77.1 ☑
          streetcar (traffic) V76.6 ☑
            nontraffic V76.1 ☑
          three wheeled motor vehicle (traffic)
            V72.6 ☑
            nontraffic V72.1 ☑
          truck (traffic) V74.6 ☑
            nontraffic V74.1 ☑
          two wheeled motor vehicle (traffic)
            V72.6 ☑
            nontraffic V72.1 ☑
          van (traffic) V73.6 ☑
            nontraffic V73.1 ☑
        noncollision accident (traffic) V78.6 ☑
          nontraffic V78.1 ☑
      specified type NEC V79.88 ☑
      military vehicle V79.81 ☑
    cable car, not on rails V98.0 ☑
      on rails — *see* Accident, transport, streetcar
        occupant
    car occupant V49.9 ☑
      ambulance occupant — *see* Accident, transport,
        ambulance occupant
      collision (with)
        animal (traffic) V40.9 ☑
          being ridden (traffic) V46.9 ☑
            nontraffic V46.3 ☑
            while boarding or alighting V46.4 ☑
          nontraffic V40.3 ☑
          while boarding or alighting V40.4 ☑
        animal-drawn vehicle (traffic) V46.9 ☑
          nontraffic V46.3 ☑
          while boarding or alighting V46.4 ☑
        bus (traffic) V44.9 ☑
          nontraffic V44.3 ☑
          while boarding or alighting V44.4 ☑
        car (traffic) V43.92 ☑
          nontraffic V43.32 ☑
          while boarding or alighting V43.42 ☑
        motor vehicle NOS (traffic) V49.60 ☑
          nontraffic V49.20 ☑
          specified type NEC (traffic) V49.69 ☑
            nontraffic V49.29 ☑
        pedal cycle (traffic) V41.9 ☑
          nontraffic V41.3 ☑
          while boarding or alighting V41.4 ☑
        pickup truck (traffic) V43.93 ☑
          nontraffic V43.33 ☑
          while boarding or alighting V43.43 ☑
        railway vehicle (traffic) V45.9 ☑
          nontraffic V45.3 ☑
          while boarding or alighting V45.4 ☑
        specified vehicle NEC (traffic) V46.9 ☑
          nontraffic V46.3 ☑

Accident — *continued*
  transport — *continued*
    car occupant — *continued*
      collision — *continued*
        specified vehicle — *continued*
          while boarding or alighting V46.4 ☑
        sport utility vehicle (traffic) V43.91 ☑
          nontraffic V43.31 ☑
          while boarding or alighting V43.41 ☑
        stationary object (traffic) V47.9 ☑
          nontraffic V47.3 ☑
          while boarding or alighting V47.4 ☑
        streetcar (traffic) V46.9 ☑
          nontraffic V46.3 ☑
          while boarding or alighting V46.4 ☑
        three wheeled motor vehicle (traffic)
          V42.9 ☑
          nontraffic V42.3 ☑
          while boarding or alighting V42.4 ☑
        truck (traffic) V44.9 ☑
          nontraffic V44.3 ☑
          while boarding or alighting V44.4 ☑
        two wheeled motor vehicle (traffic) V42.9 ☑
          nontraffic V42.3 ☑
          while boarding or alighting V42.4 ☑
        van (traffic) V43.94 ☑
          nontraffic V43.34 ☑
          while boarding or alighting V43.44 ☑
      driver
        collision (with)
          animal (traffic) V40.5 ☑
            being ridden (traffic) V46.5 ☑
              nontraffic V46.0 ☑
            nontraffic V40.0 ☑
          animal-drawn vehicle (traffic) V46.5 ☑
            nontraffic V46.0 ☑
          bus (traffic) V44.5 ☑
            nontraffic V44.0 ☑
          car (traffic) V43.52 ☑
            nontraffic V43.02 ☑
          motor vehicle NOS (traffic) V49.40 ☑
            nontraffic V49.00 ☑
            specified type NEC (traffic) V49.49 ☑
              nontraffic V49.09 ☑
          pedal cycle (traffic) V41.5 ☑
            nontraffic V41.0 ☑
          pickup truck (traffic) V43.53 ☑
            nontraffic V43.03 ☑
          railway vehicle (traffic) V45.5 ☑
            nontraffic V45.0 ☑
          specified vehicle NEC (traffic) V46.5 ☑
            nontraffic V46.0 ☑
          sport utility vehicle (traffic) V43.51 ☑
            nontraffic V43.01 ☑
          stationary object (traffic) V47.5 ☑
            nontraffic V47.0 ☑
          streetcar (traffic) V46.5 ☑
            nontraffic V46.0 ☑
          three wheeled motor vehicle (traffic)
            V42.5 ☑
            nontraffic V42.0 ☑
          truck (traffic) V44.5 ☑
            nontraffic V44.0 ☑
          two wheeled motor vehicle (traffic)
            V42.5 ☑
            nontraffic V42.0 ☑
          van (traffic) V43.54 ☑
            nontraffic V43.04 ☑
        noncollision accident (traffic) V48.5 ☑
          nontraffic V48.0 ☑
      hanger-on
        collision (with)
          animal (traffic) V40.7 ☑
            being ridden (traffic) V46.7 ☑
              nontraffic V46.2 ☑
            nontraffic V40.2 ☑
          animal-drawn vehicle (traffic) V46.7 ☑
            nontraffic V46.2 ☑
          bus (traffic) V44.7 ☑
            nontraffic V44.2 ☑
          car (traffic) V43.72 ☑
            nontraffic V43.22 ☑
          pedal cycle (traffic) V41.7 ☑
            nontraffic V41.2 ☑
          pickup truck (traffic) V43.73 ☑
            nontraffic V43.23 ☑

Accident — *continued*
  transport — *continued*
    car occupant — *continued*
      hanger-on — *continued*
        collision — *continued*
          railway vehicle (traffic) V45.7 ☑
            nontraffic V45.2 ☑
          specified vehicle NEC (traffic) V46.7 ☑
            nontraffic V46.2 ☑
          sport utility vehicle (traffic) V43.71 ☑
            nontraffic V43.21 ☑
          stationary object (traffic) V47.7 ☑
            nontraffic V47.2 ☑
          streetcar (traffic) V46.7 ☑
            nontraffic V46.2 ☑
          three wheeled motor vehicle (traffic)
            V42.7 ☑
            nontraffic V42.2 ☑
          truck (traffic) V44.7 ☑
            nontraffic V44.2 ☑
          two wheeled motor vehicle (traffic)
            V42.7 ☑
            nontraffic V42.2 ☑
          van (traffic) V43.74 ☑
            nontraffic V43.24 ☑
        noncollision accident (traffic) V48.7 ☑
          nontraffic V48.2 ☑
      noncollision accident (traffic) V48.9 ☑
        nontraffic V48.3 ☑
        while boarding or alighting V48.4 ☑
      nontraffic V49.3 ☑
      passenger
        collision (with)
          animal (traffic) V40.6 ☑
            being ridden (traffic) V46.6 ☑
              nontraffic V46.1 ☑
            nontraffic V40.1 ☑
          animal-drawn vehicle (traffic) V46.6 ☑
            nontraffic V46.1 ☑
          bus (traffic) V44.6 ☑
            nontraffic V44.1 ☑
          car (traffic) V43.62 ☑
            nontraffic V43.12 ☑
          motor vehicle NOS (traffic) V49.50 ☑
            nontraffic V49.10 ☑
            specified type NEC (traffic) V49.59 ☑
              nontraffic V49.19 ☑
          pedal cycle (traffic) V41.6 ☑
            nontraffic V41.1 ☑
          pickup truck (traffic) V43.63 ☑
            nontraffic V43.13 ☑
          railway vehicle (traffic) V45.6 ☑
            nontraffic V45.1 ☑
          specified vehicle NEC (traffic) V46.6 ☑
            nontraffic V46.1 ☑
          sport utility vehicle (traffic) V43.61 ☑
            nontraffic V43.11 ☑
          stationary object (traffic) V47.6 ☑
            nontraffic V47.1 ☑
          streetcar (traffic) V46.6 ☑
            nontraffic V46.1 ☑
          three wheeled motor vehicle (traffic)
            V42.6 ☑
            nontraffic V42.1 ☑
          truck (traffic) V44.6 ☑
            nontraffic V44.1 ☑
          two wheeled motor vehicle (traffic)
            V42.6 ☑
            nontraffic V42.1 ☑
          van (traffic) V43.64 ☑
            nontraffic V43.14 ☑
        noncollision accident (traffic) V48.6 ☑
          nontraffic V48.1 ☑
      specified type NEC V49.88 ☑
      military vehicle V49.81 ☑
    coal car — *see* Accident, transport, industrial vehi-
      cle occupant
    construction vehicle occupant (nontraffic) V85.9 ☑
      driver V85.5 ☑
      hanger-on V85.7 ☑
      passenger V85.6 ☑
      traffic V85.3 ☑
        driver V85.0 ☑
        hanger-on V85.2 ☑
        passenger V85.1 ☑
      while boarding or alighting V85.4 ☑

Accident — *continued*
  transport — *continued*
    dirt bike rider (nontraffic) V86.96 ☑
      driver V86.56 ☑
      hanger-on V86.76 ☑
      passenger V86.66 ☑
      traffic V86.36 ☑
        driver V86.06 ☑
        hanger-on V86.26 ☑
        passenger V86.16 ☑
      while boarding or alighting V86.46 ☑
    due to cataclysm — *see* Forces of nature, by type
    dune buggy occupant (nontraffic) V86.93 ☑
      driver V86.53 ☑
      hanger-on V86.73 ☑
      passenger V86.63 ☑
      traffic V86.33 ☑
        driver V86.03 ☑
        hanger-on V86.23 ☑
        passenger V86.13 ☑
      while boarding or alighting V86.43 ☑
    forklift — *see* Accident, transport, industrial vehicle occupant
    go cart — *see* Accident, transport, all-terrain vehicle occupant
    golf cart — *see* Accident, transport, all-terrain vehicle occupant
    heavy transport vehicle occupant — *see* Accident, transport, truck occupant
    ice yacht V98.2 ☑
    industrial vehicle occupant (nontraffic) V83.9 ☑
      driver V83.5 ☑
      hanger-on V83.7 ☑
      passenger V83.6 ☑
      traffic V83.3 ☑
        driver V83.0 ☑
        hanger-on V83.2 ☑
        passenger V83.1 ☑
      while boarding or alighting V83.4 ☑
    interurban electric car — *see* Accident, transport, streetcar
    land yacht V98.1 ☑
    logging car — *see* Accident, transport, industrial vehicle occupant
    military vehicle occupant (traffic) V86.34 ☑
      driver V86.04 ☑
      hanger-on V86.24 ☑
      nontraffic V86.94 ☑
        driver V86.54 ☑
        hanger-on V86.74 ☑
        passenger V86.64 ☑
      passenger V86.14 ☑
      while boarding or alighting V86.44 ☑
    mine tram — *see* Accident, transport, industrial vehicle occupant
    motor vehicle NEC occupant (traffic) V89.2 ☑
    motorcoach — *see* Accident, transport, bus occupant
    motor/cross bike rider (*see also* Accident, transport, dirt bike rider) V86.96 ☑
    motorcyclist V29.9 ☑
      collision (with)
        animal (traffic) V20.9 ☑
          being ridden (traffic) V26.9 ☑
            nontraffic V26.2 ☑
            while boarding or alighting V26.3 ☑
          nontraffic V20.2 ☑
          while boarding or alighting V20.3 ☑
        animal-drawn vehicle (traffic) V26.9 ☑
          nontraffic V26.2 ☑
          while boarding or alighting V26.3 ☑
        bus (traffic) V24.9 ☑
          nontraffic V24.2 ☑
          while boarding or alighting V24.3 ☑
        car (traffic) V23.9 ☑
          nontraffic V23.2 ☑
          while boarding or alighting V23.3 ☑
        motor vehicle NOS (traffic) V29.60 ☑
          nontraffic V29.20 ☑
          specified type NEC (traffic) V29.69 ☑
            nontraffic V29.29 ☑
        pedal cycle (traffic) V21.9 ☑
          nontraffic V21.2 ☑
          while boarding or alighting V21.3 ☑
        pickup truck (traffic) V23.9 ☑
          nontraffic V23.2 ☑

Accident — *continued*
  transport — *continued*
    motorcyclist — *continued*
      collision — *continued*
        pickup truck — *continued*
          while boarding or alighting V23.3 ☑
        railway vehicle (traffic) V25.9 ☑
          nontraffic V25.2 ☑
          while boarding or alighting V25.3 ☑
        specified vehicle NEC (traffic) V26.9 ☑
          nontraffic V26.2 ☑
          while boarding or alighting V26.3 ☑
        stationary object (traffic) V27.9 ☑
          nontraffic V27.2 ☑
          while boarding or alighting V27.3 ☑
        streetcar (traffic) V26.9 ☑
          nontraffic V26.2 ☑
          while boarding or alighting V26.3 ☑
        three wheeled motor vehicle (traffic) V22.9 ☑
          nontraffic V22.2 ☑
          while boarding or alighting V22.3 ☑
        truck (traffic) V24.9 ☑
          nontraffic V24.2 ☑
          while boarding or alighting V24.3 ☑
        two wheeled motor vehicle (traffic) V22.9 ☑
          nontraffic V22.2 ☑
          while boarding or alighting V22.3 ☑
        van (traffic) V23.9 ☑
          nontraffic V23.2 ☑
          while boarding or alighting V23.3 ☑
      driver
        collision (with)
          animal (traffic) V20.4 ☑
            being ridden (traffic) V26.4 ☑
              nontraffic V26.0 ☑
            nontraffic V20.0 ☑
          animal-drawn vehicle (traffic) V26.4 ☑
            nontraffic V26.0 ☑
          bus (traffic) V24.4 ☑
            nontraffic V24.0 ☑
          car (traffic) V23.4 ☑
            nontraffic V23.0 ☑
          motor vehicle NOS (traffic) V29.40 ☑
            nontraffic V29.00 ☑
            specified type NEC (traffic) V29.49 ☑
              nontraffic V29.09 ☑
          pedal cycle (traffic) V21.4 ☑
            nontraffic V21.0 ☑
          pickup truck (traffic) V23.4 ☑
            nontraffic V23.0 ☑
          railway vehicle (traffic) V25.4 ☑
            nontraffic V25.0 ☑
          specified vehicle NEC (traffic) V26.4 ☑
            nontraffic V26.0 ☑
          stationary object (traffic) V27.4 ☑
            nontraffic V27.0 ☑
          streetcar (traffic) V26.4 ☑
            nontraffic V26.0 ☑
          three wheeled motor vehicle (traffic) V22.4 ☑
            nontraffic V22.0 ☑
          truck (traffic) V24.4 ☑
            nontraffic V24.0 ☑
          two wheeled motor vehicle (traffic) V22.4 ☑
            nontraffic V22.0 ☑
          van (traffic) V23.4 ☑
            nontraffic V23.0 ☑
          noncollision accident (traffic) V28.4 ☑
            nontraffic V28.0 ☑
      noncollision accident (traffic) V28.9 ☑
        nontraffic V28.2 ☑
        while boarding or alighting V28.3 ☑
      nontraffic V29.3 ☑
      passenger
        collision (with)
          animal (traffic) V20.5 ☑
            being ridden (traffic) V26.5 ☑
              nontraffic V26.1 ☑
            nontraffic V20.1 ☑
          animal-drawn vehicle (traffic) V26.5 ☑
            nontraffic V26.1 ☑
          bus (traffic) V24.5 ☑
            nontraffic V24.1 ☑
          car (traffic) V23.5 ☑

Accident — *continued*
  transport — *continued*
    motorcyclist — *continued*
      passenger — *continued*
        collision — *continued*
          car — *continued*
            nontraffic V23.1 ☑
          motor vehicle NOS (traffic) V29.50 ☑
            nontraffic V29.10 ☑
            specified type NEC (traffic) V29.59 ☑
              nontraffic V29.19 ☑
          pedal cycle (traffic) V21.5 ☑
            nontraffic V21.1 ☑
          pickup truck (traffic) V23.5 ☑
            nontraffic V23.1 ☑
          railway vehicle (traffic) V25.5 ☑
            nontraffic V25.1 ☑
          specified vehicle NEC (traffic) V26.5 ☑
            nontraffic V26.1 ☑
          stationary object (traffic) V27.5 ☑
            nontraffic V27.1 ☑
          streetcar (traffic) V26.5 ☑
            nontraffic V26.1 ☑
          three wheeled motor vehicle (traffic) V22.5 ☑
            nontraffic V22.1 ☑
          truck (traffic) V24.5 ☑
            nontraffic V24.1 ☑
          two wheeled motor vehicle (traffic) V22.5 ☑
            nontraffic V22.1 ☑
          van (traffic) V23.5 ☑
            nontraffic V23.1 ☑
        noncollision accident (traffic) V28.5 ☑
          nontraffic V28.1 ☑
      specified type NEC V29.88 ☑
      military vehicle V29.81 ☑
    occupant (of)
      aircraft (powered) V95.9 ☑
        fixed wing
          commercial — *see* Accident, transport, aircraft, occupant, powered, fixed wing, commercial
          private — *see* Accident, transport, aircraft, occupant, powered, fixed wing, private
        nonpowered V96.9 ☑
        specified NEC V95.8 ☑
      airport battery-powered vehicle — *see* Accident, transport, industrial vehicle occupant
      all-terrain vehicle (ATV) — *see* Accident, transport, all-terrain vehicle occupant
      animal-drawn vehicle — *see* Accident, transport, animal-drawn vehicle occupant
      automobile — *see* Accident, transport, car occupant
      balloon V96.00 ☑
      battery-powered vehicle — *see* Accident, transport, industrial vehicle occupant
      bicycle — *see* Accident, transport, pedal cyclist
        motorized — *see* Accident, transport, motorcycle rider
      boat NEC — *see* Accident, watercraft
      bulldozer — *see* Accident, transport, construction vehicle occupant
      bus — *see* Accident, transport, bus occupant
      cable car (on rails) (*see also* Accident, transport, streetcar occupant)
        not on rails V98.0 ☑
      car (*see also* Accident, transport, car occupant)
        cable (on rails) (*see also* Accident, transport, streetcar occupant)
          not on rails V98.0 ☑
      coach — *see* Accident, transport, bus occupant
      coal-car — *see* Accident, transport, industrial vehicle occupant
      digger — *see* Accident, transport, construction vehicle occupant
      dump truck — *see* Accident, transport, construction vehicle occupant
      earth-leveler — *see* Accident, transport, construction vehicle occupant
      farm machinery (self-propelled) — *see* Accident, transport, agricultural vehicle occupant

☑ Additional Character Required — Refer to the Tabular List for Character Selection   ▽ Subterms under main terms may continue to next column or page

Accident — *continued*
  transport — *continued*
    occupant — *continued*
      forklift — *see* Accident, transport, industrial vehicle occupant
      glider (unpowered) V96.20 ☑
        hang V96.10 ☑
        powered (microlight) (ultralight) — *see* Accident, transport, aircraft, occupant, powered, glider
      glider (unpowered) NEC V96.20 ☑
      hang-glider V96.10 ☑
      harvester — *see* Accident, transport, agricultural vehicle occupant
      heavy (transport) vehicle — *see* Accident, transport, truck occupant
      helicopter — *see* Accident, transport, aircraft, occupant, helicopter
      ice-yacht V98.2 ☑
      kite (carrying person) V96.8 ☑
      land-yacht V98.1 ☑
      logging car — *see* Accident, transport, industrial vehicle occupant
      mechanical shovel — *see* Accident, transport, construction vehicle occupant
      microlight — *see* Accident, transport, aircraft, occupant, powered, glider
      minibus — *see* Accident, transport, pickup truck occupant
      minivan — *see* Accident, transport, pickup truck occupant
      moped — *see* Accident, transport, motorcycle
      motor scooter — *see* Accident, transport, motorcycle
      motorcycle (with sidecar) — *see* Accident, transport, motorcycle
      off-road motor-vehicle (*see also* Accident, transport, all-terrain vehicle occupant) V86.99 ☑
      pedal cycle (*see also* Accident, transport, pedal cyclist)
      pick-up (truck) — *see* Accident, transport, pickup truck occupant
      railway (train) (vehicle) (subterranean) (elevated) — *see* Accident, transport, railway vehicle occupant
      rickshaw — *see* Accident, transport, pedal cycle
        motorized — *see* Accident, transport, three-wheeled motor vehicle
        pedal driven — *see* Accident, transport, pedal cyclist
      road-roller — *see* Accident, transport, construction vehicle occupant
      ship NOS V94.9 ☑
      ski-lift (chair) (gondola) V98.3 ☑
      snowmobile — *see* Accident, transport, snowmobile occupant
      spacecraft, spaceship — *see* Accident, transport, aircraft, occupant, spacecraft
      sport utility vehicle — *see* Accident, transport, pickup truck occupant
      streetcar (interurban) (operating on public street or highway) — *see* Accident, transport, streetcar occupant
      SUV — *see* Accident, transport, pickup truck occupant
      téléférique V98.0 ☑
      three-wheeled vehicle (motorized) (*see also* Accident, transport, three-wheeled motor vehicle occupant)
        nonmotorized — *see* Accident, transport, pedal cycle
      tractor (farm) (and trailer) — *see* Accident, transport, agricultural vehicle occupant
      train — *see* Accident, transport, railway vehicle occupant
      tram — *see* Accident, transport, streetcar occupant
        in mine or quarry — *see* Accident, transport, industrial vehicle occupant
      tricycle — *see* Accident, transport, pedal cycle
        motorized — *see* Accident, transport, three-wheeled motor vehicle
      trolley — *see* Accident, transport, streetcar occupant
        in mine or quarry — *see* Accident, transport, industrial vehicle occupant

Accident — *continued*
  transport — *continued*
    occupant — *continued*
      tub, in mine or quarry — *see* Accident, transport, industrial vehicle occupant
      ultralight — *see* Accident, transport, aircraft, occupant, powered, glider
      van — *see* Accident, transport, van occupant
      vehicle NEC V89.9 ☑
        heavy transport — *see* Accident, transport, truck occupant
        motor (traffic) NEC V89.2 ☑
        nontraffic NEC V89.0 ☑
      watercraft NOS V94.9 ☑
        causing drowning — *see* Drowning, resulting from accident to boat
    off-road motor-vehicle (*see also* Accident, transport, all-terrain vehicle occupant) V86.99 ☑
    parachutist V97.29 ☑
      after accident to aircraft — *see* Accident, transport, aircraft
      entangled in object V97.21 ☑
      injured on landing V97.22 ☑
    pedal cyclist V19.9 ☑
      collision (with)
        animal (traffic) V10.9 ☑
          being ridden (traffic) V16.9 ☑
            nontraffic V16.2 ☑
            while boarding or alighting V16.3 ☑
          nontraffic V10.2 ☑
          while boarding or alighting V10.3 ☑
        animal-drawn vehicle (traffic) V16.9 ☑
          nontraffic V16.2 ☑
          while boarding or alighting V16.3 ☑
        bus (traffic) V14.9 ☑
          nontraffic V14.2 ☑
          while boarding or alighting V14.3 ☑
        car (traffic) V13.9 ☑
          nontraffic V13.2 ☑
          while boarding or alighting V13.3 ☑
        motor vehicle NOS (traffic) V19.60 ☑
          nontraffic V19.20 ☑
          specified type NEC (traffic) V19.69 ☑
            nontraffic V19.29 ☑
        pedal cycle (traffic) V11.9 ☑
          nontraffic V11.2 ☑
          while boarding or alighting V11.3 ☑
        pickup truck (traffic) V13.9 ☑
          nontraffic V13.2 ☑
          while boarding or alighting V13.3 ☑
        railway vehicle (traffic) V15.9 ☑
          nontraffic V15.2 ☑
          while boarding or alighting V15.3 ☑
        specified vehicle NEC (traffic) V16.9 ☑
          nontraffic V16.2 ☑
          while boarding or alighting V16.3 ☑
        stationary object (traffic) V17.9 ☑
          nontraffic V17.2 ☑
          while boarding or alighting V17.3 ☑
        streetcar (traffic) V16.9 ☑
          nontraffic V16.2 ☑
          while boarding or alighting V16.3 ☑
        three wheeled motor vehicle (traffic) V12.9 ☑
          nontraffic V12.2 ☑
          while boarding or alighting V12.3 ☑
        truck (traffic) V14.9 ☑
          nontraffic V14.2 ☑
          while boarding or alighting V14.3 ☑
        two wheeled motor vehicle (traffic) V12.9 ☑
          nontraffic V12.2 ☑
          while boarding or alighting V12.3 ☑
        van (traffic) V13.9 ☑
          nontraffic V13.2 ☑
          while boarding or alighting V13.3 ☑
      driver
        collision (with)
          animal (traffic) V10.4 ☑
            being ridden (traffic) V16.4 ☑
              nontraffic V16.0 ☑
            nontraffic V10.0 ☑
          animal-drawn vehicle (traffic) V16.4 ☑
            nontraffic V16.0 ☑
          bus (traffic) V14.4 ☑
            nontraffic V14.0 ☑
          car (traffic) V13.4 ☑

Accident — *continued*
  transport — *continued*
    pedal cyclist — *continued*
      driver — *continued*
        collision — *continued*
          car — *continued*
            nontraffic V13.0 ☑
            motor vehicle NOS (traffic) V19.40 ☑
              nontraffic V19.00 ☑
              specified type NEC (traffic) V19.49 ☑
                nontraffic V19.09 ☑
            pedal cycle (traffic) V11.4 ☑
              nontraffic V11.0 ☑
            pickup truck (traffic) V13.4 ☑
              nontraffic V13.0 ☑
            railway vehicle (traffic) V15.4 ☑
              nontraffic V15.0 ☑
            specified vehicle NEC (traffic) V16.4 ☑
              nontraffic V16.0 ☑
            stationary object (traffic) V17.4 ☑
              nontraffic V17.0 ☑
            streetcar (traffic) V16.4 ☑
              nontraffic V16.0 ☑
            three wheeled motor vehicle (traffic) V12.4 ☑
              nontraffic V12.0 ☑
            truck (traffic) V14.4 ☑
              nontraffic V14.0 ☑
            two wheeled motor vehicle (traffic) V12.4 ☑
              nontraffic V12.0 ☑
            van (traffic) V13.4 ☑
              nontraffic V13.0 ☑
          noncollision accident (traffic) V18.4 ☑
            nontraffic V18.0 ☑
        noncollision accident (traffic) V18.9 ☑
          nontraffic V18.2 ☑
          while boarding or alighting V18.3 ☑
      nontraffic V19.3 ☑
      passenger
        collision (with)
          animal (traffic) V10.5 ☑
            being ridden (traffic) V16.5 ☑
              nontraffic V16.1 ☑
            nontraffic V10.1 ☑
          animal-drawn vehicle (traffic) V16.5 ☑
            nontraffic V16.1 ☑
          bus (traffic) V14.5 ☑
            nontraffic V14.1 ☑
          car (traffic) V13.5 ☑
            nontraffic V13.1 ☑
          motor vehicle NOS (traffic) V19.50 ☑
            nontraffic V19.10 ☑
            specified type NEC (traffic) V19.59 ☑
              nontraffic V19.19 ☑
          pedal cycle (traffic) V11.5 ☑
            nontraffic V11.1 ☑
          pickup truck (traffic) V13.5 ☑
            nontraffic V13.1 ☑
          railway vehicle (traffic) V15.5 ☑
            nontraffic V15.1 ☑
          specified vehicle NEC (traffic) V16.5 ☑
            nontraffic V16.1 ☑
          stationary object (traffic) V17.5 ☑
            nontraffic V17.1 ☑
          streetcar (traffic) V16.5 ☑
            nontraffic V16.1 ☑
          three wheeled motor vehicle (traffic) V12.5 ☑
            nontraffic V12.1 ☑
          truck (traffic) V14.5 ☑
            nontraffic V14.1 ☑
          two wheeled motor vehicle (traffic) V12.5 ☑
            nontraffic V12.1 ☑
          van (traffic) V13.5 ☑
            nontraffic V13.1 ☑
        noncollision accident (traffic) V18.5 ☑
          nontraffic V18.1 ☑
      specified type NEC V19.88 ☑
        military vehicle V19.81 ☑
    pedestrian
      conveyance (occupant) V09.9 ☑
        babystroller V00.828 ☑
          collision (with) V09.9 ☑

Accident — *continued*
  transport — *continued*
    pedestrian — *continued*
      conveyance — *continued*
        babystroller — *continued*
          collision — *continued*
            animal being ridden or animal drawn vehicle V06.99 ☑
              nontraffic V06.09 ☑
              traffic V06.19 ☑
            bus or heavy transport V04.99 ☑
              nontraffic V04.09 ☑
              traffic V04.19 ☑
            car V03.99 ☑
              nontraffic V03.09 ☑
              traffic V03.19 ☑
            pedal cycle V01.99 ☑
              nontraffic V01.09 ☑
              traffic V01.19 ☑
            pick-up truck or van V03.99 ☑
              nontraffic V03.09 ☑
              traffic V03.19 ☑
            railway (train) (vehicle) V05.99 ☑
              nontraffic V05.09 ☑
              traffic V05.19 ☑
            stationary object V00.822 ☑
            streetcar V06.99 ☑
              nontraffic V06.09 ☑
              traffic V06.19 ☑
            two- or three-wheeled motor vehicle V02.99 ☑
              nontraffic V02.09 ☑
              traffic V02.19 ☑
            vehicle V09.9 ☑
              animal-drawn V06.99 ☑
                nontraffic V06.09 ☑
                traffic V06.19 ☑
              motor
                nontraffic V09.00 ☑
                traffic V09.20 ☑
           fall V00.821 ☑
          nontraffic V09.1 ☑
            involving motor vehicle NEC V09.00 ☑
          traffic V09.3 ☑
            involving motor vehicle NEC V09.20 ☑
         flat-bottomed NEC V00.388 ☑
          collision (with) V09.9 ☑
            animal being ridden or animal drawn vehicle V06.99 ☑
              nontraffic V06.09 ☑
              traffic V06.19 ☑
            bus or heavy transport V04.99 ☑
              nontraffic V04.09 ☑
              traffic V04.19 ☑
            car V03.99 ☑
              nontraffic V03.09 ☑
              traffic V03.19 ☑
            pedal cycle V01.99 ☑
              nontraffic V01.09 ☑
              traffic V01.19 ☑
            pick-up truck or van V03.99 ☑
              nontraffic V03.09 ☑
              traffic V03.19 ☑
            railway (train) (vehicle) V05.99 ☑
              nontraffic V05.09 ☑
              traffic V05.19 ☑
            stationary object V00.382 ☑
            streetcar V06.99 ☑
              nontraffic V06.09 ☑
              traffic V06.19 ☑
            two- or three-wheeled motor vehicle V02.99 ☑
              nontraffic V02.09 ☑
              traffic V02.19 ☑
            vehicle V09.9 ☑
              animal-drawn V06.99 ☑
                nontraffic V06.09 ☑
                traffic V06.19 ☑
              motor
                nontraffic V09.00 ☑
                traffic V09.20 ☑
           fall V00.381 ☑
          nontraffic V09.1 ☑

Accident — *continued*
  transport — *continued*
    pedestrian — *continued*
      conveyance — *continued*
        flat-bottomed — *continued*
          nontraffic — *continued*
            involving motor vehicle NEC V09.00 ☑
          snow
            board — *see* Accident, transport, pedestrian, conveyance, snow board
            ski — *see* Accident, transport, pedestrian, conveyance, skis (snow)
          traffic V09.3 ☑
            involving motor vehicle NEC V09.20 ☑
        gliding type NEC V00.288 ☑
          collision (with) V09.9 ☑
            animal being ridden or animal drawn vehicle V06.99 ☑
              nontraffic V06.09 ☑
              traffic V06.19 ☑
            bus or heavy transport V04.99 ☑
              nontraffic V04.09 ☑
              traffic V04.19 ☑
            car V03.99 ☑
              nontraffic V03.09 ☑
              traffic V03.19 ☑
            pedal cycle V01.99 ☑
              nontraffic V01.09 ☑
              traffic V01.19 ☑
            pick-up truck or van V03.99 ☑
              nontraffic V03.09 ☑
              traffic V03.19 ☑
            railway (train) (vehicle) V05.99 ☑
              nontraffic V05.09 ☑
              traffic V05.19 ☑
            stationary object V00.282 ☑
            streetcar V06.99 ☑
              nontraffic V06.09 ☑
              traffic V02.19 ☑
            two- or three-wheeled motor vehicle V02.99 ☑
              nontraffic V02.09 ☑
              traffic V02.19 ☑
            vehicle V09.9 ☑
              animal-drawn V06.99 ☑
                nontraffic V06.09 ☑
                traffic V06.19 ☑
              motor
                nontraffic V09.00 ☑
                traffic V09.20 ☑
          fall V00.281 ☑
         heelies — *see* Accident, transport, pedestrian, conveyance, heelies
        ice skate — *see* Accident, transport, pedestrian, conveyance, ice skate
        nontraffic V09.1 ☑
          involving motor vehicle NEC V09.00 ☑
        sled — *see* Accident, transport, pedestrian, conveyance, sled
        traffic V09.3 ☑
          involving motor vehicle NEC V09.20 ☑
          wheelies — *see* Accident, transport, pedestrian, conveyance, heelies
        heelies V00.158 ☑
          colliding with stationary object V00.152 ☑
          fall V00.151 ☑
        ice skates V00.218 ☑
          collision (with) V09.9 ☑
            animal being ridden or animal drawn vehicle V06.99 ☑
              nontraffic V06.09 ☑
              traffic V06.19 ☑
            bus or heavy transport V04.99 ☑
              nontraffic V04.09 ☑
              traffic V04.19 ☑
            car V03.99 ☑
              nontraffic V03.09 ☑
              traffic V03.19 ☑

Accident — *continued*
  transport — *continued*
    pedestrian — *continued*
      conveyance — *continued*
        ice skates — *continued*
          collision — *continued*
            pedal cycle V01.99 ☑
              nontraffic V01.09 ☑
              traffic V01.19 ☑
            pick-up truck or van V03.99 ☑
              nontraffic V03.09 ☑
              traffic V03.19 ☑
            railway (train) (vehicle) V05.99 ☑
              nontraffic V05.09 ☑
              traffic V05.19 ☑
            stationary object V00.212 ☑
            streetcar V06.99 ☑
              nontraffic V06.09 ☑
              traffic V06.19 ☑
            two- or three-wheeled motor vehicle V02.99 ☑
              nontraffic V02.09 ☑
              traffic V02.19 ☑
            vehicle V09.9 ☑
              animal-drawn V06.99 ☑
                nontraffic V06.09 ☑
                traffic V06.19 ☑
              motor
                nontraffic V09.00 ☑
                traffic V09.20 ☑
          fall V00.211 ☑
         nontraffic V09.1 ☑
          involving motor vehicle NEC V09.00 ☑
        traffic V09.3 ☑
          involving motor vehicle NEC V09.20 ☑
        motorized mobility scooter V00.838 ☑
          collision with stationary object V00.832 ☑
          fall from V00.831 ☑
          nontraffic V09.1 ☑
            involving motor vehicle V09.00 ☑
              military V09.01 ☑
              specified type NEC V09.09 ☑
        roller skates (non in-line) V00.128 ☑
          collision (with) V09.9 ☑
            animal being ridden or animal drawn vehicle V06.91 ☑
              nontraffic V06.01 ☑
              traffic V06.11 ☑
            bus or heavy transport V04.91 ☑
              nontraffic V04.01 ☑
              traffic V04.11 ☑
            car V03.91 ☑
              nontraffic V03.01 ☑
              traffic V03.11 ☑
            pedal cycle V01.91 ☑
              nontraffic V01.01 ☑
              traffic V01.11 ☑
            pick-up truck or van V03.91 ☑
              nontraffic V03.01 ☑
              traffic V03.11 ☑
            railway (train) (vehicle) V05.91 ☑
              nontraffic V05.01 ☑
              traffic V05.11 ☑
            stationary object V00.122 ☑
            streetcar V06.91 ☑
              nontraffic V06.01 ☑
              traffic V06.11 ☑
            two- or three-wheeled motor vehicle V02.91 ☑
              nontraffic V02.01 ☑
              traffic V02.11 ☑
            vehicle V09.9 ☑
              animal-drawn V06.91 ☑
                nontraffic V06.01 ☑
                traffic V06.11 ☑
              motor
                nontraffic V09.00 ☑
                traffic V09.20 ☑
          fall V00.121 ☑
        in-line V00.118 ☑

☑ **Additional Character Required** — Refer to the Tabular List for Character Selection   ⍐ Subterms under main terms may continue to next column or page

Accident — *continued*
  transport — *continued*
    pedestrian — *continued*
      conveyance — *continued*
        roller skates — *continued*
          in-line — *continued*
            collision — *see also* Accident, transport, pedestrian, conveyance occupant, roller skates, collision
              with stationary object V00.112 ☑
            fall V00.111 ☑
          nontraffic V09.1 ☑
            involving motor vehicle NEC V09.00 ☑
          traffic V09.3 ☑
            involving motor vehicle NEC V09.20 ☑
        rolling shoes V00.158 ☑
          colliding with stationary object V00.152 ☑
          fall V00.151 ☑
        rolling type NEC V00.188 ☑
          collision (with) V09.9
            animal being ridden or animal drawn vehicle V06.99 ☑
              nontraffic V06.09 ☑
              traffic V06.19 ☑
            bus or heavy transport V04.99 ☑
              nontraffic V04.09 ☑
              traffic V04.19 ☑
            car V03.99 ☑
              nontraffic V03.09 ☑
              traffic V03.19 ☑
            pedal cycle V01.99 ☑
              nontraffic V01.09 ☑
              traffic V01.19 ☑
            pick-up truck or van V03.99 ☑
              nontraffic V03.09 ☑
              traffic V03.19 ☑
            railway (train) (vehicle) V05.99 ☑
              nontraffic V05.09 ☑
              traffic V05.19 ☑
            stationary object V00.182 ☑
            streetcar V06.99 ☑
              nontraffic V06.09 ☑
              traffic V06.19 ☑
            two- or three-wheeled motor vehicle V02.99 ☑
              nontraffic V02.09 ☑
              traffic V02.19 ☑
            vehicle V09.9 ☑
              animal-drawn V06.99 ☑
                nontraffic V06.09 ☑
                traffic V06.19 ☑
              motor
                nontraffic V09.00 ☑
                traffic V09.20 ☑
          fall V00.181 ☑
          in-line roller skate — *see* Accident, transport, pedestrian, conveyance, roller skate, in-line
          nontraffic V09.1 ☑
            involving motor vehicle NEC V09.00 ☑
          roller skate — *see* Accident, transport, pedestrian, conveyance, roller skate
          scooter (non-motorized) — *see* Accident, transport, pedestrian, conveyance, scooter
          skateboard — *see* Accident, transport, pedestrian, conveyance, skateboard
          traffic V09.3 ☑
            involving motor vehicle NEC V09.20 ☑
        scooter (non-motorized) V00.148 ☑
          collision (with) V09.9
            animal being ridden or animal drawn vehicle V06.99 ☑
              nontraffic V06.09 ☑
              traffic V06.19 ☑
            bus or heavy transport V04.99 ☑
              nontraffic V04.09 ☑
              traffic V04.19 ☑

Accident — *continued*
  transport — *continued*
    pedestrian — *continued*
      conveyance — *continued*
        scooter — *continued*
          collision — *continued*
            car V03.99 ☑
              nontraffic V03.09 ☑
              traffic V03.19 ☑
            pedal cycle V01.99 ☑
              nontraffic V01.09 ☑
              traffic V01.19 ☑
            pick-up truck or van V03.99 ☑
              nontraffic V03.09 ☑
              traffic V03.19 ☑
            railway (train) (vehicle) V05.99 ☑
              nontraffic V05.09 ☑
              traffic V05.19 ☑
            stationary object V00.142 ☑
            streetcar V06.99 ☑
              nontraffic V06.09 ☑
              traffic V06.19 ☑
            two- or three-wheeled motor vehicle V02.99 ☑
              nontraffic V02.09 ☑
              traffic V02.19 ☑
            vehicle V09.9 ☑
              animal-drawn V06.99 ☑
                nontraffic V06.09 ☑
                traffic V06.19 ☑
              motor
                nontraffic V09.00 ☑
                traffic V09.20 ☑
          fall V00.141 ☑
          nontraffic V09.1 ☑
            involving motor vehicle NEC V09.00 ☑
          traffic V09.3 ☑
            involving motor vehicle NEC V09.20 ☑
        skate board V00.138 ☑
          collision (with) V09.9 ☑
            animal being ridden or animal drawn vehicle V06.92 ☑
              nontraffic V06.02 ☑
              traffic V06.12 ☑
            bus or heavy transport V04.92 ☑
              nontraffic V04.02 ☑
              traffic V04.12 ☑
            car V03.92 ☑
              nontraffic V03.02 ☑
              traffic V03.12 ☑
            pedal cycle V01.92 ☑
              nontraffic V01.02 ☑
              traffic V01.12 ☑
            pick-up truck or van V03.92 ☑
              nontraffic V03.02 ☑
              traffic V03.12 ☑
            railway (train) (vehicle) V05.92 ☑
              nontraffic V05.02 ☑
              traffic V05.12 ☑
            stationary object V00.132 ☑
            streetcar V06.92 ☑
              nontraffic V06.02 ☑
              traffic V06.12 ☑
            two- or three-wheeled motor vehicle V02.92 ☑
              nontraffic V02.02 ☑
              traffic V02.12 ☑
            vehicle V09.9 ☑
              animal-drawn V06.92 ☑
                nontraffic V06.02 ☑
                traffic V06.12 ☑
              motor
                nontraffic V09.00 ☑
                traffic V09.20 ☑
          fall V00.131 ☑
          nontraffic V09.1 ☑
            involving motor vehicle NEC V09.00 ☑
          traffic V09.3 ☑
            involving motor vehicle NEC V09.20 ☑
        skis (snow) V00.328 ☑
          collision (with) V09.9 ☑

Accident — *continued*
  transport — *continued*
    pedestrian — *continued*
      conveyance — *continued*
        skis — *continued*
          collision — *continued*
            animal being ridden or animal drawn vehicle V06.99 ☑
              nontraffic V06.09 ☑
              traffic V06.19 ☑
            bus or heavy transport V04.99 ☑
              nontraffic V04.09 ☑
              traffic V04.19 ☑
            car V03.99 ☑
              nontraffic V03.09 ☑
              traffic V03.19 ☑
            pedal cycle V01.99 ☑
              nontraffic V01.09 ☑
              traffic V01.19 ☑
            pick-up truck or van V03.99 ☑
              nontraffic V03.09 ☑
              traffic V03.19 ☑
            railway (train) (vehicle) V05.99 ☑
              nontraffic V05.09 ☑
              traffic V05.19 ☑
            stationary object V00.322 ☑
            streetcar V06.99 ☑
              nontraffic V06.09 ☑
              traffic V06.19 ☑
            two- or three-wheeled motor vehicle V02.99 ☑
              nontraffic V02.09 ☑
              traffic V02.19 ☑
            vehicle V09.9 ☑
              animal-drawn V06.99 ☑
                nontraffic V06.09 ☑
                traffic V06.19 ☑
              motor
                nontraffic V09.00 ☑
                traffic V09.20 ☑
          fall V00.321 ☑
          nontraffic V09.1 ☑
            involving motor vehicle NEC V09.00 ☑
          traffic V09.3 ☑
            involving motor vehicle NEC V09.20 ☑
        sled V00.228 ☑
          collision (with) V09.9 ☑
            animal being ridden or animal drawn vehicle V06.99 ☑
              nontraffic V06.09 ☑
              traffic V06.19 ☑
            bus or heavy transport V04.99 ☑
              nontraffic V04.09 ☑
              traffic V04.19 ☑
            car V03.99 ☑
              nontraffic V03.09 ☑
              traffic V03.19 ☑
            pedal cycle V01.99 ☑
              nontraffic V01.09 ☑
              traffic V01.19 ☑
            pick-up truck or van V03.99 ☑
              nontraffic V03.09 ☑
              traffic V03.19 ☑
            railway (train) (vehicle) V05.99 ☑
              nontraffic V05.09 ☑
              traffic V05.19 ☑
            stationary object V00.222 ☑
            streetcar V06.99 ☑
              nontraffic V06.09 ☑
              traffic V06.19 ☑
            two- or three-wheeled motor vehicle V02.99 ☑
              nontraffic V02.09 ☑
              traffic V02.19 ☑
            vehicle V09.9 ☑
              animal-drawn V06.99 ☑
                nontraffic V06.09 ☑
                traffic V06.19 ☑
              motor
                nontraffic V09.00 ☑
                traffic V09.20 ☑
          fall V00.221 ☑
          nontraffic V09.1 ☑

Accident — *continued*
  transport — *continued*
    pedestrian — *continued*
      conveyance — *continued*
        sled — *continued*
          nontraffic — *continued*
            involving motor vehicle NEC V09.00 ☑
          traffic V09.3 ☑
            involving motor vehicle NEC V09.20 ☑
        snow board V00.318 ☑
          collision (with) V09.9 ☑
            animal being ridden or animal drawn vehicle V06.99 ☑
              nontraffic V06.09 ☑
              traffic V06.19 ☑
            bus or heavy transport V04.99 ☑
              nontraffic V04.09 ☑
              traffic V04.19 ☑
            car V03.99 ☑
              nontraffic V03.09 ☑
              traffic V03.19 ☑
            pedal cycle V01.99 ☑
              nontraffic V01.09 ☑
              traffic V01.19 ☑
            pick-up truck or van V03.99 ☑
              nontraffic V03.09 ☑
              traffic V03.19 ☑
            railway (train) (vehicle) V05.99 ☑
              nontraffic V05.09 ☑
              traffic V05.19 ☑
            stationary object V00.312 ☑
            streetcar V06.99 ☑
              nontraffic V06.09 ☑
              traffic V06.19 ☑
            two- or three-wheeled motor vehicle V02.99 ☑
              nontraffic V02.09 ☑
              traffic V02.19 ☑
            vehicle V09.9 ☑
              animal-drawn V06.99 ☑
                nontraffic V06.09 ☑
                traffic V06.19 ☑
              motor
                nontraffic V09.00 ☑
                traffic V09.20 ☑
           fall V00.311 ☑
          nontraffic V09.1 ☑
            involving motor vehicle NEC V09.00 ☑
          traffic V09.3 ☑
            involving motor vehicle NEC V09.20 ☑
        specified type NEC V00.898 ☑
          collision (with) V09.9 ☑
            animal being ridden or animal drawn vehicle V06.99 ☑
              nontraffic V06.09 ☑
              traffic V06.19 ☑
            bus or heavy transport V04.99 ☑
              nontraffic V04.09 ☑
              traffic V04.19 ☑
            car V03.99 ☑
              nontraffic V03.09 ☑
              traffic V03.19 ☑
            pedal cycle V01.99 ☑
              nontraffic V01.09 ☑
              traffic V01.19 ☑
            pick-up truck or van V03.99 ☑
              nontraffic V03.09 ☑
              traffic V03.19 ☑
            railway (train) (vehicle) V05.99 ☑
              nontraffic V05.09 ☑
              traffic V05.19 ☑
            stationary object V00.892 ☑
            streetcar V06.99 ☑
              nontraffic V06.09 ☑
              traffic V06.19 ☑
            two- or three-wheeled motor vehicle V02.99 ☑
              nontraffic V02.09 ☑
              traffic V02.19 ☑
            vehicle V09.9 ☑
              animal-drawn V06.99 ☑
                nontraffic V06.09 ☑

Accident — *continued*
  transport — *continued*
    pedestrian — *continued*
      conveyance — *continued*
        specified type — *continued*
          collision — *continued*
            vehicle — *continued*
              animal-drawn — *continued*
                traffic V06.19 ☑
              motor
                nontraffic V09.00 ☑
                traffic V09.20 ☑
          fall V00.891 ☑
          nontraffic V09.1 ☑
            involving motor vehicle NEC V09.00 ☑
          traffic V09.3 ☑
            involving motor vehicle NEC V09.20 ☑
        traffic V09.3 ☑
          involving motor vehicle V09.20 ☑
            military V09.21 ☑
            specified type NEC V09.29 ☑
        wheelchair (powered) V00.818 ☑
          collision (with) V09.9 ☑
            animal being ridden or animal drawn vehicle V06.99 ☑
              nontraffic V06.09 ☑
              traffic V06.19 ☑
            bus or heavy transport V04.99 ☑
              nontraffic V04.09 ☑
              traffic V04.19 ☑
            car V03.99 ☑
              nontraffic V03.09 ☑
              traffic V03.19 ☑
            pedal cycle V01.99 ☑
              nontraffic V01.09 ☑
              traffic V01.19 ☑
            pick-up truck or van V03.99 ☑
              nontraffic V03.09 ☑
              traffic V03.19 ☑
            railway (train) (vehicle) V05.99 ☑
              nontraffic V05.09 ☑
              traffic V05.19 ☑
            stationary object V00.812 ☑
            streetcar V06.99 ☑
              nontraffic V06.09 ☑
              traffic V06.19 ☑
            two- or three-wheeled motor vehicle V02.99 ☑
              nontraffic V02.09 ☑
              traffic V02.19 ☑
            vehicle V09.9 ☑
              animal-drawn V06.99 ☑
                nontraffic V06.09 ☑
                traffic V06.19 ☑
              motor
                nontraffic V09.00 ☑
                traffic V09.20 ☑
          fall V00.811 ☑
          nontraffic V09.1 ☑
            involving motor vehicle NEC V09.00 ☑
          traffic V09.3 ☑
            involving motor vehicle NEC V09.20 ☑
        wheeled shoe V00.158 ☑
          colliding with stationary object V00.152 ☑
          fall V00.151 ☑
      on foot (*see also* Accident, pedestrian)
        collision (with)
          animal being ridden or animal drawn vehicle V06.90 ☑
            nontraffic V06.00 ☑
            traffic V06.10 ☑
          bus or heavy transport V04.90 ☑
            nontraffic V04.00 ☑
            traffic V04.10 ☑
          car V03.90 ☑
            nontraffic V03.00 ☑
            traffic V03.10 ☑
          pedal cycle V01.90 ☑
            nontraffic V01.00 ☑
            traffic V01.10 ☑
          pick-up truck or van V03.90 ☑

Accident — *continued*
  transport — *continued*
    pedestrian — *continued*
      on foot (*see also* Accident, pedestrian) — *continued*
        collision — *continued*
          pick-up truck or van — *continued*
            nontraffic V03.00 ☑
            traffic V03.10 ☑
          railway (train) (vehicle) V05.90 ☑
            nontraffic V05.00 ☑
            traffic V05.10 ☑
          streetcar V06.90 ☑
            nontraffic V06.00 ☑
            traffic V06.10 ☑
          two- or three-wheeled motor vehicle V02.90 ☑
            nontraffic V02.00 ☑
            traffic V02.10 ☑
          vehicle V09.9 ☑
            animal-drawn V06.90 ☑
              nontraffic V06.00 ☑
              traffic V06.10 ☑
            motor
          nontraffic V09.1 ☑
            involving motor vehicle V09.00 ☑
              military V09.01 ☑
              specified type NEC V09.09 ☑
          traffic V09.3 ☑
            involving motor vehicle V09.20 ☑
              military V09.21 ☑
              specified type NEC V09.29 ☑
      person NEC (unknown way or transportation) V99 ☑
      collision (between)
        bus (with)
          heavy transport vehicle (traffic) V87.5 ☑
            nontraffic V88.5 ☑
        car (with)
          bus (traffic) V87.3 ☑
            nontraffic V88.3 ☑
          heavy transport vehicle (traffic) V87.4 ☑
            nontraffic V88.4 ☑
          nontraffic V88.5 ☑
          pick-up truck or van (traffic) V87.2 ☑
            nontraffic V88.2 ☑
          train or railway vehicle (traffic) V87.6 ☑
            nontraffic V88.6 ☑
          two- or three-wheeled motor vehicle (traffic) V87.0 ☑
            nontraffic V88.0 ☑
        motor vehicle (traffic) NEC V87.7 ☑
          nontraffic V88.7 ☑
        two- or three-wheeled vehicle (with) (traffic) motor vehicle NEC V87.1 ☑
          nontraffic V88.1 ☑
        nonmotor vehicle (collision) (noncollision) (traffic) V87.9 ☑
        nontraffic V88.9 ☑
      pickup truck occupant V59.9 ☑
        collision (with)
          animal (traffic) V50.9 ☑
            being ridden (traffic) V56.9 ☑
              nontraffic V56.3 ☑
              while boarding or alighting V56.4 ☑
            nontraffic V50.3 ☑
            while boarding or alighting V50.4 ☑
          animal-drawn vehicle (traffic) V56.9 ☑
            nontraffic V56.3 ☑
            while boarding or alighting V56.4 ☑
          bus (traffic) V54.9 ☑
            nontraffic V54.3 ☑
            while boarding or alighting V54.4 ☑
          car (traffic) V53.9 ☑
            nontraffic V53.3 ☑
            while boarding or alighting V53.4 ☑
          motor vehicle NOS (traffic) V59.60 ☑
            nontraffic V59.20 ☑
            specified type NEC (traffic) V59.69 ☑
              nontraffic V59.29 ☑
          pedal cycle (traffic) V51.9 ☑
            nontraffic V51.3 ☑
            while boarding or alighting V51.4 ☑
          pickup truck (traffic) V53.9 ☑
            nontraffic V53.3 ☑
            while boarding or alighting V53.4 ☑

☑ **Additional Character Required — Refer to the Tabular List for Character Selection** ▽ **Subterms under main terms may continue to next column or page**

Accident — *continued*
  transport — *continued*
    pickup truck occupant — *continued*
      collision — *continued*
        railway vehicle (traffic) V55.9 ☑
          nontraffic V55.3 ☑
          while boarding or alighting V55.4 ☑
        specified vehicle NEC (traffic) V56.9 ☑
          nontraffic V56.3 ☑
          while boarding or alighting V56.4 ☑
        stationary object (traffic) V57.9 ☑
          nontraffic V57.3 ☑
          while boarding or alighting V57.4 ☑
        streetcar (traffic) V56.9 ☑
          nontraffic V56.3 ☑
          while boarding or alighting V56.4 ☑
        three wheeled motor vehicle (traffic) V52.9 ☑
          nontraffic V52.3 ☑
          while boarding or alighting V52.4 ☑
         truck (traffic) V54.9 ☑
          nontraffic V54.3 ☑
          while boarding or alighting V54.4 ☑
        two wheeled motor vehicle (traffic) V52.9 ☑
          nontraffic V52.3 ☑
          while boarding or alighting V52.4 ☑
        van (traffic) V53.9 ☑
          nontraffic V53.3 ☑
          while boarding or alighting V53.4 ☑
      driver
        collision (with)
          animal (traffic) V50.5 ☑
            being ridden (traffic) V56.5 ☑
              nontraffic V56.0 ☑
            nontraffic V50.0 ☑
          animal-drawn vehicle (traffic) V56.5 ☑
            nontraffic V56.0 ☑
          bus (traffic) V54.5 ☑
            nontraffic V54.0 ☑
          car (traffic) V53.5 ☑
            nontraffic V53.0 ☑
          motor vehicle NOS (traffic) V59.40 ☑
            nontraffic V59.00 ☑
            specified type NEC (traffic) V59.49 ☑
              nontraffic V59.09 ☑
          pedal cycle (traffic) V51.5 ☑
            nontraffic V51.0 ☑
          pickup truck (traffic) V53.5 ☑
            nontraffic V53.0 ☑
          railway vehicle (traffic) V55.5 ☑
            nontraffic V55.0 ☑
          specified vehicle NEC (traffic) V56.5 ☑
            nontraffic V56.0 ☑
          stationary object (traffic) V57.5 ☑
            nontraffic V57.0 ☑
          streetcar (traffic) V56.5 ☑
            nontraffic V56.0 ☑
          three wheeled motor vehicle (traffic) V52.5 ☑
            nontraffic V52.0 ☑
          truck (traffic) V54.5 ☑
            nontraffic V54.0 ☑
          two wheeled motor vehicle (traffic) V52.5 ☑
            nontraffic V52.0 ☑
          van (traffic) V53.5 ☑
            nontraffic V53.0 ☑
        noncollision accident (traffic) V58.5 ☑
          nontraffic V58.0 ☑
      hanger-on
        collision (with)
          animal (traffic) V50.7 ☑
            being ridden (traffic) V56.7 ☑
              nontraffic V56.2 ☑
            nontraffic V50.2 ☑
          animal-drawn vehicle (traffic) V56.7 ☑
            nontraffic V56.2 ☑
          bus (traffic) V54.7 ☑
            nontraffic V54.2 ☑
          car (traffic) V53.7 ☑
            nontraffic V53.2 ☑
          pedal cycle (traffic) V51.7 ☑
            nontraffic V51.2 ☑
          pickup truck (traffic) V53.7 ☑
            nontraffic V53.2 ☑
          railway vehicle (traffic) V55.7 ☑

Accident — *continued*
  transport — *continued*
    pickup truck occupant — *continued*
      hanger-on — *continued*
        collision — *continued*
          railway vehicle — *continued*
            nontraffic V55.2 ☑
          specified vehicle NEC (traffic) V56.7 ☑
            nontraffic V56.2 ☑
          stationary object (traffic) V57.7 ☑
            nontraffic V57.2 ☑
          streetcar (traffic) V56.7 ☑
            nontraffic V56.2 ☑
          three wheeled motor vehicle (traffic) V52.7 ☑
            nontraffic V52.2 ☑
          truck (traffic) V54.7 ☑
            nontraffic V54.2 ☑
          two wheeled motor vehicle (traffic) V52.7 ☑
            nontraffic V52.2 ☑
          van (traffic) V53.7 ☑
            nontraffic V53.2 ☑
        noncollision accident (traffic) V58.7 ☑
          nontraffic V58.2 ☑
      noncollision accident (traffic) V58.9 ☑
        nontraffic V58.3 ☑
        while boarding or alighting V58.4 ☑
      nontraffic V59.3 ☑
      passenger
        collision (with)
          animal (traffic) V50.6 ☑
            being ridden (traffic) V56.6 ☑
              nontraffic V50.1 ☑
            nontraffic V50.1 ☑
          animal-drawn vehicle (traffic) V56.6 ☑
            nontraffic V56.1 ☑
          bus (traffic) V54.6 ☑
            nontraffic V54.1 ☑
          car (traffic) V53.6 ☑
            nontraffic V53.1 ☑
          motor vehicle NOS (traffic) V59.50 ☑
            nontraffic V59.10 ☑
            specified type NEC (traffic) V59.59 ☑
              nontraffic V59.19 ☑
          pedal cycle (traffic) V51.6 ☑
            nontraffic V51.1 ☑
          pickup truck (traffic) V53.6 ☑
            nontraffic V53.1 ☑
          railway vehicle (traffic) V55.6 ☑
            nontraffic V55.1 ☑
          specified vehicle NEC (traffic) V56.6 ☑
            nontraffic V56.1 ☑
          stationary object (traffic) V57.6 ☑
            nontraffic V57.1 ☑
          streetcar (traffic) V56.6 ☑
            nontraffic V56.1 ☑
          three wheeled motor vehicle (traffic) V52.6 ☑
            nontraffic V52.1 ☑
          truck (traffic) V54.6 ☑
            nontraffic V54.1 ☑
          two wheeled motor vehicle (traffic) V52.6 ☑
            nontraffic V52.1 ☑
          van (traffic) V53.6 ☑
            nontraffic V53.1 ☑
        noncollision accident (traffic) V58.6 ☑
          nontraffic V58.1 ☑
      specified type NEC V59.88 ☑
      military vehicle V59.81 ☑
    quarry truck — *see* Accident, transport, industrial vehicle occupant
    race car — *see* Accident, transport, motor vehicle NEC occupant
    railway vehicle occupant V81.9 ☑
      collision (with) V81.3 ☑
        motor vehicle (non-military) (traffic) V81.1 ☑
          military V81.83 ☑
          nontraffic V81.0 ☑
        rolling stock V81.2 ☑
        specified object NEC V81.3 ☑
      during derailment V81.7 ☑

Accident — *continued*
  transport — *continued*
    railway vehicle occupant — *continued*
      during derailment — *continued*
        with antecedent collision — *see* Accident, transport, railway vehicle occupant, collision
      explosion V81.81 ☑
      fall (in railway vehicle) V81.5 ☑
        during derailment V81.7 ☑
          with antecedent collision — *see* Accident, transport, railway vehicle occupant, collision
        from railway vehicle V81.6 ☑
          during derailment V81.7 ☑
            with antecedent collision — *see* Accident, transport, railway vehicle occupant, collision
        while boarding or alighting V81.4 ☑
      fire V81.81 ☑
      object falling onto train V81.82 ☑
      specified type NEC V81.89 ☑
      while boarding or alighting V81.4 ☑
    ski lift V98.3 ☑
    snowmobile occupant (nontraffic) V86.92 ☑
      driver V86.52 ☑
      hanger-on V86.72 ☑
      passenger V86.62 ☑
      traffic V86.32 ☑
        driver V86.02 ☑
        hanger-on V86.22 ☑
        passenger V86.12 ☑
      while boarding or alighting V86.42 ☑
    specified NEC V98.8 ☑
    sport utility vehicle occupant (*see also* Accident, transport, pickup truck occupant)
    streetcar occupant V82.9 ☑
      collision (with) V82.3 ☑
        motor vehicle (traffic) V82.1 ☑
          nontraffic V82.0 ☑
        rolling stock V82.2 ☑
      during derailment V82.7 ☑
        with antecedent collision — *see* Accident, transport, streetcar occupant, collision
      fall (in streetcar) V82.5 ☑
        during derailment V82.7 ☑
          with antecedent collision — *see* Accident, transport, streetcar occupant, collision
        from streetcar V82.6 ☑
          during derailment V82.7 ☑
            with antecedent collision — *see* Accident, transport, streetcar occupant, collision
        while boarding or alighting V82.4 ☑
      while boarding or alighting V82.4 ☑
      specified type NEC V82.8 ☑
      while boarding or alighting V82.4 ☑
    three-wheeled motor vehicle occupant V39.9 ☑
      collision (with)
        animal (traffic) V30.9 ☑
          being ridden (traffic) V36.9 ☑
            nontraffic V36.3 ☑
            while boarding or alighting V36.4 ☑
          nontraffic V30.3 ☑
          while boarding or alighting V30.4 ☑
        animal-drawn vehicle (traffic) V36.9 ☑
          nontraffic V36.3 ☑
          while boarding or alighting V36.4 ☑
        bus (traffic) V34.9 ☑
          nontraffic V34.3 ☑
          while boarding or alighting V34.4 ☑
        car (traffic) V33.9 ☑
          nontraffic V33.3 ☑
          while boarding or alighting V33.4 ☑
        motor vehicle NOS (traffic) V39.60 ☑
          nontraffic V39.20 ☑
          specified type NEC (traffic) V39.69 ☑
            nontraffic V39.29 ☑
        pedal cycle (traffic) V31.9 ☑
          nontraffic V31.3 ☑
          while boarding or alighting V31.4 ☑
        pickup truck (traffic) V33.9 ☑
          nontraffic V33.3 ☑
          while boarding or alighting V33.4 ☑
        railway vehicle (traffic) V35.9 ☑

Accident — *continued*
  transport — *continued*
    three-wheeled motor vehicle occupant — *continued*
      collision — *continued*
        railway vehicle — *continued*
          nontraffic V35.3 ☑
          while boarding or alighting V35.4 ☑
        specified vehicle NEC (traffic) V36.9 ☑
          nontraffic V36.3 ☑
          while boarding or alighting V36.4 ☑
        stationary object (traffic) V37.9 ☑
          nontraffic V37.3 ☑
          while boarding or alighting V37.4 ☑
        streetcar (traffic) V36.9 ☑
          nontraffic V36.3 ☑
          while boarding or alighting V36.4 ☑
        three wheeled motor vehicle (traffic) V32.9 ☑
          nontraffic V32.3 ☑
          while boarding or alighting V32.4 ☑
        truck (traffic) V34.9 ☑
          nontraffic V34.3 ☑
          while boarding or alighting V34.4 ☑
        two wheeled motor vehicle (traffic) V32.9 ☑
          nontraffic V32.3 ☑
          while boarding or alighting V32.4 ☑
        van (traffic) V33.9 ☑
          nontraffic V33.3 ☑
          while boarding or alighting V33.4 ☑
     driver
      collision (with)
        animal (traffic) V30.5 ☑
          being ridden (traffic) V36.5 ☑
            nontraffic V36.0 ☑
          nontraffic V30.0 ☑
        animal-drawn vehicle (traffic) V36.5 ☑
          nontraffic V36.0 ☑
        bus (traffic) V34.5 ☑
          nontraffic V34.0 ☑
        car (traffic) V33.5 ☑
          nontraffic V33.0 ☑
        motor vehicle NOS (traffic) V39.40 ☑
          nontraffic V39.00 ☑
          specified type NEC (traffic) V39.49 ☑
            nontraffic V39.09 ☑
        pedal cycle (traffic) V31.5 ☑
          nontraffic V31.0 ☑
        pickup truck (traffic) V33.5 ☑
          nontraffic V33.0 ☑
        railway vehicle (traffic) V35.5 ☑
          nontraffic V35.0 ☑
        specified vehicle NEC (traffic) V36.5 ☑
          nontraffic V36.0 ☑
        stationary object (traffic) V37.5 ☑
          nontraffic V37.0 ☑
        streetcar (traffic) V36.5 ☑
          nontraffic V36.0 ☑
        three wheeled motor vehicle (traffic) V32.5 ☑
          nontraffic V32.0 ☑
        truck (traffic) V34.5 ☑
          nontraffic V34.0 ☑
        two wheeled motor vehicle (traffic) V32.5 ☑
          nontraffic V32.0 ☑
        van (traffic) V33.5 ☑
          nontraffic V33.0 ☑
      noncollision accident (traffic) V38.5 ☑
        nontraffic V38.0 ☑
     hanger-on
      collision (with)
        animal (traffic) V30.7 ☑
          being ridden (traffic) V36.7 ☑
            nontraffic V36.2 ☑
          nontraffic V30.2 ☑
        animal-drawn vehicle (traffic) V36.7 ☑
          nontraffic V36.2 ☑
        bus (traffic) V34.7 ☑
          nontraffic V34.2 ☑
        car (traffic) V33.7 ☑
          nontraffic V33.2 ☑
        pedal cycle (traffic) V31.7 ☑
          nontraffic V31.2 ☑
        pickup truck (traffic) V33.7 ☑
          nontraffic V33.2 ☑

Accident — *continued*
  transport — *continued*
    three-wheeled motor vehicle occupant — *continued*
     hanger-on — *continued*
      collision — *continued*
        railway vehicle (traffic) V35.7 ☑
          nontraffic V35.2 ☑
        specified vehicle NEC (traffic) V36.7 ☑
          nontraffic V36.2 ☑
        stationary object (traffic) V37.7 ☑
          nontraffic V37.2 ☑
        streetcar (traffic) V36.7 ☑
          nontraffic V36.2 ☑
        three wheeled motor vehicle (traffic) V32.7 ☑
          nontraffic V32.2 ☑
        truck (traffic) V34.7 ☑
          nontraffic V34.2 ☑
        two wheeled motor vehicle (traffic) V32.7 ☑
          nontraffic V32.2 ☑
        van (traffic) V33.7 ☑
          nontraffic V33.2 ☑
      noncollision accident (traffic) V38.7 ☑
        nontraffic V38.2 ☑
    noncollision accident (traffic) V38.9 ☑
      nontraffic V38.3 ☑
      while boarding or alighting V38.4 ☑
    nontraffic V39.3 ☑
    passenger
      collision (with)
        animal (traffic) V30.6 ☑
          being ridden (traffic) V36.6 ☑
            nontraffic V36.1 ☑
          nontraffic V30.1 ☑
        animal-drawn vehicle (traffic) V36.6 ☑
          nontraffic V36.1 ☑
        bus (traffic) V34.6 ☑
          nontraffic V34.1 ☑
        car (traffic) V33.6 ☑
          nontraffic V33.1 ☑
        motor vehicle NOS (traffic) V39.50 ☑
          nontraffic V39.10 ☑
          specified type NEC (traffic) V39.59 ☑
            nontraffic V39.19 ☑
        pedal cycle (traffic) V31.6 ☑
          nontraffic V31.1 ☑
        pickup truck (traffic) V33.6 ☑
          nontraffic V33.1 ☑
        railway vehicle (traffic) V35.6 ☑
          nontraffic V35.1 ☑
        specified vehicle NEC (traffic) V36.6 ☑
          nontraffic V36.1 ☑
        stationary object (traffic) V37.6 ☑
          nontraffic V37.1 ☑
        streetcar (traffic) V36.6 ☑
          nontraffic V36.1 ☑
        three wheeled motor vehicle (traffic) V32.6 ☑
          nontraffic V32.1 ☑
        truck (traffic) V34.6 ☑
          nontraffic V34.1 ☑
        two wheeled motor vehicle (traffic) V32.6 ☑
          nontraffic V32.1 ☑
        van (traffic) V33.6 ☑
          nontraffic V33.1 ☑
      noncollision accident (traffic) V38.6 ☑
        nontraffic V38.1 ☑
    specified type NEC V39.89 ☑
    military vehicle V39.81 ☑
    tractor (farm) (and trailer) — *see* Accident, transport, agricultural vehicle occupant
    tram — *see* Accident, transport, streetcar
      in mine or quarry — *see* Accident, transport, industrial vehicle occupant
    trolley — *see* Accident, transport, streetcar
      in mine or quarry — *see* Accident, transport, industrial vehicle occupant
    truck (heavy) occupant V69.9 ☑
     collision (with)
      animal (traffic) V60.9 ☑
        being ridden (traffic) V66.9 ☑
          nontraffic V66.3 ☑
          while boarding or alighting V66.4 ☑

Accident — *continued*
  transport — *continued*
    truck occupant — *continued*
     collision — *continued*
      animal — *continued*
        nontraffic V60.3 ☑
        while boarding or alighting V60.4 ☑
      animal-drawn vehicle (traffic) V66.9 ☑
        nontraffic V66.3 ☑
        while boarding or alighting V66.4 ☑
      bus (traffic) V64.9 ☑
        nontraffic V64.3 ☑
        while boarding or alighting V64.4 ☑
      car (traffic) V63.9 ☑
        nontraffic V63.3 ☑
        while boarding or alighting V63.4 ☑
      motor vehicle NOS (traffic) V69.60 ☑
        nontraffic V69.20 ☑
        specified type NEC (traffic) V69.69 ☑
          nontraffic V69.29 ☑
      pedal cycle (traffic) V61.9 ☑
        nontraffic V61.3 ☑
        while boarding or alighting V61.4 ☑
      pickup truck (traffic) V63.9 ☑
        nontraffic V63.3 ☑
        while boarding or alighting V63.4 ☑
      railway vehicle (traffic) V65.9 ☑
        nontraffic V65.3 ☑
        while boarding or alighting V65.4 ☑
      specified vehicle NEC (traffic) V66.9 ☑
        nontraffic V66.3 ☑
        while boarding or alighting V66.4 ☑
      stationary object (traffic) V67.9 ☑
        nontraffic V67.3 ☑
        while boarding or alighting V67.4 ☑
      streetcar (traffic) V66.9 ☑
        nontraffic V66.3 ☑
        while boarding or alighting V66.4 ☑
      three wheeled motor vehicle (traffic) V62.9 ☑
        nontraffic V62.3 ☑
        while boarding or alighting V62.4 ☑
      truck (traffic) V64.9 ☑
        nontraffic V64.3 ☑
        while boarding or alighting V64.4 ☑
      two wheeled motor vehicle (traffic) V62.9 ☑
        nontraffic V62.3 ☑
        while boarding or alighting V62.4 ☑
      van (traffic) V63.9 ☑
        nontraffic V63.3 ☑
        while boarding or alighting V63.4 ☑
     driver
      collision (with)
        animal (traffic) V60.5 ☑
          being ridden (traffic) V66.5 ☑
            nontraffic V66.0 ☑
          nontraffic V60.0 ☑
        animal-drawn vehicle (traffic) V66.5 ☑
          nontraffic V66.0 ☑
        bus (traffic) V64.5 ☑
          nontraffic V64.0 ☑
        car (traffic) V63.5 ☑
          nontraffic V63.0 ☑
        motor vehicle NOS (traffic) V69.40 ☑
          nontraffic V69.00 ☑
          specified type NEC (traffic) V69.49 ☑
            nontraffic V69.09 ☑
        pedal cycle (traffic) V61.5 ☑
          nontraffic V61.0 ☑
        pickup truck (traffic) V63.5 ☑
          nontraffic V63.0 ☑
        railway vehicle (traffic) V65.5 ☑
          nontraffic V65.0 ☑
        specified vehicle NEC (traffic) V66.5 ☑
          nontraffic V66.0 ☑
        stationary object (traffic) V67.5 ☑
          nontraffic V67.0 ☑
        streetcar (traffic) V66.5 ☑
          nontraffic V66.0 ☑
        three wheeled motor vehicle (traffic) V62.5 ☑
          nontraffic V62.0 ☑
        truck (traffic) V64.5 ☑
          nontraffic V64.0 ☑
        two wheeled motor vehicle (traffic) V62.5 ☑

Accident — *continued*
  transport — *continued*
    truck occupant — *continued*
      driver — *continued*
        collision — *continued*
          two wheeled motor vehicle — *continued*
            nontraffic V62.0 ☑
          van (traffic) V63.5 ☑
            nontraffic V63.0 ☑
        noncollision accident (traffic) V68.5 ☑
          nontraffic V68.0 ☑
      dump — *see* Accident, transport, construction vehicle occupant
      hanger-on
        collision (with)
          animal (traffic) V60.7 ☑
            being ridden (traffic) V66.7 ☑
              nontraffic V66.2 ☑
            nontraffic V60.2 ☑
          animal-drawn vehicle (traffic) V66.7 ☑
            nontraffic V66.2 ☑
          bus (traffic) V64.7 ☑
            nontraffic V64.2 ☑
          car (traffic) V63.7 ☑
            nontraffic V63.2 ☑
          pedal cycle (traffic) V61.7 ☑
            nontraffic V61.2 ☑
          pickup truck (traffic) V63.7 ☑
            nontraffic V63.2 ☑
          railway vehicle (traffic) V65.7 ☑
            nontraffic V65.2 ☑
          specified vehicle NEC (traffic) V66.7 ☑
            nontraffic V66.2 ☑
          stationary object (traffic) V67.7 ☑
            nontraffic V67.2 ☑
          streetcar (traffic) V66.7 ☑
            nontraffic V66.2 ☑
          three wheeled motor vehicle (traffic) V62.7 ☑
            nontraffic V62.2 ☑
          truck (traffic) V64.7 ☑
            nontraffic V64.2 ☑
          two wheeled motor vehicle (traffic) V62.7 ☑
            nontraffic V62.2 ☑
          van (traffic) V63.7 ☑
            nontraffic V63.2 ☑
        noncollision accident (traffic) V68.7 ☑
          nontraffic V68.2 ☑
      noncollision accident (traffic) V68.9 ☑
        nontraffic V68.3 ☑
        while boarding or alighting V68.4 ☑
      nontraffic V69.3 ☑
      passenger
        collision (with)
          animal (traffic) V60.6 ☑
            being ridden (traffic) V66.6 ☑
              nontraffic V66.1- ☑
            nontraffic V60.1 ☑
          animal-drawn vehicle (traffic) V66.6 ☑
            nontraffic V66.1 ☑
          bus (traffic) V64.6 ☑
            nontraffic V64.1 ☑
          car (traffic) V63.6 ☑
            nontraffic V63.1 ☑
          motor vehicle NOS (traffic) V69.50 ☑
            nontraffic V69.10 ☑
            specified type NEC (traffic) V69.59 ☑
              nontraffic V69.19 ☑
          pedal cycle (traffic) V61.6 ☑
            nontraffic V61.1 ☑
          pickup truck (traffic) V63.6 ☑
            nontraffic V63.1 ☑
          railway vehicle (traffic) V65.6 ☑
            nontraffic V65.1 ☑
          specified vehicle NEC (traffic) V66.6 ☑
            nontraffic V66.1 ☑
          stationary object (traffic) V67.6 ☑
            nontraffic V67.1 ☑
          streetcar (traffic) V66.6 ☑
            nontraffic V66.1 ☑
          three wheeled motor vehicle (traffic) V62.6 ☑
            nontraffic V62.1 ☑
          truck (traffic) V64.6 ☑

Accident — *continued*
  transport — *continued*
    truck occupant — *continued*
      passenger — *continued*
        collision — *continued*
          truck — *continued*
            nontraffic V64.1 ☑
          two wheeled motor vehicle (traffic) V62.6 ☑
            nontraffic V62.1 ☑
          van (traffic) V63.6 ☑
            nontraffic V63.1 ☑
        noncollision accident (traffic) V68.6 ☑
          nontraffic V68.1 ☑
      pickup — *see* Accident, transport, pickup truck occupant
      specified type NEC V69.88 ☑
      military vehicle V69.81 ☑
    van occupant V59.9 ☑
      collision (with)
        animal (traffic) V50.9 ☑
          being ridden (traffic) V56.9 ☑
            nontraffic V56.3 ☑
            while boarding or alighting V56.4 ☑
          nontraffic V50.3 ☑
          while boarding or alighting V50.4 ☑
        animal-drawn vehicle (traffic) V56.9 ☑
          nontraffic V56.3 ☑
          while boarding or alighting V56.4 ☑
        bus (traffic) V54.9 ☑
          nontraffic V54.3 ☑
          while boarding or alighting V54.4 ☑
        car (traffic) V53.9 ☑
          nontraffic V53.3 ☑
          while boarding or alighting V53.4 ☑
        motor vehicle NOS (traffic) V59.60 ☑
          nontraffic V59.20 ☑
          specified type NEC (traffic) V59.69 ☑
            nontraffic V59.29 ☑
        pedal cycle (traffic) V51.9 ☑
          nontraffic V51.3 ☑
          while boarding or alighting V51.4 ☑
        pickup truck (traffic) V53.9 ☑
          nontraffic V53.3 ☑
          while boarding or alighting V53.4 ☑
        railway vehicle (traffic) V55.9 ☑
          nontraffic V55.3 ☑
          while boarding or alighting V55.4 ☑
        specified vehicle NEC (traffic) V56.9 ☑
          nontraffic V56.3 ☑
          while boarding or alighting V56.4 ☑
        stationary object (traffic) V57.9 ☑
          nontraffic V57.3 ☑
          while boarding or alighting V57.4 ☑
        streetcar (traffic) V56.9 ☑
          nontraffic V56.3 ☑
          while boarding or alighting V56.4 ☑
        three wheeled motor vehicle (traffic) V52.9 ☑
          nontraffic V52.3 ☑
          while boarding or alighting V52.4 ☑
        truck (traffic) V54.9 ☑
          nontraffic V54.3 ☑
          while boarding or alighting V54.4 ☑
        two wheeled motor vehicle (traffic) V52.9 ☑
          nontraffic V52.3 ☑
          while boarding or alighting V52.4 ☑
        van (traffic) V53.9 ☑
          nontraffic V53.3 ☑
          while boarding or alighting V53.4 ☑
      driver
        collision (with)
          animal (traffic) V50.5 ☑
            being ridden (traffic) V56.5 ☑
              nontraffic V56.0 ☑
            nontraffic V50.0 ☑
          animal-drawn vehicle (traffic) V56.5 ☑
            nontraffic V56.0 ☑
          bus (traffic) V54.5 ☑
            nontraffic V54.0 ☑
          car (traffic) V53.5 ☑
            nontraffic V53.0 ☑
          motor vehicle NOS (traffic) V59.40 ☑
            nontraffic V59.00 ☑
            specified type NEC (traffic) V59.49 ☑
              nontraffic V59.09 ☑

Accident — *continued*
  transport — *continued*
    van occupant — *continued*
      driver — *continued*
        collision — *continued*
          pedal cycle (traffic) V51.5 ☑
            nontraffic V51.0 ☑
          pickup truck (traffic) V53.5 ☑
            nontraffic V53.0 ☑
          railway vehicle (traffic) V55.5 ☑
            nontraffic V55.0 ☑
          specified vehicle NEC (traffic) V56.5 ☑
            nontraffic V56.0 ☑
          stationary object (traffic) V57.5 ☑
            nontraffic V57.0 ☑
          streetcar (traffic) V56.5 ☑
            nontraffic V56.0 ☑
          three wheeled motor vehicle (traffic) V52.5 ☑
            nontraffic V52.0 ☑
          truck (traffic) V54.5 ☑
            nontraffic V54.0 ☑
          two wheeled motor vehicle (traffic) V52.5 ☑
            nontraffic V52.0 ☑
          van (traffic) V53.5 ☑
            nontraffic V53.0 ☑
        noncollision accident (traffic) V58.5 ☑
          nontraffic V58.0 ☑
      hanger-on
        collision (with)
          animal (traffic) V50.7 ☑
            being ridden (traffic) V56.7 ☑
              nontraffic V56.2 ☑
            nontraffic V50.2 ☑
          animal-drawn vehicle (traffic) V56.7 ☑
            nontraffic V56.2 ☑
          bus (traffic) V54.7 ☑
            nontraffic V54.2 ☑
          car (traffic) V53.7 ☑
            nontraffic V53.2 ☑
          pedal cycle (traffic) V51.7 ☑
            nontraffic V51.2 ☑
          pickup truck (traffic) V53.7 ☑
            nontraffic V53.2 ☑
          railway vehicle (traffic) V55.7 ☑
            nontraffic V55.2 ☑
          specified vehicle NEC (traffic) V56.7 ☑
            nontraffic V56.2 ☑
          stationary object (traffic) V57.7 ☑
            nontraffic V57.2 ☑
          streetcar (traffic) V56.7 ☑
            nontraffic V56.2 ☑
          three wheeled motor vehicle (traffic) V52.7 ☑
            nontraffic V52.2 ☑
          truck (traffic) V54.7 ☑
            nontraffic V54.2 ☑
          two wheeled motor vehicle (traffic) V52.7 ☑
            nontraffic V52.2 ☑
          van (traffic) V53.7 ☑
            nontraffic V53.2 ☑
        noncollision accident (traffic) V58.7 ☑
          nontraffic V58.2 ☑
      noncollision accident (traffic) V58.9 ☑
        nontraffic V58.3 ☑
        while boarding or alighting V58.4 ☑
      nontraffic V59.3 ☑
      passenger
        collision (with)
          animal (traffic) V50.6 ☑
            being ridden (traffic) V56.6 ☑
              nontraffic V56.1 ☑
            nontraffic V50.1 ☑
          animal-drawn vehicle (traffic) V56.6 ☑
            nontraffic V56.1 ☑
          bus (traffic) V54.6 ☑
            nontraffic V54.1 ☑
          car (traffic) V53.6 ☑
            nontraffic V53.1 ☑
          motor vehicle NOS (traffic) V59.50 ☑
            nontraffic V59.10 ☑
            specified type NEC (traffic) V59.59 ☑
              nontraffic V59.19 ☑
          pedal cycle (traffic) V51.6 ☑

Accident — *continued*
  transport — *continued*
    van occupant — *continued*
      passenger — *continued*
        collision — *continued*
          pedal cycle — *continued*
            nontraffic V51.1 ☑
          pickup truck (traffic) V53.6 ☑
            nontraffic V53.1 ☑
          railway vehicle (traffic) V55.6 ☑
            nontraffic V55.1 ☑
          specified vehicle NEC (traffic) V56.6 ☑
            nontraffic V56.1 ☑
          stationary object (traffic) V57.6 ☑
            nontraffic V57.1 ☑
          streetcar (traffic) V56.6 ☑
            nontraffic V56.1 ☑
          three wheeled motor vehicle (traffic)
            V52.6 ☑
            nontraffic V52.1 ☑
          truck (traffic) V54.6 ☑
            nontraffic V54.1 ☑
          two wheeled motor vehicle (traffic)
            V52.6 ☑
            nontraffic V52.1 ☑
          van (traffic) V53.6 ☑
            nontraffic V53.1 ☑
        noncollision accident (traffic) V58.6 ☑
          nontraffic V58.1 ☑
        specified type NEC V59.88 ☑
          military vehicle V59.81 ☑
    watercraft occupant — *see* Accident, watercraft
   vehicle NEC V89.9 ☑
    animal-drawn NEC — *see* Accident, transport, animal-drawn vehicle occupant
   special
    agricultural — *see* Accident, transport, agricultural vehicle occupant
    construction — *see* Accident, transport, construction vehicle occupant
    industrial — *see* Accident, transport, industrial vehicle occupant
    three-wheeled NEC (motorized) — *see* Accident, transport, three-wheeled motor vehicle occupant
  watercraft V94.9 ☑
   causing
    drowning — *see* Drowning, due to, accident to, watercraft
    injury NEC V91.89 ☑
      crushed between craft and object V91.19 ☑
        powered craft V91.13 ☑
          ferry boat V91.11 ☑
          fishing boat V91.12 ☑
          jetskis V91.13 ☑
          liner V91.11 ☑
          merchant ship V91.10 ☑
          passenger ship V91.11 ☑
        unpowered craft V91.18 ☑
          canoe V91.15 ☑
          inflatable V91.16 ☑
          kayak V91.15 ☑
          sailboat V91.14 ☑
          surf-board V91.18 ☑
          windsurfer V91.18 ☑
      fall on board V91.29 ☑
        powered craft V91.23 ☑
          ferry boat V91.21 ☑
          fishing boat V91.22 ☑
          jetskis V91.23 ☑
          liner V91.21 ☑
          merchant ship V91.20 ☑
          passenger ship V91.21 ☑
        unpowered craft
          canoe V91.25 ☑
          inflatable V91.26 ☑
          kayak V91.25 ☑
          sailboat V91.24 ☑
      fire on board causing burn V91.09 ☑
        powered craft V91.03 ☑
          ferry boat V91.01 ☑
          fishing boat V91.02 ☑
          jetskis V91.03 ☑
          liner V91.01 ☑
          merchant ship V91.00 ☑
          passenger ship V91.01 ☑

Accident — *continued*
  watercraft — *continued*
   causing — *continued*
    injury — *continued*
      fire on board causing burn — *continued*
        unpowered craft V91.08 ☑
          canoe V91.05 ☑
          inflatable V91.06 ☑
          kayak V91.05 ☑
          sailboat V91.04 ☑
          surf-board V91.08 ☑
          water skis V91.07 ☑
          windsurfer V91.08 ☑
      hit by falling object V91.39 ☑
        powered craft V91.33 ☑
          ferry boat V91.31 ☑
          fishing boat V91.32 ☑
          jetskis V91.33 ☑
          liner V91.31 ☑
          merchant ship V91.30 ☑
          passenger ship V91.31 ☑
        unpowered craft V91.38 ☑
          canoe V91.35 ☑
          inflatable V91.36 ☑
          kayak V91.35 ☑
          sailboat V91.34 ☑
          surf-board V91.38 ☑
          water skis V91.37 ☑
          windsurfer V91.38 ☑
      specified type NEC V91.89 ☑
        powered craft V91.83 ☑
          ferry boat V91.81 ☑
          fishing boat V91.82 ☑
          jetskis V91.83 ☑
          liner V91.81 ☑
          merchant ship V91.80 ☑
          passenger ship V91.81 ☑
        unpowered craft V91.88 ☑
          canoe V91.85 ☑
          inflatable V91.86 ☑
          kayak V91.85 ☑
          sailboat V91.84 ☑
          surf-board V91.88 ☑
          water skis V91.87 ☑
          windsurfer V91.88 ☑
    due to, caused by cataclysm — *see* Forces of nature, by type
    military NEC V94.818 ☑
      with civilian watercraft V94.810 ☑
      civilian in water injured by V94.811 ☑
    nonpowered, struck by
      nonpowered vessel V94.22 ☑
      powered vessel V94.21 ☑
    specified type NEC V94.89 ☑
    striking swimmer
      powered V94.11 ☑
      unpowered V94.12 ☑
Acid throwing (assault) Y08.89 ☑
Activity (involving) (of victim at time of event) Y93.9
  aerobic and step exercise (class) Y93.A3 (*following* Y93.7)
  alpine skiing Y93.23
  animal care NEC Y93.K9 (*following* Y93.7)
  arts and handcrafts NEC Y93.D9 (*following* Y93.7)
  athletics played as a team or group NEC Y93.69
  athletics played individually NEC Y93.59
  athletics NEC Y93.79
  baking Y93.G3 (*following* Y93.7)
  ballet Y93.41
  barbells Y93.B3 (*following* Y93.7)
  BASE (Building, Antenna, Span, Earth) jumping Y93.33
  baseball Y93.64
  basketball Y93.67
  bathing (personal) Y93.E1 (*following* Y93.7)
  beach volleyball Y93.68
  bike riding Y93.55
  blackout game Y93.85
  boogie boarding Y93.18
  bowling Y93.54
  boxing Y93.71
  brass instrument playing Y93.J4 (*following* Y93.7)
  building construction Y93.H3 (*following* Y93.7)
  bungee jumping Y93.34
  calisthenics Y93.A2 (*following* Y93.7)
  canoeing (in calm and turbulent water) Y93.16
  capture the flag Y93.6A
  cardiorespiratory exercise NEC Y93.A9 (*following* Y93.7)

Activity — *continued*
  caregiving (providing) NEC Y93.F9 (*following* Y93.7)
    bathing Y93.F1 (*following* Y93.7)
    lifting Y93.F2 (*following* Y93.7)
  cellular
    communication device Y93.C2 (*following* Y93.7)
    telephone Y93.C2 (*following* Y93.7)
  challenge course Y93.A5 (*following* Y93.7)
  cheerleading Y93.45
  choking game Y93.85
  circuit training Y93.A4 (*following* Y93.7)
  cleaning
    floor Y93.E5 (*following* Y93.7)
  climbing NEC Y93.39
    mountain Y93.31
    rock Y93.31
    wall Y93.31
  clothing care and maintenance NEC Y93.E9 (*following* Y93.7)
  combatives Y93.75
  computer
    keyboarding Y93.C1 (*following* Y93.7)
    technology NEC Y93.C9 (*following* Y93.7)
  confidence course Y93.A5 (*following* Y93.7)
  construction (building) Y93.H3 (*following* Y93.7)
  cooking and baking Y93.G3 (*following* Y93.7)
  cool down exercises Y93.A2 (*following* Y93.7)
  cricket Y93.69
  crocheting Y93.D1 (*following* Y93.7)
  cross country skiing Y93.24
  dancing (all types) Y93.41
  digging
    dirt Y93.H1 (*following* Y93.7)
  dirt digging Y93.H1 (*following* Y93.7)
  dishwashing Y93.G1 (*following* Y93.7)
  diving (platform) (springboard) Y93.12
    underwater Y93.15
  dodge ball Y93.6A
  downhill skiing Y93.23
  drum playing Y93.J2 (*following* Y93.7)
  dumbbells Y93.B3 (*following* Y93.7)
  electronic
    devices NEC Y93.C9 (*following* Y93.7)
      hand held interactive Y93.C2 (*following* Y93.7)
    game playing (using) (with)
      interactive device Y93.C2 (*following* Y93.7)
      keyboard or other stationary device Y93.C1 (*following* Y93.7)
  elliptical machine Y93.A1 (*following* Y93.7)
  exercise(s)
    machines ((primarily) for)
      cardiorespiratory conditioning Y93.A1 (*following* Y93.7)
      muscle strengthening Y93.B1 (*following* Y93.7)
    muscle strengthening (non-machine) NEC Y93.B9 (*following* Y93.7)
  external motion NEC Y93.I9 (*following* Y93.7)
    rollercoaster Y93.I1 (*following* Y93.7)
  fainting game Y93.85
  field hockey Y93.65
  figure skating (pairs) (singles) Y93.21
  flag football Y93.62
  floor mopping and cleaning Y93.E5 (*following* Y93.7)
  food preparation and clean up Y93.G1 (*following* Y93.7)
  football (American) NOS Y93.61
    flag Y93.62
    tackle Y93.61
    touch Y93.62
  four square Y93.6A
  free weights Y93.B3 (*following* Y93.7)
  frisbee (ultimate) Y93.74
  furniture
    building Y93.D3 (*following* Y93.7)
    finishing Y93.D3 (*following* Y93.7)
    repair Y93.D3 (*following* Y93.7)
  game playing (electronic)
    using interactive device Y93.C2 (*following* Y93.7)
    using keyboard or other stationary device Y93.C1 (*following* Y93.7)
  gardening Y93.H2 (*following* Y93.7)
  golf Y93.53
  grass drills Y93.A6 (*following* Y93.7)
  grilling and smoking food Y93.G2 (*following* Y93.7)
  grooming and shearing an animal Y93.K3 (*following* Y93.7)
  guerilla drills Y93.A6 (*following* Y93.7)
  gymnastics (rhythmic) Y93.43
  hand held interactive electronic device Y93.C2 (*following* Y93.7)

☑ Additional Character Required — Refer to the Tabular List for Character Selection   ▼ Subterms under main terms may continue to next column or page

Activity — *continued*
handball Y93.73
handcrafts NEC Y93.D9 (*following* Y93.7)
hang gliding Y93.35
hiking (on level or elevated terrain) Y93.01
hockey (ice) Y93.22
 field Y93.65
horseback riding Y93.52
household (interior) maintenance NEC Y93.E9 (*following* Y93.7)
ice NEC Y93.29
 dancing Y93.21
 hockey Y93.22
 skating Y93.21
inline roller skating Y93.51
ironing Y93.E4 (*following* Y93.7)
judo Y93.75
jumping jacks Y93.A2 (*following* Y93.7)
jumping rope Y93.56
jumping (off) NEC Y93.39
 BASE (Building, Antenna, Span, Earth) Y93.33
 bungee Y93.34
 jacks Y93.A2 (*following* Y93.7)
 rope Y93.56
karate Y93.75
kayaking (in calm and turbulent water) Y93.16
keyboarding (computer) Y93.C1 (*following* Y93.7)
kickball Y93.6A
knitting Y93.D1 (*following* Y93.7)
lacrosse Y93.65
land maintenance NEC Y93.H9 (*following* Y93.7)
landscaping Y93.H2 (*following* Y93.7)
laundry Y93.E2 (*following* Y93.7)
machines (exercise)
 primarily for cardiorespiratory conditioning Y93.A1 (*following* Y93.7)
 primarily for muscle strengthening Y93.B1 (*following* Y93.7)
maintenance
 exterior building NEC Y93.H9 (*following* Y93.7)
 household (interior) NEC Y93.E9 (*following* Y93.7)
 land Y93.H9 (*following* Y93.7)
 property Y93.H9 (*following* Y93.7)
marching (on level or elevated terrain) Y93.01
martial arts Y93.75
microwave oven Y93.G3 (*following* Y93.7)
milking an animal Y93.K2 (*following* Y93.7)
mopping (floor) Y93.E5 (*following* Y93.7)
mountain climbing Y93.31
muscle strengthening
 exercises (non-machine) NEC Y93.B9 (*following* Y93.7)
 machines Y93.B1 (*following* Y93.7)
musical keyboard (electronic) playing Y93.J1 (*following* Y93.7)
nordic skiing Y93.24
obstacle course Y93.A5 (*following* Y93.7)
oven (microwave) Y93.G3 (*following* Y93.7)
packing up and unpacking in moving to a new residence Y93.E6 (*following* Y93.7)
parasailing Y93.19
pass out game Y93.85
percussion instrument playing NEC Y93.J2 (*following* Y93.7)
personal
 bathing and showering Y93.E1 (*following* Y93.7)
 hygiene NEC Y93.E8 (*following* Y93.7)
 showering Y93.E1 (*following* Y93.7)
physical games generally associated with school recess, summer camp and children Y93.6A
physical training NEC Y93.A9 (*following* Y93.7)
piano playing Y93.J1 (*following* Y93.7)
pilates Y93.B4 (*following* Y93.7)
platform diving Y93.12
playing musical instrument
 brass instrument Y93.J4 (*following* Y93.7)
 drum Y93.J2 (*following* Y93.7)
 musical keyboard (electronic) Y93.J1 (*following* Y93.7)
 percussion instrument NEC Y93.J2 (*following* Y93.7)
 piano Y93.J1 (*following* Y93.7)
 string instrument Y93.J3 (*following* Y93.7)
 winds instrument Y93.J4 (*following* Y93.7)
property maintenance
 exterior NEC Y93.H9 (*following* Y93.7)
 interior NEC Y93.E9 (*following* Y93.7)
pruning (garden and lawn) Y93.H2 (*following* Y93.7)
pull-ups Y93.B2 (*following* Y93.7)
push-ups Y93.B2 (*following* Y93.7)

Activity — *continued*
racquetball Y93.73
rafting (in calm and turbulent water) Y93.16
raking (leaves) Y93.H1 (*following* Y93.7)
rappelling Y93.32
refereeing a sports activity Y93.81
residential relocation Y93.E6 (*following* Y93.7)
rhythmic gymnastics Y93.43
rhythmic movement NEC Y93.49
riding
 horseback Y93.52
 rollercoaster Y93.I1 (*following* Y93.7)
rock climbing Y93.31
roller skating (inline) Y93.51
rollercoaster riding Y93.I1 (*following* Y93.7)
rough housing and horseplay Y93.83
rowing (in calm and turbulent water) Y93.16
rugby Y93.63
running Y93.02
SCUBA diving Y93.15
sewing Y93.D2 (*following* Y93.7)
shoveling Y93.H1 (*following* Y93.7)
 dirt Y93.H1 (*following* Y93.7)
 snow Y93.H1 (*following* Y93.7)
showering (personal) Y93.E1 (*following* Y93.7)
sit-ups Y93.B2 (*following* Y93.7)
skateboarding Y93.51
skating (ice) Y93.21
 roller Y93.51
skiing (alpine) (downhill) Y93.23
 cross country Y93.24
 nordic Y93.24
 water Y93.17
sledding (snow) Y93.23
sleeping (sleep) Y93.84
smoking and grilling food Y93.G2 (*following* Y93.7)
snorkeling Y93.15
snow NEC Y93.29
 boarding Y93.23
 shoveling Y93.H1 (*following* Y93.7)
 sledding Y93.23
 tubing Y93.23
soccer Y93.66
softball Y93.64
specified NEC Y93.89
spectator at an event Y93.82
sports NEC Y93.79
 sports played as a team or group NEC Y93.69
 sports played individually NEC Y93.59
springboard diving Y93.12
squash Y93.73
stationary bike Y93.A1 (*following* Y93.7)
step (stepping) exercise (class) Y93.A3 (*following* Y93.7)
stepper machine Y93.A1 (*following* Y93.7)
stove Y93.G3 (*following* Y93.7)
string instrument playing Y93.J3 (*following* Y93.7)
surfing Y93.18
 wind Y93.18
swimming Y93.11
tackle football Y93.61
tap dancing Y93.41
tennis Y93.73
tobogganing Y93.23
touch football Y93.62
track and field events (non-running) Y93.57
 running Y93.02
trampoline Y93.44
treadmill Y93.A1 (*following* Y93.7)
trimming shrubs Y93.H2 (*following* Y93.7)
tubing (in calm and turbulent water) Y93.16
 snow Y93.23
ultimate frisbee Y93.74
underwater diving Y93.15
unpacking in moving to a new residence Y93.E6 (*following* Y93.7)
use of stove, oven and microwave oven Y93.G3 (*following* Y93.7)
vacuuming Y93.E3 (*following* Y93.7)
volleyball (beach) (court) Y93.68
wake boarding Y93.17
walking (on level or elevated terrain) Y93.01
 an animal Y93.K1 (*following* Y93.7)
walking an animal Y93.K1 (*following* Y93.7)
wall climbing Y93.31
warm up and cool down exercises Y93.A2 (*following* Y93.7)
water NEC Y93.19
 aerobics Y93.14
 craft NEC Y93.19

Activity — *continued*
 water — *continued*
 exercise Y93.14
 polo Y93.13
 skiing Y93.17
 sliding Y93.18
 survival training and testing Y93.19
 weeding (garden and lawn) Y93.H2 (*following* Y93.7)
 wind instrument playing Y93.J4 (*following* Y93.7)
 windsurfing Y93.18
 wrestling Y93.72
 yoga Y93.42
Adverse effect of drugs — *see* Table of Drugs and Chemicals
Aerosinusitis — *see* Air, pressure
After-effect, late — *see* Sequelae
Air
 blast in war operations — *see* War operations, air blast
 pressure
 change, rapid
 during
 ascent W94.29 ☑
 while (in) (surfacing from)
 aircraft W94.23 ☑
 deep water diving W94.21 ☑
 underground W94.22 ☑
 descent W94.39 ☑
 in
 aircraft W94.31 ☑
 water W94.32 ☑
 high, prolonged W94.0 ☑
 low, prolonged W94.12 ☑
 due to residence or long visit at high altitude W94.11 ☑
Alpine sickness W94.11 ☑
Altitude sickness W94.11 ☑
Anaphylactic shock, anaphylaxis — *see* Table of Drugs and Chemicals
Andes disease W94.11 ☑
Arachnidism, arachnoidism X58 ☑
Arson (with intent to injure or kill) X97 ☑
Asphyxia, asphyxiation
 by
 food (bone) (seed) — *see* categories T17 and T18 ☑
 gas (*see also* Table of Drugs and Chemicals)
 legal
 execution — *see* Legal, intervention, gas
 intervention — *see* Legal, intervention, gas
 from
 fire (*see also* Exposure, fire)
 in war operations — *see* War operations, fire
 ignition — *see* Ignition
 vomitus T17.81 ☑
 in war operations — *see* War operations, restriction of airway
Aspiration
 food (any type) (into respiratory tract) (with asphyxia, obstruction respiratory tract, suffocation) — *see* categories T17 and T18 ☑
 foreign body — *see* Foreign body, aspiration
 vomitus (with asphyxia, obstruction respiratory tract, suffocation) T17.81 ☑
Assassination (attempt) — *see* Assault
Assault (homicidal) (by) (in) Y09
 arson X97 ☑
 bite (of human being) Y04.1 ☑
 bodily force Y04.8 ☑
 bite Y04.1 ☑
 bumping into Y04.2 ☑
 sexual — *see* subcategories T74.0, T76.0 ☑
 unarmed fight Y04.0 ☑
 bomb X96.9 ☑
 antipersonnel X96.0 ☑
 fertilizer X96.3 ☑
 gasoline X96.1 ☑
 letter X96.2 ☑
 petrol X96.1 ☑
 pipe X96.3 ☑
 specified NEC X96.8 ☑
 brawl (hand) (fists) (foot) (unarmed) Y04.0 ☑
 burning, burns (by fire) NEC X97 ☑
 acid Y08.89 ☑
 caustic, corrosive substance Y08.89 ☑
 chemical from swallowing caustic, corrosive substance — *see* Table of Drugs and Chemicals

Assault — *continued*
  burning, burns — *continued*
    cigarette(s) X97 ☑
    hot object X98.9 ☑
      fluid NEC X98.2 ☑
      household appliance X98.3 ☑
      specified NEC X98.8 ☑
      steam X98.0 ☑
      tap water X98.1 ☑
      vapors X98.0 ☑
    scalding — *see* Assault, burning
    steam X98.0 ☑
    vitriol Y08.89 ☑
  caustic, corrosive substance (gas) Y08.89 ☑
  crashing of
    aircraft Y08.81 ☑
    motor vehicle Y03.8 ☑
      pushed in front of Y02.0 ☑
      run over Y03.0 ☑
      specified NEC Y03.8 ☑
  cutting or piercing instrument X99.9 ☑
    dagger X99.2 ☑
    glass X99.0 ☑
    knife X99.1 ☑
    specified NEC X99.8 ☑
    sword X99.2 ☑
  dagger X99.2 ☑
  drowning (in) X92.9 ☑
    bathtub X92.0 ☑
    natural water X92.3 ☑
    specified NEC X92.8 ☑
    swimming pool X92.1 ☑
      following fall X92.2 ☑
  dynamite X96.8 ☑
  explosive(s) (material) X96.9 ☑
  fight (hand) (fists) (foot) (unarmed) Y04.0 ☑
    with weapon — *see* Assault, by type of weapon
  fire X97 ☑
  firearm X95.9 ☑
    airgun X95.01 ☑
    handgun X93 ☑
    hunting rifle X94.1 ☑
    larger X94.9 ☑
      specified NEC X94.8 ☑
    machine gun X94.2 ☑
    shotgun X94.0 ☑
    specified NEC X95.8 ☑
  from high place Y01 ☑
  gunshot (wound) NEC — *see* Assault, firearm, by type
  incendiary device X97 ☑
  injury Y09
    to child due to criminal abortion attempt NEC Y08.89 ☑
  knife X99.1 ☑
  late effect of — *see* categories X92-Y08 with 7th character S
  placing before moving object NEC Y02.8 ☑
    motor vehicle Y02.0 ☑
  poisoning — *see* categories T36-T65 with 7th character S
  puncture, any part of body — *see* Assault, cutting or piercing instrument
  pushing
    before moving object NEC Y02.8 ☑
      motor vehicle Y02.0 ☑
      subway train Y02.1 ☑
      train Y02.1 ☑
    from high place Y01 ☑
  rape T74.2- ☑
  scalding — *see* Assault, burning
  sequelae of — *see* categories X92-Y08 with 7th character S
  sexual (by bodily force) T74.2- ☑
  shooting — *see* Assault, firearm
  specified means NEC Y08.89 ☑
  stab, any part of body — *see* Assault, cutting or piercing instrument
  steam X98.0 ☑
  striking against
    other person Y04.2 ☑
    sports equipment Y08.09 ☑
      baseball bat Y08.02 ☑
      hockey stick Y08.01 ☑
  struck by
    sports equipment Y08.09 ☑
      baseball bat Y08.02 ☑

Assault — *continued*
  struck by — *continued*
    sports equipment — *continued*
      hockey stick Y08.01 ☑
  submersion — *see* Assault, drowning
  violence Y09
  weapon Y09
    blunt Y00 ☑
    cutting or piercing — *see* Assault, cutting or piercing instrument
    firearm — *see* Assault, firearm
  wound Y09
    cutting — *see* Assault, cutting or piercing instrument
    gunshot — *see* Assault, firearm
    knife X99.1 ☑
    piercing — *see* Assault, cutting or piercing instrument
    puncture — *see* Assault, cutting or piercing instrument
    stab — *see* Assault, cutting or piercing instrument
Attack by mammals NEC W55.89 ☑
Avalanche — *see* Landslide
Aviator's disease — *see* Air, pressure

B

Barotitis, barodontalgia, barosinusitis, barotrauma (otitic) (sinus) — *see* Air, pressure
Battered (baby) (child) (person) (syndrome) X58 ☑
Bayonet wound W26.1 ☑
  in
    legal intervention — *see* Legal, intervention, sharp object, bayonet
    war operations — *see* War operations, combat
  stated as undetermined whether accidental or intentional Y28.8 ☑
  suicide (attempt) X78.2 ☑
Bean in nose — *see* categories T17 and T18 ☑
Bed set on fire NEC — *see* Exposure, fire, uncontrolled, building, bed
Beheading (by guillotine)
  homicide X99.9 ☑
  legal execution — *see* Legal, intervention
Bending, injury in (prolonged) (static) X50.1 ☑
Bends — *see* Air, pressure, change
Bite, bitten by
  alligator W58.01 ☑
  arthropod (nonvenomous) NEC W57 ☑
  bull W55.21 ☑
  cat W55.01 ☑
  cow W55.21 ☑
  crocodile W58.11 ☑
  dog W54.0 ☑
  goat W55.31 ☑
  hoof stock NEC W55.31 ☑
  horse W55.11 ☑
  human being (accidentally) W50.3 ☑
    with intent to injure or kill Y04.1 ☑
    as, or caused by, a crowd or human stampede (with fall) W52 ☑
    assault Y04.1 ☑
    homicide (attempt) Y04.1 ☑
    in
      fight Y04.1 ☑
  insect (nonvenomous) W57 ☑
  lizard (nonvenomous) W59.01 ☑
  mammal NEC W55.81 ☑
    marine W56.31 ☑
  marine animal (nonvenomous) W56.81 ☑
  millipede W57 ☑
  moray eel W56.51 ☑
  mouse W53.01 ☑
  person(s) (accidentally) W50.3 ☑
    with intent to injure or kill Y04.1 ☑
    as, or caused by, a crowd or human stampede (with fall) W52 ☑
    assault Y04.1 ☑
    homicide (attempt) Y04.1 ☑
    in
      fight Y04.1 ☑
  pig W55.41 ☑
  raccoon W55.51 ☑
  rat W53.11 ☑
  reptile W59.81 ☑
    lizard W59.01 ☑

Bite, bitten by — *continued*
  reptile — *continued*
    snake W59.11 ☑
    turtle W59.21 ☑
      terrestrial W59.81 ☑
  rodent W53.81 ☑
    mouse W53.01 ☑
    rat W53.11 ☑
    specified NEC W53.81 ☑
    squirrel W53.21 ☑
  shark W56.41 ☑
  sheep W55.31 ☑
  snake (nonvenomous) W59.11 ☑
  spider (nonvenomous) W57 ☑
  squirrel W53.21 ☑
Blast (air) in war operations — *see* War operations, blast
Blizzard X37.2 ☑
Blood alcohol level Y90.9
  less than 20mg/100ml Y90.0
  20-39mg/100ml Y90.1
  40-59mg/100ml Y90.2
  60-79mg/100ml Y90.3
  80-99mg/100ml Y90.4
  100-119mg/100ml Y90.5
  120-199mg/100ml Y90.6
  200-239mg/100ml Y90.7
  presence in blood, level not specified Y90.9
Blow X58 ☑
  by law-enforcing agent, police (on duty) — *see* Legal, intervention, manhandling
    blunt object — *see* Legal, intervention, blunt object
Blowing up — *see* Explosion
Brawl (hand) (fists) (foot) Y04.0 ☑
Breakage (accidental) (part of)
  ladder (causing fall) W11 ☑
  scaffolding (causing fall) W12 ☑
Broken
  glass, contact with — *see* Contact, with, glass
  power line (causing electric shock) W85 ☑
Bumping against, into (accidentally)
  object NEC W22.8 ☑
    with fall — *see* Fall, due to, bumping against, object
    caused by crowd or human stampede (with fall) W52 ☑
    sports equipment W21.9 ☑
  person(s) W51 ☑
    with fall W03 ☑
      due to ice or snow W00.0 ☑
    assault Y04.2 ☑
    caused by, a crowd or human stampede (with fall) W52 ☑
    homicide (attempt) Y04.2 ☑
    sports equipment W21.9 ☑
Burn, burned, burning (accidental) (by) (from) (on)
  acid NEC — *see* Table of Drugs and Chemicals
  bed linen — *see* Exposure, fire, uncontrolled, in building, bed
  blowtorch X08.8 ☑
    with ignition of clothing NEC X06.2 ☑
      nightwear X05 ☑
  bonfire, campfire (controlled) (*see also* Exposure, fire, controlled, not in building)
    uncontrolled — *see* Exposure, fire, uncontrolled, not in building
  candle X08.8 ☑
    with ignition of clothing NEC X06.2 ☑
      nightwear X05 ☑
  caustic liquid, substance (external) (internal) NEC — *see* Table of Drugs and Chemicals
  chemical (external) (internal) (*see also* Table of Drugs and Chemicals)
    in war operations — *see* War operations. fire
  cigar(s) or cigarette(s) X08.8 ☑
    with ignition of clothing NEC X06.2 ☑
      nightwear X05 ☑
  clothes, clothing NEC (from controlled fire) X06.2 ☑
    with conflagration — *see* Exposure, fire, uncontrolled, building
    not in building or structure — *see* Exposure, fire, uncontrolled, not in building
  cooker (hot) X15.8 ☑
    stated as undetermined whether accidental or intentional Y27.3 ☑
    suicide (attempt) X77.3 ☑
  electric blanket X16 ☑

☑ Additional Character Required — Refer to the Tabular List for Character Selection   ▽ Subterms under main terms may continue to next column or page

Burn, burned, burning — *continued*
- engine (hot) X17 ☑
- fire, flames — *see* Exposure, fire
- flare, Very pistol — *see* Discharge, firearm NEC
- heat
  - from appliance (electrical) (household) X15.8 ☑
    - cooker X15.8 ☑
    - hotplate X15.2 ☑
    - kettle X15.8 ☑
    - light bulb X15.8 ☑
    - saucepan X15.3 ☑
    - skillet X15.3 ☑
    - stated as undetermined whether accidental or intentional Y27.3 ☑
    - stove X15.0 ☑
    - suicide (attempt) X77.3 ☑
    - toaster X15.1 ☑
  - in local application or packing during medical or surgical procedure Y63.5
- heating
  - appliance, radiator or pipe X16 ☑
- homicide (attempt) — *see* Assault, burning
- hot
  - air X14.1 ☑
  - cooker X15.8 ☑
  - drink X10.0 ☑
  - engine X17 ☑
  - fat X10.2 ☑
  - fluid NEC X12 ☑
  - food X10.1 ☑
  - gases X14.1 ☑
  - heating appliance X16 ☑
  - household appliance NEC X15.8 ☑
  - kettle X15.8 ☑
  - liquid NEC X12 ☑
  - machinery X17 ☑
  - metal (molten) (liquid) NEC X18 ☑
  - object (not producing fire or flames) NEC X19 ☑
  - oil (cooking) X10.2 ☑
  - pipe(s) X16 ☑
  - radiator X16 ☑
  - saucepan (glass) (metal) X15.3 ☑
  - stove (kitchen) X15.0 ☑
  - substance NEC X19 ☑
    - caustic or corrosive NEC — *see* Table of Drugs and Chemicals
  - toaster X15.1 ☑
  - tool X17 ☑
  - vapor X13.1 ☑
  - water (tap) — *see* Contact, with, hot, tap water
- hotplate X15.2 ☑
  - suicide (attempt) X77.3 ☑
- ignition — *see* Ignition
- in war operations — *see* War operations, fire
- inflicted by other person X97 ☑
  - by hot objects, hot vapor, and steam — *see* Assault, burning, hot object
- internal, from swallowed caustic, corrosive liquid, substance — *see* Table of Drugs and Chemicals
- iron (hot) X15.8 ☑
  - stated as undetermined whether accidental or intentional Y27.3 ☑
  - suicide (attempt) X77.3 ☑
- kettle (hot) X15.8 ☑
  - stated as undetermined whether accidental or intentional Y27.3 ☑
  - suicide (attempt) X77.3 ☑
- lamp (flame) X08.8 ☑
  - with ignition of clothing NEC X06.2 ☑
    - nightwear X05 ☑
- lighter (cigar) (cigarette) X08.8 ☑
  - with ignition of clothing NEC X06.2 ☑
    - nightwear X05 ☑
- lightning — *see* subcategory T75.0 ☑
  - causing fire — *see* Exposure, fire
- liquid (boiling) (hot) NEC X12 ☑
  - stated as undetermined whether accidental or intentional Y27.2 ☑
  - suicide (attempt) X77.2 ☑
- local application of externally applied substance in medical or surgical care Y63.5
- machinery (hot) X17 ☑
- matches X08.8 ☑
  - with ignition of clothing NEC X06.2 ☑
    - nightwear X05 ☑

Burn, burned, burning — *continued*
- mattress — *see* Exposure, fire, uncontrolled, building, bed
- medicament, externally applied Y63.5
- metal (hot) (liquid) (molten) NEC X18 ☑
- nightwear (nightclothes, nightdress, gown, pajamas, robe) X05 ☑
- object (hot) NEC X19 ☑
- on board watercraft
  - due to
    - accident to watercraft V91.09 ☑
      - powered craft V91.03 ☑
        - ferry boat V91.01 ☑
        - fishing boat V91.02 ☑
        - jetskis V91.03 ☑
        - liner V91.01 ☑
        - merchant ship V91.00 ☑
        - passenger ship V91.01 ☑
      - unpowered craft V91.08 ☑
        - canoe V91.05 ☑
        - inflatable V91.06 ☑
        - kayak V91.05 ☑
        - sailboat V91.04 ☑
        - surf-board V91.08 ☑
        - water skis V91.07 ☑
        - windsurfer V91.08 ☑
    - fire on board V93.09 ☑
      - ferry boat V93.01 ☑
      - fishing boat V93.02 ☑
      - jetskis V93.03 ☑
      - liner V93.01 ☑
      - merchant ship V93.00 ☑
      - passenger ship V93.01 ☑
      - powered craft NEC V93.03 ☑
      - sailboat V93.04 ☑
    - specified heat source NEC on board V93.19 ☑
      - ferry boat V93.11 ☑
      - fishing boat V93.12 ☑
      - jetskis V93.13 ☑
      - liner V93.11 ☑
      - merchant ship V93.10 ☑
      - passenger ship V93.11 ☑
      - powered craft NEC V93.13 ☑
      - sailboat V93.14 ☑
- pipe (hot) X16 ☑
- smoking X08.8 ☑
  - with ignition of clothing NEC X06.2 ☑
    - nightwear X05 ☑
- powder — *see* Powder burn
- radiator (hot) X16 ☑
- saucepan (hot) (glass) (metal) X15.3 ☑
  - stated as undetermined whether accidental or intentional Y27.3 ☑
  - suicide (attempt) X77.3 ☑
- self-inflicted X76 ☑
  - stated as undetermined whether accidental or intentional Y26 ☑
- stated as undetermined whether accidental or intentional Y27.0 ☑
- steam X13.1 ☑
  - pipe X16 ☑
    - stated as undetermined whether accidental or intentional Y27.8 ☑
  - stated as undetermined whether accidental or intentional Y27.0 ☑
  - suicide (attempt) X77.0 ☑
- stove (hot) (kitchen) X15.0 ☑
  - stated as undetermined whether accidental or intentional Y27.3 ☑
  - suicide (attempt) X77.3 ☑
- substance (hot) NEC X19 ☑
  - boiling X12 ☑
    - stated as undetermined whether accidental or intentional Y27.2 ☑
    - suicide (attempt) X77.2 ☑
  - molten (metal) X18 ☑
- suicide (attempt) NEC X76 ☑
  - hot
    - household appliance X77.3 ☑
    - object X77.9 ☑
- therapeutic misadventure
  - heat in local application or packing during medical or surgical procedure Y63.5
  - overdose of radiation Y63.2
- toaster (hot) X15.1 ☑

Burn, burned, burning — *continued*
- toaster — *continued*
  - stated as undetermined whether accidental or intentional Y27.3 ☑
  - suicide (attempt) X77.3 ☑
- tool (hot) X17 ☑
- torch, welding X08.8 ☑
  - with ignition of clothing NEC X06.2 ☑
    - nightwear X05 ☑
- trash fire (controlled) — *see* Exposure, fire, controlled, not in building
  - uncontrolled — *see* Exposure, fire, uncontrolled, not in building
- vapor (hot) X13.1 ☑
  - stated as undetermined whether accidental or intentional Y27.0 ☑
  - suicide (attempt) X77.0 ☑
- Very pistol — *see* Discharge, firearm NEC
Butted by animal W55.82 ☑
- bull W55.22 ☑
- cow W55.22 ☑
- goat W55.32 ☑
- horse W55.12 ☑
- pig W55.42 ☑
- sheep W55.32 ☑

C

Caisson disease — *see* Air, pressure, change
Campfire (exposure to) (controlled) (*see also* Exposure, fire, controlled, not in building)
- uncontrolled — *see* Exposure, fire, uncontrolled, not in building
Capital punishment (any means) — *see* Legal, intervention
Car sickness T75.3 ☑
Casualty (not due to war) NEC X58 ☑
- war — *see* War operations
Cat
- bite W55.01 ☑
- scratch W55.03 ☑
Cataclysm, cataclysmic (any injury) NEC — *see* Forces of nature
Catching fire — *see* Exposure, fire
Caught
- between
  - folding object W23.0 ☑
  - objects (moving) (stationary and moving) W23.0 ☑
    - and machinery — *see* Contact, with, by type of machine
    - stationary W23.1 ☑
  - sliding door and door frame W23.0 ☑
- by, in
  - machinery (moving parts of) — *see* Contact, with, by type of machine
  - washing-machine wringer W23.0 ☑
- under packing crate (due to losing grip) W23.1 ☑
Cave-in caused by cataclysmic earth surface movement or eruption — *see* Landslide
Change(s) in air pressure — *see* Air, pressure, change
Choked, choking (on) (any object except food or vomitus)
- food (bone) (seed) — *see* categories T17 and T18 ☑
- vomitus T17.81- ☑
Civil insurrection — *see* War operations
Cloudburst (any injury) X37.8 ☑
Cold, exposure to (accidental) (excessive) (extreme) (natural) (place) NEC — *see* Exposure, cold
Collapse
- building W20.1 ☑
  - burning (uncontrolled fire) X00.2 ☑
- dam or man-made structure (causing earth movement) X36.0 ☑
- machinery — *see* Contact, with, by type of machine
- structure W20.1 ☑
  - burning (uncontrolled fire) X00.2 ☑
Collision (accidental) NEC (*see also* Accident, transport) V89.9 ☑
- pedestrian W51 ☑
  - with fall W03 ☑
    - due to ice or snow W00.0 ☑
    - involving pedestrian conveyance — *see* Accident, transport, pedestrian, conveyance
  - and
    - crowd or human stampede (with fall) W52 ☑
    - object W22.8 ☑

Collision — *continued*
  pedestrian — *continued*
    and — *continued*
      object — *continued*
        with fall — *see* Fall, due to, bumping
          against, object
    person(s) — *see* Collision, pedestrian
  transport vehicle NEC V89.9 ☑
    and
      avalanche, fallen or not moving — *see* Accident,
        transport
        falling or moving — *see* Landslide
      landslide, fallen or not moving — *see* Accident,
        transport
        falling or moving — *see* Landslide
    due to cataclysm — *see* Forces of nature, by type
    intentional, purposeful suicide (attempt) — *see*
      Suicide, collision
Combustion, spontaneous — *see* Ignition
Complication (delayed) **of or following** (medical or
  surgical procedure) Y84.9
  with misadventure — *see* Misadventure
  amputation of limb(s) Y83.5
  anastomosis (arteriovenous) (blood vessel) (gastroje-
    junal) (tendon) (natural or artificial material)
    Y83.2
  aspiration (of fluid) Y84.4
    tissue Y84.8
  biopsy Y84.8
  blood
    sampling Y84.7
    transfusion
      procedure Y84.8
  bypass Y83.2
  catheterization (urinary) Y84.6
    cardiac Y84.0
  colostomy Y83.3
  cystostomy Y83.3
  dialysis (kidney) Y84.1
  drug — *see* Table of Drugs and Chemicals
  due to misadventure — *see* Misadventure
  duodenostomy Y83.3
  electroshock therapy Y84.3
  external stoma, creation of Y83.3
  formation of external stoma Y83.3
  gastrostomy Y83.3
  graft Y83.2
  hypothermia (medically-induced) Y84.8
  implant, implantation (of)
    artificial
      internal device (cardiac pacemaker) (electrodes
        in brain) (heart valve prosthesis) (ortho-
        pedic) Y83.1
      material or tissue (for anastomosis or bypass)
        Y83.2
        with creation of external stoma Y83.3
      natural tissues (for anastomosis or bypass) Y83.2
        with creation of external stoma Y83.3
  infusion
    procedure Y84.8
  injection — *see* Table of Drugs and Chemicals
    procedure Y84.8
  insertion of gastric or duodenal sound Y84.5
  insulin-shock therapy Y84.3
  paracentesis (abdominal) (thoracic) (aspirative) Y84.4
  procedures other than surgical operation — *see*
    Complication of or following, by type of proce-
    dure
  radiological procedure or therapy Y84.2
  removal of organ (partial) (total) NEC Y83.6
  sampling
    blood Y84.7
    fluid NEC Y84.4
    tissue Y84.8
  shock therapy Y84.3
  surgical operation NEC (*see also* Complication of or
    following, by type of operation) Y83.9
    reconstructive NEC Y83.4
      with
        anastomosis, bypass or graft Y83.2
        formation of external stoma Y83.3
    specified NEC Y83.8
  transfusion (*see also* Table of Drugs and Chemicals)
    procedure Y84.8
  transplant, transplantation (heart) (kidney) (liver)
    (whole organ, any) Y83.0
    partial organ Y83.4
  ureterostomy Y83.3

Complication (delayed) **of or following** —
  continued
  vaccination (*see also* Table of Drugs and Chemicals)
    procedure Y84.8
Compression
  divers' squeeze — *see* Air, pressure, change
  trachea by
    food (lodged in esophagus) — *see* categories T17
      and T18 ☑
    vomitus (lodged in esophagus) T17.81- ☑
Conflagration — *see* Exposure, fire, uncontrolled
Constriction (external)
  hair W49.01 ☑
  jewelry W49.04 ☑
  ring W49.04 ☑
  rubber band W49.03 ☑
  specified item NEC W49.09 ☑
  string W49.02 ☑
  thread W49.02 ☑
Contact (accidental)
  with
    abrasive wheel (metalworking) W31.1 ☑
    alligator W58.09 ☑
      bite W58.01 ☑
      crushing W58.03 ☑
      strike W58.02 ☑
    amphibian W62.9 ☑
      frog W62.0 ☑
      toad W62.1 ☑
    animal (nonvenomous) NEC W64 ☑
      marine W56.89 ☑
        bite W56.81 ☑
        dolphin — *see* Contact, with, dolphin
        fish NEC — *see* Contact, with, fish
        mammal — *see* Contact, with, mammal,
          marine
        orca — *see* Contact, with, orca
        sea lion — *see* Contact, with, sea lion
        shark — *see* Contact, with, shark
        strike W56.82 ☑
    animate mechanical force NEC W64 ☑
    arrow W21.89 ☑
      not thrown, projected or falling W45.8 ☑
    arthropods (nonvenomous) W57 ☑
    axe W27.0 ☑
    band-saw (industrial) W31.2 ☑
    bayonet — *see* Bayonet wound
    bee(s) X58 ☑
    bench-saw (industrial) W31.2 ☑
    bird W61.99 ☑
      bite W61.91 ☑
      chicken — *see* Contact, with, chicken
      duck — *see* Contact, with, duck
      goose — *see* Contact, with, goose
      macaw — *see* Contact, with, macaw
      parrot — *see* Contact, with, parrot
      psittacine — *see* Contact, with, psittacine
      strike W61.92 ☑
      turkey — *see* Contact, with, turkey
    blender W29.0 ☑
    boiling water X12 ☑
      stated as undetermined whether accidental or
        intentional Y27.2 ☑
      suicide (attempt) X77.2 ☑
    bore, earth-drilling or mining (land) (seabed)
      W31.0 ☑
    buffalo — *see* Contact, with, hoof stock NEC
    bull W55.29 ☑
      bite W55.21 ☑
      gored W55.22 ☑
      strike W55.22 ☑
    bumper cars W31.81 ☑
    camel — *see* Contact, with, hoof stock NEC
    can
      lid W26.8 ☑
      opener W27.4 ☑
        powered W29.0 ☑
    cat W55.09 ☑
      bite W55.01 ☑
      scratch W55.03 ☑
    caterpillar (venomous) X58 ☑
    centipede (venomous) X58 ☑
    chain
      hoist W24.0 ☑
        agricultural operations W30.89 ☑
      saw W29.3 ☑

Contact — *continued*
  with — *continued*
    chicken W61.39 ☑
      peck W61.33 ☑
      strike W61.32 ☑
    chisel W27.0 ☑
    circular saw W31.2 ☑
    cobra X58 ☑
    combine (harvester) W30.0 ☑
    conveyer belt W24.1 ☑
    cooker (hot) X15.8 ☑
      stated as undetermined whether accidental or
        intentional Y27.3 ☑
      suicide (attempt) X77.3 ☑
    coral X58 ☑
    cotton gin W31.82 ☑
    cow W55.29 ☑
      bite W55.21 ☑
      strike W55.22 ☑
    crane W24.0 ☑
      agricultural operations W30.89 ☑
    crocodile W58.19 ☑
      bite W58.11 ☑
      crushing W58.13 ☑
      strike W58.12 ☑
    dagger W26.1 ☑
      stated as undetermined whether accidental or
        intentional Y28.2 ☑
      suicide (attempt) X78.2 ☑
    dairy equipment W31.82 ☑
    dart W21.89 ☑
      not thrown, projected or falling W45.8 ☑
    deer — *see* Contact, with, hoof stock NEC
    derrick W24.0 ☑
      agricultural operations W30.89 ☑
        hay W30.2 ☑
    dog W54.8 ☑
      bite W54.0 ☑
      strike W54.1 ☑
    dolphin W56.09 ☑
      bite W56.01 ☑
      strike W56.02 ☑
    donkey — *see* Contact, with, hoof stock NEC
    drill (powered) W29.8 ☑
      earth (land) (seabed) W31.0 ☑
      nonpowered W27.8 ☑
    drive belt W24.0 ☑
      agricultural operations W30.89 ☑
    dry ice — *see* Exposure, cold, man-made
    dryer (clothes) (powered) (spin) W29.2 ☑
    duck W61.69 ☑
      bite W61.61 ☑
      strike W61.62 ☑
    earth (-)
      drilling machine (industrial) W31.0 ☑
      scraping machine in stationary use W31.83 ☑
    edge of stiff paper W26.2 ☑
    electric
      beater W29.0 ☑
      blanket X16 ☑
      fan W29.2 ☑
        commercial W31.82 ☑
      knife W29.1 ☑
      mixer W29.0 ☑
    elevator (building) W24.0 ☑
      agricultural operations W30.89 ☑
        grain W30.3 ☑
    engine(s), hot NEC X17 ☑
    excavating machine W31.0 ☑
    farm machine W30.9 ☑
    feces — *see* Contact, with, by type of animal
    fer de lance X58 ☑
    fish W56.59 ☑
      bite W56.51 ☑
      shark — *see* Contact, with, shark
      strike W56.52 ☑
    flying horses W31.81 ☑
    forging (metalworking) machine W31.1 ☑
    fork W27.4 ☑
    forklift (truck) W24.0 ☑
      agricultural operations W30.89 ☑
    frog W62.0 ☑
    garden
      cultivator (powered) W29.3 ☑
        riding W30.89 ☑
      fork W27.1 ☑

☑ Additional Character Required — Refer to the Tabular List for Character Selection   🔻 Subterms under main terms may continue to next column or page

Contact — *continued*
  with — *continued*
    gas turbine W31.3 ☑
    Gila monster X58 ☑
    giraffe — *see* Contact, with, hoof stock NEC
    glass (sharp) (broken) W25 ☑
      with subsequent fall W18.02 ☑
      assault X99.0 ☑
      due to fall — *see* Fall, by type
      stated as undetermined whether accidental or
        intentional Y28.0 ☑
      suicide (attempt) X78.0 ☑
    goat W55.39 ☑
      bite W55.31 ☑
      strike W55.32 ☑
    goose W61.59 ☑
      bite W61.51 ☑
      strike W61.52 ☑
    hand
      saw W27.0 ☑
      tool (not powered) NEC W27.8 ☑
        powered W29.8 ☑
    harvester W30.0 ☑
    hay-derrick W30.2 ☑
    heating
      appliance (hot) X16 ☑
      pad (electric) X16 ☑
    heat NEC X19 ☑
      from appliance (electrical) (household) — *see*
        Contact, with, hot, household appliance
        heating appliance X16 ☑
    hedge-trimmer (powered) W29.3 ☑
    hoe W27.1 ☑
    hoist (chain) (shaft) NEC W24.0 ☑
      agricultural W30.89 ☑
    hoof stock NEC W55.39 ☑
      bite W55.31 ☑
      strike W55.32 ☑
    hornet(s) X58 ☑
    horse W55.19 ☑
      bite W55.11 ☑
      strike W55.12 ☑
    hot
      air X14.1 ☑
        inhalation X14.0 ☑
      cooker X15.8 ☑
      drinks X10.0 ☑
      engine X17 ☑
      fats X10.2 ☑
      fluids NEC X12 ☑
        assault X98.2 ☑
        suicide (attempt) X77.2 ☑
        undetermined whether accidental or inten-
          tional Y27.2 ☑
      food X10.1 ☑
      gases X14.1 ☑
        inhalation X14.0 ☑
      heating appliance X16 ☑
      household appliance X15.8 ☑
        assault X98.3 ☑
        cooker X15.8 ☑
        hotplate X15.2 ☑
        kettle X15.8 ☑
        light bulb X15.8 ☑
        object NEC X19 ☑
          assault X98.8 ☑
          stated as undetermined whether acciden-
            tal or intentional Y27.9 ☑
          suicide (attempt) X77.8 ☑
        saucepan X15.3 ☑
        skillet X15.3 ☑
        stated as undetermined whether accidental
          or intentional Y27.3 ☑
        stove X15.0 ☑
        suicide (attempt) X77.3 ☑
        toaster X15.1 ☑
      kettle X15.8 ☑
      light bulb X15.8 ☑
      liquid NEC (*see also* Burn) X12 ☑
        drinks X10.0 ☑
        stated as undetermined whether accidental
          or intentional Y27.2 ☑
        suicide (attempt) X77.2 ☑
        tap water X11.8 ☑
          stated as undetermined whether acciden-
            tal or intentional Y27.1 ☑

Contact — *continued*
  with — *continued*
    hot — *continued*
      liquid (*see also* Burn) — *continued*
        tap water — *continued*
          suicide (attempt) X77.1 ☑
      machinery X17 ☑
      metal (molten) (liquid) NEC X18 ☑
      object (not producing fire or flames) NEC X19 ☑
      oil (cooking) X10.2 ☑
      pipe X16 ☑
      plate X15.2 ☑
      radiator X16 ☑
      saucepan (glass) (metal) X15.3 ☑
      skillet X15.3 ☑
      stove (kitchen) X15.0 ☑
      substance NEC X19 ☑
      tap-water X11.8 ☑
        assault X98.1 ☑
        heated on stove X12 ☑
          stated as undetermined whether acciden-
            tal or intentional Y27.2 ☑
          suicide (attempt) X77.2 ☑
        in bathtub X11.0 ☑
        running X11.1 ☑
        stated as undetermined whether accidental
          or intentional Y27.1 ☑
        suicide (attempt) X77.1 ☑
      toaster X15.1 ☑
      tool X17 ☑
      vapors X13.1 ☑
        inhalation X13.0 ☑
      water (tap) X11.8 ☑
        boiling X12 ☑
          stated as undetermined whether acciden-
            tal or intentional Y27.2 ☑
          suicide (attempt) X77.2 ☑
        heated on stove X12 ☑
          stated as undetermined whether acciden-
            tal or intentional Y27.2 ☑
          suicide (attempt) X77.2 ☑
        in bathtub X11.0 ☑
        running X11.1 ☑
        stated as undetermined whether accidental
          or intentional Y27.1 ☑
        suicide (attempt) X77.1 ☑
    hotplate X15.2 ☑
    ice-pick W27.4 ☑
    insect (nonvenomous) NEC W57 ☑
    kettle (hot) X15.8 ☑
    knife W26.0 ☑
      assault X99.1 ☑
      electric W29.1 ☑
      stated as undetermined whether accidental or
        intentional Y28.1 ☑
      suicide (attempt) X78.1 ☑
    lathe (metalworking) W31.1 ☑
      turnings W45.8 ☑
      woodworking W31.2 ☑
    lawnmower (powered) (ridden) W28 ☑
      causing electrocution W86.8 ☑
        suicide (attempt) X83.1 ☑
      unpowered W27.1 ☑
    lift, lifting (devices) W24.0 ☑
      agricultural operations W30.89 ☑
      shaft W24.0 ☑
    liquefied gas — *see* Exposure, cold, man-made
    liquid air, hydrogen, nitrogen — *see* Exposure, cold,
      man-made
    lizard (nonvenomous) W59.09 ☑
      bite W59.01 ☑
      strike W59.02 ☑
    llama — *see* Contact, with, hoof stock NEC
    macaw W61.19 ☑
      bite W61.11 ☑
      strike W61.12 ☑
    machine, machinery W31.9 ☑
      abrasive wheel W31.1 ☑
      agricultural including animal-powered
        W30.9 ☑
        combine harvester W30.0 ☑
        grain storage elevator W30.3 ☑
        hay derrick W30.2 ☑
        power take-off device W30.1 ☑
        reaper W30.0 ☑
        specified NEC W30.89 ☑

Contact — *continued*
  with — *continued*
    machine, machinery — *continued*
      agricultural including animal-powered — *con-*
        tinued
        thresher W30.0 ☑
        transport vehicle, stationary W30.81 ☑
      band saw W31.2 ☑
      bench saw W31.2 ☑
      circular saw W31.2 ☑
      commercial NEC W31.82 ☑
      drilling, metal (industrial) W31.1 ☑
      earth-drilling W31.0 ☑
      earthmoving or scraping W31.89 ☑
      excavating W31.89 ☑
      forging machine W31.1 ☑
      gas turbine W31.3 ☑
      hot X17 ☑
      internal combustion engine W31.3 ☑
      land drill W31.0 ☑
      lathe W31.1 ☑
      lifting (devices) W24.0 ☑
      metal drill W31.1 ☑
      metalworking (industrial) W31.1 ☑
      milling, metal W31.1 ☑
      mining W31.0 ☑
      molding W31.2 ☑
      overhead plane W31.2 ☑
      power press, metal W31.1 ☑
      prime mover W31.3 ☑
      printing W31.89 ☑
      radial saw W31.2 ☑
      recreational W31.81 ☑
      roller-coaster W31.81 ☑
      rolling mill, metal W31.1 ☑
      sander W31.2 ☑
      seabed drill W31.0 ☑
      shaft
        hoist W31.0 ☑
        lift W31.0 ☑
      specified NEC W31.89 ☑
      spinning W31.89 ☑
      steam engine W31.3 ☑
      transmission W24.1 ☑
      undercutter W31.0 ☑
      water driven turbine W31.3 ☑
      weaving W31.89 ☑
      woodworking or forming (industrial) W31.2 ☑
    mammal (feces) (urine) W55.89 ☑
      bull — *see* Contact, with, bull
      cat — *see* Contact, with, cat
      cow — *see* Contact, with, cow
      goat — *see* Contact, with, goat
      hoof stock — *see* Contact, with, hoof stock
      horse — *see* Contact, with, horse
      marine W56.39 ☑
        dolphin — *see* Contact, with, dolphin
        orca — *see* Contact, with, orca
        sea lion — *see* Contact, with, sea lion
        specified NEC W56.39 ☑
          bite W56.31 ☑
          strike W56.32 ☑
      pig — *see* Contact, with, pig
      raccoon — *see* Contact, with, raccoon
      rodent — *see* Contact, with, rodent
      sheep — *see* Contact, with, sheep
      specified NEC W55.89 ☑
        bite W55.81 ☑
        strike W55.82 ☑
    marine
      animal W56.89 ☑
        bite W56.81 ☑
        dolphin — *see* Contact, with, dolphin
        fish NEC — *see* Contact, with, fish
        mammal — *see* Contact, with, mammal,
          marine
        orca — *see* Contact, with, orca
        sea lion — *see* Contact, with, sea lion
        shark — *see* Contact, with, shark
        strike W56.82 ☑
    meat
      grinder (domestic) W29.0 ☑
        industrial W31.82 ☑
        nonpowered W27.4 ☑
      slicer (domestic) W29.0 ☑
        industrial W31.82 ☑

Contact — *continued*
with — *continued*
merry go round W31.81 ☑
metal, hot (liquid) (molten) NEC X18 ☑
millipede W57 ☑
nail W45.0 ☑
gun W29.4 ☑
needle (sewing) W27.3 ☑
hypodermic W46.0 ☑
contaminated W46.1 ☑
object (blunt) NEC
hot NEC X19 ☑
legal intervention — *see* Legal, intervention,
blunt object
sharp NEC W45.8 ☑
inflicted by other person NEC W45.8 ☑
stated as
intentional homicide (attempt) —
see Assault, cutting or piercing
instrument
legal intervention — *see* Legal, intervention,
sharp object
self-inflicted X78.9 ☑
orca W56.29 ☑
bite W56.21 ☑
strike W56.22 ☑
overhead plane W31.2 ☑
paper (as sharp object) W26.2 ☑
paper-cutter W27.5 ☑
parrot W61.09 ☑
bite W61.01 ☑
strike W61.02 ☑
pig W55.49 ☑
bite W55.41 ☑
strike W55.42 ☑
pipe, hot X16 ☑
pitchfork W27.1 ☑
plane (metal) (wood) W27.0 ☑
overhead W31.2 ☑
plant thorns, spines, sharp leaves or other mechanisms W60 ☑
powered
garden cultivator W29.3 ☑
household appliance, implement, or machine
W29.8 ☑
saw (industrial) W31.2 ☑
hand W29.8 ☑
printing machine W31.89 ☑
psittacine bird W61.29 ☑
bite W61.21 ☑
macaw — *see* Contact, with, macaw
parrot — *see* Contact, with, parrot
strike W61.22 ☑
pulley (block) (transmission) W24.0 ☑
agricultural operations W30.89 ☑
raccoon W55.59 ☑
bite W55.51 ☑
strike W55.52 ☑
radial-saw (industrial) W31.2 ☑
radiator (hot) X16 ☑
rake W27.1 ☑
rattlesnake X58 ☑
reaper W30.0 ☑
reptile W59.89 ☑
lizard — *see* Contact, with, lizard
snake — *see* Contact, with, snake
specified NEC W59.89 ☑
bite W59.81 ☑
crushing W59.83 ☑
strike W59.82 ☑
turtle — *see* Contact, with, turtle
rivet gun (powered) W29.4 ☑
road scraper — *see* Accident, transport, construction vehicle
rodent (feces) (urine) W53.89 ☑
bite W53.81 ☑
mouse W53.09 ☑
bite W53.01 ☑
rat W53.19 ☑
bite W53.11 ☑
specified NEC W53.89 ☑
bite W53.81 ☑
squirrel W53.29 ☑
bite W53.21 ☑
roller coaster W31.81 ☑
rope NEC W24.0 ☑

Contact — *continued*
with — *continued*
rope — *continued*
agricultural operations W30.89 ☑
saliva — *see* Contact, with, by type of animal
sander W29.8 ☑
industrial W31.2 ☑
saucepan (hot) (glass) (metal) X15.3 ☑
saw W27.0 ☑
band (industrial) W31.2 ☑
bench (industrial) W31.2 ☑
chain W29.3 ☑
hand W27.0 ☑
sawing machine, metal W31.1 ☑
scissors W27.2 ☑
scorpion X58 ☑
screwdriver W27.0 ☑
powered W29.8 ☑
sea
anemone, cucumber or urchin (spine) X58 ☑
lion W56.19 ☑
bite W56.11 ☑
strike W56.12 ☑
serpent — *see* Contact, with, snake, by type
sewing-machine (electric) (powered) W29.2 ☑
not powered W27.8 ☑
shaft (hoist) (lift) (transmission) NEC W24.0 ☑
agricultural W30.89 ☑
shark W56.49 ☑
bite W56.41 ☑
strike W56.42 ☑
sharp object(s) W26.9 ☑
specified NEC W26.8 ☑
shears (hand) W27.2 ☑
powered (industrial) W31.1 ☑
domestic W29.2 ☑
sheep W55.39 ☑
bite W55.31 ☑
strike W55.32 ☑
shovel W27.8 ☑
steam — *see* Accident, transport, construction
vehicle
snake (nonvenomous) W59.19 ☑
bite W59.11 ☑
crushing W59.13 ☑
strike W59.12 ☑
spade W27.1 ☑
spider (venomous) X58 ☑
spin-drier W29.2 ☑
spinning machine W31.89 ☑
splinter W45.8 ☑
sports equipment W21.9 ☑
staple gun (powered) W29.8 ☑
steam X13.1 ☑
engine W31.3 ☑
inhalation X13.0 ☑
pipe X16 ☑
shovel W31.89 ☑
stove (hot) (kitchen) X15.0 ☑
substance, hot NEC X19 ☑
molten (metal) X18 ☑
sword W26.1 ☑
assault X99.2 ☑
stated as undetermined whether accidental or
intentional Y28.2 ☑
suicide (attempt) X78.2 ☑
tarantula X58 ☑
thresher W30.0 ☑
tin can lid W26.8 ☑
toad W62.1 ☑
toaster (hot) X15.1 ☑
tool W27.8 ☑
hand (not powered) W27.8 ☑
auger W27.0 ☑
axe W27.0 ☑
can opener W27.4 ☑
chisel W27.0 ☑
fork W27.4 ☑
garden W27.1 ☑
handsaw W27.0 ☑
hoe W27.1 ☑
ice-pick W27.4 ☑
kitchen utensil W27.4 ☑
manual
lawn mower W27.1 ☑
sewing machine W27.8 ☑

Contact — *continued*
with — *continued*
tool — *continued*
hand — *continued*
meat grinder W27.4 ☑
needle (sewing) W27.3 ☑
hypodermic W46.0 ☑
contaminated W46.1 ☑
paper cutter W27.5 ☑
pitchfork W27.1 ☑
rake W27.1 ☑
scissors W27.2 ☑
screwdriver W27.0 ☑
specified NEC W27.8 ☑
workbench W27.0 ☑
hot X17 ☑
powered W29.8 ☑
blender W29.0 ☑
commercial W31.82 ☑
can opener W29.0 ☑
commercial W31.82 ☑
chainsaw W29.3 ☑
clothes dryer W29.2 ☑
commercial W31.82 ☑
dishwasher W29.2 ☑
commercial W31.82 ☑
edger W29.3 ☑
electric fan W29.2 ☑
commercial W31.82 ☑
electric knife W29.1 ☑
food processor W29.0 ☑
commercial W31.82 ☑
garbage disposal W29.0 ☑
commercial W31.82 ☑
garden tool W29.3 ☑
hedge trimmer W29.3 ☑
ice maker W29.0 ☑
commercial W31.82 ☑
kitchen appliance W29.0 ☑
commercial W31.82 ☑
lawn mower W28 ☑
meat grinder W29.0 ☑
commercial W31.82 ☑
mixer W29.0 ☑
commercial W31.82 ☑
rototiller W29.3 ☑
sewing machine W29.2 ☑
commercial W31.82 ☑
washing machine W29.2 ☑
commercial W31.82 ☑
transmission device (belt, cable, chain, gear, pinion,
shaft) W24.1 ☑
agricultural operations W30.89 ☑
turbine (gas) (water-driven) W31.3 ☑
turkey W61.49 ☑
peck W61.43 ☑
strike W61.42 ☑
turtle (nonvenomous) W59.29 ☑
bite W59.21 ☑
strike W59.22 ☑
terrestrial W59.89 ☑
bite W59.81 ☑
crushing W59.83 ☑
strike W59.82 ☑
under-cutter W31.0 ☑
urine — *see* Contact, with, by type of animal
vehicle
agricultural use (transport) — *see* Accident,
transport, agricultural vehicle
not on public highway W30.81 ☑
industrial use (transport) — *see* Accident,
transport, industrial vehicle
not on public highway W31.83 ☑
off-road use (transport) — *see* Accident, transport, all-terrain or off-road vehicle
not on public highway W31.83 ☑
special construction use (transport) — *see* Accident, transport, construction vehicle
not on public highway W31.83 ☑
venomous
animal X58 ☑
arthropods X58 ☑
lizard X58 ☑
marine animal NEC X58 ☑
marine plant NEC X58 ☑
millipedes (tropical) X58 ☑

Contact — *continued*
  with — *continued*
    venomous — *continued*
      plant(s) X58 ☑
      snake X58 ☑
      spider X58 ☑
      viper X58 ☑
      washing-machine (powered) W29.2 ☑
      wasp X58 ☑
      weaving-machine W31.89 ☑
      winch W24.0 ☑
        agricultural operations W30.89 ☑
      wire NEC W24.0 ☑
        agricultural operations W30.89 ☑
      wood slivers W45.8 ☑
      yellow jacket X58 ☑
      zebra — *see* Contact, with, hoof stock NEC
    pressure X50.9 ☑
    stress X50.9 ☑
Coup de soleil X32 ☑
Crash
  aircraft (in transit) (powered) V95.9 ☑
    balloon V96.01 ☑
    fixed wing NEC (private) V95.21 ☑
      commercial V95.31 ☑
    glider V96.21 ☑
      hang V96.11 ☑
      powered V95.11 ☑
    helicopter V95.01 ☑
    in war operations — *see* War operations, destruction of aircraft
    microlight V95.11 ☑
    nonpowered V96.9 ☑
      specified NEC V96.8 ☑
    powered NEC V95.8 ☑
    stated as
      homicide (attempt) Y08.81 ☑
      suicide (attempt) X83.0 ☑
    ultralight V95.11 ☑
  spacecraft V95.41 ☑
  transport vehicle NEC (*see also* Accident, transport) V89.9 ☑
    homicide (attempt) Y03.8 ☑
    motor NEC (traffic) V89.2 ☑
      homicide (attempt) Y03.8 ☑
    suicide (attempt) — *see* Suicide, collision
Cruelty (mental) (physical) (sexual) X58 ☑
Crushed (accidentally) X58 ☑
  between objects (moving) (stationary and moving) W23.0 ☑
    stationary W23.1 ☑
  by
    alligator W58.03 ☑
    avalanche NEC — *see* Landslide
    cave-in W20.0 ☑
      caused by cataclysmic earth surface movement — *see* Landslide
    crocodile W58.13 ☑
    crowd or human stampede W52 ☑
    falling
      aircraft V97.39 ☑
        in war operations — *see* War operations, destruction of aircraft
      earth, material W20.0 ☑
        caused by cataclysmic earth surface movement — *see* Landslide
      object NEC W20.8 ☑
    landslide NEC — *see* Landslide
    lizard (nonvenomous) W59.09 ☑
    machinery — *see* Contact, with, by type of machine
    reptile NEC W59.89 ☑
    snake (nonvenomous) W59.13 ☑
  in
    machinery — *see* Contact, with, by type of machine
Cut, cutting (any part of body) (accidental) (*see also* Contact, with, by object or machine)
  during medical or surgical treatment as misadventure — *see* Index to Diseases and Injuries, Complications
  homicide (attempt) — *see* Assault, cutting or piercing instrument
  inflicted by other person — *see* Assault, cutting or piercing instrument
  legal
    execution — *see* Legal, intervention

Cut, cutting — *continued*
  legal — *continued*
    intervention — *see* Legal, intervention, sharp object
  machine NEC (*see also* Contact, with, by type of machine) W31.9 ☑
  self-inflicted — *see* Suicide, cutting or piercing instrument
  suicide (attempt) — *see* Suicide, cutting or piercing instrument
Cyclone (any injury) X37.1 ☑

D

Decapitation (accidental circumstances) NEC X58 ☑
  homicide X99.9 ☑
  legal execution — *see* Legal, intervention
Dehydration from lack of water X58 ☑
Deprivation X58 ☑
Derailment (accidental)
  railway (rolling stock) (train) (vehicle) (without antecedent collision) V81.7 ☑
    with antecedent collision — *see* Accident, transport, railway vehicle occupant
  streetcar (without antecedent collision) V82.7 ☑
    with antecedent collision — *see* Accident, transport, streetcar occupant
Descent
  parachute (voluntary) (without accident to aircraft) V97.29 ☑
    due to accident to aircraft — *see* Accident, transport, aircraft
Desertion X58 ☑
Destitution X58 ☑
Disability, late effect or sequela of injury — *see* Sequelae
Discharge (accidental)
  airgun W34.010 ☑
    assault X95.01 ☑
    homicide (attempt) X95.01 ☑
    stated as undetermined whether accidental or intentional Y24.0 ☑
    suicide (attempt) X74.01 ☑
  BB gun — *see* Discharge, airgun
  firearm (accidental) W34.00 ☑
    assault X95.9 ☑
    handgun (pistol) (revolver) W32.0 ☑
      assault X93 ☑
      homicide (attempt) X93 ☑
      legal intervention — *see* Legal, intervention, firearm, handgun
      stated as undetermined whether accidental or intentional Y22 ☑
      suicide (attempt) X72 ☑
    homicide (attempt) X95.9 ☑
    hunting rifle W33.02 ☑
      assault X94.1 ☑
      homicide (attempt) X94.1 ☑
      legal intervention
        injuring
          bystander Y35.032 ☑
          law enforcement personnel Y35.031 ☑
          suspect Y35.033 ☑
      stated as undetermined whether accidental or intentional Y23.1 ☑
      suicide (attempt) X73.1 ☑
    larger W33.00 ☑
      assault X94.9 ☑
      homicide (attempt) X94.9 ☑
      hunting rifle — *see* Discharge, firearm, hunting rifle
      legal intervention — *see* Legal, intervention, firearm by type of firearm
      machine gun — *see* Discharge, firearm, machine gun
      shotgun — *see* Discharge, firearm, shotgun
      specified NEC W33.09 ☑
        assault X94.8 ☑
        homicide (attempt) X94.8 ☑
        legal intervention
          injuring
            bystander Y35.092 ☑
            law enforcement personnel Y35.091 ☑
            suspect Y35.093 ☑

Discharge — *continued*
  firearm — *continued*
    larger — *continued*
      specified — *continued*
        stated as undetermined whether accidental or intentional Y23.8 ☑
        suicide (attempt) X73.8 ☑
      stated as undetermined whether accidental or intentional Y23.9 ☑
      suicide (attempt) X73.9 ☑
    legal intervention
      injuring
        bystander Y35.002 ☑
        law enforcement personnel Y35.001 ☑
        suspect Y35.03 ☑
      using rubber bullet
        injuring
          bystander Y35.042 ☑
          law enforcement personnel Y35.041 ☑
          suspect Y35.043 ☑
    machine gun W33.03 ☑
      assault X94.2 ☑
      homicide (attempt) X94.2 ☑
      legal intervention — *see* Legal, intervention, firearm, machine gun
      stated as undetermined whether accidental or intentional Y23.3 ☑
      suicide (attempt) X73.2 ☑
    pellet gun — *see* Discharge, airgun
    shotgun W33.01 ☑
      assault X94.0 ☑
      homicide (attempt) X94.0 ☑
      legal intervention — *see* Legal, intervention, firearm, specified NEC
      stated as undetermined whether accidental or intentional Y23.0 ☑
      suicide (attempt) X73.0 ☑
    specified NEC W34.09 ☑
      assault X95.8 ☑
      homicide (attempt) X95.8 ☑
      legal intervention — *see* Legal, intervention, firearm, specified NEC
      stated as undetermined whether accidental or intentional Y24.8 ☑
      suicide (attempt) X74.8 ☑
    stated as undetermined whether accidental or intentional Y24.9 ☑
    suicide (attempt) X74.9 ☑
    Very pistol W34.09 ☑
      assault X95.8 ☑
      homicide (attempt) X95.8 ☑
      stated as undetermined whether accidental or intentional Y24.8 ☑
      suicide (attempt) X74.8 ☑
  firework(s) W39 ☑
    stated as undetermined whether accidental or intentional Y25 ☑
  gas-operated gun NEC W34.018 ☑
    airgun — *see* Discharge, airgun
    assault X95.09 ☑
    homicide (attempt) X95.09 ☑
    paintball gun — *see* Discharge, paintball gun
    stated as undetermined whether accidental or intentional Y24.8 ☑
    suicide (attempt) X74.09 ☑
  gun NEC (*see also* Discharge, firearm NEC)
    air — *see* Discharge, airgun
    BB — *see* Discharge, airgun
    for single hand use — *see* Discharge, firearm, handgun
    hand — *see* Discharge, firearm, handgun
    machine — *see* Discharge, firearm, machine gun
    other specified — *see* Discharge, firearm NEC
    paintball — *see* Discharge, paintball gun
    pellet — *see* Discharge, airgun
  handgun — *see* Discharge, firearm, handgun
  machine gun — *see* Discharge, firearm, machine gun
  paintball gun W34.011 ☑
    assault X95.02 ☑
    homicide (attempt) X95.02 ☑
    stated as undetermined whether accidental or intentional Y24.8 ☑
    suicide (attempt) X74.02 ☑
  pistol — *see* Discharge, firearm, handgun
    flare — *see* Discharge, firearm, Very pistol
    pellet — *see* Discharge, airgun

Discharge — *continued*
  pistol — *see* Discharge, firearm, handgun — *continued*
    Very — *see* Discharge, firearm, Very pistol
  revolver — *see* Discharge, firearm, handgun
  rifle (hunting) — *see* Discharge, firearm, hunting rifle
  shotgun — *see* Discharge, firearm, shotgun
  spring-operated gun NEC W34.018 ☑
    assault X95.09 ☑
    homicide (attempt) X95.09 ☑
    stated as undetermined whether accidental or intentional Y24.8 ☑
    suicide (attempt) X74.09 ☑
Disease
  Andes W94.11 ☑
  aviator's — *see* Air, pressure
  range W94.11 ☑
Diver's disease, palsy, paralysis, squeeze — *see* Air, pressure
Diving (into water) — *see* Accident, diving
Dog bite W54.0 ☑
Dragged by transport vehicle NEC (*see also* Accident, transport) V09.9 ☑
Drinking poison (accidental) — *see* Table of Drugs and Chemicals
Dropped (accidentally) **while being carried or supported by other person** W04 ☑
Drowning (accidental) W74 ☑
  assault X92.9 ☑
  due to
    accident (to)
      machinery — *see* Contact, with, by type of machine
      watercraft V90.89 ☑
        burning V90.29 ☑
          powered V90.23 ☑
            fishing boat V90.22 ☑
            jetskis V90.23 ☑
            merchant ship V90.20 ☑
            passenger ship V90.21 ☑
          unpowered V90.28 ☑
            canoe V90.25 ☑
            inflatable V90.26 ☑
            kayak V90.25 ☑
            sailboat V90.24 ☑
            water skis V90.27 ☑
        crushed V90.39 ☑
          powered V90.33 ☑
            fishing boat V90.32 ☑
            jetskis V90.33 ☑
            merchant ship V90.30 ☑
            passenger ship V90.31 ☑
          unpowered V90.38 ☑
            canoe V90.35 ☑
            inflatable V90.36 ☑
            kayak V90.35 ☑
            sailboat V90.34 ☑
            water skis V90.37 ☑
        overturning V90.09 ☑
          powered V90.03 ☑
            fishing boat V90.02 ☑
            jetskis V90.03 ☑
            merchant ship V90.00 ☑
            passenger ship V90.01 ☑
          unpowered V90.08 ☑
            canoe V90.05 ☑
            inflatable V90.06 ☑
            kayak V90.05 ☑
            sailboat V90.04 ☑
        sinking V90.19 ☑
          powered V90.13 ☑
            fishing boat V90.12 ☑
            jetskis V90.13 ☑
            merchant ship V90.10 ☑
            passenger ship V90.11 ☑
          unpowered V90.18 ☑
            canoe V90.15 ☑
            inflatable V90.16 ☑
            kayak V90.15 ☑
            sailboat V90.14 ☑
        specified type NEC V90.89 ☑
          powered V90.83 ☑
            fishing boat V90.82 ☑
            jetskis V90.83 ☑
            merchant ship V90.80 ☑
            passenger ship V90.81 ☑

Drowning — *continued*
  due to — *continued*
    accident — *continued*
      watercraft — *continued*
        specified type — *continued*
          unpowered V90.88 ☑
            canoe V90.85 ☑
            inflatable V90.86 ☑
            kayak V90.85 ☑
            sailboat V90.84 ☑
            water skis V90.87 ☑
    avalanche — *see* Landslide
    cataclysmic
      earth surface movement NEC — *see* Forces of nature, earth movement
      storm — *see* Forces of nature, cataclysmic storm
    cloudburst X37.8 ☑
    cyclone X37.1 ☑
    fall overboard (from) V92.09 ☑
      powered craft V92.03 ☑
        ferry boat V92.01 ☑
        fishing boat V92.02 ☑
        jetskis V92.03 ☑
        liner V92.01 ☑
        merchant ship V92.00 ☑
        passenger ship V92.01 ☑
      resulting from
        accident to watercraft — *see* Drowning, due to, accident to, watercraft
        being washed overboard (from) V92.29 ☑
          powered craft V92.23 ☑
            ferry boat V92.21 ☑
            fishing boat V92.22 ☑
            jetskis V92.23 ☑
            liner V92.21 ☑
            merchant ship V92.20 ☑
            passenger ship V92.21 ☑
          unpowered craft V92.28 ☑
            canoe V92.25 ☑
            inflatable V92.26 ☑
            kayak V92.25 ☑
            sailboat V92.24 ☑
            surf-board V92.28 ☑
            water skis V92.27 ☑
            windsurfer V92.28 ☑
        motion of watercraft V92.19 ☑
          powered craft V92.13 ☑
            ferry boat V92.11 ☑
            fishing boat V92.12 ☑
            jetskis V92.13 ☑
            liner V92.11 ☑
            merchant ship V92.10 ☑
            passenger ship V92.11 ☑
          unpowered craft
            canoe V92.15 ☑
            inflatable V92.16 ☑
            kayak V92.15 ☑
            sailboat V92.14 ☑
      unpowered craft V92.08 ☑
        canoe V92.05 ☑
        inflatable V92.06 ☑
        kayak V92.05 ☑
        sailboat V92.04 ☑
        surf-board V92.08 ☑
        water skis V92.07 ☑
        windsurfer V92.08 ☑
    hurricane X37.0 ☑
    jumping into water from watercraft (involved in accident) (*see also* Drowning, due to, accident to, watercraft)
      without accident to or on watercraft W16.711 ☑
    tidal wave NEC — *see* Forces of nature, tidal wave
    torrential rain X37.8 ☑
  following
    fall
      into
        bathtub W16.211 ☑
        bucket W16.221 ☑
        fountain — *see* Drowning, following, fall, into, water, specified NEC
        quarry — *see* Drowning, following, fall, into, water, specified NEC
        reservoir — *see* Drowning, following, fall, into, water, specified NEC

Drowning — *continued*
  following — *continued*
    fall — *continued*
      into — *continued*
        swimming-pool W16.011 ☑
          stated as undetermined whether accidental or intentional Y21.3 ☑
          striking
            bottom W16.021 ☑
            wall W16.031 ☑
          suicide (attempt) X71.2 ☑
        water NOS W16.41 ☑
          natural (lake) (open sea) (river) (stream) (pond) W16.111 ☑
            striking
              bottom W16.121 ☑
              side W16.131 ☑
          specified NEC W16.311 ☑
            striking
              bottom W16.321 ☑
              wall W16.331 ☑
      overboard NEC — *see* Drowning, due to, fall overboard
    jump or dive
      from boat W16.711 ☑
        striking bottom W16.721 ☑
      into
        fountain — *see* Drowning, following, jump or dive, into, water, specified NEC
        quarry — *see* Drowning, following, jump or dive, into, water, specified NEC
        reservoir — *see* Drowning, following, jump or dive, into, water, specified NEC
        swimming-pool W16.511 ☑
          striking
            bottom W16.521 ☑
            wall W16.531 ☑
          suicide (attempt) X71.2 ☑
        water NOS W16.91 ☑
          natural (lake) (open sea) (river) (stream) (pond) W16.611 ☑
          specified NEC W16.811 ☑
            bottom W16.821 ☑
            striking
              bottom W16.821 ☑
              wall W16.831 ☑
          striking
            bottom W16.821 ☑
            wall W16.831 ☑
          striking bottom W16.621 ☑
  homicide (attempt) X92.9 ☑
  in
    bathtub (accidental) W65 ☑
      assault X92.0 ☑
      following fall W16.211 ☑
        stated as undetermined whether accidental or intentional Y21.1 ☑
      stated as undetermined whether accidental or intentional Y21.0 ☑
      suicide (attempt) X71.0 ☑
    lake — *see* Drowning, in, natural water
    natural water (lake) (open sea) (river) (stream) (pond) W69
      assault X92.3 ☑
      following
        dive or jump W16.611 ☑
          striking bottom W16.621 ☑
        fall W16.111 ☑
          striking
            bottom W16.121 ☑
            side W16.131 ☑
      stated as undetermined whether accidental or intentional Y21.4 ☑
      suicide (attempt) X71.3 ☑
    quarry — *see* Drowning, in, specified place NEC
    quenching tank — *see* Drowning, in, specified place NEC
    reservoir — *see* Drowning, in, specified place NEC
    river — *see* Drowning, in, natural water
    sea — *see* Drowning, in, natural water
    specified place NEC W73 ☑
      assault X92.8 ☑
      following
        dive or jump W16.811 ☑
          striking
            bottom W16.821 ☑
            wall W16.831 ☑

☑ **Additional Character Required — Refer to the Tabular List for Character Selection** ▼ **Subterms under main terms may continue to next column or page**

Drowning — continued
  in — continued
    specified place — continued
      following — continued
        fall W16.311 ☑
          striking
            bottom W16.321 ☑
            wall W16.331 ☑
      stated as undetermined whether accidental or intentional Y21.8 ☑
      suicide (attempt) X71.8 ☑
    stream — see Drowning, in, natural water
    swimming-pool W67 ☑
      assault X92.1 ☑
        following fall X92.2 ☑
      following
        dive or jump W16.511 ☑
          striking
            bottom W16.521 ☑
            wall W16.531 ☑
        fall W16.011 ☑
          striking
            bottom W16.021 ☑
            wall W16.031 ☑
      stated as undetermined whether accidental or intentional Y21.2 ☑
        following fall Y21.3 ☑
      suicide (attempt) X71.1 ☑
        following fall X71.2 ☑
    war operations — see War operations, restriction of airway
  resulting from accident to watercraft — see Drowning, due to, accident, watercraft
  self-inflicted X71.9 ☑
  stated as undetermined whether accidental or intentional Y21.9 ☑
  suicide (attempt) X71.9 ☑

E

Earth falling (on) W20.0 ☑
  caused by cataclysmic earth surface movement or eruption — see Landslide
Earth (surface) **movement NEC** — see Forces of nature, earth movement
Earthquake (any injury) X34 ☑
Effect(s) (adverse) **of**
  air pressure (any) — see Air, pressure
  cold, excessive (exposure to) — see Exposure, cold
  heat (excessive) — see Heat
  hot place (weather) — see Heat
  insolation X30 ☑
  late — see Sequelae
  motion — see Motion
  nuclear explosion or weapon in war operations — see War operations, nuclear weapon
  radiation — see Radiation
  travel — see Travel
Electric shock (accidental) (by) (in) — see Exposure, electric current
Electrocution (accidental) — see Exposure, electric current
Endotracheal tube wrongly placed during anesthetic procedure
Entanglement
  in
    bed linen, causing suffocation T71 ☑
    wheel of pedal cycle V19.88 ☑
Entry of foreign body or material — see Foreign body
Environmental pollution related condition — see category Z57
Execution, legal (any method) — see Legal, intervention
Exhaustion
  cold — see Exposure, cold
  due to excessive exertion (see also Overexertion) X50.9 ☑
  heat — see Heat
Explosion (accidental) (of) (with secondary fire) W40.9 ☑
  acetylene W40.1 ☑
  aerosol can W36.1 ☑
  air tank (compressed) (in machinery) W36.2 ☑
  aircraft (in transit) (powered) NEC V95.9 ☑
    balloon V96.05 ☑
    fixed wing NEC (private) V95.25 ☑
      commercial V95.35 ☑
    glider V96.25 ☑

Explosion — continued
  aircraft — continued
    glider — continued
      hang V96.15 ☑
      powered V95.15 ☑
    helicopter V95.05 ☑
    in war operations — see War operations, destruction of aircraft
    microlight V95.15 ☑
    nonpowered V96.9 ☑
      specified NEC V96.8 ☑
    powered NEC V95.8 ☑
    stated as
      homicide (attempt) Y03.8 ☑
      suicide (attempt) X83.0 ☑
    ultralight V95.15 ☑
  anesthetic gas in operating room W40.1 ☑
  antipersonnel bomb W40.8 ☑
    assault X96.0 ☑
    homicide (attempt) X96.0 ☑
    suicide (attempt) X75 ☑
  assault X96.9 ☑
  bicycle tire W37.0 ☑
  blasting (cap) (materials) W40.0 ☑
  boiler (machinery), not on transport vehicle W35 ☑
    on watercraft — see Explosion, in, watercraft
  butane W40.1 ☑
  caused by other person X96.9 ☑
  coal gas W40.1 ☑
  detonator W40.0 ☑
  dump (munitions) W40.8 ☑
  dynamite W40.0 ☑
    in
      assault X96.8 ☑
      homicide (attempt) X96.8 ☑
      legal intervention
        injuring
          bystander Y35.112 ☑
          law enforcement personnel Y35.111 ☑
          suspect Y35.113 ☑
      suicide (attempt) X75 ☑
  explosive (material) W40.9 ☑
    gas W40.1 ☑
    in blasting operation W40.0 ☑
    specified NEC W40.8 ☑
      in
        assault X96.8 ☑
        homicide (attempt) X96.8 ☑
        legal intervention
          injuring
            bystander Y35.192 ☑
            law enforcement personnel Y35.191 ☑
            suspect Y35.193 ☑
        suicide (attempt) X75 ☑
  factory (munitions) W40.8 ☑
  fertilizer bomb W40.8 ☑
    assault X96.3 ☑
    homicide (attempt) X96.3 ☑
    suicide (attempt) X75 ☑
  firearm (parts) NEC W34.19 ☑
    airgun W34.110 ☑
    BB gun W34.110 ☑
    gas, air or spring-operated gun NEC W34.118 ☑
    hangun W32.1 ☑
    hunting rifle W33.12 ☑
    larger firearm W33.10 ☑
      specified NEC W33.19 ☑
    machine gun W33.13 ☑
    paintball gun W34.111 ☑
    pellet gun W34.110 ☑
    shotgun W33.11 ☑
    Very pistol [flare] W34.19 ☑
  fire-damp W40.1 ☑
  fireworks W39 ☑
  gas (coal) (explosive) W40.1 ☑
    cylinder W36.9 ☑
      aerosol can W36.1 ☑
      air tank W36.2 ☑
      pressurized W36.3 ☑
      specified NEC W36.8 ☑
  gasoline (fumes) (tank) not in moving motor vehicle W40.1 ☑
    bomb W40.8 ☑
      assault X96.1 ☑
      homicide (attempt) X96.1 ☑

Explosion — continued
  gasoline not in moving motor vehicle — continued
    bomb — continued
      suicide (attempt) X75 ☑
    in motor vehicle — see Accident, transport, by type of vehicle
  grain store W40.8 ☑
  grenade W40.8 ☑
    in
      assault X96.8 ☑
      homicide (attempt) X96.8 ☑
      legal intervention
        injuring
          bystander Y35.192 ☑
          law enforcement personnel Y35.191 ☑
          suspect Y35.193 ☑
      suicide (attempt) X75 ☑
  handgun (parts) — see Explosion, firearm, hangun (parts)
  homicide (attempt) X96.9 ☑
    antipersonnel bomb — see Explosion, antipersonnel bomb
    fertilizer bomb — see Explosion, fertilizer bomb
    gasoline bomb — see Explosion, gasoline bomb
    letter bomb — see Explosion, letter bomb
    pipe bomb — see Explosion, pipe bomb
    specified NEC X96.8 ☑
  hose, pressurized W37.8 ☑
  hot water heater, tank (in machinery) W35 ☑
    on watercraft — see Explosion, in, watercraft
  in, on
    dump W40.8 ☑
    factory W40.8 ☑
    mine (of explosive gases) NEC W40.1 ☑
    watercraft V93.59 ☑
      powered craft V93.53 ☑
        ferry boat V93.51 ☑
        fishing boat V93.52 ☑
        jetskis V93.53 ☑
        liner V93.51 ☑
        merchant ship V93.50 ☑
        passenger ship V93.51 ☑
        sailboat V93.54 ☑
  letter bomb W40.8 ☑
    assault X96.2 ☑
    homicide (attempt) X96.2 ☑
    suicide (attempt) X75 ☑
  machinery (see also Contact, with, by type of machine)
    on board watercraft — see Explosion, in, watercraft
    pressure vessel — see Explosion, by type of vessel
  methane W40.1 ☑
  mine W40.1 ☑
  missile NEC W40.8 ☑
  mortar bomb W40.8 ☑
    in
      assault X96.8 ☑
      homicide (attempt) X96.8 ☑
      legal intervention
        injuring
          bystander Y35.192 ☑
          law enforcement personnel Y35.191 ☑
          suspect Y35.193 ☑
      suicide (attempt) X75 ☑
  munitions (dump) (factory) W40.8 ☑
  pipe, pressurized W37.8 ☑
    bomb W40.8 ☑
      assault X96.4 ☑
      homicide (attempt) X96.4 ☑
      suicide (attempt) X75 ☑
  pressure, pressurized
    cooker W38 ☑
    gas tank (in machinery) W36.3 ☑
    hose W37.8 ☑
    pipe W37.8 ☑
    specified device NEC W38 ☑
    tire W37.8 ☑
      bicycle W37.0 ☑
    vessel (in machinery) W38 ☑
  propane W40.1 ☑
  self-inflicted X75 ☑
  shell (artillery) NEC W40.8 ☑
    during war operations — see War operations, explosion

Explosion — continued
  shell — continued
    in
      legal intervention
        injuring
          bystander Y35.122 ☑
          law enforcement personnel Y35.121 ☑
          suspect Y35.123 ☑
      war — see War operations, explosion
  spacecraft V95.45 ☑
  stated as undetermined whether accidental or intentional Y25 ☑
  steam or water lines (in machinery) W37.8 ☑
  stove W40.9 ☑
  suicide (attempt) X75 ☑
  tire, pressurized W37.8 ☑
    bicycle W37.0 ☑
  undetermined whether accidental or intentional Y25 ☑
  vehicle tire NEC W37.8 ☑
    bicycle W37.0 ☑
  war operations — see War operations, explosion
Exposure (to) X58 ☑
  air pressure change — see Air, pressure
  cold (accidental) (excessive) (extreme) (natural) (place) X31 ☑
    assault Y08.89 ☑
    due to
      man-made conditions W93.8 ☑
        dry ice (contact) W93.01 ☑
          inhalation W93.02 ☑
        liquid air (contact) (hydrogen) (nitrogen) W93.11 ☑
          inhalation W93.12 ☑
        refrigeration unit (deep freeze) W93.2 ☑
        suicide (attempt) X83.2 ☑
      weather (conditions) X31 ☑
    homicide (attempt) Y08.89 ☑
    self-inflicted X83.2 ☑
  due to abandonment or neglect X58 ☑
  electric current W86.8 ☑
    appliance (faulty) W86.8 ☑
      domestic W86.0 ☑
    caused by other person Y08.89 ☑
    conductor (faulty) W86.1 ☑
    control apparatus (faulty) W86.1 ☑
    electric power generating plant, distribution station W86.1 ☑
    electroshock gun — see Exposure, electric current, taser
    high-voltage cable W85 ☑
    homicide (attempt) Y08.89 ☑
    legal execution — see Legal, intervention, specified means NEC
    lightning — see subcategory T75.0 ☑
    live rail W86.8 ☑
    misadventure in medical or surgical procedure in electroshock therapy Y63.4
    motor (electric) (faulty) W86.8 ☑
      domestic W86.0 ☑
    self-inflicted X83.1 ☑
    specified NEC W86.8 ☑
      domestic W86.0 ☑
    stun gun — see Exposure, electric current, taser
    suicide (attempt) X83.1 ☑
    taser W86.8 ☑
      assault Y08.89 ☑
      legal intervention — see category Y35 ☑
      self-harm (intentional) X83.8 ☑
      undetermined intent Y33 ☑
    third rail W86.8 ☑
    transformer (faulty) W86.1 ☑
    transmission lines W85 ☑
  environmental tobacco smoke X58 ☑
  excessive
    cold — see Exposure, cold
    heat (natural) NEC X30 ☑
      man-made W92 ☑
  factor(s) NOS X58 ☑
    environmental NEC X58 ☑
      man-made NEC W99 ☑
    natural NEC — see Forces of nature
    specified NEC X58 ☑
  fire, flames (accidental) X08.8 ☑
    assault X97 ☑

Exposure — continued
  fire, flames — continued
    campfire — see Exposure, fire, controlled, not in building
    controlled (in)
      with ignition (of) clothing (see also Ignition, clothes) X06.2 ☑
        nightwear X05 ☑
      bonfire — see Exposure, fire, controlled, not in building
      brazier (in building or structure) (see also Exposure, fire, controlled, building)
        not in building or structure — see Exposure, fire, controlled, not in building
      building or structure X02.0 ☑
        with
          fall from building X02.3 ☑
          from building X02.5 ☑
          injury due to building collapse X02.2 ☑
          smoke inhalation X02.1 ☑
        hit by object from building X02.4 ☑
        specified mode of injury NEC X02.8 ☑
      fireplace, furnace or stove — see Exposure, fire, controlled, building
      not in building or structure X03.0 ☑
        with
          fall X03.3 ☑
          smoke inhalation X03.1 ☑
        hit by object X03.4 ☑
        specified mode of injury NEC X03.8 ☑
      trash — see Exposure, fire, controlled, not in building
    fireplace — see Exposure, fire, controlled, building
    fittings or furniture (in building or structure) (uncontrolled) — see Exposure, fire, uncontrolled, building
    forest (uncontrolled) — see Exposure, fire, uncontrolled, not in building
    grass (uncontrolled) — see Exposure, fire, uncontrolled, not in building
    hay (uncontrolled) — see Exposure, fire, uncontrolled, not in building
    homicide (attempt) X97 ☑
    ignition of highly flammable material X04 ☑
    in, of, on, starting in
      machinery — see Contact, with, by type of machine
      motor vehicle (in motion) (see also Accident, transport, occupant by type of vehicle) V87.8 ☑
        with collision — see Collision
      railway rolling stock, train, vehicle V81.81 ☑
        with collision — see Accident, transport, railway vehicle occupant
      street car (in motion) V82.8 ☑
        with collision — see Accident, transport, streetcar occupant
      transport vehicle NEC (see also Accident, transport)
        with collision — see Collision
      war operations (see also War operations, fire)
        from nuclear explosion — see War operations, nuclear weapons
      watercraft (in transit) (not in transit) V91.09 ☑
        localized — see Burn, on board watercraft, due to, fire on board
        powered craft V91.03 ☑
          ferry boat V91.01 ☑
          fishing boat V91.02 ☑
          jet skis V91.03 ☑
          liner V91.01 ☑
          merchant ship V91.00 ☑
          passenger ship V91.01 ☑
        unpowered craft V91.08 ☑
          canoe V91.05 ☑
          inflatable V91.06 ☑
          kayak V91.05 ☑
          sailboat V91.04 ☑
          surf-board V91.08 ☑
          waterskis V91.07 ☑
          windsurfer V91.08 ☑
    lumber (uncontrolled) — see Exposure, fire, uncontrolled, not in building
    mine (uncontrolled) — see Exposure, fire, uncontrolled, not in building
    prairie (uncontrolled) — see Exposure, fire, uncontrolled, not in building

Exposure — continued
  fire, flames — continued
    resulting from
      explosion — see Explosion
      lightning X08.8 ☑
    self-inflicted X76 ☑
    specified NEC X08.8 ☑
    started by other person X97 ☑
    stated as undetermined whether accidental or intentional Y26 ☑
    stove — see Exposure, fire, controlled, building
    suicide (attempt) X76 ☑
    tunnel (uncontrolled) — see Exposure, fire, uncontrolled, not in building
    uncontrolled
      in building or structure X00.0 ☑
        with
          fall from building X00.3 ☑
          injury due to building collapse X00.2 ☑
          jump from building X00.5 ☑
          smoke inhalation X00.1 ☑
        bed X08.00 ☑
          due to
            cigarette X08.01 ☑
            specified material NEC X08.09 ☑
        furniture NEC X08.20 ☑
          due to
            cigarette X08.21 ☑
            specified material NEC X08.29 ☑
        hit by object from building X00.4 ☑
        sofa X08.10 ☑
          due to
            cigarette X08.11 ☑
            specified material NEC X08.19 ☑
        specified mode of injury NEC X00.8 ☑
      not in building or structure (any) X01.0 ☑
        with
          fall X01.3 ☑
          smoke inhalation X01.1 ☑
        hit by object X01.4 ☑
        specified mode of injury NEC X01.8 ☑
    undetermined whether accidental or intentional Y26 ☑
  forces of nature NEC — see Forces of nature
  G-forces (abnormal) W49.9 ☑
  gravitational forces (abnormal) W49.9 ☑
  heat (natural) NEC — see Heat
  high-pressure jet (hydraulic) (pneumatic) W49.9 ☑
  hydraulic jet W49.9 ☑
  inanimate mechanical force W49.9 ☑
  jet, high-pressure (hydraulic) (pneumatic) W49.9 ☑
  lightning — see subcategory T75.0 ☑
    causing fire — see Exposure, fire
  mechanical forces NEC W49.9 ☑
    animate NEC W64 ☑
    inanimate NEC W49.9 ☑
  noise W42.9 ☑
    supersonic W42.0 ☑
  noxious substance — see Table of Drugs and Chemicals
  pneumatic jet W49.9 ☑
  prolonged in deep-freeze unit or refrigerator W93.2 ☑
  radiation — see Radiation
  smoke (see also Exposure, fire)
    tobacco, second hand Z77.22
  specified factors NEC X58 ☑
  sunlight X32 ☑
    man-made (sun lamp) W89.8 ☑
      tanning bed W89.1 ☑
  supersonic waves W42.0 ☑
  transmission line(s), electric W85 ☑
  vibration W49.9 ☑
  waves
    infrasound W49.9 ☑
    sound W42.9 ☑
    supersonic W42.0 ☑
  weather NEC — see Forces of nature
External cause status Y99.9
  child assisting in compensated work for family Y99.8
  civilian activity done for financial or other compensation Y99.0
  civilian activity done for income or pay Y99.0
  family member assisting in compensated work for other family member Y99.8
  hobby not done for income Y99.8
  leisure activity Y99.8

External cause status — *continued*
  military activity Y99.1
  off-duty activity of military personnel Y99.8
  recreation or sport not for income or while a student
    Y99.8
  specified NEC Y99.8
  student activity Y99.8
  volunteer activity Y99.2

F

Factors, supplemental
  alcohol
    blood level
      less than 20mg/100ml Y90.0
      20-39mg/100ml Y90.1
      40-59mg/100ml Y90.2
      60-79mg/100ml Y90.3
      80-99mg/100ml Y90.4
      100-119mg/100ml Y90.5
      120-199mg/100ml Y90.6
      200-239mg/100ml Y90.7
      240mg/100ml or more Y90.8
      presence in blood, level not specified Y90.9
    presence in blood, but level not specified Y90.9
  environmental-pollution-related condition- see Z57 ☑
  nosocomial condition Y95
  work-related condition Y99.0
Failure
  in suture or ligature during surgical procedure Y65.2
  mechanical, of instrument or apparatus (any) (during
    any medical or surgical procedure) Y65.8
  sterile precautions (during medical and surgical care)
    — *see* Misadventure, failure, sterile precautions,
    by type of procedure
  to
    introduce tube or instrument Y65.4
    endotracheal tube during anesthesia Y65.3
    make curve (transport vehicle) NEC — *see* Accident,
      transport
    remove tube or instrument Y65.4
Fall, falling (accidental) W19 ☑
  building W20.1 ☑
    burning (uncontrolled fire) X00.3 ☑
  down
    embankment W17.81 ☑
    escalator W10.0 ☑
    hill W17.81 ☑
    ladder W11 ☑
    ramp W10.2 ☑
    stairs, steps W10.9 ☑
  due to
    bumping against
      object W18.00 ☑
        sharp glass W18.02 ☑
        specified NEC W18.09 ☑
        sports equipment W18.01 ☑
      person W03 ☑
        due to ice or snow W00.0 ☑
        on pedestrian conveyance — *see* Accident,
          transport, pedestrian, conveyance
    collision with another person W03 ☑
      due to ice or snow W00.0 ☑
      involving pedestrian conveyance — *see* Acci-
        dent, transport, pedestrian, conveyance
    grocery cart tipping over W17.82 ☑
    ice or snow W00.9 ☑
      from one level to another W00.2 ☑
      on stairs or steps W00.1 ☑
    involving pedestrian conveyance — *see* Acci-
      dent, transport, pedestrian, conveyance
    on same level W00.0 ☑
    slipping (on moving sidewalk) W01.0 ☑
      with subsequent striking against object
        W01.10 ☑
        furniture W01.190 ☑
        sharp object W01.119 ☑
          glass W01.110 ☑
          power tool or machine W01.111 ☑
          specified NEC W01.118 ☑
        specified NEC W01.198 ☑
    striking against
      object W18.00 ☑
        sharp glass W18.02 ☑
        specified NEC W18.09 ☑
        sports equipment W18.01 ☑
      person W03 ☑

Fall, falling — *continued*
  due to — *continued*
    striking against — *continued*
      person — *continued*
        due to ice or snow W00.0 ☑
        on pedestrian conveyance — *see* Accident,
          transport, pedestrian, conveyance
  earth (with asphyxia or suffocation (by pressure)) —
    see Earth, falling
  from, off, out of
    aircraft NEC (with accident to aircraft NEC) V97.0 ☑
      while boarding or alighting V97.1 ☑
    balcony W13.0 ☑
    bed W06 ☑
    boat, ship, watercraft NEC (with drowning or sub-
      mersion) — *see* Drowning, due to, fall over-
      board
      with hitting bottom or object V94.0 ☑
    bridge W13.1 ☑
    building W13.9 ☑
      burning (uncontrolled fire) X00.3 ☑
    cavity W17.2 ☑
    chair W07 ☑
    cherry picker W17.89 ☑
    cliff W15 ☑
    dock W17.4 ☑
    embankment W17.81 ☑
    escalator W10.0 ☑
    flagpole W13.8 ☑
    furniture NEC W08 ☑
    grocery cart W17.82 ☑
    haystack W17.89 ☑
    high place NEC W17.89 ☑
      stated as undetermined whether accidental or
        intentional Y30 ☑
    hole W17.2 ☑
    incline W10.2 ☑
    ladder W11 ☑
    lifting device W17.89 ☑
    machine, machinery (*see also* Contact, with, by
      type of machine)
      not in operation W17.89 ☑
    manhole W17.1 ☑
    mobile elevated work platform [MEWP] W17.89 ☑
    motorized mobility scooter W05.2 ☑
    one level to another NEC W17.89 ☑
      intentional, purposeful, suicide (attempt)
        X80 ☑
      stated as undetermined whether accidental or
        intentional Y30 ☑
    pit W17.2 ☑
    playground equipment W09.8 ☑
      jungle gym W09.2 ☑
      slide W09.0 ☑
      swing W09.1 ☑
    quarry W17.89 ☑
    railing W13.9 ☑
    ramp W10.2 ☑
    roof W13.2 ☑
    scaffolding W12 ☑
    scooter (nonmotorized) W05.1 ☑
      motorized mobility W05.2 ☑
    sky lift W17.89 ☑
    stairs, steps W10.9 ☑
      curb W10.1 ☑
      due to ice or snow W00.1 ☑
      escalator W10.0 ☑
      incline W10.2 ☑
      ramp W10.2 ☑
      sidewalk curb W10.1 ☑
      specified NEC W10.8 ☑
    stepladder W11 ☑
    storm drain W17.1 ☑
    streetcar NEC V82.6 ☑
      with antecedent collision — *see* Accident,
        transport, streetcar occupant
      while boarding or alighting V82.4 ☑
    structure NEC W13.8 ☑
      burning (uncontrolled fire) X00.3 ☑
    table W08 ☑
    toilet W18.11 ☑
      with subsequent striking against object
        W18.12 ☑
    train NEC V81.6 ☑
      during derailment (without antecedent colli-
        sion) V81.7 ☑

Fall, falling — *continued*
  from, off, out of — *continued*
    train — *continued*
      during derailment — *continued*
        with antecedent collision — *see* Accident,
          transport, railway vehicle occupant
      while boarding or alighting V81.4 ☑
    transport vehicle after collision — *see* Accident,
      transport, by type of vehicle, collision
    tree W14 ☑
    vehicle (in motion) NEC (*see also* Accident, trans-
      port) V89.9 ☑
      motor NEC (*see also* Accident, transport, occu-
        pant, by type of vehicle) V87.8 ☑
      stationary W17.89 ☑
        while boarding or alighting — *see* Accident,
          transport, by type of vehicle, while
          boarding or alighting
    viaduct W13.8 ☑
    wall W13.8 ☑
    watercraft (*see also* Drowning, due to, fall over-
      board)
      with hitting bottom or object V94.0 ☑
    well W17.0 ☑
    wheelchair, non-moving W05.0 ☑
      powered — *see* Accident, transport, pedestrian,
        conveyance occupant, specified type NEC
    window W13.4 ☑
  in, on
    aircraft NEC V97.0 ☑
      with accident to aircraft V97.0 ☑
      while boarding or alighting V97.1 ☑
    bathtub (empty) W18.2 ☑
      filled W16.212 ☑
        causing drowning W16.211 ☑
    escalator W10.0 ☑
    incline W10.2 ☑
    ladder W11 ☑
    machine, machinery — *see* Contact, with, by type
      of machine
    object, edged, pointed or sharp (with cut) — *see*
      Fall, by type
    playground equipment W09.8 ☑
      jungle gym W09.2 ☑
      slide W09.0 ☑
      swing W09.1 ☑
    ramp W10.2 ☑
    scaffolding W12 ☑
    shower W18.2 ☑
      causing drowning W16.211 ☑
    staircase, stairs, steps W10.9 ☑
      curb W10.1 ☑
      due to ice or snow W00.1 ☑
      escalator W10.0 ☑
      incline W10.2 ☑
      specified NEC W10.8 ☑
    streetcar (without antecedent collision) V82.5 ☑
      with antecedent collision — *see* Accident,
        transport, streetcar occupant
      while boarding or alighting V82.4 ☑
    train (without antecedent collision) V81.5 ☑
      with antecedent collision — *see* Accident,
        transport, railway vehicle occupant
      during derailment (without antecedent colli-
        sion) V81.7 ☑
        with antecedent collision — *see* Accident,
          transport, railway vehicle occupant
      while boarding or alighting V81.4 ☑
    transport vehicle after collision — *see* Accident,
      transport, by type of vehicle, collision
    watercraft V93.39 ☑
      due to
        accident to craft V91.29 ☑
          powered craft V91.23 ☑
            ferry boat V91.21 ☑
            fishing boat V91.22 ☑
            jetskis V91.23 ☑
            liner V91.21 ☑
            merchant ship V91.20 ☑
            passenger ship V91.21 ☑
          unpowered craft
            canoe V91.25 ☑
            inflatable V91.26 ☑
            kayak V91.25 ☑
            sailboat V91.24 ☑
        powered craft V93.33 ☑

Fall, falling — *continued*
  in, on — *continued*
    watercraft — *continued*
      powered craft — *continued*
        ferry boat V93.31 ☑
        fishing boat V93.32 ☑
        jetskis V93.33 ☑
        liner V93.31 ☑
        merchant ship V93.30 ☑
        passenger ship V93.31 ☑
      unpowered craft V93.38 ☑
        canoe V93.35 ☑
        inflatable V93.36 ☑
        kayak V93.35 ☑
        sailboat V93.34 ☑
        surf-board V93.38 ☑
        windsurfer V93.38 ☑
  into
    cavity W17.2 ☑
    dock W17.4 ☑
    fire — *see* Exposure, fire, by type
    haystack W17.89 ☑
    hole W17.2 ☑
    lake — *see* Fall, into, water
    manhole W17.1 ☑
    moving part of machinery — *see* Contact, with, by
      type of machine
    ocean — *see* Fall, into, water
    opening in surface NEC W17.89 ☑
    pit W17.2 ☑
    pond — *see* Fall, into, water
    quarry W17.89 ☑
    river — *see* Fall, into, water
    shaft W17.89 ☑
    storm drain W17.1 ☑
    stream — *see* Fall, into, water
    swimming pool (*see also* Fall, into, water, in,
      swimming pool)
      empty W17.3 ☑
    tank W17.89 ☑
    water W16.42 ☑
      causing drowning W16.41 ☑
      from watercraft — *see* Drowning, due to, fall
        overboard
      hitting diving board W21.4 ☑
      in
        bathtub W16.212 ☑
          causing drowning W16.211 ☑
        bucket W16.222 ☑
          causing drowning W16.221 ☑
        natural body of water W16.112 ☑
          causing drowning W16.111 ☑
          striking
            bottom W16.122 ☑
              causing drowning W16.121 ☑
            side W16.132 ☑
              causing drowning W16.131 ☑
        specified water NEC W16.312 ☑
          causing drowning W16.311 ☑
          striking
            bottom W16.322 ☑
              causing drowning W16.321 ☑
            wall W16.332 ☑
              causing drowning W16.331 ☑
        swimming pool W16.012 ☑
          causing drowning W16.011 ☑
          striking
            bottom W16.022 ☑
              causing drowning W16.031 ☑
            wall W16.032 ☑
              causing drowning W16.021 ☑
        utility bucket W16.222 ☑
          causing drowning W16.221 ☑
    well W17.0 ☑
  involving
    bed W06 ☑
    chair W07 ☑
    furniture NEC W08 ☑
    glass — *see* Fall, by type
    playground equipment W09.8 ☑
      jungle gym W09.2 ☑
      slide W09.0 ☑
      swing W09.1 ☑
    roller blades — *see* Accident, transport, pedestrian,
      conveyance

Fall, falling — *continued*
  involving — *continued*
    skateboard(s) — *see* Accident, transport, pedestri-
      an, conveyance
    skates (ice) (in line) (roller) — *see* Accident, trans-
      port, pedestrian, conveyance
    skis — *see* Accident, transport, pedestrian, con-
      veyance
    table W08 ☑
    wheelchair, non-moving W05.0 ☑
      powered — *see* Accident, transport, pedestrian,
        conveyance, specified type NEC
  object — *see* Struck by, object, falling
  off
    toilet W18.11 ☑
      with subsequent striking against object
        W18.12 ☑
  on same level W18.30 ☑
    due to
      specified NEC W18.39 ☑
      stepping on an object W18.31 ☑
  out of
    bed W06 ☑
    building NEC W13.8 ☑
    chair W07 ☑
    furniture NEC W08 ☑
    wheelchair, non-moving W05.0 ☑
      powered — *see* Accident, transport, pedestrian,
        conveyance, specified type NEC
    window W13.4 ☑
  over
    animal W01.0 ☑
    cliff W15 ☑
    embankment W17.81 ☑
    small object W01.0 ☑
  rock W20.8 ☑
  same level W18.30 ☑
    from
      being crushed, pushed, or stepped on by a
        crowd or human stampede W52 ☑
      collision, pushing, shoving, by or with other
        person W03 ☑
      slipping, stumbling, tripping W01.0 ☑
    involving ice or snow W00.0 ☑
      involving skates (ice) (roller), skateboard, skis
        — *see* Accident, transport, pedestrian,
        conveyance
  snowslide (avalanche) — *see* Landslide
  stone W20.8 ☑
  structure W20.1 ☑
    burning (uncontrolled fire) X00.3 ☑
  through
    bridge W13.1 ☑
    floor W13.3 ☑
    roof W13.2 ☑
    wall W13.8 ☑
    window W13.4 ☑
  timber W20.8 ☑
  tree (caused by lightning) W20.8 ☑
  while being carried or supported by other person(s)
    W04 ☑

Fallen on by
  animal (not being ridden) NEC W55.89 ☑
Felo-de-se — *see* Suicide
Fight (hand) (fists) (foot) — *see* Assault, fight
Fire (accidental) — *see* Exposure, fire
Firearm discharge — *see* Discharge, firearm
**Fireball effects from nuclear explosion in war oper-
  ations** — *see* War operations, nuclear weapons
Fireworks (explosion) W39 ☑
Flash burns from explosion — *see* Explosion
Flood (any injury) (caused by) X38 ☑
  collapse of man-made structure causing earth move-
    ment X36.0 ☑
  tidal wave — *see* Forces of nature, tidal wave
Food (any type) **in**
  air passages (with asphyxia, obstruction, or suffoca-
    tion) — *see* categories T17 and T18 ☑
  alimentary tract causing asphyxia (due to compression
    of trachea) — *see* categories T17 and T18 ☑
Forces of nature X39.8 ☑
  avalanche X36.1 ☑
    causing transport accident — *see* Accident, trans-
      port, by type of vehicle
  blizzard X37.2 ☑
  cataclysmic storm X37.9 ☑

Forces of nature — *continued*
  cataclysmic storm — *continued*
    with flood X38 ☑
    blizzard X37.2 ☑
    cloudburst X37.8 ☑
    cyclone X37.1 ☑
    dust storm X37.3 ☑
    hurricane X37.0 ☑
    specified storm NEC X37.8 ☑
    storm surge X37.0 ☑
    tornado X37.1 ☑
    twister X37.1 ☑
    typhoon X37.0 ☑
  cloudburst X37.8 ☑
  cold (natural) X31 ☑
  cyclone X37.1 ☑
  dam collapse causing earth movement X36.0 ☑
  dust storm X37.3 ☑
  earth movement X36.1 ☑
    caused by dam or structure collapse X36.0 ☑
    earthquake X34 ☑
  earthquake X34 ☑
  flood (caused by) X38 ☑
    dam collapse X36.0 ☑
    tidal wave — *see* Forces of nature, tidal wave
  heat (natural) X30 ☑
  hurricane X37.0 ☑
  landslide X36.1 ☑
    causing transport accident — *see* Accident, trans-
      port, by type of vehicle
  lightning — *see* subcategory T75.0 ☑
    causing fire — *see* Exposure, fire
  mudslide X36.1 ☑
    causing transport accident — *see* Accident, trans-
      port, by type of vehicle
  radiation (natural) X39.08 ☑
    radon X39.01 ☑
  radon X39.01 ☑
  specified force NEC X39.8 ☑
  storm surge X37.0 ☑
  structure collapse causing earth movement X36.0 ☑
  sunlight X32 ☑
  tidal wave X37.41 ☑
    due to
      earthquake X37.41 ☑
      landslide X37.43 ☑
      storm X37.42 ☑
      volcanic eruption X37.41 ☑
  tornado X37.1 ☑
  tsunami X37.41 ☑
  twister X37.1 ☑
  typhoon X37.0 ☑
  volcanic eruption X35 ☑
Foreign body
  aspiration — *see* Index to Diseases and Injuries, For-
    eign body, respiratory tract
  embedded in skin W45 ☑
  entering through skin W45.8 ☑
    can lid W26.8 ☑
    nail W45.0 ☑
    paper W26.2 ☑
    specified NEC W45.8 ☑
    splinter W45.8 ☑
Forest fire (exposure to) — *see* Exposure, fire, uncontrolled, not in building
Found injured X58 ☑
  from exposure (to) — *see* Exposure
  on
    highway, road(way), street V89.9 ☑
    railway right of way V81.9 ☑
Fracture (circumstances unknown or unspecified) X58 ☑
  due to specified cause NEC X58 ☑
Freezing — *see* Exposure, cold
Frostbite X31 ☑
  due to man-made conditions — *see* Exposure, cold,
    man-made
Frozen — *see* Exposure, cold

G

Gored by bull W55.22 ☑
Gunshot wound W34.00 ☑

H

Hailstones, injured by X39.8 ☑

Hanged herself or himself — *see* Hanging, self-inflicted
Hanging (accidental) (*see also* category) T71 ☑
   legal execution — *see* Legal, intervention, specified
      means NEC
Heat (effects of) (excessive) X30 ☑
   due to
      man-made conditions W92 ☑
         on board watercraft V93.29 ☑
           fishing boat V93.22 ☑
           merchant ship V93.20 ☑
           passenger ship V93.21 ☑
           sailboat V93.24 ☑
           specified powered craft NEC V93.23 ☑
      weather (conditions) X30 ☑
   from
      electric heating apparatus causing burning X16 ☑
      nuclear explosion in war operations — *see* War
         operations, nuclear weapons
   inappropriate in local application or packing in medical
      or surgical procedure Y63.5
Hemorrhage
   delayed following medical or surgical treatment
      without mention of misadventure — *see* Index
         to Diseases and Injuries, Complication(s)
   during medical or surgical treatment as misadventure
      — *see* Index to Diseases and Injuries, Complica-
      tion(s)
High
   altitude (effects) — *see* Air, pressure, low
   level of radioactivity, effects — *see* Radiation
   pressure (effects) — *see* Air, pressure, high
   temperature, effects — *see* Heat
Hit, hitting (accidental) by — *see* Struck by
Hitting against — *see* Striking against
Homicide (attempt) (justifiable) — *see* Assault
Hot
   place, effects (*see also* Heat)
   weather, effects X30 ☑
House fire (uncontrolled) — *see* Exposure, fire, uncon-
   trolled, building
Humidity, causing problem X39.8 ☑
Hunger X58 ☑
Hurricane (any injury) X37.0 ☑
Hypobarism, hypobaropathy — *see* Air, pressure, low

I

Ictus
   caloris (*see also* Heat)
   solaris X30 ☑
Ignition (accidental) (*see also* Exposure, fire) X08.8 ☑
   anesthetic gas in operating room W40.1 ☑
   apparel X06.2 ☑
      from highly flammable material X04 ☑
      nightwear X05 ☑
   bed linen (sheets) (spreads) (pillows) (mattress) — *see*
      Exposure, fire, uncontrolled, building, bed
   benzine X04 ☑
   clothes, clothing NEC (from controlled fire) X06.2 ☑
      from
         highly flammable material X04 ☑
   ether X04 ☑
      in operating room W40.1 ☑
   explosive material — *see* Explosion
   gasoline X04 ☑
   jewelry (plastic) (any) X06.0 ☑
   kerosene X04 ☑
   material
      explosive — *see* Explosion
      highly flammable with secondary explosion X04 ☑
   nightwear X05 ☑
   paraffin X04 ☑
   petrol X04 ☑
Immersion (accidental) (*see also* Drowning)
   hand or foot due to cold (excessive) X31 ☑
Implantation of quills of porcupine W55.89 ☑
Inanition (from) (hunger) X58 ☑
   thirst X58 ☑
Inappropriate operation performed
   correct operation on wrong side or body part (wrong
      side) (wrong site) Y65.53
   operation intended for another patient done on wrong
      patient Y65.52
   wrong operation performed on correct patient Y65.51
Inattention after, at birth (homicidal intent) (infantici-
   dal intent) X58 ☑

Incident, adverse
   device
      anesthesiology Y70.8
         accessory Y70.2
         diagnostic Y70.0
         miscellaneous Y70.8
         monitoring Y70.0
         prosthetic Y70.2
         rehabilitative Y70.1
         surgical Y70.3
         therapeutic Y70.1
      cardiovascular Y71.8
         accessory Y71.2
         diagnostic Y71.0
         miscellaneous Y71.8
         monitoring Y71.0
         prosthetic Y71.2
         rehabilitative Y71.1
         surgical Y71.3
         therapeutic Y71.1
      gastroenterology Y73.8
         accessory Y73.2
         diagnostic Y73.0
         miscellaneous Y73.8
         monitoring Y73.0
         prosthetic Y73.2
         rehabilitative Y73.1
         surgical Y73.3
         therapeutic Y73.1
      general
         hospital Y74.8
           accessory Y74.2
           diagnostic Y74.0
           miscellaneous Y74.8
           monitoring Y74.0
           prosthetic Y74.2
           rehabilitative Y74.1
           surgical Y74.3
           therapeutic Y74.1
         surgical Y81.8
           accessory Y81.2
           diagnostic Y81.0
           miscellaneous Y81.8
           monitoring Y81.0
           prosthetic Y81.2
           rehabilitative Y81.1
           surgical Y81.3
           therapeutic Y81.1
      gynecological Y76.8
         accessory Y76.2
         diagnostic Y76.0
         miscellaneous Y76.8
         monitoring Y76.0
         prosthetic Y76.2
         rehabilitative Y76.1
         surgical Y76.3
         therapeutic Y76.1
      medical Y82.9
         specified type NEC Y82.8
      neurological Y75.8
         accessory Y75.2
         diagnostic Y75.0
         miscellaneous Y75.8
         monitoring Y75.0
         prosthetic Y75.2
         rehabilitative Y75.1
         surgical Y75.3
         therapeutic Y75.1
      obstetrical Y76.8
         accessory Y76.2
         diagnostic Y76.0
         miscellaneous Y76.8
         monitoring Y76.0
         prosthetic Y76.2
         rehabilitative Y76.1
         surgical Y76.3
         therapeutic Y76.1
      ophthalmic Y77.8
         accessory Y77.2
         diagnostic Y77.0
         miscellaneous Y77.8
         monitoring Y77.0
         prosthetic Y77.2
         rehabilitative Y77.1
         surgical Y77.3
         therapeutic Y77.1
      orthopedic Y79.8
         accessory Y79.2
         diagnostic Y79.0

Incident, adverse — *continued*
   device — *continued*
      orthopedic — *continued*
         miscellaneous Y79.8
         monitoring Y79.0
         prosthetic Y79.2
         rehabilitative Y79.1
         surgical Y79.3
         therapeutic Y79.1
      otorhinolaryngological Y72.8
         accessory Y72.2
         diagnostic Y72.0
         miscellaneous Y72.8
         monitoring Y72.0
         prosthetic Y72.2
         rehabilitative Y72.1
         surgical Y72.3
         therapeutic Y72.1
      personal use Y74.8
         accessory Y74.2
         diagnostic Y74.0
         miscellaneous Y74.8
         monitoring Y74.0
         prosthetic Y74.2
         rehabilitative Y74.1
         surgical Y74.3
         therapeutic Y74.1
      physical medicine Y80.8
         accessory Y80.2
         diagnostic Y80.0
         miscellaneous Y80.8
         monitoring Y80.0
         prosthetic Y80.2
         rehabilitative Y80.1
         surgical Y80.3
         therapeutic Y80.1
      plastic surgical Y81.8
         accessory Y81.2
         diagnostic Y81.0
         miscellaneous Y81.8
         monitoring Y81.0
         prosthetic Y81.2
         rehabilitative Y81.1
         surgical Y81.3
         therapeutic Y81.1
      radiological Y78.8
         accessory Y78.2
         diagnostic Y78.0
         miscellaneous Y78.8
         monitoring Y78.0
         prosthetic Y78.2
         rehabilitative Y78.1
         surgical Y78.3
         therapeutic Y78.1
      urology Y73.8
         accessory Y73.2
         diagnostic Y73.0
         miscellaneous Y73.8
         monitoring Y73.0
         prosthetic Y73.2
         rehabilitative Y73.1
         surgical Y73.3
         therapeutic Y73.1
Incineration (accidental) — *see* Exposure, fire
Infanticide — *see* Assault
Infrasound waves (causing injury) W49.9 ☑
Ingestion
   foreign body (causing injury) (with obstruction) — *see*
      Foreign body, alimentary canal
   poisonous
      plant(s) X58 ☑
      substance NEC — *see* Table of Drugs and Chemicals
Inhalation
   excessively cold substance, man-made — *see* Expo-
      sure, cold, man-made
   food (any type) (into respiratory tract) (with asphyxia,
      obstruction respiratory tract, suffocation) — *see*
      categories T17 and T18
   foreign body — *see* Foreign body, aspiration
   gastric contents (with asphyxia, obstruction respiratory
      passage, suffocation) T17.81- ☑
   hot air or gases X14.0 ☑
   liquid air, hydrogen, nitrogen W93.12 ☑
      suicide (attempt) X83.2 ☑
   steam X13.0 ☑
      assault X98.0 ☑
      stated as undetermined whether accidental or in-
         tentional Y27.0 ☑

Inhalation — *continued*
  steam — *continued*
    suicide (attempt) X77.0 ☑
  toxic gas — *see* Table of Drugs and Chemicals
  vomitus (with asphyxia, obstruction respiratory passage, suffocation) T17.81- ☑
Injury, injured (accidental(ly)) NOS X58 ☑
  by, caused by, from
    assault — *see* Assault
    law-enforcing agent, police, in course of legal intervention — *see* Legal intervention
    suicide (attempt) X83.8 ☑
  due to, in
    civil insurrection — *see* War operations
    fight (*see also* Assault, fight) Y04.0 ☑
    war operations — *see* War operations
  homicide (*see also* Assault) Y09
  inflicted (by)
    in course of arrest (attempted), suppression of disturbance, maintenance of order, by law-enforcing agents — *see* Legal intervention
    other person
      stated as
        accidental X58 ☑
        intentional, homicide (attempt) — *see* Assault
        undetermined whether accidental or intentional Y33 ☑
    purposely (inflicted) by other person(s) — *see* Assault
    self-inflicted X83.8 ☑
      stated as accidental X58 ☑
    specified cause NEC X58 ☑
    undetermined whether accidental or intentional Y33 ☑
Insolation, effects X30 ☑
Insufficient nourishment X58 ☑
Interruption of respiration (by)
  food (lodged in esophagus) — *see* categories T17 and T18 ☑
  vomitus (lodged in esophagus) T17.81- ☑
Intervention, legal — *see* Legal intervention
Intoxication
  drug — *see* Table of Drugs and Chemicals
  poison — *see* Table of Drugs and Chemicals

J

Jammed (accidentally)
  between objects (moving) (stationary and moving) W23.0 ☑
    stationary W23.1 ☑
Jumped, jumping
  before moving object NEC X81.8 ☑
    motor vehicle X81.0 ☑
    subway train X81.1 ☑
    train X81.1 ☑
    undetermined whether accidental or intentional Y31 ☑
  from
    boat (into water) voluntarily, without accident (to or on boat) W16.712 ☑
      with
        accident to or on boat — *see* Accident, watercraft
        drowning or submersion W16.711 ☑
          suicide (attempt) X71.3 ☑
        striking bottom W16.722 ☑
          causing drowning W16.721 ☑
    building (*see also* Jumped, from, high place) W13.9 ☑
      burning (uncontrolled fire) X00.5 ☑
    high place NEC W17.89 ☑
      suicide (attempt) X80 ☑
      undetermined whether accidental or intentional Y30 ☑
    structure (*see also* Jumped, from, high place) W13.9 ☑
      burning (uncontrolled fire) X00.5 ☑
  into water W16.92 ☑
    causing drowning W16.91 ☑
    from, off watercraft — *see* Jumped, from, boat
    in
      natural body W16.612 ☑
        causing drowning W16.611 ☑
        striking bottom W16.622 ☑
          causing drowning W16.621 ☑

Jumped, jumping — *continued*
  into water — *continued*
    in — *continued*
      specified place NEC W16.812 ☑
        causing drowning W16.811 ☑
        striking
          bottom W16.822 ☑
            causing drowning W16.821 ☑
          wall W16.832 ☑
            causing drowning W16.831 ☑
      swimming pool W16.512 ☑
        causing drowning W16.511 ☑
        striking
          bottom W16.522 ☑
            causing drowning W16.521 ☑
          wall W16.532 ☑
            causing drowning W16.531 ☑
    suicide (attempt) X71.3 ☑

K

Kicked by
  animal NEC W55.82 ☑
  person(s) (accidentally) W50.1 ☑
    with intent to injure or kill Y04.0 ☑
    as, or caused by, a crowd or human stampede (with fall) W52 ☑
    assault Y04.0 ☑
    homicide (attempt) Y04.0 ☑
    in
      fight Y04.0 ☑
      legal intervention
        injuring
          bystander Y35.812 ☑
          law enforcement personnel Y35.811 ☑
          suspect Y35.813 ☑
Kicking
  against
    object W22.8 ☑
      sports equipment W21.9 ☑
      stationary W22.09 ☑
        sports equipment W21.89 ☑
    person — *see* Striking against, person
    sports equipment W21.9 ☑
  carpet stretcher with knee X50.3 ☑
Killed, killing (accidentally) NOS (*see also* Injury) X58 ☑
  in
    action — *see* War operations
    brawl, fight (hand) (fists) (foot) Y04.0 ☑
      by weapon (*see also* Assault)
        cutting, piercing — *see* Assault, cutting or piercing instrument
        firearm — *see* Discharge, firearm, by type, homicide
  self
    stated as
      accident NOS X58 ☑
      suicide — *see* Suicide
      undetermined whether accidental or intentional Y33 ☑
Kneeling (prolonged (static)) X50.1 ☑
Knocked down (accidentally) (by) NOS X58 ☑
  animal (not being ridden) NEC (*see also* Struck by, by type of animal)
  crowd or human stampede W52 ☑
  person W51 ☑
    in brawl, fight Y04.0 ☑
  transport vehicle NEC (*see also* Accident, transport) V09.9 ☑

L

Laceration NEC — *see* Injury
Lack of
  care (helpless person) (infant) (newborn) X58 ☑
  food except as result of abandonment or neglect X58 ☑
    due to abandonment or neglect X58 ☑
  water except as result of transport accident X58 ☑
    due to transport accident — *see* Accident, transport, by type
  helpless person, infant, newborn X58 ☑
Landslide (falling on transport vehicle) X36.1 ☑
  caused by collapse of man-made structure X36.0 ☑
Late effect — *see* Sequelae

Legal
  execution (any method) — *see* Legal, intervention
  intervention (by)
    baton — *see* Legal, intervention, blunt object, baton
    bayonet — *see* Legal, intervention, sharp object, bayonet
    blow — *see* Legal, intervention, manhandling
    blunt object
      baton
        injuring
          bystander Y35.312 ☑
          law enforcement personnel Y35.311 ☑
          suspect Y35.313 ☑
      injuring
        bystander Y35.302 ☑
        law enforcement personnel Y35.301 ☑
        suspect Y35.303 ☑
      specified NEC
        injuring
          bystander Y35.392 ☑
          law enforcement personnel Y35.391 ☑
          suspect Y35.393 ☑
      stave
        injuring
          bystander Y35.392 ☑
          law enforcement personnel Y35.391 ☑
          suspect Y35.393 ☑
    bomb — *see* Legal, intervention, explosive
    cutting or piercing instrument — *see* Legal, intervention, sharp object
    dynamite — *see* Legal, intervention, explosive, dynamite
    explosive(s)
      dynamite
        injuring
          bystander Y35.112 ☑
          law enforcement personnel Y35.111 ☑
          suspect Y35.113 ☑
      grenade
        injuring
          bystander Y35.192 ☑
          law enforcement personnel Y35.191 ☑
          suspect Y35.193 ☑
      injuring
        bystander Y35.102 ☑
        law enforcement personnel Y35.101 ☑
        suspect Y35.103 ☑
      mortar bomb
        injuring
          bystander Y35.192 ☑
          law enforcement personnel Y35.191 ☑
          suspect Y35.193 ☑
      shell
        injuring
          bystander Y35.122 ☑
          law enforcement personnel Y35.121 ☑
          suspect Y35.123 ☑
      specified NEC
        injuring
          bystander Y35.192 ☑
          law enforcement personnel Y35.191 ☑
          suspect Y35.193 ☑
    firearm(s) (discharge)
      handgun
        injuring
          bystander Y35.022 ☑
          law enforcement personnel Y35.021 ☑
          suspect Y35.023 ☑
      injuring
        bystander Y35.002 ☑
        law enforcement personnel Y35.001 ☑
        suspect Y35.003 ☑
      machine gun
        injuring
          bystander Y35.012 ☑
          law enforcement personnel Y35.011 ☑
          suspect Y35.013 ☑
      rifle pellet
        injuring
          bystander Y35.032 ☑
          law enforcement personnel Y35.031 ☑
          suspect Y35.033 ☑
      rubber bullet
        injuring
          bystander Y35.042 ☑
          law enforcement personnel Y35.041 ☑

☑ Additional Character Required — Refer to the Tabular List for Character Selection   ▽ Subterms under main terms may continue to next column or page

Legal — *continued*
  intervention — *continued*
    firearm(s) — *continued*
      rubber bullet — *continued*
        injuring — *continued*
          suspect Y35.043 ☑
      shotgun — *see* Legal, intervention, firearm, specified NEC
      specified NEC
        injuring
          bystander Y35.092 ☑
          law enforcement personnel Y35.091 ☑
          suspect Y35.093 ☑
    gas (asphyxiation) (poisoning)
      injuring
        bystander Y35.202 ☑
        law enforcement personnel Y35.201 ☑
        suspect Y35.203 ☑
      specified NEC
        injuring
          bystander Y35.292 ☑
          law enforcement personnel Y35.291 ☑
          suspect Y35.293 ☑
      tear gas
        injuring
          bystander Y35.212 ☑
          law enforcement personnel Y35.211 ☑
          suspect Y35.213 ☑
    grenade — *see* Legal, intervention, explosive, grenade
    injuring
      bystander Y35.92 ☑
      law enforcement personnel Y35.91 ☑
      suspect Y35.93 ☑
    late effect (of) — *see* with 7th character S Y35 ☑
    manhandling
      injuring
        bystander Y35.812 ☑
        law enforcement personnel Y35.811 ☑
        suspect Y35.813 ☑
    sequelae (of) — *see* with 7th character S Y35 ☑
    sharp objects
      bayonet
        injuring
          bystander Y35.412 ☑
          law enforcement personnel Y35.411 ☑
          suspect Y35.413 ☑
      injuring
        bystander Y35.402 ☑
        law enforcement personnel Y35.401 ☑
        suspect Y35.403 ☑
      specified NEC
        injuring
          bystander Y35.492 ☑
          law enforcement personnel Y35.491 ☑
          suspect Y35.493 ☑
    specified means NEC
      injuring
        bystander Y35.892 ☑
        law enforcement personnel Y35.891 ☑
        suspect Y35.893 ☑
    stabbing — *see* Legal, intervention, sharp object
    stave — *see* Legal, intervention, blunt object, stave
    tear gas — *see* Legal, intervention, gas, tear gas
    truncheon — *see* Legal, intervention, blunt object, stave

Lifting — *see also* Overexertion
  heavy objects X50.0 ☑
  weights X50.0 ☑
Lightning (shock) (stroke) (struck by) — *see* subcategory T75.0 ☑
  causing fire — *see* Exposure, fire
Loss of control (transport vehicle) NEC — *see* Accident, transport
Lost at sea NOS — *see* Drowning, due to, fall overboard
Low
  pressure (effects) — *see* Air, pressure, low
  temperature (effects) — *see* Exposure, cold
Lying before train, vehicle or other moving object X81.8 ☑
  subway train X81.1 ☑
  train X81.1 ☑
  undetermined whether accidental or intentional Y31 ☑
Lynching — *see* Assault

M

Malfunction (mechanism or component) (of)
  firearm W34.10 ☑
    airgun W34.110 ☑
    BB gun W34.110 ☑
    gas, air or spring-operated gun NEC W34.118 ☑
    handgun W32.1 ☑
    hunting rifle W33.12 ☑
    larger firearm W33.10 ☑
      specified NEC W33.19 ☑
    machine gun W33.13 ☑
    paintball gun W34.111 ☑
    pellet gun W34.110 ☑
    shotgun W33.11 ☑
    specified NEC W34.19 ☑
    Very pistol [flare] W34.19 ☑
  handgun — *see* Malfunction, firearm, handgun
Maltreatment — *see* Perpetrator
Mangled (accidentally) NOS X58 ☑
Manhandling (in brawl, fight) Y04.0 ☑
  legal intervention — *see* Legal, intervention, manhandling
Manslaughter (nonaccidental) — *see* Assault
Mauled by animal NEC W55.89 ☑
Medical procedure, complication of (delayed or as an abnormal reaction without mention of misadventure) — *see* Complication of or following, by specified type of procedure
  due to or as a result of misadventure — *see* Misadventure
Melting (due to fire) (*see also* Exposure, fire)
  apparel NEC X06.3 ☑
  clothes, clothing NEC X06.3 ☑
    nightwear X05 ☑
  fittings or furniture (burning building) (uncontrolled fire) X00.8 ☑
  nightwear X05 ☑
  plastic jewelry X06.1 ☑
Mental cruelty X58 ☑
Military operations (injuries to military and civilians occuring during peacetime on military property and during routine military exercises and operations) (by) (from) (involving) Y37.90- ☑
  air blast Y37.20- ☑
  aircraft
    destruction — *see* Military operations, destruction of aircraft
  airway restriction — *see* Military operations, restriction of airways
  asphyxiation — *see* Military operations, restriction of airways
  biological weapons Y37.6X- ☑
  blast Y37.20- ☑
  blast fragments Y37.20- ☑
  blast wave Y37.20- ☑
  blast wind Y37.20- ☑
  bomb Y37.20- ☑
    dirty Y37.50- ☑
    gasoline Y37.31- ☑
    incendiary Y37.31- ☑
    petrol Y37.31- ☑
  bullet Y37.43- ☑
    incendiary Y37.32- ☑
    rubber Y37.41- ☑
  chemical weapons Y37.7X- ☑
  combat
    hand to hand (unarmed) combat Y37.44- ☑
    using blunt or piercing object Y37.45- ☑
  conflagration — *see* Military operations, fire
  conventional warfare NEC Y37.49- ☑
  depth-charge Y37.01- ☑
  destruction of aircraft Y37.10- ☑
    due to
      air to air missile Y37.11- ☑
      collision with other aircraft Y37.12- ☑
      detonation (accidental) of onboard munitions and explosives Y37.14- ☑
      enemy fire or explosives Y37.11- ☑
      explosive placed on aircraft Y37.11- ☑
      onboard fire Y37.13- ☑
      rocket propelled grenade [RPG] Y37.11- ☑
      small arms fire Y37.11- ☑
      surface to air missile Y37.11- ☑
    specified NEC Y37.19- ☑

Military operations — *continued*
  detonation (accidental) of
    onboard marine weapons Y37.05- ☑
    own munitions or munitions launch device Y37.24- ☑
  dirty bomb Y37.50- ☑
  explosion (of) Y37.20- ☑
    aerial bomb Y37.21- ☑
    bomb NOS (*see also* Military operations, bomb(s)) Y37.20- ☑
    fragments Y37.20- ☑
    grenade Y37.29- ☑
    guided missile Y37.22- ☑
    improvised explosive device [IED] (person-borne) (roadside) (vehicle-borne) Y37.23- ☑
    land mine Y37.29- ☑
    marine mine (at sea) (in harbor) Y37.02- ☑
    marine weapon Y37.00- ☑
      specified NEC Y37.09- ☑
    own munitions or munitions launch device (accidental) Y37.24- ☑
    sea-based artillery shell Y37.03- ☑
    specified NEC Y37.29- ☑
    torpedo Y37.04- ☑
  fire Y37.30- ☑
    specified NEC Y37.39- ☑
  firearms
    discharge Y37.43- ☑
    pellets Y37.42- ☑
  flamethrower Y37.33- ☑
  fragments (from) (of)
    improvised explosive device [IED] (person-borne) (roadside) (vehicle-borne) Y37.26- ☑
    munitions Y37.25- ☑
    specified NEC Y37.29- ☑
    weapons Y37.27- ☑
  friendly fire Y37.92- ☑
  hand to hand (unarmed) combat Y37.44- ☑
  hot substances — *see* Military operations, fire
  incendiary bullet Y37.32- ☑
  nuclear weapon (effects of) Y37.50- ☑
    acute radiation exposure Y37.54- ☑
    blast pressure Y37.51- ☑
    direct blast Y37.51- ☑
    direct heat Y37.53- ☑
    fallout exposure Y37.54- ☑
    fireball Y37.53- ☑
    indirect blast (struck or crushed by blast debris) (being thrown by blast) Y37.52- ☑
    ionizing radiation (immediate exposure) Y37.54- ☑
    nuclear radiation Y37.54- ☑
    radiation
      ionizing (immediate exposure) Y37.54- ☑
      nuclear Y37.54- ☑
      thermal Y37.53- ☑
    secondary effects Y37.54- ☑
    specified NEC Y37.59- ☑
    thermal radiation Y37.53- ☑
  restriction of air (airway)
    intentional Y37.46- ☑
    unintentional Y37.47- ☑
  rubber bullets Y37.41- ☑
  shrapnel NOS Y37.29- ☑
  suffocation — *see* Military operations, restriction of airways
  unconventional warfare NEC Y37.7X- ☑
  underwater blast NOS Y37.00- ☑
  warfare
    conventional NEC Y37.49- ☑
    unconventional NEC Y37.7X- ☑
  weapon of mass destruction [WMD] Y37.91- ☑
  weapons
    biological weapons Y37.6X- ☑
    chemical Y37.7X- ☑
    nuclear (effects of) Y37.50- ☑
      acute radiation exposure Y37.54- ☑
      blast pressure Y37.51- ☑
      direct blast Y37.51- ☑
      direct heat Y37.53- ☑
      fallout exposure Y37.54- ☑
      fireball Y37.53- ☑
      radiation
        ionizing (immediate exposure) Y37.54- ☑
        nuclear Y37.54- ☑
        thermal Y37.53- ☑
      secondary effects Y37.54- ☑

Military operations — *continued*
  weapons — *continued*
    nuclear — *continued*
      specified NEC Y37.59- ☑
    of mass destruction [WMD] Y37.91- ☑
Misadventure(s) to patient(s) during surgical or
    medical care Y69
  contaminated medical or biological substance (blood,
    drug, fluid) Y64.9
    administered (by) NEC Y64.9
      immunization Y64.1
      infusion Y64.0
      injection Y64.1
      specified means NEC Y64.8
      transfusion Y64.0
      vaccination Y64.1
  excessive amount of blood or other fluid during
    transfusion or infusion Y63.0
  failure
    in dosage Y63.9
      electroshock therapy Y63.4
      inappropriate temperature (too hot or too cold)
        in local application and packing Y63.5
      infusion
        excessive amount of fluid Y63.0
        incorrect dilution of fluid Y63.1
      insulin-shock therapy Y63.4
      nonadministration of necessary drug or biolog-
        ical substance Y63.6
      overdose — *see* Table of Drugs and Chemicals
        radiation, in therapy Y63.2
      radiation
        overdose Y63.2
      specified procedure NEC Y63.8
      transfusion
        excessive amount of blood Y63.0
  mechanical, of instrument or apparatus (any)
    (during any procedure) Y65.8
  sterile precautions (during procedure) Y62.9
    aspiration of fluid or tissue (by puncture or
      catheterization, except heart) Y62.6
    biopsy (except needle aspiration) Y62.8
      needle (aspirating) Y62.6
    blood sampling Y62.6
    catheterization Y62.6
      heart Y62.5
    dialysis (kidney) Y62.2
    endoscopic examination Y62.4
    enema Y62.8
    immunization Y62.3
    infusion Y62.1
    injection Y62.3
    needle biopsy Y62.6
    paracentesis (abdominal) (thoracic) Y62.6
    perfusion Y62.2
    puncture (lumbar) Y62.6
    removal of catheter or packing Y62.8
    specified procedure NEC Y62.8
    surgical operation Y62.0
    transfusion Y62.1
    vaccination Y62.3
  suture or ligature during surgical procedure Y65.2
  to introduce or to remove tube or instrument —
    see Failure, to
  hemorrhage — *see* Index to Diseases and Injuries,
    Complication(s)
  inadvertent exposure of patient to radiation Y63.3
  inappropriate
    operation performed — *see* Inappropriate opera-
      tion performed
    temperature (too hot or too cold) in local applica-
      tion or packing Y63.5
  infusion (*see also* Misadventure, by type, infusion) Y69
    excessive amount of fluid Y63.0
    incorrect dilution of fluid Y63.1
    wrong fluid Y65.1
  mismatched blood in transfusion Y65.0
  nonadministration of necessary drug or biological
    substance Y63.6
  overdose — *see* Table of Drugs and Chemicals
    radiation (in therapy) Y63.2
  perforation — *see* Index to Diseases and Injuries,
    Complication(s)
  performance of inappropriate operation — *see* Inap-
    propriate operation performed
  puncture — *see* Index to Diseases and Injuries, Com-
    plication(s)
  specified type NEC Y65.8

Misadventure(s) to patient(s) during surgical or
    medical care — *continued*
  specified type — *continued*
    failure
      suture or ligature during surgical operation
        Y65.2
      to introduce or to remove tube or instrument
        — *see* Failure, to
    infusion of wrong fluid Y65.1
    performance of inappropriate operation — *see* In-
      appropriate operation performed
    transfusion of mismatched blood Y65.0
    wrong
      fluid in infusion Y65.1
      placement of endotracheal tube during anes-
        thetic procedure Y65.3
  transfusion — *see* Misadventure, by type, transfusion
    excessive amount of blood Y63.0
    mismatched blood Y65.0
  wrong
    drug given in error — *see* Table of Drugs and
      Chemicals
    fluid in infusion Y65.1
    placement of endotracheal tube during anesthetic
      procedure Y65.3
Mismatched blood in transfusion Y65.0
Motion sickness T75.3
Mountain sickness W94.11 ☑
Mudslide (of cataclysmic nature) — *see* Landslide
Murder (attempt) — *see* Assault

N

Nail
  contact with W45.0 ☑
    gun W29.4 ☑
  embedded in skin W45.0 ☑
Neglect (criminal) (homicidal intent) X58 ☑
Noise (causing injury) (pollution) W42.9 ☑
  supersonic W42.0 ☑
Nonadministration (of)
  drug or biological substance (necessary) Y63.6
  surgical and medical care Y66
Nosocomial condition Y95

O

Object
  falling
    from, in, on, hitting
      machinery — *see* Contact, with, by type of
        machine
  set in motion by
    accidental explosion or rupture of pressure vessel
      W38 ☑
    firearm — *see* Discharge, firearm, by type
    machine(ry) — *see* Contact, with, by type of ma-
      chine
Overdose (drug) — *see* Table of Drugs and Chemicals
  radiation Y63.2
Overexertion X50.9 ☑
  from
    prolonged static or awkward postures X50.1 ☑
    repetitive movements X50.3 ☑
    specified strenuous movements or postures NEC
      X50.9 ☑
    strenuous movement or load X50.0 ☑
Overexposure (accidental) (to)
  cold (*see also* Exposure, cold) X31 ☑
    due to man-made conditions — *see* Exposure, cold,
      man-made
  heat (*see also* Heat) X30 ☑
  radiation — *see* Radiation
  radioactivity W88.0 ☑
  sun (sunburn) X32 ☑
  weather NEC — *see* Forces of nature
  wind NEC — *see* Forces of nature
Overheated — *see* Heat
Overturning (accidental)
  machinery — *see* Contact, with, by type of machine
  transport vehicle NEC (*see also* Accident, transport)
    V89.9 ☑
  watercraft (causing drowning, submersion) (*see also*
    Drowning, due to, accident to, watercraft, over-
    turning)
    causing injury except drowning or submersion —
      see Accident, watercraft, causing, injury NEC

P

Parachute descent (voluntary) (without accident to
    aircraft) V97.29 ☑
  due to accident to aircraft — *see* Accident, transport
    aircraft
Pecked by bird W61.99 ☑
Perforation during medical or surgical treatment
    as misadventure — *see* Index to Diseases and In
    juries, Complication(s)
Perpetrator, perpetration, of assault, maltreatmen
    and neglect (by) Y07.9
  boyfriend Y07.03
  brother Y07.410
    stepbrother Y07.435
  coach Y07.53
  cousin
    female Y07.491
    male Y07.490
  daycare provider Y07.519
    at-home
      adult care Y07.512
      childcare Y07.510
    care center
      adult care Y07.513
      childcare Y07.511
  family member NEC Y07.499
  father Y07.11
    adoptive Y07.13
    foster Y07.420
    stepfather Y07.430
  foster father Y07.420
  foster mother Y07.421
  girl friend Y07.04
  healthcare provider Y07.529
    mental health Y07.521
    specified NEC Y07.528
  husband Y07.01
  instructor Y07.53
  mother Y07.12
    adoptive Y07.14
    foster Y07.421
    stepmother Y07.433
  nonfamily member Y07.50
    specified NEC Y07.59
  nurse Y07.528
  occupational therapist Y07.528
  partner of parent
    female Y07.434
    male Y07.432
  physical therapist Y07.528
  sister Y07.411
  speech therapist Y07.528
  stepbrother Y07.435
  stepfather Y07.430
  stepmother Y07.433
  stepsister Y07.436
  teacher Y07.53
  wife Y07.02
Piercing — *see* Contact, with, by type of object or ma-
    chine
Pinched
  between objects (moving) (stationary and moving)
    W23.0 ☑
  stationary W23.1 ☑
Pinned under machine(ry) — *see* Contact, with, by typ
    of machine
Place of occurrence Y92.9
  abandoned house Y92.89
  airplane Y92.813
  airport Y92.520
  ambulatory health services establishment NEC Y92.538
  ambulatory surgery center Y92.530
  amusement park Y92.831
  apartment (co-op) — *see* Place of occurrence, resi-
    dence, apartment
  assembly hall Y92.29
  bank Y92.510
  barn Y92.71
  baseball field Y92.320
  basketball court Y92.310
  beach Y92.832
  boarding house — *see* Place of occurrence, residence
    boarding house
  boat Y92.814
  bowling alley Y92.39
  bridge Y92.89

Place of occurrence — continued
  building under construction Y92.61
  bus Y92.811
    station Y92.521
  cafe Y92.511
  campsite Y92.833
  campus — see Place of occurrence, school
  canal Y92.89
  car Y92.810
  casino Y92.59
  children's home — see Place of occurrence, residence,
      institutional, orphanage
  church Y92.22
  cinema Y92.26
  clubhouse Y92.29
  coal pit Y92.64
  college (community) Y92.214
  condominium — see Place of occurrence, residence,
      apartment
  construction area — see Place of occurrence, industrial
      and construction area
  convalescent home — see Place of occurrence, resi-
      dence, institutional, nursing home
  court-house Y92.240
  cricket ground Y92.328
  cultural building Y92.258
    art gallery Y92.250
    museum Y92.251
    music hall Y92.252
    opera house Y92.253
    specified NEC Y92.258
    theater Y92.254
  dancehall Y92.252
  day nursery Y92.210
  dentist office Y92.531
  derelict house Y92.89
  desert Y92.820
  dockyard Y92.62
  dock NOS Y92.89
  doctor's office Y92.531
  dormitory — see Place of occurrence, residence, insti-
      tutional, school dormitory
  dry dock Y92.62
  factory (building) (premises) Y92.63
  farm (land under cultivation) (outbuildings) Y92.79
    barn Y92.71
    chicken coop Y92.72
    field Y92.73
    hen house Y92.72
    house — see Place of occurrence, residence, house
    orchard Y92.74
    specified NEC Y92.79
  football field Y92.321
  forest Y92.821
  freeway Y92.411
  gallery Y92.250
  garage (commercial) Y92.59
    boarding house Y92.044
    military base Y92.135
    mobile home Y92.025
    nursing home Y92.124
    orphanage Y92.114
    private house Y92.015
    reform school Y92.155
  gas station Y92.524
  gasworks Y92.69
  golf course Y92.39
  gravel pit Y92.64
  grocery Y92.512
  gymnasium Y92.39
  handball court Y92.318
  harbor Y92.89
  harness racing course Y92.39
  healthcare provider office Y92.531
  highway (interstate) Y92.411
  hill Y92.828
  hockey rink Y92.330
  home — see Place of occurrence, residence
  hospice — see Place of occurrence, residence, institu-
      tional, nursing home
  hospital Y92.239
    cafeteria Y92.233
    corridor Y92.232
    operating room Y92.234
    patient
      bathroom Y92.231
      room Y92.230
    specified NEC Y92.238

Place of occurrence — continued
  hotel Y92.59
  house (see also Place of occurrence, residence)
    abandoned Y92.89
    under construction Y92.61
  industrial and construction area (yard) Y92.69
    building under construction Y92.61
    dock Y92.62
    dry dock Y92.62
    factory Y92.63
    gasworks Y92.69
    mine Y92.64
    oil rig Y92.65
    pit Y92.64
    power station Y92.69
    shipyard Y92.62
    specified NEC Y92.69
    tunnel under construction Y92.69
    workshop Y92.69
  kindergarten Y92.211
  lacrosse field Y92.328
  lake Y92.828
  library Y92.241
  mall Y92.59
  market Y92.512
  marsh Y92.828
  military
    base — see Place of occurrence, residence, institu-
        tional, military base
    training ground Y92.84
  mine Y92.64
  mosque Y92.22
  motel Y92.59
  motorway (interstate) Y92.411
  mountain Y92.828
  movie-house Y92.26
  museum Y92.251
  music-hall Y92.252
  not applicable Y92.9
  nuclear power station Y92.69
  nursing home — see Place of occurrence, residence,
      institutional, nursing home
  office building Y92.59
  offshore installation Y92.65
  oil rig Y92.65
  old people's home — see Place of occurrence, resi-
      dence, institutional, specified NEC
  opera-house Y92.253
  orphanage — see Place of occurrence, residence, insti-
      tutional, orphanage
  outpatient surgery center Y92.530
  park (public) Y92.830
    amusement Y92.831
  parking garage Y92.89
    lot Y92.481
  pavement Y92.480
  physician office Y92.531
  polo field Y92.328
  pond Y92.828
  post office Y92.242
  power station Y92.69
  prairie Y92.828
  prison — see Place of occurrence, residence, institu-
      tional, prison
  public
    administration building Y92.248
      city hall Y92.243
      courthouse Y92.240
      library Y92.241
      post office Y92.242
      specified NEC Y92.248
    building NEC Y92.29
    hall Y92.29
    place NOS Y92.89
  race course Y92.39
  radio station Y92.59
  railway line (bridge) Y92.85
  ranch (outbuildings) — see Place of occurrence, farm
  recreation area Y92.838
    amusement park Y92.831
    beach Y92.832
    campsite Y92.833
    park (public) Y92.830
    seashore Y92.832
    specified NEC Y92.838
  reform school - — see Place of occurrence, residence,
      institutional, reform school
  religious institution Y92.22

Place of occurrence — continued
  residence (non-institutional) (private) Y92.009
    apartment Y92.039
      bathroom Y92.031
      bedroom Y92.032
      kitchen Y92.030
      specified NEC Y92.038
    bathroom Y92.002
    bedroom Y92.003
    boarding house Y92.049
      bathroom Y92.041
      bedroom Y92.042
      driveway Y92.043
      garage Y92.044
      garden Y92.046
      kitchen Y92.040
      specified NEC Y92.048
      swimming pool Y92.045
      yard Y92.046
    dining room Y92.001
    garden Y92.007
    home Y92.009
    house, single family Y92.019
      bathroom Y92.012
      bedroom Y92.013
      dining room Y92.011
      driveway Y92.014
      garage Y92.015
      garden Y92.017
      kitchen Y92.010
      specified NEC Y92.018
      swimming pool Y92.016
      yard Y92.017
    institutional Y92.10
      children's home — see Place of occurrence,
          residence, institutional, orphanage
      hospice — see Place of occurrence, residence,
          institutional, nursing home
      military base Y92.139
        barracks Y92.133
        garage Y92.135
        garden Y92.137
        kitchen Y92.130
        mess hall Y92.131
        specified NEC Y92.138
        swimming pool Y92.136
        yard Y92.137
      nursing home Y92.129
        bathroom Y92.121
        bedroom Y92.122
        driveway Y92.123
        garage Y92.124
        garden Y92.126
        kitchen Y92.120
        specified NEC Y92.128
        swimming pool Y92.125
        yard Y92.126
      orphanage Y92.119
        bathroom Y92.111
        bedroom Y92.112
        driveway Y92.113
        garage Y92.114
        garden Y92.116
        kitchen Y92.110
        specified NEC Y92.118
        swimming pool Y92.115
        yard Y92.116
      prison Y92.149
        bathroom Y92.142
        cell Y92.143
        courtyard Y92.147
        dining room Y92.141
        kitchen Y92.140
        specified NEC Y92.148
        swimming pool Y92.146
      reform school Y92.159
        bathroom Y92.152
        bedroom Y92.153
        dining room Y92.151
        driveway Y92.154
        garage Y92.155
        garden Y92.157
        kitchen Y92.150
        specified NEC Y92.158
        swimming pool Y92.156
        yard Y92.157
      school dormitory Y92.169
        bathroom Y92.162
        bedroom Y92.163

Place of occurrence — *continued*
  residence — *continued*
    institutional — *continued*
      school dormitory — *continued*
        dining room Y92.161
        kitchen Y92.160
        specified NEC Y92.168
      specified NEC Y92.199
        bathroom Y92.192
        bedroom Y92.193
        dining room Y92.191
        driveway Y92.194
        garage Y92.195
        garden Y92.197
        kitchen Y92.190
        specified NEC Y92.198
        swimming pool Y92.196
        yard Y92.197
    kitchen Y92.000
    mobile home Y92.029
      bathroom Y92.022
      bedroom Y92.023
      dining room Y92.021
      driveway Y92.024
      garage Y92.025
      garden Y92.027
      kitchen Y92.020
      specified NEC Y92.028
      swimming pool Y92.026
      yard Y92.027
    specified place in residence NEC Y92.008
    specified residence type NEC Y92.099
      bathroom Y92.091
      bedroom Y92.092
      driveway Y92.093
      garage Y92.094
      garden Y92.096
      kitchen Y92.090
      specified NEC Y92.098
      swimming pool Y92.095
      yard Y92.096
  restaurant Y92.511
  riding school Y92.39
  river Y92.828
  road Y92.488
  rodeo ring Y92.39
  rugby field Y92.328
  same day surgery center Y92.530
  sand pit Y92.64
  school (private) (public) (state) Y92.219
    college Y92.214
    daycare center Y92.210
    elementary school Y92.211
    high school Y92.213
    kindergarten Y92.211
    middle school Y92.212
    specified NEC Y92.218
    trace school Y92.215
    university Y92.214
    vocational school Y92.215
  sea (shore) Y92.832
  senior citizen center Y92.29
  service area
    airport Y92.520
    bus station Y92.521
    gas station Y92.524
    highway rest stop Y92.523
    railway station Y92.522
  shipyard Y92.62
  shop (commercial) Y92.513
  sidewalk Y92.480
  silo Y92.79
  skating rink (roller) Y92.331
    ice Y92.330
  slaughter house Y92.86
  soccer field Y92.322
  specified place NEC Y92.89
  sports area Y92.39
    athletic
      court Y92.318
        basketball Y92.310
        specified NEC Y92.318
        squash Y92.311
        tennis Y92.312
      field Y92.328
        baseball Y92.320
        cricket ground Y92.328
        football Y92.321
        hockey Y92.328

Place of occurrence — *continued*
  sports area — *continued*
    athletic — *continued*
      field — *continued*
        soccer Y92.322
        specified NEC Y92.328
    golf course Y92.39
    gymnasium Y92.39
    riding school Y92.39
    skating rink (roller) Y92.331
      ice Y92.330
    stadium Y92.39
    swimming pool Y92.34
  squash court Y92.311
  stadium Y92.39
  steeplechasing course Y92.39
  store Y92.512
  stream Y92.828
  street and highway Y92.410
    bike path Y92.482
    freeway Y92.411
    highway ramp Y92.415
    interstate highway Y92.411
    local residential or business street Y92.414
    motorway Y92.411
    parking lot Y92.481
    parkway Y92.412
    sidewalk Y92.480
    specified NEC Y92.488
    state road Y92.413
  subway car Y92.816
  supermarket Y92.512
  swamp Y92.828
  swimming pool (public) Y92.34
    private (at) Y92.095
      boarding house Y92.045
      military base Y92.136
      mobile home Y92.026
      nursing home Y92.125
      orphanage Y92.115
      prison Y92.146
      reform school Y92.156
      single family residence Y92.016
  synagogue Y92.22
  television station Y92.59
  tennis court Y92.312
  theater Y92.254
  trade area Y92.59
    bank Y92.510
    cafe Y92.511
    casino Y92.59
    garage Y92.59
    hotel Y92.59
    market Y92.512
    office building Y92.59
    radio station Y92.59
    restaurant Y92.511
    shop Y92.513
    shopping mall Y92.59
    store Y92.512
    supermarket Y92.512
    television station Y92.59
    warehouse Y92.59
  trailer park, residential — *see* Place of occurrence, residence, mobile home
  trailer site NOS Y92.89
  train Y92.815
    station Y92.522
  truck Y92.812
  tunnel under construction Y92.69
  university Y92.214
  urgent (health) care center Y92.532
  vehicle (transport) Y92.818
    airplane Y92.813
    boat Y92.814
    bus Y92.811
    car Y92.810
    specified NEC Y92.818
    subway car Y92.816
    train Y92.815
    truck Y92.812
  warehouse Y92.59
  water reservoir Y92.89
  wilderness area Y92.828
    desert Y92.820
    forest Y92.821
    marsh Y92.828
    mountain Y92.828
    prairie Y92.828

Place of occurrence — *continued*
  wilderness area — *continued*
    specified NEC Y92.828
    swamp Y92.828
  workshop Y92.69
  yard, private Y92.096
    boarding house Y92.046
    mobile home Y92.027
    single family house Y92.017
  youth center Y92.29
  zoo (zoological garden) Y92.834
Plumbism — *see* Table of Drugs and Chemicals, lead
Poisoning (accidental) (by) (*see also* Table of Drugs and Chemicals)
  by plant, thorns, spines, sharp leaves or other mechanisms NEC X58 ☑
  carbon monoxide
    generated by
      motor vehicle — *see* Accident, transport
      watercraft (in transit) (not in transit) V93.89 ☑
        ferry boat V93.81 ☑
        fishing boat V93.82 ☑
        jet skis V93.83 ☑
        liner V93.81 ☑
        merchant ship V93.80 ☑
        passenger ship V93.81 ☑
        powered craft NEC V93.83 ☑
  caused by injection of poisons into skin by plant thorns, spines, sharp leaves X58 ☑
  marine or sea plants (venomous) X58 ☑
  execution — *see* Legal, intervention, gas
  intervention
    by gas — *see* Legal, intervention, gas
    other specified means — *see* Legal, intervention, specified means NEC
  exhaust gas
    generated by
      motor vehicle — *see* Accident, transport
      watercraft (in transit) (not in transit) V93.89 ☑
        ferry boat V93.81 ☑
        fishing boat V93.82 ☑
        jet skis V93.83 ☑
        liner V93.81 ☑
        merchant ship V93.80 ☑
        passenger ship V93.81 ☑
        powered craft NEC V93.83 ☑
  fumes or smoke due to
    explosion (*see also* Explosion) W40.9 ☑
    fire — *see* Exposure, fire
    ignition — *see* Ignition
  gas
    in legal intervention — *see* Legal, intervention, gas
    legal execution — *see* Legal, intervention, gas
  in war operations — *see* War operations
  legal
Powder burn (by) (from)
  airgun W34.110 ☑
  BB gun W34.110 ☑
  firearm NEC W34.19 ☑
  gas, air or spring-operated gun NEC W34.118 ☑
  handgun W32.1 ☑
  hunting rifle W33.12 ☑
  larger firearm W33.10 ☑
    specified NEC W33.19 ☑
  machine gun W33.13 ☑
  paintball gun W34.111 ☑
  pellet gun W34.110 ☑
  shotgun W33.11 ☑
  Very pistol [flare] W34.19 ☑
Premature cessation (of) **surgical and medical care** Y66
Privation (food) (water) X58 ☑
Procedure (operation)
  correct, on wrong side or body part (wrong side) (wrong site) Y65.53
  intended for another patient done on wrong patient Y65.52
  performed on patient not scheduled for surgery Y65.52
  performed on wrong patient Y65.52
  wrong, performed on correct patient Y65.51
Prolonged
  sitting in transport vehicle — *see* Travel, by type of vehicle
  stay in
    high altitude as cause of anoxia, barodontalgia, barotitis or hypoxia W94.11 ☑
    weightless environment X52 ☑

Pulling, excessive (see also Overexertion) X50.9- ☑
Puncture, puncturing (see also Contact, with, by type
 of object or machine)
 by
  plant thorns, spines, sharp leaves or other mechanisms NEC W60 ☑
 during medical or surgical treatment as misadventure
  — see Index to Diseases and Injuries, Complica-
  tion(s)
Pushed, pushing (accidental) (injury in)
 by other person(s) (accidental) W51 ☑
  with fall W03 ☑
   due to ice or snow W00.0 ☑
  as, or caused by, a crowd or human stampede (with
   fall) W52 ☑
  before moving object NEC Y02.8 ☑
   motor vehicle Y02.0 ☑
   subway train Y02.1 ☑
   train Y02.1 ☑
  from
   high place NEC
    in accidental circumstances W17.89 ☑
    stated as
     intentional, homicide (attempt) Y01 ☑
     undetermined whether accidental or
      intentional Y30 ☑
   transport vehicle NEC (see also Accident, trans-
    port) V89.9 ☑
    stated as
     intentional, homicide (attempt)
      Y08.89 ☑
 overexertion X50.9 ☑

R

Radiation (exposure to)
 arc lamps W89.0 ☑
 atomic power plant (malfunction) NEC W88.1 ☑
 complication of or abnormal reaction to medical radiotherapy Y84.2
 electromagnetic, ionizing W88.0 ☑
 gamma rays W88.1 ☑
 in
  war operations (from or following nuclear explosion) — see War operations
 inadvertent exposure of patient (receiving test or
  therapy) Y63.3
 infrared (heaters and lamps) W90.1 ☑
  excessive heat from W92 ☑
 ionized, ionizing (particles, artificially accelerated)
  radioisotopes W88.1 ☑
  specified NEC W88.8 ☑
  x-rays W88.0 ☑
 isotopes, radioactive — see Radiation, radioactive
  isotopes
 laser(s) W90.2 ☑
  in war operations — see War operations
  misadventure in medical care Y63.2
 light sources (man-made visible and ultraviolet)
  W89.9 ☑
  natural X32 ☑
  specified NEC W89.8 ☑
  tanning bed W89.1 ☑
  welding light W89.0 ☑
 man-made visible light W89.9 ☑
  specified NEC W89.8 ☑
  tanning bed W89.1 ☑
  welding light W89.0 ☑
 microwave W90.8 ☑
 misadventure in medical or surgical procedure Y63.2
 natural NEC X39.08 ☑
  radon X39.01 ☑
 overdose (in medical or surgical procedure) Y63.2
 radar W90.0 ☑
 radioactive isotopes (any) W88.1 ☑
  atomic power plant malfunction W88.1 ☑
  misadventure in medical or surgical treatment
   Y63.2
 radiofrequency W90.0 ☑
 radium NEC W88.1 ☑
 sun X32 ☑
 ultraviolet (light) (man-made) W89.9 ☑
  natural X32 ☑
  specified NEC W89.8 ☑
  tanning bed W89.1 ☑
  welding light W89.0 ☑

Radiation — continued
 welding arc, torch, or light W89.0 ☑
  excessive heat from W92 ☑
 x-rays (hard) (soft) W88.0 ☑
Range disease W94.11 ☑
Rape (attempted) T74.2- ☑
Rat bite W53.11 ☑
Reaching (prolonged) (static) X50.1 ☑
Reaction, abnormal to medical procedure (see also
 Complication of or following, by type of procedure)
 Y84.9
 with misadventure — see Misadventure
 biologicals — see Table of Drugs and Chemicals
 drugs — see Table of Drugs and Chemicals
 vaccine — see Table of Drugs and Chemicals
Recoil
 airgun W34.110 ☑
 BB gun W34.110 ☑
 firearm NEC W34.19 ☑
 gas, air or spring-operated gun NEC W34.118 ☑
 handgun W32.1 ☑
 hunting rifle W33.12 ☑
 larger firearm W33.10 ☑
  specified NEC W33.19 ☑
 machine gun W33.13 ☑
 paintball gun W34.111 ☑
 pellet W34.110 ☑
 shotgun W33.11 ☑
 Very pistol [flare] W34.19 ☑
Reduction in
 atmospheric pressure — see Air, pressure, change
Rock falling on or hitting (accidentally) (person)
 W20.8 ☑
 in cave-in W20.0 ☑
Run over (accidentally) (by)
 animal (not being ridden) NEC W55.89 ☑
 machinery — see Contact, with, by specified type of
  machine
 transport vehicle NEC (see also Accident, transport)
  V09.9 ☑
  intentional homicide (attempt) Y03.0 ☑
  motor NEC V09.20 ☑
   intentional homicide (attempt) Y03.0 ☑
Running
 before moving object X81.8 ☑
  motor vehicle X81.0 ☑
Running off, away
 animal (being ridden) (see also Accident, transport)
  V80.918 ☑
  not being ridden W55.89 ☑
 animal-drawn vehicle NEC (see also Accident, transport) V80.928 ☑
 highway, road(way), street
  transport vehicle NEC (see also Accident, transport)
   V89.9 ☑
Rupture pressurized devices — see Explosion, by type
 of device

S

Saturnism — see Table of Drugs and Chemicals, lead
Scald, scalding (accidental) (by) (from) (in) X19 ☑
 air (hot) X14.1 ☑
 gases (hot) X14.1 ☑
 homicide (attempt) — see Assault, burning, hot object
 inflicted by other person
  stated as intentional, homicide (attempt) — see
   Assault, burning, hot object
 liquid (boiling) (hot) NEC X12 ☑
  stated as undetermined whether accidental or intentional Y27.2 ☑
  suicide (attempt) X77.2 ☑
 local application of externally applied substance in
  medical or surgical care Y63.5
 metal (molten) (liquid) (hot) NEC X18 ☑
 self-inflicted X77.9 ☑
 stated as undetermined whether accidental or intentional Y27.8 ☑
 steam X13.1 ☑
  assault X98.0 ☑
  stated as undetermined whether accidental or intentional Y27.0 ☑
  suicide (attempt) X77.0 ☑
 suicide (attempt) X77.9 ☑
 vapor (hot) X13.1 ☑
  assault X98.0 ☑

Scald, scalding — continued
 vapor — continued
  stated as undetermined whether accidental or intentional Y27.0 ☑
  suicide (attempt) X77.0 ☑
Scratched by
 cat W55.03 ☑
 person(s) (accidentally) W50.4 ☑
  with intent to injure or kill Y04.0 ☑
  as, or caused by, a crowd or human stampede (with
   fall) W52 ☑
  assault Y04.0 ☑
  homicide (attempt) Y04.0 ☑
  in
   fight Y04.0 ☑
   legal intervention
    injuring
     bystander Y35.892 ☑
     law enforcement personnel Y35.891 ☑
     suspect Y35.893 ☑
Seasickness T75.3 ☑
Self-harm NEC (see also External cause by type, undetermined whether accidental or intentional)
 intentional — see Suicide
 poisoning NEC — see Table of Drugs and Chemicals,
  poisoning, accidental
Self-inflicted (injury) **NEC** (see also External cause by
 type, undetermined whether accidental or intentional)
 intentional — see Suicide
 poisoning NEC — see Table of Drugs and Chemicals,
  poisoning, accidental
Sequelae (of)
 accident NEC — see W00-X58 with 7th character S
 assault (homicidal) (any means) — see X92-Y08 with
  7th character S
 homicide, attempt (any means) — see X92-Y08 with
  7th character S
 injury undetermined whether accidentally or purposely
  inflicted — see Y21-Y33 with 7th character S
 intentional self-harm (classifiable to X71-X83) — see
  X71-X83 with 7th character S
 legal intervention — see with 7th character S Y35 ☑
 motor vehicle accident — see V00-V99 with 7th character S
 suicide, attempt (any means) — see X71-X83 with 7th
  character S
 transport accident — see V00-V99 with 7th character
  S
 war operations — see War operations
Shock
 electric — see Exposure, electric current
 from electric appliance (any) (faulty) W86.8 ☑
  domestic W86.0 ☑
  suicide (attempt) X83.1 ☑
Shooting, shot (accidental(ly)) (see also Discharge,
 firearm, by type)
 herself or himself — see Discharge, firearm by type,
  self-inflicted
 homicide (attempt) — see Discharge, firearm by type,
  homicide
 in war operations — see War operations
 inflicted by other person — see Discharge, firearm by
  type, homicide
  accidental — see Discharge, firearm, by type of
   firearm
 legal
  execution — see Legal, intervention, firearm
  intervention — see Legal, intervention, firearm
 self-inflicted — see Discharge, firearm by type, suicide
  accidental — see Discharge, firearm, by type of
   firearm
 suicide (attempt) — see Discharge, firearm by type,
  suicide
Shoving (accidentally) **by other person** — see Pushed,
 by other person
Sickness
 alpine W94.11 ☑
 motion — see Motion
 mountain W94.11 ☑
Sinking (accidental)
 watercraft (causing drowning, submersion) (see also
  Drowning, due to, accident to, watercraft, sinking)
  causing injury except drowning or submersion —
   see Accident, watercraft, causing, injury NEC
Siriasis X32 ☑

Sitting (prolonged) (static) X50.1 ☑
Slashed wrists — *see* Cut, self-inflicted
Slipping (accidental) (on same level) (with fall) W01.0 ☑
  without fall W18.40 ☑
    due to
      specified NEC W18.49 ☑
      stepping from one level to another W18.43 ☑
      stepping into hole or opening W18.42 ☑
      stepping on object W18.41 ☑
  on
    ice W00.0 ☑
      with skates — *see* Accident, transport, pedestrian, conveyance
    mud W01.0 ☑
    oil W01.0 ☑
    snow W00.0 ☑
      with skis — *see* Accident, transport, pedestrian, conveyance
    surface (slippery) (wet) NEC W01.0 ☑
Sliver, wood, contact with W45.8 ☑
Smoldering (due to fire) — *see* Exposure, fire
Sodomy (attempted) **by force** T74.2 ☑
Sound waves (causing injury) W42.9 ☑
  supersonic W42.0 ☑
Splinter, contact with W45.8 ☑
Stab, stabbing — *see* Cut
Standing (prolonged) (static) X50.1 ☑
Starvation X58 ☑
Status of external cause Y99.9
  child assisting in compensated work for family Y99.8
  civilian activity done for financial or other compensation Y99.0
  civilian activity done for income or pay Y99.0
  family member assisting in compensated work for other family member Y99.8
  hobby not done for income Y99.8
  leisure activity Y99.8
  military activity Y99.1
  off-duty activity of military personnel Y99.8
  recreation or sport not for income or while a student Y99.8
  specified NEC Y99.8
  student activity Y99.8
  volunteer activity Y99.2
Stepped on
  by
    animal (not being ridden) NEC W55.89 ☑
    crowd or human stampede W52 ☑
    person W50.0 ☑
Stepping on
  object W22.8 ☑
    with fall W18.31 ☑
    sports equipment W21.9 ☑
    stationary W22.09 ☑
      sports equipment W21.89 ☑
  person W51 ☑
    by crowd or human stampede W52 ☑
  sports equipment W21.9 ☑
Sting
  arthropod, nonvenomous W57 ☑
  insect, nonvenomous W57 ☑
Storm (cataclysmic) — *see* Forces of nature, cataclysmic storm
Straining, excessive (*see also* Overexertion) X50.9 ☑
Strangling — *see* Strangulation
Strangulation (accidental) T71 ☑
Strenuous movements (*see also* Overexertion) X50.9 ☑
Striking against
  airbag (automobile) W22.10 ☑
    driver side W22.11 ☑
    front passenger side W22.12 ☑
    specified NEC W22.19 ☑
  bottom when
    diving or jumping into water (in) W16.822 ☑
      causing drowning W16.821 ☑
      from boat W16.722 ☑
        causing drowning W16.721 ☑
      natural body W16.622 ☑
        causing drowning W16.821 ☑
      swimming pool W16.522 ☑
        causing drowning W16.521 ☑
    falling into water (in) W16.322 ☑
      causing drowning W16.321 ☑
      fountain — *see* Striking against, bottom when, falling into water, specified NEC
      natural body W16.122 ☑

Striking against — *continued*
  bottom when — *continued*
    falling into water — *continued*
      natural body — *continued*
        causing drowning W16.121 ☑
      reservoir — *see* Striking against, bottom when, falling into water, specified NEC
      specified NEC W16.322 ☑
        causing drowning W16.321 ☑
      swimming pool W16.022 ☑
        causing drowning W16.021 ☑
  diving board (swimming-pool) W21.4 ☑
  object W22.8 ☑
    with
      drowning or submersion — *see* Drowning
      fall — *see* Fall, due to, bumping against, object
    caused by crowd or human stampede (with fall) W52 ☑
    furniture W22.03 ☑
    lamppost W22.02 ☑
    sports equipment W21.9 ☑
    stationary W22.09 ☑
      sports equipment W21.89 ☑
    wall W22.01 ☑
  person(s) W51 ☑
    with fall W03 ☑
      due to ice or snow W00.0 ☑
    as, or caused by, a crowd or human stampede (with fall) W52 ☑
    assault Y04.2 ☑
    homicide (attempt) Y04.2 ☑
  sports equipment W21.9 ☑
  wall (when) W22.01 ☑
    diving or jumping into water (in) W16.832 ☑
      causing drowning W16.831 ☑
      swimming pool W16.532 ☑
        causing drowning W16.531 ☑
    falling into water (in) W16.332 ☑
      causing drowning W16.331 ☑
      fountain — *see* Striking against, wall when, falling into water, specified NEC
      natural body W16.132 ☑
        causing drowning W16.131 ☑
      reservoir — *see* Striking against, wall when, falling into water, specified NEC
      specified NEC W16.332 ☑
        causing drowning W16.331 ☑
      swimming pool W16.032 ☑
        causing drowning W16.031 ☑
    swimming pool (when) W22.042 ☑
      causing drowning W22.041 ☑
      diving or jumping into water W16.532 ☑
        causing drowning W16.531 ☑
      falling into water W16.032 ☑
        causing drowning W16.031 ☑
Struck (accidentally) **by**
  airbag (automobile) W22.10 ☑
    driver side W22.11 ☑
    front passenger side W22.12 ☑
    specified NEC W22.19 ☑
  alligator W58.02 ☑
  animal (not being ridden) NEC W55.89 ☑
  avalanche — *see* Landslide
  ball (hit) (thrown) W21.00 ☑
    assault Y08.09 ☑
    baseball W21.03 ☑
    basketball W21.05 ☑
    football W21.01 ☑
    golf ball W21.04 ☑
    soccer W21.02 ☑
    softball W21.07 ☑
    specified NEC W21.09 ☑
    volleyball W21.06 ☑
  bat or racquet
    baseball bat W21.11 ☑
      assault Y08.02 ☑
    golf club W21.13 ☑
      assault Y08.09 ☑
    specified NEC W21.19 ☑
      assault Y08.09 ☑
    tennis racquet W21.12 ☑
      assault Y08.09 ☑
  bullet (*see also* Discharge, firearm by type)
    in war operations — *see* War operations
  crocodile W58.12 ☑
  dog W54.1 ☑

Struck (accidentally) **by** — *continued*
  flare, Very pistol — *see* Discharge, firearm NEC
  hailstones X39.8 ☑
  hockey (ice)
    field
      puck W21.221 ☑
      stick W21.211 ☑
    puck W21.220 ☑
    stick W21.210 ☑
      assault Y08.01 ☑
  landslide — *see* Landslide
  law-enforcement agent (on duty) — *see* Legal, intervention, manhandling
    with blunt object — *see* Legal, intervention, blunt object
  lightning T75.0 ☑
    causing fire — *see* Exposure, fire
  machine — *see* Contact, with, by type of machine
  mammal NEC W55.89 ☑
    marine W56.32 ☑
  marine animal W56.82 ☑
  missile
    firearm — *see* Discharge, firearm by type
    in war operations — *see* War operations, missile
  object W22.8 ☑
    blunt W22.8 ☑
      assault Y00 ☑
      suicide (attempt) X79 ☑
      undetermined whether accidental or intentional Y29 ☑
    falling W20.8 ☑
      from, in, on
        building W20.1 ☑
          burning (uncontrolled fire) X00.4 ☑
        cataclysmic
          earth surface movement NEC — *see* Landslide
          storm — *see* Forces of nature, cataclysmic storm
        cave-in W20.0 ☑
        earthquake X34 ☑
        machine (in operation) — *see* Contact, with, by type of machine
        structure W20.1 ☑
          burning X00.4 ☑
        transport vehicle (in motion) — *see* Accident, transport, by type of vehicle
        watercraft V93.49 ☑
          due to
            accident to craft V91.39 ☑
              powered craft V91.33 ☑
                ferry boat V91.31 ☑
                fishing boat V91.32 ☑
                jetskis V91.33 ☑
                liner V91.31 ☑
                merchant ship V91.30 ☑
                passenger ship V91.31 ☑
              unpowered craft V91.38 ☑
                canoe V91.35 ☑
                inflatable V91.36 ☑
                kayak V91.35 ☑
                sailboat V91.34 ☑
                surf-board V91.38 ☑
                windsurfer V91.38 ☑
            powered craft V93.43 ☑
              ferry boat V93.41 ☑
              fishing boat V93.42 ☑
              jetskis V93.43 ☑
              liner V93.41 ☑
              merchant ship V93.40 ☑
              passenger ship V93.41 ☑
            unpowered craft V93.48 ☑
              sailboat V93.44 ☑
              surf-board V93.48 ☑
              windsurfer V93.48 ☑
    moving NEC W20.8 ☑
    projected W20.8 ☑
      assault Y00 ☑
      in sports W21.9 ☑
        assault Y08.09 ☑
        ball W21.00 ☑
          baseball W21.03 ☑
          basketball W21.05 ☑
          football W21.01 ☑
          golf ball W21.04 ☑
          soccer W21.02 ☑

☑ **Additional Character Required** — Refer to the Tabular List for Character Selection   🔻 Subterms under main terms may continue to next column or page

Struck (accidentally) **by** — *continued*
  object — *continued*
    projected — *continued*
      in sports — *continued*
        ball — *continued*
          softball W21.07 ☑
          specified NEC W21.09 ☑
          volleyball W21.06 ☑
        bat or racquet
          baseball bat W21.11 ☑
            assault Y08.02 ☑
          golf club W21.13 ☑
            assault Y08.09 ☑
          specified NEC W21.19 ☑
            assault Y08.09 ☑
          tennis racquet W21.12 ☑
            assault Y08.09 ☑
        hockey (ice)
          field
            puck W21.221 ☑
            stick W21.211 ☑
          puck W21.220 ☑
          stick W21.210 ☑
            assault Y08.01 ☑
        specified NEC W21.89 ☑
    set in motion by explosion — *see* Explosion
    thrown W20.8 ☑
      assault Y00 ☑
      in sports W21.9 ☑
        assault Y08.09 ☑
        ball W21.00 ☑
          baseball W21.03 ☑
          basketball W21.05 ☑
          football W21.01 ☑
          golf ball W21.04 ☑
          soccer W21.02 ☑
          soft ball W21.07 ☑
          specified NEC W21.09 ☑
          volleyball W21.06 ☑
        bat or racquet
          baseball bat W21.11 ☑
            assault Y08.02 ☑
          golf club W21.13 ☑
            assault Y08.09 ☑
          specified NEC W21.19 ☑
            assault Y08.09 ☑
          tennis racquet W21.12 ☑
            assault Y08.09 ☑
        hockey (ice)
          field
            puck W21.221 ☑
            stick W21.211 ☑
          puck W21.220 ☑
          stick W21.210 ☑
            assault Y08.01 ☑
        specified NEC W21.89 ☑
  other person(s) W50.0 ☑
    with
      blunt object W22.8 ☑
      intentional, homicide (attempt) Y00 ☑
      sports equipment W21.9 ☑
      undetermined whether accidental or intentional Y29 ☑
    fall W03 ☑
      due to ice or snow W00.0 ☑
    as, or caused by, a crowd or human stampede (with fall) W52 ☑
    assault Y04.2 ☑
    homicide (attempt) Y04.2 ☑
    in legal intervention
      injuring
        bystander Y35.812 ☑
        law enforcement personnel Y35.811 ☑
        suspect Y35.813 ☑
    sports equipment W21.9 ☑
  police (on duty) — *see* Legal, intervention, manhandling
    with blunt object — *see* Legal, intervention, blunt object
  sports equipment W21.9 ☑
    assault Y08.09 ☑
    ball W21.00 ☑
      baseball W21.03 ☑
      basketball W21.05 ☑
      football W21.01 ☑
      golf ball W21.04 ☑

Struck (accidentally) **by** — *continued*
  sports equipment — *continued*
    ball — *continued*
      soccer W21.02 ☑
      soft ball W21.07 ☑
      specified NEC W21.09 ☑
      volleyball W21.06 ☑
    bat or racquet
      baseball bat W21.11 ☑
        assault Y08.02 ☑
      golf club W21.13 ☑
        assault Y08.09 ☑
      specified NEC W21.19 ☑
      tennis racquet W21.12 ☑
        assault Y08.09 ☑
    cleats (shoe) W21.31 ☑
    foot wear NEC W21.39 ☑
    football helmet W21.81 ☑
    hockey (ice)
      field
        puck W21.221 ☑
        stick W21.211 ☑
      puck W21.220 ☑
      stick W21.210 ☑
        assault Y08.01 ☑
    skate blades W21.32 ☑
    specified NEC W21.89 ☑
      assault Y08.09 ☑
  thunderbolt — *see* subcategory T75.0 ☑
    causing fire — *see* Exposure, fire
  transport vehicle NEC (*see also* Accident, transport) V09.9 ☑
    intentional, homicide (attempt) Y03.0 ☑
    motor NEC (*see also* Accident, transport) V09.20 ☑
      homicide Y03.0 ☑
  vehicle (transport) NEC — *see* Accident, transport, by type of vehicle
    stationary (falling from jack, hydraulic lift, ramp) W20.8 ☑

Stumbling
  without fall W18.40 ☑
    due to
      specified NEC W18.49 ☑
      stepping from one level to another W18.43 ☑
      stepping into hole or opening W18.42 ☑
      stepping on object W18.41 ☑
  over
    animal NEC W01.0 ☑
      with fall W18.09 ☑
    carpet, rug or (small) object W22.8 ☑
      with fall W18.09 ☑
    person W51 ☑
      with fall W03 ☑
        due to ice or snow W00.0 ☑

Submersion (accidental) — *see* Drowning
Suffocation (accidental) (by external means) (by pressure) (mechanical) (*see also* category) T71 ☑
  due to, by
    avalanche — *see* Landslide
    explosion — *see* Explosion
    fire — *see* Exposure, fire
    food, any type (aspiration) (ingestion) (inhalation) — *see* categories T17 and T18
    ignition — *see* Ignition
    landslide — *see* Landslide
    machine(ry) — *see* Contact, with, by type of machine
    vomitus (aspiration) (inhalation) T17.81- ☑
  in
    burning building X00.8 ☑
Suicide, suicidal (attempted) (by) X83.8 ☑
  blunt object X79 ☑
  burning, burns X76 ☑
    hot object X77.9 ☑
      fluid NEC X77.2 ☑
      household appliance X77.3 ☑
      specified NEC X77.8 ☑
      steam X77.0 ☑
      tap water X77.1 ☑
      vapors X77.0 ☑
  caustic substance — *see* Table of Drugs and Chemicals
  cold, extreme X83.2 ☑
  collision of motor vehicle with
    motor vehicle X82.0 ☑
    specified NEC X82.8 ☑
    train X82.1 ☑

Suicide, suicidal — *continued*
  collision of motor vehicle with — *continued*
    tree X82.2 ☑
  crashing of aircraft X83.0 ☑
  cut (any part of body) X78.9 ☑
  cutting or piercing instrument X78.9 ☑
    dagger X78.2 ☑
    glass X78.0 ☑
    knife X78.1 ☑
    specified NEC X78.8 ☑
    sword X78.2 ☑
  drowning (in) X71.9 ☑
    bathtub X71.0 ☑
    natural water X71.3 ☑
    specified NEC X71.8 ☑
    swimming pool X71.1 ☑
      following fall X71.2 ☑
  electrocution X83.1 ☑
  explosive(s) (material) X75 ☑
  fire, flames X76 ☑
  firearm X74.9 ☑
    airgun X74.01 ☑
    handgun X72 ☑
    hunting rifle X73.1 ☑
    larger X73.9 ☑
      specified NEC X73.8 ☑
    machine gun X73.2 ☑
    shotgun X73.0 ☑
    specified NEC X74.8 ☑
  hanging X83.8 ☑
  hot object — *see* Suicide, burning, hot object
  jumping
    before moving object X81.8 ☑
      motor vehicle X81.0 ☑
      subway train X81.1 ☑
      train X81.1 ☑
    from high place X80 ☑
  late effect of attempt — *see* X71-X83 with 7th character S
  lying before moving object, train, vehicle X81.8 ☑
  poisoning — *see* Table of Drugs and Chemicals
  puncture (any part of body) — *see* Suicide, cutting or piercing instrument
  scald — *see* Suicide, burning, hot object
  sequelae of attempt — *see* X71-X83 with 7th character S
  sharp object (any) — *see* Suicide, cutting or piercing instrument
  shooting — *see* Suicide, firearm
  specified means NEC X83.8 ☑
  stab (any part of body) — *see* Suicide, cutting or piercing instrument
  steam, hot vapors X77.0 ☑
  strangulation X83.8 ☑
  submersion — *see* Suicide, drowning
  suffocation X83.8 ☑
  wound NEC X83.8 ☑
Sunstroke X32 ☑
Supersonic waves (causing injury) W42.0 ☑
Surgical procedure, complication of (delayed or as an abnormal reaction without mention of misadventure) (*see also* Complication of or following, by type of procedure)
  due to or as a result of misadventure — *see* Misadventure
Swallowed, swallowing
  foreign body — *see* Foreign body, alimentary canal
  poison — *see* Table of Drugs and Chemicals
  substance
    caustic or corrosive — *see* Table of Drugs and Chemicals
    poisonous — *see* Table of Drugs and Chemicals

T

Tackle in sport W03 ☑
Terrorism (involving) Y38.80 ☑
  biological weapons Y38.6X- ☑
  chemical weapons Y38.7X- ☑
  conflagration Y38.3X- ☑
  drowning and submersion Y38.89- ☑
  explosion Y38.2X- ☑
    destruction of aircraft Y38.1X- ☑
    marine weapons Y38.0X- ☑
  fire Y38.3X- ☑
  firearms Y38.4X- ☑

Terrorism — *continued*
- hot substances Y38.3X- ☑
- lasers Y38.89- ☑
- nuclear weapons Y38.5X- ☑
- piercing or stabbing instruments Y38.89- ☑
- secondary effects Y38.9X- ☑
- specified method NEC Y38.89- ☑
- suicide bomber Y38.81- ☑

Thirst X58 ☑

Threat to breathing
- aspiration — *see* Aspiration
- due to cave-in, falling earth or substance NEC T71 ☑

Thrown (accidentally)
- against part (any) of or object in transport vehicle (in motion) NEC (*see also* Accident, transport)
- from
  - high place, homicide (attempt) Y01 ☑
  - machinery — *see* Contact, with, by type of machine
  - transport vehicle NEC (*see also* Accident, transport) V89.9 ☑
- off — *see* Thrown, from

Thunderbolt — *see* subcategory T75.0 ☑
- causing fire — *see* Exposure, fire

Tidal wave (any injury) **NEC** — *see* Forces of nature, tidal wave

Took
- overdose (drug) — *see* Table of Drugs and Chemicals
- poison — *see* Table of Drugs and Chemicals

Tornado (any injury) X37.1 ☑

Torrential rain (any injury) X37.8 ☑

Torture X58 ☑

Trampled by animal NEC W55.89 ☑

Trapped (accidentally)
- between objects (moving) (stationary and moving) — *see* Caught
- by part (any) of
  - motorcycle V29.88 ☑
  - pedal cycle V19.88 ☑
  - transport vehicle NEC (*see also* Accident, transport) V89.9 ☑

Travel (effects) (sickness) T75.3 ☑

Tree falling on or hitting (accidentally) (person) W20.8 ☑

Tripping
- without fall W18.40 ☑
  - due to
    - specified NEC W18.49 ☑
    - stepping from one level to another W18.43 ☑
    - stepping into hole or opening W18.42 ☑
    - stepping on object W18.41 ☑
  - over
    - animal W01.0 ☑
      - with fall W01.0 ☑
    - carpet, rug or (small) object W22.8 ☑
      - with fall W18.09 ☑
    - person W51 ☑
      - with fall W03 ☑
      - due to ice or snow W00.0 ☑

Twisted by person(s) (accidentally) W50.2 ☑
- with intent to injure or kill Y04.0 ☑
- as, or caused by, a crowd or human stampede (with fall) W52 ☑
- assault Y04.0 ☑
- homicide (attempt) Y04.0 ☑
- in
  - fight Y04.0 ☑
  - legal intervention — *see* Legal, intervention, manhandling

Twisting (prolonged) (static) X50.1- ☑

U

Underdosing of necessary drugs, medicaments or biological substances Y63.6

Undetermined intent (contact) (exposure)
- automobile collision Y32 ☑
- blunt object Y29 ☑
- drowning (submersion) (in) Y21.9 ☑
  - bathtub Y21.0 ☑
    - after fall Y21.1 ☑
  - natural water (lake) (ocean) (pond) (river) (stream) Y21.4 ☑
  - specified place NEC Y21.8 ☑
  - swimming pool Y21.2 ☑
    - after fall Y21.3 ☑
- explosive material Y25 ☑

Undetermined intent — *continued*
- fall, jump or push from high place Y30 ☑
- falling, lying or running before moving object Y31 ☑
- fire Y26 ☑
- firearm discharge Y24.9 ☑
  - airgun (BB) (pellet) Y24.0 ☑
  - handgun (pistol) (revolver) Y22 ☑
  - hunting rifle Y23.1 ☑
  - larger Y23.9 ☑
    - hunting rifle Y23.1 ☑
    - machine gun Y23.3 ☑
    - military Y23.2 ☑
    - shotgun Y23.0 ☑
    - specified type NEC Y23.8 ☑
  - machine gun Y23.3 ☑
  - military Y23.2 ☑
  - shotgun Y23.0 ☑
  - specified type NEC Y24.8 ☑
  - Very pistol Y24.8 ☑
- hot object Y27.9 ☑
  - fluid NEC Y27.2 ☑
  - household appliance Y27.3 ☑
  - specified object NEC Y27.8 ☑
  - steam Y27.0 ☑
  - tap water Y27.1 ☑
  - vapor Y27.0 ☑
- jump, fall or push from high place Y30 ☑
- lying, falling or running before moving object Y31 ☑
- motor vehicle crash Y32 ☑
- push, fall or jump from high place Y30 ☑
- running, falling or lying before moving object Y31 ☑
- sharp object Y28.9 ☑
  - dagger Y28.2 ☑
  - glass Y28.0 ☑
  - knife Y28.1 ☑
  - specified object NEC Y28.8 ☑
  - sword Y28.2 ☑
- smoke Y26 ☑
- specified event NEC Y33 ☑

Use of hand as hammer X50.3 ☑

V

Vibration (causing injury) W49.9 ☑

Victim (of)
- avalanche — *see* Landslide
- earth movements NEC — *see* Forces of nature, earth movement
- earthquake X34 ☑
- flood — *see* Flood
- landslide — *see* Landslide
- lightning — *see* subcategory T75.0 ☑
  - causing fire — *see* Exposure, fire
- storm (cataclysmic) NEC — *see* Forces of nature, cataclysmic storm
- volcanic eruption X35 ☑

Volcanic eruption (any injury) X35 ☑

Vomitus, gastric contents in air passages (with asphyxia, obstruction or suffocation) T17.81- ☑

W

Walked into stationary object (any) W22.09 ☑
- furniture W22.03 ☑
- lamppost W22.02 ☑
- wall W22.01 ☑

War operations (injuries to military personnel and civilians during war, civil insurrection and peacekeeping missions) (by) (from) (involving) Y36.90 ☑
- after cessation of hostilities Y36.89- ☑
  - explosion (of)
    - bomb placed during war operations Y36.82- ☑
    - mine placed during war operations Y36.81- ☑
    - specified NEC Y36.88- ☑
- air blast Y36.20- ☑
- aircraft
  - destruction — *see* War operations, destruction of aircraft
  - airway restriction — *see* War operations, restriction of airways
  - asphyxiation — *see* War operations, restriction of airways
- biological weapons Y36.6X- ☑
- blast Y36.20- ☑
- blast fragments Y36.20- ☑
- blast wave Y36.20- ☑

War operations — *continued*
- blast wind Y36.20- ☑
- bomb Y36.20- ☑
  - dirty Y36.50- ☑
  - gasoline Y36.31- ☑
  - incendiary Y36.31- ☑
  - petrol Y36.31- ☑
- bullet Y36.43- ☑
  - incendiary Y36.32- ☑
  - rubber Y36.41- ☑
- chemical weapons Y36.7X- ☑
- combat
  - hand to hand (unarmed) combat Y36.44- ☑
  - using blunt or piercing object Y36.45- ☑
- conflagration — *see* War operations, fire
- conventional warfare NEC Y36.49- ☑
- depth-charge Y36.01- ☑
- destruction of aircraft Y36.10- ☑
  - due to
    - air to air missile Y36.11- ☑
    - collision with other aircraft Y36.12- ☑
    - detonation (accidental) of onboard munitions and explosives Y36.14- ☑
    - enemy fire or explosives Y36.11- ☑
    - explosive placed on aircraft Y36.11- ☑
    - onboard fire Y36.13- ☑
    - rocket propelled grenade [RPG] Y36.11- ☑
    - small arms fire Y36.11- ☑
    - surface to air missile Y36.11- ☑
    - specified NEC Y36.19- ☑
- detonation (accidental) of
  - onboard marine weapons Y36.05- ☑
  - own munitions or munitions launch device Y36.24- ☑
- dirty bomb Y36.50- ☑
- explosion (of) Y36.20- ☑
  - aerial bomb Y36.21- ☑
  - after cessation of hostilities
    - bomb placed during war operations Y36.82- ☑
    - mine placed during war operations Y36.81- ☑
  - bomb NOS (*see also* War operations, bomb(s)) Y36.20- ☑
  - fragments Y36.20- ☑
  - grenade Y36.29- ☑
  - guided missile Y36.22- ☑
  - improvised explosive device [IED] (person-borne) (roadside) (vehicle-borne) Y36.23- ☑
  - land mine Y36.29- ☑
  - marine mine (at sea) (in harbor) Y36.02- ☑
  - marine weapon Y36.00- ☑
    - specified NEC Y36.09- ☑
  - own munitions or munitions launch device (accidental) Y36.24- ☑
  - sea-based artillery shell Y36.03- ☑
  - specified NEC Y36.29- ☑
  - torpedo Y36.04- ☑
- fire Y36.30- ☑
  - specified NEC Y36.39- ☑
- firearms
  - discharge Y36.43- ☑
  - pellets Y36.42- ☑
- flamethrower Y36.33- ☑
- fragments (from) (of)
  - improvised explosive device [IED] (person-borne) (roadside) (vehicle-borne) Y36.26- ☑
  - munitions Y36.25- ☑
  - specified NEC Y36.29- ☑
  - weapons Y36.27- ☑
- friendly fire Y36.92 ☑
- hand to hand (unarmed) combat Y36.44- ☑
- hot substances — *see* War operations, fire
- incendiary bullet Y36.32- ☑
- nuclear weapon (effects of) Y36.50- ☑
  - acute radiation exposure Y36.54- ☑
  - blast pressure Y36.51- ☑
  - direct blast Y36.51- ☑
  - direct heat Y36.53- ☑
  - fallout exposure Y36.54- ☑
  - fireball Y36.53- ☑
  - indirect blast (struck or crushed by blast debris) (being thrown by blast) Y36.52- ☑
  - ionizing radiation (immediate exposure) Y36.54- ☑
  - nuclear radiation Y36.54- ☑
  - radiation
    - ionizing (immediate exposure) Y36.54- ☑
    - nuclear Y36.54- ☑

War operations — *continued*
  nuclear weapon — *continued*
    radiation — *continued*
      thermal Y36.53- ☑
    secondary effects Y36.54- ☑
    specified NEC Y36.59- ☑
    thermal radiation Y36.53- ☑
  restriction of air (airway)
    intentional Y36.46- ☑
    unintentional Y36.47- ☑
  rubber bullets Y36.41- ☑
  shrapnel NOS Y36.29- ☑
  suffocation — *see* War operations, restriction of airways
  unconventional warfare NEC Y36.7X- ☑
  underwater blast NOS Y36.00- ☑
  warfare
    conventional NEC Y36.49- ☑
    unconventional NEC Y36.7X- ☑

War operations — *continued*
  weapon of mass destruction [WMD] Y36.91 ☑
  weapons
    biological weapons Y36.6X- ☑
    chemical Y36.7X- ☑
    nuclear (effects of) Y36.50- ☑
      acute radiation exposure Y36.54- ☑
      blast pressure Y36.51- ☑
      direct blast Y36.51- ☑
      direct heat Y36.53- ☑
      fallout exposure Y36.54- ☑
      fireball Y36.53- ☑
      radiation
        ionizing (immediate exposure) Y36.54- ☑
        nuclear Y36.54- ☑
        thermal Y36.53- ☑
      secondary effects Y36.54- ☑
      specified NEC Y36.59- ☑
    of mass destruction [WMD] Y36.91 ☑

Washed
  away by flood — *see* Flood
  off road by storm (transport vehicle) — *see* Forces of nature, cataclysmic storm
Weather exposure NEC — *see* Forces of nature
Weightlessness (causing injury) (effects of) (in spacecraft, real or simulated) X52 ☑
Work related condition Y99.0
Wound (accidental) NEC (*see also* Injury) X58 ☑
  battle (*see also* War operations) Y36.90 ☑
  gunshot — *see* Discharge, firearm by type
Wreck transport vehicle NEC (*see also* Accident, transport) V89.9 ☑
Wrong
  device implanted into correct surgical site Y65.51
  fluid in infusion Y65.1
  patient, procedure performed on Y65.52
  procedure (operation) on correct patient Y65.51

Chapter 1. Certain Infectious and Parasitic Diseases (AØØ–B99)

Chapter Specific Guidelines with Coding Examples

The chapter specific guidelines from the ICD-10-CM Official Guidelines for Coding and Reporting have been provided below. Along with these guidelines are coding examples, contained in the shaded boxes, that have been developed to help illustrate the coding and/or sequencing guidance found in these guidelines.

a. Human immunodeficiency virus (HIV) infections

1) Code only confirmed cases

Code only confirmed cases of HIV infection/illness. This is an exception to the hospital inpatient guideline Section II, H.

In this context, "confirmation" does not require documentation of positive serology or culture for HIV; the provider's diagnostic statement that the patient is HIV positive, or has an HIV-related illness is sufficient.

> Patient being seen for hypothyroidism with possible HIV infection
>
> **EØ3.9   Hypothyroidism, unspecified**
>
> *Explanation:* Only the hypothyroidism is coded in this scenario because it has not been confirmed that an HIV infection is present.

2) Selection and sequencing of HIV codes

(a) Patient admitted for HIV-related condition

If a patient is admitted for an HIV-related condition, the principal diagnosis should be B2Ø, Human immunodeficiency virus [HIV] disease followed by additional diagnosis codes for all reported HIV-related conditions.

> HIV with CMV
>
> **B2Ø   Human immunodeficiency virus [HIV] disease**
>
> **B25.9   Cytomegaloviral disease, unspecified**
>
> *Explanation:* Cytomegaloviral infection is an HIV related condition, so the HIV diagnosis code is reported first, followed by the code for the CMV.

(b) Patient with HIV disease admitted for unrelated condition

If a patient with HIV disease is admitted for an unrelated condition (such as a traumatic injury), the code for the unrelated condition (e.g., the nature of injury code) should be the principal diagnosis. Other diagnoses would be B2Ø followed by additional diagnosis codes for all reported HIV-related conditions.

> Sprain of the internal collateral ligament, right ankle; HIV
>
> **S93.491A   Sprain of other ligament of right ankle, initial encounter**
>
> **B2Ø   Human immunodeficiency virus [HIV] disease**
>
> *Explanation:* The ankle sprain is not related to HIV, so it is the first-listed diagnosis code, and HIV is reported secondarily.

(c) Whether the patient is newly diagnosed

Whether the patient is newly diagnosed or has had previous admissions/encounters for HIV conditions is irrelevant to the sequencing decision.

> Newly diagnosed multiple cutaneous Kaposi's sarcoma lesions in previously diagnosed HIV disease
>
> **B2Ø   Human immunodeficiency virus [HIV] disease**
>
> **C46.Ø   Kaposi's sarcoma of skin**
>
> *Explanation:* Even though the HIV was diagnosed on a previous encounter, it is still sequenced first when coded with an HIV related condition. Kaposi's sarcoma is an HIV-related condition.

(d) Asymptomatic human immunodeficiency virus

Z21, Asymptomatic human immunodeficiency virus [HIV] infection status, is to be applied when the patient without any documentation of symptoms is listed as being "HIV positive," "known HIV," "HIV test positive," or similar terminology. Do not use this code if the term "AIDS" is used or if the patient is treated for any HIV-related illness or is described as having any condition(s) resulting from his/her HIV positive status; use B2Ø in these cases.

> Patient is being seen for iron deficiency anemia. Status positive HIV test on Atripla, with no prior symptoms
>
> **D5Ø.9   Iron deficiency anemia, unspecified**
>
> **Z21   Asymptomatic human immunodeficiency virus [HIV] infection status**
>
> *Explanation:* Code Z21 is sequenced second since documentation indicates that the patient has had a positive HIV test but has been asymptomatic. Being on medication for HIV is not an indication that code B2Ø is used instead of Z21. Unless there has been documentation that the patient has had current or prior symptoms or HIV-related complications, code B2Ø is not used. The anemia is not an AIDS-related complication and is sequenced first.

(e) Patients with inconclusive HIV serology

Patients with inconclusive HIV serology, but no definitive diagnosis or manifestations of the illness, may be assigned code R75, Inconclusive laboratory evidence of human immunodeficiency virus [HIV].

(f) Previously diagnosed HIV-related illness

Patients with any known prior diagnosis of an HIV-related illness should be coded to B2Ø. Once a patient has developed an HIV-related illness, the patient should always be assigned code B2Ø on every subsequent admission/encounter. Patients previously diagnosed with any HIV illness (B2Ø) should never be assigned to R75 or Z21, Asymptomatic human immunodeficiency virus [HIV] infection status.

(g) HIV infection in pregnancy, childbirth and the puerperium

During pregnancy, childbirth or the puerperium, a patient admitted (or presenting for a health care encounter) because of an HIV-related illness should receive a principal diagnosis code of O98.7-, Human immunodeficiency [HIV] disease complicating pregnancy, childbirth and the puerperium, followed by B2Ø and the code(s) for the HIV-related illness(es). Codes from Chapter 15 always take sequencing priority.

Patients with asymptomatic HIV infection status admitted (or presenting for a health care encounter) during pregnancy, childbirth, or the puerperium should receive codes of O98.7- and Z21.

(h) Encounters for testing for HIV

If a patient is being seen to determine his/her HIV status, use code Z11.4, Encounter for screening for human immunodeficiency virus [HIV]. Use additional codes for any associated high risk behavior.

If a patient with signs or symptoms is being seen for HIV testing, code the signs and symptoms. An additional counseling code Z71.7, Human immunodeficiency virus [HIV] counseling, may be used if counseling is provided during the encounter for the test.

When a patient returns to be informed of his/her HIV test results and the test result is negative, use code Z71.7, Human immunodeficiency virus [HIV] counseling.

If the results are positive, see previous guidelines and assign codes as appropriate.

b. Infectious agents as the cause of diseases classified to other chapters

Certain infections are classified in chapters other than Chapter 1 and no organism is identified as part of the infection code. In these instances, it is necessary to use an additional code from Chapter 1 to identify the organism. A code from category B95, Streptococcus, Staphylococcus, and Enterococcus as the cause of diseases classified to other chapters, B96, Other bacterial agents as the cause of diseases classified to other chapters, or B97, Viral agents as the cause of diseases classified to other chapters, is to be used as an additional code to identify the organism. An instructional note will be found at the infection code advising that an additional organism code is required.

Acute *E. coli* cystitis

N30.00	**Acute cystitis without hematuria**
B96.20	**Unspecified Escherichia coli [E.coli] as the cause of diseases classified elsewhere**

Explanation: An instructional note under the category for the cystitis indicates to code also the specific organism.

c. Infections resistant to antibiotics

Many bacterial infections are resistant to current antibiotics. It is necessary to identify all infections documented as antibiotic resistant. Assign a code from category Z16, Resistance to antimicrobial drugs, following the infection code only if the infection code does not identify drug resistance.

Penicillin-resistant *Streptococcus pneumoniae* pneumonia

J13	**Pneumonia due to Streptococcus pneumoniae**
Z16.11	**Resistance to penicillins**

Explanation: Code Z16.11 is assigned as a secondary code to represent the penicillin resistance. This code includes resistance to amoxicillin and ampicillin.

d. Sepsis, severe sepsis, and septic shock

1) Coding of Sepsis and Severe Sepsis

(a) Sepsis

For a diagnosis of sepsis, assign the appropriate code for the underlying systemic infection. If the type of infection or causal organism is not further specified, assign code A41.9, Sepsis, unspecified organism.

A code from subcategory R65.2, Severe sepsis, should not be assigned unless severe sepsis or an associated acute organ dysfunction is documented.

Gram-negative sepsis

A41.50	**Gram-negative sepsis, unspecified**

Staphylococcal sepsis

A41.2	**Sepsis due to unspecified staphylococcus**

Explanation: In both examples above the organism causing the sepsis is identified, therefore A41.9 Sepsis, unspecified organism, would not be appropriate as this code would not capture the highest degree of specificity found in the documentation. Do not use an additional code for severe sepsis unless an acute organ dysfunction was also documented as "associated with" or "due to" the sepsis or the sepsis was documented as "severe."

(i) Negative or inconclusive blood cultures and sepsis

Negative or inconclusive blood cultures do not preclude a diagnosis of sepsis in patients with clinical evidence of the condition; however, the provider should be queried.

(ii) Urosepsis

The term urosepsis is a nonspecific term. It is not to be considered synonymous with sepsis. It has no default code in the Alphabetic Index. Should a provider use this term, he/she must be queried for clarification.

(iii) Sepsis with organ dysfunction

If a patient has sepsis and associated acute organ dysfunction or multiple organ dysfunction (MOD), follow the instructions for coding severe sepsis.

(iv) Acute organ dysfunction that is not clearly associated with the sepsis

If a patient has sepsis and an acute organ dysfunction, but the medical record documentation indicates that the acute organ dysfunction is related to a medical condition other than the sepsis, do not assign a code from subcategory R65.2, Severe sepsis. An acute organ dysfunction must be associated with the sepsis in order to assign the severe sepsis code. If the documentation is not clear as to whether an acute organ dysfunction is related to the sepsis or another medical condition, query the provider.

Sepsis and acute respiratory failure due to COPD exacerbation

A41.9	**Sepsis, unspecified organism**
J44.1	**Chronic obstructive pulmonary disease with (acute) exacerbation**
J96.00	**Acute respiratory failure, unspecified whether with hypoxia or hypercapnia**

Explanation: Although acute organ dysfunction is present in the form of acute respiratory failure, severe sepsis (R65.2) is not coded in this example, as the acute respiratory failure is attributed to the COPD exacerbation rather than the sepsis. Sequencing of these codes would be determined by the reason for the encounter.

(b) Severe sepsis

The coding of severe sepsis requires a minimum of 2 codes: first a code for the underlying systemic infection, followed by a code from subcategory R65.2, Severe sepsis. If the causal organism is not documented, assign code A41.9, Sepsis, unspecified organism, for the infection. Additional code(s) for the associated acute organ dysfunction are also required.

Due to the complex nature of severe sepsis, some cases may require querying the provider prior to assignment of the codes.

2) Septic shock

(a) Septic shock generally refers to circulatory failure associated with severe sepsis, and therefore, it represents a type of acute organ dysfunction.

For cases of septic shock, the code for the systemic infection should be sequenced first, followed by code R65.21, Severe sepsis with septic shock or code T81.12, Postprocedural septic shock. Any additional codes for the other acute organ dysfunctions should also be assigned. As noted in the sequencing instructions in the Tabular List, the code for septic shock cannot be assigned as a principal diagnosis.

Sepsis with septic shock

A41.9	**Sepsis, unspecified organism**
R65.21	**Severe sepsis with septic shock**

Explanation: Documentation of septic shock automatically implies severe sepsis as it is a form of acute organ dysfunction. Septic shock is not coded as the first-listed diagnosis; it is always preceded by the code for the systemic infection.

3) Sequencing of severe sepsis

If severe sepsis is present on admission, and meets the definition of principal diagnosis, the underlying systemic infection should be assigned as principal diagnosis followed by the appropriate code from subcategory R65.2 as required by the sequencing rules in the Tabular List. A code from subcategory R65.2 can never be assigned as a principal diagnosis.

When severe sepsis develops during an encounter (it was not present on admission), the underlying systemic infection and the appropriate code from subcategory R65.2 should be assigned as secondary diagnoses.

Severe sepsis may be present on admission, but the diagnosis may not be confirmed until sometime after admission. If the documentation is not clear whether severe sepsis was present on admission, the provider should be queried.

4) Sepsis and severe sepsis with a localized infection

If the reason for admission is both sepsis or severe sepsis and a localized infection, such as pneumonia or cellulitis, a code(s) for the underlying systemic infection should be assigned first and the code for the localized infection should be assigned as a secondary diagnosis. If the patient has severe sepsis, a code from subcategory R65.2 should also be assigned as a secondary diagnosis. If the patient is admitted with a localized infection, such as pneumonia, and sepsis/severe sepsis doesn't develop until after admission, the localized infection should be assigned first, followed by the appropriate sepsis/severe sepsis codes.

Patient presents with acute renal failure due to severe sepsis from *Pseudomonas pneumonia*

A41.52	**Sepsis, due to Pseudomonas**
J15.1	**Pneumonia due to Pseudomonas**
R65.2Ø	**Severe sepsis without septic shock**
N17.9	**Acute kidney failure, unspecified**

Explanation: If all conditions are present, the systemic infection (sepsis) is sequenced first followed by the codes for the localized infection (pneumonia), severe sepsis and any organ dysfunction.

5) Sepsis due to a postprocedural infection

(a) Documentation of causal relationship

As with all postprocedural complications, code assignment is based on the provider's documentation of the relationship between the infection and the procedure.

(b) Sepsis due to a postprocedural infection

For such cases, the postprocedural infection code, such as T8Ø.2, Infections following infusion, transfusion, and therapeutic injection, T81.4, Infection following a procedure, T88.Ø, Infection following immunization, or O86.Ø, Infection of obstetric surgical wound, should be coded first, followed by the code for the specific infection. If the patient has severe sepsis, the appropriate code from subcategory R65.2 should also be assigned with the additional code(s) for any acute organ dysfunction.

(c) Postprocedural infection and postprocedural septic shock

In cases where a postprocedural infection has occurred and has resulted in severe sepsis the code for the precipitating complication such as code T81.4, Infection following a procedure, or O86.Ø, Infection of obstetrical surgical wound should be coded first followed by code R65.2Ø, Severe sepsis without septic shock. A code for the systemic infection should also be assigned.

If a postprocedural infection has resulted in postprocedural septic shock, the code for the precipitating complication such as code T81.4, Infection following a procedure, or O86.Ø, Infection of obstetrical surgical wound should be coded first followed by code T81.12-, Postprocedural septic shock. A code for the systemic infection should also be assigned.

6) Sepsis and severe sepsis associated with a noninfectious process (condition)

In some cases a noninfectious process (condition), such as trauma, may lead to an infection which can result in sepsis or severe sepsis. If sepsis or severe sepsis is documented as associated with a noninfectious condition, such as a burn or serious injury, and this condition meets the definition for principal diagnosis, the code for the noninfectious condition should be sequenced first, followed by the code for the resulting infection. If severe sepsis is present, a code from subcategory R65.2 should also be assigned with any associated organ dysfunction(s) codes. It is not necessary to assign a code from subcategory R65.1, Systemic inflammatory response syndrome (SIRS) of non-infectious origin, for these cases.

If the infection meets the definition of principal diagnosis, it should be sequenced before the non-infectious condition. When both the associated non-infectious condition and the infection meet the definition of principal diagnosis, either may be assigned as principal diagnosis.

Only one code from category R65, Symptoms and signs specifically associated with systemic inflammation and infection, should be assigned. Therefore, when a non-infectious condition leads to an infection resulting in severe sepsis, assign the appropriate code from subcategory R65.2, Severe sepsis. Do not additionally assign a code from subcategory R65.1, Systemic inflammatory response syndrome (SIRS) of non-infectious origin.

See Section I.C.18. SIRS due to non-infectious process

7) Sepsis and septic shock complicating abortion, pregnancy, childbirth, and the puerperium

See Section I.C.15. Sepsis and septic shock complicating abortion, pregnancy, childbirth and the puerperium

8) Newborn sepsis

See Section I.C.16. f. Bacterial sepsis of Newborn

e. Methicillin resistant *Staphylococcus aureus* (MRSA) conditions

1) Selection and sequencing of MRSA codes

(a) Combination codes for MRSA infection

When a patient is diagnosed with an infection that is due to methicillin resistant *Staphylococcus aureus* (MRSA), and that infection has a combination code that includes the causal organism (e.g., sepsis, pneumonia) assign the appropriate combination code for the condition (e.g., code A41.Ø2, Sepsis due to Methicillin resistant Staphylococcus aureus or code J15.212, Pneumonia due to Methicillin resistant Staphylococcus aureus). Do not assign code B95.62, Methicillin resistant Staphylococcus aureus infection as the cause of diseases classified elsewhere, as an additional code, because the combination code includes the type of infection and the MRSA organism. Do not assign a code from subcategory Z16.11, Resistance to penicillins, as an additional diagnosis.

See Section C.1. for instructions on coding and sequencing of sepsis and severe sepsis.

(b) Other codes for MRSA infection

When there is documentation of a current infection (e.g., wound infection, stitch abscess, urinary tract infection) due to MRSA, and that infection does not have a combination code that includes the causal organism, assign the appropriate code to identify the condition along with code B95.62, Methicillin resistant Staphylococcus aureus infection as the cause of diseases classified elsewhere for the MRSA infection. Do not assign a code from subcategory Z16.11, Resistance to penicillins.

(c) Methicillin susceptible Staphylococcus aureus (MSSA) and MRSA colonization

The condition or state of being colonized or carrying MSSA or MRSA is called colonization or carriage, while an individual person is described as being colonized or being a carrier. Colonization means that MSSA or MSRA is present on or in the body without necessarily causing illness. A positive MRSA colonization test might be documented by the provider as "MRSA screen positive" or "MRSA nasal swab positive".

Assign code Z22.322, Carrier or suspected carrier of Methicillin resistant Staphylococcus aureus, for patients documented as having MRSA colonization. Assign code Z22.321, Carrier or suspected carrier of Methicillin susceptible Staphylococcus aureus, for patient documented as having MSSA colonization. Colonization is not necessarily indicative of a disease process or as the cause of a specific condition the patient may have unless documented as such by the provider.

(d) MRSA colonization and infection

If a patient is documented as having both MRSA colonization and infection during a hospital admission, code Z22.322, Carrier or suspected carrier of Methicillin resistant Staphylococcus aureus, and a code for the MRSA infection may both be assigned.

f. Zika virus infections

1) Code only confirmed cases

Code only a confirmed diagnosis of Zika virus (A92.5, Zika virus disease) as documented by the provider. This is an exception to the hospital inpatient guideline Section II, H.

In this context, "confirmation" does not require documentation of the type of test performed; the physician's diagnostic statement that the condition is confirmed is sufficient. This code should be assigned regardless of the stated mode of transmission.

If the provider documents "suspected", "possible" or "probable" Zika, do not assign code A92.5. Assign a code(s) explaining the reason for encounter (such as fever, rash, or joint pain) or Z20.828, Contact with and (suspected) exposure to other viral communicable diseases.

Chapter 1. Certain Infectious and Parasitic Diseases (A00-B99)

INCLUDES diseases generally recognized as communicable or transmissible

Use additional code to identify resistance to antimicrobial drugs (Z16.-)

EXCLUDES 1 certain localized infections—see body system-related chapters

EXCLUDES 2 carrier or suspected carrier of infectious disease (Z22.-)

infectious and parasitic diseases specific to the perinatal period (P35-P39)

infectious and parasitic diseases complicating pregnancy, childbirth and the puerperium (O98.-)

influenza and other acute respiratory infections (J00-J22)

This chapter contains the following blocks:

A00-A09 Intestinal infectious diseases
A15-A19 Tuberculosis
A20-A28 Certain zoonotic bacterial diseases
A30-A49 Other bacterial diseases
A50-A64 Infections with a predominantly sexual mode of transmission
A65-A69 Other spirochetal diseases
A70-A74 Other diseases caused by chlamydiae
A75-A79 Rickettsioses
A80-A89 Viral infections of the central nervous system
A90-A99 Arthropod-borne viral fevers and viral hemorrhagic fevers
B00-B09 Viral infections characterized by skin and mucous membrane lesions
B10   Other human herpesviruses
B15-B19 Viral hepatitis
B20   Human immunodeficiency virus [HIV] disease
B25-B34 Other viral diseases
B35-B49 Mycoses
B50-B64 Protozoal diseases
B65-B83 Helminthiases
B85-B89 Pediculosis, acariasis and other infestations
B90-B94 Sequelae of infectious and parasitic diseases
B95-B97 Bacterial and viral infectious agents
B99   Other infectious diseases

Intestinal Infectious Diseases (A00-A09)

✓4ᵗʰ **A00 Cholera**

A00.0 Cholera due to Vibrio cholerae 01, biovar cholerae
Classical cholera

A00.1 Cholera due to Vibrio cholerae 01, biovar eltor
Cholera eltor

A00.9 Cholera, unspecified ▽

✓4ᵗʰ **A01 Typhoid and paratyphoid fevers**
DEF: Typhoid fever: An acute generalized illness caused by *Salmonella typhi*; clinical features are fever, headache, abdominal pain, cough, toxemia, leukopenia, abnormal pulse, rose spots on the skin, bacteremia, hyperplasia of intestinal lymph nodes, mesenteric lymphadenopathy, and Peyer's patches in the intestines.
DEF: Paratyphoid fever: A prolonged febrile illness, caused by *Salmonella* serotypes other than *S. typhi*, especially *S. enterica* serotypes paratyphi A, B, and C.

✓5ᵗʰ **A01.0 Typhoid fever**
Infection due to Salmonella typhi

A01.00 Typhoid fever, unspecified ▽

A01.01 Typhoid meningitis

A01.02 Typhoid fever with heart involvement
Typhoid endocarditis
Typhoid myocarditis

A01.03 Typhoid pneumonia HCC

A01.04 Typhoid arthritis HCC

A01.05 Typhoid osteomyelitis HCC

A01.09 Typhoid fever with other complications

A01.1 Paratyphoid fever A

A01.2 Paratyphoid fever B

A01.3 Paratyphoid fever C

A01.4 Paratyphoid fever, unspecified ▽
Infection due to Salmonella paratyphi NOS

✓4ᵗʰ **A02 Other salmonella infections**
INCLUDES infection or foodborne intoxication due to any Salmonella species other than S. typhi and S. paratyphi

A02.0 Salmonella enteritis
Salmonellosis

A02.1 Salmonella sepsis HCC

✓5ᵗʰ **A02.2 Localized salmonella infections**

A02.20 Localized salmonella infection, unspecified ▽

A02.21 Salmonella meningitis

A02.22 Salmonella pneumonia HCC

A02.23 Salmonella arthritis HCC

A02.24 Salmonella osteomyelitis HCC

A02.25 Salmonella pyelonephritis
Salmonella tubulo-interstitial nephropathy

A02.29 Salmonella with other localized infection

A02.8 Other specified salmonella infections

A02.9 Salmonella infection, unspecified ▽

✓4ᵗʰ **A03 Shigellosis**
DEF: Infection caused by the genus *Shigella*, of the family *Enterobacteriaceae*; known to cause an acute dysenteric infection of the bowel with fever, drowsiness, anorexia, nausea, vomiting, bloody diarrhea, abdominal cramps, and distention.

A03.0 Shigellosis due to Shigella dysenteriae
Group A shigellosis [Shiga-Kruse dysentery]

A03.1 Shigellosis due to Shigella flexneri
Group B shigellosis

A03.2 Shigellosis due to Shigella boydii
Group C shigellosis

A03.3 Shigellosis due to Shigella sonnei
Group D shigellosis

A03.8 Other shigellosis

A03.9 Shigellosis, unspecified ▽
Bacillary dysentery NOS

✓4ᵗʰ **A04 Other bacterial intestinal infections**
EXCLUDES 1 bacterial foodborne intoxications, NEC (A05.-)
tuberculous enteritis (A18.32)

A04.0 Enteropathogenic Escherichia coli infection

A04.1 Enterotoxigenic Escherichia coli infection

A04.2 Enteroinvasive Escherichia coli infection

A04.3 Enterohemorrhagic Escherichia coli infection
DEF: *E. coli* infection penetrating the intestinal mucosa, producing microscopic ulceration and bleeding.

A04.4 Other intestinal Escherichia coli infections
Escherichia coli enteritis NOS

A04.5 Campylobacter enteritis

A04.6 Enteritis due to Yersinia enterocolitica
EXCLUDES 1 extraintestinal yersiniosis (A28.2)

✓5ᵗʰ **A04.7 Enterocolitis due to Clostridium difficile**
Foodborne intoxication by Clostridium difficile
Pseudomembraneous colitis

● **A04.71 Enterocolitis due to Clostridium difficile, recurrent**

● **A04.72 Enterocolitis due to Clostridium difficile, not specified as recurrent**

A04.8 Other specified bacterial intestinal infections

A04.9 Bacterial intestinal infection, unspecified ▽
Bacterial enteritis NOS

✓4ᵗʰ **A05 Other bacterial foodborne intoxications, not elsewhere classified**
EXCLUDES 1 Clostridium difficile foodborne intoxication and infection ►(A04.7-)◄
Escherichia coli infection (A04.0-A04.4)
listeriosis (A32.-)
salmonella foodborne intoxication and infection (A02.-)
toxic effect of noxious foodstuffs (T61-T62)

A05.0 Foodborne staphylococcal intoxication

A05.1 Botulism food poisoning
Botulism NOS
Classical foodborne intoxication due to Clostridium botulinum
EXCLUDES 1 infant botulism (A48.51)
wound botulism (A48.52)

A05.2 Foodborne Clostridium perfringens [Clostridium welchii] intoxication
Enteritis necroticans
Pig-bel

A05.3 Foodborne Vibrio parahaemolyticus intoxication

A05.4 Foodborne Bacillus cereus intoxication

A05.5 Foodborne Vibrio vulnificus intoxication

A05.8 Other specified bacterial foodborne intoxications

A05.9 Bacterial foodborne intoxication, unspecified ▽

EXCLUDES 1 Not coded here   EXCLUDES 2 Not included here   N Newborn Age: 0   P Pediatric Age: 0-17   M Maternity Age: 12-55   A Adult Age: 15-124

436   ICD-10-CM 2018

☑4ᵗʰ **A06 Amebiasis**

    INCLUDES   infection due to Entamoeba histolytica
    EXCLUDES 1   *other protozoal intestinal diseases (A07.-)*
    EXCLUDES 2   *acanthamebiasis (B60.1-)*
         Naegleriasis (B60.2)

A06.0 Acute amebic dysentery
     Acute amebiasis
     Intestinal amebiasis NOS

A06.1 Chronic intestinal amebiasis

A06.2 Amebic nondysenteric colitis

A06.3 Ameboma of intestine
     Ameboma NOS

A06.4 Amebic liver abscess
     Hepatic amebiasis

A06.5 Amebic lung abscess   HCC
     Amebic abscess of lung (and liver)

A06.6 Amebic brain abscess
     Amebic abscess of brain (and liver) (and lung)

A06.7 Cutaneous amebiasis

☑5ᵗʰ **A06.8 Amebic infection of other sites**

    A06.81 Amebic cystitis

    A06.82 Other amebic genitourinary infections
         Amebic balanitis
         Amebic vesiculitis
         Amebic vulvovaginitis

    A06.89 Other amebic infections
         Amebic appendicitis
         Amebic splenic abscess

A06.9 Amebiasis, unspecified ▽

☑4ᵗʰ **A07 Other protozoal intestinal diseases**

A07.0 Balantidiasis
     Balantidial dysentery

A07.1 Giardiasis [lambliasis]

A07.2 Cryptosporidiosis   HCC

A07.3 Isosporiasis
     Infection due to Isospora belli and Isospora hominis
     Intestinal coccidiosis
     Isosporosis

A07.4 Cyclosporiasis

A07.8 Other specified protozoal intestinal diseases
     Intestinal microsporidiosis
     Intestinal trichomoniasis
     Sarcocystosis
     Sarcosporidiosis

A07.9 Protozoal intestinal disease, unspecified ▽
     Flagellate diarrhea
     Protozoal colitis
     Protozoal diarrhea
     Protozoal dysentery

☑4ᵗʰ **A08 Viral and other specified intestinal infections**

    EXCLUDES 1   *influenza with involvement of gastrointestinal tract (J09.X3, J10.2, J11.2)*

A08.0 Rotaviral enteritis

☑5ᵗʰ **A08.1 Acute gastroenteropathy due to Norwalk agent and other small round viruses**

    A08.11 Acute gastroenteropathy due to Norwalk agent
         Acute gastroenteropathy due to Norovirus
         Acute gastroenteropathy due to Norwalk-like agent

    A08.19 Acute gastroenteropathy due to other small round viruses
         Acute gastroenteropathy due to small round virus [SRV] NOS

A08.2 Adenoviral enteritis

☑5ᵗʰ **A08.3 Other viral enteritis**

    A08.31 Calicivirus enteritis

    A08.32 Astrovirus enteritis

    A08.39 Other viral enteritis
         Coxsackie virus enteritis
         Echovirus enteritis
         Enterovirus enteritis NEC
         Torovirus enteritis

A08.4 Viral intestinal infection, unspecified ▽
     Viral enteritis NOS
     Viral gastroenteritis NOS
     Viral gastroenteropathy NOS
     AHA: 2016, 3Q, 12

A08.8 Other specified intestinal infections

A09 Infectious gastroenteritis and colitis, unspecified ▽
     Infectious colitis NOS
     Infectious enteritis NOS
     Infectious gastroenteritis NOS
    EXCLUDES 1   *colitis NOS (K52.9)*
         diarrhea NOS (R19.7)
         enteritis NOS (K52.9)
         gastroenteritis NOS (K52.9)
         noninfective gastroenteritis and colitis, unspecified (K52.9)
DEF: Colitis: An inflammation of mucous membranes of the colon.
DEF: Enteritis: An inflammation of mucous membranes of the small intestine.
DEF: Gastroenteritis: An inflammation of mucous membranes of stomach and intestines.

Tuberculosis (A15-A19)

    INCLUDES   infections due to Mycobacterium tuberculosis and Mycobacterium bovis
    EXCLUDES 1   *congenital tuberculosis (P37.0)*
         nonspecific reaction to test for tuberculosis without active tuberculosis (R76.1-)
         pneumoconiosis associated with tuberculosis, any type in A15 (J65)
         positive PPD (R76.11)
         positive tuberculin skin test without active tuberculosis (R76.11)
         sequelae of tuberculosis (B90.-)
         silicotuberculosis (J65)

☑4ᵗʰ **A15 Respiratory tuberculosis**

A15.0 Tuberculosis of lung
     Tuberculous bronchiectasis
     Tuberculous fibrosis of lung
     Tuberculous pneumonia
     Tuberculous pneumothorax

A15.4 Tuberculosis of intrathoracic lymph nodes
     Tuberculosis of hilar lymph nodes
     Tuberculosis of mediastinal lymph nodes
     Tuberculosis of tracheobronchial lymph nodes
    EXCLUDES 1   *tuberculosis specified as primary (A15.7)*

A15.5 Tuberculosis of larynx, trachea and bronchus
     Tuberculosis of bronchus   Tuberculosis of larynx
     Tuberculosis of glottis   Tuberculosis of trachea

A15.6 Tuberculous pleurisy
     Tuberculosis of pleura   Tuberculous empyema
    EXCLUDES 1   *primary respiratory tuberculosis (A15.7)*

A15.7 Primary respiratory tuberculosis

A15.8 Other respiratory tuberculosis
     Mediastinal tuberculosis
     Nasopharyngeal tuberculosis
     Tuberculosis of nose
     Tuberculosis of sinus [any nasal]

A15.9 Respiratory tuberculosis unspecified ▽

☑4ᵗʰ **A17 Tuberculosis of nervous system**

A17.0 Tuberculous meningitis
     Tuberculosis of meninges (cerebral) (spinal)
     Tuberculous leptomeningitis
    EXCLUDES 1   *tuberculous meningoencephalitis (A17.82)*

A17.1 Meningeal tuberculoma
     Tuberculoma of meninges (cerebral) (spinal)
    EXCLUDES 2   *tuberculoma of brain and spinal cord (A17.81)*

Tuberculosis of Lung

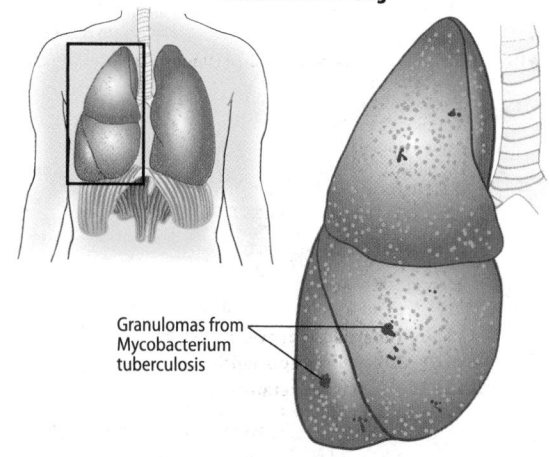

Granulomas from Mycobacterium tuberculosis

☑ Additional Character Req   ✔x7ᵗʰ Placeholder Alert   Manifestation   HCC CMS-HCC Condition   ▽ Unspecified Code   ▶◀ Revised Text   ● New Code   ▲ Revised Code Title

✓5ᵗʰ A17.8 Other tuberculosis of nervous system

A17.81 Tuberculoma of brain and spinal cord
Tuberculous abscess of brain and spinal cord

A17.82 Tuberculous meningoencephalitis
Tuberculous myelitis

A17.83 Tuberculous neuritis
Tuberculous mononeuropathy

A17.89 Other tuberculosis of nervous system
Tuberculous polyneuropathy

A17.9 Tuberculosis of nervous system, unspecified ▽

✓4ᵗʰ A18 Tuberculosis of other organs

✓5ᵗʰ A18.0 Tuberculosis of bones and joints

A18.01 Tuberculosis of spine
Pott's disease or curvature of spine
Tuberculous arthritis
Tuberculous osteomyelitis of spine
Tuberculous spondylitis

A18.02 Tuberculous arthritis of other joints
Tuberculosis of hip (joint)
Tuberculosis of knee (joint)

A18.03 Tuberculosis of other bones
Tuberculous mastoiditis
Tuberculous osteomyelitis

A18.09 Other musculoskeletal tuberculosis
Tuberculous myositis
Tuberculous synovitis
Tuberculous tenosynovitis

✓5ᵗʰ A18.1 Tuberculosis of genitourinary system

A18.10 Tuberculosis of genitourinary system, unspecified ▽

A18.11 Tuberculosis of kidney and ureter

A18.12 Tuberculosis of bladder

A18.13 Tuberculosis of other urinary organs
Tuberculous urethritis

A18.14 Tuberculosis of prostate Ⓐ♂

A18.15 Tuberculosis of other male genital organs ♂

A18.16 Tuberculosis of cervix ♀

A18.17 Tuberculous female pelvic inflammatory disease ♀
Tuberculous endometritis
Tuberculous oophoritis and salpingitis

A18.18 Tuberculosis of other female genital organs ♀
Tuberculous ulceration of vulva

A18.2 Tuberculous peripheral lymphadenopathy
Tuberculous adenitis
EXCLUDES 2 tuberculosis of bronchial and mediastinal lymph nodes (A15.4)
tuberculosis of mesenteric and retroperitoneal lymph nodes (A18.39)
tuberculous tracheobronchial adenopathy (A15.4)

✓5ᵗʰ A18.3 Tuberculosis of intestines, peritoneum and mesenteric glands

A18.31 Tuberculous peritonitis
Tuberculous ascites
DEF: Tuberculous inflammation of the membrane lining the abdomen.

A18.32 Tuberculous enteritis
Tuberculosis of anus and rectum
Tuberculosis of intestine (large) (small)

A18.39 Retroperitoneal tuberculosis
Tuberculosis of mesenteric glands
Tuberculosis of retroperitoneal (lymph glands)

A18.4 Tuberculosis of skin and subcutaneous tissue
Erythema induratum, tuberculous
Lupus excedens
Lupus vulgaris NOS
Lupus vulgaris of eyelid
Scrofuloderma
Tuberculosis of external ear
EXCLUDES 2 lupus erythematosus (L93.-)
lupus NOS (M32.9)
systemic (M32.-)

✓5ᵗʰ A18.5 Tuberculosis of eye
EXCLUDES 2 lupus vulgaris of eyelid (A18.4)

A18.50 Tuberculosis of eye, unspecified ▽

A18.51 Tuberculous episcleritis

A18.52 Tuberculous keratitis
Tuberculous interstitial keratitis
Tuberculous keratoconjunctivitis (interstitial) (phlyctenular)

A18.53 Tuberculous chorioretinitis

A18.54 Tuberculous iridocyclitis

A18.59 Other tuberculosis of eye
Tuberculous conjunctivitis

A18.6 Tuberculosis of (inner) (middle) ear
Tuberculous otitis media
EXCLUDES 2 tuberculosis of external ear (A18.4)
tuberculous mastoiditis (A18.03)

A18.7 Tuberculosis of adrenal glands
Tuberculous Addison's disease

✓5ᵗʰ A18.8 Tuberculosis of other specified organs

A18.81 Tuberculosis of thyroid gland

A18.82 Tuberculosis of other endocrine glands
Tuberculosis of pituitary gland
Tuberculosis of thymus gland

A18.83 Tuberculosis of digestive tract organs, not elsewhere classified
EXCLUDES 1 tuberculosis of intestine (A18.32)

A18.84 Tuberculosis of heart
Tuberculous cardiomyopathy
Tuberculous endocarditis
Tuberculous myocarditis
Tuberculous pericarditis

A18.85 Tuberculosis of spleen

A18.89 Tuberculosis of other sites
Tuberculosis of muscle
Tuberculous cerebral arteritis

✓4ᵗʰ A19 Miliary tuberculosis
INCLUDES disseminated tuberculosis
generalized tuberculosis
tuberculous polyserositis

A19.0 Acute miliary tuberculosis of a single specified site

A19.1 Acute miliary tuberculosis of multiple sites

A19.2 Acute miliary tuberculosis, unspecified ▽

A19.8 Other miliary tuberculosis

A19.9 Miliary tuberculosis, unspecified ▽

Certain zoonotic bacterial diseases (A20-A28)

✓4ᵗʰ A20 Plague
INCLUDES infection due to Yersinia pestis

A20.0 Bubonic plague

A20.1 Cellulocutaneous plague

A20.2 Pneumonic plague HCC

A20.3 Plague meningitis

A20.7 Septicemic plague HCC

A20.8 Other forms of plague
Abortive plague
Asymptomatic plague
Pestis minor

A20.9 Plague, unspecified ▽

✓4ᵗʰ A21 Tularemia
INCLUDES deer-fly fever
infection due to Francisella tularensis
rabbit fever
DEF: A febrile disease transmitted to humans by the bites of deer flies, fleas, and ticks; by inhaling aerosolized *F. tularensis*; or by ingesting contaminated food or water. Patients quickly develop fever, chills, weakness, headache, backache, and malaise.

A21.0 Ulceroglandular tularemia

A21.1 Oculoglandular tularemia
Ophthalmic tularemia

A21.2 Pulmonary tularemia HCC

A21.3 Gastrointestinal tularemia
Abdominal tularemia

A21.7 Generalized tularemia

A21.8 Other forms of tularemia

A21.9 Tularemia, unspecified ▽

✓4ᵗʰ A22 Anthrax
INCLUDES infection due to Bacillus anthracis

A22.0 Cutaneous anthrax
Malignant carbuncle
Malignant pustule

A22.1 Pulmonary anthrax HCC
Inhalation anthrax
Ragpicker's disease
Woolsorter's disease

EXCLUDES 1 Not coded here   EXCLUDES 2 Not included here   Ⓝ Newborn Age: 0   Ⓟ Pediatric Age: 0-17   Ⓜ Maternity Age: 12-55   Ⓐ Adult Age: 15-124

438   ICD-10-CM 2018

A22.2 **Gastrointestinal anthrax**

A22.7 **Anthrax** sepsis   `HCC`

A22.8 **Other forms of anthrax**
Anthrax meningitis

A22.9 **Anthrax, unspecified**   ▽

✓4ᵗʰ **A23 Brucellosis**
`INCLUDES`   Malta fever
Mediterranean fever
undulant fever

A23.0 **Brucellosis due to** Brucella melitensis

A23.1 **Brucellosis due to** Brucella abortus

A23.2 **Brucellosis due to** Brucella suis

A23.3 **Brucellosis due to** Brucella canis

A23.8 **Other brucellosis**

A23.9 **Brucellosis, unspecified**   ▽

✓4ᵗʰ **A24 Glanders and melioidosis**

A24.0 **Glanders**
Infection due to Pseudomonas mallei
Malleus

A24.1 **Acute and fulminating melioidosis**
Melioidosis pneumonia
Melioidosis sepsis

A24.2 **Subacute and chronic melioidosis**

A24.3 **Other melioidosis**

A24.9 **Melioidosis, unspecified**   ▽
Infection due to Pseudomonas pseudomallei NOS
Whitmore's disease

✓4ᵗʰ **A25 Rat-bite fevers**

A25.0 **Spirillosis**
Sodoku

A25.1 **Streptobacillosis**
Epidemic arthritic erythema
Haverhill fever
Streptobacillary rat-bite fever

A25.9 **Rat-bite fever, unspecified**   ▽

✓4ᵗʰ **A26 Erysipeloid**

A26.0 **Cutaneous erysipeloid**
Erythema migrans

A26.7 **Erysipelothrix sepsis**   `HCC`

A26.8 **Other forms of erysipeloid**

A26.9 **Erysipeloid, unspecified**   ▽

✓4ᵗʰ **A27 Leptospirosis**

A27.0 **Leptospirosis icterohemorrhagica**
Leptospiral or spirochetal jaundice (hemorrhagic)
Weil's disease

✓5ᵗʰ A27.8 **Other forms of leptospirosis**

A27.81 **Aseptic meningitis in leptospirosis**

A27.89 **Other forms of leptospirosis**

A27.9 **Leptospirosis, unspecified**   ▽

✓4ᵗʰ **A28 Other zoonotic bacterial diseases, not elsewhere classified**

A28.0 **Pasteurellosis**

A28.1 **Cat-scratch disease**
Cat-scratch fever

A28.2 **Extraintestinal yersiniosis**
`EXCLUDES 1`   enteritis due to Yersinia enterocolitica (A04.6)
plague (A20.-)

A28.8 **Other specified zoonotic bacterial diseases, not elsewhere classified**

A28.9 **Zoonotic bacterial disease, unspecified**   ▽

Other bacterial diseases (A30-A49)
AHA: 2016, 3Q, 8-14

✓4ᵗʰ **A30 Leprosy [Hansen's disease]**
`INCLUDES`   infection due to Mycobacterium leprae
`EXCLUDES 1`   sequelae of leprosy (B92)

A30.0 **Indeterminate leprosy**
I leprosy

A30.1 **Tuberculoid leprosy**
TT leprosy

A30.2 **Borderline tuberculoid leprosy**
BT leprosy

A30.3 **Borderline leprosy**
BB leprosy

A30.4 **Borderline lepromatous leprosy**
BL leprosy

A30.5 **Lepromatous leprosy**
LL leprosy

A30.8 **Other forms of leprosy**

A30.9 **Leprosy, unspecified**   ▽

✓4ᵗʰ **A31 Infection due to other mycobacteria**
`EXCLUDES 2`   leprosy (A30.-)
tuberculosis (A15-A19)

A31.0 **Pulmonary mycobacterial infection**   `HCC`
Infection due to Mycobacterium avium
Infection due to Mycobacterium intracellulare [Battey bacillus]
Infection due to Mycobacterium kansasii

A31.1 **Cutaneous mycobacterial infection**
Buruli ulcer
Infection due to Mycobacterium marinum
Infection due to Mycobacterium ulcerans

A31.2 **Disseminated mycobacterium avium-intracellulare complex (DMAC)**   `HCC`
MAC sepsis

A31.8 **Other mycobacterial infections**

A31.9 **Mycobacterial infection, unspecified**   ▽
Atypical mycobacterial infection NOS
Mycobacteriosis NOS

✓4ᵗʰ **A32 Listeriosis**
`INCLUDES`   listerial foodborne infection
`EXCLUDES 1`   neonatal (disseminated) listeriosis (P37.2)

A32.0 **Cutaneous listeriosis**

✓5ᵗʰ A32.1 **Listerial meningitis and meningoencephalitis**

A32.11 **Listerial meningitis**

A32.12 **Listerial meningoencephalitis**

A32.7 **Listerial sepsis**   `HCC`

✓5ᵗʰ A32.8 **Other forms of listeriosis**

A32.81 **Oculoglandular listeriosis**

A32.82 **Listerial endocarditis**

A32.89 **Other forms of listeriosis**
Listerial cerebral arteritis

A32.9 **Listeriosis, unspecified**   ▽

A33 Tetanus neonatorum   `N`

A34 Obstetrical tetanus   `M` ♀

A35 Other tetanus
Tetanus NOS
`EXCLUDES 1`   obstetrical tetanus (A34)
tetanus neonatorum (A33)

✓4ᵗʰ **A36 Diphtheria**

A36.0 **Pharyngeal diphtheria**
Diphtheritic membranous angina
Tonsillar diphtheria

A36.1 **Nasopharyngeal diphtheria**

A36.2 **Laryngeal diphtheria**
Diphtheritic laryngotracheitis

A36.3 **Cutaneous diphtheria**
`EXCLUDES 2`   erythrasma (L08.1)

✓5ᵗʰ A36.8 **Other diphtheria**

A36.81 **Diphtheritic cardiomyopathy**   `HCC`
Diphtheritic myocarditis

A36.82 **Diphtheritic radiculomyelitis**

A36.83 **Diphtheritic polyneuritis**

A36.84 **Diphtheritic tubulo-interstitial nephropathy**

A36.85 **Diphtheritic cystitis**

A36.86 **Diphtheritic conjunctivitis**

A36.89 **Other diphtheritic complications**
Diphtheritic peritonitis

A36.9 **Diphtheria, unspecified**   ▽

✓4ᵗʰ **A37 Whooping cough**

✓5ᵗʰ A37.0 **Whooping cough due to** Bordetella pertussis

A37.00 **Whooping cough due to Bordetella pertussis without pneumonia**

A37.01 **Whooping cough due to Bordetella pertussis with pneumonia**

✓5ᵗʰ A37.1 **Whooping cough due to** Bordetella parapertussis

A37.10 **Whooping cough due to Bordetella parapertussis without pneumonia**

✓ Additional Character Req   `x7ᵗʰ` Placeholder Alert   Manifestation   `HCC` CMS-HCC Condition   ▽ Unspecified Code   ►◄ Revised Text   ● New Code   ▲ Revised Code Title

A37.11   **Whooping cough due to Bordetella parapertussis with pneumonia**

✓5ᵗʰ **A37.8**   **Whooping cough due to other Bordetella species**

     A37.80   **Whooping cough due to other Bordetella species without pneumonia**

     A37.81   **Whooping cough due to other Bordetella species with pneumonia**

✓5ᵗʰ **A37.9**   **Whooping cough, unspecified species**

     A37.90   **Whooping cough, unspecified species without pneumonia** ▽

     A37.91   **Whooping cough, unspecified species with pneumonia** ▽

✓4ᵗʰ **A38**   **Scarlet fever**
> INCLUDES   scarlatina
> EXCLUDES 2   streptococcal sore throat (J02.0)

   A38.0   **Scarlet fever with otitis media**

   A38.1   **Scarlet fever with myocarditis**

   A38.8   **Scarlet fever with other complications**

   A38.9   **Scarlet fever, uncomplicated** ▽
> Scarlet fever, NOS

✓4ᵗʰ **A39**   **Meningococcal infection**

   A39.0   **Meningococcal meningitis**

   A39.1   **Waterhouse-Friderichsen syndrome**   HCC
> Meningococcal hemorrhagic adrenalitis
> Meningococcic adrenal syndrome

   A39.2   **Acute meningococcemia**   HCC

   A39.3   **Chronic meningococcemia**   HCC

   A39.4   **Meningococcemia, unspecified**   HCC ▽

✓5ᵗʰ **A39.5**   **Meningococcal heart disease**

     A39.50   **Meningococcal carditis, unspecified** ▽

     A39.51   **Meningococcal endocarditis**

     A39.52   **Meningococcal myocarditis**

     A39.53   **Meningococcal pericarditis**

✓5ᵗʰ **A39.8**   **Other meningococcal infections**

     A39.81   **Meningococcal encephalitis**

     A39.82   **Meningococcal retrobulbar neuritis**

     A39.83   **Meningococcal arthritis**   HCC

     A39.84   **Postmeningococcal arthritis**   HCC

     A39.89   **Other meningococcal infections**
> Meningococcal conjunctivitis

   A39.9   **Meningococcal infection, unspecified** ▽
> Meningococcal disease NOS

✓4ᵗʰ **A40**   **Streptococcal sepsis**
> Code first: postprocedural streptococcal sepsis (T81.4-)
>   streptococcal sepsis during labor (O75.3)
>   streptococcal sepsis following abortion or ectopic or molar pregnancy (O03-O07, O08.0)
>   streptococcal sepsis following immunization (T88.0)
>   streptococcal sepsis following infusion, transfusion or therapeutic injection (T80.2-)
> EXCLUDES 1   neonatal (P36.0-P36.1)
>   puerperal sepsis (O85)
>   sepsis due to Streptococcus, group D (A41.81)
> AHA: 2016, 1Q, 32

   A40.0   **Sepsis due to streptococcus, group A**   HCC

   A40.1   **Sepsis due to streptococcus, group B**   HCC

   A40.3   **Sepsis due to Streptococcus pneumoniae**   HCC
> Pneumococcal sepsis

   A40.8   **Other streptococcal sepsis**   HCC

   A40.9   **Streptococcal sepsis, unspecified**   HCC ▽

✓4ᵗʰ **A41**   **Other sepsis**
> Code first: postprocedural sepsis (T81.4-)
>   sepsis during labor (O75.3)
>   sepsis following abortion, ectopic or molar pregnancy (O03-O07, O08.0)
>   sepsis following immunization (T88.0)
>   sepsis following infusion, transfusion or therapeutic injection (T80.2-)
> EXCLUDES 1   bacteremia NOS (R78.81)
>   neonatal (P36.-)
>   puerperal sepsis (O85)
>   streptococcal sepsis (A40.-)
> EXCLUDES 2   sepsis (due to) (in) actinomycotic (A42.7)
>   sepsis (due to) (in) anthrax (A22.7)
>   sepsis (due to) (in) candidal (B37.7)
>   sepsis (due to) (in) Erysipelothrix (A26.7)
>   sepsis (due to) (in) extraintestinal yersiniosis (A28.2)
>   sepsis (due to) (in) gonococcal (A54.86)
>   sepsis (due to) (in) herpesviral (B00.7)
>   sepsis (due to) (in) listerial (A32.7)
>   sepsis (due to) (in) melioidosis (A24.1)
>   sepsis (due to) (in) meningococcal (A39.2-A39.4)
>   sepsis (due to) (in) plague (A20.7)
>   sepsis (due to) (in) tularemia (A21.7)
>   toxic shock syndrome (A48.3)
> AHA: 2016, 1Q, 32; 2014, 2Q, 13

✓5ᵗʰ **A41.0**   **Sepsis due to Staphylococcus aureus**

     A41.01   **Sepsis due to Methicillin susceptible Staphylococcus aureus**   HCC
> MSSA sepsis
> Staphylococcus aureus sepsis NOS

     A41.02   **Sepsis due to Methicillin resistant Staphylococcus aureus**   HCC

   A41.1   **Sepsis due to other specified staphylococcus**   HCC
> Coagulase negative staphylococcus sepsis

   A41.2   **Sepsis due to unspecified staphylococcus**   HCC ▽

   A41.3   **Sepsis due to Hemophilus influenzae**   HCC

   A41.4   **Sepsis due to anaerobes**   HCC
> EXCLUDES 1   gas gangrene (A48.0)

✓5ᵗʰ **A41.5**   **Sepsis due to other Gram-negative organisms**

     A41.50   **Gram-negative sepsis, unspecified**   HCC ▽
> Gram-negative sepsis NOS

     A41.51   **Sepsis due to Escherichia coli [E. coli]**   HCC

     A41.52   **Sepsis due to Pseudomonas**   HCC
> Pseudomonas aeroginosa

     A41.53   **Sepsis due to Serratia**   HCC

     A41.59   **Other Gram-negative sepsis**   HCC

✓5ᵗʰ **A41.8**   **Other specified sepsis**

     A41.81   **Sepsis due to Enterococcus**   HCC

     A41.89   **Other specified sepsis**   HCC
> AHA: 2017, 1Q, 51; 2016, 3Q, 8-14

   A41.9   **Sepsis, unspecified organism**   HCC ▽
> Septicemia NOS

✓4ᵗʰ **A42**   **Actinomycosis**
> EXCLUDES 1   actinomycetoma (B47.1)

   A42.0   **Pulmonary actinomycosis**   HCC

   A42.1   **Abdominal actinomycosis**

   A42.2   **Cervicofacial actinomycosis**

   A42.7   **Actinomycotic sepsis**   HCC

✓5ᵗʰ **A42.8**   **Other forms of actinomycosis**

     A42.81   **Actinomycotic meningitis**

     A42.82   **Actinomycotic encephalitis**

     A42.89   **Other forms of actinomycosis**

   A42.9   **Actinomycosis, unspecified** ▽

✓4ᵗʰ **A43**   **Nocardiosis**

   A43.0   **Pulmonary nocardiosis**   HCC

   A43.1   **Cutaneous nocardiosis**

   A43.8   **Other forms of nocardiosis**

   A43.9   **Nocardiosis, unspecified** ▽

✓4ᵗʰ **A44**   **Bartonellosis**

   A44.0   **Systemic bartonellosis**
> Oroya fever

   A44.1   **Cutaneous and mucocutaneous bartonellosis**
> Verruga peruana

   A44.8   **Other forms of bartonellosis**

EXCLUDES 1 Not coded here   EXCLUDES 2 Not included here   N Newborn Age: 0   P Pediatric Age: 0-17   M Maternity Age: 12-55   A Adult Age: 15-124

440   ICD-10-CM 2018

A44.9   Bartonellosis, unspecified   ▽

A46   Erysipelas
EXCLUDES 1   *postpartum or puerperal erysipelas (O86.89)*
DEF: A skin infection affecting the upper dermis and superficial dermal lymphatics; lesion edges are well-demarcated with distinct raised borders; it is often caused by group A *Streptococci.*

✓4th A48   Other bacterial diseases, not elsewhere classified
EXCLUDES 1   *actinomycetoma (B47.1)*

A48.0   Gas gangrene   HCC
Clostridial cellulitis
Clostridial myonecrosis

A48.1   Legionnaires' disease   HCC
DEF: Severe and often fatal infection by *Legionella pneumophila;* symptoms include high fever, gastrointestinal pain, headache, myalgia, dry cough, and pneumonia; usually transmitted through airborne water droplets via air conditioning systems or hot tubs.

A48.2   Nonpneumonic Legionnaires' disease [Pontiac fever]

A48.3   Toxic shock syndrome   HCC
Use additional code to identify the organism (B95, B96)
EXCLUDES 1   *endotoxic shock NOS (R57.8)*
sepsis NOS (A41.9)

A48.4   Brazilian purpuric fever
Systemic Hemophilus aegyptius infection

✓5th A48.5   Other specified botulism
Non-foodborne intoxication due to toxins of Clostridium botulinum [C. botulinum]
EXCLUDES 1   *food poisoning due to toxins of Clostridium botulinum (A05.1)*

A48.51   Infant botulism   P

A48.52   Wound botulism
Non-foodborne botulism NOS
Use additional code for associated wound

A48.8   Other specified bacterial diseases

✓4th A49   Bacterial infection of unspecified site
EXCLUDES 1   *bacterial agents as the cause of diseases classified elsewhere (B95-B96)*
chlamydial infection NOS (A74.9)
meningococcal infection NOS (A39.9)
rickettsial infection NOS (A79.9)
spirochetal infection NOS (A69.9)

✓5th A49.0   Staphylococcal infection, unspecified site

A49.01   Methicillin susceptible Staphylococcus aureus infection, unspecified site
Methicillin susceptible Staphylococcus aureus (MSSA) infection
Staphylococcus aureus infection NOS

A49.02   Methicillin resistant Staphylococcus aureus infection, unspecified site
Methicillin resistant Staphylococcus aureus (MRSA) infection

A49.1   Streptococcal infection, unspecified site

A49.2   Hemophilus influenzae infection, unspecified site

A49.3   Mycoplasma infection, unspecified site

A49.8   Other bacterial infections of unspecified site

A49.9   Bacterial infection, unspecified   ▽
EXCLUDES 1   *bacteremia NOS (R78.81)*

Infections with a predominantly sexual mode of transmission (A50-A64)
EXCLUDES 1   *human immunodeficiency virus [HIV] disease (B20)*
nonspecific and nongonococcal urethritis (N34.1)
Reiter's disease (M02.3-)

✓4th A50   Congenital syphilis

✓5th A50.0   Early congenital syphilis, symptomatic
Any congenital syphilitic condition specified as early or manifest less than two years after birth.

A50.01   Early congenital syphilitic oculopathy

A50.02   Early congenital syphilitic osteochondropathy

A50.03   Early congenital syphilitic pharyngitis
Early congenital syphilitic laryngitis

A50.04   Early congenital syphilitic pneumonia

A50.05   Early congenital syphilitic rhinitis

A50.06   Early cutaneous congenital syphilis

A50.07   Early mucocutaneous congenital syphilis

A50.08   Early visceral congenital syphilis

A50.09   Other early congenital syphilis, symptomatic

A50.1   Early congenital syphilis, latent
Congenital syphilis without clinical manifestations, with positive serological reaction and negative spinal fluid test, less than two years after birth.

A50.2   Early congenital syphilis, unspecified   ▽
Congenital syphilis NOS less than two years after birth.

✓5th A50.3   Late congenital syphilitic oculopathy
EXCLUDES 1   *Hutchinson's triad (A50.53)*

A50.30   Late congenital syphilitic oculopathy, unspecified ▽

A50.31   Late congenital syphilitic interstitial keratitis

A50.32   Late congenital syphilitic chorioretinitis

A50.39   Other late congenital syphilitic oculopathy

✓5th A50.4   Late congenital neurosyphilis [juvenile neurosyphilis]
Use additional code to identify any associated mental disorder
EXCLUDES 1   *Hutchinson's triad (A50.53)*

A50.40   Late congenital neurosyphilis, unspecified   ▽
Juvenile neurosyphilis NOS

A50.41   Late congenital syphilitic meningitis

A50.42   Late congenital syphilitic encephalitis

A50.43   Late congenital syphilitic polyneuropathy

A50.44   Late congenital syphilitic optic nerve atrophy

A50.45   Juvenile general paresis
Dementia paralytica juvenilis
Juvenile tabetoparetic neurosyphilis

A50.49   Other late congenital neurosyphilis
Juvenile tabes dorsalis

✓5th A50.5   Other late congenital syphilis, symptomatic
Any congenital syphilitic condition specified as late or manifest two years or more after birth.

A50.51   Clutton's joints

A50.52   Hutchinson's teeth

A50.53   Hutchinson's triad

A50.54   Late congenital cardiovascular syphilis

A50.55   Late congenital syphilitic arthropathy   HCC

A50.56   Late congenital syphilitic osteochondropathy

A50.57   Syphilitic saddle nose

A50.59   Other late congenital syphilis, symptomatic

A50.6   Late congenital syphilis, latent
Congenital syphilis without clinical manifestations, with positive serological reaction and negative spinal fluid test, two years or more after birth.

A50.7   Late congenital syphilis, unspecified   ▽
Congenital syphilis NOS two years or more after birth.

A50.9   Congenital syphilis, unspecified   ▽

✓4th A51   Early syphilis

A51.0   Primary genital syphilis
Syphilitic chancre NOS

A51.1   Primary anal syphilis

A51.2   Primary syphilis of other sites

✓5th A51.3   Secondary syphilis of skin and mucous membranes
DEF: Transitory or chronic cutaneous eruptions that present within two to 10 weeks following initial syphilis infection that may include nontender lymphadenopathy along with alopecia and condylomata lata.

A51.31   Condyloma latum

A51.32   Syphilitic alopecia

A51.39   Other secondary syphilis of skin
Syphilitic leukoderma
Syphilitic mucous patch
EXCLUDES 1   *late syphilitic leukoderma (A52.79)*

✓5th A51.4   Other secondary syphilis

A51.41   Secondary syphilitic meningitis

A51.42   Secondary syphilitic female pelvic disease   ♀

A51.43   Secondary syphilitic oculopathy
Secondary syphilitic chorioretinitis
Secondary syphilitic iridocyclitis, iritis
Secondary syphilitic uveitis

A51.44   Secondary syphilitic nephritis

A51.45   Secondary syphilitic hepatitis

A51.46   Secondary syphilitic osteopathy

A51.49   Other secondary syphilitic conditions
Secondary syphilitic lymphadenopathy
Secondary syphilitic myositis

✓ Additional Character Req   ✓x7th Placeholder Alert   Manifestation   HCC CMS-HCC Condition   ▽ Unspecified Code   ►◄ Revised Text   ● New Code   ▲ Revised Code Title

A51.5   **Early syphilis, latent**
Syphilis (acquired) without clinical manifestations, with positive serological reaction and negative spinal fluid test, less than two years after infection.

A51.9   **Early syphilis, unspecified** ▽

✓4th A52   **Late syphilis**

   ✓5th A52.0   **Cardiovascular and cerebrovascular syphilis**

     A52.00   **Cardiovascular syphilis, unspecified** ▽

     A52.01   **Syphilitic aneurysm of aorta**

     A52.02   **Syphilitic aortitis**

     A52.03   **Syphilitic endocarditis**
       Syphilitic aortic valve incompetence or stenosis
       Syphilitic mitral valve stenosis
       Syphilitic pulmonary valve regurgitation

     A52.04   **Syphilitic cerebral arteritis**

     A52.05   **Other cerebrovascular syphilis**
       Syphilitic cerebral aneurysm (ruptured) (non-ruptured)
       Syphilitic cerebral thrombosis

     A52.06   **Other syphilitic heart involvement**
       Syphilitic coronary artery disease
       Syphilitic myocarditis
       Syphilitic pericarditis

     A52.09   **Other cardiovascular syphilis**

   ✓5th A52.1   **Symptomatic neurosyphilis**

     A52.10   **Symptomatic neurosyphilis, unspecified** ▽

     A52.11   **Tabes dorsalis**
       Locomotor ataxia (progressive)
       Tabetic neurosyphilis

     A52.12   **Other cerebrospinal syphilis**

     A52.13   **Late syphilitic meningitis**

     A52.14   **Late syphilitic encephalitis**

     A52.15   **Late syphilitic neuropathy**
       Late syphilitic acoustic neuritis
       Late syphilitic optic (nerve) atrophy
       Late syphilitic polyneuropathy
       Late syphilitic retrobulbar neuritis

     A52.16   **Charcôt's arthropathy (tabetic)**

     A52.17   **General paresis**
       Dementia paralytica

     A52.19   **Other symptomatic neurosyphilis**
       Syphilitic parkinsonism

   A52.2   **Asymptomatic neurosyphilis**

   A52.3   **Neurosyphilis, unspecified** ▽
     Gumma (syphilitic)
     Syphilis (late)
     Syphiloma

   ✓5th A52.7   **Other symptomatic late syphilis**

     A52.71   **Late syphilitic oculopathy**
       Late syphilitic chorioretinitis
       Late syphilitic episcleritis

     A52.72   **Syphilis of lung and bronchus**

     A52.73   **Symptomatic late syphilis of other respiratory organs**

     A52.74   **Syphilis of liver and other viscera**
       Late syphilitic peritonitis

     A52.75   **Syphilis of kidney and ureter**
       Syphilitic glomerular disease

     A52.76   **Other genitourinary symptomatic late syphilis**
       Late syphilitic female pelvic inflammatory disease

     A52.77   **Syphilis of bone and joint**

     A52.78   **Syphilis of other musculoskeletal tissue**
       Late syphilitic bursitis
       Syphilis [stage unspecified] of bursa
       Syphilis [stage unspecified] of muscle
       Syphilis [stage unspecified] of synovium
       Syphilis [stage unspecified] of tendon

     A52.79   **Other symptomatic late syphilis**
       Late syphilitic leukoderma
       Syphilis of adrenal gland
       Syphilis of pituitary gland
       Syphilis of thyroid gland
       Syphilitic splenomegaly
       EXCLUDES 1   *syphilitic leukoderma (secondary) (A51.39)*

   A52.8   **Late syphilis, latent**
     Syphilis (acquired) without clinical manifestations, with positive serological reaction and negative spinal fluid test, two years or more after infection

A52.9   **Late syphilis, unspecified** ▽

✓4th A53   **Other and unspecified syphilis**

   A53.0   **Latent syphilis, unspecified as early or late**
     Latent syphilis NOS
     Positive serological reaction for syphilis

   A53.9   **Syphilis, unspecified** ▽
     Infection due to Treponema pallidum NOS
     Syphilis (acquired) NOS
     EXCLUDES 1   *syphilis NOS under two years of age (A50.2)*

✓4th A54   **Gonococcal infection**

   ✓5th A54.0   **Gonococcal infection of lower genitourinary tract without periurethral or accessory gland abscess**
     EXCLUDES 1   *gonococcal infection with genitourinary gland abscess (A54.1)*
             gonococcal infection with periurethral abscess (A54.1)

     A54.00   **Gonococcal infection of lower genitourinary tract, unspecified** ▽

     A54.01   **Gonococcal cystitis and urethritis, unspecified** ▽

     A54.02   **Gonococcal vulvovaginitis, unspecified** ♀▽

     A54.03   **Gonococcal cervicitis, unspecified** ♀▽

     A54.09   **Other gonococcal infection of lower genitourinary tract**

   A54.1   **Gonococcal infection of lower genitourinary tract with periurethral and accessory gland abscess**
     Gonococcal Bartholin's gland abscess

   ✓5th A54.2   **Gonococcal pelviperitonitis and other gonococcal genitourinary infection**

     A54.21   **Gonococcal infection of kidney and ureter**

     A54.22   **Gonococcal prostatitis** ♂

     A54.23   **Gonococcal infection of other male genital organs** ♂
       Gonococcal epididymitis
       Gonococcal orchitis

     A54.24   **Gonococcal female pelvic inflammatory disease** ♀
       Gonococcal pelviperitonitis
       EXCLUDES 1   *gonococcal peritonitis (A54.85)*

     A54.29   **Other gonococcal genitourinary infections**

   ✓5th A54.3   **Gonococcal infection of eye**

     A54.30   **Gonococcal infection of eye, unspecified** ▽

     A54.31   **Gonococcal conjunctivitis**
       Ophthalmia neonatorum due to gonococcus

     A54.32   **Gonococcal iridocyclitis**

     A54.33   **Gonococcal keratitis**

     A54.39   **Other gonococcal eye infection**
       Gonococcal endophthalmia

   ✓5th A54.4   **Gonococcal infection of musculoskeletal system**

     A54.40   **Gonococcal infection of musculoskeletal system, unspecified** `HCC` ▽

     A54.41   **Gonococcal spondylopathy** `HCC`

     A54.42   **Gonococcal arthritis** `HCC`
       EXCLUDES 2   *gonococcal infection of spine (A54.41)*

     A54.43   **Gonococcal osteomyelitis** `HCC`
       EXCLUDES 2   *gonococcal infection of spine (A54.41)*

     A54.49   **Gonococcal infection of other musculoskeletal tissue** `HCC`
       Gonococcal bursitis
       Gonococcal myositis
       Gonococcal synovitis
       Gonococcal tenosynovitis

   A54.5   **Gonococcal pharyngitis**

   A54.6   **Gonococcal infection of anus and rectum**

   ✓5th A54.8   **Other gonococcal infections**

     A54.81   **Gonococcal meningitis**

     A54.82   **Gonococcal brain abscess**

     A54.83   **Gonococcal heart infection**
       Gonococcal endocarditis
       Gonococcal myocarditis
       Gonococcal pericarditis

     A54.84   **Gonococcal pneumonia** `HCC`

     A54.85   **Gonococcal peritonitis** `HCC`
       EXCLUDES 1   *gonococcal pelviperitonitis (A54.24)*

     A54.86   **Gonococcal sepsis** `HCC`

     A54.89   **Other gonococcal infections**
       Gonococcal keratoderma
       Gonococcal lymphadenitis

   A54.9   **Gonococcal infection, unspecified** ▽

EXCLUDES 1 Not coded here   **EXCLUDES 2** Not included here   **N** Newborn Age: 0   **P** Pediatric Age: 0-17   **M** Maternity Age: 12-55   **A** Adult Age: 15-124

A55 Chlamydial lymphogranuloma (venereum)
Climatic or tropical bubo
Durand-Nicolas-Favre disease
Esthiomene
Lymphogranuloma inguinale

✓4ᵗʰ A56 Other sexually transmitted chlamydial diseases
INCLUDES   sexually transmitted diseases due to Chlamydia
trachomatis
EXCLUDES 1   neonatal chlamydial conjunctivitis (P39.1)
neonatal chlamydial pneumonia (P23.1)
EXCLUDES 2   chlamydial lymphogranuloma (A55)
conditions classified to A74-

   ✓5ᵗʰ A56.0 Chlamydial infection of lower genitourinary tract
     A56.00 Chlamydial infection of lower genitourinary ▽
         tract, unspecified
     A56.01 Chlamydial cystitis and urethritis
     A56.02 Chlamydial vulvovaginitis ♀
     A56.09 Other chlamydial infection of lower genitourinary
         tract
         Chlamydial cervicitis

   ✓5ᵗʰ A56.1 Chlamydial infection of pelviperitoneum and other
     genitourinary organs
     A56.11 Chlamydial female pelvic inflammatory disease ♀
     A56.19 Other chlamydial genitourinary infection
         Chlamydial epididymitis
         Chlamydial orchitis
   A56.2 Chlamydial infection of genitourinary tract, unspecified ▽
   A56.3 Chlamydial infection of anus and rectum
   A56.4 Chlamydial infection of pharynx
   A56.8 Sexually transmitted chlamydial infection of other sites

A57 Chancroid
Ulcus molle

A58 Granuloma inguinale
Donovanosis

✓4ᵗʰ A59 Trichomoniasis
EXCLUDES 2   intestinal trichomoniasis (A07.8)

   ✓5ᵗʰ A59.0 Urogenital trichomoniasis
     A59.00 Urogenital trichomoniasis, unspecified ▽
         Fluor (vaginalis) due to Trichomonas
         Leukorrhea (vaginalis) due to Trichomonas
     A59.01 Trichomonal vulvovaginitis ♀
     A59.02 Trichomonal prostatitis ♂
     A59.03 Trichomonal cystitis and urethritis
     A59.09 Other urogenital trichomoniasis
         Trichomonas cervicitis
   A59.8 Trichomoniasis of other sites
   A59.9 Trichomoniasis, unspecified ▽

✓4ᵗʰ A60 Anogenital herpesviral [herpes simplex] infections
   ✓5ᵗʰ A60.0 Herpesviral infection of genitalia and urogenital tract
     A60.00 Herpesviral infection of urogenital system, ▽
         unspecified
     A60.01 Herpesviral infection of penis ♂
     A60.02 Herpesviral infection of other male genital ♂
         organs
     A60.03 Herpesviral cervicitis ♀
     A60.04 Herpesviral vulvovaginitis ♀
         Herpesviral [herpes simplex] ulceration
         Herpesviral [herpes simplex] vaginitis
         Herpesviral [herpes simplex] vulvitis
     A60.09 Herpesviral infection of other urogenital tract
   A60.1 Herpesviral infection of perianal skin and rectum
   A60.9 Anogenital herpesviral infection, unspecified ▽

✓4ᵗʰ A63 Other predominantly sexually transmitted diseases, not
elsewhere classified
EXCLUDES 2   molluscum contagiosum (B08.1)
papilloma of cervix (D26.0)

   A63.0 Anogenital (venereal) warts
     Anogenital warts due to (human) papillomavirus [HPV]
     Condyloma acuminatum
   A63.8 Other specified predominantly sexually transmitted diseases

A64 Unspecified sexually transmitted disease ▽

Other spirochetal diseases (A65-A69)
EXCLUDES 2   leptospirosis (A27.-)
syphilis (A50-A53)

A65 Nonvenereal syphilis
Bejel   Njovera
Endemic syphilis

✓4ᵗʰ A66 Yaws
INCLUDES   bouba
frambesia (tropica)
pian

   A66.0 Initial lesions of yaws
     Chancre of yaws
     Frambesia, initial or primary
     Initial frambesial ulcer
     Mother yaw
   A66.1 Multiple papillomata and wet crab yaws
     Frambesioma
     Pianoma
     Plantar or palmar papilloma of yaws
   A66.2 Other early skin lesions of yaws
     Cutaneous yaws, less than five years after infection
     Early yaws (cutaneous) (macular) (maculopapular)
       (micropapular) (papular)
     Frambeside of early yaws
   A66.3 Hyperkeratosis of yaws
     Ghoul hand
     Hyperkeratosis, palmar or plantar (early) (late) due to yaws
     Worm-eaten soles
   A66.4 Gummata and ulcers of yaws
     Gummatous frambeside
     Nodular late yaws (ulcerated)
   A66.5 Gangosa
     Rhinopharyngitis mutilans
   A66.6 Bone and joint lesions of yaws   HCC
     Yaws ganglion   Yaws hydrarthrosis
     Yaws goundou   Yaws osteitis
     Yaws gumma, bone   Yaws periostitis (hypertrophic)
     Yaws gummatous osteitis
       or periostitis
   A66.7 Other manifestations of yaws
     Juxta-articular nodules of yaws
     Mucosal yaws
   A66.8 Latent yaws
     Yaws without clinical manifestations, with positive serology
   A66.9 Yaws, unspecified ▽

✓4ᵗʰ A67 Pinta [carate]
   A67.0 Primary lesions of pinta
     Chancre (primary) of pinta
     Papule (primary) of pinta
   A67.1 Intermediate lesions of pinta
     Erythematous plaques of pinta
     Hyperchromic lesions of pinta
     Hyperkeratosis of pinta
     Pintids
   A67.2 Late lesions of pinta
     Achromic skin lesions of pinta
     Cicatricial skin lesions of pinta
     Dyschromic skin lesions of pinta
   A67.3 Mixed lesions of pinta
     Achromic with hyperchromic skin lesions of pinta [carate]
   A67.9 Pinta, unspecified ▽

✓4ᵗʰ A68 Relapsing fevers
INCLUDES   recurrent fever
EXCLUDES 2   Lyme disease (A69.2-)

   A68.0 Louse-borne relapsing fever
     Relapsing fever due to Borrelia recurrentis
   A68.1 Tick-borne relapsing fever
     Relapsing fever due to any Borrelia species other than Borrelia
       recurrentis
   A68.9 Relapsing fever, unspecified ▽

✓4ᵗʰ A69 Other spirochetal infections
   A69.0 Necrotizing ulcerative stomatitis
     Cancrum oris
     Fusospirochetal gangrene
     Noma
     Stomatitis gangrenosa

☑ Additional Character Req   ✓x7ᵗʰ Placeholder Alert   Manifestation   HCC CMS-HCC Condition   ▽ Unspecified Code   ▶◀ Revised Text   ● New Code   ▲ Revised Code Title

ICD-10-CM 2018   **443**

A69.1 Other Vincent's infections
Fusospirochetal pharyngitis
Necrotizing ulcerative (acute) gingivitis
Necrotizing ulcerative (acute) gingivostomatitis
Spirochetal stomatitis
Trench mouth
Vincent's angina
Vincent's gingivitis

✓5ᵗʰ **A69.2 Lyme disease**
Erythema chronicum migrans due to Borrelia burgdorferi
DEF: A recurrent multisystem disorder through tick bites; begins
with lesions of erythema chronicum migrans; followed by arthritis
of the large joints, myalgia, malaise, and neurological and cardiac
manifestations.

  A69.20   Lyme disease, unspecified   ▽
  A69.21   Meningitis due to Lyme disease
  A69.22   Other neurologic disorders in Lyme disease
    Cranial neuritis
    Meningoencephalitis
    Polyneuropathy
  A69.23   Arthritis due to Lyme disease   HCC
  A69.29   Other conditions associated with Lyme disease
    Myopericarditis due to Lyme disease
    AHA: 2016, 3Q, 12

A69.8 Other specified spirochetal infections
A69.9 Spirochetal infection, unspecified   ▽

Other diseases caused by chlamydiae (A70-A74)
EXCLUDES 1 *sexually transmitted chlamydial diseases (A55-A56)*

A70 Chlamydia psittaci infections
Ornithosis
Parrot fever
Psittacosis

✓4ᵗʰ **A71 Trachoma**
EXCLUDES 1 *sequelae of trachoma (B94.0)*

  A71.0   Initial stage of trachoma
    Trachoma dubium
  A71.1   Active stage of trachoma
    Granular conjunctivitis (trachomatous)
    Trachomatous follicular conjunctivitis
    Trachomatous pannus
  A71.9   Trachoma, unspecified   ▽

✓4ᵗʰ **A74 Other diseases caused by chlamydiae**
EXCLUDES 1 *neonatal chlamydial conjunctivitis (P39.1)*
           neonatal chlamydial pneumonia (P23.1)
           Reiter's disease (M02.3-)
           sexually transmitted chlamydial diseases (A55-A56)
EXCLUDES 2 *chlamydial pneumonia (J16.0)*

  A74.0   Chlamydial conjunctivitis
    Paratrachoma
  ✓5ᵗʰ **A74.8   Other chlamydial diseases**
    A74.81   Chlamydial peritonitis
    A74.89   Other chlamydial diseases
  A74.9   Chlamydial infection, unspecified   ▽
    Chlamydiosis NOS

Rickettsioses (A75-A79)

✓4ᵗʰ **A75 Typhus fever**
EXCLUDES 1 *rickettsiosis due to Ehrlichia sennetsu (A79.81)*

  **A75.0   Epidemic louse-borne typhus fever due to Rickettsia
           prowazekii**
    Classical typhus (fever)
    Epidemic (louse-borne) typhus
  A75.1   Recrudescent typhus [Brill's disease]
    Brill-Zinsser disease
  A75.2   Typhus fever due to Rickettsia typhi
    Murine (flea-borne) typhus
  A75.3   Typhus fever due to Rickettsia tsutsugamushi
    Scrub (mite-borne) typhus
    Tsutsugamushi fever
  A75.9   Typhus fever, unspecified   ▽
    Typhus (fever) NOS

✓4ᵗʰ **A77 Spotted fever [tick-borne rickettsioses]**

  A77.0   Spotted fever due to Rickettsia rickettsii
    Rocky Mountain spotted fever
    Sao Paulo fever
  A77.1   Spotted fever due to Rickettsia conorii
    African tick typhus
    Boutonneuse fever
    India tick typhus
    Kenya tick typhus
    Marseilles fever
    Mediterranean tick fever
  A77.2   Spotted fever due to Rickettsia siberica
    North Asian tick fever
    Siberian tick typhus
  A77.3   Spotted fever due to Rickettsia australis
    Queensland tick typhus
  ✓5ᵗʰ **A77.4   Ehrlichiosis**
    EXCLUDES 1 *Rickettsiosis due to Ehrlichia sennetsu (A79.81)*
    A77.40   Ehrlichiosis, unspecified   ▽
    A77.41   Ehrlichiosis chafeensis [E. chafeensis]
    A77.49   Other ehrlichiosis
  A77.8   Other spotted fevers
  A77.9   Spotted fever, unspecified   ▽
    Tick-borne typhus NOS

A78 Q fever
Infection due to Coxiella burnetii
Nine Mile fever
Quadrilateral fever

✓4ᵗʰ **A79 Other rickettsioses**

  A79.0   Trench fever
    Quintan fever
    Wolhynian fever
  A79.1   Rickettsialpox due to Rickettsia akari
    Kew Garden fever
    Vesicular rickettsiosis
  ✓5ᵗʰ **A79.8   Other specified rickettsioses**
    A79.81   Rickettsiosis due to Ehrlichia sennetsu
    A79.89   Other specified rickettsioses
  A79.9   Rickettsiosis, unspecified   ▽
    Rickettsial infection NOS

Viral and prion infections of the central nervous system (A80-A89)
EXCLUDES 1 *postpolio syndrome (G14)*
           sequelae of poliomyelitis (B91)
           sequelae of viral encephalitis (B94.1)

✓4ᵗʰ **A80 Acute poliomyelitis**
  A80.0   Acute paralytic poliomyelitis, vaccine-associated
  A80.1   Acute paralytic poliomyelitis, wild virus, imported
  A80.2   Acute paralytic poliomyelitis, wild virus, indigenous
  ✓5ᵗʰ **A80.3   Acute paralytic poliomyelitis, other and unspecified**
    A80.30   Acute paralytic poliomyelitis, unspecified   ▽
    A80.39   Other acute paralytic poliomyelitis
  A80.4   Acute nonparalytic poliomyelitis
  A80.9   Acute poliomyelitis, unspecified   ▽

✓4ᵗʰ **A81 Atypical virus infections of central nervous system**
  INCLUDES diseases of the central nervous system caused by prions
  Use additional code to identify:
    dementia with behavioral disturbance (F02.81)
    dementia without behavioral disturbance (F02.80)
  ✓5ᵗʰ **A81.0   Creutzfeldt-Jakob disease**
    A81.00   Creutzfeldt-Jakob disease, unspecified   ▽
      Jakob-Creutzfeldt disease, unspecified
    A81.01   Variant Creutzfeldt-Jakob disease
      vCJD
    A81.09   Other Creutzfeldt-Jakob disease
      CJD
      Familial Creutzfeldt-Jakob disease
      Iatrogenic Creutzfeldt-Jakob disease
      Sporadic Creutzfeldt-Jakob disease
      Subacute spongiform encephalopathy (with
        dementia)
  A81.1   Subacute sclerosing panencephalitis
    Dawson's inclusion body encephalitis
    Van Bogaert's sclerosing leukoencephalopathy
  A81.2   Progressive multifocal leukoencephalopathy
    Multifocal leukoencephalopathy NOS

EXCLUDES 1 Not coded here   EXCLUDES 2 Not included here   N Newborn Age: 0   P Pediatric Age: 0-17   M Maternity Age: 12-55   A Adult Age: 15-124

☑5ᵗʰ **A81.8** **Other atypical virus infections of central nervous system**

     A81.81 **Kuru**

     A81.82 **Gerstmann-Sträussler-Scheinker syndrome**
         GSS syndrome

     A81.83 **Fatal familial insomnia**
         FFI

     A81.89 **Other atypical virus infections of central nervous system**

A81.9 **Atypical virus infection of central nervous system, unspecified** ▽
     Prion diseases of the central nervous system NOS

☑4ᵗʰ **A82** **Rabies**

A82.0 **Sylvatic rabies**

A82.1 **Urban rabies**

A82.9 **Rabies, unspecified** ▽

☑4ᵗʰ **A83** **Mosquito-borne viral encephalitis**
     INCLUDES mosquito-borne viral meningoencephalitis
     EXCLUDES 2 *Venezuelan equine encephalitis (A92.2)*
         West Nile fever (A92.3-)
         West Nile virus (A92.3-)

A83.0 **Japanese encephalitis**

A83.1 **Western equine encephalitis**

A83.2 **Eastern equine encephalitis**

A83.3 **St Louis encephalitis**

A83.4 **Australian encephalitis**
     Kunjin virus disease

A83.5 **California encephalitis**
     California meningoencephalitis
     La Crosse encephalitis

A83.6 **Rocio virus disease**

A83.8 **Other mosquito-borne viral encephalitis**

A83.9 **Mosquito-borne viral encephalitis, unspecified** ▽

☑4ᵗʰ **A84** **Tick-borne viral encephalitis**
     INCLUDES tick-borne viral meningoencephalitis

A84.0 **Far Eastern tick-borne encephalitis [Russian spring-summer encephalitis]**

A84.1 **Central European tick-borne encephalitis**

A84.8 **Other tick-borne viral encephalitis**
     Louping ill
     Powassan virus disease

A84.9 **Tick-borne viral encephalitis, unspecified** ▽

☑4ᵗʰ **A85** **Other viral encephalitis, not elsewhere classified**
     INCLUDES specified viral encephalomyelitis NEC
         specified viral meningoencephalitis NEC
     EXCLUDES 1 *benign myalgic encephalomyelitis (G93.3)*
         encephalitis due to cytomegalovirus (B25.8)
         encephalitis due to herpesvirus NEC (B10.0-)
         encephalitis due to herpesvirus [herpes simplex] (B00.4)
         encephalitis due to measles virus (B05.0)
         encephalitis due to mumps virus (B26.2)
         encephalitis due to poliomyelitis virus (A80.-)
         encephalitis due to zoster (B02.0)
         lymphocytic choriomeningitis (A87.2)

A85.0 **Enteroviral encephalitis**
     Enteroviral encephalomyelitis

A85.1 **Adenoviral encephalitis**
     Adenoviral meningoencephalitis

A85.2 **Arthropod-borne viral encephalitis, unspecified** ▽
     EXCLUDES 1 *West nile virus with encephalitis (A92.31)*

A85.8 **Other specified viral encephalitis**
     Encephalitis lethargica
     Von Economo-Cruchet disease

A86 **Unspecified viral encephalitis** ▽
     Viral encephalomyelitis NOS
     Viral meningoencephalitis NOS

☑4ᵗʰ **A87** **Viral meningitis**
     EXCLUDES 1 *meningitis due to herpesvirus [herpes simplex] (B00.3)*
         meningitis due to measles virus (B05.1)
         meningitis due to mumps virus (B26.1)
         meningitis due to poliomyelitis virus (A80.-)
         meningitis due to zoster (B02.1)

A87.0 **Enteroviral meningitis**
     Coxsackievirus meningitis
     Echovirus meningitis

A87.1 **Adenoviral meningitis**

A87.2 **Lymphocytic choriomeningitis**
     Lymphocytic meningoencephalitis

A87.8 **Other viral meningitis**

A87.9 **Viral meningitis, unspecified** ▽

☑4ᵗʰ **A88** **Other viral infections of central nervous system, not elsewhere classified**
     EXCLUDES 1 *viral encephalitis NOS (A86)*
         viral meningitis NOS (A87.9)

A88.0 **Enteroviral exanthematous fever [Boston exanthem]**

A88.1 **Epidemic vertigo**

A88.8 **Other specified viral infections of central nervous system**

A89 **Unspecified viral infection of central nervous system** ▽

Arthropod-borne viral fevers and viral hemorrhagic fevers (A90-A99)

A90 **Dengue fever [classical dengue]**
     EXCLUDES 1 *dengue hemorrhagic fever (A91)*
     AHA: 2016, 3Q, 13

A91 **Dengue hemorrhagic fever**

☑4ᵗʰ **A92** **Other mosquito-borne viral fevers**
     EXCLUDES 1 *Ross River disease (B33.1)*

A92.0 **Chikungunya virus disease**
     Chikungunya (hemorrhagic) fever

A92.1 **O'nyong-nyong fever**

A92.2 **Venezuelan equine fever**
     Venezuelan equine encephalitis
     Venezuelan equine encephalomyelitis virus disease

☑5ᵗʰ **A92.3** **West Nile virus infection**
     West Nile fever
     AHA: 2016, 3Q, 12

     A92.30 **West Nile virus infection, unspecified** ▽
         West Nile fever NOS
         West Nile fever without complications
         West Nile virus NOS

     A92.31 **West Nile virus infection with encephalitis**
         West Nile encephalitis
         West Nile encephalomyelitis

     A92.32 **West Nile virus infection with other neurologic manifestation**
         Use additional code to specify the neurologic manifestation

     A92.39 **West Nile virus infection with other complications**
         Use additional code to specify the other conditions

A92.4 **Rift Valley fever**

A92.5 **Zika virus disease**
     Zika virus fever
     Zika virus infection
     Zika NOS

A92.8 **Other specified mosquito-borne viral fevers**

A92.9 **Mosquito-borne viral fever, unspecified** ▽

☑4ᵗʰ **A93** **Other arthropod-borne viral fevers, not elsewhere classified**

A93.0 **Oropouche virus disease**
     Oropouche fever

A93.1 **Sandfly fever**
     Pappataci fever
     Phlebotomus fever

A93.2 **Colorado tick fever**

A93.8 **Other specified arthropod-borne viral fevers**
     Piry virus disease
     Vesicular stomatitis virus disease [Indiana fever]

A94 **Unspecified arthropod-borne viral fever** ▽
     Arboviral fever NOS
     Arbovirus infection NOS

☑4ᵗʰ **A95** **Yellow fever**

A95.0 **Sylvatic yellow fever**
     Jungle yellow fever

A95.1 **Urban yellow fever**

A95.9 **Yellow fever, unspecified** ▽

☑4ᵗʰ **A96** **Arenaviral hemorrhagic fever**

A96.0 **Junin hemorrhagic fever**
     Argentinian hemorrhagic fever

A96.1 **Machupo hemorrhagic fever**
     Bolivian hemorrhagic fever

A96.2 **Lassa fever**

☑ Additional Character Req   ☑7ᵗʰ Placeholder Alert   Manifestation   **HCC** CMS-HCC Condition   ▽ Unspecified Code   ►◄ Revised Text   ● New Code   ▲ Revised Code Title

A96.8 **Other arenaviral hemorrhagic fevers**

A96.9 **Arenaviral hemorrhagic fever, unspecified** ▽

✓4ᵗʰ **A98 Other viral hemorrhagic fevers, not elsewhere classified**
     EXCLUDES 1 *chikungunya hemorrhagic fever (A92.0)*
               dengue hemorrhagic fever (A91)

A98.0 **Crimean-Congo hemorrhagic fever**
     Central Asian hemorrhagic fever

A98.1 **Omsk hemorrhagic fever**

A98.2 **Kyasanur Forest disease**

A98.3 **Marburg virus disease**

A98.4 **Ebola virus disease**

A98.5 **Hemorrhagic fever with renal syndrome**
     Epidemic hemorrhagic fever
     Korean hemorrhagic fever
     Russian hemorrhagic fever
     Hantaan virus disease
     Hantavirus disease with renal manifestations
     Nephropathia epidemica
     Songo fever
     EXCLUDES 1 *hantavirus (cardio)-pulmonary syndrome (B33.4)*

A98.8 **Other specified viral hemorrhagic fevers**

A99 **Unspecified viral hemorrhagic fever** ▽

Viral infections characterized by skin and mucous membrane lesions (B00-B09)

✓4ᵗʰ **B00 Herpesviral [herpes simplex] infections**
     EXCLUDES 1 *congenital herpesviral infections (P35.2)*
     EXCLUDES 2 *anogenital herpesviral infection (A60.-)*
               gammaherpesviral mononucleosis (B27.0-)
               herpangina (B08.5)

B00.0 **Eczema herpeticum**
     Kaposi's varicelliform eruption

B00.1 **Herpesviral vesicular dermatitis**
     Herpes simplex facialis
     Herpes simplex labialis
     Herpes simplex otitis externa
     Vesicular dermatitis of ear
     Vesicular dermatitis of lip

B00.2 **Herpesviral gingivostomatitis and pharyngotonsillitis**
     Herpesviral pharyngitis

B00.3 **Herpesviral meningitis**

B00.4 **Herpesviral encephalitis**
     Herpesviral meningoencephalitis
     Simian B disease
     EXCLUDES 1 *herpesviral encephalitis due to herpesvirus 6 and 7 (B10.01, B10.09)*
               non-simplex herpesviral encephalitis (B10.0-)

✓5ᵗʰ B00.5 **Herpesviral ocular disease**

     B00.50 **Herpesviral ocular disease, unspecified** ▽

     B00.51 **Herpesviral iridocyclitis**
         Herpesviral iritis
         Herpesviral uveitis, anterior

     B00.52 **Herpesviral keratitis**
         Herpesviral keratoconjunctivitis

     B00.53 **Herpesviral conjunctivitis**

     B00.59 **Other herpesviral disease of eye**
         Herpesviral dermatitis of eyelid

B00.7 **Disseminated herpesviral disease** HCC
     Herpesviral sepsis

✓5ᵗʰ B00.8 **Other forms of herpesviral infections**
     B00.81 **Herpesviral hepatitis**
     B00.82 **Herpes simplex myelitis** HCC
     B00.89 **Other herpesviral infection**
         Herpesviral whitlow

B00.9 **Herpesviral infection, unspecified** ▽
     Herpes simplex infection NOS

✓4ᵗʰ **B01 Varicella [chickenpox]**

B01.0 **Varicella meningitis**

✓5ᵗʰ B01.1 **Varicella encephalitis, myelitis and encephalomyelitis**
     Postchickenpox encephalitis, myelitis and encephalomyelitis

     B01.11 **Varicella encephalitis and encephalomyelitis**
         Postchickenpox encephalitis and encephalomyelitis

     B01.12 **Varicella myelitis** HCC
         Postchickenpox myelitis

B01.2 **Varicella pneumonia**

✓5ᵗʰ B01.8 **Varicella with other complications**
     B01.81 **Varicella keratitis**
     B01.89 **Other varicella complications**

B01.9 **Varicella without complication** ▽
     Varicella NOS

✓4ᵗʰ **B02 Zoster [herpes zoster]**
     INCLUDES shingles
               zona

B02.0 **Zoster encephalitis**
     Zoster meningoencephalitis

B02.1 **Zoster meningitis**

✓5ᵗʰ B02.2 **Zoster with other nervous system involvement**

     B02.21 **Postherpetic geniculate ganglionitis**

     B02.22 **Postherpetic trigeminal neuralgia**

     B02.23 **Postherpetic polyneuropathy**

     B02.24 **Postherpetic myelitis** HCC
         Herpes zoster myelitis

     B02.29 **Other postherpetic nervous system involvement**
         Postherpetic radiculopathy

✓5ᵗʰ B02.3 **Zoster ocular disease**

     B02.30 **Zoster ocular disease, unspecified** ▽

     B02.31 **Zoster conjunctivitis**

     B02.32 **Zoster iridocyclitis**

     B02.33 **Zoster keratitis**
         Herpes zoster keratoconjunctivitis

     B02.34 **Zoster scleritis**

     B02.39 **Other herpes zoster eye disease**
         Zoster blepharitis

B02.7 **Disseminated zoster**

B02.8 **Zoster with other complications**
     Herpes zoster otitis externa

B02.9 **Zoster without complications** ▽
     Zoster NOS

B03 Smallpox
     NOTE   In 1980 the 33rd World Health Assembly declared that smallpox had been eradicated.
               The classification is maintained for surveillance purposes.

B04 Monkeypox

✓4ᵗʰ **B05 Measles**
     INCLUDES morbilli
     EXCLUDES 1 *subacute sclerosing panencephalitis (A81.1)*

B05.0 **Measles complicated by encephalitis**
     Postmeasles encephalitis

B05.1 **Measles complicated by meningitis**
     Postmeasles meningitis

B05.2 **Measles complicated by pneumonia**
     Postmeasles pneumonia

B05.3 **Measles complicated by otitis media**
     Postmeasles otitis media

B05.4 **Measles with intestinal complications**

✓5ᵗʰ B05.8 **Measles with other complications**
     B05.81 **Measles keratitis and keratoconjunctivitis**
     B05.89 **Other measles complications**

B05.9 **Measles without complication** ▽
     Measles NOS

✓4ᵗʰ **B06 Rubella [German measles]**
     EXCLUDES 1 *congenital rubella (P35.0)*

✓5ᵗʰ B06.0 **Rubella with neurological complications**

     B06.00 **Rubella with neurological complication, unspecified** ▽

     B06.01 **Rubella encephalitis**
         Rubella meningoencephalitis

     B06.02 **Rubella meningitis**

     B06.09 **Other neurological complications of rubella**

✓5ᵗʰ B06.8 **Rubella with other complications**

     B06.81 **Rubella pneumonia**

     B06.82 **Rubella arthritis** HCC

     B06.89 **Other rubella complications**

B06.9 **Rubella without complication** ▽
     Rubella NOS

EXCLUDES 1 Not coded here   EXCLUDES 2 Not included here   N Newborn Age: 0   P Pediatric Age: 0-17   M Maternity Age: 12-55   A Adult Age: 15-124

446   ICD-10-CM 2018

☑4ᵗʰ **B07 Viral warts**

INCLUDES   verruca simplex
     verruca vulgaris
     viral warts due to human papillomavirus

EXCLUDES 2   *anogenital (venereal) warts (A63.0)*
     papilloma of bladder (D41.4)
     papilloma of cervix (D26.0)
     papilloma larynx (D14.1)

B07.0 Plantar wart
     Verruca plantaris

B07.8 Other viral warts
     Common wart
     Flat wart
     Verruca plana

B07.9 Viral wart, unspecified ▽

☑4ᵗʰ **B08 Other viral infections characterized by skin and mucous membrane lesions, not elsewhere classified**

EXCLUDES 1   *vesicular stomatitis virus disease (A93.8)*

☑5ᵗʰ **B08.0 Other orthopoxvirus infections**

EXCLUDES 2   *monkeypox (B04)*

☑6ᵗʰ **B08.01 Cowpox and vaccinia not from vaccine**

B08.010 Cowpox
     DEF: A disease contracted by milking infected cows; vesicles usually appear on the fingers, hands, and adjacent areas and usually disappear without scarring; other symptoms: local edema, lymphangitis, and regional lymphadenitis with or without fever.

B08.011 Vaccinia not from vaccine
     EXCLUDES 1   *vaccinia (from vaccination) (generalized) (T88.1)*

B08.02 Orf virus disease
     Contagious pustular dermatitis
     Ecthyma contagiosum

B08.03 Pseudocowpox [milker's node]

B08.04 Paravaccinia, unspecified ▽

B08.09 Other orthopoxvirus infections
     Orthopoxvirus infection NOS

B08.1 Molluscum contagiosum
     DEF: Benign poxvirus infection causing small bumps on the skin or conjunctiva; transmitted by close contact.

☑5ᵗʰ **B08.2 Exanthema subitum [sixth disease]**
     Roseola infantum

B08.20 Exanthema subitum [sixth disease], unspecified 🅿 ▽
     Roseola infantum, unspecified

B08.21 Exanthema subitum [sixth disease] due to human herpesvirus 6 🅿
     Roseola infantum due to human herpesvirus 6

B08.22 Exanthema subitum [sixth disease] due to human herpesvirus 7 🅿
     Roseola infantum due to human herpesvirus 7

B08.3 Erythema infectiosum [fifth disease]

B08.4 Enteroviral vesicular stomatitis with exanthem
     Hand, foot and mouth disease

B08.5 Enteroviral vesicular pharyngitis
     Herpangina
     DEF: Acute infectious Coxsackie virus infection causing throat lesions, fever, and vomiting; generally affects children in summer.

☑5ᵗʰ **B08.6 Parapoxvirus infections**

B08.60 Parapoxvirus infection, unspecified ▽

B08.61 Bovine stomatitis

B08.62 Sealpox

B08.69 Other parapoxvirus infections

☑5ᵗʰ **B08.7 Yatapoxvirus infections**

B08.70 Yatapoxvirus infection, unspecified ▽

B08.71 Tanapox virus disease

B08.72 Yaba pox virus disease
     Yaba monkey tumor disease

B08.79 Other yatapoxvirus infections

B08.8 Other specified viral infections characterized by skin and mucous membrane lesions
     Enteroviral lymphonodular pharyngitis
     Foot-and-mouth disease
     Poxvirus NEC

B09 Unspecified viral infection characterized by skin and mucous membrane lesions ▽
     Viral enanthema NOS
     Viral exanthema NOS

Other human herpesviruses (B10)

☑4ᵗʰ **B10 Other human herpesviruses**

EXCLUDES 2   *cytomegalovirus (B25.9)*
     Epstein-Barr virus (B27.0-)
     herpes NOS (B00.9)
     herpes simplex (B00.-)
     herpes zoster (B02.-)
     human herpesvirus NOS (B00.-)
     human herpesvirus 1 and 2 (B00.-)
     human herpesvirus 3 (B01.-, B02.-)
     human herpesvirus 4 (B27.0-)
     human herpesvirus (B25.-)
     varicella (B01.-)
     zoster (B02.-)

☑5ᵗʰ **B10.0 Other human herpesvirus encephalitis**

EXCLUDES 2   *herpes encephalitis NOS (B00.4)*
     herpes simplex encephalitis (B00.4)
     human herpesvirus encephalitis (B00.4)
     simian B herpes virus encephalitis (B00.4)

B10.01 Human herpesvirus 6 encephalitis

B10.09 Other human herpesvirus encephalitis
     Human herpesvirus 7 encephalitis

☑5ᵗʰ **B10.8 Other human herpesvirus infection**

B10.81 Human herpesvirus 6 infection

B10.82 Human herpesvirus 7 infection

B10.89 Other human herpesvirus infection
     Human herpesvirus 8 infection
     Kaposi's sarcoma-associated herpesvirus infection

Viral hepatitis (B15-B19)

EXCLUDES 1   *sequelae of viral hepatitis (B94.2)*
EXCLUDES 2   *cytomegaloviral hepatitis (B25.1)*
     herpesviral [herpes simplex] hepatitis (B00.81)

DEF: Hepatitis A: HAV infection is self-limiting with flulike symptoms; transmission, fecal-oral.
DEF: Hepatitis B: HBV infection can be chronic and systemic; transmission, bodily fluids.
DEF: Hepatitis C: HCV infection can be chronic and systemic; transmission, blood transfusion and unidentified agents.
DEF: Hepatitis D (delta): HDV occurs only in the presence of hepatitis B virus; transmission, contaminated blood in contact with mucous membranes.
DEF: Hepatitis E: HEV is epidemic form; transmission, fecal-oral, most often from contaminated water.

☑4ᵗʰ **B15 Acute hepatitis A**

B15.0 Hepatitis A with hepatic coma

B15.9 Hepatitis A without hepatic coma
     Hepatitis A (acute)(viral) NOS

☑4ᵗʰ **B16 Acute hepatitis B**
     AHA: 2016, 3Q, 13

B16.0 Acute hepatitis B with delta-agent with hepatic coma

B16.1 Acute hepatitis B with delta-agent without hepatic coma

B16.2 Acute hepatitis B without delta-agent with hepatic coma

B16.9 Acute hepatitis B without delta-agent and without hepatic coma
     Hepatitis B (acute) (viral) NOS

☑4ᵗʰ **B17 Other acute viral hepatitis**

B17.0 Acute delta-(super) infection of hepatitis B carrier

☑5ᵗʰ **B17.1 Acute hepatitis C**

B17.10 Acute hepatitis C without hepatic coma
     Acute hepatitis C NOS

B17.11 Acute hepatitis C with hepatic coma

B17.2 Acute hepatitis E

B17.8 Other specified acute viral hepatitis
     Hepatitis non-A non-B (acute) (viral) NEC

B17.9 Acute viral hepatitis, unspecified ▽
     Acute hepatitis NOS
     Acute infectious hepatitis NOS

☑4ᵗʰ **B18 Chronic viral hepatitis**

INCLUDES   carrier of viral hepatitis
AHA: 2017, 1Q, 41

B18.0 Chronic viral hepatitis B with delta-agent HCC

☑ Additional Character Req   ✓ˣ˙⁷ᵗʰ Placeholder Alert   Manifestation   HCC CMS-HCC Condition   ▽ Unspecified Code   ▶◀ Revised Text   ● New Code   ▲ Revised Code Title

 ICD-10-CM 2018   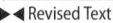 447

B18.1   **Chronic viral hepatitis B** without delta-agent   HCC
Carrier of viral hepatitis B
Chronic (viral) hepatitis B

B18.2   **Chronic viral** hepatitis C   HCC
Carrier of viral hepatitis C

B18.8   **Other chronic viral hepatitis**   HCC
Carrier of other viral hepatitis

B18.9   **Chronic viral hepatitis, unspecified**   HCC ▽
Carrier of unspecified viral hepatitis

✓4th **B19**   **Unspecified viral hepatitis**

B19.0   **Unspecified viral hepatitis** with hepatic coma   ▽

✓5th **B19.1**   **Unspecified viral** hepatitis B

    B19.10   **Unspecified viral hepatitis B** without hepatic coma   ▽
Unspecified viral hepatitis B NOS

    B19.11   **Unspecified viral hepatitis B** with hepatic coma   ▽

✓5th **B19.2**   **Unspecified viral** hepatitis C

    B19.20   **Unspecified viral hepatitis C** without hepatic coma   ▽
Viral hepatitis C NOS

    B19.21   **Unspecified viral hepatitis C** with hepatic coma   ▽

B19.9   **Unspecified viral hepatitis** without hepatic coma   ▽
Viral hepatitis NOS

Human immunodeficiency virus [HIV] disease (B20)

B20   **Human immunodeficiency virus [HIV] disease**   HCC
INCLUDES   acquired immune deficiency syndrome [AIDS]
AIDS-related complex [ARC]
HIV infection, symptomatic
Code first human immunodeficiency virus [HIV] disease complicating pregnancy, childbirth and the puerperium, if applicable (O98.7-)
Use additional code(s) to identify all manifestations of HIV infection
EXCLUDES 1   asymptomatic human immunodeficiency virus [HIV] infection status (Z21)
exposure to HIV virus (Z20.6)
inconclusive serologic evidence of HIV (R75)

Other viral diseases (B25-B34)

✓4th **B25**   **Cytomegaloviral disease**
EXCLUDES 1   congenital cytomegalovirus infection (P35.1)
cytomegaloviral mononucleosis (B27.1-)

B25.0   **Cytomegaloviral** pneumonitis   HCC

B25.1   **Cytomegaloviral** hepatitis   HCC

B25.2   **Cytomegaloviral** pancreatitis   HCC

B25.8   **Other cytomegaloviral diseases**   HCC
Cytomegaloviral encephalitis

B25.9   **Cytomegaloviral disease, unspecified**   HCC ▽

✓4th **B26**   **Mumps**
INCLUDES   epidemic parotitis
infectious parotitis

B26.0   **Mumps** orchitis   ♂

B26.1   **Mumps** meningitis

B26.2   **Mumps** encephalitis

B26.3   **Mumps** pancreatitis

✓5th **B26.8**   **Mumps with other complications**

    B26.81   **Mumps** hepatitis

    B26.82   **Mumps** myocarditis

    B26.83   **Mumps** nephritis

    B26.84   **Mumps** polyneuropathy

    B26.85   **Mumps** arthritis   HCC

    B26.89   **Other mumps complications**

B26.9   **Mumps without complication**   ▽
Mumps NOS
Mumps parotitis NOS

✓4th **B27**   **Infectious mononucleosis**
INCLUDES   glandular fever
monocytic angina
Pfeiffer's disease

✓5th **B27.0**   **Gammaherpesviral** mononucleosis
Mononucleosis due to Epstein-Barr virus

    B27.00   **Gammaherpesviral mononucleosis** without complication

    B27.01   **Gammaherpesviral mononucleosis** with polyneuropathy

    B27.02   **Gammaherpesviral mononucleosis** with meningitis

    B27.09   **Gammaherpesviral mononucleosis with other complications**
Hepatomegaly in gammaherpesviral mononucleosis

✓5th **B27.1**   **Cytomegaloviral** mononucleosis

    B27.10   **Cytomegaloviral mononucleosis** without complications

    B27.11   **Cytomegaloviral mononucleosis** with polyneuropathy

    B27.12   **Cytomegaloviral mononucleosis** with meningitis

    B27.19   **Cytomegaloviral mononucleosis with other complication**
Hepatomegaly in cytomegaloviral mononucleosis

✓5th **B27.8**   **Other infectious mononucleosis**

    B27.80   **Other infectious mononucleosis** without complication

    B27.81   **Other infectious mononucleosis** with polyneuropathy

    B27.82   **Other infectious mononucleosis** with meningitis

    B27.89   **Other infectious mononucleosis with other complication**
Hepatomegaly in other infectious mononucleosis

✓5th **B27.9**   **Infectious mononucleosis, unspecified**

    B27.90   **Infectious mononucleosis, unspecified** without complication   ▽

    B27.91   **Infectious mononucleosis, unspecified** with polyneuropathy   ▽

    B27.92   **Infectious mononucleosis, unspecified** with meningitis   ▽

    B27.99   **Infectious mononucleosis, unspecified with other complication**   ▽
Hepatomegaly in unspecified infectious mononucleosis

✓4th **B30**   **Viral conjunctivitis**
EXCLUDES 1   herpesviral [herpes simplex] ocular disease (B00.5)
ocular zoster (B02.3)

B30.0   **Keratoconjunctivitis** due to adenovirus
Epidemic keratoconjunctivitis
Shipyard eye

B30.1   **Conjunctivitis** due to adenovirus
Acute adenoviral follicular conjunctivitis
Swimming-pool conjunctivitis

B30.2   **Viral** pharyngoconjunctivitis

B30.3   **Acute epidemic hemorrhagic conjunctivitis (enteroviral)**
Conjunctivitis due to coxsackievirus 24
Conjunctivitis due to enterovirus 70
Hemorrhagic conjunctivitis (acute)(epidemic)

B30.8   **Other viral conjunctivitis**
Newcastle conjunctivitis

B30.9   **Viral conjunctivitis, unspecified**   ▽

✓4th **B33**   **Other viral diseases, not elsewhere classified**

B33.0   **Epidemic myalgia**
Bornholm disease

B33.1   **Ross River disease**
Epidemic polyarthritis and exanthema
Ross River fever

Viral Conjunctivitis

Normal conjunctiva

Inflamed conjunctiva

✓5ᵗʰ **B33.2 Viral carditis**
  Coxsackie (virus) carditis

    B33.20 Viral carditis, unspecified ▽

    B33.21 Viral endocarditis

    B33.22 Viral myocarditis

    B33.23 Viral pericarditis

    B33.24 Viral cardiomyopathy HCC

B33.3 Retrovirus infections, not elsewhere classified
  Retrovirus infection NOS

B33.4 Hantavirus (cardio)-pulmonary syndrome [HPS] [HCPS]
  Hantavirus disease with pulmonary manifestations
  Sin nombre virus disease
  Use additional code to identify any associated acute kidney
    failure (N17.9)
  EXCLUDES 1 *hantavirus disease with renal manifestations (A98.5)*
    hemorrhagic fever with renal manifestations (A98.5)

B33.8 Other specified viral diseases
  EXCLUDES 1 *anogenital human papillomavirus infection (A63.0)*
    viral warts due to human papillomavirus infection
    (B07)

✓4ᵗʰ **B34 Viral infection of unspecified site**
  EXCLUDES 1 *anogenital human papillomavirus infection (A63.0)*
    cytomegaloviral disease NOS (B25.9)
    herpesvirus [herpes simplex] infection NOS (B00.9)
    retrovirus infection NOS (B33.3)
    viral agents as the cause of diseases classified elsewhere (B97.-)
    viral warts due to human papillomavirus infection (B07)

B34.0 Adenovirus infection, unspecified ▽

B34.1 Enterovirus infection, unspecified ▽
  Coxsackievirus infection NOS
  Echovirus infection NOS

B34.2 Coronavirus infection, unspecified ▽
  EXCLUDES 1 *pneumonia due to SARS-associated coronavirus*
    (J12.81)

B34.3 Parvovirus infection, unspecified ▽

B34.4 Papovavirus infection, unspecified ▽

B34.8 Other viral infections of unspecified site ▽

B34.9 Viral infection, unspecified ▽
  Viremia NOS
  AHA: 2016, 3Q, 10

Mycoses (B35-B49)

EXCLUDES 2 *hypersensitivity pneumonitis due to organic dust (J67.-)*
  mycosis fungoides (C84.0-)

✓4ᵗʰ **B35 Dermatophytosis**
  INCLUDES favus
    infections due to species of Epidermophyton, Micro-sporum
      and Trichophyton
    tinea, any type except those in B36-
  DEF: Contagious superficial fungal infection of the skin that invades and
  grows in dead keratin.

B35.0 Tinea barbae and tinea capitis
  Beard ringworm
  Kerion
  Scalp ringworm
  Sycosis, mycotic

B35.1 Tinea unguium
  Dermatophytic onychia
  Dermatophytosis of nail
  Onychomycosis
  Ringworm of nails

B35.2 Tinea manuum
  Dermatophytosis of hand
  Hand ringworm

B35.3 Tinea pedis
  Athlete's foot
  Dermatophytosis of foot
  Foot ringworm

B35.4 Tinea corporis
  Ringworm of the body

B35.5 Tinea imbricata
  Tokelau

B35.6 Tinea cruris
  Dhobi itch
  Groin ringworm
  Jock itch

B35.8 Other dermatophytoses
  Disseminated dermatophytosis
  Granulomatous dermatophytosis ▽

B35.9 Dermatophytosis, unspecified ▽
  Ringworm NOS

✓4ᵗʰ **B36 Other superficial mycoses**

B36.0 Pityriasis versicolor
  Tinea flava
  Tinea versicolor

B36.1 Tinea nigra
  Keratomycosis nigricans palmaris
  Microsporosis nigra
  Pityriasis nigra

B36.2 White piedra
  Tinea blanca

B36.3 Black piedra

B36.8 Other specified superficial mycoses

B36.9 Superficial mycosis, unspecified ▽

✓4ᵗʰ **B37 Candidiasis**
  INCLUDES candidosis
    moniliasis
  EXCLUDES 1 *neonatal candidiasis (P37.5)*

B37.0 Candidal stomatitis
  Oral thrush

B37.1 Pulmonary candidiasis HCC
  Candidal bronchitis
  Candidal pneumonia

B37.2 Candidiasis of skin and nail
  Candidal onychia
  Candidal paronychia
  EXCLUDES 2 *diaper dermatitis (L22)*

B37.3 Candidiasis of vulva and vagina ♀
  Candidal vulvovaginitis
  Monilial vulvovaginitis
  Vaginal thrush

✓5ᵗʰ **B37.4 Candidiasis of other urogenital sites**

    B37.41 Candidal cystitis and urethritis

    B37.42 Candidal balanitis

    B37.49 Other urogenital candidiasis
      Candidal pyelonephritis

B37.5 Candidal meningitis

B37.6 Candidal endocarditis

B37.7 Candidal sepsis HCC
  Disseminated candidiasis
  Systemic candidiasis
  AHA: 2014, 4Q, 46

✓5ᵗʰ **B37.8 Candidiasis of other sites**

    B37.81 Candidal esophagitis HCC

    B37.82 Candidal enteritis
      Candidal proctitis

    B37.83 Candidal cheilitis

    B37.84 Candidal otitis externa

    B37.89 Other sites of candidiasis
      Candidal osteomyelitis

B37.9 Candidiasis, unspecified ▽
  Thrush NOS

✓4ᵗʰ **B38 Coccidioidomycosis**

B38.0 Acute pulmonary coccidioidomycosis HCC

B38.1 Chronic pulmonary coccidioidomycosis HCC

B38.2 Pulmonary coccidioidomycosis, unspecified HCC ▽

B38.3 Cutaneous coccidioidomycosis

B38.4 Coccidioidomycosis meningitis
  DEF: *Coccidioides immitis* infection of the lining of the brain and/or
  spinal cord.

B38.7 Disseminated coccidioidomycosis
  Generalized coccidioidomycosis

✓5ᵗʰ **B38.8 Other forms of coccidioidomycosis**

    B38.81 Prostatic coccidioidomycosis ♂

    B38.89 Other forms of coccidioidomycosis

B38.9 Coccidioidomycosis, unspecified ▽

☑ Additional Character Req   ✓x7ᵗʰ Placeholder Alert   Manifestation   HCC CMS-HCC Condition   ▽ Unspecified Code   ►◄ Revised Text   ● New Code   ▲ Revised Code Title

ICD-10-CM 2018   449

Chapter 1. Certain Infectious and Parasitic Diseases

B33.2–B38.9

Histoplasmosis

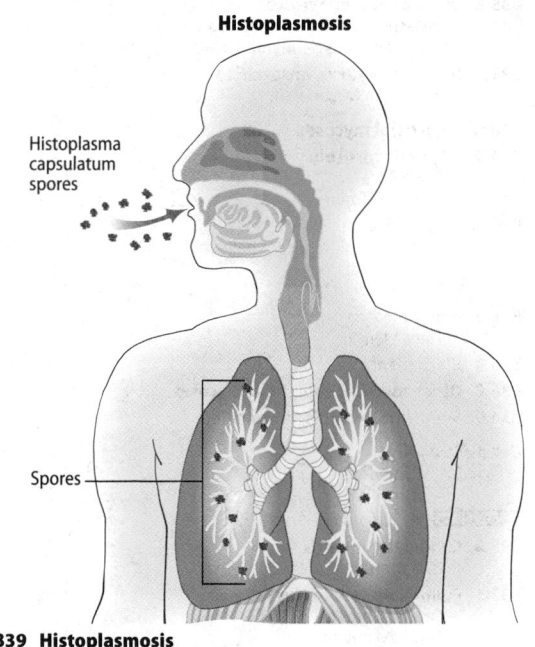

Histoplasma capsulatum spores

Spores

☑4ᵗʰ **B39 Histoplasmosis**
Code first associated AIDS (B20)
Use additional code for any associated manifestations, such as:
    endocarditis (I39)
    meningitis (G02)
    pericarditis (I32)
    retinitits (H32)
DEF: Type of lung infection caused by breathing in fungal spores often found in the droppings of bats and birds or soil contaminated by their droppings.

  B39.0 Acute pulmonary histoplasmosis capsulati   HCC
  B39.1 Chronic pulmonary histoplasmosis capsulati   HCC
  B39.2 Pulmonary histoplasmosis capsulati, unspecified   HCC ▽
  B39.3 Disseminated histoplasmosis capsulati
      Generalized histoplasmosis capsulati
  B39.4 Histoplasmosis capsulati, unspecified   ▽
      American histoplasmosis
  B39.5 Histoplasmosis duboisii
      African histoplasmosis
  B39.9 Histoplasmosis, unspecified   ▽

☑4ᵗʰ **B40 Blastomycosis**
    EXCLUDES 1 Brazilian blastomycosis (B41.-)
             keloidal blastomycosis (B48.0)
  B40.0 Acute pulmonary blastomycosis   HCC
  B40.1 Chronic pulmonary blastomycosis   HCC
  B40.2 Pulmonary blastomycosis, unspecified   HCC ▽
  B40.3 Cutaneous blastomycosis
  B40.7 Disseminated blastomycosis
      Generalized blastomycosis
  ☑5ᵗʰ **B40.8** Other forms of blastomycosis
      B40.81 Blastomycotic meningoencephalitis
          Meningomyelitis due to blastomycosis
      B40.89 Other forms of blastomycosis
  B40.9 Blastomycosis, unspecified   ▽

☑4ᵗʰ **B41 Paracoccidioidomycosis**
    INCLUDES Brazilian blastomycosis
             Lutz' disease
  B41.0 Pulmonary paracoccidioidomycosis   HCC
  B41.7 Disseminated paracoccidioidomycosis
      Generalized paracoccidioidomycosis
  B41.8 Other forms of paracoccidioidomycosis
  B41.9 Paracoccidioidomycosis, unspecified   ▽

☑4ᵗʰ **B42 Sporotrichosis**
  B42.0 Pulmonary sporotrichosis
  B42.1 Lymphocutaneous sporotrichosis
  B42.7 Disseminated sporotrichosis
      Generalized sporotrichosis

  ☑5ᵗʰ **B42.8** Other forms of sporotrichosis
      B42.81 Cerebral sporotrichosis
          Meningitis due to sporotrichosis
      B42.82 Sporotrichosis arthritis   HCC
      B42.89 Other forms of sporotrichosis
  B42.9 Sporotrichosis, unspecified   ▽

☑4ᵗʰ **B43 Chromomycosis and pheomycotic abscess**
  B43.0 Cutaneous chromomycosis
      Dermatitis verrucosa
  B43.1 Pheomycotic brain abscess
      Cerebral chromomycosis
  B43.2 Subcutaneous pheomycotic abscess and cyst
  B43.8 Other forms of chromomycosis
  B43.9 Chromomycosis, unspecified   ▽

☑4ᵗʰ **B44 Aspergillosis**
    INCLUDES aspergilloma
  B44.0 Invasive pulmonary aspergillosis   HCC
  B44.1 Other pulmonary aspergillosis   HCC
  B44.2 Tonsillar aspergillosis   HCC
  B44.7 Disseminated aspergillosis   HCC
      Generalized aspergillosis
  ☑5ᵗʰ **B44.8** Other forms of aspergillosis
      B44.81 Allergic bronchopulmonary aspergillosis   HCC
      B44.89 Other forms of aspergillosis   HCC
  B44.9 Aspergillosis, unspecified   HCC ▽

☑4ᵗʰ **B45 Cryptococcosis**
  B45.0 Pulmonary cryptococcosis   HCC
  B45.1 Cerebral cryptococcosis   HCC
      Cryptococcal meningitis
      Cryptococcosis meningocerebralis
  B45.2 Cutaneous cryptococcosis   HCC
  B45.3 Osseous cryptococcosis   HCC
  B45.7 Disseminated cryptococcosis   HCC
      Generalized cryptococcosis
  B45.8 Other forms of cryptococcosis   HCC
  B45.9 Cryptococcosis, unspecified   HCC ▽

☑4ᵗʰ **B46 Zygomycosis**
  B46.0 Pulmonary mucormycosis   HCC
  B46.1 Rhinocerebral mucormycosis   HCC
  B46.2 Gastrointestinal mucormycosis   HCC
  B46.3 Cutaneous mucormycosis   HCC
      Subcutaneous mucormycosis
  B46.4 Disseminated mucormycosis   HCC
      Generalized mucormycosis
  B46.5 Mucormycosis, unspecified   HCC ▽
  B46.8 Other zygomycoses   HCC
      Entomophthoromycosis
  B46.9 Zygomycosis, unspecified   HCC ▽
      Phycomycosis NOS

☑4ᵗʰ **B47 Mycetoma**
  B47.0 Eumycetoma
      Madura foot, mycotic
      Maduromycosis
  B47.1 Actinomycetoma
  B47.9 Mycetoma, unspecified   ▽
      Madura foot NOS

☑4ᵗʰ **B48 Other mycoses, not elsewhere classified**
  B48.0 Lobomycosis
      Keloidal blastomycosis
      Lobo's disease
  B48.1 Rhinosporidiosis
  B48.2 Allescheriasis
      Infection due to Pseudallescheria boydii
      EXCLUDES 1 eumycetoma (B47.0)
  B48.3 Geotrichosis
      Geotrichum stomatitis
  B48.4 Penicillosis   HCC

EXCLUDES 1 Not coded here   **EXCLUDES 2** Not included here   N Newborn Age: 0   P Pediatric Age: 0-17   M Maternity Age: 12-55   A Adult Age: 15-124

450   ICD-10-CM 2018

B48.8 Other specified mycoses `HCC`
  Adiaspiromycosis
  Infection of tissue and organs by Alternaria
  Infection of tissue and organs by Drechslera
  Infection of tissue and organs by Fusarium
  Infection of tissue and organs by saprophytic fungi NEC
  AHA: 2014, 4Q, 46; 2014, 2Q, 13

B49 Unspecified mycosis ▽
  Fungemia NOS

Protozoal diseases (B50-B64)

EXCLUDES 1 amebiasis (A06.-)
  other protozoal intestinal diseases (A07.-)

✓4ᵗʰ B50 Plasmodium falciparum malaria
  INCLUDES mixed infections of Plasmodium falciparum with any other Plasmodium species

  B50.0 Plasmodium falciparum malaria with cerebral complications
    Cerebral malaria NOS

  B50.8 Other severe and complicated Plasmodium falciparum malaria
    Severe or complicated Plasmodium falciparum malaria NOS

  B50.9 Plasmodium falciparum malaria, unspecified ▽

✓4ᵗʰ B51 Plasmodium vivax malaria
  INCLUDES mixed infections of Plasmodium vivax with other Plasmodium species, except Plasmodium falciparum
  EXCLUDES 1 plasmodium vivax with Plasmodium falciparum (B50.-)

  B51.0 Plasmodium vivax malaria with rupture of spleen
  B51.8 Plasmodium vivax malaria with other complications
  B51.9 Plasmodium vivax malaria without complication ▽
    Plasmodium vivax malaria NOS

✓4ᵗʰ B52 Plasmodium malariae malaria
  INCLUDES mixed infections of Plasmodium malariae with other Plasmodium species, except Plasmodium falciparum and Plasmodium vivax
  EXCLUDES 1 Plasmodium falciparum (B50.-)
    Plasmodium vivax (B51.-)

  B52.0 Plasmodium malariae malaria with nephropathy
  B52.8 Plasmodium malariae malaria with other complications
  B52.9 Plasmodium malariae malaria without complication ▽
    Plasmodium malariae malaria NOS

✓4ᵗʰ B53 Other specified malaria
  B53.0 Plasmodium ovale malaria
    EXCLUDES 1 Plasmodium ovale with Plasmodium falciparum (B50.-)
      Plasmodium ovale with Plasmodium malariae (B52.-)
      Plasmodium ovale with Plasmodium vivax (B51.-)

  B53.1 Malaria due to simian plasmodia
    EXCLUDES 1 Malaria due to simian plasmodia with Plasmodium falciparum (B50.-)
      Malaria due to simian plasmodia with Plasmodium malariae (B52.-)
      Malaria due to simian plasmodia with Plasmodium ovale (B53.0)
      Malaria due to simian plasmodia with Plasmodium vivax (B51.-)

  B53.8 Other malaria, not elsewhere classified

B54 Unspecified malaria ▽

✓4ᵗʰ B55 Leishmaniasis
  B55.0 Visceral leishmaniasis
    Kala-azar
    Post-kala-azar dermal leishmaniasis
  B55.1 Cutaneous leishmaniasis
  B55.2 Mucocutaneous leishmaniasis
  B55.9 Leishmaniasis, unspecified ▽

✓4ᵗʰ B56 African trypanosomiasis
  B56.0 Gambiense trypanosomiasis
    Infection due to Trypanosoma brucei gambiense
    West African sleeping sickness
  B56.1 Rhodesiense trypanosomiasis
    East African sleeping sickness
    Infection due to Trypanosoma brucei rhodesiense
  B56.9 African trypanosomiasis, unspecified ▽
    Sleeping sickness NOS

✓4ᵗʰ B57 Chagas' disease
  INCLUDES American trypanosomiasis
    infection due to Trypanosoma cruzi

  B57.0 Acute Chagas' disease with heart involvement
    Acute Chagas' disease with myocarditis
  B57.1 Acute Chagas' disease without heart involvement
    Acute Chagas' disease NOS
  B57.2 Chagas' disease (chronic) with heart involvement
    American trypanosomiasis NOS
    Chagas' disease (chronic) NOS
    Chagas' disease (chronic) with myocarditis
    Trypanosomiasis NOS

  ✓5ᵗʰ B57.3 Chagas' disease (chronic) with digestive system involvement
    B57.30 Chagas' disease with digestive system involvement, unspecified ▽
    B57.31 Megaesophagus in Chagas' disease
    B57.32 Megacolon in Chagas' disease
    B57.39 Other digestive system involvement in Chagas' disease

  ✓5ᵗʰ B57.4 Chagas' disease (chronic) with nervous system involvement
    B57.40 Chagas' disease with nervous system involvement, unspecified ▽
    B57.41 Meningitis in Chagas' disease
    B57.42 Meningoencephalitis in Chagas' disease
    B57.49 Other nervous system involvement in Chagas' disease

  B57.5 Chagas' disease (chronic) with other organ involvement

✓4ᵗʰ B58 Toxoplasmosis
  INCLUDES infection due to Toxoplasma gondii
  EXCLUDES 1 congenital toxoplasmosis (P37.1)

  ✓5ᵗʰ B58.0 Toxoplasma oculopathy
    B58.00 Toxoplasma oculopathy, unspecified ▽
    B58.01 Toxoplasma chorioretinitis
    B58.09 Other toxoplasma oculopathy
      Toxoplasma uveitis
  B58.1 Toxoplasma hepatitis
  B58.2 Toxoplasma meningoencephalitis `HCC`
  B58.3 Pulmonary toxoplasmosis `HCC`
  ✓5ᵗʰ B58.8 Toxoplasmosis with other organ involvement
    B58.81 Toxoplasma myocarditis
    B58.82 Toxoplasma myositis
    B58.83 Toxoplasma tubulo-interstitial nephropathy
      Toxoplasma pyelonephritis
    B58.89 Toxoplasmosis with other organ involvement
  B58.9 Toxoplasmosis, unspecified ▽

B59 Pneumocystosis `HCC`
  Pneumonia due to Pneumocystis carinii
  Pneumonia due to Pneumocystis jiroveci

✓4ᵗʰ B60 Other protozoal diseases, not elsewhere classified
  EXCLUDES 1 cryptosporidiosis (A07.2)
    intestinal microsporidiosis (A07.8)
    isosporiasis (A07.3)

  B60.0 Babesiosis
    Piroplasmosis
  ✓5ᵗʰ B60.1 Acanthamebiasis
    B60.10 Acanthamebiasis, unspecified ▽
    B60.11 Meningoencephalitis due to Acanthamoeba (culbertsoni)
    B60.12 Conjunctivitis due to Acanthamoeba
    B60.13 Keratoconjunctivitis due to Acanthamoeba
    B60.19 Other acanthamebic disease
  B60.2 Naegleriasis
    Primary amebic meningoencephalitis
  B60.8 Other specified protozoal diseases
    Microsporidiosis

B64 Unspecified protozoal disease ▽

☑ Additional Character Req   ✓x7ᵗʰ Placeholder Alert   Manifestation   `HCC` CMS-HCC Condition   ▽ Unspecified Code   ▶◀ Revised Text   ● New Code   ▲ Revised Code Title

ICD-10-CM 2018   451

Helminthiases (B65-B83)

✓4th B65 Schistosomiasis [bilharziasis]
INCLUDES snail fever

B65.0 Schistosomiasis due to Schistosoma haematobium [urinary schistosomiasis]

B65.1 Schistosomiasis due to Schistosoma mansoni [intestinal schistosomiasis]

B65.2 Schistosomiasis due to Schistosoma japonicum
Asiatic schistosomiasis

B65.3 Cercarial dermatitis
Swimmer's itch

B65.8 Other schistosomiasis
Infection due to Schistosoma intercalatum
Infection due to Schistosoma mattheei
Infection due to Schistosoma mekongi

B65.9 Schistosomiasis, unspecified ▽

✓4th B66 Other fluke infections

B66.0 Opisthorchiasis
Infection due to cat liver fluke
Infection due to Opisthorchis (felineus)(viverrini)

B66.1 Clonorchiasis
Chinese liver fluke disease
Infection due to Clonorchis sinensis
Oriental liver fluke disease

B66.2 Dicroceliasis
Infection due to Dicrocoelium dendriticum
Lancet fluke infection

B66.3 Fascioliasis
Infection due to Fasciola gigantica
Infection due to Fasciola hepatica
Infection due to Fasciola indica
Sheep liver fluke disease

B66.4 Paragonimiasis HCC
Infection due to Paragonimus species
Lung fluke disease
Pulmonary distomiasis

B66.5 Fasciolopsiasis
Infection due to Fasciolopsis buski
Intestinal distomiasis

B66.8 Other specified fluke infections
Echinostomiasis
Heterophyiasis
Metagonimiasis
Nanophyetiasis
Watsoniasis

B66.9 Fluke infection, unspecified ▽

✓4th B67 Echinococcosis
INCLUDES hydatidosis

B67.0 Echinococcus granulosus infection of liver

B67.1 Echinococcus granulosus infection of lung HCC

B67.2 Echinococcus granulosus infection of bone

✓5th B67.3 Echinococcus granulosus infection, other and multiple sites

B67.31 Echinococcus granulosus infection, thyroid gland

B67.32 Echinococcus granulosus infection, multiple sites

B67.39 Echinococcus granulosus infection, other sites

B67.4 Echinococcus granulosus infection, unspecified ▽
Dog tapeworm (infection)

B67.5 Echinococcus multilocularis infection of liver

✓5th B67.6 Echinococcus multilocularis infection, other and multiple sites

B67.61 Echinococcus multilocularis infection, multiple sites

B67.69 Echinococcus multilocularis infection, other sites

B67.7 Echinococcus multilocularis infection, unspecified ▽

B67.8 Echinococcosis, unspecified, of liver ▽

✓5th B67.9 Echinococcosis, other and unspecified

B67.90 Echinococcosis, unspecified ▽
Echinococcosis NOS

B67.99 Other echinococcosis

✓4th B68 Taeniasis
EXCLUDES 1 cysticercosis (B69.-)

B68.0 Taenia solium taeniasis
Pork tapeworm (infection)

B68.1 Taenia saginata taeniasis
Beef tapeworm (infection)
Infection due to adult tapeworm Taenia saginata

B68.9 Taeniasis, unspecified ▽

✓4th B69 Cysticercosis
INCLUDES cysticerciasis infection due to larval form of Taenia solium

B69.0 Cysticercosis of central nervous system

B69.1 Cysticercosis of eye

✓5th B69.8 Cysticercosis of other sites

B69.81 Myositis in cysticercosis

B69.89 Cysticercosis of other sites

B69.9 Cysticercosis, unspecified ▽

✓4th B70 Diphyllobothriasis and sparganosis

B70.0 Diphyllobothriasis
Diphyllobothrium (adult) (latum) (pacificum) infection
Fish tapeworm (infection)
EXCLUDES 2 larval diphyllobothriasis (B70.1)

B70.1 Sparganosis
Infection due to Sparganum (mansoni) (proliferum)
Infection due to Spirometra larva
Larval diphyllobothriasis
Spirometrosis

✓4th B71 Other cestode infections

B71.0 Hymenolepiasis
Dwarf tapeworm infection
Rat tapeworm (infection)

B71.1 Dipylidiasis

B71.8 Other specified cestode infections
Coenurosis

B71.9 Cestode infection, unspecified ▽
Tapeworm (infection) NOS

B72 Dracunculiasis
INCLUDES guinea worm infection
infection due to Dracunculus medinensis

✓4th B73 Onchocerciasis
INCLUDES onchocerca volvulus infection
onchocercosis
river blindness

✓5th B73.0 Onchocerciasis with eye disease

B73.00 Onchocerciasis with eye involvement, unspecified ▽

B73.01 Onchocerciasis with endophthalmitis

B73.02 Onchocerciasis with glaucoma

B73.09 Onchocerciasis with other eye involvement
Infestation of eyelid due to onchocerciasis

B73.1 Onchocerciasis without eye disease

✓4th B74 Filariasis
EXCLUDES 2 onchocerciasis (B73)
tropical (pulmonary) eosinophilia NOS (J82)

B74.0 Filariasis due to Wuchereria bancrofti
Bancroftian elephantiasis
Bancroftian filariasis

B74.1 Filariasis due to Brugia malayi

B74.2 Filariasis due to Brugia timori

B74.3 Loiasis
Calabar swelling
Eyeworm disease of Africa
Loa loa infection

B74.4 Mansonelliasis
Infection due to Mansonella ozzardi
Infection due to Mansonella perstans
Infection due to Mansonella streptocerca

B74.8 Other filariases
Dirofilariasis

B74.9 Filariasis, unspecified ▽

B75 Trichinellosis
INCLUDES infection due to Trichinella species
trichiniasis

✓4th B76 Hookworm diseases
INCLUDES uncinariasis

B76.0 Ancylostomiasis
Infection due to Ancylostoma species

B76.1 Necatoriasis
Infection due to Necator americanus

B76.8 Other hookworm diseases

B76.9 Hookworm disease, unspecified ▽
Cutaneous larva migrans NOS

☑4ᵗʰ **B77 Ascariasis**
     INCLUDES   ascaridiasis
             roundworm infection

     B77.0 Ascariasis with intestinal complications

     ☑5ᵗʰ **B77.8 Ascariasis with other complications**

         B77.81 Ascariasis pneumonia

         B77.89 Ascariasis with other complications

     B77.9 Ascariasis, unspecified ▽

☑4ᵗʰ **B78 Strongyloidiasis**
     EXCLUDES 1   trichostrongyliasis (B81.2)

     B78.0 Intestinal strongyloidiasis

     B78.1 Cutaneous strongyloidiasis

     B78.7 Disseminated strongyloidiasis

     B78.9 Strongyloidiasis, unspecified ▽

B79 Trichuriasis
     INCLUDES   trichocephaliasis
             whipworm (disease)(infection)

B80 Enterobiasis
     INCLUDES   oxyuriasis
             pinworm infection
             threadworm infection

☑4ᵗʰ **B81 Other intestinal helminthiases, not elsewhere classified**
     EXCLUDES 1 ▶angiostrongyliasis due to:
         angiostrongylus cantonensis (B83.2)
         parastrongylus cantonensis (B83.2) ◀

     B81.0 Anisakiasis
         Infection due to Anisakis larva

     B81.1 Intestinal capillariasis
         Capillariasis NOS
         Infection due to Capillaria philippinensis
         EXCLUDES 2   hepatic capillariasis (B83.8)

     B81.2 Trichostrongyliasis

     B81.3 Intestinal angiostrongyliasis
         ▶Angiostrongyliasis due to:
         angiostrongylus costaricensis
         parastrongylus costaricensis◀

     B81.4 Mixed intestinal helminthiases
         Infection due to intestinal helminths classified to more than one
             of the categories B65.0-B81.3 and B81.8
         Mixed helminthiasis NOS

     B81.8 Other specified intestinal helminthiases
         Infection due to Oesophagostomum species
             [esophagostomiasis]
         Infection due to Ternidens diminutus [ternidensiasis]

☑4ᵗʰ **B82 Unspecified intestinal parasitism**

     B82.0 Intestinal helminthiasis, unspecified ▽

     B82.9 Intestinal parasitism, unspecified ▽

☑4ᵗʰ **B83 Other helminthiases**
     EXCLUDES 1   capillariasis NOS (B81.1)
     EXCLUDES 2   intestinal capillariasis (B81.1)

     B83.0 Visceral larva migrans
         Toxocariasis

     B83.1 Gnathostomiasis
         Wandering swelling

     B83.2 Angiostrongyliasis due to Parastrongylus cantonensis
         Eosinophilic meningoencephalitis due to Parastrongylus
             cantonensis
         EXCLUDES 2   intestinal angiostrongyliasis (B81.3)

     B83.3 Syngamiasis
         Syngamosis

     B83.4 Internal hirudiniasis
         EXCLUDES 2   external hirudiniasis (B88.3)

     B83.8 Other specified helminthiases
         Acanthocephaliasis
         Gongylonemiasis
         Hepatic capillariasis
         Metastrongyliasis
         Thelaziasis

     B83.9 Helminthiasis, unspecified ▽
         Worms NOS
         EXCLUDES 1   intestinal helminthiasis NOS (B82.0)

Pediculosis, acariasis and other infestations (B85-B89)

☑4ᵗʰ **B85 Pediculosis and phthiriasis**

     B85.0 Pediculosis due to Pediculus humanus capitis
         Head-louse infestation

     B85.1 Pediculosis due to Pediculus humanus corporis
         Body-louse infestation

     B85.2 Pediculosis, unspecified ▽

     B85.3 Phthiriasis
         Infestation by crab-louse
         Infestation by Phthirus pubis

     B85.4 Mixed pediculosis and phthiriasis
         Infestation classifiable to more than one of the categories
             B85.0- B85.3

B86 Scabies
     Sarcoptic itch

☑4ᵗʰ **B87 Myiasis**
     INCLUDES   infestation by larva of flies

     B87.0 Cutaneous myiasis
         Creeping myiasis

     B87.1 Wound myiasis
         Traumatic myiasis

     B87.2 Ocular myiasis

     B87.3 Nasopharyngeal myiasis
         Laryngeal myiasis

     B87.4 Aural myiasis

     ☑5ᵗʰ **B87.8 Myiasis of other sites**

         B87.81 Genitourinary myiasis

         B87.82 Intestinal myiasis

         B87.89 Myiasis of other sites

     B87.9 Myiasis, unspecified ▽

☑4ᵗʰ **B88 Other infestations**

     B88.0 Other acariasis
         Acarine dermatitis
         Dermatitis due to Demodex species
         Dermatitis due to Dermanyssus gallinae
         Dermatitis due to Liponyssoides sanguineus
         Trombiculosis
         EXCLUDES 2   scabies (B86)

     B88.1 Tungiasis [sandflea infestation]

     B88.2 Other arthropod infestations
         Scarabiasis

     B88.3 External hirudiniasis
         Leech infestation NOS
         EXCLUDES 2   internal hirudiniasis (B83.4)

     B88.8 Other specified infestations
         Ichthyoparasitism due to Vandellia cirrhosa
         Linguatulosis
         Porocephaliasis

     B88.9 Infestation, unspecified ▽
         Infestation (skin) NOS
         Infestation by mites NOS
         Skin parasites NOS

B89 Unspecified parasitic disease ▽

Sequelae of infectious and parasitic diseases (B90-B94)

     NOTE   Categories B90-B94 are to be used to indicate conditions in
         categories A00-B89 as the cause of sequelae, which are themselves
         classified elsewhere. The "sequelae" include conditions specified as
         such; they also include residuals of diseases classifiable to the above
         categories if there is no evidence that the disease itself is no longer
         present. Codes from these categories are not to be used for chronic
         infections. Code chronic current infections to active infectious
         disease as appropriate.
     Code first condition resulting from (sequela) the infectious or parasitic disease

☑4ᵗʰ **B90 Sequelae of tuberculosis**

     B90.0 Sequelae of central nervous system tuberculosis

     B90.1 Sequelae of genitourinary tuberculosis

     B90.2 Sequelae of tuberculosis of bones and joints

     B90.8 Sequelae of tuberculosis of other organs
         EXCLUDES 2   sequelae of respiratory tuberculosis (B90.9)

     B90.9 Sequelae of respiratory and unspecified tuberculosis ▽
         Sequelae of tuberculosis NOS

☑ Additional Character Req   ✓x7ᵗʰ Placeholder Alert   Manifestation   HCC CMS-HCC Condition   ▽ Unspecified Code   ▶◀ Revised Text   ● New Code   ▲ Revised Code Title

B91 Sequelae of poliomyelitis
     EXCLUDES 1   postpolio syndrome (G14)

B92 Sequelae of leprosy

✓4th **B94 Sequelae of other and unspecified infectious and parasitic diseases**

     B94.0 Sequelae of trachoma

     B94.1 Sequelae of viral encephalitis

     B94.2 Sequelae of viral hepatitis

     B94.8 Sequelae of other specified infectious and parasitic diseases

     B94.9 Sequelae of unspecified infectious and parasitic disease ▽

Bacterial and viral infectious agents (B95-B97)

> **NOTE**   These categories are provided for use as supplementary or additional codes to identify the infectious agent(s) in diseases classified elsewhere.

✓4th **B95 Streptococcus, Staphylococcus, and Enterococcus as the cause of diseases classified elsewhere**

     B95.0 Streptococcus, group A, as the cause of diseases classified elsewhere

     B95.1 Streptococcus, group B, as the cause of diseases classified elsewhere

     B95.2 Enterococcus as the cause of diseases classified elsewhere

     B95.3 Streptococcus pneumoniae as the cause of diseases classified elsewhere

     B95.4 Other streptococcus as the cause of diseases classified elsewhere

     B95.5 Unspecified streptococcus as the cause of diseases classified elsewhere ▽

✓5th   **B95.6 Staphylococcus aureus as the cause of diseases classified elsewhere**

         B95.61 Methicillin susceptible Staphylococcus aureus infection as the cause of diseases classified elsewhere
            Methicillin susceptible Staphylococcus aureus (MSSA) infection as the cause of diseases classified elsewhere
            Staphylococcus aureus infection NOS as the cause of diseases classified elsewhere

         B95.62 Methicillin resistant Staphylococcus aureus infection as the cause of diseases classified elsewhere
            Methicillin resistant Staphylococcus aureus (MRSA) infection as the cause of diseases classified elsewhere
            AHA: 2016, 1Q, 12

     B95.7 Other staphylococcus as the cause of diseases classified elsewhere

     B95.8 Unspecified staphylococcus as the cause of diseases classified elsewhere ▽

✓4th **B96 Other bacterial agents as the cause of diseases classified elsewhere**

     B96.0 Mycoplasma pneumoniae [M. pneumoniae] as the cause of diseases classified elsewhere
         Pleuro-pneumonia-like-organism [PPLO]

     B96.1 Klebsiella pneumoniae [K. pneumoniae] as the cause of diseases classified elsewhere

✓5th   **B96.2 Escherichia coli [E. coli] as the cause of diseases classified elsewhere**

         B96.20 Unspecified Escherichia coli [E. coli] as the cause of diseases classified elsewhere ▽
            Escherichia coli [E. coli] NOS

         B96.21 Shiga toxin-producing Escherichia coli [E. coli] (STEC) O157 as the cause of diseases classified elsewhere
            E. coli O157:H- (nonmotile) with confirmation of Shiga toxin
            E. coli O157 with confirmation of Shiga toxin when H antigen is unknown, or is not H7
            O157:H7 Escherichia coli [E.coli] with or without confirmation of Shiga toxin-production
            Shiga toxin-producing Escherichia coli [E.coli] O157:H7 with or without confirmation of Shiga toxin-production
            STEC O157:H7 with or without confirmation of Shiga toxin-production

         B96.22 Other specified Shiga toxin-producing Escherichia coli [E. coli] (STEC) as the cause of diseases classified elsewhere
            Non-O157 Shiga toxin-producing Escherichia coli [E.coli]
            Non-O157 Shiga toxin-producing Escherichia coli [E.coli] with known O group

         B96.23 Unspecified Shiga toxin-producing Escherichia coli [E. coli] (STEC) as the cause of diseases classified elsewhere ▽
            Shiga toxin-producing Escherichia coli [E. coli] with unspecified O group
            STEC NOS

         B96.29 Other Escherichia coli [E. coli] as the cause of diseases classified elsewhere
            Non-Shiga toxin-producing E. coli

     B96.3 Hemophilus influenzae [H. influenzae] as the cause of diseases classified elsewhere

     B96.4 Proteus (mirabilis) (morganii) as the cause of diseases classified elsewhere

     B96.5 Pseudomonas (aeruginosa) (mallei) (pseudomallei) as the cause of diseases classified elsewhere
         AHA: 2015, 1Q, 18

     B96.6 Bacteroides fragilis [B. fragilis] as the cause of diseases classified elsewhere

     B96.7 Clostridium perfringens [C. perfringens] as the cause of diseases classified elsewhere

✓5th   **B96.8 Other specified bacterial agents as the cause of diseases classified elsewhere**

         B96.81 Helicobacter pylori [H. pylori] as the cause of diseases classified elsewhere

         B96.82 Vibrio vulnificus as the cause of diseases classified elsewhere

         B96.89 Other specified bacterial agents as the cause of diseases classified elsewhere

✓4th **B97 Viral agents as the cause of diseases classified elsewhere**
     AHA: 2016, 3Q, 8-10, 14

     B97.0 Adenovirus as the cause of diseases classified elsewhere

✓5th   **B97.1 Enterovirus as the cause of diseases classified elsewhere**

         B97.10 Unspecified enterovirus as the cause of diseases classified elsewhere ▽

         B97.11 Coxsackievirus as the cause of diseases classified elsewhere

         B97.12 Echovirus as the cause of diseases classified elsewhere

         B97.19 Other enterovirus as the cause of diseases classified elsewhere

✓5th   **B97.2 Coronavirus as the cause of diseases classified elsewhere**

         B97.21 SARS-associated coronavirus as the cause of diseases classified elsewhere
            EXCLUDES 1   pneumonia due to SARS-associated coronavirus (J12.81)

         B97.29 Other coronavirus as the cause of diseases classified elsewhere

✓5th   **B97.3 Retrovirus as the cause of diseases classified elsewhere**
         EXCLUDES 1   human immunodeficiency virus [HIV} disease (B20)

         B97.30 Unspecified retrovirus as the cause of diseases classified elsewhere ▽

         B97.31 Lentivirus as the cause of diseases classified elsewhere

         B97.32 Oncovirus as the cause of diseases classified elsewhere

         B97.33 Human T-cell lymphotrophic virus, type I [HTLV-I] as the cause of diseases classified elsewhere

         B97.34 Human T-cell lymphotrophic virus, type II [HTLV-II] as the cause of diseases classified elsewhere

         B97.35 Human immunodeficiency virus, type 2 [HIV 2] HCC **as the cause of diseases classified elsewhere**

         B97.39 Other retrovirus as the cause of diseases classified elsewhere

     B97.4 Respiratory syncytial virus as the cause of diseases classified elsewhere

     B97.5 Reovirus as the cause of diseases classified elsewhere

     B97.6 Parvovirus as the cause of diseases classified elsewhere

     B97.7 Papillomavirus as the cause of diseases classified elsewhere

EXCLUDES 1 Not coded here   *EXCLUDES 2* Not included here   N Newborn Age: 0   P Pediatric Age: 0-17   M Maternity Age: 12-55   A Adult Age: 15-124

454   ICD-10-CM 2018

✓5ᵗʰ **B97.8** **Other viral agents as the cause of diseases classified elsewhere**

    B97.81 Human metapneumovirus as the cause of diseases classified elsewhere

    B97.89 Other viral agents as the cause of diseases classified elsewhere

Other infectious diseases (B99)

✓4ᵗʰ **B99** **Other and unspecified infectious diseases**

    B99.8 Other infectious disease

    B99.9 Unspecified infectious disease   ▽

☑ Additional Character Req   ✓7ᵗʰ Placeholder Alert   Manifestation   HCC CMS-HCC Condition   ▽ Unspecified Code   ►◄ Revised Text   ● New Code   ▲ Revised Code Title

ICD-10-CM 2018   **455**

Chapter 2. Neoplasms (C00–D49)

Chapter Specific Guidelines with Coding Examples

The chapter specific guidelines from the ICD-10-CM Official Guidelines for Coding and Reporting have been provided below. Along with these guidelines are coding examples, contained in the shaded boxes, that have been developed to help illustrate the coding and/or sequencing guidance found in these guidelines.

General guidelines

Chapter 2 of the ICD-10-CM contains the codes for most benign and all malignant neoplasms. Certain benign neoplasms, such as prostatic adenomas, may be found in the specific body system chapters. To properly code a neoplasm it is necessary to determine from the record if the neoplasm is benign, in-situ, malignant, or of uncertain histologic behavior. If malignant, any secondary (metastatic) sites should also be determined.

Primary malignant neoplasms overlapping site boundaries

A primary malignant neoplasm that overlaps two or more contiguous (next to each other) sites should be classified to the subcategory/code .8 ('overlapping lesion'), unless the combination is specifically indexed elsewhere. For multiple neoplasms of the same site that are not contiguous such as tumors in different quadrants of the same breast, codes for each site should be assigned.

> A 62-year-old female with a malignant lesion of the upper lip that extends from the lipstick area to the labial frenulum
>
> **C00.8**   **Malignant neoplasm of overlapping sites of lip**
>
> *Explanation*: Because this is a single lesion that overlaps two contiguous sites, a single code for overlapping sites is assigned.

> A 74-year-old male is treated for two distinct malignant lesions, one in the mucosa of the upper lip and a second in the mucosa of the lower lip.
>
> **C00.3**   **Malignant neoplasm of upper lip, inner aspect**
>
> **C00.4**   **Malignant neoplasm of lower lip, inner aspect**
>
> *Explanation*: This patient has two distinct malignant lesions of the upper and lower lips. Because the lesions are not contiguous, two codes are reported.

Malignant neoplasm of ectopic tissue

Malignant neoplasms of ectopic tissue are to be coded to the site of origin mentioned, e.g., ectopic pancreatic malignant neoplasms involving the stomach are coded to pancreas, unspecified (C25.9).

The neoplasm table in the Alphabetic Index should be referenced first. However, if the histological term is documented, that term should be referenced first, rather than going immediately to the Neoplasm Table, in order to determine which column in the Neoplasm Table is appropriate. For example, if the documentation indicates "adenoma," refer to the term in the Alphabetic Index to review the entries under this term and the instructional note to "see also neoplasm, by site, benign." The table provides the proper code based on the type of neoplasm and the site. It is important to select the proper column in the table that corresponds to the type of neoplasm. The Tabular List should then be referenced to verify that the correct code has been selected from the table and that a more specific site code does not exist.

See Section I.C.21. Factors influencing health status and contact with health services, Status, for information regarding Z15.0, codes for genetic susceptibility to cancer.

a. Treatment directed at the malignancy

If the treatment is directed at the malignancy, designate the malignancy as the principal diagnosis.

The only exception to this guideline is if a patient admission/encounter is solely for the administration of chemotherapy, immunotherapy or radiation therapy, assign the appropriate Z51.-- code as the first-listed or principal diagnosis, and the diagnosis or problem for which the service is being performed as a secondary diagnosis.

b. Treatment of secondary site

When a patient is admitted because of a primary neoplasm with metastasis and treatment is directed toward the secondary site only, the secondary neoplasm is designated as the principal diagnosis even though the primary malignancy is still present.

> Patient with primary prostate cancer with metastasis to lungs presents for wedge resection of mass in right lung
>
> **C78.01**   **Secondary malignant neoplasm of right lung**
>
> **C61**   **Malignant neoplasm of prostate**
>
> *Explanation*: Since the encounter is for treatment of the lung metastasis, the secondary lung metastasis is sequenced before the primary prostate cancer.

c. Coding and sequencing of complications

Coding and sequencing of complications associated with the malignancies or with the therapy thereof are subject to the following guidelines:

1) Anemia associated with malignancy

When admission/encounter is for management of an anemia associated with the malignancy, and the treatment is only for anemia, the appropriate code for the malignancy is sequenced as the principal or first-listed diagnosis followed by the appropriate code for the anemia (such as code D63.0, Anemia in neoplastic disease).

> Patient is seen for treatment of anemia in advanced primary liver cancer
>
> **C22.8**   **Malignant neoplasm of liver, primary, unspecified as to type**
>
> **D63.0**   **Anemia in neoplastic disease**
>
> *Explanation*: Even though the admission was solely to treat the anemia, this guideline indicates that the code for the malignancy is sequenced first.

2) Anemia associated with chemotherapy, immunotherapy and radiation therapy

When the admission/encounter is for management of an anemia associated with an adverse effect of the administration of chemotherapy or immunotherapy and the only treatment is for the anemia, the anemia code is sequenced first followed by the appropriate codes for the neoplasm and the adverse effect (T45.1X5, Adverse effect of antineoplastic and immunosuppressive drugs).

> A 56-year-old Hispanic male with grade II follicular lymphoma involving multiple lymph node sites referred for blood transfusion to treat anemia due to chemotherapy
>
> **D64.81**   **Anemia due to antineoplastic chemotherapy**
>
> **C82.18**   **Follicular lymphoma grade II, lymph nodes of multiple sites**
>
> **T45.1X5A**   **Adverse effect of antineoplastic and immunosuppressive drugs, initial encounter**
>
> *Explanation*: The code for the anemia is sequenced first followed by the code for the malignant neoplasm and lastly the code for the adverse effect.

When the admission/encounter is for management of an anemia associated with an adverse effect of radiotherapy, the anemia code should be sequenced first, followed by the appropriate neoplasm code and code Y84.2, Radiological procedure and radiotherapy as the cause of abnormal reaction of the patient, or of later complication, without mention of misadventure at the time of the procedure.

Chapter 2. Neoplasms

A 55-year-old male with a large malignant rectal tumor has been receiving external radiation therapy to shrink the tumor prior to planned surgery. He is referred today for a blood transfusion to treat anemia related to radiation therapy.

D64.89	**Other specified anemias**
C20	**Malignant neoplasm of rectum**
Y84.2	**Radiological procedure and radiotherapy as the cause of abnormal reaction of the patient, or of later complication, without mention of misadventure at the time of the procedure**

Explanation: The code for the anemia is sequenced first, followed by the code for the malignancy, and lastly the code for the abnormal reaction due to radiotherapy.

3) Management of dehydration due to the malignancy

When the admission/encounter is for management of dehydration due to the malignancy and only the dehydration is being treated (intravenous rehydration), the dehydration is sequenced first, followed by the code(s) for the malignancy.

4) Treatment of a complication resulting from a surgical procedure

When the admission/encounter is for treatment of a complication resulting from a surgical procedure, designate the complication as the principal or first-listed diagnosis if treatment is directed at resolving the complication.

d. Primary malignancy previously excised

When a primary malignancy has been previously excised or eradicated from its site and there is no further treatment directed to that site and there is no evidence of any existing primary malignancy, a code from category Z85, Personal history of malignant neoplasm, should be used to indicate the former site of the malignancy. Any mention of extension, invasion, or metastasis to another site is coded as a secondary malignant neoplasm to that site. The secondary site may be the principal or first-listed with the Z85 code used as a secondary code.

History of lung cancer, left upper lobectomy 18 months ago with no current treatment; MRI of the brain shows metastatic disease in the brain

C79.31	**Secondary malignant neoplasm of brain**
Z85.118	**Personal history of other other malignant neoplasm of bronchifus and bronchfuls and lung**

Explanation: The patient has undergone a diagnostic procedure that revealed metastatic lung cancer in the brain. The code for the secondary (metastatic) site is sequenced first, followed by a personal history code to identify the former site of the primary malignancy.

e. Admissions/encounters involving chemotherapy, immunotherapy and radiation therapy

1) Episode of care involves surgical removal of neoplasm

When an episode of care involves the surgical removal of a neoplasm, primary or secondary site, followed by adjunct chemotherapy or radiation treatment during the same episode of care, the code for the neoplasm should be assigned as principal or first-listed diagnosis.

2) Patient admission/encounter solely for administration of chemotherapy, immunotherapy and radiation therapy

If a patient admission/encounter is solely for the administration of chemotherapy, immunotherapy or radiation therapy assign code Z51.0, Encounter for antineoplastic radiation therapy, or Z51.11, Encounter for antineoplastic chemotherapy, or Z51.12, Encounter for antineoplastic immunotherapy as the first-listed or principal diagnosis. If a patient receives more than one of these therapies during the same admission more than one of these codes may be assigned, in any sequence.

The malignancy for which the therapy is being administered should be assigned as a secondary diagnosis.

Patient presents for second round of rituximab and fludarabine for his chronic B cell lymphocytic leukemia

Z51.11	**Encounter for antineoplastic chemotherapy**
Z51.12	**Encounter for antineoplastic immunotherapy**
C91.10	**Chronic lymphocytic leukemia of B-cell type not having achieved remission**

Explanation: Rituximab is an antineoplastic immunotherapy while fludarabine is an antineoplastic chemotherapy. The two treatments are often used together. The encounter was solely for the purpose of administering this treatment and either can be sequenced first, before the neoplastic condition.

3) Patient admitted for radiation therapy, chemotherapy or immunotherapy and develops complications

When a patient is admitted for the purpose of radiotherapy, immunotherapy or chemotherapy and develops complications such as uncontrolled nausea and vomiting or dehydration, the principal or first-listed diagnosis is Z51.0, Encounter for antineoplastic radiation therapy, or Z51.11, Encounter for antineoplastic chemotherapy, or Z51.12, Encounter for antineoplastic immunotherapy followed by any codes for the complications.

f. Admission/encounter to determine extent of malignancy

When the reason for admission/encounter is to determine the extent of the malignancy, or for a procedure such as paracentesis or thoracentesis, the primary malignancy or appropriate metastatic site is designated as the principal or first-listed diagnosis, even though chemotherapy or radiotherapy is administered.

Patient with left lung cancer with malignant pleural effusion being seen for paracentesis and initiation/administration of chemotherapy

C34.92	**Malignant neoplasm of unspecified part of left bronchus or lung**
J91.0	**Malignant pleural effusion**
Z51.11	**Encounter for antineoplastic chemotherapy**

Explanation: The lung cancer is sequenced before the chemotherapy in this instance because the paracentesis for the malignant effusion is also being performed. An instructional note under the malignant effusion instructs that the lung cancer be sequenced first.

g. Symptoms, signs, and abnormal findings listed in Chapter 18 associated with neoplasms

Symptoms, signs, and ill-defined conditions listed in Chapter 18 characteristic of, or associated with, an existing primary or secondary site malignancy cannot be used to replace the malignancy as principal or first-listed diagnosis, regardless of the number of admissions or encounters for treatment and care of the neoplasm.

See Section I.C.21. Factors influencing health status and contact with health services, Encounter for prophylactic organ removal.

h. Admission/encounter for pain control/management

See Section I.C.6. for information on coding admission/encounter for pain control/management.

i. Malignancy in two or more noncontiguous sites

A patient may have more than one malignant tumor in the same organ. These tumors may represent different primaries or metastatic disease, depending on the site. Should the documentation be unclear, the provider should be queried as to the status of each tumor so that the correct codes can be assigned.

j. Disseminated malignant neoplasm, unspecified

Code C80.0, Disseminated malignant neoplasm, unspecified, is for use only in those cases where the patient has advanced metastatic disease and no known primary or secondary sites are specified. It should not be used in place of assigning codes for the primary site and all known secondary sites.

Patient who has had no medical care for many years is seen today and diagnosed with carcinomatosis

C80.0	**Disseminated malignant neoplasm, unspecified**

Explanation: Carcinomatosis NOS is an "includes" note under this code. Should seldom be used but is available for use in cases such as this.

k. Malignant neoplasm without specification of site

Code C80.1, Malignant (primary) neoplasm, unspecified, equates to Cancer, unspecified. This code should only be used when no determination can be made as to the primary site of a malignancy. This code should rarely be used in the inpatient setting.

Evaluation of painful hip leads to diagnosis of a metastatic bone lesion from an unknown primary neoplasm source

C79.51   **Secondary malignant neoplasm of bone**

C80.1   **Malignant (primary) neoplasm, unspecified**

Explanation: If only the secondary site is known, use code C80.1 for the unknown primary site.

---

l. Sequencing of neoplasm codes

1) Encounter for treatment of primary malignancy

If the reason for the encounter is for treatment of a primary malignancy, assign the malignancy as the principal/first-listed diagnosis. The primary site is to be sequenced first, followed by any metastatic sites.

2) Encounter for treatment of secondary malignancy

When an encounter is for a primary malignancy with metastasis and treatment is directed toward the metastatic (secondary) site(s) only, the metastatic site(s) is designated as the principal/first-listed diagnosis. The primary malignancy is coded as an additional code.

Patient has primary colon cancer with metastasis to rib and is evaluated for possible excision of portion of rib bone

C79.51   **Secondary malignant neoplasm of bone**

C18.9   **Malignant neoplasm of colon, unspecified**

Explanation: The treatment for this encounter is focused on the metastasis to the rib bone rather than the primary colon cancer, thus indicating that the bone metastasis is sequenced as the first-listed code.

---

3) Malignant neoplasm in a pregnant patient

When a pregnant woman has a malignant neoplasm, a code from subcategory O9A.1-, Malignant neoplasm complicating pregnancy, childbirth, and the puerperium, should be sequenced first, followed by the appropriate code from Chapter 2 to indicate the type of neoplasm.

A 30-year-old pregnant female in first trimester evaluated for pituitary gland malignancy

O9A.111   **Malignant neoplasm complicating pregnancy, first trimester**

C75.1   **Malignant neoplasm of pituitary gland**

Explanation: Codes from chapter 15 describing complications of pregnancy are sequenced as first-listed codes, further specified by codes from other chapters such as neoplastic, unless the pregnancy is documented as incidental to the condition. See also guideline 1.C.15.a.1.

---

4) Encounter for complication associated with a neoplasm

When an encounter is for management of a complication associated with a neoplasm, such as dehydration, and the treatment is only for the complication, the complication is coded first, followed by the appropriate code(s) for the neoplasm.

The exception to this guideline is anemia. When the admission/encounter is for management of an anemia associated with the malignancy, and the treatment is only for anemia, the appropriate code for the malignancy is sequenced as the principal or first-listed diagnosis followed by code D63.0, Anemia in neoplastic disease.

Patient with pancreatic cancer is seen for initiation of TPN for cancer-related moderate protein-calorie malnutrition

E44.0   **Moderate protein-calorie malnutrition**

C25.9   **Malignant neoplasm of pancreas, unspecified**

Explanation: The encounter is to initiate treatment for malnutrition, a common complication of many types of neoplasms, and is sequenced first.

---

5) Complication from surgical procedure for treatment of a neoplasm

When an encounter is for treatment of a complication resulting from a surgical procedure performed for the treatment of the neoplasm, designate the complication as the principal/first-listed diagnosis. See guideline regarding the coding of a current malignancy versus personal history to determine if the code for the neoplasm should also be assigned.

6) Pathologic fracture due to a neoplasm

When an encounter is for a pathological fracture due to a neoplasm, and the focus of treatment is the fracture, a code from subcategory M84.5, Pathological fracture in neoplastic disease, should be sequenced first, followed by the code for the neoplasm.

If the focus of treatment is the neoplasm with an associated pathological fracture, the neoplasm code should be sequenced first, followed by a code from M84.5 for the pathological fracture.

m. Current malignancy versus personal history of malignancy

When a primary malignancy has been excised but further treatment, such as an additional surgery for the malignancy, radiation therapy or chemotherapy is directed to that site, the primary malignancy code should be used until treatment is completed.

When a primary malignancy has been previously excised or eradicated from its site, there is no further treatment (of the malignancy) directed to that site, and there is no evidence of any existing primary malignancy, a code from category Z85, Personal history of malignant neoplasm, should be used to indicate the former site of the malignancy.

See Section I.C.21. Factors influencing health status and contact with health services, History (of)

Female patient with ongoing chemotherapy after right mastectomy for breast cancer

C50.911   **Malignant neoplasm of unspecified site of right female breast**

Z90.11   **Acquired absence of right breast and nipple**

Explanation: Even though the breast has been removed, the breast cancer is still being treated with chemotherapy and therefore is still coded as a current condition rather than personal history.

---

n. Leukemia, multiple myeloma, and malignant plasma cell neoplasms in remission versus personal history

The categories for leukemia, and category C90, Multiple myeloma and malignant plasma cell neoplasms, have codes indicating whether or not the leukemia has achieved remission. There are also codes Z85.6, Personal history of leukemia, and Z85.79, Personal history of other malignant neoplasms of lymphoid, hematopoietic and related tissues. If the documentation is unclear as to whether the leukemia has achieved remission, the provider should be queried.

See Section I.C.21. Factors influencing health status and contact with health services, History (of)

o. Aftercare following surgery for neoplasm

See Section I.C.21. Factors influencing health status and contact with health services, Aftercare

p. Follow-up care for completed treatment of a malignancy

See Section I.C.21. Factors influencing health status and contact with health services, Follow-up

q. Prophylactic organ removal for prevention of malignancy

See Section I.C. 21, Factors influencing health status and contact with health services, Prophylactic organ removal

r. Malignant neoplasm associated with transplanted organ

A malignant neoplasm of a transplanted organ should be coded as a transplant complication. Assign first the appropriate code from category T86.-, Complications of transplanted organs and tissue, followed by code C80.2, Malignant neoplasm associated with transplanted organ. Use an additional code for the specific malignancy.

Chapter 2. Neoplasms

Chapter 2. Neoplasms (C00-D49)

NOTE

Functional activity

All neoplasms are classified in this chapter, whether they are functionally active or not. An additional code from Chapter 4 may be used, to identify functional activity associated with any neoplasm.

Morphology [Histology]

Chapter 2 classifies neoplasms primarily by site (topography), with broad groupings for behavior, malignant, in situ, benign, etc. The Table of Neoplasms should be used to identify the correct topography code. In a few cases, such as for malignant melanoma and certain neuroendocrine tumors, the morphology (histologic type) is included in the category and codes.

Primary malignant neoplasms overlapping site boundaries

A primary malignant neoplasm that overlaps two or more contiguous (next to each other) sites should be classified to the subcategory/code .8 ("overlapping lesion"), unless the combination is specifically indexed elsewhere. For multiple neoplasms of the same site that are not contiguous, such as tumors in different quadrants of the same breast, codes for each site should be assigned.

Malignant neoplasm of ectopic tissue

Malignant neoplasms of ectopic tissue are to be coded to the site mentioned, e.g., ectopic pancreatic malignant neoplasms are coded to pancreas, unspecified (C25.9).

AHA: 2017, 1Q, 4, 5-6, 8

This chapter contains the following blocks:

C00-C14	Malignant neoplasms of lip, oral cavity and pharynx
C15-C26	Malignant neoplasms of digestive organs
C30-C39	Malignant neoplasms of respiratory and intrathoracic organs
C40-C41	Malignant neoplasms of bone and articular cartilage
C43-C44	Melanoma and other malignant neoplasms of skin
C45-C49	Malignant neoplasms of mesothelial and soft tissue
C50	Malignant neoplasms of breast
C51-C58	Malignant neoplasms of female genital organs
C60-C63	Malignant neoplasms of male genital organs
C64-C68	Malignant neoplasms of urinary tract
C69-C72	Malignant neoplasms of eye, brain and other parts of central nervous system
C73-C75	Malignant neoplasms of thyroid and other endocrine glands
C7A	Malignant neuroendocrine tumors
C7B	Secondary neuroendocrine tumors
C76-C80	Malignant neoplasms of ill-defined, other secondary and unspecified sites
C81-C96	Malignant neoplasms of lymphoid, hematopoietic and related tissue
D00-D09	In situ neoplasms
D10-D36	Benign neoplasms, except benign neuroendocrine tumors
D3A	Benign neuroendocrine tumors
D37-D48	Neoplasms of uncertain behavior, polycythemia vera and myelodysplastic syndromes
D49	Neoplasms of unspecified behavior

MALIGNANT NEOPLASMS (C00-C96)

Malignant neoplasms, stated or presumed to be primary (of specified sites), and certain specified histologies, except neuroendocrine, and of lymphoid, hematopoietic and related tissue (C00-C75)

Malignant neoplasms of lip, oral cavity and pharynx (C00-C14)

✓4ᵗʰ **C00**   **Malignant neoplasm of lip**

Use additional code to identify:
    alcohol abuse and dependence (F10.-)
    history of tobacco dependence (Z87.891)
    tobacco dependence (F17.-)
    tobacco use (Z72.0)

    EXCLUDES 1   *malignant melanoma of lip (C43.0)*
              Merkel cell carcinoma of lip (C4A.0)
              other and unspecified malignant neoplasm of skin of lip (C44.0-)

  C00.0   **Malignant neoplasm of external upper lip**
      Malignant neoplasm of lipstick area of upper lip
      Malignant neoplasm of upper lip NOS
      Malignant neoplasm of vermilion border of upper lip

  C00.1   **Malignant neoplasm of external lower lip**
      Malignant neoplasm of lower lip NOS
      Malignant neoplasm of lipstick area of lower lip
      Malignant neoplasm of vermilion border of lower lip

  C00.2   **Malignant neoplasm of external lip, unspecified**   ▽
      Malignant neoplasm of vermilion border of lip NOS

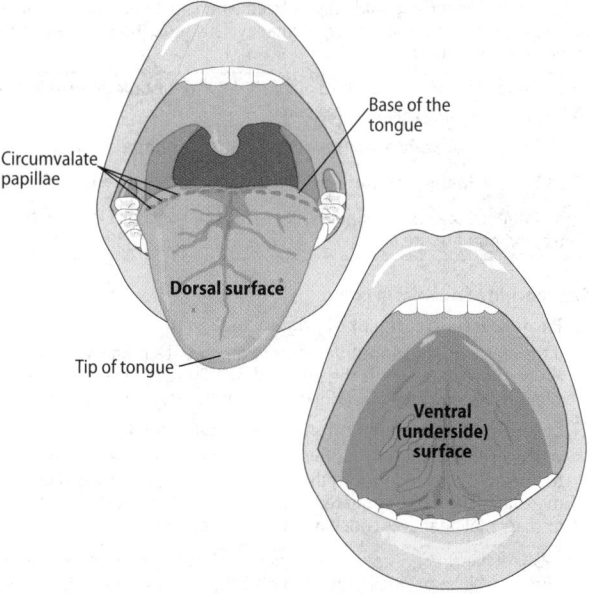

Malignant Neoplasm of Tongue

Base of the tongue
Circumvallate papillae
Dorsal surface
Tip of tongue
Ventral (underside) surface

  C00.3   **Malignant neoplasm of upper lip, inner aspect**
      Malignant neoplasm of buccal aspect of upper lip
      Malignant neoplasm of frenulum of upper lip
      Malignant neoplasm of mucosa of upper lip
      Malignant neoplasm of oral aspect of upper lip

  C00.4   **Malignant neoplasm of lower lip, inner aspect**
      Malignant neoplasm of buccal aspect of lower lip
      Malignant neoplasm of frenulum of lower lip
      Malignant neoplasm of mucosa of lower lip
      Malignant neoplasm of oral aspect of lower lip

  C00.5   **Malignant neoplasm of lip, unspecified, inner aspect** ▽
      Malignant neoplasm of buccal aspect of lip, unspecified
      Malignant neoplasm of frenulum of lip, unspecified
      Malignant neoplasm of mucosa of lip, unspecified
      Malignant neoplasm of oral aspect of lip, unspecified

  C00.6   **Malignant neoplasm of commissure of lip, unspecified** ▽

  C00.8   **Malignant neoplasm of overlapping sites of lip**

  C00.9   **Malignant neoplasm of lip, unspecified**   ▽

C01   **Malignant neoplasm of base of tongue**   HCC
    Malignant neoplasm of dorsal surface of base of tongue
    Malignant neoplasm of fixed part of tongue NOS
    Malignant neoplasm of posterior third of tongue
    Use additional code to identify:
      alcohol abuse and dependence (F10.-)
      history of tobacco dependence (Z87.891)
      tobacco dependence (F17.-)
      tobacco use (Z72.0)

✓4ᵗʰ **C02**   **Malignant neoplasm of other and unspecified parts of tongue**
    Use additional code to identify:
      alcohol abuse and dependence (F10.-)
      history of tobacco dependence (Z87.891)
      tobacco dependence (F17.-)
      tobacco use (Z72.0)

  C02.0   **Malignant neoplasm of dorsal surface of tongue** HCC
      Malignant neoplasm of anterior two-thirds of tongue, dorsal surface
      EXCLUDES 2   *malignant neoplasm of dorsal surface of base of tongue (C01)*

  C02.1   **Malignant neoplasm of border of tongue**   HCC
      Malignant neoplasm of tip of tongue

  C02.2   **Malignant neoplasm of ventral surface of tongue** HCC
      Malignant neoplasm of anterior two-thirds of tongue, ventral surface
      Malignant neoplasm of frenulum linguae

  C02.3   **Malignant neoplasm of anterior two-thirds of tongue, part unspecified** HCC
      Malignant neoplasm of middle third of tongue NOS
      Malignant neoplasm of mobile part of tongue NOS

  C02.4   **Malignant neoplasm of lingual tonsil**   HCC
      EXCLUDES 2   *malignant neoplasm of tonsil NOS (C09.9)*

  C02.8   **Malignant neoplasm of overlapping sites of tongue** HCC
      Malignant neoplasm of two or more contiguous sites of tongue

EXCLUDES 1 Not coded here   EXCLUDES 2 Not included here   N Newborn Age: 0   P Pediatric Age: 0-17   M Maternity Age: 12-55   A Adult Age: 15-124

460   ICD-10-CM 2018

C02.9   **Malignant neoplasm of tongue, unspecified**   HCC ▽

✓4ᵗʰ **C03**   **Malignant neoplasm of gum**
> INCLUDES   malignant neoplasm of alveolar (ridge) mucosa
> malignant neoplasm of gingiva
>
> Use additional code to identify:
> alcohol abuse and dependence (F10.-)
> history of tobacco dependence (Z87.891)
> tobacco dependence (F17.-)
> tobacco use (Z72.0)
>
> EXCLUDES 2   *malignant odontogenic neoplasms (C41.0-C41.1)*

C03.0   **Malignant neoplasm of upper gum**   HCC

C03.1   **Malignant neoplasm of lower gum**   HCC

C03.9   **Malignant neoplasm of gum, unspecified**   HCC ▽

✓4ᵗʰ **C04**   **Malignant neoplasm of floor of mouth**
> Use additional code to identify:
> alcohol abuse and dependence (F10.-)
> history of tobacco dependence (Z87.891)
> tobacco dependence (F17.-)
> tobacco use (Z72.0)

C04.0   **Malignant neoplasm of anterior floor of mouth**   HCC
> Malignant neoplasm of anterior to the premolar-canine junction

C04.1   **Malignant neoplasm of lateral floor of mouth**   HCC

C04.8   **Malignant neoplasm of overlapping sites of floor of mouth**   HCC

C04.9   **Malignant neoplasm of floor of mouth, unspecified**   HCC ▽

✓4ᵗʰ **C05**   **Malignant neoplasm of palate**
> Use additional code to identify:
> alcohol abuse and dependence (F10.-)
> history of tobacco dependence (Z87.891)
> tobacco dependence (F17.-)
> tobacco use (Z72.0)
>
> EXCLUDES 1   *Kaposi's sarcoma of palate (C46.2)*

C05.0   **Malignant neoplasm of hard palate**   HCC

C05.1   **Malignant neoplasm of soft palate**   HCC
> EXCLUDES 2   *malignant neoplasm of nasopharyngeal surface of soft palate (C11.3)*

C05.2   **Malignant neoplasm of uvula**   HCC

C05.8   **Malignant neoplasm of overlapping sites of palate**   HCC

C05.9   **Malignant neoplasm of palate, unspecified**   HCC ▽
> Malignant neoplasm of roof of mouth

✓4ᵗʰ **C06**   **Malignant neoplasm of other and unspecified parts of mouth**
> Use additional code to identify:
> alcohol abuse and dependence (F10.-)
> history of tobacco dependence (Z87.891)
> tobacco dependence (F17.-)
> tobacco use (Z72.0)

C06.0   **Malignant neoplasm of cheek mucosa**   HCC
> Malignant neoplasm of buccal mucosa NOS
> Malignant neoplasm of internal cheek

C06.1   **Malignant neoplasm of vestibule of mouth**
> Malignant neoplasm of buccal sulcus (upper) (lower)
> Malignant neoplasm of labial sulcus (upper) (lower)

C06.2   **Malignant neoplasm of retromolar area**   HCC

✓5ᵗʰ **C06.8**   **Malignant neoplasm of overlapping sites of other and unspecified parts of mouth**

    C06.80   **Malignant neoplasm of overlapping sites of unspecified parts of mouth**   HCC ▽

    C06.89   **Malignant neoplasm of overlapping sites of other parts of mouth**   HCC
> "book leaf" neoplasm [ventral surface of tongue and floor of mouth]

C06.9   **Malignant neoplasm of mouth, unspecified**   HCC ▽
> Malignant neoplasm of minor salivary gland, unspecified site
> Malignant neoplasm of oral cavity NOS

C07   **Malignant neoplasm of parotid gland**   HCC
> Use additional code to identify:
> alcohol abuse and dependence (F10.-)
> exposure to environmental tobacco smoke (Z77.22)
> exposure to tobacco smoke in the perinatal period (P96.81)
> history of tobacco dependence (Z87.891)
> occupational exposure to environmental tobacco smoke (Z57.31)
> tobacco dependence (F17.-)
> tobacco use (Z72.0)

✓4ᵗʰ **C08**   **Malignant neoplasm of other and unspecified major salivary glands**
> INCLUDES   malignant neoplasm of salivary ducts
>
> Use additional code to identify:
> alcohol abuse and dependence (F10.-)
> exposure to environmental tobacco smoke (Z77.22)
> exposure to tobacco smoke in the perinatal period (P96.81)
> history of tobacco dependence (Z87.891)
> occupational exposure to environmental tobacco smoke (Z57.31)
> tobacco dependence (F17.-)
> tobacco use (Z72.0)
>
> EXCLUDES 1   *malignant neoplasms of specified minor salivary glands which are classified according to their anatomical location*
>
> EXCLUDES 2   *malignant neoplasms of minor salivary glands NOS (C06.9)*
> *malignant neoplasm of parotid gland (C07)*

C08.0   **Malignant neoplasm of submandibular gland**   HCC
> Malignant neoplasm of submaxillary gland

C08.1   **Malignant neoplasm of sublingual gland**   HCC

C08.9   **Malignant neoplasm of major salivary gland, unspecified**   HCC ▽
> Malignant neoplasm of salivary gland (major) NOS

✓4ᵗʰ **C09**   **Malignant neoplasm of tonsil**
> Use additional code to identify:
> alcohol abuse and dependence (F10.-)
> exposure to environmental tobacco smoke (Z77.22)
> exposure to tobacco smoke in the perinatal period (P96.81)
> history of tobacco dependence (Z87.891)
> occupational exposure to environmental tobacco smoke (Z57.31)
> tobacco dependence (F17.-)
> tobacco use (Z72.0)
>
> EXCLUDES 2   *malignant neoplasm of lingual tonsil (C02.4)*
> *malignant neoplasm of pharyngeal tonsil (C11.1)*

C09.0   **Malignant neoplasm of tonsillar fossa**   HCC

C09.1   **Malignant neoplasm of tonsillar pillar (anterior) (posterior)**   HCC

C09.8   **Malignant neoplasm of overlapping sites of tonsil**   HCC

C09.9   **Malignant neoplasm of tonsil, unspecified**   HCC ▽
> Malignant neoplasm of tonsil NOS
> Malignant neoplasm of faucial tonsils
> Malignant neoplasm of palatine tonsils

✓4ᵗʰ **C10**   **Malignant neoplasm of oropharynx**
> Use additional code to identify:
> alcohol abuse and dependence (F10.-)
> exposure to environmental tobacco smoke (Z77.22)
> exposure to tobacco smoke in the perinatal period (P96.81)
> history of tobacco dependence (Z87.891)
> occupational exposure to environmental tobacco smoke (Z57.31)
> tobacco dependence (F17.-)
> tobacco use (Z72.0)
>
> EXCLUDES 2   *malignant neoplasm of tonsil (C09.-)*

C10.0   **Malignant neoplasm of vallecula**   HCC

C10.1   **Malignant neoplasm of anterior surface of epiglottis**   HCC
> Malignant neoplasm of epiglottis, free border [margin]
> Malignant neoplasm of glossoepiglottic fold(s)
>
> EXCLUDES 2   *malignant neoplasm of epiglottis (suprahyoid portion) NOS (C32.1)*

C10.2   **Malignant neoplasm of lateral wall of oropharynx**   HCC

C10.3   **Malignant neoplasm of posterior wall of oropharynx**   HCC

C10.4   **Malignant neoplasm of branchial cleft**   HCC
> Malignant neoplasm of branchial cyst [site of neoplasm]

C10.8   **Malignant neoplasm of overlapping sites of oropharynx**   HCC
> Malignant neoplasm of junctional region of oropharynx

C10.9   **Malignant neoplasm of oropharynx, unspecified**   HCC ▽

✓4ᵗʰ **C11**   **Malignant neoplasm of nasopharynx**
> Use additional code to identify:
> exposure to environmental tobacco smoke (Z77.22)
> exposure to tobacco smoke in the perinatal period (P96.81)
> history of tobacco dependence (Z87.891)
> occupational exposure to environmental tobacco smoke (Z57.31)
> tobacco dependence (F17.-)
> tobacco use (Z72.0)

C11.0   **Malignant neoplasm of superior wall of nasopharynx**   HCC
> Malignant neoplasm of roof of nasopharynx

C11.1   **Malignant neoplasm of posterior wall of nasopharynx**   HCC
> Malignant neoplasm of adenoid
> Malignant neoplasm of pharyngeal tonsil

✓ Additional Character Req   ✓x7ᵗʰ Placeholder Alert   Manifestation   HCC CMS-HCC Condition   ▽ Unspecified Code   ►◄ Revised Text   ● New Code   ▲ Revised Code Title

C11.2 Malignant neoplasm of lateral wall of nasopharynx HCC
Malignant neoplasm of fossa of Rosenmüller
Malignant neoplasm of opening of auditory tube
Malignant neoplasm of pharyngeal recess

C11.3 Malignant neoplasm of anterior wall of nasopharynx HCC
Malignant neoplasm of floor of nasopharynx
Malignant neoplasm of nasopharyngeal (anterior) (posterior) surface of soft palate
Malignant neoplasm of posterior margin of nasal choana
Malignant neoplasm of posterior margin of nasal septum

C11.8 Malignant neoplasm of overlapping sites of nasopharynx HCC

C11.9 Malignant neoplasm of nasopharynx, unspecified HCC ▽
Malignant neoplasm of nasopharyngeal wall NOS

C12 Malignant neoplasm of pyriform sinus HCC
Malignant neoplasm of pyriform fossa
Use additional code to identify:
exposure to environmental tobacco smoke (Z77.22)
exposure to tobacco smoke in the perinatal period (P96.81)
history of tobacco dependence (Z87.891)
occupational exposure to environmental tobacco smoke (Z57.31)
tobacco dependence (F17.-)
tobacco use (Z72.0)

✓4th **C13 Malignant neoplasm of hypopharynx**
Use additional code to identify:
exposure to environmental tobacco smoke (Z77.22)
exposure to tobacco smoke in the perinatal period (P96.81)
history of tobacco dependence (Z87.891)
occupational exposure to environmental tobacco smoke (Z57.31)
tobacco dependence (F17.-)
tobacco use (Z72.0)
EXCLUDES 2 malignant neoplasm of pyriform sinus (C12)

C13.0 Malignant neoplasm of postcricoid region HCC

C13.1 Malignant neoplasm of aryepiglottic fold, hypopharyngeal aspect HCC
Malignant neoplasm of aryepiglottic fold, marginal zone
Malignant neoplasm of aryepiglottic fold NOS
Malignant neoplasm of interarytenoid fold, marginal zone
Malignant neoplasm of interarytenoid fold NOS
EXCLUDES 2 malignant neoplasm of aryepiglottic fold or interarytenoid fold, laryngeal aspect (C32.1)

C13.2 Malignant neoplasm of posterior wall of hypopharynx HCC

C13.8 Malignant neoplasm of overlapping sites of hypopharynx HCC

C13.9 Malignant neoplasm of hypopharynx, unspecified HCC ▽
Malignant neoplasm of hypopharyngeal wall NOS

✓4th **C14 Malignant neoplasm of other and ill-defined sites in the lip, oral cavity and pharynx**
Use additional code to identify:
alcohol abuse and dependence (F10.-)
exposure to environmental tobacco smoke (Z77.22)
exposure to tobacco smoke in the perinatal period (P96.81)
history of tobacco dependence (Z87.891)
occupational exposure to environmental tobacco smoke (Z57.31)
tobacco dependence (F17.-)
tobacco use (Z72.0)
EXCLUDES 1 malignant neoplasm of oral cavity NOS (C06.9)

C14.0 Malignant neoplasm of pharynx, unspecified HCC ▽

C14.2 Malignant neoplasm of Waldeyer's ring HCC

C14.8 Malignant neoplasm of overlapping sites of lip, oral cavity and pharynx HCC
Primary malignant neoplasm of two or more contiguous sites of lip, oral cavity and pharynx
EXCLUDES 1 "book leaf" neoplasm [ventral surface of tongue and floor of mouth] (C06.89)

Malignant neoplasms of digestive organs (C15-C26)

EXCLUDES 1 Kaposi's sarcoma of gastrointestinal sites (C46.4)
EXCLUDES 2 gastrointestinal stromal tumors (C49.A-)

✓4th **C15 Malignant neoplasm of esophagus**
Use additional code to identify:
alcohol abuse and dependence (F10.-)

C15.3 Malignant neoplasm of upper third of esophagus HCC

C15.4 Malignant neoplasm of middle third of esophagus HCC

C15.5 Malignant neoplasm of lower third of esophagus HCC
EXCLUDES 1 malignant neoplasm of cardio-esophageal junction (C16.0)

C15.8 Malignant neoplasm of overlapping sites of esophagus HCC

C15.9 Malignant neoplasm of esophagus, unspecified HCC ▽

✓4th **C16 Malignant neoplasm of stomach**
Use additional code to identify:
alcohol abuse and dependence (F10.-)
EXCLUDES 2 malignant carcinoid tumor of the stomach (C7A.092)

C16.0 Malignant neoplasm of cardia HCC
Malignant neoplasm of cardiac orifice
Malignant neoplasm of cardio-esophageal junction
Malignant neoplasm of esophagus and stomach
Malignant neoplasm of gastro-esophageal junction

C16.1 Malignant neoplasm of fundus of stomach HCC

C16.2 Malignant neoplasm of body of stomach HCC

C16.3 Malignant neoplasm of pyloric antrum HCC
Malignant neoplasm of gastric antrum

C16.4 Malignant neoplasm of pylorus HCC
Malignant neoplasm of prepylorus
Malignant neoplasm of pyloric canal

C16.5 Malignant neoplasm of lesser curvature of stomach, unspecified HCC ▽
Malignant neoplasm of lesser curvature of stomach, not classifiable to C16.1-C16.4

C16.6 Malignant neoplasm of greater curvature of stomach, unspecified HCC ▽
Malignant neoplasm of greater curvature of stomach, not classifiable to C16.0-C16.4

C16.8 Malignant neoplasm of overlapping sites of stomach HCC

C16.9 Malignant neoplasm of stomach, unspecified HCC ▽
Gastric cancer NOS

✓4th **C17 Malignant neoplasm of small intestine**
EXCLUDES 1 malignant carcinoid tumors of the small intestine (C7A.01)
AHA: 2016, 1Q, 19

C17.0 Malignant neoplasm of duodenum HCC

C17.1 Malignant neoplasm of jejunum HCC

C17.2 Malignant neoplasm of ileum HCC
EXCLUDES 1 malignant neoplasm of ileocecal valve (C18.0)

C17.3 Meckel's diverticulum, malignant HCC
EXCLUDES 1 Meckel's diverticulum, congenital (Q43.0)

C17.8 Malignant neoplasm of overlapping sites of small intestine HCC

C17.9 Malignant neoplasm of small intestine, unspecified HCC ▽

✓4th **C18 Malignant neoplasm of colon**
EXCLUDES 1 malignant carcinoid tumors of the colon (C7A.02-)

C18.0 Malignant neoplasm of cecum HCC
Malignant neoplasm of ileocecal valve

C18.1 Malignant neoplasm of appendix HCC

C18.2 Malignant neoplasm of ascending colon HCC

C18.3 Malignant neoplasm of hepatic flexure HCC

C18.4 Malignant neoplasm of transverse colon HCC

C18.5 Malignant neoplasm of splenic flexure HCC

C18.6 Malignant neoplasm of descending colon HCC

C18.7 Malignant neoplasm of sigmoid colon HCC
Malignant neoplasm of sigmoid (flexure)
EXCLUDES 1 malignant neoplasm of rectosigmoid junction (C19)

C18.8 Malignant neoplasm of overlapping sites of colon HCC

C18.9 Malignant neoplasm of colon, unspecified HCC ▽
Malignant neoplasm of large intestine NOS

C19 Malignant neoplasm of rectosigmoid junction HCC
Malignant neoplasm of colon with rectum
Malignant neoplasm of rectosigmoid (colon)
EXCLUDES 1 malignant carcinoid tumors of the colon (C7A.02-)

C20 Malignant neoplasm of rectum HCC
Malignant neoplasm of rectal ampulla
EXCLUDES 1 malignant carcinoid tumor of the rectum (C7A.026)

✓4th **C21 Malignant neoplasm of anus and anal canal**
EXCLUDES 2 malignant carcinoid tumors of the colon (C7A.02-)
malignant melanoma of anal margin (C43.51)
malignant melanoma of anal skin (C43.51)
malignant melanoma of perianal skin (C43.51)
other and unspecified malignant neoplasm of anal margin (C44.500, C44.510, C44.520, C44.590)
other and unspecified malignant neoplasm of anal skin (C44.500, C44.510, C44.520, C44.590)
other and unspecified malignant neoplasm of perianal skin (C44.500, C44.510, C44.520, C44.590)

C21.0 Malignant neoplasm of anus, unspecified HCC ▽

EXCLUDES 1 Not coded here   EXCLUDES 2 Not included here   N Newborn Age: 0   P Pediatric Age: 0-17   M Maternity Age: 12-55   A Adult Age: 15-124

Colon

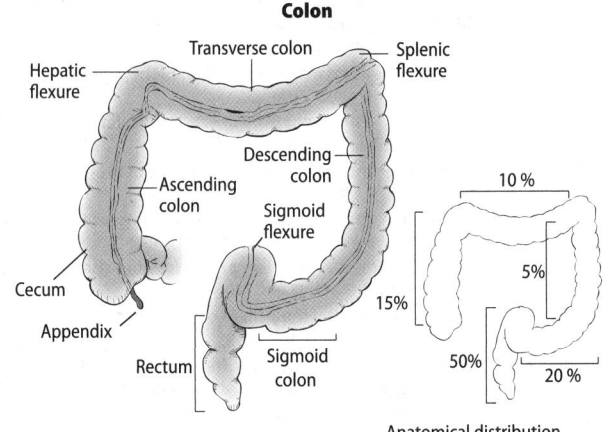

Anatomical distribution
of large bowel cancers

Pancreas

C21.1 Malignant neoplasm of anal canal   `HCC`
Malignant neoplasm of anal sphincter

C21.2 Malignant neoplasm of cloacogenic zone   `HCC`

C21.8 Malignant neoplasm of overlapping sites of rectum, anus and anal canal   `HCC`
Malignant neoplasm of anorectal junction
Malignant neoplasm of anorectum
Primary malignant neoplasm of two or more contiguous sites of rectum, anus and anal canal

`✓4ᵗʰ` **C22 Malignant neoplasm of liver and intrahepatic bile ducts**
Use additional code to identify:
alcohol abuse and dependence (F10.-)
hepatitis B (B16.-, B18.0-B18.1)
hepatitis C (B17.1-, B18.2)
`EXCLUDES 1`   *malignant neoplasm of biliary tract NOS (C24.9)*
secondary malignant neoplasm of liver and intrahepatic bile duct (C78.7)

C22.0 Liver cell carcinoma   `HCC`
Hepatocellular carcinoma   Hepatoma
AHA: 2016, 1Q, 18

C22.1 Intrahepatic bile duct carcinoma   `HCC`
Cholangiocarcinoma
`EXCLUDES 1`   *malignant neoplasm of hepatic duct (C24.0)*

C22.2 Hepatoblastoma   `HCC`

C22.3 Angiosarcoma of liver   `HCC`
Kupffer cell sarcoma

C22.4 Other sarcomas of liver   `HCC`

C22.7 Other specified carcinomas of liver   `HCC`

C22.8 Malignant neoplasm of liver, primary, unspecified as to type   `HCC` ▽

C22.9 Malignant neoplasm of liver, not specified as primary or secondary   `HCC` ▽

C23 Malignant neoplasm of gallbladder   `HCC`

`✓4ᵗʰ` **C24 Malignant neoplasm of other and unspecified parts of biliary tract**
`EXCLUDES 1`   *malignant neoplasm of intrahepatic bile duct (C22.1)*

C24.0 Malignant neoplasm of extrahepatic bile duct   `HCC`
Malignant neoplasm of biliary duct or passage NOS
Malignant neoplasm of common bile duct
Malignant neoplasm of cystic duct
Malignant neoplasm of hepatic duct

C24.1 Malignant neoplasm of ampulla of Vater   `HCC`
DEF: Malignant neoplasm in the area of dilation at the juncture of the common bile and pancreatic ducts near the opening into the lumen of the duodenum.

C24.8 Malignant neoplasm of overlapping sites of biliary tract   `HCC`
Malignant neoplasm involving both intrahepatic and extrahepatic bile ducts
Primary malignant neoplasm of two or more contiguous sites of biliary tract

C24.9 Malignant neoplasm of biliary tract, unspecified   `HCC` ▽

`✓4ᵗʰ` **C25 Malignant neoplasm of pancreas**
Code also exocrine pancreatic insufficiency (K86.81)
Use additional code to identify:
alcohol abuse and dependence (F10.-)

C25.0 Malignant neoplasm of head of pancreas   `HCC`

C25.1 Malignant neoplasm of body of pancreas   `HCC`

C25.2 Malignant neoplasm of tail of pancreas   `HCC`

C25.3 Malignant neoplasm of pancreatic duct   `HCC`

C25.4 Malignant neoplasm of endocrine pancreas   `HCC`
Malignant neoplasm of islets of Langerhans
Use additional code to identify any functional activity

C25.7 Malignant neoplasm of other parts of pancreas   `HCC`
Malignant neoplasm of neck of pancreas

C25.8 Malignant neoplasm of overlapping sites of pancreas   `HCC`

C25.9 Malignant neoplasm of pancreas, unspecified   `HCC` ▽

`✓4ᵗʰ` **C26 Malignant neoplasm of other and ill-defined digestive organs**
`EXCLUDES 1`   *malignant neoplasm of peritoneum and retroperitoneum (C48.-)*

C26.0 Malignant neoplasm of intestinal tract, part unspecified   `HCC` ▽
Malignant neoplasm of intestine NOS

C26.1 Malignant neoplasm of spleen   `HCC`
`EXCLUDES 1`   *Hodgkin lymphoma (C81.-)*
non-Hodgkin lymphoma (C82-C85)

C26.9 Malignant neoplasm of ill-defined sites within the digestive system   `HCC` ▽
Malignant neoplasm of alimentary canal or tract NOS
Malignant neoplasm of gastrointestinal tract NOS
`EXCLUDES 1`   *malignant neoplasm of abdominal NOS (C76.2)*
malignant neoplasm of intra-abdominal NOS (C76.2)

Malignant neoplasms of respiratory and intrathoracic organs (C30-C39)

`INCLUDES`   malignant neoplasm of middle ear
`EXCLUDES 1`   *mesothelioma (C45.-)*

`✓4ᵗʰ` **C30 Malignant neoplasm of nasal cavity and middle ear**

C30.0 Malignant neoplasm of nasal cavity   `HCC`
Malignant neoplasm of cartilage of nose
Malignant neoplasm of nasal concha
Malignant neoplasm of internal nose
Malignant neoplasm of septum of nose
Malignant neoplasm of vestibule of nose
`EXCLUDES 1`   *malignant melanoma of skin of nose (C43.31)*
malignant neoplasm of nasal bone (C41.0)
malignant neoplasm of nose NOS (C76.0)
malignant neoplasm of olfactory bulb (C72.2-)
malignant neoplasm of posterior margin of nasal septum and choana (C11.3)
malignant neoplasm of turbinates (C41.0)
other and unspecified malignant neoplasm of skin of nose (C44.301, C44.311, C44.321, C44.391)

C30.1 Malignant neoplasm of middle ear   `HCC`
Malignant neoplasm of antrum tympanicum
Malignant neoplasm of auditory tube
Malignant neoplasm of eustachian tube
Malignant neoplasm of inner ear
Malignant neoplasm of mastoid air cells
Malignant neoplasm of tympanic cavity
`EXCLUDES 1`   *malignant melanoma of skin of (external) ear (C43.2-)*
malignant neoplasm of auricular canal (external) (C43.2-,C44.2-)
malignant neoplasm of bone of ear (meatus) (C41.0)
malignant neoplasm of cartilage of ear (C49.0)
other and unspecified malignant neoplasm of skin of (external) ear (C44.2-)

☑ Additional Character Req   `✓x7ᵗʰ` Placeholder Alert   Manifestation   `HCC` CMS-HCC Condition   ▽ Unspecified Code   ▶◀ Revised Text   ● New Code   ▲ Revised Code Title

ICD-10-CM 2018   **463**

✓4ᵗʰ **C31 Malignant neoplasm of** accessory sinuses

C31.0 Malignant neoplasm of maxillary sinus �⃞HCC
　　　Malignant neoplasm of antrum (Highmore) (maxillary)

C31.1 Malignant neoplasm of ethmoidal sinus �⃞HCC

C31.2 Malignant neoplasm of frontal sinus ▮HCC

C31.3 Malignant neoplasm of sphenoid sinus ▮HCC

C31.8 Malignant neoplasm of overlapping sites of ▮HCC
　　　accessory sinuses

C31.9 Malignant neoplasm of accessory sinus, unspecified ▮HCC ▽

✓4ᵗʰ **C32 Malignant neoplasm of** larynx
　　Use additional code to identify:
　　　alcohol abuse and dependence (F10.-)
　　　exposure to environmental tobacco smoke (Z77.22)
　　　exposure to tobacco smoke in the perinatal period (P96.81)
　　　history of tobacco dependence (Z87.891)
　　　occupational exposure to environmental tobacco smoke (Z57.31)
　　　tobacco dependence (F17.-)
　　　tobacco use (Z72.0)

C32.0 Malignant neoplasm of glottis ▮HCC
　　　Malignant neoplasm of intrinsic larynx
　　　Malignant neoplasm of laryngeal commissure
　　　　(anterior)(posterior)
　　　Malignant neoplasm of vocal cord (true) NOS

C32.1 Malignant neoplasm of supraglottis ▮HCC
　　　Malignant neoplasm of aryepiglottic fold or interarytenoid fold,
　　　　laryngeal aspect
　　　Malignant neoplasm of epiglottis (suprahyoid portion) NOS
　　　Malignant neoplasm of extrinsic larynx
　　　Malignant neoplasm of false vocal cord
　　　Malignant neoplasm of posterior (laryngeal) surface of epiglottis
　　　Malignant neoplasm of ventricular bands
　　　　EXCLUDES 2 malignant neoplasm of anterior surface of epiglottis
　　　　　　　　　　(C10.1)
　　　　　　　　malignant neoplasm of aryepiglottic fold or
　　　　　　　　　interarytenoid fold, hypopharyngeal aspect
　　　　　　　　　(C13.1)
　　　　　　　　malignant neoplasm of aryepiglottic fold or
　　　　　　　　　interarytenoid fold, marginal zone (C13.1)
　　　　　　　　malignant neoplasm of aryepiglottic fold or
　　　　　　　　　interarytenoid fold NOS (C13.1)

C32.2 Malignant neoplasm of subglottis ▮HCC

C32.3 Malignant neoplasm of laryngeal cartilage ▮HCC

C32.8 Malignant neoplasm of overlapping sites **of larynx** ▮HCC

C32.9 Malignant neoplasm of larynx, unspecified ▮HCC ▽

C33 Malignant neoplasm of trachea ▮HCC
　　Use additional code to identify:
　　　exposure to environmental tobacco smoke (Z77.22)
　　　exposure to tobacco smoke in the perinatal period (P96.81)
　　　history of tobacco dependence (Z87.891)
　　　occupational exposure to environmental tobacco smoke (Z57.31)
　　　tobacco dependence (F17.-)
　　　tobacco use (Z72.0)

✓4ᵗʰ **C34 Malignant neoplasm of** bronchus and lung
　　Use additional code to identify:
　　　exposure to environmental tobacco smoke (Z77.22)
　　　exposure to tobacco smoke in the perinatal period (P96.81)
　　　history of tobacco dependence (Z87.891)
　　　occupational exposure to environmental tobacco smoke (Z57.31)
　　　tobacco dependence (F17.-)
　　　tobacco use (Z72.0)
　　　EXCLUDES 1 Kaposi's sarcoma of lung (C46.5-)
　　　　　　　　malignant carcinoid tumor of the bronchus and lung (C7A.090)

✓5ᵗʰ **C34.0 Malignant neoplasm of** main bronchus
　　　Malignant neoplasm of carina
　　　Malignant neoplasm of hilus (of lung)

　　　C34.00 Malignant neoplasm of unspecified main ▮HCC ▽
　　　　　bronchus

　　　C34.01 Malignant neoplasm of right **main bronchus** ▮HCC

　　　C34.02 Malignant neoplasm of left **main bronchus** ▮HCC

✓5ᵗʰ **C34.1 Malignant neoplasm of** upper lobe, bronchus or lung

　　　C34.10 Malignant neoplasm of upper lobe, ▮HCC ▽
　　　　　unspecified bronchus or lung

　　　C34.11 Malignant neoplasm of upper lobe, right ▮HCC
　　　　　bronchus or lung

　　　C34.12 Malignant neoplasm of upper lobe, left ▮HCC
　　　　　bronchus or lung

C34.2 Malignant neoplasm of middle lobe, bronchus or lung ▮HCC

✓5ᵗʰ **C34.3 Malignant neoplasm of** lower lobe, bronchus or lung

　　　C34.30 Malignant neoplasm of lower lobe, ▮HCC ▽
　　　　　unspecified bronchus or lung

　　　C34.31 Malignant neoplasm of lower lobe, right ▮HCC
　　　　　bronchus or lung

　　　C34.32 Malignant neoplasm of lower lobe, left ▮HCC
　　　　　bronchus or lung

✓5ᵗʰ **C34.8 Malignant neoplasm of** overlapping sites **of bronchus and**
　　　lung

　　　C34.80 Malignant neoplasm of overlapping sites ▮HCC ▽
　　　　　of unspecified bronchus and lung

　　　C34.81 Malignant neoplasm of overlapping sites of ▮HCC
　　　　　right **bronchus and lung**

　　　C34.82 Malignant neoplasm of overlapping sites of ▮HCC
　　　　　left **bronchus and lung**

✓5ᵗʰ **C34.9 Malignant neoplasm of unspecified part of bronchus or lung**

　　　C34.90 Malignant neoplasm of unspecified part of ▮HCC ▽
　　　　　unspecified bronchus or lung
　　　　　Lung cancer NOS

　　　C34.91 Malignant neoplasm of unspecified part of ▮HCC ▽
　　　　　right **bronchus or lung**

　　　C34.92 Malignant neoplasm of unspecified part of ▮HCC ▽
　　　　　left **bronchus or lung**

C37 Malignant neoplasm of thymus ▮HCC
　　　EXCLUDES 1 malignant carcinoid tumor of the thymus (C7A.091)

✓4ᵗʰ **C38 Malignant neoplasm of** heart, mediastinum and pleura
　　　EXCLUDES 1 mesothelioma (C45.-)

C38.0 Malignant neoplasm of heart ▮HCC
　　　Malignant neoplasm of pericardium
　　　EXCLUDES 1 malignant neoplasm of great vessels (C49.3)

C38.1 Malignant neoplasm of anterior mediastinum ▮HCC

C38.2 Malignant neoplasm of posterior mediastinum ▮HCC

C38.3 Malignant neoplasm of mediastinum, ▮HCC ▽
　　　part unspecified

C38.4 Malignant neoplasm of pleura ▮HCC

C38.8 Malignant neoplasm of overlapping sites **of heart,** ▮HCC
　　　mediastinum and pleura

✓4ᵗʰ **C39 Malignant neoplasm of other and ill-defined sites in the**
　　　respiratory system and intrathoracic organs
　　Use additional code to identify:
　　　exposure to environmental tobacco smoke (Z77.22)
　　　exposure to tobacco smoke in the perinatal period (P96.81)
　　　history of tobacco dependence (Z87.891)
　　　occupational exposure to environmental tobacco smoke (Z57.31)
　　　tobacco dependence (F17.-)
　　　tobacco use (Z72.0)
　　　EXCLUDES 1 intrathoracic malignant neoplasm NOS (C76.1)
　　　　　　　　thoracic malignant neoplasm NOS (C76.1)

C39.0 Malignant neoplasm of upper **respiratory tract, part** ▮HCC ▽
　　　unspecified

C39.9 Malignant neoplasm of lower **respiratory tract, part** ▮HCC ▽
　　　unspecified
　　　Malignant neoplasm of respiratory tract NOS

Malignant neoplasms of bone and articular cartilage (C40-C41)

　　INCLUDES malignant neoplasm of cartilage (articular) (joint)
　　　　　malignant neoplasm of periosteum
　　EXCLUDES 1 malignant neoplasm of bone marrow NOS (C96.9)
　　　　　malignant neoplasm of synovia (C49.-)

✓4ᵗʰ **C40 Malignant neoplasm of** bone and articular cartilage of limbs
　　Use additional code to identify major osseous defect, if applicable
　　　(M89.7-)

✓5ᵗʰ **C40.0 Malignant neoplasm of** scapula and long bones of upper limb

　　　C40.00 Malignant neoplasm of scapula and long ▮HCC ▽
　　　　　bones of unspecified upper limb

　　　C40.01 Malignant neoplasm of scapula and long bones ▮HCC
　　　　　of right **upper limb**

　　　C40.02 Malignant neoplasm of scapula and long bones ▮HCC
　　　　　of left **upper limb**

✓5ᵗʰ **C40.1 Malignant neoplasm of** short bones of upper limb

　　　C40.10 Malignant neoplasm of short bones of ▮HCC ▽
　　　　　unspecified upper limb

　　　C40.11 Malignant neoplasm of short bones of right ▮HCC
　　　　　upper limb

　　　C40.12 Malignant neoplasm of short bones of left ▮HCC
　　　　　upper limb

EXCLUDES 1 Not coded here　　　*EXCLUDES 2* Not included here　　　Ⓝ Newborn Age: 0　　　Ⓟ Pediatric Age: 0-17　　　Ⓜ Maternity Age: 12-55　　　Ⓐ Adult Age: 15-124

464　　　　　ICD-10-CM 2018

✓5ᵗʰ **C40.2** Malignant neoplasm of long bones of lower limb

  C40.20 Malignant neoplasm of long bones of unspecified lower limb   HCC ▽

  C40.21 Malignant neoplasm of long bones of right lower limb   HCC

  C40.22 Malignant neoplasm of long bones of left lower limb   HCC

✓5ᵗʰ **C40.3** Malignant neoplasm of short bones of lower limb

  C40.30 Malignant neoplasm of short bones of unspecified lower limb   HCC ▽

  C40.31 Malignant neoplasm of short bones of right lower limb   HCC

  C40.32 Malignant neoplasm of short bones of left lower limb   HCC

✓5ᵗʰ **C40.8** Malignant neoplasm of overlapping sites of bone and articular cartilage of limb

  C40.80 Malignant neoplasm of overlapping sites of bone and articular cartilage of unspecified limb   HCC ▽

  C40.81 Malignant neoplasm of overlapping sites of bone and articular cartilage of right limb   HCC

  C40.82 Malignant neoplasm of overlapping sites of bone and articular cartilage of left limb   HCC

✓5ᵗʰ **C40.9** Malignant neoplasm of unspecified bones and articular cartilage of limb

  C40.90 Malignant neoplasm of unspecified bones and articular cartilage of unspecified limb   HCC ▽

  C40.91 Malignant neoplasm of unspecified bones and articular cartilage of right limb   HCC ▽

  C40.92 Malignant neoplasm of unspecified bones and articular cartilage of left limb   HCC ▽

✓4ᵗʰ **C41** **Malignant neoplasm of bone and articular cartilage of other and unspecified sites**

  EXCLUDES 1   *malignant neoplasm of bones of limbs (C40.-)*
     malignant neoplasm of cartilage of ear (C49.0)
     malignant neoplasm of cartilage of eyelid (C49.0)
     malignant neoplasm of cartilage of larynx (C32.3)
     malignant neoplasm of cartilage of limbs (C40.-)
     malignant neoplasm of cartilage of nose (C30.0)

  C41.0 Malignant neoplasm of bones of skull and face   HCC

    Malignant neoplasm of maxilla (superior)
    Malignant neoplasm of orbital bone

    EXCLUDES 2   *carcinoma, any type except intraosseous or odontogenic of:*
      maxillary sinus (C31.0)
      upper jaw (C03.0)
      malignant neoplasm of jaw bone (lower) (C41.1)

  C41.1 Malignant neoplasm of mandible   HCC

    Malignant neoplasm of inferior maxilla
    Malignant neoplasm of lower jaw bone

    EXCLUDES 2   *carcinoma, any type except intraosseous or odontogenic of:*
      jaw NOS (C03.9)
      lower (C03.1)
      malignant neoplasm of upper jaw bone (C41.0)

  C41.2 Malignant neoplasm of vertebral column   HCC

    EXCLUDES 1   *malignant neoplasm of sacrum and coccyx (C41.4)*

  C41.3 Malignant neoplasm of ribs, sternum and clavicle   HCC

  C41.4 Malignant neoplasm of pelvic bones, sacrum and coccyx   HCC

  C41.9 Malignant neoplasm of bone and articular cartilage, unspecified   HCC ▽

Melanoma and other malignant neoplasms of skin (C43-C44)

✓4ᵗʰ **C43** **Malignant melanoma of skin**

  EXCLUDES 1   *melanoma in situ (D03.-)*

  EXCLUDES 2   *malignant melanoma of skin of genital organs (C51-C52, C60.-, C63.-)*
     Merkel cell carcinoma (C4A.-)
     sites other than skin—code to malignant neoplasm of the site

  C43.0 Malignant melanoma of lip   HCC

    EXCLUDES 1   *malignant neoplasm of vermilion border of lip (C00.0-C00.2)*

✓5ᵗʰ **C43.1** Malignant melanoma of eyelid, including canthus

  C43.10 Malignant melanoma of unspecified eyelid, including canthus   HCC ▽

  C43.11 Malignant melanoma of right eyelid, including canthus   HCC

  C43.12 Malignant melanoma of left eyelid, including canthus   HCC

✓5ᵗʰ **C43.2** Malignant melanoma of ear and external auricular canal

  C43.20 Malignant melanoma of unspecified ear and external auricular canal   HCC ▽

  C43.21 Malignant melanoma of right ear and external auricular canal   HCC

  C43.22 Malignant melanoma of left ear and external auricular canal   HCC

✓5ᵗʰ **C43.3** Malignant melanoma of other and unspecified parts of face

  C43.30 Malignant melanoma of unspecified part of face   HCC ▽

  C43.31 Malignant melanoma of nose   HCC

  C43.39 Malignant melanoma of other parts of face   HCC

  C43.4 Malignant melanoma of scalp and neck   HCC

✓5ᵗʰ **C43.5** Malignant melanoma of trunk

  EXCLUDES 2   *malignant neoplasm of anus NOS (C21.0)*
     malignant neoplasm of scrotum (C63.2)

  C43.51 Malignant melanoma of anal skin   HCC

    Malignant melanoma of anal margin
    Malignant melanoma of perianal skin

  C43.52 Malignant melanoma of skin of breast   HCC

  C43.59 Malignant melanoma of other part of trunk   HCC

✓5ᵗʰ **C43.6** Malignant melanoma of upper limb, including shoulder

  C43.60 Malignant melanoma of unspecified upper limb, including shoulder   HCC ▽

  C43.61 Malignant melanoma of right upper limb, including shoulder   HCC

  C43.62 Malignant melanoma of left upper limb, including shoulder   HCC

✓5ᵗʰ **C43.7** Malignant melanoma of lower limb, including hip

  C43.70 Malignant melanoma of unspecified lower limb, including hip   HCC ▽

  C43.71 Malignant melanoma of right lower limb, including hip   HCC

  C43.72 Malignant melanoma of left lower limb, including hip   HCC

  C43.8 Malignant melanoma of overlapping sites of skin   HCC

  C43.9 Malignant melanoma of skin, unspecified   HCC ▽

    Malignant melanoma of unspecified site of skin
    Melanoma (malignant) NOS

✓4ᵗʰ **C4A** **Merkel cell carcinoma**

  DEF: Malignant cutaneous cancer predominantly found in elderly patients with sun exposure that usually presents as a flesh-colored or bluish-red lump typically seen on the neck, head and face.

  C4A.0 Merkel cell carcinoma of lip   HCC

    EXCLUDES 1   *malignant neoplasm of vermilion border of lip (C00.0-C00.2)*

✓5ᵗʰ **C4A.1** Merkel cell carcinoma of eyelid, including canthus

  C4A.10 Merkel cell carcinoma of unspecified eyelid, including canthus   HCC ▽

  C4A.11 Merkel cell carcinoma of right eyelid, including canthus   HCC

  C4A.12 Merkel cell carcinoma of left eyelid, including canthus   HCC

✓5ᵗʰ **C4A.2** Merkel cell carcinoma of ear and external auricular canal

  C4A.20 Merkel cell carcinoma of unspecified ear and external auricular canal   HCC ▽

  C4A.21 Merkel cell carcinoma of right ear and external auricular canal   HCC

  C4A.22 Merkel cell carcinoma of left ear and external auricular canal   HCC

✓5ᵗʰ **C4A.3** Merkel cell carcinoma of other and unspecified parts of face

  C4A.30 Merkel cell carcinoma of unspecified part of face   HCC ▽

  C4A.31 Merkel cell carcinoma of nose   HCC

  C4A.39 Merkel cell carcinoma of other parts of face   HCC

  C4A.4 Merkel cell carcinoma of scalp and neck   HCC

✓5ᵗʰ **C4A.5** Merkel cell carcinoma of trunk

  EXCLUDES 2   *malignant neoplasm of anus NOS (C21.0)*
     malignant neoplasm of scrotum (C63.2)

  C4A.51 Merkel cell carcinoma of anal skin   HCC

    Merkel cell carcinoma of anal margin
    Merkel cell carcinoma of perianal skin

✓ Additional Character Req   ✓ₓ7ᵗʰ Placeholder Alert   Manifestation   HCC CMS-HCC Condition   ▽ Unspecified Code   ▶◀ Revised Text   ● New Code   ▲ Revised Code Title

ICD-10-CM 2018   465

C4A.52   Merkel cell carcinoma of skin of breast   **HCC**
C4A.59   Merkel cell carcinoma of other part of trunk   **HCC**

√5ᵗʰ   **C4A.6   Merkel cell carcinoma of upper limb, including shoulder**
C4A.6Ø   Merkel cell carcinoma of unspecified upper limb, including shoulder   **HCC** ▽
C4A.61   Merkel cell carcinoma of right upper limb, including shoulder   **HCC**
C4A.62   Merkel cell carcinoma of left upper limb, including shoulder   **HCC**

√5ᵗʰ   **C4A.7   Merkel cell carcinoma of lower limb, including hip**
C4A.7Ø   Merkel cell carcinoma of unspecified lower limb, including hip   **HCC** ▽
C4A.71   Merkel cell carcinoma of right lower limb, including hip   **HCC**
C4A.72   Merkel cell carcinoma of left lower limb, including hip   **HCC**

C4A.8   Merkel cell carcinoma of overlapping sites   **HCC**
C4A.9   Merkel cell carcinoma, unspecified   **HCC** ▽
Merkel cell carcinoma of unspecified site

√4ᵗʰ   **C44   Other and unspecified malignant neoplasm of skin**
INCLUDES   malignant neoplasm of sebaceous glands
malignant neoplasm of sweat glands
EXCLUDES 1   Kaposi's sarcoma of skin (C46.Ø)
malignant melanoma of skin (C43.-)
malignant neoplasm of skin of genital organs (C51-C52, C6Ø-, C63.2)
Merkel cell carcinoma (C4A.-)
DEF: Basal cell carcinoma: An abnormal growth of skin cells that arises from the deepest layer of the epidermis and may present as an open sore, red patches, pink growth, or scar. One of the most common forms of skin cancer, typically caused by sun exposure.
DEF: Squamous cell carcinoma: An uncontrolled growth of abnormal skin cells that arises from the skin's outer layers (epidermis) and may present as an open sore; firm, red nodule; elevated growth with a central depression; or flat sore with a scaly crust.

√5ᵗʰ   **C44.Ø   Other and unspecified malignant neoplasm of skin of lip**
EXCLUDES 1   malignant neoplasm of lip (CØØ.-)
C44.ØØ   Unspecified malignant neoplasm of skin of lip   ▽
C44.Ø1   Basal cell carcinoma of skin of lip
C44.Ø2   Squamous cell carcinoma of skin of lip
C44.Ø9   Other specified malignant neoplasm of skin of lip

√5ᵗʰ   **C44.1   Other and unspecified malignant neoplasm of skin of eyelid, including canthus**
EXCLUDES 1   connective tissue of eyelid (C49.Ø)

√6ᵗʰ   **C44.1Ø   Unspecified malignant neoplasm of skin of eyelid, including canthus**
C44.1Ø1   Unspecified malignant neoplasm of skin of unspecified eyelid, including canthus   ▽
C44.1Ø2   Unspecified malignant neoplasm of skin of right eyelid, including canthus   ▽
C44.1Ø9   Unspecified malignant neoplasm of skin of left eyelid, including canthus   ▽

√6ᵗʰ   **C44.11   Basal cell carcinoma of skin of eyelid, including canthus**
C44.111   Basal cell carcinoma of skin of unspecified eyelid, including canthus   ▽
C44.112   Basal cell carcinoma of skin of right eyelid, including canthus
C44.119   Basal cell carcinoma of skin of left eyelid, including canthus

√6ᵗʰ   **C44.12   Squamous cell carcinoma of skin of eyelid, including canthus**
C44.121   Squamous cell carcinoma of skin of unspecified eyelid, including canthus   ▽
C44.122   Squamous cell carcinoma of skin of right eyelid, including canthus
C44.129   Squamous cell carcinoma of skin of left eyelid, including canthus

√6ᵗʰ   **C44.19   Other specified malignant neoplasm of skin of eyelid, including canthus**
C44.191   Other specified malignant neoplasm of skin of unspecified eyelid, including canthus   ▽
C44.192   Other specified malignant neoplasm of skin of right eyelid, including canthus
C44.199   Other specified malignant neoplasm of skin of left eyelid, including canthus

√5ᵗʰ   **C44.2   Other and unspecified malignant neoplasm of skin of ear and external auricular canal**
EXCLUDES 1   connective tissue of ear (C49.Ø)

√6ᵗʰ   **C44.2Ø   Unspecified malignant neoplasm of skin of ear and external auricular canal**
C44.2Ø1   Unspecified malignant neoplasm of skin of unspecified ear and external auricular canal   ▽
C44.2Ø2   Unspecified malignant neoplasm of skin of right ear and external auricular canal   ▽
C44.2Ø9   Unspecified malignant neoplasm of skin of left ear and external auricular canal   ▽

√6ᵗʰ   **C44.21   Basal cell carcinoma of skin of ear and external auricular canal**
C44.211   Basal cell carcinoma of skin of unspecified ear and external auricular canal   ▽
C44.212   Basal cell carcinoma of skin of right ear and external auricular canal
C44.219   Basal cell carcinoma of skin of left ear and external auricular canal

√6ᵗʰ   **C44.22   Squamous cell carcinoma of skin of ear and external auricular canal**
C44.221   Squamous cell carcinoma of skin of unspecified ear and external auricular canal   ▽
C44.222   Squamous cell carcinoma of skin of right ear and external auricular canal
C44.229   Squamous cell carcinoma of skin of left ear and external auricular canal

√6ᵗʰ   **C44.29   Other specified malignant neoplasm of skin of ear and external auricular canal**
C44.291   Other specified malignant neoplasm of skin of unspecified ear and external auricular canal   ▽
C44.292   Other specified malignant neoplasm of skin of right ear and external auricular canal
C44.299   Other specified malignant neoplasm of skin of left ear and external auricular canal

√5ᵗʰ   **C44.3   Other and unspecified malignant neoplasm of skin of other and unspecified parts of face**

√6ᵗʰ   **C44.3Ø   Unspecified malignant neoplasm of skin of other and unspecified parts of face**
C44.3ØØ   Unspecified malignant neoplasm of skin of unspecified part of face   ▽
C44.3Ø1   Unspecified malignant neoplasm of skin of nose   ▽
C44.3Ø9   Unspecified malignant neoplasm of skin of other parts of face   ▽

√6ᵗʰ   **C44.31   Basal cell carcinoma of skin of other and unspecified parts of face**
C44.31Ø   Basal cell carcinoma of skin of unspecified parts of face   ▽
C44.311   Basal cell carcinoma of skin of nose
C44.319   Basal cell carcinoma of skin of other parts of face

√6ᵗʰ   **C44.32   Squamous cell carcinoma of skin of other and unspecified parts of face**
C44.32Ø   Squamous cell carcinoma of skin of unspecified parts of face   ▽
C44.321   Squamous cell carcinoma of skin of nose
C44.329   Squamous cell carcinoma of skin of other parts of face

√6ᵗʰ   **C44.39   Other specified malignant neoplasm of skin of other and unspecified parts of face**
C44.39Ø   Other specified malignant neoplasm of skin of unspecified parts of face   ▽
C44.391   Other specified malignant neoplasm of skin of nose
C44.399   Other specified malignant neoplasm of skin of other parts of face

√5ᵗʰ   **C44.4   Other and unspecified malignant neoplasm of skin of scalp and neck**
C44.4Ø   Unspecified malignant neoplasm of skin of scalp and neck   ▽

EXCLUDES 1 Not coded here   **EXCLUDES 2** Not included here   **N** Newborn Age: 0   **P** Pediatric Age: 0-17   **M** Maternity Age: 12-55   **A** Adult Age: 15-124

C44.41 Basal cell carcinoma of skin of scalp and neck

C44.42 Squamous cell carcinoma of skin of scalp and neck

C44.49 Other specified malignant neoplasm of skin of scalp and neck

☑5ᵗʰ **C44.5** Other and unspecified malignant neoplasm of skin of trunk

> EXCLUDES 1   anus NOS (C21.0)
> scrotum (C63.2)

☑6ᵗʰ **C44.50** Unspecified malignant neoplasm of trunk

C44.500 Unspecified malignant neoplasm of anal skin ▽
> Unspecified malignant neoplasm of anal margin
> Unspecified malignant neoplasm of perianal skin

C44.501 Unspecified malignant neoplasm of skin of breast ▽

C44.509 Unspecified malignant neoplasm of skin of other part of trunk ▽

☑6ᵗʰ **C44.51** Basal cell carcinoma of skin of trunk

C44.510 Basal cell carcinoma of anal skin
> Basal cell carcinoma of anal margin
> Basal cell carcinoma of perianal skin

C44.511 Basal cell carcinoma of skin of breast

C44.519 Basal cell carcinoma of skin of other part of trunk

☑6ᵗʰ **C44.52** Squamous cell carcinoma of skin of trunk

C44.520 Squamous cell carcinoma of anal skin
> Squamous cell carcinoma of anal margin
> Squamous cell carcinoma of perianal skin

C44.521 Squamous cell carcinoma of skin of breast

C44.529 Squamous cell carcinoma of skin of other part of trunk

☑6ᵗʰ **C44.59** Other specified malignant neoplasm of skin of trunk

C44.590 Other specified malignant neoplasm of anal skin
> Other specified malignant neoplasm of anal margin
> Other specified malignant neoplasm of perianal skin

C44.591 Other specified malignant neoplasm of skin of breast

C44.599 Other specified malignant neoplasm of skin of other part of trunk

☑5ᵗʰ **C44.6** Other and unspecified malignant neoplasm of skin of upper limb, including shoulder

☑6ᵗʰ **C44.60** Unspecified malignant neoplasm of skin of upper limb, including shoulder

C44.601 Unspecified malignant neoplasm of skin of unspecified upper limb, including shoulder ▽

C44.602 Unspecified malignant neoplasm of skin of right upper limb, including shoulder ▽

C44.609 Unspecified malignant neoplasm of skin of left upper limb, including shoulder ▽

☑6ᵗʰ **C44.61** Basal cell carcinoma of skin of upper limb, including shoulder

C44.611 Basal cell carcinoma of skin of unspecified upper limb, including shoulder ▽

C44.612 Basal cell carcinoma of skin of right upper limb, including shoulder

C44.619 Basal cell carcinoma of skin of left upper limb, including shoulder

☑6ᵗʰ **C44.62** Squamous cell carcinoma of skin of upper limb, including shoulder

C44.621 Squamous cell carcinoma of skin of unspecified upper limb, including shoulder ▽

C44.622 Squamous cell carcinoma of skin of right upper limb, including shoulder

C44.629 Squamous cell carcinoma of skin of left upper limb, including shoulder

☑6ᵗʰ **C44.69** Other specified malignant neoplasm of skin of upper limb, including shoulder

C44.691 Other specified malignant neoplasm of skin of unspecified upper limb, including shoulder ▽

C44.692 Other specified malignant neoplasm of skin of right upper limb, including shoulder

C44.699 Other specified malignant neoplasm of skin of left upper limb, including shoulder

☑5ᵗʰ **C44.7** Other and unspecified malignant neoplasm of skin of lower limb, including hip

☑6ᵗʰ **C44.70** Unspecified malignant neoplasm of skin of lower limb, including hip

C44.701 Unspecified malignant neoplasm of skin of unspecified lower limb, including hip ▽

C44.702 Unspecified malignant neoplasm of skin of right lower limb, including hip ▽

C44.709 Unspecified malignant neoplasm of skin of left lower limb, including hip ▽

☑6ᵗʰ **C44.71** Basal cell carcinoma of skin of lower limb, including hip

C44.711 Basal cell carcinoma of skin of unspecified lower limb, including hip ▽

C44.712 Basal cell carcinoma of skin of right lower limb, including hip

C44.719 Basal cell carcinoma of skin of left lower limb, including hip

☑6ᵗʰ **C44.72** Squamous cell carcinoma of skin of lower limb, including hip

C44.721 Squamous cell carcinoma of skin of unspecified lower limb, including hip ▽

C44.722 Squamous cell carcinoma of skin of right lower limb, including hip

C44.729 Squamous cell carcinoma of skin of left lower limb, including hip

☑6ᵗʰ **C44.79** Other specified malignant neoplasm of skin of lower limb, including hip

C44.791 Other specified malignant neoplasm of skin of unspecified lower limb, including hip ▽

C44.792 Other specified malignant neoplasm of skin of right lower limb, including hip

C44.799 Other specified malignant neoplasm of skin of left lower limb, including hip

☑5ᵗʰ **C44.8** Other and unspecified malignant neoplasm of overlapping sites of skin

C44.80 Unspecified malignant neoplasm of overlapping sites of skin ▽

C44.81 Basal cell carcinoma of overlapping sites of skin

C44.82 Squamous cell carcinoma of overlapping sites of skin

C44.89 Other specified malignant neoplasm of overlapping sites of skin

☑5ᵗʰ **C44.9** Other and unspecified malignant neoplasm of skin, unspecified

C44.90 Unspecified malignant neoplasm of skin, unspecified ▽
> Malignant neoplasm of unspecified site of skin

C44.91 Basal cell carcinoma of skin, unspecified ▽

C44.92 Squamous cell carcinoma of skin, unspecified ▽

C44.99 Other specified malignant neoplasm of skin, unspecified ▽

Malignant neoplasms of mesothelial and soft tissue (C45-C49)

☑4ᵗʰ **C45** Mesothelioma
> **DEF:** Rare type of cancer that forms in the thin layer of protective tissue that covers the majority of internal organs (mesothelium).

C45.0 Mesothelioma of pleura   HCC
> EXCLUDES 1   other malignant neoplasm of pleura (C38.4)
> **AHA:** 2017, 2Q, 11

C45.1 Mesothelioma of peritoneum   HCC
> Mesothelioma of cul-de-sac   Mesothelioma of omentum
> Mesothelioma of mesentery   Mesothelioma of peritoneum
> Mesothelioma of mesocolon   (parietal) (pelvic)
> EXCLUDES 1   other malignant neoplasm of soft tissue of peritoneum (C48.-)

C45.2 Mesothelioma of pericardium   HCC
> EXCLUDES 1   other malignant neoplasm of pericardium (C38.0)

C45.7 Mesothelioma of other sites   HCC

C45.9 Mesothelioma, unspecified   HCC ▽

☑ Additional Character Req   ☑x7ᵗʰ Placeholder Alert   Manifestation   HCC CMS-HCC Condition   ▽ Unspecified Code   ▶◀ Revised Text   ● New Code   ▲ Revised Code Title

ICD-10-CM 2018   467

C44.41–C45.9

Chapter 2. Neoplasms

☑4ᵗʰ **C46 Kaposi's sarcoma**

Code first any human immunodeficiency virus [HIV] disease (B20)

DEF: Malignant neoplasm that causes patches of abnormal tissue to grow under the skin, in the lining of the mouth, nose, and throat, in lymph nodes, or in other visceral organs. Kaposi's sarcoma is caused by human herpesvirus8 (HHV8).

C46.0 Kaposi's sarcoma of skin   HCC

C46.1 Kaposi's sarcoma of soft tissue   HCC
    Kaposi's sarcoma of blood vessel
    Kaposi's sarcoma of connective tissue
    Kaposi's sarcoma of fascia
    Kaposi's sarcoma of ligament
    Kaposi's sarcoma of lymphatic(s) NEC
    Kaposi's sarcoma of muscle
    EXCLUDES 2   Kaposi's sarcoma of lymph glands and nodes (C46.3)

C46.2 Kaposi's sarcoma of palate   HCC

C46.3 Kaposi's sarcoma of lymph nodes   HCC

C46.4 Kaposi's sarcoma of gastrointestinal sites   HCC

☑5ᵗʰ **C46.5 Kaposi's sarcoma of lung**

    C46.50 Kaposi's sarcoma of unspecified lung   HCC ▽

    C46.51 Kaposi's sarcoma of right lung   HCC

    C46.52 Kaposi's sarcoma of left lung   HCC

C46.7 Kaposi's sarcoma of other sites   HCC

C46.9 Kaposi's sarcoma, unspecified   HCC ▽
    Kaposi's sarcoma of unspecified site

☑4ᵗʰ **C47 Malignant neoplasm of peripheral nerves and autonomic nervous system**

    INCLUDES   malignant neoplasm of sympathetic and parasympathetic nerves and ganglia

    EXCLUDES 1   Kaposi's sarcoma of soft tissue (C46.1)

C47.0 Malignant neoplasm of peripheral nerves of head, face and neck   HCC

    EXCLUDES 1   malignant neoplasm of peripheral nerves of orbit (C69.6-)

☑5ᵗʰ **C47.1 Malignant neoplasm of peripheral nerves of upper limb, including shoulder**

    C47.10 Malignant neoplasm of peripheral nerves of unspecified upper limb, including shoulder   HCC ▽

    C47.11 Malignant neoplasm of peripheral nerves of right upper limb, including shoulder   HCC

    C47.12 Malignant neoplasm of peripheral nerves of left upper limb, including shoulder   HCC

☑5ᵗʰ **C47.2 Malignant neoplasm of peripheral nerves of lower limb, including hip**

    C47.20 Malignant neoplasm of peripheral nerves of unspecified lower limb, including hip   HCC ▽

    C47.21 Malignant neoplasm of peripheral nerves of right lower limb, including hip   HCC

    C47.22 Malignant neoplasm of peripheral nerves of left lower limb, including hip   HCC

C47.3 Malignant neoplasm of peripheral nerves of thorax   HCC

C47.4 Malignant neoplasm of peripheral nerves of abdomen   HCC

C47.5 Malignant neoplasm of peripheral nerves of pelvis   HCC

C47.6 Malignant neoplasm of peripheral nerves of trunk, unspecified   HCC ▽
    Malignant neoplasm of peripheral nerves of unspecified part of trunk

C47.8 Malignant neoplasm of overlapping sites of peripheral nerves and autonomic nervous system   HCC

C47.9 Malignant neoplasm of peripheral nerves and autonomic nervous system, unspecified   HCC ▽
    Malignant neoplasm of unspecified site of peripheral nerves and autonomic nervous system

☑4ᵗʰ **C48 Malignant neoplasm of retroperitoneum and peritoneum**

    EXCLUDES 1   Kaposi's sarcoma of connective tissue (C46.1)
              mesothelioma (C45.-)

C48.0 Malignant neoplasm of retroperitoneum   HCC

C48.1 Malignant neoplasm of specified parts of peritoneum   HCC
    Malignant neoplasm of cul-de-sac
    Malignant neoplasm of mesentery
    Malignant neoplasm of mesocolon
    Malignant neoplasm of omentum
    Malignant neoplasm of parietal peritoneum
    Malignant neoplasm of pelvic peritoneum

C48.2 Malignant neoplasm of peritoneum, unspecified   HCC ▽

C48.8 Malignant neoplasm of overlapping sites of retroperitoneum and peritoneum   HCC

☑4ᵗʰ **C49 Malignant neoplasm of other connective and soft tissue**

    INCLUDES   malignant neoplasm of blood vessel
              malignant neoplasm of bursa
              malignant neoplasm of cartilage
              malignant neoplasm of fascia
              malignant neoplasm of fat
              malignant neoplasm of ligament, except uterine
              malignant neoplasm of lymphatic vessel
              malignant neoplasm of muscle
              malignant neoplasm of synovia
              malignant neoplasm of tendon (sheath)

    EXCLUDES 1   malignant neoplasm of cartilage (of):
              articular (C40-C41)
              larynx (C32.3)
              nose (C30.0)
            malignant neoplasm of connective tissue of breast (C50.-)

    EXCLUDES 2   Kaposi's sarcoma of soft tissue (C46.1)
            malignant neoplasm of heart (C38.0)
            malignant neoplasm of peripheral nerves and autonomic nervous system (C47.-)
            malignant neoplasm of peritoneum (C48.2)
            malignant neoplasm of retroperitoneum (C48.0)
            malignant neoplasm of uterine ligament (C57.3)
            mesothelioma (C45.-)

C49.0 Malignant neoplasm of connective and soft tissue of head, face and neck   HCC
    Malignant neoplasm of connective tissue of ear
    Malignant neoplasm of connective tissue of eyelid
    EXCLUDES 1   connective tissue of orbit (C69.6-)

☑5ᵗʰ **C49.1 Malignant neoplasm of connective and soft tissue of upper limb, including shoulder**

    C49.10 Malignant neoplasm of connective and soft tissue of unspecified upper limb, including shoulder   HCC ▽

    C49.11 Malignant neoplasm of connective and soft tissue of right upper limb, including shoulder   HCC

    C49.12 Malignant neoplasm of connective and soft tissue of left upper limb, including shoulder   HCC

☑5ᵗʰ **C49.2 Malignant neoplasm of connective and soft tissue of lower limb, including hip**

    C49.20 Malignant neoplasm of connective and soft tissue of unspecified lower limb, including hip   HCC ▽

    C49.21 Malignant neoplasm of connective and soft tissue of right lower limb, including hip   HCC

    C49.22 Malignant neoplasm of connective and soft tissue of left lower limb, including hip   HCC

C49.3 Malignant neoplasm of connective and soft tissue of thorax   HCC
    Malignant neoplasm of axilla
    Malignant neoplasm of diaphragm
    Malignant neoplasm of great vessels
    EXCLUDES 1   malignant neoplasm of breast (C50.-)
              malignant neoplasm of heart (C38.0)
              malignant neoplasm of mediastinum (C38.1-C38.3)
              malignant neoplasm of thymus (C37)
    AHA: 2015, 3Q, 19

C49.4 Malignant neoplasm of connective and soft tissue of abdomen   HCC
    Malignant neoplasm of abdominal wall
    Malignant neoplasm of hypochondrium

C49.5 Malignant neoplasm of connective and soft tissue of pelvis   HCC
    Malignant neoplasm of buttock
    Malignant neoplasm of groin
    Malignant neoplasm of perineum

C49.6 Malignant neoplasm of connective and soft tissue of trunk, unspecified   HCC ▽
    Malignant neoplasm of back NOS

C49.8 Malignant neoplasm of overlapping sites of connective and soft tissue   HCC
    Primary malignant neoplasm of two or more contiguous sites of connective and soft tissue

C49.9 Malignant neoplasm of connective and soft tissue, unspecified   HCC ▽

☑5ᵗʰ **C49.A Gastrointestinal stromal tumor**

    C49.A0 Gastrointestinal stromal tumor, unspecified site   HCC ▽

    C49.A1 Gastrointestinal stromal tumor of esophagus   HCC

    C49.A2 Gastrointestinal stromal tumor of stomach   HCC

    C49.A3 Gastrointestinal stromal tumor of small intestine   HCC

EXCLUDES 1 Not coded here   *EXCLUDES 2* Not included here   N Newborn Age: 0   P Pediatric Age: 0-17   M Maternity Age: 12-55   A Adult Age: 15-124

C49.A4   Gastrointestinal stromal tumor of large intestine HCC

C49.A5   Gastrointestinal stromal tumor of rectum   HCC

C49.A9   Gastrointestinal stromal tumor of other sites   HCC

Malignant neoplasms of breast (C50)

✓4ᵗʰ **C50**   **Malignant neoplasm of breast**
     INCLUDES   connective tissue of breast
                 Paget's disease of breast
                 Paget's disease of nipple
     Use additional code to identify estrogen receptor status (Z17.0, Z17.1)
     EXCLUDES 1   *skin of breast (C44.501, C44.511, C44.521, C44.591)*

✓5ᵗʰ   **C50.0**   **Malignant neoplasm of nipple and areola**

     ✓6ᵗʰ   **C50.01**   **Malignant neoplasm of nipple and areola, female**

         C50.011   Malignant neoplasm of nipple and   HCC ♀
                    areola, right female breast

         C50.012   Malignant neoplasm of nipple and   HCC ♀
                    areola, left female breast

         C50.019   Malignant neoplasm of nipple   HCC ♀ ▽
                    and areola, unspecified female breast

     ✓6ᵗʰ   **C50.02**   **Malignant neoplasm of nipple and areola, male**

         C50.021   Malignant neoplasm of nipple and   HCC ♂
                    areola, right male breast

         C50.022   Malignant neoplasm of nipple and   HCC ♂
                    areola, left male breast

         C50.029   Malignant neoplasm of nipple   HCC ♂ ▽
                    and areola, unspecified male breast

✓5ᵗʰ   **C50.1**   **Malignant neoplasm of central portion of breast**

     ✓6ᵗʰ   **C50.11**   **Malignant neoplasm of central portion of breast, female**

         C50.111   Malignant neoplasm of central   HCC ♀
                    portion of right female breast

         C50.112   Malignant neoplasm of central   HCC ♀
                    portion of left female breast

         C50.119   Malignant neoplasm of central   HCC ♀ ▽
                    portion of unspecified female breast

     ✓6ᵗʰ   **C50.12**   **Malignant neoplasm of central portion of breast, male**

         C50.121   Malignant neoplasm of central   HCC ♂
                    portion of right male breast

         C50.122   Malignant neoplasm of central   HCC ♂
                    portion of left male breast

         C50.129   Malignant neoplasm of central   HCC ♂ ▽
                    portion of unspecified male breast

✓5ᵗʰ   **C50.2**   **Malignant neoplasm of upper-inner quadrant of breast**

     ✓6ᵗʰ   **C50.21**   **Malignant neoplasm of upper-inner quadrant of breast, female**

         C50.211   Malignant neoplasm of upper-inner   HCC ♀
                    quadrant of right female breast

         C50.212   Malignant neoplasm of upper-inner   HCC ♀
                    quadrant of left female breast

         C50.219   Malignant neoplasm of   HCC ♀ ▽
                    upper-inner quadrant of unspecified
                    female breast

     ✓6ᵗʰ   **C50.22**   **Malignant neoplasm of upper-inner quadrant of breast, male**

         C50.221   Malignant neoplasm of upper-inner   HCC ♂
                    quadrant of right male breast

         C50.222   Malignant neoplasm of upper-inner   HCC ♂
                    quadrant of left male breast

         C50.229   Malignant neoplasm of   HCC ♂ ▽
                    upper-inner quadrant of unspecified
                    male breast

✓5ᵗʰ   **C50.3**   **Malignant neoplasm of lower-inner quadrant of breast**

     ✓6ᵗʰ   **C50.31**   **Malignant neoplasm of lower-inner quadrant of breast, female**

         C50.311   Malignant neoplasm of lower-inner   HCC ♀
                    quadrant of right female breast

         C50.312   Malignant neoplasm of lower-inner   HCC ♀
                    quadrant of left female breast

         C50.319   Malignant neoplasm of   HCC ♀ ▽
                    lower-inner quadrant of unspecified
                    female breast

     ✓6ᵗʰ   **C50.32**   **Malignant neoplasm of lower-inner quadrant of breast, male**

         C50.321   Malignant neoplasm of lower-inner   HCC ♂
                    quadrant of right male breast

Female Breast

C50.322   Malignant neoplasm of lower-inner   HCC ♂
            quadrant of left male breast

C50.329   Malignant neoplasm of lower-   HCC ♂ ▽
            inner quadrant of unspecified male breast

✓5ᵗʰ   **C50.4**   **Malignant neoplasm of upper-outer quadrant of breast**

     ✓6ᵗʰ   **C50.41**   **Malignant neoplasm of upper-outer quadrant of breast, female**

         C50.411   Malignant neoplasm of upper-outer   HCC ♀
                    quadrant of right female breast

         C50.412   Malignant neoplasm of upper-outer   HCC ♀
                    quadrant of left female breast

         C50.419   Malignant neoplasm of   HCC ♀ ▽
                    upper-outer quadrant of unspecified
                    female breast

     ✓6ᵗʰ   **C50.42**   **Malignant neoplasm of upper-outer quadrant of breast, male**

         C50.421   Malignant neoplasm of upper-outer   HCC ♂
                    quadrant of right male breast

         C50.422   Malignant neoplasm of upper-outer   HCC ♂
                    quadrant of left male breast

         C50.429   Malignant neoplasm of   HCC ♂ ▽
                    upper-outer quadrant of unspecified
                    male breast

✓5ᵗʰ   **C50.5**   **Malignant neoplasm of lower-outer quadrant of breast**

     ✓6ᵗʰ   **C50.51**   **Malignant neoplasm of lower-outer quadrant of breast, female**

         C50.511   Malignant neoplasm of lower-outer   HCC ♀
                    quadrant of right female breast

         C50.512   Malignant neoplasm of lower-outer   HCC ♀
                    quadrant of left female breast

         C50.519   Malignant neoplasm of   HCC ♀ ▽
                    lower-outer quadrant of unspecified
                    female breast

     ✓6ᵗʰ   **C50.52**   **Malignant neoplasm of lower-outer quadrant of breast, male**

         C50.521   Malignant neoplasm of lower-outer   HCC ♂
                    quadrant of right male breast

         C50.522   Malignant neoplasm of lower-outer   HCC ♂
                    quadrant of left male breast

         C50.529   Malignant neoplasm of   HCC ♂ ▽
                    lower-outer quadrant of unspecified
                    male breast

✓5ᵗʰ   **C50.6**   **Malignant neoplasm of axillary tail of breast**

     ✓6ᵗʰ   **C50.61**   **Malignant neoplasm of axillary tail of breast, female**

         C50.611   Malignant neoplasm of axillary tail   HCC ♀
                    of right female breast

         C50.612   Malignant neoplasm of axillary tail   HCC ♀
                    of left female breast

         C50.619   Malignant neoplasm of axillary   HCC ♀ ▽
                    tail of unspecified female breast

     ✓6ᵗʰ   **C50.62**   **Malignant neoplasm of axillary tail of breast, male**

         C50.621   Malignant neoplasm of axillary tail   HCC ♂
                    of right male breast

☑ Additional Character Req   ✓x7ᵗʰ Placeholder Alert   Manifestation   HCC CMS-HCC Condition   ▽ Unspecified Code   ►◄ Revised Text   ● New Code   ▲ Revised Code Title

ICD-10-CM 2018   469

Chapter 2. Neoplasms

C50.622–C61

C50.622 Malignant neoplasm of axillary tail of left male breast   HCC ♂

C50.629 Malignant neoplasm of axillary tail of unspecified male breast   HCC ♂

✓5th **C50.8** **Malignant neoplasm of overlapping sites of breast**

  ✓6th **C50.81** Malignant neoplasm of overlapping sites of breast, female

C50.811 Malignant neoplasm of overlapping sites of right female breast   HCC ♀

C50.812 Malignant neoplasm of overlapping sites of left female breast   HCC ♀

C50.819 Malignant neoplasm of overlapping sites of unspecified female breast   HCC ♀ ▽

  ✓6th **C50.82** Malignant neoplasm of overlapping sites of breast, male

C50.821 Malignant neoplasm of overlapping sites of right male breast   HCC ♂

C50.822 Malignant neoplasm of overlapping sites of left male breast   HCC ♂

C50.829 Malignant neoplasm of overlapping sites of unspecified male breast   HCC ♂ ▽

✓5th **C50.9** **Malignant neoplasm of breast of unspecified site**

  ✓6th **C50.91** Malignant neoplasm of breast of unspecified site, female

C50.911 Malignant neoplasm of unspecified site of right female breast   HCC ♀

C50.912 Malignant neoplasm of unspecified site of left female breast   HCC ♀

C50.919 Malignant neoplasm of unspecified site of unspecified female breast   HCC ♀ ▽

  ✓6th **C50.92** Malignant neoplasm of breast of unspecified site, male

C50.921 Malignant neoplasm of unspecified site of right male breast   HCC ♂

C50.922 Malignant neoplasm of unspecified site of left male breast   HCC ♂

C50.929 Malignant neoplasm of unspecified site of unspecified male breast   HCC ♂ ▽

Malignant neoplasms of female genital organs (C51-C58)

INCLUDES   malignant neoplasm of skin of female genital organs

✓4th **C51** **Malignant neoplasm of vulva**

EXCLUDES 1   carcinoma in situ of vulva (D07.1)

C51.0 **Malignant neoplasm of labium majus**   HCC ♀
Malignant neoplasm of Bartholin's [greater vestibular] gland

C51.1 **Malignant neoplasm of labium minus**   HCC ♀

C51.2 **Malignant neoplasm of clitoris**   HCC ♀

C51.8 **Malignant neoplasm of overlapping sites of vulva**   HCC ♀

C51.9 **Malignant neoplasm of vulva, unspecified**   HCC ♀ ▽
Malignant neoplasm of external female genitalia NOS
Malignant neoplasm of pudendum

C52 **Malignant neoplasm of vagina**   HCC ♀
EXCLUDES 1   carcinoma in situ of vagina (D07.2)

✓4th **C53** **Malignant neoplasm of cervix uteri**
EXCLUDES 1   carcinoma in situ of cervix uteri (D06.-)

C53.0 **Malignant neoplasm of endocervix**   HCC ♀

C53.1 **Malignant neoplasm of exocervix**   HCC ♀

C53.8 **Malignant neoplasm of overlapping sites of cervix uteri**   HCC ♀

C53.9 **Malignant neoplasm of cervix uteri, unspecified**   HCC ♀ ▽

✓4th **C54** **Malignant neoplasm of corpus uteri**

C54.0 **Malignant neoplasm of isthmus uteri**   HCC ♀
Malignant neoplasm of lower uterine segment

C54.1 **Malignant neoplasm of endometrium**   HCC ♀

C54.2 **Malignant neoplasm of myometrium**   HCC ♀

C54.3 **Malignant neoplasm of fundus uteri**   HCC ♀

C54.8 **Malignant neoplasm of overlapping sites of corpus uteri**   HCC ♀

C54.9 **Malignant neoplasm of corpus uteri, unspecified**   HCC ♀ ▽

C55 **Malignant neoplasm of uterus, part unspecified**   HCC ♀ ▽

✓4th **C56** **Malignant neoplasm of ovary**
Use additional code to identify any functional activity

C56.1 **Malignant neoplasm of right ovary**   HCC ♀

C56.2 **Malignant neoplasm of left ovary**   HCC ♀

C56.9 **Malignant neoplasm of unspecified ovary**   HCC ♀ ▽

✓4th **C57** **Malignant neoplasm of other and unspecified female genital organs**

  ✓5th **C57.0** **Malignant neoplasm of fallopian tube**
Malignant neoplasm of oviduct
Malignant neoplasm of uterine tube

C57.00 Malignant neoplasm of unspecified fallopiantube   HCC ♀ ▽

C57.01 Malignant neoplasm of right fallopian tube   HCC ♀

C57.02 Malignant neoplasm of left fallopian tube   HCC ♀

  ✓5th **C57.1** **Malignant neoplasm of broad ligament**

C57.10 Malignant neoplasm of unspecified broad ligament   HCC ♀ ▽

C57.11 Malignant neoplasm of right broad ligament   HCC ♀

C57.12 Malignant neoplasm of left broad ligament   HCC ♀

  ✓5th **C57.2** **Malignant neoplasm of round ligament**

C57.20 Malignant neoplasm of unspecified round ligament   HCC ♀ ▽

C57.21 Malignant neoplasm of right round ligament   HCC ♀

C57.22 Malignant neoplasm of left round ligament   HCC ♀

C57.3 **Malignant neoplasm of parametrium**   HCC ♀
Malignant neoplasm of uterine ligament NOS

C57.4 **Malignant neoplasm of uterine adnexa, unspecified**   HCC ♀

C57.7 **Malignant neoplasm of other specified female genital organs**   HCC ♀
Malignant neoplasm of wolffian body or duct

C57.8 **Malignant neoplasm of overlapping sites of female genital organs**   HCC ♀
Primary malignant neoplasm of two or more contiguous sites of the female genital organs whose point of origin cannot be determined
Primary tubo-ovarian malignant neoplasm whose point of origin cannot be determined
Primary utero-ovarian malignant neoplasm whose point of origin cannot be determined

C57.9 **Malignant neoplasm of female genital organ, unspecified**   HCC ♀ ▽
Malignant neoplasm of female genitourinary tract NOS

C58 **Malignant neoplasm of placenta**   HCC M ♀
INCLUDES   choriocarcinoma NOS
      chorionepithelioma NOS
EXCLUDES 1   chorioadenoma (destruens) (D39.2)
      hydatidiform mole NOS (O01.9)
      invasive hydatidiform mole (D39.2)
      male choriocarcinoma NOS (C62.9-)
      malignant hydatidiform mole (D39.2)

Malignant neoplasms of male genital organs (C60-C63)

INCLUDES   malignant neoplasm of skin of male genital organs

✓4th **C60** **Malignant neoplasm of penis**

C60.0 **Malignant neoplasm of prepuce**   HCC ♂
Malignant neoplasm of foreskin

C60.1 **Malignant neoplasm of glans penis**   HCC ♂

C60.2 **Malignant neoplasm of body of penis**   HCC ♂
Malignant neoplasm of corpus cavernosum

C60.8 **Malignant neoplasm of overlapping sites of penis**   HCC ♂

C60.9 **Malignant neoplasm of penis, unspecified**   HCC ♂ ▽
Malignant neoplasm of skin of penis NOS

C61 **Malignant neoplasm of prostate**   HCC ♂
Use additional code to identify:
   hormone sensitivity status (Z19.1-Z19.2)
   rising PSA following treatment for malignant neoplasm of prostate (R97.21)
EXCLUDES 1   malignant neoplasm of seminal vesicle (C63.7)
AHA: 2017, 1Q, 17

☑4ᵗʰ C62 Malignant neoplasm of testis
Use additional code to identify any functional activity

☑5ᵗʰ C62.0 Malignant neoplasm of undescended testis
Malignant neoplasm of ectopic testis
Malignant neoplasm of retained testis

C62.00 **Malignant neoplasm of unspecified undescended testis**   HCC ♂ ▽

C62.01 **Malignant neoplasm of undescended right testis**   HCC ♂

C62.02 **Malignant neoplasm of undescended left testis**   HCC ♂

☑5ᵗʰ C62.1 Malignant neoplasm of descended testis
Malignant neoplasm of scrotal testis

C62.10 **Malignant neoplasm of unspecified descended testis**   HCC ♂ ▽

C62.11 **Malignant neoplasm of descended right testis**   HCC ♂

C62.12 **Malignant neoplasm of descended left testis**   HCC ♂

☑5ᵗʰ C62.9 Malignant neoplasm of testis, unspecified whether descended or undescended

C62.90 **Malignant neoplasm of unspecified testis, unspecified whether descended or undescended**   HCC ♂ ▽
Malignant neoplasm of testis NOS

C62.91 **Malignant neoplasm of right testis, unspecified whether descended or undescended**   HCC ♂ ▽

C62.92 **Malignant neoplasm of left testis, unspecified whether descended or undescended**   HCC ♂ ▽

☑4ᵗʰ C63 Malignant neoplasm of other and unspecified male genital organs

☑5ᵗʰ C63.0 Malignant neoplasm of epididymis

C63.00 **Malignant neoplasm of unspecified epididymis**   HCC ♂ ▽

C63.01 **Malignant neoplasm of right epididymis**   HCC ♂

C63.02 **Malignant neoplasm of left epididymis**   HCC ♂

☑5ᵗʰ C63.1 Malignant neoplasm of spermatic cord

C63.10 **Malignant neoplasm of unspecified spermatic cord**   HCC ♂ ▽

C63.11 **Malignant neoplasm of right spermatic cord**   HCC ♂

C63.12 **Malignant neoplasm of left spermatic cord**   HCC ♂

C63.2 **Malignant neoplasm of scrotum**   HCC ♂
Malignant neoplasm of skin of scrotum

C63.7 **Malignant neoplasm of other specified male genital organs**   HCC ♂
Malignant neoplasm of seminal vesicle
Malignant neoplasm of tunica vaginalis

C63.8 **Malignant neoplasm of overlapping sites of male genital organs**   HCC ♂
Primary malignant neoplasm of two or more contiguous sites of male genital organs whose point of origin cannot be determined

C63.9 **Malignant neoplasm of male genital organ, unspecified**   HCC ♂ ▽
Malignant neoplasm of male genitourinary tract NOS

Malignant neoplasms of urinary tract (C64-C68)

☑4ᵗʰ C64 Malignant neoplasm of kidney, except renal pelvis
EXCLUDES 1   *malignant carcinoid tumor of the kidney (C7A.093)*
malignant neoplasm of renal calyces (C65.-)
malignant neoplasm of renal pelvis (C65.-)

C64.1 **Malignant neoplasm of right kidney, except renal pelvis**   HCC

C64.2 **Malignant neoplasm of left kidney, except renal pelvis**   HCC

C64.9 **Malignant neoplasm of unspecified kidney, except renal pelvis**   HCC ▽

☑4ᵗʰ C65 Malignant neoplasm of renal pelvis
INCLUDES   malignant neoplasm of pelviureteric junction
malignant neoplasm of renal calyces

C65.1 **Malignant neoplasm of right renal pelvis**   HCC

C65.2 **Malignant neoplasm of left renal pelvis**   HCC

C65.9 **Malignant neoplasm of unspecified renal pelvis**   HCC ▽

☑4ᵗʰ C66 Malignant neoplasm of ureter
EXCLUDES 1   *malignant neoplasm of ureteric orifice of bladder (C67.6)*

C66.1 **Malignant neoplasm of right ureter**   HCC

C66.2 **Malignant neoplasm of left ureter**   HCC

C66.9 **Malignant neoplasm of unspecified ureter**   HCC ▽

☑4ᵗʰ C67 Malignant neoplasm of bladder

C67.0 **Malignant neoplasm of trigone of bladder**   HCC

C67.1 **Malignant neoplasm of dome of bladder**   HCC

C67.2 **Malignant neoplasm of lateral wall of bladder**   HCC

C67.3 **Malignant neoplasm of anterior wall of bladder**   HCC

C67.4 **Malignant neoplasm of posterior wall of bladder**   HCC

C67.5 **Malignant neoplasm of bladder neck**   HCC
Malignant neoplasm of internal urethral orifice

C67.6 **Malignant neoplasm of ureteric orifice**   HCC

C67.7 **Malignant neoplasm of urachus**   HCC

C67.8 **Malignant neoplasm of overlapping sites of bladder**   HCC

C67.9 **Malignant neoplasm of bladder, unspecified**   HCC ▽
AHA: 2016, 1Q, 19

☑4ᵗʰ C68 Malignant neoplasm of other and unspecified urinary organs
EXCLUDES 1   *malignant neoplasm of female genitourinary tract NOS (C57.9)*
malignant neoplasm of male genitourinary tract NOS (C63.9)

C68.0 **Malignant neoplasm of urethra**   HCC
EXCLUDES 1   *malignant neoplasm of urethral orifice of bladder (C67.5)*

C68.1 **Malignant neoplasm of paraurethral glands**   HCC

C68.8 **Malignant neoplasm of overlapping sites of urinary organs**   HCC
Primary malignant neoplasm of two or more contiguous sites of urinary organs whose point of origin cannot be determined

C68.9 **Malignant neoplasm of urinary organ, unspecified**   HCC ▽
Malignant neoplasm of urinary system NOS

Malignant neoplasms of eye, brain and other parts of central nervous system (C69-C72)

☑4ᵗʰ C69 Malignant neoplasm of eye and adnexa
EXCLUDES 1   *malignant neoplasm of connective tissue of eyelid (C49.0)*
malignant neoplasm of eyelid (skin) (C43.1-, C44.1-)
malignant neoplasm of optic nerve (C72.3-)

☑5ᵗʰ C69.0 Malignant neoplasm of conjunctiva

C69.00 **Malignant neoplasm of unspecified conjunctiva**   HCC ▽

C69.01 **Malignant neoplasm of right conjunctiva**   HCC

C69.02 **Malignant neoplasm of left conjunctiva**   HCC

☑5ᵗʰ C69.1 Malignant neoplasm of cornea

C69.10 **Malignant neoplasm of unspecified cornea**   HCC ▽

C69.11 **Malignant neoplasm of right cornea**   HCC

C69.12 **Malignant neoplasm of left cornea**   HCC

☑5ᵗʰ C69.2 Malignant neoplasm of retina
EXCLUDES 1   *dark area on retina (D49.81)*
neoplasm of unspecified behavior of retina and choroid (D49.81)
retinal freckle (D49.81)

C69.20 **Malignant neoplasm of unspecified retina**   HCC ▽

C69.21 **Malignant neoplasm of right retina**   HCC

C69.22 **Malignant neoplasm of left retina**   HCC

☑5ᵗʰ C69.3 Malignant neoplasm of choroid

C69.30 **Malignant neoplasm of unspecified choroid**   HCC ▽

C69.31 **Malignant neoplasm of right choroid**   HCC

C69.32 **Malignant neoplasm of left choroid**   HCC

☑5ᵗʰ C69.4 Malignant neoplasm of ciliary body

C69.40 **Malignant neoplasm of unspecified ciliary body**   HCC ▽

C69.41 **Malignant neoplasm of right ciliary body**   HCC

C69.42 **Malignant neoplasm of left ciliary body**   HCC

☑5ᵗʰ C69.5 Malignant neoplasm of lacrimal gland and duct
Malignant neoplasm of lacrimal sac
Malignant neoplasm of nasolacrimal duct

C69.50 **Malignant neoplasm of unspecified lacrimal gland and duct**   HCC ▽

C69.51 **Malignant neoplasm of right lacrimal gland and duct**   HCC

C69.52 **Malignant neoplasm of left lacrimal gland and duct**   HCC

☑ Additional Character Req   ✓x7ᵗʰ Placeholder Alert   Manifestation   HCC CMS-HCC Condition   ▽ Unspecified Code   ▶◀ Revised Text   ● New Code   ▲ Revised Code Title

√5th **C69.6** **Malignant neoplasm of orbit**
     Malignant neoplasm of connective tissue of orbit
     Malignant neoplasm of extraocular muscle
     Malignant neoplasm of peripheral nerves of orbit
     Malignant neoplasm of retrobulbar tissue
     Malignant neoplasm of retro-ocular tissue
     EXCLUDES 1   malignant neoplasm of orbital bone (C41.0)

     C69.60 **Malignant neoplasm of unspecified orbit**   HCC ▽
     C69.61 **Malignant neoplasm of right orbit**   HCC
     C69.62 **Malignant neoplasm of left orbit**   HCC

√5th **C69.8** **Malignant neoplasm of overlapping sites of eye and adnexa**
     C69.80 **Malignant neoplasm of overlapping sites of**   HCC ▽
     unspecified eye and adnexa
     C69.81 **Malignant neoplasm of overlapping sites of**   HCC
     right eye and adnexa
     C69.82 **Malignant neoplasm of overlapping sites of**   HCC
     left eye and adnexa

√5th **C69.9** **Malignant neoplasm of unspecified site of eye**
     Malignant neoplasm of eyeball
     C69.90 **Malignant neoplasm of unspecified site of**   HCC ▽
     unspecified eye
     C69.91 **Malignant neoplasm of unspecified site of**   HCC ▽
     right eye
     C69.92 **Malignant neoplasm of unspecified site of**   HCC ▽
     left eye

√4th **C70** **Malignant neoplasm of meninges**
     C70.0 **Malignant neoplasm of cerebral meninges**   HCC
     C70.1 **Malignant neoplasm of spinal meninges**   HCC
     C70.9 **Malignant neoplasm of meninges, unspecified**   HCC ▽

√4th **C71** **Malignant neoplasm of brain**
     EXCLUDES 1   malignant neoplasm of cranial nerves (C72.2-C72.5)
              retrobulbar malignant neoplasm (C69.6-)

     C71.0 **Malignant neoplasm of cerebrum, except lobes and**   HCC
     ventricles
     Malignant neoplasm of supratentorial NOS
     C71.1 **Malignant neoplasm of frontal lobe**   HCC
     C71.2 **Malignant neoplasm of temporal lobe**   HCC
     C71.3 **Malignant neoplasm of parietal lobe**   HCC
     C71.4 **Malignant neoplasm of occipital lobe**   HCC
     C71.5 **Malignant neoplasm of cerebral ventricle**   HCC
         EXCLUDES 1   malignant neoplasm of fourth cerebral ventricle
                 (C71.7)
     C71.6 **Malignant neoplasm of cerebellum**   HCC
     C71.7 **Malignant neoplasm of brain stem**   HCC
     Malignant neoplasm of fourth cerebral ventricle
     Infratentorial malignant neoplasm NOS
     C71.8 **Malignant neoplasm of overlapping sites of brain**   HCC
     C71.9 **Malignant neoplasm of brain, unspecified**   HCC ▽
     AHA: 2014, 3Q, 3

√4th **C72** **Malignant neoplasm of spinal cord, cranial nerves and other parts of central nervous system**
     EXCLUDES 1   malignant neoplasm of meninges (C70.-)
              malignant neoplasm of peripheral nerves and autonomic
                 nervous system (C47.-)

     C72.0 **Malignant neoplasm of spinal cord**   HCC
     C72.1 **Malignant neoplasm of cauda equina**   HCC
√5th   **C72.2** **Malignant neoplasm of olfactory nerve**
     Malignant neoplasm of olfactory bulb
     C72.20 **Malignant neoplasm of unspecified olfactory**   HCC ▽
     nerve
     C72.21 **Malignant neoplasm of right olfactory nerve**   HCC
     C72.22 **Malignant neoplasm of left olfactory nerve**   HCC
√5th   **C72.3** **Malignant neoplasm of optic nerve**
     C72.30 **Malignant neoplasm of unspecified optic**   HCC ▽
     nerve
     C72.31 **Malignant neoplasm of right optic nerve**   HCC
     C72.32 **Malignant neoplasm of left optic nerve**   HCC
√5th   **C72.4** **Malignant neoplasm of acoustic nerve**
     C72.40 **Malignant neoplasm of unspecified acoustic**   HCC ▽
     nerve
     C72.41 **Malignant neoplasm of right acoustic nerve**   HCC
     C72.42 **Malignant neoplasm of left acoustic nerve**   HCC

Lobes of the Brain

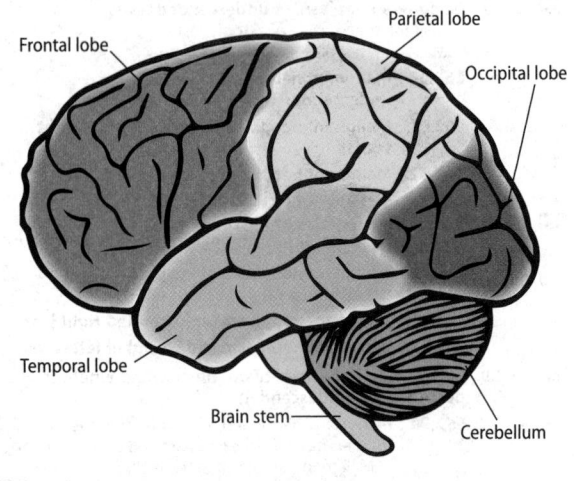

Frontal lobe   Parietal lobe   Occipital lobe   Temporal lobe   Brain stem   Cerebellum

√5th **C72.5** **Malignant neoplasm of other and unspecified cranial nerves**
     C72.50 **Malignant neoplasm of unspecified cranial**   HCC ▽
     nerve
     Malignant neoplasm of cranial nerve NOS
     C72.59 **Malignant neoplasm of other cranial nerves**   HCC
     C72.9 **Malignant neoplasm of central nervous system,**   HCC ▽
     unspecified
     Malignant neoplasm of unspecified site of central nervous
     system
     Malignant neoplasm of nervous system NOS

Malignant neoplasms of thyroid and other endocrine glands (C73-C75)

C73 **Malignant neoplasm of thyroid gland**   HCC
     Use additional code to identify any functional activity

√4th **C74** **Malignant neoplasm of adrenal gland**
√5th   **C74.0** **Malignant neoplasm of cortex of adrenal gland**
     C74.00 **Malignant neoplasm of cortex of unspecified**   HCC ▽
     adrenal gland
     C74.01 **Malignant neoplasm of cortex of right adrenal**   HCC
     gland
     C74.02 **Malignant neoplasm of cortex of left adrenal**   HCC
     gland
√5th   **C74.1** **Malignant neoplasm of medulla of adrenal gland**
     C74.10 **Malignant neoplasm of medulla of**   HCC ▽
     unspecified adrenal gland
     C74.11 **Malignant neoplasm of medulla of right**   HCC
     adrenal gland
     C74.12 **Malignant neoplasm of medulla of left**   HCC
     adrenal gland
√5th   **C74.9** **Malignant neoplasm of unspecified part of adrenal gland**
     C74.90 **Malignant neoplasm of unspecified part of**   HCC ▽
     unspecified adrenal gland
     C74.91 **Malignant neoplasm of unspecified part of**   HCC ▽
     right adrenal gland
     C74.92 **Malignant neoplasm of unspecified part of**   HCC ▽
     left adrenal gland

√4th **C75** **Malignant neoplasm of other endocrine glands and related structures**
     EXCLUDES 1   malignant carcinoid tumors (C7A.0-)
              malignant neoplasm of adrenal gland (C74.-)
              malignant neoplasm of endocrine pancreas (C25.4)
              malignant neoplasm of islets of Langerhans (C25.4)
              malignant neoplasm of ovary (C56.-)
              malignant neoplasm of testis (C62.-)
              malignant neoplasm of thymus (C37)
              malignant neoplasm of thyroid gland (C73)
              malignant neuroendocrine tumors (C7A.-)

     C75.0 **Malignant neoplasm of parathyroid gland**   HCC
     C75.1 **Malignant neoplasm of pituitary gland**   HCC
     C75.2 **Malignant neoplasm of craniopharyngeal duct**   HCC
     C75.3 **Malignant neoplasm of pineal gland**   HCC
     C75.4 **Malignant neoplasm of carotid body**   HCC

C75.5   Malignant neoplasm of aortic body and other paraganglia   `HCC`

C75.8   Malignant neoplasm with pluriglandular involvement, unspecified   `HCC` ▽

C75.9   Malignant neoplasm of endocrine gland, unspecified   `HCC` ▽

Malignant neuroendocrine tumors (C7A)

✅4ᵗʰ **C7A**   Malignant neuroendocrine tumors

Code also any associated multiple endocrine neoplasia [MEN] syndromes (E31.2-)

Use additional code to identify any associated endocrine syndrome, such as:
carcinoid syndrome (E34.0)

EXCLUDES 2   malignant pancreatic islet cell tumors (C25.4)
Merkel cell carcinoma (C4A.-)

✅5ᵗʰ **C7A.0**   Malignant carcinoid tumors

     C7A.00   Malignant carcinoid tumor of unspecified site   `HCC` ▽

     ✅6ᵗʰ **C7A.01**   Malignant carcinoid tumors of the small intestine

         C7A.010   Malignant carcinoid tumor of the duodenum   `HCC`

         C7A.011   Malignant carcinoid tumor of the jejunum   `HCC`

         C7A.012   Malignant carcinoid tumor of the ileum   `HCC`

         C7A.019   Malignant carcinoid tumor of the small intestine, unspecified portion   `HCC` ▽

     ✅6ᵗʰ **C7A.02**   Malignant carcinoid tumors of the appendix, large intestine, and rectum

         C7A.020   Malignant carcinoid tumor of the appendix   `HCC`

         C7A.021   Malignant carcinoid tumor of the cecum   `HCC`

         C7A.022   Malignant carcinoid tumor of the ascending colon   `HCC`

         C7A.023   Malignant carcinoid tumor of the transverse colon   `HCC`

         C7A.024   Malignant carcinoid tumor of the descending colon   `HCC`

         C7A.025   Malignant carcinoid tumor of the sigmoid colon   `HCC`

         C7A.026   Malignant carcinoid tumor of the rectum   `HCC`

         C7A.029   Malignant carcinoid tumor of the large intestine, unspecified portion   `HCC` ▽
Malignant carcinoid tumor of the colon NOS

     ✅6ᵗʰ **C7A.09**   Malignant carcinoid tumors of other sites

         C7A.090   Malignant carcinoid tumor of the bronchus and lung   `HCC`

         C7A.091   Malignant carcinoid tumor of the thymus   `HCC`

         C7A.092   Malignant carcinoid tumor of the stomach   `HCC`

         C7A.093   Malignant carcinoid tumor of the kidney   `HCC`

         C7A.094   Malignant carcinoid tumor of the foregut unspecified   `HCC` ▽

         C7A.095   Malignant carcinoid tumor of the midgut unspecified   `HCC` ▽

         C7A.096   Malignant carcinoid tumor of the hindgut unspecified   `HCC` ▽

         C7A.098   Malignant carcinoid tumors of other sites   `HCC`

C7A.1   Malignant poorly differentiated neuroendocrine tumors   `HCC`
High grade neuroendocrine carcinoma, any site
Malignant poorly differentiated neuroendocrine tumor NOS
Malignant poorly differentiated neuroendocrine carcinoma, any site

C7A.8   Other malignant neuroendocrine tumors   `HCC`

Secondary neuroendocrine tumors (C7B)

✅4ᵗʰ **C7B**   Secondary neuroendocrine tumors

Use additional code to identify any functional activity

✅5ᵗʰ **C7B.0**   Secondary carcinoid tumors

     C7B.00   Secondary carcinoid tumors, unspecified site   `HCC` ▽

     C7B.01   Secondary carcinoid tumors of distant lymph nodes   `HCC`

     C7B.02   Secondary carcinoid tumors of liver   `HCC`

     C7B.03   Secondary carcinoid tumors of bone   `HCC`

     C7B.04   Secondary carcinoid tumors of peritoneum   `HCC`
Mesentery metastasis of carcinoid tumor

     C7B.09   Secondary carcinoid tumors of other sites   `HCC`

C7B.1   Secondary Merkel cell carcinoma   `HCC`
Merkel cell carcinoma nodal presentation
Merkel cell carcinoma visceral metastatic presentation

C7B.8   Other secondary neuroendocrine tumors   `HCC`

Malignant neoplasms of ill-defined, other secondary and unspecified sites (C76-C80)

✅4ᵗʰ **C76**   Malignant neoplasm of other and ill-defined sites

EXCLUDES 1   malignant neoplasm of female genitourinary tract NOS (C57.9)
malignant neoplasm of male genitourinary tract NOS (C63.9)
malignant neoplasm of lymphoid, hematopoietic and related tissue (C81-C96)
malignant neoplasm of skin (C44.-)
malignant neoplasm of unspecified site NOS (C80.1)

C76.0   Malignant neoplasm of head, face and neck   `HCC`
Malignant neoplasm of cheek NOS
Malignant neoplasm of nose NOS

C76.1   Malignant neoplasm of thorax   `HCC`
Intrathoracic malignant neoplasm NOS
Malignant neoplasm of axilla NOS
Thoracic malignant neoplasm NOS

C76.2   Malignant neoplasm of abdomen   `HCC`

C76.3   Malignant neoplasm of pelvis   `HCC`
Malignant neoplasm of groin NOS
Malignant neoplasm of sites overlapping systems within the pelvis
Rectovaginal (septum) malignant neoplasm
Rectovesical (septum) malignant neoplasm

✅5ᵗʰ **C76.4**   Malignant neoplasm of upper limb

     C76.40   Malignant neoplasm of unspecified upper limb   `HCC` ▽

     C76.41   Malignant neoplasm of right upper limb   `HCC`

     C76.42   Malignant neoplasm of left upper limb   `HCC`

✅5ᵗʰ **C76.5**   Malignant neoplasm of lower limb

     C76.50   Malignant neoplasm of unspecified lower limb   `HCC` ▽

     C76.51   Malignant neoplasm of right lower limb   `HCC`

     C76.52   Malignant neoplasm of left lower limb   `HCC`

C76.8   Malignant neoplasm of other specified ill-defined sites   `HCC`
Malignant neoplasm of overlapping ill-defined sites

✅4ᵗʰ **C77**   Secondary and unspecified malignant neoplasm of lymph nodes

EXCLUDES 1   malignant neoplasm of lymph nodes, specified as primary (C81-C86, C88, C96.-)
mesentery metastasis of carcinoid tumor (C7B.04)
secondary carcinoid tumors of distant lymph nodes (C7B.01)

C77.0   Secondary and unspecified malignant neoplasm of lymph nodes of head, face and neck   `HCC`
Secondary and unspecified malignant neoplasm of supraclavicular lymph nodes

C77.1   Secondary and unspecified malignant neoplasm of intrathoracic lymph nodes   `HCC`

C77.2   Secondary and unspecified malignant neoplasm of intra-abdominal lymph nodes   `HCC`

C77.3   Secondary and unspecified malignant neoplasm of axilla and upper limb lymph nodes   `HCC`
Secondary and unspecified malignant neoplasm of pectoral lymph nodes

C77.4   Secondary and unspecified malignant neoplasm of inguinal and lower limb lymph nodes   `HCC`

C77.5   Secondary and unspecified malignant neoplasm of intrapelvic lymph nodes   `HCC`

C77.8   Secondary and unspecified malignant neoplasm of lymph nodes of multiple regions   `HCC`

C77.9   Secondary and unspecified malignant neoplasm of lymph node, unspecified   `HCC` ▽

✅ Additional Character Req   ✅ˣ⁷ᵗʰ Placeholder Alert   Manifestation   `HCC` CMS-HCC Condition   ▽ Unspecified Code   ▶◀ Revised Text   ● New Code   ▲ Revised Code Title

✓4th **C78** **Secondary malignant neoplasm of** respiratory and digestive organs
> EXCLUDES 1   *secondary carcinoid tumors of liver (C7B.02)*
> *secondary carcinoid tumors of peritoneum (C7B.04)*
> EXCLUDES 2   *lymph node metastases (C77.0)*

✓5th **C78.0** **Secondary malignant neoplasm of** lung
- **C78.00** **Secondary malignant neoplasm of** unspecified lung   HCC ▽
- **C78.01** **Secondary malignant neoplasm of** right lung   HCC
- **C78.02** **Secondary malignant neoplasm of** left lung   HCC

C78.1 **Secondary malignant neoplasm of** mediastinum   HCC

C78.2 **Secondary malignant neoplasm of** pleura   HCC

✓5th **C78.3** **Secondary malignant neoplasm of** other and unspecified respiratory organs
- **C78.30** **Secondary malignant neoplasm of** unspecified respiratory organ   HCC ▽
- **C78.39** **Secondary malignant neoplasm of** other respiratory organs   HCC

C78.4 **Secondary malignant neoplasm of** small intestine   HCC

C78.5 **Secondary malignant neoplasm of** large intestine and rectum   HCC

C78.6 **Secondary malignant neoplasm of** retroperitoneum and peritoneum   HCC
> AHA: 2017, 2Q, 12

C78.7 **Secondary malignant neoplasm of** liver and intrahepatic bile duct   HCC

✓5th **C78.8** **Secondary malignant neoplasm of** other and unspecified digestive organs
- **C78.80** **Secondary malignant neoplasm of** unspecified digestive organ   HCC ▽
- **C78.89** **Secondary malignant neoplasm of** other digestive organs   HCC
  > Code also exocrine pancreatic insufficiency (K86.81)

✓4th **C79** **Secondary** malignant neoplasm of other and unspecified sites
> EXCLUDES 1   *secondary carcinoid tumors (C7B.-)*
> *secondary neuroendocrine tumors (C7B.-)*
> EXCLUDES 2   ~~*lymph node metastases (C77.0)*~~

✓5th **C79.0** **Secondary malignant neoplasm of** kidney and renal pelvis
- **C79.00** **Secondary malignant neoplasm of** unspecified kidney and renal pelvis   HCC ▽
- **C79.01** **Secondary malignant neoplasm of** right kidney and renal pelvis   HCC
- **C79.02** **Secondary malignant neoplasm of** left kidney and renal pelvis   HCC

✓5th **C79.1** **Secondary malignant neoplasm of** bladder and other and unspecified urinary organs
- **C79.10** **Secondary malignant neoplasm of** unspecified urinary organs   HCC ▽
- **C79.11** **Secondary malignant neoplasm of** bladder   HCC
  > EXCLUDES 2   ►*lymph node metastases (C77.0)*◄
- **C79.19** **Secondary malignant neoplasm of** other urinary organs   HCC

C79.2 **Secondary malignant neoplasm of** skin   HCC
> EXCLUDES 1   *secondary Merkel cell carcinoma (C7B.1)*

✓5th **C79.3** **Secondary malignant neoplasm of** brain and cerebral meninges
- **C79.31** **Secondary malignant neoplasm of** brain   HCC
- **C79.32** **Secondary malignant neoplasm of** cerebral meninges   HCC

✓5th **C79.4** **Secondary malignant neoplasm of** other and unspecified parts of nervous system
- **C79.40** **Secondary malignant neoplasm of** unspecified part of nervous system   HCC ▽
- **C79.49** **Secondary malignant neoplasm of** other parts of nervous system   HCC

✓5th **C79.5** **Secondary malignant neoplasm of** bone and bone marrow
> EXCLUDES 1   *secondary carcinoid tumors of bone (C7B.03)*
- **C79.51** **Secondary malignant neoplasm of** bone   HCC
- **C79.52** **Secondary malignant neoplasm of** bone marrow   HCC

✓5th **C79.6** **Secondary malignant neoplasm of** ovary
- **C79.60** **Secondary malignant neoplasm of** unspecified ovary   HCC ♀▽
- **C79.61** **Secondary malignant neoplasm of** right ovary   HCC ♀
- **C79.62** **Secondary malignant neoplasm of** left ovary   HCC ♀

✓5th **C79.7** **Secondary malignant neoplasm of** adrenal gland
- **C79.70** **Secondary malignant neoplasm of** unspecified adrenal gland   HCC ▽
- **C79.71** **Secondary malignant neoplasm of** right adrenal gland   HCC
- **C79.72** **Secondary malignant neoplasm of** left adrenal gland   HCC

✓5th **C79.8** **Secondary malignant neoplasm of** other specified sites
- **C79.81** **Secondary malignant neoplasm of** breast   HCC
- **C79.82** **Secondary malignant neoplasm of** genital organs   HCC
- **C79.89** **Secondary malignant neoplasm of** other specified sites
  > AHA: 2017, 2Q, 11

C79.9 **Secondary malignant neoplasm of** unspecified site   HCC ▽
> Metastatic cancer NOS
> Metastatic disease NOS
> EXCLUDES 1   *carcinomatosis NOS (C80.0)*
> *generalized cancer NOS (C80.0)*
> *malignant (primary) neoplasm of unspecified site (C80.1)*

✓4th **C80** **Malignant neoplasm** without specification of site
> EXCLUDES 1   *malignant carcinoid tumor of unspecified site (C7A.00)*
> *malignant neoplasm of specified multiple sites—code to each site*

C80.0 **Disseminated malignant neoplasm, unspecified**   HCC ▽
> Carcinomatosis NOS
> Generalized cancer, unspecified site (primary) (secondary)
> Generalized malignancy, unspecified site (primary) (secondary)

C80.1 **Malignant** (primary) **neoplasm, unspecified**   HCC ▽
> Cancer NOS
> Cancer unspecified site (primary)
> Carcinoma unspecified site (primary)
> Malignancy unspecified site (primary)
> EXCLUDES 1   *secondary malignant neoplasm of unspecified site (C79.9)*

C80.2 **Malignant neoplasm associated with** transplanted organ   HCC
> Code first complication of transplanted organ (T86.-)
> Use additional code to identify the specific malignancy

Malignant neoplasms of lymphoid, hematopoietic and related tissue (C81-C96)

> EXCLUDES 2   *Kaposi's sarcoma of lymph nodes (C46.3)*
> *secondary and unspecified neoplasm of lymph nodes (C77.-)*
> *secondary neoplasm of bone marrow (C79.52)*
> *secondary neoplasm of spleen (C78.89)*

✓4th **C81** **Hodgkin lymphoma**
> EXCLUDES 1   *personal history of Hodgkin lymphoma (Z85.71)*

✓5th **C81.0** Nodular lymphocyte predominant **Hodgkin lymphoma**
- **C81.00** **Nodular lymphocyte predominant Hodgkin lymphoma, unspecified site**   HCC ▽
- **C81.01** **Nodular lymphocyte predominant Hodgkin lymphoma, lymph nodes of** head, face, and neck   HCC
- **C81.02** **Nodular lymphocyte predominant Hodgkin lymphoma,** intrathoracic **lymph nodes**   HCC
- **C81.03** **Nodular lymphocyte predominant Hodgkin lymphoma,** intra-abdominal **lymph nodes**   HCC
- **C81.04** **Nodular lymphocyte predominant Hodgkin lymphoma, lymph nodes of** axilla and upper limb   HCC
- **C81.05** **Nodular lymphocyte predominant Hodgkin lymphoma, lymph nodes of** inguinal region and lower limb   HCC
- **C81.06** **Nodular lymphocyte predominant Hodgkin lymphoma,** intrapelvic **lymph nodes**   HCC
- **C81.07** **Nodular lymphocyte predominant Hodgkin lymphoma,** spleen   HCC
- **C81.08** **Nodular lymphocyte predominant Hodgkin lymphoma, lymph nodes of** multiple sites   HCC
- **C81.09** **Nodular lymphocyte predominant Hodgkin lymphoma,** extranodal and solid organ sites   HCC

✓5th **C81.1** Nodular sclerosis **Hodgkin lymphoma**
> Nodular sclerosis classical Hodgkin lymphoma
- **C81.10** **Nodular sclerosis Hodgkin lymphoma, unspecified site**   HCC ▽
- **C81.11** **Nodular sclerosis Hodgkin lymphoma, lymph nodes of** head, face, and neck   HCC

EXCLUDES 1 Not coded here   EXCLUDES 2 Not included here   N Newborn Age: 0   P Pediatric Age: 0-17   M Maternity Age: 12-55   A Adult Age: 15-124

474   ICD-10-CM 2018

C81.12 Nodular sclerosis Hodgkin lymphoma, intrathoracic **lymph nodes** `HCC`

C81.13 Nodular sclerosis Hodgkin lymphoma, intra-abdominal **lymph nodes** `HCC`

C81.14 Nodular sclerosis Hodgkin lymphoma, lymph nodes of axilla and upper limb `HCC`

C81.15 Nodular sclerosis Hodgkin lymphoma, lymph nodes of inguinal region and lower limb `HCC`

C81.16 Nodular sclerosis Hodgkin lymphoma, intrapelvic **lymph nodes** `HCC`

C81.17 Nodular sclerosis Hodgkin lymphoma, spleen `HCC`

C81.18 Nodular sclerosis Hodgkin lymphoma, lymph nodes of multiple sites `HCC`

C81.19 Nodular sclerosis Hodgkin lymphoma, extranodal and solid organ sites `HCC`

✓5ᵗʰ **C81.2** Mixed cellularity **Hodgkin lymphoma**
Mixed cellularity classical Hodgkin lymphoma

C81.20 Mixed cellularity Hodgkin lymphoma, unspecified site `HCC` ▽

C81.21 Mixed cellularity Hodgkin lymphoma, lymph nodes of head, face, and neck `HCC`

C81.22 Mixed cellularity Hodgkin lymphoma, intrathoracic **lymph nodes** `HCC`

C81.23 Mixed cellularity Hodgkin lymphoma, intra-abdominal **lymph nodes** `HCC`

C81.24 Mixed cellularity Hodgkin lymphoma, lymph nodes of axilla and upper limb `HCC`

C81.25 Mixed cellularity Hodgkin lymphoma, lymph nodes of inguinal region and lower limb `HCC`

C81.26 Mixed cellularity Hodgkin lymphoma, intrapelvic **lymph nodes** `HCC`

C81.27 Mixed cellularity Hodgkin lymphoma, spleen `HCC`

C81.28 Mixed cellularity Hodgkin lymphoma, lymph nodes of multiple sites `HCC`

C81.29 Mixed cellularity Hodgkin lymphoma, extranodal and solid organ sites `HCC`

✓5ᵗʰ **C81.3** Lymphocyte depleted **Hodgkin lymphoma**
Lymphocyte depleted classical Hodgkin lymphoma

C81.30 Lymphocyte depleted Hodgkin lymphoma, unspecified site `HCC` ▽

C81.31 Lymphocyte depleted Hodgkin lymphoma, lymph nodes of head, face, and neck `HCC`

C81.32 Lymphocyte depleted Hodgkin lymphoma, intrathoracic **lymph nodes** `HCC`

C81.33 Lymphocyte depleted Hodgkin lymphoma, intra-abdominal **lymph nodes** `HCC`

C81.34 Lymphocyte depleted Hodgkin lymphoma, lymph nodes of axilla and upper limb `HCC`

C81.35 Lymphocyte depleted Hodgkin lymphoma, lymph nodes of inguinal region and lower limb `HCC`

C81.36 Lymphocyte depleted Hodgkin lymphoma, intrapelvic **lymph nodes** `HCC`

C81.37 Lymphocyte depleted Hodgkin lymphoma, spleen `HCC`

C81.38 Lymphocyte depleted Hodgkin lymphoma, lymph nodes of multiple sites `HCC`

C81.39 Lymphocyte depleted Hodgkin lymphoma, extranodal and solid organ sites `HCC`

✓5ᵗʰ **C81.4** Lymphocyte-rich **Hodgkin lymphoma**
Lymphocyte-rich classical Hodgkin lymphoma
EXCLUDES 1 nodular lymphocyte predominant Hodgkin lymphoma (C81.0-)

C81.40 Lymphocyte-rich Hodgkin lymphoma, unspecified site `HCC` ▽

C81.41 Lymphocyte-rich Hodgkin lymphoma, lymph nodes of head, face, and neck `HCC`

C81.42 Lymphocyte-rich Hodgkin lymphoma, intrathoracic **lymph nodes** `HCC`

C81.43 Lymphocyte-rich Hodgkin lymphoma, intra-abdominal **lymph nodes** `HCC`

C81.44 Lymphocyte-rich Hodgkin lymphoma, lymph nodes of axilla and upper limb `HCC`

C81.45 Lymphocyte-rich Hodgkin lymphoma, lymph nodes of inguinal region and lower limb `HCC`

C81.46 Lymphocyte-rich Hodgkin lymphoma, intrapelvic **lymph nodes** `HCC`

C81.47 Lymphocyte-rich Hodgkin lymphoma, spleen `HCC`

C81.48 Lymphocyte-rich Hodgkin lymphoma, lymph nodes of multiple sites `HCC`

C81.49 Lymphocyte-rich Hodgkin lymphoma, extranodal and solid organ sites `HCC`

✓5ᵗʰ **C81.7** Other Hodgkin lymphoma
Classical Hodgkin lymphoma NOS
Other classical Hodgkin lymphoma

C81.70 Other Hodgkin lymphoma, unspecified site `HCC` ▽

C81.71 Other Hodgkin lymphoma, lymph nodes of head, face, and neck `HCC`

C81.72 Other Hodgkin lymphoma, intrathoracic **lymph nodes** `HCC`

C81.73 Other Hodgkin lymphoma, intra-abdominal **lymph nodes** `HCC`

C81.74 Other Hodgkin lymphoma, lymph nodes of axilla and upper limb `HCC`

C81.75 Other Hodgkin lymphoma, lymph nodes of inguinal region and lower limb `HCC`

C81.76 Other Hodgkin lymphoma, intrapelvic **lymph nodes** `HCC`

C81.77 Other Hodgkin lymphoma, spleen `HCC`

C81.78 Other Hodgkin lymphoma, lymph nodes of multiple sites `HCC`

C81.79 Other Hodgkin lymphoma, extranodal and solid organ sites `HCC`

✓5ᵗʰ **C81.9** Hodgkin lymphoma, unspecified

C81.90 Hodgkin lymphoma, unspecified, unspecified site `HCC` ▽

C81.91 Hodgkin lymphoma, unspecified, lymph nodes of head, face, and neck `HCC` ▽

C81.92 Hodgkin lymphoma, unspecified, intrathoracic **lymph nodes** `HCC` ▽

C81.93 Hodgkin lymphoma, unspecified, intra-abdominal **lymph nodes** `HCC` ▽

C81.94 Hodgkin lymphoma, unspecified, lymph nodes of axilla and upper limb `HCC` ▽

C81.95 Hodgkin lymphoma, unspecified, lymph nodes of inguinal region and lower limb `HCC` ▽

C81.96 Hodgkin lymphoma, unspecified, intrapelvic **lymph nodes** `HCC` ▽

C81.97 Hodgkin lymphoma, unspecified, spleen `HCC` ▽

C81.98 Hodgkin lymphoma, unspecified, lymph nodes of multiple sites `HCC` ▽

C81.99 Hodgkin lymphoma, unspecified, extranodal and solid organ sites `HCC` ▽

✓4ᵗʰ **C82** Follicular **lymphoma**
INCLUDES follicular lymphoma with or without diffuse areas
EXCLUDES 1 mature T/NK-cell lymphomas (C84.-)
personal history of non-Hodgkin lymphoma (Z85.72)

✓5ᵗʰ **C82.0** Follicular lymphoma grade I

C82.00 Follicular lymphoma grade I, unspecified site `HCC` ▽

C82.01 Follicular lymphoma grade I, lymph nodes of head, face, and neck `HCC`

C82.02 Follicular lymphoma grade I, intrathoracic **lymph nodes** `HCC`

C82.03 Follicular lymphoma grade I, intra-abdominal **lymph nodes** `HCC`

C82.04 Follicular lymphoma grade I, lymph nodes of axilla and upper limb `HCC`

C82.05 Follicular lymphoma grade I, lymph nodes of inguinal region and lower limb `HCC`

C82.06 Follicular lymphoma grade I, intrapelvic **lymph nodes** `HCC`

C82.07 Follicular lymphoma grade I, spleen `HCC`

C82.08 Follicular lymphoma grade I, lymph nodes of multiple sites `HCC`

C82.09 Follicular lymphoma grade I, extranodal and solid organ sites `HCC`

✓5ᵗʰ **C82.1** Follicular lymphoma grade II

C82.10 Follicular lymphoma grade II, unspecified site `HCC` ▽

C82.11 Follicular lymphoma grade II, lymph nodes of head, face, and neck `HCC`

C82.12 Follicular lymphoma grade II, intrathoracic **lymph nodes** `HCC`

C82.13 Follicular lymphoma grade II, intra-abdominal **lymph nodes** `HCC`

☑ Additional Character Req   ✓ₓ7ᵗʰ Placeholder Alert   Manifestation   `HCC` CMS-HCC Condition   ▽ Unspecified Code   ►◄ Revised Text   ● New Code   ▲ Revised Code Title

Chapter 2. Neoplasms

C82.14 Follicular lymphoma grade II, lymph nodes of axilla and upper limb `HCC`

C82.15 Follicular lymphoma grade II, lymph nodes of inguinal region and lower limb `HCC`

C82.16 Follicular lymphoma grade II, intrapelvic lymph nodes `HCC`

C82.17 Follicular lymphoma grade II, spleen `HCC`

C82.18 Follicular lymphoma grade II, lymph nodes of multiple sites `HCC`

C82.19 Follicular lymphoma grade II, extranodal and solid organ sites `HCC`

✓5ᵗʰ **C82.2** Follicular lymphoma grade III, unspecified

C82.20 Follicular lymphoma grade III, unspecified, unspecified site `HCC` ▽

C82.21 Follicular lymphoma grade III, unspecified, lymph nodes of head, face, and neck `HCC` ▽

C82.22 Follicular lymphoma grade III, unspecified, intrathoracic lymph nodes `HCC` ▽

C82.23 Follicular lymphoma grade III, unspecified, intra-abdominal lymph nodes `HCC` ▽

C82.24 Follicular lymphoma grade III, unspecified, lymph nodes of axilla and upper limb `HCC` ▽

C82.25 Follicular lymphoma grade III, unspecified, lymph nodes of inguinal region and lower limb `HCC` ▽

C82.26 Follicular lymphoma grade III, unspecified, intrapelvic lymph nodes `HCC` ▽

C82.27 Follicular lymphoma grade III, unspecified, spleen `HCC` ▽

C82.28 Follicular lymphoma grade III, unspecified, lymph nodes of multiple sites `HCC` ▽

C82.29 Follicular lymphoma grade III, unspecified, extranodal and solid organ sites `HCC` ▽

✓5ᵗʰ **C82.3** Follicular lymphoma grade IIIa

C82.30 Follicular lymphoma grade IIIa, unspecified site `HCC` ▽

C82.31 Follicular lymphoma grade IIIa, lymph nodes of head, face, and neck `HCC`

C82.32 Follicular lymphoma grade IIIa, intrathoracic lymph nodes `HCC`

C82.33 Follicular lymphoma grade IIIa, intra-abdominal lymph nodes `HCC`

C82.34 Follicular lymphoma grade IIIa, lymph nodes of axilla and upper limb `HCC`

C82.35 Follicular lymphoma grade IIIa, lymph nodes of inguinal region and lower limb `HCC`

C82.36 Follicular lymphoma grade IIIa, intrapelvic lymph nodes `HCC`

C82.37 Follicular lymphoma grade IIIa, spleen `HCC`

C82.38 Follicular lymphoma grade IIIa, lymph nodes of multiple sites `HCC`

C82.39 Follicular lymphoma grade IIIa, extranodal and solid organ sites `HCC`

✓5ᵗʰ **C82.4** Follicular lymphoma grade IIIb

C82.40 Follicular lymphoma grade IIIb, unspecified site `HCC` ▽

C82.41 Follicular lymphoma grade IIIb, lymph nodes of head, face, and neck `HCC`

C82.42 Follicular lymphoma grade IIIb, intrathoracic lymph nodes `HCC`

C82.43 Follicular lymphoma grade IIIb, intra-abdominal lymph nodes `HCC`

C82.44 Follicular lymphoma grade IIIb, lymph nodes of axilla and upper limb `HCC`

C82.45 Follicular lymphoma grade IIIb, lymph nodes of inguinal region and lower limb `HCC`

C82.46 Follicular lymphoma grade IIIb, intrapelvic lymph nodes `HCC`

C82.47 Follicular lymphoma grade IIIb, spleen `HCC`

C82.48 Follicular lymphoma grade IIIb, lymph nodes of multiple sites `HCC`

C82.49 Follicular lymphoma grade IIIb, extranodal and solid organ sites `HCC`

✓5ᵗʰ **C82.5** Diffuse follicle center lymphoma

C82.50 Diffuse follicle center lymphoma, unspecified site `HCC` ▽

C82.51 Diffuse follicle center lymphoma, lymph nodes of head, face, and neck `HCC`

C82.52 Diffuse follicle center lymphoma, intrathoracic lymph nodes `HCC`

C82.53 Diffuse follicle center lymphoma, intra-abdominal lymph nodes `HCC`

C82.54 Diffuse follicle center lymphoma, lymph nodes of axilla and upper limb `HCC`

C82.55 Diffuse follicle center lymphoma, lymph nodes of inguinal region and lower limb `HCC`

C82.56 Diffuse follicle center lymphoma, intrapelvic lymph nodes `HCC`

C82.57 Diffuse follicle center lymphoma, spleen `HCC`

C82.58 Diffuse follicle center lymphoma, lymph nodes of multiple sites `HCC`

C82.59 Diffuse follicle center lymphoma, extranodal and solid organ sites `HCC`

✓5ᵗʰ **C82.6** Cutaneous follicle center lymphoma

C82.60 Cutaneous follicle center lymphoma, unspecified site `HCC` ▽

C82.61 Cutaneous follicle center lymphoma, lymph nodes of head, face, and neck `HCC`

C82.62 Cutaneous follicle center lymphoma, intrathoracic lymph nodes `HCC`

C82.63 Cutaneous follicle center lymphoma, intra-abdominal lymph nodes `HCC`

C82.64 Cutaneous follicle center lymphoma, lymph nodes of axilla and upper limb `HCC`

C82.65 Cutaneous follicle center lymphoma, lymph nodes of inguinal region and lower limb `HCC`

C82.66 Cutaneous follicle center lymphoma, intrapelvic lymph nodes `HCC`

C82.67 Cutaneous follicle center lymphoma, spleen `HCC`

C82.68 Cutaneous follicle center lymphoma, lymph nodes of multiple sites `HCC`

C82.69 Cutaneous follicle center lymphoma, extranodal and solid organ sites `HCC`

✓5ᵗʰ **C82.8** Other types of follicular lymphoma

C82.80 Other types of follicular lymphoma, unspecified site `HCC` ▽

C82.81 Other types of follicular lymphoma, lymph nodes of head, face, and neck `HCC`

C82.82 Other types of follicular lymphoma, intrathoracic lymph nodes `HCC`

C82.83 Other types of follicular lymphoma, intra-abdominal lymph nodes `HCC`

C82.84 Other types of follicular lymphoma, lymph nodes of axilla and upper limb `HCC`

C82.85 Other types of follicular lymphoma, lymph nodes of inguinal region and lower limb `HCC`

C82.86 Other types of follicular lymphoma, intrapelvic lymph nodes `HCC`

C82.87 Other types of follicular lymphoma, spleen `HCC`

C82.88 Other types of follicular lymphoma, lymph nodes of multiple sites `HCC`

C82.89 Other types of follicular lymphoma, extranodal and solid organ sites `HCC`

✓5ᵗʰ **C82.9** Follicular lymphoma, unspecified

C82.90 Follicular lymphoma, unspecified, unspecified site `HCC` ▽

C82.91 Follicular lymphoma, unspecified, lymph nodes of head, face, and neck `HCC` ▽

C82.92 Follicular lymphoma, unspecified, intrathoracic lymph nodes `HCC` ▽

C82.93 Follicular lymphoma, unspecified, intra-abdominal lymph nodes `HCC` ▽

C82.94 Follicular lymphoma, unspecified, lymph nodes of axilla and upper limb `HCC` ▽

C82.95 Follicular lymphoma, unspecified, lymph nodes of inguinal region and lower limb `HCC` ▽

C82.96 Follicular lymphoma, unspecified, intrapelvic lymph nodes `HCC` ▽

C82.97 Follicular lymphoma, unspecified, spleen `HCC` ▽

EXCLUDES 1 Not coded here   *EXCLUDES 2* Not included here   N Newborn Age: 0   P Pediatric Age: 0-17   M Maternity Age: 12-55   A Adult Age: 15-124

476   ICD-10-CM 2018

C82.98   Follicular lymphoma, unspecified, HCC ▽
lymph nodes of multiple sites

C82.99   Follicular lymphoma, unspecified, HCC ▽
extranodal and solid organ sites

✓4ᵗʰ **C83   Non-follicular lymphoma**
EXCLUDES 1 *personal history of non-Hodgkin lymphoma (Z85.72)*

✓5ᵗʰ **C83.0   Small cell B-cell lymphoma**
Lymphoplasmacytic lymphoma
Nodal marginal zone lymphoma
Non-leukemic variant of B-CLL
Splenic marginal zone lymphoma
EXCLUDES 1 *chronic lymphocytic leukemia (C91.1)*
mature T/NK-cell lymphomas (C84.-)
Waldenström macroglobulinemia (C88.0)

C83.00   Small cell B-cell lymphoma, unspecified site   HCC ▽

C83.01   Small cell B-cell lymphoma, lymph nodes of   HCC
head, face, and neck

C83.02   Small cell B-cell lymphoma, intrathoracic   HCC
lymph nodes

C83.03   Small cell B-cell lymphoma, intra-abdominal   HCC
lymph nodes

C83.04   Small cell B-cell lymphoma, lymph nodes of   HCC
axilla and upper limb

C83.05   Small cell B-cell lymphoma, lymph nodes of   HCC
inguinal region and lower limb

C83.06   Small cell B-cell lymphoma, intrapelvic lymph   HCC
nodes

C83.07   Small cell B-cell lymphoma, spleen   HCC

C83.08   Small cell B-cell lymphoma, lymph nodes of   HCC
multiple sites

C83.09   Small cell B-cell lymphoma, extranodal and   HCC
solid organ sites

✓5ᵗʰ **C83.1   Mantle cell lymphoma**
Centrocytic lymphoma
Malignant lymphomatous polyposis
DEF: Rare form of B-cell non-Hodgkin lymphoma named for the
location of tumor cell production, the mantle zone of the lymph
nodes.

C83.10   Mantle cell lymphoma, unspecified site   HCC ▽

C83.11   Mantle cell lymphoma, lymph nodes of head,   HCC
face, and neck

C83.12   Mantle cell lymphoma, intrathoracic lymph   HCC
nodes

C83.13   Mantle cell lymphoma, intra-abdominal lymph   HCC
nodes

C83.14   Mantle cell lymphoma, lymph nodes of axilla   HCC
and upper limb

C83.15   Mantle cell lymphoma, lymph nodes of inguinal   HCC
region and lower limb

C83.16   Mantle cell lymphoma, intrapelvic lymph nodes   HCC

C83.17   Mantle cell lymphoma, spleen   HCC

C83.18   Mantle cell lymphoma, lymph nodes of   HCC
multiple sites

C83.19   Mantle cell lymphoma, extranodal and   HCC
solid organ sites

✓5ᵗʰ **C83.3   Diffuse large B-cell lymphoma**
Anaplastic diffuse large B-cell lymphoma
CD30-positive diffuse large B-cell lymphoma
Centroblastic diffuse large B-cell lymphoma
Diffuse large B-cell lymphoma, subtype not specified
Immunoblastic diffuse large B-cell lymphoma
Plasmablastic diffuse large B-cell lymphoma
T-cell rich diffuse large B-cell lymphoma
EXCLUDES 1 *mature T/NK-cell lymphomas (C84.-)*
mediastinal (thymic) large B-cell lymphoma (C85.2-)

C83.30   Diffuse large B-cell lymphoma,   HCC ▽
unspecified site

C83.31   Diffuse large B-cell lymphoma, lymph nodes   HCC
of head, face, and neck

C83.32   Diffuse large B-cell lymphoma, intrathoracic   HCC
lymph nodes

C83.33   Diffuse large B-cell lymphoma, intra-abdominal   HCC
lymph nodes

C83.34   Diffuse large B-cell lymphoma, lymph nodes of   HCC
axilla and upper limb

C83.35   Diffuse large B-cell lymphoma, lymph nodes of   HCC
inguinal region and lower limb

C83.36   Diffuse large B-cell lymphoma, intrapelvic   HCC
lymph nodes

C83.37   Diffuse large B-cell lymphoma, spleen   HCC

C83.38   Diffuse large B-cell lymphoma, lymph nodes   HCC
of multiple sites

C83.39   Diffuse large B-cell lymphoma, extranodal   HCC
and solid organ sites

✓5ᵗʰ **C83.5   Lymphoblastic (diffuse) lymphoma**
B-precursor lymphoma
Lymphoblastic B-cell lymphoma
Lymphoblastic lymphoma NOS
Lymphoblastic T-cell lymphoma
T-precursor lymphoma

C83.50   Lymphoblastic (diffuse) lymphoma,   HCC ▽
unspecified site

C83.51   Lymphoblastic (diffuse) lymphoma, lymph   HCC
nodes of head, face, and neck

C83.52   Lymphoblastic (diffuse) lymphoma,   HCC
intrathoracic lymph nodes

C83.53   Lymphoblastic (diffuse) lymphoma,   HCC
intra-abdominal lymph nodes

C83.54   Lymphoblastic (diffuse) lymphoma, lymph   HCC
nodes of axilla and upper limb

C83.55   Lymphoblastic (diffuse) lymphoma, lymph   HCC
nodes of inguinal region and lower limb

C83.56   Lymphoblastic (diffuse) lymphoma, intrapelvic   HCC
lymph nodes

C83.57   Lymphoblastic (diffuse) lymphoma, spleen   HCC

C83.58   Lymphoblastic (diffuse) lymphoma, lymph   HCC
nodes of multiple sites

C83.59   Lymphoblastic (diffuse) lymphoma,   HCC
extranodal and solid organ sites

✓5ᵗʰ **C83.7   Burkitt lymphoma**
Atypical Burkitt lymphoma
Burkitt-like lymphoma
EXCLUDES 1 *mature B-cell leukemia Burkitt type (C91.A-)*
DEF: Malignancy of the lymphatic system, most often seen as a
large bone-deteriorating lesion within the jaw or as an abdominal
mass. It is a form of non-Hodgkin's lymphoma and is recognized as
the fastest growing human tumor.

C83.70   Burkitt lymphoma, unspecified site   HCC ▽

C83.71   Burkitt lymphoma, lymph nodes of head, face,   HCC
and neck

C83.72   Burkitt lymphoma, intrathoracic lymph nodes   HCC

C83.73   Burkitt lymphoma, intra-abdominal lymph   HCC
nodes

C83.74   Burkitt lymphoma, lymph nodes of axilla and   HCC
upper limb

C83.75   Burkitt lymphoma, lymph nodes of inguinal   HCC
region and lower limb

C83.76   Burkitt lymphoma, intrapelvic lymph nodes   HCC

C83.77   Burkitt lymphoma, spleen   HCC

C83.78   Burkitt lymphoma, lymph nodes of   HCC
multiple sites

C83.79   Burkitt lymphoma, extranodal and solid   HCC
organ sites

✓5ᵗʰ **C83.8   Other non-follicular lymphoma**
Intravascular large B-cell lymphoma
Lymphoid granulomatosis
Primary effusion B-cell lymphoma
EXCLUDES 1 *mediastinal (thymic) large B-cell lymphoma (C85.2-)*
T-cell rich B-cell lymphoma (C83.3-)

C83.80   Other non-follicular lymphoma,   HCC ▽
unspecified site

C83.81   Other non-follicular lymphoma, lymph   HCC
nodes of head, face, and neck

C83.82   Other non-follicular lymphoma, intrathoracic   HCC
lymph nodes

C83.83   Other non-follicular lymphoma,   HCC
intra-abdominal lymph nodes

C83.84   Other non-follicular lymphoma, lymph nodes   HCC
of axilla and upper limb

C83.85   Other non-follicular lymphoma, lymph nodes   HCC
of inguinal region and lower limb

C83.86 Other non-follicular lymphoma, intrapelvic lymph nodes `HCC`

C83.87 Other non-follicular lymphoma, spleen `HCC`

C83.88 Other non-follicular lymphoma, lymph nodes of multiple sites `HCC`

C83.89 Other non-follicular lymphoma, extranodal and solid organ sites `HCC`

✓5ᵗʰ **C83.9** Non-follicular (diffuse) lymphoma, unspecified

C83.90 Non-follicular (diffuse) lymphoma, unspecified, unspecified site `HCC` ▽

C83.91 Non-follicular (diffuse) lymphoma, unspecified, lymph nodes of head, face, and neck `HCC` ▽

C83.92 Non-follicular (diffuse) lymphoma, unspecified, intrathoracic lymph nodes `HCC` ▽

C83.93 Non-follicular (diffuse) lymphoma, unspecified, intra-abdominal lymph nodes `HCC` ▽

C83.94 Non-follicular (diffuse) lymphoma, unspecified, lymph nodes of axilla and upper limb `HCC` ▽

C83.95 Non-follicular (diffuse) lymphoma, unspecified, lymph nodes of inguinal region and lower limb `HCC` ▽

C83.96 Non-follicular (diffuse) lymphoma, unspecified, intrapelvic lymph nodes `HCC` ▽

C83.97 Non-follicular (diffuse) lymphoma, unspecified, spleen `HCC` ▽

C83.98 Non-follicular (diffuse) lymphoma, unspecified, lymph nodes of multiple sites `HCC` ▽

C83.99 Non-follicular (diffuse) lymphoma, unspecified, extranodal and solid organ sites `HCC` ▽

✓4ᵗʰ **C84** **Mature T/NK-cell lymphomas**

> *EXCLUDES 1* personal history of non-Hodgkin lymphoma (Z85.72)

✓5ᵗʰ **C84.0** **Mycosis fungoides**

> *EXCLUDES 1* peripheral T-cell lymphoma, not classified (C84.4-)
>
> **DEF:** Most common form of cutaneous T-cell lymphoma, also known as Alibert-Bazin syndrome. A type of non-Hodgkin lymphoma in which white blood cells become cancerous and affect the skin and sometimes internal organs.

C84.00 Mycosis fungoides, unspecified site `HCC` ▽

C84.01 Mycosis fungoides, lymph nodes of head, face, and neck `HCC`

C84.02 Mycosis fungoides, intrathoracic lymph nodes `HCC`

C84.03 Mycosis fungoides, intra-abdominal lymph nodes `HCC`

C84.04 Mycosis fungoides, lymph nodes of axilla and upper limb `HCC`

C84.05 Mycosis fungoides, lymph nodes of inguinal region and lower limb `HCC`

C84.06 Mycosis fungoides, intrapelvic lymph nodes `HCC`

C84.07 Mycosis fungoides, spleen `HCC`

C84.08 Mycosis fungoides, lymph nodes of multiple sites `HCC`

C84.09 Mycosis fungoides, extranodal and solid organ sites `HCC`

✓5ᵗʰ **C84.1** **Sézary disease**

C84.10 Sézary disease, unspecified site `HCC` ▽

C84.11 Sézary disease, lymph nodes of head, face, and neck `HCC`

C84.12 Sézary disease, intrathoracic lymph nodes `HCC`

C84.13 Sézary disease, intra-abdominal lymph nodes `HCC`

C84.14 Sézary disease, lymph nodes of axilla and upper limb `HCC`

C84.15 Sézary disease, lymph nodes of inguinal region and lower limb `HCC`

C84.16 Sézary disease, intrapelvic lymph nodes `HCC`

C84.17 Sézary disease, spleen `HCC`

C84.18 Sézary disease, lymph nodes of multiple sites `HCC`

C84.19 Sézary disease, extranodal and solid organ sites `HCC`

✓5ᵗʰ **C84.4** **Peripheral T-cell lymphoma, not classified**

> Lennert's lymphoma
> Lymphoepithelioid lymphoma
> Mature T-cell lymphoma, not elsewhere classified

C84.40 Peripheral T-cell lymphoma, not classified, unspecified site `HCC` ▽

C84.41 Peripheral T-cell lymphoma, not classified, lymph nodes of head, face, and neck `HCC`

C84.42 Peripheral T-cell lymphoma, not classified, intrathoracic lymph nodes `HCC`

C84.43 Peripheral T-cell lymphoma, not classified, intra-abdominal lymph nodes `HCC`

C84.44 Peripheral T-cell lymphoma, not classified, lymph nodes of axilla and upper limb `HCC`

C84.45 Peripheral T-cell lymphoma, not classified, lymph nodes of inguinal region and lower limb `HCC`

C84.46 Peripheral T-cell lymphoma, not classified, intrapelvic lymph nodes `HCC`

C84.47 Peripheral T-cell lymphoma, not classified, spleen `HCC`

C84.48 Peripheral T-cell lymphoma, not classified, lymph nodes of multiple sites `HCC`

C84.49 Peripheral T-cell lymphoma, not classified, extranodal and solid organ sites `HCC`

✓5ᵗʰ **C84.6** **Anaplastic large cell lymphoma, ALK-positive**

> Anaplastic large cell lymphoma, CD3Ø-positive

C84.60 Anaplastic large cell lymphoma, ALK-positive, unspecified site `HCC` ▽

C84.61 Anaplastic large cell lymphoma, ALK-positive, lymph nodes of head, face, and neck `HCC`

C84.62 Anaplastic large cell lymphoma, ALK-positive, intrathoracic lymph nodes `HCC`

C84.63 Anaplastic large cell lymphoma, ALK-positive, intra-abdominal lymph nodes `HCC`

C84.64 Anaplastic large cell lymphoma, ALK-positive, lymph nodes of axilla and upper limb `HCC`

C84.65 Anaplastic large cell lymphoma, ALK-positive, lymph nodes of inguinal region and lower limb `HCC`

C84.66 Anaplastic large cell lymphoma, ALK-positive, intrapelvic lymph nodes `HCC`

C84.67 Anaplastic large cell lymphoma, ALK-positive, spleen `HCC`

C84.68 Anaplastic large cell lymphoma, ALK-positive, lymph nodes of multiple sites `HCC`

C84.69 Anaplastic large cell lymphoma, ALK-positive, extranodal and solid organ sites `HCC`

✓5ᵗʰ **C84.7** **Anaplastic large cell lymphoma, ALK-negative**

> *EXCLUDES 1* primary cutaneous CD3Ø-positive T-cell proliferations (C86.6-)

C84.70 Anaplastic large cell lymphoma, ALK-negative, unspecified site `HCC` ▽

C84.71 Anaplastic large cell lymphoma, ALK-negative, lymph nodes of head, face, and neck `HCC`

C84.72 Anaplastic large cell lymphoma, ALK-negative, intrathoracic lymph nodes `HCC`

C84.73 Anaplastic large cell lymphoma, ALK-negative, intra-abdominal lymph nodes `HCC`

C84.74 Anaplastic large cell lymphoma, ALK-negative, lymph nodes of axilla and upper limb `HCC`

C84.75 Anaplastic large cell lymphoma, ALK-negative, lymph nodes of inguinal region and lower limb `HCC`

C84.76 Anaplastic large cell lymphoma, ALK-negative, intrapelvic lymph nodes `HCC`

C84.77 Anaplastic large cell lymphoma, ALK-negative, spleen `HCC`

C84.78 Anaplastic large cell lymphoma, ALK-negative, lymph nodes of multiple sites `HCC`

C84.79 Anaplastic large cell lymphoma, ALK-negative, extranodal and solid organ sites `HCC`

✓5ᵗʰ **C84.A** **Cutaneous T-cell lymphoma, unspecified**

C84.AØ Cutaneous T-cell lymphoma, unspecified, unspecified site `HCC` ▽

C84.A1 Cutaneous T-cell lymphoma, unspecified, lymph nodes of head, face, and neck `HCC` ▽

C84.A2 Cutaneous T-cell lymphoma, unspecified, intrathoracic lymph nodes `HCC` ▽

C84.A3 Cutaneous T-cell lymphoma, unspecified, intra-abdominal lymph nodes `HCC` ▽

C84.A4 Cutaneous T-cell lymphoma, unspecified, lymph nodes of axilla and upper limb `HCC` ▽

C84.A5 Cutaneous T-cell lymphoma, unspecified, lymph nodes of inguinal region and lower limb `HCC` ▽

C84.A6 Cutaneous T-cell lymphoma, unspecified, intrapelvic lymph nodes `HCC` ▽

EXCLUDES 1 Not coded here   *EXCLUDES 2* Not included here   N Newborn Age: 0   P Pediatric Age: 0-17   M Maternity Age: 12-55   A Adult Age: 15-124

478   ICD-10-CM 2018

C84.A7   Cutaneous T-cell lymphoma, unspecified, spleen   HCC ▽

C84.A8   Cutaneous T-cell lymphoma, unspecified, lymph nodes of multiple sites   HCC ▽

C84.A9   Cutaneous T-cell lymphoma, unspecified, extranodal and solid organ sites   HCC ▽

✓5ᵗʰ **C84.Z**   **Other mature T/NK-cell lymphomas**

> NOTE   If T-cell lineage or involvement is mentioned in conjunction with a specific lymphoma, code to the more specific description.

> EXCLUDES 1   angioimmunoblastic T-cell lymphoma (C86.5)
> blastic NK-cell lymphoma (C86.4)
> enteropathy-type T-cell lymphoma (C86.2)
> extranodal NK-cell lymphoma, nasal type (C86.0)
> hepatosplenic T-cell lymphoma (C86.1)
> primary cutaneous CD30-positive T-cell proliferations (C86.6)
> subcutaneous panniculitis-like T-cell lymphoma (C86.3)
> T-cell leukemia (C91.1-)

C84.Z0   Other mature T/NK-cell lymphomas, unspecified site   HCC ▽

C84.Z1   Other mature T/NK-cell lymphomas, lymph nodes of head, face, and neck   HCC

C84.Z2   Other mature T/NK-cell lymphomas, intrathoracic lymph nodes   HCC

C84.Z3   Other mature T/NK-cell lymphomas, intra-abdominal lymph nodes   HCC

C84.Z4   Other mature T/NK-cell lymphomas, lymph nodes of axilla and upper limb   HCC

C84.Z5   Other mature T/NK-cell lymphomas, lymph nodes of inguinal region and lower limb   HCC

C84.Z6   Other mature T/NK-cell lymphomas, intrapelvic lymph nodes   HCC

C84.Z7   Other mature T/NK-cell lymphomas, spleen   HCC

C84.Z8   Other mature T/NK-cell lymphomas, lymph nodes of multiple sites   HCC

C84.Z9   Other mature T/NK-cell lymphomas, extranodal and solid organ sites   HCC

✓5ᵗʰ **C84.9**   **Mature T/NK-cell lymphomas, unspecified**

NK/T cell lymphoma NOS

> EXCLUDES 1   mature T-cell lymphoma, not elsewhere classified (C84.4-)

C84.90   Mature T/NK-cell lymphomas, unspecified, unspecified site   HCC ▽

C84.91   Mature T/NK-cell lymphomas, unspecified, lymph nodes of head, face, and neck   HCC ▽

C84.92   Mature T/NK-cell lymphomas, unspecified, intrathoracic lymph nodes   HCC ▽

C84.93   Mature T/NK-cell lymphomas, unspecified, intra-abdominal lymph nodes   HCC ▽

C84.94   Mature T/NK-cell lymphomas, unspecified, lymph nodes of axilla and upper limb   HCC ▽

C84.95   Mature T/NK-cell lymphomas, unspecified, lymph nodes of inguinal region and lower limb   HCC ▽

C84.96   Mature T/NK-cell lymphomas, unspecified, intrapelvic lymph nodes   HCC ▽

C84.97   Mature T/NK-cell lymphomas, unspecified, spleen   HCC ▽

C84.98   Mature T/NK-cell lymphomas, unspecified, lymph nodes of multiple sites   HCC ▽

C84.99   Mature T/NK-cell lymphomas, unspecified, extranodal and solid organ sites   HCC ▽

✓4ᵗʰ **C85**   **Other specified and unspecified types of non-Hodgkin lymphoma**

> EXCLUDES 1   other specified types of T/NK-cell lymphoma (C86.-)
> personal history of non-Hodgkin lymphoma (Z85.72)

✓5ᵗʰ **C85.1**   **Unspecified B-cell lymphoma**

> NOTE   If B-cell lineage or involvement is mentioned in conjunction with a specific lymphoma, code to the more specific description.

C85.10   Unspecified B-cell lymphoma, unspecified site   HCC ▽

C85.11   Unspecified B-cell lymphoma, lymph nodes of head, face, and neck   HCC ▽

C85.12   Unspecified B-cell lymphoma, intrathoracic lymph nodes   HCC ▽

C85.13   Unspecified B-cell lymphoma, intra-abdominal lymph nodes   HCC ▽

C85.14   Unspecified B-cell lymphoma, lymph nodes of axilla and upper limb   HCC ▽

C85.15   Unspecified B-cell lymphoma, lymph nodes of inguinal region and lower limb   HCC ▽

C85.16   Unspecified B-cell lymphoma, intrapelvic lymph nodes   HCC ▽

C85.17   Unspecified B-cell lymphoma, spleen   HCC ▽

C85.18   Unspecified B-cell lymphoma, lymph nodes of multiple sites   HCC ▽

C85.19   Unspecified B-cell lymphoma, extranodal and solid organ sites   HCC ▽

✓5ᵗʰ **C85.2**   **Mediastinal (thymic) large B-cell lymphoma**

C85.20   Mediastinal (thymic) large B-cell lymphoma, unspecified site   HCC ▽

C85.21   Mediastinal (thymic) large B-cell lymphoma, lymph nodes of head, face, and neck   HCC

C85.22   Mediastinal (thymic) large B-cell lymphoma, intrathoracic lymph nodes   HCC

C85.23   Mediastinal (thymic) large B-cell lymphoma, intra-abdominal lymph nodes   HCC

C85.24   Mediastinal (thymic) large B-cell lymphoma, lymph nodes of axilla and upper limb   HCC

C85.25   Mediastinal (thymic) large B-cell lymphoma, lymph nodes of inguinal region and lower limb   HCC

C85.26   Mediastinal (thymic) large B-cell lymphoma, intrapelvic lymph nodes   HCC

C85.27   Mediastinal (thymic) large B-cell lymphoma, spleen   HCC

C85.28   Mediastinal (thymic) large B-cell lymphoma, lymph nodes of multiple sites   HCC

C85.29   Mediastinal (thymic) large B-cell lymphoma, extranodal and solid organ sites   HCC

✓5ᵗʰ **C85.8**   **Other specified types of non-Hodgkin lymphoma**

C85.80   Other specified types of non-Hodgkin lymphoma, unspecified site   HCC ▽

C85.81   Other specified types of non-Hodgkin lymphoma, lymph nodes of head, face, and neck   HCC

C85.82   Other specified types of non-Hodgkin lymphoma, intrathoracic lymph nodes   HCC

C85.83   Other specified types of non-Hodgkin lymphoma, intra-abdominal lymph nodes   HCC

C85.84   Other specified types of non-Hodgkin lymphoma, lymph nodes of axilla and upper limb   HCC

C85.85   Other specified types of non-Hodgkin lymphoma, lymph nodes of inguinal region and lower limb   HCC

C85.86   Other specified types of non-Hodgkin lymphoma, intrapelvic lymph nodes   HCC

C85.87   Other specified types of non-Hodgkin lymphoma, spleen   HCC

C85.88   Other specified types of non-Hodgkin lymphoma, lymph nodes of multiple sites   HCC

C85.89   Other specified types of non-Hodgkin lymphoma, extranodal and solid organ sites   HCC

✓5ᵗʰ **C85.9**   **Non-Hodgkin lymphoma, unspecified**

Lymphoma NOS
Malignant lymphoma NOS
Non-Hodgkin lymphoma NOS

C85.90   Non-Hodgkin lymphoma, unspecified, unspecified site   HCC ▽

C85.91   Non-Hodgkin lymphoma, unspecified, lymph nodes of head, face, and neck   HCC ▽

C85.92   Non-Hodgkin lymphoma, unspecified, intrathoracic lymph nodes   HCC ▽

C85.93   Non-Hodgkin lymphoma, unspecified, intra-abdominal lymph nodes   HCC ▽

C85.94   Non-Hodgkin lymphoma, unspecified, lymph nodes of axilla and upper limb   HCC ▽

C85.95   Non-Hodgkin lymphoma, unspecified, lymph nodes of inguinal region and lower limb   HCC ▽

C85.96   Non-Hodgkin lymphoma, unspecified, intrapelvic lymph nodes   HCC ▽

C85.97   Non-Hodgkin lymphoma, unspecified, spleen   HCC ▽

C85.98   Non-Hodgkin lymphoma, unspecified, lymph nodes of multiple sites   HCC ▽

C85.99   Non-Hodgkin lymphoma, unspecified, extranodal and solid organ sites   HCC ▽

☑ Additional Character Req   ✓x7ᵗʰ Placeholder Alert   Manifestation   HCC CMS-HCC Condition   ▽ Unspecified Code   ►◄ Revised Text   ● New Code   ▲ Revised Code Title

Chapter 2. Neoplasms

✓4ᵗʰ **C86 Other specified types of T/NK-cell lymphoma**
> **EXCLUDES 1** anaplastic large cell lymphoma, ALK negative (C84.7-)
> anaplastic large cell lymphoma, ALK positive (C84.6-)
> mature T/NK-cell lymphomas (C84.-)
> other specified types of non-Hodgkin lymphoma (C85.8-)

C86.0 Extranodal NK/T-cell lymphoma, nasal type   HCC

C86.1 Hepatosplenic T-cell lymphoma   HCC
> Alpha-beta and gamma delta types

C86.2 Enteropathy-type (intestinal) T-cell lymphoma   HCC
> Enteropathy associated T-cell lymphoma

C86.3 Subcutaneous panniculitis-like T-cell lymphoma   HCC

C86.4 Blastic NK-cell lymphoma   HCC
> ▶Blastic plasmacytoid dendritic cell neoplasm (BPDCN)◀

C86.5 Angioimmunoblastic T-cell lymphoma   HCC
> Angioimmunoblastic lymphadenopathy with dysproteinemia [AILD]

C86.6 Primary cutaneous CD30-positive T-cell proliferations   HCC
> Lymphomatoid papulosis
> Primary cutaneous anaplastic large cell lymphoma
> Primary cutaneous CD30-positive large T-cell lymphoma

✓4ᵗʰ **C88 Malignant immunoproliferative diseases and certain other B-cell lymphomas**
> **EXCLUDES 1** B-cell lymphoma, unspecified (C85.1-)
> personal history of other malignant neoplasms of lymphoid, hematopoietic and related tissues (Z85.79)

C88.0 Waldenström macroglobulinemia   HCC
> Lymphoplasmacytic lymphoma with IgM-production
> Macroglobulinemia (idiopathic) (primary)
> **EXCLUDES 1** small cell B-cell lymphoma (C83.0)

C88.2 Heavy chain disease   HCC
> Franklin disease
> Gamma heavy chain disease
> Mu heavy chain disease

C88.3 Immunoproliferative small intestinal disease   HCC
> Alpha heavy chain disease
> Mediterranean lymphoma

C88.4 Extranodal marginal zone B-cell lymphoma of mucosa-associated lymphoid tissue [MALT-lymphoma]   HCC
> Lymphoma of skin-associated lymphoid tissue [SALT-lymphoma]
> Lymphoma of bronchial-associated lymphoid tissue [BALT-lymphoma]
> **EXCLUDES 1** high malignant (diffuse large B-cell) lymphoma (C83.3-)

C88.8 Other malignant immunoproliferative diseases   HCC

C88.9 Malignant immunoproliferative disease, unspecified   HCC ▽
> Immunoproliferative disease NOS

✓4ᵗʰ **C90 Multiple myeloma and malignant plasma cell neoplasms**
> **EXCLUDES 1** personal history of other malignant neoplasms of lymphoid, hematopoietic and related tissues (Z85.79)

✓5ᵗʰ **C90.0 Multiple myeloma**
> Kahler's disease   Myelomatosis
> Medullary plasmacytoma   Plasma cell myeloma
> **EXCLUDES 1** solitary myeloma (C90.3-)
> solitary plasmactyoma (C90.3-)

C90.00 Multiple myeloma not having achieved remission   HCC
> Multiple myeloma with failed remission
> Multiple myeloma NOS

C90.01 Multiple myeloma in remission   HCC

C90.02 Multiple myeloma in relapse   HCC

✓5ᵗʰ **C90.1 Plasma cell leukemia**
> Plasmacytic leukemia

C90.10 Plasma cell leukemia not having achieved remission   HCC
> Plasma cell leukemia with failed remission
> Plasma cell leukemia NOS

C90.11 Plasma cell leukemia in remission   HCC

C90.12 Plasma cell leukemia in relapse   HCC

✓5ᵗʰ **C90.2 Extramedullary plasmacytoma**

C90.20 Extramedullary plasmacytoma not having achieved remission   HCC
> Extramedullary plasmacytoma with failed remission
> Extramedullary plasmacytoma NOS

C90.21 Extramedullary plasmacytoma in remission   HCC

C90.22 Extramedullary plasmacytoma in relapse   HCC

✓5ᵗʰ **C90.3 Solitary plasmacytoma**
> Localized malignant plasma cell tumor NOS
> Plasmacytoma NOS
> Solitary myeloma

C90.30 Solitary plasmacytoma not having achieved remission   HCC
> Solitary plasmacytoma with failed remission
> Solitary plasmacytoma NOS

C90.31 Solitary plasmacytoma in remission   HCC

C90.32 Solitary plasmacytoma in relapse   HCC

✓4ᵗʰ **C91 Lymphoid leukemia**
> **EXCLUDES 1** personal history of leukemia (Z85.6)

✓5ᵗʰ **C91.0 Acute lymphoblastic leukemia [ALL]**
> **NOTE** Code C91.0 should only be used for T-cell and B-cell precursor leukemia.

C91.00 Acute lymphoblastic leukemia not having achieved remission   HCC
> Acute lymphoblastic leukemia with failed remission
> Acute lymphoblastic leukemia NOS

C91.01 Acute lymphoblastic leukemia, in remission   HCC

C91.02 Acute lymphoblastic leukemia, in relapse   HCC

✓5ᵗʰ **C91.1 Chronic lymphocytic leukemia of B-cell type**
> Lymphoplasmacytic leukemia
> Richter syndrome
> **EXCLUDES 1** lymphoplasmacytic lymphoma (C83.0-)

C91.10 Chronic lymphocytic leukemia of B-cell type not having achieved remission   HCC
> Chronic lymphocytic leukemia of B-cell type with failed remission
> Chronic lymphocytic leukemia of B-cell type NOS

C91.11 Chronic lymphocytic leukemia of B-cell type in remission   HCC

C91.12 Chronic lymphocytic leukemia of B-cell type in relapse   HCC

✓5ᵗʰ **C91.3 Prolymphocytic leukemia of B-cell type**

C91.30 Prolymphocytic leukemia of B-cell type not having achieved remission   HCC
> Prolymphocytic leukemia of B-cell type with failed remission
> Prolymphocytic leukemia of B-cell type NOS

C91.31 Prolymphocytic leukemia of B-cell type, in remission   HCC

C91.32 Prolymphocytic leukemia of B-cell type, in relapse   HCC

✓5ᵗʰ **C91.4 Hairy cell leukemia**
> Leukemic reticuloendotheliosis

C91.40 Hairy cell leukemia not having achieved remission   HCC
> Hairy cell leukemia with failed remission
> Hairy cell leukemia NOS

C91.41 Hairy cell leukemia, in remission   HCC

C91.42 Hairy cell leukemia, in relapse   HCC

✓5ᵗʰ **C91.5 Adult T-cell lymphoma/leukemia (HTLV-1-associated)**
> Acute variant of adult T-cell lymphoma/leukemia (HTLV-1-associated)
> Chronic variant of adult T-cell lymphoma/leukemia (HTLV-1-associated)
> Lymphomatoid variant of adult T-cell lymphoma/leukemia (HTLV-1-associated)
> Smouldering variant of adult T-cell lymphoma/leukemia (HTLV-1-associated)

C91.50 Adult T-cell lymphoma/leukemia (HTLV-1-associated) not having achieved remission   HCC A
> Adult T-cell lymphoma/leukemia (HTLV-1-associated) with failed remission
> Adult T-cell lymphoma/leukemia (HTLV-1-associated) NOS

C91.51 Adult T-cell lymphoma/leukemia (HTLV-1-associated), in remission   HCC A

C91.52 Adult T-cell lymphoma/leukemia (HTLV-1-associated), in relapse   HCC A

✓5ᵗʰ **C91.6 Prolymphocytic leukemia of T-cell type**

C91.60 Prolymphocytic leukemia of T-cell type not having achieved remission   HCC
> Prolymphocytic leukemia of T-cell type with failed remission
> Prolymphocytic leukemia of T-cell type NOS

EXCLUDES 1 Not coded here   **EXCLUDES 2** Not included here   N Newborn Age: 0   P Pediatric Age: 0-17   M Maternity Age: 12-55   A Adult Age: 15-124

480   ICD-10-CM 2018

C91.61   **Prolymphocytic leukemia of T-cell type, in remission**   HCC

C91.62   **Prolymphocytic leukemia of T-cell type, in relapse**   HCC

✓5ᵗʰ **C91.A**   Mature B-cell leukemia Burkitt-type

> EXCLUDES 1   *Burkitt lymphoma (C83.7-)*

C91.A0   **Mature B-cell leukemia Burkitt-type, not having achieved remission**   HCC
> Mature B-cell leukemia Burkitt-type with failed remission
> Mature B-cell leukemia Burkitt-type NOS

C91.A1   **Mature B-cell leukemia Burkitt-type, in remission**   HCC

C91.A2   **Mature B-cell leukemia Burkitt-type, in relapse**   HCC

✓5ᵗʰ **C91.Z**   Other lymphoid leukemia

> T-cell large granular lymphocytic leukemia (associated with rheumatoid arthritis)

C91.Z0   **Other lymphoid leukemia not having achieved remission**   HCC
> Other lymphoid leukemia with failed remission
> Other lymphoid leukemia NOS

C91.Z1   **Other lymphoid leukemia, in remission**   HCC

C91.Z2   **Other lymphoid leukemia, in relapse**   HCC

✓5ᵗʰ **C91.9**   Lymphoid leukemia, unspecified

C91.90   **Lymphoid leukemia, unspecified not having achieved remission**   HCC ▽
> Lymphoid leukemia with failed remission
> Lymphoid leukemia NOS

C91.91   **Lymphoid leukemia, unspecified, in remission**   HCC ▽

C91.92   **Lymphoid leukemia, unspecified, in relapse**   HCC ▽

✓4ᵗʰ **C92**   **Myeloid leukemia**

> INCLUDES   granulocytic leukemia
> myelogenous leukemia
> EXCLUDES 1   *personal history of leukemia (Z85.6)*

✓5ᵗʰ **C92.0**   Acute myeloblastic leukemia

> Acute myeloblastic leukemia, minimal differentiation
> Acute myeloblastic leukemia (with maturation)
> Acute myeloblastic leukemia 1/ETO
> Acute myeloblastic leukemia M0
> Acute myeloblastic leukemia M1
> Acute myeloblastic leukemia M2
> Acute myeloblastic leukemia with t(8;21)
> Acute myeloblastic leukemia (without a FAB classification) NOS
> Refractory anemia with excess blasts in transformation [RAEB T]
>> EXCLUDES 1   *acute exacerbation of chronic myeloid leukemia (C92.10)*
>> *refractory anemia with excess of blasts not in transformation (D46.2-)*

C92.00   **Acute myeloblastic leukemia, not having achieved remission**   HCC
> Acute myeloblastic leukemia with failed remission
> Acute myeloblastic leukemia NOS

C92.01   **Acute myeloblastic leukemia, in remission**   HCC

C92.02   **Acute myeloblastic leukemia, in relapse**   HCC

✓5ᵗʰ **C92.1**   Chronic myeloid leukemia, BCR/ABL-positive

> Chronic myelogenous leukemia, Philadelphia chromosome (Ph1) positive
> Chronic myelogenous leukemia, t(9;22) (q34;q11)
> Chronic myelogenous leukemia with crisis of blast cells
>> EXCLUDES 1   *atypical chronic myeloid leukemia BCR/ABL-negative (C92.2-)*
>> *chronic myelomonocytic leukemia (C93.1-)*
>> *chronic myeloproliferative disease (D47.1)*

C92.10   **Chronic myeloid leukemia, BCR/ABL-positive, not having achieved remission**   HCC
> Chronic myeloid leukemia, BCR/ABL-positive with failed remission
> Chronic myeloid leukemia, BCR/ABL-positive NOS

C92.11   **Chronic myeloid leukemia, BCR/ABL-positive, in remission**   HCC

C92.12   **Chronic myeloid leukemia, BCR/ABL-positive, in relapse**   HCC

✓5ᵗʰ **C92.2**   Atypical chronic myeloid leukemia, BCR/ABL-negative

C92.20   **Atypical chronic myeloid leukemia, BCR/ABL-negative, not having achieved remission**   HCC
> Atypical chronic myeloid leukemia, BCR/ABL-negative with failed remission
> Atypical chronic myeloid leukemia, BCR/ABL-negative NOS

C92.21   **Atypical chronic myeloid leukemia, BCR/ABL-negative, in remission**   HCC

C92.22   **Atypical chronic myeloid leukemia, BCR/ABL-negative, in relapse**   HCC

✓5ᵗʰ **C92.3**   Myeloid sarcoma

> A malignant tumor of immature myeloid cells
> Chloroma
> Granulocytic sarcoma

C92.30   **Myeloid sarcoma, not having achieved remission**   HCC
> Myeloid sarcoma with failed remission
> Myeloid sarcoma NOS

C92.31   **Myeloid sarcoma, in remission**   HCC

C92.32   **Myeloid sarcoma, in relapse**   HCC

✓5ᵗʰ **C92.4**   Acute promyelocytic leukemia

> AML M3
> AML Me with t(15;17) and variants

C92.40   **Acute promyelocytic leukemia, not having achieved remission**   HCC
> Acute promyelocytic leukemia with failed remission
> Acute promyelocytic leukemia NOS

C92.41   **Acute promyelocytic leukemia, in remission**   HCC

C92.42   **Acute promyelocytic leukemia, in relapse**   HCC

✓5ᵗʰ **C92.5**   Acute myelomonocytic leukemia

> AML M4
> AML M4 Eo with inv(16) or t(16;16)

C92.50   **Acute myelomonocytic leukemia, not having achieved remission**   HCC
> Acute myelomonocytic leukemia with failed remission
> Acute myelomonocytic leukemia NOS

C92.51   **Acute myelomonocytic leukemia, in remission**   HCC

C92.52   **Acute myelomonocytic leukemia, in relapse**   HCC

✓5ᵗʰ **C92.6**   Acute myeloid leukemia with 11q23-abnormality

> Acute myeloid leukemia with variation of MLL-gene

C92.60   **Acute myeloid leukemia with 11q23-abnormality not having achieved remission**   HCC
> Acute myeloid leukemia with 11q23-abnormality with failed remission
> Acute myeloid leukemia with 11q23-abnormality NOS

C92.61   **Acute myeloid leukemia with 11q23-abnormality in remission**   HCC

C92.62   **Acute myeloid leukemia with 11q23-abnormality in relapse**   HCC

✓5ᵗʰ **C92.A**   Acute myeloid leukemia with multilineage dysplasia

> Acute myeloid leukemia with dysplasia of remaining hematopoesis and/or myelodysplastic disease in its history

C92.A0   **Acute myeloid leukemia with multilineage dysplasia, not having achieved remission**   HCC
> Acute myeloid leukemia with multilineage dysplasia with failed remission
> Acute myeloid leukemia with multilineage dysplasia NOS

C92.A1   **Acute myeloid leukemia with multilineage dysplasia, in remission**   HCC

C92.A2   **Acute myeloid leukemia with multilineage dysplasia, in relapse**   HCC

✓5ᵗʰ **C92.Z**   Other myeloid leukemia

C92.Z0   **Other myeloid leukemia not having achieved remission**   HCC
> Myeloid leukemia NEC with failed remission
> Myeloid leukemia NEC

C92.Z1   **Other myeloid leukemia, in remission**   HCC

C92.Z2   **Other myeloid leukemia, in relapse**   HCC

✓5ᵗʰ **C92.9**   Myeloid leukemia, unspecified

C92.90   **Myeloid leukemia, unspecified, not having achieved remission**   HCC ▽
> Myeloid leukemia, unspecified with failed remission
> Myeloid leukemia, unspecified NOS

C92.91   **Myeloid leukemia, unspecified in remission**   HCC ▽

C92.92   **Myeloid leukemia, unspecified in relapse**   HCC ▽

☑ Additional Character Req   ✓x7ᵗʰ Placeholder Alert   Manifestation   HCC CMS-HCC Condition   ▽ Unspecified Code   ▶◀ Revised Text   ● New Code   ▲ Revised Code Title

ICD-10-CM 2018   481

✓4th C93 Monocytic leukemia
> INCLUDES monocytoid leukemia
> EXCLUDES 1 personal history of leukemia (Z85.6)

✓5th C93.0 Acute monoblastic/monocytic leukemia
> AML M5   AML M5b
> AML M5a

> **C93.00 Acute monoblastic/monocytic leukemia,**   HCC
> **not having achieved remission**
>> Acute monoblastic/monocytic leukemia with failed remission
>> Acute monoblastic/monocytic leukemia NOS

> **C93.01 Acute monoblastic/monocytic leukemia,**   HCC
> **in remission**

> **C93.02 Acute monoblastic/monocytic leukemia,**   HCC
> **in relapse**

✓5th C93.1 Chronic myelomonocytic leukemia
> Chronic monocytic leukemia
> CMML-1
> CMML-2
> CMML with eosinophilia

> **C93.10 Chronic myelomonocytic leukemia not having**   HCC
> **achieved remission**
>> Chronic myelomonocytic leukemia with failed remission
>> Chronic myelomonocytic leukemia NOS

> **C93.11 Chronic myelomonocytic leukemia, in remission**   HCC
> **C93.12 Chronic myelomonocytic leukemia, in relapse**   HCC

✓5th C93.3 Juvenile myelomonocytic leukemia

> **C93.30 Juvenile myelomonocytic leukemia,**   HCC P
> **not having achieved remission**
>> Juvenile myelomonocytic leukemia with failed remission
>> Juvenile myelomonocytic leukemia NOS

> **C93.31 Juvenile myelomonocytic leukemia,**   HCC P
> **in remission**

> **C93.32 Juvenile myelomonocytic leukemia,**   HCC P
> **in relapse**

✓5th C93.Z Other monocytic leukemia

> **C93.Z0 Other monocytic leukemia, not having**   HCC
> **achieved remission**
>> Other monocytic leukemia NOS

> **C93.Z1 Other monocytic leukemia, in remission**   HCC
> **C93.Z2 Other monocytic leukemia, in relapse**   HCC

✓5th C93.9 Monocytic leukemia, unspecified

> **C93.90 Monocytic leukemia, unspecified, not having**   HCC ▽
> **achieved remission**
>> Monocytic leukemia, unspecified with failed remission
>> Monocytic leukemia, unspecified NOS

> **C93.91 Monocytic leukemia, unspecified in remission**   HCC ▽
> **C93.92 Monocytic leukemia, unspecified in relapse**   HCC ▽

✓4th C94 Other leukemias of specified cell type
> EXCLUDES 1 leukemic reticuloendotheliosis (C91.4-)
> myelodysplastic syndromes (D46.-)
> personal history of leukemia (Z85.6)
> plasma cell leukemia (C90.1-)

✓5th C94.0 Acute erythroid leukemia
> Acute myeloid leukemia M6(a)(b)
> Erythroleukemia
> **DEF:** Erythroleukemia: A malignant blood dyscrasia (a myeloproliferative disorder).

> **C94.00 Acute erythroid leukemia, not having achieved**   HCC
> **remission**
>> Acute erythroid leukemia with failed remission
>> Acute erythroid leukemia NOS

> **C94.01 Acute erythroid leukemia, in remission**   HCC
> **C94.02 Acute erythroid leukemia, in relapse**   HCC

✓5th C94.2 Acute megakaryoblastic leukemia
> Acute myeloid leukemia M7
> Acute megakaryocytic leukemia

> **C94.20 Acute megakaryoblastic leukemia not having**   HCC
> **achieved remission**
>> Acute megakaryoblastic leukemia with failed remission
>> Acute megakaryoblastic leukemia NOS

> **C94.21 Acute megakaryoblastic leukemia, in remission**   HCC
> **C94.22 Acute megakaryoblastic leukemia, in relapse**   HCC

✓5th C94.3 Mast cell leukemia

> **C94.30 Mast cell leukemia not having achieved**   HCC
> **remission**
>> Mast cell leukemia with failed remission
>> Mast cell leukemia NOS

> **C94.31 Mast cell leukemia, in remission**   HCC
> **C94.32 Mast cell leukemia, in relapse**   HCC

✓5th C94.4 Acute panmyelosis with myelofibrosis
> Acute myelofibrosis
> EXCLUDES 1 myelofibrosis NOS (D75.81)
> secondary myelofibrosis NOS (D75.81)

> **C94.40 Acute panmyelosis with myelofibrosis not**   HCC
> **having achieved remission**
>> Acute myelofibrosis NOS
>> Acute panmyelosis with myelofibrosis with failed remission
>> Acute panmyelosis NOS

> **C94.41 Acute panmyelosis with myelofibrosis,**   HCC
> **in remission**

> **C94.42 Acute panmyelosis with myelofibrosis,**   HCC
> **in relapse**

> **C94.6 Myelodysplastic disease, not classified**   HCC
>> Myeloproliferative disease, not classified

✓5th C94.8 Other specified leukemias
> Aggressive NK-cell leukemia
> Acute basophilic leukemia

> **C94.80 Other specified leukemias not having**   HCC
> **achieved remission**
>> Other specified leukemia with failed remission
>> Other specified leukemias NOS

> **C94.81 Other specified leukemias, in remission**   HCC
> **C94.82 Other specified leukemias, in relapse**   HCC

✓4th C95 Leukemia of unspecified cell type
> EXCLUDES 1 personal history of leukemia (Z85.6)

✓5th C95.0 Acute leukemia of unspecified cell type
> Acute bilineal leukemia
> Acute mixed lineage leukemia
> Biphenotypic acute leukemia
> Stem cell leukemia of unclear lineage
> EXCLUDES 1 acute exacerbation of unspecified chronic leukemia (C95.10)

> **C95.00 Acute leukemia of unspecified cell type**   HCC
> **not having achieved remission**
>> Acute leukemia of unspecified cell type with failed remission
>> Acute leukemia NOS

> **C95.01 Acute leukemia of unspecified cell type,**   HCC
> **in remission**

> **C95.02 Acute leukemia of unspecified cell type,**   HCC
> **in relapse**

✓5th C95.1 Chronic leukemia of unspecified cell type

> **C95.10 Chronic leukemia of unspecified cell type**   HCC
> **not having achieved remission**
>> Chronic leukemia of unspecified cell type with failed remission
>> Chronic leukemia NOS

> **C95.11 Chronic leukemia of unspecified cell type,**   HCC
> **in remission**

> **C95.12 Chronic leukemia of unspecified cell type,**   HCC
> **in relapse**

✓5th C95.9 Leukemia, unspecified

> **C95.90 Leukemia, unspecified not having achieved**   HCC ▽
> **remission**
>> Leukemia, unspecified with failed remission
>> Leukemia NOS

> **C95.91 Leukemia, unspecified, in remission**   HCC ▽
> **C95.92 Leukemia, unspecified, in relapse**   HCC ▽

EXCLUDES 1 Not coded here   EXCLUDES 2 Not included here   N Newborn Age: 0   P Pediatric Age: 0-17   M Maternity Age: 12-55   A Adult Age: 15-124

482   ICD-10-CM 2018

C93–C95.92

☑4ᵗʰ **C96** **Other and unspecified malignant neoplasms of lymphoid, hematopoietic and related tissue**
    EXCLUDES 1   *personal history of other malignant neoplasms of lymphoid, hematopoietic and related tissues (Z85.79)*

    C96.0 **Multifocal and multisystemic (disseminated)**   HCC
        Langerhans-cell histiocytosis
        Histiocytosis X, multisystemic
        Letterer-Siwe disease
        EXCLUDES 1   *adult pulmonary Langerhans cell histiocytosis (J84.82)*
                   multifocal and unisystemic Langerhans-cell histiocytosis (C96.5)
                   unifocal Langerhans-cell histiocytosis (C96.6)

▲   ☑5ᵗʰ **C96.2** **Malignant mast cell neoplasm**
        ~~Aggressive systemic mastocytosis~~
        ~~Mast cell sarcoma~~
        EXCLUDES 1   *indolent mastocytosis ▶(D47.02)◀*
                   mast cell leukemia (C94.30)
                   mastocytosis (congenital) (cutaneous) (Q82.2)

●   **C96.20** **Malignant mast cell neoplasm, unspecified**   ▽
●   **C96.21** **Aggressive systemic mastocytosis**
●   **C96.22** **Mast cell sarcoma**
●   **C96.29** **Other malignant mast cell neoplasm**

    C96.4 **Sarcoma of dendritic cells (accessory cells)**   HCC
        Follicular dendritic cell sarcoma
        Interdigitating dendritic cell sarcoma
        Langerhans cell sarcoma

    C96.5 **Multifocal and unisystemic Langerhans-cell histiocytosis**   HCC
        Hand-Schüller-Christian disease
        Histiocytosis X, multifocal
        EXCLUDES 1   *multifocal and multisystemic (disseminated) Langerhans-cell histiocytosis (C96.0)*
                   unifocal Langerhans-cell histiocytosis (C96.6)

    C96.6 **Unifocal Langerhans-cell histiocytosis**   HCC
        Eosinophilic granuloma
        Histiocytosis X, unifocal
        Histiocytosis X NOS
        Langerhans-cell histiocytosis NOS
        EXCLUDES 1   *multifocal and multisysemic (disseminated) Langerhans-cell histiocytosis (C96.0)*
                   multifocal and unisystemic Langerhans-cell histiocytosis (C96.5)

    C96.A **Histiocytic sarcoma**   HCC
        Malignant histiocytosis

    C96.Z **Other specified malignant neoplasms of lymphoid, hematopoietic and related tissue**   HCC

    C96.9 **Malignant neoplasm of lymphoid, hematopoietic and related tissue, unspecified**   HCC ▽

In situ neoplasms (D00-D09)

INCLUDES   Bowen's disease
             erythroplasia
             grade III intraepithelial neoplasia
             Queyrat's erythroplasia

☑4ᵗʰ **D00** **Carcinoma in situ of oral cavity, esophagus and stomach**
    EXCLUDES 1   *melanoma in situ (D03.-)*

    ☑5ᵗʰ **D00.0** **Carcinoma in situ of lip, oral cavity and pharynx**
        Use additional code to identify:
        exposure to environmental tobacco smoke (Z77.22)
        exposure to tobacco smoke in the perinatal period (P96.81)
        history of tobacco dependence (Z87.891)
        occupational exposure to environmental tobacco smoke (Z57.31)
        tobacco dependence (F17.-)
        tobacco use (Z72.0)
        EXCLUDES 1   *carcinoma in situ of aryepiglottic fold or interarytenoid fold, laryngeal aspect (D02.0)*
                 carcinoma in situ of epiglottis NOS (D02.0)
                 carcinoma in situ of epiglottis suprahyoid portion (D02.0)
                 carcinoma in situ of skin of lip (D03.0, D04.0)

        D00.00 **Carcinoma in situ of oral cavity, unspecified site**   ▽
        D00.01 **Carcinoma in situ of labial mucosa and vermilion border**
        D00.02 **Carcinoma in situ of buccal mucosa**
        D00.03 **Carcinoma in situ of gingiva and edentulous alveolar ridge**
        D00.04 **Carcinoma in situ of soft palate**
        D00.05 **Carcinoma in situ of hard palate**
        D00.06 **Carcinoma in situ of floor of mouth**

        D00.07 **Carcinoma in situ of tongue**
        D00.08 **Carcinoma in situ of pharynx**
            Carcinoma in situ of aryepiglottic fold NOS
            Carcinoma in situ of hypopharyngeal aspect of aryepiglottic fold
            Carcinoma in situ of marginal zone of aryepiglottic fold

    D00.1 **Carcinoma in situ of esophagus**
    D00.2 **Carcinoma in situ of stomach**

☑4ᵗʰ **D01** **Carcinoma in situ of other and unspecified digestive organs**
    EXCLUDES 1   *melanoma in situ (D03.-)*

    D01.0 **Carcinoma in situ of colon**
        EXCLUDES 1   *carcinoma in situ of rectosigmoid junction (D01.1)*

    D01.1 **Carcinoma in situ of rectosigmoid junction**
    D01.2 **Carcinoma in situ of rectum**
    D01.3 **Carcinoma in situ of anus and anal canal**
        Anal intraepithelial neoplasia III [AIN III]
        Severe dysplasia of anus
        EXCLUDES 1   *anal intraepithelial neoplasia I and II [AIN I and AIN II] (K62.82)*
                 carcinoma in situ of anal margin (D04.5)
                 carcinoma in situ of anal skin (D04.5)
                 carcinoma in situ of perianal skin (D04.5)

    ☑5ᵗʰ **D01.4** **Carcinoma in situ of other and unspecified parts of intestine**
        EXCLUDES 1   *carcinoma in situ of ampulla of Vater (D01.5)*
        D01.40 **Carcinoma in situ of unspecified part of intestine**   ▽
        D01.49 **Carcinoma in situ of other parts of intestine**

    D01.5 **Carcinoma in situ of liver, gallbladder and bile ducts**
        Carcinoma in situ of ampulla of Vater

    D01.7 **Carcinoma in situ of other specified digestive organs**
        Carcinoma in situ of pancreas

    D01.9 **Carcinoma in situ of digestive organ, unspecified**   ▽

☑4ᵗʰ **D02** **Carcinoma in situ of middle ear and respiratory system**
        Use additional code to identify:
        exposure to environmental tobacco smoke (Z77.22)
        exposure to tobacco smoke in the perinatal period (P96.81)
        history of tobacco dependence(Z87.891)
        occupational exposure to environmental tobacco smoke (Z57.31)
        tobacco dependence (F17.-)
        tobacco use (Z72.0)
        EXCLUDES 1   *melanoma in situ (D03.-)*

    D02.0 **Carcinoma in situ of larynx**
        Carcinoma in situ of aryepiglottic fold or interarytenoid fold, laryngeal aspect
        Carcinoma in situ of epiglottis (suprahyoid portion)
        EXCLUDES 1   *carcinoma in situ of aryepiglottic fold or interarytenoid fold NOS (D00.08)*
                 carcinoma in situ of hypopharyngeal aspect (D00.08)
                 carcinoma in situ of marginal zone (D00.08)

    D02.1 **Carcinoma in situ of trachea**
    ☑5ᵗʰ **D02.2** **Carcinoma in situ of bronchus and lung**
        D02.20 **Carcinoma in situ of unspecified bronchus and lung**   ▽
        D02.21 **Carcinoma in situ of right bronchus and lung**
        D02.22 **Carcinoma in situ of left bronchus and lung**

    D02.3 **Carcinoma in situ of other parts of respiratory system**
        Carcinoma in situ of accessory sinuses
        Carcinoma in situ of middle ear
        Carcinoma in situ of nasal cavities
        EXCLUDES 1   *carcinoma in situ of ear (external) (skin) (D04.2-)*
                 carcinoma in situ of nose NOS (D09.8)
                 carcinoma in situ of skin of nose (D04.3)

    D02.4 **Carcinoma in situ of respiratory system, unspecified**   ▽

☑4ᵗʰ **D03** **Melanoma in situ**
    D03.0 **Melanoma in situ of lip**   HCC
    ☑5ᵗʰ **D03.1** **Melanoma in situ of eyelid, including canthus**
        D03.10 **Melanoma in situ of unspecified eyelid, including canthus**   HCC ▽
        D03.11 **Melanoma in situ of right eyelid, including canthus**   HCC
        D03.12 **Melanoma in situ of left eyelid, including canthus**   HCC
    ☑5ᵗʰ **D03.2** **Melanoma in situ of ear and external auricular canal**
        D03.20 **Melanoma in situ of unspecified ear and external auricular canal**   HCC ▽

☑ Additional Character Req   ✓ˣ⁷ᵗʰ Placeholder Alert   Manifestation   HCC CMS-HCC Condition   ▽ Unspecified Code   ▶◀ Revised Text   ● New Code   ▲ Revised Code Title

ICD-10-CM 2018   483

D03.21 **Melanoma in situ of** right **ear and external auricular canal** `HCC`

D03.22 **Melanoma in situ of** left **ear and external auricular canal** `HCC`

√5th D03.3 **Melanoma in situ of other and unspecified** parts of face

D03.30 **Melanoma in situ of unspecified part of face** `HCC` ▽

D03.39 **Melanoma in situ of other parts of face** `HCC`

D03.4 **Melanoma in situ of** scalp and neck

√5th D03.5 **Melanoma in situ of** trunk

D03.51 **Melanoma in situ of** anal skin `HCC`
Melanoma in situ of anal margin
Melanoma in situ of perianal skin

D03.52 **Melanoma in situ of** breast (skin) (soft tissue) `HCC`

D03.59 **Melanoma in situ of other part of trunk** `HCC`

√5th D03.6 **Melanoma in situ of** upper limb, including shoulder

D03.60 **Melanoma in situ of unspecified upper limb, including shoulder** `HCC` ▽

D03.61 **Melanoma in situ of** right **upper limb, including shoulder** `HCC`

D03.62 **Melanoma in situ of** left **upper limb, including shoulder** `HCC`

√5th D03.7 **Melanoma in situ of** lower limb, including hip

D03.70 **Melanoma in situ of unspecified lower limb, including hip** `HCC` ▽

D03.71 **Melanoma in situ of** right **lower limb, including hip** `HCC`

D03.72 **Melanoma in situ of** left **lower limb, including hip** `HCC`

D03.8 **Melanoma in situ of other sites** `HCC`
Melanoma in situ of scrotum
EXCLUDES 1   *carcinoma in situ of scrotum (D07.61)*

D03.9 **Melanoma in situ, unspecified** `HCC` ▽

√4th **D04 Carcinoma in situ of** skin
EXCLUDES 1   *erythroplasia of Queyrat (penis) NOS (D07.4)*
melanoma in situ (D03.-)

D04.0 **Carcinoma in situ of skin of** lip
EXCLUDES 1   *carcinoma in situ of vermilion border of lip (D00.01)*

√5th D04.1 **Carcinoma in situ of skin of** eyelid, including canthus

D04.10 **Carcinoma in situ of skin of unspecified eyelid, including canthus** ▽

D04.11 **Carcinoma in situ of skin of** right **eyelid, including canthus**

D04.12 **Carcinoma in situ of skin of** left **eyelid, including canthus**

√5th D04.2 **Carcinoma in situ of skin of** ear and external auricular canal

D04.20 **Carcinoma in situ of skin of unspecified ear and external auricular canal** ▽

D04.21 **Carcinoma in situ of skin of** right **ear and external auricular canal**

D04.22 **Carcinoma in situ of skin of** left **ear and external auricular canal**

√5th D04.3 **Carcinoma in situ of skin of other and unspecified** parts of face

D04.30 **Carcinoma in situ of skin of unspecified part of face** ▽

D04.39 **Carcinoma in situ of skin of other parts of face**

D04.4 **Carcinoma in situ of skin of** scalp and neck

D04.5 **Carcinoma in situ of skin of** trunk
Carcinoma in situ of anal margin
Carcinoma in situ of anal skin
Carcinoma in situ of perianal skin
Carcinoma in situ of skin of breast
EXCLUDES 1   *carcinoma in situ of anus NOS (D01.3)*
carcinoma in situ of scrotum (D07.61)
carcinoma in situ of skin of genital organs (D07.-)

√5th D04.6 **Carcinoma in situ of skin of** upper limb, including shoulder

D04.60 **Carcinoma in situ of skin of unspecified upper limb, including shoulder** ▽

D04.61 **Carcinoma in situ of skin of** right **upper limb, including shoulder**

D04.62 **Carcinoma in situ of skin of** left **upper limb, including shoulder**

√5th D04.7 **Carcinoma in situ of skin of** lower limb, including hip

D04.70 **Carcinoma in situ of skin of unspecified lower limb, including hip** ▽

D04.71 **Carcinoma in situ of skin of** right **lower limb, including hip**

D04.72 **Carcinoma in situ of skin of** left **lower limb, including hip**

D04.8 **Carcinoma in situ of skin of other sites**

D04.9 **Carcinoma in situ of skin, unspecified** ▽

√4th **D05 Carcinoma in situ of** breast
EXCLUDES 1   *carcinoma in situ of skin of breast (D04.5)*
melanoma in situ of breast (skin) (D03.5)
Paget's disease of breast or nipple (C50.-)

√5th D05.0 Lobular **carcinoma in situ of breast**

D05.00 **Lobular carcinoma in situ of unspecified breast** ▽

D05.01 **Lobular carcinoma in situ of** right **breast**

D05.02 **Lobular carcinoma in situ of** left **breast**

√5th D05.1 Intraductal **carcinoma in situ of breast**

D05.10 **Intraductal carcinoma in situ of unspecified breast** ▽

D05.11 **Intraductal carcinoma in situ of** right **breast**

D05.12 **Intraductal carcinoma in situ of** left **breast**

√5th D05.8 **Other specified type of carcinoma in situ of breast**

D05.80 **Other specified type of carcinoma in situ of unspecified breast** ▽

D05.81 **Other specified type of carcinoma in situ of** right **breast**

D05.82 **Other specified type of carcinoma in situ of** left **breast**

√5th D05.9 **Unspecified type of carcinoma in situ of breast**

D05.90 **Unspecified type of carcinoma in situ of unspecified breast** ▽

D05.91 **Unspecified type of carcinoma in situ of** right **breast** ▽

D05.92 **Unspecified type of carcinoma in situ of** left **breast** ▽

√4th **D06 Carcinoma in situ of** cervix uteri
`INCLUDES`   cervical adenocarcinoma in situ
cervical intraepithelial glandular neoplasia
cervical intraepithelial neoplasia III [CIN III]
severe dysplasia of cervix uteri
EXCLUDES 1   *cervical intraepithelial neoplasia II [CIN II] (N87.1)*
cytologic evidence of malignancy of cervix without histologic confirmation (R87.614)
high grade squamous intraepithelial lesion (HGSIL) of cervix (R87.613)
melanoma in situ of cervix (D03.5)
moderate cervical dysplasia (N87.1)

D06.0 **Carcinoma in situ of** endocervix   ♀

D06.1 **Carcinoma in situ of** exocervix   ♀

D06.7 **Carcinoma in situ of other** parts **of cervix**   ♀

D06.9 **Carcinoma in situ of cervix, unspecified**   ♀▽

√4th **D07 Carcinoma in situ of other and unspecified** genital organs
EXCLUDES 1   *melanoma in situ of trunk (D03.5)*

D07.0 **Carcinoma in situ of** endometrium   ♀

D07.1 **Carcinoma in situ of** vulva   ♀
Severe dysplasia of vulva
Vulvar intraepithelial neoplasia III [VIN III]
EXCLUDES 1   *moderate dysplasia of vulva (N90.1)*
vulvar intraepithelial neoplasia II [VIN II] (N90.1)

D07.2 **Carcinoma in situ of** vagina   ♀
Severe dysplasia of vagina
Vaginal intraepithelial neoplasia III [VAIN III]
EXCLUDES 1   *moderate dysplasia of vagina (N89.1)*
vaginal intraepithelial neoplasia II [VIN II] (N89.1)

√5th D07.3 **Carcinoma in situ of other and unspecified** female genital organs

D07.30 **Carcinoma in situ of unspecified female genital organs**   ♀▽

D07.39 **Carcinoma in situ of other female genital organs**   ♀

D07.4 **Carcinoma in situ of** penis   ♂
Erythroplasia of Queyrat NOS

D07.5 **Carcinoma in situ of** prostate   ♂
Prostatic intraepithelial neoplasia III (PIN III)
Severe dysplasia of prostate
EXCLUDES 1   *dysplasia (mild) (moderate) of prostate (N42.3-)*
prostatic intraepithelial neoplasia II [PIN II] (N42.3-)

EXCLUDES 1 Not coded here   *EXCLUDES 2* Not included here   N Newborn Age: 0   P Pediatric Age: 0-17   M Maternity Age: 12-55   A Adult Age: 15-124

☑5ᵗʰ **D07.6 Carcinoma in situ of other and unspecified** male genital organs

    D07.60 Carcinoma in situ of unspecified male genital organs ♂ ▽

    D07.61 Carcinoma in situ of scrotum ♂

    D07.69 Carcinoma in situ of other male genital organs ♂

☑4ᵗʰ **D09 Carcinoma in situ of other and unspecified** sites

    EXCLUDES 1   melanoma in situ (D03.-)

    D09.0 Carcinoma in situ of bladder

☑5ᵗʰ **D09.1 Carcinoma in situ of other and unspecified** urinary organs

    D09.10 Carcinoma in situ of unspecified urinary organ ▽

    D09.19 Carcinoma in situ of other urinary organs

☑5ᵗʰ **D09.2 Carcinoma in situ of** eye

    EXCLUDES 1   carcinoma in situ of skin of eyelid (D04.1-)

    D09.20 Carcinoma in situ of unspecified eye ▽

    D09.21 Carcinoma in situ of right **eye**

    D09.22 Carcinoma in situ of left **eye**

    D09.3 Carcinoma in situ of thyroid **and other** endocrine glands

    EXCLUDES 1   carcinoma in situ of endocrine pancreas (D01.7)
           carcinoma in situ of ovary (D07.39)
           carcinoma in situ of testis (D07.69)

    D09.8 Carcinoma in situ of other specified sites

    D09.9 Carcinoma in situ, unspecified ▽

Benign neoplasms, except benign neuroendocrine tumors (D10-D36)

☑4ᵗʰ **D10 Benign neoplasm of** mouth and pharynx

    D10.0 Benign neoplasm of lip
    Benign neoplasm of lip (frenulum) (inner aspect) (mucosa) (vermilion border)
    EXCLUDES 1   benign neoplasm of skin of lip (D22.0, D23.0)

    D10.1 Benign neoplasm of tongue
    Benign neoplasm of lingual tonsil

    D10.2 Benign neoplasm of floor **of mouth**

☑5ᵗʰ **D10.3 Benign neoplasm of other and unspecified parts of mouth**

    D10.30 Benign neoplasm of unspecified part of mouth ▽

    D10.39 Benign neoplasm of other parts of mouth
    Benign neoplasm of minor salivary gland NOS
    EXCLUDES 1   benign odontogenic neoplasms (D16.4-D16.5)
           benign neoplasm of mucosa of lip (D10.0)
           benign neoplasm of nasopharyngeal surface of soft palate (D10.6)

    D10.4 Benign neoplasm of tonsil
    Benign neoplasm of tonsil (faucial) (palatine)
    EXCLUDES 1   benign neoplasm of lingual tonsil (D10.1)
           benign neoplasm of pharyngeal tonsil (D10.6)
           benign neoplasm of tonsillar fossa (D10.5)
           benign neoplasm of tonsillar pillars (D10.5)

    D10.5 Benign neoplasm of other parts of oropharynx
    Benign neoplasm of epiglottis, anterior aspect
    Benign neoplasm of tonsillar fossa
    Benign neoplasm of tonsillar pillars
    Benign neoplasm of vallecula
    EXCLUDES 1   benign neoplasm of epiglottis NOS (D14.1)
           benign neoplasm of epiglottis, suprahyoid portion (D14.1)

    D10.6 Benign neoplasm of nasopharynx
    Benign neoplasm of pharyngeal tonsil
    Benign neoplasm of posterior margin of septum and choanae

    D10.7 Benign neoplasm of hypopharynx

    D10.9 Benign neoplasm of pharynx, unspecified ▽

☑4ᵗʰ **D11 Benign neoplasm of** major salivary glands

    EXCLUDES 1   benign neoplasms of minor salivary glands NOS (D10.39)
           benign neoplasms of specified minor salivary glands which are classified according to their anatomical location

    D11.0 Benign neoplasm of parotid gland

    D11.7 Benign neoplasm of other major salivary glands
    Benign neoplasm of sublingual salivary gland
    Benign neoplasm of submandibular salivary gland

    D11.9 Benign neoplasm of major salivary gland, unspecified ▽

☑4ᵗʰ **D12 Benign neoplasm of colon, rectum, anus and anal canal**

    EXCLUDES 1   benign carcinoid tumors of the large intestine, and rectum (D3A.02-)
    AHA: 2017, 1Q, 15; 2015, 2Q, 14

    D12.0 Benign neoplasm of cecum
    Benign neoplasm of ileocecal valve

    D12.1 Benign neoplasm of appendix
    EXCLUDES 1   benign carcinoid tumor of the appendix (D3A.020)

    D12.2 Benign neoplasm of ascending colon

    D12.3 Benign neoplasm of transverse colon
    Benign neoplasm of hepatic flexure
    Benign neoplasm of splenic flexure
    AHA: 2017, 1Q, 16

    D12.4 Benign neoplasm of descending colon

    D12.5 Benign neoplasm of sigmoid colon

    D12.6 Benign neoplasm of colon, unspecified ▽
    Adenomatosis of colon
    Benign neoplasm of large intestine NOS
    Polyposis (hereditary) of colon
    EXCLUDES 1   inflammatory polyp of colon (K51.4-)
           polyp of colon NOS (K63.5)

    D12.7 Benign neoplasm of rectosigmoid junction

    D12.8 Benign neoplasm of rectum
    EXCLUDES 1   benign carcinoid tumor of the rectum (D3A.026)

    D12.9 Benign neoplasm of anus and anal canal
    Benign neoplasm of anus NOS
    EXCLUDES 1   benign neoplasm of anal margin (D22.5, D23.5)
           benign neoplasm of anal skin (D22.5, D23.5)
           benign neoplasm of perianal skin (D22.5, D23.5)

☑4ᵗʰ **D13 Benign neoplasm of other and ill-defined parts of** digestive system

    EXCLUDES 1   benign stromal tumors of digestive system (D21.4)

    D13.0 Benign neoplasm of esophagus

    D13.1 Benign neoplasm of stomach
    EXCLUDES 1   benign carcinoid tumor of the stomach (D3A.092)

    D13.2 Benign neoplasm of duodenum
    EXCLUDES 1   benign carcinoid tumor of the duodenum (D3A.010)

☑5ᵗʰ **D13.3 Benign neoplasm of other and unspecified parts of** small intestine
    EXCLUDES 1   benign carcinoid tumors of the small intestine (D3A.01-)
           benign neoplasm of ileocecal valve (D12.0)

    D13.30 Benign neoplasm of unspecified part of small intestine ▽

    D13.39 Benign neoplasm of other parts of small intestine

    D13.4 Benign neoplasm of liver
    Benign neoplasm of intrahepatic bile ducts

    D13.5 Benign neoplasm of extrahepatic bile ducts

    D13.6 Benign neoplasm of pancreas
    EXCLUDES 1   benign neoplasm of endocrine pancreas (D13.7)

    D13.7 Benign neoplasm of endocrine pancreas
    Islet cell tumor
    Benign neoplasm of islets of Langerhans
    Use additional code to identify any functional activity

    D13.9 Benign neoplasm of ill-defined sites **within the digestive system**
    Benign neoplasm of digestive system NOS
    Benign neoplasm of intestine NOS
    Benign neoplasm of spleen

☑4ᵗʰ **D14 Benign neoplasm of middle ear and respiratory system**

    D14.0 Benign neoplasm of middle ear, nasal cavity and accessory sinuses
    Benign neoplasm of cartilage of nose
    EXCLUDES 1   benign neoplasm of auricular canal (external) (D22.2-, D23.2-)
           benign neoplasm of bone of ear (D16.4)
           benign neoplasm of bone of nose (D16.4)
           benign neoplasm of cartilage of ear (D21.0)
           benign neoplasm of ear (external)(skin) (D22.2-, D23.2-)
           benign neoplasm of nose NOS (D36.7)
           benign neoplasm of skin of nose (D22.39, D23.39)
           benign neoplasm of olfactory bulb (D33.3)
           benign neoplasm of posterior margin of septum and choanae (D10.6)
           polyp of accessory sinus (J33.8)
           polyp of ear (middle) (H74.4)
           polyp of nasal (cavity) (J33.-)

☑ Additional Character Req   ✓x7ᵗʰ Placeholder Alert   Manifestation   HCC CMS-HCC Condition   ▽ Unspecified Code   ►◄ Revised Text   ● New Code   ▲ Revised Code Title

Chapter 2. Neoplasms

D14.1   **Benign neoplasm of larynx**
Adenomatous polyp of larynx
Benign neoplasm of epiglottis (suprahyoid portion)
EXCLUDES 1   *benign neoplasm of epiglottis, anterior aspect (D10.5)*
polyp (nonadenomatous) of vocal cord or larynx (J38.1)

D14.2   **Benign neoplasm of trachea**

√5th   **D14.3**   **Benign neoplasm of bronchus and lung**
EXCLUDES 1   *benign carcinoid tumor of the bronchus and lung (D3A.090)*

    D14.30   Benign neoplasm of unspecified bronchus and lung   ▽

    D14.31   Benign neoplasm of right bronchus and lung

    D14.32   Benign neoplasm of left bronchus and lung

D14.4   **Benign neoplasm of respiratory system, unspecified**   ▽

√4th   **D15**   **Benign neoplasm of other and unspecified intrathoracic organs**
EXCLUDES 1   *benign neoplasm of mesothelial tissue (D19.-)*

D15.0   **Benign neoplasm of thymus**
EXCLUDES 1   *benign carcinoid tumor of the thymus (D3A.091)*

D15.1   **Benign neoplasm of heart**
EXCLUDES 1   *benign neoplasm of great vessels (D21.3)*

D15.2   **Benign neoplasm of mediastinum**

D15.7   **Benign neoplasm of other specified intrathoracic organs**

D15.9   **Benign neoplasm of intrathoracic organ, unspecified**   ▽

√4th   **D16**   **Benign neoplasm of bone and articular cartilage**
EXCLUDES 1   *benign neoplasm of connective tissue of ear (D21.0)*
benign neoplasm of connective tissue of eyelid (D21.0)
benign neoplasm of connective tissue of larynx (D14.1)
benign neoplasm of connective tissue of nose (D14.0)
benign neoplasm of synovia (D21.-)

√5th   **D16.0**   **Benign neoplasm of scapula and long bones of upper limb**

    D16.00   Benign neoplasm of scapula and long bones of unspecified upper limb   ▽

    D16.01   Benign neoplasm of scapula and long bones of right upper limb

    D16.02   Benign neoplasm of scapula and long bones of left upper limb

√5th   **D16.1**   **Benign neoplasm of short bones of upper limb**

    D16.10   Benign neoplasm of short bones of unspecified upper limb   ▽

    D16.11   Benign neoplasm of short bones of right upper limb

    D16.12   Benign neoplasm of short bones of left upper limb

√5th   **D16.2**   **Benign neoplasm of long bones of lower limb**

    D16.20   Benign neoplasm of long bones of unspecified lower limb   ▽

    D16.21   Benign neoplasm of long bones of right lower limb

    D16.22   Benign neoplasm of long bones of left lower limb

√5th   **D16.3**   **Benign neoplasm of short bones of lower limb**

    D16.30   Benign neoplasm of short bones of unspecified lower limb   ▽

    D16.31   Benign neoplasm of short bones of right lower limb

    D16.32   Benign neoplasm of short bones of left lower limb

D16.4   **Benign neoplasm of bones of skull and face**
Benign neoplasm of maxilla (superior)
Benign neoplasm of orbital bone
Keratocyst of maxilla
Keratocystic odontogenic tumor of maxilla
EXCLUDES 2   *benign neoplasm of lower jaw bone (D16.5)*

D16.5   **Benign neoplasm of lower jaw bone**
Keratocyst of mandible
Keratocystic odontogenic tumor of mandible

D16.6   **Benign neoplasm of vertebral column**
EXCLUDES 1   *benign neoplasm of sacrum and coccyx (D16.8)*

D16.7   **Benign neoplasm of ribs, sternum and clavicle**

D16.8   **Benign neoplasm of pelvic bones, sacrum and coccyx**

D16.9   **Benign neoplasm of bone and articular cartilage, unspecified**   ▽

√4th   **D17**   **Benign lipomatous neoplasm**

D17.0   **Benign lipomatous neoplasm of skin and subcutaneous tissue of head, face and neck**

D17.1   **Benign lipomatous neoplasm of skin and subcutaneous tissue of trunk**

√5th   **D17.2**   **Benign lipomatous neoplasm of skin and subcutaneous tissue of limb**

    D17.20   Benign lipomatous neoplasm of skin and subcutaneous tissue of unspecified limb   ▽

    D17.21   Benign lipomatous neoplasm of skin and subcutaneous tissue of right arm

    D17.22   Benign lipomatous neoplasm of skin and subcutaneous tissue of left arm

    D17.23   Benign lipomatous neoplasm of skin and subcutaneous tissue of right leg

    D17.24   Benign lipomatous neoplasm of skin and subcutaneous tissue of left leg

√5th   **D17.3**   **Benign lipomatous neoplasm of skin and subcutaneous tissue of other and unspecified sites**

    D17.30   Benign lipomatous neoplasm of skin and subcutaneous tissue of unspecified sites   ▽

    D17.39   Benign lipomatous neoplasm of skin and subcutaneous tissue of other sites

D17.4   **Benign lipomatous neoplasm of intrathoracic organs**

D17.5   **Benign lipomatous neoplasm of intra-abdominal organs**
EXCLUDES 1   *benign lipomatous neoplasm of peritoneum and retroperitoneum (D17.79)*

D17.6   **Benign lipomatous neoplasm of spermatic cord**   ♂

√5th   **D17.7**   **Benign lipomatous neoplasm of other sites**

    D17.71   Benign lipomatous neoplasm of kidney

    D17.72   Benign lipomatous neoplasm of other genitourinary organ

    D17.79   Benign lipomatous neoplasm of other sites
Benign lipomatous neoplasm of peritoneum
Benign lipomatous neoplasm of retroperitoneum

D17.9   **Benign lipomatous neoplasm, unspecified**   ▽
Lipoma NOS

√4th   **D18**   **Hemangioma and lymphangioma, any site**
EXCLUDES 1   *benign neoplasm of glomus jugulare (D35.6)*
blue or pigmented nevus (D22.-)
nevus NOS (D22.-)
vascular nevus (Q82.5)

√5th   **D18.0**   **Hemangioma**
Angioma NOS
Cavernous nevus
DEF: A common benign tumor usually occurring in infancy; composed of newly formed blood vessels due to malformation of angioblastic tissue.

    D18.00   Hemangioma unspecified site   ▽

    D18.01   Hemangioma of skin and subcutaneous tissue

    D18.02   Hemangioma of intracranial structures   HCC

    D18.03   Hemangioma of intra-abdominal structures

    D18.09   Hemangioma of other sites

D18.1   **Lymphangioma, any site**

√4th   **D19**   **Benign neoplasm of mesothelial tissue**

D19.0   **Benign neoplasm of mesothelial tissue of pleura**

D19.1   **Benign neoplasm of mesothelial tissue of peritoneum**

D19.7   **Benign neoplasm of mesothelial tissue of other sites**

D19.9   **Benign neoplasm of mesothelial tissue, unspecified**   ▽
Benign mesothelioma NOS

√4th   **D20**   **Benign neoplasm of soft tissue of retroperitoneum and peritoneum**
EXCLUDES 1   *benign lipomatous neoplasm of peritoneum and retroperitoneum (D17.79)*
benign neoplasm of mesothelial tissue (D19.-)

D20.0   **Benign neoplasm of soft tissue of retroperitoneum**

D20.1   **Benign neoplasm of soft tissue of peritoneum**

☑4th **D21 Other benign neoplasms of connective and other soft tissue**

INCLUDES   benign neoplasm of blood vessel
benign neoplasm of bursa
benign neoplasm of cartilage
benign neoplasm of fascia
benign neoplasm of fat
benign neoplasm of ligament, except uterine
benign neoplasm of lymphatic channel
benign neoplasm of muscle
benign neoplasm of synovia
benign neoplasm of tendon (sheath)
benign stromal tumors

EXCLUDES 1   *benign neoplasm of articular cartilage (D16.-)*
benign neoplasm of cartilage of larynx (D14.1)
benign neoplasm of cartilage of nose (D14.0)
benign neoplasm of connective tissue of breast (D24.-)
benign neoplasm of peripheral nerves and autonomic nervous system (D36.1-)
benign neoplasm of peritoneum (D20.1)
benign neoplasm of retroperitoneum (D20.0)
benign neoplasm of uterine ligament, any (D28.2)
benign neoplasm of vascular tissue (D18.-)
hemangioma (D18.0-)
lipomatous neoplasm (D17.-)
lymphangioma (D18.1)
uterine leiomyoma (D25.-)

D21.0 Benign neoplasm of connective and other soft tissue of head, face and neck
Benign neoplasm of connective tissue of ear
Benign neoplasm of connective tissue of eyelid
EXCLUDES 1   *benign neoplasm of connective tissue of orbit (D31.6-)*

☑5th **D21.1 Benign neoplasm of connective and other soft tissue of upper limb, including shoulder**

D21.10 Benign neoplasm of connective and other soft ▽ tissue of unspecified upper limb, including shoulder

D21.11 Benign neoplasm of connective and other soft tissue of right upper limb, including shoulder

D21.12 Benign neoplasm of connective and other soft tissue of left upper limb, including shoulder

☑5th **D21.2 Benign neoplasm of connective and other soft tissue of lower limb, including hip**

D21.20 Benign neoplasm of connective and other soft ▽ tissue of unspecified lower limb, including hip

D21.21 Benign neoplasm of connective and other soft tissue of right lower limb, including hip

D21.22 Benign neoplasm of connective and other soft tissue of left lower limb, including hip

D21.3 Benign neoplasm of connective and other soft tissue of thorax
Benign neoplasm of axilla
Benign neoplasm of diaphragm
Benign neoplasm of great vessels
EXCLUDES 1   *benign neoplasm of heart (D15.1)*
benign neoplasm of mediastinum (D15.2)
benign neoplasm of thymus (D15.0)

D21.4 Benign neoplasm of connective and other soft tissue of abdomen
Benign stromal tumors of abdomen

D21.5 Benign neoplasm of connective and other soft tissue of pelvis
EXCLUDES 1   *benign neoplasm of any uterine ligament (D28.2)*
uterine leiomyoma (D25.-)

D21.6 Benign neoplasm of connective and other soft tissue of ▽ trunk, unspecified
Benign neoplasm of back NOS

D21.9 Benign neoplasm of connective and other soft tissue, ▽ unspecified

☑4th **D22 Melanocytic nevi**
INCLUDES   atypical nevus
blue hairy pigmented nevus
nevus NOS

D22.0 Melanocytic nevi of lip

☑5th **D22.1 Melanocytic nevi of eyelid, including canthus**

D22.10 Melanocytic nevi of unspecified eyelid, including ▽ canthus

D22.11 Melanocytic nevi of right eyelid, including canthus

D22.12 Melanocytic nevi of left eyelid, including canthus

☑5th **D22.2 Melanocytic nevi of ear and external auricular canal**

D22.20 Melanocytic nevi of unspecified ear and external ▽ auricular canal

D22.21 Melanocytic nevi of right ear and external auricular canal

D22.22 Melanocytic nevi of left ear and external auricular canal

☑5th **D22.3 Melanocytic nevi of other and unspecified parts of face**

D22.30 Melanocytic nevi of unspecified part of face ▽

D22.39 Melanocytic nevi of other parts of face

D22.4 Melanocytic nevi of scalp and neck

D22.5 Melanocytic nevi of trunk
Melanocytic nevi of anal margin
Melanocytic nevi of anal skin
Melanocytic nevi of perianal skin
Melanocytic nevi of skin of breast

☑5th **D22.6 Melanocytic nevi of upper limb, including shoulder**

D22.60 Melanocytic nevi of unspecified upper limb, ▽ including shoulder

D22.61 Melanocytic nevi of right upper limb, including shoulder

D22.62 Melanocytic nevi of left upper limb, including shoulder

☑5th **D22.7 Melanocytic nevi of lower limb, including hip**

D22.70 Melanocytic nevi of unspecified lower limb, ▽ including hip

D22.71 Melanocytic nevi of right lower limb, including hip

D22.72 Melanocytic nevi of left lower limb, including hip

D22.9 Melanocytic nevi, unspecified ▽

☑4th **D23 Other benign neoplasms of skin**
INCLUDES   benign neoplasm of hair follicles
benign neoplasm of sebaceous glands
benign neoplasm of sweat glands
EXCLUDES 1   *benign lipomatous neoplasms of skin (D17.0-D17.3)*
melanocytic nevi (D22.-)

D23.0 Other benign neoplasm of skin of lip
EXCLUDES 1   *benign neoplasm of vermilion border of lip (D10.0)*

☑5th **D23.1 Other benign neoplasm of skin of eyelid, including canthus**

D23.10 Other benign neoplasm of skin of unspecified ▽ eyelid, including canthus

D23.11 Other benign neoplasm of skin of right eyelid, including canthus

D23.12 Other benign neoplasm of skin of left eyelid, including canthus

☑5th **D23.2 Other benign neoplasm of skin of ear and external auricular canal**

D23.20 Other benign neoplasm of skin of unspecified ▽ ear and external auricular canal

D23.21 Other benign neoplasm of skin of right ear and external auricular canal

D23.22 Other benign neoplasm of skin of left ear and external auricular canal

☑5th **D23.3 Other benign neoplasm of skin of other and unspecified parts of face**

D23.30 Other benign neoplasm of skin of unspecified ▽ part of face

D23.39 Other benign neoplasm of skin of other parts of face

D23.4 Other benign neoplasm of skin of scalp and neck

D23.5 Other benign neoplasm of skin of trunk
Other benign neoplasm of anal margin
Other benign neoplasm of anal skin
Other benign neoplasm of perianal skin
Other benign neoplasm of skin of breast
EXCLUDES 1   *benign neoplasm of anus NOS (D12.9)*

☑5th **D23.6 Other benign neoplasm of skin of upper limb, including shoulder**

D23.60 Other benign neoplasm of skin of unspecified ▽ upper limb, including shoulder

D23.61 Other benign neoplasm of skin of right upper limb, including shoulder

D23.62 Other benign neoplasm of skin of left upper limb, including shoulder

☑5th **D23.7 Other benign neoplasm of skin of lower limb, including hip**

D23.70 Other benign neoplasm of skin of unspecified ▽ lower limb, including hip

D23.71 Other benign neoplasm of skin of right lower limb, including hip

D23.72 Other benign neoplasm of skin of left lower limb, including hip

---

☑ Additional Character Req   ☑x7th Placeholder Alert   Manifestation   HCC CMS-HCC Condition   ▽ Unspecified Code   ►◄ Revised Text   ● New Code   ▲ Revised Code Title

ICD-10-CM 2018   487

D23.9   Other benign neoplasm of skin, unspecified ▽

✓4ᵗʰ D24   **Benign neoplasm of** breast
> **INCLUDES**   benign neoplasm of connective tissue of breast
> benign neoplasm of soft parts of breast
> fibroadenoma of breast
>
> **EXCLUDES 2**   *adenofibrosis of breast (N60.2)*
> *benign cyst of breast (N60.-)*
> *benign mammary dysplasia (N60.-)*
> *benign neoplasm of skin of breast (D22.5, D23.5)*
> *fibrocystic disease of breast (N60.-)*

D24.1   Benign neoplasm of right breast
D24.2   Benign neoplasm of left breast
D24.9   Benign neoplasm of unspecified breast ▽

✓4ᵗʰ D25   **Leiomyoma of uterus**
> **INCLUDES**   uterine fibroid
> uterine fibromyoma
> uterine myoma

D25.0   Submucous leiomyoma of uterus ♀
D25.1   Intramural leiomyoma of uterus ♀
> Interstitial leiomyoma of uterus

D25.2   Subserosal leiomyoma of uterus ♀
> Subperitoneal leiomyoma of uterus

D25.9   Leiomyoma of uterus, unspecified ♀▽

✓4ᵗʰ D26   **Other benign neoplasms of** uterus
D26.0   Other benign neoplasm of cervix uteri ♀
D26.1   Other benign neoplasm of corpus uteri ♀
D26.7   Other benign neoplasm of other parts of uterus ♀
D26.9   Other benign neoplasm of uterus, unspecified ♀▽

✓4ᵗʰ D27   **Benign neoplasm of** ovary
> Use additional code to identify any functional activity
>
> **EXCLUDES 2**   *corpus albicans cyst (N83.2-)*
> *corpus luteum cyst (N83.1-)*
> *endometrial cyst (N80.1)*
> *follicular (atretic) cyst (N83.0-)*
> *graafian follicle cyst (N83.0-)*
> *ovarian cyst NEC (N83.2-)*
> *ovarian retention cyst (N83.2-)*

D27.0   Benign neoplasm of right ovary ♀
D27.1   Benign neoplasm of left ovary ♀
D27.9   Benign neoplasm of unspecified ovary ♀▽

✓4ᵗʰ D28   **Benign neoplasm of other and unspecified** female genital organs
> **INCLUDES**   adenomatous polyp
> benign neoplasm of skin of female genital organs
> benign teratoma
>
> **EXCLUDES 1**   *epoophoron cyst (Q50.5)*
> *fimbrial cyst (Q50.4)*
> *Gartner's duct cyst (Q52.4)*
> *parovarian cyst (Q50.5)*

D28.0   Benign neoplasm of vulva ♀
D28.1   Benign neoplasm of vagina ♀
D28.2   Benign neoplasm of uterine tubes and ligaments ♀
> Benign neoplasm of fallopian tube
> Benign neoplasm of uterine ligament (broad) (round)

D28.7   Benign neoplasm of other specified female genital organs ♀
D28.9   Benign neoplasm of female genital organ, unspecified ♀▽

Uterine Leiomyomas (Fibroids)

Cornual — Pedunculated
Uterine cavity — Intramural
Subserosal — Submucosal
Cervical

✓4ᵗʰ D29   **Benign neoplasm of** male genital organs
> **INCLUDES**   benign neoplasm of skin of male genital organs

D29.0   Benign neoplasm of penis ♂
D29.1   Benign neoplasm of prostate ♂
> **EXCLUDES 1**   *enlarged prostate (N40.-)*

✓5ᵗʰ D29.2   Benign neoplasm of testis
> Use additional code to identify any functional activity

D29.20   Benign neoplasm of unspecified testis ♂▽
D29.21   Benign neoplasm of right testis ♂
D29.22   Benign neoplasm of left testis ♂

✓5ᵗʰ D29.3   Benign neoplasm of epididymis
D29.30   Benign neoplasm of unspecified epididymis ♂▽
D29.31   Benign neoplasm of right epididymis ♂
D29.32   Benign neoplasm of left epididymis ♂

D29.4   Benign neoplasm of scrotum ♂
> Benign neoplasm of skin of scrotum

D29.8   Benign neoplasm of other specified male genital organs ♂
> Benign neoplasm of seminal vesicle
> Benign neoplasm of spermatic cord
> Benign neoplasm of tunica vaginalis

D29.9   Benign neoplasm of male genital organ, unspecified ♂▽

✓4ᵗʰ D30   **Benign neoplasm of** urinary organs
✓5ᵗʰ D30.0   Benign neoplasm of kidney
> **EXCLUDES 1**   *benign carcinoid tumor of the kidney (D3A.093)*
> *benign neoplasm of renal calyces (D30.1-)*
> *benign neoplasm of renal pelvis (D30.1-)*

D30.00   Benign neoplasm of unspecified kidney ▽
D30.01   Benign neoplasm of right kidney
D30.02   Benign neoplasm of left kidney

✓5ᵗʰ D30.1   Benign neoplasm of renal pelvis
D30.10   Benign neoplasm of unspecified renal pelvis ▽
D30.11   Benign neoplasm of right renal pelvis
D30.12   Benign neoplasm of left renal pelvis

✓5ᵗʰ D30.2   Benign neoplasm of ureter
> **EXCLUDES 1**   *benign neoplasm of ureteric orifice of bladder (D30.3)*

D30.20   Benign neoplasm of unspecified ureter ▽
D30.21   Benign neoplasm of right ureter
D30.22   Benign neoplasm of left ureter

D30.3   Benign neoplasm of bladder
> Benign neoplasm of ureteric orifice of bladder
> Benign neoplasm of urethral orifice of bladder

D30.4   Benign neoplasm of urethra
> **EXCLUDES 1**   *benign neoplasm of urethral orifice of bladder (D30.3)*

D30.8   Benign neoplasm of other specified urinary organs
> Benign neoplasm of paraurethral glands

D30.9   Benign neoplasm of urinary organ, unspecified ▽
> Benign neoplasm of urinary system NOS

✓4ᵗʰ D31   **Benign neoplasm of** eye and adnexa
> **EXCLUDES 1**   *benign neoplasm of connective tissue of eyelid (D21.0)*
> *benign neoplasm of optic nerve (D33.3)*
> *benign neoplasm of skin of eyelid (D22.1-, D23.1-)*

✓5ᵗʰ D31.0   Benign neoplasm of conjunctiva
D31.00   Benign neoplasm of unspecified conjunctiva ▽
D31.01   Benign neoplasm of right conjunctiva
D31.02   Benign neoplasm of left conjunctiva

✓5ᵗʰ D31.1   Benign neoplasm of cornea
D31.10   Benign neoplasm of unspecified cornea ▽
D31.11   Benign neoplasm of right cornea
D31.12   Benign neoplasm of left cornea

✓5ᵗʰ D31.2   Benign neoplasm of retina
> **EXCLUDES 1**   *dark area on retina (D49.81)*
> *hemangioma of retina (D49.81)*
> *neoplasm of unspecified behavior of retina and choroid (D49.81)*
> *retinal freckle (D49.81)*

D31.20   Benign neoplasm of unspecified retina ▽
D31.21   Benign neoplasm of right retina
D31.22   Benign neoplasm of left retina

✓5ᵗʰ D31.3   Benign neoplasm of choroid
D31.30   Benign neoplasm of unspecified choroid ▽
D31.31   Benign neoplasm of right choroid
D31.32   Benign neoplasm of left choroid

EXCLUDES 1 Not coded here   **EXCLUDES 2** Not included here   N Newborn Age: 0   P Pediatric Age: 0-17   M Maternity Age: 12-55   A Adult Age: 15-124

√5ᵗʰ **D31.4 Benign neoplasm of** ciliary body
     D31.40 Benign neoplasm of unspecified ciliary body ▽
     D31.41 Benign neoplasm of right **ciliary body**
     D31.42 Benign neoplasm of left **ciliary body**

√5ᵗʰ **D31.5 Benign neoplasm of** lacrimal gland and duct
     Benign neoplasm of lacrimal sac
     Benign neoplasm of nasolacrimal duct
     D31.50 Benign neoplasm of unspecified lacrimal gland ▽
            and duct
     D31.51 Benign neoplasm of right **lacrimal gland and duct**
     D31.52 Benign neoplasm of left **lacrimal gland and duct**

√5ᵗʰ **D31.6 Benign neoplasm of unspecified site of** orbit
     Benign neoplasm of connective tissue of orbit
     Benign neoplasm of extraocular muscle
     Benign neoplasm of peripheral nerves of orbit
     Benign neoplasm of retrobulbar tissue
     Benign neoplasm of retro-ocular tissue
     EXCLUDES 1   *benign neoplasm of orbital bone (D16.4)*
     D31.60 Benign neoplasm of unspecified site of ▽
            unspecified orbit
     D31.61 Benign neoplasm of unspecified site of right **orbit**
     D31.62 Benign neoplasm of unspecified site of left **orbit**

√5ᵗʰ **D31.9 Benign neoplasm of unspecified** part of eye
     Benign neoplasm of eyeball
     D31.90 Benign neoplasm of unspecified part of ▽
            unspecified eye
     D31.91 Benign neoplasm of unspecified part of right **eye**
     D31.92 Benign neoplasm of unspecified part of left **eye**

√4ᵗʰ **D32 Benign neoplasm of** meninges
     D32.0 Benign neoplasm of cerebral **meninges** HCC
     D32.1 Benign neoplasm of spinal **meninges** HCC
     D32.9 Benign neoplasm of meninges, unspecified HCC ▽
         Meningioma NOS

√4ᵗʰ **D33 Benign neoplasm of** brain and other parts of central nervous system
     EXCLUDES 1   *angioma (D18.0-)*
            benign neoplasm of meninges (D32.-)
            benign neoplasm of peripheral nerves and autonomic nervous
                 system (D36.1-)
            hemangioma (D18.0-)
            neurofibromatosis (Q85.0-)
            retro-ocular benign neoplasm (D31.6-)
     D33.0 Benign neoplasm of brain, supratentorial HCC
         Benign neoplasm of cerebral ventricle
         Benign neoplasm of cerebrum
         Benign neoplasm of frontal lobe
         Benign neoplasm of occipital lobe
         Benign neoplasm of parietal lobe
         Benign neoplasm of temporal lobe
         EXCLUDES 1   *benign neoplasm of fourth ventricle (D33.1)*
     D33.1 Benign neoplasm of brain, infratentorial HCC
         Benign neoplasm of brain stem
         Benign neoplasm of cerebellum
         Benign neoplasm of fourth ventricle
     D33.2 Benign neoplasm of brain, unspecified HCC ▽
     D33.3 Benign neoplasm of cranial nerves HCC
         Benign neoplasm of olfactory bulb
     D33.4 Benign neoplasm of spinal cord HCC
     D33.7 Benign neoplasm of other specified parts of HCC
         central nervous system
     D33.9 Benign neoplasm of central nervous system, HCC ▽
         unspecified
         Benign neoplasm of nervous system (central) NOS

D34 Benign neoplasm of thyroid gland
     Use additional code to identify any functional activity

√4ᵗʰ **D35 Benign neoplasm of other and unspecified** endocrine glands
     Use additional code to identify any functional activity
     EXCLUDES 1   *benign neoplasm of endocrine pancreas (D13.7)*
            benign neoplasm of ovary (D27.-)
            benign neoplasm of testis (D29.2-)
            benign neoplasm of thymus (D15.0)
√5ᵗʰ   **D35.0 Benign neoplasm of** adrenal gland
     D35.00 Benign neoplasm of unspecified adrenal gland ▽
     D35.01 Benign neoplasm of right **adrenal gland**
     D35.02 Benign neoplasm of left **adrenal gland**
     D35.1 Benign neoplasm of parathyroid gland

     D35.2 Benign neoplasm of pituitary gland HCC
         AHA: 2014, 3Q, 22
     D35.3 Benign neoplasm of craniopharyngeal duct HCC
     D35.4 Benign neoplasm of pineal gland HCC
     D35.5 Benign neoplasm of carotid body
     D35.6 Benign neoplasm of aortic body and other paraganglia
         Benign tumor of glomus jugulare
     D35.7 Benign neoplasm of other specified endocrine glands
     D35.9 Benign neoplasm of endocrine gland, unspecified ▽
         Benign neoplasm of unspecified endocrine gland

√4ᵗʰ **D36 Benign neoplasm of other and unspecified sites**
     D36.0 Benign neoplasm of lymph nodes
         EXCLUDES 1   *lymphangioma (D18.1)*
√5ᵗʰ   **D36.1 Benign neoplasm of** peripheral nerves and autonomic nervous system
         EXCLUDES 1   *benign neoplasm of peripheral nerves of orbit (D31.6-)*
                   neurofibromatosis (Q85.0-)
     D36.10 Benign neoplasm of peripheral nerves and ▽
            autonomic nervous system, unspecified
     D36.11 Benign neoplasm of peripheral nerves and
            autonomic nervous system of face, head, and neck
     D36.12 Benign neoplasm of peripheral nerves and
            autonomic nervous system, upper limb, including shoulder
     D36.13 Benign neoplasm of peripheral nerves and
            autonomic nervous system of lower limb, including hip
     D36.14 Benign neoplasm of peripheral nerves and
            autonomic nervous system of thorax
     D36.15 Benign neoplasm of peripheral nerves and
            autonomic nervous system of abdomen
     D36.16 Benign neoplasm of peripheral nerves and
            autonomic nervous system of pelvis
     D36.17 Benign neoplasm of peripheral nerves and ▽
            autonomic nervous system of trunk, unspecified
     D36.7 Benign neoplasm of other specified sites
         Benign neoplasm of nose NOS
     D36.9 Benign neoplasm, unspecified site ▽

Benign neuroendocrine tumors (D3A)

√4ᵗʰ **D3A Benign neuroendocrine tumors**
     Code also any associated multiple endocrine neoplasia [MEN]
         syndromes (E31.2-)
     Use additional code to identify any associated endocrine syndrome,
         such as:
     carcinoid syndrome (E34.0)
     EXCLUDES 2   *benign pancreatic islet cell tumors (D13.7)*
√5ᵗʰ   **D3A.0 Benign** carcinoid tumors
     D3A.00 Benign carcinoid tumor of unspecified site ▽
         Carcinoid tumor NOS
     √6ᵗʰ **D3A.01 Benign carcinoid tumors of the** small intestine
         D3A.010 Benign carcinoid tumor of the duodenum
         D3A.011 Benign carcinoid tumor of the jejunum
         D3A.012 Benign carcinoid tumor of the ileum
         D3A.019 Benign carcinoid tumor of the small ▽
             intestine, unspecified portion
     √6ᵗʰ **D3A.02 Benign carcinoid tumors of the** appendix, large intestine, and rectum
         D3A.020 Benign carcinoid tumor of the appendix
         D3A.021 Benign carcinoid tumor of the cecum
         D3A.022 Benign carcinoid tumor of the ascending colon
         D3A.023 Benign carcinoid tumor of the transverse colon
         D3A.024 Benign carcinoid tumor of the descending colon
         D3A.025 Benign carcinoid tumor of the sigmoid colon
         D3A.026 Benign carcinoid tumor of the rectum
         D3A.029 Benign carcinoid tumor of the large ▽
             intestine, unspecified portion
             Benign carcinoid tumor of the colon NOS
     √6ᵗʰ **D3A.09 Benign carcinoid tumors of other sites**
         D3A.090 Benign carcinoid tumor of the bronchus and lung
         D3A.091 Benign carcinoid tumor of the thymus

✓ Additional Character Req   ✓x7ᵗʰ Placeholder Alert   Manifestation   HCC CMS-HCC Condition   ▽ Unspecified Code   ►◄ Revised Text   ● New Code   ▲ Revised Code Title

D3A.Ø92   Benign carcinoid tumor of the stomach

D3A.Ø93   Benign carcinoid tumor of the kidney

D3A.Ø94   Benign carcinoid tumor of the foregut, ▽
     unspecified

D3A.Ø95   Benign carcinoid tumor of the midgut, ▽
     unspecified

D3A.Ø96   Benign carcinoid tumor of the hindgut, ▽
     unspecified

D3A.Ø98   Benign carcinoid tumors of other sites

D3A.8   Other benign neuroendocrine tumors
     Neuroendocrine tumor NOS

Neoplasms of uncertain behavior, polycythemia vera and myelodysplastic syndromes (D37-D48)

NOTE   Categories D37-D44, and D48 classify by site neoplasms of uncertain behavior, i.e., histologic confirmation whether the neoplasm is malignant or benign cannot be made.

EXCLUDES 1   *neoplasms of unspecified behavior (D49.-)*

☑4th **D37   Neoplasm of uncertain behavior of oral cavity and digestive organs**

EXCLUDES 1   *stromal tumors of uncertain behavior of digestive system (D48.1)*

☑5th **D37.Ø   Neoplasm of uncertain behavior of lip, oral cavity and pharynx**

EXCLUDES 1   *neoplasm of uncertain behavior of aryepiglottic fold or interarytenoid fold, laryngeal aspect (D38.Ø)*
neoplasm of uncertain behavior of epiglottis NOS (D38.Ø)
neoplasm of uncertain behavior of skin of lip (D48.5)
neoplasm of uncertain behavior of suprahyoid portion of epiglottis (D38.Ø)

D37.Ø1   Neoplasm of uncertain behavior of lip
     Neoplasm of uncertain behavior of vermilion border of lip

D37.Ø2   Neoplasm of uncertain behavior of tongue

☑6th **D37.Ø3   Neoplasm of uncertain behavior of the major salivary glands**

D37.Ø3Ø   Neoplasm of uncertain behavior of the parotid salivary glands

D37.Ø31   Neoplasm of uncertain behavior of the sublingual salivary glands

D37.Ø32   Neoplasm of uncertain behavior of the submandibular salivary glands

D37.Ø39   Neoplasm of uncertain behavior of ▽
     the major salivary glands, unspecified

D37.Ø4   Neoplasm of uncertain behavior of the minor salivary glands
     Neoplasm of uncertain behavior of submucosal salivary glands of lip
     Neoplasm of uncertain behavior of submucosal salivary glands of cheek
     Neoplasm of uncertain behavior of submucosal salivary glands of hard palate
     Neoplasm of uncertain behavior of submucosal salivary glands of soft palate

D37.Ø5   Neoplasm of uncertain behavior of pharynx
     Neoplasm of uncertain behavior of aryepiglottic fold of pharynx NOS
     Neoplasm of uncertain behavior of hypopharyngeal aspect of aryepiglottic fold of pharynx
     Neoplasm of uncertain behavior of marginal zone of aryepiglottic fold of pharynx

D37.Ø9   Neoplasm of uncertain behavior of other specified sites of the oral cavity

D37.1   Neoplasm of uncertain behavior of stomach

D37.2   Neoplasm of uncertain behavior of small intestine

D37.3   Neoplasm of uncertain behavior of appendix

D37.4   Neoplasm of uncertain behavior of colon

D37.5   Neoplasm of uncertain behavior of rectum
     Neoplasm of uncertain behavior of rectosigmoid junction

D37.6   Neoplasm of uncertain behavior of liver, gallbladder and bile ducts
     Neoplasm of uncertain behavior of ampulla of Vater

D37.8   Neoplasm of uncertain behavior of other specified digestive organs
     Neoplasm of uncertain behavior of anal canal
     Neoplasm of uncertain behavior of anal sphincter
     Neoplasm of uncertain behavior of anus NOS
     Neoplasm of uncertain behavior of esophagus
     Neoplasm of uncertain behavior of intestine NOS
     Neoplasm of uncertain behavior of pancreas

EXCLUDES 1   *neoplasm of uncertain behavior of anal margin (D48.5)*
neoplasm of uncertain behavior of anal skin (D48.5)
neoplasm of uncertain behavior of perianal skin (D48.5)

D37.9   Neoplasm of uncertain behavior of digestive organ, ▽
     unspecified

☑4th **D38   Neoplasm of uncertain behavior of middle ear and respiratory and intrathoracic organs**

EXCLUDES 1   *neoplasm of uncertain behavior of heart (D48.7)*

D38.Ø   Neoplasm of uncertain behavior of larynx
     Neoplasm of uncertain behavior of aryepiglottic fold or interarytenoid fold, laryngeal aspect
     Neoplasm of uncertain behavior of epiglottis (suprahyoid portion)

EXCLUDES 1   *neoplasm of uncertain behavior of aryepiglottic fold or interarytenoid fold NOS (D37.Ø5)*
neoplasm of uncertain behavior of hypopharyngeal aspect of aryepiglottic fold (D37.Ø5)
neoplasm of uncertain behavior of marginal zone of aryepiglottic fold (D37.Ø5)

D38.1   Neoplasm of uncertain behavior of trachea, bronchus and lung

D38.2   Neoplasm of uncertain behavior of pleura

D38.3   Neoplasm of uncertain behavior of mediastinum

D38.4   Neoplasm of uncertain behavior of thymus

D38.5   Neoplasm of uncertain behavior of other respiratory organs
     Neoplasm of uncertain behavior of accessory sinuses
     Neoplasm of uncertain behavior of cartilage of nose
     Neoplasm of uncertain behavior of middle ear
     Neoplasm of uncertain behavior of nasal cavities

EXCLUDES 1   *neoplasm of uncertain behavior of ear (external) (skin) (D48.5)*
neoplasm of uncertain behavior of nose NOS (D48.7)
neoplasm of uncertain behavior of skin of nose (D48.5)

D38.6   Neoplasm of uncertain behavior of respiratory organ, ▽
     unspecified

☑4th **D39   Neoplasm of uncertain behavior of female genital organs**

D39.Ø   Neoplasm of uncertain behavior of uterus   ♀

☑5th **D39.1   Neoplasm of uncertain behavior of ovary**
     Use additional code to identify any functional activity

D39.1Ø   Neoplasm of uncertain behavior of unspecified ovary   ♀▽

D39.11   Neoplasm of uncertain behavior of right ovary   ♀

D39.12   Neoplasm of uncertain behavior of left ovary   ♀

D39.2   Neoplasm of uncertain behavior of placenta   Ⓜ♀
     Chorioadenoma destruens
     Invasive hydatidiform mole
     Malignant hydatidiform mole

EXCLUDES 1   *hydatidiform mole NOS (OØ1.9)*

D39.8   Neoplasm of uncertain behavior of other specified   ♀
     female genital organs
     Neoplasm of uncertain behavior of skin of female genital organs

D39.9   Neoplasm of uncertain behavior of female genital organ,   ♀▽
     unspecified

☑4th **D4Ø   Neoplasm of uncertain behavior of male genital organs**

D4Ø.Ø   Neoplasm of uncertain behavior of prostate   ♂

☑5th **D4Ø.1   Neoplasm of uncertain behavior of testis**

D4Ø.1Ø   Neoplasm of uncertain behavior of unspecified   ♂▽
     testis

D4Ø.11   Neoplasm of uncertain behavior of right testis   ♂

D4Ø.12   Neoplasm of uncertain behavior of left testis   ♂

D4Ø.8   Neoplasm of uncertain behavior of other specified male   ♂
     genital organs
     Neoplasm of uncertain behavior of skin of male genital organs

D4Ø.9   Neoplasm of uncertain behavior of male genital organ,   ♂▽
     unspecified

EXCLUDES 1 Not coded here   **EXCLUDES 2** Not included here   Ⓝ Newborn Age: 0   Ⓟ Pediatric Age: 0-17   Ⓜ Maternity Age: 12-55   Ⓐ Adult Age: 15-124

490   ICD-10-CM 2018

☑4ᵗʰ **D41**   **Neoplasm of uncertain behavior of** urinary organs

    ✓5ᵗʰ **D41.0**   **Neoplasm of uncertain behavior of** kidney
       EXCLUDES 1   *neoplasm of uncertain behavior of renal pelvis (D41.1-)*

       D41.00   **Neoplasm of uncertain behavior of unspecified** ▽
             kidney

       D41.01   **Neoplasm of uncertain behavior of** right **kidney**

       D41.02   **Neoplasm of uncertain behavior of** left **kidney**

    ✓5ᵗʰ **D41.1**   **Neoplasm of uncertain behavior of** renal pelvis

       D41.10   **Neoplasm of uncertain behavior of unspecified** ▽
             renal pelvis

       D41.11   **Neoplasm of uncertain behavior of** right **renal pelvis**

       D41.12   **Neoplasm of uncertain behavior of** left **renal pelvis**

    ✓5ᵗʰ **D41.2**   **Neoplasm of uncertain behavior of** ureter

       D41.20   **Neoplasm of uncertain behavior of unspecified** ▽
             ureter

       D41.21   **Neoplasm of uncertain behavior of** right **ureter**

       D41.22   **Neoplasm of uncertain behavior of** left **ureter**

    D41.3   **Neoplasm of uncertain behavior of** urethra

    D41.4   **Neoplasm of uncertain behavior of** bladder

    D41.8   **Neoplasm of uncertain behavior of other specified urinary organs**

    D41.9   **Neoplasm of uncertain behavior of unspecified urinary** ▽
      organ

☑4ᵗʰ **D42**   **Neoplasm of uncertain behavior of** meninges

    D42.0   **Neoplasm of uncertain behavior of** cerebral **meninges** ᴴᶜᶜ

    D42.1   **Neoplasm of uncertain behavior of** spinal **meninges** ᴴᶜᶜ

    D42.9   **Neoplasm of uncertain behavior of meninges,** ᴴᶜᶜ ▽
      unspecified

☑4ᵗʰ **D43**   **Neoplasm of uncertain behavior of** brain and central nervous system
    EXCLUDES 1   *neoplasm of uncertain behavior of peripheral nerves and autonomic nervous system (D48.2)*

    D43.0   **Neoplasm of uncertain behavior of** brain, supratentorial ᴴᶜᶜ
      Neoplasm of uncertain behavior of cerebral ventricle
      Neoplasm of uncertain behavior of cerebrum
      Neoplasm of uncertain behavior of frontal lobe
      Neoplasm of uncertain behavior of occipital lobe
      Neoplasm of uncertain behavior of parietal lobe
      Neoplasm of uncertain behavior of temporal lobe
      EXCLUDES 1   *neoplasm of uncertain behavior of fourth ventricle (D43.1)*

    D43.1   **Neoplasm of uncertain behavior of** brain, infratentorial ᴴᶜᶜ
      Neoplasm of uncertain behavior of brain stem
      Neoplasm of uncertain behavior of cerebellum
      Neoplasm of uncertain behavior of fourth ventricle

    D43.2   **Neoplasm of uncertain behavior of** brain, unspecified ᴴᶜᶜ ▽

    D43.3   **Neoplasm of uncertain behavior of** cranial nerves ᴴᶜᶜ

    D43.4   **Neoplasm of uncertain behavior of** spinal cord ᴴᶜᶜ

    D43.8   **Neoplasm of uncertain behavior of other** specified ᴴᶜᶜ
      parts of central nervous system

    D43.9   **Neoplasm of uncertain behavior of central nervous** ᴴᶜᶜ ▽
      system, unspecified
      Neoplasm of uncertain behavior of nervous system (central) NOS

☑4ᵗʰ **D44**   **Neoplasm of uncertain behavior of** endocrine glands
    EXCLUDES 1   *multiple endocrine adenomatosis (E31.2-)*
           multiple endocrine neoplasia (E31.2-)
           neoplasm of uncertain behavior of endocrine pancreas (D37.8)
           neoplasm of uncertain behavior of ovary (D39.1-)
           neoplasm of uncertain behavior of testis (D40.1-)
           neoplasm of uncertain behavior of thymus (D38.4)

    D44.0   **Neoplasm of uncertain behavior of** thyroid gland

    ✓5ᵗʰ **D44.1**   **Neoplasm of uncertain behavior of** adrenal gland
      Use additional code to identify any functional activity

       D44.10   **Neoplasm of uncertain behavior of unspecified** ▽
             adrenal gland

       D44.11   **Neoplasm of uncertain behavior of** right **adrenal gland**

       D44.12   **Neoplasm of uncertain behavior of** left **adrenal gland**

    D44.2   **Neoplasm of uncertain behavior of** parathyroid gland

    D44.3   **Neoplasm of uncertain behavior of** pituitary gland ᴴᶜᶜ
      Use additional code to identify any functional activity

    D44.4   **Neoplasm of uncertain behavior of** craniopharyngeal ᴴᶜᶜ
      duct

    D44.5   **Neoplasm of uncertain behavior of** pineal gland ᴴᶜᶜ

    D44.6   **Neoplasm of uncertain behavior of** carotid body ᴴᶜᶜ

    D44.7   **Neoplasm of uncertain behavior of** aortic body and ᴴᶜᶜ
      other paraganglia

    D44.9   **Neoplasm of uncertain behavior of unspecified** ▽
      endocrine gland

D45   **Polycythemia vera** ᴴᶜᶜ
    EXCLUDES 1   *familial polycythemia (D75.0)*
           secondary polycythemia (D75.1)
    DEF: Abnormal proliferation of all bone marrow elements, increased red cell mass, and total blood volume; unknown etiology, frequently associated with splenomegaly, leukocytosis, and thrombocythemia.

☑4ᵗʰ **D46**   **Myelodysplastic syndromes**
    Use additional code for adverse effect, if applicable, to identify drug (T36-T50 with fifth or sixth character 5)
    EXCLUDES 2   *drug-induced aplastic anemia (D61.1)*

    D46.0   **Refractory anemia** without ring sideroblasts, **so stated** ᴴᶜᶜ
      Refractory anemia without sideroblasts, without excess of blasts

    D46.1   **Refractory anemia** with ring sideroblasts ᴴᶜᶜ
      RARS

    ✓5ᵗʰ **D46.2**   **Refractory anemia** with excess of blasts [RAEB]

       D46.20   **Refractory anemia with excess of blasts,** ᴴᶜᶜ ▽
             unspecified
             RAEB NOS

       D46.21   **Refractory anemia with excess of** blasts 1 ᴴᶜᶜ
             RAEB 1

       D46.22   **Refractory anemia with excess of** blasts 2 ᴴᶜᶜ
             RAEB 2

    D46.A   **Refractory** cytopenia with multilineage dysplasia ᴴᶜᶜ

    D46.B   **Refractory** cytopenia with multilineage dysplasia ᴴᶜᶜ
      and ring sideroblasts
      RCMD RS

    D46.C   **Myelodysplastic syndrome** with isolated del(5q) ᴴᶜᶜ
      chromosomal abnormality
      Myelodysplastic syndrome with 5q deletion
      5q minus syndrome NOS

    D46.4   **Refractory anemia, unspecified** ᴴᶜᶜ ▽

    D46.Z   **Other myelodysplastic syndromes** ᴴᶜᶜ
      EXCLUDES 1   *chronic myelomonocytic leukemia (C93.1-)*

    D46.9   **Myelodysplastic syndrome, unspecified** ᴴᶜᶜ ▽
      Myelodysplasia NOS

☑4ᵗʰ **D47**   **Other neoplasms of uncertain behavior of** lymphoid, hematopoietic and related tissue

▲   ✓5ᵗʰ **D47.0**   **Mast cell neoplasms of uncertain behavior**
      ~~Indolent systemic mastocytosis~~
      ~~Mast cell tumor NOS~~
      ~~Mastocytoma NOS~~
      EXCLUDES 1   ▶*congenital cutaneous mastocytosis (Q82.2-)*
             histiocytic neoplasms of uncertain behavior (D47.Z9)
             malignant mast cell neoplasm (C96.2-)◀
             ~~*mastocytosis (congenital) (cutaneous) (Q82.2)*~~

●   **D47.01**   **Cutaneous mastocytosis**
             Diffuse cutaneous mastocytosis
             Maculopapular cutaneous mastocytosis
             Solitary mastocytoma
             Telangiectasia macularis eruptiva perstans
             Urticaria pigmentosa
             EXCLUDES 1   *congenital (diffuse) (maculopapular) cutaneous mastocytosis (Q82.2)*
                       congenital urticaria pigmentosa (Q82.2)
                       extracutaneous mastocytoma (D47.09)

☑ Additional Character Req   ✓×7ᵗʰ Placeholder Alert   Manifestation   ᴴᶜᶜ CMS-HCC Condition   ▽ Unspecified Code   ▶◀ Revised Text   ● New Code   ▲ Revised Code Title

●   **D47.02**   **Systemic mastocytosis**
Indolent systemic mastocytosis
Isolated bone marrow mastocytosis
Smoldering systemic mastocytosis
Systemic mastocytosis, with an associated
    hematological non-mast cell lineage disease
    (SM-AHNMD)
Code also, if applicable, any associated hematological
    non-mast cell lineage disease, such as:
    acute myeloid leukemia (C92.6-, C92.A-)
    chronic myelomonocytic leukemia (C93.1-)
    essential thrombocytosis (D47.3)
    hypereosinophilic syndrome (D72.1)
    myelodysplastic syndrome (D46.9)
    myeloproliferative syndrome (D47.1)
    non-Hodgkin lymphoma (C82-C85)
    plasma cell myeloma (C90.0-)
    polycythemia vera (D45)
    EXCLUDES 1   *aggressive systemic mastocytosis (C96.21)*
               mast cell leukemia (C94.3-)

●   **D47.09**   **Other mast cell neoplasms of uncertain behavior**
Extracutaneous mastocytoma
Mast cell tumor NOS
Mastocytoma NOS
Mastocytosis NOS

D47.1   **Chronic myeloproliferative disease**   `HCC`
Chronic neutrophilic leukemia
Myeloproliferative disease, unspecified
    EXCLUDES 1   *atypical chronic myeloid leukemia BCR/ABL-negative*
               (C92.2-)
               chronic myeloid leukemia BCR/ABL-positive (C92.1-)
               myelofibrosis NOS (D75.81)
               myelophthisic anemia (D61.82)
               myelophthisis (D61.82)
               secondary myelofibrosis NOS (D75.81)

D47.2   **Monoclonal gammopathy**
Monoclonal gammopathy of undetermined significance [MGUS]

D47.3   **Essential (hemorrhagic) thrombocythemia**   `HCC`
Essential thrombocytosis
Idiopathic hemorrhagic thrombocythemia

D47.4   **Osteomyelofibrosis**   `HCC`
Chronic idiopathic myelofibrosis
Myelofibrosis (idiopathic) (with myeloid metaplasia)
Myelosclerosis (megakaryocytic) with myeloid metaplasia
Secondary myelofibrosis in myeloproliferative disease
    EXCLUDES 1   *acute myelofibrosis (C94.4-)*

✓5th   **D47.Z**   **Other specified neoplasms of uncertain behavior of lymphoid, hematopoietic and related tissue**

    D47.Z1   **Post-transplant lymphoproliferative**   `HCC`
               disorder (PTLD)
               Code first complications of transplanted organs and
                  tissue (T86.-)
               DEF: Excessive proliferation of B-cell lymphocytes
               following Epstein-Barr virus infection in organ
               transplant patients; may progress to non-Hodgkin
               lymphoma.

    D47.Z2   **Castleman disease**   `HCC`
               Code also if applicable human herpesvirus 8 infection
                  (B10.89)
               EXCLUDES 2   *Kaposi's sarcoma (C46-)*

    D47.Z9   **Other specified neoplasms of uncertain**   `HCC`
               behavior of lymphoid, hematopoietic and related
               tissue
               Histiocytic tumors of uncertain behavior

D47.9   **Neoplasm of uncertain behavior of lymphoid,**   `HCC` ▽
     hematopoietic and related tissue, unspecified
     Lymphoproliferative disease NOS

✓4th   **D48**   **Neoplasm of uncertain behavior of other and unspecified sites**
    EXCLUDES 1   *neurofibromatosis (nonmalignant) (Q85.0-)*

D48.0   **Neoplasm of uncertain behavior of bone and articular cartilage**
    EXCLUDES 1   *neoplasm of uncertain behavior of cartilage of ear*
               (D48.1)
               neoplasm of uncertain behavior of cartilage of larynx
               (D38.0)
               neoplasm of uncertain behavior of cartilage of nose
               (D38.5)
               neoplasm of uncertain behavior of connective tissue of
               eyelid (D48.1)
               neoplasm of uncertain behavior of synovia (D48.1)

D48.1   **Neoplasm of uncertain behavior of connective and other soft tissue**
Neoplasm of uncertain behavior of connective tissue of ear
Neoplasm of uncertain behavior of connective tissue of eyelid
Stromal tumors of uncertain behavior of digestive system
    EXCLUDES 1   *neoplasm of uncertain behavior of articular cartilage*
               (D48.0)
               neoplasm of uncertain behavior of cartilage of larynx
               (D38.0)
               neoplasm of uncertain behavior of cartilage of nose
               (D38.5)
               neoplasm of uncertain behavior of connective tissue of
               breast (D48.6-)

D48.2   **Neoplasm of uncertain behavior of peripheral nerves and autonomic nervous system**
    EXCLUDES 1   *neoplasm of uncertain behavior of peripheral nerves of*
               orbit (D48.7)

D48.3   **Neoplasm of uncertain behavior of retroperitoneum**

D48.4   **Neoplasm of uncertain behavior of peritoneum**

D48.5   **Neoplasm of uncertain behavior of skin**
Neoplasm of uncertain behavior of anal margin
Neoplasm of uncertain behavior of anal skin
Neoplasm of uncertain behavior of perianal skin
Neoplasm of uncertain behavior of skin of breast
    EXCLUDES 1   *neoplasm of uncertain behavior of anus NOS (D37.8)*
               neoplasm of uncertain behavior of skin of genital
               organs (D39.8, D40.8)
               neoplasm of uncertain behavior of vermilion border of
               lip (D37.0)

✓5th   **D48.6**   **Neoplasm of uncertain behavior of breast**
Neoplasm of uncertain behavior of connective tissue of breast
Cystosarcoma phyllodes
    EXCLUDES 1   *neoplasm of uncertain behavior of skin of breast*
               (D48.5)

    D48.60   **Neoplasm of uncertain behavior of unspecified**   ▽
               breast

    D48.61   **Neoplasm of uncertain behavior of right breast**

    D48.62   **Neoplasm of uncertain behavior of left breast**

D48.7   **Neoplasm of uncertain behavior of other specified sites**
Neoplasm of uncertain behavior of eye
Neoplasm of uncertain behavior of heart
Neoplasm of uncertain behavior of peripheral nerves of orbit
    EXCLUDES 1   *neoplasm of uncertain behavior of connective tissue*
               (D48.1)
               neoplasm of uncertain behavior of skin of eyelid
               (D48.5)

D48.9   **Neoplasm of uncertain behavior, unspecified**   ▽

Neoplasms of unspecified behavior (D49)

✓4th   **D49**   **Neoplasms of unspecified behavior**
    NOTE   Category D49 classifies by site neoplasms of unspecified
             morphology and behavior. The term "mass", unless
             otherwise stated, is not to be regarded as a neoplastic
             growth.
    INCLUDES   "growth" NOS
             neoplasm NOS
             new growth NOS
             tumor NOS
    EXCLUDES 1   *neoplasms of uncertain behavior (D37-D44, D48)*

D49.0   **Neoplasm of unspecified behavior of digestive system**
    EXCLUDES 1   *neoplasm of unspecified behavior of margin of anus*
               (D49.2)
               neoplasm of unspecified behavior of perianal skin
               (D49.2)
               neoplasm of unspecified behavior of skin of anus
               (D49.2)

D49.1   **Neoplasm of unspecified behavior of respiratory system**

EXCLUDES 1 Not coded here   **EXCLUDES 2** Not included here   N Newborn Age: 0   P Pediatric Age: 0-17   M Maternity Age: 12-55   A Adult Age: 15-124

D49.2   **Neoplasm of unspecified behavior of** bone, soft tissue, and skin

     EXCLUDES 1   *neoplasm of unspecified behavior of anal canal (D49.0)*

                     neoplasm of unspecified behavior of anus NOS (D49.0)

                     neoplasm of unspecified behavior of bone marrow (D49.89)

                     neoplasm of unspecified behavior of cartilage of larynx (D49.1)

                     neoplasm of unspecified behavior of cartilage of nose (D49.1)

                     neoplasm of unspecified behavior of connective tissue of breast (D49.3)

                     neoplasm of unspecified behavior of skin of genital organs (D49.59)

                     neoplasm of unspecified behavior of vermilion border of lip (D49.0)

D49.3   **Neoplasm of unspecified behavior of** breast

     EXCLUDES 1   *neoplasm of unspecified behavior of skin of breast (D49.2)*

D49.4   **Neoplasm of unspecified behavior of** bladder

√5ᵗʰ   **D49.5**   **Neoplasm of unspecified behavior of other** genitourinary organs

     √6ᵗʰ   **D49.51**   **Neoplasm of unspecified behavior of** kidney

           D49.511   **Neoplasm of unspecified behavior of** right kidney

           D49.512   **Neoplasm of unspecified behavior of** left kidney

           D49.519   **Neoplasm of unspecified behavior of** unspecified kidney   ▽

       D49.59   **Neoplasm of unspecified behavior of other** genitourinary organ

D49.6   **Neoplasm of unspecified behavior of** brain   HCC

     EXCLUDES 1   *neoplasm of unspecified behavior of cerebral meninges (D49.7)*

                     neoplasm of unspecified behavior of cranial nerves (D49.7)

D49.7   **Neoplasm of unspecified behavior of** endocrine glands and other parts of nervous system

     EXCLUDES 1   *neoplasm of unspecified behavior of peripheral, sympathetic, and parasympathetic nerves and ganglia (D49.2)*

√5ᵗʰ   **D49.8**   **Neoplasm of unspecified behavior of other specified sites**

     EXCLUDES 1   *neoplasm of unspecified behavior of eyelid (skin) (D49.2)*

                     neoplasm of unspecified behavior of eyelid cartilage (D49.2)

                     neoplasm of unspecified behavior of great vessels (D49.2)

                     neoplasm of unspecified behavior of optic nerve (D49.7)

       D49.81   **Neoplasm of unspecified behavior of** retina and choroid

           Dark area on retina

           Retinal freckle

       D49.89   **Neoplasm of unspecified behavior of other specified sites**

D49.9   **Neoplasm of unspecified behavior of unspecified site**   ▽

Chapter 3. Disease of the Blood and Blood-Forming Organs and Certain Disorders Involving the Immune Mechanism (D5Ø–D89)

Chapter Specific Coding Guidelines and Examples
Reserved for future guideline expansion.

Chapter 3. Diseases of the Blood and Blood-forming Organs and Certain Disorders Involving the Immune Mechanism (D50-D89)

EXCLUDES 2   autoimmune disease (systemic) NOS (M35.9)
certain conditions originating in the perinatal period (P00-P96)
complications of pregnancy, childbirth and the puerperium (O00-O9A)
congenital malformations, deformations and chromosomal
    abnormalities (Q00-Q99)
endocrine, nutritional and metabolic diseases (E00-E88)
human immunodeficiency virus [HIV] disease (B20)
injury, poisoning and certain other consequences of external causes
    (S00-T88)
neoplasms (C00-D49)
symptoms, signs and abnormal clinical and laboratory findings, not
    elsewhere classified (R00-R94)

This chapter contains the following blocks:

D50-D53	Nutritional anemias
D55-D59	Hemolytic anemias
D60-D64	Aplastic and other anemias and other bone marrow failure syndromes
D65-D69	Coagulation defects, purpura and other hemorrhagic conditions
D70-D77	Other disorders of blood and blood-forming organs
D78	Intraoperative and postprocedural complications of the spleen
D80-D89	Certain disorders involving the immune mechanism

Nutritional anemias (D50-D53)

D50   **Iron deficiency anemia**
     INCLUDES   asiderotic anemia
                hypochromic anemia

    D50.0   **Iron deficiency anemia secondary to blood loss (chronic)**
       Posthemorrhagic anemia (chronic)
       EXCLUDES 1   acute posthemorrhagic anemia (D62)
                     congenital anemia from fetal blood loss (P61.3)

    D50.1   **Sideropenic dysphagia**
       Kelly-Paterson syndrome
       Plummer-Vinson syndrome

    D50.8   **Other iron deficiency anemias**
       Iron deficiency anemia due to inadequate dietary iron intake

    D50.9   **Iron deficiency anemia, unspecified**   ▽

D51   **Vitamin B12 deficiency anemia**
     EXCLUDES 1   vitamin B12 deficiency (E53.8)

    D51.0   **Vitamin B12 deficiency anemia due to intrinsic factor deficiency**
       Addison anemia
       Biermer anemia
       Pernicious (congenital) anemia
       Congenital intrinsic factor deficiency
       DEF: Chronic progressive anemia due to vitamin B12 malabsorption; caused by lack of secretion of intrinsic factor, which is produced by the gastric mucosa of the stomach.

    D51.1   **Vitamin B12 deficiency anemia due to selective vitamin B12 malabsorption with proteinuria**
       Imerslund (Gräsbeck) syndrome
       Megaloblastic hereditary anemia

    D51.2   **Transcobalamin II deficiency**

    D51.3   **Other dietary vitamin B12 deficiency anemia**
       Vegan anemia

    D51.8   **Other vitamin B12 deficiency anemias**

    D51.9   **Vitamin B12 deficiency anemia, unspecified**   ▽

D52   **Folate deficiency anemia**
     EXCLUDES 1   folate deficiency without anemia (E53.8)

    D52.0   **Dietary folate deficiency anemia**
       Nutritional megaloblastic anemia
       DEF: The result of a poor diet with inadequate intake of folate, which is needed to produce healthy red blood cells.

    D52.1   **Drug-induced folate deficiency anemia**
       Use additional code for adverse effect, if applicable, to identify drug (T36-T50 with fifth or sixth character 5)

    D52.8   **Other folate deficiency anemias**

    D52.9   **Folate deficiency anemia, unspecified**   ▽
       Folic acid deficiency anemia NOS

D53   **Other nutritional anemias**
     INCLUDES   megaloblastic anemia unresponsive to vitamin B12 or folate therapy

    D53.0   **Protein deficiency anemia**
       Amino-acid deficiency anemia
       Orotaciduric anemia
       EXCLUDES 1   Lesch-Nyhan syndrome (E79.1)

    D53.1   **Other megaloblastic anemias, not elsewhere classified**
       Megaloblastic anemia NOS
       EXCLUDES 1   Di Guglielmo's disease (C94.0)

    D53.2   **Scorbutic anemia**
       EXCLUDES 1   scurvy (E54)

    D53.8   **Other specified nutritional anemias**
       Anemia associated with deficiency of copper
       Anemia associated with deficiency of molybdenum
       Anemia associated with deficiency of zinc
       EXCLUDES 1   nutritional deficiencies without anemia, such as:
                    copper deficiency NOS (E61.0)
                    molybdenum deficiency NOS (E61.5)
                    zinc deficiency NOS (E60)

    D53.9   **Nutritional anemia, unspecified**   ▽
       Simple chronic anemia
       EXCLUDES 1   anemia NOS (D64.9)

Hemolytic anemias (D55-D59)

D55   **Anemia due to enzyme disorders**
     EXCLUDES 1   drug-induced enzyme deficiency anemia (D59.2)

    D55.0   **Anemia due to glucose-6-phosphate dehydrogenase [G6PD] deficiency**   HCC
       Favism
       G6PD deficiency anemia

    D55.1   **Anemia due to other disorders of glutathione metabolism**   HCC
       Anemia (due to) enzyme deficiencies, except G6PD, related to the hexose monophosphate [HMP] shunt pathway
       Anemia (due to) hemolytic nonspherocytic (hereditary), type I

    D55.2   **Anemia due to disorders of glycolytic enzymes**   HCC
       Hemolytic nonspherocytic (hereditary) anemia, type II
       Hexokinase deficiency anemia
       Pyruvate kinase [PK] deficiency anemia
       Triose-phosphate isomerase deficiency anemia
       EXCLUDES 1   disorders of glycolysis not associated with anemia (E74.8)

    D55.3   **Anemia due to disorders of nucleotide metabolism**   HCC

    D55.8   **Other anemias due to enzyme disorders**   HCC

    D55.9   **Anemia due to enzyme disorder, unspecified**   HCC ▽

D56   **Thalassemia**
     EXCLUDES 1   sickle-cell thalassemia (D57.4-)

    D56.0   **Alpha thalassemia**   HCC
       Alpha thalassemia major
       Hemoglobin H Constant Spring
       Hemoglobin H disease
       Hydrops fetalis due to alpha thalassemia
       Severe alpha thalassemia
       Triple gene defect alpha thalassemia
       Use additional code, if applicable, for hydrops fetalis due to alpha thalassemia (P56.99)
       EXCLUDES 1   alpha thalassemia trait or minor (D56.3)
                    asymptomatic alpha thalassemia (D56.3)
                    hydrops fetalis due to isoimmunization (P56.0)
                    hydrops fetalis not due to immune hemolysis (P83.2)
       DEF: HBA1 and HBA2 genetic variant of chromosome 16 prevalent among those of African and Southeast Asian descent; associated with a wide spectrum of anemic presentation; includes hemoglobin H disease subtypes.

    D56.1   **Beta thalassemia**   HCC
       Beta thalassemia major
       Cooley's anemia
       Homozygous beta thalassemia
       Severe beta thalassemia
       Thalassemia intermedia
       Thalassemia major
       EXCLUDES 1   beta thalassemia minor (D56.3)
                    beta thalassemia trait (D56.3)
                    delta-beta thalassemia (D56.2)
                    hemoglobin E-beta thalassemia (D56.5)
                    sickle-cell beta thalassemia (D57.4-)

EXCLUDES 1 Not coded here   EXCLUDES 2 Not included here   N Newborn Age: 0   P Pediatric Age: 0-17   M Maternity Age: 12-55   A Adult Age: 15-124

496   ICD-10-CM 2018

Chapter 3. Disease of the Blood and Blood-Forming Organs

Thalassemia

Misshapen RBC

Misshapen RBC

Healthy RBC

Sickle cell

Sickle cells

Normal RBCs

D56.2   ~~Delta-beta~~ **thalassemia**   `HCC`
    Homozygous delta-beta thalassemia
    EXCLUDES 1   *delta-beta thalassemia minor (D56.3)*
            delta-beta thalassemia trait (D56.3)

D56.3   **Thalassemia** minor
    Alpha thalassemia minor
    Alpha thalassemia silent carrier
    Alpha thalassemia trait
    Beta thalassemia minor
    Beta thalassemia trait
    Delta-beta thalassemia minor
    Delta-beta thalassemia trait
    Thalassemia trait NOS
    EXCLUDES 1   *alpha thalassemia (D56.0)*
            beta thalassemia (D56.1)
            delta-beta thalassemia (D56.2)
            hemoglobin E-beta thalassemia (D56.5)
            sickle-cell trait (D57.3)
    DEF: Solitary abnormal gene that identifies a carrier of the disease, yet with an absence of symptoms or a clinically mild anemic presentation.

D56.4   **Hereditary persistence of fetal hemoglobin [HPFH]**   `HCC`

D56.5   **Hemoglobin E-beta** thalassemia   `HCC`
    EXCLUDES 1   *beta thalassemia (D56.1)*
            beta thalassemia minor (D56.3)
            beta thalassemia trait (D56.3)
            delta-beta thalassemia (D56.2)
            delta-beta thalassemia trait (D56.3)
            hemoglobin E disease (D58.2)
            other hemoglobinopathies (D58.2)
            sickle-cell beta thalassemia (D57.4-)

D56.8   **Other thalassemias**   `HCC`
    Dominant thalassemia
    Hemoglobin C thalassemia
    Mixed thalassemia
    Thalassemia with other hemoglobinopathy
    EXCLUDES 1   *hemoglobin C disease (D58.2)*
            hemoglobin E disease (D58.2)
            other hemoglobinopathies (D58.2)
            sickle-cell anemia (D57.-)
            sickle-cell thalassemia (D57.4)

D56.9   **Thalassemia, unspecified**   ▽
    Mediterranean anemia (with other hemoglobinopathy)

✔4ᵗʰ **D57**   **Sickle-cell disorders**
    Use additional code for any associated fever (R50.81)
    EXCLUDES 1   *other hemoglobinopathies (D58.-)*

✔5ᵗʰ   **D57.0**   **Hb-SS disease** with crisis
    Sickle-cell disease NOS with crisis
    Hb-SS disease with vasoocclusive pain
     D57.00   **Hb-SS disease with crisis, unspecified**   `HCC` ▽
     D57.01   **Hb-SS disease with** acute chest syndrome   `HCC`
     D57.02   **Hb-SS disease with** splenic sequestration   `HCC`

    D57.1   **Sickle-cell disease** without crisis   `HCC` ▽
    Hb-SS disease without crisis
    Sickle-cell anemia NOS
    Sickle-cell disease NOS
    Sickle-cell disorder NOS

✔5ᵗʰ   **D57.2**   **Sickle-cell/Hb-C disease**
    Hb-SC disease
    Hb-S/Hb-C disease
     D57.20   **Sickle-cell/Hb-C disease** without crisis   `HCC` ▽
✔6ᵗʰ   **D57.21**   **Sickle-cell/Hb-C disease** with crisis
       D57.211   **Sickle-cell/Hb-C disease with** acute chest syndrome   `HCC`
       D57.212   **Sickle-cell/Hb-C disease with** splenic sequestration   `HCC`
       D57.219   **Sickle-cell/Hb-C disease with crisis, unspecified**   `HCC` ▽
         Sickle-cell/Hb-C disease with crisis NOS

    D57.3   **Sickle-cell** trait   `HCC`
    Hb-S trait
    Heterozygous hemoglobin S
    DEF: Heterozygous genetic makeup characterized by one gene for normal hemoglobin and one for sickle-cell hemoglobin; clinical disease rarely present.

✔5ᵗʰ   **D57.4**   **Sickle-cell** thalassemia
    Sickle-cell beta thalassemia
    Thalassemia Hb-S disease
     D57.40   **Sickle-cell thalassemia** without crisis   `HCC` ▽
         Microdrepanocytosis
         Sickle-cell thalassemia NOS
✔6ᵗʰ   **D57.41**   **Sickle-cell thalassemia** with crisis
         Sickle-cell thalassemia with vasoocclusive pain
       D57.411   **Sickle-cell thalassemia with** acute chest syndrome   `HCC`
       D57.412   **Sickle-cell thalassemia with** splenic sequestration   `HCC`
       D57.419   **Sickle-cell thalassemia with crisis, unspecified**   `HCC` ▽
         Sickle-cell thalassemia with crisis NOS

✔5ᵗʰ   **D57.8**   **Other sickle-cell disorders**
    Hb-SD disease
    Hb-SE disease
     D57.80   **Other sickle-cell disorders** without crisis   `HCC` ▽
✔6ᵗʰ   **D57.81**   **Other sickle-cell disorders** with crisis
       D57.811   **Other sickle-cell disorders with** acute chest syndrome   `HCC`
       D57.812   **Other sickle-cell disorders with** splenic sequestration   `HCC`
       D57.819   **Other sickle-cell disorders with crisis, unspecified**   `HCC` ▽
         Other sickle-cell disorders with crisis NOS

✔4ᵗʰ **D58**   **Other** hereditary **hemolytic anemias**
    EXCLUDES 1   *hemolytic anemia of the newborn (P55.-)*

    D58.0   **Hereditary** spherocytosis   `HCC`
    Acholuric (familial) jaundice
    Congenital (spherocytic) hemolytic icterus
    Minkowski-Chauffard syndrome

    D58.1   **Hereditary** elliptocytosis   `HCC`
    Elliptocytosis (congenital)
    Ovalocytosis (congenital) (hereditary)

✔ Additional Character Req   ✔x7ᵗʰ Placeholder Alert   Manifestation   `HCC` CMS-HCC Condition   ▽ Unspecified Code   ►◄ Revised Text   ● New Code   ▲ Revised Code Title

ICD-10-CM 2018   **497**

D56.2–D58.1

D58.2 Other hemoglobinopathies HCC
- Abnormal hemoglobin NOS
- Congenital Heinz body anemia
- Hb-C disease
- Hb-D disease
- Hb-E disease
- Hemoglobinopathy NOS
- Unstable hemoglobin hemolytic disease
  - EXCLUDES 1 familial polycythemia (D75.0)
    - Hb-M disease (D74.0)
    - hemoglobin E-beta thalassemia (D56.5)
    - hereditary persistence of fetal hemoglobin [HPFH] (D56.4)
    - high-altitude polycythemia (D75.1)
    - methemoglobinemia (D74.-)
    - other hemoglobinopathies with thalassemia (D56.8)

D58.8 Other specified hereditary hemolytic anemias HCC
- Stomatocytosis

D58.9 Hereditary hemolytic anemia, unspecified HCC ▽

✓4ᵗʰ D59 Acquired hemolytic anemia
- DEF: Non-hereditary anemia characterized by premature destruction of red blood cells; caused by infectious organisms, poisons, and physical agents.

D59.0 Drug-induced autoimmune hemolytic anemia HCC
- Use additional code for adverse effect, if applicable, to identify drug (T36-T50 with fifth or sixth character 5)

D59.1 Other autoimmune hemolytic anemias HCC
- Autoimmune hemolytic disease (cold type) (warm type)
- Chronic cold hemagglutinin disease
- Cold agglutinin disease
- Cold agglutinin hemoglobinuria
- Cold type (secondary) (symptomatic) hemolytic anemia
- Warm type (secondary) (symptomatic) hemolytic anemia
  - EXCLUDES 1 Evans syndrome (D69.41)
    - hemolytic disease of newborn (P55.-)
    - paroxysmal cold hemoglobinuria (D59.6)

D59.2 Drug-induced nonautoimmune hemolytic anemia HCC
- Drug-induced enzyme deficiency anemia
- Use additional code for adverse effect, if applicable, to identify drug (T36-T50 with fifth or sixth character 5)

D59.3 Hemolytic-uremic syndrome HCC
- Use additional code to identify associated:
  - E. coli infection (B96.2-)
  - Pneumococcal pneumonia (J13)
  - Shigella dysenteriae (A03.9)

D59.4 Other nonautoimmune hemolytic anemias HCC
- Mechanical hemolytic anemia
- Microangiopathic hemolytic anemia
- Toxic hemolytic anemia

D59.5 Paroxysmal nocturnal hemoglobinuria [Marchiafava-Micheli] HCC
- EXCLUDES 1 hemoglobinuria NOS (R82.3)

D59.6 Hemoglobinuria due to hemolysis from other external causes HCC
- Hemoglobinuria from exertion
- March hemoglobinuria
- Paroxysmal cold hemoglobinuria
- Use additional code (Chapter 20) to identify external cause
  - EXCLUDES 1 hemoglobinuria NOS (R82.3)

D59.8 Other acquired hemolytic anemias HCC

D59.9 Acquired hemolytic anemia, unspecified HCC ▽
- Idiopathic hemolytic anemia, chronic

Aplastic and other anemias and other bone marrow failure syndromes (D60-D64)

✓4ᵗʰ D60 Acquired pure red cell aplasia [erythroblastopenia]
- INCLUDES red cell aplasia (acquired) (adult) (with thymoma)
- EXCLUDES 1 congenital red cell aplasia (D61.01)

D60.0 Chronic acquired pure red cell aplasia HCC
D60.1 Transient acquired pure red cell aplasia HCC
D60.8 Other acquired pure red cell aplasias HCC
D60.9 Acquired pure red cell aplasia, unspecified HCC ▽

✓4ᵗʰ D61 Other aplastic anemias and other bone marrow failure syndromes
- EXCLUDES 1 neutropenia (D70.-)
- AHA: 2014, 4Q, 22

✓5ᵗʰ D61.0 Constitutional aplastic anemia
- **D61.01 Constitutional (pure) red blood cell aplasia** HCC
  - Blackfan-Diamond syndrome
  - Congenital (pure) red cell aplasia
  - Familial hypoplastic anemia
  - Primary (pure) red cell aplasia
  - Red cell (pure) aplasia of infants
    - EXCLUDES 1 acquired red cell aplasia (D60.9)
- **D61.09 Other constitutional aplastic anemia**
  - Fanconi's anemia
  - Pancytopenia with malformations

D61.1 Drug-induced aplastic anemia HCC
- Use additional code for adverse effect, if applicable, to identify drug (T36-T50 with fifth or sixth character 5)

D61.2 Aplastic anemia due to other external agents HCC
- Code first, if applicable, toxic effects of substances chiefly nonmedicinal as to source (T51-T65)

D61.3 Idiopathic aplastic anemia HCC

✓5ᵗʰ D61.8 Other specified aplastic anemias and other bone marrow failure syndromes
- **✓6ᵗʰ D61.81 Pancytopenia**
  - EXCLUDES 1 pancytopenia (due to) (with) aplastic anemia (D61.9)
    - pancytopenia (due to) (with) bone marrow infiltration (D61.82)
    - pancytopenia (due to) (with) congenital (pure) red cell aplasia (D61.01)
    - pancytopenia (due to) (with) hairy cell leukemia (C91.4-)
    - pancytopenia (due to) (with) human immunodeficiency virus disease (B20)
    - pancytopenia (due to) (with) leukoerythroblastic anemia (D61.82)
    - pancytopenia (due to) (with) myeloproliferative disease (D47.1)
  - EXCLUDES 2 pancytopenia (due to) (with) myelodysplastic syndromes (D46.-)
  - DEF: Occurs when a person has a shortage of all three blood cells: white, red, and platelets.
  - **D61.810 Antineoplastic chemotherapy induced pancytopenia** HCC
    - EXCLUDES 2 aplastic anemia due to antineoplastic chemotherapy (D61.1)
  - **D61.811 Other drug-induced pancytopenia** HCC
    - EXCLUDES 2 aplastic anemia due to drugs (D61.1)
  - **D61.818 Other pancytopenia** HCC
- **D61.82 Myelophthisis** HCC
  - Leukoerythroblastic anemia
  - Myelophthisic anemia
  - Panmyelophthisis
  - Code also the underlying disorder, such as:
    - malignant neoplasm of breast (C50.-)
    - tuberculosis (A15.-)
  - EXCLUDES 1 idiopathic myelofibrosis (D47.1)
    - myelofibrosis NOS (D75.81)
    - myelofibrosis with myeloid metaplasia (D47.4)
    - primary myelofibrosis (D47.1)
    - secondary myelofibrosis (D75.81)
- **D61.89 Other specified aplastic anemias and other bone marrow failure syndromes** HCC

D61.9 Aplastic anemia, unspecified HCC ▽
- Hypoplastic anemia NOS
- Medullary hypoplasia

D62 Acute posthemorrhagic anemia
- EXCLUDES 1 anemia due to chronic blood loss (D50.0)
  - blood loss anemia NOS (D50.0)
  - congenital anemia from fetal blood loss (P61.3)

EXCLUDES 1 Not coded here   EXCLUDES 2 Not included here   N Newborn Age: 0   P Pediatric Age: 0-17   M Maternity Age: 12-55   A Adult Age: 15-124

498   ICD-10-CM 2018

☑4ᵗʰ **D63 Anemia in chronic diseases classified elsewhere**

  D63.0 *Anemia in neoplastic disease*
    Code first neoplasm (C00-D49)
    EXCLUDES 1 *anemia due to antineoplastic chemotherapy (D64.81)*
       aplastic anemia due to antineoplastic chemotherapy (D61.1)
    EXCLUDES 2 ▶*anemia due to antineoplastic chemotherapy (D64.81)*◄

  D63.1 *Anemia in chronic kidney disease*
    Erythropoietin resistant anemia (EPO resistant anemia)
    Code first underlying chronic kidney disease (CKD) (N18.-)

  D63.8 *Anemia in other chronic diseases classified elsewhere*
    Code first underlying disease, such as:
      diphyllobothriasis (B70.0)
      hookworm disease (B76.0-B76.9)
      hypothyroidism (E00.0-E03.9)
      malaria (B50.0-B54)
      symptomatic late syphilis (A52.79)
      tuberculosis (A18.89)

☑4ᵗʰ **D64 Other anemias**
    EXCLUDES 1 *refractory anemia (D46.-)*
      refractory anemia with excess blasts in transformation [RAEB T] (C92.0-)

  D64.0 **Hereditary sideroblastic anemia**   HCC
    Sex-linked hypochromic sideroblastic anemia

  D64.1 *Secondary sideroblastic anemia due to disease*   HCC
    Code first underlying disease

  D64.2 **Secondary sideroblastic anemia due to drugs and toxins**   HCC
    Code first poisoning due to drug or toxin, if applicable (T36-T65 with fifth or sixth character 1-4 or 6)
    Use additional code for adverse effect, if applicable, to identify drug (T36-T50 with fifth or sixth character 5)

  D64.3 **Other sideroblastic anemias**   HCC
    Sideroblastic anemia NOS
    Pyridoxine-responsive sideroblastic anemia NEC

  D64.4 **Congenital dyserythropoietic anemia**
    Dyshematopoietic anemia (congenital)
    EXCLUDES 1 *Blackfan-Diamond syndrome (D61.01)*
      Di Guglielmo's disease (C94.0)

☑5ᵗʰ   **D64.8** **Other specified anemias**

    D64.81 **Anemia due to antineoplastic chemotherapy**
      Antineoplastic chemotherapy induced anemia
      EXCLUDES 1 *aplastic anemia due to antineoplastic chemotherapy (D61.1)*
      EXCLUDES 2 *anemia in neoplastic disease (D63.0)*
      AHA: 2014, 4Q, 22
      DEF: Reversible adverse effect of chemotherapy, causing inhibition of bone marrow production; decrease in red blood cell production prevents adequate oxygenation of the tissues and organs causing fatigue, SOB, and exacerbation of other medical conditions.

    D64.89 **Other specified anemias**
      Infantile pseudoleukemia

  D64.9 **Anemia, unspecified**   ▽
    AHA: 2017, 1Q, 7

Coagulation defects, purpura and other hemorrhagic conditions (D65-D69)

D65 Disseminated intravascular coagulation [defibrination syndrome]   HCC
    Afibrinogenemia, acquired
    Consumption coagulopathy
    Diffuse or disseminated intravascular coagulation [DIC]
    Fibrinolytic hemorrhage, acquired
    Fibrinolytic purpura
    Purpura fulminans
    EXCLUDES 1 *disseminated intravascular coagulation (complicating):*
      abortion or ectopic or molar pregnancy (O00-O07, O08.1)
      in newborn (P60)
      pregnancy, childbirth and the puerperium (O45.0, O46.0, O67.0, O72.3)

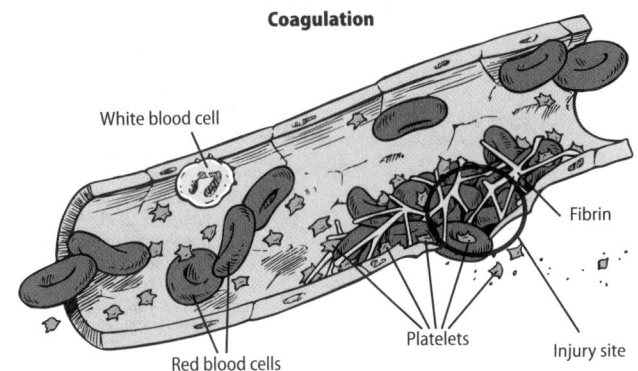

Coagulation

White blood cell

Fibrin

Platelets

Injury site

Red blood cells

D66 Hereditary factor VIII deficiency   HCC
    Classical hemophilia
    Deficiency factor VIII (with functional defect)
    Hemophilia A
    Hemophilia NOS
    EXCLUDES 1 *factor VIII deficiency with vascular defect (D68.0)*
    DEF: Hereditary, sex-linked lack of antihemophilic globulin (AHG) (factor VIII); causes abnormal coagulation characterized by increased bleeding, large bruises of skin, bleeding in mouth, nose, gastrointestinal tract; hemorrhages into joints, resulting in swelling and impaired function.

D67 Hereditary factor IX deficiency   HCC
    Christmas disease
    Factor IX deficiency (with functional defect)
    Hemophilia B
    Plasma thromboplastin component [PTC] deficiency

☑4ᵗʰ **D68 Other coagulation defects**
    EXCLUDES 1 *abnormal coagulation profile (R79.1)*
      coagulation defects complicating abortion or ectopic or molar pregnancy (O00-O07, O08.1)
      coagulation defects complicating pregnancy, childbirth and the puerperium (O45.0, O46.0, O67.0, O72.3)
    AHA: 2016, 1Q, 14

  D68.0 **Von Willebrand's disease**   HCC
    Angiohemophilia
    Factor VIII deficiency with vascular defect
    Vascular hemophilia
    EXCLUDES 1 *capillary fragility (hereditary) (D69.8)*
      factor VIII deficiency NOS (D66)
      factor VIII deficiency with functional defect (D66)
    DEF: Abnormal blood coagulation caused by deficient blood factor VII; congenital; symptoms include excess or prolonged bleeding.

  D68.1 **Hereditary factor XI deficiency**   HCC
    Hemophilia C
    Plasma thromboplastin antecedent [PTA] deficiency
    Rosenthal's disease

  D68.2 **Hereditary deficiency of other clotting factors**   HCC
    AC globulin deficiency
    Congenital afibrinogenemia
    Deficiency of factor I [fibrinogen]
    Deficiency of factor II [prothrombin]
    Deficiency of factor V [labile]
    Deficiency of factor VII [stable]
    Deficiency of factor X [Stuart-Prower]
    Deficiency of factor XII [Hageman]
    Deficiency of factor XIII [fibrin stabilizing]
    Dysfibrinogenemia (congenital)
    Hypoproconvertinemia
    Owren's disease
    Proaccelerin deficiency

☑5ᵗʰ   **D68.3** **Hemorrhagic disorder due to circulating anticoagulants**

☑6ᵗʰ   **D68.31** **Hemorrhagic disorder due to intrinsic circulating anticoagulants, antibodies, or inhibitors**

      D68.311 **Acquired hemophilia**   HCC
        Autoimmune hemophilia
        Autoimmune inhibitors to clotting factors
        Secondary hemophilia

Chapter 3. Disease of the Blood and Blood-Forming Organs

D68.312 Antiphospholipid antibody with hemorrhagic disorder `HCC`
Lupus anticoagulant (LAC) with hemorrhagic disorder
Systemic lupus erythematosus [SLE] inhibitor with hemorrhagic disorder
> EXCLUDES 1 antiphospholipid antibody, finding without diagnosis (R76.Ø)
> antiphospholipid antibody syndrome (D68.61)
> antiphospholipid antibody with hypercoagulable state (D68.61)
> lupus anticoagulant (LAC) finding without diagnosis (R76.Ø)
> lupus anticoagulant (LAC) with hypercoagulable state (D68.62)
> systemic lupus erythematosus [SLE] inhibitor finding without diagnosis (R76.Ø)
> systemic lupus erythematosus [SLE] inhibitor with hypercoagulable state (D68.62)

D68.318 Other hemorrhagic disorder due to intrinsic circulating anticoagulants, antibodies, or inhibitors `HCC`
Antithromboplastinemia
Antithromboplastinogenemia
Hemorrhagic disorder due to intrinsic increase in antithrombin
Hemorrhagic disorder due to intrinsic increase in anti-VIIIa
Hemorrhagic disorder due to intrinsic increase in anti-IXa
Hemorrhagic disorder due to intrinsic increase in anti-XIa

D68.32 Hemorrhagic disorder due to extrinsic circulating anticoagulants `HCC`
Drug-induced hemorrhagic disorder
Hemorrhagic disorder due to increase in anti-IIa
Hemorrhagic disorder due to increase in anti-Xa
Hyperheparinemia
Use additional code for adverse effect, if applicable, to identify drug (T45.515, T45.525)
AHA: 2016, 1Q, 14-15

D68.4 Acquired coagulation factor deficiency `HCC`
Deficiency of coagulation factor due to liver disease
Deficiency of coagulation factor due to vitamin K deficiency
> EXCLUDES 1 vitamin K deficiency of newborn (P53)

√5ᵗʰ **D68.5** Primary thrombophilia
Primary hypercoagulable states
> EXCLUDES 1 antiphospholipid syndrome (D68.61)
> lupus anticoagulant (D68.62)
> secondary activated protein C resistance (D68.69)
> secondary antiphospholipid antibody syndrome (D68.69)
> secondary lupus anticoagulant with hypercoagulable state (D68.69)
> secondary systemic lupus erythematosus [SLE] inhibitor with hypercoagulable state (D68.69)
> systemic lupus erythematosus [SLE] inhibitor finding without diagnosis (R76.Ø)
> systemic lupus erythematosus [SLE] inhibitor with hemorrhagic disorder (D68.312)
> thrombotic thrombocytopenic purpura (M31.1)

D68.51 Activated protein C resistance `HCC`
Factor V Leiden mutation

D68.52 Prothrombin gene mutation `HCC`

D68.59 Other primary thrombophilia `HCC`
Antithrombin III deficiency
Hypercoagulable state NOS
Primary hypercoagulable state NEC
Primary thrombophilia NEC
Protein C deficiency
Protein S deficiency
Thrombophilia NOS

√5ᵗʰ **D68.6** Other thrombophilia
Other hypercoagulable states
> EXCLUDES 1 diffuse or disseminated intravascular coagulation [DIC] (D65)
> heparin induced thrombocytopenia (HIT) (D75.82)
> hyperhomocysteinemia (E72.11)

D68.61 Antiphospholipid syndrome `HCC`
Anticardiolipin syndrome
Antiphospholipid antibody syndrome
> EXCLUDES 1 antiphospholipid antibody, finding without diagnosis (R76.Ø)
> antiphospholipid antibody with hemorrhagic disorder (D68.312)
> lupus anticoagulant syndrome (D68.62)

D68.62 Lupus anticoagulant syndrome `HCC`
Lupus anticoagulant
Presence of systemic lupus erythematosus [SLE] inhibitor
> EXCLUDES 1 anticardiolipin syndrome (D68.61)
> antiphospholipid syndrome (D68.61)
> lupus anticoagulant (LAC) finding without diagnosis (R76.Ø)
> lupus anticoagulant (LAC) with hemorrhagic disorder (D68.312)

D68.69 Other thrombophilia `HCC`
Hypercoagulable states NEC
Secondary hypercoagulable state NOS

D68.8 Other specified coagulation defects `HCC`
> EXCLUDES 1 hemorrhagic disease of newborn (P53)

D68.9 Coagulation defect, unspecified `HCC` ▽

√4ᵗʰ **D69** Purpura and other hemorrhagic conditions
> EXCLUDES 1 benign hypergammaglobulinemic purpura (D89.Ø)
> cryoglobulinemic purpura (D89.1)
> essential (hemorrhagic) thrombocythemia (D47.3)
> hemorrhagic thrombocythemia (D47.3)
> purpura fulminans (D65)
> thrombotic thrombocytopenic purpura (M31.1)
> Waldenström hypergammaglobulinemic purpura (D89.Ø)

D69.Ø Allergic purpura `HCC`
Allergic vasculitis
Nonthrombocytopenic hemorrhagic purpura
Nonthrombocytopenic idiopathic purpura
Purpura anaphylactoid
Purpura Henoch(-Schönlein)
Purpura rheumatica
Vascular purpura
> EXCLUDES 1 thrombocytopenic hemorrhagic purpura (D69.3)
DEF: Any hemorrhagic condition, thrombocytic or nonthrombocytopenic in origin, caused by a presumed allergic reaction.

D69.1 Qualitative platelet defects `HCC`
Bernard-Soulier [giant platelet] syndrome
Glanzmann's disease
Grey platelet syndrome
Thromboasthenia (hemorrhagic) (hereditary)
Thrombocytopathy
> EXCLUDES 1 von Willebrand's disease (D68.Ø)

D69.2 Other nonthrombocytopenic purpura `HCC`
Purpura NOS
Purpura simplex
Senile purpura

D69.3 Immune thrombocytopenic purpura `HCC`
Hemorrhagic (thrombocytopenic) purpura
Idiopathic thrombocytopenic purpura
Tidal platelet dysgenesis
DEF: Tidal platelet dysgenesis: Platelet counts fluctuate from normal to very low within periods of 20 to 40 days and may involve autoimmune platelet destruction.

√5ᵗʰ **D69.4** Other primary thrombocytopenia
> EXCLUDES 1 transient neonatal thrombocytopenia (P61.Ø)
> Wiskott-Aldrich syndrome (D82.Ø)

D69.41 Evans syndrome `HCC`

D69.42 Congenital and hereditary thrombocytopenia purpura `HCC`
Congenital thrombocytopenia
Hereditary thrombocytopenia
Code first congenital or hereditary disorder, such as: thrombocytopenia with absent radius (TAR syndrome) (Q87.2)

D69.49 Other primary thrombocytopenia `HCC`
Megakaryocytic hypoplasia
Primary thrombocytopenia NOS

✓5th **D69.5** **Secondary thrombocytopenia**
     EXCLUDES 1   *heparin induced thrombocytopenia (HIT) (D75.82)*
                 transient thrombocytopenia of newborn (P61.0)

     D69.51   **Posttransfusion purpura**
             Posttransfusion purpura from whole blood (fresh) or
                 blood products
             PTP

     D69.59   **Other secondary thrombocytopenia**
             AHA: 2014, 4Q, 22

D69.6 **Thrombocytopenia, unspecified**   HCC ▽

D69.8 **Other specified hemorrhagic conditions**   HCC
     Capillary fragility (hereditary)
     Vascular pseudohemophilia

D69.9 **Hemorrhagic condition, unspecified**   HCC ▽

Other disorders of blood and blood-forming organs (D70-D77)

✓4th **D70** **Neutropenia**
     INCLUDES   agranulocytosis
             decreased absolute neurophile count (ANC)
     Use additional code for any associated:
         fever (R50.81)
         mucositis (J34.81, K12.3-, K92.81, N76.81)
     EXCLUDES 1   *neutropenic splenomegaly (D73.81)*
                 transient neonatal neutropenia (P61.5)

     D70.0   **Congenital agranulocytosis**   HCC
             Congenital neutropenia   Kostmann's disease
             Infantile genetic agranulocytosis

     D70.1   **Agranulocytosis secondary to cancer chemotherapy**   HCC
             Code also underlying neoplasm
             Use additional code for adverse effect, if applicable, to identify
                 drug (T45.1X5)
             AHA: 2014, 4Q, 22

     D70.2   **Other drug-induced agranulocytosis**   HCC
             Use additional code for adverse effect, if applicable, to identify
                 drug (T36-T50 with fifth or sixth character 5)

     D70.3   **Neutropenia due to infection**   HCC

     D70.4   **Cyclic neutropenia**   HCC
             Cyclic hematopoiesis
             Periodic neutropenia

     D70.8   **Other neutropenia**   HCC

     D70.9   **Neutropenia, unspecified**   HCC ▽

D71 **Functional disorders of polymorphonuclear neutrophils**   HCC
     Cell membrane receptor complex [CR3] defect
     Chronic (childhood) granulomatous disease
     Congenital dysphagocytosis
     Progressive septic granulomatosis

✓4th **D72** **Other disorders of white blood cells**
     EXCLUDES 1   *basophilia (D72.824)*
                 immunity disorders (D80-D89)
                 neutropenia (D70)
                 preleukemia (syndrome) (D46.9)

     D72.0   **Genetic anomalies of leukocytes**   HCC
             Alder (granulation) (granulocyte) anomaly
             Alder syndrome
             Hereditary leukocytic hypersegmentation
             Hereditary leukocytic hyposegmentation
             Hereditary leukomelanopathy
             May-Hegglin (granulation) (granulocyte) anomaly
             May-Hegglin syndrome
             Pelger-Huët (granulation) (granulocyte) anomaly
             Pelger-Huët syndrome
          EXCLUDES 1   *Chédiak (-Steinbrinck)-Higashi syndrome (E70.330)*

     D72.1   **Eosinophilia**
             Allergic eosinophilia   Hereditary eosinophilia
          EXCLUDES 1   *Löffler's syndrome (J82)*
                 pulmonary eosinophilia (J82)

     ✓5th **D72.8**   **Other specified disorders of white blood cells**
          EXCLUDES 1   *leukemia (C91-C95)*

         ✓6th **D72.81**   **Decreased white blood cell count**
              EXCLUDES 1   *neutropenia (D70.-)*

             D72.810   **Lymphocytopenia**
                  Decreased lymphocytes

             D72.818   **Other decreased white blood cell count**
                  Basophilic leukopenia
                  Eosinophilic leukopenia
                  Monocytopenia
                  Other decreased leukocytes
                  Plasmacytopenia

             D72.819   **Decreased white blood cell count,** ▽
                  unspecified
                  Decreased leukocytes, unspecified
                  Leukocytopenia, unspecified
                  Leukopenia
              EXCLUDES 1   *malignant leukopenia (D70.9)*

         ✓6th **D72.82**   **Elevated white blood cell count**
              EXCLUDES 1   *eosinophilia (D72.1)*

             D72.820   **Lymphocytosis (symptomatic)**
                  Elevated lymphocytes

             D72.821   **Monocytosis (symptomatic)**
              EXCLUDES 1   *infectious mononucleosis (B27.-)*

             D72.822   **Plasmacytosis**

             D72.823   **Leukemoid reaction**
                  Basophilic leukemoid reaction
                  Leukemoid reaction NOS
                  Lymphocytic leukemoid reaction
                  Monocytic leukemoid reaction
                  Myelocytic leukemoid reaction
                  Neutrophilic leukemoid reaction

             D72.824   **Basophilia**

             D72.825   **Bandemia**
                  Bandemia without diagnosis of specific
                     infection
                  EXCLUDES 1   *confirmed infection—code to*
                         infection
                         leukemia (C91.-, C92.-, C93.-,
                           C94.-, C95.-)
                  DEF: Increase in early neutrophil cells, called
                  band cells; may indicate infection.

             D72.828   **Other elevated white blood cell count**

             D72.829   **Elevated white blood cell count,** ▽
                  unspecified
                  Elevated leukocytes, unspecified
                  Leukocytosis, unspecified

         D72.89   **Other specified disorders of white blood cells**
             Abnormality of white blood cells NEC

     D72.9   **Disorder of white blood cells, unspecified** ▽
             Abnormal leukocyte differential NOS

✓4th **D73** **Diseases of spleen**

     D73.0   **Hyposplenism**
             Atrophy of spleen
          EXCLUDES 1   *asplenia (congenital) (Q89.01)*
                 postsurgical absence of spleen (Z90.81)

     D73.1   **Hypersplenism**
          EXCLUDES 1   *neutropenic splenomegaly (D73.81)*
                 primary splenic neutropenia (D73.81)
                 splenitis, splenomegaly in late syphilis (A52.79)
                 splenitis, splenomegaly in tuberculosis (A18.85)
                 splenomegaly NOS (R16.1)
                 splenomegaly congenital (Q89.0)

     D73.2   **Chronic congestive splenomegaly**

     D73.3   **Abscess of spleen**

     D73.4   **Cyst of spleen**

     D73.5   **Infarction of spleen**
             Splenic rupture, nontraumatic
             Torsion of spleen
          EXCLUDES 1   *rupture of spleen due to Plasmodium vivax malaria*
                   (B51.0)
                 traumatic rupture of spleen (S36.03-)

     ✓5th **D73.8**   **Other diseases of spleen**

         D73.81   **Neutropenic splenomegaly**
                 Werner-Schultz disease

         D73.89   **Other diseases of spleen**
                 Fibrosis of spleen NOS
                 Perisplenitis
                 Splenitis NOS

     D73.9   **Disease of spleen, unspecified** ▽

✓4th **D74** **Methemoglobinemia**

     D74.0   **Congenital methemoglobinemia**
             Congenital NADH-methemoglobin reductase deficiency
             Hemoglobin-M [Hb-M] disease
             Methemoglobinemia, hereditary

     D74.8   **Other methemoglobinemias**
             Acquired methemoglobinemia (with sulfhemoglobinemia)
             Toxic methemoglobinemia

     D74.9   **Methemoglobinemia, unspecified** ▽

☑ Additional Character Req   ✓x7th Placeholder Alert   Manifestation   HCC CMS-HCC Condition   ▽ Unspecified Code   ►◄ Revised Text   ● New Code   ▲ Revised Code Title

☑4ᵗʰ **D75 Other and unspecified diseases of blood and blood-forming organs**
> EXCLUDES 2 acute lymphadenitis (L04.-)
> chronic lymphadenitis (I88.1)
> enlarged lymph nodes (R59.-)
> hypergammaglobulinemia NOS (D89.2)
> lymphadenitis NOS (I88.9)
> mesenteric lymphadenitis (acute) (chronic) (I88.0)

D75.0 Familial erythrocytosis
Benign polycythemia
Familial polycythemia
> EXCLUDES 1 hereditary ovalocytosis (D58.1)

D75.1 Secondary polycythemia
Acquired polycythemia
Emotional polycythemia
Erythrocytosis NOS
Hypoxemic polycythemia
Nephrogenous polycythemia
Polycythemia due to erythropoietin
Polycythemia due to fall in plasma volume
Polycythemia due to high altitude
Polycythemia due to stress
Polycythemia NOS
Relative polycythemia
> EXCLUDES 1 polycythemia neonatorum (P61.1)
> polycythemia vera (D45)

DEF: Elevated number of red blood cells in circulating blood as a result of reduced oxygen supply to the tissues.

☑5ᵗʰ **D75.8 Other specified diseases of blood and blood-forming organs**

D75.81 Myelofibrosis HCC
Myelofibrosis NOS
Secondary myelofibrosis NOS
Code first the underlying disorder, such as:
  malignant neoplasm of breast (C50.-)
Use additional code, if applicable, for associated therapy-related myelodysplastic syndrome (D46.-)
Use additional code for adverse effect, if applicable, to identify drug (T45.1X5)
> EXCLUDES 1 acute myelofibrosis (C94.4-)
> idiopathic myelofibrosis (D47.1)
> leukoerythroblastic anemia (D61.82)
> myelofibrosis with myeloid metaplasia (D47.4)
> myelophthisic anemia (D61.82)
> myelophthisis (D61.82)
> primary myelofibrosis (D47.1)

D75.82 Heparin induced thrombocytopenia (HIT) HCC
DEF: Immune-mediated reaction to heparin therapy causing an abrupt fall in platelet count and serious complications such as pulmonary embolism, stroke, AMI, or DVT.

D75.89 Other specified diseases of blood and blood-forming organs

D75.9 Disease of blood and blood-forming organs, unspecified ▽

☑4ᵗʰ **D76 Other specified diseases with participation of lymphoreticular and reticulohistiocytic tissue**
> EXCLUDES 1 (Abt-) Letterer-Siwe disease (C96.0)
> eosinophilic granuloma (C96.6)
> Hand-Schüller-Christian disease (C96.5)
> histiocytic medullary reticulosis (C96.9)
> histiocytic sarcoma (C96.A)
> histiocytosis X, multifocal (C96.5)
> histiocytosis X, unifocal (C96.6)
> Langerhans-cell histiocytosis, multifocal (C96.5)
> Langerhans-cell histiocytosis NOS (C96.6)
> Langerhans-cell histiocytosis, unifocal (C96.6)
> leukemic reticuloendotheliosis (C91.4-)
> lipomelanotic reticulosis (I89.8)
> malignant histiocytosis (C96.A)
> malignant reticulosis (C86.0)
> nonlipid reticuloendotheliosis (C96.0)

D76.1 Hemophagocytic lymphohistiocytosis HCC
Familial hemophagocytic reticulosis
Histiocytoses of mononuclear phagocytes

D76.2 Hemophagocytic syndrome, infection-associated HCC
Use additional code to identify infectious agent or disease

D76.3 Other histiocytosis syndromes HCC
Reticulohistiocytoma (giant-cell)
Sinus histiocytosis with massive lymphadenopathy
Xanthogranuloma

D77 Other disorders of blood and blood-forming organs in diseases classified elsewhere
Code first underlying disease, such as:
  amyloidosis (E85.-)
  congenital early syphilis (A50.0)
  echinococcosis (B67.0-B67.9)
  malaria (B50.0-B54)
  schistosomiasis [bilharziasis] (B65.0-B65.9)
  vitamin C deficiency (E54)
> EXCLUDES 1 rupture of spleen due to Plasmodium vivax malaria (B51.0)
> splenitis, splenomegaly in late syphilis (A52.79)
> splenitis, splenomegaly in tuberculosis (A18.85)

Intraoperative and postprocedural complications of the spleen (D78)

☑4ᵗʰ **D78 Intraoperative and postprocedural complications of the spleen**

☑5ᵗʰ **D78.0 Intraoperative hemorrhage and hematoma of the spleen complicating a procedure**
> EXCLUDES 1 intraoperative hemorrhage and hematoma of the spleen due to accidental puncture or laceration during a procedure (D78.1-)

D78.01 Intraoperative hemorrhage and hematoma of the spleen complicating a procedure on the spleen

D78.02 Intraoperative hemorrhage and hematoma of the spleen complicating other procedure

☑5ᵗʰ **D78.1 Accidental puncture and laceration of the spleen during a procedure**

D78.11 Accidental puncture and laceration of the spleen during a procedure on the spleen

D78.12 Accidental puncture and laceration of the spleen during other procedure

☑5ᵗʰ **D78.2 Postprocedural hemorrhage of the spleen following a procedure**

D78.21 Postprocedural hemorrhage of the spleen following a procedure on the spleen

D78.22 Postprocedural hemorrhage of the spleen following other procedure

☑5ᵗʰ **D78.3 Postprocedural hematoma and seroma of the spleen following a procedure**

D78.31 Postprocedural hematoma of the spleen following a procedure on the spleen

D78.32 Postprocedural hematoma of the spleen following other procedure

D78.33 Postprocedural seroma of the spleen following a procedure on the spleen

D78.34 Postprocedural seroma of the spleen following other procedure

☑5ᵗʰ **D78.8 Other intraoperative and postprocedural complications of the spleen**
Use additional code, if applicable, to further specify disorder

D78.81 Other intraoperative complications of the spleen

D78.89 Other postprocedural complications of the spleen

Certain disorders involving the immune mechanism (D80-D89)

> INCLUDES defects in the complement system
> immunodeficiency disorders, except human immunodeficiency virus [HIV] disease
> sarcoidosis
> EXCLUDES 1 autoimmune disease (systemic) NOS (M35.9)
> functional disorders of polymorphonuclear neutrophils (D71)
> human immunodeficiency virus [HIV] disease (B20)

☑4ᵗʰ **D80 Immunodeficiency with predominantly antibody defects**

D80.0 Hereditary hypogammaglobulinemia HCC
Autosomal recessive agammaglobulinemia (Swiss type)
X-linked agammaglobulinemia [Bruton] (with growth hormone deficiency)

D80.1 Nonfamilial hypogammaglobulinemia HCC
Agammaglobulinemia with immunoglobulin-bearing B-lymphocytes
Common variable agammaglobulinemia [CVAgamma]
Hypogammaglobulinemia NOS

D80.2 Selective deficiency of immunoglobulin A [IgA] HCC

D80.3 Selective deficiency of immunoglobulin G [IgG] subclasses HCC

D80.4 Selective deficiency of immunoglobulin M [IgM] HCC

D80.5 Immunodeficiency with increased immunoglobulin M [IgM] HCC

EXCLUDES 1 Not coded here   EXCLUDES 2 Not included here   N Newborn Age: 0   P Pediatric Age: 0-17   M Maternity Age: 12-55   A Adult Age: 15-124

502   ICD-10-CM 2018

D80.6 Antibody deficiency with near-normal immunoglobulins or with hyperimmunoglobulinemia   HCC

D80.7 Transient hypogammaglobulinemia of infancy   HCC

D80.8 Other immunodeficiencies with predominantly antibody defects   HCC
> Kappa light chain deficiency

D80.9 Immunodeficiency with predominantly antibody defects, unspecified   HCC ▽

☑4ᵗʰ **D81 Combined immunodeficiencies**
> EXCLUDES 1   autosomal recessive agammaglobulinemia (Swiss type) (D80.0)

D81.0 Severe combined immunodeficiency [SCID] with reticular dysgenesis   HCC

D81.1 Severe combined immunodeficiency [SCID] with low T- and B-cell numbers   HCC

D81.2 Severe combined immunodeficiency [SCID] with low or normal B-cell numbers   HCC

D81.3 Adenosine deaminase [ADA] deficiency   HCC

D81.4 Nezelof's syndrome   HCC

D81.5 Purine nucleoside phosphorylase [PNP] deficiency   HCC

D81.6 Major histocompatibility complex class I deficiency   HCC
> Bare lymphocyte syndrome

D81.7 Major histocompatibility complex class II deficiency   HCC

☑5ᵗʰ **D81.8 Other combined immunodeficiencies**

   ☑6ᵗʰ **D81.81 Biotin-dependent carboxylase deficiency**
> Multiple carboxylase deficiency
> EXCLUDES 1   biotin-dependent carboxylase deficiency due to dietary deficiency of biotin (E53.8)

     D81.810 Biotinidase deficiency

     D81.818 Other biotin-dependent carboxylase deficiency
> Holocarboxylase synthetase deficiency
> Other multiple carboxylase deficiency

     D81.819 Biotin-dependent carboxylase deficiency, unspecified ▽
> Multiple carboxylase deficiency, unspecified

   D81.89 Other combined immunodeficiencies   HCC

D81.9 Combined immunodeficiency, unspecified   HCC ▽
> Severe combined immunodeficiency disorder [SCID] NOS

☑4ᵗʰ **D82 Immunodeficiency associated with other major defects**
> EXCLUDES 1   ataxia telangiectasia [Louis-Bar] (G11.3)

D82.0 Wiskott-Aldrich syndrome   HCC
> Immunodeficiency with thrombocytopenia and eczema

D82.1 Di George's syndrome   HCC
> Pharyngeal pouch syndrome
> Thymic alymphoplasia
> Thymic aplasia or hypoplasia with immunodeficiency

D82.2 Immunodeficiency with short-limbed stature   HCC

D82.3 Immunodeficiency following hereditary defective response to Epstein-Barr virus   HCC
> X-linked lymphoproliferative disease

D82.4 Hyperimmunoglobulin E [IgE] syndrome   HCC

D82.8 Immunodeficiency associated with other specified major defects   HCC

D82.9 Immunodeficiency associated with major defect, unspecified   HCC ▽

☑4ᵗʰ **D83 Common variable immunodeficiency**

D83.0 Common variable immunodeficiency with predominant abnormalities of B-cell numbers and function   HCC

D83.1 Common variable immunodeficiency with predominant immunoregulatory T-cell disorders   HCC

D83.2 Common variable immunodeficiency with autoantibodies to B- or T-cells   HCC

D83.8 Other common variable immunodeficiencies   HCC

D83.9 Common variable immunodeficiency, unspecified   HCC ▽

☑4ᵗʰ **D84 Other immunodeficiencies**

D84.0 Lymphocyte function antigen-1 [LFA-1] defect   HCC

D84.1 Defects in the complement system   HCC
> C1 esterase inhibitor [C1-INH] deficiency

D84.8 Other specified immunodeficiencies   HCC

D84.9 Immunodeficiency, unspecified   HCC ▽

☑4ᵗʰ **D86 Sarcoidosis**

D86.0 Sarcoidosis of lung   HCC

D86.1 Sarcoidosis of lymph nodes

D86.2 Sarcoidosis of lung with sarcoidosis of lymph nodes   HCC

D86.3 Sarcoidosis of skin

☑5ᵗʰ **D86.8 Sarcoidosis of other sites**

   D86.81 Sarcoid meningitis

   D86.82 Multiple cranial nerve palsies in sarcoidosis   HCC

   D86.83 Sarcoid iridocyclitis

   D86.84 Sarcoid pyelonephritis
> Tubulo-interstitial nephropathy in sarcoidosis

   D86.85 Sarcoid myocarditis

   D86.86 Sarcoid arthropathy
> Polyarthritis in sarcoidosis

   D86.87 Sarcoid myositis

   D86.89 Sarcoidosis of other sites
> Hepatic granuloma
> Uveoparotid fever [Heerfordt]

D86.9 Sarcoidosis, unspecified ▽

☑4ᵗʰ **D89 Other disorders involving the immune mechanism, not elsewhere classified**
> EXCLUDES 1   hyperglobulinemia NOS (R77.1)
> monoclonal gammopathy (of undetermined significance) (D47.2)
> EXCLUDES 2   transplant failure and rejection (T86.-)

D89.0 Polyclonal hypergammaglobulinemia
> Benign hypergammaglobulinemic purpura
> Polyclonal gammopathy NOS

D89.1 Cryoglobulinemia   HCC
> Cryoglobulinemic purpura   Mixed cryoglobulinemia
> Cryoglobulinemic vasculitis   Primary cryoglobulinemia
> Essential cryoglobulinemia   Secondary cryoglobulinemia
> Idiopathic cryoglobulinemia

D89.2 Hypergammaglobulinemia, unspecified ▽

D89.3 Immune reconstitution syndrome   HCC
> Immune reconstitution inflammatory syndrome [IRIS]
> Use additional code for adverse effect, if applicable, to identify drug (T36-T50 with fifth or sixth character 5)

☑5ᵗʰ **D89.4 Mast cell activation syndrome and related disorders**
> EXCLUDES 1   aggressive systemic mastocytosis ▶(C96.21)◀
> ▶congenital cutaneous mastocytosis◀ (Q82.2)
> ▶(non-congenital) cutaneous mastocytosis (D47.01)
> (indolent) systemic mastocytosis (D47.02)
> malignant mast cell neoplasm (C96.2-)◀
> malignant mastocytoma ▶(C96.29)◀
> mast cell leukemia (C94.3-)
> ▶mast cell sarcoma (C96.22)
> mastocytoma NOS (D47.09)
> other mast cell neoplasms of uncertain behavior (D47.09)◀
> systemic mastocytosis associated with a clonal hematologic non-mast cell lineage disease (SM-AHNMD)▶(D47.02)◀

   D89.40 Mast cell activation, unspecified   HCC ▽
> Mast cell activation disorder, unspecified
> Mast cell activation syndrome, NOS

   D89.41 Monoclonal mast cell activation syndrome   HCC

   D89.42 Idiopathic mast cell activation syndrome   HCC

   D89.43 Secondary mast cell activation   HCC
> Secondary mast cell activation syndrome
> Code also underlying etiology, if known

   D89.49 Other mast cell activation disorder   HCC
> Other mast cell activation syndrome

☑5ᵗʰ **D89.8 Other specified disorders involving the immune mechanism, not elsewhere classified**

   ☑6ᵗʰ **D89.81 Graft-versus-host disease**
> Code first underlying cause, such as:
> complications of transplanted organs and tissue (T86.-)
> complications of blood transfusion (T80.89)
> Use additional code to identify associated manifestations, such as:
> desquamative dermatitis (L30.8)
> diarrhea (R19.7)
> elevated bilirubin (R17)
> hair loss (L65.9)

     D89.810 Acute graft-versus-host disease   HCC

     D89.811 Chronic graft-versus-host disease   HCC

     D89.812 Acute on chronic graft-versus-host disease   HCC

     D89.813 Graft-versus-host disease, unspecified   HCC ▽

☑ Additional Character Req   ☑x7ᵗʰ Placeholder Alert   Manifestation   HCC CMS-HCC Condition   ▽ Unspecified Code   ▶◀ Revised Text   ● New Code   ▲ Revised Code Title

D89.82   **Autoimmune lymphoproliferative syndrome**   HCC
[ALPS]

DEF: Rare genetic alteration of the Fas protein; impairs normal cellular apoptosis (normal cell death), causing abnormal accumulation of lymphocytes in the lymph glands, liver, and spleen; symptoms include neutropenia, anemia, and thrombocytopenia.

D89.89   **Other specified disorders involving the immune**   HCC
mechanism, not elsewhere classified

EXCLUDES 1   human immunodeficiency virus disease (B2Ø)

D89.9   **Disorder involving the immune mechanism,**   HCC ▽
unspecified

Immune disease NOS
AHA: 2015, 3Q, 22

EXCLUDES 1 Not coded here   *EXCLUDES 2* Not included here   N Newborn Age: 0   P Pediatric Age: 0-17   M Maternity Age: 12-55   A Adult Age: 15-124

504   ICD-10-CM 2018

Chapter 4. Endocrine, Nutritional, and Metabolic Diseases (E00–E89)

Chapter Specific Guidelines with Coding Examples

The chapter specific guidelines from the ICD-10-CM Official Guidelines for Coding and Reporting have been provided below. Along with these guidelines are coding examples, contained in the shaded boxes, that have been developed to help illustrate the coding and/or sequencing guidance found in these guidelines.

a. Diabetes mellitus

The diabetes mellitus codes are combination codes that include the type of diabetes mellitus, the body system affected, and the complications affecting that body system. As many codes within a particular category as are necessary to describe all of the complications of the disease may be used. They should be sequenced based on the reason for a particular encounter. Assign as many codes from categories E08–E13 as needed to identify all of the associated conditions that the patient has.

> Patient is seen for uncontrolled diabetes, type 2, with diabetic nephropathy and diabetic gastroparesis.
>
> **E11.65**   **Type 2 diabetes mellitus with hyperglycemia**
>
> **E11.21**   **Type 2 diabetes mellitus with diabetic nephropathy**
>
> **E11.43**   **Type 2 diabetes mellitus with diabetic automomic (poly)neuropathy**
>
> *Explanation*: Use as many codes to describe the diabetic complications as needed. Many are combination codes that describe more than one condition. Code first the reason for the encounter. "Uncontrolled" is described as "with hyperglycemia."

1) Type of diabetes

The age of a patient is not the sole determining factor, though most type 1 diabetics develop the condition before reaching puberty. For this reason type 1 diabetes mellitus is also referred to as juvenile diabetes.

> A 45-year-old patient is diagnosed with type 1 diabetes
>
> **E10.9**   **Type 1 diabetes mellitus without complications**
>
> *Explanation*: Although most type 1 diabetics are diagnosed in childhood or adolescence, it can also begin in adults.

2) Type of diabetes mellitus not documented

If the type of diabetes mellitus is not documented in the medical record the default is E11.-, Type 2 diabetes mellitus.

> Office visit lists diabetic retinopathy with macular edema and hypertension on patient problem list
>
> **E11.311**   **Type 2 diabetes mellitus with unspecified diabetic retinopathy with macular edema**
>
> **I10**   **Essential (primary) hypertension**
>
> *Explanation*: Since the type of diabetes was not documented, default to category E11.

3) Diabetes mellitus and the use of insulin and oral hypoglycemics

If the documentation in a medical record does not indicate the type of diabetes but does indicate that the patient uses insulin, code E11, Type 2 diabetes mellitus, should be assigned. Code Z79.4, Long-term (current) use of insulin, or Z79.84, Long term (current) use of oral hypoglycemic drugs, should also be assigned to indicate that the patient uses insulin or hypoglycemic drugs. Code Z79.4 should not be assigned if insulin is given temporarily to bring a type 2 patient's blood sugar under control during an encounter.

> Office visit lists chronic diabetes with daily insulin use on patient problem list
>
> **E11.9**   **Type 2 diabetes mellitus without complications**
>
> **Z79.4**   **Long term (current) use of insulin**
>
> *Explanation*: Do not assume that a patient on insulin must have type 1 diabetes. The default for diabetes without further specification defaults to type 2. Add the code for long term use of insulin.

4) Diabetes mellitus in pregnancy and gestational diabetes

See Section I.C.15. Diabetes mellitus in pregnancy.

See Section I.C.15. Gestational (pregnancy induced) diabetes

5) Complications due to insulin pump malfunction

(a) Underdose of insulin due to insulin pump failure

An underdose of insulin due to an insulin pump failure should be assigned to a code from subcategory T85.6, Mechanical complication of other specified internal and external prosthetic devices, implants and grafts, that specifies the type of pump malfunction, as the principal or first-listed code, followed by code T38.3X6-, Underdosing of insulin and oral hypoglycemic [antidiabetic] drugs. Additional codes for the type of diabetes mellitus and any associated complications due to the underdosing should also be assigned.

> A 24-year-old type 1 diabetic male treated in for hyperglycemia; insulin pump found to be malfunctioning and underdosing
>
> **T85.614A**   **Breakdown (mechanical) of insulin pump, initial encounter**
>
> **T38.3X6A**   **Underdosing of insulin and oral hypoglycemic [antidiabetic] drugs, initial encounter**
>
> **E10.65**   **Type 1 diabetes mellitus with hyperglycemia**
>
> *Explanation*: The complication code for the mechanical breakdown of the pump is sequenced first, followed by the underdosing code and type of diabetes with complication. Code all other diabetic complication codes necessary to describe the patient's condition.

(b) Overdose of insulin due to insulin pump failure

The principal or first-listed code for an encounter due to an insulin pump malfunction resulting in an overdose of insulin, should also be T85.6-, Mechanical complication of other specified internal and external prosthetic devices, implants and grafts, followed by code T38.3X1-, Poisoning by insulin and oral hypoglycemic [antidiabetic] drugs, accidental (unintentional).

> A 24-year-old type 1 diabetic male found down with diabetic coma, brought into ED and treated for hypoglycemia; insulin pump found to be malfunctioning and overdosing
>
> **T85.614A**   **Breakdown (mechanical) of insulin pump, initial encounter**
>
> **T38.3X1A**   **Poisoning by insulin and oral hypoglycemic [antidiabetic] drugs, accidental (unintentional), initial encounter**
>
> **E10.641**   **Type 1 diabetes mellitus with hypoglycemia with coma**
>
> *Explanation*: The complication code for the mechanical breakdown of the pump is sequenced first, followed by the poisoning code and type of diabetes with complication. All the characters in the combination code must be used to form a valid code and to fully describe the type of diabetes, the hypoglycemia, and the coma.

6) Secondary diabetes mellitus

Codes under categories E08, Diabetes mellitus due to underlying condition, E09, Drug or chemical induced diabetes mellitus, and E13, Other specified diabetes mellitus, identify complications/manifestations associated with secondary diabetes mellitus. Secondary diabetes is always caused by another condition or event (e.g., cystic fibrosis, malignant neoplasm of pancreas, pancreatectomy, adverse effect of drug, or poisoning).

(a) Secondary diabetes mellitus and the use of insulin or hypoglycemic drugs

For patients who routinely use insulin or hypoglycemic drugs, code Z79.4, Long-term (current) use of insulin, or Z79.84, Long term (current) use of oral hypoglycemic drugs should also be assigned. Code Z79.4 should not be assigned if insulin is given temporarily to bring a patient's blood sugar under control during an encounter.

Type 2 diabetic with no complications, normally only on oral metformin, is given insulin for three days to maintain glucose control while in the hospital recovering from surgery

E11.9   **Type 2 diabetes mellitus without complications**

Z79.84   **Long term (current) use of oral hypoglycemic drugs**

Explanation: Although the patient was given insulin for a short time during his hospital stay, the intent was only to maintain the patient's glucose levels while off his regular oral hypoglycemic medication, not for long term use. No code is needed for long term use of insulin, but a Z code for long term use of an oral hypoglycemic should be added to identify the chronic use of this drug.

Type 2 diabetic with diabetic polyneuropathy on insulin

E11.42   **Type 2 diabetes mellitus with diabetic polyneuropathy**

Z79.4   **Long term (current) use of insulin**

Explanation: Add the Z code for the long term use of insulin because the insulin is taken chronically.

(b) Assigning and sequencing secondary diabetes codes and its causes

The sequencing of the secondary diabetes codes in relationship to codes for the cause of the diabetes is based on the Tabular List instructions for categories E08, E09 and E13.

(i) Secondary diabetes mellitus due to pancreatectomy

For postpancreatectomy diabetes mellitus (lack of insulin due to the surgical removal of all or part of the pancreas), assign code E89.1, Postprocedural hypoinsulinemia. Assign a code from category E13 and a code from subcategory Z90.41-, Acquired absence of pancreas, as additional codes.

Patient with newly diagnosed diabetes after surgical removal of part of pancreas

E89.1   **Postprocedural hypoinsulinemia**

E13.9   **Other specified diabetes mellitus without complications**

Z90.411   **Acquired partial absence of pancreas**

Explanation: Sequence the postprocedural complication of the hypoinsulinemia due to the partial removal of the pancreas as the first-listed code, followed by the other specified diabetes (NEC) with or without complications and the partial or total acquired absence of the pancreas.

(ii) Secondary diabetes due to drugs

Secondary diabetes may be caused by an adverse effect of correctly administered medications, poisoning or sequela of poisoning.

See section I.C.19.e for coding of adverse effects and poisoning, and section I.C.20 for external cause code reporting.

Initial encounter for corticosteroid-induced diabetes mellitus

E09.9   **Drug or chemical induced diabetes mellitus without complications**

T38.0X5A   **Adverse effect of glucocorticoids and synthetic analogues, initial encounter**

Explanation: If the diabetes is caused by an adverse effect of a drug, the diabetic condition is coded first. If it occurs from a poisoning or overdose, the poisoning code causing the diabetes is sequenced first.

Chapter 4. Endocrine, Nutritional and Metabolic Diseases (E00-E89)

NOTE All neoplasms, whether functionally active or not, are classified in Chapter 2. Appropriate codes in this chapter (i.e. E05.8, E07.0, E16-E31, E34-) may be used as additional codes to indicate either functional activity by neoplasms and ectopic endocrine tissue or hyperfunction and hypofunction of endocrine glands associated with neoplasms and other conditions classified elsewhere.

EXCLUDES 1 *transitory endocrine and metabolic disorders specific to newborn (P70-P74)*

This chapter contains the following blocks:

E00-E07	Disorders of thyroid gland
E08-E13	Diabetes mellitus
E15-E16	Other disorders of glucose regulation and pancreatic internal secretion
E20-E35	Disorders of other endocrine glands
E36	Intraoperative complications of endocrine system
E40-E46	Malnutrition
E50-E64	Other nutritional deficiencies
E65-E68	Overweight, obesity and other hyperalimentation
E70-E88	Metabolic disorders
E89	Postprocedural endocrine and metabolic complications and disorders, not elsewhere classified

Disorders of thyroid gland (E00-E07)

☑4ᵗʰ **E00 Congenital iodine-deficiency syndrome**
Use additional code (F70-F79) to identify associated intellectual disabilities
EXCLUDES 1 *subclinical iodine-deficiency hypothyroidism (E02)*

E00.0 Congenital iodine-deficiency syndrome, neurological type
Endemic cretinism, neurological type

E00.1 Congenital iodine-deficiency syndrome, myxedematous type
Endemic hypothyroid cretinism
Endemic cretinism, myxedematous type

E00.2 Congenital iodine-deficiency syndrome, mixed type
Endemic cretinism, mixed type

E00.9 Congenital iodine-deficiency syndrome, unspecified ▽
Congenital iodine-deficiency hypothyroidism NOS
Endemic cretinism NOS

☑4ᵗʰ **E01 Iodine-deficiency related thyroid disorders and allied conditions**
EXCLUDES 1 *congenital iodine-deficiency syndrome (E00.-)*
subclinical iodine-deficiency hypothyroidism (E02)

E01.0 Iodine-deficiency related diffuse (endemic) goiter

E01.1 Iodine-deficiency related multinodular (endemic) goiter
Iodine-deficiency related nodular goiter

E01.2 Iodine-deficiency related (endemic) goiter, unspecified ▽
Endemic goiter NOS

E01.8 Other iodine-deficiency related thyroid disorders and allied conditions
Acquired iodine-deficiency hypothyroidism NOS

E02 Subclinical iodine-deficiency hypothyroidism

☑4ᵗʰ **E03 Other hypothyroidism**
EXCLUDES 1 *iodine-deficiency related hypothyroidism (E00-E02)*
postprocedural hypothyroidism (E89.0)

E03.0 Congenital hypothyroidism with diffuse goiter
Congenital parenchymatous goiter (nontoxic)
Congenital goiter (nontoxic) NOS
EXCLUDES 1 *transitory congenital goiter with normal function (P72.0)*

E03.1 Congenital hypothyroidism without goiter
Aplasia of thyroid (with myxedema)
Congenital atrophy of thyroid
Congenital hypothyroidism NOS

E03.2 Hypothyroidism due to medicaments and other exogenous substances
Code first poisoning due to drug or toxin, if applicable (T36-T65 with fifth or sixth character 1-4 or 6)
Use additional code for adverse effect, if applicable, to identify drug (T36-T50 with fifth or sixth character 5)

E03.3 Postinfectious hypothyroidism

E03.4 Atrophy of thyroid (acquired)
EXCLUDES 1 *congenital atrophy of thyroid (E03.1)*

E03.5 Myxedema coma **HCC**

E03.8 Other specified hypothyroidism

E03.9 Hypothyroidism, unspecified ▽
Myxedema NOS

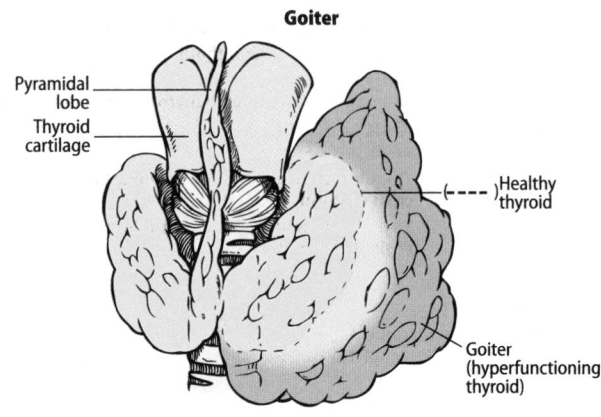

Goiter

Pyramidal lobe

Thyroid cartilage

Healthy thyroid

Goiter (hyperfunctioning thyroid)

☑4ᵗʰ **E04 Other nontoxic goiter**
EXCLUDES 1 *congenital goiter (NOS) (diffuse) (parenchymatous) (E03.0)*
iodine-deficiency related goiter (E00-E02)

E04.0 Nontoxic diffuse goiter
Diffuse (colloid) nontoxic goiter
Simple nontoxic goiter

E04.1 Nontoxic single thyroid nodule
Colloid nodule (cystic) (thyroid)
Nontoxic uninodular goiter
Thyroid (cystic) nodule NOS
DEF: Enlarged thyroid, commonly due to decreased thyroid production, with single nodule; no clinical hypothyroidism.

E04.2 Nontoxic multinodular goiter
Cystic goiter NOS
Multinodular (cystic) goiter NOS
DEF: Enlarged thyroid, commonly due to decreased thyroid production with multiple nodules; no clinical hypothyroidism.

E04.8 Other specified nontoxic goiter

E04.9 Nontoxic goiter, unspecified ▽
Goiter NOS
Nodular goiter (nontoxic) NOS

☑4ᵗʰ **E05 Thyrotoxicosis [hyperthyroidism]**
EXCLUDES 1 *chronic thyroiditis with transient thyrotoxicosis (E06.2)*
neonatal thyrotoxicosis (P72.1)c

☑5ᵗʰ **E05.0 Thyrotoxicosis with diffuse goiter**
Exophthalmic or toxic goiter NOS   Graves' disease
     Toxic diffuse goiter
DEF: Diffuse thyroid enlargement accompanied by hyperthyroidism, bulging eyes, and dermopathy.

E05.00 Thyrotoxicosis with diffuse goiter without thyrotoxic crisis or storm

E05.01 Thyrotoxicosis with diffuse goiter with thyrotoxic crisis or storm

☑5ᵗʰ **E05.1 Thyrotoxicosis with toxic single thyroid nodule**
Thyrotoxicosis with toxic uninodular goiter
DEF: Symptomatic hyperthyroidism with a single nodule on the enlarged thyroid gland. Abrupt onset of symptoms include extreme nervousness, insomnia, weight loss, tremors, and psychosis or coma.

E05.10 Thyrotoxicosis with toxic single thyroid nodule without thyrotoxic crisis or storm

E05.11 Thyrotoxicosis with toxic single thyroid nodule with thyrotoxic crisis or storm

☑5ᵗʰ **E05.2 Thyrotoxicosis with toxic multinodular goiter**
Toxic nodular goiter NOS

E05.20 Thyrotoxicosis with toxic multinodular goiter without thyrotoxic crisis or storm

E05.21 Thyrotoxicosis with toxic multinodular goiter with thyrotoxic crisis or storm

☑5ᵗʰ **E05.3 Thyrotoxicosis from ectopic thyroid tissue**

E05.30 Thyrotoxicosis from ectopic thyroid tissue without thyrotoxic crisis or storm

E05.31 Thyrotoxicosis from ectopic thyroid tissue with thyrotoxic crisis or storm

☑5ᵗʰ **E05.4 Thyrotoxicosis factitia**

E05.40 Thyrotoxicosis factitia without thyrotoxic crisis or storm

E05.41 Thyrotoxicosis factitia with thyrotoxic crisis or storm

---

☑ Additional Character Req   ✓x7ᵗʰ Placeholder Alert   Manifestation   **HCC** CMS-HCC Condition   ▽ Unspecified Code   ▶◀ Revised Text   ● New Code   ▲ Revised Code Title

☑5th **E05.8** **Other thyrotoxicosis**
     Overproduction of thyroid-stimulating hormone

     E05.80 **Other thyrotoxicosis** without thyrotoxic crisis or storm

     E05.81 **Other thyrotoxicosis** with thyrotoxic crisis or storm

☑5th **E05.9** **Thyrotoxicosis, unspecified**
     Hyperthyroidism NOS

     E05.90 **Thyrotoxicosis, unspecified** without thyrotoxic crisis or storm   ▽

     E05.91 **Thyrotoxicosis, unspecified** with thyrotoxic crisis or storm   ▽

☑4th **E06** **Thyroiditis**
     EXCLUDES 1 *postpartum thyroiditis (O90.5)*

     E06.0 **Acute thyroiditis**
         Abscess of thyroid
         Pyogenic thyroiditis
         Suppurative thyroiditis
         Use additional code (B95-B97) to identify infectious agent

     E06.1 **Subacute thyroiditis**
         de Quervain thyroiditis
         Giant-cell thyroiditis
         Granulomatous thyroiditis
         Nonsuppurative thyroiditis
         Viral thyroiditis
         EXCLUDES 1 *autoimmune thyroiditis (E06.3)*

     E06.2 **Chronic thyroiditis with transient thyrotoxicosis**
         EXCLUDES 1 *autoimmune thyroiditis (E06.3)*

     E06.3 **Autoimmune thyroiditis**
         Hashimoto's thyroiditis
         Hashitoxicosis (transient)
         Lymphadenoid goiter
         Lymphocytic thyroiditis
         Struma lymphomatosa

     E06.4 **Drug-induced thyroiditis**
         Use additional code for adverse effect, if applicable, to identify drug (T36-T50 with fifth or sixth character 5)

     E06.5 **Other chronic thyroiditis**
         Chronic fibrous thyroiditis
         Chronic thyroiditis NOS
         Ligneous thyroiditis
         Riedel thyroiditis

     E06.9 **Thyroiditis, unspecified**   ▽

☑4th **E07** **Other disorders of thyroid**

     E07.0 **Hypersecretion of calcitonin**
         C-cell hyperplasia of thyroid
         Hypersecretion of thyrocalcitonin

     E07.1 **Dyshormogenetic goiter**
         Familial dyshormogenetic goiter
         Pendred's syndrome
         EXCLUDES 1 *transitory congenital goiter with normal function (P72.0)*

☑5th **E07.8** **Other specified disorders of thyroid**

     E07.81 **Sick-euthyroid syndrome**
         Euthyroid sick-syndrome

     E07.89 **Other specified disorders of thyroid**
         Abnormality of thyroid-binding globulin
         Hemorrhage of thyroid
         Infarction of thyroid

     E07.9 **Disorder of thyroid, unspecified**   ▽

Diabetes mellitus (E08-E13)

AHA: 2017, 1Q, 42; 2016, 2Q, 36; 2016, 1Q, 11-13

☑4th **E08** **Diabetes mellitus** due to underlying condition
     Code first the underlying condition, such as:
         congenital rubella (P35.0)
         Cushing's syndrome (E24.-)
         cystic fibrosis (E84.-)
         malignant neoplasm (C00-C96)
         malnutrition (E40-E46)
         pancreatitis and other diseases of the pancreas (K85.-, K86.-)
     Use additional code to identify control using:
         insulin (Z79.4)
         oral antidiabetic drugs (Z79.84)
         oral hypoglycemic drugs (Z79.84)
     EXCLUDES 1 *drug or chemical induced diabetes mellitus (E09.-)*
         gestational diabetes (O24.4-)
         neonatal diabetes mellitus (P70.2)
         postpancreatectomy diabetes mellitus (E13.-)
         postprocedural diabetes mellitus (E13.-)
         secondary diabetes mellitus NEC (E13.-)
         type 1 diabetes mellitus (E10.-)
         type 2 diabetes mellitus (E11.-)
     AHA: 2013, 4Q, 114; 2013, 3Q, 20

☑5th **E08.0** **Diabetes mellitus due to underlying condition with hyperosmolarity**

     E08.00 *Diabetes mellitus due to underlying condition with hyperosmolarity without nonketotic hyperglycemic-hyperosmolar coma (NKHHC)*   HCC

     E08.01 *Diabetes mellitus due to underlying condition with hyperosmolarity with coma*   HCC

☑5th **E08.1** **Diabetes mellitus due to underlying condition with ketoacidosis**

     E08.10 *Diabetes mellitus due to underlying condition with ketoacidosis without coma*   HCC

     E08.11 *Diabetes mellitus due to underlying condition with ketoacidosis with coma*   HCC

☑5th **E08.2** **Diabetes mellitus due to underlying condition with kidney complications**

     E08.21 *Diabetes mellitus due to underlying condition with diabetic nephropathy*   HCC
         Diabetes mellitus due to underlying condition with intercapillary glomerulosclerosis
         Diabetes mellitus due to underlying condition with intracapillary glomerulonephrosis
         Diabetes mellitus due to underlying condition with Kimmelstiel-Wilson disease

     E08.22 *Diabetes mellitus due to underlying condition with diabetic chronic kidney disease*   HCC
         Use additional code to identify stage of chronic kidney disease (N18.1-N18.6)

     E08.29 *Diabetes mellitus due to underlying condition with other diabetic kidney complication*   HCC
         Renal tubular degeneration in diabetes mellitus due to underlying condition

☑5th **E08.3** **Diabetes mellitus due to underlying condition with ophthalmic complications**

     One of the following 7th characters is to be assigned to codes in subcategories E08.32, E08.33, E08.34, E08.35, and E08.37 to designate laterality of the disease:
     1   right eye
     2   left eye
     3   bilateral
     9   unspecified eye

     ☑6th **E08.31** **Diabetes mellitus due to underlying condition with unspecified diabetic retinopathy**

         E08.311 *Diabetes mellitus due to underlying condition with unspecified diabetic retinopathy with macular edema*   HCC ▽

         E08.319 *Diabetes mellitus due to underlying condition with unspecified diabetic retinopathy without macular edema*   HCC ▽

     ☑6th **E08.32** **Diabetes mellitus due to underlying condition with mild nonproliferative diabetic retinopathy**
         Diabetes mellitus due to underlying condition with nonproliferative diabetic retinopathy NOS

         ☑7th *E08.321* *Diabetes mellitus due to underlying condition with mild nonproliferative diabetic retinopathy with macular edema*   HCC

EXCLUDES 1 Not coded here   **EXCLUDES 2** Not included here   N Newborn Age: 0   P Pediatric Age: 0-17   M Maternity Age: 12-55   A Adult Age: 15-124

508   ICD-10-CM 2018

✓7ᵗʰ **E08.329** *Diabetes mellitus due to underlying condition with mild nonproliferative diabetic retinopathy without macular edema* [HCC]

✓6ᵗʰ **E08.33** **Diabetes mellitus due to underlying condition with** moderate nonproliferative diabetic retinopathy

   ✓7ᵗʰ **E08.331** *Diabetes mellitus due to underlying condition with moderate nonproliferative diabetic retinopathy with macular edema* [HCC]

   ✓7ᵗʰ **E08.339** *Diabetes mellitus due to underlying condition with moderate nonproliferative diabetic retinopathy without macular edema* [HCC]

✓6ᵗʰ **E08.34** **Diabetes mellitus due to underlying condition with** severe nonproliferative diabetic retinopathy

   ✓7ᵗʰ **E08.341** *Diabetes mellitus due to underlying condition with severe nonproliferative diabetic retinopathy with macular edema* [HCC]

   ✓7ᵗʰ **E08.349** *Diabetes mellitus due to underlying condition with severe nonproliferative diabetic retinopathy without macular edema* [HCC]

✓6ᵗʰ **E08.35** **Diabetes mellitus due to underlying condition with** proliferative diabetic retinopathy

   ✓7ᵗʰ **E08.351** *Diabetes mellitus due to underlying condition with proliferative diabetic retinopathy with macular edema* [HCC]

   ✓7ᵗʰ **E08.352** *Diabetes mellitus due to underlying condition with proliferative diabetic retinopathy with traction retinal detachment involving the macula* [HCC]

   ✓7ᵗʰ **E08.353** *Diabetes mellitus due to underlying condition with proliferative diabetic retinopathy with traction retinal detachment not involving the macula* [HCC]

   ✓7ᵗʰ **E08.354** *Diabetes mellitus due to underlying condition with proliferative diabetic retinopathy with combined traction retinal detachment and rhegmatogenous retinal detachment* [HCC]

   ✓7ᵗʰ **E08.355** *Diabetes mellitus due to underlying condition with stable proliferative diabetic retinopathy* [HCC]

   ✓7ᵗʰ **E08.359** *Diabetes mellitus due to underlying condition with proliferative diabetic retinopathy without macular edema* [HCC]

E08.36 *Diabetes mellitus due to underlying condition with diabetic cataract* [HCC]
   AHA: 2016, 4Q, 142

✓x7ᵗʰ **E08.37** *Diabetes mellitus due to underlying condition with diabetic macular edema, resolved following treatment* [HCC]

E08.39 *Diabetes mellitus due to underlying condition with other diabetic ophthalmic complication* [HCC]
   Use additional code to identify manifestation, such as: diabetic glaucoma (H40-H42)

✓5ᵗʰ **E08.4** **Diabetes mellitus due to underlying condition with** neurological complications

   E08.40 *Diabetes mellitus due to underlying condition with diabetic neuropathy, unspecified* [HCC] ▽

   E08.41 *Diabetes mellitus due to underlying condition with diabetic mononeuropathy* [HCC]

   E08.42 *Diabetes mellitus due to underlying condition with diabetic polyneuropathy* [HCC]
      Diabetes mellitus due to underlying condition with diabetic neuralgia

   E08.43 *Diabetes mellitus due to underlying condition with diabetic autonomic (poly)neuropathy* [HCC]
      Diabetes mellitus due to underlying condition with diabetic gastroparesis
      AHA: 2013, 4Q, 114

   E08.44 *Diabetes mellitus due to underlying condition with diabetic amyotrophy* [HCC]

   E08.49 *Diabetes mellitus due to underlying condition with other diabetic neurological complication* [HCC]

✓5ᵗʰ **E08.5** **Diabetes mellitus due to underlying condition with** circulatory complications

   E08.51 *Diabetes mellitus due to underlying condition with diabetic peripheral angiopathy without gangrene* [HCC]

E08.52 *Diabetes mellitus due to underlying condition with diabetic peripheral angiopathy with gangrene* [HCC]
   Diabetes mellitus due to underlying condition with diabetic gangrene

E08.59 *Diabetes mellitus due to underlying condition with other circulatory complications* [HCC]

✓5ᵗʰ **E08.6** **Diabetes mellitus due to underlying condition with other specified complications**

✓6ᵗʰ **E08.61** **Diabetes mellitus due to underlying condition with** diabetic arthropathy

   E08.610 *Diabetes mellitus due to underlying condition with diabetic neuropathic arthropathy* [HCC]
      Diabetes mellitus due to underlying condition with Charcôt's joints

   E08.618 *Diabetes mellitus due to underlying condition with other diabetic arthropathy* [HCC]

✓6ᵗʰ **E08.62** **Diabetes mellitus due to underlying condition with** skin complications

   E08.620 *Diabetes mellitus due to underlying condition with diabetic dermatitis* [HCC]
      Diabetes mellitus due to underlying condition with diabetic necrobiosis lipoidica

   E08.621 *Diabetes mellitus due to underlying condition with foot ulcer* [HCC]
      Use additional code to identify site of ulcer (L97.4-, L97.5-)

   E08.622 *Diabetes mellitus due to underlying condition with other skin ulcer* [HCC]
      Use additional code to identify site of ulcer (L97.1-L97.9, L98.41-L98.49)

   E08.628 *Diabetes mellitus due to underlying condition with other skin complications* [HCC]

✓6ᵗʰ **E08.63** **Diabetes mellitus due to underlying condition with** oral complications

   E08.630 *Diabetes mellitus due to underlying condition with periodontal disease* [HCC]

   E08.638 *Diabetes mellitus due to underlying condition with other oral complications* [HCC]

✓6ᵗʰ **E08.64** **Diabetes mellitus due to underlying condition with** hypoglycemia

   E08.641 *Diabetes mellitus due to underlying condition with hypoglycemia with coma* [HCC]

   E08.649 *Diabetes mellitus due to underlying condition with hypoglycemia without coma* [HCC]
      AHA: 2016, 3Q, 42; 2015, 3Q, 21

E08.65 *Diabetes mellitus due to underlying condition with hyperglycemia* [HCC]

E08.69 *Diabetes mellitus due to underlying condition with other specified complication* [HCC]
   Use additional code to identify complication
   AHA: 2016, 4Q, 141; 2016, 1Q, 13

E08.8 *Diabetes mellitus due to underlying condition with unspecified complications* [HCC] ▽

E08.9 *Diabetes mellitus due to underlying condition without complications* [HCC]

✓4ᵗʰ **E09** **Drug or chemical induced diabetes mellitus**
   Code first poisoning due to drug or toxin, if applicable (T36-T65 with fifth or sixth character 1-4 or 6)
   Use additional code for adverse effect, if applicable, to identify drug (T36-T50 with fifth or sixth character 5)
   Use additional code to identify control using:
      insulin (Z79.4)
      oral antidiabetic drugs (Z79.84)
      oral hypoglycemic drugs (Z79.84)
   EXCLUDES 1 *diabetes mellitus due to underlying condition (E08.-)*
      gestational diabetes (O24.4-)
      neonatal diabetes mellitus (P70.2)
      postpancreatectomy diabetes mellitus (E13.-)
      postprocedural diabetes mellitus (E13.-)
      secondary diabetes mellitus NEC (E13.-)
      type 1 diabetes mellitus (E10.-)
      type 2 diabetes mellitus (E11.-)
   AHA: 2013, 4Q, 114; 2013, 3Q, 20

✓5ᵗʰ **E09.0** **Drug or chemical induced diabetes mellitus with** hyperosmolarity

   E09.00 **Drug or chemical induced diabetes mellitus with hyperosmolarity** without nonketotic hyperglycemic-hyperosmolar coma **(NKHHC)** [HCC]

✓ Additional Character Req   ✓x7ᵗʰ Placeholder Alert   Manifestation   [HCC] CMS-HCC Condition   ▽ Unspecified Code   ►◄ Revised Text   ● New Code   ▲ Revised Code Title

Chapter 4. Endocrine, Nutritional, and Metabolic Diseases

E09.01   **Drug or chemical induced diabetes mellitus with hyperosmolarity with coma**   HCC

√5ᵗʰ **E09.1**   **Drug or chemical induced diabetes mellitus with ketoacidosis**

     E09.10   **Drug or chemical induced diabetes mellitus with ketoacidosis without coma**   HCC

     E09.11   **Drug or chemical induced diabetes mellitus with ketoacidosis with coma**   HCC

√5ᵗʰ **E09.2**   **Drug or chemical induced diabetes mellitus with kidney complications**

     E09.21   **Drug or chemical induced diabetes mellitus with diabetic nephropathy**   HCC
         Drug or chemical induced diabetes mellitus with intercapillary glomerulosclerosis
         Drug or chemical induced diabetes mellitus with intracapillary glomerulonephrosis
         Drug or chemical induced diabetes mellitus with Kimmelstiel-Wilson disease

     E09.22   **Drug or chemical induced diabetes mellitus with diabetic chronic kidney disease**   HCC
         Use additional code to identify stage of chronic kidney disease (N18.1-N18.6)

     E09.29   **Drug or chemical induced diabetes mellitus with other diabetic kidney complication**   HCC
         Drug or chemical induced diabetes mellitus with renal tubular degeneration

√5ᵗʰ **E09.3**   **Drug or chemical induced diabetes mellitus with ophthalmic complications**

> One of the following 7th characters is to be assigned to codes in subcategories E09.32, E09.33, E09.34, E09.35, and E09.37 to designate laterality of the disease:
> 1   right eye
> 2   left eye
> 3   bilateral
> 9   unspecified eye

   √6ᵗʰ **E09.31**   **Drug or chemical induced diabetes mellitus with unspecified diabetic retinopathy**

       E09.311   **Drug or chemical induced diabetes mellitus with unspecified diabetic retinopathy with macular edema**   HCC ▽

       E09.319   **Drug or chemical induced diabetes mellitus with unspecified diabetic retinopathy without macular edema**   HCC ▽

   √6ᵗʰ **E09.32**   **Drug or chemical induced diabetes mellitus with mild nonproliferative diabetic retinopathy**
         Drug or chemical induced diabetes mellitus with nonproliferative diabetic retinopathy NOS

       √7ᵗʰ **E09.321**   **Drug or chemical induced diabetes mellitus with mild nonproliferative diabetic retinopathy with macular edema**   HCC

       √7ᵗʰ **E09.329**   **Drug or chemical induced diabetes mellitus with mild nonproliferative diabetic retinopathy without macular edema**   HCC

   √6ᵗʰ **E09.33**   **Drug or chemical induced diabetes mellitus with moderate nonproliferative diabetic retinopathy**

       √7ᵗʰ **E09.331**   **Drug or chemical induced diabetes mellitus with moderate nonproliferative diabetic retinopathy with macular edema**   HCC

       √7ᵗʰ **E09.339**   **Drug or chemical induced diabetes mellitus with moderate nonproliferative diabetic retinopathy without macular edema**   HCC

   √6ᵗʰ **E09.34**   **Drug or chemical induced diabetes mellitus with severe nonproliferative diabetic retinopathy**

       √7ᵗʰ **E09.341**   **Drug or chemical induced diabetes mellitus with severe nonproliferative diabetic retinopathy with macular edema**   HCC

       √7ᵗʰ **E09.349**   **Drug or chemical induced diabetes mellitus with severe nonproliferative diabetic retinopathy without macular edema**   HCC

   √6ᵗʰ **E09.35**   **Drug or chemical induced diabetes mellitus with proliferative diabetic retinopathy**

       √7ᵗʰ **E09.351**   **Drug or chemical induced diabetes mellitus with proliferative diabetic retinopathy with macular edema**   HCC

       √7ᵗʰ **E09.352**   **Drug or chemical induced diabetes mellitus with proliferative diabetic retinopathy with traction retinal detachment involving the macula**   HCC

       √7ᵗʰ **E09.353**   **Drug or chemical induced diabetes mellitus with proliferative diabetic retinopathy with traction retinal detachment not involving the macula**   HCC

       √7ᵗʰ **E09.354**   **Drug or chemical induced diabetes mellitus with proliferative diabetic retinopathy with combined traction retinal detachment and rhegmatogenous retinal detachment**   HCC

       √7ᵗʰ **E09.355**   **Drug or chemical induced diabetes mellitus with stable proliferative diabetic retinopathy**   HCC

       √7ᵗʰ **E09.359**   **Drug or chemical induced diabetes mellitus with proliferative diabetic retinopathy without macular edema**   HCC

     E09.36   **Drug or chemical induced diabetes mellitus with diabetic cataract**   HCC
         AHA: 2016, 4Q, 142

   √x7ᵗʰ **E09.37**   **Drug or chemical induced diabetes mellitus with diabetic macular edema, resolved following treatment**   HCC

     E09.39   **Drug or chemical induced diabetes mellitus with other diabetic ophthalmic complication**   HCC
         Use additional code to identify manifestation, such as: diabetic glaucoma (H40-H42)

√5ᵗʰ **E09.4**   **Drug or chemical induced diabetes mellitus with neurological complications**

     E09.40   **Drug or chemical induced diabetes mellitus with neurological complications with diabetic neuropathy, unspecified**   HCC ▽

     E09.41   **Drug or chemical induced diabetes mellitus with neurological complications with diabetic mononeuropathy**   HCC

     E09.42   **Drug or chemical induced diabetes mellitus with neurological complications with diabetic polyneuropathy**   HCC
         Drug or chemical induced diabetes mellitus with diabetic neuralgia

     E09.43   **Drug or chemical induced diabetes mellitus with neurological complications with diabetic autonomic (poly)neuropathy**   HCC
         Drug or chemical induced diabetes mellitus with diabetic gastroparesis
         AHA: 2013, 4Q, 114

     E09.44   **Drug or chemical induced diabetes mellitus with neurological complications with diabetic amyotrophy**   HCC

     E09.49   **Drug or chemical induced diabetes mellitus with neurological complications with other diabetic neurological complication**   HCC

√5ᵗʰ **E09.5**   **Drug or chemical induced diabetes mellitus with circulatory complications**

     E09.51   **Drug or chemical induced diabetes mellitus with diabetic peripheral angiopathy without gangrene**   HCC

     E09.52   **Drug or chemical induced diabetes mellitus with diabetic peripheral angiopathy with gangrene**   HCC
         Drug or chemical induced diabetes mellitus with diabetic gangrene

     E09.59   **Drug or chemical induced diabetes mellitus with other circulatory complications**   HCC

√5ᵗʰ **E09.6**   **Drug or chemical induced diabetes mellitus with other specified complications**

   √6ᵗʰ **E09.61**   **Drug or chemical induced diabetes mellitus with diabetic arthropathy**

       E09.610   **Drug or chemical induced diabetes mellitus with diabetic neuropathic arthropathy**   HCC
         Drug or chemical induced diabetes mellitus with Charcôt's joints

       E09.618   **Drug or chemical induced diabetes mellitus with other diabetic arthropathy**   HCC

EXCLUDES 1 Not coded here   **EXCLUDES 2** Not included here   N Newborn Age: 0   P Pediatric Age: 0-17   M Maternity Age: 12-55   A Adult Age: 15-124

510   ICD-10-CM 2018

✓6ᵗʰ **E09.62 Drug or chemical induced diabetes mellitus with skin complications**

     E09.620 Drug or chemical induced diabetes   HCC
            mellitus with diabetic dermatitis
               Drug or chemical induced diabetes mellitus
                 with diabetic necrobiosis lipoidica

     E09.621 Drug or chemical induced diabetes   HCC
            mellitus with foot ulcer
               Use additional code to identify site of ulcer
                 (L97.4-, L97.5-)

     E09.622 Drug or chemical induced diabetes   HCC
            mellitus with other skin ulcer
               Use additional code to identify site of ulcer
                 (L97.1-L97.9, L98.41-L98.49)

     E09.628 Drug or chemical induced diabetes   HCC
            mellitus with other skin complications

✓6ᵗʰ **E09.63 Drug or chemical induced diabetes mellitus with oral complications**

     E09.630 Drug or chemical induced diabetes   HCC
            mellitus with periodontal disease

     E09.638 Drug or chemical induced diabetes   HCC
            mellitus with other oral complications

✓6ᵗʰ **E09.64 Drug or chemical induced diabetes mellitus with hypoglycemia**

     E09.641 Drug or chemical induced diabetes   HCC
            mellitus with hypoglycemia with coma

     E09.649 Drug or chemical induced diabetes   HCC
            mellitus with hypoglycemia without coma
               AHA: 2016, 3Q, 42; 2015, 3Q, 21

     E09.65 Drug or chemical induced diabetes mellitus   HCC
            with hyperglycemia

     E09.69 Drug or chemical induced diabetes mellitus   HCC
            with other specified complication
               Use additional code to identify complication
               AHA: 2016, 4Q, 141; 2016, 1Q, 13

E09.8 Drug or chemical induced diabetes mellitus with   HCC ▽
unspecified complications

E09.9 Drug or chemical induced diabetes mellitus without   HCC
complications

✓4ᵗʰ **E10 Type 1 diabetes mellitus**

     INCLUDES   brittle diabetes (mellitus)
            diabetes (mellitus) due to autoimmune process
            diabetes (mellitus) due to immune mediated pancreatic islet
               beta-cell destruction
            idiopathic diabetes (mellitus)
            juvenile onset diabetes (mellitus)
            ketosis-prone diabetes (mellitus)

     EXCLUDES 1   *diabetes mellitus due to underlying condition (E08.-)*
            drug or chemical induced diabetes mellitus (E09.-)
            gestational diabetes (O24.4-)
            hyperglycemia NOS (R73.9)
            neonatal diabetes mellitus (P70.2)
            postpancreatectomy diabetes mellitus (E13.-)
            postprocedural diabetes mellitus (E13.-)
            secondary diabetes mellitus NEC (E13.-)
            type 2 diabetes mellitus (E11.-)

   AHA: 2013, 4Q, 114; 2013, 3Q, 20

✓5ᵗʰ **E10.1 Type 1 diabetes mellitus with ketoacidosis**
       AHA: 2013, 3Q, 20

     E10.10 Type 1 diabetes mellitus with ketoacidosis   HCC
            without coma

     E10.11 Type 1 diabetes mellitus with ketoacidosis   HCC
            with coma

✓5ᵗʰ **E10.2 Type 1 diabetes mellitus with kidney complications**

     E10.21 Type 1 diabetes mellitus with diabetic   HCC
            nephropathy
               Type 1 diabetes mellitus with intercapillary
                 glomerulosclerosis
               Type 1 diabetes mellitus with intracapillary
                 glomerulonephrosis
               Type 1 diabetes mellitus with Kimmelstiel-Wilson
                 disease

     E10.22 Type 1 diabetes mellitus with diabetic chronic   HCC
            kidney disease
               Use additional code to identify stage of chronic kidney
                 disease (N18.1-N18.6)

     E10.29 Type 1 diabetes mellitus with other diabetic   HCC
            kidney complication
               Type 1 diabetes mellitus with renal tubular
                 degeneration
               AHA: 2016, 1Q, 13

✓5ᵗʰ **E10.3 Type 1 diabetes mellitus with ophthalmic complications**

     One of the following 7th characters is to be assigned to codes
     in subcategories E10.32, E10.33, E10.34, E10.35, and E10.37 to
     designate laterality of the disease:
     1   right eye
     2   left eye
     3   bilateral
     9   unspecified eye

✓6ᵗʰ **E10.31 Type 1 diabetes mellitus with unspecified diabetic retinopathy**

     E10.311 Type 1 diabetes mellitus with   HCC ▽
            unspecified diabetic retinopathy
            with macular edema

     E10.319 Type 1 diabetes mellitus with   HCC ▽
            unspecified diabetic retinopathy
            without macular edema

✓6ᵗʰ **E10.32 Type 1 diabetes mellitus with mild nonproliferative diabetic retinopathy**
       Type 1 diabetes mellitus with nonproliferative diabetic
       retinopathy NOS

     ✓7ᵗʰ **E10.321 Type 1 diabetes mellitus with mild**   HCC
            nonproliferative diabetic retinopathy
            with macular edema

     ✓7ᵗʰ **E10.329 Type 1 diabetes mellitus with mild**   HCC
            nonproliferative diabetic retinopathy
            without macular edema

✓6ᵗʰ **E10.33 Type 1 diabetes mellitus with moderate nonproliferative diabetic retinopathy**

     ✓7ᵗʰ **E10.331 Type 1 diabetes mellitus with**   HCC
            moderate nonproliferative diabetic
            retinopathy with macular edema

     ✓7ᵗʰ **E10.339 Type 1 diabetes mellitus with**   HCC
            moderate nonproliferative diabetic
            retinopathy without macular edema

✓6ᵗʰ **E10.34 Type 1 diabetes mellitus with severe nonproliferative diabetic retinopathy**

     ✓7ᵗʰ **E10.341 Type 1 diabetes mellitus with severe**   HCC
            nonproliferative diabetic retinopathy
            with macular edema

     ✓7ᵗʰ **E10.349 Type 1 diabetes mellitus with severe**   HCC
            nonproliferative diabetic retinopathy
            without macular edema

✓6ᵗʰ **E10.35 Type 1 diabetes mellitus with proliferative diabetic retinopathy**

     ✓7ᵗʰ **E10.351 Type 1 diabetes mellitus with**   HCC
            proliferative diabetic retinopathy
            with macular edema

     ✓7ᵗʰ **E10.352 Type 1 diabetes mellitus with**   HCC
            proliferative diabetic retinopathy
            with traction retinal detachment
            involving the macula

     ✓7ᵗʰ **E10.353 Type 1 diabetes mellitus with**   HCC
            proliferative diabetic retinopathy
            with traction retinal detachment not
            involving the macula

     ✓7ᵗʰ **E10.354 Type 1 diabetes mellitus with**   HCC
            proliferative diabetic retinopathy with
            combined traction retinal detachment and
            rhegmatogenous retinal detachment

     ✓7ᵗʰ **E10.355 Type 1 diabetes mellitus with stable**   HCC
            proliferative diabetic retinopathy

     ✓7ᵗʰ **E10.359 Type 1 diabetes mellitus with**   HCC
            proliferative diabetic retinopathy
            without macular edema

     E10.36 Type 1 diabetes mellitus with diabetic cataract   HCC
               AHA: 2016, 4Q, 142

     ✓x7ᵗʰ **E10.37 Type 1 diabetes mellitus with diabetic macular**   HCC
            edema, resolved following treatment

     E10.39 Type 1 diabetes mellitus with other diabetic   HCC
            ophthalmic complication
               Use additional code to identify manifestation, such as:
                 diabetic glaucoma (H40-H42)

✓5ᵗʰ **E10.4 Type 1 diabetes mellitus with neurological complications**

     E10.40 Type 1 diabetes mellitus with diabetic   HCC ▽
            neuropathy, unspecified

     E10.41 Type 1 diabetes mellitus with diabetic   HCC
            mononeuropathy

✓ Additional Character Req   ✓x7ᵗʰ Placeholder Alert   Manifestation   HCC CMS-HCC Condition   ▽ Unspecified Code   ▶◀ Revised Text   ● New Code   ▲ Revised Code Title

Chapter 4. Endocrine, Nutritional, and Metabolic Diseases

E10.42   **Type 1 diabetes mellitus with diabetic polyneuropathy**   HCC
Type 1 diabetes mellitus with diabetic neuralgia

E10.43   **Type 1 diabetes mellitus with diabetic autonomic (poly)neuropathy**   HCC
Type 1 diabetes mellitus with diabetic gastroparesis
AHA: 2013, 4Q, 114

E10.44   **Type 1 diabetes mellitus with diabetic amyotrophy**   HCC

E10.49   **Type 1 diabetes mellitus with other diabetic neurological complication**   HCC

√5ᵗʰ **E10.5**   **Type 1 diabetes mellitus with circulatory complications**

E10.51   **Type 1 diabetes mellitus with diabetic peripheral angiopathy without gangrene**   HCC

E10.52   **Type 1 diabetes mellitus with diabetic peripheral angiopathy with gangrene**   HCC
Type 1 diabetes mellitus with diabetic gangrene

E10.59   **Type 1 diabetes mellitus with other circulatory complications**   HCC

√5ᵗʰ **E10.6**   **Type 1 diabetes mellitus with other specified complications**

√6ᵗʰ **E10.61**   **Type 1 diabetes mellitus with diabetic arthropathy**

E10.610   **Type 1 diabetes mellitus with diabetic neuropathic arthropathy**   HCC
Type 1 diabetes mellitus with Charcôt's joints

E10.618   **Type 1 diabetes mellitus with other diabetic arthropathy**   HCC

√6ᵗʰ **E10.62**   **Type 1 diabetes mellitus with skin complications**

E10.620   **Type 1 diabetes mellitus with diabetic dermatitis**   HCC
Type 1 diabetes mellitus with diabetic necrobiosis lipoidica

E10.621   **Type 1 diabetes mellitus with foot ulcer**   HCC
Use additional code to identify site of ulcer (L97.4-, L97.5-)

E10.622   **Type 1 diabetes mellitus with other skin ulcer**   HCC
Use additional code to identify site of ulcer (L97.1-L97.9, L98.41-L98.49)

E10.628   **Type 1 diabetes mellitus with other skin complications**   HCC

√6ᵗʰ **E10.63**   **Type 1 diabetes mellitus with oral complications**

E10.630   **Type 1 diabetes mellitus with periodontal disease**   HCC

E10.638   **Type 1 diabetes mellitus with other oral complications**   HCC

√6ᵗʰ **E10.64**   **Type 1 diabetes mellitus with hypoglycemia**

E10.641   **Type 1 diabetes mellitus with hypoglycemia with coma**   HCC

E10.649   **Type 1 diabetes mellitus with hypoglycemia without coma**   HCC
AHA: 2016, 3Q, 42; 2016, 1Q, 13; 2015, 3Q, 21

E10.65   **Type 1 diabetes mellitus with hyperglycemia**   HCC
AHA: 2013, 3Q, 20

E10.69   **Type 1 diabetes mellitus with other specified complication**   HCC
Use additional code to identify complication
AHA: 2016, 4Q, 141; 2016, 1Q, 13

E10.8   **Type 1 diabetes mellitus with unspecified complications**   HCC ▽

E10.9   **Type 1 diabetes mellitus without complications**   HCC

√4ᵗʰ **E11**   **Type 2 diabetes mellitus**
   INCLUDES   diabetes (mellitus) due to insulin secretory defect
       diabetes NOS
       insulin resistant diabetes (mellitus)
Use additional code to identify control using:
   insulin (Z79.4)
   oral antidiabetic drugs (Z79.84)
   oral hypoglycemic drugs (Z79.84)
   EXCLUDES 1   *diabetes mellitus due to underlying condition (E08.-)*
       drug or chemical induced diabetes mellitus (E09.-)
       gestational diabetes (O24.4-)
       neonatal diabetes mellitus (P70.2)
       postpancreatectomy diabetes mellitus (E13.-)
       postprocedural diabetes mellitus (E13.-)
       secondary diabetes mellitus NEC (E13.-)
       type 1 diabetes mellitus (E10.-)
  AHA: 2016, 2Q, 10; 2013, 4Q, 114; 2013, 3Q, 20; 2013, 1Q, 26

√5ᵗʰ **E11.0**   **Type 2 diabetes mellitus with hyperosmolarity**

E11.00   **Type 2 diabetes mellitus with hyperosmolarity without nonketotic hyperglycemic-hyperosmolar coma (NKHHC)**   HCC

E11.01   **Type 2 diabetes mellitus with hyperosmolarity with coma**   HCC

● √5ᵗʰ **E11.1**   **Type 2 diabetes mellitus with ketoacidosis**

●   **E11.10**   **Type 2 diabetes mellitus with ketoacidosis without coma**

●   **E11.11**   **Type 2 diabetes mellitus with ketoacidosis with coma**

√5ᵗʰ **E11.2**   **Type 2 diabetes mellitus with kidney complications**

E11.21   **Type 2 diabetes mellitus with diabetic nephropathy**   HCC
Type 2 diabetes mellitus with intercapillary glomerulosclerosis
Type 2 diabetes mellitus with intracapillary glomerulonephrosis
Type 2 diabetes mellitus with Kimmelstiel-Wilson disease

E11.22   **Type 2 diabetes mellitus with diabetic chronic kidney disease**   HCC
Use additional code to identify stage of chronic kidney disease (N18.1-N18.6)
AHA: 2016, 1Q, 12

E11.29   **Type 2 diabetes mellitus with other diabetic kidney complication**   HCC
Type 2 diabetes mellitus with renal tubular degeneration

√5ᵗʰ **E11.3**   **Type 2 diabetes mellitus with ophthalmic complications**

One of the following 7th characters is to be assigned to codes in subcategories E11.32, E11.33, E11.34, E11.35, and E11.37 to designate laterality of the disease:
1   right eye
2   left eye
3   bilateral
9   unspecified eye

√6ᵗʰ **E11.31**   **Type 2 diabetes mellitus with unspecified diabetic retinopathy**

E11.311   **Type 2 diabetes mellitus with unspecified diabetic retinopathy with macular edema**   HCC ▽

E11.319   **Type 2 diabetes mellitus with unspecified diabetic retinopathy without macular edema**   HCC ▽

√6ᵗʰ **E11.32**   **Type 2 diabetes mellitus with mild nonproliferative diabetic retinopathy**
Type 2 diabetes mellitus with nonproliferative diabetic retinopathy NOS

√7ᵗʰ **E11.321**   **Type 2 diabetes mellitus with mild nonproliferative diabetic retinopathy with macular edema**   HCC

√7ᵗʰ **E11.329**   **Type 2 diabetes mellitus with mild nonproliferative diabetic retinopathy without macular edema**   HCC

√6ᵗʰ **E11.33**   **Type 2 diabetes mellitus with moderate nonproliferative diabetic retinopathy**

√7ᵗʰ **E11.331**   **Type 2 diabetes mellitus with moderate nonproliferative diabetic retinopathy with macular edema**   HCC

√7ᵗʰ **E11.339**   **Type 2 diabetes mellitus with moderate nonproliferative diabetic retinopathy without macular edema**   HCC

✓6th **E11.34 Type 2 diabetes mellitus with** severe nonproliferative **diabetic** retinopathy

  ✓7th **E11.341 Type 2 diabetes mellitus with severe** HCC **nonproliferative diabetic retinopathy with macular edema**

  ✓7th **E11.349 Type 2 diabetes mellitus with severe** HCC **nonproliferative diabetic retinopathy without macular edema**

✓6th **E11.35 Type 2 diabetes mellitus with** proliferative diabetic retinopathy

  ✓7th **E11.351 Type 2 diabetes mellitus with** HCC **proliferative diabetic retinopathy with macular edema**

  ✓7th **E11.352 Type 2 diabetes mellitus with** HCC **proliferative diabetic retinopathy with traction retinal detachment involving the macula**

  ✓7th **E11.353 Type 2 diabetes mellitus with** HCC **proliferative diabetic retinopathy** with traction retinal detachment not involving the macula

  ✓7th **E11.354 Type 2 diabetes mellitus with** HCC **proliferative diabetic retinopathy** with combined traction retinal detachment and rhegmatogenous retinal detachment

  ✓7th **E11.355 Type 2 diabetes mellitus with** stable HCC **proliferative diabetic retinopathy**

  ✓7th **E11.359 Type 2 diabetes mellitus with** HCC **proliferative diabetic retinopathy** without macular edema

E11.36 Type 2 diabetes mellitus with diabetic cataract HCC
  AHA: 2016, 4Q, 142

✓x7th **E11.37 Type 2 diabetes mellitus with diabetic** macular HCC edema, resolved following treatment

E11.39 Type 2 diabetes mellitus with other diabetic HCC **ophthalmic complication**
  Use additional code to identify manifestation, such as: diabetic glaucoma (H40-H42)

✓5th **E11.4 Type 2 diabetes mellitus with** neurological complications

E11.40 Type 2 diabetes mellitus with diabetic HCC ▽ neuropathy, unspecified
  AHA: 2013, 4Q, 129

E11.41 Type 2 diabetes mellitus with diabetic HCC **mononeuropathy**

E11.42 Type 2 diabetes mellitus with diabetic HCC **polyneuropathy**
  Type 2 diabetes mellitus with diabetic neuralgia
  AHA: 2016, 1Q, 12

E11.43 Type 2 diabetes mellitus with diabetic HCC **autonomic (poly)neuropathy**
  Type 2 diabetes mellitus with diabetic gastroparesis
  AHA: 2013, 4Q, 114

E11.44 Type 2 diabetes mellitus with diabetic HCC **amyotrophy**

E11.49 Type 2 diabetes mellitus with other diabetic HCC **neurological complication**

✓5th **E11.5 Type 2 diabetes mellitus with** circulatory complications

E11.51 Type 2 diabetes mellitus with diabetic HCC **peripheral angiopathy without gangrene**

E11.52 Type 2 diabetes mellitus with diabetic HCC **peripheral angiopathy with gangrene**
  Type 2 diabetes mellitus with diabetic gangrene

E11.59 Type 2 diabetes mellitus with other HCC **circulatory complications**

✓5th **E11.6 Type 2 diabetes mellitus with other specified complications**

✓6th **E11.61 Type 2 diabetes mellitus with diabetic** arthropathy

  E11.610 Type 2 diabetes mellitus with diabetic HCC **neuropathic arthropathy**
    Type 2 diabetes mellitus with Charcôt's joints

  E11.618 Type 2 diabetes mellitus with other HCC **diabetic arthropathy**

✓6th **E11.62 Type 2 diabetes mellitus with** skin complications

  E11.620 Type 2 diabetes mellitus with diabetic HCC dermatitis
    Type 2 diabetes mellitus with diabetic necrobiosis lipoidica

E11.621 Type 2 diabetes mellitus with HCC foot ulcer
  Use additional code to identify site of ulcer (L97.4-, L97.5-)
  AHA: 2016, 1Q, 12

E11.622 Type 2 diabetes mellitus with other HCC skin ulcer
  Use additional code to identify site of ulcer (L97.1-L97.9, L98.41-L98.49)

E11.628 Type 2 diabetes mellitus with other HCC **skin complications**

✓6th **E11.63 Type 2 diabetes mellitus with** oral complications

E11.630 Type 2 diabetes mellitus with HCC **periodontal disease**

E11.638 Type 2 diabetes mellitus with other HCC **oral complications**

✓6th **E11.64 Type 2 diabetes mellitus with** hypoglycemia

E11.641 Type 2 diabetes mellitus with HCC **hypoglycemia with coma**

E11.649 Type 2 diabetes mellitus with HCC **hypoglycemia** without coma
  AHA: 2016, 3Q, 42; 2015, 3Q, 21

E11.65 Type 2 diabetes mellitus with hyperglycemia HCC
  AHA: 2013, 3Q, 20

E11.69 Type 2 diabetes mellitus with other specified HCC **complication**
  Use additional code to identify complication
  AHA: 2016, 4Q, 141; 2016, 1Q, 13

E11.8 Type 2 diabetes mellitus with unspecified HCC ▽ **complications**

E11.9 Type 2 diabetes mellitus without complications HCC

✓4th **E13 Other specified diabetes mellitus**
  INCLUDES diabetes mellitus due to genetic defects of beta-cell function
    diabetes mellitus due to genetic defects in insulin action
    postpancreatectomy diabetes mellitus
    postprocedural diabetes mellitus
    secondary diabetes mellitus NEC
  Use additional code to identify control using:
    insulin (Z79.4)
    oral antidiabetic drugs (Z79.84)
    oral hypoglycemic drugs (Z79.84)
  EXCLUDES 1 diabetes (mellitus) due to autoimmune process (E10.-)
    diabetes (mellitus) due to immune mediated pancreatic islet beta-cell destruction (E10.-)
    diabetes mellitus due to underlying condition (E08.-)
    drug or chemical induced diabetes mellitus (E09.-)
    gestational diabetes (O24.4-)
    neonatal diabetes mellitus (P70.2)
    type 1 diabetes mellitus (E10.-)
    ~~type 2 diabetes mellitus (E11.-)~~
  AHA: 2013, 4Q, 114; 2013, 3Q, 20

✓5th **E13.0 Other specified diabetes mellitus with** hyperosmolarity

E13.00 Other specified diabetes mellitus with HCC **hyperosmolarity** without nonketotic **hyperglycemic-hyperosmolar coma (NKHHC)**
  EXCLUDES 2 ▶type 2 diabetes mellitus (E11.-)◀

E13.01 Other specified diabetes mellitus with HCC **hyperosmolarity** with coma

✓5th **E13.1 Other specified diabetes mellitus with** ketoacidosis
  AHA: 2016, 2Q, 10; 2013, 1Q, 26

E13.10 Other specified diabetes mellitus with HCC **ketoacidosis** without coma

E13.11 Other specified diabetes mellitus with HCC **ketoacidosis** with coma

✓5th **E13.2 Other specified diabetes mellitus with** kidney complications

E13.21 Other specified diabetes mellitus with diabetic HCC **nephropathy**
  Other specified diabetes mellitus with intercapillary glomerulosclerosis
  Other specified diabetes mellitus with intracapillary glomerulonephrosis
  Other specified diabetes mellitus with Kimmelstiel-Wilson disease

E13.22 Other specified diabetes mellitus with diabetic HCC **chronic kidney disease**
  Use additional code to identify stage of chronic kidney disease (N18.1-N18.6)

✓ Additional Character Req   ✓x7th Placeholder Alert   Manifestation   HCC CMS-HCC Condition   ▽ Unspecified Code   ▶◀ Revised Text   ● New Code   ▲ Revised Code Title

E13.29 **Other specified diabetes mellitus with other** `HCC`
diabetic kidney complication
Other specified diabetes mellitus with renal tubular
degeneration

✓5th **E13.3** **Other specified diabetes mellitus with ophthalmic**
complications

> One of the following 7th characters is to be assigned to codes
> in subcategories E13.32, E13.33, E13.34, E13.35, and E13.37 to
> designate laterality of the disease:
> 1   right eye
> 2   left eye
> 3   bilateral
> 9   unspecified eye

✓6th **E13.31** **Other specified diabetes mellitus with unspecified**
diabetic retinopathy

E13.311 **Other specified diabetes mellitus** `HCC` ▽
with unspecified diabetic retinopathy
with macular edema

E13.319 **Other specified diabetes mellitus** `HCC` ▽
with unspecified diabetic retinopathy
without macular edema

✓6th **E13.32** **Other specified diabetes mellitus with mild**
nonproliferative diabetic retinopathy
Other specified diabetes mellitus with nonproliferative
diabetic retinopathy NOS

✓7th **E13.321** **Other specified diabetes mellitus** `HCC`
with mild nonproliferative diabetic
retinopathy with macular edema

✓7th **E13.329** **Other specified diabetes mellitus** `HCC`
with mild nonproliferative diabetic
retinopathy without macular edema

✓6th **E13.33** **Other specified diabetes mellitus with moderate**
nonproliferative diabetic retinopathy

✓7th **E13.331** **Other specified diabetes mellitus** `HCC`
with moderate nonproliferative diabetic
retinopathy with macular edema

✓7th **E13.339** **Other specified diabetes mellitus** `HCC`
with moderate nonproliferative diabetic
retinopathy without macular edema

✓6th **E13.34** **Other specified diabetes mellitus with severe**
nonproliferative diabetic retinopathy

✓7th **E13.341** **Other specified diabetes mellitus** `HCC`
with severe nonproliferative diabetic
retinopathy with macular edema

✓7th **E13.349** **Other specified diabetes mellitus** `HCC`
with severe nonproliferative diabetic
retinopathy without macular edema

✓6th **E13.35** **Other specified diabetes mellitus with proliferative**
diabetic retinopathy

✓7th **E13.351** **Other specified diabetes mellitus with** `HCC`
proliferative diabetic retinopathy with
macular edema

✓7th **E13.352** **Other specified diabetes mellitus with** `HCC`
proliferative diabetic retinopathy with
traction retinal detachment involving the
macula

✓7th **E13.353** **Other specified diabetes mellitus with** `HCC`
proliferative diabetic retinopathy with
traction retinal detachment not involving
the macula

✓7th **E13.354** **Other specified diabetes mellitus with** `HCC`
proliferative diabetic retinopathy with
combined traction retinal detachment and
rhegmatogenous retinal detachment

✓7th **E13.355** **Other specified diabetes mellitus with** `HCC`
stable proliferative diabetic retinopathy

✓7th **E13.359** **Other specified diabetes mellitus with** `HCC`
proliferative diabetic retinopathy without
macular edema

E13.36 **Other specified diabetes mellitus with diabetic** `HCC`
cataract
AHA: 2016, 4Q, 142

✓x7th **E13.37** **Other specified diabetes mellitus with diabetic** `HCC`
macular edema, resolved following treatment

E13.39 **Other specified diabetes mellitus with other** `HCC`
diabetic ophthalmic complication
Use additional code to identify manifestation, such as:
diabetic glaucoma (H40-H42)

✓5th **E13.4** **Other specified diabetes mellitus with neurological**
complications

E13.40 **Other specified diabetes mellitus with** `HCC` ▽
diabetic neuropathy, unspecified

E13.41 **Other specified diabetes mellitus with diabetic** `HCC`
mononeuropathy

E13.42 **Other specified diabetes mellitus with diabetic** `HCC`
polyneuropathy
Other specified diabetes mellitus with diabetic
neuralgia

E13.43 **Other specified diabetes mellitus with diabetic** `HCC`
autonomic (poly)neuropathy
Other specified diabetes mellitus with diabetic
gastroparesis
AHA: 2013, 4Q, 114

E13.44 **Other specified diabetes mellitus with diabetic** `HCC`
amyotrophy

E13.49 **Other specified diabetes mellitus with other** `HCC`
diabetic neurological complication

✓5th **E13.5** **Other specified diabetes mellitus with circulatory**
complications

E13.51 **Other specified diabetes mellitus with diabetic** `HCC`
peripheral angiopathy without gangrene

E13.52 **Other specified diabetes mellitus with diabetic** `HCC`
peripheral angiopathy with gangrene
Other specified diabetes mellitus with diabetic
gangrene

E13.59 **Other specified diabetes mellitus with other** `HCC`
circulatory complications

✓5th **E13.6** **Other specified diabetes mellitus with other specified**
complications

✓6th **E13.61** **Other specified diabetes mellitus with diabetic**
arthropathy

E13.610 **Other specified diabetes mellitus** `HCC`
with diabetic neuropathic arthropathy
Other specified diabetes mellitus with
Charcôt's joints

E13.618 **Other specified diabetes mellitus** `HCC`
with other diabetic arthropathy

✓6th **E13.62** **Other specified diabetes mellitus with skin**
complications

E13.620 **Other specified diabetes mellitus** `HCC`
with diabetic dermatitis
Other specified diabetes mellitus with
diabetic necrobiosis lipoidica

E13.621 **Other specified diabetes mellitus** `HCC`
with foot ulcer
Use additional code to identify site of ulcer
(L97.4-, L97.5-)

E13.622 **Other specified diabetes mellitus** `HCC`
with other skin ulcer
Use additional code to identify site of ulcer
(L97.1-L97.9, L98.41-L98.49)

E13.628 **Other specified diabetes mellitus** `HCC`
with other skin complications

✓6th **E13.63** **Other specified diabetes mellitus with oral**
complications

E13.630 **Other specified diabetes mellitus** `HCC`
with periodontal disease

E13.638 **Other specified diabetes mellitus** `HCC`
with other oral complications

✓6th **E13.64** **Other specified diabetes mellitus with hypoglycemia**

E13.641 **Other specified diabetes mellitus** `HCC`
with hypoglycemia with coma

E13.649 **Other specified diabetes mellitus** `HCC`
with hypoglycemia without coma
AHA: 2016, 3Q, 42; 2015, 3Q, 21

E13.65 **Other specified diabetes mellitus with** `HCC`
hyperglycemia

E13.69 **Other specified diabetes mellitus with other** `HCC`
specified complication
Use additional code to identify complication
AHA: 2016, 4Q, 141; 2016, 1Q, 13

E13.8 **Other specified diabetes mellitus with unspecified** `HCC` ▽
complications

E13.9 **Other specified diabetes mellitus without complications** `HCC`

`EXCLUDES 1` Not coded here   `EXCLUDES 2` Not included here   N Newborn Age: 0   P Pediatric Age: 0-17   M Maternity Age: 12-55   A Adult Age: 15-124

514   ICD-10-CM 2018

Other disorders of glucose regulation and pancreatic internal secretion (E15-E16)

E15   **Nondiabetic hypoglycemic coma**   HCC
INCLUDES   drug-induced insulin coma in nondiabetic
hyperinsulinism with hypoglycemic coma
hypoglycemic coma NOS

☑4th **E16**   **Other disorders of pancreatic internal secretion**

E16.0   **Drug-induced hypoglycemia without coma**
Use additional code for adverse effect, if applicable, to identify
drug (T36-T50 with fifth or sixth character 5)
EXCLUDES1   diabetes with hypoglycemia without coma
▶(E09.649)◀

E16.1   **Other hypoglycemia**
Functional hyperinsulinism
Functional nonhyperinsulinemic hypoglycemia
Hyperinsulinism NOS
Hyperplasia of pancreatic islet beta cells NOS
EXCLUDES1   diabetes with hypoglycemia (E08.649, E10.649,
E11.649, E13.649)
hypoglycemia in infant of diabetic mother (P70.1)
neonatal hypoglycemia (P70.4)

E16.2   **Hypoglycemia, unspecified**   ▽
EXCLUDES1   diabetes with hypoglycemia (E08.649, E10.649,
E11.649, E13.649)
AHA: 2016, 3Q, 42

E16.3   **Increased secretion of glucagon**
Hyperplasia of pancreatic endocrine cells with glucagon excess

E16.4   **Increased secretion of gastrin**
Hypergastrinemia
Hyperplasia of pancreatic endocrine cells with gastrin excess
Zollinger-Ellison syndrome

E16.8   **Other specified disorders of pancreatic internal secretion**
Increased secretion from endocrine pancreas of growth
hormone-releasing hormone
Increased secretion from endocrine pancreas of pancreatic
polypeptide
Increased secretion from endocrine pancreas of somatostatin
Increased secretion from endocrine pancreas of
vasoactive-intestinal polypeptide

E16.9   **Disorder of pancreatic internal secretion, unspecified**   ▽
Islet-cell hyperplasia NOS
Pancreatic endocrine cell hyperplasia NOS

Disorders of other endocrine glands (E20-E35)

EXCLUDES1   galactorrhea (N64.3)
gynecomastia (N62)

☑4th **E20**   **Hypoparathyroidism**
EXCLUDES1   Di George's syndrome (D82.1)
postprocedural hypoparathyroidism (E89.2)
tetany NOS (R29.0)
transitory neonatal hypoparathyroidism (P71.4)

E20.0   **Idiopathic hypoparathyroidism**   HCC
DEF: Abnormally low secretion of parathyroid hormones, with
unknown cause, which causes decreased calcium and increased
phosphorus in the blood, resulting in muscle cramps, tetany,
tingling, or burning in lips, fingers, and toes, and cataracts.

E20.1   **Pseudohypoparathyroidism**

E20.8   **Other hypoparathyroidism**   HCC

E20.9   **Hypoparathyroidism, unspecified**   HCC ▽
Parathyroid tetany

☑4th **E21**   **Hyperparathyroidism and other disorders of parathyroid gland**
EXCLUDES1   adult osteomalacia (M83.-)
ectopic hyperparathyroidism (E34.2)
familial hypocalciuric hypercalcemia (E83.52)
hungry bone syndrome (E83.81)
infantile and juvenile osteomalacia (E55.0)

E21.0   **Primary hyperparathyroidism**   HCC
Hyperplasia of parathyroid
Osteitis fibrosa cystica generalisata [von Recklinghausen's
disease of bone]
DEF: Parathyroid dysfunction commonly caused by hyperplasia of
two or more glands; characteristic hypercalcemia and increased
parathyroid hormone levels.

E21.1   **Secondary hyperparathyroidism, not elsewhere classified** HCC
EXCLUDES1   secondary hyperparathyroidism of renal origin
(N25.81)

E21.2   **Other hyperparathyroidism**   HCC
Tertiary hyperparathyroidism
EXCLUDES1   familial hypocalciuric hypercalcemia (E83.52)

E21.3   **Hyperparathyroidism, unspecified**   HCC ▽
E21.4   **Other specified disorders of parathyroid gland**   HCC
E21.5   **Disorder of parathyroid gland, unspecified**   HCC ▽

☑4th **E22**   **Hyperfunction of pituitary gland**
EXCLUDES1   Cushing's syndrome (E24.-)
Nelson's syndrome (E24.1)
overproduction of ACTH not associated with Cushing's disease
(E27.0)
overproduction of pituitary ACTH (E24.0)
overproduction of thyroid-stimulating hormone (E05.8-)

E22.0   **Acromegaly and pituitary gigantism**   HCC
Overproduction of growth hormone
EXCLUDES1   constitutional gigantism (E34.4)
constitutional tall stature (E34.4)
increased secretion from endocrine pancreas of growth
hormone-releasing hormone (E16.8)

E22.1   **Hyperprolactinemia**   HCC
Use additional code for adverse effect, if applicable, to identify
drug (T36-T50 with fifth or sixth character 5)

E22.2   **Syndrome of inappropriate secretion of antidiuretic** HCC
hormone

E22.8   **Other hyperfunction of pituitary gland**   HCC
Central precocious puberty

E22.9   **Hyperfunction of pituitary gland, unspecified**   HCC ▽

☑4th **E23**   **Hypofunction and other disorders of the pituitary gland**
INCLUDES   the listed conditions whether the disorder is in the pituitary
or the hypothalamus
EXCLUDES1   postprocedural hypopituitarism (E89.3)

E23.0   **Hypopituitarism**   HCC
Fertile eunuch syndrome
Hypogonadotropic hypogonadism
Idiopathic growth hormone deficiency
Isolated deficiency of gonadotropin
Isolated deficiency of growth hormone
Isolated deficiency of pituitary hormone
Kallmann's syndrome
Lorain-Levi short stature
Necrosis of pituitary gland (postpartum)
Panhypopituitarism
Pituitary cachexia
Pituitary insufficiency NOS
Pituitary short stature
Sheehan's syndrome
Simmonds' disease

E23.1   **Drug-induced hypopituitarism**   HCC
Use additional code for adverse effect, if applicable, to identify
drug (T36-T50 with fifth or sixth character 5)

E23.2   **Diabetes insipidus**   HCC
EXCLUDES1   nephrogenic diabetes insipidus (N25.1)

E23.3   **Hypothalamic dysfunction, not elsewhere classified** HCC
EXCLUDES1   Prader-Willi syndrome (Q87.1)
Russell-Silver syndrome (Q87.1)

E23.6   **Other disorders of pituitary gland**   HCC
Abscess of pituitary   Adiposogenital dystrophy

E23.7   **Disorder of pituitary gland, unspecified**   HCC ▽

☑4th **E24**   **Cushing's syndrome**
EXCLUDES1   congenital adrenal hyperplasia (E25.0)

E24.0   **Pituitary-dependent Cushing's disease**   HCC
Overproduction of pituitary ACTH
Pituitary-dependent hypercorticalism

E24.1   **Nelson's syndrome**   HCC

E24.2   **Drug-induced Cushing's syndrome**   HCC
Use additional code for adverse effect, if applicable, to identify
drug (T36-T50 with fifth or sixth character 5)

E24.3   **Ectopic ACTH syndrome**   HCC
E24.4   **Alcohol-induced pseudo-Cushing's syndrome**   HCC
E24.8   **Other Cushing's syndrome**   HCC
E24.9   **Cushing's syndrome, unspecified**   HCC ▽

Chapter 4. Endocrine, Nutritional, and Metabolic Diseases

E25–E31.1

✓4th **E25** **Adrenogenital disorders**

INCLUDES   adrenogenital syndromes, virilizing or feminizing, whether acquired or due to adrenal hyperplasia

consequent on inborn enzyme defects in hormone synthesis

female adrenal pseudohermaphroditism

female heterosexual precocious pseudopuberty

male isosexual precocious pseudopuberty

male macrogenitosomia praecox

male sexual precocity with adrenal hyperplasia

male virilization (female)

EXCLUDES 1   *indeterminate sex and pseudohermaphroditism (Q56)*
chromosomal abnormalities (Q90-Q99)

E25.0 **Congenital** **adrenogenital disorders** associated with enzyme deficiency   HCC

Congenital adrenal hyperplasia

21-Hydroxylase deficiency

Salt-losing congenital adrenal hyperplasia

E25.8 **Other adrenogenital disorders**   HCC

Idiopathic adrenogenital disorder

Use additional code for adverse effect, if applicable, to identify drug (T36-T50 with fifth or sixth character 5)

E25.9 **Adrenogenital disorder, unspecified**   HCC ▽

Adrenogenital syndrome NOS

✓4th **E26** **Hyperaldosteronism**

✓5th **E26.0** **Primary** **hyperaldosteronism**

E26.01 **Conn's syndrome**   HCC

Code also adrenal adenoma (D35.0-)

E26.02 **Glucocorticoid-remediable aldosteronism**   HCC

Familial aldosteronism type I

DEF: Rare autosomal dominant familial form of primary aldosteronism in which the secretion of aldosterone is under the influence of adrenocorticotrophic hormone (ACTH) rather than the renin-angiotensin mechanism; moderate hypersecretion of aldosterone and suppressed plasma renin activity that are rapidly reversed by administration of glucosteroids; symptoms include hypertension and mild hypokalemia.

E26.09 **Other primary hyperaldosteronism**   HCC

Primary aldosteronism due to adrenal hyperplasia (bilateral)

E26.1 **Secondary hyperaldosteronism**   HCC

✓5th **E26.8** **Other hyperaldosteronism**

E26.81 **Bartter's syndrome**   HCC

E26.89 **Other hyperaldosteronism**   HCC

E26.9 **Hyperaldosteronism, unspecified**   HCC ▽

Aldosteronism NOS

Hyperaldosteronism NOS

✓4th **E27** **Other disorders of adrenal gland**

E27.0 **Other adrenocortical overactivity**   HCC

Overproduction of ACTH, not associated with Cushing's disease

Premature adrenarche

EXCLUDES 1   *Cushing's syndrome (E24.-)*

E27.1 **Primary adrenocortical insufficiency**   HCC

Addison's disease

Autoimmune adrenalitis

EXCLUDES 1   *Addison only phenotype adrenoleukodystrophy (E71.528)*
amyloidosis (E85.-)
tuberculous Addison's disease (A18.7)
Waterhouse-Friderichsen syndrome (A39.1)

E27.2 **Addisonian crisis**   HCC

Adrenal crisis

Adrenocortical crisis

E27.3 **Drug-induced adrenocortical insufficiency**   HCC

Use additional code for adverse effect, if applicable, to identify drug (T36-T50 with fifth or sixth character 5)

✓5th **E27.4** **Other and unspecified adrenocortical insufficiency**

EXCLUDES 1   *adrenoleukodystrophy [Addison-Schilder] (E71.528)*
Waterhouse-Friderichsen syndrome (A39.1)

E27.40 **Unspecified adrenocortical insufficiency**   HCC ▽

Adrenocortical insufficiency NOS

Hypoaldosteronism

E27.49 **Other adrenocortical insufficiency**   HCC

Adrenal hemorrhage

Adrenal infarction

E27.5 **Adrenomedullary hyperfunction**   HCC

Adrenomedullary hyperplasia

Catecholamine hypersecretion

E27.8 **Other specified disorders of adrenal gland**   HCC

Abnormality of cortisol-binding globulin

E27.9 **Disorder of adrenal gland, unspecified**   HCC ▽

✓4th **E28** **Ovarian dysfunction**

EXCLUDES 1   *isolated gonadotropin deficiency (E23.0)*
postprocedural ovarian failure (E89.4-)

E28.0 **Estrogen excess**   ♀

Use additional code for adverse effect, if applicable, to identify drug (T36-T50 with fifth or sixth character 5)

E28.1 **Androgen excess**   ♀

Hypersecretion of ovarian androgens

Use additional code for adverse effect, if applicable, to identify drug (T36-T50 with fifth or sixth character 5)

E28.2 **Polycystic ovarian syndrome**   ♀

Sclerocystic ovary syndrome

Stein-Leventhal syndrome

✓5th **E28.3** **Primary ovarian failure**

EXCLUDES 1   *pure gonadal dysgenesis (Q99.1)*
Turner's syndrome (Q96.-)

✓6th **E28.31** **Premature** **menopause**

E28.310 **Symptomatic** **premature menopause**   Ⓐ♀

Symptoms such as flushing, sleeplessness, headache, lack of concentration, associated with premature menopause

E28.319 **Asymptomatic** **premature menopause**   Ⓐ♀

Premature menopause NOS

E28.39 **Other primary ovarian failure**   ♀

Decreased estrogen

Resistant ovary syndrome

E28.8 **Other ovarian dysfunction**   ♀

Ovarian hyperfunction NOS

EXCLUDES 1   *postprocedural ovarian failure (E89.4-)*

E28.9 **Ovarian dysfunction, unspecified**   ♀▽

✓4th **E29** **Testicular dysfunction**

EXCLUDES 1   *androgen insensitivity syndrome (E34.5-)*
azoospermia or oligospermia NOS (N46.0-N46.1)
isolated gonadotropin deficiency (E23.0)
Klinefelter's syndrome (Q98.0-Q98.1, Q98.4)

E29.0 **Testicular** **hyperfunction**   ♂

Hypersecretion of testicular hormones

E29.1 **Testicular** **hypofunction**   ♂

Defective biosynthesis of testicular androgen NOS

5-delta-Reductase deficiency (with male pseudohermaphroditism)

Testicular hypogonadism NOS

Use additional code for adverse effect, if applicable, to identify drug (T36-T50 with fifth or sixth character 5)

EXCLUDES 1   *postprocedural testicular hypofunction (E89.5)*

E29.8 **Other testicular dysfunction**   ♂

E29.9 **Testicular dysfunction, unspecified**   ♂▽

✓4th **E30** **Disorders of puberty, not elsewhere classified**

E30.0 **Delayed** **puberty**

Constitutional delay of puberty

Delayed sexual development

E30.1 **Precocious** **puberty**   Ⓟ

Precocious menstruation

EXCLUDES 1   *Albright (-McCune) (-Sternberg) syndrome (Q78.1)*
central precocious puberty (E22.8)
congenital adrenal hyperplasia (E25.0)
female heterosexual precocious pseudopuberty (E25.-)
male isosexual precocious pseudopuberty (E25.-)

E30.8 **Other disorders of puberty**   Ⓟ

Premature thelarche

E30.9 **Disorder of puberty, unspecified**   ▽

✓4th **E31** **Polyglandular dysfunction**

EXCLUDES 1   *ataxia telangiectasia [Louis-Bar] (G11.3)*
dystrophia myotonica [Steinert] (G71.11)
pseudohypoparathyroidism (E20.1)

E31.0 **Autoimmune polyglandular** **failure**   HCC

Schmidt's syndrome

E31.1 **Polyglandular** **hyperfunction**   HCC

EXCLUDES 1   *multiple endocrine adenomatosis (E31.2-)*
multiple endocrine neoplasia (E31.2-)

EXCLUDES 1 Not coded here   EXCLUDES 2 Not included here   Ⓝ Newborn Age: 0   Ⓟ Pediatric Age: 0-17   Ⓜ Maternity Age: 12-55   Ⓐ Adult Age: 15-124

516   ICD-10-CM 2018

☑5ᵗʰ E31.2 Multiple endocrine neoplasia [MEN] syndromes
Multiple endocrine adenomatosis
Code also any associated malignancies and other conditions associated with the syndromes

E31.20 Multiple endocrine neoplasia [MEN] syndrome, unspecified HCC ▽
Multiple endocrine adenomatosis NOS
Multiple endocrine neoplasia [MEN] syndrome NOS

E31.21 Multiple endocrine neoplasia [MEN] type I HCC
Wermer's syndrome

E31.22 Multiple endocrine neoplasia [MEN] type IIA HCC
Sipple's syndrome

E31.23 Multiple endocrine neoplasia [MEN] type IIB HCC

E31.8 Other polyglandular dysfunction HCC

E31.9 Polyglandular dysfunction, unspecified HCC ▽

☑4ᵗʰ E32 Diseases of thymus
EXCLUDES 1   aplasia or hypoplasia of thymus with immunodeficiency (D82.1)
myasthenia gravis (G70.0)

E32.0 Persistent hyperplasia of thymus HCC
Hypertrophy of thymus

E32.1 Abscess of thymus HCC

E32.8 Other diseases of thymus HCC
EXCLUDES 1   aplasia or hypoplasia with immunodeficiency (D82.1)
thymoma (D15.0)

E32.9 Disease of thymus, unspecified HCC ▽

☑4ᵗʰ E34 Other endocrine disorders
EXCLUDES 1   pseudohypoparathyroidism (E20.1)

E34.0 Carcinoid syndrome HCC
NOTE   May be used as an additional code to identify functional activity associated with a carcinoid tumor.

E34.1 Other hypersecretion of intestinal hormones

E34.2 Ectopic hormone secretion, not elsewhere classified
EXCLUDES 1   ectopic ACTH syndrome (E24.3)

E34.3 Short stature due to endocrine disorder
Constitutional short stature
Laron-type short stature
EXCLUDES 1   achondroplastic short stature (Q77.4)
hypochondroplastic short stature (Q77.4)
nutritional short stature (E45)
pituitary short stature (E23.0)
progeria (E34.8)
renal short stature (N25.0)
Russell-Silver syndrome (Q87.1)
short-limbed stature with immunodeficiency (D82.2)
short stature in specific dysmorphic syndromes— code to syndrome—see Alphabetical Index
short stature NOS (R62.52)

E34.4 Constitutional tall stature HCC
Constitutional gigantism

☑5ᵗʰ E34.5 Androgen insensitivity syndrome

E34.50 Androgen insensitivity syndrome, unspecified ▽
Androgen insensitivity NOS

E34.51 Complete androgen insensitivity syndrome
Complete androgen insensitivity
de Quervain syndrome
Goldberg-Maxwell syndrome

E34.52 Partial androgen insensitivity syndrome
Partial androgen insensitivity
Reifenstein syndrome

E34.8 Other specified endocrine disorders
Pineal gland dysfunction
Progeria
EXCLUDES 2   pseudohypoparathyroidism (E20.1)

E34.9 Endocrine disorder, unspecified ▽
Endocrine disturbance NOS
Hormone disturbance NOS

E35 Disorders of endocrine glands in diseases classified elsewhere
Code first underlying disease, such as:
late congenital syphilis of thymus gland [Dubois disease] (A50.5)
Use additional code, if applicable, to identify:
sequelae of tuberculosis of other organs (B90.8)
EXCLUDES 1   Echinococcus granulosus infection of thyroid gland (B67.3)
meningococcal hemorrhagic adrenalitis (A39.1)
syphilis of endocrine gland (A52.79)
tuberculosis of adrenal gland, except calcification (A18.7)
tuberculosis of endocrine gland NEC (A18.82)
tuberculosis of thyroid gland (A18.81)
Waterhouse-Friderichsen syndrome (A39.1)

Intraoperative complications of endocrine system (E36)

☑4ᵗʰ E36 Intraoperative complications of endocrine system
EXCLUDES 2   postprocedural endocrine and metabolic complications and disorders, not elsewhere classified (E89.-)

☑5ᵗʰ E36.0 Intraoperative hemorrhage and hematoma of an endocrine system organ or structure complicating a procedure
EXCLUDES 1   intraoperative hemorrhage and hematoma of an endocrine system organ or structure due to accidental puncture or laceration during a procedure (E36.1-)

E36.01 Intraoperative hemorrhage and hematoma of an endocrine system organ or structure complicating an endocrine system procedure

E36.02 Intraoperative hemorrhage and hematoma of an endocrine system organ or structure complicating other procedure

☑5ᵗʰ E36.1 Accidental puncture and laceration of an endocrine system organ or structure during a procedure

E36.11 Accidental puncture and laceration of an endocrine system organ or structure during an endocrine system procedure

E36.12 Accidental puncture and laceration of an endocrine system organ or structure during other procedure

E36.8 Other intraoperative complications of endocrine system
Use additional code, if applicable, to further specify disorder

Malnutrition (E40-E46)
EXCLUDES 1   intestinal malabsorption (K90.-)
sequelae of protein-calorie malnutrition (E64.0)
EXCLUDES 2   nutritional anemias (D50-D53)
starvation (T73.0)

E40 Kwashiorkor HCC
Severe malnutrition with nutritional edema with dyspigmentation of skin and hair
EXCLUDES 1   marasmic kwashiorkor (E42)

E41 Nutritional marasmus HCC
Severe malnutrition with marasmus
EXCLUDES 1   marasmic kwashiorkor (E42)
DEF: Protein-calorie malabsorption or malnutrition in children; characterized by tissue wasting, dehydration, and subcutaneous fat depletion; may occur with infectious disease; also called infantile atrophy.

E42 Marasmic kwashiorkor HCC
Intermediate form severe protein-calorie malnutrition
Severe protein-calorie malnutrition with signs of both kwashiorkor and marasmus

E43 Unspecified severe protein-calorie malnutrition HCC ▽
Starvation edema

☑4ᵗʰ E44 Protein-calorie malnutrition of moderate and mild degree
E44.0 Moderate protein-calorie malnutrition HCC
E44.1 Mild protein-calorie malnutrition HCC

E45 Retarded development following protein-calorie malnutrition HCC
Nutritional short stature
Nutritional stunting
Physical retardation due to malnutrition

E46 Unspecified protein-calorie malnutrition HCC ▽
Malnutrition NOS
Protein-calorie imbalance NOS
EXCLUDES 1   nutritional deficiency NOS (E63.9)

Other nutritional deficiencies (E50-E64)
EXCLUDES 2   nutritional anemias (D50-D53)

☑4ᵗʰ E50 Vitamin A deficiency
EXCLUDES 1   sequelae of vitamin A deficiency (E64.1)

E50.0 Vitamin A deficiency with conjunctival xerosis

E50.1 Vitamin A deficiency with Bitot's spot and conjunctival xerosis
Bitot's spot in the young child
DEF: Vitamin A deficiency with conjunctival dryness, superficial spots of keratinized epithelium.

E50.2 Vitamin A deficiency with corneal xerosis

E50.3 Vitamin A deficiency with corneal ulceration and xerosis

E50.4 Vitamin A deficiency with keratomalacia
DEF: Vitamin A deficiency creating corneal dryness; progresses to corneal insensitivity, softness, and necrosis; usually bilateral.

☑ Additional Character Req   ✕ 7ᵗʰ Placeholder Alert   Manifestation   HCC CMS-HCC Condition   ▽ Unspecified Code   ►◄ Revised Text   ● New Code   ▲ Revised Code Title

Chapter 4. Endocrine, Nutritional, and Metabolic Diseases

E50.5–E66.1

E50.5   **Vitamin A deficiency with night blindness**

E50.6   **Vitamin A deficiency with xerophthalmic scars of cornea**

E50.7   **Other ocular manifestations of vitamin A deficiency**
Xerophthalmia NOS

E50.8   **Other manifestations of vitamin A deficiency**
Follicular keratosis
Xeroderma

E50.9   **Vitamin A deficiency, unspecified** ▽
Hypovitaminosis A NOS

✓4ᵗʰ **E51**   **Thiamine deficiency**
EXCLUDES 1   *sequelae of thiamine deficiency (E64.8)*

  ✓5ᵗʰ **E51.1**   **Beriberi**

     E51.11   **Dry beriberi**
Beriberi NOS
Beriberi with polyneuropathy

     E51.12   **Wet beriberi**
Beriberi with cardiovascular manifestations
Cardiovascular beriberi
Shoshin disease

E51.2   **Wernicke's encephalopathy**

E51.8   **Other manifestations of thiamine deficiency**

E51.9   **Thiamine deficiency, unspecified** ▽

E52   **Niacin deficiency [pellagra]**
Niacin (-tryptophan) deficiency
Nicotinamide deficiency
Pellagra (alcoholic)
EXCLUDES 1   *sequelae of niacin deficiency (E64.8)*

✓4ᵗʰ **E53**   **Deficiency of other B group vitamins**
EXCLUDES 1   *sequelae of vitamin B deficiency (E64.8)*

E53.0   **Riboflavin deficiency**
Ariboflavinosis
Vitamin B2 deficiency

E53.1   **Pyridoxine deficiency**
Vitamin B6 deficiency
EXCLUDES 1   *pyridoxine-responsive sideroblastic anemia (D64.3)*

E53.8   **Deficiency of other specified B group vitamins**
Biotin deficiency
Cyanocobalamin deficiency
Folate deficiency
Folic acid deficiency
Pantothenic acid deficiency
Vitamin B12 deficiency
EXCLUDES 1   *folate deficiency anemia (D52.-)*
            vitamin B12 deficiency anemia (D51.-)

E53.9   **Vitamin B deficiency, unspecified** ▽

E54   **Ascorbic acid deficiency**
Deficiency of vitamin C
Scurvy
EXCLUDES 1   *scorbutic anemia (D53.2)*
            sequelae of vitamin C deficiency (E64.2)
DEF: Vitamin C deficiency causing swollen gums, myalgia, weight loss, and weakness.

✓4ᵗʰ **E55**   **Vitamin D deficiency**
EXCLUDES 1   *adult osteomalacia (M83.-)*
            osteoporosis (M80.-)
            sequelae of rickets (E64.3)

E55.0   **Rickets, active**
Infantile osteomalacia
Juvenile osteomalacia
EXCLUDES 1   *celiac rickets (K90.0)*
            Crohn's rickets (K50.-)
            hereditary vitamin D-dependent rickets (E83.32)
            inactive rickets (E64.3)
            renal rickets (N25.0)
            sequelae of rickets (E64.3)
            vitamin D-resistant rickets (E83.31)

E55.9   **Vitamin D deficiency, unspecified** ▽
Avitaminosis D

✓4ᵗʰ **E56**   **Other vitamin deficiencies**
EXCLUDES 1   *sequelae of other vitamin deficiencies (E64.8)*

E56.0   **Deficiency of vitamin E**

E56.1   **Deficiency of vitamin K**
EXCLUDES 1   *deficiency of coagulation factor due to vitamin K deficiency (D68.4)*
            vitamin K deficiency of newborn (P53)

E56.8   **Deficiency of other vitamins**

E56.9   **Vitamin deficiency, unspecified** ▽

E58   **Dietary calcium deficiency**
EXCLUDES 1   *disorders of calcium metabolism (E83.5-)*
            sequelae of calcium deficiency (E64.8)

E59   **Dietary selenium deficiency**
Keshan disease
EXCLUDES 1   *sequelae of selenium deficiency (E64.8)*

E60   **Dietary zinc deficiency**

✓4ᵗʰ **E61**   **Deficiency of other nutrient elements**
Use additional code for adverse effect, if applicable, to identify drug (T36-T50 with fifth or sixth character 5)
EXCLUDES 1   *disorders of mineral metabolism (E83.-)*
            iodine deficiency related thyroid disorders (E00-E02)
            sequelae of malnutrition and other nutritional deficiencies (E64.-)

E61.0   **Copper deficiency**

E61.1   **Iron deficiency**
EXCLUDES 1   *iron deficiency anemia (D50.-)*

E61.2   **Magnesium deficiency**

E61.3   **Manganese deficiency**

E61.4   **Chromium deficiency**

E61.5   **Molybdenum deficiency**

E61.6   **Vanadium deficiency**

E61.7   **Deficiency of multiple nutrient elements**

E61.8   **Deficiency of other specified nutrient elements**

E61.9   **Deficiency of nutrient element, unspecified** ▽

✓4ᵗʰ **E63**   **Other nutritional deficiencies**
EXCLUDES 1   *dehydration (E86.0)*
            failure to thrive, adult (R62.7)
            failure to thrive, child (R62.51)
            feeding problems in newborn (P92.-)
            sequelae of malnutrition and other nutritional deficiencies (E64.-)

E63.0   **Essential fatty acid [EFA] deficiency**

E63.1   **Imbalance of constituents of food intake**

E63.8   **Other specified nutritional deficiencies**

E63.9   **Nutritional deficiency, unspecified** ▽

✓4ᵗʰ **E64**   **Sequelae of malnutrition and other nutritional deficiencies**
NOTE   This category is to be used to indicate conditions in categories E43, E44, E46, E50-E63 as the cause of sequelae, which are themselves classified elsewhere. The 'sequelae' include conditions specified as such; they also include the late effects of diseases classifiable to the above categories if the disease itself is no longer present.
Code first condition resulting from (sequela) of malnutrition and other nutritional deficiencies

E64.0   **Sequelae of protein-calorie malnutrition**   HCC
EXCLUDES 2   *retarded development following protein-calorie malnutrition (E45)*

E64.1   **Sequelae of vitamin A deficiency**

E64.2   **Sequelae of vitamin C deficiency**

E64.3   **Sequelae of rickets**

E64.8   **Sequelae of other nutritional deficiencies**

E64.9   **Sequelae of unspecified nutritional deficiency** ▽

Overweight, obesity and other hyperalimentation (E65-E68)

E65   **Localized adiposity**
Fat pad

✓4ᵗʰ **E66**   **Overweight and obesity**
Code first obesity complicating pregnancy, childbirth and the puerperium, if applicable (O99.21-)
Use additional code to identify body mass index (BMI), if known (Z68.-)
EXCLUDES 1   *adiposogenital dystrophy (E23.6)*
            lipomatosis NOS (E88.2)
            lipomatosis dolorosa [Dercum] (E88.2)
            Prader-Willi syndrome (Q87.1)

  ✓5ᵗʰ **E66.0**   **Obesity due to excess calories**

     E66.01   **Morbid (severe) obesity due to excess calories**   HCC
EXCLUDES 1   *morbid (severe) obesity with alveolar hypoventilation (E66.2)*

     E66.09   **Other obesity due to excess calories**

E66.1   **Drug-induced obesity**
Use additional code for adverse effect, if applicable, to identify drug (T36-T50 with fifth or sixth character 5)

EXCLUDES 1 Not coded here   EXCLUDES 2 Not included here   N Newborn Age: 0   P Pediatric Age: 0-17   M Maternity Age: 12-55   A Adult Age: 15-124

518   ICD-10-CM 2018

Chapter 4. Endocrine, Nutritional, and Metabolic Diseases

E66.2   **Morbid (severe) obesity with alveolar hypoventilation** `HCC`
     Obesity hypoventilation syndrome (OHS)
     Pickwickian syndrome

E66.3   **Overweight**

E66.8   **Other obesity**

E66.9   **Obesity, unspecified**   ▽
     Obesity NOS

✓4ᵗʰ **E67**   **Other hyperalimentation**
   EXCLUDES 1   *hyperalimentation NOS (R63.2)*
          sequelae of hyperalimentation (E68)

E67.0   **Hypervitaminosis A**

E67.1   **Hypercarotinemia**

E67.2   **Megavitamin-B6 syndrome**

E67.3   **Hypervitaminosis D**

E67.8   **Other specified hyperalimentation**

E68   **Sequelae of hyperalimentation**
     Code first condition resulting from (sequela) of hyperalimentation

Metabolic disorders (E70-E88)

EXCLUDES 1   *androgen insensitivity syndrome (E34.5-)*
     congenital adrenal hyperplasia (E25.0)
     Ehlers-Danlos syndrome (Q79.6)
     hemolytic anemias attributable to enzyme disorders (D55.-)
     Marfan's syndrome (Q87.4)
     5-alpha-reductase deficiency (E29.1)

✓4ᵗʰ **E70**   **Disorders of aromatic amino-acid metabolism**

E70.0   **Classical phenylketonuria**   `HCC`

E70.1   **Other hyperphenylalaninemias**   `HCC`

✓5ᵗʰ **E70.2**   **Disorders of tyrosine metabolism**
   EXCLUDES 1   *transitory tyrosinemia of newborn (P74.5)*

     E70.20   **Disorder of tyrosine metabolism, unspecified** `HCC` ▽

     E70.21   **Tyrosinemia**   `HCC`
          Hypertyrosinemia

     E70.29   **Other disorders of tyrosine metabolism**   `HCC`
          Alkaptonuria
          Ochronosis

✓5ᵗʰ **E70.3**   **Albinism**

     E70.30   **Albinism, unspecified**   `HCC` ▽

     ✓6ᵗʰ **E70.31**   **Ocular albinism**

         E70.310   **X-linked ocular albinism**   `HCC`

         E70.311   **Autosomal recessive ocular albinism**   `HCC`

         E70.318   **Other ocular albinism**   `HCC`

         E70.319   **Ocular albinism, unspecified**   `HCC` ▽

     ✓6ᵗʰ **E70.32**   **Oculocutaneous albinism**
       EXCLUDES 1   *Chediak-Higashi syndrome (E70.330)*
            Hermansky-Pudlak syndrome (E70.331)

         E70.320   **Tyrosinase negative oculocutaneous albinism**   `HCC`
            Albinism I
            Oculocutaneous albinism ty-neg

         E70.321   **Tyrosinase positive oculocutaneous albinism**   `HCC`
            Albinism II
            Oculocutaneous albinism ty-pos

         E70.328   **Other oculocutaneous albinism**   `HCC`
            Cross syndrome

         E70.329   **Oculocutaneous albinism, unspecified**   `HCC` ▽

     ✓6ᵗʰ **E70.33**   **Albinism with hematologic abnormality**

         E70.330   **Chediak-Higashi syndrome**   `HCC`

         E70.331   **Hermansky-Pudlak syndrome**   `HCC`

         E70.338   **Other albinism with hematologic abnormality**   `HCC`

         E70.339   **Albinism with hematologic abnormality, unspecified**   `HCC` ▽

     E70.39   **Other specified albinism**   `HCC`
          Piebaldism

✓5ᵗʰ **E70.4**   **Disorders of histidine metabolism**

     E70.40   **Disorders of histidine metabolism, unspecified**   `HCC` ▽

     E70.41   **Histidinemia**   `HCC`

     E70.49   **Other disorders of histidine metabolism**   `HCC`

E70.5   **Disorders of tryptophan metabolism**   `HCC`

E70.8   **Other disorders of aromatic amino-acid metabolism**   `HCC`

E70.9   **Disorder of aromatic amino-acid metabolism, unspecified**   `HCC` ▽

✓4ᵗʰ **E71**   **Disorders of branched-chain amino-acid metabolism and fatty-acid metabolism**

E71.0   **Maple-syrup-urine disease**   `HCC`

✓5ᵗʰ **E71.1**   **Other disorders of branched-chain amino-acid metabolism**

     ✓6ᵗʰ **E71.11**   **Branched-chain organic acidurias**

         E71.110   **Isovaleric acidemia**   `HCC`

         E71.111   **3-methylglutaconic aciduria**   `HCC`

         E71.118   **Other branched-chain organic acidurias**   `HCC`

     ✓6ᵗʰ **E71.12**   **Disorders of propionate metabolism**

         E71.120   **Methylmalonic acidemia**   `HCC`

         E71.121   **Propionic acidemia**   `HCC`

         E71.128   **Other disorders of propionate metabolism**   `HCC`

     E71.19   **Other disorders of branched-chain amino-acid metabolism**   `HCC`
          Hyperleucine-isoleucinemia
          Hypervalinemia

E71.2   **Disorder of branched-chain amino-acid metabolism, unspecified**   `HCC` ▽

✓5ᵗʰ **E71.3**   **Disorders of fatty-acid metabolism**
   EXCLUDES 1   *peroxisomal disorders (E71.5)*
          Refsum's disease (G60.1)
          Schilder's disease (G37.0)
   EXCLUDES 2   *carnitine deficiency due to inborn error of metabolism (E71.42)*

     E71.30   **Disorder of fatty-acid metabolism, unspecified**   ▽

     ✓6ᵗʰ **E71.31**   **Disorders of fatty-acid oxidation**

         E71.310   **Long chain/very long chain acyl CoA dehydrogenase deficiency**   `HCC`
            LCAD   VLCAD

         E71.311   **Medium chain acyl CoA dehydrogenase deficiency**   `HCC`
            MCAD

         E71.312   **Short chain acyl CoA dehydrogenase deficiency**   `HCC`
            SCAD

         E71.313   **Glutaric aciduria type II**   `HCC`
            Glutaric aciduria type II A
            Glutaric aciduria type II B
            Glutaric aciduria type II C
          EXCLUDES 1   *glutaric aciduria (type 1) NOS (E72.3)*

         E71.314   **Muscle carnitine palmitoyltransferase deficiency**   `HCC`

         E71.318   **Other disorders of fatty-acid oxidation**   `HCC`

     E71.32   **Disorders of ketone metabolism**   `HCC`

     E71.39   **Other disorders of fatty-acid metabolism**   `HCC`

✓5ᵗʰ **E71.4**   **Disorders of carnitine metabolism**
   EXCLUDES 1   *muscle carnitine palmitoyltransferase deficiency (E71.314)*

     E71.40   **Disorder of carnitine metabolism, unspecified**   `HCC` ▽

     E71.41   **Primary carnitine deficiency**   `HCC`

     E71.42   **Carnitine deficiency due to inborn errors of metabolism**   `HCC`
          Code also associated inborn error or metabolism

     E71.43   **Iatrogenic carnitine deficiency**   `HCC`
          Carnitine deficiency due to hemodialysis
          Carnitine deficiency due to Valproic acid therapy

     ✓6ᵗʰ **E71.44**   **Other secondary carnitine deficiency**

         E71.440   **Ruvalcaba-Myhre-Smith syndrome**   `HCC`

         E71.448   **Other secondary carnitine deficiency**   `HCC`

✓5ᵗʰ **E71.5**   **Peroxisomal disorders**
   EXCLUDES 1   *Schilder's disease (G37.0)*

     E71.50   **Peroxisomal disorder, unspecified**   `HCC` ▽

     ✓6ᵗʰ **E71.51**   **Disorders of peroxisome biogenesis**
         Group 1 peroxisomal disorders
       EXCLUDES 1   *Refsum's disease (G60.1)*

         E71.510   **Zellweger syndrome**   `HCC`

         E71.511   **Neonatal adrenoleukodystrophy**   `HCC`
          EXCLUDES 1   *X-linked adrenoleuko- dystrophy (E71.52-)*

         E71.518   **Other disorders of peroxisome biogenesis**   `HCC`

✓ Additional Character Req   ✓x7ᵗʰ Placeholder Alert   Manifestation   `HCC` CMS-HCC Condition   ▽ Unspecified Code   ►◄ Revised Text   ● New Code   ▲ Revised Code Title

ICD-10-CM 2018   **519**

✓6th **E71.52 X-linked adrenoleukodystrophy**

    E71.520 Childhood cerebral X-linked adrenoleukodystrophy `HCC`

    E71.521 Adolescent X-linked adrenoleukodystrophy `HCC`

    E71.522 Adrenomyeloneuropathy `HCC`

    E71.528 Other X-linked adrenoleukodystrophy `HCC`
        Addison only phenotype adrenoleukodystrophy
        Addison-Schilder adrenoleukodystrophy

    E71.529 X-linked adrenoleukodystrophy, unspecified type `HCC` ▽

E71.53 Other group 2 peroxisomal disorders `HCC`

✓6th **E71.54 Other peroxisomal disorders**

    E71.540 Rhizomelic chondrodysplasia punctata
        EXCLUDES 1 chondrodysplasia punctata NOS (Q77.3)

    E71.541 Zellweger-like syndrome `HCC`

    E71.542 Other group 3 peroxisomal disorders `HCC`

    E71.548 Other peroxisomal disorders `HCC`

✓4th **E72 Other disorders of amino-acid metabolism**
    EXCLUDES 1 disorders of:
        aromatic amino-acid metabolism (E70.-)
        branched-chain amino-acid metabolism (E71.0-E71.2)
        fatty-acid metabolism (E71.3)
        purine and pyrimidine metabolism (E79.-)
        gout (M1A.-, M10.-)

✓5th **E72.0 Disorders of amino-acid transport**
    EXCLUDES 1 disorders of tryptophan metabolism (E70.5)

    E72.00 Disorders of amino-acid transport, unspecified `HCC` ▽

    E72.01 Cystinuria `HCC`

    E72.02 Hartnup's disease `HCC`

    E72.03 Lowe's syndrome `HCC`
        Use additional code for associated glaucoma (H42)

    E72.04 Cystinosis `HCC`
        Fanconi (-de Toni) (-Debré) syndrome with cystinosis
        EXCLUDES 1 Fanconi (-de Toni) (-Debré) syndrome without cystinosis (E72.09)

    E72.09 Other disorders of amino-acid transport `HCC`
        Fanconi (-de Toni) (-Debré) syndrome, unspecified

✓5th **E72.1 Disorders of sulfur-bearing amino-acid metabolism**
    EXCLUDES 1 cystinosis (E72.04)
        cystinuria (E72.01)
        transcobalamin II deficiency (D51.2)

    E72.10 Disorders of sulfur-bearing amino-acid metabolism, unspecified `HCC` ▽

    E72.11 Homocystinuria `HCC`
        Cystathionine synthase deficiency

    E72.12 Methylenetetrahydrofolate reductase deficiency `HCC`

    E72.19 Other disorders of sulfur-bearing amino-acid metabolism `HCC`
        Cystathioninuria
        Methioninemia
        Sulfite oxidase deficiency

✓5th **E72.2 Disorders of urea cycle metabolism**
    EXCLUDES 1 disorders of ornithine metabolism (E72.4)

    E72.20 Disorder of urea cycle metabolism, unspecified `HCC` ▽
        Hyperammonemia
        EXCLUDES 1 hyperammonemia- hyperornithinemia-homocitrullinemia syndrome (E72.4)
            transient hyperammonemia of newborn (P74.6)

    E72.21 Argininemia `HCC`

    E72.22 Arginosuccinic aciduria `HCC`

    E72.23 Citrullinemia `HCC`

    E72.29 Other disorders of urea cycle metabolism `HCC`

E72.3 Disorders of lysine and hydroxylysine metabolism `HCC`
    Glutaric aciduria NOS   Hydroxylysinemia
    Glutaric aciduria (type I)   Hyperlysinemia
    EXCLUDES 1 glutaric aciduria type II (E71.313)
        Refsum's disease (G60.1)
        Zellweger syndrome (E71.510)

E72.4 Disorders of ornithine metabolism `HCC`
    Hyperammonemia-hyperornithinemia-homocitrullinemia syndrome
    Ornithinemia (types I, II)
    Ornithine transcarbamylase deficiency
    EXCLUDES 1 hereditary choroidal dystrophy (H31.2-)

✓5th **E72.5 Disorders of glycine metabolism**

    E72.50 Disorder of glycine metabolism, unspecified `HCC` ▽

    E72.51 Non-ketotic hyperglycinemia `HCC`

    E72.52 Trimethylaminuria `HCC`

    E72.53 Hyperoxaluria `HCC`
        Oxalosis
        Oxaluria

    E72.59 Other disorders of glycine metabolism `HCC`
        D-glycericacidemia
        Hyperhydroxyprolinemia
        Hyperprolinemia (types I, II)
        Sarcosinemia

E72.8 Other specified disorders of amino-acid metabolism `HCC`
    Disorders of beta-amino-acid metabolism
    Disorders of gamma-glutamyl cycle

E72.9 Disorder of amino-acid metabolism, unspecified `HCC` ▽

✓4th **E73 Lactose intolerance**

E73.0 Congenital lactase deficiency

E73.1 Secondary lactase deficiency

E73.8 Other lactose intolerance

E73.9 Lactose intolerance, unspecified ▽

✓4th **E74 Other disorders of carbohydrate metabolism**
    EXCLUDES 1 diabetes mellitus (E08-E13)
        hypoglycemia NOS (E16.2)
        increased secretion of glucagon (E16.3)
        mucopolysaccharidosis (E76.0-E76.3)

✓5th **E74.0 Glycogen storage disease**

    E74.00 Glycogen storage disease, unspecified `HCC` ▽

    E74.01 von Gierke disease `HCC`
        Type I glycogen storage disease

    E74.02 Pompe disease `HCC`
        Cardiac glycogenosis
        Type II glycogen storage disease

    E74.03 Cori disease `HCC`
        Forbes disease
        Type III glycogen storage disease

    E74.04 McArdle disease `HCC`
        Type V glycogen storage disease

    E74.09 Other glycogen storage disease `HCC`
        Andersen disease
        Hers disease
        Tauri disease
        Glycogen storage disease, types 0, IV, VI-XI
        Liver phosphorylase deficiency
        Muscle phosphofructokinase deficiency

✓5th **E74.1 Disorders of fructose metabolism**
    EXCLUDES 1 muscle phosphofructokinase deficiency (E74.09)

    E74.10 Disorder of fructose metabolism, unspecified ▽

    E74.11 Essential fructosuria
        Fructokinase deficiency

    E74.12 Hereditary fructose intolerance
        Fructosemia

    E74.19 Other disorders of fructose metabolism
        Fructose-1, 6-diphosphatase deficiency

✓5th **E74.2 Disorders of galactose metabolism**

    E74.20 Disorders of galactose metabolism, unspecified `HCC` ▽

    E74.21 Galactosemia `HCC`
        DEF: Any of three genetic disorders due to defective galactose metabolism; symptoms include failure to thrive in infancy, jaundice, liver and spleen damage, cataracts, and mental retardation.

    E74.29 Other disorders of galactose metabolism `HCC`
        Galactokinase deficiency

✓5th **E74.3 Other disorders of intestinal carbohydrate absorption**
    EXCLUDES 2 lactose intolerance (E73.-)

    E74.31 Sucrase-isomaltase deficiency

EXCLUDES 1 Not coded here   *EXCLUDES 2* Not included here   N Newborn Age: 0   P Pediatric Age: 0-17   M Maternity Age: 12-55   A Adult Age: 15-124

520   ICD-10-CM 2018

Tay-Sachs Disease

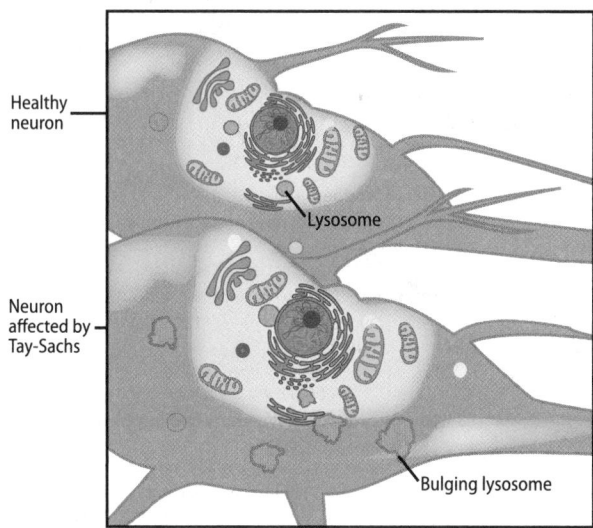

Healthy neuron

Lysosome

Neuron affected by Tay-Sachs

Bulging lysosome

E74.39   **Other disorders of intestinal carbohydrate absorption**
Disorder of intestinal carbohydrate absorption NOS
Glucose-galactose malabsorption
Sucrase deficiency

E74.4   **Disorders of pyruvate metabolism and gluconeogenesis** [HCC]
Deficiency of phosphoenolpyruvate carboxykinase
Deficiency of pyruvate carboxylase
Deficiency of pyruvate dehydrogenase
> **EXCLUDES 1**   disorders of pyruvate metabolism and gluconeogenesis with anemia (D55.-)
> Leigh's syndrome (G31.82)

E74.8   **Other specified disorders of carbohydrate metabolism** [HCC]
Essential pentosuria
Renal glycosuria

E74.9   **Disorder of carbohydrate metabolism, unspecified** [HCC] ▽

✓4th **E75**   **Disorders of sphingolipid metabolism and other lipid storage disorders**
> **EXCLUDES 1**   mucolipidosis, types I-III (E77.0-E77.1)
> Refsum's disease (G60.1)

✓5th **E75.0**   **GM2 gangliosidosis**

    E75.00   **GM2 gangliosidosis, unspecified**   ▽

    E75.01   **Sandhoff disease**

    E75.02   **Tay-Sachs disease**
      DEF: Genetic mutation of the HEXA gene that inhibits the breakdown of a toxic substance called ganglioside. The accumulation of ganglioside results in destruction of the neurons in the brain and spinal cord.

    E75.09   **Other GM2 gangliosidosis**
      Adult GM2 gangliosidosis
      Juvenile GM2 gangliosidosis

✓5th **E75.1**   **Other and unspecified gangliosidosis**

    E75.10   **Unspecified gangliosidosis**   ▽
      Gangliosidosis NOS

    E75.11   **Mucolipidosis IV**

    E75.19   **Other gangliosidosis**
      GM1 gangliosidosis
      GM3 gangliosidosis

✓5th **E75.2**   **Other sphingolipidosis**
> **EXCLUDES 1**   adrenoleukodystrophy [Addison-Schilder] (E71.528)

    E75.21   **Fabry (-Anderson) disease** [HCC]

    E75.22   **Gaucher disease** [HCC]

    E75.23   **Krabbe disease**

✓6th   **E75.24**   **Niemann-Pick disease**
      E75.240   **Niemann-Pick disease type A** [HCC]
      E75.241   **Niemann-Pick disease type B** [HCC]
      E75.242   **Niemann-Pick disease type C** [HCC]
      E75.243   **Niemann-Pick disease type D** [HCC]
      E75.248   **Other Niemann-Pick disease** [HCC]
      E75.249   **Niemann-Pick disease, unspecified** [HCC] ▽

    E75.25   **Metachromatic leukodystrophy**

    E75.29   **Other sphingolipidosis**
      Farber's syndrome
      Sulfatase deficiency
      Sulfatide lipidosis

E75.3   **Sphingolipidosis, unspecified**   [HCC] ▽

E75.4   **Neuronal ceroid lipofuscinosis**
      Batten disease   Kufs disease
      Bielschowsky-Jansky disease   Spielmeyer-Vogt disease

E75.5   **Other lipid storage disorders**
      Cerebrotendinous cholesterosis [van Bogaert-Scherer-Epstein]
      Wolman's disease

E75.6   **Lipid storage disorder, unspecified**   ▽

✓4th **E76**   **Disorders of glycosaminoglycan metabolism**

✓5th   **E76.0**   **Mucopolysaccharidosis, type I**

    E76.01   **Hurler's syndrome** [HCC]

    E76.02   **Hurler-Scheie syndrome** [HCC]

    E76.03   **Scheie's syndrome** [HCC]

  E76.1   **Mucopolysaccharidosis, type II** [HCC]
      Hunter's syndrome

✓5th   **E76.2**   **Other mucopolysaccharidoses**

✓6th   **E76.21**   **Morquio mucopolysaccharidoses**
      E76.210   **Morquio A mucopolysaccharidoses** [HCC]
         Classic Morquio syndrome
         Morquio syndrome A
         Mucopolysaccharidosis, type IVA
      E76.211   **Morquio B mucopolysaccharidoses** [HCC]
         Morquio-like mucopolysaccharidoses
         Morquio-like syndrome
         Morquio syndrome B
         Mucopolysaccharidosis, type IVB
      E76.219   **Morquio mucopolysaccharidoses, unspecified** [HCC] ▽
         Morquio syndrome
         Mucopolysaccharidosis, type IV

    E76.22   **Sanfilippo mucopolysaccharidoses** [HCC]
      Mucopolysaccharidosis, type III (A) (B) (C) (D)
      Sanfilippo A syndrome
      Sanfilippo B syndrome
      Sanfilippo C syndrome
      Sanfilippo D syndrome

    E76.29   **Other mucopolysaccharidoses** [HCC]
      beta-Glucuronidase deficiency
      Maroteaux-Lamy (mild) (severe) syndrome
      Mucopolysaccharidosis, types VI, VII

  E76.3   **Mucopolysaccharidosis, unspecified** [HCC] ▽

  E76.8   **Other disorders of glucosaminoglycan metabolism** [HCC]

  E76.9   **Glucosaminoglycan metabolism disorder, unspecified** [HCC] ▽

✓4th **E77**   **Disorders of glycoprotein metabolism**

  E77.0   **Defects in post-translational modification of lysosomal enzymes** [HCC]
      Mucolipidosis II [I-cell disease]
      Mucolipidosis III [pseudo-Hurler polydystrophy]

  E77.1   **Defects in glycoprotein degradation** [HCC]
      Aspartylglucosaminuria
      Fucosidosis
      Mannosidosis
      Sialidosis [mucolipidosis I]

  E77.8   **Other disorders of glycoprotein metabolism** [HCC]

  E77.9   **Disorder of glycoprotein metabolism, unspecified** [HCC] ▽

✓4th **E78**   **Disorders of lipoprotein metabolism and other lipidemias**
> **EXCLUDES 1**   sphingolipidosis (E75.0-E75.3)

✓5th   **E78.0**   **Pure hypercholesterolemia**

    E78.00   **Pure hypercholesterolemia, unspecified**   ▽
      Fredrickson's hyperlipoproteinemia, type IIa
      Hyperbetalipoproteinemia
      Low-density-lipoprotein-type [LDL] hyperlipoproteinemia
      ▶(Pure) hypercholesterolemia NOS◀

    E78.01   **Familial hypercholesterolemia**

  E78.1   **Pure hyperglyceridemia**
      Elevated fasting triglycerides
      Endogenous hyperglyceridemia
      Fredrickson's hyperlipoproteinemia, type IV
      Hyperlipidemia, group B
      Hyperprebetalipoproteinemia
      Very-low-density-lipoprotein-type [VLDL] hyperlipoproteinemia

✓ Additional Character Req   ✓x7th Placeholder Alert   Manifestation   HCC CMS-HCC Condition   ▽ Unspecified Code   ▶◀ Revised Text   ● New Code   ▲ Revised Code Title

ICD-10-CM 2018   521

E78.2   **Mixed hyperlipidemia**
  Broad- or floating-betalipoproteinemia
  Combined hyperlipidemia NOS
  Elevated cholesterol with elevated triglycerides NEC
  Fredrickson's hyperlipoproteinemia, type IIb or III
  Hyperbetalipoproteinemia with prebetalipoproteinemia
  Hypercholesteremia with endogenous hyperglyceridemia
  Hyperlipidemia, group C
  Tubo-eruptive xanthoma
  Xanthoma tuberosum
  EXCLUDES 1   *cerebrotendinous cholesterosis [van Bogaert-Scherer-Epstein] (E75.5)*
       familial combined hyperlipidemia (E78.4)

E78.3   **Hyperchylomicronemia**
  Chylomicron retention disease
  Fredrickson's hyperlipoproteinemia, type I or V
  Hyperlipidemia, group D
  Mixed hyperglyceridemia

E78.4   **Other hyperlipidemia**
  Familial combined hyperlipidemia

E78.5   **Hyperlipidemia, unspecified**   ▽

E78.6   **Lipoprotein deficiency**
  Abetalipoproteinemia
  Depressed HDL cholesterol
  High-density lipoprotein deficiency
  Hypoalphalipoproteinemia
  Hypobetalipoproteinemia (familial)
  Lecithin cholesterol acyltransferase deficiency
  Tangier disease

✓5ᵗʰ **E78.7**   **Disorders of bile acid and cholesterol metabolism**
  EXCLUDES 1   *Niemann-Pick disease type C (E75.242)*

     E78.70   **Disorder of bile acid and cholesterol metabolism, unspecified** ▽

     E78.71   **Barth syndrome**

     E78.72   **Smith-Lemli-Opitz syndrome**

     E78.79   **Other disorders of bile acid and cholesterol metabolism**

✓5ᵗʰ **E78.8**   **Other disorders of lipoprotein metabolism**

     E78.81   **Lipoid dermatoarthritis**

     E78.89   **Other lipoprotein metabolism disorders**

E78.9   **Disorder of lipoprotein metabolism, unspecified**   ▽

✓4ᵗʰ **E79**   **Disorders of purine and pyrimidine metabolism**
  EXCLUDES 1   *Ataxia-telangiectasia (Q87.1)*
     Bloom's syndrome (Q82.8)
     Cockayne's syndrome (Q87.1)
     calculus of kidney (N20.0)
     combined immunodeficiency disorders (D81.-)
     Fanconi's anemia (D61.09)
     gout (M1A.-, M10.-)
     orotaciduric anemia (D53.0)
     progeria (E34.8)
     Werner's syndrome (E34.8)
     xeroderma pigmentosum (Q82.1)

E79.0   **Hyperuricemia without signs of inflammatory arthritis and tophaceous disease**
  Asymptomatic hyperuricemia

E79.1   **Lesch-Nyhan syndrome**   HCC
  HGPRT deficiency

E79.2   **Myoadenylate deaminase deficiency**   HCC

E79.8   **Other disorders of purine and pyrimidine metabolism**   HCC
  Hereditary xanthinuria

E79.9   **Disorder of purine and pyrimidine metabolism, unspecified**   HCC ▽

✓4ᵗʰ **E80**   **Disorders of porphyrin and bilirubin metabolism**
  INCLUDES   defects of catalase and peroxidase

E80.0   **Hereditary erythropoietic porphyria**   HCC
  Congenital erythropoietic porphyria
  Erythropoietic protoporphyria

E80.1   **Porphyria cutanea tarda**   HCC

✓5ᵗʰ **E80.2**   **Other and unspecified porphyria**

     E80.20   **Unspecified porphyria**   HCC ▽
  Porphyria NOS

     E80.21   **Acute intermittent (hepatic) porphyria**   HCC

     E80.29   **Other porphyria**   HCC
  Hereditary coproporphyria

E80.3   **Defects of catalase and peroxidase**   HCC
  Acatalasia [Takahara]

E80.4   **Gilbert syndrome**

E80.5   **Crigler-Najjar syndrome**

E80.6   **Other disorders of bilirubin metabolism**
  Dubin-Johnson syndrome
  Rotor's syndrome

E80.7   **Disorder of bilirubin metabolism, unspecified**   ▽

✓4ᵗʰ **E83**   **Disorders of mineral metabolism**
  EXCLUDES 1   *dietary mineral deficiency (E58-E61)*
     parathyroid disorders (E20-E21)
     vitamin D deficiency (E55.-)

✓5ᵗʰ **E83.0**   **Disorders of copper metabolism**

     E83.00   **Disorder of copper metabolism, unspecified** ▽

     E83.01   **Wilson's disease**
  Code also associated Kayser Fleischer ring (H18.04-)

     E83.09   **Other disorders of copper metabolism**
  Menkes' (kinky hair) (steely hair) disease

✓5ᵗʰ **E83.1**   **Disorders of iron metabolism**
  EXCLUDES 1   *iron deficiency anemia (D50.-)*
     sideroblastic anemia (D64.0-D64.3)

     E83.10   **Disorder of iron metabolism, unspecified** ▽

     ✓6ᵗʰ **E83.11**   **Hemochromatosis**
  EXCLUDES 1   ▶*GALD (P78.84)*
     gestational alloimmune liver disease (P78.84)
     neonatal hemochromatosis (P78.84)◀

       E83.110   **Hereditary hemochromatosis**   HCC
  Bronzed diabetes
  Pigmentary cirrhosis (of liver)
  Primary (hereditary) hemochromatosis

       E83.111   **Hemochromatosis due to repeated red blood cell transfusions**
  Iron overload due to repeated red blood cell transfusions
  Transfusion (red blood cell) associated hemochromatosis

       E83.118   **Other hemochromatosis**

       E83.119   **Hemochromatosis, unspecified**   ▽

     E83.19   **Other disorders of iron metabolism**
  Use additional code, if applicable, for idiopathic pulmonary hemosiderosis (J84.03)

E83.2   **Disorders of zinc metabolism**
  Acrodermatitis enteropathica

✓5ᵗʰ **E83.3**   **Disorders of phosphorus metabolism and phosphatases**
  EXCLUDES 1   *adult osteomalacia (M83.-)*
     osteoporosis (M80.-)

     E83.30   **Disorder of phosphorus metabolism, unspecified** ▽

     E83.31   **Familial hypophosphatemia**
  Vitamin D-resistant osteomalacia
  Vitamin D-resistant rickets
  EXCLUDES 1   *vitamin D-deficiency rickets (E55.0)*

     E83.32   **Hereditary vitamin D-dependent rickets (type 1) (type 2)**
  25-hydroxyvitamin D 1-alpha-hydroxylase deficiency
  Pseudovitamin D deficiency
  Vitamin D receptor defect

     E83.39   **Other disorders of phosphorus metabolism**
  Acid phosphatase deficiency
  Hypophosphatasia

✓5ᵗʰ **E83.4**   **Disorders of magnesium metabolism**

     E83.40   **Disorders of magnesium metabolism, unspecified** ▽

     E83.41   **Hypermagnesemia**

     E83.42   **Hypomagnesemia**

     E83.49   **Other disorders of magnesium metabolism**

✓5ᵗʰ **E83.5**   **Disorders of calcium metabolism**
  EXCLUDES 1   *chondrocalcinosis (M11.1-M11.2)*
     hungry bone syndrome (E83.81)
     hyperparathyroidism (E21.0-E21.3)

     E83.50   **Unspecified disorder of calcium metabolism** ▽

     E83.51   **Hypocalcemia**

     E83.52   **Hypercalcemia**
  Familial hypocalciuric hypercalcemia

     E83.59   **Other disorders of calcium metabolism**
  Idiopathic hypercalciuria

✓5ᵗʰ **E83.8**   **Other disorders of mineral metabolism**

     E83.81   **Hungry bone syndrome**

     E83.89   **Other disorders of mineral metabolism**

E83.9   **Disorder of mineral metabolism, unspecified**   ▽

EXCLUDES 1 Not coded here   EXCLUDES 2 Not included here   N Newborn Age: 0   P Pediatric Age: 0-17   M Maternity Age: 12-55   A Adult Age: 15-124

522   ICD-10-CM 2018

☑4ᵗʰ **E84 Cystic fibrosis**
  INCLUDES mucoviscidosis
  Code also exocrine pancreatic insufficiency (K86.81)

  E84.0 Cystic fibrosis with pulmonary manifestations   HCC
    Use additional code to identify any infectious organism present, such as:
    Pseudomonas (B96.5)

☑5ᵗʰ **E84.1 Cystic fibrosis with intestinal manifestations**
    E84.11 Meconium ileus in cystic fibrosis   HCC N
      EXCLUDES 1 meconium ileus not due to cystic fibrosis (P76.0)
    E84.19 Cystic fibrosis with other intestinal manifestations   HCC
      Distal intestinal obstruction syndrome

  E84.8 Cystic fibrosis with other manifestations   HCC
  E84.9 Cystic fibrosis, unspecified   HCC ▽

☑4ᵗʰ **E85 Amyloidosis**
  EXCLUDES 1 Alzheimer's disease (G30.0-)
  EXCLUDES 2 ►Alzheimer's disease (G30.0-)◄
  DEF: Conditions of diverse etiologies characterized by the accumulation of insoluble fibrillar proteins (amyloid) in various organs and tissues of the body, compromising vital functions.

  E85.0 Non-neuropathic heredofamilial amyloidosis   HCC
    Hereditary amyloid nephropathy
    ►Code also associated disorders, such as:
      autoinflammatory syndromes (M04.-)◄
      EXCLUDES 2 ►transthyretin-related (ATTR) familial amyloid cardiomyopathy (E85.4)◄

  E85.1 Neuropathic heredofamilial amyloidosis   HCC
    Amyloid polyneuropathy (Portuguese)
    ►Transthyretin-related (ATTR) familial amyloid polyneuropathy◄
    AHA: 2012, 4Q, 99

  E85.2 Heredofamilial amyloidosis, unspecified   HCC ▽
  E85.3 Secondary systemic amyloidosis   HCC
    Hemodialysis-associated amyloidosis
  E85.4 Organ-limited amyloidosis   HCC
    Localized amyloidosis
    ►Transthyretin-related (ATTR) familial amyloid cardiomyopathy◄

☑5ᵗʰ **E85.8 Other amyloidosis**
●   **E85.81 Light chain (AL) amyloidosis**
●   **E85.82 Wild-type transthyretin-related (ATTR) amyloidosis**
    Senile systemic amyloidosis (SSA)
  E85.89 Other amyloidosis
  E85.9 Amyloidosis, unspecified   HCC

☑4ᵗʰ **E86 Volume depletion**
  Use additional code(s) for any associated disorders of electrolyte and acid-base balance (E87.-)
  EXCLUDES 1 dehydration of newborn (P74.1)
    hypovolemic shock NOS (R57.1)
    postprocedural hypovolemic shock (T81.19)
    traumatic hypovolemic shock (T79.4)

  E86.0 Dehydration
    AHA: 2014, 1Q, 7
  E86.1 Hypovolemia
    Depletion of volume of plasma
  E86.9 Volume depletion, unspecified   ▽
    DEF: Depletion of total body water (dehydration) and/or contraction of total intravascular plasma (hypovolemia).

☑4ᵗʰ **E87 Other disorders of fluid, electrolyte and acid-base balance**
  EXCLUDES 1 diabetes insipidus (E23.2)
    electrolyte imbalance associated with hyperemesis gravidarum (O21.1)
    electrolyte imbalance following ectopic or molar pregnancy (O08.5)
    familial periodic paralysis (G72.3)

  E87.0 Hyperosmolality and hypernatremia
    Sodium [Na] excess
    Sodium [Na] overload
    AHA: 2014, 1Q, 7
  E87.1 Hypo-osmolality and hyponatremia
    Sodium [Na] deficiency
    EXCLUDES 1 syndrome of inappropriate secretion of antidiuretic hormone (E22.2)
    AHA: 2014, 1Q, 7

E87.2 Acidosis
  Acidosis NOS   Metabolic acidosis
  Lactic acidosis   Respiratory acidosis
  EXCLUDES 1 diabetic acidosis—see categories E08-E10, E13 with ketoacidosis

E87.3 Alkalosis
  Alkalosis NOS   Respiratory alkalosis
  Metabolic alkalosis

E87.4 Mixed disorder of acid-base balance
E87.5 Hyperkalemia
  Potassium [K] excess   Potassium [K] overload
E87.6 Hypokalemia
  Potassium [K] deficiency

☑5ᵗʰ **E87.7 Fluid overload**
  EXCLUDES 1 edema NOS (R60.9)
    fluid retention (R60.9)
  E87.70 Fluid overload, unspecified   ▽
  E87.71 Transfusion associated circulatory overload
    Fluid overload due to transfusion (blood) (blood components)
    TACO
  E87.79 Other fluid overload

E87.8 Other disorders of electrolyte and fluid balance, not elsewhere classified
  Electrolyte imbalance NOS
  Hyperchloremia
  Hypochloremia

☑4ᵗʰ **E88 Other and unspecified metabolic disorders**
  Use additional codes for associated conditions
  EXCLUDES 1 histiocytosis X (chronic) (C96.6)

☑5ᵗʰ **E88.0 Disorders of plasma-protein metabolism, not elsewhere classified**
  EXCLUDES 1 disorder of lipoprotein metabolism (E78.-)
    monoclonal gammopathy (of undetermined significance) (D47.2)
    polyclonal hypergammaglobulinemia (D89.0)
    Waldenström's macroglobulinemia (C88.0)
  E88.01 Alpha-1-antitrypsin deficiency   HCC
    AAT deficiency
  E88.09 Other disorders of plasma-protein metabolism, not elsewhere classified
    Bisalbuminemia

E88.1 Lipodystrophy, not elsewhere classified
  Lipodystrophy NOS
  EXCLUDES 1 Whipple's disease (K90.81)

E88.2 Lipomatosis, not elsewhere classified
  Lipomatosis NOS
  Lipomatosis (Check) dolorosa [Dercum]

E88.3 Tumor lysis syndrome
  Tumor lysis syndrome (spontaneous)
  Tumor lysis syndrome following antineoplastic drug chemotherapy
  Use additional code for adverse effect, if applicable, to identify drug (T45.1X5)
  DEF: A potentially fatal metabolic complication of tumor necrosis caused by either spontaneous or treatment-related accumulation of byproducts from dying cancer cells; symptoms include hyperkalemia, hyperphosphatemia, hypocalcemia, hyperuricemia, and hyperuricosuria.

☑5ᵗʰ **E88.4 Mitochondrial metabolism disorders**
  EXCLUDES 1 disorders of pyruvate metabolism (E74.4)
    Kearns-Sayre syndrome (H49.81)
    Leber's disease (H47.22)
    Leigh's encephalopathy (G31.82)
    Mitochondrial myopathy, NEC (G71.3)
    Reye's syndrome (G93.7)
  E88.40 Mitochondrial metabolism disorder, unspecified   HCC ▽
  E88.41 MELAS syndrome   HCC
    Mitochondrial myopathy, encephalopathy, lactic acidosis and stroke-like episodes
  E88.42 MERRF syndrome   HCC
    Myoclonic epilepsy associated with ragged-red fibers
    Code also progressive myoclonic epilepsy (G40.3-)
  E88.49 Other mitochondrial metabolism disorders   HCC

Chapter 4. Endocrine, Nutritional, and Metabolic Diseases

E88.8–E89.89

✓5ᵗʰ **E88.8 Other specified metabolic disorders**

    E88.81 Metabolic syndrome
        Dysmetabolic syndrome X
        Use additional codes for associated manifestations,
          such as:
          obesity (E66.-)

    E88.89 Other specified metabolic disorders   HCC
        Launois-Bensaude adenolipomatosis
        EXCLUDES 1   adult pulmonary Langerhans cell
            histiocytosis (J84.82)

E88.9 Metabolic disorder, unspecified   ▽

Postprocedural endocrine and metabolic complications and disorders, not elsewhere classified (E89)

✓4ᵗʰ **E89 Postprocedural endocrine and metabolic complications and disorders, not elsewhere classified**
    EXCLUDES 2   intraoperative complications of endocrine system organ or
        structure (E36.0-, E36.1-, E36.8)

E89.0 Postprocedural hypothyroidism
    Postirradiation hypothyroidism
    Postsurgical hypothyroidism

E89.1 Postprocedural hypoinsulinemia
    Postpancreatectomy hyperglycemia
    Postsurgical hypoinsulinemia
    Use additional code, if applicable, to identify:
        acquired absence of pancreas (Z90.41-)
        diabetes mellitus (postpancreatectomy) (postprocedural)
          (E13.-)
        insulin use (Z79.4)
        EXCLUDES 1   transient postprocedural hyperglycemia (R73.9)
            transient postprocedural hypoglycemia (E16.2)

E89.2 Postprocedural hypoparathyroidism   HCC
    Parathyroprival tetany

E89.3 Postprocedural hypopituitarism   HCC
    Postirradiation hypopituitarism

✓5ᵗʰ **E89.4 Postprocedural ovarian failure**

    E89.40 Asymptomatic postprocedural ovarian failure   ♀
        Postprocedural ovarian failure NOS

    E89.41 Symptomatic postprocedural ovarian failure   ♀
        Symptoms such as flushing, sleeplessness, headache,
          lack of concentration, associated with
          postprocedural menopause

E89.5 Postprocedural testicular hypofunction   ♂

E89.6 Postprocedural adrenocortical (-medullary) hypofunction HCC

✓5ᵗʰ **E89.8 Other postprocedural endocrine and metabolic complications and disorders**

    ✓6ᵗʰ **E89.81 Postprocedural hemorrhage of an endocrine system organ or structure following a procedure**

        E89.810 Postprocedural hemorrhage of an endocrine system organ or structure following an endocrine system procedure

        E89.811 Postprocedural hemorrhage of an endocrine system organ or structure following other procedure

    ✓6ᵗʰ **E89.82 Postprocedural hematoma and seroma of an endocrine system organ or structure following a procedure**

        E89.820 Postprocedural hematoma of an endocrine system organ or structure following an endocrine system procedure

        E89.821 Postprocedural hematoma of an endocrine system organ or structure following other procedure

        E89.822 Postprocedural seroma of an endocrine system organ or structure following an endocrine system procedure

        E89.823 Postprocedural seroma of an endocrine system organ or structure following other procedure

    E89.89 Other postprocedural endocrine and metabolic complications and disorders
        Use additional code, if applicable, to further specify
          disorder

EXCLUDES 1 Not coded here   EXCLUDES 2 Not included here   N Newborn Age: 0   P Pediatric Age: 0-17   M Maternity Age: 12-55   A Adult Age: 15-124

524   ICD-10-CM 2018

Chapter 5. Mental, Behavioral and Neurodevelopmental Disorders (F01–F99)

Chapter Specific Guidelines with Coding Examples

The chapter specific guidelines from the ICD-10-CM Official Guidelines for Coding and Reporting have been provided below. Along with these guidelines are coding examples, contained in the shaded boxes, that have been developed to help illustrate the coding and/or sequencing guidance found in these guidelines.

a. Pain disorders related to psychological factors

Assign code F45.41, for pain that is exclusively related to psychological disorders. As indicated by the Excludes 1 note under category G89, a code from category G89 should not be assigned with code F45.41.

> Chest pain determined to be persistent somatoform pain disorder
>
> **F45.41   Pain disorder exclusively related to psychological factors**
>
> *Explanation*: This pain was diagnosed as being exclusively psychological; therefore, no code from category G89 is added.

Code F45.42, Pain disorders with related psychological factors, should be used with a code from category G89, Pain, not elsewhere classified, if there is documentation of a psychological component for a patient with acute or chronic pain.

See Section I.C.6. Pain

b. Mental and behavioral disorders due to psychoactive substance use

1) In remission

Selection of codes for "in remission" for categories F10-F19, Mental and behavioral disorders due to psychoactive substance use (categories F10-F19 with -.21) requires the provider's clinical judgment. The appropriate codes for "in remission" are assigned only on the basis of provider documentation (as defined in the Official Guidelines for Coding and Reporting).

> Medical history: Alcohol dependence in remission
>
> **F10.21   Alcohol dependence, in remission**
>
> *Explanation*: The "in remission" codes are assigned when the provider documents the remission.

2) Psychoactive substance use, abuse and dependence

When the provider documentation refers to use, abuse and dependence of the same substance (e.g. alcohol, opioid, cannabis, etc.), only one code should be assigned to identify the pattern of use based on the following hierarchy:

- If both use and abuse are documented, assign only the code for abuse

    If both abuse and dependence are documented, assign only the code for dependence
- If use, abuse and dependence are all documented, assign only the code for dependence
- If both use and dependence are documented, assign only the code for dependence.

> History and physical notes cannabis dependence and ongoing cannabis abuse
>
> **F12.20   Cannabis dependence, uncomplicated**
>
> *Explanation*: In the hierarchy, the dependence code is used if both abuse and dependence are documented.

> Current problem list indicates daily opioid use with opioid abuse.
>
> **F11.10   Opioid abuse, uncomplicated**
>
> *Explanation*: In the hierarchy, the abuse code is used if both abuse and use are documented.

3) Psychoactive substance use

As with all other diagnoses, the codes for psychoactive substance use (F10.9-, F11.9-, F12.9-, F13.9-, F14.9-, F15.9-, F16.9-) should only be assigned based on provider documentation and when they meet the definition of a reportable diagnosis (see Section III, Reporting Additional Diagnoses). The codes are to be used only when the psychoactive substance use is associated with a mental or behavioral disorder, and such a relationship is documented by the provider.

> ED reports that a 27-year-old female tripped and twisted and broke her right ankle. Her friends reported that they were drinking and dancing at a nightclub.
>
> **S82.891A   Other fracture of right lower leg, initial encounter for closed fracture**
>
> **W18.40XA   Slipping, tripping and stumbling without falling, unspecified, initial encounter**
>
> **Y92.252   Music hall as the place of occurrence of the external cause**
>
> **Y93.41   Activity, dancing**
>
> *Explanation*: Note that no code was added for alcohol use or abuse. Unless it is specifically associated with a diagnosis by provider documentation and meets the definition of a reportable diagnosis, it is not assigned. However, if the documentation from the provider stated: "The patient tripped, and twisted and fractured her right ankle while dancing due to her elevated blood alcohol, consistent with her ongoing alcohol abuse," the following code would be added:
>
> **F10.10   Alcohol abuse, uncomplicated**

Chapter 5. Mental, Behavioral, and Neurodevelopmental Disorders (F01-F99)

INCLUDES disorders of psychological development
EXCLUDES 2 *symptoms, signs and abnormal clinical laboratory findings, not elsewhere classified (R00-R99)*

This chapter contains the following blocks:

F01-F09	Mental disorders due to known physiological conditions
F10-F19	Mental and behavioral disorders due to psychoactive substance use
F20-F29	Schizophrenia, schizotypal, delusional, and other non-mood psychotic disorders
F30-F39	Mood [affective] disorders
F40-F48	Anxiety, dissociative, stress-related, somatoform and other nonpsychotic mental disorders
F50-F59	Behavioral syndromes associated with physiological disturbances and physical factors
F60-F69	Disorders of adult personality and behavior
F70-F79	Intellectual disabilities
F80-F89	Pervasive and specific developmental disorders
F90-F98	Behavioral and emotional disorders with onset usually occurring in childhood and adolescence
F99	Unspecified mental disorder

Mental disorders due to known physiological conditions (F01-F09)

NOTE This block comprises a range of mental disorders grouped together on the basis of their having in common a demonstrable etiology in cerebral disease, brain injury, or other insult leading to cerebral dysfunction. The dysfunction may be primary, as in diseases, injuries, and insults that affect the brain directly and selectively; or secondary, as in systemic diseases and disorders that attack the brain only as one of the multiple organs or systems of the body that are involved.

✓4th F01   Vascular dementia

Vascular dementia as a result of infarction of the brain due to vascular disease, including hypertensive cerebrovascular disease.

INCLUDES arteriosclerotic dementia

Code first the underlying physiological condition or sequelae of cerebrovascular disease.

✓5th F01.5   Vascular dementia

F01.50   Vascular dementia without behavioral disturbance   A

Major neurocognitive disorder without behavioral disturbance

F01.51   Vascular dementia with behavioral disturbance   A

Major neurocognitive disorder due to vascular disease, with behavioral disturbance

Major neurocognitive disorder with aggressive behavior

Major neurocognitive disorder with combative behavior

Major neurocognitive disorder with violent behavior

Vascular dementia with aggressive behavior

Vascular dementia with combative behavior

Vascular dementia with violent behavior

Use additional code, if applicable, to identify wandering in vascular dementia (Z91.83)

✓4th F02   Dementia in other diseases classified elsewhere

INCLUDES major neurocognitive disorder in other diseases classified elsewhere

Code first the underlying physiological condition, such as:
Alzheimer's (G30.-)
cerebral lipidosis (E75.4)
Creutzfeldt-Jakob disease (A81.0-)
dementia with Lewy bodies (G31.83)
dementia with Parkinsonism (G31.83)
epilepsy and recurrent seizures (G40.-)
frontotemporal dementia (G31.09)
hepatolenticular degeneration (E83.0)
human immunodeficiency virus [HIV] disease (B20)
Huntington's disease (G10)
hypercalcemia (E83.52)
hypothyroidism, acquired (E00-E03.-)
intoxications (T36-T65)
Jakob-Creutzfeldt disease (A81.0-)
multiple sclerosis (G35)
neurosyphilis (A52.17)
niacin deficiency [pellagra] (E52)
Parkinson's disease (G20)
Pick's disease (G31.01)
polyarteritis nodosa (M30.0)
prion disease (A81.9)
systemic lupus erythematosus (M32.-)
traumatic brain injury (S06.-)
trypanosomiasis (B56.-, B57.-)
vitamin B deficiency (E53.8)

EXCLUDES 2 *dementia in alcohol and psychoactive substance disorders (F10-F19, with .17, .27, .97)*
vascular dementia (F01.5-)

✓5th F02.8   Dementia in other diseases classified elsewhere

AHA: 2017, 2Q, 7; 2016, 4Q, 141; 2016, 2Q, 6

F02.80   Dementia in other diseases classified elsewhere without behavioral disturbance

Dementia in other diseases classified elsewhere NOS

Major neurocognitive disorder in other diseases classified elsewhere

F02.81   Dementia in other diseases classified elsewhere with behavioral disturbance

Dementia in other diseases classified elsewhere with aggressive behavior

Dementia in other diseases classified elsewhere with combative behavior

Dementia in other diseases classified elsewhere with violent behavior

Major neurocognitive disorder in other diseases classified elsewhere with aggressive behavior

Major neurocognitive disorder in other diseases classified elsewhere with combative behavior

Major neurocognitive disorder in other diseases classified elsewhere with violent behavior

Use additional code, if applicable, to identify wandering in dementia in conditions classified elsewhere (Z91.83)

✓4th F03   Unspecified dementia

Presenile dementia NOS
Presenile psychosis NOS
Primary degenerative dementia NOS
Senile dementia NOS
Senile dementia depressed or paranoid type
Senile psychosis NOS

EXCLUDES 1 *senility NOS (R41.81)*

EXCLUDES 2 *mild memory disturbance due to known physiological condition (F06.8)*
senile dementia with delirium or acute confusional state (F05)

✓5th F03.9   Unspecified dementia

F03.90   Unspecified dementia without behavioral disturbance   A▽

Dementia NOS
AHA: 2012, 4Q, 92

F03.91   Unspecified dementia with behavioral disturbance   A▽

Unspecified dementia with aggressive behavior
Unspecified dementia with combative behavior
Unspecified dementia with violent behavior
Use additional code, if applicable, to identify wandering in unspecified dementia (Z91.83)

EXCLUDES 1 Not coded here   **EXCLUDES 2** Not included here   N Newborn Age: 0   P Pediatric Age: 0-17   M Maternity Age: 12-55   A Adult Age: 15-124

526   ICD-10-CM 2018

F04   Amnestic disorder due to known physiological condition
Korsakov's psychosis or syndrome, nonalcoholic
Code first the underlying physiological condition
> *EXCLUDES 1*   *amnesia NOS (R41.3)*
> *anterograde amnesia (R41.1)*
> *dissociative amnesia (F44.0)*
> *retrograde amnesia (R41.2)*
> *EXCLUDES 2*   *alcohol-induced or unspecified Korsakov's syndrome (F10.26, F10.96)*
> *Korsakov's syndrome induced by other psychoactive substances (F13.26, F13.96, F19.16, F19.26, F19.96)*

F05   Delirium due to known physiological condition
Acute or subacute brain syndrome
Acute or subacute confusional state (nonalcoholic)
Acute or subacute infective psychosis
Acute or subacute organic reaction
Acute or subacute psycho-organic syndrome
Delirium of mixed etiology
Delirium superimposed on dementia
Sundowning
Code first the underlying physiological condition
> *EXCLUDES 1*   *delirium NOS (R41.0)*
> *EXCLUDES 2*   *delirium tremens alcohol-induced or unspecified (F10.231, F10.921)*

✓4ᵗʰ F06   Other mental disorders due to known physiological condition
> *INCLUDES*   mental disorders due to endocrine disorder
> mental disorders due to exogenous hormone
> mental disorders due to exogenous toxic substance
> mental disorders due to primary cerebral disease
> mental disorders due to somatic illness
> mental disorders due to systemic disease affecting the brain

Code first the underlying physiological condition
> *EXCLUDES 1*   *unspecified dementia (F03)*
> *EXCLUDES 2*   *delirium due to known physiological condition (F05)*
> *dementia as classified in F01-F02*
> *other mental disorders associated with alcohol and other psychoactive substances (F10-F19)*

F06.0   Psychotic disorder with hallucinations due to known physiological condition
Organic hallucinatory state (nonalcoholic)
> *EXCLUDES 2*   *hallucinations and perceptual disturbance induced by alcohol and other psychoactive substances (F10-F19 with .151, .251, .951)*
> *schizophrenia (F20.-)*

F06.1   Catatonic disorder due to known physiological condition
Catatonia associated with another mental disorder
Catatonia NOS
> *EXCLUDES 1*   *catatonic stupor (R40.1)*
> *stupor NOS (R40.1)*
> *EXCLUDES 2*   *catatonic schizophrenia (F20.2)*
> *dissociative stupor (F44.2)*

F06.2   Psychotic disorder with delusions due to known physiological condition
Paranoid and paranoid-hallucinatory organic states
Schizophrenia-like psychosis in epilepsy
> *EXCLUDES 2*   *alcohol and drug-induced psychotic disorder (F10-F19 with .150, .250, .950)*
> *brief psychotic disorder (F23)*
> *delusional disorder (F22)*
> *schizophrenia (F20.-)*

✓5ᵗʰ F06.3   Mood disorder due to known physiological condition
> *EXCLUDES 2*   *mood disorders due to alcohol and other psychoactive substances (F10-F19 with .14, .24, .94)*
> *mood disorders, not due to known physiological condition or unspecified (F30-F39)*

> **F06.30   Mood disorder due to known physiological condition, unspecified**   ▽

> **F06.31   Mood disorder due to known physiological condition with depressive features**
> ▶Depressive disorder due to known physiological condition, with depressive features◀

> **F06.32   Mood disorder due to known physiological condition with major depressive-like episode**
> ▶Depressive disorder due to known physiological condition, with major depressive–like episode◀

F06.33   Mood disorder due to known physiological condition with manic features
> ▶Bipolar and related disorder due to a known physiological condition, with manic features
> Bipolar and related disorder due to known physiological condition, with manic- or hypomanic-like episodes◀

F06.34   Mood disorder due to known physiological condition with mixed features
> ▶Bipolar and related disorder due to known physiological condition, with mixed features
> Depressive disorder due to known physiological condition, with mixed features◀

F06.4   Anxiety disorder due to known physiological condition
> *EXCLUDES 2*   *anxiety disorders due to alcohol and other psychoactive substances (F10-F19 with .180, .280, .980)*
> *anxiety disorders, not due to known physiological condition or unspecified (F40.-, F41.-)*

F06.8   Other specified mental disorders due to known physiological condition
Epileptic psychosis NOS
▶Obsessive-compulsive and related disorder due to a known physiological condition◀
Organic dissociative disorder
Organic emotionally labile [asthenic] disorder

✓4ᵗʰ F07   Personality and behavioral disorders due to known physiological condition
Code first the underlying physiological condition

F07.0   Personality change due to known physiological condition
Frontal lobe syndrome
Limbic epilepsy personality syndrome
Lobotomy syndrome
Organic personality disorder
Organic pseudopsychopathic personality
Organic pseudoretarded personality
Postleucotomy syndrome
Code first underlying physiological condition
> *EXCLUDES 1*   *mild cognitive impairment (G31.84)*
> *postconcussional syndrome (F07.81)*
> *postencephalitic syndrome (F07.89)*
> *signs and symptoms involving emotional state (R45.-)*
> *EXCLUDES 2*   *specific personality disorder (F60.-)*

✓5ᵗʰ F07.8   Other personality and behavioral disorders due to known physiological condition

> **F07.81   Postconcussional syndrome**
> Postcontusional syndrome (encephalopathy)
> Post-traumatic brain syndrome, nonpsychotic
> Use additional code to identify associated post-traumatic headache, if applicable (G44.3-)
> > *EXCLUDES 1*   *current concussion (brain) (S06.0-)*
> > *postencephalitic syndrome (F07.89)*

> **F07.89   Other personality and behavioral disorders due to known physiological condition**
> Postencephalitic syndrome
> Right hemispheric organic affective disorder

F07.9   Unspecified personality and behavioral disorder due to known physiological condition   ▽
Organic psychosyndrome

F09   Unspecified mental disorder due to known physiological condition   ▽
Mental disorder NOS due to known physiological condition
Organic brain syndrome NOS
Organic mental disorder NOS
Organic psychosis NOS
Symptomatic psychosis NOS
Code first the underlying physiological condition
> *EXCLUDES 1*   *psychosis NOS (F29)*

Mental and behavioral disorders due to psychoactive substance use (F10-F19)
AHA: 2017, 2Q, 27

✓4ᵗʰ F10   Alcohol related disorders
Use additional code for blood alcohol level, if applicable (Y90.-)

✓5ᵗʰ F10.1   Alcohol abuse
> *EXCLUDES 1*   *alcohol dependence (F10.2-)*
> *alcohol use, unspecified (F10.9-)*
> AHA: 2015, 2Q, 15

> **F10.10   Alcohol abuse, uncomplicated**
> Alcohol use disorder, mild

☑ Additional Character Req   ✓7ᵗʰ Placeholder Alert   Manifestation   HCC CMS-HCC Condition   ▽ Unspecified Code   ▶◀ Revised Text   ● New Code   ▲ Revised Code Title

●   **F10.11**   **Alcohol abuse, in remission**
Alcohol use disorder, mild, in early remission
Alcohol use disorder, mild, in sustained remission

✓6ᵗʰ   **F10.12**   **Alcohol abuse with intoxication**

     F10.120   **Alcohol abuse with intoxication,**   HCC
                  uncomplicated

     F10.121   **Alcohol abuse with intoxication**   HCC
                  delirium

     F10.129   **Alcohol abuse with intoxication,**   HCC ▽
                  unspecified

   F10.14   **Alcohol abuse with alcohol-induced mood**   HCC
          disorder
Alcohol use disorder, mild, with alcohol-induced
    bipolar or related disorder
Alcohol use disorder, mild, with alcohol-induced
    depressive disorder

✓6ᵗʰ   **F10.15**   **Alcohol abuse with alcohol-induced psychotic disorder**

     F10.150   **Alcohol abuse with alcohol-induced**   HCC
                  psychotic disorder with delusions

     F10.151   **Alcohol abuse with alcohol-induced**   HCC
                  psychotic disorder with hallucinations
                  DEF: Psychosis lasting less than six months
                  with slight or no clouding of consciousness
                  in which auditory hallucinations
                  predominate.

     F10.159   **Alcohol abuse with alcohol-induced**   HCC ▽
                  psychotic disorder, unspecified

✓6ᵗʰ   **F10.18**   **Alcohol abuse with other alcohol-induced disorders**

     F10.180   **Alcohol abuse with alcohol-induced**   HCC
                  anxiety disorder

     F10.181   **Alcohol abuse with alcohol-induced**   HCC
                  sexual dysfunction

     F10.182   **Alcohol abuse with alcohol-induced**   HCC
                  sleep disorder

     F10.188   **Alcohol abuse with other**   HCC
                  alcohol-induced disorder

   F10.19   **Alcohol abuse with unspecified**   HCC ▽
          alcohol-induced disorder

✓5ᵗʰ   **F10.2**   **Alcohol dependence**

     EXCLUDES 1   *alcohol abuse (F10.1-)*
               alcohol use, unspecified (F10.9-)
     EXCLUDES 2   *toxic effect of alcohol (T51.0-)*

   F10.20   **Alcohol dependence, uncomplicated**   HCC
Alcohol use disorder, moderate
Alcohol use disorder, severe

   F10.21   **Alcohol dependence, in remission**   HCC
▶Alcohol use disorder, moderate, in early remission
Alcohol use disorder, moderate, in sustained remission
Alcohol use disorder, severe, in early remission
Alcohol use disorder, severe, in sustained remission◀

✓6ᵗʰ   **F10.22**   **Alcohol dependence with intoxication**
Acute drunkenness (in alcoholism)
     EXCLUDES 2   *alcohol dependence with withdrawal*
               (F10.23-)

     F10.220   **Alcohol dependence with**   HCC
                  intoxication, uncomplicated

     F10.221   **Alcohol dependence with**   HCC
                  intoxication delirium

     F10.229   **Alcohol dependence with**   HCC ▽
                  intoxication, unspecified

✓6ᵗʰ   **F10.23**   **Alcohol dependence with withdrawal**
     EXCLUDES 2   *alcohol dependence with withdrawal*
               (F10.22-)
     AHA: 2015, 2Q, 15

     F10.230   **Alcohol dependence with**   HCC
                  withdrawal, uncomplicated

     F10.231   **Alcohol dependence with**   HCC
                  withdrawal delirium

     F10.232   **Alcohol dependence with**   HCC
                  withdrawal with perceptual disturbance

     F10.239   **Alcohol dependence with**   HCC ▽
                  withdrawal, unspecified

   F10.24   **Alcohol dependence with alcohol-induced**   HCC
          mood disorder
Alcohol use disorder, moderate, with alcohol-induced
    bipolar or related disorder
Alcohol use disorder, moderate, with alcohol-induced
    depressive disorder
Alcohol use disorder, severe, with alcohol-induced
    bipolar or related disorder
Alcohol use disorder, severe, with alcohol-induced
    depressive disorder

✓6ᵗʰ   **F10.25**   **Alcohol dependence with alcohol-induced psychotic disorder**

     F10.250   **Alcohol dependence with alcohol-**   HCC
                  induced psychotic disorder with delusions

     F10.251   **Alcohol dependence with**   HCC
                  alcohol-induced psychotic disorder with hallucinations

     F10.259   **Alcohol dependence with alcohol-**   HCC ▽
                  induced psychotic disorder, unspecified

   F10.26   **Alcohol dependence with alcohol-induced**   HCC
          persisting amnestic disorder
Alcohol use disorder, moderate, with alcohol-induced
    major neurocognitive disorder,
    amnestic-confabulatory type
Alcohol use disorder, severe, with alcohol-induced
    major neurocognitive disorder,
    amnestic-confabulatory type
    DEF: Prominent and lasting reduced memory span,
    disordered time appreciation and confabulation, occurs
    in alcoholics as sequel to acute alcoholic psychosis.

   F10.27   **Alcohol dependence with alcohol-induced**   HCC
          persisting dementia
Alcohol use disorder, moderate, with alcohol-induced
    major neurocognitive disorder,
    nonamnestic-confabulatory type
Alcohol use disorder, severe, with alcohol-induced
    major neurocognitive disorder,
    nonamnestic-confabulatory type

✓6ᵗʰ   **F10.28**   **Alcohol dependence with other alcohol-induced disorders**

     F10.280   **Alcohol dependence with**   HCC
                  alcohol-induced anxiety disorder

     F10.281   **Alcohol dependence with**   HCC
                  alcohol-induced sexual dysfunction

     F10.282   **Alcohol dependence with**   HCC
                  alcohol-induced sleep disorder

     F10.288   **Alcohol dependence with other**   HCC
                  alcohol-induced disorder
                  Alcohol use disorder, moderate, with
                  alcohol-induced mild neurocognitive
                  disorder
                  Alcohol use disorder, severe, with
                  alcohol-induced mild neurocognitive
                  disorder

   F10.29   **Alcohol dependence with unspecified**   HCC ▽
          alcohol-induced disorder

✓5ᵗʰ   **F10.9**   **Alcohol use, unspecified**
     EXCLUDES 1   *alcohol abuse (F10.1-)*
               alcohol dependence (F10.2-)

✓6ᵗʰ   **F10.92**   **Alcohol use, unspecified with intoxication**

     F10.920   **Alcohol use, unspecified with**   HCC
                  intoxication, uncomplicated

     F10.921   **Alcohol use, unspecified with**   HCC
                  intoxication delirium

     F10.929   **Alcohol use, unspecified with**   HCC ▽
                  intoxication, unspecified

   F10.94   **Alcohol use, unspecified with alcohol-induced**   HCC
          mood disorder
Alcohol induced bipolar or related disorder, without
    use disorder
Alcohol induced depressive disorder, without use
    disorder

✓6ᵗʰ   **F10.95**   **Alcohol use, unspecified with alcohol-induced psychotic disorder**

     F10.950   **Alcohol use, unspecified with**   HCC
                  alcohol-induced psychotic disorder with delusions

     F10.951   **Alcohol use, unspecified with**   HCC
                  alcohol-induced psychotic disorder with hallucinations

---

EXCLUDES 1 Not coded here   EXCLUDES 2 Not included here   N Newborn Age: 0   P Pediatric Age: 0-17   M Maternity Age: 12-55   A Adult Age: 15-124

528   ICD-10-CM 2018

F10.959   **Alcohol use, unspecified with alcohol-induced psychotic disorder, unspecified**   HCC ▽
  Alcohol-induced psychotic disorder without use disorder

F10.96   **Alcohol use, unspecified with alcohol-induced persisting amnestic disorder**   HCC
  Alcohol-induced major neurocognitive disorder, amnestic-confabulatory type, without use disorder

F10.97   **Alcohol use, unspecified with alcohol-induced persisting dementia**   HCC
  Alcohol-induced major neurocognitive disorder, amnestic-confabulatory type, without use disorder

✓6th **F10.98**   **Alcohol use, unspecified with other alcohol-induced disorders**

   F10.980   **Alcohol use, unspecified with alcohol-induced anxiety disorder**   HCC
  Alcohol induced anxiety disorder, without use disorder

   F10.981   **Alcohol use, unspecified with alcohol-induced sexual dysfunction**   HCC
  Alcohol induced sexual dysfunction, without use disorder

   F10.982   **Alcohol use, unspecified with alcohol-induced sleep disorder**   HCC
  Alcohol induced sleep disorder, without use disorder

   F10.988   **Alcohol use, unspecified with other alcohol-induced disorder**   HCC
  Alcohol induced mild neurocognitive disorder, without use disorder

F10.99   **Alcohol use, unspecified with unspecified alcohol-induced disorder**   HCC ▽

✓4th **F11**   **Opioid related disorders**

✓5th **F11.1**   **Opioid abuse**
  EXCLUDES 1   *opioid dependence (F11.2-)*
       opioid use, unspecified (F11.9-)

   F11.10   **Opioid abuse, uncomplicated**
  Opioid use disorder, mild

●   **F11.11**   **Opioid abuse, in remission**
  Opioid use disorder, mild, in early remission
  Opioid use disorder, mild, in sustained remission

✓6th **F11.12**   **Opioid abuse with intoxication**

   F11.120   **Opioid abuse with intoxication, uncomplicated**   HCC

   F11.121   **Opioid abuse with intoxication delirium**   HCC

   F11.122   **Opioid abuse with intoxication with perceptual disturbance**   HCC

   F11.129   **Opioid abuse with intoxication, unspecified**   HCC ▽

   F11.14   **Opioid abuse with opioid-induced mood disorder**   HCC
  Opioid use disorder, mild, with opioid-induced depressive disorder

✓6th **F11.15**   **Opioid abuse with opioid-induced psychotic disorder**

   F11.150   **Opioid abuse with opioid-induced psychotic disorder with delusions**   HCC

   F11.151   **Opioid abuse with opioid-induced psychotic disorder with hallucinations**   HCC

   F11.159   **Opioid abuse with opioid-induced psychotic disorder, unspecified**   HCC ▽

✓6th **F11.18**   **Opioid abuse with other opioid-induced disorder**

   F11.181   **Opioid abuse with opioid-induced sexual dysfunction**   HCC

   F11.182   **Opioid abuse with opioid-induced sleep disorder**   HCC

   F11.188   **Opioid abuse with other opioid-induced disorder**   HCC

   F11.19   **Opioid abuse with unspecified opioid-induced disorder**   HCC ▽

✓5th **F11.2**   **Opioid dependence**
  EXCLUDES 1   *opioid abuse (F11.1-)*
       opioid use, unspecified (F11.9-)
  EXCLUDES 2   *opioid poisoning (T40.0-T40.2-)*

   F11.20   **Opioid dependence, uncomplicated**   HCC
  Opioid use disorder, moderate
  Opioid use disorder, severe

   F11.21   **Opioid dependence, in remission**   HCC
  ▶Opioid use disorder, moderate, in early remission
  Opioid use disorder, moderate, in sustained remission
  Opioid use disorder, severe, in early remission
  Opioid use disorder, severe, in sustained remission◀

✓6th **F11.22**   **Opioid dependence with intoxication**
  EXCLUDES 1   *opioid dependence with withdrawal (F11.23)*

   F11.220   **Opioid dependence with intoxication, uncomplicated**   HCC

   F11.221   **Opioid dependence with intoxication delirium**   HCC

   F11.222   **Opioid dependence with intoxication with perceptual disturbance**   HCC

   F11.229   **Opioid dependence with intoxication, unspecified**   HCC ▽

   F11.23   **Opioid dependence with withdrawal**   HCC
  EXCLUDES 1   *opioid dependence with intoxication (F11.22-)*

   F11.24   **Opioid dependence with opioid-induced mood disorder**   HCC
  Opioid use disorder, moderate, with opioid induced depressive disorder

✓6th **F11.25**   **Opioid dependence with opioid-induced psychotic disorder**

   F11.250   **Opioid dependence with opioid-induced psychotic disorder with delusions**   HCC

   F11.251   **Opioid dependence with opioid-induced psychotic disorder with hallucinations**   HCC

   F11.259   **Opioid dependence with opioid-induced psychotic disorder, unspecified**   HCC ▽

✓6th **F11.28**   **Opioid dependence with other opioid-induced disorder**

   F11.281   **Opioid dependence with opioid-induced sexual dysfunction**   HCC

   F11.282   **Opioid dependence with opioid-induced sleep disorder**   HCC

   F11.288   **Opioid dependence with other opioid-induced disorder**   HCC

   F11.29   **Opioid dependence with unspecified opioid-induced disorder**   HCC ▽

✓5th **F11.9**   **Opioid use, unspecified**
  EXCLUDES 1   *opioid abuse (F11.1-)*
       opioid dependence (F11.2-)

   F11.90   **Opioid use, unspecified, uncomplicated**

✓6th **F11.92**   **Opioid use, unspecified with intoxication**
  EXCLUDES 1   *opioid use, unspecified with withdrawal (F11.93)*

   F11.920   **Opioid use, unspecified with intoxication, uncomplicated**   HCC

   F11.921   **Opioid use, unspecified with intoxication delirium**   HCC
  Opioid-induced delirium

   F11.922   **Opioid use, unspecified with intoxication with perceptual disturbance**   HCC

   F11.929   **Opioid use, unspecified with intoxication, unspecified**   HCC ▽

   F11.93   **Opioid use, unspecified with withdrawal**   HCC
  EXCLUDES 1   *opioid use, unspecified with intoxication (F11.92-)*

   F11.94   **Opioid use, unspecified with opioid-induced mood disorder**   HCC
  Opioid induced depressive disorder, without use disorder

✓6th **F11.95**   **Opioid use, unspecified with opioid-induced psychotic disorder**

   F11.950   **Opioid use, unspecified with opioid-induced psychotic disorder with delusions**   HCC

✓ Additional Character Req   ✓x7th Placeholder Alert   Manifestation   HCC CMS-HCC Condition   ▽ Unspecified Code   ▶◀ Revised Text   ● New Code   ▲ Revised Code Title

F11.951   **Opioid use, unspecified with opioid-induced psychotic disorder with** hallucinations   HCC

F11.959   **Opioid use, unspecified with opioid-induced psychotic disorder,** unspecified   HCC ▽

✓6ᵗʰ **F11.98 Opioid use, unspecified with other specified opioid-induced disorder**

F11.981   **Opioid use, unspecified with opioid-induced** sexual dysfunction   HCC
    Opioid induced sexual dysfunction, without use disorder

F11.982   **Opioid use, unspecified with opioid-induced** sleep disorder   HCC
    Opioid induced sleep disorder, without use disorder

F11.988   **Opioid use, unspecified with other opioid-induced disorder**   HCC
    Opioid induced anxiety disorder, without use disorder

F11.99   **Opioid use, unspecified with unspecified opioid-induced disorder**   HCC ▽

✓4ᵗʰ **F12 Cannabis related disorders**
    INCLUDES   marijuana

✓5ᵗʰ **F12.1 Cannabis** abuse
    EXCLUDES 1   cannabis dependence (F12.2-)
          cannabis use, unspecified (F12.9-)

F12.10   **Cannabis abuse,** uncomplicated
    Cannabis use disorder, mild

●   F12.11   **Cannabis abuse,** in remission
    Cannabis use disorder, mild, in early remission
    Cannabis use disorder, mild, in sustained remission

✓6ᵗʰ **F12.12 Cannabis abuse with** intoxication

F12.120   **Cannabis abuse with intoxication,** uncomplicated   HCC

F12.121   **Cannabis abuse with intoxication** delirium   HCC

F12.122   **Cannabis abuse with intoxication with** perceptual disturbance   HCC

F12.129   **Cannabis abuse with intoxication,** unspecified   HCC ▽

✓6ᵗʰ **F12.15 Cannabis abuse with** psychotic disorder

F12.150   **Cannabis abuse with psychotic disorder with** delusions   HCC

F12.151   **Cannabis abuse with psychotic disorder with** hallucinations   HCC

F12.159   **Cannabis abuse with psychotic disorder, unspecified**   HCC ▽

✓6ᵗʰ **F12.18 Cannabis abuse with other cannabis-induced disorder**

F12.180   **Cannabis abuse with cannabis-induced** anxiety disorder   HCC

F12.188   **Cannabis abuse with other cannabis-induced disorder**   HCC
    Cannabis use disorder, mild, with cannabis-induced sleep disorder

F12.19   **Cannabis abuse with unspecified cannabis-induced disorder**   HCC ▽

✓5ᵗʰ **F12.2 Cannabis** dependence
    EXCLUDES 1   cannabis abuse (F12.1-)
          cannabis use, unspecified (F12.9-)
    EXCLUDES 2   cannabis poisoning (T40.7-)

F12.20   **Cannabis dependence, uncomplicated**   HCC
    Cannabis use disorder, moderate
    Cannabis use disorder, severe

F12.21   **Cannabis dependence,** in remission   HCC
    ▶Cannabis use disorder, moderate, in early remission
    Cannabis use disorder, moderate, in sustained remission
    Cannabis use disorder, severe, in early remission
    Cannabis use disorder, severe, in sustained remission◀

✓6ᵗʰ **F12.22 Cannabis dependence with** intoxication

F12.220   **Cannabis dependence with intoxication, uncomplicated**   HCC

F12.221   **Cannabis dependence with intoxication** delirium   HCC

F12.222   **Cannabis dependence with intoxication with** perceptual disturbance   HCC

F12.229   **Cannabis dependence with intoxication, unspecified**   HCC ▽

✓6ᵗʰ **F12.25 Cannabis dependence with** psychotic disorder

F12.250   **Cannabis dependence with psychotic disorder with** delusions   HCC

F12.251   **Cannabis dependence with psychotic disorder with** hallucinations   HCC

F12.259   **Cannabis dependence with psychotic disorder, unspecified**   HCC ▽

✓6ᵗʰ **F12.28 Cannabis dependence with other cannabis-induced disorder**

F12.280   **Cannabis dependence with cannabis-induced** anxiety disorder   HCC

F12.288   **Cannabis dependence with other cannabis-induced disorder**   HCC
    Cannabis use disorder, moderate, with cannabis-induced sleep disorder
    Cannabis use disorder, severe, with cannabis-induced sleep disorder
    Cannabis withdrawal

F12.29   **Cannabis dependence with unspecified cannabis-induced disorder**   HCC ▽

✓5ᵗʰ **F12.9 Cannabis use, unspecified**
    EXCLUDES 1   cannabis abuse (F12.1-)
          cannabis dependence (F12.2-)

F12.90   **Cannabis use, unspecified,** uncomplicated

✓6ᵗʰ **F12.92 Cannabis use, unspecified with** intoxication

F12.920   **Cannabis use, unspecified with intoxication,** uncomplicated   HCC

F12.921   **Cannabis use, unspecified with intoxication** delirium   HCC

F12.922   **Cannabis use, unspecified with intoxication with** perceptual disturbance   HCC

F12.929   **Cannabis use, unspecified with intoxication, unspecified**   HCC ▽

✓6ᵗʰ **F12.95 Cannabis use, unspecified with** psychotic disorder

F12.950   **Cannabis use, unspecified with psychotic disorder with** delusions   HCC

F12.951   **Cannabis use, unspecified with psychotic disorder with** hallucinations   HCC

F12.959   **Cannabis use, unspecified with psychotic disorder, unspecified**   HCC ▽
    Cannabis induced psychotic disorder, without use disorder

✓6ᵗʰ **F12.98 Cannabis use, unspecified with other cannabis-induced disorder**

F12.980   **Cannabis use, unspecified with** anxiety disorder   HCC
    Cannabis induced anxiety disorder, without use disorder

F12.988   **Cannabis use, unspecified with other cannabis-induced disorder**   HCC
    Cannabis induced sleep disorder, without use disorder

F12.99   **Cannabis use, unspecified with unspecified cannabis-induced disorder**   HCC ▽

✓4ᵗʰ **F13 Sedative, hypnotic, or anxiolytic related disorders**

✓5ᵗʰ **F13.1 Sedative, hypnotic or anxiolytic-related** abuse
    EXCLUDES 1   sedative, hypnotic or anxiolytic-related dependence (F13.2-)
          sedative, hypnotic, or anxiolytic use, unspecified (F13.9-)

F13.10   **Sedative, hypnotic or anxiolytic abuse,** uncomplicated
    Sedative, hypnotic, or anxiolytic use disorder, mild

●   F13.11   **Sedative, hypnotic or anxiolytic abuse,** in remission
    Sedative, hypnotic or anxiolytic use disorder, mild, in early remission
    Sedative, hypnotic or anxiolytic use disorder, mild, in sustained remission

✓6ᵗʰ **F13.12 Sedative, hypnotic or anxiolytic abuse with** intoxication

F13.120   **Sedative, hypnotic or anxiolytic abuse with intoxication,** uncomplicated   HCC

F13.121   **Sedative, hypnotic or anxiolytic abuse with intoxication** delirium   HCC

F13.129   **Sedative, hypnotic or anxiolytic abuse with intoxication, unspecified**   HCC ▽

EXCLUDES 1 Not coded here   EXCLUDES 2 Not included here   N Newborn Age: 0   P Pediatric Age: 0-17   M Maternity Age: 12-55   A Adult Age: 15-124

530   ICD-10-CM 2018

F13.14 **Sedative, hypnotic or anxiolytic abuse with sedative, hypnotic or anxiolytic-induced mood disorder** `HCC`
▶Sedative, hypnotic, or anxiolytic use disorder, mild, with sedative, hypnotic, or anxiolytic-induced bipolar or related disorder
Sedative, hypnotic, or anxiolytic use disorder, mild, with sedative, hypnotic, or anxiolytic-induced depressive disorder◀

√6ᵗʰ F13.15 **Sedative, hypnotic or anxiolytic abuse with sedative, hypnotic or anxiolytic-induced psychotic disorder**

     F13.150 **Sedative, hypnotic or anxiolytic abuse with sedative, hypnotic or anxiolytic-induced psychotic disorder with delusions** `HCC`

     F13.151 **Sedative, hypnotic or anxiolytic abuse with sedative, hypnotic or anxiolytic-induced psychotic disorder with hallucinations** `HCC`

     F13.159 **Sedative, hypnotic or anxiolytic abuse with sedative, hypnotic or anxiolytic-induced psychotic disorder, unspecified** `HCC` ▽

√6ᵗʰ F13.18 **Sedative, hypnotic or anxiolytic abuse with other sedative, hypnotic or anxiolytic-induced disorders**

     F13.180 **Sedative, hypnotic or anxiolytic abuse with sedative, hypnotic or anxiolytic-induced anxiety disorder** `HCC`

     F13.181 **Sedative, hypnotic or anxiolytic abuse with sedative, hypnotic or anxiolytic-induced sexual dysfunction** `HCC`

     F13.182 **Sedative, hypnotic or anxiolytic abuse with sedative, hypnotic or anxiolytic-induced sleep disorder** `HCC`

     F13.188 **Sedative, hypnotic or anxiolytic abuse with other sedative, hypnotic or anxiolytic-induced disorder** `HCC`

F13.19 **Sedative, hypnotic or anxiolytic abuse with unspecified sedative, hypnotic or anxiolytic-induced disorder** `HCC` ▽

√5ᵗʰ F13.2 **Sedative, hypnotic or anxiolytic-related dependence**
     EXCLUDES 1   *sedative, hypnotic or anxiolytic-related abuse (F13.1-)*
                 sedative, hypnotic, or anxiolytic use, unspecified (F13.9-)
     EXCLUDES 2   *sedative, hypnotic, or anxiolytic poisoning (T42.-)*

     F13.20 **Sedative, hypnotic or anxiolytic dependence, uncomplicated** `HCC`

     F13.21 **Sedative, hypnotic or anxiolytic dependence, in remission** `HCC`
▶Sedative, hypnotic or anxiolytic use disorder, moderate, in early remission
Sedative, hypnotic or anxiolytic use disorder, moderate, in sustained remission
Sedative, hypnotic or anxiolytic use disorder, severe, in early remission
Sedative, hypnotic or anxiolytic use disorder, severe, in sustained remission◀

√6ᵗʰ F13.22 **Sedative, hypnotic or anxiolytic dependence with intoxication**
     EXCLUDES 1   *sedative, hypnotic or anxiolytic dependence with withdrawal (F13.23-)*

     F13.220 **Sedative, hypnotic or anxiolytic dependence with intoxication, uncomplicated** `HCC`

     F13.221 **Sedative, hypnotic or anxiolytic dependence with intoxication delirium** `HCC`

     F13.229 **Sedative, hypnotic or anxiolytic dependence with intoxication, unspecified** `HCC` ▽

√6ᵗʰ F13.23 **Sedative, hypnotic or anxiolytic dependence with withdrawal**
Sedative, hypnotic, or anxiolytic use disorder, moderate
Sedative, hypnotic, or anxiolytic use disorder, severe
     EXCLUDES 1   *sedative, hypnotic or anxiolytic dependence with intoxication (F13.22-)*

     F13.230 **Sedative, hypnotic or anxiolytic dependence with withdrawal, uncomplicated** `HCC`

     F13.231 **Sedative, hypnotic or anxiolytic dependence with withdrawal delirium** `HCC`

     F13.232 **Sedative, hypnotic or anxiolytic dependence with withdrawal with perceptual disturbance** `HCC`
Sedative, hypnotic, or anxiolytic withdrawal with perceptual disturbances

     F13.239 **Sedative, hypnotic or anxiolytic dependence with withdrawal, unspecified** `HCC` ▽
Sedative, hypnotic, or anxiolytic withdrawal without perceptual disturbances

F13.24 **Sedative, hypnotic or anxiolytic dependence with sedative, hypnotic or anxiolytic-induced mood disorder** `HCC`
▶Sedative, hypnotic, or anxiolytic use disorder, moderate, with sedative, hypnotic, or anxiolytic-induced bipolar or related disorder
Sedative, hypnotic, or anxiolytic use disorder, moderate, with sedative, hypnotic, or anxiolytic-induced depressive disorder◀
Sedative, hypnotic, or anxiolytic use disorder, severe, with sedative, hypnotic, or anxiolytic-induced bipolar or related disorder
▶Sedative, hypnotic, or anxiolytic use disorder, severe, with sedative, hypnotic, or anxiolytic-induced depressive disorder◀

√6ᵗʰ F13.25 **Sedative, hypnotic or anxiolytic dependence with sedative, hypnotic or anxiolytic-induced psychotic disorder**

     F13.250 **Sedative, hypnotic or anxiolytic dependence with sedative, hypnotic or anxiolytic-induced psychotic disorder with delusions** `HCC`

     F13.251 **Sedative, hypnotic or anxiolytic dependence with sedative, hypnotic or anxiolytic-induced psychotic disorder with hallucinations** `HCC`

     F13.259 **Sedative, hypnotic or anxiolytic dependence with sedative, hypnotic or anxiolytic-induced psychotic disorder, unspecified** `HCC` ▽

F13.26 **Sedative, hypnotic or anxiolytic dependence with sedative, hypnotic or anxiolytic-induced persisting amnestic disorder** `HCC`

F13.27 **Sedative, hypnotic or anxiolytic dependence with sedative, hypnotic or anxiolytic-induced persisting dementia** `HCC`
▶Sedative, hypnotic, or anxiolytic use disorder, moderate, with sedative, hypnotic, or anxiolytic-induced major neurocognitive disorder◀
Sedative, hypnotic, or anxiolytic use disorder, severe, with sedative, hypnotic, or anxiolytic-induced major neurocognitive disorder

√6ᵗʰ F13.28 **Sedative, hypnotic or anxiolytic dependence with other sedative, hypnotic or anxiolytic-induced disorders**

     F13.280 **Sedative, hypnotic or anxiolytic dependence with sedative, hypnotic or anxiolytic-induced anxiety disorder** `HCC`

     F13.281 **Sedative, hypnotic or anxiolytic dependence with sedative, hypnotic or anxiolytic-induced sexual dysfunction** `HCC`

     F13.282 **Sedative, hypnotic or anxiolytic dependence with sedative, hypnotic or anxiolytic-induced sleep disorder** `HCC`

     F13.288 **Sedative, hypnotic or anxiolytic dependence with other sedative, hypnotic or anxiolytic-induced disorder** `HCC`
▶Sedative, hypnotic, or anxiolytic use disorder, moderate, with sedative, hypnotic, or anxiolytic-induced mild neurocognitive disorder
Sedative, hypnotic, or anxiolytic use disorder, severe, with sedative, hypnotic, or anxiolytic-induced mild neurocognitive disorder◀

F13.29 **Sedative, hypnotic or anxiolytic dependence with unspecified sedative, hypnotic or anxiolytic-induced disorder** `HCC` ▽

☑ Additional Character Req   ⁷ˣ⁷ᵗʰ Placeholder Alert   Manifestation   `HCC` CMS-HCC Condition   ▽ Unspecified Code   ▶◀ Revised Text   ● New Code   ▲ Revised Code Title

✓5ᵗʰ **F13.9 Sedative, hypnotic or anxiolytic-related use, unspecified**
  EXCLUDES 1 *sedative, hypnotic or anxiolytic-related abuse (F13.1-)*
  sedative, hypnotic or anxiolytic-related dependence (F13.2-)

F13.90 Sedative, hypnotic, or anxiolytic use, unspecified, uncomplicated

✓6ᵗʰ **F13.92 Sedative, hypnotic or anxiolytic use, unspecified with intoxication**
  EXCLUDES 1 *sedative, hypnotic or anxiolytic use, unspecified with withdrawal (F13.93-)*

  F13.920 Sedative, hypnotic or anxiolytic use, HCC unspecified with intoxication, uncomplicated
  F13.921 Sedative, hypnotic or anxiolytic use, HCC unspecified with intoxication delirium
    Sedative, hypnotic, or anxiolytic-induced delirium
  F13.929 Sedative, hypnotic or anxiolytic use, HCC ▽ unspecified with intoxication, unspecified

✓6ᵗʰ **F13.93 Sedative, hypnotic or anxiolytic use, unspecified with withdrawal**
  EXCLUDES 1 *sedative, hypnotic or anxiolytic use, unspecified with intoxication (F13.92-)*

  F13.930 Sedative, hypnotic or anxiolytic use, HCC unspecified with withdrawal, uncomplicated
  F13.931 Sedative, hypnotic or anxiolytic use, HCC unspecified with withdrawal delirium
  F13.932 Sedative, hypnotic or anxiolytic use, HCC unspecified with withdrawal with perceptual disturbances
  F13.939 Sedative, hypnotic or anxiolytic use, HCC ▽ unspecified with withdrawal, unspecified

F13.94 Sedative, hypnotic or anxiolytic use, HCC ▽ unspecified with sedative, hypnotic or anxiolytic-induced mood disorder
  Sedative, hypnotic, or anxiolytic-induced bipolar or related disorder, without use disorder
  Sedative, hypnotic, or anxiolytic-induced depressive disorder, without use disorder

✓6ᵗʰ **F13.95 Sedative, hypnotic or anxiolytic use, unspecified with sedative, hypnotic or anxiolytic-induced psychotic disorder**

  F13.950 Sedative, hypnotic or anxiolytic use, HCC unspecified with sedative, hypnotic or anxiolytic-induced psychotic disorder with delusions
  F13.951 Sedative, hypnotic or anxiolytic use, HCC unspecified with sedative, hypnotic or anxiolytic-induced psychotic disorder with hallucinations
  F13.959 Sedative, hypnotic or anxiolytic use, HCC ▽ unspecified with sedative, hypnotic or anxiolytic-induced psychotic disorder, unspecified
    ▶Sedative, hypnotic, or anxiolytic-induced psychotic disorder, without use disorder◄

F13.96 Sedative, hypnotic or anxiolytic use, unspecified HCC with sedative, hypnotic or anxiolytic-induced persisting amnestic disorder

F13.97 Sedative, hypnotic or anxiolytic use, unspecified HCC with sedative, hypnotic or anxiolytic-induced persisting dementia
  ▶Sedative, hypnotic, or anxiolytic-induced major neurocognitive disorder, without use disorder◄

✓6ᵗʰ **F13.98 Sedative, hypnotic or anxiolytic use, unspecified with other sedative, hypnotic or anxiolytic-induced disorders**

  F13.980 Sedative, hypnotic or anxiolytic use, HCC unspecified with sedative, hypnotic or anxiolytic-induced anxiety disorder
    ▶Sedative, hypnotic, or anxiolytic-induced anxiety disorder, without use disorder◄
  F13.981 Sedative, hypnotic or anxiolytic use, HCC unspecified with sedative, hypnotic or anxiolytic-induced sexual dysfunction
    ▶Sedative, hypnotic, or anxiolytic-induced sexual dysfunction, without use disorder◄

F13.982 Sedative, hypnotic or anxiolytic use, HCC unspecified with sedative, hypnotic or anxiolytic-induced sleep disorder
  ▶Sedative, hypnotic, or anxiolytic-induced sleep disorder, without use disorder◄
F13.988 Sedative, hypnotic or anxiolytic use, HCC unspecified with other sedative, hypnotic or anxiolytic-induced disorder
  ▶Sedative, hypnotic, or anxiolytic-induced mild neurocognitive disorder◄
F13.99 Sedative, hypnotic or anxiolytic use, HCC ▽ unspecified with unspecified sedative, hypnotic or anxiolytic-induced disorder

✓4ᵗʰ **F14 Cocaine related disorders**
  EXCLUDES 2 *other stimulant-related disorders (F15.-)*

✓5ᵗʰ **F14.1 Cocaine abuse**
  EXCLUDES 1 *cocaine dependence (F14.2-)*
  cocaine use, unspecified (F14.9-)

  F14.10 Cocaine abuse, uncomplicated
    Cocaine use disorder, mild
  • **F14.11 Cocaine abuse, in remission**
    Cocaine use disorder, mild, in early remission
    Cocaine use disorder, mild, in sustained remission

✓6ᵗʰ **F14.12 Cocaine abuse with intoxication**
  F14.120 Cocaine abuse with intoxication, HCC uncomplicated
  F14.121 Cocaine abuse with intoxication with HCC delirium
  F14.122 Cocaine abuse with intoxication with HCC perceptual disturbance
  F14.129 Cocaine abuse with intoxication, HCC ▽ unspecified

  F14.14 Cocaine abuse with cocaine-induced HCC mood disorder
    Cocaine use disorder, mild, with cocaine-induced bipolar or related disorder
    Cocaine use disorder, mild, with cocaine-induced depressive disorder

✓6ᵗʰ **F14.15 Cocaine abuse with cocaine-induced psychotic disorder**
  F14.150 Cocaine abuse with cocaine-induced HCC psychotic disorder with delusions
  F14.151 Cocaine abuse with cocaine-induced HCC psychotic disorder with hallucinations
  F14.159 Cocaine abuse with cocaine- HCC ▽ induced psychotic disorder, unspecified

✓6ᵗʰ **F14.18 Cocaine abuse with other cocaine-induced disorder**
  F14.180 Cocaine abuse with cocaine-induced HCC anxiety disorder
  F14.181 Cocaine abuse with cocaine-induced HCC sexual dysfunction
  F14.182 Cocaine abuse with cocaine-induced HCC sleep disorder
  F14.188 Cocaine abuse with other cocaine- HCC induced disorder
    Cocaine use disorder, mild, with cocaine-induced obsessive compulsive or related disorder

  F14.19 Cocaine abuse with unspecified cocaine- HCC ▽ induced disorder

✓5ᵗʰ **F14.2 Cocaine dependence**
  EXCLUDES 1 *cocaine abuse (F14.1-)*
  cocaine use, unspecified (F14.9-)
  EXCLUDES 2 *cocaine poisoning (T40.5-)*

  F14.20 Cocaine dependence, uncomplicated HCC
    Cocaine use disorder, moderate
    Cocaine use disorder, severe
  F14.21 Cocaine dependence, in remission HCC
    ▶Cocaine use disorder, moderate, in early remission
    Cocaine use disorder, moderate, in sustained remission
    Cocaine use disorder, severe, in early remission
    Cocaine use disorder, severe, in sustained remission◄

✓6ᵗʰ **F14.22 Cocaine dependence with intoxication**
  EXCLUDES 1 *cocaine dependence with withdrawal (F14.23)*

  F14.220 Cocaine dependence with HCC intoxication, uncomplicated

EXCLUDES 1 Not coded here   EXCLUDES 2 Not included here   N Newborn Age: 0   P Pediatric Age: 0-17   M Maternity Age: 12-55   A Adult Age: 15-124

532   ICD-10-CM 2018

F14.221 **Cocaine dependence with intoxication** delirium `HCC`

F14.222 **Cocaine dependence with intoxication with** perceptual disturbance `HCC`

F14.229 **Cocaine dependence with intoxication, unspecified** `HCC` ▽

F14.23 **Cocaine dependence with** withdrawal `HCC`
> *EXCLUDES 1* cocaine dependence with intoxication (F14.22-)

F14.24 **Cocaine dependence with cocaine-induced** mood disorder `HCC`
Cocaine use disorder, moderate, with cocaine-induced bipolar or related disorder
Cocaine use disorder, moderate, with cocaine-induced depressive disorder
Cocaine use disorder, severe, with cocaine-induced bipolar or related disorder
Cocaine use disorder, severe, with cocaine-induced depressive disorder

✓6ᵗʰ F14.25 **Cocaine dependence with cocaine-induced** psychotic disorder

F14.250 **Cocaine dependence with cocaine-induced psychotic disorder with** delusions `HCC`

F14.251 **Cocaine dependence with cocaine-induced psychotic disorder with** hallucinations `HCC`

F14.259 **Cocaine dependence with cocaine-induced psychotic disorder, unspecified** `HCC` ▽

✓6ᵗʰ F14.28 **Cocaine dependence with other cocaine-induced disorder**

F14.280 **Cocaine dependence with cocaine-induced** anxiety disorder `HCC`

F14.281 **Cocaine dependence with cocaine-induced** sexual dysfunction `HCC`

F14.282 **Cocaine dependence with cocaine-induced** sleep disorder `HCC`

F14.288 **Cocaine dependence with other cocaine-induced disorder** `HCC`
Cocaine use disorder, moderate, with cocaine-induced obsessive compulsive or related disorder
Cocaine use disorder, severe, with cocaine-induced obsessive compulsive or related disorder

F14.29 **Cocaine dependence with unspecified cocaine-induced disorder** `HCC` ▽

✓5ᵗʰ F14.9 **Cocaine use, unspecified**
> *EXCLUDES 1* cocaine abuse (F14.1-)
> cocaine dependence (F14.2-)

F14.90 **Cocaine use, unspecified,** uncomplicated

✓6ᵗʰ F14.92 **Cocaine use, unspecified with** intoxication

F14.920 **Cocaine use, unspecified with intoxication,** uncomplicated `HCC`

F14.921 **Cocaine use, unspecified with intoxication** delirium `HCC`

F14.922 **Cocaine use, unspecified with intoxication with** perceptual disturbance `HCC`

F14.929 **Cocaine use, unspecified with intoxication, unspecified** `HCC` ▽

F14.94 **Cocaine use, unspecified with cocaine-induced** mood disorder `HCC`
Cocaine induced bipolar or related disorder, without use disorder
Cocaine induced depressive disorder, without use disorder

✓6ᵗʰ F14.95 **Cocaine use, unspecified with cocaine-induced** psychotic disorder

F14.950 **Cocaine use, unspecified with cocaine-induced psychotic disorder with** delusions `HCC`

F14.951 **Cocaine use, unspecified with cocaine-induced psychotic disorder with** hallucinations `HCC`

F14.959 **Cocaine use, unspecified with cocaine-induced psychotic disorder, unspecified** `HCC` ▽
Cocaine induced psychotic disorder, without use disorder

✓6ᵗʰ F14.98 **Cocaine use, unspecified with other specified cocaine-induced disorder**

F14.980 **Cocaine use, unspecified with cocaine-induced** anxiety disorder `HCC`
Cocaine induced anxiety disorder, without use disorder

F14.981 **Cocaine use, unspecified with cocaine-induced** sexual dysfunction `HCC`
Cocaine induced sexual dysfunction, without use disorder

F14.982 **Cocaine use, unspecified with cocaine-induced** sleep disorder `HCC`
Cocaine induced sleep disorder, without use disorder

F14.988 **Cocaine use, unspecified with other cocaine-induced disorder** `HCC`
Cocaine induced obsessive compulsive or related disorder

F14.99 **Cocaine use, unspecified with unspecified cocaine-induced disorder** `HCC` ▽

✓4ᵗʰ F15 **Other** stimulant **related disorders**
> *INCLUDES* amphetamine-related disorders
> caffeine
> *EXCLUDES 2* cocaine-related disorders (F14.-)

✓5ᵗʰ F15.1 **Other stimulant** abuse
> *EXCLUDES 1* other stimulant dependence (F15.2-)
> other stimulant use, unspecified (F15.9-)

F15.10 **Other stimulant abuse,** uncomplicated
Amphetamine type substance use disorder, mild
Other or unspecified stimulant use disorder, mild

● F15.11 **Other stimulant abuse,** in remission
Amphetamine type substance use disorder, mild, in early remission
Amphetamine type substance use disorder, mild, in sustained remission
Other or unspecified stimulant use disorder, mild, in early remission
Other or unspecified stimulant use disorder, mild, in sustained remission

✓6ᵗʰ F15.12 **Other stimulant abuse with** intoxication

F15.120 **Other stimulant abuse with intoxication,** uncomplicated `HCC`

F15.121 **Other stimulant abuse with intoxication** delirium `HCC`

F15.122 **Other stimulant abuse with intoxication with** perceptual disturbance `HCC`
Amphetamine or other stimulant use disorder, mild, with amphetamine or other stimulant intoxication, with perceptual disturbances

F15.129 **Other stimulant abuse with intoxication, unspecified** `HCC` ▽
Amphetamine or other stimulant use disorder, mild, with amphetamine or other stimulant intoxication, without perceptual disturbances

F15.14 **Other stimulant abuse with stimulant-induced** mood disorder `HCC`
Amphetamine or other stimulant use disorder, mild, with amphetamine or other stimulant induced bipolar or related disorder
Amphetamine or other stimulant use disorder, mild, with amphetamine or other stimulant induced depressive disorder

✓6ᵗʰ F15.15 **Other stimulant abuse with stimulant-induced** psychotic disorder

F15.150 **Other stimulant abuse with stimulant-induced psychotic disorder with** delusions `HCC`

F15.151 **Other stimulant abuse with stimulant-induced psychotic disorder with** hallucinations `HCC`

F15.159 **Other stimulant abuse with stimulant-induced psychotic disorder, unspecified** `HCC` ▽

✓6ᵗʰ F15.18 **Other stimulant abuse with other stimulant-induced disorder**

F15.180 **Other stimulant abuse with stimulant-induced** anxiety disorder `HCC`

F15.181 **Other stimulant abuse with stimulant-induced** sexual dysfunction `HCC`

☑ Additional Character Req   ⌐x7ᵗʰ Placeholder Alert   Manifestation   `HCC` CMS-HCC Condition   ▽ Unspecified Code   ►◄ Revised Text   ● New Code   ▲ Revised Code Title

F15.182 Other stimulant abuse with stimulant-induced sleep disorder `HCC`

F15.188 Other stimulant abuse with other stimulant-induced disorder `HCC`
Amphetamine or other stimulant use disorder, mild, with amphetamine or other stimulant induced obsessive-compulsive or related disorder

F15.19 Other stimulant abuse with unspecified stimulant-induced disorder `HCC` ▽

F15.2 Other stimulant dependence ✓5th
EXCLUDES 1 other stimulant abuse (F15.1-)
other stimulant use, unspecified (F15.9-)

F15.20 Other stimulant dependence, uncomplicated `HCC`
Amphetamine type substance use disorder, moderate
Amphetamine type substance use disorder, severe
Other or unspecified stimulant use disorder, moderate
Other or unspecified stimulant use disorder, severe

F15.21 Other stimulant dependence, in remission `HCC`
▶Amphetamine type substance use disorder, moderate, in early remission
Amphetamine type substance use disorder, moderate, in sustained remission
Amphetamine type substance use disorder, severe, in early remission
Amphetamine type substance use disorder, severe, in sustained remission
Other or unspecified stimulant use disorder, moderate, in early remission
Other or unspecified stimulant use disorder, moderate, in sustained remission
Other or unspecified stimulant use disorder, severe, in early remission
Other or unspecified stimulant use disorder, severe, in sustained remission◀

F15.22 Other stimulant dependence with intoxication ✓6th
EXCLUDES 1 other stimulant dependence with withdrawal (F15.23)

F15.220 Other stimulant dependence with intoxication, uncomplicated `HCC`

F15.221 Other stimulant dependence with intoxication delirium `HCC`

F15.222 Other stimulant dependence with intoxication with perceptual disturbance `HCC`
Amphetamine or other stimulant use disorder, moderate, with amphetamine or other stimulant intoxication, with perceptual disturbances
Amphetamine or other stimulant use disorder, severe, with amphetamine or other stimulant intoxication, with perceptual disturbances

F15.229 Other stimulant dependence with intoxication, unspecified `HCC` ▽
Amphetamine or other stimulant use disorder, moderate, with amphetamine or other stimulant intoxication, without perceptual disturbances
Amphetamine or other stimulant use disorder, severe, with amphetamine or other stimulant intoxication, without perceptual disturbances

F15.23 Other stimulant dependence with withdrawal `HCC`
Amphetamine or other stimulant withdrawal
EXCLUDES 1 other stimulant dependence with intoxication (F15.22-)

F15.24 Other stimulant dependence with stimulant-induced mood disorder `HCC`
Amphetamine or other stimulant use disorder, moderate, with amphetamine or other stimulant-induced bipolar or related disorder
Amphetamine or other stimulant use disorder, moderate, with amphetamine or other stimulant induced depressive disorder
Amphetamine or other stimulant use disorder, severe, with amphetamine or other stimulant-induced bipolar or related disorder
Amphetamine or other stimulant use disorder, severe, with amphetamine or other stimulant-induced depressive disorder

F15.25 Other stimulant dependence with stimulant-induced psychotic disorder ✓6th

F15.250 Other stimulant dependence with stimulant-induced psychotic disorder with delusions `HCC`

F15.251 Other stimulant dependence with stimulant-induced psychotic disorder with hallucinations `HCC`

F15.259 Other stimulant dependence with stimulant-induced psychotic disorder, unspecified `HCC` ▽

F15.28 Other stimulant dependence with other stimulant-induced disorder ✓6th

F15.280 Other stimulant dependence with stimulant-induced anxiety disorder `HCC`

F15.281 Other stimulant dependence with stimulant-induced sexual dysfunction `HCC`

F15.282 Other stimulant dependence with stimulant-induced sleep disorder `HCC`

F15.288 Other stimulant dependence with other stimulant-induced disorder `HCC`
▶Amphetamine or other stimulant use disorder, moderate, with amphetamine or other stimulant induced obsessive compulsive or related disorder
Amphetamine or other stimulant use disorder, severe, with amphetamine or other stimulant induced obsessive compulsive or related disorder◀

F15.29 Other stimulant dependence with unspecified stimulant-induced disorder `HCC` ▽

F15.9 Other stimulant use, unspecified ✓5th
EXCLUDES 1 other stimulant abuse (F15.1-)
other stimulant dependence (F15.2-)

F15.90 Other stimulant use, unspecified, uncomplicated

F15.92 Other stimulant use, unspecified with intoxication ✓6th
EXCLUDES 1 other stimulant use, unspecified with withdrawal (F15.93)

F15.920 Other stimulant use, unspecified with intoxication, uncomplicated `HCC`

F15.921 Other stimulant use, unspecified with intoxication delirium `HCC`
Amphetamine or other stimulant-induced delirium

F15.922 Other stimulant use, unspecified with intoxication with perceptual disturbance `HCC`

F15.929 Other stimulant use, unspecified with intoxication, unspecified `HCC` ▽
Caffeine intoxication

F15.93 Other stimulant use, unspecified with withdrawal `HCC`
Caffeine withdrawal
EXCLUDES 1 other stimulant use, unspecified with intoxication (F15.92-)

F15.94 Other stimulant use, unspecified with stimulant-induced mood disorder `HCC`
Amphetamine or other stimulant-induced bipolar or related disorder, without use disorder
Amphetamine or other stimulant-induced depressive disorder, without use disorder

F15.95 Other stimulant use, unspecified with stimulant-induced psychotic disorder ✓6th

F15.950 Other stimulant use, unspecified with stimulant-induced psychotic disorder with delusions `HCC`

F15.951 Other stimulant use, unspecified with stimulant-induced psychotic disorder with hallucinations `HCC`

F15.959 Other stimulant use, unspecified with stimulant-induced psychotic disorder, unspecified `HCC` ▽
▶Amphetamine or other stimulant-induced psychotic disorder, without use disorder◀

✓6ᵗʰ **F15.98　Other stimulant use, unspecified with other stimulant-induced disorder**

F15.980　Other stimulant use, unspecified with HCC **stimulant-induced anxiety disorder**
Amphetamine or other stimulant-induced anxiety disorder, without use disorder
Caffeine induced anxiety disorder, without use disorder

F15.981　Other stimulant use, unspecified with HCC **stimulant-induced sexual dysfunction**
Amphetamine or other stimulant-induced sexual dysfunction, without use disorder

F15.982　Other stimulant use, unspecified with HCC **stimulant-induced sleep disorder**
Amphetamine or other stimulant-induced sleep disorder, without use disorder
Caffeine induced sleep disorder, without use disorder

F15.988　Other stimulant use, unspecified with HCC **other stimulant-induced disorder**
Amphetamine or other stimulant-induced obsessive compulsive or related disorder, without use disorder

F15.99　Other stimulant use, unspecified with HCC ▽ **unspecified stimulant-induced disorder**

✓4ᵗʰ **F16　Hallucinogen related disorders**
INCLUDES　ecstasy
PCP
phencyclidine

✓5ᵗʰ **F16.1　Hallucinogen abuse**
EXCLUDES 1　*hallucinogen dependence (F16.2-)*
hallucinogen use, unspecified (F16.9-)

F16.10　Hallucinogen abuse, uncomplicated
Other hallucinogen use disorder, mild
Phencyclidine use disorder, mild

● **F16.11　Hallucinogen abuse, in remission**
Other hallucinogen use disorder, mild, in early remission
Other hallucinogen use disorder, mild, in sustained remission
Phencyclidine use disorder, mild, in early remission
Phencyclidine use disorder, mild, in sustained remission

✓6ᵗʰ **F16.12　Hallucinogen abuse with intoxication**

F16.120　Hallucinogen abuse with intoxication, HCC **uncomplicated**

F16.121　Hallucinogen abuse with intoxication HCC **with delirium**

F16.122　Hallucinogen abuse with intoxication HCC **with perceptual disturbance**

F16.129　Hallucinogen abuse with HCC ▽ **intoxication, unspecified**

F16.14　Hallucinogen abuse with hallucinogen-induced mood disorder
Other hallucinogen use disorder, mild, with other hallucinogen induced bipolar or related disorder
Other hallucinogen use disorder, mild, with other hallucinogen induced depressive disorder
Phencyclidine use disorder, mild, with phencyclidine induced bipolar or related disorder
Phencyclidine use disorder, mild, with phencyclidine induced depressive disorder

✓6ᵗʰ **F16.15　Hallucinogen abuse with hallucinogen-induced psychotic disorder**

F16.150　Hallucinogen abuse with HCC **hallucinogen-induced psychotic disorder with delusions**

F16.151　Hallucinogen abuse with HCC **hallucinogen-induced psychotic disorder with hallucinations**

F16.159　Hallucinogen abuse with HCC ▽ **hallucinogen-induced psychotic disorder, unspecified**

✓6ᵗʰ **F16.18　Hallucinogen abuse with other hallucinogen-induced disorder**

F16.180　Hallucinogen abuse with HCC **hallucinogen-induced anxiety disorder**

F16.183　Hallucinogen abuse with HCC **hallucinogen persisting perception disorder (flashbacks)**

F16.188　Hallucinogen abuse with other HCC **hallucinogen-induced disorder**

F16.19　Hallucinogen abuse with unspecified HCC ▽ **hallucinogen-induced disorder**

✓5ᵗʰ **F16.2　Hallucinogen dependence**
EXCLUDES 1　*hallucinogen abuse (F16.1-)*
hallucinogen use, unspecified (F16.9-)

F16.20　Hallucinogen dependence, uncomplicated HCC
Other hallucinogen use disorder, moderate
Other hallucinogen use disorder, severe
Phencyclidine use disorder, moderate
Phencyclidine use disorder, severe

F16.21　Hallucinogen dependence, in remission HCC
▶Other hallucinogen use disorder, moderate, in early remission
Other hallucinogen use disorder, moderate, in sustained remission
Other hallucinogen use disorder, severe, in early remission
Other hallucinogen use disorder, severe, in sustained remission
Phencyclidine use disorder, moderate, in early remission
Phencyclidine use disorder, moderate, in sustained remission
Phencyclidine use disorder, severe, in early remission
Phencyclidine use disorder, severe, in sustained remission◀

✓6ᵗʰ **F16.22　Hallucinogen dependence with intoxication**

F16.220　Hallucinogen dependence with HCC **intoxication, uncomplicated**

F16.221　Hallucinogen dependence with HCC **intoxication with delirium**

F16.229　Hallucinogen dependence with HCC ▽ **intoxication, unspecified**

F16.24　Hallucinogen dependence with HCC **hallucinogen-induced mood disorder**
Other hallucinogen use disorder, moderate, with other hallucinogen induced bipolar or related disorder
Other hallucinogen use disorder, moderate, with other hallucinogen induced depressive disorder
Other hallucinogen use disorder, severe, with other hallucinogen-induced bipolar or related disorder
Other hallucinogen use disorder, severe, with other hallucinogen-induced depressive disorder
Phencyclidine use disorder, moderate, with phencyclidine induced bipolar or related disorder
Phencyclidine use disorder, moderate, with phencyclidine induced depressive disorder
Phencyclidine use disorder, severe, with phencyclidine induced bipolar or related disorder
Phencyclidine use disorder, severe, with phencyclidine-induced depressive disorder

✓6ᵗʰ **F16.25　Hallucinogen dependence with hallucinogen-induced psychotic disorder**

F16.250　Hallucinogen dependence with HCC **hallucinogen-induced psychotic disorder with delusions**

F16.251　Hallucinogen dependence with HCC **hallucinogen-induced psychotic disorder with hallucinations**

F16.259　Hallucinogen dependence with HCC ▽ **hallucinogen-induced psychotic disorder, unspecified**

✓6ᵗʰ **F16.28　Hallucinogen dependence with other hallucinogen-induced disorder**

F16.280　Hallucinogen dependence with HCC **hallucinogen-induced anxiety disorder**

F16.283　Hallucinogen dependence with HCC **hallucinogen persisting perception disorder (flashbacks)**

F16.288　Hallucinogen dependence with other HCC **hallucinogen-induced disorder**

F16.29　Hallucinogen dependence with unspecified HCC ▽ **hallucinogen-induced disorder**

✓5ᵗʰ **F16.9　Hallucinogen use, unspecified**
EXCLUDES 1　*hallucinogen abuse (F16.1-)*
hallucinogen dependence (F16.2-)

F16.90　Hallucinogen use, unspecified, uncomplicated

✓ Additional Character Req　　✓ˣ⁷ᵗʰ Placeholder Alert　　Manifestation　　HCC CMS-HCC Condition　　▽ Unspecified Code　　▶◀ Revised Text　　● New Code　　▲ Revised Code Title

Chapter 5. Mental, Behavioral and Neurodevelopmental Disorders

✓6ᵗʰ **F16.92 Hallucinogen use, unspecified with** intoxication

F16.920 **Hallucinogen use, unspecified with** HCC **intoxication,** uncomplicated

F16.921 **Hallucinogen use, unspecified with** HCC **intoxication with** delirium
  Other hallucinogen intoxication delirium

F16.929 **Hallucinogen use, unspecified with** HCC ▽ **intoxication, unspecified**

F16.94 Hallucinogen use, unspecified with HCC **hallucinogen-induced** mood disorder
  Other hallucinogen induced bipolar or related disorder, without use disorder
  Other hallucinogen induced depressive disorder, without use disorder
  Phencyclidine induced bipolar or related disorder, without use disorder
  Phencyclidine induced depressive disorder, without use disorder

✓6ᵗʰ **F16.95 Hallucinogen use, unspecified with hallucinogen-induced** psychotic disorder

F16.950 **Hallucinogen use, unspecified with** HCC **hallucinogen-induced psychotic disorder with** delusions

F16.951 **Hallucinogen use, unspecified with** HCC **hallucinogen-induced psychotic disorder with** hallucinations

F16.959 **Hallucinogen use, unspecified with** HCC ▽ **hallucinogen-induced psychotic disorder, unspecified**
  Other hallucinogen induced psychotic disorder, without use disorder
  Phencyclidine induced psychotic disorder, without use disorder

✓6ᵗʰ **F16.98 Hallucinogen use, unspecified with other specified hallucinogen-induced disorder**

F16.980 **Hallucinogen use, unspecified with** HCC **hallucinogen-induced** anxiety disorder
  Other hallucinogen-induced anxiety disorder, without use disorder
  Phencyclidine induced anxiety disorder, without use disorder

F16.983 **Hallucinogen use, unspecified with** HCC **hallucinogen** persisting perception disorder (flashbacks)

F16.988 **Hallucinogen use, unspecified with** HCC **other hallucinogen-induced disorder**

F16.99 Hallucinogen use, unspecified with HCC ▽ **unspecified hallucinogen-induced disorder**

✓4ᵗʰ **F17** Nicotine dependence

EXCLUDES 1   history of tobacco dependence (Z87.891)
  tobacco use NOS (Z72.0)

EXCLUDES 2   tobacco use (smoking) during pregnancy, childbirth and the puerperium (O99.33-)
  toxic effect of nicotine (T65.2-)

AHA: 2013, 4Q, 108-109

✓5ᵗʰ **F17.2** Nicotine dependence

✓6ᵗʰ **F17.20 Nicotine dependence, unspecified**

F17.200 **Nicotine dependence, unspecified,** ▽ uncomplicated
  Tobacco use disorder, mild
  Tobacco use disorder, moderate
  Tobacco use disorder, severe
  AHA: 2016, 1Q, 36

F17.201 **Nicotine dependence, unspecified, in** ▽ remission
  ▶Tobacco use disorder, mild, in early remission
  Tobacco use disorder, mild, in sustained remission
  Tobacco use disorder, moderate, in early remission
  Tobacco use disorder, moderate, in sustained remission
  Tobacco use disorder, severe, in early remission
  Tobacco use disorder, severe, in sustained remission◀

F17.203 **Nicotine dependence unspecified,** ▽ **with** withdrawal
  Tobacco withdrawal

F17.208 **Nicotine dependence, unspecified,** ▽ **with other nicotine-induced disorders**

F17.209 **Nicotine dependence, unspecified,** ▽ **with unspecified nicotine-induced disorders**

✓6ᵗʰ **F17.21 Nicotine dependence,** cigarettes

F17.210 **Nicotine dependence, cigarettes,** uncomplicated
  AHA: 2017, 2Q, 28-29

F17.211 **Nicotine dependence, cigarettes, in** remission
  ▶Tobacco use disorder, cigarettes, mild, in early remission
  Tobacco use disorder, cigarettes, mild, in sustained remission
  Tobacco use disorder, cigarettes, moderate, in early remission
  Tobacco use disorder, cigarettes, moderate, in sustained remission
  Tobacco use disorder, cigarettes, severe, in early remission
  Tobacco use disorder, cigarettes, severe, in sustained remission◀

F17.213 **Nicotine dependence, cigarettes, with** withdrawal

F17.218 **Nicotine dependence, cigarettes, with other nicotine-induced disorders**

F17.219 **Nicotine dependence, cigarettes, with** ▽ **unspecified nicotine-induced disorders**

✓6ᵗʰ **F17.22 Nicotine dependence,** chewing tobacco

F17.220 **Nicotine dependence, chewing tobacco,** uncomplicated

F17.221 **Nicotine dependence, chewing tobacco, in** remission
  ▶Tobacco use disorder, chewing tobacco, mild, in early remission
  Tobacco use disorder, chewing tobacco, mild, in sustained remission
  Tobacco use disorder, chewing tobacco, moderate, in early remission
  Tobacco use disorder, chewing tobacco, moderate, in sustained remission
  Tobacco use disorder, chewing tobacco, severe, in early remission
  Tobacco use disorder, chewing tobacco, severe, in sustained remission◀

F17.223 **Nicotine dependence, chewing tobacco, with** withdrawal

F17.228 **Nicotine dependence, chewing tobacco, with other nicotine-induced disorders**

F17.229 **Nicotine dependence, chewing** ▽ **tobacco, with unspecified nicotine-induced disorders**

✓6ᵗʰ **F17.29 Nicotine dependence, other tobacco product**

F17.290 **Nicotine dependence, other tobacco product,** uncomplicated
  AHA: 2017, 2Q, 28-29

F17.291 **Nicotine dependence, other tobacco product,** in remission
  ▶Tobacco use disorder, other tobacco product, mild, in early remission
  Tobacco use disorder, other tobacco product, mild, in sustained remission
  Tobacco use disorder, other tobacco product, moderate, in early remission
  Tobacco use disorder, other tobacco product, moderate, in sustained remission
  Tobacco use disorder, other tobacco product, severe, in early remission
  Tobacco use disorder, other tobacco product, severe, in sustained remission◀

F17.293 **Nicotine dependence, other tobacco product, with** withdrawal

F17.298 **Nicotine dependence, other tobacco product, with other nicotine-induced disorders**

F17.299 **Nicotine dependence, other tobacco** ▽ **product, with unspecified nicotine-induced disorders**

EXCLUDES 1 Not coded here   EXCLUDES 2 Not included here   N Newborn Age: 0   P Pediatric Age: 0-17   M Maternity Age: 12-55   A Adult Age: 15-124

536   ICD-10-CM 2018

✓4th **F18** Inhalant related disorders

    INCLUDES volatile solvents

   ✓5th **F18.1** Inhalant abuse

       EXCLUDES1 inhalant dependence (F18.2-)

            inhalant use, unspecified (F18.9-)

      F18.10 Inhalant abuse, uncomplicated

          Inhalant use disorder, mild

•   **F18.11** Inhalant abuse, in remission

          Inhalant use disorder, mild, in early remission

          Inhalant use disorder, mild, in sustained remission

  ✓6th **F18.12** Inhalant abuse with intoxication

        F18.120 Inhalant abuse with intoxication, uncomplicated HCC

        F18.121 Inhalant abuse with intoxication delirium HCC

        F18.129 Inhalant abuse with intoxication, unspecified HCC ▽

      F18.14 Inhalant abuse with inhalant-induced mood disorder HCC

          Inhalant use disorder, mild, with inhalant induced depressive disorder

  ✓6th **F18.15** Inhalant abuse with inhalant-induced psychotic disorder

        F18.150 Inhalant abuse with inhalant-induced psychotic disorder with delusions HCC

        F18.151 Inhalant abuse with inhalant-induced psychotic disorder with hallucinations HCC

        F18.159 Inhalant abuse with inhalant-induced psychotic disorder, unspecified HCC ▽

      F18.17 Inhalant abuse with inhalant-induced dementia HCC

          Inhalant use disorder, mild, with inhalant induced major neurocognitive disorder

  ✓6th **F18.18** Inhalant abuse with other inhalant-induced disorders

        F18.180 Inhalant abuse with inhalant-induced anxiety disorder HCC

        F18.188 Inhalant abuse with other inhalant-induced disorder HCC

           Inhalant use disorder, mild, with inhalant induced mild neurocognitive disorder

      F18.19 Inhalant abuse with unspecified inhalant-induced disorder HCC ▽

   ✓5th **F18.2** Inhalant dependence

       EXCLUDES1 inhalant abuse (F18.1-)

            inhalant use, unspecified (F18.9-)

      F18.20 Inhalant dependence, uncomplicated HCC

          Inhalant use disorder, moderate

          Inhalant use disorder, severe

      F18.21 Inhalant dependence, in remission HCC

         ▶Inhalant use disorder, moderate, in early remission

         Inhalant use disorder, moderate, in sustained remission

         Inhalant use disorder, severe, in early remission

         Inhalant use disorder, severe, in sustained remission◀

  ✓6th **F18.22** Inhalant dependence with intoxication

        F18.220 Inhalant dependence with intoxication, uncomplicated HCC

        F18.221 Inhalant dependence with intoxication delirium HCC

        F18.229 Inhalant dependence with intoxication, unspecified HCC ▽

      F18.24 Inhalant dependence with inhalant-induced mood disorder HCC

          Inhalant use disorder, moderate, with inhalant induced depressive disorder

          Inhalant use disorder, severe, with inhalant induced depressive disorder

  ✓6th **F18.25** Inhalant dependence with inhalant-induced psychotic disorder

        F18.250 Inhalant dependence with inhalant-induced psychotic disorder with delusions HCC

        F18.251 Inhalant dependence with inhalant-induced psychotic disorder with hallucinations HCC

        F18.259 Inhalant dependence with inhalant-induced psychotic disorder, unspecified HCC ▽

      F18.27 Inhalant dependence with inhalant-induced dementia HCC

          Inhalant use disorder, moderate, with inhalant induced major neurocognitive disorder

          Inhalant use disorder, severe, with inhalant induced major neurocognitive disorder

  ✓6th **F18.28** Inhalant dependence with other inhalant-induced disorders

        F18.280 Inhalant dependence with inhalant-induced anxiety disorder HCC

        F18.288 Inhalant dependence with other inhalant-induced disorder HCC

           Inhalant use disorder, moderate, with inhalant-induced mild neurocognitive disorder

           Inhalant use disorder, severe, with inhalant-induced mild neurocognitive disorder

      F18.29 Inhalant dependence with unspecified inhalant-induced disorder HCC ▽

   ✓5th **F18.9** Inhalant use, unspecified

       EXCLUDES1 inhalant abuse (F18.1-)

            inhalant dependence (F18.2-)

      F18.90 Inhalant use, unspecified, uncomplicated

  ✓6th **F18.92** Inhalant use, unspecified with intoxication

        F18.920 Inhalant use, unspecified with intoxication, uncomplicated HCC

        F18.921 Inhalant use, unspecified with intoxication with delirium HCC

        F18.929 Inhalant use, unspecified with intoxication, unspecified HCC ▽

      F18.94 Inhalant use, unspecified with inhalant-induced mood disorder HCC

          Inhalant induced depressive disorder

  ✓6th **F18.95** Inhalant use, unspecified with inhalant-induced psychotic disorder

        F18.950 Inhalant use, unspecified with inhalant-induced psychotic disorder with delusions HCC

        F18.951 Inhalant use, unspecified with inhalant-induced psychotic disorder with hallucinations HCC

        F18.959 Inhalant use, unspecified with inhalant-induced psychotic disorder, unspecified HCC ▽

      F18.97 Inhalant use, unspecified with inhalant-induced persisting dementia HCC

          Inhalant-induced major neurocognitive disorder

  ✓6th **F18.98** Inhalant use, unspecified with other inhalant-induced disorders

        F18.980 Inhalant use, unspecified with inhalant-induced anxiety disorder HCC

        F18.988 Inhalant use, unspecified with other inhalant-induced disorder HCC

           Inhalant-induced mild neurocognitive disorder

      F18.99 Inhalant use, unspecified with unspecified inhalant-induced disorder HCC ▽

✓4th **F19** Other psychoactive substance related disorders

    INCLUDES polysubstance drug use (indiscriminate drug use)

   ✓5th **F19.1** Other psychoactive substance abuse

       EXCLUDES1 other psychoactive substance dependence (F19.2-)

            other psychoactive substance use, unspecified (F19.9-)

      F19.10 Other psychoactive substance abuse, uncomplicated

          Other (or unknown) substance use disorder, mild

•   **F19.11** Other psychoactive substance abuse, in remission

          Other (or unknown) substance use disorder, mild, in early remission

          Other (or unknown) substance use disorder, mild, in sustained remission

  ✓6th **F19.12** Other psychoactive substance abuse with intoxication

        F19.120 Other psychoactive substance abuse with intoxication, uncomplicated

        F19.121 Other psychoactive substance abuse with intoxication delirium HCC

✓ Additional Character Req   ✓x7th Placeholder Alert   Manifestation   HCC CMS-HCC Condition   ▽ Unspecified Code   ▶◀ Revised Text   ● New Code   ▲ Revised Code Title

ICD-10-CM 2018   537

Chapter 5. Mental, Behavioral and Neurodevelopmental Disorders

F19.122–F19.282

F19.122 Other psychoactive substance abuse with intoxication with perceptual disturbances HCC

F19.129 Other psychoactive substance abuse with intoxication, unspecified HCC ▽

F19.14 Other psychoactive substance abuse with psychoactive substance-induced mood disorder HCC
Other (or unknown) substance use disorder, mild, with other (or unknown) substance-induced bipolar or related disorder
Other (or unknown) substance use disorder, mild, with other (or unknown) substance-induced depressive disorder

✓6ᵗʰ **F19.15** Other psychoactive substance abuse with psychoactive substance-induced psychotic disorder

F19.150 Other psychoactive substance abuse with psychoactive substance-induced psychotic disorder with delusions HCC

F19.151 Other psychoactive substance abuse with psychoactive substance-induced psychotic disorder with hallucinations HCC

F19.159 Other psychoactive substance abuse with psychoactive substance-induced psychotic disorder, unspecified HCC ▽

F19.16 Other psychoactive substance abuse with psychoactive substance-induced persisting amnestic disorder HCC

F19.17 Other psychoactive substance abuse with psychoactive substance-induced persisting dementia HCC
Other (or unknown) substance use disorder, mild, with other (or unknown) substance-induced major neurocognitive disorder

✓6ᵗʰ **F19.18** Other psychoactive substance abuse with other psychoactive substance-induced disorders

F19.180 Other psychoactive substance abuse with psychoactive substance-induced anxiety disorder HCC

F19.181 Other psychoactive substance abuse with psychoactive substance-induced sexual dysfunction HCC

F19.182 Other psychoactive substance abuse with psychoactive substance-induced sleep disorder HCC

F19.188 Other psychoactive substance abuse with other psychoactive substance-induced disorder HCC
Other (or unknown) substance use disorder, mild, with other (or unknown) substance induced mild neurocognitive disorder
Other (or unknown) substance use disorder, mild, with other (or unknown) substance induced obsessive-compulsive or related disorder

F19.19 Other psychoactive substance abuse with unspecified psychoactive substance-induced disorder HCC ▽

✓5ᵗʰ **F19.2** Other psychoactive substance dependence
EXCLUDES1 other psychoactive substance abuse (F19.1-)
other psychoactive substance use, unspecified (F19.9-)

F19.20 Other psychoactive substance dependence, uncomplicated HCC
Other (or unknown) substance use disorder, moderate
Other (or unknown) substance use disorder, severe

F19.21 Other psychoactive substance dependence, in remission HCC
▶Other (or unknown) substance use disorder, moderate, in early remission
Other (or unknown) substance use disorder, moderate, in sustained remission
Other (or unknown) substance use disorder, severe, in early remission
Other (or unknown) substance use, severe, in sustained remission◀

✓6ᵗʰ **F19.22** Other psychoactive substance dependence with intoxication
EXCLUDES1 other psychoactive substance dependence with withdrawal (F19.23-)

F19.220 Other psychoactive substance dependence with intoxication, uncomplicated HCC

F19.221 Other psychoactive substance dependence with intoxication delirium HCC

F19.222 Other psychoactive substance dependence with intoxication with perceptual disturbance HCC

F19.229 Other psychoactive substance dependence with intoxication, unspecified HCC ▽

✓6ᵗʰ **F19.23** Other psychoactive substance dependence with withdrawal
EXCLUDES1 other psychoactive substance dependence with intoxication (F19.22-)

F19.230 Other psychoactive substance dependence with withdrawal, uncomplicated HCC

F19.231 Other psychoactive substance dependence with withdrawal delirium HCC

F19.232 Other psychoactive substance dependence with withdrawal with perceptual disturbance HCC

F19.239 Other psychoactive substance dependence with withdrawal, unspecified HCC ▽

F19.24 Other psychoactive substance dependence with psychoactive substance-induced mood disorder HCC
Other (or unknown) substance use disorder, moderate, with other (or unknown) substance induced bipolar or related disorder
Other (or unknown) substance use disorder, moderate, with other (or unknown) substance induced depressive disorder
Other (or unknown) use disorder, severe, with other (or unknown) substance induced bipolar or related disorder
Other (or unknown) substance use disorder, severe, with other (or unknown) substance induced depressive disorder

✓6ᵗʰ **F19.25** Other psychoactive substance dependence with psychoactive substance-induced psychotic disorder

F19.250 Other psychoactive substance dependence with psychoactive substance-induced psychotic disorder with delusions HCC

F19.251 Other psychoactive substance dependence with psychoactive substance-induced psychotic disorder with hallucinations HCC

F19.259 Other psychoactive substance dependence with psychoactive substance-induce d psychotic disorder, unspecified HCC ▽

F19.26 Other psychoactive substance dependence with psychoactive substance-induced persisting amnestic disorder HCC

F19.27 Other psychoactive substance dependence with psychoactive substance-induced persisting dementia HCC
Other (or unknown) substance use disorder, moderate, with other (or unknown) substance induced major neurocognitive disorder
Other (or unknown) substance use disorder, severe, with other (or unknown) substance induced major neurocognitive disorder

✓6ᵗʰ **F19.28** Other psychoactive substance dependence with other psychoactive substance-induced disorders

F19.280 Other psychoactive substance dependence with psychoactive substance-induced anxiety disorder HCC

F19.281 Other psychoactive substance dependence with psychoactive substance-induced sexual dysfunction HCC

F19.282 Other psychoactive substance dependence with psychoactive substance-induced sleep disorder HCC

F19.288 Other psychoactive substance dependence with other psychoactive substance-induced disorder `HCC`
> Other (or unknown) substance use disorder, moderate, with other (or unknown) substance induced mild neurocognitive disorder
> Other (or unknown) substance use disorder, severe, with other (or unknown) substance induced mild neurocognitive disorder
> Other (or unknown) substance use disorder, moderate, with other (or unknown) substance induced obsessive compulsive or related disorder
> Other (or unknown) substance use disorder, severe, with other (or unknown) substance induced obsessive-compulsive or related disorder

F19.29 Other psychoactive substance dependence with unspecified psychoactive substance-induced disorder `HCC` ▽

✓5th **F19.9 Other psychoactive substance use, unspecified**
> `EXCLUDES 1` other psychoactive substance abuse (F19.1-)
> other psychoactive substance dependence (F19.2-)

F19.90 Other psychoactive substance use, unspecified, uncomplicated

✓6th **F19.92 Other psychoactive substance use, unspecified with intoxication**
> `EXCLUDES 1` other psychoactive substance use, unspecified with withdrawal (F19.93)

F19.920 Other psychoactive substance use, unspecified with intoxication, uncomplicated `HCC`

F19.921 Other psychoactive substance use, unspecified with intoxication with delirium `HCC`
> Other (or unknown) substance-induced delirium

F19.922 Other psychoactive substance use, unspecified with intoxication with perceptual disturbance `HCC`

F19.929 Other psychoactive substance use, unspecified with intoxication, unspecified `HCC` ▽

✓6th **F19.93 Other psychoactive substance use, unspecified with withdrawal**
> `EXCLUDES 1` other psychoactive substance use, unspecified with intoxication (F19.92-)

F19.930 Other psychoactive substance use, unspecified with withdrawal, uncomplicated `HCC`

F19.931 Other psychoactive substance use, unspecified with withdrawal delirium `HCC`

F19.932 Other psychoactive substance use, unspecified with withdrawal with perceptual disturbance `HCC`

F19.939 Other psychoactive substance use, unspecified with withdrawal, unspecified `HCC` ▽

F19.94 Other psychoactive substance use, unspecified with psychoactive substance-induced mood disorder `HCC`
> Other (or unknown) substance-induced bipolar or related disorder, without use disorder
> Other (or unknown) substance-induced depressive disorder, without use disorder

✓6th **F19.95 Other psychoactive substance use, unspecified with psychoactive substance-induced psychotic disorder**

F19.950 Other psychoactive substance use, unspecified with psychoactive substance-induced psychotic disorder with delusions `HCC`

F19.951 Other psychoactive substance use, unspecified with psychoactive substance-induced psychotic disorder with hallucinations `HCC`

F19.959 Other psychoactive substance use, unspecified with psychoactive substance-induced psychotic disorder, unspecified `HCC` ▽
> Other or unknown substance-induced psychotic disorder, without use disorder

F19.96 Other psychoactive substance use, unspecified with psychoactive substance-induced persisting amnestic disorder `HCC`

F19.97 Other psychoactive substance use, unspecified with psychoactive substance-induced persisting dementia `HCC`
> Other (or unknown) substance-induced major neurocognitive disorder, without use disorder

✓6th **F19.98 Other psychoactive substance use, unspecified with other psychoactive substance-induced disorders**

F19.980 Other psychoactive substance use, unspecified with psychoactive substance-induced anxiety disorder `HCC`
> Other (or unknown) substance-induced anxiety disorder, without use disorder

F19.981 Other psychoactive substance use, unspecified with psychoactive substance-induced sexual dysfunction `HCC`
> Other (or unknown) substance-induced sexual dysfunction, without use disorder

F19.982 Other psychoactive substance use, unspecified with psychoactive substance-induced sleep disorder `HCC`
> Other (or unknown) substance-induced sleep disorder, without use disorder

F19.988 Other psychoactive substance use, unspecified with other psychoactive substance-induced disorder `HCC`
> Other (or unknown) substance-induced mild neurocognitive disorder, without use disorder
> Other (or unknown) substance-induced obsessive-compulsive or related disorder, without use disorder

F19.99 Other psychoactive substance use, unspecified with unspecified psychoactive substance-induced disorder `HCC` ▽

Schizophrenia, schizotypal, delusional, and other non-mood psychotic disorders (F20-F29)

✓4th **F20 Schizophrenia**
> `EXCLUDES 1` brief psychotic disorder (F23)
> cyclic schizophrenia (F25.0)
> mood [affective] disorders with psychotic symptoms (F30.2, F31.2, F31.5, F31.64, F32.3, F33.3)
> schizoaffective disorder (F25.-)
> schizophrenic reaction NOS (F23)
> `EXCLUDES 2` schizophrenic reaction in:
> alcoholism (F10.15-, F10.25-, F10.95-)
> brain disease (F06.2)
> epilepsy (F06.2)
> psychoactive drug use (F11-F19 with .15, .25, .95)
> schizotypal disorder (F21)

DEF: Group of disorders with disturbances in thought (delusions, hallucinations), mood (blunted, flattened, inappropriate affect), sense of self; also bizarre, purposeless behavior, repetitious activity, or inactivity.

F20.0 Paranoid schizophrenia `HCC`
> Paraphrenic schizophrenia
> `EXCLUDES 1` involutional paranoid state (F22)
> paranoia (F22)

DEF: Preoccupied with delusional suspicions and auditory hallucinations related to single theme; usually hostile, grandiose, threatening, persecutory, occasionally hypochondriacal.

F20.1 Disorganized schizophrenia `HCC`
> Hebephrenic schizophrenia
> Hebephrenia

F20.2 Catatonic schizophrenia `HCC`
> Schizophrenic catalepsy
> Schizophrenic catatonia
> Schizophrenic flexibilitas cerea
> `EXCLUDES 1` catatonic stupor (R40.1)

DEF: Extreme changes in motor activity; one extreme is decreased response or reaction to the environment and the other is spontaneous activity.

✓ Additional Character Req   ✓x7th Placeholder Alert   Manifestation   HCC CMS-HCC Condition   ▽ Unspecified Code   ►◄ Revised Text   ● New Code   ▲ Revised Code Title

ICD-10-CM 2018   539

Chapter 5. Mental, Behavioral and Neurodevelopmental Disorders

F19.288–F20.2

F20.3　Undifferentiated schizophrenia　`HCC`
Atypical schizophrenia
　　EXCLUDES 1　*acute schizophrenia-like psychotic disorder (F23)*
　　EXCLUDES 2　*post-schizophrenic depression (F32.89)*

F20.5　Residual schizophrenia　`HCC`
Restzustand (schizophrenic)
Schizophrenic residual state

✓5th **F20.8　Other schizophrenia**
　F20.81　Schizophreniform disorder　`HCC`
　　Schizophreniform psychosis NOS
　F20.89　Other schizophrenia　`HCC`
　　Cenesthopathic schizophrenia
　　Simple schizophrenia

F20.9　Schizophrenia, unspecified　`HCC` ▽

F21　Schizotypal disorder
Borderline schizophrenia　　　Prodromal schizophrenia
Latent schizophrenia　　　　　Pseudoneurotic schizophrenia
Latent schizophrenic reaction　Pseudopsychopathic schizophrenia
Prepsychotic schizophrenia　　Schizotypal personality disorder
　EXCLUDES 2　*Asperger's syndrome (F84.5)*
　　　　　　　schizoid personality disorder (F60.1)

F22　Delusional disorders　`HCC`
Delusional dysmorphophobia　　Paranoid psychosis
Involutional paranoid state　　Paranoid state
Paranoia　　　　　　　　　　Paraphrenia (late)
Paranoia querulans　　　　　　Sensitiver Beziehungswahn
　EXCLUDES 1　*mood [affective] disorders with psychotic symptoms (F30.2,*
　　　　　　　F31.2, F31.5, F31.64, F32.3, F33.3)
　　　　　　　paranoid schizophrenia (F20.0)
　EXCLUDES 2　*paranoid personality disorder (F60.0)*
　　　　　　　paranoid psychosis, psychogenic (F23)
　　　　　　　paranoid reaction (F23)

F23　Brief psychotic disorder
Paranoid reaction
Psychogenic paranoid psychosis
　EXCLUDES 2　*mood [affective] disorders with psychotic symptoms (F30.2,*
　　　　　　　F31.2, F31.5, F31.64, F32.3, F33.3)

F24　Shared psychotic disorder　`HCC`
Folie à deux
Induced paranoid disorder
Induced psychotic disorder

✓4th **F25　Schizoaffective disorders**
　EXCLUDES 1　*mood [affective] disorders with psychotic symptoms (F30.2,*
　　　　　　　F31.2, F31.5, F31.64, F32.3, F33.3)
　　　　　　　schizophrenia (F20.-)
　F25.0　Schizoaffective disorder, bipolar type　`HCC`
　　Cyclic schizophrenia
　　Schizoaffective disorder, manic type
　　Schizoaffective disorder, mixed type
　　Schizoaffective psychosis, bipolar type
　　~~Schizophreniform psychosis, manic type~~
　F25.1　Schizoaffective disorder, depressive type　`HCC`
　　Schizoaffective psychosis, depressive type
　　~~Schizophreniform psychosis, depressive type~~
　F25.8　Other schizoaffective disorders　`HCC`
　F25.9　Schizoaffective disorder, unspecified　`HCC` ▽
　　Schizoaffective psychosis NOS

F28　Other psychotic disorder not due to a substance or known physiological condition
Chronic hallucinatory psychosis
▶Other specified schizophrenia spectrum and other psychotic disorder◀

F29　Unspecified psychosis not due to a substance or known physiological condition　▽
Psychosis NOS
▶Unspecified schizophrenia spectrum and other psychotic disorder◀
　EXCLUDES 1　*mental disorder NOS (F99)*
　　　　　　　unspecified mental disorder due to known physiological condition (F09)

Mood [affective] disorders (F30-F39)

✓4th **F30　Manic episode**
　INCLUDES　bipolar disorder, single manic episode
　　　　　　mixed affective episode
　EXCLUDES 1　*bipolar disorder (F31.-)*
　　　　　　　major depressive disorder, recurrent (F33.-)
　　　　　　　major depressive disorder, single episode (F32.-)

✓5th **F30.1　Manic episode without psychotic symptoms**
　F30.10　Manic episode without psychotic symptoms, unspecified　`HCC` ▽
　F30.11　Manic episode without psychotic symptoms, mild　`HCC`
　F30.12　Manic episode without psychotic symptoms, moderate　`HCC`
　F30.13　Manic episode, severe, without psychotic symptoms　`HCC`

F30.2　Manic episode, severe with psychotic symptoms　`HCC`
Manic stupor
Mania with mood-congruent psychotic symptoms
Mania with mood-incongruent psychotic symptoms

F30.3　Manic episode in partial remission　`HCC`

F30.4　Manic episode in full remission　`HCC`

F30.8　Other manic episodes　`HCC`
Hypomania

F30.9　Manic episode, unspecified　`HCC` ▽
Mania NOS

✓4th **F31　Bipolar disorder**
　INCLUDES　▶bipolar I disorder
　　　　　　bipolar type I disorder◀
　　　　　　manic-depressive illness
　　　　　　manic-depressive psychosis
　　　　　　manic-depressive reaction
　EXCLUDES 1　*bipolar disorder, single manic episode (F30.-)*
　　　　　　　major depressive disorder, single episode (F32.-)
　　　　　　　major depressive disorder, recurrent (F33.-)
　EXCLUDES 2　*cyclothymia (F34.0)*

F31.0　Bipolar disorder, current episode hypomanic　`HCC`

✓5th **F31.1　Bipolar disorder, current episode manic without psychotic features**
　F31.10　Bipolar disorder, current episode manic without psychotic features, unspecified　`HCC` ▽
　F31.11　Bipolar disorder, current episode manic without psychotic features, mild　`HCC`
　F31.12　Bipolar disorder, current episode manic without psychotic features, moderate　`HCC`
　F31.13　Bipolar disorder, current episode manic without psychotic features, severe　`HCC`

F31.2　Bipolar disorder, current episode manic severe with psychotic features　`HCC`
Bipolar disorder, current episode manic with mood-congruent psychotic symptoms
Bipolar disorder, current episode manic with mood-incongruent psychotic symptoms
▶Bipolar I disorder, current or most recent episode manic with psychotic features◀

✓5th **F31.3　Bipolar disorder, current episode depressed, mild or moderate severity**
　F31.30　Bipolar disorder, current episode depressed, mild or moderate severity, unspecified　`HCC` ▽
　F31.31　Bipolar disorder, current episode depressed, mild　`HCC`
　F31.32　Bipolar disorder, current episode depressed, moderate　`HCC`

F31.4　Bipolar disorder, current episode depressed, severe, without psychotic features　`HCC`

F31.5　Bipolar disorder, current episode depressed, severe, with psychotic features　`HCC`
Bipolar disorder, current episode depressed with mood-incongruent psychotic symptoms
Bipolar disorder, current episode depressed with mood-congruent psychotic symptoms
▶Bipolar I disorder, current or most recent episode depressed, with psychotic features◀

✓5th **F31.6　Bipolar disorder, current episode mixed**
　F31.60　Bipolar disorder, current episode mixed, unspecified　`HCC` ▽
　F31.61　Bipolar disorder, current episode mixed, mild　`HCC`

F31.62   **Bipolar disorder, current episode mixed, moderate**   `HCC`

F31.63   **Bipolar disorder, current episode mixed, severe, without psychotic features**   `HCC`

F31.64   **Bipolar disorder, current episode mixed, severe, with psychotic features**   `HCC`
Bipolar disorder, current episode mixed with mood-congruent psychotic symptoms
Bipolar disorder, current episode mixed with mood-incongruent psychotic symptoms

✓5ᵗʰ **F31.7**   **Bipolar disorder, currently in remission**

F31.70   **Bipolar disorder, currently in remission, most recent episode unspecified**   `HCC` ▽

F31.71   **Bipolar disorder, in partial remission, most recent episode hypomanic**   `HCC`

F31.72   **Bipolar disorder, in full remission, most recent episode hypomanic**   `HCC`

F31.73   **Bipolar disorder, in partial remission, most recent episode manic**   `HCC`

F31.74   **Bipolar disorder, in full remission, most recent episode manic**   `HCC`

F31.75   **Bipolar disorder, in partial remission, most recent episode depressed**   `HCC`

F31.76   **Bipolar disorder, in full remission, most recent episode depressed**   `HCC`

F31.77   **Bipolar disorder, in partial remission, most recent episode mixed**   `HCC`

F31.78   **Bipolar disorder, in full remission, most recent episode mixed**   `HCC`

✓5ᵗʰ **F31.8**   **Other bipolar disorders**

F31.81   **Bipolar II disorder**   `HCC`
▶Bipolar disorder, type 2◀

F31.89   **Other bipolar disorder**   `HCC`
Recurrent manic episodes NOS

F31.9   **Bipolar disorder, unspecified**   `HCC` ▽
▶Manic depression◀

✓4ᵗʰ **F32**   **Major depressive disorder, single episode**
`INCLUDES` single episode of agitated depression
single episode of depressive reaction
single episode of major depression
single episode of psychogenic depression
single episode of reactive depression
single episode of vital depression
`EXCLUDES 1` bipolar disorder (F31.-)
manic episode (F30.-)
recurrent depressive disorder (F33.-)
`EXCLUDES 2` adjustment disorder (F43.2)
DEF: Mood disorder that produces depression; may exhibit as sadness, low self-esteem, or guilt feelings; other manifestations may be withdrawal from friends and family and interrupted sleep.

F32.0   **Major depressive disorder, single episode, mild**   `HCC`

F32.1   **Major depressive disorder, single episode, moderate**   `HCC`

F32.2   **Major depressive disorder, single episode, severe without psychotic features**   `HCC`

F32.3   **Major depressive disorder, single episode, severe with psychotic features**   `HCC`
Single episode of major depression with mood-congruent psychotic symptoms
Single episode of major depression with mood-incongruent psychotic symptoms
Single episode of major depression with psychotic symptoms
Single episode of psychogenic depressive psychosis
Single episode of psychotic depression
Single episode of reactive depressive psychosis

F32.4   **Major depressive disorder, single episode, in partial remission**   `HCC`

F32.5   **Major depressive disorder, single episode, in full remission**   `HCC`

✓5ᵗʰ **F32.8**   **Other depressive episodes**

F32.81   **Premenstrual dysphoric disorder**   ♀
`EXCLUDES 1` premenstrual tension syndrome (N94.3)

F32.89   **Other specified depressive episodes**
Atypical depression
Post-schizophrenic depression
Single episode of 'masked' depression NOS

F32.9   **Major depressive disorder, single episode, unspecified**   ▽
Depression NOS
Depressive disorder NOS
Major depression NOS
AHA: 2013, 4Q, 107

✓4ᵗʰ **F33**   **Major depressive disorder, recurrent**
Recurrent episodes of depressive reaction
Recurrent episodes of endogenous depression
Recurrent episodes of major depression
Recurrent episodes of psychogenic depression
Recurrent episodes of reactive depression
Recurrent episodes of seasonal depressive disorder
Recurrent episodes of vital depression
`EXCLUDES 1` bipolar disorder (F31.-)
manic episode (F30.-)

F33.0   **Major depressive disorder, recurrent, mild**   `HCC`

F33.1   **Major depressive disorder, recurrent, moderate**   `HCC`

F33.2   **Major depressive disorder, recurrent, severe without psychotic features**   `HCC`

F33.3   **Major depressive disorder, recurrent, severe with psychotic symptoms**   `HCC`
Endogenous depression with psychotic symptoms
▶Major depressive disorder, recurrent, with psychotic features◀
Recurrent severe episodes of major depression with mood-congruent psychotic symptoms
Recurrent severe episodes of major depression with mood-incongruent psychotic symptoms
Recurrent severe episodes of major depression with psychotic symptoms
Recurrent severe episodes of psychogenic depressive psychosis
Recurrent severe episodes of psychotic depression
Recurrent severe episodes of reactive depressive psychosis

✓5ᵗʰ **F33.4**   **Major depressive disorder, recurrent, in remission**

F33.40   **Major depressive disorder, recurrent, in remission, unspecified**   `HCC` ▽

F33.41   **Major depressive disorder, recurrent, in partial remission**   `HCC`

F33.42   **Major depressive disorder, recurrent, in full remission**   `HCC`

F33.8   **Other recurrent depressive disorders**   `HCC`
Recurrent brief depressive episodes

F33.9   **Major depressive disorder, recurrent, unspecified**   `HCC` ▽
Monopolar depression NOS

✓4ᵗʰ **F34**   **Persistent mood [affective] disorders**

F34.0   **Cyclothymic disorder**
Affective personality disorder
Cycloid personality
Cyclothymia
Cyclothymic personality

F34.1   **Dysthymic disorder**
Depressive neurosis
Depressive personality disorder
Dysthymia
Neurotic depression
Persistent anxiety depression
Persistent depressive disorder
`EXCLUDES 2` anxiety depression (mild or not persistent) (F41.8)
DEF: Depression without psychosis; less severe but persistent depression; is considered a mild to moderate chronic form of depression.

✓5ᵗʰ **F34.8**   **Other persistent mood [affective] disorders**

F34.81   **Disruptive mood dysregulation disorder**   `HCC`

F34.89   **Other specified persistent mood disorders**   `HCC`

F34.9   **Persistent mood [affective] disorder, unspecified**   `HCC` ▽

F39   **Unspecified mood [affective] disorder**   `HCC` ▽
Affective psychosis NOS

Anxiety, dissociative, stress-related, somatoform and other nonpsychotic mental disorders (F40-F48)

✓4ᵗʰ **F40**   **Phobic anxiety disorders**

✓5ᵗʰ **F40.0**   **Agoraphobia**
DEF: Profound anxiety or fear of leaving familiar settings like home, or being in unfamiliar locations or with strangers or crowds; may or may not be preceded by recurrent panic attacks.

F40.00   **Agoraphobia, unspecified**   ▽

F40.01   **Agoraphobia with panic disorder**
Panic disorder with agoraphobia
`EXCLUDES 1` panic disorder without agoraphobia (F41.0)

☑ Additional Character Req   `✓x7ᵗʰ` Placeholder Alert   Manifestation   `HCC` CMS-HCC Condition   ▽ Unspecified Code   ▶◀ Revised Text   ● New Code   ▲ Revised Code Title

F40.02   Agoraphobia without panic disorder

✓5th **F40.1   Social phobias**
Anthropophobia
▶Social anxiety disorder◀
Social anxiety disorder of childhood
Social neurosis

    F40.10   Social phobia, unspecified   ▽

    F40.11   Social phobia, generalized

✓5th **F40.2   Specific (isolated) phobias**
    EXCLUDES 2   *dysmorphophobia (nondelusional) (F45.22)*
             nosophobia (F45.22)

   ✓6th **F40.21   Animal type phobia**

       F40.210   Arachnophobia
              Fear of spiders

       F40.218   Other animal type phobia

   ✓6th **F40.22   Natural environment type phobia**

       F40.220   Fear of thunderstorms

       F40.228   Other natural environment type phobia

   ✓6th **F40.23   Blood, injection, injury type phobia**

       F40.230   Fear of blood

       F40.231   Fear of injections and transfusions

       F40.232   Fear of other medical care

       F40.233   Fear of injury

   ✓6th **F40.24   Situational type phobia**

       F40.240   Claustrophobia

       F40.241   Acrophobia

       F40.242   Fear of bridges

       F40.243   Fear of flying

       F40.248   Other situational type phobia

   ✓6th **F40.29   Other specified phobia**

       F40.290   Androphobia
              Fear of men

       F40.291   Gynephobia
              Fear of women

       F40.298   Other specified phobia

F40.8   Other phobic anxiety disorders
Phobic anxiety disorder of childhood

F40.9   Phobic anxiety disorder, unspecified   ▽
Phobia NOS
Phobic state NOS

✓4th **F41   Other anxiety disorders**
    EXCLUDES 2   *anxiety in:*
             acute stress reaction (F43.0)
             transient adjustment reaction (F43.2)
             neurasthenia (F48.8)
             psychophysiologic disorders (F45.-)
             separation anxiety (F93.0)

▲ **F41.0   Panic disorder [episodic paroxysmal anxiety]**
Panic attack
Panic state
    EXCLUDES 1   *panic disorder with agoraphobia (F40.01)*
DEF: Neurotic disorder characterized by recurrent panic or anxiety, apprehension, fear, or terror; symptoms include shortness of breath, palpitations, dizziness, shakiness; fear of dying may persist.

F41.1   Generalized anxiety disorder
Anxiety neurosis   Anxiety state
Anxiety reaction   Overanxious disorder
    EXCLUDES 2   *neurasthenia (F48.8)*

F41.3   Other mixed anxiety disorders

F41.8   Other specified anxiety disorders
Anxiety depression (mild or not persistent)
Anxiety hysteria
Mixed anxiety and depressive disorder

F41.9   Anxiety disorder, unspecified   ▽
Anxiety NOS

✓4th **F42   Obsessive-compulsive disorder**
    EXCLUDES 2   *obsessive-compulsive personality (disorder) (F60.5)*
             obsessive-compulsive symptoms occurring in depression (F32-F33)
             obsessive-compulsive symptoms occurring in schizophrenia (F20.-)

F42.2   Mixed obsessional thoughts and acts

F42.3   Hoarding disorder

F42.4   Excoriation (skin-picking) disorder
    EXCLUDES 1   *factitial dermatitis (L98.1)*
             other specified behavioral and emotional disorders with onset usually occurring in early childhood and adolescence (F98.8)

F42.8   Other obsessive-compulsive disorder
Anancastic neurosis
Obsessive-compulsive neurosis

F42.9   Obsessive-compulsive disorder, unspecified   ▽

✓4th **F43   Reaction to severe stress, and adjustment disorders**

F43.0   Acute stress reaction
Acute crisis reaction
Acute reaction to stress
Combat and operational stress reaction
Combat fatigue
Crisis state
Psychic shock

✓5th **F43.1   Post-traumatic stress disorder (PTSD)**
Traumatic neurosis
DEF: Preoccupation with traumatic events beyond normal experience; i.e., rape, personal assault, etc.; also recurring flashbacks of trauma; symptoms include difficulty remembering, sleeping, or concentrating, and guilt feelings for surviving.   ▽

    F43.10   Post-traumatic stress disorder, unspecified   ▽

    F43.11   Post-traumatic stress disorder, acute

    F43.12   Post-traumatic stress disorder, chronic

✓5th **F43.2   Adjustment disorders**
Culture shock
Grief reaction
Hospitalism in children
    EXCLUDES 2   *separation anxiety disorder of childhood (F93.0)*

    F43.20   Adjustment disorder, unspecified   ▽

    F43.21   Adjustment disorder with depressed mood
           AHA: 2014, 1Q, 25

    F43.22   Adjustment disorder with anxiety

    F43.23   Adjustment disorder with mixed anxiety and depressed mood

    F43.24   Adjustment disorder with disturbance of conduct

    F43.25   Adjustment disorder with mixed disturbance of emotions and conduct

    F43.29   Adjustment disorder with other symptoms

F43.8   Other reactions to severe stress
Other specified trauma and stressor-related disorder

F43.9   Reaction to severe stress, unspecified   ▽
Trauma and stressor-related disorder, NOS

✓4th **F44   Dissociative and conversion disorders**
    INCLUDES   conversion hysteria
             conversion reaction
             hysteria
             hysterical psychosis
    EXCLUDES 2   *malingering [conscious simulation] (Z76.5)*

F44.0   Dissociative amnesia
    EXCLUDES 1   *amnesia NOS (R41.3)*
             anterograde amnesia (R41.1)
             dissociative amnesia with dissociative fugue (F44.1)
             retrograde amnesia (R41.2)
    EXCLUDES 2   *alcohol-or other psychoactive substance-induced amnestic disorder (F10, F13, F19 with .26, .96)*
             amnestic disorder due to known physiological condition (F04)
             postictal amnesia in epilepsy (G40.-)

F44.1   Dissociative fugue
Dissociative amnesia with dissociative fugue
    EXCLUDES 2   *postictal fugue in epilepsy (G40.-)*
DEF: Dissociative hysteria; identified by loss of memory, flight from familiar surroundings to a completely separate environment, episodes may last hours or days; conscious activity is not associated with perception of surroundings and there is no later memory of episode.

F44.2   Dissociative stupor
    EXCLUDES 1   *catatonic stupor (R40.1)*
             stupor NOS (R40.1)
    EXCLUDES 2   *catatonic disorder due to known physiological condition (F06.1)*
             depressive stupor (F32, F33)
             manic stupor (F30, F31)

EXCLUDES 1 Not coded here   EXCLUDES 2 Not included here   N Newborn Age: 0   P Pediatric Age: 0-17   M Maternity Age: 12-55   A Adult Age: 15-124

542   ICD-10-CM 2018

F44.4 **Conversion disorder with** motor symptom or deficit
▶Conversion disorder with abnormal movement
Conversion disorder with speech symptoms
Conversion disorder with swallowing symptoms
Conversion disorder with weakness/paralysis◀
Dissociative motor disorders
Psychogenic aphonia
Psychogenic dysphonia

F44.5 **Conversion disorder with** seizures or convulsions
▶Conversion disorder with attacks or seizures◀
Dissociative convulsions

F44.6 **Conversion disorder with** sensory symptom or deficit
▶Conversion disorder with anesthesia or sensory loss
Conversion disorder with special sensory symptoms◀
Dissociative anesthesia and sensory loss
Psychogenic deafness

F44.7 **Conversion disorder with** mixed symptom presentation

✓5ᵗʰ **F44.8** **Other dissociative and conversion disorders**

    F44.81 **Dissociative** identity **disorder**
        Multiple personality disorder

    F44.89 **Other dissociative and conversion disorders**
        Ganser's syndrome
        Psychogenic confusion
        Psychogenic twilight state
        Trance and possession disorders

F44.9 **Dissociative and conversion disorder, unspecified** ▽
Dissociative disorder NOS

✓4ᵗʰ **F45** **Somatoform disorders**
    EXCLUDES 2   dissociative and conversion disorders (F44.-)
            factitious disorders (F68.1-)
            hair-plucking (F63.3)
            lalling (F80.0)
            lisping (F80.0)
            malingering [conscious simulation] (Z76.5)
            nail-biting (F98.8)
            psychological or behavioral factors associated with disorders or
                diseases classified elsewhere (F54)
            sexual dysfunction, not due to a substance or known
                physiological condition (F52.-)
            thumb-sucking (F98.8)
            tic disorders (in childhood and adolescence) (F95.-)
            Tourette's syndrome (F95.2)
            trichotillomania (F63.3)

    F45.0 **Somatization disorder**
        Briquet's disorder
        Multiple psychosomatic disorder

    F45.1 **Undifferentiated somatoform disorder**
        Somatic symptom disorder
        Undifferentiated psychosomatic disorder

✓5ᵗʰ **F45.2** **Hypochondriacal disorders**
        EXCLUDES 2   delusional dysmorphophobia (F22)
                fixed delusions about bodily functions or shape (F22)

    F45.20 **Hypochondriacal disorder, unspecified** ▽

    F45.21 **Hypochondriasis**
        Hypochondriacal neurosis
        Illness anxiety disorder

    F45.22 **Body dysmorphic disorder**
        Dysmorphophobia (nondelusional)
        Nosophobia

    F45.29 **Other hypochondriacal disorders**

✓5ᵗʰ **F45.4** **Pain disorders related to psychological factors**
        EXCLUDES 1   pain NOS (R52)

    F45.41 **Pain disorder exclusively related to psychological factors**
        Somatoform pain disorder (persistent)

    F45.42 **Pain disorder with related psychological factors**
        Code also associated acute or chronic pain (G89.-)

    F45.8 **Other somatoform disorders**
        Psychogenic dysmenorrhea
        Psychogenic dysphagia, including "globus hystericus"
        Psychogenic pruritus
        Psychogenic torticollis
        Somatoform autonomic dysfunction
        Teeth grinding
        EXCLUDES 1   sleep related teeth grinding (G47.63)

    F45.9 **Somatoform disorder, unspecified** ▽
        Psychosomatic disorder NOS

✓4ᵗʰ **F48** **Other nonpsychotic mental disorders**

    F48.1 **Depersonalization-derealization syndrome**

    F48.2 **Pseudobulbar affect**
        Involuntary emotional expression disorder
        Code first underlying cause, if known, such as:
            amyotrophic lateral sclerosis (G12.21)
            multiple sclerosis (G35)
            sequelae of cerebrovascular disease (I69.-)
            sequelae of traumatic intracranial injury (S06.-)

    F48.8 **Other specified nonpsychotic mental disorders**
        Dhat syndrome
        Neurasthenia
        Occupational neurosis, including writer's cramp
        Psychasthenia
        Psychasthenic neurosis
        Psychogenic syncope

    F48.9 **Nonpsychotic mental disorder, unspecified** ▽
        Neurosis NOS

Behavioral syndromes associated with physiological disturbances and physical factors (F50-F59)

✓4ᵗʰ **F50** **Eating disorders**
    EXCLUDES 1   anorexia NOS (R63.0)
            feeding difficulties (R63.3)
            ▶feeding problems of newborn (P92.-)◀
            polyphagia (R63.2)
    EXCLUDES 2   feeding disorder in infancy or childhood (F98.2-)

✓5ᵗʰ **F50.0** **Anorexia nervosa**
        EXCLUDES 1   loss of appetite (R63.0)
                psychogenic loss of appetite (F50.89)

    F50.00 **Anorexia nervosa, unspecified** ▽

    F50.01 **Anorexia nervosa,** restricting type

    F50.02 **Anorexia nervosa,** binge eating/purging type
        EXCLUDES 1   bulimia nervosa (F50.2)

    F50.2 **Bulimia nervosa**
        Bulimia NOS
        Hyperorexia nervosa
        EXCLUDES 1   anorexia nervosa, binge eating/purging type (F50.02)

✓5ᵗʰ **F50.8** **Other eating disorders**
        EXCLUDES 2   pica of infancy and childhood (F98.3)

    F50.81 **Binge eating disorder**

    ● **F50.82** **Avoidant/restrictive food intake disorder**

    F50.89 **Other specified eating disorder**
        Pica in adults
        Psychogenic loss of appetite

    F50.9 **Eating disorder, unspecified** ▽
        Atypical anorexia nervosa
        Atypical bulimia nervosa
        ▶Feeding or eating disorder, unspecified
        Other specified feeding disorder ◀

✓4ᵗʰ **F51** **Sleep disorders not due to a substance or known physiological condition**
    EXCLUDES 2   organic sleep disorders (G47.-)

✓5ᵗʰ **F51.0** **Insomnia** not due to a substance or known physiological condition
        EXCLUDES 2   alcohol related insomnia (F10.182, F10.282, F10.982)
                drug-related insomnia (F11.182, F11.282, F11.982,
                    F13.182, F13.282, F13.982, F14.182, F14.282,
                    F14.982, F15.182, F15.282, F15.982, F19.182,
                    F19.282, F19.982)
                insomnia NOS (G47.0-)
                insomnia due to known physiological condition
                    (G47.0-)
                organic insomnia (G47.0-)
                sleep deprivation (Z72.820)

    F51.01 **Primary insomnia**
        Idiopathic insomnia

    F51.02 **Adjustment insomnia**

    F51.03 **Paradoxical insomnia**

    F51.04 **Psychophysiologic insomnia**

    F51.05 **Insomnia due to other** mental disorder
        Code also associated mental disorder

    F51.09 **Other insomnia not due to a substance or known physiological condition**

☑ Additional Character Req   √x7ᵗʰ Placeholder Alert   Manifestation   HCC CMS-HCC Condition   ▽ Unspecified Code   ▶◀ Revised Text   ● New Code   ▲ Revised Code Title

ICD-10-CM 2018   **543**

✓5ᵗʰ **F51.1 Hypersomnia not due to a substance or known physiological condition**
> EXCLUDES 2   alcohol related hypersomnia (F10.182, F10.282, F10.982)
> drug-related hypersomnia (F11.182, F11.282, F11.982, F13.182, F13.282, F13.982, F14.182, F14.282, F14.982, F15.182, F15.282, F15.982, F19.182, F19.282, F19.982)
> hypersomnia NOS (G47.10)
> hypersomnia due to known physiological condition (G47.10)
> idiopathic hypersomnia (G47.11, G47.12)
> narcolepsy (G47.4-)

F51.11 Primary hypersomnia

F51.12 Insufficient sleep syndrome
> EXCLUDES 1   sleep deprivation (Z72.820)

F51.13 Hypersomnia due to other mental disorder
> Code also associated mental disorder

F51.19 Other hypersomnia not due to a substance or known physiological condition

F51.3 Sleepwalking [somnambulism]
> ▶Non–rapid eye movement sleep arousal disorders, sleepwalking type◀

F51.4 Sleep terrors [night terrors]
> ▶Non–rapid eye movement sleep arousal disorders, sleep terror type◀

F51.5 Nightmare disorder
> Dream anxiety disorder

F51.8 Other sleep disorders not due to a substance or known physiological condition

F51.9 Sleep disorder not due to a substance or known physiological condition, unspecified   ▽
> Emotional sleep disorder NOS

✓4ᵗʰ **F52 Sexual dysfunction not due to a substance or known physiological condition**
> EXCLUDES 2   Dhat syndrome (F48.8)

F52.0 Hypoactive sexual desire disorder
> Lack or loss of sexual desire
> ▶Male hypoactive sexual desire disorder◀
> Sexual anhedonia
> EXCLUDES 1   decreased libido (R68.82)

F52.1 Sexual aversion disorder
> Sexual aversion and lack of sexual enjoyment

✓5ᵗʰ **F52.2 Sexual arousal disorders**
> Failure of genital response

F52.21 Male erectile disorder   ♂
> ▶Erectile disorder◀
> Psychogenic impotence
> EXCLUDES 1   impotence of organic origin (N52.-)
> impotence NOS (N52.-)

F52.22 Female sexual arousal disorder   ♀
> ▶Female sexual interest/arousal disorder◀

✓5ᵗʰ **F52.3 Orgasmic disorder**
> Inhibited orgasm
> Psychogenic anorgasmy

F52.31 Female orgasmic disorder   ♀

F52.32 Male orgasmic disorder   ♂
> Delayed ejaculation

F52.4 Premature ejaculation   ♂

F52.5 Vaginismus not due to a substance or known physiological condition   ♀
> Psychogenic vaginismus
> EXCLUDES 2   vaginismus (due to a known physiological condition) (N94.2)
>
> **DEF:** Psychogenic response resulting in painful contractions of vaginal canal muscles; can be severe enough to prevent sexual intercourse.

F52.6 Dyspareunia not due to a substance or known physiological condition   ♀
> Genito-pelvic pain or penetration disorder
> Psychogenic dyspareunia
> EXCLUDES 2   dyspareunia (due to a known physiological condition) (N94.1-)

F52.8 Other sexual dysfunction not due to a substance or known physiological condition
> Excessive sexual drive
> Nymphomania
> Satyriasis

F52.9 Unspecified sexual dysfunction not due to a substance or known physiological condition   ▽
> Sexual dysfunction NOS

F53 Puerperal psychosis   Ⓜ♀
> Postpartum depression
> EXCLUDES 1   mood disorders with psychotic features (F30.2, F31.2, F31.5, F31.64, F32.3, F33.3)
> postpartum dysphoria (O90.6)
> psychosis in schizophrenia, schizotypal, delusional, and other psychotic disorders (F20-F29)

F54 _Psychological and behavioral factors associated with disorders or diseases classified elsewhere_
> Psychological factors affecting physical conditions
> Code first the associated physical disorder, such as:
> asthma (J45.-)
> dermatitis (L23-L25)
> gastric ulcer (K25.-)
> mucous colitis (K58.-)
> ulcerative colitis (K51.-)
> urticaria (L50.-)
> EXCLUDES 2   tension-type headache (G44.2)

✓4ᵗʰ **F55 Abuse of non-psychoactive substances**
> EXCLUDES 2   abuse of psychoactive substances (F10-F19)

F55.0 Abuse of antacids

F55.1 Abuse of herbal or folk remedies

F55.2 Abuse of laxatives

F55.3 Abuse of steroids or hormones

F55.4 Abuse of vitamins

F55.8 Abuse of other non-psychoactive substances

F59 Unspecified behavioral syndromes associated with physiological disturbances and physical factors   ▽
> Psychogenic physiological dysfunction NOS

Disorders of adult personality and behavior (F60-F69)

✓4ᵗʰ **F60 Specific personality disorders**

F60.0 Paranoid personality disorder
> Expansive paranoid personality (disorder)
> Fanatic personality (disorder)
> Paranoid personality (disorder)
> Querulant personality (disorder)
> Sensitive paranoid personality (disorder)
> EXCLUDES 2   paranoia (F22)
> paranoia querulans (F22)
> paranoid psychosis (F22)
> paranoid schizophrenia (F20.0)
> paranoid state (F22)

F60.1 Schizoid personality disorder
> EXCLUDES 2   Asperger's syndrome (F84.5)
> delusional disorder (F22)
> schizoid disorder of childhood (F84.5)
> schizophrenia (F20.-)
> schizotypal disorder (F21)

F60.2 Antisocial personality disorder
> Amoral personality (disorder)
> Asocial personality (disorder)
> Dissocial personality disorder
> Psychopathic personality (disorder)
> Sociopathic personality (disorder)
> EXCLUDES 1   conduct disorders (F91.-)
> EXCLUDES 2   borderline personality disorder (F60.3)

F60.3 Borderline personality disorder
> Aggressive personality (disorder)
> Emotionally unstable personality disorder
> Explosive personality (disorder)
> EXCLUDES 2   antisocial personality disorder (F60.2)

F60.4 Histrionic personality disorder
> Hysterical personality (disorder)
> Psychoinfantile personality (disorder)

F60.5 Obsessive-compulsive personality disorder
> Anankastic personality (disorder)
> Compulsive personality (disorder)
> Obsessional personality (disorder)
> EXCLUDES 2   obsessive-compulsive disorder (F42-)

F60.6 Avoidant personality disorder
> Anxious personality disorder

F60.7 Dependent personality disorder
> Asthenic personality (disorder)
> Inadequate personality (disorder)
> Passive personality (disorder)

EXCLUDES 1 Not coded here   EXCLUDES 2 Not included here   Ⓝ Newborn Age: 0   Ⓟ Pediatric Age: 0-17   Ⓜ Maternity Age: 12-55   Ⓐ Adult Age: 15-124

544

ICD-10-CM 2018

☑️5ᵗʰ **F60.8 Other specific personality disorders**

    F60.81 Narcissistic personality disorder

    F60.89 Other specific personality disorders
        Eccentric personality disorder
        "Haltlose" type personality disorder
        Immature personality disorder
        Passive-aggressive personality disorder
        Psychoneurotic personality disorder
        Self-defeating personality disorder

F60.9 Personality disorder, unspecified ▽
    Character disorder NOS
    Character neurosis NOS
    Pathological personality NOS

☑️4ᵗʰ **F63 Impulse disorders**
    EXCLUDES 2   habitual excessive use of alcohol or psychoactive substances (F10-F19)
               impulse disorders involving sexual behavior (F65.-)

F63.0 Pathological gambling
    Compulsive gambling
    ▶Gambling disorder◀
    EXCLUDES 1   gambling and betting NOS (Z72.6)
    EXCLUDES 2   excessive gambling by manic patients (F30, F31)
               gambling in antisocial personality disorder (F60.2)

F63.1 Pyromania
    Pathological fire-setting
    EXCLUDES 2   fire-setting (by) (in):
               adult with antisocial personality disorder (F60.2)
               alcohol or psychoactive substance intoxication (F10-F19)
               conduct disorders (F91.-)
               mental disorders due to known physiological condition (F01-F09)
               schizophrenia (F20.-)

F63.2 Kleptomania
    Pathological stealing
    EXCLUDES 1   shoplifting as the reason for observation for suspected mental disorder (Z03.8)
    EXCLUDES 2   depressive disorder with stealing (F31-F33)
               stealing due to underlying mental condition—code to mental condition
               stealing in mental disorders due to known physiological condition (F01-F09)

F63.3 Trichotillomania
    Hair plucking
    EXCLUDES 2   other stereotyped movement disorder (F98.4)

☑️5ᵗʰ **F63.8 Other impulse disorders**
    F63.81 Intermittent explosive disorder
    F63.89 Other impulse disorders

F63.9 Impulse disorder, unspecified ▽
    Impulse control disorder NOS

☑️4ᵗʰ **F64 Gender identity disorders**

F64.0 Transsexualism
    Gender identity disorder in adolescence and adulthood
    Gender dysphoria in adolescents and adults

F64.1 Dual role transvestism
    Use additional code to identify sex reassignment status (Z87.890)
    EXCLUDES 1   gender identity disorder in childhood (F64.2)
    EXCLUDES 2   fetishistic transvestism (F65.1)

F64.2 Gender identity disorder of childhood 🅿
    Gender dysphoria in children
    EXCLUDES 1   gender identity disorder in adolescence and adulthood (F64.0)
    EXCLUDES 2   sexual maturation disorder (F66)

F64.8 Other gender identity disorders
    ▶Other specified gender dysphoria◀

F64.9 Gender identity disorder, unspecified ▽
    ▶Gender dysphoria, unspecified◀
    Gender-role disorder NOS

☑️4ᵗʰ **F65 Paraphilias**

F65.0 Fetishism
    ▶Fetishistic disorder◀

F65.1 Transvestic fetishism
    Fetishistic transvestism
    ▶Transvestic disorder◀

F65.2 Exhibitionism
    ▶Exhibitionistic disorder◀

F65.3 Voyeurism
    ▶Voyeuristic disorder◀

F65.4 Pedophilia
    ▶Pedophilic disorder◀

☑️5ᵗʰ **F65.5 Sadomasochism**

    F65.50 Sadomasochism, unspecified ▽

    F65.51 Sexual masochism
        ▶Sexual masochism disorder◀

    F65.52 Sexual sadism
        ▶Sexual sadism disorder◀

☑️5ᵗʰ **F65.8 Other paraphilias**

    F65.81 Frotteurism
        ▶Frotteuristic disorder◀

    F65.89 Other paraphilias
        Necrophilia
        ▶Other specified paraphilic disorder◀

F65.9 Paraphilia, unspecified ▽
    ▶Paraphilic disorder, unspecified◀
    Sexual deviation NOS

F66 Other sexual disorders
    Sexual maturation disorder
    Sexual relationship disorder

☑️4ᵗʰ **F68 Other disorders of adult personality and behavior**

☑️5ᵗʰ **F68.1 Factitious disorder**
    Compensation neurosis
    Elaboration of physical symptoms for psychological reasons
    Hospital hopper syndrome
    Münchhausen's syndrome
    Peregrinating patient
    EXCLUDES 2   factitial dermatitis (L98.1)
               person feigning illness (with obvious motivation) (Z76.5)

    F68.10 Factitious disorder, unspecified ▽

    F68.11 Factitious disorder with predominantly psychological signs and symptoms

    F68.12 Factitious disorder with predominantly physical signs and symptoms

    F68.13 Factitious disorder with combined psychological and physical signs and symptoms

F68.8 Other specified disorders of adult personality and behavior

F69 Unspecified disorder of adult personality and behavior 🅰▽

Intellectual Disabilities (F70-F79)

Code first any associated physical or developmental disorders
EXCLUDES 1   borderline intellectual functioning, IQ above 70 to 84 (R41.83)

F70 Mild intellectual disabilities
    IQ level 50-55 to approximately 70
    Mild mental subnormality

F71 Moderate intellectual disabilities
    IQ level 35-40 to 50-55
    Moderate mental subnormality

F72 Severe intellectual disabilities
    IQ 20-25 to 35-40
    Severe mental subnormality

F73 Profound intellectual disabilities
    IQ level below 20-25
    Profound mental subnormality

F78 Other intellectual disabilities

F79 Unspecified intellectual disabilities ▽
    Mental deficiency NOS
    Mental subnormality NOS

☑️ Additional Character Req   ✓x7ᵗʰ Placeholder Alert   Manifestation   HCC CMS-HCC Condition   ▽ Unspecified Code   ▶◀ Revised Text   ● New Code   ▲ Revised Code Title

Chapter 5. Mental, Behavioral and Neurodevelopmental Disorders

Pervasive and specific developmental disorders (F80-F89)

✓4ᵗʰ F80   Specific developmental disorders of speech and language

F80.0   Phonological disorder
Dyslalia
Functional speech articulation disorder
Lalling
Lisping
Phonological developmental disorder
Speech articulation developmental disorder
Speech-sound disorder

> *EXCLUDES 1*   speech articulation impairment due to aphasia NOS (R47.01)
>   speech articulation impairment due to apraxia (R48.2)
>
> *EXCLUDES 2*   speech articulation impairment due to hearing loss (F80.4)
>   speech articulation impairment due to intellectual disabilities (F70-F79)
>   speech articulation impairment with expressive language developmental disorder (F80.1)
>   speech articulation impairment with mixed receptive expressive language developmental disorder (F80.2)

F80.1   Expressive language disorder
Developmental dysphasia or aphasia, expressive type

> *EXCLUDES 1*   dysphasia and aphasia NOS (R47.-)
>   mixed receptive-expressive language disorder (F80.2)
>
> *EXCLUDES 2*   acquired aphasia with epilepsy [Landau-Kleffner] (G40.80-)
>   intellectual disabilities (F70-F79)
>   pervasive developmental disorders (F84.-)
>   selective mutism (F94.0)

F80.2   Mixed receptive-expressive language disorder
Developmental dysphasia or aphasia, receptive type
Developmental Wernicke's aphasia

> *EXCLUDES 1*   central auditory processing disorder (H93.25)
>   dysphasia or aphasia NOS (R47.-)
>   expressive language disorder (F80.1)
>   expressive type dysphasia or aphasia (F80.1)
>   word deafness (H93.25)
>
> *EXCLUDES 2*   acquired aphasia with epilepsy [Landau-Kleffner] (G40.80-)
>   intellectual disabilities (F70-F79)
>   pervasive developmental disorders (F84.-)
>   selective mutism (F94.0)

F80.4   Speech and language development delay due to hearing loss
Code also type of hearing loss (H90.-, H91.-)

✓5ᵗʰ F80.8   Other developmental disorders of speech and language
AHA: 2017, 1Q, 27

F80.81   Childhood onset fluency disorder
Cluttering NOS
Stuttering NOS

> *EXCLUDES 1*   adult onset fluency disorder (F98.5)
>   fluency disorder in conditions classified elsewhere (R47.82)
>   fluency disorder (stuttering) following cerebrovascular disease (I69. with final characters-23)

F80.82   Social pragmatic communication disorder

> *EXCLUDES 1*   Asperger's syndrome (F84.5)
>   autistic disorder (F84.0)

F80.89   Other developmental disorders of speech and language

F80.9   Developmental disorder of speech and language, unspecified   ▽
Communication disorder NOS
Language disorder NOS

✓4ᵗʰ F81   Specific developmental disorders of scholastic skills

F81.0   Specific reading disorder
"Backward reading"
Developmental dyslexia
▶Specific learning disorder, with impairment in reading◀
Specific reading retardation

> *EXCLUDES 1*   alexia NOS (R48.0)
>   dyslexia NOS (R48.0)

DEF: Serious impairment of reading skills unexplained in relation to general intelligence and teaching processes.

F81.2   Mathematics disorder
Developmental acalculia
Developmental arithmetical disorder
Developmental Gerstmann's syndrome
▶Specific learning disorder, with impairment in mathmatics◀

> *EXCLUDES 1*   acalculia NOS (R48.8)
>
> *EXCLUDES 2*   arithmetical difficulties associated with a reading disorder (F81.0)
>   arithmetical difficulties associated with a spelling disorder (F81.81)
>   arithmetical difficulties due to inadequate teaching (Z55.8)

✓5ᵗʰ F81.8   Other developmental disorders of scholastic skills

F81.81   Disorder of written expression
▶Specific learning disorder, with impairment in written expression◀
Specific spelling disorder

F81.89   Other developmental disorders of scholastic skills

F81.9   Developmental disorder of scholastic skills, unspecified   ▽
Knowledge acquisition disability NOS
Learning disability NOS
Learning disorder NOS

F82   Specific developmental disorder of motor function
Clumsy child syndrome
Developmental coordination disorder
Developmental dyspraxia

> *EXCLUDES 1*   abnormalities of gait and mobility (R26.-)
>   lack of coordination (R27.-)
>
> *EXCLUDES 2*   lack of coordination secondary to intellectual disabilities (F70-F79)

✓4ᵗʰ F84   Pervasive developmental disorders
Use additional code to identify any associated medical condition and intellectual disabilities

F84.0   Autistic disorder
Autism spectrum disorder
Infantile autism
Infantile psychosis
Kanner's syndrome

> *EXCLUDES 1*   Asperger's syndrome (F84.5)

AHA: 2017, 1Q, 27

F84.2   Rett's syndrome

> *EXCLUDES 1*   Asperger's syndrome (F84.5)
>   Autistic disorder (F84.0)
>   Other childhood disintegrative disorder (F84.3)

F84.3   Other childhood disintegrative disorder   P
Dementia infantilis
Disintegrative psychosis
Heller's syndrome
Symbiotic psychosis
Use additional code to identify any associated neurological condition

> *EXCLUDES 1*   Asperger's syndrome (F84.5)
>   Autistic disorder (F84.0)
>   Rett's syndrome (F84.2)

F84.5   Asperger's syndrome
Asperger's disorder
Autistic psychopathy
Schizoid disorder of childhood

F84.8   Other pervasive developmental disorders
Overactive disorder associated with intellectual disabilities and stereotyped movements

F84.9   Pervasive developmental disorder, unspecified   ▽
Atypical autism

F88   Other disorders of psychological development
Developmental agnosia
Global development delay
Other specified neurodevelopmental disorder

F89   Unspecified disorder of psychological development   ▽
Developmental disorder NOS
Neurodevelopmental disorder NOS

EXCLUDES 1 Not coded here   *EXCLUDES 2* Not included here   N Newborn Age: 0   P Pediatric Age: 0-17   M Maternity Age: 12-55   A Adult Age: 15-124

546   ICD-10-CM 2018

Behavioral and emotional disorders with onset usually occurring in childhood and adolescence (F90-F98)

NOTE   Codes within categories F90-F98 may be used regardless of the age of a patient. These disorders generally have onset within the childhood or adolescent years, but may continue throughout life or not be diagnosed until adulthood.

✓4th **F90 Attention-deficit hyperactivity disorders**

   INCLUDES   attention deficit disorder with hyperactivity
              attention deficit syndrome with hyperactivity

   EXCLUDES 2   *anxiety disorders (F40.-, F41.-)*
              mood [affective] disorders (F30-F39)
              pervasive developmental disorders (F84.-)
              schizophrenia (F20.-)

   F90.0 Attention-deficit hyperactivity disorder, predominantly inattentive type
        ▶Attention-deficit/hyperactivity disorder, predominantly inattentive presentation◀

   F90.1 Attention-deficit hyperactivity disorder, predominantly hyperactive type
        ▶Attention-deficit/hyperactivity disorder, predominantly hyperactive impulsive presentation◀

   F90.2 Attention-deficit hyperactivity disorder, combined type
        ▶Attention-deficit/hyperactivity disorder, combined presentation◀

   F90.8 Attention-deficit hyperactivity disorder, other type

   F90.9 Attention-deficit hyperactivity disorder, unspecified type   ▽
        Attention-deficit hyperactivity disorder of childhood or adolescence NOS
        Attention-deficit hyperactivity disorder NOS

✓4th **F91 Conduct disorders**

   EXCLUDES 1   *antisocial behavior (Z72.81-)*
              antisocial personality disorder (F60.2)

   EXCLUDES 2   *conduct problems associated with attention-deficit hyperactivity disorder (F90.-)*
              mood [affective] disorders (F30-F39)
              pervasive developmental disorders (F84.-)
              schizophrenia (F20.-)

   F91.0 Conduct disorder confined to family context

   F91.1 Conduct disorder, childhood-onset type
        Unsocialized conduct disorder
        Conduct disorder, solitary aggressive type
        Unsocialized aggressive disorder

   F91.2 Conduct disorder, adolescent-onset type
        Socialized conduct disorder
        Conduct disorder, group type

   F91.3 Oppositional defiant disorder

   F91.8 Other conduct disorders
        Other specified conduct disorder
        Other specified disruptive disorder

   F91.9 Conduct disorder, unspecified   ▽
        Behavioral disorder NOS
        Conduct disorder NOS
        Disruptive behavior disorder NOS
        Disruptive disorder NOS

✓4th **F93 Emotional disorders with onset specific to childhood**

   F93.0 Separation anxiety disorder of childhood
       EXCLUDES 2   *mood [affective] disorders (F30-F39)*
                 nonpsychotic mental disorders (F40-F48)
                 phobic anxiety disorder of childhood (F40.8)
                 social phobia (F40.1)

   F93.8 Other childhood emotional disorders
        Identity disorder
       EXCLUDES 2   *gender identity disorder of childhood (F64.2)*

   F93.9 Childhood emotional disorder, unspecified   ▽

✓4th **F94 Disorders of social functioning with onset specific to childhood and adolescence**

   F94.0 Selective mutism
        Elective mutism
       EXCLUDES 2   *pervasive developmental disorders (F84.-)*
                 schizophrenia (F20.-)
                 specific developmental disorders of speech and language (F80.-)
                 transient mutism as part of separation anxiety in young children (F93.0)

   F94.1 Reactive attachment disorder of childhood
        Use additional code to identify any associated failure to thrive or growth retardation
       EXCLUDES 1   *disinhibited attachment disorder of childhood (F94.1)*
                 normal variation in pattern of selective attachment
       EXCLUDES 2   *Asperger's syndrome (F84.5)*
                 maltreatment syndromes (T74.-)
                 sexual or physical abuse in childhood, resulting in psychosocial problems (Z62.81-)

   F94.2 Disinhibited attachment disorder of childhood
        Affectionless psychopathy
        Institutional syndrome
       EXCLUDES 1   *reactive attachment disorder of childhood (F94.1)*
       EXCLUDES 2   *Asperger's syndrome (F84.5)*
                 attention-deficit hyperactivity disorders (F90.-)
                 hospitalism in children (F43.2-)

   F94.8 Other childhood disorders of social functioning

   F94.9 Childhood disorder of social functioning, unspecified   ▽

✓4th **F95 Tic disorder**

   F95.0 Transient tic disorder
        Provisional tic disorder

   F95.1 Chronic motor or vocal tic disorder

   F95.2 Tourette's disorder
        Combined vocal and multiple motor tic disorder [de la Tourette]
        Tourette's syndrome

   F95.8 Other tic disorders

   F95.9 Tic disorder, unspecified   ▽
        Tic NOS

✓4th **F98 Other behavioral and emotional disorders with onset usually occurring in childhood and adolescence**

   EXCLUDES 2   *breath-holding spells (R06.89)*
              gender identity disorder of childhood (F64.2)
              Kleine-Levin syndrome (G47.13)
              obsessive-compulsive disorder (F42-)
              sleep disorders not due to a substance or known physiological condition (F51.-)

   F98.0 Enuresis not due to a substance or known physiological condition
        Enuresis (primary) (secondary) of nonorganic origin
        Functional enuresis
        Psychogenic enuresis
        Urinary incontinence of nonorganic origin
       EXCLUDES 1   *enuresis NOS (R32)*

   F98.1 Encopresis not due to a substance or known physiological condition
        Functional encopresis
        Incontinence of feces of nonorganic origin
        Psychogenic encopresis
        Use additional code to identify the cause of any coexisting constipation
       EXCLUDES 1   *encopresis NOS (R15.-)*

✓5th   **F98.2 Other feeding disorders of infancy and childhood**
       EXCLUDES 1   *feeding difficulties (R63.3)*
       EXCLUDES 2   *anorexia nervosa and other eating disorders (F50.-)*
                 feeding problems of newborn (P92.-)
                 pica of infancy or childhood (F98.3)

     F98.21 Rumination disorder of infancy

     F98.29 Other feeding disorders of infancy and early childhood

   F98.3 Pica of infancy and childhood

   F98.4 Stereotyped movement disorders
        Stereotype/habit disorder
       EXCLUDES 1   *abnormal involuntary movements (R25.-)*
       EXCLUDES 2   *compulsions in obsessive-compulsive disorder (F42-)*
                 hair plucking (F63.3)
                 movement disorders of organic origin (G20-G25)
                 nail-biting (F98.8)
                 nose-picking (F98.8)
                 stereotypies that are part of a broader psychiatric condition (F01-F95)
                 thumb-sucking (F98.8)
                 tic disorders (F95.-)
                 trichotillomania (F63.3)

✓ Additional Character Req   ✓x7th Placeholder Alert   **Manifestation**   **HCC** CMS-HCC Condition   ▽ Unspecified Code   ▶◀ Revised Text   ● New Code   ▲ Revised Code Title

F98.5 Adult onset fluency disorder

EXCLUDES 1   *childhood onset fluency disorder (F80.81)*
         dysphasia (R47.02)
         fluency disorder in conditions classified elsewhere
             (R47.82)
         fluency disorder (stuttering) following cerebrovascular
             disease (I69. with final characters -23)
         tic disorders (F95.-)

F98.8 Other specified behavioral and emotional disorders with onset usually occurring in childhood and adolescence

Excessive masturbation
Nail-biting
Nose-picking
Thumb-sucking

F98.9 Unspecified behavioral and emotional disorders with onset usually occurring in childhood and adolescence   ▽

Unspecified mental disorder (F99)

F99 Mental disorder, not otherwise specified

Mental illness NOS

EXCLUDES 1   *unspecified mental disorder due to known physiological condition (F09)*

Chapter 6. Diseases of the Nervous System (GØØ-G99)

Chapter Specific Guidelines with Coding Examples

The chapter specific guidelines from the ICD-10-CM Official Guidelines for Coding and Reporting have been provided below. Along with these guidelines are coding examples, contained in the shaded boxes, that have been developed to help illustrate the coding and/or sequencing guidance found in these guidelines.

a. Dominant/nondominant side

Codes from category G81, Hemiplegia and hemiparesis, and subcategories G83.1, Monoplegia of lower limb, G83.2, Monoplegia of upper limb, and G83.3, Monoplegia, unspecified, identify whether the dominant or nondominant side is affected. Should the affected side be documented, but not specified as dominant or nondominant, and the classification system does not indicate a default, code selection is as follows:

- For ambidextrous patients, the default should be dominant.
- If the left side is affected, the default is non-dominant.
- If the right side is affected, the default is dominant.

Hemiplegia affecting left side of ambidextrous patient

G81.92   Hemiplegia, unspecified affecting left dominant side

Explanation: Documentation states that the left side is affected and dominant is used for ambidextrous persons.

Right spastic hemiplegia, unknown whether patient is right- or left-handed

G81.11   Spastic hemiplegia affecting right dominant side

Explanation: Since it is unknown whether the patient is right- or left-handed, if the right side is affected, the default is dominant.

---

b. Pain—Category G89

1) General coding information

Codes in category G89, Pain, not elsewhere classified, may be used in conjunction with codes from other categories and chapters to provide more detail about acute or chronic pain and neoplasm-related pain, unless otherwise indicated below.

If the pain is not specified as acute or chronic, post-thoracotomy, postprocedural, or neoplasm-related, do not assign codes from category G89.

A code from category G89 should not be assigned if the underlying (definitive) diagnosis is known, unless the reason for the encounter is pain control/ management and not management of the underlying condition.

When an admission or encounter is for a procedure aimed at treating the underlying condition (e.g., spinal fusion, kyphoplasty), a code for the underlying condition (e.g., vertebral fracture, spinal stenosis) should be assigned as the principal diagnosis. No code from category G89 should be assigned.

Elderly patient with back pain is admitted for outpatient kyphoplasty for age-related osteopathic compression fracture at vertebra T3

M80.08XA   Age-related osteoporosis with current pathological fracture, vertebra(e), initial encounter for fracture

Explanation: No code is assigned for the pain as it is inherent in the underlying condition being treated.

(a) Category G89 codes as principal or first-listed diagnosis

Category G89 codes are acceptable as principal diagnosis or the first-listed code:

- When pain control or pain management is the reason for the admission/encounter (e.g., a patient with displaced intervertebral disc, nerve impingement and severe back pain presents for injection of steroid into the spinal canal). The underlying cause of the pain should be reported as an additional diagnosis, if known.

Patient presents for steroid injection in the right elbow due to chronic pain associated with primary degenerative joint disease.

G89.29   Other chronic pain

M19.021   Primary osteoarthritis, right elbow

Explanation: Since the encounter is for control of pain, not treating the underlying condition, the pain code is sequenced first followed by the underlying condition. The M25 pain code is not necessary as the underlying condition code represents the specific site.

- When a patient is admitted for the insertion of a neurostimulator for pain control, assign the appropriate pain code as the principal or first-listed diagnosis. When an admission or encounter is for a procedure aimed at treating the underlying condition and a neurostimulator is inserted for pain control during the same admission/encounter, a code for the underlying condition should be assigned as the principal diagnosis and the appropriate pain code should be assigned as a secondary diagnosis.

(b) Use of category G89 codes in conjunction with site specific pain codes

(i) Assigning category G89 and site-specific pain codes

Codes from category G89 may be used in conjunction with codes that identify the site of pain (including codes from chapter 18) if the category G89 code provides additional information. For example, if the code describes the site of the pain, but does not fully describe whether the pain is acute or chronic, then both codes should be assigned.

Patient is seen to evaluate chronic right knee pain

M25.561   Pain in right knee

G89.29   Other chronic pain

Explanation: No underlying condition has been determined yet so the pain would be the reason for the visit. The M25 pain code in this instance does not fully describe the condition as it does not represent that the pain is chronic. The G89 chronic pain code is assigned to provide specificity.

(ii) Sequencing of category G89 codes with site-specific pain codes

The sequencing of category G89 codes with site-specific pain codes (including chapter 18 codes), is dependent on the circumstances of the encounter/admission as follows:

- If the encounter is for pain control or pain management, assign the code from category G89 followed by the code identifying the specific site of pain (e.g., encounter for pain management for acute neck pain from trauma is assigned code G89.11, Acute pain due to trauma, followed by code M54.2, Cervicalgia, to identify the site of pain).

Management of acute, traumatic left shoulder pain

G89.11   Acute pain due to trauma

M25.512   Pain in left shoulder

Explanation: The reason for the encounter is to manage or control the pain, not to treat or evaluate an underlying condition. The G89 pain code is assigned as the first-listed diagnosis but in this instance does not fully describe the condition as it does not include the site and laterality. The M25 pain code is added to provide this information.

- If the encounter is for any other reason except pain control or pain management, and a related definitive diagnosis has not been established (confirmed) by the provider, assign the code for the specific site of pain first, followed by the appropriate code from category G89.

Tests are performed to investigate the source of the patient's chronic epigastric abdominal pain

R10.13   **Epigastric pain**

G89.29   **Other chronic pain**

Explanation: In this instance the patient's epigastric pain is not being treated; rather the source of the pain is being investigated. A code from chapter 18 for epigastric pain is sequenced before the additional specificity of the G89 code for the chronic pain.

2) Pain due to devices, implants and grafts

See Section I.C.19. Pain due to medical devices

3) Postoperative Pain

The provider's documentation should be used to guide the coding of postoperative pain, as well as *Section III. Reporting Additional Diagnoses* and *Section IV. Diagnostic Coding and Reporting in the Outpatient Setting*.

The default for post-thoracotomy and other postoperative pain not specified as acute or chronic is the code for the acute form.

Routine or expected postoperative pain immediately after surgery should not be coded.

Pain pump dose is increased for the patient's unexpected, extreme pain post-thoracotomy

G89.12   **Acute post-thoracotomy pain**

Explanation: When acute or chronic is not documented, default to acute. The use of "unexpected, extreme" and the increase of medication dosage indicate that the pain was more than routine or expected.

(a) Postoperative pain not associated with specific postoperative complication

Postoperative pain not associated with a specific postoperative complication is assigned to the appropriate postoperative pain code in category G89.

(b) Postoperative pain associated with specific postoperative complication

Postoperative pain associated with a specific postoperative complication (such as painful wire sutures) is assigned to the appropriate code(s) found in Chapter 19, Injury, poisoning, and certain other consequences of external causes. If appropriate, use additional code(s) from category G89 to identify acute or chronic pain (G89.18 or G89.28).

4) Chronic pain

Chronic pain is classified to subcategory G89.2. There is no time frame defining when pain becomes chronic pain. The provider's documentation should be used to guide use of these codes.

5) Neoplasm related pain

Code G89.3 is assigned to pain documented as being related, associated or due to cancer, primary or secondary malignancy, or tumor. This code is assigned regardless of whether the pain is acute or chronic.

This code may be assigned as the principal or first-listed code when the stated reason for the admission/encounter is documented as pain control/pain management. The underlying neoplasm should be reported as an additional diagnosis.

Patient referred today for pain management due to acute pain related to malignancy of the right breast.

G89.3   **Neoplasm related pain (acute)(chronic)**

C50.911   **Malignant neoplasm of unspecified site of right female breast**

Explanation: Since the encounter was for pain medication management, the pain, rather than the neoplasm, was the reason for the encounter and is sequenced first. This "neoplasm-related pain" code includes both acute and chronic pain.

When the reason for the admission/encounter is management of the neoplasm and the pain associated with the neoplasm is also documented, code G89.3 may be assigned as an additional diagnosis. It is not necessary to assign an additional code for the site of the pain.

See Section I.C.2 for instructions on the sequencing of neoplasms for all other stated reasons for the admission/encounter (except for pain control/pain management).

Patient with lung cancer presents with acute hip pain and is evaluated and found to have iliac bone metastasis

C79.51   **Secondary malignant neoplasm of bone**

C34.90   **Malignant neoplasm of unspecified part of unspecified bronchus or lung**

G89.3   **Neoplasm related pain (acute)(chronic)**

Explanation: The reason for the encounter was the evaluation and diagnosis of the bone metastasis, whose code would be assigned as first-listed, followed by codes for the primary neoplasm and the pain due to the iliac bone metastasis.

6) Chronic pain syndrome

Central pain syndrome (G89.0) and chronic pain syndrome (G89.4) are different than the term "chronic pain," and therefore codes should only be used when the provider has specifically documented this condition.

See Section I.C.5. Pain disorders related to psychological factors

Chapter 6. Diseases of the Nervous System (G00-G99)

EXCLUDES 2   *certain conditions originating in the perinatal period (P04-P96)*
certain infectious and parasitic diseases (A00-B99)
complications of pregnancy, childbirth and the puerperium (O00-O9A)
congenital malformations, deformations, and chromosomal abnormalities (Q00-Q99)
endocrine, nutritional and metabolic diseases (E00-E88)
injury, poisoning and certain other consequences of external causes (S00-T88)
neoplasms (C00-D49)
symptoms, signs and abnormal clinical and laboratory findings, not elsewhere classified (R00-R94)

This chapter contains the following blocks:

G00-G09   Inflammatory diseases of the central nervous system
G10-G14   Systemic atrophies primarily affecting the central nervous system
G20-G26   Extrapyramidal and movement disorders
G30-G32   Other degenerative diseases of the nervous system
G35-G37   Demyelinating diseases of the central nervous system
G40-G47   Episodic and paroxysmal disorders
G50-G59   Nerve, nerve root and plexus disorders
G60-G65   Polyneuropathies and other disorders of the peripheral nervous system
G70-G73   Diseases of myoneural junction and muscle
G80-G83   Cerebral palsy and other paralytic syndromes
G89-G99   Other disorders of the nervous system

Inflammatory diseases of the central nervous system (G00-G09)

☑4ᵗʰ G00 Bacterial meningitis, not elsewhere classified
     INCLUDES   bacterial arachnoiditis
               bacterial leptomeningitis
               bacterial meningitis
               bacterial pachymeningitis
     EXCLUDES 1   ▶*bacterial meningoencephalitis*◀ *(G04.2)*
            ▶*bacterial meningomyelitis*◀ *(G04.2)*

G00.0 Hemophilus meningitis
     Meningitis due to Hemophilus influenzae

G00.1 Pneumococcal meningitis
     Meningtitis due to Streptococcal pneumoniae

G00.2 Streptococcal meningitis
     Use additional code to further identify organism (B95.0-B95.5)

G00.3 Staphylococcal meningitis
     Use additional code to further identify organism (B95.61-B95.8)

G00.8 Other bacterial meningitis
     Meningitis due to Escherichia coli
     Meningitis due to Friedländer's bacillus
     Meningitis due to Klebsiella
     Use additional code to further identify organism (B96.-)

G00.9 Bacterial meningitis, unspecified   ▽
     Meningitis due to gram-negative bacteria, unspecified
     Purulent meningitis NOS
     Pyogenic meningitis NOS
     Suppurative meningitis NOS

G01 *Meningitis in bacterial diseases classified elsewhere*
     Code first underlying disease
     EXCLUDES 1   *meningitis (in):*
            gonococcal (A54.81)
            leptospirosis (A27.81)
            listeriosis (A32.11)
            Lyme disease (A69.21)
            meningococcal (A39.0)
            neurosyphilis (A52.13)
            tuberculosis (A17.0)
         meningoencephalitis and meningomyelitis in bacterial diseases classified elsewhere (G05)

G02 *Meningitis in other infectious and parasitic diseases classified elsewhere*
     Code first underlying disease, such as:
     African trypanosomiasis (B56.-)
     poliovirus infection (A80.-)
     EXCLUDES 1   *candidal meningitis (B37.5)*
            coccidioidomycosis meningitis (B38.4)
            cryptococcal meningitis (B45.1)
            herpesviral [herpes simplex] meningitis (B00.3)
            infectious mononucleosis complicated by meningitis (B27.- with fourth character 2)
            measles complicated by meningitis (B05.1)
            meningoencephalitis and meningomyelitis in other infectious and parasitic diseases classified elsewhere (G05)
            mumps meningitis (B26.1)
            rubella meningitis (B06.02)
            varicella [chickenpox] meningitis (B01.0)
            zoster meningitis (B02.1)

☑4ᵗʰ G03 Meningitis due to other and unspecified causes
     INCLUDES   arachnoiditis NOS
            leptomeningitis NOS
            meningitis NOS
            pachymeningitis NOS
     EXCLUDES 1   *meningoencephalitis (G04.-)*
            meningomyelitis (G04.-)

G03.0 Nonpyogenic meningitis
     Aseptic meningitis
     Nonbacterial meningitis

G03.1 Chronic meningitis

G03.2 Benign recurrent meningitis [Mollaret]

G03.8 Meningitis due to other specified causes

G03.9 Meningitis, unspecified   ▽
     Arachnoiditis (spinal) NOS

☑4ᵗʰ G04 Encephalitis, myelitis and encephalomyelitis
     INCLUDES   acute ascending myelitis
            meningoencephalitis
            meningomyelitis
     EXCLUDES 1   *encephalopathy NOS (G93.40)*
     EXCLUDES 2   *acute transverse myelitis (G37.3-)*
            alcoholic encephalopathy (G31.2)
            benign myalgic encephalomyelitis (G93.3)
            multiple sclerosis (G35)
            subacute necrotizing myelitis (G37.4)
            toxic encephalitis (G92)
            toxic encephalopathy (G92)

☑5ᵗʰ G04.0 Acute disseminated encephalitis and encephalomyelitis (ADEM)
     EXCLUDES 1   *acute necrotizing hemorrhagic encephalopathy (G04.3-)*
            other noninfectious acute disseminated encephalomyelitis (noninfectious ADEM) (G04.81)

     G04.00 Acute disseminated encephalitis and encephalomyelitis, unspecified   ▽

     G04.01 Postinfectious acute disseminated encephalitis and encephalomyelitis (postinfectious ADEM)
         EXCLUDES 1   *post chickenpox encephalitis (B01.1)*
                post measles encephalitis (B05.0)
                post measles myelitis (B05.1)

     G04.02 Postimmunization acute disseminated encephalitis, myelitis and encephalomyelitis
         Encephalitis, postimmunization
         Encephalomyelitis, postimmunization
         Use additional code to identify the vaccine (T50.A-, T50.B-, T50.Z-)

G04.1 Tropical spastic paraplegia   HCC

G04.2 Bacterial meningoencephalitis and meningomyelitis, not elsewhere classified

☑5ᵗʰ G04.3 Acute necrotizing hemorrhagic encephalopathy
     EXCLUDES 1   *acute disseminated encephalitis and encephalomyelitis (G04.0-)*

     G04.30 Acute necrotizing hemorrhagic encephalopathy, unspecified   ▽

     G04.31 Postinfectious acute necrotizing hemorrhagic encephalopathy

     G04.32 Postimmunization acute necrotizing hemorrhagic encephalopathy
         Use additional code to identify the vaccine (T50.A-, T50.B-, T50.Z-)

☑ Additional Character Req   ☑x7ᵗʰ Placeholder Alert   Manifestation   HCC CMS-HCC Condition   ▽ Unspecified Code   ▶◀ Revised Text   ● New Code   ▲ Revised Code Title

G04.39   Other acute necrotizing hemorrhagic encephalopathy
   Code also underlying etiology, if applicable

✓5th **G04.8   Other encephalitis, myelitis and encephalomyelitis**
   Code also any associated seizure (G40.-, R56.9)

G04.81   Other encephalitis and encephalomyelitis
   Noninfectious acute disseminated encephalomyelitis (noninfectious ADEM)

G04.89   Other myelitis   HCC

✓5th **G04.9   Encephalitis, myelitis and encephalomyelitis, unspecified**

G04.90   Encephalitis and encephalomyelitis, unspecified   ▽
   Ventriculitis (cerebral) NOS

G04.91   Myelitis, unspecified   HCC ▽

✓4th **G05   Encephalitis, myelitis and encephalomyelitis in diseases classified elsewhere**
   Code first underlying disease, such as:
      human immunodeficiency virus [HIV] disease (B20)
      poliovirus (A80.-)
      suppurative otitis media (H66.01-H66.4)
      trichinellosis (B75)

   EXCLUDES 1   adenoviral encephalitis, myelitis and encephalomyelitis (A85.1)
      congenital toxoplasmosis encephalitis, myelitis and encephalomyelitis (P37.1)
      cytomegaloviral encephalitis, myelitis and encephalomyelitis (B25.8)
      encephalitis, myelitis and encephalomyelitis (in) measles (B05.0)
      encephalitis, myelitis and encephalomyelitis (in) systemic lupus erythematosus (M32.19)
      enteroviral encephalitis, myelitis and encephalomyelitis (A85.0)
      eosinophilic meningoencephalitis (B83.2)
      herpesviral [herpes simplex] encephalitis, myelitis and encephalomyelitis (B00.4)
      listerial encephalitis, myelitis and encephalomyelitis (A32.12)
      meningococcal encephalitis, myelitis and encephalomyelitis (A39.81)
      mumps encephalitis, myelitis and encephalomyelitis (B26.2)
      postchickenpox encephalitis, myelitis and encephalomyelitis (B01.1-)
      rubella encephalitis, myelitis and encephalomyelitis (B06.01)
      toxoplasmosis encephalitis, myelitis and encephalomyelitis (B58.2)
      zoster encephalitis, myelitis and encephalomyelitis (B02.0)

G05.3   Encephalitis and encephalomyelitis in diseases classified elsewhere
   Meningoencephalitis in diseases classified elsewhere

G05.4   Myelitis in diseases classified elsewhere   HCC
   Meningomyelitis in diseases classified elsewhere

✓4th **G06   Intracranial and intraspinal abscess and granuloma**
   Use additional code (B95-B97) to identify infectious agent

G06.0   Intracranial abscess and granuloma
   Brain [any part] abscess (embolic)
   Cerebellar abscess (embolic)
   Cerebral abscess (embolic)
   Intracranial epidural abscess or granuloma
   Intracranial extradural abscess or granuloma
   Intracranial subdural abscess or granuloma
   Otogenic abscess (embolic)
   EXCLUDES 1   tuberculous intracranial abscess and granuloma (A17.81)

G06.1   Intraspinal abscess and granuloma
   Abscess (embolic) of spinal cord [any part]
   Intraspinal epidural abscess or granuloma
   Intraspinal extradural abscess or granuloma
   Intraspinal subdural abscess or granuloma
   EXCLUDES 1   tuberculous intraspinal abscess and granuloma (A17.81)

G06.2   Extradural and subdural abscess, unspecified   ▽

G07   Intracranial and intraspinal abscess and granuloma in diseases classified elsewhere
   Code first underlying disease, such as:
      schistosomiasis granuloma of brain (B65.-)
   EXCLUDES 1   abscess of brain:
      amebic (A06.6)
      chromomycotic (B43.1)
      gonococcal (A54.82)
      tuberculous (A17.81)
      tuberculoma of meninges (A17.1)

G08   Intracranial and intraspinal phlebitis and thrombophlebitis
   Septic embolism of intracranial or intraspinal venous sinuses and veins
   Septic endophlebitis of intracranial or intraspinal venous sinuses and veins
   Septic phlebitis of intracranial or intraspinal venous sinuses and veins
   Septic thrombophlebitis of intracranial or intraspinal venous sinuses and veins
   Septic thrombosis of intracranial or intraspinal venous sinuses and veins
   EXCLUDES 1   intracranial phlebitis and thrombophlebitis complicating:
      abortion, ectopic or molar pregnancy (O00-O07, O08.7)
      pregnancy, childbirth and the puerperium (O22.5, O87.3)
      nonpyogenic intracranial phlebitis and thrombophlebitis (I67.6)
   EXCLUDES 2   intracranial phlebitis and thrombophlebitis complicating nonpyogenic intraspinal phlebitis and thrombophlebitis (G95.1)
   DEF: Inflammation and formation of blood clot in a vein within the brain or spine, or their linings.

G09   Sequelae of inflammatory diseases of central nervous system
   NOTE   Category G09 is to be used to indicate conditions whose primary classification is to G00-G08 as the cause of sequelae, themselves classifiable elsewhere. The "sequelae" include conditions specified as residuals.
   Code first condition resulting from (sequela) of inflammatory diseases of central nervous system

Systemic atrophies primarily affecting the central nervous system (G10-G14)

G10   Huntington's disease   HCC
   Huntington's chorea
   Huntington's dementia
   ▶Code also dementia in other diseases classified elsewhere without behavioral disturbance (F02.80)◀
   DEF: Genetic disease caused by degeneration of nerve cells in the brain, characterized by chronic progressive mental deterioration; dementia and death within 15 to 20 years of onset.

✓4th **G11   Hereditary ataxia**
   EXCLUDES 2   cerebral palsy (G80.-)
      hereditary and idiopathic neuropathy (G60.-)
      metabolic disorders (E70-E88)

G11.0   Congenital nonprogressive ataxia   HCC

G11.1   Early-onset cerebellar ataxia   HCC
   Early-onset cerebellar ataxia with essential tremor
   Early-onset cerebellar ataxia with myoclonus [Hunt's ataxia]
   Early-onset cerebellar ataxia with retained tendon reflexes
   Friedreich's ataxia (autosomal recessive)
   X-linked recessive spinocerebellar ataxia

G11.2   Late-onset cerebellar ataxia   HCC A

G11.3   Cerebellar ataxia with defective DNA repair   HCC
   Ataxia telangiectasia [Louis-Bar]
   EXCLUDES 2   Cockayne's syndrome (Q87.1)
      other disorders of purine and pyrimidine metabolism (E79.-)
      xeroderma pigmentosum (Q82.1)

G11.4   Hereditary spastic paraplegia   HCC

G11.8   Other hereditary ataxias   HCC

G11.9   Hereditary ataxia, unspecified   HCC ▽
   Hereditary cerebellar ataxia NOS
   Hereditary cerebellar degeneration
   Hereditary cerebellar disease
   Hereditary cerebellar syndrome

✓4th **G12   Spinal muscular atrophy and related syndromes**

G12.0   Infantile spinal muscular atrophy, type I [Werdnig-Hoffman]   HCC

G12.1   Other inherited spinal muscular atrophy   HCC
   Adult form spinal muscular atrophy
   Childhood form, type II spinal muscular atrophy
   Distal spinal muscular atrophy
   Juvenile form, type III spinal muscular atrophy [Kugelberg-Welander]
   Progressive bulbar palsy of childhood [Fazio-Londe]
   Scapuloperoneal form spinal muscular atrophy

✓5th **G12.2   Motor neuron disease**

G12.20   Motor neuron disease, unspecified   HCC ▽

G12.21   Amyotrophic lateral sclerosis   HCC A
   ~~Progressive spinal muscle atrophy~~

G12.22   Progressive bulbar palsy   HCC

● **G12.23   Primary lateral sclerosis**

● **G12.24   Familial motor neuron disease**

● **G12.25   Progressive spinal muscle atrophy**

EXCLUDES 1   Not coded here   EXCLUDES 2   Not included here   N Newborn Age: 0   P Pediatric Age: 0-17   M Maternity Age: 12-55   A Adult Age: 15-124

552   ICD-10-CM 2018

G12.29   **Other motor neuron disease**   HCC
     ~~Familial motor neuron disease~~
     ~~Primary lateral sclerosis~~

G12.8   **Other spinal muscular atrophies and related syndromes**   HCC

G12.9   **Spinal muscular atrophy, unspecified**   HCC ▽

✓4ᵗʰ **G13**   **Systemic atrophies primarily affecting central nervous system in diseases classified elsewhere**

G13.0   *Paraneoplastic neuromyopathy and neuropathy*   HCC
     Carcinomatous neuromyopathy
     Sensorial paraneoplastic neuropathy [Denny Brown]
     Code first underlying neoplasm (C00-D49)

G13.1   *Other systemic atrophy primarily affecting central nervous*   HCC
     system in neoplastic disease
     Paraneoplastic limbic encephalopathy
     Code first underlying neoplasm (C00-D49)

G13.2   *Systemic atrophy primarily affecting the central nervous*
     system in myxedema
     Code first underlying disease, such as:
       hypothyroidism (E03.-)
       myxedematous congenital iodine deficiency (E00.1)

G13.8   *Systemic atrophy primarily affecting central nervous system in*
     other diseases classified elsewhere
     Code first underlying disease

G14   **Postpolio syndrome**
     Postpolio myelitic syndrome
     EXCLUDES 1   *sequelae of poliomyelitis (B91)*

Extrapyramidal and movement disorders (G20-G26)

G20   **Parkinson's disease**   HCC
     Hemiparkinsonism
     Idiopathic Parkinsonism or Parkinson's disease
     Paralysis agitans
     Parkinsonism or Parkinson's disease NOS
     Primary Parkinsonism or Parkinson's disease
     EXCLUDES 1   *dementia with Parkinsonism (G31.83)*
     AHA: 2017, 2Q, 7; 2016, 2Q, 6

✓4ᵗʰ **G21**   **Secondary parkinsonism**
     EXCLUDES 1   *dementia with Parkinsonism (G31.83)*
       Huntington's disease (G10)
       Shy-Drager syndrome (G90.3)
       syphilitic Parkinsonism (A52.19)

G21.0   **Malignant neuroleptic syndrome**
     Use additional code for adverse effect, if applicable, to identify
     drug (T43.3X5, T43.4X5, T43.505, T43.595)
     EXCLUDES 1   *neuroleptic induced parkinsonism (G21.11)*

✓5ᵗʰ G21.1   **Other drug-induced secondary parkinsonism**

     G21.11   **Neuroleptic induced parkinsonism**   HCC
       Use additional code for adverse effect, if applicable, to
       identify drug (T43.3X5, T43.4X5, T43.505,
       T43.595)
       EXCLUDES 1   *malignant neuroleptic syndrome (G21.0)*

     G21.19   **Other drug induced secondary parkinsonism**   HCC
       ►Other medication-induced parkinsonism◄
       Use additional code for adverse effect, if applicable, to
       identify drug (T36-T50 with fifth or sixth
       character 5)

G21.2   **Secondary parkinsonism due to other external agents**   HCC
     Code first (T51-T65) to identify external agent

G21.3   **Postencephalitic parkinsonism**   HCC

G21.4   **Vascular parkinsonism**   HCC

G21.8   **Other secondary parkinsonism**   HCC

G21.9   **Secondary parkinsonism, unspecified**   HCC ▽

✓4ᵗʰ **G23**   **Other degenerative diseases of basal ganglia**
     EXCLUDES 2   *multi-system degeneration of the autonomic nervous system*
       (G90.3)

G23.0   **Hallervorden-Spatz disease**   HCC
     Pigmentary pallidal degeneration

G23.1   **Progressive supranuclear ophthalmoplegia**
     [Steele-Richardson-Olszewski]
     Progressive supranuclear palsy

G23.2   **Striatonigral degeneration**   HCC

G23.8   **Other specified degenerative diseases of basal ganglia**   HCC
     Calcification of basal ganglia

G23.9   **Degenerative disease of basal ganglia, unspecified**   HCC ▽

✓4ᵗʰ **G24**   **Dystonia**
     INCLUDES   dyskinesia
     EXCLUDES 2   *athetoid cerebral palsy (G80.3)*

✓5ᵗʰ G24.0   **Drug induced dystonia**
     Use additional code for adverse effect, if applicable, to identify
     drug (T36-T50 with fifth or sixth character5)

     G24.01   **Drug induced subacute dyskinesia**
       Drug induced blepharospasm
       Drug induced orofacial dyskinesia
       Neuroleptic induced tardive dyskinesia
       Tardive dyskinesia

     G24.02   **Drug induced acute dystonia**
       Acute dystonic reaction to drugs
       Neuroleptic induced acute dystonia

     G24.09   **Other drug induced dystonia**

G24.1   **Genetic torsion dystonia**
     Dystonia deformans progressiva
     Dystonia musculorum deformans
     Familial torsion dystonia
     Idiopathic familial dystonia
     Idiopathic (torsion) dystonia NOS
     (Schwalbe-) Ziehen-Oppenheim disease

G24.2   **Idiopathic nonfamilial dystonia**

G24.3   **Spasmodic torticollis**
     EXCLUDES 1   *congenital torticollis (Q68.0)*
       hysterical torticollis (F44.4)
       ocular torticollis (R29.891)
       psychogenic torticollis (F45.8)
       torticollis NOS (M43.6)
       traumatic recurrent torticollis (S13.4)

G24.4   **Idiopathic orofacial dystonia**
     Orofacial dyskinesia
     EXCLUDES 1   *drug induced orofacial dyskinesia (G24.01)*

G24.5   **Blepharospasm**
     EXCLUDES 1   *drug induced blepharospasm (G24.01)*

G24.8   **Other dystonia**
     Acquired torsion dystonia NOS

G24.9   **Dystonia, unspecified**   ▽
     Dyskinesia NOS

✓4ᵗʰ **G25**   **Other extrapyramidal and movement disorders**
     EXCLUDES 2   *sleep related movement disorders (G47.6-)*

G25.0   **Essential tremor**
     Familial tremor
     EXCLUDES 1   *tremor NOS (R25.1)*

G25.1   **Drug-induced tremor**
     Use additional code for adverse effect, if applicable, to identify
     drug (T36-T50 with fifth or sixth character 5)

G25.2   **Other specified forms of tremor**
     Intention tremor

G25.3   **Myoclonus**
     Drug-induced myoclonus
     Palatal myoclonus
     Use additional code for adverse effect, if applicable, to identify
     drug (T36-T50 with fifth or sixth character 5)
     EXCLUDES 1   *facial myokymia (G51.4)*
       myoclonic epilepsy (G40.-)

G25.4   **Drug-induced chorea**
     Use additional code for adverse effect, if applicable, to identify
     drug (T36-T50 with fifth or sixth character 5)

G25.5   **Other chorea**
     Chorea NOS
     EXCLUDES 1   *chorea NOS with heart involvement (I02.0)*
       Huntington's chorea (G10)
       rheumatic chorea (I02.-)
       Sydenham's chorea (I02.-)

✓5ᵗʰ G25.6   **Drug induced tics and other tics of organic origin**

     G25.61   **Drug induced tics**
       Use additional code for adverse effect, if applicable, to
       identify drug (T36-T50 with fifth or sixth
       character 5)

     G25.69   **Other tics of organic origin**
       EXCLUDES 1   *habit spasm (F95.9)*
       tic NOS (F95.9)
       Tourette's syndrome (F95.2)

✓5ᵗʰ G25.7   **Other and unspecified drug induced movement disorders**
     Use additional code for adverse effect, if applicable, to identify
     drug (T36-T50 with fifth or sixth character 5)

     G25.70   **Drug induced movement disorder, unspecified**   ▽

☑ Additional Character Req   ✓x7ᵗʰ Placeholder Alert   Manifestation   HCC CMS-HCC Condition   ▽ Unspecified Code   ►◄ Revised Text   ● New Code   ▲ Revised Code Title

G25.71 Drug induced akathisia
Drug induced acathisia
Neuroleptic induced acute akathisia
►Tardive akathisia◄

G25.79 Other drug induced movement disorders

✓5ᵗʰ **G25.8 Other specified extrapyramidal and movement disorders**

G25.81 Restless legs syndrome
DEF: Neurological disorder of unknown etiology creating an irresistible urge to move the legs, which may temporarily relieve the symptoms; is accompanied by motor restlessness and sensations of pain, burning, prickling, or tingling.

G25.82 Stiff-man syndrome

G25.83 Benign shuddering attacks

G25.89 Other specified extrapyramidal and movement disorders

G25.9 Extrapyramidal and movement disorder, unspecified   ▽

G26 Extrapyramidal and movement disorders in diseases classified elsewhere
Code first underlying disease

Other degenerative diseases of the nervous system (G30-G32)

✓4ᵗʰ **G30 Alzheimer's disease**
INCLUDES Alzheimer's dementia senile and presenile forms
Use additional code to identify:
delirium, if applicable (F05)
dementia with behavioral disturbance (F02.81)
dementia without behavioral disturbance (F02.80)
EXCLUDES 1 senile degeneration of brain NEC (G31.1)
senile dementia NOS (F03)
senility NOS (R41.81)
AHA: 2017, 1Q, 43

G30.0 Alzheimer's disease with early onset

G30.1 Alzheimer's disease with late onset   Ⓐ

G30.8 Other Alzheimer's disease

G30.9 Alzheimer's disease, unspecified   ▽
AHA: 2016, 2Q, 6; 2012, 4Q, 95

✓4ᵗʰ **G31 Other degenerative diseases of nervous system, not elsewhere classified**
Use additional code to identify:
dementia with behavioral disturbance (F02.81)
dementia without behavioral disturbance (F02.80)
EXCLUDES 2 Reye's syndrome (G93.7)

✓5ᵗʰ **G31.0 Frontotemporal dementia**

G31.01 Pick's disease
Primary progressive aphasia
Progressive isolated aphasia
DEF: A progressive frontotemporal dementia with asymmetrical atrophy of the frontal and temporal regions of the cerebral cortex, abnormal rounded brain cells called Pick cells with the presence of abnormal staining of protein (called tau); symptoms include prominent apathy, behavioral changes such as disinhibition and restlessness, echolalia, impairment of language, memory, and intellect, increased carelessness, poor personal hygiene, and decreased attention span.

G31.09 Other frontotemporal dementia
Frontal dementia

G31.1 Senile degeneration of brain, not elsewhere classified
EXCLUDES 1 Alzheimer's disease (G30.-)
senility NOS (R41.81)

G31.2 Degeneration of nervous system due to alcohol
Alcoholic cerebellar ataxia
Alcoholic cerebellar degeneration
Alcoholic cerebral degeneration
Alcoholic encephalopathy
Dysfunction of the autonomic nervous system due to alcohol
Code also associated alcoholism (F10.-)

✓5ᵗʰ **G31.8 Other specified degenerative diseases of nervous system**

G31.81 Alpers disease
Grey-matter degeneration

G31.82 Leigh's disease
Subacute necrotizing encephalopathy

G31.83 Dementia with Lewy bodies
Dementia with Parkinsonism
Lewy body dementia
Lewy body disease
AHA: 2017, 2Q, 7; 2016, 4Q, 141
DEF: A cerebral dementia with neurophysiologic changes, increased hippocampal volume, hypoperfusion in the occipital lobes, beta amyloid deposits with neurofibrillary tangles, and atrophy of cortex and brainstem. Hallmark neuropsychological characteristics include fluctuating cognition with pronounced variation in attention and alertness; recurrent hallucinations; and Parkinsonism.

G31.84 Mild cognitive impairment, so stated
►Mild neurocognitive disorder◄
EXCLUDES 1 age related cognitive decline (R41.81)
altered mental status (R41.82)
cerebral degeneration (G31.9)
change in mental status (R41.82)
cognitive deficits following (sequelae of) cerebral hemorrhage or infarction (I69.01-, I69.11-, I69.21-, I69.31-, I69.81-, I69.91-)
cognitive impairment due to intracranial or head injury (S06.-)
dementia (F01.-, F02.-, F03)
mild memory disturbance (F06.8)
neurologic neglect syndrome (R41.4)
personality change, nonpsychotic (F68.8)

G31.85 Corticobasal degeneration

G31.89 Other specified degenerative diseases of nervous system

G31.9 Degenerative disease of nervous system, unspecified   ▽

✓4ᵗʰ **G32 Other degenerative disorders of nervous system in diseases classified elsewhere**

G32.0 Subacute combined degeneration of spinal cord in diseases HCC **classified elsewhere**
Dana-Putnam syndrome
Sclerosis of spinal cord (combined) (dorsolateral) (posterolateral)
Code first underlying disease, such as:
vitamin B12 deficiency (E53.8)
vitamin B12 deficiency:
anemia (D51.9)
dietary (D51.3)
pernicious (D51.0)
EXCLUDES 1 syphilitic combined degeneration of spinal cord (A52.11)

✓5ᵗʰ **G32.8 Other specified degenerative disorders of nervous system in diseases classified elsewhere**
Code first underlying disease, such as:
amyloidosis cerebral degeneration (E85.-)
cerebral degeneration (due to) hypothyroidism (E00.0-E03.9)
cerebral degeneration (due to) neoplasm (C00-D49)
cerebral degeneration (due to) vitamin B deficiency, except thiamine (E52-E53.-)
EXCLUDES 1 superior hemorrhagic polioencephalitis [Wernicke's encephalopathy] (E51.2)

G32.81 Cerebellar ataxia in diseases classified elsewhere HCC
Code first underlying disease, such as:
celiac disease (with gluten ataxia) (K90.0)
cerebellar ataxia (in) neoplastic disease (paraneoplastic cerebellar degeneration) (C00-D49)
non-celiac gluten ataxia (M35.9)
EXCLUDES 1 systemic atrophy primarily affecting the central nervous system in alcoholic cerebellar ataxia (G31.2)
systemic atrophy primarily affecting the central nervous system in myxedema (G13.2)

G32.89 Other specified degenerative disorders of nervous system in diseases classified elsewhere
Degenerative encephalopathy in diseases classified elsewhere

Demyelinating diseases of the central nervous system (G35-G37)

G35 Multiple sclerosis   HCC
Disseminated multiple sclerosis
Generalized multiple sclerosis
Multiple sclerosis NOS
Multiple sclerosis of brain stem
Multiple sclerosis of cord

EXCLUDES 1 Not coded here   EXCLUDES 2 Not included here   Ⓝ Newborn Age: 0   Ⓟ Pediatric Age: 0-17   Ⓜ Maternity Age: 12-55   Ⓐ Adult Age: 15-124

554   ICD-10-CM 2018

G36 Other acute disseminated demyelination
> **EXCLUDES 1** *postinfectious encephalitis and encephalomyelitis NOS (G04.01)*

G36.0 Neuromyelitis optica [Devic]   HCC
> Demyelination in optic neuritis
> **EXCLUDES 1** *optic neuritis NOS (H46)*

G36.1 Acute and subacute hemorrhagic leukoencephalitis [Hurst]   HCC

G36.8 Other specified acute disseminated demyelination   HCC

G36.9 Acute disseminated demyelination, unspecified   HCC ▽

G37 Other demyelinating diseases of central nervous system

G37.0 Diffuse sclerosis of central nervous system   HCC
> Periaxial encephalitis
> Schilder's disease
> **EXCLUDES 1** *X linked adrenoleukodystrophy (E71.52-)*

G37.1 Central demyelination of corpus callosum   HCC

G37.2 Central pontine myelinolysis   HCC

G37.3 Acute transverse myelitis in demyelinating disease of central nervous system   HCC
> Acute transverse myelitis NOS
> Acute transverse myelopathy
> **EXCLUDES 1** *multiple sclerosis (G35)*
> *neuromyelitis optica [Devic] (G36.0)*

G37.4 Subacute necrotizing myelitis of central nervous system   HCC

G37.5 Concentric sclerosis [Balo] of central nervous system   HCC

G37.8 Other specified demyelinating diseases of central nervous system   HCC

G37.9 Demyelinating disease of central nervous system, unspecified   HCC ▽

Episodic and paroxysmal disorders (G40-G47)

G40 Epilepsy and recurrent seizures
> **NOTE** The following terms are to be considered equivalent to intractable: pharmacoresistant (pharmacologically resistant), treatment resistant, refractory (medically) and poorly controlled
> **EXCLUDES 1** *conversion disorder with seizures (F44.5)*
> *convulsions NOS (R56.9)*
> *post traumatic seizures (R56.1)*
> *seizure (convulsive) NOS (R56.9)*
> *seizure of newborn (P90)*
> **EXCLUDES 2** *hippocampal sclerosis (G93.81)*
> *mesial temporal sclerosis (G93.81)*
> *temporal sclerosis (G93.81)*
> *Todd's paralysis (G83.84)*

G40.0 Localization-related (focal) (partial) idiopathic epilepsy and epileptic syndromes with seizures of localized onset
> Benign childhood epilepsy with centrotemporal EEG spikes
> Childhood epilepsy with occipital EEG paroxysms
> **EXCLUDES 1** *adult onset localization-related epilepsy (G40.1-, G40.2-)*

G40.00 Localization-related (focal) (partial) idiopathic epilepsy and epileptic syndromes with seizures of localized onset, not intractable
> Localization-related (focal) (partial) idiopathic epilepsy and epileptic syndromes with seizures of localized onset without intractability

G40.001 Localization-related (focal) (partial) idiopathic epilepsy and epileptic syndromes with seizures of localized onset, not intractable, with status epilepticus   HCC

G40.009 Localization-related (focal) (partial) idiopathic epilepsy and epileptic syndromes with seizures of localized onset, not intractable, without status epilepticus   HCC
> Localization-related (focal) (partial) idiopathic epilepsy and epileptic syndromes with seizures of localized onset NOS

G40.01 Localization-related (focal) (partial) idiopathic epilepsy and epileptic syndromes with seizures of localized onset, intractable

G40.011 Localization-related (focal) (partial) idiopathic epilepsy and epileptic syndromes with seizures of localized onset, intractable, with status epilepticus   HCC

G40.019 Localization-related (focal) (partial) idiopathic epilepsy and epileptic syndromes with seizures of localized onset, intractable, without status epilepticus   HCC

G40.1 Localization-related (focal) (partial) symptomatic epilepsy and epileptic syndromes with simple partial seizures
> Attacks without alteration of consciousness
> Epilepsia partialis continua [Kozhevnikof]
> Simple partial seizures developing into secondarily generalized seizures

G40.10 Localization-related (focal) (partial) symptomatic epilepsy and epileptic syndromes with simple partial seizures, not intractable
> Localization-related (focal) (partial) symptomatic epilepsy and epileptic syndromes with simple partial seizures without intractability

G40.101 Localization-related (focal) (partial) symptomatic epilepsy and epileptic syndromes with simple partial seizures, not intractable, with status epilepticus   HCC

G40.109 Localization-related (focal) (partial) symptomatic epilepsy and epileptic syndromes with simple partial seizures, not intractable, without status epilepticus   HCC
> Localization-related (focal) (partial) symptomatic epilepsy and epileptic syndromes with simple partial seizures NOS

G40.11 Localization-related (focal) (partial) symptomatic epilepsy and epileptic syndromes with simple partial seizures, intractable

G40.111 Localization-related (focal) (partial) symptomatic epilepsy and epileptic syndromes with simple partial seizures, intractable, with status epilepticus   HCC

G40.119 Localization-related (focal) (partial) symptomatic epilepsy and epileptic syndromes with simple partial seizures, intractable, without status epilepticus   HCC

G40.2 Localization-related (focal) (partial) symptomatic epilepsy and epileptic syndromes with complex partial seizures
> Attacks with alteration of consciousness, often with automatisms
> Complex partial seizures developing into secondarily generalized seizures

G40.20 Localization-related (focal) (partial) symptomatic epilepsy and epileptic syndromes with complex partial seizures, not intractable
> Localization-related (focal) (partial) symptomatic epilepsy and epileptic syndromes with complex partial seizures without intractability

G40.201 Localization-related (focal) (partial) symptomatic epilepsy and epileptic syndromes with complex partial seizures, not intractable, with status epilepticus   HCC

G40.209 Localization-related (focal) (partial) symptomatic epilepsy and epileptic syndromes with complex partial seizures, not intractable, without status epilepticus   HCC
> Localization-related (focal) (partial) symptomatic epilepsy and epileptic syndromes with complex partial seizures NOS

G40.21 Localization-related (focal) (partial) symptomatic epilepsy and epileptic syndromes with complex partial seizures, intractable

G40.211 Localization-related (focal) (partial) symptomatic epilepsy and epileptic syndromes with complex partial seizures, intractable, with status epilepticus   HCC

G40.219 Localization-related (focal) (partial) symptomatic epilepsy and epileptic syndromes with complex partial seizures, intractable, without status epilepticus   HCC

G40.3 Generalized idiopathic epilepsy and epileptic syndromes
> Code also MERRF syndrome, if applicable (E88.42)

G40.30 Generalized idiopathic epilepsy and epileptic syndromes, not intractable
> Generalized idiopathic epilepsy and epileptic syndromes without intractability

---

☑ Additional Character Req   ☑x7ᵗʰ Placeholder Alert   Manifestation   HCC CMS-HCC Condition   ▽ Unspecified Code   ►◄ Revised Text   ● New Code   ▲ Revised Code Title

G40.301   Generalized idiopathic epilepsy and epileptic syndromes, not intractable, with status epilepticus   HCC

G40.309   Generalized idiopathic epilepsy and epileptic syndromes, not intractable, without status epilepticus   HCC
    Generalized idiopathic epilepsy and epileptic syndromes NOS

✓6th **G40.31**   Generalized idiopathic epilepsy and epileptic syndromes, intractable

G40.311   Generalized idiopathic epilepsy and epileptic syndromes, intractable, with status epilepticus   HCC

G40.319   Generalized idiopathic epilepsy and epileptic syndromes, intractable, without status epilepticus   HCC

✓5th **G40.A**   Absence epileptic syndrome
    Childhood absence epilepsy [pyknolepsy]
    Juvenile absence epilepsy
    Absence epileptic syndrome, NOS

✓6th **G40.A0**   Absence epileptic syndrome, not intractable

G40.A01   Absence epileptic syndrome, not intractable, with status epilepticus   HCC

G40.A09   Absence epileptic syndrome, not intractable, without status epilepticus   HCC

✓6th **G40.A1**   Absence epileptic syndrome, intractable

G40.A11   Absence epileptic syndrome, intractable, with status epilepticus   HCC

G40.A19   Absence epileptic syndrome, intractable, without status epilepticus   HCC

✓5th **G40.B**   Juvenile myoclonic epilepsy [impulsive petit mal]

✓6th **G40.B0**   Juvenile myoclonic epilepsy, not intractable

G40.B01   Juvenile myoclonic epilepsy, not intractable, with status epilepticus   HCC

G40.B09   Juvenile myoclonic epilepsy, not intractable, without status epilepticus   HCC

✓6th **G40.B1**   Juvenile myoclonic epilepsy, intractable

G40.B11   Juvenile myoclonic epilepsy, intractable, with status epilepticus   HCC

G40.B19   Juvenile myoclonic epilepsy, intractable, without status epilepticus   HCC

✓5th **G40.4**   Other generalized epilepsy and epileptic syndromes
    Epilepsy with grand mal seizures on awakening
    Epilepsy with myoclonic absences
    Epilepsy with myoclonic-astatic seizures
    Grand mal seizure NOS
    Nonspecific atonic epileptic seizures
    Nonspecific clonic epileptic seizures
    Nonspecific myoclonic epileptic seizures
    Nonspecific tonic epileptic seizures
    Nonspecific tonic-clonic epileptic seizures
    Symptomatic early myoclonic encephalopathy

✓6th **G40.40**   Other generalized epilepsy and epileptic syndromes, not intractable
    Other generalized epilepsy and epileptic syndromes without intractability
    Other generalized epilepsy and epileptic syndromes NOS

G40.401   Other generalized epilepsy and epileptic syndromes, not intractable, with status epilepticus   HCC

G40.409   Other generalized epilepsy and epileptic syndromes, not intractable, without status epilepticus   HCC

✓6th **G40.41**   Other generalized epilepsy and epileptic syndromes, intractable

G40.411   Other generalized epilepsy and epileptic syndromes, intractable, with status epilepticus   HCC

G40.419   Other generalized epilepsy and epileptic syndromes, intractable, without status epilepticus   HCC

✓5th **G40.5**   Epileptic seizures related to external causes
    Epileptic seizures related to alcohol
    Epileptic seizures related to drugs
    Epileptic seizures related to hormonal changes
    Epileptic seizures related to sleep deprivation
    Epileptic seizures related to stress
    Code also, if applicable, associated epilepsy and recurrent seizures (G40.-)
    Use additional code for adverse effect, if applicable, to identify drug (T36-T50 with fifth or sixth character 5)

✓6th **G40.50**   Epileptic seizures related to external causes, not intractable

G40.501   Epileptic seizures related to external causes, not intractable, with status epilepticus   HCC

G40.509   Epileptic seizures related to external causes, not intractable, without status epilepticus   HCC
    Epileptic seizures related to external causes, NOS

✓5th **G40.8**   Other epilepsy and recurrent seizures
    Epilepsies and epileptic syndromes undetermined as to whether they are focal or generalized
    Landau-Kleffner syndrome

✓6th **G40.80**   Other epilepsy

G40.801   Other epilepsy, not intractable, with status epilepticus   HCC
    Other epilepsy without intractability with status epilepticus

G40.802   Other epilepsy, not intractable, without status epilepticus   HCC
    Other epilepsy NOS
    Other epilepsy without intractability without status epilepticus

G40.803   Other epilepsy, intractable, with status epilepticus   HCC

G40.804   Other epilepsy, intractable, without status epilepticus   HCC

✓6th **G40.81**   Lennox-Gastaut syndrome

G40.811   Lennox-Gastaut syndrome, not intractable, with status epilepticus   HCC

G40.812   Lennox-Gastaut syndrome, not intractable, without status epilepticus   HCC

G40.813   Lennox-Gastaut syndrome, intractable, with status epilepticus   HCC

G40.814   Lennox-Gastaut syndrome, intractable, without status epilepticus   HCC

✓6th **G40.82**   Epileptic spasms
    Infantile spasms
    Salaam attacks
    West's syndrome

G40.821   Epileptic spasms, not intractable, with status epilepticus   HCC

G40.822   Epileptic spasms, not intractable, without status epilepticus   HCC

G40.823   Epileptic spasms, intractable, with status epilepticus   HCC

G40.824   Epileptic spasms, intractable, without status epilepticus   HCC

G40.89   Other seizures   HCC
    EXCLUDES 1   post traumatic seizures (R56.1)
                recurrent seizures NOS (G40.909)
                seizure NOS (R56.9)

✓5th **G40.9**   Epilepsy, unspecified

✓6th **G40.90**   Epilepsy, unspecified, not intractable
    Epilepsy, unspecified, without intractability

G40.901   Epilepsy, unspecified, not intractable, with status epilepticus   HCC ▽

G40.909   Epilepsy, unspecified, not intractable, without status epilepticus   HCC ▽
    Epilepsy NOS
    Epileptic convulsions NOS
    Epileptic fits NOS
    Epileptic seizures NOS
    Recurrent seizures NOS
    Seizure disorder NOS

EXCLUDES 1 Not coded here   EXCLUDES 2 Not included here   N Newborn Age: 0   P Pediatric Age: 0-17   M Maternity Age: 12-55   A Adult Age: 15-124

556   ICD-10-CM 2018

✓6ᵗʰ **G40.91** **Epilepsy, unspecified,** intractable
         Intractable seizure disorder NOS

     G40.911 **Epilepsy, unspecified, intractable,** HCC ▽
             with status epilepticus

     G40.919 **Epilepsy, unspecified, intractable,** HCC ▽
             without status epilepticus

✓4ᵗʰ **G43** **Migraine**
   NOTE   The following terms are to be considered equivalent to intractable: pharmacoresistant (pharmacologically resistant), treatment resistant, refractory (medically) and poorly controlled.
   Use additional code for adverse effect, if applicable, to identify drug (T36-T50 with fifth or sixth character 5)
   EXCLUDES 1   headache NOS (R51)
                 lower half migraine (G44.00)
   EXCLUDES 2   headache syndromes (G44.-)

✓5ᵗʰ **G43.0** **Migraine** without aura
     Common migraine
     EXCLUDES 1   chronic migraine without aura (G43.7-)

   ✓6ᵗʰ **G43.00** **Migraine without aura,** not intractable
       Migraine without aura without mention of refractory migraine

     G43.001 **Migraine without aura, not intractable, with status migrainosus**

     G43.009 **Migraine without aura, not intractable, without status migrainosus**
         Migraine without aura NOS

   ✓6ᵗʰ **G43.01** **Migraine without aura,** intractable
       Migraine without aura with refractory migraine

     G43.011 **Migraine without aura, intractable, with status migrainosus**

     G43.019 **Migraine without aura, intractable, without status migrainosus**

✓5ᵗʰ **G43.1** **Migraine** with aura
     Basilar migraine
     Classical migraine
     Migraine equivalents
     Migraine preceded or accompanied by transient focal neurological phenomena
     Migraine triggered seizures
     Migraine with acute-onset aura
     Migraine with aura without headache (migraine equivalents)
     Migraine with prolonged aura
     Migraine with typical aura
     Retinal migraine
     Code also any associated seizure (G40.-, R56.9)
     EXCLUDES 1   persistent migraine aura (G43.5-, G43.6-)

   ✓6ᵗʰ **G43.10** **Migraine with aura,** not intractable
       Migraine with aura without mention of refractory migraine

     G43.101 **Migraine with aura, not intractable, with status migrainosus**

     G43.109 **Migraine with aura, not intractable, without status migrainosus**
         Migraine with aura NOS

   ✓6ᵗʰ **G43.11** **Migraine with aura,** intractable
       Migraine with aura with refractory migraine

     G43.111 **Migraine with aura, intractable, with status migrainosus**

     G43.119 **Migraine with aura, intractable, without status migrainosus**

✓5ᵗʰ **G43.4** **Hemiplegic migraine**
     Familial migraine
     Sporadic migraine

   ✓6ᵗʰ **G43.40** **Hemiplegic migraine,** not intractable
       Hemiplegic migraine without refractory migraine

     G43.401 **Hemiplegic migraine, not intractable, with status migrainosus**

     G43.409 **Hemiplegic migraine, not intractable, without status migrainosus**
         Hemiplegic migraine NOS

   ✓6ᵗʰ **G43.41** **Hemiplegic migraine,** intractable
       Hemiplegic migraine with refractory migraine

     G43.411 **Hemiplegic migraine, intractable, with status migrainosus**

     G43.419 **Hemiplegic migraine, intractable, without status migrainosus**

✓5ᵗʰ **G43.5** Persistent **migraine** aura without cerebral infarction

   ✓6ᵗʰ **G43.50** **Persistent migraine aura without cerebral infarction,** not intractable
       Persistent migraine aura without cerebral infarction, without refractory migraine

     G43.501 **Persistent migraine aura without cerebral infarction, not intractable, with status migrainosus**

     G43.509 **Persistent migraine aura without cerebral infarction, not intractable, without status migrainosus**
         Persistent migraine aura NOS

   ✓6ᵗʰ **G43.51** **Persistent migraine aura without cerebral infarction,** intractable
       Persistent migraine aura without cerebral infarction, with refractory migraine

     G43.511 **Persistent migraine aura without cerebral infarction, intractable, with status migrainosus**

     G43.519 **Persistent migraine aura without cerebral infarction, intractable, without status migrainosus**

✓5ᵗʰ **G43.6** Persistent **migraine** aura with cerebral infarction
     Code also the type of cerebral infarction (I63.-)

   ✓6ᵗʰ **G43.60** **Persistent migraine aura with cerebral infarction,** not intractable
       Persistent migraine aura with cerebral infarction, without refractory migraine

     G43.601 **Persistent migraine aura with cerebral infarction, not intractable, with status migrainosus**

     G43.609 **Persistent migraine aura with cerebral infarction, not intractable, without status migrainosus**

   ✓6ᵗʰ **G43.61** **Persistent migraine aura with cerebral infarction,** intractable
       Persistent migraine aura with cerebral infarction, with refractory migraine

     G43.611 **Persistent migraine aura with cerebral infarction, intractable, with status migrainosus**

     G43.619 **Persistent migraine aura with cerebral infarction, intractable, without status migrainosus**

✓5ᵗʰ **G43.7** Chronic **migraine** without aura
     Transformed migraine
     EXCLUDES 1   migraine without aura (G43.0-)

   ✓6ᵗʰ **G43.70** **Chronic migraine without aura,** not intractable
       Chronic migraine without aura, without refractory migraine

     G43.701 **Chronic migraine without aura, not intractable, with status migrainosus**

     G43.709 **Chronic migraine without aura, not intractable, without status migrainosus**
         Chronic migraine without aura NOS

   ✓6ᵗʰ **G43.71** **Chronic migraine without aura,** intractable
       Chronic migraine without aura, with refractory migraine

     G43.711 **Chronic migraine without aura, intractable, with status migrainosus**

     G43.719 **Chronic migraine without aura, intractable, without status migrainosus**

✓5ᵗʰ **G43.A** Cyclical vomiting

     G43.A0 **Cyclical vomiting,** not intractable
         Cyclical vomiting, without refractory migraine

     G43.A1 **Cyclical vomiting,** intractable
         Cyclical vomiting, with refractory migraine

✓5ᵗʰ **G43.B** Ophthalmoplegic **migraine**

     G43.B0 **Ophthalmoplegic migraine,** not intractable
         Ophthalmoplegic migraine, without refractory migraine

     G43.B1 **Ophthalmoplegic migraine,** intractable
         Ophthalmoplegic migraine, with refractory migraine

✓5ᵗʰ **G43.C** Periodic headache **syndromes in child or adult**

     G43.C0 **Periodic headache syndromes in child or adult,** not intractable
         Periodic headache syndromes in child or adult, without refractory migraine

---

☑ Additional Character Req   ✓ᴬ7ᵗʰ Placeholder Alert   Manifestation   HCC CMS-HCC Condition   ▽ Unspecified Code   ►◄ Revised Text   ● New Code   ▲ Revised Code Title

    G43.C1   **Periodic headache syndromes in child or adult, intractable**
          Periodic headache syndromes in child or adult, with refractory migraine

✓5ᵗʰ **G43.D**   Abdominal **migraine**

    G43.D0   **Abdominal migraine,** not intractable
          Abdominal migraine, without refractory migraine

    G43.D1   **Abdominal migraine,** intractable
          Abdominal migraine, with refractory migraine

✓5ᵗʰ **G43.8**   **Other migraine**

    ✓6ᵗʰ **G43.80**   **Other migraine,** not intractable
          Other migraine, without refractory migraine

        G43.801   **Other migraine, not intractable, with status migrainosus**

        G43.809   **Other migraine, not intractable, without status migrainosus**

    ✓6ᵗʰ **G43.81**   **Other migraine,** intractable
          Other migraine, with refractory migraine

        G43.811   **Other migraine, intractable, with status migrainosus**

        G43.819   **Other migraine, intractable, without status migrainosus**

    ✓6ᵗʰ **G43.82**   **Menstrual migraine,** not intractable
          Menstrual headache, not intractable
          Menstrual migraine, without refractory migraine
          Menstrually related migraine, not intractable
          Pre-menstrual headache, not intractable
          Pre-menstrual migraine, not intractable
          Pure menstrual migraine, not intractable
          Code also associated premenstrual tension syndrome (N94.3)

        G43.821   **Menstrual migraine, not intractable, with status migrainosus**   ♀

        G43.829   **Menstrual migraine, not intractable, without status migrainosus**   ♀
            Menstrual migraine NOS

    ✓6ᵗʰ **G43.83**   Menstrual **migraine,** intractable
          Menstrual headache, intractable
          Menstrual migraine, with refractory migraine
          Menstrually related migraine, intractable
          Pre-menstrual headache, intractable
          Pre-menstrual migraine, intractable
          Pure menstrual migraine, intractable
          Code also associated premenstrual tension syndrome (N94.3)

        G43.831   **Menstrual migraine, intractable, with status migrainosus**   ♀

        G43.839   **Menstrual migraine, intractable, without status migrainosus**   ♀

✓5ᵗʰ **G43.9**   **Migraine, unspecified**

    ✓6ᵗʰ **G43.90**   **Migraine, unspecified,** not intractable
          Migraine, unspecified, without refractory migraine

        G43.901   **Migraine, unspecified, not intractable, with status migrainosus**   ▽
            Status migrainosus NOS

        G43.909   **Migraine, unspecified, not intractable, without status migrainosus**   ▽
            Migraine NOS

    ✓6ᵗʰ **G43.91**   **Migraine, unspecified,** intractable
          Migraine, unspecified, with refractory migraine

        G43.911   **Migraine, unspecified, intractable, with status migrainosus**   ▽

        G43.919   **Migraine, unspecified, intractable, without status migrainosus**   ▽

✓4ᵗʰ **G44**   **Other** headache **syndromes**
    EXCLUDES 1   *headache NOS (R51)*
    EXCLUDES 2   *atypical facial pain (G50.1)*
           headache due to lumbar puncture (G97.1)
           migraines (G43.-)
           trigeminal neuralgia (G50.0)

✓5ᵗʰ **G44.0**   Cluster headaches **and other trigeminal autonomic cephalgias (TAC)**

    ✓6ᵗʰ **G44.00**   **Cluster headache syndrome, unspecified**
          Ciliary neuralgia
          Cluster headache NOS
          Histamine cephalgia
          Lower half migraine
          Migrainous neuralgia

        G44.001   **Cluster headache syndrome, unspecified,** intractable   ▽

        G44.009   **Cluster headache syndrome, unspecified,** not intractable   ▽
            Cluster headache syndrome NOS

    ✓6ᵗʰ **G44.01**   Episodic **cluster headache**

        G44.011   **Episodic cluster headache,** intractable

        G44.019   **Episodic cluster headache,** not intractable
            Episodic cluster headache NOS

    ✓6ᵗʰ **G44.02**   Chronic **cluster headache**

        G44.021   **Chronic cluster headache,** intractable

        G44.029   **Chronic cluster headache,** not intractable
            Chronic cluster headache NOS

    ✓6ᵗʰ **G44.03**   Episodic **paroxysmal hemicrania**
          Paroxysmal hemicrania NOS

        G44.031   **Episodic paroxysmal hemicrania,** intractable

        G44.039   **Episodic paroxysmal hemicrania,** not intractable
            Episodic paroxysmal hemicrania NOS

    ✓6ᵗʰ **G44.04**   Chronic **paroxysmal hemicrania**

        G44.041   **Chronic paroxysmal hemicrania,** intractable

        G44.049   **Chronic paroxysmal hemicrania,** not intractable
            Chronic paroxysmal hemicrania NOS

    ✓6ᵗʰ **G44.05**   Short lasting unilateral **neuralgiform headache with conjunctival injection and tearing (SUNCT)**

        G44.051   **Short lasting unilateral neuralgiform headache with conjunctival injection and tearing (SUNCT),** intractable

        G44.059   **Short lasting unilateral neuralgiform headache with conjunctival injection and tearing (SUNCT),** not intractable
            Short lasting unilateral neuralgiform headache with conjunctival injection and tearing (SUNCT) NOS

    ✓6ᵗʰ **G44.09**   **Other** trigeminal autonomic cephalgias **(TAC)**

        G44.091   **Other trigeminal autonomic cephalgias (TAC),** intractable

        G44.099   **Other trigeminal autonomic cephalgias syndrome (TAC),** not intractable

    G44.1   Vascular **headache, not elsewhere classified**
        EXCLUDES 2   *cluster headache (G44.0)*
           complicated headache syndromes (G44.5-)
           drug-induced headache (G44.4-)
           migraine (G43.-)
           other specified headache syndromes (G44.8-)
           post-traumatic headache (G44.3-)
           tension-type headache (G44.2-)

✓5ᵗʰ **G44.2**   Tension-type **headache**

    ✓6ᵗʰ **G44.20**   **Tension-type headache, unspecified**

        G44.201   **Tension-type headache, unspecified,** intractable   ▽

        G44.209   **Tension-type headache, unspecified,** not intractable   ▽
            Tension headache NOS

    ✓6ᵗʰ **G44.21**   Episodic **tension-type headache**

        G44.211   **Episodic tension-type headache,** intractable

        G44.219   **Episodic tension-type headache,** not intractable
            Episodic tension-type headache NOS

EXCLUDES 1 Not coded here   **EXCLUDES 2** Not included here   **N** Newborn Age: 0   **P** Pediatric Age: 0-17   **M** Maternity Age: 12-55   **A** Adult Age: 15-124

558   ICD-10-CM 2018

✔6th **G44.22**   **Chronic tension-type headache**

     G44.221   **Chronic tension-type headache, intractable**

     G44.229   **Chronic tension-type headache, not intractable**
         Chronic tension-type headache NOS

✔5th **G44.3**   **Post-traumatic headache**

   ✔6th **G44.30**   **Post-traumatic headache, unspecified**

     G44.301   **Post-traumatic headache, unspecified, intractable** ▽

     G44.309   **Post-traumatic headache, unspecified, not intractable** ▽
         Post-traumatic headache NOS

   ✔6th **G44.31**   **Acute post-traumatic headache**

     G44.311   **Acute post-traumatic headache, intractable**

     G44.319   **Acute post-traumatic headache, not intractable**
         Acute post-traumatic headache NOS

   ✔6th **G44.32**   **Chronic post-traumatic headache**

     G44.321   **Chronic post-traumatic headache, intractable**

     G44.329   **Chronic post-traumatic headache, not intractable**
         Chronic post-traumatic headache NOS

✔5th **G44.4**   **Drug-induced headache, not elsewhere classified**
     Medication overuse headache
     Use additional code for adverse effect, if applicable, to identify drug (T36-T50 with fifth or sixth character 5)

     G44.40   **Drug-induced headache, not elsewhere classified, not intractable**

     G44.41   **Drug-induced headache, not elsewhere classified, intractable**

✔5th **G44.5**   **Complicated headache syndromes**

     G44.51   **Hemicrania continua**

     G44.52   **New daily persistent headache (NDPH)**

     G44.53   **Primary thunderclap headache**

     G44.59   **Other complicated headache syndrome**

✔5th **G44.8**   **Other specified headache syndromes**

     G44.81   **Hypnic headache**

     G44.82   **Headache associated with sexual activity**
         Orgasmic headache
         Preorgasmic headache

     G44.83   **Primary cough headache**

     G44.84   **Primary exertional headache**

     G44.85   **Primary stabbing headache**

     G44.89   **Other headache syndrome**

✔4th **G45**   **Transient cerebral ischemic attacks and related syndromes**
     EXCLUDES 1   neonatal cerebral ischemia (P91.0)
         transient retinal artery occlusion (H34.0-)

   G45.0   **Vertebro-basilar artery syndrome**

   G45.1   **Carotid artery syndrome (hemispheric)**

   G45.2   **Multiple and bilateral precerebral artery syndromes**

   G45.3   **Amaurosis fugax**

   G45.4   **Transient global amnesia**
     EXCLUDES 1   amnesia NOS (R41.3)

   G45.8   **Other transient cerebral ischemic attacks and related syndromes**

   G45.9   **Transient cerebral ischemic attack, unspecified** ▽
     Spasm of cerebral artery
     TIA
     Transient cerebral ischemia NOS

✔4th **G46**   **Vascular syndromes of brain in cerebrovascular diseases**
     Code first underlying cerebrovascular disease (I60-I69)

   G46.0   **Middle cerebral artery syndrome**

   G46.1   **Anterior cerebral artery syndrome**

   G46.2   **Posterior cerebral artery syndrome**

   G46.3   **Brain stem stroke syndrome**
     Benedikt syndrome
     Claude syndrome
     Foville syndrome
     Millard-Gubler syndrome
     Wallenberg syndrome
     Weber syndrome

   G46.4   **Cerebellar stroke syndrome**

   G46.5   **Pure motor lacunar syndrome**

   G46.6   **Pure sensory lacunar syndrome**

   G46.7   **Other lacunar syndromes**

   G46.8   **Other vascular syndromes of brain in cerebrovascular diseases**

✔4th **G47**   **Sleep disorders**
     EXCLUDES 2   nightmares (F51.5)
         nonorganic sleep disorders (F51.-)
         sleep terrors (F51.4)
         sleepwalking (F51.3)

   ✔5th **G47.0**   **Insomnia**
     EXCLUDES 2   alcohol related insomnia (F10.182, F10.282, F10.982)
         drug-related insomnia (F11.182, F11.282, F11.982, F13.182, F13.282, F13.982, F14.182, F14.282,F14.982, F15.182, F15.282, F15.982, F19.182, F19.282, F19.982)
         idiopathic insomnia (F51.01)
         insomnia due to a mental disorder (F51.05)
         insomnia not due to a substance or known physiological condition (F51.0-)
         nonorganic insomnia (F51.0-)
         primary insomnia (F51.01)
         sleep apnea (G47.3-)

     G47.00   **Insomnia, unspecified** ▽
         Insomnia NOS

     G47.01   **Insomnia due to medical condition**
         Code also associated medical condition

     G47.09   **Other insomnia**

   ✔5th **G47.1**   **Hypersomnia**
     EXCLUDES 2   alcohol-related hypersomnia (F10.182, F10.282, F10.982)
         drug-related hypersomnia (F11.182, F11.282, F11.982, F13.182, F13.282, F13.982, F14.182,F14.282, F14.982, F15.182, F15.282, F15.982, F19.182, F19.282, F19.982)
         hypersomnia due to a mental disorder (F51.13)
         hypersomnia not due to a substance or known physiological condition (F51.1-)
         primary hypersomnia (F51.11)
         sleep apnea (G47.3-)

     G47.10   **Hypersomnia, unspecified** ▽
         Hypersomnia NOS

     G47.11   **Idiopathic hypersomnia with long sleep time**
         Idiopathic hypersomnia NOS

     G47.12   **Idiopathic hypersomnia without long sleep time**

     G47.13   **Recurrent hypersomnia**
         Kleine-Levin syndrome
         Menstrual related hypersomnia

     G47.14   **Hypersomnia due to medical condition**
         Code also associated medical condition

     G47.19   **Other hypersomnia**

   ✔5th **G47.2**   **Circadian rhythm sleep disorders**
     Disorders of the sleep wake schedule
     Inversion of nyctohemeral rhythm
     Inversion of sleep rhythm

     G47.20   **Circadian rhythm sleep disorder, unspecified type** ▽
         Sleep wake schedule disorder NOS

     G47.21   **Circadian rhythm sleep disorder, delayed sleep phase type**
         Delayed sleep phase syndrome

     G47.22   **Circadian rhythm sleep disorder, advanced sleep phase type**

     G47.23   **Circadian rhythm sleep disorder, irregular sleep wake type**
         Irregular sleep-wake pattern

     G47.24   **Circadian rhythm sleep disorder, free running type**
         ►Circadian rhythm sleep disorder, non-24-hour sleep-wake type◄

     G47.25   **Circadian rhythm sleep disorder, jet lag type**

     G47.26   **Circadian rhythm sleep disorder, shift work type**

     G47.27   *Circadian rhythm sleep disorder in conditions classified elsewhere*
         Code first underlying condition

     G47.29   **Other circadian rhythm sleep disorder**

✔ Additional Character Req   vx7th Placeholder Alert   Manifestation   HCC CMS-HCC Condition   ▽ Unspecified Code   ►◄ Revised Text   ● New Code   ▲ Revised Code Title

Chapter 6. Diseases of the Nervous System

✓5ᵗʰ G47.3 Sleep apnea
Code also any associated underlying condition
EXCLUDES 1 apnea NOS (R06.81)
Cheyne-Stokes breathing (R06.3)
pickwickian syndrome (E66.2)
sleep apnea of newborn (P28.3)

G47.30 Sleep apnea, unspecified ▽
Sleep apnea NOS

G47.31 Primary central sleep apnea
▶Idiopathic central sleep apnea◀

G47.32 High altitude periodic breathing

G47.33 Obstructive sleep apnea (adult) (pediatric)
▶Obstructive sleep apnea hypopnea◀
EXCLUDES 1 obstructive sleep apnea of newborn (P28.3)

G47.34 Idiopathic sleep related nonobstructive alveolar hypoventilation
Sleep related hypoxia

G47.35 Congenital central alveolar hypoventilation syndrome

G47.36 Sleep related hypoventilation in conditions classified elsewhere
Sleep related hypoxemia in conditions classified elsewhere
Code first underlying condition

G47.37 Central sleep apnea in conditions classified elsewhere
Code first underlying condition

G47.39 Other sleep apnea

✓5ᵗʰ G47.4 Narcolepsy and cataplexy

✓6ᵗʰ G47.41 Narcolepsy
G47.411 Narcolepsy with cataplexy
G47.419 Narcolepsy without cataplexy
Narcolepsy NOS

✓6ᵗʰ G47.42 Narcolepsy in conditions classified elsewhere
Code first underlying condition
G47.421 Narcolepsy in conditions classified elsewhere with cataplexy
G47.429 Narcolepsy in conditions classified elsewhere without cataplexy

✓5ᵗʰ G47.5 Parasomnia
EXCLUDES 1 alcohol induced parasomnia (F10.182, F10.282, F10.982)
drug induced parasomnia (F11.182, F11.282, F11.982, F13.182, F13.282, F13.982, F14.182, F14.282, F14.982, F15.182, F15.282, F15.982, F19.182, F19.282, F19.982)
parasomnia not due to a substance or known physiological condition (F51.8)

G47.50 Parasomnia, unspecified ▽
Parasomnia NOS

G47.51 Confusional arousals

G47.52 REM sleep behavior disorder

G47.53 Recurrent isolated sleep paralysis

G47.54 Parasomnia in conditions classified elsewhere
Code first underlying condition

G47.59 Other parasomnia

✓5ᵗʰ G47.6 Sleep related movement disorders
EXCLUDES 2 restless legs syndrome (G25.81)

G47.61 Periodic limb movement disorder
Periodic limb movement disorder

G47.62 Sleep related leg cramps

G47.63 Sleep related bruxism
EXCLUDES 1 psychogenic bruxism (F45.8)

G47.69 Other sleep related movement disorders

G47.8 Other sleep disorders
▶Other specified sleep-wake disorder◀

G47.9 Sleep disorder, unspecified ▽
Sleep disorder NOS
▶Unspecified sleep-wake disorder◀

Trigeminal and Facial Nerve Branches

Nerve, nerve root and plexus disorders (G50-G59)
EXCLUDES 1 current traumatic nerve, nerve root and plexus disorders—see Injury, nerve by body region
neuralgia NOS (M79.2)
neuritis NOS (M79.2)
peripheral neuritis in pregnancy (O26.82-)
radiculitis NOS (M54.1-)

✓4ᵗʰ G50 Disorders of trigeminal nerve
INCLUDES disorders of 5th cranial nerve

G50.0 Trigeminal neuralgia
Syndrome of paroxysmal facial pain
Tic douloureux

G50.1 Atypical facial pain

G50.8 Other disorders of trigeminal nerve

G50.9 Disorder of trigeminal nerve, unspecified ▽

✓4ᵗʰ G51 Facial nerve disorders
INCLUDES disorders of 7th cranial nerve

G51.0 Bell's palsy
Facial palsy

G51.1 Geniculate ganglionitis
EXCLUDES 1 postherpetic geniculate ganglionitis (B02.21)

G51.2 Melkersson's syndrome
Melkersson-Rosenthal syndrome

G51.3 Clonic hemifacial spasm

G51.4 Facial myokymia

G51.8 Other disorders of facial nerve

G51.9 Disorder of facial nerve, unspecified ▽

✓4ᵗʰ G52 Disorders of other cranial nerves
EXCLUDES 2 disorders of acoustic [8th] nerve (H93.3)
disorders of optic [2nd] nerve (H46, H47.0)
paralytic strabismus due to nerve palsy (H49.0-H49.2)

G52.0 Disorders of olfactory nerve
Disorders of 1st cranial nerve

G52.1 Disorders of glossopharyngeal nerve
Disorder of 9th cranial nerve
Glossopharyngeal neuralgia

G52.2 Disorders of vagus nerve
Disorders of pneumogastric [10th] nerve

G52.3 Disorders of hypoglossal nerve
Disorders of 12th cranial nerve

G52.7 Disorders of multiple cranial nerves
Polyneuritis cranialis

G52.8 Disorders of other specified cranial nerves

G52.9 Cranial nerve disorder, unspecified ▽

G53 Cranial nerve disorders in diseases classified elsewhere
Code first underlying disease, such as:
neoplasm (C00-D49)
EXCLUDES 1 multiple cranial nerve palsy in sarcoidosis (D86.82)
multiple cranial nerve palsy in syphilis (A52.15)
postherpetic geniculate ganglionitis (B02.21)
postherpetic trigeminal neuralgia (B02.22)

✓4ᵗʰ **G54** Nerve root and plexus **disorders**

    EXCLUDES 1   *current traumatic nerve root and plexus disorders—see nerve*
          injury by body region
          intervertebral disc disorders (M50-M51)
          neuralgia or neuritis NOS (M79.2)
          neuritis or radiculitis brachial NOS (M54.13)
          neuritis or radiculitis lumbar NOS (M54.16)
          neuritis or radiculitis lumbosacral NOS (M54.17)
          neuritis or radiculitis thoracic NOS (M54.14)
          radiculitis NOS (M54.10)
          radiculopathy NOS (M54.10)
          spondylosis (M47.-)

  G54.0 Brachial plexus **disorders**
      Thoracic outlet syndrome
      DEF: Acquired disorder affecting the spinal nerves that send
      signals to the shoulder, arm, and hand; causes corresponding
      motor and sensory dysfunction; characterized by regional
      paresthesia, pain, and muscle weakness, and in severe cases
      paralysis.

  G54.1 Lumbosacral plexus **disorders**

  G54.2 Cervical root **disorders, not elsewhere classified**

  G54.3 Thoracic root **disorders, not elsewhere classified**

  G54.4 Lumbosacral root **disorders, not elsewhere classified**

  G54.5 Neuralgic amyotrophy
      Parsonage-Aldren-Turner syndrome
      Shoulder-girdle neuritis
      EXCLUDES 1   *neuralgic amyotrophy in diabetes mellitus (E08-E13
            with .44)*

  G54.6 Phantom limb **syndrome with pain**   HCC

  G54.7 Phantom limb **syndrome without pain**   HCC
      Phantom limb syndrome NOS

  G54.8 Other nerve root and plexus disorders

  G54.9 Nerve root and plexus disorder, unspecified   ▽

G55 *Nerve root and plexus compressions in diseases classified
elsewhere*
    Code first underlying disease, such as:
      neoplasm (C00-D49)
    EXCLUDES 1   *nerve root compression (due to) (in) ankylosing spondylitis
           (M45.-)*
          nerve root compression (due to) (in) dorsopathies (M53.-, M54.-)
          *nerve root compression (due to) (in) intervertebral disc
            disorders (M50.1-, M51.1-)*
          *nerve root compression (due to) (in) spondylopathies
            (M46.-, M48.-)*

✓4ᵗʰ **G56** Mononeuropathies of **upper limb**
    EXCLUDES 1   *current traumatic nerve disorder—see nerve injury by body
          region*

  ✓5ᵗʰ **G56.0** Carpal tunnel **syndrome**
      G56.00 Carpal tunnel syndrome, unspecified upper limb ▽
      G56.01 Carpal tunnel syndrome, right upper limb
      G56.02 Carpal tunnel syndrome, left upper limb
      G56.03 Carpal tunnel syndrome, bilateral upper limbs

  ✓5ᵗʰ **G56.1** Other lesions of median nerve
      G56.10 Other lesions of median nerve, unspecified ▽
         upper limb
      G56.11 Other lesions of median nerve, right upper limb
      G56.12 Other lesions of median nerve, left upper limb
      G56.13 Other lesions of median nerve, bilateral upper limbs

  ✓5ᵗʰ **G56.2** Lesion of ulnar nerve
      Tardy ulnar nerve palsy
      G56.20 Lesion of ulnar nerve, unspecified upper limb ▽
      G56.21 Lesion of ulnar nerve, right upper limb
      G56.22 Lesion of ulnar nerve, left upper limb
      G56.23 Lesion of ulnar nerve, bilateral upper limbs

  ✓5ᵗʰ **G56.3** Lesion of radial nerve
      G56.30 Lesion of radial nerve, unspecified upper limb ▽
      G56.31 Lesion of radial nerve, right upper limb
      G56.32 Lesion of radial nerve, left upper limb
      G56.33 Lesion of radial nerve, bilateral upper limbs

Nerves of Upper Limb

Radial

Deep branch of radial
Ulnar
Superficial branch of radial
Median

  ✓5ᵗʰ **G56.4** Causalgia **of upper limb**
      Complex regional pain syndrome II of upper limb
      EXCLUDES 1   *complex regional pain syndrome I of lower limb (G90.52-)*
            complex regional pain syndrome I of upper limb (G90.51-)
            complex regional pain syndrome II of lower limb (G57.7-)
            reflex sympathetic dystrophy of lower limb (G90.52-)
            reflex sympathetic dystrophy of upper limb (G90.51-)
      G56.40 Causalgia of unspecified upper limb ▽
      G56.41 Causalgia of right upper limb
      G56.42 Causalgia of left upper limb
      G56.43 Causalgia of bilateral upper limbs

  ✓5ᵗʰ **G56.8** Other specified mononeuropathies of upper limb
      Interdigital neuroma of upper limb
      G56.80 Other specified mononeuropathies of ▽
         unspecified upper limb
      G56.81 Other specified mononeuropathies of right upper
         limb
      G56.82 Other specified mononeuropathies of left upper
         limb
      G56.83 Other specified mononeuropathies of bilateral
         upper limbs

  ✓5ᵗʰ **G56.9** Unspecified mononeuropathy of upper limb
      G56.90 Unspecified mononeuropathy of unspecified ▽
         upper limb
      G56.91 Unspecified mononeuropathy of right upper ▽
         limb
      G56.92 Unspecified mononeuropathy of left upper ▽
         limb
      G56.93 Unspecified mononeuropathy of bilateral ▽
         upper limbs

✓4ᵗʰ **G57** Mononeuropathies of **lower limb**
    EXCLUDES 1   *current traumatic nerve disorder—see nerve injury by body
          region*

  ✓5ᵗʰ **G57.0** Lesion of sciatic nerve
      EXCLUDES 1   *sciatica NOS (M54.3-)*
      EXCLUDES 2   *sciatica attributed to intervertebral disc disorder
           (M51.1-)*
      G57.00 Lesion of sciatic nerve, unspecified lower limb ▽
      G57.01 Lesion of sciatic nerve, right lower limb
      G57.02 Lesion of sciatic nerve, left lower limb
      G57.03 Lesion of sciatic nerve, bilateral lower limbs

  ✓5ᵗʰ **G57.1** Meralgia paresthetica
      Lateral cutaneous nerve of thigh syndrome
      G57.10 Meralgia paresthetica, unspecified lower limb ▽
      G57.11 Meralgia paresthetica, right lower limb
      G57.12 Meralgia paresthetica, left lower limb
      G57.13 Meralgia paresthetica, bilateral lower limbs

☑ Additional Character Req   √×7ᵗʰ Placeholder Alert   Manifestation   HCC CMS-HCC Condition   ▽ Unspecified Code   ►◄ Revised Text   ● New Code   ▲ Revised Code Title

Chapter 6. Diseases of the Nervous System

Nerves of Lower Limb

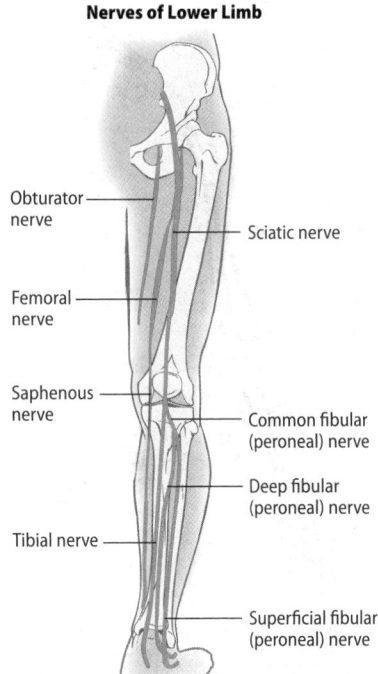

Obturator nerve

Sciatic nerve

Femoral nerve

Saphenous nerve

Common fibular (peroneal) nerve

Deep fibular (peroneal) nerve

Tibial nerve

Superficial fibular (peroneal) nerve

√5ᵗʰ **G57.2 Lesion of** femoral nerve
- **G57.20 Lesion of femoral nerve, unspecified lower limb** ▽
- **G57.21 Lesion of femoral nerve, right lower limb**
- **G57.22 Lesion of femoral nerve, left lower limb**
- **G57.23 Lesion of femoral nerve, bilateral lower limbs**

√5ᵗʰ **G57.3 Lesion of** lateral popliteal nerve
Peroneal nerve palsy
- **G57.30 Lesion of lateral popliteal nerve, unspecified lower limb** ▽
- **G57.31 Lesion of lateral popliteal nerve, right lower limb**
- **G57.32 Lesion of lateral popliteal nerve, left lower limb**
- **G57.33 Lesion of lateral popliteal nerve, bilateral lower limbs**

√5ᵗʰ **G57.4 Lesion of** medial popliteal nerve
- **G57.40 Lesion of medial popliteal nerve, unspecified lower limb** ▽
- **G57.41 Lesion of medial popliteal nerve, right lower limb**
- **G57.42 Lesion of medial popliteal nerve, left lower limb**
- **G57.43 Lesion of medial popliteal nerve, bilateral lower limbs**

√5ᵗʰ **G57.5 Tarsal tunnel syndrome**
- **G57.50 Tarsal tunnel syndrome, unspecified lower limb** ▽
- **G57.51 Tarsal tunnel syndrome, right lower limb**
- **G57.52 Tarsal tunnel syndrome, left lower limb**
- **G57.53 Tarsal tunnel syndrome, bilateral lower limbs**

√5ᵗʰ **G57.6 Lesion of** plantar nerve
Morton's metatarsalgia
- **G57.60 Lesion of plantar nerve, unspecified lower limb** ▽
- **G57.61 Lesion of plantar nerve, right lower limb**
- **G57.62 Lesion of plantar nerve, left lower limb**
- **G57.63 Lesion of plantar nerve, bilateral lower limbs**

√5ᵗʰ **G57.7 Causalgia of** lower limb
Complex regional pain syndrome II of lower limb
  - **EXCLUDES 1** complex regional pain syndrome I of lower limb (G90.52-)
  complex regional pain syndrome I of upper limb (G90.51-)
  complex regional pain syndrome II of upper limb (G56.4-)
  reflex sympathetic dystrophy of lower limb (G90.52-)
  reflex sympathetic dystrophy of upper limb (G90.51-)
- **G57.70 Causalgia of unspecified lower limb** ▽
- **G57.71 Causalgia of right lower limb**
- **G57.72 Causalgia of left lower limb**
- **G57.73 Causalgia of bilateral lower limbs**

√5ᵗʰ **G57.8 Other specified mononeuropathies of lower limb**
Interdigital neuroma of lower limb
- **G57.80 Other specified mononeuropathies of unspecified lower limb** ▽
- **G57.81 Other specified mononeuropathies of right lower limb**
- **G57.82 Other specified mononeuropathies of left lower limb**
- **G57.83 Other specified mononeuropathies of bilateral lower limbs**

√5ᵗʰ **G57.9 Unspecified mononeuropathy of lower limb**
- **G57.90 Unspecified mononeuropathy of unspecified lower limb** ▽
- **G57.91 Unspecified mononeuropathy of right lower limb** ▽
- **G57.92 Unspecified mononeuropathy of left lower limb** ▽
- **G57.93 Unspecified mononeuropathy of bilateral lower limbs** ▽

√4ᵗʰ **G58 Other mononeuropathies**
- **G58.0 Intercostal neuropathy**
- **G58.7 Mononeuritis multiplex**
- **G58.8 Other specified mononeuropathies**
- **G58.9 Mononeuropathy, unspecified** ▽

G59 Mononeuropathy in diseases classified elsewhere
Code first underlying disease
EXCLUDES 1 diabetic mononeuropathy (E08-E13 with .41)
syphilitic nerve paralysis (A52.19)
syphilitic neuritis (A52.15)
tuberculous mononeuropathy (A17.83)

Polyneuropathies and other disorders of the peripheral nervous system (G60-G65)

EXCLUDES 1 neuralgia NOS (M79.2)
neuritis NOS (M79.2)
peripheral neuritis in pregnancy (O26.82-)
radiculitis NOS (M54.10)

√4ᵗʰ **G60 Hereditary and idiopathic neuropathy**
- **G60.0 Hereditary motor and sensory neuropathy**
  Charcôt-Marie-Tooth disease
  Déjérine-Sottas disease
  Hereditary motor and sensory neuropathy, types I-IV
  Hypertrophic neuropathy of infancy
  Peroneal muscular atrophy (axonal type) (hypertrophic type)
  Roussy-Levy syndrome
- **G60.1 Refsum's disease**
  Infantile Refsum disease
  DEF: Genetic disorder of lipid metabolism; characterized by retinitis pigmentosa, degenerative nerve disease, ataxia, and dry, rough, scaly skin.
- **G60.2 Neuropathy in association with hereditary ataxia**
- **G60.3 Idiopathic progressive neuropathy**
- **G60.8 Other hereditary and idiopathic neuropathies**
  Dominantly inherited sensory neuropathy
  Morvan's disease
  Nelaton's syndrome
  Recessively inherited sensory neuropathy
- **G60.9 Hereditary and idiopathic neuropathy, unspecified** ▽

√4ᵗʰ **G61 Inflammatory polyneuropathy**
- **G61.0 Guillain-Barre syndrome**   HCC
  Acute (post-)infective polyneuritis
  Miller Fisher syndrome
  AHA: 2014, 2Q, 4
- **G61.1 Serum neuropathy**   HCC
  Use additional code for adverse effect, if applicable, to identify serum (T50.-)
√5ᵗʰ **G61.8 Other inflammatory polyneuropathies**
- **G61.81 Chronic inflammatory demyelinating polyneuritis**   HCC
- **G61.82 Multifocal motor neuropathy**   HCC
  MMN
- **G61.89 Other inflammatory polyneuropathies**   HCC
- **G61.9 Inflammatory polyneuropathy, unspecified**   HCC ▽

EXCLUDES 1 Not coded here   **EXCLUDES 2** Not included here   N Newborn Age: 0   P Pediatric Age: 0-17   M Maternity Age: 12-55   A Adult Age: 15-124

562   ICD-10-CM 2018

☑4th **G62 Other and unspecified polyneuropathies**

G62.0 Drug-induced polyneuropathy
Use additional code for adverse effect, if applicable, to identify drug (T36-T50 with fifth or sixth character 5)

G62.1 Alcoholic polyneuropathy `HCC`

G62.2 Polyneuropathy due to other toxic agents `HCC`
Code first (T51-T65) to identify toxic agent

☑5th **G62.8 Other specified polyneuropathies**

G62.81 Critical illness polyneuropathy `HCC`
Acute motor neuropathy

G62.82 Radiation-induced polyneuropathy `HCC`
Use additional external cause code (W88-W90, X39.0-) to identify cause

G62.89 Other specified polyneuropathies
AHA: 2016, 2Q, 11

G62.9 Polyneuropathy, unspecified ▽
Neuropathy NOS

G63 *Polyneuropathy in diseases classified elsewhere* `HCC`
Code first underlying disease, such as:
amyloidosis (E85.-)
endocrine disease, except diabetes (E00-E07, E15-E16, E20-E34)
metabolic diseases (E70-E88)
neoplasm (C00-D49)
nutritional deficiency (E40-E64)
EXCLUDES 1 *polyneuropathy (in):*
diabetes mellitus (E08-E13 with .42)
diphtheria (A36.83)
infectious mononucleosis (B27.0-B27.9 with 1)
Lyme disease (A69.22)
mumps (B26.84)
postherpetic (B02.23)
rheumatoid arthritis (M05.33)
scleroderma (M34.83)
systemic lupus erythematosus (M32.19)
AHA: 2012, 4Q, 99

G64 Other disorders of peripheral nervous system
Disorder of peripheral nervous system NOS

☑4th **G65 Sequelae of inflammatory and toxic polyneuropathies**
Code first condition resulting from (sequela) of inflammatory and toxic polyneuropathies

G65.0 Sequelae of Guillain-Barré syndrome `HCC`

G65.1 Sequelae of other inflammatory polyneuropathy `HCC`

G65.2 Sequelae of toxic polyneuropathy `HCC`

Diseases of myoneural junction and muscle (G70-G73)

☑4th **G70 Myasthenia gravis and other myoneural disorders**
EXCLUDES 1 *botulism (A05.1, A48.51-A48.52)*
transient neonatal myasthenia gravis (P94.0)

☑5th **G70.0 Myasthenia gravis**

G70.00 Myasthenia gravis without (acute) exacerbation `HCC`
Myasthenia gravis NOS

G70.01 Myasthenia gravis with (acute) exacerbation `HCC`
Myasthenia gravis in crisis

G70.1 Toxic myoneural disorders `HCC`
Code first (T51-T65) to identify toxic agent

G70.2 Congenital and developmental myasthenia `HCC`

☑5th **G70.8 Other specified myoneural disorders**

G70.80 Lambert-Eaton syndrome, unspecified `HCC` ▽
Lambert-Eaton syndrome NOS

G70.81 *Lambert-Eaton syndrome in disease classified elsewhere* `HCC`
Code first underlying disease
EXCLUDES 1 *Lambert-Eaton syndrome in neoplastic disease (G73.1)*

G70.89 Other specified myoneural disorders `HCC`

G70.9 Myoneural disorder, unspecified `HCC` ▽

☑4th **G71 Primary disorders of muscles**
EXCLUDES 2 *arthrogryposis multiplex congenita (Q74.3)*
metabolic disorders (E70-E88)
myositis (M60.-)

G71.0 Muscular dystrophy `HCC`
Autosomal recessive, childhood type, muscular dystrophy resembling Duchenne or Becker muscular dystrophy
Benign [Becker] muscular dystrophy
Benign scapuloperoneal muscular dystrophy with early contractures [Emery-Dreifuss]
Congenital muscular dystrophy NOS
Congenital muscular dystrophy with specific morphological abnormalities of the muscle fiber
Distal muscular dystrophy
Facioscapulohumeral muscular dystrophy
Limb-girdle muscular dystrophy
Ocular muscular dystrophy
Oculopharyngeal muscular dystrophy
Scapuloperoneal muscular dystrophy
Severe [Duchenne] muscular dystrophy

☑5th **G71.1 Myotonic disorders**

G71.11 Myotonic muscular dystrophy `HCC`
Dystrophia myotonica [Steinert]
Myotonia atrophica
Myotonic dystrophy
Proximal myotonic myopathy (PROMM)
Steinert disease

G71.12 Myotonia congenita
Acetazolamide responsive myotonia congenita
Dominant myotonia congenita [Thomsen disease]
Myotonia levior
Recessive myotonia congenita [Becker disease]

G71.13 Myotonic chondrodystrophy
Chondrodystrophic myotonia
Congenital myotonic chondrodystrophy
Schwartz-Jampel disease

G71.14 Drug induced myotonia
Use additional code for adverse effect, if applicable, to identify drug (T36-T50 with fifth or sixth character 5)

G71.19 Other specified myotonic disorders
Myotonia fluctuans
Myotonia permanens
Neuromyotonia [Isaacs]
Paramyotonia congenita (of von Eulenburg)
Pseudomyotonia
Symptomatic myotonia

G71.2 Congenital myopathies `HCC`
Central core disease
Fiber-type disproportion
Minicore disease
Multicore disease
Myotubular (centronuclear) myopathy
Nemaline myopathy
EXCLUDES 1 *arthrogryposis multiplex congenita (Q74.3)*

G71.3 Mitochondrial myopathy, not elsewhere classified
EXCLUDES 1 *Kearns-Sayre syndrome (H49.81)*
Leber's disease (H47.21)
Leigh's encephalopathy (G31.82)
mitochondrial metabolism disorders (E88.4-)
Reye's syndrome (G93.7)

G71.8 Other primary disorders of muscles

G71.9 Primary disorder of muscle, unspecified ▽
Hereditary myopathy NOS

☑4th **G72 Other and unspecified myopathies**
EXCLUDES 1 *arthrogryposis multiplex congenita (Q74.3)*
dermatopolymyositis (M33.-)
ischemic infarction of muscle (M62.2-)
myositis (M60.-)
polymyositis (M33.2-)

G72.0 Drug-induced myopathy
Use additional code for adverse effect, if applicable, to identify drug (T36-T50 with fifth or sixth character 5)

G72.1 Alcoholic myopathy
Use additional code to identify alcoholism (F10.-)

G72.2 Myopathy due to other toxic agents
Code first (T51-T65) to identify toxic agent

☑ Additional Character Req   ☑7th Placeholder Alert   Manifestation   `HCC` CMS-HCC Condition   ▽ Unspecified Code   ▶◀ Revised Text   ● New Code   ▲ Revised Code Title

G72.3 Periodic paralysis
Familial periodic paralysis
Hyperkalemic periodic paralysis (familial)
Hypokalemic periodic paralysis (familial)
Myotonic periodic paralysis (familial)
Normokalemic paralysis (familial)
Potassium sensitive periodic paralysis
> **EXCLUDES 1**   paramyotonia congenita (of von Eulenburg) (G71.19)

✓5ᵗʰ **G72.4** Inflammatory and immune **myopathies, not elsewhere classified**

     G72.41 Inclusion body myositis **[IBM]**

     G72.49 **Other inflammatory and immune myopathies, not elsewhere classified**
         Inflammatory myopathy NOS

✓5ᵗʰ **G72.8** **Other specified myopathies**

     G72.81 Critical illness **myopathy**
         Acute necrotizing myopathy
         Acute quadriplegic myopathy
         Intensive care (ICU) myopathy
         Myopathy of critical illness

     G72.89 **Other specified myopathies**

G72.9 **Myopathy, unspecified** ▽

✓4ᵗʰ **G73** **Disorders of myoneural junction and muscle in diseases classified elsewhere**

     G73.1 *Lambert-Eaton syndrome in neoplastic disease*   HCC
         Code first underlying neoplasm (C00-D49)
         > **EXCLUDES 1**   Lambert-Eaton syndrome not associated with neoplasm (G70.80-G70.81)

     G73.3 *Myasthenic syndromes in other diseases classified elsewhere*   HCC
         Code first underlying disease, such as:
           neoplasm (C00-D49)
           thyrotoxicosis (E05.-)

     G73.7 *Myopathy in diseases classified elsewhere*
         Code first underlying disease, such as:
           hyperparathyroidism (E21.0, E21.3)
           hypoparathyroidism (E20.-)
           glycogen storage disease (E74.0)
           lipid storage disorders (E75.-)
         > **EXCLUDES 1**   myopathy in:
             rheumatoid arthritis (M05.4-)
             sarcoidosis (D86.87)
             scleroderma (M34.82)
             sicca syndrome [Sjögren] (M35.03)
             systemic lupus erythematosus (M32.19)

Cerebral palsy and other paralytic syndromes (G80-G83)

✓4ᵗʰ **G80** **Cerebral palsy**
     > **EXCLUDES 1**   hereditary spastic paraplegia (G11.4)

     G80.0 Spastic quadriplegic **cerebral palsy**   HCC
         Congenital spastic paralysis (cerebral)

     G80.1 Spastic diplegic **cerebral palsy**   HCC
         Spastic cerebral palsy NOS

     G80.2 Spastic hemiplegic **cerebral palsy**   HCC

     G80.3 Athetoid **cerebral palsy**   HCC
         Double athetosis (syndrome)
         Dyskinetic cerebral palsy
         Dystonic cerebral palsy
         Vogt disease

     G80.4 Ataxic **cerebral palsy**   HCC

     G80.8 **Other cerebral palsy**   HCC
         Mixed cerebral palsy syndromes

     G80.9 **Cerebral palsy, unspecified**   HCC ▽
         Cerebral palsy NOS

✓4ᵗʰ **G81** **Hemiplegia and hemiparesis**
     NOTE   This category is to be used only when hemiplegia (complete)(incomplete) is reported without further specification, or is stated to be old or longstanding but of unspecified cause. The category is also for use in multiple coding to identify these types of hemiplegia resulting from any cause.
     > **EXCLUDES 1**   congenital cerebral palsy (G80.-)
          hemiplegia and hemiparesis due to sequela of cerebrovascular disease (I69.05-, I69.15-, I69.25-, I69.35-, I69.85-, I69.95-)
     AHA: 2015, 1Q, 25

✓5ᵗʰ **G81.0** **Flaccid** hemiplegia

     G81.00 **Flaccid hemiplegia affecting unspecified side**   HCC ▽

     G81.01 **Flaccid hemiplegia affecting** right dominant **side** HCC

     G81.02 **Flaccid hemiplegia affecting** left dominant **side** HCC

     G81.03 **Flaccid hemiplegia affecting** right nondominant **side**   HCC

     G81.04 **Flaccid hemiplegia affecting** left nondominant **side**   HCC

✓5ᵗʰ **G81.1** **Spastic** hemiplegia

     G81.10 **Spastic hemiplegia affecting unspecified side**   HCC ▽

     G81.11 **Spastic hemiplegia affecting** right dominant **side** HCC

     G81.12 **Spastic hemiplegia affecting** left dominant **side**   HCC

     G81.13 **Spastic hemiplegia affecting** right nondominant **side**   HCC

     G81.14 **Spastic hemiplegia affecting** left nondominant **side**   HCC

✓5ᵗʰ **G81.9** Hemiplegia, **unspecified**
     AHA: 2014, 1Q, 23

     G81.90 **Hemiplegia, unspecified affecting unspecified side**   HCC ▽

     G81.91 **Hemiplegia, unspecified affecting** right dominant **side**   HCC ▽

     G81.92 **Hemiplegia, unspecified affecting** left dominant **side**   HCC ▽

     G81.93 **Hemiplegia, unspecified affecting** right nondominant **side**   HCC ▽

     G81.94 **Hemiplegia, unspecified affecting** left nondominant **side**   HCC ▽

✓4ᵗʰ **G82** **Paraplegia (paraparesis) and quadriplegia (quadriparesis)**
     NOTE   This category is to be used only when the listed conditions are reported without further specification, or are stated to be old or longstanding but of unspecified cause. The category is also for use in multiple coding to identify these conditions resulting from any cause
     > **EXCLUDES 1**   congenital cerebral palsy (G80.-)
          functional quadriplegia (R53.2)
          hysterical paralysis (F44.4)

✓5ᵗʰ **G82.2** Paraplegia
     Paralysis of both lower limbs NOS
     Paraparesis (lower) NOS
     Paraplegia (lower) NOS

     G82.20 **Paraplegia, unspecified**   HCC ▽

     G82.21 **Paraplegia,** complete   HCC

     G82.22 **Paraplegia,** incomplete   HCC

✓5ᵗʰ **G82.5** Quadriplegia

     G82.50 **Quadriplegia, unspecified**   HCC ▽

     G82.51 **Quadriplegia,** C1-C4 complete   HCC

     G82.52 **Quadriplegia,** C1-C4 incomplete   HCC

     G82.53 **Quadriplegia,** C5-C7 complete   HCC

     G82.54 **Quadriplegia,** C5-C7 incomplete   HCC

✓4ᵗʰ **G83** **Other paralytic syndromes**
     NOTE   This category is to be used only when the listed conditions are reported without further specification, or are stated to be old or longstanding but of unspecified cause. The category is also for use in multiple coding to identify these conditions resulting from any cause.
     INCLUDES   paralysis (complete) (incomplete), except as in G80-G82

     G83.0 Diplegia **of upper limbs**   HCC
         Diplegia (upper)
         Paralysis of both upper limbs

✓5ᵗʰ **G83.1** Monoplegia **of lower limb**
     Paralysis of lower limb
     > **EXCLUDES 1**   monoplegia of lower limbs due to sequela of cerebrovascular disease (I69.04-, I69.14-, I69.24-, I69.34-, I69.84-, I69.94-)

     G83.10 **Monoplegia of lower limb affecting unspecified side**   HCC ▽

     G83.11 **Monoplegia of lower limb affecting** right dominant **side**   HCC

     G83.12 **Monoplegia of lower limb affecting** left dominant **side**   HCC

     G83.13 **Monoplegia of lower limb affecting** right nondominant **side**   HCC

     G83.14 **Monoplegia of lower limb affecting** left nondominant **side**   HCC

EXCLUDES 1 Not coded here   **EXCLUDES 2** Not included here   N Newborn Age: 0   P Pediatric Age: 0-17   M Maternity Age: 12-55   A Adult Age: 15-124

564   ICD-10-CM 2018

✓6th **G83.2** Monoplegia **of** upper limb
Paralysis of upper limb
> **EXCLUDES 1**   *monoplegia of upper limbs due to sequela of*
> *cerebrovascular disease (I69.03-, I69.13-, I69.23-,*
> *I69.33-, I69.83-, I69.93-)*

    G83.20   **Monoplegia of upper limb affecting**   HCC ▽
            unspecified side

    G83.21   **Monoplegia of upper limb affecting** right   HCC
            dominant side

    G83.22   **Monoplegia of upper limb affecting** left   HCC
            dominant side

    G83.23   **Monoplegia of upper limb affecting** right   HCC
            nondominant side

    G83.24   **Monoplegia of upper limb affecting** left   HCC
            nondominant side

✓5th **G83.3** **Monoplegia, unspecified**

    G83.30   **Monoplegia, unspecified affecting**   HCC ▽
            unspecified side

    G83.31   **Monoplegia, unspecified affecting** right   HCC ▽
            dominant side

    G83.32   **Monoplegia, unspecified affecting** left   HCC ▽
            dominant side

    G83.33   **Monoplegia, unspecified affecting** right   HCC ▽
            nondominant side

    G83.34   **Monoplegia, unspecified affecting** left   HCC ▽
            nondominant side

G83.4   **Cauda equina syndrome**   HCC
     Neurogenic bladder due to cauda equina syndrome
> **EXCLUDES 1**   *cord bladder NOS (G95.89)*
> *neurogenic bladder NOS (N31.9)*

G83.5   **Locked-in state**   HCC

✓5th **G83.8** **Other specified paralytic syndromes**
> **EXCLUDES 1**   *paralytic syndromes due to current spinal cord*
> *injury—code to spinal cord injury (S14, S24, S34)*

    G83.81   **Brown-Séquard syndrome**   HCC
    G83.82   **Anterior cord syndrome**   HCC
    G83.83   **Posterior cord syndrome**   HCC
    G83.84   **Todd's paralysis (postepileptic)**   HCC
    G83.89   **Other specified paralytic syndromes**   HCC

G83.9   **Paralytic syndrome, unspecified**   HCC ▽

Other disorders of the nervous system (G89-G99)

✓4th **G89**   **Pain, not elsewhere classified**
     Code also related psychological factors associated with pain (F45.42)
> **EXCLUDES 1**   *generalized pain NOS (R52)*
> *pain disorders exclusively related to psychological factors*
> *(F45.41)*
> *pain NOS (R52)*
>
> **EXCLUDES 2**   *atypical face pain (G50.1)*
> *headache syndromes (G44.-)*
> *localized pain, unspecified type—code to pain by site, such as:*
>   *abdomen pain (R10.-)*
>   *back pain (M54.9)*
>   *breast pain (N64.4)*
>   *chest pain (R07.1-R07.9)*
>   *ear pain (H92.0-)*
>   *eye pain (H57.1)*
>   *headache (R51)*
>   *joint pain (M25.5-)*
>   *limb pain (M79.6-)*
>   *lumbar region pain (M54.5)*
>   *painful urination (R30.9)*
>   *pelvic and perineal pain (R10.2)*
>   *renal colic (N23)*
>   *shoulder pain (M25.51-)*
>   *spine pain (M54.-)*
>   *throat pain (R07.0)*
>   *tongue pain (K14.6)*
>   *tooth pain (K08.8)*
> *migraines (G43.-)*
> *myalgia (M79.1)*
> *pain from prosthetic devices, implants, and grafts (T82.84,*
>   *T83.84, T84.84, T85.84-)*
> *phantom limb syndrome with pain (G54.6)*
> *vulvar vestibulitis (N94.810)*
> *vulvodynia (N94.81-)*

G89.0   **Central pain** **syndrome**
     Déjérine-Roussy syndrome
     Myelopathic pain syndrome
     Thalamic pain syndrome (hyperesthetic)

✓5th **G89.1** **Acute pain,** **not elsewhere classified**

    G89.11   **Acute pain** due to trauma
    G89.12   **Acute** post-thoracotomy **pain**
            Post-thoracotomy pain NOS
    G89.18   **Other acute** postprocedural **pain**
            Postoperative pain NOS
            Postprocedural pain NOS

✓5th **G89.2** **Chronic pain,** **not elsewhere classified**
> **EXCLUDES 1**   *causalgia, lower limb (G57.7-)*
> *causalgia, upper limb (G56.4-)*
> *central pain syndrome (G89.0)*
> *chronic pain syndrome (G89.4)*
> *complex regional pain syndrome II, lower limb (G57.7-)*
> *complex regional pain syndrome II, upper limb (G56.4-)*
> *neoplasm related chronic pain (G89.3)*
> *reflex sympathetic dystrophy (G90.5-)*

    G89.21   **Chronic pain due to** trauma
    G89.22   **Chronic** post-thoracotomy **pain**
    G89.28   **Other chronic** postprocedural **pain**
            Other chronic postoperative pain
    G89.29   **Other chronic pain**

G89.3   **Neoplasm related pain (acute) (chronic)**
     Cancer associated pain
     Pain due to malignancy (primary) (secondary)
     Tumor associated pain

G89.4   **Chronic pain syndrome**
     Chronic pain associated with significant psychosocial
     dysfunction

✓4th **G90**   **Disorders of autonomic nervous system**
> **EXCLUDES 1**   *dysfunction of the autonomic nervous system due to alcohol*
> *(G31.2)*

✓5th **G90.0** **Idiopathic peripheral autonomic neuropathy**

    G90.01   **Carotid sinus syncope**
            Carotid sinus syndrome
            DEF: Vagal activation caused by pressure on the carotid
            sinus baroreceptors; sympathetic nerve impulses may
            cause sinus arrest or AV block.
    G90.09   **Other idiopathic peripheral autonomic neuropathy**
            Idiopathic peripheral autonomic neuropathy NOS

G90.1   **Familial dysautonomia [Riley-Day]**   HCC

G90.2   **Horner's syndrome**
     Bernard(-Horner) syndrome
     Cervical sympathetic dystrophy or paralysis

G90.3   **Multi-system degeneration of the autonomic nervous**   HCC
     system
     Neurogenic orthostatic hypotension [Shy-Drager]
> **EXCLUDES 1**   *orthostatic hypotension NOS (I95.1)*

G90.4   **Autonomic dysreflexia**
     Use additional code to identify the cause, such as:
         fecal impaction (K56.41)
         pressure ulcer (pressure area) (L89.-)
         urinary tract infection (N39.0)

✓5th **G90.5** **Complex regional pain syndrome I (CRPS I)**
     Reflex sympathetic dystrophy
> **EXCLUDES 1**   *causalgia of lower limb (G57.7-)*
> *causalgia of upper limb (G56.4-)*
> *complex regional pain syndrome II of lower limb*
>   *(G57.7-)*
> *complex regional pain syndrome II of upper limb*
>   *(G56.4-)*

    G90.50   **Complex regional pain syndrome I, unspecified**   ▽

✓6th   **G90.51**   **Complex regional pain syndrome I of** upper limb

        G90.511   **Complex regional pain syndrome I of**
                 right **upper limb**

        G90.512   **Complex regional pain syndrome I of**
                 left **upper limb**

        G90.513   **Complex regional pain syndrome I of**
                 upper limb, bilateral

        G90.519   **Complex regional pain syndrome I of**   ▽
                 unspecified upper limb

✓6th   **G90.52**   **Complex regional pain syndrome I of** lower limb

        G90.521   **Complex regional pain syndrome I of**
                 right **lower limb**

☑ Additional Character Req   ✓x7th Placeholder Alert   Manifestation   HCC CMS-HCC Condition   ▽ Unspecified Code   ►◄ Revised Text   ● New Code   ▲ Revised Code Title

ICD-10-CM 2018   565

Chapter 6. Diseases of the Nervous System

G90.522–G95.81

Hydrocephalus (Acquired)

Normal ventricles   Hydrocephalic ventricles

G90.522   **Complex regional pain syndrome I of left lower limb**

G90.523   **Complex regional pain syndrome I of lower limb, bilateral**

G90.529   **Complex regional pain syndrome I of unspecified lower limb** ▽

G90.59   **Complex regional pain syndrome I of other specified site**

G90.8   **Other disorders of autonomic nervous system**

G90.9   **Disorder of the autonomic nervous system, unspecified** ▽

☑4ᵗʰ **G91**   **Hydrocephalus**
   INCLUDES   acquired hydrocephalus
   EXCLUDES 1   *Arnold-Chiari syndrome with hydrocephalus (Q07.-)*
      congenital hydrocephalus (Q03.-)
      spina bifida with hydrocephalus (Q05.-)

G91.0   **Communicating hydrocephalus**
   Secondary normal pressure hydrocephalus

G91.1   **Obstructive hydrocephalus**
   DEF: Obstruction of cerebrospinal fluid passage from brain into spinal canal; characterized by headaches, drowsiness, poor coordination, urinary incontinence, nausea, vomiting, and papilledema.

G91.2   **(Idiopathic) normal pressure hydrocephalus**
   Normal pressure hydrocephalus NOS

G91.3   **Post-traumatic hydrocephalus, unspecified**

G91.4   *Hydrocephalus in diseases classified elsewhere*
   Code first underlying condition, such as:
     congenital syphilis (A50.4-)
     neoplasm (C00-D49)
   EXCLUDES 1   *hydrocephalus due to congenital toxoplasmosis (P37.1)*
   AHA: 2014, 3Q, 3

G91.8   **Other hydrocephalus**

G91.9   **Hydrocephalus, unspecified** ▽

G92   **Toxic encephalopathy**
   Toxic encephalitis
   Toxic metabolic encephalopathy
   ▶Code first, if applicable, drug induced (T36-T50)◀
   Code first (T51-T65) to identify toxic agent
   AHA: 2017, 1Q, 39-40
   DEF: Brain tissue degeneration due to toxic substance.

☑4ᵗʰ **G93**   **Other disorders of brain**

G93.0   **Cerebral cysts**
   Arachnoid cyst
   Porencephalic cyst, acquired
   EXCLUDES 1   *acquired periventricular cysts of newborn (P91.1)*
      congenital cerebral cysts (Q04.6)

G93.1   **Anoxic brain damage, not elsewhere classified** HCC
   EXCLUDES 1   *cerebral anoxia due to anesthesia during labor and delivery (O74.3)*
      cerebral anoxia due to anesthesia during the puerperium (O89.2)
      neonatal anoxia (P84)
   DEF: Brain injury not resulting from birth trauma that is due to lack of oxygen. Brain cells, when deprived of oxygen, begin to expire after 4 minutes.

G93.2   **Benign intracranial hypertension**
   EXCLUDES 1   *hypertensive encephalopathy (I67.4)*

G93.3   **Postviral fatigue syndrome**
   Benign myalgic encephalomyelitis
   EXCLUDES 1   *chronic fatigue syndrome NOS (R53.82)*

☑5ᵗʰ **G93.4**   **Other and unspecified encephalopathy**
   EXCLUDES 1   *alcoholic encephalopathy (G31.2)*
      encephalopathy in diseases classified elsewhere (G94)
      hypertensive encephalopathy (I67.4)
      toxic (metabolic) encephalopathy (G92)

   G93.40   **Encephalopathy, unspecified** ▽
     AHA: 2017, 2Q, 8

   G93.41   **Metabolic encephalopathy**
     Septic encephalopathy
     AHA: 2017, 2Q, 8; 2016, 3Q, 42; 2015, 3Q, 21

   G93.49   **Other encephalopathy**
     Encephalopathy NEC
     AHA: 2017, 2Q, 9

G93.5   **Compression of brain** HCC
   Arnold-Chiari type 1 compression of brain
   Compression of brain (stem)
   Herniation of brain (stem)
   EXCLUDES 1   *diffuse traumatic compression of brain (S06.2-)*
      focal traumatic compression of brain (S06.3-)

G93.6   **Cerebral edema** HCC
   EXCLUDES 1   *cerebral edema due to birth injury (P11.0)*
      traumatic cerebral edema (S06.1-)

G93.7   **Reye's syndrome** P
   ~~Code first (T39.0-), if salicylates-induced~~
   ▶Code first poisoning due to salicylates, if applicable (T39.0-, with sixth character 1-4)◀
   ▶Use additional code for adverse effect due to salicylates, if applicable (T39.0-, with sixth character 5)◀
   DEF: Rare childhood illness often developed after a viral upper respiratory infection; characterized by vomiting, elevated serum transaminase, brain swelling, disturbances of consciousness, seizures, and changes in liver and other viscera; can be fatal.

☑5ᵗʰ **G93.8**   **Other specified disorders of brain**

   G93.81   **Temporal sclerosis**
     Hippocampal sclerosis
     Mesial temporal sclerosis

   G93.82   **Brain death**

   G93.89   **Other specified disorders of brain**
     Postradiation encephalopathy

G93.9   **Disorder of brain, unspecified** ▽

G94   *Other disorders of brain in diseases classified elsewhere*
   Code first underlying disease
   EXCLUDES 1   *encephalopathy in congenital syphilis (A50.49)*
      encephalopathy in influenza (J09.X9, J10.81, J11.81)
      encephalopathy in syphilis (A52.19)
      hydrocephalus in diseases classified elsewhere (G91.4)

☑4ᵗʰ **G95**   **Other and unspecified diseases of spinal cord**
   EXCLUDES 2   *myelitis (G04.-)*

G95.0   **Syringomyelia and syringobulbia** HCC

☑5ᵗʰ **G95.1**   **Vascular myelopathies**
   EXCLUDES 2   *intraspinal phlebitis and thrombophlebitis, except non-pyogenic (G08)*

   G95.11   **Acute infarction of spinal cord (embolic) (nonembolic)** HCC
     Anoxia of spinal cord
     Arterial thrombosis of spinal cord

   G95.19   **Other vascular myelopathies** HCC
     Edema of spinal cord
     Hematomyelia
     Nonpyogenic intraspinal phlebitis and thrombophlebitis
     Subacute necrotic myelopathy

☑5ᵗʰ **G95.2**   **Other and unspecified cord compression**

   G95.20   **Unspecified cord compression** HCC ▽

   G95.29   **Other cord compression** HCC

☑5ᵗʰ **G95.8**   **Other specified diseases of spinal cord**
   EXCLUDES 1   *neurogenic bladder NOS (N31.9)*
      neurogenic bladder due to cauda equina syndrome (G83.4)
      neuromuscular dysfunction of bladder without spinal cord lesion (N31.-)

   G95.81   **Conus medullaris syndrome** HCC

EXCLUDES 1 Not coded here   EXCLUDES 2 Not included here   N Newborn Age: 0   P Pediatric Age: 0-17   M Maternity Age: 12-55   A Adult Age: 15-124

566   ICD-10-CM 2018

G95.89   Other specified diseases of spinal cord   HCC
Cord bladder NOS
Drug-induced myelopathy
Radiation-induced myelopathy
EXCLUDES 1   *myelopathy NOS (G95.9)*

G95.9   Disease of spinal cord, unspecified   HCC ▽
Myelopathy NOS

✓4ᵗʰ **G96   Other disorders of central nervous system**

G96.0   Cerebrospinal fluid leak
EXCLUDES 1   *cerebrospinal fluid leak from spinal puncture (G97.0)*
DEF: Cerebrospinal fluid discharging from the nose or the ear;
caused by fracture of frontal bone with tearing of dura mater and
arachnoid; characterized by watery drainage usually from only one
side of the nose or one ear, headache, vision changes, and hearing
loss.

✓5ᵗʰ **G96.1   Disorders of meninges, not elsewhere classified**

G96.11   Dural tear
EXCLUDES 1   *accidental puncture or laceration of dura*
during a procedure (G97.41)
AHA: 2014, 4Q, 24

G96.12   Meningeal adhesions (cerebral) (spinal)

G96.19   Other disorders of meninges, not elsewhere classified

G96.8   Other specified disorders of central nervous system

G96.9   Disorder of central nervous system, unspecified   ▽

✓4ᵗʰ **G97   Intraoperative and postprocedural complications and disorders of nervous system, not elsewhere classified**
EXCLUDES 2   *intraoperative and postprocedural cerebrovascular infarction (I97.81-, I97.82-)*

G97.0   Cerebrospinal fluid leak from spinal puncture

G97.1   Other reaction to spinal and lumbar puncture
Headache due to lumbar puncture

G97.2   Intracranial hypotension following ventricular shunting

✓5ᵗʰ **G97.3   Intraoperative hemorrhage and hematoma of a nervous system organ or structure complicating a procedure**
EXCLUDES 1   *intraoperative hemorrhage and hematoma of a nervous system organ or structure due to accidental puncture and laceration during a procedure (G97.4-)*

G97.31   Intraoperative hemorrhage and hematoma of a nervous system organ or structure complicating a nervous system procedure

G97.32   Intraoperative hemorrhage and hematoma of a nervous system organ or structure complicating other procedure

✓5ᵗʰ **G97.4   Accidental puncture and laceration of a nervous system organ or structure during a procedure**

G97.41   Accidental puncture or laceration of dura during a procedure
Incidental (inadvertent) durotomy
AHA: 2014, 4Q, 24

G97.48   Accidental puncture and laceration of other nervous system organ or structure during a nervous system procedure

G97.49   Accidental puncture and laceration of other nervous system organ or structure during other procedure

✓5ᵗʰ **G97.5   Postprocedural hemorrhage of a nervous system organ or structure following a procedure**

G97.51   Postprocedural hemorrhage of a nervous system organ or structure following a nervous system procedure

G97.52   Postprocedural hemorrhage of a nervous system organ or structure following other procedure

✓5ᵗʰ **G97.6   Postprocedural hematoma and seroma of a nervous system organ or structure following a procedure**

G97.61   Postprocedural hematoma of a nervous system organ or structure following a nervous system procedure

G97.62   Postprocedural hematoma of a nervous system organ or structure following other procedure

G97.63   Postprocedural seroma of a nervous system organ or structure following a nervous system procedure

G97.64   Postprocedural seroma of a nervous system organ or structure following other procedure

✓5ᵗʰ **G97.8   Other intraoperative and postprocedural complications and disorders of nervous system**
Use additional code to further specify disorder

G97.81   Other intraoperative complications of nervous system

G97.82   Other postprocedural complications and disorders of nervous system

✓4ᵗʰ **G98   Other disorders of nervous system not elsewhere classified**
INCLUDES   nervous system disorder NOS

G98.0   Neurogenic arthritis, not elsewhere classified
Nonsyphilitic neurogenic arthropathy NEC
Nonsyphilitic neurogenic spondylopathy NEC
EXCLUDES 1   *spondylopathy (in):*
syringomyelia and syringobulbia (G95.0)
tabes dorsalis (A52.11)

G98.8   Other disorders of nervous system
Nervous system disorder NOS

✓4ᵗʰ **G99   Other disorders of nervous system in diseases classified elsewhere**

G99.0   *Autonomic neuropathy in diseases classified elsewhere*
Code first underlying disease, such as:
amyloidosis (E85.-)
gout (M1A.-, M10.-)
hyperthyroidism (E05.-)
EXCLUDES 1   *diabetic autonomic neuropathy (E08-E13 with .43)*

G99.2   *Myelopathy in diseases classified elsewhere*   HCC
Code first underlying disease, such as:
neoplasm (C00-D49)
EXCLUDES 1   *myelopathy in:*
intervertebral disease (M50.0-, M51.0-)
spondylosis (M47.0-, M47.1-)

G99.8   *Other specified disorders of nervous system in diseases classified elsewhere*
Code first underlying disorder, such as:
amyloidosis (E85.-)
avitaminosis (E56.9)
EXCLUDES 1   *nervous system involvement in:*
cysticercosis (B69.0)
rubella (B06.0-)
syphilis (A52.1-)

Spinal Puncture

Spinal cord
Epidural space
Subarachnoid space
Vertebra
Spinal needle

Lumbar area

Chapter 7. Diseases of the Eye and Adnexa (H00–H59)

Chapter Specific Guidelines with Coding Examples

The chapter specific guidelines from the ICD-10-CM Official Guidelines for Coding and Reporting have been provided below. Along with these guidelines are coding examples, contained in the shaded boxes, that have been developed to help illustrate the coding and/or sequencing guidance found in these guidelines.

a. Glaucoma

1) Assigning glaucoma codes

Assign as many codes from category H40, Glaucoma, as needed to identify the type of glaucoma, the affected eye, and the glaucoma stage.

2) Bilateral glaucoma with same type and stage

When a patient has bilateral glaucoma and both eyes are documented as being the same type and stage, and there is a code for bilateral glaucoma, report only the code for the type of glaucoma, bilateral, with the seventh character for the stage.

> Bilateral mild stage primary open-angle glaucoma
>
> **H40.1131   Primary open-angle glaucoma, bilateral, mild stage**
>
> *Explanation*: In this scenario, the patient has the same type and stage of glaucoma in both eyes. As this type of glaucoma has a code for bilateral, assign only the code for the bilateral glaucoma with the seventh character for the stage.

When a patient has bilateral glaucoma and both eyes are documented as being the same type and stage, and the classification does not provide a code for bilateral glaucoma (i.e. subcategories H40.10, H40.11 and H40.20) report only one code for the type of glaucoma with the appropriate seventh character for the stage.

> Bilateral open-angle glaucoma, severe stage; not specified as to type
>
> **H40.10X3   Unspecified open-angle glaucoma, severe stage**
>
> *Explanation*: In this scenario, the patient has glaucoma of the same type and stage of both eyes, but there is no code specifically for bilateral glaucoma. Only one code is assigned with the appropriate seventh character for the stage.

3) Bilateral glaucoma stage with different types or stages

When a patient has bilateral glaucoma and each eye is documented as having a different type or stage, and the classification distinguishes laterality, assign the appropriate code for each eye rather than the code for bilateral glaucoma.

> Bilateral chronic angle-closure glaucoma; right eye is documented as mild stage and left eye as moderate stage
>
> **H40.2211   Chronic angle-closure glaucoma, right eye, mild stage**
>
> **H40.2222   Chronic angle-closure glaucoma, left eye, moderate stage**
>
> *Explanation*: In this scenario the patient has the same type of glaucoma in both eyes, but each eye is at a different stage. Because the subcategory for this condition identifies laterality, one code is assigned for the right eye and one code is assigned for the left eye, each with the appropriate seventh character for the stage appended.

When a patient has bilateral glaucoma and each eye is documented as having a different type, and the classification does not distinguish laterality (i.e. subcategories H40.10, H40.11 and H40.20), assign one code for each type of glaucoma with the appropriate seventh character for the stage.

> Documentation relates mild, unspecified primary angle-closure glaucoma of the left eye with mild unspecified open-angle glaucoma of the right eye
>
> **H40.20X1   Unspecified primary angle-closure glaucoma, mild stage**
>
> **H40.10X1   Unspecified open-angle glaucoma, mild stage**
>
> *Explanation*: In this scenario the patient has a different type of glaucoma in each eye and the classification does not distinguish laterality. A code for each type of glaucoma is assigned, each with the appropriate seventh character for the stage.

When a patient has bilateral glaucoma and each eye is documented as having the same type, but different stage, and the classification does not distinguish laterality (i.e. subcategories H40.10, H40.11 and H40.20), assign a code for the type of glaucoma for each eye with the seventh character for the specific glaucoma stage documented for each eye.

> Bilateral open-angle glaucoma, not specified as to type; the right eye is documented to be in mild stage and the left eye as being in moderate stage
>
> **H40.10X1   Unspecified open-angle glaucoma, mild stage**
>
> **H40.10X2   Unspecified open-angle glaucoma, moderate stage**
>
> *Explanation*: In this scenario the patient has the same type of glaucoma in each eye but each eye is at a different stage, and the classification does not distinguish laterality at this subcategory level. Two codes are assigned; both codes represent the same type of glaucoma but each has a different seventh character identifying the appropriate stage for each eye.

4) Patient admitted with glaucoma and stage evolves during the admission

If a patient is admitted with glaucoma and the stage progresses during the admission, assign the code for highest stage documented.

5) Indeterminate stage glaucoma

Assignment of the seventh character "4" for "indeterminate stage" should be based on the clinical documentation. The seventh character "4" is used for glaucomas whose stage cannot be clinically determined. This seventh character should not be confused with the seventh character "0", unspecified, which should be assigned when there is no documentation regarding the stage of the glaucoma.

Chapter 7. Diseases of the Eye and Adnexa (H00-H59)

NOTE   Use an external cause code following the code for the eye condition, if applicable, to identify the cause of the eye condition.

EXCLUDES 2   certain conditions originating in the perinatal period (P04-P96)
certain infectious and parasitic diseases (A00-B99)
complications of pregnancy, childbirth and the puerperium (O00-O9A)
congenital malformations, deformations, and chromosomal abnormalities (Q00-Q99)
diabetes mellitus related eye conditions (E09.3-, E10.3-, E11.3-, E13.3-)
endocrine, nutritional and metabolic diseases (E00-E88)
injury (trauma) of eye and orbit (S05.-)
injury, poisoning and certain other consequences of external causes (S00-T88)
neoplasms (C00-D49)
symptoms, signs and abnormal clinical and laboratory findings, not elsewhere classified (R00-R94)
syphilis related eye disorders (A50.01, A50.3-, A51.43, A52.71)

This chapter contains the following blocks:

H00-H05   Disorders of eyelid, lacrimal system and orbit
H10-H11   Disorders of conjunctiva
H15-H22   Disorders of sclera, cornea, iris and ciliary body
H25-H28   Disorders of lens
H30-H36   Disorders of choroid and retina
H40-H42   Glaucoma
H43-H44   Disorders of vitreous body and globe
H46-H47   Disorders of optic nerve and visual pathways
H49-H52   Disorders of ocular muscles, binocular movement, accommodation and refraction
H53-H54   Visual disturbances and blindness
H55-H57   Other disorders of eye and adnexa
H59   Intraoperative and postprocedural complications and disorders of eye and adnexa, not elsewhere classified

Disorders of eyelid, lacrimal system and orbit (H00-H05)

EXCLUDES 2   open wound of eyelid (S01.1-)
superficial injury of eyelid (S00.1-, S00.2-)

✓4ᵗʰ H00   Hordeolum and chalazion

✓5ᵗʰ H00.0   Hordeolum (externum) (internum) of eyelid

✓6ᵗʰ H00.01   **Hordeolum externum**
Hordeolum NOS
Stye
    H00.011   **Hordeolum externum right upper eyelid**
    H00.012   **Hordeolum externum right lower eyelid**
    H00.013   **Hordeolum externum right eye, unspecified eyelid** ▽
    H00.014   **Hordeolum externum left upper eyelid**
    H00.015   **Hordeolum externum left lower eyelid**
    H00.016   **Hordeolum externum left eye, unspecified eyelid** ▽
    H00.019   **Hordeolum externum unspecified eye, unspecified eyelid** ▽

✓6ᵗʰ H00.02   **Hordeolum internum**
Infection of meibomian gland
    H00.021   **Hordeolum internum right upper eyelid**
    H00.022   **Hordeolum internum right lower eyelid**
    H00.023   **Hordeolum internum right eye, unspecified eyelid** ▽
    H00.024   **Hordeolum internum left upper eyelid**
    H00.025   **Hordeolum internum left lower eyelid**
    H00.026   **Hordeolum internum left eye, unspecified eyelid** ▽
    H00.029   **Hordeolum internum unspecified eye, unspecified eyelid** ▽

✓6ᵗʰ H00.03   **Abscess of eyelid**
Furuncle of eyelid
    H00.031   **Abscess of right upper eyelid**
    H00.032   **Abscess of right lower eyelid**
    H00.033   **Abscess of eyelid right eye, unspecified eyelid** ▽
    H00.034   **Abscess of left upper eyelid**
    H00.035   **Abscess of left lower eyelid**
    H00.036   **Abscess of eyelid left eye, unspecified eyelid** ▽
    H00.039   **Abscess of eyelid unspecified eye, unspecified eyelid** ▽

✓5ᵗʰ H00.1   **Chalazion**
Meibomian (gland) cyst
   EXCLUDES 2   infected meibomian gland (H00.02-)
    H00.11   **Chalazion right upper eyelid**
    H00.12   **Chalazion right lower eyelid**
    H00.13   **Chalazion right eye, unspecified eyelid** ▽
    H00.14   **Chalazion left upper eyelid**
    H00.15   **Chalazion left lower eyelid**
    H00.16   **Chalazion left eye, unspecified eyelid** ▽
    H00.19   **Chalazion unspecified eye, unspecified eyelid** ▽

✓4ᵗʰ H01   Other inflammation of eyelid

✓5ᵗʰ H01.0   **Blepharitis**
   EXCLUDES 1   blepharoconjunctivitis (H10.5-)

✓6ᵗʰ H01.00   **Unspecified blepharitis**
    H01.001   **Unspecified blepharitis right upper eyelid** ▽
    H01.002   **Unspecified blepharitis right lower eyelid** ▽
    H01.003   **Unspecified blepharitis right eye, unspecified eyelid** ▽
    H01.004   **Unspecified blepharitis left upper eyelid** ▽
    H01.005   **Unspecified blepharitis left lower eyelid** ▽
    H01.006   **Unspecified blepharitis left eye, unspecified eyelid** ▽
    H01.009   **Unspecified blepharitis unspecified eye, unspecified eyelid** ▽

✓6ᵗʰ H01.01   **Ulcerative blepharitis**
    H01.011   **Ulcerative blepharitis right upper eyelid**
    H01.012   **Ulcerative blepharitis right lower eyelid**
    H01.013   **Ulcerative blepharitis right eye, unspecified eyelid** ▽
    H01.014   **Ulcerative blepharitis left upper eyelid**
    H01.015   **Ulcerative blepharitis left lower eyelid**
    H01.016   **Ulcerative blepharitis left eye, unspecified eyelid** ▽
    H01.019   **Ulcerative blepharitis unspecified eye, unspecified eyelid** ▽

✓6ᵗʰ H01.02   **Squamous blepharitis**
    H01.021   **Squamous blepharitis right upper eyelid**
    H01.022   **Squamous blepharitis right lower eyelid**
    H01.023   **Squamous blepharitis right eye, unspecified eyelid** ▽
    H01.024   **Squamous blepharitis left upper eyelid**
    H01.025   **Squamous blepharitis left lower eyelid**
    H01.026   **Squamous blepharitis left eye, unspecified eyelid** ▽
    H01.029   **Squamous blepharitis unspecified eye, unspecified eyelid** ▽

✓5ᵗʰ H01.1   **Noninfectious dermatoses of eyelid**

✓6ᵗʰ H01.11   **Allergic dermatitis of eyelid**
Contact dermatitis of eyelid
    H01.111   **Allergic dermatitis of right upper eyelid**
    H01.112   **Allergic dermatitis of right lower eyelid**
    H01.113   **Allergic dermatitis of right eye, unspecified eyelid** ▽
    H01.114   **Allergic dermatitis of left upper eyelid**
    H01.115   **Allergic dermatitis of left lower eyelid**
    H01.116   **Allergic dermatitis of left eye, unspecified eyelid** ▽
    H01.119   **Allergic dermatitis of unspecified eye, unspecified eyelid** ▽

✓6ᵗʰ H01.12   **Discoid lupus erythematosus of eyelid**
    H01.121   **Discoid lupus erythematosus of right upper eyelid**
    H01.122   **Discoid lupus erythematosus of right lower eyelid**
    H01.123   **Discoid lupus erythematosus of right eye, unspecified eyelid** ▽
    H01.124   **Discoid lupus erythematosus of left upper eyelid**
    H01.125   **Discoid lupus erythematosus of left lower eyelid**

H01.126   **Discoid lupus erythematosus of** left eye, unspecified eyelid   ▽

H01.129   **Discoid lupus erythematosus of unspecified eye, unspecified eyelid**   ▽

✓6th **H01.13 Eczematous dermatitis of eyelid**

H01.131   **Eczematous dermatitis of** right upper eyelid

H01.132   **Eczematous dermatitis of** right lower eyelid

H01.133   **Eczematous dermatitis of** right eye, unspecified eyelid   ▽

H01.134   **Eczematous dermatitis of** left upper **eyelid**

H01.135   **Eczematous dermatitis of** left lower **eyelid**

H01.136   **Eczematous dermatitis of** left eye, unspecified eyelid   ▽

H01.139   **Eczematous dermatitis of unspecified eye, unspecified eyelid**   ▽

✓6th **H01.14 Xeroderma of eyelid**

H01.141   **Xeroderma of** right upper **eyelid**

H01.142   **Xeroderma of** right lower **eyelid**

H01.143   **Xeroderma of** right eye, **unspecified eyelid**   ▽

H01.144   **Xeroderma of** left upper **eyelid**

H01.145   **Xeroderma of** left lower **eyelid**

H01.146   **Xeroderma of** left eye, unspecified eyelid   ▽

H01.149   **Xeroderma of unspecified eye, unspecified eyelid**   ▽

H01.8 Other specified inflammations of eyelid

H01.9 Unspecified inflammation of eyelid   ▽
    Inflammation of eyelid NOS

✓4th **H02 Other disorders of eyelid**

   EXCLUDES 1   *congenital malformations of eyelid (Q10.0-Q10.3)*

✓5th **H02.0 Entropion and trichiasis of eyelid**

✓6th **H02.00 Unspecified entropion of eyelid**

H02.001   **Unspecified entropion of** right upper **eyelid**   ▽

H02.002   **Unspecified entropion of** right lower **eyelid**   ▽

H02.003   **Unspecified entropion of** right eye, unspecified eyelid   ▽

H02.004   **Unspecified entropion of** left upper **eyelid**   ▽

H02.005   **Unspecified entropion of** left lower **eyelid**   ▽

H02.006   **Unspecified entropion of** left eye, unspecified eyelid   ▽

H02.009   **Unspecified entropion of unspecified eye, unspecified eyelid**   ▽

✓6th **H02.01 Cicatricial entropion of eyelid**

H02.011   **Cicatricial entropion of** right upper **eyelid**

H02.012   **Cicatricial entropion of** right lower **eyelid**

H02.013   **Cicatricial entropion of** right eye, unspecified eyelid   ▽

H02.014   **Cicatricial entropion of** left upper **eyelid**

H02.015   **Cicatricial entropion of** left lower **eyelid**

H02.016   **Cicatricial entropion of** left eye, unspecified eyelid   ▽

H02.019   **Cicatricial entropion of unspecified eye, unspecified eyelid**   ▽

✓6th **H02.02 Mechanical entropion of eyelid**

H02.021   **Mechanical entropion of** right upper eyelid

H02.022   **Mechanical entropion of** right lower **eyelid**

H02.023   **Mechanical entropion of** right eye, unspecified eyelid   ▽

H02.024   **Mechanical entropion of** left upper **eyelid**

H02.025   **Mechanical entropion of** left lower **eyelid**

H02.026   **Mechanical entropion of** left eye, unspecified eyelid   ▽

H02.029   **Mechanical entropion of unspecified eye, unspecified eyelid**   ▽

✓6th **H02.03 Senile entropion of eyelid**

H02.031   **Senile entropion of** right upper **eyelid**   A

H02.032   **Senile entropion of** right lower **eyelid**   A

H02.033   **Senile entropion of** right eye, unspecified eyelid   A ▽

H02.034   **Senile entropion of** left upper **eyelid**   A

H02.035   **Senile entropion of** left lower **eyelid**   A

H02.036   **Senile entropion of** left eye, unspecified eyelid   A ▽

H02.039   **Senile entropion of unspecified eye, unspecified eyelid**   A ▽

✓6th **H02.04 Spastic entropion of eyelid**

H02.041   **Spastic entropion of** right upper **eyelid**

H02.042   **Spastic entropion of** right lower **eyelid**

H02.043   **Spastic entropion of** right eye, unspecified eyelid   ▽

H02.044   **Spastic entropion of** left upper **eyelid**

H02.045   **Spastic entropion of** left lower **eyelid**

H02.046   **Spastic entropion of** left eye, unspecified eyelid   ▽

H02.049   **Spastic entropion of unspecified eye, unspecified eyelid**   ▽

✓6th **H02.05 Trichiasis without entropion**

▲   H02.051   **Trichiasis without entropion** right upper eyelid

▲   H02.052   **Trichiasis without entropion** right lower **eyelid**

▲   H02.053   **Trichiasis without entropion** right eye, unspecified eyelid   ▽

▲   H02.054   **Trichiasis without entropion** left upper **eyelid**

▲   H02.055   **Trichiasis without entropion** left lower **eyelid**

▲   H02.056   **Trichiasis without entropion** left eye, unspecified eyelid   ▽

▲   H02.059   **Trichiasis without entropion unspecified eye, unspecified eyelid**   ▽

✓5th **H02.1 Ectropion of eyelid**

✓6th **H02.10 Unspecified ectropion of eyelid**

H02.101   **Unspecified ectropion of** right upper eyelid   ▽

H02.102   **Unspecified ectropion of** right lower eyelid   ▽

H02.103   **Unspecified ectropion of** right eye, unspecified eyelid   ▽

H02.104   **Unspecified ectropion of** left upper eyelid   ▽

H02.105   **Unspecified ectropion of** left lower eyelid   ▽

H02.106   **Unspecified ectropion of** left eye, unspecified eyelid   ▽

H02.109   **Unspecified ectropion of unspecified eye, unspecified eyelid**   ▽

✓6th **H02.11 Cicatricial ectropion of eyelid**

H02.111   **Cicatricial ectropion of** right upper **eyelid**

H02.112   **Cicatricial ectropion of** right lower **eyelid**

H02.113   **Cicatricial ectropion of** right eye, unspecified eyelid   ▽

H02.114   **Cicatricial ectropion of** left upper **eyelid**

H02.115   **Cicatricial ectropion of** left lower **eyelid**

H02.116   **Cicatricial ectropion of** left eye, unspecified eyelid   ▽

H02.119   **Cicatricial ectropion of unspecified eye, unspecified eyelid**   ▽

Entropion and Ectropion

Normal eyelid   Entropion   Ectropion

☑ Additional Character Req   ✓x7th Placeholder Alert   Manifestation   HCC CMS-HCC Condition   ▽ Unspecified Code   ►◄ Revised Text   ● New Code   ▲ Revised Code Title

✓6ᵗʰ **H02.12** Mechanical **ectropion of eyelid**
- H02.121 Mechanical ectropion of right upper eyelid
- H02.122 Mechanical ectropion of right lower eyelid
- H02.123 Mechanical ectropion of right eye, unspecified eyelid ▽
- H02.124 Mechanical ectropion of left upper eyelid
- H02.125 Mechanical ectropion of left lower eyelid
- H02.126 Mechanical ectropion of left eye, unspecified eyelid ▽
- H02.129 Mechanical ectropion of unspecified eye, unspecified eyelid ▽

✓6ᵗʰ **H02.13** Senile **ectropion of eyelid**
- H02.131 Senile ectropion of right upper eyelid Ⓐ
- H02.132 Senile ectropion of right lower eyelid Ⓐ
- H02.133 Senile ectropion of right eye, unspecified eyelid Ⓐ▽
- H02.134 Senile ectropion of left upper eyelid Ⓐ
- H02.135 Senile ectropion of left lower eyelid Ⓐ
- H02.136 Senile ectropion of left eye, unspecified eyelid Ⓐ▽
- H02.139 Senile ectropion of unspecified eye, unspecified eyelid Ⓐ▽

✓6ᵗʰ **H02.14** Spastic **ectropion of eyelid**
- H02.141 Spastic ectropion of right upper eyelid
- H02.142 Spastic ectropion of right lower eyelid
- H02.143 Spastic ectropion of right eye, unspecified eyelid ▽
- H02.144 Spastic ectropion of left upper eyelid
- H02.145 Spastic ectropion of left lower eyelid
- H02.146 Spastic ectropion of left eye, unspecified eyelid ▽
- H02.149 Spastic ectropion of unspecified eye, unspecified eyelid ▽

✓5ᵗʰ **H02.2 Lagophthalmos**

✓6ᵗʰ **H02.20** Unspecified **lagophthalmos**
- H02.201 Unspecified lagophthalmos right upper eyelid ▽
- H02.202 Unspecified lagophthalmos right lower eyelid ▽
- H02.203 Unspecified lagophthalmos right eye, unspecified eyelid ▽
- H02.204 Unspecified lagophthalmos left upper eyelid ▽
- H02.205 Unspecified lagophthalmos left lower eyelid ▽
- H02.206 Unspecified lagophthalmos left eye, unspecified eyelid ▽
- H02.209 Unspecified lagophthalmos unspecified eye, unspecified eyelid ▽

✓6ᵗʰ **H02.21** Cicatricial **lagophthalmos**
- H02.211 Cicatricial lagophthalmos right upper eyelid
- H02.212 Cicatricial lagophthalmos right lower eyelid
- H02.213 Cicatricial lagophthalmos right eye, unspecified eyelid ▽
- H02.214 Cicatricial lagophthalmos left upper eyelid
- H02.215 Cicatricial lagophthalmos left lower eyelid
- H02.216 Cicatricial lagophthalmos left eye, unspecified eyelid ▽
- H02.219 Cicatricial lagophthalmos unspecified eye, unspecified eyelid ▽

✓6ᵗʰ **H02.22** Mechanical **lagophthalmos**
- H02.221 Mechanical lagophthalmos right upper eyelid
- H02.222 Mechanical lagophthalmos right lower eyelid
- H02.223 Mechanical lagophthalmos right eye, unspecified eyelid ▽
- H02.224 Mechanical lagophthalmos left upper eyelid
- H02.225 Mechanical lagophthalmos left lower eyelid
- H02.226 Mechanical lagophthalmos left eye, unspecified eyelid ▽
- H02.229 Mechanical lagophthalmos unspecified eye, unspecified eyelid ▽

✓6ᵗʰ **H02.23** Paralytic **lagophthalmos**
- H02.231 Paralytic lagophthalmos right upper eyelid
- H02.232 Paralytic lagophthalmos right lower eyelid
- H02.233 Paralytic lagophthalmos right eye, unspecified eyelid ▽
- H02.234 Paralytic lagophthalmos left upper eyelid
- H02.235 Paralytic lagophthalmos left lower eyelid
- H02.236 Paralytic lagophthalmos left eye, unspecified eyelid ▽
- H02.239 Paralytic lagophthalmos unspecified eye, unspecified eyelid ▽

✓5ᵗʰ **H02.3 Blepharochalasis**
Pseudoptosis
- H02.30 Blepharochalasis unspecified eye, unspecified eyelid ▽
- H02.31 Blepharochalasis right upper eyelid
- H02.32 Blepharochalasis right lower eyelid
- H02.33 Blepharochalasis right eye, unspecified eyelid ▽
- H02.34 Blepharochalasis left upper eyelid
- H02.35 Blepharochalasis left lower eyelid
- H02.36 Blepharochalasis left eye, unspecified eyelid ▽

✓5ᵗʰ **H02.4 Ptosis of eyelid**

✓6ᵗʰ **H02.40** Unspecified **ptosis of eyelid**
- H02.401 Unspecified ptosis of right eyelid ▽
- H02.402 Unspecified ptosis of left eyelid ▽
- H02.403 Unspecified ptosis of bilateral eyelids ▽
- H02.409 Unspecified ptosis of unspecified eyelid ▽

✓6ᵗʰ **H02.41** Mechanical **ptosis of eyelid**
- H02.411 Mechanical ptosis of right eyelid
- H02.412 Mechanical ptosis of left eyelid
- H02.413 Mechanical ptosis of bilateral eyelids
- H02.419 Mechanical ptosis of unspecified eyelid ▽

✓6ᵗʰ **H02.42** Myogenic **ptosis of eyelid**
- H02.421 Myogenic ptosis of right eyelid
- H02.422 Myogenic ptosis of left eyelid
- H02.423 Myogenic ptosis of bilateral eyelids
- H02.429 Myogenic ptosis of unspecified eyelid ▽

✓6ᵗʰ **H02.43** Paralytic **ptosis of eyelid**
Neurogenic ptosis of eyelid
- H02.431 Paralytic ptosis of right eyelid
- H02.432 Paralytic ptosis of left eyelid
- H02.433 Paralytic ptosis of bilateral eyelids
- H02.439 Paralytic ptosis unspecified eyelid ▽

✓5ᵗʰ **H02.5 Other disorders affecting eyelid function**
EXCLUDES 2   blepharospasm (G24.5)
    organic tic (G25.69)
    psychogenic tic (F95.-)

✓6ᵗʰ **H02.51** Abnormal **innervation syndrome**
- H02.511 Abnormal innervation syndrome right upper eyelid
- H02.512 Abnormal innervation syndrome right lower eyelid
- H02.513 Abnormal innervation syndrome right eye, unspecified eyelid ▽
- H02.514 Abnormal innervation syndrome left upper eyelid
- H02.515 Abnormal innervation syndrome left lower eyelid
- H02.516 Abnormal innervation syndrome left eye, unspecified eyelid ▽
- H02.519 Abnormal innervation syndrome unspecified eye, unspecified eyelid ▽

✓6ᵗʰ **H02.52** Blepharophimosis
Ankyloblepharon
- H02.521 Blepharophimosis right upper eyelid
- H02.522 Blepharophimosis right lower eyelid
- H02.523 Blepharophimosis right eye, unspecified eyelid ▽
- H02.524 Blepharophimosis left upper eyelid
- H02.525 Blepharophimosis left lower eyelid
- H02.526 Blepharophimosis left eye, unspecified eyelid ▽

H02.529 **Blepharophimosis unspecified eye, unspecified lid** ▽

✓6th **H02.53 Eyelid retraction**
Eyelid lag

H02.531 **Eyelid retraction** right upper **eyelid**

H02.532 **Eyelid retraction** right lower **eyelid**

H02.533 **Eyelid retraction** right eye, unspecified **eyelid** ▽

H02.534 **Eyelid retraction** left upper **eyelid**

H02.535 **Eyelid retraction** left lower **eyelid**

H02.536 **Eyelid retraction** left eye, unspecified **eyelid** ▽

H02.539 **Eyelid retraction unspecified eye, unspecified lid** ▽

H02.59 **Other disorders affecting eyelid function**
Deficient blink reflex
Sensory disorders

✓5th **H02.6 Xanthelasma of eyelid**

H02.60 **Xanthelasma of unspecified eye, unspecified eyelid** ▽

H02.61 **Xanthelasma of** right upper **eyelid**

H02.62 **Xanthelasma of** right lower **eyelid**

H02.63 **Xanthelasma of** right eye, unspecified **eyelid** ▽

H02.64 **Xanthelasma of** left upper **eyelid**

H02.65 **Xanthelasma of** left lower **eyelid**

H02.66 **Xanthelasma of** left eye, unspecified **eyelid** ▽

✓5th **H02.7 Other and unspecified degenerative disorders of eyelid and periocular area**

H02.70 **Unspecified degenerative disorders of eyelid and periocular area** ▽

✓6th **H02.71 Chloasma of eyelid and periocular area**
Dyspigmentation of eyelid
Hyperpigmentation of eyelid

H02.711 **Chloasma of** right upper **eyelid and periocular area**

H02.712 **Chloasma of** right lower **eyelid and periocular area**

H02.713 **Chloasma of** right eye, unspecified **eyelid and periocular area** ▽

H02.714 **Chloasma of** left upper **eyelid and periocular area**

H02.715 **Chloasma of** left lower **eyelid and periocular area**

H02.716 **Chloasma of** left eye, unspecified **eyelid and periocular area** ▽

H02.719 **Chloasma of unspecified eye, unspecified eyelid and periocular area** ▽

✓6th **H02.72 Madarosis of eyelid and periocular area**
Hypotrichosis of eyelid

H02.721 **Madarosis of** right upper **eyelid and periocular area**

H02.722 **Madarosis of** right lower **eyelid and periocular area**

H02.723 **Madarosis of** right eye, unspecified **eyelid and periocular area** ▽

H02.724 **Madarosis of** left upper **eyelid and periocular area**

H02.725 **Madarosis of** left lower **eyelid and periocular area**

H02.726 **Madarosis of** left eye, unspecified **eyelid and periocular area** ▽

H02.729 **Madarosis of unspecified eye, unspecified eyelid and periocular area** ▽

✓6th **H02.73 Vitiligo of eyelid and periocular area**
Hypopigmentation of eyelid

H02.731 **Vitiligo of** right upper **eyelid and periocular area**

H02.732 **Vitiligo of** right lower **eyelid and periocular area**

H02.733 **Vitiligo of** right eye, unspecified **eyelid and periocular area** ▽

H02.734 **Vitiligo of** left upper **eyelid and periocular area**

H02.735 **Vitiligo of** left lower **eyelid and periocular area**

H02.736 **Vitiligo of** left eye, unspecified **eyelid and periocular area** ▽

H02.739 **Vitiligo of unspecified eye, unspecified eyelid and periocular area** ▽

H02.79 **Other degenerative disorders of eyelid and periocular area**

✓5th **H02.8 Other specified disorders of eyelid**

✓6th **H02.81 Retained foreign body in eyelid**
Use additional code to identify the type of retained foreign body (Z18.-)
EXCLUDES 1 *laceration of eyelid with foreign body (S01.12-)*
retained intraocular foreign body (H44.6-, H44.7-)
superficial foreign body of eyelid and periocular area (S00.25-)

H02.811 **Retained foreign body in** right upper **eyelid**

H02.812 **Retained foreign body in** right lower **eyelid**

H02.813 **Retained foreign body in** right eye, unspecified **eyelid** ▽

H02.814 **Retained foreign body in** left upper **eyelid**

H02.815 **Retained foreign body in** left lower **eyelid**

H02.816 **Retained foreign body in** left eye, unspecified **eyelid** ▽

H02.819 **Retained foreign body in unspecified eye, unspecified eyelid** ▽

✓6th **H02.82 Cysts of eyelid**
Sebaceous cyst of eyelid

H02.821 **Cysts of** right upper **eyelid**

H02.822 **Cysts of** right lower **eyelid**

H02.823 **Cysts of** right eye, unspecified **eyelid** ▽

H02.824 **Cysts of** left upper **eyelid**

H02.825 **Cysts of** left lower **eyelid**

H02.826 **Cysts of** left eye, unspecified **eyelid** ▽

H02.829 **Cysts of unspecified eye, unspecified eyelid** ▽

✓6th **H02.83 Dermatochalasis of eyelid**
DEF: Acquired form of connective tissue disorder associated with decreased elastic tissue and abnormal elastin formation, resulting in loss of elasticity of the skin of the eyelid; generally associated with aging.

H02.831 **Dermatochalasis of** right upper **eyelid**

H02.832 **Dermatochalasis of** right lower **eyelid**

H02.833 **Dermatochalasis of** right eye, unspecified **eyelid** ▽

H02.834 **Dermatochalasis of** left upper **eyelid**

H02.835 **Dermatochalasis of** left lower **eyelid**

H02.836 **Dermatochalasis of** left eye, unspecified **eyelid** ▽

H02.839 **Dermatochalasis of unspecified eye, unspecified eyelid** ▽

✓6th **H02.84 Edema of eyelid**
Hyperemia of eyelid

H02.841 **Edema of** right upper **eyelid**

H02.842 **Edema of** right lower **eyelid**

H02.843 **Edema of** right eye, unspecified **eyelid** ▽

H02.844 **Edema of** left upper **eyelid**

H02.845 **Edema of** left lower **eyelid**

H02.846 **Edema of** left eye, unspecified **eyelid** ▽

H02.849 **Edema of unspecified eye, unspecified eyelid** ▽

✓6th **H02.85 Elephantiasis of eyelid**

H02.851 **Elephantiasis of** right upper **eyelid**

H02.852 **Elephantiasis of** right lower **eyelid**

H02.853 **Elephantiasis of** right eye, unspecified **eyelid** ▽

H02.854 **Elephantiasis of** left upper **eyelid**

H02.855 **Elephantiasis of** left lower **eyelid**

H02.856 **Elephantiasis of** left eye, unspecified **eyelid** ▽

H02.859 **Elephantiasis of unspecified eye, unspecified eyelid** ▽

✓6th **H02.86 Hypertrichosis of eyelid**

H02.861 **Hypertrichosis of** right upper **eyelid**

H02.862 **Hypertrichosis of** right lower **eyelid**

H02.863 **Hypertrichosis of** right eye, unspecified **eyelid** ▽

✓ Additional Character Req   ✓x7th Placeholder Alert   Manifestation   HCC CMS-HCC Condition   ▽ Unspecified Code   ►◄ Revised Text   ● New Code   ▲ Revised Code Title

H02.864 Hypertrichosis of left upper eyelid

H02.865 Hypertrichosis of left lower eyelid

H02.866 Hypertrichosis of left eye, unspecified eyelid ▽

H02.869 Hypertrichosis of unspecified eye, unspecified eyelid ▽

✓6th **H02.87** Vascular anomalies of eyelid

H02.871 Vascular anomalies of right upper eyelid

H02.872 Vascular anomalies of right lower eyelid

H02.873 Vascular anomalies of right eye, unspecified eyelid ▽

H02.874 Vascular anomalies of left upper eyelid

H02.875 Vascular anomalies of left lower eyelid

H02.876 Vascular anomalies of left eye, unspecified eyelid ▽

H02.879 Vascular anomalies of unspecified eye, unspecified eyelid ▽

H02.89 Other specified disorders of eyelid
Hemorrhage of eyelid

H02.9 Unspecified disorder of eyelid ▽
Disorder of eyelid NOS

✓4th **H04** Disorders of lacrimal system
EXCLUDES 1 congenital malformations of lacrimal system (Q10.4-Q10.6)

✓5th **H04.0** Dacryoadenitis

✓6th **H04.00** Unspecified dacryoadenitis

H04.001 Unspecified dacryoadenitis, right lacrimal gland ▽

H04.002 Unspecified dacryoadenitis, left lacrimal gland ▽

H04.003 Unspecified dacryoadenitis, bilateral lacrimal glands ▽

H04.009 Unspecified dacryoadenitis, unspecified lacrimal gland ▽

✓6th **H04.01** Acute dacryoadenitis

H04.011 Acute dacryoadenitis, right lacrimal gland

H04.012 Acute dacryoadenitis, left lacrimal gland

H04.013 Acute dacryoadenitis, bilateral lacrimal glands

H04.019 Acute dacryoadenitis, unspecified lacrimal gland ▽

✓6th **H04.02** Chronic dacryoadenitis

H04.021 Chronic dacryoadenitis, right lacrimal gland

H04.022 Chronic dacryoadenitis, left lacrimal gland

H04.023 Chronic dacryoadenitis, bilateral lacrimal glands

H04.029 Chronic dacryoadenitis, unspecified lacrimal gland ▽

✓6th **H04.03** Chronic enlargement of lacrimal gland

H04.031 Chronic enlargement of right lacrimal gland

H04.032 Chronic enlargement of left lacrimal gland

H04.033 Chronic enlargement of bilateral lacrimal glands

H04.039 Chronic enlargement of unspecified lacrimal gland ▽

✓5th **H04.1** Other disorders of lacrimal gland

✓6th **H04.11** Dacryops

H04.111 Dacryops of right lacrimal gland

H04.112 Dacryops of left lacrimal gland

H04.113 Dacryops of bilateral lacrimal glands

H04.119 Dacryops of unspecified lacrimal gland ▽

✓6th **H04.12** Dry eye syndrome
Tear film insufficiency, NOS

H04.121 Dry eye syndrome of right lacrimal gland

H04.122 Dry eye syndrome of left lacrimal gland

H04.123 Dry eye syndrome of bilateral lacrimal glands

H04.129 Dry eye syndrome of unspecified lacrimal gland ▽

✓6th **H04.13** Lacrimal cyst
Lacrimal cystic degeneration

H04.131 Lacrimal cyst, right lacrimal gland

H04.132 Lacrimal cyst, left lacrimal gland

H04.133 Lacrimal cyst, bilateral lacrimal glands

H04.139 Lacrimal cyst, unspecified lacrimal gland ▽

✓6th **H04.14** Primary lacrimal gland atrophy

H04.141 Primary lacrimal gland atrophy, right lacrimal gland

H04.142 Primary lacrimal gland atrophy, left lacrimal gland

H04.143 Primary lacrimal gland atrophy, bilateral lacrimal glands

H04.149 Primary lacrimal gland atrophy, unspecified lacrimal gland ▽

✓6th **H04.15** Secondary lacrimal gland atrophy

H04.151 Secondary lacrimal gland atrophy, right lacrimal gland

H04.152 Secondary lacrimal gland atrophy, left lacrimal gland

H04.153 Secondary lacrimal gland atrophy, bilateral lacrimal glands

H04.159 Secondary lacrimal gland atrophy, unspecified lacrimal gland ▽

✓6th **H04.16** Lacrimal gland dislocation

H04.161 Lacrimal gland dislocation, right lacrimal gland

H04.162 Lacrimal gland dislocation, left lacrimal gland

H04.163 Lacrimal gland dislocation, bilateral lacrimal glands

H04.169 Lacrimal gland dislocation, unspecified lacrimal gland ▽

H04.19 Other specified disorders of lacrimal gland

✓5th **H04.2** Epiphora

✓6th **H04.20** Unspecified epiphora

H04.201 Unspecified epiphora, right lacrimal gland ▽

H04.202 Unspecified epiphora, left lacrimal gland ▽

H04.203 Unspecified epiphora, bilateral lacrimal glands ▽

H04.209 Unspecified epiphora, unspecified lacrimal gland ▽

✓6th **H04.21** Epiphora due to excess lacrimation

H04.211 Epiphora due to excess lacrimation, right lacrimal gland

H04.212 Epiphora due to excess lacrimation, left lacrimal gland

H04.213 Epiphora due to excess lacrimation, bilateral lacrimal glands

H04.219 Epiphora due to excess lacrimation, unspecified lacrimal gland ▽

✓6th **H04.22** Epiphora due to insufficient drainage

H04.221 Epiphora due to insufficient drainage, right lacrimal gland

H04.222 Epiphora due to insufficient drainage, left lacrimal gland

H04.223 Epiphora due to insufficient drainage, bilateral lacrimal glands

H04.229 Epiphora due to insufficient drainage, unspecified lacrimal gland ▽

✓5th **H04.3** Acute and unspecified inflammation of lacrimal passages
EXCLUDES 1 neonatal dacryocystitis (P39.1)

✓6th **H04.30** Unspecified dacryocystitis

H04.301 Unspecified dacryocystitis of right lacrimal passage ▽

H04.302 Unspecified dacryocystitis of left lacrimal passage ▽

H04.303 Unspecified dacryocystitis of bilateral lacrimal passages ▽

H04.309 Unspecified dacryocystitis of unspecified lacrimal passage ▽

✓6th **H04.31** Phlegmonous dacryocystitis

H04.311 Phlegmonous dacryocystitis of right lacrimal passage

H04.312 Phlegmonous dacryocystitis of left lacrimal passage

H04.313 Phlegmonous dacryocystitis of bilateral lacrimal passages

EXCLUDES 1 Not coded here   EXCLUDES 2 Not included here   N Newborn Age: 0   P Pediatric Age: 0-17   M Maternity Age: 12-55   A Adult Age: 15-124

574   ICD-10-CM 2018

H04.319   Phlegmonous dacryocystitis of unspecified lacrimal passage ▽

✓6ᵗʰ **H04.32**   Acute **dacryocystitis**
Acute dacryopericystitis
H04.321   Acute dacryocystitis of right lacrimal passage
H04.322   Acute dacryocystitis of left lacrimal passage
H04.323   Acute dacryocystitis of bilateral lacrimal passages
H04.329   Acute dacryocystitis of unspecified lacrimal passage ▽

✓6ᵗʰ **H04.33**   Acute lacrimal canaliculitis
H04.331   Acute lacrimal canaliculitis of right lacrimal passage
H04.332   Acute lacrimal canaliculitis of left lacrimal passage
H04.333   Acute lacrimal canaliculitis of bilateral lacrimal passages
H04.339   Acute lacrimal canaliculitis of unspecified lacrimal passage ▽

✓5ᵗʰ **H04.4**   Chronic inflammation of lacrimal passages
✓6ᵗʰ **H04.41**   Chronic dacryocystitis
H04.411   Chronic dacryocystitis of right lacrimal passage
H04.412   Chronic dacryocystitis of left lacrimal passage
H04.413   Chronic dacryocystitis of bilateral lacrimal passages
H04.419   Chronic dacryocystitis of unspecified lacrimal passage ▽

✓6ᵗʰ **H04.42**   Chronic lacrimal canaliculitis
H04.421   Chronic lacrimal canaliculitis of right lacrimal passage
H04.422   Chronic lacrimal canaliculitis of left lacrimal passage
H04.423   Chronic lacrimal canaliculitis of bilateral lacrimal passages
H04.429   Chronic lacrimal canaliculitis of unspecified lacrimal passage ▽

✓6ᵗʰ **H04.43**   Chronic lacrimal mucocele
H04.431   Chronic lacrimal mucocele of right lacrimal passage
H04.432   Chronic lacrimal mucocele of left lacrimal passage
H04.433   Chronic lacrimal mucocele of bilateral lacrimal passages
H04.439   Chronic lacrimal mucocele of unspecified lacrimal passage ▽

✓5ᵗʰ **H04.5**   Stenosis and insufficiency of lacrimal passages
✓6ᵗʰ **H04.51**   Dacryolith
H04.511   Dacryolith of right lacrimal passage
H04.512   Dacryolith of left lacrimal passage
H04.513   Dacryolith of bilateral lacrimal passages
H04.519   Dacryolith of unspecified lacrimal passage ▽

✓6ᵗʰ **H04.52**   Eversion of lacrimal punctum
H04.521   Eversion of right lacrimal punctum
H04.522   Eversion of left lacrimal punctum
H04.523   Eversion of bilateral lacrimal punctum
H04.529   Eversion of unspecified lacrimal punctum ▽

✓6ᵗʰ **H04.53**   Neonatal obstruction of nasolacrimal duct
EXCLUDES1   congenital stenosis and stricture of lacrimal duct (Q10.5)
H04.531   Neonatal obstruction of right nasolacrimal duct N
H04.532   Neonatal obstruction of left nasolacrimal duct N
H04.533   Neonatal obstruction of bilateral nasolacrimal duct N
H04.539   Neonatal obstruction of unspecified nasolacrimal duct N ▽

✓6ᵗʰ **H04.54**   Stenosis of lacrimal canaliculi
H04.541   Stenosis of right lacrimal canaliculi
H04.542   Stenosis of left lacrimal canaliculi

H04.543   Stenosis of bilateral lacrimal canaliculi
H04.549   Stenosis of unspecified lacrimal canaliculi ▽

✓6ᵗʰ **H04.55**   Acquired stenosis of nasolacrimal duct
H04.551   Acquired stenosis of right nasolacrimal duct
H04.552   Acquired stenosis of left nasolacrimal duct
H04.553   Acquired stenosis of bilateral nasolacrimal duct
H04.559   Acquired stenosis of unspecified nasolacrimal duct ▽

✓6ᵗʰ **H04.56**   Stenosis of lacrimal punctum
H04.561   Stenosis of right lacrimal punctum
H04.562   Stenosis of left lacrimal punctum
H04.563   Stenosis of bilateral lacrimal punctum
H04.569   Stenosis of unspecified lacrimal punctum ▽

✓6ᵗʰ **H04.57**   Stenosis of lacrimal sac
H04.571   Stenosis of right lacrimal sac
H04.572   Stenosis of left lacrimal sac
H04.573   Stenosis of bilateral lacrimal sac
H04.579   Stenosis of unspecified lacrimal sac ▽

✓5ᵗʰ **H04.6**   Other changes of lacrimal passages
✓6ᵗʰ **H04.61**   Lacrimal fistula
H04.611   Lacrimal fistula right lacrimal passage
H04.612   Lacrimal fistula left lacrimal passage
H04.613   Lacrimal fistula bilateral lacrimal passages
H04.619   Lacrimal fistula unspecified lacrimal passage ▽

H04.69   Other changes of lacrimal passages

✓5ᵗʰ **H04.8**   Other disorders of lacrimal system
✓6ᵗʰ **H04.81**   Granuloma of lacrimal passages
H04.811   Granuloma of right lacrimal passage
H04.812   Granuloma of left lacrimal passage
H04.813   Granuloma of bilateral lacrimal passages
H04.819   Granuloma of unspecified lacrimal passage ▽

H04.89   Other disorders of lacrimal system
H04.9   Disorder of lacrimal system, unspecified ▽

✓4ᵗʰ **H05**   **Disorders of orbit**
EXCLUDES1   congenital malformation of orbit (Q10.7)
✓5ᵗʰ **H05.0**   Acute inflammation of orbit
H05.00   Unspecified acute inflammation of orbit ▽
✓6ᵗʰ **H05.01**   Cellulitis of orbit
Abscess of orbit
H05.011   Cellulitis of right orbit
H05.012   Cellulitis of left orbit
H05.013   Cellulitis of bilateral orbits
H05.019   Cellulitis of unspecified orbit ▽
✓6ᵗʰ **H05.02**   Osteomyelitis of orbit
H05.021   Osteomyelitis of right orbit
H05.022   Osteomyelitis of left orbit
H05.023   Osteomyelitis of bilateral orbits
H05.029   Osteomyelitis of unspecified orbit ▽
✓6ᵗʰ **H05.03**   Periostitis of orbit
H05.031   Periostitis of right orbit
H05.032   Periostitis of left orbit
H05.033   Periostitis of bilateral orbits
H05.039   Periostitis of unspecified orbit ▽
✓6ᵗʰ **H05.04**   Tenonitis of orbit
H05.041   Tenonitis of right orbit
H05.042   Tenonitis of left orbit
H05.043   Tenonitis of bilateral orbits
H05.049   Tenonitis of unspecified orbit ▽

✓5ᵗʰ **H05.1**   Chronic inflammatory disorders of orbit
H05.10   Unspecified chronic inflammatory disorders of orbit ▽
✓6ᵗʰ **H05.11**   Granuloma of orbit
Pseudotumor (inflammatory) of orbit
H05.111   Granuloma of right orbit
H05.112   Granuloma of left orbit
H05.113   Granuloma of bilateral orbits

H05.119   Granuloma of unspecified orbit ▽

✓6ᵗʰ **H05.12**   **Orbital** myositis
   H05.121   Orbital myositis, right orbit
   H05.122   Orbital myositis, left orbit
   H05.123   Orbital myositis, bilateral
   H05.129   Orbital myositis, unspecified orbit ▽

✓5ᵗʰ **H05.2**   **Exophthalmic conditions**
   H05.20   Unspecified exophthalmos ▽
✓6ᵗʰ **H05.21**   **Displacement (lateral) of globe**
   H05.211   Displacement (lateral) of globe, right eye
   H05.212   Displacement (lateral) of globe, left eye
   H05.213   Displacement (lateral) of globe, bilateral
   H05.219   Displacement (lateral) of globe, unspecified eye ▽

✓6ᵗʰ **H05.22**   **Edema of orbit**
     Orbital congestion
   H05.221   Edema of right orbit
   H05.222   Edema of left orbit
   H05.223   Edema of bilateral orbit
   H05.229   Edema of unspecified orbit ▽

✓6ᵗʰ **H05.23**   **Hemorrhage of orbit**
   H05.231   Hemorrhage of right orbit
   H05.232   Hemorrhage of left orbit
   H05.233   Hemorrhage of bilateral orbit
   H05.239   Hemorrhage of unspecified orbit ▽

✓6ᵗʰ **H05.24**   **Constant** exophthalmos
   H05.241   Constant exophthalmos, right eye
   H05.242   Constant exophthalmos, left eye
   H05.243   Constant exophthalmos, bilateral
   H05.249   Constant exophthalmos, unspecified eye ▽

✓6ᵗʰ **H05.25**   **Intermittent** exophthalmos
   H05.251   Intermittent exophthalmos, right eye
   H05.252   Intermittent exophthalmos, left eye
   H05.253   Intermittent exophthalmos, bilateral
   H05.259   Intermittent exophthalmos, unspecified eye ▽

✓6ᵗʰ **H05.26**   **Pulsating** exophthalmos
   H05.261   Pulsating exophthalmos, right eye
   H05.262   Pulsating exophthalmos, left eye
   H05.263   Pulsating exophthalmos, bilateral
   H05.269   Pulsating exophthalmos, unspecified eye ▽

✓5ᵗʰ **H05.3**   **Deformity of orbit**
    EXCLUDES 1   *congenital deformity of orbit (Q10.7)*
           hypertelorism (Q75.2)
   H05.30   Unspecified deformity of orbit ▽
✓6ᵗʰ **H05.31**   **Atrophy** of orbit
   H05.311   Atrophy of right orbit
   H05.312   Atrophy of left orbit
   H05.313   Atrophy of bilateral orbit
   H05.319   Atrophy of unspecified orbit ▽

✓6ᵗʰ **H05.32**   **Deformity of orbit** due to bone disease
     Code also associated bone disease
   H05.321   Deformity of right orbit due to bone disease
   H05.322   Deformity of left orbit due to bone disease
   H05.323   Deformity of bilateral orbits due to bone disease
   H05.329   Deformity of unspecified orbit due to bone disease ▽

✓6ᵗʰ **H05.33**   **Deformity of orbit** due to trauma or surgery
   H05.331   Deformity of right orbit due to trauma or surgery
   H05.332   Deformity of left orbit due to trauma or surgery
   H05.333   Deformity of bilateral orbits due to trauma or surgery
   H05.339   Deformity of unspecified orbit due to trauma or surgery ▽

✓6ᵗʰ **H05.34**   **Enlargement** of orbit
   H05.341   Enlargement of right orbit
   H05.342   Enlargement of left orbit
   H05.343   Enlargement of bilateral orbits

H05.349   Enlargement of unspecified orbit ▽

✓6ᵗʰ **H05.35**   **Exostosis** of orbit
   H05.351   Exostosis of right orbit
   H05.352   Exostosis of left orbit
   H05.353   Exostosis of bilateral orbits
   H05.359   Exostosis of unspecified orbit ▽

✓5ᵗʰ **H05.4**   **Enophthalmos**
✓6ᵗʰ **H05.40**   **Unspecified enophthalmos**
   H05.401   Unspecified enophthalmos, right eye ▽
   H05.402   Unspecified enophthalmos, left eye ▽
   H05.403   Unspecified enophthalmos, bilateral ▽
   H05.409   Unspecified enophthalmos, unspecified eye ▽

✓6ᵗʰ **H05.41**   **Enophthalmos** due to atrophy of orbital tissue
   H05.411   Enophthalmos due to atrophy of orbital tissue, right eye
   H05.412   Enophthalmos due to atrophy of orbital tissue, left eye
   H05.413   Enophthalmos due to atrophy of orbital tissue, bilateral
   H05.419   Enophthalmos due to atrophy of orbital tissue, unspecified eye ▽

✓6ᵗʰ **H05.42**   **Enophthalmos** due to trauma or surgery
   H05.421   Enophthalmos due to trauma or surgery, right eye
   H05.422   Enophthalmos due to trauma or surgery, left eye
   H05.423   Enophthalmos due to trauma or surgery, bilateral
   H05.429   Enophthalmos due to trauma or surgery, unspecified eye ▽

✓5ᵗʰ **H05.5**   **Retained (old) foreign body following penetrating wound of orbit**
     Retrobulbar foreign body
     Use additional code to identify the type of retained foreign body (Z18.-)
    EXCLUDES 1   *current penetrating wound of orbit (S05.4-)*
    EXCLUDES 2   *retained foreign body of eyelid (H02.81-)*
            retained intraocular foreign body (H44.6-, H44.7-)
   H05.50   Retained (old) foreign body following penetrating wound of unspecified orbit ▽
   H05.51   Retained (old) foreign body following penetrating wound of right orbit
   H05.52   Retained (old) foreign body following penetrating wound of left orbit
   H05.53   Retained (old) foreign body following penetrating wound of bilateral orbits

✓5ᵗʰ **H05.8**   **Other disorders of orbit**
✓6ᵗʰ **H05.81**   **Cyst of orbit**
     Encephalocele of orbit
   H05.811   Cyst of right orbit
   H05.812   Cyst of left orbit
   H05.813   Cyst of bilateral orbits
   H05.819   Cyst of unspecified orbit ▽

✓6ᵗʰ **H05.82**   **Myopathy of extraocular muscles**
   H05.821   Myopathy of extraocular muscles, right orbit
   H05.822   Myopathy of extraocular muscles, left orbit
   H05.823   Myopathy of extraocular muscles, bilateral
   H05.829   Myopathy of extraocular muscles, unspecified orbit ▽

   H05.89   Other disorders of orbit
H05.9   Unspecified disorder of orbit ▽

Disorders of conjunctiva (H10-H11)

✓4ᵗʰ **H10**   **Conjunctivitis**
    EXCLUDES 1   *keratoconjunctivitis (H16.2-)*
✓5ᵗʰ **H10.0**   **Mucopurulent** conjunctivitis
✓6ᵗʰ **H10.01**   **Acute follicular conjunctivitis**
   H10.011   Acute follicular conjunctivitis, right eye
   H10.012   Acute follicular conjunctivitis, left eye
   H10.013   Acute follicular conjunctivitis, bilateral

EXCLUDES 1 Not coded here   *EXCLUDES 2* Not included here   N Newborn Age: 0   P Pediatric Age: 0-17   M Maternity Age: 12-55   A Adult Age: 15-124

576   ICD-10-CM 2018

      H10.019   **Acute follicular conjunctivitis, unspecified eye** ▽

✓6ᵗʰ **H10.02**   **Other mucopurulent conjunctivitis**
      H10.021   **Other mucopurulent conjunctivitis, right eye**
      H10.022   **Other mucopurulent conjunctivitis, left eye**
      H10.023   **Other mucopurulent conjunctivitis, bilateral**
      H10.029   **Other mucopurulent conjunctivitis, unspecified eye** ▽

✓5ᵗʰ **H10.1**   **Acute atopic conjunctivitis**
    Acute papillary conjunctivitis
    H10.10   **Acute atopic conjunctivitis, unspecified eye** ▽
    H10.11   **Acute atopic conjunctivitis, right eye**
    H10.12   **Acute atopic conjunctivitis, left eye**
    H10.13   **Acute atopic conjunctivitis, bilateral**

✓5ᵗʰ **H10.2**   **Other acute conjunctivitis**
    ✓6ᵗʰ **H10.21**   **Acute toxic conjunctivitis**
      Acute chemical conjunctivitis
      Code first (T51-T65) to identify chemical and intent
      EXCLUDES 1   *burn and corrosion of eye and adnexa (T26.-)*
      H10.211   **Acute toxic conjunctivitis, right eye**
      H10.212   **Acute toxic conjunctivitis, left eye**
      H10.213   **Acute toxic conjunctivitis, bilateral**
      H10.219   **Acute toxic conjunctivitis, unspecified eye** ▽

    ✓6ᵗʰ **H10.22**   **Pseudomembranous conjunctivitis**
      H10.221   **Pseudomembranous conjunctivitis, right eye**
      H10.222   **Pseudomembranous conjunctivitis, left eye**
      H10.223   **Pseudomembranous conjunctivitis, bilateral**
      H10.229   **Pseudomembranous conjunctivitis, unspecified eye** ▽

    ✓6ᵗʰ **H10.23**   **Serous conjunctivitis, except viral**
      EXCLUDES 1   *viral conjunctivitis (B30.-)*
      H10.231   **Serous conjunctivitis, except viral, right eye**
      H10.232   **Serous conjunctivitis, except viral, left eye**
      H10.233   **Serous conjunctivitis, except viral, bilateral**
      H10.239   **Serous conjunctivitis, except viral, unspecified eye** ▽

✓5ᵗʰ **H10.3**   **Unspecified acute conjunctivitis**
    EXCLUDES 1   *ophthalmia neonatorum NOS (P39.1)*
    H10.30   **Unspecified acute conjunctivitis, unspecified eye** ▽
    H10.31   **Unspecified acute conjunctivitis, right eye** ▽
    H10.32   **Unspecified acute conjunctivitis, left eye** ▽
    H10.33   **Unspecified acute conjunctivitis, bilateral** ▽

✓5ᵗʰ **H10.4**   **Chronic conjunctivitis**
    ✓6ᵗʰ **H10.40**   **Unspecified chronic conjunctivitis**
      H10.401   **Unspecified chronic conjunctivitis, right eye** ▽
      H10.402   **Unspecified chronic conjunctivitis, left eye** ▽
      H10.403   **Unspecified chronic conjunctivitis, bilateral** ▽
      H10.409   **Unspecified chronic conjunctivitis, unspecified eye** ▽

    ✓6ᵗʰ **H10.41**   **Chronic giant papillary conjunctivitis**
      H10.411   **Chronic giant papillary conjunctivitis, right eye**
      H10.412   **Chronic giant papillary conjunctivitis, left eye**
      H10.413   **Chronic giant papillary conjunctivitis, bilateral**
      H10.419   **Chronic giant papillary conjunctivitis, unspecified eye** ▽

    ✓6ᵗʰ **H10.42**   **Simple chronic conjunctivitis**
      H10.421   **Simple chronic conjunctivitis, right eye**
      H10.422   **Simple chronic conjunctivitis, left eye**
      H10.423   **Simple chronic conjunctivitis, bilateral**
      H10.429   **Simple chronic conjunctivitis, unspecified eye** ▽

    ✓6ᵗʰ **H10.43**   **Chronic follicular conjunctivitis**
      H10.431   **Chronic follicular conjunctivitis, right eye**
      H10.432   **Chronic follicular conjunctivitis, left eye**
      H10.433   **Chronic follicular conjunctivitis, bilateral**
      H10.439   **Chronic follicular conjunctivitis, unspecified eye** ▽

    H10.44   **Vernal conjunctivitis**
      EXCLUDES 1   *vernal keratoconjunctivitis with limbar and corneal involvement (H16.26-)*

    H10.45   **Other chronic allergic conjunctivitis**

✓5ᵗʰ **H10.5**   **Blepharoconjunctivitis**
    ✓6ᵗʰ **H10.50**   **Unspecified blepharoconjunctivitis**
      H10.501   **Unspecified blepharoconjunctivitis, right eye** ▽
      H10.502   **Unspecified blepharoconjunctivitis, left eye** ▽
      H10.503   **Unspecified blepharoconjunctivitis, bilateral** ▽
      H10.509   **Unspecified blepharoconjunctivitis, unspecified eye** ▽

    ✓6ᵗʰ **H10.51**   **Ligneous conjunctivitis**
      H10.511   **Ligneous conjunctivitis, right eye**
      H10.512   **Ligneous conjunctivitis, left eye**
      H10.513   **Ligneous conjunctivitis, bilateral**
      H10.519   **Ligneous conjunctivitis, unspecified eye** ▽

    ✓6ᵗʰ **H10.52**   **Angular blepharoconjunctivitis**
      H10.521   **Angular blepharoconjunctivitis, right eye**
      H10.522   **Angular blepharoconjunctivitis, left eye**
      H10.523   **Angular blepharoconjunctivitis, bilateral**
      H10.529   **Angular blepharoconjunctivitis, unspecified eye** ▽

    ✓6ᵗʰ **H10.53**   **Contact blepharoconjunctivitis**
      H10.531   **Contact blepharoconjunctivitis, right eye**
      H10.532   **Contact blepharoconjunctivitis, left eye**
      H10.533   **Contact blepharoconjunctivitis, bilateral**
      H10.539   **Contact blepharoconjunctivitis, unspecified eye** ▽

✓5ᵗʰ **H10.8**   **Other conjunctivitis**
    ✓6ᵗʰ **H10.81**   **Pingueculitis**
      EXCLUDES 1   *pinguecula (H11.15-)*
      H10.811   **Pingueculitis, right eye**
      H10.812   **Pingueculitis, left eye**
      H10.813   **Pingueculitis, bilateral**
      H10.819   **Pingueculitis, unspecified eye** ▽

    H10.89   **Other conjunctivitis**
    H10.9   **Unspecified conjunctivitis** ▽

✓4ᵗʰ **H11**   **Other disorders of conjunctiva**
    EXCLUDES 1   *keratoconjunctivitis (H16.2-)*

    ✓5ᵗʰ **H11.0**   **Pterygium of eye**
      EXCLUDES 1   *pseudopterygium (H11.81-)*
      ✓6ᵗʰ **H11.00**   **Unspecified pterygium of eye**
        H11.001   **Unspecified pterygium of right eye** ▽
        H11.002   **Unspecified pterygium of left eye** ▽
        H11.003   **Unspecified pterygium of eye, bilateral** ▽
        H11.009   **Unspecified pterygium of unspecified eye** ▽

Pterygium

Pterygium

☑ Additional Character Req   ✓x7ᵗʰ Placeholder Alert   Manifestation   HCC CMS-HCC Condition   ▽ Unspecified Code   ▶◀ Revised Text   ● New Code   ▲ Revised Code Title

Chapter 7. Diseases of the Eye and Adnexa

H11.01–H11.439

√6ᵗʰ H11.01 Amyloid pterygium
　　H11.011 Amyloid pterygium of right eye
　　H11.012 Amyloid pterygium of left eye
　　H11.013 Amyloid pterygium of eye, bilateral
　　H11.019 Amyloid pterygium of unspecified eye ▽

√6ᵗʰ H11.02 Central pterygium of eye
　　H11.021 Central pterygium of right eye
　　H11.022 Central pterygium of left eye
　　H11.023 Central pterygium of eye, bilateral
　　H11.029 Central pterygium of unspecified eye ▽

√6ᵗʰ H11.03 Double pterygium of eye
　　H11.031 Double pterygium of right eye
　　H11.032 Double pterygium of left eye
　　H11.033 Double pterygium of eye, bilateral
　　H11.039 Double pterygium of unspecified eye ▽

√6ᵗʰ H11.04 Peripheral pterygium of eye, stationary
　　H11.041 Peripheral pterygium, stationary, right eye
　　H11.042 Peripheral pterygium, stationary, left eye
　　H11.043 Peripheral pterygium, stationary, bilateral
　　H11.049 Peripheral pterygium, stationary, unspecified eye ▽

√6ᵗʰ H11.05 Peripheral pterygium of eye, progressive
　　H11.051 Peripheral pterygium, progressive, right eye
　　H11.052 Peripheral pterygium, progressive, left eye
　　H11.053 Peripheral pterygium, progressive, bilateral
　　H11.059 Peripheral pterygium, progressive, unspecified eye ▽

√6ᵗʰ H11.06 Recurrent pterygium of eye
　　H11.061 Recurrent pterygium of right eye
　　H11.062 Recurrent pterygium of left eye
　　H11.063 Recurrent pterygium of eye, bilateral
　　H11.069 Recurrent pterygium of unspecified eye ▽

√5ᵗʰ H11.1 Conjunctival degenerations and deposits
　　EXCLUDES 2 pseudopterygium (H11.81)
　　H11.10 Unspecified conjunctival degenerations ▽

√6ᵗʰ H11.11 Conjunctival deposits
　　H11.111 Conjunctival deposits, right eye
　　H11.112 Conjunctival deposits, left eye
　　H11.113 Conjunctival deposits, bilateral
　　H11.119 Conjunctival deposits, unspecified eye ▽

√6ᵗʰ H11.12 Conjunctival concretions
　　H11.121 Conjunctival concretions, right eye
　　H11.122 Conjunctival concretions, left eye
　　H11.123 Conjunctival concretions, bilateral
　　H11.129 Conjunctival concretions, unspecified eye ▽

√6ᵗʰ H11.13 Conjunctival pigmentations
　　Conjunctival argyrosis [argyria]
　　H11.131 Conjunctival pigmentations, right eye
　　H11.132 Conjunctival pigmentations, left eye
　　H11.133 Conjunctival pigmentations, bilateral
　　H11.139 Conjunctival pigmentations, unspecified eye ▽

√6ᵗʰ H11.14 Conjunctival xerosis, unspecified
　　EXCLUDES 1 xerosis of conjunctiva due to vitamin A deficiency (E50.0, E50.1)
　　DEF: Abnormal dryness of conjunctiva due to lack of insufficient tears or conjunctival secretions.
　　H11.141 Conjunctival xerosis, unspecified, right eye ▽
　　H11.142 Conjunctival xerosis , unspecified, left eye ▽
　　H11.143 Conjunctival xerosis, unspecified, bilateral ▽
　　H11.149 Conjunctival xerosis, unspecified, unspecified eye ▽

√6ᵗʰ H11.15 Pinguecula
　　EXCLUDES 1 pingueculitis (H10.81-)
　　H11.151 Pinguecula, right eye

Pinguecula

Pinguecula

　　H11.152 Pinguecula, left eye
　　H11.153 Pinguecula, bilateral
　　H11.159 Pinguecula, unspecified eye ▽

√5ᵗʰ H11.2 Conjunctival scars
√6ᵗʰ H11.21 Conjunctival adhesions and strands (localized)
　　H11.211 Conjunctival adhesions and strands (localized), right eye
　　H11.212 Conjunctival adhesions and strands (localized), left eye
　　H11.213 Conjunctival adhesions and strands (localized), bilateral
　　H11.219 Conjunctival adhesions and strands (localized), unspecified eye ▽

√6ᵗʰ H11.22 Conjunctival granuloma
　　H11.221 Conjunctival granuloma, right eye
　　H11.222 Conjunctival granuloma, left eye
　　H11.223 Conjunctival granuloma, bilateral
　　H11.229 Conjunctival granuloma, unspecified ▽

√6ᵗʰ H11.23 Symblepharon
　　H11.231 Symblepharon, right eye
　　H11.232 Symblepharon, left eye
　　H11.233 Symblepharon, bilateral
　　H11.239 Symblepharon, unspecified eye ▽

√6ᵗʰ H11.24 Scarring of conjunctiva
　　H11.241 Scarring of conjunctiva, right eye
　　H11.242 Scarring of conjunctiva, left eye
　　H11.243 Scarring of conjunctiva, bilateral
　　H11.249 Scarring of conjunctiva, unspecified eye ▽

√5ᵗʰ H11.3 Conjunctival hemorrhage
　　Subconjunctival hemorrhage
　　H11.30 Conjunctival hemorrhage, unspecified eye ▽
　　H11.31 Conjunctival hemorrhage, right eye
　　H11.32 Conjunctival hemorrhage, left eye
　　H11.33 Conjunctival hemorrhage, bilateral

√5ᵗʰ H11.4 Other conjunctival vascular disorders and cysts
√6ᵗʰ H11.41 Vascular abnormalities of conjunctiva
　　Conjunctival aneurysm
　　H11.411 Vascular abnormalities of conjunctiva, right eye
　　H11.412 Vascular abnormalities of conjunctiva, left eye
　　H11.413 Vascular abnormalities of conjunctiva, bilateral
　　H11.419 Vascular abnormalities of conjunctiva, unspecified eye ▽

√6ᵗʰ H11.42 Conjunctival edema
　　H11.421 Conjunctival edema, right eye
　　H11.422 Conjunctival edema, left eye
　　H11.423 Conjunctival edema, bilateral
　　H11.429 Conjunctival edema, unspecified eye ▽

√6ᵗʰ H11.43 Conjunctival hyperemia
　　H11.431 Conjunctival hyperemia, right eye
　　H11.432 Conjunctival hyperemia, left eye
　　H11.433 Conjunctival hyperemia, bilateral
　　H11.439 Conjunctival hyperemia, unspecified eye ▽

EXCLUDES 1 Not coded here   EXCLUDES 2 Not included here   N Newborn Age: 0   P Pediatric Age: 0-17   M Maternity Age: 12-55   A Adult Age: 15-124

578   ICD-10-CM 2018

✓6ᵗʰ H11.44 **Conjunctival** cysts
　　　H11.441 **Conjunctival cysts, right eye**
　　　H11.442 **Conjunctival cysts, left eye**
　　　H11.443 **Conjunctival cysts, bilateral**
　　　H11.449 **Conjunctival cysts, unspecified eye** ▽

✓5ᵗʰ H11.8 **Other specified disorders of conjunctiva**
　✓6ᵗʰ H11.81 **Pseudopterygium of conjunctiva**
　　　H11.811 **Pseudopterygium of conjunctiva, right eye**
　　　H11.812 **Pseudopterygium of conjunctiva, left eye**
　　　H11.813 **Pseudopterygium of conjunctiva, bilateral**
　　　H11.819 **Pseudopterygium of conjunctiva, unspecified eye** ▽

　✓6ᵗʰ H11.82 **Conjunctivochalasis**
　　　H11.821 **Conjunctivochalasis, right eye**
　　　H11.822 **Conjunctivochalasis, left eye**
　　　H11.823 **Conjunctivochalasis, bilateral**
　　　H11.829 **Conjunctivochalasis, unspecified eye** ▽
　　H11.89 **Other specified disorders of conjunctiva**
　H11.9 **Unspecified disorder of conjunctiva** ▽

Disorders of sclera, cornea, iris and ciliary body (H15-H22)

✓4ᵗʰ **H15 Disorders of sclera**
　✓5ᵗʰ H15.0 **Scleritis**
　　✓6ᵗʰ H15.00 **Unspecified scleritis**
　　　H15.001 **Unspecified scleritis, right eye** ▽
　　　H15.002 **Unspecified scleritis, left eye** ▽
　　　H15.003 **Unspecified scleritis, bilateral** ▽
　　　H15.009 **Unspecified scleritis, unspecified eye** ▽

　　✓6ᵗʰ H15.01 **Anterior scleritis**
　　　H15.011 **Anterior scleritis, right eye**
　　　H15.012 **Anterior scleritis, left eye**
　　　H15.013 **Anterior scleritis, bilateral**
　　　H15.019 **Anterior scleritis, unspecified eye** ▽

　　✓6ᵗʰ H15.02 **Brawny scleritis**
　　　H15.021 **Brawny scleritis, right eye**
　　　H15.022 **Brawny scleritis, left eye**
　　　H15.023 **Brawny scleritis, bilateral**
　　　H15.029 **Brawny scleritis, unspecified eye** ▽

　　✓6ᵗʰ H15.03 **Posterior scleritis**
　　　　Sclerotenonitis
　　　H15.031 **Posterior scleritis, right eye**
　　　H15.032 **Posterior scleritis, left eye**
　　　H15.033 **Posterior scleritis, bilateral**
　　　H15.039 **Posterior scleritis, unspecified eye** ▽

　　✓6ᵗʰ H15.04 **Scleritis with corneal involvement**
　　　H15.041 **Scleritis with corneal involvement, right eye**
　　　H15.042 **Scleritis with corneal involvement, left eye**
　　　H15.043 **Scleritis with corneal involvement, bilateral**
　　　H15.049 **Scleritis with corneal involvement, unspecified eye** ▽

　　✓6ᵗʰ H15.05 **Scleromalacia perforans**
　　　H15.051 **Scleromalacia perforans, right eye**
　　　H15.052 **Scleromalacia perforans, left eye**
　　　H15.053 **Scleromalacia perforans, bilateral**
　　　H15.059 **Scleromalacia perforans, unspecified eye** ▽

　　✓6ᵗʰ H15.09 **Other scleritis**
　　　　Scleral abscess
　　　H15.091 **Other scleritis, right eye**
　　　H15.092 **Other scleritis, left eye**
　　　H15.093 **Other scleritis, bilateral**
　　　H15.099 **Other scleritis, unspecified eye** ▽

　✓5ᵗʰ H15.1 **Episcleritis**
　　✓6ᵗʰ H15.10 **Unspecified episcleritis**
　　　H15.101 **Unspecified episcleritis, right eye** ▽
　　　H15.102 **Unspecified episcleritis, left eye** ▽
　　　H15.103 **Unspecified episcleritis, bilateral** ▽
　　　H15.109 **Unspecified episcleritis, unspecified eye** ▽

　　✓6ᵗʰ H15.11 **Episcleritis** periodica fugax
　　　H15.111 **Episcleritis periodica fugax, right eye**
　　　H15.112 **Episcleritis periodica fugax, left eye**
　　　H15.113 **Episcleritis periodica fugax, bilateral**
　　　H15.119 **Episcleritis periodica fugax, unspecified eye** ▽

　　✓6ᵗʰ H15.12 **Nodular episcleritis**
　　　H15.121 **Nodular episcleritis, right eye**
　　　H15.122 **Nodular episcleritis, left eye**
　　　H15.123 **Nodular episcleritis, bilateral**
　　　H15.129 **Nodular episcleritis, unspecified eye** ▽

　✓5ᵗʰ H15.8 **Other disorders of sclera**
　　　EXCLUDES 2　blue sclera (Q13.5)
　　　　　　degenerative myopia (H44.2-)
　　✓6ᵗʰ H15.81 **Equatorial staphyloma**
　　　H15.811 **Equatorial staphyloma, right eye**
　　　H15.812 **Equatorial staphyloma, left eye**
　　　H15.813 **Equatorial staphyloma, bilateral**
　　　H15.819 **Equatorial staphyloma, unspecified eye** ▽

　　✓6ᵗʰ H15.82 **Localized anterior staphyloma**
　　　H15.821 **Localized anterior staphyloma, right eye**
　　　H15.822 **Localized anterior staphyloma, left eye**
　　　H15.823 **Localized anterior staphyloma, bilateral**
　　　H15.829 **Localized anterior staphyloma, unspecified eye** ▽

　　✓6ᵗʰ H15.83 **Staphyloma posticum**
　　　H15.831 **Staphyloma posticum, right eye**
　　　H15.832 **Staphyloma posticum, left eye**
　　　H15.833 **Staphyloma posticum, bilateral**
　　　H15.839 **Staphyloma posticum, unspecified eye** ▽

　　✓6ᵗʰ H15.84 **Scleral ectasia**
　　　H15.841 **Scleral ectasia, right eye**
　　　H15.842 **Scleral ectasia, left eye**
　　　H15.843 **Scleral ectasia, bilateral**
　　　H15.849 **Scleral ectasia, unspecified eye** ▽

　　✓6ᵗʰ H15.85 **Ring staphyloma**
　　　H15.851 **Ring staphyloma, right eye**
　　　H15.852 **Ring staphyloma, left eye**
　　　H15.853 **Ring staphyloma, bilateral**
　　　H15.859 **Ring staphyloma, unspecified eye** ▽
　　H15.89 **Other disorders of sclera**
　H15.9 **Unspecified disorder of sclera** ▽

✓4ᵗʰ **H16 Keratitis**
　✓5ᵗʰ H16.0 **Corneal ulcer**
　　✓6ᵗʰ H16.00 **Unspecified corneal ulcer**
　　　H16.001 **Unspecified corneal ulcer, right eye** ▽
　　　H16.002 **Unspecified corneal ulcer, left eye** ▽
　　　H16.003 **Unspecified corneal ulcer, bilateral** ▽
　　　H16.009 **Unspecified corneal ulcer, unspecified eye** ▽

　　✓6ᵗʰ H16.01 **Central corneal ulcer**
　　　H16.011 **Central corneal ulcer, right eye**
　　　H16.012 **Central corneal ulcer, left eye**
　　　H16.013 **Central corneal ulcer, bilateral**
　　　H16.019 **Central corneal ulcer, unspecified eye** ▽

　　✓6ᵗʰ H16.02 **Ring corneal ulcer**
　　　H16.021 **Ring corneal ulcer, right eye**
　　　H16.022 **Ring corneal ulcer, left eye**
　　　H16.023 **Ring corneal ulcer, bilateral**
　　　H16.029 **Ring corneal ulcer, unspecified eye** ▽

　　✓6ᵗʰ H16.03 **Corneal ulcer** with hypopyon
　　　H16.031 **Corneal ulcer with hypopyon, right eye**
　　　H16.032 **Corneal ulcer with hypopyon, left eye**
　　　H16.033 **Corneal ulcer with hypopyon, bilateral**
　　　H16.039 **Corneal ulcer with hypopyon, unspecified eye** ▽

　　✓6ᵗʰ H16.04 **Marginal corneal ulcer**
　　　H16.041 **Marginal corneal ulcer, right eye**
　　　H16.042 **Marginal corneal ulcer, left eye**
　　　H16.043 **Marginal corneal ulcer, bilateral**
　　　H16.049 **Marginal corneal ulcer, unspecified eye** ▽

☑ Additional Character Req　　✓ˣ7ᵗʰ Placeholder Alert　　Manifestation　　HCC CMS-HCC Condition　　▽ Unspecified Code　　►◄ Revised Text　　● New Code　　▲ Revised Code Title

Chapter 7. Diseases of the Eye and Adnexa

H16.05–H16.339

√6ᵗʰ **H16.05** Mooren's corneal ulcer
    H16.051 Mooren's corneal ulcer, right eye
    H16.052 Mooren's corneal ulcer, left eye
    H16.053 Mooren's corneal ulcer, bilateral
    H16.059 Mooren's corneal ulcer, unspecified eye ▽

√6ᵗʰ **H16.06** Mycotic corneal ulcer
    H16.061 Mycotic corneal ulcer, right eye
    H16.062 Mycotic corneal ulcer, left eye
    H16.063 Mycotic corneal ulcer, bilateral
    H16.069 Mycotic corneal ulcer, unspecified eye ▽

√6ᵗʰ **H16.07** Perforated corneal ulcer
    H16.071 Perforated corneal ulcer, right eye
    H16.072 Perforated corneal ulcer, left eye
    H16.073 Perforated corneal ulcer, bilateral
    H16.079 Perforated corneal ulcer, unspecified eye ▽

√5ᵗʰ **H16.1** Other and unspecified superficial keratitis without conjunctivitis

√6ᵗʰ **H16.10** Unspecified superficial keratitis
    H16.101 Unspecified superficial keratitis, right eye ▽
    H16.102 Unspecified superficial keratitis, left eye ▽
    H16.103 Unspecified superficial keratitis, bilateral ▽
    H16.109 Unspecified superficial keratitis, unspecified eye ▽

√6ᵗʰ **H16.11** Macular keratitis
    Areolar keratitis
    Nummular keratitis
    Stellate keratitis
    Striate keratitis
    H16.111 Macular keratitis, right eye
    H16.112 Macular keratitis, left eye
    H16.113 Macular keratitis, bilateral
    H16.119 Macular keratitis, unspecified eye ▽

√6ᵗʰ **H16.12** Filamentary keratitis
    H16.121 Filamentary keratitis, right eye
    H16.122 Filamentary keratitis, left eye
    H16.123 Filamentary keratitis, bilateral
    H16.129 Filamentary keratitis, unspecified eye ▽

√6ᵗʰ **H16.13** Photokeratitis
    Snow blindness
    Welders keratitis
    H16.131 Photokeratitis, right eye
    H16.132 Photokeratitis, left eye
    H16.133 Photokeratitis, bilateral
    H16.139 Photokeratitis, unspecified eye ▽

√6ᵗʰ **H16.14** Punctate keratitis
    H16.141 Punctate keratitis, right eye
    H16.142 Punctate keratitis, left eye
    H16.143 Punctate keratitis, bilateral
    H16.149 Punctate keratitis, unspecified eye ▽

√5ᵗʰ **H16.2** Keratoconjunctivitis

√6ᵗʰ **H16.20** Unspecified keratoconjunctivitis
    Superficial keratitis with conjunctivitis NOS
    H16.201 Unspecified keratoconjunctivitis, right eye ▽
    H16.202 Unspecified keratoconjunctivitis, left eye ▽
    H16.203 Unspecified keratoconjunctivitis, bilateral ▽
    H16.209 Unspecified keratoconjunctivitis, unspecified eye ▽

√6ᵗʰ **H16.21** Exposure keratoconjunctivitis
    H16.211 Exposure keratoconjunctivitis, right eye
    H16.212 Exposure keratoconjunctivitis, left eye
    H16.213 Exposure keratoconjunctivitis, bilateral
    H16.219 Exposure keratoconjunctivitis, unspecified eye ▽

√6ᵗʰ **H16.22** Keratoconjunctivitis sicca, not specified as Sjögren's
    EXCLUDES 1 Sjögren's syndrome (M35.01)
    H16.221 Keratoconjunctivitis sicca, not specified as Sjögren's, right eye

    H16.222 Keratoconjunctivitis sicca, not specified as Sjögren's, left eye
    H16.223 Keratoconjunctivitis sicca, not specified as Sjögren's, bilateral
    H16.229 Keratoconjunctivitis sicca, not specified as Sjögren's, unspecified eye ▽

√6ᵗʰ **H16.23** Neurotrophic keratoconjunctivitis
    H16.231 Neurotrophic keratoconjunctivitis, right eye
    H16.232 Neurotrophic keratoconjunctivitis, left eye
    H16.233 Neurotrophic keratoconjunctivitis, bilateral
    H16.239 Neurotrophic keratoconjunctivitis, unspecified eye ▽

√6ᵗʰ **H16.24** Ophthalmia nodosa
    H16.241 Ophthalmia nodosa, right eye
    H16.242 Ophthalmia nodosa, left eye
    H16.243 Ophthalmia nodosa, bilateral
    H16.249 Ophthalmia nodosa, unspecified eye ▽

√6ᵗʰ **H16.25** Phlyctenular keratoconjunctivitis
    H16.251 Phlyctenular keratoconjunctivitis, right eye
    H16.252 Phlyctenular keratoconjunctivitis, left eye
    H16.253 Phlyctenular keratoconjunctivitis, bilateral
    H16.259 Phlyctenular keratoconjunctivitis, unspecified eye ▽

√6ᵗʰ **H16.26** Vernal keratoconjunctivitis, with limbar and corneal involvement
    EXCLUDES 1 vernal conjunctivitis without limbar and corneal involvement (H10.44)
    H16.261 Vernal keratoconjunctivitis, with limbar and corneal involvement, right eye
    H16.262 Vernal keratoconjunctivitis, with limbar and corneal involvement, left eye
    H16.263 Vernal keratoconjunctivitis, with limbar and corneal involvement, bilateral
    H16.269 Vernal keratoconjunctivitis, with limbar and corneal involvement, unspecified eye ▽

√6ᵗʰ **H16.29** Other keratoconjunctivitis
    H16.291 Other keratoconjunctivitis, right eye
    H16.292 Other keratoconjunctivitis, left eye
    H16.293 Other keratoconjunctivitis, bilateral
    H16.299 Other keratoconjunctivitis, unspecified eye ▽

√5ᵗʰ **H16.3** Interstitial and deep keratitis

√6ᵗʰ **H16.30** Unspecified interstitial keratitis
    H16.301 Unspecified interstitial keratitis, right eye ▽
    H16.302 Unspecified interstitial keratitis, left eye ▽
    H16.303 Unspecified interstitial keratitis, bilateral ▽
    H16.309 Unspecified interstitial keratitis, unspecified eye ▽

√6ᵗʰ **H16.31** Corneal abscess
    H16.311 Corneal abscess, right eye
    H16.312 Corneal abscess, left eye
    H16.313 Corneal abscess, bilateral
    H16.319 Corneal abscess, unspecified eye ▽

√6ᵗʰ **H16.32** Diffuse interstitial keratitis
    Cogan's syndrome
    H16.321 Diffuse interstitial keratitis, right eye
    H16.322 Diffuse interstitial keratitis, left eye
    H16.323 Diffuse interstitial keratitis, bilateral
    H16.329 Diffuse interstitial keratitis, unspecified eye ▽

√6ᵗʰ **H16.33** Sclerosing keratitis
    H16.331 Sclerosing keratitis, right eye
    H16.332 Sclerosing keratitis, left eye
    H16.333 Sclerosing keratitis, bilateral
    H16.339 Sclerosing keratitis, unspecified eye ▽

EXCLUDES 1 Not coded here   **EXCLUDES 2** Not included here   N Newborn Age: 0   P Pediatric Age: 0-17   M Maternity Age: 12-55   A Adult Age: 15-124

580   ICD-10-CM 2018

✓6ᵗʰ **H16.39 Other interstitial and deep keratitis**

    H16.391 Other interstitial and deep keratitis, right eye

    H16.392 Other interstitial and deep keratitis, left eye

    H16.393 Other interstitial and deep keratitis, bilateral

    H16.399 Other interstitial and deep keratitis, unspecified eye ▽

✓5ᵗʰ **H16.4 Corneal neovascularization**

  ✓6ᵗʰ **H16.40 Unspecified corneal neovascularization**

    H16.401 Unspecified corneal neovascularization, right eye ▽

    H16.402 Unspecified corneal neovascularization, left eye ▽

    H16.403 Unspecified corneal neovascularization, bilateral ▽

    H16.409 Unspecified corneal neovascularization, unspecified eye ▽

  ✓6ᵗʰ **H16.41 Ghost vessels (corneal)**

    H16.411 Ghost vessels (corneal), right eye

    H16.412 Ghost vessels (corneal), left eye

    H16.413 Ghost vessels (corneal), bilateral

    H16.419 Ghost vessels (corneal), unspecified eye ▽

  ✓6ᵗʰ **H16.42 Pannus (corneal)**

    H16.421 Pannus (corneal), right eye

    H16.422 Pannus (corneal), left eye

    H16.423 Pannus (corneal), bilateral

    H16.429 Pannus (corneal), unspecified eye ▽

  ✓6ᵗʰ **H16.43 Localized vascularization of cornea**

    H16.431 Localized vascularization of cornea, right eye

    H16.432 Localized vascularization of cornea, left eye

    H16.433 Localized vascularization of cornea, bilateral

    H16.439 Localized vascularization of cornea, unspecified eye ▽

  ✓6ᵗʰ **H16.44 Deep vascularization of cornea**

    H16.441 Deep vascularization of cornea, right eye

    H16.442 Deep vascularization of cornea, left eye

    H16.443 Deep vascularization of cornea, bilateral

    H16.449 Deep vascularization of cornea, unspecified eye ▽

H16.8 Other keratitis

H16.9 Unspecified keratitis ▽

✓4ᵗʰ **H17 Corneal scars and opacities**

  ✓5ᵗʰ **H17.0 Adherent leukoma**

    H17.00 Adherent leukoma, unspecified eye ▽

    H17.01 Adherent leukoma, right eye

    H17.02 Adherent leukoma, left eye

    H17.03 Adherent leukoma, bilateral

  ✓5ᵗʰ **H17.1 Central corneal opacity**

    H17.10 Central corneal opacity, unspecified eye ▽

    H17.11 Central corneal opacity, right eye

    H17.12 Central corneal opacity, left eye

    H17.13 Central corneal opacity, bilateral

  ✓5ᵗʰ **H17.8 Other corneal scars and opacities**

  ✓6ᵗʰ **H17.81 Minor opacity of cornea**
    Corneal nebula

    H17.811 Minor opacity of cornea, right eye

    H17.812 Minor opacity of cornea, left eye

    H17.813 Minor opacity of cornea, bilateral

    H17.819 Minor opacity of cornea, unspecified eye ▽

  ✓6ᵗʰ **H17.82 Peripheral opacity of cornea**

    H17.821 Peripheral opacity of cornea, right eye

    H17.822 Peripheral opacity of cornea, left eye

    H17.823 Peripheral opacity of cornea, bilateral

    H17.829 Peripheral opacity of cornea, unspecified eye ▽

    H17.89 Other corneal scars and opacities

H17.9 Unspecified corneal scar and opacity ▽

✓4ᵗʰ **H18 Other disorders of cornea**

  ✓5ᵗʰ **H18.0 Corneal pigmentations and deposits**

  ✓6ᵗʰ **H18.00 Unspecified corneal deposit**

    H18.001 Unspecified corneal deposit, right eye ▽

    H18.002 Unspecified corneal deposit, left eye ▽

    H18.003 Unspecified corneal deposit, bilateral ▽

    H18.009 Unspecified corneal deposit, unspecified eye ▽

  ✓6ᵗʰ **H18.01 Anterior corneal pigmentations**
    Staehli's line

    H18.011 Anterior corneal pigmentations, right eye

    H18.012 Anterior corneal pigmentations, left eye

    H18.013 Anterior corneal pigmentations, bilateral

    H18.019 Anterior corneal pigmentations, unspecified eye ▽

  ✓6ᵗʰ **H18.02 Argentous corneal deposits**

    H18.021 Argentous corneal deposits, right eye

    H18.022 Argentous corneal deposits, left eye

    H18.023 Argentous corneal deposits, bilateral

    H18.029 Argentous corneal deposits, unspecified eye ▽

  ✓6ᵗʰ **H18.03 Corneal deposits in metabolic disorders**
    Code also associated metabolic disorder

    H18.031 Corneal deposits in metabolic disorders, right eye

    H18.032 Corneal deposits in metabolic disorders, left eye

    H18.033 Corneal deposits in metabolic disorders, bilateral

    H18.039 Corneal deposits in metabolic disorders, unspecified eye ▽

  ✓6ᵗʰ **H18.04 Kayser-Fleischer ring**
    Code also associated Wilson's disease (E83.01)

    H18.041 Kayser-Fleischer ring, right eye

    H18.042 Kayser-Fleischer ring, left eye

    H18.043 Kayser-Fleischer ring, bilateral

    H18.049 Kayser-Fleischer ring, unspecified eye ▽

  ✓6ᵗʰ **H18.05 Posterior corneal pigmentations**
    Krukenberg's spindle

    H18.051 Posterior corneal pigmentations, right eye

    H18.052 Posterior corneal pigmentations, left eye

    H18.053 Posterior corneal pigmentations, bilateral

    H18.059 Posterior corneal pigmentations, unspecified eye ▽

  ✓6ᵗʰ **H18.06 Stromal corneal pigmentations**
    Hematocornea

    H18.061 Stromal corneal pigmentations, right eye

    H18.062 Stromal corneal pigmentations, left eye

    H18.063 Stromal corneal pigmentations, bilateral

    H18.069 Stromal corneal pigmentations, unspecified eye ▽

  ✓5ᵗʰ **H18.1 Bullous keratopathy**
    DEF: Corneal swelling due to damaged corneal endothelium; characterized by recurring, rupturing epithelial "blisters"; occurs in glaucoma, iridocyclitis and Fuchs dystrophy.

    H18.10 Bullous keratopathy, unspecified eye ▽

    H18.11 Bullous keratopathy, right eye

    H18.12 Bullous keratopathy, left eye

    H18.13 Bullous keratopathy, bilateral

  ✓5ᵗʰ **H18.2 Other and unspecified corneal edema**

    H18.20 Unspecified corneal edema ▽

  ✓6ᵗʰ **H18.21 Corneal edema secondary to contact lens**
    EXCLUDES 2 other corneal disorders due to contact lens (H18.82-)

    H18.211 Corneal edema secondary to contact lens, right eye

    H18.212 Corneal edema secondary to contact lens, left eye

    H18.213 Corneal edema secondary to contact lens, bilateral

    H18.219 Corneal edema secondary to contact lens, unspecified eye ▽

✓ Additional Character Req   ✓x7ᵗʰ Placeholder Alert   Manifestation   HCC CMS-HCC Condition   ▽ Unspecified Code   ►◄ Revised Text   ● New Code   ▲ Revised Code Title

Chapter 7. Diseases of the Eye and Adnexa

H18.22–H18.829

✓6th **H18.22** **Idiopathic** corneal edema
    H18.221 Idiopathic corneal edema, right eye
    H18.222 Idiopathic corneal edema, left eye
    H18.223 Idiopathic corneal edema, bilateral
    H18.229 Idiopathic corneal edema, unspecified ▽
          eye

✓6th **H18.23** **Secondary** corneal edema
    H18.231 Secondary corneal edema, right eye
    H18.232 Secondary corneal edema, left eye
    H18.233 Secondary corneal edema, bilateral
    H18.239 Secondary corneal edema, unspecified ▽
          eye

✓5th **H18.3** **Changes of corneal membranes**
    H18.30 Unspecified corneal membrane change ▽

  ✓6th **H18.31** Folds and rupture in Bowman's membrane
    H18.311 Folds and rupture in Bowman's
          membrane, right eye
    H18.312 Folds and rupture in Bowman's
          membrane, left eye
    H18.313 Folds and rupture in Bowman's
          membrane, bilateral
    H18.319 Folds and rupture in Bowman's ▽
          membrane, unspecified eye

  ✓6th **H18.32** Folds in Descemet's membrane
    H18.321 Folds in Descemet's membrane, right eye
    H18.322 Folds in Descemet's membrane, left eye
    H18.323 Folds in Descemet's membrane, bilateral
    H18.329 Folds in Descemet's membrane, ▽
          unspecified eye

  ✓6th **H18.33** Rupture in Descemet's membrane
    H18.331 Rupture in Descemet's membrane, right
          eye
    H18.332 Rupture in Descemet's membrane, left eye
    H18.333 Rupture in Descemet's membrane,
          bilateral
    H18.339 Rupture in Descemet's membrane, ▽
          unspecified eye

✓5th **H18.4** **Corneal degeneration**
    EXCLUDES 1   *Mooren's ulcer (H16.0-)*
          recurrent erosion of cornea (H18.83-)
    H18.40 Unspecified corneal degeneration ▽

  ✓6th **H18.41** Arcus senilis
        Senile corneal changes
    H18.411 Arcus senilis, right eye
    H18.412 Arcus senilis, left eye
    H18.413 Arcus senilis, bilateral
    H18.419 Arcus senilis, unspecified eye ▽

  ✓6th **H18.42** Band keratopathy
    H18.421 Band keratopathy, right eye
    H18.422 Band keratopathy, left eye
    H18.423 Band keratopathy, bilateral
    H18.429 Band keratopathy, unspecified eye ▽
    H18.43 Other calcerous corneal degeneration

  ✓6th **H18.44** Keratomalacia
    EXCLUDES 1   *keratomalacia due to vitamin A deficiency*
          (E50.4)
    H18.441 Keratomalacia, right eye
    H18.442 Keratomalacia, left eye
    H18.443 Keratomalacia, bilateral
    H18.449 Keratomalacia, unspecified eye ▽

  ✓6th **H18.45** Nodular corneal degeneration
    H18.451 Nodular corneal degeneration, right eye
    H18.452 Nodular corneal degeneration, left eye
    H18.453 Nodular corneal degeneration, bilateral
    H18.459 Nodular corneal degeneration, ▽
          unspecified eye

  ✓6th **H18.46** Peripheral corneal degeneration
    H18.461 Peripheral corneal degeneration, right
          eye
    H18.462 Peripheral corneal degeneration, left eye
    H18.463 Peripheral corneal degeneration, bilateral
    H18.469 Peripheral corneal degeneration, ▽
          unspecified eye
    H18.49 Other corneal degeneration

✓5th **H18.5** **Hereditary corneal dystrophies**
    H18.50 Unspecified hereditary corneal dystrophies ▽
    H18.51 Endothelial corneal dystrophy
        Fuchs' dystrophy
    H18.52 Epithelial (juvenile) corneal dystrophy
    H18.53 Granular corneal dystrophy
    H18.54 Lattice corneal dystrophy
    H18.55 Macular corneal dystrophy
    H18.59 Other hereditary corneal dystrophies

✓5th **H18.6** **Keratoconus**
  ✓6th **H18.60** Keratoconus, unspecified
    H18.601 Keratoconus, unspecified, right eye ▽
    H18.602 Keratoconus, unspecified, left eye ▽
    H18.603 Keratoconus, unspecified, bilateral ▽
    H18.609 Keratoconus, unspecified, ▽
          unspecified eye

  ✓6th **H18.61** Keratoconus, stable
    H18.611 Keratoconus, stable, right eye
    H18.612 Keratoconus, stable, left eye
    H18.613 Keratoconus, stable, bilateral
    H18.619 Keratoconus, stable, unspecified eye ▽

  ✓6th **H18.62** Keratoconus, unstable
        Acute hydrops
    H18.621 Keratoconus, unstable, right eye
    H18.622 Keratoconus, unstable, left eye
    H18.623 Keratoconus, unstable, bilateral
    H18.629 Keratoconus, unstable, unspecified eye ▽

✓5th **H18.7** **Other and unspecified corneal deformities**
    EXCLUDES 1   *congenital malformations of cornea (Q13.3-Q13.4)*
    H18.70 Unspecified corneal deformity ▽

  ✓6th **H18.71** Corneal ectasia
    H18.711 Corneal ectasia, right eye
    H18.712 Corneal ectasia, left eye
    H18.713 Corneal ectasia, bilateral
    H18.719 Corneal ectasia, unspecified eye ▽

  ✓6th **H18.72** Corneal staphyloma
    H18.721 Corneal staphyloma, right eye
    H18.722 Corneal staphyloma, left eye
    H18.723 Corneal staphyloma, bilateral
    H18.729 Corneal staphyloma, unspecified eye ▽

  ✓6th **H18.73** Descemetocele
    H18.731 Descemetocele, right eye
    H18.732 Descemetocele, left eye
    H18.733 Descemetocele, bilateral
    H18.739 Descemetocele, unspecified eye ▽

  ✓6th **H18.79** Other corneal deformities
    H18.791 Other corneal deformities, right eye
    H18.792 Other corneal deformities, left eye
    H18.793 Other corneal deformities, bilateral
    H18.799 Other corneal deformities, ▽
          unspecified eye

✓5th **H18.8** **Other specified disorders of cornea**
  ✓6th **H18.81** Anesthesia and hypoesthesia of cornea
    H18.811 Anesthesia and hypoesthesia of cornea,
          right eye
    H18.812 Anesthesia and hypoesthesia of cornea,
          left eye
    H18.813 Anesthesia and hypoesthesia of cornea,
          bilateral
    H18.819 Anesthesia and hypoesthesia of ▽
          cornea, unspecified eye

  ✓6th **H18.82** Corneal disorder due to contact lens
    EXCLUDES 2   *corneal edema due to contact lens (H18.21-)*
    H18.821 Corneal disorder due to contact lens, right
          eye
    H18.822 Corneal disorder due to contact lens, left
          eye
    H18.823 Corneal disorder due to contact lens,
          bilateral
    H18.829 Corneal disorder due to contact lens, ▽
          unspecified eye

EXCLUDES 1 Not coded here   **EXCLUDES 2** Not included here   N Newborn Age: 0   P Pediatric Age: 0-17   M Maternity Age: 12-55   A Adult Age: 15-124

582   ICD-10-CM 2018

✓6ᵗʰ **H18.83** **Recurrent erosion of cornea**
     H18.831 **Recurrent erosion of cornea,** right **eye**
     H18.832 **Recurrent erosion of cornea,** left **eye**
     H18.833 **Recurrent erosion of cornea,** bilateral
     H18.839 **Recurrent erosion of cornea, unspecified eye** ▽

✓6ᵗʰ **H18.89** **Other specified disorders of cornea**
     H18.891 **Other specified disorders of cornea,** right **eye**
     H18.892 **Other specified disorders of cornea,** left **eye**
     H18.893 **Other specified disorders of cornea,** bilateral
     H18.899 **Other specified disorders of cornea, unspecified eye** ▽

H18.9 **Unspecified disorder of cornea** ▽

✓4ᵗʰ **H20** **Iridocyclitis**

✓5ᵗʰ **H20.0** Acute **and** subacute **iridocyclitis**
     Acute anterior uveitis
     Acute cyclitis
     Acute iritis
     Subacute anterior uveitis
     Subacute cyclitis
     Subacute iritis
     EXCLUDES 1   *iridocyclitis, iritis, uveitis (due to) (in) diabetes mellitus (E08-E13 with .39)*
         iridocyclitis, iritis, uveitis (due to) (in) diphtheria (A36.89)
         iridocyclitis, iritis, uveitis (due to) (in) gonococcal (A54.32)
         iridocyclitis, iritis, uveitis (due to) (in) herpes (simplex) (B00.51)
         iridocyclitis, iritis, uveitis (due to) (in) herpes zoster (B02.32)
         iridocyclitis, iritis, uveitis (due to) (in) late congenital syphilis (A50.39)
         iridocyclitis, iritis, uveitis (due to) (in) late syphilis (A52.71)
         iridocyclitis, iritis, uveitis (due to) (in) sarcoidosis (D86.83)
         iridocyclitis, iritis, uveitis (due to) (in) syphilis (A51.43)
         iridocyclitis, iritis, uveitis (due to) (in) toxoplasmosis (B58.09)
         iridocyclitis, iritis, uveitis (due to) (in) tuberculosis (A18.54)

     H20.00 **Unspecified acute and subacute iridocyclitis** ▽

✓6ᵗʰ **H20.01** Primary **iridocyclitis**
     H20.011 **Primary iridocyclitis,** right **eye**
     H20.012 **Primary iridocyclitis,** left **eye**
     H20.013 **Primary iridocyclitis,** bilateral
     H20.019 **Primary iridocyclitis, unspecified eye** ▽

✓6ᵗʰ **H20.02** Recurrent acute **iridocyclitis**
     H20.021 **Recurrent acute iridocyclitis,** right **eye**
     H20.022 **Recurrent acute iridocyclitis,** left **eye**
     H20.023 **Recurrent acute iridocyclitis,** bilateral
     H20.029 **Recurrent acute iridocyclitis, unspecified eye** ▽

✓6ᵗʰ **H20.03** Secondary infectious **iridocyclitis**
     H20.031 **Secondary infectious iridocyclitis,** right **eye**
     H20.032 **Secondary infectious iridocyclitis,** left **eye**
     H20.033 **Secondary infectious iridocyclitis,** bilateral
     H20.039 **Secondary infectious iridocyclitis, unspecified eye** ▽

✓6ᵗʰ **H20.04** Secondary noninfectious **iridocyclitis**
     H20.041 **Secondary noninfectious iridocyclitis,** right **eye**
     H20.042 **Secondary noninfectious iridocyclitis,** left **eye**
     H20.043 **Secondary noninfectious iridocyclitis,** bilateral
     H20.049 **Secondary noninfectious iridocyclitis, unspecified eye** ▽

✓6ᵗʰ **H20.05** Hypopyon
     H20.051 **Hypopyon,** right **eye**
     H20.052 **Hypopyon,** left **eye**
     H20.053 **Hypopyon,** bilateral

     H20.059 **Hypopyon, unspecified eye** ▽

✓5ᵗʰ **H20.1** Chronic **iridocyclitis**
     Use additional code for any associated cataract (H26.21-)
     EXCLUDES 2   *posterior cyclitis (H30.2-)*
     H20.10 **Chronic iridocyclitis, unspecified eye** ▽
     H20.11 **Chronic iridocyclitis,** right **eye**
     H20.12 **Chronic iridocyclitis,** left **eye**
     H20.13 **Chronic iridocyclitis,** bilateral

✓5ᵗʰ **H20.2** Lens-induced **iridocyclitis**
     H20.20 **Lens-induced iridocyclitis, unspecified eye** ▽
     H20.21 **Lens-induced iridocyclitis,** right **eye**
     H20.22 **Lens-induced iridocyclitis,** left **eye**
     H20.23 **Lens-induced iridocyclitis, bilateral**

✓5ᵗʰ **H20.8** **Other iridocyclitis**
     EXCLUDES 2   *glaucomatocyclitis crises (H40.4-)*
         posterior cyclitis (H30.2-)
         sympathetic uveitis (H44.13-)

     ✓6ᵗʰ **H20.81** **Fuchs' heterochromic cyclitis**
         H20.811 **Fuchs' heterochromic cyclitis,** right **eye**
         H20.812 **Fuchs' heterochromic cyclitis,** left **eye**
         H20.813 **Fuchs' heterochromic cyclitis,** bilateral
         H20.819 **Fuchs' heterochromic cyclitis, unspecified eye** ▽

     ✓6ᵗʰ **H20.82** **Vogt-Koyanagi syndrome**
         H20.821 **Vogt-Koyanagi syndrome,** right **eye**
         H20.822 **Vogt-Koyanagi syndrome,** left **eye**
         H20.823 **Vogt-Koyanagi syndrome,** bilateral
         H20.829 **Vogt-Koyanagi syndrome, unspecified eye** ▽

H20.9 **Unspecified iridocyclitis** ▽
     Uveitis NOS

✓4ᵗʰ **H21** **Other disorders of iris and ciliary body**
     EXCLUDES 2   *sympathetic uveitis (H44.1-)*

✓5ᵗʰ **H21.0** **Hyphema**
     EXCLUDES 1   *traumatic hyphema (S05.1-)*
     H21.00 **Hyphema, unspecified eye** ▽
     H21.01 **Hyphema,** right **eye**
     H21.02 **Hyphema,** left **eye**
     H21.03 **Hyphema,** bilateral

✓5ᵗʰ **H21.1** **Other vascular disorders of iris and ciliary body**
     Neovascularization of iris or ciliary body
     Rubeosis iridis
     Rubeosis of iris

     ✓6ᵗʰ **H21.1X** **Other vascular disorders of iris and ciliary body**
         H21.1X1 **Other vascular disorders of iris and ciliary body,** right **eye**
         H21.1X2 **Other vascular disorders of iris and ciliary body,** left **eye**
         H21.1X3 **Other vascular disorders of iris and ciliary body,** bilateral
         H21.1X9 **Other vascular disorders of iris and ciliary body, unspecified eye** ▽

✓5ᵗʰ **H21.2** **Degeneration of iris and ciliary body**

     ✓6ᵗʰ **H21.21** **Degeneration of** chamber angle
         H21.211 **Degeneration of chamber angle,** right **eye**
         H21.212 **Degeneration of chamber angle,** left **eye**
         H21.213 **Degeneration of chamber angle,** bilateral
         H21.219 **Degeneration of chamber angle, unspecified eye** ▽

Hyphema

Iris
Cornea
Hyphema

☑ Additional Character Req	ᵛˣ⁷ᵗʰ Placeholder Alert	Manifestation	HCC CMS-HCC Condition	▽ Unspecified Code	►◄ Revised Text ● New Code ▲ Revised Code Title

✓6ᵗʰ **H21.22 Degeneration of ciliary body**
- H21.221 Degeneration of ciliary body, right eye
- H21.222 Degeneration of ciliary body, left eye
- H21.223 Degeneration of ciliary body, bilateral
- H21.229 Degeneration of ciliary body, unspecified eye ▽

✓6ᵗʰ **H21.23 Degeneration of iris (pigmentary)**
Translucency of iris
- H21.231 Degeneration of iris (pigmentary), right eye
- H21.232 Degeneration of iris (pigmentary), left eye
- H21.233 Degeneration of iris (pigmentary), bilateral
- H21.239 Degeneration of iris (pigmentary), unspecified eye ▽

✓6ᵗʰ **H21.24 Degeneration of pupillary margin**
- H21.241 Degeneration of pupillary margin, right eye
- H21.242 Degeneration of pupillary margin, left eye
- H21.243 Degeneration of pupillary margin, bilateral
- H21.249 Degeneration of pupillary margin, unspecified eye ▽

✓6ᵗʰ **H21.25 Iridoschisis**
- H21.251 Iridoschisis, right eye
- H21.252 Iridoschisis, left eye
- H21.253 Iridoschisis, bilateral
- H21.259 Iridoschisis, unspecified eye ▽

✓6ᵗʰ **H21.26 Iris atrophy (essential) (progressive)**
- H21.261 Iris atrophy (essential) (progressive), right eye
- H21.262 Iris atrophy (essential) (progressive), left eye
- H21.263 Iris atrophy (essential) (progressive), bilateral
- H21.269 Iris atrophy (essential) (progressive), unspecified eye ▽

✓6ᵗʰ **H21.27 Miotic pupillary cyst**
- H21.271 Miotic pupillary cyst, right eye
- H21.272 Miotic pupillary cyst, left eye
- H21.273 Miotic pupillary cyst, bilateral
- H21.279 Miotic pupillary cyst, unspecified eye ▽

H21.29 Other iris atrophy

✓5ᵗʰ **H21.3 Cyst of iris, ciliary body and anterior chamber**
EXCLUDES 2 miotic pupillary cyst (H21.27-)

✓6ᵗʰ **H21.30 Idiopathic cysts of iris, ciliary body or anterior chamber**
Cyst of iris, ciliary body or anterior chamber NOS
- H21.301 Idiopathic cysts of iris, ciliary body or anterior chamber, right eye
- H21.302 Idiopathic cysts of iris, ciliary body or anterior chamber, left eye
- H21.303 Idiopathic cysts of iris, ciliary body or anterior chamber, bilateral
- H21.309 Idiopathic cysts of iris, ciliary body or anterior chamber, unspecified eye ▽

✓6ᵗʰ **H21.31 Exudative cysts of iris or anterior chamber**
- H21.311 Exudative cysts of iris or anterior chamber, right eye
- H21.312 Exudative cysts of iris or anterior chamber, left eye
- H21.313 Exudative cysts of iris or anterior chamber, bilateral
- H21.319 Exudative cysts of iris or anterior chamber, unspecified eye ▽

✓6ᵗʰ **H21.32 Implantation cysts of iris, ciliary body or anterior chamber**
- H21.321 Implantation cysts of iris, ciliary body or anterior chamber, right eye
- H21.322 Implantation cysts of iris, ciliary body or anterior chamber, left eye
- H21.323 Implantation cysts of iris, ciliary body or anterior chamber, bilateral
- H21.329 Implantation cysts of iris, ciliary body or anterior chamber, unspecified eye ▽

✓6ᵗʰ **H21.33 Parasitic cyst of iris, ciliary body or anterior chamber**
- H21.331 Parasitic cyst of iris, ciliary body or anterior chamber, right eye
- H21.332 Parasitic cyst of iris, ciliary body or anterior chamber, left eye
- H21.333 Parasitic cyst of iris, ciliary body or anterior chamber, bilateral
- H21.339 Parasitic cyst of iris, ciliary body or anterior chamber, unspecified eye ▽

✓6ᵗʰ **H21.34 Primary cyst of pars plana**
- H21.341 Primary cyst of pars plana, right eye
- H21.342 Primary cyst of pars plana, left eye
- H21.343 Primary cyst of pars plana, bilateral
- H21.349 Primary cyst of pars plana, unspecified eye ▽

✓6ᵗʰ **H21.35 Exudative cyst of pars plana**
DEF: Protein, fatty-filled bullous elevation of nonpigmented outermost ciliary body epithelium of pars plana; due to fluid leak from blood vessels.
- H21.351 Exudative cyst of pars plana, right eye
- H21.352 Exudative cyst of pars plana, left eye
- H21.353 Exudative cyst of pars plana, bilateral
- H21.359 Exudative cyst of pars plana, unspecified eye ▽

✓5ᵗʰ **H21.4 Pupillary membranes**
Iris bombé
Pupillary occlusion
Pupillary seclusion
EXCLUDES 1 congenital pupillary membranes (Q13.8)
- H21.40 Pupillary membranes, unspecified eye ▽
- H21.41 Pupillary membranes, right eye
- H21.42 Pupillary membranes, left eye
- H21.43 Pupillary membranes, bilateral

✓5ᵗʰ **H21.5 Other and unspecified adhesions and disruptions of iris and ciliary body**
EXCLUDES 1 corectopia (Q13.2)

✓6ᵗʰ **H21.50 Unspecified adhesions of iris**
Synechia (iris) NOS
- H21.501 Unspecified adhesions of iris, right eye ▽
- H21.502 Unspecified adhesions of iris, left eye ▽
- H21.503 Unspecified adhesions of iris, bilateral ▽
- H21.509 Unspecified adhesions of iris and ciliary body, unspecified eye ▽

✓6ᵗʰ **H21.51 Anterior synechiae (iris)**
- H21.511 Anterior synechiae (iris), right eye
- H21.512 Anterior synechiae (iris), left eye
- H21.513 Anterior synechiae (iris), bilateral
- H21.519 Anterior synechiae (iris), unspecified eye ▽

✓6ᵗʰ **H21.52 Goniosynechiae**
- H21.521 Goniosynechiae, right eye
- H21.522 Goniosynechiae, left eye
- H21.523 Goniosynechiae, bilateral
- H21.529 Goniosynechiae, unspecified eye ▽

✓6ᵗʰ **H21.53 Iridodialysis**
- H21.531 Iridodialysis, right eye
- H21.532 Iridodialysis, left eye
- H21.533 Iridodialysis, bilateral
- H21.539 Iridodialysis, unspecified eye ▽

✓6ᵗʰ **H21.54 Posterior synechiae (iris)**
- H21.541 Posterior synechiae (iris), right eye
- H21.542 Posterior synechiae (iris), left eye
- H21.543 Posterior synechiae (iris), bilateral
- H21.549 Posterior synechiae (iris), unspecified eye ▽

✓6ᵗʰ **H21.55 Recession of chamber angle**
- H21.551 Recession of chamber angle, right eye
- H21.552 Recession of chamber angle, left eye
- H21.553 Recession of chamber angle, bilateral
- H21.559 Recession of chamber angle, unspecified eye ▽

EXCLUDES 1 Not coded here   EXCLUDES 2 Not included here   N Newborn Age: 0   P Pediatric Age: 0-17   M Maternity Age: 12-55   A Adult Age: 15-124

584 ICD-10-CM 2018

✓6ᵗʰ **H21.56 Pupillary abnormalities**
Deformed pupil
Ectopic pupil
Rupture of sphincter, pupil
EXCLUDES 1   *congenital deformity of pupil (Q13.2-)*

     H21.561 Pupillary abnormality, right eye
     H21.562 Pupillary abnormality, left eye
     H21.563 Pupillary abnormality, bilateral
     H21.569 Pupillary abnormality, unspecified eye ▽

✓5ᵗʰ **H21.8 Other specified disorders of iris and ciliary body**

     H21.81 Floppy iris syndrome
         Intraoperative floppy iris syndrome (IFIS)
         Use additional code for adverse effect, if applicable, to identify drug (T36-T50 with fifth or sixth character 5)

     H21.82 Plateau iris syndrome (post-iridectomy) (postprocedural)

     H21.89 Other specified disorders of iris and ciliary body

H21.9 Unspecified disorder of iris and ciliary body ▽

H22 *Disorders of iris and ciliary body in diseases classified elsewhere*
Code first underlying disease, such as:
     gout (M1A.-, M10.-)
     leprosy (A30.-)
     parasitic disease (B89)

Disorders of lens (H25-H28)

✓4ᵗʰ **H25 Age-related cataract**
Senile cataract
EXCLUDES 2   *capsular glaucoma with pseudoexfoliation of lens (H40.1-)*

✓5ᵗʰ **H25.0 Age-related incipient cataract**

     ✓6ᵗʰ **H25.01 Cortical age-related cataract**
         H25.011 Cortical age-related cataract, right eye Ⓐ
         H25.012 Cortical age-related cataract, left eye Ⓐ
         H25.013 Cortical age-related cataract, bilateral Ⓐ
         H25.019 Cortical age-related cataract, unspecified eye Ⓐ▽

     ✓6ᵗʰ **H25.03 Anterior subcapsular polar age-related cataract**
         H25.031 Anterior subcapsular polar age-related cataract, right eye Ⓐ
         H25.032 Anterior subcapsular polar age-related cataract, left eye Ⓐ
         H25.033 Anterior subcapsular polar age-related cataract, bilateral Ⓐ
         H25.039 Anterior subcapsular polar age-related cataract, unspecified eye Ⓐ▽

     ✓6ᵗʰ **H25.04 Posterior subcapsular polar age-related cataract**
         H25.041 Posterior subcapsular polar age-related cataract, right eye Ⓐ
         H25.042 Posterior subcapsular polar age-related cataract, left eye Ⓐ
         H25.043 Posterior subcapsular polar age-related cataract, bilateral Ⓐ
         H25.049 Posterior subcapsular polar age-related cataract, unspecified eye Ⓐ▽

     ✓6ᵗʰ **H25.09 Other age-related incipient cataract**
         Coronary age-related cataract
         Punctate age-related cataract
         Water clefts
         H25.091 Other age-related incipient cataract, right eye Ⓐ
         H25.092 Other age-related incipient cataract, left eye Ⓐ
         H25.093 Other age-related incipient cataract, bilateral Ⓐ
         H25.099 Other age-related incipient cataract, unspecified eye Ⓐ▽

✓5ᵗʰ **H25.1 Age-related nuclear cataract**
Cataracta brunescens
Nuclear sclerosis cataract
AHA: 2016, 1Q, 36

     H25.10 Age-related nuclear cataract, unspecified eye Ⓐ▽
     H25.11 Age-related nuclear cataract, right eye Ⓐ
     H25.12 Age-related nuclear cataract, left eye Ⓐ
     H25.13 Age-related nuclear cataract, bilateral Ⓐ

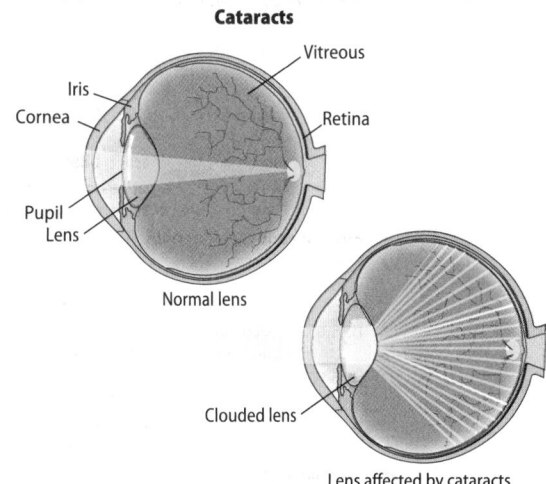

Cataracts

Vitreous
Iris
Cornea
Retina
Pupil
Lens
Normal lens
Clouded lens

Lens affected by cataracts

✓5ᵗʰ **H25.2 Age-related cataract, morgagnian type**
Age-related hypermature cataract

     H25.20 Age-related cataract, morgagnian type, unspecified eye Ⓐ▽
     H25.21 Age-related cataract, morgagnian type, right eye Ⓐ
     H25.22 Age-related cataract, morgagnian type, left eye Ⓐ
     H25.23 Age-related cataract, morgagnian type, bilateral Ⓐ

✓5ᵗʰ **H25.8 Other age-related cataract**

     ✓6ᵗʰ **H25.81 Combined forms of age-related cataract**
         H25.811 Combined forms of age-related cataract, right eye Ⓐ
         H25.812 Combined forms of age-related cataract, left eye Ⓐ
         H25.813 Combined forms of age-related cataract, bilateral Ⓐ
         H25.819 Combined forms of age-related cataract, unspecified eye Ⓐ▽

     H25.89 Other age-related cataract Ⓐ

H25.9 Unspecified age-related cataract Ⓐ▽

✓4ᵗʰ **H26 Other cataract**
EXCLUDES 1   *congenital cataract (Q12.0)*

✓5ᵗʰ **H26.0 Infantile and juvenile cataract**

     ✓6ᵗʰ **H26.00 Unspecified infantile and juvenile cataract**
         H26.001 Unspecified infantile and juvenile cataract, right eye Ⓟ▽
         H26.002 Unspecified infantile and juvenile cataract, left eye Ⓟ▽
         H26.003 Unspecified infantile and juvenile cataract, bilateral Ⓟ▽
         H26.009 Unspecified infantile and juvenile cataract, unspecified eye Ⓟ▽

     ✓6ᵗʰ **H26.01 Infantile and juvenile cortical, lamellar, or zonular cataract**
         H26.011 Infantile and juvenile cortical, lamellar, or zonular cataract, right eye Ⓟ
         H26.012 Infantile and juvenile cortical, lamellar, or zonular cataract, left eye Ⓟ
         H26.013 Infantile and juvenile cortical, lamellar, or zonular cataract, bilateral Ⓟ
         H26.019 Infantile and juvenile cortical, lamellar, or zonular cataract, unspecified eye Ⓟ▽

     ✓6ᵗʰ **H26.03 Infantile and juvenile nuclear cataract**
         H26.031 Infantile and juvenile nuclear cataract, right eye Ⓟ
         H26.032 Infantile and juvenile nuclear cataract, left eye Ⓟ
         H26.033 Infantile and juvenile nuclear cataract, bilateral Ⓟ
         H26.039 Infantile and juvenile nuclear cataract, unspecified eye Ⓟ▽

☑ Additional Character Req   ✓ˣ7ᵗʰ Placeholder Alert   Manifestation   ᴴᶜᶜ CMS-HCC Condition   ▽ Unspecified Code   ►◄ Revised Text   ● New Code   ▲ Revised Code Title

√6th **H26.04** Anterior subcapsular polar **infantile and juvenile cataract**
- **H26.041** **Anterior subcapsular polar infantile and juvenile cataract,** right **eye** P
- **H26.042** **Anterior subcapsular polar infantile and juvenile cataract,** left **eye** P
- **H26.043** **Anterior subcapsular polar infantile and juvenile cataract,** bilateral P
- **H26.049** **Anterior subcapsular polar infantile and juvenile cataract, unspecified eye** P ▽

√6th **H26.05** Posterior subcapsular polar **infantile and juvenile cataract**
- **H26.051** **Posterior subcapsular polar infantile and juvenile cataract,** right **eye** P
- **H26.052** **Posterior subcapsular polar infantile and juvenile cataract,** left **eye** P
- **H26.053** **Posterior subcapsular polar infantile and juvenile cataract,** bilateral P
- **H26.059** **Posterior subcapsular polar infantile and juvenile cataract, unspecified eye** P ▽

√6th **H26.06** Combined forms **of infantile and juvenile cataract**
- **H26.061** **Combined forms of infantile and juvenile cataract,** right **eye** P
- **H26.062** **Combined forms of infantile and juvenile cataract,** left **eye** P
- **H26.063** **Combined forms of infantile and juvenile cataract,** bilateral P
- **H26.069** **Combined forms of infantile and juvenile cataract, unspecified eye** P ▽

H26.09 **Other infantile and juvenile cataract** P

√5th **H26.1** Traumatic **cataract**
    Use additional code (Chapter 20) to identify external cause

√6th **H26.10** **Unspecified traumatic cataract**
- **H26.101** **Unspecified traumatic cataract,** right **eye** ▽
- **H26.102** **Unspecified traumatic cataract,** left **eye** ▽
- **H26.103** **Unspecified traumatic cataract, bilateral** ▽
- **H26.109** **Unspecified traumatic cataract, unspecified eye** ▽

√6th **H26.11** Localized **traumatic opacities**
- **H26.111** **Localized traumatic opacities,** right **eye**
- **H26.112** **Localized traumatic opacities,** left **eye**
- **H26.113** **Localized traumatic opacities,** bilateral
- **H26.119** **Localized traumatic opacities, unspecified eye** ▽

√6th **H26.12** Partially resolved **traumatic cataract**
- **H26.121** **Partially resolved traumatic cataract,** right **eye**
- **H26.122** **Partially resolved traumatic cataract,** left **eye**
- **H26.123** **Partially resolved traumatic cataract, bilateral**
- **H26.129** **Partially resolved traumatic cataract, unspecified eye** ▽

√6th **H26.13** Total **traumatic cataract**
- **H26.131** **Total traumatic cataract,** right **eye**
- **H26.132** **Total traumatic cataract,** left **eye**
- **H26.133** **Total traumatic cataract,** bilateral
- **H26.139** **Total traumatic cataract, unspecified eye** ▽

√5th **H26.2** Complicated **cataract**

H26.20 **Unspecified complicated cataract** ▽
    Cataracta complicata NOS

√6th **H26.21** **Cataract** with neovascularization
    Code also associated condition, such as:
      chronic iridocyclitis (H20.1-)
- **H26.211** **Cataract with neovascularization,** right **eye**
- **H26.212** **Cataract with neovascularization,** left **eye**
- **H26.213** **Cataract with neovascularization,** bilateral
- **H26.219** **Cataract with neovascularization, unspecified eye** ▽

√6th **H26.22** Cataract secondary to ocular disorders **(degenerative) (inflammatory)**
    Code also associated ocular disorder
- **H26.221** **Cataract secondary to ocular disorders (degenerative) (inflammatory),** right **eye**
- **H26.222** **Cataract secondary to ocular disorders (degenerative) (inflammatory),** left **eye**
- **H26.223** **Cataract secondary to ocular disorders (degenerative) (inflammatory),** bilateral
- **H26.229** **Cataract secondary to ocular disorders (degenerative) (inflammatory), unspecified eye** ▽

√6th **H26.23** Glaucomatous flecks (subcapsular)
    Code first underlying glaucoma (H40-H42)
- **H26.231** **Glaucomatous flecks (subcapsular),** right **eye**
- **H26.232** **Glaucomatous flecks (subcapsular),** left **eye**
- **H26.233** **Glaucomatous flecks (subcapsular),** bilateral
- **H26.239** **Glaucomatous flecks (subcapsular), unspecified eye** ▽

√5th **H26.3** Drug-induced **cataract**
    Toxic cataract
    Use additional code for adverse effect, if applicable, to identify drug (T36-T50 with fifth or sixth character 5)
- **H26.30** **Drug-induced cataract, unspecified eye** ▽
- **H26.31** **Drug-induced cataract,** right **eye**
- **H26.32** **Drug-induced cataract,** left **eye**
- **H26.33** **Drug-induced cataract,** bilateral

√5th **H26.4** Secondary **cataract**
- **H26.40** **Unspecified secondary cataract** ▽

√6th **H26.41** Soemmering's ring
- **H26.411** **Soemmering's ring,** right **eye**
- **H26.412** **Soemmering's ring,** left **eye**
- **H26.413** **Soemmering's ring,** bilateral
- **H26.419** **Soemmering's ring, unspecified eye** ▽

√6th **H26.49** **Other secondary cataract**
- **H26.491** **Other secondary cataract,** right **eye**
- **H26.492** **Other secondary cataract,** left **eye**
- **H26.493** **Other secondary cataract,** bilateral
- **H26.499** **Other secondary cataract, unspecified eye** ▽

H26.8 **Other specified cataract**

H26.9 **Unspecified cataract** ▽

√4th **H27** **Other disorders of lens**
    EXCLUDES 1   *congenital lens malformations (Q12.-)*
       mechanical complications of intraocular lens implant (T85.2)
       pseudophakia (Z96.1)

√5th **H27.0** Aphakia
    Acquired absence of lens
    Acquired aphakia
    Aphakia due to trauma
    EXCLUDES 1   *cataract extraction status (Z98.4-)*
       congenital absence of lens (Q12.3)
       congenital aphakia (Q12.3)
- **H27.00** **Aphakia, unspecified eye** ▽
- **H27.01** **Aphakia,** right **eye**
- **H27.02** **Aphakia,** left **eye**
- **H27.03** **Aphakia,** bilateral

√5th **H27.1** Dislocation of lens
- **H27.10** **Unspecified dislocation of lens** ▽

√6th **H27.11** Subluxation of lens
- **H27.111** **Subluxation of lens,** right **eye**
- **H27.112** **Subluxation of lens,** left **eye**
- **H27.113** **Subluxation of lens,** bilateral
- **H27.119** **Subluxation of lens, unspecified eye** ▽

√6th **H27.12** Anterior dislocation of lens
- **H27.121** **Anterior dislocation of lens,** right **eye**
- **H27.122** **Anterior dislocation of lens,** left **eye**
- **H27.123** **Anterior dislocation of lens,** bilateral
- **H27.129** **Anterior dislocation of lens, unspecified eye** ▽

☑6ᵗʰ **H27.13 Posterior dislocation of lens**
     H27.131 Posterior dislocation of lens, right eye
     H27.132 Posterior dislocation of lens, left eye
     H27.133 Posterior dislocation of lens, bilateral
     H27.139 Posterior dislocation of lens, unspecified eye ▽

H27.8 Other specified disorders of lens
H27.9 Unspecified disorder of lens ▽

H28 ***Cataract in diseases classified elsewhere***
Code first underlying disease, such as:
     hypoparathyroidism (E20.-)
     myotonia (G71.1-)
     myxedema (E03.-)
     protein-calorie malnutrition (E40-E46)
     EXCLUDES 1 *cataract in diabetes mellitus (E08.36, E09.36, E10.36, E11.36, E13.36)*

Disorders of choroid and retina (H30-H36)

☑4ᵗʰ **H30 Chorioretinal inflammation**

☑5ᵗʰ **H30.0 Focal chorioretinal inflammation**
     Focal chorioretinitis
     Focal choroiditis
     Focal retinitis
     Focal retinochoroiditis

  ☑6ᵗʰ **H30.00 Unspecified focal chorioretinal inflammation**
     Focal chorioretinitis NOS
     Focal choroiditis NOS
     Focal retinitis NOS
     Focal retinochoroiditis NOS
     H30.001 Unspecified focal chorioretinal inflammation, right eye ▽
     H30.002 Unspecified focal chorioretinal inflammation, left eye ▽
     H30.003 Unspecified focal chorioretinal inflammation, bilateral ▽
     H30.009 Unspecified focal chorioretinal inflammation, unspecified eye ▽

  ☑6ᵗʰ **H30.01 Focal chorioretinal inflammation, juxtapapillary**
     H30.011 Focal chorioretinal inflammation, juxtapapillary, right eye
     H30.012 Focal chorioretinal inflammation, juxtapapillary, left eye
     H30.013 Focal chorioretinal inflammation, juxtapapillary, bilateral
     H30.019 Focal chorioretinal inflammation, juxtapapillary, unspecified eye ▽

  ☑6ᵗʰ **H30.02 Focal chorioretinal inflammation of posterior pole**
     H30.021 Focal chorioretinal inflammation of posterior pole, right eye
     H30.022 Focal chorioretinal inflammation of posterior pole, left eye
     H30.023 Focal chorioretinal inflammation of posterior pole, bilateral
     H30.029 Focal chorioretinal inflammation of posterior pole, unspecified eye ▽

  ☑6ᵗʰ **H30.03 Focal chorioretinal inflammation, peripheral**
     H30.031 Focal chorioretinal inflammation, peripheral, right eye
     H30.032 Focal chorioretinal inflammation, peripheral, left eye
     H30.033 Focal chorioretinal inflammation, peripheral, bilateral
     H30.039 Focal chorioretinal inflammation, peripheral, unspecified eye ▽

  ☑6ᵗʰ **H30.04 Focal chorioretinal inflammation, macular or paramacular**
     H30.041 Focal chorioretinal inflammation, macular or paramacular, right eye
     H30.042 Focal chorioretinal inflammation, macular or paramacular, left eye
     H30.043 Focal chorioretinal inflammation, macular or paramacular, bilateral
     H30.049 Focal chorioretinal inflammation, macular or paramacular, unspecified eye ▽

☑5ᵗʰ **H30.1 Disseminated chorioretinal inflammation**
     Disseminated chorioretinitis
     Disseminated choroiditis
     Disseminated retinitis
     Disseminated retinochoroiditis
     EXCLUDES 2 *exudative retinopathy (H35.02-)*

  ☑6ᵗʰ **H30.10 Unspecified disseminated chorioretinal inflammation**
     Disseminated chorioretinitis NOS
     Disseminated choroiditis NOS
     Disseminated retinitis NOS
     Disseminated retinochoroiditis NOS
     H30.101 Unspecified disseminated chorioretinal inflammation, right eye ▽
     H30.102 Unspecified disseminated chorioretinal inflammation, left eye ▽
     H30.103 Unspecified disseminated chorioretinal inflammation, bilateral ▽
     H30.109 Unspecified disseminated chorioretinal inflammation, unspecified eye ▽

  ☑6ᵗʰ **H30.11 Disseminated chorioretinal inflammation of posterior pole**
     H30.111 Disseminated chorioretinal inflammation of posterior pole, right eye
     H30.112 Disseminated chorioretinal inflammation of posterior pole, left eye
     H30.113 Disseminated chorioretinal inflammation of posterior pole, bilateral
     H30.119 Disseminated chorioretinal inflammation of posterior pole, unspecified eye ▽

  ☑6ᵗʰ **H30.12 Disseminated chorioretinal inflammation, peripheral**
     H30.121 Disseminated chorioretinal inflammation, peripheral right eye
     H30.122 Disseminated chorioretinal inflammation, peripheral, left eye
     H30.123 Disseminated chorioretinal inflammation, peripheral, bilateral
     H30.129 Disseminated chorioretinal inflammation, peripheral, unspecified eye ▽

  ☑6ᵗʰ **H30.13 Disseminated chorioretinal inflammation, generalized**
     H30.131 Disseminated chorioretinal inflammation, generalized, right eye
     H30.132 Disseminated chorioretinal inflammation, generalized, left eye
     H30.133 Disseminated chorioretinal inflammation, generalized, bilateral
     H30.139 Disseminated chorioretinal inflammation, generalized, unspecified eye ▽

  ☑6ᵗʰ **H30.14 Acute posterior multifocal placoid pigment epitheliopathy**
     H30.141 Acute posterior multifocal placoid pigment epitheliopathy, right eye
     H30.142 Acute posterior multifocal placoid pigment epitheliopathy, left eye
     H30.143 Acute posterior multifocal placoid pigment epitheliopathy, bilateral
     H30.149 Acute posterior multifocal placoid pigment epitheliopathy, unspecified eye ▽

☑5ᵗʰ **H30.2 Posterior cyclitis**
     Pars planitis
     H30.20 Posterior cyclitis, unspecified eye ▽
     H30.21 Posterior cyclitis, right eye
     H30.22 Posterior cyclitis, left eye
     H30.23 Posterior cyclitis, bilateral

☑5ᵗʰ **H30.8 Other chorioretinal inflammations**

  ☑6ᵗʰ **H30.81 Harada's disease**
     H30.811 Harada's disease, right eye
     H30.812 Harada's disease, left eye
     H30.813 Harada's disease, bilateral
     H30.819 Harada's disease, unspecified eye ▽

☑ Additional Character Req   ☑×7ᵗʰ Placeholder Alert   Manifestation   **HCC** CMS-HCC Condition   ▽ Unspecified Code   ►◄ Revised Text   ● New Code   ▲ Revised Code Title

Chapter 7. Diseases of the Eye and Adnexa

√6ᵗʰ **H30.89** **Other chorioretinal inflammations**
    H30.891 **Other chorioretinal inflammations, right eye**
    H30.892 **Other chorioretinal inflammations, left eye**
    H30.893 **Other chorioretinal inflammations, bilateral**
    H30.899 **Other chorioretinal inflammations, unspecified eye** ▽

√5ᵗʰ **H30.9** **Unspecified chorioretinal inflammation**
    Chorioretinitis NOS   Retinitis NOS
    Choroiditis NOS   Retinochoroiditis NOS
    Neuroretinitis NOS
    H30.90 **Unspecified chorioretinal inflammation, unspecified eye** ▽
    H30.91 **Unspecified chorioretinal inflammation, right eye** ▽
    H30.92 **Unspecified chorioretinal inflammation, left eye** ▽
    H30.93 **Unspecified chorioretinal inflammation, bilateral** ▽

√4ᵗʰ **H31** **Other disorders of choroid**

√5ᵗʰ **H31.0** **Chorioretinal scars**
    EXCLUDES 2   *postsurgical chorioretinal scars (H59.81-)*

    √6ᵗʰ **H31.00** **Unspecified chorioretinal scars**
        H31.001 **Unspecified chorioretinal scars, right eye** ▽
        H31.002 **Unspecified chorioretinal scars, left eye** ▽
        H31.003 **Unspecified chorioretinal scars, bilateral** ▽
        H31.009 **Unspecified chorioretinal scars, unspecified eye** ▽

    √6ᵗʰ **H31.01** **Macula scars of posterior pole (postinflammatory) (post-traumatic)**
        EXCLUDES 1   *postprocedural chorioretinal scar (H59.81-)*
        H31.011 **Macula scars of posterior pole (postinflammatory) (post-traumatic), right eye**
        H31.012 **Macula scars of posterior pole (postinflammatory) (post-traumatic), left eye**
        H31.013 **Macula scars of posterior pole (postinflammatory) (post-traumatic), bilateral**
        H31.019 **Macula scars of posterior pole (postinflammatory) (post-traumatic), unspecified eye** ▽

    √6ᵗʰ **H31.02** **Solar retinopathy**
        H31.021 **Solar retinopathy, right eye**
        H31.022 **Solar retinopathy, left eye**
        H31.023 **Solar retinopathy, bilateral**
        H31.029 **Solar retinopathy, unspecified eye** ▽

    √6ᵗʰ **H31.09** **Other chorioretinal scars**
        H31.091 **Other chorioretinal scars, right eye**
        H31.092 **Other chorioretinal scars, left eye**
        H31.093 **Other chorioretinal scars, bilateral**
        H31.099 **Other chorioretinal scars, unspecified eye** ▽

√5ᵗʰ **H31.1** **Choroidal degeneration**
    EXCLUDES 2   *angioid streaks of macula (H35.33)*

    √6ᵗʰ **H31.10** **Unspecified choroidal degeneration**
        Choroidal sclerosis NOS
        H31.101 **Choroidal degeneration, unspecified, right eye** ▽
        H31.102 **Choroidal degeneration, unspecified, left eye** ▽
        H31.103 **Choroidal degeneration, unspecified, bilateral** ▽
        H31.109 **Choroidal degeneration, unspecified, unspecified eye** ▽

    √6ᵗʰ **H31.11** **Age-related choroidal atrophy**
        H31.111 **Age-related choroidal atrophy, right eye** 🅰
        H31.112 **Age-related choroidal atrophy, left eye** 🅰
        H31.113 **Age-related choroidal atrophy, bilateral** 🅰
        H31.119 **Age-related choroidal atrophy, unspecified eye** 🅰▽

√6ᵗʰ **H31.12** **Diffuse secondary atrophy of choroid**
    H31.121 **Diffuse secondary atrophy of choroid, right eye**
    H31.122 **Diffuse secondary atrophy of choroid, left eye**
    H31.123 **Diffuse secondary atrophy of choroid, bilateral**
    H31.129 **Diffuse secondary atrophy of choroid, unspecified eye** ▽

√5ᵗʰ **H31.2** **Hereditary choroidal dystrophy**
    EXCLUDES 2   *hyperornithinemia (E72.4)*
                  ornithinemia (E72.4)
    H31.20 **Hereditary choroidal dystrophy, unspecified** ▽
    H31.21 **Choroideremia**
    H31.22 **Choroidal dystrophy (central areolar) (generalized) (peripapillary)**
    H31.23 **Gyrate atrophy, choroid**
    H31.29 **Other hereditary choroidal dystrophy**

√5ᵗʰ **H31.3** **Choroidal hemorrhage and rupture**
    √6ᵗʰ **H31.30** **Unspecified choroidal hemorrhage**
        H31.301 **Unspecified choroidal hemorrhage, right eye** ▽
        H31.302 **Unspecified choroidal hemorrhage, left eye** ▽
        H31.303 **Unspecified choroidal hemorrhage, bilateral** ▽
        H31.309 **Unspecified choroidal hemorrhage, unspecified eye** ▽

    √6ᵗʰ **H31.31** **Expulsive choroidal hemorrhage**
        H31.311 **Expulsive choroidal hemorrhage, right eye**
        H31.312 **Expulsive choroidal hemorrhage, left eye**
        H31.313 **Expulsive choroidal hemorrhage, bilateral**
        H31.319 **Expulsive choroidal hemorrhage, unspecified eye** ▽

    √6ᵗʰ **H31.32** **Choroidal rupture**
        H31.321 **Choroidal rupture, right eye**
        H31.322 **Choroidal rupture, left eye**
        H31.323 **Choroidal rupture, bilateral**
        H31.329 **Choroidal rupture, unspecified eye** ▽

√5ᵗʰ **H31.4** **Choroidal detachment**
    √6ᵗʰ **H31.40** **Unspecified choroidal detachment**
        H31.401 **Unspecified choroidal detachment, right eye** ▽
        H31.402 **Unspecified choroidal detachment, left eye** ▽
        H31.403 **Unspecified choroidal detachment, bilateral** ▽
        H31.409 **Unspecified choroidal detachment, unspecified eye** ▽

    √6ᵗʰ **H31.41** **Hemorrhagic choroidal detachment**
        H31.411 **Hemorrhagic choroidal detachment, right eye**
        H31.412 **Hemorrhagic choroidal detachment, left eye**
        H31.413 **Hemorrhagic choroidal detachment, bilateral**
        H31.419 **Hemorrhagic choroidal detachment, unspecified eye** ▽

    √6ᵗʰ **H31.42** **Serous choroidal detachment**
        H31.421 **Serous choroidal detachment, right eye**
        H31.422 **Serous choroidal detachment, left eye**
        H31.423 **Serous choroidal detachment, bilateral**
        H31.429 **Serous choroidal detachment, unspecified eye** ▽

H31.8 **Other specified disorders of choroid**
H31.9 **Unspecified disorder of choroid** ▽

H32 *Chorioretinal disorders in diseases classified elsewhere*
    Code first underlying disease, such as:
        congenital toxoplasmosis (P37.1)
        histoplasmosis (B39.-)
        leprosy (A30.-)
    EXCLUDES 1   *chorioretinitis (in):*
        toxoplasmosis (acquired) (B58.01)
        tuberculosis (A18.53)

EXCLUDES 1 Not coded here   *EXCLUDES 2* Not included here   🅽 Newborn Age: 0   🅿 Pediatric Age: 0-17   🅼 Maternity Age: 12-55   🅰 Adult Age: 15-124

588   ICD-10-CM 2018

Retinal Detachment

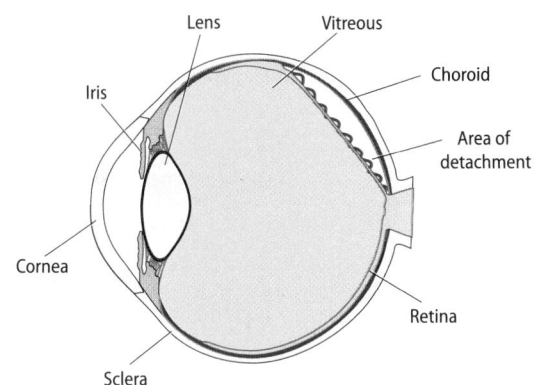

H33 **Retinal detachments and breaks**

EXCLUDES 1   *detachment of retinal pigment epithelium (H35.72-, H35.73-)*

√5ᵗʰ H33.0 **Retinal detachment** with retinal break
Rhegmatogenous retinal detachment
EXCLUDES 1   *serous retinal detachment (without retinal break) (H33.2-)*

√6ᵗʰ H33.00 **Unspecified retinal detachment with retinal break**
H33.001 **Unspecified retinal detachment with retinal break, right eye** ▽
H33.002 **Unspecified retinal detachment with retinal break, left eye** ▽
H33.003 **Unspecified retinal detachment with retinal break, bilateral** ▽
H33.009 **Unspecified retinal detachment with retinal break, unspecified eye** ▽

√6ᵗʰ H33.01 **Retinal detachment with** single break
H33.011 **Retinal detachment with single break, right eye**
H33.012 **Retinal detachment with single break, left eye**
H33.013 **Retinal detachment with single break, bilateral**
H33.019 **Retinal detachment with single break, unspecified eye** ▽

√6ᵗʰ H33.02 **Retinal detachment with** multiple breaks
H33.021 **Retinal detachment with multiple breaks, right eye**
H33.022 **Retinal detachment with multiple breaks, left eye**
H33.023 **Retinal detachment with multiple breaks, bilateral**
H33.029 **Retinal detachment with multiple breaks, unspecified eye** ▽

√6ᵗʰ H33.03 **Retinal detachment with** giant retinal tear
H33.031 **Retinal detachment with giant retinal tear, right eye**
H33.032 **Retinal detachment with giant retinal tear, left eye**
H33.033 **Retinal detachment with giant retinal tear, bilateral**
H33.039 **Retinal detachment with giant retinal tear, unspecified eye** ▽

√6ᵗʰ H33.04 **Retinal detachment with** retinal dialysis
H33.041 **Retinal detachment with retinal dialysis, right eye**
H33.042 **Retinal detachment with retinal dialysis, left eye**
H33.043 **Retinal detachment with retinal dialysis, bilateral**
H33.049 **Retinal detachment with retinal dialysis, unspecified eye** ▽

√6ᵗʰ H33.05 **Total retinal detachment**
H33.051 **Total retinal detachment, right eye**
H33.052 **Total retinal detachment, left eye**
H33.053 **Total retinal detachment, bilateral**

H33.059 **Total retinal detachment, unspecified eye** ▽

√5ᵗʰ H33.1 **Retinoschisis and retinal cysts**
EXCLUDES 1   *congenital retinoschisis (Q14.1)*
microcystoid degeneration of retina (H35.42-)

√6ᵗʰ H33.10 **Unspecified retinoschisis**
H33.101 **Unspecified retinoschisis, right eye** ▽
H33.102 **Unspecified retinoschisis, left eye** ▽
H33.103 **Unspecified retinoschisis, bilateral** ▽
H33.109 **Unspecified retinoschisis, unspecified eye** ▽

√6ᵗʰ H33.11 **Cyst of ora serrata**
H33.111 **Cyst of ora serrata, right eye**
H33.112 **Cyst of ora serrata, left eye**
H33.113 **Cyst of ora serrata, bilateral**
H33.119 **Cyst of ora serrata, unspecified eye** ▽

√6ᵗʰ H33.12 **Parasitic cyst of retina**
H33.121 **Parasitic cyst of retina, right eye**
H33.122 **Parasitic cyst of retina, left eye**
H33.123 **Parasitic cyst of retina, bilateral**
H33.129 **Parasitic cyst of retina, unspecified eye** ▽

√6ᵗʰ H33.19 **Other retinoschisis and retinal cysts**
Pseudocyst of retina
H33.191 **Other retinoschisis and retinal cysts, right eye**
H33.192 **Other retinoschisis and retinal cysts, left eye**
H33.193 **Other retinoschisis and retinal cysts, bilateral**
H33.199 **Other retinoschisis and retinal cysts, unspecified eye** ▽

√5ᵗʰ H33.2 **Serous** retinal detachment
Retinal detachment NOS
Retinal detachment without retinal break
EXCLUDES 1   *central serous chorioretinopathy (H35.71-)*
H33.20 **Serous retinal detachment, unspecified eye** ▽
H33.21 **Serous retinal detachment, right eye**
H33.22 **Serous retinal detachment, left eye**
H33.23 **Serous retinal detachment, bilateral**

√5ᵗʰ H33.3 **Retinal breaks** without detachment
EXCLUDES 1   *chorioretinal scars after surgery for detachment (H59.81-)*
peripheral retinal degeneration without break (H35.4-)

√6ᵗʰ H33.30 **Unspecified retinal break**
H33.301 **Unspecified retinal break, right eye** ▽
H33.302 **Unspecified retinal break, left eye** ▽
H33.303 **Unspecified retinal break, bilateral** ▽
H33.309 **Unspecified retinal break, unspecified eye** ▽

√6ᵗʰ H33.31 **Horseshoe tear** of retina without detachment
Operculum of retina without detachment
H33.311 **Horseshoe tear of retina without detachment, right eye**
H33.312 **Horseshoe tear of retina without detachment, left eye**
H33.313 **Horseshoe tear of retina without detachment, bilateral**
H33.319 **Horseshoe tear of retina without detachment, unspecified eye** ▽

√6ᵗʰ H33.32 **Round hole** of retina without detachment
H33.321 **Round hole, right eye**
H33.322 **Round hole, left eye**
H33.323 **Round hole, bilateral**
H33.329 **Round hole, unspecified eye** ▽

√6ᵗʰ H33.33 **Multiple defects** of retina without detachment
H33.331 **Multiple defects of retina without detachment, right eye**
H33.332 **Multiple defects of retina without detachment, left eye**
H33.333 **Multiple defects of retina without detachment, bilateral**
H33.339 **Multiple defects of retina without detachment, unspecified eye** ▽

☑ Additional Character Req   √x7ᵗʰ Placeholder Alert   Manifestation   HCC CMS-HCC Condition   ▽ Unspecified Code   ►◄ Revised Text   ● New Code   ▲ Revised Code Title

Chapter 7. Diseases of the Eye and Adnexa

✓5ᵗʰ **H33.4** Traction detachment of retina
Proliferative vitreo-retinopathy with retinal detachment

    H33.40 **Traction detachment of retina, unspecified eye** ▽

    H33.41 **Traction detachment of retina, right eye**

    H33.42 **Traction detachment of retina, left eye**

    H33.43 **Traction detachment of retina, bilateral**

H33.8 **Other retinal detachments**

✓4ᵗʰ **H34** **Retinal vascular occlusions**
    EXCLUDES 1   amaurosis fugax (G45.3)

✓5ᵗʰ **H34.Ø** **Transient retinal artery occlusion**

    H34.00 **Transient retinal artery occlusion, unspecified eye** ▽

    H34.01 **Transient retinal artery occlusion, right eye**

    H34.02 **Transient retinal artery occlusion, left eye**

    H34.03 **Transient retinal artery occlusion, bilateral**

✓5ᵗʰ **H34.1** **Central retinal artery occlusion**

    H34.10 **Central retinal artery occlusion, unspecified eye** ▽

    H34.11 **Central retinal artery occlusion, right eye**

    H34.12 **Central retinal artery occlusion, left eye**

    H34.13 **Central retinal artery occlusion, bilateral**

✓5ᵗʰ **H34.2** **Other retinal artery occlusions**

    ✓6ᵗʰ **H34.21** Partial **retinal artery occlusion**
        Hollenhorst's plaque
        Retinal microembolism

        H34.211 **Partial retinal artery occlusion, right eye**

        H34.212 **Partial retinal artery occlusion, left eye**

        H34.213 **Partial retinal artery occlusion, bilateral**

        H34.219 **Partial retinal artery occlusion, unspecified eye** ▽

    ✓6ᵗʰ **H34.23** **Retinal artery branch occlusion**

        H34.231 **Retinal artery branch occlusion, right eye**

        H34.232 **Retinal artery branch occlusion, left eye**

        H34.233 **Retinal artery branch occlusion, bilateral**

        H34.239 **Retinal artery branch occlusion, unspecified eye** ▽

✓5ᵗʰ **H34.8** **Other retinal vascular occlusions**

    ✓6ᵗʰ **H34.81** **Central retinal vein occlusion**

> One of the following 7th characters is to be assigned to codes in subcategory H34.81 to designate the severity of the occlusion:
> Ø   with macular edema
> 1   with retinal neovascularization
> 2   stable
>   old central retinal vein occlusion

        ✓7ᵗʰ **H34.811** **Central retinal vein occlusion, right eye**

        ✓7ᵗʰ **H34.812** **Central retinal vein occlusion, left eye**

        ✓7ᵗʰ **H34.813** **Central retinal vein occlusion, bilateral**

        ✓7ᵗʰ **H34.819** **Central retinal vein occlusion, unspecified eye** ▽

    ✓6ᵗʰ **H34.82** **Venous engorgement**
        Incipient retinal vein occlusion
        Partial retinal vein occlusion

        H34.821 **Venous engorgement, right eye**

        H34.822 **Venous engorgement, left eye**

        H34.823 **Venous engorgement, bilateral**

        H34.829 **Venous engorgement, unspecified eye** ▽

    ✓6ᵗʰ **H34.83** **Tributary (branch) retinal vein occlusion**

> One of the following 7th characters is to be assigned to codes in subcategory H34.83 to designate the severity of the occlusion:
> Ø   with macular edema
> 1   with retinal neovascularization
> 2   stable
>   old tributary (branch) retinal vein occlusion

        ✓7ᵗʰ **H34.831** **Tributary (branch) retinal vein occlusion, right eye**

        ✓7ᵗʰ **H34.832** **Tributary (branch) retinal vein occlusion, left eye**

        ✓7ᵗʰ **H34.833** **Tributary (branch) retinal vein occlusion, bilateral**

        ✓7ᵗʰ **H34.839** **Tributary (branch) retinal vein occlusion, unspecified eye** ▽

H34.9 **Unspecified retinal vascular occlusion** ▽

✓4ᵗʰ **H35** **Other retinal disorders**
    EXCLUDES 2   diabetic retinal disorders (EØ8.311- EØ8.359, EØ9.311- EØ9.359, E1Ø.311- E1Ø.359, E11.311- E11.359, E13.311- E13.359)

✓5ᵗʰ **H35.Ø** **Background retinopathy and retinal vascular changes**
Code also any associated hypertension (I1Ø.-)

    H35.00 **Unspecified background retinopathy** ▽

    ✓6ᵗʰ **H35.01** **Changes in retinal vascular appearance**
        Retinal vascular sheathing

        H35.011 **Changes in retinal vascular appearance, right eye**

        H35.012 **Changes in retinal vascular appearance, left eye**

        H35.013 **Changes in retinal vascular appearance, bilateral**

        H35.019 **Changes in retinal vascular appearance, unspecified eye** ▽

    ✓6ᵗʰ **H35.02** Exudative **retinopathy**
        Coats retinopathy

        H35.021 **Exudative retinopathy, right eye**

        H35.022 **Exudative retinopathy, left eye**

        H35.023 **Exudative retinopathy, bilateral**

        H35.029 **Exudative retinopathy, unspecified eye** ▽

    ✓6ᵗʰ **H35.03** Hypertensive **retinopathy**

        H35.031 **Hypertensive retinopathy, right eye**

        H35.032 **Hypertensive retinopathy, left eye**

        H35.033 **Hypertensive retinopathy, bilateral**

        H35.039 **Hypertensive retinopathy, unspecified eye** ▽

    ✓6ᵗʰ **H35.04** **Retinal** micro-aneurysms, **unspecified**

        H35.041 **Retinal micro-aneurysms, unspecified, right eye**

        H35.042 **Retinal micro-aneurysms, unspecified, left eye**

        H35.043 **Retinal micro-aneurysms, unspecified, bilateral** ▽

        H35.049 **Retinal micro-aneurysms, unspecified, unspecified eye** ▽

    ✓6ᵗʰ **H35.05** **Retinal** neovascularization, **unspecified**

        H35.051 **Retinal neovascularization, unspecified, right eye** ▽

        H35.052 **Retinal neovascularization, unspecified, left eye** ▽

        H35.053 **Retinal neovascularization, unspecified, bilateral** ▽

        H35.059 **Retinal neovascularization, unspecified, unspecified eye** ▽

    ✓6ᵗʰ **H35.06** **Retinal** vasculitis
        Eales disease
        Retinal perivasculitis
        DEF: Sight-threatening intraocular inflammation of the retinal blood vessels; causes minimal, partial, or even complete blindness.

        H35.061 **Retinal vasculitis, right eye**

        H35.062 **Retinal vasculitis, left eye**

        H35.063 **Retinal vasculitis, bilateral**

        H35.069 **Retinal vasculitis, unspecified eye** ▽

    ✓6ᵗʰ **H35.07** **Retinal** telangiectasis

        H35.071 **Retinal telangiectasis, right eye**

        H35.072 **Retinal telangiectasis, left eye**

        H35.073 **Retinal telangiectasis, bilateral**

        H35.079 **Retinal telangiectasis, unspecified eye** ▽

    H35.09 **Other intraretinal microvascular abnormalities**
        Retinal varices

✓5ᵗʰ **H35.1** **Retinopathy of prematurity**

    ✓6ᵗʰ **H35.10** **Retinopathy of prematurity, unspecified**
        Retinopathy of prematurity NOS

        H35.101 **Retinopathy of prematurity, unspecified, right eye** ▽

        H35.102 **Retinopathy of prematurity, unspecified, left eye** ▽

        H35.103 **Retinopathy of prematurity, unspecified, bilateral** ▽

        H35.109 **Retinopathy of prematurity, unspecified, unspecified eye** ▽

EXCLUDES 1 Not coded here   EXCLUDES 2 Not included here   N Newborn Age: 0   P Pediatric Age: 0-17   M Maternity Age: 12-55   A Adult Age: 15-124

590   ICD-10-CM 2018

✓6ᵗʰ H35.11 Retinopathy of prematurity, stage 0
- **H35.111 Retinopathy of prematurity, stage 0, right eye**
- **H35.112 Retinopathy of prematurity, stage 0, left eye**
- **H35.113 Retinopathy of prematurity, stage 0, bilateral**
- **H35.119 Retinopathy of prematurity, stage 0, unspecified eye** ▽

✓6ᵗʰ H35.12 Retinopathy of prematurity, stage 1
- **H35.121 Retinopathy of prematurity, stage 1, right eye**
- **H35.122 Retinopathy of prematurity, stage 1, left eye**
- **H35.123 Retinopathy of prematurity, stage 1, bilateral**
- **H35.129 Retinopathy of prematurity, stage 1, unspecified eye** ▽

✓6ᵗʰ H35.13 Retinopathy of prematurity, stage 2
- **H35.131 Retinopathy of prematurity, stage 2, right eye**
- **H35.132 Retinopathy of prematurity, stage 2, left eye**
- **H35.133 Retinopathy of prematurity, stage 2, bilateral**
- **H35.139 Retinopathy of prematurity, stage 2, unspecified eye** ▽

✓6ᵗʰ H35.14 Retinopathy of prematurity, stage 3
- **H35.141 Retinopathy of prematurity, stage 3, right eye**
- **H35.142 Retinopathy of prematurity, stage 3, left eye**
- **H35.143 Retinopathy of prematurity, stage 3, bilateral**
- **H35.149 Retinopathy of prematurity, stage 3, unspecified eye** ▽

✓6ᵗʰ H35.15 Retinopathy of prematurity, stage 4
- **H35.151 Retinopathy of prematurity, stage 4, right eye**
- **H35.152 Retinopathy of prematurity, stage 4, left eye**
- **H35.153 Retinopathy of prematurity, stage 4, bilateral**
- **H35.159 Retinopathy of prematurity, stage 4, unspecified eye** ▽

✓6ᵗʰ H35.16 Retinopathy of prematurity, stage 5
- **H35.161 Retinopathy of prematurity, stage 5, right eye**
- **H35.162 Retinopathy of prematurity, stage 5, left eye**
- **H35.163 Retinopathy of prematurity, stage 5, bilateral**
- **H35.169 Retinopathy of prematurity, stage 5, unspecified eye** ▽

✓6ᵗʰ H35.17 Retrolental fibroplasia
- **H35.171 Retrolental fibroplasia, right eye**
- **H35.172 Retrolental fibroplasia, left eye**
- **H35.173 Retrolental fibroplasia, bilateral**
- **H35.179 Retrolental fibroplasia, unspecified eye** ▽

✓5ᵗʰ H35.2 Other non-diabetic proliferative retinopathy
Proliferative vitreo-retinopathy
EXCLUDES 1 *proliferative vitreo-retinopathy with retinal detachment (H33.4-)*
- **H35.20 Other non-diabetic proliferative retinopathy, unspecified eye** ▽
- **H35.21 Other non-diabetic proliferative retinopathy, right eye**
- **H35.22 Other non-diabetic proliferative retinopathy, left eye**
- **H35.23 Other non-diabetic proliferative retinopathy, bilateral**

✓5ᵗʰ H35.3 Degeneration of macula and posterior pole
- **H35.30 Unspecified macular degeneration** Ⓐ▽
  Age-related macular degeneration

✓6ᵗʰ H35.31 Nonexudative age-related macular degeneration
Atrophic age-related macular degeneration
Dry age-related macular degeneration
AHA: 2016, 4Q, 21

One of the following 7th characters is to be assigned to codes in subcategory H35.31 to designate the stage of the disease:
0   stage unspecified
1   early dry stage
2   intermediate dry stage
3   advanced atrophic without subfoveal involvement
    advanced dry stage
4   advanced atrophic with subfoveal involvement

- **✓7ᵗʰ H35.311 Nonexudative age-related macular degeneration, right eye** Ⓐ
- **✓7ᵗʰ H35.312 Nonexudative age-related macular degeneration, left eye** Ⓐ
- **✓7ᵗʰ H35.313 Nonexudative age-related macular degeneration, bilateral** Ⓐ
- **✓7ᵗʰ H35.319 Nonexudative age-related macular degeneration, unspecified eye** Ⓐ▽

✓6ᵗʰ H35.32 Exudative age-related macular degeneration
Wet age-related macular degeneration

One of the following 7th characters is to be assigned to codes in subcategory H35.32 to designate the stage of the disease:
0   stage unspecified
1   with active choroidal neovascularization
2   with inactive choroidal neovascularization
    with involuted or regressed neovascularization
3   with inactive scar

- **✓7ᵗʰ H35.321 Exudative age-related macular degeneration, right eye** HCC Ⓐ
- **✓7ᵗʰ H35.322 Exudative age-related macular degeneration, left eye** HCC Ⓐ
- **✓7ᵗʰ H35.323 Exudative age-related macular degeneration, bilateral** HCC Ⓐ
- **✓7ᵗʰ H35.329 Exudative age-related macular degeneration, unspecified eye** HCC Ⓐ▽

- **H35.33 Angioid streaks of macula**
  DEF: Degeneration of choroid; characterized by broad, irregular, dark brown streaks radiating from optic disc; occurs with pseudoxanthoma elasticum or Paget's disease.

✓6ᵗʰ H35.34 Macular cyst, hole, or pseudohole
- **H35.341 Macular cyst, hole, or pseudohole, right eye**
- **H35.342 Macular cyst, hole, or pseudohole, left eye**
- **H35.343 Macular cyst, hole, or pseudohole, bilateral**
- **H35.349 Macular cyst, hole, or pseudohole, unspecified eye** ▽

✓6ᵗʰ H35.35 Cystoid macular degeneration
EXCLUDES 1 *cystoid macular edema following cataract surgery (H59.03-)*
- **H35.351 Cystoid macular degeneration, right eye**
- **H35.352 Cystoid macular degeneration, left eye**
- **H35.353 Cystoid macular degeneration, bilateral**
- **H35.359 Cystoid macular degeneration, unspecified eye** ▽

✓6ᵗʰ H35.36 Drusen (degenerative) of macula
AHA: 2017, 1Q, 51; 2016, 4Q, 21
- **H35.361 Drusen (degenerative) of macula, right eye**
- **H35.362 Drusen (degenerative) of macula, left eye**
- **H35.363 Drusen (degenerative) of macula, bilateral**
- **H35.369 Drusen (degenerative) of macula, unspecified eye** ▽

✓6ᵗʰ H35.37 Puckering of macula
- **H35.371 Puckering of macula, right eye**
- **H35.372 Puckering of macula, left eye**
- **H35.373 Puckering of macula, bilateral**
- **H35.379 Puckering of macula, unspecified eye** ▽

☑ Additional Character Req   ✓ₓ7ᵗʰ Placeholder Alert   Manifestation   HCC CMS-HCC Condition   ▽ Unspecified Code   ►◄ Revised Text   ● New Code   ▲ Revised Code Title

ICD-10-CM 2018   591

✓6th **H35.38 Toxic maculopathy**
Code first poisoning due to drug or toxin, if applicable (T36-T65 with fifth or sixth character 1-4 or 6)
Use additional code for adverse effect, if applicable, to identify drug (T36-T50 with fifth or sixth character 5)

     H35.381 Toxic maculopathy, right eye
     H35.382 Toxic maculopathy, left eye
     H35.383 Toxic maculopathy, bilateral
     H35.389 Toxic maculopathy, unspecified eye ▽

✓5th **H35.4 Peripheral retinal degeneration**
     EXCLUDES 1   hereditary retinal degeneration (dystrophy) (H35.5-)
        peripheral retinal degeneration with retinal break (H33.3-)

    H35.40 Unspecified peripheral retinal degeneration ▽

✓6th **H35.41 Lattice degeneration of retina**
Palisade degeneration of retina
DEF: Degeneration of retina; often bilateral, usually benign; characterized by lines intersecting at irregular intervals in peripheral retina; retinal thinning and retinal holes may occur.

     H35.411 Lattice degeneration of retina, right eye
     H35.412 Lattice degeneration of retina, left eye
     H35.413 Lattice degeneration of retina, bilateral
     H35.419 Lattice degeneration of retina, unspecified eye ▽

✓6th **H35.42 Microcystoid degeneration of retina**
     H35.421 Microcystoid degeneration of retina, right eye
     H35.422 Microcystoid degeneration of retina, left eye
     H35.423 Microcystoid degeneration of retina, bilateral
     H35.429 Microcystoid degeneration of retina, unspecified eye ▽

✓6th **H35.43 Paving stone degeneration of retina**
     H35.431 Paving stone degeneration of retina, right eye
     H35.432 Paving stone degeneration of retina, left eye
     H35.433 Paving stone degeneration of retina, bilateral
     H35.439 Paving stone degeneration of retina, unspecified eye ▽

✓6th **H35.44 Age-related reticular degeneration of retina**
     H35.441 Age-related reticular degeneration of retina, right eye A
     H35.442 Age-related reticular degeneration of retina, left eye A
     H35.443 Age-related reticular degeneration of retina, bilateral A
     H35.449 Age-related reticular degeneration of retina, unspecified eye A ▽

✓6th **H35.45 Secondary pigmentary degeneration**
     H35.451 Secondary pigmentary degeneration, right eye
     H35.452 Secondary pigmentary degeneration, left eye
     H35.453 Secondary pigmentary degeneration, bilateral
     H35.459 Secondary pigmentary degeneration, unspecified eye ▽

✓6th **H35.46 Secondary vitreoretinal degeneration**
     H35.461 Secondary vitreoretinal degeneration, right eye
     H35.462 Secondary vitreoretinal degeneration, left eye
     H35.463 Secondary vitreoretinal degeneration, bilateral
     H35.469 Secondary vitreoretinal degeneration, unspecified eye ▽

✓5th **H35.5 Hereditary retinal dystrophy**
     EXCLUDES 1   dystrophies primarily involving Bruch's membrane (H31.1-)

    H35.50 Unspecified hereditary retinal dystrophy ▽
    H35.51 Vitreoretinal dystrophy

H35.52 Pigmentary retinal dystrophy
Albipunctate retinal dystrophy
Retinitis pigmentosa
Tapetoretinal dystrophy

H35.53 Other dystrophies primarily involving the sensory retina
Stargardt's disease

H35.54 Dystrophies primarily involving the retinal pigment epithelium
Vitelliform retinal dystrophy

✓5th **H35.6 Retinal hemorrhage**
    H35.60 Retinal hemorrhage, unspecified eye ▽
    H35.61 Retinal hemorrhage, right eye
    H35.62 Retinal hemorrhage, left eye
    H35.63 Retinal hemorrhage, bilateral

✓5th **H35.7 Separation of retinal layers**
     EXCLUDES 1   retinal detachment (serous) (H33.2-)
        rhegmatogenous retinal detachment (H33.0-)

    H35.70 Unspecified separation of retinal layers ▽

✓6th **H35.71 Central serous chorioretinopathy**
     H35.711 Central serous chorioretinopathy, right eye
     H35.712 Central serous chorioretinopathy, left eye
     H35.713 Central serous chorioretinopathy, bilateral
     H35.719 Central serous chorioretinopathy, unspecified eye ▽

✓6th **H35.72 Serous detachment of retinal pigment epithelium**
     H35.721 Serous detachment of retinal pigment epithelium, right eye
     H35.722 Serous detachment of retinal pigment epithelium, left eye
     H35.723 Serous detachment of retinal pigment epithelium, bilateral
     H35.729 Serous detachment of retinal pigment epithelium, unspecified eye ▽

✓6th **H35.73 Hemorrhagic detachment of retinal pigment epithelium**
     H35.731 Hemorrhagic detachment of retinal pigment epithelium, right eye
     H35.732 Hemorrhagic detachment of retinal pigment epithelium, left eye
     H35.733 Hemorrhagic detachment of retinal pigment epithelium, bilateral
     H35.739 Hemorrhagic detachment of retinal pigment epithelium, unspecified eye ▽

✓5th **H35.8 Other specified retinal disorders**
     EXCLUDES 2   retinal hemorrhage (H35.6-)

    H35.81 Retinal edema
Retinal cotton wool spots
    H35.82 Retinal ischemia
    H35.89 Other specified retinal disorders

H35.9 Unspecified retinal disorder ▽

H36 Retinal disorders in diseases classified elsewhere
Code first underlying disease, such as:
lipid storage disorders (E75.-)
sickle-cell disorders (D57.-)
     EXCLUDES 1   arteriosclerotic retinopathy (H35.0-)
        diabetic retinopathy (E08.3-, E09.3-, E10.3-, E11.3-, E13.3-)

Glaucoma (H40-H42)

✓4th **H40 Glaucoma**
     EXCLUDES 1   absolute glaucoma (H44.51-)
        congenital glaucoma (Q15.0)
        traumatic glaucoma due to birth injury (P15.3)

✓5th **H40.0 Glaucoma suspect**
   ✓6th **H40.00 Preglaucoma, unspecified**
     H40.001 Preglaucoma, unspecified, right eye ▽
     H40.002 Preglaucoma, unspecified, left eye ▽
     H40.003 Preglaucoma, unspecified, bilateral ▽
     H40.009 Preglaucoma, unspecified, unspecified eye ▽

EXCLUDES 1 Not coded here   *EXCLUDES 2* Not included here   N Newborn Age: 0   P Pediatric Age: 0-17   M Maternity Age: 12-55   A Adult Age: 15-124

592   ICD-10-CM 2018

Chapter 7. Diseases of the Eye and Adnexa

✓6ᵗʰ H40.01 Open angle with borderline findings, low risk
     Open angle, low risk
- **H40.011** Open angle with borderline findings, low risk, **right** eye
- **H40.012** Open angle with borderline findings, low risk, **left** eye
- **H40.013** Open angle with borderline findings, low risk, **bilateral**
- **H40.019** Open angle with borderline findings, low risk, unspecified eye ▽

✓6ᵗʰ H40.02 Open angle with borderline findings, high risk
     Open angle, high risk
- **H40.021** Open angle with borderline findings, high risk, **right** eye
- **H40.022** Open angle with borderline findings, high risk, **left** eye
- **H40.023** Open angle with borderline findings, high risk, **bilateral**
- **H40.029** Open angle with borderline findings, high risk, unspecified eye ▽

✓6ᵗʰ H40.03 Anatomical narrow angle
     Primary angle closure suspect
- **H40.031** Anatomical narrow angle, **right** eye
- **H40.032** Anatomical narrow angle, **left** eye
- **H40.033** Anatomical narrow angle, **bilateral**
- **H40.039** Anatomical narrow angle, unspecified eye ▽

✓6ᵗʰ H40.04 Steroid responder
- **H40.041** Steroid responder, **right** eye
- **H40.042** Steroid responder, **left** eye
- **H40.043** Steroid responder, **bilateral**
- **H40.049** Steroid responder, unspecified eye ▽

✓6ᵗʰ H40.05 Ocular hypertension
- **H40.051** Ocular hypertension, **right** eye
- **H40.052** Ocular hypertension, **left** eye
- **H40.053** Ocular hypertension, **bilateral**
- **H40.059** Ocular hypertension, unspecified eye ▽

✓6ᵗʰ H40.06 Primary angle closure without glaucoma damage
- **H40.061** Primary angle closure without glaucoma damage, **right** eye
- **H40.062** Primary angle closure without glaucoma damage, **left** eye
- **H40.063** Primary angle closure without glaucoma damage, **bilateral**
- **H40.069** Primary angle closure without glaucoma damage, unspecified eye ▽

✓5ᵗʰ H40.1 Open-angle glaucoma

One of the following 7th characters is to be assigned to each code in subcategories H40.10, H40.11-, H40.12-, H40.13-, and H40.14- to designate the stage of glaucoma.
- 0   stage unspecified
- 1   mild stage
- 2   moderate stage
- 3   severe stage
- 4   indeterminate stage

✓x7ᵗʰ H40.10 Unspecified open-angle glaucoma ▽

✓6ᵗʰ H40.11 Primary open-angle glaucoma
     Chronic simple glaucoma
- **✓7ᵗʰ H40.111** Primary open-angle glaucoma, **right** eye
- **✓7ᵗʰ H40.112** Primary open-angle glaucoma, **left** eye
- **✓7ᵗʰ H40.113** Primary open-angle glaucoma, **bilateral**
- **✓7ᵗʰ H40.119** Primary open-angle glaucoma, unspecified eye ▽

✓6ᵗʰ H40.12 Low-tension glaucoma
- **✓7ᵗʰ H40.121** Low-tension glaucoma, **right** eye
- **✓7ᵗʰ H40.122** Low-tension glaucoma, **left** eye
- **✓7ᵗʰ H40.123** Low-tension glaucoma, **bilateral**
- **✓7ᵗʰ H40.129** Low-tension glaucoma, unspecified eye ▽

✓6ᵗʰ H40.13 Pigmentary glaucoma
- **✓7ᵗʰ H40.131** Pigmentary glaucoma, **right** eye
- **✓7ᵗʰ H40.132** Pigmentary glaucoma, **left** eye
- **✓7ᵗʰ H40.133** Pigmentary glaucoma, **bilateral**
- **✓7ᵗʰ H40.139** Pigmentary glaucoma, unspecified eye ▽

Open Angle/Angle Closure Glaucoma

✓6ᵗʰ H40.14 Capsular glaucoma with pseudoexfoliation of lens
- **✓7ᵗʰ H40.141** Capsular glaucoma with pseudoexfoliation of lens, **right** eye
- **✓7ᵗʰ H40.142** Capsular glaucoma with pseudoexfoliation of lens, **left** eye
- **✓7ᵗʰ H40.143** Capsular glaucoma with pseudoexfoliation of lens, **bilateral**
- **✓7ᵗʰ H40.149** Capsular glaucoma with pseudoexfoliation of lens, unspecified eye ▽

✓6ᵗʰ H40.15 Residual stage of open-angle glaucoma
- **H40.151** Residual stage of open-angle glaucoma, **right** eye
- **H40.152** Residual stage of open-angle glaucoma, **left** eye
- **H40.153** Residual stage of open-angle glaucoma, **bilateral**
- **H40.159** Residual stage of open-angle glaucoma, unspecified eye ▽

✓5ᵗʰ H40.2 Primary angle-closure glaucoma
> **EXCLUDES 1**   aqueous misdirection (H40.83-)
>   malignant glaucoma (H40.83-)

One of the following 7th characters is to be assigned to each code in subcategories H40.20 and H40.22- to designate the stage of glaucoma.
- 0   stage unspecified
- 1   mild stage
- 2   moderate stage
- 3   severe stage
- 4   indeterminate stage

✓x7ᵗʰ H40.20 Unspecified primary angle-closure glaucoma ▽

✓6ᵗʰ H40.21 Acute angle-closure glaucoma
     Acute angle-closure glaucoma attack
     Acute angle-closure glaucoma crisis
- **H40.211** Acute angle-closure glaucoma, **right** eye
- **H40.212** Acute angle-closure glaucoma, **left** eye
- **H40.213** Acute angle-closure glaucoma, **bilateral**
- **H40.219** Acute angle-closure glaucoma, unspecified eye ▽

✓6ᵗʰ H40.22 Chronic angle-closure glaucoma
     Chronic primary angle-closure glaucoma
- **✓7ᵗʰ H40.221** Chronic angle-closure glaucoma, **right** eye
- **✓7ᵗʰ H40.222** Chronic angle-closure glaucoma, **left** eye
- **✓7ᵗʰ H40.223** Chronic angle-closure glaucoma, **bilateral**
- **✓7ᵗʰ H40.229** Chronic angle-closure glaucoma, unspecified eye ▽

✓6ᵗʰ H40.23 Intermittent angle-closure glaucoma
- **H40.231** Intermittent angle-closure glaucoma, **right** eye
- **H40.232** Intermittent angle-closure glaucoma, **left** eye
- **H40.233** Intermittent angle-closure glaucoma, **bilateral**
- **H40.239** Intermittent angle-closure glaucoma, unspecified eye ▽

✓6ᵗʰ H40.24 Residual stage of angle-closure glaucoma
- **H40.241** Residual stage of angle-closure glaucoma, **right** eye
- **H40.242** Residual stage of angle-closure glaucoma, **left** eye

---

✓ Additional Character Req   ✓x7ᵗʰ Placeholder Alert   Manifestation   HCC CMS-HCC Condition   ▽ Unspecified Code   ▶◀ Revised Text   ● New Code   ▲ Revised Code Title

Chapter 7. Diseases of the Eye and Adnexa

H40.243   Residual stage of angle-closure glaucoma, bilateral

H40.249   Residual stage of angle-closure glaucoma, unspecified eye ▽

✓5ᵗʰ **H40.3**   Glaucoma secondary to eye trauma

Code also underlying condition

One of the following 7th characters is to be assigned to each code in subcategory H40.3- to designate the stage of glaucoma.
- 0   stage unspecified
- 1   mild stage
- 2   moderate stage
- 3   severe stage
- 4   indeterminate stage

✓x7ᵗʰ **H40.30**   Glaucoma secondary to eye trauma, unspecified eye ▽

✓x7ᵗʰ **H40.31**   Glaucoma secondary to eye trauma, right eye

✓x7ᵗʰ **H40.32**   Glaucoma secondary to eye trauma, left eye

✓x7ᵗʰ **H40.33**   Glaucoma secondary to eye trauma, bilateral

✓5ᵗʰ **H40.4**   Glaucoma secondary to eye inflammation

Code also underlying condition

One of the following 7th characters is to be assigned to each code in subcategory H40.4- to designate the stage of glaucoma.
- 0   stage unspecified
- 1   mild stage
- 2   moderate stage
- 3   severe stage
- 4   indeterminate stage

✓x7ᵗʰ **H40.40**   Glaucoma secondary to eye inflammation, unspecified eye ▽

✓x7ᵗʰ **H40.41**   Glaucoma secondary to eye inflammation, right eye

✓x7ᵗʰ **H40.42**   Glaucoma secondary to eye inflammation, left eye

✓x7ᵗʰ **H40.43**   Glaucoma secondary to eye inflammation, bilateral

✓5ᵗʰ **H40.5**   Glaucoma secondary to other eye disorders

Code also underlying eye disorder

One of the following 7th characters is to be assigned to each code in subcategory H40.5- to designate the stage of glaucoma.
- 0   stage unspecified
- 1   mild stage
- 2   moderate stage
- 3   severe stage
- 4   indeterminate stage

✓x7ᵗʰ **H40.50**   Glaucoma secondary to other eye disorders, unspecified eye ▽

✓x7ᵗʰ **H40.51**   Glaucoma secondary to other eye disorders, right eye

✓x7ᵗʰ **H40.52**   Glaucoma secondary to other eye disorders, left eye

✓x7ᵗʰ **H40.53**   Glaucoma secondary to other eye disorders, bilateral

✓5ᵗʰ **H40.6**   Glaucoma secondary to drugs

Use additional code for adverse effect, if applicable, to identify drug (T36-T50 with fifth or sixth character 5)

One of the following 7th characters is to be assigned to each code in subcategory H40.6- to designate the stage of glaucoma.
- 0   stage unspecified
- 1   mild stage
- 2   moderate stage
- 3   severe stage
- 4   indeterminate stage

✓x7ᵗʰ **H40.60**   Glaucoma secondary to drugs, unspecified eye ▽

✓x7ᵗʰ **H40.61**   Glaucoma secondary to drugs, right eye

✓x7ᵗʰ **H40.62**   Glaucoma secondary to drugs, left eye

✓x7ᵗʰ **H40.63**   Glaucoma secondary to drugs, bilateral

✓5ᵗʰ **H40.8**   Other glaucoma

✓6ᵗʰ **H40.81**   Glaucoma with increased episcleral venous pressure

H40.811   Glaucoma with increased episcleral venous pressure, right eye

H40.812   Glaucoma with increased episcleral venous pressure, left eye

H40.813   Glaucoma with increased episcleral venous pressure, bilateral

H40.819   Glaucoma with increased episcleral venous pressure, unspecified eye ▽

✓6ᵗʰ **H40.82**   Hypersecretion glaucoma

H40.821   Hypersecretion glaucoma, right eye

H40.822   Hypersecretion glaucoma, left eye

H40.823   Hypersecretion glaucoma, bilateral

H40.829   Hypersecretion glaucoma, unspecified eye ▽

✓6ᵗʰ **H40.83**   Aqueous misdirection

Malignant glaucoma

H40.831   Aqueous misdirection, right eye

H40.832   Aqueous misdirection, left eye

H40.833   Aqueous misdirection, bilateral

H40.839   Aqueous misdirection, unspecified eye ▽

H40.89   Other specified glaucoma

H40.9   Unspecified glaucoma ▽

H42   *Glaucoma in diseases classified elsewhere*

Code first underlying condition, such as:
- amyloidosis (E85.-)
- aniridia (Q13.1)
- ▶glaucoma (in) diabetes mellitus (E08.39, E09.39, E10.39, E11.39, E13.39)◀
- Lowe's syndrome (E72.03)
- Reiger's anomaly (Q13.81)
- specified metabolic disorder (E70-E88)

EXCLUDES 1   glaucoma (in) onchocerciasis (B73.02)
glaucoma (in) syphilis (A52.71)
glaucoma (in) tuberculous (A18.59)

EXCLUDES 2   ~~glaucoma (in) diabetes mellitus (E08.39, E09.39, E10.39, E11.39, E13.39)~~

Disorders of vitreous body and globe (H43-H44)

✓4ᵗʰ **H43**   Disorders of vitreous body

✓5ᵗʰ **H43.0**   Vitreous prolapse

EXCLUDES 1   traumatic vitreous prolapse (S05.2-)
vitreous syndrome following cataract surgery (H59.0-)

H43.00   Vitreous prolapse, unspecified eye ▽

H43.01   Vitreous prolapse, right eye

H43.02   Vitreous prolapse, left eye

H43.03   Vitreous prolapse, bilateral

✓5ᵗʰ **H43.1**   Vitreous hemorrhage

H43.10   Vitreous hemorrhage, unspecified eye   HCC ▽

H43.11   Vitreous hemorrhage, right eye   HCC

H43.12   Vitreous hemorrhage, left eye   HCC

H43.13   Vitreous hemorrhage, bilateral   HCC

✓5ᵗʰ **H43.2**   Crystalline deposits in vitreous body

H43.20   Crystalline deposits in vitreous body, unspecified eye ▽

H43.21   Crystalline deposits in vitreous body, right eye

H43.22   Crystalline deposits in vitreous body, left eye

H43.23   Crystalline deposits in vitreous body, bilateral

✓5ᵗʰ **H43.3**   Other vitreous opacities

✓6ᵗʰ **H43.31**   Vitreous membranes and strands

H43.311   Vitreous membranes and strands, right eye

H43.312   Vitreous membranes and strands, left eye

H43.313   Vitreous membranes and strands, bilateral

H43.319   Vitreous membranes and strands, unspecified eye ▽

✓6ᵗʰ **H43.39**   Other vitreous opacities

Vitreous floaters

H43.391   Other vitreous opacities, right eye

H43.392   Other vitreous opacities, left eye

H43.393   Other vitreous opacities, bilateral

H43.399   Other vitreous opacities, unspecified eye ▽

✓5ᵗʰ **H43.8**   Other disorders of vitreous body

EXCLUDES 1   proliferative vitreo-retinopathy with retinal detachment (H33.4-)

EXCLUDES 2   vitreous abscess (H44.02-)

✓6ᵗʰ **H43.81**   Vitreous degeneration

Vitreous detachment

H43.811   Vitreous degeneration, right eye

EXCLUDES 1 Not coded here   *EXCLUDES 2* Not included here   N Newborn Age: 0   P Pediatric Age: 0-17   M Maternity Age: 12-55   A Adult Age: 15-124

594   ICD-10-CM 2018

H43.812   Vitreous degeneration, left eye
H43.813   Vitreous degeneration, bilateral
H43.819   Vitreous degeneration, unspecified eye ▽

✓6th **H43.82**   **Vitreomacular** adhesion
Vitreomacular traction
H43.821   Vitreomacular adhesion, right eye Ⓐ
H43.822   Vitreomacular adhesion, left eye Ⓐ
H43.823   Vitreomacular adhesion, bilateral Ⓐ
H43.829   Vitreomacular adhesion, unspecified Ⓐ ▽
eye

H43.89   **Other disorders of vitreous body**

H43.9   **Unspecified disorder of vitreous body** ▽

✓4th **H44**   **Disorders of globe**
INCLUDES   disorders affecting multiple structures of eye

✓5th **H44.0**   **Purulent endophthalmitis**
Use additional code to identify organism
EXCLUDES 1   bleb associated endophthalmitis (H59.4-)

✓6th **H44.00**   **Unspecified purulent endophthalmitis**
H44.001   Unspecified purulent endophthalmitis, ▽
right eye
H44.002   Unspecified purulent endophthalmitis, ▽
left eye
H44.003   Unspecified purulent endophthalmitis, ▽
bilateral
H44.009   Unspecified purulent endophthalmitis, ▽
unspecified eye

✓6th **H44.01**   **Panophthalmitis (acute)**
H44.011   Panophthalmitis (acute), right eye
H44.012   Panophthalmitis (acute), left eye
H44.013   Panophthalmitis (acute), bilateral
H44.019   Panophthalmitis (acute), unspecified ▽
eye

✓6th **H44.02**   **Vitreous abscess (chronic)**
H44.021   Vitreous abscess (chronic), right eye
H44.022   Vitreous abscess (chronic), left eye
H44.023   Vitreous abscess (chronic), bilateral
H44.029   Vitreous abscess (chronic), unspecified ▽
eye

✓5th **H44.1**   **Other endophthalmitis**
EXCLUDES 1   bleb associated endophthalmitis (H59.4-)
EXCLUDES 2   ophthalmia nodosa (H16.2-)

✓6th **H44.11**   **Panuveitis**
DEF: Inflammation of all layers of uvea of eye, including
choroid, iris, and ciliary body; also typically involves lens,
retina, optic nerve, and vitreous; causes reduced vision
or blindness.
H44.111   Panuveitis, right eye
H44.112   Panuveitis, left eye
H44.113   Panuveitis, bilateral
H44.119   Panuveitis, unspecified eye ▽

✓6th **H44.12**   **Parasitic endophthalmitis, unspecified**
H44.121   Parasitic endophthalmitis, unspecified, ▽
right eye
H44.122   Parasitic endophthalmitis, unspecified, ▽
left eye
H44.123   Parasitic endophthalmitis, unspecified, ▽
bilateral
H44.129   Parasitic endophthalmitis, unspecified, ▽
unspecified eye

✓6th **H44.13**   **Sympathetic uveitis**
H44.131   Sympathetic uveitis, right eye
H44.132   Sympathetic uveitis, left eye
H44.133   Sympathetic uveitis, bilateral
H44.139   Sympathetic uveitis, unspecified eye ▽

H44.19   **Other endophthalmitis**

✓5th **H44.2**   **Degenerative myopia**
Malignant myopia
H44.20   Degenerative myopia, unspecified eye ▽
H44.21   Degenerative myopia, right eye
H44.22   Degenerative myopia, left eye
H44.23   Degenerative myopia, bilateral

✓6th **H44.2A**   **Degenerative myopia** with choroidal
neovascularization
Use additional code for any associated choroid
disorders (H31.-)
H44.2A1   Degenerative myopia with choroidal
neovascularization, right eye
H44.2A2   Degenerative myopia with choroidal
neovascularization, left eye
H44.2A3   Degenerative myopia with choroidal
neovascularization, bilateral
H44.2A9   Degenerative myopia with choroidal ▽
neovascularization, unspecified eye

✓6th **H44.2B**   **Degenerative myopia** with macular hole
H44.2B1   Degenerative myopia with macular hole,
right eye
H44.2B2   Degenerative myopia with macular hole,
left eye
H44.2B3   Degenerative myopia with macular hole,
bilateral eye
H44.2B9   Degenerative myopia with macular ▽
hole, unspecified eye

✓6th **H44.2C**   **Degenerative myopia** with retinal detachment
Use additional code to identify the retinal detachment
(H33.-)
H44.2C1   Degenerative myopia with retinal
detachment, right eye
H44.2C2   Degenerative myopia with retinal
detachment, left eye
H44.2C3   Degenerative myopia with retinal
detachment, bilateral eye
H44.2C9   Degenerative myopia with retinal ▽
detachment, unspecified eye

✓6th **H44.2D**   **Degenerative myopia** with foveoschisis
H44.2D1   Degenerative myopia with foveoschisis,
right eye
H44.2D2   Degenerative myopia with foveoschisis,
left eye
H44.2D3   Degenerative myopia with foveoschisis,
bilateral eye
H44.2D9   Degenerative myopia with ▽
foveoschisis, unspecified eye

✓6th **H44.2E**   **Degenerative myopia** with other maculopathy
H44.2E1   Degenerative myopia with other
maculopathy, right eye
H44.2E2   Degenerative myopia with other
maculopathy, left eye
H44.2E3   Degenerative myopia with other
maculopathy, bilateral eye
H44.2E9   Degenerative myopia with other ▽
maculopathy, unspecified eye

✓5th **H44.3**   **Other and unspecified degenerative disorders of globe**
H44.30   Unspecified degenerative disorder of globe ▽

✓6th **H44.31**   **Chalcosis**
H44.311   Chalcosis, right eye
H44.312   Chalcosis, left eye
H44.313   Chalcosis, bilateral
H44.319   Chalcosis, unspecified eye ▽

✓6th **H44.32**   **Siderosis of eye**
DEF: Iron pigment deposits within tissue of eyeball;
caused by high iron content of blood; characterized by
cataract, rust-colored anterior subcapsular deposits, iris
heterochromia, pupillary mydriasis, and depressed
electroretinogram amplitudes.
H44.321   Siderosis of eye, right eye
H44.322   Siderosis of eye, left eye
H44.323   Siderosis of eye, bilateral
H44.329   Siderosis of eye, unspecified eye ▽

✓6th **H44.39**   **Other degenerative disorders of globe**
H44.391   Other degenerative disorders of globe,
right eye
H44.392   Other degenerative disorders of globe,
left eye
H44.393   Other degenerative disorders of globe,
bilateral
H44.399   Other degenerative disorders of globe, ▽
unspecified eye

☑ Additional Character Req   ✓x7th Placeholder Alert   Manifestation   HCC CMS-HCC Condition   ▽ Unspecified Code   ▶◀ Revised Text   ● New Code   ▲ Revised Code Title

Chapter 7. Diseases of the Eye and Adnexa

✓5ᵗʰ **H44.4** **Hypotony of eye**

    H44.40 Unspecified hypotony of eye ▽

    ✓6ᵗʰ **H44.41** Flat anterior chamber hypotony of eye

        H44.411 Flat anterior chamber hypotony of right eye

        H44.412 Flat anterior chamber hypotony of left eye

        H44.413 Flat anterior chamber hypotony of eye, bilateral

        H44.419 Flat anterior chamber hypotony of unspecified eye ▽

    ✓6ᵗʰ **H44.42** Hypotony of eye due to ocular fistula

        H44.421 Hypotony of right eye due to ocular fistula

        H44.422 Hypotony of left eye due to ocular fistula

        H44.423 Hypotony of eye due to ocular fistula, bilateral

        H44.429 Hypotony of unspecified eye due to ocular fistula ▽

    ✓6ᵗʰ **H44.43** Hypotony of eye due to other ocular disorders

        H44.431 Hypotony of eye due to other ocular disorders, right eye

        H44.432 Hypotony of eye due to other ocular disorders, left eye

        H44.433 Hypotony of eye due to other ocular disorders, bilateral

        H44.439 Hypotony of eye due to other ocular disorders, unspecified eye ▽

    ✓6ᵗʰ **H44.44** Primary hypotony of eye

        H44.441 Primary hypotony of right eye

        H44.442 Primary hypotony of left eye

        H44.443 Primary hypotony of eye, bilateral

        H44.449 Primary hypotony of unspecified eye ▽

✓5ᵗʰ **H44.5** **Degenerated conditions of globe**

    H44.50 Unspecified degenerated conditions of globe ▽

    ✓6ᵗʰ **H44.51** Absolute glaucoma

        H44.511 Absolute glaucoma, right eye

        H44.512 Absolute glaucoma, left eye

        H44.513 Absolute glaucoma, bilateral

        H44.519 Absolute glaucoma, unspecified eye ▽

    ✓6ᵗʰ **H44.52** Atrophy of globe

        Phthisis bulbi

        H44.521 Atrophy of globe, right eye

        H44.522 Atrophy of globe, left eye

        H44.523 Atrophy of globe, bilateral

        H44.529 Atrophy of globe, unspecified eye ▽

    ✓6ᵗʰ **H44.53** Leucocoria

        H44.531 Leucocoria, right eye

        H44.532 Leucocoria, left eye

        H44.533 Leucocoria, bilateral

        H44.539 Leucocoria, unspecified eye ▽

✓5ᵗʰ **H44.6** **Retained (old) intraocular foreign body, magnetic**

    Use additional code to identify magnetic foreign body (Z18.11)

    EXCLUDES 1 current intraocular foreign body (S05.-)

    EXCLUDES 2 retained foreign body in eyelid (H02.81-)

        retained (old) foreign body following penetrating wound of orbit (H05.5-)

        retained (old) intraocular foreign body, nonmagnetic (H44.7-)

    ✓6ᵗʰ **H44.60** Unspecified retained (old) intraocular foreign body, magnetic

        H44.601 Unspecified retained (old) intraocular foreign body, magnetic, right eye ▽

        H44.602 Unspecified retained (old) intraocular foreign body, magnetic, left eye ▽

        H44.603 Unspecified retained (old) intraocular foreign body, magnetic, bilateral ▽

        H44.609 Unspecified retained (old) intraocular foreign body, magnetic, unspecified eye ▽

    ✓6ᵗʰ **H44.61** Retained (old) magnetic foreign body in anterior chamber

        H44.611 Retained (old) magnetic foreign body in anterior chamber, right eye

        H44.612 Retained (old) magnetic foreign body in anterior chamber, left eye

        H44.613 Retained (old) magnetic foreign body in anterior chamber, bilateral

        H44.619 Retained (old) magnetic foreign body in anterior chamber, unspecified eye ▽

    ✓6ᵗʰ **H44.62** Retained (old) magnetic foreign body in iris or ciliary body

        H44.621 Retained (old) magnetic foreign body in iris or ciliary body, right eye

        H44.622 Retained (old) magnetic foreign body in iris or ciliary body, left eye

        H44.623 Retained (old) magnetic foreign body in iris or ciliary body, bilateral

        H44.629 Retained (old) magnetic foreign body in iris or ciliary body, unspecified eye ▽

    ✓6ᵗʰ **H44.63** Retained (old) magnetic foreign body in lens

        H44.631 Retained (old) magnetic foreign body in lens, right eye

        H44.632 Retained (old) magnetic foreign body in lens, left eye

        H44.633 Retained (old) magnetic foreign body in lens, bilateral

        H44.639 Retained (old) magnetic foreign body in lens, unspecified eye ▽

    ✓6ᵗʰ **H44.64** Retained (old) magnetic foreign body in posterior wall of globe

        H44.641 Retained (old) magnetic foreign body in posterior wall of globe, right eye

        H44.642 Retained (old) magnetic foreign body in posterior wall of globe, left eye

        H44.643 Retained (old) magnetic foreign body in posterior wall of globe, bilateral

        H44.649 Retained (old) magnetic foreign body in posterior wall of globe, unspecified eye ▽

    ✓6ᵗʰ **H44.65** Retained (old) magnetic foreign body in vitreous body

        H44.651 Retained (old) magnetic foreign body in vitreous body, right eye

        H44.652 Retained (old) magnetic foreign body in vitreous body, left eye

        H44.653 Retained (old) magnetic foreign body in vitreous body, bilateral

        H44.659 Retained (old) magnetic foreign body in vitreous body, unspecified eye ▽

    ✓6ᵗʰ **H44.69** Retained (old) intraocular foreign body, magnetic, in other or multiple sites

        H44.691 Retained (old) intraocular foreign body, magnetic, in other or multiple sites, right eye

        H44.692 Retained (old) intraocular foreign body, magnetic, in other or multiple sites, left eye

        H44.693 Retained (old) intraocular foreign body, magnetic, in other or multiple sites, bilateral

        H44.699 Retained (old) intraocular foreign body, magnetic, in other or multiple sites, unspecified eye ▽

✓5ᵗʰ **H44.7** **Retained (old) intraocular foreign body, nonmagnetic**

    Use additional code to identify nonmagnetic foreign body (Z18.01-Z18.10, Z18.12, Z18.2-Z18.9)

    EXCLUDES 1 current intraocular foreign body (S05.-)

    EXCLUDES 2 retained foreign body in eyelid (H02.81-)

        retained (old) foreign body following penetrating wound of orbit (H05.5-)

        retained (old) intraocular foreign body, magnetic (H44.6-)

    ✓6ᵗʰ **H44.70** Unspecified retained (old) intraocular foreign body, nonmagnetic

        H44.701 Unspecified retained (old) intraocular foreign body, nonmagnetic, right eye ▽

        H44.702 Unspecified retained (old) intraocular foreign body, nonmagnetic, left eye ▽

        H44.703 Unspecified retained (old) intraocular foreign body, nonmagnetic, bilateral ▽

        H44.709 Unspecified retained (old) intraocular foreign body, nonmagnetic, unspecified eye ▽

            Retained (old) intraocular foreign body NOS

EXCLUDES 1 Not coded here   **EXCLUDES 2** Not included here   N Newborn Age: 0   P Pediatric Age: 0-17   M Maternity Age: 12-55   A Adult Age: 15-124

596   ICD-10-CM 2018

✓6th **H44.71** Retained (nonmagnetic) (old) foreign body in anterior chamber

     H44.711 Retained (nonmagnetic) (old) foreign body in anterior chamber, right eye

     H44.712 Retained (nonmagnetic) (old) foreign body in anterior chamber, left eye

     H44.713 Retained (nonmagnetic) (old) foreign body in anterior chamber, bilateral

     H44.719 Retained (nonmagnetic) (old) foreign ▽ body in anterior chamber, unspecified eye

✓6th **H44.72** Retained (nonmagnetic) (old) foreign body in iris or ciliary body

     H44.721 Retained (nonmagnetic) (old) foreign body in iris or ciliary body, right eye

     H44.722 Retained (nonmagnetic) (old) foreign body in iris or ciliary body, left eye

     H44.723 Retained (nonmagnetic) (old) foreign body in iris or ciliary body, bilateral

     H44.729 Retained (nonmagnetic) (old) foreign ▽ body in iris or ciliary body, unspecified eye

✓6th **H44.73** Retained (nonmagnetic) (old) foreign body in lens

     H44.731 Retained (nonmagnetic) (old) foreign body in lens, right eye

     H44.732 Retained (nonmagnetic) (old) foreign body in lens, left eye

     H44.733 Retained (nonmagnetic) (old) foreign body in lens, bilateral

     H44.739 Retained (nonmagnetic) (old) foreign ▽ body in lens, unspecified eye

✓6th **H44.74** Retained (nonmagnetic) (old) foreign body in posterior wall of globe

     H44.741 Retained (nonmagnetic) (old) foreign body in posterior wall of globe, right eye

     H44.742 Retained (nonmagnetic) (old) foreign body in posterior wall of globe, left eye

     H44.743 Retained (nonmagnetic) (old) foreign body in posterior wall of globe, bilateral

     H44.749 Retained (nonmagnetic) (old) foreign ▽ body in posterior wall of globe, unspecified eye

✓6th **H44.75** Retained (nonmagnetic) (old) foreign body in vitreous body

     H44.751 Retained (nonmagnetic) (old) foreign body in vitreous body, right eye

     H44.752 Retained (nonmagnetic) (old) foreign body in vitreous body, left eye

     H44.753 Retained (nonmagnetic) (old) foreign body in vitreous body, bilateral

     H44.759 Retained (nonmagnetic) (old) foreign ▽ body in vitreous body, unspecified eye

✓6th **H44.79** Retained (old) intraocular foreign body, nonmagnetic, in other or multiple sites

     H44.791 Retained (old) intraocular foreign body, nonmagnetic, in other or multiple sites, right eye

     H44.792 Retained (old) intraocular foreign body, nonmagnetic, in other or multiple sites, left eye

     H44.793 Retained (old) intraocular foreign body, nonmagnetic, in other or multiple sites, bilateral

     H44.799 Retained (old) intraocular foreign ▽ body, nonmagnetic, in other or multiple sites, unspecified eye

✓5th **H44.8** Other disorders of globe

✓6th **H44.81** Hemophthalmos
     DEF: Pool of blood within eyeball, not from current injury.

     H44.811 Hemophthalmos, right eye

     H44.812 Hemophthalmos, left eye

     H44.813 Hemophthalmos, bilateral

     H44.819 Hemophthalmos, unspecified eye ▽

✓6th **H44.82** Luxation of globe

     H44.821 Luxation of globe, right eye

     H44.822 Luxation of globe, left eye

     H44.823 Luxation of globe, bilateral

     H44.829 Luxation of globe, unspecified eye ▽

     H44.89 Other disorders of globe

H44.9 Unspecified disorder of globe ▽

Disorders of optic nerve and visual pathways (H46-H47)

✓4th **H46** Optic neuritis
     EXCLUDES 2   ischemic optic neuropathy (H47.01-)
         neuromyelitis optica [Devic] (G36.0)

✓5th **H46.0** Optic papillitis

     H46.00 Optic papillitis, unspecified eye ▽

     H46.01 Optic papillitis, right eye

     H46.02 Optic papillitis, left eye

     H46.03 Optic papillitis, bilateral

✓5th **H46.1** Retrobulbar neuritis
     Retrobulbar neuritis NOS
     EXCLUDES 1   syphilitic retrobulbar neuritis (A52.15)

     H46.10 Retrobulbar neuritis, unspecified eye ▽

     H46.11 Retrobulbar neuritis, right eye

     H46.12 Retrobulbar neuritis, left eye

     H46.13 Retrobulbar neuritis, bilateral

H46.2 Nutritional optic neuropathy

H46.3 Toxic optic neuropathy
     Code first (T51-T65) to identify cause

H46.8 Other optic neuritis

H46.9 Unspecified optic neuritis ▽

✓4th **H47** Other disorders of optic [2nd] nerve and visual pathways

✓5th **H47.0** Disorders of optic nerve, not elsewhere classified

✓6th **H47.01** Ischemic optic neuropathy

     H47.011 Ischemic optic neuropathy, right eye

     H47.012 Ischemic optic neuropathy, left eye

     H47.013 Ischemic optic neuropathy, bilateral

     H47.019 Ischemic optic neuropathy, ▽ unspecified eye

✓6th **H47.02** Hemorrhage in optic nerve sheath

     H47.021 Hemorrhage in optic nerve sheath, right eye

     H47.022 Hemorrhage in optic nerve sheath, left eye

     H47.023 Hemorrhage in optic nerve sheath, bilateral

     H47.029 Hemorrhage in optic nerve sheath, ▽ unspecified eye

✓6th **H47.03** Optic nerve hypoplasia

     H47.031 Optic nerve hypoplasia, right eye

     H47.032 Optic nerve hypoplasia, left eye

     H47.033 Optic nerve hypoplasia, bilateral

     H47.039 Optic nerve hypoplasia, ▽ unspecified eye

✓6th **H47.09** Other disorders of optic nerve, not elsewhere classified
     Compression of optic nerve

     H47.091 Other disorders of optic nerve, not elsewhere classified, right eye

     H47.092 Other disorders of optic nerve, not elsewhere classified, left eye

     H47.093 Other disorders of optic nerve, not elsewhere classified, bilateral

     H47.099 Other disorders of optic nerve, not ▽ elsewhere classified, unspecified eye

✓5th **H47.1** Papilledema

     H47.10 Unspecified papilledema ▽

     H47.11 Papilledema associated with increased intracranial pressure

     H47.12 Papilledema associated with decreased ocular pressure

     H47.13 Papilledema associated with retinal disorder

✓6th **H47.14** Foster-Kennedy syndrome

     H47.141 Foster-Kennedy syndrome, right eye

     H47.142 Foster-Kennedy syndrome, left eye

     H47.143 Foster-Kennedy syndrome, bilateral

     H47.149 Foster-Kennedy syndrome, ▽ unspecified eye

✓5th **H47.2** Optic atrophy

     H47.20 Unspecified optic atrophy ▽

✓ Additional Character Req   √x7th Placeholder Alert   Manifestation   HCC CMS-HCC Condition   ▽ Unspecified Code   ►◄ Revised Text   ● New Code   ▲ Revised Code Title

✓6th **H47.21 Primary** optic atrophy
  H47.211 Primary optic atrophy, **right** eye
  H47.212 Primary optic atrophy, **left** eye
  H47.213 Primary optic atrophy, **bilateral**
  H47.219 Primary optic atrophy, unspecified eye ▽

 H47.22 **Hereditary** optic atrophy
  Leber's optic atrophy

✓6th **H47.23 Glaucomatous** optic atrophy
  H47.231 Glaucomatous optic atrophy, **right** eye
  H47.232 Glaucomatous optic atrophy, **left** eye
  H47.233 Glaucomatous optic atrophy, **bilateral**
  H47.239 Glaucomatous optic atrophy, ▽
   unspecified eye

✓6th **H47.29 Other** optic atrophy
  Temporal pallor of optic disc
  H47.291 Other optic atrophy, **right** eye
  H47.292 Other optic atrophy, **left** eye
  H47.293 Other optic atrophy, **bilateral**
  H47.299 Other optic atrophy, unspecified eye ▽

✓5th **H47.3 Other disorders of optic disc**

✓6th **H47.31 Coloboma** of optic disc
  H47.311 Coloboma of optic disc, **right** eye
  H47.312 Coloboma of optic disc, **left** eye
  H47.313 Coloboma of optic disc, **bilateral**
  H47.319 Coloboma of optic disc, unspecified eye ▽

✓6th **H47.32 Drusen** of optic disc
  H47.321 Drusen of optic disc, **right** eye
  H47.322 Drusen of optic disc, **left** eye
  H47.323 Drusen of optic disc, **bilateral**
  H47.329 Drusen of optic disc, unspecified eye ▽

✓6th **H47.33 Pseudopapilledema** of optic disc
  H47.331 Pseudopapilledema of optic disc, **right** eye
  H47.332 Pseudopapilledema of optic disc, **left** eye
  H47.333 Pseudopapilledema of optic disc, **bilateral**
  H47.339 Pseudopapilledema of optic disc, ▽
   unspecified eye

✓6th **H47.39 Other disorders of optic disc**
  H47.391 Other disorders of optic disc, **right** eye
  H47.392 Other disorders of optic disc, **left** eye
  H47.393 Other disorders of optic disc, **bilateral**
  H47.399 Other disorders of optic disc, ▽
   unspecified eye

✓5th **H47.4 Disorders of optic chiasm**
  Code also underlying condition
  H47.41 Disorders of optic chiasm in (due to) **inflammatory disorders**
  H47.42 Disorders of optic chiasm in (due to) **neoplasm**
  H47.43 Disorders of optic chiasm in (due to) **vascular disorders**
  H47.49 Disorders of optic chiasm in (due to) other **disorders**

✓5th **H47.5 Disorders of other visual pathways**
  Disorders of optic tracts, geniculate nuclei and optic radiations
  Code also underlying condition

✓6th **H47.51 Disorders of visual pathways in (due to) inflammatory disorders**
  H47.511 Disorders of visual pathways in (due to) inflammatory disorders, **right** side
  H47.512 Disorders of visual pathways in (due to) inflammatory disorders, **left** side
  H47.519 Disorders of visual pathways in (due to) ▽ inflammatory disorders, unspecified side

✓6th **H47.52 Disorders of visual pathways in (due to) neoplasm**
  H47.521 Disorders of visual pathways in (due to) neoplasm, **right** side
  H47.522 Disorders of visual pathways in (due to) neoplasm, **left** side
  H47.529 Disorders of visual pathways in (due to) ▽ neoplasm, unspecified side

✓6th **H47.53 Disorders of visual pathways in (due to) vascular disorders**
  H47.531 Disorders of visual pathways in (due to) vascular disorders, **right** side
  H47.532 Disorders of visual pathways in (due to) vascular disorders, **left** side

  H47.539 Disorders of visual pathways in (due to) ▽ vascular disorders, unspecified side

✓5th **H47.6 Disorders of visual cortex**
  Code also underlying condition
  EXCLUDES 1 injury to visual cortex S04.04

✓6th **H47.61 Cortical blindness**
  H47.611 Cortical blindness, **right** side of brain
  H47.612 Cortical blindness, **left** side of brain
  H47.619 Cortical blindness, unspecified side of ▽ brain

✓6th **H47.62 Disorders of visual cortex in (due to) inflammatory disorders**
  H47.621 Disorders of visual cortex in (due to) inflammatory disorders, **right** side of brain
  H47.622 Disorders of visual cortex in (due to) inflammatory disorders, **left** side of brain
  H47.629 Disorders of visual cortex in (due to) ▽ inflammatory disorders, unspecified side of brain

✓6th **H47.63 Disorders of visual cortex in (due to) neoplasm**
  H47.631 Disorders of visual cortex in (due to) neoplasm, **right** side of brain
  H47.632 Disorders of visual cortex in (due to) neoplasm, **left** side of brain
  H47.639 Disorders of visual cortex in (due to) ▽ neoplasm, unspecified side of brain

✓6th **H47.64 Disorders of visual cortex in (due to) vascular disorders**
  H47.641 Disorders of visual cortex in (due to) vascular disorders, **right** side of brain
  H47.642 Disorders of visual cortex in (due to) vascular disorders, **left** side of brain
  H47.649 Disorders of visual cortex in (due to) ▽ vascular disorders, unspecified side of brain

 H47.9 Unspecified disorder of visual pathways ▽

Disorders of ocular muscles, binocular movement, accommodation and refraction (H49-H52)

EXCLUDES 2 nystagmus and other irregular eye movements (H55)

✓4th **H49 Paralytic strabismus**
  EXCLUDES 2 internal ophthalmoplegia (H52.51-)
   internuclear ophthalmoplegia (H51.2-)
   progressive supranuclear ophthalmoplegia (G23.1)

✓5th **H49.0 Third [oculomotor] nerve palsy**
  H49.00 Third [oculomotor] nerve palsy, unspecified eye ▽
  H49.01 Third [oculomotor] nerve palsy, **right** eye
  H49.02 Third [oculomotor] nerve palsy, **left** eye
  H49.03 Third [oculomotor] nerve palsy, **bilateral**

✓5th **H49.1 Fourth [trochlear] nerve palsy**
  H49.10 Fourth [trochlear] nerve palsy, unspecified eye ▽
  H49.11 Fourth [trochlear] nerve palsy, **right** eye
  H49.12 Fourth [trochlear] nerve palsy, **left** eye
  H49.13 Fourth [trochlear] nerve palsy, **bilateral**

✓5th **H49.2 Sixth [abducent] nerve palsy**
  H49.20 Sixth [abducent] nerve palsy, unspecified eye ▽
  H49.21 Sixth [abducent] nerve palsy, **right** eye
  H49.22 Sixth [abducent] nerve palsy, **left** eye
  H49.23 Sixth [abducent] nerve palsy, **bilateral**

✓5th **H49.3 Total (external) ophthalmoplegia**
  H49.30 Total (external) ophthalmoplegia, unspecified eye ▽
  H49.31 Total (external) ophthalmoplegia, **right** eye
  H49.32 Total (external) ophthalmoplegia, **left** eye
  H49.33 Total (external) ophthalmoplegia, **bilateral**

✓6th **H49.4 Progressive external ophthalmoplegia**
  EXCLUDES 1 Kearns-Sayre syndrome (H49.81-)
  H49.40 Progressive external ophthalmoplegia, ▽ unspecified eye
  H49.41 Progressive external ophthalmoplegia, **right** eye
  H49.42 Progressive external ophthalmoplegia, **left** eye
  H49.43 Progressive external ophthalmoplegia, **bilateral**

EXCLUDES 1 Not coded here _EXCLUDES 2_ Not included here **N** Newborn Age: 0 **P** Pediatric Age: 0-17 **M** Maternity Age: 12-55 **A** Adult Age: 15-124

✓5ᵗʰ H49.8 Other paralytic strabismus

    ✓6ᵗʰ H49.81 Kearns-Sayre syndrome
         Progressive external ophthalmoplegia with pigmentary retinopathy
         Use additional code for other manifestation, such as: heart block (I45.9)

         H49.811 Kearns-Sayre syndrome, right eye `HCC`
         H49.812 Kearns-Sayre syndrome, left eye `HCC`
         H49.813 Kearns-Sayre syndrome, bilateral `HCC`
         H49.819 Kearns-Sayre syndrome, unspecified eye `HCC` ▽

    ✓6ᵗʰ H49.88 Other paralytic strabismus
         External ophthalmoplegia NOS
         H49.881 Other paralytic strabismus, right eye
         H49.882 Other paralytic strabismus, left eye
         H49.883 Other paralytic strabismus, bilateral
         H49.889 Other paralytic strabismus, unspecified eye ▽

H49.9 Unspecified paralytic strabismus ▽

✓4ᵗʰ H50 Other strabismus

    ✓5ᵗʰ H50.0 Esotropia
         Convergent concomitant strabismus
         EXCLUDES 1 intermittent esotropia (H50.31-, H50.32)

         H50.00 Unspecified esotropia ▽

    ✓6ᵗʰ H50.01 Monocular esotropia
         H50.011 Monocular esotropia, right eye
         H50.012 Monocular esotropia, left eye

    ✓6ᵗʰ H50.02 Monocular esotropia with A pattern
         H50.021 Monocular esotropia with A pattern, right eye
         H50.022 Monocular esotropia with A pattern, left eye

    ✓6ᵗʰ H50.03 Monocular esotropia with V pattern
         H50.031 Monocular esotropia with V pattern, right eye
         H50.032 Monocular esotropia with V pattern, left eye

    ✓6ᵗʰ H50.04 Monocular esotropia with other noncomitancies
         H50.041 Monocular esotropia with other noncomitancies, right eye
         H50.042 Monocular esotropia with other noncomitancies, left eye

     H50.05 Alternating esotropia
     H50.06 Alternating esotropia with A pattern
     H50.07 Alternating esotropia with V pattern
     H50.08 Alternating esotropia with other noncomitancies

    ✓5ᵗʰ H50.1 Exotropia
         Divergent concomitant strabismus
         EXCLUDES 1 intermittent exotropia (H50.33-, H50.34)

         H50.10 Unspecified exotropia ▽

Eye Muscle Diseases

R.   L.
Monocular (one eye only) esotropia (inward)

Monocular exotropia (outward)

Monocular hypertropia (upward)

✓6ᵗʰ H50.11 Monocular exotropia
     H50.111 Monocular exotropia, right eye
     H50.112 Monocular exotropia, left eye

✓6ᵗʰ H50.12 Monocular exotropia with A pattern
     H50.121 Monocular exotropia with A pattern, right eye
     H50.122 Monocular exotropia with A pattern, left eye

✓6ᵗʰ H50.13 Monocular exotropia with V pattern
     H50.131 Monocular exotropia with V pattern, right eye
     H50.132 Monocular exotropia with V pattern, left eye

✓6ᵗʰ H50.14 Monocular exotropia with other noncomitancies
     H50.141 Monocular exotropia with other noncomitancies, right eye
     H50.142 Monocular exotropia with other noncomitancies, left eye

     H50.15 Alternating exotropia
     H50.16 Alternating exotropia with A pattern
     H50.17 Alternating exotropia with V pattern
     H50.18 Alternating exotropia with other noncomitancies

✓5ᵗʰ H50.2 Vertical strabismus
     Hypertropia
     H50.21 Vertical strabismus, right eye
     H50.22 Vertical strabismus, left eye

✓5ᵗʰ H50.3 Intermittent heterotropia
     H50.30 Unspecified intermittent heterotropia ▽

    ✓6ᵗʰ H50.31 Intermittent monocular esotropia
         H50.311 Intermittent monocular esotropia, right eye
         H50.312 Intermittent monocular esotropia, left eye

     H50.32 Intermittent alternating esotropia

    ✓6ᵗʰ H50.33 Intermittent monocular exotropia
         H50.331 Intermittent monocular exotropia, right eye
         H50.332 Intermittent monocular exotropia, left eye

     H50.34 Intermittent alternating exotropia

✓5ᵗʰ H50.4 Other and unspecified heterotropia
     H50.40 Unspecified heterotropia ▽

    ✓6ᵗʰ H50.41 Cyclotropia
         H50.411 Cyclotropia, right eye
         H50.412 Cyclotropia, left eye

     H50.42 Monofixation syndrome
     H50.43 Accommodative component in esotropia

✓5ᵗʰ H50.5 Heterophoria
     H50.50 Unspecified heterophoria ▽
     H50.51 Esophoria
     H50.52 Exophoria
     H50.53 Vertical heterophoria
     H50.54 Cyclophoria
     H50.55 Alternating heterophoria

✓5ᵗʰ H50.6 Mechanical strabismus
     H50.60 Mechanical strabismus, unspecified ▽

    ✓6ᵗʰ H50.61 Brown's sheath syndrome
         H50.611 Brown's sheath syndrome, right eye
         H50.612 Brown's sheath syndrome, left eye

     H50.69 Other mechanical strabismus
         Strabismus due to adhesions
         Traumatic limitation of duction of eye muscle

✓5ᵗʰ H50.8 Other specified strabismus

    ✓6ᵗʰ H50.81 Duane's syndrome
         H50.811 Duane's syndrome, right eye
         H50.812 Duane's syndrome, left eye

     H50.89 Other specified strabismus

H50.9 Unspecified strabismus ▽

✓4ᵗʰ H51 Other disorders of binocular movement
     H51.0 Palsy (spasm) of conjugate gaze

    ✓5ᵗʰ H51.1 Convergence insufficiency and excess
         H51.11 Convergence insufficiency
         H51.12 Convergence excess

☑ Additional Character Req   ✓x7ᵗʰ Placeholder Alert   Manifestation   `HCC` CMS-HCC Condition   ▽ Unspecified Code   ►◄ Revised Text   ● New Code   ▲ Revised Code Title

✓5th **H51.2 Internuclear ophthalmoplegia**
    H51.20 Internuclear ophthalmoplegia, unspecified eye ▽
    H51.21 Internuclear ophthalmoplegia, right eye
    H51.22 Internuclear ophthalmoplegia, left eye
    H51.23 Internuclear ophthalmoplegia, bilateral
H51.8 Other specified disorders of binocular movement
H51.9 Unspecified disorder of binocular movement ▽

✓4th **H52 Disorders of refraction and accommodation**
  ✓5th **H52.0 Hypermetropia**
    H52.00 Hypermetropia, unspecified eye ▽
    H52.01 Hypermetropia, right eye
    H52.02 Hypermetropia, left eye
    H52.03 Hypermetropia, bilateral
  ✓5th **H52.1 Myopia**
    EXCLUDES1 *degenerative myopia (H44.2-)*
    H52.10 Myopia, unspecified eye ▽
    H52.11 Myopia, right eye
    H52.12 Myopia, left eye
    H52.13 Myopia, bilateral
  ✓5th **H52.2 Astigmatism**
   ✓6th H52.20 Unspecified astigmatism
    H52.201 Unspecified astigmatism, right eye ▽
    H52.202 Unspecified astigmatism, left eye ▽
    H52.203 Unspecified astigmatism, bilateral ▽
    H52.209 Unspecified astigmatism, unspecified eye ▽
   ✓6th H52.21 Irregular astigmatism
    H52.211 Irregular astigmatism, right eye
    H52.212 Irregular astigmatism, left eye
    H52.213 Irregular astigmatism, bilateral
    H52.219 Irregular astigmatism, unspecified eye ▽
   ✓6th H52.22 Regular astigmatism
    H52.221 Regular astigmatism, right eye
    H52.222 Regular astigmatism, left eye
    H52.223 Regular astigmatism, bilateral
    H52.229 Regular astigmatism, unspecified eye ▽
  ✓5th **H52.3 Anisometropia and aniseikonia**
    H52.31 Anisometropia
    H52.32 Aniseikonia
  H52.4 Presbyopia
  ✓5th **H52.5 Disorders of accommodation**
   ✓6th H52.51 Internal ophthalmoplegia (complete) (total)
    H52.511 Internal ophthalmoplegia (complete) (total), right eye
    H52.512 Internal ophthalmoplegia (complete) (total), left eye
    H52.513 Internal ophthalmoplegia (complete) (total), bilateral
    H52.519 Internal ophthalmoplegia (complete) (total), unspecified eye ▽
   ✓6th H52.52 Paresis of accommodation
    H52.521 Paresis of accommodation, right eye
    H52.522 Paresis of accommodation, left eye
    H52.523 Paresis of accommodation, bilateral
    H52.529 Paresis of accommodation, unspecified eye ▽
   ✓6th H52.53 Spasm of accommodation
    H52.531 Spasm of accommodation, right eye
    H52.532 Spasm of accommodation, left eye
    H52.533 Spasm of accommodation, bilateral
    H52.539 Spasm of accommodation, unspecified eye ▽
  H52.6 Other disorders of refraction
  H52.7 Unspecified disorder of refraction ▽

Visual disturbances and blindness (H53-H54)

✓4th **H53 Visual disturbances**
  ✓5th **H53.0 Amblyopia ex anopsia**
    EXCLUDES1 *amblyopia due to vitamin A deficiency (E50.5)*
   ✓6th H53.00 Unspecified amblyopia
    H53.001 Unspecified amblyopia, right eye ▽

    H53.002 Unspecified amblyopia, left eye ▽
    H53.003 Unspecified amblyopia, bilateral ▽
    H53.009 Unspecified amblyopia, unspecified eye ▽
   ✓6th H53.01 Deprivation amblyopia
    H53.011 Deprivation amblyopia, right eye
    H53.012 Deprivation amblyopia, left eye
    H53.013 Deprivation amblyopia, bilateral
    H53.019 Deprivation amblyopia, unspecified eye ▽
   ✓6th H53.02 Refractive amblyopia
    H53.021 Refractive amblyopia, right eye
    H53.022 Refractive amblyopia, left eye
    H53.023 Refractive amblyopia, bilateral
    H53.029 Refractive amblyopia, unspecified eye ▽
   ✓6th H53.03 Strabismic amblyopia
    EXCLUDES1 *strabismus (H50.-)*
    H53.031 Strabismic amblyopia, right eye
    H53.032 Strabismic amblyopia, left eye
    H53.033 Strabismic amblyopia, bilateral
    H53.039 Strabismic amblyopia, unspecified eye ▽
   ✓6th H53.04 Amblyopia suspect
    H53.041 Amblyopia suspect, right eye
    H53.042 Amblyopia suspect, left eye
    H53.043 Amblyopia suspect, bilateral
    H53.049 Amblyopia suspect, unspecified eye ▽
  ✓5th **H53.1 Subjective visual disturbances**
    EXCLUDES1 *subjective visual disturbances due to vitamin A deficiency (E50.5)*
    visual hallucinations (R44.1)
    H53.10 Unspecified subjective visual disturbances ▽
    H53.11 Day blindness
      Hemeralopia
   ✓6th H53.12 Transient visual loss
      Scintillating scotoma
    EXCLUDES1 *amaurosis fugax (G45.3-)*
    transient retinal artery occlusion (H34.0-)
    H53.121 Transient visual loss, right eye
    H53.122 Transient visual loss, left eye
    H53.123 Transient visual loss, bilateral
    H53.129 Transient visual loss, unspecified eye ▽
   ✓6th H53.13 Sudden visual loss
    H53.131 Sudden visual loss, right eye
    H53.132 Sudden visual loss, left eye
    H53.133 Sudden visual loss, bilateral
    H53.139 Sudden visual loss, unspecified eye ▽
   ✓6th H53.14 Visual discomfort
      Asthenopia   Photophobia
    H53.141 Visual discomfort, right eye
    H53.142 Visual discomfort, left eye
    H53.143 Visual discomfort, bilateral
    H53.149 Visual discomfort, unspecified ▽
    H53.15 Visual distortions of shape and size
      Metamorphopsia
    H53.16 Psychophysical visual disturbances
    H53.19 Other subjective visual disturbances
      Visual halos
  H53.2 Diplopia
    Double vision
  ✓5th **H53.3 Other and unspecified disorders of binocular vision**
    H53.30 Unspecified disorder of binocular vision ▽
    H53.31 Abnormal retinal correspondence
    H53.32 Fusion with defective stereopsis
    H53.33 Simultaneous visual perception without fusion
    H53.34 Suppression of binocular vision
  ✓5th **H53.4 Visual field defects**
    H53.40 Unspecified visual field defects ▽
   ✓6th H53.41 Scotoma involving central area
      Central scotoma
    H53.411 Scotoma involving central area, right eye
    H53.412 Scotoma involving central area, left eye
    H53.413 Scotoma involving central area, bilateral

H53.419   Scotoma involving central area, unspecified eye ▽

✓6ᵗʰ **H53.42**   Scotoma of blind spot area
Enlarged blind spot

    H53.421   Scotoma of blind spot area, right eye
    H53.422   Scotoma of blind spot area, left eye
    H53.423   Scotoma of blind spot area, bilateral
    H53.429   Scotoma of blind spot area, unspecified eye ▽

✓6ᵗʰ **H53.43**   Sector or arcuate defects
Arcuate scotoma
Bjerrum scotoma

    H53.431   Sector or arcuate defects, right eye
    H53.432   Sector or arcuate defects, left eye
    H53.433   Sector or arcuate defects, bilateral
    H53.439   Sector or arcuate defects, unspecified eye ▽

✓6ᵗʰ **H53.45**   Other localized visual field defect
Peripheral visual field defect
Ring scotoma NOS
Scotoma NOS

    H53.451   Other localized visual field defect, right eye
    H53.452   Other localized visual field defect, left eye
    H53.453   Other localized visual field defect, bilateral
    H53.459   Other localized visual field defect, unspecified eye ▽

✓6ᵗʰ **H53.46**   Homonymous bilateral field defects
Homonymous hemianopia
Homonymous hemianopsia
Quadrant anopia
Quadrant anopsia

    H53.461   Homonymous bilateral field defects, right side
    H53.462   Homonymous bilateral field defects, left side
    H53.469   Homonymous bilateral field defects, unspecified side ▽
       Homonymous bilateral field defects NOS

H53.47   Heteronymous bilateral field defects
Heteronymous hemianop(s)ia

✓6ᵗʰ **H53.48**   Generalized contraction of visual field

    H53.481   Generalized contraction of visual field, right eye
    H53.482   Generalized contraction of visual field, left eye
    H53.483   Generalized contraction of visual field, bilateral
    H53.489   Generalized contraction of visual field, unspecified eye ▽

✓5ᵗʰ **H53.5**   Color vision deficiencies
Color blindness
EXCLUDES 2   day blindness (H53.11)

H53.50   Unspecified color vision deficiencies ▽
Color blindness NOS

H53.51   Achromatopsia
DEF: Nonprogressive genetic visual disorder; characterized by complete color blindness, decreased vision, and light sensitivity.

H53.52   Acquired color vision deficiency

H53.53   Deuteranomaly
Deuteranopia
DEF: Male-only genetic disorder; difficulty in distinguishing green and red, no shortened spectrum.

H53.54   Protanomaly
Protanopia

H53.55   Tritanomaly
Tritanopia

H53.59   Other color vision deficiencies

✓5ᵗʰ **H53.6**   Night blindness
EXCLUDES 1   night blindness due to vitamin A deficiency (E50.5)

H53.60   Unspecified night blindness ▽
H53.61   Abnormal dark adaptation curve
H53.62   Acquired night blindness
H53.63   Congenital night blindness
H53.69   Other night blindness

✓5ᵗʰ **H53.7**   Vision sensitivity deficiencies
H53.71   Glare sensitivity
H53.72   Impaired contrast sensitivity

H53.8   Other visual disturbances
H53.9   Unspecified visual disturbance ▽

✓4ᵗʰ **H54**   **Blindness and low vision**
NOTE   For definition of visual impairment categories see table below
Code first any associated underlying cause of the blindness
EXCLUDES 1   amaurosis fugax (G45.3)

✓5ᵗʰ **H54.0**   Blindness, both eyes
Visual impairment categories 3, 4, 5 in both eyes

   ● ✓6ᵗʰ **H54.0X**   Blindness, both eyes, different category levels

     ● ✓7ᵗʰ **H54.0X3**   Blindness right eye, category 3
       ● **H54.0X33**   Blindness right eye category 3, blindness left eye category 3
       H54.0X34   Blindness right eye category 3, blindness left eye category 4
       H54.0X35   Blindness right eye category 3, blindness left eye category 5

     ● ✓7ᵗʰ **H54.0X4**   Blindness right eye, category 4
       ● **H54.0X43**   Blindness right eye category 4, blindness left eye category 3
       H54.0X44   Blindness right eye category 4, blindness left eye category 4
       H54.0X45   Blindness right eye category 4, blindness left eye category 5

     ● ✓7ᵗʰ **H54.0X5**   Blindness right eye, category 5
       ● **H54.0X53**   Blindness right eye category 5, blindness left eye category 3
       H54.0X54   Blindness right eye category 5, blindness left eye category 4
       H54.0X55   Blindness right eye category 5, blindness left eye category 5

✓5ᵗʰ **H54.1**   Blindness, one eye, low vision other eye
Visual impairment categories 3, 4, 5 in one eye, with categories 1 or 2 in the other eye.

H54.10   Blindness, one eye, low vision other eye, unspecified eyes ▽

   ● ✓6ᵗʰ **H54.11**   Blindness, right eye, low vision left eye

     ● ✓7ᵗʰ **H54.113**   Blindness right eye category 3, low vision left eye
       ● **H54.1131**   Blindness right eye category 3, low vision left eye category 1
       H54.1132   Blindness right eye category 3, low vision left eye category 2

     ● ✓7ᵗʰ **H54.114**   Blindness right eye category 4, low vision left eye
       ● **H54.1141**   Blindness right eye category 4, low vision left eye category 1
       H54.1142   Blindness right eye category 4, low vision left eye category 2

     ● ✓7ᵗʰ **H54.115**   Blindness right eye category 5, low vision left eye
       ● **H54.1151**   Blindness right eye category 5, low vision left eye category 1
       H54.1152   Blindness right eye category 5, low vision left eye category 2

   ● ✓6ᵗʰ **H54.12**   Blindness, left eye, low vision right eye

     ● ✓7ᵗʰ **H54.121**   Low vision right eye category 1, blindness left eye
       ● **H54.1213**   Low vision right eye category 1, blindness left eye category 3
       H54.1214   Low vision right eye category 1, blindness left eye category 4
       H54.1215   Low vision right eye category 1, blindness left eye category 5

☑ Additional Character Req   ✓ₓ7ᵗʰ Placeholder Alert   Manifestation   **HCC** CMS-HCC Condition   ▽ Unspecified Code   ▶◀ Revised Text   ● New Code   ▲ Revised Code Title

Chapter 7. Diseases of the Eye and Adnexa

√7th **H54.122** Low vision right eye category 2, blindness left eye

     H54.1223 Low vision right eye category 2, blindness left eye category 3

     H54.1224 Low vision right eye category 2, blindness left eye category 4

     H54.1225 Low vision right eye category 2, blindness left eye category 5

√5th **H54.2** Low vision, both eyes
Visual impairment categories 1 or 2 in both eyes

√6th **H54.2X** Low vision, both eyes, different category levels

√7th **H54.2X1** Low vision, right eye, category 1

     H54.2X11 Low vision right eye category 1, low vision left eye category 1

     H54.2X12 Low vision right eye category 1, low vision left eye category 2

√7th **H54.2X2** Low vision, right eye, category 2

     H54.2X21 Low vision right eye category 2, low vision left eye category 1

     H54.2X22 Low vision right eye category 2, low vision left eye category 2

H54.3 Unqualified visual loss, both eyes
Visual impairment category 9 in both eyes.

√5th **H54.4** Blindness, one eye
Visual impairment categories 3, 4, 5 in one eye [normal vision in other eye]

     H54.40 Blindness, one eye, unspecified eye ▽

√6th **H54.41** Blindness, right eye, normal vision left eye

√7th **H54.413** Blindness, right eye, category 3

     H54.413A Blindness right eye category 3, normal vision left eye

√7th **H54.414** Blindness, right eye, category 4

     H54.414A Blindness right eye category 4, normal vision left eye

√7th **H54.415** Blindness, right eye, category 5

     H54.415A Blindness right eye category 5, normal vision left eye

√6th **H54.42** Blindness, left eye, normal vision right eye

√7th **H54.42A** Blindness, left eye, category 3-5

     H54.42A3 Blindness left eye category 3, normal vision right eye

     H54.42A4 Blindness left eye category 4, normal vision right eye

     H54.42A5 Blindness left eye category 5, normal vision right eye

√5th **H54.5** Low vision, one eye
Visual impairment categories 1 or 2 in one eye [normal vision in other eye]

     H54.50 Low vision, one eye, unspecified eye ▽

√6th **H54.51** Low vision, right eye, normal vision left eye

√7th **H54.511** Low vision, right eye, category 1-2

     H54.511A Low vision right eye category 1, normal vision left eye

     H54.512A Low vision right eye category 2, normal vision left eye

√6th **H54.52** Low vision, left eye, normal vision right eye

√7th **H54.52A** Low vision, left eye, category 1-2

     H54.52A1 Low vision left eye category 1, normal vision right eye

     H54.52A2 Low vision left eye category 2, normal vision right eye

√5th **H54.6** Unqualified visual loss, one eye
Visual impairment category 9 in one eye [normal vision in other eye].

     H54.60 Unqualified visual loss, one eye, unspecified ▽

     H54.61 Unqualified visual loss, right eye, normal vision left eye

     H54.62 Unqualified visual loss, left eye, normal vision right eye

H54.7 Unspecified visual loss ▽
Visual impairment category 9 NOS

H54.8 Legal blindness, as defined in USA
Blindness NOS according to USA definition
EXCLUDES 1   legal blindness with specification of impairment level (H54.0-H54.7)

NOTE   The table below gives a classification of severity of visual impairment recommended by a WHO Study Group on the Prevention of Blindness, Geneva, 6-10 November l972.

The term "low vision" in category H54 comprises categories 1 and 2 of the table, the term "blindness" categories 3, 4 and 5, and the term "unqualified visual loss" category 9.

If the extent of the visual field is taken into account, patients with a field no greater than 10 but greater than 5 around central fixation should be placed in category 3 and patients with a field greater than 5 around central fixation should be placed in category 4, even if the central acuity is not impaired.

Category of visual impairment	Visual acuity with best possible correction	
	Maximum less than:	**Minimum equal to or better than:**
1	6/18 3/10 (0.3) 20/70	6/60 1/10 (0.1) 20/200
2	6/60 1/10 (0.1) 20/200	3/60 1/20 (0.05) 20/400
3	3/60 1/200 (0.05) 20/400	1/60 (finger counting at one meter) 1/50 (0.02) 5/300 (20/1200)
4	1/60 (finger counting at one meter) 1/50 (0.02) 5/300	Light perception
5	No light perception	
9	Undetermined or unspecified	

Other disorders of eye and adnexa (H55-H57)

√4th **H55** Nystagmus and other irregular eye movements

√5th **H55.0** Nystagmus

     H55.00 Unspecified nystagmus ▽

     H55.01 Congenital nystagmus

     H55.02 Latent nystagmus

     H55.03 Visual deprivation nystagmus

     H55.04 Dissociated nystagmus

     H55.09 Other forms of nystagmus

√5th **H55.8** Other irregular eye movements

     H55.81 Saccadic eye movements

     H55.89 Other irregular eye movements

√4th **H57** Other disorders of eye and adnexa

√5th **H57.0** Anomalies of pupillary function

     H57.00 Unspecified anomaly of pupillary function ▽

     H57.01 Argyll Robertson pupil, atypical
     EXCLUDES 1   syphilitic Argyll Robertson pupil (A52.19)

     H57.02 Anisocoria

     H57.03 Miosis

     H57.04 Mydriasis

√6th **H57.05** Tonic pupil

     H57.051 Tonic pupil, right eye

     H57.052 Tonic pupil, left eye

     H57.053 Tonic pupil, bilateral

     H57.059 Tonic pupil, unspecified eye ▽

     H57.09 Other anomalies of pupillary function

√5th **H57.1** Ocular pain

     H57.10 Ocular pain, unspecified eye ▽

     H57.11 Ocular pain, right eye

     H57.12 Ocular pain, left eye

     H57.13 Ocular pain, bilateral

EXCLUDES 1 Not coded here   EXCLUDES 2 Not included here   N Newborn Age: 0   P Pediatric Age: 0-17   M Maternity Age: 12-55   A Adult Age: 15-124

602   ICD-10-CM 2018

H57.8   Other specified disorders of eye and adnexa

H57.9   Unspecified disorder of eye and adnexa ▽

Intraoperative and postprocedural complications and disorders of eye and adnexa, not elsewhere classified (H59)

✓4th H59 Intraoperative and postprocedural complications and disorders of eye and adnexa, not elsewhere classified

> *EXCLUDES 1*   *mechanical complication of intraocular lens (T85.2)*
> *mechanical complication of other ocular prosthetic devices, implants and grafts (T85.3)*
> *pseudophakia (Z96.1)*
> *secondary cataracts (H26.4-)*

✓5th H59.0 Disorders of the eye following cataract surgery

   ✓6th H59.01 Keratopathy (bullous aphakic) following cataract surgery
     Vitreal corneal syndrome
     Vitreous (touch) syndrome

     H59.011   Keratopathy (bullous aphakic) following cataract surgery, right eye
     H59.012   Keratopathy (bullous aphakic) following cataract surgery, left eye
     H59.013   Keratopathy (bullous aphakic) following cataract surgery, bilateral
     H59.019   Keratopathy (bullous aphakic) following cataract surgery, unspecified eye ▽

   ✓6th H59.02 Cataract (lens) fragments in eye following cataract surgery

     H59.021   Cataract (lens) fragments in eye following cataract surgery, right eye
     H59.022   Cataract (lens) fragments in eye following cataract surgery, left eye
     H59.023   Cataract (lens) fragments in eye following cataract surgery, bilateral
     H59.029   Cataract (lens) fragments in eye following cataract surgery, unspecified eye ▽

   ✓6th H59.03 Cystoid macular edema following cataract surgery

     H59.031   Cystoid macular edema following cataract surgery, right eye
     H59.032   Cystoid macular edema following cataract surgery, left eye
     H59.033   Cystoid macular edema following cataract surgery, bilateral
     H59.039   Cystoid macular edema following cataract surgery, unspecified eye ▽

   ✓6th H59.09 Other disorders of the eye following cataract surgery

     H59.091   Other disorders of the right eye following cataract surgery
     H59.092   Other disorders of the left eye following cataract surgery
     H59.093   Other disorders of the eye following cataract surgery, bilateral
     H59.099   Other disorders of unspecified eye following cataract surgery ▽

✓5th H59.1 Intraoperative hemorrhage and hematoma of eye and adnexa complicating a procedure

> *EXCLUDES 1*   *intraoperative hemorrhage and hematoma of eye and adnexa due to accidental puncture or laceration during a procedure (H59.2-)*

   ✓6th H59.11 Intraoperative hemorrhage and hematoma of eye and adnexa complicating an ophthalmic procedure

     H59.111   Intraoperative hemorrhage and hematoma of right eye and adnexa complicating an ophthalmic procedure
     H59.112   Intraoperative hemorrhage and hematoma of left eye and adnexa complicating an ophthalmic procedure
     H59.113   Intraoperative hemorrhage and hematoma of eye and adnexa complicating an ophthalmic procedure, bilateral
     H59.119   Intraoperative hemorrhage and hematoma of unspecified eye and adnexa complicating an ophthalmic procedure ▽

   ✓6th H59.12 Intraoperative hemorrhage and hematoma of eye and adnexa complicating other procedure

     H59.121   Intraoperative hemorrhage and hematoma of right eye and adnexa complicating other procedure
     H59.122   Intraoperative hemorrhage and hematoma of left eye and adnexa complicating other procedure
     H59.123   Intraoperative hemorrhage and hematoma of eye and adnexa complicating other procedure, bilateral
     H59.129   Intraoperative hemorrhage and hematoma of unspecified eye and adnexa complicating other procedure ▽

✓5th H59.2 Accidental puncture and laceration of eye and adnexa during a procedure

   ✓6th H59.21 Accidental puncture and laceration of eye and adnexa during an ophthalmic procedure

     H59.211   Accidental puncture and laceration of right eye and adnexa during an ophthalmic procedure
     H59.212   Accidental puncture and laceration of left eye and adnexa during an ophthalmic procedure
     H59.213   Accidental puncture and laceration of eye and adnexa during an ophthalmic procedure, bilateral
     H59.219   Accidental puncture and laceration of unspecified eye and adnexa during an ophthalmic procedure ▽

   ✓6th H59.22 Accidental puncture and laceration of eye and adnexa during other procedure

     H59.221   Accidental puncture and laceration of right eye and adnexa during other procedure
     H59.222   Accidental puncture and laceration of left eye and adnexa during other procedure
     H59.223   Accidental puncture and laceration of eye and adnexa during other procedure, bilateral
     H59.229   Accidental puncture and laceration of unspecified eye and adnexa during other procedure ▽

✓5th H59.3 Postprocedural hemorrhage, hematoma, and seroma of eye and adnexa following a procedure

   ✓6th H59.31 Postprocedural hemorrhage of eye and adnexa following an ophthalmic procedure

     H59.311   Postprocedural hemorrhage of right eye and adnexa following an ophthalmic procedure
     H59.312   Postprocedural hemorrhage of left eye and adnexa following an ophthalmic procedure
     H59.313   Postprocedural hemorrhage of eye and adnexa following an ophthalmic procedure, bilateral
     H59.319   Postprocedural hemorrhage of unspecified eye and adnexa following an ophthalmic procedure ▽

   ✓6th H59.32 Postprocedural hemorrhage of eye and adnexa following other procedure

     H59.321   Postprocedural hemorrhage of right eye and adnexa following other procedure
     H59.322   Postprocedural hemorrhage of left eye and adnexa following other procedure
     H59.323   Postprocedural hemorrhage of eye and adnexa following other procedure, bilateral
     H59.329   Postprocedural hemorrhage of unspecified eye and adnexa following other procedure ▽

   ✓6th H59.33 Postprocedural hematoma of eye and adnexa following an ophthalmic procedure

     H59.331   Postprocedural hematoma of right eye and adnexa following an ophthalmic procedure
     H59.332   Postprocedural hematoma of left eye and adnexa following an ophthalmic procedure

---

✓ Additional Character Req   ✓x7th Placeholder Alert   Manifestation   HCC CMS-HCC Condition   ▽ Unspecified Code   ►◄ Revised Text   ● New Code   ▲ Revised Code Title

H59.333 Postprocedural hematoma of eye and adnexa following an ophthalmic procedure, **bilateral**

H59.339 Postprocedural hematoma of ▽ unspecified eye and adnexa following an ophthalmic procedure

✓6ᵗʰ **H59.34** Postprocedural **hematoma** of eye and adnexa following **other procedure**

H59.341 Postprocedural hematoma of **right** eye and adnexa following other procedure

H59.342 Postprocedural hematoma of **left** eye and adnexa following other procedure

H59.343 Postprocedural hematoma of eye and adnexa following other procedure, **bilateral**

H59.349 Postprocedural hematoma of ▽ unspecified eye and adnexa following other procedure

✓6ᵗʰ **H59.35** Postprocedural **seroma** of eye and adnexa following an **ophthalmic procedure**

H59.351 Postprocedural seroma of **right** eye and adnexa following an ophthalmic procedure

H59.352 Postprocedural seroma of **left** eye and adnexa following an ophthalmic procedure

H59.353 Postprocedural seroma of eye and adnexa following an ophthalmic procedure, **bilateral**

H59.359 Postprocedural seroma of unspecified ▽ eye and adnexa following an ophthalmic procedure

✓6ᵗʰ **H59.36** Postprocedural **seroma** of eye and adnexa following **other procedure**

H59.361 Postprocedural seroma of **right** eye and adnexa following other procedure

H59.362 Postprocedural seroma of **left** eye and adnexa following other procedure

H59.363 Postprocedural seroma of eye and adnexa following other procedure, **bilateral**

H59.369 Postprocedural seroma of unspecified ▽ eye and adnexa following other procedure

✓5ᵗʰ **H59.4** **Inflammation (infection) of postprocedural bleb**
Postprocedural blebitis
EXCLUDES 1   *filtering (vitreous) bleb after glaucoma surgery status (Z98.83)*

H59.40 Inflammation (infection) of postprocedural bleb, ▽ unspecified

H59.41 Inflammation (infection) of postprocedural bleb, **stage 1**

H59.42 Inflammation (infection) of postprocedural bleb, **stage 2**

H59.43 Inflammation (infection) of postprocedural bleb, **stage 3**
Bleb endophthalmitis

✓5ᵗʰ **H59.8** **Other intraoperative and postprocedural complications and disorders of eye and adnexa, not elsewhere classified**

✓6ᵗʰ **H59.81** **Chorioretinal scars after surgery for detachment**

H59.811 Chorioretinal scars after surgery for detachment, **right** eye

H59.812 Chorioretinal scars after surgery for detachment, **left** eye

H59.813 Chorioretinal scars after surgery for detachment, **bilateral**

H59.819 Chorioretinal scars after surgery for ▽ detachment, unspecified eye

H59.88 Other intraoperative complications of eye and adnexa, not elsewhere classified

H59.89 Other postprocedural complications and disorders of eye and adnexa, not elsewhere classified

Chapter 8. Diseases of the Ear and Mastoid Process (H6Ø–H95)

Chapter Specific Coding Guidelines and Examples
Reserved for future guideline expansion.

Chapter 8. Diseases of the Ear and Mastoid Process (H60-H95)

NOTE Use an external cause code following the code for the ear condition, if applicable, to identify the cause of the ear condition.

EXCLUDES 2 *certain conditions originating in the perinatal period (P04-P96)*
certain infectious and parasitic diseases (A00-B99)
complications of pregnancy, childbirth and the puerperium (O00-O9A)
congenital malformations, deformations and chromosomal abnormalities (Q00-Q99)
endocrine, nutritional and metabolic diseases (E00-E88)
injury, poisoning and certain other consequences of external causes (S00-T88)
neoplasms (C00-D49)
symptoms, signs and abnormal clinical and laboratory findings, not elsewhere classified (R00-R94)

This chapter contains the following blocks:

H60-H62 Diseases of external ear
H65-H75 Diseases of middle ear and mastoid
H80-H83 Diseases of inner ear
H90-H94 Other disorders of ear
H95 Intraoperative and postprocedural complications and disorders of ear and mastoid process, not elsewhere classified

Diseases of external ear (H60-H62)

H60 Otitis externa

H60.0 Abscess of external ear
Boil of external ear
Carbuncle of auricle or external auditory canal
Furuncle of external ear
- H60.00 Abscess of external ear, unspecified ear ▽
- H60.01 Abscess of right external ear
- H60.02 Abscess of left external ear
- H60.03 Abscess of external ear, bilateral

H60.1 Cellulitis of external ear
Cellulitis of auricle
Cellulitis of external auditory canal
- H60.10 Cellulitis of external ear, unspecified ear ▽
- H60.11 Cellulitis of right external ear
- H60.12 Cellulitis of left external ear
- H60.13 Cellulitis of external ear, bilateral

H60.2 Malignant otitis externa
- H60.20 Malignant otitis externa, unspecified ear ▽
- H60.21 Malignant otitis externa, right ear
- H60.22 Malignant otitis externa, left ear
- H60.23 Malignant otitis externa, bilateral

H60.3 Other infective otitis externa

H60.31 Diffuse otitis externa
- H60.311 Diffuse otitis externa, right ear
- H60.312 Diffuse otitis externa, left ear
- H60.313 Diffuse otitis externa, bilateral
- H60.319 Diffuse otitis externa, unspecified ear ▽

H60.32 Hemorrhagic otitis externa
- H60.321 Hemorrhagic otitis externa, right ear
- H60.322 Hemorrhagic otitis externa, left ear
- H60.323 Hemorrhagic otitis externa, bilateral
- H60.329 Hemorrhagic otitis externa, unspecified ear ▽

H60.33 Swimmer's ear
DEF: Otitis externa; commonly occurs when water gets trapped in the ear after swimming.
- H60.331 Swimmer's ear, right ear
- H60.332 Swimmer's ear, left ear
- H60.333 Swimmer's ear, bilateral
- H60.339 Swimmer's ear, unspecified ear ▽

H60.39 Other infective otitis externa
- H60.391 Other infective otitis externa, right ear
- H60.392 Other infective otitis externa, left ear
- H60.393 Other infective otitis externa, bilateral
- H60.399 Other infective otitis externa, unspecified ear ▽

H60.4 Cholesteatoma of external ear
Keratosis obturans of external ear (canal)
EXCLUDES 2 *cholesteatoma of middle ear (H71.-)*
recurrent cholesteatoma of postmastoidectomy cavity (H95.0-)
- H60.40 Cholesteatoma of external ear, unspecified ear ▽
- H60.41 Cholesteatoma of right external ear
- H60.42 Cholesteatoma of left external ear
- H60.43 Cholesteatoma of external ear, bilateral

H60.5 Acute noninfective otitis externa

H60.50 Unspecified acute noninfective otitis externa
Acute otitis externa NOS
- H60.501 Unspecified acute noninfective otitis externa, right ear ▽
- H60.502 Unspecified acute noninfective otitis externa, left ear ▽
- H60.503 Unspecified acute noninfective otitis externa, bilateral ▽
- H60.509 Unspecified acute noninfective otitis externa, unspecified ear ▽

H60.51 Acute actinic otitis externa
- H60.511 Acute actinic otitis externa, right ear
- H60.512 Acute actinic otitis externa, left ear
- H60.513 Acute actinic otitis externa, bilateral
- H60.519 Acute actinic otitis externa, unspecified ear ▽

H60.52 Acute chemical otitis externa
- H60.521 Acute chemical otitis externa, right ear
- H60.522 Acute chemical otitis externa, left ear
- H60.523 Acute chemical otitis externa, bilateral
- H60.529 Acute chemical otitis externa, unspecified ear ▽

H60.53 Acute contact otitis externa
- H60.531 Acute contact otitis externa, right ear
- H60.532 Acute contact otitis externa, left ear
- H60.533 Acute contact otitis externa, bilateral
- H60.539 Acute contact otitis externa, unspecified ear ▽

H60.54 Acute eczematoid otitis externa
- H60.541 Acute eczematoid otitis externa, right ear
- H60.542 Acute eczematoid otitis externa, left ear
- H60.543 Acute eczematoid otitis externa, bilateral
- H60.549 Acute eczematoid otitis externa, unspecified ear ▽

H60.55 Acute reactive otitis externa
- H60.551 Acute reactive otitis externa, right ear
- H60.552 Acute reactive otitis externa, left ear
- H60.553 Acute reactive otitis externa, bilateral
- H60.559 Acute reactive otitis externa, unspecified ear ▽

H60.59 Other noninfective acute otitis externa
- H60.591 Other noninfective acute otitis externa, right ear
- H60.592 Other noninfective acute otitis externa, left ear
- H60.593 Other noninfective acute otitis externa, bilateral
- H60.599 Other noninfective acute otitis externa, unspecified ear ▽

H60.6 Unspecified chronic otitis externa
- H60.60 Unspecified chronic otitis externa, unspecified ear ▽
- H60.61 Unspecified chronic otitis externa, right ear ▽
- H60.62 Unspecified chronic otitis externa, left ear ▽
- H60.63 Unspecified chronic otitis externa, bilateral ▽

H60.8 Other otitis externa

H60.8X Other otitis externa
- H60.8X1 Other otitis externa, right ear
- H60.8X2 Other otitis externa, left ear
- H60.8X3 Other otitis externa, bilateral
- H60.8X9 Other otitis externa, unspecified ear ▽

H60.9 Unspecified otitis externa
- H60.90 Unspecified otitis externa, unspecified ear ▽
- H60.91 Unspecified otitis externa, right ear ▽

H60.92 Unspecified otitis externa, left ear ▽
H60.93 Unspecified otitis externa, bilateral ▽

✓4ᵗʰ **H61 Other disorders of external ear**

  ✓5ᵗʰ **H61.0 Chondritis and perichondritis of external ear**
    Chondrodermatitis nodularis chronica helicis
    Perichondritis of auricle
    Perichondritis of pinna

    ✓6ᵗʰ **H61.00 Unspecified perichondritis of external ear**
      H61.001 Unspecified perichondritis of right external ear ▽
      H61.002 Unspecified perichondritis of left external ear ▽
      H61.003 Unspecified perichondritis of external ear, bilateral ▽
      H61.009 Unspecified perichondritis of external ear, unspecified ear ▽

    ✓6ᵗʰ **H61.01 Acute perichondritis of external ear**
      H61.011 Acute perichondritis of right external ear
      H61.012 Acute perichondritis of left external ear
      H61.013 Acute perichondritis of external ear, bilateral
      H61.019 Acute perichondritis of external ear, unspecified ear ▽

    ✓6ᵗʰ **H61.02 Chronic perichondritis of external ear**
      H61.021 Chronic perichondritis of right external ear
      H61.022 Chronic perichondritis of left external ear
      H61.023 Chronic perichondritis of external ear, bilateral
      H61.029 Chronic perichondritis of external ear, unspecified ear ▽

    ✓6ᵗʰ **H61.03 Chondritis of external ear**
      Chondritis of auricle
      Chondritis of pinna
      AHA: 2015, 1Q, 18
      DEF: Infection that has progressed into the cartilage; presents as indurated and edematous skin over the pinna; vascular compromise occurs with tissue necrosis and deformity.
      H61.031 Chondritis of right external ear
      H61.032 Chondritis of left external ear
      H61.033 Chondritis of external ear, bilateral
      H61.039 Chondritis of external ear, unspecified ear ▽

  ✓5ᵗʰ **H61.1 Noninfective disorders of pinna**
    EXCLUDES 2 *cauliflower ear (M95.1-)*
                gouty tophi of ear (M1A.-)

    ✓6ᵗʰ **H61.10 Unspecified noninfective disorders of pinna**
      Disorder of pinna NOS
      H61.101 Unspecified noninfective disorders of pinna, right ear ▽
      H61.102 Unspecified noninfective disorders of pinna, left ear ▽
      H61.103 Unspecified noninfective disorders of pinna, bilateral ▽
      H61.109 Unspecified noninfective disorders of pinna, unspecified ear ▽

    ✓6ᵗʰ **H61.11 Acquired deformity of pinna**
      Acquired deformity of auricle
      EXCLUDES 2 *cauliflower ear (M95.1-)*
      H61.111 Acquired deformity of pinna, right ear
      H61.112 Acquired deformity of pinna, left ear
      H61.113 Acquired deformity of pinna, bilateral
      H61.119 Acquired deformity of pinna, unspecified ear ▽

    ✓6ᵗʰ **H61.12 Hematoma of pinna**
      Hematoma of auricle
      H61.121 Hematoma of pinna, right ear
      H61.122 Hematoma of pinna, left ear
      H61.123 Hematoma of pinna, bilateral
      H61.129 Hematoma of pinna, unspecified ear ▽

    ✓6ᵗʰ **H61.19 Other noninfective disorders of pinna**
      H61.191 Noninfective disorders of pinna, right ear
      H61.192 Noninfective disorders of pinna, left ear
      H61.193 Noninfective disorders of pinna, bilateral
      H61.199 Noninfective disorders of pinna, unspecified ear ▽

  ✓5ᵗʰ **H61.2 Impacted cerumen**
    Wax in ear
    H61.20 Impacted cerumen, unspecified ear ▽
    H61.21 Impacted cerumen, right ear
    H61.22 Impacted cerumen, left ear
    H61.23 Impacted cerumen, bilateral

  ✓5ᵗʰ **H61.3 Acquired stenosis of external ear canal**
    Collapse of external ear canal
    EXCLUDES 1 *postprocedural stenosis of external ear canal (H95.81-)*

    ✓6ᵗʰ **H61.30 Acquired stenosis of external ear canal, unspecified**
      H61.301 Acquired stenosis of right external ear canal, unspecified ▽
      H61.302 Acquired stenosis of left external ear canal, unspecified ▽
      H61.303 Acquired stenosis of external ear canal, unspecified, bilateral ▽
      H61.309 Acquired stenosis of external ear canal, unspecified, unspecified ear ▽

    ✓6ᵗʰ **H61.31 Acquired stenosis of external ear canal secondary to trauma**
      H61.311 Acquired stenosis of right external ear canal secondary to trauma
      H61.312 Acquired stenosis of left external ear canal secondary to trauma
      H61.313 Acquired stenosis of external ear canal secondary to trauma, bilateral
      H61.319 Acquired stenosis of external ear canal secondary to trauma, unspecified ear ▽

    ✓6ᵗʰ **H61.32 Acquired stenosis of external ear canal secondary to inflammation and infection**
      DEF: Narrowing of the external ear canal; due to chronic inflammation or infection.
      H61.321 Acquired stenosis of right external ear canal secondary to inflammation and infection
      H61.322 Acquired stenosis of left external ear canal secondary to inflammation and infection
      H61.323 Acquired stenosis of external ear canal secondary to inflammation and infection, bilateral
      H61.329 Acquired stenosis of external ear canal secondary to inflammation and infection, unspecified ear ▽

    ✓6ᵗʰ **H61.39 Other acquired stenosis of external ear canal**
      H61.391 Other acquired stenosis of right external ear canal
      H61.392 Other acquired stenosis of left external ear canal
      H61.393 Other acquired stenosis of external ear canal, bilateral
      H61.399 Other acquired stenosis of external ear canal, unspecified ear ▽

  ✓5ᵗʰ **H61.8 Other specified disorders of external ear**

    ✓6ᵗʰ **H61.81 Exostosis of external canal**
      H61.811 Exostosis of right external canal
      H61.812 Exostosis of left external canal
      H61.813 Exostosis of external canal, bilateral
      H61.819 Exostosis of external canal, unspecified ear ▽

    ✓6ᵗʰ **H61.89 Other specified disorders of external ear**
      H61.891 Other specified disorders of right external ear
      H61.892 Other specified disorders of left external ear
      H61.893 Other specified disorders of external ear, bilateral
      H61.899 Other specified disorders of external ear, unspecified ear ▽

  ✓5ᵗʰ **H61.9 Disorder of external ear, unspecified**
    H61.90 Disorder of external ear, unspecified, unspecified ear ▽
    H61.91 Disorder of right external ear, unspecified ▽
    H61.92 Disorder of left external ear, unspecified ▽
    H61.93 Disorder of external ear, unspecified, bilateral ▽

✔ Additional Character Req   v x 7ᵗʰ Placeholder Alert   Manifestation   HCC CMS-HCC Condition   ▽ Unspecified Code   ▶◀ Revised Text   ● New Code   ▲ Revised Code Title

Chapter 8. Diseases of the Ear and Mastoid Process

☑4ᵗʰ **H62 Disorders of external ear in diseases classified elsewhere**

☑5ᵗʰ **H62.4 Otitis externa in other diseases classified elsewhere**

Code first underlying disease, such as:
 erysipelas (A46)
 impetigo (L01.0)

EXCLUDES 1 otitis externa (in):
 candidiasis (B37.84)
 herpes viral [herpes simplex] (B00.1)
 herpes zoster (B02.8)

H62.40 *Otitis externa in other diseases classified elsewhere, unspecified ear* ▽

H62.41 *Otitis externa in other diseases classified elsewhere, right ear*

H62.42 *Otitis externa in other diseases classified elsewhere, left ear*

H62.43 *Otitis externa in other diseases classified elsewhere, bilateral*

☑5ᵗʰ **H62.8 Other disorders of external ear in diseases classified elsewhere**

Code first underlying disease, such as:
 gout (M1A.-, M10.-)

☑6ᵗʰ **H62.8X Other disorders of external ear in diseases classified elsewhere**

H62.8X1 *Other disorders of right external ear in diseases classified elsewhere*

H62.8X2 *Other disorders of left external ear in diseases classified elsewhere*

H62.8X3 *Other disorders of external ear in diseases classified elsewhere, bilateral*

H62.8X9 *Other disorders of external ear in diseases classified elsewhere, unspecified ear* ▽

Diseases of middle ear and mastoid (H65-H75)

☑4ᵗʰ **H65 Nonsuppurative otitis media**

INCLUDES nonsuppurative otitis media with myringitis

Use additional code for any associated perforated tympanic membrane (H72.-)

Use additional code to identify:
 exposure to environmental tobacco smoke (Z77.22)
 exposure to tobacco smoke in the perinatal period (P96.81)
 history of tobacco dependence (Z87.891)
 occupational exposure to environmental tobacco smoke (Z57.31)
 tobacco dependence (F17.-)
 tobacco use (Z72.0)

☑5ᵗʰ **H65.0 Acute serous otitis media**

Acute and subacute secretory otitis

H65.00 Acute serous otitis media, unspecified ear ▽

H65.01 Acute serous otitis media, right ear

H65.02 Acute serous otitis media, left ear

H65.03 Acute serous otitis media, bilateral

H65.04 Acute serous otitis media, recurrent, right ear

H65.05 Acute serous otitis media, recurrent, left ear

H65.06 Acute serous otitis media, recurrent, bilateral

H65.07 Acute serous otitis media, recurrent, unspecified ear ▽

☑5ᵗʰ **H65.1 Other acute nonsuppurative otitis media**

EXCLUDES 1 otitic barotrauma (T70.0)
 otitis media (acute) NOS (H66.9)

☑6ᵗʰ **H65.11 Acute and subacute allergic otitis media (mucoid) (sanguinous) (serous)**

H65.111 Acute and subacute allergic otitis media (mucoid) (sanguinous) (serous), right ear

H65.112 Acute and subacute allergic otitis media (mucoid) (sanguinous) (serous), left ear

H65.113 Acute and subacute allergic otitis media (mucoid) (sanguinous) (serous), bilateral

H65.114 Acute and subacute allergic otitis media (mucoid) (sanguinous) (serous), recurrent, right ear

H65.115 Acute and subacute allergic otitis media (mucoid) (sanguinous) (serous), recurrent, left ear

H65.116 Acute and subacute allergic otitis media (mucoid) (sanguinous) (serous), recurrent, bilateral

H65.117 Acute and subacute allergic otitis media (mucoid) (sanguinous) (serous), recurrent, unspecified ear ▽

H65.119 Acute and subacute allergic otitis media (mucoid) (sanguinous) (serous), unspecified ear ▽

☑6ᵗʰ **H65.19 Other acute nonsuppurative otitis media**

Acute and subacute mucoid otitis media
Acute and subacute nonsuppurative otitis media NOS
Acute and subacute sanguinous otitis media
Acute and subacute seromucinous otitis media

H65.191 Other acute nonsuppurative otitis media, right ear

H65.192 Other acute nonsuppurative otitis media, left ear

H65.193 Other acute nonsuppurative otitis media, bilateral

H65.194 Other acute nonsuppurative otitis media, recurrent, right ear

H65.195 Other acute nonsuppurative otitis media, recurrent, left ear

H65.196 Other acute nonsuppurative otitis media, recurrent, bilateral

H65.197 Other acute nonsuppurative otitis media recurrent, unspecified ear ▽

H65.199 Other acute nonsuppurative otitis media, unspecified ear ▽

☑5ᵗʰ **H65.2 Chronic serous otitis media**

Chronic tubotympanal catarrh

H65.20 Chronic serous otitis media, unspecified ear ▽

H65.21 Chronic serous otitis media, right ear

H65.22 Chronic serous otitis media, left ear

H65.23 Chronic serous otitis media, bilateral

☑5ᵗʰ **H65.3 Chronic mucoid otitis media**

Chronic mucinous otitis media
Chronic secretory otitis media
Chronic transudative otitis media
Glue ear

EXCLUDES 1 adhesive middle ear disease (H74.1)

H65.30 Chronic mucoid otitis media, unspecified ear ▽

H65.31 Chronic mucoid otitis media, right ear

H65.32 Chronic mucoid otitis media, left ear

H65.33 Chronic mucoid otitis media, bilateral

☑5ᵗʰ **H65.4 Other chronic nonsuppurative otitis media**

☑6ᵗʰ **H65.41 Chronic allergic otitis media**

H65.411 Chronic allergic otitis media, right ear

H65.412 Chronic allergic otitis media, left ear

H65.413 Chronic allergic otitis media, bilateral

H65.419 Chronic allergic otitis media, unspecified ear ▽

☑6ᵗʰ **H65.49 Other chronic nonsuppurative otitis media**

Chronic exudative otitis media
Chronic nonsuppurative otitis media NOS
Chronic otitis media with effusion (nonpurulent)
Chronic seromucinous otitis media

H65.491 Other chronic nonsuppurative otitis media, right ear

H65.492 Other chronic nonsuppurative otitis media, left ear

H65.493 Other chronic nonsuppurative otitis media, bilateral

H65.499 Other chronic nonsuppurative otitis media, unspecified ear ▽

☑5ᵗʰ **H65.9 Unspecified nonsuppurative otitis media**

Allergic otitis media NOS
Catarrhal otitis media NOS
Exudative otitis media NOS
Mucoid otitis media NOS
Otitis media with effusion (nonpurulent) NOS

Secretory otitis media NOS
Seromucinous otitis media NOS
Serous otitis media NOS
Transudative otitis media NOS

H65.90 Unspecified nonsuppurative otitis media, unspecified ear ▽

H65.91 Unspecified nonsuppurative otitis media, right ear ▽

H65.92 Unspecified nonsuppurative otitis media, left ear ▽

H65.93 Unspecified nonsuppurative otitis media, bilateral ▽

EXCLUDES 1 Not coded here   EXCLUDES 2 Not included here   N Newborn Age: 0   P Pediatric Age: 0-17   M Maternity Age: 12-55   A Adult Age: 15-124

608   ICD-10-CM 2018

☑4ᵗʰ **H66 Suppurative and unspecified otitis media**

    INCLUDES   suppurative and unspecified otitis media with myringitis

    Use additional code to identify:
      exposure to environmental tobacco smoke (Z77.22)
      exposure to tobacco smoke in the perinatal period (P96.81)
      history of tobacco dependence (Z87.891)
      occupational exposure to environmental tobacco smoke (Z57.31)
      tobacco dependence (F17.-)
      tobacco use (Z72.0)
    AHA: 2016, 1Q, 34

☑5ᵗʰ **H66.0** Acute suppurative otitis media

    ☑6ᵗʰ **H66.00** **Acute suppurative otitis media** without spontaneous rupture of ear drum

      H66.001 **Acute suppurative otitis media without spontaneous rupture of ear drum, right ear**

      H66.002 **Acute suppurative otitis media without spontaneous rupture of ear drum, left ear**

      H66.003 **Acute suppurative otitis media without spontaneous rupture of ear drum, bilateral**

      H66.004 **Acute suppurative otitis media without spontaneous rupture of ear drum, recurrent, right ear**

      H66.005 **Acute suppurative otitis media without spontaneous rupture of ear drum, recurrent, left ear**

      H66.006 **Acute suppurative otitis media without spontaneous rupture of ear drum, recurrent, bilateral**

      H66.007 **Acute suppurative otitis media without spontaneous rupture of ear drum, recurrent, unspecified ear** ▽

      H66.009 **Acute suppurative otitis media without spontaneous rupture of ear drum, unspecified ear** ▽

    ☑6ᵗʰ **H66.01** **Acute suppurative otitis media** with spontaneous rupture of ear drum
      DEF: Sudden, severe inflammation of middle ear, with pressure causing the perforation of ear drum tissue.

      H66.011 **Acute suppurative otitis media with spontaneous rupture of ear drum, right ear**

      H66.012 **Acute suppurative otitis media with spontaneous rupture of ear drum, left ear**

      H66.013 **Acute suppurative otitis media with spontaneous rupture of ear drum, bilateral**

      H66.014 **Acute suppurative otitis media with spontaneous rupture of ear drum, recurrent, right ear**

      H66.015 **Acute suppurative otitis media with spontaneous rupture of ear drum, recurrent, left ear**

      H66.016 **Acute suppurative otitis media with spontaneous rupture of ear drum, recurrent, bilateral**

      H66.017 **Acute suppurative otitis media with spontaneous rupture of ear drum, recurrent, unspecified ear** ▽

      H66.019 **Acute suppurative otitis media with spontaneous rupture of ear drum, unspecified ear** ▽

☑5ᵗʰ **H66.1** Chronic tubotympanic suppurative otitis media
    Benign chronic suppurative otitis media
    Chronic tubotympanic disease
    Use additional code for any associated perforated tympanic membrane (H72.-)

    H66.10 **Chronic tubotympanic suppurative otitis media, unspecified** ▽

    H66.11 **Chronic tubotympanic suppurative otitis media, right ear**

    H66.12 **Chronic tubotympanic suppurative otitis media, left ear**

    H66.13 **Chronic tubotympanic suppurative otitis media, bilateral**

☑5ᵗʰ **H66.2** Chronic atticoantral suppurative otitis media
    Chronic atticoantral disease
    Use additional code for any associated perforated tympanic membrane (H72.-)

    H66.20 **Chronic atticoantral suppurative otitis media, unspecified ear** ▽

    H66.21 **Chronic atticoantral suppurative otitis media, right ear**

    H66.22 **Chronic atticoantral suppurative otitis media, left ear**

    H66.23 **Chronic atticoantral suppurative otitis media, bilateral**

☑5ᵗʰ **H66.3** Other chronic suppurative otitis media
    Chronic suppurative otitis media NOS
    Use additional code for any associated perforated tympanic membrane (H72.-)
    EXCLUDES 1   tuberculous otitis media (A18.6)

    ☑6ᵗʰ **H66.3X** **Other chronic suppurative otitis media**

      H66.3X1 **Other chronic suppurative otitis media, right ear**

      H66.3X2 **Other chronic suppurative otitis media, left ear**

      H66.3X3 **Other chronic suppurative otitis media, bilateral**

      H66.3X9 **Other chronic suppurative otitis media, unspecified ear** ▽

☑5ᵗʰ **H66.4** Suppurative otitis media, unspecified
    Purulent otitis media NOS
    Use additional code for any associated perforated tympanic membrane (H72.-)

    H66.40 **Suppurative otitis media, unspecified, unspecified ear** ▽

    H66.41 **Suppurative otitis media, unspecified, right ear**

    H66.42 **Suppurative otitis media, unspecified, left ear**

    H66.43 **Suppurative otitis media, unspecified, bilateral**

☑5ᵗʰ **H66.9** Otitis media, unspecified
    Otitis media NOS
    Acute otitis media NOS
    Chronic otitis media NOS
    Use additional code for any associated perforated tympanic membrane (H72.-)

    H66.90 **Otitis media, unspecified, unspecified ear** ▽

    H66.91 **Otitis media, unspecified, right ear** ▽

    H66.92 **Otitis media, unspecified, left ear** ▽

    H66.93 **Otitis media, unspecified, bilateral** ▽

☑4ᵗʰ **H67 Otitis media in diseases classified elsewhere**
    Code first underlying disease, such as:
      viral disease NEC (B00-B34)
    Use additional code for any associated perforated tympanic membrane (H72.-)
    EXCLUDES 1   otitis media in:
       influenza (J09.X9, J10.83, J11.83)
       measles (B05.3)
       scarlet fever (A38.0)
       tuberculosis (A18.6)

    H67.1 *Otitis media in diseases classified elsewhere, right ear*

    H67.2 *Otitis media in diseases classified elsewhere, left ear*

    H67.3 *Otitis media in diseases classified elsewhere, bilateral*

    H67.9 *Otitis media in diseases classified elsewhere, unspecified ear* ▽

☑4ᵗʰ **H68 Eustachian salpingitis and obstruction**

    ☑5ᵗʰ **H68.0** Eustachian salpingitis

      ☑6ᵗʰ **H68.00** **Unspecified Eustachian salpingitis**

        H68.001 **Unspecified Eustachian salpingitis, right ear** ▽

        H68.002 **Unspecified Eustachian salpingitis, left ear** ▽

        H68.003 **Unspecified Eustachian salpingitis, bilateral** ▽

        H68.009 **Unspecified Eustachian salpingitis, unspecified ear** ▽

      ☑6ᵗʰ **H68.01** Acute Eustachian salpingitis

        H68.011 **Acute Eustachian salpingitis, right ear**

        H68.012 **Acute Eustachian salpingitis, left ear**

        H68.013 **Acute Eustachian salpingitis, bilateral**

☑ Additional Character Req   ☑x7ᵗʰ Placeholder Alert   Manifestation   HCC CMS-HCC Condition   ▽ Unspecified Code   ►◄ Revised Text   ● New Code   ▲ Revised Code Title

H68.019   Acute Eustachian salpingitis, unspecified ear ▽

✓6th **H68.02** Chronic Eustachian salpingitis
    H68.021   Chronic Eustachian salpingitis, right ear
    H68.022   Chronic Eustachian salpingitis, left ear
    H68.023   Chronic Eustachian salpingitis, bilateral
    H68.029   Chronic Eustachian salpingitis, unspecified ear ▽

✓5th **H68.1** Obstruction of Eustachian tube
    Stenosis of Eustachian tube   Stricture of Eustachian tube
   ✓6th **H68.10** Unspecified obstruction of Eustachian tube
      H68.101   Unspecified obstruction of Eustachian tube, right ear ▽
      H68.102   Unspecified obstruction of Eustachian tube, left ear ▽
      H68.103   Unspecified obstruction of Eustachian tube, bilateral ▽
      H68.109   Unspecified obstruction of Eustachian tube, unspecified ear ▽
   ✓6th **H68.11** Osseous obstruction of Eustachian tube
      H68.111   Osseous obstruction of Eustachian tube, right ear
      H68.112   Osseous obstruction of Eustachian tube, left ear
      H68.113   Osseous obstruction of Eustachian tube, bilateral
      H68.119   Osseous obstruction of Eustachian tube, unspecified ear ▽
   ✓6th **H68.12** Intrinsic cartilagenous obstruction of Eustachian tube
      H68.121   Intrinsic cartilagenous obstruction of Eustachian tube, right ear
      H68.122   Intrinsic cartilagenous obstruction of Eustachian tube, left ear
      H68.123   Intrinsic cartilagenous obstruction of Eustachian tube, bilateral
      H68.129   Intrinsic cartilagenous obstruction of Eustachian tube, unspecified ear ▽
   ✓6th **H68.13** Extrinsic cartilagenous obstruction of Eustachian tube
      Compression of Eustachian tube
      H68.131   Extrinsic cartilagenous obstruction of Eustachian tube, right ear
      H68.132   Extrinsic cartilagenous obstruction of Eustachian tube, left ear
      H68.133   Extrinsic cartilagenous obstruction of Eustachian tube, bilateral
      H68.139   Extrinsic cartilagenous obstruction of Eustachian tube, unspecified ear ▽

✓4th **H69** Other and unspecified disorders of Eustachian tube
   ✓5th **H69.0** Patulous Eustachian tube
      H69.00   Patulous Eustachian tube, unspecified ear ▽
      H69.01   Patulous Eustachian tube, right ear
      H69.02   Patulous Eustachian tube, left ear
      H69.03   Patulous Eustachian tube, bilateral
   ✓5th **H69.8** Other specified disorders of Eustachian tube
      H69.80   Other specified disorders of Eustachian tube, unspecified ear ▽
      H69.81   Other specified disorders of Eustachian tube, right ear
      H69.82   Other specified disorders of Eustachian tube, left ear
      H69.83   Other specified disorders of Eustachian tube, bilateral
   ✓5th **H69.9** Unspecified Eustachian tube disorder
      H69.90   Unspecified Eustachian tube disorder, unspecified ear ▽
      H69.91   Unspecified Eustachian tube disorder, right ear ▽
      H69.92   Unspecified Eustachian tube disorder, left ear ▽
      H69.93   Unspecified Eustachian tube disorder, bilateral ▽

✓4th **H70** Mastoiditis and related conditions
   ✓5th **H70.0** Acute mastoiditis
      Abscess of mastoid
      Empyema of mastoid
   ✓6th **H70.00** Acute mastoiditis without complications
      H70.001   Acute mastoiditis without complications, right ear
      H70.002   Acute mastoiditis without complications, left ear
      H70.003   Acute mastoiditis without complications, bilateral
      H70.009   Acute mastoiditis without complications, unspecified ear ▽
   ✓6th **H70.01** Subperiosteal abscess of mastoid
      H70.011   Subperiosteal abscess of mastoid, right ear
      H70.012   Subperiosteal abscess of mastoid, left ear
      H70.013   Subperiosteal abscess of mastoid, bilateral
      H70.019   Subperiosteal abscess of mastoid, unspecified ear ▽
   ✓6th **H70.09** Acute mastoiditis with other complications
      H70.091   Acute mastoiditis with other complications, right ear
      H70.092   Acute mastoiditis with other complications, left ear
      H70.093   Acute mastoiditis with other complications, bilateral
      H70.099   Acute mastoiditis with other complications, unspecified ear ▽
   ✓5th **H70.1** Chronic mastoiditis
      Caries of mastoid
      Fistula of mastoid
      EXCLUDES 1   *tuberculous mastoiditis (A18.03)*
      H70.10   Chronic mastoiditis, unspecified ear ▽
      H70.11   Chronic mastoiditis, right ear
      H70.12   Chronic mastoiditis, left ear
      H70.13   Chronic mastoiditis, bilateral
   ✓5th **H70.2** Petrositis
      Inflammation of petrous bone
   ✓6th **H70.20** Unspecified petrositis
      H70.201   Unspecified petrositis, right ear ▽
      H70.202   Unspecified petrositis, left ear ▽
      H70.203   Unspecified petrositis, bilateral ▽
      H70.209   Unspecified petrositis, unspecified ear ▽
   ✓6th **H70.21** Acute petrositis
      DEF: Sudden, severe inflammation of petrous temporal bone behind the ear; associated with middle ear infection.
      H70.211   Acute petrositis, right ear
      H70.212   Acute petrositis, left ear
      H70.213   Acute petrositis, bilateral
      H70.219   Acute petrositis, unspecified ear ▽
   ✓6th **H70.22** Chronic petrositis
      H70.221   Chronic petrositis, right ear
      H70.222   Chronic petrositis, left ear
      H70.223   Chronic petrositis, bilateral
      H70.229   Chronic petrositis, unspecified ear ▽
   ✓5th **H70.8** Other mastoiditis and related conditions
      EXCLUDES 1   *preauricular sinus and cyst (Q18.1)*
               sinus, fistula, and cyst of branchial cleft (Q18.0)
   ✓6th **H70.81** Postauricular fistula
      H70.811   Postauricular fistula, right ear
      H70.812   Postauricular fistula, left ear
      H70.813   Postauricular fistula, bilateral
      H70.819   Postauricular fistula, unspecified ear ▽
   ✓6th **H70.89** Other mastoiditis and related conditions
      H70.891   Other mastoiditis and related conditions, right ear
      H70.892   Other mastoiditis and related conditions, left ear
      H70.893   Other mastoiditis and related conditions, bilateral
      H70.899   Other mastoiditis and related conditions, unspecified ear ▽

EXCLUDES 1 Not coded here   **EXCLUDES 2** Not included here   N Newborn Age: 0   P Pediatric Age: 0-17   M Maternity Age: 12-55   A Adult Age: 15-124

610   ICD-10-CM 2018

Cholesteatoma of Middle Ear

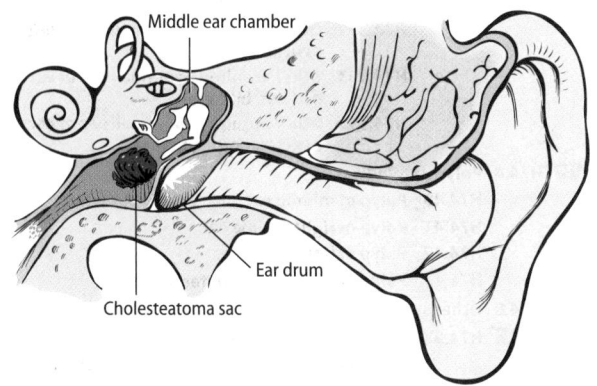

- Middle ear chamber
- Ear drum
- Cholesteatoma sac

✓5th H70.9 Unspecified mastoiditis
- H70.90 Unspecified mastoiditis, unspecified ear ▽
- H70.91 Unspecified mastoiditis, right ear ▽
- H70.92 Unspecified mastoiditis, left ear ▽
- H70.93 Unspecified mastoiditis, bilateral ▽

✓4th H71 Cholesteatoma of middle ear
> EXCLUDES 2   cholesteatoma of external ear (H60.4-)
> recurrent cholesteatoma of postmastoidectomy cavity (H95.0-)

✓5th H71.0 Cholesteatoma of attic
- H71.00 Cholesteatoma of attic, unspecified ear ▽
- H71.01 Cholesteatoma of attic, right ear
- H71.02 Cholesteatoma of attic, left ear
- H71.03 Cholesteatoma of attic, bilateral

✓5th H71.1 Cholesteatoma of tympanum
- H71.10 Cholesteatoma of tympanum, unspecified ear ▽
- H71.11 Cholesteatoma of tympanum, right ear
- H71.12 Cholesteatoma of tympanum, left ear
- H71.13 Cholesteatoma of tympanum, bilateral

✓5th H71.2 Cholesteatoma of mastoid
- H71.20 Cholesteatoma of mastoid, unspecified ear ▽
- H71.21 Cholesteatoma of mastoid, right ear
- H71.22 Cholesteatoma of mastoid, left ear
- H71.23 Cholesteatoma of mastoid, bilateral

✓5th H71.3 Diffuse cholesteatosis
- H71.30 Diffuse cholesteatosis, unspecified ear ▽
- H71.31 Diffuse cholesteatosis, right ear
- H71.32 Diffuse cholesteatosis, left ear
- H71.33 Diffuse cholesteatosis, bilateral

✓5th H71.9 Unspecified cholesteatoma
- H71.90 Unspecified cholesteatoma, unspecified ear ▽
- H71.91 Unspecified cholesteatoma, right ear ▽
- H71.92 Unspecified cholesteatoma, left ear ▽
- H71.93 Unspecified cholesteatoma, bilateral ▽

✓4th H72 Perforation of tympanic membrane
> INCLUDES   persistent post-traumatic perforation of ear drum
> postinflammatory perforation of ear drum
>
> Code first any associated otitis media (H65.-, H66.1-, H66.2-, H66.3-, H66.4-, H66.9-, H67.-)
>
> EXCLUDES 1   acute suppurative otitis media with rupture of the tympanic membrane (H66.01-)
> traumatic rupture of ear drum (S09.2-)

✓5th H72.0 Central perforation of tympanic membrane
- H72.00 Central perforation of tympanic membrane, unspecified ear ▽
- H72.01 Central perforation of tympanic membrane, right ear
- H72.02 Central perforation of tympanic membrane, left ear
- H72.03 Central perforation of tympanic membrane, bilateral

✓5th H72.1 Attic perforation of tympanic membrane
> Perforation of pars flaccida
- H72.10 Attic perforation of tympanic membrane, unspecified ear ▽

- H72.11 Attic perforation of tympanic membrane, right ear
- H72.12 Attic perforation of tympanic membrane, left ear
- H72.13 Attic perforation of tympanic membrane, bilateral

✓5th H72.2 Other marginal perforations of tympanic membrane
- **✓6th H72.2X Other marginal perforations of tympanic membrane**
  - H72.2X1 Other marginal perforations of tympanic membrane, right ear
  - H72.2X2 Other marginal perforations of tympanic membrane, left ear
  - H72.2X3 Other marginal perforations of tympanic membrane, bilateral
  - H72.2X9 Other marginal perforations of tympanic membrane, unspecified ear ▽

✓5th H72.8 Other perforations of tympanic membrane
- **✓6th H72.81 Multiple perforations of tympanic membrane**
  - H72.811 Multiple perforations of tympanic membrane, right ear
  - H72.812 Multiple perforations of tympanic membrane, left ear
  - H72.813 Multiple perforations of tympanic membrane, bilateral
  - H72.819 Multiple perforations of tympanic membrane, unspecified ear ▽
- **✓6th H72.82 Total perforations of tympanic membrane**
  - H72.821 Total perforations of tympanic membrane, right ear
  - H72.822 Total perforations of tympanic membrane, left ear
  - H72.823 Total perforations of tympanic membrane, bilateral
  - H72.829 Total perforations of tympanic membrane, unspecified ear ▽

✓5th H72.9 Unspecified perforation of tympanic membrane
- H72.90 Unspecified perforation of tympanic membrane, unspecified ear ▽
- H72.91 Unspecified perforation of tympanic membrane, right ear ▽
- H72.92 Unspecified perforation of tympanic membrane, left ear ▽
- H72.93 Unspecified perforation of tympanic membrane, bilateral ▽

✓4th H73 Other disorders of tympanic membrane
✓5th H73.0 Acute myringitis
> EXCLUDES 1   acute myringitis with otitis media (H65, H66)
- **✓6th H73.00 Unspecified acute myringitis**
  > Acute tympanitis NOS
  - H73.001 Acute myringitis, right ear
  - H73.002 Acute myringitis, left ear
  - H73.003 Acute myringitis, bilateral
  - H73.009 Acute myringitis, unspecified ear ▽
- **✓6th H73.01 Bullous myringitis**
  > DEF: Bacterial or viral otitis media; characterized by the appearance of serous or hemorrhagic blebs on the ear drum and sudden onset of severe pain in ear.
  - H73.011 Bullous myringitis, right ear
  - H73.012 Bullous myringitis, left ear
  - H73.013 Bullous myringitis, bilateral
  - H73.019 Bullous myringitis, unspecified ear ▽
- **✓6th H73.09 Other acute myringitis**
  - H73.091 Other acute myringitis, right ear
  - H73.092 Other acute myringitis, left ear
  - H73.093 Other acute myringitis, bilateral
  - H73.099 Other acute myringitis, unspecified ear ▽

✓5th H73.1 Chronic myringitis
> Chronic tympanitis
> EXCLUDES 1   chronic myringitis with otitis media (H65, H66)
- H73.10 Chronic myringitis, unspecified ear ▽
- H73.11 Chronic myringitis, right ear
- H73.12 Chronic myringitis, left ear
- H73.13 Chronic myringitis, bilateral

✓5th H73.2 Unspecified myringitis
- H73.20 Unspecified myringitis, unspecified ear ▽
- H73.21 Unspecified myringitis, right ear ▽
- H73.22 Unspecified myringitis, left ear ▽

☑ Additional Character Req   ✓x7th Placeholder Alert   Manifestation   HCC CMS-HCC Condition   ▽ Unspecified Code   ►◄ Revised Text   ● New Code   ▲ Revised Code Title

H73.23 Unspecified myringitis, bilateral ▽

✓5ᵗʰ H73.8 Other specified disorders of tympanic membrane

✓6ᵗʰ H73.81 Atrophic flaccid tympanic membrane
- H73.811 Atrophic flaccid tympanic membrane, right ear
- H73.812 Atrophic flaccid tympanic membrane, left ear
- H73.813 Atrophic flaccid tympanic membrane, bilateral
- H73.819 Atrophic flaccid tympanic membrane, unspecified ear ▽

✓6ᵗʰ H73.82 Atrophic nonflaccid tympanic membrane
- H73.821 Atrophic nonflaccid tympanic membrane, right ear
- H73.822 Atrophic nonflaccid tympanic membrane, left ear
- H73.823 Atrophic nonflaccid tympanic membrane, bilateral
- H73.829 Atrophic nonflaccid tympanic membrane, unspecified ear ▽

✓6ᵗʰ H73.89 Other specified disorders of tympanic membrane
- H73.891 Other specified disorders of tympanic membrane, right ear
- H73.892 Other specified disorders of tympanic membrane, left ear
- H73.893 Other specified disorders of tympanic membrane, bilateral
- H73.899 Other specified disorders of tympanic membrane, unspecified ear ▽

✓5ᵗʰ H73.9 Unspecified disorder of tympanic membrane
- H73.90 Unspecified disorder of tympanic membrane, unspecified ear ▽
- H73.91 Unspecified disorder of tympanic membrane, right ear ▽
- H73.92 Unspecified disorder of tympanic membrane, left ear ▽
- H73.93 Unspecified disorder of tympanic membrane, bilateral ▽

✓4ᵗʰ H74 Other disorders of middle ear mastoid
EXCLUDES 2 mastoiditis (H70.-)

✓5ᵗʰ H74.0 Tympanosclerosis
DEF: Calcification of tissue in the ear drum, middle ear bones, and middle ear canal.
- H74.01 Tympanosclerosis, right ear
- H74.02 Tympanosclerosis, left ear
- H74.03 Tympanosclerosis, bilateral
- H74.09 Tympanosclerosis, unspecified ear ▽

✓5ᵗʰ H74.1 Adhesive middle ear disease
Adhesive otitis
EXCLUDES 1 glue ear (H65.3-)
- H74.11 Adhesive right middle ear disease
- H74.12 Adhesive left middle ear disease
- H74.13 Adhesive middle ear disease, bilateral
- H74.19 Adhesive middle ear disease, unspecified ear ▽

✓5ᵗʰ H74.2 Discontinuity and dislocation of ear ossicles
- H74.20 Discontinuity and dislocation of ear ossicles, unspecified ear ▽
- H74.21 Discontinuity and dislocation of right ear ossicles
- H74.22 Discontinuity and dislocation of left ear ossicles
- H74.23 Discontinuity and dislocation of ear ossicles, bilateral

✓5ᵗʰ H74.3 Other acquired abnormalities of ear ossicles

✓6ᵗʰ H74.31 Ankylosis of ear ossicles
- H74.311 Ankylosis of ear ossicles, right ear
- H74.312 Ankylosis of ear ossicles, left ear
- H74.313 Ankylosis of ear ossicles, bilateral
- H74.319 Ankylosis of ear ossicles, unspecified ear ▽

✓6ᵗʰ H74.32 Partial loss of ear ossicles
- H74.321 Partial loss of ear ossicles, right ear
- H74.322 Partial loss of ear ossicles, left ear
- H74.323 Partial loss of ear ossicles, bilateral
- H74.329 Partial loss of ear ossicles, unspecified ear ▽

✓6ᵗʰ H74.39 Other acquired abnormalities of ear ossicles
- H74.391 Other acquired abnormalities of right ear ossicles
- H74.392 Other acquired abnormalities of left ear ossicles
- H74.393 Other acquired abnormalities of ear ossicles, bilateral
- H74.399 Other acquired abnormalities of ear ossicles, unspecified ear ▽

✓5ᵗʰ H74.4 Polyp of middle ear
- H74.40 Polyp of middle ear, unspecified ear ▽
- H74.41 Polyp of right middle ear
- H74.42 Polyp of left middle ear
- H74.43 Polyp of middle ear, bilateral

✓5ᵗʰ H74.8 Other specified disorders of middle ear and mastoid

✓6ᵗʰ H74.8X Other specified disorders of middle ear and mastoid
- H74.8X1 Other specified disorders of right middle ear and mastoid
- H74.8X2 Other specified disorders of left middle ear and mastoid
- H74.8X3 Other specified disorders of middle ear and mastoid, bilateral
- H74.8X9 Other specified disorders of middle ear and mastoid, unspecified ear ▽

✓5ᵗʰ H74.9 Unspecified disorder of middle ear and mastoid
- H74.90 Unspecified disorder of middle ear and mastoid, unspecified ear ▽
- H74.91 Unspecified disorder of right middle ear and mastoid ▽
- H74.92 Unspecified disorder of left middle ear and mastoid ▽
- H74.93 Unspecified disorder of middle ear and mastoid, bilateral ▽

✓4ᵗʰ H75 Other disorders of middle ear and mastoid in diseases classified elsewhere
Code first underlying disease

✓5ᵗʰ H75.0 Mastoiditis in infectious and parasitic diseases classified elsewhere
EXCLUDES 1 mastoiditis (in):
syphilis (A52.77)
tuberculosis (A18.03)
- H75.00 Mastoiditis in infectious and parasitic diseases classified elsewhere, unspecified ear ▽
- H75.01 Mastoiditis in infectious and parasitic diseases classified elsewhere, right ear
- H75.02 Mastoiditis in infectious and parasitic diseases classified elsewhere, left ear
- H75.03 Mastoiditis in infectious and parasitic diseases classified elsewhere, bilateral

✓5ᵗʰ H75.8 Other specified disorders of middle ear and mastoid in diseases classified elsewhere
- H75.80 Other specified disorders of middle ear and mastoid in diseases classified elsewhere, unspecified ear ▽
- H75.81 Other specified disorders of right middle ear and mastoid in diseases classified elsewhere
- H75.82 Other specified disorders of left middle ear and mastoid in diseases classified elsewhere
- H75.83 Other specified disorders of middle ear and mastoid in diseases classified elsewhere, bilateral

Diseases of inner ear (H80-H83)

✓4ᵗʰ H80 Otosclerosis
INCLUDES otospongiosis

✓5ᵗʰ H80.0 Otosclerosis involving oval window, nonobliterative
- H80.00 Otosclerosis involving oval window, nonobliterative, unspecified ear ▽
- H80.01 Otosclerosis involving oval window, nonobliterative, right ear
- H80.02 Otosclerosis involving oval window, nonobliterative, left ear
- H80.03 Otosclerosis involving oval window, nonobliterative, bilateral

✓5th **H80.1** **Otosclerosis involving oval window, obliterative**

    H80.10 **Otosclerosis involving oval window, obliterative, unspecified ear** ▽

    H80.11 **Otosclerosis involving oval window, obliterative, right ear**

    H80.12 **Otosclerosis involving oval window, obliterative, left ear**

    H80.13 **Otosclerosis involving oval window, obliterative, bilateral**

✓5th **H80.2** **Cochlear otosclerosis**
Otosclerosis involving otic capsule
Otosclerosis involving round window

    H80.20 **Cochlear otosclerosis, unspecified ear** ▽

    H80.21 **Cochlear otosclerosis, right ear**

    H80.22 **Cochlear otosclerosis, left ear**

    H80.23 **Cochlear otosclerosis, bilateral**

✓5th **H80.8** **Other otosclerosis**

    H80.80 **Other otosclerosis, unspecified ear** ▽

    H80.81 **Other otosclerosis, right ear**

    H80.82 **Other otosclerosis, left ear**

    H80.83 **Other otosclerosis, bilateral**

✓5th **H80.9** **Unspecified otosclerosis**

    H80.90 **Unspecified otosclerosis, unspecified ear** ▽

    H80.91 **Unspecified otosclerosis, right ear** ▽

    H80.92 **Unspecified otosclerosis, left ear** ▽

    H80.93 **Unspecified otosclerosis, bilateral** ▽

✓4th **H81** **Disorders of vestibular function**
     EXCLUDES 1   epidemic vertigo (A88.1)
              vertigo NOS (R42)

✓5th **H81.0** **Ménière's disease**
Labyrinthine hydrops
Ménière's syndrome or vertigo

    H81.01 **Ménière's disease, right ear**

    H81.02 **Ménière's disease, left ear**

    H81.03 **Ménière's disease, bilateral**

    H81.09 **Ménière's disease, unspecified ear** ▽

✓5th **H81.1** **Benign paroxysmal vertigo**

    H81.10 **Benign paroxysmal vertigo, unspecified ear** ▽

    H81.11 **Benign paroxysmal vertigo, right ear**

    H81.12 **Benign paroxysmal vertigo, left ear**

    H81.13 **Benign paroxysmal vertigo, bilateral**

✓5th **H81.2** **Vestibular neuronitis**
DEF: Transient benign vertigo, caused by inflammation of the vestibular nerve; characterized by response to caloric stimulation on one side, nystagmus with rhythmic movement of eyes; normal auditory function present.

    H81.20 **Vestibular neuronitis, unspecified ear** ▽

    H81.21 **Vestibular neuronitis, right ear**

    H81.22 **Vestibular neuronitis, left ear**

    H81.23 **Vestibular neuronitis, bilateral**

✓5th **H81.3** **Other peripheral vertigo**

    ✓6th **H81.31** **Aural vertigo**

        H81.311 **Aural vertigo, right ear**

        H81.312 **Aural vertigo, left ear**

        H81.313 **Aural vertigo, bilateral**

        H81.319 **Aural vertigo, unspecified ear** ▽

    ✓6th **H81.39** **Other peripheral vertigo**
             Lermoyez' syndrome
             Otogenic vertigo
             Peripheral vertigo NOS

        H81.391 **Other peripheral vertigo, right ear**

        H81.392 **Other peripheral vertigo, left ear**

        H81.393 **Other peripheral vertigo, bilateral**

        H81.399 **Other peripheral vertigo, unspecified ear** ▽

✓5th **H81.4** **Vertigo of central origin**
Central positional nystagmus

    H81.41 **Vertigo of central origin, right ear**

    H81.42 **Vertigo of central origin, left ear**

    H81.43 **Vertigo of central origin, bilateral**

    H81.49 **Vertigo of central origin, unspecified ear** ▽

✓5th **H81.8** **Other disorders of vestibular function**

    ✓6th **H81.8X** **Other disorders of vestibular function**

        H81.8X1 **Other disorders of vestibular function, right ear**

        H81.8X2 **Other disorders of vestibular function, left ear**

        H81.8X3 **Other disorders of vestibular function, bilateral**

        H81.8X9 **Other disorders of vestibular function, unspecified ear** ▽

✓5th **H81.9** **Unspecified disorder of vestibular function**
Vertiginous syndrome NOS

    H81.90 **Unspecified disorder of vestibular function, unspecified ear** ▽

    H81.91 **Unspecified disorder of vestibular function, right ear** ▽

    H81.92 **Unspecified disorder of vestibular function, left ear** ▽

    H81.93 **Unspecified disorder of vestibular function, bilateral** ▽

✓4th **H82** **Vertiginous syndromes in diseases classified elsewhere**
Code first underlying disease
     EXCLUDES 1   epidemic vertigo (A88.1)

    H82.1 *Vertiginous syndromes in diseases classified elsewhere, right ear*

    H82.2 *Vertiginous syndromes in diseases classified elsewhere, left ear*

    H82.3 *Vertiginous syndromes in diseases classified elsewhere, bilateral*

    H82.9 *Vertiginous syndromes in diseases classified elsewhere, unspecified ear* ▽

✓4th **H83** **Other diseases of inner ear**

✓5th **H83.0** **Labyrinthitis**
DEF: Inflammation of the inner ear, or labyrinth; characterized by pus, vertigo, dizziness, nausea, and hearing loss.

    H83.01 **Labyrinthitis, right ear**

    H83.02 **Labyrinthitis, left ear**

    H83.03 **Labyrinthitis, bilateral**

    H83.09 **Labyrinthitis, unspecified ear** ▽

✓5th **H83.1** **Labyrinthine fistula**

    H83.11 **Labyrinthine fistula, right ear**

    H83.12 **Labyrinthine fistula, left ear**

    H83.13 **Labyrinthine fistula, bilateral**

    H83.19 **Labyrinthine fistula, unspecified ear** ▽

✓5th **H83.2** **Labyrinthine dysfunction**
Labyrinthine hypersensitivity
Labyrinthine hypofunction
Labyrinthine loss of function
DEF: Decreased function of the labyrinth sensors.

    ✓6th **H83.2X** **Labyrinthine dysfunction**

        H83.2X1 **Labyrinthine dysfunction, right ear**

        H83.2X2 **Labyrinthine dysfunction, left ear**

        H83.2X3 **Labyrinthine dysfunction, bilateral**

        H83.2X9 **Labyrinthine dysfunction, unspecified ear** ▽

✓5th **H83.3** **Noise effects on inner ear**
Acoustic trauma of inner ear
Noise-induced hearing loss of inner ear

    ✓6th **H83.3X** **Noise effects on inner ear**

        H83.3X1 **Noise effects on right inner ear**

        H83.3X2 **Noise effects on left inner ear**

        H83.3X3 **Noise effects on inner ear, bilateral**

        H83.3X9 **Noise effects on inner ear, unspecified ear** ▽

✓5th **H83.8** **Other specified diseases of inner ear**

    ✓6th **H83.8X** **Other specified diseases of inner ear**

        H83.8X1 **Other specified diseases of right inner ear**

        H83.8X2 **Other specified diseases of left inner ear**

        H83.8X3 **Other specified diseases of inner ear, bilateral**

        H83.8X9 **Other specified diseases of inner ear, unspecified ear** ▽

✓ Additional Character Req   ✓x7th Placeholder Alert   Manifestation   HCC CMS-HCC Condition   ▽ Unspecified Code   ►◄ Revised Text   ● New Code   ▲ Revised Code Title

ICD-10-CM 2018   613

Chapter 8. Diseases of the Ear and Mastoid Process *(left margin)*

✓5ᵗʰ **H83.9　Unspecified disease of inner ear**
　　H83.9Ø　Unspecified disease of inner ear, unspecified ear ▽
　　H83.91　Unspecified disease of right inner ear ▽
　　H83.92　Unspecified disease of left inner ear ▽
　　H83.93　Unspecified disease of inner ear, bilateral ▽

Other disorders of ear (H9Ø-H94)

✓4ᵗʰ **H9Ø　Conductive and sensorineural hearing loss**
　　EXCLUDES 1　*deaf nonspeaking NEC (H91.3)*
　　　　　　deafness NOS (H91.9-)
　　　　　　hearing loss NOS (H91.9-)
　　　　　　noise-induced hearing loss (H83.3-)
　　　　　　ototoxic hearing loss (H91.Ø-)
　　　　　　sudden (idiopathic) hearing loss (H91.2-)
　　AHA: 2015, 2Q, 7
　　H9Ø.Ø　Conductive hearing loss, bilateral
✓5ᵗʰ **H9Ø.1　Conductive hearing loss, unilateral with unrestricted hearing on the contralateral side**
　　H9Ø.11　Conductive hearing loss, unilateral, right ear, with unrestricted hearing on the contralateral side
　　H9Ø.12　Conductive hearing loss, unilateral, left ear, with unrestricted hearing on the contralateral side
　　H9Ø.2　Conductive hearing loss, unspecified ▽
　　　　Conductive deafness NOS
　　H9Ø.3　Sensorineural hearing loss, bilateral
✓5ᵗʰ **H9Ø.4　Sensorineural hearing loss, unilateral with unrestricted hearing on the contralateral side**
　　H9Ø.41　Sensorineural hearing loss, unilateral, right ear, with unrestricted hearing on the contralateral side
　　H9Ø.42　Sensorineural hearing loss, unilateral, left ear, with unrestricted hearing on the contralateral side
　　H9Ø.5　Unspecified sensorineural hearing loss ▽
　　　　Central hearing loss NOS
　　　　Congenital deafness NOS
　　　　Neural hearing loss NOS
　　　　Perceptive hearing loss NOS
　　　　Sensorineural deafness NOS
　　　　Sensory hearing loss NOS
　　　　EXCLUDES 1　*abnormal auditory perception (H93.2-)*
　　　　　　　psychogenic deafness (F44.6)
　　H9Ø.6　Mixed conductive and sensorineural hearing loss, bilateral
　　　　AHA: 2015, 2Q, 7
✓5ᵗʰ **H9Ø.7　Mixed conductive and sensorineural hearing loss, unilateral with unrestricted hearing on the contralateral side**
　　H9Ø.71　Mixed conductive and sensorineural hearing loss, unilateral, right ear, with unrestricted hearing on the contralateral side
　　H9Ø.72　Mixed conductive and sensorineural hearing loss, unilateral, left ear, with unrestricted hearing on the contralateral side
　　H9Ø.8　Mixed conductive and sensorineural hearing loss, unspecified ▽
✓5ᵗʰ **H9Ø.A　Conductive and sensorineural hearing loss with restricted hearing on the contralateral side**
　　✓6ᵗʰ **H9Ø.A1　Conductive hearing loss, unilateral, with restricted hearing on the contralateral side**
　　　　H9Ø.A11　Conductive hearing loss, unilateral, right ear with restricted hearing on the contralateral side
　　　　H9Ø.A12　Conductive hearing loss, unilateral, left ear with restricted hearing on the contralateral side
　　✓6ᵗʰ **H9Ø.A2　Sensorineural hearing loss, unilateral, with restricted hearing on the contralateral side**
　　　　H9Ø.A21　Sensorineural hearing loss, unilateral, right ear, with restricted hearing on the contralateral side
　　　　H9Ø.A22　Sensorineural hearing loss, unilateral, left ear, with restricted hearing on the contralateral side
　　✓6ᵗʰ **H9Ø.A3　Mixed conductive and sensorineural hearing loss, unilateral with restricted hearing on the contralateral side**
　　　　H9Ø.A31　Mixed conductive and sensorineural hearing loss, unilateral, right ear with restricted hearing on the contralateral side

H9Ø.A32　Mixed conductive and sensorineural hearing loss, unilateral, left ear with restricted hearing on the contralateral side

✓4ᵗʰ **H91　Other and unspecified hearing loss**
　　EXCLUDES 1　*abnormal auditory perception (H93.2-)*
　　　　　　hearing loss as classified in H9Ø-
　　　　　　impacted cerumen (H61.2-)
　　　　　　noise-induced hearing loss (H83.3-)
　　　　　　psychogenic deafness (F44.6)
　　　　　　transient ischemic deafness (H93.Ø1-)
✓5ᵗʰ **H91.Ø　Ototoxic hearing loss**
　　　　Code first poisoning due to drug or toxin, if applicable (T36-T65 with fifth or sixth character 1-4 or 6)
　　　　Use additional code for adverse effect, if applicable, to identify drug (T36-T5Ø with fifth or sixth character 5)
　　H91.Ø1　Ototoxic hearing loss, right ear
　　H91.Ø2　Ototoxic hearing loss, left ear
　　H91.Ø3　Ototoxic hearing loss, bilateral
　　H91.Ø9　Ototoxic hearing loss, unspecified ear ▽
✓5ᵗʰ **H91.1　Presbycusis**
　　　　Presbyacusia
　　H91.1Ø　Presbycusis, unspecified ear ▽
　　H91.11　Presbycusis, right ear
　　H91.12　Presbycusis, left ear
　　H91.13　Presbycusis, bilateral
✓5ᵗʰ **H91.2　Sudden idiopathic hearing loss**
　　　　Sudden hearing loss NOS
　　H91.2Ø　Sudden idiopathic hearing loss, unspecified ear ▽
　　H91.21　Sudden idiopathic hearing loss, right ear
　　H91.22　Sudden idiopathic hearing loss, left ear
　　H91.23　Sudden idiopathic hearing loss, bilateral
　　H91.3　Deaf nonspeaking, not elsewhere classified
✓5ᵗʰ **H91.8　Other specified hearing loss**
　　✓6ᵗʰ **H91.8X　Other specified hearing loss**
　　　　H91.8X1　Other specified hearing loss, right ear
　　　　H91.8X2　Other specified hearing loss, left ear
　　　　H91.8X3　Other specified hearing loss, bilateral
　　　　H91.8X9　Other specified hearing loss, unspecified ear ▽
✓5ᵗʰ **H91.9　Unspecified hearing loss**
　　　　Deafness NOS
　　　　High frequency deafness
　　　　Low frequency deafness
　　H91.9Ø　Unspecified hearing loss, unspecified ear ▽
　　H91.91　Unspecified hearing loss, right ear ▽
　　H91.92　Unspecified hearing loss, left ear ▽
　　H91.93　Unspecified hearing loss, bilateral ▽

✓4ᵗʰ **H92　Otalgia and effusion of ear**
✓5ᵗʰ **H92.Ø　Otalgia**
　　H92.Ø1　Otalgia, right ear
　　H92.Ø2　Otalgia, left ear
　　H92.Ø3　Otalgia, bilateral
　　H92.Ø9　Otalgia, unspecified ear ▽
✓5ᵗʰ **H92.1　Otorrhea**
　　EXCLUDES 1　*leakage of cerebrospinal fluid through ear (G96.Ø)*
　　H92.1Ø　Otorrhea, unspecified ear ▽
　　H92.11　Otorrhea, right ear
　　H92.12　Otorrhea, left ear
　　H92.13　Otorrhea, bilateral
✓5ᵗʰ **H92.2　Otorrhagia**
　　EXCLUDES 1　*traumatic otorrhagia—code to injury*
　　H92.2Ø　Otorrhagia, unspecified ear ▽
　　H92.21　Otorrhagia, right ear
　　H92.22　Otorrhagia, left ear
　　H92.23　Otorrhagia, bilateral

✓4ᵗʰ **H93　Other disorders of ear, not elsewhere classified**
✓5ᵗʰ **H93.Ø　Degenerative and vascular disorders of ear**
　　EXCLUDES 1　*presbycusis (H91.1)*
　　✓6ᵗʰ **H93.Ø1　Transient ischemic deafness**
　　　　H93.Ø11　Transient ischemic deafness, right ear
　　　　H93.Ø12　Transient ischemic deafness, left ear

EXCLUDES 1 Not coded here　　　EXCLUDES 2 Not included here　　　N Newborn Age: 0　　P Pediatric Age: 0-17　　M Maternity Age: 12-55　　A Adult Age: 15-124

614　　　　　　　　　　　　　　　　　　　　　　　　　　　　　　　ICD-10-CM 2018

H93.013   Transient ischemic deafness, bilateral

H93.019   Transient ischemic deafness, ▽
unspecified ear

✓6ᵗʰ H93.09   **Unspecified degenerative and vascular disorders of ear**

H93.091   Unspecified degenerative and vascular ▽
disorders of right ear

H93.092   Unspecified degenerative and vascular ▽
disorders of left ear

H93.093   Unspecified degenerative and vascular ▽
disorders of ear, bilateral

H93.099   Unspecified degenerative and vascular ▽
disorders of unspecified ear

✓5ᵗʰ **H93.1   Tinnitus**

H93.11   Tinnitus, right ear

H93.12   Tinnitus, left ear

H93.13   Tinnitus, bilateral

H93.19   Tinnitus, unspecified ear ▽

✓5ᵗʰ **H93.A   Pulsatile Tinnitus**

H93.A1   Pulsatile tinnitus, right ear

H93.A2   Pulsatile tinnitus, left ear

H93.A3   Pulsatile tinnitus, bilateral

H93.A9   Pulsatile tinnitus, unspecified ear ▽

✓5ᵗʰ **H93.2   Other abnormal auditory perceptions**

EXCLUDES 2   auditory hallucinations (R44.0)

✓6ᵗʰ H93.21   **Auditory recruitment**

H93.211   Auditory recruitment, right ear

H93.212   Auditory recruitment, left ear

H93.213   Auditory recruitment, bilateral

H93.219   Auditory recruitment, unspecified ear ▽

✓6ᵗʰ H93.22   **Diplacusis**

H93.221   Diplacusis, right ear

H93.222   Diplacusis, left ear

H93.223   Diplacusis, bilateral

H93.229   Diplacusis, unspecified ear ▽

✓6ᵗʰ H93.23   **Hyperacusis**

DEF: Exceptionally acute sense of hearing caused by such conditions as Bell's palsy; this term may also refer to painful sensitivity to sounds.

H93.231   Hyperacusis, right ear

H93.232   Hyperacusis, left ear

H93.233   Hyperacusis, bilateral

H93.239   Hyperacusis, unspecified ear ▽

✓6ᵗʰ H93.24   **Temporary auditory threshold shift**

H93.241   Temporary auditory threshold shift, right ear

H93.242   Temporary auditory threshold shift, left ear

H93.243   Temporary auditory threshold shift, bilateral

H93.249   Temporary auditory threshold shift, ▽
unspecified ear

H93.25   **Central auditory processing disorder**

Congenital auditory imperception

Word deafness

EXCLUDES 1   mixed receptive-expressive language disorder (F80.2)

✓6ᵗʰ H93.29   **Other abnormal auditory perceptions**

H93.291   Other abnormal auditory perceptions, right ear

H93.292   Other abnormal auditory perceptions, left ear

H93.293   Other abnormal auditory perceptions, bilateral

H93.299   Other abnormal auditory perceptions, ▽
unspecified ear

✓5ᵗʰ **H93.3   Disorders of acoustic nerve**

Disorder of 8th cranial nerve

EXCLUDES 1   acoustic neuroma (D33.3)
syphilitic acoustic neuritis (A52.15)

✓6ᵗʰ H93.3X   **Disorders of acoustic nerve**

H93.3X1   Disorders of right acoustic nerve

H93.3X2   Disorders of left acoustic nerve

H93.3X3   Disorders of bilateral acoustic nerves

H93.3X9   Disorders of unspecified acoustic nerve ▽

✓5ᵗʰ **H93.8   Other specified disorders of ear**

✓6ᵗʰ H93.8X   **Other specified disorders of ear**

H93.8X1   Other specified disorders of right ear

H93.8X2   Other specified disorders of left ear

H93.8X3   Other specified disorders of ear, bilateral

H93.8X9   Other specified disorders of ear, ▽
unspecified ear

✓5ᵗʰ **H93.9   Unspecified disorder of ear**

H93.90   Unspecified disorder of ear, unspecified ear ▽

H93.91   Unspecified disorder of right ear ▽

H93.92   Unspecified disorder of left ear ▽

H93.93   Unspecified disorder of ear, bilateral ▽

✓4ᵗʰ **H94   Other disorders of ear in diseases classified elsewhere**

✓5ᵗʰ **H94.0   Acoustic neuritis in infectious and parasitic diseases classified elsewhere**

Code first underlying disease, such as:

parasitic disease (B65-B89)

EXCLUDES 1   acoustic neuritis (in):
herpes zoster (B02.29)
syphilis (A52.15)

*H94.00   Acoustic neuritis in infectious and parasitic ▽
diseases classified elsewhere, unspecified ear*

H94.01   Acoustic neuritis in infectious and parasitic diseases classified elsewhere, right ear

H94.02   Acoustic neuritis in infectious and parasitic diseases classified elsewhere, left ear

H94.03   Acoustic neuritis in infectious and parasitic diseases classified elsewhere, bilateral

✓5ᵗʰ **H94.8   Other specified disorders of ear in diseases classified elsewhere**

Code first underlying disease, such as:

congenital syphilis (A50.0)

EXCLUDES 1   aural myiasis (B87.4)
syphilitic labyrinthitis (A52.79)

*H94.80   Other specified disorders of ear in diseases ▽
classified elsewhere, unspecified ear*

H94.81   Other specified disorders of right ear in diseases classified elsewhere

H94.82   Other specified disorders of left ear in diseases classified elsewhere

H94.83   Other specified disorders of ear in diseases classified elsewhere, bilateral

Intraoperative and postprocedural complications and disorders of ear and mastoid process, not elsewhere classified (H95)

✓4ᵗʰ **H95   Intraoperative and postprocedural complications and disorders of ear and mastoid process, not elsewhere classified**

✓5ᵗʰ **H95.0   Recurrent cholesteatoma of postmastoidectomy cavity**

H95.00   Recurrent cholesteatoma of postmastoidectomy ▽
cavity, unspecified

H95.01   Recurrent cholesteatoma of postmastoidectomy cavity, right ear

H95.02   Recurrent cholesteatoma of postmastoidectomy cavity, left ear

H95.03   Recurrent cholesteatoma of postmastoidectomy cavity, bilateral ears

✓5ᵗʰ **H95.1   Other disorders of ear and mastoid process following mastoidectomy**

✓6ᵗʰ H95.11   **Chronic inflammation of postmastoidectomy cavity**

H95.111   Chronic inflammation of postmastoidectomy cavity, right ear

H95.112   Chronic inflammation of postmastoidectomy cavity, left ear

H95.113   Chronic inflammation of postmastoidectomy cavity, bilateral ears

H95.119   Chronic inflammation of ▽
postmastoidectomy cavity, unspecified ear

✓6ᵗʰ H95.12   **Granulation of postmastoidectomy cavity**

H95.121   Granulation of postmastoidectomy cavity, right ear

H95.122   Granulation of postmastoidectomy cavity, left ear

H95.123   Granulation of postmastoidectomy cavity, bilateral ears

☑ Additional Character Req   ✓×7ᵗʰ Placeholder Alert   Manifestation   **HCC** CMS-HCC Condition   ▽ Unspecified Code   ►◄ Revised Text   ● New Code   ▲ Revised Code Title

ICD-10-CM 2018   **615**

Chapter 8. Diseases of the Ear and Mastoid Process

                H95.129 Granulation of postmastoidectomy ▽
                        cavity, unspecified ear

     ✓6ᵗʰ **H95.13** Mucosal cyst of postmastoidectomy cavity

                H95.131 Mucosal cyst of postmastoidectomy
                        cavity, right ear

                H95.132 Mucosal cyst of postmastoidectomy
                        cavity, left ear

                H95.133 Mucosal cyst of postmastoidectomy
                        cavity, bilateral ears

                H95.139 Mucosal cyst of postmastoidectomy ▽
                        cavity, unspecified ear

     ✓6ᵗʰ **H95.19** Other disorders following mastoidectomy

                H95.191 Other disorders following mastoidectomy,
                        right ear

                H95.192 Other disorders following mastoidectomy,
                        left ear

                H95.193 Other disorders following mastoidectomy,
                        bilateral ears

                H95.199 Other disorders following ▽
                        mastoidectomy, unspecified ear

✓5ᵗʰ **H95.2** Intraoperative hemorrhage and hematoma of ear and
        mastoid process complicating a procedure

         EXCLUDES 1   *intraoperative hemorrhage and hematoma of ear and*
                      mastoid process due to accidental puncture or
                      laceration during a procedure (H95.3-)

        H95.21 Intraoperative hemorrhage and hematoma of ear
                and mastoid process complicating a procedure on
                the ear and mastoid process

        H95.22 Intraoperative hemorrhage and hematoma of ear
                and mastoid process complicating other procedure

✓5ᵗʰ **H95.3** Accidental puncture and laceration of ear and mastoid
        process during a procedure

        H95.31 Accidental puncture and laceration of the ear and
                mastoid process during a procedure on the ear and
                mastoid process

        H95.32 Accidental puncture and laceration of the ear and
                mastoid process during other procedure

✓5ᵗʰ **H95.4** Postprocedural hemorrhage of ear and mastoid process
        following a procedure

        H95.41 Postprocedural hemorrhage of ear and mastoid
                process following a procedure on
                the ear and mastoid process

        H95.42 Postprocedural hemorrhage of ear and mastoid
                process following other procedure

✓5ᵗʰ **H95.5** Postprocedural hematoma and seroma of ear and mastoid
        process following a procedure

        H95.51 Postprocedural hematoma of ear and mastoid
                process following a procedure on the ear and
                mastoid process

        H95.52 Postprocedural hematoma of ear and mastoid
                process following other procedure

        H95.53 Postprocedural seroma of ear and mastoid process
                following a procedure on the ear and mastoid
                process

        H95.54 Postprocedural seroma of ear and mastoid process
                following other procedure

✓5ᵗʰ **H95.8** Other intraoperative and postprocedural complications and
        disorders of the ear and mastoid process, not elsewhere
        classified

         EXCLUDES 2   *postprocedural complications and disorders following*
                      mastoidectomy (H95.0-, H95.1-)

     ✓6ᵗʰ **H95.81** Postprocedural stenosis of external ear canal

                H95.811 Postprocedural stenosis of right external
                        ear canal

                H95.812 Postprocedural stenosis of left external
                        ear canal

                H95.813 Postprocedural stenosis of external ear
                        canal, bilateral

                H95.819 Postprocedural stenosis of unspecified ▽
                        external ear canal

        H95.88 Other intraoperative complications and disorders of
                the ear and mastoid process, not elsewhere
                classified

                Use additional code, if applicable, to further specify
                disorder

        H95.89 Other postprocedural complications and disorders
                of the ear and mastoid process, not elsewhere
                classified

                Use additional code, if applicable, to further specify
                disorder

EXCLUDES 1 Not coded here   EXCLUDES 2 Not included here   N Newborn Age: 0   P Pediatric Age: 0-17   M Maternity Age: 12-55   A Adult Age: 15-124

616   ICD-10-CM 2018

H95.129–H95.89

Chapter 9. Diseases of the Circulatory System (I00–I99)

Chapter Specific Guidelines with Coding Examples

The chapter specific guidelines from the ICD-10-CM Official Guidelines for Coding and Reporting have been provided below. Along with these guidelines are coding examples, contained in the shaded boxes, that have been developed to help illustrate the coding and/or sequencing guidance found in these guidelines.

a. Hypertension

The classification presumes a causal relationship between hypertension and heart involvement and between hypertension and kidney involvement, as the two conditions are linked by the term "with" in the Alphabetic Index. These conditions should be coded as related even in the absence of provider documentation explicitly linking them, unless the documentation clearly states the conditions are unrelated.

For hypertension and conditions not specifically linked by relational terms such as "with," "associated with" or "due to" in the classification, provider documentation must link the conditions in order to code them as related.

1) Hypertension with heart disease

Hypertension with heart conditions classified to I50.- or I51.4-I51.9, are assigned to a code from category I11, Hypertensive heart disease. Use an additional code from category I50, Heart failure, to identify the type of heart failure in those patients with heart failure.

The same heart conditions (I50.-, I51.4-I51.9) with hypertension are coded separately if the provider has specifically documented a different cause. Sequence according to the circumstances of the admission/encounter.

> Patient is treated for left heart failure. Patient also has a history of hypertension managed by medication.
>
> **I11.Ø**   **Hypertensive heart disease with heart failure**
>
> **I5Ø.1**   **Left ventricular failure, unspecified**
>
> *Explanation*: Without a diagnostic statement to the contrary, hypertension and heart failure have an assumed causal relationship, and a combination code should be used. An additional code to identify the type of heart failure (I50.-) should also be provided.

2) Hypertensive chronic kidney disease

Assign codes from category I12, Hypertensive chronic kidney disease, when both hypertension and a condition classifiable to category N18, Chronic kidney disease (CKD), are present. CKD should not be coded as hypertensive if the physician has specifically documented a different cause.

The appropriate code from category N18 should be used as a secondary code with a code from category I12 to identify the stage of chronic kidney disease.

See Section I.C.14. Chronic kidney disease.

If a patient has hypertensive chronic kidney disease and acute renal failure, an additional code for the acute renal failure is required.

> Patient presents with stage IV chronic kidney disease (CKD). The patient also has documented hypertension secondary to primary hyperparathyroidism.
>
> **N18.4**   **Chronic kidney disease, stage 4 (severe)**
>
> **I1Ø**   **Essential (primary) hypertension**
>
> **E21.Ø**   **Primary hyperparathyroidism**
>
> *Explanation*: A combination code describing a relationship between hypertension and CKD is not used due to the physician documentation identifying the primary hyperparathyroidism as the cause for the hypertension.

3) Hypertensive heart and chronic kidney disease

Assign codes from combination category I13, Hypertensive heart and chronic kidney disease, when there is hypertension with both heart and kidney involvement. If heart failure is present, assign an additional code from category I50 to identify the type of heart failure.

The appropriate code from category N18, Chronic kidney disease, should be used as a secondary code with a code from category I13 to identify the stage of chronic kidney disease.

See Section I.C.14. Chronic kidney disease.

The codes in category I13, Hypertensive heart and chronic kidney disease, are combination codes that include hypertension, heart disease and chronic kidney disease. The Includes note at I13 specifies that the conditions included at I11 and I12 are included together in I13. If a patient has hypertension, heart disease and chronic kidney disease, then a code from I13 should be used, not individual codes for hypertension, heart disease and chronic kidney disease, or codes from I11 or I12.

For patients with both acute renal failure and chronic kidney disease, an additional code for acute renal failure is required.

> Hypertensive heart and kidney disease with congestive heart failure and stage 2 chronic kidney disease
>
> **I13.Ø**   **Hypertensive heart and chronic kidney disease with heart failure and stage 1 through stage 4 chronic kidney disease, or unspecified chronic kidney disease**
>
> **I5Ø.9**   **Heart failure, unspecified**
>
> **N18.2**   **Chronic kidney disease, stage 2 (mild)**
>
> *Explanation*: Combination codes in category I13 are used to report conditions classifiable to *both* categories I11 and I12. Do not report conditions classifiable to I11 and I12 separately. Use additional codes to report type of heart failure and stage of CKD.

4) Hypertensive cerebrovascular disease

For hypertensive cerebrovascular disease, first assign the appropriate code from categories I60-I69, followed by the appropriate hypertension code.

> Rupture of cerebral aneurysm caused by malignant hypertension
>
> **I6Ø.7**   **Nontraumatic subarachnoid hemorrhage from unspecified introcranial artery**
>
> **I1Ø**   **Essential (primary) hypertension**
>
> *Explanation*: Hypertensive cerebrovascular disease requires two codes: the appropriate I60–I69 code followed by the appropriate hypertension code.

5) Hypertensive retinopathy

Subcategory H35.Ø, Background retinopathy and retinal vascular changes, should be used with a code from category I10 – I15, Hypertensive disease to include the systemic hypertension. The sequencing is based on the reason for the encounter.

> Hypertensive retinopathy of the right eye
>
> **H35.Ø31**   **Hypertensive retinopathy, right eye**
>
> **I1Ø**   **Essential (primary) hypertension**
>
> *Explanation*: Hypertensive retinopathy requires two codes: the appropriate subcategory H35.Ø code and a code for the hypertension.

6) Hypertension, secondary

Secondary hypertension is due to an underlying condition. Two codes are required: one to identify the underlying etiology and one from category I15 to identify the hypertension. Sequencing of codes is determined by the reason for admission/encounter.

> Renovascular hypertension due to renal artery atherosclerosis
>
> **I15.Ø**   **Renovascular hypertension**
>
> **I7Ø.1**   **Atherosclerosis of renal artery**
>
> *Explanation*: Secondary hypertension requires two codes: a code to identify the etiology and the appropriate I15 code.

7) Hypertension, transient

Assign code R03.Ø, Elevated blood pressure reading without diagnosis of hypertension, unless patient has an established diagnosis of hypertension. Assign code O13.-, Gestational [pregnancy-induced] hypertension without significant proteinuria, or O14.-, Pre-eclampsia, for transient hypertension of pregnancy.

8) Hypertension, controlled

This diagnostic statement usually refers to an existing state of hypertension under control by therapy. Assign the appropriate code from categories I10-I15, Hypertensive diseases.

9) Hypertension, uncontrolled

Uncontrolled hypertension may refer to untreated hypertension or hypertension not responding to current therapeutic regimen. In either case, assign the appropriate code from categories I10-I15, Hypertensive diseases.

10) Hypertensive Crisis

Assign a code from category I16, Hypertensive crisis, for documented hypertensive urgency, hypertensive emergency or unspecified hypertensive crisis. Code also any identified hypertensive disease (I10-I15). The sequencing is based on the reason for the encounter.

b. Atherosclerotic coronary artery disease and angina

ICD-10-CM has combination codes for atherosclerotic heart disease with angina pectoris. The subcategories for these codes are I25.11, Atherosclerotic heart disease of native coronary artery with angina pectoris and I25.7, Atherosclerosis of coronary artery bypass graft(s) and coronary artery of transplanted heart with angina pectoris.

When using one of these combination codes it is not necessary to use an additional code for angina pectoris. A causal relationship can be assumed in a patient with both atherosclerosis and angina pectoris, unless the documentation indicates the angina is due to something other than the atherosclerosis.

If a patient with coronary artery disease is admitted due to an acute myocardial infarction (AMI), the AMI should be sequenced before the coronary artery disease.

See Section I.C.9. Acute myocardial infarction (AMI)

Patient is being seen for spastic angina pectoris. She also has a documented history of progressive coronary artery disease of the native vessels.	
I25.111	**Atherosclerotic heart disease of native coronary artery with angina pectoris with documented spasm**

Explanation: Report the combination code for atherosclerotic heart disease (coronary artery disease) with angina pectoris. A causal relationship is assumed in a patient with both atherosclerosis and angina pectoris, unless the documentation indicates the angina is due to something other than the atherosclerosis. When using one of these combination codes, it is not necessary to use an additional code for angina pectoris.

c. Intraoperative and postprocedural cerebrovascular accident

Medical record documentation should clearly specify the cause- and- effect relationship between the medical intervention and the cerebrovascular accident in order to assign a code for intraoperative or postprocedural cerebrovascular accident.

Proper code assignment depends on whether it was an infarction or hemorrhage and whether it occurred intraoperatively or postoperatively. If it was a cerebral hemorrhage, code assignment depends on the type of procedure performed.

Embolic cerebral infarction of the right middle cerebral artery that occurred during hip replacement surgery. The surgeon documented as due to the surgery.	
I97.811	**Intraoperative cerebrovascular infarction during other surgery**
I63.411	**Cerebral infarction due to embolism of right middle cerebral artery**

Explanation: Code assignment for intraoperative or postprocedural cerebrovascular accident is based on the provider's documentation of a cause-and-effect relationship between the condition and the procedure. Proper code assignment also depends on whether the cerebrovascular accident was an infarction or hemorrhage, occurred intraoperatively or postoperatively, and the type of procedure performed.

d. Sequelae of cerebrovascular disease

1) Category I69, Sequelae of cerebrovascular disease

Category I69 is used to indicate conditions classifiable to categories I60-I67 as the causes of sequela (neurologic deficits), themselves classified elsewhere. These "late effects" include neurologic deficits that persist after initial onset of conditions classifiable to categories I60-I67. The neurologic deficits caused by cerebrovascular disease may be present from the onset or may arise at any time after the onset of the condition classifiable to categories I60-I67.

Codes from category I69, Sequelae of cerebrovascular disease, that specify hemiplegia, hemiparesis and monoplegia identify whether the dominant or nondominant side is affected. Should the affected side be documented, but not specified as dominant or nondominant, and the classification system does not indicate a default, code selection is as follows:

- For ambidextrous patients, the default should be dominant.

- If the left side is affected, the default is non-dominant.
- If the right side is affected, the default is dominant.

2) Codes from category I69 with codes from I60-I67

Codes from category I69 may be assigned on a health care record with codes from I60-I67, if the patient has a current cerebrovascular disease and deficits from an old cerebrovascular disease.

3) Codes from category I69 and personal history of transient ischemic attack (TIA) and cerebral infarction (Z86.73)

Codes from category I69 should not be assigned if the patient does not have neurologic deficits.

See Section I.C.21. 4. History (of) for use of personal history codes

e. Acute myocardial infarction (AMI)

1) ST elevation myocardial infarction (STEMI) and non ST elevation myocardial infarction (NSTEMI)

The ICD-10-CM codes for acute myocardial infarction (AMI) identify the site, such as anterolateral wall or true posterior wall. Subcategories I21.0-I21.2 and code I21.3 are used for ST elevation myocardial infarction (STEMI). Code I21.4, Non-ST elevation (NSTEMI) myocardial infarction, is used for non ST elevation myocardial infarction (NSTEMI) and nontransmural MIs.

If NSTEMI evolves to STEMI, assign the STEMI code. If STEMI converts to NSTEMI due to thrombolytic therapy, it is still coded as STEMI.

Acute inferior NSTEMI evolved into STEMI	
I21.19	**ST elevation (STEMI) myocardial infarction involving other coronary artery of inferior wall**

Explanation: If an NSTEMI converts to a STEMI, report only the STEMI code.

For encounters occurring while the myocardial infarction is equal to, or less than, four weeks old, including transfers to another acute setting or a postacute setting, and the myocardial infarction meets the definition for "other diagnoses" (see Section III, Reporting Additional Diagnoses), codes from category I21 may continue to be reported. For encounters after the 4 week time frame and the patient is still receiving care related to the myocardial infarction, the appropriate aftercare code should be assigned, rather than a code from category I21. For old or healed myocardial infarctions not requiring further care, code I25.2, Old myocardial infarction, may be assigned.

2) Acute myocardial infarction, unspecified

Code I21.3, ST elevation (STEMI) myocardial infarction of unspecified site, is the default for unspecified acute myocardial infarction. If only STEMI or transmural MI without the site is documented, assign code I21.3.

3) AMI documented as nontransmural or subendocardial but site provided

If an AMI is documented as nontransmural or subendocardial, but the site is provided, it is still coded as a subendocardial AMI.

See Section I.C.21.3 for information on coding status post administration of tPA in a different facility within the last 24 hours.

Acute inferior subendocardial myocardial infarction (NSTEMI)	
I21.4	**Non-ST elevation (NSTEMI) myocardial infarction**

Explanation: An AMI documented as subendocardial or nontransmural is coded as such (I21.4, I22.2), even if the site of infarction is specified.

4) Subsequent acute myocardial infarction

A code from category I22, Subsequent ST elevation (STEMI) and non ST elevation (NSTEMI) myocardial infarction, is to be used when a patient who has suffered an AMI has a new AMI within the 4 week time frame of the initial AMI. A code from category I22 must be used in conjunction with a code from category I21. The sequencing of the I22 and I21 codes depends on the circumstances of the encounter.

Acute inferior STEMI status post acute NSTEMI two weeks ago.	
I22.1	**Subsequent ST elevation (STEMI) myocardial infarction of inferior wall**
I21.4	**Non-ST elevation (NSTEMI) myocardial infarction**

Explanation: A code from I22 must be used in conjunction with a code from I21 when a patient who has suffered an AMI has a new AMI within four weeks of the initial one. Category I22 is never reported alone. The guidelines for assigning the correct I22 code are the same as those for reporting the initial MI (I21). Sequencing is determined by the circumstances of the encounter.

Chapter 9. Diseases of the Circulatory System (I00-I99)

EXCLUDES 2   certain conditions originating in the perinatal period (P04-P96)
certain infectious and parasitic diseases (A00-B99)
complications of pregnancy, childbirth and the puerperium (O00-O9A)
congenital malformations, deformations, and chromosomal abnormalities (Q00-Q99)
endocrine, nutritional and metabolic diseases (E00-E88)
injury, poisoning and certain other consequences of external causes (S00-T88)
neoplasms (C00-D49)
symptoms, signs and abnormal clinical and laboratory findings, not elsewhere classified (R00-R94)
systemic connective tissue disorders (M30-M36)
transient cerebral ischemic attacks and related syndromes (G45.-)

This chapter contains the following blocks:

I00-I02	Acute rheumatic fever
I05-I09	Chronic rheumatic heart diseases
I10-I16	Hypertensive diseases
I20-I25	Ischemic heart diseases
I26-I28	Pulmonary heart disease and diseases of pulmonary circulation
I30-I52	Other forms of heart disease
I60-I69	Cerebrovascular diseases
I70-I79	Diseases of arteries, arterioles and capillaries
I80-I89	Diseases of veins, lymphatic vessels and lymph nodes, not elsewhere classified
I95-I99	Other and unspecified disorders of the circulatory system

Acute rheumatic fever (I00-I02)

I00   Rheumatic fever without heart involvement
   INCLUDES   arthritis, rheumatic, acute or subacute
   EXCLUDES 1   rheumatic fever with heart involvement (I01.0-I01.9)

✓4ᵗʰ **I01   Rheumatic fever with heart involvement**
   EXCLUDES 1   chronic diseases of rheumatic origin (I05-I09) unless rheumatic fever is also present or there is evidence of reactivation or activity of the rheumatic process.

   I01.0   Acute rheumatic pericarditis
     Any condition in I00 with pericarditis
     Rheumatic pericarditis (acute)
     EXCLUDES 1   acute pericarditis not specified as rheumatic (I30.-)

   I01.1   Acute rheumatic endocarditis
     Any condition in I00 with endocarditis or valvulitis
     Acute rheumatic valvulitis

   I01.2   Acute rheumatic myocarditis
     Any condition in I00 with myocarditis

   I01.8   Other acute rheumatic heart disease
     Any condition in I00 with other or multiple types of heart involvement
     Acute rheumatic pancarditis

   I01.9   Acute rheumatic heart disease, unspecified   ▽
     Any condition in I00 with unspecified type of heart involvement
     Rheumatic carditis, acute
     Rheumatic heart disease, active or acute

✓4ᵗʰ **I02   Rheumatic chorea**
   INCLUDES   Sydenham's chorea
   EXCLUDES 1   chorea NOS (G25.5)
             Huntington's chorea (G10)

   I02.0   Rheumatic chorea with heart involvement
     Chorea NOS with heart involvement
     Rheumatic chorea with heart involvement of any type classifiable under I01-

   I02.9   Rheumatic chorea without heart involvement
     Rheumatic chorea NOS

Chronic rheumatic heart diseases (I05-I09)

✓4ᵗʰ **I05   Rheumatic mitral valve diseases**
   INCLUDES   conditions classifiable to both I05.0 and I05.2-I05.9, whether specified as rheumatic or not
   EXCLUDES 1   mitral valve disease specified as nonrheumatic (I34.-)
             mitral valve disease with aortic and/or tricuspid valve involvement (I08.-)

   I05.0   Rheumatic mitral stenosis
     Mitral (valve) obstruction (rheumatic)
     DEF: Narrowing of mitral valve between left atrium and left ventricle; due to rheumatic fever; characterized by shortness of breath during or after exercise, fatigue, palpitations, chest discomfort, and swelling of feet or legs.

   I05.1   Rheumatic mitral insufficiency
     Rheumatic mitral incompetence
     Rheumatic mitral regurgitation
     EXCLUDES 1   mitral insufficiency not specified as rheumatic (I34.0)

   I05.2   Rheumatic mitral stenosis with insufficiency
     Rheumatic mitral stenosis with incompetence or regurgitation

   I05.8   Other rheumatic mitral valve diseases
     Rheumatic mitral (valve) failure

   I05.9   Rheumatic mitral valve disease, unspecified   ▽
     Rheumatic mitral (valve) disorder (chronic) NOS

✓4ᵗʰ **I06   Rheumatic aortic valve diseases**
   EXCLUDES 1   aortic valve disease not specified as rheumatic (I35.-)
             aortic valve disease with mitral and/or tricuspid valve involvement (I08.-)

   I06.0   Rheumatic aortic stenosis
     Rheumatic aortic (valve) obstruction

   I06.1   Rheumatic aortic insufficiency
     Rheumatic aortic incompetence
     Rheumatic aortic regurgitation

   I06.2   Rheumatic aortic stenosis with insufficiency
     Rheumatic aortic stenosis with incompetence or regurgitation

   I06.8   Other rheumatic aortic valve diseases

   I06.9   Rheumatic aortic valve disease, unspecified   ▽
     Rheumatic aortic (valve) disease NOS

✓4ᵗʰ **I07   Rheumatic tricuspid valve diseases**
   INCLUDES   rheumatic tricuspid valve diseases specified as rheumatic or unspecified
   EXCLUDES 1   tricuspid valve disease specified as nonrheumatic (I36.-)
             tricuspid valve disease with aortic and/or mitral valve involvement (I08.-)

   I07.0   Rheumatic tricuspid stenosis
     Tricuspid (valve) stenosis (rheumatic)

   I07.1   Rheumatic tricuspid insufficiency
     Tricuspid (valve) insufficiency (rheumatic)

   I07.2   Rheumatic tricuspid stenosis and insufficiency

   I07.8   Other rheumatic tricuspid valve diseases

   I07.9   Rheumatic tricuspid valve disease, unspecified   ▽
     Rheumatic tricuspid valve disorder NOS

✓4ᵗʰ **I08   Multiple valve diseases**
   INCLUDES   multiple valve diseases specified as rheumatic or unspecified
   EXCLUDES 1   endocarditis, valve unspecified (I38)
             multiple valve disease specified a nonrheumatic (I34.-, I35.-, I36.-, I37.-, I38.-, Q22.-, Q23.-, Q24.8-)
             rheumatic valve disease NOS (I09.1)

   I08.0   Rheumatic disorders of both mitral and aortic valves
     Involvement of both mitral and aortic valves specified as rheumatic or unspecified

   I08.1   Rheumatic disorders of both mitral and tricuspid valves

   I08.2   Rheumatic disorders of both aortic and tricuspid valves

   I08.3   Combined rheumatic disorders of mitral, aortic and tricuspid valves

   I08.8   Other rheumatic multiple valve diseases

   I08.9   Rheumatic multiple valve disease, unspecified   ▽

✓4ᵗʰ **I09   Other rheumatic heart diseases**

   I09.0   Rheumatic myocarditis
     EXCLUDES 1   myocarditis not specified as rheumatic (I51.4)

   I09.1   Rheumatic diseases of endocardium, valve unspecified   ▽
     Rheumatic endocarditis (chronic)
     Rheumatic valvulitis (chronic)
     EXCLUDES 1   endocarditis, valve unspecified (I38)

   I09.2   Chronic rheumatic pericarditis
     Adherent pericardium, rheumatic
     Chronic rheumatic mediastinopericarditis
     Chronic rheumatic myopericarditis
     EXCLUDES 1   chronic pericarditis not specified as rheumatic (I31.-)

✓5ᵗʰ   **I09.8   Other specified rheumatic heart diseases**

     I09.81   Rheumatic heart failure   HCC
        Use additional code to identify type of heart failure (I50.-)
        DEF: Decreased cardiac output, edema, and hypertension; due to rheumatic heart disease.

     I09.89   Other specified rheumatic heart diseases
        Rheumatic disease of pulmonary valve

   I09.9   Rheumatic heart disease, unspecified   ▽
     Rheumatic carditis
     EXCLUDES 1   rheumatoid carditis (M05.31)

☑ Additional Character Req   ✓x7ᵗʰ Placeholder Alert   Manifestation   HCC CMS-HCC Condition   ▽ Unspecified Code   ►◄ Revised Text   ● New Code   ▲ Revised Code Title

Hypertensive diseases (I10-I16)

Use additional code to identify:
  exposure to environmental tobacco smoke (Z77.22)
  history of tobacco dependence (Z87.891)
  occupational exposure to environmental tobacco smoke (Z57.31)
  tobacco dependence (F17.-)
  tobacco use (Z72.Ø)

  EXCLUDES 1   neonatal hypertension (P29.2)
        primary pulmonary hypertension (I27.Ø)

  EXCLUDES 2   hypertensive disease complicating pregnancy, childbirth and the
        puerperium (O1Ø-O11, O13-O16)

I10   Essential (primary) hypertension
  INCLUDES   high blood pressure
        hypertension (arterial) (benign) (essential) (malignant)
        (primary) (systemic)

  EXCLUDES 1   hypertensive disease complicating pregnancy, childbirth and
        the puerperium (O1Ø-O11, O13-O16)

  EXCLUDES 2   essential (primary) hypertension involving vessels of brain
        (I6Ø-I69)
        essential (primary) hypertension involving vessels of eye
        (H35.Ø-)

  AHA: 2016, 4Q, 27

✓4ᵗʰ I11   Hypertensive heart disease
  INCLUDES ▶any condition in I5Ø.-, I51.4-I51.9 due to hypertension◄

  I11.Ø   Hypertensive heart disease with heart failure   HCC
        Hypertensive heart failure
        Use additional code to identify type of heart failure (I5Ø.-)
        AHA: 2017, 1Q, 47

  I11.9   Hypertensive heart disease without heart failure   ▽
        Hypertensive heart disease NOS

✓4ᵗʰ I12   Hypertensive chronic kidney disease
  INCLUDES   any condition in N18- and N26- due to hypertension
        arteriosclerosis of kidney
        arteriosclerotic nephritis (chronic) (interstitial)
        hypertensive nephropathy
        nephrosclerosis

  EXCLUDES 1   hypertension due to kidney disease (I15.Ø, I15.1)
        renovascular hypertension (I15.Ø)
        secondary hypertension (I15.-)

  EXCLUDES 2   acute kidney failure (N17.-)

  AHA: 2016, 3Q, 22

  I12.Ø   Hypertensive chronic kidney disease with stage 5   HCC
  chronic kidney disease or end stage renal disease
        Use additional code to identify the stage of chronic kidney
        disease (N18.5, N18.6)

  I12.9   Hypertensive chronic kidney disease with stage 1 through ▽
  **stage 4 chronic kidney disease, or unspecified chronic kidney
  disease**
        Hypertensive chronic kidney disease NOS
        Hypertensive renal disease NOS
        Use additional code to identify the stage of chronic kidney
        disease (N18.1-N18.4, N18.9)

✓4ᵗʰ I13   Hypertensive heart and chronic kidney disease
  INCLUDES   any condition in I11- with any condition in I12-
        cardiorenal disease
        cardiovascular renal disease

  I13.Ø   Hypertensive heart and chronic kidney disease with   HCC
  **heart failure and stage 1 through stage 4 chronic kidney
  disease, or unspecified chronic kidney disease**
        Use additional code to identify type of heart failure (I5Ø.-)
        Use additional code to identify stage of chronic kidney disease
        (N18.1-N18.4, N18.9)

  **✓5ᵗʰ I13.1   Hypertensive heart and chronic kidney disease without heart
  failure**

     I13.10   Hypertensive heart and chronic kidney disease ▽
  **without heart failure, with stage 1 through stage 4
  chronic kidney disease, or unspecified chronic
  kidney disease**
        Hypertensive heart disease and hypertensive chronic
        kidney disease NOS
        Use additional code to identify the stage of chronic
        kidney disease (N18.1-N18.4, N18.9)

     I13.11   Hypertensive heart and chronic kidney disease   HCC
  **without heart failure, with stage 5 chronic kidney
  disease, or end stage renal disease**
        Use additional code to identify the stage of chronic
        kidney disease (N18.5, N18.6)

  I13.2   Hypertensive heart and chronic kidney disease with   HCC
  **heart failure and with stage 5 chronic kidney disease,
  or end stage renal disease**
        Use additional code to identify type of heart failure (I5Ø.-)
        Use additional code to identify the stage of chronic kidney
        disease (N18.5, N18.6)

✓4ᵗʰ I15   Secondary hypertension
  Code also underlying condition

  EXCLUDES 1   postprocedural hypertension (I97.3)

  EXCLUDES 2   secondary hypertension involving vessels of brain (I6Ø-I69)
        secondary hypertension involving vessels of eye (H35.Ø-)

  I15.Ø   Renovascular hypertension

  I15.1   Hypertension secondary to other renal disorders
        AHA: 2016, 3Q, 22

  I15.2   Hypertension secondary to endocrine disorders

  I15.8   Other secondary hypertension

  I15.9   Secondary hypertension, unspecified   ▽

✓4ᵗʰ I16   Hypertensive crisis
  Code also any identified hypertensive disease (I10-I15)
  AHA: 2016, 4Q, 27

  I16.Ø   Hypertensive urgency

  I16.1   Hypertensive emergency

  I16.9   Hypertensive crisis, unspecified   ▽

Ischemic heart diseases (I2Ø-I25)

Use additional code to identify presence of hypertension (I10-I16)

✓4ᵗʰ I2Ø   Angina pectoris
  Use additional code to identify:
        exposure to environmental tobacco smoke (Z77.22)
        history of tobacco dependence (Z87.891)
        occupational exposure to environmental tobacco smoke (Z57.31)
        tobacco dependence (F17.-)
        tobacco use (Z72.Ø)

  EXCLUDES 1   angina pectoris with atherosclerotic heart disease of native
        coronary arteries (I25.1-)
        atherosclerosis of coronary artery bypass graft(s) and coronary
        artery of transplanted heart with angina pectoris (I25.7-)
        postinfarction angina (I23.7)

  I2Ø.Ø   Unstable angina   HCC
        Accelerated angina
        Crescendo angina
        De novo effort angina
        Intermediate coronary syndrome
        Preinfarction syndrome
        Worsening effort angina
        DEF: A condition representing an intermediate stage between
        angina of effort and acute myocardial infarction.

  I2Ø.1   Angina pectoris with documented spasm   HCC
        Angiospastic angina
        Prinzmetal angina
        Spasm-induced angina
        Variant angina

  I2Ø.8   Other forms of angina pectoris   HCC
        Angina equivalent
        Angina of effort
        Coronary slow flow syndrome
        Stable angina
        Stenocardia
        Use additional code(s) for symptoms associated with angina
        equivalent

  I2Ø.9   Angina pectoris, unspecified   HCC ▽
        Angina NOS
        Anginal syndrome
        Cardiac angina
        Ischemic chest pain

EXCLUDES 1 Not coded here   EXCLUDES 2 Not included here   N Newborn Age: 0   P Pediatric Age: 0-17   M Maternity Age: 12-55   A Adult Age: 15-124

620   ICD-10-CM 2018

▲ ✓4ᵗʰ **I21 Acute myocardial infarction**

INCLUDES   cardiac infarction
coronary (artery) embolism
coronary (artery) occlusion
coronary (artery) rupture
coronary (artery) thrombosis
infarction of heart, myocardium, or ventricle
myocardial infarction specified as acute or with a stated
duration of 4 weeks (28 days) or less from onset

Use additional code, if applicable, to identify:
exposure to environmental tobacco smoke (Z77.22)
history of tobacco dependence (Z87.891)
occupational exposure to environmental tobacco smoke (Z57.31)
status post administration of tPA (rtPA) in a different facility within
the last 24 hours prior to admission to current facility (Z92.82)
tobacco dependence (F17.-)
tobacco use (Z72.0)

EXCLUDES 2   old myocardial infarction (I25.2)
postmyocardial infarction syndrome (I24.1)
▶subsequent type 1 myocardial infarction◀ (I22.-)

AHA: 2017, 1Q, 44-45; 2016, 4Q, 140; 2015, 2Q, 16; 2013, 1Q, 25; 2012, 4Q, 96, 102-103

✓5ᵗʰ **I21.0 ST elevation (STEMI) myocardial infarction of anterior wall**
▶Type 1 ST elevation myocardial infarction of anterior wall◀

     I21.01   **ST elevation (STEMI) myocardial infarction**   HCC
involving left main coronary artery

     I21.02   **ST elevation (STEMI) myocardial infarction**   HCC
involving left anterior descending coronary artery
ST elevation (STEMI) myocardial infarction involving
diagonal coronary artery
AHA: 2013, 1Q, 25

     I21.09   **ST elevation (STEMI) myocardial infarction**   HCC
involving other coronary artery of anterior wall
Acute transmural myocardial infarction of anterior wall
Anteroapical transmural (Q wave) infarction (acute)
Anterolateral transmural (Q wave) infarction (acute)
Anteroseptal transmural (Q wave) infarction (acute)
Transmural (Q wave) infarction (acute) (of) anterior
(wall) NOS
AHA: 2012, 4Q, 102-103

✓5ᵗʰ **I21.1 ST elevation (STEMI) myocardial infarction of inferior wall**
▶Type 1 ST elevation myocardial infarction of inferior wall◀

     I21.11   **ST elevation (STEMI) myocardial infarction**   HCC
involving right coronary artery
Inferoposterior transmural (Q wave) infarction (acute)

     I21.19   **ST elevation (STEMI) myocardial infarction**   HCC
involving other coronary artery of inferior wall
Acute transmural myocardial infarction of inferior wall
Inferolateral transmural (Q wave) infarction (acute)
Transmural (Q wave) infarction (acute) (of)
diaphragmatic wall
Transmural (Q wave) infarction (acute) (of) inferior
(wall) NOS
EXCLUDES 2   ST elevation (STEMI) myocardial infarction
involving left circumflex coronary artery
(I21.21)
AHA: 2012, 4Q, 96

✓5ᵗʰ **I21.2 ST elevation (STEMI) myocardial infarction of other sites**
▶Type 1 ST elevation myocardial infarction of other sites◀

     I21.21   **ST elevation (STEMI) myocardial infarction**   HCC
involving left circumflex coronary artery
ST elevation (STEMI) myocardial infarction involving
oblique marginal coronary artery

     I21.29   **ST elevation (STEMI) myocardial infarction**   HCC
involving other sites
Acute transmural myocardial infarction of other sites
Apical-lateral transmural (Q wave) infarction (acute)
Basal-lateral transmural (Q wave) infarction (acute)
High lateral transmural (Q wave) infarction (acute)
Lateral (wall) NOS transmural (Q wave) infarction
(acute)
Posterior (true) transmural (Q wave) infarction (acute)
Posterobasal transmural (Q wave) infarction (acute)
Posterolateral transmural (Q wave) infarction (acute)
Posteroseptal transmural (Q wave) infarction (acute)
Septal transmural (Q wave) infarction (acute) NOS

     I21.3   **ST elevation (STEMI) myocardial infarction of**   HCC ▽
unspecified site
Acute transmural myocardial infarction of unspecified site
~~Myocardial infarction (acute) NOS~~
Transmural (Q wave) myocardial infarction NOS
▶Type 1 ST elevation myocardial infarction of unspecified site◀

     I21.4   **Non-ST elevation (NSTEMI) myocardial infarction**   HCC
Acute subendocardial myocardial infarction
Non-Q wave myocardial infarction NOS
Nontransmural myocardial infarction NOS
▶Type 1 non-ST elevation myocardial infarction◀
AHA: 2017, 1Q, 44-45

●   **I21.9**   **Acute myocardial infarction, unspecified**   ▽
Myocardial infarction (acute) NOS

●   ✓5ᵗʰ **I21.A**   **Other type of myocardial infarction**

●   **I21.A1**   **Myocardial infarction type 2**
Myocardial infarction due to demand ischemia
Myocardial infarction secondary to ischemic
imbalance
Code also the underlying cause, if known and
applicable, such as:
anemia (D50.0-D64.9)
chronic obstructive pulmonary disease (J44.-)
heart failure (I50.-)
paroxysmal tachycardia (I47.0-I47.9)
renal failure (N17.0-N19)
shock (R57.0-R57.9)

●   **I21.A9**   **Other myocardial infarction type**
Myocardial infarction associated with
revascularization procedure
Myocardial infarction type 3
Myocardial infarction type 4a
Myocardial infarction type 4b
Myocardial infarction type 4c
Myocardial infarction type 5
Code first, if applicable, postprocedural myocardial
infarction following cardiac surgery (I97.190), or
postprocedural myocardial infarction during
cardiac surgery (I97.790)
Code also complication, if known and applicable, such
as:
(acute) stent occlusion (T82.897-)
(acute) stent stenosis (T82.857-)
(acute) stent thrombosis (T82.867-)
cardiac arrest due to underlying cardiac condition
(I46.2)
complication of percutaneous coronary
intervention (PCI) (I97.89)
occlusion of coronary artery bypass graft (T82.218-)

✓4ᵗʰ **I22 Subsequent ST elevation (STEMI) and non-ST elevation (NSTEMI) myocardial infarction**

INCLUDES   acute myocardial infarction occurring within four weeks (28
days) of a previous acute myocardial infarction,
regardless of site
cardiac infarction
coronary (artery) embolism
coronary (artery) occlusion
coronary (artery) rupture
coronary (artery) thrombosis
infarction of heart, myocardium, or ventricle
recurrent myocardial infarction
reinfarction of myocardium
rupture of heart, myocardium, or ventricle
▶subsequent type 1 myocardial infarction◀

Use additional code, if applicable, to identify:
exposure to environmental tobacco smoke (Z77.22)
history of tobacco dependence (Z87.891)
occupational exposure to environmental tobacco smoke (Z57.31)
status post administration of tPA (rtPA) in a different facility within
the last 24 hours prior to admission to current facility (Z92.82)
tobacco dependence (F17.-)
tobacco use (Z72.0)

EXCLUDES 1 ▶subsequent myocardial infarction, type 2 (I21.A1)
subsequent myocardial infarction of other type (type 3) (type 4)
(type 5) (I21.A9)◀

AHA: 2017, 2Q, 11; 2013, 1Q, 25; 2012, 4Q, 97, 102-103

     I22.0   **Subsequent ST elevation (STEMI) myocardial infarction**   HCC
of anterior wall
Subsequent acute transmural myocardial infarction of anterior
wall
Subsequent transmural (Q wave) infarction (acute)(of) anterior
(wall) NOS
Subsequent anteroapical transmural (Q wave) infarction (acute)
Subsequent anterolateral transmural (Q wave) infarction (acute)
Subsequent anteroseptal transmural (Q wave) infarction (acute)

✓ Additional Character Req   ✓x7ᵗʰ Placeholder Alert   Manifestation   HCC CMS-HCC Condition   ▽ Unspecified Code   ▶◀ Revised Text   ● New Code   ▲ Revised Code Title

I22.1   **Subsequent ST elevation (STEMI) myocardial infarction** HCC
of inferior wall
    Subsequent acute transmural myocardial infarction of inferior wall
    Subsequent transmural (Q wave) infarction (acute)(of) diaphragmatic wall
    Subsequent transmural (Q wave) infarction (acute)(of) inferior (wall) NOS
    Subsequent inferolateral transmural (Q wave) infarction (acute)
    Subsequent inferoposterior transmural (Q wave) infarction (acute)
    AHA: 2012, 4Q, 102

I22.2   **Subsequent non-ST elevation (NSTEMI) myocardial** HCC
infarction
    Subsequent acute subendocardial myocardial infarction
    Subsequent non-Q wave myocardial infarction NOS
    Subsequent nontransmural myocardial infarction NOS

I22.8   **Subsequent ST elevation (STEMI) myocardial infarction** HCC
of other sites
    Subsequent acute transmural myocardial infarction of other sites
    Subsequent apical-lateral transmural (Q wave) myocardial infarction (acute)
    Subsequent basal-lateral transmural (Q wave) myocardial infarction (acute)
    Subsequent high lateral transmural (Q wave) myocardial infarction (acute)
    Subsequent transmural (Q wave) myocardial infarction (acute)(of) lateral (wall) NOS
    Subsequent posterior (true)transmural (Q wave) myocardial infarction (acute)
    Subsequent posterobasal transmural (Q wave) myocardial infarction (acute)
    Subsequent posterolateral transmural (Q wave) myocardial infarction (acute)
    Subsequent posteroseptal transmural (Q wave) myocardial infarction (acute)
    Subsequent septal NOS transmural (Q wave) myocardial infarction (acute)

I22.9   **Subsequent ST elevation (STEMI) myocardial infarction** HCC ▽
of unspecified site
    Subsequent acute myocardial infarction of unspecified site
    Subsequent myocardial infarction (acute) NOS

✓4th **I23**   **Certain current complications following ST elevation (STEMI)**
and non-ST elevation (NSTEMI) myocardial infarction (within the
28 day period)
    AHA: 2017, 2Q, 11

I23.0   **Hemopericardium as current complication following** HCC
acute myocardial infarction
    EXCLUDES 1   hemopericardium not specified as current complication following acute myocardial infarction (I31.2)

I23.1   **Atrial septal defect as current complication following** HCC A
acute myocardial infarction
    EXCLUDES 1   acquired atrial septal defect not specified as current complication following acute myocardial infarction (I51.0)

I23.2   **Ventricular septal defect as current complication** HCC A
following acute myocardial infarction
    EXCLUDES 1   acquired ventricular septal defect not specified as current complication following acute myocardial infarction (I51.0)

I23.3   **Rupture of cardiac wall without hemopericardium as** HCC A
current complication following acute myocardial infarction

I23.4   **Rupture of chordae tendineae as current complication** HCC
following acute myocardial infarction
    EXCLUDES 1   rupture of chordae tendineae not specified as current complication following acute myocardial infarction (I51.1)

I23.5   **Rupture of papillary muscle as current complication** HCC
following acute myocardial infarction
    EXCLUDES 1   rupture of papillary muscle not specified as current complication following acute myocardial infarction (I51.2)

I23.6   **Thrombosis of atrium, auricular appendage, and** HCC A
ventricle as current complications following acute
myocardial infarction
    EXCLUDES 1   thrombosis of atrium, auricular appendage, and ventricle not specified as current complication following acute myocardial infarction (I51.3)

I23.7   **Postinfarction angina** HCC A
    AHA: 2015, 2Q, 16

I23.8   **Other current complications following acute** HCC A
myocardial infarction

✓4th **I24**   **Other acute ischemic heart diseases**
    EXCLUDES 1   angina pectoris (I20.-)
           transient myocardial ischemia in newborn (P29.4)

I24.0   **Acute coronary thrombosis not resulting in myocardial** HCC
infarction
    Acute coronary (artery) (vein) embolism not resulting in myocardial infarction
    Acute coronary (artery) (vein) occlusion not resulting in myocardial infarction
    Acute coronary (artery) (vein) thromboembolism not resulting in myocardial infarction
    EXCLUDES 1   atherosclerotic heart disease (I25.1-)
    AHA: 2013, 1Q, 24

I24.1   **Dressler's syndrome** HCC
    Postmyocardial infarction syndrome
    EXCLUDES 1   postinfarction angina (I23.7)

I24.8   **Other forms of acute ischemic heart disease** HCC
    EXCLUDES 1   ►myocardial infarction due to demand ischemia (I21.A1)◄

I24.9   **Acute ischemic heart disease, unspecified** HCC ▽
    EXCLUDES 1   ischemic heart disease (chronic) NOS (I25.9)

✓4th **I25**   **Chronic ischemic heart disease**
    Use additional code to identify:
    chronic total occlusion of coronary artery (I25.82)
    exposure to environmental tobacco smoke (Z77.22)
    history of tobacco dependence (Z87.891)
    occupational exposure to environmental tobacco smoke (Z57.31)
    tobacco dependence (F17.-)
    tobacco use (Z72.0)

✓5th **I25.1**   **Atherosclerotic heart disease of native coronary artery**
    Atherosclerotic cardiovascular disease
    Coronary (artery) atheroma
    Coronary (artery) atherosclerosis
    Coronary (artery) disease
    Coronary (artery) sclerosis
    Use additional code, if applicable, to identify:
    coronary atherosclerosis due to calcified coronary lesion (I25.84)
    coronary atherosclerosis due to lipid rich plaque (I25.83)
    EXCLUDES 2   atheroembolism (I75.-)
           atherosclerosis of coronary artery bypass graft(s) and transplanted heart (I25.7-)

I25.10   **Atherosclerotic heart disease of native coronary** A
artery without angina pectoris
    Atherosclerotic heart disease NOS
    AHA: 2015, 2Q, 16; 2012, 4Q, 92

✓6th **I25.11**   **Atherosclerotic heart disease of native coronary**
artery with angina pectoris

    I25.110   **Atherosclerotic heart disease of** HCC A
        native coronary artery with unstable
        angina pectoris
        EXCLUDES 1   unstable angina without atherosclerotic heart disease (I20.0)

    I25.111   **Atherosclerotic heart disease of** HCC A
        native coronary artery with angina
        pectoris
        with documented spasm
        EXCLUDES 1   angina pectoris with documented spasm without atherosclerotic heart disease (I20.1)

Atheromas

Atheromas (fatty tissue and/or plaque)
Lumen

EXCLUDES 1 Not coded here   EXCLUDES 2 Not included here   N Newborn Age: 0   P Pediatric Age: 0-17   M Maternity Age: 12-55   A Adult Age: 15-124

622   ICD-10-CM 2018

I25.118 Atherosclerotic heart disease of HCC A
native coronary artery with other forms of
angina pectoris
> EXCLUDES 1   other forms of angina pectoris
> without atherosclerotic
> heart disease (I20.8)
>
> AHA: 2015, 2Q, 16

I25.119 Atherosclerotic heart disease of HCC A ▽
native coronary artery with unspecified
angina pectoris
> Atherosclerotic heart disease with angina
> NOS
> Atherosclerotic heart disease with ischemic
> chest pain
> EXCLUDES 1   unspecified angina pectoris
> without atherosclerotic
> heart disease (I20.9)

I25.2 Old myocardial infarction
> Healed myocardial infarction
> Past myocardial infarction diagnosed by ECG or other
> investigation, but currently presenting no symptoms

I25.3 Aneurysm of heart
> Mural aneurysm
> Ventricular aneurysm

✓5ᵗʰ **I25.4 Coronary artery aneurysm and dissection**

I25.41 Coronary artery aneurysm
> Coronary arteriovenous fistula, acquired
> EXCLUDES 1   congenital coronary (artery) aneurysm
> (Q24.5)

I25.42 Coronary artery dissection
> **DEF:** A tear in the intimal arterial wall of a coronary
> artery resulting in the sudden intrusion of blood within
> the layers of the wall.

I25.5 Ischemic cardiomyopathy
> EXCLUDES 2   coronary atherosclerosis (I25.1-, I25.7-)

I25.6 Silent myocardial ischemia

✓5ᵗʰ **I25.7 Atherosclerosis of coronary artery** bypass graft(s) **and**
coronary artery of transplanted heart with angina pectoris
> Use additional code, if applicable, to identify:
> coronary atherosclerosis due to calcified coronary lesion
> (I25.84)
> coronary atherosclerosis due to lipid rich plaque (I25.83)
> EXCLUDES 1   atherosclerosis of bypass graft(s) of transplanted heart
> without angina pectoris (I25.812)
> atherosclerosis of coronary artery bypass graft(s)
> without angina pectoris (I25.810)
> atherosclerosis of native coronary artery of
> transplanted heart without angina pectoris
> (I25.811)
> ~~embolism or thrombus of coronary artery bypass~~
> ~~graft(s) (T82.8-)~~

✓6ᵗʰ **I25.70 Atherosclerosis of coronary artery** bypass graft(s),
unspecified, with angina pectoris

I25.700 Atherosclerosis of coronary HCC A ▽
artery bypass graft(s), unspecified, with
unstable **angina pectoris**
> EXCLUDES 1   unstable angina pectoris without
> atherosclerosis of coronary
> artery bypass graft (I20.0)

I25.701 Atherosclerosis of coronary HCC A ▽
artery bypass graft(s), unspecified, with
angina pectoris with documented spasm
> EXCLUDES 1   angina pectoris with documented
> spasm without
> atherosclerosis of coronary
> artery bypass graft (I20.1)

I25.708 Atherosclerosis of coronary HCC A ▽
artery bypass graft(s), unspecified, with
other forms of angina pectoris
> EXCLUDES 1   other forms of angina pectoris
> without atherosclerosis of
> coronary artery bypass graft
> (I20.8)

I25.709 Atherosclerosis of coronary HCC A ▽
artery bypass graft(s), unspecified, with
unspecified angina pectoris
> EXCLUDES 1   unspecified angina pectoris
> without atherosclerosis of
> coronary artery bypass graft
> (I20.9)

✓6ᵗʰ **I25.71 Atherosclerosis of** autologous vein **coronary artery**
bypass graft(s) with angina pectoris

I25.710 Atherosclerosis of autologous vein HCC A
coronary artery bypass graft(s) with
unstable **angina pectoris**
> EXCLUDES 1   unstable angina without
> atherosclerosis of
> autologous vein coronary
> artery bypass graft(s) (I20.0)
> EXCLUDES 2 ►embolism or thrombus of
> coronary artery bypass
> graft(s) (T82.8-)◄

I25.711 Atherosclerosis of autologous vein HCC A
coronary artery bypass graft(s) with
angina pectoris with documented spasm
> EXCLUDES 1   angina pectoris with documented
> spasm without
> atherosclerosis of
> autologous vein coronary
> artery bypass graft(s) (I20.1)

I25.718 Atherosclerosis of autologous vein HCC A
coronary artery bypass graft(s) with
other forms of angina pectoris
> EXCLUDES 1   other forms of angina pectoris
> without atherosclerosis of
> autologous vein coronary
> artery bypass graft(s) (I20.8)

I25.719 Atherosclerosis of autologous HCC A ▽
vein coronary artery bypass graft(s) with
unspecified angina pectoris
> EXCLUDES 1   unspecified angina pectoris
> without atherosclerosis of
> autologous vein coronary
> artery bypass graft(s) (I20.9)

✓6ᵗʰ **I25.72 Atherosclerosis of** autologous artery **coronary artery**
bypass graft(s) with angina pectoris
> Atherosclerosis of internal mammary artery graft with
> angina pectoris

I25.720 Atherosclerosis of autologous artery HCC A
coronary artery bypass graft(s) with
unstable **angina pectoris**
> EXCLUDES 1   unstable angina without
> atherosclerosis of
> autologous artery coronary
> artery bypass graft(s) (I20.0)

I25.721 Atherosclerosis of autologous artery HCC A
coronary artery bypass graft(s) with
angina pectoris with documented spasm
> EXCLUDES 1   angina pectoris with documented
> spasm without
> atherosclerosis of
> autologous artery coronary
> artery bypass graft(s) (I20.1)

I25.728 Atherosclerosis of autologous artery HCC A
coronary artery bypass graft(s) with
other forms of angina pectoris
> EXCLUDES 1   other forms of angina pectoris
> without atherosclerosis of
> autologous artery coronary
> artery bypass graft(s) (I20.8)

I25.729 Atherosclerosis of autologous HCC A ▽
artery coronary artery bypass graft(s)
with unspecified angina pectoris
> EXCLUDES 1   unspecified angina pectoris
> without atherosclerosis of
> autologous artery coronary
> artery bypass graft(s) (I20.9)

✓6ᵗʰ **I25.73 Atherosclerosis of** nonautologous biological
coronary artery bypass graft(s) with angina pectoris

I25.730 Atherosclerosis of nonautologous HCC A
biological coronary artery bypass graft(s)
with unstable **angina pectoris**
> EXCLUDES 1   unstable angina without
> atherosclerosis of
> nonautologous biological
> coronary artery bypass
> graft(s) (I20.0)

✓ Additional Character Req   ✓x7ᵗʰ Placeholder Alert   Manifestation   HCC CMS-HCC Condition   ▽ Unspecified Code   ►◄ Revised Text   ● New Code   ▲ Revised Code Title

I25.731 Atherosclerosis of nonautologous [HCC] [A]
biological coronary artery bypass graft(s)
with angina pectoris with documented
spasm
> **EXCLUDES 1** angina pectoris with documented
> spasm without
> atherosclerosis of
> nonautologous biological
> coronary artery bypass
> graft(s) (I20.1)

I25.738 Atherosclerosis of nonautologous [HCC] [A]
biological coronary artery bypass graft(s)
with other forms of angina pectoris
> **EXCLUDES 1** other forms of angina pectoris
> without atherosclerosis of
> nonautologous biological
> coronary artery bypass
> graft(s) (I20.8)

I25.739 Atherosclerosis of nonautologous [HCC] [A] ▽
biological coronary artery bypass graft(s)
with unspecified angina pectoris
> **EXCLUDES 1** unspecified angina pectoris
> without atherosclerosis of
> nonautologous biological
> coronary artery bypass
> graft(s) (I20.9)

✓6th **I25.75** Atherosclerosis of native coronary artery of
transplanted heart with angina pectoris
> **EXCLUDES 1** atherosclerosis of native coronary artery of
> transplanted heart without angina
> pectoris (I25.811)

I25.750 Atherosclerosis of native coronary [HCC]
artery of transplanted heart with
unstable angina

I25.751 Atherosclerosis of native coronary [HCC]
artery of transplanted heart with
angina pectoris with documented
spasm

I25.758 Atherosclerosis of native coronary [HCC]
artery of transplanted heart with
other forms of angina pectoris

I25.759 Atherosclerosis of native coronary [HCC] ▽
artery of transplanted heart with
unspecified angina pectoris

✓6th **I25.76** Atherosclerosis of bypass graft of coronary artery of
transplanted heart with angina pectoris
> **EXCLUDES 1** atherosclerosis of bypass graft of coronary
> artery of transplanted heart without
> angina pectoris (I25.812)

I25.760 Atherosclerosis of bypass graft of [HCC] [A]
coronary artery of transplanted heart
with unstable angina

I25.761 Atherosclerosis of bypass graft of [HCC] [A]
coronary artery of transplanted heart
with angina pectoris with documented
spasm

I25.768 Atherosclerosis of bypass graft of [HCC] [A]
coronary artery of transplanted heart
with other forms of angina pectoris

I25.769 Atherosclerosis of bypass graft of [HCC] [A] ▽
coronary artery of transplanted heart
with unspecified angina pectoris

✓6th **I25.79** Atherosclerosis of other coronary artery bypass
graft(s) with angina pectoris

I25.790 Atherosclerosis of other coronary [HCC] [A]
artery bypass graft(s) with unstable
angina pectoris
> **EXCLUDES 1** unstable angina without
> atherosclerosis of other
> coronary artery bypass
> graft(s) (I20.0)

I25.791 Atherosclerosis of other coronary [HCC] [A]
artery bypass graft(s) with angina
pectoris with documented spasm
> **EXCLUDES 1** angina pectoris with documented
> spasm without
> atherosclerosis of other
> coronary artery bypass
> graft(s) (I20.1)

I25.798 Atherosclerosis of other coronary [HCC] [A]
artery bypass graft(s) with other
forms of angina pectoris
> **EXCLUDES 1** other forms of angina pectoris
> without atherosclerosis of
> other coronary artery bypass
> graft(s) (I20.8)

I25.799 Atherosclerosis of other coronary [HCC] [A] ▽
artery bypass graft(s) with unspecified
angina pectoris
> **EXCLUDES 1** unspecified angina pectoris
> without atherosclerosis of
> other coronary artery bypass
> graft(s) (I20.9)

✓5th **I25.8** Other forms of chronic ischemic heart disease

✓6th **I25.81** Atherosclerosis of other coronary vessels without
angina pectoris
Use additional code, if applicable, to identify:
coronary atherosclerosis due to calcified coronary
lesion (I25.84)
coronary atherosclerosis due to lipid rich plaque
(I25.83)
> **EXCLUDES 1** atherosclerotic heart disease of native
> coronary artery without angina pectoris
> (I25.10)

I25.810 Atherosclerosis of coronary artery [A]
bypass graft(s) without angina pectoris
Atherosclerosis of coronary artery bypass
graft NOS
> **EXCLUDES 1** atherosclerosis of coronary
> bypass graft(s) with angina
> pectoris (I25.70--I25.73-,
> I25.79-)

I25.811 Atherosclerosis of native coronary
artery of transplanted heart without
angina pectoris
Atherosclerosis of native coronary artery of
transplanted heart NOS
> **EXCLUDES 1** atherosclerosis of native coronary
> artery of transplanted heart
> with angina pectoris
> (I25.75-)

I25.812 Atherosclerosis of bypass graft of [A]
coronary artery of transplanted heart
without angina pectoris
Atherosclerosis of bypass graft of
transplanted heart NOS
> **EXCLUDES 1** atherosclerosis of bypass graft of
> transplanted heart with
> angina pectoris (I25.76)

I25.82 Chronic total occlusion of coronary artery
Complete occlusion of coronary artery
Total occlusion of coronary artery
Code first coronary atherosclerosis (I25.1-, I25.7-,
I25.81-)
> **EXCLUDES 1** ▶acute coronary occlusion with myocardial
> infarction (I21.0-I21.9, I22.-)◀
> ▶acute coronary occlusion without
> myocardial infarction◀ (I24.0)

DEF: Complete blockage of coronary artery due to
plaque accumulation over an extended period of time;
results in substantial reduction of blood flow;
characterized by angina or chest pain.

I25.83 Coronary atherosclerosis due to lipid rich plaque [A]
Code first coronary atherosclerosis (I25.1-, I25.7-,
I25.81-)

I25.84 Coronary atherosclerosis due to calcified coronary
lesion
Coronary atherosclerosis due to severely calcified
coronary lesion
Code first coronary atherosclerosis (I25.1-, I25.7-,
I25.81-)

I25.89 Other forms of chronic ischemic heart disease

I25.9 Chronic ischemic heart disease, unspecified ▽
Ischemic heart disease (chronic) NOS

EXCLUDES 1 Not coded here   **EXCLUDES 2** Not included here   [N] Newborn Age: 0   [P] Pediatric Age: 0-17   [M] Maternity Age: 12-55   [A] Adult Age: 15-124

I25.731–I25.9

624   ICD-10-CM 2018

Pulmonary heart disease and diseases of pulmonary circulation (I26-I28)

☑4ᵗʰ **I26**   **Pulmonary embolism**
INCLUDES   pulmonary (acute) (artery)(vein) infarction
     pulmonary (acute) (artery)(vein) thromboembolism
     pulmonary (acute) (artery)(vein) thrombosis
EXCLUDES 2   *chronic pulmonary embolism (I27.82)*
     personal history of pulmonary embolism (Z86.711)
     pulmonary embolism complicating abortion, ectopic or molar
       pregnancy (O00-O07, O08.2)
     pulmonary embolism complicating pregnancy, childbirth and
       the puerperium (O88.-)
     pulmonary embolism due to complications of surgical and
       medical care (T80.0, T81.7-, T82.8-)
     pulmonary embolism due to trauma (T79.0, T79.1)
     septic (non-pulmonary) arterial embolism (I76)

   ☑5ᵗʰ **I26.0**   **Pulmonary embolism** with acute cor pulmonale
     I26.01   **Septic pulmonary embolism with acute cor**   HCC
       pulmonale
         Code first underlying infection
     I26.02   **Saddle embolus of pulmonary artery with**   HCC
       acute cor pulmonale
     I26.09   **Other pulmonary embolism with acute cor**   HCC
       pulmonale
         Acute cor pulmonale NOS
         AHA: 2014, 4Q, 21

   ☑5ᵗʰ **I26.9**   **Pulmonary embolism** without acute cor pulmonale
     I26.90   **Septic pulmonary embolism without acute**   HCC
       cor pulmonale
         Code first underlying infection
     I26.92   **Saddle embolus of pulmonary artery without**   HCC
       acute cor pulmonale
     I26.99   **Other pulmonary embolism without acute**   HCC
       cor pulmonale
         Acute pulmonary embolism NOS
         Pulmonary embolism NOS

☑4ᵗʰ **I27**   **Other pulmonary heart diseases**
     I27.0   **Primary pulmonary hypertension**   HCC
       ▶Heritable pulmonary arterial hypertension
       Idiopathic pulmonary arterial hypertension
       Primary group 1 pulmonary hypertension
       Primary pulmonary arterial hypertension◀
       EXCLUDES 1 ▶*persistent pulmonary hypertension of newborn*
         (P29.30)◀
         pulmonary hypertension NOS ▶*(I27.20)*◀
         ▶*secondary pulmonary arterial hypertension (I27.21)*◀
         secondary pulmonary hypertension ▶*(I27.29)*◀

     I27.1   **Kyphoscoliotic heart disease**   HCC

   ☑5ᵗʰ **I27.2**   **Other** secondary pulmonary hypertension
       ~~Pulmonary hypertension NOS~~
       Code also associated underlying condition
       EXCLUDES 1 ▶*Eisenmenger's syndrome (I27.83)*◀
       AHA: 2014, 4Q, 21

●   **I27.20**   **Pulmonary hypertension, unspecified**   ▽
         Pulmonary hypertension NOS

●   **I27.21**   **Secondary pulmonary arterial hypertension**
         (Associated) (drug-induced) (toxin-induced)
           pulmonary arterial hypertension NOS
         (Associated) (drug-induced) (toxin-induced)
           (secondary) group 1 pulmonary hypertension
         Code also associated conditions if applicable, or
           adverse effects of drugs or toxins, such as:
           adverse effect of appetite depressants (T50.5X5)
           congenital heart disease (Q20-Q28)
           human immunodeficiency virus [HIV] disease (B20)
           polymyositis (M33.2-)
           portal hypertension (K76.6)
           rheumatoid arthritis (M05.-)
           schistosomiasis (B65.-)
           Sjögren syndrome (M35.0-)
           systemic sclerosis (M34.-)

●   **I27.22**   **Pulmonary hypertension** due to left heart disease
         Group 2 pulmonary hypertension
         Code also associated left heart disease, if known, such
           as:
           multiple valve disease (I08.-)
           rheumatic mitral valve diseases (I05.-)
           rheumatic aortic valve diseases (I06.-)

●   **I27.23**   **Pulmonary hypertension** due to lung diseases and
       hypoxia
         Group 3 pulmonary hypertension
         Code also associated lung disease, if known, such as:
           bronchiectasis (J47.-)
           cystic fibrosis with pulmonary manifestations
             (E84.0)
           interstitial lung disease (J84.-)
           pleural effusion (J90)
           sleep apnea (G47.3-)

●   **I27.24**   Chronic thromboembolic **pulmonary hypertension**
         Group 4 pulmonary hypertension
         Code also associated pulmonary embolism, if
           applicable (I26.-, I27.82)

●   **I27.29**   **Other secondary pulmonary hypertension**
         Group 5 pulmonary hypertension
         Pulmonary hypertension with unclear multifactorial
           mechanisms
         Pulmonary hypertension due to hematologic
           disorders
         Pulmonary hypertension due to metabolic disorders
         Pulmonary hypertension due to other systemic
           disorders
         Code also other associated disorders, if known, such
           as:
           chronic myeloid leukemia (C92.10- C92.22)
           essential thrombocythemia (D47.3)
           Gaucher disease (E75.22)
           hypertensive chronic kidney disease with end stage
             renal disease (I12.0, I12.11, I13.2)
           hyperthyroidism (E05.-)
           hypothyroidism (E00-E03)
           polycythemia vera (D45)
           sarcoidosis (D86.-)
         AHA: 2016, 2Q, 8

   ☑5ᵗʰ **I27.8**   **Other specified pulmonary heart diseases**
     I27.81   **Cor pulmonale (chronic)**   HCC
         Cor pulmonale NOS
         EXCLUDES 1 *acute cor pulmonale (I26.0-)*
         AHA: 2014, 4Q, 21
     I27.82   **Chronic pulmonary embolism**   HCC
         Use additional code, if applicable, for associated
           long-term (current) use of anticoagulants
           (Z79.01)
         EXCLUDES 1 *personal history of pulmonary embolism*
           (Z86.711)
         DEF: A long-standing condition commonly associated
         with pulmonary hypertension in which small blood clots
         travel to the lungs repeatedly over many weeks,
         months, or years, requiring continuation of established
         anticoagulant or thrombolytic therapy.

●   **I27.83**   **Eisenmenger's syndrome**
         Eisenmenger's complex
         (Irreversible) Eisenmenger's disease
         Pulmonary hypertension with right to left shunt
           related to congenital heart disease
         Code also underlying heart defect, if known, such as:
           atrial septal defect (Q21.1)
           Eisenmenger's defect (Q21.8)
           patent ductus arteriosus (Q25.0)
           ventricular septal defect (Q21.0)
     I27.89   **Other specified pulmonary heart diseases**   HCC
         ~~Eisenmenger's complex~~
         ~~Eisenmenger's syndrome~~
         EXCLUDES 1 *Eisenmenger's defect (Q21.8)*

     I27.9   **Pulmonary heart disease, unspecified**   HCC ▽
       Chronic cardiopulmonary disease

☑4ᵗʰ **I28**   **Other diseases of pulmonary vessels**
     I28.0   **Arteriovenous fistula of pulmonary vessels**   HCC
       EXCLUDES 1 *congenital arteriovenous fistula (Q25.72)*
     I28.1   **Aneurysm of pulmonary artery**   HCC
       EXCLUDES 1 *congenital aneurysm (Q25.79)*
               congenital arteriovenous aneurysm (Q25.72)
     I28.8   **Other diseases of pulmonary vessels**   HCC
       Pulmonary arteritis
       Pulmonary endarteritis
       Rupture of pulmonary vessels
       Stenosis of pulmonary vessels
       Stricture of pulmonary vessels
     I28.9   **Disease of pulmonary vessels, unspecified**   HCC ▽

☑ Additional Character Req   ☑7ᵗʰ Placeholder Alert   Manifestation   HCC CMS-HCC Condition   ▽ Unspecified Code   ▶◀ Revised Text   ● New Code   ▲ Revised Code Title

Other forms of heart disease (I30-I52)

✓4th I30 Acute pericarditis
> **INCLUDES** acute mediastinopericarditis
> acute myopericarditis
> acute pericardial effusion
> acute pleuropericarditis
> acute pneumopericarditis
> **EXCLUDES 1** Dressler's syndrome (I24.1)
> rheumatic pericarditis (acute) (I01.0)
> ►viral pericarditis due to Coxsakie virus (B33.23)◄

I30.0 Acute nonspecific idiopathic pericarditis

I30.1 Infective pericarditis
> Pneumococcal pericarditis
> Pneumopyopericardium
> Purulent pericarditis
> Pyopericarditis
> Pyopericardium
> Pyopneumopericardium
> Staphylococcal pericarditis
> Streptococcal pericarditis
> Suppurative pericarditis
> Viral pericarditis
> Use additional code (B95-B97) to identify infectious agent

I30.8 Other forms of acute pericarditis

I30.9 Acute pericarditis, unspecified ▽

✓4th I31 Other diseases of pericardium
> **EXCLUDES 1** diseases of pericardium specified as rheumatic (I09.2)
> postcardiotomy syndrome (I97.0)
> traumatic injury to pericardium (S26.-)

I31.0 Chronic adhesive pericarditis
> Accretio cordis
> Adherent pericardium
> Adhesive mediastinopericarditis

I31.1 Chronic constrictive pericarditis
> Concretio cordis
> Pericardial calcification

I31.2 Hemopericardium, not elsewhere classified
> **EXCLUDES 1** hemopericardium as current complication following
> acute myocardial infarction (I23.0)
> **DEF:** Presence of blood in the pericardial sac (pericardium). It can
> lead to potentially fatal cardiac tamponade if enough blood enters
> the pericardial cavity.

I31.3 Pericardial effusion (noninflammatory)
> Chylopericardium
> **EXCLUDES 1** acute pericardial effusion (I30.9)

I31.4 Cardiac tamponade
> Code first underlying cause

I31.8 Other specified diseases of pericardium
> Epicardial plaques
> Focal pericardial adhesions

I31.9 Disease of pericardium, unspecified ▽
> Pericarditis (chronic) NOS

Cardiac Tamponade

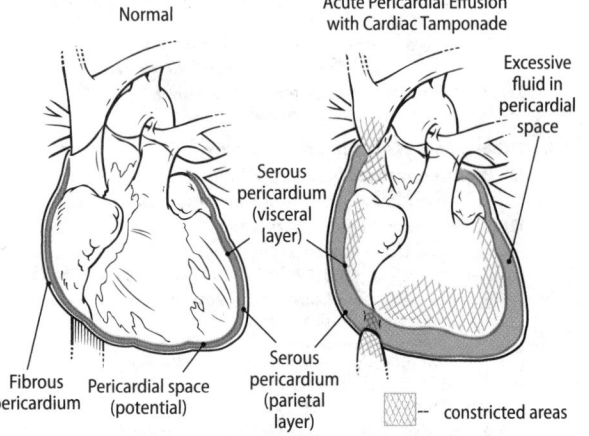

Normal

Acute Pericardial Effusion with Cardiac Tamponade

Excessive fluid in pericardial space

Serous pericardium (visceral layer)

Fibrous pericardium

Pericardial space (potential)

Serous pericardium (parietal layer)

⬚ — constricted areas

I32 Pericarditis in diseases classified elsewhere
> Code first underlying disease
> **EXCLUDES 1** pericarditis (in):
> coxsackie (virus) (B33.23)
> gonococcal (A54.83)
> meningococcal (A39.53)
> rheumatoid (arthritis) (M05.31)
> syphilitic (A52.06)
> systemic lupus erythematosus (M32.12)
> tuberculosis (A18.84)

✓4th I33 Acute and subacute endocarditis
> **EXCLUDES 1** acute rheumatic endocarditis (I01.1)
> endocarditis NOS (I38)

I33.0 Acute and subacute infective endocarditis
> Bacterial endocarditis (acute) (subacute)
> Infective endocarditis (acute) (subacute) NOS
> Endocarditis lenta (acute) (subacute)
> Malignant endocarditis (acute) (subacute)
> Purulent endocarditis (acute) (subacute)
> Septic endocarditis (acute) (subacute)
> Ulcerative endocarditis (acute) (subacute)
> Vegetative endocarditis (acute) (subacute)
> Use additional code (B95-B97) to identify infectious agent

I33.9 Acute and subacute endocarditis, unspecified ▽
> Acute endocarditis NOS
> Acute myoendocarditis NOS
> Acute periendocarditis NOS
> Subacute endocarditis NOS
> Subacute myoendocarditis NOS
> Subacute periendocarditis NOS

✓4th I34 Nonrheumatic mitral valve disorders
> **EXCLUDES 1** mitral valve disease (I05.9)
> mitral valve failure (I05.8)
> mitral valve stenosis (I05.0)
> mitral valve disorder of unspecified cause with diseases of aortic
> and/or tricuspid valve(s) (I08.-)
> mitral valve disorder of unspecified cause with mitral stenosis or
> obstruction (I05.0)
> mitral valve disorder specified as congenital ►(Q23.2, Q23.9)◄
> mitral valve disorder specified as rheumatic (I05.-)

I34.0 Nonrheumatic mitral (valve) insufficiency
> Nonrheumatic mitral (valve) incompetence NOS
> Nonrheumatic mitral (valve) regurgitation NOS

I34.1 Nonrheumatic mitral (valve) prolapse
> Floppy nonrheumatic mitral valve syndrome
> **EXCLUDES 1** Marfan's syndrome (Q87.4-)

I34.2 Nonrheumatic mitral (valve) stenosis

I34.8 Other nonrheumatic mitral valve disorders

I34.9 Nonrheumatic mitral valve disorder, unspecified ▽

✓4th I35 Nonrheumatic aortic valve disorders
> **EXCLUDES 1** aortic valve disorder of unspecified cause but with diseases of
> mitral and/or tricuspid valve(s) (I08.-)
> aortic valve disorder specified as congenital (Q23.0, Q23.1)
> aortic valve disorder specified as rheumatic (I06.-)
> hypertrophic subaortic stenosis (I42.1)

I35.0 Nonrheumatic aortic (valve) stenosis

I35.1 Nonrheumatic aortic (valve) insufficiency
> Nonrheumatic aortic (valve) incompetence NOS
> Nonrheumatic aortic (valve) regurgitation NOS

I35.2 Nonrheumatic aortic (valve) stenosis with insufficiency

I35.8 Other nonrheumatic aortic valve disorders

I35.9 Nonrheumatic aortic valve disorder, unspecified ▽

✓4th I36 Nonrheumatic tricuspid valve disorders
> **EXCLUDES 1** tricuspid valve disorders of unspecified cause (I07.-)
> tricuspid valve disorders specified as congenital (Q22.4, Q22.8,
> Q22.9)
> tricuspid valve disorders specified as rheumatic (I07.-)
> tricuspid valve disorders with aortic and/or mitral valve
> involvement (I08.-)

I36.0 Nonrheumatic tricuspid (valve) stenosis

I36.1 Nonrheumatic tricuspid (valve) insufficiency
> Nonrheumatic tricuspid (valve) incompetence
> Nonrheumatic tricuspid (valve) regurgitation

I36.2 Nonrheumatic tricuspid (valve) stenosis with insufficiency

I36.8 Other nonrheumatic tricuspid valve disorders

I36.9 Nonrheumatic tricuspid valve disorder, unspecified ▽

EXCLUDES 1 Not coded here — **EXCLUDES 2** Not included here — N Newborn Age: 0 — P Pediatric Age: 0-17 — M Maternity Age: 12-55 — A Adult Age: 15-124

626 — ICD-10-CM 2018

Chapter 9. Diseases of the Circulatory System

✓4ᵗʰ **I37** **Nonrheumatic pulmonary valve disorders**

EXCLUDES 1   pulmonary valve disorder specified as congenital (Q22.1, Q22.2, Q22.3)
    pulmonary valve disorder specified as rheumatic (I09.89)

I37.0 **Nonrheumatic pulmonary valve stenosis**

I37.1 **Nonrheumatic pulmonary valve insufficiency**
    Nonrheumatic pulmonary valve incompetence
    Nonrheumatic pulmonary valve regurgitation

I37.2 **Nonrheumatic pulmonary valve stenosis with insufficiency**

I37.8 **Other nonrheumatic pulmonary valve disorders**

I37.9 **Nonrheumatic pulmonary valve disorder, unspecified** ▽

✓4ᵗʰ **I38** **Endocarditis, valve unspecified** ▽

INCLUDES   endocarditis (chronic) NOS
    valvular incompetence NOS
    valvular insufficiency NOS
    valvular regurgitation NOS
    valvular stenosis NOS
    valvulitis (chronic) NOS

EXCLUDES 1   congenital insufficiency of cardiac valve NOS (Q24.8)
    congenital stenosis of cardiac valve NOS (Q24.8)
    endocardial fibroelastosis (I42.4)
    endocarditis specified as rheumatic (I09.1)

I39 *Endocarditis and heart valve disorders in diseases classified elsewhere*

Code first underlying disease, such as:
    Q fever (A78)

EXCLUDES 1   endocardial involvement in:
    candidiasis (B37.6)
    gonococcal infection (A54.83)
    Libman-Sacks disease (M32.11)
    listerosis (A32.82)
    meningococcal infection (A39.51)
    rheumatoid arthritis (M05.31)
    syphilis (A52.03)
    tuberculosis (A18.84)
    typhoid fever (A01.02)

✓4ᵗʰ **I40** **Acute myocarditis**

INCLUDES   subacute myocarditis
EXCLUDES 1   acute rheumatic myocarditis (I01.2)

I40.0 **Infective myocarditis**
    Septic myocarditis
    Use additional code (B95-B97) to identify infectious agent

I40.1 **Isolated myocarditis**
    Fiedler's myocarditis
    Giant cell myocarditis
    Idiopathic myocarditis

I40.8 **Other acute myocarditis**

I40.9 **Acute myocarditis, unspecified** ▽

I41 *Myocarditis in diseases classified elsewhere*

Code first underlying disease, such as:
    typhus (A75.0-A75.9)

EXCLUDES 1   myocarditis (in):
    Chagas' disease (chronic) (B57.2)
      acute (B57.0)
    coxsackie (virus) infection (B33.22)
    diphtheritic (A36.81)
    gonococcal (A54.83)
    influenzal (J09.X9, J10.82, J11.82)
    meningococcal (A39.52)
    mumps (B26.82)
    rheumatoid arthritis (M05.31)
    sarcoid (D86.85)
    syphilis (A52.06)
    toxoplasmosis (B58.81)
    tuberculous (A18.84)

✓4ᵗʰ **I42** **Cardiomyopathy**

INCLUDES   myocardiopathy
Code first pre-existing cardiomyopathy complicating pregnancy and puerperium (O99.4)

EXCLUDES 2   ischemic cardiomyopathy (I25.5)
    peripartum cardiomyopathy (O90.3)
    ventricular hypertrophy (I51.7)

I42.0 **Dilated cardiomyopathy** HCC
    Congestive cardiomyopathy

I42.1 **Obstructive hypertrophic cardiomyopathy** HCC
    Hypertrophic subaortic stenosis (idiopathic)
    DEF: Cardiomyopathy marked by left ventricle hypertrophy, enlarged septum; results in obstructed blood flow, arrhythmias, mitral regurgitation, and sudden cardiac death.

I42.2 **Other hypertrophic cardiomyopathy** HCC
    Nonobstructive hypertrophic cardiomyopathy

I42.3 **Endomyocardial (eosinophilic) disease** HCC
    Endomyocardial (tropical) fibrosis
    Löffler's endocarditis

I42.4 **Endocardial fibroelastosis** HCC
    Congenital cardiomyopathy
    Elastomyofibrosis

I42.5 **Other restrictive cardiomyopathy** HCC
    Constrictive cardiomyopathy NOS

I42.6 **Alcoholic cardiomyopathy** HCC
    Code also presence of alcoholism (F10.-)

I42.7 **Cardiomyopathy due to drug and external agent** HCC
    Code first poisoning due to drug or toxin, if applicable (T36-T65 with fifth or sixth character 1-4 or 6)
    Use additional code for adverse effect, if applicable, to identify drug (T36-T50 with fifth or sixth character 5)

I42.8 **Other cardiomyopathies** HCC

I42.9 **Cardiomyopathy, unspecified** HCC ▽
    Cardiomyopathy (primary) (secondary) NOS

I43 *Cardiomyopathy in diseases classified elsewhere* HCC

Code first underlying disease, such as:
    amyloidosis (E85.-)
    glycogen storage disease (E74.0)
    gout (M10.0-)
    thyrotoxicosis (E05.0-E05.9-)

EXCLUDES 1   cardiomyopathy (in):
    coxsackie (virus) (B33.24)
    diphtheria (A36.81)
    sarcoidosis (D86.85)
    tuberculosis (A18.84)

✓4ᵗʰ **I44** **Atrioventricular and left bundle-branch block**

I44.0 **Atrioventricular block, first degree**

I44.1 **Atrioventricular block, second degree**
    Atrioventricular block, type I and II
    Möbitz block, type I and II
    Second degree block, type I and II
    Wenckebach's block

I44.2 **Atrioventricular block, complete** HCC
    Complete heart block NOS
    Third degree block

✓5ᵗʰ **I44.3** **Other and unspecified atrioventricular block**
    Atrioventricular block NOS

   I44.30 **Unspecified atrioventricular block** ▽

   I44.39 **Other atrioventricular block**

I44.4 **Left anterior fascicular block**

I44.5 **Left posterior fascicular block**

✓5ᵗʰ **I44.6** **Other and unspecified fascicular block**

   I44.60 **Unspecified fascicular block** ▽
      Left bundle-branch hemiblock NOS

   I44.69 **Other fascicular block**

I44.7 **Left bundle-branch block, unspecified** ▽

✓4ᵗʰ **I45** **Other conduction disorders**

I45.0 **Right fascicular block**

✓5ᵗʰ **I45.1** **Other and unspecified right bundle-branch block**

   I45.10 **Unspecified right bundle-branch block** ▽
      Right bundle-branch block NOS

   I45.19 **Other right bundle-branch block**

I45.2 **Bifascicular block**

I45.3 **Trifascicular block**

I45.4 **Nonspecific intraventricular block**
    Bundle-branch block NOS

I45.5 **Other specified heart block**
    Sinoatrial block
    Sinoauricular block
    EXCLUDES 1   heart block NOS (I45.9)

I45.6 **Pre-excitation syndrome**
    Accelerated atrioventricular conduction
    Accessory atrioventricular conduction
    Anomalous atrioventricular excitation
    Lown-Ganong-Levine syndrome
    Pre-excitation atrioventricular conduction
    Wolff-Parkinson-White syndrome

Chapter 9. Diseases of the Circulatory System

Conduction Disorders

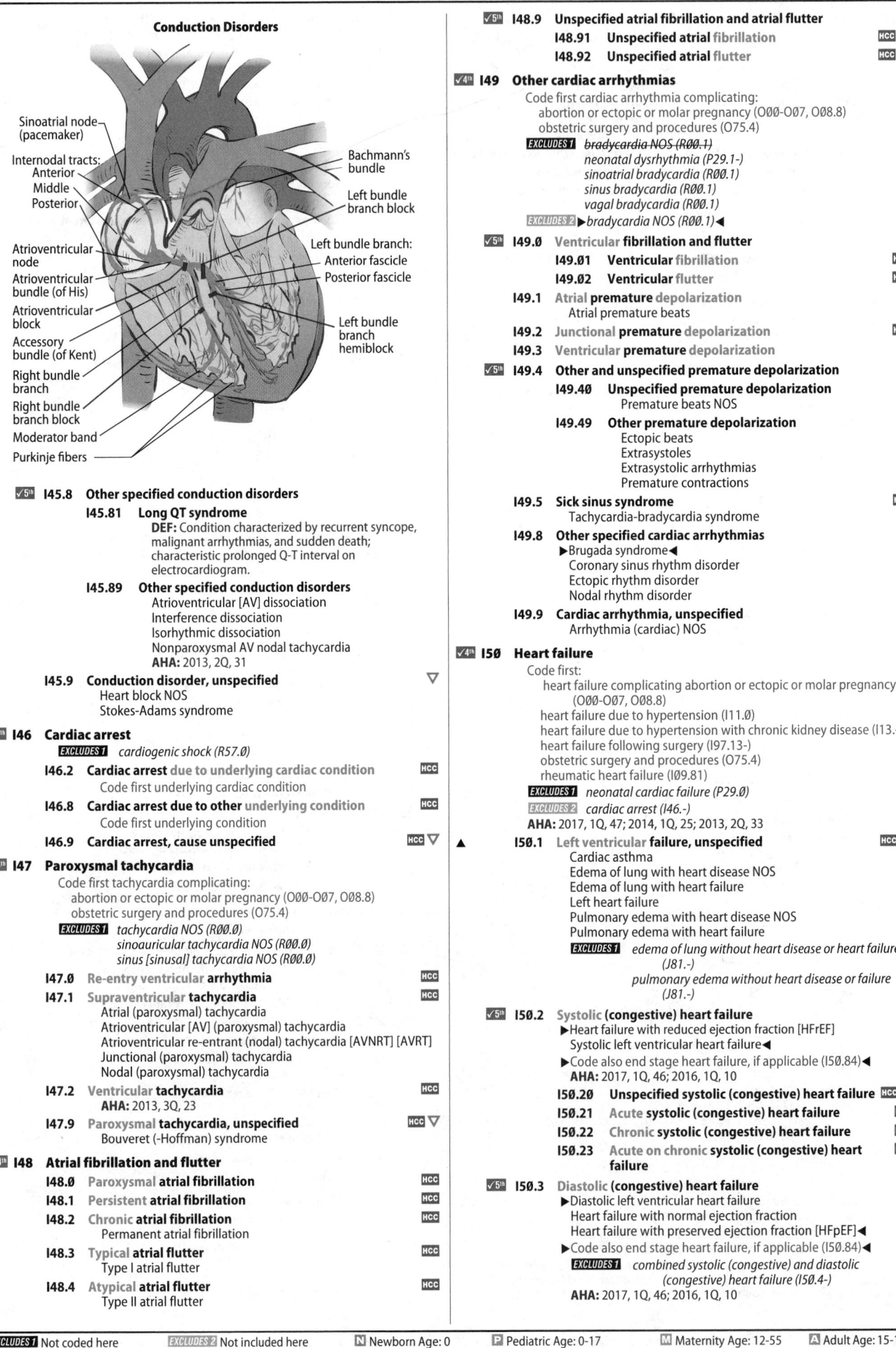

Sinoatrial node (pacemaker)
Internodal tracts: Anterior, Middle, Posterior
Atrioventricular node
Atrioventricular bundle (of His)
Atrioventricular block
Accessory bundle (of Kent)
Right bundle branch
Right bundle branch block
Moderator band
Purkinje fibers
Bachmann's bundle
Left bundle branch block
Left bundle branch: Anterior fascicle, Posterior fascicle
Left bundle branch hemiblock

✓5ᵗʰ I45.8 Other specified conduction disorders

I45.81 Long QT syndrome
DEF: Condition characterized by recurrent syncope, malignant arrhythmias, and sudden death; characteristic prolonged Q-T interval on electrocardiogram.

I45.89 Other specified conduction disorders
Atrioventricular [AV] dissociation
Interference dissociation
Isorhythmic dissociation
Nonparoxysmal AV nodal tachycardia
AHA: 2013, 2Q, 31

I45.9 Conduction disorder, unspecified ▽
Heart block NOS
Stokes-Adams syndrome

✓4ᵗʰ I46 Cardiac arrest
EXCLUDES 1 cardiogenic shock (R57.0)

I46.2 Cardiac arrest due to underlying cardiac condition HCC
Code first underlying cardiac condition

I46.8 Cardiac arrest due to other underlying condition HCC
Code first underlying condition

I46.9 Cardiac arrest, cause unspecified HCC ▽

✓4ᵗʰ I47 Paroxysmal tachycardia
Code first tachycardia complicating:
  abortion or ectopic or molar pregnancy (O00-O07, O08.8)
  obstetric surgery and procedures (O75.4)
EXCLUDES 1 tachycardia NOS (R00.0)
  sinoauricular tachycardia NOS (R00.0)
  sinus [sinusal] tachycardia NOS (R00.0)

I47.0 Re-entry ventricular arrhythmia HCC

I47.1 Supraventricular tachycardia HCC
Atrial (paroxysmal) tachycardia
Atrioventricular [AV] (paroxysmal) tachycardia
Atrioventricular re-entrant (nodal) tachycardia [AVNRT] [AVRT]
Junctional (paroxysmal) tachycardia
Nodal (paroxysmal) tachycardia

I47.2 Ventricular tachycardia HCC
AHA: 2013, 3Q, 23

I47.9 Paroxysmal tachycardia, unspecified HCC ▽
Bouveret (-Hoffman) syndrome

✓4ᵗʰ I48 Atrial fibrillation and flutter

I48.0 Paroxysmal atrial fibrillation HCC

I48.1 Persistent atrial fibrillation HCC

I48.2 Chronic atrial fibrillation HCC
Permanent atrial fibrillation

I48.3 Typical atrial flutter HCC
Type I atrial flutter

I48.4 Atypical atrial flutter HCC
Type II atrial flutter

✓5ᵗʰ I48.9 Unspecified atrial fibrillation and atrial flutter

I48.91 Unspecified atrial fibrillation HCC ▽

I48.92 Unspecified atrial flutter HCC ▽

✓4ᵗʰ I49 Other cardiac arrhythmias
Code first cardiac arrhythmia complicating:
  abortion or ectopic or molar pregnancy (O00-O07, O08.8)
  obstetric surgery and procedures (O75.4)
EXCLUDES 1 *bradycardia NOS (R00.1)*
  neonatal dysrhythmia (P29.1-)
  sinoatrial bradycardia (R00.1)
  sinus bradycardia (R00.1)
  vagal bradycardia (R00.1)
EXCLUDES 2 ▶*bradycardia NOS (R00.1)*◀

✓5ᵗʰ I49.0 Ventricular fibrillation and flutter

I49.01 Ventricular fibrillation HCC

I49.02 Ventricular flutter HCC

I49.1 Atrial premature depolarization
Atrial premature beats

I49.2 Junctional premature depolarization HCC

I49.3 Ventricular premature depolarization

✓5ᵗʰ I49.4 Other and unspecified premature depolarization

I49.40 Unspecified premature depolarization ▽
Premature beats NOS

I49.49 Other premature depolarization
Ectopic beats
Extrasystoles
Extrasystolic arrhythmias
Premature contractions

I49.5 Sick sinus syndrome HCC
Tachycardia-bradycardia syndrome

I49.8 Other specified cardiac arrhythmias
▶Brugada syndrome◀
Coronary sinus rhythm disorder
Ectopic rhythm disorder
Nodal rhythm disorder

I49.9 Cardiac arrhythmia, unspecified ▽
Arrhythmia (cardiac) NOS

✓4ᵗʰ I50 Heart failure
Code first:
  heart failure complicating abortion or ectopic or molar pregnancy (O00-O07, O08.8)
  heart failure due to hypertension (I11.0)
  heart failure due to hypertension with chronic kidney disease (I13.-)
  heart failure following surgery (I97.13-)
  obstetric surgery and procedures (O75.4)
  rheumatic heart failure (I09.81)
EXCLUDES 1 *neonatal cardiac failure (P29.0)*
EXCLUDES 2 *cardiac arrest (I46.-)*
AHA: 2017, 1Q, 47; 2014, 1Q, 25; 2013, 2Q, 33

▲ **I50.1 Left ventricular failure, unspecified** HCC ▽
Cardiac asthma
Edema of lung with heart disease NOS
Edema of lung with heart failure
Left heart failure
Pulmonary edema with heart disease NOS
Pulmonary edema with heart failure
EXCLUDES 1 *edema of lung without heart disease or heart failure (J81.-)*
  pulmonary edema without heart disease or failure (J81.-)

✓5ᵗʰ I50.2 Systolic (congestive) heart failure
▶Heart failure with reduced ejection fraction [HFrEF]
Systolic left ventricular heart failure◀
▶Code also end stage heart failure, if applicable (I50.84)◀
AHA: 2017, 1Q, 46; 2016, 1Q, 10

I50.20 Unspecified systolic (congestive) heart failure HCC ▽

I50.21 Acute systolic (congestive) heart failure HCC

I50.22 Chronic systolic (congestive) heart failure HCC

I50.23 Acute on chronic systolic (congestive) heart failure HCC

✓5ᵗʰ I50.3 Diastolic (congestive) heart failure
▶Diastolic left ventricular heart failure
Heart failure with normal ejection fraction
Heart failure with preserved ejection fraction [HFpEF]◀
▶Code also end stage heart failure, if applicable (I50.84)◀
EXCLUDES 1 *combined systolic (congestive) and diastolic (congestive) heart failure (I50.4-)*
AHA: 2017, 1Q, 46; 2016, 1Q, 10

EXCLUDES 1 Not coded here   **EXCLUDES 2** Not included here   N Newborn Age: 0   P Pediatric Age: 0-17   M Maternity Age: 12-55   A Adult Age: 15-124

628   ICD-10-CM 2018

I50.30   Unspecified diastolic (congestive) heart failure   HCC ▽

I50.31   Acute diastolic (congestive) heart failure   HCC

I50.32   Chronic diastolic (congestive) heart failure   HCC

I50.33   Acute on chronic diastolic (congestive) heart failure   HCC

✓5th **I50.4**   Combined systolic (congestive) and diastolic (congestive) heart failure

▶Combined systolic and diastolic left ventricular heart failure
Heart failure with reduced ejection fraction and diastolic dysfunction◀

▶Code also end stage heart failure, if applicable (I50.84)◀
AHA: 2017, 1Q, 46; 2016, 1Q, 10

I50.40   Unspecified combined systolic (congestive) and diastolic (congestive) heart failure   HCC ▽

I50.41   Acute combined systolic (congestive) and diastolic (congestive) heart failure   HCC

I50.42   Chronic combined systolic (congestive) and diastolic (congestive) heart failure   HCC

I50.43   Acute on chronic combined systolic (congestive) and diastolic (congestive) heart failure   HCC

● ✓5th **I50.8**   Other heart failure

● ✓6th **I50.81**   Right heart failure
Right ventricular failure

● **I50.810**   Right heart failure, unspecified   ▽
Right heart failure without mention of left heart failure
Right ventricular failure NOS

● **I50.811**   Acute right heart failure
Acute isolated right heart failure
Acute (isolated) right ventricular failure

● **I50.812**   Chronic right heart failure
Chronic isolated right heart failure
Chronic (isolated) right ventricular failure

● **I50.813**   Acute on chronic right heart failure
Acute on chronic isolated right heart failure
Acute on chronic (isolated) right ventricular failure
Acute decompensation of chronic (isolated) right ventricular failure
Acute exacerbation of chronic (isolated) right ventricular failure

● **I50.814**   Right heart failure due to left heart failure
Right ventricular failure secondary to left ventricular failure
Code also the type of left ventricular failure, if known (I50.2-I50.43)
EXCLUDES 1   right heart failure with but not due to left heart failure (I50.82)

● **I50.82**   Biventricular heart failure
Code also the type of left ventricular failure as systolic, diastolic, or combined, if known (I50.2-I50.43)

● **I50.83**   High output heart failure

● **I50.84**   End stage heart failure
Stage D heart failure
Code also the type of heart failure as systolic, diastolic, or combined, if known (I50.2-I50.43)

● **I50.89**   Other heart failure

I50.9   Heart failure, unspecified   HCC ▽
Biventricular (heart) failure NOS
Cardiac, heart or myocardial failure NOS
Congestive heart disease
Congestive heart failure NOS
Right ventricular failure (secondary to left heart failure)
EXCLUDES 2   fluid overload (E87.70)
AHA: 2017, 1Q, 45-46; 2014, 4Q, 21; 2012, 4Q, 92

✓4th **I51**   Complications and ill-defined descriptions of heart disease
EXCLUDES 1   any condition in I51.4-I51.9 due to hypertension (I11.-)
any condition in I51.4-I51.9 due to hypertension and chronic kidney disease (I13.-)
heart disease specified as rheumatic (I00-I09)

I51.0   Cardiac septal defect, acquired   A
Acquired septal atrial defect (old)
Acquired septal auricular defect (old)
Acquired septal ventricular defect (old)
EXCLUDES 1   cardiac septal defect as current complication following acute myocardial infarction (I23.1, I23.2)
DEF: Abnormal communication between opposite heart chambers due to defect of septum; not present at birth.

I51.1   Rupture of chordae tendineae, not elsewhere classified   HCC
EXCLUDES 1   rupture of chordae tendineae as current complication following acute myocardial infarction (I23.4)

I51.2   Rupture of papillary muscle, not elsewhere classified   HCC
EXCLUDES 1   rupture of papillary muscle as current complication following acute myocardial infarction (I23.5)

I51.3   Intracardiac thrombosis, not elsewhere classified
Apical thrombosis (old)   Mural thrombosis (old)
Atrial thrombosis (old)   Ventricular thrombosis (old)
Auricular thrombosis (old)
EXCLUDES 1   intracardiac thrombosis as current complication following acute myocardial infarction (I23.6)
AHA: 2013, 1Q, 24

I51.4   Myocarditis, unspecified   HCC ▽
Chronic (interstitial) myocarditis
Myocardial fibrosis
Myocarditis NOS
EXCLUDES 1   acute or subacute myocarditis (I40.-)

I51.5   Myocardial degeneration   HCC
Fatty degeneration of heart or myocardium
Myocardial disease
Senile degeneration of heart or myocardium

I51.7   Cardiomegaly
Cardiac dilatation
Cardiac hypertrophy
Ventricular dilatation

✓5th **I51.8**   Other ill-defined heart diseases

I51.81   Takotsubo syndrome
Reversible left ventricular dysfunction following sudden emotional stress
Stress induced cardiomyopathy
Takotsubo cardiomyopathy
Transient left ventricular apical ballooning syndrome

I51.89   Other ill-defined heart diseases
Carditis (acute)(chronic)
Pancarditis (acute)(chronic)

I51.9   Heart disease, unspecified   ▽

I52   *Other heart disorders in diseases classified elsewhere*
Code first underlying disease, such as:
congenital syphilis (A50.5)
mucopolysaccharidosis (E76.3)
schistosomiasis (B65.0-B65.9)
EXCLUDES 1   heart disease (in):
gonococcal infection (A54.83)
meningococcal infection (A39.50)
rheumatoid arthritis (M05.31)
syphilis (A52.06)

Cerebrovascular diseases (I60-I69)

Use additional code to identify presence of:
alcohol abuse and dependence (F10.-)
exposure to environmental tobacco smoke (Z77.22)
history of tobacco dependence (Z87.891)
hypertension (I10-I15)
occupational exposure to environmental tobacco smoke (Z57.31)
tobacco dependence (F17.-)
tobacco use (Z72.0)
EXCLUDES 1   transient cerebral ischemic attacks and related syndromes (G45.-)
traumatic intracranial hemorrhage (S06.-)
AHA: 2014, 3Q, 5; 2012, 4Q, 91-92

✓4th **I60**   Nontraumatic subarachnoid hemorrhage
INCLUDES   ruptured cerebral aneurysm
EXCLUDES 1   syphilitic ruptured cerebral aneurysm (A52.05)
EXCLUDES 2   sequelae of subarachnoid hemorrhage (I69.0-)

✓5th **I60.0**   Nontraumatic subarachnoid hemorrhage from carotid siphon and bifurcation

I60.00   Nontraumatic subarachnoid hemorrhage from unspecified carotid siphon and bifurcation   HCC ▽

I60.01   Nontraumatic subarachnoid hemorrhage from right carotid siphon and bifurcation   HCC

I60.02   Nontraumatic subarachnoid hemorrhage from left carotid siphon and bifurcation   HCC

✓ Additional Character Req   ✓x7th Placeholder Alert   Manifestation   HCC CMS-HCC Condition   ▽ Unspecified Code   ▶◀ Revised Text   ● New Code   ▲ Revised Code Title

✓5ᵗʰ I60.1 Nontraumatic subarachnoid hemorrhage from middle cerebral artery

- **I60.10** Nontraumatic subarachnoid hemorrhage from unspecified middle cerebral artery HCC ▽
- **I60.11** Nontraumatic subarachnoid hemorrhage from right middle cerebral artery HCC
- **I60.12** Nontraumatic subarachnoid hemorrhage from left middle cerebral artery HCC

I60.2 Nontraumatic subarachnoid hemorrhage from anterior communicating artery HCC

✓5ᵗʰ I60.3 Nontraumatic subarachnoid hemorrhage from posterior communicating artery

- **I60.30** Nontraumatic subarachnoid hemorrhage from unspecified posterior communicating artery HCC ▽
- **I60.31** Nontraumatic subarachnoid hemorrhage from right posterior communicating artery HCC
- **I60.32** Nontraumatic subarachnoid hemorrhage from left posterior communicating artery HCC

I60.4 Nontraumatic subarachnoid hemorrhage from basilar artery HCC

✓5ᵗʰ I60.5 Nontraumatic subarachnoid hemorrhage from vertebral artery

- **I60.50** Nontraumatic subarachnoid hemorrhage from unspecified vertebral artery HCC ▽
- **I60.51** Nontraumatic subarachnoid hemorrhage from right vertebral artery HCC
- **I60.52** Nontraumatic subarachnoid hemorrhage from left vertebral artery HCC

I60.6 Nontraumatic subarachnoid hemorrhage from other intracranial arteries HCC

I60.7 Nontraumatic subarachnoid hemorrhage from unspecified intracranial artery HCC ▽
Ruptured (congenital) berry aneurysm
Ruptured (congenital) cerebral aneurysm
Subarachnoid hemorrhage (nontraumatic) from cerebral artery NOS
Subarachnoid hemorrhage (nontraumatic) from communicating artery NOS
> EXCLUDES 1 berry aneurysm, nonruptured (I67.1)

I60.8 Other nontraumatic subarachnoid hemorrhage HCC
Meningeal hemorrhage
Rupture of cerebral arteriovenous malformation

I60.9 Nontraumatic subarachnoid hemorrhage, unspecified HCC ▽

✓4ᵗʰ I61 Nontraumatic intracerebral hemorrhage
> EXCLUDES 2 sequelae of intracerebral hemorrhage (I69.1-)
AHA: 2017, 2Q, 9-10

I61.0 Nontraumatic intracerebral hemorrhage in hemisphere, subcortical HCC
Deep intracerebral hemorrhage (nontraumatic)

I61.1 Nontraumatic intracerebral hemorrhage in hemisphere, cortical HCC
Cerebral lobe hemorrhage (nontraumatic)
Superficial intracerebral hemorrhage (nontraumatic)

I61.2 Nontraumatic intracerebral hemorrhage in hemisphere, unspecified HCC ▽

I61.3 Nontraumatic intracerebral hemorrhage in brain stem HCC

I61.4 Nontraumatic intracerebral hemorrhage in cerebellum HCC

I61.5 Nontraumatic intracerebral hemorrhage, intraventricular HCC

I61.6 Nontraumatic intracerebral hemorrhage, multiple localized HCC

I61.8 Other nontraumatic intracerebral hemorrhage HCC

I61.9 Nontraumatic intracerebral hemorrhage, unspecified HCC ▽

✓4ᵗʰ I62 Other and unspecified nontraumatic intracranial hemorrhage
> EXCLUDES 2 sequelae of intracranial hemorrhage (I69.2)

✓5ᵗʰ I62.0 Nontraumatic subdural hemorrhage

- **I62.00** Nontraumatic subdural hemorrhage, unspecified HCC ▽
- **I62.01** Nontraumatic acute subdural hemorrhage HCC
- **I62.02** Nontraumatic subacute subdural hemorrhage HCC
- **I62.03** Nontraumatic chronic subdural hemorrhage HCC

I62.1 Nontraumatic extradural hemorrhage HCC
Nontraumatic epidural hemorrhage

I62.9 Nontraumatic intracranial hemorrhage, unspecified HCC ▽

✓4ᵗʰ I63 Cerebral infarction
> INCLUDES occlusion and stenosis of cerebral and precerebral arteries, resulting in cerebral infarction
Use additional code, if applicable, to identify status post administration of tPA (rtPA) in a different facility within the last 24 hours prior to admission to current facility (Z92.82)
Use additional code, if known, to indicate National Institutes of Health Stroke Scale (NIHSS) score (R29.7-)
> EXCLUDES 2 sequelae of cerebral infarction (I69.3-)
AHA: 2017, 2Q, 9-10; 2014, 1Q, 23

✓5ᵗʰ I63.0 Cerebral infarction due to thrombosis of precerebral arteries

- **I63.00** Cerebral infarction due to thrombosis of unspecified precerebral artery HCC ▽
- **✓6ᵗʰ I63.01** Cerebral infarction due to thrombosis of vertebral artery
  - **I63.011** Cerebral infarction due to thrombosis of right vertebral artery HCC
  - **I63.012** Cerebral infarction due to thrombosis of left vertebral artery HCC
  - **I63.013** Cerebral infarction due to thrombosis of bilateral vertebral arteries HCC
  - **I63.019** Cerebral infarction due to thrombosis of unspecified vertebral artery HCC ▽
- **I63.02** Cerebral infarction due to thrombosis of basilar artery HCC
- **✓6ᵗʰ I63.03** Cerebral infarction due to thrombosis of carotid artery
  - **I63.031** Cerebral infarction due to thrombosis of right carotid artery HCC
  - **I63.032** Cerebral infarction due to thrombosis of left carotid artery HCC
  - **I63.033** Cerebral infarction due to thrombosis of bilateral carotid arteries HCC
  - **I63.039** Cerebral infarction due to thrombosis of unspecified carotid artery HCC ▽
- **I63.09** Cerebral infarction due to thrombosis of other precerebral artery HCC

✓5ᵗʰ I63.1 Cerebral infarction due to embolism of precerebral arteries

- **I63.10** Cerebral infarction due to embolism of unspecified precerebral artery HCC ▽
- **✓6ᵗʰ I63.11** Cerebral infarction due to embolism of vertebral artery
  - **I63.111** Cerebral infarction due to embolism of right vertebral artery HCC
  - **I63.112** Cerebral infarction due to embolism of left vertebral artery HCC
  - **I63.113** Cerebral infarction due to embolism of bilateral vertebral arteries HCC
  - **I63.119** Cerebral infarction due to embolism of unspecified vertebral artery HCC ▽
- **I63.12** Cerebral infarction due to embolism of basilar artery HCC
- **✓6ᵗʰ I63.13** Cerebral infarction due to embolism of carotid artery
  - **I63.131** Cerebral infarction due to embolism of right carotid artery HCC
  - **I63.132** Cerebral infarction due to embolism of left carotid artery HCC
  - **I63.133** Cerebral infarction due to embolism of bilateral carotid arteries HCC
  - **I63.139** Cerebral infarction due to embolism of unspecified carotid artery HCC ▽
- **I63.19** Cerebral infarction due to embolism of other precerebral artery HCC

✓5ᵗʰ I63.2 Cerebral infarction due to unspecified occlusion or stenosis of precerebral arteries

- **I63.20** Cerebral infarction due to unspecified occlusion or stenosis of unspecified precerebral arteries HCC ▽
- **✓6ᵗʰ I63.21** Cerebral infarction due to unspecified occlusion or stenosis of vertebral arteries
  - ▲ **I63.211** Cerebral infarction due to unspecified occlusion or stenosis of right vertebral artery HCC
  - ▲ **I63.212** Cerebral infarction due to unspecified occlusion or stenosis of left vertebral artery HCC

I63.213   Cerebral infarction due to unspecified HCC occlusion or stenosis of bilateral vertebral arteries

I63.219   Cerebral infarction due to HCC ▽ unspecified occlusion or stenosis of unspecified vertebral arteries

▲ I63.22   Cerebral infarction due to unspecified HCC occlusion or stenosis of basilar artery

✓6th I63.23   Cerebral infarction due to unspecified occlusion or stenosis of carotid arteries

I63.231   Cerebral infarction due to unspecified HCC occlusion or stenosis of right carotid arteries

I63.232   Cerebral infarction due to unspecified HCC occlusion or stenosis of left carotid arteries

I63.233   Cerebral infarction due to unspecified HCC occlusion or stenosis of bilateral carotid arteries

I63.239   Cerebral infarction due to HCC ▽ unspecified occlusion or stenosis of unspecified carotid arteries

I63.29   Cerebral infarction due to unspecified HCC ▽ occlusion or stenosis of other precerebral arteries

✓5th I63.3   Cerebral infarction due to thrombosis of cerebral arteries

I63.30   Cerebral infarction due to thrombosis of HCC ▽ unspecified cerebral artery

✓6th I63.31   Cerebral infarction due to thrombosis of middle cerebral artery

I63.311   Cerebral infarction due to thrombosis HCC of right middle cerebral artery

I63.312   Cerebral infarction due to thrombosis HCC of left middle cerebral artery

I63.313   Cerebral infarction due to thrombosis HCC of bilateral middle cerebral arteries

I63.319   Cerebral infarction due to HCC ▽ thrombosis of unspecified middle cerebral artery

✓6th I63.32   Cerebral infarction due to thrombosis of anterior cerebral artery

I63.321   Cerebral infarction due to thrombosis HCC of right anterior cerebral artery

I63.322   Cerebral infarction due to thrombosis HCC of left anterior cerebral artery

▲ I63.323   Cerebral infarction due to thrombosis HCC of bilateral anterior cerebral arteries

I63.329   Cerebral infarction due to HCC ▽ thrombosis of unspecified anterior cerebral artery

✓6th I63.33   Cerebral infarction due to thrombosis of posterior cerebral artery

I63.331   Cerebral infarction due to thrombosis HCC of right posterior cerebral artery

I63.332   Cerebral infarction due to thrombosis HCC of left posterior cerebral artery

▲ I63.333   Cerebral infarction to thrombosis of HCC bilateral posterior cerebral arteries

I63.339   Cerebral infarction due to HCC ▽ thrombosis of unspecified posterior cerebral artery

✓6th I63.34   Cerebral infarction due to thrombosis of cerebellar artery

I63.341   Cerebral infarction due to thrombosis HCC of right cerebellar artery

I63.342   Cerebral infarction due to thrombosis HCC of left cerebellar artery

I63.343   Cerebral infarction to thrombosis of HCC bilateral cerebellar arteries

I63.349   Cerebral infarction due to HCC ▽ thrombosis of unspecified cerebellar artery

I63.39   Cerebral infarction due to thrombosis of other HCC cerebral artery

✓5th I63.4   Cerebral infarction due to embolism of cerebral arteries

I63.40   Cerebral infarction due to embolism of HCC ▽ unspecified cerebral artery

✓6th I63.41   Cerebral infarction due to embolism of middle cerebral artery

I63.411   Cerebral infarction due to embolism HCC of right middle cerebral artery

I63.412   Cerebral infarction due to embolism HCC of left middle cerebral artery

I63.413   Cerebral infarction due to embolism HCC of bilateral middle cerebral arteries

I63.419   Cerebral infarction due to embolism HCC ▽ of unspecified middle cerebral artery

✓6th I63.42   Cerebral infarction due to embolism of anterior cerebral artery

I63.421   Cerebral infarction due to embolism HCC of right anterior cerebral artery

I63.422   Cerebral infarction due to embolism HCC of left anterior cerebral artery

I63.423   Cerebral infarction due to embolism HCC of bilateral anterior cerebral arteries

I63.429   Cerebral infarction due to HCC ▽ embolismof unspecified anterior cerebral artery

✓6th I63.43   Cerebral infarction due to embolism of posterior cerebral artery

I63.431   Cerebral infarction due to embolism HCC of right posterior cerebral artery

I63.432   Cerebral infarction due to embolism HCC of left posterior cerebral artery

I63.433   Cerebral infarction due to embolism HCC of bilateral posterior cerebral arteries

I63.439   Cerebral infarction due to HCC ▽ embolism of unspecified posterior cerebral artery

✓6th I63.44   Cerebral infarction due to embolism of cerebellar artery

I63.441   Cerebral infarction due to embolism HCC of right cerebellar artery

I63.442   Cerebral infarction due to embolism HCC of left cerebellar artery

I63.443   Cerebral infarction due to embolism HCC of bilateral cerebellar arteries

I63.449   Cerebral infarction due to HCC ▽ embolism of unspecified cerebellar artery

I63.49   Cerebral infarction due to embolism of other HCC cerebral artery

✓5th I63.5   Cerebral infarction due to unspecified occlusion or stenosis of cerebral arteries

I63.50   Cerebral infarction due to unspecified HCC ▽ occlusion or stenosis of unspecified cerebral artery

✓6th I63.51   Cerebral infarction due to unspecified occlusion or stenosis of middle cerebral artery

I63.511   Cerebral infarction due to unspecified HCC occlusion or stenosis of right middle cerebral artery

I63.512   Cerebral infarction due to unspecified HCC occlusion or stenosis of left middle cerebral artery

I63.513   Cerebral infarction due to unspecified HCC occlusion or stenosis of bilateral middle cerebral arteries

I63.519   Cerebral infarction due to HCC ▽ unspecified occlusion or stenosis of unspecified middle cerebral artery

✓6th I63.52   Cerebral infarction due to unspecified occlusion or stenosis of anterior cerebral artery

I63.521   Cerebral infarction due to unspecified HCC occlusion or stenosis of right anterior cerebral artery

I63.522   Cerebral infarction due to unspecified HCC occlusion or stenosis of left anterior cerebral artery

▲ I63.523   Cerebral infarction due to unspecified HCC occlusion or stenosis of bilateral anterior cerebral arteries

I63.529   Cerebral infarction due to HCC ▽ unspecified occlusion or stenosis of unspecified anterior cerebral artery

---

☑ Additional Character Req   ✓×7th Placeholder Alert   Manifestation   HCC CMS-HCC Condition   ▽ Unspecified Code   ▶◀ Revised Text   ● New Code   ▲ Revised Code Title

ICD-10-CM 2018   631

✓6th I63.53 Cerebral infarction due to unspecified occlusion or stenosis of posterior cerebral artery

    I63.531 Cerebral infarction due to unspecified occlusion or stenosis of right posterior cerebral artery HCC

    I63.532 Cerebral infarction due to unspecified occlusion or stenosis of left posterior cerebral artery HCC

    I63.533 Cerebral infarction due to unspecified occlusion or stenosis of bilateral posterior cerebral arteries HCC

    I63.539 Cerebral infarction due to unspecified occlusion or stenosis of unspecified posterior cerebral artery HCC ▽

✓6th I63.54 Cerebral infarction due to unspecified occlusion or stenosis of cerebellar artery

    I63.541 Cerebral infarction due to unspecified occlusion or stenosis of right cerebellar artery HCC

    I63.542 Cerebral infarction due to unspecified occlusion or stenosis of left cerebellar artery HCC

    I63.543 Cerebral infarction due to unspecified occlusion or stenosis of bilateral cerebellar arteries HCC

    I63.549 Cerebral infarction due to unspecified occlusion or stenosis of unspecified cerebellar artery HCC ▽

I63.59 Cerebral infarction due to unspecified occlusion or stenosis of other cerebral artery HCC ▽

I63.6 Cerebral infarction due to cerebral venous thrombosis, nonpyogenic HCC

I63.8 Other cerebral infarction HCC

I63.9 Cerebral infarction, unspecified HCC ▽
Stroke NOS
    EXCLUDES 2 ▶transient cerebral ischemic attacks and related syndromes (G45.-)◀
    AHA: 2015, 1Q, 25

✓4th I65 Occlusion and stenosis of precerebral arteries, not resulting in cerebral infarction
    INCLUDES embolism of precerebral artery
        narrowing of precerebral artery
        obstruction (complete) (partial) of precerebral artery
        thrombosis of precerebral artery
    EXCLUDES 1 insufficiency, NOS, of precerebral artery (G45.-)
        insufficiency of precerebral arteries causing cerebral infarction (I63.0-I63.2)

✓5th I65.0 Occlusion and stenosis of vertebral artery

    I65.01 Occlusion and stenosis of right vertebral artery

    I65.02 Occlusion and stenosis of left vertebral artery

    I65.03 Occlusion and stenosis of bilateral vertebral arteries

    I65.09 Occlusion and stenosis of unspecified vertebral artery ▽

I65.1 Occlusion and stenosis of basilar artery

✓5th I65.2 Occlusion and stenosis of carotid artery

    I65.21 Occlusion and stenosis of right carotid artery

    I65.22 Occlusion and stenosis of left carotid artery

    I65.23 Occlusion and stenosis of bilateral carotid arteries

    I65.29 Occlusion and stenosis of unspecified carotid artery ▽

I65.8 Occlusion and stenosis of other precerebral arteries

I65.9 Occlusion and stenosis of unspecified precerebral artery ▽
Occlusion and stenosis of precerebral artery NOS

✓4th I66 Occlusion and stenosis of cerebral arteries, not resulting in cerebral infarction
    INCLUDES embolism of cerebral artery
        narrowing of cerebral artery
        obstruction (complete) (partial) of cerebral artery
        thrombosis of cerebral artery
    EXCLUDES 1 occlusion and stenosis of cerebral artery causing cerebral infarction (I63.3-I63.5)

✓5th I66.0 Occlusion and stenosis of middle cerebral artery

    I66.01 Occlusion and stenosis of right middle cerebral artery

    I66.02 Occlusion and stenosis of left middle cerebral artery

    I66.03 Occlusion and stenosis of bilateral middle cerebral arteries

    I66.09 Occlusion and stenosis of unspecified middle cerebral artery ▽

✓5th I66.1 Occlusion and stenosis of anterior cerebral artery

    I66.11 Occlusion and stenosis of right anterior cerebral artery

    I66.12 Occlusion and stenosis of left anterior cerebral artery

    I66.13 Occlusion and stenosis of bilateral anterior cerebral arteries

    I66.19 Occlusion and stenosis of unspecified anterior cerebral artery ▽

✓5th I66.2 Occlusion and stenosis of posterior cerebral artery

    I66.21 Occlusion and stenosis of right posterior cerebral artery

    I66.22 Occlusion and stenosis of left posterior cerebral artery

    I66.23 Occlusion and stenosis of bilateral posterior cerebral arteries

    I66.29 Occlusion and stenosis of unspecified posterior cerebral artery ▽

I66.3 Occlusion and stenosis of cerebellar arteries

I66.8 Occlusion and stenosis of other cerebral arteries
Occlusion and stenosis of perforating arteries

I66.9 Occlusion and stenosis of unspecified cerebral artery ▽

✓4th I67 Other cerebrovascular diseases
    EXCLUDES 2 sequelae of the listed conditions (I69.8)

I67.0 Dissection of cerebral arteries, nonruptured HCC
    EXCLUDES 1 ruptured cerebral arteries (I60.7)

I67.1 Cerebral aneurysm, nonruptured
Cerebral aneurysm NOS
Cerebral arteriovenous fistula, acquired
Internal carotid artery aneurysm, intracranial portion
Internal carotid artery aneurysm, NOS
    EXCLUDES 1 congenital cerebral aneurysm, nonruptured (Q28.-)
        ruptured cerebral aneurysm (I60.7)

I67.2 Cerebral atherosclerosis A
Atheroma of cerebral and precerebral arteries

I67.3 Progressive vascular leukoencephalopathy
Binswanger's disease

I67.4 Hypertensive encephalopathy
    EXCLUDES 2 ▶insufficiency, NOS, of precerebral arteries (G45.2)◀

Berry Aneurysm

Berry aneurysms form at the site of a weakness in an arterial wall, often at a junction

Berry aneurysm

Anterior communicating artery — 40%
Anterior cerebral artery
34%
Internal carotid
20%
Middle cerebral artery
4%
Posterior communicating artery
Posterior cerebral artery
Basilar artery

Common sites of berry aneurysms in the circle of Willis arteries

EXCLUDES 1 Not coded here   EXCLUDES 2 Not included here   N Newborn Age: 0   P Pediatric Age: 0-17   M Maternity Age: 12-55   A Adult Age: 15-124

632   ICD-10-CM 2018

I67.5   **Moyamoya disease**
> **DEF:** Cerebrovascular ischemia; vessels occlude and rupture, causing tiny hemorrhages at base of brain; affects predominantly Japanese people.

I67.6   **Nonpyogenic thrombosis of intracranial venous system**
> Nonpyogenic thrombosis of cerebral vein
> Nonpyogenic thrombosis of intracranial venous sinus
> *EXCLUDES 1*   nonpyogenic thrombosis of intracranial venous system causing infarction (I63.6)

I67.7   **Cerebral arteritis, not elsewhere classified**
> Granulomatous angiitis of the nervous system
> *EXCLUDES 1*   allergic granulomatous angiitis (M3Ø.1)

✓5ᵗʰ **I67.8**   **Other specified cerebrovascular diseases**

     I67.81   **Acute cerebrovascular insufficiency**
> Acute cerebrovascular insufficiency unspecified as to location or reversibility

     I67.82   **Cerebral ischemia**
> Chronic cerebral ischemia

     I67.83   **Posterior reversible encephalopathy syndrome**
> PRES

     ✓6ᵗʰ **I67.84**   **Cerebral vasospasm and vasoconstriction**

         I67.841   **Reversible cerebrovascular vasoconstriction syndrome**
> Call-Fleming syndrome
> Code first underlying condition, if applicable, such as eclampsia (O15.ØØ-O15.9)

         I67.848   **Other cerebrovascular vasospasm and vasoconstriction**

     I67.89   **Other cerebrovascular disease**

I67.9   **Cerebrovascular disease, unspecified**   ▽

✓4ᵗʰ **I68**   **Cerebrovascular disorders in diseases classified elsewhere**

I68.Ø   *Cerebral amyloid angiopathy*
> Code first underlying amyloidosis (E85.-)

I68.2   *Cerebral arteritis in other diseases classified elsewhere*
> Code first underlying disease
> *EXCLUDES 1*   cerebral arteritis (in):
> > listerosis (A32.89)
> > systemic lupus erythematosus (M32.19)
> > syphilis (A52.Ø4)
> > tuberculosis (A18.89)

I68.8   *Other cerebrovascular disorders in diseases classified elsewhere*
> Code first underlying disease
> *EXCLUDES 1*   syphilitic cerebral aneurysm (A52.Ø5)

✓4ᵗʰ **I69**   **Sequelae of cerebrovascular disease**
> **NOTE**   Category I69 is to be used to indicate conditions in I6Ø-I67 as the cause of sequelae. The "sequelae" include conditions specified as such or as residuals which may occur at any time after the onset of the causal condition
> *EXCLUDES 1*   personal history of cerebral infarction without residual deficit (Z86.73)
> > personal history of prolonged reversible ischemic neurologic deficit (PRIND) (Z86.73)
> > personal history of reversible ischemic neurologcial deficit (RIND) (Z86.73)
> > sequelae of traumatic intracranial injury (SØ6.-)
> > ~~transient ischemic attack (TIA) (G45.9)~~
> **AHA:** 2017, 1Q, 47; 2015, 1Q, 25; 2012, 4Q, 106

✓5ᵗʰ **I69.Ø**   **Sequelae of nontraumatic subarachnoid hemorrhage**

     I69.ØØ   **Unspecified sequelae of nontraumatic subarachnoid hemorrhage**   ▽

     ✓6ᵗʰ **I69.Ø1**   Cognitive deficits following nontraumatic subarachnoid hemorrhage

         I69.Ø1Ø   Attention and concentration deficit following nontraumatic subarachnoid hemorrhage

         I69.Ø11   Memory deficit following nontraumatic subarachnoid hemorrhage

         I69.Ø12   Visuospatial deficit and spatial neglect following nontraumatic subarachnoid hemorrhage

         I69.Ø13   Psychomotor deficit following nontraumatic subarachnoid hemorrhage

         I69.Ø14   Frontal lobe and executive function deficit following nontraumatic subarachnoid hemorrhage

         I69.Ø15   Cognitive social or emotional deficit following nontraumatic subarachnoid hemorrhage

         I69.Ø18   **Other symptoms and signs involving cognitive functions following nontraumatic subarachnoid hemorrhage**

         I69.Ø19   **Unspecified symptoms and signs** ▽ **involving cognitive functions following nontraumatic subarachnoid hemorrhage**

     ✓6ᵗʰ **I69.Ø2**   Speech and language deficits following nontraumatic subarachnoid hemorrhage

         I69.Ø2Ø   Aphasia following nontraumatic subarachnoid hemorrhage

         I69.Ø21   Dysphasia following nontraumatic subarachnoid hemorrhage

         I69.Ø22   Dysarthria following nontraumatic subarachnoid hemorrhage

         I69.Ø23   Fluency disorder following nontraumatic subarachnoid hemorrhage
> Stuttering following nontraumatic subarachnoid hemorrhage

         I69.Ø28   **Other speech and language deficits following nontraumatic subarachnoid hemorrhage**

     ✓6ᵗʰ **I69.Ø3**   Monoplegia of upper limb following nontraumatic subarachnoid hemorrhage
> **AHA:** 2017, 1Q, 47

         I69.Ø31   **Monoplegia of upper limb following** HCC **nontraumatic subarachnoid hemorrhage affecting** right dominant **side**

         I69.Ø32   **Monoplegia of upper limb following** HCC **nontraumatic subarachnoid hemorrhage affecting** left dominant **side**

         I69.Ø33   **Monoplegia of upper limb following** HCC **nontraumatic subarachnoid hemorrhage affecting** right non-dominant **side**

         I69.Ø34   **Monoplegia of upper limb following** HCC **nontraumatic subarachnoid hemorrhage affecting** left non-dominant **side**

         I69.Ø39   **Monoplegia of upper limb** HCC ▽ **following nontraumatic subarachnoid hemorrhage affecting unspecified side**

     ✓6ᵗʰ **I69.Ø4**   Monoplegia of lower limb following nontraumatic subarachnoid hemorrhage
> **AHA:** 2017, 1Q, 47

         I69.Ø41   **Monoplegia of lower limb following** HCC **nontraumatic subarachnoid hemorrhage affecting** right dominant **side**

         I69.Ø42   **Monoplegia of lower limb following** HCC **nontraumatic subarachnoid hemorrhage affecting** left dominant **side**

         I69.Ø43   **Monoplegia of lower limb following** HCC **nontraumatic subarachnoid hemorrhage affecting** right non-dominant **side**

         I69.Ø44   **Monoplegia of lower limb following** HCC **nontraumatic subarachnoid hemorrhage affecting** left non-dominant **side**

         I69.Ø49   **Monoplegia of lower limb following** HCC ▽ **nontraumatic subarachnoid hemorrhage affecting unspecified side**

     ✓6ᵗʰ **I69.Ø5**   Hemiplegia and hemiparesis following nontraumatic subarachnoid hemorrhage
> **AHA:** 2015, 1Q, 25

         I69.Ø51   **Hemiplegia and hemiparesis following** HCC **nontraumatic subarachnoid hemorrhage affecting** right dominant **side**

         I69.Ø52   **Hemiplegia and hemiparesis following** HCC **nontraumatic subarachnoid hemorrhage affecting** left dominant **side**

         I69.Ø53   **Hemiplegia and hemiparesis following** HCC **nontraumatic subarachnoid hemorrhage affecting** right non-dominant **side**

         I69.Ø54   **Hemiplegia and hemiparesis following** HCC **nontraumatic subarachnoid hemorrhage affecting** left non-dominant **side**

         I69.Ø59   **Hemiplegia and hemiparesis** HCC ▽ **following nontraumatic subarachnoid hemorrhage affecting unspecified side**

✔ Additional Character Req   ✔x7ᵗʰ Placeholder Alert   Manifestation   HCC CMS-HCC Condition   ▽ Unspecified Code   ▶◀ Revised Text   ● New Code   ▲ Revised Code Title

ICD-10-CM 2018   633

✓6ᵗʰ I69.06 Other paralytic syndrome following nontraumatic subarachnoid hemorrhage
Use additional code to identify type of paralytic syndrome, such as:
locked-in state (G83.5)
quadriplegia (G82.5-)
EXCLUDES 1 hemiplegia/hemiparesis following nontraumatic subarachnoid hemorrhage (I69.05-)
monoplegia of lower limb following nontraumatic subarachnoid hemorrhage (I69.04-)
monoplegia of upper limb following nontraumatic subarachnoid hemorrhage (I69.03-)

I69.061 Other paralytic syndrome following nontraumatic subarachnoid hemorrhage affecting right dominant side HCC
I69.062 Other paralytic syndrome following nontraumatic subarachnoid hemorrhage affecting left dominant side HCC
I69.063 Other paralytic syndrome following nontraumatic subarachnoid hemorrhage affecting right non-dominant side HCC
I69.064 Other paralytic syndrome following nontraumatic subarachnoid hemorrhage affecting left non-dominant side HCC
I69.065 Other paralytic syndrome following nontraumatic subarachnoid hemorrhage, bilateral HCC
I69.069 Other paralytic syndrome following nontraumatic subarachnoid hemorrhage affecting unspecified side HCC ▽

✓6ᵗʰ I69.09 Other sequelae of nontraumatic subarachnoid hemorrhage
I69.090 Apraxia following nontraumatic subarachnoid hemorrhage
I69.091 Dysphagia following nontraumatic subarachnoid hemorrhage
Use additional code to identify the type of dysphagia, if known (R13.1-)
I69.092 Facial weakness following nontraumatic subarachnoid hemorrhage
Facial droop following nontraumatic subarachnoid hemorrhage
I69.093 Ataxia following nontraumatic subarachnoid hemorrhage
I69.098 Other sequelae following nontraumatic subarachnoid hemorrhage
Alterations of sensation following nontraumatic subarachnoid hemorrhage
Disturbance of vision following nontraumatic subarachnoid hemorrhage
Use additional code to identify the sequelae

✓5ᵗʰ I69.1 Sequelae of nontraumatic intracerebral hemorrhage
I69.10 Unspecified sequelae of nontraumatic intracerebral hemorrhage ▽

✓6ᵗʰ I69.11 Cognitive deficits following nontraumatic intracerebral hemorrhage
I69.110 Attention and concentration deficit following nontraumatic intracerebral hemorrhage
I69.111 Memory deficit following nontraumatic intracerebral hemorrhage
I69.112 Visuospatial deficit and spatial neglect following nontraumatic intracerebral hemorrhage
I69.113 Psychomotor deficit following nontraumatic intracerebral hemorrhage
I69.114 Frontal lobe and executive function deficit following nontraumatic intracerebral hemorrhage
I69.115 Cognitive social or emotional deficit following nontraumatic intracerebral hemorrhage
I69.118 Other symptoms and signs involving cognitive functions following nontraumatic intracerebral hemorrhage
I69.119 Unspecified symptoms and signs involving cognitive functions following nontraumatic intracerebral hemorrhage ▽

✓6ᵗʰ I69.12 Speech and language deficits following nontraumatic intracerebral hemorrhage
I69.120 Aphasia following nontraumatic intracerebral hemorrhage
I69.121 Dysphasia following nontraumatic intracerebral hemorrhage
I69.122 Dysarthria following nontraumatic intracerebral hemorrhage
I69.123 Fluency disorder following nontraumatic intracerebral hemorrhage
Stuttering following nontraumatic intracerebral hemorrhage
I69.128 Other speech and language deficits following nontraumatic intracerebral hemorrhage

✓6ᵗʰ I69.13 Monoplegia of upper limb following nontraumatic intracerebral hemorrhage
AHA: 2017, 1Q, 47
I69.131 Monoplegia of upper limb following nontraumatic intracerebral hemorrhage affecting right dominant side HCC
I69.132 Monoplegia of upper limb following nontraumatic intracerebral hemorrhage affecting left dominant side HCC
I69.133 Monoplegia of upper limb following nontraumatic intracerebral hemorrhage affecting right non-dominant side HCC
I69.134 Monoplegia of upper limb following nontraumatic intracerebral hemorrhage affecting left non-dominant side HCC
I69.139 Monoplegia of upper limb following nontraumatic intracerebral hemorrhage affecting unspecified side HCC ▽

✓6ᵗʰ I69.14 Monoplegia of lower limb following nontraumatic intracerebral hemorrhage
AHA: 2017, 1Q, 47
I69.141 Monoplegia of lower limb following nontraumatic intracerebral hemorrhage affecting right dominant side HCC
I69.142 Monoplegia of lower limb following nontraumatic intracerebral hemorrhage affecting left dominant side HCC
I69.143 Monoplegia of lower limb following nontraumatic intracerebral hemorrhage affecting right non-dominant side HCC
I69.144 Monoplegia of lower limb following nontraumatic intracerebral hemorrhage affecting left non-dominant side HCC
I69.149 Monoplegia of lower limb following nontraumatic intracerebral hemorrhage affecting unspecified side HCC ▽

✓6ᵗʰ I69.15 Hemiplegia and hemiparesis following nontraumatic intracerebral hemorrhage
AHA: 2015, 1Q, 25
I69.151 Hemiplegia and hemiparesis following nontraumatic intracerebral hemorrhage affecting right dominant side HCC
I69.152 Hemiplegia and hemiparesis following nontraumatic intracerebral hemorrhage affecting left dominant side HCC
I69.153 Hemiplegia and hemiparesis following nontraumatic intracerebral hemorrhage affecting right non-dominant side HCC
I69.154 Hemiplegia and hemiparesis following nontraumatic intracerebral hemorrhage affecting left non-dominant side HCC
I69.159 Hemiplegia and hemiparesis following nontraumatic intracerebral hemorrhage affecting unspecified side HCC ▽

✓6ᵗʰ **I69.16**   **Other** paralytic syndrome **following nontraumatic intracerebral hemorrhage**

Use additional code to identify type of paralytic syndrome, such as:
locked-in state (G83.5)
quadriplegia (G82.5-)

EXCLUDES 1   *hemiplegia/hemiparesis following nontraumatic intracerebral hemorrhage (I69.15-)*
monoplegia of lower limb following nontraumatic intracerebral hemorrhage (I69.14-)
monoplegia of upper limb following nontraumatic intracerebral hemorrhage (I69.13-)

I69.161   **Other paralytic syndrome following** HCC **nontraumatic intracerebral hemorrhage affecting** right dominant **side**

I69.162   **Other paralytic syndrome following** HCC **nontraumatic intracerebral hemorrhage affecting** left dominant **side**

I69.163   **Other paralytic syndrome following** HCC **nontraumatic intracerebral hemorrhage affecting** right non-dominant **side**

I69.164   **Other paralytic syndrome following** HCC **nontraumatic intracerebral hemorrhage affecting** left non-dominant **side**

I69.165   **Other paralytic syndrome following** HCC **nontraumatic intracerebral hemorrhage, bilateral**

I69.169   **Other paralytic syndrome** HCC ▽ **following nontraumatic intracerebral hemorrhage affecting unspecified side**

✓6ᵗʰ **I69.19**   **Other sequelae of nontraumatic intracerebral hemorrhage**

I69.190   Apraxia **following nontraumatic intracerebral hemorrhage**

I69.191   Dysphagia **following nontraumatic intracerebral hemorrhage**

Use additional code to identify the type of dysphagia, if known (R13.1-)

I69.192   Facial weakness **following nontraumatic intracerebral hemorrhage**

Facial droop following nontraumatic intracerebral hemorrhage

I69.193   Ataxia **following nontraumatic intracerebral hemorrhage**

I69.198   **Other sequelae of nontraumatic intracerebral hemorrhage**

Alteration of sensations following nontraumatic intracerebral hemorrhage
Disturbance of vision following nontraumatic intracerebral hemorrhage
Use additional code to identify the sequelae

✓5ᵗʰ **I69.2**   **Sequelae of other nontraumatic** intracranial **hemorrhage**

I69.20   **Unspecified sequelae of other nontraumatic** ▽ **intracranial hemorrhage**

✓6ᵗʰ **I69.21**   Cognitive deficits **following other nontraumatic intracranial hemorrhage**

I69.210   Attention and concentration **deficit following other nontraumatic intracranial hemorrhage**

I69.211   Memory **deficit following other nontraumatic intracranial hemorrhage**

I69.212   Visuospatial **deficit and** spatial neglect **following other nontraumatic intracranial hemorrhage**

I69.213   Psychomotor **deficit following other nontraumatic intracranial hemorrhage**

I69.214   Frontal lobe and executive function **deficit following other nontraumatic intracranial hemorrhage**

I69.215   Cognitive social or emotional **deficit following other nontraumatic intracranial hemorrhage**

I69.218   **Other symptoms and signs involving cognitive functions following other nontraumatic intracranial hemorrhage**

I69.219   **Unspecified symptoms and signs** ▽ **involving cognitive functions following other nontraumatic intracranial hemorrhage**

✓6ᵗʰ **I69.22**   Speech **and** language deficits **following other nontraumatic intracranial hemorrhage**

I69.220   Aphasia **following other nontraumatic intracranial hemorrhage**

I69.221   Dysphasia **following other nontraumatic intracranial hemorrhage**

I69.222   Dysarthria **following other nontraumatic intracranial hemorrhage**

I69.223   Fluency **disorder following other nontraumatic intracranial hemorrhage**

Stuttering following nontraumatic intracerebral hemorrhage

I69.228   **Other speech and language deficits following other nontraumatic intracranial hemorrhage**

✓6ᵗʰ **I69.23**   Monoplegia **of** upper limb **following other nontraumatic intracranial hemorrhage**

AHA: 2017, 1Q, 47

I69.231   **Monoplegia of upper limb following** HCC **other nontraumatic intracranial hemorrhage affecting** right dominant **side**

I69.232   **Monoplegia of upper limb following** HCC **other nontraumatic intracranial hemorrhage affecting** left dominant **side**

I69.233   **Monoplegia of upper limb following** HCC **other nontraumatic intracranial hemorrhage affecting** right non-dominant **side**

I69.234   **Monoplegia of upper limb following** HCC **other nontraumatic intracranial hemorrhage affecting** left non-dominant **side**

I69.239   **Monoplegia of upper limb** HCC ▽ **following other nontraumatic intracranial hemorrhage affecting unspecified side**

✓6ᵗʰ **I69.24**   Monoplegia **of** lower limb **following other nontraumatic intracranial hemorrhage**

AHA: 2017, 1Q, 47

I69.241   **Monoplegia of lower limb following** HCC **other nontraumatic intracranial hemorrhage affecting** right dominant **side**

I69.242   **Monoplegia of lower limb following** HCC **other nontraumatic intracranial hemorrhage affecting** left dominant **side**

I69.243   **Monoplegia of lower limb following** HCC **other nontraumatic intracranial hemorrhage affecting** right non-dominant **side**

I69.244   **Monoplegia of lower limb following** HCC **other nontraumatic intracranial hemorrhage affecting** left non-dominant **side**

I69.249   **Monoplegia of lower limb following** HCC ▽ **other nontraumatic intracranial hemorrhage affecting unspecified side**

✓6ᵗʰ **I69.25**   Hemiplegia **and** hemiparesis **following other nontraumatic intracranial hemorrhage**

AHA: 2015, 1Q, 25

I69.251   **Hemiplegia and hemiparesis following** HCC **other nontraumatic intracranial hemorrhage affecting** right dominant **side**

I69.252   **Hemiplegia and hemiparesis following** HCC **other nontraumatic intracranial hemorrhage affecting** left dominant **side**

I69.253   **Hemiplegia and hemiparesis following** HCC **other nontraumatic intracranial hemorrhage affecting** right non-dominant **side**

I69.254   **Hemiplegia and hemiparesis following** HCC **other nontraumatic intracranial hemorrhage affecting** left non-dominant **side**

I69.259   **Hemiplegia and hemiparesis** HCC ▽ **following other nontraumatic intracranial hemorrhage affecting unspecified side**

✓ Additional Character Req   ✓7ᵗʰ Placeholder Alert   Manifestation   HCC CMS-HCC Condition   ▽ Unspecified Code   ►◄ Revised Text   ● New Code   ▲ Revised Code Title

Chapter 9. Diseases of the Circulatory System

I69.26–I69.36

√6ᵗʰ **I69.26** **Other paralytic syndrome following other nontraumatic intracranial hemorrhage**
Use additional code to identify type of paralytic syndrome, such as:
locked-in state (G83.5)
quadriplegia (G82.5-)

EXCLUDES 1   *hemiplegia/hemiparesis following other nontraumatic intracranial hemorrhage (I69.25-)*
monoplegia of lower limb following other nontraumatic intracranial hemorrhage (I69.24-)
monoplegia of upper limb following other nontraumatic intracranial hemorrhage (I69.23-)

   I69.261 **Other paralytic syndrome following other nontraumatic intracranial hemorrhage affecting right dominant side** HCC

   I69.262 **Other paralytic syndrome following other nontraumatic intracranial hemorrhage affecting left dominant side** HCC

   I69.263 **Other paralytic syndrome following other nontraumatic intracranial hemorrhage affecting right non-dominant side** HCC

   I69.264 **Other paralytic syndrome following other nontraumatic intracranial hemorrhage affecting left non-dominant side** HCC

   I69.265 **Other paralytic syndrome following other nontraumatic intracranial hemorrhage, bilateral** HCC

   I69.269 **Other paralytic syndrome following other nontraumatic intracranial hemorrhage affecting unspecified side** HCC ▽

√6ᵗʰ **I69.29** **Other sequelae of other nontraumatic intracranial hemorrhage**

   I69.290 **Apraxia following other nontraumatic intracranial hemorrhage**

   I69.291 **Dysphagia following other nontraumatic intracranial hemorrhage**
Use additional code to identify the type of dysphagia, if known (R13.1-)

   I69.292 **Facial weakness following other nontraumatic intracranial hemorrhage**
Facial droop following other nontraumatic intracranial hemorrhage

   I69.293 **Ataxia following other nontraumatic intracranial hemorrhage**

   I69.298 **Other sequelae of other nontraumatic intracranial hemorrhage**
Alteration of sensation following other nontraumatic intracranial hemorrhage
Disturbance of vision following other nontraumatic intracranial hemorrhage
Use additional code to identify the sequelae

√5ᵗʰ **I69.3** **Sequelae of cerebral infarction**
Sequelae of stroke NOS
AHA: 2013, 4Q, 127-128; 2012, 4Q, 92, 94

   I69.30 **Unspecified sequelae of cerebral infarction** ▽

√6ᵗʰ **I69.31** **Cognitive deficits following cerebral infarction**

   I69.310 **Attention and concentration deficit following cerebral infarction**

   I69.311 **Memory deficit following cerebral infarction**

   I69.312 **Visuospatial deficit and spatial neglect following cerebral infarction**

   I69.313 **Psychomotor deficit following cerebral infarction**

   I69.314 **Frontal lobe and executive function deficit following cerebral infarction**

   I69.315 **Cognitive social or emotional deficit following cerebral infarction**

   I69.318 **Other symptoms and signs involving cognitive functions following cerebral infarction**

   I69.319 **Unspecified symptoms and signs involving cognitive functions following cerebral infarction** ▽

√6ᵗʰ **I69.32** **Speech and language deficits following cerebral infarction**

   I69.320 **Aphasia following cerebral infarction**

   I69.321 **Dysphasia following cerebral infarction**
AHA: 2012, 4Q, 91

   I69.322 **Dysarthria following cerebral infarction**
EXCLUDES 2 ▶*transient ischemic attack (TIA) (G45.9)*◀

   I69.323 **Fluency disorder following cerebral infarction**
Stuttering following cerebral infarction

   I69.328 **Other speech and language deficits following cerebral infarction**

√6ᵗʰ **I69.33** **Monoplegia of upper limb following cerebral infarction**
AHA: 2017, 1Q, 47

   I69.331 **Monoplegia of upper limb following cerebral infarction affecting right dominant side** HCC

   I69.332 **Monoplegia of upper limb following cerebral infarction affecting left dominant side** HCC

   I69.333 **Monoplegia of upper limb following cerebral infarction affecting right non-dominant side** HCC

   I69.334 **Monoplegia of upper limb following cerebral infarction affecting left non-dominant side** HCC

   I69.339 **Monoplegia of upper limb following cerebral infarction affecting unspecified side** HCC ▽

√6ᵗʰ **I69.34** **Monoplegia of lower limb following cerebral infarction**
AHA: 2017, 1Q, 47

   I69.341 **Monoplegia of lower limb following cerebral infarction affecting right dominant side** HCC

   I69.342 **Monoplegia of lower limb following cerebral infarction affecting left dominant side** HCC

   I69.343 **Monoplegia of lower limb following cerebral infarction affecting right non-dominant side** HCC

   I69.344 **Monoplegia of lower limb following cerebral infarction affecting left non-dominant side** HCC

   I69.349 **Monoplegia of lower limb following cerebral infarction affecting unspecified side** HCC ▽

√6ᵗʰ **I69.35** **Hemiplegia and hemiparesis following cerebral infarction**
AHA: 2015, 1Q, 25

   I69.351 **Hemiplegia and hemiparesis following cerebral infarction affecting right dominant side** HCC
EXCLUDES 2 ▶*transient ischemic attack (TIA) (G45.9)*◀

   I69.352 **Hemiplegia and hemiparesis following cerebral infarction affecting left dominant side** HCC

   I69.353 **Hemiplegia and hemiparesis following cerebral infarction affecting right non-dominant side** HCC

   I69.354 **Hemiplegia and hemiparesis following cerebral infarction affecting left non-dominant side** HCC
AHA: 2012, 4Q, 91

   I69.359 **Hemiplegia and hemiparesis following cerebral infarction affecting unspecified side** HCC ▽

√6ᵗʰ **I69.36** **Other paralytic syndrome following cerebral infarction**
Use additional code to identify type of paralytic syndrome, such as:
locked-in state (G83.5)
quadriplegia (G82.5-)

EXCLUDES 1   *hemiplegia/hemiparesis following cerebral infarction (I69.35-)*
monoplegia of lower limb following cerebral infarction (I69.34-)
monoplegia of upper limb following cerebral infarction (I69.33-)

EXCLUDES 1 Not coded here   EXCLUDES 2 Not included here   N Newborn Age: 0   P Pediatric Age: 0-17   M Maternity Age: 12-55   A Adult Age: 15-124

636   ICD-10-CM 2018

I69.361 **Other paralytic syndrome following cerebral infarction affecting** right **dominant** side HCC

I69.362 **Other paralytic syndrome following cerebral infarction affecting** left **dominant** side HCC

I69.363 **Other paralytic syndrome following cerebral infarction affecting** right **non-dominant** side HCC

I69.364 **Other paralytic syndrome following cerebral infarction affecting** left **non-dominant** side HCC

I69.365 **Other paralytic syndrome following cerebral infarction,** bilateral HCC

I69.369 **Other paralytic syndrome following cerebral infarction affecting unspecified side** HCC ▽

✓6ᵗʰ **I69.39 Other sequelae of cerebral infarction**

I69.390 Apraxia **following cerebral infarction**

I69.391 Dysphagia **following cerebral infarction**
Use additional code to identify the type of dysphagia, if known (R13.1-)

I69.392 Facial weakness **following cerebral infarction**
Facial droop following cerebral infarction

I69.393 Ataxia **following cerebral infarction**

I69.398 **Other sequelae of cerebral infarction**
Alteration of sensation following cerebral infarction
Disturbance of vision following cerebral infarction
Use additional code to identify the sequelae

✓5ᵗʰ **I69.8 Sequelae of other** cerebrovascular diseases
EXCLUDES 1 sequelae of traumatic intracranial injury (S06.-)

I69.80 **Unspecified sequelae of other cerebrovascular disease** ▽

✓6ᵗʰ **I69.81 Cognitive deficits following other cerebrovascular disease**

I69.810 Attention and concentration **deficit following other cerebrovascular disease**

I69.811 Memory **deficit following other cerebrovascular disease**

I69.812 Visuospatial **deficit and** spatial neglect **following other cerebrovascular disease**

I69.813 Psychomotor **deficit following other cerebrovascular disease**

I69.814 Frontal lobe and executive function **deficit following other cerebrovascular disease**

I69.815 Cognitive social or emotional **deficit following other cerebrovascular disease**

I69.818 **Other symptoms and signs involving cognitive functions following other cerebrovascular disease**

I69.819 **Unspecified symptoms and signs involving cognitive functions following other cerebrovascular disease** ▽

✓6ᵗʰ **I69.82 Speech and** language deficits **following other cerebrovascular disease**

I69.820 Aphasia **following other cerebrovascular disease**

I69.821 Dysphasia **following other cerebrovascular disease**

I69.822 Dysarthria **following other cerebrovascular disease**

I69.823 Fluency **disorder following other cerebrovascular disease**
Stuttering following other cerebrovascular disease

I69.828 **Other speech and language deficits following other cerebrovascular disease**

✓6ᵗʰ **I69.83** Monoplegia **of** upper limb **following other cerebrovascular disease**
AHA: 2017, 1Q, 47

I69.831 **Monoplegia of upper limb following other cerebrovascular disease affecting** right dominant **side** HCC

I69.832 **Monoplegia of upper limb following other cerebrovascular disease affecting** left dominant **side** HCC

I69.833 **Monoplegia of upper limb following other cerebrovascular disease affecting** right non-dominant **side** HCC

I69.834 **Monoplegia of upper limb following other cerebrovascular disease affecting** left non-dominant **side** HCC

I69.839 **Monoplegia of upper limb following other cerebrovascular disease affecting unspecified side** HCC ▽

✓6ᵗʰ **I69.84** Monoplegia **of** lower limb **following other cerebrovascular disease**
AHA: 2017, 1Q, 47

I69.841 **Monoplegia of lower limb following other cerebrovascular disease affecting** right dominant **side** HCC

I69.842 **Monoplegia of lower limb following other cerebrovascular disease affecting** left dominant **side** HCC

I69.843 **Monoplegia of lower limb following other cerebrovascular disease affecting** right non-dominant **side** HCC

I69.844 **Monoplegia of lower limb following other cerebrovascular disease affecting** left non-dominant **side** HCC

I69.849 **Monoplegia of lower limb following other cerebrovascular disease affecting unspecified side** HCC ▽

✓6ᵗʰ **I69.85** Hemiplegia **and** hemiparesis **following other cerebrovascular disease**
AHA: 2015, 1Q, 25

I69.851 **Hemiplegia and hemiparesis following other cerebrovascular disease affecting** right dominant **side** HCC

I69.852 **Hemiplegia and hemiparesis following other cerebrovascular disease affecting** left dominant **side** HCC

I69.853 **Hemiplegia and hemiparesis following other cerebrovascular disease affecting** right non-dominant **side** HCC

I69.854 **Hemiplegia and hemiparesis following other cerebrovascular disease affecting** left non-dominant **side** HCC

I69.859 **Hemiplegia and hemiparesis following other cerebrovascular disease affecting unspecified side** HCC ▽

✓6ᵗʰ **I69.86 Other** paralytic syndrome **following other cerebrovascular disease**
Use additional code to identify type of paralytic syndrome, such as:
locked-in state (G83.5)
quadriplegia (G82.5-)
EXCLUDES 1 hemiplegia/hemiparesis following other cerebrovascular disease (I69.85-)
monoplegia of lower limb following other cerebrovascular disease (I69.84-)
monoplegia of upper limb following other cerebrovascular disease (I69.83-)

I69.861 **Other paralytic syndrome following other cerebrovascular disease affecting** right dominant **side** HCC

I69.862 **Other paralytic syndrome following other cerebrovascular disease affecting** left dominant **side** HCC

I69.863 **Other paralytic syndrome following other cerebrovascular disease affecting** right non-dominant **side** HCC

I69.864 **Other paralytic syndrome following other cerebrovascular disease affecting** left non-dominant **side** HCC

I69.865 **Other paralytic syndrome following other cerebrovascular disease,** bilateral HCC

I69.869 **Other paralytic syndrome following other cerebrovascular disease affecting unspecified side** HCC ▽

✓6ᵗʰ **I69.89 Other sequelae of other cerebrovascular disease**

I69.890 Apraxia **following other cerebrovascular disease**

I69.891 Dysphagia **following other cerebrovascular disease**
Use additional code to identify the type of dysphagia, if known (R13.1-)

☑ Additional Character Req   ✓ˣ⁷ᵗʰ Placeholder Alert   Manifestation   HCC CMS-HCC Condition   ▽ Unspecified Code   ►◄ Revised Text   ● New Code   ▲ Revised Code Title

Chapter 9. Diseases of the Circulatory System

I69.892   **Facial weakness** following other cerebrovascular disease
     Facial droop following other cerebrovascular disease

I69.893   **Ataxia** following other cerebrovascular disease

I69.898   **Other sequelae of other cerebrovascular disease**
     Alteration of sensation following other cerebrovascular disease
     Disturbance of vision following other cerebrovascular disease
     Use additional code to identify the sequelae

✓5ᵗʰ **I69.9**   **Sequelae of unspecified** cerebrovascular diseases
     EXCLUDES 1   sequelae of stroke (I69.3)
                  sequelae of traumatic intracranial injury (S06.-)

I69.90   **Unspecified sequelae of unspecified cerebrovascular disease** ▽

✓6ᵗʰ **I69.91**   **Cognitive deficits** following unspecified cerebrovascular disease

     I69.910   **Attention and concentration** deficit following unspecified cerebrovascular disease ▽

     I69.911   **Memory** deficit following unspecified cerebrovascular disease ▽

     I69.912   **Visuospatial** deficit and spatial neglect following unspecified cerebrovascular disease ▽

     I69.913   **Psychomotor** deficit following unspecified cerebrovascular disease ▽

     I69.914   **Frontal lobe and executive function** deficit following unspecified cerebrovascular disease ▽

     I69.915   **Cognitive social or emotional** deficit following unspecified cerebrovascular disease ▽

     I69.918   **Other symptoms and signs involving cognitive functions following unspecified cerebrovascular disease** ▽

     I69.919   **Unspecified symptoms and signs involving cognitive functions following unspecified cerebrovascular disease** ▽

✓6ᵗʰ **I69.92**   **Speech and language deficits** following unspecified cerebrovascular disease

     I69.920   **Aphasia** following unspecified cerebrovascular disease ▽

     I69.921   **Dysphasia** following unspecified cerebrovascular disease ▽

     I69.922   **Dysarthria** following unspecified cerebrovascular disease ▽

     I69.923   **Fluency disorder** following unspecified cerebrovascular disease ▽
         Stuttering following unspecified cerebrovascular disease

     I69.928   **Other speech and language deficits following unspecified cerebrovascular disease** ▽

✓6ᵗʰ **I69.93**   **Monoplegia of upper limb** following unspecified cerebrovascular disease
     AHA: 2017, 1Q, 47

     I69.931   **Monoplegia of upper limb following** unspecified cerebrovascular disease affecting right dominant side HCC ▽

     I69.932   **Monoplegia of upper limb following** unspecified cerebrovascular disease affecting left dominant side HCC ▽

     I69.933   **Monoplegia of upper limb following** unspecified cerebrovascular disease affecting right non-dominant side HCC ▽

     I69.934   **Monoplegia of upper limb following** unspecified cerebrovascular disease affecting left non-dominant side HCC ▽

     I69.939   **Monoplegia of upper limb following** unspecified cerebrovascular disease affecting unspecified side HCC ▽

✓6ᵗʰ **I69.94**   **Monoplegia of** lower limb following unspecified cerebrovascular disease
     AHA: 2017, 1Q, 47

     I69.941   **Monoplegia of lower limb following** unspecified cerebrovascular disease affecting right dominant side HCC ▽

     I69.942   **Monoplegia of lower limb following** unspecified cerebrovascular disease affecting left dominant side HCC ▽

     I69.943   **Monoplegia of lower limb following** unspecified cerebrovascular disease affecting right non-dominant side HCC ▽

     I69.944   **Monoplegia of lower limb following** unspecified cerebrovascular disease affecting left non-dominant side HCC ▽

     I69.949   **Monoplegia of lower limb following** unspecified cerebrovascular disease affecting unspecified side HCC ▽

✓6ᵗʰ **I69.95**   **Hemiplegia** and hemiparesis following unspecified cerebrovascular disease
     AHA: 2015, 1Q, 25

     I69.951   **Hemiplegia and hemiparesis** following unspecified cerebrovascular disease affecting right dominant side HCC ▽

     I69.952   **Hemiplegia and hemiparesis** following unspecified cerebrovascular disease affecting left dominant side HCC ▽

     I69.953   **Hemiplegia and hemiparesis** following unspecified cerebrovascular disease affecting right non-dominant side HCC ▽

     I69.954   **Hemiplegia and hemiparesis** following unspecified cerebrovascular disease affecting left non-dominant side HCC ▽

     I69.959   **Hemiplegia and hemiparesis** following unspecified cerebrovascular disease affecting unspecified side HCC ▽

✓6ᵗʰ **I69.96**   **Other** paralytic syndrome following unspecified cerebrovascular disease
     Use additional code to identify type of paralytic syndrome, such as:
         locked-in state (G83.5)
         quadriplegia (G82.5-)
     EXCLUDES 1   hemiplegia/hemiparesis following unspecified cerebrovascular disease (I69.95-)
                  monoplegia of lower limb following unspecified cerebrovascular disease (I69.94-)
                  monoplegia of upper limb following unspecified cerebrovascular disease (I69.93-)

     I69.961   **Other paralytic syndrome following** unspecified cerebrovascular disease affecting right dominant side HCC ▽

     I69.962   **Other paralytic syndrome following** unspecified cerebrovascular disease affecting left dominant side HCC ▽

     I69.963   **Other paralytic syndrome following** unspecified cerebrovascular disease affecting right non-dominant side HCC ▽

     I69.964   **Other paralytic syndrome following** unspecified cerebrovascular disease affecting left non-dominant side HCC ▽

     I69.965   **Other paralytic syndrome following** unspecified cerebrovascular disease, bilateral HCC ▽

     I69.969   **Other paralytic syndrome following** unspecified cerebrovascular disease affecting unspecified side HCC ▽

✓6ᵗʰ **I69.99**   **Other sequelae of unspecified cerebrovascular disease**

     I69.990   **Apraxia** following unspecified cerebrovascular disease ▽

     I69.991   **Dysphagia** following unspecified cerebrovascular disease ▽
         Use additional code to identify the type of dysphagia, if known (R13.1-)

     I69.992   **Facial weakness** following unspecified cerebrovascular disease ▽
         Facial droop following unspecified cerebrovascular disease

---

EXCLUDES 1 Not coded here   EXCLUDES 2 Not included here   N Newborn Age: 0   P Pediatric Age: 0-17   M Maternity Age: 12-55   A Adult Age: 15-124

I69.993   **Ataxia following unspecified cerebrovascular disease** ▽

I69.998   **Other sequelae following unspecified cerebrovascular disease** ▽
> Alteration in sensation following unspecified cerebrovascular disease
> Disturbance of vision following unspecified cerebrovascular disease
> Use additional code to identify the sequelae

Diseases of arteries, arterioles and capillaries (I70-I79)

☑4th **I70   Atherosclerosis**

    INCLUDES   arteriolosclerosis
          arterial degeneration
          arteriosclerosis
          arteriosclerotic vascular disease
          arteriovascular degeneration
          atheroma
          endarteritis deformans or obliterans
          senile arteritis
          senile endarteritis
          vascular degeneration

Use additional code to identify:
    exposure to environmental tobacco smoke (Z77.22)
    history of tobacco dependence (Z87.891)
    occupational exposure to environmental tobacco smoke (Z57.31)
    tobacco dependence (F17.-)
    tobacco use (Z72.0)

    EXCLUDES 2   *arteriosclerotic cardiovascular disease (I25.1-)*
          arteriosclerotic heart disease (I25.1-)
          atheroembolism (I75.-)
          cerebral atherosclerosis (I67.2)
          coronary atherosclerosis (I25.1-)
          mesenteric atherosclerosis (K55.1)
          precerebral atherosclerosis (I67.2)
          primary pulmonary atherosclerosis (I27.0)

I70.0   **Atherosclerosis of aorta**   HCC A

I70.1   **Atherosclerosis of renal artery**   HCC A
> Goldblatt's kidney
> EXCLUDES 2   *atherosclerosis of renal arterioles (I12.-)*

☑5th **I70.2   Atherosclerosis of native arteries of the extremities**
> Mönckeberg's (medial) sclerosis
> Use additional code, if applicable, to identify chronic total occlusion of artery of extremity (I70.92)
> EXCLUDES 2   *atherosclerosis of bypass graft of extremities (I70.30-I70.79)*

    ☑6th **I70.20   Unspecified atherosclerosis of native arteries of extremities**

       I70.201   **Unspecified atherosclerosis of native arteries of extremities, right leg**   HCC A ▽

       I70.202   **Unspecified atherosclerosis of native arteries of extremities, left leg**   HCC A ▽

       I70.203   **Unspecified atherosclerosis of native arteries of extremities, bilateral legs**   HCC A ▽

       I70.208   **Unspecified atherosclerosis of native arteries of extremities, other extremity**   HCC A ▽

       I70.209   **Unspecified atherosclerosis of nativearteries of extremities, unspecified extremity**   HCC A ▽

    ☑6th **I70.21   Atherosclerosis of native arteries of extremities with intermittent claudication**

       I70.211   **Atherosclerosis of native arteries of extremities with intermittent claudication, right leg**   HCC A

       I70.212   **Atherosclerosis of native arteries of extremities with intermittent claudication, left leg**   HCC A

       I70.213   **Atherosclerosis of native arteries of extremities with intermittent claudication, bilateral legs**   HCC A

       I70.218   **Atherosclerosis of native arteries of extremities with intermittent claudication, other extremity**   HCC A

       I70.219   **Atherosclerosis of native arteries of extremities with intermittent claudication, unspecified extremity**   HCC A ▽

☑6th **I70.22   Atherosclerosis of native arteries of extremities with rest pain**
> INCLUDES   any condition classifiable to I70.21-

    I70.221   **Atherosclerosis of native arteries of extremities with rest pain, right leg**   HCC A

    I70.222   **Atherosclerosis of native arteries of extremities with rest pain, left leg**   HCC A

    I70.223   **Atherosclerosis of native arteries of extremities with rest pain, bilateral legs**   HCC A

    I70.228   **Atherosclerosis of native arteries of extremities with rest pain, other extremity**   HCC A

    I70.229   **Atherosclerosis of native arteries of extremities with rest pain, unspecified extremity**   HCC A ▽

☑6th **I70.23   Atherosclerosis of native arteries of right leg with ulceration**
> INCLUDES   any condition classifiable to I70.211 and I70.221
> Use additional code to identify severity of ulcer (L97.-)

    I70.231   **Atherosclerosis of native arteries of right leg with ulceration of thigh**   HCC A

    I70.232   **Atherosclerosis of native arteries of right leg with ulceration of calf**   HCC A

    I70.233   **Atherosclerosis of native arteries of right leg with ulceration of ankle**   HCC A

    I70.234   **Atherosclerosis of native arteries of right leg with ulceration of heel and midfoot**   HCC A
> Atherosclerosis of native arteries of right leg with ulceration of plantar surface of midfoot

    I70.235   **Atherosclerosis of native arteries of right leg with ulceration of other part of foot**   HCC A
> Atherosclerosis of native arteries of right leg extremities with ulceration of toe

    I70.238   **Atherosclerosis of native arteries of right leg with ulceration of other part of lower right leg**   HCC A

    I70.239   **Atherosclerosis of native arteries of right leg with ulceration of unspecified site**   HCC A ▽

☑6th **I70.24   Atherosclerosis of native arteries of left leg with ulceration**
> INCLUDES   any condition classifiable to I70.212 and I70.222
> Use additional code to identify severity of ulcer (L97.-)

    I70.241   **Atherosclerosis of native arteries of left leg with ulceration of thigh**   HCC A

    I70.242   **Atherosclerosis of native arteries of left leg with ulceration of calf**   HCC A

    I70.243   **Atherosclerosis of native arteries of left leg with ulceration of ankle**   HCC A

    I70.244   **Atherosclerosis of native arteries of left leg with ulceration of heel and midfoot**   HCC A
> Atherosclerosis of native arteries of left leg with ulceration of plantar surface of midfoot

    I70.245   **Atherosclerosis of native arteries of left leg with ulceration of other part of foot**   HCC A
> Atherosclerosis of native arteries of left leg extremities with ulceration of toe

    I70.248   **Atherosclerosis of native arteries of left leg with ulceration of other part of lower left leg**   HCC A

    I70.249   **Atherosclerosis of native arteries of left leg with ulceration of unspecified site**   HCC A ▽

    I70.25   **Atherosclerosis of native arteries of other extremities with ulceration**   HCC A
> INCLUDES   an y condition classifiable to I70.218 and I70.228
> Use additional code to identify the severity of the ulcer (L98.49-)

☑ Additional Character Req   v x 7th Placeholder Alert   Manifestation   HCC CMS-HCC Condition   ▽ Unspecified Code   ►◄ Revised Text   ● New Code   ▲ Revised Code Title

Chapter 9. Diseases of the Circulatory System

I70.26-I70.349

✓6ᵗʰ **I70.26 Atherosclerosis of native arteries of extremities with gangrene**
INCLUDES any condition classifiable to I70.21-, I70.22-, I70.23-, I70.24-, and I70.25-
Use additional code to identify the severity of any ulcer (L97.-, L98.49-), if applicable

I70.261 Atherosclerosis of native arteries of HCC A extremities with gangrene, right leg

I70.262 Atherosclerosis of native arteries of HCC A extremities with gangrene, left leg

I70.263 Atherosclerosis of native arteries of HCC A extremities with gangrene, bilateral legs

I70.268 Atherosclerosis of native arteries of HCC A extremities with gangrene, other extremity

I70.269 Atherosclerosis of native arteries HCC A ▽ of extremities with gangrene, unspecified extremity

✓6ᵗʰ **I70.29 Other atherosclerosis of native arteries of extremities**

I70.291 Other atherosclerosis of native HCC A arteries of extremities, right leg

I70.292 Other atherosclerosis of native HCC A arteries of extremities, left leg

I70.293 Other atherosclerosis of native HCC A arteries of extremities, bilateral legs

I70.298 Other atherosclerosis of native HCC A arteries of extremities, other extremity

I70.299 Other atherosclerosis of native HCC A ▽ arteries of extremities, unspecified extremity

✓5ᵗʰ **I70.3 Atherosclerosis of unspecified type of bypass graft(s) of the extremities**
Use additional code, if applicable, to identify chronic total occlusion of artery of extremity (I70.92)
EXCLUDES 1 embolism or thrombus of bypass graft(s) of extremities (T82.8-)

✓6ᵗʰ **I70.30 Unspecified atherosclerosis of unspecified type of bypass graft(s) of the extremities**

I70.301 Unspecified atherosclerosis of HCC A ▽ unspecified type of bypass graft(s) of the extremities, right leg

I70.302 Unspecified atherosclerosis of HCC A ▽ unspecified type of bypass graft(s) of the extremities, left leg

I70.303 Unspecified atherosclerosis of HCC A ▽ unspecified type of bypass graft(s) of the extremities, bilateral legs

I70.308 Unspecified atherosclerosis of HCC A ▽ unspecified type of bypass graft(s) of the extremities, other extremity

I70.309 Unspecified atherosclerosis of HCC A ▽ unspecified type of bypass graft(s) of the extremities, unspecified extremity

✓6ᵗʰ **I70.31 Atherosclerosis of unspecified type of bypass graft(s) of the extremities with intermittent claudication**

I70.311 Atherosclerosis of unspecified type HCC A of bypass graft(s) of the extremities with intermittent claudication, right leg

I70.312 Atherosclerosis of unspecified type HCC A of bypass graft(s) of the extremities with intermittent claudication, left leg

I70.313 Atherosclerosis of unspecified type HCC A of bypass graft(s) of the extremities with intermittent claudication, bilateral legs

I70.318 Atherosclerosis of unspecified type HCC A of bypass graft(s) of the extremities with intermittent claudication, other extremity

I70.319 Atherosclerosis of unspecified HCC A ▽ type of bypass graft(s) of the extremities with intermittent claudication, unspecified extremity

✓6ᵗʰ **I70.32 Atherosclerosis of unspecified type of bypass graft(s) of the extremities with rest pain**
INCLUDES any condition classifiable to I70.31-

I70.321 Atherosclerosis of unspecified type HCC A of bypass graft(s) of the extremities with rest pain, right leg

I70.322 Atherosclerosis of unspecified type HCC A of bypass graft(s) of the extremities with rest pain, left leg

I70.323 Atherosclerosis of unspecified type HCC A of bypass graft(s) of the extremities with rest pain, bilateral legs

I70.328 Atherosclerosis of unspecified type HCC A of bypass graft(s) of the extremities with rest pain, other extremity

I70.329 Atherosclerosis of unspecified HCC A ▽ type of bypass graft(s) of the extremities with rest pain, unspecified extremity

✓6ᵗʰ **I70.33 Atherosclerosis of unspecified type of bypass graft(s) of the right leg with ulceration**
INCLUDES any condition classifiable to I70.311 and I70.321
Use additional code to identify severity of ulcer (L97.-)

I70.331 Atherosclerosis of unspecified type HCC A of bypass graft(s) of the right leg with ulceration of thigh

I70.332 Atherosclerosis of unspecified type HCC A of bypass graft(s) of the right leg with ulceration of calf

I70.333 Atherosclerosis of unspecified type HCC A of bypass graft(s) of the right leg with ulceration of ankle

I70.334 Atherosclerosis of unspecified type HCC A of bypass graft(s) of the right leg with ulceration of heel and midfoot
Atherosclerosis of unspecified type of bypass graft(s) of right leg with ulceration of plantar surface of midfoot

I70.335 Atherosclerosis of unspecified type HCC A of bypass graft(s) of the right leg with ulceration of other part of foot
Atherosclerosis of unspecified type of bypass graft(s) of the right leg with ulceration of toe

I70.338 Atherosclerosis of unspecified type HCC A of bypass graft(s) of the right leg with ulceration of other part of lower leg

I70.339 Atherosclerosis of unspecified HCC A ▽ type of bypass graft(s) of the right leg with ulceration of unspecified site

✓6ᵗʰ **I70.34 Atherosclerosis of unspecified type of bypass graft(s) of the left leg with ulceration**
INCLUDES any condition classifiable to I70.312 and I70.322
Use additional code to identify severity of ulcer (L97.-)

I70.341 Atherosclerosis of unspecified type HCC A of bypass graft(s) of the left leg with ulceration of thigh

I70.342 Atherosclerosis of unspecified type HCC A of bypass graft(s) of the left leg with ulceration of calf

I70.343 Atherosclerosis of unspecified type HCC A of bypass graft(s) of the left leg with ulceration of ankle

I70.344 Atherosclerosis of unspecified type HCC A of bypass graft(s) of the left leg with ulceration of heel and midfoot
Atherosclerosis of unspecified type of bypass graft(s) of left leg with ulceration of plantar surface of midfoot

I70.345 Atherosclerosis of unspecified type HCC A of bypass graft(s) of the left leg with ulceration of other part of foot
Atherosclerosis of unspecified type of bypass graft(s) of the left leg with ulceration of toe

I70.348 Atherosclerosis of unspecified type HCC A of bypass graft(s) of the left leg with ulceration of other part of lower leg

I70.349 Atherosclerosis of unspecified HCC A ▽ type of bypass graft(s) of the left leg with ulceration of unspecified site

I70.35   Atherosclerosis of unspecified type of bypass HCC A graft(s) of other extremity with ulceration
> INCLUDES   any condition classifiable to I70.318 and I70.328
> Use additional code to identify severity of ulcer (L98.49-)

✓6ᵗʰ **I70.36**   Atherosclerosis of unspecified type of bypass graft(s) of the extremities with gangrene
> INCLUDES   any condition classifiable to I70.31-, I70.32-, I70.33-, I70.34-, I70.35
> Use additional code to identify the severity of any ulcer (L97.-, L98.49-), if applicable

     I70.361   Atherosclerosis of unspecified type HCC A of bypass graft(s) of the extremities with gangrene, right leg

     I70.362   Atherosclerosis of unspecified type HCC A of bypass graft(s) of the extremities with gangrene, left leg

     I70.363   Atherosclerosis of unspecified type HCC A of bypass graft(s) of the extremities with gangrene, bilateral legs

     I70.368   Atherosclerosis of unspecified type HCC A of bypass graft(s) of the extremities with gangrene, other extremity

     I70.369   Atherosclerosis of unspecified HCC A ▽ type of bypass graft(s) of the extremities with gangrene, unspecified extremity

✓6ᵗʰ **I70.39**   Other atherosclerosis of unspecified type of bypass graft(s) of the extremities

     I70.391   Other atherosclerosis of HCC A unspecified type of bypass graft(s) of the extremities, right leg

     I70.392   Other atherosclerosis of HCC A unspecified type of bypass graft(s) of the extremities, left leg

     I70.393   Other atherosclerosis of HCC A unspecified type of bypass graft(s) of the extremities, bilateral legs

     I70.398   Other atherosclerosis of HCC A unspecified type of bypass graft(s) of the extremities, other extremity

     I70.399   Other atherosclerosis of HCC A ▽ unspecified type of bypass graft(s) of the extremities, unspecified extremity

✓5ᵗʰ **I70.4**   Atherosclerosis of autologous vein bypass graft(s) of the extremities
> Use additional code, if applicable, to identify chronic total occlusion of artery of extremity (I70.92)

✓6ᵗʰ **I70.40**   Unspecified atherosclerosis of autologous vein bypass graft(s) of the extremities

     I70.401   Unspecified atherosclerosis of HCC A ▽ autologous vein bypass graft(s) of the extremities, right leg

     I70.402   Unspecified atherosclerosis of HCC A ▽ autologous vein bypass graft(s) of the extremities, left leg

     I70.403   Unspecified atherosclerosis of HCC A ▽ autologous vein bypass graft(s) of the extremities, bilateral legs

     I70.408   Unspecified atherosclerosis of HCC A ▽ autologous vein bypass graft(s) of the extremities, other extremity

     I70.409   Unspecified atherosclerosis of HCC A ▽ autologous vein bypass graft(s) of the extremities, unspecified extremity

✓6ᵗʰ **I70.41**   Atherosclerosis of autologous vein bypass graft(s) of the extremities with intermittent claudication

     I70.411   Atherosclerosis of autologous vein HCC A bypass graft(s) of the extremities with intermittent claudication, right leg

     I70.412   Atherosclerosis of autologous vein HCC A bypass graft(s) of the extremities with intermittent claudication, left leg

     I70.413   Atherosclerosis of autologous vein HCC A bypass graft(s) of the extremities with intermittent claudication, bilateral legs

     I70.418   Atherosclerosis of autologous vein HCC A bypass graft(s) of the extremities with intermittent claudication, other extremity

     I70.419   Atherosclerosis of autologous HCC A ▽ vein bypass graft(s) of the extremities with intermittent claudication, unspecified extremity

✓6ᵗʰ **I70.42**   Atherosclerosis of autologous vein bypass graft(s) of the extremities with rest pain
> INCLUDES   any condition classifiable to I70.41-

     I70.421   Atherosclerosis of autologous vein HCC A bypass graft(s) of the extremities with rest pain, right leg

     I70.422   Atherosclerosis of autologous vein HCC A bypass graft(s) of the extremities with rest pain, left leg

     I70.423   Atherosclerosis of autologous vein HCC A bypass graft(s) of the extremities with rest pain, bilateral legs

     I70.428   Atherosclerosis of autologous vein HCC A bypass graft(s) of the extremities with rest pain, other extremity

     I70.429   Atherosclerosis of autologous HCC A ▽ vein bypass graft(s) of the extremities with rest pain, unspecified extremity

✓6ᵗʰ **I70.43**   Atherosclerosis of autologous vein bypass graft(s) of the right leg with ulceration
> INCLUDES   any condition classifiable to I70.411 and I70.421
> Use additional code to identify severity of ulcer (L97.-)

     I70.431   Atherosclerosis of autologous vein HCC A bypass graft(s) of the right leg with ulceration of thigh

     I70.432   Atherosclerosis of autologous vein HCC A bypass graft(s) of the right leg with ulceration of calf

     I70.433   Atherosclerosis of autologous vein HCC A bypass graft(s) of the right leg with ulceration of ankle

     I70.434   Atherosclerosis of autologous vein HCC A bypass graft(s) of the right leg with ulceration of heel and midfoot
> Atherosclerosis of autologous vein bypass graft(s) of right leg with ulceration of plantar surface of midfoot

     I70.435   Atherosclerosis of autologous vein HCC A bypass graft(s) of the right leg with ulceration of other part of foot
> Atherosclerosis of autologous vein bypass graft(s) of right leg with ulceration of toe

     I70.438   Atherosclerosis of autologous vein HCC A bypass graft(s) of the right leg with ulceration of other part of lower leg

     I70.439   Atherosclerosis of autologous HCC A ▽ vein bypass graft(s) of the right leg with ulceration of unspecified site

✓6ᵗʰ **I70.44**   Atherosclerosis of autologous vein bypass graft(s) of the left leg with ulceration
> INCLUDES   any condition classifiable to I70.412 and I70.422
> Use additional code to identify severity of ulcer (L97.-)

     I70.441   Atherosclerosis of autologous vein HCC A bypass graft(s) of the left leg with ulceration of thigh

     I70.442   Atherosclerosis of autologous vein HCC A bypass graft(s) of the left leg with ulceration of calf

     I70.443   Atherosclerosis of autologous vein HCC A bypass graft(s) of the left leg with ulceration of ankle

     I70.444   Atherosclerosis of autologous vein HCC A bypass graft(s) of the left leg with ulceration of heel and midfoot
> Atherosclerosis of autologous vein bypass graft(s) of left leg with ulceration of plantar surface of midfoot

     I70.445   Atherosclerosis of autologous vein HCC A bypass graft(s) of the left leg with ulceration of other part of foot
> Atherosclerosis of autologous vein bypass graft(s) of left leg with ulceration of toe

---

☑ Additional Character Req   ✓x7ᵗʰ Placeholder Alert   Manifestation   HCC CMS-HCC Condition   ▽ Unspecified Code   ►◄ Revised Text   ● New Code   ▲ Revised Code Title

ICD-10-CM 2018   **641**

I70.448 Atherosclerosis of autologous vein `HCC` `A` bypass graft(s) of the left leg with ulceration of other part of lower leg

I70.449 Atherosclerosis of autologous `HCC` `A` `▽` vein bypass graft(s) of the left leg with ulceration of unspecified site

I70.45 Atherosclerosis of autologous vein bypass `HCC` `A` graft(s) of other extremity with ulceration
> INCLUDES any condition classifiable to I70.418, I70.428, and I70.438
> Use additional code to identify severity of ulcer (L98.49)

`✓6ᵗʰ` **I70.46** Atherosclerosis of autologous vein bypass graft(s) of the extremities with gangrene
> INCLUDES any condition classifiable to I70.41-, I70.42-, and I70.43-, I70.44-, I70.45
> Use additional code to identify the severity of any ulcer (L97.-, L98.49-), if applicable

I70.461 Atherosclerosis of autologous vein `HCC` `A` bypass graft(s) of the extremities with gangrene, right leg

I70.462 Atherosclerosis of autologous vein `HCC` `A` bypass graft(s) of the extremities with gangrene, left leg

I70.463 Atherosclerosis of autologous vein `HCC` `A` bypass graft(s) of the extremities with gangrene, bilateral legs

I70.468 Atherosclerosis of autologous vein `HCC` `A` bypass graft(s) of the extremities with gangrene, other extremity

I70.469 Atherosclerosis of autologous `HCC` `A` `▽` vein bypass graft(s) of the extremities with gangrene, unspecified extremity

`✓6ᵗʰ` **I70.49** Other atherosclerosis of autologous vein bypass graft(s) of the extremities

I70.491 Other atherosclerosis of autologous `HCC` `A` vein bypass graft(s) of the extremities, right leg

I70.492 Other atherosclerosis of autologous `HCC` `A` vein bypass graft(s) of the extremities, left leg

I70.493 Other atherosclerosis of autologous `HCC` `A` vein bypass graft(s) of the extremities, bilateral legs

I70.498 Other atherosclerosis of autologous `HCC` `A` vein bypass graft(s) of the extremities, other extremity

I70.499 Other atherosclerosis of `HCC` `A` `▽` autologous vein bypass graft(s) of the extremities, unspecified extremity

`✓5ᵗʰ` **I70.5** Atherosclerosis of nonautologous biological bypass graft(s) of the extremities
> Use additional code, if applicable, to identify chronic total occlusion of artery of extremity (I70.92)

`✓6ᵗʰ` **I70.50** Unspecified atherosclerosis of nonautologous biological bypass graft(s) of the extremities

I70.501 Unspecified atherosclerosis of `HCC` `A` `▽` nonautologous biological bypass graft(s) of the extremities, right leg

I70.502 Unspecified atherosclerosis of `HCC` `A` `▽` nonautologous biological bypass graft(s) of the extremities, left leg

I70.503 Unspecified atherosclerosis of `HCC` `A` `▽` nonautologous biological bypass graft(s) of the extremities, bilateral legs

I70.508 Unspecified atherosclerosis of `HCC` `A` `▽` nonautologous biological bypass graft(s) of the extremities, other extremity

I70.509 Unspecified atherosclerosis of `HCC` `A` `▽` nonautologous biological bypass graft(s) of the extremities, unspecified extremity

`✓6ᵗʰ` **I70.51** Atherosclerosis of nonautologous biological bypass graft(s) of the extremities with intermittent claudication

I70.511 Atherosclerosis of nonautologous `HCC` `A` biological bypass graft(s) of the extremities with intermittent claudication, right leg

I70.512 Atherosclerosis of nonautologous `HCC` `A` biological bypass graft(s) of the extremities with intermittent claudication, left leg

I70.513 Atherosclerosis of nonautologous `HCC` `A` biological bypass graft(s) of the extremities with intermittent claudication, bilateral legs

I70.518 Atherosclerosis of nonautologous `HCC` `A` biological bypass graft(s) of the extremities with intermittent claudication, other extremity

I70.519 Atherosclerosis of nonautologous `HCC` `A` `▽` biological bypass graft(s) of the extremities with intermittent claudication, unspecified extremity

`✓6ᵗʰ` **I70.52** Atherosclerosis of nonautologous biological bypass graft(s) of the extremities with rest pain
> INCLUDES any condition classifiable to I70.51-

I70.521 Atherosclerosis of nonautologous `HCC` `A` biological bypass graft(s) of the extremities with rest pain, right leg

I70.522 Atherosclerosis of nonautologous `HCC` `A` biological bypass graft(s) of the extremities with rest pain, left leg

I70.523 Atherosclerosis of nonautologous `HCC` `A` biological bypass graft(s) of the extremities with rest pain, bilateral legs

I70.528 Atherosclerosis of nonautologous `HCC` `A` biological bypass graft(s) of the extremities with rest pain, other extremity

I70.529 Atherosclerosis of nonautologous `HCC` `A` `▽` biological bypass graft(s) of the extremities with rest pain, unspecified extremity

`✓6ᵗʰ` **I70.53** Atherosclerosis of nonautologous biological bypass graft(s) of the right leg with ulceration
> INCLUDES any condition classifiable to I70.511 and I70.521
> Use additional code to identify severity of ulcer (L97.-)

I70.531 Atherosclerosis of nonautologous `HCC` `A` biological bypass graft(s) of the right leg with ulceration of thigh

I70.532 Atherosclerosis of nonautologous `HCC` `A` biological bypass graft(s) of the right leg with ulceration of calf

I70.533 Atherosclerosis of nonautologous `HCC` `A` biological bypass graft(s) of the right leg with ulceration of ankle

I70.534 Atherosclerosis of nonautologous `HCC` `A` biological bypass graft(s) of the right leg with ulceration of heel and midfoot
> Atherosclerosis of nonautologous biological bypass graft(s) of right leg with ulceration of plantar surface of midfoot

I70.535 Atherosclerosis of nonautologous `HCC` `A` biological bypass graft(s) of the right leg with ulceration of other part of foot
> Atherosclerosis of nonautologous biological bypass graft(s) of the right leg with ulceration of toe

I70.538 Atherosclerosis of nonautologous `HCC` `A` biological bypass graft(s) of the right leg with ulceration of other part of lower leg

I70.539 Atherosclerosis of nonautologous `HCC` `A` `▽` biological bypass graft(s) of the right leg with ulceration of unspecified site

`✓6ᵗʰ` **I70.54** Atherosclerosis of nonautologous biological bypass graft(s) of the left leg with ulceration
> INCLUDES any condition classifiable to I70.512 and I70.522
> Use additional code to identify severity of ulcer (L97.-)

I70.541 Atherosclerosis of nonautologous `HCC` `A` biological bypass graft(s) of the left leg with ulceration of thigh

I70.542 Atherosclerosis of nonautologous `HCC` `A` biological bypass graft(s) of the left leg with ulceration of calf

I70.543 Atherosclerosis of nonautologous `HCC` `A` biological bypass graft(s) of the left leg with ulceration of ankle

EXCLUDES 1 Not coded here   EXCLUDES 2 Not included here   N Newborn Age: 0   P Pediatric Age: 0-17   M Maternity Age: 12-55   A Adult Age: 15-124

642   ICD-10-CM 2018

I70.544 **Atherosclerosis of nonautologous** HCC A
biological bypass graft(s) of the left leg
with ulceration of heel and midfoot
Atherosclerosis of nonautologous
biological bypass graft(s) of left leg
with ulceration of plantar surface of
midfoot

I70.545 **Atherosclerosis of nonautologous** HCC A
biological bypass graft(s) of the left leg
with ulceration of other part of foot
Atherosclerosis of nonautologous
biological bypass graft(s) of the left leg
with ulceration of toe

I70.548 **Atherosclerosis of nonautologous** HCC A
biological bypass graft(s) of the left leg
with ulceration of other part of lower leg

I70.549 **Atherosclerosis of nonautologous** HCC A ▽
biological bypass graft(s) of the left
leg with ulceration of unspecified site

I70.55 **Atherosclerosis of nonautologous biological** HCC A
bypass graft(s) of other extremity with ulceration
[INCLUDES] any condition classifiable to I70.518,
I70.528, and I70.538
Use additional code to identify severity of ulcer
(L98.49)

✓6ᵗʰ **I70.56** **Atherosclerosis of nonautologous biological bypass**
graft(s) of the extremities with gangrene
[INCLUDES] any condition classifiable to I70.51-, I70.52-,
and I70.53-, I70.54-, I70.55
Use additional code to identify the severity of any
ulcer (L97.-, L98.49-), if applicable

I70.561 **Atherosclerosis of nonautologous** HCC A
biological bypass graft(s) of the
extremities with gangrene, right leg

I70.562 **Atherosclerosis of nonautologous** HCC A
biological bypass graft(s) of the
extremities with gangrene, left leg

I70.563 **Atherosclerosis of nonautologous** HCC A
biological bypass graft(s) of the
extremities with gangrene, bilateral legs

I70.568 **Atherosclerosis of nonautologous** HCC A
biological bypass graft(s) of the
extremities with gangrene, other
extremity

I70.569 **Atherosclerosis of nonautologous** HCC A ▽
biological bypass graft(s) of the
extremities with gangrene, unspecified
extremity

✓6ᵗʰ **I70.59** **Other atherosclerosis of nonautologous biological**
bypass graft(s) of the extremities

I70.591 **Other atherosclerosis of** HCC A
nonautologous biological bypass graft(s)
of the extremities, right leg

I70.592 **Other atherosclerosis of** HCC A
nonautologous biological bypass graft(s)
of the extremities, left leg

I70.593 **Other atherosclerosis of** HCC A
nonautologous biological bypass graft(s)
of the extremities, bilateral legs

I70.598 **Other atherosclerosis of** HCC A
nonautologous biological bypass graft(s)
of the extremities, other extremity

I70.599 **Other atherosclerosis of non-** HCC A ▽
autologous biological bypass graft(s) of
the extremities, unspecified extremity

✓5ᵗʰ **I70.6** **Atherosclerosis of** nonbiological bypass graft(s) of the
extremities
Use additional code, if applicable, to identify chronic total
occlusion of artery of extremity (I70.92)

✓6ᵗʰ **I70.60** **Unspecified atherosclerosis of nonbiological bypass**
graft(s) of the extremities

I70.601 **Unspecified atherosclerosis of** HCC A ▽
nonbiological bypass graft(s) of the
extremities, right leg

I70.602 **Unspecified atherosclerosis of** HCC A ▽
nonbiological bypass graft(s) of the
extremities, left leg

I70.603 **Unspecified atherosclerosis of** HCC A ▽
nonbiological bypass graft(s) of the
extremities, bilateral legs

I70.608 **Unspecified atherosclerosis of** HCC A ▽
nonbiological bypass graft(s) of the
extremities, other extremity

I70.609 **Unspecified atherosclerosis of** HCC A ▽
nonbiological bypass graft(s) of the
extremities, unspecified extremity

✓6ᵗʰ **I70.61** **Atherosclerosis of nonbiological bypass graft(s) of**
the extremities with intermittent claudication

I70.611 **Atherosclerosis of nonbiological** HCC A
bypass graft(s) of the extremities with
intermittent claudication, right leg

I70.612 **Atherosclerosis of nonbiological** HCC A
bypass graft(s) of the extremities with
intermittent claudication, left leg

I70.613 **Atherosclerosis of nonbiological** HCC A
bypass graft(s) of the extremities with
intermittent claudication, bilateral legs

I70.618 **Atherosclerosis of nonbiological** HCC A
bypass graft(s) of the extremities
with intermittent claudication, other
extremity

I70.619 **Atherosclerosis of nonbiological** HCC A ▽
bypass graft(s) of the extremities with
intermittent claudication, unspecified
extremity

✓6ᵗʰ **I70.62** **Atherosclerosis of nonbiological bypass graft(s) of**
the extremities with rest pain
[INCLUDES] any condition classifiable to I70.61-

I70.621 **Atherosclerosis of nonbiological** HCC A
bypass graft(s) of the extremities
with rest pain, right leg

I70.622 **Atherosclerosis of nonbiological** HCC A
bypass graft(s) of the extremities
with rest pain, left leg

I70.623 **Atherosclerosis of nonbiological** HCC A
bypass graft(s) of the extremities
with rest pain, bilateral legs

I70.628 **Atherosclerosis of nonbiological** HCC A
bypass graft(s) of the extremities
with rest pain, other extremity

I70.629 **Atherosclerosis of nonbiological** HCC A ▽
bypass graft(s) of the extremities
with rest pain, unspecified extremity

✓6ᵗʰ **I70.63** **Atherosclerosis of nonbiological bypass graft(s) of**
the right leg with ulceration
[INCLUDES] any condition classifiable to I70.611 and
I70.621
Use additional code to identify severity of ulcer (L97.-)

I70.631 **Atherosclerosis of nonbiological** HCC A
bypass graft(s) of the right leg with
ulceration of thigh

I70.632 **Atherosclerosis of nonbiological** HCC A
bypass graft(s) of the right leg with
ulceration of calf

I70.633 **Atherosclerosis of nonbiological** HCC A
bypass graft(s) of the right leg with
ulceration of ankle

I70.634 **Atherosclerosis of nonbiological** HCC A
bypass graft(s) of the right leg with
ulceration of heel and midfoot
Atherosclerosis of nonbiological bypass
graft(s) of right leg with ulceration of
plantar surface of midfoot

I70.635 **Atherosclerosis of nonbiological** HCC A
bypass graft(s) of the right leg with
ulceration of other part of foot
Atherosclerosis of nonbiological bypass
graft(s) of the right leg with ulceration
of toe

I70.638 **Atherosclerosis of nonbiological** HCC A
bypass graft(s) of the right leg with
ulceration of other part of lower leg

I70.639 **Atherosclerosis of nonbiological** HCC A ▽
bypass graft(s) of the right leg with
ulceration of unspecified site

☑ Additional Character Req   ✓ˣ⁷ᵗʰ Placeholder Alert   Manifestation   HCC CMS-HCC Condition   ▽ Unspecified Code   ►◄ Revised Text   ● New Code   ▲ Revised Code Title

✓6ᵗʰ **I70.64** **Atherosclerosis of nonbiological bypass graft(s) of the** left leg with ulceration
> INCLUDES   any condition classifiable to I70.612 and I70.622
> Use additional code to identify severity of ulcer (L97.-)

- I70.641 **Atherosclerosis of nonbiological bypass graft(s) of the left leg with ulceration of** thigh   HCC A
- I70.642 **Atherosclerosis of nonbiological bypass graft(s) of the left leg with ulceration of** calf   HCC A
- I70.643 **Atherosclerosis of nonbiological bypass graft(s) of the left leg with ulceration of** ankle   HCC A
- I70.644 **Atherosclerosis of nonbiological bypass graft(s) of the left leg with ulceration of** heel and midfoot   HCC A
  > Atherosclerosis of nonbiological bypass graft(s) of left leg with ulceration of plantar surface of midfoot
- I70.645 **Atherosclerosis of nonbiological bypassgraft(s) of the left leg with ulceration of other** part of foot   HCC A
  > Atherosclerosis of nonbiological bypass graft(s) of the left leg with ulceration of toe
- I70.648 **Atherosclerosis of nonbiological bypass graft(s) of the left leg with ulceration of other** part of lower leg   HCC A
- I70.649 **Atherosclerosis of nonbiological bypass graft(s) of the left leg with ulceration of unspecified site**   HCC A ▽

I70.65 **Atherosclerosis of nonbiological bypass graft(s) of other extremity with** ulceration   HCC A
> INCLUDES   any condition classifiable to I70.618 and I70.628
> Use additional code to identify severity of ulcer (L98.49)

✓6ᵗʰ **I70.66** **Atherosclerosis of nonbiological bypass graft(s) of the extremities with** gangrene
> INCLUDES   any condition classifiable to I70.61-, I70.62-, I70.63-, I70.64-, I70.65
> Use additional code to identify the severity of any ulcer (L97.-, L98.49-), if applicable

- I70.661 **Atherosclerosis of nonbiological bypass graft(s) of the extremities with gangrene,** right leg   HCC A
- I70.662 **Atherosclerosis of nonbiological bypass graft(s) of the extremities with gangrene,** left leg   HCC A
- I70.663 **Atherosclerosis of nonbiological bypass graft(s) of the extremities with gangrene,** bilateral legs   HCC A
- I70.668 **Atherosclerosis of nonbiological bypass graft(s) of the extremities with gangrene, other extremity**   HCC A
- I70.669 **Atherosclerosis of nonbiological bypass graft(s) of the extremities with gangrene, unspecified extremity**   HCC A ▽

✓6ᵗʰ **I70.69** **Other atherosclerosis of nonbiological bypass graft(s) of the extremities**

- I70.691 **Other atherosclerosis of nonbiological bypass graft(s) of the extremities,** right leg   HCC A
- I70.692 **Other atherosclerosis of nonbiological bypass graft(s) of the extremities,** left leg   HCC A
- I70.693 **Other atherosclerosis of nonbiological bypass graft(s) of the extremities,** bilateral legs   HCC A
- I70.698 **Other atherosclerosis of nonbiological bypass graft(s) of the extremities, other extremity**   HCC A
- I70.699 **Other atherosclerosis of non-biological bypass graft(s) of the extremities, unspecified extremity**   HCC A ▽

✓5ᵗʰ **I70.7** **Atherosclerosis of other type of** bypass graft(s) of the extremities
> Use additional code, if applicable, to identify chronic total occlusion of artery of extremity (I70.92)

✓6ᵗʰ **I70.70** **Unspecified atherosclerosis of other type of bypass graft(s) of the extremities**

- I70.701 **Unspecified atherosclerosis of other type of bypass graft(s) of the extremities,** right leg   HCC A ▽
- I70.702 **Unspecified atherosclerosis of other type of bypass graft(s) of the extremities,** left leg   HCC A ▽
- I70.703 **Unspecified atherosclerosis of other type of bypass graft(s) of the extremities,** bilateral legs   HCC A ▽
- I70.708 **Unspecified atherosclerosis of other type of bypass graft(s) of the extremities, other extremity**   HCC A ▽
- I70.709 **Unspecified atherosclerosis of other type of bypass graft(s) of the extremities, unspecified extremity**   HCC A ▽

✓6ᵗʰ **I70.71** **Atherosclerosis of other type of bypass graft(s) of the extremities with** intermittent claudication

- I70.711 **Atherosclerosis of other type of bypass graft(s) of the extremities with intermittent claudication,** right leg   HCC A
- I70.712 **Atherosclerosis of other type of bypass graft(s) of the extremities with intermittent claudication,** left leg   HCC A
- I70.713 **Atherosclerosis of other type of bypass graft(s) of the extremities with intermittent claudication,** bilateral legs   HCC A
- I70.718 **Atherosclerosis of other type of bypass graft(s) of the extremities with intermittent claudication, other extremity**   HCC A
- I70.719 **Atherosclerosis of other type of bypass graft(s) of the extremities withintermittent claudication, unspecified extremity**   HCC A ▽

✓6ᵗʰ **I70.72** **Atherosclerosis of other type of bypass graft(s) of the extremities with** rest pain
> INCLUDES   any condition classifiable to I70.71-

- I70.721 **Atherosclerosis of other type of bypass graft(s) of the extremities with rest pain,** right leg   HCC A
- I70.722 **Atherosclerosis of other type of bypass graft(s) of the extremities with rest pain,** left leg   HCC A
- I70.723 **Atherosclerosis of other type of bypass graft(s) of the extremities with rest pain,** bilateral legs   HCC A
- I70.728 **Atherosclerosis of other type of bypass graft(s) of the extremities with rest pain, other extremity**   HCC A
- I70.729 **Atherosclerosis of other type of bypass graft(s) of the extremities with rest pain, unspecified extremity**   HCC A ▽

✓6ᵗʰ **I70.73** **Atherosclerosis of other type of bypass graft(s) of the** right leg with ulceration
> INCLUDES   any condition classifiable to I70.711 and I70.721
> Use additional code to identify severity of ulcer (L97.-)

- I70.731 **Atherosclerosis of other type of bypass graft(s) of the right leg with ulceration of** thigh   HCC A
- I70.732 **Atherosclerosis of other type of bypass graft(s) of the right leg with ulceration of** calf   HCC A
- I70.733 **Atherosclerosis of other type of bypass graft(s) of the right leg with ulceration of** ankle   HCC A
- I70.734 **Atherosclerosis of other type of bypass graft(s) of the right leg with ulceration of** heel and midfoot   HCC A
  > Atherosclerosis of other type of bypass graft(s) of right leg with ulceration of plantar surface of midfoot

EXCLUDES 1 Not coded here   **EXCLUDES 2** Not included here   N Newborn Age: 0   P Pediatric Age: 0-17   M Maternity Age: 12-55   A Adult Age: 15-124

644   ICD-10-CM 2018

I70.735 **Atherosclerosis of other type of** HCC A
bypass graft(s) of the right leg with
ulceration of other part of foot
Atherosclerosis of other type of bypass
graft(s) of right leg with ulceration of
toe

I70.738 **Atherosclerosis of other type of** HCC A
bypass graft(s) of the right leg with
ulceration of other part of lower leg

I70.739 **Atherosclerosis of other type of** HCC A ▽
bypass graft(s) of the right leg with
ulceration of unspecified site

✓6th **I70.74** **Atherosclerosis of other type of bypass graft(s) of**
the left leg with ulceration
INCLUDES   any condition classifiable to I70.712 and
I70.722
Use additional code to identify severity of ulcer (L97.-)

I70.741 **Atherosclerosis of other type of** HCC A
bypass graft(s) of the left leg with
ulceration of thigh

I70.742 **Atherosclerosis of other type of** HCC A
bypass graft(s) of the left leg with
ulceration of calf

I70.743 **Atherosclerosis of other type of** HCC A
bypass raft(s) of the left leg with
ulceration of ankle

I70.744 **Atherosclerosis of other type of** HCC A
bypass graft(s) of the left leg with
ulceration of heel and midfoot
Atherosclerosis of other type of bypass
graft(s) of left leg with ulceration of
plantar surface of midfoot

I70.745 **Atherosclerosis of other type of** HCC A
bypass graft(s) of the left leg with
ulceration of other part of foot
Atherosclerosis of other type of bypass
graft(s) of left leg with ulceration of
toe

I70.748 **Atherosclerosis of other type of** HCC A
bypass graft(s) of the left leg with
ulceration of other part of lower leg

I70.749 **Atherosclerosis of other type of** HCC A ▽
bypass graft(s) of the left leg with
ulceration of unspecified site

I70.75 **Atherosclerosis of other type of bypass** HCC A
graft(s) of other extremity with ulceration
INCLUDES   any condition classifiable to I70.718 and
I70.728
Use additional code to identify severity of ulcer
(L98.49)

✓6th **I70.76** **Atherosclerosis of other type of bypass graft(s) of**
the extremities with gangrene
INCLUDES   any condition classifiable to I70.71-, I70.72-,
I70.73-, I70.74-, I70.75
Use additional code to identify the severity of any
ulcer (L97.-, L98.49-), if applicable

I70.761 **Atherosclerosis of other type of** HCC A
bypass graft(s) of the extremities
with gangrene, right leg

I70.762 **Atherosclerosis of other type of** HCC A
bypass graft(s) of the extremities
with gangrene, left leg

I70.763 **Atherosclerosis of other type of** HCC A
bypass graft(s) of the extremities
with gangrene, bilateral legs

I70.768 **Atherosclerosis of other type of** HCC A
bypass graft(s) of the extremities
with gangrene, other extremity

I70.769 **Atherosclerosis of other type of** HCC A ▽
bypass graft(s) of the extremities
with gangrene, unspecified extremity

✓6th **I70.79** **Other atherosclerosis of other type of bypass graft(s)**
of the extremities

I70.791 **Other atherosclerosis of other type** HCC A
of bypass graft(s) of the extremities,
right leg

I70.792 **Other atherosclerosis of other type** HCC A
of bypass graft(s) of the extremities, left
leg

I70.793 **Other atherosclerosis of other type** HCC A
of bypass graft(s) of the extremities,
bilateral legs

I70.798 **Other atherosclerosis of other type** HCC A
of bypass graft(s) of the extremities,
other extremity

I70.799 **Other atherosclerosis of other** HCC A ▽
typeof bypass graft(s) of the extremities,
unspecified extremity

I70.8 **Atherosclerosis of other arteries** A
TIP: Arteriosclerosis of the iliac arteries is coded here.

✓5th **I70.9** **Other and unspecified atherosclerosis**

I70.90 **Unspecified atherosclerosis** A ▽

I70.91 Generalized **atherosclerosis** A

I70.92 Chronic total occlusion **of artery of the** HCC A
extremities
Complete occlusion of artery of the extremities
Total occlusion of artery of the extremities
Code first atherosclerosis of arteries of the extremities
(I70.2-, I70.3-, I70.4-, I70.5-, I70.6-, I70.7-)

✓4th **I71** **Aortic aneurysm and dissection**
EXCLUDES 1   aortic ectasia (I77.81-)
syphilitic aortic aneurysm (A52.01)
traumatic aortic aneurysm (S25.09, S35.09)

✓5th **I71.0** Dissection of aorta

I71.00 **Dissection of unspecified site of aorta** HCC ▽

I71.01 **Dissection of** thoracic **aorta** HCC

I71.02 **Dissection of** abdominal **aorta** HCC

I71.03 **Dissection of** thoracoabdominal **aorta** HCC

I71.1 Thoracic **aortic aneurysm,** ruptured HCC

I71.2 Thoracic **aortic aneurysm,** without rupture HCC

I71.3 Abdominal **aortic aneurysm,** ruptured HCC

I71.4 Abdominal **aortic aneurysm,** without rupture HCC

I71.5 Thoracoabdominal **aortic aneurysm,** ruptured HCC

I71.6 Thoracoabdominal **aortic aneurysm,** without rupture HCC

I71.8 **Aortic aneurysm of unspecified site,** ruptured HCC ▽
Rupture of aorta NOS

I71.9 **Aortic aneurysm of unspecified site,** without rupture HCC ▽
Aneurysm of aorta
Dilatation of aorta
Hyaline necrosis of aorta

✓4th **I72** **Other aneurysm**
INCLUDES   aneurysm (cirsoid) (false) (ruptured)
EXCLUDES 2   acquired aneurysm (I77.0)
aneurysm (of) aorta (I71.-)
aneurysm (of) arteriovenous NOS (Q27.3-)
carotid artery dissection (I77.71)
cerebral (nonruptured) aneurysm (I67.1)
coronary aneurysm (I25.4)
coronary artery dissection (I25.42)
dissection of artery NEC (I77.79)
dissection of precerebral artery, congenital (nonruptured)
(Q28.1)
heart aneurysm (I25.3)
iliac artery dissection (I77.72)
▶precerebral artery, congenital (nonruptured) (Q28.1)◀
pulmonary artery aneurysm (I28.1)
renal artery dissection (I77.73)
retinal aneurysm (H35.0)
ruptured cerebral aneurysm (I60.7)
varicose aneurysm (I77.0)
vertebral artery dissection (I77.74)

I72.0 **Aneurysm of** carotid artery HCC
Aneurysm of common carotid artery
Aneurysm of external carotid artery
Aneurysm of internal carotid artery, extracranial portion
EXCLUDES 1   aneurysm of internal carotid artery, intracranial
portion (I67.1)
aneurysm of internal carotid artery NOS (I67.1)

I72.1 **Aneurysm of artery of** upper extremity HCC

I72.2 **Aneurysm of** renal artery HCC

I72.3 **Aneurysm of** iliac artery HCC

I72.4 **Aneurysm of artery of** lower extremity HCC

I72.5 **Aneurysm of other** precerebral **arteries** HCC
Aneurysm of basilar artery (trunk)
EXCLUDES 2   aneurysm of carotid artery (I72.0)
aneurysm of vertebral artery (I72.6)
dissection of carotid artery (I77.71)
dissection of other precerebral arteries (I77.75)
dissection of vertebral artery (I77.74)

☑ Additional Character Req   √x7th Placeholder Alert   Manifestation   HCC CMS-HCC Condition   ▽ Unspecified Code   ▶◀ Revised Text   ● New Code   ▲ Revised Code Title

ICD-10-CM 2018   **645**

Chapter 9. Diseases of the Circulatory System *(vertical side tab)*

Aneurysm

Outer layer

Layers of muscular and elastic tissue

Inner layer

Aneurysm

I72.6 **Aneurysm of** vertebral artery   `HCC`
     EXCLUDES 2   dissection of vertebral artery (I77.74)

I72.8 **Aneurysm of other specified arteries**   `HCC`

I72.9 **Aneurysm of unspecified site**   `HCC` ▽

✓4ᵗʰ I73 **Other peripheral vascular diseases**
     EXCLUDES 2   chilblains (T69.1)
               frostbite (T33- T34)
               immersion hand or foot (T69.0-)
               spasm of cerebral artery (G45.9)

   ✓5ᵗʰ I73.0 **Raynaud's syndrome**
           Raynaud's disease
           Raynaud's phenomenon (secondary)

      I73.00 **Raynaud's syndrome** without gangrene

      I73.01 **Raynaud's syndrome** with gangrene   `HCC`

   I73.1 **Thromboangiitis obliterans [Buerger's disease]**   `HCC`
        DEF: Inflammatory disease of extremity blood vessels, mainly the lower; associated with heavy tobacco use; arteries are more affected than veins; occurs primarily in young men and leads to tissue ischemia and gangrene.

   ✓5ᵗʰ I73.8 **Other specified peripheral vascular diseases**
       EXCLUDES 1   diabetic (peripheral) angiopathy (E08-E13 with .51-.52)

      I73.81 **Erythromelalgia**   `HCC`

      I73.89 **Other specified peripheral vascular diseases**   `HCC`
           Acrocyanosis
           Erythrocyanosis
           Simple acroparesthesia [Schultze's type]
           Vasomotor acroparesthesia [Nothnagel's type]

   I73.9 **Peripheral vascular disease, unspecified**   `HCC` ▽
        Intermittent claudication
        Peripheral angiopathy NOS
        Spasm of artery
        EXCLUDES 1   atherosclerosis of the extremities (I70.2--I70.7-)

✓4ᵗʰ I74 **Arterial embolism and thrombosis**
     INCLUDES   embolic infarction
              embolic occlusion
              thrombotic infarction
              thrombotic occlusion

   Code first:
     embolism and thrombosis complicating abortion or ectopic or molar pregnancy (O00-O07, O08.2)
     embolism and thrombosis complicating pregnancy, childbirth and the puerperium (O88.-)
     EXCLUDES 2   atheroembolism (I75.-)
               basilar embolism and thrombosis (I63.0-I63.2, I65.1)
               carotid embolism and thrombosis (I63.0-I63.2, I65.2)
               cerebral embolism and thrombosis (I63.3-I63.5, I66-)
               coronary embolism and thrombosis (I21-I25)
               mesenteric embolism and thrombosis (K55.0-)
               ophthalmic embolism and thrombosis (H34.-)
               precerebral embolism and thrombosis NOS (I63.0-I63.2, I65.9)
               pulmonary embolism and thrombosis (I26.-)
               renal embolism and thrombosis (N28.0)
               retinal embolism and thrombosis (H34.-)
               septic embolism and thrombosis (I76)
               vertebral embolism and thrombosis (I63.0-I63.2, I65.0)

   ✓5ᵗʰ I74.0 **Embolism and thrombosis of** abdominal aorta

      I74.01 **Saddle embolus of abdominal aorta**   `HCC`

      I74.09 **Other** arterial **embolism and thrombosis of abdominal aorta**   `HCC`
           Aortic bifurcation syndrome
           Aortoiliac obstruction
           Leriche's syndrome

   ✓5ᵗʰ I74.1 **Embolism and thrombosis of other and unspecified** parts of aorta

      I74.10 **Embolism and thrombosis of unspecified parts of aorta**   `HCC` ▽

      I74.11 **Embolism and thrombosis of** thoracic **aorta**   `HCC`

      I74.19 **Embolism and thrombosis of other** parts of aorta   `HCC`

   I74.2 **Embolism and thrombosis of arteries of the** upper extremities   `HCC`

   I74.3 **Embolism and thrombosis of arteries of the** lower extremities   `HCC`

   I74.4 **Embolism and thrombosis of arteries of extremities, unspecified**   `HCC` ▽
        Peripheral arterial embolism NOS

   I74.5 **Embolism and thrombosis of** iliac **artery**   `HCC`

   I74.8 **Embolism and thrombosis of other arteries**   `HCC`

   I74.9 **Embolism and thrombosis of unspecified artery**   `HCC` ▽

✓4ᵗʰ I75 **Atheroembolism**
     INCLUDES   atherothrombotic microembolism
              cholesterol embolism

   ✓5ᵗʰ I75.0 **Atheroembolism of** extremities

     ✓6ᵗʰ I75.01 **Atheroembolism of** upper **extremity**

        I75.011 **Atheroembolism of** right **upper extremity**   `HCC`

        I75.012 **Atheroembolism of** left **upper extremity**   `HCC`

        I75.013 **Atheroembolism of** bilateral **upper extremities**   `HCC`

        I75.019 **Atheroembolism of unspecified upper extremity**   `HCC` ▽

     ✓6ᵗʰ I75.02 **Atheroembolism of** lower **extremity**

        I75.021 **Atheroembolism of** right **lower extremity**   `HCC`

        I75.022 **Atheroembolism of** left **lower extremity**   `HCC`

        I75.023 **Atheroembolism of** bilateral **lower extremities**   `HCC`

        I75.029 **Atheroembolism of unspecified lower extremity**   `HCC` ▽

   ✓5ᵗʰ I75.8 **Atheroembolism of other sites**

      I75.81 **Atheroembolism of** kidney   `HCC`
           Use additional code for any associated acute kidney failure and chronic kidney disease (N17.-, N18.-)

      I75.89 **Atheroembolism of other site**   `HCC`

I76 **Septic arterial embolism**   `HCC`
     Code first underlying infection, such as:
       infective endocarditis (I33.0)
       lung abscess (J85.-)
     Use additional code to identify the site of the embolism (I74.-)
     EXCLUDES 2   septic pulmonary embolism (I26.01, I26.90)

✓4ᵗʰ I77 **Other disorders of arteries and arterioles**
     EXCLUDES 2   collagen (vascular) diseases (M30-M36)
              hypersensitivity angiitis (M31.0)
              pulmonary artery (I28.-)

   I77.0 **Arteriovenous fistula, acquired**   `HCC`
        Aneurysmal varix
        Arteriovenous aneurysm, acquired
        EXCLUDES 1   arteriovenous aneurysm NOS (Q27.3-)
               presence of arteriovenous shunt (fistula) for dialysis (Z99.2)
               traumatic—see injury of blood vessel by body region
        EXCLUDES 2   cerebral (I67.1)
               coronary (I25.4)
        DEF: Communication between an artery and vein; caused by trauma or invasive procedures.

   I77.1 **Stricture of artery**   `HCC`
        Narrowing of artery

   I77.2 **Rupture of artery**   `HCC`
        Erosion of artery
        Fistula of artery
        Ulcer of artery
        EXCLUDES 1   traumatic rupture of artery—see injury of blood vessel by body region

   I77.3 **Arterial fibromuscular dysplasia**   `HCC`
        Fibromuscular hyperplasia (of) carotid artery
        Fibromuscular hyperplasia (of) renal artery

   I77.4 **Celiac artery compression syndrome**   `HCC`

EXCLUDES 1 Not coded here   *EXCLUDES 2* Not included here   **N** Newborn Age: 0   **P** Pediatric Age: 0-17   **M** Maternity Age: 12-55   **A** Adult Age: 15-124

646   ICD-10-CM 2018

I72.6–I77.4 *(vertical side tab)*

I77.5 **Necrosis of artery** `HCC`

I77.6 **Arteritis, unspecified** `HCC` ▽
    Aortitis NOS
    Endarteritis NOS
      EXCLUDES 1 *arteritis or endarteritis:*
          aortic arch (M31.4)
          cerebral NEC (I67.7)
          coronary (I25.89)
          deformans (I70.-)
          giant cell (M31.5., M31.6)
          obliterans (I70.-)
          senile (I70.-)

✓5th I77.7 **Other arterial dissection**
      EXCLUDES 2 *dissection of aorta (I71.0-)*
          dissection of coronary artery (I25.42)

    I77.70 **Dissection of unspecified artery** `HCC` ▽

    I77.71 **Dissection of** carotid **artery** `HCC`

    I77.72 **Dissection of** iliac **artery** `HCC`

    I77.73 **Dissection of** renal **artery** `HCC`

    I77.74 **Dissection of** vertebral **artery** `HCC`
        EXCLUDES 2 *aneurysm of vertebral artery (I72.6)*

    I77.75 **Dissection of other** precerebral **arteries** `HCC`
        Dissection of basilar artery (trunk)
          EXCLUDES 2 *aneurysm of carotid artery (I72.0)*
              aneurysm of other precerebral arteries (I72.5)
              aneurysm of vertebral artery (I72.6)
              dissection of carotid artery (I77.71)
              dissection of vertebral artery (I77.74)

    I77.76 **Dissection of artery of** upper extremity `HCC`

    I77.77 **Dissection of artery of** lower extremity `HCC`

    I77.79 **Dissection of other specified artery** `HCC`

✓5th I77.8 **Other specified disorders of arteries and arterioles**
    ✓6th I77.81 **Aortic ectasia**
        Ectasis aorta
          EXCLUDES 1 *aortic aneurysm and dissection (I71.0-)*

        I77.810 Thoracic **aortic ectasia** `HCC`

        I77.811 Abdominal **aortic ectasia** `HCC`

        I77.812 Thoracoabdominal **aortic ectasia** `HCC`

        I77.819 **Aortic ectasia, unspecified site** `HCC` ▽

    I77.89 **Other specified disorders of arteries and arterioles** `HCC`

I77.9 **Disorder of arteries and arterioles, unspecified** `HCC` ▽

✓4th **I78 Diseases of capillaries**

    I78.0 **Hereditary hemorrhagic telangiectasia** `HCC`
        Rendu-Osler-Weber disease

    I78.1 **Nevus, non-neoplastic**
        Araneus nevus
        Senile nevus
        Spider nevus
        Stellar nevus
          EXCLUDES 1 *nevus NOS (D22.-)*
              vascular NOS (Q82.5)
          EXCLUDES 2 *blue nevus (D22.-)*
              flammeus nevus (Q82.5)
              hairy nevus (D22.-)
              melanocytic nevus (D22.-)
              pigmented nevus (D22.-)
              portwine nevus (Q82.5)
              sanguineous nevus (Q82.5)
              strawberry nevus (Q82.5)
              verrucous nevus (Q82.5)

    I78.8 **Other diseases of capillaries**

    I78.9 **Disease of capillaries, unspecified** ▽

✓4th **I79 Disorders of arteries, arterioles and capillaries in diseases classified elsewhere**

    I79.0 *Aneurysm of aorta in diseases classified elsewhere* `HCC`
        Code first underlying disease
          EXCLUDES 1 *syphilitic aneurysm (A52.01)*

    I79.1 *Aortitis in diseases classified elsewhere* `HCC`
        Code first underlying disease
          EXCLUDES 1 *syphilitic aortitis (A52.02)*

I79.8 *Other disorders of arteries, arterioles and capillaries in diseases classified elsewhere* `HCC`
    Code first underlying disease, such as:
      amyloidosis (E85.-)
      EXCLUDES 1 *diabetic (peripheral) angiopathy (E08-E13 with .51-.52)*
          syphilitic endarteritis (A52.09)
          tuberculous endarteritis (A18.89)

Diseases of veins, lymphatic vessels and lymph nodes, not elsewhere classified (I80-I89)

✓4th **I80 Phlebitis and thrombophlebitis**
    INCLUDES endophlebitis
        inflammation, vein
        periphlebitis
        suppurative phlebitis
    Code first:
      phlebitis and thrombophlebitis complicating abortion, ectopic or molar pregnancy (O00-O07, O08.7)
      phlebitis and thrombophlebitis complicating pregnancy, childbirth and the puerperium (O22.-, O87.-)
      EXCLUDES 1 *venous embolism and thrombosis of lower extremities ((I82.4-, I82.5-, I82.81-)*

✓5th I80.0 **Phlebitis and thrombophlebitis of** superficial vessels **of** lower extremities
    Phlebitis and thrombophlebitis of femoropopliteal vein

    I80.00 **Phlebitis and thrombophlebitis of superficial vessels of unspecified lower extremity** ▽

    I80.01 **Phlebitis and thrombophlebitis of superficial vessels of** right **lower extremity**

    I80.02 **Phlebitis and thrombophlebitis of superficial vessels of** left **lower extremity**

    I80.03 **Phlebitis and thrombophlebitis of superficial vessels of lower extremities,** bilateral

✓5th I80.1 **Phlebitis and thrombophlebitis of** femoral vein

    I80.10 **Phlebitis and thrombophlebitis of unspecified femoral vein** `HCC` ▽

    I80.11 **Phlebitis and thrombophlebitis of** right **femoral vein** `HCC`

    I80.12 **Phlebitis and thrombophlebitis of** left **femoral vein** `HCC`

    I80.13 **Phlebitis and thrombophlebitis of femoral vein,** bilateral `HCC`

✓5th I80.2 **Phlebitis and thrombophlebitis of other and unspecified** deep vessels **of** lower extremities

    ✓6th I80.20 **Phlebitis and thrombophlebitis of unspecified deep vessels of lower extremities**

        I80.201 **Phlebitis and thrombophlebitis of unspecified deep vessels of** right **lower extremity** `HCC`

        I80.202 **Phlebitis and thrombophlebitis of unspecified deep vessels of** left **lower extremity** `HCC`

        I80.203 **Phlebitis and thrombophlebitis of unspecified deep vessels of lower extremities,** bilateral `HCC`

        I80.209 **Phlebitis and thrombophlebitis of unspecified deep vessels of unspecified lower extremity** `HCC` ▽

    ✓6th I80.21 **Phlebitis and thrombophlebitis of** iliac vein

        I80.211 **Phlebitis and thrombophlebitis of** right **iliac vein** `HCC`

        I80.212 **Phlebitis and thrombophlebitis of** left **iliac vein** `HCC`

        I80.213 **Phlebitis and thrombophlebitis of iliac vein,** bilateral `HCC`

        I80.219 **Phlebitis and thrombophlebitis of unspecified iliac vein** `HCC` ▽

    ✓6th I80.22 **Phlebitis and thrombophlebitis of** popliteal vein

        I80.221 **Phlebitis and thrombophlebitis of** right **popliteal vein** `HCC`

        I80.222 **Phlebitis and thrombophlebitis of** left **popliteal vein** `HCC`

        I80.223 **Phlebitis and thrombophlebitis of popliteal vein,** bilateral `HCC`

        I80.229 **Phlebitis and thrombophlebitis of unspecified popliteal vein** `HCC` ▽

✓ Additional Character Req   ✓x7th Placeholder Alert   Manifestation   `HCC` CMS-HCC Condition   ▽ Unspecified Code   ►◄ Revised Text   ● New Code   ▲ Revised Code Title

ICD-10-CM 2018   647

✓6ᵗʰ **I80.23**   **Phlebitis and thrombophlebitis of** tibial vein

I80.231   **Phlebitis and thrombophlebitis of** right **tibial vein**   HCC

I80.232   **Phlebitis and thrombophlebitis of** left **tibial vein**   HCC

I80.233   **Phlebitis and thrombophlebitis of tibial vein,** bilateral   HCC

I80.239   **Phlebitis and thrombophlebitis of unspecified tibial vein**   HCC ▽

✓6ᵗʰ **I80.29**   **Phlebitis and thrombophlebitis of other deep vessels of lower extremities**

I80.291   **Phlebitis and thrombophlebitis of other deep vessels of** right **lower extremity**   HCC

I80.292   **Phlebitis and thrombophlebitis of other deep vessels of** left **lower extremity**   HCC

I80.293   **Phlebitis and thrombophlebitis of other deep vessels of lower extremity,** bilateral   HCC

I80.299   **Phlebitis and thrombophlebitis of other deep vessels of unspecified lower extremity**   HCC ▽

I80.3   **Phlebitis and thrombophlebitis of lower extremities, unspecified**   ▽

I80.8   **Phlebitis and thrombophlebitis of other sites**

I80.9   **Phlebitis and thrombophlebitis of unspecified site**   ▽

I81   **Portal vein thrombosis**
Portal (vein) obstruction
EXCLUDES 2   hepatic vein thrombosis (I82.0)
phlebitis of portal vein (K75.1)

✓4ᵗʰ **I82**   **Other venous embolism and thrombosis**
Code first venous embolism and thrombosis complicating:
abortion, ectopic or molar pregnancy (O00-O07, O08.7)
pregnancy, childbirth and the puerperium (O22.-, O87.-)
EXCLUDES 2   venous embolism and thrombosis (of):
cerebral (I63.6, I67.6)
coronary (I21-I25)
intracranial and intraspinal, septic or NOS (G08)
intracranial, nonpyogenic (I67.6)
intraspinal, nonpyogenic (G95.1)
mesenteric (K55.0-)
portal (I81)
pulmonary (I26.-)

I82.0   **Budd-Chiari syndrome**   HCC
Hepatic vein thrombosis
DEF: Thrombosis or other obstruction of hepatic veins; symptoms include enlarged liver, extensive collateral vessels, intractable ascites, and severe portal hypertension.

I82.1   **Thrombophlebitis migrans**

✓5ᵗʰ **I82.2**   **Embolism and thrombosis of** vena cava **and other** thoracic veins

✓6ᵗʰ **I82.21**   **Embolism and thrombosis of** superior vena cava

I82.210   **Acute embolism and thrombosis of superior vena cava**   HCC
Embolism and thrombosis of superior vena cava NOS

I82.211   **Chronic embolism and thrombosis of superior vena cava**   HCC

✓6ᵗʰ **I82.22**   **Embolism and thrombosis of** inferior vena cava

I82.220   **Acute embolism and thrombosis of inferior vena cava**   HCC
Embolism and thrombosis of inferior vena cava NOS

I82.221   **Chronic embolism and thrombosis of inferior vena cava**   HCC

✓6ᵗʰ **I82.29**   **Embolism and thrombosis of other** thoracic veins
Embolism and thrombosis of brachiocephalic (innominate) vein

I82.290   **Acute embolism and thrombosis of other thoracic veins**   HCC

I82.291   **Chronic embolism and thrombosis of other thoracic veins**   HCC

I82.3   **Embolism and thrombosis of** renal vein   HCC

✓5ᵗʰ **I82.4**   Acute **embolism and thrombosis of** deep veins of lower extremity

✓6ᵗʰ **I82.40**   **Acute embolism and thrombosis of** unspecified deep veins of lower extremity
Deep vein thrombosis NOS
DVT NOS
EXCLUDES 1   acute embolism and thrombosis of unspecified deep veins of distal lower extremity (I82.4Z-)
acute embolism and thrombosis of unspecified deep veins of proximal lower extremity (I82.4Y-)

I82.401   **Acute embolism and thrombosis of unspecified deep veins of** right **lower extremity**   HCC ▽

I82.402   **Acute embolism and thrombosis of unspecified deep veins of** left **lower extremity**   HCC ▽

I82.403   **Acute embolism and thrombosis of unspecified deep veins of lower extremity,** bilateral   HCC ▽

I82.409   **Acute embolism and thrombosis of unspecified deep veins of unspecified lower extremity**   HCC ▽

✓6ᵗʰ **I82.41**   **Acute embolism and thrombosis of** femoral vein

I82.411   **Acute embolism and thrombosis of** right **femoral vein**   HCC

I82.412   **Acute embolism and thrombosis of** left **femoral vein**   HCC

I82.413   **Acute embolism and thrombosis of femoral vein,** bilateral   HCC

I82.419   **Acute embolism and thrombosis of unspecified femoral vein**   HCC ▽

✓6ᵗʰ **I82.42**   **Acute embolism and thrombosis of** iliac vein

I82.421   **Acute embolism and thrombosis of** right **iliac vein**   HCC

I82.422   **Acute embolism and thrombosis of** left **iliac vein**   HCC

I82.423   **Acute embolism and thrombosis of iliac vein,** bilateral   HCC

I82.429   **Acute embolism and thrombosis of unspecified iliac vein**   HCC ▽

✓6ᵗʰ **I82.43**   **Acute embolism and thrombosis of** popliteal vein

I82.431   **Acute embolism and thrombosis of** right **popliteal vein**   HCC

I82.432   **Acute embolism and thrombosis of** left **popliteal vein**   HCC

I82.433   **Acute embolism and thrombosis of popliteal vein,** bilateral   HCC

I82.439   **Acute embolism and thrombosis of unspecified popliteal vein**   HCC ▽

✓6ᵗʰ **I82.44**   **Acute embolism and thrombosis of** tibial vein

I82.441   **Acute embolism and thrombosis of** right **tibial vein**   HCC

I82.442   **Acute embolism and thrombosis of** left **tibial vein**   HCC

I82.443   **Acute embolism and thrombosis of tibial vein,** bilateral   HCC

I82.449   **Acute embolism and thrombosis of unspecified tibial vein**   HCC ▽

✓6ᵗʰ **I82.49**   **Acute embolism and thrombosis of other specified deep vein of lower extremity**

I82.491   **Acute embolism and thrombosis of other specified deep vein of** right **lower extremity**   HCC

I82.492   **Acute embolism and thrombosis of other specified deep vein of** left **lower extremity**   HCC

I82.493   **Acute embolism and thrombosis of other specified deep vein of lower extremity,** bilateral   HCC

I82.499   **Acute embolism and thrombosis of other specified deep vein of unspecified lower extremity**   HCC ▽

✓6th **I82.4Y** **Acute embolism and thrombosis of unspecified deep veins of** proximal lower extremity
Acute embolism and thrombosis of deep vein of thigh NOS
Acute embolism and thrombosis of deep vein of upper leg NOS

I82.4Y1 Acute embolism and thrombosis of HCC ▽ unspecified deep veins of right proximal lower extremity

I82.4Y2 Acute embolism and thrombosis of HCC ▽ unspecified deep veins of left proximal lower extremity

I82.4Y3 Acute embolism and thrombosis of HCC ▽ unspecified deep veins of proximal lower extremity, bilateral

I82.4Y9 Acute embolism and thrombosis of HCC ▽ unspecified deep veins of unspecified proximal lower extremity

✓6th **I82.4Z** **Acute embolism and thrombosis of unspecified deep veins of** distal lower extremity
Acute embolism and thrombosis of deep vein of calf NOS
Acute embolism and thrombosis of deep vein of lower leg NOS

I82.4Z1 Acute embolism and thrombosis of HCC ▽ unspecified deep veins of right distal lower extremity

I82.4Z2 Acute embolism and thrombosis of HCC ▽ unspecified deep veins of left distal lower extremity

I82.4Z3 Acute embolism and thrombosis of HCC ▽ unspecified deep veins of distal lower extremity, bilateral

I82.4Z9 Acute embolism and thrombosis of HCC ▽ unspecified deep veins of unspecified distal lower extremity

✓5th **I82.5** Chronic **embolism and thrombosis of** deep veins of lower extremity
Use additional code, if applicable, for associated long-term (current) use of anticoagulants (Z79.01)
EXCLUDES 1   personal history of venous embolism and thrombosis (Z86.718)

✓6th **I82.50** **Chronic embolism and thrombosis of unspecified deep veins of** lower extremity
EXCLUDES 1   chronic embolism and thrombosis of unspecified deep veins of distal lower extremity (I82.5Z-)
chronic embolism and thrombosis of unspecified deep veins of proximal lower extremity (I82.5Y-)

I82.501 Chronic embolism and thrombosis HCC ▽ of unspecified deep veins of right lower extremity

I82.502 Chronic embolism and thrombosis HCC ▽ of unspecified deep veins of left lower extremity

I82.503 Chronic embolism and thrombosis HCC ▽ of unspecified deep veins of lower extremity, bilateral

I82.509 Chronic embolism and thrombosis HCC ▽ of unspecified deep veins of unspecified lower extremity

✓6th **I82.51** **Chronic embolism and thrombosis of** femoral vein

I82.511 Chronic embolism and thrombosis of HCC right femoral vein

I82.512 Chronic embolism and thrombosis of HCC left femoral vein

I82.513 Chronic embolism and thrombosis of HCC femoral vein, bilateral

I82.519 Chronic embolism and thrombosis HCC ▽ of unspecified femoral vein

✓6th **I82.52** **Chronic embolism and thrombosis of** iliac vein

I82.521 Chronic embolism and thrombosis of HCC right iliac vein

I82.522 Chronic embolism and thrombosis of HCC left iliac vein

I82.523 Chronic embolism and thrombosis of HCC iliac vein, bilateral

I82.529 Chronic embolism and thrombosis HCC ▽ of unspecified iliac vein

✓6th **I82.53** **Chronic embolism and thrombosis of** popliteal vein

I82.531 Chronic embolism and thrombosis of HCC right popliteal vein

I82.532 Chronic embolism and thrombosis of HCC left popliteal vein

I82.533 Chronic embolism and thrombosis of HCC popliteal vein, bilateral

I82.539 Chronic embolism and thrombosis HCC ▽ of unspecified popliteal vein

✓6th **I82.54** **Chronic embolism and thrombosis of** tibial vein

I82.541 Chronic embolism and thrombosis of HCC right tibial vein

I82.542 Chronic embolism and thrombosis of HCC left tibial vein

I82.543 Chronic embolism and thrombosis of HCC tibial vein, bilateral

I82.549 Chronic embolism and thrombosis HCC ▽ of unspecified tibial vein

✓6th **I82.59** **Chronic embolism and thrombosis of other specified deep vein of** lower extremity

I82.591 Chronic embolism and thrombosis of HCC other specified deep vein of right lower extremity

I82.592 Chronic embolism and thrombosis of HCC other specified deep vein of left lower extremity

I82.593 Chronic embolism and thrombosis of HCC other specified deep vein of lower extremity, bilateral

I82.599 Chronic embolism and thrombosis HCC ▽ of other specified deep vein of unspecified lower extremity

✓6th **I82.5Y** **Chronic embolism and thrombosis of unspecified deep veins of** proximal lower extremity
Chronic embolism and thrombosis of deep veins of thigh NOS
Chronic embolism and thrombosis of deep veins of upper leg NOS

I82.5Y1 Chronic embolism and thrombosis HCC ▽ of unspecified deep veins of right proximal lower extremity

I82.5Y2 Chronic embolism and thrombosis HCC ▽ of unspecified deep veins of left proximal lower extremity

I82.5Y3 Chronic embolism and thrombosis HCC ▽ of unspecified deep veins of proximal lower extremity, bilateral

I82.5Y9 Chronic embolism and thrombosis HCC ▽ of unspecified deep veins of unspecified proximal lower extremity

✓6th **I82.5Z** **Chronic embolism and thrombosis of unspecified deep veins of** distal lower extremity
Chronic embolism and thrombosis of deep veins of calf NOS
Chronic embolism and thrombosis of deep veins of lower leg NOS

I82.5Z1 Chronic embolism and thrombosis HCC ▽ of unspecified deep veins of right distal lower extremity

I82.5Z2 Chronic embolism and thrombosis HCC ▽ of unspecified deep veins of left distal lower extremity

I82.5Z3 Chronic embolism and thrombosis HCC ▽ of unspecified deep veins of distal lower extremity, bilateral

I82.5Z9 Chronic embolism and thrombosis HCC ▽ of unspecified deep veins of unspecified distal lower extremity

✓5th **I82.6** Acute **embolism and thrombosis of veins of** upper extremity

✓6th **I82.60** **Acute embolism and thrombosis of unspecified veins of upper extremity**

I82.601 Acute embolism and thrombosis of ▽ unspecified veins of right upper extremity

I82.602 Acute embolism and thrombosis of ▽ unspecified veins of left upper extremity

I82.603 Acute embolism and thrombosis of ▽ unspecified veins of upper extremity, bilateral

---

✓ Additional Character Req   ✓x7th Placeholder Alert   Manifestation   HCC CMS-HCC Condition   ▽ Unspecified Code   ►◄ Revised Text   ● New Code   ▲ Revised Code Title

Chapter 9. Diseases of the Circulatory System

I82.609   **Acute embolism and thrombosis of** ▽
unspecified veins of unspecified upper
extremity

✓6ᵗʰ   **I82.61**   **Acute embolism and thrombosis of** superficial veins
of upper extremity
Acute embolism and thrombosis of antecubital vein
Acute embolism and thrombosis of basilic vein
Acute embolism and thrombosis of cephalic vein

I82.611   **Acute embolism and thrombosis of
superficial veins of** right **upper extremity**

I82.612   **Acute embolism and thrombosis of
superficial veins of** left **upper extremity**

I82.613   **Acute embolism and thrombosis of
superficial veins of upper extremity,**
bilateral

I82.619   **Acute embolism and thrombosis of** ▽
superficial veins of unspecified upper
extremity

✓6ᵗʰ   **I82.62**   **Acute embolism and thrombosis of** deep veins of
upper extremity
Acute embolism and thrombosis of brachial vein
Acute embolism and thrombosis of radial vein
Acute embolism and thrombosis of ulnar vein

I82.621   **Acute embolism and thrombosis of** ᴴᶜᶜ
deep veins of right **upper extremity**

I82.622   **Acute embolism and thrombosis of** ᴴᶜᶜ
deep veins of left **upper extremity**

I82.623   **Acute embolism and thrombosis of** ᴴᶜᶜ
deep veins of upper extremity, bilateral

I82.629   **Acute embolism and thrombosis of** ᴴᶜᶜ ▽
deep veins of unspecified upper extremity

✓5ᵗʰ   **I82.7**   Chronic **embolism and thrombosis of veins of** upper extremity
Use additional code, if applicable, for associated long-term
(current) use of anticoagulants (Z79.01)
EXCLUDES 1   *personal history of venous embolism and thrombosis
(Z86.718)*

✓6ᵗʰ   **I82.70**   **Chronic embolism and thrombosis of unspecified
veins of upper extremity**

I82.701   **Chronic embolism and thrombosis of** ▽
unspecified veins of right **upper extremity**

I82.702   **Chronic embolism and thrombosis of** ▽
unspecified veins of left **upper extremity**

I82.703   **Chronic embolism and thrombosis of** ▽
unspecified veins of upper extremity,
bilateral

I82.709   **Chronic embolism and thrombosis of** ▽
**unspecified veins of unspecified upper
extremity**

✓6ᵗʰ   **I82.71**   **Chronic embolism and thrombosis of** superficial
veins **of upper extremity**
Chronic embolism and thrombosis of antecubital vein
Chronic embolism and thrombosis of basilic vein
Chronic embolism and thrombosis of cephalic vein

I82.711   **Chronic embolism and thrombosis of
superficial veins of** right **upper extremity**

I82.712   **Chronic embolism and thrombosis of
superficial veins of** left **upper extremity**

I82.713   **Chronic embolism and thrombosis of
superficial veins of upper extremity,**
bilateral

I82.719   **Chronic embolism and thrombosis of** ▽
**superficial veins of unspecified upper
extremity**

✓6ᵗʰ   **I82.72**   **Chronic embolism and thrombosis of** deep veins **of
upper extremity**
Chronic embolism and thrombosis of brachial vein
Chronic embolism and thrombosis of radial vein
Chronic embolism and thrombosis of ulnar vein

I82.721   **Chronic embolism and thrombosis of** ᴴᶜᶜ
deep veins of right **upper extremity**

▲ **I82.722**   **Chronic embolism and thrombosis of** ᴴᶜᶜ
deep veins of left **upper extremity**

I82.723   **Chronic embolism and thrombosis of** ᴴᶜᶜ
deep veins of upper **extremity, bilateral**

I82.729   **Chronic embolism and thrombosis** ᴴᶜᶜ ▽
**of deep veins of unspecified upper
extremity**

✓5ᵗʰ   **I82.A**   **Embolism and thrombosis of** axillary vein

✓6ᵗʰ   **I82.A1**   Acute **embolism and thrombosis of axillary vein**

I82.A11   **Acute embolism and thrombosis of** ᴴᶜᶜ
right **axillary vein**

I82.A12   **Acute embolism and thrombosis of** ᴴᶜᶜ
left **axillary vein**

I82.A13   **Acute embolism and thrombosis of** ᴴᶜᶜ
axillary vein, bilateral

I82.A19   **Acute embolism and thrombosis of** ᴴᶜᶜ ▽
unspecified axillary vein

✓6ᵗʰ   **I82.A2**   Chronic **embolism and thrombosis of axillary vein**

I82.A21   **Chronic embolism and thrombosis of** ᴴᶜᶜ
right **axillary vein**

I82.A22   **Chronic embolism and thrombosis of** ᴴᶜᶜ
left **axillary vein**

I82.A23   **Chronic embolism and thrombosis of** ᴴᶜᶜ
axillary vein, bilateral

I82.A29   **Chronic embolism and thrombosis** ᴴᶜᶜ ▽
of unspecified axillary vein

✓5ᵗʰ   **I82.B**   **Embolism and thrombosis of** subclavian vein

✓6ᵗʰ   **I82.B1**   Acute **embolism and thrombosis of subclavian vein**

I82.B11   **Acute embolism and thrombosis of** ᴴᶜᶜ
right **subclavian vein**

I82.B12   **Acute embolism and thrombosis of** ᴴᶜᶜ
left **subclavian vein**

I82.B13   **Acute embolism and thrombosis of** ᴴᶜᶜ
subclavian vein, bilateral

I82.B19   **Acute embolism and thrombosis of** ᴴᶜᶜ ▽
unspecified subclavian vein

✓6ᵗʰ   **I82.B2**   Chronic **embolism and thrombosis of subclavian
vein**

I82.B21   **Chronic embolism and thrombosis of** ᴴᶜᶜ
right **subclavian vein**

I82.B22   **Chronic embolism and thrombosis of** ᴴᶜᶜ
left **subclavian vein**

I82.B23   **Chronic embolism and thrombosis of** ᴴᶜᶜ
subclavian vein, bilateral

I82.B29   **Chronic embolism and thrombosis** ᴴᶜᶜ ▽
of unspecified subclavian vein

✓5ᵗʰ   **I82.C**   **Embolism and thrombosis of** internal jugular vein

✓6ᵗʰ   **I82.C1**   Acute **embolism and thrombosis of internal jugular
vein**

I82.C11   **Acute embolism and thrombosis of** ᴴᶜᶜ
right **internal jugular vein**

I82.C12   **Acute embolism and thrombosis of** ᴴᶜᶜ
left **internal jugular vein**

I82.C13   **Acute embolism and thrombosis of** ᴴᶜᶜ
internal jugular vein, bilateral

I82.C19   **Acute embolism and thrombosis of** ᴴᶜᶜ ▽
unspecified internal jugular vein

✓6ᵗʰ   **I82.C2**   Chronic **embolism and thrombosis of internal
jugular vein**

I82.C21   **Chronic embolism and thrombosis of** ᴴᶜᶜ
right **internal jugular vein**

I82.C22   **Chronic embolism and thrombosis of** ᴴᶜᶜ
left **internal jugular vein**

I82.C23   **Chronic embolism and thrombosis of** ᴴᶜᶜ
internal jugular vein, bilateral

I82.C29   **Chronic embolism and thrombosis** ᴴᶜᶜ ▽
of unspecified internal jugular vein

✓5ᵗʰ   **I82.8**   **Embolism and thrombosis of other** specified veins
Use additional code, if applicable, for associated long-term
(current) use of anticoagulants (Z79.01)

✓6ᵗʰ   **I82.81**   **Embolism and thrombosis of superficial veins of**
lower extremities
Embolism and thrombosis of saphenous vein (greater)
(lesser)

I82.811   **Embolism and thrombosis of superficial
veins of** right lower **extremity**

▲ **I82.812**   **Embolism and thrombosis of superficial
veins of** left lower **extremity**

I82.813   **Embolism and thrombosis of superficial
veins of lower extremities,** bilateral

▲ **I82.819**   **Embolism and thrombosis of superficial** ▽
veins of unspecified lower extremity

✓6ᵗʰ I82.89   Embolism and thrombosis of other specified veins

    I82.890   Acute embolism and thrombosis of other specified veins

    I82.891   Chronic embolism and thrombosis of other specified veins

✓5ᵗʰ I82.9   Embolism and thrombosis of unspecified vein

    I82.90   Acute embolism and thrombosis of unspecified vein   ▽

        Embolism of vein NOS
        Thrombosis (vein) NOS

    I82.91   Chronic embolism and thrombosis of unspecified vein   ▽

✓4ᵗʰ I83   Varicose veins of lower extremities

    EXCLUDES 1   varicose veins complicating pregnancy (O22.0-)
                varicose veins complicating the puerperium (O87.4)

✓5ᵗʰ I83.0   Varicose veins of lower extremities with ulcer

    Use additional code to identify severity of ulcer (L97.-)

✓6ᵗʰ I83.00   Varicose veins of unspecified lower extremity with ulcer

    I83.001   Varicose veins of unspecified lower extremity with ulcer of thigh   HCC A ▽

    I83.002   Varicose veins of unspecified lower extremity with ulcer of calf   HCC A ▽

    I83.003   Varicose veins of unspecified lower extremity with ulcer of ankle   HCC A ▽

    I83.004   Varicose veins of unspecified lower extremity with ulcer of heel and midfoot   HCC A ▽
        Varicose veins of unspecified lower extremity with ulcer of plantar surface of midfoot

    I83.005   Varicose veins of unspecified lower extremity with ulcer other part of foot   HCC A ▽
        Varicose veins of unspecified lower extremity with ulcer of toe

    I83.008   Varicose veins of unspecified lower extremity with ulcer other part of lower leg   HCC A ▽

    I83.009   Varicose veins of unspecified lower extremity with ulcer of unspecified site   HCC A ▽

✓6ᵗʰ I83.01   Varicose veins of right lower extremity with ulcer

    I83.011   Varicose veins of right lower extremity with ulcer of thigh   HCC A

    I83.012   Varicose veins of right lower extremity with ulcer of calf   HCC A

    I83.013   Varicose veins of right lower extremity with ulcer of ankle   HCC A

    I83.014   Varicose veins of right lower extremity with ulcer of heel and midfoot   HCC A
        Varicose veins of right lower extremity with ulcer of plantar surface of midfoot

    I83.015   Varicose veins of right lower extremity with ulcer other part of foot   HCC A
        Varicose veins of right lower extremity with ulcer of toe

    I83.018   Varicose veins of right lower extremity with ulcer other part of lower leg   HCC A

    I83.019   Varicose veins of right lower extremity with ulcer of unspecified site   HCC A ▽

✓6ᵗʰ I83.02   Varicose veins of left lower extremity with ulcer

    I83.021   Varicose veins of left lower extremity with ulcer of thigh   HCC A

    I83.022   Varicose veins of left lower extremity with ulcer of calf   HCC A

    I83.023   Varicose veins of left lower extremity with ulcer of ankle   HCC A

    I83.024   Varicose veins of left lower extremity with ulcer of heel and midfoot   HCC A
        Varicose veins of left lower extremity with ulcer of plantar surface of midfoot

    I83.025   Varicose veins of left lower extremity with ulcer other part of foot   HCC A
        Varicose veins of left lower extremity with ulcer of toe

    I83.028   Varicose veins of left lower extremity with ulcer other part of lower leg   HCC A

    I83.029   Varicose veins of left lower extremity with ulcer of unspecified site   HCC A ▽

✓5ᵗʰ I83.1   Varicose veins of lower extremities with inflammation

    I83.10   Varicose veins of unspecified lower extremity with inflammation   A ▽

    I83.11   Varicose veins of right lower extremity with inflammation   A

    I83.12   Varicose veins of left lower extremity with inflammation   A

✓5ᵗʰ I83.2   Varicose veins of lower extremities with both ulcer and inflammation

    Use additional code to identify severity of ulcer (L97.-)

✓6ᵗʰ I83.20   Varicose veins of unspecified lower extremity with both ulcer and inflammation

    I83.201   Varicose veins of unspecified lower extremity with both ulcer of thigh and inflammation   HCC A ▽

    I83.202   Varicose veins of unspecified lower extremity with both ulcer of calf and inflammation   HCC A ▽

    I83.203   Varicose veins of unspecified lower extremity with both ulcer of ankle and inflammation   HCC A ▽

    I83.204   Varicose veins of unspecified lower extremity with both ulcer of heel and midfoot and inflammation   HCC A ▽
        Varicose veins of unspecified lower extremity with both ulcer of plantar surface of midfoot and inflammation

    I83.205   Varicose veins of unspecified lower extremity with both ulcer of other part of foot and inflammation   HCC A ▽
        Varicose veins of unspecified lower extremity with both ulcer of toe and inflammation

    I83.208   Varicose veins of unspecified lower extremity with both ulcer of other part of lower extremity and inflammation   HCC A ▽

    I83.209   Varicose veins of unspecified lower extremity with both ulcer of unspecified site and inflammation   HCC A ▽

✓6ᵗʰ I83.21   Varicose veins of right lower extremity with both ulcer and inflammation

    I83.211   Varicose veins of right lower extremity with both ulcer of thigh and inflammation   HCC A

    I83.212   Varicose veins of right lower extremity with both ulcer of calf and inflammation   HCC A

    I83.213   Varicose veins of right lower extremity with both ulcer of ankle and inflammation   HCC A

    I83.214   Varicose veins of right lower extremity with both ulcer of heel and midfoot and inflammation   HCC A
        Varicose veins of right lower extremity with both ulcer of plantar surface of midfoot and inflammation

    I83.215   Varicose veins of right lower extremity with both ulcer other part of foot and inflammation   HCC A
        Varicose veins of right lower extremity with both ulcer of toe and inflammation

    I83.218   Varicose veins of right lower extremity with both ulcer of other part of lower extremity and inflammation   HCC A

    I83.219   Varicose veins of right lower extremity with both ulcer of unspecified site and inflammation   HCC A ▽

✓6ᵗʰ I83.22   Varicose veins of left lower extremity with both ulcer and inflammation

    I83.221   Varicose veins of left lower extremity with both ulcer of thigh and inflammation   HCC A

    I83.222   Varicose veins of left lower extremity with both ulcer of calf and inflammation   HCC A

☑ Additional Character Req   ✓ˣ7ᵗʰ Placeholder Alert   Manifestation   HCC CMS-HCC Condition   ▽ Unspecified Code   ▶◀ Revised Text   ● New Code   ▲ Revised Code Title

ICD-10-CM 2018   651

I83.223   **Varicose veins of left lower** HCC A
extremity with both ulcer of ankle **and**
inflammation

I83.224   **Varicose veins of left lower** HCC A
extremity with both ulcer of heel and
midfoot **and inflammation**
Varicose veins of left lower extremity with
both ulcer of plantar surface of
midfoot and inflammation

I83.225   **Varicose veins of left lower** HCC A
extremity with both ulcer other part of
foot **and inflammation**
Varicose veins of left lower extremity with
both ulcer of toe and inflammation

I83.228   **Varicose veins of left lower** HCC A
extremity with both ulcer of other part of
lower extremity **and inflammation**

I83.229   **Varicose veins of left lower** HCC A ▽
extremity with both ulcer of unspecified
site and inflammation

✓5th **I83.8**   **Varicose veins of lower extremities with other complications**

  ✓6th **I83.81**   **Varicose veins of lower extremities with** pain

▲   **I83.811**   **Varicose veins of** right **lower** A
extremity with pain

▲   **I83.812**   **Varicose veins of** left **lower extremity** A
with pain

     I83.813   **Varicose veins of** bilateral **lower** A
extremities with pain

▲   **I83.819**   **Varicose veins of unspecified lower** A ▽
extremity with pain

  ✓6th **I83.89**   **Varicose veins of lower extremities with other**
complications
Varicose veins of lower extremities with edema
Varicose veins of lower extremities with swelling

▲   **I83.891**   **Varicose veins of** right **lower** A
extremity with other complications

▲   **I83.892**   **Varicose veins of** left **lower extremity** A
with other complications

     I83.893   **Varicose veins of** bilateral **lower** A
extremities with other complications

▲   **I83.899**   **Varicose veins of unspecified lower** A ▽
extremity with other complications

✓5th **I83.9**   **Asymptomatic** varicose veins of lower extremities
Phlebectasia of lower extremities
Varicose veins of lower extremities
Varix of lower extremities

     I83.90   **Asymptomatic varicose veins of unspecified** A ▽
lower extremity
Varicose veins NOS

     I83.91   **Asymptomatic varicose veins of** right **lower** A
extremity

     I83.92   **Asymptomatic varicose veins of** left **lower** A
extremity

     I83.93   **Asymptomatic varicose veins of** bilateral **lower** A
extremities

✓4th **I85**   **Esophageal varices**
Use additional code to identify:
alcohol abuse and dependence (F10.-)

✓5th **I85.0**   **Esophageal varices**
Idiopathic esophageal varices
Primary esophageal varices

     I85.00   **Esophageal varices** without bleeding HCC
Esophageal varices NOS

     I85.01   **Esophageal varices** with bleeding HCC

✓5th **I85.1**   **Secondary esophageal varices**
Esophageal varices secondary to alcoholic liver disease
Esophageal varices secondary to cirrhosis of liver
Esophageal varices secondary to schistosomiasis
Esophageal varices secondary to toxic liver disease
Code first underlying disease

     I85.10   **Secondary esophageal varices** without bleeding HCC

     I85.11   **Secondary esophageal varices** with bleeding HCC

✓4th **I86**   **Varicose veins of other sites**
EXCLUDES 1   *varicose veins of unspecified site (I83.9-)*
EXCLUDES 2   *retinal varices (H35.0-)*

     I86.0   **Sublingual varices**
DEF: Distended, tortuous veins beneath tongue.

I86.1   **Scrotal varices** ♂
Varicocele

I86.2   **Pelvic varices**

I86.3   **Vulval varices** ♀
EXCLUDES 1   *vulval varices complicating childbirth and the*
puerperium (O87.8)
vulval varices complicating pregnancy (O22.1-)

I86.4   **Gastric varices**

I86.8   **Varicose veins of other specified sites** A
Varicose ulcer of nasal septum

✓4th **I87**   **Other disorders of veins**

  ✓5th **I87.0**   **Postthrombotic syndrome**
Chronic venous hypertension due to deep vein thrombosis
Postphlebitic syndrome
EXCLUDES 1   *chronic venous hypertension without deep vein*
thrombosis (I87.3-)

    ✓6th **I87.00**   **Postthrombotic syndrome** without complications
Asymptomatic postthrombotic syndrome

       I87.001   **Postthrombotic syndrome without**
complications of right lower **extremity**

       I87.002   **Postthrombotic syndrome without**
complications of left lower **extremity**

       I87.003   **Postthrombotic syndrome without**
complications of bilateral lower **extremity**

       I87.009   **Postthrombotic syndrome without** ▽
complications of unspecified extremity
Postthrombotic syndrome NOS

    ✓6th **I87.01**   **Postthrombotic syndrome with** ulcer
Use additional code to specify site and severity of ulcer
(L97.-)

       I87.011   **Postthrombotic syndrome with ulcer** HCC
of right lower **extremity**

       I87.012   **Postthrombotic syndrome with ulcer** HCC
of left lower **extremity**

       I87.013   **Postthrombotic syndrome with ulcer** HCC
of bilateral lower **extremity**

       I87.019   **Postthrombotic syndrome with** HCC ▽
ulcer of unspecified lower extremity

    ✓6th **I87.02**   **Postthrombotic syndrome with** inflammation

       I87.021   **Postthrombotic syndrome with**
inflammation of right lower **extremity**

       I87.022   **Postthrombotic syndrome with**
inflammation of left lower **extremity**

       I87.023   **Postthrombotic syndrome with**
inflammation of bilateral lower **extremity**

       I87.029   **Postthrombotic syndrome with** ▽
inflammation of unspecified lower
extremity

    ✓6th **I87.03**   **Postthrombotic syndrome with** ulcer and
inflammation
Use additional code to specify site and severity of ulcer
(L97.-)

       I87.031   **Postthrombotic syndrome with ulcer** HCC
and inflammation of right lower **extremity**

       I87.032   **Postthrombotic syndrome with ulcer** HCC
and inflammation of left lower **extremity**

       I87.033   **Postthrombotic syndrome with ulcer** HCC
and inflammation of bilateral lower
extremity

       I87.039   **Postthrombotic syndrome with** HCC ▽
ulcer and inflammation of unspecified
lower extremity

    ✓6th **I87.09**   **Postthrombotic syndrome with other complications**

       I87.091   **Postthrombotic syndrome with other**
complications of right lower **extremity**

       I87.092   **Postthrombotic syndrome with other**
complications of left lower **extremity**

       I87.093   **Postthrombotic syndrome with other**
complications of bilateral lower **extremity**

       I87.099   **Postthrombotic syndrome with other** ▽
complications of unspecified lower
extremity

I87.1   **Compression of vein**
Stricture of vein
Vena cava syndrome (inferior) (superior)
EXCLUDES 2   *compression of pulmonary vein (I28.8)*

EXCLUDES 1 Not coded here   EXCLUDES 2 Not included here   N Newborn Age: 0   P Pediatric Age: 0-17   M Maternity Age: 12-55   A Adult Age: 15-124

652   ICD-10-CM 2018

I87.2　Venous insufficiency (chronic) (peripheral)
Stasis dermatitis
EXCLUDES 1　*stasis dermatitis with varicose veins of lower extremities (I83.1-, I83.2-)*
DEF: Insufficient drainage of venous blood in any part of body; results in edema or dermatosis.

✓5th **I87.3　Chronic venous hypertension (idiopathic)**
Stasis edema
EXCLUDES 1　*chronic venous hypertension due to deep vein thrombosis (I87.0-)*
varicose veins of lower extremities (I83.-)

✓6th **I87.30　Chronic venous hypertension (idiopathic) without complications**
Asymptomatic chronic venous hypertension (idiopathic)

I87.301　Chronic venous hypertension (idiopathic) without complications of right lower extremity

I87.302　Chronic venous hypertension (idiopathic) without complications of left lower extremity

I87.303　Chronic venous hypertension (idiopathic) without complications of bilateral lower extremity

I87.309　Chronic venous hypertension (idiopathic) without complications of unspecified lower extremity ▽
Chronic venous hypertension NOS

✓6th **I87.31　Chronic venous hypertension (idiopathic) with ulcer**
Use additional code to specify site and severity of ulcer (L97.-)

I87.311　Chronic venous hypertension (idiopathic) with ulcer of right lower extremity HCC

I87.312　Chronic venous hypertension (idiopathic) with ulcer of left lower extremity HCC

I87.313　Chronic venous hypertension (idiopathic) with ulcer of bilateral lower extremity HCC

I87.319　Chronic venous hypertension (idiopathic) with ulcer of unspecified lower extremity HCC ▽

✓6th **I87.32　Chronic venous hypertension (idiopathic) with inflammation**

I87.321　Chronic venous hypertension (idiopathic) with inflammation of right lower extremity

I87.322　Chronic venous hypertension (idiopathic) with inflammation of left lower extremity

I87.323　Chronic venous hypertension (idiopathic) with inflammation of bilateral lower extremity

I87.329　Chronic venous hypertension (idiopathic) with inflammation of unspecified lower extremity ▽

✓6th **I87.33　Chronic venous hypertension (idiopathic) with ulcer and inflammation**
Use additional code to specify site and severity of ulcer (L97.-)

I87.331　Chronic venous hypertension (idiopathic) with ulcer and inflammation of right lower extremity HCC

I87.332　Chronic venous hypertension (idiopathic) with ulcer and inflammation of left lower extremity HCC

I87.333　Chronic venous hypertension (idiopathic) with ulcer and inflammation of bilateral lower extremity HCC

I87.339　Chronic venous hypertension (idiopathic) with ulcer and inflammation of unspecified lower extremity HCC ▽

✓6th **I87.39　Chronic venous hypertension (idiopathic) with other complications**

I87.391　Chronic venous hypertension (idiopathic) with other complications of right lower extremity

I87.392　Chronic venous hypertension (idiopathic) with other complications of left lower extremity

I87.393　Chronic venous hypertension (idiopathic) with other complications of bilateral lower extremity

I87.399　Chronic venous hypertension (idiopathic) with other complications of unspecified lower extremity ▽

I87.8　Other specified disorders of veins
Phlebosclerosis
Venofibrosis

I87.9　Disorder of vein, unspecified ▽

✓4th **I88　Nonspecific lymphadenitis**
EXCLUDES 1　*acute lymphadenitis, except mesenteric (L04.-)*
enlarged lymph nodes NOS (R59.-)
human immunodeficiency virus [HIV] disease resulting in generalized lymphadenopathy (B20)

I88.0　Nonspecific mesenteric lymphadenitis
Mesenteric lymphadenitis (acute)(chronic)

I88.1　Chronic lymphadenitis, except mesenteric
Adenitis
Lymphadenitis

I88.8　Other nonspecific lymphadenitis

I88.9　Nonspecific lymphadenitis, unspecified ▽
Lymphadenitis NOS

✓4th **I89　Other noninfective disorders of lymphatic vessels and lymph nodes**
EXCLUDES 1　*chylocele, tunica vaginalis (nonfilarial) NOS (N50.89)*
enlarged lymph nodes NOS (R59.-)
filarial chylocele (B74.-)
hereditary lymphedema (Q82.0)

I89.0　Lymphedema, not elsewhere classified
Elephantiasis (nonfilarial) NOS
Lymphangiectasis
Obliteration, lymphatic vessel
Praecox lymphedema
Secondary lymphedema
EXCLUDES 1　*postmastectomy lymphedema (I97.2)*

I89.1　Lymphangitis
Chronic lymphangitis
Lymphangitis NOS
Subacute lymphangitis
EXCLUDES 1　*acute lymphangitis (L03.-)*

I89.8　Other specified noninfective disorders of lymphatic vessels and lymph nodes
Chylocele (nonfilarial)
Chylous ascites
Chylous cyst
Lipomelanotic reticulosis
Lymph node or vessel fistula
Lymph node or vessel infarction
Lymph node or vessel rupture

I89.9　Noninfective disorder of lymphatic vessels and lymph nodes, unspecified ▽
Disease of lymphatic vessels NOS

Other and unspecified disorders of the circulatory system (I95-I99)

✓4th **I95　Hypotension**
EXCLUDES 1　*cardiovascular collapse (R57.9)*
maternal hypotension syndrome (O26.5-)
nonspecific low blood pressure reading NOS (R03.1)

I95.0　Idiopathic hypotension

I95.1　Orthostatic hypotension
Hypotension, postural
EXCLUDES 1　*neurogenic orthostatic hypotension [Shy-Drager] (G90.3)*
orthostatic hypotension due to drugs (I95.2)

I95.2　Hypotension due to drugs
Orthostatic hypotension due to drugs
Use additional code for adverse effect, if applicable, to identify drug (T36-T50 with fifth or sixth character 5)

I95.3　Hypotension of hemodialysis
Intra-dialytic hypotension

✓5th **I95.8　Other hypotension**

I95.81　Postprocedural hypotension

I95.89　Other hypotension
Chronic hypotension

I95.9　Hypotension, unspecified ▽

✓ Additional Character Req　✓x7th Placeholder Alert　Manifestation　HCC CMS-HCC Condition　▽ Unspecified Code　▶◀ Revised Text　● New Code　▲ Revised Code Title

Chapter 9. Diseases of the Circulatory System

I96   Gangrene, not elsewhere classified   `HCC`
Gangrenous cellulitis
EXCLUDES1   *gangrene in atherosclerosis of native arteries of the extremities (I70.26)*
gangrene in diabetes mellitus (E08-E13 with .52)
gangrene in hernia (K40.1, K40.4, K41.1, K41.4, K42.1, K43.1-, K44.1, K45.1, K46.1)
gangrene in other peripheral vascular diseases (I73.-)
gangrene of certain specified sites—see Alphabetical Index
gas gangrene (A48.0)
pyoderma gangrenosum (L88)
EXCLUDES2 ▶*gangrene in diabetes mellitus (E08-E13 with .52)*◀
AHA: 2013, 2Q, 34

✓4th **I97   Intraoperative and postprocedural complications and disorders of circulatory system, not elsewhere classified**
EXCLUDES2   *postprocedural shock (T81.1-)*

I97.0   Postcardiotomy syndrome

✓5th **I97.1   Other postprocedural cardiac** functional disturbances
EXCLUDES2   *acute pulmonary insufficiency following thoracic surgery (J95.1)*
intraoperative cardiac functional disturbances (I97.7-)

✓6th **I97.11   Postprocedural** cardiac insufficiency
I97.110   Postprocedural cardiac insufficiency following cardiac surgery
I97.111   Postprocedural cardiac insufficiency following other surgery

✓6th **I97.12   Postprocedural** cardiac arrest
I97.120   Postprocedural cardiac arrest following cardiac surgery
I97.121   Postprocedural cardiac arrest following other surgery

✓6th **I97.13   Postprocedural** heart failure
Use additional code to identify the heart failure (I50.-)
I97.130   Postprocedural heart failure following cardiac surgery
I97.131   Postprocedural heart failure following other surgery

✓6th **I97.19   Other postprocedural cardiac** functional disturbances
Use additional code, if applicable, to further specify disorder
I97.190   Other postprocedural cardiac functional disturbances following cardiac surgery
▶Use additional code, if applicable, for type 4 or type 5 myocardial infarction, to further specify disorder◀
I97.191   Other postprocedural cardiac functional disturbances following other surgery

I97.2   Postmastectomy lymphedema syndrome   `A`
Elephantiasis due to mastectomy
Obliteration of lymphatic vessels

I97.3   Postprocedural hypertension

✓5th **I97.4   Intraoperative hemorrhage and hematoma** of a circulatory system organ or structure complicating a procedure
EXCLUDES1   *intraoperative hemorrhage and hematoma of a circulatory system organ or structure due to accidental puncture and laceration during a procedure (I97.5-)*
EXCLUDES2   *intraoperative cerebrovascular hemorrhage complicating a procedure (G97.3-)*

✓6th **I97.41   Intraoperative hemorrhage and hematoma of a circulatory system organ or structure complicating a** circulatory system procedure
I97.410   Intraoperative hemorrhage and hematoma of a circulatory system organ or structure complicating a cardiac catheterization
I97.411   Intraoperative hemorrhage and hematoma of a circulatory system organ or structure complicating a cardiac bypass
I97.418   Intraoperative hemorrhage and hematoma of a circulatory system organ or structure complicating other circulatory system procedure

I97.42   Intraoperative hemorrhage and hematoma of a circulatory system organ or structure complicating other procedure

✓5th **I97.5   Accidental puncture and laceration** of a circulatory system organ or structure during a procedure
EXCLUDES2   *accidental puncture and laceration of brain during a procedure (G97.4-)*

I97.51   Accidental puncture and laceration of a circulatory system organ or structure during a circulatory system procedure
I97.52   Accidental puncture and laceration of a circulatory system organ or structure during other procedure

✓5th **I97.6   Postprocedural hemorrhage, hematoma and seroma** of a circulatory system organ or structure following a procedure
EXCLUDES2   *postprocedural cerebrovascular hemorrhage complicating a procedure (G97.5-)*

✓6th **I97.61   Postprocedural** hemorrhage of a circulatory system organ or structure following a circulatory system procedure
I97.610   Postprocedural hemorrhage of a circulatory system organ or structure following a cardiac catheterization
I97.611   Postprocedural hemorrhage of a circulatory system organ or structure following cardiac bypass
I97.618   Postprocedural hemorrhage of a circulatory system organ or structure following other circulatory system procedure

✓6th **I97.62   Postprocedural hemorrhage, hematoma and seroma of a circulatory system organ or structure following** other procedure
I97.620   Postprocedural hemorrhage of a circulatory system organ or structure following other procedure
I97.621   Postprocedural hematoma of a circulatory system organ or structure following other procedure
I97.622   Postprocedural seroma of a circulatory system organ or structure following procedure

✓6th **I97.63   Postprocedural hematoma** of a circulatory system organ or structure following a circulatory system procedure
I97.630   Postprocedural hematoma of a circulatory system organ or structure following a cardiac catheterization
I97.631   Postprocedural hematoma of a circulatory system organ or structure following cardiac bypass
I97.638   Postprocedural hematoma of a circulatory system organ or structure following other circulatory system procedure

✓6th **I97.64   Postprocedural seroma** of a circulatory system organ or structure following a circulatory system procedure
I97.640   Postprocedural seroma of a circulatory system organ or structure following a cardiac catheterization
I97.641   Postprocedural seroma of a circulatory system organ or structure following cardiac bypass
I97.648   Postprocedural seroma of a circulatory system organ or structure following other circulatory system procedure

✓5th **I97.7   Intraoperative cardiac** functional disturbances
EXCLUDES2   *acute pulmonary insufficiency following thoracic surgery (J95.1)*
postprocedural cardiac functional disturbances (I97.1-)

✓6th **I97.71   Intraoperative** cardiac arrest
I97.710   Intraoperative cardiac arrest during cardiac surgery
I97.711   Intraoperative cardiac arrest during other surgery

✓6th **I97.79   Other intraoperative cardiac functional disturbances**
Use additional code, if applicable, to further specify disorder
I97.790   Other intraoperative cardiac functional disturbances during cardiac surgery
I97.791   Other intraoperative cardiac functional disturbances during other surgery

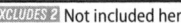

EXCLUDES1 Not coded here   *EXCLUDES2* Not included here   `N` Newborn Age: 0   `P` Pediatric Age: 0-17   `M` Maternity Age: 12-55   `A` Adult Age: 15-124

☑5ᵗʰ **I97.8**   **Other intraoperative and postprocedural complications and disorders of the circulatory system, not elsewhere classified**
Use additional code, if applicable, to further specify disorder

    ☑6ᵗʰ **I97.81**   Intraoperative **cerebrovascular infarction**

        I97.810   **Intraoperative cerebrovascular infarction during** cardiac surgery   `HCC`

        I97.811   **Intraoperative cerebrovascular infarction during** other surgery   `HCC`

    ☑6ᵗʰ **I97.82**   Postprocedural **cerebrovascular infarction**

        I97.820   **Postprocedural cerebrovascular infarction following** cardiac surgery   `HCC`

        I97.821   **Postprocedural cerebrovascular infarction following** other surgery   `HCC`

    I97.88   **Other intraoperative complications of the circulatory system, not elsewhere classified**

    I97.89   **Other postprocedural complications and disorders of the circulatory system, not elsewhere classified**

☑4ᵗʰ **I99**   **Other and unspecified disorders of circulatory system**

    I99.8   **Other disorder of circulatory system**

    I99.9   **Unspecified disorder of circulatory system**   ▽

☑ Additional Character Req   ☑ⁿᵗʰ Placeholder Alert   Manifestation   `HCC` CMS-HCC Condition   ▽ Unspecified Code   ▶◀ Revised Text   ● New Code   ▲ Revised Code Title

ICD-10-CM 2018   **655**

Chapter 10. Diseases of the Respiratory System (J00–J99)

Chapter Specific Guidelines with Coding Examples

The chapter specific guidelines from the ICD-10-CM Official Guidelines for Coding and Reporting have been provided below. Along with these guidelines are coding examples, contained in the shaded boxes, that have been developed to help illustrate the coding and/or sequencing guidance found in these guidelines.

a. Chronic obstructive pulmonary disease [COPD] and asthma

1) Acute exacerbation of chronic obstructive bronchitis and asthma

The codes in categories J44 and J45 distinguish between uncomplicated cases and those in acute exacerbation. An acute exacerbation is a worsening or a decompensation of a chronic condition. An acute exacerbation is not equivalent to an infection superimposed on a chronic condition, though an exacerbation may be triggered by an infection.

Acute streptococcal bronchitis with acute exacerbation of COPD

J20.2	**Acute bronchitis due to streptococcus**
J44.0	**Chronic obstructive pulmonary disease with acute lower respiratory infection**
J44.1	**Chronic obstructive pulmonary disease with (acute) exacerbation**

Explanation: ICD-10-CM uses combination codes to create organism-specific classifications for acute bronchitis. Category J44 codes include combination codes with severity components, which differentiate between COPD with acute lower respiratory infection (acute bronchitis), COPD with acute exacerbation, and COPD without mention of a complication (unspecified).

An acute exacerbation is a worsening or a decompensation of a chronic condition. An acute exacerbation is not equivalent to an infection superimposed on a chronic condition, though an exacerbation may be triggered by an infection, as in this example.

Exacerbation of moderate persistent asthma with status asthmaticus

J45.42	**Moderate persistent asthma with status asthmaticus**

Explanation: Category J45 Asthma includes severity-specific subcategories and fifth-character codes to distinguish between uncomplicated cases, those in acute exacerbation, and those with status asthmaticus.

---

b. Acute respiratory failure

1) Acute respiratory failure as principal diagnosis

A code from subcategory J96.0, Acute respiratory failure, or subcategory J96.2, Acute and chronic respiratory failure, may be assigned as a principal diagnosis when it is the condition established after study to be chiefly responsible for occasioning the admission to the hospital, and the selection is supported by the Alphabetic Index and Tabular List. However, chapter-specific coding guidelines (such as obstetrics, poisoning, HIV, newborn) that provide sequencing direction take precedence.

Acute hypoxic respiratory failure due to exacerbation of chronic obstructive bronchitis

J96.01	**Acute respiratory failure with hypoxia**
J44.1	**Chronic obstructive pulmonary disease with (acute) exacerbation**

Explanation: Category J96 classifies respiratory failure with combination codes that designate the severity and the presence of hypoxia and hypercapnia. Code J96.01 is sequenced as the first-listed diagnosis, as the reason for the encounter. Respiratory failure may be assigned as a principal diagnosis when it is the condition established after study to be chiefly responsible for occasioning the encounter and the selection is supported by the Alphabetic Index and Tabular List.

---

2) Acute respiratory failure as secondary diagnosis

Respiratory failure may be listed as a secondary diagnosis if it occurs after admission, or if it is present on admission, but does not meet the definition of principal diagnosis.

Acute respiratory failure due to accidental oxycodone overdose

T40.2X1A	**Poisoning by other opioids, accidental (unintentional), initial encounter**
J96.00	**Acute respiratory failure, unspecified whether with hypoxia or hypercapnia**

Explanation: Respiratory failure may be assigned as a principal diagnosis when it is the condition established after study to be chiefly responsible for occasioning the encounter, and the selection is supported by the Alphabetic Index and Tabular List. However, chapter-specific coding guidelines, such as poisoning, that provide sequencing direction take precedence. When coding a poisoning or reaction to the improper use of a medication (e.g. overdose, wrong substance given or taken in error, wrong route of administration), first assign the appropriate code from categories T36–T50. Use additional code(s) for all manifestations of the poisoning. In this instance, the respiratory failure is a manifestation of the poisoning and is sequenced as a secondary diagnosis.

---

3) Sequencing of acute respiratory failure and another acute condition

When a patient is admitted with respiratory failure and another acute condition, (e.g., myocardial infarction, cerebrovascular accident, aspiration pneumonia), the principal diagnosis will not be the same in every situation. This applies whether the other acute condition is a respiratory or nonrespiratory condition. Selection of the principal diagnosis will be dependent on the circumstances of admission. If both the respiratory failure and the other acute condition are equally responsible for occasioning the admission to the hospital, and there are no chapter-specific sequencing rules, the guideline regarding two or more diagnoses that equally meet the definition for principal diagnosis (*Section II, C.*) may be applied in these situations.

If the documentation is not clear as to whether acute respiratory failure and another condition are equally responsible for occasioning the admission, query the provider for clarification.

Patient presents with acute pneumococcal pneumonia and acute respiratory failure

J96.00	**Acute respiratory failure, unspecified whether with hypoxia or hypercapnia**
J13	**Pneumonia due to Streptococcus pneumoniae**

Explanation: When a patient is seen for respiratory failure and another acute condition, such as a bacterial pneumonia, the principal or first-listed diagnosis is not the same in every situation. This applies whether the other acute condition is a respiratory or nonrespiratory condition. The principal diagnosis depends on the problem chiefly responsible for the encounter.

---

c. Influenza due to certain identified influenza viruses

Code only confirmed cases of influenza due to certain identified influenza viruses (category J09), and due to other identified influenza virus (category J10). This is an exception to the hospital inpatient guideline Section II, H. (Uncertain Diagnosis).

In this context, "confirmation" does not require documentation of positive laboratory testing specific for avian or other novel influenza A or other identified influenza virus. However, coding should be based on the provider's diagnostic statement that the patient has avian influenza, or other novel influenza A, for category J09, or has another particular identified strain of influenza, such as H1N1 or H3N2, but not identified as novel or variant, for category J10.

If the provider records "suspected" or "possible" or "probable" avian influenza, or novel influenza, or other identified influenza, then the appropriate influenza code from category J11, Influenza due to unidentified influenza virus, should be assigned. A code from category J09, Influenza due to certain identified influenza viruses, should not be assigned nor should a code from category J10, Influenza due to other identified influenza virus.

Influenza due to avian influenza virus with pneumonia

J09.X1   **Influenza due to identified novel influenza A virus with pneumonia**

Explanation: Codes in category J09 Influenza due to certain identified influenza viruses should be assigned only for confirmed cases. "Confirmation" does not require positive laboratory testing of a specific influenza virus but does need to be based on the provider's diagnostic statement, which should not include terms such as "possible," "probable," or "suspected."

d. Ventilator associated pneumonia

1) Documentation of ventilator associated pneumonia

As with all procedural or postprocedural complications, code assignment is based on the provider's documentation of the relationship between the condition and the procedure.

Code J95.851, Ventilator associated pneumonia, should be assigned only when the provider has documented ventilator associated pneumonia (VAP). An additional code to identify the organism (e.g., Pseudomonas aeruginosa, code B96.5) should also be assigned. Do not assign an additional code from categories J12-J18 to identify the type of pneumonia.

Code J95.851 should not be assigned for cases where the patient has pneumonia and is on a mechanical ventilator and the provider has not specifically stated that the pneumonia is ventilator-associated pneumonia. If the documentation is unclear as to whether the patient has a pneumonia that is a complication attributable to the mechanical ventilator, query the provider.

2) Ventilator associated pneumonia develops after admission

A patient may be admitted with one type of pneumonia (e.g., code J13, Pneumonia due to Streptococcus pneumonia) and subsequently develop VAP. In this instance, the principal diagnosis would be the appropriate code from categories J12-J18 for the pneumonia diagnosed at the time of admission. Code J95.851, Ventilator associated pneumonia, would be assigned as an additional diagnosis when the provider has also documented the presence of ventilator associated pneumonia.

Chapter 10. Diseases of the Respiratory System (J00-J99)

NOTE   When a respiratory condition is described as occurring in more than one site and is not specifically indexed, it should be classified to the lower anatomic site (e.g. tracheobronchitis to bronchitis in J40).

Use additional code, where applicable, to identify:
exposure to environmental tobacco smoke (Z77.22)
exposure to tobacco smoke in the perinatal period (P96.81)
history of tobacco dependence (Z87.891)
occupational exposure to environmental tobacco smoke (Z57.31)
tobacco dependence (F17.-)
tobacco use (Z72.0)

EXCLUDES 2   *certain conditions originating in the perinatal period (P04-P96)*
certain infectious and parasitic diseases (A00-B99)
complications of pregnancy, childbirth and the puerperium (O00-O9A)
congenital malformations, deformations and chromosomal abnormalities (Q00-Q99)
endocrine, nutritional and metabolic diseases (E00-E88)
injury, poisoning and certain other consequences of external causes (S00-T88)
neoplasms (C00-D49)
smoke inhalation (T59.81-)
symptoms, signs and abnormal clinical and laboratory findings, not elsewhere classified (R00-R94)

This chapter contains the following blocks:

J00-J06	Acute upper respiratory infections
J09-J18	Influenza and pneumonia
J20-J22	Other acute lower respiratory infections
J30-J39	Other diseases of upper respiratory tract
J40-J47	Chronic lower respiratory diseases
J60-J70	Lung diseases due to external agents
J80-J84	Other respiratory diseases principally affecting the interstitium
J85-J86	Suppurative and necrotic conditions of the lower respiratory tract
J90-J94	Other diseases of the pleura
J95	Intraoperative and postprocedural complications and disorders of respiratory system, not elsewhere classified
J96-J99	Other diseases of the respiratory system

Acute upper respiratory infections (J00-J06)

EXCLUDES 1   *chronic obstructive pulmonary disease with acute lower respiratory infection (J44.0)*
influenza virus with other respiratory manifestations (J09.X2, J10.1, J11.1)

J00   Acute nasopharyngitis (common cold)
Acute rhinitis
Coryza (acute)
Infective nasopharyngitis NOS
Infective rhinitis
Nasal catarrh, acute
Nasopharyngitis NOS

EXCLUDES 1   *acute pharyngitis (J02.-)*
acute sore throat NOS (J02.9)
pharyngitis NOS (J02.9)
rhinitis NOS (J31.0)
sore throat NOS (J02.9)

EXCLUDES 2   *allergic rhinitis (J30.1-J30.9)*
chronic pharyngitis (J31.2)
chronic rhinitis (J31.0)
chronic sore throat (J31.2)
nasopharyngitis, chronic (J31.1)
vasomotor rhinitis (J30.0)

DEF: Acute inflammation of mucous membranes; extends from nares to pharynx; characterized by nasal obstruction, sneezing, runny nose, and sore throat.

√4th J01   Acute sinusitis
INCLUDES   acute abscess of sinus
acute empyema of sinus
acute infection of sinus
acute inflammation of sinus
acute suppuration of sinus

Use additional code (B95-B97) to identify infectious agent

EXCLUDES 1   *sinusitis NOS (J32.9)*
EXCLUDES 2   *chronic sinusitis (J32.0-J32.8)*

   √5th J01.0   Acute maxillary sinusitis
Acute antritis
     J01.00   Acute maxillary sinusitis, unspecified ▽
     J01.01   Acute recurrent maxillary sinusitis

   √5th J01.1   Acute frontal sinusitis
     J01.10   Acute frontal sinusitis, unspecified ▽
     J01.11   Acute recurrent frontal sinusitis

   √5th J01.2   Acute ethmoidal sinusitis
     J01.20   Acute ethmoidal sinusitis, unspecified ▽
     J01.21   Acute recurrent ethmoidal sinusitis

   √5th J01.3   Acute sphenoidal sinusitis
     J01.30   Acute sphenoidal sinusitis, unspecified ▽
     J01.31   Acute recurrent sphenoidal sinusitis

   √5th J01.4   Acute pansinusitis
     J01.40   Acute pansinusitis, unspecified ▽
     J01.41   Acute recurrent pansinusitis

   √5th J01.8   Other acute sinusitis
     J01.80   Other acute sinusitis
Acute sinusitis involving more than one sinus but not pansinusitis
     J01.81   Other acute recurrent sinusitis
Acute recurrent sinusitis involving more than one sinus but not pansinusitis

   √5th J01.9   Acute sinusitis, unspecified
     J01.90   Acute sinusitis, unspecified ▽
     J01.91   Acute recurrent sinusitis, unspecified ▽

√4th J02   Acute pharyngitis
INCLUDES   acute sore throat
EXCLUDES 1   *acute laryngopharyngitis (J06.0)*
peritonsillar abscess (J36)
pharyngeal abscess (J39.1)
retropharyngeal abscess (J39.0)
EXCLUDES 2   *chronic pharyngitis (J31.2)*

   J02.0   Streptococcal pharyngitis
Septic pharyngitis
Streptococcal sore throat
EXCLUDES 2   *scarlet fever (A38.-)*

   J02.8   Acute pharyngitis due to other specified organisms
Use additional code (B95-B97) to identify infectious agent
EXCLUDES 1   *acute pharyngitis due to coxsackie virus (B08.5)*
acute pharyngitis due to gonococcus (A54.5)
acute pharyngitis due to herpes [simplex] virus (B00.2)
acute pharyngitis due to infectious mononucleosis (B27.-)
enteroviral vesicular pharyngitis (B08.5)

   J02.9   Acute pharyngitis, unspecified ▽
Gangrenous pharyngitis (acute)
Infective pharyngitis (acute) NOS
Pharyngitis (acute) NOS
Sore throat (acute) NOS
Suppurative pharyngitis (acute)
Ulcerative pharyngitis (acute)

√4th J03   Acute tonsillitis
EXCLUDES 1   *acute sore throat (J02.-)*
hypertrophy of tonsils (J35.1)
peritonsillar abscess (J36)
sore throat NOS (J02.9)
streptococcal sore throat (J02.0)
EXCLUDES 2   *chronic tonsillitis (J35.0)*

   √5th J03.0   Streptococcal tonsillitis
     J03.00   Acute streptococcal tonsillitis, unspecified ▽
     J03.01   Acute recurrent streptococcal tonsillitis

   √5th J03.8   Acute tonsillitis due to other specified organisms
Use additional code (B95-B97) to identify infectious agent
EXCLUDES 1   *diphtheritic tonsillitis (A36.0)*
herpesviral pharyngotonsillitis (B00.2)
streptococcal tonsillitis (J03.0)
tuberculous tonsillitis (A15.8)
Vincent's tonsillitis (A69.1)
     J03.80   Acute tonsillitis due to other specified organisms
     J03.81   Acute recurrent tonsillitis due to other specified organisms

   √5th J03.9   Acute tonsillitis, unspecified
Follicular tonsillitis (acute)
Gangrenous tonsillitis (acute)
Infective tonsillitis (acute)
Tonsillitis (acute) NOS
Ulcerative tonsillitis (acute)
     J03.90   Acute tonsillitis, unspecified ▽
     J03.91   Acute recurrent tonsillitis, unspecified ▽

✔ Additional Character Req   *√x7th* Placeholder Alert   Manifestation   **HCC** CMS-HCC Condition   ▽ Unspecified Code   ►◄ Revised Text   ● New Code   ▲ Revised Code Title

ICD-10-CM 2018   **659**

Chapter 10. Diseases of the Respiratory System

✓4ᵗʰ J04   Acute laryngitis and tracheitis

     Use additional code (B95-B97) to identify infectious agent

     EXCLUDES 1   *acute obstructive laryngitis [croup] and epiglottitis (J05.-)*

     EXCLUDES 2   *laryngismus (stridulus) (J38.5)*

     J04.0   Acute laryngitis

         Edematous laryngitis (acute)

         Laryngitis (acute) NOS

         Subglottic laryngitis (acute)

         Suppurative laryngitis (acute)

         Ulcerative laryngitis (acute)

         EXCLUDES 1   *acute obstructive laryngitis (J05.0)*

         EXCLUDES 2   *chronic laryngitis (J37.0)*

     ✓5ᵗʰ J04.1   Acute tracheitis

         Acute viral tracheitis

         Catarrhal tracheitis (acute)

         Tracheitis (acute) NOS

         EXCLUDES 2   *chronic tracheitis (J42)*

         J04.10   Acute tracheitis without obstruction

         J04.11   Acute tracheitis with obstruction

     J04.2   Acute laryngotracheitis

         Laryngotracheitis NOS

         Tracheitis (acute) with laryngitis (acute)

         EXCLUDES 1   *acute obstructive laryngotracheitis (J05.0)*

         EXCLUDES 2   *chronic laryngotracheitis (J37.1)*

     ✓5ᵗʰ J04.3   Supraglottitis, unspecified

         J04.30   Supraglottitis, unspecified, without obstruction ▽

         J04.31   Supraglottitis, unspecified, with obstruction ▽

✓4ᵗʰ J05   Acute obstructive laryngitis [croup] and epiglottitis

     Use additional code (B95-B97) to identify infectious agent

     J05.0   Acute obstructive laryngitis [croup]

         Obstructive laryngitis (acute) NOS

         Obstructive laryngotracheitis NOS

         DEF: Acute laryngeal obstruction due to allergy, foreign body, or in the majority of cases a viral infection; symptoms include harsh, barking cough, hoarseness, and persistent high-pitched respiratory sound (stridor).

     ✓5ᵗʰ J05.1   Acute epiglottitis

         EXCLUDES 2   *epiglottitis, chronic (J37.0)*

         J05.10   Acute epiglottitis without obstruction

              Epiglottitis NOS

         J05.11   Acute epiglottitis with obstruction

✓4ᵗʰ J06   Acute upper respiratory infections of multiple and unspecified sites

     EXCLUDES 1   *acute respiratory infection NOS (J22)*

                streptococcal pharyngitis (J02.0)3

     J06.0   Acute laryngopharyngitis

     J06.9   Acute upper respiratory infection, unspecified ▽

         Upper respiratory disease, acute

         Upper respiratory infection NOS

Influenza and pneumonia (J09-J18)

     EXCLUDES 2   *allergic or eosinophilic pneumonia (J82)*

                aspiration pneumonia NOS (J69.0)

                congenital pneumonia (P23.9)

                lipid pneumonia (J69.1)

                meconium pneumonia (P24.01)

                neonatal aspiration pneumonia (P24.-)

                pneumonia due to solids and liquids (J69.-)

                rheumatic pneumonia (I00)

                ventilator associated pneumonia (J95.851)

✓4ᵗʰ J09   Influenza due to certain identified influenza viruses

     EXCLUDES 1   ►*influenza A/H1N1 (J10.-)*◄

                influenza due to other identified influenza virus (J10.-)

                influenza due to unidentified influenza virus (J11.-)

                seasonal influenza due to other identified influenza virus (J10.-)

                seasonal influenza due to unidentified influenza virus (J11.-)

     ✓5ᵗʰ J09.X   Influenza due to identified novel influenza A virus

         Avian influenza

         Bird influenza

         Influenza A/H5N1

         Influenza of other animal origin, not bird or swine

         Swine influenza virus (viruses that normally cause infections in pigs)

         AHA: 2016, 3Q, 10

         J09.X1   Influenza due to identified novel influenza A virus with pneumonia

                Code also, if applicable, associated:

                lung abscess (J85.1)

                other specified type of pneumonia

         J09.X2   Influenza due to identified novel influenza A virus with other respiratory manifestations

                Influenza due to identified novel influenza A virus NOS

                Influenza due to identified novel influenza A virus with laryngitis

                Influenza due to identified novel influenza A virus with pharyngitis

                Influenza due to identified novel influenza A virus with upper respiratory symptoms

                Use additional code, if applicable, for associated:

                pleural effusion (J91.8)

                sinusitis (J01.-)

         J09.X3   Influenza due to identified novel influenza A virus with gastrointestinal manifestations

                Influenza due to identified novel influenza A virus gastroenteritis

                EXCLUDES 1   *'intestinal flu' [viral gastroenteritis] (A08.-)*

         J09.X9   Influenza due to identified novel influenza A virus with other manifestations

                Influenza due to identified novel influenza A virus with encephalopathy

                Influenza due to identified novel influenza A virus with myocarditis

                Influenza due to identified novel influenza A virus with otitis media

                Use additional code to identify manifestation

✓4ᵗʰ J10   Influenza due to other identified influenza virus

     EXCLUDES 1   *influenza due to avian influenza virus (J09.X-)*

                influenza due to swine flu (J09.X-)

                influenza due to unidentifed influenza virus (J11.-)

     ✓5ᵗʰ J10.0   Influenza due to other identified influenza virus with pneumonia

         Code also associated lung abscess, if applicable (J85.1)

         J10.00   Influenza due to other identified influenza virus with unspecified type of pneumonia ▽

         J10.01   Influenza due to other identified influenza virus with the same other identified influenza virus pneumonia

         J10.08   Influenza due to other identified influenza virus with other specified pneumonia

                Code also other specified type of pneumonia

     J10.1   Influenza due to other identified influenza virus with other respiratory manifestations

         Influenza due to other identified influenza virus NOS

         Influenza due to other identified influenza virus with laryngitis

         Influenza due to other identified influenza virus with pharyngitis

         Influenza due to other identified influenza virus with upper respiratory symptoms

         Use additional code for associated pleural effusion, if applicable (J91.8)

         Use additional code for associated sinusitis, if applicable (J01.-)

         AHA: 2016, 3Q, 10-11

     J10.2   Influenza due to other identified influenza virus with gastrointestinal manifestations

         Influenza due to other identified influenza virus gastroenteritis

         EXCLUDES 1   *'intestinal flu' [viral gastroenteritis] (A08.-)*

     ✓5ᵗʰ J10.8   Influenza due to other identified influenza virus with other manifestations

         J10.81   Influenza due to other identified influenza virus with encephalopathy

         J10.82   Influenza due to other identified influenza virus with myocarditis

         J10.83   Influenza due to other identified influenza virus with otitis media

                Use additional code for any associated perforated tympanic membrane (H72.-)

         J10.89   Influenza due to other identified influenza virus with other manifestations

                Use additional codes to identify the manifestations

✓4ᵗʰ J11   Influenza due to unidentified influenza virus

     ✓5ᵗʰ J11.0   Influenza due to unidentified influenza virus with pneumonia

         Code also associated lung abscess, if applicable (J85.1)

         AHA: 2016, 3Q, 11

         J11.00   Influenza due to unidentified influenza virus with unspecified type of pneumonia ▽

                Influenza with pneumonia NOS

EXCLUDES 1 Not coded here   *EXCLUDES 2* Not included here   N Newborn Age: 0   P Pediatric Age: 0-17   M Maternity Age: 12-55   A Adult Age: 15-124

660   ICD-10-CM 2018

J11.Ø8 **Influenza due to unidentified influenza virus with** specified **pneumonia**
Code also other specified type of pneumonia

J11.1 **Influenza due to unidentified influenza virus with other respiratory manifestations**
Influenza NOS
Influenzal laryngitis NOS
Influenzal pharyngitis NOS
Influenza with upper respiratory symptoms NOS
Use additional code for associated pleural effusion, if applicable (J91.8)
Use additional code for associated sinusitis, if applicable (J01.-)

J11.2 **Influenza due to unidentified influenza virus with gastrointestinal manifestations**
Influenza gastroenteritis NOS
EXCLUDES 1 'intestinal flu' [viral gastroenteritis] (A08.-)

☑5ᵗʰ **J11.8** **Influenza due to unidentified influenza virus with other manifestations**

J11.81 **Influenza due to unidentified influenza virus with** encephalopathy
Influenzal encephalopathy NOS

J11.82 **Influenza due to unidentified influenza virus with** myocarditis
Influenzal myocarditis NOS

J11.83 **Influenza due to unidentified influenza virus with** otitis media
Influenzal otitis media NOS
Use additional code for any associated perforated tympanic membrane (H72.-)

J11.89 **Influenza due to unidentified influenza virus with other manifestations**
Use additional codes to identify the manifestations

☑4ᵗʰ **J12** **Viral pneumonia, not elsewhere classified**
INCLUDES bronchopneumonia due to viruses other than influenza viruses
Code first associated influenza, if applicable (J09.X1, J10.0-, J11.0-)
Code also associated abscess, if applicable (J85.1)
EXCLUDES 1 aspiration pneumonia due to anesthesia during labor and delivery (O74.0)
aspiration pneumonia due to anesthesia during pregnancy (O29)
aspiration pneumonia due to anesthesia during puerperium (O89.0)
aspiration pneumonia due to solids and liquids (J69.-)
aspiration pneumonia NOS (J69.0)
congenital pneumonia (P23.0)
congenital rubella pneumonitis (P35.0)
interstitial pneumonia NOS (J84.9)
lipid pneumonia (J69.1)
neonatal aspiration pneumonia (P24.-)
AHA: 2016, 3Q, 15; 2013, 4Q, 118

J12.0 Adenoviral **pneumonia**

J12.1 Respiratory syncytial **virus pneumonia**

J12.2 Parainfluenza **virus pneumonia**

J12.3 Human metapneumovirus **pneumonia**

☑5ᵗʰ **J12.8** **Other viral pneumonia**

J12.81 **Pneumonia due to SARS-associated coronavirus**
Severe acute respiratory syndrome NOS
DEF: A severe adult respiratory syndrome caused by the coronavirus, specified as inflammation of the lungs with consolidation.

J12.89 **Other viral pneumonia**

J12.9 **Viral pneumonia, unspecified** ▽

J13 **Pneumonia due to** Streptococcus pneumoniae HCC
Bronchopneumonia due to S. pneumoniae
Code first associated influenza, if applicable (J09.X1, J10.0-, J11.0-)
Code also associated lung abscess, if applicable (J85.1)
EXCLUDES 1 congenital pneumonia due to S. pneumoniae (P23.6)
lobar pneumonia, unspecified organism (J18.1)
pneumonia due to other streptococci (J15.3-J15.4)
AHA: 2016, 3Q, 15; 2013, 4Q, 118

J14 **Pneumonia due to** Hemophilus influenzae HCC
Bronchopneumonia due to H. influenzae
Code first associated influenza, if applicable (J09.X1, J10.0-, J11.0-)
Code also associated lung abscess, if applicable (J85.1)
EXCLUDES 1 congenital pneumonia due to H. influenzae (P23.6)
AHA: 2016, 3Q, 15; 2013, 4Q, 118

☑4ᵗʰ **J15** Bacterial **pneumonia, not elsewhere classified**
INCLUDES bronchopneumonia due to bacteria other than S. pneumoniae and H. influenzae
Code first associated influenza, if applicable (J09.X1, J10.0-, J11.0-)
Code also associated lung abscess, if applicable (J85.1)
EXCLUDES 1 chlamydial pneumonia (J16.0)
congenital pneumonia (P23.-)
Legionnaires' disease (A48.1)
spirochetal pneumonia (A69.8)
AHA: 2016, 3Q, 15; 2013, 4Q, 118

J15.0 **Pneumonia due to** Klebsiella pneumoniae HCC

J15.1 **Pneumonia due to** Pseudomonas HCC

☑5ᵗʰ **J15.2** **Pneumonia due to** staphylococcus

J15.20 **Pneumonia due to staphylococcus, unspecified** HCC ▽

☑6ᵗʰ **J15.21** **Pneumonia due to Staphylococcus** aureus

J15.211 **Pneumonia due to** Methicillin susceptible **Staphylococcus aureus** HCC
MSSA pneumonia
Pneumonia due to Staphylococcus aureus NOS

J15.212 **Pneumonia due to** Methicillin resistant **Staphylococcus aureus** HCC

J15.29 **Pneumonia due to other staphylococcus** HCC

J15.3 **Pneumonia due to streptococcus,** group B HCC

J15.4 **Pneumonia due to other streptococci** HCC
EXCLUDES 1 pneumonia due to streptococcus, group B (J15.3)
pneumonia due to Streptococcus pneumoniae (J13)

J15.5 **Pneumonia due to** Escherichia coli HCC

▲ **J15.6** **Pneumonia due to** other Gram-negative bacteria HCC
►Pneumonia due to other aerobic Gram-negative bacteria◄
Pneumonia due to Serratia marcescens

J15.7 **Pneumonia due to** Mycoplasma pneumoniae

J15.8 **Pneumonia due to other specified bacteria** HCC

J15.9 **Unspecified bacterial pneumonia** ▽
Pneumonia due to gram-positive bacteria

☑4ᵗʰ **J16** **Pneumonia due to other infectious organisms, not elsewhere classified**
Code first associated influenza, if applicable (J09.X1, J10.0-, J11.0-)
Code also associated lung abscess, if applicable (J85.1)
EXCLUDES 1 congenital pneumonia (P23.-)
ornithosis (A70)
pneumocystosis (B59)
pneumonia NOS (J18.9)
AHA: 2016, 3Q, 15; 2013, 4Q, 118

J16.0 Chlamydial **pneumonia**

J16.8 **Pneumonia due to other** specified infectious organisms

J17 *Pneumonia in diseases classified elsewhere*
Code first underlying disease, such as:
Q fever (A78)
rheumatic fever (I00)
schistosomiasis (B65.0-B65.9)
EXCLUDES 1 candidial pneumonia (B37.1)
chlamydial pneumonia (J16.0)
gonorrheal pneumonia (A54.84)
histoplasmosis pneumonia (B39.0-B39.2)
measles pneumonia (B05.2)
nocardiosis pneumonia (A43.0)
pneumocystosis (B59)
pneumonia due to Pneumocystis carinii (B59)
pneumonia due to Pneumocystis jiroveci (B59)
pneumonia in actinomycosis (A42.0)
pneumonia in anthrax (A22.1)
pneumonia in ascariasis (B77.81)
pneumonia in aspergillosis (B44.0-B44.1)
pneumonia in coccidioidomycosis (B38.0-B38.2)
pneumonia in cytomegalovirus disease (B25.0)
pneumonia in toxoplasmosis (B58.3)
rubella pneumonia (B06.81)
salmonella pneumonia (A02.22)
spirochetal infection NEC with pneumonia (A69.8)
tularemia pneumonia (A21.2)
typhoid fever with pneumonia (A01.03)
varicella pneumonia (B01.2)
whooping cough with pneumonia (A37 with fifth-character 1)
AHA: 2016, 3Q, 15; 2013, 4Q, 118

☑ Additional Character Req ✓ₓ7ᵗʰ Placeholder Alert Manifestation HCC CMS-HCC Condition ▽ Unspecified Code ►◄ Revised Text ● New Code ▲ Revised Code Title

Chapter 10. Diseases of the Respiratory System

J18–J32.2

✓4ᵗʰ J18   Pneumonia, unspecified organism

Code first associated influenza, if applicable (J09.X1, J10.0-, J11.0-)

EXCLUDES 1   abscess of lung with pneumonia (J85.1)
aspiration pneumonia due to anesthesia during labor and delivery (O74.0)
aspiration pneumonia due to anesthesia during pregnancy (O29)
aspiration pneumonia due to anesthesia during puerperium (O89.0)
aspiration pneumonia due to solids and liquids (J69.-)
aspiration pneumonia NOS (J69.0)
congenital pneumonia (P23.0)
drug-induced interstitial lung disorder (J70.2-J70.4)
interstitial pneumonia NOS (J84.9)
lipid pneumonia (J69.1)
neonatal aspiration pneumonia (P24.-)
pneumonitis due to external agents (J67-J70)
pneumonitis due to fumes and vapors (J68.0)
usual interstitial pneumonia (J84.17)

AHA: 2016, 3Q, 15; 2013, 4Q, 118

J18.0   Bronchopneumonia, unspecified organism   ▽

EXCLUDES 1   hypostatic bronchopneumonia (J18.2)
lipid pneumonia (J69.1)

EXCLUDES 2   acute bronchiolitis (J21.-)
chronic bronchiolitis (J44.9)

J18.1   Lobar pneumonia, unspecified organism   HCC ▽

J18.2   Hypostatic pneumonia, unspecified organism   ▽
Hypostatic bronchopneumonia
Passive pneumonia

J18.8   Other pneumonia, unspecified organism   ▽

J18.9   Pneumonia, unspecified organism   ▽
AHA: 2014, 3Q, 4; 2013, 4Q, 119; 2012, 4Q, 94

Other acute lower respiratory infections (J20-J22)

EXCLUDES 2   chronic obstructive pulmonary disease with acute lower respiratory infection (J44.0)

✓4ᵗʰ J20   Acute bronchitis

INCLUDES   acute and subacute bronchitis (with) bronchospasm
acute and subacute bronchitis (with) tracheitis
acute and subacute bronchitis (with) tracheobronchitis, acute
acute and subacute fibrinous bronchitis
acute and subacute membranous bronchitis
acute and subacute purulent bronchitis
acute and subacute septic bronchitis

EXCLUDES 1   bronchitis NOS (J40)
tracheobronchitis NOS (J40)

EXCLUDES 2   acute bronchitis with bronchiectasis (J47.0)
acute bronchitis with chronic obstructive asthma (J44.0)
acute bronchitis with chronic obstructive pulmonary disease (J44.0)
allergic bronchitis NOS (J45.909)
bronchitis due to chemicals, fumes and vapors (J68.0)
chronic bronchitis NOS (J42)
chronic mucopurulent bronchitis (J41.1)
chronic obstructive bronchitis (J44.-)
chronic obstructive tracheobronchitis (J44.-)
chronic simple bronchitis (J41.0)
chronic tracheobronchitis (J42)

AHA: 2016, 3Q, 10, 16

DEF: Acute inflammation of main branches of bronchial tree due to infectious or irritant agents; symptoms include cough with a varied production of sputum, fever, substernal soreness, and lung rales; usually last for three to 10 days.

J20.0   Acute bronchitis due to Mycoplasma pneumoniae

J20.1   Acute bronchitis due to Hemophilus influenzae

J20.2   Acute bronchitis due to streptococcus

J20.3   Acute bronchitis due to coxsackievirus

J20.4   Acute bronchitis due to parainfluenza virus

J20.5   Acute bronchitis due to respiratory syncytial virus

J20.6   Acute bronchitis due to rhinovirus

J20.7   Acute bronchitis due to echovirus

J20.8   Acute bronchitis due to other specified organisms

J20.9   Acute bronchitis, unspecified   ▽

✓4ᵗʰ J21   Acute bronchiolitis

Acute bronchiolitis with bronchospasm

EXCLUDES 2   respiratory bronchiolitis interstitial lung disease (J84.115)

J21.0   Acute bronchiolitis due to respiratory syncytial virus

J21.1   Acute bronchiolitis due to human metapneumovirus

J21.8   Acute bronchiolitis due to other specified organisms

J21.9   Acute bronchiolitis, unspecified   ▽
Bronchiolitis (acute)

EXCLUDES 1   chronic bronchiolitis (J44.-)

J22   Unspecified acute lower respiratory infection   ▽
Acute (lower) respiratory (tract) infection NOS

EXCLUDES 1   upper respiratory infection (acute) (J06.9)

Other diseases of upper respiratory tract (J30-J39)

✓4ᵗʰ J30   Vasomotor and allergic rhinitis

INCLUDES   spasmodic rhinorrhea

EXCLUDES 1   allergic rhinitis with asthma (bronchial) (J45.909)
rhinitis NOS (J31.0)

J30.0   Vasomotor rhinitis

J30.1   Allergic rhinitis due to pollen
Allergy NOS due to pollen
Hay fever
Pollinosis

J30.2   Other seasonal allergic rhinitis

J30.5   Allergic rhinitis due to food

✓5ᵗʰ **J30.8   Other allergic rhinitis**

J30.81   Allergic rhinitis due to animal (cat) (dog) hair and dander

J30.89   Other allergic rhinitis
Perennial allergic rhinitis

J30.9   Allergic rhinitis, unspecified   ▽

✓4ᵗʰ J31   Chronic rhinitis, nasopharyngitis and pharyngitis

Use additional code to identify:
exposure to environmental tobacco smoke (Z77.22)
exposure to tobacco smoke in the perinatal period (P96.81)
history of tobacco dependence (Z87.891)
occupational exposure to environmental tobacco smoke (Z57.31)
tobacco dependence (F17.-)
tobacco use (Z72.0)

J31.0   Chronic rhinitis
Atrophic rhinitis (chronic)
Granulomatous rhinitis (chronic)
Hypertrophic rhinitis (chronic)
Obstructive rhinitis (chronic)
Ozena
Purulent rhinitis (chronic)
Rhinitis (chronic) NOS
Ulcerative rhinitis (chronic)

EXCLUDES 1   allergic rhinitis (J30.1-J30.9)
vasomotor rhinitis (J30.0)

DEF: Persistent inflammation of mucous membranes of nose; characterized by postnasal drip.

J31.1   Chronic nasopharyngitis

EXCLUDES 2   acute nasopharyngitis (J00)

DEF: Persistent inflammation of mucous membranes extending from nares to pharynx; characterized by constant irritation in nasopharynx and postnasal drip.

J31.2   Chronic pharyngitis
Atrophic pharyngitis (chronic)
Chronic sore throat
Granular pharyngitis (chronic)
Hypertrophic pharyngitis (chronic)

EXCLUDES 2   acute pharyngitis (J02.9)

✓4ᵗʰ J32   Chronic sinusitis

INCLUDES   sinus abscess
sinus empyema
sinus infection
sinus suppuration

Use additional code to identify:
exposure to environmental tobacco smoke (Z77.22)
exposure to tobacco smoke in the perinatal period (P96.81)
history of tobacco dependence (Z87.891)
infectious agent (B95-B97)
occupational exposure to environmental tobacco smoke (Z57.31)
tobacco dependence (F17.-)
tobacco use (Z72.0)

EXCLUDES 2   acute sinusitis (J01.-)

J32.0   Chronic maxillary sinusitis
Antritis (chronic)
Maxillary sinusitis NOS

J32.1   Chronic frontal sinusitis
Frontal sinusitis NOS

J32.2   Chronic ethmoidal sinusitis
Ethmoidal sinusitis NOS

EXCLUDES 1   Woakes' ethmoiditis (J33.1)

EXCLUDES 1 Not coded here   EXCLUDES 2 Not included here   N Newborn Age: 0   P Pediatric Age: 0-17   M Maternity Age: 12-55   A Adult Age: 15-124

662   ICD-10-CM 2018

J32.3   **Chronic** sphenoidal **sinusitis**
     Sphenoidal sinusitis NOS

J32.4   **Chronic** pansinusitis
     Pansinusitis NOS

J32.8   **Other chronic sinusitis**
     Sinusitis (chronic) involving more than one sinus but not pansinusitis

J32.9   **Chronic sinusitis, unspecified**   ▽
     Sinusitis (chronic) NOS

✓4ᵗʰ **J33**   **Nasal polyp**
Use additional code to identify:
     exposure to environmental tobacco smoke (Z77.22)
     exposure to tobacco smoke in the perinatal period (P96.81)
     history of tobacco dependence (Z87.891)
     occupational exposure to environmental tobacco smoke (Z57.31)
     tobacco dependence (F17.-)
     tobacco use (Z72.0)
   EXCLUDES 1   *adenomatous polyps (D14.0)*

J33.0   **Polyp of nasal cavity**
     Choanal polyp
     Nasopharyngeal polyp

J33.1   **Polypoid sinus degeneration**
     Woakes' syndrome or ethmoiditis

J33.8   **Other polyp of sinus**
     Accessory polyp of sinus
     Ethmoidal polyp of sinus
     Maxillary polyp of sinus
     Sphenoidal polyp of sinus

J33.9   **Nasal polyp, unspecified**   ▽

✓4ᵗʰ **J34**   **Other and unspecified disorders of nose and nasal sinuses**
   EXCLUDES 2   *varicose ulcer of nasal septum (I86.8)*

J34.0   **Abscess, furuncle and carbuncle of nose**
     Cellulitis of nose
     Necrosis of nose
     Ulceration of nose

J34.1   **Cyst and mucocele of nose and nasal sinus**

J34.2   **Deviated nasal septum**
     Deflection or deviation of septum (nasal) (acquired)
     EXCLUDES 1   *congenital deviated nasal septum (Q67.4)*

J34.3   **Hypertrophy of nasal turbinates**

✓5ᵗʰ **J34.8**   **Other specified disorders of nose and nasal sinuses**

J34.81   **Nasal mucositis (ulcerative)**
     Code also type of associated therapy, such as:
       antineoplastic and immunosuppressive drugs (T45.1X-)
       radiological procedure and radiotherapy (Y84.2)
     EXCLUDES 2   *gastrointestinal mucositis (ulcerative) (K92.81)*
         mucositis (ulcerative) of vagina and vulva (N76.81)
         oral mucositis (ulcerative) (K12.3-)

J34.89   **Other specified disorders of nose and nasal sinuses**
     Perforation of nasal septum NOS
     Rhinolith

J34.9   **Unspecified disorder of nose and nasal sinuses**   ▽

✓4ᵗʰ **J35**   **Chronic diseases of tonsils and adenoids**
Use additional code to identify:
     exposure to environmental tobacco smoke (Z77.22)
     exposure to tobacco smoke in the perinatal period (P96.81)
     history of tobacco dependence (Z87.891)
     occupational exposure to environmental tobacco smoke (Z57.31)
     tobacco dependence (F17.-)
     tobacco use (Z72.0)

✓5ᵗʰ **J35.0**   **Chronic tonsillitis and adenoiditis**
     EXCLUDES 2   *acute tonsillitis (J03.-)*

J35.01   **Chronic** tonsillitis

J35.02   **Chronic** adenoiditis

J35.03   **Chronic** tonsillitis and adenoiditis

J35.1   **Hypertrophy of** tonsils
     Enlargement of tonsils
     EXCLUDES 1   *hypertrophy of tonsils with tonsillitis (J35.0-)*

J35.2   **Hypertrophy of** adenoids
     Enlargement of adenoids
     EXCLUDES 1   *hypertrophy of adenoids with adenoiditis (J35.0-)*

J35.3   **Hypertrophy of** tonsils with hypertrophy of adenoids
     EXCLUDES 1   *hypertrophy of tonsils and adenoids with tonsillitis and adenoiditis (J35.03)*

J35.8   **Other chronic diseases of tonsils and adenoids**
     Adenoid vegetations
     Amygdalolith
     Calculus, tonsil
     Cicatrix of tonsil (and adenoid)
     Tonsillar tag
     Ulcer of tonsil

J35.9   **Chronic disease of tonsils and adenoids, unspecified**   ▽
     Disease (chronic) of tonsils and adenoids NOS

J36   **Peritonsillar abscess**
   INCLUDES   abscess of tonsil
         peritonsillar cellulitis
         quinsy
Use additional code (B95-B97) to identify infectious agent
   EXCLUDES 1   *acute tonsillitis (J03.-)*
         chronic tonsillitis (J35.0)
         retropharyngeal abscess (J39.0)
         tonsillitis NOS (J03.9-)

✓4ᵗʰ **J37**   **Chronic laryngitis and laryngotracheitis**
Use additional code to identify:
     exposure to environmental tobacco smoke (Z77.22)
     exposure to tobacco smoke in the perinatal period (P96.81)
     history of tobacco dependence (Z87.891)
     infectious agent (B95-B97)
     occupational exposure to environmental tobacco smoke (Z57.31)
     tobacco dependence (F17.-)
     tobacco use (Z72.0)

J37.0   **Chronic** laryngitis
     Catarrhal laryngitis
     Hypertrophic laryngitis
     Sicca laryngitis
     EXCLUDES 2   *acute laryngitis (J04.0)*
         obstructive (acute) laryngitis (J05.0)

J37.1   **Chronic** laryngotracheitis
     Laryngitis, chronic, with tracheitis (chronic)
     Tracheitis, chronic, with laryngitis
     EXCLUDES 1   *chronic tracheitis (J42)*
     EXCLUDES 2   *acute laryngotracheitis (J04.2)*
         acute tracheitis (J04.1)

✓4ᵗʰ **J38**   **Diseases of vocal cords and larynx, not elsewhere classified**
Use additional code to identify:
     exposure to environmental tobacco smoke (Z77.22)
     exposure to tobacco smoke in the perinatal period (P96.81)
     history of tobacco dependence (Z87.891)
     occupational exposure to environmental tobacco smoke (Z57.31)
     tobacco dependence (F17.-)
     tobacco use (Z72.0)
   EXCLUDES 1   *congenital laryngeal stridor (P28.89)*
         obstructive laryngitis (acute) (J05.0)
         postprocedural subglottic stenosis (J95.5)
         stridor (R06.1)
         ulcerative laryngitis (J04.0)

✓5ᵗʰ **J38.0**   **Paralysis of vocal cords and larynx**
     Laryngoplegia
     Paralysis of glottis

J38.00   **Paralysis of vocal cords and larynx, unspecified**   ▽

J38.01   **Paralysis of vocal cords and larynx,** unilateral

J38.02   **Paralysis of vocal cords and larynx,** bilateral

J38.1   **Polyp of vocal cord and larynx**
     EXCLUDES 1   *adenomatous polyps (D14.1)*

J38.2   **Nodules of vocal cords**
     Chorditis (fibrinous)(nodosa)(tuberosa)
     Singer's nodes
     Teacher's nodes

J38.3   **Other diseases of vocal cords**
     Abscess of vocal cords
     Cellulitis of vocal cords
     Granuloma of vocal cords
     Leukokeratosis of vocal cords
     Leukoplakia of vocal cords

J38.4   **Edema of larynx**
     Edema (of) glottis
     Subglottic edema
     Supraglottic edema
     EXCLUDES 1   *acute obstructive laryngitis [croup] (J05.0)*
         edematous laryngitis (J04.0)

J38.5   **Laryngeal** spasm
     Laryngismus (stridulus)

J38.6   **Stenosis of larynx**

☑ Additional Character Req   ✓x7ᵗʰ Placeholder Alert   Manifestation   HCC CMS-HCC Condition   ▽ Unspecified Code   ►◄ Revised Text   ● New Code   ▲ Revised Code Title

ICD-10-CM 2018   **663**

Chapter 10. Diseases of the Respiratory System

J38.7   **Other diseases of larynx**
Abscess of larynx
Cellulitis of larynx
Disease of larynx NOS
Necrosis of larynx
Pachyderma of larynx
Perichondritis of larynx
Ulcer of larynx

✓4ᵗʰ **J39**   **Other diseases of upper respiratory tract**
EXCLUDES 1   *acute respiratory infection NOS (J22)*
acute upper respiratory infection (J06.9)
upper respiratory inflammation due to chemicals, gases, fumes or vapors (J68.2)

J39.0   **Retropharyngeal and parapharyngeal abscess**
Peripharyngeal abscess
EXCLUDES 1   *peritonsillar abscess (J36)*
DEF: Purulent infection behind pharynx and front of precerebral fascia; characterized by neck stiffness, cervical lymphadenopathy, sore throat, fever, and stridor.

J39.1   **Other abscess of pharynx**
Cellulitis of pharynx
Nasopharyngeal abscess

J39.2   **Other diseases of pharynx**
Cyst of pharynx
Edema of pharynx
EXCLUDES 2   *chronic pharyngitis (J31.2)*
ulcerative pharyngitis (J02.9)

J39.3   **Upper respiratory tract hypersensitivity reaction, site unspecified**   ▽
EXCLUDES 1   *hypersensitivity reaction of upper respiratory tract, such as:*
extrinsic allergic alveolitis (J67.9)
pneumoconiosis (J60-J67.9)

J39.8   **Other specified diseases of upper respiratory tract**

J39.9   **Disease of upper respiratory tract, unspecified**   ▽

Chronic lower respiratory diseases (J40-J47)

EXCLUDES 1   *bronchitis due to chemicals, gases, fumes and vapors (J68.0)*
EXCLUDES 2   *cystic fibrosis (E84.-)*

J40   **Bronchitis, not specified as acute or chronic**   ▽
Bronchitis NOS
Bronchitis with tracheitis NOS
Catarrhal bronchitis
Tracheobronchitis NOS
Use additional code to identify:
    exposure to environmental tobacco smoke (Z77.22)
    exposure to tobacco smoke in the perinatal period (P96.81)
    history of tobacco dependence (Z87.891)
    occupational exposure to environmental tobacco smoke (Z57.31)
    tobacco dependence (F17.-)
    tobacco use (Z72.0)
EXCLUDES 1   *acute bronchitis (J20.-)*
allergic bronchitis NOS (J45.909)
asthmatic bronchitis NOS (J45.9-)
bronchitis due to chemicals, gases, fumes and vapors (J68.0)

✓4ᵗʰ **J41**   **Simple and mucopurulent chronic bronchitis**
Use additional code to identify:
    exposure to environmental tobacco smoke (Z77.22)
    exposure to tobacco smoke in the perinatal period (P96.81)
    history of tobacco dependence (Z87.891)
    occupational exposure to environmental tobacco smoke (Z57.31)
    tobacco dependence (F17.-)
    tobacco use (Z72.0)
EXCLUDES 1   *chronic bronchitis NOS (J42)*
chronic obstructive bronchitis (J44.-)

J41.0   **Simple chronic bronchitis**   HCC

J41.1   **Mucopurulent chronic bronchitis**   HCC

J41.8   **Mixed simple and mucopurulent chronic bronchitis**   HCC

Emphysema

Healthy alveoli   Alveoli w/ Emphysema

Patent bronchiole
Collapsed bronchiole
Well-vascularized
Dilated alveoli
Excess mucus
Alveolar membranes break down
Enlarged alveoli
Broken/fewer capillaries

J42   **Unspecified chronic bronchitis**   HCC ▽
Chronic bronchitis NOS
Chronic tracheitis
Chronic tracheobronchitis
Use additional code to identify:
    exposure to environmental tobacco smoke (Z77.22)
    exposure to tobacco smoke in the perinatal period (P96.81)
    history of tobacco dependence (Z87.891)
    occupational exposure to environmental tobacco smoke (Z57.31)
    tobacco dependence (F17.-)
    tobacco use (Z72.0)
EXCLUDES 1   *chronic asthmatic bronchitis (J44.-)*
chronic bronchitis with airways obstruction (J44.-)
chronic emphysematous bronchitis (J44.-)
chronic obstructive pulmonary disease NOS (J44.9)
simple and mucopurulent chronic bronchitis (J41.-)

✓4ᵗʰ **J43**   **Emphysema**
Use additional code to identify:
    exposure to environmental tobacco smoke (Z77.22)
    history of tobacco dependence (Z87.891)
    occupational exposure to environmental tobacco smoke (Z57.31)
    tobacco dependence (F17.-)
    tobacco use (Z72.0)
EXCLUDES 1   *compensatory emphysema (J98.3)*
emphysema due to inhalation of chemicals, gases, fumes or vapors (J68.4)
emphysema with chronic (obstructive) bronchitis (J44.-)
emphysematous (obstructive) bronchitis (J44.-)
interstitial emphysema (J98.2)
mediastinal emphysema (J98.2)
neonatal interstitial emphysema (P25.0)
surgical (subcutaneous) emphysema (T81.82)
traumatic subcutaneous emphysema (T79.7)

J43.0   **Unilateral pulmonary emphysema [MacLeod's syndrome]**   HCC
Swyer-James syndrome
Unilateral emphysema
Unilateral hyperlucent lung
Unilateral pulmonary artery functional hypoplasia
Unilateral transparency of lung

J43.1   **Panlobular emphysema**   HCC
Panacinar emphysema

J43.2   **Centrilobular emphysema**   HCC

J43.8   **Other emphysema**   HCC

J43.9   **Emphysema, unspecified**   HCC ▽
Bullous emphysema (lung)(pulmonary)
Emphysema (lung)(pulmonary) NOS
Emphysematous bleb
Vesicular emphysema (lung)(pulmonary)

EXCLUDES 1 Not coded here   *EXCLUDES 2* Not included here   N Newborn Age: 0   P Pediatric Age: 0-17   M Maternity Age: 12-55   A Adult Age: 15-124

664   ICD-10-CM 2018

✓4th J44   Other chronic obstructive pulmonary disease

INCLUDES   asthma with chronic obstructive pulmonary disease
chronic asthmatic (obstructive) bronchitis
chronic bronchitis with airways obstruction
chronic bronchitis with emphysema
chronic emphysematous bronchitis
chronic obstructive asthma
chronic obstructive bronchitis
chronic obstructive tracheobronchitis

Code also type of asthma, if applicable (J45.-)
Use additional code to identify:
   exposure to environmental tobacco smoke (Z77.22)
   history of tobacco dependence (Z87.891)
   occupational exposure to environmental tobacco smoke (Z57.31)
   tobacco dependence (F17.-)
   tobacco use (Z72.0)

EXCLUDES 1   *bronchiectasis (J47.-)*
   chronic bronchitis NOS (J42)
   chronic simple and mucopurulent bronchitis (J41.-)
   chronic tracheitis (J42)
   chronic tracheobronchitis (J42)
   emphysema without chronic bronchitis (J43.-)

EXCLUDES 2   ~~*lung diseases due to external agents (J60-J70)*~~

AHA: 2017, 1Q, 25-26; 2016, 3Q, 15-16; 2013, 4Q, 109

J44.0   Chronic obstructive pulmonary disease with acute lower **HCC** respiratory infection

   ►Code also to identify the infection◄
   ~~Use additional code to identify the infection~~
   AHA: 2017, 1Q, 24-25

J44.1   Chronic obstructive pulmonary disease with (acute) HCC exacerbation

   Decompensated COPD
   Decompensated COPD with (acute) exacerbation

   EXCLUDES 2   *chronic obstructive pulmonary disease [COPD] with acute bronchitis (J44.0)*
      ►*lung diseases due to external agents (J60-J70)*◄
   AHA: 2017, 1Q, 26; 2016, 1Q, 35

J44.9   Chronic obstructive pulmonary disease, unspecified HCC ▽
   Chronic obstructive airway disease NOS
   Chronic obstructive lung disease NOS

   EXCLUDES 2   ►*lung diseases due to external agents (J60-J70)*◄
   AHA: 2016, 1Q, 36; 2014, 4Q, 21; 2013, 4Q, 129

✓4th J45   Asthma

INCLUDES   allergic (predominantly) asthma
allergic bronchitis nos
allergic rhinitis with asthma
atopic asthma
extrinsic allergic asthma
hay fever with asthma
idiosyncratic asthma
intrinsic nonallergic asthma
nonallergic asthma

Use additional code to identify:
   exposure to environmental tobacco smoke (Z77.22)
   exposure to tobacco smoke in the perinatal period (P96.81)
   history of tobacco dependence (Z87.891)
   occupational exposure to environmental tobacco smoke (Z57.31)
   tobacco dependence (F17.-)
   tobacco use (Z72.0)

EXCLUDES 1   *detergent asthma (J69.8)*
   eosinophilic asthma (J82)
   ~~*lung diseases due to external agents (J60-J70)*~~
   miner's asthma (J60)
   wheezing NOS (R06.2)
   wood asthma (J67.8)

EXCLUDES 2   *asthma with chronic obstructive pulmonary disease (J44.9)*
   chronic asthmatic (obstructive) bronchitis (J44.9)
   chronic obstructive asthma (J44.9)

AHA: 2017, 1Q, 25-26; 2012, 4Q, 99
DEF: Status asthmaticus: Severe, intractable episode of asthma that is unresponsive to normal therapeutic measures.

✓5th J45.2   Mild intermittent **asthma**

J45.20   Mild intermittent asthma, uncomplicated
   Mild intermittent asthma NOS

J45.21   Mild intermittent asthma with (acute) exacerbation

J45.22   Mild intermittent asthma with status asthmaticus

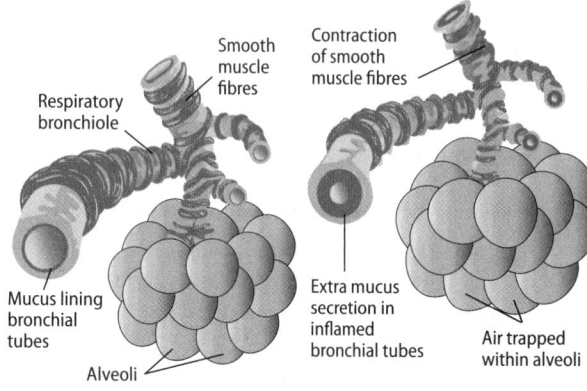

Asthma

Smooth muscle fibres
Contraction of smooth muscle fibres
Respiratory bronchiole
Mucus lining bronchial tubes
Extra mucus secretion in inflamed bronchial tubes
Air trapped within alveoli
Alveoli

Normal alveoli   Asthmatic alveoli

✓5th J45.3   Mild persistent **asthma**

J45.30   Mild persistent asthma, uncomplicated
   Mild persistent asthma NOS

J45.31   Mild persistent asthma with (acute) exacerbation
   AHA: 2016, 1Q, 35

J45.32   Mild persistent asthma with status asthmaticus

✓5th J45.4   Moderate persistent **asthma**

J45.40   Moderate persistent asthma, uncomplicated
   Moderate persistent asthma NOS

J45.41   Moderate persistent asthma with (acute) exacerbation
   AHA: 2017, 1Q, 26

J45.42   Moderate persistent asthma with status asthmaticus

✓5th J45.5   Severe persistent **asthma**

J45.50   Severe persistent asthma, uncomplicated
   Severe persistent asthma NOS

J45.51   Severe persistent asthma with (acute) exacerbation

J45.52   Severe persistent asthma with status asthmaticus

✓5th J45.9   Other and unspecified asthma

✓6th J45.90   Unspecified asthma
   Asthmatic bronchitis NOS
   Childhood asthma NOS
   Late onset asthma

J45.901   Unspecified asthma with (acute) ▽ exacerbation

J45.902   Unspecified asthma with status ▽ asthmaticus

J45.909   Unspecified asthma, uncomplicated ▽
   Asthma NOS
   EXCLUDES 2   ►*lung diseases due to external agents (J60-J70)*◄
   AHA: 2017, 1Q, 25

✓6th J45.99   Other asthma

J45.990   Exercise induced bronchospasm

J45.991   Cough variant asthma

J45.998   Other asthma

✓4th J47   Bronchiectasis

INCLUDES   bronchiolectasis

Use additional code to identify:
   exposure to environmental tobacco smoke (Z77.22)
   exposure to tobacco smoke in the perinatal period (P96.81)
   history of tobacco dependence (Z87.891)
   occupational exposure to environmental tobacco smoke (Z57.31)
   tobacco dependence (F17.-)
   tobacco use (Z72.0)

EXCLUDES 1   *congenital bronchiectasis (Q33.4)*
   tuberculous bronchiectasis (current disease) (A15.0)

J47.0   Bronchiectasis with acute lower respiratory infection **HCC**
   Bronchiectasis with acute bronchitis
   Use additional code to identify the infection

J47.1   Bronchiectasis with (acute) exacerbation **HCC**

J47.9   Bronchiectasis, uncomplicated **HCC ▽**
   Bronchiectasis NOS

✓ Additional Character Req   ✓x7th Placeholder Alert   Manifestation   **HCC** CMS-HCC Condition   ▽ Unspecified Code   ►◄ Revised Text   ● New Code   ▲ Revised Code Title

Lung diseases due to external agents (J60-J70)

EXCLUDES 2 *asthma (J45.-)*
malignant neoplasm of bronchus and lung (C34.-)

J60 Coalworker's pneumoconiosis [HCC] [A]
Anthracosilicosis
Anthracosis
Black lung disease
Coalworker's lung
EXCLUDES 1 *coalworker pneumoconiosis with tuberculosis, any type in A15 (J65)*

J61 Pneumoconiosis due to asbestos and other mineral fibers [HCC] [A]
Asbestosis
EXCLUDES 1 *pleural plaque with asbestosis (J92.0)*
pneumoconiosis with tuberculosis, any type in A15 (J65)

✓4ᵗʰ J62 Pneumoconiosis due to dust containing silica
INCLUDES silicotic fibrosis (massive) of lung
EXCLUDES 1 *pneumoconiosis with tuberculosis, any type in A15 (J65)*
   J62.0 Pneumoconiosis due to talc dust [HCC]
   J62.8 Pneumoconiosis due to other dust containing silica [HCC]
     Silicosis NOS

✓4ᵗʰ J63 Pneumoconiosis due to other inorganic dusts
EXCLUDES 1 *pneumoconiosis with tuberculosis, any type in A15 (J65)*
   J63.0 Aluminosis (of lung) [HCC]
   J63.1 Bauxite fibrosis (of lung) [HCC]
   J63.2 Berylliosis [HCC]
   J63.3 Graphite fibrosis (of lung) [HCC]
   J63.4 Siderosis [HCC]
   J63.5 Stannosis [HCC]
   J63.6 Pneumoconiosis due to other specified inorganic dusts [HCC]

J64 Unspecified pneumoconiosis [HCC] ▽
EXCLUDES 1 *pneumonoconiosis with tuberculosis, any type in A15 (J65)*

J65 Pneumoconiosis associated with tuberculosis [HCC]
Any condition in J60-J64 with tuberculosis, any type in A15
Silicotuberculosis

✓4ᵗʰ J66 Airway disease due to specific organic dust
EXCLUDES 2 *allergic alveolitis (J67.-)*
asbestosis (J61)
bagassosis (J67.1)
farmer's lung (J67.0)
hypersensitivity pneumonitis due to organic dust (J67.-)
reactive airways dysfunction syndrome (J68.3)
   J66.0 Byssinosis [HCC]
     Airway disease due to cotton dust
   J66.1 Flax-dressers' disease [HCC]
   J66.2 Cannabinosis [HCC]
   J66.8 Airway disease due to other specific organic dusts [HCC]

✓4ᵗʰ J67 Hypersensitivity pneumonitis due to organic dust
INCLUDES allergic alveolitis and pneumonitis due to inhaled organic dust and particles of fungal, actinomycetic or other origin
EXCLUDES 1 *pneumonitis due to inhalation of chemicals, gases, fumes or vapors (J68.0)*
   J67.0 Farmer's lung [HCC]
     Harvester's lung   Moldy hay disease
     Haymaker's lung
   J67.1 Bagassosis [HCC]
     Bagasse disease   Bagasse pneumonitis
   J67.2 Bird fancier's lung [HCC]
     Budgerigar fancier's disease or lung
     Pigeon fancier's disease or lung
   J67.3 Suberosis [HCC]
     Corkhandler's disease or lung
     Corkworker's disease or lung
   J67.4 Maltworker's lung [HCC]
     Alveolitis due to Aspergillus clavatus
   J67.5 Mushroom-worker's lung [HCC]
   J67.6 Maple-bark-stripper's lung [HCC]
     Alveolitis due to Cryptostroma corticale
     Cryptostromosis
   J67.7 Air conditioner and humidifier lung [HCC]
     Allergic alveolitis due to fungal, thermophilic actinomycetes and other organisms growing in ventilation [air conditioning] systems

   J67.8 Hypersensitivity pneumonitis due to other organic dusts [HCC]
     Cheese-washer's lung   Furrier's lung
     Coffee-worker's lung   Sequoiosis
     Fish-meal worker's lung
   J67.9 Hypersensitivity pneumonitis due to unspecified organic dust [HCC] ▽
     Allergic alveolitis (extrinsic) NOS
     Hypersensitivity pneumonitis NOS

✓4ᵗʰ J68 Respiratory conditions due to inhalation of chemicals, gases, fumes and vapors
Code first (T51-T65) to identify cause
Use additional code to identify associated respiratory conditions, such as:
acute respiratory failure (J96.0-)
   J68.0 Bronchitis and pneumonitis due to chemicals, gases, fumes and vapors [HCC]
     Chemical bronchitis (acute)
   J68.1 Pulmonary edema due to chemicals, gases, fumes and vapors [HCC]
     Chemical pulmonary edema (acute) (chronic)
     EXCLUDES 1 *pulmonary edema (acute) (chronic) NOS (J81.-)*
   J68.2 Upper respiratory inflammation due to chemicals, gases, fumes and vapors, not elsewhere classified [HCC]
   J68.3 Other acute and subacute respiratory conditions due to chemicals, gases, fumes and vapors [HCC]
     Reactive airways dysfunction syndrome
   J68.4 Chronic respiratory conditions due to chemicals, gases, fumes and vapors [HCC]
     Emphysema (diffuse) (chronic) due to inhalation of chemicals, gases, fumes and vapors
     Obliterative bronchiolitis (chronic) (subacute) due to inhalation of chemicals, gases, fumes and vapors
     Pulmonary fibrosis (chronic) due to inhalation of chemicals, gases, fumes and vapors
     EXCLUDES 1 *chronic pulmonary edema due to chemicals, gases, fumes and vapors (J68.1)*
   J68.8 Other respiratory conditions due to chemicals, gases, fumes and vapors [HCC]
   J68.9 Unspecified respiratory condition due to chemicals, gases, fumes and vapors [HCC] ▽

✓4ᵗʰ J69 Pneumonitis due to solids and liquids
EXCLUDES 1 *neonatal aspiration syndromes (P24.-)*
postprocedural pneumonitis (J95.4)
AHA: 2017, 1Q, 24
   J69.0 Pneumonitis due to inhalation of food and vomit [HCC]
     Aspiration pneumonia NOS
     Aspiration pneumonia (due to) food (regurgitated)
     Aspiration pneumonia (due to) gastric secretions
     Aspiration pneumonia (due to) milk
     Aspiration pneumonia (due to) vomit
     Code also any associated foreign body in respiratory tract (T17.-)
     EXCLUDES 1 *chemical pneumonitis due to anesthesia (J95.4)*
obstetric aspiration pneumonia (O74.0)
   J69.1 Pneumonitis due to inhalation of oils and essences [HCC]
     Exogenous lipoid pneumonia
     Lipid pneumonia NOS
     Code first (T51-T65) to identify substance
     EXCLUDES 1 *endogenous lipoid pneumonia (J84.89)*
   J69.8 Pneumonitis due to inhalation of other solids and liquids [HCC]
     Pneumonitis due to aspiration of blood
     Pneumonitis due to aspiration of detergent
     Code first (T51-T65) to identify substance

✓4ᵗʰ J70 Respiratory conditions due to other external agents
   J70.0 Acute pulmonary manifestations due to radiation [HCC]
     Radiation pneumonitis
     Use additional code (W88-W90, X39.0-) to identify the external cause
   J70.1 Chronic and other pulmonary manifestations due to radiation [HCC]
     Fibrosis of lung following radiation
     Use additional code (W88-W90, X39.0-) to identify the external cause
   J70.2 Acute drug-induced interstitial lung disorders [HCC]
     Use additional code for adverse effect, if applicable, to identify drug (T36-T50 with fifth or sixth character 5)
     EXCLUDES 1 *interstitial pneumonia NOS (J84.9)*
lymphoid interstitial pneumonia (J84.2)

EXCLUDES 1 Not coded here   **EXCLUDES 2** Not included here   N Newborn Age: 0   P Pediatric Age: 0-17   M Maternity Age: 12-55   A Adult Age: 15-124

666   ICD-10-CM 2018

J60–J70.2

J70.3   Chronic drug-induced interstitial **lung disorders**   HCC
    Use additional code for adverse effect, if applicable, to identify drug (T36-T50 with fifth or sixth character 5)
     EXCLUDES 1   *interstitial pneumonia NOS (J84.9)*
       lymphoid interstitial pneumonia (J84.2)

J70.4   **Drug-induced interstitial lung disorders, unspecified**   HCC ▽
    Use additional code for adverse effect, if applicable, to identify drug (T36-T50 with fifth or sixth character 5)
     EXCLUDES 1   *interstitial pneumonia NOS (J84.9)*
       lymphoid interstitial pneumonia (J84.2)

J70.5   **Respiratory conditions due to** smoke inhalation   HCC
    Smoke inhalation NOS
     EXCLUDES 1   *smoke inhalation due to chemicals, gases, fumes and vapors (J68.9)*
    AHA: 2013, 4Q, 121

J70.8   **Respiratory conditions due to other specified external agents**   HCC
    Code first (T51-T65) to identify the external agent

J70.9   **Respiratory conditions due to unspecified external agent**   HCC ▽
    Code first (T51-T65) to identify the external agent

Other respiratory diseases principally affecting the interstitium (J80-J84)

J80   **Acute respiratory distress syndrome**   HCC
    Acute respiratory distress syndrome in adult or child
    Adult hyaline membrane disease
     EXCLUDES 1   *respiratory distress syndrome in newborn (perinatal) (P22.0)*
    AHA: 2017, 1Q, 26

☑4th **J81**   **Pulmonary edema**
    Use additional code to identify:
     exposure to environmental tobacco smoke (Z77.22)
     history of tobacco dependence (Z87.891)
     occupational exposure to environmental tobacco smoke (Z57.31)
     tobacco dependence (F17.-)
     tobacco use (Z72.0)
     EXCLUDES 1   *chemical (acute) pulmonary edema (J68.1)*
       hypostatic pneumonia (J18.2)
       passive pneumonia (J18.2)
       pulmonary edema due to external agents (J60-J70)
       pulmonary edema with heart disease NOS (I50.1)
       pulmonary edema with heart failure (I50.1)

J81.0   Acute **pulmonary edema**   HCC
    Acute edema of lung

J81.1   Chronic **pulmonary edema**
    Pulmonary congestion (chronic) (passive)
    Pulmonary edema NOS

J82   **Pulmonary eosinophilia, not elsewhere classified**   HCC
    Allergic pneumonia   Löffler's pneumonia
    Eosinophilic asthma   Tropical (pulmonary)
    Eosinophilic pneumonia   eosinophilia NOS
     EXCLUDES 1   *pulmonary eosinophilia due to aspergillosis (B44.-)*
       pulmonary eosinophilia due to drugs (J70.2-J70.4)
       pulmonary eosinophilia due to specified parasitic infection (B50-B83)
       pulmonary eosinophilia due to systemic connective tissue disorders (M30-M36)
       pulmonary infiltrate NOS (R91.8)

☑4th **J84**   **Other** interstitial **pulmonary diseases**
     EXCLUDES 1   *drug-induced interstitial lung disorders (J70.2-J70.4)*
       interstitial emphysema (J98.2)
       ~~lung diseases due to external agents (J60-J70)~~
     EXCLUDES 2   ►*lung diseases due to external agents (J60-J70)*◄

☑5th **J84.0**   **Alveolar and parieto-alveolar conditions**

    J84.01   **Alveolar** proteinosis   HCC
       DEF: Reduced ventilation due to proteinaceous deposits on alveoli; symptoms include dyspnea, cough, chest pain, weakness, weight loss, and hemoptysis.

    J84.02   **Pulmonary alveolar** microlithiasis   HCC

    J84.03   *Idiopathic pulmonary* hemosiderosis   HCC
       Essential brown induration of lung
       Code first underlying disease, such as:
         disorders of iron metabolism (E83.1-)
         EXCLUDES 1   *acute idiopathic pulmonary hemorrhage in infants [AIPHI] (R04.81)*
       DEF: Fibrosis of alveolar walls; marked by abnormal accumulation of iron as hemosiderin in lungs; primarily affects children; symptoms include anemia, fluid in lungs, and blood in sputum; etiology unknown.

    J84.09   **Other alveolar and parieto-alveolar conditions**   HCC

☑5th **J84.1**   **Other interstitial pulmonary diseases with fibrosis**
     EXCLUDES 1   *pulmonary fibrosis (chronic) due to inhalation of chemicals, gases, fumes or vapors (J68.4)*
       pulmonary fibrosis (chronic) following radiation (J70.1)

    J84.10   **Pulmonary fibrosis, unspecified**   HCC ▽
       Capillary fibrosis of lung
       Cirrhosis of lung (chronic) NOS
       Fibrosis of lung (atrophic) (chronic) (confluent) (massive) (perialveolar) (peribronchial) NOS
       Induration of lung (chronic) NOS
       Postinflammatory pulmonary fibrosis

    ☑6th **J84.11**   **Idiopathic interstitial pneumonia**
       EXCLUDES 1   *lymphoid interstitial pneumonia (J84.2)*
         pneumocystis pneumonia (B59)

       J84.111   **Idiopathic interstitial** pneumonia, **not otherwise specified**   HCC ▽

       J84.112   **Idiopathic** pulmonary fibrosis   HCC
         Cryptogenic fibrosing alveolitis
         Idiopathic fibrosing alveolitis

       J84.113   **Idiopathic** non-specific interstitial **pneumonitis**   HCC
         EXCLUDES 1   *non-specific interstitial pneumonia NOS, or due to known underlying cause (J84.89)*

       J84.114   **Acute interstitial pneumonitis**   HCC
         Hamman-Rich syndrome
         EXCLUDES 1   *pneumocystis pneumonia (B59)*

       J84.115   Respiratory bronchiolitis interstitial **lung disease**   HCC

       J84.116   Cryptogenic organizing **pneumonia**   HCC
         EXCLUDES 1   *organizing pneumonia NOS, or due to known underlying cause (J84.89)*

       J84.117   Desquamative **interstitial pneumonia**   HCC

    J84.17   *Other interstitial pulmonary diseases with fibrosis*   HCC *in diseases classified elsewhere*
       Interstitial pneumonia (nonspecific) (usual) due to collagen vascular disease
       Interstitial pneumonia (nonspecific) (usual) in diseases classified elsewhere
       Organizing pneumonia due to collagen vascular disease
       Organizing pneumonia in diseases classified elsewhere
       Code first underlying disease, such as:
         progressive systemic sclerosis (M34.0)
         rheumatoid arthritis (M05.00-M06.9)
         systemic lupus erythematosis (M32.0-M32.9)

J84.2   Lymphoid **interstitial pneumonia**   HCC
    Lymphoid interstitial pneumonitis

☑5th **J84.8**   **Other specified interstitial pulmonary diseases**
     EXCLUDES 1   *exogenous lipoid pneumonia (J69.1)*
       unspecified lipoid pneumonia (J69.1)

    J84.81   **Lymphangioleiomyomatosis**   HCC ♀
       Lymphangiomyomatosis

    J84.82   **Adult pulmonary Langerhans cell histiocytosis** HCC A
       Adult PLCH

    J84.83   **Surfactant mutations of the lung**   HCC
       DEF: Genetic disorder resulting in insufficient secretion of a complex mixture of phospholipids and proteins that reduce surface tension in the alveoli following the onset of breathing to facilitate lung expansion in the newborn; leading indication for pediatric lung transplantation.

    ☑6th **J84.84**   **Other interstitial lung diseases of** childhood

       J84.841   **Neuroendocrine cell hyperplasia of infancy**   HCC

       J84.842   **Pulmonary interstitial glycogenosis**   HCC

       J84.843   **Alveolar capillary dysplasia with vein misalignment**   HCC

       J84.848   **Other interstitial lung diseases of childhood**   HCC

☑ Additional Character Req   ✓x7th Placeholder Alert   Manifestation   HCC CMS-HCC Condition   ▽ Unspecified Code   ►◄ Revised Text   ● New Code   ▲ Revised Code Title

J84.89   **Other specified interstitial pulmonary diseases** `HCC`
Endogenous lipoid pneumonia
Interstitial pneumonitis
Non-specific interstitial pneumonitis NOS
Organizing pneumonia NOS
Code first, if applicable:
   poisoning due to drug or toxin (T51-T65 with fifth or sixth character to indicate intent), for toxic pneumonopathy
   underlying cause of pneumonopathy, if known
Use additional code, for adverse effect, to identify drug (T36-T50 with fifth or sixth character 5), if drug-induced
   EXCLUDES 1   cryptogenic organizing pneumonia (J84.116)
       idiopathic non-specific interstitial pneumonitis (J84.113)
       lipoid pneumonia, exogenous or unspecified (J69.1)
       lymphoid interstitial pneumonia (J84.2)

J84.9   **Interstitial pulmonary disease, unspecified** `HCC` ▽
Interstitial pneumonia NOS

Suppurative and necrotic conditions of the lower respiratory tract (J85-J86)

✓4ᵗʰ **J85**   **Abscess of lung and mediastinum**
Use additional code (B95-B97) to identify infectious agent.

J85.0   **Gangrene and necrosis of lung** `HCC`

J85.1   **Abscess of lung with pneumonia** `HCC`
Code also the type of pneumonia

J85.2   **Abscess of lung without pneumonia** `HCC`
Abscess of lung NOS

J85.3   **Abscess of mediastinum** `HCC`

✓4ᵗʰ **J86**   **Pyothorax**
Use additional code (B95-B97) to identify infectious agent
   EXCLUDES 1   abscess of lung (J85.-)
       pyothorax due to tuberculosis (A15.6)

J86.0   **Pyothorax with fistula** `HCC`
Bronchocutaneous fistula
Bronchopleural fistula
Hepatopleural fistula
Mediastinal fistula
Pleural fistula
Thoracic fistula
Any condition classifiable to J86.9 with fistula
DEF: Purulent infection of respiratory cavity, with communication from cavity to another structure.

J86.9   **Pyothorax without fistula** `HCC`
Abscess of pleura   Pyopneumothorax
Abscess of thorax   Septic pleurisy
Empyema (chest) (lung) (pleura)   Seropurulent pleurisy
Fibrinopurulent pleurisy   Suppurative pleurisy
Purulent pleurisy

Other diseases of the pleura (J90-J94)

J90   **Pleural effusion, not elsewhere classified**
Encysted pleurisy
Pleural effusion NOS
Pleurisy with effusion (exudative) (serous)
   EXCLUDES 1   chylous (pleural) effusion (J94.0)
       malignant pleural effusion (J91.0))
       pleurisy NOS (R09.1)
       tuberculous pleural effusion (A15.6)

✓4ᵗʰ **J91**   **Pleural effusion in conditions classified elsewhere**
   EXCLUDES 2   pleural effusion in heart failure (I50.-)
       pleural effusion in systemic lupus erythematosus (M32.13)

J91.0   *Malignant pleural effusion*
Code first underlying neoplasm

J91.8   *Pleural effusion in other conditions classified elsewhere*
Code first underlying disease, such as:
   filariasis (B74.0-B74.9)
   influenza (J09.X2, J10.1, J11.1)
AHA: 2015, 2Q, 15

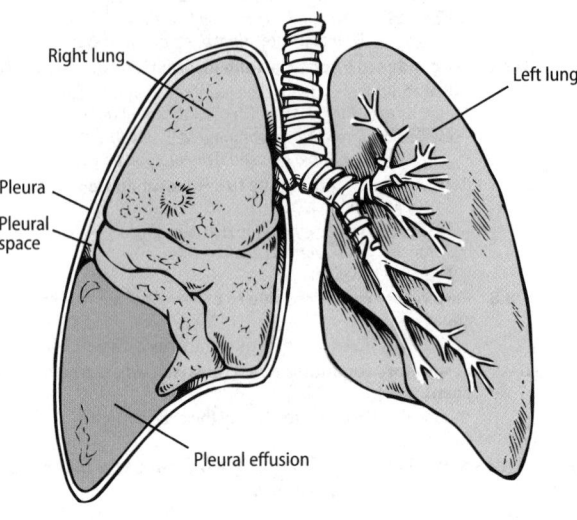

Pleural Effusion

Right lung
Left lung
Pleura
Pleural space
Pleural effusion

✓4ᵗʰ **J92**   **Pleural plaque**
   `INCLUDES`   pleural thickening

J92.0   **Pleural plaque with presence of asbestos**

J92.9   **Pleural plaque without asbestos**
Pleural plaque NOS

✓4ᵗʰ **J93**   **Pneumothorax and air leak**
   EXCLUDES 1   congenital or perinatal pneumothorax (P25.1)
       postprocedural air leak (J95.812)
       postprocedural pneumothorax (J95.811)
       traumatic pneumothorax (S27.0)
       tuberculous (current disease) pneumothorax (A15.-)
       pyopneumothorax (J86.-)

J93.0   **Spontaneous tension pneumothorax**
DEF: Leaking air from lung into lining, causing collapse.

✓5ᵗʰ **J93.1**   **Other spontaneous pneumothorax**

J93.11   **Primary spontaneous pneumothorax**

J93.12   **Secondary spontaneous pneumothorax**
Code first underlying condition, such as:
   catamenial pneumothorax due to endometriosis (N80.8)
   cystic fibrosis (E84.-)
   eosinophilic pneumonia (J82)
   lymphangioleiomyomatosis (J84.81)
   malignant neoplasm of bronchus and lung (C34.-)
   Marfan's syndrome (Q87.4)
   pneumonia due to Pneumocystis carinii (B59)
   secondary malignant neoplasm of lung (C78.0-)
   spontaneous rupture of the esophagus (K22.3)

✓5ᵗʰ **J93.8**   **Other pneumothorax and air leak**

J93.81   **Chronic pneumothorax**

J93.82   **Other air leak**
Persistent air leak

J93.83   **Other pneumothorax**
Acute pneumothorax
Spontaneous pneumothorax NOS

J93.9   **Pneumothorax, unspecified** ▽
Pneumothorax NOS

✓4ᵗʰ **J94**   **Other pleural conditions**
   EXCLUDES 1   pleurisy NOS (R09.1)
       traumatic hemopneumothorax (S27.2)
       traumatic hemothorax (S27.1)
       tuberculous pleural conditions (current disease) (A15.-)

J94.0   **Chylous effusion**
Chyliform effusion

J94.1   **Fibrothorax**

J94.2   **Hemothorax**
Hemopneumothorax

J94.8   **Other specified pleural conditions**
Hydropneumothorax
Hydrothorax

J94.9   **Pleural condition, unspecified** ▽

EXCLUDES 1 Not coded here   *EXCLUDES 2* Not included here   `N` Newborn Age: 0   `P` Pediatric Age: 0-17   `M` Maternity Age: 12-55   `A` Adult Age: 15-124

Tracheostomy

Tracheostomy
in place

Incision
in trachea

Tracheostomy
tube

Trachea

Intraoperative and postprocedural complications and disorders of respiratory system, not elsewhere classified (J95)

✓4ᵗʰ J95 Intraoperative and postprocedural complications and disorders of respiratory system, not elsewhere classified
  EXCLUDES 2 aspiration pneumonia (J69.-)
      emphysema (subcutaneous) resulting from a procedure
      (T81.82)
      hypostatic pneumonia (J18.2)
      pulmonary manifestations due to radiation (J70.0- J70.1)

✓5ᵗʰ J95.0 Tracheostomy complications
  J95.00 Unspecified tracheostomy complication HCC ▽
  J95.01 Hemorrhage from tracheostomy stoma HCC
  J95.02 Infection of tracheostomy stoma HCC
      Use additional code to identify type of infection, such as:
        cellulitis of neck ▶(L03.221)◀
        sepsis (A40, A41-)
  J95.03 Malfunction of tracheostomy stoma HCC
      Mechanical complication of tracheostomy stoma
      Obstruction of tracheostomy airway
      Tracheal stenosis due to tracheostomy
  J95.04 Tracheo-esophageal fistula following tracheostomy HCC
  J95.09 Other tracheostomy complication HCC

J95.1 Acute pulmonary insufficiency following thoracic surgery HCC
  EXCLUDES 2 functional disturbances following cardiac surgery
      (I97.0, I97.1-)
J95.2 Acute pulmonary insufficiency following nonthoracic surgery HCC
  EXCLUDES 2 functional disturbances following cardiac surgery
      (I97.0, I97.1-)
J95.3 Chronic pulmonary insufficiency following surgery HCC
  EXCLUDES 2 functional disturbances following cardiac surgery
      (I97.0, I97.1-)
J95.4 Chemical pneumonitis due to anesthesia
      Mendelson's syndrome
      Postprocedural aspiration pneumonia
      Use additional code for adverse effect, if applicable, to identify
      drug (T41.- with fifth or sixth character 5)
  EXCLUDES 1 aspiration pneumonitis due to anesthesia
        complicating labor and delivery (O74.0)
      aspiration pneumonitis due to anesthesia
        complicating pregnancy (O29)
      aspiration pneumonitis due to anesthesia
        complicating the puerperium (O89.01)
J95.5 Postprocedural subglottic stenosis

✓5ᵗʰ J95.6 Intraoperative hemorrhage and hematoma of a respiratory system organ or structure complicating a procedure
  EXCLUDES 1 intraoperative hemorrhage and hematoma of a
        respiratory system organ or structure due to
        accidental puncture and laceration during
        procedure (J95.7-)
  J95.61 Intraoperative hemorrhage and hematoma of a respiratory system organ or structure complicating a respiratory system procedure
  J95.62 Intraoperative hemorrhage and hematoma of a respiratory system organ or structure complicating other procedure

✓5ᵗʰ J95.7 Accidental puncture and laceration of a respiratory system organ or structure during a procedure
  EXCLUDES 2 postprocedural pneumothorax (J95.811)
  J95.71 Accidental puncture and laceration of a respiratory system organ or structure during a respiratory system procedure
  J95.72 Accidental puncture and laceration of a respiratory system organ or structure during other procedure

✓5ᵗʰ J95.8 Other intraoperative and postprocedural complications and disorders of respiratory system, not elsewhere classified
  ✓6ᵗʰ J95.81 Postprocedural pneumothorax and air leak
      J95.811 Postprocedural pneumothorax
      J95.812 Postprocedural air leak
  ✓6ᵗʰ J95.82 Postprocedural respiratory failure
      EXCLUDES 1 respiratory failure in other conditions (J96.-)
      J95.821 Acute postprocedural respiratory failure HCC
          Postprocedural respiratory failure NOS
      J95.822 Acute and chronic postprocedural respiratory failure HCC
  ✓6ᵗʰ J95.83 Postprocedural hemorrhage of a respiratory system organ or structure following a procedure
      J95.830 Postprocedural hemorrhage of a respiratory system organ or structure following a respiratory system procedure
      J95.831 Postprocedural hemorrhage of a respiratory system organ or structure following other procedure
  J95.84 Transfusion-related acute lung injury (TRALI)
      DEF: A relatively rare, but serious, pulmonary
      complication of blood transfusion, with acute
      respiratory distress, noncardiogenic pulmonary edema,
      cyanosis, hypoxemia, hypotension, fever, and chills.
  ✓6ᵗʰ J95.85 Complication of respirator [ventilator]
      J95.850 Mechanical complication of respirator HCC
          EXCLUDES 1 encounter for respirator
            [ventilator] dependence
            during power failure
            (Z99.12)
      J95.851 Ventilator associated pneumonia HCC
          Ventilator associated pneumonitis
          Use additional code to identify the
          organism, if known (B95.-, B96.-, B97.-)
          EXCLUDES 1 ventilator lung in newborn
            (P27.8)
          AHA: 2017, 1Q, 25
      J95.859 Other complication of respirator [ventilator] HCC
  ✓6ᵗʰ J95.86 Postprocedural hematoma and seroma of a respiratory system organ or structure following a procedure
      J95.860 Postprocedural hematoma of a respiratory system organ or structure following a respiratory system procedure
      J95.861 Postprocedural hematoma of a respiratory system organ or structure following other procedure
      J95.862 Postprocedural seroma of a respiratory system organ or structure following a respiratory system procedure
      J95.863 Postprocedural seroma of a respiratory system organ or structure following other procedure
  J95.88 Other intraoperative complications of respiratory system, not elsewhere classified

---

✔ Additional Character Req   ✓ˣ7ᵗʰ Placeholder Alert   Manifestation   HCC CMS-HCC Condition   ▽ Unspecified Code   ▶◀ Revised Text   ● New Code   ▲ Revised Code Title

J95.89   Other postprocedural complications and disorders of respiratory system, not elsewhere classified
Use additional code to identify disorder, such as:
aspiration pneumonia (J69.-)
bacterial or viral pneumonia (J12-J18)
EXCLUDES 2   acute pulmonary insufficiency following thoracic surgery (J95.1)
postprocedural subglottic stenosis (J95.5)

Other diseases of the respiratory system (J96-J99)

✓4th **J96   Respiratory failure, not elsewhere classified**
EXCLUDES 1   acute respiratory distress syndrome (J80)
cardiorespiratory failure (R09.2)
newborn respiratory distress syndrome (P22.0)
postprocedural respiratory failure (J95.82-)
respiratory arrest (R09.2)
respiratory arrest of newborn (P28.81)
respiratory failure of newborn (P28.5)

✓5th **J96.0   Acute respiratory failure**

J96.00   Acute respiratory failure, unspecified whether with hypoxia or hypercapnia   HCC ▽
AHA: 2016, 3Q, 14; 2013, 4Q, 121

J96.01   Acute respiratory failure with hypoxia   HCC

J96.02   Acute respiratory failure with hypercapnia   HCC

✓5th **J96.1   Chronic respiratory failure**

J96.10   Chronic respiratory failure, unspecified whether with hypoxia or hypercapnia   HCC ▽
AHA: 2016, 1Q, 38; 2015, 1Q, 21

J96.11   Chronic respiratory failure with hypoxia   HCC
AHA: 2013, 4Q, 129

J96.12   Chronic respiratory failure with hypercapnia   HCC

✓5th **J96.2   Acute and chronic respiratory failure**
Acute on chronic respiratory failure

J96.20   Acute and chronic respiratory failure, unspecified whether with hypoxia or hypercapnia   HCC ▽

J96.21   Acute and chronic respiratory failure with hypoxia   HCC

J96.22   Acute and chronic respiratory failure with hypercapnia   HCC

✓5th **J96.9   Respiratory failure, unspecified**

J96.90   Respiratory failure, unspecified, unspecified whether with hypoxia or hypercapnia   HCC ▽

J96.91   Respiratory failure, unspecified with hypoxia   HCC ▽

J96.92   Respiratory failure, unspecified with hypercapnia   HCC ▽

✓4th **J98   Other respiratory disorders**
Use additional code to identify:
exposure to environmental tobacco smoke (Z77.22)
exposure to tobacco smoke in the perinatal period (P96.81)
history of tobacco dependence (Z87.891)
occupational exposure to environmental tobacco smoke (Z57.31)
tobacco dependence (F17.-)
tobacco use (Z72.0)
EXCLUDES 1   newborn apnea (P28.4)
newborn sleep apnea (P28.3)
EXCLUDES 2   apnea NOS (R06.81)
sleep apnea (G47.3-)

✓5th **J98.0   Diseases of bronchus, not elsewhere classified**

J98.01   Acute bronchospasm
EXCLUDES 1   acute bronchiolitis with bronchospasm (J21.-)
acute bronchitis with bronchospasm (J20.-)
asthma (J45.-)
exercise induced bronchospasm (J45.990)

J98.09   Other diseases of bronchus, not elsewhere classified
Broncholithiasis
Calcification of bronchus
Stenosis of bronchus
Tracheobronchial collapse
Tracheobronchial dyskinesia
Ulcer of bronchus

✓5th **J98.1   Pulmonary collapse**
EXCLUDES 1   therapeutic collapse of lung status (Z98.3)

J98.11   Atelectasis
EXCLUDES 1   newborn atelectasis
tuberculous atelectasis (current disease) (A15)

J98.19   Other pulmonary collapse

J98.2   Interstitial emphysema   HCC
Mediastinal emphysema
EXCLUDES 1   emphysema NOS (J43.9)
emphysema in newborn (P25.0)
surgical emphysema (subcutaneous) (T81.82)
traumatic subcutaneous emphysema (T79.7)

J98.3   Compensatory emphysema   HCC
DEF: Distention of all or part of the lung caused by disease processes or surgical intervention that decreased volume in another part of the lung; overcompensation reaction to the loss of capacity in another part of the lung; occurs in association with pneumonias, pleural effusions, atelectasis, empyema, and pneumothorax.

J98.4   Other disorders of lung
Calcification of lung
Cystic lung disease (acquired)
Lung disease NOS
Pulmolithiasis
EXCLUDES 1   acute interstitial pneumonitis (J84.114)
pulmonary insufficiency following surgery (J95.1-J95.2)

✓5th **J98.5   Diseases of mediastinum, not elsewhere classified**
EXCLUDES 2   abscess of mediastinum (J85.3)

J98.51   Mediastinitis
Code first:
underlying condition, if applicable, such as postoperative mediastinitis (T81.-)

J98.59   Other diseases of mediastinum, not elsewhere classified
Fibrosis of mediastinum
Hernia of mediastinum
Retraction of mediastinum

J98.6   Disorders of diaphragm
Diaphragmatitis
Paralysis of diaphragm
Relaxation of diaphragm
EXCLUDES 1   congenital malformation of diaphragm NEC (Q79.1)
congenital diaphragmatic hernia (Q79.0)
EXCLUDES 2   diaphragmatic hernia (K44.-)

J98.8   Other specified respiratory disorders

J98.9   Respiratory disorder, unspecified   ▽
Respiratory disease (chronic) NOS

J99   *Respiratory disorders in diseases classified elsewhere*   HCC
Code first underlying disease, such as:
amyloidosis (E85.-)
ankylosing spondylitis (M45)
congenital syphilis (A50.5)
cryoglobulinemia (D89.1)
early congenital syphilis (A50.0)
schistosomiasis (B65.0-B65.9)
EXCLUDES 1   respiratory disorders in:
amebiasis (A06.5)
blastomycosis (B40.0-B40.2)
candidiasis (B37.1)
coccidioidomycosis (B38.0-B38.2)
cystic fibrosis with pulmonary manifestations (E84.0)
dermatomyositis (M33.01, M33.11)
histoplasmosis (B39.0-B39.2)
late syphilis (A52.72, A52.73)
polymyositis (M33.21)
sicca syndrome (M35.02)
systemic lupus erythematosus (M32.13)
systemic sclerosis (M34.81)
Wegener's granulomatosis (M31.30-M31.31)

Chapter 11. Diseases of the Digestive System (KØØ–K95)

Chapter Specific Coding Guidelines and Examples
Reserved for future guideline expansion.

Chapter 11. Diseases of the Digestive System

Chapter 11. Diseases of the Digestive System (K00-K95)

EXCLUDES 2   *certain conditions originating in the perinatal period (P04-P96)*
certain infectious and parasitic diseases (A00-B99)
complications of pregnancy, childbirth and the puerperium (O00-O9A)
congenital malformations, deformations and chromosomal abnormalities (Q00-Q99)
endocrine, nutritional and metabolic diseases (E00-E88)
injury, poisoning and certain other consequences of external causes (S00-T88)
neoplasms (C00-D49)
symptoms, signs and abnormal clinical and laboratory findings, not elsewhere classified (R00-R94)

This chapter contains the following blocks:

K00-K14	Diseases of oral cavity and salivary glands
K20-K31	Diseases of esophagus, stomach and duodenum
K35-K38	Diseases of appendix
K40-K46	Hernia
K50-K52	Noninfective enteritis and colitis
K55-K64	Other diseases of intestines
K65-K68	Diseases of peritoneum and retroperitoneum
K70-K77	Diseases of liver
K80-K87	Disorders of gallbladder, biliary tract and pancreas
K90-K95	Other diseases of the digestive system

Diseases of oral cavity and salivary glands (K00-K14)

✓4ᵗʰ K00   Disorders of tooth development and eruption
EXCLUDES 2   *embedded and impacted teeth (K01.-)*

K00.0   Anodontia
Hypodontia
Oligodontia
EXCLUDES 1   *acquired absence of teeth (K08.1-)*

K00.1   Supernumerary teeth
Distomolar
Fourth molar
Mesiodens
Paramolar
Supplementary teeth
EXCLUDES 2   *supernumerary roots (K00.2)*

K00.2   Abnormalities of size and form of teeth
Concrescence of teeth
Dens evaginatus
Dens in dente
Dens invaginatus
Enamel pearls
Fusion of teeth
Gemination of teeth
Macrodontia
Microdontia
Peg-shaped [conical] teeth
Supernumerary roots
Taurodontism
Tuberculum paramolare
EXCLUDES 1   *abnormalities of teeth due to congenital syphilis (A50.5)*
tuberculum Carabelli, which is regarded as a normal variation and should not be coded

K00.3   Mottled teeth
Dental fluorosis
Mottling of enamel
Nonfluoride enamel opacities
EXCLUDES 2   *deposits [accretions] on teeth (K03.6)*

K00.4   Disturbances in tooth formation
Aplasia and hypoplasia of cementum
Dilaceration of tooth
Enamel hypoplasia (neonatal) (postnatal) (prenatal)
Regional odontodysplasia
Turner's tooth
EXCLUDES 1   *Hutchinson's teeth and mulberry molars in congenital syphilis (A50.5)*
EXCLUDES 2   *mottled teeth (K00.3)*

K00.5   Hereditary disturbances in tooth structure, not elsewhere classified
Amelogenesis imperfecta
Dentinogenesis imperfecta
Odontogenesis imperfecta
Dentinal dysplasia
Shell teeth

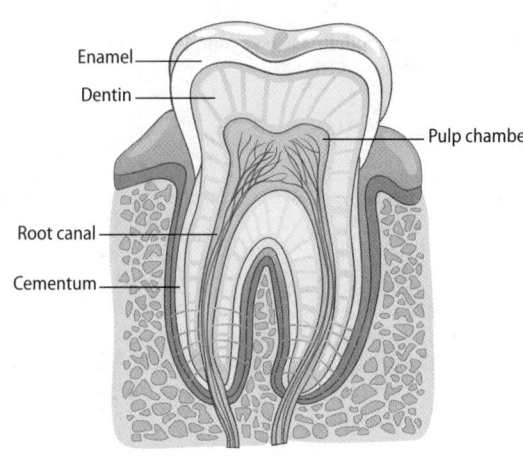

Tooth Anatomy

Enamel
Dentin
Pulp chamber
Root canal
Cementum

K00.6   Disturbances in tooth eruption
Dentia praecox
Natal tooth
Neonatal tooth
Premature eruption of tooth
Premature shedding of primary [deciduous] tooth
Prenatal teeth
Retained [persistent] primary tooth
EXCLUDES 2   *embedded and impacted teeth (K01.-)*

K00.7   Teething syndrome

K00.8   Other disorders of tooth development
Color changes during tooth formation
Intrinsic staining of teeth NOS
EXCLUDES 2   *posteruptive color changes (K03.7)*

K00.9   Disorder of tooth development, unspecified   ▽
Disorder of odontogenesis NOS

✓4ᵗʰ K01   Embedded and impacted teeth
EXCLUDES 1   *abnormal position of fully erupted teeth (M26.3-)*

K01.0   Embedded teeth

K01.1   Impacted teeth

✓4ᵗʰ K02   Dental caries
INCLUDES   caries of dentine
dental cavities
early childhood caries
pre-eruptive caries
recurrent caries (dentino enamel junction) (enamel) (to the pulp)
tooth decay

K02.3   Arrested dental caries
Arrested coronal and root caries

✓5ᵗʰ K02.5   Dental caries on pit and fissure surface
Dental caries on chewing surface of tooth

K02.51   Dental caries on pit and fissure surface limited to enamel
White spot lesions [initial caries] on pit and fissure surface of tooth

K02.52   Dental caries on pit and fissure surface penetrating into dentin
Primary dental caries, cervical origin)

K02.53   Dental caries on pit and fissure surface penetrating into pulp

✓5ᵗʰ K02.6   Dental caries on smooth surface

K02.61   Dental caries on smooth surface limited to enamel
White spot lesions [initial caries] on smooth surface of tooth

K02.62   Dental caries on smooth surface penetrating into dentin

K02.63   Dental caries on smooth surface penetrating into pulp

K02.7   Dental root caries

K02.9   Dental caries, unspecified   ▽

EXCLUDES 1   Not coded here   EXCLUDES 2   Not included here   N   Newborn Age: 0   P   Pediatric Age: 0-17   M   Maternity Age: 12-55   A   Adult Age: 15-124

672   ICD-10-CM 2018

K00-K02.9

✓4ᵗʰ **K03** **Other diseases of hard tissues of teeth**

     EXCLUDES 2   *bruxism (F45.8)*
         dental caries (K02.-)
         teeth-grinding NOS (F45.8)

     K03.0 **Excessive attrition of teeth**
         Approximal wear of teeth
         Occlusal wear of teeth

     K03.1 **Abrasion of teeth**
         Dentifrice abrasion of teeth
         Habitual abrasion of teeth
         Occupational abrasion of teeth
         Ritual abrasion of teeth
         Traditional abrasion of teeth
         Wedge defect NOS

     K03.2 **Erosion of teeth**
         Erosion of teeth due to diet
         Erosion of teeth due to drugs and medicaments
         Erosion of teeth due to persistent vomiting
         Erosion of teeth NOS
         Idiopathic erosion of teeth
         Occupational erosion of teeth

     K03.3 **Pathological resorption of teeth**
         Internal granuloma of pulp
         Resorption of teeth (external)

     K03.4 **Hypercementosis**
         Cementation hyperplasia

     K03.5 **Ankylosis of teeth**

     K03.6 **Deposits [accretions] on teeth**
         Betel deposits [accretions] on teeth
         Black deposits [accretions] on teeth
         Extrinsic staining of teeth NOS
         Green deposits [accretions] on teeth
         Materia alba deposits [accretions] on teeth
         Orange deposits [accretions] on teeth
         Staining of teeth NOS
         Subgingival dental calculus
         Supragingival dental calculus
         Tobacco deposits [accretions] on teeth

     K03.7 **Posteruptive color changes of dental hard tissues**
         EXCLUDES 2   *deposits [accretions] on teeth (K03.6)*

✓5ᵗʰ   **K03.8** **Other specified diseases of hard tissues of teeth**
     K03.81 **Cracked tooth**
         EXCLUDES 1   *asymptomatic craze lines in enamel—omit code*
             broken or fractured tooth due to trauma (S02.5)

     K03.89 **Other specified diseases of hard tissues of teeth**

     K03.9 **Disease of hard tissues of teeth, unspecified**   ▽

✓4ᵗʰ **K04** **Diseases of pulp and periapical tissues**

✓5ᵗʰ   **K04.0** **Pulpitis**
         Acute pulpitis
         Chronic (hyperplastic) (ulcerative) pulpitis

     K04.01 **Reversible pulpitis**

     K04.02 **Irreversible pulpitis**

     K04.1 **Necrosis of pulp**
         Pulpal gangrene

     K04.2 **Pulp degeneration**
         Denticles
         Pulpal calcifications
         Pulpal stones

     K04.3 **Abnormal hard tissue formation in pulp**
         Secondary or irregular dentine

     K04.4 **Acute apical periodontitis of pulpal origin**
         Acute apical periodontitis NOS
         EXCLUDES 1   *acute periodontitis (K05.2-)*
         DEF: Severe inflammation of the area surrounding the tip of a tooth's root; often secondary to infection or trauma.

     K04.5 **Chronic apical periodontitis**
         Apical or periapical granuloma
         Apical periodontitis NOS
         EXCLUDES 1   *chronic periodontitis (K05.3-)*

     K04.6 **Periapical abscess with sinus**
         Dental abscess with sinus
         Dentoalveolar abscess with sinus

     K04.7 **Periapical abscess without sinus**
         Dental abscess without sinus
         Dentoalveolar abscess without sinus
         ~~Periapical abscess without sinus~~

     K04.8 **Radicular cyst**
         Apical (periodontal) cyst
         Periapical cyst
         Residual radicular cyst
         EXCLUDES 2   *lateral periodontal cyst (K09.0)*
         DEF: Most common odontogenic cyst in tissue around tooth apex due to chronic inflammation of dental pulp.

✓5ᵗʰ   **K04.9** **Other and unspecified diseases of pulp and periapical tissues**
     K04.90 **Unspecified diseases of pulp and periapical tissues**   ▽

     K04.99 **Other diseases of pulp and periapical tissues**

✓4ᵗʰ **K05** **Gingivitis and periodontal diseases**
     Use additional code to identify:
     alcohol abuse and dependence (F10.-)
     exposure to environmental tobacco smoke (Z77.22)
     exposure to tobacco smoke in the perinatal period (P96.81)
     history of tobacco dependence (Z87.891)
     occupational exposure to environmental tobacco smoke (Z57.31)
     tobacco dependence (F17.-)
     tobacco use (Z72.0)

✓5ᵗʰ   **K05.0** **Acute gingivitis**
     EXCLUDES 1   *acute necrotizing ulcerative gingivitis (A69.1)*
         herpesviral [herpes simplex] gingivostomatitis (B00.2)

     K05.00 **Acute gingivitis, plaque induced**
         Acute gingivitis NOS
         Plaque induced gingival disease

     K05.01 **Acute gingivitis, non-plaque induced**

✓5ᵗʰ   **K05.1** **Chronic gingivitis**
         Desquamative gingivitis (chronic)
         Gingivitis (chronic) NOS
         Hyperplastic gingivitis (chronic)
         Pregnancy associated gingivitis
         Simple marginal gingivitis (chronic)
         Ulcerative gingivitis (chronic)
         Code first, if applicable, diseases of the digestive system complicating pregnancy (O99.61-)

     K05.10 **Chronic gingivitis, plaque induced**
         Chronic gingivitis NOS
         Gingivitis NOS

     K05.11 **Chronic gingivitis, non-plaque induced**

✓5ᵗʰ   **K05.2** **Aggressive periodontitis**
         Acute pericoronitis
     EXCLUDES 1   *acute apical periodontitis (K04.4)*
         periapical abscess (K04.7)
         periapical abscess with sinus (K04.6)

     K05.20 **Aggressive periodontitis, unspecified**   ▽

✓6ᵗʰ   **K05.21** **Aggressive periodontitis, localized**
         Periodontal abscess

     K05.211 **Aggressive periodontitis, localized, slight**

     K05.212 **Aggressive periodontitis, localized, moderate**

     K05.213 **Aggressive periodontitis, localized, severe**

     K05.219 **Aggressive periodontitis, localized, unspecified severity**   ▽

✓6ᵗʰ   **K05.22** **Aggressive periodontitis, generalized**

     K05.221 **Aggressive periodontitis, generalized, slight**

     K05.222 **Aggressive periodontitis, generalized, moderate**

     K05.223 **Aggressive periodontitis, generalized, severe**

     K05.229 **Aggressive periodontitis, generalized, unspecified severity**   ▽

✓5ᵗʰ   **K05.3** **Chronic periodontitis**
         Chronic pericoronitis
         Complex periodontitis
         Periodontitis NOS
         Simplex periodontitis
     EXCLUDES 1   *chronic apical periodontitis (K04.5)*

     K05.30 **Chronic periodontitis, unspecified**   ▽

✓6ᵗʰ   **K05.31** **Chronic periodontitis, localized**

     K05.311 **Chronic periodontitis, localized, slight**

     K05.312 **Chronic periodontitis, localized, moderate**

☑ Additional Character Req   ✓×7ᵗʰ Placeholder Alert   Manifestation   HCC CMS-HCC Condition   ▽ Unspecified Code   ►◄ Revised Text   ● New Code   ▲ Revised Code Title

ICD-10-CM 2018   673

      K05.313   **Chronic periodontitis, localized, severe**

      K05.319   **Chronic periodontitis, localized, unspecified severity** ▽

✓6ᵗʰ   **K05.32**   **Chronic periodontitis, generalized**

      K05.321   **Chronic periodontitis, generalized, slight**

      K05.322   **Chronic periodontitis, generalized, moderate**

      K05.323   **Chronic periodontitis, generalized, severe**

      K05.329   **Chronic periodontitis, generalized, unspecified severity** ▽

K05.4   **Periodontosis**
Juvenile periodontosis

K05.5   **Other periodontal diseases**
Combined periodontic-endodontic lesion
Narrow gingival width (of periodontal soft tissue)
  EXCLUDES 2   leukoplakia of gingiva (K13.21)

K05.6   **Periodontal disease, unspecified** ▽

✓4ᵗʰ   **K06**   **Other disorders of gingiva and edentulous alveolar ridge**
  EXCLUDES 2   acute gingivitis (K05.0)
      atrophy of edentulous alveolar ridge (K08.2)
      chronic gingivitis (K05.1)
      gingivitis NOS (K05.1)

✓5ᵗʰ   **K06.0**   **Gingival recession**
  ▶Gingival recession (postinfective) (postprocedural)◀

  ●   ✓6ᵗʰ   **K06.01**   **Gingival recession, localized**
  ●   K06.010   **Localized gingival recession, unspecified** ▽
          Localized gingival recession, NOS

  ●   K06.011   **Localized gingival recession, minimal**
  ●   K06.012   **Localized gingival recession, moderate**
  ●   K06.013   **Localized gingival recession, severe**

  ●   ✓6ᵗʰ   **K06.02**   **Gingival recession, generalized**
  ●   K06.020   **Generalized gingival recession, unspecified** ▽
          Generalized gingival recession, NOS

  ●   K06.021   **Generalized gingival recession, minimal**
  ●   K06.022   **Generalized gingival recession, moderate**
  ●   K06.023   **Generalized gingival recession, severe**

K06.1   **Gingival enlargement**
Gingival fibromatosis

K06.2   **Gingival and edentulous alveolar ridge lesions associated with trauma**
Irritative hyperplasia of edentulous ridge [denture hyperplasia]
Use additional code (Chapter 20) to identify external cause or denture status (Z97.2)

K06.3   **Horizontal alveolar bone loss**

K06.8   **Other specified disorders of gingiva and edentulous alveolar ridge**
Fibrous epulis
Flabby alveolar ridge
Giant cell epulis
Peripheral giant cell granuloma of gingiva
Pyogenic granuloma of gingiva
Vertical ridge deficiency
  EXCLUDES 2   gingival cyst (K09.0)

K06.9   **Disorder of gingiva and edentulous alveolar ridge, unspecified** ▽

✓4ᵗʰ   **K08**   **Other disorders of teeth and supporting structures**
  EXCLUDES 2   dentofacial anomalies [including malocclusion] (M26.-)
      disorders of jaw (M27.-)

K08.0   **Exfoliation of teeth due to systemic causes**
Code also underlying systemic condition

✓5ᵗʰ   **K08.1**   **Complete loss of teeth**
Acquired loss of teeth, complete
  EXCLUDES 1   congenital absence of teeth (K00.0)
      exfoliation of teeth due to systemic causes (K08.0)
      partial loss of teeth (K08.4-)

  ✓6ᵗʰ   **K08.10**   **Complete loss of teeth, unspecified cause**
      K08.101   **Complete loss of teeth, unspecified cause, class I** ▽
      K08.102   **Complete loss of teeth, unspecified cause, class II** ▽
      K08.103   **Complete loss of teeth, unspecified cause, class III** ▽

      K08.104   **Complete loss of teeth, unspecified cause, class IV** ▽
      K08.109   **Complete loss of teeth, unspecified cause, unspecified class** ▽
          Edentulism NOS

✓6ᵗʰ   **K08.11**   **Complete loss of teeth due to trauma**
      K08.111   **Complete loss of teeth due to trauma, class I**
      K08.112   **Complete loss of teeth due to trauma, class II**
      K08.113   **Complete loss of teeth due to trauma, class III**
      K08.114   **Complete loss of teeth due to trauma, class IV**
      K08.119   **Complete loss of teeth due to trauma, unspecified class** ▽

✓6ᵗʰ   **K08.12**   **Complete loss of teeth due to periodontal diseases**
      K08.121   **Complete loss of teeth due to periodontal diseases, class I**
      K08.122   **Complete loss of teeth due to periodontal diseases, class II**
      K08.123   **Complete loss of teeth due to periodontal diseases, class III**
      K08.124   **Complete loss of teeth due to periodontal diseases, class IV**
      K08.129   **Complete loss of teeth due to periodontal diseases, unspecified class** ▽

✓6ᵗʰ   **K08.13**   **Complete loss of teeth due to caries**
      K08.131   **Complete loss of teeth due to caries, class I**
      K08.132   **Complete loss of teeth due to caries, class II**
      K08.133   **Complete loss of teeth due to caries, class III**
      K08.134   **Complete loss of teeth due to caries, class IV**
      K08.139   **Complete loss of teeth due to caries, unspecified class** ▽

✓6ᵗʰ   **K08.19**   **Complete loss of teeth due to other specified cause**
      K08.191   **Complete loss of teeth due to other specified cause, class I**
      K08.192   **Complete loss of teeth due to other specified cause, class II**
      K08.193   **Complete loss of teeth due to other specified cause, class III**
      K08.194   **Complete loss of teeth due to other specified cause, class IV**
      K08.199   **Complete loss of teeth due to other specified cause, unspecified class** ▽

✓5ᵗʰ   **K08.2**   **Atrophy of edentulous alveolar ridge**
      K08.20   **Unspecified atrophy of edentulous alveolar ridge** ▽
          Atrophy of the mandible NOS
          Atrophy of the maxilla NOS

      K08.21   **Minimal atrophy of the mandible**
          Minimal atrophy of the edentulous mandible
      K08.22   **Moderate atrophy of the mandible**
          Moderate atrophy of the edentulous mandible
      K08.23   **Severe atrophy of the mandible**
          Severe atrophy of the edentulous mandible
      K08.24   **Minimal atrophy of maxilla**
          Minimal atrophy of the edentulous maxilla
      K08.25   **Moderate atrophy of the maxilla**
          Moderate atrophy of the edentulous maxilla
      K08.26   **Severe atrophy of the maxilla**
          Severe atrophy of the edentulous maxilla

K08.3   **Retained dental root**

✓5ᵗʰ   **K08.4**   **Partial loss of teeth**
Acquired loss of teeth, partial
  EXCLUDES 1   complete loss of teeth (K08.1-)
      congenital absence of teeth (K00.0)
  EXCLUDES 2   exfoliation of teeth due to systemic causes (K08.0)

  ✓6ᵗʰ   **K08.40**   **Partial loss of teeth, unspecified cause** ▽
      K08.401   **Partial loss of teeth, unspecified cause, class I** ▽
      K08.402   **Partial loss of teeth, unspecified cause, class II** ▽
      K08.403   **Partial loss of teeth, unspecified cause, class III** ▽

EXCLUDES 1 Not coded here   *EXCLUDES 2* Not included here   N Newborn Age: 0   P Pediatric Age: 0-17   M Maternity Age: 12-55   A Adult Age: 15-124

674   ICD-10-CM 2018

K08.404 Partial loss of teeth, unspecified cause, ▽
class IV

K08.409 Partial loss of teeth, unspecified ▽
cause, unspecified class
Tooth extraction status NOS

✓6ᵗʰ **K08.41 Partial loss of teeth due to** trauma
K08.411 Partial loss of teeth due to trauma, class I
K08.412 Partial loss of teeth due to trauma, class II
K08.413 Partial loss of teeth due to trauma, class III
K08.414 Partial loss of teeth due to trauma, class IV
K08.419 Partial loss of teeth due to trauma, ▽
unspecified class

✓6ᵗʰ **K08.42 Partial loss of teeth due to** periodontal diseases
K08.421 Partial loss of teeth due to periodontal
diseases, class I
K08.422 Partial loss of teeth due to periodontal
diseases, class II
K08.423 Partial loss of teeth due to periodontal
diseases, class III
K08.424 Partial loss of teeth due to periodontal
diseases, class IV
K08.429 Partial loss of teeth due to periodontal ▽
diseases, unspecified class

✓6ᵗʰ **K08.43 Partial loss of teeth due to** caries
K08.431 Partial loss of teeth due to caries, class I
K08.432 Partial loss of teeth due to caries, class II
K08.433 Partial loss of teeth due to caries, class III
K08.434 Partial loss of teeth due to caries, class IV
K08.439 Partial loss of teeth due to caries, ▽
unspecified class

✓6ᵗʰ **K08.49 Partial loss of teeth due to other specified cause**
K08.491 Partial loss of teeth due to other specified
cause, class I
K08.492 Partial loss of teeth due to other specified
cause, class II
K08.493 Partial loss of teeth due to other specified
cause, class III
K08.494 Partial loss of teeth due to other specified
cause, class IV
K08.499 Partial loss of teeth due to other ▽
specified cause, unspecified class

✓5ᵗʰ **K08.5 Unsatisfactory restoration of tooth**
Defective bridge, crown, filling
Defective dental restoration
EXCLUDES 1   dental restoration status (Z98.811)
EXCLUDES 2   endosseous dental implant failure (M27.6-)
unsatisfactory endodontic treatment (M27.5-)

K08.50 Unsatisfactory restoration of tooth, unspecified ▽
Defective dental restoration NOS

K08.51 Open restoration margins of tooth
Dental restoration failure of marginal integrity
Open margin on tooth restoration
Poor gingival margin to tooth restoration

K08.52 Unrepairable overhanging of dental restorative
materials
Overhanging of tooth restoration

✓6ᵗʰ **K08.53 Fractured dental restorative material**
EXCLUDES 1   cracked tooth (K03.81)
traumatic fracture of tooth (S02.5)
K08.530 Fractured dental restorative material
without loss of material
K08.531 Fractured dental restorative material with
loss of material
K08.539 Fractured dental restorative material, ▽
unspecified

K08.54 Contour of existing restoration of tooth biologically
incompatible with oral health
Dental restoration failure of periodontal anatomical
integrity
Unacceptable contours of existing restoration of tooth
Unacceptable morphology of existing restoration of
tooth

K08.55 Allergy to existing dental restorative material
Use additional code to identify the specific type of
allergy

K08.56 Poor aesthetic of existing restoration of tooth
Dental restoration aesthetically inadequate or
displeasing

K08.59 Other unsatisfactory restoration of tooth
Other defective dental restoration

✓5ᵗʰ **K08.8 Other specified disorders of teeth and supporting structures**
K08.81 Primary occlusal trauma
K08.82 Secondary occlusal trauma
K08.89 Other specified disorders of teeth and supporting
structures
Enlargement of alveolar ridge NOS
Insufficient anatomic crown height
Insufficient clinical crown length
Irregular alveolar process
Toothache NOS

K08.9 Disorder of teeth and supporting structures, unspecified ▽

✓4ᵗʰ **K09 Cysts of oral region, not elsewhere classified**
INCLUDES   lesions showing histological features both of aneurysmal cyst
and of another fibro-osseous lesion
EXCLUDES 2   cysts of jaw (M27.0-, M27.4-)
radicular cyst (K04.8)

K09.0 Developmental odontogenic cysts
Dentigerous cyst
Eruption cyst
Follicular cyst
Gingival cyst
Lateral periodontal cyst
Primordial cyst
EXCLUDES 2   keratocysts (D16.4, D16.5)
odontogenic keratocystic tumors (D16.4, D16.5)

K09.1 Developmental (nonodontogenic) cysts of oral region
Cyst (of) incisive canal
Cyst (of) palatine of papilla
Globulomaxillary cyst
Median palatal cyst
Nasoalveolar cyst
Nasolabial cyst
Nasopalatine duct cyst

K09.8 Other cysts of oral region, not elsewhere classified
Dermoid cyst
Epidermoid cyst
Lymphoepithelial cyst
Epstein's pearl

K09.9 Cyst of oral region, unspecified ▽

✓4ᵗʰ **K11 Diseases of salivary glands**
Use additional code to identify:
alcohol abuse and dependence (F10.-)
exposure to environmental tobacco smoke (Z77.22)
exposure to tobacco smoke in the perinatal period (P96.81)
history of tobacco dependence (Z87.891)
occupational exposure to environmental tobacco smoke (Z57.31)
tobacco dependence (F17.-)
tobacco use (Z72.0)

K11.0 Atrophy of salivary gland

K11.1 Hypertrophy of salivary gland
DEF: Overgrowth of or enlarged salivary gland tissue; caused by
infection, salivary duct blockage, autoimmune diseases, and
benign and malignant tumors.

✓5ᵗʰ **K11.2 Sialoadenitis**
Parotitis
EXCLUDES 1   epidemic parotitis (B26.-)
mumps (B26.-)
uveoparotid fever [Heerfordt] (D86.89)

K11.20 Sialoadenitis, unspecified ▽
K11.21 Acute sialoadenitis
EXCLUDES 1   acute recurrent sialoadenitis (K11.22)
K11.22 Acute recurrent sialoadenitis
K11.23 Chronic sialoadenitis

K11.3 Abscess of salivary gland

K11.4 Fistula of salivary gland
EXCLUDES 1   congenital fistula of salivary gland (Q38.4)

K11.5 Sialolithiasis
Calculus of salivary gland or duct
Stone of salivary gland or duct

K11.6 Mucocele of salivary gland
Mucous extravasation cyst of salivary gland
Mucous retention cyst of salivary gland
Ranula

☑ Additional Character Req   ✓•ᵀ• Placeholder Alert   Manifestation   HCC CMS-HCC Condition   ▽ Unspecified Code   ▶◀ Revised Text   ● New Code   ▲ Revised Code Title

Chapter 11. Diseases of the Digestive System

K11.7 Disturbances of salivary secretion
Hypoptyalism
Ptyalism
Xerostomia
EXCLUDES 2 dry mouth NOS (R68.2)

K11.8 Other diseases of salivary glands
Benign lymphoepithelial lesion of salivary gland
Mikulicz' disease
Necrotizing sialometaplasia
Sialectasia
Stenosis of salivary duct
Stricture of salivary duct
EXCLUDES 1 sicca syndrome [Sjögren] (M35.0-)

K11.9 Disease of salivary gland, unspecified ▽
Sialoadenopathy NOS

✓4th K12 Stomatitis and related lesions
Use additional code to identify:
alcohol abuse and dependence (F10.-)
exposure to environmental tobacco smoke (Z77.22)
exposure to tobacco smoke in the perinatal period (P96.81)
history of tobacco dependence (Z87.891)
occupational exposure to environmental tobacco smoke (Z57.31)
tobacco dependence (F17.-)
tobacco use (Z72.0)
EXCLUDES 1 cancrum oris (A69.0)
cheilitis (K13.0)
gangrenous stomatitis (A69.0)
herpesviral [herpes simplex] gingivostomatitis (B00.2)
noma (A69.0)

K12.0 Recurrent oral aphthae
Aphthous stomatitis (major) (minor)
Bednar's aphthae
Periadenitis mucosa necrotica recurrens
Recurrent aphthous ulcer
Stomatitis herpetiformis
DEF: Disorder of unknown etiology with small oval or round painful ulcers of the mouth marked by a grayish exudate and a red halo effect.

K12.1 Other forms of stomatitis
Stomatitis NOS   Ulcerative stomatitis
Denture stomatitis   Vesicular stomatitis
EXCLUDES 1 acute necrotizing ulcerative stomatitis (A69.1)
Vincent's stomatitis (A69.1)

K12.2 Cellulitis and abscess of mouth
Cellulitis of mouth (floor)
Submandibular abscess
EXCLUDES 2 abscess of salivary gland (K11.3)
abscess of tongue (K14.0)
periapical abscess (K04.6-K04.7)
periodontal abscess (K05.21)
peritonsillar abscess (J36)

✓5th K12.3 Oral mucositis (ulcerative)
Mucositis (oral) (oropharyneal)
EXCLUDES 2 gastrointestinal mucositis (ulcerative) (K92.81)
mucositis (ulcerative) of vagina and vulva (N76.81)
nasal mucositis (ulcerative) (J34.81)

K12.30 Oral mucositis (ulcerative), unspecified ▽

K12.31 Oral mucositis (ulcerative) due to antineoplastic therapy
Use additional code for adverse effect, if applicable, to identify antineoplastic and immunosuppressive drugs (T45.1X5)
Use additional code for other antineoplastic therapy, such as:
radiological procedure and radiotherapy (Y84.2)

K12.32 Oral mucositis (ulcerative) due to other drugs
Use additional code for adverse effect, if applicable, to identify drug (T36-T50 with fifth or sixth character 5)

K12.33 Oral mucositis (ulcerative) due to radiation
Use additional external cause code (W88-W90, X39.0-) to identify cause

K12.39 Other oral mucositis (ulcerative)
Viral oral mucositis (ulcerative)

✓4th K13 Other diseases of lip and oral mucosa
INCLUDES epithelial disturbances of tongue
Use additional code to identify:
alcohol abuse and dependence (F10.-)
exposure to environmental tobacco smoke (Z77.22)
exposure to tobacco smoke in the perinatal period (P96.81)
history of tobacco dependence (Z87.891)
occupational exposure to environmental tobacco smoke (Z57.31)
tobacco dependence (F17.-)
tobacco use (Z72.0)
EXCLUDES 2 certain disorders of gingiva and edentulous alveolar ridge (K05-K06)
cysts of oral region (K09.-)
diseases of tongue (K14.-)
stomatitis and related lesions (K12.-)

K13.0 Diseases of lips
Abscess of lips   Exfoliative cheilitis
Angular cheilitis   Fistula of lips
Cellulitis of lips   Glandular cheilitis
Cheilitis NOS   Hypertrophy of lips
Cheilodynia   Perlèche NEC
Cheilosis
EXCLUDES 1 ariboflavinosis (E53.0)
cheilitis due to radiation-related disorders (L55-L59)
congenital fistula of lips (Q38.0)
congenital hypertrophy of lips (Q18.6)
Perlèche due to candidiasis (B37.83)
Perlèche due to riboflavin deficiency (E53.0)

K13.1 Cheek and lip biting

✓5th K13.2 Leukoplakia and other disturbances of oral epithelium, including tongue
EXCLUDES 1 carcinoma in situ of oral epithelium (D00.0-)
hairy leukoplakia (K13.3)

K13.21 Leukoplakia of oral mucosa, including tongue
Leukokeratosis of oral mucosa
Leukoplakia of gingiva, lips, tongue
EXCLUDES 1 hairy leukoplakia (K13.3)
leukokeratosis nicotina palati (K13.24)

K13.22 Minimal keratinized residual ridge mucosa
Minimal keratinization of alveolar ridge mucosa

K13.23 Excessive keratinized residual ridge mucosa
Excessive keratinization of alveolar ridge mucosa

K13.24 Leukokeratosis nicotina palati
Smoker's palate

K13.29 Other disturbances of oral epithelium, including tongue
Erythroplakia of mouth or tongue
Focal epithelial hyperplasia of mouth or tongue
Leukoedema of mouth or tongue
Other oral epithelium disturbances

K13.3 Hairy leukoplakia

K13.4 Granuloma and granuloma-like lesions of oral mucosa
Eosinophilic granuloma
Granuloma pyogenicum
Verrucous xanthoma

K13.5 Oral submucous fibrosis
Submucous fibrosis of tongue

K13.6 Irritative hyperplasia of oral mucosa
EXCLUDES 2 irritative hyperplasia of edentulous ridge [denture hyperplasia] (K06.2)

✓5th K13.7 Other and unspecified lesions of oral mucosa ▽

K13.70 Unspecified lesions of oral mucosa

K13.79 Other lesions of oral mucosa
Focal oral mucinosis

EXCLUDES 1 Not coded here   EXCLUDES 2 Not included here   N Newborn Age: 0   P Pediatric Age: 0-17   M Maternity Age: 12-55   A Adult Age: 15-124

676   ICD-10-CM 2018

Chapter 11. Diseases of the Digestive System

✓4th **K14** **Diseases of tongue**

Use additional code to identify:
    alcohol abuse and dependence (F10.-)
    exposure to environmental tobacco smoke (Z77.22)
    history of tobacco dependence (Z87.891)
    occupational exposure to environmental tobacco smoke (Z57.31)
    tobacco dependence (F17.-)
    tobacco use (Z72.0)
    EXCLUDES 2   *erythroplakia (K13.29)*
             focal epithelial hyperplasia (K13.29)
             leukedema of tongue (K13.29)
             leukoplakia of tongue (K13.21)
             hairy leukoplakia (K13.3)
             macroglossia (congenital) (Q38.2)
             submucous fibrosis of tongue (K13.5)

K14.0 **Glossitis**
    Abscess of tongue
    Ulceration (traumatic) of tongue
    EXCLUDES 1   *atrophic glossitis (K14.4)*

K14.1 **Geographic tongue**
    Benign migratory glossitis
    Glossitis areata exfoliativa

K14.2 **Median rhomboid glossitis**

K14.3 **Hypertrophy of tongue papillae**
    Black hairy tongue
    Coated tongue
    Hypertrophy of foliate papillae
    Lingua villosa nigra

K14.4 **Atrophy of tongue papillae**
    Atrophic glossitis

K14.5 **Plicated tongue**
    Fissured tongue
    Furrowed tongue
    Scrotal tongue
    EXCLUDES 1   *fissured tongue, congenital (Q38.3)*

K14.6 **Glossodynia**
    Glossopyrosis
    Painful tongue

K14.8 **Other diseases of tongue**

Atrophy of tongue	Glossocele
Crenated tongue	Glossoptosis
Enlargement of tongue	Hypertrophy of tongue

K14.9 **Disease of tongue, unspecified**   ▽
    Glossopathy NOS

Diseases of esophagus, stomach and duodenum (K20-K31)

EXCLUDES 2   *hiatus hernia (K44.-)*

✓4th **K20** **Esophagitis**

Use additional code to identify:
    alcohol abuse and dependence (F10.-)
    EXCLUDES 1   *erosion of esophagus (K22.1-)*
             esophagitis with gastro-esophageal reflux disease (K21.0)
             reflux esophagitis (K21.0)
             ulcerative esophagitis (K22.1-)
    EXCLUDES 2   *eosinophilic gastritis or gastroenteritis (K52.81)*

K20.0 **Eosinophilic esophagitis**

K20.8 **Other esophagitis**
    Abscess of esophagus

K20.9 **Esophagitis, unspecified**   ▽
    Esophagitis NOS

✓4th **K21** **Gastro-esophageal reflux disease**
    EXCLUDES 1   *newborn esophageal reflux (P78.83)*

K21.0 **Gastro-esophageal reflux disease with esophagitis**
    Reflux esophagitis

K21.9 **Gastro-esophageal reflux disease without esophagitis**
    Esophageal reflux NOS
    AHA: 2016, 1Q, 18

✓4th **K22** **Other diseases of esophagus**
    EXCLUDES 2   *esophageal varices (I85.-)*

K22.0 **Achalasia of cardia**
    Achalasia NOS
    Cardiospasm
    EXCLUDES 1   *congenital cardiospasm (Q39.5)*
    DEF: Esophageal motility disorder; caused by absence of esophageal peristalsis and impaired relaxation of lower esophageal sphincter; characterized by dysphagia, regurgitation, and heartburn.

✓5th **K22.1** **Ulcer of esophagus**
    Barrett's ulcer
    Erosion of esophagus
    Fungal ulcer of esophagus
    Peptic ulcer of esophagus
    Ulcer of esophagus due to ingestion of chemicals
    Ulcer of esophagus due to ingestion of drugs and medicaments
    Ulcerative esophagitis
    Code first poisoning due to drug or toxin, if applicable (T36-T65 with fifth or sixth character 1-4 or 6)
    Use additional code for adverse effect, if applicable, to identify drug (T36-T50 with fifth or sixth character 5)
    EXCLUDES 1   *Barrett's esophagus (K22.7-)*

    K22.10 **Ulcer of esophagus without bleeding**
        Ulcer of esophagus NOS

    K22.11 **Ulcer of esophagus with bleeding**
        EXCLUDES 2   *bleeding esophageal varices (I85.01, I85.11)*

K22.2 **Esophageal obstruction**
    Compression of esophagus
    Constriction of esophagus
    Stenosis of esophagus
    Stricture of esophagus
    EXCLUDES 1   *congenital stenosis or stricture of esophagus (Q39.3)*

K22.3 **Perforation of esophagus**
    Rupture of esophagus
    EXCLUDES 1   *traumatic perforation of (thoracic) esophagus (S27.8-)*

K22.4 **Dyskinesia of esophagus**
    Corkscrew esophagus
    Diffuse esophageal spasm
    Spasm of esophagus
    EXCLUDES 1   *cardiospasm (K22.0)*

K22.5 **Diverticulum of esophagus, acquired**
    Esophageal pouch, acquired
    EXCLUDES 1   *diverticulum of esophagus (congenital) (Q39.6)*

K22.6 **Gastro-esophageal laceration-hemorrhage syndrome**
    Mallory-Weiss syndrome

✓5th **K22.7** **Barrett's esophagus**
    Barrett's disease
    Barrett's syndrome
    EXCLUDES 1   *Barrett's ulcer (K22.1)*
             malignant neoplasm of esophagus (C15.-)
    DEF: A metaplastic disorder in which specialized columnar epithelial cells replace the normal squamous epithelial cells; secondary to chronic gastroesophageal reflux damage to the mucosa; increases risk of developing adenocarcinoma.

    K22.70 **Barrett's esophagus without dysplasia**
        Barrett's esophagus NOS

    ✓6th **K22.71** **Barrett's esophagus with dysplasia**
        K22.710 **Barrett's esophagus with low grade dysplasia**
        K22.711 **Barrett's esophagus with high grade dysplasia**
        K22.719 **Barrett's esophagus with dysplasia, unspecified**   ▽

K22.8 **Other specified diseases of esophagus**
    Hemorrhage of esophagus NOS
    EXCLUDES 2   *esophageal varices (I85.-)*
             Paterson-Kelly syndrome (D50.1)

K22.9 **Disease of esophagus, unspecified**   ▽

K23 *Disorders of esophagus in diseases classified elsewhere*
    Code first underlying disease, such as:
        congenital syphilis (A50.5)
    EXCLUDES 1   *late syphilis (A52.79)*
             megaesophagus due to Chagas' disease (B57.31)
             tuberculosis (A18.83)

✓4th **K25** **Gastric ulcer**
    INCLUDES   erosion (acute) of stomach
              pylorus ulcer (peptic)
              stomach ulcer (peptic)
    Use additional code to identify:
        alcohol abuse and dependence (F10.-)
    EXCLUDES 1   *acute gastritis (K29.0-)*
             peptic ulcer NOS (K27.-)

K25.0 **Acute gastric ulcer with hemorrhage**

K25.1 **Acute gastric ulcer with perforation**   HCC

K25.2 **Acute gastric ulcer with both hemorrhage and perforation**   HCC

K25.3 **Acute gastric ulcer without hemorrhage or perforation**

✓ Additional Character Req   ✓x7th Placeholder Alert   Manifestation   HCC CMS-HCC Condition   ▽ Unspecified Code   ►◄ Revised Text   ● New Code   ▲ Revised Code Title

ICD-10-CM 2018   677

Chapter 11. Diseases of the Digestive System

K25.4–K30

Gastrointestinal Ulcers

Esophagus —
Esophageal ulcer —

Stomach

Duodenal ulcer —

Gastric ulcer

Small intestine

K25.4 Chronic or unspecified gastric ulcer with hemorrhage

K25.5 Chronic or unspecified gastric ulcer with perforation   HCC

K25.6 Chronic or unspecified gastric ulcer with both hemorrhage and perforation   HCC

K25.7 Chronic gastric ulcer without hemorrhage or perforation

K25.9 Gastric ulcer, unspecified as acute or chronic, without hemorrhage or perforation   ▽

✓4ᵗʰ **K26** Duodenal ulcer
> INCLUDES   erosion (acute) of duodenum
> duodenum ulcer (peptic)
> postpyloric ulcer (peptic)
>
> Use additional code to identify:
> alcohol abuse and dependence (F10.-)
> EXCLUDES 1   peptic ulcer NOS (K27.-)

K26.0 Acute duodenal ulcer with hemorrhage

K26.1 Acute duodenal ulcer with perforation   HCC

K26.2 Acute duodenal ulcer with both hemorrhage and perforation   HCC

K26.3 Acute duodenal ulcer without hemorrhage or perforation

K26.4 Chronic or unspecified duodenal ulcer with hemorrhage
> AHA: 2016, 1Q, 14

K26.5 Chronic or unspecified duodenal ulcer with perforation   HCC

K26.6 Chronic or unspecified duodenal ulcer with both hemorrhage and perforation   HCC

K26.7 Chronic duodenal ulcer without hemorrhage or perforation

K26.9 Duodenal ulcer, unspecified as acute or chronic, without hemorrhage or perforation   ▽

✓4ᵗʰ **K27** Peptic ulcer, site unspecified
> INCLUDES   gastroduodenal ulcer NOS
> peptic ulcer NOS
>
> Use additional code to identify:
> alcohol abuse and dependence (F10.-)
> EXCLUDES 1   peptic ulcer of newborn (P78.82)

K27.0 Acute peptic ulcer, site unspecified, with hemorrhage

K27.1 Acute peptic ulcer, site unspecified, with perforation   HCC

K27.2 Acute peptic ulcer, site unspecified, with both hemorrhage and perforation   HCC

K27.3 Acute peptic ulcer, site unspecified, without hemorrhage or perforation

K27.4 Chronic or unspecified peptic ulcer, site unspecified, with hemorrhage

K27.5 Chronic or unspecified peptic ulcer, site unspecified, with perforation   HCC

K27.6 Chronic or unspecified peptic ulcer, site unspecified, with both hemorrhage and perforation   HCC

K27.7 Chronic peptic ulcer, site unspecified, without hemorrhage or perforation

K27.9 Peptic ulcer, site unspecified, unspecified as acute or chronic, without hemorrhage or perforation   ▽

✓4ᵗʰ **K28** Gastrojejunal ulcer
> INCLUDES   anastomotic ulcer (peptic) or erosion
> gastrocolic ulcer (peptic) or erosion
> gastrointestinal ulcer (peptic) or erosion
> gastrojejunal ulcer (peptic) or erosion
> jejunal ulcer (peptic) or erosion
> marginal ulcer (peptic) or erosion
> stomal ulcer (peptic) or erosion
>
> Use additional code to identify:
> alcohol abuse and dependence (F10.-)
> EXCLUDES 1   primary ulcer of small intestine (K63.3)

K28.0 Acute gastrojejunal ulcer with hemorrhage

K28.1 Acute gastrojejunal ulcer with perforation   HCC

K28.2 Acute gastrojejunal ulcer with both hemorrhage and perforation   HCC

K28.3 Acute gastrojejunal ulcer without hemorrhage or perforation

K28.4 Chronic or unspecified gastrojejunal ulcer with hemorrhage

K28.5 Chronic or unspecified gastrojejunal ulcer with perforation   HCC

K28.6 Chronic or unspecified gastrojejunal ulcer with both hemorrhage and perforation   HCC

K28.7 Chronic gastrojejunal ulcer without hemorrhage or perforation

K28.9 Gastrojejunal ulcer, unspecified as acute or chronic, without hemorrhage or perforation   ▽

✓4ᵗʰ **K29** Gastritis and duodenitis
> EXCLUDES 1   eosinophilic gastritis or gastroenteritis (K52.81)
> Zollinger-Ellison syndrome (E16.4)

✓5ᵗʰ **K29.0** Acute gastritis
> Use additional code to identify:
> alcohol abuse and dependence (F10.-)
> EXCLUDES 1   erosion (acute) of stomach (K25.-)

K29.00 Acute gastritis without bleeding

K29.01 Acute gastritis with bleeding

✓5ᵗʰ **K29.2** Alcoholic gastritis
> Use additional code to identify:
> alcohol abuse and dependence (F10.-)

K29.20 Alcoholic gastritis without bleeding

K29.21 Alcoholic gastritis with bleeding

✓5ᵗʰ **K29.3** Chronic superficial gastritis

K29.30 Chronic superficial gastritis without bleeding

K29.31 Chronic superficial gastritis with bleeding

✓5ᵗʰ **K29.4** Chronic atrophic gastritis
> Gastric atrophy

K29.40 Chronic atrophic gastritis without bleeding

K29.41 Chronic atrophic gastritis with bleeding

✓5ᵗʰ **K29.5** Unspecified chronic gastritis
> Chronic antral gastritis
> Chronic fundal gastritis

K29.50 Unspecified chronic gastritis without bleeding   ▽

K29.51 Unspecified chronic gastritis with bleeding   ▽

✓5ᵗʰ **K29.6** Other gastritis
> Giant hypertrophic gastritis
> Granulomatous gastritis
> Ménétrier's disease

K29.60 Other gastritis without bleeding

K29.61 Other gastritis with bleeding

✓5ᵗʰ **K29.7** Gastritis, unspecified

K29.70 Gastritis, unspecified, without bleeding   ▽

K29.71 Gastritis, unspecified, with bleeding   ▽

✓5ᵗʰ **K29.8** Duodenitis

K29.80 Duodenitis without bleeding

K29.81 Duodenitis with bleeding

✓5ᵗʰ **K29.9** Gastroduodenitis, unspecified

K29.90 Gastroduodenitis, unspecified, without bleeding   ▽

K29.91 Gastroduodenitis, unspecified, with bleeding   ▽

K30 Functional dyspepsia
> Indigestion
> EXCLUDES 1   dyspepsia NOS (R10.13)
> heartburn (R12)
> nervous dyspepsia (F45.8)
> neurotic dyspepsia (F45.8)
> psychogenic dyspepsia (F45.8)

EXCLUDES 1 Not coded here   EXCLUDES 2 Not included here   N Newborn Age: 0   P Pediatric Age: 0-17   M Maternity Age: 12-55   A Adult Age: 15-124

678   ICD-10-CM 2018

✓4ᵗʰ K31 Other diseases of stomach and duodenum
> INCLUDES functional disorders of stomach
> EXCLUDES 2 *diabetic gastroparesis (E08.43, E09.43, E10.43, E11.43, E13.43)*
> *diverticulum of duodenum (K57.00-K57.13)*

K31.0 Acute dilatation of stomach
> Acute distention of stomach

K31.1 Adult hypertrophic pyloric stenosis   A
> Pyloric stenosis NOS
> EXCLUDES 1 *congenital or infantile pyloric stenosis (Q40.0)*

K31.2 Hourglass stricture and stenosis of stomach
> EXCLUDES 1 *congenital hourglass stomach (Q40.2)*
> *hourglass contraction of stomach (K31.89)*

K31.3 Pylorospasm, not elsewhere classified
> EXCLUDES 1 *congenital or infantile pylorospasm (Q40.0)*
> *neurotic pylorospasm (F45.8)*
> *psychogenic pylorospasm (F45.8)*

K31.4 Gastric diverticulum
> EXCLUDES 1 *congenital diverticulum of stomach (Q40.2)*

K31.5 Obstruction of duodenum
> Constriction of duodenum
> Duodenal ileus (chronic)
> Stenosis of duodenum
> Stricture of duodenum
> Volvulus of duodenum
> EXCLUDES 1 *congenital stenosis of duodenum (Q41.0)*

K31.6 Fistula of stomach and duodenum
> Gastrocolic fistula
> Gastrojejunocolic fistula

K31.7 Polyp of stomach and duodenum
> EXCLUDES 1 *adenomatous polyp of stomach (D13.1)*

✓5ᵗʰ K31.8 Other specified diseases of stomach and duodenum

    ✓6ᵗʰ K31.81 Angiodysplasia of stomach and duodenum

       K31.811 Angiodysplasia of stomach and duodenum with bleeding

       K31.819 Angiodysplasia of stomach and duodenum without bleeding
> Angiodysplasia of stomach and duodenum NOS

    K31.82 Dieulafoy lesion (hemorrhagic) of stomach and duodenum
> EXCLUDES 2 *Dieulafoy lesion of intestine (K63.81)*

    K31.83 Achlorhydria
> **DEF:** Absence of hydrochloric acid in gastric secretions due to gastric mucosa atrophy; unresponsive to histamines; also known as gastric anacidity.

    K31.84 Gastroparesis
> Gastroparalysis
> Code first underlying disease, if known, such as:
> anorexia nervosa (F50.0-)
> diabetes mellitus (E08.43, E09.43, E10.43, E11.43, E13.43)
> scleroderma (M34.-)
> **AHA:** 2013, 4Q, 114

    K31.89 Other diseases of stomach and duodenum
> **AHA:** 2017, 1Q, 28

K31.9 Disease of stomach and duodenum, unspecified   ▽

Diseases of appendix (K35-K38)

✓4ᵗʰ K35 Acute appendicitis

K35.2 Acute appendicitis with generalized peritonitis
> Appendicitis (acute) with generalized (diffuse) peritonitis following rupture or perforation of appendix
> Perforated appendix NOS
> Ruptured appendix NOS

K35.3 Acute appendicitis with localized peritonitis
> Acute appendicitis with or without perforation or rupture with peritonitis NOS
> Acute appendicitis with or without perforation or rupture with localized peritonitis
> Acute appendicitis with peritoneal abscess

✓5ᵗʰ K35.8 Other and unspecified acute appendicitis

    K35.80 Unspecified acute appendicitis   ▽
> Acute appendicitis NOS
> Acute appendicitis without (localized) (generalized) peritonitis

    K35.89 Other acute appendicitis

K36 Other appendicitis
> Chronic appendicitis
> Recurrent appendicitis

K37 Unspecified appendicitis   ▽
> EXCLUDES 1 *unspecified appendicitis with peritonitis (K35.2-K35.3)*

✓4ᵗʰ K38 Other diseases of appendix

K38.0 Hyperplasia of appendix

K38.1 Appendicular concretions
> Fecalith of appendix
> Stercolith of appendix

K38.2 Diverticulum of appendix

K38.3 Fistula of appendix

K38.8 Other specified diseases of appendix
> Intussusception of appendix

K38.9 Disease of appendix, unspecified   ▽

Hernia (K40-K46)

> NOTE Hernia with both gangrene and obstruction is classified to hernia with gangrene.
> INCLUDES acquired hernia
> congenital [except diaphragmatic or hiatus] hernia
> recurrent hernia

✓4ᵗʰ K40 Inguinal hernia
> INCLUDES bubonocele
> direct inguinal hernia
> double inguinal hernia
> indirect inguinal hernia
> inguinal hernia NOS
> oblique inguinal hernia
> scrotal hernia

✓5ᵗʰ K40.0 Bilateral inguinal hernia, with obstruction, without gangrene
> Inguinal hernia (bilateral) causing obstruction without gangrene
> Incarcerated inguinal hernia (bilateral) without gangrene
> Irreducible inguinal hernia (bilateral) without gangrene
> Strangulated inguinal hernia (bilateral) without gangrene

    K40.00 Bilateral inguinal hernia, with obstruction, without gangrene, not specified as recurrent
> Bilateral inguinal hernia, with obstruction, without gangrene NOS

    K40.01 Bilateral inguinal hernia, with obstruction, without gangrene, recurrent

✓5ᵗʰ K40.1 Bilateral inguinal hernia, with gangrene

    K40.10 Bilateral inguinal hernia, with gangrene, not specified as recurrent
> Bilateral inguinal hernia, with gangrene NOS

    K40.11 Bilateral inguinal hernia, with gangrene, recurrent

✓5ᵗʰ K40.2 Bilateral inguinal hernia, without obstruction or gangrene

    K40.20 Bilateral inguinal hernia, without obstruction or gangrene, not specified as recurrent
> Bilateral inguinal hernia NOS

    K40.21 Bilateral inguinal hernia, without obstruction or gangrene, recurrent

✓5ᵗʰ K40.3 Unilateral inguinal hernia, with obstruction, without gangrene
> Inguinal hernia (unilateral) causing obstruction without gangrene
> Incarcerated inguinal hernia (unilateral) without gangrene
> Irreducible inguinal hernia (unilateral) without gangrene
> Strangulated inguinal hernia (unilateral) without gangrene

    K40.30 Unilateral inguinal hernia, with obstruction, without gangrene, not specified as recurrent
> Inguinal hernia, with obstruction NOS
> Unilateral inguinal hernia, with obstruction, without gangrene NOS

    K40.31 Unilateral inguinal hernia, with obstruction, without gangrene, recurrent

✓5ᵗʰ K40.4 Unilateral inguinal hernia, with gangrene

    K40.40 Unilateral inguinal hernia, with gangrene, not specified as recurrent
> Inguinal hernia with gangrene NOS
> Unilateral inguinal hernia with gangrene NOS

    K40.41 Unilateral inguinal hernia, with gangrene, recurrent

✓5ᵗʰ K40.9 Unilateral inguinal hernia, without obstruction or gangrene

    K40.90 Unilateral inguinal hernia, without obstruction or gangrene, not specified as recurrent
> Inguinal hernia NOS
> Unilateral inguinal hernia NOS

    K40.91 Unilateral inguinal hernia, without obstruction or gangrene, recurrent

---

✓ Additional Character Req   ✓x7ᵗʰ Placeholder Alert   Manifestation   HCC CMS-HCC Condition   ▽ Unspecified Code   ►◄ Revised Text   ● New Code   ▲ Revised Code Title

Chapter 11. Diseases of the Digestive System *(left margin)*

K41–K44.1 *(left margin)*

Hernia Sites

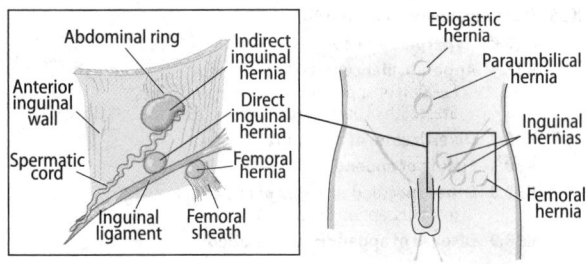

✓4ᵗʰ **K41** **Femoral hernia**

✓5ᵗʰ **K41.0** **Bilateral femoral hernia, with obstruction, without gangrene**
Femoral hernia (bilateral) causing obstruction, without gangrene
Incarcerated femoral hernia (bilateral), without gangrene
Irreducible femoral hernia (bilateral), without gangrene
Strangulated femoral hernia (bilateral), without gangrene

  K41.00 **Bilateral femoral hernia, with obstruction, without gangrene, not specified as recurrent**
Bilateral femoral hernia, with obstruction, without gangrene NOS

  K41.01 **Bilateral femoral hernia, with obstruction, without gangrene, recurrent**

✓5ᵗʰ **K41.1** **Bilateral femoral hernia, with gangrene**

  K41.10 **Bilateral femoral hernia, with gangrene, not specified as recurrent**
Bilateral femoral hernia, with gangrene NOS

  K41.11 **Bilateral femoral hernia, with gangrene, recurrent**

✓5ᵗʰ **K41.2** **Bilateral femoral hernia, without obstruction or gangrene**

  K41.20 **Bilateral femoral hernia, without obstruction or gangrene, not specified as recurrent**
Bilateral femoral hernia NOS

  K41.21 **Bilateral femoral hernia, without obstruction or gangrene, recurrent**

✓5ᵗʰ **K41.3** **Unilateral femoral hernia, with obstruction, without gangrene**
Femoral hernia (unilateral) causing obstruction, without gangrene
Incarcerated femoral hernia (unilateral), without gangrene
Irreducible femoral hernia (unilateral), without gangrene
Strangulated femoral hernia (unilateral), without gangrene

  K41.30 **Unilateral femoral hernia, with obstruction, without gangrene, not specified as recurrent**
Femoral hernia, with obstruction NOS
Unilateral femoral hernia, with obstruction NOS

  K41.31 **Unilateral femoral hernia, with obstruction, without gangrene, recurrent**

✓5ᵗʰ **K41.4** **Unilateral femoral hernia, with gangrene**

  K41.40 **Unilateral femoral hernia, with gangrene, not specified as recurrent**
Femoral hernia, with gangrene NOS
Unilateral femoral hernia, with gangrene NOS

  K41.41 **Unilateral femoral hernia, with gangrene, recurrent**

✓5ᵗʰ **K41.9** **Unilateral femoral hernia, without obstruction or gangrene**

  K41.90 **Unilateral femoral hernia, without obstruction or gangrene, not specified as recurrent**
Femoral hernia NOS
Unilateral femoral hernia NOS

  K41.91 **Unilateral femoral hernia, without obstruction or gangrene, recurrent**

✓4ᵗʰ **K42** **Umbilical hernia**
   INCLUDES   paraumbilical hernia
   EXCLUDES 1   *omphalocele (Q79.2)*

K42.0 **Umbilical hernia with obstruction, without gangrene**
Umbilical hernia causing obstruction, without gangrene
Incarcerated umbilical hernia, without gangrene
Irreducible umbilical hernia, without gangrene
Strangulated umbilical hernia, without gangrene

K42.1 **Umbilical hernia with gangrene**
Gangrenous umbilical hernia

K42.9 **Umbilical hernia without obstruction or gangrene**
Umbilical hernia NOS

✓4ᵗʰ **K43** **Ventral hernia**

K43.0 **Incisional hernia with obstruction, without gangrene**
Incisional hernia causing obstruction, without gangrene
Incarcerated incisional hernia, without gangrene
Irreducible incisional hernia, without gangrene
Strangulated incisional hernia, without gangrene

K43.1 **Incisional hernia with gangrene**
Gangrenous incisional hernia

K43.2 **Incisional hernia without obstruction or gangrene**
Incisional hernia NOS

K43.3 **Parastomal hernia with obstruction, without gangrene**
Incarcerated parastomal hernia, without gangrene
Irreducible parastomal hernia, without gangrene
Parastomal hernia causing obstruction, without gangrene
Strangulated parastomal hernia, without gangrene

K43.4 **Parastomal hernia with gangrene**
Gangrenous parastomal hernia

K43.5 **Parastomal hernia without obstruction or gangrene**
Parastomal hernia NOS

K43.6 **Other and unspecified ventral hernia with obstruction, without gangrene** ▽
Epigastric hernia causing obstruction, without gangrene
Hypogastric hernia causing obstruction, without gangrene
Incarcerated epigastric hernia without gangrene
Incarcerated hypogastric hernia without gangrene
Incarcerated midline hernia without gangrene
Incarcerated spigelian hernia without gangrene
Incarcerated subxiphoid hernia without gangrene
Irreducible epigastric hernia without gangrene
Irreducible hypogastric hernia without gangrene
Irreducible midline hernia without gangrene
Irreducible spigelian hernia without gangrene
Irreducible subxiphoid hernia without gangrene
Midline hernia causing obstruction, without gangrene
Spigelian hernia causing obstruction, without gangrene
Strangulated epigastric hernia without gangrene
Strangulated hypogastric hernia without gangrene
Strangulated midline hernia without gangrene
Strangulated spigelian hernia without gangrene
Strangulated subxiphoid hernia without gangrene
Subxiphoid hernia causing obstruction, without gangrene

K43.7 **Other and unspecified ventral hernia with gangrene** ▽
Any condition listed under K43.6 specified as gangrenous

K43.9 **Ventral hernia without obstruction or gangrene** ▽
Epigastric hernia
Ventral hernia NOS

✓4ᵗʰ **K44** **Diaphragmatic hernia**
   INCLUDES   hiatus hernia (esophageal) (sliding)
                paraesophageal hernia
   EXCLUDES 1   *congenital diaphragmatic hernia (Q79.0)*
                congenital hiatus hernia (Q40.1)

K44.0 **Diaphragmatic hernia with obstruction, without gangrene**
Diaphragmatic hernia causing obstruction
Incarcerated diaphragmatic hernia
Irreducible diaphragmatic hernia
Strangulated diaphragmatic hernia

K44.1 **Diaphragmatic hernia with gangrene**
Gangrenous diaphragmatic hernia

Hiatal Hernia

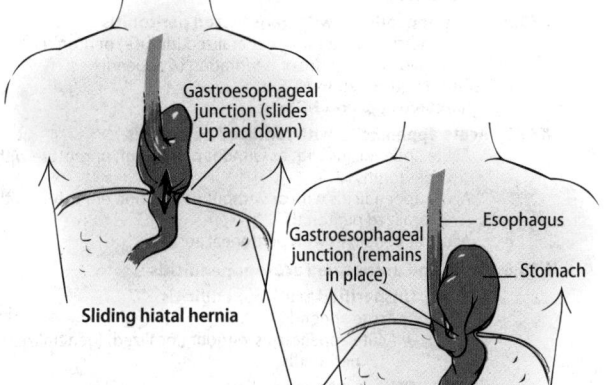

Gastroesophageal junction (slides up and down)

Gastroesophageal junction (remains in place)

Esophagus

Stomach

Sliding hiatal hernia

Diaphragm

Paraesophageal hiatal hernia

EXCLUDES 1 Not coded here   EXCLUDES 2 Not included here   N Newborn Age: 0   P Pediatric Age: 0-17   M Maternity Age: 12-55   A Adult Age: 15-124

K44.9 Diaphragmatic hernia without obstruction or gangrene
Diaphragmatic hernia NOS

✓4ᵗʰ **K45 Other abdominal hernia**
INCLUDES   abdominal hernia, specified site NEC
lumbar hernia
obturator hernia
pudendal hernia
retroperitoneal hernia
sciatic hernia

K45.0 Other specified abdominal hernia with obstruction, without gangrene
Other specified abdominal hernia causing obstruction
Other specified incarcerated abdominal hernia
Other specified irreducible abdominal hernia
Other specified strangulated abdominal hernia

K45.1 Other specified abdominal hernia with gangrene
Any condition listed under K45 specified as gangrenous

K45.8 Other specified abdominal hernia without obstruction or gangrene

✓4ᵗʰ **K46 Unspecified abdominal hernia**
INCLUDES   enterocele
epiplocele
hernia NOS
interstitial hernia
intestinal hernia
intra-abdominal hernia
EXCLUDES 1   vaginal enterocele (N81.5)

K46.0 Unspecified abdominal hernia with obstruction, without ▽
gangrene
Unspecified abdominal hernia causing obstruction
Unspecified incarcerated abdominal hernia
Unspecified irreducible abdominal hernia
Unspecified strangulated abdominal hernia

K46.1 Unspecified abdominal hernia with gangrene ▽
Any condition listed under K46 specified as gangrenous

K46.9 Unspecified abdominal hernia without obstruction or ▽
gangrene
Abdominal hernia NOS

Noninfective enteritis and colitis (K50-K52)

INCLUDES   noninfective inflammatory bowel disease
EXCLUDES 1   irritable bowel syndrome (K58.-)
megacolon (K59.3-)

✓4ᵗʰ **K50 Crohn's disease [regional enteritis]**
INCLUDES   granulomatous enteritis
Use additional code to identify manifestations, such as:
pyoderma gangrenosum (L88)
EXCLUDES 1   ulcerative colitis (K51.-)
AHA: 2012, 4Q, 104

✓5ᵗʰ **K50.0 Crohn's disease of** small intestine
Crohn's disease [regional enteritis] of duodenum
Crohn's disease [regional enteritis] of ileum
Crohn's disease [regional enteritis] of jejunum
Regional ileitis
Terminal ileitis
EXCLUDES 1   Crohn's disease of both small and large intestine
(K50.8-)

K50.00 Crohn's disease of small intestine without   HCC
complications

✓6ᵗʰ **K50.01 Crohn's disease of small intestine** with complications
K50.011 Crohn's disease of small intestine   HCC
with rectal bleeding
K50.012 Crohn's disease of small intestine   HCC
with intestinal obstruction
K50.013 Crohn's disease of small intestine   HCC
with fistula
K50.014 Crohn's disease of small intestine   HCC
with abscess
AHA: 2012, 4Q, 104
K50.018 Crohn's disease of small intestine   HCC
with other complication
K50.019 Crohn's disease of small intestine   HCC ▽
with unspecified complications

✓5ᵗʰ **K50.1 Crohn's disease of** large intestine
Crohn's disease [regional enteritis] of colon
Crohn's disease [regional enteritis] of large bowel
Crohn's disease [regional enteritis] of rectum
Granulomatous colitis
Regional colitis
EXCLUDES 1   Crohn's disease of both small and large intestine
(K50.8)

K50.10 Crohn's disease of large intestine without   HCC
complications

✓6ᵗʰ **K50.11 Crohn's disease of large intestine** with complications
K50.111 Crohn's disease of large intestine   HCC
with rectal bleeding
K50.112 Crohn's disease of large intestine   HCC
with intestinal obstruction
K50.113 Crohn's disease of large intestine   HCC
with fistula
K50.114 Crohn's disease of large intestine   HCC
with abscess
K50.118 Crohn's disease of large intestine   HCC
with other complication
K50.119 Crohn's disease of large intestine   HCC ▽
with unspecified complications

✓5ᵗʰ **K50.8 Crohn's disease of** both small and large intestine
K50.80 Crohn's disease of both small and large   HCC
intestine without complications

✓6ᵗʰ **K50.81 Crohn's disease of both small and large intestine**
with complications
K50.811 Crohn's disease of both small and   HCC
large intestine with rectal bleeding
K50.812 Crohn's disease of both small and   HCC
large intestine with intestinal obstruction
K50.813 Crohn's disease of both small and   HCC
large intestine with fistula
K50.814 Crohn's disease of both small and   HCC
large intestine with abscess
K50.818 Crohn's disease of both small and   HCC
large intestine with other complication
K50.819 Crohn's disease of both small and   HCC ▽
large intestine with unspecified
complications

✓5ᵗʰ **K50.9 Crohn's disease, unspecified**
K50.90 Crohn's disease, unspecified, without   HCC ▽
complications
Crohn's disease NOS
Regional enteritis NOS

✓6ᵗʰ **K50.91 Crohn's disease, unspecified,** with complications
K50.911 Crohn's disease, unspecified, with   HCC ▽
rectal bleeding
K50.912 Crohn's disease, unspecified, with   HCC ▽
intestinal obstruction
K50.913 Crohn's disease, unspecified, with   HCC ▽
fistula
K50.914 Crohn's disease, unspecified, with   HCC ▽
abscess
K50.918 Crohn's disease, unspecified, with   HCC ▽
other complication
K50.919 Crohn's disease, unspecified, with   HCC ▽
unspecified complications

✓4ᵗʰ **K51 Ulcerative colitis**
Use additional code to identify manifestations, such as:
pyoderma gangrenosum (L88)
EXCLUDES 1   Crohn's disease [regional enteritis] (K50.-)

✓5ᵗʰ **K51.0 Ulcerative (chronic)** pancolitis
Backwash ileitis
K51.00 Ulcerative (chronic) pancolitis without   HCC
complications
Ulcerative (chronic) pancolitis NOS

✓6ᵗʰ **K51.01 Ulcerative (chronic) pancolitis** with complications
K51.011 Ulcerative (chronic) pancolitis with   HCC
rectal bleeding
K51.012 Ulcerative (chronic) pancolitis with   HCC
intestinal obstruction
K51.013 Ulcerative (chronic) pancolitis with   HCC
fistula
K51.014 Ulcerative (chronic) pancolitis with   HCC
abscess

K51.Ø18 Ulcerative (chronic) pancolitis with other complication **HCC**

K51.Ø19 Ulcerative (chronic) pancolitis with unspecified complications **HCC** ▽

✓5ᵗʰ **K51.2 Ulcerative (chronic) proctitis**

  K51.2Ø Ulcerative (chronic) proctitis without complications **HCC**
    Ulcerative (chronic) proctitis NOS

  ✓6ᵗʰ **K51.21** Ulcerative (chronic) proctitis with complications

    K51.211 Ulcerative (chronic) proctitis with rectal bleeding **HCC**

    K51.212 Ulcerative (chronic) proctitis with intestinal obstruction **HCC**

    K51.213 Ulcerative (chronic) proctitis with fistula **HCC**

    K51.214 Ulcerative (chronic) proctitis with abscess **HCC**

    K51.218 Ulcerative (chronic) proctitis with other complication **HCC**

    K51.219 Ulcerative (chronic) proctitis with unspecified complications **HCC** ▽

✓5ᵗʰ **K51.3 Ulcerative (chronic) rectosigmoiditis**

  K51.3Ø Ulcerative (chronic) rectosigmoiditis without complications **HCC**
    Ulcerative (chronic) rectosigmoiditis NOS

  ✓6ᵗʰ **K51.31** Ulcerative (chronic) rectosigmoiditis with complications

    K51.311 Ulcerative (chronic) rectosigmoiditis with rectal bleeding **HCC**

    K51.312 Ulcerative (chronic) rectosigmoiditis with intestinal obstruction **HCC**

    K51.313 Ulcerative (chronic) rectosigmoiditis with fistula **HCC**

    K51.314 Ulcerative (chronic) rectosigmoiditis with abscess **HCC**

    K51.318 Ulcerative (chronic) rectosigmoiditis with other complication **HCC**

    K51.319 Ulcerative (chronic) rectosigmoiditis with unspecified complications **HCC** ▽

✓5ᵗʰ **K51.4 Inflammatory polyps of colon**

  EXCLUDES 1   adenomatous polyp of colon (D12.6)
      polyposis of colon (D12.6)
      polyps of colon NOS (K63.5)

  K51.4Ø Inflammatory polyps of colon without complications **HCC**
    Inflammatory polyps of colon NOS

  ✓6ᵗʰ **K51.41** Inflammatory polyps of colon with complications

    K51.411 Inflammatory polyps of colon with rectal bleeding **HCC**

    K51.412 Inflammatory polyps of colon with intestinal obstruction **HCC**

    K51.413 Inflammatory polyps of colon with fistula **HCC**

    K51.414 Inflammatory polyps of colon with abscess **HCC**

    K51.418 Inflammatory polyps of colon with other complication **HCC**

    K51.419 Inflammatory polyps of colon with unspecified complications **HCC** ▽

✓5ᵗʰ **K51.5 Left sided colitis**
  Left hemicolitis

  K51.5Ø Left sided colitis without complications **HCC**
    Left sided colitis NOS

  ✓6ᵗʰ **K51.51** Left sided colitis with complications

    K51.511 Left sided colitis with rectal bleeding **HCC**

    K51.512 Left sided colitis with intestinal obstruction **HCC**

    K51.513 Left sided colitis with fistula **HCC**

    K51.514 Left sided colitis with abscess **HCC**

    K51.518 Left sided colitis with other complication **HCC**

    K51.519 Left sided colitis with unspecified complications **HCC** ▽

✓5ᵗʰ **K51.8 Other ulcerative colitis**

  K51.8Ø Other ulcerative colitis without complications **HCC**

  ✓6ᵗʰ **K51.81** Other ulcerative colitis with complications

    K51.811 Other ulcerative colitis with rectal bleeding **HCC**

    K51.812 Other ulcerative colitis with intestinal obstruction **HCC**

    K51.813 Other ulcerative colitis with fistula **HCC**

    K51.814 Other ulcerative colitis with abscess **HCC**

    K51.818 Other ulcerative colitis with other complication **HCC**

    K51.819 Other ulcerative colitis with unspecified complications **HCC** ▽

✓5ᵗʰ **K51.9 Ulcerative colitis, unspecified**

  K51.9Ø Ulcerative colitis, unspecified, without complications **HCC** ▽

  ✓6ᵗʰ **K51.91** Ulcerative colitis, unspecified, with complications

    K51.911 Ulcerative colitis, unspecified with rectal bleeding **HCC** ▽

    K51.912 Ulcerative colitis, unspecified with intestinal obstruction **HCC** ▽

    K51.913 Ulcerative colitis, unspecified with fistula **HCC** ▽

    K51.914 Ulcerative colitis, unspecified with abscess **HCC** ▽

    K51.918 Ulcerative colitis, unspecified with other complication **HCC** ▽

    K51.919 Ulcerative colitis, unspecified with unspecified complications **HCC** ▽

✓4ᵗʰ **K52 Other and unspecified noninfective gastroenteritis and colitis**

  K52.Ø Gastroenteritis and colitis due to radiation

  K52.1 Toxic gastroenteritis and colitis
    Drug-induced gastroenteritis and colitis
    Code first (T51-T65) to identify toxic agent
    Use additional code for adverse effect, if applicable, to identify drug (T36-T5Ø with fifth or sixth character 5)

  ✓5ᵗʰ **K52.2 Allergic and dietetic gastroenteritis and colitis**
    Food hypersensitivity gastroenteritis or colitis
    Use additional code to identify type of food allergy (Z91.Ø1-, Z91.Ø2-)

    EXCLUDES 2   allergic eosinophilic colitis (K52.82)
      allergic eosinophilic esophagitis (K20.Ø)
      allergic eosinophilic gastritis (K52.81)
      allergic eosinophilic gastroenteritis (K52.81)
      food protein-induced proctocolitis (K52.82)

    DEF: True immunoglobulin E (IgE)-mediated allergic reaction of the lining of the stomach, intestines, or colon to food proteins; causes nausea, vomiting, diarrhea, and abdominal cramping.

    K52.21 Food protein-induced enterocolitis syndrome
      Use additional code for hypovolemic shock, if present (R57.1)

    K52.22 Food protein-induced enteropathy

    K52.29 Other allergic and dietetic gastroenteritis and colitis
      Food hypersensitivity gastroenteritis or colitis
      Immediate gastrointestinal hypersensitivity

  K52.3 Indeterminate colitis
    Colonic inflammatory bowel disease unclassified (IBDU)
    EXCLUDES 1 unspecified colitis (K52.9)

  ✓5ᵗʰ **K52.8 Other specified noninfective gastroenteritis and colitis**

    K52.81 Eosinophilic gastritis or gastroenteritis
      Eosinophilic enteritis
      EXCLUDES 2   eosinophilic esophagitis (K20.Ø)

    K52.82 Eosinophilic colitis
      Allergic proctocolitis
      Food-induced eosinophilic proctocolitis
      Food protein-induced proctocolitis
      Milk protein-induced proctocolitis

    ✓6ᵗʰ **K52.83** Microscopic colitis

      K52.831 Collagenous colitis

      K52.832 Lymphocytic colitis

      K52.838 Other microscopic colitis

      K52.839 Microscopic colitis, unspecified ▽

    K52.89 Other specified noninfective gastroenteritis and colitis

---

EXCLUDES 1 Not coded here   EXCLUDES 2 Not included here   N Newborn Age: 0   P Pediatric Age: 0-17   M Maternity Age: 12-55   A Adult Age: 15-124

K52.9   **Noninfective gastroenteritis and colitis, unspecified**   ▽
Colitis NOS   Ileitis NOS
Enteritis NOS   Jejunitis NOS
Gastroenteritis NOS   Sigmoiditis NOS
EXCLUDES 1   *diarrhea NOS (R19.7)*
functional diarrhea (K59.1)
infectious gastroenteritis and colitis NOS (A09)
neonatal diarrhea (noninfective) (P78.3)
psychogenic diarrhea (F45.8)

Other diseases of intestines (K55-K64)

☑4ᵗʰ **K55**   **Vascular disorders of intestine**
EXCLUDES 1   *necrotizing enterocolitis of newborn (P77.-)*

☑5ᵗʰ **K55.0**   Acute **vascular disorders of intestine**   HCC
Infarction of appendices epiploicae
Mesenteric (artery) (vein) embolism
Mesenteric (artery) (vein) infarction
Mesenteric (artery) (vein) thrombosis

   ☑6ᵗʰ **K55.01**   **Acute (reversible)** ischemia of small intestine
     K55.011   Focal **(segmental) acute (reversible)** HCC
           ischemia of small intestine
     K55.012   Diffuse **acute (reversible) ischemia of** HCC
           small intestine
     K55.019   **Acute (reversible) ischemia of small** HCC ▽
           intestine, extent unspecified

   ☑6ᵗʰ **K55.02**   **Acute** infarction of small intestine
     Gangrene of small intestine
     Necrosis of small intestine
     K55.021   Focal **(segmental) acute infarction of** HCC
           small intestine
     K55.022   Diffuse **acute infarction of small** HCC
           intestine
     K55.029   **Acute infarction of small intestine,** HCC ▽
           extent unspecified

   ☑6ᵗʰ **K55.03**   **Acute (reversible)** ischemia of large intestine
     Acute fulminant ischemic colitis
     Subacute ischemic colitis
     K55.031   Focal **(segmental) acute (reversible)** HCC
           ischemia of large intestine
     K55.032   Diffuse **acute (reversible) ischemia of** HCC
           large intestine
     K55.039   **Acute (reversible) ischemia of large** HCC ▽
           intestine, extent unspecified

   ☑6ᵗʰ **K55.04**   **Acute** infarction of large intestine
     Gangrene of small intestine
     Necrosis of small intestine
     K55.041   Focal **(segmental) acute infarction of** HCC
           large intestine
     K55.042   Diffuse **acute infarction of large** HCC
           intestine
     K55.049   **Acute infarction of large intestine,** HCC ▽
           extent unspecified

   ☑6ᵗʰ **K55.05**   **Acute (reversible)** ischemia **of intestine, part**
     unspecified
     K55.051   Focal **(segmental) acute (reversible)** HCC ▽
           ischemia of intestine, part unspecified
     K55.052   Diffuse **acute (reversible) ischemia** HCC ▽
           of intestine, part unspecified
     K55.059   **Acute (reversible) ischemia of** HCC ▽
           intestine, part and extent unspecified

   ☑6ᵗʰ **K55.06**   **Acute** infarction **of intestine, part unspecified**
     Acute intestinal infarction
     Gangrene of intestine
     Necrosis of intestine
     K55.061   Focal **(segmental) acute infarction** HCC ▽
           of intestine, part unspecified
     K55.062   Diffuse **acute infarction of** HCC ▽
           intestine, part unspecified
     K55.069   **Acute infarction of intestine, part** HCC ▽
           and extent unspecified

   K55.1   Chronic **vascular disorders of intestine**   HCC
     Chronic ischemic colitis   Mesenteric atherosclerosis
     Chronic ischemic enteritis   Mesenteric vascular
     Chronic ischemic enterocolitis   insufficiency
     Ischemic stricture of intestine

☑5ᵗʰ **K55.2**   Angiodysplasia **of colon**
   K55.20   **Angiodysplasia of colon** without hemorrhage
   K55.21   **Angiodysplasia of colon** with hemorrhage
     DEF: Small vascular abnormalities due to fragile blood
     vessels in the colon; results in blood loss from the
     gastrointestinal (GI) tract.

☑5ᵗʰ **K55.3**   **Necrotizing enterocolitis**
   EXCLUDES 1   *necrotizing enterocolitis of newborn (P77.-)*
   EXCLUDES 2   *necrotizing enterocolitis due to Clostridium difficile*
     ▶*(A04.7-)*◄
   K55.30   **Necrotizing enterocolitis, unspecified**   HCC ▽
     Necrotizing enterocolitis, NOS
   K55.31   Stage 1 **necrotizing enterocolitis**   HCC
     Necrotizing enterocolitis without pneumatosis,
     without perforation
   K55.32   Stage 2 **necrotizing enterocolitis**   HCC
     Necrotizing enterocolitis with pneumatosis, without
     perforation
   K55.33   Stage 3 **necrotizing enterocolitis**   HCC
     Necrotizing enterocolitis with perforation
     Necrotizing enterocolitis with pneumatosis and
     perforation

   K55.8   **Other vascular disorders of intestine**   HCC
   K55.9   **Vascular disorder of intestine, unspecified**   HCC ▽
     Ischemic colitis   Ischemic enterocolitis
     Ischemic enteritis

☑4ᵗʰ **K56**   **Paralytic ileus and intestinal obstruction without hernia**
   EXCLUDES 1   *congenital stricture or stenosis of intestine (Q41-Q42)*
     cystic fibrosis with meconium ileus (E84.11)
     ~~*intestinal obstruction with hernia (K40-K46)*~~
     ischemic stricture of intestine (K55.1)
     meconium ileus NOS (P76.0)
     neonatal intestinal obstructions classifiable to P76-
     obstruction of duodenum (K31.5)
     postprocedural intestinal obstruction ▶(K91.3-)◄
     stenosis of anus or rectum (K62.4)

   K56.0   **Paralytic ileus**   HCC
     Paralysis of bowel   Paralysis of intestine
     Paralysis of colon
     EXCLUDES 1   *gallstone ileus (K56.3)*
         ileus NOS (K56.7)
         obstructive ileus NOS ▶(K56.69-)◄

   K56.1   **Intussusception**   HCC
     Intussusception or invagination of bowel
     Intussusception or invagination of colon
     Intussusception or invagination of intestine
     Intussusception or invagination of rectum
     EXCLUDES 2   *intussusception of appendix (K38.8)*
     DEF: Intestinal obstruction due to prolapse of a bowel section into
     adjacent section; occurs primarily in children; symptoms include
     acute abdominal pain, vomiting, and passage of blood and mucus
     from rectum.

   K56.2   **Volvulus**   HCC
     Strangulation of colon or intestine
     Torsion of colon or intestine
     Twist of colon or intestine
     EXCLUDES 2   *volvulus of duodenum (K31.5)*

Volvulus

Knotted
intestine
(volvulus)

☑ Additional Character Req   ☑7ᵗʰ Placeholder Alert   Manifestation   HCC CMS-HCC Condition   ▽ Unspecified Code   ▶◄ Revised Text   ● New Code   ▲ Revised Code Title

ICD-10-CM 2018   683

K56.3 Gallstone ileus HCC
Obstruction of intestine by gallstone

✓5ᵗʰ **K56.4 Other impaction of intestine**

K56.41 Fecal impaction HCC
EXCLUDES 1 constipation (K59.0-)
incomplete defecation (R15.0)

K56.49 Other impaction of intestine HCC

▲ ✓5ᵗʰ **K56.5 Intestinal adhesions [bands] with obstruction (postinfection)**
Abdominal hernia due to adhesions with obstruction
▶Peritoneal adhesions [bands] with intestinal obstruction (postinfection)◀

● **K56.50 Intestinal adhesions [bands], unspecified as to partial versus complete obstruction** ▽
Intestinal adhesions with obstruction NOS

● **K56.51 Intestinal adhesions [bands], with partial obstruction**
Intestinal adhesions with incomplete obstruction

● **K56.52 Intestinal adhesions [bands] with complete obstruction**

✓5ᵗʰ **K56.6 Other and unspecified intestinal obstruction**
AHA: 2017, 2Q, 12

✓6ᵗʰ **K56.60 Unspecified intestinal obstruction**
Intestinal obstruction NOS
EXCLUDES 1 intestinal obstruction due to specified condition—code to condition

● **K56.600 Partial intestinal obstruction, unspecified as to cause** ▽
Incomplete intestinal obstruction, NOS

● **K56.601 Complete intestinal obstruction, unspecified as to cause** ▽

● **K56.609 Unspecified intestinal obstruction, unspecified as to partial versus complete obstruction** ▽
Intestinal obstruction NOS

✓6ᵗʰ **K56.69 Other intestinal obstruction**
Enterostenosis NOS
Obstructive ileus NOS
Occlusion of colon or intestine NOS
Stenosis of colon or intestine NOS
Stricture of colon or intestine NOS
EXCLUDES 1 intestinal obstruction due to specified condition—code to condition

● **K56.690 Other partial intestinal obstruction**
Other incomplete intestinal obstruction

● **K56.691 Other complete intestinal obstruction**

● **K56.699 Other intestinal obstruction unspecified as to partial versus complete obstruction** ▽
Other intestinal obstruction, NEC

K56.7 Ileus, unspecified HCC ▽
EXCLUDES 1 obstructive ileus ▶(K56.69-)◀
EXCLUDES 2 ▶intestinal obstruction with hernia (K40-K46)◀
AHA: 2017, 1Q, 40

✓4ᵗʰ **K57 Diverticular disease of intestine**
EXCLUDES 1 congenital diverticulum of intestine (Q43.8)
Meckel's diverticulum (Q43.0)
EXCLUDES 2 diverticulum of appendix (K38.2)

✓5ᵗʰ **K57.0 Diverticulitis of small intestine with perforation and abscess**
Diverticulitis of small intestine with peritonitis
EXCLUDES 1 diverticulitis of both small and large intestine with perforation and abscess (K57.4-)

K57.00 Diverticulitis of small intestine with perforation and abscess without bleeding

K57.01 Diverticulitis of small intestine with perforation and abscess with bleeding

✓5ᵗʰ **K57.1 Diverticular disease of small intestine without perforation or abscess**
EXCLUDES 1 diverticular disease of both small and large intestine without perforation or abscess (K57.5-)

K57.10 Diverticulosis of small intestine without perforation or abscess without bleeding
Diverticular disease of small intestine NOS

K57.11 Diverticulosis of small intestine without perforation or abscess with bleeding

K57.12 Diverticulitis of small intestine without perforation or abscess without bleeding

K57.13 Diverticulitis of small intestine without perforation or abscess with bleeding

✓5ᵗʰ **K57.2 Diverticulitis of large intestine with perforation and abscess**
Diverticulitis of colon with peritonitis
EXCLUDES 1 diverticulitis of both small and large intestine with perforation and abscess (K57.4-)

K57.20 Diverticulitis of large intestine with perforation and abscess without bleeding

K57.21 Diverticulitis of large intestine with perforation and abscess with bleeding

✓5ᵗʰ **K57.3 Diverticular disease of large intestine without perforation or abscess**
EXCLUDES 1 diverticular disease of both small and large intestine without perforation or abscess (K57.5-)

K57.30 Diverticulosis of large intestine without perforation or abscess without bleeding
Diverticular disease of colon NOS

K57.31 Diverticulosis of large intestine without perforation or abscess with bleeding

K57.32 Diverticulitis of large intestine without perforation or abscess without bleeding

K57.33 Diverticulitis of large intestine without perforation or abscess with bleeding

✓5ᵗʰ **K57.4 Diverticulitis of both small and large intestine with perforation and abscess**
Diverticulitis of both small and large intestine with peritonitis

K57.40 Diverticulitis of both small and large intestine with perforation and abscess without bleeding

K57.41 Diverticulitis of both small and large intestine with perforation and abscess with bleeding

✓5ᵗʰ **K57.5 Diverticular disease of both small and large intestine without perforation or abscess**

K57.50 Diverticulosis of both small and large intestine without perforation or abscess without bleeding
Diverticular disease of both small and large intestine NOS

K57.51 Diverticulosis of both small and large intestine without perforation or abscess with bleeding

K57.52 Diverticulitis of both small and large intestine without perforation or abscess without bleeding

K57.53 Diverticulitis of both small and large intestine without perforation or abscess with bleeding

✓5ᵗʰ **K57.8 Diverticulitis of intestine, part unspecified, with perforation and abscess**
Diverticulitis of intestine NOS with peritonitis

K57.80 Diverticulitis of intestine, part unspecified, with perforation and abscess without bleeding ▽

K57.81 Diverticulitis of intestine, part unspecified, with perforation and abscess with bleeding ▽

✓5ᵗʰ **K57.9 Diverticular disease of intestine, part unspecified, without perforation or abscess**

K57.90 Diverticulosis of intestine, part unspecified, without perforation or abscess without bleeding ▽
Diverticular disease of intestine NOS

K57.91 Diverticulosis of intestine, part unspecified, without perforation or abscess with bleeding ▽

K57.92 Diverticulitis of intestine, part unspecified, without perforation or abscess without bleeding ▽

K57.93 Diverticulitis of intestine, part unspecified, without perforation or abscess with bleeding ▽

✓4ᵗʰ **K58 Irritable bowel syndrome**
INCLUDES irritable colon
spastic colon

K58.0 Irritable bowel syndrome with diarrhea

K58.1 Irritable bowel syndrome with constipation

K58.2 Mixed irritable bowel syndrome

K58.8 Other irritable bowel syndrome

K58.9 Irritable bowel syndrome without diarrhea
Irritable bowel syndrome NOS

✓4ᵗʰ K59 Other functional intestinal disorders

EXCLUDES1   change in bowel habit NOS (R19.4)
     intestinal malabsorption (K90.-)
     psychogenic intestinal disorders (F45.8)
EXCLUDES2   functional disorders of stomach (K31.-)

✓5ᵗʰ K59.0 Constipation
Use additional code for adverse effect, if applicable, to identify drug (T36-T50 with fifth or sixth character 5)
EXCLUDES1   fecal impaction (K56.41)
     incomplete defecation (R15.0)

K59.00 Constipation, unspecified   ▽
K59.01 Slow transit constipation
DEF: Delay in the transit of fecal material through the colon secondary to smooth muscle dysfunction or decreased peristaltic contractions along the colon: also called colonic inertia or delayed transit.
K59.02 Outlet dysfunction constipation
K59.03 Drug induced constipation
Use additional code for adverse effect, if applicable, to identify drug (T36-T50 with fifth or sixth character 5)
K59.04 Chronic idiopathic constipation
Functional constipation
K59.09 Other constipation
Chronic constipation

K59.1 Functional diarrhea
EXCLUDES1   diarrhea NOS (R19.7)
     irritable bowel syndrome with diarrhea (K58.0)

K59.2 Neurogenic bowel, not elsewhere classified
DEF: Disorder of bowel due to spinal cord lesion due to injury or as a complication of conditions such as multiple sclerosis (MS) or spina bifida; loss of bowel control is the primary symptom, manifested as constipation or bowel incontinence.

✓5ᵗʰ K59.3 Megacolon, not elsewhere classified
Dilatation of colon
Code first, if applicable (T51-T65) to identify toxic agent
EXCLUDES1   congenital megacolon (aganglionic) (Q43.1)
     megacolon (due to) (in) Chagas' disease (B57.32)
     megacolon (due to) (in) Clostridium difficile
       ▶(A04.7-)◀
     megacolon (due to) (in) Hirschsprung's disease (Q43.1)

K59.31 Toxic megacolon   HCC
K59.39 Other megacolon
Megacolon NOS

K59.4 Anal spasm
Proctalgia fugax

K59.8 Other specified functional intestinal disorders
Atony of colon
Pseudo-obstruction (acute) (chronic) of intestine

K59.9 Functional intestinal disorder, unspecified   ▽

✓4ᵗʰ K60 Fissure and fistula of anal and rectal regions

EXCLUDES1   fissure and fistula of anal and rectal regions with abscess or cellulitis (K61.-)
EXCLUDES2   anal sphincter tear (healed) (nontraumatic) (old) (K62.81)

K60.0 Acute anal fissure
K60.1 Chronic anal fissure
K60.2 Anal fissure, unspecified   ▽
K60.3 Anal fistula
K60.4 Rectal fistula
Fistula of rectum to skin
EXCLUDES1   rectovaginal fistula (N82.3)
     vesicorectal fistual (N32.1)
K60.5 Anorectal fistula

✓4ᵗʰ K61 Abscess of anal and rectal regions

INCLUDES   abscess of anal and rectal regions
     cellulitis of anal and rectal regions

K61.0 Anal abscess
Perianal abscess
EXCLUDES1   intrasphincteric abscess (K61.4)
K61.1 Rectal abscess
Perirectal abscess
EXCLUDES1   ischiorectal abscess (K61.3)
AHA: 2012, 4Q, 104
K61.2 Anorectal abscess
K61.3 Ischiorectal abscess
Abscess of ischiorectal fossa
K61.4 Intrasphincteric abscess

✓4ᵗʰ K62 Other diseases of anus and rectum

INCLUDES   anal canal
EXCLUDES2   colostomy and enterostomy malfunction (K94.0-, K94.1-)
     fecal incontinence (R15.-)
     hemorrhoids (K64.-)

K62.0 Anal polyp
K62.1 Rectal polyp
EXCLUDES1   adenomatous polyp (D12.8)
K62.2 Anal prolapse
Prolapse of anal canal
K62.3 Rectal prolapse
Prolapse of rectal mucosa
K62.4 Stenosis of anus and rectum
Stricture of anus (sphincter)
K62.5 Hemorrhage of anus and rectum
EXCLUDES1   gastrointestinal bleeding NOS (K92.2)
     melena (K92.1)
     neonatal rectal hemorrhage (P54.2)
K62.6 Ulcer of anus and rectum
Solitary ulcer of anus and rectum
Stercoral ulcer of anus and rectum
EXCLUDES1   fissure and fistula of anus and rectum (K60.-)
     ulcerative colitis (K51.-)
K62.7 Radiation proctitis
Use additional code to identify the type of radiation (W90.-)

✓5ᵗʰ K62.8 Other specified diseases of anus and rectum
EXCLUDES2   ulcerative proctitis (K51.2)

K62.81 Anal sphincter tear (healed) (nontraumatic) (old)
Tear of anus, nontraumatic
Use additional code for any associated fecal incontinence (R15.-)
EXCLUDES2   anal fissure (K60.-)
     anal sphincter tear (healed) (old) complicating delivery (O34.7-)
     traumatic tear of anal sphincter (S31.831)

K62.82 Dysplasia of anus
Anal intraepithelial neoplasia I and II (AIN I and II) (histologically confirmed)
Dysplasia of anus NOS
Mild and moderate dysplasia of anus (histologically confirmed)
EXCLUDES1   abnormal results from anal cytologic examination without histologic confirmation (R85.61-)
     anal intraepithelial neoplasia III (D01.3)
     carcinoma in situ of anus (D01.3)
     HGSIL of anus (R85.613)
     severe dysplasia of anus (D01.3)

K62.89 Other specified diseases of anus and rectum
Proctitis NOS
Use additional code for any associated fecal incontinence (R15.-)

K62.9 Disease of anus and rectum, unspecified   ▽

✓4ᵗʰ K63 Other diseases of intestine

K63.0 Abscess of intestine
EXCLUDES1   abscess of intestine with Crohn's disease (K50.014, K50.114, K50.814, K50.914)
     abscess of intestine with diverticular disease (K57.0, K57.2, K57.4, K57.8)
     abscess of intestine with ulcerative colitis (K51.014, K51.214, K51.314, K51.414, K51.514, K51.814, K51.914)
EXCLUDES2   abscess of anal and rectal regions (K61.-)
     abscess of appendix (K35.3)

K63.1 Perforation of intestine (nontraumatic)   HCC
Perforation (nontraumatic) of rectum
EXCLUDES1   perforation (nontraumatic) of duodenum (K26.-)
     perforation (nontraumatic) of intestine with diverticular disease (K57.0, K57.2, K57.4, K57.8)
EXCLUDES2   perforation (nontraumatic) of appendix (K35.2, K35.3)

✓ Additional Character Req   ✓x7ᵗʰ Placeholder Alert   Manifestation   HCC CMS-HCC Condition   ▽ Unspecified Code   ▶◀ Revised Text   ● New Code   ▲ Revised Code Title

K63.2 Fistula of intestine
EXCLUDES 1   fistula of duodenum (K31.6)
     fistula of intestine with Crohn's disease (K5Ø.Ø13,
        K5Ø.113, K5Ø.813, K5Ø.913)
     fistula of intestine with ulcerative colitis (K51.Ø13,
        K51.213, K51.313, K51.413, K51.513, K51.813,
        K51.913)
EXCLUDES 2   fistula of anal and rectal regions (K6Ø.-)
     fistula of appendix (K38.3)
     intestinal-genital fistula, female (N82.2-N82.4)
     vesicointestinal fistula (N32.1)

K63.3 Ulcer of intestine
Primary ulcer of small intestine
EXCLUDES 1   duodenal ulcer (K26.-)
     gastrointestinal ulcer (K28.-)
     gastrojejunal ulcer (K28.-)
     jejunal ulcer (K28.-)
     peptic ulcer, site unspecified (K27.-)
     ulcer of intestine with perforation (K63.1)
     ulcer of anus or rectum (K62.6)
     ulcerative colitis (K51.-)

K63.4 Enteroptosis

K63.5 Polyp of colon
EXCLUDES 1   adenomatous polyp of colon (D12.6)
     inflammatory polyp of colon (K51.4-)
     polyposis of colon (D12.6)
AHA: 2017, 1Q, 15; 2015, 2Q, 14

✓5ᵗʰ **K63.8 Other specified diseases of intestine**

     K63.81 Dieulafoy lesion of intestine
        EXCLUDES 2   Dieulafoy lesion of stomach and duodenum
            (K31.82)

     K63.89 Other specified diseases of intestine
        AHA: 2013, 2Q, 31

K63.9 Disease of intestine, unspecified   ▽

✓4ᵗʰ **K64 Hemorrhoids and perianal venous thrombosis**
INCLUDES   piles
EXCLUDES 1   hemorrhoids complicating childbirth and the puerperium
        (O87.2)
     hemorrhoids complicating pregnancy (O22.4)

K64.Ø First degree hemorrhoids
Grade/stage I hemorrhoids
Hemorrhoids (bleeding) without prolapse outside of anal canal

K64.1 Second degree hemorrhoids
Grade/stage II hemorrhoids
Hemorrhoids (bleeding) that prolapse with straining, but retract
    spontaneously

K64.2 Third degree hemorrhoids
Grade/stage III hemorrhoids
Hemorrhoids (bleeding) that prolapse with straining and require
    manual replacement back inside anal cana

K64.3 Fourth degree hemorrhoids
Grade/stage IV hemorrhoids
Hemorrhoids (bleeding) with prolapsed tissue that cannot be
    manually replaced

K64.4 Residual hemorrhoidal skin tags
External hemorrhoids, NOS
Skin tags of anus

Hemorrhoids

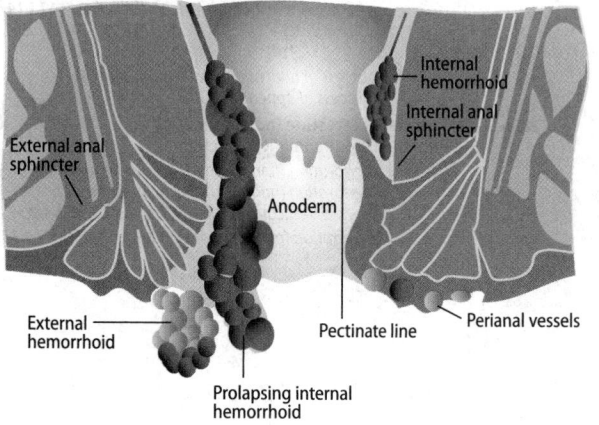

External anal sphincter
External hemorrhoid
Anoderm
Pectinate line
Prolapsing internal hemorrhoid
Internal hemorrhoid
Internal anal sphincter
Perianal vessels

K64.5 Perianal venous thrombosis
External hemorrhoids with thrombosis
Perianal hematoma
Thrombosed hemorrhoids NOS

K64.8 Other hemorrhoids
Internal hemorrhoids, without mention of degree
Prolapsed hemorrhoids, degree not specified

K64.9 Unspecified hemorrhoids   ▽
Hemorrhoids (bleeding) NOS
Hemorrhoids (bleeding) without mention of degree

Diseases of peritoneum and retroperitoneum (K65-K68)

✓4ᵗʰ **K65 Peritonitis**
Use additional code (B95-B97), to identify infectious agent
EXCLUDES 1   acute appendicitis with generalized peritonitis (K35.2)
     aseptic peritonitis (T81.6)
     benign paroxysmal peritonitis (E85.Ø)
     chemical peritonitis (T81.6)
     diverticulitis of both small and large intestine with peritonitis
        (K57.4-)
     diverticulitis of colon with peritonitis (K57.2-)
     diverticulitis of intestine, NOS, with peritonitis (K57.8-)
     diverticulitis of small intestine with peritonitis (K57.Ø-)
     gonococcal peritonitis (A54.85)
     neonatal peritonitis (P78.Ø-P78.1)
     pelvic peritonitis, female (N73.3-N73.5)
     periodic familial peritonitis (E85.Ø)
     peritonitis due to talc or other foreign substance (T81.6)
     peritonitis in chlamydia (A74.81)
     peritonitis in diphtheria (A36.89)
     peritonitis in syphilis (late) (A52.74)
     peritonitis in tuberculosis (A18.31)
     peritonitis with or following abortion or ectopic or molar
        pregnancy (OØØ-OØ7, OØ8.Ø)
     peritonitis with or following appendicitis (K35.-)
     peritonitis with or following diverticular disease of intestine
        (K57.-)
     puerperal peritonitis (O85)
     retroperitoneal infections (K68.-)

K65.Ø Generalized (acute) peritonitis   HCC
Pelvic peritonitis (acute), male
Subphrenic peritonitis (acute)
Suppurative peritonitis (acute)

K65.1 Peritoneal abscess   HCC
Abdominopelvic abscess   Subdiaphragmatic abscess
Abscess (of) omentum   Subhepatic abscess
Abscess (of) peritoneum   Subphrenic abscess
Mesenteric abscess
Retrocecal abscess

K65.2 Spontaneous bacterial peritonitis   HCC
EXCLUDES 1   bacterial peritonitis NOS (K65.9)

K65.3 Choleperitonitis   HCC
Peritonitis due to bile
DEF: Inflammation of the peritoneum due to leakage of bile into
the peritoneal cavity resulting from rupture of the bile passages or
gallbladder.

K65.4 Sclerosing mesenteritis   HCC
Fat necrosis of peritoneum
(Idiopathic) sclerosing mesenteric fibrosis
Mesenteric lipodystrophy
Mesenteric panniculitis
Retractile mesenteritis

K65.8 Other peritonitis   HCC
Chronic proliferative peritonitis
Peritonitis due to urine

K65.9 Peritonitis, unspecified   HCC ▽
Bacterial peritonitis NOS
AHA: 2013, 2Q, 31

✓4ᵗʰ **K66 Other disorders of peritoneum**
EXCLUDES 2   ascites (R18.-)
     peritoneal effusion (chronic) (R18.8)

K66.Ø Peritoneal adhesions (postprocedural) (postinfection)
Adhesions (of) abdominal (wall)   Adhesions (of) omentum
Adhesions (of) diaphragm   Adhesions (of) stomach
Adhesions (of) intestine   Adhesive bands
Adhesions (of) male pelvis   Mesenteric adhesions
    EXCLUDES 1   female pelvic adhesions [bands] (N73.6)
        peritoneal adhesions with intestinal obstruction
           ▶(K56.5-)◀

EXCLUDES 1   Not coded here   EXCLUDES 2   Not included here   N   Newborn Age: 0   P   Pediatric Age: 0-17   M   Maternity Age: 12-55   A   Adult Age: 15-124

686   ICD-10-CM 2018

K66.1   **Hemoperitoneum**
> EXCLUDES 1   *traumatic hemoperitoneum (S36.8-)*

K66.8   **Other specified disorders of peritoneum**

K66.9   **Disorder of peritoneum, unspecified**   ▽

K67   *Disorders of peritoneum in infectious diseases classified elsewhere*   HCC
> Code first underlying disease, such as:
>   congenital syphilis (A50.0)
>   helminthiasis (B65.0-B83.9)
> EXCLUDES 1   *peritonitis in chlamydia (A74.81)*
>   *peritonitis in diphtheria (A36.89)*
>   *peritonitis in gonococcal (A54.85)*
>   *peritonitis in syphilis (late) (A52.74)*
>   *peritonitis in tuberculosis (A18.31)*

✓4th **K68**   **Disorders of retroperitoneum**

   ✓5th **K68.1**   **Retroperitoneal abscess**

     K68.11   **Postprocedural** retroperitoneal abscess

     K68.12   **Psoas muscle** abscess   HCC

     K68.19   **Other retroperitoneal abscess**   HCC

   K68.9   **Other disorders of retroperitoneum**

Diseases of liver (K70-K77)

> EXCLUDES 1   *jaundice NOS (R17)*
> EXCLUDES 2   *hemochromatosis (E83.11-)*
>   *Reye's syndrome (G93.7)*
>   *viral hepatitis (B15-B19)*
>   *Wilson's disease (E83.0)*

✓4th **K70**   **Alcoholic liver disease**
> Use additional code to identify:
>   alcohol abuse and dependence (F10.-)

   K70.0   **Alcoholic** fatty liver   A

   ✓5th **K70.1**   **Alcoholic** hepatitis

     K70.10   **Alcoholic hepatitis** without ascites   A

     K70.11   **Alcoholic hepatitis** with ascites   A

   K70.2   **Alcoholic** fibrosis and sclerosis **of liver**   A

   ✓5th **K70.3**   **Alcoholic** cirrhosis **of liver**
> Alcoholic cirrhosis NOS

     K70.30   **Alcoholic cirrhosis of liver** without ascites   HCC A

     K70.31   **Alcoholic cirrhosis of liver** with ascites   HCC A

   ✓5th **K70.4**   **Alcoholic** hepatic failure
> Acute alcoholic hepatic failure
> Alcoholic hepatic failure NOS
> Chronic alcoholic hepatic failure
> Subacute alcoholic hepatic failure

     K70.40   **Alcoholic hepatic failure** without coma   HCC A

     K70.41   **Alcoholic hepatic failure** with coma   HCC A

   K70.9   **Alcoholic liver disease, unspecified**   HCC A ▽

✓4th **K71**   **Toxic liver disease**
> INCLUDES   drug-induced idiosyncratic (unpredictable) liver disease
>   drug-induced toxic (predictable) liver disease
> Code first poisoning due to drug or toxin, if applicable (T36-T65 with fifth or sixth character 1-4 or 6)
> Use additional code for adverse effect, if applicable, to identify drug (T36-T50 with fifth or sixth character 5)
> EXCLUDES 2   *alcoholic liver disease (K70.-)*
>   *Budd-Chiari syndrome (I82.0)*

   K71.0   **Toxic liver disease with** cholestasis
> Cholestasis with hepatocyte injury
> "Pure" cholestasis

   ✓5th **K71.1**   **Toxic liver disease with** hepatic necrosis
> Hepatic failure (acute) (chronic) due to drugs

     K71.10   **Toxic liver disease with hepatic necrosis, without coma**

     K71.11   **Toxic liver disease with hepatic necrosis, with coma**   HCC

   K71.2   **Toxic liver disease with** acute hepatitis

   K71.3   **Toxic liver disease with** chronic persistent hepatitis

   K71.4   **Toxic liver disease with** chronic lobular hepatitis

   ✓5th **K71.5**   **Toxic liver disease with** chronic active hepatitis
> Toxic liver disease with lupoid hepatitis

     K71.50   **Toxic liver disease with chronic active hepatitis without ascites**

     K71.51   **Toxic liver disease with chronic active hepatitis with ascites**

K71.6   **Toxic liver disease with** hepatitis, not elsewhere classified

K71.7   **Toxic liver disease with** fibrosis and cirrhosis **of liver**

K71.8   **Toxic liver disease with other disorders of liver**
> Toxic liver disease with focal nodular hyperplasia
> Toxic liver disease with hepatic granulomas
> Toxic liver disease with peliosis hepatis
> Toxic liver disease with veno-occlusive disease of liver

K71.9   **Toxic liver disease, unspecified**   ▽

✓4th **K72**   **Hepatic failure, not elsewhere classified**
> INCLUDES   fulminant hepatitis NEC, with hepatic failure
>   hepatic encephalopathy NOS
>   liver (cell) necrosis with hepatic failure
>   malignant hepatitis NEC, with hepatic failure
>   yellow liver atrophy or dystrophy
> EXCLUDES 1   *alcoholic hepatic failure (K70.4)*
>   *hepatic failure with toxic liver disease (K71.1-)*
>   *icterus of newborn (P55-P59)*
>   *postprocedural hepatic failure (K91.82)*
> EXCLUDES 2   *hepatic failure complicating abortion or ectopic or molar pregnancy (O00-O07, O08.8)*
>   *hepatic failure complicating pregnancy, childbirth and the puerperium (O26.6-)*
>   *viral hepatitis with hepatic coma (B15-B19)*
> AHA: 2017, 1Q, 41

   ✓5th **K72.0**   **Acute and subacute** hepatic failure
> Acute non-viral hepatitis NOS
> AHA: 2015, 2Q, 17; 2014, 2Q, 13

     K72.00   **Acute and subacute hepatic failure** without coma

     K72.01   **Acute and subacute hepatic failure** with coma   HCC

   ✓5th **K72.1**   **Chronic** hepatic failure

     K72.10   **Chronic hepatic failure** without coma   HCC

     K72.11   **Chronic hepatic failure** with coma   HCC

   ✓5th **K72.9**   **Hepatic failure, unspecified**

     K72.90   **Hepatic failure, unspecified** without coma   HCC ▽
> AHA: 2016, 2Q, 35

     K72.91   **Hepatic failure, unspecified** with coma   HCC ▽
> Hepatic coma NOS

✓4th **K73**   **Chronic hepatitis, not elsewhere classified**
> EXCLUDES 1   *alcoholic hepatitis (chronic) (K70.1-)*
>   *drug-induced hepatitis (chronic) (K71.-)*
>   *granulomatous hepatitis (chronic) NEC (K75.3)*
>   *reactive, nonspecific hepatitis (chronic) (K75.2)*
>   *viral hepatitis (chronic) (B15-B19)*

   K73.0   **Chronic** persistent **hepatitis, not elsewhere classified**   HCC

   K73.1   **Chronic** lobular **hepatitis, not elsewhere classified**   HCC

   K73.2   **Chronic** active **hepatitis, not elsewhere classified**   HCC

   K73.8   **Other chronic hepatitis, not elsewhere classified**   HCC

   K73.9   **Chronic hepatitis, unspecified**   HCC ▽

✓4th **K74**   **Fibrosis and cirrhosis of liver**
> Code also, if applicable, viral hepatitis (acute) (chronic) (B15-B19)
> EXCLUDES 1   *alcoholic cirrhosis (of liver) (K70.3)*
>   *alcoholic fibrosis of liver (K70.2)*
>   *cardiac sclerosis of liver (K76.1)*
>   *cirrhosis (of liver) with toxic liver disease (K71.7)*
>   *congenital cirrhosis (of liver) (P78.81)*
>   *pigmentary cirrhosis (of liver) (E83.110)*

   K74.0   **Hepatic** fibrosis

   K74.1   **Hepatic** sclerosis

   K74.2   **Hepatic** fibrosis with hepatic sclerosis

   K74.3   **Primary biliary cirrhosis**   HCC
> Chronic nonsuppurative destructive cholangitis

   K74.4   **Secondary biliary cirrhosis**   HCC

   K74.5   **Biliary cirrhosis, unspecified**   HCC ▽

   ✓5th **K74.6**   **Other and unspecified cirrhosis of liver**

     K74.60   **Unspecified cirrhosis of liver**   HCC ▽
> Cirrhosis (of liver) NOS

     K74.69   **Other cirrhosis of liver**   HCC
> Cryptogenic cirrhosis (of liver)
> Macronodular cirrhosis (of liver)
> Micronodular cirrhosis (of liver)
> Mixed type cirrhosis (of liver)
> Portal cirrhosis (of liver)
> Postnecrotic cirrhosis (of liver)

✓ Additional Character Req   ✓×7th Placeholder Alert   Manifestation   HCC CMS-HCC Condition   ▽ Unspecified Code   ►◄ Revised Text   ● New Code   ▲ Revised Code Title

ICD-10-CM 2018   687

K66.1–K74.69

Chapter 11. Diseases of the Digestive System

✓4ᵗʰ **K75** **Other inflammatory liver diseases**
> EXCLUDES 2   toxic liver disease (K71.-)

K75.0   **Abscess of liver**
Cholangitic hepatic abscess
Hematogenic hepatic abscess
Hepatic abscess NOS
Lymphogenic hepatic abscess
Pylephlebitic hepatic abscess
> EXCLUDES 1   amebic liver abscess (A06.4)
> cholangitis without liver abscess (K83.0)
> pylephlebitis without liver abscess (K75.1)

> EXCLUDES 2   acute or subacute hepatitis NOS (B17.9)
> acute or subacute non-viral hepatitis (K72.0)
> chronic hepatitis NEC (K73.8)

K75.1   **Phlebitis of portal vein**
Pylephlebitis
> EXCLUDES 1   pylephlebitic liver abscess (K75.0)

DEF: Inflammation of portal vein or branches; may be due to diverticulitis, perforated appendicitis, or peritonitis; symptoms include fever, chills, jaundice, sweating, and abscess in various body parts.

K75.2   **Nonspecific reactive hepatitis**
> EXCLUDES 1   acute or subacute hepatitis (K72.0-)
> chronic hepatitis NEC (K73.-)
> viral hepatitis (B15-B19)

K75.3   **Granulomatous hepatitis, not elsewhere classified**
> EXCLUDES 1   acute or subacute hepatitis (K72.0-)
> chronic hepatitis NEC (K73.-)
> viral hepatitis (B15-B19)

K75.4   **Autoimmune hepatitis**   HCC
Lupoid hepatitis NEC

✓5ᵗʰ **K75.8**   **Other specified inflammatory liver diseases**
    K75.81   **Nonalcoholic steatohepatitis (NASH)**
    K75.89   **Other specified inflammatory liver diseases**

K75.9   **Inflammatory liver disease, unspecified**   ▽
Hepatitis NOS
> EXCLUDES 1   acute or subacute hepatitis (K72.0-)
> chronic hepatitis NEC (K73.-)
> viral hepatitis (B15-B19)

AHA: 2015, 2Q, 17

✓4ᵗʰ **K76** **Other diseases of liver**
> EXCLUDES 2   alcoholic liver disease (K70.-)
> amyloid degeneration of liver (E85.-)
> cystic disease of liver (congenital) (Q44.6)
> hepatic vein thrombosis (I82.0)
> hepatomegaly NOS (R16.0)
> pigmentary cirrhosis (of liver) (E83.110)
> portal vein thrombosis (I81)
> toxic liver disease (K71.-)

K76.0   **Fatty (change of) liver, not elsewhere classified**
Nonalcoholic fatty liver disease (NAFLD)
> EXCLUDES 1   nonalcoholic steatohepatitis (NASH) (K75.81)

K76.1   **Chronic passive congestion of liver**
Cardiac cirrhosis
Cardiac sclerosis

K76.2   **Central hemorrhagic necrosis of liver**
> EXCLUDES 1   liver necrosis with hepatic failure (K72.-)

K76.3   **Infarction of liver**

K76.4   **Peliosis hepatis**
Hepatic angiomatosis

K76.5   **Hepatic veno-occlusive disease**
> EXCLUDES 1   Budd-Chiari syndrome (I82.0)

K76.6   **Portal hypertension**   HCC
Use additional code for any associated complications, such as:
portal hypertensive gastropathy (K31.89)

K76.7   **Hepatorenal syndrome**   HCC
> EXCLUDES 1   hepatorenal syndrome following labor and delivery (O90.4)
> postprocedural hepatorenal syndrome (K91.83)

✓5ᵗʰ **K76.8**   **Other specified diseases of liver**
    K76.81   **Hepatopulmonary syndrome**   HCC
Code first underlying liver disease, such as:
alcoholic cirrhosis of liver (K70.3-)
cirrhosis of liver without mention of alcohol (K74.6-)

    K76.89   **Other specified diseases of liver**
Cyst (simple) of liver
Focal nodular hyperplasia of liver
Hepatoptosis

K76.9   **Liver disease, unspecified**   ▽

K77   *Liver disorders in diseases classified elsewhere*
Code first underlying disease, such as:
amyloidosis (E85.-)
congenital syphilis (A50.0, A50.5)
congenital toxoplasmosis (P37.1)
schistosomiasis (B65.0-B65.9)
> EXCLUDES 1   alcoholic hepatitis (K70.1-)
> alcoholic liver disease (K70-.)
> cytomegaloviral hepatitis (B25.1)
> herpesviral [herpes simplex] hepatitis (B00.81)
> infectious mononucleosis with liver disease (B27.0-B27.9 with .9)
> mumps hepatitis (B26.81)
> sarcoidosis with liver disease (D86.89)
> secondary syphilis with liver disease (A51.45)
> syphilis (late) with liver disease (A52.74)
> toxoplasmosis (acquired) hepatitis (B58.1)
> tuberculosis with liver disease (A18.83)

Disorders of gallbladder, biliary tract and pancreas (K80-K87)

✓4ᵗʰ **K80** **Cholelithiasis**
> EXCLUDES 1   retained cholelithiasis following cholecystectomy (K91.86)

✓5ᵗʰ **K80.0**   **Calculus of gallbladder with acute cholecystitis**
Any condition listed in K80.2 with acute cholecystitis

    K80.00   **Calculus of gallbladder with acute cholecystitis without obstruction**

    K80.01   **Calculus of gallbladder with acute cholecystitis with obstruction**

✓5ᵗʰ **K80.1**   **Calculus of gallbladder with other cholecystitis**

    K80.10   **Calculus of gallbladder with chronic cholecystitis without obstruction**
Cholelithiasis with cholecystitis NOS

    K80.11   **Calculus of gallbladder with chronic cholecystitis with obstruction**

    K80.12   **Calculus of gallbladder with acute and chronic cholecystitis without obstruction**

    K80.13   **Calculus of gallbladder with acute and chronic cholecystitis with obstruction**

    K80.18   **Calculus of gallbladder with other cholecystitis without obstruction**

    K80.19   **Calculus of gallbladder with other cholecystitis with obstruction**

✓5ᵗʰ **K80.2**   **Calculus of gallbladder without cholecystitis**
Cholecystolithiasis without cholecystitis
Cholelithiasis (without cholecystitis)
Colic (recurrent) of gallbladder (without cholecystitis)
Gallstone (impacted) of cystic duct (without cholecystitis)
Gallstone (impacted) of gallbladder (without cholecystitis)

    K80.20   **Calculus of gallbladder without cholecystitis without obstruction**

    K80.21   **Calculus of gallbladder without cholecystitis with obstruction**

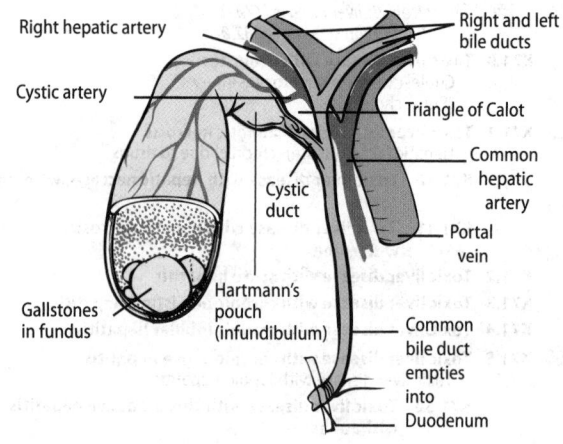

Cholelithiasis

Right hepatic artery
Cystic artery
Cystic duct
Gallstones in fundus
Hartmann's pouch (infundibulum)
Right and left bile ducts
Triangle of Calot
Common hepatic artery
Portal vein
Common bile duct empties into Duodenum

EXCLUDES 1 Not coded here   EXCLUDES 2 Not included here   N Newborn Age: 0   P Pediatric Age: 0-17   M Maternity Age: 12-55   A Adult Age: 15-124

688   ICD-10-CM 2018

✓5ᵗʰ **K80.3**　**Calculus of** bile duct with cholangitis
　　　　Any condition listed in K80.5 with cholangitis

　　　K80.30　**Calculus of bile duct with cholangitis, unspecified,** without obstruction ▽

　　　K80.31　**Calculus of bile duct with cholangitis, unspecified,** with obstruction ▽

　　　K80.32　**Calculus of bile duct with** acute **cholangitis** without obstruction

　　　K80.33　**Calculus of bile duct with** acute **cholangitis** with obstruction

　　　K80.34　**Calculus of bile duct with** chronic **cholangitis** without obstruction

　　　K80.35　**Calculus of bile duct with** chronic **cholangitis** with obstruction

　　　K80.36　**Calculus of bile duct with** acute and chronic **cholangitis** without obstruction

　　　K80.37　**Calculus of bile duct with** acute and chronic **cholangitis** with obstruction

✓5ᵗʰ **K80.4**　**Calculus of** bile duct with cholecystitis
　　　　Any condition listed in K80.5 with cholecystitis (with cholangitis)

　　　K80.40　**Calculus of bile duct with cholecystitis, unspecified,** without obstruction ▽

　　　K80.41　**Calculus of bile duct with cholecystitis, unspecified,** with obstruction ▽

　　　K80.42　**Calculus of bile duct with** acute **cholecystitis** without obstruction

　　　K80.43　**Calculus of bile duct with** acute **cholecystitis** with obstruction

　　　K80.44　**Calculus of bile duct with** chronic **cholecystitis** without obstruction

　　　K80.45　**Calculus of bile duct with** chronic **cholecystitis** with obstruction

　　　K80.46　**Calculus of bile duct with** acute and chronic **cholecystitis** without obstruction

　　　K80.47　**Calculus of bile duct with** acute and chronic **cholecystitis** with obstruction

✓5ᵗʰ **K80.5**　**Calculus of** bile duct without cholangitis or cholecystitis
　　　　Choledocholithiasis (without cholangitis or cholecystitis)
　　　　Gallstone (impacted) of bile duct NOS (without cholangitis or cholecystitis)
　　　　Gallstone (impacted) of common duct (without cholangitis or cholecystitis)
　　　　Gallstone (impacted) of hepatic duct (without cholangitis or cholecystitis)
　　　　Hepatic cholelithiasis (without cholangitis or cholecystitis)
　　　　Hepatic colic (recurrent) (without cholangitis or cholecystitis)

　　　K80.50　**Calculus of bile duct without cholangitis or cholecystitis** without obstruction

　　　K80.51　**Calculus of bile duct without cholangitis or cholecystitis** with obstruction

✓5ᵗʰ **K80.6**　**Calculus of** gallbladder and bile duct with cholecystitis

　　　K80.60　**Calculus of gallbladder and bile duct with cholecystitis, unspecified,** without obstruction ▽

　　　K80.61　**Calculus of gallbladder and bile duct with cholecystitis, unspecified,** with obstruction ▽

　　　K80.62　**Calculus of gallbladder and bile duct with** acute **cholecystitis** without obstruction

　　　K80.63　**Calculus of gallbladder and bile duct with** acute **cholecystitis** with obstruction

　　　K80.64　**Calculus of gallbladder and bile duct with** chronic **cholecystitis** without obstruction

　　　K80.65　**Calculus of gallbladder and bile duct with** chronic **cholecystitis** with obstruction

　　　K80.66　**Calculus of gallbladder and bile duct with** acute and chronic **cholecystitis** without obstruction

　　　K80.67　**Calculus of gallbladder and bile duct with** acute and chronic **cholecystitis** with obstruction

✓5ᵗʰ **K80.7**　**Calculus of** gallbladder and bile duct without cholecystitis

　　　K80.70　**Calculus of gallbladder and bile duct without cholecystitis** without obstruction

　　　K80.71　**Calculus of gallbladder and bile duct without cholecystitis** with obstruction

✓5ᵗʰ **K80.8**　**Other cholelithiasis**

　　　K80.80　**Other cholelithiasis** without obstruction

　　　K80.81　**Other cholelithiasis** with obstruction

✓4ᵗʰ **K81**　**Cholecystitis**
　　　EXCLUDES 1　cholecystitis with cholelithiasis (K80.-)

　　　K81.0　**Acute cholecystitis**
　　　　Abscess of gallbladder
　　　　Angiocholecystitis
　　　　Emphysematous (acute) cholecystitis
　　　　Empyema of gallbladder
　　　　Gangrene of gallbladder
　　　　Gangrenous cholecystitis
　　　　Suppurative cholecystitis

　　　K81.1　Chronic **cholecystitis**

　　　K81.2　Acute **cholecystitis** with chronic **cholecystitis**

　　　K81.9　**Cholecystitis, unspecified** ▽

✓4ᵗʰ **K82**　**Other diseases of gallbladder**
　　　EXCLUDES 1　nonvisualization of gallbladder (R93.2)
　　　　　　　　postcholecystectomy syndrome (K91.5)

　　　K82.0　**Obstruction of gallbladder**
　　　　Occlusion of cystic duct or gallbladder without cholelithiasis
　　　　Stenosis of cystic duct or gallbladder without cholelithiasis
　　　　Stricture of cystic duct or gallbladder without cholelithiasis
　　　　EXCLUDES 1　obstruction of gallbladder with cholelithiasis (K80.-)

　　　K82.1　**Hydrops of gallbladder**
　　　　Mucocele of gallbladder

　　　K82.2　**Perforation of gallbladder**
　　　　Rupture of cystic duct or gallbladder

　　　K82.3　**Fistula of gallbladder**
　　　　Cholecystocolic fistula
　　　　Cholecystoduodenal fistula

　　　K82.4　**Cholesterolosis of gallbladder**
　　　　Strawberry gallbladder
　　　　EXCLUDES 1　cholesterolosis of gallbladder with cholecystitis (K81.-)
　　　　　　　　cholesterolosis of gallbladder with cholelithiasis (K80.-)

　　　K82.8　**Other specified diseases of gallbladder**
　　　　Adhesions of cystic duct or gallbladder
　　　　Atrophy of cystic duct or gallbladder
　　　　Cyst of cystic duct or gallbladder
　　　　Dyskinesia of cystic duct or gallbladder
　　　　Hypertrophy of cystic duct or gallbladder
　　　　Nonfunctioning of cystic duct or gallbladder
　　　　Ulcer of cystic duct or gallbladder

　　　K82.9　**Disease of gallbladder, unspecified** ▽

✓4ᵗʰ **K83**　**Other diseases of biliary tract**
　　　EXCLUDES 1　postcholecystectomy syndrome (K91.5)
　　　EXCLUDES 2　conditions involving the gallbladder (K81-K82)
　　　　　　　　conditions involving the cystic duct (K81-K82)

　　　K83.0　**Cholangitis**
　　　　Ascending cholangitis
　　　　Cholangitis NOS
　　　　Primary cholangitis
　　　　Recurrent cholangitis
　　　　Sclerosing cholangitis
　　　　Secondary cholangitis
　　　　Stenosing cholangitis
　　　　Suppurative cholangitis
　　　　EXCLUDES 1　cholangitic liver abscess (K75.0)
　　　　　　　　cholangitis with choledocholithiasis (K80.3-, K80.4-)
　　　　　　　　chronic nonsuppurative destructive cholangitis (K74.3)

　　　K83.1　**Obstruction of bile duct**
　　　　Occlusion of bile duct without cholelithiasis
　　　　Stenosis of bile duct without cholelithiasis
　　　　Stricture of bile duct without cholelithiasis
　　　　EXCLUDES 1　congenital obstruction of bile duct (Q44.3)
　　　　　　　　obstruction of bile duct with cholelithiasis (K80.-)
　　　　AHA: 2016, 1Q, 18

　　　K83.2　**Perforation of bile duct**
　　　　Rupture of bile duct

　　　K83.3　**Fistula of bile duct**
　　　　Choledochoduodenal fistula

　　　K83.4　**Spasm of sphincter of Oddi**

　　　K83.5　**Biliary cyst**

　　　K83.8　**Other specified diseases of biliary tract**
　　　　Adhesions of biliary tract
　　　　Atrophy of biliary tract
　　　　Hypertrophy of biliary tract
　　　　Ulcer of biliary tract

　　　K83.9　**Disease of biliary tract, unspecified** ▽

✓ Additional Character Req　　✓×7ᵗʰ Placeholder Alert　　Manifestation　　HCC CMS-HCC Condition　　▽ Unspecified Code　　▶◀ Revised Text　　● New Code　　▲ Revised Code Title

✓4ᵗʰ **K85 Acute pancreatitis**
    INCLUDES acute (recurrent) pancreatitis
                 subacute pancreatitis

✓5ᵗʰ **K85.0 Idiopathic acute pancreatitis**

    K85.00 Idiopathic acute pancreatitis without necrosis or infection

    K85.01 Idiopathic acute pancreatitis with uninfected necrosis

    K85.02 Idiopathic acute pancreatitis with infected necrosis

✓5ᵗʰ **K85.1 Biliary acute pancreatitis**
    Gallstone pancreatitis

    K85.10 Biliary acute pancreatitis without necrosis or infection

    K85.11 Biliary acute pancreatitis with uninfected necrosis

    K85.12 Biliary acute pancreatitis with infected necrosis

✓5ᵗʰ **K85.2 Alcohol induced acute pancreatitis**
    EXCLUDES 2 alcohol induced chronic pancreatitis (K86.0)

    K85.20 Alcohol induced acute pancreatitis without necrosis or infection

    K85.21 Alcohol induced acute pancreatitis with uninfected necrosis

    K85.22 Alcohol induced acute pancreatitis with infected necrosis

✓5ᵗʰ **K85.3 Drug induced acute pancreatitis**
    Use additional code for adverse effect, if applicable, to identify drug (T36-T50 with fifth or sixth character 5)
    Use additional code to identify drug abuse and dependence (F11. – F17.-)

    K85.30 Drug induced acute pancreatitis without necrosis or infection

    K85.31 Drug induced acute pancreatitis with uninfected necrosis

    K85.32 Drug induced acute pancreatitis with infected necrosis

✓5ᵗʰ **K85.8 Other acute pancreatitis**

    K85.80 Other acute pancreatitis without necrosis or infection

    K85.81 Other acute pancreatitis with uninfected necrosis

    K85.82 Other acute pancreatitis with infected necrosis

✓5ᵗʰ **K85.9 Acute pancreatitis, unspecified**
    Pancreatitis NOS

    K85.90 Acute pancreatitis without necrosis or infection, unspecified ▽

    K85.91 Acute pancreatitis with uninfected necrosis, unspecified ▽

    K85.92 Acute pancreatitis with infected necrosis, unspecified ▽

✓4ᵗʰ **K86 Other diseases of pancreas**
    EXCLUDES 2 fibrocystic disease of pancreas (E84.-)
                 islet cell tumor (of pancreas) (D13.7)
                  pancreatic steatorrhea (K90.3)

    K86.0 Alcohol-induced chronic pancreatitis **HCC**
    Use additional code to identify:
       alcohol abuse and dependence (F10.-)
    Code also exocrine pancreatic insufficiency (K86.81)
    EXCLUDES 2 alcohol induced acute pancreatitis (K85.2-)

    K86.1 Other chronic pancreatitis **HCC**
    Chronic pancreatitis NOS
    Infectious chronic pancreatitis
    Recurrent chronic pancreatitis
    Relapsing chronic pancreatitis
    Code also exocrine pancreatic insufficiency (K86.81)

    K86.2 Cyst of pancreas

    K86.3 Pseudocyst of pancreas

✓5ᵗʰ **K86.8 Other specified diseases of pancreas**

    K86.81 Exocrine pancreatic insufficiency

    K86.89 Other specified diseases of pancreas
       Aseptic pancreatic necrosis, unrelated to acute pancreatitis
       Atrophy of pancreas
       Calculus of pancreas
       Cirrhosis of pancreas
       Fibrosis of pancreas
       Pancreatic fat necrosis, unrelated to acute pancreatitis
       Pancreatic infantilism
       Pancreatic necrosis NOS, unrelated to acute pancreatitis

K86.9 Disease of pancreas, unspecified ▽

K87 Disorders of gallbladder, biliary tract and pancreas in diseases classified elsewhere
    Code first underlying disease
    EXCLUDES 1 cytomegaloviral pancreatitis (B25.2)
                 mumps pancreatitis (B26.3)
                 syphilitic gallbladder (A52.74)
                 syphilitic pancreas (A52.74)
                 tuberculosis of gallbladder (A18.83)
                 tuberculosis of pancreas (A18.83)

Other diseases of the digestive system (K90-K95)

✓4ᵗʰ **K90 Intestinal malabsorption**
    EXCLUDES 1 intestinal malabsorption following gastrointestinal surgery (K91.2)

    K90.0 Celiac disease
    Celiac disease with steatorrhea
    ►Celiac gluten-sensitive enteropathy◄
    Nontropical sprue
    Use additional code for associated disorders including:
       dermatitis herpetiformis (L13.0)
       gluten ataxia (G32.81)
    Code also exocrine pancreatic insufficiency (K86.81)
    DEF: Malabsorption syndrome due to gluten consumption; symptoms include fetid, bulky, frothy, oily stools, distended abdomen, gas, asthenia, electrolyte depletion, and vitamin B, D, and K deficiency.

    K90.1 Tropical sprue
    Sprue NOS
    Tropical steatorrhea

    K90.2 Blind loop syndrome, not elsewhere classified
    Blind loop syndrome NOS
    EXCLUDES 1 congenital blind loop syndrome (Q43.8)
                 postsurgical blind loop syndrome (K91.2)

    K90.3 Pancreatic steatorrhea

✓5ᵗʰ **K90.4 Other malabsorption due to intolerance**
    EXCLUDES 2 ►celiac gluten-sensitive enteropathy◄ (K90.0)
                 lactose intolerance (E73.-)

    K90.41 Non-celiac gluten sensitivity
       Gluten sensitivity NOS
       Non-celiac gluten sensitive enteropathy

    K90.49 Malabsorption due to intolerance, not elsewhere classified
       Malabsorption due to intolerance to carbohydrate
       Malabsorption due to intolerance to fat
       Malabsorption due to intolerance to protein
       Malabsorption due to intolerance to starch

✓5ᵗʰ **K90.8 Other intestinal malabsorption**

    K90.81 Whipple's disease

    K90.89 Other intestinal malabsorption

    K90.9 Intestinal malabsorption, unspecified ▽

✓4ᵗʰ **K91 Intraoperative and postprocedural complications and disorders of digestive system, not elsewhere classified**
    EXCLUDES 2 complications of artificial opening of digestive system (K94.-)
                 complications of bariatric procedures (K95.-)
                 gastrojejunal ulcer (K28.-)
                 postprocedural (radiation) retroperitoneal abscess (K68.11)
                 radiation colitis (K52.0)
                 radiation gastroenteritis (K52.0)
                 radiation proctitis (K62.7)

    K91.0 Vomiting following gastrointestinal surgery

    K91.1 Postgastric surgery syndromes
    Dumping syndrome
    Postgastrectomy syndrome
    Postvagotomy syndrome

    K91.2 Postsurgical malabsorption, not elsewhere classified
    Postsurgical blind loop syndrome
    EXCLUDES 1 malabsorption osteomalacia in adults (M83.2)
                 malabsorption osteoporosis, postsurgical (M80.8-, M81.8)

✓5ᵗʰ **K91.3 Postprocedural intestinal obstruction**
    AHA: 2017, 1Q, 40

●   **K91.30 Postprocedural intestinal obstruction, unspecified as to partial versus complete** ▽
       Postprocedural intestinal obstruction NOS

●   **K91.31 Postprocedural partial intestinal obstruction**
       Postprocedural incomplete intestinal obstruction

●   **K91.32 Postprocedural complete intestinal obstruction**

K91.5 Postcholecystectomy syndrome

✓5ᵗʰ **K91.6 Intraoperative hemorrhage and hematoma of a digestive system organ or structure complicating a procedure**

    EXCLUDES 1   *intraoperative hemorrhage and hematoma of a digestive system organ or structure due to accidental puncture and laceration during a procedure (K91.7-)*

    K91.61 Intraoperative hemorrhage and hematoma of a digestive system organ or structure complicating a digestive system procedure

    K91.62 Intraoperative hemorrhage and hematoma of a digestive system organ or structure complicating other procedure

✓5ᵗʰ **K91.7 Accidental puncture and laceration of a digestive system organ or structure during a procedure**

    K91.71 Accidental puncture and laceration of a digestive system organ or structure during a digestive system procedure

    K91.72 Accidental puncture and laceration of a digestive system organ or structure during other procedure

✓5ᵗʰ **K91.8 Other intraoperative and postprocedural complications and disorders of digestive system**

    K91.81 Other intraoperative complications of digestive system

    K91.82 Postprocedural hepatic failure

    K91.83 Postprocedural hepatorenal syndrome

  ✓6ᵗʰ **K91.84 Postprocedural hemorrhage of a digestive system organ or structure following a procedure**

      K91.840 Postprocedural hemorrhage of a digestive system organ or structure following a digestive system procedure
        AHA: 2016, 1Q, 15

      K91.841 Postprocedural hemorrhage of a digestive system organ or structure following other procedure

  ✓6ᵗʰ **K91.85 Complications of intestinal pouch**

      K91.850 Pouchitis   HCC
        Inflammation of internal ileoanal pouch
        DEF: Inflammatory complication of an existing surgically created ileoanal pouch, resulting in multiple GI complaints, including diarrhea, abdominal pain, rectal bleeding, fecal urgency, or incontinence.

      K91.858 Other complications of intestinal pouch   HCC

    K91.86 Retained cholelithiasis following cholecystectomy

  ✓6ᵗʰ **K91.87 Postprocedural hematoma and seroma of a digestive system organ or structure following a procedure**

      K91.870 Postprocedural hematoma of a digestive system organ or structure following a digestive system procedure

      K91.871 Postprocedural hematoma of a digestive system organ or structure following other procedure

      K91.872 Postprocedural seroma of a digestive system organ or structure following a digestive system procedure

      K91.873 Postprocedural seroma of a digestive system organ or structure following other procedure

    K91.89 Other postprocedural complications and disorders of digestive system
       Use additional code, if applicable, to further specify disorder
       EXCLUDES 2 *postprocedural retroperitoneal abscess (K68.11)*
       AHA: 2017, 1Q, 40

✓4ᵗʰ **K92 Other diseases of digestive system**
    EXCLUDES 1 *neonatal gastrointestinal hemorrhage (P54.0-P54.3)*

K92.0 Hematemesis

K92.1 Melena
    EXCLUDES 1 *occult blood in feces (R19.5)*

K92.2 Gastrointestinal hemorrhage, unspecified ▽
   Gastric hemorrhage NOS
   Intestinal hemorrhage NOS
    EXCLUDES 1   *acute hemorrhagic gastritis (K29.01)*
       hemorrhage of anus and rectum (K62.5)
       angiodysplasia of stomach with hemorrhage (K31.811)
       diverticular disease with hemorrhage (K57.-)
       gastritis and duodenitis with hemorrhage (K29.-)
       peptic ulcer with hemorrhage (K25-K28)

✓5ᵗʰ **K92.8 Other specified diseases of the digestive system**

    K92.81 Gastrointestinal mucositis (ulcerative)
       Code also type of associated therapy, such as:
         antineoplastic and immunosuppressive drugs (T45.1X-)
         radiological procedure and radiotherapy (Y84.2)
       EXCLUDES 2 *mucositis (ulcerative) of vagina and vulva (N76.81)*
        nasal mucositis (ulcerative) (J34.81)
        oral mucositis (ulcerative) (K12.3-)

    K92.89 Other specified diseases of the digestive system

K92.9 Disease of digestive system, unspecified ▽

✓4ᵗʰ **K94 Complications of artificial openings of the digestive system**

  ✓5ᵗʰ **K94.0 Colostomy complications**

    K94.00 Colostomy complication, unspecified   HCC ▽

    K94.01 Colostomy hemorrhage   HCC

    K94.02 Colostomy infection   HCC
       Use additional code to specify type of infection, such as:
        cellulitis of abdominal wall (L03.311)
        sepsis (A40-, A41-)

    K94.03 Colostomy malfunction   HCC
       Mechanical complication of colostomy

    K94.09 Other complications of colostomy   HCC

  ✓5ᵗʰ **K94.1 Enterostomy complications**

    K94.10 Enterostomy complication, unspecified   HCC ▽

    K94.11 Enterostomy hemorrhage   HCC

    K94.12 Enterostomy infection   HCC
       Use additional code to specify type of infection, such as:
        cellulitis of abdominal wall (L03.311)
        sepsis (A40-, A41-)

    K94.13 Enterostomy malfunction   HCC
       Mechanical complication of enterostomy

    K94.19 Other complications of enterostomy   HCC

  ✓5ᵗʰ **K94.2 Gastrostomy complications**

    K94.20 Gastrostomy complication, unspecified   HCC ▽

    K94.21 Gastrostomy hemorrhage   HCC

    K94.22 Gastrostomy infection   HCC
       Use additional code to specify type of infection, such as:
        cellulitis of abdominal wall (L03.311)
        sepsis (A40-, A41-)

    K94.23 Gastrostomy malfunction   HCC
       Mechanical complication of gastrostomy

    K94.29 Other complications of gastrostomy   HCC

  ✓5ᵗʰ **K94.3 Esophagostomy complications**

    K94.30 Esophagostomy complications, unspecified   HCC ▽

    K94.31 Esophagostomy hemorrhage   HCC

    K94.32 Esophagostomy infection   HCC
       Use additional code to identify the infection

    K94.33 Esophagostomy malfunction   HCC
       Mechanical complication of esophagostomy

    K94.39 Other complications of esophagostomy   HCC

✓4ᵗʰ **K95 Complications of bariatric procedures**

  ✓5ᵗʰ **K95.0 Complications of gastric band procedure**

    K95.01 Infection due to gastric band procedure
       Use additional code to specify type of infection or organism, such as:
        bacterial and viral infectious agents (B95.-, B96.-)
        cellulitis of abdominal wall (L03.311)
        sepsis (A40.-, A41.-)

    K95.09 Other complications of gastric band procedure
       Use additional code, if applicable, to further specify complication

---

☑ Additional Character Req   ✓x7ᵗʰ Placeholder Alert   Manifestation   HCC CMS-HCC Condition   ▽ Unspecified Code   ►◄ Revised Text   ● New Code   ▲ Revised Code Title

√5ᵗʰ **K95.8** **Complications of other bariatric procedure**

> EXCLUDES 1   *complications of gastric band surgery (K95.Ø-)*

    K95.81 **Infection due to other bariatric procedure**

> Use additional code to specify type of infection or organism, such as:
> bacterial and viral infectious agents (B95.-, B96.-)
> cellulitis of abdominal wall (LØ3.311)
> sepsis (A4Ø.-, A41.-)

    K95.89 **Other complications of other bariatric procedure**

> Use additional code, if applicable, to further specify complication

EXCLUDES 1 Not coded here   EXCLUDES 2 Not included here   N Newborn Age: 0   P Pediatric Age: 0-17   M Maternity Age: 12-55   A Adult Age: 15-124

692   ICD-10-CM 2018

Chapter 12. Diseases of the Skin and Subcutaneous Tissue (L00–L99)

Chapter Specific Guidelines with Coding Examples

The chapter specific guidelines from the ICD-10-CM Official Guidelines for Coding and Reporting have been provided below. Along with these guidelines are coding examples, contained in the shaded boxes, that have been developed to help illustrate the coding and/or sequencing guidance found in these guidelines.

a. Pressure ulcer stage codes

1) Pressure ulcer stages

Codes from category L89, Pressure ulcer, identify the site of the pressure ulcer as well as the stage of the ulcer.

The ICD-10-CM classifies pressure ulcer stages based on severity, which is designated by stages 1-4, unspecified stage and unstageable.

Assign as many codes from category L89 as needed to identify all the pressure ulcers the patient has, if applicable.

> Stage 3 pressure ulcer left ankle, 6 x 7 cm that invades the fascia; stage 2 pressure ulcer of left hip
>
> **L89.523**   **Pressure ulcer of left ankle, stage 3**
>
> **L89.222**   **Pressure ulcer of left hip, stage 2**
>
> *Explanation:* Patient has a left ankle pressure ulcer documented as stage 3 and a left hip pressure ulcer documented as stage 2. Combination codes from category L89 Pressure ulcer, identify the site of the pressure ulcer as well as the stage. Assign as many codes from category L89 as needed to identify all the pressure ulcers the patient has.

2) Unstageable pressure ulcers

Assignment of the code for unstageable pressure ulcer (L89.--0) should be based on the clinical documentation. These codes are used for pressure ulcers whose stage cannot be clinically determined (e.g., the ulcer is covered by eschar or has been treated with a skin or muscle graft) and pressure ulcers that are documented as deep tissue injury but not documented as due to trauma. This code should not be confused with the codes for unspecified stage (L89.--9). When there is no documentation regarding the stage of the pressure ulcer, assign the appropriate code for unspecified stage (L89.--9).

> Pressure ulcer of the right lower back documented as unstageable due to the presence of thick eschar covering the ulcer
>
> **L89.130**   **Pressure ulcer of right lower back, unstageable**
>
> *Explanation:* Codes for unstageable pressure ulcers are assigned when the stage cannot be clinically determined (e.g., the ulcer is covered by eschar or has been treated with a skin or muscle graft).

3) Documented pressure ulcer stage

Assignment of the pressure ulcer stage code should be guided by clinical documentation of the stage or documentation of the terms found in the Alphabetic Index. For clinical terms describing the stage that are not found in the Alphabetic Index, and there is no documentation of the stage, the provider should be queried.

> Left heel pressure ulcer with partial thickness skin loss involving the dermis
>
> **L89.622**   **Pressure ulcer of left heel, stage 2**
>
> *Explanation:* Code assignment for the pressure ulcer stage should be guided by either the clinical documentation of the stage or the documentation of terms found in the Alphabetic Index. The clinical documentation describing the left heel pressure ulcer "partial thickness skin loss involving the dermis" matches the ICD-10-CM index parenthetical description for stage 2 "(abrasion, blister, partial thickness skin loss involving epidermis and/or dermis)."

4) Patients admitted with pressure ulcers documented as healed

No code is assigned if the documentation states that the pressure ulcer is completely healed.

> Patient receiving follow-up examination of a completely healed pressure ulcer of the foot
>
> **Z09**   **Encounter for follow-up examination after completed treatment for conditions other than malignant neoplasm**
>
> **Z87.2**   **Personal history of diseases of the skin and subcutaneous tissue**
>
> *Explanation:* Assign only codes for the reason for the encounter and the personal history of the pressure ulcer. Personal history code Z87.2 includes conditions classifiable to L00–L99 such as pressure ulcer. No code is assigned for a pressure ulcer documented as completely healed.

5) Patients admitted with pressure ulcers documented as healing

Pressure ulcers described as healing should be assigned the appropriate pressure ulcer stage code based on the documentation in the medical record. If the documentation does not provide information about the stage of the healing pressure ulcer, assign the appropriate code for unspecified stage.

If the documentation is unclear as to whether the patient has a current (new) pressure ulcer or if the patient is being treated for a healing pressure ulcer, query the provider.

For ulcers that were present on admission but healed at the time of discharge, assign the code for the site and stage of the pressure ulcer at the time of admission.

6) Patient admitted with pressure ulcer evolving into another stage during the admission

If a patient is admitted with a pressure ulcer at one stage and it progresses to a higher stage, two separate codes should be assigned: one code for the site and stage of the ulcer on admission and a second code for the same ulcer site and the highest stage reported during the stay.

Chapter 12. Diseases of the Skin and Subcutaneous Tissue (L00-L99)

EXCLUDES 2   certain conditions originating in the perinatal period (P04-P96)
certain infectious and parasitic diseases (A00-B99)
complications of pregnancy, childbirth and the puerperium (O00-O9A)
congenital malformations, deformations, and chromosomal abnormalities (Q00-Q99)
endocrine, nutritional and metabolic diseases (E00-E88)
lipomelanotic reticulosis (I89.8)
neoplasms (C00-D49)
symptoms, signs and abnormal clinical and laboratory findings, not elsewhere classified (R00-R94)
systemic connective tissue disorders (M30-M36)
viral warts (B07.-)

This chapter contains the following blocks:
L00-L08   Infections of the skin and subcutaneous tissue
L10-L14   Bullous disorders
L20-L30   Dermatitis and eczema
L40-L45   Papulosquamous disorders
L49-L54   Urticaria and erythema
L55-L59   Radiation-related disorders of the skin and subcutaneous tissue
L60-L75   Disorders of skin appendages
L76   Intraoperative and postprocedural complications of skin and subcutaneous tissue
L80-L99   Other disorders of the skin and subcutaneous tissue

Infections of the skin and subcutaneous tissue (L00-L08)

Use additional code (B95-B97) to identify infectious agent
EXCLUDES 2   hordeolum (H00.0)
infective dermatitis (L30.3)
local infections of skin classified in Chapter 1
lupus panniculitis (L93.2)
panniculitis NOS (M79.3)
panniculitis of neck and back (M54.0-)
perlèche NOS (K13.0)
perlèche due to candidiasis (B37.0)
perlèche due to riboflavin deficiency (E53.0)
pyogenic granuloma (L98.0)
relapsing panniculitis [Weber-Christian] (M35.6)
viral warts (B07.-)
zoster (B02.-)

L00   Staphylococcal scalded skin syndrome
Ritter's disease
Use additional code to identify percentage of skin exfoliation (L49.-)
EXCLUDES 1   bullous impetigo (L01.03)
pemphigus neonatorum (L01.03)
toxic epidermal necrolysis [Lyell] (L51.2)
DEF: Infectious skin disease of children younger than 5 years marked by eruptions ranging from a few localized blisters to widespread, easily ruptured, fine vesicles and bullae affecting almost the entire body; results in exfoliation of large planes of skin and leaves raw areas.

✓4ᵗʰ L01   Impetigo
EXCLUDES 1   impetigo herpetiformis (L40.1)

✓5ᵗʰ L01.0   Impetigo
Impetigo contagiosa
Impetigo vulgaris
   L01.00   Impetigo, unspecified   ▽
Impetigo NOS
   L01.01   Non-bullous impetigo
   L01.02   Bockhart's impetigo
Impetigo follicularis
Perifolliculitis NOS
Superficial pustular perifolliculitis
   L01.03   Bullous impetigo
Impetigo neonatorum
Pemphigus neonatorum
   L01.09   Other impetigo
Ulcerative impetigo
   L01.1   Impetiginization of other dermatoses

✓4ᵗʰ L02   Cutaneous abscess, furuncle and carbuncle
Use additional code to identify organism (B95-B96)
EXCLUDES 2   abscess of anus and rectal regions (K61.-)
abscess of female genital organs (external) (N76.4)
abscess of male genital organs (external) (N48.2, N49-)

✓5ᵗʰ L02.0   Cutaneous abscess, furuncle and carbuncle of face
EXCLUDES 2   abscess of ear, external (H60.0)
abscess of eyelid (H00.0)
abscess of head [any part, except face] (L02.8)
abscess of lacrimal gland (H04.0)
abscess of lacrimal passages (H04.3)
abscess of mouth (K12.2)
abscess of nose (J34.0)
abscess of orbit (H05.0)
submandibular abscess (K12.2)
   L02.01   Cutaneous abscess of face
   L02.02   Furuncle of face
Boil of face
Folliculitis of face
   L02.03   Carbuncle of face

✓5ᵗʰ L02.1   Cutaneous abscess, furuncle and carbuncle of neck
   L02.11   Cutaneous abscess of neck
   L02.12   Furuncle of neck
Boil of neck
Folliculitis of neck
   L02.13   Carbuncle of neck

✓5ᵗʰ L02.2   Cutaneous abscess, furuncle and carbuncle of trunk
EXCLUDES 1   non-newborn omphalitis (L08.82)
omphalitis of newborn (P38.-)
EXCLUDES 2   abscess of breast (N61.1)
abscess of buttocks (L02.3)
abscess of female external genital organs (N76.4)
abscess of hip (L02.4)
abscess of male external genital organs (N48.2, N49-)
   ✓6ᵗʰ L02.21   Cutaneous abscess of trunk
     L02.211   Cutaneous abscess of abdominal wall
     L02.212   Cutaneous abscess of back [any part, except buttock]
     L02.213   Cutaneous abscess of chest wall
     L02.214   Cutaneous abscess of groin
     L02.215   Cutaneous abscess of perineum
     L02.216   Cutaneous abscess of umbilicus
     L02.219   Cutaneous abscess of trunk, unspecified   ▽
   ✓6ᵗʰ L02.22   Furuncle of trunk
Boil of trunk
Folliculitis of trunk
     L02.221   Furuncle of abdominal wall
     L02.222   Furuncle of back [any part, except buttock]
     L02.223   Furuncle of chest wall
     L02.224   Furuncle of groin
     L02.225   Furuncle of perineum
     L02.226   Furuncle of umbilicus
     L02.229   Furuncle of trunk, unspecified   ▽
   ✓6ᵗʰ L02.23   Carbuncle of trunk
     L02.231   Carbuncle of abdominal wall
     L02.232   Carbuncle of back [any part, except buttock]
     L02.233   Carbuncle of chest wall
     L02.234   Carbuncle of groin
     L02.235   Carbuncle of perineum
     L02.236   Carbuncle of umbilicus
     L02.239   Carbuncle of trunk, unspecified   ▽

✓5ᵗʰ L02.3   Cutaneous abscess, furuncle and carbuncle of buttock
EXCLUDES 1   pilonidal cyst with abscess (L05.01)
   L02.31   Cutaneous abscess of buttock
Cutaneous abscess of gluteal region
   L02.32   Furuncle of buttock
Boil of buttock
Folliculitis of buttock
Furuncle of gluteal region
   L02.33   Carbuncle of buttock
Carbuncle of gluteal region

✓5ᵗʰ **L02.4 Cutaneous abscess, furuncle and carbuncle of** limb
> **EXCLUDES 2** *cutaneous abscess, furuncle and carbuncle of groin (L02.214, L02.224, L02.234)*
> *cutaneous abscess, furuncle and carbuncle of hand (L02.5-)*
> *cutaneous abscess, furuncle and carbuncle of foot (L02.6-)*

✓6ᵗʰ **L02.41 Cutaneous abscess of limb**
- **L02.411 Cutaneous abscess of** right axilla
- **L02.412 Cutaneous abscess of** left axilla
- **L02.413 Cutaneous abscess of** right upper limb
- **L02.414 Cutaneous abscess of** left upper limb
- **L02.415 Cutaneous abscess of** right lower limb
- **L02.416 Cutaneous abscess of** left lower limb
- **L02.419 Cutaneous abscess of limb, unspecified** ▽

✓6ᵗʰ **L02.42 Furuncle of limb**
> Boil of limb
> Folliculitis of limb
- **L02.421 Furuncle of** right axilla
- **L02.422 Furuncle of** left axilla
- **L02.423 Furuncle of** right upper limb
- **L02.424 Furuncle of** left upper limb
- **L02.425 Furuncle of** right lower limb
- **L02. Furuncle of** left lower limb
- **L02.429 Furuncle of limb, unspecified** ▽

✓6ᵗʰ **L02.43 Carbuncle of limb**
- **L02.431 Carbuncle of** right axilla
- **L02.432 Carbuncle of** left axilla
- **L02.433 Carbuncle of** right upper limb
- **L02.434 Carbuncle of** left upper limb
- **L02.435 Carbuncle of** right lower limb
- **L02.436 Carbuncle of** left lower limb
- **L02.439 Carbuncle of limb, unspecified** ▽

✓5ᵗʰ **L02.5 Cutaneous abscess, furuncle and carbuncle of** hand

✓6ᵗʰ **L02.51 Cutaneous abscess of hand**
- **L02.511 Cutaneous abscess of** right hand
- **L02.512 Cutaneous abscess of** left hand
- **L02.519 Cutaneous abscess of unspecified hand** ▽

✓6ᵗʰ **L02.52 Furuncle hand**
> Boil of hand
> Folliculitis of hand
- **L02.521 Furuncle** right hand
- **L02.522 Furuncle** left hand
- **L02.529 Furuncle unspecified hand** ▽

✓6ᵗʰ **L02.53 Carbuncle of hand**
- **L02.531 Carbuncle of** right hand
- **L02.532 Carbuncle of** left hand
- **L02.539 Carbuncle of unspecified hand** ▽

✓5ᵗʰ **L02.6 Cutaneous abscess, furuncle and carbuncle of** foot

✓6ᵗʰ **L02.61 Cutaneous abscess of foot**
- **L02.611 Cutaneous abscess of** right foot
- **L02.612 Cutaneous abscess of** left foot
- **L02.619 Cutaneous abscess of unspecified foot** ▽

✓6ᵗʰ **L02.62 Furuncle of foot**
> Boil of foot
> Folliculitis of foot
- **L02.621 Furuncle of** right foot
- **L02.622 Furuncle of** left foot
- **L02.629 Furuncle of unspecified foot** ▽

✓6ᵗʰ **L02.63 Carbuncle of foot**
- **L02.631 Carbuncle of** right foot
- **L02.632 Carbuncle of** left foot
- **L02.639 Carbuncle of unspecified foot** ▽

✓5ᵗʰ **L02.8 Cutaneous abscess, furuncle and carbuncle of other sites**

✓6ᵗʰ **L02.81 Cutaneous abscess of other sites**
- **L02.811 Cutaneous abscess of** head [any part, except face]
- **L02.818 Cutaneous abscess of other sites**

✓6ᵗʰ **L02.82 Furuncle of other sites**
> Boil of other sites
> Folliculitis of other sites
- **L02.821 Furuncle of** head [any part, except face]
- **L02.828 Furuncle of other sites**

✓6ᵗʰ **L02.83 Carbuncle of other sites**
- **L02.831 Carbuncle of** head [any part, except face]
- **L02.838 Carbuncle of other sites**

✓5ᵗʰ **L02.9 Cutaneous abscess, furuncle and carbuncle, unspecified**
- **L02.91 Cutaneous abscess, unspecified** ▽
- **L02.92 Furuncle, unspecified** ▽
  > Boil NOS
  > Furunculosis NOS
- **L02.93 Carbuncle, unspecified** ▽

✓4ᵗʰ **L03 Cellulitis and acute lymphangitis**
> **EXCLUDES 2** *cellulitis of anal and rectal region (K61.-)*
> *cellulitis of external auditory canal (H60.1)*
> *cellulitis of eyelid (H00.03-)*
> *cellulitis of female external genital organs (N76.4)*
> *cellulitis of lacrimal apparatus (H04.3)*
> *cellulitis of male external genital organs (N48.2, N49-)*
> *cellulitis of mouth (K12.2)*
> *cellulitis of nose (J34.0)*
> *eosinophilic cellulitis [Wells] (L98.3)*
> *febrile neutrophilic dermatosis [Sweet] (L98.2)*
> *lymphangitis (chronic) (subacute) (I89.1)*

✓5ᵗʰ **L03.0 Cellulitis and acute lymphangitis of** finger and toe
> Infection of nail
> Onychia
> Paronychia
> Perionychia

✓6ᵗʰ **L03.01 Cellulitis of** finger
> Felon
> Whitlow
> **EXCLUDES 1** *herpetic whitlow (B00.89)*
> **DEF:** Felon: Superficial bacterial skin infection at the tip of the finger.
- **L03.011 Cellulitis of** right finger
- **L03.012 Cellulitis of** left finger
- **L03.019 Cellulitis of unspecified finger** ▽

✓6ᵗʰ **L03.02 Acute lymphangitis of** finger
> Hangnail with lymphangitis of finger
- **L03.021 Acute lymphangitis of** right finger
- **L03.022 Acute lymphangitis of** left finger
- **L03.029 Acute lymphangitis of unspecified finger** ▽

✓6ᵗʰ **L03.03 Cellulitis of** toe
- **L03.031 Cellulitis of** right toe
- **L03.032 Cellulitis of** left toe
- **L03.039 Cellulitis of unspecified toe** ▽

✓6ᵗʰ **L03.04 Acute lymphangitis of** toe
> Hangnail with lymphangitis of toe
- **L03.041 Acute lymphangitis of** right toe
- **L03.042 Acute lymphangitis of** left toe
- **L03.049 Acute lymphangitis of unspecified toe** ▽

✓5ᵗʰ **L03.1 Cellulitis and acute lymphangitis of other parts of limb**

✓6ᵗʰ **L03.11 Cellulitis of other parts of limb**
> **EXCLUDES 2** *cellulitis of fingers (L03.01-)*
> *cellulitis of toes (L03.03-)*
> *groin (L03.314)*
- **L03.111 Cellulitis of** right axilla
- **L03.112 Cellulitis of** left axilla
- **L03.113 Cellulitis of** right upper limb
- **L03.114 Cellulitis of** left upper limb
- **L03.115 Cellulitis of** right lower limb
- **L03.116 Cellulitis of** left lower limb
- **L03.119 Cellulitis of unspecified part of limb** ▽

✓6ᵗʰ **L03.12 Acute lymphangitis of other parts of limb**
> **EXCLUDES 2** *acute lymphangitis of fingers (L03.02-)*
> *acute lymphangitis of groin (L03.324)*
> *acute lymphangitis of toes (L03.04-)*
- **L03.121 Acute lymphangitis of** right axilla
- **L03.122 Acute lymphangitis of** left axilla
- **L03.123 Acute lymphangitis of** right upper limb
- **L03.124 Acute lymphangitis of** left upper limb
- **L03.125 Acute lymphangitis of** right lower limb
- **L03.126 Acute lymphangitis of** left lower limb
- **L03.129 Acute lymphangitis of unspecified part of limb** ▽

✓ Additional Character Req   ✓7ᵗʰ Placeholder Alert   Manifestation   **HCC** CMS-HCC Condition   ▽ Unspecified Code   ▶◀ Revised Text   ● New Code   ▲ Revised Code Title

✓5ᵗʰ **L03.2**   **Cellulitis and acute lymphangitis of** face and neck

     ✓6ᵗʰ **L03.21**   **Cellulitis and acute lymphangitis of** face

         L03.211   **Cellulitis** of face

            EXCLUDES 2   *abscess of orbit (H05.01-)*
                 cellulitis of ear (H60.1-)
                 cellulitis of eyelid (H00.03-)
                 cellulitis of head (L03.811)
                 cellulitis of lacrimal apparatus
                     (H04.3)
                 cellulitis of lip (K13.0)
                 cellulitis of mouth (K12.2)
                 cellulitis of nose (internal) (J34.0)
                 cellulitis of orbit (H05.01-)
                 cellulitis of scalp (L03.811)

            AHA: 2013, 4Q, 123

         L03.212   **Acute lymphangitis** of face

         L03.213   **Periorbital cellulitis**
            Preseptal cellulitis

     ✓6ᵗʰ **L03.22**   **Cellulitis and acute lymphangitis of** neck

         L03.221   **Cellulitis** of neck

         L03.222   **Acute lymphangitis** of neck

✓5ᵗʰ **L03.3**   **Cellulitis and acute lymphangitis of** trunk

     ✓6ᵗʰ **L03.31**   **Cellulitis** of trunk

         EXCLUDES 2   *cellulitis of anal and rectal regions (K61.-)*
                 cellulitis of breast NOS (N61.0)
                 cellulitis of female external genital organs
                     (N76.4)
                 cellulitis of male external genital organs
                     (N48.2, N49-)
                 omphalitis of newborn (P38.-)
                 puerperal cellulitis of breast (O91.2)

         L03.311   **Cellulitis of** abdominal wall
            EXCLUDES 2   *cellulitis of umbilicus (L03.316)*
                   cellulitis of groin (L03.314)

         L03.312   **Cellulitis of** back [any part except buttock]

         L03.313   **Cellulitis of** chest wall

         L03.314   **Cellulitis of** groin

         L03.315   **Cellulitis of** perineum

         L03.316   **Cellulitis of** umbilicus

         L03.317   **Cellulitis of** buttock

         L03.319   **Cellulitis of trunk, unspecified** ▽

     ✓6ᵗʰ **L03.32**   **Acute lymphangitis** of trunk

         L03.321   **Acute lymphangitis of** abdominal wall

         L03.322   **Acute lymphangitis of** back [any part except buttock]

         L03.323   **Acute lymphangitis of** chest wall

         L03.324   **Acute lymphangitis of** groin

         L03.325   **Acute lymphangitis of** perineum

         L03.326   **Acute lymphangitis of** umbilicus

         L03.327   **Acute lymphangitis of** buttock

         L03.329   **Acute lymphangitis of trunk, unspecified** ▽

✓5ᵗʰ **L03.8**   **Cellulitis and acute lymphangitis of** other sites

     ✓6ᵗʰ **L03.81**   **Cellulitis of** other sites

         L03.811   **Cellulitis of** head [any part, except face]
            Cellulitis of scalp
            EXCLUDES 2   *cellulitis of face (L03.211)*

         L03.818   **Cellulitis of other sites**

     ✓6ᵗʰ **L03.89**   **Acute lymphangitis** of other sites

         L03.891   **Acute lymphangitis of** head [any part, except face]

         L03.898   **Acute lymphangitis of other sites**

✓5ᵗʰ **L03.9**   **Cellulitis and acute lymphangitis, unspecified**

     L03.90   **Cellulitis, unspecified** ▽

     L03.91   **Acute lymphangitis, unspecified** ▽
         EXCLUDES 1   *lymphangitis NOS (I89.1)*

✓4ᵗʰ **L04**   **Acute lymphadenitis**

     INCLUDES   abscess (acute) of lymph nodes, except mesenteric
               acute lymphadenitis, except mesenteric

     EXCLUDES 1   *chronic or subacute lymphadenitis, except mesenteric (I88.1)*
               enlarged lymph nodes (R59.-)
               human immunodeficiency virus [HIV] disease resulting in
                   generalized lymphadenopathy (B20)
               lymphadenitis NOS (I88.9)
               nonspecific mesenteric lymphadenitis (I88.0)

     L04.0   **Acute lymphadenitis of** face, head and neck

Pilonidal Cyst

- Skin
- Fistula
- Pilonidal cyst
- Fat
- Bone

     L04.1   **Acute lymphadenitis of** trunk

     L04.2   **Acute lymphadenitis of** upper limb
         Acute lymphadenitis of axilla
         Acute lymphadenitis of shoulder

     L04.3   **Acute lymphadenitis of** lower limb
         Acute lymphadenitis of hip
         EXCLUDES 2   *acute lymphadenitis of groin (L04.1)*

     L04.8   **Acute lymphadenitis of other sites**

     L04.9   **Acute lymphadenitis, unspecified** ▽

✓4ᵗʰ **L05**   **Pilonidal cyst and sinus**

     ✓5ᵗʰ **L05.0**   **Pilonidal cyst and sinus** with abscess

         L05.01   **Pilonidal** cyst with abscess
            Pilonidal abscess
            Pilonidal dimple with abscess
            Postanal dimple with abscess
            EXCLUDES 2   *congenital sacral dimple (Q82.6)*
                 parasacral dimple (Q82.6)

         L05.02   **Pilonidal** sinus with abscess
            Coccygeal fistula with abscess
            Coccygeal sinus with abscess
            Pilonidal fistula with abscess

     ✓5ᵗʰ **L05.9**   **Pilonidal cyst and sinus** without abscess

         L05.91   **Pilonidal** cyst without abscess
            Pilonidal dimple
            Postanal dimple
            Pilonidal cyst NOS
            EXCLUDES 2   *congenital sacral dimple (Q82.6)*
                 parasacral dimple (Q82.6)

         L05.92   **Pilonidal** sinus without abscess
            Coccygeal fistula
            Coccygeal sinus without abscess
            Pilonidal fistula

✓4ᵗʰ **L08**   **Other local infections of skin and subcutaneous tissue**

     L08.0   **Pyoderma**
         Dermatitis gangrenosa
         Purulent dermatitis
         Septic dermatitis
         Suppurative dermatitis
         EXCLUDES 1   *pyoderma gangrenosum (L88)*
                 pyoderma vegetans (L08.81)

     L08.1   **Erythrasma**

     ✓5ᵗʰ **L08.8**   **Other specified local infections of the skin and subcutaneous tissue**

         L08.81   **Pyoderma vegetans**
            EXCLUDES 1   *pyoderma gangrenosum (L88)*
                 pyoderma NOS (L08.0)

         L08.82   **Omphalitis not of newborn**
            EXCLUDES 1   *omphalitis of newborn (P38.-)*

         L08.89   **Other specified local infections of the skin and subcutaneous tissue**

     L08.9   **Local infection of the skin and subcutaneous tissue, unspecified** ▽

Bullous disorders (L10-L14)

EXCLUDES 1   benign familial pemphigus [Hailey-Hailey] (Q82.8)
staphylococcal scalded skin syndrome (L00)
toxic epidermal necrolysis [Lyell] (L51.2)

✓4ᵗʰ **L10 Pemphigus**
   EXCLUDES 1   pemphigus neonatorum (L01.03)
- **L10.0 Pemphigus** vulgaris
- **L10.1 Pemphigus** vegetans
- **L10.2 Pemphigus** foliaceous
- **L10.3** Brazilian **pemphigus [fogo selvagem]**
- **L10.4 Pemphigus** erythematosus
  Senear-Usher syndrome
- **L10.5** Drug-induced **pemphigus**
  Use additional code for adverse effect, if applicable, to identify drug (T36-T50 with fifth or sixth character 5)

✓5ᵗʰ **L10.8 Other pemphigus**
- **L10.81** Paraneoplastic **pemphigus**
- **L10.89 Other pemphigus**
- **L10.9 Pemphigus, unspecified** ▽

✓4ᵗʰ **L11 Other acantholytic disorders**
- **L11.0 Acquired keratosis follicularis**
  EXCLUDES 1   keratosis follicularis (congenital) [Darier-White] (Q82.8)
- **L11.1 Transient acantholytic dermatosis [Grover]**
- **L11.8 Other specified acantholytic disorders**
- **L11.9 Acantholytic disorder, unspecified** ▽

✓4ᵗʰ **L12 Pemphigoid**
   EXCLUDES 1   herpes gestationis (O26.4-)
     impetigo herpetiformis (L40.1)
- **L12.0** Bullous **pemphigoid**
- **L12.1** Cicatricial **pemphigoid**
  Benign mucous membrane pemphigoid
  DEF: Chronic autoimmune disease characterized by subepidermal blistering lesions of mucosa, including the conjunctiva; seen predominantly in the elderly; produces adhesions and scarring.
- **L12.2** Chronic **bullous disease of childhood** [P]
  Juvenile dermatitis herpetiformis

✓5ᵗʰ **L12.3** Acquired **epidermolysis bullosa**
   EXCLUDES 1   epidermolysis bullosa (congenital) (Q81.-)
- **L12.30 Acquired epidermolysis bullosa, unspecified** HCC ▽
- **L12.31 Epidermolysis bullosa** due to drug HCC
  Use additional code for adverse effect, if applicable, to identify drug (T36-T50 with fifth or sixth character 5)
- **L12.35 Other acquired epidermolysis bullosa** HCC
- **L12.8 Other pemphigoid**
- **L12.9 Pemphigoid, unspecified** ▽

✓4ᵗʰ **L13 Other bullous disorders**
- **L13.0 Dermatitis herpetiformis**
  Duhring's disease
  Hydroa herpetiformis
  EXCLUDES 1   juvenile dermatitis herpetiformis (L12.2)
       senile dermatitis herpetiformis (L12.0)
  DEF: Skin disease to which people are genetically predisposed resulting from an immunological response to gluten; seen as an extremely pruritic eruption of various lesions that frequently heal, leaving hyperpigmentation and hypopigmentation and occasionally scarring; usually associated with an asymptomatic gluten-sensitive enteropathy.
- **L13.1 Subcorneal pustular dermatitis**
  Sneddon-Wilkinson disease
- **L13.8 Other specified bullous disorders**
- **L13.9 Bullous disorder, unspecified** ▽

L14 Bullous disorders in diseases classified elsewhere
   Code first underlying disease

Dermatitis and eczema (L20-L30)

NOTE   In this block the terms dermatitis and eczema are used synonymously and interchangeably.

EXCLUDES 2   chronic (childhood) granulomatous disease (D71)
dermatitis gangrenosa (L08.0)
dermatitis herpetiformis (L13.0)
dry skin dermatitis (L85.3)
factitial dermatitis (L98.1)
perioral dermatitis (L71.0)
radiation-related disorders of the skin and subcutaneous tissue (L55-L59)
stasis dermatitis (I87.2)

✓4ᵗʰ **L20 Atopic dermatitis**
- **L20.0 Besnier's prurigo**

✓5ᵗʰ **L20.8 Other atopic dermatitis**
   EXCLUDES 2   circumscribed neurodermatitis (L28.0)
- **L20.81 Atopic** neurodermatitis
  Diffuse neurodermatitis
- **L20.82 Flexural eczema**
- **L20.83 Infantile** (acute) (chronic) **eczema** [P]
- **L20.84 Intrinsic** (allergic) **eczema**
- **L20.89 Other atopic dermatitis**
- **L20.9 Atopic dermatitis, unspecified** ▽

✓4ᵗʰ **L21 Seborrheic dermatitis**
   EXCLUDES 2   infective dermatitis (L30.3)
     seborrheic keratosis (L82.-)
- **L21.0 Seborrhea** capitis [P]
  Cradle cap
- **L21.1 Seborrheic** infantile dermatitis [P]
- **L21.8 Other seborrheic dermatitis**
- **L21.9 Seborrheic dermatitis, unspecified** ▽
  Seborrhea NOS

L22 Diaper dermatitis
   Diaper erythema
   Diaper rash
   Psoriasiform diaper rash

✓4ᵗʰ **L23 Allergic contact dermatitis**
   EXCLUDES 1   allergy NOS (T78.40)
     contact dermatitis NOS (L25.9)
     dermatitis NOS (L30.9)
   EXCLUDES 2   dermatitis due to substances taken internally (L27.-)
     dermatitis of eyelid (H01.1-)
     diaper dermatitis (L22)
     eczema of external ear (H60.5-)
     irritant contact dermatitis (L24.-)
     perioral dermatitis (L71.0)
     radiation-related disorders of the skin and subcutaneous tissue (L55-L59)
- **L23.0 Allergic contact dermatitis due to** metals
  Allergic contact dermatitis due to chromium
  Allergic contact dermatitis due to nickel
- **L23.1 Allergic contact dermatitis due to** adhesives
- **L23.2 Allergic contact dermatitis due to** cosmetics
- **L23.3 Allergic contact dermatitis due to** drugs in contact with skin
  Use additional code for adverse effect, if applicable, to identify drug (T36-T50 with fifth or sixth character 5)
  EXCLUDES 2   dermatitis due to ingested drugs and medicaments (L27.0-L27.1)
- **L23.4 Allergic contact dermatitis due to** dyes
- **L23.5 Allergic contact dermatitis due to other chemical products**
  Allergic contact dermatitis due to cement
  Allergic contact dermatitis due to insecticide
  Allergic contact dermatitis due to plastic
  Allergic contact dermatitis due to rubber
- **L23.6 Allergic contact dermatitis due to** food in contact with the skin
  EXCLUDES 2   dermatitis due to ingested food (L27.2)
- **L23.7 Allergic contact dermatitis due to** plants, except food
  EXCLUDES 2   allergy NOS due to pollen (J30.1)

✓5ᵗʰ **L23.8 Allergic contact dermatitis due to other agents**
- **L23.81 Allergic contact dermatitis due to** animal (cat) (dog) dander
  Allergic contact dermatitis due to animal (cat) (dog) hair
- **L23.89 Allergic contact dermatitis due to other agents**

☑ Additional Character Req   ✓7ᵗʰ Placeholder Alert   Manifestation   HCC CMS-HCC Condition   ▽ Unspecified Code   ►◄ Revised Text   ● New Code   ▲ Revised Code Title

L23.9 **Allergic contact dermatitis, unspecified cause** ▽
    Allergic contact eczema NOS

✓4ᵗʰ **L24** **Irritant contact dermatitis**
    EXCLUDES 1 *allergy NOS (T78.40)*
        contact dermatitis NOS (L25.9)
        dermatitis NOS (L30.9)
    EXCLUDES 2 *allergic contact dermatitis (L23.-)*
        dermatitis due to substances taken internally (L27.-)
        dermatitis of eyelid (H01.1-)
        diaper dermatitis (L22)
        eczema of external ear (H60.5-)
        perioral dermatitis (L71.0)
        radiation-related disorders of the skin and subcutaneous tissue (L55-L59)

L24.0 **Irritant contact dermatitis due to detergents**

L24.1 **Irritant contact dermatitis due to oils and greases**

L24.2 **Irritant contact dermatitis due to solvents**
    Irritant contact dermatitis due to chlorocompound
    Irritant contact dermatitis due to cyclohexane
    Irritant contact dermatitis due to ester
    Irritant contact dermatitis due to glycol
    Irritant contact dermatitis due to hydrocarbon
    Irritant contact dermatitis due to ketone

L24.3 **Irritant contact dermatitis due to cosmetics**

L24.4 **Irritant contact dermatitis due to drugs in contact with skin**
    Use additional code for adverse effect, if applicable, to identify drug (T36-T50 with fifth or sixth character 5)

L24.5 **Irritant contact dermatitis due to other chemical products**
    Irritant contact dermatitis due to cement
    Irritant contact dermatitis due to insecticide
    Irritant contact dermatitis due to plastic
    Irritant contact dermatitis due to rubber

L24.6 **Irritant contact dermatitis due to food in contact with skin**
    EXCLUDES 2 *dermatitis due to ingested food (L27.2)*

L24.7 **Irritant contact dermatitis due to plants, except food**
    EXCLUDES 2 *allergy NOS to pollen (J30.1)*

✓5ᵗʰ **L24.8** **Irritant contact dermatitis due to other agents**

    L24.81 **Irritant contact dermatitis due to metals**
        Irritant contact dermatitis due to chromium
        Irritant contact dermatitis due to nickel

    L24.89 **Irritant contact dermatitis due to other agents**
        Irritant contact dermatitis due to dyes

L24.9 **Irritant contact dermatitis, unspecified cause** ▽
    Irritant contact eczema NOS

✓4ᵗʰ **L25** **Unspecified contact dermatitis**
    EXCLUDES 1 *allergic contact dermatitis (L23.-)*
        allergy NOS (T78.40)
        dermatitis NOS (L30.9)
        irritant contact dermatitis (L24.-)
    EXCLUDES 2 *dermatitis due to ingested substances (L27.-)*
        dermatitis of eyelid (H01.1-)
        eczema of external ear (H60.5-)
        perioral dermatitis (L71.0)
        radiation-related disorders of the skin and subcutaneous tissue (L55-L59)

L25.0 **Unspecified contact dermatitis due to cosmetics** ▽

L25.1 **Unspecified contact dermatitis due to drugs in contact with skin** ▽
    Use additional code for adverse effect, if applicable, to identify drug (T36-T50 with fifth or sixth character 5)
    EXCLUDES 2 *dermatitis due to ingested drugs and medicaments (L27.0-L27.1)*

L25.2 **Unspecified contact dermatitis due to dyes** ▽

L25.3 **Unspecified contact dermatitis due to other chemical products** ▽
    Unspecified contact dermatitis due to cement
    Unspecified contact dermatitis due to insecticide

L25.4 **Unspecified contact dermatitis due to food in contact with skin** ▽
    EXCLUDES 2 *dermatitis due to ingested food (L27.2)*

L25.5 **Unspecified contact dermatitis due to plants, except food** ▽
    EXCLUDES 1 *nettle rash (L50.9)*
    EXCLUDES 2 *allergy NOS due to pollen (J30.1)*

L25.8 **Unspecified contact dermatitis due to other agents** ▽

L25.9 **Unspecified contact dermatitis, unspecified cause** ▽
    Contact dermatitis (occupational) NOS
    Contact eczema (occupational) NOS

L26 **Exfoliative dermatitis**
    Hebra's pityriasis
    EXCLUDES 1 *Ritter's disease (L00)*

✓4ᵗʰ **L27** **Dermatitis due to substances taken internally**
    EXCLUDES 1 *allergy NOS (T78.40)*
    EXCLUDES 2 *adverse food reaction, except dermatitis (T78.0-T78.1)*
        contact dermatitis (L23-L25)
        drug photoallergic response (L56.1)
        drug phototoxic response (L56.0)
        urticaria (L50.-)

L27.0 **Generalized skin eruption due to drugs and medicaments taken internally**
    Use additional code for adverse effect, if applicable, to identify drug (T36-T50 with fifth or sixth character 5)

L27.1 **Localized skin eruption due to drugs and medicaments taken internally**
    Use additional code for adverse effect, if applicable, to identify drug (T36-T50 with fifth or sixth character 5)

L27.2 **Dermatitis due to ingested food**
    EXCLUDES 2 *dermatitis due to food in contact with skin (L23.6, L24.6, L25.4)*

L27.8 **Dermatitis due to other substances taken internally**

L27.9 **Dermatitis due to unspecified substance taken internally** ▽

✓4ᵗʰ **L28** **Lichen simplex chronicus and prurigo**

L28.0 **Lichen simplex chronicus**
    Circumscribed neurodermatitis
    Lichen NOS

L28.1 **Prurigo nodularis**

L28.2 **Other prurigo**
    Prurigo NOS
    Prurigo Hebra
    Prurigo mitis
    Urticaria papulosa

✓4ᵗʰ **L29** **Pruritus**
    EXCLUDES 1 *neurotic excoriation (L98.1)*
        psychogenic pruritus (F45.8)

L29.0 **Pruritus ani**

L29.1 **Pruritus scroti** ♂

L29.2 **Pruritus vulvae** ♀

L29.3 **Anogenital pruritus, unspecified** ▽

L29.8 **Other pruritus**

L29.9 **Pruritus, unspecified** ▽
    Itch NOS

✓4ᵗʰ **L30** **Other and unspecified dermatitis**
    EXCLUDES 2 *contact dermatitis (L23-L25)*
        dry skin dermatitis (L85.3)
        small plaque parapsoriasis (L41.3)
        stasis dermatitis (I87.2)

L30.0 **Nummular dermatitis**

L30.1 **Dyshidrosis [pompholyx]**

L30.2 **Cutaneous autosensitization**
    Candidid [levurid]
    Dermatophytid
    Eczematid

L30.3 **Infective dermatitis**
    Infectious eczematoid dermatitis

L30.4 **Erythema intertrigo**

L30.5 **Pityriasis alba**

L30.8 **Other specified dermatitis**

L30.9 **Dermatitis, unspecified** ▽
    Eczema NOS

Papulosquamous disorders (L40-L45)

✓4ᵗʰ **L40** **Psoriasis**

L40.0 **Psoriasis vulgaris**
    Nummular psoriasis
    Plaque psoriasis

L40.1 **Generalized pustular psoriasis**
    Impetigo herpetiformis
    Von Zumbusch's disease

L40.2 **Acrodermatitis continua**

L40.3 **Pustulosis palmaris et plantaris**

L40.4 **Guttate psoriasis**

EXCLUDES 1 Not coded here   **EXCLUDES 2** Not included here   N Newborn Age: 0   P Pediatric Age: 0-17   M Maternity Age: 12-55   A Adult Age: 15-124

698   ICD-10-CM 2018

☑5ᵗʰ **L40.5 Arthropathic psoriasis**

    L40.50 Arthropathic psoriasis, unspecified `HCC` ▽

    L40.51 Distal interphalangeal psoriatic arthropathy `HCC`

    L40.52 Psoriatic arthritis mutilans `HCC`

    L40.53 Psoriatic spondylitis `HCC`

    L40.54 Psoriatic juvenile arthropathy `HCC`

    L40.59 Other psoriatic arthropathy `HCC`

  L40.8 Other psoriasis
    Flexural psoriasis

  L40.9 Psoriasis, unspecified ▽

☑4ᵗʰ **L41 Parapsoriasis**
    EXCLUDES1 *poikiloderma vasculare atrophicans (L94.5)*

  L41.0 Pityriasis lichenoides et varioliformis acuta
    Mucha-Habermann disease

  L41.1 Pityriasis lichenoides chronica

  L41.3 Small plaque parapsoriasis

  L41.4 Large plaque parapsoriasis

  L41.5 Retiform parapsoriasis

  L41.8 Other parapsoriasis

  L41.9 Parapsoriasis, unspecified ▽

  L42 Pityriasis rosea

☑4ᵗʰ **L43 Lichen planus**
    EXCLUDES1 *lichen planopilaris (L66.1)*

  L43.0 Hypertrophic lichen planus

  L43.1 Bullous lichen planus

  L43.2 Lichenoid drug reaction
    Use additional code for adverse effect, if applicable, to identify drug (T36-T50 with fifth or sixth character 5)

  L43.3 Subacute (active) lichen planus
    Lichen planus tropicus

  L43.8 Other lichen planus

  L43.9 Lichen planus, unspecified ▽

☑4ᵗʰ **L44 Other papulosquamous disorders**

  L44.0 Pityriasis rubra pilaris

  L44.1 Lichen nitidus
    DEF: Chronic, inflammatory, asymptomatic skin disorder, characterized by numerous glistening, flat-topped, discrete, skin-colored micropapules, most often on the penis, lower abdomen, inner thighs, wrists, forearms, breasts and buttocks.

  L44.2 Lichen striatus

  L44.3 Lichen ruber moniliformis

  L44.4 Infantile papular acrodermatitis [Gianotti-Crosti] `P`

  L44.8 Other specified papulosquamous disorders

  L44.9 Papulosquamous disorder, unspecified ▽

L45 Papulosquamous disorders in diseases classified elsewhere
    Code first underlying disease

Urticaria and erythema (L49-L54)

EXCLUDES1 *Lyme disease (A69.2-)*
    rosacea (L71.-)

☑4ᵗʰ **L49 Exfoliation due to erythematous conditions according to extent of body surface involved**
    Code first erythematous condition causing exfoliation, such as:
      Ritter's disease (L00)
      (Staphylococcal) scalded skin syndrom (L00)
      Stevens-Johnson syndrome (L51.1)
      Stevens-Johnson syndrome-toxic epidermal necrolysis overlap syndrome (L51.3)
      toxic epidermal necrolysis (L51.2)

  L49.0 Exfoliation due to erythematous condition involving less than 10 percent of body surface
    Exfoliation due to erythematous condition NOS

  L49.1 Exfoliation due to erythematous condition involving 10-19 percent of body surface

  L49.2 Exfoliation due to erythematous condition involving 20-29 percent of body surface

  L49.3 Exfoliation due to erythematous condition involving 30-39 percent of body surface

  L49.4 Exfoliation due to erythematous condition involving 40-49 percent of body surface

  L49.5 Exfoliation due to erythematous condition involving 50-59 percent of body surface

  L49.6 Exfoliation due to erythematous condition involving 60-69 percent of body surface

  L49.7 Exfoliation due to erythematous condition involving 70-79 percent of body surface

  L49.8 Exfoliation due to erythematous condition involving 80-89 percent of body surface

  L49.9 Exfoliation due to erythematous condition involving 90 or more percent of body surface

☑4ᵗʰ **L50 Urticaria**
    EXCLUDES1 *allergic contact dermatitis (L23.-)*
      angioneurotic edema (T78.3)
      giant urticaria (T78.3)
      hereditary angio-edema (D84.1)
      Quincke's edema (T78.3)
      serum urticaria (T80.6-)
      solar urticaria (L56.3)
      urticaria neonatorum (P83.8)
      urticaria papulosa (L28.2)
      urticaria pigmentosa (Q82.2)

  L50.0 Allergic urticaria

  L50.1 Idiopathic urticaria

  L50.2 Urticaria due to cold and heat
    EXCLUDES2 *familial cold urticaria (M04.2)*

  L50.3 Dermatographic urticaria

  L50.4 Vibratory urticaria

  L50.5 Cholinergic urticaria

  L50.6 Contact urticaria

  L50.8 Other urticaria
    Chronic urticaria
    Recurrent periodic urticaria

  L50.9 Urticaria, unspecified ▽

☑4ᵗʰ **L51 Erythema multiforme**
    Use additional code for adverse effect, if applicable, to identify drug (T36-T50 with fifth or sixth character 5)
    Use additional code to identify associated manifestations, such as:
      arthropathy associated with dermatological disorders (M14.8-)
      conjunctival edema (H11.42)
      conjunctivitis (H10.22-)
      corneal scars and opacities (H17.-)
      corneal ulcer (H16.0-)
      edema of eyelid (H02.84)
      inflammation of eyelid (H01.8)
      keratoconjunctivitis sicca (H16.22-)
      mechanical lagophthalmos (H02.22-)
      stomatitis (K12.-)
      symblepharon (H11.23-)
    Use additional code to identify percentage of skin exfoliation (L49.-)
    EXCLUDES1 *staphylococcal scalded skin syndrome (L00)*
      Ritter's disease (L00)

  L51.0 Nonbullous erythema multiforme

  L51.1 Stevens-Johnson syndrome `HCC`

  L51.2 Toxic epidermal necrolysis [Lyell] `HCC`

  L51.3 Stevens-Johnson syndrome-toxic epidermal necrolysis overlap syndrome `HCC`
    SJS-TEN overlap syndrome

  L51.8 Other erythema multiforme

  L51.9 Erythema multiforme, unspecified ▽
    Erythema iris
    Erythema multiforme major NOS
    Erythema multiforme minor NOS
    Herpes iris

  L52 Erythema nodosum
    EXCLUDES1 *tuberculous erythema nodosum (A18.4)*
    DEF: A form of panniculitis (inflammation of the fat layer beneath the skin) of particularly women, usually seen as a hypersensitivity reaction to infections, drugs, sarcoidosis, and specific enteropathies; the acute stage is associated with fever, malaise, and arthralgia; the lesions are pink to blue in color as tender nodules and are found on the front of the legs below the knees.

☑4ᵗʰ **L53 Other erythematous conditions**
    EXCLUDES1 *erythema ab igne (L59.0)*
      erythema due to external agents in contact with skin (L23-L25)
      erythema intertrigo (L30.4)

  L53.0 Toxic erythema
    Code first poisoning due to drug or toxin, if applicable (T36-T65 with fifth or sixth character 1-4 or 6)
    Use additional code for adverse effect, if applicable, to identify drug (T36-T50 with fifth or sixth character 5)
    EXCLUDES1 *neonatal erythema toxicum (P83.1)*

☑ Additional Character Req   ✓x7ᵗʰ Placeholder Alert   Manifestation   `HCC` CMS-HCC Condition   ▽ Unspecified Code   ►◄ Revised Text   ● New Code   ▲ Revised Code Title

Chapter 12. Diseases of the Skin and Subcutaneous Tissue

L40.5–L53.0

L53.1　**Erythema** annulare centrifugum

L53.2　**Erythema** marginatum

L53.3　**Other chronic figurate erythema**

L53.8　**Other specified erythematous conditions**

L53.9　**Erythematous condition, unspecified**　▽
　　　　Erythema NOS
　　　　Erythroderma NOS

L54　***Erythema in diseases classified elsewhere***
　　　　Code first underlying disease

Radiation-related disorders of the skin and subcutaneous tissue (L55-L59)

✓4ᵗʰ **L55**　**Sunburn**

L55.0　**Sunburn of** first degree

L55.1　**Sunburn of** second degree

L55.2　**Sunburn of** third degree

L55.9　**Sunburn, unspecified**　▽

✓4ᵗʰ **L56**　**Other acute skin changes due to ultraviolet radiation**
　　　　Use additional code to identify the source of the ultraviolet radiation (W89, X32)

L56.0　**Drug phototoxic response**
　　　　Use additional code for adverse effect, if applicable, to identify drug (T36-T50 with fifth or sixth character 5)

L56.1　**Drug photoallergic response**
　　　　Use additional code for adverse effect, if applicable, to identify drug (T36-T50 with fifth or sixth character 5)

L56.2　**Photocontact dermatitis [berloque dermatitis]**

L56.3　**Solar urticaria**

L56.4　**Polymorphous light eruption**

L56.5　**Disseminated superficial actinic porokeratosis (DSAP)**
　　　　DEF: Autosomal dominant skin condition occurring in sun-exposed areas of the skin (particularly the arms and legs); characterized by superficial annular, keratotic, brownish-red spots or thickenings with depressed centers and sharp, ridged borders; may evolve into squamous cell carcinoma.

L56.8　**Other specified acute skin changes due to ultraviolet radiation**

L56.9　**Acute skin change due to ultraviolet radiation, unspecified**　▽

✓4ᵗʰ **L57**　**Skin changes due to chronic exposure to nonionizing radiation**
　　　　Use additional code to identify the source of the ultraviolet radiation ▶(W89)◀

L57.0　**Actinic keratosis**
　　　　Keratosis NOS
　　　　Senile keratosis
　　　　Solar keratosis

L57.1　**Actinic reticuloid**

L57.2　**Cutis rhomboidalis nuchae**

L57.3　**Poikiloderma of Civatte**

L57.4　**Cutis laxa senilis**
　　　　Elastosis senilis

L57.5　**Actinic granuloma**

L57.8　**Other skin changes due to chronic exposure to nonionizing radiation**
　　　　Farmer's skin
　　　　Sailor's skin
　　　　Solar dermatitis

L57.9　**Skin changes due to chronic exposure to nonionizing radiation, unspecified**　▽

✓4ᵗʰ **L58**　**Radiodermatitis**
　　　　Use additional code to identify the source of the radiation (W88, W90)

L58.0　Acute **radiodermatitis**

L58.1　Chronic **radiodermatitis**

L58.9　**Radiodermatitis, unspecified**　▽

✓4ᵗʰ **L59**　**Other disorders of skin and subcutaneous tissue related to radiation**

L59.0　**Erythema ab igne [dermatitis ab igne]**

L59.8　**Other specified disorders of the skin and subcutaneous tissue related to radiation**
　　　　AHA: 2017, 1Q, 33

L59.9　**Disorder of the skin and subcutaneous tissue related to radiation, unspecified**　▽

Nail Disorders

Normal

Koilonychia

Beau's Lines

Disorders of skin appendages (L60-L75)

EXCLUDES 1　congenital malformations of integument (Q84.-)

✓4ᵗʰ **L60**　**Nail disorders**
　　　　EXCLUDES 2　clubbing of nails (R68.3)
　　　　　　　　　　onychia and paronychia (L03.0-)

L60.0　**Ingrowing nail**

L60.1　**Onycholysis**

L60.2　**Onychogryphosis**

L60.3　**Nail dystrophy**

L60.4　**Beau's lines**

L60.5　**Yellow nail syndrome**

L60.8　**Other nail disorders**

L60.9　**Nail disorder, unspecified**　▽

L62　***Nail disorders in diseases classified elsewhere***
　　　　Code first underlying disease, such as:
　　　　pachydermoperiostosis (M89.4-)

✓4ᵗʰ **L63**　**Alopecia areata**

L63.0　**Alopecia (capitis)** totalis

L63.1　**Alopecia** universalis

L63.2　Ophiasis

L63.8　**Other alopecia areata**

L63.9　**Alopecia areata, unspecified**　▽

✓4ᵗʰ **L64**　**Androgenic alopecia**
　　　　INCLUDES　male-pattern baldness

L64.0　Drug-induced **androgenic alopecia**
　　　　Use additional code for adverse effect, if applicable, to identify drug (T36-T50 with fifth or sixth character 5)

L64.8　**Other androgenic alopecia**

L64.9　**Androgenic alopecia, unspecified**　▽

✓4ᵗʰ **L65**　**Other nonscarring hair loss**
　　　　Use additional code for adverse effect, if applicable, to identify drug (T36-T50 with fifth or sixth character 5)
　　　　EXCLUDES 1　trichotillomania (F63.3)

L65.0　**Telogen effluvium**
　　　　DEF: A form of nonscarring alopecia characterized by shedding of hair from premature telogen development in follicles due to stress, including shock, childbirth, surgery, drugs, or weight loss.

L65.1　**Anagen effluvium**

L65.2　**Alopecia mucinosa**

L65.8　**Other specified nonscarring hair loss**

L65.9　**Nonscarring hair loss, unspecified**　▽
　　　　Alopecia NOS

✓4ᵗʰ **L66**　**Cicatricial alopecia [scarring hair loss]**

L66.0　**Pseudopelade**

L66.1　**Lichen planopilaris**
　　　　Follicular lichen planus

L66.2　**Folliculitis decalvans**

L66.3　**Perifolliculitis capitis abscedens**

L66.4　**Folliculitis ulerythematosa reticulata**

L66.8　**Other cicatricial alopecia**
　　　　AHA: 2015, 1Q, 19

L66.9　**Cicatricial alopecia, unspecified**　▽

EXCLUDES 1 Not coded here　　　EXCLUDES 2 Not included here　　　N Newborn Age: 0　　　P Pediatric Age: 0-17　　　M Maternity Age: 12-55　　　A Adult Age: 15-124

700　　ICD-10-CM 2018

☑️**4ᵗʰ** **L67** **Hair color and hair shaft abnormalities**
     EXCLUDES 1   monilethrix (Q84.1)
           pili annulati (Q84.1)
           telogen effluvium (L65.0)

     L67.0 **Trichorrhexis nodosa**

     L67.1 **Variations in hair color**
         Canities
         Greyness, hair (premature)
         Heterochromia of hair
         Poliosis circumscripta, acquired
         Poliosis NOS

     L67.8 **Other hair color and hair shaft abnormalities**
         Fragilitas crinium

     L67.9 **Hair color and hair shaft abnormality, unspecified** ▽

☑️**4ᵗʰ** **L68** **Hypertrichosis**
     INCLUDES   excess hair
     EXCLUDES 1   congenital hypertrichosis (Q84.2)
           persistent lanugo (Q84.2)

     L68.0 **Hirsutism**

     L68.1 **Acquired hypertrichosis lanuginosa**

     L68.2 **Localized hypertrichosis**

     L68.3 **Polytrichia**

     L68.8 **Other hypertrichosis**

     L68.9 **Hypertrichosis, unspecified** ▽

☑️**4ᵗʰ** **L70** **Acne**
     EXCLUDES 2   acne keloid (L73.0)

     L70.0 **Acne** vulgaris

     L70.1 **Acne** conglobata

     L70.2 **Acne** varioliformis
         Acne necrotica miliaris
         DEF: Rare form of acne characterized by development of
         persistent brown papulo-pustules followed by scar formation;
         usually on the brow and temporoparietal part of the scalp.

     L70.3 **Acne** tropica

     L70.4 Infantile **acne**   P

     L70.5 Acné excoriée
         Acné excoriée des jeunes filles
         Picker's acne

     L70.8 **Other acne**

     L70.9 **Acne, unspecified** ▽

☑️**4ᵗʰ** **L71** **Rosacea**
     Use additional code for adverse effect, if applicable, to identify drug
     (T36-T50 with fifth or sixth character 5)

     L71.0 **Perioral dermatitis**

     L71.1 **Rhinophyma**

     L71.8 **Other rosacea**

     L71.9 **Rosacea, unspecified** ▽

☑️**4ᵗʰ** **L72** **Follicular cysts of skin and subcutaneous tissue**

     L72.0 **Epidermal cyst**

     ☑️**5ᵗʰ** **L72.1** **Pilar and trichodermal cyst**

         L72.11 **Pilar cyst**

         L72.12 **Trichodermal cyst**
                Trichilemmal (proliferating) cyst

     L72.2 **Steatocystoma multiplex**

     L72.3 **Sebaceous cyst**
         EXCLUDES 2   pilar cyst (L72.11)
                trichilemmal (proliferating) cyst (L72.12)

     L72.8 **Other follicular cysts of the skin and subcutaneous tissue**

     L72.9 **Follicular cyst of the skin and subcutaneous tissue,** ▽
         unspecified

☑️**4ᵗʰ** **L73** **Other follicular disorders**

     L73.0 **Acne keloid**

     L73.1 **Pseudofolliculitis barbae**

     L73.2 **Hidradenitis suppurativa**

     L73.8 **Other specified follicular disorders**
         Sycosis barbae

     L73.9 **Follicular disorder, unspecified** ▽

☑️**4ᵗʰ** **L74** **Eccrine sweat disorders**
     EXCLUDES 2   generalized hyperhidrosis (R61)

     L74.0 **Miliaria** rubra

     L74.1 **Miliaria** crystallina

     L74.2 **Miliaria** profunda
         Miliaria tropicalis

     L74.3 **Miliaria, unspecified** ▽

     L74.4 **Anhidrosis**
         Hypohidrosis

     ☑️**5ᵗʰ** **L74.5** **Focal hyperhidrosis**

         ☑️**6ᵗʰ** **L74.51** Primary **focal hyperhidrosis**

             L74.510 **Primary focal hyperhidrosis,** axilla

             L74.511 **Primary focal hyperhidrosis,** face

             L74.512 **Primary focal hyperhidrosis,** palms

             L74.513 **Primary focal hyperhidrosis,** soles

             L74.519 **Primary focal hyperhidrosis,** ▽
                      unspecified

         L74.52 Secondary **focal hyperhidrosis**
             Frey's syndrome

     L74.8 **Other eccrine sweat disorders**

     L74.9 **Eccrine sweat disorder, unspecified** ▽
         Sweat gland disorder NOS

☑️**4ᵗʰ** **L75** **Apocrine sweat disorders**
     EXCLUDES 1   dyshidrosis (L30.1)
           hidradenitis suppurativa (L73.2)

     L75.0 **Bromhidrosis**

     L75.1 **Chromhidrosis**

     L75.2 **Apocrine miliaria**
         Fox-Fordyce disease
         DEF: Chronic, usually pruritic disease evidenced by small follicular
         papular eruptions, especially in the axillary and pubic areas;
         develops from the closure and rupture of the affected apocrine
         glands' intraepidermal portion of the ducts.

     L75.8 **Other apocrine sweat disorders**

     L75.9 **Apocrine sweat disorder, unspecified** ▽

Intraoperative and postprocedural complications of skin and subcutaneous tissue (L76)

☑️**4ᵗʰ** **L76** **Intraoperative and postprocedural complications of skin and subcutaneous tissue**

     ☑️**5ᵗʰ** **L76.0** **Intraoperative hemorrhage and hematoma** of skin and subcutaneous tissue complicating a procedure
         EXCLUDES 1   intraoperative hemorrhage and hematoma of skin and
                subcutaneous tissue due to accidental puncture
                and laceration during a procedure (L76.1-)

         L76.01 **Intraoperative hemorrhage and hematoma of skin and subcutaneous tissue complicating a** dermatologic procedure

         L76.02 **Intraoperative hemorrhage and hematoma of skin and subcutaneous tissue complicating** other procedure

     ☑️**5ᵗʰ** **L76.1** **Accidental puncture and laceration** of skin and subcutaneous tissue during a procedure

         L76.11 **Accidental puncture and laceration of skin and subcutaneous tissue during a** dermatologic procedure

         L76.12 **Accidental puncture and laceration of skin and subcutaneous tissue during** other procedure

     ☑️**5ᵗʰ** **L76.2** **Postprocedural hemorrhage** of skin and subcutaneous tissue following a procedure

         L76.21 **Postprocedural hemorrhage of skin and subcutaneous tissue following a** dermatologic procedure

         L76.22 **Postprocedural hemorrhage of skin and subcutaneous tissue following** other procedure

     ☑️**5ᵗʰ** **L76.3** **Postprocedural hematoma and seroma** of skin and subcutaneous tissue following a procedure

         L76.31 **Postprocedural** hematoma **of skin and subcutaneous tissue following a** dermatologic procedure

         L76.32 **Postprocedural** hematoma **of skin and subcutaneous tissue following** other procedure

         L76.33 **Postprocedural** seroma **of skin and subcutaneous tissue following a** dermatologic procedure

         L76.34 **Postprocedural** seroma **of skin and subcutaneous tissue following** other procedure

     ☑️**5ᵗʰ** **L76.8** **Other intraoperative and postprocedural complications of skin and subcutaneous tissue**
         Use additional code, if applicable, to further specify disorder

         L76.81 **Other intraoperative complications of skin and subcutaneous tissue**

         L76.82 **Other postprocedural complications of skin and subcutaneous tissue**

☑️ Additional Character Req   ⁷ˣ⁷ᵗʰ Placeholder Alert   *Manifestation*   **HCC** CMS-HCC Condition   ▽ Unspecified Code   ▶◀ Revised Text   ● New Code   ▲ Revised Code Title

Chapter 12. Diseases of the Skin and Subcutaneous Tissue

Other disorders of the skin and subcutaneous tissue (L80-L99)

L80 Vitiligo
> *EXCLUDES 2*   vitiligo of eyelids (H02.73-)
> vitiligo of vulva (N90.89)
> **DEF:** Persistent, progressive development of nonpigmented white patches on otherwise normal skin.

✓4ᵗʰ L81 Other disorders of pigmentation
> *EXCLUDES 1*   birthmark NOS (Q82.5)
> Peutz-Jeghers syndrome (Q85.8)
> *EXCLUDES 2*   nevus—see Alphabetical Index

L81.0 Postinflammatory hyperpigmentation

L81.1 Chloasma

L81.2 Freckles

L81.3 Café au lait spots

L81.4 Other melanin hyperpigmentation
> Lentigo

L81.5 Leukoderma, not elsewhere classified

L81.6 Other disorders of diminished melanin formation

L81.7 Pigmented purpuric dermatosis
> Angioma serpiginosum

L81.8 Other specified disorders of pigmentation
> Iron pigmentation
> Tattoo pigmentation

L81.9 Disorder of pigmentation, unspecified   ▽

✓4ᵗʰ L82 Seborrheic keratosis
> *INCLUDES*   basal cell papilloma
> dermatosis papulosa nigra
> Leser-Trélat disease
> *EXCLUDES 2*   seborrheic dermatitis (L21.-)

L82.0 Inflamed seborrheic keratosis

L82.1 Other seborrheic keratosis
> Seborrheic keratosis NOS

L83 Acanthosis nigricans
> Confluent and reticulated papillomatosis
> **DEF:** Diffuse, velvety hyperplasia of the spinous skin layer of the axilla and other body folds marked by gray, brown, or black pigmentation; in adult form often associated with malignant acanthosis nigricans in a benign, nevoid form relatively generalized.

L84 Corns and callosities
> Callus
> Clavus

✓4ᵗʰ L85 Other epidermal thickening
> *EXCLUDES 2*   hypertrophic disorders of the skin (L91.-)

L85.0 Acquired ichthyosis
> *EXCLUDES 1*   congenital ichthyosis (Q80.-)

L85.1 Acquired keratosis [keratoderma] palmaris et plantaris
> *EXCLUDES 1*   inherited keratosis palmaris et plantaris (Q82.8)

L85.2 Keratosis punctata (palmaris et plantaris)

L85.3 Xerosis cutis
> Dry skin dermatitis

L85.8 Other specified epidermal thickening
> Cutaneous horn

L85.9 Epidermal thickening, unspecified   ▽

L86 Keratoderma in diseases classified elsewhere
> Code first underlying disease, such as:
> Reiter's disease (M02.3-)
> *EXCLUDES 1*   gonococcal keratoderma (A54.89)
> gonococcal keratosis (A54.89)
> keratoderma due to vitamin A deficiency (E50.8)
> keratosis due to vitamin A deficiency (E50.8)
> xeroderma due to vitamin A deficiency (E50.8)

✓4ᵗʰ L87 Transepidermal elimination disorders
> *EXCLUDES 1*   granuloma annulare (perforating) (L92.0)

L87.0 Keratosis follicularis et parafollicularis in cutem penetrans
> Hyperkeratosis follicularis penetrans
> Kyrle disease

L87.1 Reactive perforating collagenosis

L87.2 Elastosis perforans serpiginosa

L87.8 Other transepidermal elimination disorders

L87.9 Transepidermal elimination disorder, unspecified   ▽

L88 Pyoderma gangrenosum
> Phagedenic pyoderma
> *EXCLUDES 1*   dermatitis gangrenosa (L08.0)
> **DEF:** Persistent debilitating skin disease characterized by irregular, boggy, blue-red ulcerations, with central healing and undermined edges.

Four Stages of Pressure Ulcer

Epidermis
Dermis

Stage 1
Persistent focal erythema

Subcutaneous tissue

Stage 2
Abrasion, blister, partial thickness skin loss involving epidermis and/or dermis

Superficial fascia
Muscle

Stage 3
Full thickness skin loss involving damage or necrosis of subcutaneous tissue

Deep fascia
Bone

Stage 4
Necrosis of soft tissues through to underlying muscle, tendon, or bone

✓4ᵗʰ L89 Pressure ulcer
> *INCLUDES*   bed sore
> decubitus ulcer
> plaster ulcer
> pressure area
> pressure sore
> Code first any associated gangrene (I96)
> *EXCLUDES 2*   decubitus (trophic) ulcer of cervix (uteri) (N86)
> diabetic ulcers (E08.621, E08.622, E09.621, E09.622, E10.621, E10.622, E11.621, E11.622, E13.621, E13.622)
> non-pressure chronic ulcer of skin (L97.-)
> skin infections (L00-L08)
> varicose ulcer (I83.0, I83.2)
> **AHA:** 2017, 1Q, 49; 2016, 4Q, 143

✓5ᵗʰ L89.0 Pressure ulcer of elbow

✓6ᵗʰ L89.00 Pressure ulcer of unspecified elbow

L89.000 Pressure ulcer of unspecified elbow, HCC ▽
unstageable

L89.001 Pressure ulcer of unspecified elbow, ▽
stage 1
> Healing pressure ulcer of unspecified elbow, stage 1
> Pressure pre-ulcer skin changes limited to persistent focal edema, unspecified elbow

L89.002 Pressure ulcer of unspecified elbow, ▽
stage 2
> Healing pressure ulcer of unspecified elbow, stage 2
> Pressure ulcer with abrasion, blister, partial thickness skin loss involving epidermis and/or dermis, unspecified elbow

L89.003 Pressure ulcer of unspecified HCC ▽
elbow, stage 3
> Healing pressure ulcer of unspecified elbow, stage 3
> Pressure ulcer with full thickness skin loss involving damage or necrosis of subcutaneous tissue, unspecified elbow

L89.004 Pressure ulcer of unspecified HCC ▽
elbow, stage 4
> Healing pressure ulcer of unspecified elbow, stage 4
> Pressure ulcer with necrosis of soft tissues through to underlying muscle, tendon, or bone, unspecified elbow

L89.009 Pressure ulcer of unspecified elbow, ▽
unspecified stage
> Healing pressure ulcer of elbow NOS
> Healing pressure ulcer of unspecified elbow, unspecified stage

✓6ᵗʰ L89.01 Pressure ulcer of right elbow

L89.010 Pressure ulcer of right elbow, HCC
unstageable

EXCLUDES 1 Not coded here   *EXCLUDES 2* Not included here   N Newborn Age: 0   P Pediatric Age: 0-17   M Maternity Age: 12-55   A Adult Age: 15-124

702   ICD-10-CM 2018

L89.011 Pressure ulcer of right elbow, stage 1
    Healing pressure ulcer of right elbow, stage 1
    Pressure pre-ulcer skin changes limited to persistent focal edema, right elbow

L89.012 Pressure ulcer of right elbow, stage 2
    Healing pressure ulcer of right elbow, stage 2
    Pressure ulcer with abrasion, blister, partial thickness skin loss involving epidermis and/or dermis, right elbow

L89.013 Pressure ulcer of right elbow, stage 3 HCC
    Healing pressure ulcer of right elbow, stage 3
    Pressure ulcer with full thickness skin loss involving damage or necrosis of subcutaneous tissue, right elbow

L89.014 Pressure ulcer of right elbow, stage 4 HCC
    Healing pressure ulcer of right elbow, stage 4
    Pressure ulcer with necrosis of soft tissues through to underlying muscle, tendon, or bone, right elbow

L89.019 Pressure ulcer of right elbow, unspecified stage ▽
    Healing pressure right of elbow NOS
    ►Healing pressure ulcer of right elbow, unspecified stage◄

✓6th **L89.02 Pressure ulcer of** left elbow

L89.020 Pressure ulcer of left elbow, unstageable HCC

L89.021 Pressure ulcer of left elbow, stage 1
    Healing pressure ulcer of left elbow, stage 1
    Pressure pre-ulcer skin changes limited to persistent focal edema, left elbow

L89.022 Pressure ulcer of left elbow, stage 2
    Healing pressure ulcer of left elbow, stage 2
    Pressure ulcer with abrasion, blister, partial thickness skin loss involving epidermis and/or dermis, left elbow

L89.023 Pressure ulcer of left elbow, stage 3 HCC
    Healing pressure ulcer of left elbow, stage 3
    Pressure ulcer with full thickness skin loss involving damage or necrosis of subcutaneous tissue, left elbow

L89.024 Pressure ulcer of left elbow, stage 4 HCC
    Healing pressure ulcer of left elbow, stage 4
    Pressure ulcer with necrosis of soft tissues through to underlying muscle, tendon, or bone, left elbow

L89.029 Pressure ulcer of left elbow, unspecified stage ▽
    Healing pressure ulcer of left of elbow NOS
    ►Healing pressure ulcer of left elbow, unspecified stage◄

✓5th **L89.1 Pressure ulcer of** back

✓6th **L89.10 Pressure ulcer of unspecified part of back**

L89.100 Pressure ulcer of unspecified part of back, unstageable HCC ▽

L89.101 Pressure ulcer of unspecified part of back, stage 1 ▽
    Healing pressure ulcer of unspecified part of back, stage 1
    Pressure pre-ulcer skin changes limited to persistent focal edema, unspecified part of back

L89.102 Pressure ulcer of unspecified part of back, stage 2 ▽
    Healing pressure ulcer of unspecified part of back, stage 2
    Pressure ulcer with abrasion, blister, partial thickness skin loss involving epidermis and/or dermis, unspecified part of back

L89.103 Pressure ulcer of unspecified part of back, stage 3 HCC ▽
    Healing pressure ulcer of unspecified part of back, stage 3
    Pressure ulcer with full thickness skin loss involving damage or necrosis of subcutaneous tissue, unspecified part of back

L89.104 Pressure ulcer of unspecified part of back, stage 4 HCC ▽
    Healing pressure ulcer of unspecified part of back, stage 4
    Pressure ulcer with necrosis of soft tissues through to underlying muscle, tendon, or bone, unspecified part of back

L89.109 Pressure ulcer of unspecified part of back, unspecified stage ▽
    Healing pressure ulcer of unspecified part of back NOS
    Healing pressure ulcer of unspecified part of back, unspecified stage

✓6th **L89.11 Pressure ulcer of** right upper **back**
    Pressure ulcer of right shoulder blade

L89.110 Pressure ulcer of right upper back, unstageable HCC

L89.111 Pressure ulcer of right upper back, stage 1
    Healing pressure ulcer of right upper back, stage 1
    Pressure pre-ulcer skin changes limited to persistent focal edema, right upper back

L89.112 Pressure ulcer of right upper back, stage 2
    Healing pressure ulcer of right upper back, stage 2
    Pressure ulcer with abrasion, blister, partial thickness skin loss involving epidermis and/or dermis, right upper back

L89.113 Pressure ulcer of right upper back, stage 3 HCC
    Healing pressure ulcer of right upper back, stage 3
    Pressure ulcer with full thickness skin loss involving damage or necrosis of subcutaneous tissue, right upper back

L89.114 Pressure ulcer of right upper back, stage 4 HCC
    Healing pressure ulcer of right upper back, stage 4
    Pressure ulcer with necrosis of soft tissues through to underlying muscle, tendon, or bone, right upper back

L89.119 Pressure ulcer of right upper back, unspecified stage ▽
    Healing pressure ulcer of right upper back NOS
    Healing pressure ulcer of right upper back, unspecified stage

✓6th **L89.12 Pressure ulcer of** left upper **back**
    Pressure ulcer of left shoulder blade

L89.120 Pressure ulcer of left upper back, unstageable HCC

L89.121 Pressure ulcer of left upper back, stage 1
    Healing pressure ulcer of left upper back, stage 1
    Pressure pre-ulcer skin changes limited to persistent focal edema, left upper back

L89.122 Pressure ulcer of left upper back, stage 2
    Healing pressure ulcer of left upper back, stage 2
    Pressure ulcer with abrasion, blister, partial thickness skin loss involving epidermis and/or dermis, left upper back

L89.123 Pressure ulcer of left upper back, stage 3 HCC
    Healing pressure ulcer of left upper back, stage 3
    Pressure ulcer with full thickness skin loss involving damage or necrosis of subcutaneous tissue, left upper back

L89.124 Pressure ulcer of left upper back, stage 4 HCC
    Healing pressure ulcer of left upper back, stage 4
    Pressure ulcer with necrosis of soft tissues through to underlying muscle, tendon, or bone, left upper back

---

✓ Additional Character Req   ✓x7th Placeholder Alert   Manifestation   HCC CMS-HCC Condition   ▽ Unspecified Code   ►◄ Revised Text   ● New Code   ▲ Revised Code Title

L89.129   **Pressure ulcer of left upper back,** ▽
unspecified stage
     Healing pressure ulcer of left upper back
       NOS
     Healing pressure ulcer of left upper back,
       unspecified stage

✓6ᵗʰ **L89.13**   **Pressure ulcer of right lower back**
L89.130   **Pressure ulcer of right lower back,** HCC
unstageable
L89.131   **Pressure ulcer of right lower back, stage 1**
     Healing pressure ulcer of right lower back,
       stage 1
     Pressure pre-ulcer skin changes limited to
       persistent focal edema, right lower
       back
L89.132   **Pressure ulcer of right lower back, stage 2**
     Healing pressure ulcer of right lower back,
       stage 2
     Pressure ulcer with abrasion, blister, partial
       thickness skin loss involving epidermis
       and/or dermis, right lower back
L89.133   **Pressure ulcer of right lower back,** HCC
stage 3
     Healing pressure ulcer of right lower back,
       stage 3
     Pressure ulcer with full thickness skin loss
       involving damage or necrosis of
       subcutaneous tissue, right lower back
L89.134   **Pressure ulcer of right lower back,** HCC
stage 4
     Healing pressure ulcer of right lower back,
       stage 4
     Pressure ulcer with necrosis of soft tissues
       through to underlying muscle,
       tendon, or bone, right lower back
L89.139   **Pressure ulcer of right lower back,** ▽
unspecified stage
     Healing pressure ulcer of right lower back
       NOS
     Healing pressure ulcer of right lower back,
       unspecified stage

✓6ᵗʰ **L89.14**   **Pressure ulcer of left lower back**
L89.140   **Pressure ulcer of left lower back,** HCC
unstageable
L89.141   **Pressure ulcer of left lower back, stage 1**
     Healing pressure ulcer of left lower back,
       stage 1
     Pressure pre-ulcer skin changes limited to
       persistent focal edema, left lower back
L89.142   **Pressure ulcer of left lower back, stage 2**
     Healing pressure ulcer of left lower back,
       stage 2
     Pressure ulcer with abrasion, blister, partial
       thickness skin loss involving epidermis
       and/or dermis, left lower back
L89.143   **Pressure ulcer of left lower back,** HCC
stage 3
     Healing pressure ulcer of left lower back,
       stage 3
     Pressure ulcer with full thickness skin loss
       involving damage or necrosis of
       subcutaneous tissue, left lower back
L89.144   **Pressure ulcer of left lower back,** HCC
stage 4
     Healing pressure ulcer of left lower back,
       stage 4
     Pressure ulcer with necrosis of soft tissues
       through to underlying muscle,
       tendon, or bone, left lower back
L89.149   **Pressure ulcer of left lower back,** ▽
unspecified stage
     Healing pressure ulcer of left lower back
       NOS
     Healing pressure ulcer of left lower back,
       unspecified stage

✓6ᵗʰ **L89.15**   **Pressure ulcer of sacral region**
     Pressure ulcer of coccyx
     Pressure ulcer of tailbone
L89.150   **Pressure ulcer of sacral region,** HCC
unstageable

L89.151   **Pressure ulcer of sacral region, stage 1**
     Healing pressure ulcer of sacral region,
       stage 1
     Pressure pre-ulcer skin changes limited to
       persistent focal edema, sacral region
L89.152   **Pressure ulcer of sacral region, stage 2**
     Healing pressure ulcer of sacral region,
       stage 2
     Pressure ulcer with abrasion, blister, partial
       thickness skin loss involving epidermis
       and/or dermis, sacral region
L89.153   **Pressure ulcer of sacral region, stage 3** HCC
     Healing pressure ulcer of sacral region,
       stage 3
     Pressure ulcer with full thickness skin loss
       involving damage or necrosis of
       subcutaneous tissue, sacral region
L89.154   **Pressure ulcer of sacral region, stage 4** HCC
     Healing pressure ulcer of sacral region,
       stage 4
     Pressure ulcer with necrosis of soft tissues
       through to underlying muscle,
       tendon, or bone, sacral region
L89.159   **Pressure ulcer of sacral region,** ▽
unspecified stage
     Healing pressure ulcer of sacral region NOS
     Healing pressure ulcer of sacral region,
       unspecified stage

✓5ᵗʰ **L89.2**   **Pressure ulcer of hip**
✓6ᵗʰ **L89.20**   **Pressure ulcer of unspecified hip**
L89.200   **Pressure ulcer of unspecified hip,** HCC ▽
unstageable
L89.201   **Pressure ulcer of unspecified hip,** ▽
stage 1
     Healing pressure ulcer of unspecified hip,
       stage 1
     Pressure pre-ulcer skin changes limited to
       persistent focal edema, unspecified
       hip
L89.202   **Pressure ulcer of unspecified hip,** ▽
stage 2
     Healing pressure ulcer of unspecified hip,
       stage 2
     Pressure ulcer with abrasion, blister, partial
       thickness skin loss involving epidermis
       and/or dermis, unspecified hip
L89.203   **Pressure ulcer of unspecified hip,** HCC ▽
stage 3
     Healing pressure ulcer of unspecified hip,
       stage 3
     Pressure ulcer with full thickness skin loss
       involving damage or necrosis of
       subcutaneous tissue, unspecified hip
L89.204   **Pressure ulcer of unspecified hip,** HCC ▽
stage 4
     Healing pressure ulcer of unspecified hip,
       stage 4
     Pressure ulcer with necrosis of soft tissues
       through to underlying muscle,
       tendon, or bone, unspecified hip
L89.209   **Pressure ulcer of unspecified hip,** ▽
unspecified stage
     Healing pressure ulcer of unspecified hip
       NOS
     Healing pressure ulcer of unspecified hip,
       unspecified stage

✓6ᵗʰ **L89.21**   **Pressure ulcer of right hip**
L89.210   **Pressure ulcer of right hip,** HCC
unstageable
L89.211   **Pressure ulcer of right hip, stage 1**
     Healing pressure ulcer of right hip, stage 1
     Pressure pre-ulcer skin changes limited to
       persistent focal edema, right hip
L89.212   **Pressure ulcer of right hip, stage 2**
     Healing pressure ulcer of right hip, stage 2
     Pressure ulcer with abrasion, blister, partial
       thickness skin loss involving epidermis
       and/or dermis, right hip
L89.213   **Pressure ulcer of right hip, stage 3** HCC
     Healing pressure ulcer of right hip, stage 3
     Pressure ulcer with full thickness skin loss
       involving damage or necrosis of
       subcutaneous tissue, right hip

EXCLUDES 1 Not coded here   **EXCLUDES 2** Not included here   N Newborn Age: 0   P Pediatric Age: 0-17   M Maternity Age: 12-55   A Adult Age: 15-124

704   ICD-10-CM 2018

      L89.214 **Pressure ulcer of right hip,** stage 4 HCC
            Healing pressure ulcer of right hip, stage 4
            Pressure ulcer with necrosis of soft tissues through to underlying muscle, tendon, or bone, right hip

      L89.219 **Pressure ulcer of right hip, unspecified stage** ▽
            Healing pressure ulcer of right hip NOS
            Healing pressure ulcer of right hip, unspecified stage

✓6ᵗʰ **L89.22** **Pressure ulcer of** left hip
      L89.220 **Pressure ulcer of left hip,** unstageable HCC

      L89.221 **Pressure ulcer of left hip,** stage 1
            Healing pressure ulcer of left hip, stage 1
            Pressure pre-ulcer skin changes limited to persistent focal edema, left hip

      L89.222 **Pressure ulcer of left hip,** stage 2
            Healing pressure ulcer of left hip, stage 2
            Pressure ulcer with abrasion, blister, partial thickness skin loss involving epidermis and/or dermis, left hip

      L89.223 **Pressure ulcer of left hip,** stage 3 HCC
            Healing pressure ulcer of left hip, stage 3
            Pressure ulcer with full thickness skin loss involving damage or necrosis of subcutaneous tissue, left hip

      L89.224 **Pressure ulcer of left hip,** stage 4 HCC
            Healing pressure ulcer of left hip, stage 4
            Pressure ulcer with necrosis of soft tissues through to underlying muscle, tendon, or bone, left hip

      L89.229 **Pressure ulcer of left hip, unspecified stage** ▽
            Healing pressure ulcer of left hip NOS
            Healing pressure ulcer of left hip, unspecified stage

✓5ᵗʰ **L89.3** **Pressure ulcer of** buttock
   ✓6ᵗʰ **L89.30** **Pressure ulcer of unspecified buttock**

      L89.300 **Pressure ulcer of unspecified buttock,** unstageable HCC ▽

      L89.301 **Pressure ulcer of unspecified buttock,** stage 1 ▽
            Healing pressure ulcer of unspecified buttock, stage 1
            Pressure pre-ulcer skin changes limited to persistent focal edema, unspecified buttock

      L89.302 **Pressure ulcer of unspecified buttock,** stage 2 ▽
            Healing pressure ulcer of unspecified buttock, stage 2
            Pressure ulcer with abrasion, blister, partial thickness skin loss involving epidermis and/or dermis, unspecified buttock

      L89.303 **Pressure ulcer of unspecified buttock,** stage 3 HCC ▽
            Healing pressure ulcer of unspecified buttock, stage 3
            Pressure ulcer with full thickness skin loss involving damage or necrosis of subcutaneous tissue, unspecified buttock

      L89.304 **Pressure ulcer of unspecified buttock,** stage 4 HCC ▽
            Healing pressure ulcer of unspecified buttock, stage 4
            Pressure ulcer with necrosis of soft tissues through to underlying muscle, tendon, or bone, unspecified buttock

      L89.309 **Pressure ulcer of unspecified buttock, unspecified stage** ▽
            Healing pressure ulcer of unspecified buttock NOS
            Healing pressure ulcer of unspecified buttock, unspecified stage

   ✓6ᵗʰ **L89.31** **Pressure ulcer of** right **buttock**
      L89.310 **Pressure ulcer of right buttock,** unstageable HCC

      L89.311 **Pressure ulcer of right buttock,** stage 1
            Healing pressure ulcer of right buttock, stage 1
            Pressure pre-ulcer skin changes limited to persistent focal edema, right buttock

      L89.312 **Pressure ulcer of right buttock,** stage 2
            Healing pressure ulcer of right buttock, stage 2
            Pressure ulcer with abrasion, blister, partial thickness skin loss involving epidermis and/or dermis, right buttock

      L89.313 **Pressure ulcer of right buttock,** stage 3 HCC
            Healing pressure ulcer of right buttock, stage 3
            Pressure ulcer with full thickness skin loss involving damage or necrosis of subcutaneous tissue, right buttock

      L89.314 **Pressure ulcer of right buttock,** stage 4 HCC
            Healing pressure ulcer of right buttock, stage 4
            Pressure ulcer with necrosis of soft tissues through to underlying muscle, tendon, or bone, right buttock

      L89.319 **Pressure ulcer of right buttock, unspecified stage** ▽
            Healing pressure ulcer of right buttock NOS
            Healing pressure ulcer of right buttock, unspecified stage

   ✓6ᵗʰ **L89.32** **Pressure ulcer of** left **buttock**
      L89.320 **Pressure ulcer of left buttock,** unstageable HCC

      L89.321 **Pressure ulcer of left buttock,** stage 1
            Healing pressure ulcer of left buttock, stage 1
            Pressure pre-ulcer skin changes limited to persistent focal edema, left buttock

      L89.322 **Pressure ulcer of left buttock,** stage 2
            Healing pressure ulcer of left buttock, stage 2
            Pressure ulcer with abrasion, blister, partial thickness skin loss involving epidermis and/or dermis, left buttock

      L89.323 **Pressure ulcer of left buttock,** stage 3 HCC
            Healing pressure ulcer of left buttock, stage 3
            Pressure ulcer with full thickness skin loss involving damage or necrosis of subcutaneous tissue, left buttock

      L89.324 **Pressure ulcer of left buttock,** stage 4 HCC
            Healing pressure ulcer of left buttock, stage 4
            Pressure ulcer with necrosis of soft tissues through to underlying muscle, tendon, or bone, left buttock

      L89.329 **Pressure ulcer of left buttock, unspecified stage** ▽
            Healing pressure ulcer of left buttock NOS
            Healing pressure ulcer of left buttock, unspecified stage

✓5ᵗʰ **L89.4** **Pressure ulcer of contiguous site of** back, buttock and hip
      L89.40 **Pressure ulcer of contiguous site of back, buttock and hip, unspecified stage** ▽
            Healing pressure ulcer of contiguous site of back, buttock and hip NOS
            Healing pressure ulcer of contiguous site of back, buttock and hip, unspecified stage

      L89.41 **Pressure ulcer of contiguous site of back, buttock and hip,** stage 1
            Healing pressure ulcer of contiguous site of back, buttock and hip, stage 1
            Pressure pre-ulcer skin changes limited to persistent focal edema, contiguous site of back, buttock and hip

      L89.42 **Pressure ulcer of contiguous site of back, buttock and hip,** stage 2
            Healing pressure ulcer of contiguous site of back, buttock and hip, stage 2
            Pressure ulcer with abrasion, blister, partial thickness skin loss involving epidermis and/or dermis, contiguous site of back, buttock and hip

---

☑ Additional Character Req   ✓x7ᵗʰ Placeholder Alert   Manifestation   HCC CMS-HCC Condition   ▽ Unspecified Code   ▶◀ Revised Text   ● New Code   ▲ Revised Code Title

L89.43   **Pressure ulcer of contiguous site of back,**   HCC
buttock and hip, stage 3
    Healing pressure ulcer of contiguous site of back,
    buttock and hip, stage 3
    Pressure ulcer with full thickness skin loss involving
    damage or necrosis of subcutaneous tissue,
    contiguous site of back, buttock and hip

L89.44   **Pressure ulcer of contiguous site of back,**   HCC
buttock and hip, stage 4
    Healing pressure ulcer of contiguous site of back,
    buttock and hip, stage 4
    Pressure ulcer with necrosis of soft tissues through to
    underlying muscle, tendon, or bone, contiguous
    site of back, buttock and hip

L89.45   **Pressure ulcer of contiguous site of back,**   HCC
buttock and hip, unstageable

✓5ᵗʰ **L89.5**   **Pressure ulcer of ankle**

    ✓6ᵗʰ **L89.50**   **Pressure ulcer of unspecified ankle**

      L89.500   **Pressure ulcer of unspecified ankle,**   HCC ▽
unstageable

      L89.501   **Pressure ulcer of unspecified ankle,**   ▽
stage 1
      Healing pressure ulcer of unspecified ankle,
      stage 1
      Pressure pre-ulcer skin changes limited to
      persistent focal edema, unspecified
      ankle

      L89.502   **Pressure ulcer of unspecified ankle,**   ▽
stage 2
      Healing pressure ulcer of unspecified ankle,
      stage 2
      Pressure ulcer with abrasion, blister, partial
      thickness skin loss involving epidermis
      and/or dermis, unspecified ankle

      L89.503   **Pressure ulcer of unspecified ankle,**   HCC ▽
stage 3
      Healing pressure ulcer of unspecified ankle,
      stage 3
      Pressure ulcer with full thickness skin loss
      involving damage or necrosis of
      subcutaneous tissue, unspecified
      ankle

      L89.504   **Pressure ulcer of unspecified ankle,**   HCC ▽
stage 4
      Healing pressure ulcer of unspecified ankle,
      stage 4
      Pressure ulcer with necrosis of soft tissues
      through to underlying muscle,
      tendon, or bone, unspecified ankle

      L89.509   **Pressure ulcer of unspecified ankle,**   ▽
unspecified stage
      Healing pressure ulcer of unspecified ankle
      NOS
      Healing pressure ulcer of unspecified ankle,
      unspecified stage

    ✓6ᵗʰ **L89.51**   **Pressure ulcer of right ankle**

      L89.510   **Pressure ulcer of right ankle,**   HCC
unstageable

      L89.511   **Pressure ulcer of right ankle, stage 1**
      Healing pressure ulcer of right ankle,
      stage 1
      Pressure pre-ulcer skin changes limited to
      persistent focal edema, right ankle

      L89.512   **Pressure ulcer of right ankle, stage 2**
      Healing pressure ulcer of right ankle,
      stage 2
      Pressure ulcer with abrasion, blister, partial
      thickness skin loss involving epidermis
      and/or dermis, right ankle

      L89.513   **Pressure ulcer of right ankle, stage 3**   HCC
      Healing pressure ulcer of right ankle,
      stage 3
      Pressure ulcer with full thickness skin loss
      involving damage or necrosis of
      subcutaneous tissue, right ankle

      L89.514   **Pressure ulcer of right ankle, stage 4**   HCC
      Healing pressure ulcer of right ankle,
      stage 4
      Pressure ulcer with necrosis of soft tissues
      through to underlying muscle,
      tendon, or bone, right ankle

      L89.519   **Pressure ulcer of right ankle,**   ▽
unspecified stage
      Healing pressure ulcer of right ankle NOS
      Healing pressure ulcer of right ankle,
      unspecified stage

    ✓6ᵗʰ **L89.52**   **Pressure ulcer of left ankle**

      L89.520   **Pressure ulcer of left ankle,**   HCC
unstageable

      L89.521   **Pressure ulcer of left ankle, stage 1**
      Healing pressure ulcer of left ankle, stage 1
      Pressure pre-ulcer skin changes limited to
      persistent focal edema, left ankle

      L89.522   **Pressure ulcer of left ankle, stage 2**
      Healing pressure ulcer of left ankle,
      stage 2
      Pressure ulcer with abrasion, blister, partial
      thickness skin loss involving epidermis
      and/or dermis, left ankle

      L89.523   **Pressure ulcer of left ankle, stage 3**   HCC
      Healing pressure ulcer of left ankle,
      stage 3
      Pressure ulcer with full thickness skin loss
      involving damage or necrosis of
      subcutaneous tissue, left ankle

      L89.524   **Pressure ulcer of left ankle, stage 4**   HCC
      Healing pressure ulcer of left ankle,
      stage 4
      Pressure ulcer with necrosis of soft tissues
      through to underlying muscle,
      tendon, or bone, left ankle

      L89.529   **Pressure ulcer of left ankle,**   ▽
unspecified stage
      Healing pressure ulcer of left ankle NOS
      Healing pressure ulcer of left ankle,
      unspecified stage

✓5ᵗʰ **L89.6**   **Pressure ulcer of heel**

    ✓6ᵗʰ **L89.60**   **Pressure ulcer of unspecified heel**

      L89.600   **Pressure ulcer of unspecified heel,**   HCC ▽
unstageable

      L89.601   **Pressure ulcer of unspecified heel,**   ▽
stage 1
      Healing pressure ulcer of unspecified heel,
      stage 1
      Pressure pre-ulcer skin changes limited to
      persistent focal edema, unspecified
      heel

      L89.602   **Pressure ulcer of unspecified heel,**   ▽
stage 2
      Healing pressure ulcer of unspecified heel,
      stage 2
      Pressure ulcer with abrasion, blister, partial
      thickness skin loss involving epidermis
      and/or dermis, unspecified heel

      L89.603   **Pressure ulcer of unspecified heel,**   HCC ▽
stage 3
      Healing pressure ulcer of unspecified heel,
      stage 3
      Pressure ulcer with full thickness skin loss
      involving damage or necrosis of
      subcutaneous tissue, unspecified heel

      L89.604   **Pressure ulcer of unspecified heel,**   HCC ▽
stage 4
      Healing pressure ulcer of unspecified heel,
      stage 4
      Pressure ulcer with necrosis of soft tissues
      through to underlying muscle,
      tendon, or bone, unspecified heel

      L89.609   **Pressure ulcer of unspecified heel,**   ▽
unspecified stage
      Healing pressure ulcer of unspecified heel
      NOS
      Healing pressure ulcer of unspecified heel,
      unspecified stage

    ✓6ᵗʰ **L89.61**   **Pressure ulcer of right heel**

      L89.610   **Pressure ulcer of right heel,**   HCC
unstageable

      L89.611   **Pressure ulcer of right heel, stage 1**
      Healing pressure ulcer of right heel,
      stage 1
      Pressure pre-ulcer skin changes limited to
      persistent focal edema, right heel

EXCLUDES 1 Not coded here   EXCLUDES 2 Not included here   N Newborn Age: 0   P Pediatric Age: 0-17   M Maternity Age: 12-55   A Adult Age: 15-124

706   ICD-10-CM 2018

L89.612 **Pressure ulcer of right heel,** stage 2
Healing pressure ulcer of right heel, stage 2
Pressure ulcer with abrasion, blister, partial thickness skin loss involving epidermis and/or dermis, right heel

L89.613 **Pressure ulcer of right heel,** stage 3   HCC
Healing pressure ulcer of right heel, stage 3
Pressure ulcer with full thickness skin loss involving damage or necrosis of subcutaneous tissue, right heel

L89.614 **Pressure ulcer of right heel,** stage 4   HCC
Healing pressure ulcer of right heel, stage 4
Pressure ulcer with necrosis of soft tissues through to underlying muscle, tendon, or bone, right heel

L89.619 **Pressure ulcer of right heel, unspecified stage** ▽
Healing pressure ulcer of right heel NOS
▶Healing pressure ulcer of right heel, unspecified stage◀

✓6ᵗʰ **L89.62** **Pressure ulcer of** left **heel**

L89.620 **Pressure ulcer of left heel,** unstageable   HCC

L89.621 **Pressure ulcer of left heel,** stage 1
Healing pressure ulcer of left heel, stage 1
Pressure pre-ulcer skin changes limited to persistent focal edema, left heel

L89.622 **Pressure ulcer of left heel,** stage 2
Healing pressure ulcer of left heel, stage 2
Pressure ulcer with abrasion, blister, partial thickness skin loss involving epidermis and/or dermis, left heel

L89.623 **Pressure ulcer of left heel,** stage 3   HCC
Healing pressure ulcer of left heel, stage 3
Pressure ulcer with full thickness skin loss involving damage or necrosis of subcutaneous tissue, left heel

L89.624 **Pressure ulcer of left heel,** stage 4   HCC
Healing pressure ulcer of left heel, stage 4
Pressure ulcer with necrosis of soft tissues through to underlying muscle, tendon, or bone, left heel

L89.629 **Pressure ulcer of left heel, unspecified stage** ▽
Healing pressure ulcer of left heel NOS
Healing pressure ulcer of left heel, unspecified stage

✓5ᵗʰ **L89.8** **Pressure ulcer of other site**

✓6ᵗʰ **L89.81** **Pressure ulcer of** head
Pressure ulcer of face

L89.810 **Pressure ulcer of head,** unstageable   HCC

L89.811 **Pressure ulcer of head,** stage 1
Healing pressure ulcer of head, stage 1
Pressure pre-ulcer skin changes limited to persistent focal edema, head

L89.812 **Pressure ulcer of head,** stage 2
Healing pressure ulcer of head, stage 2
Pressure ulcer with abrasion, blister, partial thickness skin loss involving epidermis and/or dermis, head

L89.813 **Pressure ulcer of head,** stage 3   HCC
Healing pressure ulcer of head, stage 3
Pressure ulcer with full thickness skin loss involving damage or necrosis of subcutaneous tissue, head

L89.814 **Pressure ulcer of head,** stage 4   HCC
Healing pressure ulcer of head, stage 4
Pressure ulcer with necrosis of soft tissues through to underlying muscle, tendon, or bone, head

L89.819 **Pressure ulcer of head, unspecified stage** ▽
Healing pressure ulcer of head NOS
Healing pressure ulcer of head, unspecified stage

✓6ᵗʰ **L89.89** **Pressure ulcer of other site**

L89.890 **Pressure ulcer of other site, unstageable**   HCC

L89.891 **Pressure ulcer of other site,** stage 1
Healing pressure ulcer of other site, stage 1
Pressure pre-ulcer skin changes limited to persistent focal edema, other site

L89.892 **Pressure ulcer of other site,** stage 2
Healing pressure ulcer of other site, stage 2
Pressure ulcer with abrasion, blister, partial thickness skin loss involving epidermis and/or dermis, other site

L89.893 **Pressure ulcer of other site,** stage 3   HCC
Healing pressure ulcer of other site, stage 3
Pressure ulcer with full thickness skin loss involving damage or necrosis of subcutaneous tissue, other site

L89.894 **Pressure ulcer of other site,** stage 4   HCC
Healing pressure ulcer of other site, stage 4
Pressure ulcer with necrosis of soft tissues through to underlying muscle, tendon, or bone, other site

L89.899 **Pressure ulcer of other site, unspecified stage** ▽
Healing pressure ulcer of other site NOS
Healing pressure ulcer of other site, unspecified stage

✓5ᵗʰ **L89.9** **Pressure ulcer of unspecified site**

L89.90 **Pressure ulcer of unspecified site, unspecified stage** ▽
Healing pressure ulcer of unspecified site NOS
Healing pressure ulcer of unspecified site, unspecified stage

L89.91 **Pressure ulcer of unspecified site,** stage 1 ▽
Healing pressure ulcer of unspecified site, stage 1
Pressure pre-ulcer skin changes limited to persistent focal edema, unspecified site

L89.92 **Pressure ulcer of unspecified site,** stage 2 ▽
Healing pressure ulcer of unspecified site, stage 2
Pressure ulcer with abrasion, blister, partial thickness skin loss involving epidermis and/or dermis, unspecified site

L89.93 **Pressure ulcer of unspecified site,** stage 3   HCC ▽
Healing pressure ulcer of unspecified site, stage 3
Pressure ulcer with full thickness skin loss involving damage or necrosis of subcutaneous tissue, unspecified site

L89.94 **Pressure ulcer of unspecified site,** stage 4   HCC ▽
Healing pressure ulcer of unspecified site, stage 4
Pressure ulcer with necrosis of soft tissues through to underlying muscle, tendon, or bone, unspecified site

L89.95 **Pressure ulcer of unspecified site, unstageable**   HCC ▽

✓4ᵗʰ **L90** **Atrophic disorders of skin**

L90.0 **Lichen sclerosus et atrophicus**
EXCLUDES 2   *lichen sclerosus of external female genital organs (N90.4)*
lichen sclerosus of external male genital organs (N48.0)

L90.1 **Anetoderma of Schweninger-Buzzi**

L90.2 **Anetoderma of Jadassohn-Pellizzari**

L90.3 **Atrophoderma of Pasini and Pierini**

L90.4 **Acrodermatitis chronica atrophicans**

L90.5 **Scar conditions and fibrosis of skin**
Adherent scar (skin)
Cicatrix
Disfigurement of skin due to scar
Fibrosis of skin NOS
Scar NOS
EXCLUDES 2   *hypertrophic scar (L91.0)*
keloid scar (L91.0)
AHA: 2016, 2Q, 5; 2015, 1Q, 19

L90.6 **Striae atrophicae**

L90.8 **Other atrophic disorders of skin**

L90.9 **Atrophic disorder of skin, unspecified** ▽

✓ Additional Character Req   ✓ˣ⁷ᵗʰ Placeholder Alert   Manifestation   HCC CMS-HCC Condition   ▽ Unspecified Code   ▶◀ Revised Text   ● New Code   ▲ Revised Code Title

✓4ᵗʰ L91 Hypertrophic disorders of skin

L91.0 Hypertrophic scar
Keloid
Keloid scar
EXCLUDES 2   *acne keloid (L73.0)*
           scar NOS (L90.5)
DEF: Overgrowth of scar tissue due to excess amounts of collagen during connective tissue repair; occurs mainly on upper trunk, face.

L91.8 Other hypertrophic disorders of the skin

L91.9 Hypertrophic disorder of the skin, unspecified ▽

✓4ᵗʰ L92 Granulomatous disorders of skin and subcutaneous tissue
EXCLUDES 2   *actinic granuloma (L57.5)*

L92.0 Granuloma annulare
Perforating granuloma annulare

L92.1 Necrobiosis lipoidica, not elsewhere classified
EXCLUDES 1   *necrobiosis lipoidica associated with diabetes mellitus (E08-E13 with .620)*

L92.2 Granuloma faciale [eosinophilic granuloma of skin]

L92.3 Foreign body granuloma of the skin and subcutaneous tissue
Use additional code to identify the type of retained foreign body (Z18.-)

L92.8 Other granulomatous disorders of the skin and subcutaneous tissue

L92.9 Granulomatous disorder of the skin and subcutaneous tissue, unspecified ▽
EXCLUDES 2   ▶*umbilical granuloma (P83.81)*◀

✓4ᵗʰ L93 Lupus erythematosus
Use additional code for adverse effect, if applicable, to identify drug (T36-T50 with fifth or sixth character 5)
EXCLUDES 1   *lupus exedens (A18.4)*
           lupus vulgaris (A18.4)
           scleroderma (M34.-)
           systemic lupus erythematosus (M32.-)

L93.0 Discoid lupus erythematosus
Lupus erythematosus NOS

L93.1 Subacute cutaneous lupus erythematosus

L93.2 Other local lupus erythematosus
Lupus erythematosus profundus
Lupus panniculitis

✓4ᵗʰ L94 Other localized connective tissue disorders
EXCLUDES 1   *systemic connective tissue disorders (M30-M36)*

L94.0 Localized scleroderma [morphea]
Circumscribed scleroderma

L94.1 Linear scleroderma
En coup de sabre lesion

L94.2 Calcinosis cutis

L94.3 Sclerodactyly

L94.4 Gottron's papules

L94.5 Poikiloderma vasculare atrophicans

L94.6 Ainhum

L94.8 Other specified localized connective tissue disorders

L94.9 Localized connective tissue disorder, unspecified ▽

✓4ᵗʰ L95 Vasculitis limited to skin, not elsewhere classified
EXCLUDES 1   *angioma serpiginosum (L81.7)*
           Henoch(-Schönlein) purpura (D69.0)
           hypersensitivity angiitis (M31.0)
           lupus panniculitis (L93.2)
           panniculitis NOS (M79.3)
           panniculitis of neck and back (M54.0-)
           polyarteritis nodosa (M30.0)
           relapsing panniculitis (M35.6)
           rheumatoid vasculitis (M05.2)
           serum sickness (T80.6-)
           urticaria (L50.-)
           Wegener's granulomatosis (M31.3-)

L95.0 Livedoid vasculitis
Atrophie blanche (en plaque)

L95.1 Erythema elevatum diutinum

L95.8 Other vasculitis limited to the skin

L95.9 Vasculitis limited to the skin, unspecified ▽

✓4ᵗʰ L97 Non-pressure chronic ulcer of lower limb, not elsewhere classified
INCLUDES   chronic ulcer of skin of lower limb NOS
           non-healing ulcer of skin
           non-infected sinus of skin
           trophic ulcer NOS
           tropical ulcer NOS
           ulcer of skin of lower limb NOS
Code first any associated underlying condition, such as:
       any associated gangrene (I96)
       atherosclerosis of the lower extremities (I70.23-, I70.24-, I70.33-, I70.34-, I70.43-, I70.44-, I70.53-, I70.54-, I70.63-, I70.64-, I70.73-, I70.74-)
       chronic venous hypertension (I87.31-, I87.33-)
       diabetic ulcers (E08.621, E08.622, E09.621, E09.622, E10.621, E10.622, E11.621, E11.622, E13.621, E13.622)
       postphlebitic syndrome (I87.01-, I87.03-)
       postthrombotic syndrome (I87.01-, I87.03-)
       varicose ulcer (I83.0-, I83.2-)
EXCLUDES 2   *pressure ulcer (pressure area) (L89.-)*
           skin infections (L00-L08)
           specific infections classified to A00-B99

✓5ᵗʰ L97.1 Non-pressure chronic ulcer of thigh

✓6ᵗʰ L97.10 Non-pressure chronic ulcer of unspecified thigh

L97.101   **Non-pressure chronic ulcer of unspecified thigh** limited to breakdown of skin   HCC ▽

L97.102   **Non-pressure chronic ulcer of unspecified thigh** with fat layer exposed   HCC ▽

L97.103   **Non-pressure chronic ulcer of unspecified thigh** with necrosis of muscle   HCC ▽

L97.104   **Non-pressure chronic ulcer of unspecified thigh** with necrosis of bone   HCC ▽

● L97.105   **Non-pressure chronic ulcer of unspecified thigh** with muscle involvement without evidence of necrosis   ▽

● L97.106   **Non-pressure chronic ulcer of unspecified thigh** with bone involvement without evidence of necrosis   ▽

● L97.108   **Non-pressure chronic ulcer of unspecified thigh with other specified severity**   ▽

L97.109   **Non-pressure chronic ulcer of unspecified thigh with unspecified severity**   HCC ▽

✓6ᵗʰ L97.11 Non-pressure chronic ulcer of right thigh

L97.111   **Non-pressure chronic ulcer of right thigh** limited to breakdown of skin   HCC

L97.112   **Non-pressure chronic ulcer of right thigh** with fat layer exposed   HCC

L97.113   **Non-pressure chronic ulcer of right high** with necrosis of muscle   HCC

L97.114   **Non-pressure chronic ulcer of right thigh** with necrosis of bone   HCC

● L97.115   **Non-pressure chronic ulcer of right thigh** with muscle involvement without evidence of necrosis

● L97.116   **Non-pressure chronic ulcer of right thigh** with bone involvement without evidence of necrosis

● L97.118   **Non-pressure chronic ulcer of right thigh with other specified severity**

L97.119   **Non-pressure chronic ulcer of right thigh with unspecified severity**   HCC ▽

✓6ᵗʰ L97.12 Non-pressure chronic ulcer of left thigh

L97.121   **Non-pressure chronic ulcer of left thigh** limited to breakdown of skin   HCC

L97.122   **Non-pressure chronic ulcer of left thigh** with fat layer exposed   HCC

L97.123   **Non-pressure chronic ulcer of left thigh** with necrosis of muscle   HCC

L97.124   **Non-pressure chronic ulcer of left thigh** with necrosis of bone   HCC

● L97.125   **Non-pressure chronic ulcer of left thigh** with muscle involvement without evidence of necrosis

EXCLUDES 1 Not coded here   EXCLUDES 2 Not included here   N Newborn Age: 0   P Pediatric Age: 0-17   M Maternity Age: 12-55   A Adult Age: 15-124

708   ICD-10-CM 2018

L97.126   **Non-pressure chronic ulcer of left thigh** with bone involvement without evidence of necrosis

L97.128   **Non-pressure chronic ulcer of left thigh with other specified severity**

L97.129   **Non-pressure chronic ulcer of left** HCC ▽ **thigh with unspecified severity**

✓5th **L97.2   Non-pressure chronic ulcer of** calf

  ✓6th **L97.20   Non-pressure chronic ulcer of unspecified calf**

L97.201   **Non-pressure chronic ulcer of** HCC ▽ **unspecified calf** limited to breakdown of skin

L97.202   **Non-pressure chronic ulcer of** HCC ▽ **unspecified calf** with fat layer exposed

L97.203   **Non-pressure chronic ulcer of** HCC ▽ **unspecified calf** with necrosis of muscle

L97.204   **Non-pressure chronic ulcer of** HCC ▽ **unspecified calf** with necrosis of bone

L97.205   **Non-pressure chronic ulcer of** ▽ **unspecified calf** with muscle involvement without evidence of necrosis

L97.206   **Non-pressure chronic ulcer of** ▽ **unspecified calf** with bone involvement without evidence of necrosis

L97.208   **Non-pressure chronic ulcer of** ▽ **unspecified calf with other specified severity**

L97.209   **Non-pressure chronic ulcer of** HCC ▽ **unspecified calf with unspecified severity**

  ✓6th **L97.21   Non-pressure chronic ulcer of** right **calf**

L97.211   **Non-pressure chronic ulcer of right** HCC **calf** limited to breakdown of skin

L97.212   **Non-pressure chronic ulcer of right** HCC **calf** with fat layer exposed

L97.213   **Non-pressure chronic ulcer of right** HCC **calf** with necrosis of muscle

L97.214   **Non-pressure chronic ulcer of right** HCC **calf** with necrosis of bone

L97.215   **Non-pressure chronic ulcer of right calf** with muscle involvement without evidence of necrosis

L97.216   **Non-pressure chronic ulcer of right calf** with bone involvement without evidence of necrosis

L97.218   **Non-pressure chronic ulcer of right calf with other specified severity**

L97.219   **Non-pressure chronic ulcer of right** HCC ▽ **calf with unspecified severity**

  ✓6th **L97.22   Non-pressure chronic ulcer of** left **calf**

L97.221   **Non-pressure chronic ulcer of left** HCC **calf** limited to breakdown of skin

L97.222   **Non-pressure chronic ulcer of left** HCC **calf** with fat layer exposed

L97.223   **Non-pressure chronic ulcer of left** HCC **calf** with necrosis of muscle

L97.224   **Non-pressure chronic ulcer of left** HCC **calf** with necrosis of bone

L97.225   **Non-pressure chronic ulcer of left calf** with muscle involvement without evidence of necrosis

L97.226   **Non-pressure chronic ulcer of left calf** with bone involvement without evidence of necrosis

L97.228   **Non-pressure chronic ulcer of left calf with other specified severity**

L97.229   **Non-pressure chronic ulcer of left** HCC ▽ **calf with unspecified severity**

✓5th **L97.3   Non-pressure chronic ulcer of** ankle

  ✓6th **L97.30   Non-pressure chronic ulcer of unspecified ankle**

L97.301   **Non-pressure chronic ulcer of** HCC ▽ **unspecified ankle** limited to breakdown of skin

L97.302   **Non-pressure chronic ulcer of** HCC ▽ **unspecified ankle** with fat layer exposed

L97.303   **Non-pressure chronic ulcer of** HCC ▽ **unspecified ankle** with necrosis of muscle

L97.304   **Non-pressure chronic ulcer of** HCC ▽ **unspecified ankle** with necrosis of bone

L97.305   **Non-pressure chronic ulcer of** ▽ **unspecified ankle** with muscle involvement without evidence of necrosis

L97.306   **Non-pressure chronic ulcer of** ▽ **unspecified ankle** with bone involvement without evidence of necrosis

L97.308   **Non-pressure chronic ulcer of** ▽ **unspecified ankle with other specified severity**

L97.309   **Non-pressure chronic ulcer of** HCC ▽ **unspecified ankle with unspecified severity**

  ✓6th **L97.31   Non-pressure chronic ulcer of** right **ankle**

L97.311   **Non-pressure chronic ulcer of right** HCC **ankle** limited to breakdown of skin

L97.312   **Non-pressure chronic ulcer of right** HCC **ankle** with fat layer exposed

L97.313   **Non-pressure chronic ulcer of right** HCC **ankle** with necrosis of muscle

L97.314   **Non-pressure chronic ulcer of right** HCC **ankle** with necrosis of bone

L97.315   **Non-pressure chronic ulcer of right ankle** with muscle involvement without evidence of necrosis

L97.316   **Non-pressure chronic ulcer of right ankle** with bone involvement without evidence of necrosis

L97.318   **Non-pressure chronic ulcer of right ankle with other specified severity**

L97.319   **Non-pressure chronic ulcer of right** HCC ▽ **ankle with unspecified severity**

  ✓6th **L97.32   Non-pressure chronic ulcer of** left **ankle**

L97.321   **Non-pressure chronic ulcer of left** HCC **ankle** limited to breakdown of skin

L97.322   **Non-pressure chronic ulcer of left** HCC **ankle** with fat layer exposed

L97.323   **Non-pressure chronic ulcer of left** HCC **ankle** with necrosis of muscle

L97.324   **Non-pressure chronic ulcer of left** HCC **ankle** with necrosis of bone

L97.325   **Non-pressure chronic ulcer of left ankle** with muscle involvement without evidence of necrosis

L97.326   **Non-pressure chronic ulcer of left ankle** with bone involvement without evidence of necrosis

L97.328   **Non-pressure chronic ulcer of left ankle with other specified severity**

L97.329   **Non-pressure chronic ulcer of left** HCC ▽ **ankle with unspecified severity**

✓5th **L97.4   Non-pressure chronic ulcer of** heel and midfoot
Non-pressure chronic ulcer of plantar surface of midfoot

  ✓6th **L97.40   Non-pressure chronic ulcer of unspecified heel and midfoot**

L97.401   **Non-pressure chronic ulcer of** HCC ▽ **unspecified heel and midfoot** limited to breakdown of skin

L97.402   **Non-pressure chronic ulcer of** HCC ▽ **unspecified heel and midfoot** with fat layer exposed

L97.403   **Non-pressure chronic ulcer of** HCC ▽ **unspecified heel and midfoot** with necrosis of muscle

L97.404   **Non-pressure chronic ulcer of** HCC ▽ **unspecified heel and midfoot** with necrosis of bone

L97.405   **Non-pressure chronic ulcer of** ▽ **unspecified heel and midfoot** with muscle involvement without evidence of necrosis

L97.406   **Non-pressure chronic ulcer of** ▽ **unspecified heel and midfoot** with bone involvement without evidence of necrosis

---

☑ Additional Character Req   ✓x7th Placeholder Alert   Manifestation   HCC CMS-HCC Condition   ▽ Unspecified Code   ▶◀ Revised Text   ● New Code   ▲ Revised Code Title

L97.408   Non-pressure chronic ulcer of unspecified heel and midfoot with other specified severity ▽

L97.409   Non-pressure chronic ulcer of unspecified heel and midfoot with unspecified severity HCC ▽

✓6th **L97.41**   Non-pressure chronic ulcer of right heel and midfoot

L97.411   Non-pressure chronic ulcer of right heel and midfoot limited to breakdown of skin HCC

L97.412   Non-pressure chronic ulcer of right heel and midfoot with fat layer exposed HCC

L97.413   Non-pressure chronic ulcer of right heel and midfoot with necrosis of muscle HCC

L97.414   Non-pressure chronic ulcer of right heel and midfoot with necrosis of bone HCC

L97.415   Non-pressure chronic ulcer of right heel and midfoot with muscle involvement without evidence of necrosis

L97.416   Non-pressure chronic ulcer of right heel and midfoot with bone involvement without evidence of necrosis

L97.418   Non-pressure chronic ulcer of right heel and midfoot with other specified severity

L97.419   Non-pressure chronic ulcer of right heel and midfoot with unspecified severity HCC ▽

✓6th **L97.42**   Non-pressure chronic ulcer of left heel and midfoot

L97.421   Non-pressure chronic ulcer of left heel and midfoot limited to breakdown of skin HCC
     AHA: 2016, 1Q, 12

L97.422   Non-pressure chronic ulcer of left heel and midfoot with fat layer exposed HCC

L97.423   Non-pressure chronic ulcer of left heel and midfoot with necrosis of muscle HCC

L97.424   Non-pressure chronic ulcer of left heel and midfoot with necrosis of bone HCC

L97.425   Non-pressure chronic ulcer of left heel and midfoot with muscle involvement without evidence of necrosis

L97.426   Non-pressure chronic ulcer of left heel and midfoot with bone involvement without evidence of necrosis

L97.428   Non-pressure chronic ulcer of left heel and midfoot with other specified severity

L97.429   Non-pressure chronic ulcer of left heel and midfoot with unspecified severity HCC ▽

✓5th **L97.5**   Non-pressure chronic ulcer of other part of foot
     Non-pressure chronic ulcer of toe

✓6th **L97.50**   Non-pressure chronic ulcer of other part of unspecified foot

L97.501   Non-pressure chronic ulcer of other part of unspecified foot limited to breakdown of skin HCC ▽

L97.502   Non-pressure chronic ulcer of other part of unspecified foot with fat layer exposed HCC ▽

L97.503   Non-pressure chronic ulcer of other part of unspecified foot with necrosis of muscle HCC ▽

L97.504   Non-pressure chronic ulcer of other part of unspecified foot with necrosis of bone HCC ▽

L97.505   Non-pressure chronic ulcer of other part of unspecified foot with muscle involvement without evidence of necrosis ▽

L97.506   Non-pressure chronic ulcer of other part of unspecified foot with bone involvement without evidence of necrosis ▽

L97.508   Non-pressure chronic ulcer of other part of unspecified foot with other specified severity ▽

L97.509   Non-pressure chronic ulcer of other part of unspecified foot with unspecified severity HCC ▽

✓6th **L97.51**   Non-pressure chronic ulcer of other part of right foot

L97.511   Non-pressure chronic ulcer of other part of right foot limited to breakdown of skin HCC

L97.512   Non-pressure chronic ulcer of other part of right foot with fat layer exposed HCC

L97.513   Non-pressure chronic ulcer of other part of right foot with necrosis of muscle HCC

L97.514   Non-pressure chronic ulcer of other part of right foot with necrosis of bone HCC

L97.515   Non-pressure chronic ulcer of other part of right foot with muscle involvement without evidence of necrosis

L97.516   Non-pressure chronic ulcer of other part of right foot with bone involvement without evidence of necrosis

L97.518   Non-pressure chronic ulcer of other part of right foot with other specified severity

L97.519   Non-pressure chronic ulcer of other part of right foot with unspecified severity HCC ▽

✓6th **L97.52**   Non-pressure chronic ulcer of other part of left foot

L97.521   Non-pressure chronic ulcer of other part of left foot limited to breakdown of skin HCC

L97.522   Non-pressure chronic ulcer of other part of left foot with fat layer exposed HCC

L97.523   Non-pressure chronic ulcer of other part of left foot with necrosis of muscle HCC

L97.524   Non-pressure chronic ulcer of other part of left foot with necrosis of bone HCC

L97.525   Non-pressure chronic ulcer of other part of left foot with muscle involvement without evidence of necrosis

L97.526   Non-pressure chronic ulcer of other part of left foot with bone involvement without evidence of necrosis

L97.528   Non-pressure chronic ulcer of other part of left foot with other specified severity

L97.529   Non-pressure chronic ulcer of other part of left foot with unspecified severity HCC ▽

✓5th **L97.8**   Non-pressure chronic ulcer of other part of lower leg

✓6th **L97.80**   Non-pressure chronic ulcer of other part of unspecified lower leg

L97.801   Non-pressure chronic ulcer of other part of unspecified lower leg limited to breakdown of skin HCC ▽

L97.802   Non-pressure chronic ulcer of other part of unspecified lower leg with fat layer exposed HCC ▽

L97.803   Non-pressure chronic ulcer of other part of unspecified lower leg with necrosis of muscle HCC ▽

L97.804   Non-pressure chronic ulcer of other part of unspecified lower leg with necrosis of bone HCC ▽

L97.805   Non-pressure chronic ulcer of other part of unspecified lower leg with muscle involvement without evidence of necrosis ▽

L97.806   Non-pressure chronic ulcer of other part of unspecified lower leg with bone involvement without evidence of necrosis ▽

L97.808   Non-pressure chronic ulcer of other part of unspecified lower leg with other specified severity ▽

L97.809   Non-pressure chronic ulcer of other part of unspecified lower leg with unspecified severity HCC ▽

✓6th **L97.81**   Non-pressure chronic ulcer of other part of right lower leg

L97.811   Non-pressure chronic ulcer of other part of right lower leg limited to breakdown of skin HCC

L97.812   Non-pressure chronic ulcer of other part of right lower leg with fat layer exposed HCC

L97.813 Non-pressure chronic ulcer of other part of right lower leg with necrosis of muscle `HCC`

L97.814 Non-pressure chronic ulcer of other part of right lower leg with necrosis of bone `HCC`

● **L97.815** Non-pressure chronic ulcer of other part of right lower leg with muscle involvement without evidence of necrosis

● **L97.816** Non-pressure chronic ulcer of other part of right lower leg with bone involvement without evidence of necrosis

● **L97.818** Non-pressure chronic ulcer of other part of right lower leg with other specified severity

L97.819 Non-pressure chronic ulcer of other part of right lower leg with unspecified severity `HCC` ▽

✓6ᵗʰ **L97.82** Non-pressure chronic ulcer of other part of left lower leg

L97.821 Non-pressure chronic ulcer of other part of left lower leg limited to breakdown of skin `HCC`

L97.822 Non-pressure chronic ulcer of other part of left lower leg with fat layer exposed `HCC`

L97.823 Non-pressure chronic ulcer of other part of left lower leg with necrosis of muscle `HCC`

L97.824 Non-pressure chronic ulcer of other part of left lower leg with necrosis of bone `HCC`

● **L97.825** Non-pressure chronic ulcer of other part of left lower leg with muscle involvement without evidence of necrosis

● **L97.826** Non-pressure chronic ulcer of other part of left lower leg with bone involvement without evidence of necrosis

L97.828 Non-pressure chronic ulcer of other part of left lower leg with other specified severity

L97.829 Non-pressure chronic ulcer of other part of left lower leg with unspecified severity `HCC` ▽

✓5ᵗʰ **L97.9** Non-pressure chronic ulcer of unspecified part of lower leg

✓6ᵗʰ **L97.90** Non-pressure chronic ulcer of unspecified part of unspecified lower leg

L97.901 Non-pressure chronic ulcer of unspecified part of unspecified lower leg limited to breakdown of skin `HCC` ▽

L97.902 Non-pressure chronic ulcer of unspecified part of unspecified lower leg with fat layer exposed `HCC` ▽

L97.903 Non-pressure chronic ulcer of unspecified part of unspecified lower leg with necrosis of muscle `HCC` ▽

L97.904 Non-pressure chronic ulcer of unspecified part of unspecified lower leg with necrosis of bone `HCC` ▽

● **L97.905** Non-pressure chronic ulcer of unspecified part of unspecified lower leg with muscle involvement without evidence of necrosis ▽

● **L97.906** Non-pressure chronic ulcer of unspecified part of unspecified lower leg with bone involvement without evidence of necrosis ▽

● **L97.908** Non-pressure chronic ulcer of unspecified part of unspecified lower leg with other specified severity ▽

L97.909 Non-pressure chronic ulcer of unspecified part of unspecified lower leg with unspecified severity `HCC` ▽

✓6ᵗʰ **L97.91** Non-pressure chronic ulcer of unspecified part of right lower leg

L97.911 Non-pressure chronic ulcer of unspecified part of right lower leg limited to breakdown of skin `HCC` ▽

L97.912 Non-pressure chronic ulcer of unspecified part of right lower leg with fat layer exposed `HCC` ▽

L97.913 Non-pressure chronic ulcer of unspecified part of right lower leg with necrosis of muscle `HCC` ▽

L97.914 Non-pressure chronic ulcer of unspecified part of right lower leg with necrosis of bone `HCC` ▽

● **L97.915** Non-pressure chronic ulcer of unspecified part of right lower leg with muscle involvement without evidence of necrosis ▽

● **L97.916** Non-pressure chronic ulcer of unspecified part of right lower leg with bone involvement without evidence of necrosis ▽

● **L97.918** Non-pressure chronic ulcer of unspecified part of right lower leg with other specified severity ▽

L97.919 Non-pressure chronic ulcer of unspecified part of right lower leg with unspecified severity `HCC` ▽

✓6ᵗʰ **L97.92** Non-pressure chronic ulcer of unspecified part of left lower leg

L97.921 Non-pressure chronic ulcer of unspecified part of left lower leg limited to breakdown of skin `HCC` ▽

L97.922 Non-pressure chronic ulcer of unspecified part of left lower leg with fat layer exposed `HCC` ▽

L97.923 Non-pressure chronic ulcer of unspecified part of left lower leg with necrosis of muscle `HCC` ▽

L97.924 Non-pressure chronic ulcer of unspecified part of left lower leg with necrosis of bone `HCC` ▽

● **L97.925** Non-pressure chronic ulcer of unspecified part of left lower leg with muscle involvement without evidence of necrosis ▽

● **L97.926** Non-pressure chronic ulcer of unspecified part of left lower leg with bone involvement without evidence of necrosis ▽

● **L97.928** Non-pressure chronic ulcer of unspecified part of left lower leg with other specified severity ▽

L97.929 Non-pressure chronic ulcer of unspecified part of left lower leg with unspecified severity `HCC` ▽

✓4ᵗʰ **L98** Other disorders of skin and subcutaneous tissue, not elsewhere classified

L98.0 Pyogenic granuloma

EXCLUDES 2 pyogenic granuloma of gingiva (K06.8)
pyogenic granuloma of maxillary alveolar ridge (K04.5)
pyogenic granuloma of oral mucosa (K13.4)

DEF: Solitary polypoid capillary hemangioma often associated with local irritation, trauma, and superimposed inflammation; located on the skin and gingival or oral mucosa; they bleed easily and may ulcerate and form crusted sores.

L98.1 Factitial dermatitis
Neurotic excoriation

EXCLUDES 1 excoriation (skin-picking) disorder (F42.4)

DEF: Self-inflicted skin lesions to satisfy an unconscious psychological or emotional need; methods used to injure the skin include deep excoriations with a sharp instrument, scarification with a knife, or the application of caustic chemicals and burning, sometimes with a cigarette.

L98.2 Febrile neutrophilic dermatosis [Sweet]

L98.3 Eosinophilic cellulitis [Wells]

✓5ᵗʰ **L98.4** Non-pressure chronic ulcer of skin, not elsewhere classified
Chronic ulcer of skin NOS
Tropical ulcer NOS
Ulcer of skin NOS

EXCLUDES 2 pressure ulcer (pressure area) (L89.-)
gangrene (I96)
skin infections (L00-L08)
specific infections classified to A00-B99
ulcer of lower limb NEC (L97.-)
varicose ulcer (I83.0-I82.2)

✓6ᵗʰ **L98.41** Non-pressure chronic ulcer of buttock

L98.411 Non-pressure chronic ulcer of buttock limited to breakdown of skin `HCC`

✓ Additional Character Req   ✓x7ᵗʰ Placeholder Alert   Manifestation   `HCC` CMS-HCC Condition   ▽ Unspecified Code   ▶◀ Revised Text   ● New Code   ▲ Revised Code Title

ICD-10-CM 2018   **711**

L98.412   **Non-pressure chronic ulcer of buttock** HCC
with fat layer exposed

L98.413   **Non-pressure chronic ulcer of buttock** HCC
with necrosis of muscle

L98.414   **Non-pressure chronic ulcer of buttock** HCC
with necrosis of bone

● **L98.415**   **Non-pressure chronic ulcer of buttock**
with muscle involvement without
evidence of necrosis

● **L98.416**   **Non-pressure chronic ulcer of buttock**
with bone involvement without evidence
of necrosis

● **L98.418**   **Non-pressure chronic ulcer of buttock**
with other specified severity

L98.419   **Non-pressure chronic ulcer of**   HCC ▽
buttock with unspecified severity

✓6ᵗʰ **L98.42**   **Non-pressure chronic ulcer of** back

L98.421   **Non-pressure chronic ulcer of back**   HCC
limited to breakdown of skin

L98.422   **Non-pressure chronic ulcer of back**   HCC
with fat layer exposed

L98.423   **Non-pressure chronic ulcer of back**   HCC
with necrosis of muscle

L98.424   **Non-pressure chronic ulcer of back**   HCC
with necrosis of bone

● **L98.425**   **Non-pressure chronic ulcer of back** with
muscle involvement without evidence of
necrosis

● **L98.426**   **Non-pressure chronic ulcer of back** with
bone involvement without evidence of
necrosis

● **L98.428**   **Non-pressure chronic ulcer of back** with
other specified severity

L98.429   **Non-pressure chronic ulcer of back** HCC ▽
with unspecified severity

✓6ᵗʰ **L98.49**   **Non-pressure chronic ulcer of skin of other sites**
Non-pressure chronic ulcer of skin NOS

L98.491   **Non-pressure chronic ulcer of skin of**   HCC
other sites limited to breakdown of skin

L98.492   **Non-pressure chronic ulcer of skin of**   HCC
other sites with fat layer exposed

L98.493   **Non-pressure chronic ulcer of skin of**   HCC
other sites with necrosis of muscle

L98.494   **Non-pressure chronic ulcer of skin of**   HCC
other sites with necrosis of bone

● **L98.495**   **Non-pressure chronic ulcer of other sites**
with muscle involvement without
evidence of necrosis

● **L98.496**   **Non-pressure chronic ulcer of other sites**
with bone involvement without evidence
of necrosis

● **L98.498**   **Non-pressure chronic ulcer of other sites**
with other specified severity

L98.499   **Non-pressure chronic ulcer of skin**   HCC ▽
of other sites with unspecified severity

L98.5   **Mucinosis of the skin**
Focal mucinosis
Lichen myxedematosus
Reticular erythematous mucinosis
EXCLUDES 1   *focal oral mucinosis (K13.79)*
myxedema (E03.9)

L98.6   **Other infiltrative disorders of the skin and subcutaneous
tissue**
EXCLUDES 1   *hyalinosis cutis et mucosae (E78.89)*

L98.7   **Excessive and redundant skin and subcutaneous tissue**
Loose or sagging skin following bariatric surgery weight loss
Loose or sagging skin following dietary weight loss
Loose or sagging skin, NOS
EXCLUDES 2   *acquired excess or redundant skin of eyelid (H02.3-)*
congenital excess or redundant skin of eyelid (Q10.3)
*skin changes due to chronic exposure to nonionizing
radiation (L57.-)*

L98.8   **Other specified disorders of the skin and subcutaneous tissue**
AHA: 2013, 2Q, 32

L98.9   **Disorder of the skin and subcutaneous tissue, unspecified** ▽

L99   ***Other disorders of skin and subcutaneous tissue in diseases
classified elsewhere***
Code first underlying disease, such as:
amyloidosis (E85.-)
EXCLUDES 1   *skin disorders in diabetes (E08-E13 with .62)*
skin disorders in gonorrhea (A54.89)
skin disorders in syphilis (A51.31, A52.79)

Chapter 13. Diseases of the Musculoskeletal System and Connective Tissue (M00–M99)

Chapter Specific Guidelines with Coding Examples

The chapter specific guidelines from the ICD-10-CM Official Guidelines for Coding and Reporting have been provided below. Along with these guidelines are coding examples, contained in the shaded boxes, that have been developed to help illustrate the coding and/or sequencing guidance found in these guidelines.

a. Site and laterality

Most of the codes within Chapter 13 have site and laterality designations. The site represents the bone, joint or the muscle involved. For some conditions where more than one bone, joint or muscle is usually involved, such as osteoarthritis, there is a "multiple sites" code available. For categories where no multiple site code is provided and more than one bone, joint or muscle is involved, multiple codes should be used to indicate the different sites involved.

Olecranon bursitis of the left elbow

M70.22   Olecranon bursitis, left elbow

Explanation: Most of the codes within chapter 13 have site and laterality designations. The site represents the bone, joint, or the muscle involved.

Rheumatoid arthritis of multiple sites without rheumatoid factor

M06.09   Rheumatoid arthritis without rheumatoid factor, multiple sites

Explanation: For some conditions where more than one bone, joint or muscle is usually involved, such as osteoarthritis, there is a "multiple sites" code available.

Adolescent scoliosis in the upper thoracic region and the lumbar vertebrae

M41.124   Adolescent idiopathic scoliosis, thoracic region

M41.126   Adolescent idiopathic scoliosis, lumbar region

Explanation: For categories without a multiple site code and more than one bone, joint, or muscle is involved, multiple codes should be used to indicate the different sites involved.

---

1) Bone versus joint

For certain conditions, the bone may be affected at the upper or lower end, (e.g., avascular necrosis of bone, M87, Osteoporosis, M80, M81). Though the portion of the bone affected may be at the joint, the site designation will be the bone, not the joint.

Idiopathic avascular necrosis of the femoral head of the left hip joint

M87.052   Idiopathic aseptic necrosis of left femur

Explanation: For certain conditions such as avascular necrosis, the bone may be affected at the joint, but the site designation is the bone, not the joint.

---

b. Acute traumatic versus chronic or recurrent musculoskeletal conditions

Many musculoskeletal conditions are a result of previous injury or trauma to a site, or are recurrent conditions. Bone, joint or muscle conditions that are the result of a healed injury are usually found in chapter 13. Recurrent bone, joint or muscle conditions are also usually found in chapter 13. Any current, acute injury should be coded to the appropriate injury code from chapter 19. Chronic or recurrent conditions should generally be coded with a code from chapter 13. If it is difficult to determine from the documentation in the record which code is best to describe a condition, query the provider.

Acute traumatic bucket handle tear of right medial meniscus

S83.211A   Bucket-handle tear of medial meniscus, current injury, right knee, initial encounter

Explanation: Any current, acute injury is not coded in chapter 13. It should instead be coded to the appropriate injury code from chapter 19.

Old bucket handle tear of right medial meniscus

M23.203   Derangement of unspecified medial meniscus due to old tear or injury, right knee

Explanation: Chronic or recurrent conditions should generally be coded with a code from chapter 13.

---

c. Coding of Pathologic Fractures

7th character A is for use as long as the patient is receiving active treatment for the fracture. Examples of active treatment are: surgical treatment, emergency department encounter, evaluation and continuing treatment by the same or a different physician. While the patient may be seen by a new or different provider over the course of treatment for a pathological fracture, assignment of the 7th character is based on whether the patient is undergoing active treatment and not whether the provider is seeing the patient for the first time.

Pathologic fracture of left foot, unknown cause, currently under active treatment by a follow-up provider

M84.475A   Pathological fracture, left foot, initial encounter for fracture

Explanation: Seventh character A is for use as long as the patient is receiving active treatment for a pathologic fracture. Examples of active treatment are surgical treatment, emergency department encounter, evaluation, and continuing treatment by the same or a different physician.

The seventh character is based on whether the patient is undergoing active treatment and not whether the provider is seeing the patient for the first time.

7th character D is to be used for encounters after the patient has completed active treatment. The other 7th characters, listed under each subcategory in the Tabular List, are to be used for subsequent encounters for routine care of fractures during the healing and recovery phase as well as treatment of problems associated with the healing, such as malunions, nonunions, and sequelae.

Care for complications of surgical treatment for fracture repairs during the healing or recovery phase should be coded with the appropriate complication codes.

See Section I.C.19. Coding of traumatic fractures.

d. Osteoporosis

Osteoporosis is a systemic condition, meaning that all bones of the musculoskeletal system are affected. Therefore, site is not a component of the codes under category M81, Osteoporosis without current pathological fracture. The site codes under category M80, Osteoporosis with current pathological fracture, identify the site of the fracture, not the osteoporosis.

1) Osteoporosis without pathological fracture

Category M81, Osteoporosis without current pathological fracture, is for use for patients with osteoporosis who do not currently have a pathologic fracture due to the osteoporosis, even if they have had a fracture in the past. For patients with a history of osteoporosis fractures, status code Z87.310, Personal history of (healed) osteoporosis fracture, should follow the code from M81.

Age-related osteoporosis with healed osteoporotic fracture of the lumbar vertebra

M81.0   Age-related osteoporosis without current pathological fracture

Z87.310   Personal history of (healed) osteoporosis fracture

Explanation: Category M81 is used for patients with osteoporosis who do not currently have a pathologic fracture due to the osteoporosis. To report a previous (healed) fracture, status code Z87.310 Personal history of (healed) osteoporosis fracture, should follow the code from M81.

---

2) Osteoporosis with current pathological fracture

Category M80, Osteoporosis with current pathological fracture, is for patients who have a current pathologic fracture at the time of an encounter. The codes under M80 identify the site of the fracture. A code from category M80, not a traumatic fracture code, should be used for any patient with known osteoporosis who suffers a fracture, even if the patient had a minor fall or trauma, if that fall or trauma would not usually break a normal, healthy bone.

Disuse osteoporosis with current fracture of right shoulder sustained lifting a grocery bag, initial encounter

M80.811A   Other osteoporosis with current pathological fracture, right shoulder, initial encounter for fracture

Explanation: A code from category M80, not a traumatic fracture code, should be used for any patient with known osteoporosis who suffers a fracture, even if the patient had a minor fall or trauma, if that fall or trauma would not usually break a normal, healthy bone.

Muscle/Tendon Table

ICD-10-CM categorizes certain muscles and tendons in the upper and lower extremities by their action (e.g., extension, flexion), their anatomical location (e.g., posterior, anterior), and/or whether they are intrinsic or extrinsic to a certain anatomical area. The Muscle/Tendon Table is provided at the beginning of chapters 13 and 19 as a resource to help users when code selection depends on one or more of these characteristics. A **TIP** has been placed at those categories and/or subcategories that relate to this table. Please note that this table is not all-inclusive, and proper code assignment should be based on the provider's documentation.

Body Region	Muscle	Extensor Tendon	Flexor Tendon	Other Tendon
Shoulder				
	Deltoid	Posterior deltoid	Anterior deltoid	
	Rotator cuff			
	Infraspinatus			Infraspinatus
	Subscapularis			Subscapularis
	Supraspinatus			Supraspinatus
	Teres minor			Teres minor
	Teres major	Teres major		
Upper arm				
	Anterior muscles			
	Biceps brachii — long head		Biceps brachii — long head	
	Biceps brachii — short head		Biceps brachii — short head	
	Brachialis		Brachialis	
	Coracobrachialis		Coracobrachialis	
	Posterior muscles			
	Triceps brachii	Triceps brachii		
Forearm				
	Anterior muscles			
	Flexors			
	Deep			
	Flexor digitorum profundus		Flexor digitorum profundus	
	Flexor pollicis longus		Flexor pollicis longus	
	Intermediate			
	Flexor digitorum superficialis		Flexor digitorum superficialis	
	Superficial			
	Flexor carpi radialis		Flexor carpi radialis	
	Flexor carpi ulnaris		Flexor carpi ulnaris	
	Palmaris longus		Palmaris longus	
	Pronators			
	Pronator quadratus			Pronator quadratus
	Pronator teres			Pronator teres
	Posterior muscles			
	Extensors			
	Deep			
	Abductor pollicis longus			Abductor pollicis longus
	Extensor indicis	Extensor indicis		
	Extensor pollicis brevis	Extensor pollicis brevis		
	Extensor pollicis longus	Extensor pollicis longus		
	Superficial			
	Brachioradialis			Brachioradialis
	Extensor carpi radialis brevis	Extensor carpi radialis brevis		
	Extensor carpi radialis longus	Extensor carpi radialis longus		
	Extensor carpi ulnaris	Extensor carpi ulnaris		
	Extensor digiti minimi	Extensor digiti minimi		
	Extensor digitorum	Extensor digitorum		
	Anconeus	Anconeus		
	Supinator			Supinator

Body Region	Muscle	Extensor Tendon	Flexor Tendon	Other Tendon
Hand				
Extrinsic — attach to a site in the forearm as well as a site in the hand with action related to hand movement at the wrist				
	Extensor carpi radialis brevis	Extensor carpi radialis brevis		
	Extensor carpi radialis longus	Extensor carpie radialis longus		
	Extensor carpi ulnaris	Extensor carpi ulnaris		
	Flexor carpi radialis		Flexor carpi radialis	
	Flexor carpi ulnaris		Flexor carpi ulnaris	
	Flexor digitorum superficialis		Flexor digitorum superficialis	
	Palmaris longus		Palmaris longus	
Extrinsic — attach to a site in the forearm as well as a site in the hand with action in the hand related to finger movement				
	Adductor pollicis longus			Adductor pollicis longus
	Extensor digiti minimi	Extensor digiti minimi		
	Extensor digitorum	Extensor digitorum		
	Extensor indicis	Extensor indicis		
	Flexor digitorum profundus		Flexor digitorum profundus	
	Flexor digitorum superficialis		Flexor digitorum superficialis	
Extrinsic — attach to a site in the forearm as well as a site in the hand with action in the hand related to thumb movement				
	Extensor pollicis brevis	Extensor pollicis brevis		
	Extensor pollicis longus	Extensor pollicis longus		
	Flexor pollicis longus		Flexor pollicis longus	
Intrinsic — found within the hand only				
	Adductor pollicis			Adductor pollicis
	Dorsal interossei	Dorsal interossei	Dorsal interossei	
	Lumbricals	Lumbricals	Lumbricals	
	Palmaris brevis			Palmaris brevis
	Palmar interossei	Palmar interossei	Palmar interossei	
	Hypothenar muscles			
	Abductor digiti minimi			Abductor digiti minimi
	Flexor digiti minimi brevis		Flexor digiti minimi brevis	
	Oppenens digiti minimi		Oppenens digiti minimi	
	Thenar muscles			
	Abductor pollicis brevis			Abductor pollicis brevis
	Flexor pollicis brevis		Flexor pollicis brevis	
	Oppenens pollicis		Oppenens pollicis	
Thigh				
	Anterior muscles			
	Iliopsoas		Iliopsoas	
	Pectineus		Pectineus	
	Quadriceps	Quadriceps		
	Rectus femoris	Rectus femoris — Extends knee	Rectus femoris — Flexes hip	
	Vastus intermedius	Vastus intermedius		
	Vastus lateralis	Vastus lateralis		
	Vastus medialis	Vastus medialis		
	Sartorius		Sartorius	
	Medial muscles			
	Adductor brevis			Adductor brevis
	Adductor longus			Adductor longus
	Adductor magnus			Adductor magnus
	Gracilis			Gracilis
	Obturator externus			Obturator externus
	Posterior muscles			
	Hamstring	Hamstring — Extends hip	Hamstring — Flexes knee	
	Biceps femoris	Biceps femoris	Biceps femoris	
	Semimembranosus	Semimembranosus	Semimembranosus	
	Semitendinosus	Semitendinosus	Semitendinosus	

Chapter 13. Diseases of the Musculoskeletal System and Connective Tissue

Body Region	Muscle	Extensor Tendon	Flexor Tendon	Other Tendon
Lower leg				
	Anterior muscles			
	Extensor digitorum longus	Extensor digitorum longus		
	Extensor hallucis longus	Extensor hallucis longus		
	Fibularis (peroneus) tertius	Fibularis (peroneus) tertius		
	Tibialis anterior	Tibialis anterior		Tibialis anterior
	Lateral muscles			
	Fibularis (peroneus) brevis		Fibularis (peroneus) brevis	
	Fibularis (peroneus) longus		Fibularis (peroneus) longus	
	Posterior muscles			
	Deep			
	Flexor digitorum longus		Flexor digitorum longus	
	Flexor hallucis longus		Flexor hallucis longus	
	Popliteus		Popliteus	
	Tibialis posterior		Tibialis posterior	
	Superficial			
	Gastrocnemius		Gastrocnemius	
	Plantaris		Plantaris	
	Soleus		Soleus	
				Calcaneal (Achilles)
Ankle/Foot				
Extrinsic — attach to a site in the lower leg as well as a site in the foot with action related to foot movement at the ankle				
	Plantaris		Plantaris	
	Soleus		Soleus	
	Tibialis anterior	Tibialis anterior		
	Tibialis posterior		Tibialis posterior	
Extrinsic — attach to a site in the lower leg as well as a site in the foot with action in the foot related to toe movement				
	Extensor digitorum longus	Extensor digitorum longus		
	Extensor hallicus longus	Extensor hallicus longus		
	Flexor digitorum longus		Flexor digitorum longus	
	Flexor hallucis longus		Flexor hallucis longus	
Intrinsic — found within the ankle/foot only				
	Dorsal muscles			
	Extensor digitorum brevis	Extensor digitorum brevis		
	Extensor hallucis brevis	Extensor hallucis brevis		
	Plantar muscles			
	Abductor digiti minimi		Abductor digiti minimi	
	Abductor hallucis		Abductor hallucis	
	Dorsal interossei	Dorsal interossei	Dorsal interossei	
	Flexor digiti minimi brevis		Flexor digiti minimi brevis	
	Flexor digitorum brevis		Flexor digitorum brevis	
	Flexor hallucis brevis		Flexor hallucis brevis	
	Lumbricals	Lumbricals	Lumbricals	
	Quadratus plantae		Quadratus plantae	
	Plantar interossei	Plantar interossei	Plantar interossei	

Chapter 13. Diseases of the Musculoskeletal System and Connective Tissue (M00-M99)

NOTE Use an external cause code following the code for the musculoskeletal condition, if applicable, to identify the cause of the musculoskeletal condition.

EXCLUDES 2 arthropathic psoriasis (L40.5-)
certain conditions originating in the perinatal period (P04-P96)
certain infectious and parasitic diseases (A00-B99)
compartment syndrome (traumatic) (T79.A-)
complications of pregnancy, childbirth and the puerperium (O00-O9A)
congenital malformations, deformations, and chromosomal abnormalities (Q00-Q99)
endocrine, nutritional and metabolic diseases (E00-E88)
injury, poisoning and certain other consequences of external causes (S00-T88)
neoplasms (C00-D49)
symptoms, signs and abnormal clinical and laboratory findings, not elsewhere classified (R00-R94)

This chapter contains the following blocks:

M00-M02   Infectious arthropathies
~~M04~~   ~~Autoinflammatory syndromes~~
M05-M14   Inflammatory polyarthropathies
M15-M19   Osteoarthritis
M20-M25   Other joint disorders
M26-M27   Dentofacial anomalies [including malocclusion] and other disorders of jaw
M30-M36   Systemic connective tissue disorders
M40-M43   Deforming dorsopathies
M45-M49   Spondylopathies
M50-M54   Other dorsopathies
M60-M63   Disorders of muscles
M65-M67   Disorders of synovium and tendon
M70-M79   Other soft tissue disorders
M80-M85   Disorders of bone density and structure
M86-M90   Other osteopathies
M91-M94   Chondropathies
M95   Other disorders of the musculoskeletal system and connective tissue
M96   Intraoperative and postprocedural complications and disorders of musculoskeletal system, not elsewhere classified
~~M97~~   ~~Periprosthetic fracture around internal prosthetic joint~~
M99   Biomechanical lesions, not elsewhere classified

ARTHROPATHIES (M00-M25)

INCLUDES disorders affecting predominantly peripheral (limb) joints

Infectious arthropathies (M00-M02)

NOTE This block comprises arthropathies due to microbiological agents. Distinction is made between the following types of etiological relationship:

a) direct infection of joint, where organisms invade synovial tissue and microbial antigen is present in the joint;

b) indirect infection, which may be of two types: a reactive arthropathy, where microbial infection of the body is established but neither organisms nor antigens can be identified in the joint, and a postinfective arthropathy, where microbial antigen is present but recovery of an organism is inconstant and evidence of local multiplication is lacking.

✓4th **M00 Pyogenic arthritis**

   ✓5th **M00.0 Staphylococcal arthritis and polyarthritis**
       Use additional code (B95.61-B95.8) to identify bacterial agent
       EXCLUDES 2 infection and inflammatory reaction due to internal joint prosthesis (T84.5-)

     M00.00 Staphylococcal arthritis, unspecified joint HCC ▽

   ✓6th **M00.01 Staphylococcal arthritis, shoulder**
       M00.011 Staphylococcal arthritis, right shoulder HCC
       M00.012 Staphylococcal arthritis, left shoulder HCC
       M00.019 Staphylococcal arthritis, unspecified shoulder HCC ▽

   ✓6th **M00.02 Staphylococcal arthritis, elbow**
       M30.021 Staphylococcal arthritis, right elbow HCC
       M00.022 Staphylococcal arthritis, left elbow HCC
       M00.029 Staphylococcal arthritis, unspecified elbow HCC ▽

   ✓6th **M00.03 Staphylococcal arthritis, wrist**
       Staphylococcal arthritis of carpal bones
       M00.031 Staphylococcal arthritis, right wrist HCC
       M00.032 Staphylococcal arthritis, left wrist HCC
       M00.039 Staphylococcal arthritis, unspecified wrist HCC ▽

   ✓6th **M00.04 Staphylococcal arthritis, hand**
       Staphylococcal arthritis of metacarpus and phalanges
       M00.041 Staphylococcal arthritis, right hand HCC
       M00.042 Staphylococcal arthritis, left hand HCC
       M00.049 Staphylococcal arthritis, unspecified hand HCC ▽

   ✓6th **M00.05 Staphylococcal arthritis, hip**
       M00.051 Staphylococcal arthritis, right hip HCC
       M00.052 Staphylococcal arthritis, left hip HCC
       M00.059 Staphylococcal arthritis, unspecified hip HCC ▽

   ✓6th **M00.06 Staphylococcal arthritis, knee**
       M00.061 Staphylococcal arthritis, right knee HCC
       M00.062 Staphylococcal arthritis, left knee HCC
       M00.069 Staphylococcal arthritis, unspecified knee HCC ▽

   ✓6th **M00.07 Staphylococcal arthritis, ankle and foot**
       Staphylococcal arthritis, tarsus, metatarsus and phalanges
       M00.071 Staphylococcal arthritis, right ankle and foot HCC
       M00.072 Staphylococcal arthritis, left ankle and foot HCC
       M00.079 Staphylococcal arthritis, unspecified ankle and foot HCC ▽

     M00.08 Staphylococcal arthritis, vertebrae HCC
     M00.09 Staphylococcal polyarthritis HCC

   ✓5th **M00.1 Pneumococcal arthritis and polyarthritis**
     M00.10 Pneumococcal arthritis, unspecified joint HCC ▽

   ✓6th **M00.11 Pneumococcal arthritis, shoulder**
       M00.111 Pneumococcal arthritis, right shoulder HCC
       M00.112 Pneumococcal arthritis, left shoulder HCC
       M00.119 Pneumococcal arthritis, unspecified shoulder HCC ▽

   ✓6th **M00.12 Pneumococcal arthritis, elbow**
       M00.121 Pneumococcal arthritis, right elbow HCC
       M00.122 Pneumococcal arthritis, left elbow HCC
       M00.129 Pneumococcal arthritis, unspecified elbow HCC ▽

   ✓6th **M00.13 Pneumococcal arthritis, wrist**
       Pneumococcal arthritis of carpal bones
       M00.131 Pneumococcal arthritis, right wrist HCC
       M00.132 Pneumococcal arthritis, left wrist HCC
       M00.139 Pneumococcal arthritis, unspecified wrist HCC ▽

   ✓6th **M00.14 Pneumococcal arthritis, hand**
       Pneumococcal arthritis of metacarpus and phalanges
       M00.141 Pneumococcal arthritis, right hand HCC
       M00.142 Pneumococcal arthritis, left hand HCC
       M00.149 Pneumococcal arthritis, unspecified hand HCC ▽

   ✓6th **M00.15 Pneumococcal arthritis, hip**
       M00.151 Pneumococcal arthritis, right hip HCC
       M00.152 Pneumococcal arthritis, left hip HCC
       M00.159 Pneumococcal arthritis, unspecified hip HCC ▽

   ✓6th **M00.16 Pneumococcal arthritis, knee**
       M00.161 Pneumococcal arthritis, right knee HCC
       M00.162 Pneumococcal arthritis, left knee HCC
       M00.169 Pneumococcal arthritis, unspecified knee HCC ▽

   ✓6th **M00.17 Pneumococcal arthritis, ankle and foot**
       Pneumococcal arthritis, tarsus, metatarsus and phalanges
       M00.171 Pneumococcal arthritis, right ankle and foot HCC
       M00.172 Pneumococcal arthritis, left ankle and foot HCC

✅ Additional Character Req   ✓7th Placeholder Alert   Manifestation   HCC CMS-HCC Condition   ▽ Unspecified Code   ►◄ Revised Text   ● New Code   ▲ Revised Code Title

          M00.179 **Pneumococcal arthritis, unspecified ankle and foot** HCC ▽

    M00.18 **Pneumococcal arthritis, vertebrae** HCC

    M00.19 **Pneumococcal polyarthritis** HCC

✓5th **M00.2** **Other streptococcal arthritis and polyarthritis**

    Use additional code (B95.0-B95.2, B95.4-B95.5) to identify bacterial agent

    M00.20 **Other streptococcal arthritis, unspecified joint** HCC ▽

    ✓6th **M00.21** **Other streptococcal arthritis, shoulder**

          M00.211 **Other streptococcal arthritis, right shoulder** HCC

          M00.212 **Other streptococcal arthritis, left shoulder** HCC

          M00.219 **Other streptococcal arthritis, unspecified shoulder** HCC ▽

    ✓6th **M00.22** **Other streptococcal arthritis, elbow**

          M00.221 **Other streptococcal arthritis, right elbow** HCC

          M00.222 **Other streptococcal arthritis, left elbow** HCC

          M00.229 **Other streptococcal arthritis, unspecified elbow** HCC ▽

    ✓6th **M00.23** **Other streptococcal arthritis, wrist**

          Other streptococcal arthritis of carpal bones

          M00.231 **Other streptococcal arthritis, right wrist** HCC

          M00.232 **Other streptococcal arthritis, left wrist** HCC

          M00.239 **Other streptococcal arthritis, unspecified wrist** HCC ▽

    ✓6th **M00.24** **Other streptococcal arthritis, hand**

          Other streptococcal arthritis metacarpus and phalanges

          M00.241 **Other streptococcal arthritis, right hand** HCC

          M00.242 **Other streptococcal arthritis, left hand** HCC

          M00.249 **Other streptococcal arthritis, unspecified hand** HCC ▽

    ✓6th **M00.25** **Other streptococcal arthritis, hip**

          M00.251 **Other streptococcal arthritis, right hip** HCC

          M00.252 **Other streptococcal arthritis, left hip** HCC

          M00.259 **Other streptococcal arthritis, unspecified hip** HCC ▽

    ✓6th **M00.26** **Other streptococcal arthritis, knee**

          M00.261 **Other streptococcal arthritis, right knee** HCC

          M00.262 **Other streptococcal arthritis, left knee** HCC

          M00.269 **Other streptococcal arthritis, unspecified knee** HCC ▽

    ✓6th **M00.27** **Other streptococcal arthritis, ankle and foot**

          Other streptococcal arthritis, tarsus, metatarsus and phalanges

          M00.271 **Other streptococcal arthritis, right ankle and foot** HCC

          M00.272 **Other streptococcal arthritis, left ankle and foot** HCC

          M00.279 **Other streptococcal arthritis, unspecified ankle and foot** HCC ▽

    M00.28 **Other streptococcal arthritis, vertebrae** HCC

    M00.29 **Other streptococcal polyarthritis** HCC

✓5th **M00.8** **Arthritis and polyarthritis due to other bacteria**

    Use additional code (B96) to identify bacteria

    M00.80 **Arthritis due to other bacteria, unspecified joint** HCC ▽

    ✓6th **M00.81** **Arthritis due to other bacteria, shoulder**

          M00.811 **Arthritis due to other bacteria, right shoulder** HCC

          M00.812 **Arthritis due to other bacteria, left shoulder** HCC

          M00.819 **Arthritis due to other bacteria, unspecified shoulder** HCC ▽

    ✓6th **M00.82** **Arthritis due to other bacteria, elbow**

          M00.821 **Arthritis due to other bacteria, right elbow** HCC

          M00.822 **Arthritis due to other bacteria, left elbow** HCC

          M00.829 **Arthritis due to other bacteria, unspecified elbow** HCC ▽

    ✓6th **M00.83** **Arthritis due to other bacteria, wrist**

          Arthritis due to other bacteria, carpal bones

          M00.831 **Arthritis due to other bacteria, right wrist** HCC

          M00.832 **Arthritis due to other bacteria, left wrist** HCC

          M00.839 **Arthritis due to other bacteria, unspecified wrist** HCC ▽

    ✓6th **M00.84** **Arthritis due to other bacteria, hand**

          Arthritis due to other bacteria, metacarpus and phalanges

          M00.841 **Arthritis due to other bacteria, right hand** HCC

          M00.842 **Arthritis due to other bacteria, left hand** HCC

          M00.849 **Arthritis due to other bacteria, unspecified hand** HCC ▽

    ✓6th **M00.85** **Arthritis due to other bacteria, hip**

          M00.851 **Arthritis due to other bacteria, right hip** HCC

          M00.852 **Arthritis due to other bacteria, left hip** HCC

          M00.859 **Arthritis due to other bacteria, unspecified hip** HCC ▽

    ✓6th **M00.86** **Arthritis due to other bacteria, knee**

          M00.861 **Arthritis due to other bacteria, right knee** HCC

          M00.862 **Arthritis due to other bacteria, left knee** HCC

          M00.869 **Arthritis due to other bacteria, unspecified knee** HCC ▽

    ✓6th **M00.87** **Arthritis due to other bacteria, ankle and foot**

          Arthritis due to other bacteria, tarsus, metatarsus, and phalanges

          M00.871 **Arthritis due to other bacteria, right ankle and foot** HCC

          M00.872 **Arthritis due to other bacteria, left ankle and foot** HCC

          M00.879 **Arthritis due to other bacteria, unspecified ankle and foot** HCC ▽

    M00.88 **Arthritis due to other bacteria, vertebrae** HCC

    M00.89 **Polyarthritis due to other bacteria** HCC

M00.9 **Pyogenic arthritis, unspecified** HCC ▽

    Infective arthritis NOS

✓4th **M01** **Direct infections of joint in infectious and parasitic diseases classified elsewhere**

    Code first underlying disease, such as:

      leprosy [Hansen's disease] (A30.-)

      mycoses (B35-B49)

      O'nyong-nyong fever (A92.1)

      paratyphoid fever (A01.1-A01.4)

      EXCLUDES 1   arthropathy in Lyme disease (A69.23)

          gonococcal arthritis (A54.42)

          meningococcal arthritis (A39.83)

          mumps arthritis (B26.85)

          postinfective arthropathy (M02.-)

          postmeningococcal arthritis (A39.84)

          reactive arthritis (M02.3)

          rubella arthritis (B06.82)

          sarcoidosis arthritis (D86.86)

          typhoid fever arthritis (A01.04)

          tuberculosis arthritis (A18.01-A18.02)

    ✓5th **M01.X** **Direct infection of joint in infectious and parasitic diseases classified elsewhere**

      M01.X0 ***Direct infection of unspecified joint in infectious and parasitic diseases classified elsewhere*** HCC ▽

      ✓6th **M01.X1** **Direct infection of shoulder joint in infectious and parasitic diseases classified elsewhere**

          M01.X11 ***Direct infection of right shoulder in infectious and parasitic diseases classified elsewhere*** HCC

EXCLUDES 1 Not coded here   **EXCLUDES 2** Not included here   N Newborn Age: 0   P Pediatric Age: 0-17   M Maternity Age: 12-55   A Adult Age: 15-124

718   ICD-10-CM 2018

M01.X12   **Direct infection of** left **shoulder in infectious and parasitic diseases classified elsewhere**   HCC

M01.X19   **Direct infection of unspecified shoulder in infectious and parasitic diseases classified elsewhere**   HCC ▽

✓6ᵗʰ   **M01.X2**   **Direct infection of** elbow **in infectious and parasitic diseases classified elsewhere**

M01.X21   **Direct infection of** right **elbow in infectious and parasitic diseases classified elsewhere**   HCC

M01.X22   **Direct infection of** left **elbow in infectious and parasitic diseases classified elsewhere**   HCC

M01.X29   **Direct infection of unspecified elbow in infectious and parasitic diseases classified elsewhere**   HCC ▽

✓6ᵗʰ   **M01.X3**   **Direct infection of** wrist **in infectious and parasitic diseases classified elsewhere**
Direct infection of carpal bones in infectious and parasitic diseases classified elsewhere

M01.X31   **Direct infection of** right **wrist in infectious and parasitic diseases classified elsewhere**   HCC

M01.X32   **Direct infection of** left **wrist in infectious and parasitic diseases classified elsewhere**   HCC

M01.X39   **Direct infection of unspecified wrist in infectious and parasitic diseases classified elsewhere**   HCC ▽

✓6ᵗʰ   **M01.X4**   **Direct infection of** hand **in infectious and parasitic diseases classified elsewhere**
Direct infection of metacarpus and phalanges in infectious and parasitic diseases classified elsewhere

M01.X41   **Direct infection of** right **hand in infectious and parasitic diseases classified elsewhere**   HCC

M01.X42   **Direct infection of** left **hand in infectious and parasitic diseases classified elsewhere**   HCC

M01.X49   **Direct infection of unspecified hand in infectious and parasitic diseases classified elsewhere**   HCC ▽

✓6ᵗʰ   **M01.X5**   **Direct infection of** hip **in infectious and parasitic diseases classified elsewhere**

M01.X51   **Direct infection of** right **hip in infectious and parasitic diseases classified elsewhere**   HCC

M01.X52   **Direct infection of** left **hip in infectious and parasitic diseases classified elsewhere**   HCC

M01.X59   **Direct infection of unspecified hip in infectious and parasitic diseases classified elsewhere**   HCC ▽

✓6ᵗʰ   **M01.X6**   **Direct infection of** knee **in infectious and parasitic diseases classified elsewhere**

M01.X61   **Direct infection of** right **knee in infectious and parasitic diseases classified elsewhere**   HCC

M01.X62   **Direct infection of** left **knee in infectious and parasitic diseases classified elsewhere**   HCC

M01.X69   **Direct infection of unspecified knee in infectious and parasitic diseases classified elsewhere**   HCC ▽

✓6ᵗʰ   **M01.X7**   **Direct infection of** ankle and foot **in infectious and parasitic diseases classified elsewhere**
Direct infection of tarsus, metatarsus and phalanges in infectious and parasitic diseases classified elsewhere

M01.X71   **Direct infection of** right **ankle and foot in infectious and parasitic diseases classified elsewhere**   HCC

M01.X72   **Direct infection of** left **ankle and foot in infectious and parasitic diseases classified elsewhere**   HCC

M01.X79   **Direct infection of unspecified ankle and foot in infectious and parasitic diseases classified elsewhere**   HCC ▽

M01.X8   **Direct infection of** vertebrae **in infectious and parasitic diseases classified elsewhere**   HCC

M01.X9   **Direct infection of** multiple joints **in infectious and parasitic diseases classified elsewhere**   HCC

✓4ᵗʰ   **M02**   **Postinfective and reactive arthropathies**
Code first underlying disease, such as:
   congenital syphilis [Clutton's joints] (A50.5)
   enteritis due to Yersinia enterocolitica (A04.6)
   infective endocarditis (I33.0)
   viral hepatitis (B15-B19)

> **EXCLUDES 1**   Behçet's disease (M35.2)
> direct infections of joint in infectious and parasitic diseases classified elsewhere (M01.-)
> postmeningococcal arthritis (A39.84)
> mumps arthritis (B26.85)
> rheumatic fever (I00)
> rubella arthritis (B06.82)
> syphilis arthritis (late) (A52.77)
> tabetic arthropathy [Charcôt's] (A52.16)

✓5ᵗʰ   **M02.0**   **Arthropathy** following intestinal bypass

M02.00   **Arthropathy following intestinal bypass, unspecified site**   ▽

✓6ᵗʰ   *M02.01*   **Arthropathy following intestinal bypass,** shoulder

M02.011   **Arthropathy following intestinal bypass,** right **shoulder**

M02.012   **Arthropathy following intestinal bypass,** left **shoulder**

M02.019   **Arthropathy following intestinal bypass, unspecified shoulder**   ▽

✓6ᵗʰ   *M02.02*   **Arthropathy following intestinal bypass,** elbow

M02.021   **Arthropathy following intestinal bypass,** right **elbow**

M02.022   **Arthropathy following intestinal bypass,** left **elbow**

M02.029   **Arthropathy following intestinal bypass, unspecified elbow**   ▽

✓6ᵗʰ   *M02.03*   **Arthropathy following intestinal bypass,** wrist
Arthropathy following intestinal bypass, carpal bones

M02.031   **Arthropathy following intestinal bypass,** right **wrist**

M02.032   **Arthropathy following intestinal bypass,** left **wrist**

M02.039   **Arthropathy following intestinal bypass, unspecified wrist**   ▽

✓6ᵗʰ   *M02.04*   **Arthropathy following intestinal bypass,** hand
Arthropathy following intestinal bypass, metacarpals and phalanges

M02.041   **Arthropathy following intestinal bypass,** right **hand**

M02.042   **Arthropathy following intestinal bypass,** left **hand**

M02.049   **Arthropathy following intestinal bypass, unspecified hand**   ▽

✓6ᵗʰ   *M02.05*   **Arthropathy following intestinal bypass,** hip

M02.051   **Arthropathy following intestinal bypass,** right **hip**

M02.052   **Arthropathy following intestinal bypass,** left **hip**

M02.059   **Arthropathy following intestinal bypass, unspecified hip**   ▽

✓6ᵗʰ   *M02.06*   **Arthropathy following intestinal bypass,** knee

M02.061   **Arthropathy following intestinal bypass,** right **knee**

M02.062   **Arthropathy following intestinal bypass,** left **knee**

M02.069   **Arthropathy following intestinal bypass, unspecified knee**   ▽

✓6ᵗʰ   *M02.07*   **Arthropathy following intestinal bypass,** ankle and foot
Arthropathy following intestinal bypass, tarsus, metatarsus and phalanges

M02.071   **Arthropathy following intestinal bypass,** right **ankle and foot**

M02.072   **Arthropathy following intestinal bypass,** left **ankle and foot**

M02.079   **Arthropathy following intestinal bypass, unspecified ankle and foot**   ▽

M02.08   **Arthropathy following intestinal bypass,** vertebrae

---

☑ Additional Character Req   ✓x7ᵗʰ Placeholder Alert   Manifestation   HCC CMS-HCC Condition   ▽ Unspecified Code   ▶◀ Revised Text   ● New Code   ▲ Revised Code Title

Chapter 13. Diseases of the Musculoskeletal System and Connective Tissue

M02.09–M02.38

    M02.09   Arthropathy following intestinal bypass, multiple sites

✓5ᵗʰ **M02.1**   Postdysenteric arthropathy
- **M02.10**   Postdysenteric arthropathy, unspecified site   HCC ▽

✓6ᵗʰ **M02.11**   Postdysenteric arthropathy, shoulder
- **M02.111**   Postdysenteric arthropathy, right shoulder   HCC
- **M02.112**   Postdysenteric arthropathy, left shoulder   HCC
- **M02.119**   Postdysenteric arthropathy, unspecified shoulder   HCC ▽

✓6ᵗʰ **M02.12**   Postdysenteric arthropathy, elbow
- **M02.121**   Postdysenteric arthropathy, right elbow   HCC
- **M02.122**   Postdysenteric arthropathy, left elbow   HCC
- **M02.129**   Postdysenteric arthropathy, unspecified elbow   HCC ▽

✓6ᵗʰ **M02.13**   Postdysenteric arthropathy, wrist
     Postdysenteric arthropathy, carpal bones
- **M02.131**   Postdysenteric arthropathy, right wrist   HCC
- **M02.132**   Postdysenteric arthropathy, left wrist   HCC
- **M02.139**   Postdysenteric arthropathy, unspecified wrist   HCC ▽

✓6ᵗʰ **M02.14**   Postdysenteric arthropathy, hand
     Postdysenteric arthropathy, metacarpus and phalanges
- **M02.141**   Postdysenteric arthropathy, right hand   HCC
- **M02.142**   Postdysenteric arthropathy, left hand   HCC
- **M02.149**   Postdysenteric arthropathy, unspecified hand   HCC ▽

✓6ᵗʰ **M02.15**   Postdysenteric arthropathy, hip
- **M02.151**   Postdysenteric arthropathy, right hip   HCC
- **M02.152**   Postdysenteric arthropathy, left hip   HCC
- **M02.159**   Postdysenteric arthropathy, unspecified hip   HCC ▽

✓6ᵗʰ **M02.16**   Postdysenteric arthropathy, knee
- **M02.161**   Postdysenteric arthropathy, right knee   HCC
- **M02.162**   Postdysenteric arthropathy, left knee   HCC
- **M02.169**   Postdysenteric arthropathy, unspecified knee   HCC ▽

✓6ᵗʰ **M02.17**   Postdysenteric arthropathy, ankle and foot
     Postdysenteric arthropathy, tarsus, metatarsus and phalanges
- **M02.171**   Postdysenteric arthropathy, right ankle and foot   HCC
- **M02.172**   Postdysenteric arthropathy, left ankle and foot   HCC
- **M02.179**   Postdysenteric arthropathy, unspecified ankle and foot   HCC ▽

    M02.18   Postdysenteric arthropathy, vertebrae   HCC
    M02.19   Postdysenteric arthropathy, multiple sites   HCC

✓5ᵗʰ **M02.2**   Postimmunization arthropathy
- **M02.20**   Postimmunization arthropathy, unspecified site   ▽

✓6ᵗʰ **M02.21**   Postimmunization arthropathy, shoulder
- **M02.211**   Postimmunization arthropathy, right shoulder
- **M02.212**   Postimmunization arthropathy, left shoulder
- **M02.219**   Postimmunization arthropathy, unspecified shoulder   ▽

✓6ᵗʰ **M02.22**   Postimmunization arthropathy, elbow
- **M02.221**   Postimmunization arthropathy, right elbow
- **M02.222**   Postimmunization arthropathy, left elbow
- **M02.229**   Postimmunization arthropathy, unspecified elbow   ▽

✓6ᵗʰ **M02.23**   Postimmunization arthropathy, wrist
     Postimmunization arthropathy, carpal bones
- **M02.231**   Postimmunization arthropathy, right wrist
- **M02.232**   Postimmunization arthropathy, left wrist
- **M02.239**   Postimmunization arthropathy, unspecified wrist   ▽

✓6ᵗʰ **M02.24**   Postimmunization arthropathy, hand
     Postimmunization arthropathy, metacarpus and phalanges
- **M02.241**   Postimmunization arthropathy, right hand
- **M02.242**   Postimmunization arthropathy, left hand
- **M02.249**   Postimmunization arthropathy, unspecified hand   ▽

✓6ᵗʰ **M02.25**   Postimmunization arthropathy, hip
- **M02.251**   Postimmunization arthropathy, right hip
- **M02.252**   Postimmunization arthropathy, left hip
- **M02.259**   Postimmunization arthropathy, unspecified hip   ▽

✓6ᵗʰ **M02.26**   Postimmunization arthropathy, knee
- **M02.261**   Postimmunization arthropathy, right knee
- **M02.262**   Postimmunization arthropathy, left knee
- **M02.269**   Postimmunization arthropathy, unspecified knee   ▽

✓6ᵗʰ **M02.27**   Postimmunization arthropathy, ankle and foot
     Postimmunization arthropathy, tarsus, metatarsus and phalanges
- **M02.271**   Postimmunization arthropathy, right ankle and foot
- **M02.272**   Postimmunization arthropathy, left ankle and foot
- **M02.279**   Postimmunization arthropathy, unspecified ankle and foot   ▽

    M02.28   Postimmunization arthropathy, vertebrae
    M02.29   Postimmunization arthropathy, multiple sites

✓5ᵗʰ **M02.3**   Reiter's disease
     Reactive arthritis
- **M02.30**   Reiter's disease, unspecified site   HCC ▽

✓6ᵗʰ **M02.31**   Reiter's disease, shoulder
- **M02.311**   Reiter's disease, right shoulder   HCC
- **M02.312**   Reiter's disease, left shoulder   HCC
- **M02.319**   Reiter's disease, unspecified shoulder   HCC ▽

✓6ᵗʰ **M02.32**   Reiter's disease, elbow
- **M02.321**   Reiter's disease, right elbow   HCC
- **M02.322**   Reiter's disease, left elbow   HCC
- **M02.329**   Reiter's disease, unspecified elbow   HCC ▽

✓6ᵗʰ **M02.33**   Reiter's disease, wrist
     Reiter's disease, carpal bones
- **M02.331**   Reiter's disease, right wrist   HCC
- **M02.332**   Reiter's disease, left wrist   HCC
- **M02.339**   Reiter's disease, unspecified wrist   HCC ▽

✓6ᵗʰ **M02.34**   Reiter's disease, hand
     Reiter's disease, metacarpus and phalanges
- **M02.341**   Reiter's disease, right hand   HCC
- **M02.342**   Reiter's disease, left hand   HCC
- **M02.349**   Reiter's disease, unspecified hand   HCC ▽

✓6ᵗʰ **M02.35**   Reiter's disease, hip
- **M02.351**   Reiter's disease, right hip   HCC
- **M02.352**   Reiter's disease, left hip   HCC
- **M02.359**   Reiter's disease, unspecified hip   HCC ▽

✓6ᵗʰ **M02.36**   Reiter's disease, knee
- **M02.361**   Reiter's disease, right knee   HCC
- **M02.362**   Reiter's disease, left knee   HCC
- **M02.369**   Reiter's disease, unspecified knee   HCC ▽

✓6ᵗʰ **M02.37**   Reiter's disease, ankle and foot
     Reiter's disease, tarsus, metatarsus and phalanges
- **M02.371**   Reiter's disease, right ankle and foot   HCC
- **M02.372**   Reiter's disease, left ankle and foot   HCC
- **M02.379**   Reiter's disease, unspecified ankle and foot   HCC ▽

    M02.38   Reiter's disease, vertebrae   HCC

EXCLUDES 1 Not coded here   EXCLUDES 2 Not included here   N Newborn Age: 0   P Pediatric Age: 0-17   M Maternity Age: 12-55   A Adult Age: 15-124

720   ICD-10-CM 2018

M02.39   Reiter's disease, multiple sites   HCC

✓5ᵗʰ **M02.8   Other** reactive **arthropathies**

   M02.80   *Other reactive arthropathies, unspecified site*   HCC ▽

   ✓6ᵗʰ **M02.81   Other reactive arthropathies,** shoulder

     M02.811   *Other reactive arthropathies, right shoulder*   HCC

     M02.812   *Other reactive arthropathies, left shoulder*   HCC

     M02.819   *Other reactive arthropathies, unspecified shoulder*   HCC ▽

   ✓6ᵗʰ **M02.82   Other reactive arthropathies,** elbow

     M02.821   *Other reactive arthropathies, right elbow*   HCC

     M02.822   *Other reactive arthropathies, left elbow*   HCC

     M02.829   *Other reactive arthropathies, unspecified elbow*   HCC ▽

   ✓6ᵗʰ **M02.83   Other reactive arthropathies,** wrist

     Other reactive arthropathies, carpal bones

     M02.831   *Other reactive arthropathies, right wrist*   HCC

     M02.832   *Other reactive arthropathies, left wrist*   HCC

     M02.839   *Other reactive arthropathies, unspecified wrist*   HCC ▽

   ✓6ᵗʰ **M02.84   Other reactive arthropathies,** hand

     Other reactive arthropathies, metacarpus and phalanges

     M02.841   *Other reactive arthropathies, right hand*   HCC

     M02.842   *Other reactive arthropathies, left hand*   HCC

     M02.849   *Other reactive arthropathies, unspecified hand*   HCC ▽

   ✓6ᵗʰ **M02.85   Other reactive arthropathies,** hip

     M02.851   *Other reactive arthropathies, right hip*   HCC

     M02.852   *Other reactive arthropathies, left hip*   HCC

     M02.859   *Other reactive arthropathies, unspecified hip*   HCC ▽

   ✓6ᵗʰ **M02.86   Other reactive arthropathies,** knee

     M02.861   *Other reactive arthropathies, right knee*   HCC

     M02.862   *Other reactive arthropathies, left knee*   HCC

     M02.869   *Other reactive arthropathies, unspecified knee*   HCC ▽

   ✓6ᵗʰ **M02.87   Other reactive arthropathies,** ankle and foot

     Other reactive arthropathies, tarsus, metatarsus and phalanges

     M02.871   *Other reactive arthropathies, right ankle and foot*   HCC

     M02.872   *Other reactive arthropathies, left ankle and foot*   HCC

     M02.879   *Other reactive arthropathies, unspecified ankle and foot*   HCC ▽

   M02.88   *Other reactive arthropathies, vertebrae*   HCC

   M02.89   *Other reactive arthropathies, multiple sites*   HCC

   M02.9   *Reactive arthropathy, unspecified*   HCC ▽

Autoinflammatory syndromes (M04)

✓4ᵗʰ **M04   Autoinflammatory syndromes**

   EXCLUDES 2   Crohn's disease (K50.-)

   M04.1   Periodic fever syndromes   HCC

     Familial Mediterranean fever

     Hyperimmunoglobin D syndrome

     Mevalonate kinase deficiency

     Tumor necrosis factor receptor associated periodic syndrome [TRAPS]

   M04.2   Cryopyrin-associated periodic syndromes   HCC

     Chronic infantile neurological, cutaneous and articular syndrome [CINCA]

     Familial cold autoinflammatory syndrome

     Familial cold urticaria

     Muckle-Wells syndrome

     Neonatal onset multisystemic inflammatory disorder [NOMID]

   M04.8   Other autoinflammatory syndromes   HCC

     Blau syndrome

     Deficiency of interleukin 1 receptor antagonist [DIRA]

     Majeed syndrome

     Periodic fever, aphthous stomatitis, pharyngitis, and adenopathy syndrome [PFAPA]

     Pyogenic arthritis, pyoderma gangrenosum, and acne syndrome [PAPA]

   M04.9   Autoinflammatory syndrome, unspecified   HCC ▽

Inflammatory polyarthropathies (M05-M14)

✓4ᵗʰ **M05   Rheumatoid arthritis with rheumatoid factor**

   EXCLUDES 1   rheumatic fever (I00)

        juvenile rheumatoid arthritis (M08.-)

        rheumatoid arthritis of spine (M45.-)

   DEF: Autoimmune systemic disease that causes chronic inflammation of joints and other areas of the body, manifested by inflammatory changes in articular structures and synovial membranes, atrophy, and loss in bone density.

   ✓5ᵗʰ **M05.0   Felty's syndrome**

     Rheumatoid arthritis with splenoadenomegaly and leukopenia

     M05.00   Felty's syndrome, unspecified site   HCC ▽

     ✓6ᵗʰ **M05.01   Felty's syndrome,** shoulder

       M05.011   Felty's syndrome, right shoulder   HCC

       M05.012   Felty's syndrome, left shoulder   HCC

       M05.019   Felty's syndrome, unspecified shoulder   HCC ▽

     ✓6ᵗʰ **M05.02   Felty's syndrome,** elbow

       M05.021   Felty's syndrome, right elbow   HCC

       M05.022   Felty's syndrome, left elbow   HCC

       M05.029   Felty's syndrome, unspecified elbow   HCC ▽

     ✓6ᵗʰ **M05.03   Felty's syndrome,** wrist

       Felty's syndrome, carpal bones

       M05.031   Felty's syndrome, right wrist   HCC

       M05.032   Felty's syndrome, left wrist   HCC

       M05.039   Felty's syndrome, unspecified wrist   HCC ▽

     ✓6ᵗʰ **M05.04   Felty's syndrome,** hand

       Felty's syndrome, metacarpus and phalanges

       M05.041   Felty's syndrome, right hand   HCC

       M05.042   Felty's syndrome, left hand   HCC

       M05.049   Felty's syndrome, unspecified hand   HCC ▽

     ✓6ᵗʰ **M05.05   Felty's syndrome,** hip

       M05.051   Felty's syndrome, right hip   HCC

       M05.052   Felty's syndrome, left hip   HCC

       M05.059   Felty's syndrome, unspecified hip   HCC ▽

     ✓6ᵗʰ **M05.06   Felty's syndrome,** knee

       M05.061   Felty's syndrome, right knee   HCC

       M05.062   Felty's syndrome, left knee   HCC

       M05.069   Felty's syndrome, unspecified knee   HCC ▽

     ✓6ᵗʰ **M05.07   Felty's syndrome,** ankle and foot

       Felty's syndrome, tarsus, metatarsus and phalanges

       M05.071   Felty's syndrome, right ankle and foot   HCC

       M05.072   Felty's syndrome, left ankle and foot   HCC

       M05.079   Felty's syndrome, unspecified ankle and foot   HCC ▽

     M05.09   Felty's syndrome, multiple sites   HCC

   ✓5ᵗʰ **M05.1   Rheumatoid lung disease with rheumatoid arthritis**

     DEF: Lung disorders associated with rheumatoid arthritis.

     M05.10   Rheumatoid lung disease with rheumatoid arthritis of unspecified site   HCC ▽

     ✓6ᵗʰ **M05.11   Rheumatoid lung disease with rheumatoid arthritis of** shoulder

       M05.111   Rheumatoid lung disease with rheumatoid arthritis of right shoulder   HCC

       M05.112   Rheumatoid lung disease with rheumatoid arthritis of left shoulder   HCC

       M05.119   Rheumatoid lung disease with rheumatoid arthritis of unspecified shoulder   HCC ▽

✓ Additional Character Req   ✓x7ᵗʰ Placeholder Alert   Manifestation   HCC CMS-HCC Condition   ▽ Unspecified Code   ►◄ Revised Text   ● New Code   ▲ Revised Code Title

✓6ᵗʰ M05.12 Rheumatoid lung disease with rheumatoid arthritis of elbow
- **M05.121** Rheumatoid lung disease with rheumatoid arthritis of right elbow   HCC
- **M05.122** Rheumatoid lung disease with rheumatoid arthritis of left elbow   HCC
- **M05.129** Rheumatoid lung disease with rheumatoid arthritis of unspecified elbow   HCC ▽

✓6ᵗʰ M05.13 Rheumatoid lung disease with rheumatoid arthritis of wrist
Rheumatoid lung disease with rheumatoid arthritis, carpal bones
- **M05.131** Rheumatoid lung disease with rheumatoid arthritis of right wrist   HCC
- **M05.132** Rheumatoid lung disease with rheumatoid arthritis of left wrist   HCC
- **M05.139** Rheumatoid lung disease with rheumatoid arthritis of unspecified wrist   HCC ▽

✓6ᵗʰ M05.14 Rheumatoid lung disease with rheumatoid arthritis of hand
Rheumatoid lung disease with rheumatoid arthritis, metacarpus and phalanges
- **M05.141** Rheumatoid lung disease with rheumatoid arthritis of right hand   HCC
- **M05.142** Rheumatoid lung disease with rheumatoid arthritis of left hand   HCC
- **M05.149** Rheumatoid lung disease with rheumatoid arthritis of unspecified hand   HCC ▽

✓6ᵗʰ M05.15 Rheumatoid lung disease with rheumatoid arthritis of hip
- **M05.151** Rheumatoid lung disease with rheumatoid arthritis of right hip   HCC
- **M05.152** Rheumatoid lung disease with rheumatoid arthritis of left hip   HCC
- **M05.159** Rheumatoid lung disease with rheumatoid arthritis of unspecified hip   HCC ▽

✓6ᵗʰ M05.16 Rheumatoid lung disease with rheumatoid arthritis of knee
- **M05.161** Rheumatoid lung disease with rheumatoid arthritis of right knee   HCC
- **M05.162** Rheumatoid lung disease with rheumatoid arthritis of left knee   HCC
- **M05.169** Rheumatoid lung disease with rheumatoid arthritis of unspecified knee   HCC ▽

✓6ᵗʰ M05.17 Rheumatoid lung disease with rheumatoid arthritis of ankle and foot
Rheumatoid lung disease with rheumatoid arthritis, tarsus, metatarsus and phalanges
- **M05.171** Rheumatoid lung disease with rheumatoid arthritis of right ankle and foot   HCC
- **M05.172** Rheumatoid lung disease with rheumatoid arthritis of left ankle and foot   HCC
- **M05.179** Rheumatoid lung disease with rheumatoid arthritis of unspecified ankle and foot   HCC ▽

M05.19 Rheumatoid lung disease with rheumatoid arthritis of multiple sites   HCC

✓5ᵗʰ M05.2 Rheumatoid vasculitis with rheumatoid arthritis
- **M05.20** Rheumatoid vasculitis with rheumatoid arthritis of unspecified site   HCC ▽

✓6ᵗʰ M05.21 Rheumatoid vasculitis with rheumatoid arthritis of shoulder
- **M05.211** Rheumatoid vasculitis with rheumatoid arthritis of right shoulder   HCC
- **M05.212** Rheumatoid vasculitis with rheumatoid arthritis of left shoulder   HCC
- **M05.219** Rheumatoid vasculitis with rheumatoid arthritis of unspecified shoulder   HCC ▽

✓6ᵗʰ M05.22 Rheumatoid vasculitis with rheumatoid arthritis of elbow
- **M05.221** Rheumatoid vasculitis with rheumatoid arthritis of right elbow   HCC
- **M05.222** Rheumatoid vasculitis with rheumatoid arthritis of left elbow   HCC
- **M05.229** Rheumatoid vasculitis with rheumatoid arthritis of unspecified elbow   HCC ▽

✓6ᵗʰ M05.23 Rheumatoid vasculitis with rheumatoid arthritis of wrist
Rheumatoid vasculitis with rheumatoid arthritis, carpal bones
- **M05.231** Rheumatoid vasculitis with rheumatoid arthritis of right wrist   HCC
- **M05.232** Rheumatoid vasculitis with rheumatoid arthritis of left wrist   HCC
- **M05.239** Rheumatoid vasculitis with rheumatoid arthritis of unspecified wrist   HCC ▽

✓6ᵗʰ M05.24 Rheumatoid vasculitis with rheumatoid arthritis of hand
Rheumatoid vasculitis with rheumatoid arthritis, metacarpus and phalanges
- **M05.241** Rheumatoid vasculitis with rheumatoid arthritis of right hand   HCC
- **M05.242** Rheumatoid vasculitis with rheumatoid arthritis of left hand   HCC
- **M05.249** Rheumatoid vasculitis with rheumatoid arthritis of unspecified hand   HCC ▽

✓6ᵗʰ M05.25 Rheumatoid vasculitis with rheumatoid arthritis of hip
- **M05.251** Rheumatoid vasculitis with rheumatoid arthritis of right hip   HCC
- **M05.252** Rheumatoid vasculitis with rheumatoid arthritis of left hip   HCC
- **M05.259** Rheumatoid vasculitis with rheumatoid arthritis of unspecified hip   HCC ▽

✓6ᵗʰ M05.26 Rheumatoid vasculitis with rheumatoid arthritis of knee
- **M05.261** Rheumatoid vasculitis with rheumatoid arthritis of right knee   HCC
- **M05.262** Rheumatoid vasculitis with rheumatoid arthritis of left knee   HCC
- **M05.269** Rheumatoid vasculitis with rheumatoid arthritis of unspecified knee   HCC ▽

✓6ᵗʰ M05.27 Rheumatoid vasculitis with rheumatoid arthritis of ankle and foot
Rheumatoid vasculitis with rheumatoid arthritis, tarsus, metatarsus and phalanges
- **M05.271** Rheumatoid vasculitis with rheumatoid arthritis of right ankle and foot   HCC
- **M05.272** Rheumatoid vasculitis with rheumatoid arthritis of left ankle and foot   HCC
- **M05.279** Rheumatoid vasculitis with rheumatoid arthritis of unspecified ankle and foot   HCC ▽

M05.29 Rheumatoid vasculitis with rheumatoid arthritis of multiple sites   HCC

✓5ᵗʰ M05.3 Rheumatoid heart disease with rheumatoid arthritis
Rheumatoid carditis   Rheumatoid myocarditis
Rheumatoid endocarditis   Rheumatoid pericarditis
- **M05.30** Rheumatoid heart disease with rheumatoid arthritis of unspecified site   HCC ▽

✓6ᵗʰ M05.31 Rheumatoid heart disease with rheumatoid arthritis of shoulder
- **M05.311** Rheumatoid heart disease with rheumatoid arthritis of right shoulder   HCC
- **M05.312** Rheumatoid heart disease with rheumatoid arthritis of left shoulder   HCC
- **M05.319** Rheumatoid heart disease with rheumatoid arthritis of unspecified shoulder   HCC ▽

EXCLUDES 1 Not coded here   EXCLUDES 2 Not included here   N Newborn Age: 0   P Pediatric Age: 0-17   M Maternity Age: 12-55   A Adult Age: 15-124

722   ICD-10-CM 2018

√6ᵗʰ M05.32 Rheumatoid heart disease with rheumatoid arthritis of elbow

     M05.321 Rheumatoid heart disease with rheumatoid arthritis of right elbow   HCC

     M05.322 Rheumatoid heart disease with rheumatoid arthritis of left elbow   HCC

     M05.329 Rheumatoid heart disease with rheumatoid arthritis of unspecified elbow   HCC ▽

√6ᵗʰ M05.33 Rheumatoid heart disease with rheumatoid arthritis of wrist
     Rheumatoid heart disease with rheumatoid arthritis, carpal bones

     M05.331 Rheumatoid heart disease with rheumatoid arthritis of right wrist   HCC

     M05.332 Rheumatoid heart disease with rheumatoid arthritis of left wrist   HCC

     M05.339 Rheumatoid heart disease with rheumatoid arthritis of unspecified wrist   HCC ▽

√6ᵗʰ M05.34 Rheumatoid heart disease with rheumatoid arthritis of hand
     Rheumatoid heart disease with rheumatoid arthritis, metacarpus and phalanges

     M05.341 Rheumatoid heart disease with rheumatoid arthritis of right hand   HCC

     M05.342 Rheumatoid heart disease with rheumatoid arthritis of left hand   HCC

     M05.349 Rheumatoid heart disease with rheumatoid arthritis of unspecified hand   HCC ▽

√6ᵗʰ M05.35 Rheumatoid heart disease with rheumatoid arthritis of hip

     M05.351 Rheumatoid heart disease with rheumatoid arthritis of right hip   HCC

     M05.352 Rheumatoid heart disease with rheumatoid arthritis of left hip   HCC

     M05.359 Rheumatoid heart disease with rheumatoid arthritis of unspecified hip   HCC ▽

√6ᵗʰ M05.36 Rheumatoid heart disease with rheumatoid arthritis of knee

     M05.361 Rheumatoid heart disease with rheumatoid arthritis of right knee   HCC

     M05.362 Rheumatoid heart disease with rheumatoid arthritis of left knee   HCC

     M05.369 Rheumatoid heart disease with rheumatoid arthritis of unspecified knee   HCC ▽

√6ᵗʰ M05.37 Rheumatoid heart disease with rheumatoid arthritis of ankle and foot
     Rheumatoid heart disease with rheumatoid arthritis, tarsus, metatarsus and phalanges

     M05.371 Rheumatoid heart disease with rheumatoid arthritis of right ankle and foot   HCC

     M05.372 Rheumatoid heart disease with rheumatoid arthritis of left ankle and foot   HCC

     M05.379 Rheumatoid heart disease with rheumatoid arthritis of unspecified ankle and foot   HCC ▽

     M05.39 Rheumatoid heart disease with rheumatoid arthritis of multiple sites   HCC

√5ᵗʰ M05.4 Rheumatoid myopathy with rheumatoid arthritis

     M05.40 Rheumatoid myopathy with rheumatoid arthritis of unspecified site   HCC ▽

√6ᵗʰ M05.41 Rheumatoid myopathy with rheumatoid arthritis of shoulder

     M05.411 Rheumatoid myopathy with rheumatoid arthritis of right shoulder   HCC

     M05.412 Rheumatoid myopathy with rheumatoid arthritis of left shoulder   HCC

     M05.419 Rheumatoid myopathy with rheumatoid arthritis of unspecified shoulder   HCC ▽

√6ᵗʰ M05.42 Rheumatoid myopathy with rheumatoid arthritis of elbow

     M05.421 Rheumatoid myopathy with rheumatoid arthritis of right elbow   HCC

     M05.422 Rheumatoid myopathy with rheumatoid arthritis of left elbow   HCC

     M05.429 Rheumatoid myopathy with rheumatoid arthritis of unspecified elbow   HCC ▽

√6ᵗʰ M05.43 Rheumatoid myopathy with rheumatoid arthritis of wrist
     Rheumatoid myopathy with rheumatoid arthritis, carpal bones

     M05.431 Rheumatoid myopathy with rheumatoid arthritis of right wrist   HCC

     M05.432 Rheumatoid myopathy with rheumatoid arthritis of left wrist   HCC

     M05.439 Rheumatoid myopathy with rheumatoid arthritis of unspecified wrist   HCC ▽

√6ᵗʰ M05.44 Rheumatoid myopathy with rheumatoid arthritis of hand
     Rheumatoid myopathy with rheumatoid arthritis, metacarpus and phalanges

     M05.441 Rheumatoid myopathy with rheumatoid arthritis of right hand   HCC

     M05.442 Rheumatoid myopathy with rheumatoid arthritis of left hand   HCC

     M05.449 Rheumatoid myopathy with rheumatoid arthritis of unspecified hand   HCC ▽

√6ᵗʰ M05.45 Rheumatoid myopathy with rheumatoid arthritis of hip

     M05.451 Rheumatoid myopathy with rheumatoid arthritis of right hip   HCC

     M05.452 Rheumatoid myopathy with rheumatoid arthritis of left hip   HCC

     M05.459 Rheumatoid myopathy with rheumatoid arthritis of unspecified hip   HCC ▽

√6ᵗʰ M05.46 Rheumatoid myopathy with rheumatoid arthritis of knee

     M05.461 Rheumatoid myopathy with rheumatoid arthritis of right knee   HCC

     M05.462 Rheumatoid myopathy with rheumatoid arthritis of left knee   HCC

     M05.469 Rheumatoid myopathy with rheumatoid arthritis of unspecified knee   HCC ▽

√6ᵗʰ M05.47 Rheumatoid myopathy with rheumatoid arthritis of ankle and foot
     Rheumatoid myopathy with rheumatoid arthritis, tarsus, metatarsus and phalanges

     M05.471 Rheumatoid myopathy with rheumatoid arthritis of right ankle and foot   HCC

     M05.472 Rheumatoid myopathy with rheumatoid arthritis of left ankle and foot   HCC

     M05.479 Rheumatoid myopathy with rheumatoid arthritis of unspecified ankle and foot   HCC ▽

     M05.49 Rheumatoid myopathy with rheumatoid arthritis of multiple sites   HCC

√5ᵗʰ M05.5 Rheumatoid polyneuropathy with rheumatoid arthritis

     M05.50 Rheumatoid polyneuropathy with rheumatoid arthritis of unspecified site   HCC ▽

√6ᵗʰ M05.51 Rheumatoid polyneuropathy with rheumatoid arthritis of shoulder

     M05.511 Rheumatoid polyneuropathy with rheumatoid arthritis of right shoulder   HCC

     M05.512 Rheumatoid polyneuropathy with rheumatoid arthritis of left shoulder   HCC

     M05.519 Rheumatoid polyneuropathy with rheumatoid arthritis of unspecified shoulder   HCC ▽

☑ Additional Character Req   √x7ᵗʰ Placeholder Alert   Manifestation   HCC CMS-HCC Condition   ▽ Unspecified Code   ►◄ Revised Text   ● New Code   ▲ Revised Code Title

✓6th **M05.52 Rheumatoid polyneuropathy with rheumatoid arthritis of** elbow

     M05.521 Rheumatoid polyneuropathy with rheumatoid arthritis of right **elbow**   HCC

     M05.522 Rheumatoid polyneuropathy with rheumatoid arthritis of left **elbow**   HCC

     M05.529 Rheumatoid polyneuropathy with rheumatoid arthritis of unspecified elbow   HCC ▽

✓6th **M05.53 Rheumatoid polyneuropathy with rheumatoid arthritis of** wrist

     Rheumatoid polyneuropathy with rheumatoid arthritis, carpal bones

     M05.531 Rheumatoid polyneuropathy with rheumatoid arthritis of right **wrist**   HCC

     M05.532 Rheumatoid polyneuropathy with rheumatoid arthritis of left **wrist**   HCC

     M05.539 Rheumatoid polyneuropathy with rheumatoid arthritis of unspecified wrist   HCC ▽

✓6th **M05.54 Rheumatoid polyneuropathy with rheumatoid arthritis of** hand

     Rheumatoid polyneuropathy with rheumatoid arthritis, metacarpus and phalanges

     M05.541 Rheumatoid polyneuropathy with rheumatoid arthritis of right **hand**   HCC

     M05.542 Rheumatoid polyneuropathy with rheumatoid arthritis of left **hand**   HCC

     M05.549 Rheumatoid polyneuropathy with rheumatoid arthritis of unspecified hand   HCC ▽

✓6th **M05.55 Rheumatoid polyneuropathy with rheumatoid arthritis of** hip

     M05.551 Rheumatoid polyneuropathy with rheumatoid arthritis of right **hip**   HCC

     M05.552 Rheumatoid polyneuropathy with rheumatoid arthritis of left **hip**   HCC

     M05.559 Rheumatoid polyneuropathy with rheumatoid arthritis of unspecified hip   HCC ▽

✓6th **M05.56 Rheumatoid polyneuropathy with rheumatoid arthritis of** knee

     M05.561 Rheumatoid polyneuropathy with rheumatoid arthritis of right **knee**   HCC

     M05.562 Rheumatoid polyneuropathy with rheumatoid arthritis of left **knee**   HCC

     M05.569 Rheumatoid polyneuropathy with rheumatoid arthritis of unspecified knee   HCC ▽

✓6th **M05.57 Rheumatoid polyneuropathy with rheumatoid arthritis of** ankle and foot

     Rheumatoid polyneuropathy with rheumatoid arthritis, tarsus, metatarsus and phalanges

     M05.571 Rheumatoid polyneuropathy with rheumatoid arthritis of right **ankle and foot**   HCC

     M05.572 Rheumatoid polyneuropathy with rheumatoid arthritis of left **ankle and foot**   HCC

     M05.579 Rheumatoid polyneuropathy with rheumatoid arthritis of unspecified ankle and foot   HCC ▽

     M05.59 Rheumatoid polyneuropathy with rheumatoid arthritis of multiple sites   HCC

✓5th **M05.6 Rheumatoid arthritis** with involvement of other organs and systems

     M05.60 Rheumatoid arthritis of unspecified site with involvement of other organs and systems   HCC ▽

✓6th **M05.61 Rheumatoid arthritis of** shoulder **with involvement of other organs and systems**

     M05.611 Rheumatoid arthritis of right **shoulder with involvement of other organs and systems**   HCC

     M05.612 Rheumatoid arthritis of left **shoulder with involvement of other organs and systems**   HCC

     M05.619 Rheumatoid arthritis of unspecified shoulder with involvement of other organs and systems   HCC ▽

✓6th **M05.62 Rheumatoid arthritis of** elbow **with involvement of other organs and systems**

     M05.621 Rheumatoid arthritis of right **elbow with involvement of other organs and systems**   HCC

     M05.622 Rheumatoid arthritis of left **elbow with involvement of other organs and systems**   HCC

     M05.629 Rheumatoid arthritis of unspecified elbow with involvement of other organs and systems   HCC ▽

✓6th **M05.63 Rheumatoid arthritis of** wrist **with involvement of other organs and systems**

     Rheumatoid arthritis of carpal bones with involvement of other organs and systems

     M05.631 Rheumatoid arthritis of right **wrist with involvement of other organs and systems**   HCC

     M05.632 Rheumatoid arthritis of left **wrist with involvement of other organs and systems**   HCC

     M05.639 Rheumatoid arthritis of unspecified wrist with involvement of other organs and systems   HCC ▽

✓6th **M05.64 Rheumatoid arthritis of** hand **with involvement of other organs and systems**

     Rheumatoid arthritis of metacarpus and phalanges with involvement of other organs and systems

     M05.641 Rheumatoid arthritis of right **hand with involvement of other organs and systems**   HCC

     M05.642 Rheumatoid arthritis of left **hand with involvement of other organs and systems**   HCC

     M05.649 Rheumatoid arthritis of unspecified hand with involvement of other organs and systems   HCC ▽

✓6th **M05.65 Rheumatoid arthritis of** hip **with involvement of other organs and systems**

     M05.651 Rheumatoid arthritis of right **hip with involvement of other organs and systems**   HCC

     M05.652 Rheumatoid arthritis of left **hip with involvement of other organs and systems**   HCC

     M05.659 Rheumatoid arthritis of unspecified hip with involvement of other organs and systems   HCC ▽

✓6th **M05.66 Rheumatoid arthritis of** knee **with involvement of other organs and systems**

     M05.661 Rheumatoid arthritis of right **knee with involvement of other organs and systems**   HCC

     M05.662 Rheumatoid arthritis of left **knee with involvement of other organs and systems**   HCC

     M05.669 Rheumatoid arthritis of unspecified knee with involvement of other organs and systems   HCC ▽

✓6th **M05.67 Rheumatoid arthritis of** ankle and foot **with involvement of other organs and systems**

     Rheumatoid arthritis of tarsus, metatarsus and phalanges with involvement of other organs and systems

     M05.671 Rheumatoid arthritis of right **ankle and foot with involvement of other organs and systems**   HCC

     M05.672 Rheumatoid arthritis of left **ankle and foot with involvement of other organs and systems**   HCC

     M05.679 Rheumatoid arthritis of unspecified ankle and foot with involvement of other organs and systems   HCC ▽

     M05.69 Rheumatoid arthritis of multiple sites **with involvement of other organs and systems**   HCC

✓5th **M05.7 Rheumatoid arthritis** with rheumatoid factor without organ or systems involvement

     M05.70 Rheumatoid arthritis with rheumatoid factor of unspecified site without organ or systems involvement   HCC ▽

EXCLUDES 1 Not coded here   **EXCLUDES 2** Not included here   N Newborn Age: 0   P Pediatric Age: 0-17   M Maternity Age: 12-55   A Adult Age: 15-124

724   ICD-10-CM 2018

✓6ᵗʰ **M05.71 Rheumatoid arthritis with rheumatoid factor of shoulder without organ or systems involvement**

     M05.711 Rheumatoid arthritis with rheumatoid factor of right shoulder without organ or systems involvement   HCC

     M05.712 Rheumatoid arthritis with rheumatoid factor of left shoulder without organ or systems involvement   HCC

     M05.719 Rheumatoid arthritis with rheumatoid factor of unspecified shoulder without organ or systems involvement   HCC ▽

✓6ᵗʰ **M05.72 Rheumatoid arthritis with rheumatoid factor of elbow without organ or systems involvement**

     M05.721 Rheumatoid arthritis with rheumatoid factor of right elbow without organ or systems involvement   HCC

     M05.722 Rheumatoid arthritis with rheumatoid factor of left elbow without organ or systems involvement   HCC

     M05.729 Rheumatoid arthritis with rheumatoid factor of unspecified elbow without organ or systems involvement   HCC ▽

✓6ᵗʰ **M05.73 Rheumatoid arthritis with rheumatoid factor of wrist without organ or systems involvement**

     M05.731 Rheumatoid arthritis with rheumatoid factor of right wrist without organ or systems involvement   HCC

     M05.732 Rheumatoid arthritis with rheumatoid factor of left wrist without organ or systems involvement   HCC

     M05.739 Rheumatoid arthritis with rheumatoid factor of unspecified wrist without organ or systems involvement   HCC ▽

✓6ᵗʰ **M05.74 Rheumatoid arthritis with rheumatoid factor of hand without organ or systems involvement**

     M05.741 Rheumatoid arthritis with rheumatoid factor of right hand without organ or systems involvement   HCC

     M05.742 Rheumatoid arthritis with rheumatoid factor of left hand without organ or systems involvement   HCC

     M05.749 Rheumatoid arthritis with factor of rheumatoid unspecified hand without organ or systems involvement   HCC ▽

✓6ᵗʰ **M05.75 Rheumatoid arthritis with rheumatoid factor of hip without organ or systems involvement**

     M05.751 Rheumatoid arthritis with rheumatoid factor of right hip without organ or systems involvement   HCC

     M05.752 Rheumatoid arthritis with rheumatoid factor of left hip without organ or systems involvement   HCC

     M05.759 Rheumatoid arthritis with rheumatoid factor of unspecified hip without organ or systems involvement   HCC ▽

✓6ᵗʰ **M05.76 Rheumatoid arthritis with rheumatoid factor of knee without organ or systems involvement**

     M05.761 Rheumatoid arthritis with rheumatoid factor of right knee without organ or systems involvement   HCC

     M05.762 Rheumatoid arthritis with rheumatoid factor of left knee without organ or systems involvement   HCC

     M05.769 Rheumatoid arthritis with rheumatoidfactor of unspecified knee without organ or systems involvement   HCC ▽

✓6ᵗʰ **M05.77 Rheumatoid arthritis with rheumatoid factor of ankle and foot without organ or systems involvement**

     M05.771 Rheumatoid arthritis with rheumatoid factor of right ankle and foot without organ or systems involvement   HCC

     M05.772 Rheumatoid arthritis with rheumatoid factor of left ankle and foot without organ or systems involvement   HCC

     M05.779 Rheumatoid arthritis with rheumatoid factor of unspecified ankle and foot without organ or systems involvement   HCC ▽

     M05.79 Rheumatoid arthritis with rheumatoid factor of multiple sites without organ or systems involvement   HCC

✓5ᵗʰ **M05.8 Other rheumatoid arthritis with rheumatoid factor**

     M05.80 Other rheumatoid arthritis with rheumatoid factor of unspecified site   HCC ▽

✓6ᵗʰ **M05.81 Other rheumatoid arthritis with rheumatoid factor of shoulder**

     M05.811 Other rheumatoid arthritis with rheumatoid factor of right shoulder   HCC

     M05.812 Other rheumatoid arthritis with rheumatoid factor of left shoulder   HCC

     M05.819 Other rheumatoid arthritis with rheumatoid factor of unspecified shoulder   HCC ▽

✓6ᵗʰ **M05.82 Other rheumatoid arthritis with rheumatoid factor of elbow**

     M05.821 Other rheumatoid arthritis with rheumatoid factor of right elbow   HCC

     M05.822 Other rheumatoid arthritis with rheumatoid factor of left elbow   HCC

     M05.829 Other rheumatoid arthritis with rheumatoid factor of unspecified elbow   HCC ▽

✓6ᵗʰ **M05.83 Other rheumatoid arthritis with rheumatoid factor of wrist**

     M05.831 Other rheumatoid arthritis with rheumatoid factor of right wrist   HCC

     M05.832 Other rheumatoid arthritis with rheumatoid factor of left wrist   HCC

     M05.839 Other rheumatoid arthritis with rheumatoid factor of unspecified wrist   HCC ▽

✓6ᵗʰ **M05.84 Other rheumatoid arthritis with rheumatoid factor of hand**

     M05.841 Other rheumatoid arthritis with rheumatoid factor of right hand   HCC

     M05.842 Other rheumatoid arthritis with rheumatoid factor of left hand   HCC

     M05.849 Other rheumatoid arthritis with rheumatoid factor of unspecified hand   HCC ▽

✓6ᵗʰ **M05.85 Other rheumatoid arthritis with rheumatoid factor of hip**

     M05.851 Other rheumatoid arthritis with rheumatoid factor of right hip   HCC

     M05.852 Other rheumatoid arthritis with rheumatoid factor of left hip   HCC

     M05.859 Other rheumatoid arthritis with rheumatoid factor of unspecified hip   HCC ▽

✓6ᵗʰ **M05.86 Other rheumatoid arthritis with rheumatoid factor of knee**

     M05.861 Other rheumatoid arthritis with rheumatoid factor of right knee   HCC

     M05.862 Other rheumatoid arthritis with rheumatoid factor of left knee   HCC

     M05.869 Other rheumatoid arthritis with rheumatoid factor of unspecified knee   HCC ▽

✓6ᵗʰ **M05.87 Other rheumatoid arthritis with rheumatoid factor of ankle and foot**

     M05.871 Other rheumatoid arthritis with rheumatoid factor of right ankle and foot   HCC

     M05.872 Other rheumatoid arthritis with rheumatoid factor of left ankle and foot   HCC

     M05.879 Other rheumatoid arthritis with rheumatoid factor of unspecified ankle and foot   HCC ▽

     M05.89 Other rheumatoid arthritis with rheumatoid factor of multiple sites   HCC

     M05.9 Rheumatoid arthritis with rheumatoid factor, unspecified   HCC ▽

✓4ᵗʰ **M06 Other rheumatoid arthritis**

     DEF: Autoimmune systemic disease that causes chronic inflammation of joints and other areas of the body, manifested by inflammatory changes in articular structures and synovial membranes, atrophy, and loss in bone density.

✓5ᵗʰ **M06.0 Rheumatoid arthritis without rheumatoid factor**

     M06.00 Rheumatoid arthritis without rheumatoid factor, unspecified site   HCC ▽

✅ Additional Character Req   ✓7ᵗʰ Placeholder Alert   Manifestation   HCC CMS-HCC Condition   ▽ Unspecified Code   ►◄ Revised Text   ● New Code   ▲ Revised Code Title

✓6ᵗʰ **M06.01** Rheumatoid arthritis without rheumatoid factor, shoulder

    M06.011 Rheumatoid arthritis without rheumatoid factor, right shoulder   HCC

    M06.012 Rheumatoid arthritis without rheumatoid factor, left shoulder   HCC

    M06.019 Rheumatoid arthritis without rheumatoid factor, unspecified shoulder   HCC ▽

✓6ᵗʰ **M06.02** Rheumatoid arthritis without rheumatoid factor, elbow

    M06.021 Rheumatoid arthritis without rheumatoid factor, right elbow   HCC

    M06.022 Rheumatoid arthritis without rheumatoid factor, left elbow   HCC

    M06.029 Rheumatoid arthritis without rheumatoid factor, unspecified elbow   HCC ▽

✓6ᵗʰ **M06.03** Rheumatoid arthritis without rheumatoid factor, wrist

    M06.031 Rheumatoid arthritis without rheumatoid factor, right wrist   HCC

    M06.032 Rheumatoid arthritis without rheumatoid factor, left wrist   HCC

    M06.039 Rheumatoid arthritis without rheumatoid factor, unspecified wrist   HCC ▽

✓6ᵗʰ **M06.04** Rheumatoid arthritis without rheumatoid factor, hand

    M06.041 Rheumatoid arthritis without rheumatoid factor, right hand   HCC

    M06.042 Rheumatoid arthritis without rheumatoid factor, left hand   HCC

    M06.049 Rheumatoid arthritis without rheumatoid factor, unspecified hand   HCC ▽

✓6ᵗʰ **M06.05** Rheumatoid arthritis without rheumatoid factor, hip

    M06.051 Rheumatoid arthritis without rheumatoid factor, right hip   HCC

    M06.052 Rheumatoid arthritis without rheumatoid factor, left hip   HCC

    M06.059 Rheumatoid arthritis without rheumatoid factor, unspecified hip   HCC ▽

✓6ᵗʰ **M06.06** Rheumatoid arthritis without rheumatoid factor, knee

    M06.061 Rheumatoid arthritis without rheumatoid factor, right knee   HCC

    M06.062 Rheumatoid arthritis without rheumatoid factor, left knee   HCC

    M06.069 Rheumatoid arthritis without rheumatoid factor, unspecified knee   HCC ▽

✓6ᵗʰ **M06.07** Rheumatoid arthritis without rheumatoid factor, ankle and foot

    M06.071 Rheumatoid arthritis without rheumatoid factor, right ankle and foot   HCC

    M06.072 Rheumatoid arthritis without rheumatoid factor, left ankle and foot   HCC

    M06.079 Rheumatoid arthritis without rheumatoid factor, unspecified ankle and foot   HCC ▽

M06.08 Rheumatoid arthritis without rheumatoid factor, vertebrae   HCC

M06.09 Rheumatoid arthritis without rheumatoid factor, multiple sites   HCC

M06.1 Adult-onset Still's disease   HCC A

    EXCLUDES 1   Still's disease NOS (M08.2-)

✓5ᵗʰ **M06.2** Rheumatoid bursitis

    M06.20 Rheumatoid bursitis, unspecified site   HCC ▽

✓6ᵗʰ   **M06.21** Rheumatoid bursitis, shoulder

        M06.211 Rheumatoid bursitis, right shoulder   HCC

        M06.212 Rheumatoid bursitis, left shoulder   HCC

        M06.219 Rheumatoid bursitis, unspecified shoulder   HCC ▽

✓6ᵗʰ   **M06.22** Rheumatoid bursitis, elbow

        M06.221 Rheumatoid bursitis, right elbow   HCC

        M06.222 Rheumatoid bursitis, left elbow   HCC

        M06.229 Rheumatoid bursitis, unspecified elbow   HCC ▽

✓6ᵗʰ **M06.23** Rheumatoid bursitis, wrist

    M06.231 Rheumatoid bursitis, right wrist   HCC

    M06.232 Rheumatoid bursitis, left wrist   HCC

    M06.239 Rheumatoid bursitis, unspecified wrist   HCC ▽

✓6ᵗʰ **M06.24** Rheumatoid bursitis, hand

    M06.241 Rheumatoid bursitis, right hand   HCC

    M06.242 Rheumatoid bursitis, left hand   HCC

    M06.249 Rheumatoid bursitis, unspecified hand   HCC ▽

✓6ᵗʰ **M06.25** Rheumatoid bursitis, hip

    M06.251 Rheumatoid bursitis, right hip   HCC

    M06.252 Rheumatoid bursitis, left hip   HCC

    M06.259 Rheumatoid bursitis, unspecified hip   HCC ▽

✓6ᵗʰ **M06.26** Rheumatoid bursitis, knee

    M06.261 Rheumatoid bursitis, right knee   HCC

    M06.262 Rheumatoid bursitis, left knee   HCC

    M06.269 Rheumatoid bursitis, unspecified knee   HCC ▽

✓6ᵗʰ **M06.27** Rheumatoid bursitis, ankle and foot

    M06.271 Rheumatoid bursitis, right ankle and foot   HCC

    M06.272 Rheumatoid bursitis, left ankle and foot   HCC

    M06.279 Rheumatoid bursitis, unspecified ankle and foot   HCC ▽

M06.28 Rheumatoid bursitis, vertebrae   HCC

M06.29 Rheumatoid bursitis, multiple sites   HCC

✓5ᵗʰ **M06.3** Rheumatoid nodule

    M06.30 Rheumatoid nodule, unspecified site   HCC ▽

✓6ᵗʰ **M06.31** Rheumatoid nodule, shoulder

    M06.311 Rheumatoid nodule, right shoulder   HCC

    M06.312 Rheumatoid nodule, left shoulder   HCC

    M06.319 Rheumatoid nodule, unspecified shoulder   HCC ▽

✓6ᵗʰ **M06.32** Rheumatoid nodule, elbow

    M06.321 Rheumatoid nodule, right elbow   HCC

    M06.322 Rheumatoid nodule, left elbow   HCC

    M06.329 Rheumatoid nodule, unspecified elbow   HCC ▽

✓6ᵗʰ **M06.33** Rheumatoid nodule, wrist

    M06.331 Rheumatoid nodule, right wrist   HCC

    M06.332 Rheumatoid nodule, left wrist   HCC

    M06.339 Rheumatoid nodule, unspecified wrist   HCC ▽

✓6ᵗʰ **M06.34** Rheumatoid nodule, hand

    M06.341 Rheumatoid nodule, right hand   HCC

    M06.342 Rheumatoid nodule, left hand   HCC

    M06.349 Rheumatoid nodule, unspecified hand   HCC ▽

✓6ᵗʰ **M06.35** Rheumatoid nodule, hip

    M06.351 Rheumatoid nodule, right hip   HCC

    M06.352 Rheumatoid nodule, left hip   HCC

    M06.359 Rheumatoid nodule, unspecified hip   HCC ▽

✓6ᵗʰ **M06.36** Rheumatoid nodule, knee

    M06.361 Rheumatoid nodule, right knee   HCC

    M06.362 Rheumatoid nodule, left knee   HCC

    M06.369 Rheumatoid nodule, unspecified knee   HCC ▽

✓6ᵗʰ **M06.37** Rheumatoid nodule, ankle and foot

    M06.371 Rheumatoid nodule, right ankle and foot   HCC

    M06.372 Rheumatoid nodule, left ankle and foot   HCC

    M06.379 Rheumatoid nodule, unspecified and ankle foot   HCC ▽

M06.38 Rheumatoid nodule, vertebrae   HCC

M06.39 Rheumatoid nodule, multiple sites   HCC

M06.4 Inflammatory polyarthropathy   HCC

    EXCLUDES 1   polyarthritis NOS (M13.0)

EXCLUDES 1 Not coded here   EXCLUDES 2 Not included here   N Newborn Age: 0   P Pediatric Age: 0-17   M Maternity Age: 12-55   A Adult Age: 15-124

✓5ᵗʰ **M06.8 Other specified rheumatoid arthritis**

   M06.80 Other specified rheumatoid arthritis, HCC ▽
      unspecified site

  ✓6ᵗʰ **M06.81 Other specified rheumatoid arthritis,** shoulder

     M06.811 Other specified rheumatoid arthritis, HCC
        right shoulder

     M06.812 Other specified rheumatoid arthritis, HCC
        left shoulder

     M06.819 Other specified rheumatoid HCC ▽
        arthritis, unspecified shoulder

  ✓6ᵗʰ **M06.82 Other specified rheumatoid arthritis,** elbow

     M06.821 Other specified rheumatoid arthritis, HCC
        right elbow

     M06.822 Other specified rheumatoid arthritis, HCC
        left elbow

     M06.829 Other specified rheumatoid HCC ▽
        arthritis, unspecified elbow

  ✓6ᵗʰ **M06.83 Other specified rheumatoid arthritis,** wrist

     M06.831 Other specified rheumatoid arthritis, HCC
        right wrist

     M06.832 Other specified rheumatoid arthritis, HCC
        left wrist

     M06.839 Other specified rheumatoid HCC ▽
        arthritis, unspecified wrist

  ✓6ᵗʰ **M06.84 Other specified rheumatoid arthritis,** hand

     M06.841 Other specified rheumatoid arthritis, HCC
        right hand

     M06.842 Other specified rheumatoid arthritis, HCC
        left hand

     M06.849 Other specified rheumatoid HCC ▽
        arthritis, unspecified hand

  ✓6ᵗʰ **M06.85 Other specified rheumatoid arthritis,** hip

     M06.851 Other specified rheumatoid arthritis, HCC
        right hip

     M06.852 Other specified rheumatoid arthritis, HCC
        left hip

     M06.859 Other specified rheumatoid HCC ▽
        arthritis, unspecified hip

  ✓6ᵗʰ **M06.86 Other specified rheumatoid arthritis,** knee

     M06.861 Other specified rheumatoid arthritis, HCC
        right knee

     M06.862 Other specified rheumatoid arthritis, HCC
        left knee

     M06.869 Other specified rheumatoid HCC ▽
        arthritis, unspecified knee

  ✓6ᵗʰ **M06.87 Other specified rheumatoid arthritis,** ankle and foot

     M06.871 Other specified rheumatoid arthritis, HCC
        right ankle and foot

     M06.872 Other specified rheumatoid arthritis, HCC
        left ankle and foot

     M06.879 Other specified rhe umatoid HCC ▽
        arthritis, unspecified ankle and foot

   M06.88 Other specified rheumatoid arthritis, HCC
      vertebrae

   M06.89 Other specified rheumatoid arthritis, HCC
      multiple sites

  M06.9 Rheumatoid arthritis, unspecified HCC ▽
   DEF: Autoimmune systemic disease that causes chronic inflammation of joints and other areas of the body, manifested by inflammatory changes in articular structures and synovial membranes, atrophy, and loss in bone density.

✓4ᵗʰ **M07 Enteropathic arthropathies**

   Code also associated enteropathy, such as:
     regional enteritis [Crohn's disease] (K50.-)
     ulcerative colitis (K51.-)
   EXCLUDES 1 psoriatic arthropathies (L40.5-)

  ✓5ᵗʰ **M07.6 Enteropathic arthropathies**

   M07.60 Enteropathic arthropathies, unspecified site ▽

  ✓6ᵗʰ **M07.61 Enteropathic arthropathies,** shoulder

     M07.611 Enteropathic arthropathies, right
        shoulder

     M07.612 Enteropathic arthropathies, left shoulder

     M07.619 Enteropathic arthropathies, ▽
        unspecified shoulder

  ✓6ᵗʰ **M07.62 Enteropathic arthropathies,** elbow

     M07.621 Enteropathic arthropathies, right elbow

     M07.622 Enteropathic arthropathies, left elbow

     M07.629 Enteropathic arthropathies, ▽
        unspecified elbow

  ✓6ᵗʰ **M07.63 Enteropathic arthropathies,** wrist

     M07.631 Enteropathic arthropathies, right wrist

     M07.632 Enteropathic arthropathies, left wrist

     M07.639 Enteropathic arthropathies, ▽
        unspecified wrist

  ✓6ᵗʰ **M07.64 Enteropathic arthropathies,** hand

     M07.641 Enteropathic arthropathies, right hand

     M07.642 Enteropathic arthropathies, left hand

     M07.649 Enteropathic arthropathies, ▽
        unspecified hand

  ✓6ᵗʰ **M07.65 Enteropathic arthropathies,** hip

     M07.651 Enteropathic arthropathies, right hip

     M07.652 Enteropathic arthropathies, left hip

     M07.659 Enteropathic arthropathies, ▽
        unspecified hip

  ✓6ᵗʰ **M07.66 Enteropathic arthropathies,** knee

     M07.661 Enteropathic arthropathies, right knee

     M07.662 Enteropathic arthropathies, left knee

     M07.669 Enteropathic arthropathies, ▽
        unspecified knee

  ✓6ᵗʰ **M07.67 Enteropathic arthropathies,** ankle and foot

     M07.671 Enteropathic arthropathies, right ankle
        and foot

     M07.672 Enteropathic arthropathies, left ankle
        and foot

     M07.679 Enteropathic arthropathies, ▽
        unspecified ankle and foot

   M07.68 Enteropathic arthropathies, vertebrae

   M07.69 Enteropathic arthropathies, multiple sites

✓4ᵗʰ **M08 Juvenile arthritis**

   Code also any associated underlying condition, such as:
     regional enteritis [Crohn's disease] (K50.-)
     ulcerative colitis (K51.-)
   EXCLUDES 1 arthropathy in Whipple's disease (M14.8)
        Felty's syndrome (M05.0)
        juvenile dermatomyositis (M33.0-)
        psoriatic juvenile arthropathy (L40.54)

  ✓5ᵗʰ **M08.0 Unspecified juvenile rheumatoid arthritis**
     Juvenile rheumatoid arthritis with or without rheumatoid factor

   M08.00 Unspecified juvenile rheumatoid arthritis of HCC ▽
      unspecified site

  ✓6ᵗʰ **M08.01 Unspecified juvenile rheumatoid arthritis,** shoulder

     M08.011 Unspecified juvenile rheumatoid HCC ▽
        arthritis, right shoulder

     M08.012 Unspecified juvenile rheumatoid HCC ▽
        arthritis, left shoulder

     M08.019 Unspecified juvenile rheumatoid HCC ▽
        arthritis, unspecified shoulder

  ✓6ᵗʰ **M08.02 Unspecified juvenile rheumatoid arthritis of** elbow

     M08.021 Unspecified juvenile rheumatoid HCC ▽
        arthritis, right elbow

     M08.022 Unspecified juvenile rheumatoid HCC ▽
        arthritis, left elbow

     M08.029 Unspecified juvenile rheumatoid HCC ▽
        arthritis, unspecified elbow

  ✓6ᵗʰ **M08.03 Unspecified juvenile rheumatoid arthritis,** wrist

     M08.031 Unspecified juvenile rheumatoid HCC ▽
        arthritis, right wrist

     M08.032 Unspecified juvenile rheumatoid HCC ▽
        arthritis, left wrist

     M08.039 Unspecified juvenile rheumatoid HCC ▽
        arthritis, unspecified wrist

  ✓6ᵗʰ **M08.04 Unspecified juvenile rheumatoid arthritis,** hand

     M08.041 Unspecified juvenile rheumatoid HCC ▽
        arthritis, right hand

     M08.042 Unspecified juvenile rheumatoid HCC ▽
        arthritis, left hand

     M08.049 Unspecified juvenile rheumatoid HCC ▽
        arthritis, unspecified hand

  ✓6ᵗʰ **M08.05 Unspecified juvenile rheumatoid arthritis,** hip

     M08.051 Unspecified juvenile rheumatoid HCC ▽
        arthritis, right hip

✅ Additional Character Req   ✓x7ᵗʰ Placeholder Alert   Manifestation   HCC CMS-HCC Condition   ▽ Unspecified Code   ►◄ Revised Text   ● New Code   ▲ Revised Code Title

Chapter 13. Diseases of the Musculoskeletal System and Connective Tissue

M08.052–M08.819

M08.052 Unspecified juvenile rheumatoid arthritis, left hip HCC ▽

M08.059 Unspecified juvenile rheumatoid arthritis, unspecified hip HCC ▽

✓6ᵗʰ M08.06 Unspecified juvenile rheumatoid arthritis, knee

M08.061 Unspecified juvenile rheumatoid arthritis, right knee HCC ▽

M08.062 Unspecified juvenile rheumatoid arthritis, left knee HCC ▽

M08.069 Unspecified juvenile rheumatoid arthritis, unspecified knee HCC ▽

✓6ᵗʰ M08.07 Unspecified juvenile rheumatoid arthritis, ankle and foot

M08.071 Unspecified juvenile rheumatoid arthritis, right ankle and foot HCC ▽

M08.072 Unspecified juvenile rheumatoid arthritis, left ankle and foot HCC ▽

M08.079 Unspecified juvenile rheumatoid arthritis, unspecified ankle and foot HCC ▽

M08.08 Unspecified juvenile rheumatoid arthritis, vertebrae HCC ▽

M08.09 Unspecified juvenile rheumatoid arthritis, multiple sites HCC ▽

M08.1 Juvenile ankylosing spondylitis HCC
    EXCLUDES 1 ankylosing spondylitis in adults (M45.0-)

✓5ᵗʰ M08.2 Juvenile rheumatoid arthritis with systemic onset
    Still's disease NOS
    EXCLUDES 1 adult-onset Still's disease (M06.1-)

M08.20 Juvenile rheumatoid arthritis with systemic onset, unspecified site HCC ▽

✓6ᵗʰ M08.21 Juvenile rheumatoid arthritis with systemic onset, shoulder

M08.211 Juvenile rheumatoid arthritis with systemic onset, right shoulder HCC

M08.212 Juvenile rheumatoid arthritis with systemic onset, left shoulder HCC

M08.219 Juvenile rheumatoid arthritis with systemic onset, unspecified shoulder HCC ▽

✓6ᵗʰ M08.22 Juvenile rheumatoid arthritis with systemic onset, elbow

M08.221 Juvenile rheumatoid arthritis with systemic onset, right elbow HCC

M08.222 Juvenile rheumatoid arthritis with systemic onset, left elbow HCC

M08.229 Juvenile rheumatoid arthritis with systemic onset, unspecified elbow HCC ▽

✓6ᵗʰ M08.23 Juvenile rheumatoid arthritis with systemic onset, wrist

M08.231 Juvenile rheumatoid arthritis with systemic onset, right wrist HCC

M08.232 Juvenile rheumatoid arthritis with systemic onset, left wrist HCC

M08.239 Juvenile rheumatoid arthritis with systemic onset, unspecified wrist HCC ▽

✓6ᵗʰ M08.24 Juvenile rheumatoid arthritis with systemic onset, hand

M08.241 Juvenile rheumatoid arthritis with systemic onset, right hand HCC

M08.242 Juvenile rheumatoid arthritis with systemic onset, left hand HCC

M08.249 Juvenile rheumatoid arthritis with systemic onset, unspecified hand HCC ▽

✓6ᵗʰ M08.25 Juvenile rheumatoid arthritis with systemic onset, hip

M08.251 Juvenile rheumatoid arthritis with systemic onset, right hip HCC

M08.252 Juvenile rheumatoid arthritis with systemic onset, left hip HCC

M08.259 Juvenile rheumatoid arthritis with systemic onset, unspecified hip HCC ▽

✓6ᵗʰ M08.26 Juvenile rheumatoid arthritis with systemic onset, knee

M08.261 Juvenile rheumatoid arthritis with systemic onset, right knee HCC

M08.262 Juvenile rheumatoid arthritis with systemic onset, left knee HCC

M08.269 Juvenile rheumatoid arthritis with systemic onset, unspecified knee HCC ▽

✓6ᵗʰ M08.27 Juvenile rheumatoid arthritis with systemic onset, ankle and foot

M08.271 Juvenile rheumatoid arthritis with systemic onset, right ankle and foot HCC

M08.272 Juvenile rheumatoid arthritis with systemic onset, left ankle and foot HCC

M08.279 Juvenile rheumatoid arthritis with systemic onset, unspecified ankle and foot HCC ▽

M08.28 Juvenile rheumatoid arthritis with systemic onset, vertebrae HCC

M08.29 Juvenile rheumatoid arthritis with systemic onset, multiple sites HCC

M08.3 Juvenile rheumatoid polyarthritis (seronegative) HCC

✓5ᵗʰ M08.4 Pauciarticular juvenile rheumatoid arthritis

M08.40 Pauciarticular juvenile rheumatoid arthritis, unspecified site HCC ▽

✓6ᵗʰ M08.41 Pauciarticular juvenile rheumatoid arthritis, shoulder

M08.411 Pauciarticular juvenile rheumatoid arthritis, right shoulder HCC

M08.412 Pauciarticular juvenile rheumatoid arthritis, left shoulder HCC

M08.419 Pauciarticular juvenile rheumatoid arthritis, unspecified shoulder HCC ▽

✓6ᵗʰ M08.42 Pauciarticular juvenile rheumatoid arthritis, elbow

M08.421 Pauciarticular juvenile rheumatoid arthritis, right elbow HCC

M08.422 Pauciarticular juvenile rheumatoid arthritis, left elbow HCC

M08.429 Pauciarticular juvenile rheumatoid arthritis, unspecified elbow HCC ▽

✓6ᵗʰ M08.43 Pauciarticular juvenile rheumatoid arthritis, wrist

M08.431 Pauciarticular juvenile rheumatoid arthritis, right wrist HCC

M08.432 Pauciarticular juvenile rheumatoid arthritis, left wrist HCC

M08.439 Pauciarticular juvenile rheumatoid arthritis, unspecified wrist HCC ▽

✓6ᵗʰ M08.44 Pauciarticular juvenile rheumatoid arthritis, hand

M08.441 Pauciarticular juvenile rheumatoid arthritis, right hand HCC

M08.442 Pauciarticular juvenile rheumatoid arthritis, left hand HCC

M08.449 Pauciarticular juvenile rheumatoid arthritis, unspecified hand HCC ▽

✓6ᵗʰ M08.45 Pauciarticular juvenile rheumatoid arthritis, hip

M08.451 Pauciarticular juvenile rheumatoid arthritis, right hip HCC

M08.452 Pauciarticular juvenile rheumatoid arthritis, left hip HCC

M08.459 Pauciarticular juvenile rheumatoid arthritis, unspecified hip HCC ▽

✓6ᵗʰ M08.46 Pauciarticular juvenile rheumatoid arthritis, knee

M08.461 Pauciarticular juvenile rheumatoid arthritis, right knee HCC

M08.462 Pauciarticular juvenile rheumatoid arthritis, left knee HCC

M08.469 Pauciarticular juvenile rheumatoid arthritis, unspecified knee HCC ▽

✓6ᵗʰ M08.47 Pauciarticular juvenile rheumatoid arthritis, ankle and foot

M08.471 Pauciarticular juvenile rheumatoid arthritis, right ankle and foot HCC

M08.472 Pauciarticular juvenile rheumatoid arthritis, left ankle and foot HCC

M08.479 Pauciarticular juvenile rheumatoid arthritis, unspecified ankle and foot HCC ▽

M08.48 Pauciarticular juvenile rheumatoid arthritis, vertebrae HCC

✓5ᵗʰ M08.8 Other juvenile arthritis

M08.80 Other juvenile arthritis, unspecified site HCC ▽

✓6ᵗʰ M08.81 Other juvenile arthritis, shoulder

M08.811 Other juvenile arthritis, right shoulder HCC

M08.812 Other juvenile arthritis, left shoulder HCC

M08.819 Other juvenile arthritis, unspecified shoulder HCC ▽

EXCLUDES 1 Not coded here   EXCLUDES 2 Not included here   N Newborn Age: 0   P Pediatric Age: 0-17   M Maternity Age: 12-55   A Adult Age: 15-124

728   ICD-10-CM 2018

√6ᵗʰ **M08.82 Other juvenile arthritis,** elbow

     M08.821 Other juvenile arthritis, right **elbow** HCC
     M08.822 Other juvenile arthritis, left **elbow** HCC
     M08.829 Other juvenile arthritis, unspecified HCC ▽
     elbow

√6ᵗʰ **M08.83 Other juvenile arthritis,** wrist

     M08.831 Other juvenile arthritis, right **wrist** HCC
     M08.832 Other juvenile arthritis, left **wrist** HCC
     M08.839 Other juvenile arthritis, unspecified HCC ▽
     wrist

√6ᵗʰ **M08.84 Other juvenile arthritis,** hand

     M08.841 Other juvenile arthritis, right **hand** HCC
     M08.842 Other juvenile arthritis, left **hand** HCC
     M08.849 Other juvenile arthritis, unspecified HCC ▽
     hand

√6ᵗʰ **M08.85 Other juvenile arthritis,** hip

     M08.851 Other juvenile arthritis, right **hip** HCC
     M08.852 Other juvenile arthritis, left **hip** HCC
     M08.859 Other juvenile arthritis, HCC ▽
     unspecified hip

√6ᵗʰ **M08.86 Other juvenile arthritis,** knee

     M08.861 Other juvenile arthritis, right **knee** HCC
     M08.862 Other juvenile arthritis, left **knee** HCC
     M08.869 Other juvenile arthritis, HCC ▽
     unspecified knee

√6ᵗʰ **M08.87 Other juvenile arthritis,** ankle and foot

     M08.871 Other juvenile arthritis, right **ankle** HCC
     and foot
     M08.872 Other juvenile arthritis, left **ankle** HCC
     and foot
     M08.879 Other juvenile arthritis, HCC ▽
     unspecified ankle and foot

     M08.88 Other juvenile arthritis, other specified site HCC
     Other juvenile arthritis, vertebrae

     M08.89 Other juvenile arthritis, multiple sites HCC

√5ᵗʰ **M08.9 Juvenile arthritis, unspecified**

     EXCLUDES 1   juvenile rheumatoid arthritis, unspecified (M08.0-)

     M08.90 Juvenile arthritis, unspecified, HCC ▽
     unspecified site

√6ᵗʰ **M08.91 Juvenile arthritis, unspecified,** shoulder

     M08.911 Juvenile arthritis, unspecified, right HCC ▽
     shoulder
     M08.912 Juvenile arthritis, unspecified, left HCC ▽
     shoulder
     M08.919 Juvenile arthritis, unspecified, HCC ▽
     unspecified shoulder

√6ᵗʰ **M08.92 Juvenile arthritis, unspecified,** elbow

     M08.921 Juvenile arthritis, unspecified, HCC ▽
     right **elbow**
     M08.922 Juvenile arthritis, unspecified, HCC ▽
     left **elbow**
     M08.929 Juvenile arthritis, unspecified, HCC ▽
     unspecified elbow

√6ᵗʰ **M08.93 Juvenile arthritis, unspecified,** wrist

     M08.931 Juvenile arthritis, unspecified, HCC ▽
     right **wrist**
     M08.932 Juvenile arthritis, unspecified, HCC ▽
     left **wrist**
     M08.939 Juvenile arthritis, unspecified, HCC ▽
     unspecified **wrist**

√6ᵗʰ **M08.94 Juvenile arthritis, unspecified,** hand

     M08.941 Juvenile arthritis, unspecified, HCC ▽
     right **hand**
     M08.942 Juvenile arthritis, unspecified, HCC ▽
     left **hand**
     M08.949 Juvenile arthritis, unspecified, HCC ▽
     unspecified hand

√6ᵗʰ **M08.95 Juvenile arthritis, unspecified,** hip

     M08.951 Juvenile arthritis, unspecified, HCC ▽
     right **hip**
     M08.952 Juvenile arthritis, unspecified, HCC ▽
     left **hip**
     M08.959 Juvenile arthritis, unspecified, HCC ▽
     unspecified **hip**

√6ᵗʰ **M08.96 Juvenile arthritis, unspecified,** knee

     M08.961 Juvenile arthritis, unspecified, HCC ▽
     right **knee**
     M08.962 Juvenile arthritis, unspecified, HCC ▽
     left **knee**
     M08.969 Juvenile arthritis, unspecified, HCC ▽
     unspecified knee

√6ᵗʰ **M08.97 Juvenile arthritis, unspecified,** ankle and foot

     M08.971 Juvenile arthritis, unspecified, HCC ▽
     right **ankle and foot**
     M08.972 Juvenile arthritis, unspecified, HCC ▽
     left **ankle and foot**
     M08.979 Juvenile arthritis, unspecified, HCC ▽
     unspecified ankle and foot

     M08.98 Juvenile arthritis, unspecified, vertebrae HCC ▽

     M08.99 Juvenile arthritis, unspecified, multiple sites HCC ▽

√4ᵗʰ **M1A Chronic gout**

     Use additional code to identify:
        autonomic neuropathy in diseases classified elsewhere (G99.0)
        calculus of urinary tract in diseases classified elsewhere (N22)
        cardiomyopathy in diseases classified elsewhere (I43)
        disorders of external ear in diseases classified elsewhere (H61.1-,
          H62.8-)
        disorders of iris and ciliary body in diseases classified elsewhere (H22)
        glomerular disorders in diseases classified elsewhere (N08)
     EXCLUDES 1   gout NOS (M10.-)
     EXCLUDES 2   acute gout (M10.-)

     The appropriate 7th character is to be added to each code
     from category M1A.
     0   without tophus (tophi)
     1   with tophus (tophi)

√5ᵗʰ **M1A.0** Idiopathic **chronic gout**
     Chronic gouty bursitis   Primary chronic gout

√x7ᵗʰ **M1A.00 Idiopathic chronic gout, unspecified site** ▽

√6ᵗʰ **M1A.01 Idiopathic chronic gout,** shoulder

     √7ᵗʰ **M1A.011 Idiopathic chronic gout,** right **shoulder**
     √7ᵗʰ **M1A.012 Idiopathic chronic gout,** left **shoulder**
     √7ᵗʰ **M1A.019 Idiopathic chronic gout, unspecified** ▽
     shoulder

√6ᵗʰ **M1A.02 Idiopathic chronic gout,** elbow

     √7ᵗʰ **M1A.021 Idiopathic chronic gout,** right **elbow**
     √7ᵗʰ **M1A.022 Idiopathic chronic gout,** left **elbow**
     √7ᵗʰ **M1A.029 Idiopathic chronic gout, unspecified** ▽
     elbow

√6ᵗʰ **M1A.03 Idiopathic chronic gout,** wrist

     √7ᵗʰ **M1A.031 Idiopathic chronic gout,** right **wrist**
     √7ᵗʰ **M1A.032 Idiopathic chronic gout,** left **wrist**
     √7ᵗʰ **M1A.039 Idiopathic chronic gout, unspecified** ▽
     wrist

√6ᵗʰ **M1A.04 Idiopathic chronic gout,** hand

     √7ᵗʰ **M1A.041 Idiopathic chronic gout,** right **hand**
     √7ᵗʰ **M1A.042 Idiopathic chronic gout,** left **hand**
     √7ᵗʰ **M1A.049 Idiopathic chronic gout, unspecified** ▽
     hand

√6ᵗʰ **M1A.05 Idiopathic chronic gout,** hip

     √7ᵗʰ **M1A.051 Idiopathic chronic gout,** right **hip**
     √7ᵗʰ **M1A.052 Idiopathic chronic gout,** left **hip**
     √7ᵗʰ **M1A.059 Idiopathic chronic gout, unspecified hip** ▽

√6ᵗʰ **M1A.06 Idiopathic chronic gout,** knee

     √7ᵗʰ **M1A.061 Idiopathic chronic gout,** right **knee**
     √7ᵗʰ **M1A.062 Idiopathic chronic gout,** left **knee**
     √7ᵗʰ **M1A.069 Idiopathic chronic gout, unspecified** ▽
     knee

√6ᵗʰ **M1A.07 Idiopathic chronic gout,** ankle and foot

     √7ᵗʰ **M1A.071 Idiopathic chronic gout,** right **ankle and**
     foot
     √7ᵗʰ **M1A.072 Idiopathic chronic gout,** left **ankle and**
     foot
     √7ᵗʰ **M1A.079 Idiopathic chronic gout, unspecified** ▽
     ankle and foot

√x7ᵗʰ **M1A.08 Idiopathic chronic gout,** vertebrae

√x7ᵗʰ **M1A.09 Idiopathic chronic gout,** multiple sites

☑ Additional Character Req   √x7ᵗʰ Placeholder Alert   Manifestation   HCC CMS-HCC Condition   ▽ Unspecified Code   ►◄ Revised Text   ● New Code   ▲ Revised Code Title

ICD-10-CM 2018   729

☑5ᵗʰ **M1A.1** Lead-induced **chronic gout**

  Code first toxic effects of lead and its compounds (T56.0-)

☑x7ᵗʰ **M1A.10** **Lead-induced chronic gout, unspecified site** ▽

☑6ᵗʰ **M1A.11** **Lead-induced chronic gout,** shoulder

  ☑7ᵗʰ **M1A.111** **Lead-induced chronic gout,** right **shoulder**

  ☑7ᵗʰ **M1A.112** **Lead-induced chronic gout,** left **shoulder**

  ☑7ᵗʰ **M1A.119** **Lead-induced chronic gout, unspecified shoulder** ▽

☑6ᵗʰ **M1A.12** **Lead-induced chronic gout,** elbow

  ☑7ᵗʰ **M1A.121** **Lead-induced chronic gout,** right **elbow**

  ☑7ᵗʰ **M1A.122** **Lead-induced chronic gout,** left **elbow**

  ☑7ᵗʰ **M1A.129** **Lead-induced chronic gout, unspecified elbow** ▽

☑6ᵗʰ **M1A.13** **Lead-induced chronic gout,** wrist

  ☑7ᵗʰ **M1A.131** **Lead-induced chronic gout,** right **wrist**

  ☑7ᵗʰ **M1A.132** **Lead-induced chronic gout,** left **wrist**

  ☑7ᵗʰ **M1A.139** **Lead-induced chronic gout, unspecified wrist** ▽

☑6ᵗʰ **M1A.14** **Lead-induced chronic gout,** hand

  ☑7ᵗʰ **M1A.141** **Lead-induced chronic gout,** right **hand**

  ☑7ᵗʰ **M1A.142** **Lead-induced chronic gout,** left **hand**

  ☑7ᵗʰ **M1A.149** **Lead-induced chronic gout, unspecified hand** ▽

☑6ᵗʰ **M1A.15** **Lead-induced chronic gout,** hip

  ☑7ᵗʰ **M1A.151** **Lead-induced chronic gout,** right **hip**

  ☑7ᵗʰ **M1A.152** **Lead-induced chronic gout,** left **hip**

  ☑7ᵗʰ **M1A.159** **Lead-induced chronic gout, unspecified hip** ▽

☑6ᵗʰ **M1A.16** **Lead-induced chronic gout,** knee

  ☑7ᵗʰ **M1A.161** **Lead-induced chronic gout,** right **knee**

  ☑7ᵗʰ **M1A.162** **Lead-induced chronic gout,** left **knee**

  ☑7ᵗʰ **M1A.169** **Lead-induced chronic gout, unspecified knee** ▽

☑6ᵗʰ **M1A.17** **Lead-induced chronic gout,** ankle and foot

  ☑7ᵗʰ **M1A.171** **Lead-induced chronic gout,** right **ankle and foot**

  ☑7ᵗʰ **M1A.172** **Lead-induced chronic gout,** left **ankle and foot**

  ☑7ᵗʰ **M1A.179** **Lead-induced chronic gout, unspecified ankle and foot** ▽

☑x7ᵗʰ **M1A.18** **Lead-induced chronic gout,** vertebrae

☑x7ᵗʰ **M1A.19** **Lead-induced chronic gout,** multiple sites

☑5ᵗʰ **M1A.2** Drug-induced **chronic gout**

  Use additional code for adverse effect, if applicable, to identify drug (T36-T50 with fifth or sixth character 5)

☑x7ᵗʰ **M1A.20** **Drug-induced chronic gout, unspecified site** ▽

☑6ᵗʰ **M1A.21** **Drug-induced chronic gout,** shoulder

  ☑7ᵗʰ **M1A.211** **Drug-induced chronic gout,** right **shoulder**

  ☑7ᵗʰ **M1A.212** **Drug-induced chronic gout,** left **shoulder**

  ☑7ᵗʰ **M1A.219** **Drug-induced chronic gout, unspecified shoulder** ▽

☑6ᵗʰ **M1A.22** **Drug-induced chronic gout,** elbow

  ☑7ᵗʰ **M1A.221** **Drug-induced chronic gout,** right **elbow**

  ☑7ᵗʰ **M1A.222** **Drug-induced chronic gout,** left **elbow**

  ☑7ᵗʰ **M1A.229** **Drug-induced chronic gout, unspecified elbow** ▽

☑6ᵗʰ **M1A.23** **Drug-induced chronic gout,** wrist

  ☑7ᵗʰ **M1A.231** **Drug-induced chronic gout,** right **wrist**

  ☑7ᵗʰ **M1A.232** **Drug-induced chronic gout,** left **wrist**

  ☑7ᵗʰ **M1A.239** **Drug-induced chronic gout, unspecified wrist** ▽

☑6ᵗʰ **M1A.24** **Drug-induced chronic gout,** hand

  ☑7ᵗʰ **M1A.241** **Drug-induced chronic gout,** right **hand**

  ☑7ᵗʰ **M1A.242** **Drug-induced chronic gout,** left **hand**

  ☑7ᵗʰ **M1A.249** **Drug-induced chronic gout, unspecified hand** ▽

☑6ᵗʰ **M1A.25** **Drug-induced chronic gout,** hip

  ☑7ᵗʰ **M1A.251** **Drug-induced chronic gout,** right **hip**

  ☑7ᵗʰ **M1A.252** **Drug-induced chronic gout,** left **hip**

☑7ᵗʰ **M1A.259** **Drug-induced chronic gout, unspecified hip** ▽

☑6ᵗʰ **M1A.26** **Drug-induced chronic gout,** knee

  ☑7ᵗʰ **M1A.261** **Drug-induced chronic gout,** right **knee**

  ☑7ᵗʰ **M1A.262** **Drug-induced chronic gout,** left **knee**

  ☑7ᵗʰ **M1A.269** **Drug-induced chronic gout, unspecified knee** ▽

☑6ᵗʰ **M1A.27** **Drug-induced chronic gout,** ankle and foot

  ☑7ᵗʰ **M1A.271** **Drug-induced chronic gout,** right **ankle and foot**

  ☑7ᵗʰ **M1A.272** **Drug-induced chronic gout,** left **ankle and foot**

  ☑7ᵗʰ **M1A.279** **Drug-induced chronic gout, unspecified ankle and foot** ▽

☑x7ᵗʰ **M1A.28** **Drug-induced chronic gout,** vertebrae

☑x7ᵗʰ **M1A.29** **Drug-induced chronic gout,** multiple sites

☑5ᵗʰ **M1A.3** Chronic gout due to renal impairment

  Code first associated renal disease

☑x7ᵗʰ **M1A.30** **Chronic gout due to renal impairment, unspecified site** ▽

☑6ᵗʰ **M1A.31** **Chronic gout due to renal impairment,** shoulder

  ☑7ᵗʰ **M1A.311** **Chronic gout due to renal impairment,** right **shoulder**

  ☑7ᵗʰ **M1A.312** **Chronic gout due to renal impairment,** left **shoulder**

  ☑7ᵗʰ **M1A.319** **Chronic gout due to renal impairment, unspecified shoulder** ▽

☑6ᵗʰ **M1A.32** **Chronic gout due to renal impairment,** elbow

  ☑7ᵗʰ **M1A.321** **Chronic gout due to renal impairment,** right **elbow**

  ☑7ᵗʰ **M1A.322** **Chronic gout due to renal impairment,** left **elbow**

  ☑7ᵗʰ **M1A.329** **Chronic gout due to renal impairment, unspecified elbow** ▽

☑6ᵗʰ **M1A.33** **Chronic gout due to renal impairment,** wrist

  ☑7ᵗʰ **M1A.331** **Chronic gout due to renal impairment,** right **wrist**

  ☑7ᵗʰ **M1A.332** **Chronic gout due to renal impairment,** left **wrist**

  ☑7ᵗʰ **M1A.339** **Chronic gout due to renal impairment, unspecified wrist** ▽

☑6ᵗʰ **M1A.34** **Chronic gout due to renal impairment,** hand

  ☑7ᵗʰ **M1A.341** **Chronic gout due to renal impairment,** right **hand**

  ☑7ᵗʰ **M1A.342** **Chronic gout due to renal impairment,** left **hand**

  ☑7ᵗʰ **M1A.349** **Chronic gout due to renal impairment, unspecified hand** ▽

☑6ᵗʰ **M1A.35** **Chronic gout due to renal impairment,** hip

  ☑7ᵗʰ **M1A.351** **Chronic gout due to renal impairment,** right **hip**

  ☑7ᵗʰ **M1A.352** **Chronic gout due to renal impairment,** left **hip**

  ☑7ᵗʰ **M1A.359** **Chronic gout due to renal impairment, unspecified hip** ▽

☑6ᵗʰ **M1A.36** **Chronic gout due to renal impairment,** knee

  ☑7ᵗʰ **M1A.361** **Chronic gout due to renal impairment,** right **knee**

  ☑7ᵗʰ **M1A.362** **Chronic gout due to renal impairment,** left **knee**

  ☑7ᵗʰ **M1A.369** **Chronic gout due to renal impairment, unspecified knee** ▽

☑6ᵗʰ **M1A.37** **Chronic gout due to renal impairment,** ankle and foot

  ☑7ᵗʰ **M1A.371** **Chronic gout due to renal impairment,** right **ankle and foot**

  ☑7ᵗʰ **M1A.372** **Chronic gout due to renal impairment,** left **ankle and foot**

  ☑7ᵗʰ **M1A.379** **Chronic gout due to renal impairment, unspecified ankle and foot** ▽

☑x7ᵗʰ **M1A.38** **Chronic gout due to renal impairment,** vertebrae

☑x7ᵗʰ **M1A.39** **Chronic gout due to renal impairment,** multiple sites

EXCLUDES 1 Not coded here   **EXCLUDES 2** Not included here   **N** Newborn Age: 0   **P** Pediatric Age: 0-17   **M** Maternity Age: 12-55   **A** Adult Age: 15-124

730   ICD-10-CM 2018

✓5ᵗʰ **M1A.4 Other** secondary chronic gout
     Code first associated condition

✓x7ᵗʰ **M1A.40 Other secondary chronic gout, unspecified site** ▽

✓6ᵗʰ **M1A.41 Other secondary chronic gout,** shoulder

     ✓7ᵗʰ **M1A.411 Other secondary chronic gout,** right shoulder

     ✓7ᵗʰ **M1A.412 Other secondary chronic gout,** left shoulder

     ✓7ᵗʰ **M1A.419 Other secondary chronic gout,** unspecified shoulder ▽

✓6ᵗʰ **M1A.42 Other secondary chronic gout,** elbow

     ✓7ᵗʰ **M1A.421 Other secondary chronic gout,** right elbow

     ✓7ᵗʰ **M1A.422 Other secondary chronic gout,** left elbow

     ✓7ᵗʰ **M1A.429 Other secondary chronic gout,** unspecified elbow ▽

✓6ᵗʰ **M1A.43 Other secondary chronic gout,** wrist

     ✓7ᵗʰ **M1A.431 Other secondary chronic gout,** right wrist

     ✓7ᵗʰ **M1A.432 Other secondary chronic gout,** left wrist

     ✓7ᵗʰ **M1A.439 Other secondary chronic gout,** unspecified wrist ▽

✓6ᵗʰ **M1A.44 Other secondary chronic gout,** hand

     ✓7ᵗʰ **M1A.441 Other secondary chronic gout,** right hand

     ✓7ᵗʰ **M1A.442 Other secondary chronic gout,** left hand

     ✓7ᵗʰ **M1A.449 Other secondary chronic gout,** unspecified hand

✓6ᵗʰ **M1A.45 Other secondary chronic gout,** hip

     ✓7ᵗʰ **M1A.451 Other secondary chronic gout,** right hip

     ✓7ᵗʰ **M1A.452 Other secondary chronic gout,** left hip

     ✓7ᵗʰ **M1A.459 Other secondary chronic gout,** unspecified hip ▽

✓6ᵗʰ **M1A.46 Other secondary chronic gout,** knee

     ✓7ᵗʰ **M1A.461 Other secondary chronic gout,** right knee

     ✓7ᵗʰ **M1A.462 Other secondary chronic gout,** left knee

     ✓7ᵗʰ **M1A.469 Other secondary chronic gout,** unspecified knee ▽

✓6ᵗʰ **M1A.47 Other secondary chronic gout,** ankle and foot

     ✓7ᵗʰ **M1A.471 Other secondary chronic gout,** right ankle and foot

     ✓7ᵗʰ **M1A.472 Other secondary chronic gout,** left ankle and foot

     ✓7ᵗʰ **M1A.479 Other secondary chronic gout,** unspecified ankle and foot ▽

✓x7ᵗʰ **M1A.48 Other secondary chronic gout,** vertebrae

✓x7ᵗʰ **M1A.49 Other secondary chronic gout,** multiple sites

✓x7ᵗʰ **M1A.9 Chronic gout, unspecified** ▽

✓4ᵗʰ **M10 Gout**
     Acute gout   Gout flare
     Gout attack   Podagra
     Use additional code to identify:
       autonomic neuropathy in diseases classified elsewhere (G99.0)
       calculus of urinary tract in diseases classified elsewhere (N22)
       cardiomyopathy in diseases classified elsewhere (I43)
       disorders of external ear in diseases classified elsewhere (H61.1-, H62.8-)
       disorders of iris and ciliary body in diseases classified elsewhere (H22)
       glomerular disorders in diseases classified elsewhere (N08)
     EXCLUDES 2   chronic gout (M1A.-)
     DEF: Purine and pyrimidine metabolic disorders; manifested by hyperuricemia and recurrent acute inflammatory arthritis; monosodium urate or monohydrate crystals may be deposited in and around the joints, leading to joint destruction and severe crippling.

✓5ᵗʰ **M10.0 Idiopathic gout**
     Gouty bursitis
     Primary gout

M10.00 Idiopathic gout, unspecified site ▽

✓6ᵗʰ **M10.01 Idiopathic gout,** shoulder

     M10.011 Idiopathic gout, right shoulder

     M10.012 Idiopathic gout, left shoulder

     M10.019 Idiopathic gout, unspecified shoulder ▽

✓6ᵗʰ **M10.02 Idiopathic gout,** elbow

     M10.021 Idiopathic gout, right elbow

     M10.022 Idiopathic gout, left elbow

     M10.029 Idiopathic gout, unspecified elbow ▽

✓6ᵗʰ **M10.03 Idiopathic gout,** wrist

     M10.031 Idiopathic gout, right wrist

     M10.032 Idiopathic gout, left wrist

     M10.039 Idiopathic gout, unspecified wrist ▽

✓6ᵗʰ **M10.04 Idiopathic gout,** hand

     M10.041 Idiopathic gout, right hand

     M10.042 Idiopathic gout, left hand

     M10.049 Idiopathic gout, unspecified hand ▽

✓6ᵗʰ **M10.05 Idiopathic gout,** hip

     M10.051 Idiopathic gout, right hip

     M10.052 Idiopathic gout, left hip

     M10.059 Idiopathic gout, unspecified hip ▽

✓6ᵗʰ **M10.06 Idiopathic gout,** knee

     M10.061 Idiopathic gout, right knee

     M10.062 Idiopathic gout, left knee

     M10.069 Idiopathic gout, unspecified knee ▽

✓6ᵗʰ **M10.07 Idiopathic gout,** ankle and foot

     M10.071 Idiopathic gout, right ankle and foot

     M10.072 Idiopathic gout, left ankle and foot

     M10.079 Idiopathic gout, unspecified ankle and foot ▽

M10.08 Idiopathic gout, vertebrae

M10.09 Idiopathic gout, multiple sites

✓5ᵗʰ **M10.1 Lead-induced gout**
     Code first toxic effects of lead and its compounds (T56.0-)

M10.10 Lead-induced gout, unspecified site ▽

✓6ᵗʰ **M10.11 Lead-induced gout,** shoulder

     M10.111 Lead-induced gout, right shoulder

     M10.112 Lead-induced gout, left shoulder

     M10.119 Lead-induced gout, unspecified shoulder ▽

✓6ᵗʰ **M10.12 Lead-induced gout,** elbow

     M10.121 Lead-induced gout, right elbow

     M10.122 Lead-induced gout, left elbow

     M10.129 Lead-induced gout, unspecified elbow ▽

✓6ᵗʰ **M10.13 Lead-induced gout,** wrist

     M10.131 Lead-induced gout, right wrist

     M10.132 Lead-induced gout, left wrist

     M10.139 Lead-induced gout, unspecified wrist ▽

✓6ᵗʰ **M10.14 Lead-induced gout,** hand

     M10.141 Lead-induced gout, right hand

     M10.142 Lead-induced gout, left hand

     M10.149 Lead-induced gout, unspecified hand ▽

✓6ᵗʰ **M10.15 Lead-induced gout,** hip

     M10.151 Lead-induced gout, right hip

     M10.152 Lead-induced gout, left hip

     M10.159 Lead-induced gout, unspecified hip ▽

✓6ᵗʰ **M10.16 Lead-induced gout,** knee

     M10.161 Lead-induced gout, right knee

     M10.162 Lead-induced gout, left knee

     M10.169 Lead-induced gout, unspecified knee ▽

✓6ᵗʰ **M10.17 Lead-induced gout,** ankle and foot

     M10.171 Lead-induced gout, right ankle and foot

     M10.172 Lead-induced gout, left ankle and foot

     M10.179 Lead-induced gout, unspecified ankle and foot ▽

M10.18 Lead-induced gout, vertebrae

M10.19 Lead-induced gout, multiple sites

✓5ᵗʰ **M10.2 Drug-induced gout**
     Use additional code for adverse effect, if applicable, to identify drug (T36-T50 with fifth or sixth character 5)

M10.20 Drug-induced gout, unspecified site ▽

✓6ᵗʰ **M10.21 Drug-induced gout,** shoulder

     M10.211 Drug-induced gout, right shoulder

     M10.212 Drug-induced gout, left shoulder

     M10.219 Drug-induced gout, unspecified shoulder ▽

✓6ᵗʰ **M10.22 Drug-induced gout,** elbow

     M10.221 Drug-induced gout, right elbow

     M10.222 Drug-induced gout, left elbow

     M10.229 Drug-induced gout, unspecified elbow

☑ Additional Character Req   ✓x7ᵗʰ Placeholder Alert   Manifestation   **HCC** CMS-HCC Condition   ▽ Unspecified Code   ►◄ Revised Text   ● New Code   ▲ Revised Code Title

✓6ᵗʰ **M10.23** Drug-induced gout, wrist
     M10.231 Drug-induced gout, right wrist
     M10.232 Drug-induced gout, left wrist
     M10.239 Drug-induced gout, unspecified wrist ▽

✓6ᵗʰ **M10.24** Drug-induced gout, hand
     M10.241 Drug-induced gout, right hand
     M10.242 Drug-induced gout, left hand
     M10.249 Drug-induced gout, unspecified hand ▽

✓6ᵗʰ **M10.25** Drug-induced gout, hip
     M10.251 Drug-induced gout, right hip
     M10.252 Drug-induced gout, left hip
     M10.259 Drug-induced gout, unspecified hip ▽

✓6ᵗʰ **M10.26** Drug-induced gout, knee
     M10.261 Drug-induced gout, right knee
     M10.262 Drug-induced gout, left knee
     M10.269 Drug-induced gout, unspecified knee ▽

✓6ᵗʰ **M10.27** Drug-induced gout, ankle and foot
     M10.271 Drug-induced gout, right ankle and foot
     M10.272 Drug-induced gout, left ankle and foot
     M10.279 Drug-induced gout, unspecified ankle and foot

M10.28 Drug-induced gout, vertebrae
M10.29 Drug-induced gout, multiple sites

✓5ᵗʰ **M10.3** Gout due to renal impairment
     Code first associated renal disease

M10.30 Gout due to renal impairment, unspecified site ▽

✓6ᵗʰ **M10.31** Gout due to renal impairment, shoulder
     M10.311 Gout due to renal impairment, right shoulder
     M10.312 Gout due to renal impairment, left shoulder
     M10.319 Gout due to renal impairment, unspecified shoulder ▽

✓6ᵗʰ **M10.32** Gout due to renal impairment, elbow
     M10.321 Gout due to renal impairment, right elbow
     M10.322 Gout due to renal impairment, left elbow
     M10.329 Gout due to renal impairment, unspecified elbow ▽

✓6ᵗʰ **M10.33** Gout due to renal impairment, wrist
     M10.331 Gout due to renal impairment, right wrist
     M10.332 Gout due to renal impairment, left wrist
     M10.339 Gout due to renal impairment, unspecified wrist ▽

✓6ᵗʰ **M10.34** Gout due to renal impairment, hand
     M10.341 Gout due to renal impairment, right hand
     M10.342 Gout due to renal impairment, left hand
     M10.349 Gout due to renal impairment, unspecified hand ▽

✓6ᵗʰ **M10.35** Gout due to renal impairment, hip
     M10.351 Gout due to renal impairment, right hip
     M10.352 Gout due to renal impairment, left hip
     M10.359 Gout due to renal impairment, unspecified hip ▽

✓6ᵗʰ **M10.36** Gout due to renal impairment, knee
     M10.361 Gout due to renal impairment, right knee
     M10.362 Gout due to renal impairment, left knee
     M10.369 Gout due to renal impairment, unspecified knee ▽

✓6ᵗʰ **M10.37** Gout due to renal impairment, ankle and foot
     M10.371 Gout due to renal impairment, right ankle and foot
     M10.372 Gout due to renal impairment, left ankle and foot
     M10.379 Gout due to renal impairment, unspecified ankle and foot ▽

M10.38 Gout due to renal impairment, vertebrae
M10.39 Gout due to renal impairment, multiple sites

✓5ᵗʰ **M10.4** Other secondary gout
     Code first associated condition

M10.40 Other secondary gout, unspecified site ▽

✓6ᵗʰ **M10.41** Other secondary gout, shoulder
     M10.411 Other secondary gout, right shoulder
     M10.412 Other secondary gout, left shoulder

     M10.419 Other secondary gout, unspecified shoulder ▽

✓6ᵗʰ **M10.42** Other secondary gout, elbow
     M10.421 Other secondary gout, right elbow
     M10.422 Other secondary gout, left elbow
     M10.429 Other secondary gout, unspecified elbow ▽

✓6ᵗʰ **M10.43** Other secondary gout, wrist
     M10.431 Other secondary gout, right wrist
     M10.432 Other secondary gout, left wrist
     M10.439 Other secondary gout, unspecified wrist ▽

✓6ᵗʰ **M10.44** Other secondary gout, hand
     M10.441 Other secondary gout, right hand
     M10.442 Other secondary gout, left hand
     M10.449 Other secondary gout, unspecified hand ▽

✓6ᵗʰ **M10.45** Other secondary gout, hip
     M10.451 Other secondary gout, right hip
     M10.452 Other secondary gout, left hip
     M10.459 Other secondary gout, unspecified hip ▽

✓6ᵗʰ **M10.46** Other secondary gout, knee
     M10.461 Other secondary gout, right knee
     M10.462 Other secondary gout, left knee
     M10.469 Other secondary gout, unspecified knee ▽

✓6ᵗʰ **M10.47** Other secondary gout, ankle and foot
     M10.471 Other secondary gout, right ankle and foot
     M10.472 Other secondary gout, left ankle and foot
     M10.479 Other secondary gout, unspecified ankle and foot ▽

M10.48 Other secondary gout, vertebrae
M10.49 Other secondary gout, multiple sites

M10.9 Gout, unspecified ▽
     Gout NOS

✓4ᵗʰ **M11 Other crystal arthropathies**

✓5ᵗʰ **M11.0** Hydroxyapatite deposition disease

M11.00 Hydroxyapatite deposition disease, unspecified site ▽

✓6ᵗʰ **M11.01** Hydroxyapatite deposition disease, shoulder
     M11.011 Hydroxyapatite deposition disease, right shoulder
     M11.012 Hydroxyapatite deposition disease, left shoulder
     M11.019 Hydroxyapatite deposition disease, unspecified shoulder ▽

✓6ᵗʰ **M11.02** Hydroxyapatite deposition disease, elbow
     M11.021 Hydroxyapatite deposition disease, right elbow
     M11.022 Hydroxyapatite deposition disease, left elbow
     M11.029 Hydroxyapatite deposition disease, unspecified elbow ▽

✓6ᵗʰ **M11.03** Hydroxyapatite deposition disease, wrist
     M11.031 Hydroxyapatite deposition disease, right wrist
     M11.032 Hydroxyapatite deposition disease, left wrist
     M11.039 Hydroxyapatite deposition disease, unspecified wrist ▽

✓6ᵗʰ **M11.04** Hydroxyapatite deposition disease, hand
     M11.041 Hydroxyapatite deposition disease, right hand
     M11.042 Hydroxyapatite deposition disease, left hand
     M11.049 Hydroxyapatite deposition disease, unspecified hand ▽

✓6ᵗʰ **M11.05** Hydroxyapatite deposition disease, hip
     M11.051 Hydroxyapatite deposition disease, right hip
     M11.052 Hydroxyapatite deposition disease, left hip
     M11.059 Hydroxyapatite deposition disease, unspecified hip ▽

EXCLUDES 1 Not coded here   **EXCLUDES 2** Not included here   **N** Newborn Age: 0   **P** Pediatric Age: 0-17   **M** Maternity Age: 12-55   **A** Adult Age: 15-124

✓6th **M11.06** Hydroxyapatite deposition disease, knee
     M11.061 Hydroxyapatite deposition disease, right knee
     M11.062 Hydroxyapatite deposition disease, left knee
     M11.069 Hydroxyapatite deposition disease, unspecified knee ▽

✓6th **M11.07** Hydroxyapatite deposition disease, ankle and foot
     M11.071 Hydroxyapatite deposition disease, right ankle and foot
     M11.072 Hydroxyapatite deposition disease, left ankle and foot
     M11.079 Hydroxyapatite deposition disease, unspecified ankle and foot ▽

M11.08 Hydroxyapatite deposition disease, vertebrae
M11.09 Hydroxyapatite deposition disease, multiple sites

✓5th **M11.1** Familial chondrocalcinosis
M11.10 Familial chondrocalcinosis, unspecified site ▽

✓6th **M11.11** Familial chondrocalcinosis, shoulder
     M11.111 Familial chondrocalcinosis, right shoulder
     M11.112 Familial chondrocalcinosis, left shoulder
     M11.119 Familial chondrocalcinosis, unspecified shoulder ▽

✓6th **M11.12** Familial chondrocalcinosis, elbow
     M11.121 Familial chondrocalcinosis, right elbow
     M11.122 Familial chondrocalcinosis, left elbow
     M11.129 Familial chondrocalcinosis, unspecified elbow ▽

✓6th **M11.13** Familial chondrocalcinosis, wrist
     M11.131 Familial chondrocalcinosis, right wrist
     M11.132 Familial chondrocalcinosis, left wrist
     M11.139 Familial chondrocalcinosis, unspecified wrist ▽

✓6th **M11.14** Familial chondrocalcinosis, hand
     M11.141 Familial chondrocalcinosis, right hand
     M11.142 Familial chondrocalcinosis, left hand
     M11.149 Familial chondrocalcinosis, unspecified hand ▽

✓6th **M11.15** Familial chondrocalcinosis, hip
     M11.151 Familial chondrocalcinosis, right hip
     M11.152 Familial chondrocalcinosis, left hip
     M11.159 Familial chondrocalcinosis, unspecified hip ▽

✓6th **M11.16** Familial chondrocalcinosis, knee
     M11.161 Familial chondrocalcinosis, right knee
     M11.162 Familial chondrocalcinosis, left knee
     M11.169 Familial chondrocalcinosis, unspecified knee ▽

✓6th **M11.17** Familial chondrocalcinosis, ankle and foot
     M11.171 Familial chondrocalcinosis, right ankle and foot
     M11.172 Familial chondrocalcinosis, left ankle and foot
     M11.179 Familial chondrocalcinosis, unspecified ankle and foot ▽

M11.18 Familial chondrocalcinosis, vertebrae
M11.19 Familial chondrocalcinosis, multiple sites

✓5th **M11.2** Other chondrocalcinosis
     Chondrocalcinosis NOS
M11.20 Other chondrocalcinosis, unspecified site ▽

✓6th **M11.21** Other chondrocalcinosis, shoulder
     M11.211 Other chondrocalcinosis, right shoulder
     M11.212 Other chondrocalcinosis, left shoulder
     M11.219 Other chondrocalcinosis, unspecified shoulder ▽

✓6th **M11.22** Other chondrocalcinosis, elbow
     M11.221 Other chondrocalcinosis, right elbow
     M11.222 Other chondrocalcinosis, left elbow
     M11.229 Other chondrocalcinosis, unspecified elbow ▽

✓6th **M11.23** Other chondrocalcinosis, wrist
     M11.231 Other chondrocalcinosis, right wrist
     M11.232 Other chondrocalcinosis, left wrist

     M11.239 Other chondrocalcinosis, unspecified wrist ▽

✓6th **M11.24** Other chondrocalcinosis, hand
     M11.241 Other chondrocalcinosis, right hand
     M11.242 Other chondrocalcinosis, left hand
     M11.249 Other chondrocalcinosis, unspecified hand ▽

✓6th **M11.25** Other chondrocalcinosis, hip
     M11.251 Other chondrocalcinosis, right hip
     M11.252 Other chondrocalcinosis, left hip
     M11.259 Other chondrocalcinosis, unspecified hip ▽

✓6th **M11.26** Other chondrocalcinosis, knee
     M11.261 Other chondrocalcinosis, right knee
     M11.262 Other chondrocalcinosis, left knee
     M11.269 Other chondrocalcinosis, unspecified knee ▽

✓6th **M11.27** Other chondrocalcinosis, ankle and foot
     M11.271 Other chondrocalcinosis, right ankle and foot
     M11.272 Other chondrocalcinosis, left ankle and foot
     M11.279 Other chondrocalcinosis, unspecified ankle and foot ▽

M11.28 Other chondrocalcinosis, vertebrae
M11.29 Other chondrocalcinosis, multiple sites

✓5th **M11.8** Other specified crystal arthropathies
M11.80 Other specified crystal arthropathies, unspecified site ▽

✓6th **M11.81** Other specified crystal arthropathies, shoulder
     M11.811 Other specified crystal arthropathies, right shoulder
     M11.812 Other specified crystal arthropathies, left shoulder
     M11.819 Other specified crystal arthropathies, unspecified shoulder ▽

✓6th **M11.82** Other specified crystal arthropathies, elbow
     M11.821 Other specified crystal arthropathies, right elbow
     M11.822 Other specified crystal arthropathies, left elbow
     M11.829 Other specified crystal arthropathies, unspecified elbow ▽

✓6th **M11.83** Other specified crystal arthropathies, wrist
     M11.831 Other specified crystal arthropathies, right wrist
     M11.832 Other specified crystal arthropathies, left wrist
     M11.839 Other specified crystal arthropathies, unspecified wrist ▽

✓6th **M11.84** Other specified crystal arthropathies, hand
     M11.841 Other specified crystal arthropathies, right hand
     M11.842 Other specified crystal arthropathies, left hand
     M11.849 Other specified crystal arthropathies, unspecified hand ▽

✓6th **M11.85** Other specified crystal arthropathies, hip
     M11.851 Other specified crystal arthropathies, right hip
     M11.852 Other specified crystal arthropathies, left hip
     M11.859 Other specified crystal arthropathies, unspecified hip ▽

✓6th **M11.86** Other specified crystal arthropathies, knee
     M11.861 Other specified crystal arthropathies, right knee
     M11.862 Other specified crystal arthropathies, left knee
     M11.869 Other specified crystal arthropathies, unspecified knee ▽

✓6th **M11.87** Other specified crystal arthropathies, ankle and foot
     M11.871 Other specified crystal arthropathies, right ankle and foot
     M11.872 Other specified crystal arthropathies, left ankle and foot

✓ Additional Character Req   ✓x7th Placeholder Alert   Manifestation   HCC CMS-HCC Condition   ▽ Unspecified Code   ▶◀ Revised Text   ● New Code   ▲ Revised Code Title

ICD-10-CM 2018   **733**

Chapter 13. Diseases of the Musculoskeletal System and Connective Tissue

M11.879–M12.269

M11.879　Other specified crystal arthropathies, ▽
　　　　　unspecified ankle and foot

M11.88　Other specified crystal arthropathies, vertebrae

M11.89　Other specified crystal arthropathies, multiple sites

M11.9　Crystal arthropathy, unspecified ▽

✓4th **M12　Other and unspecified arthropathy**
　　EXCLUDES 1　arthrosis (M15-M19)
　　　　　　　cricoarytenoid arthropathy (J38.7)

✓5th M12.0　Chronic postrheumatic arthropathy [Jaccoud]

M12.00　Chronic postrheumatic arthropathy [Jaccoud], HCC ▽
　　　　　unspecified site

✓6th M12.01　Chronic postrheumatic arthropathy [Jaccoud],
　　　　　shoulder

M12.011　Chronic postrheumatic arthropathy HCC
　　　　　[Jaccoud], right shoulder

M12.012　Chronic postrheumatic arthropathy HCC
　　　　　[Jaccoud], left shoulder

M12.019　Chronic postrheumatic arthropathy HCC ▽
　　　　　[Jaccoud], unspecified shoulder

✓6th M12.02　Chronic postrheumatic arthropathy [Jaccoud], elbow

M12.021　Chronic postrheumatic arthropathy HCC
　　　　　[Jaccoud], right elbow

M12.022　Chronic postrheumatic arthropathy HCC
　　　　　[Jaccoud], left elbow

M12.029　Chronic postrheumatic arthropathy HCC ▽
　　　　　[Jaccoud], unspecified elbow

✓6th M12.03　Chronic postrheumatic arthropathy [Jaccoud], wrist

M12.031　Chronic postrheumatic arthropathy HCC
　　　　　[Jaccoud], right wrist

M12.032　Chronic postrheumatic arthropathy HCC
　　　　　[Jaccoud], left wrist

M12.039　Chronic postrheumatic arthropathy HCC ▽
　　　　　[Jaccoud], unspecified wrist

✓6th M12.04　Chronic postrheumatic arthropathy [Jaccoud], hand

M12.041　Chronic postrheumatic arthropathy HCC
　　　　　[Jaccoud], right hand

M12.042　Chronic postrheumatic arthropathy HCC
　　　　　[Jaccoud], left hand

M12.049　Chronic postrheumatic arthropathy HCC ▽
　　　　　[Jaccoud], unspecified hand

✓6th M12.05　Chronic postrheumatic arthropathy [Jaccoud], hip

M12.051　Chronic postrheumatic arthropathy HCC
　　　　　[Jaccoud], right hip

M12.052　Chronic postrheumatic arthropathy HCC
　　　　　[Jaccoud], left hip

M12.059　Chronic postrheumatic arthropathy HCC ▽
　　　　　[Jaccoud], unspecified hip

✓6th M12.06　Chronic postrheumatic arthropathy [Jaccoud], knee

M12.061　Chronic postrheumatic arthropathy HCC
　　　　　[Jaccoud], right knee

M12.062　Chronic postrheumatic arthropathy HCC
　　　　　[Jaccoud], left knee

M12.069　Chronic postrheumatic arthropathy HCC ▽
　　　　　[Jaccoud], unspecified knee

✓6th M12.07　Chronic postrheumatic arthropathy [Jaccoud],
　　　　　ankle and foot

M12.071　Chronic postrheumatic arthropathy HCC
　　　　　[Jaccoud], right ankle and foot

M12.072　Chronic postrheumatic arthropathy HCC
　　　　　[Jaccoud], left ankle and foot

M12.079　Chronic postrheumatic arthropathy HCC ▽
　　　　　[Jaccoud], unspecified ankle and foot

M12.08　Chronic postrheumatic arthropathy [Jaccoud], HCC
　　　　　other specified site
　　　　　Chronic postrheumatic arthropathy [Jaccoud],
　　　　　　vertebrae

M12.09　Chronic postrheumatic arthropathy [Jaccoud], HCC
　　　　　multiple sites

✓5th M12.1　Kaschin-Beck disease
　　　　　Osteochondroarthrosis deformans endemica

M12.10　Kaschin-Beck disease, unspecified site ▽

✓6th M12.11　Kaschin-Beck disease, shoulder

M12.111　Kaschin-Beck disease, right shoulder

M12.112　Kaschin-Beck disease, left shoulder

M12.119　Kaschin-Beck disease, unspecified ▽
　　　　　shoulder

✓6th M12.12　Kaschin-Beck disease, elbow

M12.121　Kaschin-Beck disease, right elbow

M12.122　Kaschin-Beck disease, left elbow

M12.129　Kaschin-Beck disease, unspecified ▽
　　　　　elbow

✓6th M12.13　Kaschin-Beck disease, wrist

M12.131　Kaschin-Beck disease, right wrist

M12.132　Kaschin-Beck disease, left wrist

M12.139　Kaschin-Beck disease, unspecified wrist ▽

✓6th M12.14　Kaschin-Beck disease, hand

M12.141　Kaschin-Beck disease, right hand

M12.142　Kaschin-Beck disease, left hand

M12.149　Kaschin-Beck disease, unspecified hand ▽

✓6th M12.15　Kaschin-Beck disease, hip

M12.151　Kaschin-Beck disease, right hip

M12.152　Kaschin-Beck disease, left hip

M12.159　Kaschin-Beck disease, unspecified hip ▽

✓6th M12.16　Kaschin-Beck disease, knee

M12.161　Kaschin-Beck disease, right knee

M12.162　Kaschin-Beck disease, left knee

M12.169　Kaschin-Beck disease, unspecified ▽
　　　　　knee

✓6th M12.17　Kaschin-Beck disease, ankle and foot

M12.171　Kaschin-Beck disease, right ankle and foot

M12.172　Kaschin-Beck disease, left ankle and foot

M12.179　Kaschin-Beck disease, unspecified a ▽
　　　　　nkle and foot

M12.18　Kaschin-Beck disease, vertebrae

M12.19　Kaschin-Beck disease, multiple sites

✓5th M12.2　Villonodular synovitis (pigmented)

M12.20　Villonodular synovitis (pigmented), unspecified ▽
　　　　　site

✓6th M12.21　Villonodular synovitis (pigmented), shoulder

M12.211　Villonodular synovitis (pigmented), right
　　　　　shoulder

M12.212　Villonodular synovitis (pigmented), left
　　　　　shoulder

M12.219　Villonodular synovitis (pigmented), ▽
　　　　　unspecified shoulder

✓6th M12.22　Villonodular synovitis (pigmented), elbow

M12.221　Villonodular synovitis (pigmented), right
　　　　　elbow

M12.222　Villonodular synovitis (pigmented), left
　　　　　elbow

M12.229　Villonodular synovitis (pigmented), ▽
　　　　　unspecified elbow

✓6th M12.23　Villonodular synovitis (pigmented), wrist

M12.231　Villonodular synovitis (pigmented), right
　　　　　wrist

M12.232　Villonodular synovitis (pigmented), left
　　　　　wrist

M12.239　Villonodular synovitis (pigmented), ▽
　　　　　unspecified wrist

✓6th M12.24　Villonodular synovitis (pigmented), hand

M12.241　Villonodular synovitis (pigmented), right
　　　　　hand

M12.242　Villonodular synovitis (pigmented), left
　　　　　hand

M12.249　Villonodular synovitis (pigmented), ▽
　　　　　unspecified hand

✓6th M12.25　Villonodular synovitis (pigmented), hip

M12.251　Villonodular synovitis (pigmented), right
　　　　　hip

M12.252　Villonodular synovitis (pigmented), left
　　　　　hip

M12.259　Villonodular synovitis (pigmented), ▽
　　　　　unspecified hip

✓6th M12.26　Villonodular synovitis (pigmented), knee

M12.261　Villonodular synovitis (pigmented), right
　　　　　knee

M12.262　Villonodular synovitis (pigmented), left
　　　　　knee

M12.269　Villonodular synovitis (pigmented), ▽
　　　　　unspecified knee

EXCLUDES 1 Not coded here　　EXCLUDES 2 Not included here　　N Newborn Age: 0　　P Pediatric Age: 0-17　　M Maternity Age: 12-55　　A Adult Age: 15-124

734　　　　　　　　　　　　　　　　　　　　　　　　　　　　　　　　　　　　　　　ICD-10-CM 2018

√6ᵗʰ **M12.27 Villonodular synovitis (pigmented)**, ankle and foot
     M12.271 Villonodular synovitis (pigmented), right ankle and foot
     M12.272 Villonodular synovitis (pigmented), left ankle and foot
     M12.279 Villonodular synovitis (pigmented), unspecified ankle and foot ▽
   M12.28 Villonodular synovitis (pigmented), other specified site
     Villonodular synovitis (pigmented), vertebrae
   M12.29 Villonodular synovitis (pigmented), multiple sites

√5ᵗʰ **M12.3 Palindromic rheumatism**
   M12.30 Palindromic rheumatism, unspecified site ▽
√6ᵗʰ **M12.31 Palindromic rheumatism**, shoulder
     M12.311 Palindromic rheumatism, right shoulder
     M12.312 Palindromic rheumatism, left shoulder
     M12.319 Palindromic rheumatism, unspecified shoulder ▽
√6ᵗʰ **M12.32 Palindromic rheumatism**, elbow
     M12.321 Palindromic rheumatism, right elbow
     M12.322 Palindromic rheumatism, left elbow
     M12.329 Palindromic rheumatism, unspecified elbow ▽
√6ᵗʰ **M12.33 Palindromic rheumatism**, wrist
     M12.331 Palindromic rheumatism, right wrist
     M12.332 Palindromic rheumatism, left wrist
     M12.339 Palindromic rheumatism, unspecified wrist ▽
√6ᵗʰ **M12.34 Palindromic rheumatism**, hand
     M12.341 Palindromic rheumatism, right hand
     M12.342 Palindromic rheumatism, left hand
     M12.349 Palindromic rheumatism, unspecified hand ▽
√6ᵗʰ **M12.35 Palindromic rheumatism**, hip
     M12.351 Palindromic rheumatism, right hip
     M12.352 Palindromic rheumatism, left hip
     M12.359 Palindromic rheumatism, unspecified hip ▽
√6ᵗʰ **M12.36 Palindromic rheumatism**, knee
     M12.361 Palindromic rheumatism, right knee
     M12.362 Palindromic rheumatism, left knee
     M12.369 Palindromic rheumatism, unspecified knee ▽
√6ᵗʰ **M12.37 Palindromic rheumatism**, ankle and foot
     M12.371 Palindromic rheumatism, right ankle and foot
     M12.372 Palindromic rheumatism, left ankle and foot
     M12.379 Palindromic rheumatism, unspecified ankle and foot ▽
   M12.38 Palindromic rheumatism, other specified site
     Palindromic rheumatism, vertebrae
   M12.39 Palindromic rheumatism, multiple sites

√5ᵗʰ **M12.4 Intermittent hydrarthrosis**
   M12.40 Intermittent hydrarthrosis, unspecified site ▽
√6ᵗʰ **M12.41 Intermittent hydrarthrosis**, shoulder
     M12.411 Intermittent hydrarthrosis, right shoulder
     M12.412 Intermittent hydrarthrosis, left shoulder
     M12.419 Intermittent hydrarthrosis, unspecified shoulder ▽
√6ᵗʰ **M12.42 Intermittent hydrarthrosis**, elbow
     M12.421 Intermittent hydrarthrosis, right elbow
     M12.422 Intermittent hydrarthrosis, left elbow
     M12.429 Intermittent hydrarthrosis, unspecified elbow ▽
√6ᵗʰ **M12.43 Intermittent hydrarthrosis**, wrist
     M12.431 Intermittent hydrarthrosis, right wrist
     M12.432 Intermittent hydrarthrosis, left wrist
     M12.439 Intermittent hydrarthrosis, unspecified wrist ▽
√6ᵗʰ **M12.44 Intermittent hydrarthrosis**, hand
     M12.441 Intermittent hydrarthrosis, right hand
     M12.442 Intermittent hydrarthrosis, left hand

     M12.449 Intermittent hydrarthrosis, unspecified hand
√6ᵗʰ **M12.45 Intermittent hydrarthrosis**, hip
     M12.451 Intermittent hydrarthrosis, right hip
     M12.452 Intermittent hydrarthrosis, left hip
     M12.459 Intermittent hydrarthrosis, unspecified hip ▽
√6ᵗʰ **M12.46 Intermittent hydrarthrosis**, knee
     M12.461 Intermittent hydrarthrosis, right knee
     M12.462 Intermittent hydrarthrosis, left knee
     M12.469 Intermittent hydrarthrosis, unspecified knee ▽
√6ᵗʰ **M12.47 Intermittent hydrarthrosis**, ankle and foot
     M12.471 Intermittent hydrarthrosis, right ankle and foot
     M12.472 Intermittent hydrarthrosis, left ankle and foot
     M12.479 Intermittent hydrarthrosis, unspecified ankle and foot ▽
   M12.48 Intermittent hydrarthrosis, other site
   M12.49 Intermittent hydrarthrosis, multiple sites

√5ᵗʰ **M12.5 Traumatic arthropathy**
     EXCLUDES 1   *current injury-see Alphabetic Index*
     post-traumatic osteoarthritis NOS (M19.1-)
     post-traumatic osteoarthritis of first carpometacarpal joint (M18.2-M18.3)
     post-traumatic osteoarthritis of hip (M16.4-M16.5)
     post-traumatic osteoarthritis of knee (M17.2-M17.3)
     post-traumatic osteoarthritis of other single joints (M19.1-)
     AHA: 2015, 1Q, 17
   M12.50 Traumatic arthropathy, unspecified site ▽
√6ᵗʰ **M12.51 Traumatic arthropathy**, shoulder
     M12.511 Traumatic arthropathy, right shoulder
     M12.512 Traumatic arthropathy, left shoulder
     M12.519 Traumatic arthropathy, unspecified shoulder ▽
√6ᵗʰ **M12.52 Traumatic arthropathy**, elbow
     M12.521 Traumatic arthropathy, right elbow
     M12.522 Traumatic arthropathy, left elbow
     M12.529 Traumatic arthropathy, unspecified elbow ▽
√6ᵗʰ **M12.53 Traumatic arthropathy**, wrist
     M12.531 Traumatic arthropathy, right wrist
     M12.532 Traumatic arthropathy, left wrist
     M12.539 Traumatic arthropathy, unspecified wrist ▽
√6ᵗʰ **M12.54 Traumatic arthropathy**, hand
     M12.541 Traumatic arthropathy, right hand
     M12.542 Traumatic arthropathy, left hand
     M12.549 Traumatic arthropathy, unspecified hand ▽
√6ᵗʰ **M12.55 Traumatic arthropathy**, hip
     M12.551 Traumatic arthropathy, right hip
     M12.552 Traumatic arthropathy, left hip
     M12.559 Traumatic arthropathy, unspecified hip ▽
√6ᵗʰ **M12.56 Traumatic arthropathy**, knee
     M12.561 Traumatic arthropathy, right knee
     M12.562 Traumatic arthropathy, left knee
     M12.569 Traumatic arthropathy, unspecified knee ▽
√6ᵗʰ **M12.57 Traumatic arthropathy**, ankle and foot
     M12.571 Traumatic arthropathy, right ankle and foot
     M12.572 Traumatic arthropathy, left ankle and foot
     M12.579 Traumatic arthropathy, unspecified ankle and foot ▽
   M12.58 Traumatic arthropathy, other specified site
     Traumatic arthropathy, vertebrae
   M12.59 Traumatic arthropathy, multiple sites
√5ᵗʰ **M12.8 Other specific arthropathies, not elsewhere classified**
     Transient arthropathy
   M12.80 Other specific arthropathies, not elsewhere classified, unspecified site ▽

✓ Additional Character Req   √ˣ7ᵗʰ Placeholder Alert   Manifestation   ᴴᶜᶜ CMS-HCC Condition   ▽ Unspecified Code   ▶◀ Revised Text   ● New Code   ▲ Revised Code Title

ICD-10-CM 2018   735

√6ᵗʰ **M12.81** **Other specific arthropathies, not elsewhere classified,** shoulder
     M12.811 **Other specific arthropathies, not elsewhere classified,** right **shoulder**
     M12.812 **Other specific arthropathies, not elsewhere classified,** left **shoulder**
     M12.819 **Other specific arthropathies, not elsewhere classified, unspecified shoulder** ▽

√6ᵗʰ **M12.82** **Other specific arthropathies, not elsewhere classified,** elbow
     M12.821 **Other specific arthropathies, not elsewhere classified,** right **elbow**
     M12.822 **Other specific arthropathies, not elsewhere classified,** left **elbow**
     M12.829 **Other specific arthropathies, not elsewhere classified, unspecified elbow** ▽

√6ᵗʰ **M12.83** **Other specific arthropathies, not elsewhere classified,** wrist
     M12.831 **Other specific arthropathies, not elsewhere classified,** right **wrist**
     M12.832 **Other specific arthropathies, not elsewhere classified,** left **wrist**
     M12.839 **Other specific arthropathies, not elsewhere classified, unspecified wrist** ▽

√6ᵗʰ **M12.84** **Other specific arthropathies, not elsewhere classified,** hand
     M12.841 **Other specific arthropathies, not elsewhere classified,** right **hand**
     M12.842 **Other specific arthropathies, not elsewhere classified,** left **hand**
     M12.849 **Other specific arthropathies, not elsewhere classified, unspecified hand** ▽

√6ᵗʰ **M12.85** **Other specific arthropathies, not elsewhere classified,** hip
     M12.851 **Other specific arthropathies, not elsewhere classified,** right **hip**
     M12.852 **Other specific arthropathies, not elsewhere classified,** left **hip**
     M12.859 **Other specific arthropathies, not elsewhere classified, unspecified hip** ▽

√6ᵗʰ **M12.86** **Other specific arthropathies, not elsewhere classified,** knee
     M12.861 **Other specific arthropathies, not elsewhere classified,** right **knee**
     M12.862 **Other specific arthropathies, not elsewhere classified,** left **knee**
     M12.869 **Other specific arthropathies, not elsewhere classified, unspecified knee** ▽

√6ᵗʰ **M12.87** **Other specific arthropathies, not elsewhere classified,** ankle and foot
     M12.871 **Other specific arthropathies, not elsewhere classified,** right **ankle and foot**
     M12.872 **Other specific arthropathies, not elsewhere classified,** left **ankle and foot**
     M12.879 **Other specific arthropathies, not elsewhere classified, unspecified ankle and foot** ▽

M12.88 **Other specific arthropathies, not elsewhere classified, other specified site**
     Other specific arthropathies, not elsewhere classified, vertebrae

M12.89 **Other specific arthropathies, not elsewhere classified,** multiple sites

M12.9 **Arthropathy, unspecified** ▽

√4ᵗʰ **M13** **Other arthritis**
     EXCLUDES 1   arthrosis (M15-M19)
             osteoarthritis (M15-M19)

M13.0 **Polyarthritis, unspecified** ▽

√5ᵗʰ **M13.1** **Monoarthritis, not elsewhere classified**
     M13.10 **Monoarthritis, not elsewhere classified, unspecified site** ▽

√6ᵗʰ **M13.11** **Monoarthritis, not elsewhere classified,** shoulder
     M13.111 **Monoarthritis, not elsewhere classified,** right **shoulder**
     M13.112 **Monoarthritis, not elsewhere classified,** left **shoulder**
     M13.119 **Monoarthritis, not elsewhere classified, unspecified shoulder** ▽

√6ᵗʰ **M13.12** **Monoarthritis, not elsewhere classified,** elbow
     M13.121 **Monoarthritis, not elsewhere classified,** right **elbow**
     M13.122 **Monoarthritis, not elsewhere classified,** left **elbow**
     M13.129 **Monoarthritis, not elsewhere classified, unspecified elbow** ▽

√6ᵗʰ **M13.13** **Monoarthritis, not elsewhere classified,** wrist
     M13.131 **Monoarthritis, not elsewhere classified,** right **wrist**
     M13.132 **Monoarthritis, not elsewhere classified,** left **wrist**
     M13.139 **Monoarthritis, not elsewhere classified, unspecified wrist** ▽

√6ᵗʰ **M13.14** **Monoarthritis, not elsewhere classified,** hand
     M13.141 **Monoarthritis, not elsewhere classified,** right **hand**
     M13.142 **Monoarthritis, not elsewhere classified,** left **hand**
     M13.149 **Monoarthritis, not elsewhere classified, unspecified hand** ▽

√6ᵗʰ **M13.15** **Monoarthritis, not elsewhere classified,** hip
     M13.151 **Monoarthritis, not elsewhere classified,** right **hip**
     M13.152 **Monoarthritis, not elsewhere classified,** left **hip**
     M13.159 **Monoarthritis, not elsewhere classified, unspecified hip** ▽

√6ᵗʰ **M13.16** **Monoarthritis, not elsewhere classified,** knee
     M13.161 **Monoarthritis, not elsewhere classified,** right **knee**
     M13.162 **Monoarthritis, not elsewhere classified,** left **knee**
     M13.169 **Monoarthritis, not elsewhere classified, unspecified knee** ▽

√6ᵗʰ **M13.17** **Monoarthritis, not elsewhere classified,** ankle and foot
     M13.171 **Monoarthritis, not elsewhere classified,** right **ankle and foot**
     M13.172 **Monoarthritis, not elsewhere classified,** left **ankle and foot**
     M13.179 **Monoarthritis, not elsewhere classified, unspecified ankle and foot** ▽

√5ᵗʰ **M13.8** **Other specified arthritis**
     Allergic arthritis
     EXCLUDES 1   osteoarthritis (M15-M19)

M13.80 **Other specified arthritis, unspecified site** ▽

√6ᵗʰ **M13.81** **Other specified arthritis,** shoulder
     M13.811 **Other specified arthritis,** right **shoulder**
     M13.812 **Other specified arthritis,** left **shoulder**
     M13.819 **Other specified arthritis, unspecified shoulder** ▽

√6ᵗʰ **M13.82** **Other specified arthritis,** elbow
     M13.821 **Other specified arthritis,** right **elbow**
     M13.822 **Other specified arthritis,** left **elbow**
     M13.829 **Other specified arthritis, unspecified elbow** ▽

√6ᵗʰ **M13.83** **Other specified arthritis,** wrist
     M13.831 **Other specified arthritis,** right **wrist**
     M13.832 **Other specified arthritis,** left **wrist**
     M13.839 **Other specified arthritis, unspecified wrist** ▽

√6ᵗʰ **M13.84** **Other specified arthritis,** hand
     M13.841 **Other specified arthritis,** right **hand**
     M13.842 **Other specified arthritis,** left **hand**
     M13.849 **Other specified arthritis, unspecified hand** ▽

√6ᵗʰ **M13.85** **Other specified arthritis,** hip
     M13.851 **Other specified arthritis,** right **hip**
     M13.852 **Other specified arthritis,** left **hip**
     M13.859 **Other specified arthritis, unspecified hip** ▽

EXCLUDES 1 Not coded here   EXCLUDES 2 Not included here   N Newborn Age: 0   P Pediatric Age: 0-17   M Maternity Age: 12-55   A Adult Age: 15-124

736   ICD-10-CM 2018

☑6ᵗʰ **M13.86** Other specified arthritis, knee

     M13.861 Other specified arthritis, right knee

     M13.862 Other specified arthritis, left knee

     M13.869 Other specified arthritis, unspecified knee ▽

☑6ᵗʰ **M13.87** Other specified arthritis, ankle and foot

     M13.871 Other specified arthritis, right ankle and foot

     M13.872 Other specified arthritis, left ankle and foot

     M13.879 Other specified arthritis, unspecified ankle and foot ▽

M13.88 Other specified arthritis, other site

M13.89 Other specified arthritis, multiple sites

☑4ᵗʰ **M14 Arthropathies in other diseases classified elsewhere**

   EXCLUDES 1   *arthropathy in:*
     diabetes mellitus (E08-E13 with .61-)
     hematological disorders (M36.2-M36.3)
     hypersensitivity reactions (M36.4)
     neoplastic disease (M36.1)
     neurosyphillis (A52.16)
     sarcoidosis (D86.86)
   enteropathic arthropathies (M07.-)
   juvenile psoriatic arthropathy (L40.54)
   lipoid dermatoarthritis (E78.81)

☑5ᵗʰ **M14.6 Charcôt's joint**

   Neuropathic arthropathy

   EXCLUDES 1   *Charcôt's joint in diabetes mellitus (E08-E13 with .610)*
     Charcôt's joint in tabes dorsalis (A52.16)

M14.60 Charcôt's joint, unspecified site ▽

☑6ᵗʰ **M14.61** Charcôt's joint, shoulder

     M14.611 Charcôt's joint, right shoulder

     M14.612 Charcôt's joint, left shoulder

     M14.619 Charcôt's joint, unspecified shoulder ▽

☑6ᵗʰ **M14.62** Charcôt's joint, elbow

     M14.621 Charcôt's joint, right elbow

     M14.622 Charcôt's joint, left elbow

     M14.629 Charcôt's joint, unspecified elbow ▽

☑6ᵗʰ **M14.63** Charcôt's joint, wrist

     M14.631 Charcôt's joint, right wrist

     M14.632 Charcôt's joint, left wrist

     M14.639 Charcôt's joint, unspecified wrist ▽

☑6ᵗʰ **M14.64** Charcôt's joint, hand

     M14.641 Charcôt's joint, right hand

     M14.642 Charcôt's joint, left hand

     M14.649 Charcôt's joint, unspecified hand ▽

☑6ᵗʰ **M14.65** Charcôt's joint, hip

     M14.651 Charcôt's joint, right hip

     M14.652 Charcôt's joint, left hip

     M14.659 Charcôt's joint, unspecified hip ▽

☑6ᵗʰ **M14.66** Charcôt's joint, knee

     M14.661 Charcôt's joint, right knee

     M14.662 Charcôt's joint, left knee

     M14.669 Charcôt's joint, unspecified knee ▽

☑6ᵗʰ **M14.67** Charcôt's joint, ankle and foot

     M14.671 Charcôt's joint, right ankle and foot

     M14.672 Charcôt's joint, left ankle and foot

     M14.679 Charcôt's joint, unspecified ankle and foot ▽

M14.68 Charcôt's joint, vertebrae

M14.69 Charcôt's joint, multiple sites

☑5ᵗʰ **M14.8 Arthropathies in other specified diseases classified elsewhere**

   Code first underlying disease, such as:
     amyloidosis (E85.-)
     erythema multiforme (L51.-)
     erythema nodosum (L52)
     hemochromatosis (E83.11-)
     hyperparathyroidism (E21.-)
     hypothyroidism (E00-E03)
     sickle-cell disorders (D57.-)
     thyrotoxicosis [hyperthyroidism] (E05.-)
     Whipple's disease (K90.81)

     M14.80   *Arthropathies in other specified diseases classified elsewhere, unspecified site* ▽

☑6ᵗʰ **M14.81** Arthropathies in other specified diseases classified elsewhere, shoulder

     M14.811   *Arthropathies in other specified diseases classified elsewhere, right shoulder*

     M14.812   *Arthropathies in other specified diseases classified elsewhere, left shoulder*

     M14.819   *Arthropathies in other specified diseases classified elsewhere, unspecified shoulder* ▽

☑6ᵗʰ **M14.82** Arthropathies in other specified diseases classified elsewhere, elbow

     M14.821   *Arthropathies in other specified diseases classified elsewhere, right elbow*

     M14.822   *Arthropathies in other specified diseases classified elsewhere, left elbow*

     M14.829   *Arthropathies in other specified diseases classified elsewhere, unspecified elbow* ▽

☑6ᵗʰ **M14.83** Arthropathies in other specified diseases classified elsewhere, wrist

     M14.831   *Arthropathies in other specified diseases classified elsewhere, right wrist*

     M14.832   *Arthropathies in other specified diseases classified elsewhere, left wrist*

     M14.839   *Arthropathies in other specified diseases classified elsewhere, unspecified wrist* ▽

☑6ᵗʰ **M14.84** Arthropathies in other specified diseases classified elsewhere, hand

     M14.841   *Arthropathies in other specified diseases classified elsewhere, right hand*

     M14.842   *Arthropathies in other specified diseases classified elsewhere, left hand*

     M14.849   *Arthropathies in other specified diseases classified elsewhere, unspecified hand* ▽

☑6ᵗʰ **M14.85** Arthropathies in other specified diseases classified elsewhere, hip

     M14.851   *Arthropathies in other specified diseases classified elsewhere, right hip*

     M14.852   *Arthropathies in other specified diseases classified elsewhere, left hip*

     M14.859   *Arthropathies in other specified diseases classified elsewhere, unspecified hip* ▽

☑6ᵗʰ **M14.86** Arthropathies in other specified diseases classified elsewhere, knee

     M14.861   *Arthropathies in other specified diseases classified elsewhere, right knee*

     M14.862   *Arthropathies in other specified diseases classified elsewhere, left knee*

     M14.869   *Arthropathies in other specified diseases classified elsewhere, unspecified knee* ▽

☑6ᵗʰ **M14.87** Arthropathies in other specified diseases classified elsewhere, ankle and foot

     M14.871   *Arthropathies in other specified diseases classified elsewhere, right ankle and foot*

     M14.872   *Arthropathies in other specified diseases classified elsewhere, left ankle and foot*

     M14.879   *Arthropathies in other specified diseases classified elsewhere, unspecified ankle and foot* ▽

     M14.88   *Arthropathies in other specified diseases classified elsewhere, vertebrae*

     M14.89   *Arthropathies in other specified diseases classified elsewhere, multiple sites*

Osteoarthritis (M15-M19)

   EXCLUDES 2   osteoarthritis of spine (M47.-)

☑4ᵗʰ **M15 Polyosteoarthritis**

   INCLUDES   arthritis of multiple sites

   EXCLUDES 1   *bilateral involvement of single joint (M16-M19)*

M15.0 Primary generalized (osteo)arthritis

M15.1 Heberden's nodes (with arthropathy)

   Interphalangeal distal osteoarthritis

M15.2 Bouchard's nodes (with arthropathy)

   Juxtaphalangeal distal osteoarthritis

M15.3 Secondary multiple arthritis

   Post-traumatic polyosteoarthritis

M15.4 Erosive (osteo)arthritis

M15.8 Other polyosteoarthritis

☑ Additional Character Req   ☑×7ᵗʰ Placeholder Alert   Manifestation   HCC CMS-HCC Condition   ▽ Unspecified Code   ▶◀ Revised Text   ● New Code   ▲ Revised Code Title

Chapter 13. Diseases of the Musculoskeletal System and Connective Tissue

M15.9   Polyosteoarthritis, unspecified   ▽
Generalized osteoarthritis NOS

✓4ᵗʰ **M16**   Osteoarthritis of hip
AHA: 2016, 4Q, 146

M16.0   Bilateral primary osteoarthritis of hip

✓5ᵗʰ **M16.1**   Unilateral primary osteoarthritis of hip
Primary osteoarthritis of hip NOS

M16.10   Unilateral primary osteoarthritis, unspecified hip   ▽

M16.11   Unilateral primary osteoarthritis, right hip

M16.12   Unilateral primary osteoarthritis, left hip

M16.2   Bilateral osteoarthritis resulting from hip dysplasia

✓5ᵗʰ **M16.3**   Unilateral osteoarthritis resulting from hip dysplasia
Dysplastic osteoarthritis of hip NOS

M16.30   Unilateral osteoarthritis resulting from hip dysplasia, unspecified hip   ▽

M16.31   Unilateral osteoarthritis resulting from hip dysplasia, right hip

M16.32   Unilateral osteoarthritis resulting from hip dysplasia, left hip

M16.4   Bilateral post-traumatic osteoarthritis of hip

✓5ᵗʰ **M16.5**   Unilateral post-traumatic osteoarthritis of hip
Post-traumatic osteoarthritis of hip NOS

M16.50   Unilateral post-traumatic osteoarthritis, unspecified hip   ▽

M16.51   Unilateral post-traumatic osteoarthritis, right hip

M16.52   Unilateral post-traumatic osteoarthritis, left hip

M16.6   Other bilateral secondary osteoarthritis of hip

M16.7   Other unilateral secondary osteoarthritis of hip
Secondary osteoarthritis of hip NOS

M16.9   Osteoarthritis of hip, unspecified   ▽

✓4ᵗʰ **M17**   Osteoarthritis of knee
AHA: 2016, 4Q, 146-147

M17.0   Bilateral primary osteoarthritis of knee

✓5ᵗʰ **M17.1**   Unilateral primary osteoarthritis of knee
Primary osteoarthritis of knee NOS

M17.10   Unilateral primary osteoarthritis, unspecified knee   ▽

M17.11   Unilateral primary osteoarthritis, right knee

M17.12   Unilateral primary osteoarthritis, left knee

M17.2   Bilateral post-traumatic osteoarthritis of knee

✓5ᵗʰ **M17.3**   Unilateral post-traumatic osteoarthritis of knee
Post-traumatic osteoarthritis of knee NOS

M17.30   Unilateral post-traumatic osteoarthritis, unspecified knee   ▽

M17.31   Unilateral post-traumatic osteoarthritis, right knee

M17.32   Unilateral post-traumatic osteoarthritis, left knee

M17.4   Other bilateral secondary osteoarthritis of knee

M17.5   Other unilateral secondary osteoarthritis of knee
Secondary osteoarthritis of knee NOS

M17.9   Osteoarthritis of knee, unspecified   ▽

✓4ᵗʰ **M18**   Osteoarthritis of first carpometacarpal joint

M18.0   Bilateral primary osteoarthritis of first carpometacarpal joints

✓5ᵗʰ **M18.1**   Unilateral primary osteoarthritis of first carpometacarpal joint
Primary osteoarthritis of first carpometacarpal joint NOS

M18.10   Unilateral primary osteoarthritis of first carpometacarpal joint, unspecified hand   ▽

M18.11   Unilateral primary osteoarthritis of first carpometacarpal joint, right hand

M18.12   Unilateral primary osteoarthritis of first carpometacarpal joint, left hand

M18.2   Bilateral post-traumatic osteoarthritis of first carpometacarpal joints

✓5ᵗʰ **M18.3**   Unilateral post-traumatic osteoarthritis of first carpometacarpal joint
Post-traumatic osteoarthritis of first carpometacarpal joint NOS

M18.30   Unilateral post-traumatic osteoarthritis of first carpometacarpal joint, unspecified hand   ▽

M18.31   Unilateral post-traumatic osteoarthritis of first carpometacarpal joint, right hand

M18.32   Unilateral post-traumatic osteoarthritis of first carpometacarpal joint, left hand

M18.4   Other bilateral secondary osteoarthritis of first carpometacarpal joints

✓5ᵗʰ **M18.5**   Other unilateral secondary osteoarthritis of first carpometacarpal joint
Secondary osteoarthritis of first carpometacarpal joint NOS

M18.50   Other unilateral secondary osteoarthritis of first carpometacarpal joint, unspecified hand   ▽

M18.51   Other unilateral secondary osteoarthritis of first carpometacarpal joint, right hand

M18.52   Other unilateral secondary osteoarthritis of first carpometacarpal joint, left hand

M18.9   Osteoarthritis of first carpometacarpal joint, unspecified   ▽

✓4ᵗʰ **M19**   Other and unspecified osteoarthritis
EXCLUDES 1   polyarthritis (M15.-)
EXCLUDES 2   arthrosis of spine (M47.-)
hallux rigidus (M20.2)
osteoarthritis of spine (M47.-)

✓5ᵗʰ **M19.0**   Primary osteoarthritis of other joints
AHA: 2016, 4Q, 145

✓6ᵗʰ **M19.01**   Primary osteoarthritis, shoulder

M19.011   Primary osteoarthritis, right shoulder

M19.012   Primary osteoarthritis, left shoulder

M19.019   Primary osteoarthritis, unspecified shoulder   ▽

✓6ᵗʰ **M19.02**   Primary osteoarthritis, elbow

M19.021   Primary osteoarthritis, right elbow

M19.022   Primary osteoarthritis, left elbow

M19.029   Primary osteoarthritis, unspecified elbow   ▽

✓6ᵗʰ **M19.03**   Primary osteoarthritis, wrist

M19.031   Primary osteoarthritis, right wrist

M19.032   Primary osteoarthritis, left wrist

M19.039   Primary osteoarthritis, unspecified wrist   ▽

✓6ᵗʰ **M19.04**   Primary osteoarthritis, hand
EXCLUDES 2   primary osteoarthritis of first carpometacarpal joint (M18.0-, M18.1-)

M19.041   Primary osteoarthritis, right hand

M19.042   Primary osteoarthritis, left hand

M19.049   Primary osteoarthritis, unspecified hand   ▽

✓6ᵗʰ **M19.07**   Primary osteoarthritis ankle and foot

M19.071   Primary osteoarthritis, right ankle and foot

M19.072   Primary osteoarthritis, left ankle and foot

M19.079   Primary osteoarthritis, unspecified ankle and foot   ▽

✓5ᵗʰ **M19.1**   Post-traumatic osteoarthritis of other joints

✓6ᵗʰ **M19.11**   Post-traumatic osteoarthritis, shoulder

M19.111   Post-traumatic osteoarthritis, right shoulder

M19.112   Post-traumatic osteoarthritis, left shoulder

M19.119   Post-traumatic osteoarthritis, unspecified shoulder   ▽

✓6ᵗʰ **M19.12**   Post-traumatic osteoarthritis, elbow

M19.121   Post-traumatic osteoarthritis, right elbow

M19.122   Post-traumatic osteoarthritis, left elbow

M19.129   Post-traumatic osteoarthritis, unspecified elbow   ▽

✓6ᵗʰ **M19.13**   Post-traumatic osteoarthritis, wrist

M19.131   Post-traumatic osteoarthritis, right wrist

M19.132   Post-traumatic osteoarthritis, left wrist

M19.139   Post-traumatic osteoarthritis, unspecified wrist   ▽

✓6ᵗʰ **M19.14**   Post-traumatic osteoarthritis, hand
EXCLUDES 2   post-traumatic osteoarthritis of first carpometacarpal joint (M18.2-, M18.3-)

M19.141   Post-traumatic osteoarthritis, right hand

M19.142   Post-traumatic osteoarthritis, left hand

M19.149   Post-traumatic osteoarthritis, unspecified hand   ▽

EXCLUDES 1 Not coded here   EXCLUDES 2 Not included here   N Newborn Age: 0   P Pediatric Age: 0-17   M Maternity Age: 12-55   A Adult Age: 15-124

738   ICD-10-CM 2018

✓6ᵗʰ **M19.17** Post-traumatic osteoarthritis, ankle and foot
- **M19.171** Post-traumatic osteoarthritis, right ankle and foot
- **M19.172** Post-traumatic osteoarthritis, left ankle and foot
- **M19.179** Post-traumatic osteoarthritis, unspecified ankle and foot ▽

✓5ᵗʰ **M19.2** Secondary osteoarthritis of other joints

✓6ᵗʰ **M19.21** Secondary osteoarthritis, shoulder
- **M19.211** Secondary osteoarthritis, right shoulder
- **M19.212** Secondary osteoarthritis, left shoulder
- **M19.219** Secondary osteoarthritis, unspecified shoulder ▽

✓6ᵗʰ **M19.22** Secondary osteoarthritis, elbow
- **M19.221** Secondary osteoarthritis, right elbow
- **M19.222** Secondary osteoarthritis, left elbow
- **M19.229** Secondary osteoarthritis, unspecified elbow ▽

✓6ᵗʰ **M19.23** Secondary osteoarthritis, wrist
- **M19.231** Secondary osteoarthritis, right wrist
- **M19.232** Secondary osteoarthritis, left wrist
- **M19.239** Secondary osteoarthritis, unspecified wrist ▽

✓6ᵗʰ **M19.24** Secondary osteoarthritis, hand
- **M19.241** Secondary osteoarthritis, right hand
- **M19.242** Secondary osteoarthritis, left hand
- **M19.249** Secondary osteoarthritis, unspecified hand ▽

✓6ᵗʰ **M19.27** Secondary osteoarthritis, ankle and foot
- **M19.271** Secondary osteoarthritis, right ankle and foot
- **M19.272** Secondary osteoarthritis, left ankle and foot
- **M19.279** Secondary osteoarthritis, unspecified ankle and foot ▽

✓5ᵗʰ **M19.9** Osteoarthritis, unspecified site
- **M19.90** Unspecified osteoarthritis, unspecified site ▽
  Arthrosis NOS Osteoarthritis NOS
  Arthritis NOS
  AHA: 2016, 4Q, 147
- **M19.91** Primary osteoarthritis, unspecified site ▽
  Primary osteoarthritis NOS
- **M19.92** Post-traumatic osteoarthritis, unspecified site ▽
  Post-traumatic osteoarthritis NOS
- **M19.93** Secondary osteoarthritis, unspecified site ▽
  Secondary osteoarthritis NOS

Other joint disorders (M20-M25)

EXCLUDES 2   joints of the spine (M40-M54)

✓4ᵗʰ **M20 Acquired deformities of fingers and toes**
EXCLUDES 1   acquired absence of fingers and toes (Z89.-)
congenital absence of fingers and toes (Q71.3-, Q72.3-)
congenital deformities and malformations of fingers and toes (Q66-, Q68-Q70, Q74-)

✓5ᵗʰ **M20.0** Deformity of finger(s)
EXCLUDES 1   clubbing of fingers (R68.3)
palmar fascial fibromatosis [Dupuytren] (M72.0)
trigger finger (M65.3)

✓6ᵗʰ **M20.00** Unspecified deformity of finger(s)
- **M20.001** Unspecified deformity of right finger(s) ▽
- **M20.002** Unspecified deformity of left finger(s) ▽
- **M20.009** Unspecified deformity of unspecified finger(s) ▽

✓6ᵗʰ **M20.01** Mallet finger
- **M20.011** Mallet finger of right finger(s)
- **M20.012** Mallet finger of left finger(s)
- **M20.019** Mallet finger of unspecified finger(s) ▽

✓6ᵗʰ **M20.02** Boutonnière deformity
DEF: A deformity of the finger caused by flexion of the proximal interphalangeal joint and hyperextension of the distal joint; results from rheumatoid arthritis, osteoarthritis, or injury; also called buttonhole deformity.
- **M20.021** Boutonnière deformity of right finger(s)
- **M20.022** Boutonnière deformity of left finger(s)

- **M20.029** Boutonnière deformity of unspecified finger(s) ▽

✓6ᵗʰ **M20.03** Swan-neck deformity
DEF: Flexed distal and hyperextended proximal interphalangeal joint; most commonly caused by rheumatoid arthritis.
- **M20.031** Swan-neck deformity of right finger(s)
- **M20.032** Swan-neck deformity of left finger(s)
- **M20.039** Swan-neck deformity of unspecified finger(s) ▽

✓6ᵗʰ **M20.09** Other deformity of finger(s)
- **M20.091** Other deformity of right finger(s)
- **M20.092** Other deformity of left finger(s)
- **M20.099** Other deformity of finger(s), unspecified finger(s) ▽

✓5ᵗʰ **M20.1** Hallux valgus (acquired)
EXCLUDES 2   bunion (M21.6-)
- **M20.10** Hallux valgus (acquired), unspecified foot ▽
- **M20.11** Hallux valgus (acquired), right foot
- **M20.12** Hallux valgus (acquired), left foot

✓5ᵗʰ **M20.2** Hallux rigidus
- **M20.20** Hallux rigidus, unspecified foot ▽
- **M20.21** Hallux rigidus, right foot
- **M20.22** Hallux rigidus, left foot

✓5ᵗʰ **M20.3** Hallux varus (acquired)
- **M20.30** Hallux varus (acquired), unspecified foot ▽
- **M20.31** Hallux varus (acquired), right foot
- **M20.32** Hallux varus (acquired), left foot

✓5ᵗʰ **M20.4** Other hammer toe(s) (acquired)
- **M20.40** Other hammer toe(s) (acquired), unspecified foot ▽
- **M20.41** Other hammer toe(s) (acquired), right foot
- **M20.42** Other hammer toe(s) (acquired), left foot

✓5ᵗʰ **M20.5** Other deformities of toe(s) (acquired)
✓6ᵗʰ **M20.5X** Other deformities of toe(s) (acquired)
- **M20.5X1** Other deformities of toe(s) (acquired), right foot
- **M20.5X2** Other deformities of toe(s) (acquired), left foot
- **M20.5X9** Other deformities of toe(s) (acquired), unspecified foot ▽

✓5ᵗʰ **M20.6** Acquired deformities of toe(s), unspecified
- **M20.60** Acquired deformities of toe(s), unspecified, unspecified foot ▽
- **M20.61** Acquired deformities of toe(s), unspecified, right foot ▽
- **M20.62** Acquired deformities of toe(s), unspecified, left foot ▽

Hallux Valgus

Hallux valgus

Medial eminence of metatarsal bone

Right foot

☑ Additional Character Req   ✓x7ᵗʰ Placeholder Alert   Manifestation   HCC CMS-HCC Condition   ▽ Unspecified Code   ▶◀ Revised Text   ● New Code   ▲ Revised Code Title

Genu Valga (knock-knee)

Genu Varus (bowleg)

✓4th **M21 Other acquired deformities of limbs**
> EXCLUDES 1   acquired absence of limb (Z89.-)
> congenital absence of limbs (Q71-Q73)
> congenital deformities and malformations of limbs (Q65-Q66, Q68-Q74)
>
> EXCLUDES 2   acquired deformities of fingers or toes (M20.-)
> coxa plana (M91.2)

✓5th **M21.0 Valgus deformity, not elsewhere classified**
> EXCLUDES 1   metatarsus valgus (Q66.6)
> talipes calcaneovalgus (Q66.4)

     M21.00 Valgus deformity, not elsewhere classified, unspecified site ▽

✓6th   **M21.02 Valgus deformity, not elsewhere classified, elbow**
     Cubitus valgus
     M21.021 Valgus deformity, not elsewhere classified, right elbow
     M21.022 Valgus deformity, not elsewhere classified, left elbow
     M21.029 Valgus deformity, not elsewhere classified, unspecified elbow ▽

✓6th   **M21.05 Valgus deformity, not elsewhere classified, hip**
     M21.051 Valgus deformity, not elsewhere classified, right hip
     M21.052 Valgus deformity, not elsewhere classified, left hip
     M21.059 Valgus deformity, not elsewhere classified, unspecified hip ▽

✓6th   **M21.06 Valgus deformity, not elsewhere classified, knee**
     Genu valgum
     Knock knee
     M21.061 Valgus deformity, not elsewhere classified, right knee
     M21.062 Valgus deformity, not elsewhere classified, left knee
     M21.069 Valgus deformity, not elsewhere classified, unspecified knee ▽

✓6th   **M21.07 Valgus deformity, not elsewhere classified, ankle**
     M21.071 Valgus deformity, not elsewhere classified, right ankle
     M21.072 Valgus deformity, not elsewhere classified, left ankle
     M21.079 Valgus deformity, not elsewhere classified, unspecified ankle ▽

✓5th **M21.1 Varus deformity, not elsewhere classified**
> EXCLUDES 1   metatarsus varus (Q66.22)
> tibia vara (M92.5)

     M21.10 Varus deformity, not elsewhere classified, unspecified site ▽

✓6th   **M21.12 Varus deformity, not elsewhere classified, elbow**
     Cubitus varus, elbow
     M21.121 Varus deformity, not elsewhere classified, right elbow

     M21.122 Varus deformity, not elsewhere classified, left elbow
     M21.129 Varus deformity, not elsewhere classified, unspecified elbow ▽

✓6th **M21.15 Varus deformity, not elsewhere classified, hip**
     M21.151 Varus deformity, not elsewhere classified, right hip
     M21.152 Varus deformity, not elsewhere classified, left hip
     M21.159 Varus deformity, not elsewhere classified, unspecified ▽

✓6th **M21.16 Varus deformity, not elsewhere classified, knee**
     Bow leg
     Genu varum
     M21.161 Varus deformity, not elsewhere classified, right knee
     M21.162 Varus deformity, not elsewhere classified, left knee
     M21.169 Varus deformity, not elsewhere classified, unspecified knee ▽

✓6th **M21.17 Varus deformity, not elsewhere classified, ankle**
     M21.171 Varus deformity, not elsewhere classified, right ankle
     M21.172 Varus deformity, not elsewhere classified, left ankle
     M21.179 Varus deformity, not elsewhere classified, unspecified ankle ▽

✓5th **M21.2 Flexion deformity**
     M21.20 Flexion deformity, unspecified site ▽

✓6th **M21.21 Flexion deformity, shoulder**
     M21.211 Flexion deformity, right shoulder
     M21.212 Flexion deformity, left shoulder
     M21.219 Flexion deformity, unspecified shoulder ▽

✓6th **M21.22 Flexion deformity, elbow**
     M21.221 Flexion deformity, right elbow
     M21.222 Flexion deformity, left elbow
     M21.229 Flexion deformity, unspecified elbow ▽

✓6th **M21.23 Flexion deformity, wrist**
     M21.231 Flexion deformity, right wrist
     M21.232 Flexion deformity, left wrist
     M21.239 Flexion deformity, unspecified wrist ▽

✓6th **M21.24 Flexion deformity, finger joints**
     M21.241 Flexion deformity, right finger joints
     M21.242 Flexion deformity, left finger joints
     M21.249 Flexion deformity, unspecified finger joints ▽

✓6th **M21.25 Flexion deformity, hip**
     M21.251 Flexion deformity, right hip
     M21.252 Flexion deformity, left hip
     M21.259 Flexion deformity, unspecified hip ▽

✓6ᵗʰ **M21.26** Flexion deformity, knee
    M21.261 Flexion deformity, right knee
    M21.262 Flexion deformity, left knee
    M21.269 Flexion deformity, unspecified knee ▽

✓6ᵗʰ **M21.27** Flexion deformity, ankle and toes
    M21.271 Flexion deformity, right ankle and toes
    M21.272 Flexion deformity, left ankle and toes
    M21.279 Flexion deformity, unspecified ankle and toes ▽

✓5ᵗʰ **M21.3** Wrist or foot drop (acquired)

    ✓6ᵗʰ **M21.33** Wrist drop (acquired)
      M21.331 Wrist drop, right wrist
      M21.332 Wrist drop, left wrist
      M21.339 Wrist drop, unspecified wrist ▽

    ✓6ᵗʰ **M21.37** Foot drop (acquired)
      M21.371 Foot drop, right foot
      M21.372 Foot drop, left foot
      M21.379 Foot drop, unspecified foot ▽

✓5ᵗʰ **M21.4** Flat foot [pes planus] (acquired)
    EXCLUDES 1   congenital pes planus (Q66.5-)
    M21.40 Flat foot [pes planus] (acquired), unspecified foot ▽
    M21.41 Flat foot [pes planus] (acquired), right foot
    M21.42 Flat foot [pes planus] (acquired), left foot

✓5ᵗʰ **M21.5** Acquired clawhand, clubhand, clawfoot and clubfoot
    EXCLUDES 1   clubfoot, not specified as acquired (Q66.89)

    ✓6ᵗʰ **M21.51** Acquired clawhand
      M21.511 Acquired clawhand, right hand
      M21.512 Acquired clawhand, left hand
      M21.519 Acquired clawhand, unspecified hand ▽

    ✓6ᵗʰ **M21.52** Acquired clubhand
      M21.521 Acquired clubhand, right hand
      M21.522 Acquired clubhand, left hand
      M21.529 Acquired clubhand, unspecified hand ▽

    ✓6ᵗʰ **M21.53** Acquired clawfoot
      DEF: High foot arch with hyperextended toes at metatarsophalangeal joint and flexed toes at distal joints.
      M21.531 Acquired clawfoot, right foot
      M21.532 Acquired clawfoot, left foot
      M21.539 Acquired clawfoot, unspecified foot ▽

    ✓6ᵗʰ **M21.54** Acquired clubfoot
      M21.541 Acquired clubfoot, right foot
      M21.542 Acquired clubfoot, left foot
      M21.549 Acquired clubfoot, unspecified foot ▽

✓5ᵗʰ **M21.6** Other acquired deformities of foot
    EXCLUDES 2   deformities of toe (acquired) (M20.1-M20.6-)

    ✓6ᵗʰ **M21.61** Bunion
      M21.611 Bunion of right foot
      M21.612 Bunion of left foot
      M21.619 Bunion of unspecified foot ▽

    ✓6ᵗʰ **M21.62** Bunionette
      M21.621 Bunionette of right foot
      M21.622 Bunionette of left foot
      M21.629 Bunionette of unspecified foot ▽

    ✓6ᵗʰ **M21.6X** Other acquired deformities of foot
      M21.6X1 Other acquired deformities of right foot
      M21.6X2 Other acquired deformities of left foot
      M21.6X9 Other acquired deformities of unspecified foot ▽

✓5ᵗʰ **M21.7** Unequal limb length (acquired)
    NOTE   The site used should correspond to the shorter limb.
    M21.70 Unequal limb length (acquired), unspecified site ▽

    ✓6ᵗʰ **M21.72** Unequal limb length (acquired), humerus
      M21.721 Unequal limb length (acquired), right humerus
      M21.722 Unequal limb length (acquired), left humerus
      M21.729 Unequal limb length (acquired), unspecified humerus ▽

    ✓6ᵗʰ **M21.73** Unequal limb length (acquired), ulna and radius
      M21.731 Unequal limb length (acquired), right ulna
      M21.732 Unequal limb length (acquired), left ulna
      M21.733 Unequal limb length (acquired), right radius
      M21.734 Unequal limb length (acquired), left radius
      M21.739 Unequal limb length (acquired), unspecified ulna and radius ▽

    ✓6ᵗʰ **M21.75** Unequal limb length (acquired), femur
      M21.751 Unequal limb length (acquired), right femur
      M21.752 Unequal limb length (acquired), left femur
      M21.759 Unequal limb length (acquired), unspecified femur ▽

    ✓6ᵗʰ **M21.76** Unequal limb length (acquired), tibia and fibula
      M21.761 Unequal limb length (acquired), right tibia
      M21.762 Unequal limb length (acquired), left tibia
      M21.763 Unequal limb length (acquired), right fibula
      M21.764 Unequal limb length (acquired), left fibula
      M21.769 Unequal limb length (acquired), unspecified tibia and fibula ▽

✓5ᵗʰ **M21.8** Other specified acquired deformities of limbs
    EXCLUDES 2   coxa plana (M91.2)
    M21.80 Other specified acquired deformities of unspecified limb ▽

    ✓6ᵗʰ **M21.82** Other specified acquired deformities of upper arm
      M21.821 Other specified acquired deformities of right upper arm
      M21.822 Other specified acquired deformities of left upper arm
      M21.829 Other specified acquired deformities of unspecified upper arm ▽

    ✓6ᵗʰ **M21.83** Other specified acquired deformities of forearm
      M21.831 Other specified acquired deformities of right forearm
      M21.832 Other specified acquired deformities of left forearm
      M21.839 Other specified acquired deformities of unspecified forearm ▽

    ✓6ᵗʰ **M21.85** Other specified acquired deformities of thigh
      M21.851 Other specified acquired deformities of right thigh
      M21.852 Other specified acquired deformities of left thigh
      M21.859 Other specified acquired deformities of unspecified thigh ▽

    ✓6ᵗʰ **M21.86** Other specified acquired deformities of lower leg
      M21.861 Other specified acquired deformities of right lower leg
      M21.862 Other specified acquired deformities of left lower leg
      M21.869 Other specified acquired deformities of unspecified lower leg ▽

✓5ᵗʰ **M21.9** Unspecified acquired deformity of limb and hand
    M21.90 Unspecified acquired deformity of unspecified limb ▽

    ✓6ᵗʰ **M21.92** Unspecified acquired deformity of upper arm
      M21.921 Unspecified acquired deformity of right upper arm ▽
      M21.922 Unspecified acquired deformity of left upper arm ▽
      M21.929 Unspecified acquired deformity of unspecified upper arm ▽

    ✓6ᵗʰ **M21.93** Unspecified acquired deformity of forearm
      M21.931 Unspecified acquired deformity of right forearm ▽
      M21.932 Unspecified acquired deformity of left forearm ▽
      M21.939 Unspecified acquired deformity of unspecified forearm ▽

    ✓6ᵗʰ **M21.94** Unspecified acquired deformity of hand
      M21.941 Unspecified acquired deformity of hand, right hand ▽
      M21.942 Unspecified acquired deformity of hand, left hand ▽
      M21.949 Unspecified acquired deformity of hand, unspecified hand ▽

✓ Additional Character Req   ✗7ᵗʰ Placeholder Alert   Manifestation   **HCC** CMS-HCC Condition   ▽ Unspecified Code   ▶◀ Revised Text   ● New Code   ▲ Revised Code Title

ICD-10-CM 2018   **741**

√6ᵗʰ **M21.95** Unspecified acquired deformity of thigh

     M21.951 Unspecified acquired deformity of right thigh ▽

     M21.952 Unspecified acquired deformity of left thigh ▽

     M21.959 Unspecified acquired deformity of unspecified thigh ▽

√6ᵗʰ **M21.96** Unspecified acquired deformity of lower leg

     M21.961 Unspecified acquired deformity of right lower leg ▽

     M21.962 Unspecified acquired deformity of left lower leg ▽

     M21.969 Unspecified acquired deformity of unspecified lower leg ▽

√4ᵗʰ **M22** **Disorder of patella**

     EXCLUDES 1   traumatic dislocation of patella (S83.0-)

√5ᵗʰ **M22.0** Recurrent dislocation of patella

     M22.00 Recurrent dislocation of patella, unspecified knee ▽

     M22.01 Recurrent dislocation of patella, right knee

     M22.02 Recurrent dislocation of patella, left knee

√5ᵗʰ **M22.1** Recurrent subluxation of patella

     Incomplete dislocation of patella

     M22.10 Recurrent subluxation of patella, unspecified knee ▽

     M22.11 Recurrent subluxation of patella, right knee

     M22.12 Recurrent subluxation of patella, left knee

√5ᵗʰ **M22.2** Patellofemoral disorders

     √6ᵗʰ **M22.2X** Patellofemoral disorders

         M22.2X1 Patellofemoral disorders, right knee

         M22.2X2 Patellofemoral disorders, left knee

         M22.2X9 Patellofemoral disorders, unspecified knee ▽

√5ᵗʰ **M22.3** Other derangements of patella

     √6ᵗʰ **M22.3X** Other derangements of patella

         M22.3X1 Other derangements of patella, right knee

         M22.3X2 Other derangements of patella, left knee

         M22.3X9 Other derangements of patella, unspecified knee ▽

√5ᵗʰ **M22.4** Chondromalacia patellae

     M22.40 Chondromalacia patellae, unspecified knee ▽

     M22.41 Chondromalacia patellae, right knee

     M22.42 Chondromalacia patellae, left knee

√5ᵗʰ **M22.8** Other disorders of patella

     √6ᵗʰ **M22.8X** Other disorders of patella

         M22.8X1 Other disorders of patella, right knee

         M22.8X2 Other disorders of patella, left knee

         M22.8X9 Other disorders of patella, unspecified knee ▽

√5ᵗʰ **M22.9** Unspecified disorder of patella

     M22.90 Unspecified disorder of patella, unspecified knee ▽

     M22.91 Unspecified disorder of patella, right knee ▽

     M22.92 Unspecified disorder of patella, left knee ▽

√4ᵗʰ **M23** **Internal derangement of knee**

     EXCLUDES 1   ankylosis (M24.66)

         current injury—see injury of knee and lower leg (S80-S89)

         deformity of knee (M21.-)

         osteochondritis dissecans (M93.2)

         recurrent dislocation or subluxation of joints (M24.4)

         recurrent dislocation or subluxation of patella (M22.0-M22.1)

√5ᵗʰ **M23.0** Cystic meniscus

     √6ᵗʰ **M23.00** Cystic meniscus, unspecified meniscus

         Cystic meniscus, unspecified lateral meniscus

         Cystic meniscus, unspecified medial meniscus

         M23.000 Cystic meniscus, unspecified lateral meniscus, right knee

         M23.001 Cystic meniscus, unspecified lateral meniscus, left knee

         M23.002 Cystic meniscus, unspecified lateral meniscus, unspecified knee ▽

         M23.003 Cystic meniscus, unspecified medial meniscus, right knee

         M23.004 Cystic meniscus, unspecified medial meniscus, left knee

         M23.005 Cystic meniscus, unspecified medial meniscus, unspecified knee ▽

         M23.006 Cystic meniscus, unspecified meniscus, right knee

         M23.007 Cystic meniscus, unspecified meniscus, left knee

         M23.009 Cystic meniscus, unspecified meniscus, unspecified knee ▽

     √6ᵗʰ **M23.01** Cystic meniscus, anterior horn of medial meniscus

         M23.011 Cystic meniscus, anterior horn of medial meniscus, right knee

         M23.012 Cystic meniscus, anterior horn of medial meniscus, left knee

         M23.019 Cystic meniscus, anterior horn of medial meniscus, unspecified knee ▽

     √6ᵗʰ **M23.02** Cystic meniscus, posterior horn of medial meniscus

         M23.021 Cystic meniscus, posterior horn of medial meniscus, right knee

         M23.022 Cystic meniscus, posterior horn of medial meniscus, left knee

         M23.029 Cystic meniscus, posterior horn of medial meniscus, unspecified knee ▽

     √6ᵗʰ **M23.03** Cystic meniscus, other medial meniscus

         M23.031 Cystic meniscus, other medial meniscus, right knee

         M23.032 Cystic meniscus, other medial meniscus, left knee

         M23.039 Cystic meniscus, other medial meniscus, unspecified knee ▽

     √6ᵗʰ **M23.04** Cystic meniscus, anterior horn of lateral meniscus

         M23.041 Cystic meniscus, anterior horn of lateral meniscus, right knee

         M23.042 Cystic meniscus, anterior horn of lateral meniscus, left knee

         M23.049 Cystic meniscus, anterior horn of lateral meniscus, unspecified knee ▽

     √6ᵗʰ **M23.05** Cystic meniscus, posterior horn of lateral meniscus

         M23.051 Cystic meniscus, posterior horn of lateral meniscus, right knee

         M23.052 Cystic meniscus, posterior horn of lateral meniscus, left knee

         M23.059 Cystic meniscus, posterior horn of lateral meniscus, unspecified knee ▽

     √6ᵗʰ **M23.06** Cystic meniscus, other lateral meniscus

         M23.061 Cystic meniscus, other lateral meniscus, right knee

         M23.062 Cystic meniscus, other lateral meniscus, left knee

         M23.069 Cystic meniscus, other lateral meniscus, unspecified knee ▽

√5ᵗʰ **M23.2** Derangement of meniscus due to old tear or injury

     Old bucket-handle tear

     √6ᵗʰ **M23.20** Derangement of unspecified meniscus due to old tear or injury

         Derangement of unspecified lateral meniscus due to old tear or injury

         Derangement of unspecified medial meniscus due to old tear or injury

         M23.200 Derangement of unspecified lateral meniscus due to old tear or injury, right knee ▽

         M23.201 Derangement of unspecified lateral meniscus due to old tear or injury, left knee ▽

         M23.202 Derangement of unspecified lateral meniscus due to old tear or injury, unspecified knee ▽

         M23.203 Derangement of unspecified medial meniscus due to old tear or injury, right knee ▽

         M23.204 Derangement of unspecified medial meniscus due to old tear or injury, left knee ▽

EXCLUDES 1 Not coded here   *EXCLUDES 2* Not included here   N Newborn Age: 0   P Pediatric Age: 0-17   M Maternity Age: 12-55   A Adult Age: 15-124

742   ICD-10-CM 2018

Derangement of Meniscus

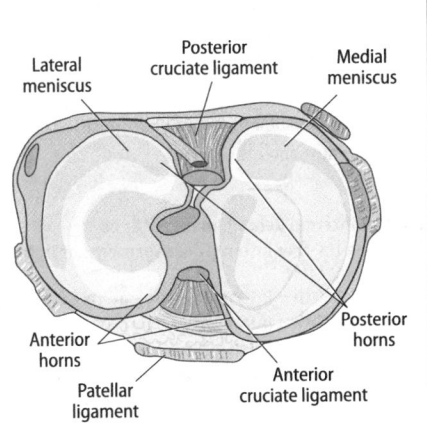

Lateral meniscus | Posterior cruciate ligament | Medial meniscus

Anterior horns

Patellar ligament

Posterior horns

Anterior cruciate ligament

Overhead view of right knee

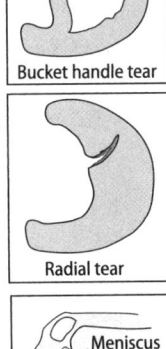

Bucket handle tear

Radial tear

Meniscus

M23.205 Derangement of unspecified medial meniscus due to old tear or injury, unspecified knee ▽

M23.206 Derangement of unspecified meniscus due to old tear or injury, right knee ▽

M23.207 Derangement of unspecified meniscus due to old tear or injury, left knee ▽

M23.209 Derangement of unspecified meniscus due to old tear or injury, unspecified knee ▽

✓6th **M23.21** Derangement of anterior horn of medial meniscus due to old tear or injury

   M23.211 Derangement of anterior horn of medial meniscus due to old tear or injury, right knee

   M23.212 Derangement of anterior horn of medial meniscus due to old tear or injury, left knee

   M23.219 Derangement of anterior horn of medial meniscus due to old tear or injury, unspecified knee ▽

✓6th **M23.22** Derangement of posterior horn of medial meniscus due to old tear or injury

   M23.221 Derangement of posterior horn of medial meniscus due to old tear or injury, right knee

   M23.222 Derangement of posterior horn of medial meniscus due to old tear or injury, left knee

   M23.229 Derangement of posterior horn of medial meniscus due to old tear or injury, unspecified knee ▽

✓6th **M23.23** Derangement of other medial meniscus due to old tear or injury

   M23.231 Derangement of other medial meniscus due to old tear or injury, right knee

   M23.232 Derangement of other medial meniscus due to old tear or injury, left knee

   M23.239 Derangement of other medial meniscus due to old tear or injury, unspecified knee ▽

✓6th **M23.24** Derangement of anterior horn of lateral meniscus due to old tear or injury

   M23.241 Derangement of anterior horn of lateral meniscus due to old tear or injury, right knee

   M23.242 Derangement of anterior horn of lateral meniscus due to old tear or injury, left knee

   M23.249 Derangement of anterior horn of lateral meniscus due to old tear or injury, unspecified knee ▽

✓6th **M23.25** Derangement of posterior horn of lateral meniscus due to old tear or injury

   M23.251 Derangement of posterior horn of lateral meniscus due to old tear or injury, right knee

   M23.252 Derangement of posterior horn of lateral meniscus due to old tear or injury, left knee

   M23.259 Derangement of posterior horn of lateral meniscus due to old tear or injury, unspecified knee ▽

✓6th **M23.26** Derangement of other lateral meniscus due to old tear or injury

   M23.261 Derangement of other lateral meniscus due to old tear or injury, right knee

   M23.262 Derangement of other lateral meniscus due to old tear or injury, left knee

   M23.269 Derangement of other lateral meniscus due to old tear or injury, unspecified knee ▽

✓5th **M23.3 Other meniscus derangements**
   Degenerate meniscus
   Detached meniscus
   Retained meniscus

✓6th **M23.30** Other meniscus derangements, unspecified meniscus
   Other meniscus derangements, unspecified lateral meniscus
   Other meniscus derangements, unspecified medial meniscus

   M23.300 Other meniscus derangements, unspecified lateral meniscus, right knee ▽

   M23.301 Other meniscus derangements, unspecified lateral meniscus, left knee ▽

   M23.302 Other meniscus derangements, unspecified lateral meniscus, unspecified knee ▽

   M23.303 Other meniscus derangements, unspecified medial meniscus, right knee ▽

   M23.304 Other meniscus derangements, unspecified medial meniscus, left knee ▽

   M23.305 Other meniscus derangements, unspecified medial meniscus, unspecified knee ▽

   M23.306 Other meniscus derangements, unspecified meniscus, right knee ▽

   M23.307 Other meniscus derangements, unspecified meniscus, left knee ▽

   M23.309 Other meniscus derangements, unspecified meniscus, unspecified knee ▽

✓6th **M23.31** Other meniscus derangements, anterior horn of medial meniscus

   M23.311 Other meniscus derangements, anterior horn of medial meniscus, right knee

   M23.312 Other meniscus derangements, anterior horn of medial meniscus, left knee

   M23.319 Other meniscus derangements, anterior horn of medial meniscus, unspecified knee ▽

✓6th **M23.32** Other meniscus derangements, posterior horn of medial meniscus

   M23.321 Other meniscus derangements, posterior horn of medial meniscus, right knee

   M23.322 Other meniscus derangements, posterior horn of medial meniscus, left knee

   M23.329 Other meniscus derangements, posterior horn of medial meniscus, unspecified knee ▽

✓6th **M23.33** Other meniscus derangements, other medial meniscus

   M23.331 Other meniscus derangements, other medial meniscus, right knee

   M23.332 Other meniscus derangements, other medial meniscus, left knee

   M23.339 Other meniscus derangements, other medial meniscus, unspecified knee ▽

✓6th **M23.34** Other meniscus derangements, anterior horn of lateral meniscus

   M23.341 Other meniscus derangements, anterior horn of lateral meniscus, right knee

☑ Additional Character Req   ✓7th Placeholder Alert   Manifestation   HCC CMS-HCC Condition   ▽ Unspecified Code   ▶◀ Revised Text   ● New Code   ▲ Revised Code Title

ICD-10-CM 2018   **743**

M23.342　Other meniscus derangements, anterior horn of lateral meniscus, **left** knee

M23.349　Other meniscus derangements, anterior horn of lateral meniscus, unspecified knee ▽

✓6th **M23.35**　Other meniscus derangements, posterior horn of lateral meniscus

M23.351　Other meniscus derangements, posterior horn of lateral meniscus, **right** knee

M23.352　Other meniscus derangements, posterior horn of lateral meniscus, **left** knee

M23.359　Other meniscus derangements, posterior horn of lateral meniscus, unspecified knee ▽

✓6th **M23.36**　Other meniscus derangements, other lateral meniscus

M23.361　Other meniscus derangements, other lateral meniscus, **right** knee

M23.362　Other meniscus derangements, other lateral meniscus, **left** knee

M23.369　Other meniscus derangements, other lateral meniscus, unspecified knee ▽

✓5th **M23.4**　Loose body in knee

M23.40　Loose body in knee, unspecified knee ▽

M23.41　Loose body in knee, **right** knee

M23.42　Loose body in knee, **left** knee

✓5th **M23.5**　Chronic instability of knee

M23.50　Chronic instability of knee, unspecified knee ▽

M23.51　Chronic instability of knee, **right** knee

M23.52　Chronic instability of knee, **left** knee

✓5th **M23.6**　Other spontaneous disruption of ligament(s) of knee

✓6th **M23.60**　Other spontaneous disruption of unspecified ligament of knee

M23.601　Other spontaneous disruption of unspecified ligament of **right** knee ▽

M23.602　Other spontaneous disruption of unspecified ligament of **left** knee ▽

M23.609　Other spontaneous disruption of unspecified ligament of unspecified knee ▽

✓6th **M23.61**　Other spontaneous disruption of anterior cruciate ligament of knee

M23.611　Other spontaneous disruption of anterior cruciate ligament of **right** knee

M23.612　Other spontaneous disruption of anterior cruciate ligament of **left** knee

M23.619　Other spontaneous disruption of anterior cruciate ligament of unspecified knee ▽

✓6th **M23.62**　Other spontaneous disruption of posterior cruciate ligament of knee

M23.621　Other spontaneous disruption of posterior cruciate ligament of **right** knee

M23.622　Other spontaneous disruption of posterior cruciate ligament of **left** knee

M23.629　Other spontaneous disruption of posterior cruciate ligament of unspecified knee ▽

✓6th **M23.63**　Other spontaneous disruption of medial collateral ligament of knee

M23.631　Other spontaneous disruption of medial collateral ligament of **right** knee

M23.632　Other spontaneous disruption of medial collateral ligament of **left** knee

M23.639　Other spontaneous disruption of medial collateral ligament of unspecified knee ▽

✓6th **M23.64**　Other spontaneous disruption of lateral collateral ligament of knee

M23.641　Other spontaneous disruption of lateral collateral ligament of **right** knee

M23.642　Other spontaneous disruption of lateral collateral ligament of **left** knee

M23.649　Other spontaneous disruption of lateral collateral ligament of unspecified knee ▽

✓6th **M23.67**　Other spontaneous disruption of capsular ligament of knee

M23.671　Other spontaneous disruption of capsular ligament of **right** knee

M23.672　Other spontaneous disruption of capsular ligament of **left** knee

M23.679　Other spontaneous disruption of capsular ligament of unspecified knee ▽

✓5th **M23.8**　Other internal derangements of knee
Laxity of ligament of knee
Snapping knee

✓6th **M23.8X**　Other internal derangements of knee

M23.8X1　Other internal derangements of **right** knee

M23.8X2　Other internal derangements of **left** knee

M23.8X9　Other internal derangements of unspecified knee ▽

✓5th **M23.9**　Unspecified internal derangement of knee

M23.90　Unspecified internal derangement of unspecified knee ▽

M23.91　Unspecified internal derangement of **right** knee ▽

M23.92　Unspecified internal derangement of **left** knee ▽

✓4th **M24**　Other specific joint derangements
EXCLUDES 1　current injury—see injury of joint by body region
EXCLUDES 2　ganglion (M67.4)
snapping knee (M23.8-)
temporomandibular joint disorders (M26.6-)

✓5th **M24.0**　Loose body in joint
EXCLUDES 2　loose body in knee (M23.4)

M24.00　Loose body in unspecified joint ▽

✓6th **M24.01**　Loose body in shoulder

M24.011　Loose body in **right** shoulder

M24.012　Loose body in **left** shoulder

M24.019　Loose body in unspecified shoulder ▽

✓6th **M24.02**　Loose body in elbow

M24.021　Loose body in **right** elbow

M24.022　Loose body in **left** elbow

M24.029　Loose body in unspecified elbow ▽

✓6th **M24.03**　Loose body in wrist

M24.031　Loose body in **right** wrist

M24.032　Loose body in **left** wrist

M24.039　Loose body in unspecified wrist ▽

✓6th **M24.04**　Loose body in finger joints

M24.041　Loose body in **right** finger joint(s)

M24.042　Loose body in **left** finger joint(s)

M24.049　Loose body in unspecified finger joint(s) ▽

✓6th **M24.05**　Loose body in hip

M24.051　Loose body in **right** hip

M24.052　Loose body in **left** hip

M24.059　Loose body in unspecified hip ▽

✓6th **M24.07**　Loose body in ankle and toe joints

M24.071　Loose body in **right** ankle

M24.072　Loose body in **left** ankle

M24.073　Loose body in unspecified ankle ▽

M24.074　Loose body in **right** toe joint(s)

M24.075　Loose body in **left** toe joint(s)

M24.076　Loose body in unspecified toe joints ▽

M24.08　Loose body, other site

✓5th **M24.1**　Other articular cartilage disorders
EXCLUDES 2　chondrocalcinosis (M11.1, M11.2-)
internal derangement of knee (M23.-)
metastatic calcification (E83.5)
ochronosis (E70.2)

M24.10　Other articular cartilage disorders, unspecified site ▽

✓6th **M24.11**　Other articular cartilage disorders, shoulder

M24.111　Other articular cartilage disorders, **right** shoulder

M24.112　Other articular cartilage disorders, **left** shoulder

M24.119　Other articular cartilage disorders, unspecified shoulder ▽

EXCLUDES 1 Not coded here　　EXCLUDES 2 Not included here　　N Newborn Age: 0　　P Pediatric Age: 0-17　　M Maternity Age: 12-55　　A Adult Age: 15-124

744
ICD-10-CM 2018

✓6ᵗʰ **M24.12** **Other articular cartilage disorders,** elbow

     M24.121 **Other articular cartilage disorders,** right elbow

     M24.122 **Other articular cartilage disorders,** left elbow

     M24.129 **Other articular cartilage disorders,** ▽ unspecified elbow

✓6ᵗʰ **M24.13** **Other articular cartilage disorders,** wrist

     M24.131 **Other articular cartilage disorders,** right wrist

     M24.132 **Other articular cartilage disorders,** left wrist

     M24.139 **Other articular cartilage disorders,** ▽ unspecified wrist

✓6ᵗʰ **M24.14** **Other articular cartilage disorders,** hand

     M24.141 **Other articular cartilage disorders,** right hand

     M24.142 **Other articular cartilage disorders,** left hand

     M24.149 **Other articular cartilage disorders,** ▽ unspecified hand

✓6ᵗʰ **M24.15** **Other articular cartilage disorders,** hip

     M24.151 **Other articular cartilage disorders,** right hip

     M24.152 **Other articular cartilage disorders,** left hip

     M24.159 **Other articular cartilage disorders,** ▽ unspecified hip

✓6ᵗʰ **M24.17** **Other articular cartilage disorders,** ankle and foot

     M24.171 **Other articular cartilage disorders,** right ankle

     M24.172 **Other articular cartilage disorders,** left ankle

     M24.173 **Other articular cartilage disorders,** ▽ unspecified ankle

     M24.174 **Other articular cartilage disorders,** right foot

     M24.175 **Other articular cartilage disorders,** left foot

     M24.176 **Other articular cartilage disorders,** ▽ unspecified foot

✓5ᵗʰ **M24.2** **Disorder of ligament**

     Instability secondary to old ligament injury

     Ligamentous laxity NOS

     EXCLUDES 1   familial ligamentous laxity (M35.7)

     EXCLUDES 2   internal derangement of knee (M23.5-M23.89)

     M24.20 **Disorder of ligament, unspecified site** ▽

✓6ᵗʰ **M24.21** **Disorder of ligament,** shoulder

     M24.211 **Disorder of ligament,** right shoulder

     M24.212 **Disorder of ligament,** left shoulder

     M24.219 **Disorder of ligament, unspecified** ▽ shoulder

✓6ᵗʰ **M24.22** **Disorder of ligament,** elbow

     M24.221 **Disorder of ligament,** right elbow

     M24.222 **Disorder of ligament,** left elbow

     M24.229 **Disorder of ligament, unspecified** ▽ elbow

✓6ᵗʰ **M24.23** **Disorder of ligament,** wrist

     M24.231 **Disorder of ligament,** right wrist

     M24.232 **Disorder of ligament,** left wrist

     M24.239 **Disorder of ligament, unspecified wrist** ▽

✓6ᵗʰ **M24.24** **Disorder of ligament,** hand

     M24.241 **Disorder of ligament,** right hand

     M24.242 **Disorder of ligament,** left hand

     M24.249 **Disorder of ligament, unspecified hand** ▽

✓6ᵗʰ **M24.25** **Disorder of ligament,** hip

     M24.251 **Disorder of ligament,** right hip

     M24.252 **Disorder of ligament,** left hip

     M24.259 **Disorder of ligament, unspecified hip** ▽

✓6ᵗʰ **M24.27** **Disorder of ligament,** ankle and foot

     M24.271 **Disorder of ligament,** right ankle

     M24.272 **Disorder of ligament,** left ankle

     M24.273 **Disorder of ligament, unspecified ankle** ▽

     M24.274 **Disorder of ligament,** right foot

     M24.275 **Disorder of ligament,** left foot

     M24.276 **Disorder of ligament, unspecified foot** ▽

M24.28 **Disorder of ligament,** vertebrae

✓5ᵗʰ **M24.3** **Pathological dislocation of joint, not elsewhere classified**

     EXCLUDES 1   congenital dislocation or displacement of joint—see congenital malformations and deformations of the musculoskeletal system (Q65-Q79)

                 current injury—see injury of joints and ligaments by body region

                 recurrent dislocation of joint (M24.4-)

     M24.30 **Pathological dislocation of unspecified joint,** ▽ **not elsewhere classified**

✓6ᵗʰ **M24.31** **Pathological dislocation of** shoulder, **not elsewhere classified**

     M24.311 **Pathological dislocation of** right **shoulder, not elsewhere classified**

     M24.312 **Pathological dislocation of** left **shoulder, not elsewhere classified**

     M24.319 **Pathological dislocation of unspecified** ▽ **shoulder, not elsewhere classified**

✓6ᵗʰ **M24.32** **Pathological dislocation of** elbow, **not elsewhere classified**

     M24.321 **Pathological dislocation of** right **elbow, not elsewhere classified**

     M24.322 **Pathological dislocation of** left **elbow, not elsewhere classified**

     M24.329 **Pathological dislocation of unspecified** ▽ **elbow, not elsewhere classified**

✓6ᵗʰ **M24.33** **Pathological dislocation of** wrist, **not elsewhere classified**

     M24.331 **Pathological dislocation of** right **wrist, not elsewhere classified**

     M24.332 **Pathological dislocation of** left **wrist, not elsewhere classified**

     M24.339 **Pathological dislocation of unspecified** ▽ **wrist, not elsewhere classified**

✓6ᵗʰ **M24.34** **Pathological dislocation of** hand, **not elsewhere classified**

     M24.341 **Pathological dislocation of** right **hand, not elsewhere classified**

     M24.342 **Pathological dislocation of** left **hand, not elsewhere classified**

     M24.349 **Pathological dislocation of unspecified** ▽ **hand, not elsewhere classified**

✓6ᵗʰ **M24.35** **Pathological dislocation of** hip, **not elsewhere classified**

     M24.351 **Pathological dislocation of** right **hip, not elsewhere classified**

     M24.352 **Pathological dislocation of** left **hip, not elsewhere classified**

     M24.359 **Pathological dislocation of unspecified** ▽ **hip, not elsewhere classified**

✓6ᵗʰ **M24.36** **Pathological dislocation of** knee, **not elsewhere classified**

     M24.361 **Pathological dislocation of** right **knee, not elsewhere classified**

     M24.362 **Pathological dislocation of** left **knee, not elsewhere classified**

     M24.369 **Pathological dislocation of unspecified** ▽ **knee, not elsewhere classified**

✓6ᵗʰ **M24.37** **Pathological dislocation of** ankle and foot, **not elsewhere classified**

     M24.371 **Pathological dislocation of** right **ankle, not elsewhere classified**

     M24.372 **Pathological dislocation of** left **ankle, not elsewhere classified**

     M24.373 **Pathological dislocation of unspecified** ▽ **ankle, not elsewhere classified**

     M24.374 **Pathological dislocation of** right **foot, not elsewhere classified**

     M24.375 **Pathological dislocation of** left **foot, not elsewhere classified**

     M24.376 **Pathological dislocation of unspecified** ▽ **foot, not elsewhere classified**

☑ Additional Character Req   ✓7ᵗʰ Placeholder Alert   Manifestation   ᴴᶜᶜ CMS-HCC Condition   ▽ Unspecified Code   ▶◀ Revised Text   ● New Code   ▲ Revised Code Title

Chapter 13. Diseases of the Musculoskeletal System and Connective Tissue

M24.4–M24.829

✓5ᵗʰ M24.4 Recurrent dislocation of joint
　　　Recurrent subluxation of joint
　　　EXCLUDES 2　recurrent dislocation of patella (M22.0-M22.1)
　　　　　　　　recurrent vertebral dislocation (M43.3-, M43.4, M43.5-)
　　M24.40　Recurrent dislocation, unspecified joint ▽
　　✓6ᵗʰ M24.41　Recurrent dislocation, shoulder
　　　　M24.411　Recurrent dislocation, right shoulder
　　　　M24.412　Recurrent dislocation, left shoulder
　　　　M24.419　Recurrent dislocation, unspecified ▽
　　　　　　　　shoulder
　　✓6ᵗʰ M24.42　Recurrent dislocation, elbow
　　　　M24.421　Recurrent dislocation, right elbow
　　　　M24.422　Recurrent dislocation, left elbow
　　　　M24.429　Recurrent dislocation, unspecified ▽
　　　　　　　　elbow
　　✓6ᵗʰ M24.43　Recurrent dislocation, wrist
　　　　M24.431　Recurrent dislocation, right wrist
　　　　M24.432　Recurrent dislocation, left wrist
　　　　M24.439　Recurrent dislocation, unspecified wrist ▽
　　✓6ᵗʰ M24.44　Recurrent dislocation, hand and finger(s)
　　　　M24.441　Recurrent dislocation, right hand
　　　　M24.442　Recurrent dislocation, left hand
　　　　M24.443　Recurrent dislocation, unspecified hand ▽
　　　　M24.444　Recurrent dislocation, right finger
　　　　M24.445　Recurrent dislocation, left finger
　　　　M24.446　Recurrent dislocation, unspecified ▽
　　　　　　　　finger
　　✓6ᵗʰ M24.45　Recurrent dislocation, hip
　　　　M24.451　Recurrent dislocation, right hip
　　　　M24.452　Recurrent dislocation, left hip
　　　　M24.459　Recurrent dislocation, unspecified hip ▽
　　✓6ᵗʰ M24.46　Recurrent dislocation, knee
　　　　M24.461　Recurrent dislocation, right knee
　　　　M24.462　Recurrent dislocation, left knee
　　　　M24.469　Recurrent dislocation, unspecified knee ▽
　　✓6ᵗʰ M24.47　Recurrent dislocation, ankle, foot and toes
　　　　M24.471　Recurrent dislocation, right ankle
　　　　M24.472　Recurrent dislocation, left ankle
　　　　M24.473　Recurrent dislocation, unspecified ▽
　　　　　　　　ankle
　　　　M24.474　Recurrent dislocation, right foot
　　　　M24.475　Recurrent dislocation, left foot
　　　　M24.476　Recurrent dislocation, unspecified foot ▽
　　　　M24.477　Recurrent dislocation, right toe(s)
　　　　M24.478　Recurrent dislocation, left toe(s)
　　　　M24.479　Recurrent dislocation, unspecified ▽
　　　　　　　　toe(s)

✓5ᵗʰ M24.5 Contracture of joint
　　　EXCLUDES 1　contracture of muscle without contracture of joint
　　　　　　　　(M62.4-)
　　　　　　　contracture of tendon (sheath) without contracture of
　　　　　　　joint (M62.4-)
　　　　　　　Dupuytren's contracture (M72.0)
　　　EXCLUDES 2　acquired deformities of limbs (M20-M21)
　　　AHA: 2016, 2Q, 6
　　M24.50　Contracture, unspecified joint ▽
　　✓6ᵗʰ M24.51　Contracture, shoulder
　　　　M24.511　Contracture, right shoulder
　　　　M24.512　Contracture, left shoulder
　　　　M24.519　Contracture, unspecified shoulder ▽
　　✓6ᵗʰ M24.52　Contracture, elbow
　　　　M24.521　Contracture, right elbow
　　　　M24.522　Contracture, left elbow
　　　　M24.529　Contracture, unspecified elbow ▽
　　✓6ᵗʰ M24.53　Contracture, wrist
　　　　M24.531　Contracture, right wrist
　　　　M24.532　Contracture, left wrist
　　　　M24.539　Contracture, unspecified wrist ▽
　　✓6ᵗʰ M24.54　Contracture, hand
　　　　M24.541　Contracture, right hand
　　　　M24.542　Contracture, left hand
　　　　M24.549　Contracture, unspecified hand ▽

✓6ᵗʰ M24.55　Contracture, hip
　　　M24.551　Contracture, right hip
　　　M24.552　Contracture, left hip
　　　M24.559　Contracture, unspecified hip ▽
✓6ᵗʰ M24.56　Contracture, knee
　　　M24.561　Contracture, right knee
　　　M24.562　Contracture, left knee
　　　M24.569　Contracture, unspecified knee ▽
✓6ᵗʰ M24.57　Contracture, ankle and foot
　　　M24.571　Contracture, right ankle
　　　M24.572　Contracture, left ankle
　　　M24.573　Contracture, unspecified ankle ▽
　　　M24.574　Contracture, right foot
　　　M24.575　Contracture, left foot
　　　M24.576　Contracture, unspecified foot ▽

✓5ᵗʰ M24.6 Ankylosis of joint
　　　EXCLUDES 1　stiffness of joint without ankylosis (M25.6-)
　　　EXCLUDES 2　spine (M43.2-)
　　M24.60　Ankylosis, unspecified joint ▽
　　✓6ᵗʰ M24.61　Ankylosis, shoulder
　　　　M24.611　Ankylosis, right shoulder
　　　　M24.612　Ankylosis, left shoulder
　　　　M24.619　Ankylosis, unspecified shoulder ▽
　　✓6ᵗʰ M24.62　Ankylosis, elbow
　　　　M24.621　Ankylosis, right elbow
　　　　M24.622　Ankylosis, left elbow
　　　　M24.629　Ankylosis, unspecified elbow ▽
　　✓6ᵗʰ M24.63　Ankylosis, wrist
　　　　M24.631　Ankylosis, right wrist
　　　　M24.632　Ankylosis, left wrist
　　　　M24.639　Ankylosis, unspecified wrist ▽
　　✓6ᵗʰ M24.64　Ankylosis, hand
　　　　M24.641　Ankylosis, right hand
　　　　M24.642　Ankylosis, left hand
　　　　M24.649　Ankylosis, unspecified hand ▽
　　✓6ᵗʰ M24.65　Ankylosis, hip
　　　　M24.651　Ankylosis, right hip
　　　　M24.652　Ankylosis, left hip
　　　　M24.659　Ankylosis, unspecified hip ▽
　　✓6ᵗʰ M24.66　Ankylosis, knee
　　　　M24.661　Ankylosis, right knee
　　　　M24.662　Ankylosis, left knee
　　　　M24.669　Ankylosis, unspecified knee ▽
　　✓6ᵗʰ M24.67　Ankylosis, ankle and foot
　　　　M24.671　Ankylosis, right ankle
　　　　M24.672　Ankylosis, left ankle
　　　　M24.673　Ankylosis, unspecified ankle ▽
　　　　M24.674　Ankylosis, right foot
　　　　M24.675　Ankylosis, left foot
　　　　M24.676　Ankylosis, unspecified foot ▽

M24.7 Protrusio acetabuli

✓5ᵗʰ M24.8 Other specific joint derangements, not elsewhere classified
　　　EXCLUDES 2　iliotibial band syndrome (M76.3)
　　M24.80　Other specific joint derangements of unspecified ▽
　　　　　　joint, not elsewhere classified
　　✓6ᵗʰ M24.81　Other specific joint derangements of shoulder, not
　　　　　　elsewhere classified
　　　　M24.811　Other specific joint derangements of right
　　　　　　　　shoulder, not elsewhere classified
　　　　M24.812　Other specific joint derangements of left
　　　　　　　　shoulder, not elsewhere classified
　　　　M24.819　Other specific joint derangements of ▽
　　　　　　　　unspecified shoulder, not elsewhere
　　　　　　　　classified
　　✓6ᵗʰ M24.82　Other specific joint derangements of elbow, not
　　　　　　elsewhere classified
　　　　M24.821　Other specific joint derangements of
　　　　　　　　right elbow, not elsewhere classified
　　　　M24.822　Other specific joint derangements of
　　　　　　　　left elbow, not elsewhere classified
　　　　M24.829　Other specific joint derangements of ▽
　　　　　　　　unspecified elbow, not elsewhere
　　　　　　　　classified

✓6ᵗʰ **M24.83** **Other specific joint derangements of wrist, not elsewhere classified**

    M24.831 **Other specific joint derangements of right wrist, not elsewhere classified**

    M24.832 **Other specific joint derangements of left wrist, not elsewhere classified**

    M24.839 **Other specific joint derangements of unspecified wrist, not elsewhere classified** ▽

✓6ᵗʰ **M24.84** **Other specific joint derangements of hand, not elsewhere classified**

    M24.841 **Other specific joint derangements of right hand, not elsewhere classified**

    M24.842 **Other specific joint derangements of left hand, not elsewhere classified**

    M24.849 **Other specific joint derangements of unspecified hand, not elsewhere classified** ▽

✓6ᵗʰ **M24.85** **Other specific joint derangements of hip, not elsewhere classified**
    Irritable hip

    M24.851 **Other specific joint derangements of right hip, not elsewhere classified**

    M24.852 **Other specific joint derangements of left hip, not elsewhere classified**

    M24.859 **Other specific joint derangements of unspecified hip, not elsewhere classified** ▽

✓6ᵗʰ **M24.87** **Other specific joint derangements of ankle and foot, not elsewhere classified**

    M24.871 **Other specific joint derangements of right ankle, not elsewhere classified**

    M24.872 **Other specific joint derangements of left ankle, not elsewhere classified**

    M24.873 **Other specific joint derangements of unspecified ankle, not elsewhere classified** ▽

    M24.874 **Other specific joint derangements of right foot, not elsewhere classified**

    M24.875 **Other specific joint derangements left foot, not elsewhere classified**

    M24.876 **Other specific joint derangements of unspecified foot, not elsewhere classified** ▽

M24.9 **Joint derangement, unspecified** ▽

✓4ᵗʰ **M25** **Other joint disorder, not elsewhere classified**
    EXCLUDES 2 *abnormality of gait and mobility (R26.-)*
        acquired deformities of limb (M20-M21)
        calcification of bursa (M71.4-)
        calcification of shoulder (joint) (M75.3)
        calcification of tendon (M65.2-)
        difficulty in walking (R26.2)
        temporomandibular joint disorder (M26.6-)

✓5ᵗʰ **M25.0** **Hemarthrosis**
    EXCLUDES 1 *current injury—see injury of joint by body region*
        hemophilic arthropathy (M36.2)

    M25.00 **Hemarthrosis, unspecified joint** ▽

✓6ᵗʰ **M25.01** **Hemarthrosis, shoulder**
    M25.011 **Hemarthrosis, right shoulder**
    M25.012 **Hemarthrosis, left shoulder**
    M25.019 **Hemarthrosis, unspecified shoulder** ▽

✓6ᵗʰ **M25.02** **Hemarthrosis, elbow**
    M25.021 **Hemarthrosis, right elbow**
    M25.022 **Hemarthrosis, left elbow**
    M25.029 **Hemarthrosis, unspecified elbow** ▽

✓6ᵗʰ **M25.03** **Hemarthrosis, wrist**
    M25.031 **Hemarthrosis, right wrist**
    M25.032 **Hemarthrosis, left wrist**
    M25.039 **Hemarthrosis, unspecified wrist** ▽

✓6ᵗʰ **M25.04** **Hemarthrosis, hand**
    M25.041 **Hemarthrosis, right hand**
    M25.042 **Hemarthrosis, left hand**
    M25.049 **Hemarthrosis, unspecified hand** ▽

✓6ᵗʰ **M25.05** **Hemarthrosis, hip**
    M25.051 **Hemarthrosis, right hip**
    M25.052 **Hemarthrosis, left hip**
    M25.059 **Hemarthrosis, unspecified hip** ▽

✓6ᵗʰ **M25.06** **Hemarthrosis, knee**
    M25.061 **Hemarthrosis, right knee**
    M25.062 **Hemarthrosis, left knee**

    M25.069 **Hemarthrosis, unspecified knee** ▽

✓6ᵗʰ **M25.07** **Hemarthrosis, ankle and foot**
    M25.071 **Hemarthrosis, right ankle**
    M25.072 **Hemarthrosis, left ankle**
    M25.073 **Hemarthrosis, unspecified ankle** ▽
    M25.074 **Hemarthrosis, right foot**
    M25.075 **Hemarthrosis, left foot**
    M25.076 **Hemarthrosis, unspecified foot** ▽

    M25.08 **Hemarthrosis, other specified site**
        Hemarthrosis, vertebrae

✓5ᵗʰ **M25.1** **Fistula of joint**
    M25.10 **Fistula, unspecified joint** ▽

✓6ᵗʰ **M25.11** **Fistula, shoulder**
    M25.111 **Fistula, right shoulder**
    M25.112 **Fistula, left shoulder**
    M25.119 **Fistula, unspecified shoulder** ▽

✓6ᵗʰ **M25.12** **Fistula, elbow**
    M25.121 **Fistula, right elbow**
    M25.122 **Fistula, left elbow**
    M25.129 **Fistula, unspecified elbow** ▽

✓6ᵗʰ **M25.13** **Fistula, wrist**
    M25.131 **Fistula, right wrist**
    M25.132 **Fistula, left wrist**
    M25.139 **Fistula, unspecified wrist** ▽

✓6ᵗʰ **M25.14** **Fistula, hand**
    M25.141 **Fistula, right hand**
    M25.142 **Fistula, left hand**
    M25.149 **Fistula, unspecified hand** ▽

✓6ᵗʰ **M25.15** **Fistula, hip**
    M25.151 **Fistula, right hip**
    M25.152 **Fistula, left hip**
    M25.159 **Fistula, unspecified hip** ▽

✓6ᵗʰ **M25.16** **Fistula, knee**
    M25.161 **Fistula, right knee**
    M25.162 **Fistula, left knee**
    M25.169 **Fistula, unspecified knee** ▽

✓6ᵗʰ **M25.17** **Fistula, ankle and foot**
    M25.171 **Fistula, right ankle**
    M25.172 **Fistula, left ankle**
    M25.173 **Fistula, unspecified ankle** ▽
    M25.174 **Fistula, right foot**
    M25.175 **Fistula, left foot**
    M25.176 **Fistula, unspecified foot** ▽

    M25.18 **Fistula, other specified site**
        Fistula, vertebrae

✓5ᵗʰ **M25.2** **Flail joint**
    M25.20 **Flail joint, unspecified joint** ▽

✓6ᵗʰ **M25.21** **Flail joint, shoulder**
    M25.211 **Flail joint, right shoulder**
    M25.212 **Flail joint, left shoulder**
    M25.219 **Flail joint, unspecified shoulder** ▽

✓6ᵗʰ **M25.22** **Flail joint, elbow**
    M25.221 **Flail joint, right elbow**
    M25.222 **Flail joint, left elbow**
    M25.229 **Flail joint, unspecified elbow** ▽

✓6ᵗʰ **M25.23** **Flail joint, wrist**
    M25.231 **Flail joint, right wrist**
    M25.232 **Flail joint, left wrist**
    M25.239 **Flail joint, unspecified wrist** ▽

✓6ᵗʰ **M25.24** **Flail joint, hand**
    M25.241 **Flail joint, right hand**
    M25.242 **Flail joint, left hand**
    M25.249 **Flail joint, unspecified hand** ▽

✓6ᵗʰ **M25.25** **Flail joint, hip**
    M25.251 **Flail joint, right hip**
    M25.252 **Flail joint, left hip**
    M25.259 **Flail joint, unspecified hip** ▽

✓6ᵗʰ **M25.26** **Flail joint, knee**
    M25.261 **Flail joint, right knee**
    M25.262 **Flail joint, left knee**
    M25.269 **Flail joint, unspecified knee** ▽

✓ Additional Character Req   ✓x7ᵗʰ Placeholder Alert   Manifestation   HCC CMS-HCC Condition   ▽ Unspecified Code   ►◄ Revised Text   ● New Code   ▲ Revised Code Title

ICD-10-CM 2018   747

✓6ᵗʰ **M25.27 Flail joint,** ankle and foot
     M25.271 Flail joint, right **ankle and foot**
     M25.272 Flail joint, left **ankle and foot**
     M25.279 Flail joint, unspecified ankle and foot ▽
M25.28 Flail joint, other site

✓5ᵗʰ **M25.3 Other instability of joint**
     EXCLUDES 1   *instability of joint secondary to old ligament injury (M24.2-)*
               instability of joint secondary to removal of joint prosthesis (M96.8-)
     EXCLUDES 2   *spinal instabilities (M53.2-)*
     M25.30 Other instability, unspecified joint ▽
✓6ᵗʰ **M25.31 Other instability,** shoulder
     M25.311 Other instability, right **shoulder**
     M25.312 Other instability, left **shoulder**
     M25.319 Other instability, unspecified shoulder ▽
✓6ᵗʰ **M25.32 Other instability,** elbow
     M25.321 Other instability, right **elbow**
     M25.322 Other instability, left **elbow**
     M25.329 Other instability, unspecified elbow ▽
✓6ᵗʰ **M25.33 Other instability,** wrist
     M25.331 Other instability, right **wrist**
     M25.332 Other instability, left **wrist**
     M25.339 Other instability, unspecified wrist ▽
✓6ᵗʰ **M25.34 Other instability,** hand
     M25.341 Other instability, right **hand**
     M25.342 Other instability, left **hand**
     M25.349 Other instability, unspecified hand ▽
✓6ᵗʰ **M25.35 Other instability,** hip
     M25.351 Other instability, right **hip**
     M25.352 Other instability, left **hip**
     M25.359 Other instability, unspecified hip ▽
✓6ᵗʰ **M25.36 Other instability,** knee
     M25.361 Other instability, right **knee**
     M25.362 Other instability, left **knee**
     M25.369 Other instability, unspecified knee ▽
✓6ᵗʰ **M25.37 Other instability,** ankle and foot
     M25.371 Other instability, right **ankle**
     M25.372 Other instability, left **ankle**
     M25.373 Other instability, unspecified ankle ▽
     M25.374 Other instability, right **foot**
     M25.375 Other instability, left **foot**
     M25.376 Other instability, unspecified foot ▽

✓5ᵗʰ **M25.4 Effusion of joint**
     EXCLUDES 1   *hydrarthrosis in yaws (A66.6)*
               intermittent hydrarthrosis (M12.4-)
               other infective (teno)synovitis (M65.1-)
     M25.40 Effusion, unspecified joint ▽
✓6ᵗʰ **M25.41 Effusion,** shoulder
     M25.411 Effusion, right **shoulder**
     M25.412 Effusion, left **shoulder**
     M25.419 Effusion, unspecified shoulder ▽
✓6ᵗʰ **M25.42 Effusion,** elbow
     M25.421 Effusion, right **elbow**
     M25.422 Effusion, left **elbow**
     M25.429 Effusion, unspecified elbow ▽
✓6ᵗʰ **M25.43 Effusion,** wrist
     M25.431 Effusion, right **wrist**
     M25.432 Effusion, left **wrist**
     M25.439 Effusion, unspecified wrist ▽
✓6ᵗʰ **M25.44 Effusion,** hand
     M25.441 Effusion, right **hand**
     M25.442 Effusion, left **hand**
     M25.449 Effusion, unspecified hand ▽
✓6ᵗʰ **M25.45 Effusion,** hip
     M25.451 Effusion, right **hip**
     M25.452 Effusion, left **hip**
     M25.459 Effusion, unspecified hip ▽
✓6ᵗʰ **M25.46 Effusion,** knee
     M25.461 Effusion, right **knee**
     M25.462 Effusion, left **knee**
     M25.469 Effusion, unspecified knee ▽

✓6ᵗʰ **M25.47 Effusion,** ankle and foot
     M25.471 Effusion, right **ankle**
     M25.472 Effusion, left **ankle**
     M25.473 Effusion, unspecified ankle ▽
     M25.474 Effusion, right **foot**
     M25.475 Effusion, left **foot**
     M25.476 Effusion, unspecified foot ▽
M25.48 Effusion, other site

✓5ᵗʰ **M25.5 Pain in joint**
     EXCLUDES 2   *pain in hand (M79.64-)*
               pain in fingers (M79.64-)
               pain in foot (M79.67-)
               pain in limb (M79.6-)
               pain in toes (M79.67-)
     M25.50 Pain in unspecified joint ▽
✓6ᵗʰ **M25.51 Pain in** shoulder
     M25.511 Pain in right **shoulder**
     M25.512 Pain in left **shoulder**
     M25.519 Pain in unspecified shoulder ▽
✓6ᵗʰ **M25.52 Pain in** elbow
     M25.521 Pain in right **elbow**
     M25.522 Pain in left **elbow**
     M25.529 Pain in unspecified elbow ▽
✓6ᵗʰ **M25.53 Pain in** wrist
     M25.531 Pain in right **wrist**
     M25.532 Pain in left **wrist**
     M25.539 Pain in unspecified wrist ▽
✓6ᵗʰ **M25.54 Pain in** joints of hand
     M25.541 Pain in joints of right **hand**
     M25.542 Pain in joints of left **hand**
     M25.549 Pain in joints of unspecified hand ▽
               Pain in joints of hand NOS
✓6ᵗʰ **M25.55 Pain in** hip
     M25.551 Pain in right **hip**
     M25.552 Pain in left **hip**
     M25.559 Pain in unspecified hip ▽
✓6ᵗʰ **M25.56 Pain in** knee
     M25.561 Pain in right **knee**
     M25.562 Pain in left **knee**
     M25.569 Pain in unspecified knee ▽
✓6ᵗʰ **M25.57 Pain in** ankle and joints of foot
     M25.571 Pain in right **ankle and joints of right foot**
     M25.572 Pain in left **ankle and joints of left foot**
     M25.579 Pain in unspecified ankle and joints of ▽ **unspecified foot**

✓5ᵗʰ **M25.6 Stiffness of joint, not elsewhere classified**
     EXCLUDES 1   *ankylosis of joint (M24.6-)*
               contracture of joint (M24.5-)
     M25.60 Stiffness of unspecified joint, not elsewhere ▽ **classified**
✓6ᵗʰ **M25.61 Stiffness of** shoulder, **not elsewhere classified**
     M25.611 Stiffness of right **shoulder, not elsewhere classified**
     M25.612 Stiffness of left **shoulder, not elsewhere classified**
     M25.619 Stiffness of unspecified shoulder, not ▽ **elsewhere classified**
✓6ᵗʰ **M25.62 Stiffness of** elbow, **not elsewhere classified**
     M25.621 Stiffness of right **elbow, not elsewhere classified**
     M25.622 Stiffness of left **elbow, not elsewhere classified**
     M25.629 Stiffness of unspecified elbow, not ▽ **elsewhere classified**
✓6ᵗʰ **M25.63 Stiffness of** wrist, **not elsewhere classified**
     M25.631 Stiffness of right **wrist, not elsewhere classified**
     M25.632 Stiffness of left **wrist, not elsewhere classified**
     M25.639 Stiffness of unspecified wrist, not ▽ **elsewhere classified**

✓6ᵗʰ **M25.64** Stiffness of hand, not elsewhere classified

    M25.641 Stiffness of right hand, not elsewhere classified

    M25.642 Stiffness of left hand, not elsewhere classified

    M25.649 Stiffness of unspecified hand, not elsewhere classified ▽

✓6ᵗʰ **M25.65** Stiffness of hip, not elsewhere classified

    M25.651 Stiffness of right hip, not elsewhere classified

    M25.652 Stiffness of left hip, not elsewhere classified

    M25.659 Stiffness of unspecified hip, not elsewhere classified ▽

✓6ᵗʰ **M25.66** Stiffness of knee, not elsewhere classified

    M25.661 Stiffness of right knee, not elsewhere classified

    M25.662 Stiffness of left knee, not elsewhere classified

    M25.669 Stiffness of unspecified knee, not elsewhere classified ▽

✓6ᵗʰ **M25.67** Stiffness of ankle and foot, not elsewhere classified

    M25.671 Stiffness of right ankle, not elsewhere classified

    M25.672 Stiffness of left ankle, not elsewhere classified

    M25.673 Stiffness of unspecified ankle, not elsewhere classified ▽

    M25.674 Stiffness of right foot, not elsewhere classified

    M25.675 Stiffness of left foot, not elsewhere classified

    M25.676 Stiffness of unspecified foot, not elsewhere classified ▽

✓5ᵗʰ **M25.7** Osteophyte

    M25.70 Osteophyte, unspecified joint ▽

✓6ᵗʰ **M25.71** Osteophyte, shoulder

    M25.711 Osteophyte, right shoulder

    M25.712 Osteophyte, left shoulder

    M25.719 Osteophyte, unspecified shoulder ▽

✓6ᵗʰ **M25.72** Osteophyte, elbow

    M25.721 Osteophyte, right elbow

    M25.722 Osteophyte, left elbow

    M25.729 Osteophyte, unspecified elbow ▽

✓6ᵗʰ **M25.73** Osteophyte, wrist

    M25.731 Osteophyte, right wrist

    M25.732 Osteophyte, left wrist

    M25.739 Osteophyte, unspecified wrist ▽

✓6ᵗʰ **M25.74** Osteophyte, hand

    M25.741 Osteophyte, right hand

    M25.742 Osteophyte, left hand

    M25.749 Osteophyte, unspecified hand ▽

✓6ᵗʰ **M25.75** Osteophyte, hip

    M25.751 Osteophyte, right hip

    M25.752 Osteophyte, left hip

    M25.759 Osteophyte, unspecified hip ▽

✓6ᵗʰ **M25.76** Osteophyte, knee

    M25.761 Osteophyte, right knee

    M25.762 Osteophyte, left knee

    M25.769 Osteophyte, unspecified knee ▽

✓6ᵗʰ **M25.77** Osteophyte, ankle and foot

    M25.771 Osteophyte, right ankle

    M25.772 Osteophyte, left ankle

    M25.773 Osteophyte, unspecified ankle ▽

    M25.774 Osteophyte, right foot

    M25.775 Osteophyte, left foot

    M25.776 Osteophyte, unspecified foot ▽

    M25.78 Osteophyte, vertebrae

✓5ᵗʰ **M25.8** Other specified joint disorders

    M25.80 Other specified joint disorders, unspecified joint ▽

✓6ᵗʰ **M25.81** Other specified joint disorders, shoulder

    M25.811 Other specified joint disorders, right shoulder

    M25.812 Other specified joint disorders, left shoulder

    M25.819 Other specified joint disorders, unspecified shoulder ▽

✓6ᵗʰ **M25.82** Other specified joint disorders, elbow

    M25.821 Other specified joint disorders, right elbow

    M25.822 Other specified joint disorders, left elbow

    M25.829 Other specified joint disorders, unspecified elbow ▽

✓6ᵗʰ **M25.83** Other specified joint disorders, wrist

    M25.831 Other specified joint disorders, right wrist

    M25.832 Other specified joint disorders, left wrist

    M25.839 Other specified joint disorders, unspecifiedwrist ▽

✓6ᵗʰ **M25.84** Other specified joint disorders, hand

    M25.841 Other specified joint disorders, right hand

    M25.842 Other specified joint disorders, left hand

    M25.849 Other specified joint disorders, unspecified hand ▽

✓6ᵗʰ **M25.85** Other specified joint disorders, hip

    AHA: 2014, 4Q, 25

    M25.851 Other specified joint disorders, right hip

    M25.852 Other specified joint disorders, left hip

    M25.859 Other specified joint disorders, unspecified hip ▽

✓6ᵗʰ **M25.86** Other specified joint disorders, knee

    M25.861 Other specified joint disorders, right knee

    M25.862 Other specified joint disorders, left knee

    M25.869 Other specified joint disorders, unspecified knee ▽

✓6ᵗʰ **M25.87** Other specified joint disorders, ankle and foot

    M25.871 Other specified joint disorders, right ankle and foot

    M25.872 Other specified joint disorders, left ankle and foot

    M25.879 Other specified joint disorders, unspecified ankle and foot ▽

M25.9 Joint disorder, unspecified ▽

Dentofacial anomalies [including malocclusion] and other disorders of jaw (M26-M27)

EXCLUDES 1   hemifacial atrophy or hypertrophy (Q67.4)
          unilateral condylar hyperplasia or hypoplasia (M27.8)

✓4ᵗʰ **M26 Dentofacial anomalies [including malocclusion]**

✓5ᵗʰ **M26.0** Major anomalies of jaw size

    EXCLUDES 1   acromegaly (E22.0)
             Robin's syndrome (Q87.0)

    M26.00 Unspecified anomaly of jaw size ▽

    M26.01 Maxillary hyperplasia

    M26.02 Maxillary hypoplasia
         AHA: 2014, 3Q, 23

    M26.03 Mandibular hyperplasia

    M26.04 Mandibular hypoplasia

    M26.05 Macrogenia

    M26.06 Microgenia

    M26.07 Excessive tuberosity of jaw
         Entire maxillary tuberosity

    M26.09 Other specified anomalies of jaw size

✓5ᵗʰ **M26.1** Anomalies of jaw-cranial base relationship

    M26.10 Unspecified anomaly of jaw-cranial base relationship ▽

    M26.11 Maxillary asymmetry

    M26.12 Other jaw asymmetry

    M26.19 Other specified anomalies of jaw-cranial base relationship

✓5ᵗʰ **M26.2** Anomalies of dental arch relationship

    M26.20 Unspecified anomaly of dental arch relationship ▽

✓6ᵗʰ **M26.21** Malocclusion, Angle's class

    M26.211 Malocclusion, Angle's class I
         Neutro-occlusion

    M26.212 Malocclusion, Angle's class II
         Disto-occlusion Division I
         Disto-occlusion Division II

☑ Additional Character Req   ✓x7ᵗʰ Placeholder Alert   Manifestation   HCC CMS-HCC Condition   ▽ Unspecified Code   ►◄ Revised Text   ● New Code   ▲ Revised Code Title

M26.213 Malocclusion, Angle's class III
Mesio-occlusion

M26.219 Malocclusion, Angle's class, unspecified ▽

✓6ᵗʰ **M26.22 Open occlusal relationship**

M26.220 Open anterior occlusal relationship
Anterior openbite

M26.221 Open posterior occlusal relationship
Posterior openbite

M26.23 Excessive horizontal overlap
Excessive horizontal overjet

M26.24 Reverse articulation
Crossbite (anterior) (posterior)

M26.25 Anomalies of interarch distance

M26.29 Other anomalies of dental arch relationship
Midline deviation of dental arch
Overbite (excessive) deep
Overbite (excessive) horizontal
Overbite (excessive) vertical
Posterior lingual occlusion of mandibular teeth

✓5ᵗʰ **M26.3 Anomalies of tooth position of fully erupted tooth or teeth**
EXCLUDES 2   embedded and impacted teeth (K01.-)

M26.30 Unspecified anomaly of tooth position of fully ▽
erupted tooth or teeth
Abnormal spacing of fully erupted tooth or teeth NOS
Displacement of fully erupted tooth or teeth NOS
Transposition of fully erupted tooth or teeth NOS

M26.31 Crowding of fully erupted teeth

M26.32 Excessive spacing of fully erupted teeth
Diastema of fully erupted tooth or teeth NOS

M26.33 Horizontal displacement of fully erupted tooth or
teeth
Tipped tooth or teeth
Tipping of fully erupted tooth

M26.34 Vertical displacement of fully erupted tooth or teeth
Extruded tooth
Infraeruption of tooth or teeth
Supraeruption of tooth or teeth

M26.35 Rotation of fully erupted tooth or teeth

M26.36 Insufficient interocclusal distance of fully erupted
teeth (ridge)
Lack of adequate intermaxillary vertical dimension of
fully erupted teeth

M26.37 Excessive interocclusal distance of fully erupted
teeth
Excessive intermaxillary vertical dimension of fully
erupted teeth
Loss of occlusal vertical dimension of fully erupted
teeth

M26.39 Other anomalies of tooth position of fully erupted
tooth or teeth

M26.4 Malocclusion, unspecified ▽

✓5ᵗʰ **M26.5 Dentofacial functional abnormalities**
EXCLUDES 1   bruxism (F45.8)
teeth-grinding NOS (F45.8)

M26.50 Dentofacial functional abnormalities, unspecified ▽

M26.51 Abnormal jaw closure

M26.52 Limited mandibular range of motion

M26.53 Deviation in opening and closing of the mandible

M26.54 Insufficient anterior guidance
Insufficient anterior occlusal guidance

M26.55 Centric occlusion maximum intercuspation
discrepancy
EXCLUDES 1   centric occlusion NOS (M26.59)

M26.56 Non-working side interference
Balancing side interference

M26.57 Lack of posterior occlusal support

M26.59 Other dentofacial functional abnormalities
Centric occlusion (of teeth) NOS
Malocclusion due to abnormal swallowing
Malocclusion due to mouth breathing
Malocclusion due to tongue, lip or finger habits

Temporomandibular Joint

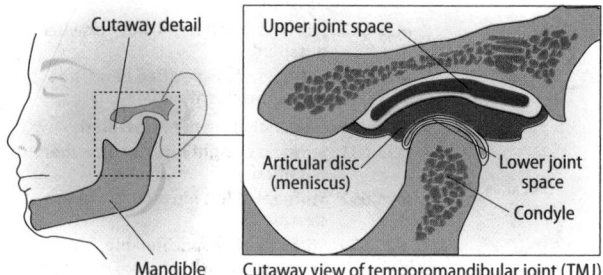

Cutaway view of temporomandibular joint (TMJ)

✓5ᵗʰ **M26.6 Temporomandibular joint disorders**
EXCLUDES 2   current temporomandibular joint dislocation (S03.0)
current temporomandibular joint sprain (S03.4)

✓6ᵗʰ **M26.60 Temporomandibular joint disorder, unspecified**

M26.601 Right temporomandibular joint ▽
disorder, unspecified

M26.602 Left temporomandibular joint ▽
disorder, unspecified

M26.603 Bilateral temporomandibular joint ▽
disorder, unspecified

M26.609 Unspecified temporomandibular joint ▽
disorder, unspecified side
Temporomandibular joint disorder NOS

✓6ᵗʰ **M26.61 Adhesions and ankylosis of temporomandibular**
joint

M26.611 Adhesions and ankylosis of right
temporomandibular joint

M26.612 Adhesions and ankylosis of left
temporomandibular joint

M26.613 Adhesions and ankylosis of bilateral
temporomandibular joint

M26.619 Adhesions and ankylosis of ▽
temporomandibular joint,
unspecified side

✓6ᵗʰ **M26.62 Arthralgia of temporomandibular joint**

M26.621 Arthralgia of right temporomandibular
joint

M26.622 Arthralgia of left temporomandibular
joint

M26.623 Arthralgia of bilateral
temporomandibular joint

M26.629 Arthralgia of temporomandibular ▽
joint, unspecified side

✓6ᵗʰ **M26.63 Articular disc disorder of temporomandibular joint**

M26.631 Articular disc disorder of right
temporomandibular joint

M26.632 Articular disc disorder of left
temporomandibular joint

M26.633 Articular disc disorder of bilateral
temporomandibular joint

M26.639 Articular disc disorder of ▽
temporomandibular joint,
unspecified side

M26.69 Other specified disorders of temporomandibular
joint

✓5ᵗʰ **M26.7 Dental alveolar anomalies**

M26.70 Unspecified alveolar anomaly ▽

M26.71 Alveolar maxillary hyperplasia

M26.72 Alveolar mandibular hyperplasia

M26.73 Alveolar maxillary hypoplasia

M26.74 Alveolar mandibular hypoplasia

M26.79 Other specified alveolar anomalies

✓5ᵗʰ **M26.8 Other dentofacial anomalies**

M26.81 Anterior soft tissue impingement
Anterior soft tissue impingement on teeth

M26.82 Posterior soft tissue impingement
Posterior soft tissue impingement on teeth

M26.89 Other dentofacial anomalies

M26.9 Dentofacial anomaly, unspecified ▽

☑️4ᵗʰ **M27 Other diseases of jaws**

  M27.0 Developmental disorders of jaws
    Latent bone cyst of jaw   Torus mandibularis
    Stafne's cyst   Torus palatinus

  M27.1 Giant cell granuloma, central
    Giant cell granuloma NOS
    EXCLUDES 1   peripheral giant cell granuloma (K06.8)

  M27.2 Inflammatory conditions of jaws
    Osteitis of jaw(s)   Periostitis jaw(s)
    Osteomyelitis (neonatal) jaw(s)   Sequestrum of jaw bone
    Osteoradionecrosis jaw(s)
    Use additional code (W88-W90, X39.0) to identify radiation, if radiation-induced
    EXCLUDES 2   osteonecrosis of jaw due to drug (M87.180)

  M27.3 Alveolitis of jaws
    Alveolar osteitis   Dry socket

☑️5ᵗʰ **M27.4 Other and unspecified cysts of jaw**
    EXCLUDES 1   cysts of oral region (K09.-)
             latent bone cyst of jaw (M27.0)
             Stafne's cyst (M27.0)

    M27.40 Unspecified cyst of jaw ▽
      Cyst of jaw NOS

    M27.49 Other cysts of jaw
      Aneurysmal cyst of jaw
      Hemorrhagic cyst of jaw
      Traumatic cyst of jaw

☑️5ᵗʰ **M27.5 Periradicular pathology associated with previous endodontic treatment**

    M27.51 Perforation of root canal space due to endodontic treatment

    M27.52 Endodontic overfill

    M27.53 Endodontic underfill

    M27.59 Other periradicular pathology associated with previous endodontic treatment

☑️5ᵗʰ **M27.6 Endosseous dental implant failure**

    M27.61 Osseointegration failure of dental implant
      Hemorrhagic complications of dental implant placement
      Iatrogenic osseointegration failure of dental implant
      Osseointegration failure of dental implant due to complications of systemic disease
      Osseointegration failure of dental implant due to poor bone quality
      Pre-integration failure of dental implant NOS
      Pre-osseointegration failure of dental implant

    M27.62 Post-osseointegration biological failure of dental implant
      Failure of dental implant due to lack of attached gingiva
      Failure of dental implant due to occlusal trauma (caused by poor prosthetic design)
      Failure of dental implant due to parafunctional habits
      Failure of dental implant due to periodontal infection (peri-implantitis)
      Failure of dental implant due to poor oral hygiene
      Iatrogenic post-osseointegration failure of dental implant
      Post-osseointegration failure of dental implant due to complications of systemic disease

    M27.63 Post-osseointegration mechanical failure of dental implant
      Failure of dental prosthesis causing loss of dental implant
      Fracture of dental implant
      EXCLUDES 2   cracked tooth (K03.81)
             fractured dental restorative material with loss of material (K08.531)
             fractured dental restorative material without loss of material (K08.530)
             fractured tooth (S02.5)

    M27.69 Other endosseous dental implant failure
      Dental implant failure NOS

  M27.8 Other specified diseases of jaws
    Cherubism   Unilateral condylar hyperplasia
    Exostosis   Unilateral condylar hypoplasia
    Fibrous dysplasia
    EXCLUDES 1   jaw pain (R68.84)

  M27.9 Disease of jaws, unspecified ▽

Systemic connective tissue disorders (M30-M36)

INCLUDES   autoimmune disease NOS
    collagen (vascular) disease NOS
    systemic autoimmune disease
    systemic collagen (vascular) disease
EXCLUDES 1   autoimmune disease, single organ or single cell-type—code to relevant condition category

☑️4ᵗʰ **M30 Polyarteritis nodosa and related conditions**
  EXCLUDES 1   microscopic polyarteritis (M31.7)

  M30.0 Polyarteritis nodosa ᴴᶜᶜ

  M30.1 Polyarteritis with lung involvement [Churg-Strauss] ᴴᶜᶜ
    Allergic granulomatous angiitis

  M30.2 Juvenile polyarteritis ᴴᶜᶜ

  M30.3 Mucocutaneous lymph node syndrome [Kawasaki] ᴴᶜᶜ

  M30.8 Other conditions related to polyarteritis nodosa ᴴᶜᶜ
    Polyangiitis overlap syndrome

☑️4ᵗʰ **M31 Other necrotizing vasculopathies**

  M31.0 Hypersensitivity angiitis ᴴᶜᶜ
    Goodpasture's syndrome

  M31.1 Thrombotic microangiopathy ᴴᶜᶜ
    Thrombotic thrombocytopenic purpura

  M31.2 Lethal midline granuloma ᴴᶜᶜ

☑️5ᵗʰ **M31.3 Wegener's granulomatosis**
    Necrotizing respiratory granulomatosis

    M31.30 Wegener's granulomatosis without renal involvement ᴴᶜᶜ
      Wegener's granulomatosis NOS

    M31.31 Wegener's granulomatosis with renal involvement ᴴᶜᶜ

  M31.4 Aortic arch syndrome [Takayasu] ᴴᶜᶜ

  M31.5 Giant cell arteritis with polymyalgia rheumatica ᴴᶜᶜ

  M31.6 Other giant cell arteritis ᴴᶜᶜ

  M31.7 Microscopic polyangiitis ᴴᶜᶜ
    Microscopic polyarteritis
    EXCLUDES 1   polyarteritis nodosa (M30.0)

  M31.8 Other specified necrotizing vasculopathies ᴴᶜᶜ
    Hypocomplementemic vasculitis
    Septic vasculitis

  M31.9 Necrotizing vasculopathy, unspecified ᴴᶜᶜ ▽

☑️4ᵗʰ **M32 Systemic lupus erythematosus (SLE)**
  EXCLUDES 1   lupus erythematosus (discoid) (NOS) (L93.0)

  M32.0 Drug-induced systemic lupus erythematosus ᴴᶜᶜ
    Use additional code for adverse effect, if applicable, to identify drug (T36-T50 with fifth or sixth character 5)

☑️5ᵗʰ **M32.1 Systemic lupus erythematosus with organ or system involvement**

    M32.10 Systemic lupus erythematosus, organ or system involvement unspecified ᴴᶜᶜ ▽

    M32.11 Endocarditis in systemic lupus erythematosus ᴴᶜᶜ
      Libman-Sacks disease

    M32.12 Pericarditis in systemic lupus erythematosus ᴴᶜᶜ
      Lupus pericarditis

    M32.13 Lung involvement in systemic lupus erythematosus ᴴᶜᶜ
      Pleural effusion due to systemic lupus erythematosus

    M32.14 Glomerular disease in systemic lupus erythematosus ᴴᶜᶜ
      Lupus renal disease NOS
      AHA: 2013, 4Q, 125

    M32.15 Tubulo-interstitial nephropathy in systemic lupus erythematosus ᴴᶜᶜ

    M32.19 Other organ or system involvement in systemic lupus erythematosus ᴴᶜᶜ

  M32.8 Other forms of systemic lupus erythematosus ᴴᶜᶜ

  M32.9 Systemic lupus erythematosus, unspecified ᴴᶜᶜ ▽
    SLE NOS
    Systemic lupus erythematosus NOS
    Systemic lupus erythematosus without organ involvement

☑️4ᵗʰ **M33 Dermatopolymyositis**

▲ ☑️5ᵗʰ **M33.0 Juvenile dermatomyositis**

▲   **M33.00 Juvenile dermatomyositis, organ involvement unspecified** ᴴᶜᶜ ▽

▲   **M33.01 Juvenile dermatomyositis with respiratory involvement** ᴴᶜᶜ

▲   **M33.02 Juvenile dermatomyositis with myopathy** ᴴᶜᶜ

☑️ Additional Character Req   ✓✗7ᵗʰ Placeholder Alert   Manifestation   ᴴᶜᶜ CMS-HCC Condition   ▽ Unspecified Code   ►◄ Revised Text   ● New Code   ▲ Revised Code Title

ICD-10-CM 2018   **751**

●   M33.03   **Juvenile dermatomyositis without myopathy**

▲   M33.09   **Juvenile dermatomyositis with other organ involvement**   HCC

▲ ✓5ᵗʰ   **M33.1 Other dermatomyositis**
▶Adult dermatomyositis◀

▲   M33.10   **Other dermatomyositis, organ involvement unspecified**   HCC ▽

▲   M33.11   **Other dermatomyositis with respiratory involvement**   HCC

▲   M33.12   **Other dermatomyositis with myopathy**   HCC

●   M33.13   **Other dermatomyositis without myopathy**
Dermatomyositis NOS

▲   M33.19   **Other dermatomyositis with other organ involvement**   HCC

✓5ᵗʰ   **M33.2 Polymyositis**

   M33.20   **Polymyositis, organ involvement unspecified**   HCC ▽

   M33.21   **Polymyositis with respiratory involvement**   HCC

   M33.22   **Polymyositis with myopathy**   HCC

   M33.29   **Polymyositis with other organ involvement**   HCC

✓5ᵗʰ   **M33.9 Dermatopolymyositis, unspecified**

   M33.90   **Dermatopolymyositis, unspecified, organ involvement unspecified**   HCC ▽

   M33.91   **Dermatopolymyositis, unspecified with respiratory involvement**   HCC ▽

   M33.92   **Dermatopolymyositis, unspecified with myopathy**   HCC ▽

●   M33.93   **Dermatopolymyositis, unspecified without myopathy**   ▽

   M33.99   **Dermatopolymyositis, unspecified with other organ involvement**   HCC ▽

✓4ᵗʰ   **M34 Systemic sclerosis [scleroderma]**
   EXCLUDES 1   circumscribed scleroderma (L94.0)
       neonatal scleroderma (P83.8)

   M34.0 Progressive systemic sclerosis   HCC

   M34.1 CR(E)ST syndrome   HCC
Combination of calcinosis, Raynaud's phenomenon, esophageal dysfunction, sclerodactyly, telangiectasia

   M34.2 Systemic sclerosis induced by drug and chemical   HCC
Code first poisoning due to drug or toxin, if applicable (T36-T65 with fifth or sixth character 1-4 or 6)
Use additional code for adverse effect, if applicable, to identify drug (T36-T50 with fifth or sixth character 5)

✓5ᵗʰ   **M34.8 Other forms of systemic sclerosis**

   M34.81   **Systemic sclerosis with lung involvement**   HCC

   M34.82   **Systemic sclerosis with myopathy**   HCC

   M34.83   **Systemic sclerosis with polyneuropathy**   HCC

   M34.89   **Other systemic sclerosis**   HCC

   M34.9 Systemic sclerosis, unspecified   HCC ▽

✓4ᵗʰ   **M35 Other systemic involvement of connective tissue**
   EXCLUDES 1   reactive perforating collagenosis (L87.1)

✓5ᵗʰ   **M35.0 Sicca syndrome [Sjögren]**
   DEF: Autoimmune disease; associated with keratoconjunctivitis, laryngopharyngitis, rhinitis, dry mouth, enlarged parotid gland, and chronic polyarthritis.

   M35.00   **Sicca syndrome, unspecified**   HCC ▽

   M35.01   **Sicca syndrome with keratoconjunctivitis**   HCC

   M35.02   **Sicca syndrome with lung involvement**   HCC

   M35.03   **Sicca syndrome with myopathy**   HCC

   M35.04   **Sicca syndrome with tubulo-interstitial nephropathy**   HCC
Renal tubular acidosis in sicca syndrome

   M35.09   **Sicca syndrome with other organ involvement**   HCC

   M35.1 Other overlap syndromes   HCC
Mixed connective tissue disease
   EXCLUDES 1   polyangiitis overlap syndrome (M30.8)

   M35.2 Behçet's disease   HCC

   M35.3 Polymyalgia rheumatica   HCC
   EXCLUDES 1   polymyalgia rheumatica with giant cell arteritis (M31.5)

   M35.4 Diffuse (eosinophilic) fasciitis

   M35.5 Multifocal fibrosclerosis   HCC

   M35.6 Relapsing panniculitis [Weber-Christian]
   EXCLUDES 1   lupus panniculitis (L93.2)
       panniculitis NOS (M79.3-)

   M35.7 Hypermobility syndrome
Familial ligamentous laxity
   EXCLUDES 1   Ehlers-Danlos syndrome (Q79.6)
       ligamentous laxity, NOS (M24.2-)

   M35.8 Other specified systemic involvement of connective tissue   HCC

   M35.9 Systemic involvement of connective tissue, unspecified   HCC ▽
Autoimmune disease (systemic) NOS
Collagen (vascular) disease NOS

✓4ᵗʰ   **M36 Systemic disorders of connective tissue in diseases classified elsewhere**
   EXCLUDES 2   arthropathies in diseases classified elsewhere (M14.-)

   M36.0 Dermato(poly)myositis in neoplastic disease   HCC
Code first underlying neoplasm (C00-D49)

   M36.1 Arthropathy in neoplastic disease
Code first underlying neoplasm, such as:
leukemia (C91-C95)
malignant histiocytosis (C96.A)
multiple myeloma (C90.0)

   M36.2 Hemophilic arthropathy
Hemarthrosis in hemophilic arthropathy
Code first underlying disease, such as:
factor VIII deficiency (D66)
   with vascular defect (D68.0)
factor IX deficiency (D67)
hemophilia (classical) (D66)
hemophilia B (D67)
hemophilia C (D68.1)

   M36.3 Arthropathy in other blood disorders

   M36.4 Arthropathy in hypersensitivity reactions classified elsewhere
Code first underlying disease, such as:
Henoch (-Schönlein) purpura (D69.0)
serum sickness (T80.6-)

   M36.8 Systemic disorders of connective tissue in other diseases classified elsewhere   HCC
Code first underlying disease, such as:
alkaptonuria (E70.2)
hypogammaglobulinemia (D80.-)
ochronosis (E70.2)

Dorsopathies (M40-M54)

Deforming dorsopathies (M40-M43)

✓4ᵗʰ   **M40 Kyphosis and lordosis**
   EXCLUDES 1   congenital kyphosis and lordosis (Q76.4)
       kyphoscoliosis (M41.-)
       postprocedural kyphosis and lordosis (M96.-)

✓5ᵗʰ   **M40.0 Postural kyphosis**
   EXCLUDES 1   osteochondrosis of spine (M42.-)

   M40.00   **Postural kyphosis, site unspecified**   ▽

   M40.03   **Postural kyphosis, cervicothoracic region**

   M40.04   **Postural kyphosis, thoracic region**

   M40.05   **Postural kyphosis, thoracolumbar region**

✓5ᵗʰ   **M40.1 Other secondary kyphosis**

   M40.10   **Other secondary kyphosis, site unspecified**   ▽

   M40.12   **Other secondary kyphosis, cervical region**

   M40.13   **Other secondary kyphosis, cervicothoracic region**

   M40.14   **Other secondary kyphosis, thoracic region**

   M40.15   **Other secondary kyphosis, thoracolumbar region**

✓5ᵗʰ   **M40.2 Other and unspecified kyphosis**

   ✓6ᵗʰ   M40.20   **Unspecified kyphosis**

     M40.202   **Unspecified kyphosis, cervical region**   ▽

     M40.203   **Unspecified kyphosis, cervicothoracic region**   ▽

     M40.204   **Unspecified kyphosis, thoracic region**   ▽

     M40.205   **Unspecified kyphosis, thoracolumbar region**   ▽

     M40.209   **Unspecified kyphosis, site unspecified**   ▽

   ✓6ᵗʰ   M40.29   **Other kyphosis**

     M40.292   **Other kyphosis, cervical region**

     M40.293   **Other kyphosis, cervicothoracic region**

     M40.294   **Other kyphosis, thoracic region**

     M40.295   **Other kyphosis, thoracolumbar region**

     M40.299   **Other kyphosis, site unspecified**   ▽

EXCLUDES 1 Not coded here   *EXCLUDES 2* Not included here   N Newborn Age: 0   P Pediatric Age: 0-17   M Maternity Age: 12-55   A Adult Age: 15-124

Kyphosis and Lordosis

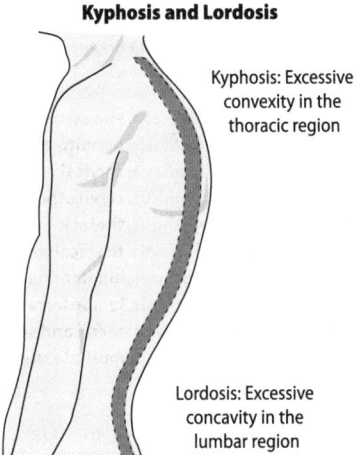

Kyphosis: Excessive convexity in the thoracic region

Lordosis: Excessive concavity in the lumbar region

Scoliosis

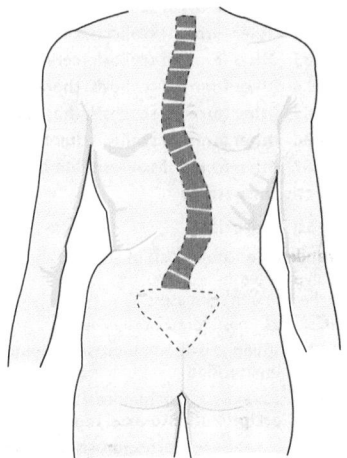

Lateral curvature of spine

✓5ᵗʰ **M40.3** Flatback syndrome
    M40.30 Flatback syndrome, site unspecified ▽
    M40.35 Flatback syndrome, thoracolumbar region
    M40.36 Flatback syndrome, lumbar region
    M40.37 Flatback syndrome, lumbosacral region

✓5ᵗʰ **M40.4** Postural lordosis
    Acquired lordosis
    M40.40 Postural lordosis, site unspecified ▽
    M40.45 Postural lordosis, thoracolumbar region
    M40.46 Postural lordosis, lumbar region
    M40.47 Postural lordosis, lumbosacral region

✓5ᵗʰ **M40.5** Lordosis, unspecified
    M40.50 Lordosis, unspecified, site unspecified ▽
    M40.55 Lordosis, unspecified, thoracolumbar region
    M40.56 Lordosis, unspecified, lumbar region
    M40.57 Lordosis, unspecified, lumbosacral region

✓4ᵗʰ **M41 Scoliosis**
    INCLUDES kyphoscoliosis
    EXCLUDES 1 congenital scoliosis due to bony malformation (Q76.3)
        congenital scoliosis NOS (Q67.5)
        kyphoscoliotic heart disease (I27.1)
        postprocedural scoliosis (M96.-)
        postural congenital scoliosis (Q67.5)

✓5ᵗʰ **M41.0** Infantile idiopathic scoliosis
    AHA: 2014, 4Q, 26
    M41.00 Infantile idiopathic scoliosis, site unspecified ▽
    M41.02 Infantile idiopathic scoliosis, cervical region
    M41.03 Infantile idiopathic scoliosis, cervicothoracic region
    M41.04 Infantile idiopathic scoliosis, thoracic region
    M41.05 Infantile idiopathic scoliosis, thoracolumbar region
    M41.06 Infantile idiopathic scoliosis, lumbar region
    M41.07 Infantile idiopathic scoliosis, lumbosacral region
    M41.08 Infantile idiopathic scoliosis, sacral and sacrococcygeal region

✓5ᵗʰ **M41.1** Juvenile and adolescent idiopathic scoliosis
    ✓6ᵗʰ **M41.11** Juvenile idiopathic scoliosis
        AHA: 2014, 4Q, 28
        M41.112 Juvenile idiopathic scoliosis, cervical region
        M41.113 Juvenile idiopathic scoliosis, cervicothoracic region
        M41.114 Juvenile idiopathic scoliosis, thoracic region
        M41.115 Juvenile idiopathic scoliosis, thoracolumbar region
        M41.116 Juvenile idiopathic scoliosis, lumbar region
        M41.117 Juvenile idiopathic scoliosis, lumbosacral region
        M41.119 Juvenile idiopathic scoliosis, site unspecified ▽

✓6ᵗʰ **M41.12** Adolescent scoliosis
    M41.122 Adolescent idiopathic scoliosis, cervical region
    M41.123 Adolescent idiopathic scoliosis, cervicothoracic region
    M41.124 Adolescent idiopathic scoliosis, thoracic region
    M41.125 Adolescent idiopathic scoliosis, thoracolumbar region
    M41.126 Adolescent idiopathic scoliosis, lumbar region
    M41.127 Adolescent idiopathic scoliosis, lumbosacral region
    M41.129 Adolescent idiopathic scoliosis, site unspecified ▽

✓5ᵗʰ **M41.2** Other idiopathic scoliosis
    M41.20 Other idiopathic scoliosis, site unspecified ▽
    M41.22 Other idiopathic scoliosis, cervical region
    M41.23 Other idiopathic scoliosis, cervicothoracic region
    M41.24 Other idiopathic scoliosis, thoracic region
    M41.25 Other idiopathic scoliosis, thoracolumbar region
    M41.26 Other idiopathic scoliosis, lumbar region
    M41.27 Other idiopathic scoliosis, lumbosacral region

✓5ᵗʰ **M41.3** Thoracogenic scoliosis
    M41.30 Thoracogenic scoliosis, site unspecified ▽
    M41.34 Thoracogenic scoliosis, thoracic region
    M41.35 Thoracogenic scoliosis, thoracolumbar region

✓5ᵗʰ **M41.4** Neuromuscular scoliosis
    Scoliosis secondary to cerebral palsy, Friedreich's ataxia, poliomyelitis and other neuromuscular disorders
    Code also underlying condition
    AHA: 2014, 4Q, 27
    M41.40 Neuromuscular scoliosis, site unspecified ▽
    M41.41 Neuromuscular scoliosis, occipito-atlanto-axial region
    M41.42 Neuromuscular scoliosis, cervical region
    M41.43 Neuromuscular scoliosis, cervicothoracic region
    M41.44 Neuromuscular scoliosis, thoracic region
    M41.45 Neuromuscular scoliosis, thoracolumbar region
    M41.46 Neuromuscular scoliosis, lumbar region
    M41.47 Neuromuscular scoliosis, lumbosacral region

✓5ᵗʰ **M41.5** Other secondary scoliosis
    M41.50 Other secondary scoliosis, site unspecified ▽
    M41.52 Other secondary scoliosis, cervical region
    M41.53 Other secondary scoliosis, cervicothoracic region
    M41.54 Other secondary scoliosis, thoracic region
    M41.55 Other secondary scoliosis, thoracolumbar region
    M41.56 Other secondary scoliosis, lumbar region
    M41.57 Other secondary scoliosis, lumbosacral region

✓5ᵗʰ M41.8 Other forms of scoliosis

     M41.80 Other forms of scoliosis, site unspecified ▽

     M41.82 Other forms of scoliosis, cervical region

     M41.83 Other forms of scoliosis, cervicothoracic region

     M41.84 Other forms of scoliosis, thoracic region

     M41.85 Other forms of scoliosis, thoracolumbar region

     M41.86 Other forms of scoliosis, lumbar region

     M41.87 Other forms of scoliosis, lumbosacral region

M41.9 Scoliosis, unspecified ▽

✓4ᵗʰ M42 Spinal osteochondrosis

✓5ᵗʰ M42.0 Juvenile osteochondrosis of spine

     Calvé's disease

     Scheuermann's disease

     EXCLUDES 1   *postural kyphosis (M40.0)*

     M42.00 Juvenile osteochondrosis of spine, site unspecified ▽

     M42.01 Juvenile osteochondrosis of spine, occipito-atlanto-axial region

     M42.02 Juvenile osteochondrosis of spine, cervical region

     M42.03 Juvenile osteochondrosis of spine, cervicothoracic region

     M42.04 Juvenile osteochondrosis of spine, thoracic region

     M42.05 Juvenile osteochondrosis of spine, thoracolumbar region

     M42.06 Juvenile osteochondrosis of spine, lumbar region

     M42.07 Juvenile osteochondrosis of spine, lumbosacral region

     M42.08 Juvenile osteochondrosis of spine, sacral and sacrococcygeal region

     M42.09 Juvenile osteochondrosis of spine, multiple sites in spine

✓5ᵗʰ M42.1 Adult osteochondrosis of spine

     M42.10 Adult osteochondrosis of spine, site unspecified 🅐▽

     M42.11 Adult osteochondrosis of spine, occipito-atlanto-axial region 🅐

     M42.12 Adult osteochondrosis of spine, cervical region 🅐

     M42.13 Adult osteochondrosis of spine, cervicothoracic region 🅐

     M42.14 Adult osteochondrosis of spine, thoracic region 🅐

     M42.15 Adult osteochondrosis of spine, thoracolumbar region 🅐

     M42.16 Adult osteochondrosis of spine, lumbar region 🅐

     M42.17 Adult osteochondrosis of spine, lumbosacral region 🅐

     M42.18 Adult osteochondrosis of spine, sacral and sacrococcygeal region 🅐

     M42.19 Adult osteochondrosis of spine, multiple sites in spine 🅐

M42.9 Spinal osteochondrosis, unspecified ▽

✓4ᵗʰ M43 Other deforming dorsopathies

     EXCLUDES 1   *congenital spondylolysis and spondylolisthesis (Q76.2)*

     hemivertebra (Q76.3-Q76.4)

     Klippel-Feil syndrome (Q76.1)

     lumbarization and sacralization (Q76.4)

     platyspondylisis (Q76.4)

     spina bifida occulta (Q76.0)

     spinal curvature in osteoporosis (M80.-)

     spinal curvature in Paget's disease of bone [osteitis deformans] (M88.-)

✓5ᵗʰ M43.0 Spondylolysis

     EXCLUDES 1   *congenital spondylolysis (Q76.2)*

     spondylolisthesis (M43.1)

     M43.00 Spondylolysis, site unspecified ▽

     M43.01 Spondylolysis, occipito-atlanto-axial region

     M43.02 Spondylolysis, cervical region

     M43.03 Spondylolysis, cervicothoracic region

     M43.04 Spondylolysis, thoracic region

     M43.05 Spondylolysis, thoracolumbar region

     M43.06 Spondylolysis, lumbar region

     M43.07 Spondylolysis, lumbosacral region

     M43.08 Spondylolysis, sacral and sacrococcygeal region

     M43.09 Spondylolysis, multiple sites in spine

✓5ᵗʰ M43.1 Spondylolisthesis

     EXCLUDES 1   *acute traumatic of lumbosacral region (S33.1)*

     acute traumatic of sites other than lumbosacral— code to Fracture, vertebra, by region

     congenital spondylolisthesis (Q76.2)

     M43.10 Spondylolisthesis, site unspecified ▽

     M43.11 Spondylolisthesis, occipito-atlanto-axial region

     M43.12 Spondylolisthesis, cervical region

     M43.13 Spondylolisthesis, cervicothoracic region

     M43.14 Spondylolisthesis, thoracic region

     M43.15 Spondylolisthesis, thoracolumbar region

     M43.16 Spondylolisthesis, lumbar region

     M43.17 Spondylolisthesis, lumbosacral region

     M43.18 Spondylolisthesis, sacral and sacrococcygeal region

     M43.19 Spondylolisthesis, multiple sites in spine

✓5ᵗʰ M43.2 Fusion of spine

     Ankylosis of spinal joint

     EXCLUDES 1   *ankylosing spondylitis (M45.0-)*

     congenital fusion of spine (Q76.4)

     EXCLUDES 2   *arthrodesis status (Z98.1)*

     pseudoarthrosis after fusion or arthrodesis (M96.0)

     M43.20 Fusion of spine, site unspecified ▽

     M43.21 Fusion of spine, occipito-atlanto-axial region

     M43.22 Fusion of spine, cervical region

     M43.23 Fusion of spine, cervicothoracic region

     M43.24 Fusion of spine, thoracic region

     M43.25 Fusion of spine, thoracolumbar region

     M43.26 Fusion of spine, lumbar region

     M43.27 Fusion of spine, lumbosacral region

     M43.28 Fusion of spine, sacral and sacrococcygeal region

M43.3 Recurrent atlantoaxial dislocation with myelopathy

M43.4 Other recurrent atlantoaxial dislocation

✓5ᵗʰ M43.5 Other recurrent vertebral dislocation

     EXCLUDES 1   *biomechanical lesions NEC (M99.-)*

     ✓6ᵗʰ M43.5X Other recurrent vertebral dislocation

         M43.5X2 Other recurrent vertebral dislocation, cervical region

         M43.5X3 Other recurrent vertebral dislocation, cervicothoracic region

         M43.5X4 Other recurrent vertebral dislocation, thoracic region

         M43.5X5 Other recurrent vertebral dislocation, thoracolumbar region

         M43.5X6 Other recurrent vertebral dislocation, lumbar region

         M43.5X7 Other recurrent vertebral dislocation, lumbosacral region

         M43.5X8 Other recurrent vertebral dislocation, sacral and sacrococcygeal region

         M43.5X9 Other recurrent vertebral dislocation, site unspecified ▽

M43.6 Torticollis

     EXCLUDES 1   *congenital (sternomastoid) torticollis (Q68.0)*

     current injury—see Injury, of spine, by body region

     ocular torticollis (R29.891)

     psychogenic torticollis (F45.8)

     spasmodic torticollis (G24.3)

     torticollis due to birth injury (P15.2)

✓5ᵗʰ M43.8 Other specified deforming dorsopathies

     EXCLUDES 2   *kyphosis and lordosis (M40.-)*

     scoliosis (M41.-)

     ✓6ᵗʰ M43.8X Other specified deforming dorsopathies

         M43.8X1 Other specified deforming dorsopathies, occipito-atlanto-axial region

         M43.8X2 Other specified deforming dorsopathies, cervical region

         M43.8X3 Other specified deforming dorsopathies, cervicothoracic region

         M43.8X4 Other specified deforming dorsopathies, thoracic region

         M43.8X5 Other specified deforming dorsopathies, thoracolumbar region

         M43.8X6 Other specified deforming dorsopathies, lumbar region

         M43.8X7 Other specified deforming dorsopathies, lumbosacral region

---

EXCLUDES 1 Not coded here   *EXCLUDES 2* Not included here   🅝 Newborn Age: 0   🅟 Pediatric Age: 0-17   🅜 Maternity Age: 12-55   🅐 Adult Age: 15-124

M43.8X8   **Other specified deforming dorsopathies, sacral and sacrococcygeal region**

M43.8X9   **Other specified deforming dorsopathies, site unspecified** ▽

M43.9   **Deforming dorsopathy, unspecified** ▽
Curvature of spine NOS

Spondylopathies (M45-M49)

☑4ᵗʰ **M45 Ankylosing spondylitis**
Rheumatoid arthritis of spine
EXCLUDES 1   arthropathy in Reiter's disease (M02.3-)
juvenile (ankylosing) spondylitis (M08.1)
EXCLUDES 2   Behçet's disease (M35.2)

M45.0   **Ankylosing spondylitis of multiple sites in spine**   HCC

M45.1   **Ankylosing spondylitis of occipito-atlanto-axial region**   HCC

M45.2   **Ankylosing spondylitis of cervical region**   HCC

M45.3   **Ankylosing spondylitis of cervicothoracic region**   HCC

M45.4   **Ankylosing spondylitis of thoracic region**   HCC

M45.5   **Ankylosing spondylitis of thoracolumbar region**   HCC

M45.6   **Ankylosing spondylitis lumbar region**   HCC

M45.7   **Ankylosing spondylitis of lumbosacral region**   HCC

M45.8   **Ankylosing spondylitis sacral and sacrococcygeal region**   HCC

M45.9   **Ankylosing spondylitis of unspecified sites in spine**   HCC ▽

☑4ᵗʰ **M46 Other inflammatory spondylopathies**

☑5ᵗʰ   M46.0   **Spinal enthesopathy**
Disorder of ligamentous or muscular attachments of spine

M46.00   **Spinal enthesopathy, site unspecified**   HCC ▽

M46.01   **Spinal enthesopathy, occipito-atlanto-axial region**   HCC

M46.02   **Spinal enthesopathy, cervical region**   HCC

M46.03   **Spinal enthesopathy, cervicothoracic region**   HCC

M46.04   **Spinal enthesopathy, thoracic region**   HCC

M46.05   **Spinal enthesopathy, thoracolumbar region**   HCC

M46.06   **Spinal enthesopathy, lumbar region**   HCC

M46.07   **Spinal enthesopathy, lumbosacral region**   HCC

M46.08   **Spinal enthesopathy, sacral and sacrococcygeal region**   HCC

M46.09   **Spinal enthesopathy, multiple sites in spine**   HCC

M46.1   **Sacroiliitis, not elsewhere classified**   HCC
DEF: Inflammation of sacroiliac joint (situated at juncture of sacrum and hip); characterized by pain in buttocks or lower back that can extend down one or both legs.

☑5ᵗʰ   M46.2   **Osteomyelitis of vertebra**

M46.20   **Osteomyelitis of vertebra, site unspecified**   HCC ▽

M46.21   **Osteomyelitis of vertebra, occipito-atlanto-axial region**   HCC

M46.22   **Osteomyelitis of vertebra, cervical region**   HCC

M46.23   **Osteomyelitis of vertebra, cervicothoracic region**   HCC

M46.24   **Osteomyelitis of vertebra, thoracic region**   HCC

M46.25   **Osteomyelitis of vertebra, thoracolumbar region**   HCC

M46.26   **Osteomyelitis of vertebra, lumbar region**   HCC

M46.27   **Osteomyelitis of vertebra, lumbosacral region**   HCC

M46.28   **Osteomyelitis of vertebra, sacral and sacrococcygeal region**   HCC

☑5ᵗʰ   M46.3   **Infection of intervertebral disc (pyogenic)**
Use additional code (B95-B97) to identify infectious agent

M46.30   **Infection of intervertebral disc (pyogenic), site unspecified**   HCC ▽

M46.31   **Infection of intervertebral disc (pyogenic), occipito-atlanto-axial region**   HCC

M46.32   **Infection of intervertebral disc (pyogenic), cervical region**   HCC

M46.33   **Infection of intervertebral disc (pyogenic), cervicothoracic region**   HCC

M46.34   **Infection of intervertebral disc (pyogenic), thoracic region**   HCC

M46.35   **Infection of intervertebral disc (pyogenic), thoracolumbar region**   HCC

M46.36   **Infection of intervertebral disc (pyogenic), lumbar region**   HCC

M46.37   **Infection of intervertebral disc (pyogenic), lumbosacral region**   HCC

M46.38   **Infection of intervertebral disc (pyogenic), sacral and sacrococcygeal region**   HCC

M46.39   **Infection of intervertebral disc (pyogenic), multiple sites in spine**   HCC

☑5ᵗʰ   M46.4   **Discitis, unspecified**

M46.40   **Discitis, unspecified, site unspecified** ▽

M46.41   **Discitis, unspecified, occipito-atlanto-axial region** ▽

M46.42   **Discitis, unspecified, cervical region** ▽

M46.43   **Discitis, unspecified, cervicothoracic region** ▽

M46.44   **Discitis, unspecified, thoracic region** ▽

M46.45   **Discitis, unspecified, thoracolumbar region** ▽

M46.46   **Discitis, unspecified, lumbar region** ▽

M46.47   **Discitis, unspecified, lumbosacral region** ▽

M46.48   **Discitis, unspecified, sacral and sacrococcygeal region** ▽

M46.49   **Discitis, unspecified, multiple sites in spine** ▽

☑5ᵗʰ   M46.5   **Other infective spondylopathies**

M46.50   **Other infective spondylopathies, site unspecified**   HCC ▽

M46.51   **Other infective spondylopathies, occipito-atlanto-axial region**   HCC

M46.52   **Other infective spondylopathies, cervical region**   HCC

M46.53   **Other infective spondylopathies, cervicothoracic region**   HCC

M46.54   **Other infective spondylopathies, thoracic region**   HCC

M46.55   **Other infective spondylopathies, thoracolumbar region**   HCC

M46.56   **Other infective spondylopathies, lumbar region**   HCC

M46.57   **Other infective spondylopathies, lumbosacral region**   HCC

M46.58   **Other infective spondylopathies, sacral and sacrococcygeal region**   HCC

M46.59   **Other infective spondylopathies, multiple sites in spine**   HCC

☑5ᵗʰ   M46.8   **Other specified inflammatory spondylopathies**

M46.80   **Other specified inflammatory spondylopathies, site unspecified**   HCC ▽

M46.81   **Other specified inflammatory spondylopathies, occipito-atlanto-axial region**   HCC

M46.82   **Other specified inflammatory spondylopathies, cervical region**   HCC

M46.83   **Other specified inflammatory spondylopathies, cervicothoracic region**   HCC

M46.84   **Other specified inflammatory spondylopathies, thoracic region**   HCC

M46.85   **Other specified inflammatory spondylopathies, thoracolumbar region**   HCC

M46.86   **Other specified inflammatory spondylopathies, lumbar region**   HCC

M46.87   **Other specified inflammatory spondylopathies, lumbosacral region**   HCC

M46.88   **Other specified inflammatory spondylopathies, sacral and sacrococcygeal region**   HCC

M46.89   **Other specified inflammatory spondylopathies, multiple sites in spine**   HCC

☑5ᵗʰ   M46.9   **Unspecified inflammatory spondylopathy**

M46.90   **Unspecified inflammatory spondylopathy, site unspecified**   HCC ▽

M46.91   **Unspecified inflammatory spondylopathy, occipito-atlanto-axial region**   HCC ▽

M46.92   **Unspecified inflammatory spondylopathy, cervical region**   HCC ▽

M46.93   **Unspecified inflammatory spondylopathy, cervicothoracic region**   HCC ▽

M46.94   **Unspecified inflammatory spondylopathy, thoracic region**   HCC ▽

M46.95   **Unspecified inflammatory spondylopathy, thoracolumbar region**   HCC ▽

M46.96   **Unspecified inflammatory spondylopathy, lumbar region**   HCC ▽

M46.97   **Unspecified inflammatory spondylopathy, lumbosacral region**   HCC ▽

☑ Additional Character Req   ✓ˣ⁷ Placeholder Alert   Manifestation   HCC CMS-HCC Condition   ▽ Unspecified Code   ►◄ Revised Text   ● New Code   ▲ Revised Code Title

M46.98   Unspecified inflammatory spondylopathy, sacral and sacrococcygeal region   HCC ▽

M46.99   Unspecified inflammatory spondylopathy, multiple sites in spine   HCC ▽

✓4th **M47 Spondylosis**
>   INCLUDES   arthrosis or osteoarthritis of spine
>   degeneration of facet joints

✓5th **M47.0 Anterior spinal and vertebral artery compression syndromes**

✓6th **M47.01 Anterior spinal artery compression syndromes**

M47.011   Anterior spinal artery compression syndromes, occipito-atlanto-axial region

M47.012   Anterior spinal artery compression syndromes, cervical region

M47.013   Anterior spinal artery compression syndromes, cervicothoracic region

M47.014   Anterior spinal artery compression syndromes, thoracic region

M47.015   Anterior spinal artery compression syndromes, thoracolumbar region

M47.016   Anterior spinal artery compression syndromes, lumbar region

M47.019   Anterior spinal artery compression syndromes, site unspecified ▽

✓6th **M47.02 Vertebral artery compression syndromes**

M47.021   Vertebral artery compression syndromes, occipito-atlanto-axial region

M47.022   Vertebral artery compression syndromes, cervical region

M47.029   Vertebral artery compression syndromes, site unspecified ▽

✓5th **M47.1 Other spondylosis with myelopathy**
>   Spondylogenic compression of spinal cord
>   EXCLUDES 1   vertebral subluxation (M43.3-M43.5X9)

M47.10   Other spondylosis with myelopathy, site unspecified ▽

M47.11   Other spondylosis with myelopathy, occipito-atlanto-axial region

M47.12   Other spondylosis with myelopathy, cervical region

M47.13   Other spondylosis with myelopathy, cervicothoracic region

M47.14   Other spondylosis with myelopathy, thoracic region

M47.15   Other spondylosis with myelopathy, thoracolumbar region

M47.16   Other spondylosis with myelopathy, lumbar region

✓5th **M47.2 Other spondylosis with radiculopathy**

M47.20   Other spondylosis with radiculopathy, site unspecified ▽

M47.21   Other spondylosis with radiculopathy, occipito-atlanto-axial region

M47.22   Other spondylosis with radiculopathy, cervical region

M47.23   Other spondylosis with radiculopathy, cervicothoracic region

M47.24   Other spondylosis with radiculopathy, thoracic region

M47.25   Other spondylosis with radiculopathy, thoracolumbar region

M47.26   Other spondylosis with radiculopathy, lumbar region

M47.27   Other spondylosis with radiculopathy, lumbosacral region

M47.28   Other spondylosis with radiculopathy, sacral and sacrococcygeal region

✓5th **M47.8 Other spondylosis**

✓6th **M47.81 Spondylosis without myelopathy or radiculopathy**

M47.811   Spondylosis without myelopathy or radiculopathy, occipito-atlanto-axial region

M47.812   Spondylosis without myelopathy or radiculopathy, cervical region

M47.813   Spondylosis without myelopathy or radiculopathy, cervicothoracic region

M47.814   Spondylosis without myelopathy or radiculopathy, thoracic region

M47.815   Spondylosis without myelopathy or radiculopathy, thoracolumbar region

M47.816   Spondylosis without myelopathy or radiculopathy, lumbar region

M47.817   Spondylosis without myelopathy or radiculopathy, lumbosacral region

M47.818   Spondylosis without myelopathy or radiculopathy, sacral and sacrococcygeal region

M47.819   Spondylosis without myelopathy or radiculopathy, site unspecified ▽

✓6th **M47.89 Other spondylosis**

M47.891   Other spondylosis, occipito-atlanto-axial region

M47.892   Other spondylosis, cervical region

M47.893   Other spondylosis, cervicothoracic region

M47.894   Other spondylosis, thoracic region

M47.895   Other spondylosis, thoracolumbar region

M47.896   Other spondylosis, lumbar region

M47.897   Other spondylosis, lumbosacral region

M47.898   Other spondylosis, sacral and sacrococcygeal region

M47.899   Other spondylosis, site unspecified ▽

M47.9   Spondylosis, unspecified ▽

✓4th **M48 Other spondylopathies**

✓5th **M48.0 Spinal stenosis**
>   Caudal stenosis

M48.00   Spinal stenosis, site unspecified ▽

M48.01   Spinal stenosis, occipito-atlanto-axial region

M48.02   Spinal stenosis, cervical region

M48.03   Spinal stenosis, cervicothoracic region

M48.04   Spinal stenosis, thoracic region

M48.05   Spinal stenosis, thoracolumbar region

✓6th **M48.06 Spinal stenosis, lumbar region**
>   DEF: Spinal canal narrowing in the lumbar area with nerve root compression, causing muscle pain, fatigue, and weakness during extension of the lumbar spine; pain is relieved by sitting or bending.

● M48.061   Spinal stenosis, lumbar region without neurogenic claudication
>   Spinal stenosis, lumbar region NOS

● M48.062   Spinal stenosis, lumbar region with neurogenic claudication

M48.07   Spinal stenosis, lumbosacral region

M48.08   Spinal stenosis, sacral and sacrococcygeal region

✓5th **M48.1 Ankylosing hyperostosis [Forestier]**
>   Diffuse idiopathic skeletal hyperostosis [DISH]

M48.10   Ankylosing hyperostosis [Forestier], site unspecified ▽

M48.11   Ankylosing hyperostosis [Forestier], occipito-atlanto-axial region

M48.12   Ankylosing hyperostosis [Forestier], cervical region

M48.13   Ankylosing hyperostosis [Forestier], cervicothoracic region

M48.14   Ankylosing hyperostosis [Forestier], thoracic region

M48.15   Ankylosing hyperostosis [Forestier], thoracolumbar region

M48.16   Ankylosing hyperostosis [Forestier], lumbar region

M48.17   Ankylosing hyperostosis [Forestier], lumbosacral region

M48.18   Ankylosing hyperostosis [Forestier], sacral and sacrococcygeal region

M48.19   Ankylosing hyperostosis [Forestier], multiple sites in spine

✓5th **M48.2 Kissing spine**

M48.20   Kissing spine, site unspecified ▽

M48.21   Kissing spine, occipito-atlanto-axial region

M48.22   Kissing spine, cervical region

M48.23   Kissing spine, cervicothoracic region

M48.24   Kissing spine, thoracic region

M48.25   Kissing spine, thoracolumbar region

M48.26   Kissing spine, lumbar region

M48.27   Kissing spine, lumbosacral region

√5ᵗʰ **M48.3 Traumatic spondylopathy**

M48.30 Traumatic spondylopathy, site unspecified ▽

M48.31 Traumatic spondylopathy, occipito-atlanto-axial region

M48.32 Traumatic spondylopathy, cervical region

M48.33 Traumatic spondylopathy, cervicothoracic region

M48.34 Traumatic spondylopathy, thoracic region

M48.35 Traumatic spondylopathy, thoracolumbar region

M48.36 Traumatic spondylopathy, lumbar region

M48.37 Traumatic spondylopathy, lumbosacral region

M48.38 Traumatic spondylopathy, sacral and sacrococcygeal region

√5ᵗʰ **M48.4 Fatigue fracture of vertebra**
Stress fracture of vertebra

EXCLUDES 1 *pathological fracture NOS (M84.4-)*
pathological fracture of vertebra due to neoplasm (M84.58)
pathological fracture of vertebra due to other diagnosis (M84.68)
pathological fracture due to osteoporosis (M80.-)
traumatic fracture of vertebrae (S12.0-S12.3-, S22.0-, S32.0-)

The appropriate 7th character is to be added to each code from subcategory M48.4.
A	initial encounter for fracture
D	subsequent encounter for fracture with routine healing
G	subsequent encounter for fracture with delayed healing
S	sequela of fracture

√x 7ᵗʰ **M48.40** Fatigue fracture of vertebra, site unspecified ▽

√x 7ᵗʰ **M48.41** Fatigue fracture of vertebra, occipito-atlanto-axial region

√x 7ᵗʰ **M48.42** Fatigue fracture of vertebra, cervical region

√x 7ᵗʰ **M48.43** Fatigue fracture of vertebra, cervicothoracic region

√x 7ᵗʰ **M48.44** Fatigue fracture of vertebra, thoracic region

√x 7ᵗʰ **M48.45** Fatigue fracture of vertebra, thoracolumbar region

√x 7ᵗʰ **M48.46** Fatigue fracture of vertebra, lumbar region

√x 7ᵗʰ **M48.47** Fatigue fracture of vertebra, lumbosacral region

√x 7ᵗʰ **M48.48** Fatigue fracture of vertebra, sacral and sacrococcygeal region

√5ᵗʰ **M48.5 Collapsed vertebra, not elsewhere classified**
Collapsed vertebra NOS
Compression fracture of vertebra NOS
Wedging of vertebra NOS

EXCLUDES 1 *current injury—see Injury of spine, by body region*
fatigue fracture of vertebra (M48.4)
pathological fracture of vertebra due to neoplasm (M84.58)
pathological fracture of vertebra due to other diagnosis (M84.68)
pathological fracture due to osteoporosis (M80.-)
pathological fracture NOS (M84.4-)
stress fracture of vertebra (M48.4-)
traumatic fracture of vertebra (S12-, S22-, S32-)

The appropriate 7th character is to be added to each code from subcategory M48.5.
A	initial encounter for fracture
D	subsequent encounter for fracture with routine healing
G	subsequent encounter for fracture with delayed healing
S	sequela of fracture

¹ √x 7ᵗʰ **M48.50** Collapsed vertebra, not elsewhere classified, HCC ▽ site unspecified

¹ √x 7ᵗʰ **M48.51** Collapsed vertebra, not elsewhere classified, HCC occipito-atlanto-axial region

¹ √x 7ᵗʰ **M48.52** Collapsed vertebra, not elsewhere classified, HCC cervical region

¹ √x 7ᵗʰ **M48.53** Collapsed vertebra, not elsewhere classified, HCC cervicothoracic region

¹ √x 7ᵗʰ **M48.54** Collapsed vertebra, not elsewhere classified, HCC thoracic region

¹ √x 7ᵗʰ **M48.55** Collapsed vertebra, not elsewhere classified, HCC thoracolumbar region

¹ √x 7ᵗʰ **M48.56** Collapsed vertebra, not elsewhere classified, HCC lumbar region

¹ √x 7ᵗʰ **M48.57** Collapsed vertebra, not elsewhere classified, HCC lumbosacral region

¹ √x 7ᵗʰ **M48.58** Collapsed vertebra, not elsewhere classified, HCC sacral and sacrococcygeal region

√5ᵗʰ **M48.8 Other specified spondylopathies**
Ossification of posterior longitudinal ligament

√6ᵗʰ **M48.8X** Other specified spondylopathies

M48.8X1 Other specified spondylopathies, HCC occipito-atlanto-axial region

M48.8X2 Other specified spondylopathies, HCC cervical region

M48.8X3 Other specified spondylopathies, HCC cervicothoracic region

M48.8X4 Other specified spondylopathies, HCC thoracic region

M48.8X5 Other specified spondylopathies, HCC thoracolumbar region

M48.8X6 Other specified spondylopathies, HCC lumbar region

M48.8X7 Other specified spondylopathies, HCC lumbosacral region

M48.8X8 Other specified spondylopathies, HCC sacral and sacrococcygeal region

M48.8X9 Other specified spondylopathies, HCC ▽ site unspecified

M48.9 Spondylopathy, unspecified ▽

√4ᵗʰ **M49 Spondylopathies in diseases classified elsewhere**

INCLUDES	curvature of spine in diseases classified elsewhere
deformity of spine in diseases classified elsewhere
kyphosis in diseases classified elsewhere
scoliosis in diseases classified elsewhere
spondylopathy in diseases classified elsewhere

Code first underlying disease, such as:
brucellosis (A23.-)
Charcôt-Marie-Tooth disease (G60.0)
enterobacterial infections (A01-A04)
osteitis fibrosa cystica (E21.0)

EXCLUDES 1 *curvature of spine in tuberculosis [Pott's] (A18.01)*
enteropathic arthropathies (M07.-)
gonococcal spondylitis (A54.41)
neuropathic [tabes dorsalis] spondylitis (A52.11)
neuropathic spondylopathy in syringomyelia (G95.0)
neuropathic spondylopathy in tabes dorsalis (A52.11)
nonsyphilitic neuropathic spondylopathy NEC (G98.0)
spondylitis in syphilis (acquired) (A52.77)
tuberculous spondylitis (A18.01)
typhoid fever spondylitis (A01.05)

√5ᵗʰ **M49.8 Spondylopathy in diseases classified elsewhere**

M49.80 *Spondylopathy in diseases classified elsewhere,* HCC ▽ *site unspecified*

M49.81 *Spondylopathy in diseases classified elsewhere,* HCC *occipito-atlanto-axial region*

M49.82 *Spondylopathy in diseases classified elsewhere,* HCC *cervical region*

M49.83 *Spondylopathy in diseases classified elsewhere,* HCC *cervicothoracic region*

M49.84 *Spondylopathy in diseases classified elsewhere,* HCC *thoracic region*

M49.85 *Spondylopathy in diseases classified elsewhere,* HCC *thoracolumbar region*

M49.86 *Spondylopathy in diseases classified elsewhere,* HCC *lumbar region*

M49.87 *Spondylopathy in diseases classified elsewhere,* HCC *lumbosacral region*

M49.88 *Spondylopathy in diseases classified elsewhere,* HCC *sacral and sacrococcygeal region*

M49.89 *Spondylopathy in diseases classified elsewhere,* HCC *multiple sites in spine*

---

¹ HCC with 7th character indicating initial encounter (A, B or C - specific to category).

☑ Additional Character Req	√x 7ᵗʰ Placeholder Alert	Manifestation	HCC CMS-HCC Condition	▽ Unspecified Code	►◄ Revised Text	● New Code	▲ Revised Code Title

Other dorsopathies (M50-M54)

EXCLUDES 1   current injury—see injury of spine by body region
discitis NOS (M46.4-)

✓4th M50 Cervical disc disorders

> **NOTE**   Code to the most superior level of disorder.
> **INCLUDES**   cervicothoracic disc disorders with cervicalgia
> cervicothoracic disc disorders
> **AHA:** 2016, 1Q, 17

✓5th M50.0 Cervical disc disorder with myelopathy

- **M50.00 Cervical disc disorder with myelopathy, unspecified cervical region** ▽
- **M50.01 Cervical disc disorder with myelopathy, high cervical region**
  - C2-C3 disc disorder with myelopathy
  - C3-C4 disc disorder with myelopathy

✓6th M50.02 Cervical disc disorder with myelopathy, mid-cervical region
- **M50.020 Cervical disc disorder with myelopathy, mid-cervical region, unspecified level** ▽
- **M50.021 Cervical disc disorder at C4-C5 level with myelopathy**
  - C4-C5 disc disorder with myelopathy
- **M50.022 Cervical disc disorder at C5-C6 level with myelopathy**
  - C5-C6 disc disorder with myelopathy
- **M50.023 Cervical disc disorder at C6-C7 level with myelopathy**
  - C6-C7 disc disorder with myelopathy

- **M50.03 Cervical disc disorder with myelopathy, cervicothoracic region**
  - C7-T1 disc disorder with myelopathy

✓5th M50.1 Cervical disc disorder with radiculopathy

> **EXCLUDES 2**   brachial radiculitis NOS (M54.13)

- **M50.10 Cervical disc disorder with radiculopathy, unspecified cervical region** ▽
- **M50.11 Cervical disc disorder with radiculopathy, high cervical region**
  - C2-C3 disc disorder with radiculopathy
  - C3 radiculopathy due to disc disorder
  - C3-C4 disc disorder with radiculopathy
  - C4 radiculopathy due to disc disorder

✓6th M50.12 Cervical disc disorder with radiculopathy, mid-cervical region
- **M50.120 Mid-cervical disc disorder, unspecified** ▽
- **M50.121 Cervical disc disorder at C4-C5 level with radiculopathy**
  - C4-C5 disc disorder with radiculopathy
  - C5 radiculopathy due to disc disorder
- **M50.122 Cervical disc disorder at C5-C6 level with radiculopathy**
  - C5-C6 disc disorder with radiculopathy
  - C6 radiculopathy due to disc disorder
- **M50.123 Cervical disc disorder at C6-C7 level with radiculopathy**
  - C6-C7 disc disorder with radiculopathy
  - C7 radiculopathy due to disc disorder

- **M50.13 Cervical disc disorder with radiculopathy, cervicothoracic region**
  - C7-T1 disc disorder with radiculopathy
  - C8 radiculopathy due to disc disorder

✓5th M50.2 Other cervical disc displacement

- **M50.20 Other cervical disc displacement, unspecified cervical region** ▽
- **M50.21 Other cervical disc displacement, high cervical region**
  - Other C2-C3 cervical disc displacement
  - Other C3-C4 cervical disc displacement

✓6th M50.22 Other cervical disc displacement, mid-cervical region
- **M50.220 Other cervical disc displacement, mid-cervical region, unspecified level** ▽
- **M50.221 Other cervical disc displacement at C4-C5 level**
  - Other C4-C5 cervical disc displacement
- **M50.222 Other cervical disc displacement at C5-C6 level**
  - Other C5-C6 cervical disc displacement

- **M50.223 Other cervical disc displacement at C6-C7 level**
  - Other C6-C7 cervical disc displacement

- **M50.23 Other cervical disc displacement, cervicothoracic region**
  - Other C7-T1 cervical disc displacement

✓5th M50.3 Other cervical disc degeneration

- **M50.30 Other cervical disc degeneration, unspecified cervical region** ▽
- **M50.31 Other cervical disc degeneration, high cervical region**
  - Other C2-C3 cervical disc degeneration
  - Other C3-C4 cervical disc degeneration

✓6th M50.32 Other cervical disc degeneration, mid-cervical region
- **M50.320 Other cervical disc degeneration, mid-cervical region, unspecified level** ▽
- **M50.321 Other cervical disc degeneration at C4-C5 level**
  - Other C4-C5 cervical disc degeneration
- **M50.322 Other cervical disc degeneration at C5-C6 level**
  - Other C5-C6 cervical disc degeneration
- **M50.323 Other cervical disc degeneration at C6-C7 level**
  - Other C6-C7 cervical disc degeneration

- **M50.33 Other cervical disc degeneration, cervicothoracic region**
  - Other C7-T1 cervical disc degeneration

✓5th M50.8 Other cervical disc disorders

- **M50.80 Other cervical disc disorders, unspecified cervical region** ▽
- **M50.81 Other cervical disc disorders, high cervical region**
  - Other C2-C3 cervical disc disorders
  - Other C3-C4 cervical disc disorders

✓6th M50.82 Other cervical disc disorders, mid-cervical region
- **M50.820 Other cervical disc disorders, mid-cervical region, unspecified level** ▽
- **M50.821 Other cervical disc disorders at C4-C5 level**
  - Other C4-C5 cervical disc disorders
- **M50.822 Other cervical disc disorders at C5-C6 level**
  - Other C5-C6 cervical disc disorders
- **M50.823 Other cervical disc disorders at C6-C7 level**
  - Other C6-C7 cervical disc disorders

- **M50.83 Other cervical disc disorders, cervicothoracic region**
  - Other C7-T1 cervical disc disorders

✓5th M50.9 Cervical disc disorder, unspecified

- **M50.90 Cervical disc disorder, unspecified, unspecified cervical region** ▽
- **M50.91 Cervical disc disorder, unspecified, high cervical region** ▽
  - C2-C3 cervical disc disorder, unspecified
  - C3-C4 cervical disc disorder, unspecified

✓6th M50.92 Cervical disc disorder, unspecified, mid-cervical region
- **M50.920 Unspecified cervical disc disorder, mid-cervical region, unspecified level** ▽
- **M50.921 Unspecified cervical disc disorder at C4-C5 level** ▽
  - Unspecified C4-C5 cervical disc disorder
- **M50.922 Unspecified cervical disc disorder at C5-C6 level** ▽
  - Unspecified C5-C6 cervical disc disorder
- **M50.923 Unspecified cervical disc disorder at C6-C7 level** ▽
  - Unspecified C6-C7 cervical disc disorder

- **M50.93 Cervical disc disorder, unspecified, cervicothoracic region** ▽
  - C7-T1 cervical disc disorder, unspecified

✓4th M51 Thoracic, thoracolumbar, and lumbosacral intervertebral disc disorders

> **EXCLUDES 2**   cervical and cervicothoracic disc disorders (M50.-)
> sacral and sacrococcygeal disorders (M53.3)

✓5th M51.0 Thoracic, thoracolumbar and lumbosacral intervertebral disc disorders with myelopathy
- **M51.04 Intervertebral disc disorders with myelopathy, thoracic region**

| **EXCLUDES 1** Not coded here | **EXCLUDES 2** Not included here | **N** Newborn Age: 0 | **P** Pediatric Age: 0-17 | **M** Maternity Age: 12-55 | **A** Adult Age: 15-124 |

M51.Ø5   **Intervertebral disc disorders with myelopathy, thoracolumbar region**

M51.Ø6   **Intervertebral disc disorders with myelopathy, lumbar region**

✓5ᵗʰ **M51.1 Thoracic, thoracolumbar and lumbosacral intervertebral disc disorders** with radiculopathy
Sciatica due to intervertebral disc disorder
   EXCLUDES 1   lumbar radiculitis NOS (M54.16)
           sciatica NOS (M54.3)

M51.14   **Intervertebral disc with radiculopathy, thoracic region**

M51.15   **Intervertebral disc disorders with radiculopathy, thoracolumbar region**

M51.16   **Intervertebral disc disorders with radiculopathy, lumbar region**

M51.17   **Intervertebral disc disorders with radiculopathy, lumbosacral region**

✓5ᵗʰ **M51.2 Other thoracic, thoracolumbar and lumbosacral intervertebral disc** displacement
Lumbago due to displacement of intervertebral disc

M51.24   **Other intervertebral disc displacement, thoracic region**

M51.25   **Other intervertebral disc displacement, thoracolumbar region**

M51.26   **Other intervertebral disc displacement, lumbar region**

M51.27   **Other intervertebral disc displacement, lumbosacral region**

✓5ᵗʰ **M51.3 Other thoracic, thoracolumbar and lumbosacral intervertebral disc** degeneration
AHA: 2013, 3Q, 22

M51.34   **Other intervertebral disc degeneration, thoracic region**

M51.35   **Other intervertebral disc degeneration, thoracolumbar region**

M51.36   **Other intervertebral disc degeneration, lumbar region**

M51.37   **Other intervertebral disc degeneration, lumbosacral region**

✓5ᵗʰ **M51.4 Schmorl's nodes**
DEF: Irregular bone defect in the margin of the vertebral body; causes herniation into end plate of vertebral body.

M51.44   **Schmorl's nodes, thoracic region**

M51.45   **Schmorl's nodes, thoracolumbar region**

M51.46   **Schmorl's nodes, lumbar region**

M51.47   **Schmorl's nodes, lumbosacral region**

✓5ᵗʰ **M51.8 Other thoracic, thoracolumbar and lumbosacral intervertebral disc disorders**

M51.84   **Other intervertebral disc disorders, thoracic region**

M51.85   **Other intervertebral disc disorders, thoracolumbar region**

M51.86   **Other intervertebral disc disorders, lumbar region**

M51.87   **Other intervertebral disc disorders, lumbosacral region**

M51.9   **Unspecified thoracic, thoracolumbar and lumbosacral intervertebral disc disorder** ▽

✓4ᵗʰ **M53 Other and unspecified dorsopathies, not elsewhere classified**

M53.Ø   **Cervicocranial syndrome**
Posterior cervical sympathetic syndrome

M53.1   **Cervicobrachial syndrome**
   EXCLUDES 2   cervical disc disorder (M5Ø.-)
           thoracic outlet syndrome (G54.Ø)

✓5ᵗʰ **M53.2 Spinal instabilities**

   ✓6ᵗʰ **M53.2X Spinal** instabilities

M53.2X1   **Spinal instabilities, occipito-atlanto-axial region**

M53.2X2   **Spinal instabilities, cervical region**

M53.2X3   **Spinal instabilities, cervicothoracic region**

M53.2X4   **Spinal instabilities, thoracic region**

M53.2X5   **Spinal instabilities, thoracolumbar region**

M53.2X6   **Spinal instabilities, lumbar region**

M53.2X7   **Spinal instabilities, lumbosacral region**

M53.2X8   **Spinal instabilities, sacral and sacrococcygeal region**

Displacement Intervertebral Disc

Normal Top View   Herniated Top View

M53.2X9   **Spinal instabilities, site unspecified** ▽

M53.3   **Sacrococcygeal disorders, not elsewhere classified**
Coccygodynia

✓5ᵗʰ **M53.8 Other specified** dorsopathies

M53.8Ø   **Other specified dorsopathies, site unspecified** ▽

M53.81   **Other specified dorsopathies, occipito-atlanto-axial region**

M53.82   **Other specified dorsopathies, cervical region**

M53.83   **Other specified dorsopathies, cervicothoracic region**

M53.84   **Other specified dorsopathies, thoracic region**

M53.85   **Other specified dorsopathies, thoracolumbar region**

M53.86   **Other specified dorsopathies, lumbar region**

M53.87   **Other specified dorsopathies, lumbosacral region**

M53.88   **Other specified dorsopathies, sacral and sacrococcygeal region**

M53.9   **Dorsopathy, unspecified** ▽

✓4ᵗʰ **M54 Dorsalgia**
   EXCLUDES 1   psychogenic dorsalgia (F45.41)

✓5ᵗʰ **M54.Ø Panniculitis affecting regions of neck and back**
   EXCLUDES 1   lupus panniculitis (L93.2)
           panniculitis NOS (M79.3)
           relapsing [Weber-Christian] panniculitis (M35.6)

M54.ØØ   **Panniculitis affecting regions of neck and back, site unspecified** ▽

M54.Ø1   **Panniculitis affecting regions of neck and back, occipito-atlanto-axial region**

M54.Ø2   **Panniculitis affecting regions of neck and back, cervical region**

M54.Ø3   **Panniculitis affecting regions of neck and back, cervicothoracic region**

M54.Ø4   **Panniculitis affecting regions of neck and back, thoracic region**

M54.Ø5   **Panniculitis affecting regions of neck and back, thoracolumbar region**

M54.Ø6   **Panniculitis affecting regions of neck and back, lumbar region**

M54.Ø7   **Panniculitis affecting regions of neck and back, lumbosacral region**

M54.Ø8   **Panniculitis affecting regions of neck and back, sacral and sacrococcygeal region**

M54.Ø9   **Panniculitis affecting regions, neck and back, multiple sites in spine**

✓5ᵗʰ **M54.1 Radiculopathy**
Brachial neuritis or radiculitis NOS
Lumbar neuritis or radiculitis NOS
Lumbosacral neuritis or radiculitis NOS
Thoracic neuritis or radiculitis NOS
Radiculitis NOS
   EXCLUDES 1   neuralgia and neuritis NOS (M79.2)
           radiculopathy with cervical disc disorder (M5Ø.1)
           radiculopathy with lumbar and other intervertebral disc disorder (M51.1-)
           radiculopathy with spondylosis (M47.2-)

M54.1Ø   **Radiculopathy, site unspecified** ▽

M54.11   **Radiculopathy, occipito-atlanto-axial region**

M54.12   **Radiculopathy, cervical region**

M54.13   **Radiculopathy, cervicothoracic region**

M54.14   **Radiculopathy, thoracic region**

☑ Additional Character Req   ✓x7ᵗʰ Placeholder Alert   Manifestation   HCC CMS-HCC Condition   ▽ Unspecified Code   ►◄ Revised Text   ● New Code   ▲ Revised Code Title

ICD-10-CM 2018   759

M54.15   Radiculopathy, **thoracolumbar** region

M54.16   Radiculopathy, **lumbar** region

M54.17   Radiculopathy, **lumbosacral** region

M54.18   Radiculopathy, **sacral and sacrococcygeal** region

M54.2 Cervicalgia
> EXCLUDES 1   cervicalgia due to intervertebral cervical disc disorder (M50.-)

✓5ᵗʰ M54.3 Sciatica
> EXCLUDES 1   lesion of sciatic nerve (G57.0)
> sciatica due to intervertebral disc disorder (M51.1-)
> sciatica with lumbago (M54.4-)

M54.30   Sciatica, unspecified side   ▽

M54.31   Sciatica, **right** side

M54.32   Sciatica, **left** side

✓5ᵗʰ M54.4 Lumbago with sciatica
> EXCLUDES 1   lumbago with sciatica due to intervertebral disc disorder (M51.1-)
>
> **AHA:** 2016, 2Q, 7

M54.40   Lumbago with sciatica, unspecified side   ▽

M54.41   Lumbago with sciatica, **right** side

M54.42   Lumbago with sciatica, **left** side

M54.5 Low back pain
> Loin pain
> Lumbago NOS
> EXCLUDES 1   low back strain (S39.012)
> lumbago due to intervertebral disc displacement (M51.2-)
> lumbago with sciatica (M54.4-)

M54.6 Pain in thoracic spine
> EXCLUDES 1   pain in thoracic spine due to intervertebral disc disorder (M51.-)

✓5ᵗʰ M54.8 Other dorsalgia
> EXCLUDES 1   dorsalgia in thoracic region (M54.6)
> low back pain (M54.5)

M54.81   Occipital neuralgia

M54.89   Other dorsalgia

M54.9 Dorsalgia, unspecified   ▽
> Backache NOS   Back pain NOS

SOFT TISSUE DISORDERS (M60-M79)

Disorders of muscles (M60-M63)
> EXCLUDES 1   dermatopolymyositis (M33.-)
> muscular dystrophies and myopathies (G71-G72)
> myopathy in amyloidosis (E85.-)
> myopathy in polyarteritis nodosa (M30.0)
> myopathy in rheumatoid arthritis (M05.32)
> myopathy in scleroderma (M34.-)
> myopathy in Sjögren's syndrome (M35.03)
> myopathy in systemic lupus erythematosus (M32.-)

✓4ᵗʰ M60 Myositis
> EXCLUDES 2   inclusion body myositis [IBM] (G72.41)

✓5ᵗʰ M60.0 Infective myositis
> Tropical pyomyositis
> Use additional code (B95-B97) to identify infectious agent

✓6ᵗʰ M60.00 Infective myositis, unspecified site

M60.000   **Infective myositis, unspecified right arm**
> Infective myositis, right upper limb NOS

M60.001   **Infective myositis, unspecified left arm**
> Infective myositis, left upper limb NOS

M60.002   **Infective myositis, unspecified arm**   ▽
> Infective myositis, upper limb NOS

M60.003   **Infective myositis, unspecified right leg**
> Infective myositis, right lower limb NOS

M60.004   **Infective myositis, unspecified left leg**
> Infective myositis, left lower limb NOS

M60.005   **Infective myositis, unspecified leg**   ▽
> Infective myositis, lower limb NOS

M60.009   **Infective myositis, unspecified site**   ▽

✓6ᵗʰ M60.01 Infective myositis, shoulder

M60.011   Infective myositis, **right** shoulder

M60.012   Infective myositis, **left** shoulder

M60.019   Infective myositis, **unspecified** shoulder ▽

✓6ᵗʰ M60.02 Infective myositis, upper arm

M60.021   Infective myositis, **right upper arm**

M60.022   Infective myositis, **left upper arm**

M60.029   **Infective myositis, unspecified**   ▽
> **upper arm**

✓6ᵗʰ M60.03 Infective myositis, forearm

M60.031   Infective myositis, **right forearm**

M60.032   Infective myositis, **left forearm**

M60.039   Infective myositis, **unspecified forearm** ▽

✓6ᵗʰ M60.04 Infective myositis, hand and fingers

M60.041   Infective myositis, **right hand**

M60.042   Infective myositis, **left hand**

M60.043   Infective myositis, **unspecified hand**   ▽

M60.044   Infective myositis, **right finger(s)**

M60.045   Infective myositis, **left finger(s)**

M60.046   Infective myositis, **unspecified finger(s)** ▽

✓6ᵗʰ M60.05 Infective myositis, thigh

M60.051   Infective myositis, **right thigh**

M60.052   Infective myositis, **left thigh**

M60.059   Infective myositis, **unspecified thigh**   ▽

✓6ᵗʰ M60.06 Infective myositis, lower leg

M60.061   Infective myositis, **right lower leg**

M60.062   Infective myositis, **left lower leg**

M60.069   **Infective myositis, unspecified**   ▽
> **lower leg**

✓6ᵗʰ M60.07 Infective myositis, ankle, foot and toes

M60.070   Infective myositis, **right ankle**

M60.071   Infective myositis, **left ankle**

M60.072   Infective myositis, **unspecified ankle**   ▽

M60.073   Infective myositis, **right foot**

M60.074   Infective myositis, **left foot**

M60.075   Infective myositis, **unspecified foot**   ▽

M60.076   Infective myositis, **right toe(s)**

M60.077   Infective myositis, **left toe(s)**

M60.078   Infective myositis, **unspecified toe(s)**   ▽

M60.08   Infective myositis, other site

M60.09   Infective myositis, **multiple sites**

✓5ᵗʰ M60.1 Interstitial myositis

M60.10   Interstitial myositis of unspecified site   ▽

✓6ᵗʰ M60.11 Interstitial myositis, shoulder

M60.111   Interstitial myositis, **right shoulder**

M60.112   Interstitial myositis, **left shoulder**

M60.119   **Interstitial myositis, unspecified**   ▽
> **shoulder**

✓6ᵗʰ M60.12 Interstitial myositis, upper arm

M60.121   Interstitial myositis, **right upper arm**

M60.122   Interstitial myositis, **left upper arm**

M60.129   **Interstitial myositis, unspecified**   ▽
> **upper arm**

✓6ᵗʰ M60.13 Interstitial myositis, forearm

M60.131   Interstitial myositis, **right forearm**

M60.132   Interstitial myositis, **left forearm**

M60.139   **Interstitial myositis, unspecified**   ▽
> **forearm**

✓6ᵗʰ M60.14 Interstitial myositis, hand

M60.141   Interstitial myositis, **right hand**

M60.142   Interstitial myositis, **left hand**

M60.149   Interstitial myositis, **unspecified hand**   ▽

✓6ᵗʰ M60.15 Interstitial myositis, thigh

M60.151   Interstitial myositis, **right thigh**

M60.152   Interstitial myositis, **left thigh**

M60.159   Interstitial myositis, **unspecified thigh** ▽

✓6ᵗʰ M60.16 Interstitial myositis, lower leg

M60.161   Interstitial myositis, **right lower leg**

M60.162   Interstitial myositis, **left lower leg**

M60.169   **Interstitial myositis, unspecified**   ▽
> **lower leg**

✓6ᵗʰ M60.17 Interstitial myositis, ankle and foot

M60.171   Interstitial myositis, **right ankle and foot**

M60.172   Interstitial myositis, **left ankle and foot**

M60.179   **Interstitial myositis, unspecified**   ▽
> **ankle and foot**

M60.18   Interstitial myositis, other site

M60.19   Interstitial myositis, **multiple sites**

EXCLUDES 1 Not coded here   EXCLUDES 2 Not included here   N Newborn Age: 0   P Pediatric Age: 0-17   M Maternity Age: 12-55   A Adult Age: 15-124

760   ICD-10-CM 2018

✓5ᵗʰ **M60.2 Foreign body granuloma of soft tissue, not elsewhere classified**
> Use additional code to identify the type of retained foreign body (Z18.-)
> EXCLUDES 1   *foreign body granuloma of skin and subcutaneous tissue (L92.3)*

   M60.20 Foreign body granuloma of soft tissue, not elsewhere classified, unspecified site ▽

   ✓6ᵗʰ M60.21 Foreign body granuloma of soft tissue, not elsewhere classified, shoulder
     M60.211 Foreign body granuloma of soft tissue, not elsewhere classified, right shoulder
     M60.212 Foreign body granuloma of soft tissue, not elsewhere classified, left shoulder
     M60.219 Foreign body granuloma of soft tissue, not elsewhere classified, unspecified shoulder ▽

   ✓6ᵗʰ M60.22 Foreign body granuloma of soft tissue, not elsewhere classified, upper arm
     M60.221 Foreign body granuloma of soft tissue, not elsewhere classified, right upper arm
     M60.222 Foreign body granuloma of soft tissue, not elsewhere classified, left upper arm
     M60.229 Foreign body granuloma of soft tissue, not elsewhere classified, unspecified upper arm ▽

   ✓6ᵗʰ M60.23 Foreign body granuloma of soft tissue, not elsewhere classified, forearm
     M60.231 Foreign body granuloma of soft tissue, not elsewhere classified, right forearm
     M60.232 Foreign body granuloma of soft tissue, not elsewhere classified, left forearm
     M60.239 Foreign body granuloma of soft tissue, not elsewhere classified, unspecified forearm ▽

   ✓6ᵗʰ M60.24 Foreign body granuloma of soft tissue, not elsewhere classified, hand
     M60.241 Foreign body granuloma of soft tissue, not elsewhere classified, right hand
     M60.242 Foreign body granuloma of soft tissue, not elsewhere classified, left hand
     M60.249 Foreign body granuloma of soft tissue, not elsewhere classified, unspecified hand ▽

   ✓6ᵗʰ M60.25 Foreign body granuloma of soft tissue, not elsewhere classified, thigh
     M60.251 Foreign body granuloma of soft tissue, not elsewhere classified, right thigh
     M60.252 Foreign body granuloma of soft tissue, not elsewhere classified, left thigh
     M60.259 Foreign body granuloma of soft tissue, not elsewhere classified, unspecified thigh ▽

   ✓6ᵗʰ M60.26 Foreign body granuloma of soft tissue, not elsewhere classified, lower leg
     M60.261 Foreign body granuloma of soft tissue, not elsewhere classified, right lower leg
     M60.262 Foreign body granuloma of soft tissue, not elsewhere classified, left lower leg
     M60.269 Foreign body granuloma of soft tissue, not elsewhere classified, unspecified lower leg ▽

   ✓6ᵗʰ M60.27 Foreign body granuloma of soft tissue, not elsewhere classified, ankle and foot
     M60.271 Foreign body granuloma of soft tissue, not elsewhere classified, right ankle and foot
     M60.272 Foreign body granuloma of soft tissue, not elsewhere classified, left ankle and foot
     M60.279 Foreign body granuloma of soft tissue, not elsewhere classified, unspecified ankle and foot ▽

   M60.28 Foreign body granuloma of soft tissue, not elsewhere classified, other site

✓5ᵗʰ **M60.8 Other myositis**
   M60.80 Other myositis, unspecified site ▽
   ✓6ᵗʰ M60.81 Other myositis shoulder
     M60.811 Other myositis, right shoulder
     M60.812 Other myositis, left shoulder
     M60.819 Other myositis, unspecified shoulder ▽

   ✓6ᵗʰ M60.82 Other myositis, upper arm
     M60.821 Other myositis, right upper arm
     M60.822 Other myositis, left upper arm
     M60.829 Other myositis, unspecified upper arm ▽

   ✓6ᵗʰ M60.83 Other myositis, forearm
     M60.831 Other myositis, right forearm
     M60.832 Other myositis, left forearm
     M60.839 Other myositis, unspecified forearm ▽

   ✓6ᵗʰ M60.84 Other myositis, hand
     M60.841 Other myositis, right hand
     M60.842 Other myositis, left hand
     M60.849 Other myositis, unspecified hand ▽

   ✓6ᵗʰ M60.85 Other myositis, thigh
     M60.851 Other myositis, right thigh
     M60.852 Other myositis, left thigh
     M60.859 Other myositis, unspecified thigh ▽

   ✓6ᵗʰ M60.86 Other myositis, lower leg
     M60.861 Other myositis, right lower leg
     M60.862 Other myositis, left lower leg
     M60.869 Other myositis, unspecified lower leg ▽

   ✓6ᵗʰ M60.87 Other myositis, ankle and foot
     M60.871 Other myositis, right ankle and foot
     M60.872 Other myositis, left ankle and foot
     M60.879 Other myositis, unspecified ankle and foot ▽

   M60.88 Other myositis, other site
   M60.89 Other myositis, multiple sites

   M60.9 Myositis, unspecified ▽

✓4ᵗʰ **M61 Calcification and ossification of muscle**

✓5ᵗʰ **M61.0 Myositis ossificans traumatica**
   M61.00 Myositis ossificans traumatica, unspecified site ▽

   ✓6ᵗʰ M61.01 Myositis ossificans traumatica, shoulder
     M61.011 Myositis ossificans traumatica, right shoulder
     M61.012 Myositis ossificans traumatica, left shoulder
     M61.019 Myositis ossificans traumatica, unspecified shoulder ▽

   ✓6ᵗʰ M61.02 Myositis ossificans traumatica, upper arm
     M61.021 Myositis ossificans traumatica, right upper arm
     M61.022 Myositis ossificans traumatica, left upper arm
     M61.029 Myositis ossificans traumatica, unspecified upper arm ▽

   ✓6ᵗʰ M61.03 Myositis ossificans traumatica, forearm
     M61.031 Myositis ossificans traumatica, right forearm
     M61.032 Myositis ossificans traumatica, left forearm
     M61.039 Myositis ossificans traumatica, unspecified forearm ▽

   ✓6ᵗʰ M61.04 Myositis ossificans traumatica, hand
     M61.041 Myositis ossificans traumatica, right hand
     M61.042 Myositis ossificans traumatica, left hand
     M61.049 Myositis ossificans traumatica, unspecified hand ▽

   ✓6ᵗʰ M61.05 Myositis ossificans traumatica, thigh
     M61.051 Myositis ossificans traumatica, right thigh
     M61.052 Myositis ossificans traumatica, left thigh
     M61.059 Myositis ossificans traumatica, unspecified thigh ▽

   ✓6ᵗʰ M61.06 Myositis ossificans traumatica, lower leg
     M61.061 Myositis ossificans traumatica, right lower leg
     M61.062 Myositis ossificans traumatica, left lower leg
     M61.069 Myositis ossificans traumatica, unspecified lower leg ▽

   ✓6ᵗʰ M61.07 Myositis ossificans traumatica, ankle and foot
     M61.071 Myositis ossificans traumatica, right ankle and foot

---

☑ Additional Character Req   ✓x7ᵗʰ Placeholder Alert   Manifestation   HCC CMS-HCC Condition   ▽ Unspecified Code   ►◄ Revised Text   ● New Code   ▲ Revised Code Title

M61.072 **Myositis ossificans traumatica, left ankle and foot**

M61.079 **Myositis ossificans traumatica, unspecified ankle and foot** ▽

M61.08 **Myositis ossificans traumatica, other site**

M61.09 **Myositis ossificans traumatica, multiple sites**

✓5ᵗʰ M61.1 **Myositis ossificans progressiva**
Fibrodysplasia ossificans progressiva

M61.10 **Myositis ossificans progressiva, unspecified site** ▽

✓6ᵗʰ M61.11 **Myositis ossificans progressiva, shoulder**

M61.111 **Myositis ossificans progressiva, right shoulder**

M61.112 **Myositis ossificans progressiva, left shoulder**

M61.119 **Myositis ossificans progressiva, unspecified shoulder** ▽

✓6ᵗʰ M61.12 **Myositis ossificans progressiva, upper arm**

M61.121 **Myositis ossificans progressiva, right upper arm**

M61.122 **Myositis ossificans progressiva, left upper arm**

M61.129 **Myositis ossificans progressiva, unspecified arm** ▽

✓6ᵗʰ M61.13 **Myositis ossificans progressiva, forearm**

M61.131 **Myositis ossificans progressiva, right forearm**

M61.132 **Myositis ossificans progressiva, left forearm**

M61.139 **Myositis ossificans progressiva, unspecified forearm** ▽

✓6ᵗʰ M61.14 **Myositis ossificans progressiva, hand and finger(s)**

M61.141 **Myositis ossificans progressiva, right hand**

M61.142 **Myositis ossificans progressiva, left hand**

M61.143 **Myositis ossificans progressiva, unspecified hand** ▽

M61.144 **Myositis ossificans progressiva, right finger(s)**

M61.145 **Myositis ossificans progressiva, left finger(s)**

M61.146 **Myositis ossificans progressiva, unspecified finger(s)** ▽

✓6ᵗʰ M61.15 **Myositis ossificans progressiva, thigh**

M61.151 **Myositis ossificans progressiva, right thigh**

M61.152 **Myositis ossificans progressiva, left thigh**

M61.159 **Myositis ossificans progressiva, unspecified thigh** ▽

✓6ᵗʰ M61.16 **Myositis ossificans progressiva, lower leg**

M61.161 **Myositis ossificans progressiva, right lower leg**

M61.162 **Myositis ossificans progressiva, left lower leg**

M61.169 **Myositis ossificans progressiva, unspecified lower leg** ▽

✓6ᵗʰ M61.17 **Myositis ossificans progressiva, ankle, foot and toe(s)**

M61.171 **Myositis ossificans progressiva, right ankle**

M61.172 **Myositis ossificans progressiva, left ankle**

M61.173 **Myositis ossificans progressiva, unspecified ankle** ▽

M61.174 **Myositis ossificans progressiva, right foot**

M61.175 **Myositis ossificans progressiva, left foot**

M61.176 **Myositis ossificans progressiva, unspecified foot** ▽

M61.177 **Myositis ossificans progressiva, right toe(s)**

M61.178 **Myositis ossificans progressiva, left toe(s)**

M61.179 **Myositis ossificans progressiva, unspecified toe(s)** ▽

M61.18 **Myositis ossificans progressiva, other site**

M61.19 **Myositis ossificans progressiva, multiple sites**

✓5ᵗʰ M61.2 **Paralytic calcification and ossification of muscle**
Myositis ossificans associated with quadriplegia or paraplegia

M61.20 **Paralytic calcification and ossification of muscle, unspecified site** ▽

✓6ᵗʰ M61.21 **Paralytic calcification and ossification of muscle, shoulder**

M61.211 **Paralytic calcification and ossification of muscle, right shoulder**

M61.212 **Paralytic calcification and ossification of muscle, left shoulder**

M61.219 **Paralytic calcification and ossification of muscle, unspecified shoulder** ▽

✓6ᵗʰ M61.22 **Paralytic calcification and ossification of muscle, upper arm**

M61.221 **Paralytic calcification and ossification of muscle, right upper arm**

M61.222 **Paralytic calcification and ossification of muscle, left upper arm**

M61.229 **Paralytic calcification and ossification of muscle, unspecified upper arm** ▽

✓6ᵗʰ M61.23 **Paralytic calcification and ossification of muscle, forearm**

M61.231 **Paralytic calcification and ossification of muscle, right forearm**

M61.232 **Paralytic calcification and ossification of muscle, left forearm**

M61.239 **Paralytic calcification and ossification of muscle, unspecified forearm** ▽

✓6ᵗʰ M61.24 **Paralytic calcification and ossification of muscle, hand**

M61.241 **Paralytic calcification and ossification of muscle, right hand**

M61.242 **Paralytic calcification and ossification of muscle, left hand**

M61.249 **Paralytic calcification and ossification of muscle, unspecified hand** ▽

✓6ᵗʰ M61.25 **Paralytic calcification and ossification of muscle, thigh**

M61.251 **Paralytic calcification and ossification of muscle, right thigh**

M61.252 **Paralytic calcification and ossification of muscle, left thigh**

M61.259 **Paralytic calcification and ossification of muscle, unspecified thigh** ▽

✓6ᵗʰ M61.26 **Paralytic calcification and ossification of muscle, lower leg**

M61.261 **Paralytic calcification and ossification of muscle, right lower leg**

M61.262 **Paralytic calcification and ossification of muscle, left lower leg**

M61.269 **Paralytic calcification and ossification of muscle, unspecified lower leg** ▽

✓6ᵗʰ M61.27 **Paralytic calcification and ossification of muscle, ankle and foot**

M61.271 **Paralytic calcification and ossification of muscle, right ankle and foot**

M61.272 **Paralytic calcification and ossification of muscle, left ankle and foot**

M61.279 **Paralytic calcification and ossification of muscle, unspecified ankle and foot** ▽

M61.28 **Paralytic calcification and ossification of muscle, other site**

M61.29 **Paralytic calcification and ossification of muscle, multiple sites**

✓5ᵗʰ M61.3 **Calcification and ossification of muscles associated with burns**
Myositis ossificans associated with burns

M61.30 **Calcification and ossification of muscles associated with burns, unspecified site** ▽

✓6ᵗʰ M61.31 **Calcification and ossification of muscles associated with burns, shoulder**

M61.311 **Calcification and ossification of muscles associated with burns, right shoulder**

M61.312 **Calcification and ossification of muscles associated with burns, left shoulder**

M61.319 **Calcification and ossification of muscles associated with burns, unspecified shoulder** ▽

✓6ᵗʰ M61.32 **Calcification and ossification of muscles associated with burns, upper arm**

M61.321 **Calcification and ossification of muscles associated with burns, right upper arm**

EXCLUDES 1 Not coded here   EXCLUDES 2 Not included here   N Newborn Age: 0   P Pediatric Age: 0-17   M Maternity Age: 12-55   A Adult Age: 15-124

762   ICD-10-CM 2018

    M61.322   Calcification and ossification of muscles associated with burns, left upper arm

    M61.329   Calcification and ossification of muscles associated with burns, unspecified upper arm ▽

✓6ᵗʰ M61.33   Calcification and ossification of muscles associated with burns, forearm

    M61.331   Calcification and ossification of muscles associated with burns, right forearm

    M61.332   Calcification and ossification of muscles associated with burns, left forearm

    M61.339   Calcification and ossification of muscles associated with burns, unspecified forearm ▽

✓6ᵗʰ M61.34   Calcification and ossification of muscles associated with burns, hand

    M61.341   Calcification and ossification of muscles associated with burns, right hand

    M61.342   Calcification and ossification of muscles associated with burns, left hand

    M61.349   Calcification and ossification of muscles associated with burns, unspecified hand ▽

✓6ᵗʰ M61.35   Calcification and ossification of muscles associated with burns, thigh

    M61.351   Calcification and ossification of muscles associated with burns, right thigh

    M61.352   Calcification and ossification of muscles associated with burns, left thigh

    M61.359   Calcification and ossification of muscles associated with burns, unspecified thigh ▽

✓6ᵗʰ M61.36   Calcification and ossification of muscles associated with burns, lower leg

    M61.361   Calcification and ossification of muscles associated with burns, right lower leg

    M61.362   Calcification and ossification of muscles associated with burns, left lower leg

    M61.369   Calcification and ossification of muscles associated with burns, unspecified lower leg ▽

✓6ᵗʰ M61.37   Calcification and ossification of muscles associated with burns, ankle and foot

    M61.371   Calcification and ossification of muscles associated with burns, right ankle and foot

    M61.372   Calcification and ossification of muscles associated with burns, left ankle and foot

    M61.379   Calcification and ossification of muscles associated with burns, unspecified ankle and foot ▽

  M61.38   Calcification and ossification of muscles associated with burns, other site

  M61.39   Calcification and ossification of muscles associated with burns, multiple sites

✓5ᵗʰ M61.4   Other calcification of muscle

    EXCLUDES 1   calcific tendinitis NOS (M65.2-)
            calcific tendinitis of shoulder (M75.3)

  M61.40   Other calcification of muscle, unspecified site ▽

✓6ᵗʰ M61.41   Other calcification of muscle, shoulder

    M61.411   Other calcification of muscle, right shoulder

    M61.412   Other calcification of muscle, left shoulder

    M61.419   Other calcification of muscle, unspecified shoulder ▽

✓6ᵗʰ M61.42   Other calcification of muscle, upper arm

    M61.421   Other calcification of muscle, right upper arm

    M61.422   Other calcification of muscle, left upper arm

    M61.429   Other calcification of muscle, unspecified upper arm ▽

✓6ᵗʰ M61.43   Other calcification of muscle, forearm

    M61.431   Other calcification of muscle, right forearm

    M61.432   Other calcification of muscle, left forearm

    M61.439   Other calcification of muscle, unspecified forearm ▽

✓6ᵗʰ M61.44   Other calcification of muscle, hand

    M61.441   Other calcification of muscle, right hand

    M61.442   Other calcification of muscle, left hand

    M61.449   Other calcification of muscle, unspecified hand ▽

✓6ᵗʰ M61.45   Other calcification of muscle, thigh

    M61.451   Other calcification of muscle, right thigh

    M61.452   Other calcification of muscle, left thigh

    M61.459   Other calcification of muscle, unspecified thigh ▽

✓6ᵗʰ M61.46   Other calcification of muscle, lower leg

    M61.461   Other calcification of muscle, right lower leg

    M61.462   Other calcification of muscle, left lower leg

    M61.469   Other calcification of muscle, unspecified lower leg ▽

✓6ᵗʰ M61.47   Other calcification of muscle, ankle and foot

    M61.471   Other calcification of muscle, right ankle and foot

    M61.472   Other calcification of muscle, left ankle and foot

    M61.479   Other calcification of muscle, unspecified ankle and foot ▽

  M61.48   Other calcification of muscle, other site

  M61.49   Other calcification of muscle, multiple sites

✓5ᵗʰ M61.5   Other ossification of muscle

  M61.50   Other ossification of muscle, unspecified site ▽

✓6ᵗʰ M61.51   Other ossification of muscle, shoulder

    M61.511   Other ossification of muscle, right shoulder

    M61.512   Other ossification of muscle, left shoulder

    M61.519   Other ossification of muscle, unspecified shoulder ▽

✓6ᵗʰ M61.52   Other ossification of muscle, upper arm

    M61.521   Other ossification of muscle, right upper arm

    M61.522   Other ossification of muscle, left upper arm

    M61.529   Other ossification of muscle, unspecified upper arm ▽

✓6ᵗʰ M61.53   Other ossification of muscle, forearm

    M61.531   Other ossification of muscle, right forearm

    M61.532   Other ossification of muscle, left forearm

    M61.539   Other ossification of muscle, unspecified forearm ▽

✓6ᵗʰ M61.54   Other ossification of muscle, hand

    M61.541   Other ossification of muscle, right hand

    M61.542   Other ossification of muscle, left hand

    M61.549   Other ossification of muscle, unspecified hand ▽

✓6ᵗʰ M61.55   Other ossification of muscle, thigh

    M61.551   Other ossification of muscle, right thigh

    M61.552   Other ossification of muscle, left thigh

    M61.559   Other ossification of muscle, unspecified thigh ▽

✓6ᵗʰ M61.56   Other ossification of muscle, lower leg

    M61.561   Other ossification of muscle, right lower leg

    M61.562   Other ossification of muscle, left lower leg

    M61.569   Other ossification of muscle, unspecified lower leg ▽

✓6ᵗʰ M61.57   Other ossification of muscle, ankle and foot

    M61.571   Other ossification of muscle, right ankle and foot

    M61.572   Other ossification of muscle, left ankle and foot

    M61.579   Other ossification of muscle, unspecified ankle and foot ▽

  M61.58   Other ossification of muscle, other site

  M61.59   Other ossification of muscle, multiple sites

  M61.9   Calcification and ossification of muscle, unspecified ▽

☑ Additional Character Req   ⓥₓ⁷ᵗʰ Placeholder Alert   Manifestation   HCC CMS-HCC Condition   ▽ Unspecified Code   ▶◀ Revised Text   ● New Code   ▲ Revised Code Title

✓4ᵗʰ **M62 Other disorders of muscle**

    EXCLUDES 1   alcoholic myopathy (G72.1)
                cramp and spasm (R25.2)
                drug-induced myopathy (G72.0)
                myalgia (M79.1)
                stiff-man syndrome (G25.82)
    EXCLUDES 2   nontraumatic hematoma of muscle (M79.81)

✓5ᵗʰ **M62.0 Separation of muscle (nontraumatic)**

    Diastasis of muscle
    EXCLUDES 1   diastasis recti complicating pregnancy, labor and
                delivery (O71.8)
                traumatic separation of muscle—see strain of muscle
                by body region

    **M62.00 Separation of muscle (nontraumatic), ▽
                unspecified site**

✓6ᵗʰ **M62.01 Separation of muscle (nontraumatic), shoulder**
      M62.011 Separation of muscle (nontraumatic), right shoulder
      M62.012 Separation of muscle (nontraumatic), left shoulder
      M62.019 Separation of muscle (nontraumatic), ▽ unspecified shoulder

✓6ᵗʰ **M62.02 Separation of muscle (nontraumatic), upper arm**
      M62.021 Separation of muscle (nontraumatic), right upper arm
      M62.022 Separation of muscle (nontraumatic), left upper arm
      M62.029 Separation of muscle (nontraumatic), ▽ unspecified upper arm

✓6ᵗʰ **M62.03 Separation of muscle (nontraumatic), forearm**
      M62.031 Separation of muscle (nontraumatic), right forearm
      M62.032 Separation of muscle (nontraumatic), left forearm
      M62.039 Separation of muscle (nontraumatic), ▽ unspecified forearm

✓6ᵗʰ **M62.04 Separation of muscle (nontraumatic), hand**
      M62.041 Separation of muscle (nontraumatic), right hand
      M62.042 Separation of muscle (nontraumatic), left hand
      M62.049 Separation of muscle (nontraumatic), ▽ unspecified hand

✓6ᵗʰ **M62.05 Separation of muscle (nontraumatic), thigh**
      M62.051 Separation of muscle (nontraumatic), right thigh
      M62.052 Separation of muscle (nontraumatic), left thigh
      M62.059 Separation of muscle (nontraumatic), ▽ unspecified thigh

✓6ᵗʰ **M62.06 Separation of muscle (nontraumatic), lower leg**
      M62.061 Separation of muscle (nontraumatic), right lower leg
      M62.062 Separation of muscle (nontraumatic), left lower leg
      M62.069 Separation of muscle (nontraumatic), ▽ unspecified lower leg

✓6ᵗʰ **M62.07 Separation of muscle (nontraumatic), ankle and foot**
      M62.071 Separation of muscle (nontraumatic), right ankle and foot
      M62.072 Separation of muscle (nontraumatic), left ankle and foot
      M62.079 Separation of muscle (nontraumatic), ▽ unspecified ankle and foot

    M62.08 Separation of muscle (nontraumatic), other site

✓5ᵗʰ **M62.1 Other rupture of muscle (nontraumatic)**
    EXCLUDES 1   traumatic rupture of muscle—see strain of muscle by
                body region
    EXCLUDES 2   rupture of tendon (M66.-)

    M62.10 Other rupture of muscle (nontraumatic), ▽ unspecified site

✓6ᵗʰ **M62.11 Other rupture of muscle (nontraumatic), shoulder**
      M62.111 Other rupture of muscle (nontraumatic), right shoulder
      M62.112 Other rupture of muscle (nontraumatic), left shoulder

      M62.119 Other rupture of muscle ▽ (nontraumatic), unspecified shoulder

✓6ᵗʰ **M62.12 Other rupture of muscle (nontraumatic), upper arm**
      M62.121 Other rupture of muscle (nontraumatic), right upper arm
      M62.122 Other rupture of muscle (nontraumatic), left upper arm
      M62.129 Other rupture of muscle ▽ (nontraumatic), unspecified upper arm

✓6ᵗʰ **M62.13 Other rupture of muscle (nontraumatic), forearm**
      M62.131 Other rupture of muscle (nontraumatic), right forearm
      M62.132 Other rupture of muscle (nontraumatic), left forearm
      M62.139 Other rupture of muscle ▽ (nontraumatic), unspecified forearm

✓6ᵗʰ **M62.14 Other rupture of muscle (nontraumatic), hand**
      M62.141 Other rupture of muscle (nontraumatic), right hand
      M62.142 Other rupture of muscle (nontraumatic), left hand
      M62.149 Other rupture of muscle ▽ (nontraumatic), unspecified hand

✓6ᵗʰ **M62.15 Other rupture of muscle (nontraumatic), thigh**
      M62.151 Other rupture of muscle (nontraumatic), right thigh
      M62.152 Other rupture of muscle (nontraumatic), left thigh
      M62.159 Other rupture of muscle ▽ (nontraumatic), unspecified thigh

✓6ᵗʰ **M62.16 Other rupture of muscle (nontraumatic), lower leg**
      M62.161 Other rupture of muscle (nontraumatic), right lower leg
      M62.162 Other rupture of muscle (nontraumatic), left lower leg
      M62.169 Other rupture of muscle ▽ (nontraumatic), unspecified lower leg

✓6ᵗʰ **M62.17 Other rupture of muscle (nontraumatic), ankle and foot**
      M62.171 Other rupture of muscle (nontraumatic), right ankle and foot
      M62.172 Other rupture of muscle (nontraumatic), left ankle and foot
      M62.179 Other rupture of muscle ▽ (nontraumatic), unspecified ankle and foot

    M62.18 Other rupture of muscle (nontraumatic), other site

✓5ᵗʰ **M62.2 Nontraumatic ischemic infarction of muscle**
    EXCLUDES 1   compartment syndrome (traumatic) (T79.A-)
                nontraumatic compartment syndrome (M79.A-)
                rhabdomyolysis (M62.82)
                traumatic ischemia of muscle (T79.6)
                Volkmann's ischemic contracture (T79.6)

    M62.20 Nontraumatic ischemic infarction of muscle, ▽ unspecified site

✓6ᵗʰ **M62.21 Nontraumatic ischemic infarction of muscle, shoulder**
      M62.211 Nontraumatic ischemic infarction of muscle, right shoulder
      M62.212 Nontraumatic ischemic infarction of muscle, left shoulder
      M62.219 Nontraumatic ischemic infarction of ▽ muscle, unspecified shoulder

✓6ᵗʰ **M62.22 Nontraumatic ischemic infarction of muscle, upper arm**
      M62.221 Nontraumatic ischemic infarction of muscle, right upper arm
      M62.222 Nontraumatic ischemic infarction of muscle, left upper arm
      M62.229 Nontraumatic ischemic infarction of ▽ muscle, unspecified upper arm

✓6ᵗʰ **M62.23 Nontraumatic ischemic infarction of muscle, forearm**
      M62.231 Nontraumatic ischemic infarction of muscle, right forearm
      M62.232 Nontraumatic ischemic infarction of muscle, left forearm
      M62.239 Nontraumatic ischemic infarction of ▽ muscle, unspecified forearm

EXCLUDES 1 Not coded here   *EXCLUDES 2* Not included here   N Newborn Age: 0   P Pediatric Age: 0-17   M Maternity Age: 12-55   A Adult Age: 15-124

764   ICD-10-CM 2018

✓6ᵗʰ **M62.24 Nontraumatic ischemic infarction of muscle,** hand

    M62.241 Nontraumatic ischemic infarction of muscle, right **hand**

    M62.242 Nontraumatic ischemic infarction of muscle, left **hand**

    M62.249 Nontraumatic ischemic infarction of muscle, unspecified hand ▽

✓6ᵗʰ **M62.25 Nontraumatic ischemic infarction of muscle,** thigh

    M62.251 Nontraumatic ischemic infarction of muscle, right **thigh**

    M62.252 Nontraumatic ischemic infarction of muscle, left **thigh**

    M62.259 Nontraumatic ischemic infarction of muscle, unspecified thigh ▽

✓6ᵗʰ **M62.26 Nontraumatic ischemic infarction of muscle,** lower leg

    M62.261 Nontraumatic ischemic infarction of muscle, right **lower leg**

    M62.262 Nontraumatic ischemic infarction of muscle, left **lower leg**

    M62.269 Nontraumatic ischemic infarction of muscle, unspecified lower leg ▽

✓6ᵗʰ **M62.27 Nontraumatic ischemic infarction of muscle,** ankle and foot

    M62.271 Nontraumatic ischemic infarction of muscle, right **ankle and foot**

    M62.272 Nontraumatic ischemic infarction of muscle, left **ankle and foot**

    M62.279 Nontraumatic ischemic infarction of muscle, unspecified ankle and foot ▽

    M62.28 Nontraumatic ischemic infarction of muscle, other site

M62.3 Immobility syndrome (paraplegic)

✓5ᵗʰ **M62.4 Contracture of muscle**

    Contracture of tendon (sheath)

    EXCLUDES 1   *contracture of joint (M24.5-)*

    M62.40 Contracture of muscle, unspecified site ▽

  ✓6ᵗʰ **M62.41 Contracture of muscle,** shoulder

    M62.411 Contracture of muscle, right **shoulder**

    M62.412 Contracture of muscle, left **shoulder**

    M62.419 Contracture of muscle, unspecified shoulder ▽

  ✓6ᵗʰ **M62.42 Contracture of muscle,** upper arm

    M62.421 Contracture of muscle, right **upper arm**

    M62.422 Contracture of muscle, left **upper arm**

    M62.429 Contracture of muscle, unspecified upper arm ▽

  ✓6ᵗʰ **M62.43 Contracture of muscle,** forearm

    M62.431 Contracture of muscle, right **forearm**

    M62.432 Contracture of muscle, left **forearm**

    M62.439 Contracture of muscle, unspecified forearm ▽

  ✓6ᵗʰ **M62.44 Contracture of muscle,** hand

    M62.441 Contracture of muscle, right **hand**

    M62.442 Contracture of muscle, left **hand**

    M62.449 Contracture of muscle, unspecified hand ▽

  ✓6ᵗʰ **M62.45 Contracture of muscle,** thigh

    M62.451 Contracture of muscle, right **thigh**

    M62.452 Contracture of muscle, left **thigh**

    M62.459 Contracture of muscle, unspecified thigh ▽

  ✓6ᵗʰ **M62.46 Contracture of muscle,** lower leg

    M62.461 Contracture of muscle, right **lower leg**

    M62.462 Contracture of muscle, left **lower leg**

    M62.469 Contracture of muscle, unspecified lower leg ▽

  ✓6ᵗʰ **M62.47 Contracture of muscle,** ankle and foot

    M62.471 Contracture of muscle, right **ankle and foot**

    M62.472 Contracture of muscle, left **ankle and foot**

    M62.479 Contracture of muscle, unspecified ankle and foot ▽

    M62.48 Contracture of muscle, other site

    M62.49 Contracture of muscle, multiple sites

✓5ᵗʰ **M62.5 Muscle wasting and atrophy, not elsewhere classified**

    Disuse atrophy NEC

    EXCLUDES 1   *neuralgic amyotrophy (G54.5)*

        progressive muscular atrophy ▶(G12.21)◀

        sarcopenia (M62.84)

    EXCLUDES 2   *pelvic muscle wasting (N81.84)*

    M62.50 Muscle wasting and atrophy, not elsewhere classified, unspecified site ▽

  ✓6ᵗʰ **M62.51 Muscle wasting and atrophy, not elsewhere classified,** shoulder

    M62.511 Muscle wasting and atrophy, not elsewhere classified, right **shoulder**

    M62.512 Muscle wasting and atrophy, not elsewhere classified, left **shoulder**

    M62.519 Muscle wasting and atrophy, not elsewhere classified, unspecified shoulder ▽

  ✓6ᵗʰ **M62.52 Muscle wasting and atrophy, not elsewhere classified,** upper arm

    M62.521 Muscle wasting and atrophy, not elsewhere classified, right **upper arm**

    M62.522 Muscle wasting and atrophy, not elsewhere classified, left **upper arm**

    M62.529 Muscle wasting and atrophy, not elsewhere classified, unspecified upper arm ▽

  ✓6ᵗʰ **M62.53 Muscle wasting and atrophy, not elsewhere classified,** forearm

    M62.531 Muscle wasting and atrophy, not elsewhere classified, right **forearm**

    M62.532 Muscle wasting and atrophy, not elsewhere classified, left **forearm**

    M62.539 Muscle wasting and atrophy, not elsewhere classified, unspecified forearm ▽

  ✓6ᵗʰ **M62.54 Muscle wasting and atrophy, not elsewhere classified,** hand

    M62.541 Muscle wasting and atrophy, not elsewhere classified, right **hand**

    M62.542 Muscle wasting and atrophy, not elsewhere classified, left **hand**

    M62.549 Muscle wasting and atrophy, not elsewhere classified, unspecified hand ▽

  ✓6ᵗʰ **M62.55 Muscle wasting and atrophy, not elsewhere classified,** thigh

    M62.551 Muscle wasting and atrophy, not elsewhere classified, right **thigh**

    M62.552 Muscle wasting and atrophy, not elsewhere classified, left **thigh**

    M62.559 Muscle wasting and atrophy, not elsewhere classified, unspecified thigh ▽

  ✓6ᵗʰ **M62.56 Muscle wasting and atrophy, not elsewhere classified,** lower leg

    M62.561 Muscle wasting and atrophy, not elsewhere classified, right **lower leg**

    M62.562 Muscle wasting and atrophy, not elsewhere classified, left **lower leg**

    M62.569 Muscle wasting and atrophy, not elsewhere classified, unspecified lower leg ▽

  ✓6ᵗʰ **M62.57 Muscle wasting and atrophy, not elsewhere classified,** ankle and foot

    M62.571 Muscle wasting and atrophy, not elsewhere classified, right **ankle and foot**

    M62.572 Muscle wasting and atrophy, not elsewhere classified, left **ankle and foot**

    M62.579 Muscle wasting and atrophy, not elsewhere classified, unspecified ankle and foot ▽

    M62.58 Muscle wasting and atrophy, not elsewhere classified, other site

    M62.59 Muscle wasting and atrophy, not elsewhere classified, multiple sites

✓5ᵗʰ **M62.8 Other specified disorders of muscle**

    EXCLUDES 2   *nontraumatic hematoma of muscle (M79.81)*

    M62.81 Muscle weakness (generalized)

        EXCLUDES 1   *muscle weakness in sarcopenia (M62.84)*

☑ Additional Character Req   ᵛˣ⁷ᵗʰ Placeholder Alert   Manifestation   HCC CMS-HCC Condition   ▽ Unspecified Code   ▶◀ Revised Text   ● New Code   ▲ Revised Code Title

Chapter 13. Diseases of the Musculoskeletal System and Connective Tissue

M62.82 Rhabdomyolysis

> **EXCLUDES 1**   *traumatic rhabdomyolysis (T79.6)*
> **DEF:** Rapid disintegration or destruction of skeletal muscle caused by direct or indirect injury; resulting in the excretion of muscle protein myoglobin into the urine.

√6ᵗʰ **M62.83 Muscle spasm**

M62.830 Muscle spasm of back
M62.831 Muscle spasm of calf
> Charley-horse
M62.838 Other muscle spasm

M62.84 Sarcopenia
> Age-related sarcopenia
> Code first underlying disease, if applicable, such as:
>   disorders of myoneural junction and muscle disease
>   in diseases classified elsewhere (G73.-)
>   other and unspecified myopathies (G72.-)
>   primary disorders of muscles (G71.-)

M62.89 Other specified disorders of muscle
> Muscle (sheath) hernia

M62.9 Disorder of muscle, unspecified ▽

√4ᵗʰ **M63 Disorders of muscle in diseases classified elsewhere**
> Code first underlying disease, such as:
>   leprosy (A30.-)
>   neoplasm (C49-, C79.89, D21-, D48.1)
>   schistosomiasis (B65.-)
>   trichinellosis (B75)
> **EXCLUDES 1**   *myopathy in cysticercosis (B69.81)*
>   *myopathy in endocrine diseases (G73.7)*
>   *myopathy in metabolic diseases (G73.7)*
>   *myopathy in sarcoidosis (D86.87)*
>   *myopathy in secondary syphilis (A51.49)*
>   *myopathy in syphilis (late) (A52.78)*
>   *myopathy in toxoplasmosis (B58.82)*
>   *myopathy in tuberculosis (A18.09)*

√5ᵗʰ **M63.8 Disorders of muscle in diseases classified elsewhere**

M63.80 *Disorders of muscle in diseases classified* ▽
elsewhere, unspecified site

√6ᵗʰ **M63.81** *Disorders of muscle in diseases classified elsewhere,*
shoulder
M63.811 *Disorders of muscle in diseases classified*
elsewhere, right shoulder
M63.812 *Disorders of muscle in diseases classified*
elsewhere, left shoulder
M63.819 *Disorders of muscle in diseases classified* ▽
elsewhere, unspecified shoulder

√6ᵗʰ **M63.82** *Disorders of muscle in diseases classified elsewhere,*
upper arm
M63.821 *Disorders of muscle in diseases classified*
elsewhere, right upper arm
M63.822 *Disorders of muscle in diseases classified*
elsewhere, left upper arm
M63.829 *Disorders of muscle in diseases classified* ▽
elsewhere, unspecified upper arm

√6ᵗʰ **M63.83** *Disorders of muscle in diseases classified elsewhere,*
forearm
M63.831 *Disorders of muscle in diseases classified*
elsewhere, right forearm
M63.832 *Disorders of muscle in diseases classified*
elsewhere, left forearm
M63.839 *Disorders of muscle in diseases classified* ▽
elsewhere, unspecified forearm

√6ᵗʰ **M63.84** *Disorders of muscle in diseases classified elsewhere,*
hand
M63.841 *Disorders of muscle in diseases classified*
elsewhere, right hand
M63.842 *Disorders of muscle in diseases classified*
elsewhere, left hand
M63.849 *Disorders of muscle in diseases* ▽
classified elsewhere, unspecified hand

√6ᵗʰ **M63.85** *Disorders of muscle in diseases classified elsewhere,*
thigh
M63.851 *Disorders of muscle in diseases classified*
elsewhere, right thigh
M63.852 *Disorders of muscle in diseases classified*
elsewhere, left thigh
M63.859 *Disorders of muscle in diseases classified* ▽
elsewhere, unspecified thigh

√6ᵗʰ **M63.86** *Disorders of muscle in diseases classified elsewhere,*
lower leg
M63.861 *Disorders of muscle in diseases classified*
elsewhere, right lower leg
M63.862 *Disorders of muscle in diseases classified*
elsewhere, left lower leg
M63.869 *Disorders of muscle in diseases classified* ▽
elsewhere, unspecified lower leg

√6ᵗʰ **M63.87** *Disorders of muscle in diseases classified elsewhere,*
ankle and foot
M63.871 *Disorders of muscle in diseases classified*
elsewhere, right ankle and foot
M63.872 *Disorders of muscle in diseases classified*
elsewhere, left ankle and foot
M63.879 *Disorders of muscle in diseases classified* ▽
elsewhere, unspecified ankle and foot

M63.88 *Disorders of muscle in diseases classified elsewhere,*
other site

M63.89 *Disorders of muscle in diseases classified elsewhere,*
multiple sites

Disorders of synovium and tendon (M65-M67)

√4ᵗʰ **M65 Synovitis and tenosynovitis**
> **EXCLUDES 1**   *chronic crepitant synovitis of hand and wrist (M70.0-)*
>   *current injury—see injury of ligament or tendon by body region*
>   *soft tissue disorders related to use, overuse and pressure (M70.-)*

√5ᵗʰ **M65.0 Abscess of tendon sheath**
> Use additional code (B95-B96) to identify bacterial agent.

M65.00 Abscess of tendon sheath, unspecified site ▽

√6ᵗʰ **M65.01 Abscess of tendon sheath,** shoulder
M65.011 Abscess of tendon sheath, right shoulder
M65.012 Abscess of tendon sheath, left shoulder
M65.019 Abscess of tendon sheath, ▽
unspecified shoulder

√6ᵗʰ **M65.02 Abscess of tendon sheath,** upper arm
M65.021 Abscess of tendon sheath, right upper arm
M65.022 Abscess of tendon sheath, left upper arm
M65.029 Abscess of tendon sheath, ▽
unspecified upper arm

√6ᵗʰ **M65.03 Abscess of tendon sheath,** forearm
M65.031 Abscess of tendon sheath, right forearm
M65.032 Abscess of tendon sheath, left forearm
M65.039 Abscess of tendon sheath, ▽
unspecified forearm

√6ᵗʰ **M65.04 Abscess of tendon sheath,** hand
M65.041 Abscess of tendon sheath, right hand
M65.042 Abscess of tendon sheath, left hand
M65.049 Abscess of tendon sheath, ▽
unspecified hand

√6ᵗʰ **M65.05 Abscess of tendon sheath,** thigh
M65.051 Abscess of tendon sheath, right thigh
M65.052 Abscess of tendon sheath, left thigh
M65.059 Abscess of tendon sheath, ▽
unspecified thigh

√6ᵗʰ **M65.06 Abscess of tendon sheath,** lower leg
M65.061 Abscess of tendon sheath, right lower leg
M65.062 Abscess of tendon sheath, left lower leg
M65.069 Abscess of tendon sheath, ▽
unspecified lower leg

√6ᵗʰ **M65.07 Abscess of tendon sheath,** ankle and foot
M65.071 Abscess of tendon sheath, right ankle and
foot
M65.072 Abscess of tendon sheath, left ankle and
foot
M65.079 Abscess of tendon sheath, ▽
unspecified ankle and foot

M65.08 Abscess of tendon sheath, other site

√5ᵗʰ **M65.1 Other infective (teno)synovitis**

M65.10 Other infective (teno)synovitis, unspecified site ▽

√6ᵗʰ **M65.11 Other infective (teno)synovitis,** shoulder
M65.111 Other infective (teno)synovitis, right
shoulder
M65.112 Other infective (teno)synovitis, left
shoulder

EXCLUDES 1 Not coded here   **EXCLUDES 2** Not included here   N Newborn Age: 0   P Pediatric Age: 0-17   M Maternity Age: 12-55   A Adult Age: 15-124

766   **ICD-10-CM 2018**

M65.119   Other infective (teno)synovitis, unspecified shoulder ▽

✓6ᵗʰ **M65.12**   Other infective (teno)synovitis, elbow
    M65.121   Other infective (teno)synovitis, right elbow
    M65.122   Other infective (teno)synovitis, left elbow
    M65.129   Other infective (teno)synovitis, unspecified elbow ▽

✓6ᵗʰ **M65.13**   Other infective (teno)synovitis, wrist
    M65.131   Other infective (teno)synovitis, right wrist
    M65.132   Other infective (teno)synovitis, left wrist
    M65.139   Other infective (teno)synovitis, unspecified wrist ▽

✓6ᵗʰ **M65.14**   Other infective (teno)synovitis, hand
    M65.141   Other infective (teno)synovitis, right hand
    M65.142   Other infective (teno)synovitis, left hand
    M65.149   Other infective (teno)synovitis, unspecified hand ▽

✓6ᵗʰ **M65.15**   Other infective (teno)synovitis, hip
    M65.151   Other infective (teno)synovitis, right hip
    M65.152   Other infective (teno)synovitis, left hip
    M65.159   Other infective (teno)synovitis, unspecified hip ▽

✓6ᵗʰ **M65.16**   Other infective (teno)synovitis, knee
    M65.161   Other infective (teno)synovitis, right knee
    M65.162   Other infective (teno)synovitis, left knee
    M65.169   Other infective (teno)synovitis, unspecified knee ▽

✓6ᵗʰ **M65.17**   Other infective (teno)synovitis, ankle and foot
    M65.171   Other infective (teno)synovitis, right ankle and foot
    M65.172   Other infective (teno)synovitis, left ankle and foot
    M65.179   Other infective (teno)synovitis, unspecified ankle and foot ▽

   M65.18   Other infective (teno)synovitis, other site
   M65.19   Other infective (teno)synovitis, multiple sites

✓5ᵗʰ **M65.2**   **Calcific tendinitis**
    EXCLUDES 1   tendinitis as classified in M75-M77
              calcified tendinitis of shoulder (M75.3)

   M65.20   Calcific tendinitis, unspecified site ▽

✓6ᵗʰ **M65.22**   Calcific tendinitis, upper arm
    M65.221   Calcific tendinitis, right upper arm
    M65.222   Calcific tendinitis, left upper arm
    M65.229   Calcific tendinitis, unspecified upper arm ▽

✓6ᵗʰ **M65.23**   Calcific tendinitis, forearm
    M65.231   Calcific tendinitis, right forearm
    M65.232   Calcific tendinitis, left forearm
    M65.239   Calcific tendinitis, unspecified forearm ▽

✓6ᵗʰ **M65.24**   Calcific tendinitis, hand
    M65.241   Calcific tendinitis, right hand
    M65.242   Calcific tendinitis, left hand
    M65.249   Calcific tendinitis, unspecified hand ▽

✓6ᵗʰ **M65.25**   Calcific tendinitis, thigh
    M65.251   Calcific tendinitis, right thigh
    M65.252   Calcific tendinitis, left thigh
    M65.259   Calcific tendinitis, unspecified thigh ▽

✓6ᵗʰ **M65.26**   Calcific tendinitis, lower leg
    M65.261   Calcific tendinitis, right lower leg
    M65.262   Calcific tendinitis, left lower leg
    M65.269   Calcific tendinitis, unspecified lower leg ▽

✓6ᵗʰ **M65.27**   Calcific tendinitis, ankle and foot
    M65.271   Calcific tendinitis, right ankle and foot
    M65.272   Calcific tendinitis, left ankle and foot
    M65.279   Calcific tendinitis, unspecified ankle and foot ▽

   M65.28   Calcific tendinitis, other site
   M65.29   Calcific tendinitis, multiple sites

✓5ᵗʰ **M65.3**   **Trigger finger**
    Nodular tendinous disease

   M65.30   Trigger finger, unspecified finger ▽

✓6ᵗʰ **M65.31**   Trigger thumb
    M65.311   Trigger thumb, right thumb
    M65.312   Trigger thumb, left thumb
    M65.319   Trigger thumb, unspecified thumb ▽

✓6ᵗʰ **M65.32**   Trigger finger, index finger
    M65.321   Trigger finger, right index finger
    M65.322   Trigger finger, left index finger
    M65.329   Trigger finger, unspecified index finger ▽

✓6ᵗʰ **M65.33**   Trigger finger, middle finger
    M65.331   Trigger finger, right middle finger
    M65.332   Trigger finger, left middle finger
    M65.339   Trigger finger, unspecified middle finger ▽

✓6ᵗʰ **M65.34**   Trigger finger, ring finger
    M65.341   Trigger finger, right ring finger
    M65.342   Trigger finger, left ring finger
    M65.349   Trigger finger, unspecified ring finger ▽

✓6ᵗʰ **M65.35**   Trigger finger, little finger
    M65.351   Trigger finger, right little finger
    M65.352   Trigger finger, left little finger
    M65.359   Trigger finger, unspecified little finger ▽

   M65.4   **Radial styloid tenosynovitis [de Quervain]**

✓5ᵗʰ **M65.8**   **Other synovitis and tenosynovitis**
    M65.80   Other synovitis and tenosynovitis, unspecified site ▽

✓6ᵗʰ **M65.81**   Other synovitis and tenosynovitis, shoulder
    M65.811   Other synovitis and tenosynovitis, right shoulder
    M65.812   Other synovitis and tenosynovitis, left shoulder
    M65.819   Other synovitis and tenosynovitis, unspecified shoulder ▽

✓6ᵗʰ **M65.82**   Other synovitis and tenosynovitis, upper arm
    M65.821   Other synovitis and tenosynovitis, right upper arm
    M65.822   Other synovitis and tenosynovitis, left upper arm
    M65.829   Other synovitis and tenosynovitis, unspecified upper arm ▽

✓6ᵗʰ **M65.83**   Other synovitis and tenosynovitis, forearm
    M65.831   Other synovitis and tenosynovitis, right forearm
    M65.832   Other synovitis and tenosynovitis, left forearm
    M65.839   Other synovitis and tenosynovitis, unspecified forearm ▽

✓6ᵗʰ **M65.84**   Other synovitis and tenosynovitis, hand
    M65.841   Other synovitis and tenosynovitis, right hand
    M65.842   Other synovitis and tenosynovitis, left hand
    M65.849   Other synovitis and tenosynovitis, unspecified hand ▽

✓6ᵗʰ **M65.85**   Other synovitis and tenosynovitis, thigh
    M65.851   Other synovitis and tenosynovitis, right thigh
    M65.852   Other synovitis and tenosynovitis, left thigh
    M65.859   Other synovitis and tenosynovitis, unspecified thigh ▽

✓6ᵗʰ **M65.86**   Other synovitis and tenosynovitis, lower leg
    M65.861   Other synovitis and tenosynovitis, right lower leg
    M65.862   Other synovitis and tenosynovitis, left lower leg
    M65.869   Other synovitis and tenosynovitis, unspecified lower leg ▽

✓6ᵗʰ **M65.87**   Other synovitis and tenosynovitis, ankle and foot
    M65.871   Other synovitis and tenosynovitis, right ankle and foot
    M65.872   Other synovitis and tenosynovitis, left ankle and foot
    M65.879   Other synovitis and tenosynovitis, unspecified ankle and foot ▽

☑ Additional Character Req   ✓7ᵗʰ Placeholder Alert   Manifestation   HCC CMS-HCC Condition   ▽ Unspecified Code   ▶◀ Revised Text   ● New Code   ▲ Revised Code Title

M65.88   **Other synovitis and tenosynovitis, other site**

M65.89   **Other synovitis and tenosynovitis,** multiple sites

M65.9 Synovitis and tenosynovitis, unspecified   ▽

☑4ᵗʰ **M66 Spontaneous rupture of synovium and tendon**

> INCLUDES   rupture that occurs when a normal force is applied to tissues that are inferred to have less than normal strength
>
> EXCLUDES 2   *rotator cuff syndrome (M75.1-)*
> *rupture where an abnormal force is applied to normal tissue—see injury of tendon by body region*

M66.0 Rupture of popliteal cyst

☑5ᵗʰ **M66.1 Rupture of** synovium

> Rupture of synovial cyst
>
> EXCLUDES 2   *rupture of popliteal cyst (M66.0)*

   M66.10 Rupture of synovium, unspecified joint   ▽

   ☑6ᵗʰ **M66.11 Rupture of synovium,** shoulder

     M66.111   **Rupture of synovium,** right **shoulder**

     M66.112   **Rupture of synovium,** left **shoulder**

     M66.119   **Rupture of synovium, unspecified shoulder**   ▽

   ☑6ᵗʰ **M66.12 Rupture of synovium,** elbow

     M66.121   **Rupture of synovium,** right **elbow**

     M66.122   **Rupture of synovium,** left **elbow**

     M66.129   **Rupture of synovium, unspecified elbow**   ▽

   ☑6ᵗʰ **M66.13 Rupture of synovium,** wrist

     M66.131   **Rupture of synovium,** right **wrist**

     M66.132   **Rupture of synovium,** left **wrist**

     M66.139   **Rupture of synovium, unspecified wrist** ▽

   ☑6ᵗʰ **M66.14 Rupture of synovium, hand and fingers**

     M66.141   **Rupture of synovium,** right **hand**

     M66.142   **Rupture of synovium,** left **hand**

     M66.143   **Rupture of synovium, unspecified hand** ▽

     M66.144   **Rupture of synovium,** right **finger(s)**

     M66.145   **Rupture of synovium,** left **finger(s)**

     M66.146   **Rupture of synovium, unspecified finger(s)**   ▽

   ☑6ᵗʰ **M66.15 Rupture of synovium,** hip

     M66.151   **Rupture of synovium,** right **hip**

     M66.152   **Rupture of synovium,** left **hip**

     M66.159   **Rupture of synovium, unspecified hip**   ▽

   ☑6ᵗʰ **M66.17 Rupture of synovium, ankle, foot and toes**

     M66.171   **Rupture of synovium,** right **ankle**

     M66.172   **Rupture of synovium,** left **ankle**

     M66.173   **Rupture of synovium, unspecified ankle** ▽

     M66.174   **Rupture of synovium,** right **foot**

     M66.175   **Rupture of synovium,** left **foot**

     M66.176   **Rupture of synovium, unspecified foot** ▽

     M66.177   **Rupture of synovium,** right **toe(s)**

     M66.178   **Rupture of synovium,** left **toe(s)**

     M66.179   **Rupture of synovium, unspecified toe(s)**   ▽

   M66.18 Rupture of synovium, other site

☑5ᵗʰ **M66.2 Spontaneous rupture of** extensor tendons

> **TIP:** Refer to the Muscle/Tendon table at the beginning of this chapter.

   M66.20 Spontaneous rupture of extensor tendons, unspecified site   ▽

   ☑6ᵗʰ **M66.21 Spontaneous rupture of extensor tendons,** shoulder

     M66.211   **Spontaneous rupture of extensor tendons,** right **shoulder**

     M66.212   **Spontaneous rupture of extensor tendons,** left **shoulder**

     M66.219   **Spontaneous rupture of extensor tendons, unspecified shoulder**   ▽

   ☑6ᵗʰ **M66.22 Spontaneous rupture of extensor tendons,** upper arm

     M66.221   **Spontaneous rupture of extensor tendons,** right **upper arm**

     M66.222   **Spontaneous rupture of extensor tendons,** left **upper arm**

     M66.229   **Spontaneous rupture of extensor tendons, unspecified upper arm**   ▽

   ☑6ᵗʰ **M66.23 Spontaneous rupture of extensor tendons,** forearm

     M66.231   **Spontaneous rupture of extensor tendons,** right **forearm**

     M66.232   **Spontaneous rupture of extensor tendons,** left **forearm**

     M66.239   **Spontaneous rupture of extensor tendons, unspecified forearm**   ▽

   ☑6ᵗʰ **M66.24 Spontaneous rupture of extensor tendons,** hand

     M66.241   **Spontaneous rupture of extensor tendons,** right **hand**

     M66.242   **Spontaneous rupture of extensor tendons,** left **hand**

     M66.249   **Spontaneous rupture of extensor tendons, unspecified hand**   ▽

   ☑6ᵗʰ **M66.25 Spontaneous rupture of extensor tendons,** thigh

     M66.251   **Spontaneous rupture of extensor tendons,** right **thigh**

     M66.252   **Spontaneous rupture of extensor tendons,** left **thigh**

     M66.259   **Spontaneous rupture of extensor tendons, unspecified thigh**   ▽

   ☑6ᵗʰ **M66.26 Spontaneous rupture of extensor tendons,** lower leg

     M66.261   **Spontaneous rupture of extensor tendons,** right **lower leg**

     M66.262   **Spontaneous rupture of extensor tendons,** left **lower leg**

     M66.269   **Spontaneous rupture of extensor tendons, unspecified lower leg**   ▽

   ☑6ᵗʰ **M66.27 Spontaneous rupture of extensor tendons,** ankle and foot

     M66.271   **Spontaneous rupture of extensor tendons,** right **ankle and foot**

     M66.272   **Spontaneous rupture of extensor tendons,** left **ankle and foot**

     M66.279   **Spontaneous rupture of extensor tendons, unspecified ankle and foot**   ▽

   M66.28 Spontaneous rupture of extensor tendons, other site

   M66.29 Spontaneous rupture of extensor tendons, multiple sites

☑5ᵗʰ **M66.3 Spontaneous rupture of** flexor tendons

> **TIP:** Refer to the Muscle/Tendon table at the beginning of this chapter.

   M66.30 Spontaneous rupture of flexor tendons, unspecified site   ▽

   ☑6ᵗʰ **M66.31 Spontaneous rupture of flexor tendons,** shoulder

     M66.311   **Spontaneous rupture of flexor tendons,** right **shoulder**

     M66.312   **Spontaneous rupture of flexor tendons,** left **shoulder**

     M66.319   **Spontaneous rupture of flexor tendons, unspecified shoulder**   ▽

   ☑6ᵗʰ **M66.32 Spontaneous rupture of flexor tendons,** upper arm

     M66.321   **Spontaneous rupture of flexor tendons,** right **upper arm**

     M66.322   **Spontaneous rupture of flexor tendons,** left **upper arm**

     M66.329   **Spontaneous rupture of flexor tendons, unspecified upper arm**   ▽

   ☑6ᵗʰ **M66.33 Spontaneous rupture of flexor tendons,** forearm

     M66.331   **Spontaneous rupture of flexor tendons,** right **forearm**

     M66.332   **Spontaneous rupture of flexor tendons,** left **forearm**

     M66.339   **Spontaneous rupture of flexor tendons, unspecified forearm**   ▽

   ☑6ᵗʰ **M66.34 Spontaneous rupture of flexor tendons,** hand

     M66.341   **Spontaneous rupture of flexor tendons,** right **hand**

     M66.342   **Spontaneous rupture of flexor tendons,** left **hand**

     M66.349   **Spontaneous rupture of flexor tendons, unspecified hand**   ▽

   ☑6ᵗʰ **M66.35 Spontaneous rupture of flexor tendons,** thigh

     M66.351   **Spontaneous rupture of flexor tendons,** right **thigh**

     M66.352   **Spontaneous rupture of flexor tendons,** left **thigh**

EXCLUDES 1 Not coded here   EXCLUDES 2 Not included here   N Newborn Age: 0   P Pediatric Age: 0-17   M Maternity Age: 12-55   A Adult Age: 15-124

768   ICD-10-CM 2018

M66.359   Spontaneous rupture of flexor tendons, unspecified thigh ▽

✓6ᵗʰ **M66.36**   Spontaneous rupture of flexor tendons, lower leg

    M66.361   Spontaneous rupture of flexor tendons, right lower leg

    M66.362   Spontaneous rupture of flexor tendons, left lower leg

    M66.369   Spontaneous rupture of flexor tendons, unspecified lower leg ▽

✓6ᵗʰ **M66.37**   Spontaneous rupture of flexor tendons, ankle and foot

    M66.371   Spontaneous rupture of flexor tendons, right ankle and foot

    M66.372   Spontaneous rupture of flexor tendons, left ankle and foot

    M66.379   Spontaneous rupture of flexor tendons, unspecified ankle and foot ▽

    M66.38   Spontaneous rupture of flexor tendons, other site

    M66.39   Spontaneous rupture of flexor tendons, multiple sites

✓5ᵗʰ **M66.8**   Spontaneous rupture of other tendons

    TIP: Refer to the Muscle/Tendon table at the beginning of this chapter.

    M66.80   Spontaneous rupture of other tendons, unspecified site ▽

✓6ᵗʰ **M66.81**   Spontaneous rupture of other tendons, shoulder

    M66.811   Spontaneous rupture of other tendons, right shoulder

    M66.812   Spontaneous rupture of other tendons, left shoulder

    M66.819   Spontaneous rupture of other tendons, unspecified shoulder ▽

✓6ᵗʰ **M66.82**   Spontaneous rupture of other tendons, upper arm

    M66.821   Spontaneous rupture of other tendons, right upper arm

    M66.822   Spontaneous rupture of other tendons, left upper arm

    M66.829   Spontaneous rupture of other tendons, unspecified upper arm ▽

✓6ᵗʰ **M66.83**   Spontaneous rupture of other tendons, forearm

    M66.831   Spontaneous rupture of other tendons, right forearm

    M66.832   Spontaneous rupture of other tendons, left forearm

    M66.839   Spontaneous rupture of other tendons, unspecified forearm ▽

✓6ᵗʰ **M66.84**   Spontaneous rupture of other tendons, hand

    M66.841   Spontaneous rupture of other tendons, right hand

    M66.842   Spontaneous rupture of other tendons, left hand

    M66.849   Spontaneous rupture of other tendons, unspecified hand ▽

✓6ᵗʰ **M66.85**   Spontaneous rupture of other tendons, thigh

    M66.851   Spontaneous rupture of other tendons, right thigh

    M66.852   Spontaneous rupture of other tendons, left thigh

    M66.859   Spontaneous rupture of other tendons, unspecified thigh ▽

✓6ᵗʰ **M66.86**   Spontaneous rupture of other tendons, lower leg

    M66.861   Spontaneous rupture of other tendons, right lower leg

    M66.862   Spontaneous rupture of other tendons, left lower leg

    M66.869   Spontaneous rupture of other tendons, unspecified lower leg ▽

✓6ᵗʰ **M66.87**   Spontaneous rupture of other tendons, ankle and foot

    M66.871   Spontaneous rupture of other tendons, right ankle and foot

    M66.872   Spontaneous rupture of other tendons, left ankle and foot

    M66.879   Spontaneous rupture of other tendons, unspecified ankle and foot ▽

    M66.88   Spontaneous rupture of other tendons, other

    M66.89   Spontaneous rupture of other tendons, multiple sites

M66.9   Spontaneous rupture of unspecified tendon ▽

    Rupture at musculotendinous junction, nontraumatic

✓4ᵗʰ **M67**   **Other disorders of synovium and tendon**

    EXCLUDES 1   *palmar fascial fibromatosis [Dupuytren] (M72.0)*

            tendinitis NOS (M77.9-)

            xanthomatosis localized to tendons (E78.2)

✓5ᵗʰ **M67.0**   Short Achilles tendon (acquired)

    M67.00   Short Achilles tendon (acquired), unspecified ankle ▽

    M67.01   Short Achilles tendon (acquired), right ankle

    M67.02   Short Achilles tendon (acquired), left ankle

✓5ᵗʰ **M67.2**   Synovial hypertrophy, not elsewhere classified

    EXCLUDES 1   *villonodular synovitis (pigmented) (M12.2-)*

    M67.20   Synovial hypertrophy, not elsewhere classified, unspecified site ▽

✓6ᵗʰ **M67.21**   Synovial hypertrophy, not elsewhere classified, shoulder

    M67.211   Synovial hypertrophy, not elsewhere classified, right shoulder

    M67.212   Synovial hypertrophy, not elsewhere classified, left shoulder

    M67.219   Synovial hypertrophy, not elsewhere classified, unspecified shoulder ▽

✓6ᵗʰ **M67.22**   Synovial hypertrophy, not elsewhere classified, upper arm

    M67.221   Synovial hypertrophy, not elsewhere classified, right upper arm

    M67.222   Synovial hypertrophy, not elsewhere classified, left upper arm

    M67.229   Synovial hypertrophy, not elsewhere classified, unspecified upper arm ▽

✓6ᵗʰ **M67.23**   Synovial hypertrophy, not elsewhere classified, forearm

    M67.231   Synovial hypertrophy, not elsewhere classified, right forearm

    M67.232   Synovial hypertrophy, not elsewhere classified, left forearm

    M67.239   Synovial hypertrophy, not elsewhere classified, unspecified forearm ▽

✓6ᵗʰ **M67.24**   Synovial hypertrophy, not elsewhere classified, hand

    M67.241   Synovial hypertrophy, not elsewhere classified, right hand

    M67.242   Synovial hypertrophy, not elsewhere classified, left hand

    M67.249   Synovial hypertrophy, not elsewhere classified, unspecified hand ▽

✓6ᵗʰ **M67.25**   Synovial hypertrophy, not elsewhere classified, thigh

    M67.251   Synovial hypertrophy, not elsewhere classified, right thigh

    M67.252   Synovial hypertrophy, not elsewhere classified, left thigh

    M67.259   Synovial hypertrophy, not elsewhere classified, unspecified thigh ▽

✓6ᵗʰ **M67.26**   Synovial hypertrophy, not elsewhere classified, lower leg

    M67.261   Synovial hypertrophy, not elsewhere classified, right lower leg

    M67.262   Synovial hypertrophy, not elsewhere classified, left lower leg

    M67.269   Synovial hypertrophy, not elsewhere classified, unspecified lower leg ▽

✓6ᵗʰ **M67.27**   Synovial hypertrophy, not elsewhere classified, ankle and foot

    M67.271   Synovial hypertrophy, not elsewhere classified, right ankle and foot

    M67.272   Synovial hypertrophy, not elsewhere classified, left ankle and foot

    M67.279   Synovial hypertrophy, not elsewhere classified, unspecified ankle and foot ▽

    M67.28   Synovial hypertrophy, not elsewhere classified, other site

    M67.29   Synovial hypertrophy, not elsewhere classified, multiple sites

---

☑ Additional Character Req   ✓7ᵗʰ Placeholder Alert   Manifestation   HCC CMS-HCC Condition   ▽ Unspecified Code   ▶◀ Revised Text   ● New Code   ▲ Revised Code Title

✓5ᵗʰ M67.3 Transient synovitis
Toxic synovitis
EXCLUDES 1   palindromic rheumatism (M12.3-)
M67.3Ø Transient synovitis, unspecified site ▽
✓6ᵗʰ M67.31 Transient synovitis, shoulder
M67.311 Transient synovitis, right shoulder
M67.312 Transient synovitis, left shoulder
M67.319 Transient synovitis, unspecified ▽
shoulder
✓6ᵗʰ M67.32 Transient synovitis, elbow
M67.321 Transient synovitis, right elbow
M67.322 Transient synovitis, left elbow
M67.329 Transient synovitis, unspecified elbow ▽
✓6ᵗʰ M67.33 Transient synovitis, wrist
M67.331 Transient synovitis, right wrist
M67.332 Transient synovitis, left wrist
M67.339 Transient synovitis, unspecified wrist ▽
✓6ᵗʰ M67.34 Transient synovitis, hand
M67.341 Transient synovitis, right hand
M67.342 Transient synovitis, left hand
M67.349 Transient synovitis, unspecified hand ▽
✓6ᵗʰ M67.35 Transient synovitis, hip
M67.351 Transient synovitis, right hip
M67.352 Transient synovitis, left hip
M67.359 Transient synovitis, unspecified hip ▽
✓6ᵗʰ M67.36 Transient synovitis, knee
M67.361 Transient synovitis, right knee
M67.362 Transient synovitis, left knee
M67.369 Transient synovitis, unspecified knee ▽
✓6ᵗʰ M67.37 Transient synovitis, ankle and foot
M67.371 Transient synovitis, right ankle and foot
M67.372 Transient synovitis, left ankle and foot
M67.379 Transient synovitis, unspecified ▽
ankle and foot
M67.38 Transient synovitis, other site
M67.39 Transient synovitis, multiple sites
✓5ᵗʰ M67.4 Ganglion
Ganglion of joint or tendon (sheath)
EXCLUDES 1   ganglion in yaws (A66.6)
EXCLUDES 2   cyst of bursa (M71.2-M71.3)
cyst of synovium (M71.2-M71.3)
M67.4Ø Ganglion, unspecified site ▽
✓6ᵗʰ M67.41 Ganglion, shoulder
M67.411 Ganglion, right shoulder
M67.412 Ganglion, left shoulder
M67.419 Ganglion, unspecified shoulder ▽
✓6ᵗʰ M67.42 Ganglion, elbow
M67.421 Ganglion, right elbow
M67.422 Ganglion, left elbow
M67.429 Ganglion, unspecified elbow ▽
✓6ᵗʰ M67.43 Ganglion, wrist
M67.431 Ganglion, right wrist
M67.432 Ganglion, left wrist
M67.439 Ganglion, unspecified wrist ▽
✓6ᵗʰ M67.44 Ganglion, hand
M67.441 Ganglion, right hand
M67.442 Ganglion, left hand
M67.449 Ganglion, unspecified hand ▽
✓6ᵗʰ M67.45 Ganglion, hip
M67.451 Ganglion, right hip
M67.452 Ganglion, left hip
M67.459 Ganglion, unspecified hip ▽
✓6ᵗʰ M67.46 Ganglion, knee
M67.461 Ganglion, right knee
M67.462 Ganglion, left knee
M67.469 Ganglion, unspecified knee ▽

Ganglion of Wrist

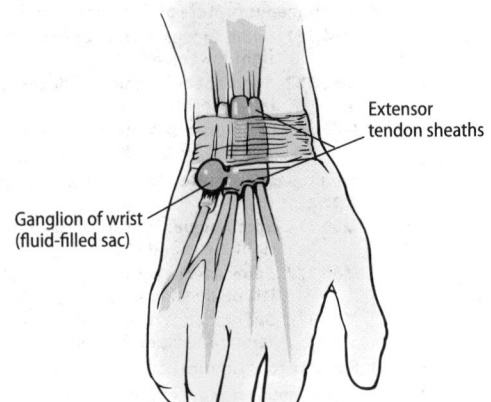

Extensor
tendon sheaths

Ganglion of wrist
(fluid-filled sac)

✓6ᵗʰ M67.47 Ganglion, ankle and foot
M67.471 Ganglion, right ankle and foot
M67.472 Ganglion, left ankle and foot
M67.479 Ganglion, unspecified ankle and foot ▽
M67.48 Ganglion, other site
M67.49 Ganglion, multiple sites
✓5ᵗʰ M67.5 Plica syndrome
Plica knee
M67.5Ø Plica syndrome, unspecified knee ▽
M67.51 Plica syndrome, right knee
M67.52 Plica syndrome, left knee
✓5ᵗʰ M67.8 Other specified disorders of synovium and tendon
M67.8Ø Other specified disorders of synovium and ▽
tendon, unspecified site
✓6ᵗʰ M67.81 Other specified disorders of synovium and tendon, shoulder
M67.811 Other specified disorders of synovium, right shoulder
M67.812 Other specified disorders of synovium, left shoulder
M67.813 Other specified disorders of tendon, right shoulder
M67.814 Other specified disorders of tendon, left shoulder
M67.819 Other specified disorders of synovium ▽
and tendon, unspecified shoulder
✓6ᵗʰ M67.82 Other specified disorders of synovium and tendon, elbow
M67.821 Other specified disorders of synovium, right elbow
M67.822 Other specified disorders of synovium, left elbow
M67.823 Other specified disorders of tendon, right elbow
M67.824 Other specified disorders of tendon, left elbow
M67.829 Other specified disorders of synovium ▽
and tendon, unspecified elbow
✓6ᵗʰ M67.83 Other specified disorders of synovium and tendon, wrist
M67.831 Other specified disorders of synovium, right wrist
M67.832 Other specified disorders of synovium, left wrist
M67.833 Other specified disorders of tendon, right wrist
M67.834 Other specified disorders of tendon, left wrist
M67.839 Other specified disorders of synovium ▽
and tendon, unspecified forearm

✓6ᵗʰ **M67.84 Other specified disorders of synovium and tendon, hand**

     M67.841 Other specified disorders of synovium, right hand

     M67.842 Other specified disorders of synovium, left hand

     M67.843 Other specified disorders of tendon, right hand

     M67.844 Other specified disorders of tendon, left hand

     M67.849 Other specified disorders of synovium and tendon, unspecified hand ▽

✓6ᵗʰ **M67.85 Other specified disorders of synovium and tendon, hip**

     M67.851 Other specified disorders of synovium, right hip

     M67.852 Other specified disorders of synovium, left hip

     M67.853 Other specified disorders of tendon, right hip

     M67.854 Other specified disorders of tendon, left hip

     M67.859 Other specified disorders of synovium and tendon, unspecified hip ▽

✓6ᵗʰ **M67.86 Other specified disorders of synovium and tendon, knee**

     M67.861 Other specified disorders of synovium, right knee

     M67.862 Other specified disorders of synovium, left knee

     M67.863 Other specified disorders of tendon, right knee

     M67.864 Other specified disorders of tendon, left knee

     M67.869 Other specified disorders of synovium and tendon, unspecified knee ▽

✓6ᵗʰ **M67.87 Other specified disorders of synovium and tendon, ankle and foot**

     M67.871 Other specified disorders of synovium, right ankle and foot

     M67.872 Other specified disorders of synovium, left ankle and foot

     M67.873 Other specified disorders of tendon, right ankle and foot

     M67.874 Other specified disorders of tendon, left ankle and foot

     M67.879 Other specified disorders of synovium and tendon, unspecified ankle and foot ▽

     M67.88 Other specified disorders of synovium and tendon, other site

     M67.89 Other specified disorders of synovium and tendon, multiple sites

✓5ᵗʰ **M67.9 Unspecified disorder of synovium and tendon**

     M67.90 Unspecified disorder of synovium and tendon, unspecified site ▽

✓6ᵗʰ **M67.91 Unspecified disorder of synovium and tendon, shoulder**

     M67.911 Unspecified disorder of synovium and tendon, right shoulder ▽

     M67.912 Unspecified disorder of synovium and tendon, left shoulder ▽

     M67.919 Unspecified disorder of synovium and tendon, unspecified shoulder ▽

✓6ᵗʰ **M67.92 Unspecified disorder of synovium and tendon, upper arm**

     M67.921 Unspecified disorder of synovium and tendon, right upper arm ▽

     M67.922 Unspecified disorder of synovium and tendon, left upper arm ▽

     M67.929 Unspecified disorder of synovium and tendon, unspecified upper arm ▽

✓6ᵗʰ **M67.93 Unspecified disorder of synovium and tendon, forearm**

     M67.931 Unspecified disorder of synovium and tendon, right forearm ▽

     M67.932 Unspecified disorder of synovium and tendon, left forearm ▽

     M67.939 Unspecified disorder of synovium and tendon, unspecified forearm ▽

✓6ᵗʰ **M67.94 Unspecified disorder of synovium and tendon, hand**

     M67.941 Unspecified disorder of synovium and tendon, right hand ▽

     M67.942 Unspecified disorder of synovium and tendon, left hand ▽

     M67.949 Unspecified disorder of synovium and tendon, unspecified hand ▽

✓6ᵗʰ **M67.95 Unspecified disorder of synovium and tendon, thigh**

     M67.951 Unspecified disorder of synovium and tendon, right thigh ▽

     M67.952 Unspecified disorder of synovium and tendon, left thigh ▽

     M67.959 Unspecified disorder of synovium and tendon, unspecified thigh ▽

✓6ᵗʰ **M67.96 Unspecified disorder of synovium and tendon, lower leg**

     M67.961 Unspecified disorder of synovium and tendon, right lower leg ▽

     M67.962 Unspecified disorder of synovium and tendon, left lower leg ▽

     M67.969 Unspecified disorder of synovium and tendon, unspecified lower leg ▽

✓6ᵗʰ **M67.97 Unspecified disorder of synovium and tendon, ankle and foot**

     M67.971 Unspecified disorder of synovium and tendon, right ankle and foot ▽

     M67.972 Unspecified disorder of synovium and tendon, left ankle and foot ▽

     M67.979 Unspecified disorder of synovium and tendon, unspecified ankle and foot ▽

     M67.98 Unspecified disorder of synovium and tendon, other site ▽

     M67.99 Unspecified disorder of synovium and tendon, multiple sites ▽

Other soft tissue disorders (M70-M79)

✓4ᵗʰ **M70 Soft tissue disorders related to use, overuse and pressure**

     INCLUDES   soft tissue disorders of occupational origin

     Use additional external cause code to identify activity causing disorder (Y93.-)

     EXCLUDES 1   bursitis NOS (M71.9-)

     EXCLUDES 2   bursitis of shoulder (M75.5)

             enthesopathies (M76-M77)

             pressure ulcer (pressure area) (L89.-)

✓5ᵗʰ **M70.0 Crepitant synovitis (acute) (chronic) of hand and wrist**

     ✓6ᵗʰ **M70.03 Crepitant synovitis (acute) (chronic), wrist**

         M70.031 Crepitant synovitis (acute) (chronic), right wrist

         M70.032 Crepitant synovitis (acute) (chronic), left wrist

         M70.039 Crepitant synovitis (acute) (chronic), unspecified wrist ▽

     ✓6ᵗʰ **M70.04 Crepitant synovitis (acute) (chronic), hand**

         M70.041 Crepitant synovitis (acute) (chronic), right hand

         M70.042 Crepitant synovitis (acute) (chronic), left hand

         M70.049 Crepitant synovitis (acute) (chronic), unspecified hand ▽

✓5ᵗʰ **M70.1 Bursitis of hand**

     M70.10 Bursitis, unspecified hand ▽

     M70.11 Bursitis, right hand

     M70.12 Bursitis, left hand

✓5ᵗʰ **M70.2 Olecranon bursitis**

     M70.20 Olecranon bursitis, unspecified elbow ▽

     M70.21 Olecranon bursitis, right elbow

     M70.22 Olecranon bursitis, left elbow

✓5ᵗʰ **M70.3 Other bursitis of elbow**

     M70.30 Other bursitis of elbow, unspecified elbow ▽

     M70.31 Other bursitis of elbow, right elbow

     M70.32 Other bursitis of elbow, left elbow

☑ Additional Character Req   **✓x7ᵗʰ** Placeholder Alert   Manifestation   **HCC** CMS-HCC Condition   ▽ Unspecified Code   ▶◀ Revised Text   ● New Code   ▲ Revised Code Title

✓5ᵗʰ M70.4 Prepatellar bursitis
     M70.40 Prepatellar bursitis, unspecified knee ▽
     M70.41 Prepatellar bursitis, right knee
     M70.42 Prepatellar bursitis, left knee

✓5ᵗʰ M70.5 Other bursitis of knee
     M70.50 Other bursitis of knee, unspecified knee ▽
     M70.51 Other bursitis of knee, right knee
     M70.52 Other bursitis of knee, left knee

✓5ᵗʰ M70.6 Trochanteric bursitis
     Trochanteric tendinitis
     M70.60 Trochanteric bursitis, unspecified hip ▽
     M70.61 Trochanteric bursitis, right hip
     M70.62 Trochanteric bursitis, left hip

✓5ᵗʰ M70.7 Other bursitis of hip
     Ischial bursitis
     M70.70 Other bursitis of hip, unspecified hip ▽
     M70.71 Other bursitis of hip, right hip
     M70.72 Other bursitis of hip, left hip

✓5ᵗʰ M70.8 Other soft tissue disorders related to use, overuse and pressure
     M70.80 Other soft tissue disorders related to use, overuse and pressure of unspecified site ▽

     ✓6ᵗʰ M70.81 Other soft tissue disorders related to use, overuse and pressure of shoulder
       M70.811 Other soft tissue disorders related to use, overuse and pressure, right shoulder
       M70.812 Other soft tissue disorders related to use, overuse and pressure, left shoulder
       M70.819 Other soft tissue disorders related to use, overuse and pressure, unspecified shoulder ▽

     ✓6ᵗʰ M70.82 Other soft tissue disorders related to use, overuse and pressure of upper arm
       M70.821 Other soft tissue disorders related to use, overuse and pressure, right upper arm
       M70.822 Other soft tissue disorders related to use, overuse and pressure, left upper arm
       M70.829 Other soft tissue disorders related to use, overuse and pressure, unspecified upper arms ▽

     ✓6ᵗʰ M70.83 Other soft tissue disorders related to use, overuse and pressure of forearm
       M70.831 Other soft tissue disorders related to use, overuse and pressure, right forearm
       M70.832 Other soft tissue disorders related to use, overuse and pressure, left forearm
       M70.839 Other soft tissue disorders related to use, overuse and pressure, unspecified forearm ▽

     ✓6ᵗʰ M70.84 Other soft tissue disorders related to use, overuse and pressure of hand
       M70.841 Other soft tissue disorders related to use, overuse and pressure, right hand
       M70.842 Other soft tissue disorders related to use, overuse and pressure, left hand
       M70.849 Other soft tissue disorders related to use, overuse and pressure, unspecified hand ▽

     ✓6ᵗʰ M70.85 Other soft tissue disorders related to use, overuse and pressure of thigh
       M70.851 Other soft tissue disorders related to use, overuse and pressure, right thigh
       M70.852 Other soft tissue disorders related to use, overuse and pressure, left thigh
       M70.859 Other soft tissue disorders related to use, overuse and pressure, unspecified thigh ▽

     ✓6ᵗʰ M70.86 Other soft tissue disorders related to use, overuse and pressure lower leg
       M70.861 Other soft tissue disorders related to use, overuse and pressure, right lower leg
       M70.862 Other soft tissue disorders related to use, overuse and pressure, left lower leg
       M70.869 Other soft tissue disorders related to use, overuse and pressure, unspecified leg ▽

     ✓6ᵗʰ M70.87 Other soft tissue disorders related to use, overuse and pressure of ankle and foot
       M70.871 Other soft tissue disorders related to use, overuse and pressure, right ankle and foot
       M70.872 Other soft tissue disorders related to use, overuse and pressure, left ankle and foot
       M70.879 Other soft tissue disorders related to use, overuse and pressure, unspecified ankle and foot

     M70.88 Other soft tissue disorders related to use, overuse and pressure other site
     M70.89 Other soft tissue disorders related to use, overuse and pressure multiple sites

✓5ᵗʰ M70.9 Unspecified soft tissue disorder related to use, overuse and pressure
     M70.90 Unspecified soft tissue disorder related to use, overuse and pressure of unspecified site ▽

     ✓6ᵗʰ M70.91 Unspecified soft tissue disorder related to use, overuse and pressure of shoulder
       M70.911 Unspecified soft tissue disorder related to use, overuse and pressure, right shoulder ▽
       M70.912 Unspecified soft tissue disorder related to use, overuse and pressure, left shoulder ▽
       M70.919 Unspecified soft tissue disorder related to use, overuse and pressure, unspecified shoulder ▽

     ✓6ᵗʰ M70.92 Unspecified soft tissue disorder related to use, overuse and pressure of upper arm
       M70.921 Unspecified soft tissue disorder related to use, overuse and pressure, right upper arm ▽
       M70.922 Unspecified soft tissue disorder related to use, overuse and pressure, left upper arm ▽
       M70.929 Unspecified soft tissue disorder related to use, overuse and pressure, unspecified upper arm ▽

     ✓6ᵗʰ M70.93 Unspecified soft tissue disorder related to use, overuse and pressure of forearm
       M70.931 Unspecified soft tissue disorder related to use, overuse and pressure, right forearm ▽
       M70.932 Unspecified soft tissue disorder related to use, overuse and pressure, left forearm ▽
       M70.939 Unspecified soft tissue disorder related to use, overuse and pressure, unspecified forearm ▽

     ✓6ᵗʰ M70.94 Unspecified soft tissue disorder related to use, overuse and pressure of hand
       M70.941 Unspecified soft tissue disorder related to use, overuse and pressure, right hand ▽
       M70.942 Unspecified soft tissue disorder related to use, overuse and pressure, left hand ▽
       M70.949 Unspecified soft tissue disorder related to use, overuse and pressure, unspecified hand ▽

     ✓6ᵗʰ M70.95 Unspecified soft tissue disorder related to use, overuse and pressure of thigh
       M70.951 Unspecified soft tissue disorder related to use, overuse and pressure, right thigh ▽
       M70.952 Unspecified soft tissue disorder related to use, overuse and pressure, left thigh ▽
       M70.959 Unspecified soft tissue disorder related to use, overuse and pressure, unspecified thigh ▽

     ✓6ᵗʰ M70.96 Unspecified soft tissue disorder related to use, overuse and pressure lower leg
       M70.961 Unspecified soft tissue disorder related to use, overuse and pressure, right lower leg ▽
       M70.962 Unspecified soft tissue disorder related to use, overuse and pressure, left lower leg ▽
       M70.969 Unspecified soft tissue disorder related to use, overuse and pressure, unspecified lower leg ▽

EXCLUDES 1 Not coded here   **EXCLUDES 2** Not included here   **N** Newborn Age: 0   **P** Pediatric Age: 0-17   **M** Maternity Age: 12-55   **A** Adult Age: 15-124

772   ICD-10-CM 2018

√6ᵗʰ **M70.97** Unspecified soft tissue disorder related to use, overuse and pressure of ankle and foot ▽

     M70.971 Unspecified soft tissue disorder related to use, overuse and pressure, right ankle and foot ▽

     M70.972 Unspecified soft tissue disorder related to use, overuse and pressure, left ankle and foot ▽

     M70.979 Unspecified soft tissue disorder related to use, overuse and pressure, unspecified ankle and foot ▽

M70.98 Unspecified soft tissue disorder related to use, overuse and pressure other ▽

M70.99 Unspecified soft tissue disorder related to use, overuse and pressure multiple sites ▽

√4ᵗʰ **M71 Other bursopathies**

     EXCLUDES 1   bunion (M20.1)
                   bursitis related to use, overuse or pressure (M70.-)
                   enthesopathies (M76-M77)

√5ᵗʰ **M71.0 Abscess of bursa**

     Use additional code (B95.-, B96.-) to identify causative organism

     M71.00 Abscess of bursa, unspecified site ▽

√6ᵗʰ **M71.01** Abscess of bursa, shoulder

     M71.011 Abscess of bursa, right shoulder
     M71.012 Abscess of bursa, left shoulder
     M71.019 Abscess of bursa, unspecified shoulder ▽

√6ᵗʰ **M71.02** Abscess of bursa, elbow

     M71.021 Abscess of bursa, right elbow
     M71.022 Abscess of bursa, left elbow
     M71.029 Abscess of bursa, unspecified elbow ▽

√6ᵗʰ **M71.03** Abscess of bursa, wrist

     M71.031 Abscess of bursa, right wrist
     M71.032 Abscess of bursa, left wrist
     M71.039 Abscess of bursa, unspecified wrist ▽

√6ᵗʰ **M71.04** Abscess of bursa, hand

     M71.041 Abscess of bursa, right hand
     M71.042 Abscess of bursa, left hand
     M71.049 Abscess of bursa, unspecified hand ▽

√6ᵗʰ **M71.05** Abscess of bursa, hip

     M71.051 Abscess of bursa, right hip
     M71.052 Abscess of bursa, left hip
     M71.059 Abscess of bursa, unspecified hip ▽

√6ᵗʰ **M71.06** Abscess of bursa, knee

     M71.061 Abscess of bursa, right knee
     M71.062 Abscess of bursa, left knee
     M71.069 Abscess of bursa, unspecified knee ▽

√6ᵗʰ **M71.07** Abscess of bursa, ankle and foot

     M71.071 Abscess of bursa, right ankle and foot
     M71.072 Abscess of bursa, left ankle and foot
     M71.079 Abscess of bursa, unspecified ankle and foot ▽

     M71.08 Abscess of bursa, other site

     M71.09 Abscess of bursa, multiple sites

√5ᵗʰ **M71.1 Other infective bursitis**

     Use additional code (B95.-, B96.-) to identify causative organism

     M71.10 Other infective bursitis, unspecified site ▽

√6ᵗʰ **M71.11** Other infective bursitis, shoulder

     M71.111 Other infective bursitis, right shoulder
     M71.112 Other infective bursitis, left shoulder
     M71.119 Other infective bursitis, unspecified shoulder ▽

√6ᵗʰ **M71.12** Other infective bursitis, elbow

     M71.121 Other infective bursitis, right elbow
     M71.122 Other infective bursitis, left elbow
     M71.129 Other infective bursitis, unspecified elbow ▽

√6ᵗʰ **M71.13** Other infective bursitis, wrist

     M71.131 Other infective bursitis, right wrist
     M71.132 Other infective bursitis, left wrist
     M71.139 Other infective bursitis, unspecified wrist ▽

√6ᵗʰ **M71.14** Other infective bursitis, hand

     M71.141 Other infective bursitis, right hand
     M71.142 Other infective bursitis, left hand
     M71.149 Other infective bursitis, unspecified hand ▽

√6ᵗʰ **M71.15** Other infective bursitis, hip

     M71.151 Other infective bursitis, right hip
     M71.152 Other infective bursitis, left hip
     M71.159 Other infective bursitis, unspecified hip ▽

√6ᵗʰ **M71.16** Other infective bursitis, knee

     M71.161 Other infective bursitis, right knee
     M71.162 Other infective bursitis, left knee
     M71.169 Other infective bursitis, unspecified knee ▽

√6ᵗʰ **M71.17** Other infective bursitis, ankle and foot

     M71.171 Other infective bursitis, right ankle and foot
     M71.172 Other infective bursitis, left ankle and foot
     M71.179 Other infective bursitis, unspecified ankle and foot ▽

     M71.18 Other infective bursitis, other site

     M71.19 Other infective bursitis, multiple sites

√5ᵗʰ **M71.2 Synovial cyst of popliteal space [Baker]**

     EXCLUDES 1   synovial cyst of popliteal space with rupture (M66.0)

     M71.20 Synovial cyst of popliteal space [Baker], unspecified knee ▽

     M71.21 Synovial cyst of popliteal space [Baker], right knee

     M71.22 Synovial cyst of popliteal space [Baker], left knee

√5ᵗʰ **M71.3 Other bursal cyst**

     Synovial cyst NOS

     EXCLUDES 1   synovial cyst with rupture (M66.1-)

     M71.30 Other bursal cyst, unspecified site ▽

√6ᵗʰ **M71.31** Other bursal cyst, shoulder

     M71.311 Other bursal cyst, right shoulder
     M71.312 Other bursal cyst, left shoulder
     M71.319 Other bursal cyst, unspecified shoulder ▽

√6ᵗʰ **M71.32** Other bursal cyst, elbow

     M71.321 Other bursal cyst, right elbow
     M71.322 Other bursal cyst, left elbow
     M71.329 Other bursal cyst, unspecified elbow ▽

√6ᵗʰ **M71.33** Other bursal cyst, wrist

     M71.331 Other bursal cyst, right wrist
     M71.332 Other bursal cyst, left wrist
     M71.339 Other bursal cyst, unspecified wrist ▽

√6ᵗʰ **M71.34** Other bursal cyst, hand

     M71.341 Other bursal cyst, right hand
     M71.342 Other bursal cyst, left hand
     M71.349 Other bursal cyst, unspecified hand ▽

Baker's Cyst

Baker's cyst connected to knee joint synovial cavity

✔ Additional Character Req   ✔x7ᵗʰ Placeholder Alert   Manifestation   HCC CMS-HCC Condition   ▽ Unspecified Code   ▶◀ Revised Text   ● New Code   ▲ Revised Code Title

ICD-10-CM 2018   **773**

M70.97–M71.349

✓6ᵗʰ **M71.35 Other bursal cyst, hip**
     M71.351 Other bursal cyst, right hip
     M71.352 Other bursal cyst, left hip
     M71.359 Other bursal cyst, unspecified hip ▽

✓6ᵗʰ **M71.37 Other bursal cyst, ankle and foot**
     M71.371 Other bursal cyst, right ankle and foot
     M71.372 Other bursal cyst, left ankle and foot
     M71.379 Other bursal cyst, unspecified ankle and foot ▽

M71.38 Other bursal cyst, other site
M71.39 Other bursal cyst, multiple sites

✓5ᵗʰ **M71.4 Calcium deposit in bursa**
     EXCLUDES 2   calcium deposit in bursa of shoulder (M75.3)
     M71.40 Calcium deposit in bursa, unspecified site ▽

✓6ᵗʰ **M71.42 Calcium deposit in bursa, elbow**
     M71.421 Calcium deposit in bursa, right elbow
     M71.422 Calcium deposit in bursa, left elbow
     M71.429 Calcium deposit in bursa, unspecified elbow ▽

✓6ᵗʰ **M71.43 Calcium deposit in bursa, wrist**
     M71.431 Calcium deposit in bursa, right wrist
     M71.432 Calcium deposit in bursa, left wrist
     M71.439 Calcium deposit in bursa, unspecified wrist ▽

✓6ᵗʰ **M71.44 Calcium deposit in bursa, hand**
     M71.441 Calcium deposit in bursa, right hand
     M71.442 Calcium deposit in bursa, left hand
     M71.449 Calcium deposit in bursa, unspecified hand ▽

✓6ᵗʰ **M71.45 Calcium deposit in bursa, hip**
     M71.451 Calcium deposit in bursa, right hip
     M71.452 Calcium deposit in bursa, left hip
     M71.459 Calcium deposit in bursa, unspecified hip ▽

✓6ᵗʰ **M71.46 Calcium deposit in bursa, knee**
     M71.461 Calcium deposit in bursa, right knee
     M71.462 Calcium deposit in bursa, left knee
     M71.469 Calcium deposit in bursa, unspecified knee ▽

✓6ᵗʰ **M71.47 Calcium deposit in bursa, ankle and foot**
     M71.471 Calcium deposit in bursa, right ankle and foot
     M71.472 Calcium deposit in bursa, left ankle and foot
     M71.479 Calcium deposit in bursa, unspecified ankle and foot ▽

M71.48 Calcium deposit in bursa, other site
M71.49 Calcium deposit in bursa, multiple sites

✓5ᵗʰ **M71.5 Other bursitis, not elsewhere classified**
     EXCLUDES 1   bursitis NOS (M71.9-)
     EXCLUDES 2   bursitis of shoulder (M75.5)
                bursitis of tibial collateral [Pellegrini-Stieda] (M76.4-)
     M71.50 Other bursitis, not elsewhere classified, unspecified site ▽

✓6ᵗʰ **M71.52 Other bursitis, not elsewhere classified, elbow**
     M71.521 Other bursitis, not elsewhere classified, right elbow
     M71.522 Other bursitis, not elsewhere classified, left elbow
     M71.529 Other bursitis, not elsewhere classified, unspecified elbow ▽

✓6ᵗʰ **M71.53 Other bursitis, not elsewhere classified, wrist**
     M71.531 Other bursitis, not elsewhere classified, right wrist
     M71.532 Other bursitis, not elsewhere classified, left wrist
     M71.539 Other bursitis, not elsewhere classified, unspecified wrist ▽

✓6ᵗʰ **M71.54 Other bursitis, not elsewhere classified, hand**
     M71.541 Other bursitis, not elsewhere classified, right hand
     M71.542 Other bursitis, not elsewhere classified, left hand

M71.549 Other bursitis, not elsewhere classified, unspecified hand ▽

✓6ᵗʰ **M71.55 Other bursitis, not elsewhere classified, hip**
     M71.551 Other bursitis, not elsewhere classified, right hip
     M71.552 Other bursitis, not elsewhere classified, left hip
     M71.559 Other bursitis, not elsewhere classified, unspecified hip ▽

✓6ᵗʰ **M71.56 Other bursitis, not elsewhere classified, knee**
     M71.561 Other bursitis, not elsewhere classified, right knee
     M71.562 Other bursitis, not elsewhere classified, left knee
     M71.569 Other bursitis, not elsewhere classified, unspecified knee ▽

✓6ᵗʰ **M71.57 Other bursitis, not elsewhere classified, ankle and foot**
     M71.571 Other bursitis, not elsewhere classified, right ankle and foot
     M71.572 Other bursitis, not elsewhere classified, left ankle and foot
     M71.579 Other bursitis, not elsewhere classified, unspecified ankle and foot ▽

M71.58 Other bursitis, not elsewhere classified, other site

✓5ᵗʰ **M71.8 Other specified bursopathies**
     M71.80 Other specified bursopathies, unspecified site ▽

✓6ᵗʰ **M71.81 Other specified bursopathies, shoulder**
     M71.811 Other specified bursopathies, right shoulder
     M71.812 Other specified bursopathies, left shoulder
     M71.819 Other specified bursopathies, unspecified shoulder ▽

✓6ᵗʰ **M71.82 Other specified bursopathies, elbow**
     M71.821 Other specified bursopathies, right elbow
     M71.822 Other specified bursopathies, left elbow
     M71.829 Other specified bursopathies, unspecified elbow ▽

✓6ᵗʰ **M71.83 Other specified bursopathies, wrist**
     M71.831 Other specified bursopathies, right wrist
     M71.832 Other specified bursopathies, left wrist
     M71.839 Other specified bursopathies, unspecified wrist ▽

✓6ᵗʰ **M71.84 Other specified bursopathies, hand**
     M71.841 Other specified bursopathies, right hand
     M71.842 Other specified bursopathies, left hand
     M71.849 Other specified bursopathies, unspecified hand ▽

✓6ᵗʰ **M71.85 Other specified bursopathies, hip**
     M71.851 Other specified bursopathies, right hip
     M71.852 Other specified bursopathies, left hip
     M71.859 Other specified bursopathies, unspecified hip ▽

✓6ᵗʰ **M71.86 Other specified bursopathies, knee**
     M71.861 Other specified bursopathies, right knee
     M71.862 Other specified bursopathies, left knee
     M71.869 Other specified bursopathies, unspecified knee ▽

✓6ᵗʰ **M71.87 Other specified bursopathies, ankle and foot**
     M71.871 Other specified bursopathies, right ankle and foot
     M71.872 Other specified bursopathies, left ankle and foot
     M71.879 Other specified bursopathies, unspecified ankle and foot ▽

M71.88 Other specified bursopathies, other site
M71.89 Other specified bursopathies, multiple sites

M71.9 Bursopathy, unspecified ▽
     Bursitis NOS

EXCLUDES 1 Not coded here   EXCLUDES 2 Not included here   N Newborn Age: 0   P Pediatric Age: 0-17   M Maternity Age: 12-55   A Adult Age: 15-124

774   ICD-10-CM 2018

M71.35–M71.9

✓4ᵗʰ **M72 Fibroblastic disorders**

     EXCLUDES 2   *retroperitoneal fibromatosis (D48.3)*

    M72.0 Palmar fascial fibromatosis [Dupuytren]   A

      DEF: Dupuytren's contracture: Flexion deformity of finger, due to shortened, thickened fibrosing of palmar fascia; cause unknown; associated with long-standing epilepsy.

    M72.1 Knuckle pads

    M72.2 Plantar fascial fibromatosis

      Plantar fasciitis

      DEF: Rapid-growing and multiplanar nodular swellings and pain in the foot; not associated with contractures.

    M72.4 Pseudosarcomatous fibromatosis

      Nodular fasciitis

    M72.6 Necrotizing fasciitis   HCC

      Use additional code (B95.-, B96.-) to identify causative organism

    M72.8 Other fibroblastic disorders

      Abscess of fascia

      Fasciitis NEC

      Other infective fasciitis

      Use additional code to (B95.-, B96.-) identify causative organism

      EXCLUDES 1   *diffuse (eosinophilic) fasciitis (M35.4)*
              necrotizing fasciitis (M72.6)
              nodular fasciitis (M72.4)
              perirenal fasciitis NOS (N13.5)
              perirenal fasciitis with infection (N13.6)
              plantar fasciitis (M72.2)

    M72.9 Fibroblastic disorder, unspecified   ▽

      Fasciitis NOS

      Fibromatosis NOS

✓4ᵗʰ **M75 Shoulder lesions**

     EXCLUDES 2   *shoulder-hand syndrome (M89.0-)*

   ✓6ᵗʰ **M75.0 Adhesive capsulitis of shoulder**

      Frozen shoulder

      Periarthritis of shoulder

      AHA: 2015, 2Q, 23

     M75.00 Adhesive capsulitis of unspecified shoulder   ▽

     M75.01 Adhesive capsulitis of right shoulder

     M75.02 Adhesive capsulitis of left shoulder

   ✓5ᵗʰ **M75.1 Rotator cuff tear or rupture, not specified as traumatic**

      Rotator cuff syndrome

      Supraspinatus syndrome

      Supraspinatus tear or rupture, not specified as traumatic

      EXCLUDES 1   *tear of rotator cuff, traumatic (S46.01-)*

    ✓6ᵗʰ **M75.10 Unspecified rotator cuff tear or rupture, not specified as traumatic**

      M75.100 Unspecified rotator cuff tear or rupture ▽ **of unspecified shoulder, not specified as traumatic**

      M75.101 Unspecified rotator cuff tear or rupture ▽ **of right shoulder, not specified as traumatic**

      M75.102 Unspecified rotator cuff tear or rupture ▽ **of left shoulder, not specified as traumatic**

    ✓6ᵗʰ **M75.11 Incomplete rotator cuff tear or rupture not specified as traumatic**

      M75.110 Incomplete rotator cuff tear or rupture ▽ **of unspecified shoulder, not specified as traumatic**

      M75.111 Incomplete rotator cuff tear or rupture of right shoulder, not specified as traumatic

      M75.112 Incomplete rotator cuff tear or rupture of left shoulder, not specified as traumatic

    ✓6ᵗʰ **M75.12 Complete rotator cuff tear or rupture not specified as traumatic**

      M75.120 Complete rotator cuff tear or rupture ▽ **of unspecified shoulder, not specified as traumatic**

      M75.121 Complete rotator cuff tear or rupture of right shoulder, not specified as traumatic

      M75.122 Complete rotator cuff tear or rupture of left shoulder, not specified as traumatic

   ✓5ᵗʰ **M75.2 Bicipital tendinitis**

     M75.20 Bicipital tendinitis, unspecified shoulder   ▽

     M75.21 Bicipital tendinitis, right shoulder

     M75.22 Bicipital tendinitis, left shoulder

   ✓5ᵗʰ **M75.3 Calcific tendinitis of shoulder**

      Calcified bursa of shoulder

     M75.30 Calcific tendinitis of unspecified shoulder   ▽

     M75.31 Calcific tendinitis of right shoulder

     M75.32 Calcific tendinitis of left shoulder

   ✓5ᵗʰ **M75.4 Impingement syndrome of shoulder**

     M75.40 Impingement syndrome of unspecified shoulder   ▽

     M75.41 Impingement syndrome of right shoulder

     M75.42 Impingement syndrome of left shoulder

   ✓5ᵗʰ **M75.5 Bursitis of shoulder**

     M75.50 Bursitis of unspecified shoulder   ▽

     M75.51 Bursitis of right shoulder

     M75.52 Bursitis of left shoulder

   ✓5ᵗʰ **M75.8 Other shoulder lesions**

     M75.80 Other shoulder lesions, unspecified shoulder   ▽

     M75.81 Other shoulder lesions, right shoulder

     M75.82 Other shoulder lesions, left shoulder

   ✓5ᵗʰ **M75.9 Shoulder lesion, unspecified**

     M75.90 Shoulder lesion, unspecified, unspecified shoulder   ▽

     M75.91 Shoulder lesion, unspecified, right shoulder   ▽

     M75.92 Shoulder lesion, unspecified, left shoulder   ▽

✓4ᵗʰ **M76 Enthesopathies, lower limb, excluding foot**

     EXCLUDES 2   *bursitis due to use, overuse and pressure (M70.-)*
              enthesopathies of ankle and foot (M77.5-)

   ✓5ᵗʰ **M76.0 Gluteal tendinitis**

     M76.00 Gluteal tendinitis, unspecified hip   ▽

     M76.01 Gluteal tendinitis, right hip

     M76.02 Gluteal tendinitis, left hip

   ✓5ᵗʰ **M76.1 Psoas tendinitis**

     M76.10 Psoas tendinitis, unspecified hip   ▽

     M76.11 Psoas tendinitis, right hip

     M76.12 Psoas tendinitis, left hip

   ✓5ᵗʰ **M76.2 Iliac crest spur**

     M76.20 Iliac crest spur, unspecified hip   ▽

     M76.21 Iliac crest spur, right hip

     M76.22 Iliac crest spur, left hip

   ✓5ᵗʰ **M76.3 Iliotibial band syndrome**

     M76.30 Iliotibial band syndrome, unspecified leg   ▽

     M76.31 Iliotibial band syndrome, right leg

     M76.32 Iliotibial band syndrome, left leg

   ✓5ᵗʰ **M76.4 Tibial collateral bursitis [Pellegrini-Stieda]**

     M76.40 Tibial collateral bursitis [Pellegrini-Stieda], unspecified leg   ▽

     M76.41 Tibial collateral bursitis [Pellegrini-Stieda], right leg

     M76.42 Tibial collateral bursitis [Pellegrini-Stieda], left leg

   ✓5ᵗʰ **M76.5 Patellar tendinitis**

     M76.50 Patellar tendinitis, unspecified knee   ▽

     M76.51 Patellar tendinitis, right knee

     M76.52 Patellar tendinitis, left knee

   ✓5ᵗʰ **M76.6 Achilles tendinitis**

      Achilles bursitis

     M76.60 Achilles tendinitis, unspecified leg   ▽

     M76.61 Achilles tendinitis, right leg

     M76.62 Achilles tendinitis, left leg

   ✓5ᵗʰ **M76.7 Peroneal tendinitis**

     M76.70 Peroneal tendinitis, unspecified leg   ▽

     M76.71 Peroneal tendinitis, right leg

     M76.72 Peroneal tendinitis, left leg

   ✓5ᵗʰ **M76.8 Other specified enthesopathies of lower limb, excluding foot**

    ✓6ᵗʰ **M76.81 Anterior tibial syndrome**

      M76.811 Anterior tibial syndrome, right leg

      M76.812 Anterior tibial syndrome, left leg

      M76.819 Anterior tibial syndrome, unspecified ▽ **leg**

    ✓6ᵗʰ **M76.82 Posterior tibial tendinitis**

      M76.821 Posterior tibial tendinitis, right leg

      M76.822 Posterior tibial tendinitis, left leg

      M76.829 Posterior tibial tendinitis, unspecified ▽ **leg**

✓ Additional Character Req   ✓x7ᵗʰ Placeholder Alert   Manifestation   HCC CMS-HCC Condition   ▽ Unspecified Code   ►◄ Revised Text   ● New Code   ▲ Revised Code Title

ICD-10-CM 2018   775

✓6ᵗʰ M76.89 Other specified enthesopathies of lower limb, excluding foot

     M76.891 Other specified enthesopathies of right lower limb, excluding foot

     M76.892 Other specified enthesopathies of left lower limb, excluding foot

     M76.899 Other specified enthesopathies of unspecified lower limb, excluding foot ▽

M76.9 Unspecified enthesopathy, lower limb, excluding foot ▽

✓4ᵗʰ M77 Other enthesopathies

     EXCLUDES 1   bursitis NOS (M71.9-)

     EXCLUDES 2   bursitis due to use, overuse and pressure (M70.-)
              osteophyte (M25.7)
              spinal enthesopathy (M46.0-)

✓5ᵗʰ M77.0 Medial epicondylitis

     M77.00 Medial epicondylitis, unspecified elbow ▽

     M77.01 Medial epicondylitis, right elbow

     M77.02 Medial epicondylitis, left elbow

✓5ᵗʰ M77.1 Lateral epicondylitis
     Tennis elbow

     M77.10 Lateral epicondylitis, unspecified elbow ▽

     M77.11 Lateral epicondylitis, right elbow

     M77.12 Lateral epicondylitis, left elbow

✓5ᵗʰ M77.2 Periarthritis of wrist

     M77.20 Periarthritis, unspecified wrist ▽

     M77.21 Periarthritis, right wrist

     M77.22 Periarthritis, left wrist

✓5ᵗʰ M77.3 Calcaneal spur
     DEF: Overgrowth of calcaneus bone on underside of the heel; causes pain on walking; due to chronic avulsion injury of plantar fascia from calcaneus.

     M77.30 Calcaneal spur, unspecified foot ▽

     M77.31 Calcaneal spur, right foot

     M77.32 Calcaneal spur, left foot

✓5ᵗʰ M77.4 Metatarsalgia

     EXCLUDES 1   Morton's metatarsalgia (G57.6)

     M77.40 Metatarsalgia, unspecified foot ▽

     M77.41 Metatarsalgia, right foot

     M77.42 Metatarsalgia, left foot

✓5ᵗʰ M77.5 Other enthesopathy of foot

     M77.50 Other enthesopathy of unspecified foot ▽

     M77.51 Other enthesopathy of right foot

     M77.52 Other enthesopathy of left foot

M77.8 Other enthesopathies, not elsewhere classified

M77.9 Enthesopathy, unspecified ▽

     Bone spur NOS   Periarthritis NOS
     Capsulitis NOS   Tendinitis NOS

✓4ᵗʰ M79 Other and unspecified soft tissue disorders, not elsewhere classified

     EXCLUDES 1   psychogenic rheumatism (F45.8)
              soft tissue pain, psychogenic (F45.41)

M79.0 Rheumatism, unspecified ▽

     EXCLUDES 1   fibromyalgia (M79.7)
              palindromic rheumatism (M12.3-)

M79.1 Myalgia
     Myofascial pain syndrome

     EXCLUDES 1   fibromyalgia (M79.7)
              myositis (M60.-)

M79.2 Neuralgia and neuritis, unspecified ▽

     EXCLUDES 1   brachial radiculitis NOS (M54.1)
              lumbosacral radiculitis NOS (M54.1)
              mononeuropathies (G56-G58)
              radiculitis NOS (M54.1)
              sciatica (M54.3-M54.4)

M79.3 Panniculitis, unspecified ▽

     EXCLUDES 1   lupus panniculitis (L93.2)
              neck and back panniculitis (M54.0-)
              relapsing [Weber-Christian] panniculitis (M35.6)

M79.4 Hypertrophy of (infrapatellar) fat pad

M79.5 Residual foreign body in soft tissue

     EXCLUDES 1   foreign body granuloma of skin and subcutaneous tissue (L92.3)
              foreign body granuloma of soft tissue (M60.2-)

✓5ᵗʰ M79.6 Pain in limb, hand, foot, fingers and toes

     EXCLUDES 2   pain in joint (M25.5-)

✓6ᵗʰ M79.60 Pain in limb, unspecified

     M79.601 Pain in right arm
              Pain in right upper limb NOS

     M79.602 Pain in left arm
              Pain in left upper limb NOS

     M79.603 Pain in arm, unspecified ▽
              Pain in upper limb NOS

     M79.604 Pain in right leg
              Pain in right lower limb NOS

     M79.605 Pain in left leg
              Pain in left lower limb NOS

     M79.606 Pain in leg, unspecified ▽
              Pain in lower limb NOS

     M79.609 Pain in unspecified limb ▽
              Pain in limb NOS

✓6ᵗʰ M79.62 Pain in upper arm
     Pain in axillary region

     M79.621 Pain in right upper arm

     M79.622 Pain in left upper arm

     M79.629 Pain in unspecified upper arm ▽

✓6ᵗʰ M79.63 Pain in forearm

     M79.631 Pain in right forearm

     M79.632 Pain in left forearm

     M79.639 Pain in unspecified forearm ▽

✓6ᵗʰ M79.64 Pain in hand and fingers

     M79.641 Pain in right hand

     M79.642 Pain in left hand

     M79.643 Pain in unspecified hand ▽

     M79.644 Pain in right finger(s)

     M79.645 Pain in left finger(s)

     M79.646 Pain in unspecified finger(s) ▽

✓6ᵗʰ M79.65 Pain in thigh

     M79.651 Pain in right thigh

     M79.652 Pain in left thigh

     M79.659 Pain in unspecified thigh ▽

✓6ᵗʰ M79.66 Pain in lower leg

     M79.661 Pain in right lower leg

     M79.662 Pain in left lower leg

     M79.669 Pain in unspecified lower leg ▽

✓6ᵗʰ M79.67 Pain in foot and toes

     M79.671 Pain in right foot

     M79.672 Pain in left foot

     M79.673 Pain in unspecified foot ▽

     M79.674 Pain in right toe(s)

     M79.675 Pain in left toe(s)

     M79.676 Pain in unspecified toe(s) ▽

M79.7 Fibromyalgia
     Fibromyositis   Myofibrositis
     Fibrositis

✓5ᵗʰ M79.A Nontraumatic compartment syndrome
     Code first, if applicable, associated postprocedural complication

     EXCLUDES 1   compartment syndrome NOS (T79.A-)
              fibromyalgia (M79.7)
              nontraumatic ischemic infarction of muscle (M62.2-)
              traumatic compartment syndrome (T79.A-)

✓6ᵗʰ M79.A1 Nontraumatic compartment syndrome of upper extremity
     Nontraumatic compartment syndrome of shoulder, arm, forearm, wrist, hand, and fingers

     M79.A11 Nontraumatic compartment syndrome of right upper extremity

     M79.A12 Nontraumatic compartment syndrome of left upper extremity

     M79.A19 Nontraumatic compartment syndrome ▽ **of unspecified upper extremity**

✓6ᵗʰ M79.A2 Nontraumatic compartment syndrome of lower extremity
     Nontraumatic compartment syndrome of hip, buttock, thigh, leg, foot, and toes

     M79.A21 Nontraumatic compartment syndrome of right lower extremity

     M79.A22 Nontraumatic compartment syndrome of left lower extremity

---

EXCLUDES 1 Not coded here   *EXCLUDES 2* Not included here   N Newborn Age: 0   P Pediatric Age: 0-17   M Maternity Age: 12-55   A Adult Age: 15-124

776   ICD-10-CM 2018

M79.A29   **Nontraumatic compartment syndrome** ▽
of unspecified lower extremity

M79.A3   **Nontraumatic compartment syndrome of** abdomen

M79.A9   **Nontraumatic compartment syndrome of other sites**

✓5ᵗʰ **M79.8**   **Other specified soft tissue disorders**

M79.81   **Nontraumatic hematoma of soft tissue**
Nontraumatic hematoma of muscle
Nontraumatic seroma of muscle and soft tissue

M79.89   **Other specified soft tissue disorders**
Polyalgia

M79.9   **Soft tissue disorder, unspecified**   ▽

OSTEOPATHIES AND CHONDROPATHIES (M80-M94)

Disorders of bone density and structure (M80-M85)

✓4ᵗʰ **M80**   **Osteoporosis** with current pathological fracture
INCLUDES   osteoporosis with current fragility fracture
Use additional code to identify major osseous defect, if applicable (M89.7-)
EXCLUDES 1   collapsed vertebra NOS (M48.5)
pathological fracture NOS (M84.4)
wedging of vertebra NOS (M48.5)
EXCLUDES 2   personal history of (healed) osteoporosis fracture (Z87.310)

The appropriate 7th character is to be added to each code from category M80.
A   initial encounter for fracture
D   subsequent encounter for fracture with routine healing
G   subsequent encounter for fracture with delayed healing
K   subsequent encounter for fracture with nonunion
P   subsequent encounter for fracture with malunion
S   sequela

✓5ᵗʰ **M80.0**   **Age-related osteoporosis with current pathological fracture**
Involutional osteoporosis with current pathological fracture
Osteoporosis NOS with current pathological fracture
Postmenopausal osteoporosis with current pathological fracture
Senile osteoporosis with current pathological fracture

✓x7ᵗʰ **M80.00**   **Age-related osteoporosis with current** Ⓐ ▽
pathological fracture, unspecified site

✓6ᵗʰ **M80.01**   **Age-related osteoporosis with current pathological fracture,** shoulder

✓7ᵗʰ **M80.011**   **Age-related osteoporosis with current** Ⓐ
pathological fracture, right shoulder

✓7ᵗʰ **M80.012**   **Age-related osteoporosis with current** Ⓐ
pathological fracture, left shoulder

✓7ᵗʰ **M80.019**   **Age-related osteoporosis with** Ⓐ ▽
current pathological fracture,
unspecified shoulder

✓6ᵗʰ **M80.02**   **Age-related osteoporosis with current pathological fracture,** humerus

✓7ᵗʰ **M80.021**   **Age-related osteoporosis with current** Ⓐ
pathological fracture, right humerus

✓7ᵗʰ **M80.022**   **Age-related osteoporosis with current** Ⓐ
pathological fracture, left humerus

✓7ᵗʰ **M80.029**   **Age-related osteoporosis with** Ⓐ ▽
current pathological fracture,
unspecified humerus

✓6ᵗʰ **M80.03**   **Age-related osteoporosis with current pathological fracture,** forearm
Age-related osteoporosis with current pathological
fracture of wrist

✓7ᵗʰ **M80.031**   **Age-related osteoporosis with current** Ⓐ
pathological fracture, right forearm

✓7ᵗʰ **M80.032**   **Age-related osteoporosis with current** Ⓐ
pathological fracture, left forearm

✓7ᵗʰ **M80.039**   **Age-related osteoporosis with** Ⓐ ▽
current pathological fracture,
unspecified forearm

✓6ᵗʰ **M80.04**   **Age-related osteoporosis with current pathological fracture,** hand

✓7ᵗʰ **M80.041**   **Age-related osteoporosis with current** Ⓐ
pathological fracture, right hand

✓7ᵗʰ **M80.042**   **Age-related osteoporosis with current** Ⓐ
pathological fracture, left hand

✓7ᵗʰ **M80.049**   **Age-related osteoporosis with** Ⓐ ▽
current pathological fracture,
unspecified hand

✓6ᵗʰ **M80.05**   **Age-related osteoporosis with current pathological fracture,** femur
Age-related osteoporosis with current pathological
fracture of hip

¹ ✓7ᵗʰ **M80.051**   **Age-related osteoporosis with** ᴴᶜᶜ Ⓐ
current pathological fracture,
right femur

¹ ✓7ᵗʰ **M80.052**   **Age-related osteoporosis with** ᴴᶜᶜ Ⓐ
current pathological fracture,
left femur

¹ ✓7ᵗʰ **M80.059**   **Age-related osteoporosis with** ᴴᶜᶜ Ⓐ ▽
current pathological fracture,
unspecified femur

✓6ᵗʰ **M80.06**   **Age-related osteoporosis with current pathological fracture,** lower leg

✓7ᵗʰ **M80.061**   **Age-related osteoporosis with current** Ⓐ
pathological fracture, right lower leg

✓7ᵗʰ **M80.062**   **Age-related osteoporosis with current** Ⓐ
pathological fracture, left lower leg

✓7ᵗʰ **M80.069**   **Age-related osteoporosis with** Ⓐ ▽
current pathological fracture,
unspecified lower leg

✓6ᵗʰ **M80.07**   **Age-related osteoporosis with current pathological fracture,** ankle and foot

✓7ᵗʰ **M80.071**   **Age-related osteoporosis with current** Ⓐ
pathological fracture, right ankle and foot

✓7ᵗʰ **M80.072**   **Age-related osteoporosis with current** Ⓐ
pathological fracture, left ankle and foot

✓7ᵗʰ **M80.079**   **Age-related osteoporosis with** Ⓐ ▽
current pathological fracture,
unspecified ankle and foot

¹ ✓x7ᵗʰ **M80.08**   **Age-related osteoporosis with current** ᴴᶜᶜ Ⓐ
pathological fracture, vertebra(e)

✓5ᵗʰ **M80.8**   **Other osteoporosis with current pathological fracture**
Drug-induced osteoporosis with current pathological fracture
Idiopathic osteoporosis with current pathological fracture
Osteoporosis of disuse with current pathological fracture
Postoophorectomy osteoporosis with current pathological
fracture
Postsurgical malabsorption osteoporosis with current
pathological fracture
Post-traumatic osteoporosis with current pathological fracture
Use additional code for adverse effect, if applicable, to identify
drug (T36-T50 with fifth or sixth character 5)

✓x7ᵗʰ **M80.80**   **Other osteoporosis with current pathological** ▽
fracture, unspecified site

✓6ᵗʰ **M80.81**   **Other osteoporosis with pathological fracture,** shoulder

✓7ᵗʰ **M80.811**   **Other osteoporosis with current**
pathological fracture, right shoulder

✓7ᵗʰ **M80.812**   **Other osteoporosis with current**
pathological fracture, left shoulder

✓7ᵗʰ **M80.819**   **Other osteoporosis with current** ▽
pathological fracture, unspecified
shoulder

✓6ᵗʰ **M80.82**   **Other osteoporosis with current pathological fracture,** humerus

✓7ᵗʰ **M80.821**   **Other osteoporosis with current**
pathological fracture, right humerus

✓7ᵗʰ **M80.822**   **Other osteoporosis with current**
pathological fracture, left humerus

✓7ᵗʰ **M80.829**   **Other osteoporosis with current** ▽
pathological fracture, unspecified
humerus

✓6ᵗʰ **M80.83**   **Other osteoporosis with current pathological fracture,** forearm
Other osteoporosis with current pathological fracture
of wrist

✓7ᵗʰ **M80.831**   **Other osteoporosis with current**
pathological fracture, right forearm

✓7ᵗʰ **M80.832**   **Other osteoporosis with current**
pathological fracture, left forearm

✓7ᵗʰ **M80.839**   **Other osteoporosis with current** ▽
pathological fracture, unspecified forearm

---

¹   HCC with 7th character indicating initial encounter (A, B or C - specific to category).

☑ Additional Character Req   ✓x7ᵗʰ Placeholder Alert   Manifestation   ᴴᶜᶜ CMS-HCC Condition   ▽ Unspecified Code   ►◄ Revised Text   ● New Code   ▲ Revised Code Title

✓6ᵗʰ **M80.84 Other osteoporosis with current pathological fracture, hand**

  ✓7ᵗʰ **M80.841 Other osteoporosis with current pathological fracture, right hand**

  ✓7ᵗʰ **M80.842 Other osteoporosis with current pathological fracture, left hand**

  ✓7ᵗʰ **M80.849 Other osteoporosis with current pathological fracture, unspecified hand** ▽

✓6ᵗʰ **M80.85 Other osteoporosis with current pathological fracture, femur**

  Other osteoporosis with current pathological fracture of hip

  ¹ ✓7ᵗʰ **M80.851 Other osteoporosis with current pathological fracture, right femur** HCC

  ¹ ✓7ᵗʰ **M80.852 Other osteoporosis with current pathological fracture, left femur** HCC

  ¹ ✓7ᵗʰ **M80.859 Other osteoporosis with current pathological fracture, unspecified femur** HCC ▽

✓6ᵗʰ **M80.86 Other osteoporosis with current pathological fracture, lower leg**

  ✓7ᵗʰ **M80.861 Other osteoporosis with current pathological fracture, right lower leg**

  ✓7ᵗʰ **M80.862 Other osteoporosis with current pathological fracture, left lower leg**

  ✓7ᵗʰ **M80.869 Other osteoporosis with current pathological fracture, unspecified lower leg** ▽

✓6ᵗʰ **M80.87 Other osteoporosis with current pathological fracture, ankle and foot**

  ✓7ᵗʰ **M80.871 Other osteoporosis with current pathological fracture, right ankle and foot**

  ✓7ᵗʰ **M80.872 Other osteoporosis with current pathological fracture, left ankle and foot**

  ✓7ᵗʰ **M80.879 Other osteoporosis with current pathological fracture, unspecified ankle and foot** ▽

¹ ✓x7ᵗʰ **M80.88 Other osteoporosis with current pathological fracture, vertebra(e)** HCC

✓4ᵗʰ **M81 Osteoporosis without current pathological fracture**

  Use additional code to identify:
    major osseous defect, if applicable (M89.7-)
    personal history of (healed) osteoporosis fracture, if applicable (Z87.310)
  EXCLUDES 1 *osteoporosis with current pathological fracture (M80.-)*
  Sudeck's atrophy (M89.0)

  M81.0 Age-related osteoporosis without current pathological fracture Ⓐ
    Involutional osteoporosis without current pathological fracture
    Osteoporosis NOS
    Postmenopausal osteoporosis without current pathological fracture
    Senile osteoporosis without current pathological fracture

  M81.6 Localized osteoporosis [Lequesne]
    EXCLUDES 1 *Sudeck's atrophy (M89.0)*

  M81.8 Other osteoporosis without current pathological fracture
    Drug-induced osteoporosis without current pathological fracture
    Idiopathic osteoporosis without current pathological fracture
    Osteoporosis of disuse without current pathological fracture
    Postoophorectomy osteoporosis without current pathological fracture
    Postsurgical malabsorption osteoporosis without current pathological fracture
    Post-traumatic osteoporosis without current pathological fracture
    Use additional code for adverse effect, if applicable, to identify drug (T36-T50 with fifth or sixth character 5)

✓4ᵗʰ **M83 Adult osteomalacia**
  EXCLUDES 1 *infantile and juvenile osteomalacia (E55.0)*
  renal osteodystrophy (N25.0)
  rickets (active) (E55.0)
  rickets (active) sequelae (E64.3)
  vitamin D-resistant osteomalacia (E83.3)
  vitamin D-resistant rickets (active) (E83.3)

  M83.0 Puerperal osteomalacia Ⓜ♀

  M83.1 Senile osteomalacia Ⓐ

M83.2 Adult osteomalacia due to malabsorption Ⓐ
  Postsurgical malabsorption osteomalacia in adults

M83.3 Adult osteomalacia due to malnutrition Ⓐ

M83.4 Aluminum bone disease

M83.5 Other drug-induced osteomalacia in adults Ⓐ
  Use additional code for adverse effect, if applicable, to identify drug (T36-T50 with fifth or sixth character 5)

M83.8 Other adult osteomalacia Ⓐ

M83.9 Adult osteomalacia, unspecified Ⓐ▽

✓4ᵗʰ **M84 Disorder of continuity of bone**
  EXCLUDES 2 *traumatic fracture of bone-see fracture, by site*

✓5ᵗʰ **M84.3 Stress fracture**
  Fatigue fracture   Stress fracture NOS
  March fracture   Stress reaction
  Use additional external cause code(s) to identify the cause of the stress fracture
  EXCLUDES 1 *pathological fracture NOS (M84.4-)*
  pathological fracture due to osteoporosis (M80.-)
  traumatic fracture (S12-, S22-, S32-, S42-, S52-, S62-, S72-, S82-, S92-)
  EXCLUDES 2 *personal history of (healed) stress (fatigue) fracture (Z87.312)*
  stress fracture of vertebra (M48.4-)

  The appropriate 7th character is to be added to each code from subcategory M84.3.
  A   initial encounter for fracture
  D   subsequent encounter for fracture with routine healing
  G   subsequent encounter for fracture with delayed healing
  K   subsequent encounter for fracture with nonunion
  P   subsequent encounter for fracture with malunion
  S   sequela

  ✓x7ᵗʰ **M84.30 Stress fracture, unspecified site** ▽

  ✓6ᵗʰ **M84.31 Stress fracture, shoulder**
    ✓7ᵗʰ **M84.311 Stress fracture, right shoulder**
    ✓7ᵗʰ **M84.312 Stress fracture, left shoulder**
    ✓7ᵗʰ **M84.319 Stress fracture, unspecified shoulder** ▽

  ✓6ᵗʰ **M84.32 Stress fracture, humerus**
    ✓7ᵗʰ **M84.321 Stress fracture, right humerus**
    ✓7ᵗʰ **M84.322 Stress fracture, left humerus**
    ✓7ᵗʰ **M84.329 Stress fracture, unspecified humerus** ▽

  ✓6ᵗʰ **M84.33 Stress fracture, ulna and radius**
    ✓7ᵗʰ **M84.331 Stress fracture, right ulna**
    ✓7ᵗʰ **M84.332 Stress fracture, left ulna**
    ✓7ᵗʰ **M84.333 Stress fracture, right radius**
    ✓7ᵗʰ **M84.334 Stress fracture, left radius**
    ✓7ᵗʰ **M84.339 Stress fracture, unspecified ulna and radius** ▽

  ✓6ᵗʰ **M84.34 Stress fracture, hand and fingers**
    ✓7ᵗʰ **M84.341 Stress fracture, right hand**
    ✓7ᵗʰ **M84.342 Stress fracture, left hand**
    ✓7ᵗʰ **M84.343 Stress fracture, unspecified hand** ▽
    ✓7ᵗʰ **M84.344 Stress fracture, right finger(s)**
    ✓7ᵗʰ **M84.345 Stress fracture, left finger(s)**
    ✓7ᵗʰ **M84.346 Stress fracture, unspecified finger(s)** ▽

  ✓6ᵗʰ **M84.35 Stress fracture, pelvis and femur**
    Stress fracture, hip
    ✓7ᵗʰ **M84.350 Stress fracture, pelvis**
    ✓7ᵗʰ **M84.351 Stress fracture, right femur**
    ✓7ᵗʰ **M84.352 Stress fracture, left femur**
    ✓7ᵗʰ **M84.353 Stress fracture, unspecified femur** ▽
    ✓7ᵗʰ **M84.359 Stress fracture, hip, unspecified** ▽

  ✓6ᵗʰ **M84.36 Stress fracture, tibia and fibula**
    ✓7ᵗʰ **M84.361 Stress fracture, right tibia**
    ✓7ᵗʰ **M84.362 Stress fracture, left tibia**
    ✓7ᵗʰ **M84.363 Stress fracture, right fibula**
    ✓7ᵗʰ **M84.364 Stress fracture, left fibula**
    ✓7ᵗʰ **M84.369 Stress fracture, unspecified tibia and fibula** ▽

---

¹ HCC with 7th character indicating initial encounter (A, B or C - specific to category).

EXCLUDES 1 Not coded here   *EXCLUDES 2* Not included here   Ⓝ Newborn Age: 0   Ⓟ Pediatric Age: 0-17   Ⓜ Maternity Age: 12-55   Ⓐ Adult Age: 15-124

778   ICD-10-CM 2018

✓6ᵗʰ M84.37 Stress fracture, ankle, foot and toes

    ✓7ᵗʰ **M84.371 Stress fracture,** right ankle

    ✓7ᵗʰ **M84.372 Stress fracture,** left ankle

    ✓7ᵗʰ **M84.373 Stress fracture, unspecified ankle** ▽

    ✓7ᵗʰ **M84.374 Stress fracture,** right foot

    ✓7ᵗʰ **M84.375 Stress fracture,** left foot

    ✓7ᵗʰ **M84.376 Stress fracture, unspecified foot** ▽

    ✓7ᵗʰ **M84.377 Stress fracture,** right toe(s)

    ✓7ᵗʰ **M84.378 Stress fracture,** left toe(s)

    ✓7ᵗʰ **M84.379 Stress fracture, unspecified toe(s)** ▽

✓x7ᵗʰ M84.38 Stress fracture, other site

    EXCLUDES 2   stress fracture of vertebra (M48.4-)

✓5ᵗʰ M84.4 Pathological fracture, not elsewhere classified

    Chronic fracture

    Pathological fracture NOS

    EXCLUDES 1   collapsed vertebra NEC (M48.5)

         pathological fracture in neoplastic disease (M84.5-)

         pathological fracture in osteoporosis (M80.-)

         pathological fracture in other disease (M84.6-)

         stress fracture (M84.3-)

         traumatic fracture (S12.-, S22.-, S32.-, S42.-, S52.-, S62.-, S72.-, S82.-, S92.-)

    EXCLUDES 2   personal history of (healed) pathological fracture (Z87.311)

    The appropriate 7th character is to be added to each code from subcategory M84.4.

    A   initial encounter for fracture

    D   subsequent encounter for fracture with routine healing

    G   subsequent encounter for fracture with delayed healing

    K   subsequent encounter for fracture with nonunion

    P   subsequent encounter for fracture with malunion

    S   sequela

✓x7ᵗʰ M84.40 Pathological fracture, unspecified site ▽

✓6ᵗʰ M84.41 Pathological fracture, shoulder

    ✓7ᵗʰ **M84.411 Pathological fracture,** right shoulder

    ✓7ᵗʰ **M84.412 Pathological fracture,** left shoulder

    ✓7ᵗʰ **M84.419 Pathological fracture, unspecified shoulder** ▽

✓6ᵗʰ M84.42 Pathological fracture, humerus

    ✓7ᵗʰ **M84.421 Pathological fracture,** right humerus

    ✓7ᵗʰ **M84.422 Pathological fracture,** left humerus

    ✓7ᵗʰ **M84.429 Pathological fracture, unspecified humerus** ▽

✓6ᵗʰ M84.43 Pathological fracture, ulna and radius

    ✓7ᵗʰ **M84.431 Pathological fracture,** right ulna

    ✓7ᵗʰ **M84.432 Pathological fracture,** left ulna

    ✓7ᵗʰ **M84.433 Pathological fracture,** right radius

    ✓7ᵗʰ **M84.434 Pathological fracture,** left radius

    ✓7ᵗʰ **M84.439 Pathological fracture, unspecified ulna and radius** ▽

✓6ᵗʰ M84.44 Pathological fracture, hand and fingers

    ✓7ᵗʰ **M84.441 Pathological fracture,** right hand

    ✓7ᵗʰ **M84.442 Pathological fracture,** left hand

    ✓7ᵗʰ **M84.443 Pathological fracture, unspecified hand** ▽

    ✓7ᵗʰ **M84.444 Pathological fracture,** right finger(s)

    ✓7ᵗʰ **M84.445 Pathological fracture,** left finger(s)

    ✓7ᵗʰ **M84.446 Pathological fracture, unspecified finger(s)** ▽

✓6ᵗʰ M84.45 Pathological fracture, femur and pelvis

    [1] ✓7ᵗʰ **M84.451 Pathological fracture,** right femur   **HCC**

    [1] ✓7ᵗʰ **M84.452 Pathological fracture,** left femur   **HCC**

    [1] ✓7ᵗʰ **M84.453 Pathological fracture, unspecified femur**   **HCC** ▽

    ✓7ᵗʰ **M84.454 Pathological fracture,** pelvis

    [1] ✓7ᵗʰ **M84.459 Pathological fracture, hip, unspecified**   **HCC** ▽

✓6ᵗʰ M84.46 Pathological fracture, tibia and fibula

    ✓7ᵗʰ **M84.461 Pathological fracture,** right tibia

    ✓7ᵗʰ **M84.462 Pathological fracture,** left tibia

    ✓7ᵗʰ **M84.463 Pathological fracture,** right fibula

    ✓7ᵗʰ **M84.464 Pathological fracture,** left fibula

    ✓7ᵗʰ **M84.469 Pathological fracture, unspecified tibia and fibula** ▽

✓6ᵗʰ M84.47 Pathological fracture, ankle, foot and toes

    ✓7ᵗʰ **M84.471 Pathological fracture,** right ankle

    ✓7ᵗʰ **M84.472 Pathological fracture,** left ankle

    ✓7ᵗʰ **M84.473 Pathological fracture, unspecified ankle** ▽

    ✓7ᵗʰ **M84.474 Pathological fracture,** right foot

    ✓7ᵗʰ **M84.475 Pathological fracture,** left foot

    ✓7ᵗʰ **M84.476 Pathological fracture, unspecified foot** ▽

    ✓7ᵗʰ **M84.477 Pathological fracture,** right toe(s)

    ✓7ᵗʰ **M84.478 Pathological fracture,** left toe(s)

    ✓7ᵗʰ **M84.479 Pathological fracture, unspecified toe(s)** ▽

✓x7ᵗʰ M84.48 Pathological fracture, other site

✓5ᵗʰ M84.5 Pathological fracture in neoplastic disease

    Code also underlying neoplasm

    The appropriate 7th character is to be added to each code from subcategory M84.5.

    A   initial encounter for fracture

    D   subsequent encounter for fracture with routine healing

    G   subsequent encounter for fracture with delayed healing

    K   subsequent encounter for fracture with nonunion

    P   subsequent encounter for fracture with malunion

    S   sequela

✓x7ᵗʰ M84.50 Pathological fracture in neoplastic disease, unspecified site ▽

✓6ᵗʰ M84.51 Pathological fracture in neoplastic disease, shoulder

    ✓7ᵗʰ **M84.511 Pathological fracture in neoplastic disease,** right shoulder

    ✓7ᵗʰ **M84.512 Pathological fracture in neoplastic disease,** left shoulder

    ✓7ᵗʰ **M84.519 Pathological fracture in neoplastic disease, unspecified shoulder** ▽

✓6ᵗʰ M84.52 Pathological fracture in neoplastic disease, humerus

    ✓7ᵗʰ **M84.521 Pathological fracture in neoplastic disease,** right humerus

    ✓7ᵗʰ **M84.522 Pathological fracture in neoplastic disease,** left humerus

    ✓7ᵗʰ **M84.529 Pathological fracture in neoplastic disease, unspecified humerus** ▽

✓6ᵗʰ M84.53 Pathological fracture in neoplastic disease, ulna and radius

    ✓7ᵗʰ **M84.531 Pathological fracture in neoplastic disease,** right ulna

    ✓7ᵗʰ **M84.532 Pathological fracture in neoplastic disease,** left ulna

    ✓7ᵗʰ **M84.533 Pathological fracture in neoplastic disease,** right radius

    ✓7ᵗʰ **M84.534 Pathological fracture in neoplastic disease,** left radius

    ✓7ᵗʰ **M84.539 Pathological fracture in neoplastic disease, unspecified ulna and radius** ▽

✓6ᵗʰ M84.54 Pathological fracture in neoplastic disease, hand

    ✓7ᵗʰ **M84.541 Pathological fracture in neoplastic disease,** right hand

    ✓7ᵗʰ **M84.542 Pathological fracture in neoplastic disease,** left hand

    ✓7ᵗʰ **M84.549 Pathological fracture in neoplastic disease, unspecified hand** ▽

✓6ᵗʰ M84.55 Pathological fracture in neoplastic disease, pelvis and femur

    ✓7ᵗʰ **M84.550 Pathological fracture in neoplastic disease,** pelvis

    [1] ✓7ᵗʰ **M84.551 Pathological fracture in neoplastic disease,** right femur   **HCC**

    [1] ✓7ᵗʰ **M84.552 Pathological fracture in neoplastic disease,** left femur   **HCC**

    [1] ✓7ᵗʰ **M84.553 Pathological fracture in neoplastic disease, unspecified femur**   **HCC** ▽

    [1] ✓7ᵗʰ **M84.559 Pathological fracture in neoplastic disease, hip, unspecified**   **HCC** ▽

---

[1]   HCC with 7th character indicating initial encounter (A, B or C - specific to category).

☑ Additional Character Req   ✓x7ᵗʰ Placeholder Alert   Manifestation   **HCC** CMS-HCC Condition   ▽ Unspecified Code   ►◄ Revised Text   ● New Code   ▲ Revised Code Title

Chapter 13. Diseases of the Musculoskeletal System and Connective Tissue

M84.56–M84.759

✓6ᵗʰ **M84.56** Pathological fracture in neoplastic disease, tibia and fibula

    ✓7ᵗʰ **M84.561** Pathological fracture in neoplastic disease, right tibia

    ✓7ᵗʰ **M84.562** Pathological fracture in neoplastic disease, left tibia

    ✓7ᵗʰ **M84.563** Pathological fracture in neoplastic disease, right fibula

    ✓7ᵗʰ **M84.564** Pathological fracture in neoplastic disease, left fibula

    ✓7ᵗʰ **M84.569** Pathological fracture in neoplastic disease, unspecified tibia and fibula ▽

✓6ᵗʰ **M84.57** Pathological fracture in neoplastic disease, ankle and foot

    ✓7ᵗʰ **M84.571** Pathological fracture in neoplastic disease, right ankle

    ✓7ᵗʰ **M84.572** Pathological fracture in neoplastic disease, left ankle

    ✓7ᵗʰ **M84.573** Pathological fracture in neoplastic disease, unspecified ankle ▽

    ✓7ᵗʰ **M84.574** Pathological fracture in neoplastic disease, right foot

    ✓7ᵗʰ **M84.575** Pathological fracture in neoplastic disease, left foot

    ✓7ᵗʰ **M84.576** Pathological fracture in neoplastic disease, unspecified foot ▽

✓x7ᵗʰ **M84.58** Pathological fracture in neoplastic disease, other specified site

       Pathological fracture in neoplastic disease, vertebrae

✓5ᵗʰ **M84.6** Pathological fracture in other disease

    Code also underlying condition

    EXCLUDES 1 pathological fracture in osteoporosis (M80.-)

    The appropriate 7th character is to be added to each code from subcategory M84.6.
    A   initial encounter for fracture
    D   subsequent encounter for fracture with routine healing
    G   subsequent encounter for fracture with delayed healing
    K   subsequent encounter for fracture with nonunion
    P   subsequent encounter for fracture with malunion
    S   sequela

✓x7ᵗʰ **M84.60** Pathological fracture in other disease, unspecified site ▽

✓6ᵗʰ **M84.61** Pathological fracture in other disease, shoulder

    ✓7ᵗʰ **M84.611** Pathological fracture in other disease, right shoulder

    ✓7ᵗʰ **M84.612** Pathological fracture in other disease, left shoulder

    ✓7ᵗʰ **M84.619** Pathological fracture in other disease, unspecified shoulder ▽

✓6ᵗʰ **M84.62** Pathological fracture in other disease, humerus

    ✓7ᵗʰ **M84.621** Pathological fracture in other disease, right humerus

    ✓7ᵗʰ **M84.622** Pathological fracture in other disease, left humerus

    ✓7ᵗʰ **M84.629** Pathological fracture in other disease, unspecified humerus ▽

✓6ᵗʰ **M84.63** Pathological fracture in other disease, ulna and radius

    ✓7ᵗʰ **M84.631** Pathological fracture in other disease, right ulna

    ✓7ᵗʰ **M84.632** Pathological fracture in other disease, left ulna

    ✓7ᵗʰ **M84.633** Pathological fracture in other disease, right radius

    ✓7ᵗʰ **M84.634** Pathological fracture in other disease, left radius

    ✓7ᵗʰ **M84.639** Pathological fracture in other disease, unspecified ulna and radius ▽

✓6ᵗʰ **M84.64** Pathological fracture in other disease, hand

    ✓7ᵗʰ **M84.641** Pathological fracture in other disease, right hand

    ✓7ᵗʰ **M84.642** Pathological fracture in other disease, left hand

    ✓7ᵗʰ **M84.649** Pathological fracture in other disease, unspecified hand ▽

✓6ᵗʰ **M84.65** Pathological fracture in other disease, pelvis and femur

    ✓7ᵗʰ **M84.650** Pathological fracture in other disease, pelvis

    1 ✓7ᵗʰ **M84.651** Pathological fracture in other disease, right femur   HCC

    1 ✓7ᵗʰ **M84.652** Pathological fracture in other disease, left femur   HCC

    1 ✓7ᵗʰ **M84.653** Pathological fracture in other disease, unspecified femur   HCC ▽

    1 ✓7ᵗʰ **M84.659** Pathological fracture in other disease, hip, unspecified   HCC ▽

✓6ᵗʰ **M84.66** Pathological fracture in other disease, tibia and fibula

    ✓7ᵗʰ **M84.661** Pathological fracture in other disease, right tibia

    ✓7ᵗʰ **M84.662** Pathological fracture in other disease, left tibia

    ✓7ᵗʰ **M84.663** Pathological fracture in other disease, right fibula

    ✓7ᵗʰ **M84.664** Pathological fracture in other disease, left fibula

    ✓7ᵗʰ **M84.669** Pathological fracture in other disease, unspecified tibia and fibula ▽

✓6ᵗʰ **M84.67** Pathological fracture in other disease, ankle and foot

    ✓7ᵗʰ **M84.671** Pathological fracture in other disease, right ankle

    ✓7ᵗʰ **M84.672** Pathological fracture in other disease, left ankle

    ✓7ᵗʰ **M84.673** Pathological fracture in other disease, unspecified ankle ▽

    ✓7ᵗʰ **M84.674** Pathological fracture in other disease, right foot

    ✓7ᵗʰ **M84.675** Pathological fracture in other disease, left foot

    ✓7ᵗʰ **M84.676** Pathological fracture in other disease, unspecified foot ▽

✓x7ᵗʰ **M84.68** Pathological fracture in other disease, other site

✓5ᵗʰ **M84.7** Nontraumatic fracture, not elsewhere classified

    ✓6ᵗʰ **M84.75** Atypical femoral fracture

    The appropriate 7th character is to be added to each code from subcategory M84.75.
    A   initial encounter for fracture
    D   subsequent encounter for fracture with routine healing
    G   subsequent encounter for fracture with delayed healing
    K   subsequent encounter for fracture with nonunion
    P   subsequent encounter for fracture with malunion
    S   sequela

    ✓7ᵗʰ **M84.750** Atypical femoral fracture, unspecified ▽

    ✓7ᵗʰ **M84.751** Incomplete atypical femoral fracture, right leg

    ✓7ᵗʰ **M84.752** Incomplete atypical femoral fracture, left leg

    ✓7ᵗʰ **M84.753** Incomplete atypical femoral fracture, unspecified leg ▽

    1 ✓7ᵗʰ **M84.754** Complete transverse atypical femoral fracture, right leg   HCC

    1 ✓7ᵗʰ **M84.755** Complete transverse atypical femoral fracture, left leg   HCC

    1 ✓7ᵗʰ **M84.756** Complete transverse atypical femoral fracture, unspecified leg   HCC ▽

    1 ✓7ᵗʰ **M84.757** Complete oblique atypical femoral fracture, right leg   HCC

    1 ✓7ᵗʰ **M84.758** Complete oblique atypical femoral fracture, left leg   HCC

    1 ✓7ᵗʰ **M84.759** Complete oblique atypical femoral fracture, unspecified leg   HCC ▽

---

1   HCC with 7th character indicating initial encounter (A, B or C - specific to category).

EXCLUDES 1 Not coded here   **EXCLUDES 2** Not included here   N Newborn Age: 0   P Pediatric Age: 0-17   M Maternity Age: 12-55   A Adult Age: 15-124

780   ICD-10-CM 2018

☑5ᵗʰ **M84.8** **Other disorders of continuity of bone**

     M84.80 Other disorders of continuity of bone, unspecified site ▽

     ☑6ᵗʰ **M84.81** Other disorders of continuity of bone, shoulder

        M84.811 Other disorders of continuity of bone, right shoulder

        M84.812 Other disorders of continuity of bone, left shoulder

        M84.819 Other disorders of continuity of bone, unspecified shoulder ▽

     ☑6ᵗʰ **M84.82** Other disorders of continuity of bone, humerus

        M84.821 Other disorders of continuity of bone, right humerus

        M84.822 Other disorders of continuity of bone, left humerus

        M84.829 Other disorders of continuity of bone, unspecified humerus ▽

     ☑6ᵗʰ **M84.83** Other disorders of continuity of bone, ulna and radius

        M84.831 Other disorders of continuity of bone, right ulna

        M84.832 Other disorders of continuity of bone, left ulna

        M84.833 Other disorders of continuity of bone, right radius

        M84.834 Other disorders of continuity of bone, left radius

        M84.839 Other disorders of continuity of bone, unspecified ulna and radius ▽

     ☑6ᵗʰ **M84.84** Other disorders of continuity of bone, hand

        M84.841 Other disorders of continuity of bone, right hand

        M84.842 Other disorders of continuity of bone, left hand

        M84.849 Other disorders of continuity of bone, unspecified hand ▽

     ☑6ᵗʰ **M84.85** Other disorders of continuity of bone, pelvic region and thigh

        M84.851 Other disorders of continuity of bone, right pelvic region and thigh

        M84.852 Other disorders of continuity of bone, left pelvic region and thigh

        M84.859 Other disorders of continuity of bone, unspecified pelvic region and thigh ▽

     ☑6ᵗʰ **M84.86** Other disorders of continuity of bone, tibia and fibula

        M84.861 Other disorders of continuity of bone, right tibia

        M84.862 Other disorders of continuity of bone, left tibia

        M84.863 Other disorders of continuity of bone, right fibula

        M84.864 Other disorders of continuity of bone, left fibula

        M84.869 Other disorders of continuity of bone, unspecified tibia and fibula ▽

     ☑6ᵗʰ **M84.87** Other disorders of continuity of bone, ankle and foot

        M84.871 Other disorders of continuity of bone, right ankle and foot

        M84.872 Other disorders of continuity of bone, left ankle and foot

        M84.879 Other disorders of continuity of bone, unspecified ankle and foot ▽

     M84.88 Other disorders of continuity of bone, other site

     M84.9 Disorder of continuity of bone, unspecified ▽

☑4ᵗʰ **M85** **Other disorders of bone density and structure**

     EXCLUDES 1   osteogenesis imperfecta (Q78.0)
              osteopetrosis (Q78.2)
              osteopoikilosis (Q78.8)
              polyostotic fibrous dysplasia (Q78.1)

     ☑5ᵗʰ **M85.0** **Fibrous dysplasia (monostotic)**

        EXCLUDES 2   fibrous dysplasia of jaw (M27.8)

        M85.00 Fibrous dysplasia (monostotic), unspecified site ▽

        ☑6ᵗʰ **M85.01** Fibrous dysplasia (monostotic), shoulder

            M85.011 Fibrous dysplasia (monostotic), right shoulder

            M85.012 Fibrous dysplasia (monostotic), left shoulder

            M85.019 Fibrous dysplasia (monostotic), unspecified shoulder ▽

        ☑6ᵗʰ **M85.02** Fibrous dysplasia (monostotic), upper arm

            M85.021 Fibrous dysplasia (monostotic), right upper arm

            M85.022 Fibrous dysplasia (monostotic), left upper arm

            M85.029 Fibrous dysplasia (monostotic), unspecified upper arm ▽

        ☑6ᵗʰ **M85.03** Fibrous dysplasia (monostotic), forearm

            M85.031 Fibrous dysplasia (monostotic), right forearm

            M85.032 Fibrous dysplasia (monostotic), left forearm

            M85.039 Fibrous dysplasia (monostotic), unspecified forearm ▽

        ☑6ᵗʰ **M85.04** Fibrous dysplasia (monostotic), hand

            M85.041 Fibrous dysplasia (monostotic), right hand

            M85.042 Fibrous dysplasia (monostotic), left hand

            M85.049 Fibrous dysplasia (monostotic), unspecified hand ▽

        ☑6ᵗʰ **M85.05** Fibrous dysplasia (monostotic), thigh

            M85.051 Fibrous dysplasia (monostotic), right thigh

            M85.052 Fibrous dysplasia (monostotic), left thigh

            M85.059 Fibrous dysplasia (monostotic), unspecified thigh ▽

        ☑6ᵗʰ **M85.06** Fibrous dysplasia (monostotic), lower leg

            M85.061 Fibrous dysplasia (monostotic), right lower leg

            M85.062 Fibrous dysplasia (monostotic), left lower leg

            M85.069 Fibrous dysplasia (monostotic), unspecified lower leg ▽

        ☑6ᵗʰ **M85.07** Fibrous dysplasia (monostotic), ankle and foot

            M85.071 Fibrous dysplasia (monostotic), right ankle and foot

            M85.072 Fibrous dysplasia (monostotic), left ankle and foot

            M85.079 Fibrous dysplasia (monostotic), unspecified ankle and foot ▽

        M85.08 Fibrous dysplasia (monostotic), other site

        M85.09 Fibrous dysplasia (monostotic), multiple sites

     ☑5ᵗʰ **M85.1** **Skeletal fluorosis**

        M85.10 Skeletal fluorosis, unspecified site ▽

        ☑6ᵗʰ **M85.11** Skeletal fluorosis, shoulder

            M85.111 Skeletal fluorosis, right shoulder

            M85.112 Skeletal fluorosis, left shoulder

            M85.119 Skeletal fluorosis, unspecified shoulder ▽

        ☑6ᵗʰ **M85.12** Skeletal fluorosis, upper arm

            M85.121 Skeletal fluorosis, right upper arm

            M85.122 Skeletal fluorosis, left upper arm

            M85.129 Skeletal fluorosis, unspecified upper arm ▽

        ☑6ᵗʰ **M85.13** Skeletal fluorosis, forearm

            M85.131 Skeletal fluorosis, right forearm

            M85.132 Skeletal fluorosis, left forearm

            M85.139 Skeletal fluorosis, unspecified forearm ▽

        ☑6ᵗʰ **M85.14** Skeletal fluorosis, hand

            M85.141 Skeletal fluorosis, right hand

            M85.142 Skeletal fluorosis, left hand

            M85.149 Skeletal fluorosis, unspecified hand ▽

        ☑6ᵗʰ **M85.15** Skeletal fluorosis, thigh

            M85.151 Skeletal fluorosis, right thigh

            M85.152 Skeletal fluorosis, left thigh

            M85.159 Skeletal fluorosis, unspecified thigh ▽

        ☑6ᵗʰ **M85.16** Skeletal fluorosis, lower leg

            M85.161 Skeletal fluorosis, right lower leg

            M85.162 Skeletal fluorosis, left lower leg

            M85.169 Skeletal fluorosis, unspecified lower leg ▽

☑ Additional Character Req   ✓x7ᵗʰ Placeholder Alert   Manifestation   HCC CMS-HCC Condition   ▽ Unspecified Code   ►◄ Revised Text   ● New Code   ▲ Revised Code Title

Chapter 13. Diseases of the Musculoskeletal System and Connective Tissue

✓6ᵗʰ **M85.17 Skeletal fluorosis,** ankle and foot
     M85.171 Skeletal fluorosis, right **ankle and foot**
     M85.172 Skeletal fluorosis, left **ankle and foot**
     M85.179 Skeletal fluorosis, unspecified ankle ▽
              and foot

   M85.18 Skeletal fluorosis, other site
   M85.19 Skeletal fluorosis, multiple sites

M85.2 Hyperostosis of skull
     DEF: Abnormal bone growth on inner aspect of cranial bones.

✓5ᵗʰ **M85.3 Osteitis condensans**
   M85.30 Osteitis condensans, unspecified site ▽
   ✓6ᵗʰ **M85.31 Osteitis condensans,** shoulder
     M85.311 Osteitis condensans, right **shoulder**
     M85.312 Osteitis condensans, left **shoulder**
     M85.319 Osteitis condensans, unspecified ▽
              shoulder
   ✓6ᵗʰ **M85.32 Osteitis condensans,** upper arm
     M85.321 Osteitis condensans, right **upper arm**
     M85.322 Osteitis condensans, left **upper arm**
     M85.329 Osteitis condensans, unspecified ▽
              upper arm
   ✓6ᵗʰ **M85.33 Osteitis condensans,** forearm
     M85.331 Osteitis condensans, right **forearm**
     M85.332 Osteitis condensans, left **forearm**
     M85.339 Osteitis condensans, unspecified ▽
              forearm
   ✓6ᵗʰ **M85.34 Osteitis condensans,** hand
     M85.341 Osteitis condensans, right **hand**
     M85.342 Osteitis condensans, left **hand**
     M85.349 Osteitis condensans, unspecified hand ▽
   ✓6ᵗʰ **M85.35 Osteitis condensans,** thigh
     M85.351 Osteitis condensans, right **thigh**
     M85.352 Osteitis condensans, left **thigh**
     M85.359 Osteitis condensans, unspecified thigh ▽
   ✓6ᵗʰ **M85.36 Osteitis condensans,** lower leg
     M85.361 Osteitis condensans, right **lower leg**
     M85.362 Osteitis condensans, left **lower leg**
     M85.369 Osteitis condensans, unspecified ▽
              lower leg
   ✓6ᵗʰ **M85.37 Osteitis condensans,** ankle and foot
     M85.371 Osteitis condensans, right **ankle and foot**
     M85.372 Osteitis condensans, left **ankle and foot**
     M85.379 Osteitis condensans, unspecified ▽
              ankle and foot
   M85.38 Osteitis condensans, other site
   M85.39 Osteitis condensans, multiple sites

✓5ᵗʰ **M85.4 Solitary bone cyst**
     EXCLUDES 2 solitary cyst of jaw (M27.4)
   M85.40 Solitary bone cyst, unspecified site ▽
   ✓6ᵗʰ **M85.41 Solitary bone cyst,** shoulder
     M85.411 Solitary bone cyst, right **shoulder**
     M85.412 Solitary bone cyst, left **shoulder**
     M85.419 Solitary bone cyst, unspecified ▽
              shoulder
   ✓6ᵗʰ **M85.42 Solitary bone cyst,** humerus
     M85.421 Solitary bone cyst, right **humerus**
     M85.422 Solitary bone cyst, left **humerus**
     M85.429 Solitary bone cyst, unspecified humerus ▽
   ✓6ᵗʰ **M85.43 Solitary bone cyst,** ulna and radius
     M85.431 Solitary bone cyst, right **ulna and radius**
     M85.432 Solitary bone cyst, left **ulna and radius**
     M85.439 Solitary bone cyst, unspecified ulna ▽
              and radius
   ✓6ᵗʰ **M85.44 Solitary bone cyst,** hand
     M85.441 Solitary bone cyst, right **hand**
     M85.442 Solitary bone cyst, left **hand**
     M85.449 Solitary bone cyst, unspecified hand ▽
   ✓6ᵗʰ **M85.45 Solitary bone cyst,** pelvis
     M85.451 Solitary bone cyst, right **pelvis**
     M85.452 Solitary bone cyst, left **pelvis**
     M85.459 Solitary bone cyst, unspecified pelvis ▽

✓6ᵗʰ **M85.46 Solitary bone cyst,** tibia and fibula
     M85.461 Solitary bone cyst, right **tibia and fibula**
     M85.462 Solitary bone cyst, left **tibia and fibula**
     M85.469 Solitary bone cyst, unspecified tibia ▽
              and fibula
   ✓6ᵗʰ **M85.47 Solitary bone cyst,** ankle and foot
     M85.471 Solitary bone cyst, right **ankle and foot**
     M85.472 Solitary bone cyst, left **ankle and foot**
     M85.479 Solitary bone cyst, unspecified ankle ▽
              and foot
   M85.48 Solitary bone cyst, other site

✓5ᵗʰ **M85.5 Aneurysmal bone cyst**
     EXCLUDES 2 aneurysmal cyst of jaw (M27.4)
     DEF: Solitary bone lesion, bulges into periosteum; marked by calcified rim.
   M85.50 Aneurysmal bone cyst, unspecified site ▽
   ✓6ᵗʰ **M85.51 Aneurysmal bone cyst,** shoulder
     M85.511 Aneurysmal bone cyst, right **shoulder**
     M85.512 Aneurysmal bone cyst, left **shoulder**
     M85.519 Aneurysmal bone cyst, unspecified ▽
              shoulder
   ✓6ᵗʰ **M85.52 Aneurysmal bone cyst,** upper arm
     M85.521 Aneurysmal bone cyst, right **upper arm**
     M85.522 Aneurysmal bone cyst, left **upper arm**
     M85.529 Aneurysmal bone cyst, unspecified ▽
              upper arm
   ✓6ᵗʰ **M85.53 Aneurysmal bone cyst,** forearm
     M85.531 Aneurysmal bone cyst, right **forearm**
     M85.532 Aneurysmal bone cyst, left **forearm**
     M85.539 Aneurysmal bone cyst, unspecified ▽
              forearm
   ✓6ᵗʰ **M85.54 Aneurysmal bone cyst,** hand
     M85.541 Aneurysmal bone cyst, right **hand**
     M85.542 Aneurysmal bone cyst, left **hand**
     M85.549 Aneurysmal bone cyst, unspecified ▽
              hand
   ✓6ᵗʰ **M85.55 Aneurysmal bone cyst,** thigh
     M85.551 Aneurysmal bone cyst, right **thigh**
     M85.552 Aneurysmal bone cyst, left **thigh**
     M85.559 Aneurysmal bone cyst, unspecified ▽
              thigh
   ✓6ᵗʰ **M85.56 Aneurysmal bone cyst,** lower leg
     M85.561 Aneurysmal bone cyst, right **lower leg**
     M85.562 Aneurysmal bone cyst, left **lower leg**
     M85.569 Aneurysmal bone cyst, unspecified ▽
              lower leg
   ✓6ᵗʰ **M85.57 Aneurysmal bone cyst,** ankle and foot
     M85.571 Aneurysmal bone cyst, right **ankle and foot**
     M85.572 Aneurysmal bone cyst, left **ankle and foot**
     M85.579 Aneurysmal bone cyst, unspecified ▽
              ankle and foot
   M85.58 Aneurysmal bone cyst, other site
   M85.59 Aneurysmal bone cyst, multiple sites

✓5ᵗʰ **M85.6 Other cyst of bone**
     EXCLUDES 1 cyst of jaw NEC (M27.4)
               osteitis fibrosa cystica generalisata [von Recklinghausen's disease of bone] (E21.Ø)
   M85.60 Other cyst of bone, unspecified site ▽
   ✓6ᵗʰ **M85.61 Other cyst of bone,** shoulder
     M85.611 Other cyst of bone, right **shoulder**
     M85.612 Other cyst of bone, left **shoulder**
     M85.619 Other cyst of bone, unspecified ▽
              shoulder
   ✓6ᵗʰ **M85.62 Other cyst of bone,** upper arm
     M85.621 Other cyst of bone, right **upper arm**
     M85.622 Other cyst of bone, left **upper arm**
     M85.629 Other cyst of bone, unspecified upper ▽
              arm
   ✓6ᵗʰ **M85.63 Other cyst of bone,** forearm
     M85.631 Other cyst of bone, right **forearm**
     M85.632 Other cyst of bone, left **forearm**
     M85.639 Other cyst of bone, unspecified forearm ▽

EXCLUDES 1 Not coded here   **EXCLUDES 2** Not included here   N Newborn Age: 0   P Pediatric Age: 0-17   M Maternity Age: 12-55   A Adult Age: 15-124

782   ICD-10-CM 2018

✓6th **M85.64** Other cyst of bone, hand
     M85.641 Other cyst of bone, right hand
     M85.642 Other cyst of bone, left hand
     M85.649 Other cyst of bone, unspecified hand ▽

✓6th **M85.65** Other cyst of bone, thigh
     M85.651 Other cyst of bone, right thigh
     M85.652 Other cyst of bone, left thigh
     M85.659 Other cyst of bone, unspecified thigh ▽

✓6th **M85.66** Other cyst of bone, lower leg
     M85.661 Other cyst of bone, right lower leg
     M85.662 Other cyst of bone, left lower leg
     M85.669 Other cyst of bone, unspecified lower leg ▽

✓6th **M85.67** Other cyst of bone, ankle and foot
     M85.671 Other cyst of bone, right ankle and foot
     M85.672 Other cyst of bone, left ankle and foot
     M85.679 Other cyst of bone, unspecified ankle and foot ▽

   M85.68 Other cyst of bone, other site
   M85.69 Other cyst of bone, multiple sites

✓5th **M85.8** Other specified disorders of bone density and structure
Hyperostosis of bones, except skull
Osteosclerosis, acquired
    EXCLUDES 1   diffuse idiopathic skeletal hyperostosis [DISH] (M48.1)
          osteosclerosis congenita (Q77.4)
          osteosclerosis fragilitas (generalista) (Q78.2)
          osteosclerosis myelofibrosis (D75.81)

     M85.80 Other specified disorders of bone density and structure, unspecified site ▽

✓6th **M85.81** Other specified disorders of bone density and structure, shoulder
     M85.811 Other specified disorders of bone density and structure, right shoulder
     M85.812 Other specified disorders of bone density and structure, left shoulder
     M85.819 Other specified disorders of bone density and structure, unspecified shoulder ▽

✓6th **M85.82** Other specified disorders of bone density and structure, upper arm
     M85.821 Other specified disorders of bone density and structure, right upper arm
     M85.822 Other specified disorders of bone density and structure, left upper arm
     M85.829 Other specified disorders of bone density and structure, unspecified upper arm ▽

✓6th **M85.83** Other specified disorders of bone density and structure, forearm
     M85.831 Other specified disorders of bone density and structure, right forearm
     M85.832 Other specified disorders of bone density and structure, left forearm
     M85.839 Other specified disorders of bone density and structure, unspecified forearm ▽

✓6th **M85.84** Other specified disorders of bone density and structure, hand
     M85.841 Other specified disorders of bone density and structure, right hand
     M85.842 Other specified disorders of bone density and structure, left hand
     M85.849 Other specified disorders of bone density and structure, unspecified hand ▽

✓6th **M85.85** Other specified disorders of bone density and structure, thigh
     M85.851 Other specified disorders of bone density and structure, right thigh
     M85.852 Other specified disorders of bone density and structure, left thigh
     M85.859 Other specified disorders of bone density and structure, unspecified thigh ▽

✓6th **M85.86** Other specified disorders of bone density and structure, lower leg
     M85.861 Other specified disorders of bone density and structure, right lower leg

     M85.862 Other specified disorders of bone density and structure, left lower leg
     M85.869 Other specified disorders of bone density and structure, unspecified lower leg ▽

✓6th **M85.87** Other specified disorders of bone density and structure, ankle and foot
     M85.871 Other specified disorders of bone density and structure, right ankle and foot
     M85.872 Other specified disorders of bone density and structure, left ankle and foot
     M85.879 Other specified disorders of bone density and structure, unspecified ankle and foot ▽

     M85.88 Other specified disorders of bone density and structure, other site
     M85.89 Other specified disorders of bone density and structure, multiple sites

   M85.9 Disorder of bone density and structure, unspecified ▽

Other osteopathies (M86-M90)

EXCLUDES 1   postprocedural osteopathies (M96.-)

✓4th **M86 Osteomyelitis**
Use additional code (B95-B97) to identify infectious agent
Use additional code to identify major osseous defect, if applicable (M89.7-)
    EXCLUDES 1   osteomyelitis due to:
          echinococcus (B67.2)
          gonococcus (A54.43)
          salmonella (A02.24)
    EXCLUDES 2   ostemyelitis of:
          orbit (H05.0-)
          petrous bone (H70.2-)
          vertebra (M46.2-)

✓5th **M86.0** Acute hematogenous osteomyelitis
     M86.00 Acute hematogenous osteomyelitis, unspecified site   HCC ▽

✓6th **M86.01** Acute hematogenous osteomyelitis, shoulder
     M86.011 Acute hematogenous osteomyelitis, right shoulder   HCC
     M86.012 Acute hematogenous osteomyelitis, left shoulder   HCC
     M86.019 Acute hematogenous osteomyelitis, unspecified shoulder   HCC ▽

✓6th **M86.02** Acute hematogenous osteomyelitis, humerus
     M86.021 Acute hematogenous osteomyelitis, right humerus   HCC
     M86.022 Acute hematogenous osteomyelitis, left humerus   HCC
     M86.029 Acute hematogenous osteomyelitis, unspecified humerus   HCC ▽

✓6th **M86.03** Acute hematogenous osteomyelitis, radius and ulna
     M86.031 Acute hematogenous osteomyelitis, right radius and ulna   HCC
     M86.032 Acute hematogenous osteomyelitis, left radius and ulna   HCC
     M86.039 Acute hematogenous osteomyelitis, unspecified radius and ulna   HCC ▽

✓6th **M86.04** Acute hematogenous osteomyelitis, hand
     M86.041 Acute hematogenous osteomyelitis, right hand   HCC
     M86.042 Acute hematogenous osteomyelitis, left hand   HCC
     M86.049 Acute hematogenous osteomyelitis, unspecified hand   HCC ▽

✓6th **M86.05** Acute hematogenous osteomyelitis, femur
     M86.051 Acute hematogenous osteomyelitis, right femur   HCC
     M86.052 Acute hematogenous osteomyelitis, left femur   HCC
     M86.059 Acute hematogenous osteomyelitis, unspecified femur   HCC ▽

✓ Additional Character Req   ✓x7th Placeholder Alert   Manifestation   HCC CMS-HCC Condition   ▽ Unspecified Code   ►◄ Revised Text   ● New Code   ▲ Revised Code Title

√6ᵗʰ **M86.06 Acute hematogenous osteomyelitis, tibia and fibula**
    M86.061 Acute hematogenous osteomyelitis, right tibia and fibula HCC
    M86.062 Acute hematogenous osteomyelitis, left tibia and fibula HCC
    M86.069 Acute hematogenous osteomyelitis, unspecified tibia and fibula HCC ▽

√6ᵗʰ **M86.07 Acute hematogenous osteomyelitis, ankle and foot**
    M86.071 Acute hematogenous osteomyelitis, right ankle and foot HCC
    M86.072 Acute hematogenous osteomyelitis, left ankle and foot HCC
    M86.079 Acute hematogenous osteomyelitis, unspecified ankle and foot HCC ▽

M86.08 Acute hematogenous osteomyelitis, other sites HCC

M86.09 Acute hematogenous osteomyelitis, multiple sites HCC

√5ᵗʰ **M86.1 Other acute osteomyelitis**
    M86.10 Other acute osteomyelitis, unspecified site HCC ▽

√6ᵗʰ **M86.11 Other acute osteomyelitis, shoulder**
    M86.111 Other acute osteomyelitis, right shoulder HCC
    M86.112 Other acute osteomyelitis, left shoulder HCC
    M86.119 Other acute osteomyelitis, unspecified shoulder HCC ▽

√6ᵗʰ **M86.12 Other acute osteomyelitis, humerus**
    M86.121 Other acute osteomyelitis, right humerus HCC
    M86.122 Other acute osteomyelitis, left humerus HCC
    M86.129 Other acute osteomyelitis, unspecified humerus HCC ▽

√6ᵗʰ **M86.13 Other acute osteomyelitis, radius and ulna**
    M86.131 Other acute osteomyelitis, right radius and ulna HCC
    M86.132 Other acute osteomyelitis, left radius and ulna HCC
    M86.139 Other acute osteomyelitis, unspecified radius and ulna HCC ▽

√6ᵗʰ **M86.14 Other acute osteomyelitis, hand**
    M86.141 Other acute osteomyelitis, right hand HCC
    M86.142 Other acute osteomyelitis, left hand HCC
    M86.149 Other acute osteomyelitis, unspecified hand HCC ▽

√6ᵗʰ **M86.15 Other acute osteomyelitis, femur**
    M86.151 Other acute osteomyelitis, right femur HCC
    M86.152 Other acute osteomyelitis, left femur HCC
    M86.159 Other acute osteomyelitis, unspecified femur HCC ▽

√6ᵗʰ **M86.16 Other acute osteomyelitis, tibia and fibula**
    M86.161 Other acute osteomyelitis, right tibia and fibula HCC
    M86.162 Other acute osteomyelitis, left tibia and fibula HCC
    M86.169 Other acute osteomyelitis, unspecified tibia and fibula HCC ▽

√6ᵗʰ **M86.17 Other acute osteomyelitis, ankle and foot**
    M86.171 Other acute osteomyelitis, right ankle and foot HCC
    M86.172 Other acute osteomyelitis, left ankle and foot HCC
    M86.179 Other acute osteomyelitis, unspecified ankle and foot HCC ▽

M86.18 Other acute osteomyelitis, other site HCC

M86.19 Other acute osteomyelitis, multiple sites HCC

√5ᵗʰ **M86.2 Subacute osteomyelitis**
    M86.20 Subacute osteomyelitis, unspecified site HCC ▽

√6ᵗʰ **M86.21 Subacute osteomyelitis, shoulder**
    M86.211 Subacute osteomyelitis, right shoulder HCC
    M86.212 Subacute osteomyelitis, left shoulder HCC
    M86.219 Subacute osteomyelitis, unspecified shoulder HCC ▽

√6ᵗʰ **M86.22 Subacute osteomyelitis, humerus**
    M86.221 Subacute osteomyelitis, right humerus HCC
    M86.222 Subacute osteomyelitis, left humerus HCC
    M86.229 Subacute osteomyelitis, unspecified humerus HCC ▽

√6ᵗʰ **M86.23 Subacute osteomyelitis, radius and ulna**
    M86.231 Subacute osteomyelitis, right radius and ulna HCC
    M86.232 Subacute osteomyelitis, left radius and ulna HCC
    M86.239 Subacute osteomyelitis, unspecified radius and ulna HCC ▽

√6ᵗʰ **M86.24 Subacute osteomyelitis, hand**
    M86.241 Subacute osteomyelitis, right hand HCC
    M86.242 Subacute osteomyelitis, left hand HCC
    M86.249 Subacute osteomyelitis, unspecified hand HCC ▽

√6ᵗʰ **M86.25 Subacute osteomyelitis, femur**
    M86.251 Subacute osteomyelitis, right femur HCC
    M86.252 Subacute osteomyelitis, left femur HCC
    M86.259 Subacute osteomyelitis, unspecified femur HCC ▽

√6ᵗʰ **M86.26 Subacute osteomyelitis, tibia and fibula**
    M86.261 Subacute osteomyelitis, right tibia and fibula HCC
    M86.262 Subacute osteomyelitis, left tibia and fibula HCC
    M86.269 Subacute osteomyelitis, unspecified tibia and fibula HCC ▽

√6ᵗʰ **M86.27 Subacute osteomyelitis, ankle and foot**
    M86.271 Subacute osteomyelitis, right ankle and foot HCC
    M86.272 Subacute osteomyelitis, left ankle and foot HCC
    M86.279 Subacute osteomyelitis, unspecified ankle and foot HCC ▽

M86.28 Subacute osteomyelitis, other site HCC

M86.29 Subacute osteomyelitis, multiple sites HCC

√5ᵗʰ **M86.3 Chronic multifocal osteomyelitis**
    M86.30 Chronic multifocal osteomyelitis, unspecified site HCC ▽

√6ᵗʰ **M86.31 Chronic multifocal osteomyelitis, shoulder**
    M86.311 Chronic multifocal osteomyelitis, right shoulder HCC
    M86.312 Chronic multifocal osteomyelitis, left shoulder HCC
    M86.319 Chronic multifocal osteomyelitis, unspecified shoulder HCC ▽

√6ᵗʰ **M86.32 Chronic multifocal osteomyelitis, humerus**
    M86.321 Chronic multifocal osteomyelitis, right humerus HCC
    M86.322 Chronic multifocal osteomyelitis, left humerus HCC
    M86.329 Chronic multifocal osteomyelitis, unspecified humerus HCC ▽

√6ᵗʰ **M86.33 Chronic multifocal osteomyelitis, radius and ulna**
    M86.331 Chronic multifocal osteomyelitis, right radius and ulna HCC
    M86.332 Chronic multifocal osteomyelitis, left radius and ulna HCC
    M86.339 Chronic multifocal osteomyelitis, unspecified radius and ulna HCC ▽

√6ᵗʰ **M86.34 Chronic multifocal osteomyelitis, hand**
    M86.341 Chronic multifocal osteomyelitis, right hand HCC
    M86.342 Chronic multifocal osteomyelitis, left hand HCC
    M86.349 Chronic multifocal osteomyelitis, unspecified hand HCC ▽

EXCLUDES 1 Not coded here   EXCLUDES 2 Not included here   N Newborn Age: 0   P Pediatric Age: 0-17   M Maternity Age: 12-55   A Adult Age: 15-124

784   ICD-10-CM 2018

√6ᵗʰ **M86.35** **Chronic multifocal osteomyelitis,** femur

     M86.351 **Chronic multifocal osteomyelitis,** `HCC` **right** femur

     M86.352 **Chronic multifocal osteomyelitis,** `HCC` **left** femur

     M86.359 **Chronic multifocal osteomyelitis,** `HCC` ▽ **unspecified femur**

√6ᵗʰ **M86.36** **Chronic multifocal osteomyelitis,** tibia and fibula

     M86.361 **Chronic multifocal osteomyelitis,** `HCC` **right** tibia and fibula

     M86.362 **Chronic multifocal osteomyelitis,** `HCC` **left** tibia and fibula

     M86.369 **Chronic multifocal osteomyelitis,** `HCC` ▽ **unspecified tibia and fibula**

√6ᵗʰ **M86.37** **Chronic multifocal osteomyelitis,** ankle and foot

     M86.371 **Chronic multifocal osteomyelitis,** `HCC` **right** ankle and foot

     M86.372 **Chronic multifocal osteomyelitis,** `HCC` **left** ankle and foot

     M86.379 **Chronic multifocal osteomyelitis,** `HCC` ▽ **unspecified ankle and foot**

     M86.38 **Chronic multifocal osteomyelitis, other site** `HCC`

     M86.39 **Chronic multifocal osteomyelitis,** multiple sites `HCC`

√5ᵗʰ **M86.4** Chronic **osteomyelitis** with draining sinus

     M86.40 **Chronic osteomyelitis with draining sinus,** `HCC` ▽ **unspecified site**

√6ᵗʰ **M86.41** **Chronic osteomyelitis with draining sinus,** shoulder

     M86.411 **Chronic osteomyelitis with draining** `HCC` **sinus, right** shoulder

     M86.412 **Chronic osteomyelitis with draining** `HCC` **sinus, left** shoulder

     M86.419 **Chronic osteomyelitis with draining** `HCC` ▽ **sinus, unspecified shoulder**

√6ᵗʰ **M86.42** **Chronic osteomyelitis with draining sinus,** humerus

     M86.421 **Chronic osteomyelitis with draining** `HCC` **sinus, right** humerus

     M86.422 **Chronic osteomyelitis with draining** `HCC` **sinus, left** humerus

     M86.429 **Chronic osteomyelitis with draining** `HCC` ▽ **sinus, unspecified humerus**

√6ᵗʰ **M86.43** **Chronic osteomyelitis with draining sinus,** radius and ulna

     M86.431 **Chronic osteomyelitis with draining** `HCC` **sinus, right** radius and ulna

     M86.432 **Chronic osteomyelitis with draining** `HCC` **sinus, left** radius and ulna

     M86.439 **Chronic osteomyelitis with draining** `HCC` ▽ **sinus, unspecified radius and ulna**

√6ᵗʰ **M86.44** **Chronic osteomyelitis with draining sinus,** hand

     M86.441 **Chronic osteomyelitis with draining** `HCC` **sinus, right** hand

     M86.442 **Chronic osteomyelitis with draining** `HCC` **sinus, left** hand

     M86.449 **Chronic osteomyelitis with draining** `HCC` ▽ **sinus, unspecified hand**

√6ᵗʰ **M86.45** **Chronic osteomyelitis with draining sinus,** femur

     M86.451 **Chronic osteomyelitis with draining** `HCC` **sinus, right** femur

     M86.452 **Chronic osteomyelitis with draining** `HCC` **sinus, left** femur

     M86.459 **Chronic osteomyelitis with draining** `HCC` ▽ **sinus, unspecified femur**

√6ᵗʰ **M86.46** **Chronic osteomyelitis with draining sinus,** tibia and fibula

     M86.461 **Chronic osteomyelitis with draining** `HCC` **sinus, right** tibia and fibula

     M86.462 **Chronic osteomyelitis with draining** `HCC` **sinus, left** tibia and fibula

     M86.469 **Chronic osteomyelitis with draining** `HCC` ▽ **sinus, unspecified tibia and fibula**

√6ᵗʰ **M86.47** **Chronic osteomyelitis with draining sinus,** ankle and foot

     M86.471 **Chronic osteomyelitis with draining** `HCC` **sinus, right** ankle and foot

     M86.472 **Chronic osteomyelitis with draining** `HCC` **sinus, left** ankle and foot

     M86.479 **Chronic osteomyelitis with draining** `HCC` ▽ **sinus, unspecified ankle and foot**

     M86.48 **Chronic osteomyelitis with draining sinus,** `HCC` **other site**

     M86.49 **Chronic osteomyelitis with draining sinus,** `HCC` **multiple sites**

√5ᵗʰ **M86.5** **Other** chronic hematogenous **osteomyelitis**

     M86.50 **Other chronic hematogenous osteomyelitis,** `HCC` ▽ **unspecified site**

√6ᵗʰ **M86.51** **Other chronic hematogenous osteomyelitis,** shoulder

     M86.511 **Other chronic hematogenous** `HCC` **osteomyelitis, right** shoulder

     M86.512 **Other chronic hematogenous** `HCC` **osteomyelitis, left** shoulder

     M86.519 **Other chronic hematogenous** `HCC` ▽ **osteomyelitis, unspecified shoulder**

√6ᵗʰ **M86.52** **Other chronic hematogenous osteomyelitis,** humerus

     M86.521 **Other chronic hematogenous** `HCC` **osteomyelitis, right** humerus

     M86.522 **Other chronic hematogenous** `HCC` **osteomyelitis, left** humerus

     M86.529 **Other chronic hematogenous** `HCC` ▽ **osteomyelitis, unspecified humerus**

√6ᵗʰ **M86.53** **Other chronic hematogenous osteomyelitis,** radius and ulna

     M86.531 **Other chronic hematogenous** `HCC` **osteomyelitis, right** radius and ulna

     M86.532 **Other chronic hematogenous** `HCC` **osteomyelitis, left** radius and ulna

     M86.539 **Other chronic hematogenous** `HCC` ▽ **osteomyelitis, unspecified radius and ulna**

√6ᵗʰ **M86.54** **Other chronic hematogenous osteomyelitis,** hand

     M86.541 **Other chronic hematogenous** `HCC` **osteomyelitis, right** hand

     M86.542 **Other chronic hematogenous** `HCC` **osteomyelitis, left** hand

     M86.549 **Other chronic hematogenous** `HCC` ▽ **osteomyelitis, unspecified hand**

√6ᵗʰ **M86.55** **Other chronic hematogenous osteomyelitis,** femur

     M86.551 **Other chronic hematogenous** `HCC` **osteomyelitis, right** femur

     M86.552 **Other chronic hematogenous** `HCC` **osteomyelitis, left** femur

     M86.559 **Other chronic hematogenous** `HCC` ▽ **osteomyelitis, unspecified femur**

√6ᵗʰ **M86.56** **Other chronic hematogenous osteomyelitis,** tibia and fibula

     M86.561 **Other chronic hematogenous** `HCC` **osteomyelitis, right** tibia and fibula

     M86.562 **Other chronic hematogenous** `HCC` **osteomyelitis, left** tibia and fibula

     M86.569 **Other chronic hematogenous** `HCC` ▽ **osteomyelitis, unspecified tibia and fibula**

√6ᵗʰ **M86.57** **Other chronic hematogenous osteomyelitis,** ankle and foot

     M86.571 **Other chronic hematogenous** `HCC` **osteomyelitis, right** ankle and foot

     M86.572 **Other chronic hematogenous** `HCC` **osteomyelitis, left** ankle and foot

     M86.579 **Other chronic hematogenous** `HCC` ▽ **osteomyelitis, unspecified ankle and foot**

     M86.58 **Other chronic hematogenous osteomyelitis,** `HCC` **other site**

     M86.59 **Other chronic hematogenous osteomyelitis,** `HCC` **multiple sites**

√5ᵗʰ **M86.6** **Other** chronic **osteomyelitis**

     M86.60 **Other chronic osteomyelitis, unspecified site** `HCC` ▽

√6ᵗʰ **M86.61** **Other chronic osteomyelitis,** shoulder

     M86.611 **Other chronic osteomyelitis, right** `HCC` **shoulder**

     M86.612 **Other chronic osteomyelitis, left** `HCC` **shoulder**

     M86.619 **Other chronic osteomyelitis,** `HCC` ▽ **unspecified shoulder**

☑ Additional Character Req   √x7ᵗʰ Placeholder Alert   Manifestation   `HCC` CMS-HCC Condition   ▽ Unspecified Code   ►◄ Revised Text   ● New Code   ▲ Revised Code Title

Chapter 13. Diseases of the Musculoskeletal System and Connective Tissue

✓6ᵗʰ **M86.62 Other chronic osteomyelitis, humerus**
- **M86.621 Other chronic osteomyelitis, right humerus** `HCC`
- **M86.622 Other chronic osteomyelitis, left humerus** `HCC`
- **M86.629 Other chronic osteomyelitis, unspecified humerus** `HCC` ▽

✓6ᵗʰ **M86.63 Other chronic osteomyelitis, radius and ulna**
- **M86.631 Other chronic osteomyelitis, right radius and ulna** `HCC`
- **M86.632 Other chronic osteomyelitis, left radius and ulna** `HCC`
- **M86.639 Other chronic osteomyelitis, unspecified radius and ulna** `HCC` ▽

✓6ᵗʰ **M86.64 Other chronic osteomyelitis, hand**
- **M86.641 Other chronic osteomyelitis, right hand** `HCC`
- **M86.642 Other chronic osteomyelitis, left hand** `HCC`
- **M86.649 Other chronic osteomyelitis, unspecified hand** `HCC` ▽

✓6ᵗʰ **M86.65 Other chronic osteomyelitis, thigh**
- **M86.651 Other chronic osteomyelitis, right thigh** `HCC`
- **M86.652 Other chronic osteomyelitis, left thigh** `HCC`
- **M86.659 Other chronic osteomyelitis, unspecified thigh** `HCC` ▽

✓6ᵗʰ **M86.66 Other chronic osteomyelitis, tibia and fibula**
- **M86.661 Other chronic osteomyelitis, right tibia and fibula** `HCC`
- **M86.662 Other chronic osteomyelitis, left tibia and fibula** `HCC`
- **M86.669 Other chronic osteomyelitis, unspecified tibia and fibula** `HCC` ▽

✓6ᵗʰ **M86.67 Other chronic osteomyelitis, ankle and foot**
- **M86.671 Other chronic osteomyelitis, right ankle and foot** `HCC`
  - **AHA:** 2016, 1Q, 13
- **M86.672 Other chronic osteomyelitis, left ankle and foot** `HCC`
- **M86.679 Other chronic osteomyelitis, unspecified ankle and foot** `HCC` ▽

- **M86.68 Other chronic osteomyelitis, other site** `HCC`
- **M86.69 Other chronic osteomyelitis, multiple sites** `HCC`

✓5ᵗʰ **M86.8 Other osteomyelitis**
    Brodie's abscess

✓6ᵗʰ **M86.8X Other osteomyelitis**
- **M86.8X0 Other osteomyelitis, multiple sites** `HCC`
- **M86.8X1 Other osteomyelitis, shoulder** `HCC`
- **M86.8X2 Other osteomyelitis, upper arm** `HCC`
- **M86.8X3 Other osteomyelitis, forearm** `HCC`
- **M86.8X4 Other osteomyelitis, hand** `HCC`
- **M86.8X5 Other osteomyelitis, thigh** `HCC`
- **M86.8X6 Other osteomyelitis, lower leg** `HCC`
- **M86.8X7 Other osteomyelitis, ankle and foot** `HCC`
- **M86.8X8 Other osteomyelitis, other site** `HCC`
- **M86.8X9 Other osteomyelitis, unspecified sites** `HCC` ▽

M86.9 Osteomyelitis, unspecified `HCC` ▽
    Infection of bone NOS
    Periostitis without osteomyelitis

✓4ᵗʰ **M87 Osteonecrosis**
    INCLUDES avascular necrosis of bone
    Use additional code to identify major osseous defect, if applicable (M89.7-)
    EXCLUDES 1 juvenile osteonecrosis (M91-M92)
    osteochondropathies (M90-M93)

✓5ᵗʰ **M87.0 Idiopathic aseptic necrosis of bone**
- **M87.00 Idiopathic aseptic necrosis of unspecified bone** `HCC` ▽

✓6ᵗʰ **M87.01 Idiopathic aseptic necrosis of shoulder**
    Idiopathic aseptic necrosis of clavicle and scapula
- **M87.011 Idiopathic aseptic necrosis of right shoulder** `HCC`
- **M87.012 Idiopathic aseptic necrosis of left shoulder** `HCC`
- **M87.019 Idiopathic aseptic necrosis of unspecified shoulder** `HCC` ▽

✓6ᵗʰ **M87.02 Idiopathic aseptic necrosis of humerus**
- **M87.021 Idiopathic aseptic necrosis of right humerus** `HCC`
- **M87.022 Idiopathic aseptic necrosis of left humerus** `HCC`
- **M87.029 Idiopathic aseptic necrosis of unspecified humerus** `HCC` ▽

✓6ᵗʰ **M87.03 Idiopathic aseptic necrosis of radius, ulna and carpus**
- **M87.031 Idiopathic aseptic necrosis of right radius** `HCC`
- **M87.032 Idiopathic aseptic necrosis of left radius** `HCC`
- **M87.033 Idiopathic aseptic necrosis of unspecified radius** `HCC` ▽
- **M87.034 Idiopathic aseptic necrosis of right ulna** `HCC`
- **M87.035 Idiopathic aseptic necrosis of left ulna** `HCC`
- **M87.036 Idiopathic aseptic necrosis of unspecified ulna** `HCC` ▽
- **M87.037 Idiopathic aseptic necrosis of right carpus** `HCC`
- **M87.038 Idiopathic aseptic necrosis of left carpus** `HCC`
- **M87.039 Idiopathic aseptic necrosis of unspecified carpus** `HCC` ▽

✓6ᵗʰ **M87.04 Idiopathic aseptic necrosis of hand and fingers**
    Idiopathic aseptic necrosis of metacarpals and phalanges of hands
- **M87.041 Idiopathic aseptic necrosis of right hand** `HCC`
- **M87.042 Idiopathic aseptic necrosis of left hand** `HCC`
- **M87.043 Idiopathic aseptic necrosis of unspecified hand** `HCC` ▽
- **M87.044 Idiopathic aseptic necrosis of right finger(s)** `HCC`
- **M87.045 Idiopathic aseptic necrosis of left finger(s)** `HCC`
- **M87.046 Idiopathic aseptic necrosis of unspecified finger(s)** `HCC` ▽

✓6ᵗʰ **M87.05 Idiopathic aseptic necrosis of pelvis and femur**
- **M87.050 Idiopathic aseptic necrosis of pelvis** `HCC`
- **M87.051 Idiopathic aseptic necrosis of right femur** `HCC`
- **M87.052 Idiopathic aseptic necrosis of left femur** `HCC`
- **M87.059 Idiopathic aseptic necrosis of unspecified femur** `HCC` ▽
  - Idiopathic aseptic necrosis of hip NOS

✓6ᵗʰ **M87.06 Idiopathic aseptic necrosis of tibia and fibula**
- **M87.061 Idiopathic aseptic necrosis of right tibia** `HCC`
- **M87.062 Idiopathic aseptic necrosis of left tibia** `HCC`
- **M87.063 Idiopathic aseptic necrosis of unspecified tibia** `HCC` ▽
- **M87.064 Idiopathic aseptic necrosis of right fibula** `HCC`
- **M87.065 Idiopathic aseptic necrosis of left fibula** `HCC`
- **M87.066 Idiopathic aseptic necrosis of unspecified fibula** `HCC` ▽

✓6ᵗʰ **M87.07 Idiopathic aseptic necrosis of ankle, foot and toes**
    Idiopathic aseptic necrosis of metatarsus, tarsus, and phalanges of toes
- **M87.071 Idiopathic aseptic necrosis of right ankle** `HCC`
- **M87.072 Idiopathic aseptic necrosis of left ankle** `HCC`
- **M87.073 Idiopathic aseptic necrosis of unspecified ankle** `HCC` ▽
- **M87.074 Idiopathic aseptic necrosis of right foot** `HCC`

EXCLUDES 1 Not coded here   **EXCLUDES 2** Not included here   N Newborn Age: 0   P Pediatric Age: 0-17   M Maternity Age: 12-55   A Adult Age: 15-124

786   ICD-10-CM 2018

M87.075 **Idiopathic aseptic necrosis of left foot** `HCC`

M87.076 **Idiopathic aseptic necrosis of unspecified foot** `HCC` ▽

M87.077 **Idiopathic aseptic necrosis of right toe(s)** `HCC`

M87.078 **Idiopathic aseptic necrosis of left toe(s)** `HCC`

M87.079 **Idiopathic aseptic necrosis of unspecified toe(s)** `HCC` ▽

M87.08 **Idiopathic aseptic necrosis of bone, other site'** `HCC`

M87.09 **Idiopathic aseptic necrosis of bone, multiple sites** `HCC`

✓5ᵗʰ **M87.1 Osteonecrosis due to drugs**

Use additional code for adverse effect, if applicable, to identify drug (T36-T50 with fifth or sixth character 5)

M87.10 **Osteonecrosis due to drugs, unspecified bone** `HCC` ▽

✓6ᵗʰ **M87.11 Osteonecrosis due to drugs, shoulder**

M87.111 **Osteonecrosis due to drugs, right shoulder** `HCC`

M87.112 **Osteonecrosis due to drugs, left shoulder** `HCC`

M87.119 **Osteonecrosis due to drugs, unspecified shoulder** `HCC` ▽

✓6ᵗʰ **M87.12 Osteonecrosis due to drugs, humerus**

M87.121 **Osteonecrosis due to drugs, right humerus** `HCC`

M87.122 **Osteonecrosis due to drugs, left humerus** `HCC`

M87.129 **Osteonecrosis due to drugs, unspecified humerus** `HCC` ▽

✓6ᵗʰ **M87.13 Osteonecrosis due to drugs of radius, ulna and carpus**

M87.131 **Osteonecrosis due to drugs of right radius** `HCC`

M87.132 **Osteonecrosis due to drugs of left radius** `HCC`

M87.133 **Osteonecrosis due to drugs of unspecified radius** `HCC` ▽

M87.134 **Osteonecrosis due to drugs of right ulna** `HCC`

M87.135 **Osteonecrosis due to drugs of left ulna** `HCC`

M87.136 **Osteonecrosis due to drugs of unspecified ulna** `HCC` ▽

M87.137 **Osteonecrosis due to drugs of right carpus** `HCC`

M87.138 **Osteonecrosis due to drugs of left carpus** `HCC`

M87.139 **Osteonecrosis due to drugs of unspecified carpus** `HCC` ▽

✓6ᵗʰ **M87.14 Osteonecrosis due to drugs, hand and fingers**

M87.141 **Osteonecrosis due to drugs, right hand** `HCC`

M87.142 **Osteonecrosis due to drugs, left hand** `HCC`

M87.143 **Osteonecrosis due to drugs, unspecified hand** `HCC` ▽

M87.144 **Osteonecrosis due to drugs, right finger(s)** `HCC`

M87.145 **Osteonecrosis due to drugs, left finger(s)** `HCC`

M87.146 **Osteonecrosis due to drugs, unspecified finger(s)** `HCC` ▽

✓6ᵗʰ **M87.15 Osteonecrosis due to drugs, pelvis and femur**

M87.150 **Osteonecrosis due to drugs, pelvis** `HCC`

M87.151 **Osteonecrosis due to drugs, right femur** `HCC`

M87.152 **Osteonecrosis due to drugs, left femur** `HCC`

M87.159 **Osteonecrosis due to drugs, unspecified femur** `HCC` ▽

✓6ᵗʰ **M87.16 Osteonecrosis due to drugs, tibia and fibula**

M87.161 **Osteonecrosis due to drugs, right tibia** `HCC`

M87.162 **Osteonecrosis due to drugs, left tibia** `HCC`

M87.163 **Osteonecrosis due to drugs, unspecified tibia** `HCC` ▽

M87.164 **Osteonecrosis due to drugs, right fibula** `HCC`

M87.165 **Osteonecrosis due to drugs, left fibula** `HCC`

M87.166 **Osteonecrosis due to drugs, unspecified fibula** `HCC` ▽

✓6ᵗʰ **M87.17 Osteonecrosis due to drugs, ankle, foot and toes**

M87.171 **Osteonecrosis due to drugs, right ankle** `HCC`

M87.172 **Osteonecrosis due to drugs, left ankle** `HCC`

M87.173 **Osteonecrosis due to drugs, unspecified ankle** `HCC` ▽

M87.174 **Osteonecrosis due to drugs, right foot** `HCC`

M87.175 **Osteonecrosis due to drugs, left foot** `HCC`

M87.176 **Osteonecrosis due to drugs, unspecified foot** `HCC` ▽

M87.177 **Osteonecrosis due to drugs, right toe(s)** `HCC`

M87.178 **Osteonecrosis due to drugs, left toe(s)** `HCC`

M87.179 **Osteonecrosis due to drugs, unspecified toe(s)** `HCC` ▽

✓6ᵗʰ **M87.18 Osteonecrosis due to drugs, other site**

M87.180 **Osteonecrosis due to drugs, jaw** `HCC`

M87.188 **Osteonecrosis due to drugs, other site** `HCC`

M87.19 **Osteonecrosis due to drugs, multiple sites** `HCC`

✓5ᵗʰ **M87.2 Osteonecrosis due to previous trauma**

M87.20 **Osteonecrosis due to previous trauma, unspecified bone** `HCC` ▽

✓6ᵗʰ **M87.21 Osteonecrosis due to previous trauma, shoulder**

M87.211 **Osteonecrosis due to previous trauma, right shoulder** `HCC`

M87.212 **Osteonecrosis due to previous trauma, left shoulder** `HCC`

M87.219 **Osteonecrosis due to previous trauma, unspecified shoulder** `HCC` ▽

✓6ᵗʰ **M87.22 Osteonecrosis due to previous trauma, humerus**

M87.221 **Osteonecrosis due to previous trauma, right humerus** `HCC`

M87.222 **Osteonecrosis due to previous trauma, left humerus** `HCC`

M87.229 **Osteonecrosis due to previous trauma, unspecified humerus** `HCC` ▽

✓6ᵗʰ **M87.23 Osteonecrosis due to previous trauma of radius, ulna and carpus**

M87.231 **Osteonecrosis due to previous trauma of right radius** `HCC`

M87.232 **Osteonecrosis due to previous trauma of left radius** `HCC`

M87.233 **Osteonecrosis due to previous trauma of unspecified radius** `HCC` ▽

M87.234 **Osteonecrosis due to previous trauma of right ulna** `HCC`

M87.235 **Osteonecrosis due to previous trauma of left ulna** `HCC`

M87.236 **Osteonecrosis due to previous trauma of unspecified ulna** `HCC` ▽

M87.237 **Osteonecrosis due to previous trauma of right carpus** `HCC`

M87.238 **Osteonecrosis due to previous trauma of left carpus** `HCC`

M87.239 **Osteonecrosis due to previous trauma of unspecified carpus** `HCC` ▽

✓6ᵗʰ **M87.24 Osteonecrosis due to previous trauma, hand and fingers**

M87.241 **Osteonecrosis due to previous trauma, right hand** `HCC`

M87.242 **Osteonecrosis due to previous trauma, left hand** `HCC`

M87.243 **Osteonecrosis due to previous trauma, unspecified hand** `HCC` ▽

☑ Additional Character Req   ✓x7ᵗʰ Placeholder Alert   Manifestation   `HCC` CMS-HCC Condition   ▽ Unspecified Code   ►◄ Revised Text   ● New Code   ▲ Revised Code Title

ICD-10-CM 2018   787

M87.244   Osteonecrosis due to previous trauma, right finger(s)   `HCC`

M87.245   Osteonecrosis due to previous trauma, left finger(s)   `HCC`

M87.246   Osteonecrosis due to previous trauma, unspecified finger(s)   `HCC` ▽

✓6ᵗʰ   **M87.25**   Osteonecrosis due to previous trauma, pelvis and femur

M87.250   Osteonecrosis due to previous trauma, pelvis   `HCC`

M87.251   Osteonecrosis due to previous trauma, right femur   `HCC`

M87.252   Osteonecrosis due to previous trauma, left femur   `HCC`

M87.256   Osteonecrosis due to previous trauma, unspecified femur   `HCC` ▽

✓6ᵗʰ   **M87.26**   Osteonecrosis due to previous trauma, tibia and fibula

M87.261   Osteonecrosis due to previous trauma, right tibia   `HCC`

M87.262   Osteonecrosis due to previous trauma, left tibia   `HCC`

M87.263   Osteonecrosis due to previous trauma, unspecified tibia   `HCC` ▽

M87.264   Osteonecrosis due to previous trauma, right fibula   `HCC`

M87.265   Osteonecrosis due to previous trauma, left fibula   `HCC`

M87.266   Osteonecrosis due to previous trauma, unspecified fibula   `HCC` ▽

✓6ᵗʰ   **M87.27**   Osteonecrosis due to previous trauma, ankle, foot and toes

M87.271   Osteonecrosis due to previous trauma, right ankle   `HCC`

M87.272   Osteonecrosis due to previous trauma, left ankle   `HCC`

M87.273   Osteonecrosis due to previous trauma, unspecified ankle   `HCC` ▽

M87.274   Osteonecrosis due to previous trauma, right foot   `HCC`

M87.275   Osteonecrosis due to previous trauma, left foot   `HCC`

M87.276   Osteonecrosis due to previous trauma, unspecified foot   `HCC` ▽

M87.277   Osteonecrosis due to previous trauma, right toe(s)   `HCC`

M87.278   Osteonecrosis due to previous trauma, left toe(s)   `HCC`

M87.279   Osteonecrosis due to previous trauma, unspecified toe(s)   `HCC` ▽

M87.28   Osteonecrosis due to previous trauma, other site   `HCC`

M87.29   Osteonecrosis due to previous trauma, multiple sites   `HCC`

✓5ᵗʰ   **M87.3**   Other secondary osteonecrosis

M87.30   Other secondary osteonecrosis, unspecified bone   `HCC` ▽

✓6ᵗʰ   **M87.31**   Other secondary osteonecrosis, shoulder

M87.311   Other secondary osteonecrosis, right shoulder   `HCC`

M87.312   Other secondary osteonecrosis, left shoulder   `HCC`

M87.319   Other secondary osteonecrosis, unspecified shoulder   `HCC` ▽

✓6ᵗʰ   **M87.32**   Other secondary osteonecrosis, humerus

M87.321   Other secondary osteonecrosis, right humerus   `HCC`

M87.322   Other secondary osteonecrosis, left humerus   `HCC`

M87.329   Other secondary osteonecrosis, unspecified humerus   `HCC` ▽

✓6ᵗʰ   **M87.33**   Other secondary osteonecrosis of radius, ulna and carpus

M87.331   Other secondary osteonecrosis of right radius   `HCC`

M87.332   Other secondary osteonecrosis of left radius   `HCC`

M87.333   Other secondary osteonecrosis of unspecified radius   `HCC` ▽

M87.334   Other secondary osteonecrosis of right ulna   `HCC`

M87.335   Other secondary osteonecrosis of left ulna   `HCC`

M87.336   Other secondary osteonecrosis of unspecified ulna   `HCC` ▽

M87.337   Other secondary osteonecrosis of right carpus   `HCC`

M87.338   Other secondary osteonecrosis of left carpus   `HCC`

M87.339   Other secondary osteonecrosis of unspecified carpus   `HCC` ▽

✓6ᵗʰ   **M87.34**   Other secondary osteonecrosis, hand and fingers

M87.341   Other secondary osteonecrosis, right hand   `HCC`

M87.342   Other secondary osteonecrosis, left hand   `HCC`

M87.343   Other secondary osteonecrosis, unspecified hand   `HCC` ▽

M87.344   Other secondary osteonecrosis, right finger(s)   `HCC`

M87.345   Other secondary osteonecrosis, left finger(s)   `HCC`

M87.346   Other secondary osteonecrosis, unspecified finger(s)   `HCC` ▽

✓6ᵗʰ   **M87.35**   Other secondary osteonecrosis, pelvis and femur

M87.350   Other secondary osteonecrosis, pelvis   `HCC`

M87.351   Other secondary osteonecrosis, right femur   `HCC`

M87.352   Other secondary osteonecrosis, left femur   `HCC`

M87.353   Other secondary osteonecrosis, unspecified femur   `HCC` ▽

✓6ᵗʰ   **M87.36**   Other secondary osteonecrosis, tibia and fibula

M87.361   Other secondary osteonecrosis, right tibia   `HCC`

M87.362   Other secondary osteonecrosis, left tibia   `HCC`

M87.363   Other secondary osteonecrosis, unspecified tibia   `HCC` ▽

M87.364   Other secondary osteonecrosis, right fibula   `HCC`

M87.365   Other secondary osteonecrosis, left fibula   `HCC`

M87.366   Other secondary osteonecrosis, unspecified fibula   `HCC` ▽

✓6ᵗʰ   **M87.37**   Other secondary osteonecrosis, ankle and foot

M87.371   Other secondary osteonecrosis, right ankle   `HCC`

M87.372   Other secondary osteonecrosis, left ankle   `HCC`

M87.373   Other secondary osteonecrosis, unspecified ankle   `HCC` ▽

M87.374   Other secondary osteonecrosis, right foot   `HCC`

M87.375   Other secondary osteonecrosis, left foot   `HCC`

M87.376   Other secondary osteonecrosis, unspecified foot   `HCC` ▽

M87.377   Other secondary osteonecrosis, right toe(s)   `HCC`

M87.378   Other secondary osteonecrosis, left toe(s)   `HCC`

M87.379   Other secondary osteonecrosis, unspecified toe(s)   `HCC` ▽

M87.38   Other secondary osteonecrosis, other site   `HCC`

M87.39   Other secondary osteonecrosis, multiple sites   `HCC`

✓5ᵗʰ   **M87.8**   Other osteonecrosis

M87.80   Other osteonecrosis, unspecified bone   `HCC` ▽

✓6ᵗʰ   **M87.81**   Other osteonecrosis, shoulder

M87.811   Other osteonecrosis, right shoulder   `HCC`

M87.812   Other osteonecrosis, left shoulder   `HCC`

M87.819   Other osteonecrosis, unspecified shoulder   `HCC` ▽

`EXCLUDES 1` Not coded here   `EXCLUDES 2` Not included here   N Newborn Age: 0   P Pediatric Age: 0-17   M Maternity Age: 12-55   A Adult Age: 15-124

788   ICD-10-CM 2018

✓6th **M87.82 Other osteonecrosis, humerus**
M87.821 Other osteonecrosis, right humerus HCC
M87.822 Other osteonecrosis, left humerus HCC
M87.829 Other osteonecrosis, unspecified humerus HCC ▽

✓6th **M87.83 Other osteonecrosis of radius, ulna and carpus**
M87.831 Other osteonecrosis of right radius HCC
M87.832 Other osteonecrosis of left radius HCC
M87.833 Other osteonecrosis of unspecified radius HCC ▽
M87.834 Other osteonecrosis of right ulna HCC
M87.835 Other osteonecrosis of left ulna HCC
M87.836 Other osteonecrosis of unspecified ulna HCC ▽
M87.837 Other osteonecrosis of right carpus HCC
M87.838 Other osteonecrosis of left carpus HCC
M87.839 Other osteonecrosis of unspecified carpus HCC ▽

✓6th **M87.84 Other osteonecrosis, hand and fingers**
M87.841 Other osteonecrosis, right hand HCC
M87.842 Other osteonecrosis, left hand HCC
M87.843 Other osteonecrosis, unspecified hand HCC ▽
M87.844 Other osteonecrosis, right finger(s) HCC
M87.845 Other osteonecrosis, left finger(s) HCC
M87.849 Other osteonecrosis, unspecified finger(s) HCC ▽

✓6th **M87.85 Other osteonecrosis, pelvis and femur**
M87.850 Other osteonecrosis, pelvis HCC
M87.851 Other osteonecrosis, right femur HCC
M87.852 Other osteonecrosis, left femur HCC
M87.859 Other osteonecrosis, unspecified femur HCC ▽

✓6th **M87.86 Other osteonecrosis, tibia and fibula**
M87.861 Other osteonecrosis, right tibia HCC
M87.862 Other osteonecrosis, left tibia HCC
M87.863 Other osteonecrosis, unspecified tibia HCC ▽
M87.864 Other osteonecrosis, right fibula HCC
M87.865 Other osteonecrosis, left fibula HCC
M87.869 Other osteonecrosis, unspecified fibula HCC ▽

✓6th **M87.87 Other osteonecrosis, ankle, foot and toes**
M87.871 Other osteonecrosis, right ankle HCC
M87.872 Other osteonecrosis, left ankle HCC
M87.873 Other osteonecrosis, unspecified ankle HCC ▽
M87.874 Other osteonecrosis, right foot HCC
M87.875 Other osteonecrosis, left foot HCC
M87.876 Other osteonecrosis, unspecified foot HCC ▽
M87.877 Other osteonecrosis, right toe(s) HCC
M87.878 Other osteonecrosis, left toe(s) HCC
M87.879 Other osteonecrosis, unspecified toe(s) HCC ▽

M87.88 Other osteonecrosis, other site HCC
M87.89 Other osteonecrosis, multiple sites HCC

M87.9 Osteonecrosis, unspecified HCC ▽
Necrosis of bone NOS

✓4th **M88 Osteitis deformans [Paget's disease of bone]**
EXCLUDES 1 osteitis deformans in neoplastic disease (M90.6)

M88.0 Osteitis deformans of skull
M88.1 Osteitis deformans of vertebrae
✓5th **M88.8 Osteitis deformans of other bones**
✓6th **M88.81 Osteitis deformans of shoulder**
M88.811 Osteitis deformans of right shoulder
M88.812 Osteitis deformans of left shoulder
M88.819 Osteitis deformans of unspecified shoulder ▽

✓6th **M88.82 Osteitis deformans of upper arm**
M88.821 Osteitis deformans of right upper arm
M88.822 Osteitis deformans of left upper arm
M88.829 Osteitis deformans of unspecified upper arm ▽

✓6th **M88.83 Osteitis deformans of forearm**
M88.831 Osteitis deformans of right forearm
M88.832 Osteitis deformans of left forearm
M88.839 Osteitis deformans of unspecified forearm ▽

✓6th **M88.84 Osteitis deformans of hand**
M88.841 Osteitis deformans of right hand
M88.842 Osteitis deformans of left hand
M88.849 Osteitis deformans of unspecified hand ▽

✓6th **M88.85 Osteitis deformans of thigh**
M88.851 Osteitis deformans of right thigh
M88.852 Osteitis deformans of left thigh
M88.859 Osteitis deformans of unspecified thigh ▽

✓6th **M88.86 Osteitis deformans of lower leg**
M88.861 Osteitis deformans of right lower leg
M88.862 Osteitis deformans of left lower leg
M88.869 Osteitis deformans of unspecified lower leg ▽

✓6th **M88.87 Osteitis deformans of ankle and foot**
M88.871 Osteitis deformans of right ankle and foot
M88.872 Osteitis deformans of left ankle and foot
M88.879 Osteitis deformans of unspecified ankle and foot ▽

M88.88 Osteitis deformans of other bones
EXCLUDES 2 osteitis deformans of skull (M88.0)
osteitis deformans of vertebrae (M88.1)

M88.89 Osteitis deformans of multiple sites

M88.9 Osteitis deformans of unspecified bone ▽

✓4th **M89 Other disorders of bone**
✓5th **M89.0 Algoneurodystrophy**
Shoulder-hand syndrome
Sudeck's atrophy
EXCLUDES 1 causalgia, lower limb (G57.7-)
causalgia, upper limb (G56.4-)
complex regional pain syndrome II, lower limb (G57.7-)
complex regional pain syndrome II, upper limb (G56.4-)
reflex sympathetic dystrophy (G90.5-)

M89.00 Algoneurodystrophy, unspecified site ▽
✓6th **M89.01 Algoneurodystrophy, shoulder**
M89.011 Algoneurodystrophy, right shoulder
M89.012 Algoneurodystrophy, left shoulder
M89.019 Algoneurodystrophy, unspecified shoulder ▽

✓6th **M89.02 Algoneurodystrophy, upper arm**
M89.021 Algoneurodystrophy, right upper arm
M89.022 Algoneurodystrophy, left upper arm
M89.029 Algoneurodystrophy, unspecified upper arm ▽

✓6th **M89.03 Algoneurodystrophy, forearm**
M89.031 Algoneurodystrophy, right forearm
M89.032 Algoneurodystrophy, left forearm
M89.039 Algoneurodystrophy, unspecified forearm ▽

✓6th **M89.04 Algoneurodystrophy, hand**
M89.041 Algoneurodystrophy, right hand
M89.042 Algoneurodystrophy, left hand
M89.049 Algoneurodystrophy, unspecified hand ▽

✓6th **M89.05 Algoneurodystrophy, thigh**
M89.051 Algoneurodystrophy, right thigh
M89.052 Algoneurodystrophy, left thigh
M89.059 Algoneurodystrophy, unspecified thigh ▽

✓6th **M89.06 Algoneurodystrophy, lower leg**
M89.061 Algoneurodystrophy, right lower leg
M89.062 Algoneurodystrophy, left lower leg
M89.069 Algoneurodystrophy, unspecified lower leg ▽

✓6th **M89.07 Algoneurodystrophy, ankle and foot**
M89.071 Algoneurodystrophy, right ankle and foot
M89.072 Algoneurodystrophy, left ankle and foot
M89.079 Algoneurodystrophy, unspecified ankle and foot ▽

M89.08 Algoneurodystrophy, other site
M89.09 Algoneurodystrophy, multiple sites

✓ Additional Character Req   ✓x7th Placeholder Alert   Manifestation   HCC CMS-HCC Condition   ▽ Unspecified Code   ►◄ Revised Text   ● New Code   ▲ Revised Code Title

Chapter 13. Diseases of the Musculoskeletal System and Connective Tissue

✓5ᵗʰ **M89.1 Physeal arrest**
- Arrest of growth plate
- Epiphyseal arrest
- Growth plate arrest

✓6ᵗʰ **M89.12 Physeal arrest, humerus**
- M89.121 Complete physeal arrest, right proximal humerus
- M89.122 Complete physeal arrest, left proximal humerus
- M89.123 Partial physeal arrest, right proximal humerus
- M89.124 Partial physeal arrest, left proximal humerus
- M89.125 Complete physeal arrest, right distal humerus
- M89.126 Complete physeal arrest, left distal humerus
- M89.127 Partial physeal arrest, right distal humerus
- M89.128 Partial physeal arrest, left distal humerus
- M89.129 Physeal arrest, humerus, unspecified ▽

✓6ᵗʰ **M89.13 Physeal arrest, forearm**
- M89.131 Complete physeal arrest, right distal radius
- M89.132 Complete physeal arrest, left distal radius
- M89.133 Partial physeal arrest, right distal radius
- M89.134 Partial physeal arrest, left distal radius
- M89.138 Other physeal arrest of forearm
- M89.139 Physeal arrest, forearm, unspecified ▽

✓6ᵗʰ **M89.15 Physeal arrest, femur**
- M89.151 Complete physeal arrest, right proximal femur
- M89.152 Complete physeal arrest, left proximal femur
- M89.153 Partial physeal arrest, right proximal femur
- M89.154 Partial physeal arrest, left proximal femur
- M89.155 Complete physeal arrest, right distal femur
- M89.156 Complete physeal arrest, left distal femur
- M89.157 Partial physeal arrest, right distal femur
- M89.158 Partial physeal arrest, left distal femur
- M89.159 Physeal arrest, femur, unspecified ▽

✓6ᵗʰ **M89.16 Physeal arrest, lower leg**
- M89.160 Complete physeal arrest, right proximal tibia
- M89.161 Complete physeal arrest, left proximal tibia
- M89.162 Partial physeal arrest, right proximal tibia
- M89.163 Partial physeal arrest, left proximal tibia
- M89.164 Complete physeal arrest, right distal tibia
- M89.165 Complete physeal arrest, left distal tibia
- M89.166 Partial physeal arrest, right distal tibia
- M89.167 Partial physeal arrest, left distal tibia
- M89.168 Other physeal arrest of lower leg
- M89.169 Physeal arrest, lower leg, unspecified ▽

M89.18 Physeal arrest, other site

✓5ᵗʰ **M89.2 Other disorders of bone development and growth**
- M89.20 Other disorders of bone development and growth, unspecified site ▽

✓6ᵗʰ **M89.21 Other disorders of bone development and growth, shoulder**
- M89.211 Other disorders of bone development and growth, right shoulder
- M89.212 Other disorders of bone development and growth, left shoulder
- M89.219 Other disorders of bone development and growth, unspecified shoulder ▽

✓6ᵗʰ **M89.22 Other disorders of bone development and growth, humerus**
- M89.221 Other disorders of bone development and growth, right humerus
- M89.222 Other disorders of bone development and growth, left humerus
- M89.229 Other disorders of bone development and growth, unspecified humerus ▽

✓6ᵗʰ **M89.23 Other disorders of bone development and growth, ulna and radius**
- M89.231 Other disorders of bone development and growth, right ulna
- M89.232 Other disorders of bone development and growth, left ulna
- M89.233 Other disorders of bone development and growth, right radius
- M89.234 Other disorders of bone development and growth, left radius
- M89.239 Other disorders of bone development and growth, unspecified ulna and radius ▽

✓6ᵗʰ **M89.24 Other disorders of bone development and growth, hand**
- M89.241 Other disorders of bone development and growth, right hand
- M89.242 Other disorders of bone development and growth, left hand
- M89.249 Other disorders of bone development and growth, unspecified hand ▽

✓6ᵗʰ **M89.25 Other disorders of bone development and growth, femur**
- M89.251 Other disorders of bone development and growth, right femur
- M89.252 Other disorders of bone development and growth, left femur
- M89.259 Other disorders of bone development and growth, unspecified femur ▽

✓6ᵗʰ **M89.26 Other disorders of bone development and growth, tibia and fibula**
- M89.261 Other disorders of bone development and growth, right tibia
- M89.262 Other disorders of bone development and growth, left tibia
- M89.263 Other disorders of bone development and growth, right fibula
- M89.264 Other disorders of bone development and growth, left fibula
- M89.269 Other disorders of bone development and growth, unspecified lower leg ▽

✓6ᵗʰ **M89.27 Other disorders of bone development and growth, ankle and foot**
- M89.271 Other disorders of bone development and growth, right ankle and foot
- M89.272 Other disorders of bone development and growth, left ankle and foot
- M89.279 Other disorders of bone development and growth, unspecified ankle and foot ▽

M89.28 Other disorders of bone development and growth, other site

M89.29 Other disorders of bone development and growth, multiple sites

✓5ᵗʰ **M89.3 Hypertrophy of bone**
- M89.30 Hypertrophy of bone, unspecified site ▽

✓6ᵗʰ **M89.31 Hypertrophy of bone, shoulder**
- M89.311 Hypertrophy of bone, right shoulder
- M89.312 Hypertrophy of bone, left shoulder
- M89.319 Hypertrophy of bone, unspecified shoulder ▽

✓6ᵗʰ **M89.32 Hypertrophy of bone, humerus**
- M89.321 Hypertrophy of bone, right humerus
- M89.322 Hypertrophy of bone, left humerus
- M89.329 Hypertrophy of bone, unspecified humerus ▽

✓6ᵗʰ **M89.33 Hypertrophy of bone, ulna and radius**
- M89.331 Hypertrophy of bone, right ulna
- M89.332 Hypertrophy of bone, left ulna
- M89.333 Hypertrophy of bone, right radius
- M89.334 Hypertrophy of bone, left radius
- M89.339 Hypertrophy of bone, unspecified ulna and radius ▽

✓6ᵗʰ **M89.34 Hypertrophy of bone, hand**
- M89.341 Hypertrophy of bone, right hand
- M89.342 Hypertrophy of bone, left hand
- M89.349 Hypertrophy of bone, unspecified hand ▽

EXCLUDES 1 Not coded here   EXCLUDES 2 Not included here   N Newborn Age: 0   P Pediatric Age: 0-17   M Maternity Age: 12-55   A Adult Age: 15-124

790   ICD-10-CM 2018

√6ᵗʰ **M89.35 Hypertrophy of bone,** femur
    M89.351 Hypertrophy of bone, right **femur**
    M89.352 Hypertrophy of bone, left **femur**
    M89.359 Hypertrophy of bone, unspecified ▽
          femur

√6ᵗʰ **M89.36 Hypertrophy of bone,** tibia and fibula
    M89.361 Hypertrophy of bone, right **tibia**
    M89.362 Hypertrophy of bone, left **tibia**
    M89.363 Hypertrophy of bone, right **fibula**
    M89.364 Hypertrophy of bone, left **fibula**
    M89.369 Hypertrophy of bone, unspecified ▽
          tibia and fibula

√6ᵗʰ **M89.37 Hypertrophy of bone,** ankle and foot
    M89.371 Hypertrophy of bone, right **ankle and foot**
    M89.372 Hypertrophy of bone, left **ankle and foot**
    M89.379 Hypertrophy of bone, unspecified ▽
          ankle and foot

    M89.38 Hypertrophy of bone, other site
    M89.39 Hypertrophy of bone, multiple sites

√5ᵗʰ **M89.4 Other hypertrophic osteoarthropathy**
    Marie-Bamberger disease   Pachydermoperiostosis
    M89.40 Other hypertrophic osteoarthropathy, ▽
         unspecified site

√6ᵗʰ **M89.41 Other hypertrophic osteoarthropathy,** shoulder
    M89.411 Other hypertrophic osteoarthropathy,
          right **shoulder**
    M89.412 Other hypertrophic osteoarthropathy,
          left **shoulder**
    M89.419 Other hypertrophic osteoarthropathy, ▽
          unspecified shoulder

√6ᵗʰ **M89.42 Other hypertrophic osteoarthropathy,** upper arm
    M89.421 Other hypertrophic osteoarthropathy,
          right **upper arm**
    M89.422 Other hypertrophic osteoarthropathy,
          left **upper arm**
    M89.429 Other hypertrophic osteoarthropathy, ▽
          unspecified upper arm

√6ᵗʰ **M89.43 Other hypertrophic osteoarthropathy,** forearm
    M89.431 Other hypertrophic osteoarthropathy,
          right **forearm**
    M89.432 Other hypertrophic osteoarthropathy,
          left **forearm**
    M89.439 Other hypertrophic osteoarthropathy, ▽
          unspecified forearm

√6ᵗʰ **M89.44 Other hypertrophic osteoarthropathy,** hand
    M89.441 Other hypertrophic osteoarthropathy,
          right **hand**
    M89.442 Other hypertrophic osteoarthropathy,
          left **hand**
    M89.449 Other hypertrophic osteoarthropathy, ▽
          unspecified hand

√6ᵗʰ **M89.45 Other hypertrophic osteoarthropathy,** thigh
    M89.451 Other hypertrophic osteoarthropathy,
          right **thigh**
    M89.452 Other hypertrophic osteoarthropathy,
          left **thigh**
    M89.459 Other hypertrophic osteoarthropathy, ▽
          unspecified thigh

√6ᵗʰ **M89.46 Other hypertrophic osteoarthropathy,** lower leg
    M89.461 Other hypertrophic osteoarthropathy,
          right **lower leg**
    M89.462 Other hypertrophic osteoarthropathy,
          left **lower leg**
    M89.469 Other hypertrophic osteoarthropathy, ▽
          unspecified lower leg

√6ᵗʰ **M89.47 Other hypertrophic osteoarthropathy,** ankle and foot
    M89.471 Other hypertrophic osteoarthropathy,
          right **ankle and foot**
    M89.472 Other hypertrophic osteoarthropathy,
          left **ankle and foot**
    M89.479 Other hypertrophic osteoarthropathy, ▽
          unspecified ankle and foot

    M89.48 Other hypertrophic osteoarthropathy, other site
    M89.49 Other hypertrophic osteoarthropathy, multiple sites

√5ᵗʰ **M89.5 Osteolysis**
    Use additional code to identify major osseous defect, if
    applicable (M89.7-)
    EXCLUDES 2   periprosthetic osteolysis of internal prosthetic joint
          (T84.05-)
    M89.50 Osteolysis, unspecified site ▽

√6ᵗʰ **M89.51 Osteolysis,** shoulder
    M89.511 Osteolysis, right **shoulder**
    M89.512 Osteolysis, left **shoulder**
    M89.519 Osteolysis, unspecified shoulder ▽

√6ᵗʰ **M89.52 Osteolysis,** upper arm
    M89.521 Osteolysis, right **upper arm**
    M89.522 Osteolysis, left **upper arm**
    M89.529 Osteolysis, unspecified upper arm ▽

√6ᵗʰ **M89.53 Osteolysis,** forearm
    M89.531 Osteolysis, right **forearm**
    M89.532 Osteolysis, left **forearm**
    M89.539 Osteolysis, unspecified forearm ▽

√6ᵗʰ **M89.54 Osteolysis,** hand
    M89.541 Osteolysis, right **hand**
    M89.542 Osteolysis, left **hand**
    M89.549 Osteolysis, unspecified hand ▽

√6ᵗʰ **M89.55 Osteolysis,** thigh
    M89.551 Osteolysis, right **thigh**
    M89.552 Osteolysis, left **thigh**
    M89.559 Osteolysis, unspecified thigh ▽

√6ᵗʰ **M89.56 Osteolysis,** lower leg
    M89.561 Osteolysis, right **lower leg**
    M89.562 Osteolysis, left **lower leg**
    M89.569 Osteolysis, unspecified lower leg ▽

√6ᵗʰ **M89.57 Osteolysis,** ankle and foot
    M89.571 Osteolysis, right **ankle and foot**
    M89.572 Osteolysis, left **ankle and foot**
    M89.579 Osteolysis, unspecified ankle and foot ▽

    M89.58 Osteolysis, other site
    M89.59 Osteolysis, multiple sites

√5ᵗʰ **M89.6 Osteopathy after poliomyelitis**
    Use additional code (B91) to identify previous poliomyelitis
    EXCLUDES 1   postpolio syndrome (G14)
    M89.60 Osteopathy after poliomyelitis, unspecified HCC ▽
         site

√6ᵗʰ **M89.61 Osteopathy after poliomyelitis,** shoulder
    M89.611 Osteopathy after poliomyelitis, right   HCC
          shoulder
    M89.612 Osteopathy after poliomyelitis, left   HCC
          shoulder
    M89.619 Osteopathy after poliomyelitis,   HCC ▽
          unspecified shoulder

√6ᵗʰ **M89.62 Osteopathy after poliomyelitis,** upper arm
    M89.621 Osteopathy after poliomyelitis, right   HCC
          upper arm
    M89.622 Osteopathy after poliomyelitis, left   HCC
          upper arm
    M89.629 Osteopathy after poliomyelitis,   HCC ▽
          unspecified upper arm

√6ᵗʰ **M89.63 Osteopathy after poliomyelitis,** forearm
    M89.631 Osteopathy after poliomyelitis, right   HCC
          forearm
    M89.632 Osteopathy after poliomyelitis, left   HCC
          forearm
    M89.639 Osteopathy after poliomyelitis,   HCC ▽
          unspecified forearm

√6ᵗʰ **M89.64 Osteopathy after poliomyelitis,** hand
    M89.641 Osteopathy after poliomyelitis,   HCC
          right hand
    M89.642 Osteopathy after poliomyelitis,   HCC
          left hand
    M89.649 Osteopathy after poliomyelitis,   HCC ▽
          unspecified hand

√6ᵗʰ **M89.65 Osteopathy after poliomyelitis,** thigh
    M89.651 Osteopathy after poliomyelitis,   HCC
          right thigh
    M89.652 Osteopathy after poliomyelitis,   HCC
          left thigh

☑ Additional Character Req   ✓x7ᵗʰ Placeholder Alert   Manifestation   HCC CMS-HCC Condition   ▽ Unspecified Code   ►◄ Revised Text   ● New Code   ▲ Revised Code Title

Chapter 13. Diseases of the Musculoskeletal System and Connective Tissue

       M89.659   Osteopathy after poliomyelitis, unspecified thigh   HCC ▽

✓6ᵗʰ   M89.66   Osteopathy after poliomyelitis, lower leg

       M89.661   Osteopathy after poliomyelitis, right lower leg   HCC

       M89.662   Osteopathy after poliomyelitis, left lower leg   HCC

       M89.669   Osteopathy after poliomyelitis, unspecified lower leg   HCC ▽

✓6ᵗʰ   M89.67   Osteopathy after poliomyelitis, ankle and foot

       M89.671   Osteopathy after poliomyelitis, right ankle and foot   HCC

       M89.672   Osteopathy after poliomyelitis, left ankle and foot   HCC

       M89.679   Osteopathy after poliomyelitis, unspecified ankle and foot   HCC ▽

    M89.68   Osteopathy after poliomyelitis, other site   HCC

    M89.69   Osteopathy after poliomyelitis, multiple sites   HCC

✓5ᵗʰ   M89.7   Major osseous defect

       Code first underlying disease, if known, such as:
       aseptic necrosis of bone (M87.-)
       malignant neoplasm of bone (C40.-)
       osteolysis (M89.5)
       osteomyelitis (M86.-)
       osteonecrosis (M87.-)
       osteoporosis (M80.-, M81.-)
       periprosthetic osteolysis (T84.05-)

    M89.70   Major osseous defect, unspecified site   ▽

✓6ᵗʰ   M89.71   Major osseous defect, shoulder region
       Major osseous defect clavicle or scapula

       M89.711   Major osseous defect, right shoulder region

       M89.712   Major osseous defect, left shoulder region

       M89.719   Major osseous defect, unspecified shoulder region   ▽

✓6ᵗʰ   M89.72   Major osseous defect, humerus

       M89.721   Major osseous defect, right humerus

       M89.722   Major osseous defect, left humerus

       M89.729   Major osseous defect, unspecified humerus   ▽

✓6ᵗʰ   M89.73   Major osseous defect, forearm
       Major osseous defect of radius and ulna

       M89.731   Major osseous defect, right forearm

       M89.732   Major osseous defect, left forearm

       M89.739   Major osseous defect, unspecified forearm   ▽

✓6ᵗʰ   M89.74   Major osseous defect, hand
       Major osseous defect of carpus, fingers, metacarpus

       M89.741   Major osseous defect, right hand

       M89.742   Major osseous defect, left hand

       M89.749   Major osseous defect, unspecified hand ▽

✓6ᵗʰ   M89.75   Major osseous defect, pelvic region and thigh
       Major osseous defect of femur and pelvis

       M89.751   Major osseous defect, right pelvic region and thigh

       M89.752   Major osseous defect, left pelvic region and thigh

       M89.759   Major osseous defect, unspecified pelvic region and thigh   ▽

✓6ᵗʰ   M89.76   Major osseous defect, lower leg
       Major osseous defect of fibula and tibia

       M89.761   Major osseous defect, right lower leg

       M89.762   Major osseous defect, left lower leg

       M89.769   Major osseous defect, unspecified lower leg   ▽

✓6ᵗʰ   M89.77   Major osseous defect, ankle and foot
       Major osseous defect of metatarsus, tarsus, toes

       M89.771   Major osseous defect, right ankle and foot

       M89.772   Major osseous defect, left ankle and foot

       M89.779   Major osseous defect, unspecified ankle and foot   ▽

    M89.78   Major osseous defect, other site

    M89.79   Major osseous defect, multiple sites

✓5ᵗʰ   M89.8   Other specified disorders of bone
       Infantile cortical hyperostoses
       Post-traumatic subperiosteal ossification

✓6ᵗʰ   M89.8X   Other specified disorders of bone

       M89.8X0   Other specified disorders of bone, multiple sites

       M89.8X1   Other specified disorders of bone, shoulder

       M89.8X2   Other specified disorders of bone, upper arm

       M89.8X3   Other specified disorders of bone, forearm

       M89.8X4   Other specified disorders of bone, hand

       M89.8X5   Other specified disorders of bone, thigh

       M89.8X6   Other specified disorders of bone, lower leg

       M89.8X7   Other specified disorders of bone, ankle and foot

       M89.8X8   Other specified disorders of bone, other site

       M89.8X9   Other specified disorders of bone, unspecified site   ▽

    M89.9   Disorder of bone, unspecified   ▽

✓4ᵗʰ   **M90   Osteopathies in diseases classified elsewhere**

       EXCLUDES 1   osteochondritis, osteomyelitis, and osteopathy (in):
             cryptococcosis (B45.3)
             diabetes mellitus (E08-E13 with .69-)
             gonococcal (A54.43)
             neurogenic syphilis (A52.11)
             renal osteodystrophy (N25.0)
             salmonellosis (A02.24)
             secondary syphilis (A51.46)
             syphilis (late) (A52.77)

✓5ᵗʰ   M90.5   Osteonecrosis in diseases classified elsewhere
       Code first underlying disease, such as:
       caisson disease (T70.3)
       hemoglobinopathy (D50-D64)

    M90.50   *Osteonecrosis in diseases classified elsewhere, unspecified site*   HCC ▽

✓6ᵗʰ   *M90.51*   *Osteonecrosis in diseases classified elsewhere, shoulder*

       M90.511   *Osteonecrosis in diseases classified elsewhere, right shoulder*   HCC

       M90.512   *Osteonecrosis in diseases classified elsewhere, left shoulder*   HCC

       M90.519   *Osteonecrosis in diseases classified elsewhere, unspecified shoulder*   HCC ▽

✓6ᵗʰ   *M90.52*   *Osteonecrosis in diseases classified elsewhere, upper arm*

       M90.521   *Osteonecrosis in diseases classified elsewhere, right upper arm*   HCC

       M90.522   *Osteonecrosis in diseases classified elsewhere, left upper arm*   HCC

       M90.529   *Osteonecrosis in diseases classified elsewhere, unspecified upper arm*   HCC ▽

✓6ᵗʰ   *M90.53*   *Osteonecrosis in diseases classified elsewhere, forearm*

       M90.531   *Osteonecrosis in diseases classified elsewhere, right forearm*   HCC

       M90.532   *Osteonecrosis in diseases classified elsewhere, left forearm*   HCC

       M90.539   *Osteonecrosis in diseases classified elsewhere, unspecified forearm*   HCC ▽

✓6ᵗʰ   *M90.54*   *Osteonecrosis in diseases classified elsewhere, hand*

       M90.541   *Osteonecrosis in diseases classified elsewhere, right hand*   HCC

       M90.542   *Osteonecrosis in diseases classified elsewhere, left hand*   HCC

       M90.549   *Osteonecrosis in diseases classified elsewhere, unspecified hand*   HCC ▽

✓6ᵗʰ   *M90.55*   *Osteonecrosis in diseases classified elsewhere, thigh*

       M90.551   *Osteonecrosis in diseases classified elsewhere, right thigh*   HCC

       M90.552   *Osteonecrosis in diseases classified elsewhere, left thigh*   HCC

       M90.559   *Osteonecrosis in diseases classified elsewhere, unspecified thigh*   HCC ▽

EXCLUDES 1 Not coded here   EXCLUDES 2 Not included here   N Newborn Age: 0   P Pediatric Age: 0-17   M Maternity Age: 12-55   A Adult Age: 15-124

792   ICD-10-CM 2018

☑6ᵗʰ **M90.56** Osteonecrosis in diseases classified elsewhere, lower leg

    M90.561 Osteonecrosis in diseases classified elsewhere, *right lower leg* **HCC**

    M90.562 Osteonecrosis in diseases classified elsewhere, *left lower leg* **HCC**

    M90.569 Osteonecrosis in diseases classified elsewhere, *unspecified lower leg* **HCC** ▽

☑6ᵗʰ **M90.57** Osteonecrosis in diseases classified elsewhere, ankle and foot

    M90.571 Osteonecrosis in diseases classified elsewhere, *right ankle and foot* **HCC**

    M90.572 Osteonecrosis in diseases classified elsewhere, *left ankle and foot* **HCC**

    M90.579 Osteonecrosis in diseases classified elsewhere, *unspecified ankle and foot* **HCC** ▽

M90.58 Osteonecrosis in diseases classified elsewhere, other site **HCC**

M90.59 Osteonecrosis in diseases classified elsewhere, *multiple sites* **HCC**

☑5ᵗʰ **M90.6 Osteitis deformans in neoplastic diseases**
Osteitis deformans in malignant neoplasm of bone
Code first the neoplasm (C40-, C41-)
EXCLUDES 1   osteitis deformans [Paget's disease of bone] (M88.-)

M90.60 Osteitis deformans in neoplastic diseases, unspecified site ▽

☑6ᵗʰ **M90.61** Osteitis deformans in neoplastic diseases, shoulder

    M90.611 Osteitis deformans in neoplastic diseases, *right shoulder*

    M90.612 Osteitis deformans in neoplastic diseases, *left shoulder*

    M90.619 Osteitis deformans in neoplastic diseases, unspecified shoulder ▽

☑6ᵗʰ **M90.62** Osteitis deformans in neoplastic diseases, upper arm

    M90.621 Osteitis deformans in neoplastic diseases, *right upper arm*

    M90.622 Osteitis deformans in neoplastic diseases, *left upper arm*

    M90.629 Osteitis deformans in neoplastic diseases, unspecified upper arm ▽

☑6ᵗʰ **M90.63** Osteitis deformans in neoplastic diseases, forearm

    M90.631 Osteitis deformans in neoplastic diseases, *right forearm*

    M90.632 Osteitis deformans in neoplastic diseases, *left forearm*

    M90.639 Osteitis deformans in neoplastic diseases, unspecified forearm ▽

☑6ᵗʰ **M90.64** Osteitis deformans in neoplastic diseases, hand

    M90.641 Osteitis deformans in neoplastic diseases, *right hand*

    M90.642 Osteitis deformans in neoplastic diseases, *left hand*

    M90.649 Osteitis deformans in neoplastic diseases, unspecified hand ▽

☑6ᵗʰ **M90.65** Osteitis deformans in neoplastic diseases, thigh

    M90.651 Osteitis deformans in neoplastic diseases, *right thigh*

    M90.652 Osteitis deformans in neoplastic diseases, *left thigh*

    M90.659 Osteitis deformans in neoplastic diseases, unspecified thigh ▽

☑6ᵗʰ **M90.66** Osteitis deformans in neoplastic diseases, lower leg

    M90.661 Osteitis deformans in neoplastic diseases, *right lower leg*

    M90.662 Osteitis deformans in neoplastic diseases, *left lower leg*

    M90.669 Osteitis deformans in neoplastic diseases, unspecified lower leg ▽

☑6ᵗʰ **M90.67** Osteitis deformans in neoplastic diseases, ankle and foot

    M90.671 Osteitis deformans in neoplastic diseases, *right ankle and foot*

    M90.672 Osteitis deformans in neoplastic diseases, *left ankle and foot*

    M90.679 Osteitis deformans in neoplastic diseases, unspecified ankle and foot ▽

M90.68 Osteitis deformans in neoplastic diseases, other site

M90.69 Osteitis deformans in neoplastic diseases, *multiple sites*

☑5ᵗʰ **M90.8 Osteopathy in diseases classified elsewhere**
Code first underlying disease, such as:
    rickets (E55.0)
    vitamin-D-resistant rickets (E83.3)

M90.80 Osteopathy in diseases classified elsewhere, unspecified site ▽

☑6ᵗʰ **M90.81** Osteopathy in diseases classified elsewhere, shoulder

    M90.811 Osteopathy in diseases classified elsewhere, *right shoulder*

    M90.812 Osteopathy in diseases classified elsewhere, *left shoulder*

    M90.819 Osteopathy in diseases classified elsewhere, unspecified shoulder ▽

☑6ᵗʰ **M90.82** Osteopathy in diseases classified elsewhere, upper arm

    M90.821 Osteopathy in diseases classified elsewhere, *right upper arm*

    M90.822 Osteopathy in diseases classified elsewhere, *left upper arm*

    M90.829 Osteopathy in diseases classified elsewhere, unspecified upper arm ▽

☑6ᵗʰ **M90.83** Osteopathy in diseases classified elsewhere, forearm

    M90.831 Osteopathy in diseases classified elsewhere, *right forearm*

    M90.832 Osteopathy in diseases classified elsewhere, *left forearm*

    M90.839 Osteopathy in diseases classified elsewhere, unspecified forearm ▽

☑6ᵗʰ **M90.84** Osteopathy in diseases classified elsewhere, hand

    M90.841 Osteopathy in diseases classified elsewhere, *right hand*

    M90.842 Osteopathy in diseases classified elsewhere, *left hand*

    M90.849 Osteopathy in diseases classified elsewhere, unspecified hand ▽

☑6ᵗʰ **M90.85** Osteopathy in diseases classified elsewhere, thigh

    M90.851 Osteopathy in diseases classified elsewhere, *right thigh*

    M90.852 Osteopathy in diseases classified elsewhere, *left thigh*

    M90.859 Osteopathy in diseases classified elsewhere, unspecified thigh ▽

☑6ᵗʰ **M90.86** Osteopathy in diseases classified elsewhere, lower leg

    M90.861 Osteopathy in diseases classified elsewhere, *right lower leg*

    M90.862 Osteopathy in diseases classified elsewhere, *left lower leg*

    M90.869 Osteopathy in diseases classified elsewhere, unspecified lower leg ▽

☑6ᵗʰ **M90.87** Osteopathy in diseases classified elsewhere, ankle and foot

    M90.871 Osteopathy in diseases classified elsewhere, *right ankle and foot*

    M90.872 Osteopathy in diseases classified elsewhere, *left ankle and foot*

    M90.879 Osteopathy in diseases classified elsewhere, unspecified ankle and foot ▽

M90.88 Osteopathy in diseases classified elsewhere, other site

M90.89 Osteopathy in diseases classified elsewhere, *multiple sites*

Chondropathies (M91-M94)

EXCLUDES 1   postprocedural chondropathies (M96.-)

☑4ᵗʰ **M91 Juvenile osteochondrosis of hip and pelvis**
EXCLUDES 1   slipped upper femoral epiphysis (nontraumatic) (M93.0)

M91.0 Juvenile osteochondrosis of pelvis
Osteochondrosis (juvenile) of acetabulum
Osteochondrosis (juvenile) of iliac crest [Buchanan]
Osteochondrosis (juvenile) of ischiopubic synchondrosis [van Neck]
Osteochondrosis (juvenile) of symphysis pubis [Pierson]

✓5ᵗʰ **M91.1** **Juvenile osteochondrosis of** head of femur **[Legg-Calvé-Perthes]**

     M91.10 Juvenile osteochondrosis of head of femur [Legg-Calvé-Perthes], unspecified leg ▽

     M91.11 Juvenile osteochondrosis of head of femur [Legg-Calvé-Perthes], right leg

     M91.12 Juvenile osteochondrosis of head of femur [Legg-Calvé-Perthes], left leg

✓5ᵗʰ **M91.2** Coxa plana
     Hip deformity due to previous juvenile osteochondrosis

     M91.20 Coxa plana, unspecified hip ▽

     M91.21 Coxa plana, right hip

     M91.22 Coxa plana, left hip

✓5ᵗʰ **M91.3** Pseudocoxalgia

     M91.30 Pseudocoxalgia, unspecified hip ▽

     M91.31 Pseudocoxalgia, right hip

     M91.32 Pseudocoxalgia, left hip

✓5ᵗʰ **M91.4** Coxa magna

     M91.40 Coxa magna, unspecified hip ▽

     M91.41 Coxa magna, right hip

     M91.42 Coxa magna, left hip

✓5ᵗʰ **M91.8** **Other juvenile osteochondrosis of hip and pelvis**
     Juvenile osteochondrosis after reduction of congenital dislocation of hip

     M91.80 Other juvenile osteochondrosis of hip and pelvis, unspecified leg ▽

     M91.81 Other juvenile osteochondrosis of hip and pelvis, right leg

     M91.82 Other juvenile osteochondrosis of hip and pelvis, left leg

✓5ᵗʰ **M91.9** **Juvenile osteochondrosis of hip and pelvis, unspecified**

     M91.90 Juvenile osteochondrosis of hip and pelvis, unspecified, unspecified leg ▽

     M91.91 Juvenile osteochondrosis of hip and pelvis, unspecified, right leg ▽

     M91.92 Juvenile osteochondrosis of hip and pelvis, unspecified, left leg ▽

✓4ᵗʰ **M92** **Other juvenile osteochondrosis**

✓5ᵗʰ **M92.0** **Juvenile osteochondrosis of** humerus
     Osteochondrosis (juvenile) of capitulum of humerus [Panner]
     Osteochondrosis (juvenile) of head of humerus [Haas]

     M92.00 Juvenile osteochondrosis of humerus, unspecified arm ▽

     M92.01 Juvenile osteochondrosis of humerus, right arm

     M92.02 Juvenile osteochondrosis of humerus, left arm

✓5ᵗʰ **M92.1** **Juvenile osteochondrosis of** radius and ulna
     Osteochondrosis (juvenile) of lower ulna [Burns]
     Osteochondrosis (juvenile) of radial head [Brailsford]

     M92.10 Juvenile osteochondrosis of radius and ulna, unspecified arm ▽

     M92.11 Juvenile osteochondrosis of radius and ulna, right arm

     M92.12 Juvenile osteochondrosis of radius and ulna, left arm

✓5ᵗʰ **M92.2** **Juvenile osteochondrosis,** hand

     ✓6ᵗʰ **M92.20** Unspecified juvenile osteochondrosis, hand

         M92.201 Unspecified juvenile osteochondrosis, right hand ▽

         M92.202 Unspecified juvenile osteochondrosis, left hand ▽

         M92.209 Unspecified juvenile osteochondrosis, unspecified hand ▽

     ✓6ᵗʰ **M92.21** Osteochondrosis (juvenile) of carpal lunate [Kienböck]

         M92.211 Osteochondrosis (juvenile) of carpal lunate [Kienböck], right hand

         M92.212 Osteochondrosis (juvenile) of carpal lunate [Kienböck], left hand

         M92.219 Osteochondrosis (juvenile) of carpal lunate [Kienböck], unspecified hand ▽

     ✓6ᵗʰ **M92.22** Osteochondrosis (juvenile) of metacarpal heads [Mauclaire]

         M92.221 Osteochondrosis (juvenile) of metacarpal heads [Mauclaire], right hand

         M92.222 Osteochondrosis (juvenile) of metacarpal heads [Mauclaire], left hand

         M92.229 Osteochondrosis (juvenile) of metacarpal heads [Mauclaire], unspecified hand ▽

     ✓6ᵗʰ **M92.29** Other juvenile osteochondrosis, hand

         M92.291 Other juvenile osteochondrosis, right hand

         M92.292 Other juvenile osteochondrosis, left hand

         M92.299 Other juvenile osteochondrosis, unspecified hand ▽

✓5ᵗʰ **M92.3** **Other juvenile osteochondrosis,** upper limb

     M92.30 Other juvenile osteochondrosis, unspecified upper limb ▽

     M92.31 Other juvenile osteochondrosis, right upper limb

     M92.32 Other juvenile osteochondrosis, left upper limb

✓5ᵗʰ **M92.4** **Juvenile osteochondrosis of** patella
     Osteochondrosis (juvenile) of primary patellar center [Köhler]
     Osteochondrosis (juvenile) of secondary patellar centre [Sinding Larsen]

     M92.40 Juvenile osteochondrosis of patella, unspecified knee ▽

     M92.41 Juvenile osteochondrosis of patella, right knee

     M92.42 Juvenile osteochondrosis of patella, left knee

✓5ᵗʰ **M92.5** **Juvenile osteochondrosis of** tibia and fibula
     Osteochondrosis (juvenile) of proximal tibia [Blount]
     Osteochondrosis (juvenile) of tibial tubercle [Osgood-Schlatter]
     Tibia vara

     M92.50 Juvenile osteochondrosis of tibia and fibula, unspecified leg ▽

     M92.51 Juvenile osteochondrosis of tibia and fibula, right leg

     M92.52 Juvenile osteochondrosis of tibia and fibula, left leg

✓5ᵗʰ **M92.6** **Juvenile osteochondrosis of** tarsus
     Osteochondrosis (juvenile) of calcaneum [Sever]
     Osteochondrosis (juvenile) of os tibiale externum [Haglund]
     Osteochondrosis (juvenile) of talus [Diaz]
     Osteochondrosis (juvenile) of tarsal navicular [Köhler]

     M92.60 Juvenile osteochondrosis of tarsus, unspecified ankle ▽

     M92.61 Juvenile osteochondrosis of tarsus, right ankle

     M92.62 Juvenile osteochondrosis of tarsus, left ankle

✓5ᵗʰ **M92.7** **Juvenile osteochondrosis of** metatarsus
     Osteochondrosis (juvenile) of fifth metatarsus [Iselin]
     Osteochondrosis (juvenile) of second metatarsus [Freiberg]

     M92.70 Juvenile osteochondrosis of metatarsus, unspecified foot ▽

     M92.71 Juvenile osteochondrosis of metatarsus, right foot

     M92.72 Juvenile osteochondrosis of metatarsus, left foot

     M92.8 **Other specified juvenile osteochondrosis**
     Calcaneal apophysitis

     M92.9 **Juvenile osteochondrosis, unspecified** ▽
     Juvenile apophysitis NOS
     Juvenile epiphysitis NOS
     Juvenile osteochondritis NOS
     Juvenile osteochondrosis NOS

✓4ᵗʰ **M93** **Other osteochondropathies**
     EXCLUDES 2 osteochondrosis of spine (M42.-)

✓5ᵗʰ **M93.0** **Slipped upper femoral epiphysis (nontraumatic)**
     Use additional code for associated chondrolysis (M94.3)

     ✓6ᵗʰ **M93.00** Unspecified slipped upper femoral epiphysis (nontraumatic)

         M93.001 Unspecified slipped upper femoral epiphysis (nontraumatic), right hip ▽

         M93.002 Unspecified slipped upper femoral epiphysis (nontraumatic), left hip ▽

         M93.003 Unspecified slipped upper femoral epiphysis (nontraumatic), unspecified hip ▽

     ✓6ᵗʰ **M93.01** Acute slipped upper femoral epiphysis (nontraumatic)

         M93.011 Acute slipped upper femoral epiphysis (nontraumatic), right hip

         M93.012 Acute slipped upper femoral epiphysis (nontraumatic), left hip

         M93.013 Acute slipped upper femoral epiphysis (nontraumatic), unspecified hip ▽

EXCLUDES 1 Not coded here   *EXCLUDES 2* Not included here   N Newborn Age: 0   P Pediatric Age: 0-17   M Maternity Age: 12-55   A Adult Age: 15-124

794   ICD-10-CM 2018

✓6th **M93.02** Chronic slipped upper femoral epiphysis (nontraumatic)

    M93.021 Chronic slipped upper femoral epiphysis (nontraumatic), right hip

    M93.022 Chronic slipped upper femoral epiphysis (nontraumatic), left hip

    M93.023 Chronic slipped upper femoral epiphysis (nontraumatic), unspecified hip ▽

✓6th **M93.03** Acute on chronic slipped upper femoral epiphysis (nontraumatic)

    M93.031 Acute on chronic slipped upper femoral epiphysis (nontraumatic), right hip

    M93.032 Acute on chronic slipped upper femoral epiphysis (nontraumatic), left hip

    M93.033 Acute on chronic slipped upper femoral epiphysis (nontraumatic), unspecified hip ▽

M93.1 Kienböck's disease of adults   △

    Adult osteochondrosis of carpal lunates

✓5th **M93.2** Osteochondritis dissecans

    M93.20 Osteochondritis dissecans of unspecified site ▽

  ✓6th **M93.21** Osteochondritis dissecans of shoulder

    M93.211 Osteochondritis dissecans, right shoulder

    M93.212 Osteochondritis dissecans, left shoulder

    M93.219 Osteochondritis dissecans, unspecified shoulder ▽

  ✓6th **M93.22** Osteochondritis dissecans of elbow

    M93.221 Osteochondritis dissecans, right elbow

    M93.222 Osteochondritis dissecans, left elbow

    M93.229 Osteochondritis dissecans, unspecified elbow ▽

  ✓6th **M93.23** Osteochondritis dissecans of wrist

    M93.231 Osteochondritis dissecans, right wrist

    M93.232 Osteochondritis dissecans, left wrist

    M93.239 Osteochondritis dissecans, unspecified wrist ▽

  ✓6th **M93.24** Osteochondritis dissecans of joints of hand

    M93.241 Osteochondritis dissecans, joints of right hand

    M93.242 Osteochondritis dissecans, joints of left hand

    M93.249 Osteochondritis dissecans, joints of unspecified hand ▽

  ✓6th **M93.25** Osteochondritis dissecans of hip

    M93.251 Osteochondritis dissecans, right hip

    M93.252 Osteochondritis dissecans, left hip

    M93.259 Osteochondritis dissecans, unspecified hip ▽

  ✓6th **M93.26** Osteochondritis dissecans knee

    M93.261 Osteochondritis dissecans, right knee

    M93.262 Osteochondritis dissecans, left knee

    M93.269 Osteochondritis dissecans, unspecified knee ▽

  ✓6th **M93.27** Osteochondritis dissecans of ankle and joints of foot

    M93.271 Osteochondritis dissecans, right ankle and joints of right foot

    M93.272 Osteochondritis dissecans, left ankle and joints of left foot

    M93.279 Osteochondritis dissecans, unspecified ankle and joints of foot ▽

    M93.28 Osteochondritis dissecans other site

    M93.29 Osteochondritis dissecans multiple sites

✓5th **M93.8** Other specified osteochondropathies

    M93.80 Other specified osteochondropathies of unspecified site ▽

  ✓6th **M93.81** Other specified osteochondropathies of shoulder

    M93.811 Other specified osteochondropathies, right shoulder

    M93.812 Other specified osteochondropathies, left shoulder

    M93.819 Other specified osteochondropathies, unspecified shoulder ▽

  ✓6th **M93.82** Other specified osteochondropathies of upper arm

    M93.821 Other specified osteochondropathies, right upper arm

    M93.822 Other specified osteochondropathies, left upper arm

    M93.829 Other specified osteochondropathies, unspecified upper arm ▽

  ✓6th **M93.83** Other specified osteochondropathies of forearm

    M93.831 Other specified osteochondropathies, right forearm

    M93.832 Other specified osteochondropathies, left forearm

    M93.839 Other specified osteochondropathies, unspecified forearm ▽

  ✓6th **M93.84** Other specified osteochondropathies of hand

    M93.841 Other specified osteochondropathies, right hand

    M93.842 Other specified osteochondropathies, left hand

    M93.849 Other specified osteochondropathies, unspecified hand ▽

  ✓6th **M93.85** Other specified osteochondropathies of thigh

    M93.851 Other specified osteochondropathies, right thigh

    M93.852 Other specified osteochondropathies, left thigh

    M93.859 Other specified osteochondropathies, unspecified thigh ▽

  ✓6th **M93.86** Other specified osteochondropathies lower leg

    M93.861 Other specified osteochondropathies, right lower leg

    M93.862 Other specified osteochondropathies, left lower leg

    M93.869 Other specified osteochondropathies, unspecified lower leg ▽

  ✓6th **M93.87** Other specified osteochondropathies of ankle and foot

    M93.871 Other specified osteochondropathies, right ankle and foot

    M93.872 Other specified osteochondropathies, left ankle and foot

    M93.879 Other specified osteochondropathies, unspecified ankle and foot ▽

    M93.88 Other specified osteochondropathies other site

    M93.89 Other specified osteochondropathies multiple sites

✓5th **M93.9** Osteochondropathy, unspecified

    Apophysitis NOS   Osteochondritis NOS

    Epiphysitis NOS   Osteochondrosis NOS

    M93.90 Osteochondropathy, unspecified of unspecified site ▽

  ✓6th **M93.91** Osteochondropathy, unspecified of shoulder

    M93.911 Osteochondropathy, unspecified, right shoulder ▽

    M93.912 Osteochondropathy, unspecified, left shoulder ▽

    M93.919 Osteochondropathy, unspecified, unspecified shoulder ▽

  ✓6th **M93.92** Osteochondropathy, unspecified of upper arm

    M93.921 Osteochondropathy, unspecified, right upper arm ▽

    M93.922 Osteochondropathy, unspecified, left upper arm ▽

    M93.929 Osteochondropathy, unspecified, unspecified upper arm ▽

  ✓6th **M93.93** Osteochondropathy, unspecified of forearm

    M93.931 Osteochondropathy, unspecified, right forearm ▽

    M93.932 Osteochondropathy, unspecified, left forearm ▽

    M93.939 Osteochondropathy, unspecified, unspecified forearm ▽

  ✓6th **M93.94** Osteochondropathy, unspecified of hand

    M93.941 Osteochondropathy, unspecified, right hand ▽

    M93.942 Osteochondropathy, unspecified, left hand ▽

    M93.949 Osteochondropathy, unspecified, unspecified hand ▽

☑ Additional Character Req   ✓x7th Placeholder Alert   Manifestation   HCC CMS-HCC Condition   ▽ Unspecified Code   ▶◀ Revised Text   ● New Code   ▲ Revised Code Title

✓6ᵗʰ **M93.95 Osteochondropathy, unspecified of thigh**
    M93.951 Osteochondropathy, unspecified, right thigh ▽
    M93.952 Osteochondropathy, unspecified, left thigh ▽
    M93.959 Osteochondropathy, unspecified, unspecified thigh ▽

✓6ᵗʰ **M93.96 Osteochondropathy, unspecified lower leg**
    M93.961 Osteochondropathy, unspecified, right lower leg ▽
    M93.962 Osteochondropathy, unspecified, left lower leg ▽
    M93.969 Osteochondropathy, unspecified, unspecified lower leg ▽

✓6ᵗʰ **M93.97 Osteochondropathy, unspecified of ankle and foot**
    M93.971 Osteochondropathy, unspecified, right ankle and foot ▽
    M93.972 Osteochondropathy, unspecified, left ankle and foot ▽
    M93.979 Osteochondropathy, unspecified, unspecified ankle and foot ▽

M93.98 Osteochondropathy, unspecified other site ▽
M93.99 Osteochondropathy, unspecified multiple sites ▽

✓4ᵗʰ **M94 Other disorders of cartilage**

M94.0 Chondrocostal junction syndrome [Tietze]
    Costochondritis

M94.1 Relapsing polychondritis

✓5ᵗʰ **M94.2 Chondromalacia**
    EXCLUDES 1 chondromalacia patellae (M22.4)

    M94.20 Chondromalacia, unspecified site ▽

    ✓6ᵗʰ **M94.21 Chondromalacia, shoulder**
        M94.211 Chondromalacia, right shoulder
        M94.212 Chondromalacia, left shoulder
        M94.219 Chondromalacia, unspecified shoulder ▽

    ✓6ᵗʰ **M94.22 Chondromalacia, elbow**
        M94.221 Chondromalacia, right elbow
        M94.222 Chondromalacia, left elbow
        M94.229 Chondromalacia, unspecified elbow ▽

    ✓6ᵗʰ **M94.23 Chondromalacia, wrist**
        M94.231 Chondromalacia, right wrist
        M94.232 Chondromalacia, left wrist
        M94.239 Chondromalacia, unspecified wrist ▽

    ✓6ᵗʰ **M94.24 Chondromalacia, joints of hand**
        M94.241 Chondromalacia, joints of right hand
        M94.242 Chondromalacia, joints of left hand
        M94.249 Chondromalacia, joints of unspecified hand ▽

    ✓6ᵗʰ **M94.25 Chondromalacia, hip**
        M94.251 Chondromalacia, right hip
        M94.252 Chondromalacia, left hip
        M94.259 Chondromalacia, unspecified hip ▽

    ✓6ᵗʰ **M94.26 Chondromalacia, knee**
        M94.261 Chondromalacia, right knee
        M94.262 Chondromalacia, left knee
        M94.269 Chondromalacia, unspecified knee ▽

    ✓6ᵗʰ **M94.27 Chondromalacia, ankle and joints of foot**
        M94.271 Chondromalacia, right ankle and joints of right foot
        M94.272 Chondromalacia, left ankle and joints of left foot
        M94.279 Chondromalacia, unspecified ankle and joints of foot ▽

    M94.28 Chondromalacia, other site
    M94.29 Chondromalacia, multiple sites

✓5ᵗʰ **M94.3 Chondrolysis**
    Code first any associated slipped upper femoral epiphysis (nontraumatic) (M93.0-)

    ✓6ᵗʰ **M94.35 Chondrolysis, hip**
        M94.351 Chondrolysis, right hip
        M94.352 Chondrolysis, left hip
        M94.359 Chondrolysis, unspecified hip ▽

✓5ᵗʰ **M94.8 Other specified disorders of cartilage**

    ✓6ᵗʰ **M94.8X Other specified disorders of cartilage**
        M94.8X0 Other specified disorders of cartilage, multiple sites
        M94.8X1 Other specified disorders of cartilage, shoulder
        M94.8X2 Other specified disorders of cartilage, upper arm
        M94.8X3 Other specified disorders of cartilage, forearm
        M94.8X4 Other specified disorders of cartilage, hand
        M94.8X5 Other specified disorders of cartilage, thigh
        M94.8X6 Other specified disorders of cartilage, lower leg
        M94.8X7 Other specified disorders of cartilage, ankle and foot
        M94.8X8 Other specified disorders of cartilage, other site
        M94.8X9 Other specified disorders of cartilage, unspecified sites ▽

M94.9 Disorder of cartilage, unspecified ▽

Other disorders of the musculoskeletal system and connective tissue (M95)

✓4ᵗʰ **M95 Other acquired deformities of musculoskeletal system and connective tissue**
    EXCLUDES 2 acquired absence of limbs and organs (Z89-Z90)
        acquired deformities of limbs (M20-M21)
        congenital malformations and deformations of the musculoskeletal system (Q65-Q79)
        deforming dorsopathies (M40-M43)
        dentofacial anomalies [including malocclusion] (M26.-)
        postprocedural musculoskeletal disorders (M96.-)

    M95.0 Acquired deformity of nose
        EXCLUDES 2 deviated nasal septum (J34.2)

    ✓5ᵗʰ **M95.1 Cauliflower ear**
        EXCLUDES 2 other acquired deformities of ear (H61.1)
        DEF: Acquired deformity of the external ear; due to injury, subsequent perichondritis.

        M95.10 Cauliflower ear, unspecified ear ▽
        M95.11 Cauliflower ear, right ear
        M95.12 Cauliflower ear, left ear

    M95.2 Other acquired deformity of head
    M95.3 Acquired deformity of neck
    M95.4 Acquired deformity of chest and rib
        AHA: 2014, 4Q, 26-27
    M95.5 Acquired deformity of pelvis
        EXCLUDES 1 maternal care for known or suspected disproportion (O33.-)

    M95.8 Other specified acquired deformities of musculoskeletal system
    M95.9 Acquired deformity of musculoskeletal system, unspecified ▽

Intraoperative and postprocedural complications and disorders of musculoskeletal system, not elsewhere classified (M96)

✓4ᵗʰ **M96 Intraoperative and postprocedural complications and disorders of musculoskeletal system, not elsewhere classified**
    EXCLUDES 2 arthropathy following intestinal bypass (M02.0-)
        complications of internal orthopedic prosthetic devices, implants and grafts (T84.-)
        disorders associated with osteoporosis (M80)
        periprosthetic fracture around internal prosthetic joint (M97.-)
        presence of functional implants and other devices (Z96-Z97)

    M96.0 Pseudarthrosis after fusion or arthrodesis
    M96.1 Postlaminectomy syndrome, not elsewhere classified
    M96.2 Postradiation kyphosis
    M96.3 Postlaminectomy kyphosis
    M96.4 Postsurgical lordosis
    M96.5 Postradiation scoliosis

EXCLUDES 1 Not coded here   *EXCLUDES 2* Not included here   N Newborn Age: 0   P Pediatric Age: 0-17   M Maternity Age: 12-55   A Adult Age: 15-124

796   ICD-10-CM 2018

✓5ᵗʰ **M96.6 Fracture of bone following insertion of orthopedic implant, joint prosthesis, or bone plate**
    Intraoperative fracture of bone during insertion of orthopedic implant, joint prosthesis, or bone plate
    EXCLUDES 2   complication of internal orthopedic devices, implants or grafts (T84.-)

   ✓6ᵗʰ **M96.62 Fracture of humerus following insertion of orthopedic implant, joint prosthesis, or bone plate**

     M96.621 Fracture of humerus following insertion of orthopedic implant, joint prosthesis, or bone plate, right arm   HCC

     M96.622 Fracture of humerus following insertion of orthopedic implant, joint prosthesis, or bone plate, left arm   HCC

     M96.629 Fracture of humerus following insertion of orthopedic implant, joint prosthesis, or bone plate, unspecified arm   HCC ▽

   ✓6ᵗʰ **M96.63 Fracture of radius or ulna following insertion of orthopedic implant, joint prosthesis, or bone plate**

     M96.631 Fracture of radius or ulna following insertion of orthopedic implant, joint prosthesis, or bone plate, right arm   HCC

     M96.632 Fracture of radius or ulna following insertion of orthopedic implant, joint prosthesis, or bone plate, left arm   HCC

     M96.639 Fracture of radius or ulna following insertion of orthopedic implant, joint prosthesis, or bone plate, unspecified arm   HCC ▽

   M96.65 Fracture of pelvis following insertion of orthopedic implant, joint prosthesis, or bone plate   HCC

   ✓6ᵗʰ **M96.66 Fracture of femur following insertion of orthopedic implant, joint prosthesis, or bone plate**

     M96.661 Fracture of femur following insertion of orthopedic implant, joint prosthesis, or bone plate, right leg   HCC

     M96.662 Fracture of femur following insertion of orthopedic implant, joint prosthesis, or bone plate, left leg   HCC

     M96.669 Fracture of femur following insertion of orthopedic implant, joint prosthesis, or bone plate, unspecified leg   HCC ▽

   ✓6ᵗʰ **M96.67 Fracture of tibia or fibula following insertion of orthopedic implant, joint prosthesis, or bone plate**

     M96.671 Fracture of tibia or fibula following insertion of orthopedic implant, joint prosthesis, or bone plate, right leg   HCC

     M96.672 Fracture of tibia or fibula following insertion of orthopedic implant, joint prosthesis, or bone plate, left leg   HCC

     M96.679 Fracture of tibia or fibula following insertion of orthopedic implant, joint prosthesis, or bone plate, unspecified leg   HCC ▽

   M96.69 Fracture of other bone following insertion of orthopedic implant, joint prosthesis, or bone plate   HCC

✓5ᵗʰ **M96.8 Other intraoperative and postprocedural complications and disorders of musculoskeletal system, not elsewhere classified**

   ✓6ᵗʰ **M96.81 Intraoperative hemorrhage and hematoma of a musculoskeletal structure complicating a procedure**
    EXCLUDES 1   intraoperative hemorrhage and hematoma of a musculoskeletal structure due to accidental puncture and laceration during a procedure (M96.82-)

     M96.810 Intraoperative hemorrhage and hematoma of a musculoskeletal structure complicating a musculoskeletal system procedure

     M96.811 Intraoperative hemorrhage and hematoma of a musculoskeletal structure complicating other procedure

   ✓6ᵗʰ **M96.82 Accidental puncture and laceration of a musculoskeletal structure during a procedure**

     M96.820 Accidental puncture and laceration of a musculoskeletal structure during a musculoskeletal system procedure

     M96.821 Accidental puncture and laceration of a musculoskeletal structure during other procedure

   ✓6ᵗʰ **M96.83 Postprocedural hemorrhage of a musculoskeletal structure following a procedure**

     M96.830 Postprocedural hemorrhage of a musculoskeletal structure following a musculoskeletal system procedure

     M96.831 Postprocedural hemorrhage of a musculoskeletal structure following other procedure

   ✓6ᵗʰ **M96.84 Postprocedural hematoma and seroma of a musculoskeletal structure following a procedure**

     M96.840 Postprocedural hematoma of a musculoskeletal structure following a musculoskeletal system procedure

     M96.841 Postprocedural hematoma of a musculoskeletal structure following other procedure

     M96.842 Postprocedural seroma of a musculoskeletal structure following a musculoskeletal system procedure

     M96.843 Postprocedural seroma of a musculoskeletal structure following other procedure

   M96.89 Other intraoperative and postprocedural complications and disorders of the musculoskeletal system
    Instability of joint secondary to removal of joint prosthesis
    Use additional code, if applicable, to further specify disorder

Periprosthetic fracture around internal prosthetic joint (M97)

✓4ᵗʰ **M97 Periprosthetic fracture around internal prosthetic joint**
    EXCLUDES 2   breakage (fracture) of prosthetic joint (T84.01-)
    fracture of bone following insertion of orthopedic implant, joint prosthesis or bone plate (M96.6-)

> The appropriate 7th character is to be added to each code from category M97.
> A   initial encounter
> D   subsequent encounter
> S   sequela

✓5ᵗʰ **M97.0 Periprosthetic fracture around internal prosthetic hip joint**

   [1] ✓x7ᵗʰ **M97.01** Periprosthetic fracture around internal prosthetic right hip joint   HCC

   [1] ✓x7ᵗʰ **M97.02** Periprosthetic fracture around internal prosthetic left hip joint   HCC

✓5ᵗʰ **M97.1 Periprosthetic fracture around internal prosthetic knee joint**

   ✓x7ᵗʰ **M97.11** Periprosthetic fracture around internal prosthetic right knee joint

   ✓x7ᵗʰ **M97.12** Periprosthetic fracture around internal prosthetic left knee joint

✓5ᵗʰ **M97.2 Periprosthetic fracture around internal prosthetic ankle joint**

   ✓x7ᵗʰ **M97.21** Periprosthetic fracture around internal prosthetic right ankle joint

   ✓x7ᵗʰ **M97.22** Periprosthetic fracture around internal prosthetic left ankle joint

✓5ᵗʰ **M97.3 Periprosthetic fracture around internal prosthetic shoulder joint**

   ✓x7ᵗʰ **M97.31** Periprosthetic fracture around internal prosthetic right shoulder joint

   ✓x7ᵗʰ **M97.32** Periprosthetic fracture around internal prosthetic left shoulder joint

✓5ᵗʰ **M97.4 Periprosthetic fracture around internal prosthetic elbow joint**

   ✓x7ᵗʰ **M97.41** Periprosthetic fracture around internal prosthetic right elbow joint

   ✓x7ᵗʰ **M97.42** Periprosthetic fracture around internal prosthetic left elbow joint

✓x7ᵗʰ **M97.8 Periprosthetic fracture around other internal prosthetic joint**
    Periprosthetic fracture around internal prosthetic finger joint
    Periprosthetic fracture around internal prosthetic spinal joint
    Periprosthetic fracture around internal prosthetic toe joint
    Periprosthetic fracture around internal prosthetic wrist joint
    Use additional code to identify the joint (Z96.6-)

✓x7ᵗʰ **M97.9 Periprosthetic fracture around unspecified internal prosthetic joint** ▽

---

[1]   HCC with 7th character indicating initial encounter (A, B or C - specific to category).

☑ Additional Character Req   ✓x7ᵗʰ Placeholder Alert   Manifestation   HCC CMS-HCC Condition   ▽ Unspecified Code   ▶◀ Revised Text   ● New Code   ▲ Revised Code Title

Biomechanical lesions, not elsewhere classified (M99)

✓4ᵗʰ M99   Biomechanical lesions, not elsewhere classified
> **NOTE**   This category should not be used if the condition can be classified elsewhere.

✓5ᵗʰ   M99.0   Segmental and somatic dysfunction
- M99.00   Segmental and somatic dysfunction of head region
- M99.01   Segmental and somatic dysfunction of cervical region
- M99.02   Segmental and somatic dysfunction of thoracic region
- M99.03   Segmental and somatic dysfunction of lumbar region
- M99.04   Segmental and somatic dysfunction of sacral region
- M99.05   Segmental and somatic dysfunction of pelvic region
- M99.06   Segmental and somatic dysfunction of lower extremity
- M99.07   Segmental and somatic dysfunction of upper extremity
- M99.08   Segmental and somatic dysfunction of rib cage
- M99.09   Segmental and somatic dysfunction of abdomen and other regions

✓5ᵗʰ   M99.1   Subluxation complex (vertebral)
- M99.10   Subluxation complex (vertebral) of head region
- M99.11   Subluxation complex (vertebral) of cervical region
- M99.12   Subluxation complex (vertebral) of thoracic region
- M99.13   Subluxation complex (vertebral) of lumbar region
- M99.14   Subluxation complex (vertebral) of sacral region
- M99.15   Subluxation complex (vertebral) of pelvic region
- M99.16   Subluxation complex (vertebral) of lower extremity
- M99.17   Subluxation complex (vertebral) of upper extremity
- M99.18   Subluxation complex (vertebral) of rib cage
- M99.19   Subluxation complex (vertebral) of abdomen and other regions

✓5ᵗʰ   M99.2   Subluxation stenosis of neural canal
- M99.20   Subluxation stenosis of neural canal of head region
- M99.21   Subluxation stenosis of neural canal of cervical region
- M99.22   Subluxation stenosis of neural canal of thoracic region
- M99.23   Subluxation stenosis of neural canal of lumbar region
- M99.24   Subluxation stenosis of neural canal of sacral region
- M99.25   Subluxation stenosis of neural canal of pelvic region
- M99.26   Subluxation stenosis of neural canal of lower extremity
- M99.27   Subluxation stenosis of neural canal of upper extremity
- M99.28   Subluxation stenosis of neural canal of rib cage
- M99.29   Subluxation stenosis of neural canal of abdomen and other regions

✓5ᵗʰ   M99.3   Osseous stenosis of neural canal
- M99.30   Osseous stenosis of neural canal of head region
- M99.31   Osseous stenosis of neural canal of cervical region
- M99.32   Osseous stenosis of neural canal of thoracic region
- M99.33   Osseous stenosis of neural canal of lumbar region
- M99.34   Osseous stenosis of neural canal of sacral region
- M99.35   Osseous stenosis of neural canal of pelvic region
- M99.36   Osseous stenosis of neural canal of lower extremity
- M99.37   Osseous stenosis of neural canal of upper extremity
- M99.38   Osseous stenosis of neural canal of rib cage
- M99.39   Osseous stenosis of neural canal of abdomen and other regions

✓5ᵗʰ   M99.4   Connective tissue stenosis of neural canal
- M99.40   Connective tissue stenosis of neural canal of head region
- M99.41   Connective tissue stenosis of neural canal of cervical region
- M99.42   Connective tissue stenosis of neural canal of thoracic region
- M99.43   Connective tissue stenosis of neural canal of lumbar region
- M99.44   Connective tissue stenosis of neural canal of sacral region
- M99.45   Connective tissue stenosis of neural canal of pelvic region
- M99.46   Connective tissue stenosis of neural canal of lower extremity
- M99.47   Connective tissue stenosis of neural canal of upper extremity
- M99.48   Connective tissue stenosis of neural canal of rib cage
- M99.49   Connective tissue stenosis of neural canal of abdomen and other regions

✓5ᵗʰ   M99.5   Intervertebral disc stenosis of neural canal
- M99.50   Intervertebral disc stenosis of neural canal of head region
- M99.51   Intervertebral disc stenosis of neural canal of cervical region
- M99.52   Intervertebral disc stenosis of neural canal of thoracic region
- M99.53   Intervertebral disc stenosis of neural canal of lumbar region
- M99.54   Intervertebral disc stenosis of neural canal of sacral region
- M99.55   Intervertebral disc stenosis of neural canal of pelvic region
- M99.56   Intervertebral disc stenosis of neural canal of lower extremity
- M99.57   Intervertebral disc stenosis of neural canal of upper extremity
- M99.58   Intervertebral disc stenosis of neural canal of rib cage
- M99.59   Intervertebral disc stenosis of neural canal of abdomen and other regions

✓5ᵗʰ   M99.6   Osseous and subluxation stenosis of intervertebral foramina
- M99.60   Osseous and subluxation stenosis of intervertebral foramina of head region
- M99.61   Osseous and subluxation stenosis of intervertebral foramina of cervical region
- M99.62   Osseous and subluxation stenosis of intervertebral foramina of thoracic region
- M99.63   Osseous and subluxation stenosis of intervertebral foramina of lumbar region
- M99.64   Osseous and subluxation stenosis of intervertebral foramina of sacral region
- M99.65   Osseous and subluxation stenosis of intervertebral foramina of pelvic region
- M99.66   Osseous and subluxation stenosis of intervertebral foramina of lower extremity
- M99.67   Osseous and subluxation stenosis of intervertebral foramina of upper extremity
- M99.68   Osseous and subluxation stenosis of intervertebral foramina of rib cage
- M99.69   Osseous and subluxation stenosis of intervertebral foramina of abdomen and other regions

✓5ᵗʰ   M99.7   Connective tissue and disc stenosis of intervertebral foramina
- M99.70   Connective tissue and disc stenosis of intervertebral foramina of head region
- M99.71   Connective tissue and disc stenosis of intervertebral foramina of cervical region
- M99.72   Connective tissue and disc stenosis of intervertebral foramina of thoracic region
- M99.73   Connective tissue and disc stenosis of intervertebral foramina of lumbar region
- M99.74   Connective tissue and disc stenosis of intervertebral foramina of sacral region
- M99.75   Connective tissue and disc stenosis of intervertebral foramina of pelvic region

EXCLUDES 1 Not coded here   EXCLUDES 2 Not included here   N Newborn Age: 0   P Pediatric Age: 0-17   M Maternity Age: 12-55   A Adult Age: 15-124

798   ICD-10-CM 2018

M99.76 **Connective tissue and disc stenosis of intervertebral foramina of** lower extremity

M99.77 **Connective tissue and disc stenosis of intervertebral foramina of** upper extremity

M99.78 **Connective tissue and disc stenosis of intervertebral foramina of** rib cage

M99.79 **Connective tissue and disc stenosis of intervertebral foramina of** abdomen and other regions

 M99.8 Other biomechanical lesions

M99.80 **Other biomechanical lesions of** head region

M99.81 **Other biomechanical lesions of** cervical region

M99.82 **Other biomechanical lesions of** thoracic region

M99.83 **Other biomechanical lesions of** lumbar region

M99.84 **Other biomechanical lesions of** sacral region

M99.85 **Other biomechanical lesions of** pelvic region

M99.86 **Other biomechanical lesions of** lower extremity

M99.87 **Other biomechanical lesions of** upper extremity

M99.88 **Other biomechanical lesions of** rib cage

M99.89 **Other biomechanical lesions of** abdomen and other regions

M99.9 **Biomechanical lesion, unspecified** ▽

☑ Additional Character Req   Placeholder Alert   Manifestation   HCC CMS-HCC Condition   ▽ Unspecified Code   ▶◀ Revised Text   ● New Code   ▲ Revised Code Title

Chapter 14. Diseases of Genitourinary System (N00–N99)

Chapter Specific Guidelines with Coding Examples

The chapter specific guidelines from the ICD-10-CM Official Guidelines for Coding and Reporting have been provided below. Along with these guidelines are coding examples, contained in the shaded boxes, that have been developed to help illustrate the coding and/or sequencing guidance found in these guidelines.

a. Chronic kidney disease

1) Stages of chronic kidney disease (CKD)

The ICD-10-CM classifies CKD based on severity. The severity of CKD is designated by stages 1-5. Stage 2, code N18.2, equates to mild CKD; stage 3, code N18.3, equates to moderate CKD; and stage 4, code N18.4, equates to severe CKD. Code N18.6, End stage renal disease (ESRD), is assigned when the provider has documented end-stage-renal disease (ESRD).

If both a stage of CKD and ESRD are documented, assign code N18.6 only.

Stage 5 chronic kidney disease with ESRD requiring chronic dialysis

N18.6   **End stage renal disease**

Z99.2   **Dependence on renal dialysis**

Explanation: The diagnostic statement indicates the patient has chronic kidney disease, documented both as stage 5 and as ESRD requiring chronic dialysis. Code N18.6 End stage renal disease (ESRD), is assigned when the provider has documented end-stage-renal disease (ESRD). If both a stage of CKD and ESRD are documented, assign code N18.6 only.

---

2) Chronic kidney disease and kidney transplant status

Patients who have undergone kidney transplant may still have some form of chronic kidney disease (CKD) because the kidney transplant may not fully restore kidney function. Therefore, the presence of CKD alone does not constitute a transplant complication. Assign the appropriate N18 code for the patient's stage of CKD and code Z94.0, Kidney transplant status. If a transplant complication such as failure or rejection or other transplant complication is documented, see section I.C.19.g for information on coding complications of a kidney transplant. If the documentation is unclear as to whether the patient has a complication of the transplant, query the provider.

Patient with residual chronic kidney disease stage 1 after kidney transplant

N18.1   **Chronic kidney disease, stage 1**

Z94.0   **Kidney transplant status**

Explanation: Patients who have undergone kidney transplant may still have some form of chronic kidney disease (CKD) because the kidney transplant may not fully restore kidney function. The presence of CKD alone does not constitute a transplant complication. Assign the appropriate N18 code for the patient's stage of CKD and code Z94.0 Kidney transplant status.

---

3) Chronic kidney disease with other conditions

Patients with CKD may also suffer from other serious conditions, most commonly diabetes mellitus and hypertension. The sequencing of the CKD code in relationship to codes for other contributing conditions is based on the conventions in the Tabular List.

See I.C.9. Hypertensive chronic kidney disease.

See I.C.19. Chronic kidney disease and kidney transplant complications.

Type 1 diabetic chronic kidney disease, stage 2

E10.22   **Type 1 diabetes mellitus with diabetic chronic kidney disease**

N18.2   **Chronic kidney disease, stage 2 (mild)**

Explanation: Patients with CKD may also suffer from other serious conditions such as diabetes mellitus. The sequencing of the CKD code in relationship to codes for other contributing conditions is based on the conventions in the Tabular List. Diabetic CKD code E10.22 includes an instructional note to "Use additional code to identify stage of chronic kidney disease (N18.1–N18.6)," thus providing sequencing direction.

Chapter 14. Diseases of the Genitourinary System (N00-N99)

EXCLUDES 2   certain conditions originating in the perinatal period (P04-P96)
certain infectious and parasitic diseases (A00-B99)
complications of pregnancy, childbirth and the puerperium (O00-O9A)
congenital malformations, deformations and chromosomal abnormalities (Q00-Q99)
endocrine, nutritional and metabolic diseases (E00-E88)
injury, poisoning and certain other consequences of external causes (S00-T88)
neoplasms (C00-D49)
symptoms, signs and abnormal clinical and laboratory findings, not elsewhere classified (R00-R94)

This chapter contains the following blocks:

N00-N08   Glomerular diseases
N10-N16   Renal tubulo-interstitial diseases
N17-N19   Acute kidney failure and chronic kidney disease
N20-N23   Urolithiasis
N25-N29   Other disorders of kidney and ureter
N30-N39   Other diseases of the urinary system
N40-N53   Diseases of male genital organs
N60-N65   Disorders of breast
N70-N77   Inflammatory diseases of female pelvic organs
N80-N98   Noninflammatory disorders of female genital tract
N99   Intraoperative and postprocedural complications and disorders of genitourinary system, not elsewhere classified

Glomerular diseases (N00-N08)

Code also any associated kidney failure (N17-N19)
EXCLUDES 1   hypertensive chronic kidney disease (I12.-)

✓4th N00   Acute nephritic syndrome
    INCLUDES   acute glomerular disease
acute glomerulonephritis
acute nephritis
    EXCLUDES 1   acute tubulo-interstitial nephritis (N10)
nephritic syndrome NOS (N05.-)

  N00.0   Acute nephritic syndrome with minor glomerular abnormality
Acute nephritic syndrome with minimal change lesion

  N00.1   Acute nephritic syndrome with focal and segmental glomerular lesions
Acute nephritic syndrome with focal and segmental hyalinosis
Acute nephritic syndrome with focal and segmental sclerosis
Acute nephritic syndrome with focal glomerulonephritis

  N00.2   Acute nephritic syndrome with diffuse membranous glomerulonephritis

  N00.3   Acute nephritic syndrome with diffuse mesangial proliferative glomerulonephritis

  N00.4   Acute nephritic syndrome with diffuse endocapillary proliferative glomerulonephritis

  N00.5   Acute nephritic syndrome with diffuse mesangiocapillary glomerulonephritis
Acute nephritic syndrome with membranoproliferative glomerulonephritis, types 1 and 3, or NOS

  N00.6   Acute nephritic syndrome with dense deposit disease
Acute nephritic syndrome with membranoproliferative glomerulonephritis, type 2

  N00.7   Acute nephritic syndrome with diffuse crescentic glomerulonephritis
Acute nephritic syndrome with extracapillary glomerulonephritis

  N00.8   Acute nephritic syndrome with other morphologic changes
Acute nephritic syndrome with proliferative glomerulonephritis NOS

  N00.9   Acute nephritic syndrome with unspecified morphologic changes ▽

✓4th N01   Rapidly progressive nephritic syndrome
    INCLUDES   rapidly progressive glomerular disease
rapidly progressive glomerulonephritis
rapidly progressive nephritis
    EXCLUDES 1   nephritic syndrome NOS (N05.-)

  N01.0   Rapidly progressive nephritic syndrome with minor glomerular abnormality
Rapidly progressive nephritic syndrome with minimal change lesion

  N01.1   Rapidly progressive nephritic syndrome with focal and segmental glomerular lesions
Rapidly progressive nephritic syndrome with focal and segmental hyalinosis
Rapidly progressive nephritic syndrome with focal and segmental sclerosis
Rapidly progressive nephritic syndrome with focal glomerulonephritis

  N01.2   Rapidly progressive nephritic syndrome with diffuse membranous glomerulonephritis

  N01.3   Rapidly progressive nephritic syndrome with diffuse mesangial proliferative glomerulonephritis

  N01.4   Rapidly progressive nephritic syndrome with diffuse endocapillary proliferative glomerulonephritis

  N01.5   Rapidly progressive nephritic syndrome with diffuse mesangiocapillary glomerulonephritis
Rapidly progressive nephritic syndrome with membranoproliferative glomerulonephritis, types 1 and 3, or NOS

  N01.6   Rapidly progressive nephritic syndrome with dense deposit disease
Rapidly progressive nephritic syndrome with membranoproliferative glomerulonephritis, type 2

  N01.7   Rapidly progressive nephritic syndrome with diffuse crescentic glomerulonephritis
Rapidly progressive nephritic syndrome with extracapillary glomerulonephritis

  N01.8   Rapidly progressive nephritic syndrome with other morphologic changes
Rapidly progressive nephritic syndrome with proliferative glomerulonephritis NOS

  N01.9   Rapidly progressive nephritic syndrome with unspecified morphologic changes ▽

✓4th N02   Recurrent and persistent hematuria
    EXCLUDES 1   acute cystitis with hematuria (N30.01)
hematuria NOS (R31.9)
hematuria not associated with specified morphologic lesions (R31.-)

  N02.0   Recurrent and persistent hematuria with minor glomerular abnormality
Recurrent and persistent hematuria with minimal change lesion

  N02.1   Recurrent and persistent hematuria with focal and segmental glomerular lesions
Recurrent and persistent hematuria with focal and segmental hyalinosis
Recurrent and persistent hematuria with focal and segmental sclerosis
Recurrent and persistent hematuria with focal glomerulonephritis

  N02.2   Recurrent and persistent hematuria with diffuse membranous glomerulonephritis

  N02.3   Recurrent and persistent hematuria with diffuse mesangial proliferative glomerulonephritis

  N02.4   Recurrent and persistent hematuria with diffuse endocapillary proliferative glomerulonephritis

  N02.5   Recurrent and persistent hematuria with diffuse mesangiocapillary glomerulonephritis
Recurrent and persistent hematuria with membranoproliferative glomerulonephritis, types 1 and 3, or NOS

  N02.6   Recurrent and persistent hematuria with dense deposit disease
Recurrent and persistent hematuria with membranoproliferative glomerulonephritis, type 2

  N02.7   Recurrent and persistent hematuria with diffuse crescentic glomerulonephritis
Recurrent and persistent hematuria with extracapillary glomerulonephritis

  N02.8   Recurrent and persistent hematuria with other morphologic changes
Recurrent and persistent hematuria with proliferative glomerulonephritis NOS

  N02.9   Recurrent and persistent hematuria with unspecified morphologic changes ▽
    AHA: 2017, 2Q, 5

EXCLUDES 1 Not coded here   **EXCLUDES 2** Not included here   N Newborn Age: 0   P Pediatric Age: 0-17   M Maternity Age: 12-55   A Adult Age: 15-124

802   ICD-10-CM 2018

☑4ᵗʰ **N03 Chronic nephritic syndrome**

INCLUDES   chronic glomerular disease
chronic glomerulonephritis
chronic nephritis

EXCLUDES 1   *chronic tubulo-interstitial nephritis (N11.-)*
diffuse sclerosing glomerulonephritis (N05.8-)
nephritic syndrome NOS (N05.-)

DEF: Slow, progressive type of nephritis characterized by inflammation of the capillary loops in the glomeruli of the kidney, which leads to renal failure.

N03.0 Chronic nephritic syndrome with minor glomerular abnormality
Chronic nephritic syndrome with minimal change lesion

N03.1 Chronic nephritic syndrome with focal and segmental glomerular lesions
Chronic nephritic syndrome with focal and segmental hyalinosis
Chronic nephritic syndrome with focal and segmental sclerosis
Chronic nephritic syndrome with focal glomerulonephritis

N03.2 Chronic nephritic syndrome with diffuse membranous glomerulonephritis

N03.3 Chronic nephritic syndrome with diffuse mesangial proliferative glomerulonephritis

N03.4 Chronic nephritic syndrome with diffuse endocapillary proliferative glomerulonephritis

N03.5 Chronic nephritic syndrome with diffuse mesangiocapillary glomerulonephritis
Chronic nephritic syndrome with membranoproliferative glomerulonephritis, types 1 and 3, or NOS

N03.6 Chronic nephritic syndrome with dense deposit disease
Chronic nephritic syndrome with membranoproliferative glomerulonephritis, type 2

N03.7 Chronic nephritic syndrome with diffuse crescentic glomerulonephritis
Chronic nephritic syndrome with extracapillary glomerulonephritis

N03.8 Chronic nephritic syndrome with other morphologic changes
Chronic nephritic syndrome with proliferative glomerulonephritis NOS

N03.9 Chronic nephritic syndrome with unspecified morphologic changes ▽

☑4ᵗʰ **N04 Nephrotic syndrome**

INCLUDES   congenital nephrotic syndrome
lipoid nephrosis

N04.0 Nephrotic syndrome with minor glomerular abnormality
Nephrotic syndrome with minimal change lesion

N04.1 Nephrotic syndrome with focal and segmental glomerular lesions
Nephrotic syndrome with focal and segmental hyalinosis
Nephrotic syndrome with focal and segmental sclerosis
Nephrotic syndrome with focal glomerulonephritis

N04.2 Nephrotic syndrome with diffuse membranous glomerulonephritis

N04.3 Nephrotic syndrome with diffuse mesangial proliferative glomerulonephritis

N04.4 Nephrotic syndrome with diffuse endocapillary proliferative glomerulonephritis

N04.5 Nephrotic syndrome with diffuse mesangiocapillary glomerulonephritis
Nephrotic syndrome with membranoproliferative glomerulonephritis, types 1 and 3, or NOS

N04.6 Nephrotic syndrome with dense deposit disease
Nephrotic syndrome with membranoproliferative glomerulonephritis, type 2

N04.7 Nephrotic syndrome with diffuse crescentic glomerulonephritis
Nephrotic syndrome with extracapillary glomerulonephritis

N04.8 Nephrotic syndrome with other morphologic changes
Nephrotic syndrome with proliferative glomerulonephritis NOS

N04.9 Nephrotic syndrome with unspecified morphologic changes ▽

☑4ᵗʰ **N05 Unspecified nephritic syndrome**

INCLUDES   glomerular disease NOS
glomerulonephritis NOS
nephritis NOS
nephropathy NOS and renal disease NOS with morphological lesion specified in .0-.8

EXCLUDES 1   *nephropathy NOS with no stated morphological lesion (N28.9)*
renal disease NOS with no stated morphological lesion (N28.9)
tubulo-interstitial nephritis NOS (N12)

N05.0 Unspecified nephritic syndrome with minor glomerular abnormality ▽
Unspecified nephritic syndrome with minimal change lesion

N05.1 Unspecified nephritic syndrome with focal and segmental glomerular lesions ▽
Unspecified nephritic syndrome with focal and segmental hyalinosis
Unspecified nephritic syndrome with focal and segmental sclerosis
Unspecified nephritic syndrome with focal glomerulonephritis

N05.2 Unspecified nephritic syndrome with diffuse membranous glomerulonephritis ▽

N05.3 Unspecified nephritic syndrome with diffuse mesangial proliferative glomerulonephritis ▽

N05.4 Unspecified nephritic syndrome with diffuse endocapillary proliferative glomerulonephritis ▽

N05.5 Unspecified nephritic syndrome with diffuse mesangiocapillary glomerulonephritis ▽
Unspecified nephritic syndrome with membranoproliferative glomerulonephritis, types 1 and 3, or NOS

N05.6 Unspecified nephritic syndrome with dense deposit disease ▽
Unspecified nephritic syndrome with membranoproliferative glomerulonephritis, type 2

N05.7 Unspecified nephritic syndrome with diffuse crescentic glomerulonephritis ▽
Unspecified nephritic syndrome with extracapillary glomerulonephritis

N05.8 Unspecified nephritic syndrome with other morphologic changes ▽
Unspecified nephritic syndrome with proliferative glomerulonephritis NOS

N05.9 Unspecified nephritic syndrome with unspecified morphologic changes ▽

☑4ᵗʰ **N06 Isolated proteinuria with specified morphological lesion**

EXCLUDES 1   *proteinuria not associated with specific morphologic lesions (R80.0)*

N06.0 Isolated proteinuria with minor glomerular abnormality
Isolated proteinuria with minimal change lesion

N06.1 Isolated proteinuria with focal and segmental glomerular lesions
Isolated proteinuria with focal and segmental hyalinosis
Isolated proteinuria with focal and segmental sclerosis
Isolated proteinuria with focal glomerulonephritis

N06.2 Isolated proteinuria with diffuse membranous glomerulonephritis

N06.3 Isolated proteinuria with diffuse mesangial proliferative glomerulonephritis

N06.4 Isolated proteinuria with diffuse endocapillary proliferative glomerulonephritis

N06.5 Isolated proteinuria with diffuse mesangiocapillary glomerulonephritis
Isolated proteinuria with membranoproliferative glomerulonephritis, types 1 and 3, or NOS

N06.6 Isolated proteinuria with dense deposit disease
Isolated proteinuria with membranoproliferative glomerulonephritis, type 2

N06.7 Isolated proteinuria with diffuse crescentic glomerulonephritis
Isolated proteinuria with extracapillary glomerulonephritis

N06.8 Isolated proteinuria with other morphologic lesion
Isolated proteinuria with proliferative glomerulonephritis NOS

N06.9 Isolated proteinuria with unspecified morphologic lesion ▽

☑ Additional Character Req   ☑x7ᵗʰ Placeholder Alert   Manifestation   HCC CMS-HCC Condition   ▽ Unspecified Code   ►◄ Revised Text   ● New Code   ▲ Revised Code Title

✓4ᵗʰ N07 Hereditary nephropathy, not elsewhere classified

    EXCLUDES 2   *Alport's syndrome (Q87.81-)*
                 hereditary amyloid nephropathy (E85.-)
                 nail patella syndrome (Q87.2)
                 non-neuropathic heredofamilial amyloidosis (E85.-)

N07.0 Hereditary nephropathy, not elsewhere classified with minor glomerular abnormality

     Hereditary nephropathy, not elsewhere classified with minimal change lesion

N07.1 Hereditary nephropathy, not elsewhere classified with focal and segmental glomerular lesions

     Hereditary nephropathy, not elsewhere classified with focal and segmental hyalinosis
     Hereditary nephropathy, not elsewhere classified with focal and segmental sclerosis
     Hereditary nephropathy, not elsewhere classified with focal glomerulonephritis

N07.2 Hereditary nephropathy, not elsewhere classified with diffuse membranous glomerulonephritis

N07.3 Hereditary nephropathy, not elsewhere classified with diffuse mesangial proliferative glomerulonephritis

N07.4 Hereditary nephropathy, not elsewhere classified with diffuse endocapillary proliferative glomerulonephritis

N07.5 Hereditary nephropathy, not elsewhere classified with diffuse mesangiocapillary glomerulonephritis

     Hereditary nephropathy, not elsewhere classified with membranoproliferative glomerulonephritis, types 1 and 3, or NOS

N07.6 Hereditary nephropathy, not elsewhere classified with dense deposit disease

     Hereditary nephropathy, not elsewhere classified with membranoproliferative glomerulonephritis, type 2

N07.7 Hereditary nephropathy, not elsewhere classified with diffuse crescentic glomerulonephritis

     Hereditary nephropathy, not elsewhere classified with extracapillary glomerulonephritis

N07.8 Hereditary nephropathy, not elsewhere classified with other morphologic lesions

     Hereditary nephropathy, not elsewhere classified with proliferative glomerulonephritis NOS

N07.9 Hereditary nephropathy, not elsewhere classified with unspecified morphologic lesions   ▽

N08 *Glomerular disorders in diseases classified elsewhere*

     Glomerulonephritis
     Nephritis
     Nephropathy
     Code first underlying disease, such as:
         amyloidosis (E85.-)
         congenital syphilis (A50.5)
         cryoglobulinemia (D89.1)
         disseminated intravascular coagulation (D65)
         gout (M1A.-, M10.-)
         microscopic polyangiitis (M31.7)
         multiple myeloma (C90.0-)
         sepsis (A40.0-A41.9)
         sickle-cell disease (D57.0-D57.8)

    EXCLUDES 1   *glomerulonephritis, nephritis and nephropathy (in):*
         antiglomerular basement membrane disease (M31.0)
         diabetes (E08-E13 with .21)
         gonococcal (A54.21)
         Goodpasture's syndrome (M31.0)
         hemolytic-uremic syndrome (D59.3)
         lupus (M32.14)
         mumps (B26.83)
         syphilis (A52.75)
         systemic lupus erythematosus (M32.14)
         Wegener's granulomatosis (M31.31)
       pyelonephritis in diseases classified elsewhere (N16)
       renal tubulo-interstitial disorders classified elsewhere (N16)

Renal tubulo-interstitial diseases (N10-N16)

    INCLUDES   pyelonephritis
    EXCLUDES 1   *pyeloureteritis cystica (N28.85)*

N10 Acute pyelonephritis

     Acute infectious interstitial nephritis
     Acute pyelitis
     Acute tubulo-interstitial nephritis
     Hemoglobin nephrosis
     Myoglobin nephrosis
     Use additional code (B95-B97), to identify infectious agent

✓4ᵗʰ N11 Chronic tubulo-interstitial nephritis

    INCLUDES   chronic infectious interstitial nephritis
              chronic pyelitis
              chronic pyelonephritis
     Use additional code (B95-B97), to identify infectious agent

N11.0 Nonobstructive reflux-associated chronic pyelonephritis

     Pyelonephritis (chronic) associated with (vesicoureteral) reflux
    EXCLUDES 1   *vesicoureteral reflux NOS (N13.70)*

N11.1 Chronic obstructive pyelonephritis

     Pyelonephritis (chronic) associated with anomaly of pelviureteric junction
     Pyelonephritis (chronic) associated with anomaly of pyeloureteric junction
     Pyelonephritis (chronic) associated with crossing of vessel
     Pyelonephritis (chronic) associated with kinking of ureter
     Pyelonephritis (chronic) associated with obstruction of ureter
     Pyelonephritis (chronic) associated with stricture of pelviureteric junction
     Pyelonephritis (chronic) associated with stricture of ureter
    EXCLUDES 1   *calculous pyelonephritis (N20.9)*
               obstructive uropathy (N13.-)

N11.8 Other chronic tubulo-interstitial nephritis

     Nonobstructive chronic pyelonephritis NOS

N11.9 Chronic tubulo-interstitial nephritis, unspecified   ▽

     Chronic interstitial nephritis NOS
     Chronic pyelitis NOS
     Chronic pyelonephritis NOS

N12 Tubulo-interstitial nephritis, not specified as acute or chronic

     Interstitial nephritis NOS
     Pyelitis NOS
     Pyelonephritis NOS
    EXCLUDES 1   *calculous pyelonephritis (N20.9)*

✓4ᵗʰ N13 Obstructive and reflux uropathy

    EXCLUDES 2   *calculus of kidney and ureter without hydronephrosis (N20.-)*
               congenital obstructive defects of renal pelvis and ureter (Q62.0-Q62.3)
               hydronephrosis with ureteropelvic junction obstruction ▶(Q62.11)◀
               obstructive pyelonephritis (N11.1)

N13.0 Hydronephrosis with ureteropelvic junction obstruction

     Hydronephrosis due to acquired occlusion of ureteropelvic junction
    EXCLUDES 2   *hydronephrosis with ureteropelvic junction obstruction due to calculus (N13.2)*

N13.1 Hydronephrosis with ureteral stricture, not elsewhere classified

    EXCLUDES 1   *hydronephrosis with ureteral stricture with infection (N13.6)*

N13.2 Hydronephrosis with renal and ureteral calculous obstruction

    EXCLUDES 1   *hydronephrosis with renal and ureteral calculous obstruction with infection (N13.6)*

Hydronephrosis/UPJ Obstruction

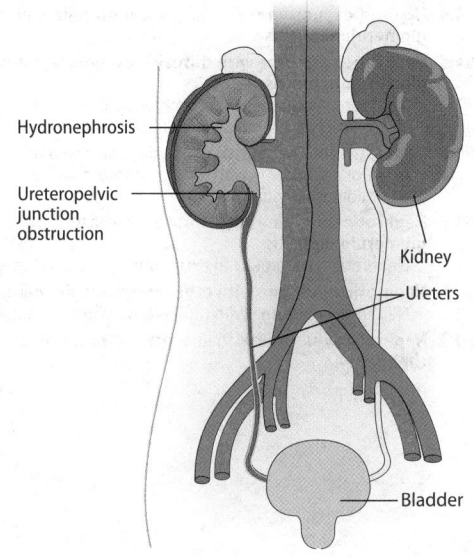

Hydronephrosis

Ureteropelvic junction obstruction

Kidney

Ureters

Bladder

EXCLUDES 1 Not coded here   *EXCLUDES 2* Not included here   N Newborn Age: 0   P Pediatric Age: 0-17   M Maternity Age: 12-55   A Adult Age: 15-124

804   ICD-10-CM 2018

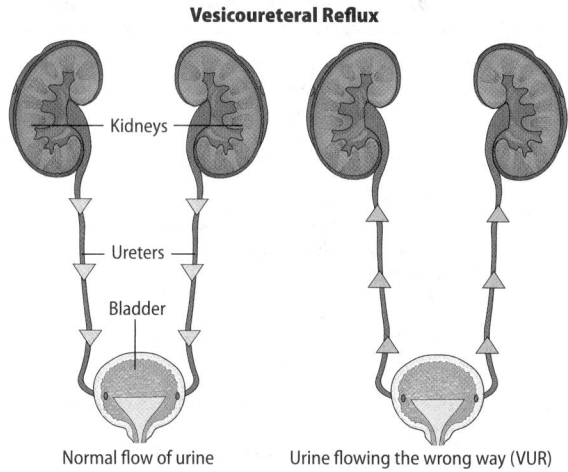

Vesicoureteral Reflux

Kidneys

Ureters

Bladder

Normal flow of urine   Urine flowing the wrong way (VUR)

✓5ᵗʰ **N13.3 Other and unspecified hydronephrosis**
     EXCLUDES 1   *hydronephrosis with infection (N13.6)*

     N13.30 Unspecified hydronephrosis ▽

     N13.39 Other hydronephrosis

N13.4 Hydroureter
     EXCLUDES 1   *congenital hydroureter (Q62.3-)*
              hydroureter with infection (N13.6)
              vesicoureteral-reflux with hydroureter (N13.73-)

N13.5 Crossing vessel and stricture of ureter without hydronephrosis
     Kinking and stricture of ureter without hydronephrosis
     EXCLUDES 1   *crossing vessel and stricture of ureter without hydronephrosis with infection (N13.6)*

N13.6 Pyonephrosis
     Conditions in N13.0-N13.5 with infection
     Obstructive uropathy with infection
     Use additional code (B95-B97), to identify infectious agent

✓5ᵗʰ **N13.7 Vesicoureteral-reflux**
     EXCLUDES 1   *reflux-associated pyelonephritis (N11.0)*

     N13.70 Vesicoureteral-reflux, unspecified ▽
              Vesicoureteral-reflux NOS

     N13.71 Vesicoureteral-reflux without reflux nephropathy

     ✓6ᵗʰ **N13.72 Vesicoureteral-reflux with reflux nephropathy without hydroureter**

         N13.721 Vesicoureteral-reflux with reflux nephropathy without hydroureter, unilateral

         N13.722 Vesicoureteral-reflux with reflux nephropathy without hydroureter, bilateral

         N13.729 Vesicoureteral-reflux with reflux nephropathy without hydroureter, unspecified ▽

     ✓6ᵗʰ **N13.73 Vesicoureteral-reflux with reflux nephropathy with hydroureter**

         N13.731 Vesicoureteral-reflux with reflux nephropathy with hydroureter, unilateral

         N13.732 Vesicoureteral-reflux with reflux nephropathy with hydroureter, bilateral

         N13.739 Vesicoureteral-reflux with reflux nephropathy with hydroureter, unspecified ▽

N13.8 Other obstructive and reflux uropathy
     Urinary tract obstruction due to specified cause
     Code first, if applicable, any causal condition, such as:
        enlarged prostate (N40.1)

N13.9 Obstructive and reflux uropathy, unspecified ▽
     Urinary tract obstruction NOS

✓4ᵗʰ **N14 Drug- and heavy-metal-induced tubulo-interstitial and tubular conditions**
     Code first poisoning due to drug or toxin, if applicable (T36-T65 with fifth or sixth character 1-4 or 6)
     Use additional code for adverse effect, if applicable, to identify drug (T36-T50 with fifth or sixth character 5)

N14.0 Analgesic nephropathy

N14.1 Nephropathy induced by other drugs, medicaments and biological substances

N14.2 Nephropathy induced by unspecified drug, medicament or biological substance ▽

N14.3 Nephropathy induced by heavy metals

N14.4 Toxic nephropathy, not elsewhere classified

✓4ᵗʰ **N15 Other renal tubulo-interstitial diseases**

     N15.0 Balkan nephropathy
         Balkan endemic nephropathy

     N15.1 Renal and perinephric abscess

     N15.8 Other specified renal tubulo-interstitial diseases

     N15.9 Renal tubulo-interstitial disease, unspecified ▽
         Infection of kidney NOS
         EXCLUDES 1   *urinary tract infection NOS (N39.0)*

N16 Renal tubulo-interstitial disorders in diseases classified elsewhere
     Pyelonephritis
     Tubulo-interstitial nephritis
     Code first underlying disease, such as:
        brucellosis (A23.0-A23.9)
        cryoglobulinemia (D89.1)
        glycogen storage disease (E74.0)
        leukemia (C91-C95)
        lymphoma (C81.0-C85.9, C96.0-C96.9)
        multiple myeloma (C90.0-)
        sepsis (A40.0-A41.9)
        Wilson's disease (E83.0)
     EXCLUDES 1   *diphtheritic pyelonephritis and tubulo-interstitial nephritis (A36.84)*
           pyelonephritis and tubulo-interstitial nephritis in candidiasis (B37.49)
           pyelonephritis and tubulo-interstitial nephritis in cystinosis (E72.04)
           pyelonephritis and tubulo-interstitial nephritis in salmonella infection (A02.25)
           pyelonephritis and tubulo-interstitial nephritis in sarcoidosis (D86.84)
           pyelonephritis and tubulo-interstitial nephritis in sicca syndrome [Sjogren's] (M35.04)
           pyelonephritis and tubulo-interstitial nephritis in systemic lupus erythematosus (M32.15)
           pyelonephritis and tubulo-interstitial nephritis in toxoplasmosis (B58.83)
           renal tubular degeneration in diabetes (E08-E13 with .29)
           syphilitic pyelonephritis and tubulo-interstitial nephritis (A52.75)

Acute kidney failure and chronic kidney disease (N17-N19)

     EXCLUDES 2   *congenital renal failure (P96.0)*
           drug- and heavy-metal-induced tubulo-interstitial and tubular conditions (N14.-)
           extrarenal uremia (R39.2)
           hemolytic-uremic syndrome (D59.3)
           hepatorenal syndrome (K76.7)
           postpartum hepatorenal syndrome (O90.4)
           posttraumatic renal failure (T79.5)
           prerenal uremia (R39.2)
           renal failure complicating abortion or ectopic or molar pregnancy (O00-O07, O08.4)
           renal failure following labor and delivery (O90.4)
           renal failure postprocedural (N99.0)

✓4ᵗʰ **N17 Acute kidney failure**
     Code also associated underlying condition
     EXCLUDES 1   *posttraumatic renal failure (T79.5)*
     AHA: 2013, 4Q, 124

     N17.0 Acute kidney failure with tubular necrosis   HCC
         Acute tubular necrosis
         Renal tubular necrosis
         Tubular necrosis NOS

     N17.1 Acute kidney failure with acute cortical necrosis   HCC
         Acute cortical necrosis
         Cortical necrosis NOS
         Renal cortical necrosis

     N17.2 Acute kidney failure with medullary necrosis   HCC
         Medullary [papillary] necrosis NOS
         Acute medullary [papillary] necrosis
         Renal medullary [papillary] necrosis

     N17.8 Other acute kidney failure   HCC

     N17.9 Acute kidney failure, unspecified   HCC ▽
         Acute kidney injury (nontraumatic)
         EXCLUDES 2   *traumatic kidney injury (S37.0-)*

✓ Additional Character Req   ✓x7ᵗʰ Placeholder Alert   Manifestation   HCC CMS-HCC Condition   ▽ Unspecified Code   ►◄ Revised Text   ● New Code   ▲ Revised Code Title

ICD-10-CM 2018   805

✓4ᵗʰ N18 Chronic kidney disease (CKD)

Code first any associated:
diabetic chronic kidney disease (E08.22, E09.22, E10.22, E11.22, E13.22)
hypertensive chronic kidney disease (I12-, I13-)
Use additional code to identify kidney transplant status, if applicable, (Z94.0)
AHA: 2013, 1Q, 24

N18.1 Chronic kidney disease, stage 1

N18.2 Chronic kidney disease, stage 2 (mild)

N18.3 Chronic kidney disease, stage 3 (moderate)

N18.4 Chronic kidney disease, stage 4 (severe)   HCC

N18.5 Chronic kidney disease, stage 5   HCC

> EXCLUDES 1   chronic kidney disease, stage 5 requiring chronic dialysis (N18.6)
>
> **DEF:** End-stage renal disease (ESRD) with GFR value of 15 ml/min or less not yet requiring chronic dialysis.

N18.6 End stage renal disease   HCC
Chronic kidney disease requiring chronic dialysis
Use additional code to identify dialysis status (Z99.2)
AHA: 2016, 3Q, 22; 2016, 1Q, 12; 2013, 4Q, 124-125

N18.9 Chronic kidney disease, unspecified ▽
Chronic renal disease
Chronic renal failure NOS
Chronic renal insufficiency
▶Chronic uremia NOS
Diffuse sclerosing glomerulonephritis NOS◀

N19 Unspecified kidney failure ▽

Uremia NOS

> EXCLUDES 1   acute kidney failure (N17.-)
> chronic kidney disease (N18.-)
> chronic uremia (N18.9)
> extrarenal uremia (R39.2)
> prerenal uremia (R39.2)
> renal insufficiency (acute) (N28.9)
> uremia of newborn (P96.0)

Urolithiasis (N20-N23)

AHA: 2017, 1Q, 5; 2015, 2Q, 8

✓4ᵗʰ N20 Calculus of kidney and ureter

Calculous pyelonephritis

> EXCLUDES 1   nephrocalcinosis (E83.5)
> that with hydronephrosis (N13.2)

N20.0 Calculus of kidney
Nephrolithiasis NOS
Renal calculus
Renal stone
Staghorn calculus
Stone in kidney

N20.1 Calculus of ureter
Ureteric stone
AHA: 2016, 3Q, 22

N20.2 Calculus of kidney with calculus of ureter

N20.9 Urinary calculus, unspecified ▽

✓4ᵗʰ N21 Calculus of lower urinary tract

Calculus of lower urinary tract with cystitis and urethritis

N21.0 Calculus in bladder
Calculus in diverticulum of bladder
Urinary bladder stone

> EXCLUDES 2   staghorn calculus (N20.0)

N21.1 Calculus in urethra

> EXCLUDES 2   calculus of prostate (N42.0)

N21.8 Other lower urinary tract calculus

N21.9 Calculus of lower urinary tract, unspecified ▽

> EXCLUDES 1   calculus of urinary tract NOS (N20.9)

N22 Calculus of urinary tract in diseases classified elsewhere

Code first underlying disease, such as:
gout (M1A.-, M10.-)
schistosomiasis (B65.0-B65.9)

N23 Unspecified renal colic ▽

Other disorders of kidney and ureter (N25-N29)

> EXCLUDES 2   disorders of kidney and ureter with urolithiasis (N20-N23)

✓4ᵗʰ N25 Disorders resulting from impaired renal tubular function

> EXCLUDES 1   metabolic disorders classifiable to E70-E88

N25.0 Renal osteodystrophy
Azotemic osteodystrophy
Phosphate-losing tubular disorders
Renal rickets
Renal short stature

> EXCLUDES 2   ▶metabolic disorders classifiable to E70-E88◀

N25.1 Nephrogenic diabetes insipidus   HCC

> EXCLUDES 1   diabetes insipidus NOS (E23.2)
>
> **DEF:** Type of diabetes due to inability of renal tubules to reabsorb water back into the body; not responsive to vasopressin (antidiuretic hormone); characterized by excessive thirst and excessive urine production; may develop into chronic renal insufficiency.

✓5ᵗʰ N25.8 Other disorders resulting from impaired renal tubular function

N25.81 Secondary hyperparathyroidism of renal origin   HCC

> EXCLUDES 1   secondary hyperparathyroidism, non-renal (E21.1)
>
> EXCLUDES 2   ▶metabolic disorders classifiable to E70-E88◀
>
> **DEF:** Parathyroid dysfunction caused by chronic renal failure; phosphate clearance is impaired, phosphate is released from bone, vitamin D is not produced, intestinal calcium absorption is low, and blood levels of calcium are lowered, causing excessive production of parathyroid hormone.

N25.89 Other disorders resulting from impaired renal tubular function
Hypokalemic nephropathy
Lightwood-Albright syndrome
Renal tubular acidosis NOS

N25.9 Disorder resulting from impaired renal tubular function, unspecified ▽

✓4ᵗʰ N26 Unspecified contracted kidney

> EXCLUDES 1   contracted kidney due to hypertension (I12.-)
> diffuse sclerosing glomerulonephritis (N05.8-)
> hypertensive nephrosclerosis (arteriolar) (arteriosclerotic) (I12.-)
> small kidney of unknown cause (N27.-)

N26.1 Atrophy of kidney (terminal)

N26.2 Page kidney

N26.9 Renal sclerosis, unspecified ▽

✓4ᵗʰ N27 Small kidney of unknown cause

> INCLUDES   oligonephronia

N27.0 Small kidney, unilateral

N27.1 Small kidney, bilateral

N27.9 Small kidney, unspecified ▽

✓4ᵗʰ N28 Other disorders of kidney and ureter, not elsewhere classified

N28.0 Ischemia and infarction of kidney   HCC
Renal artery embolism   Renal artery thrombosis
Renal artery obstruction   Renal infarct
Renal artery occlusion

> EXCLUDES 1   atherosclerosis of renal artery (extrarenal part) (I70.1)
> congenital stenosis of renal artery (Q27.1)
> Goldblatt's kidney (I70.1)

N28.1 Cyst of kidney, acquired
▶Cyst (multiple) (solitary) of kidney (acquired)◀

> EXCLUDES 1   cystic kidney disease (congenital) (Q61.-)

✓5ᵗʰ N28.8 Other specified disorders of kidney and ureter

> EXCLUDES 1   hydroureter (N13.4)
> ureteric stricture with hydronephrosis (N13.1)
> ureteric stricture without hydronephrosis (N13.5)

N28.81 Hypertrophy of kidney

N28.82 Megaloureter

N28.83 Nephroptosis

N28.84 Pyelitis cystica

N28.85 Pyeloureteritis cystica

N28.86 Ureteritis cystica

N28.89 Other specified disorders of kidney and ureter

N28.9 Disorder of kidney and ureter, unspecified ▽
Nephropathy NOS
Renal disease (acute) NOS
Renal insufficiency (acute)
EXCLUDES 1 *chronic renal insufficiency (N18.9)*
unspecified nephritic syndrome (N05.-)
AHA: 2016, 1Q, 13

N29 *Other disorders of kidney and ureter in diseases classified elsewhere*
Code first underlying disease, such as:
amyloidosis (E85.-)
nephrocalcinosis (E83.5)
schistosomiasis (B65.0-B65.9)
EXCLUDES 1 *disorders of kidney and ureter in:*
cystinosis (E72.0)
gonorrhea (A54.21)
syphilis (A52.75)
tuberculosis (A18.11)

Other diseases of the urinary system (N30-N39)
EXCLUDES 1 *urinary infection (complicating):*
abortion or ectopic or molar pregnancy (-O07, O08.8)
pregnancy, childbirth and the puerperium (O23-, O75.3, O86.2-)

√4th **N30 Cystitis**
Use additional code to identify infectious agent (B95-B97)
EXCLUDES 1 *prostatocystitis (N41.3)*
AHA: 2017, 1Q, 6

√5th **N30.0 Acute cystitis**
EXCLUDES 1 *irradiation cystitis (N30.4-)*
trigonitis (N30.3-)
N30.00 Acute cystitis without hematuria
N30.01 Acute cystitis with hematuria

√5th **N30.1 Interstitial cystitis (chronic)**
N30.10 Interstitial cystitis (chronic) without hematuria
N30.11 Interstitial cystitis (chronic) with hematuria

√5th **N30.2 Other chronic cystitis**
N30.20 Other chronic cystitis without hematuria
N30.21 Other chronic cystitis with hematuria

√5th **N30.3 Trigonitis**
Urethrotrigonitis
N30.30 Trigonitis without hematuria
N30.31 Trigonitis with hematuria

√5th **N30.4 Irradiation cystitis**
N30.40 Irradiation cystitis without hematuria
N30.41 Irradiation cystitis with hematuria

√5th **N30.8 Other cystitis**
Abscess of bladder
N30.80 Other cystitis without hematuria
N30.81 Other cystitis with hematuria

√5th **N30.9 Cystitis, unspecified**
N30.90 Cystitis, unspecified without hematuria ▽
N30.91 Cystitis, unspecified with hematuria ▽

√4th **N31 Neuromuscular dysfunction of bladder, not elsewhere classified**
Use additional code to identify any associated urinary incontinence (N39.3-N39.4-)
EXCLUDES 1 *cord bladder NOS (G95.89)*
neurogenic bladder due to cauda equina syndrome (G83.4)
neuromuscular dysfunction due to spinal cord lesion (G95.89)
N31.0 Uninhibited neuropathic bladder, not elsewhere classified
N31.1 Reflex neuropathic bladder, not elsewhere classified
N31.2 Flaccid neuropathic bladder, not elsewhere classified
Atonic (motor) (sensory) neuropathic bladder
Autonomous neuropathic bladder
Nonreflex neuropathic bladder
N31.8 Other neuromuscular dysfunction of bladder
N31.9 Neuromuscular dysfunction of bladder, unspecified ▽
Neurogenic bladder dysfunction NOS

√4th **N32 Other disorders of bladder**
EXCLUDES 2 *calculus of bladder (N21.0)*
cystocele (N81.1-)
hernia or prolapse of bladder, female (N81.1-)

N32.0 Bladder-neck obstruction
Bladder-neck stenosis (acquired)
EXCLUDES 1 *congenital bladder-neck obstruction (Q64.3-)*
DEF: Bladder outlet and vesicourethral obstruction; occurs as a consequence of benign prostatic hypertrophy or prostatic cancer; may also occur in either sex due to strictures, radiation, cystoscopy, catheterization, injury, infection, blood clots, bladder cancer, impaction, or other disease that compresses the bladder neck.

N32.1 Vesicointestinal fistula
Vesicorectal fistula

N32.2 Vesical fistula, not elsewhere classified
EXCLUDES 1 *fistula between bladder and female genital tract (N82.0-N82.1)*

N32.3 Diverticulum of bladder
EXCLUDES 1 *congenital diverticulum of bladder (Q64.6)*
diverticulitis of bladder (N30.8-)

√5th **N32.8 Other specified disorders of bladder**
N32.81 Overactive bladder
Detrusor muscle hyperactivity
EXCLUDES 1 *frequent urination due to specified bladder condition—code to condition*
DEF: Sudden involuntary contractions of the muscular wall of bladder; results in sudden, strong urge to urinate.
N32.89 Other specified disorders of bladder
Bladder hemorrhage
Bladder hypertrophy
Calcified bladder
Contracted bladder

N32.9 Bladder disorder, unspecified ▽

N33 *Bladder disorders in diseases classified elsewhere*
Code first underlying disease, such as:
schistosomiasis (B65.0-B65.9)
EXCLUDES 1 *bladder disorder in syphilis (A52.76)*
bladder disorder in tuberculosis (A18.12)
candidal cystitis (B37.41)
chlamydial cystitis (A56.01)
cystitis in gonorrhea (A54.01)
cystitis in neurogenic bladder (N31.-)
diphtheritic cystitis (A36.85)
neurogenic bladder (N31.-)
syphilitic cystitis (A52.76)
trichomonal cystitis (A59.03)

√4th **N34 Urethritis and urethral syndrome**
Use additional code (B95-B97), to identify infectious agent
EXCLUDES 2 *Reiter's disease (M02.3-)*
urethritis in diseases with a predominantly sexual mode of transmission (A50-A64)
urethrotrigonitis (N30.3-)
AHA: 2017, 1Q, 6
N34.0 Urethral abscess
Abscess (of) Cowper's gland
Abscess (of) Littrés gland
Abscess (of) urethral (gland)
Periurethral abscess
EXCLUDES 1 *urethral caruncle (N36.2)*
N34.1 Nonspecific urethritis
Nongonococcal urethritis
Nonvenereal urethritis
N34.2 Other urethritis
Meatitis, urethral
Postmenopausal urethritis
Ulcer of urethra (meatus)
Urethritis NOS
N34.3 Urethral syndrome, unspecified ▽

√4th **N35 Urethral stricture**
EXCLUDES 1 *congenital urethral stricture (Q64.3-)*
postprocedural urethral stricture (N99.1-)

√5th **N35.0 Post-traumatic urethral stricture**
Urethral stricture due to injury
EXCLUDES 1 *postprocedural urethral stricture (N99.1-)*
√6th **N35.01 Post-traumatic urethral stricture, male**
N35.010 Post-traumatic urethral stricture, male, meatal ♂
N35.011 Post-traumatic bulbous urethral stricture
N35.012 Post-traumatic membranous urethral stricture
N35.013 Post-traumatic anterior urethral stricture

☑ Additional Character Req   vx7th Placeholder Alert   Manifestation   HCC CMS-HCC Condition   ▽ Unspecified Code   ►◄ Revised Text   ● New Code   ▲ Revised Code Title

ICD-10-CM 2018   807

N35.014   **Post-traumatic urethral stricture, male, unspecified** ♂▽

✓6ᵗʰ N35.02   **Post-traumatic urethral stricture, female**
N35.021   **Urethral stricture** due to childbirth ♀
N35.028   **Other post-traumatic urethral stricture, female** ♀

✓5ᵗʰ N35.1   **Postinfective urethral stricture, not elsewhere classified**
EXCLUDES 1   urethral stricture associated with schistosomiasis (B65-, N29)
gonococcal urethral stricture (A54.01)
syphilitic urethral stricture (A52.76)

✓6ᵗʰ N35.11   **Postinfective urethral stricture, not elsewhere classified,** male
N35.111   **Postinfective urethral stricture, not** ♂ **elsewhere classified, male,** meatal
▲ N35.112   **Postinfective** bulbous **urethral stricture, not elsewhere classified, male**
▲ N35.113   **Postinfective** membranous **urethral stricture, not elsewhere classified, male**
▲ N35.114   **Postinfective** anterior **urethral stricture, not elsewhere classified, male**
N35.119   **Postinfective urethral stricture, not** ♂▽ **elsewhere classified, male, unspecified**
N35.12   **Postinfective urethral stricture, not elsewhere** ♀ **classified,** female

N35.8   **Other urethral stricture**
EXCLUDES 1   postprocedural urethral stricture (N99.1-)
N35.9   **Urethral stricture, unspecified** ▽

✓4ᵗʰ N36   **Other disorders of urethra**
N36.0   **Urethral** fistula
Urethroperineal fistula
Urethrorectal fistula
Urinary fistula NOS
EXCLUDES 1   urethroscrotal fistula (N50.89)
urethrovaginal fistula (N82.1)
urethrovesicovaginal fistula (N82.1)

N36.1   **Urethral** diverticulum
N36.2   **Urethral** caruncle

✓5ᵗʰ N36.4   **Urethral** functional and muscular disorders
Use additional code to identify associated urinary stress incontinence (N39.3)
N36.41   **Hypermobility** of urethra
N36.42   **Intrinsic sphincter deficiency (ISD)**
N36.43   **Combined hypermobility** of urethra and intrinsic sphincter deficiency
N36.44   **Muscular disorders** of urethra
Bladder sphincter dyssynergy

N36.5   **Urethral** false passage
N36.8   **Other specified disorders of urethra**
EXCLUDES 1   congenital urethrocele (Q64.7)
female urethrocele (N81.0)

N36.9   **Urethral disorder, unspecified** ▽

N37   Urethral disorders in diseases classified elsewhere
Code first underlying disease
EXCLUDES 1   urethritis (in):
candidal infection (B37.41)
chlamydial (A56.01)
gonorrhea (A54.01)
syphilis (A52.76)
trichomonal infection (A59.03)
tuberculosis (A18.13)

✓4ᵗʰ N39   **Other disorders of urinary system**
EXCLUDES 2   hematuria NOS (R31.-)
recurrent or persistent hematuria (N02.-)
recurrent or persistent hematuria with specified morphological lesion (N02.-)
proteinuria NOS (R80.-)

N39.0   **Urinary tract infection, site not specified** ▽
Use additional code (B95-B97), to identify infectious agent
EXCLUDES 1   candidiasis of urinary tract (B37.4-)
neonatal urinary tract infection (P39.3)
urinary tract infection of specified site, such as:
cystitis (N30.-)
urethritis (N34.-)
AHA: 2017, 1Q, 6; 2012, 4Q, 94

N39.3   **Stress incontinence (female) (male)**
Code also any associated overactive bladder (N32.81)
EXCLUDES 1   mixed incontinence (N39.46)

✓5ᵗʰ N39.4   **Other specified urinary incontinence**
Code also any associated overactive bladder (N32.81)
EXCLUDES 1   enuresis NOS (R32)
functional urinary incontinence (R39.81)
urinary incontinence associated with cognitive impairment (R39.81)
urinary incontinence NOS (R32)
urinary incontinence of nonorganic origin (F98.0)

N39.41   **Urge incontinence**
EXCLUDES 1   mixed incontinence (N39.46)

N39.42   **Incontinence without sensory awareness**
Insensible (urinary) incontinence
N39.43   **Post-void dribbling**
N39.44   **Nocturnal enuresis**
N39.45   **Continuous leakage**
N39.46   **Mixed incontinence**
Urge and stress incontinence

✓6ᵗʰ N39.49   **Other specified urinary incontinence**
N39.490   **Overflow incontinence**
N39.491   **Coital incontinence**
N39.492   **Postural (urinary) incontinence**
N39.498   **Other specified urinary incontinence**
Reflex incontinence
Total incontinence

N39.8   **Other specified disorders of urinary system**
N39.9   **Disorder of urinary system, unspecified** ▽

Diseases of male genital organs (N40-N53)

✓4ᵗʰ N40   **Benign prostatic hyperplasia**
INCLUDES   adenofibromatous hypertrophy of prostate
benign hypertrophy of the prostate
benign prostatic hypertrophy
BPH
enlarged prostate
nodular prostate
polyp of prostate
EXCLUDES 1   benign neoplasms of prostate (adenoma, benign) (fibroadenoma) (fibroma) (myoma) (D29.1)
EXCLUDES 2   malignant neoplasm of prostate (C61)

N40.0   **Benign prostatic hyperplasia** without lower urinary tract 🅐♂ symptoms
Enlarged prostate NOS
Enlarged prostate without LUTS

N40.1   **Benign prostatic hyperplasia** with lower urinary tract 🅐♂ symptoms
Enlarged prostate with LUTS
Use additional code for associated symptoms, when specified:
incomplete bladder emptying (R39.14)
nocturia (R35.1)
straining on urination (R39.16)
urinary frequency (R35.0)
urinary hesitancy (R39.11)
urinary incontinence (N39.4-)
urinary obstruction (N13.8)
urinary retention (R33.8)
urinary urgency (R39.15)
weak urinary stream (R39.12)

N40.2   **Nodular** prostate without lower urinary tract symptoms 🅐♂
Nodular prostate without LUTS

N40.3   **Nodular** prostate with lower urinary tract symptoms 🅐♂
Use additional code for associated symptoms, when specified:
incomplete bladder emptying (R39.14)
nocturia (R35.1)
straining on urination (R39.16)
urinary frequency (R35.0)
urinary hesitancy (R39.11)
urinary incontinence (N39.4-)
urinary obstruction (N13.8)
urinary retention (R33.8)
urinary urgency (R39.15)
weak urinary stream (R39.12)

✓4ᵗʰ N41   **Inflammatory diseases of prostate**
Use additional code (B95-B97), to identify infectious agent
N41.0   **Acute prostatitis** 🅐♂
N41.1   **Chronic prostatitis** 🅐♂

N41.2   **Abscess of prostate**   A♂

N41.3   **Prostatocystitis**   A♂

N41.4   **Granulomatous prostatitis**   A♂

N41.8   **Other inflammatory diseases of prostate**   A♂

N41.9   **Inflammatory disease of prostate, unspecified**   A♂▽
     Prostatitis NOS

✓4ᵗʰ **N42**   **Other and unspecified disorders of prostate**

   N42.0   **Calculus of prostate**   A♂
     Prostatic stone
     DEF: Formation of small, solid stone often composed of calcium carbonate or calcium phosphate in the prostate gland.

   N42.1   **Congestion and hemorrhage of prostate**   A♂
     EXCLUDES 1   enlarged prostate (N40.-)
             hematuria (R31.-)
             hyperplasia of prostate (N40.-)
             inflammatory diseases of prostate (N41.-)

   ✓5ᵗʰ **N42.3**   **Dysplasia of prostate**

     N42.30   **Unspecified dysplasia of prostate**   ♂▽

     N42.31   **Prostatic intraepithelial neoplasia**   ♂
          PIN
          Prostatic intraepithelial neoplasia I (PIN I)
          Prostatic intraepithelial neoplasia II (PIN II)
          EXCLUDES 1   prostatic intraepithelial neoplasia III (PIN III) (D07.5)
          DEF: Abnormality of shape and size of the intraepithelial tissues of the prostate; premalignant condition characterized by stalks and absence of a basilar cell layer; synonyms are intraductal dysplasia, large acinar atypical hyperplasia, atypical primary hyperplasia, hyperplasia with malignant changes, marked atypia, or duct-acinar dysplasia.

     N42.32   **Atypical small acinar proliferation of prostate**   ♂

     N42.39   **Other dysplasia of prostate**   ♂

   ✓5ᵗʰ **N42.8**   **Other specified disorders of prostate**

     N42.81   **Prostatodynia syndrome**   A♂
          Painful prostate syndrome

     N42.82   **Prostatosis syndrome**   A♂

     N42.83   **Cyst of prostate**   A♂

     N42.89   **Other specified disorders of prostate**   A♂

   N42.9   **Disorder of prostate, unspecified**   A♂▽

✓4ᵗʰ **N43**   **Hydrocele and spermatocele**
     INCLUDES   hydrocele of spermatic cord, testis or tunica vaginalis
     EXCLUDES 1   congenital hydrocele (P83.5)

   N43.0   **Encysted hydrocele**   ♂

   N43.1   **Infected hydrocele**   ♂
     Use additional code (B95-B97), to identify infectious agent

   N43.2   **Other hydrocele**   ♂

   N43.3   **Hydrocele, unspecified**   ♂▽

   ✓5ᵗʰ **N43.4**   **Spermatocele of epididymis**
     Spermatic cyst

     N43.40   **Spermatocele of epididymis, unspecified**   ♂▽

     N43.41   **Spermatocele of epididymis, single**   ♂

     N43.42   **Spermatocele of epididymis, multiple**   ♂

Hydrocele

Normal   Noncommunicating hydrocele   Communicating hydrocele   Hydrocele of the cord

---

✓4ᵗʰ **N44**   **Noninflammatory disorders of testis**

   ✓5ᵗʰ **N44.0**   **Torsion of testis**

     N44.00   **Torsion of testis, unspecified**   ♂▽

     N44.01   **Extravaginal torsion of spermatic cord**   ♂
          DEF: Torsion of the spermatic cord just below the tunica vaginalis attachments.

     N44.02   **Intravaginal torsion of spermatic cord**   ♂
          Torsion of spermatic cord NOS

     N44.03   **Torsion of appendix testis**   ♂

     N44.04   **Torsion of appendix epididymis**   ♂

   N44.1   **Cyst of tunica albuginea testis**   ♂

   N44.2   **Benign cyst of testis**   ♂

   N44.8   **Other noninflammatory disorders of the testis**   ♂

✓4ᵗʰ **N45**   **Orchitis and epididymitis**
     Use additional code (B95-B97), to identify infectious agent

   N45.1   **Epididymitis**   ♂

   N45.2   **Orchitis**   ♂

   N45.3   **Epididymo-orchitis**   ♂

   N45.4   **Abscess of epididymis or testis**   ♂

✓4ᵗʰ **N46**   **Male infertility**
     EXCLUDES 1   vasectomy status (Z98.52)

   ✓5ᵗʰ **N46.0**   **Azoospermia**
     Absolute male infertility
     Male infertility due to germinal (cell) aplasia
     Male infertility due to spermatogenic arrest (complete)

     N46.01   **Organic azoospermia**   A♂
          Azoospermia NOS

     ✓6ᵗʰ **N46.02**   **Azoospermia due to extratesticular causes**
          Code also associated cause

       N46.021   **Azoospermia due to drug therapy**   A♂

       N46.022   **Azoospermia due to infection**   A♂

       N46.023   **Azoospermia due to obstruction of efferent ducts**   A♂

       N46.024   **Azoospermia due to radiation**   A♂

       N46.025   **Azoospermia due to systemic disease**   A♂

       N46.029   **Azoospermia due to other extratesticular causes**   A♂

   ✓5ᵗʰ **N46.1**   **Oligospermia**
     Male infertility due to germinal cell desquamation
     Male infertility due to hypospermatogenesis
     Male infertility due to incomplete spermatogenic arrest

     N46.11   **Organic oligospermia**   A♂
          Oligospermia NOS

     ✓6ᵗʰ **N46.12**   **Oligospermia due to extratesticular causes**
          Code also associated cause

       N46.121   **Oligospermia due to drug therapy**   A♂

       N46.122   **Oligospermia due to infection**   A♂

       N46.123   **Oligospermia due to obstruction of efferent ducts**   A♂

       N46.124   **Oligospermia due to radiation**   A♂

       N46.125   **Oligospermia due to systemic disease**   A♂

       N46.129   **Oligospermia due to other extratesticular causes**   A♂

   N46.8   **Other male infertility**   A♂

   N46.9   **Male infertility, unspecified**   A♂▽

✓4ᵗʰ **N47**   **Disorders of prepuce**

   N47.0   **Adherent prepuce, newborn**   N♂

   N47.1   **Phimosis**   ♂

   N47.2   **Paraphimosis**   ♂

   N47.3   **Deficient foreskin**   ♂

   N47.4   **Benign cyst of prepuce**   ♂

   N47.5   **Adhesions of prepuce and glans penis**   ♂

   N47.6   **Balanoposthitis**   ♂
     Use additional code (B95-B97), to identify infectious agent
     EXCLUDES 1   balanitis (N48.1)

   N47.7   **Other inflammatory diseases of prepuce**   ♂
     Use additional code (B95-B97), to identify infectious agent

   N47.8   **Other disorders of prepuce**   ♂

☑ Additional Character Req   ✓x7ᵗʰ Placeholder Alert   Manifestation   HCC CMS-HCC Condition   ▽ Unspecified Code   ►◄ Revised Text   ● New Code   ▲ Revised Code Title

ICD-10-CM 2018   809

✓4th N48 Other disorders of penis

N48.0 Leukoplakia of penis ♂
Balanitis xerotica obliterans
Kraurosis of penis
Lichen sclerosus of external male genital organs
EXCLUDES 1   *carcinoma in situ of penis (D07.4)*

N48.1 Balanitis ♂
Use additional code (B95-B97), to identify infectious agent
EXCLUDES 1   *amebic balanitis (A06.8)*
balanitis xerotica obliterans (N48.0)
candidal balanitis (B37.42)
gonococcal balanitis (A54.23)
herpesviral [herpes simplex] balanitis (A60.01)

✓5th N48.2 Other inflammatory disorders of penis
Use additional code (B95-B97), to identify infectious agent
EXCLUDES 1   *balanitis (N48.1)*
balanitis xerotica obliterans (N48.0)
balanoposthitis (N47.6)

    N48.21 Abscess of corpus cavernosum and penis ♂
    N48.22 Cellulitis of corpus cavernosum and penis ♂
    N48.29 Other inflammatory disorders of penis ♂

✓5th N48.3 Priapism
Painful erection
Code first underlying cause
    N48.30 Priapism, unspecified ♂▽
    N48.31 Priapism due to trauma ♂
    N48.32 Priapism due to disease classified elsewhere ♂
    N48.33 Priapism, drug-induced ♂
    N48.39 Other priapism ♂

N48.5 Ulcer of penis ♂

N48.6 Induration penis plastica ♂
Peyronie's disease
Plastic induration of penis

✓5th N48.8 Other specified disorders of penis
    N48.81 Thrombosis of superficial vein of penis ♂
    N48.82 Acquired torsion of penis ♂
    Acquired torsion of penis NOS
    EXCLUDES 1   *congenital torsion of penis (Q55.63)*
    N48.83 Acquired buried penis ♂
    EXCLUDES 1   *congenital hidden penis (Q55.64)*
    N48.89 Other specified disorders of penis ♂

N48.9 Disorder of penis, unspecified ♂▽

✓4th N49 Inflammatory disorders of male genital organs, not elsewhere classified

Use additional code (B95-B97), to identify infectious agent
EXCLUDES 1   *inflammation of penis (N48.1, N48.2-)*
orchitis and epididymitis (N45.-)

N49.0 Inflammatory disorders of seminal vesicle ♂
Vesiculitis NOS

N49.1 Inflammatory disorders of spermatic cord, tunica vaginalis and vas deferens ♂
Vasitis

N49.2 Inflammatory disorders of scrotum ♂

N49.3 Fournier gangrene ♂

N49.8 Inflammatory disorders of other specified male genital organs ♂
Inflammation of multiple sites in male genital organs

N49.9 Inflammatory disorder of unspecified male genital organ ♂▽
Abscess of unspecified male genital organ
Boil of unspecified male genital organ
Carbuncle of unspecified male genital organ
Cellulitis of unspecified male genital organ

✓4th N50 Other and unspecified disorders of male genital organs

EXCLUDES 2   *torsion of testis (N44.0-)*

N50.0 Atrophy of testis ♂

N50.1 Vascular disorders of male genital organs ♂
Hematocele, NOS, of male genital organs
Hemorrhage of male genital organs
Thrombosis of male genital organs

N50.3 Cyst of epididymis ♂

✓5th N50.8 Other specified disorders of male genital organs
    ✓6th N50.81 Testicular pain
       N50.811 Right testicular pain ♂
       N50.812 Left testicular pain ♂

       N50.819 Testicular pain, unspecified ♂▽
    N50.82 Scrotal pain ♂
    N50.89 Other specified disorders of the male genital organs ♂
Atrophy of scrotum, seminal vesicle, spermatic cord, tunica vaginalis and vas deferens
Chylocele, tunica vaginalis (nonfilarial) NOS
Edema of scrotum, seminal vesicle, spermatic cord, testis, tunica vaginalis and vas deferens
Hypertrophy of scrotum, seminal vesicle, spermatic cord, testis, tunica vaginalis and vas deferens
Stricture of spermatic cord, tunica vaginalis, and vas deferens
Ulcer of scrotum, seminal vesicle, spermatic cord, testis, tunica vaginalis and vas deferens
Urethroscrotal fistula

N50.9 Disorder of male genital organs, unspecified ♂▽

N51 *Disorders of male genital organs in diseases classified elsewhere* ♂

Code first underlying disease, such as:
filariasis (B74.0-B74.9)
EXCLUDES 1   *amebic balanitis (A06.8)*
candidal balanitis (B37.42)
gonococcal balanitis (A54.23)
gonococcal prostatitis (A54.22)
herpesviral [herpes simplex] balanitis (A60.01)
trichomonal prostatitis (A59.02)
tuberculous prostatitis (A18.14)

✓4th N52 Male erectile dysfunction

EXCLUDES 1   *psychogenic impotence (F52.21)*

✓5th N52.0 Vasculogenic erectile dysfunction
    N52.01 Erectile dysfunction due to arterial insufficiency 🅐♂
    N52.02 Corporo-venous occlusive erectile dysfunction 🅐♂
    N52.03 Combined arterial insufficiency and corporo-venous occlusive erectile dysfunction 🅐♂

N52.1 *Erectile dysfunction due to diseases classified elsewhere* 🅐♂
Code first underlying disease

N52.2 Drug-induced erectile dysfunction 🅐♂

✓5th N52.3 Postprocedural erectile dysfunction
    N52.31 Erectile dysfunction following radical prostatectomy 🅐♂
    N52.32 Erectile dysfunction following radical cystectomy 🅐♂
    N52.33 Erectile dysfunction following urethral surgery 🅐♂
    N52.34 Erectile dysfunction following simple prostatectomy 🅐♂
    N52.35 Erectile dysfunction following radiation therapy 🅐♂
    N52.36 Erectile dysfunction following interstitial seed therapy 🅐♂
    N52.37 Erectile dysfunction following prostate ablative therapy 🅐♂
Erectile dysfunction following cryotherapy
Erectile dysfunction following other prostate ablative therapies
Erectile dysfunction following ultrasound ablative therapies
    N52.39 Other and unspecified postprocedural erectile dysfunction 🅐♂▽

N52.8 Other male erectile dysfunction 🅐♂

N52.9 Male erectile dysfunction, unspecified 🅐♂▽
Impotence NOS

✓4th N53 Other male sexual dysfunction

EXCLUDES 1   *psychogenic sexual dysfunction (F52.-)*

✓5th N53.1 Ejaculatory dysfunction
EXCLUDES 1   *premature ejaculation (F52.4)*
    N53.11 Retarded ejaculation ♂
    N53.12 Painful ejaculation ♂
    N53.13 Anejaculatory orgasm ♂
    N53.14 Retrograde ejaculation ♂
DEF: A form of male sexual dysfunction in which the semen enters the bladder instead of going out through the urethra during ejaculation.
    N53.19 Other ejaculatory dysfunction ♂
Ejaculatory dysfunction NOS

N53.8 Other male sexual dysfunction ♂

N53.9 Unspecified male sexual dysfunction ♂▽

EXCLUDES 1 Not coded here   EXCLUDES 2 Not included here   N Newborn Age: 0   P Pediatric Age: 0-17   M Maternity Age: 12-55   🅐 Adult Age: 15-124

810   ICD-10-CM 2018

Disorders of breast (N60-N65)

EXCLUDES 1　disorders of breast associated with childbirth (O91-O92)

✓4th **N60　Benign mammary dysplasia**
　　INCLUDES　fibrocystic mastopathy

　✓5th **N60.0　Solitary cyst of breast**
　　　　Cyst of breast
　　　N60.01　Solitary cyst of right breast
　　　N60.02　Solitary cyst of left breast
　　　N60.09　Solitary cyst of unspecified breast ▽

　✓5th **N60.1　Diffuse cystic mastopathy**
　　　　Cystic breast
　　　　Fibrocystic disease of breast
　　　　EXCLUDES 1　diffuse cystic mastopathy with epithelial proliferation
　　　　　　　(N60.3-)
　　　N60.11　Diffuse cystic mastopathy of right breast 🅰
　　　N60.12　Diffuse cystic mastopathy of left breast 🅰
　　　N60.19　Diffuse cystic mastopathy of unspecified breast 🅰▽

　✓5th **N60.2　Fibroadenosis of breast**
　　　　Adenofibrosis of breast
　　　　EXCLUDES 2　fibroadenoma of breast (D24.-)
　　　N60.21　Fibroadenosis of right breast
　　　N60.22　Fibroadenosis of left breast
　　　N60.29　Fibroadenosis of unspecified breast ▽

　✓5th **N60.3　Fibrosclerosis of breast**
　　　　Cystic mastopathy with epithelial proliferation
　　　N60.31　Fibrosclerosis of right breast
　　　N60.32　Fibrosclerosis of left breast
　　　N60.39　Fibrosclerosis of unspecified breast ▽

　✓5th **N60.4　Mammary duct ectasia**
　　　N60.41　Mammary duct ectasia of right breast
　　　N60.42　Mammary duct ectasia of left breast
　　　N60.49　Mammary duct ectasia of unspecified breast ▽

　✓5th **N60.8　Other benign mammary dysplasias**
　　　N60.81　Other benign mammary dysplasias of right breast
　　　N60.82　Other benign mammary dysplasias of left breast
　　　N60.89　Other benign mammary dysplasias of unspecified ▽
　　　　　　breast

　✓5th **N60.9　Unspecified benign mammary dysplasia**
　　　N60.91　Unspecified benign mammary dysplasia of right ▽
　　　　　　breast
　　　N60.92　Unspecified benign mammary dysplasia of left ▽
　　　　　　breast
　　　N60.99　Unspecified benign mammary dysplasia of ▽
　　　　　　unspecified breast

✓4th **N61　Inflammatory disorders of breast**
　　　EXCLUDES 1　inflammatory carcinoma of breast (C50.9)
　　　　　　inflammatory disorder of breast associated with childbirth
　　　　　　　(O91.-)
　　　　　　neonatal infective mastitis (P39.0)
　　　　　　thrombophlebitis of breast [Mondor's disease] (I80.8)

　　N61.0　Mastitis without abscess
　　　　Infective mastitis (acute) (nonpuerperal) (subacute)
　　　　Mastitis (acute) (nonpuerperal) (subacute) NOS
　　　　Cellulitis (acute) (nonpuerperal) (subacute) of breast NOS
　　　　Cellulitis (acute) (nonpuerperal) (subacute) of nipple NOS

　　N61.1　Abscess of the breast and nipple
　　　　Abscess (acute) (chronic) (nonpuerperal) of areola
　　　　Abscess (acute) (chronic) (nonpuerperal) of breast
　　　　Carbuncle of breast
　　　　Mastitis with abscess

N62　Hypertrophy of breast
　　　Gynecomastia
　　　Hypertrophy of breast NOS
　　　Massive pubertal hypertrophy of breast
　　　EXCLUDES 1　breast engorgement of newborn (P83.4)
　　　　　　disproportion of reconstructed breast (N65.1)

✓4th **N63　Unspecified lump in** breast
　　　　Nodule(s) NOS in breast
● 　　**N63.0　Unspecified lump in unspecified breast** ▽
● ✓5th **N63.1　Unspecified lump in the right breast**
● 　　　**N63.10　Unspecified lump in the right breast, unspecified** ▽
　　　　　　quadrant
● 　　　**N63.11　Unspecified lump in the right breast, upper outer** ▽
　　　　　　quadrant
● 　　　**N63.12　Unspecified lump in the right breast, upper inner** ▽
　　　　　　quadrant
● 　　　**N63.13　Unspecified lump in the right breast, lower outer** ▽
　　　　　　quadrant
● 　　　**N63.14　Unspecified lump in the right breast, lower inner** ▽
　　　　　　quadrant
● ✓5th **N63.2　Unspecified lump in the left breast**
● 　　　**N63.20　Unspecified lump in the left breast, unspecified** ▽
　　　　　　quadrant
● 　　　**N63.21　Unspecified lump in the left breast, upper outer** ▽
　　　　　　quadrant
● 　　　**N63.22　Unspecified lump in the left breast, upper inner** ▽
　　　　　　quadrant
● 　　　**N63.23　Unspecified lump in the left breast, lower outer** ▽
　　　　　　quadrant
● 　　　**N63.24　Unspecified lump in the left breast, lower inner** ▽
　　　　　　quadrant
● ✓5th **N63.3　Unspecified lump in axillary tail**
● 　　　**N63.31　Unspecified lump in axillary tail of the right** ▽
　　　　　　breast
● 　　　**N63.32　Unspecified lump in axillary tail of the left** ▽
　　　　　　breast
● ✓5th **N63.4　Unspecified lump in breast, subareolar**
● 　　　**N63.41　Unspecified lump in right breast, subareolar** ▽
● 　　　**N63.42　Unspecified lump in left breast, subareolar** ▽

✓4th **N64　Other disorders of breast**
　　　EXCLUDES 2　mechanical complication of breast prosthesis and implant
　　　　　　(T85.4-)

　　N64.0　Fissure and fistula of nipple

　　N64.1　Fat necrosis of breast
　　　　Fat necrosis (segmental) of breast
　　　　Code first breast necrosis due to breast graft (T85.898)

　　N64.2　Atrophy of breast

　　N64.3　Galactorrhea not associated with childbirth

　　N64.4　Mastodynia

　✓5th **N64.5　Other signs and symptoms in breast**
　　　　EXCLUDES 2　abnormal findings on diagnostic imaging of breast
　　　　　　(R92.-)
　　　N64.51　Induration of breast
　　　N64.52　Nipple discharge
　　　　　　EXCLUDES 1　abnormal findings in nipple discharge
　　　　　　　　(R89.-)
　　　N64.53　Retraction of nipple
　　　N64.59　Other signs and symptoms in breast

　✓5th **N64.8　Other specified disorders of breast**
　　　N64.81　Ptosis of breast 🅰
　　　　　　EXCLUDES 1　ptosis of native breast in relation to
　　　　　　　　reconstructed breast (N65.1)
　　　N64.82　Hypoplasia of breast 🅰
　　　　　　Micromastia
　　　　　　EXCLUDES 1　congenital absence of breast (Q83.0)
　　　　　　　　hypoplasia of native breast in relation to
　　　　　　　　reconstructed breast (N65.1)
　　　N64.89　Other specified disorders of breast
　　　　　　Galactocele
　　　　　　Subinvolution of breast (postlactational)

　　N64.9　Disorder of breast, unspecified ▽

✓4th **N65　Deformity and disproportion of reconstructed breast**
　　N65.0　Deformity of reconstructed breast 🅰
　　　　Contour irregularity in reconstructed breast
　　　　Excess tissue in reconstructed breast
　　　　Misshapen reconstructed breast

　　N65.1　Disproportion of reconstructed breast 🅰
　　　　Breast asymmetry between native breast and reconstructed
　　　　　breast
　　　　Disproportion between native breast and reconstructed breast

✔ Additional Character Req　　vx7th Placeholder Alert　　Manifestation　　HCC CMS-HCC Condition　　▽ Unspecified Code　　►◄ Revised Text　　● New Code　　▲ Revised Code Title

ICD-10-CM 2018　　　　　　　　　　　　　　　　　　　　　　　　　　　　　　　　　　　811

Chapter 14. Diseases of Genitourinary System

Inflammatory diseases of female pelvic organs (N70-N77)

EXCLUDES1   inflammatory diseases of female pelvic organs complicating:
    abortion or ectopic or molar pregnancy (O00-O07, O08.0)
    pregnancy, childbirth and the puerperium (O23-, O75.3, O85, O86-)

✓4th N70 Salpingitis and oophoritis

INCLUDES   abscess (of) fallopian tube
    abscess (of) ovary
    pyosalpinx
    salpingo-oophoritis
    tubo-ovarian abscess
    tubo-ovarian inflammatory disease

Use additional code (B95-B97), to identify infectious agent

EXCLUDES1   gonococcal infection (A54.24)
    tuberculous infection (A18.17)

    ✓5th **N70.0**   Acute **salpingitis and oophoritis**
       N70.01   **Acute** salpingitis   ♀
       N70.02   **Acute** oophoritis   ♀
       N70.03   **Acute** salpingitis and oophoritis   ♀

    ✓5th **N70.1**   Chronic **salpingitis and oophoritis**
       Hydrosalpinx
       N70.11   **Chronic** salpingitis   ♀
       N70.12   **Chronic** oophoritis   ♀
       N70.13   **Chronic** salpingitis and oophoritis   ♀

    ✓5th **N70.9**   **Salpingitis and oophoritis, unspecified**
       N70.91   **Salpingitis, unspecified**   ♀ ▽
       N70.92   **Oophoritis, unspecified**   ♀▽
       N70.93   **Salpingitis and oophoritis, unspecified**   ♀ ▽

✓4th N71 Inflammatory disease of uterus, except cervix

INCLUDES   endo (myo) metritis   pyometra
    metritis   uterine abscess
    myometritis

Use additional code (B95-B97), to identify infectious agent

EXCLUDES1   hyperplastic endometritis (N85.0-)
    infection of uterus following delivery (O85, O86.-)

    N71.0   Acute **inflammatory disease of uterus**   ♀
    N71.1   Chronic **inflammatory disease of uterus**   ♀
    N71.9   **Inflammatory disease of uterus, unspecified**   ♀ ▽

N72 Inflammatory disease of cervix uteri   ♀

INCLUDES   cervicitis (with or without erosion or ectropion)
    endocervicitis (with or without erosion or ectropion)
    exocervicitis (with or without erosion or ectropion)

Use additional code (B95-B97), to identify infectious agent

EXCLUDES1   erosion and ectropion of cervix without cervicitis (N86)

✓4th N73 Other female pelvic inflammatory diseases

Use additional code (B95-B97), to identify infectious agent

    N73.0   Acute **parametritis and pelvic cellulitis**   ♀
       Abscess of broad ligament
       Abscess of parametrium
       Pelvic cellulitis, female
       DEF: Parametritis: Inflammation of the parametrium; pelvic cellulitis is a synonym for parametritis.

    N73.1   Chronic **parametritis and pelvic cellulitis**   ♀
       Any condition in N73.0 specified as chronic
       EXCLUDES1   tuberculous parametritis and pelvic cellulitis (A18.17)

    N73.2   **Unspecified parametritis and pelvic cellulitis**   ♀ ▽
       Any condition in N73.0 unspecified whether acute or chronic

    N73.3   Female acute **pelvic peritonitis**   ♀
    N73.4   Female chronic **pelvic peritonitis**   ♀
       EXCLUDES1   tuberculous pelvic (female) peritonitis (A18.17)

    N73.5   **Female pelvic peritonitis, unspecified**   ♀▽
    N73.6   **Female pelvic** peritoneal adhesions **(postinfective)**   ♀
       EXCLUDES2   postprocedural pelvic peritoneal adhesions (N99.4)
       AHA: 2014, 1Q, 6

    N73.8   Other specified **female pelvic inflammatory diseases**   ♀
    N73.9   **Female pelvic inflammatory disease, unspecified**   ♀ ▽
       Female pelvic infection or inflammation NOS

N74 Female pelvic inflammatory disorders in diseases classified elsewhere   ♀

Code first underlying disease

EXCLUDES1   chlamydial cervicitis (A56.02)
    chlamydial pelvic inflammatory disease (A56.11)
    gonococcal cervicitis (A54.03)
    gonococcal pelvic inflammatory disease (A54.24)
    herpesviral [herpes simplex] cervicitis (A60.03)
    herpesviral [herpes simplex] pelvic inflammatory disease
       (A60.09)
    syphilitic cervicitis (A52.76)
    syphilitic pelvic inflammatory disease (A52.76)
    trichomonal cervicitis (A59.09)
    tuberculous cervicitis (A18.16)
    tuberculous pelvic inflammatory disease (A18.17)

✓4th N75 Diseases of Bartholin's gland

    N75.0   **Cyst** of Bartholin's gland   ♀
    N75.1   **Abscess** of Bartholin's gland   ♀
    N75.8   Other diseases of Bartholin's gland   ♀
       Bartholinitis
    N75.9   **Disease of Bartholin's gland, unspecified**   ♀ ▽

✓4th N76 Other inflammation of vagina and vulva

Use additional code (B95-B97), to identify infectious agent

EXCLUDES2   senile (atrophic) vaginitis (N95.2)
    vulvar vestibulitis (N94.810)

    N76.0   **Acute vaginitis**   ♀
       Acute vulvovaginitis
       Vaginitis NOS
       Vulvovaginitis NOS

    N76.1   **Subacute and chronic vaginitis**   ♀
       Chronic vulvovaginitis
       Subacute vulvovaginitis

    N76.2   **Acute vulvitis**   ♀
       Vulvitis NOS

    N76.3   **Subacute and chronic vulvitis**   ♀
    N76.4   **Abscess of vulva**   ♀
       Furuncle of vulva

    N76.5   **Ulceration of vagina**   ♀
    N76.6   **Ulceration of vulva**   ♀

    ✓5th **N76.8**   **Other specified inflammation of vagina and vulva**
       N76.81   **Mucositis (ulcerative) of vagina and vulva**   ♀
          Code also type of associated therapy, such as:
            antineoplastic and immunosuppressive drugs
              (T45.1X-)
            radiological procedure and radiotherapy (Y84.2)
            EXCLUDES2   gastrointestinal mucositis (ulcerative)
                (K92.81)
                nasal mucositis (ulcerative) (J34.81)
                oral mucositis (ulcerative) (K12.3-)

       N76.89   **Other specified inflammation of vagina and vulva**   ♀

✓4th N77 Vulvovaginal ulceration and inflammation in diseases classified elsewhere

    N77.0   *Ulceration of vulva in diseases classified elsewhere*   ♀
       Code first underlying disease, such as:
       Behçet's disease (M35.2)
       EXCLUDES1   ulceration of vulva in gonococcal infection (A54.02)
          ulceration of vulva in herpesviral [herpes simplex]
            infection (A60.04)
          ulceration of vulva in syphilis (A51.0)
          ulceration of vulva in tuberculosis (A18.18)

    N77.1   *Vaginitis, vulvitis and vulvovaginitis in diseases classified*   ♀
       elsewhere
       Code first underlying disease, such as:
       pinworm (B80)
       EXCLUDES1   candidal vulvovaginitis (B37.3)
          chlamydial vulvovaginitis (A56.02)
          gonococcal vulvovaginitis (A54.02)
          herpesviral [herpes simplex] vulvovaginitis (A60.04)
          trichomonal vulvovaginitis (A59.01)
          tuberculous vulvovaginitis (A18.18)
          vulvovaginitis in early syphilis (A51.0)
          vulvovaginitis in late syphilis (A52.76)

EXCLUDES1 Not coded here   EXCLUDES2 Not included here   N Newborn Age: 0   P Pediatric Age: 0-17   M Maternity Age: 12-55   A Adult Age: 15-124

812   ICD-10-CM 2018

Types of Pelvic Organ Prolapse

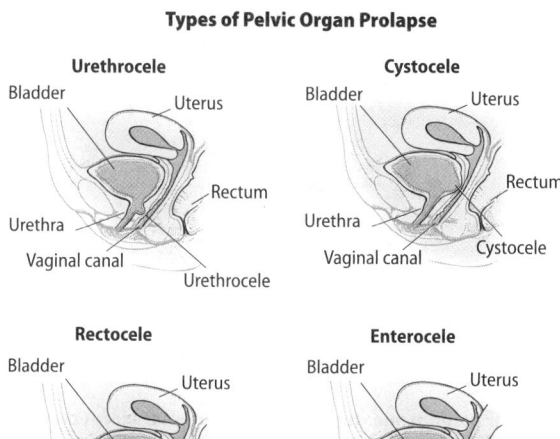

Urethrocele — Bladder, Uterus, Rectum, Urethra, Vaginal canal, Urethrocele

Cystocele — Bladder, Uterus, Rectum, Urethra, Cystocele, Vaginal canal

Rectocele — Bladder, Uterus, Rectum, Urethra, Rectocele, Vaginal canal

Enterocele — Bladder, Uterus, Enterocele, Terminal ileum, Urethra, Vaginal canal

Noninflammatory disorders of female genital tract (N80–N98)

✓4ᵗʰ N80 Endometriosis

N80.0 Endometriosis of uterus ♀
Adenomyosis
EXCLUDES 1 *stromal endometriosis (D39.0)*

N80.1 Endometriosis of ovary ♀

N80.2 Endometriosis of fallopian tube ♀

N80.3 Endometriosis of pelvic peritoneum ♀

N80.4 Endometriosis of rectovaginal septum and vagina ♀

N80.5 Endometriosis of intestine ♀

N80.6 Endometriosis in cutaneous scar ♀

N80.8 Other endometriosis ♀
►Endometriosis of thorax◄

N80.9 Endometriosis, unspecified ♀ ▽

✓4ᵗʰ N81 Female genital prolapse
EXCLUDES 1 *genital prolapse complicating pregnancy, labor or delivery (O34.5-)*
prolapse and hernia of ovary and fallopian tube (N83.4-)
prolapse of vaginal vault after hysterectomy (N99.3)

N81.0 Urethrocele ♀
EXCLUDES 1 *urethrocele with cystocele (N81.1-)*
urethrocele with prolapse of uterus (N81.2-N81.4)

✓5ᵗʰ N81.1 Cystocele
Cystocele with urethrocele
Cystourethrocele
EXCLUDES 1 *cystocele with prolapse of uterus (N81.2-N81.4)*

N81.10 Cystocele, unspecified ♀ ▽
Prolapse of (anterior) vaginal wall NOS

N81.11 Cystocele, midline ♀

N81.12 Cystocele, lateral ♀
Paravaginal cystocele
DEF: Detachment of the lateral support connections of the vagina at the arcus tendineus fasciae pelvis (ATFP) results in bladder drop; bladder herniates into the vagina laterally.

N81.2 Incomplete uterovaginal prolapse ♀
First degree uterine prolapse
Prolapse of cervix NOS
Second degree uterine prolapse
EXCLUDES 1 ►*cervical stump prolapse◄ (N81.85)*

N81.3 Complete uterovaginal prolapse ♀
Procidentia (uteri) NOS
Third degree uterine prolapse

N81.4 Uterovaginal prolapse, unspecified ♀ ▽
Prolapse of uterus NOS

N81.5 Vaginal enterocele ♀
EXCLUDES 1 *enterocele with prolapse of uterus (N81.2-N81.4)*

N81.6 Rectocele ♀
Prolapse of posterior vaginal wall
Use additional code for any associated fecal incontinence, if applicable (R15.-)
EXCLUDES 2 *perineocele (N81.81)*
rectal prolapse (K62.3)
rectocele with prolapse of uterus (N81.2-N81.4)

✓5ᵗʰ N81.8 Other female genital prolapse

N81.81 Perineocele ♀

N81.82 Incompetence or weakening of pubocervical tissue ♀

N81.83 Incompetence or weakening of rectovaginal tissue ♀

N81.84 Pelvic muscle wasting ♀
Disuse atrophy of pelvic muscles and anal sphincter

N81.85 Cervical stump prolapse ♀

N81.89 Other female genital prolapse ♀
Deficient perineum
Old laceration of muscles of pelvic floor

N81.9 Female genital prolapse, unspecified ♀ ▽

✓4ᵗʰ N82 Fistulae involving female genital tract
EXCLUDES 1 *vesicointestinal fistulae (N32.1)*

N82.0 Vesicovaginal fistula ♀

N82.1 Other female urinary-genital tract fistulae ♀
Cervicovesical fistula
Ureterovaginal fistula
Urethrovaginal fistula
Uteroureteric fistula
Uterovesical fistula

N82.2 Fistula of vagina to small intestine ♀

N82.3 Fistula of vagina to large intestine ♀
Rectovaginal fistula

N82.4 Other female intestinal-genital tract fistulae ♀
Intestinouterine fistula

N82.5 Female genital tract-skin fistulae ♀
Uterus to abdominal wall fistula
Vaginoperineal fistula

N82.8 Other female genital tract fistulae ♀

N82.9 Female genital tract fistula, unspecified ♀ ▽

✓4ᵗʰ N83 Noninflammatory disorders of ovary, fallopian tube and broad ligament
EXCLUDES 2 *hydrosalpinx (N70.1-)*

✓5ᵗʰ N83.0 Follicular cyst of ovary
Cyst of graafian follicle
Hemorrhagic follicular cyst (of ovary)

N83.00 Follicular cyst of ovary, unspecified side ♀ ▽

N83.01 Follicular cyst of right ovary ♀

N83.02 Follicular cyst of left ovary ♀

✓5ᵗʰ N83.1 Corpus luteum cyst
Hemorrhagic corpus luteum cyst

N83.10 Corpus luteum cyst of ovary, unspecified side ♀ ▽

N83.11 Corpus luteum cyst of right ovary ♀

N83.12 Corpus luteum cyst of left ovary ♀

✓5ᵗʰ N83.2 Other and unspecified ovarian cysts
EXCLUDES 1 *developmental ovarian cyst (Q50.1)*
neoplastic ovarian cyst (D27.-)
polycystic ovarian syndrome (E28.2)
Stein-Leventhal syndrome (E28.2)

✓6ᵗʰ N83.20 Unspecified ovarian cysts

N83.201 Unspecified ovarian cyst, right side ♀ ▽

N83.202 Unspecified ovarian cyst, left side ♀ ▽

N83.209 Unspecified ovarian cyst, unspecified side ♀ ▽
Ovarian cyst, NOS

✓6ᵗʰ N83.29 Other ovarian cysts
Retention cyst of ovary
Simple cyst of ovary

N83.291 Other ovarian cyst, right side ♀

N83.292 Other ovarian cyst, left side ♀

N83.299 Other ovarian cyst, unspecified side ♀ ▽

✓5ᵗʰ N83.3 Acquired atrophy of ovary and fallopian tube

✓6ᵗʰ N83.31 Acquired atrophy of ovary

N83.311 Acquired atrophy of right ovary ♀

N83.312 Acquired atrophy of left ovary ♀

N83.319   **Acquired atrophy of ovary, unspecified side** ♀▽
Acquired atrophy of ovary, NOS

✓6ᵗʰ **N83.32**   **Acquired atrophy of fallopian tube**

N83.321   **Acquired atrophy of right fallopian tube** ♀

N83.322   **Acquired atrophy of left fallopian tube** ♀

N83.329   **Acquired atrophy of fallopian tube, unspecified side** ♀▽
Acquired atrophy of fallopian tube, NOS

✓6ᵗʰ **N83.33**   **Acquired atrophy of ovary and fallopian tube**

N83.331   **Acquired atrophy of right ovary and fallopian tube** ♀

N83.332   **Acquired atrophy of left ovary and fallopian tube** ♀

N83.339   **Acquired atrophy of ovary and fallopian tube, unspecified side** ♀▽
Acquired atrophy of ovary and fallopian tube, NOS

✓5ᵗʰ **N83.4**   **Prolapse and hernia of ovary and fallopian tube**

N83.40   **Prolapse and hernia of ovary and fallopian tube, unspecified side** ♀▽
Prolapse and hernia of ovary and fallopian tube, NOS

N83.41   **Prolapse and hernia of right ovary and fallopian tube** ♀

N83.42   **Prolapse and hernia of left ovary and fallopian tube** ♀

✓5ᵗʰ **N83.5**   **Torsion of ovary, ovarian pedicle and fallopian tube**
Torsion of accessory tube

✓6ᵗʰ **N83.51**   **Torsion of ovary and ovarian pedicle**

N83.511   **Torsion of right ovary and ovarian pedicle** ♀

N83.512   **Torsion of left ovary and ovarian pedicle** ♀

N83.519   **Torsion of ovary and ovarian pedicle, unspecified side** ♀▽
Torsion of ovary and ovarian pedicle, NOS

✓6ᵗʰ **N83.52**   **Torsion of fallopian tube**
Torsion of hydatid of Morgagni

N83.521   **Torsion of right fallopian tube** ♀

N83.522   **Torsion of left fallopian tube** ♀

N83.529   **Torsion of fallopian tube, unspecified side** ♀▽
Torsion of fallopian tube, NOS

N83.53   **Torsion of ovary, ovarian pedicle and fallopian tube** ♀

N83.6   **Hematosalpinx** ♀
EXCLUDES 1   hematosalpinx (with) (in):
hematocolpos (N89.7)
hematometra (N85.7)
tubal pregnancy (O00.1-)

N83.7   **Hematoma of broad ligament** ♀

N83.8   **Other noninflammatory disorders of ovary, fallopian tube and broad ligament** ♀
Broad ligament laceration syndrome [Allen-Masters]

N83.9   **Noninflammatory disorder of ovary, fallopian tube and broad ligament, unspecified** ♀▽

✓4ᵗʰ **N84**   **Polyp of female genital tract**
EXCLUDES 1   adenomatous polyp (D28.-)
placental polyp (O90.89)

N84.0   **Polyp of corpus uteri** ♀
Polyp of endometrium
Polyp of uterus NOS
EXCLUDES 1   polypoid endometrial hyperplasia (N85.0-)

N84.1   **Polyp of cervix uteri** ♀
Mucous polyp of cervix

N84.2   **Polyp of vagina** ♀

N84.3   **Polyp of vulva** ♀
Polyp of labia

N84.8   **Polyp of other parts of female genital tract** ♀

N84.9   **Polyp of female genital tract, unspecified** ♀▽

Inversion of Uterus

Uterus

✓4ᵗʰ **N85**   **Other noninflammatory disorders of uterus, except cervix**
EXCLUDES 1   endometriosis (N80.-)
inflammatory diseases of uterus (N71.-)
noninflammatory disorders of cervix, except malposition (N86-N88)
polyp of corpus uteri (N84.0)
uterine prolapse (N81.-)

✓5ᵗʰ **N85.0**   **Endometrial hyperplasia**

N85.00   **Endometrial hyperplasia, unspecified** ♀▽
Hyperplasia (adenomatous) (cystic) (glandular) of endometrium
Hyperplastic endometritis

N85.01   **Benign endometrial hyperplasia** ♀
Endometrial hyperplasia (complex) (simple) without atypia

N85.02   **Endometrial intraepithelial neoplasia [EIN]** ♀
Endometrial hyperplasia with atypia
EXCLUDES 1   malignant neoplasm of endometrium (with endometrial intraepithelial neoplasia [EIN]) (C54.1)

N85.2   **Hypertrophy of uterus** ♀
Bulky or enlarged uterus
EXCLUDES 1   puerperal hypertrophy of uterus (O90.89)

N85.3   **Subinvolution of uterus** ♀
EXCLUDES 1   puerperal subinvolution of uterus (O90.89)

N85.4   **Malposition of uterus** ♀
Anteversion of uterus   Retroversion of uterus
Retroflexion of uterus
EXCLUDES 1   malposition of uterus complicating pregnancy, labor or delivery (O34.5-, O65.5)

N85.5   **Inversion of uterus** ♀
EXCLUDES 1   current obstetric trauma (O71.2)
postpartum inversion of uterus (O71.2)

N85.6   **Intrauterine synechiae** ♀

N85.7   **Hematometra** ♀
Hematosalpinx with hematometra
EXCLUDES 1   hematometra with hematocolpos (N89.7)
DEF: Accumulation of blood within the uterus.

N85.8   **Other specified noninflammatory disorders of uterus** ♀
Atrophy of uterus, acquired
Fibrosis of uterus NOS

N85.9   **Noninflammatory disorder of uterus, unspecified** ♀▽
Disorder of uterus NOS

N86   **Erosion and ectropion of cervix uteri** ♀
Decubitus (trophic) ulcer of cervix
Eversion of cervix
EXCLUDES 1   erosion and ectropion of cervix with cervicitis (N72)

✓4ᵗʰ **N87**   **Dysplasia of cervix uteri**
EXCLUDES 1   abnormal results from cervical cytologic examination without histologic confirmation (R87.61-)
carcinoma in situ of cervix uteri (D06.-)
cervical intraepithelial neoplasia III [CIN III] (D06.-)
HGSIL of cervix (R87.613)
severe dysplasia of cervix uteri (D06.-)

N87.0   **Mild cervical dysplasia** ♀
Cervical intraepithelial neoplasia I [CIN I]

N87.1   **Moderate cervical dysplasia** ♀
Cervical intraepithelial neoplasia II [CIN II]

N87.9   **Dysplasia of cervix uteri, unspecified** ♀▽
Anaplasia of cervix   Cervical dysplasia NOS
Cervical atypism

EXCLUDES 1 Not coded here   EXCLUDES 2 Not included here   N Newborn Age: 0   P Pediatric Age: 0-17   M Maternity Age: 12-55   A Adult Age: 15-124

✓4ᵗʰ **N88** **Other noninflammatory disorders of cervix uteri**
     EXCLUDES 2   *inflammatory disease of cervix (N72)*
                 polyp of cervix (N84.1)

     N88.0 **Leukoplakia of cervix uteri**   ♀

     N88.1 **Old laceration of cervix uteri**   ♀
          Adhesions of cervix
          EXCLUDES 1   *current obstetric trauma (O71.3)*

     N88.2 **Stricture and stenosis of cervix uteri**   ♀
          EXCLUDES 1   *stricture and stenosis of cervix uteri complicating labor (O65.5)*

     N88.3 **Incompetence of cervix uteri**   ♀
          Investigation and management of (suspected) cervical incompetence in a nonpregnant woman
          EXCLUDES 1   *cervical incompetence complicating pregnancy (O34.3-)*

     N88.4 **Hypertrophic elongation of cervix uteri**   ♀

     N88.8 **Other specified noninflammatory disorders of cervix uteri**   ♀
          EXCLUDES 1   *current obstetric trauma (O71.3)*

     N88.9 **Noninflammatory disorder of cervix uteri, unspecified**   ♀ ▽

✓4ᵗʰ **N89** **Other noninflammatory disorders of vagina**
     EXCLUDES 1   *abnormal results from vaginal cytologic examination without histologic confirmation (R87.62-)*
               carcinoma in situ of vagina (D07.2)
               HGSIL of vagina (R87.623)
               inflammation of vagina (N76.-)
               senile (atrophic) vaginitis (N95.2)
               severe dysplasia of vagina (D07.2)
               trichomonal leukorrhea (A59.00)
               vaginal intraepithelial neoplasia [VAIN], grade III (D07.2)

     N89.0 **Mild vaginal dysplasia**   ♀
          Vaginal intraepithelial neoplasia [VAIN], grade I

     N89.1 **Moderate vaginal dysplasia**   ♀
          Vaginal intraepithelial neoplasia [VAIN], grade II

     N89.3 **Dysplasia of vagina, unspecified**   ♀ ▽

     N89.4 **Leukoplakia of vagina**   ♀

     N89.5 **Stricture and atresia of vagina**   ♀
          Vaginal adhesions
          Vaginal stenosis
          EXCLUDES 1   *congenital atresia or stricture (Q52.4)*
                  postprocedural adhesions of vagina (N99.2)

     N89.6 **Tight hymenal ring**   ♀
          Rigid hymen
          Tight introitus
          EXCLUDES 1   *imperforate hymen (Q52.3)*

     N89.7 **Hematocolpos**   ♀
          Hematocolpos with hematometra or hematosalpinx

     N89.8 **Other specified noninflammatory disorders of vagina**   ♀
          Leukorrhea NOS
          Old vaginal laceration
          Pessary ulcer of vagina
          EXCLUDES 1   *current obstetric trauma (O70-, O71.4, O71.7-O71.8)*
                  old laceration involving muscles of pelvic floor (N81.8)

     N89.9 **Noninflammatory disorder of vagina, unspecified**   ♀ ▽

✓4ᵗʰ **N90** **Other noninflammatory disorders of vulva and perineum**
     EXCLUDES 1   *anogenital (venereal) warts (A63.0)*
               carcinoma in situ of vulva (D07.1)
               condyloma acuminatum (A63.0)
               current obstetric trauma (O70-, O71.7-O71.8)
               inflammation of vulva (N76.-)
               severe dysplasia of vulva (D07.1)
               vulvar intraepithelial neoplasm III [VIN III] (D07.1)

     N90.0 **Mild vulvar dysplasia**   ♀
          Vulvar intraepithelial neoplasia [VIN], grade I

     N90.1 **Moderate vulvar dysplasia**   ♀
          Vulvar intraepithelial neoplasia [VIN], grade II

     N90.3 **Dysplasia of vulva, unspecified**   ♀ ▽

     N90.4 **Leukoplakia of vulva**   ♀
          Dystrophy of vulva
          Kraurosis of vulva
          Lichen sclerosus of external female genital organs

     N90.5 **Atrophy of vulva**   ♀
          Stenosis of vulva

✓5ᵗʰ **N90.6** **Hypertrophy of vulva**   ♀

     N90.60 **Unspecified hypertrophy of vulva**   ♀ ▽
          Unspecified hypertrophy of labia

     N90.61 **Childhood asymmetric labium majus enlargement**   ♀
          CALME

     N90.69 **Other specified hypertrophy of vulva**   ♀
          Other specified hypertrophy of labia

     N90.7 **Vulvar cyst**   ♀

✓5ᵗʰ **N90.8** **Other specified noninflammatory disorders of vulva and perineum**

     ✓6ᵗʰ **N90.81** **Female genital mutilation status**
          Female genital cutting status

          N90.810 **Female genital mutilation status, unspecified**   ♀ ▽
               Female genital cutting status, unspecified
               Female genital mutilation status NOS

          N90.811 **Female genital mutilation Type I status**   ♀
               Clitorectomy status
               Female genital cutting Type I status

          N90.812 **Female genital mutilation Type II status**   ♀
               Clitorectomy with excision of labia minora status
               Female genital cutting Type II status

          N90.813 **Female genital mutilation Type III status**   ♀
               Female genital cutting Type III status
               Infibulation status

          N90.818 **Other female genital mutilation status**   ♀
               Female genital cutting Type IV status
               Female genital mutilation Type IV status
               Other female genital cutting status

     N90.89 **Other specified noninflammatory disorders of vulva and perineum**   ♀
          Adhesions of vulva   Hypertrophy of clitoris

     N90.9 **Noninflammatory disorder of vulva and perineum, unspecified**   ♀ ▽

✓4ᵗʰ **N91** **Absent, scanty and rare menstruation**
     EXCLUDES 1   *ovarian dysfunction (E28.-)*

     N91.0 **Primary amenorrhea**   ♀

     N91.1 **Secondary amenorrhea**   ♀

     N91.2 **Amenorrhea, unspecified**   ♀ ▽

     N91.3 **Primary oligomenorrhea**   ♀

     N91.4 **Secondary oligomenorrhea**   ♀

     N91.5 **Oligomenorrhea, unspecified**   ♀ ▽
          Hypomenorrhea NOS

✓4ᵗʰ **N92** **Excessive, frequent and irregular menstruation**
     EXCLUDES 1   *postmenopausal bleeding (N95.0)*
               precocious puberty (menstruation) (E30.1)

     N92.0 **Excessive and frequent menstruation with regular cycle**   ♀
          Heavy periods NOS
          Menorrhagia NOS
          Polymenorrhea

     N92.1 **Excessive and frequent menstruation with irregular cycle**   ♀
          Irregular intermenstrual bleeding
          Irregular, shortened intervals between menstrual bleeding
          Menometrorrhagia
          Metrorrhagia

     N92.2 **Excessive menstruation at puberty**   P ♀
          Excessive bleeding associated with onset of menstrual periods
          Pubertal menorrhagia
          Puberty bleeding

     N92.3 **Ovulation bleeding**   ♀
          Regular intermenstrual bleeding

     N92.4 **Excessive bleeding in the premenopausal period**   ♀
          Climacteric menorrhagia or metrorrhagia
          Menopausal menorrhagia or metrorrhagia
          Preclimacteric menorrhagia or metrorrhagia
          Premenopausal menorrhagia or metrorrhagia

     N92.5 **Other specified irregular menstruation**   ♀

     N92.6 **Irregular menstruation, unspecified**   ♀ ▽
          Irregular bleeding NOS
          Irregular periods NOS
          EXCLUDES 1   *irregular menstruation with:*
                 lengthened intervals or scanty bleeding (N91.3-N91.5)
                 shortened intervals or excessive bleeding (N92.1)

☑ Additional Character Req   ✗7ᵗʰ Placeholder Alert   Manifestation   HCC CMS-HCC Condition   ▽ Unspecified Code   ▶◀ Revised Text   ● New Code   ▲ Revised Code Title

✓4th N93 Other abnormal uterine and vaginal bleeding

EXCLUDES 1   neonatal vaginal hemorrhage (P54.6)
precocious puberty (menstruation) (E30.1)
pseudomenses (P54.6)

N93.0 Postcoital and contact bleeding ♀
N93.1 Pre-pubertal vaginal bleeding ♀
N93.8 Other specified abnormal uterine and vaginal bleeding ♀
     Dysfunctional or functional uterine or vaginal bleeding NOS
N93.9 Abnormal uterine and vaginal bleeding, unspecified ♀▽

✓4th N94 Pain and other conditions associated with female genital organs and menstrual cycle

N94.0 Mittelschmerz ♀
     DEF: One-sided, lower abdominal pain occurring between menstrual periods; associated with ovulation.

✓5th N94.1 Dyspareunia
EXCLUDES 1   psychogenic dyspareunia (F52.6)
     N94.10 Unspecified dyspareunia ♀▽
     N94.11 Superficial (introital) dyspareunia ♀
     N94.12 Deep dyspareunia ♀
     N94.19 Other specified dyspareunia ♀

N94.2 Vaginismus ♀
EXCLUDES 1   psychogenic vaginismus (F52.5)

N94.3 Premenstrual tension syndrome ♀
     ~~Premenstrual dysphoric disorder~~
     Code also associated menstrual migraine (G43.82-, G43.83-)
EXCLUDES 1   premenstrual dysphoric disorder (F32.81)

N94.4 Primary dysmenorrhea ♀
N94.5 Secondary dysmenorrhea ♀
N94.6 Dysmenorrhea, unspecified ♀▽
EXCLUDES 1   psychogenic dysmenorrhea (F45.8)

✓5th N94.8 Other specified conditions associated with female genital organs and menstrual cycle

✓6th N94.81 Vulvodynia
     N94.810 Vulvar vestibulitis ♀
     N94.818 Other vulvodynia ♀
     N94.819 Vulvodynia, unspecified ♀▽
       Vulvodynia NOS

     N94.89 Other specified conditions associated with female ♀ **genital organs and menstrual cycle**

N94.9 Unspecified condition associated with female genital ♀▽ **organs and menstrual cycle**

✓4th N95 Menopausal and other perimenopausal disorders

Menopausal and other perimenopausal disorders due to naturally occurring (age-related) menopause and perimenopause
EXCLUDES 1   excessive bleeding in the premenopausal period (N92.4)
menopausal and perimenopausal disorders due to artificial or premature menopause (E89.4-, E28.31-)
premature menopause (E28.31-)
EXCLUDES 2   postmenopausal osteoporosis (M81.0-)
postmenopausal osteoporosis with current pathological fracture (M80.0-)
postmenopausal urethritis (N34.2)

N95.0 Postmenopausal bleeding ♀
N95.1 Menopausal and female climacteric states ♀
     Symptoms such as flushing, sleeplessness, headache, lack of concentration, associated with natural (age-related) menopause
     Use additional code for associated symptoms
EXCLUDES 1   asymptomatic menopausal state (Z78.0)
symptoms associated with artificial menopause (E89.41)
symptoms associated with premature menopause (E28.310)

N95.2 Postmenopausal atrophic vaginitis ♀
     Senile (atrophic) vaginitis
N95.8 Other specified menopausal and perimenopausal ♀ **disorders**
N95.9 Unspecified menopausal and perimenopausal disorder ♀▽

N96 Recurrent pregnancy loss ♀
Investigation or care in a nonpregnant woman with history of recurrent pregnancy loss
EXCLUDES 1   recurrent pregnancy loss with current pregnancy (O26.2-)

✓4th N97 Female infertility

INCLUDES   inability to achieve a pregnancy
sterility, female NOS
EXCLUDES 1   female infertility associated with:
hypopituitarism (E23.0)
Stein-Leventhal syndrome (E28.2)
EXCLUDES 2   incompetence of cervix uteri (N88.3)
DEF: Infertility: Inability to conceive for at least one year with regular intercourse.
DEF: Primary infertility: Infertility occurring in patients who have never conceived.
DEF: Secondary infertility: Infertility occurring in patients who have previously conceived.

N97.0 Female infertility associated with anovulation ♀
N97.1 Female infertility of tubal origin ♀
     Female infertility associated with congenital anomaly of tube
     Female infertility due to tubal block
     Female infertility due to tubal occlusion
     Female infertility due to tubal stenosis

N97.2 Female infertility of uterine origin ♀
     Female infertility associated with congenital anomaly of uterus
     Female infertility due to nonimplantation of ovum

N97.8 Female infertility of other origin ♀
N97.9 Female infertility, unspecified ♀▽

✓4th N98 Complications associated with artificial fertilization

N98.0 Infection associated with artificial insemination ♀
N98.1 Hyperstimulation of ovaries ♀
     Hyperstimulation of ovaries NOS
     Hyperstimulation of ovaries associated with induced ovulation

N98.2 Complications of attempted introduction of fertilized ♀ **ovum following in vitro fertilization**
N98.3 Complications of attempted introduction of embryo in ♀ **embryo transfer**
N98.8 Other complications associated with artificial fertilization ♀
N98.9 Complication associated with artificial fertilization, ♀▽ **unspecified**

Intraoperative and postprocedural complications and disorders of genitourinary system, not elsewhere classified (N99)

✓4th N99 Intraoperative and postprocedural complications and disorders of genitourinary system, not elsewhere classified

EXCLUDES 2   irradiation cystitis (N30.4-)
postoophorectomy osteoporosis with current pathological fracture (M80.8-)
postoophorectomy osteoporosis without current pathological fracture (M81.8)

N99.0 Postprocedural (acute) (chronic) kidney failure
     Use additional code to type of kidney disease

✓5th N99.1 Postprocedural urethral stricture
Postcatheterization urethral stricture

✓6th N99.11 Postprocedural urethral stricture, male
     N99.110 Postprocedural urethral stricture, male, ♂ **meatal**
▲   **N99.111 Postprocedural bulbous urethral** ♂ **stricture, male**
▲   **N99.112 Postprocedural membranous urethral** ♂ **stricture, male**
▲   **N99.113 Postprocedural anterior bulbous** ♂ **urethral stricture, male**
     N99.114 Postprocedural urethral stricture, ♂▽ **male, unspecified**
     N99.115 Postprocedural fossa navicularis ♂ **urethral stricture**

     N99.12 Postprocedural urethral stricture, female ♀

N99.2 Postprocedural adhesions of vagina ♀
N99.3 Prolapse of vaginal vault after hysterectomy ♀
N99.4 Postprocedural pelvic peritoneal adhesions
EXCLUDES 2   pelvic peritoneal adhesions NOS (N73.6)
postinfective pelvic peritoneal adhesions (N73.6)

EXCLUDES 1 Not coded here   **EXCLUDES 2** Not included here   N Newborn Age: 0   P Pediatric Age: 0-17   M Maternity Age: 12-55   A Adult Age: 15-124

✓5ᵗʰ N99.5 Complications of stoma of urinary tract

> **EXCLUDES 2**   mechanical complication of urinary catheter (T83.Ø-)

     ✓6ᵗʰ N99.51 Complication of cystostomy

         N99.51Ø Cystostomy hemorrhage   `HCC`

         N99.511 Cystostomy infection   `HCC`

         N99.512 Cystostomy malfunction   `HCC`

         N99.518 Other cystostomy complication   `HCC`

     ✓6ᵗʰ N99.52 Complication of incontinent external stoma of urinary tract

         N99.52Ø Hemorrhage **of incontinent external stoma of urinary tract**   `HCC`

         N99.521 Infection **of incontinent external stoma of urinary tract**   `HCC`

         N99.522 Malfunction **of incontinent external stoma of urinary tract**   `HCC`

         N99.523 Herniation **of incontinent stoma of urinary tract**   `HCC`

         N99.524 Stenosis **of incontinent stoma of urinary tract**   `HCC`

         N99.528 Other complication of incontinent external stoma of urinary tract   `HCC`

     ✓6ᵗʰ N99.53 Complication of continent stoma of urinary tract

         N99.53Ø Hemorrhage **of continent stoma of urinary tract**   `HCC`

         N99.531 Infection **of continent stoma of urinary tract**   `HCC`

         N99.532 Malfunction **of continent stoma of urinary tract**   `HCC`

         N99.533 Herniation **of continent stoma of urinary tract**   `HCC`

         N99.534 Stenosis **of continent stoma of urinary tract**   `HCC`

         N99.538 Other complication of continent stoma of urinary tract   `HCC`

✓5ᵗʰ N99.6 Intraoperative hemorrhage and hematoma **of a genitourinary system organ or structure complicating a procedure**

> **EXCLUDES 1**   intraoperative hemorrhage and hematoma of a genitourinary system organ or structure due to accidental puncture or laceration during a procedure (N99.7-)

     N99.61 Intraoperative hemorrhage and hematoma of a genitourinary system organ or structure complicating a genitourinary system procedure

     N99.62 Intraoperative hemorrhage and hematoma of a genitourinary system organ or structure complicating other procedure

✓5ᵗʰ N99.7 Accidental puncture and laceration **of a genitourinary system organ or structure during a procedure**

     N99.71 Accidental puncture and laceration of a genitourinary system organ or structure during a genitourinary system procedure

     N99.72 Accidental puncture and laceration of a genitourinary system organ or structure during other procedure

✓5ᵗʰ N99.8 Other intraoperative and postprocedural complications and disorders of genitourinary system

     N99.81 Other intraoperative complications **of genitourinary system**

     ✓6ᵗʰ N99.82 Postprocedural hemorrhage **of a genitourinary system organ or structure following a procedure**

         N99.82Ø Postprocedural hemorrhage of a genitourinary system organ or structure following a genitourinary system procedure

         N99.821 Postprocedural hemorrhage of a genitourinary system organ or structure following other procedure

     N99.83 Residual ovary syndrome   ♀

     ✓6ᵗʰ N99.84 Postprocedural hematoma and seroma **of a genitourinary system organ or structure following a procedure**

         N99.84Ø Postprocedural hematoma **of a genitourinary system organ or structure following a** genitourinary system procedure

         N99.841 Postprocedural hematoma **of a genitourinary system organ or structure following** other procedure

         N99.842 Postprocedural seroma **of a genitourinary system organ or structure following a** genitourinary system procedure

         N99.843 Postprocedural seroma **of a genitourinary system organ or structure following** other procedure

     N99.89 Other postprocedural complications and disorders of genitourinary system

---

☑ Additional Character Req   ✓ˣ⁷ᵗʰ Placeholder Alert   Manifestation   `HCC` CMS-HCC Condition   ▽ Unspecified Code   ►◄ Revised Text   ● New Code   ▲ Revised Code Title

Chapter 15. Pregnancy, Childbirth, and the Puerperium (O00–O9A)

Chapter Specific Guidelines with Coding Examples

The chapter specific guidelines from the ICD-10-CM Official Guidelines for Coding and Reporting have been provided below. Along with these guidelines are coding examples, contained in the shaded boxes, that have been developed to help illustrate the coding and/or sequencing guidance found in these guidelines.

a. General rules for obstetric cases

1) Codes from Chapter 15 and sequencing priority

Obstetric cases require codes from chapter 15, codes in the range O00-O9A, Pregnancy, Childbirth, and the Puerperium. Chapter 15 codes have sequencing priority over codes from other chapters. Additional codes from other chapters may be used in conjunction with chapter 15 codes to further specify conditions. Should the provider document that the pregnancy is incidental to the encounter, then code Z33.1, Pregnant state, incidental, should be used in place of any chapter 15 codes. It is the provider's responsibility to state that the condition being treated is not affecting the pregnancy.

> Bladder abscess in pregnant patient at 25 weeks' gestation
>
> **O23.12** **Infections of bladder in pregnancy, second trimester**
>
> **N30.80** **Other cystitis without hematuria**
>
> **Z3A.25** **25 weeks gestation of pregnancy**
>
> *Explanation:* The documentation does not indicate that the pregnancy is incidental or in any way unaffected by the bladder abscess; therefore, an obstetrics code should be sequenced first. An additional code was provided to identify the specific bladder condition as this information is not called out specifically in the obstetrics code.

2) Chapter 15 codes used only on the maternal record

Chapter 15 codes are to be used only on the maternal record, never on the record of the newborn.

3) Final character for trimester

The majority of codes in Chapter 15 have a final character indicating the trimester of pregnancy. The timeframes for the trimesters are indicated at the beginning of the chapter. If trimester is not a component of a code, it is because the condition always occurs in a specific trimester, or the concept of trimester of pregnancy is not applicable. Certain codes have characters for only certain trimesters because the condition does not occur in all trimesters, but it may occur in more than just one. Assignment of the final character for trimester should be based on the provider's documentation of the trimester (or number of weeks) for the current admission/encounter. This applies to the assignment of trimester for pre-existing conditions as well as those that develop during or are due to the pregnancy. The provider's documentation of the number of weeks may be used to assign the appropriate code identifying the trimester.

Whenever delivery occurs during the current admission, and there is an "in childbirth" option for the obstetric complication being coded, the "in childbirth" code should be assigned.

> Pregnant patient at 21 weeks' gestation admitted with excessive vomiting
>
> **O21.2** **Late vomiting of pregnancy**
>
> **Z3A.21** **21 weeks gestation of pregnancy**
>
> *Explanation:* Category O21 classifies vomiting in pregnancy. Although code selection is based on whether the vomiting is before or after 20 completed weeks, these codes are not further classified by trimester. If vomiting only in the second trimester was documented, the provider should be queried for the specific week of gestation, as this will affect code selection.

4) Selection of trimester for inpatient admissions that encompass more than one trimester

In instances when a patient is admitted to a hospital for complications of pregnancy during one trimester and remains in the hospital into a subsequent trimester, the trimester character for the antepartum complication code should be assigned on the basis of the trimester when the complication developed, not the trimester of the discharge. If the condition developed prior to the current admission/encounter or represents a pre-existing condition, the trimester character for the trimester at the time of the admission/encounter should be assigned.

5) Unspecified trimester

Each category that includes codes for trimester has a code for "unspecified trimester." The "unspecified trimester" code should rarely be used, such as when the documentation in the record is insufficient to determine the trimester and it is not possible to obtain clarification.

6) 7th character for fetus identification

Where applicable, a 7th character is to be assigned for certain categories (O31, O32, O33.3 - O33.6, O35, O36, O40, O41, O60.1, O60.2, O64, and O69) to identify the fetus for which the complication code applies.

Assign 7th character "0":

- For single gestations
- When the documentation in the record is insufficient to determine the fetus affected and it is not possible to obtain clarification.
- When it is not possible to clinically determine which fetus is affected.

> Maternal patient with twin gestations is seen after ultrasound identifies fetus B to be in breech presentation
>
> **O32.1XX2** **Maternal care for breech presentation, fetus 2**
>
> *Explanation:* The documentation indicates that although there are two fetuses, only one fetus is determined to be in breech presentation. Whether fetus 2 or fetus B is used, the coder can assign the seventh character of 2 to identify the second fetus as the one in breech.

b. Selection of OB principal or first-listed diagnosis

1) Routine outpatient prenatal visits

For routine outpatient prenatal visits when no complications are present, a code from category Z34, Encounter for supervision of normal pregnancy, should be used as the first-listed diagnosis. These codes should not be used in conjunction with chapter 15 codes.

2) *Supervision of high-risk pregnancy*

Codes from category O09, Supervision of high-risk pregnancy, are intended for use only during the prenatal period. For complications during the labor or delivery episode as a result of a high-risk pregnancy, assign the applicable complication codes from Chapter 15. If there are no complications during the labor or delivery episode, assign code O80, Encounter for full-term uncomplicated delivery.

For routine prenatal outpatient visits for patients with high-risk pregnancies, a code from category O09, Supervision of high-risk pregnancy, should be used as the first-listed diagnosis. Secondary chapter 15 codes may be used in conjunction with these codes if appropriate.

> 36-year-old seen in labor with second child at 39 weeks' gestation, delivered a healthy baby, delivery complicated by tear of fourchette that was repaired
>
> **O70.0** **First degree perineal laceration during delivery**
>
> **Z3A.39** **39 weeks gestation of pregnancy**
>
> **Z37.0** **Single live birth**
>
> Explanation: Although this patient is over 35 and having her second child (elderly multigravida), do not append a code from subcategory O09.52-. A code describing the tear of the fourchette, which complicated the delivery, should be used in addition to the applicable Z codes.

3) Episodes when no delivery occurs

In episodes when no delivery occurs, the principal diagnosis should correspond to the principal complication of the pregnancy which necessitated the encounter. Should more than one complication exist, all of which are treated or monitored, any of the complications codes may be sequenced first.

4) When a delivery occurs

When an obstetric patient is admitted and delivers during that admission, the condition that prompted the admission should be sequenced as the principal diagnosis. If multiple conditions prompted the admission, sequence the one most related to the delivery as the principal diagnosis. A code for any complication of the delivery should be assigned as an additional diagnosis. In cases of cesarean delivery, if the patient was admitted with a condition that resulted in the performance of a cesarean procedure, that condition should be selected as the principal diagnosis. If the reason for the admission was unrelated to the condition resulting in the cesarean delivery, the condition related to the reason for the admission should be selected as the principal diagnosis.

> Maternal patient with diet-controlled gestational diabetes was seen at 38 weeks' gestation in obstructed labor due to footling presentation; cesarean performed for the malpresentation
>
> | O64.8XXØ | Obstructed labor due to other malposition and malpresentation, not applicable or unspecified |
> |---|---|
> | O24.42Ø | Gestational diabetes mellitus in childbirth, diet controlled |
> | Z3A.38 | 38 weeks gestation of pregnancy |
> | Z37.Ø | Single live birth |
>
> *Explanation:* The obstructed labor necessitated the cesarean procedure.

5) Outcome of delivery

A code from category Z37, Outcome of delivery, should be included on every maternal record when a delivery has occurred. These codes are not to be used on subsequent records or on the newborn record.

c. Pre-existing conditions versus conditions due to the pregnancy

Certain categories in Chapter 15 distinguish between conditions of the mother that existed prior to pregnancy (pre-existing) and those that are a direct result of pregnancy. When assigning codes from Chapter 15, it is important to assess if a condition was pre-existing prior to pregnancy or developed during or due to the pregnancy in order to assign the correct code.

Categories that do not distinguish between pre-existing and pregnancy-related conditions may be used for either. It is acceptable to use codes specifically for the puerperium with codes complicating pregnancy and childbirth if a condition arises postpartum during the delivery encounter.

d. Pre-existing hypertension in pregnancy

Category O1Ø, Pre-existing hypertension complicating pregnancy, childbirth and the puerperium, includes codes for hypertensive heart and hypertensive chronic kidney disease. When assigning one of the O1Ø codes that includes hypertensive heart disease or hypertensive chronic kidney disease, it is necessary to add a secondary code from the appropriate hypertension category to specify the type of heart failure or chronic kidney disease.

See Section I.C.9. Hypertension.

e. Fetal conditions affecting the management of the mother

1) Codes from categories O35 and O36

Codes from categories O35, Maternal care for known or suspected fetal abnormality and damage, and O36, Maternal care for other fetal problems, are assigned only when the fetal condition is actually responsible for modifying the management of the mother, i.e., by requiring diagnostic studies, additional observation, special care, or termination of pregnancy. The fact that the fetal condition exists does not justify assigning a code from this series to the mother's record.

> A patient with twin gestation is seen for spotting 15 weeks into her pregnancy; the doctors also suspect fetal hydrocephalus. Patient is instructed to return in one week for additional diagnostic testing, sooner if the problem worsens.
>
> | O35.ØXXØ | Maternal care for (suspected) central nervous system malformation in fetus, not applicable or unspecified |
> |---|---|
> | O26.852 | Spotting complicating pregnancy, second trimester |
> | Z3A.15 | 15 weeks gestation of pregnancy |
>
> *Explanation:* Whether the fetal hydrocephalus was suspected or confirmed, an additional code is warranted for this condition since documentation indicates the patient is to return sooner than her routine visit for further testing.

2) In utero surgery

In cases when surgery is performed on the fetus, a diagnosis code from category O35, Maternal care for known or suspected fetal abnormality and damage, should be assigned identifying the fetal condition. Assign the appropriate procedure code for the procedure performed.

No code from Chapter 16, the perinatal codes, should be used on the mother's record to identify fetal conditions. Surgery performed in utero on a fetus is still to be coded as an obstetric encounter.

f. HIV infection in pregnancy, childbirth and the puerperium

During pregnancy, childbirth or the puerperium, a patient admitted because of an HIV-related illness should receive a principal diagnosis from subcategory O98.7-, Human immunodeficiency [HIV] disease complicating pregnancy, childbirth and the puerperium, followed by the code(s) for the HIV-related illness(es).

Patients with asymptomatic HIV infection status admitted during pregnancy, childbirth, or the puerperium should receive codes of O98.7- and Z21, Asymptomatic human immunodeficiency virus [HIV] infection status.

> A previously asymptomatic HIV patient who is 13 weeks pregnant is evaluated for HIV-related candidal bronchitis
>
> | O98.711 | Human immunodeficiency virus [HIV] disease complicating pregnancy, first trimester |
> |---|---|
> | B2Ø | Human immunodeficiency virus [HIV] disease |
> | B37.1 | Candidal bronchitis |
> | Z3A.13 | 13 weeks gestation of pregnancy |
>
> *Explanation:* Because candidal bronchitis is an AIDS-related condition, this patient is now considered to have HIV disease. An obstetrics code indicating that HIV is complicating the pregnancy is coded first, followed by B2Ø for HIV disease as well as a code for the candidal bronchitis.

g. Diabetes mellitus in pregnancy

Diabetes mellitus is a significant complicating factor in pregnancy. Pregnant women who are diabetic should be assigned a code from category O24, Diabetes mellitus in pregnancy, childbirth, and the puerperium, first, followed by the appropriate diabetes code(s) (E08-E13) from Chapter 4.

h. Long term use of insulin and oral hypoglycemics

Code Z79.4, Long-term (current) use of insulin, or code Z79.84, Long-term (current) use of oral hypoglycemic drugs, should also be assigned if the diabetes mellitus is being treated with insulin or oral medications. If the patient is treated with both oral medications and insulin, only the code for insulin-controlled should be assigned.

i. Gestational (pregnancy induced) diabetes

Gestational (pregnancy induced) diabetes can occur during the second and third trimester of pregnancy in women who were not diabetic prior to pregnancy. Gestational diabetes can cause complications in the pregnancy similar to those of pre-existing diabetes mellitus. It also puts the woman at greater risk of developing diabetes after the pregnancy. Codes for gestational diabetes are in subcategory O24.4, Gestational diabetes mellitus. No other code from category O24, Diabetes mellitus in pregnancy, childbirth, and the puerperium, should be used with a code from O24.4.

The codes under subcategory O24.4 include diet controlled, insulin controlled, and controlled by oral hypoglycemic drugs. If a patient with gestational diabetes is treated with both diet and insulin, only the code for insulin-controlled is required. If a patient with gestational diabetes is treated with both diet and oral hypoglycemic medications, only the code for "controlled by oral hypoglycemic drugs" is required. Code Z79.4, Long-term (current) use of insulin or code Z79.84, Long-term (current) use of oral hypoglycemic drugs, should not be assigned with codes from subcategory O24.4.

An abnormal glucose tolerance in pregnancy is assigned a code from subcategory O99.81, Abnormal glucose complicating pregnancy, childbirth, and the puerperium.

j. Sepsis and septic shock complicating abortion, pregnancy, childbirth and the puerperium

When assigning a chapter 15 code for sepsis complicating abortion, pregnancy, childbirth, and the puerperium, a code for the specific type of infection should be assigned as an additional diagnosis. If severe sepsis is present, a code from subcategory R65.2, Severe sepsis, and code(s) for associated organ dysfunction(s) should also be assigned as additional diagnoses.

Patient is seen several days after a miscarriage with sepsis; cultures return MSSA

O03.87	Sepsis following complete or unspecified spontaneous abortion
B95.61	Methicillin susceptible Staphylococcus aureus infection as the cause of diseases classified elsewhere

Explanation: The type of infection that caused this patient to become septic was methicillin susceptible *Staphylococcus aureus* (MSSA), which as a secondary code helps capture all aspects related to this patient's septic condition.

k. Puerperal sepsis

Code O85, Puerperal sepsis, should be assigned with a secondary code to identify the causal organism (e.g., for a bacterial infection, assign a code from category B95-B96, Bacterial infections in conditions classified elsewhere). A code from category A40, Streptococcal sepsis, or A41, Other sepsis, should not be used for puerperal sepsis. If applicable, use additional codes to identify severe sepsis (R65.2-) and any associated acute organ dysfunction.

l. Alcohol and tobacco use during pregnancy, childbirth and the puerperium

1) Alcohol use during pregnancy, childbirth and the puerperium

Codes under subcategory O99.31, Alcohol use complicating pregnancy, childbirth, and the puerperium, should be assigned for any pregnancy case when a mother uses alcohol during the pregnancy or postpartum. A secondary code from category F10, Alcohol related disorders, should also be assigned to identify manifestations of the alcohol use.

2) Tobacco use during pregnancy, childbirth and the puerperium

Codes under subcategory O99.33, Smoking (tobacco) complicating pregnancy, childbirth, and the puerperium, should be assigned for any pregnancy case when a mother uses any type of tobacco product during the pregnancy or postpartum. A secondary code from category F17, Nicotine dependence, should also be assigned to identify the type of nicotine dependence.

m. Poisoning, toxic effects, adverse effects and underdosing in a pregnant patient

A code from subcategory O9A.2, Injury, poisoning and certain other consequences of external causes complicating pregnancy, childbirth, and the puerperium, should be sequenced first, followed by the appropriate injury, poisoning, toxic effect, adverse effect or underdosing code, and then the additional code(s) that specifies the condition caused by the poisoning, toxic effect, adverse effect or underdosing.

See Section I.C.19. Adverse effects, poisoning, underdosing and toxic effects.

Patient treated for accidental carbon monoxide poisoning from a gas heating implement; the patient is 18 weeks' pregnant

O9A.212	Injury, poisoning and certain other consequences of external causes complicating pregnancy, second trimester
T58.11XA	Toxic effect of carbon monoxide from utility gas, accidental (unintentional), initial encounter
Z3A.18	18 weeks gestation of pregnancy

Explanation: Although the carbon monoxide poisoning is the reason for the encounter, a code from the obstetrics chapter must be sequenced first. Chapter 15 codes have sequencing priority over codes from other chapters.

n. Normal delivery, code O80

1) Encounter for full term uncomplicated delivery

Code O80 should be assigned when a woman is admitted for a full-term normal delivery and delivers a single, healthy infant without any complications antepartum, during the delivery, or postpartum during the delivery episode. Code O80 is always a principal diagnosis. It is not to be used if any other code from chapter 15 is needed to describe a current complication of the antenatal, delivery, or perinatal period. Additional codes from other chapters may be used with code O80 if they are not related to or are in any way complicating the pregnancy.

2) Uncomplicated delivery with resolved antepartum complication

Code O80 may be used if the patient had a complication at some point during the pregnancy, but the complication is not present at the time of the admission for delivery.

Patient presents in labor at 39 weeks' gestation and delivers a healthy newborn; patient had abnormal glucose levels in her first trimester, which have since resolved

O80	Encounter for full-term uncomplicated delivery
Z37.0	Single live birth

Explanation: The abnormal glucose levels during the first trimester cannot be coded if they are not affecting the patient's current trimester. Without additional complications associated with the pregnancy, fetus, or mother, code O80 is appropriate.

3) Outcome of delivery for O80

Z37.0, Single live birth, is the only outcome of delivery code appropriate for use with O80.

o. The peripartum and postpartum periods

1) Peripartum and postpartum periods

The postpartum period begins immediately after delivery and continues for six weeks following delivery. The peripartum period is defined as the last month of pregnancy to five months postpartum.

2) Peripartum and postpartum complication

A postpartum complication is any complication occurring within the six-week period.

3) Pregnancy-related complications after 6 week period

Chapter 15 codes may also be used to describe pregnancy-related complications after the peripartum or postpartum period if the provider documents that a condition is pregnancy related.

Patient referred for varicose veins. She had a baby boy three months ago; the varicose veins started to appear one month ago. The doctor attributes the patient's pregnancy as the cause of the varicose veins, which continue to be painful and bother the patient. She is seeking surgical relief.

O87.4	Varicose veins of the lower extremity in the puerperium

Explanation: Although the varicose veins occurred several months after the delivery of the newborn, the doctor attributed the varicose veins to pregnancy and therefore a code from chapter 15 is appropriate.

4) Admission for routine postpartum care following delivery outside hospital

When the mother delivers outside the hospital prior to admission and is admitted for routine postpartum care and no complications are noted, code Z39.0, Encounter for care and examination of mother immediately after delivery, should be assigned as the principal diagnosis.

5) Pregnancy associated cardiomyopathy

Pregnancy associated cardiomyopathy, code O90.3, is unique in that it may be diagnosed in the third trimester of pregnancy but may continue to progress months after delivery. For this reason, it is referred to as peripartum cardiomyopathy. Code O90.3 is only for use when the cardiomyopathy develops as a result of pregnancy in a woman who did not have pre-existing heart disease.

p. Code O94, Sequelae of complication of pregnancy, childbirth, and the puerperium

1) Code O94

Code O94, Sequelae of complication of pregnancy, childbirth, and the puerperium, is for use in those cases when an initial complication of a pregnancy develops a sequelae requiring care or treatment at a future date.

2) After the initial postpartum period

This code may be used at any time after the initial postpartum period.

3) Sequencing of code O94

This code, like all sequela codes, is to be sequenced following the code describing the sequelae of the complication.

q. Termination of pregnancy and spontaneous abortions

1) Abortion with liveborn fetus

When an attempted termination of pregnancy results in a liveborn fetus, assign code Z33.2, Encounter for elective termination of pregnancy and a code from category Z37, Outcome of Delivery.

2) Retained products of conception following an abortion

Subsequent encounters for retained products of conception following a spontaneous abortion or elective termination of pregnancy are assigned the appropriate code from category O03, Spontaneous abortion, or codes O07.4, Failed attempted termination of pregnancy without complication and Z33.2, Encounter for elective termination of pregnancy. This advice is appropriate even when the patient was discharged previously with a discharge diagnosis of complete abortion.

> Patient was seen two days ago for complete spontaneous abortion but returns today for urinary tract infection (UTI) with ultrasound showing retained products of conception
>
> **O03.38   Urinary tract infection following incomplete spontaneous abortion**
>
> *Explanation:* Although the diagnosis from the patient's previous stay indicated that the patient had a complete abortion, it is now determined that there were actually retained products of conception (POC). An abortion with retained POC is considered incomplete and in this case resulted in the patient developing a UTI.

3) Complications leading to abortion

Codes from Chapter 15 may be used as additional codes to identify any documented complications of the pregnancy in conjunction with codes in categories in O07 and O08.

r. Abuse in a pregnant patient

For suspected or confirmed cases of abuse of a pregnant patient, a code(s) from subcategories O9A.3, Physical abuse complicating pregnancy, childbirth, and the puerperium, O9A.4, Sexual abuse complicating pregnancy, childbirth, and the puerperium, and O9A.5, Psychological abuse complicating pregnancy, childbirth, and the puerperium, should be sequenced first, followed by the appropriate codes (if applicable) to identify any associated current injury due to physical abuse, sexual abuse, and the perpetrator of abuse.

See Section I.C.19. Adult and child abuse, neglect and other maltreatment.

Chapter 15. Pregnancy, Childbirth and the Puerperium (O00-O9A)

NOTE CODES FROM THIS CHAPTER ARE FOR USE ONLY ON MATERNAL RECORDS, NEVER ON NEWBORN RECORDS.

Codes from this chapter are for use for conditions related to or aggravated by the pregnancy, childbirth, or by the puerperium (maternal causes or obstetric causes).

NOTE Trimesters are counted from the first day of the last menstrual period. They are defined as follows:

     1st trimester- less than 14 weeks 0 days
     2nd trimester- 14 weeks 0 days to less than 28 weeks 0 days
     3rd trimester- 28 weeks 0 days until delivery.

Use additional code from category Z3A, Weeks of gestation, to identify the specific week of the pregnancy, if known

EXCLUDES 1 *supervision of normal pregnancy (Z34.-)*
EXCLUDES 2 *mental and behavioral disorders associated with the puerperium (F53)*
     obstetrical tetanus (A34)
     postpartum necrosis of pituitary gland (E23.0)
     puerperal osteomalacia (M83.0)

AHA: 2016, 1Q, 3-5; 2014, 3Q, 17

This chapter contains the following blocks:

O00-O08	Pregnancy with abortive outcome
O09	Supervision of high risk pregnancy
O10-O16	Edema, proteinuria and hypertensive disorders in pregnancy, childbirth and the puerperium
O20-O29	Other maternal disorders predominantly related to pregnancy
O30-O48	Maternal care related to the fetus and amniotic cavity and possible delivery problems
O60-O77	Complications of labor and delivery
O80, O82	Encounter for delivery
O85-O92	Complications predominantly related to the puerperium
O94-O9A	Other obstetric conditions, not elsewhere classified

Pregnancy with abortive outcome (O00-O08)

EXCLUDES 1 *continuing pregnancy in multiple gestation after abortion of one fetus or more (O31.1-, O31.3-)*

✓4ᵗʰ O00 Ectopic pregnancy
     INCLUDES ruptured ectopic pregnancy
     Use additional code from category O08 to identify any associated complication
     AHA: 2014, 3Q, 17
     DEF: Implantation of fertilized egg outside the uterus, usually in fallopian tube or abdomen; requires emergency treatment.

   ✓5ᵗʰ O00.0 Abdominal pregnancy
     EXCLUDES 1 *maternal care for viable fetus in abdominal pregnancy (O36.7-)*

     O00.00 Abdominal pregnancy without intrauterine pregnancy   Ⓜ♀
        Abdominal pregnancy NOS

     O00.01 Abdominal pregnancy with intrauterine pregnancy   Ⓜ♀

   ✓5ᵗʰ O00.1 Tubal pregnancy
     Fallopian pregnancy
     Rupture of (fallopian) tube due to pregnancy
     Tubal abortion

     ✓6ᵗʰ O00.10 Tubal pregnancy without intrauterine pregnancy
        Tubal pregnancy NOS

●   **O00.101 Right tubal pregnancy without intrauterine pregnancy**

●   **O00.102 Left tubal pregnancy without intrauterine pregnancy**

●   **O00.109 Unspecified tubal pregnancy without intrauterine pregnancy** ▽

     ✓6ᵗʰ O00.11 Tubal pregnancy with intrauterine pregnancy

●   **O00.111 Right tubal pregnancy with intrauterine pregnancy**

●   **O00.112 Left tubal pregnancy with intrauterine pregnancy**

●   **O00.119 Unspecified tubal pregnancy with intrauterine pregnancy** ▽

   ✓5ᵗʰ O00.2 Ovarian pregnancy

     ✓6ᵗʰ O00.20 Ovarian pregnancy without intrauterine pregnancy
        Ovarian pregnancy NOS

●   **O00.201 Right ovarian pregnancy without intrauterine pregnancy**

●   **O00.202 Left ovarian pregnancy without intrauterine pregnancy**

Ectopic Pregnancy

●   **O00.209 Unspecified ovarian pregnancy without intrauterine pregnancy** ▽

     ✓6ᵗʰ O00.21 Ovarian pregnancy with intrauterine pregnancy

     O00.211 Right ovarian pregnancy with intrauterine pregnancy

     O00.212 Left ovarian pregnancy with intrauterine pregnancy

●   **O00.219 Unspecified ovarian pregnancy with intrauterine pregnancy** ▽

   ✓5ᵗʰ O00.8 Other ectopic pregnancy
     Cervical pregnancy
     Cornual pregnancy
     Intraligamentous pregnancy
     Mural pregnancy

     O00.80 Other ectopic pregnancy without intrauterine pregnancy   Ⓜ♀
        Other ectopic pregnancy NOS

     O00.81 Other ectopic pregnancy with intrauterine pregnancy   Ⓜ♀

   ✓5ᵗʰ O00.9 Ectopic pregnancy, unspecified

     O00.90 Unspecified ectopic pregnancy without intrauterine pregnancy   Ⓜ♀▽
        Ectopic pregnancy NOS

     O00.91 Unspecified ectopic pregnancy with intrauterine pregnancy   Ⓜ♀▽

✓4ᵗʰ O01 Hydatidiform mole
     Use additional code from category O08 to identify any associated complication
     EXCLUDES 1 *chorioadenoma (destruens) (D39.2)*
        malignant hydatidiform mole (D39.2)
     AHA: 2014, 3Q, 17
     DEF: Abnormal product of pregnancy; marked by mass of cysts resembling bunch of grapes due to chorionic villi proliferation and dissolution; must be surgically removed.

   O01.0 Classical hydatidiform mole   Ⓜ♀
     Complete hydatidiform mole

   O01.1 Incomplete and partial hydatidiform mole   Ⓜ♀

   O01.9 Hydatidiform mole, unspecified   Ⓜ♀▽
     Trophoblastic disease NOS
     Vesicular mole NOS

✓4ᵗʰ O02 Other abnormal products of conception
     Use additional code from category O08 to identify any associated complication
     EXCLUDES 1 *papyraceous fetus (O31.0-)*
     AHA: 2014, 3Q, 17

   O02.0 Blighted ovum and nonhydatidiform mole   Ⓜ♀
     Carneous mole
     Fleshy mole
     Intrauterine mole NOS
     Molar pregnancy NEC
     Pathological ovum

☑ Additional Character Req   ✓x7ᵗʰ Placeholder Alert   Manifestation   ℍᴄᴄ CMS-HCC Condition   ▽ Unspecified Code   ►◄ Revised Text   ● New Code   ▲ Revised Code Title

O02.1 Missed abortion Ⓜ♀
Early fetal death, before completion of 20 weeks of gestation, with retention of dead fetus
> *EXCLUDES1*   *failed induced abortion (O07.-)*
> *fetal death (intrauterine) (late) (O36.4)*
> *missed abortion with blighted ovum (O02.0)*
> *missed abortion with hydatidiform mole (O01.-)*
> *missed abortion with nonhydatidiform (O02.0)*
> *missed abortion with other abnormal products of*
>   *conception (O02.8-)*
> *missed delivery (O36.4)*
> *stillbirth (P95)*

✓5ᵗʰ **O02.8 Other specified abnormal products of conception**
> *EXCLUDES1*   *abnormal products of conception with blighted ovum*
>   *(O02.0)*
> *abnormal products of conception with hydatidiform*
>   *mole (O01.-)*
> *abnormal products of conception with*
>   *nonhydatidiform mole (O02.0)*

O02.81 Inappropriate change in quantitative human Ⓜ♀
chorionic gonadotropin (hCG) in early pregnancy
Biochemical pregnancy
Chemical pregnancy
Inappropriate level of quantitative human chorionic gonadotropin (hCG) for gestational age in early pregnancy

O02.89 Other abnormal products of conception Ⓜ♀

O02.9 Abnormal product of conception, unspecified Ⓜ♀▽

✓4ᵗʰ **O03 Spontaneous abortion**
> **NOTE**   Incomplete abortion includes retained products of conception following spontaneous abortion
> **INCLUDES**   miscarriage

O03.0 Genital tract and pelvic infection following incomplete Ⓜ♀
spontaneous abortion
Endometritis following incomplete spontaneous abortion
Oophoritis following incomplete spontaneous abortion
Parametritis following incomplete spontaneous abortion
Pelvic peritonitis following incomplete spontaneous abortion
Salpingitis following incomplete spontaneous abortion
Salpingo-oophoritis following incomplete spontaneous abortion
> *EXCLUDES1*   *sepsis following incomplete spontaneous abortion*
>   *(O03.37)*
> *urinary tract infection following incomplete*
>   *spontaneous abortion (O03.38)*

O03.1 Delayed or excessive hemorrhage following incomplete Ⓜ♀
spontaneous abortion
Afibrinogenemia following incomplete spontaneous abortion
Defibrination syndrome following incomplete spontaneous abortion
Hemolysis following incomplete spontaneous abortion
Intravascular coagulation following incomplete spontaneous abortion

O03.2 Embolism following incomplete spontaneous abortion Ⓜ♀
Air embolism following incomplete spontaneous abortion
Amniotic fluid embolism following incomplete spontaneous abortion
Blood-clot embolism following incomplete spontaneous abortion
Embolism NOS following incomplete spontaneous abortion
Fat embolism following incomplete spontaneous abortion
Pulmonary embolism following incomplete spontaneous abortion
Pyemic embolism following incomplete spontaneous abortion
Septic or septicopyemic embolism following incomplete spontaneous abortion
Soap embolism following incomplete spontaneous abortion

✓5ᵗʰ **O03.3 Other and unspecified complications following incomplete spontaneous abortion**

O03.30 Unspecified complication following Ⓜ♀▽
incomplete spontaneous abortion

O03.31 Shock following incomplete spontaneous Ⓜ♀
abortion
Circulatory collapse following incomplete spontaneous abortion
Shock (postprocedural) following incomplete spontaneous abortion
> *EXCLUDES1*   *shock due to infection following incomplete*
>   *spontaneous abortion (O03.37)*

O03.32 Renal failure following incomplete spontaneous Ⓜ♀
abortion
Kidney failure (acute) following incomplete spontaneous abortion
Oliguria following incomplete spontaneous abortion
Renal shutdown following incomplete spontaneous abortion
Renal tubular necrosis following incomplete spontaneous abortion
Uremia following incomplete spontaneous abortion

O03.33 Metabolic disorder following incomplete Ⓜ♀
spontaneous abortion

O03.34 Damage to pelvic organs following incomplete Ⓜ♀
spontaneous abortion
Laceration, perforation, tear or chemical damage of bladder following incomplete spontaneous abortion
Laceration, perforation, tear or chemical damage of bowel following incomplete spontaneous abortion
Laceration, perforation, tear or chemical damage of broad ligament following incomplete spontaneous abortion
Laceration, perforation, tear or chemical damage of cervix following incomplete spontaneous abortion
Laceration, perforation, tear or chemical damage of periurethral tissue following incomplete spontaneous abortion
Laceration, perforation, tear or chemical damage of uterus following incomplete spontaneous abortion
Laceration, perforation, tear or chemical damage of vagina following incomplete spontaneous abortion

O03.35 Other venous complications following Ⓜ♀
incomplete spontaneous abortion

O03.36 Cardiac arrest following incomplete Ⓜ♀
spontaneousabortion

O03.37 Sepsis following incomplete spontaneous Ⓜ♀
abortion
Use additional code to identify infectious agent (B95-B97)
Use additional code to identify severe sepsis, if applicable (R65.2-)
> *EXCLUDES1*   *septic or septicopyemic embolism following*
>   *incomplete spontaneous abortion*
>   *(O03.2)*

O03.38 Urinary tract infection following incomplete Ⓜ♀
spontaneous abortion
Cystitis following incomplete spontaneous abortion

O03.39 Incomplete spontaneous abortion with other Ⓜ♀
complications

O03.4 Incomplete spontaneous abortion without complication Ⓜ♀

O03.5 Genital tract and pelvic infection following complete or Ⓜ♀
unspecified spontaneous abortion
Endometritis following complete or unspecified spontaneous abortion
Oophoritis following complete or unspecified spontaneous abortion
Parametritis following complete or unspecified spontaneous abortion
Pelvic peritonitis following complete or unspecified spontaneous abortion
Salpingitis following complete or unspecified spontaneous abortion
Salpingo-oophoritis following complete or unspecified spontaneous abortion
> *EXCLUDES1*   *sepsis following complete or unspecified spontaneous*
>   *abortion (O03.87)*
> *urinary tract infection following complete or*
>   *unspecified spontaneous abortion (O03.88)*

O03.6 Delayed or excessive hemorrhage following complete or Ⓜ♀
unspecified spontaneous abortion
Afibrinogenemia following complete or unspecified spontaneous abortion
Defibrination syndrome following complete or unspecified spontaneous abortion
Hemolysis following complete or unspecified spontaneous abortion
Intravascular coagulation following complete or unspecified spontaneous abortion

---

O03.7   Embolism **following** complete or unspecified   Ⓜ♀
spontaneous abortion

Air embolism following complete or unspecified spontaneous abortion

Amniotic fluid embolism following complete or unspecified spontaneous abortion

Blood-clot embolism following complete or unspecified spontaneous abortion

Embolism NOS following complete or unspecified spontaneous abortion

Fat embolism following complete or unspecified spontaneous abortion

Pulmonary embolism following complete or unspecified spontaneous abortion

Pyemic embolism following complete or unspecified spontaneous abortion

Septic or septicopyemic embolism following complete or unspecified spontaneous abortion

Soap embolism following complete or unspecified spontaneous abortion

✓5ᵗʰ **O03.8**   **Other and unspecified complications following complete or unspecified spontaneous abortion**

O03.80   **Unspecified complication following**   Ⓜ♀▽
complete or unspecified spontaneous abortion

O03.81   **Shock following** complete or unspecified   Ⓜ♀
spontaneous abortion

Circulatory collapse following complete or unspecified spontaneous abortion

Shock (postprocedural) following complete or unspecified spontaneous abortion

EXCLUDES 1   *shock due to infection following complete or unspecified spontaneous abortion (O03.87)*

O03.82   **Renal failure following** complete or unspecified   Ⓜ♀
spontaneous abortion

Kidney failure (acute) following complete or unspecified spontaneous abortion

Oliguria following complete or unspecified spontaneous abortion

Renal shutdown following complete or unspecified spontaneous abortion

Renal tubular necrosis following complete or unspecified spontaneous abortion

Uremia following complete or unspecified spontaneous abortion

O03.83   **Metabolic disorder following** complete or   Ⓜ♀
unspecified spontaneous abortion

O03.84   **Damage to pelvic organs following** complete or   Ⓜ♀
unspecified spontaneous abortion

Laceration, perforation, tear or chemical damage of bladder following complete or unspecified spontaneous abortion

Laceration, perforation, tear or chemical damage of bowel following complete or unspecified spontaneous abortion

Laceration, perforation, tear or chemical damage of broad ligament following complete or unspecified spontaneous abortion

Laceration, perforation, tear or chemical damage of cervix following complete or unspecified spontaneous abortion

Laceration, perforation, tear or chemical damage of periurethral tissue following complete or unspecified spontaneous abortion

Laceration, perforation, tear or chemical damage of uterus following complete or unspecified spontaneous abortion

Laceration, perforation, tear or chemical damage of vagina following complete or unspecified spontaneous abortion

O03.85   **Other venous complications following** complete   Ⓜ♀
or unspecified spontaneous abortion

O03.86   **Cardiac arrest following** complete or unspecified   Ⓜ♀
spontaneous abortion

O03.87   **Sepsis following** complete or unspecified   Ⓜ♀
spontaneous abortion

Use additional code to identify infectious agent (B95-B97)

Use additional code to identify severe sepsis, if applicable (R65.2-)

EXCLUDES 1   *septic or septicopyemic embolism following complete or unspecified spontaneous abortion (O03.7)*

O03.88   **Urinary tract infection following** complete or   Ⓜ♀
unspecified spontaneous abortion

Cystitis following complete or unspecified spontaneous abortion

O03.89   **Complete or unspecified spontaneous abortion**   Ⓜ♀
with other complications

O03.9   **Complete or unspecified spontaneous abortion**   Ⓜ♀▽
without complication

Miscarriage NOS

Spontaneous abortion NOS

✓4ᵗʰ **O04**   **Complications following (induced) termination of pregnancy**

INCLUDES   complications following (induced) termination of pregnancy

EXCLUDES 1   *encounter for elective termination of pregnancy, uncomplicated (Z33.2)*

failed attempted termination of pregnancy (O07.-)

O04.5   **Genital tract and pelvic infection following (induced)**   Ⓜ♀
termination of pregnancy

Endometritis following (induced) termination of pregnancy

Oophoritis following (induced) termination of pregnancy

Parametritis following (induced) termination of pregnancy

Pelvic peritonitis following (induced) termination of pregnancy

Salpingitis following (induced) termination of pregnancy

Salpingo-oophoritis following (induced) termination of pregnancy

EXCLUDES 1   *sepsis following (induced) termination of pregnancy (O04.87)*

urinary tract infection following (induced) termination of pregnancy (O04.88)

O04.6   **Delayed or excessive hemorrhage following (induced)**   Ⓜ♀
termination of pregnancy

Afibrinogenemia following (induced) termination of pregnancy

Defibrination syndrome following (induced) termination of pregnancy

Hemolysis following (induced) termination of pregnancy

Intravascular coagulation following (induced) termination of pregnancy

O04.7   **Embolism following (induced) termination of pregnancy**   Ⓜ♀

Air embolism following (induced) termination of pregnancy

Amniotic fluid embolism following (induced) termination of pregnancy

Blood-clot embolism following (induced) termination of pregnancy

Embolism NOS following (induced) termination of pregnancy

Fat embolism following (induced) termination of pregnancy

Pulmonary embolism following (induced) termination of pregnancy

Pyemic embolism following (induced) termination of pregnancy

Septic or septicopyemic embolism following (induced) termination of pregnancy

Soap embolism following (induced) termination of pregnancy

✓5ᵗʰ **O04.8**   **(Induced) termination of pregnancy with other and unspecified complications**

O04.80   **(Induced) termination of pregnancy with**   Ⓜ♀▽
unspecified complications

O04.81   **Shock following (induced) termination of**   Ⓜ♀
pregnancy

Circulatory collapse following (induced) termination of pregnancy

Shock (postprocedural) following (induced) termination of pregnancy

EXCLUDES 1   *shock due to infection following (induced) termination of pregnancy (O04.87)*

O04.82   **Renal failure following (induced) termination**   Ⓜ♀
of pregnancy

Kidney failure (acute) following (induced) termination of pregnancy

Oliguria following (induced) termination of pregnancy

Renal shutdown following (induced) termination of pregnancy

Renal tubular necrosis following (induced) termination of pregnancy

Uremia following (induced) termination of pregnancy

O04.83   **Metabolic disorder following (induced)**   Ⓜ♀
termination of pregnancy

☑ Additional Character Req   ✓ˣ⁷ᵗʰ Placeholder Alert   Manifestation   ᴴᶜᶜ CMS-HCC Condition   ▽ Unspecified Code   ►◄ Revised Text   ● New Code   ▲ Revised Code Title

Chapter 15. Pregnancy, Childbirth, and the Puerperium

O04.84   **Damage to pelvic organs following (induced) termination of pregnancy**   Ⓜ♀

Laceration, perforation, tear or chemical damage of bladder following (induced) termination of pregnancy

Laceration, perforation, tear or chemical damage of bowel following (induced) termination of pregnancy

Laceration, perforation, tear or chemical damage of broad ligament following (induced) termination of pregnancy

Laceration, perforation, tear or chemical damage of cervix following (induced) termination of pregnancy

Laceration, perforation, tear or chemical damage of periurethral tissue following (induced) termination of pregnancy

Laceration, perforation, tear or chemical damage of uterus following (induced) termination of pregnancy

Laceration, perforation, tear or chemical damage of vagina following (induced) termination of pregnancy

O04.85   **Other venous complications following (induced) termination of pregnancy**   Ⓜ♀

O04.86   **Cardiac arrest following (induced) termination of pregnancy**   Ⓜ♀

O04.87   **Sepsis following (induced) termination of pregnancy**   Ⓜ♀

Use additional code to identify infectious agent (B95-B97)

Use additional code to identify severe sepsis, if applicable (R65.2-)

> **EXCLUDES 1**   *septic or septicopyemic embolism following (induced) termination of pregnancy (O04.7)*

O04.88   **Urinary tract infection following (induced) termination of pregnancy**   Ⓜ♀

Cystitis following (induced) termination of pregnancy

O04.89   **(Induced) termination of pregnancy with other complications**   Ⓜ♀

✓4ᵗʰ **O07**   **Failed attempted termination of pregnancy**

> **INCLUDES**   failure of attempted induction of termination of pregnancy
> incomplete elective abortion

> **EXCLUDES 1**   *incomplete spontaneous abortion (O03.0-)*

O07.0   **Genital tract and pelvic infection following failed attempted termination of pregnancy**   Ⓜ♀

Endometritis following failed attempted termination of pregnancy

Oophoritis following failed attempted termination of pregnancy

Parametritis following failed attempted termination of pregnancy

Pelvic peritonitis following failed attempted termination of pregnancy

Salpingitis following failed attempted termination of pregnancy

Salpingo-oophoritis following failed attempted termination of pregnancy

> **EXCLUDES 1**   *sepsis following failed attempted termination of pregnancy (O07.37)*
> *urinary tract infection following failed attempted termination of pregnancy (O07.38)*

O07.1   **Delayed or excessive hemorrhage following failed attempted termination of pregnancy**   Ⓜ♀

Afibrinogenemia following failed attempted termination of pregnancy

Defibrination syndrome following failed attempted termination of pregnancy

Hemolysis following failed attempted termination of pregnancy

Intravascular coagulation following failed attempted termination of pregnancy

O07.2   **Embolism following failed attempted termination of pregnancy**   Ⓜ♀

Air embolism following failed attempted termination of pregnancy

Amniotic fluid embolism following failed attempted termination of pregnancy

Blood-clot embolism following failed attempted termination of pregnancy

Embolism NOS following failed attempted termination of pregnancy

Fat embolism following failed attempted termination of pregnancy

Pulmonary embolism following failed attempted termination of pregnancy

Pyemic embolism following failed attempted termination of pregnancy

Septic or septicopyemic embolism following failed attempted termination of pregnancy

Soap embolism following failed attempted termination of pregnancy

✓5ᵗʰ **O07.3**   **Failed attempted termination of pregnancy with other and unspecified complications**

O07.30   **Failed attempted termination of pregnancy with unspecified complications**   Ⓜ♀▽

O07.31   **Shock following failed attempted termination of pregnancy**   Ⓜ♀

Circulatory collapse following failed attempted termination of pregnancy

Shock (postprocedural) following failed attempted termination of pregnancy

> **EXCLUDES 1**   *shock due to infection following failed attempted termination of pregnancy (O07.37)*

O07.32   **Renal failure following failed attempted termination of pregnancy**   Ⓜ♀

Kidney failure (acute) following failed attempted termination of pregnancy

Oliguria following failed attempted termination of pregnancy

Renal shutdown following failed attempted termination of pregnancy

Renal tubular necrosis following failed attempted termination of pregnancy

Uremia following failed attempted termination of pregnancy

O07.33   **Metabolic disorder following failed attempted termination of pregnancy**   Ⓜ♀

O07.34   **Damage to pelvic organs following failed attempted termination of pregnancy**   Ⓜ♀

Laceration, perforation, tear or chemical damage of bladder following failed attempted termination of pregnancy

Laceration, perforation, tear or chemical damage of bowel following failed attempted termination of pregnancy

Laceration, perforation, tear or chemical damage of broad ligament following failed attempted termination of pregnancy

Laceration, perforation, tear or chemical damage of cervix following failed attempted termination of pregnancy

Laceration, perforation, tear or chemical damage of periurethral tissue following failed attempted termination of pregnancy

Laceration, perforation, tear or chemical damage of uterus following failed attempted termination of pregnancy

Laceration, perforation, tear or chemical damage of vagina following failed attempted termination of pregnancy

O07.35   **Other venous complications following failed attempted termination of pregnancy**   Ⓜ♀

O07.36   **Cardiac arrest following failed attempted termination of pregnancy**   Ⓜ♀

O07.37   **Sepsis following failed attempted termination of pregnancy**   Ⓜ♀

Use additional code to identify infectious agent (B95-B97)

Use additional code to identify severe sepsis, if applicable (R65.2-)

> **EXCLUDES 1**   *septic or septicopyemic embolism following failed attempted termination of pregnancy (O07.2)*

EXCLUDES 1 Not coded here   **EXCLUDES 2** Not included here   Ⓝ Newborn Age: 0   Ⓟ Pediatric Age: 0-17   Ⓜ Maternity Age: 12-55   Ⓐ Adult Age: 15-124

826   ICD-10-CM 2018

O07.38 Urinary tract infection following failed attempted termination of pregnancy Ⓜ♀
  Cystitis following failed attempted termination of pregnancy

O07.39 Failed attempted termination of pregnancy with other complications Ⓜ♀

O07.4 Failed attempted termination of pregnancy without complication Ⓜ♀

☑4ᵗʰ **O08 Complications following ectopic and molar pregnancy**
  This category is for use with categories O00-O02 to identify any associated complications

O08.0 Genital tract and pelvic infection following ectopic and molar pregnancy Ⓜ♀
  Endometritis following ectopic and molar pregnancy
  Oophoritis following ectopic and molar pregnancy
  Parametritis following ectopic and molar pregnancy
  Pelvic peritonitis following ectopic and molar pregnancy
  Salpingitis following ectopic and molar pregnancy
  Salpingo-oophoritis following ectopic and molar pregnancy
  EXCLUDES 1 *sepsis following ectopic and molar pregnancy (O08.82)*
    urinary tract infection (O08.83)

O08.1 Delayed or excessive hemorrhage following ectopic and molar pregnancy Ⓜ♀
  Afibrinogenemia following ectopic and molar pregnancy
  Defibrination syndrome following ectopic and molar pregnancy
  Hemolysis following ectopic and molar pregnancy
  Intravascular coagulation following ectopic and molar pregnancy
  EXCLUDES 1 *delayed or excessive hemorrhage due to incomplete abortion (O03.1)*

O08.2 Embolism following ectopic and molar pregnancy Ⓜ♀
  Air embolism following ectopic and molar pregnancy
  Amniotic fluid embolism following ectopic and molar pregnancy
  Blood-clot embolism following ectopic and molar pregnancy
  Embolism NOS following ectopic and molar pregnancy
  Fat embolism following ectopic and molar pregnancy
  Pulmonary embolism following ectopic and molar pregnancy
  Pyemic embolism following ectopic and molar pregnancy
  Septic or septicopyemic embolism following ectopic and molar pregnancy
  Soap embolism following ectopic and molar pregnancy

O08.3 Shock following ectopic and molar pregnancy Ⓜ♀
  Circulatory collapse following ectopic and molar pregnancy
  Shock (postprocedural) following ectopic and molar pregnancy
  EXCLUDES 1 *shock due to infection following ectopic and molar pregnancy (O08.82)*

O08.4 Renal failure following ectopic and molar pregnancy Ⓜ♀
  Kidney failure (acute) following ectopic and molar pregnancy
  Oliguria following ectopic and molar pregnancy
  Renal shutdown following ectopic and molar pregnancy
  Renal tubular necrosis following ectopic and molar pregnancy
  Uremia following ectopic and molar pregnancy

O08.5 Metabolic disorders following an ectopic and molar pregnancy Ⓜ♀

O08.6 Damage to pelvic organs and tissues following an ectopic and molar pregnancy Ⓜ♀
  Laceration, perforation, tear or chemical damage of bladder following an ectopic and molar pregnancy
  Laceration, perforation, tear or chemical damage of bowel following an ectopic and molar pregnancy
  Laceration, perforation, tear or chemical damage of broad ligament following an ectopic and molar pregnancy
  Laceration, perforation, tear or chemical damage of cervix following an ectopic and molar pregnancy
  Laceration, perforation, tear or chemical damage of periurethral tissue following an ectopic and molar pregnancy
  Laceration, perforation, tear or chemical damage of uterus following an ectopic and molar pregnancy
  Laceration, perforation, tear or chemical damage of vagina following an ectopic and molar pregnancy

O08.7 Other venous complications following an ectopic and molar pregnancy Ⓜ♀

☑5ᵗʰ **O08.8 Other complications following an ectopic and molar pregnancy**
  O08.81 Cardiac arrest following an ectopic and molar pregnancy Ⓜ♀
  O08.82 Sepsis following ectopic and molar pregnancy Ⓜ♀
    Use additional code to identify infectious agent (B95-B97)
    Use additional code to identify severe sepsis, if applicable (R65.2-)
    EXCLUDES 1 *septic or septicopyemic embolism following ectopic and molar pregnancy (O08.2)*

O08.83 Urinary tract infection following an ectopic and molar pregnancy Ⓜ♀
  Cystitis following an ectopic and molar pregnancy

O08.89 Other complications following an ectopic and molar pregnancy Ⓜ♀

O08.9 Unspecified complication following an ectopic and molar pregnancy Ⓜ♀▽

Supervision of high risk pregnancy (O09)

☑4ᵗʰ **O09 Supervision of** high risk **pregnancy**
  AHA: 2016, 4Q, 150

☑5ᵗʰ **O09.0 Supervision of pregnancy with** history of infertility
  O09.00 Supervision of pregnancy with history of infertility, unspecified trimester Ⓜ♀▽
  O09.01 Supervision of pregnancy with history of infertility, first trimester Ⓜ♀
  O09.02 Supervision of pregnancy with history of infertility, second trimester Ⓜ♀
  O09.03 Supervision of pregnancy with history of infertility, third trimester Ⓜ♀

☑5ᵗʰ **O09.1 Supervision of pregnancy with** history of ectopic **pregnancy**
  O09.10 Supervision of pregnancy with history of ectopic pregnancy, unspecified trimester Ⓜ♀▽
  O09.11 Supervision of pregnancy with history of ectopic pregnancy, first trimester Ⓜ♀
  O09.12 Supervision of pregnancy with history of ectopic pregnancy, second trimester Ⓜ♀
  O09.13 Supervision of pregnancy with history of ectopic pregnancy, third trimester Ⓜ♀

☑5ᵗʰ **O09.A Supervision of pregnancy with** history of molar **pregnancy**
  O09.A0 Supervision of pregnancy with history of molar pregnancy, unspecified trimester Ⓜ♀▽
  O09.A1 Supervision of pregnancy with history of molar pregnancy, first trimester Ⓜ♀
  O09.A2 Supervision of pregnancy with history of molar pregnancy, second trimester Ⓜ♀
  O09.A3 Supervision of pregnancy with history of molar pregnancy, third trimester Ⓜ♀

☑5ᵗʰ **O09.2 Supervision of pregnancy with other poor reproductive or obstetric history**
  EXCLUDES 2 *pregnancy care for patient with history of recurrent pregnancy loss (O26.2-)*

  ☑6ᵗʰ **O09.21 Supervision of pregnancy with history of** pre-term labor
    O09.211 Supervision of pregnancy with history of pre-term labor, first trimester Ⓜ♀
    O09.212 Supervision of pregnancy with history of pre-term labor, second trimester Ⓜ♀
    O09.213 Supervision of pregnancy with history of pre-term labor, third trimester Ⓜ♀
    O09.219 Supervision of pregnancy with history of pre-term labor, unspecified trimester Ⓜ♀▽

  ☑6ᵗʰ **O09.29 Supervision of pregnancy with other poor reproductive or obstetric history**
    Supervision of pregnancy with history of neonatal death
    Supervision of pregnancy with history of stillbirth
    O09.291 Supervision of pregnancy with other poor reproductive or obstetric history, first trimester Ⓜ♀
    O09.292 Supervision of pregnancy with other poor reproductive or obstetric history, second trimester Ⓜ♀
    O09.293 Supervision of pregnancy with other poor reproductive or obstetric history, third trimester Ⓜ♀
    O09.299 Supervision of pregnancy with other poor reproductive or obstetric history, unspecified trimester Ⓜ♀▽

☑5ᵗʰ **O09.3 Supervision of pregnancy with** insufficient antenatal care
  Supervision of concealed pregnancy
  Supervision of hidden pregnancy
  O09.30 Supervision of pregnancy with insufficient antenatal care, unspecified trimester Ⓜ♀▽
  O09.31 Supervision of pregnancy with insufficient antenatal care, first trimester Ⓜ♀

☑ Additional Character Req   ᵥₓ7ᵗʰ Placeholder Alert   Manifestation   ℍℂℂ CMS-HCC Condition   ▽ Unspecified Code   ▶◀ Revised Text   ● New Code   ▲ Revised Code Title

O09.32   **Supervision of pregnancy with insufficient antenatal care, second trimester** Ⓜ♀

O09.33   **Supervision of pregnancy with insufficient antenatal care, third trimester** Ⓜ♀

√5ᵗʰ **O09.4 Supervision of pregnancy with** grand multiparity

O09.40   **Supervision of pregnancy with grand multiparity, unspecified trimester** Ⓜ♀▽

O09.41   **Supervision of pregnancy with grand multiparity, first trimester** Ⓜ♀

O09.42   **Supervision of pregnancy with grand multiparity, second trimester** Ⓜ♀

O09.43   **Supervision of pregnancy with grand multiparity, third trimester** Ⓜ♀

√5ᵗʰ **O09.5 Supervision of** elderly primigravida and multigravida
Pregnancy for a female 35 years and older at expected date of delivery

√6ᵗʰ **O09.51 Supervision of** elderly primigravida

O09.511   **Supervision of elderly primigravida, first trimester** Ⓜ♀

O09.512   **Supervision of elderly primigravida, second trimester** Ⓜ♀

O09.513   **Supervision of elderly primigravida, third trimester** Ⓜ♀

O09.519   **Supervision of elderly primigravida, unspecified trimester** Ⓜ♀▽

√6ᵗʰ **O09.52 Supervision of** elderly multigravida

O09.521   **Supervision of elderly multigravida, first trimester** Ⓜ♀

O09.522   **Supervision of elderly multigravida, second trimester** Ⓜ♀

O09.523   **Supervision of elderly multigravida, third trimester** Ⓜ♀

O09.529   **Supervision of elderly multigravida, unspecified trimester** Ⓜ♀▽

√5ᵗʰ **O09.6 Supervision of** young primigravida and multigravida
Supervision of pregnancy for a female less than 16 years old at expected date of delivery

√6ᵗʰ **O09.61 Supervision of** young primigravida

O09.611   **Supervision of young primigravida, first trimester** Ⓜ♀

O09.612   **Supervision of young primigravida, second trimester** Ⓜ♀

O09.613   **Supervision of young primigravida, third trimester** Ⓜ♀

O09.619   **Supervision of young primigravida, unspecified trimester** Ⓜ♀▽

√6ᵗʰ **O09.62 Supervision of** young multigravida

O09.621   **Supervision of young multigravida, first trimester** Ⓜ♀

O09.622   **Supervision of young multigravida, second trimester** Ⓜ♀

O09.623   **Supervision of young multigravida, third trimester** Ⓜ♀

O09.629   **Supervision of young multigravida, unspecified trimester** Ⓜ♀▽

√5ᵗʰ **O09.7 Supervision of high risk pregnancy due to** social problems

O09.70   **Supervision of high risk pregnancy due to social problems, unspecified trimester** Ⓜ♀▽

O09.71   **Supervision of high risk pregnancy due to social problems, first trimester** Ⓜ♀

O09.72   **Supervision of high risk pregnancy due to social problems, second trimester** Ⓜ♀

O09.73   **Supervision of high risk pregnancy due to social problems, third trimester** Ⓜ♀

√5ᵗʰ **O09.8 Supervision of other high risk pregnancies**

√6ᵗʰ **O09.81 Supervision of pregnancy** resulting from assisted reproductive technology
Supervision of pregnancy resulting from in-vitro fertilization
EXCLUDES 2   *gestational carrier status (Z33.3)*

O09.811   **Supervision of pregnancy resulting from assisted reproductive technology, first trimester** Ⓜ♀

O09.812   **Supervision of pregnancy resulting from assisted reproductive technology, second trimester** Ⓜ♀

O09.813   **Supervision of pregnancy resulting from assisted reproductive technology, third trimester** Ⓜ♀

O09.819   **Supervision of pregnancy resulting from assisted reproductive technology, unspecified trimester** Ⓜ♀▽

√6ᵗʰ **O09.82 Supervision of pregnancy with** history of in utero procedure during previous pregnancy

O09.821   **Supervision of pregnancy with history of in utero procedure during previous pregnancy, first trimester** Ⓜ♀

O09.822   **Supervision of pregnancy with history of in utero procedure during previous pregnancy, second trimester** Ⓜ♀

O09.823   **Supervision of pregnancy with history of in utero procedure during previous pregnancy, third trimester** Ⓜ♀

O09.829   **Supervision of pregnancy with history of in utero procedure during previous pregnancy, unspecified trimester** Ⓜ♀▽
EXCLUDES 1   *supervision of pregnancy affected by in utero procedure during current pregnancy (O35.7)*

√6ᵗʰ **O09.89 Supervision of other high risk pregnancies**

O09.891   **Supervision of other high risk pregnancies, first trimester** Ⓜ♀

O09.892   **Supervision of other high risk pregnancies, second trimester** Ⓜ♀

O09.893   **Supervision of other high risk pregnancies, third trimester** Ⓜ♀

O09.899   **Supervision of other high risk pregnancies, unspecified trimester** Ⓜ♀

√5ᵗʰ **O09.9 Supervision of high risk pregnancy, unspecified**

O09.90   **Supervision of high risk pregnancy, unspecified, unspecified trimester** Ⓜ♀▽

O09.91   **Supervision of high risk pregnancy, unspecified, first trimester** Ⓜ♀▽

O09.92   **Supervision of high risk pregnancy, unspecified, second trimester** Ⓜ♀▽

O09.93   **Supervision of high risk pregnancy, unspecified, third trimester** Ⓜ♀▽

Edema, proteinuria and hypertensive disorders in pregnancy, childbirth and the puerperium (O10-O16)

√4ᵗʰ **O10 Pre-existing hypertension complicating pregnancy, childbirth and the puerperium**
Pre-existing hypertension with pre-existing proteinuria complicating pregnancy, childbirth and the puerperium
EXCLUDES 2   *pre-existing hypertension with superimposed pre-eclampsia complicating pregnancy, childbirth and the puerperium (O11.-)*

√5ᵗʰ **O10.0 Pre-existing essential hypertension complicating pregnancy, childbirth and the puerperium**
Any condition in I10 specified as a reason for obstetric care during pregnancy, childbirth or the puerperium

√6ᵗʰ **O10.01 Pre-existing essential hypertension complicating pregnancy**

O10.011   **Pre-existing essential hypertension complicating pregnancy, first trimester** Ⓜ♀

O10.012   **Pre-existing essential hypertension complicating pregnancy, second trimester** Ⓜ♀

O10.013   **Pre-existing essential hypertension complicating pregnancy, third trimester** Ⓜ♀

O10.019   **Pre-existing essential hypertension complicating pregnancy, unspecified trimester** Ⓜ♀▽

O10.02   **Pre-existing essential hypertension complicating childbirth** Ⓜ♀

O10.03   **Pre-existing essential hypertension complicating the puerperium** Ⓜ♀

EXCLUDES 1 Not coded here   *EXCLUDES 2* Not included here   Ⓝ Newborn Age: 0   Ⓟ Pediatric Age: 0-17   Ⓜ Maternity Age: 12-55   Ⓐ Adult Age: 15-124

828   ICD-10-CM 2018

☑5ᵗʰ **O10.1** **Pre-existing hypertensive** heart disease **complicating pregnancy, childbirth and the puerperium**
Any condition in I11 specified as a reason for obstetric care during pregnancy, childbirth or the puerperium
Use additional code from I11 to identify the type of hypertensive heart disease

     ☑6ᵗʰ **O10.11** **Pre-existing hypertensive heart disease complicating** pregnancy

         O10.111 **Pre-existing hypertensive heart disease complicating pregnancy,** first trimester   Ⓜ♀

         O10.112 **Pre-existing hypertensive heart disease complicating pregnancy,** second trimester   Ⓜ♀

         O10.113 **Pre-existing hypertensive heart disease complicating pregnancy,** third trimester   Ⓜ♀

         O10.119 **Pre-existing hypertensive heart disease complicating pregnancy,** unspecified trimester   Ⓜ♀▽

     O10.12 **Pre-existing hypertensive heart disease complicating** childbirth   Ⓜ♀

     O10.13 **Pre-existing hypertensive heart disease complicating the** puerperium   Ⓜ♀

☑5ᵗʰ **O10.2** **Pre-existing hypertensive** chronic kidney disease **complicating pregnancy, childbirth and the puerperium**
Any condition in I12 specified as a reason for obstetric care during pregnancy, childbirth or the puerperium
Use additional code from I12 to identify the type of hypertensive chronic kidney disease

     ☑6ᵗʰ **O10.21** **Pre-existing hypertensive chronic kidney disease complicating** pregnancy

         O10.211 **Pre-existing hypertensive chronic kidney disease complicating pregnancy,** first trimester   Ⓜ♀

         O10.212 **Pre-existing hypertensive chronic kidney disease complicating pregnancy,** second trimester   Ⓜ♀

         O10.213 **Pre-existing hypertensive chronic kidney disease complicating pregnancy,** third trimester   Ⓜ♀

         O10.219 **Pre-existing hypertensive chronic kidney disease complicating pregnancy,** unspecified trimester   Ⓜ♀▽

     O10.22 **Pre-existing hypertensive chronic kidney disease complicating** childbirth   Ⓜ♀

     O10.23 **Pre-existing hypertensive chronic kidney disease complicating the** puerperium   Ⓜ♀

☑5ᵗʰ **O10.3** **Pre-existing hypertensive** heart and chronic kidney disease **complicating pregnancy, childbirth and the puerperium**
Any condition in I13 specified as a reason for obstetric care during pregnancy, childbirth or the puerperium
Use additional code from I13 to identify the type of hypertensive heart and chronic kidney disease

     ☑6ᵗʰ **O10.31** **Pre-existing hypertensive heart and chronic kidney disease complicating** pregnancy

         O10.311 **Pre-existing hypertensive heart and chronic kidney disease complicating pregnancy,** first trimester   Ⓜ♀

         O10.312 **Pre-existing hypertensive heart and chronic kidney disease complicating pregnancy,** second trimester   Ⓜ♀

         O10.313 **Pre-existing hypertensive heart and chronic kidney disease complicating pregnancy,** third trimester   Ⓜ♀

         O10.319 **Pre-existing hypertensive heart and chronic kidney disease complicating pregnancy,** unspecified trimester   Ⓜ♀▽

     O10.32 **Pre-existing hypertensive heart and chronic kidney disease complicating** childbirth   Ⓜ♀

     O10.33 **Pre-existing hypertensive heart and chronic kidney disease complicating the** puerperium   Ⓜ♀

☑5ᵗʰ **O10.4** **Pre-existing** secondary hypertension **complicating pregnancy, childbirth and the puerperium**
Any condition in I15 specified as a reason for obstetric care during pregnancy, childbirth or the puerperium
Use additional code from I15 to identify the type of secondary hypertension

     ☑6ᵗʰ **O10.41** **Pre-existing secondary hypertension complicating** pregnancy

         O10.411 **Pre-existing secondary hypertension complicating pregnancy,** first trimester   Ⓜ♀

         O10.412 **Pre-existing secondary hypertension complicating pregnancy,** second trimester   Ⓜ♀

         O10.413 **Pre-existing secondary hypertension complicating pregnancy,** third trimester   Ⓜ♀

         O10.419 **Pre-existing secondary hypertension complicating pregnancy, unspecified trimester**   Ⓜ♀▽

     O10.42 **Pre-existing secondary hypertension complicating** childbirth   Ⓜ♀

     O10.43 **Pre-existing secondary hypertension complicating the** puerperium   Ⓜ♀

☑5ᵗʰ **O10.9** **Unspecified pre-existing hypertension complicating pregnancy, childbirth and the puerperium**

     ☑6ᵗʰ **O10.91** **Unspecified pre-existing hypertension complicating** pregnancy

         O10.911 **Unspecified pre-existing hypertension complicating pregnancy,** first trimester   Ⓜ♀▽

         O10.912 **Unspecified pre-existing hypertension complicating pregnancy,** second trimester   Ⓜ♀▽

         O10.913 **Unspecified pre-existing hypertension complicating pregnancy,** third trimester   Ⓜ♀▽

         O10.919 **Unspecified pre-existing hypertension complicating pregnancy, unspecified trimester**   Ⓜ♀▽

     O10.92 **Unspecified pre-existing hypertension complicating** childbirth   Ⓜ♀▽

     O10.93 **Unspecified pre-existing hypertension complicating the** puerperium   Ⓜ♀▽

☑4ᵗʰ **O11** Pre-existing **hypertension** with pre-eclampsia
   INCLUDES   conditions in O10 complicated by pre-eclampsia
pre-eclampsia superimposed pre-existing hypertension
Use additional code from O10 to identify the type of hypertension

     O11.1 **Pre-existing hypertension with pre-eclampsia,** first trimester   Ⓜ♀

     O11.2 **Pre-existing hypertension with pre-eclampsia,** second trimester   Ⓜ♀

     O11.3 **Pre-existing hypertension with pre-eclampsia,** third trimester   Ⓜ♀

     O11.4 **Pre-existing hypertension with pre-eclampsia, complicating** childbirth   Ⓜ♀

     O11.5 **Pre-existing hypertension with pre-eclampsia, complicating the** puerperium   Ⓜ♀

     O11.9 **Pre-existing hypertension with pre-eclampsia, unspecified trimester**   Ⓜ♀▽

☑4ᵗʰ **O12** Gestational [pregnancy-induced] edema and proteinuria without hypertension

     ☑5ᵗʰ **O12.0** **Gestational** edema

         O12.00 **Gestational edema, unspecified trimester**   Ⓜ♀▽

         O12.01 **Gestational edema,** first trimester   Ⓜ♀

         O12.02 **Gestational edema,** second trimester   Ⓜ♀

         O12.03 **Gestational edema,** third trimester   Ⓜ♀

         O12.04 **Gestational edema, complicating** childbirth   Ⓜ♀

         O12.05 **Gestational edema, complicating the** puerperium   Ⓜ♀

     ☑5ᵗʰ **O12.1** **Gestational** proteinuria

         O12.10 **Gestational proteinuria, unspecified trimester**   Ⓜ♀▽

         O12.11 **Gestational proteinuria,** first trimester   Ⓜ♀

         O12.12 **Gestational proteinuria,** second trimester   Ⓜ♀

         O12.13 **Gestational proteinuria,** third trimester   Ⓜ♀

         O12.14 **Gestational proteinuria, complicating** childbirth   Ⓜ♀

☑ Additional Character Req   ✓x7ᵗʰ Placeholder Alert   Manifestation   **HCC** CMS-HCC Condition   ▽ Unspecified Code   ▶◀ Revised Text   ● New Code   ▲ Revised Code Title

Chapter 15. Pregnancy, Childbirth, and the Puerperium

O12.15–O22.00

    O12.15 Gestational proteinuria, complicating the puerperium Ⓜ♀

✓5ᵗʰ **O12.2 Gestational edema with proteinuria**

    O12.20 Gestational edema with proteinuria, unspecified trimester Ⓜ♀▽

    O12.21 Gestational edema with proteinuria, first trimester Ⓜ♀

    O12.22 Gestational edema with proteinuria, second trimester Ⓜ♀

    O12.23 Gestational edema with proteinuria, third trimester Ⓜ♀

    O12.24 Gestational edema with proteinuria, complicating childbirth Ⓜ♀

    O12.25 Gestational edema with proteinuria, complicating the puerperium Ⓜ♀

✓4ᵗʰ **O13 Gestational [pregnancy-induced] hypertension without significant proteinuria**

    INCLUDES   gestational hypertension NOS
          transient hypertension of pregnancy

    AHA: 2016, 1Q, 5

    O13.1 Gestational [pregnancy-induced] hypertension without significant proteinuria, first trimester Ⓜ♀

    O13.2 Gestational [pregnancy-induced] hypertension without significant proteinuria, second trimester Ⓜ♀

    O13.3 Gestational [pregnancy-induced] hypertension without significant proteinuria, third trimester Ⓜ♀

    O13.4 Gestational [pregnancy-induced] hypertension without significant proteinuria, complicating childbirth Ⓜ♀

    O13.5 Gestational [pregnancy-induced] hypertension without significant proteinuria, complicating the puerperium Ⓜ♀

    O13.9 Gestational [pregnancy-induced] hypertension without significant proteinuria, unspecified trimester Ⓜ♀▽

✓4ᵗʰ **O14 Pre-eclampsia**

    EXCLUDES 1   pre-existing hypertension with pre-eclampsia (O11)

✓5ᵗʰ **O14.0 Mild to moderate pre-eclampsia**

    O14.00 Mild to moderate pre-eclampsia, unspecified trimester Ⓜ♀▽

    O14.02 Mild to moderate pre-eclampsia, second trimester Ⓜ♀

    O14.03 Mild to moderate pre-eclampsia, third trimester Ⓜ♀

    O14.04 Mild to moderate pre-eclampsia, complicating childbirth Ⓜ♀

    O14.05 Mild to moderate pre-eclampsia, complicating the puerperium Ⓜ♀

✓5ᵗʰ **O14.1 Severe pre-eclampsia**

    EXCLUDES 1   HELLP syndrome (O14.2-)

    O14.10 Severe pre-eclampsia, unspecified trimester Ⓜ♀▽

    O14.12 Severe pre-eclampsia, second trimester Ⓜ♀

    O14.13 Severe pre-eclampsia, third trimester Ⓜ♀

    O14.14 Severe pre-eclampsia complicating childbirth Ⓜ♀

    O14.15 Severe pre-eclampsia, complicating the puerperium Ⓜ♀

✓5ᵗʰ **O14.2 HELLP syndrome**

    Severe pre-eclampsia with hemolysis, elevated liver enzymes and low platelet count (HELLP)

    O14.20 HELLP syndrome (HELLP), unspecified trimester Ⓜ♀▽

    O14.22 HELLP syndrome (HELLP), second trimester Ⓜ♀

    O14.23 HELLP syndrome (HELLP), third trimester Ⓜ♀

    O14.24 HELLP syndrome, complicating childbirth Ⓜ♀

    O14.25 HELLP syndrome, complicating the puerperium Ⓜ♀

✓5ᵗʰ **O14.9 Unspecified pre-eclampsia**

    O14.90 Unspecified pre-eclampsia, unspecified trimester Ⓜ♀▽

    O14.92 Unspecified pre-eclampsia, second trimester Ⓜ♀▽

    O14.93 Unspecified pre-eclampsia, third trimester Ⓜ♀▽

    O14.94 Unspecified pre-eclampsia, complicating childbirth Ⓜ♀▽

    O14.95 Unspecified pre-eclampsia, complicating the puerperium Ⓜ♀▽

✓4ᵗʰ **O15 Eclampsia**

    INCLUDES   convulsions following conditions in O10-O14 and O16

✓5ᵗʰ **O15.0 Eclampsia complicating pregnancy**

    O15.00 Eclampsia complicating pregnancy, unspecified trimester Ⓜ♀▽

    O15.02 Eclampsia complicating pregnancy, second trimester Ⓜ♀

    O15.03 Eclampsia complicating pregnancy, third trimester Ⓜ♀

    O15.1 Eclampsia complicating labor Ⓜ♀

    O15.2 Eclampsia complicating the puerperium Ⓜ♀

    O15.9 Eclampsia, unspecified as to time period Ⓜ♀▽
         Eclampsia NOS

✓4ᵗʰ **O16 Unspecified maternal hypertension**

    O16.1 Unspecified maternal hypertension, first trimester Ⓜ♀▽

    O16.2 Unspecified maternal hypertension, second trimester Ⓜ♀▽

    O16.3 Unspecified maternal hypertension, third trimester Ⓜ♀▽

    O16.4 Unspecified maternal hypertension, complicating childbirth Ⓜ♀▽

    O16.5 Unspecified maternal hypertension, complicating the puerperium Ⓜ♀▽

    O16.9 Unspecified maternal hypertension, unspecified trimester Ⓜ♀▽

Other maternal disorders predominantly related to pregnancy (O20-O29)

    EXCLUDES 2   maternal care related to the fetus and amniotic cavity and possible delivery problems (O30-O48)
          maternal diseases classifiable elsewhere but complicating pregnancy, labor and delivery, and the puerperium (O98-O99)

✓4ᵗʰ **O20 Hemorrhage in early pregnancy**

    INCLUDES   hemorrhage before completion of 20 weeks gestation
    EXCLUDES 1   pregnancy with abortive outcome (O00-O08)

    O20.0 Threatened abortion Ⓜ♀
         Hemorrhage specified as due to threatened abortion
         DEF: Bloody discharge during pregnancy; cervix may be dilated and pregnancy threatened, but the pregnancy is not terminated.

    O20.8 Other hemorrhage in early pregnancy Ⓜ♀

    O20.9 Hemorrhage in early pregnancy, unspecified Ⓜ♀▽

✓4ᵗʰ **O21 Excessive vomiting in pregnancy**

    O21.0 Mild hyperemesis gravidarum Ⓜ♀
         Hyperemesis gravidarum, mild or unspecified, starting before the end of the 20th week of gestation

    O21.1 Hyperemesis gravidarum with metabolic disturbance Ⓜ♀
         Hyperemesis gravidarum, starting before the end of the 20th week of gestation, with metabolic disturbance such as carbohydrate depletion
         Hyperemesis gravidarum, starting before the end of the 20th week of gestation, with metabolic disturbance such as dehydration
         Hyperemesis gravidarum, starting before the end of the 20th week of gestation, with metabolic disturbance such as electrolyte imbalance

    O21.2 Late vomiting of pregnancy Ⓜ♀
         Excessive vomiting starting after 20 completed weeks of gestation

    O21.8 Other vomiting complicating pregnancy Ⓜ♀
         Vomiting due to diseases classified elsewhere, complicating pregnancy
         Use additional code, to identify cause

    O21.9 Vomiting of pregnancy, unspecified Ⓜ♀▽

✓4ᵗʰ **O22 Venous complications and hemorrhoids in pregnancy**

    EXCLUDES 1   venous complications of:
          abortion NOS (O03.9)
          ectopic or molar pregnancy (O08.7)
          failed attempted abortion (O07.35)
          induced abortion (O04.85)
          spontaneous abortion (O03.89)
    EXCLUDES 2   obstetric pulmonary embolism (O88.-)
          venous complications and hemorrhoids of childbirth and the puerperium (O87.-)

✓5ᵗʰ **O22.0 Varicose veins of lower extremity in pregnancy**
         Varicose veins NOS in pregnancy
         DEF: Distended, tortuous veins of lower extremities associated with pregnancy.

    O22.00 Varicose veins of lower extremity in pregnancy, unspecified trimester Ⓜ♀▽

EXCLUDES 1 Not coded here   EXCLUDES 2 Not included here   Ⓝ Newborn Age: 0   Ⓟ Pediatric Age: 0-17   Ⓜ Maternity Age: 12-55   Ⓐ Adult Age: 15-124

O22.01 Varicose veins of lower extremity in pregnancy, Ⓜ♀
first trimester

O22.02 Varicose veins of lower extremity in pregnancy, Ⓜ♀
second trimester

O22.03 Varicose veins of lower extremity in pregnancy, Ⓜ♀
third trimester

✓5ᵗʰ **O22.1** Genital varices in pregnancy
Perineal varices in pregnancy
Vaginal varices in pregnancy
Vulval varices in pregnancy

O22.10 Genital varices in pregnancy, unspecified Ⓜ♀▽
trimester

O22.11 Genital varices in pregnancy, first trimester Ⓜ♀

O22.12 Genital varices in pregnancy, second trimester Ⓜ♀

O22.13 Genital varices in pregnancy, third trimester Ⓜ♀

✓5ᵗʰ **O22.2** Superficial thrombophlebitis in pregnancy
Phlebitis in pregnancy NOS
Thrombophlebitis of legs in pregnancy
Thrombosis in pregnancy NOS
Use additional code to identify the superficial thrombophlebitis
(I80.0-)

O22.20 Superficial thrombophlebitis in pregnancy, Ⓜ♀▽
unspecified trimester

O22.21 Superficial thrombophlebitis in pregnancy, Ⓜ♀
first trimester

O22.22 Superficial thrombophlebitis in pregnancy, Ⓜ♀
second trimester

O22.23 Superficial thrombophlebitis in pregnancy, Ⓜ♀
third trimester

✓5ᵗʰ **O22.3** Deep phlebothrombosis in pregnancy
Deep vein thrombosis, antepartum
Use additional code to identify the deep vein thrombosis (I82.4-,
I82.5-, I82.62-. I82.72-)
Use additional code, if applicable, for associated long-term
(current) use of anticoagulants (Z79.01)

O22.30 Deep phlebothrombosis in pregnancy, Ⓜ♀▽
unspecified trimester

O22.31 Deep phlebothrombosis in pregnancy, Ⓜ♀
first trimester

O22.32 Deep phlebothrombosis in pregnancy, Ⓜ♀
second trimester

O22.33 Deep phlebothrombosis in pregnancy, Ⓜ♀
third trimester

✓5ᵗʰ **O22.4** Hemorrhoids in pregnancy

O22.40 Hemorrhoids in pregnancy, unspecified Ⓜ♀▽
trimester

O22.41 Hemorrhoids in pregnancy, first trimester Ⓜ♀

O22.42 Hemorrhoids in pregnancy, second trimester Ⓜ♀

O22.43 Hemorrhoids in pregnancy, third trimester Ⓜ♀

✓5ᵗʰ **O22.5** Cerebral venous thrombosis in pregnancy
Cerebrovenous sinus thrombosis in pregnancy

O22.50 Cerebral venous thrombosis in pregnancy, Ⓜ♀▽
unspecified trimester

O22.51 Cerebral venous thrombosis in pregnancy, Ⓜ♀
first trimester

O22.52 Cerebral venous thrombosis in pregnancy, Ⓜ♀
second trimester

O22.53 Cerebral venous thrombosis in pregnancy, Ⓜ♀
third trimester

✓5ᵗʰ **O22.8** Other venous complications in pregnancy

✓6ᵗʰ **O22.8X** Other venous complications in pregnancy

O22.8X1 Other venous complications in Ⓜ♀
pregnancy, first trimester

O22.8X2 Other venous complications in Ⓜ♀
pregnancy, second trimester

O22.8X3 Other venous complications in Ⓜ♀
pregnancy, third trimester

O22.8X9 Other venous complications in Ⓜ♀▽
pregnancy, unspecified trimester

✓5ᵗʰ **O22.9** Venous complication in pregnancy, unspecified
Gestational phlebitis NOS
Gestational phlebopathy NOS
Gestational thrombosis NOS

O22.90 Venous complication in pregnancy, Ⓜ♀▽
unspecified, unspecified trimester

O22.91 Venous complication in pregnancy, Ⓜ♀▽
unspecified, first trimester

O22.92 Venous complication in pregnancy, Ⓜ♀▽
unspecified, second trimester

O22.93 Venous complication in pregnancy, Ⓜ♀▽
unspecified, third trimester

✓4ᵗʰ **O23** Infections of genitourinary tract in pregnancy
Use additional code to identify organism (B95.-, B96.-)
EXCLUDES 2 gonococcal infections complicating pregnancy, childbirth and
the puerperium (O98.2)
infections with a predominantly sexual mode of transmission
NOS complicating pregnancy, childbirth and the
puerperium (O98.3)
syphilis complicating pregnancy, childbirth and the puerperium
(O98.1)
tuberculosis of genitourinary system complicating pregnancy,
childbirth and the puerperium (O98.0)
venereal disease NOS complicating pregnancy, childbirth and
the puerperium (O98.3)

✓5ᵗʰ **O23.0** Infections of kidney in pregnancy
Pyelonephritis in pregnancy

O23.00 Infections of kidney in pregnancy, unspecifiedⓂ♀▽
trimester

O23.01 Infections of kidney in pregnancy, first trimester Ⓜ♀

O23.02 Infections of kidney in pregnancy, second Ⓜ♀
trimester

O23.03 Infections of kidney in pregnancy, third Ⓜ♀
trimester

✓5ᵗʰ **O23.1** Infections of bladder in pregnancy

O23.10 Infections of bladder in pregnancy, Ⓜ♀
unspecified trimester

O23.11 Infections of bladder in pregnancy, Ⓜ♀
first trimester

O23.12 Infections of bladder in pregnancy, Ⓜ♀
second trimester

O23.13 Infections of bladder in pregnancy, Ⓜ♀
third trimester

✓5ᵗʰ **O23.2** Infections of urethra in pregnancy

O23.20 Infections of urethra in pregnancy, Ⓜ♀
unspecified trimester

O23.21 Infections of urethra in pregnancy, Ⓜ♀
first trimester

O23.22 Infections of urethra in pregnancy, Ⓜ♀
second trimester

O23.23 Infections of urethra in pregnancy, Ⓜ♀
third trimester

✓5ᵗʰ **O23.3** Infections of other parts of urinary tract in pregnancy

O23.30 Infections of other parts of urinary tract in Ⓜ♀
pregnancy, unspecified trimester

O23.31 Infections of other parts of urinary tract in Ⓜ♀
pregnancy, first trimester

O23.32 Infections of other parts of urinary tract in Ⓜ♀
pregnancy, second trimester

O23.33 Infections of other parts of urinary tract in Ⓜ♀
pregnancy, third trimester

✓5ᵗʰ **O23.4** Unspecified infection of urinary tract in pregnancy

O23.40 Unspecified infection of urinary tract in Ⓜ♀▽
pregnancy, unspecified trimester

O23.41 Unspecified infection of urinary tract in Ⓜ♀▽
pregnancy, first trimester

O23.42 Unspecified infection of urinary tract in Ⓜ♀▽
pregnancy, second trimester

O23.43 Unspecified infection of urinary tract in Ⓜ♀▽
pregnancy, third trimester

✓5ᵗʰ **O23.5** Infections of the genital tract in pregnancy

✓6ᵗʰ **O23.51** Infection of cervix in pregnancy

O23.511 Infections of cervix in pregnancy, Ⓜ♀
first trimester

O23.512 Infections of cervix in pregnancy, Ⓜ♀
second trimester

O23.513 Infections of cervix in pregnancy, Ⓜ♀
third trimester

O23.519 Infections of cervix in pregnancy, Ⓜ♀▽
unspecified trimester

☑ Additional Character Req   ✓7ᵗʰ Placeholder Alert   Manifestation   **HCC** CMS-HCC Condition   ▽ Unspecified Code   ►◄ Revised Text   ● New Code   ▲ Revised Code Title

✓6ᵗʰ **O23.52** Salpingo-oophoritis in pregnancy
Oophoritis in pregnancy
Salpingitis in pregnancy

O23.521 Salpingo-oophoritis in pregnancy, first trimester Ⓜ♀

O23.522 Salpingo-oophoritis in pregnancy, second trimester Ⓜ♀

O23.523 Salpingo-oophoritis in pregnancy, third trimester Ⓜ♀

O23.529 Salpingo-oophoritis in pregnancy, unspecified trimester Ⓜ♀▽

✓6ᵗʰ **O23.59** Infection of other part of genital tract in pregnancy

O23.591 Infection of other part of genital tract in pregnancy, first trimester Ⓜ♀

O23.592 Infection of other part of genital tract in pregnancy, second trimester Ⓜ♀

O23.593 Infection of other part of genital tract in pregnancy, third trimester Ⓜ♀

O23.599 Infection of other part of genital tract in pregnancy, unspecified trimester Ⓜ♀▽

✓5ᵗʰ **O23.9** Unspecified genitourinary tract infection in pregnancy
Genitourinary tract infection in pregnancy NOS

O23.90 Unspecified genitourinary tract infection in pregnancy, unspecified trimester Ⓜ♀▽

O23.91 Unspecified genitourinary tract infection in pregnancy, first trimester Ⓜ♀▽

O23.92 Unspecified genitourinary tract infection in pregnancy, second trimester Ⓜ♀▽

O23.93 Unspecified genitourinary tract infection in pregnancy, third trimester Ⓜ♀▽

✓4ᵗʰ **O24** Diabetes mellitus in pregnancy, childbirth and the puerperium

✓5ᵗʰ **O24.0** Pre-existing type 1 diabetes mellitus, in pregnancy, childbirth and the puerperium
Juvenile onset diabetes mellitus, in pregnancy, childbirth and the puerperium
Ketosis-prone diabetes mellitus in pregnancy, childbirth and the puerperium
Use additional code from category E10 to further identify any manifestations

✓6ᵗʰ **O24.01** Pre-existing type 1 diabetes mellitus, in pregnancy

O24.011 Pre-existing type 1 diabetes mellitus, in pregnancy, first trimester Ⓜ♀

O24.012 Pre-existing type 1 diabetes mellitus, in pregnancy, second trimester Ⓜ♀

O24.013 Pre-existing type 1 diabetes mellitus, in pregnancy, third trimester Ⓜ♀

O24.019 Pre-existing type 1 diabetes mellitus, in pregnancy, unspecified trimester Ⓜ♀▽

O24.02 Pre-existing type 1 diabetes mellitus, in childbirth Ⓜ♀

O24.03 Pre-existing type 1 diabetes mellitus, in the puerperium Ⓜ♀

✓5ᵗʰ **O24.1** Pre-existing type 2 diabetes mellitus, in pregnancy, childbirth and the puerperium
Insulin-resistant diabetes mellitus in pregnancy, childbirth and the puerperium
Use additional code (for):
from category E11 to further identify any manifestations
long-term (current) use of insulin (Z79.4)

✓6ᵗʰ **O24.11** Pre-existing type 2 diabetes mellitus, in pregnancy

O24.111 Pre-existing type 2 diabetes mellitus, in pregnancy, first trimester Ⓜ♀

O24.112 Pre-existing type 2 diabetes mellitus, in pregnancy, second trimester Ⓜ♀

O24.113 Pre-existing type 2 diabetes mellitus, in pregnancy, third trimester Ⓜ♀

O24.119 Pre-existing type 2 diabetes mellitus, in pregnancy, unspecified trimester Ⓜ♀▽

O24.12 Pre-existing type 2 diabetes mellitus, in childbirth Ⓜ♀

O24.13 Pre-existing type 2 diabetes mellitus, in the puerperium Ⓜ♀

✓5ᵗʰ **O24.3** Unspecified pre-existing diabetes mellitus in pregnancy, childbirth and the puerperium
Use additional code (for):
from category E11 to further identify any manifestation
long-term (current) use of insulin (Z79.4)

✓6ᵗʰ **O24.31** Unspecified pre-existing diabetes mellitus in pregnancy

O24.311 Unspecified pre-existing diabetes mellitus in pregnancy, first trimester Ⓜ♀▽

O24.312 Unspecified pre-existing diabetes mellitus in pregnancy, second trimester Ⓜ♀▽

O24.313 Unspecified pre-existing diabetes mellitus in pregnancy, third trimester Ⓜ♀▽

O24.319 Unspecified pre-existing diabetes mellitus in pregnancy, unspecified trimester Ⓜ♀▽

O24.32 Unspecified pre-existing diabetes mellitus in childbirth Ⓜ♀▽

O24.33 Unspecified pre-existing diabetes mellitus in the puerperium Ⓜ♀▽

✓5ᵗʰ **O24.4** Gestational diabetes mellitus
Diabetes mellitus arising in pregnancy
Gestational diabetes mellitus NOS

✓6ᵗʰ **O24.41** Gestational diabetes mellitus in pregnancy

O24.410 Gestational diabetes mellitus in pregnancy, diet controlled Ⓜ♀

O24.414 Gestational diabetes mellitus in pregnancy, insulin controlled Ⓜ♀

O24.415 Gestational diabetes mellitus in pregnancy, controlled by oral hypoglycemic drugs Ⓜ♀
Gestational diabetes mellitus in pregnancy, controlled by oral antidiabetic drugs

O24.419 Gestational diabetes mellitus in pregnancy, unspecified control Ⓜ♀▽
AHA: 2015, 4Q, 34

✓6ᵗʰ **O24.42** Gestational diabetes mellitus in childbirth
AHA: 2016, 1Q, 5

O24.420 Gestational diabetes mellitus in childbirth, diet controlled Ⓜ♀

O24.424 Gestational diabetes mellitus in childbirth, insulin controlled Ⓜ♀

O24.425 Gestational diabetes mellitus in childbirth, controlled by oral hypoglycemic drugs Ⓜ♀
Gestational diabetes mellitus in childbirth, controlled by oral antidiabetic drugs

O24.429 Gestational diabetes mellitus in childbirth, unspecified control Ⓜ♀▽
AHA: 2015, 4Q, 34

✓6ᵗʰ **O24.43** Gestational diabetes mellitus in the puerperium

O24.430 Gestational diabetes mellitus in the puerperium, diet controlled Ⓜ♀

O24.434 Gestational diabetes mellitus in the puerperium, insulin controlled Ⓜ♀

O24.435 Gestational diabetes mellitus in the puerperium, controlled by oral hypoglycemic drugs Ⓜ♀
Gestational diabetes mellitus in puerperium, controlled by oral antidiabetic drugs

O24.439 Gestational diabetes mellitus in the puerperium, unspecified control Ⓜ♀▽
AHA: 2015, 4Q, 34

✓5ᵗʰ **O24.8** Other pre-existing diabetes mellitus in pregnancy, childbirth, and the puerperium
Use additional code (for):
from categories E08, E09 and E13 to further identify any manifestation
long-term (current) use of insulin (Z79.4)

✓6ᵗʰ **O24.81** Other pre-existing diabetes mellitus in pregnancy

O24.811 Other pre-existing diabetes mellitus in pregnancy, first trimester Ⓜ♀

O24.812 Other pre-existing diabetes mellitus in pregnancy, second trimester Ⓜ♀

O24.813 Other pre-existing diabetes mellitus in pregnancy, third trimester Ⓜ♀

O24.819 Other pre-existing diabetes mellitus in pregnancy, unspecified trimester Ⓜ♀▽

EXCLUDES1 Not coded here   EXCLUDES2 Not included here   Ⓝ Newborn Age: 0   Ⓟ Pediatric Age: 0-17   Ⓜ Maternity Age: 12-55   Ⓐ Adult Age: 15-124

832   ICD-10-CM 2018

O24.82 **Other pre-existing diabetes mellitus in** childbirth   M♀

O24.83 **Other pre-existing diabetes mellitus in the** puerperium   M♀

✓5ᵗʰ O24.9 **Unspecified diabetes mellitus in pregnancy, childbirth and the puerperium**
Use additional code for long-term (current) use of insulin (Z79.4)

  ✓6ᵗʰ O24.91 **Unspecified diabetes mellitus in** pregnancy

    O24.911 **Unspecified diabetes mellitus in pregnancy,** first trimester   M♀▽

    O24.912 **Unspecified diabetes mellitus in pregnancy,** second trimester   M♀▽

    O24.913 **Unspecified diabetes mellitus in pregnancy,** third trimester   M♀▽

    O24.919 **Unspecified diabetes mellitus in pregnancy, unspecified trimester**   M♀▽

  O24.92 **Unspecified diabetes mellitus in** childbirth   M♀▽

  O24.93 **Unspecified diabetes mellitus in the** puerperium   M♀▽

✓4ᵗʰ **O25 Malnutrition in pregnancy, childbirth and the puerperium**

  ✓5ᵗʰ O25.1 **Malnutrition in** pregnancy

    O25.10 **Malnutrition in pregnancy, unspecified trimester**   M♀▽

    O25.11 **Malnutrition in pregnancy,** first trimester   M♀

    O25.12 **Malnutrition in pregnancy,** second trimester   M♀

    O25.13 **Malnutrition in pregnancy,** third trimester   M♀

  O25.2 **Malnutrition in** childbirth   M♀

  O25.3 **Malnutrition in the** puerperium   M♀

✓4ᵗʰ **O26 Maternal care for other conditions predominantly related to pregnancy**

  ✓5ᵗʰ O26.0 **Excessive weight gain in pregnancy**
    EXCLUDES 2   gestational edema (O12.0, O12.2)

    O26.00 **Excessive weight gain in pregnancy, unspecified trimester**   M♀▽

    O26.01 **Excessive weight gain in pregnancy,** first trimester   M♀

    O26.02 **Excessive weight gain in pregnancy,** second trimester   M♀

    O26.03 **Excessive weight gain in pregnancy,** third trimester   M♀

  ✓5ᵗʰ O26.1 **Low weight gain in pregnancy**

    O26.10 **Low weight gain in pregnancy, unspecified trimester**   M♀▽

    O26.11 **Low weight gain in pregnancy,** first trimester   M♀

    O26.12 **Low weight gain in pregnancy,** second trimester   M♀

    O26.13 **Low weight gain in pregnancy,** third trimester   M♀

  ✓5ᵗʰ O26.2 **Pregnancy care for patient with recurrent pregnancy loss**

    O26.20 **Pregnancy care for patient with recurrent pregnancy loss, unspecified trimester**   M♀▽

    O26.21 **Pregnancy care for patient with recurrent pregnancy loss,** first trimester   M♀

    O26.22 **Pregnancy care for patient with recurrent pregnancy loss,** second trimester   M♀

    O26.23 **Pregnancy care for patient with recurrent pregnancy loss,** third trimester   M♀

  ✓5ᵗʰ O26.3 **Retained intrauterine contraceptive device in pregnancy**

    O26.30 **Retained intrauterine contraceptive device in pregnancy, unspecified trimester**   M♀▽

    O26.31 **Retained intrauterine contraceptive device in pregnancy,** first trimester   M♀

    O26.32 **Retained intrauterine contraceptive device in pregnancy,** second trimester   M♀

    O26.33 **Retained intrauterine contraceptive device in pregnancy,** third trimester   M♀

  ✓5ᵗʰ O26.4 **Herpes gestationis**

    O26.40 **Herpes gestationis, unspecified trimester**   M♀▽

    O26.41 **Herpes gestationis,** first trimester   M♀

    O26.42 **Herpes gestationis,** second trimester   M♀

    O26.43 **Herpes gestationis,** third trimester   M♀

✓5ᵗʰ O26.5 **Maternal hypotension syndrome**
Supine hypotensive syndrome

  O26.50 **Maternal hypotension syndrome, unspecified trimester**   M♀▽

  O26.51 **Maternal hypotension syndrome,** first trimester   M♀

  O26.52 **Maternal hypotension syndrome,** second trimester   M♀

  O26.53 **Maternal hypotension syndrome,** third trimester   M♀

✓5ᵗʰ O26.6 **Liver and biliary tract disorders in pregnancy, childbirth and the puerperium**
Use additional code to identify the specific disorder
  EXCLUDES 2   hepatorenal syndrome following labor and delivery (O90.4)

  ✓6ᵗʰ O26.61 **Liver and biliary tract disorders in** pregnancy

    O26.611 **Liver and biliary tract disorders in pregnancy,** first trimester   M♀

    O26.612 **Liver and biliary tract disorders in pregnancy,** second trimester   M♀

    O26.613 **Liver and biliary tract disorders in pregnancy,** third trimester   M♀

    O26.619 **Liver and biliary tract disorders in pregnancy, unspecified trimester**   M♀▽

  O26.62 **Liver and biliary tract disorders in** childbirth   M♀

  O26.63 **Liver and biliary tract disorders in the** puerperium   M♀

✓5ᵗʰ O26.7 **Subluxation of symphysis (pubis) in pregnancy, childbirth and the puerperium**
  EXCLUDES 1   traumatic separation of symphysis (pubis) during childbirth (O71.6)

  ✓6ᵗʰ O26.71 **Subluxation of symphysis (pubis) in** pregnancy

    O26.711 **Subluxation of symphysis (pubis) in pregnancy,** first trimester   M♀

    O26.712 **Subluxation of symphysis (pubis) in pregnancy,** second trimester   M♀

    O26.713 **Subluxation of symphysis (pubis) in pregnancy,** third trimester   M♀

    O26.719 **Subluxation of symphysis (pubis) in pregnancy, unspecified trimester**   M♀▽

  O26.72 **Subluxation of symphysis (pubis) in** childbirth   M♀

  O26.73 **Subluxation of symphysis (pubis) in the** puerperium   M♀

✓5ᵗʰ O26.8 **Other specified pregnancy related conditions**

  ✓6ᵗʰ O26.81 **Pregnancy related exhaustion and fatigue**

    O26.811 **Pregnancy related exhaustion and fatigue,** first trimester   M♀

    O26.812 **Pregnancy related exhaustion and fatigue,** second trimester   M♀

    O26.813 **Pregnancy related exhaustion and fatigue,** third trimester   M♀

    O26.819 **Pregnancy related exhaustion and fatigue, unspecified trimester**   M♀▽

  ✓6ᵗʰ O26.82 **Pregnancy related peripheral neuritis**

    O26.821 **Pregnancy related peripheral neuritis,** first trimester   M♀

    O26.822 **Pregnancy related peripheral neuritis,** second trimester   M♀

    O26.823 **Pregnancy related peripheral neuritis,** third trimester   M♀

    O26.829 **Pregnancy related peripheral neuritis, unspecified trimester**   M♀▽

  ✓6ᵗʰ O26.83 **Pregnancy related renal disease**
Use additional code to identify the specific disorder

    O26.831 **Pregnancy related renal disease,** first trimester   M♀

    O26.832 **Pregnancy related renal disease,** second trimester   M♀

    O26.833 **Pregnancy related renal disease,** third trimester   M♀

    O26.839 **Pregnancy related renal disease, unspecified trimester**   M♀▽

☑ Additional Character Req   ✓x7ᵗʰ Placeholder Alert   Manifestation   HCC CMS-HCC Condition   ▽ Unspecified Code   ►◄ Revised Text   ● New Code   ▲ Revised Code Title

✓6ᵗʰ O26.84 Uterine size-date discrepancy complicating pregnancy
EXCLUDES 1 encounter for suspected problem with fetal growth ruled out (Z03.74)

O26.841 Uterine size-date discrepancy, first trimester Ⓜ♀

O26.842 Uterine size-date discrepancy, second trimester Ⓜ♀

O26.843 Uterine size-date discrepancy, third trimester Ⓜ♀

O26.849 Uterine size-date discrepancy, unspecified trimester Ⓜ♀▽

✓6ᵗʰ O26.85 Spotting complicating pregnancy

O26.851 Spotting complicating pregnancy, first trimester Ⓜ♀

O26.852 Spotting complicating pregnancy, second trimester Ⓜ♀

O26.853 Spotting complicating pregnancy, third trimester Ⓜ♀

O26.859 Spotting complicating pregnancy, unspecified trimester Ⓜ♀▽

O26.86 Pruritic urticarial papules and plaques of pregnancy (PUPPP) Ⓜ♀
Polymorphic eruption of pregnancy

✓6ᵗʰ O26.87 Cervical shortening
EXCLUDES 1 encounter for suspected cervical shortening ruled out (Z03.75)
DEF: A cervix that has shortened to < 25 mm before the 24th week of pregnancy; warning sign for impending premature delivery; treated by cervical cerclage placement or progesterone.

O26.872 Cervical shortening, second trimester Ⓜ♀

O26.873 Cervical shortening, third trimester Ⓜ♀

O26.879 Cervical shortening, unspecified trimester Ⓜ♀▽

✓6ᵗʰ O26.89 Other specified pregnancy related conditions
AHA: 2015, 3Q, 40

O26.891 Other specified pregnancy related conditions, first trimester Ⓜ♀

O26.892 Other specified pregnancy related conditions, second trimester Ⓜ♀

O26.893 Other specified pregnancy related conditions, third trimester Ⓜ♀

O26.899 Other specified pregnancy related conditions, unspecified trimester Ⓜ♀▽

✓5ᵗʰ O26.9 Pregnancy related conditions, unspecified

O26.90 Pregnancy related conditions, unspecified, unspecified trimester Ⓜ♀▽

O26.91 Pregnancy related conditions, unspecified, first trimester Ⓜ♀▽

O26.92 Pregnancy related conditions, unspecified, second trimester Ⓜ♀▽

O26.93 Pregnancy related conditions, unspecified, third trimester Ⓜ♀▽

✓4ᵗʰ O28 Abnormal findings on antenatal screening of mother
EXCLUDES 1 diagnostic findings classified elsewhere—see Alphabetical Index

O28.0 Abnormal hematological finding on antenatal screening of mother Ⓜ♀

O28.1 Abnormal biochemical finding on antenatal screening of mother Ⓜ♀

O28.2 Abnormal cytological finding on antenatal screening of mother Ⓜ♀

O28.3 Abnormal ultrasonic finding on antenatal screening of mother Ⓜ♀

O28.4 Abnormal radiological finding on antenatal screening of mother Ⓜ♀

O28.5 Abnormal chromosomal and genetic finding on antenatal screening of mother Ⓜ♀

O28.8 Other abnormal findings on antenatal screening of mother Ⓜ♀

O28.9 Unspecified abnormal findings on antenatal screening of mother Ⓜ♀▽

✓4ᵗʰ O29 Complications of anesthesia during pregnancy
INCLUDES maternal complications arising from the administration of a general, regional or local anesthetic, analgesic or other sedation during pregnancy
Use additional code, if necessary, to identify the complication
EXCLUDES 2 complications of anesthesia during labor and delivery (O74.-)
complications of anesthesia during the puerperium (O89.-)

✓5ᵗʰ O29.0 Pulmonary complications of anesthesia during pregnancy

✓6ᵗʰ O29.01 Aspiration pneumonitis due to anesthesia during pregnancy
Inhalation of stomach contents or secretions NOS due to anesthesia during pregnancy
Mendelson's syndrome due to anesthesia during pregnancy

O29.011 Aspiration pneumonitis due to anesthesia during pregnancy, first trimester Ⓜ♀

O29.012 Aspiration pneumonitis due to anesthesia during pregnancy, second trimester Ⓜ♀

O29.013 Aspiration pneumonitis due to anesthesia during pregnancy, third trimester Ⓜ♀

O29.019 Aspiration pneumonitis due to anesthesia during pregnancy, unspecified trimester Ⓜ♀▽

✓6ᵗʰ O29.02 Pressure collapse of lung due to anesthesia during pregnancy

O29.021 Pressure collapse of lung due to anesthesia during pregnancy, first trimester Ⓜ♀

O29.022 Pressure collapse of lung due to anesthesia during pregnancy, second trimester Ⓜ♀

O29.023 Pressure collapse of lung due to anesthesia during pregnancy, third trimester Ⓜ♀

O29.029 Pressure collapse of lung due to anesthesia during pregnancy, unspecified trimester Ⓜ♀▽

✓6ᵗʰ O29.09 Other pulmonary complications of anesthesia during pregnancy

O29.091 Other pulmonary complications of anesthesia during pregnancy, first trimester Ⓜ♀

O29.092 Other pulmonary complications of anesthesia during pregnancy, second trimester Ⓜ♀

O29.093 Other pulmonary complications of anesthesia during pregnancy, third trimester Ⓜ♀

O29.099 Other pulmonary complications of anesthesia during pregnancy, unspecified trimester Ⓜ♀▽

✓5ᵗʰ O29.1 Cardiac complications of anesthesia during pregnancy

✓6ᵗʰ O29.11 Cardiac arrest due to anesthesia during pregnancy

O29.111 Cardiac arrest due to anesthesia during pregnancy, first trimester Ⓜ♀

O29.112 Cardiac arrest due to anesthesia during pregnancy, second trimester Ⓜ♀

O29.113 Cardiac arrest due to anesthesia during pregnancy, third trimester Ⓜ♀

O29.119 Cardiac arrest due to anesthesia during pregnancy, unspecified trimester Ⓜ♀▽

✓6ᵗʰ O29.12 Cardiac failure due to anesthesia during pregnancy

O29.121 Cardiac failure due to anesthesia during pregnancy, first trimester Ⓜ♀

O29.122 Cardiac failure due to anesthesia during pregnancy, second trimester Ⓜ♀

O29.123 Cardiac failure due to anesthesia during pregnancy, third trimester Ⓜ♀

O29.129 Cardiac failure due to anesthesia during pregnancy, unspecified trimester Ⓜ♀▽

EXCLUDES 1 Not coded here　　EXCLUDES 2 Not included here　　Ⓝ Newborn Age: 0　　Ⓟ Pediatric Age: 0-17　　Ⓜ Maternity Age: 12-55　　Ⓐ Adult Age: 15-124

834　　ICD-10-CM 2018

✓6ᵗʰ **O29.19** **Other cardiac complications of anesthesia during pregnancy**

　　O29.191 Other cardiac complications of Ⓜ♀ anesthesia during pregnancy, first trimester

　　O29.192 Other cardiac complications of Ⓜ♀ anesthesia during pregnancy, second trimester

　　O29.193 Other cardiac complications of Ⓜ♀ anesthesia during pregnancy, third trimester

　　O29.199 Other cardiac complications of Ⓜ♀▽ anesthesia during pregnancy, unspecified trimester

✓5ᵗʰ **O29.2** Central nervous system **complications of anesthesia during pregnancy**

✓6ᵗʰ **O29.21** Cerebral anoxia **due to anesthesia during pregnancy**

　　O29.211 Cerebral anoxia due to anesthesia Ⓜ♀ during pregnancy, first trimester

　　O29.212 Cerebral anoxia due to anesthesia Ⓜ♀ during pregnancy, second trimester

　　O29.213 Cerebral anoxia due to anesthesia Ⓜ♀ during pregnancy, third trimester

　　O29.219 Cerebral anoxia due to anesthesia Ⓜ♀▽ during pregnancy, unspecified trimester

✓6ᵗʰ **O29.29** **Other central nervous system complications of anesthesia during pregnancy**

　　O29.291 Other central nervous system Ⓜ♀ complications of anesthesia during pregnancy, first trimester

　　O29.292 Other central nervous system Ⓜ♀ complications of anesthesia during pregnancy, second trimester

　　O29.293 Other central nervous system Ⓜ♀ complications of anesthesia during pregnancy, third trimester

　　O29.299 Other central nervous system Ⓜ♀▽ complications of anesthesia during pregnancy, unspecified trimester

✓5ᵗʰ **O29.3** Toxic reaction **to local anesthesia during pregnancy**

✓6ᵗʰ **O29.3X** **Toxic reaction to local anesthesia during pregnancy**

　　O29.3X1 Toxic reaction to local anesthesia Ⓜ♀ during pregnancy, first trimester

　　O29.3X2 Toxic reaction to local anesthesia Ⓜ♀ during pregnancy, second trimester

　　O29.3X3 Toxic reaction to local anesthesia Ⓜ♀ during pregnancy, third trimester

　　O29.3X9 Toxic reaction to local anesthesia Ⓜ♀▽ during pregnancy, unspecified trimester

✓5ᵗʰ **O29.4** Spinal and epidural anesthesia induced headache **during pregnancy**

　　O29.40 Spinal and epidural anesthesia induced Ⓜ♀▽ headacheduring pregnancy, unspecified trimester

　　O29.41 Spinal and epidural anesthesia induced Ⓜ♀ headache during pregnancy, first trimester

　　O29.42 Spinal and epidural anesthesia induced Ⓜ♀ headache during pregnancy, second trimester

　　O29.43 Spinal and epidural anesthesia induced Ⓜ♀ headache during pregnancy, third trimester

✓5ᵗʰ **O29.5** **Other complications of** spinal and epidural anesthesia **during pregnancy**

✓6ᵗʰ **O29.5X** **Other complications of spinal and epidural anesthesia during pregnancy**

　　O29.5X1 Other complications of spinal and Ⓜ♀ epidural anesthesia during pregnancy, first trimester

　　O29.5X2 Other complications of spinal and Ⓜ♀ epidural anesthesia during pregnancy, second trimester

　　O29.5X3 Other complications of spinal and Ⓜ♀ epidural anesthesia during pregnancy, third trimester

　　O29.5X9 Other complications of spinal and Ⓜ♀▽ epidural anesthesia during pregnancy, unspecified trimester

✓5ᵗʰ **O29.6** Failed or difficult intubation **for anesthesia during pregnancy**

　　O29.60 Failed or difficult intubation for anesthesia Ⓜ♀▽ during pregnancy, unspecified trimester

　　O29.61 Failed or difficult intubation for anesthesia Ⓜ♀ during pregnancy, first trimester

　　O29.62 Failed or difficult intubation for anesthesia Ⓜ♀ during pregnancy, second trimester

　　O29.63 Failed or difficult intubation for anesthesia Ⓜ♀ during pregnancy, third trimester

✓5ᵗʰ **O29.8** **Other complications of anesthesia during pregnancy**

✓6ᵗʰ **O29.8X** **Other complications of anesthesia during pregnancy**

　　O29.8X1 Other complications of anesthesia Ⓜ♀ during pregnancy, first trimester

　　O29.8X2 Other complications of anesthesia Ⓜ♀ during pregnancy, second trimester

　　O29.8X3 Other complications of anesthesia Ⓜ♀ during pregnancy, third trimester

　　O29.8X9 Other complications of anesthesia Ⓜ♀▽ during pregnancy, unspecified trimester

✓5ᵗʰ **O29.9** **Unspecified complication of anesthesia during pregnancy**

　　O29.90 Unspecified complication of anesthesia Ⓜ♀▽ during pregnancy, unspecified trimester

　　O29.91 Unspecified complication of anesthesia Ⓜ♀▽ during pregnancy, first trimester

　　O29.92 Unspecified complication of anesthesia Ⓜ♀▽ during pregnancy, second trimester

　　O29.93 Unspecified complication of anesthesia Ⓜ♀▽ during pregnancy, third trimester

Maternal care related to the fetus and amniotic cavity and possible delivery problems (O30-O48)

✓4ᵗʰ **O30** **Multiple gestation**

　　Code also any complications specific to multiple gestation

✓5ᵗʰ **O30.0** Twin **pregnancy**

✓6ᵗʰ **O30.00** **Twin pregnancy, unspecified number of placenta and unspecified number of amniotic sacs**

　　O30.001 Twin pregnancy, unspecified Ⓜ♀▽ number of placenta and unspecified number of amniotic sacs, first trimester

　　O30.002 Twin pregnancy, unspecified Ⓜ♀▽ number of placenta and unspecified number of amniotic sacs, second trimester

　　O30.003 Twin pregnancy, unspecified Ⓜ♀▽ number of placenta and unspecified number of amniotic sacs, third trimester

　　O30.009 Twin pregnancy, unspecified Ⓜ♀▽ number of placenta and unspecified number of amniotic sacs, unspecified trimester

✓6ᵗʰ **O30.01** **Twin pregnancy,** monochorionic/monoamniotic

　　Twin pregnancy, one placenta, one amniotic sac

　　EXCLUDES 1 conjoined twins (O30.02-)

　　O30.011 Twin pregnancy, monochorionic/ Ⓜ♀ monoamniotic, first trimester

　　O30.012 Twin pregnancy, monochorionic/ Ⓜ♀ monoamniotic, second trimester

　　O30.013 Twin pregnancy, monochorionic/ Ⓜ♀ monoamniotic, third trimester

　　O30.019 Twin pregnancy, monochorionic/ Ⓜ♀▽ monoamniotic, unspecified trimester

Twin Gestation – Monochorionic/Monoamniotic

- 1 Chorionic sac
- 1 Amniotic sac
- 2 Fetuses
- 2 Umbilical cords
- 1 Placenta

☑ Additional Character Req　　✓ˣ⁷ᵗʰ Placeholder Alert　　Manifestation　　ᴴᶜᶜ CMS-HCC Condition　　▽ Unspecified Code　　▶◀ Revised Text　　● New Code　　▲ Revised Code Title

Chapter 15. Pregnancy, Childbirth, and the Puerperium

O30.02–O30.202

Twin Gestation – Monochorionic/Diamniotic

- 1 Chorionic sac
- 2 Amniotic sacs
- 2 Fetuses
- 2 Umbilical cords
- 1 Placenta

Twin Gestation – Dichorionic/Diamniotic

- 2 Chorionic sacs
- 2 Amniotic sacs
- 2 Fetuses
- 2 Umbilical cords
- 2 Placentas

✓6th **O30.02** Conjoined twin pregnancy
- O30.021 Conjoined twin pregnancy, first trimester   Ⓜ♀
- O30.022 Conjoined twin pregnancy, second trimester   Ⓜ♀
- O30.023 Conjoined twin pregnancy, third trimester   Ⓜ♀
- O30.029 Conjoined twin pregnancy, unspecified trimester   Ⓜ♀▽

✓6th **O30.03** Twin pregnancy, monochorionic/diamniotic
Twin pregnancy, one placenta, two amniotic sacs
- O30.031 Twin pregnancy, monochorionic/diamniotic, first trimester   Ⓜ♀
- O30.032 Twin pregnancy, monochorionic/diamniotic, second trimester   Ⓜ♀
- O30.033 Twin pregnancy, monochorionic/diamniotic, third trimester   Ⓜ♀
- O30.039 Twin pregnancy, monochorionic/diamniotic, unspecified trimester   Ⓜ♀▽

✓6th **O30.04** Twin pregnancy, dichorionic/diamniotic
Twin pregnancy, two placentae, two amniotic sacs
- O30.041 Twin pregnancy, dichorionic/diamniotic, first trimester   Ⓜ♀
- O30.042 Twin pregnancy, dichorionic/diamniotic, second trimester   Ⓜ♀
- O30.043 Twin pregnancy, dichorionic/diamniotic, third trimester   Ⓜ♀
- O30.049 Twin pregnancy, dichorionic/diamniotic, unspecified trimester   Ⓜ♀▽

✓6th **O30.09** Twin pregnancy, unable to determine number of placenta and number of amniotic sacs
- O30.091 Twin pregnancy, unable to determine number of placenta and number of amniotic sacs, first trimester   Ⓜ♀
- O30.092 Twin pregnancy, unable to determine number of placenta and number of amniotic sacs, second trimester   Ⓜ♀
- O30.093 Twin pregnancy, unable to determine number of placenta and number of amniotic sacs, third trimester   Ⓜ♀

- O30.099 Twin pregnancy, unable to determine number of placenta and number of amniotic sacs, unspecified trimester   Ⓜ♀▽

✓5th **O30.1** Triplet pregnancy
  ✓6th **O30.10** Triplet pregnancy, unspecified number of placenta and unspecified number of amniotic sacs
    AHA: 2016, 2Q, 8
- O30.101 Triplet pregnancy, unspecified number of placenta and unspecified number of amniotic sacs, first trimester   Ⓜ♀▽
- O30.102 Triplet pregnancy, unspecified number of placenta and unspecified number of amniotic sacs, second trimester   Ⓜ♀▽
- O30.103 Triplet pregnancy, unspecified number of placenta and unspecified number of amniotic sacs, third trimester   Ⓜ♀▽
- O30.109 Triplet pregnancy, unspecified number of placenta and unspecified number of amniotic sacs, unspecified trimester   Ⓜ♀▽

  ✓6th **O30.11** Triplet pregnancy with two or more monochorionic fetuses
- O30.111 Triplet pregnancy with two or more monochorionic fetuses, first trimester   Ⓜ♀
- O30.112 Triplet pregnancy with two or more monochorionic fetuses, second trimester   Ⓜ♀
- O30.113 Triplet pregnancy with two or more monochorionic fetuses, third trimester   Ⓜ♀
- O30.119 Triplet pregnancy with two or more monochorionic fetuses, unspecified trimester   Ⓜ♀▽

  ✓6th **O30.12** Triplet pregnancy with two or more monoamniotic fetuses
- O30.121 Triplet pregnancy with two or more monoamniotic fetuses, first trimester   Ⓜ♀
- O30.122 Triplet pregnancy with two or more monoamniotic fetuses, second trimester   Ⓜ♀
- O30.123 Triplet pregnancy with two or more monoamniotic fetuses, third trimester   Ⓜ♀
- O30.129 Triplet pregnancy with two or more monoamniotic fetuses, unspecified trimester   Ⓜ♀▽

  ✓6th **O30.19** Triplet pregnancy, unable to determine number of placenta and number of amniotic sacs
- O30.191 Triplet pregnancy, unable to determine number of placenta and number of amniotic sacs, first trimester   Ⓜ♀
- O30.192 Triplet pregnancy, unable to determine number of placenta and number of amniotic sacs, second trimester   Ⓜ♀
- O30.193 Triplet pregnancy, unable to determine number of placenta and number of amniotic sacs, third trimester   Ⓜ♀
- O30.199 Triplet pregnancy, unable to determine number of placenta and number of amniotic sacs, unspecified trimester   Ⓜ♀▽

✓5th **O30.2** Quadruplet pregnancy
  ✓6th **O30.20** Quadruplet pregnancy, unspecified number of placenta and unspecified number of amniotic sacs
- O30.201 Quadruplet pregnancy, unspecified number of placenta and unspecified number of amniotic sacs, first trimester   Ⓜ♀▽
- O30.202 Quadruplet pregnancy, unspecified number of placenta and unspecified number of amniotic sacs, second trimester   Ⓜ♀▽

EXCLUDES 1 Not coded here   EXCLUDES 2 Not included here   Ⓝ Newborn Age: 0   Ⓟ Pediatric Age: 0-17   Ⓜ Maternity Age: 12-55   Ⓐ Adult Age: 15-124

836   ICD-10-CM 2018

O30.203 **Quadruplet pregnancy, unspecified** Ⓜ♀▽
number of placenta and unspecified
number of amniotic sacs, third trimester

O30.209 **Quadruplet pregnancy, unspecified** Ⓜ♀▽
number of placenta and unspecified
number of amniotic sacs, unspecified
trimester

✓6ᵗʰ O30.21 **Quadruplet pregnancy with** two or more
monochorionic fetuses

O30.211 **Quadruplet pregnancy with two or** Ⓜ♀
more monochorionic fetuses, first
trimester

O30.212 **Quadruplet pregnancy with two or** Ⓜ♀
more monochorionic fetuses, second
trimester

O30.213 **Quadruplet pregnancy with two or** Ⓜ♀
more monochorionic fetuses, third
trimester

O30.219 **Quadruplet pregnancy with two or** Ⓜ♀▽
more monochorionic fetuses,
unspecified trimester

✓6ᵗʰ O30.22 **Quadruplet pregnancy with** two or more
monoamniotic fetuses

O30.221 **Quadruplet pregnancy with two or** Ⓜ ♀
more monoamniotic fetuses, first
trimester

O30.222 **Quadruplet pregnancy with two or** Ⓜ♀
more monoamniotic fetuses, second
trimester

O30.223 **Quadruplet pregnancy with two or** Ⓜ♀
more monoamniotic fetuses, third
trimester

O30.229 **Quadruplet pregnancy with two or** Ⓜ♀▽
more monoamniotic fetuses,
unspecified trimester

✓6ᵗʰ O30.29 **Quadruplet pregnancy,** unable to determine number
of placenta and number of amniotic sacs

O30.291 **Quadruplet pregnancy, unable to** Ⓜ♀
determine number of placenta and
number of amniotic sacs, first
trimester

O30.292 **Quadruplet pregnancy, unable to** Ⓜ♀
determine number of placenta and
number of amniotic sacs, second
trimester

O30.293 **Quadruplet pregnancy, unable to** Ⓜ♀
determine number of placenta and
number of amniotic sacs, third
trimester

O30.299 **Quadruplet pregnancy, unable to** Ⓜ♀▽
determine number of placenta and
number of amniotic sacs, unspecified

✓5ᵗʰ O30.8 **Other specified multiple gestation**
Multiple gestation pregnancy greater than quadruplets

✓6ᵗʰ O30.80 **Other specified multiple gestation, unspecified**
number of placenta and unspecified number of
amniotic sacs

O30.801 **Other specified multiple gestation,** Ⓜ♀▽
unspecified number of placenta and
unspecified number of amniotic sacs,
first trimester

O30.802 **Other specified multiple gestation,** Ⓜ♀▽
unspecified number of placenta and
unspecified number of amniotic sacs,
second trimester

O30.803 **Other specified multiple gestation,** Ⓜ♀▽
unspecified number of placenta and
unspecified number of amniotic sacs,
third trimester

O30.809 **Other specified multiple** Ⓜ♀▽
gestation,unspecified number of placenta
and unspecified number of amniotic sacs,
unspecified trimester

✓6ᵗʰ O30.81 **Other specified multiple gestation with** two or more
monochorionic fetuses

O30.811 **Other specified multiple gestation** Ⓜ♀
with two or more monochorionic
fetuses, first trimester

O30.812 **Other specified multiple gestation** Ⓜ♀
with two or more monochorionic
fetuses, second trimester

O30.813 **Other specified multiple gestation** Ⓜ♀
with two or more monochorionic
fetuses, third trimester

O30.819 **Other specified multiple gestation** Ⓜ♀▽
with two or more monochorionic
fetuses, unspecified trimester

✓6ᵗʰ O30.82 **Other specified multiple gestation with** two or more
monoamniotic fetuses

O30.821 **Other specified multiple gestation** Ⓜ♀
with two or more monoamniotic
fetuses, first trimester

O30.822 **Other specified multiple gestation** Ⓜ♀
with two or more monoamniotic
fetuses, second trimester

O30.823 **Other specified multiple gestation** Ⓜ♀
with two or more monoamniotic
fetuses, third trimester

O30.829 **Other specified multiple gestation** Ⓜ♀▽
with two or more monoamniotic
fetuses, unspecified trimester

✓6ᵗʰ O30.89 **Other specified multiple gestation,** unable to
determine number of placenta and number of
amniotic sacs

O30.891 **Other specified multiple gestation,** Ⓜ♀
unable to determine number of
placenta and number of amniotic sacs,
first trimester

O30.892 **Other specified multiple gestation,** Ⓜ♀
unable to determine number of placenta
and number of amniotic sacs, second
trimester

O30.893 **Other specified multiple gestation,** Ⓜ♀
unable to determine number of placenta
and number of amniotic sacs, third
trimester

O30.899 **Other specified multiple gestation,** Ⓜ♀▽
unable to determine number of
placenta and number of amniotic
sacs, unspecified trimester

✓5ᵗʰ O30.9 **Multiple gestation, unspecified**
Multiple pregnancy NOS

O30.90 **Multiple gestation, unspecified, unspecified** Ⓜ♀▽
trimester

O30.91 **Multiple gestation, unspecified,** first trimester Ⓜ♀▽

O30.92 **Multiple gestation, unspecified,** second Ⓜ♀▽
trimester

O30.93 **Multiple gestation, unspecified,** third Ⓜ♀▽
trimester

✓4ᵗʰ **O31 Complications specific to multiple gestation**

EXCLUDES 2   delayed delivery of second twin, triplet, etc. (O63.2)
     malpresentation of one fetus or more (O32.9)
     placental transfusion syndromes (O43.0-)

AHA: 2012, 4Q, 107

> One of the following 7th characters is to be assigned to each code
> under category O31. 7th character 0 is for single gestations and
> multiple gestations where the fetus is unspecified. 7th characters 1
> through 9 are for cases of multiple gestations to identify the fetus for
> which the code applies. The appropriate code from category O30,
> Multiple gestation, must also be assigned when assigning a code
> from category O31 that has a 7th character of 1 through 9.
> 0   not applicable or unspecified   4   fetus 4
> 1   fetus 1   5   fetus 5
> 2   fetus 2   9   other fetus
> 3   fetus 3

✓5ᵗʰ O31.0 **Papyraceous fetus**
Fetus compressus

✓x7ᵗʰ O31.00 **Papyraceous fetus, unspecified trimester** Ⓜ♀▽

✓x7ᵗʰ O31.01 **Papyraceous fetus,** first trimester Ⓜ♀

✓x7ᵗʰ O31.02 **Papyraceous fetus,** second trimester Ⓜ♀

✓x7ᵗʰ O31.03 **Papyraceous fetus,** third trimester Ⓜ♀

✓5ᵗʰ O31.1 **Continuing pregnancy** after spontaneous abortion of one
fetus or more

✓x7ᵗʰ O31.10 **Continuing pregnancy after spontaneous** Ⓜ♀▽
abortion of one fetus or more, unspecified
trimester

✓x7ᵗʰ O31.11 **Continuing pregnancy after spontaneous** Ⓜ♀
abortion of one fetus or more, first trimester

☑ Additional Character Req   ✓x7ᵗʰ Placeholder Alert   Manifestation   ᴴᶜᶜ CMS-HCC Condition   ▽ Unspecified Code   ▶◀ Revised Text   ● New Code   ▲ Revised Code Title

ICD-10-CM 2018   837

√x7ᵗʰ **O31.12** **Continuing pregnancy after spontaneous abortion of one fetus or more, second trimester** Ⓜ♀

√x7ᵗʰ **O31.13** **Continuing pregnancy after spontaneous abortion of one fetus or more, third trimester** Ⓜ♀

√5ᵗʰ **O31.2** Continuing pregnancy after intrauterine death of one fetus or more

√x7ᵗʰ **O31.20** **Continuing pregnancy after intrauterine death of one fetus or more, unspecified trimester** Ⓜ♀▽

√x7ᵗʰ **O31.21** **Continuing pregnancy after intrauterine death of one fetus or more, first trimester** Ⓜ♀

√x7ᵗʰ **O31.22** **Continuing pregnancy after intrauterine death of one fetus or more, second trimester** Ⓜ♀

√x7ᵗʰ **O31.23** **Continuing pregnancy after intrauterine death of one fetus or more, third trimester** Ⓜ♀

√5ᵗʰ **O31.3** Continuing pregnancy after elective fetal reduction of one fetus or more

Continuing pregnancy after selective termination of one fetus or more

√x7ᵗʰ **O31.30** **Continuing pregnancy after elective fetal reduction of one fetus or more, unspecified trimester** Ⓜ♀▽

√x7ᵗʰ **O31.31** **Continuing pregnancy after elective fetal reduction of one fetus or more, first trimester** Ⓜ♀

√x7ᵗʰ **O31.32** **Continuing pregnancy after elective fetal reduction of one fetus or more, second trimester** Ⓜ♀

√x7ᵗʰ **O31.33** **Continuing pregnancy after elective fetal reduction of one fetus or more, third trimester** Ⓜ♀

√5ᵗʰ **O31.8** Other complications specific to multiple gestation

√6ᵗʰ **O31.8X** Other complications specific to multiple gestation

√7ᵗʰ **O31.8X1** **Other complications specific to multiple gestation, first trimester** Ⓜ♀

√7ᵗʰ **O31.8X2** **Other complications specific to multiple gestation, second trimester** Ⓜ♀

√7ᵗʰ **O31.8X3** **Other complications specific to multiple gestation, third trimester** Ⓜ♀

√7ᵗʰ **O31.8X9** **Other complications specific to multiple gestation, unspecified trimester** Ⓜ♀▽

√4ᵗʰ **O32** **Maternal care for malpresentation of fetus**

INCLUDES the listed conditions as a reason for observation, hospitalization or other obstetric care of the mother, or for cesarean delivery before onset of labor

EXCLUDES 1 malpresentation of fetus with obstructed labor (O64.-)

AHA: 2012, 4Q, 107

One of the following 7th characters is to be assigned to each code under category O32. 7th character 0 is for single gestations and multiple gestations where the fetus is unspecified. 7th characters 1 through 9 are for cases of multiple gestations to identify the fetus for which the code applies. The appropriate code from category O30, Multiple gestation, must also be assigned when assigning a code from category O32 that has a 7th character of 1 through 9.

0	not applicable or unspecified	4	fetus 4
1	fetus 1	5	fetus 5
2	fetus 2	9	other fetus
3	fetus 3		

Fetal Malpresentation

Breech

Shoulder (arm prolapse)

Mother's pelvis

Compound (extremity together with head)

Face (mentum)

Oblique

√x7ᵗʰ **O32.0** **Maternal care for** unstable lie Ⓜ♀

√x7ᵗʰ **O32.1** **Maternal care for** breech presentation Ⓜ♀

Maternal care for buttocks presentation
Maternal care for complete breech
Maternal care for frank breech

EXCLUDES 1 footling presentation (O32.8)
          incomplete breech (O32.8)

DEF: Fetus presentation in a longitudinal lie with the buttocks or feet closest to birth canal; may require external cephalic version or cesarean delivery.

√x7ᵗʰ **O32.2** **Maternal care for** transverse and oblique lie Ⓜ♀

Maternal care for oblique presentation
Maternal care for transverse presentation

√x7ᵗʰ **O32.3** **Maternal care for** face, brow and chin presentation Ⓜ♀

√x7ᵗʰ **O32.4** **Maternal care for** high head at term Ⓜ♀

Maternal care for failure of head to enter pelvic brim

√x7ᵗʰ **O32.6** **Maternal care for** compound presentation Ⓜ♀

√x7ᵗʰ **O32.8** **Maternal care for** other malpresentation of fetus Ⓜ♀

Maternal care for footling presentation
Maternal care for incomplete breech

√x7ᵗʰ **O32.9** **Maternal care for malpresentation of fetus, unspecified** Ⓜ♀▽

√4ᵗʰ **O33** **Maternal care for disproportion**

INCLUDES the listed conditions as a reason for observation, hospitalization or other obstetric care of the mother, or for cesarean delivery before onset of labor

EXCLUDES 1 disproportion with obstructed labor (O65-O66)

O33.0 **Maternal care for disproportion due to** deformity of maternal pelvic bones Ⓜ♀

Maternal care for disproportion due to pelvic deformity causing disproportion NOS

O33.1 **Maternal care for disproportion due to** generally contracted pelvis Ⓜ♀

Maternal care for disproportion due to contracted pelvis NOS causing disproportion

O33.2 **Maternal care for disproportion due to** inlet contraction of pelvis Ⓜ♀

Maternal care for disproportion due to inlet contraction (pelvis) causing disproportion

√x7ᵗʰ **O33.3** **Maternal care for disproportion due to** outlet contraction of pelvis Ⓜ♀

Maternal care for disproportion due to mid-cavity contraction (pelvis)
Maternal care for disproportion due to outlet contraction (pelvis)

One of the following 7th characters is to be assigned to code O33.3. 7th character 0 is for single gestations and multiple gestations where the fetus is unspecified. 7th characters 1 through 9 are for cases of multiple gestations to identify the fetus for which the code applies. The appropriate code from category O30, Multiple gestation, must also be assigned when assigning code O33.3 with a 7th character of 1 through 9.

0	not applicable or unspecified	4	fetus 4
1	fetus 1	5	fetus 5
2	fetus 2	9	other fetus
3	fetus 3		

√x7ᵗʰ **O33.4** **Maternal care for disproportion of mixed maternal and fetal origin** Ⓜ♀

One of the following 7th characters is to be assigned to code O33.4. 7th character 0 is for single gestations and multiple gestations where the fetus is unspecified. 7th characters 1 through 9 are for cases of multiple gestations to identify the fetus for which the code applies. The appropriate code from category O30, Multiple gestation, must also be assigned when assigning code O33.4 with a 7th character of 1 through 9.

0	not applicable or unspecified	4	fetus 4
1	fetus 1	5	fetus 5
2	fetus 2	9	other fetus
3	fetus 3		

EXCLUDES 1 Not coded here   EXCLUDES 2 Not included here   Ⓝ Newborn Age: 0   Ⓟ Pediatric Age: 0-17   Ⓜ Maternity Age: 12-55   Ⓐ Adult Age: 15-124

838   ICD-10-CM 2018

√x7ᵗʰ O33.5 **Maternal care for disproportion due to unusually large** Ⓜ♀
fetus
Maternal care for disproportion due to disproportion of fetal
origin with normally formed fetus
Maternal care for disproportion due to fetal disproportion NOS

> One of the following 7th characters is to be assigned to code
> O33.5. 7th character Ø is for single gestations and multiple
> gestations where the fetus is unspecified. 7th characters 1
> through 9 are for cases of multiple gestations to identify the
> fetus for which the code applies. The appropriate code from
> category O3Ø, Multiple gestation, must also be assigned when
> assigning code O33.5 with a 7th character of 1 through 9.
> Ø   not applicable or unspecified   4   fetus 4
> 1   fetus 1   5   fetus 5
> 2   fetus 2   9   other fetus
> 3   fetus 3

√x7ᵗʰ O33.6 **Maternal care for disproportion due to hydrocephalic** Ⓜ♀
fetus

> One of the following 7th characters is to be assigned to code
> O33.6. 7th character Ø is for single gestations and multiple
> gestations where the fetus is unspecified. 7th characters 1
> through 9 are for cases of multiple gestations to identify the
> fetus for which the code applies. The appropriate code from
> category O3Ø, Multiple gestation, must also be assigned when
> assigning code O33.6 with a 7th character of 1 through 9.
> Ø   not applicable or unspecified   4   fetus 4
> 1   fetus 1   5   fetus 5
> 2   fetus 2   9   other fetus
> 3   fetus 3

√x7ᵗʰ O33.7 **Maternal care for disproportion due to other fetal** Ⓜ♀
deformities
Maternal care for disproportion due to fetal ascites
Maternal care for disproportion due to fetal hydrops
Maternal care for disproportion due to fetal meningomyelocele
Maternal care for disproportion due to fetal sacral teratoma
Maternal care for disproportion due to fetal tumor
EXCLUDES 1   obstructed labor due to other fetal deformities (O66.3)

> One of the following 7th characters is to be assigned to code
> O33.7. 7th character Ø is for single gestations and multiple
> gestations where the fetus is unspecified. 7th characters 1
> through 9 are for cases of multiple gestations to identify the
> fetus for which the code applies. The appropriate code from
> category O3Ø, Multiple gestation, must also be assigned when
> assigning code O33.7 with a 7th character of 1 through 9.
> Ø   not applicable or unspecified   4   fetus 4
> 1   fetus 1   5   fetus 5
> 2   fetus 2   9   other fetus
> 3   fetus 3

O33.8 **Maternal care for disproportion of other origin** Ⓜ♀

O33.9 **Maternal care for disproportion, unspecified** Ⓜ♀▽
Maternal care for disproportion due to cephalopelvic
disproportion NOS
Maternal care for disproportion due to fetopelvic disproportion
NOS

√4ᵗʰ O34 **Maternal care for abnormality of pelvic organs**
INCLUDES   the listed conditions as a reason for hospitalization or other
obstetric care of the mother, or for cesarean delivery
before onset of labor
Code first any associated obstructed labor (O65.5)
Use additional code for specific condition

√5ᵗʰ O34.Ø **Maternal care for** congenital malformation of uterus
Maternal care for double uterus
Maternal care for uterus bicornis
    O34.ØØ **Maternal care for unspecified congenital** Ⓜ♀▽
malformation of uterus, unspecified trimester
    O34.Ø1 **Maternal care for unspecified congenital** Ⓜ♀▽
malformation of uterus, first trimester
    O34.Ø2 **Maternal care for unspecified congenital** Ⓜ♀▽
malformation of uterus, second trimester
    O34.Ø3 **Maternal care for unspecified congenital** Ⓜ♀▽
malformation of uterus, third trimester

√5ᵗʰ O34.1 **Maternal care for** benign tumor of corpus uteri
EXCLUDES 2   maternal care for benign tumor of cervix (O34.4-)
maternal care for malignant neoplasm of uterus
(O9A.1-)
    O34.1Ø **Maternal care for benign tumor of corpus** Ⓜ♀▽
uteri, unspecified trimester
    O34.11 **Maternal care for benign tumor of corpus uteri,** Ⓜ♀
first trimester

    O34.12 **Maternal care for benign tumor of corpus uteri,** Ⓜ♀
second trimester
    O34.13 **Maternal care for benign tumor of corpus uteri,** Ⓜ♀
third trimester

√5ᵗʰ O34.2 **Maternal care due to** uterine scar from previous surgery
    √6ᵗʰ O34.21 **Maternal care for scar** from previous cesarean
delivery
        O34.211 **Maternal care for** low transverse scar Ⓜ♀
from previous cesarean delivery
        O34.212 **Maternal care for** vertical scar **from** Ⓜ♀
previous cesarean delivery
Maternal care for classical scar from
previous cesarean delivery
        O34.219 **Maternal care for unspecified type** Ⓜ♀▽
scar from previous cesarean delivery
Maternal care due to uterine scar from
other transmural uterine incision
    O34.29 **Maternal care due to uterine** scar from other Ⓜ♀
previous surgery
Maternal care due to uterine scar from other
transmural uterine incision

√5ᵗʰ O34.3 **Maternal care for** cervical incompetence
Maternal care for cerclage with or without cervical
incompetence
Maternal care for Shirodkar suture with or without cervical
incompetence
DEF: Inadequate functioning of cervix marked by abnormal
widening during pregnancy and causing premature birth or
miscarriage.
    O34.3Ø **Maternal care for cervical incompetence,** Ⓜ♀▽
unspecified trimester
    O34.31 **Maternal care for cervical incompetence, first** Ⓜ♀
trimester
    O34.32 **Maternal care for cervical incompetence, second** Ⓜ♀
trimester
    O34.33 **Maternal care for cervical incompetence, third** Ⓜ♀
trimester

√5ᵗʰ O34.4 **Maternal care for other** abnormalities of cervix
    O34.4Ø **Maternal care for other abnormalities of** Ⓜ♀▽
cervix, unspecified trimester
    O34.41 **Maternal care for other abnormalities of cervix,** Ⓜ♀
first trimester
    O34.42 **Maternal care for other abnormalities of cervix,** Ⓜ♀
second trimester
    O34.43 **Maternal care for other abnormalities of cervix,** Ⓜ♀
third trimester

√5ᵗʰ O34.5 **Maternal care for other** abnormalities of gravid uterus
    √6ᵗʰ O34.51 **Maternal care for** incarceration of gravid uterus
        O34.511 **Maternal care for incarceration of** Ⓜ♀
gravid uterus, first trimester
        O34.512 **Maternal care for incarceration of** Ⓜ♀
gravid uterus, second trimester
        O34.513 **Maternal care for incarceration of** Ⓜ♀
gravid uterus, third trimester
        O34.519 **Maternal care for incarceration of** Ⓜ♀▽
gravid uterus, unspecified trimester
    √6ᵗʰ O34.52 **Maternal care for** prolapse of gravid uterus
        O34.521 **Maternal care for prolapse of gravid** Ⓜ♀
uterus, first trimester
        O34.522 **Maternal care for prolapse of gravid** Ⓜ♀
uterus, second trimester
        O34.523 **Maternal care for prolapse of gravid** Ⓜ♀
uterus, third trimester
        O34.529 **Maternal care for prolapse of gravid** Ⓜ♀▽
uterus, unspecified trimester
    √6ᵗʰ O34.53 **Maternal care for** retroversion of gravid uterus
        O34.531 **Maternal care for retroversion of** Ⓜ♀
gravid uterus, first trimester
        O34.532 **Maternal care for retroversion of** Ⓜ♀
gravid uterus, second trimester
        O34.533 **Maternal care for retroversion of** Ⓜ♀
gravid uterus, third trimester
        O34.539 **Maternal care for retroversion of** Ⓜ♀▽
gravid uterus, unspecified trimester
    √6ᵗʰ O34.59 **Maternal care for other abnormalities of gravid**
uterus
        O34.591 **Maternal care for other abnormalities** Ⓜ♀
of gravid uterus, first trimester

☑ Additional Character Req   √7ᵗʰ Placeholder Alert   Manifestation   **HCC** CMS-HCC Condition   ▽ Unspecified Code   ▶◀ Revised Text   ● New Code   ▲ Revised Code Title

Chapter 15. Pregnancy, Childbirth, and the Puerperium

O34.592   **Maternal care for other abnormalities** Ⓜ♀
of gravid uterus, **second trimester**

O34.593   **Maternal care for other abnormalities** Ⓜ♀
of gravid uterus, **third trimester**

O34.599   **Maternal care for other** Ⓜ♀▽
**abnormalities of gravid uterus,
unspecified trimester**

✓5ᵗʰ **O34.6**   **Maternal care for** abnormality of vagina
EXCLUDES 2   *maternal care for vaginal varices in pregnancy
(O22.1-)*

O34.60   **Maternal care for abnormality of vagina,
unspecified trimester** Ⓜ♀▽

O34.61   **Maternal care for abnormality of vagina, first
trimester** Ⓜ♀

O34.62   **Maternal care for abnormality of vagina, second
trimester** Ⓜ♀

O34.63   **Maternal care for abnormality of vagina, third
trimester** Ⓜ♀

✓5ᵗʰ **O34.7**   **Maternal care for** abnormality of vulva and perineum
EXCLUDES 2   *maternal care for perineal and vulval varices in
pregnancy (O22.1-)*

O34.70   **Maternal care for abnormality of vulva and
perineum, unspecified trimester** Ⓜ♀▽

O34.71   **Maternal care for abnormality of vulva and
perineum, first trimester** Ⓜ♀

O34.72   **Maternal care for abnormality of vulva and
perineum, second trimester** Ⓜ♀

O34.73   **Maternal care for abnormality of vulva and
perineum, third trimester** Ⓜ♀

✓5ᵗʰ **O34.8**   **Maternal care for other** abnormalities of pelvic organs

O34.80   **Maternal care for other abnormalities of
pelvic organs, unspecified trimester** Ⓜ♀▽

O34.81   **Maternal care for other abnormalities of pelvic
organs, first trimester** Ⓜ♀

O34.82   **Maternal care for other abnormalities of pelvic
organs, second trimester** Ⓜ♀

O34.83   **Maternal care for other abnormalities of pelvic
organs, third trimester** Ⓜ♀

✓5ᵗʰ **O34.9**   **Maternal care for abnormality of pelvic organ, unspecified**

O34.90   **Maternal care for abnormality of pelvic
organ,unspecified, unspecified trimester** Ⓜ♀▽

O34.91   **Maternal care for abnormality of pelvic
organ, unspecified, first trimester** Ⓜ♀▽

O34.92   **Maternal care for abnormality of pelvic
organ, unspecified, second trimester** Ⓜ♀▽

O34.93   **Maternal care for abnormality of pelvic
organ, unspecified, third trimester** Ⓜ♀▽

✓4ᵗʰ **O35**   **Maternal care for known or suspected fetal abnormality and
damage**
INCLUDES   the listed conditions in the fetus as a reason for
hospitalization or other obstetric care to the mother,
or for termination of pregnancy
Code also any associated maternal condition
EXCLUDES 1   *encounter for suspected maternal and fetal conditions ruled out
(Z03.7-)*

One of the following 7th characters is to be assigned to each code
under category O35. 7th character Ø is for single gestations and
multiple gestations where the fetus is unspecified. 7th characters 1
through 9 are for cases of multiple gestations to identify the fetus for
which the code applies. The appropriate code from category O30,
Multiple gestation, must also be assigned when assigning a code
from category O35 that has a 7th character of 1 through 9.

Ø	not applicable or unspecified	4	fetus 4
1	fetus 1	5	fetus 5
2	fetus 2	9	other fetus
3	fetus 3		

✓x7ᵗʰ **O35.0**   **Maternal care for (suspected)** central nervous system Ⓜ♀
malformation in fetus
Maternal care for fetal anencephaly
Maternal care for fetal hydrocephalus
Maternal care for fetal spina bifida
EXCLUDES 2   *chromosomal abnormality in fetus (O35.1)*

✓x7ᵗʰ **O35.1**   **Maternal care for (suspected)** chromosomal abnormality Ⓜ♀
in fetus

✓x7ᵗʰ **O35.2**   **Maternal care for (suspected)** hereditary disease in fetus Ⓜ♀
EXCLUDES 2   *chromosomal abnormality in fetus (O35.1)*

✓x7ᵗʰ **O35.3**   **Maternal care for (suspected)** damage to fetus from viral Ⓜ♀
disease in mother
Maternal care for damage to fetus from maternal
cytomegalovirus infection
Maternal care for damage to fetus from maternal rubella

✓x7ᵗʰ **O35.4**   **Maternal care for (suspected)** damage to fetus from Ⓜ♀
alcohol

✓x7ᵗʰ **O35.5**   **Maternal care for (suspected)** damage to fetus by drugs Ⓜ♀
Maternal care for damage to fetus from drug addiction

✓x7ᵗʰ **O35.6**   **Maternal care for (suspected)** damage to fetus by Ⓜ♀
radiation

✓x7ᵗʰ **O35.7**   **Maternal care for (suspected)** damage to fetus by other Ⓜ♀
medical procedures
Maternal care for damage to fetus by amniocentesis
Maternal care for damage to fetus by biopsy procedures
Maternal care for damage to fetus by hematological
investigation
Maternal care for damage to fetus by intrauterine contraceptive
device
Maternal care for damage to fetus by intrauterine surgery

✓x7ᵗʰ **O35.8**   **Maternal care for other (suspected) fetal abnormality** Ⓜ♀
and damage
Maternal care for damage to fetus from maternal listeriosis
Maternal care for damage to fetus from maternal toxoplasmosis

✓x7ᵗʰ **O35.9**   **Maternal care for (suspected) fetal abnormality and** Ⓜ♀▽
damage, unspecified

✓4ᵗʰ **O36**   **Maternal care for other fetal problems**
INCLUDES   the listed conditions in the fetus as a reason for
hospitalization or other obstetric care of the mother, or
for termination of pregnancy
EXCLUDES 1   *encounter for suspected maternal and fetal conditions ruled out
(Z03.7-)*
placental transfusion syndromes (O43.0-)
EXCLUDES 2   *labor and delivery complicated by fetal stress (O77.-)*
AHA: 2015, 3Q, 40

One of the following 7th characters is to be assigned to each code
under category O36. 7th character Ø is for single gestations and
multiple gestations where the fetus is unspecified. 7th characters 1
through 9 are for cases of multiple gestations to identify the fetus for
which the code applies. The appropriate code from category O30,
Multiple gestation, must also be assigned when assigning a code
from category O36 that has a 7th character of 1 through 9.

Ø	not applicable or unspecified	4	fetus 4
1	fetus 1	5	fetus 5
2	fetus 2	9	other fetus
3	fetus 3		

✓5ᵗʰ **O36.0**   **Maternal care for rhesus isoimmunization**
Maternal care for Rh incompatibility (with hydrops fetalis)

✓6ᵗʰ **O36.01**   **Maternal care for** anti-D [Rh] antibodies
AHA: 2014, 4Q, 17

✓7ᵗʰ **O36.011**   **Maternal care for anti-D [Rh]** Ⓜ♀
antibodies, first trimester

✓7ᵗʰ **O36.012**   **Maternal care for anti-D [Rh]** Ⓜ♀
antibodies, second trimester

✓7ᵗʰ **O36.013**   **Maternal care for anti-D [Rh]** Ⓜ♀
antibodies, third trimester

✓7ᵗʰ **O36.019**   **Maternal care for anti-D [Rh]** Ⓜ♀▽
antibodies, unspecified trimester

✓6ᵗʰ **O36.09**   **Maternal care for other rhesus isoimmunization**

✓7ᵗʰ **O36.091**   **Maternal care for other rhesus** Ⓜ♀
isoimmunization, first trimester

✓7ᵗʰ **O36.092**   **Maternal care for other rhesus** Ⓜ♀
isoimmunization, second trimester

✓7ᵗʰ **O36.093**   **Maternal care for other rhesus** Ⓜ♀
isoimmunization, third trimester

✓7ᵗʰ **O36.099**   **Maternal care for other rhesus** Ⓜ♀▽
isoimmunization, unspecified trimester

✓5ᵗʰ **O36.1**   **Maternal care for other isoimmunization**
Maternal care for ABO isoimmunization

✓6ᵗʰ **O36.11**   **Maternal care for** Anti-A sensitization
Maternal care for isoimmunization NOS (with hydrops
fetalis)

✓7ᵗʰ **O36.111**   **Maternal care for Anti-A sensitization,** Ⓜ♀
first trimester

✓7ᵗʰ **O36.112**   **Maternal care for Anti-A sensitization,** Ⓜ♀
second trimester

✓7ᵗʰ **O36.113**   **Maternal care for Anti-A sensitization,** Ⓜ♀
third trimester

EXCLUDES 1 Not coded here   EXCLUDES 2 Not included here   Ⓝ Newborn Age: 0   Ⓟ Pediatric Age: 0-17   Ⓜ Maternity Age: 12-55   Ⓐ Adult Age: 15-124

840   ICD-10-CM 2018

√7ᵗʰ **O36.119** Maternal care for Anti-A ♂♀ ▽
sensitization, unspecified trimester

√6ᵗʰ **O36.19** **Maternal care for other isoimmunization**
Maternal care for Anti-B sensitization

√7ᵗʰ **O36.191** Maternal care for other ♂♀
isoimmunization, first trimester

√7ᵗʰ **O36.192** Maternal care for other ♂♀
isoimmunization, second trimester

√7ᵗʰ **O36.193** Maternal care for other ♂♀
isoimmunization, third trimester

√7ᵗʰ **O36.199** Maternal care for other ♂♀ ▽
isoimmunization, unspecified trimester

√5ᵗʰ **O36.2** **Maternal care for hydrops fetalis**
Maternal care for hydrops fetalis NOS
Maternal care for hydrops fetalis not associated with
isoimmunization
EXCLUDES 1 *hydrops fetalis associated with ABO isoimmunization (O36.1-)*
hydrops fetalis associated with rhesus isoimmunization (O36.0-)

√x7ᵗʰ **O36.20** Maternal care for hydrops fetalis, unspecified ♂♀ ▽
trimester

√x7ᵗʰ **O36.21** Maternal care for hydrops fetalis, first ♂♀
trimester

√x7ᵗʰ **O36.22** Maternal care for hydrops fetalis, second ♂♀
trimester

√x7ᵗʰ **O36.23** Maternal care for hydrops fetalis, third ♂♀
trimester

√x7ᵗʰ **O36.4** **Maternal care for intrauterine death** ♂♀
Maternal care for intrauterine fetal death NOS
Maternal care for intrauterine fetal death after completion of 20
weeks of gestation
Maternal care for late fetal death
Maternal care for missed delivery
EXCLUDES 1 *missed abortion (O02.1)*
stillbirth (P95)

√5ᵗʰ **O36.5** **Maternal care for known or suspected poor fetal growth**

√6ᵗʰ **O36.51** **Maternal care for known or suspected placental insufficiency**

√7ᵗʰ **O36.511** Maternal care for known or suspected ♂♀
placental insufficiency, first trimester

√7ᵗʰ **O36.512** Maternal care for known or suspected ♂♀
placental insufficiency, second trimester

√7ᵗʰ **O36.513** Maternal care for known or suspected ♂♀
placental insufficiency, third trimester

√7ᵗʰ **O36.519** Maternal care for known or ♂♀ ▽
suspected placental insufficiency,
unspecified trimester

√6ᵗʰ **O36.59** **Maternal care for other known or suspected poor fetal growth**
Maternal care for known or suspected light-for-dates NOS
Maternal care for known or suspected small-for-dates NOS

√7ᵗʰ **O36.591** Maternal care for other known or ♂♀
suspected poor fetal growth, first
trimester

√7ᵗʰ **O36.592** Maternal care for other known or ♂♀
suspected poor fetal growth, second
trimester

√7ᵗʰ **O36.593** Maternal care for other known or ♂♀
suspected poor fetal growth, third
trimester

√7ᵗʰ **O36.599** Maternal care for other known or ♂♀ ▽
suspected poor fetal growth,
unspecified trimester

√5ᵗʰ **O36.6** **Maternal care for excessive fetal growth**
Maternal care for known or suspected large-for-dates

√x7ᵗʰ **O36.60** Maternal care for excessive fetal growth, ♂♀ ▽
unspecified trimester

√x7ᵗʰ **O36.61** Maternal care for excessive fetal growth, ♂♀
first trimester

√x7ᵗʰ **O36.62** Maternal care for excessive fetal growth, ♂♀
second trimester

√x7ᵗʰ **O36.63** Maternal care for excessive fetal growth, ♂♀
third trimester

√5ᵗʰ **O36.7** **Maternal care for viable fetus in abdominal pregnancy**

√x7ᵗʰ **O36.70** Maternal care for viable fetus in abdominal ♂♀ ▽
pregnancy, unspecified trimester

√x7ᵗʰ **O36.71** Maternal care for viable fetus in abdominal ♂♀
pregnancy, first trimester

√x7ᵗʰ **O36.72** Maternal care for viable fetus in abdominal ♂♀
pregnancy, second trimester

√x7ᵗʰ **O36.73** Maternal care for viable fetus in abdominal ♂♀
pregnancy, third trimester

√5ᵗʰ **O36.8** **Maternal care for other specified fetal problems**

√x7ᵗʰ **O36.80** **Pregnancy with inconclusive fetal viability** ♂♀
Encounter to determine fetal viability of pregnancy

√6ᵗʰ **O36.81** **Decreased fetal movements**

√7ᵗʰ **O36.812** Decreased fetal movements, second ♂♀
trimester

√7ᵗʰ **O36.813** Decreased fetal movements, third ♂♀
trimester

√7ᵗʰ **O36.819** Decreased fetal movements, ♂♀
unspecified trimester

√6ᵗʰ **O36.82** **Fetal anemia and thrombocytopenia**

√7ᵗʰ **O36.821** Fetal anemia and thrombocytopenia, ♂♀
first trimester

√7ᵗʰ **O36.822** Fetal anemia and thrombocytopenia, ♂♀
second trimester

√7ᵗʰ **O36.823** Fetal anemia and thrombocytopenia, ♂♀
third trimester

√7ᵗʰ **O36.829** Fetal anemia and ♂♀ ▽
thrombocytopenia, unspecified trimester

√6ᵗʰ **O36.83** **Maternal care for abnormalities of the fetal heart rate or rhythm**

√7ᵗʰ **O36.831** Maternal care for abnormalities of the
fetal heart rate or rhythm, first trimester

√7ᵗʰ **O36.832** Maternal care for abnormalities of the
fetal heart rate or rhythm, second
trimester

√7ᵗʰ **O36.833** Maternal care for abnormalities of the
fetal heart rate or rhythm, third trimester

√7ᵗʰ **O36.839** Maternal care for abnormalities of the ▽
fetal heart rate or rhythm, unspecified
trimester

√6ᵗʰ **O36.89** **Maternal care for other specified fetal problems**

√7ᵗʰ **O36.891** Maternal care for other specified fetal ♂♀
problems, first trimester

√7ᵗʰ **O36.892** Maternal care for other specified fetal ♂♀
problems, second trimester

√7ᵗʰ **O36.893** Maternal care for other specified fetal ♂♀
problems, third trimester

√7ᵗʰ **O36.899** Maternal care for other specified ♂♀ ▽
fetal problems, unspecified trimester

√5ᵗʰ **O36.9** **Maternal care for fetal problem, unspecified**

√x7ᵗʰ **O36.90** Maternal care for fetal problem, unspecified, ♂♀ ▽
unspecified trimester

√x7ᵗʰ **O36.91** Maternal care for fetal problem, unspecified, ♂♀ ▽
first trimester

√x7ᵗʰ **O36.92** Maternal care for fetal problem, unspecified, ♂♀ ▽
second trimester

√x7ᵗʰ **O36.93** Maternal care for fetal problem, unspecified, ♂♀ ▽
third trimester

√4ᵗʰ **O40** **Polyhydramnios**
Hydramnios
EXCLUDES 1 *encounter for suspected maternal and fetal conditions ruled out (Z03.7-)*
AHA: 2016, 1Q, 4

One of the following 7th characters is to be assigned to each code
under category O40. 7th character 0 is for single gestations and
multiple gestations where the fetus is unspecified. 7th characters 1
through 9 are for cases of multiple gestations to identify the fetus
for which the code applies. The appropriate code from category
O30, Multiple gestation, must also be assigned when assigning a
code from category O40 that has a 7th character of 1 through 9.

0	not applicable or unspecified	4	fetus 4
1	fetus 1	5	fetus 5
2	fetus 2	9	other fetus
3	fetus 3		

√x7ᵗʰ **O40.1** **Polyhydramnios,** first trimester ♂♀

√x 7ᵗʰ **O40.2 Polyhydramnios,** second trimester   Ⓜ♀

√x 7ᵗʰ **O40.3 Polyhydramnios,** third trimester   Ⓜ♀

√x 7ᵗʰ **O40.9 Polyhydramnios, unspecified trimester**   Ⓜ♀▽

√4ᵗʰ **O41 Other disorders of amniotic fluid and membranes**

> EXCLUDES 1   encounter for suspected maternal and fetal conditions ruled out (Z03.7-)

> One of the following 7th characters is to be assigned to each code under category O41. 7th character Ø is for single gestations and multiple gestations where the fetus is unspecified. 7th characters 1 through 9 are for cases of multiple gestations to identify the fetus for which the code applies. The appropriate code from category O3Ø, Multiple gestation, must also be assigned when assigning a code from category O41 that has a 7th character of 1 through 9.
> Ø   not applicable or unspecified   4   fetus 4
> 1   fetus 1   5   fetus 5
> 2   fetus 2   9   other fetus
> 3   fetus 3

√5ᵗʰ **O41.Ø Oligohydramnios**
> Oligohydramnios without rupture of membranes

√x 7ᵗʰ **O41.ØØ Oligohydramnios, unspecified trimester**   Ⓜ♀▽

√x 7ᵗʰ **O41.Ø1 Oligohydramnios,** first trimester   Ⓜ♀

√x 7ᵗʰ **O41.Ø2 Oligohydramnios,** second trimester   Ⓜ♀

√x 7ᵗʰ **O41.Ø3 Oligohydramnios,** third trimester   Ⓜ♀

√5ᵗʰ **O41.1 Infection of amniotic sac and membranes**

√6ᵗʰ **O41.10 Infection of amniotic sac and membranes, unspecified**

√7ᵗʰ **O41.101 Infection of amniotic sac and membranes, unspecified,** first trimester   Ⓜ♀▽

√7ᵗʰ **O41.102 Infection of amniotic sac and membranes, unspecified,** second trimester   Ⓜ♀▽

√7ᵗʰ **O41.103 Infection of amniotic sac and membranes, unspecified,** third trimester   Ⓜ♀▽

√7ᵗʰ **O41.109 Infection of amniotic sac and membranes, unspecified, unspecified trimester**   Ⓜ♀▽

√6ᵗʰ **O41.12 Chorioamnionitis**

√7ᵗʰ **O41.121 Chorioamnionitis,** first trimester   Ⓜ♀

√7ᵗʰ **O41.122 Chorioamnionitis,** second trimester   Ⓜ♀

√7ᵗʰ **O41.123 Chorioamnionitis,** third trimester   Ⓜ♀

√7ᵗʰ **O41.129 Chorioamnionitis, unspecified trimester**   Ⓜ♀▽

√6ᵗʰ **O41.14 Placentitis**

√7ᵗʰ **O41.141 Placentitis,** first trimester   Ⓜ♀

√7ᵗʰ **O41.142 Placentitis,** second trimester   Ⓜ♀

√7ᵗʰ **O41.143 Placentitis,** third trimester   Ⓜ♀

√7ᵗʰ **O41.149 Placentitis, unspecified trimester**   Ⓜ♀▽

√5ᵗʰ **O41.8 Other specified disorders of amniotic fluid and membranes**

√6ᵗʰ **O41.8X Other specified disorders of amniotic fluid and membranes**

√7ᵗʰ **O41.8X1 Other specified disorders of amniotic fluid and membranes,** first trimester   Ⓜ♀

√7ᵗʰ **O41.8X2 Other specified disorders of amniotic fluid and membranes,** second trimester   Ⓜ♀

√7ᵗʰ **O41.8X3 Other specified disorders of amniotic fluid and membranes,** third trimester   Ⓜ♀

√7ᵗʰ **O41.8X9 Other specified disorders of amniotic fluid and membranes, unspecified trimester**   Ⓜ♀▽

√5ᵗʰ **O41.9 Disorder of amniotic fluid and membranes, unspecified**

√x 7ᵗʰ **O41.90 Disorder of amniotic fluid and membranes, unspecified, unspecified trimester**   Ⓜ♀▽

√x 7ᵗʰ **O41.91 Disorder of amniotic fluid and membranes, unspecified,** first trimester   Ⓜ♀▽

√x 7ᵗʰ **O41.92 Disorder of amniotic fluid and membranes, unspecified,** second trimester   Ⓜ♀▽

√x 7ᵗʰ **O41.93 Disorder of amniotic fluid and membranes, unspecified,** third trimester   Ⓜ♀▽

√4ᵗʰ **O42 Premature rupture of membranes**
> AHA: 2016, 1Q, 3

√5ᵗʰ **O42.Ø Premature rupture of membranes,** onset of labor within 24 hours of rupture

O42.ØØ Premature rupture of membranes, onset of labor within 24 hours of rupture, unspecified weeks of gestation   Ⓜ♀▽

√6ᵗʰ **O42.Ø1** Preterm **premature rupture of membranes, onset of labor within 24 hours of rupture**
> Premature rupture of membranes before 37 completed weeks of gestation

O42.Ø11 Preterm premature rupture of membranes, onset of labor within 24 hours of rupture, first trimester   Ⓜ♀

O42.Ø12 Preterm premature rupture of membranes, onset of labor within 24 hours of rupture, second trimester   Ⓜ♀

O42.Ø13 Preterm premature rupture of membranes, onset of labor within 24 hours of rupture, third trimester   Ⓜ♀

O42.Ø19 Preterm premature rupture of membranes, onset of labor within 24 hours of rupture, unspecified trimester   Ⓜ♀▽

O42.Ø2 Full-term **premature rupture of membranes, onset of labor within 24 hours of rupture**   Ⓜ♀
> Premature rupture of membranes at or after 37 completed weeks of gestation, onset of labor within 24 hours of rupture

√5ᵗʰ **O42.1 Premature rupture of membranes,** onset of labor more than 24 hours following rupture
> AHA: 2016, 1Q, 5

O42.10 Premature rupture of membranes, onset of labor more than 24 hours following rupture, unspecified weeks of gestation   Ⓜ♀▽

√6ᵗʰ **O42.11** Preterm **premature rupture of membranes, onset of labor more than 24 hours following rupture**
> Premature rupture of membranes before 37 completed weeks of gestation

O42.111 Preterm premature rupture of membranes, onset of labor more than 24 hours following rupture, first trimester   Ⓜ♀

O42.112 Preterm premature rupture of membranes, onset of labor more than 24 hours following rupture, second trimester   Ⓜ♀

O42.113 Preterm premature rupture of membranes, onset of labor more than 24 hours following rupture, third trimester   Ⓜ♀

O42.119 Preterm premature rupture of membranes, onset of labor more than 24 hours following rupture, unspecified trimester   Ⓜ♀▽

O42.12 Full-term **premature rupture of membranes, onset of labor more than 24 hours following rupture**   Ⓜ♀
> Premature rupture of membranes at or after 37 completed weeks of gestation, onset of labor within 24 hours of rupture

√5ᵗʰ **O42.9 Premature rupture of membranes,** unspecified as to length of time between rupture and onset of labor

O42.90 Premature rupture of membranes, unspecified as to length of time between rupture and onset of labor, unspecified weeks of gestation   Ⓜ♀▽

√6ᵗʰ **O42.91** Preterm **premature rupture of membranes, unspecified as to length of time between rupture and onset of labor**
> Premature rupture of membranes before 37 completed weeks of gestation

O42.911 Preterm premature rupture of membranes, unspecified as to length of time between rupture and onset of labor, first trimester   Ⓜ♀▽

O42.912 Preterm premature rupture of membranes, unspecified as to length of time between rupture and onset of labor, second trimester   Ⓜ♀▽

O42.913 Preterm premature rupture of membranes, unspecified as to length of time between rupture and onset of labor, third trimester   Ⓜ♀▽

EXCLUDES 1 Not coded here   EXCLUDES 2 Not included here   Ⓝ Newborn Age: 0   Ⓟ Pediatric Age: 0-17   Ⓜ Maternity Age: 12-55   Ⓐ Adult Age: 15-124

842   ICD-10-CM 2018

Twin to Twin Transfusion Syndrome (TTTS)

Healthy twins   Twins with TTTS

     O42.919   **Preterm premature rupture of membranes, unspecified as to length of time between rupture and onset of labor, unspecified trimester**   M♀▽

     O42.92   **Full-term premature rupture of membranes, unspecified as to length of time between rupture and onset of labor**   M♀▽
          Premature rupture of membranes at or after 37 completed weeks of gestation, unspecified as to length of time between rupture and onset of labor

✓4ᵗʰ **O43**   **Placental disorders**
     EXCLUDES 2   *maternal care for poor fetal growth due to placental insufficiency (O36.5-)*
          placenta previa (O44.-)
          placental polyp (O90.89)
          placentitis (O41.14-)
          premature separation of placenta [abruptio placentae] (O45.-)

✓5ᵗʰ **O43.0**   **Placental transfusion syndromes**

     ✓6ᵗʰ **O43.01**   **Fetomaternal** placental transfusion syndrome
          Maternofetal placental transfusion syndrome
          O43.011   **Fetomaternal placental transfusion syndrome, first trimester**   M♀
          O43.012   **Fetomaternal placental transfusion syndrome, second trimester**   M♀
          O43.013   **Fetomaternal placental transfusion syndrome, third trimester**   M♀
          O43.019   **Fetomaternal placental transfusion syndrome, unspecified trimester**   M♀▽

     ✓6ᵗʰ **O43.02**   **Fetus-to-fetus** placental transfusion syndrome
          O43.021   **Fetus-to-fetus placental transfusion syndrome, first trimester**   M♀
          O43.022   **Fetus-to-fetus placental transfusion syndrome, second trimester**   M♀
          O43.023   **Fetus-to-fetus placental transfusion syndrome, third trimester**   M♀
          O43.029   **Fetus-to-fetus placental transfusion syndrome, unspecified trimester**   M♀▽

✓5ᵗʰ **O43.1**   **Malformation of placenta**

     ✓6ᵗʰ **O43.10**   **Malformation of placenta, unspecified**
          Abnormal placenta NOS
          O43.101   **Malformation of placenta, unspecified, first trimester**   M♀▽
          O43.102   **Malformation of placenta, unspecified, second trimester**   M♀▽
          O43.103   **Malformation of placenta, unspecified, third trimester**   M♀▽
          O43.109   **Malformation of placenta, unspecified, unspecified trimester**   M♀▽

     ✓6ᵗʰ **O43.11**   **Circumvallate** placenta
          O43.111   **Circumvallate placenta, first trimester**   M♀
          O43.112   **Circumvallate placenta, second trimester**   M♀
          O43.113   **Circumvallate placenta, third trimester**   M♀
          O43.119   **Circumvallate placenta, unspecified trimester**   M♀▽

     ✓6ᵗʰ **O43.12**   **Velamentous insertion of umbilical cord**
          O43.121   **Velamentous insertion of umbilical cord, first trimester**   M♀
          O43.122   **Velamentous insertion of umbilical cord, second trimester**   M♀
          O43.123   **Velamentous insertion of umbilical cord, third trimester**   M♀
          O43.129   **Velamentous insertion of umbilical cord, unspecified trimester**   M♀▽

     ✓6ᵗʰ **O43.19**   **Other malformation of placenta**
          O43.191   **Other malformation of placenta, first trimester**   M♀
          O43.192   **Other malformation of placenta, second trimester**   M♀
          O43.193   **Other malformation of placenta, third trimester**   M♀
          O43.199   **Other malformation of placenta, unspecified trimester**   M♀▽

✓5ᵗʰ **O43.2**   **Morbidly adherent placenta**
          Code also associated third stage postpartum hemorrhage, if applicable (O72.0)
     EXCLUDES 1   *retained placenta (O73.-)*

     ✓6ᵗʰ **O43.21**   **Placenta accreta**
          O43.211   **Placenta accreta, first trimester**   M♀
          O43.212   **Placenta accreta, second trimester**   M♀
          O43.213   **Placenta accreta, third trimester**   M♀
          O43.219   **Placenta accreta, unspecified trimester**   M♀▽

     ✓6ᵗʰ **O43.22**   **Placenta increta**
          O43.221   **Placenta increta, first trimester**   M♀
          O43.222   **Placenta increta, second trimester**   M♀
          O43.223   **Placenta increta, third trimester**   M♀
          O43.229   **Placenta increta, unspecified trimester**   M♀▽

     ✓6ᵗʰ **O43.23**   **Placenta percreta**
          O43.231   **Placenta percreta, first trimester**   M♀
          O43.232   **Placenta percreta, second trimester**   M♀
          O43.233   **Placenta percreta, third trimester**   M♀
          O43.239   **Placenta percreta, unspecified trimester**   M♀▽

✓5ᵗʰ **O43.8**   **Other placental disorders**

     ✓6ᵗʰ **O43.81**   **Placental infarction**
          O43.811   **Placental infarction, first trimester**   M♀
          O43.812   **Placental infarction, second trimester**   M♀
          O43.813   **Placental infarction, third trimester**   M♀
          O43.819   **Placental infarction, unspecified trimester**   M♀▽

     ✓6ᵗʰ **O43.89**   **Other placental disorders**
          Placental dysfunction
          O43.891   **Other placental disorders, first trimester**   M♀
          O43.892   **Other placental disorders, second trimester**   M♀
          O43.893   **Other placental disorders, third trimester**   M♀
          O43.899   **Other placental disorders, unspecified trimester**   M♀▽

✓5ᵗʰ **O43.9**   **Unspecified placental disorder**
     O43.90   **Unspecified placental disorder, unspecified trimester**   M♀▽
     O43.91   **Unspecified placental disorder, first trimester**   M♀▽
     O43.92   **Unspecified placental disorder, second trimester**   M♀▽
     O43.93   **Unspecified placental disorder, third trimester**   M♀▽

✓4ᵗʰ **O44**   **Placenta previa**
     DEF: Placenta implanted in lower segment of uterus; commonly causes hemorrhage in the last trimester of pregnancy.

     ✓5ᵗʰ **O44.0**   **Complete placenta previa NOS or without hemorrhage**
          Placenta previa NOS
          O44.00   **Complete placenta previa NOS or without hemorrhage, unspecified trimester**   M♀▽
          O44.01   **Complete placenta previa NOS or without hemorrhage, first trimester**   M♀

✓ Additional Character Req   ✓x7ᵗʰ Placeholder Alert   Manifestation   HCC CMS-HCC Condition   ▽ Unspecified Code   ►◄ Revised Text   ● New Code   ▲ Revised Code Title

ICD-10-CM 2018   843

Chapter 15. Pregnancy, Childbirth, and the Puerperium

O42.919–O44.01

O44.02   Complete placenta previa NOS or without hemorrhage, second trimester   Ⓜ♀

O44.03   Complete placenta previa NOS or without hemorrhage, third trimester   Ⓜ♀

✓5ᵗʰ **O44.1**   Complete placenta previa with hemorrhage
> EXCLUDES 1   labor and delivery complicated by hemorrhage from vasa previa (O69.4)

O44.10   Complete placenta previa with hemorrhage, unspecified trimester   Ⓜ♀▽

O44.11   Complete placenta previa with hemorrhage, first trimester   Ⓜ♀

O44.12   Complete placenta previa with hemorrhage, second trimester   Ⓜ♀

O44.13   Complete placenta previa with hemorrhage, third trimester   Ⓜ♀

✓5ᵗʰ **O44.2**   Partial placenta previa without hemorrhage
> Marginal placenta previa, NOS or without hemorrhage

O44.20   Partial placenta previa NOS or without hemorrhage, unspecified trimester   Ⓜ♀▽

O44.21   Partial placenta previa NOS or without hemorrhage, first trimester   Ⓜ♀

O44.22   Partial placenta previa NOS or without hemorrhage, second trimester   Ⓜ♀

O44.23   Partial placenta previa NOS or without hemorrhage, third trimester   Ⓜ♀

✓5ᵗʰ **O44.3**   Partial placenta previa with hemorrhage
> Marginal placenta previa with hemorrhage

O44.30   Partial placenta previa with hemorrhage, unspecified trimester   Ⓜ♀▽

O44.31   Partial placenta previa with hemorrhage, first trimester   Ⓜ♀

O44.32   Partial placenta previa with hemorrhage, second trimester   Ⓜ♀

O44.33   Partial placenta previa with hemorrhage, third trimester   Ⓜ♀

✓5ᵗʰ **O44.4**   Low lying placenta NOS or without hemorrhage
> Low implantation of placenta NOS or without hemorrhage

O44.40   Low lying placenta NOS or without hemorrhage, unspecified trimester   Ⓜ♀▽

O44.41   Low lying placenta NOS or without hemorrhage, first trimester   Ⓜ♀

O44.42   Low lying placenta NOS or without hemorrhage, second trimester   Ⓜ♀

O44.43   Low lying placenta NOS or without hemorrhage, third trimester   Ⓜ♀

✓5ᵗʰ **O44.5**   Low lying placenta with hemorrhage
> Low implantation of placenta with hemorrhage

O44.50   Low lying placenta with hemorrhage, unspecified trimester   Ⓜ♀▽

O44.51   Low lying placenta with hemorrhage, first trimester   Ⓜ♀

O44.52   Low lying placenta with hemorrhage, second trimester   Ⓜ♀

O44.53   Low lying placenta with hemorrhage, third trimester   Ⓜ♀

✓4ᵗʰ **O45**   **Premature separation of placenta [abruptio placentae]**

✓5ᵗʰ **O45.0**   Premature separation of placenta with coagulation defect

✓6ᵗʰ **O45.00**   Premature separation of placenta with coagulation defect, unspecified

O45.001   Premature separation of placenta with coagulation defect, unspecified, first trimester   Ⓜ♀▽

O45.002   Premature separation of placenta with coagulation defect, unspecified, second trimester   Ⓜ♀▽

O45.003   Premature separation of placenta with coagulation defect, unspecified, third trimester   Ⓜ♀▽

O45.009   Premature separation of placenta with coagulation defect, unspecified, unspecified trimester   Ⓜ♀▽

✓6ᵗʰ **O45.01**   Premature separation of placenta with afibrinogenemia
> Premature separation of placenta with hypofibrinogenemia

O45.011   Premature separation of placenta with afibrinogenemia, first trimester   Ⓜ♀

O45.012   Premature separation of placenta with afibrinogenemia, second trimester   Ⓜ♀

O45.013   Premature separation of placenta with afibrinogenemia, third trimester   Ⓜ♀

O45.019   Premature separation of placenta with afibrinogenemia, unspecified trimester   Ⓜ♀▽

✓6ᵗʰ **O45.02**   Premature separation of placenta with disseminated intravascular coagulation

O45.021   Premature separation of placenta with disseminated intravascular coagulation, first trimester   Ⓜ♀

O45.022   Premature separation of placenta with disseminated intravascular coagulation, second trimester   Ⓜ♀

O45.023   Premature separation of placenta with disseminated intravascular coagulation, third trimester   Ⓜ♀

O45.029   Premature separation of placenta with disseminated intravascular coagulation, unspecified trimester   Ⓜ♀▽

✓6ᵗʰ **O45.09**   Premature separation of placenta with other coagulation defect

O45.091   Premature separation of placenta with other coagulation defect, first trimester   Ⓜ♀

O45.092   Premature separation of placenta with other coagulation defect, second trimester   Ⓜ♀

O45.093   Premature separation of placenta with other coagulation defect, third trimester   Ⓜ♀

O45.099   Premature separation of placenta with other coagulation defect, unspecified trimester   Ⓜ♀▽

✓5ᵗʰ **O45.8**   Other premature separation of placenta

✓6ᵗʰ **O45.8X**   Other premature separation of placenta

O45.8X1   Other premature separation of placenta, first trimester   Ⓜ♀

O45.8X2   Other premature separation of placenta, second trimester   Ⓜ♀

O45.8X3   Other premature separation of placenta, third trimester   Ⓜ♀

O45.8X9   Other premature separation of placenta, unspecified trimester   Ⓜ♀▽

✓5ᵗʰ **O45.9**   Premature separation of placenta, unspecified
> Abruptio placentae NOS

O45.90   Premature separation of placenta, unspecified, unspecified trimester   Ⓜ♀▽

O45.91   Premature separation of placenta, unspecified, first trimester   Ⓜ♀▽

O45.92   Premature separation of placenta, unspecified, second trimester   Ⓜ♀▽

O45.93   Premature separation of placenta, unspecified, third trimester   Ⓜ♀▽

✓4ᵗʰ **O46**   **Antepartum hemorrhage, not elsewhere classified**
> EXCLUDES 1   hemorrhage in early pregnancy (O20.-)
> intrapartum hemorrhage NEC (O67.-)
> placenta previa (O44.-)
> premature separation of placenta [abruptio placentae] (O45.-)
>
> **DEF:** Uterine hemorrhage prior to delivery; not related to placenta previa or abruptio placentae.

✓5ᵗʰ **O46.0**   Antepartum hemorrhage with coagulation defect

✓6ᵗʰ **O46.00**   Antepartum hemorrhage with coagulation defect, unspecified

O46.001   Antepartum hemorrhage with coagulation defect, unspecified, first trimester   Ⓜ♀▽

O46.002   Antepartum hemorrhage with coagulation defect, unspecified, second trimester   Ⓜ♀▽

O46.003   Antepartum hemorrhage with coagulation defect, unspecified, third trimester   Ⓜ♀▽

O46.009   Antepartum hemorrhage with coagulation defect, unspecified, unspecified trimester   Ⓜ♀▽

EXCLUDES 1 Not coded here   EXCLUDES 2 Not included here   Ⓝ Newborn Age: 0   Ⓟ Pediatric Age: 0-17   Ⓜ Maternity Age: 12-55   Ⓐ Adult Age: 15-124

844   ICD-10-CM 2018

✓6ᵗʰ **O46.01 Antepartum hemorrhage** with afibrinogenemia
Antepartum hemorrhage with hypofibrinogenemia
- **O46.011 Antepartum hemorrhage with afibrinogenemia,** first trimester Ⓜ♀
- **O46.012 Antepartum hemorrhage with afibrinogenemia,** second trimester Ⓜ♀
- **O46.013 Antepartum hemorrhage with afibrinogenemia,** third trimester Ⓜ♀
- **O46.019 Antepartum hemorrhage with afibrinogenemia, unspecified trimester** Ⓜ♀▽

✓6ᵗʰ **O46.02 Antepartum hemorrhage** with disseminated intravascular coagulation
- **O46.021 Antepartum hemorrhage with disseminated intravascular coagulation,** first trimester Ⓜ♀
- **O46.022 Antepartum hemorrhage with disseminated intravascular coagulation,** second trimester Ⓜ♀
- **O46.023 Antepartum hemorrhage with disseminated intravascular coagulation,** third trimester Ⓜ♀
- **O46.029 Antepartum hemorrhage with disseminated intravascular coagulation, unspecified trimester** Ⓜ♀▽

✓6ᵗʰ **O46.09 Antepartum hemorrhage with other coagulation defect**
- **O46.091 Antepartum hemorrhage with other coagulation defect,** first trimester Ⓜ♀
- **O46.092 Antepartum hemorrhage with other coagulation defect,** second trimester Ⓜ♀
- **O46.093 Antepartum hemorrhage with other coagulation defect,** third trimester Ⓜ♀
- **O46.099 Antepartum hemorrhage with other coagulation defect, unspecified trimester** Ⓜ♀▽

✓5ᵗʰ **O46.8 Other antepartum hemorrhage**
✓6ᵗʰ **O46.8X Other antepartum hemorrhage**
- **O46.8X1 Other antepartum hemorrhage,** first trimester Ⓜ♀
- **O46.8X2 Other antepartum hemorrhage,** second trimester Ⓜ♀
- **O46.8X3 Other antepartum hemorrhage,** third trimester Ⓜ♀
- **O46.8X9 Other antepartum hemorrhage, unspecified trimester** Ⓜ♀▽

✓5ᵗʰ **O46.9 Antepartum hemorrhage, unspecified**
- **O46.90 Antepartum hemorrhage, unspecified, unspecified trimester** Ⓜ♀▽
- **O46.91 Antepartum hemorrhage, unspecified,** first trimester Ⓜ♀▽
- **O46.92 Antepartum hemorrhage, unspecified,** second trimester Ⓜ♀▽
- **O46.93 Antepartum hemorrhage, unspecified,** third trimester Ⓜ♀▽

✓4ᵗʰ **O47 False labor**
INCLUDES Braxton Hicks contractions
threatened labor
EXCLUDES1 preterm labor (O60.-)
✓5ᵗʰ **O47.0 False labor** before 37 completed weeks of gestation
- **O47.00 False labor before 37 completed weeks of gestation, unspecified trimester** Ⓜ♀▽
- **O47.02 False labor before 37 completed weeks of gestation,** second trimester Ⓜ♀
- **O47.03 False labor before 37 completed weeks of gestation,** third trimester Ⓜ♀
- **O47.1 False labor** at or after 37 completed weeks of gestation Ⓜ♀
- **O47.9 False labor, unspecified** Ⓜ♀▽

✓4ᵗʰ **O48 Late pregnancy**
- **O48.0 Post-term pregnancy** Ⓜ♀
Pregnancy over 40 completed weeks to 42 completed weeks gestation
- **O48.1 Prolonged pregnancy** Ⓜ♀
Pregnancy which has advanced beyond 42 completed weeks gestation
AHA: 2016, 1Q, 5

Complications of labor and delivery (O60-O77)

✓4ᵗʰ **O60 Preterm labor**
INCLUDES onset (spontaneous) of labor before 37 completed weeks of gestation
EXCLUDES1 false labor (O47.0-)
threatened labor NOS (O47.0-)
✓5ᵗʰ **O60.0 Preterm labor** without delivery
- **O60.00 Preterm labor without delivery, unspecified trimester** Ⓜ♀▽
- **O60.02 Preterm labor without delivery,** second trimester Ⓜ♀
- **O60.03 Preterm labor without delivery,** third trimester Ⓜ♀
✓5ᵗʰ **O60.1 Preterm labor** with preterm delivery
AHA: 2016, 2Q, 10

One of the following 7th characters is to be assigned to each code under subcategory O60.1. 7th character 0 is for single gestations and multiple gestations where the fetus is unspecified. 7th characters 1 through 9 are for cases of multiple gestations to identify the fetus for which the code applies. The appropriate code from category O30, Multiple gestation, must also be assigned when assigning a code from subcategory O60.1 that has a 7th character of 1 through 9.
0 not applicable or unspecified   4 fetus 4
1 fetus 1   5 fetus 5
2 fetus 2   9 other fetus
3 fetus 3

- ✓x7ᵗʰ **O60.10 Preterm labor with preterm delivery, unspecified trimester** Ⓜ♀▽
Preterm labor with delivery NOS
- ✓x7ᵗʰ **O60.12 Preterm labor** second trimester **with preterm delivery** second trimester Ⓜ♀
- ✓x7ᵗʰ **O60.13 Preterm labor** second trimester **with preterm delivery** third trimester Ⓜ♀
- ✓x7ᵗʰ **O60.14 Preterm labor** third trimester **with preterm delivery** third trimester Ⓜ♀
✓5ᵗʰ **O60.2 Term delivery with preterm labor**

One of the following 7th characters is to be assigned to each code under subcategory O60.2. 7th character 0 is for single gestations and multiple gestations where the fetus is unspecified. 7th characters 1 through 9 are for cases of multiple gestations to identify the fetus for which the code applies. The appropriate code from category O30, Multiple gestation, must also be assigned when assigning a code from subcategory O60.2 that has a 7th character of 1 through 9.
0 not applicable or unspecified   4 fetus 4
1 fetus 1   5 fetus 5
2 fetus 2   9 other fetus
3 fetus 3

- ✓x7ᵗʰ **O60.20 Term delivery with preterm labor, unspecified trimester** Ⓜ♀▽
- ✓x7ᵗʰ **O60.22 Term delivery with preterm labor,** second trimester Ⓜ♀
- ✓x7ᵗʰ **O60.23 Term delivery with preterm labor,** third trimester Ⓜ♀

✓4ᵗʰ **O61 Failed induction of labor**
- **O61.0 Failed medical induction of labor** Ⓜ♀
Failed induction (of labor) by oxytocin
Failed induction (of labor) by prostaglandins
- **O61.1 Failed instrumental induction of labor** Ⓜ♀
Failed mechanical induction (of labor)
Failed surgical induction (of labor)
- **O61.8 Other failed induction of labor** Ⓜ♀
- **O61.9 Failed induction of labor, unspecified** Ⓜ♀▽

✓4ᵗʰ **O62 Abnormalities of forces of labor**
- **O62.0 Primary inadequate contractions** Ⓜ♀
Failure of cervical dilatation
Primary hypotonic uterine dysfunction
Uterine inertia during latent phase of labor
- **O62.1 Secondary uterine inertia** Ⓜ♀
Arrested active phase of labor
Secondary hypotonic uterine dysfunction

Fetal Malposition

Breech

Shoulder
(arm prolapse)

Mother's
pelvis

Compound
(extremity
together
with head)

Oblique

Face
(mentum)

O62.2 Other uterine inertia Ⓜ♀
Atony of uterus without hemorrhage
Atony of uterus NOS
Desultory labor
Hypotonic uterine dysfunction NOS
Irregular labor
Poor contractions
Slow slope active phase of labor
Uterine inertia NOS
EXCLUDES 1 atony of uterus with hemorrhage (postpartum) (O72.1)
postpartum atony of uterus without hemorrhage
(O75.89)

O62.3 Precipitate labor Ⓜ♀

O62.4 Hypetonic, incoordinate, and prolonged uterine Ⓜ♀
contractions
Cervical spasm
Contraction ring dystocia
Dyscoordinate labor
Hour-glass contraction of uterus
Hypertonic uterine dysfunction
Incoordinate uterine action
Tetanic contractions
Uterine dystocia NOS
Uterine spasm
EXCLUDES 1 dystocia (fetal) (maternal) NOS (O66.9)

O62.8 Other abnormalities of forces of labor Ⓜ♀

O62.9 Abnormality of forces of labor, unspecified Ⓜ♀▽

✓4ᵗʰ **O63 Long labor**
O63.0 Prolonged first stage (of labor) Ⓜ♀
O63.1 Prolonged second stage (of labor) Ⓜ♀
O63.2 Delayed delivery of second twin, triplet, etc. Ⓜ♀
O63.9 Long labor, unspecified Ⓜ♀▽
Prolonged labor NOS

✓4ᵗʰ **O64 Obstructed labor due to malposition and malpresentation of
fetus**

One of the following 7th characters is to be assigned to each code
under category O64. 7th character Ø is for single gestations and
multiple gestations where the fetus is unspecified. 7th characters 1
through 9 are for cases of multiple gestations to identify the fetus for
which the code applies. The appropriate code from category O30,
Multiple gestation, must also be assigned when assigning a code
from category O64 that has a 7th character of 1 through 9.
Ø	not applicable or unspecified	4	fetus 4
1	fetus 1	5	fetus 5
2	fetus 2	9	other fetus
3	fetus 3		

✓x7ᵗʰ **O64.0 Obstructed labor due to incomplete rotation of fetal** Ⓜ♀
head
Deep transverse arrest
Obstructed labor due to persistent occipitoiliac (position)
Obstructed labor due to persistent occipitoposterior (position)
Obstructed labor due to persistent occipitosacral (position)
Obstructed labor due to persistent occipitotransverse (position)

✓x7ᵗʰ **O64.1 Obstructed labor due to breech presentation** Ⓜ♀
Obstructed labor due to buttocks presentation
Obstructed labor due to complete breech presentation
Obstructed labor due to frank breech presentation

✓x7ᵗʰ **O64.2 Obstructed labor due to face presentation** Ⓜ♀
Obstructed labor due to chin presentation

✓x7ᵗʰ **O64.3 Obstructed labor due to brow presentation** Ⓜ♀

✓x7ᵗʰ **O64.4 Obstructed labor due to shoulder presentation** Ⓜ♀
Prolapsed arm
EXCLUDES 1 impacted shoulders (O66.0)
shoulder dystocia (O66.0)

✓x7ᵗʰ **O64.5 Obstructed labor due to compound presentation** Ⓜ♀

✓x7ᵗʰ **O64.8 Obstructed labor due to other malposition and** Ⓜ♀
malpresentation
Obstructed labor due to footling presentation
Obstructed labor due to incomplete breech presentation

✓x7ᵗʰ **O64.9 Obstructed labor due to malposition and** Ⓜ♀▽
malpresentation, unspecified

✓4ᵗʰ **O65 Obstructed labor due to maternal pelvic abnormality**
O65.0 Obstructed labor due to deformed pelvis Ⓜ♀
O65.1 Obstructed labor due to generally contracted pelvis Ⓜ♀
O65.2 Obstructed labor due to pelvic inlet contraction Ⓜ♀
O65.3 Obstructed labor due to pelvic outlet and mid-cavity Ⓜ♀
contraction
O65.4 Obstructed labor due to fetopelvic disproportion, Ⓜ♀▽
unspecified
EXCLUDES 1 dystocia due to abnormality of fetus (O66.2-O66.3)
O65.5 Obstructed labor due to abnormality of maternal Ⓜ♀
pelvic organs
Obstructed labor due to conditions listed in O34-
Use additional code to identify abnormality of pelvic organs
(O34.-)
O65.8 Obstructed labor due to other maternal pelvic Ⓜ♀
abnormalities
O65.9 Obstructed labor due to maternal pelvic abnormality, Ⓜ♀▽
unspecified

✓4ᵗʰ **O66 Other obstructed labor**
O66.0 Obstructed labor due to shoulder dystocia Ⓜ♀
Impacted shoulders
DEF: Obstructed labor due to impacted fetal shoulders;
emergency condition that may require cesarean section, forceps
delivery, vacuum extraction, or simphysiotomy.
O66.1 Obstructed labor due to locked twins Ⓜ♀
O66.2 Obstructed labor due to unusually large fetus Ⓜ♀
O66.3 Obstructed labor due to other abnormalities of fetus Ⓜ♀
Dystocia due to fetal ascites
Dystocia due to fetal hydrops
Dystocia due to fetal meningomyelocele
Dystocia due to fetal sacral teratoma
Dystocia due to fetal tumor
Dystocia due to hydrocephalic fetus
Use additional code to identify cause of obstruction
✓5ᵗʰ **O66.4 Failed trial of labor**
O66.40 Failed trial of labor, unspecified Ⓜ♀▽
O66.41 Failed attempted vaginal birth after previous Ⓜ♀
cesarean delivery
Code first rupture of uterus, if applicable (O71.0-,
O71.1)
O66.5 Attempted application of vacuum extractor and forceps Ⓜ♀
Attempted application of vacuum or forceps, with subsequent
delivery by forceps or cesarean delivery
O66.6 Obstructed labor due to other multiple fetuses Ⓜ♀
O66.8 Other specified obstructed labor Ⓜ♀
Use additional code to identify cause of obstruction
O66.9 Obstructed labor, unspecified Ⓜ♀▽
Dystocia NOS
Fetal dystocia NOS
Maternal dystocia NOS

EXCLUDES 1 Not coded here   *EXCLUDES 2* Not included here   Ⓝ Newborn Age: 0   Ⓟ Pediatric Age: 0-17   Ⓜ Maternity Age: 12-55   Ⓐ Adult Age: 15-124

846   ICD-10-CM 2018

✓4th O67 Labor and delivery complicated by intrapartum hemorrhage, not elsewhere classified

EXCLUDES 1   *antepartum hemorrhage NEC (O46.-)*
placenta previa (O44.-)
premature separation of placenta [abruptio placentae] (O45.-)

EXCLUDES 2   *postpartum hemorrhage (O72.-)*

O67.0 Intrapartum hemorrhage with coagulation defect   M♀
Intrapartum hemorrhage (excessive) associated with afibrinogenemia
Intrapartum hemorrhage (excessive) associated with disseminated intravascular coagulation
Intrapartum hemorrhage (excessive) associated with hyperfibrinolysis
Intrapartum hemorrhage (excessive) associated with hypofibrinogenemia

O67.8 Other intrapartum hemorrhage   M♀
Excessive intrapartum hemorrhage

O67.9 Intrapartum hemorrhage, unspecified   M♀▽

O68 Labor and delivery complicated by abnormality of fetal acid-base balance   M♀
Fetal acidemia complicating labor and delivery
Fetal acidosis complicating labor and delivery
Fetal alkalosis complicating labor and delivery
Fetal metabolic acidemia complicating labor and delivery

EXCLUDES 1   *fetal stress NOS (O77.9)*
labor and delivery complicated by electrocardiographic evidence of fetal stress (O77.8)
labor and delivery complicated by ultrasonic evidence of fetal stress (O77.8)

EXCLUDES 2   *abnormality in fetal heart rate or rhythm (O76)*
labor and delivery complicated by meconium in amniotic fluid (O77.0)

✓4th O69 Labor and delivery complicated by umbilical cord complications
AHA: 2016, 1Q, 5

One of the following 7th characters is to be assigned to each code under category O69. 7th character 0 is for single gestations and multiple gestations where the fetus is unspecified. 7th characters 1 through 9 are for cases of multiple gestations to identify the fetus for which the code applies. The appropriate code from category O30, Multiple gestation, must also be assigned when assigning a code from category O69 that has a 7th character of 1 through 9.

0	not applicable or unspecified	4	fetus 4
1	fetus 1	5	fetus 5
2	fetus 2	9	other fetus
3	fetus 3		

✓x7th O69.0 Labor and delivery complicated by prolapse of cord   M♀
DEF: Abnormal presentation of fetus; marked by protruding umbilical cord during labor; can cause fetal death.

✓x7th O69.1 Labor and delivery complicated by cord around neck, with compression   M♀
EXCLUDES 1   *labor and delivery complicated by cord around neck, without compression (O69.81)*

✓x7th O69.2 Labor and delivery complicated by other cord entanglement, with compression   M♀
Labor and delivery complicated by compression of cord NOS
Labor and delivery complicated by entanglement of cords of twins in monoamniotic sac
Labor and delivery complicated by knot in cord

EXCLUDES 1   *labor and delivery complicated by other cord entanglement, without compression (O69.82)*

✓x7th O69.3 Labor and delivery complicated by short cord   M♀

✓x7th O69.4 Labor and delivery complicated by vasa previa   M♀
Labor and delivery complicated by hemorrhage from vasa previa

✓x7th O69.5 Labor and delivery complicated by vascular lesion of cord   M♀
Labor and delivery complicated by cord bruising
Labor and delivery complicated by cord hematoma
Labor and delivery complicated by thrombosis of umbilical vessels

✓5th O69.8 Labor and delivery complicated by other cord complications

✓x7th O69.81 Labor and delivery complicated by cord around neck, without compression   M♀
AHA: 2016, 1Q, 5

✓x7th O69.82 Labor and delivery complicated by other cord entanglement, without compression   M♀

✓x7th O69.89 Labor and delivery complicated by other cord complications   M♀

✓x7th O69.9 Labor and delivery complicated by cord complication, unspecified   M♀▽

✓4th O70 Perineal laceration during delivery
Episiotomy extended by laceration

EXCLUDES 1   *obstetric high vaginal laceration alone (O71.4)*

AHA: 2016, 2Q, 34; 2016, 1Q, 3-4, 5

O70.0 First degree perineal laceration during delivery   M♀
Perineal laceration, rupture or tear involving fourchette during delivery
Perineal laceration, rupture or tear involving labia during delivery
Perineal laceration, rupture or tear involving skin during delivery
Perineal laceration, rupture or tear involving vagina during delivery
Perineal laceration, rupture or tear involving vulva during delivery
Slight perineal laceration, rupture or tear during delivery

O70.1 Second degree perineal laceration during delivery   M♀
Perineal laceration, rupture or tear during delivery as in O70.0, also involving pelvic floor
Perineal laceration, rupture or tear during delivery as in O70.0, also involving perineal muscles
Perineal laceration, rupture or tear during delivery as in O70.0, also involving vaginal muscles

EXCLUDES 1   *perineal laceration involving anal sphincter (O70.2)*

✓5th O70.2 Third degree perineal laceration during delivery
Perineal laceration, rupture or tear during delivery as in O70.1, also involving anal sphincter
Perineal laceration, rupture or tear during delivery as in O70.1, also involving rectovaginal septum
Perineal laceration, rupture or tear during delivery as in O70.1, also involving sphincter NOS

EXCLUDES 1   *anal sphincter tear during delivery without third degree perineal laceration (O70.4)*
perineal laceration involving anal or rectal mucosa (O70.3)

O70.20 Third degree perineal laceration during delivery, unspecified   M♀▽

O70.21 Third degree perineal laceration during delivery, IIIa   M♀
Third degree perineal laceration during delivery with less than 50% of external anal sphincter (EAS) thickness torn

O70.22 Third degree perineal laceration during delivery, IIIb   M♀
Third degree perineal laceration during delivery with more than 50% external anal sphincter (EAS) thickness torn

O70.23 Third degree perineal laceration during delivery, IIIc   M♀
Third degree perineal laceration during delivery with both external anal sphincter (EAS) and internal anal sphincter (IAS) torn

O70.3 Fourth degree perineal laceration during delivery   M♀
Perineal laceration, rupture or tear during delivery as in O70.2, also involving anal mucosa
Perineal laceration, rupture or tear during delivery as in O70.2, also involving rectal mucosa

O70.4 Anal sphincter tear complicating delivery, not associated with third degree laceration   M♀
EXCLUDES 1   *anal sphincter tear with third degree perineal laceration (O70.2)*

O70.9 Perineal laceration during delivery, unspecified   M♀▽

✓4th O71 Other obstetric trauma
INCLUDES   obstetric damage from instruments

✓5th O71.0 Rupture of uterus (spontaneous) before onset of labor
EXCLUDES 1   *disruption of (current) cesarean delivery wound (O90.0)*
laceration of uterus, NEC (O71.81)

O71.00 Rupture of uterus before onset of labor, unspecified trimester   M♀▽

O71.02 Rupture of uterus before onset of labor, second trimester   M♀

O71.03 Rupture of uterus before onset of labor, third trimester   M♀

O71.1 Rupture of uterus during labor   M♀
Rupture of uterus not stated as occurring before onset of labor
EXCLUDES 1   *disruption of cesarean delivery wound (O90.0)*
laceration of uterus, NEC (O71.81)

O71.2 Postpartum inversion of uterus   M♀

O71.3 Obstetric laceration of cervix   M♀
Annular detachment of cervix

☑ Additional Character Req   ✓x7th Placeholder Alert   Manifestation   HCC CMS-HCC Condition   ▽ Unspecified Code   ►◄ Revised Text   ● New Code   ▲ Revised Code Title

ICD-10-CM 2018   847

O67–O71.3

Chapter 15. Pregnancy, Childbirth, and the Puerperium

O71.4 Obstetric high vaginal laceration alone Ⓜ♀
Laceration of vaginal wall without perineal laceration
EXCLUDES 1   obstetric high vaginal laceration with perineal laceration (O70.-)
AHA: 2016, 1Q, 5

O71.5 Other obstetric injury to pelvic organs Ⓜ♀
Obstetric injury to bladder
Obstetric injury to urethra
EXCLUDES 2   obstetric periurethral trauma (O71.82)
AHA: 2014, 4Q, 18

O71.6 Obstetric damage to pelvic joints and ligaments Ⓜ♀
Obstetric avulsion of inner symphyseal cartilage
Obstetric damage to coccyx
Obstetric traumatic separation of symphysis (pubis)

O71.7 Obstetric hematoma of pelvis Ⓜ♀
Obstetric hematoma of perineum
Obstetric hematoma of vagina
Obstetric hematoma of vulva

✓5ᵗʰ **O71.8 Other specified obstetric trauma**
     O71.81 Laceration of uterus, not elsewhere classified Ⓜ♀
     O71.82 Other specified trauma to perineum and vulva Ⓜ♀
         Obstetric periurethral trauma
         AHA: 2016, 1Q, 4; 2014, 4Q, 18
     O71.89 Other specified obstetric trauma Ⓜ♀

O71.9 Obstetric trauma, unspecified Ⓜ♀▽

✓4ᵗʰ **O72 Postpartum hemorrhage**
INCLUDES   hemorrhage after delivery of fetus or infant

O72.0 Third-stage hemorrhage Ⓜ♀
Hemorrhage associated with retained, trapped or adherent placenta
Retained placenta NOS
Code also type of adherent placenta (O43.2-)

O72.1 Other immediate postpartum hemorrhage Ⓜ♀
Hemorrhage following delivery of placenta
Postpartum hemorrhage (atonic) NOS
Uterine atony with hemorrhage
EXCLUDES 1   uterine atony NOS (O62.2)
         uterine atony without hemorrhage (O62.2)
         postpartum atony of uterus without hemorrhage (O75.89)
AHA: 2016, 1Q, 4

O72.2 Delayed and secondary postpartum hemorrhage Ⓜ♀
Hemorrhage associated with retained portions of placenta or membranes after the first 24 hours following delivery of placenta
Retained products of conception NOS, following delivery

O72.3 Postpartum coagulation defects Ⓜ♀
Postpartum afibrinogenemia
Postpartum fibrinolysis

✓4ᵗʰ **O73 Retained placenta and membranes, without hemorrhage**
EXCLUDES 1   placenta accreta (O43.21-)
         placenta increta (O43.22-)
         placenta percreta (O43.23-)
DEF: Postpartum condition resulting from failure to expel placental membrane tissues due to failed contractions of uterine wall.

O73.0 Retained placenta without hemorrhage Ⓜ♀
Adherent placenta, without hemorrhage
Trapped placenta without hemorrhage

O73.1 Retained portions of placenta and membranes, without hemorrhage Ⓜ♀
Retained products of conception following delivery, without hemorrhage

✓4ᵗʰ **O74 Complications of anesthesia during labor and delivery**
INCLUDES   maternal complications arising from the administration of a general, regional or local anesthetic, analgesic or other sedation during labor and delivery
Use additional code, if applicable, to identify specific complication

O74.0 Aspiration pneumonitis due to anesthesia during labor and delivery Ⓜ♀
Inhalation of stomach contents or secretions NOS due to anesthesia during labor and delivery
Mendelson's syndrome due to anesthesia during labor and delivery

O74.1 Other pulmonary complications of anesthesia during labor and delivery Ⓜ♀

O74.2 Cardiac complications of anesthesia during labor and delivery Ⓜ♀

O74.3 Central nervous system complications of anesthesia during labor and delivery Ⓜ♀

O74.4 Toxic reaction to local anesthesia during labor and delivery Ⓜ♀

O74.5 Spinal and epidural anesthesia-induced headache during labor and delivery Ⓜ♀

O74.6 Other complications of spinal and epidural anesthesia during labor and delivery Ⓜ♀

O74.7 Failed or difficult intubation for anesthesia during labor and delivery Ⓜ♀

O74.8 Other complications of anesthesia during labor and delivery Ⓜ♀

O74.9 Complication of anesthesia during labor and delivery, unspecified Ⓜ♀▽

✓4ᵗʰ **O75 Other complications of labor and delivery, not elsewhere classified**
EXCLUDES 2   puerperal (postpartum) infection (O86.-)
         puerperal (postpartum) sepsis (O85)

O75.0 Maternal distress during labor and delivery Ⓜ♀

O75.1 Shock during or following labor and delivery Ⓜ♀
Obstetric shock following labor and delivery

O75.2 Pyrexia during labor, not elsewhere classified Ⓜ♀

O75.3 Other infection during labor Ⓜ♀
Sepsis during labor
Use additional code (B95-B97), to identify infectious agent

O75.4 Other complications of obstetric surgery and procedures Ⓜ♀
Cardiac arrest following obstetric surgery or procedures
Cardiac failure following obstetric surgery or procedures
Cerebral anoxia following obstetric surgery or procedures
Pulmonary edema following obstetric surgery or procedures
Use additional code to identify specific complication
EXCLUDES 2   complications of anesthesia during labor and delivery (O74.-)
         disruption of obstetrical (surgical) wound (O90.0-O90.1)
         hematoma of obstetrical (surgical) wound (O90.2)
         infection of obstetrical (surgical) wound (O86.0)

O75.5 Delayed delivery after artificial rupture of membranes Ⓜ♀

✓5ᵗʰ **O75.8 Other specified complications of labor and delivery**
     O75.81 Maternal exhaustion complicating labor and delivery Ⓜ♀
     O75.82 Onset (spontaneous) of labor after 37 completed weeks of gestation but before 39 completed weeks gestation, with delivery by (planned) cesarean section Ⓜ♀
         Delivery by (planned) cesarean section occurring after 37 completed weeks of gestation but before 39 completed weeks gestation due to (spontaneous) onset of labor
         Code first to specify reason for planned cesarean section such as:
            cephalopelvic disproportion (normally formed fetus) (O33.9)
            previous cesarean delivery (O34.21)
     O75.89 Other specified complications of labor and delivery Ⓜ♀

O75.9 Complication of labor and delivery, unspecified Ⓜ♀▽

O76 Abnormality in fetal heart rate and rhythm complicating labor and delivery Ⓜ♀
Depressed fetal heart rate tones complicating labor and delivery
Fetal bradycardia complicating labor and delivery
Fetal heart rate abnormal variability complicating labor and delivery
Fetal heart rate decelerations complicating labor and delivery
Fetal heart rate irregularity complicating labor and delivery
Fetal tachycardia complicating labor and delivery
Non-reassuring fetal heart rate or rhythm complicating labor and delivery
EXCLUDES 1   fetal stress NOS (O77.9)
         labor and delivery complicated by electrocardiographic evidence of fetal stress (O77.8)
         labor and delivery complicated by ultrasonic evidence of fetal stress (O77.8)
EXCLUDES 2   fetal metabolic acidemia (O68)
         other fetal stress (O77.0-O77.1)
AHA: 2013, 4Q, 118

✓4ᵗʰ **O77 Other fetal stress complicating labor and delivery**
O77.0 Labor and delivery complicated by meconium in amniotic fluid Ⓜ♀
     AHA: 2013, 4Q, 117-118

O77.1 Fetal stress in labor or delivery due to drug administration Ⓜ♀

EXCLUDES 1 Not coded here   *EXCLUDES 2* Not included here   Ⓝ Newborn Age: 0   Ⓟ Pediatric Age: 0-17   Ⓜ Maternity Age: 12-55   Ⓐ Adult Age: 15-124

848   ICD-10-CM 2018

O77.8 Labor and delivery complicated by other evidence of fetal stress   Ⓜ♀
Labor and delivery complicated by electrocardiographic evidence of fetal stress
Labor and delivery complicated by ultrasonic evidence of fetal stress
EXCLUDES 1   *abnormality in fetal heart rate or rhythm (O76)*
abnormality of fetal acid-base balance (O68)
fetal metabolic acidemia (O68)

O77.9 Labor and delivery complicated by fetal stress, unspecified   Ⓜ♀▽
EXCLUDES 1   *abnormality in fetal heart rate or rhythm (O76)*
abnormality of fetal acid-base balance (O68)
fetal metabolic acidemia (O68)

Encounter for delivery (O80, O82)

O80 Encounter for full-term uncomplicated delivery   Ⓜ♀
NOTE   Delivery requiring minimal or no assistance, with or without episiotomy, without fetal manipulation [e.g., rotation version] or instrumentation [forceps] of a spontaneous, cephalic, vaginal, full-term, single, live-born infant. This code is for use as a single diagnosis code and is not to be used with any other code from chapter 15.
Use additional code to indicate outcome of delivery (Z37.0)
AHA: 2016, 4Q, 150; 2014, 2Q, 9

O82 Encounter for cesarean delivery without indication   Ⓜ♀
Use additional code to indicate outcome of delivery (Z37.0)

Complications predominantly related to the puerperium (O85-O92)

EXCLUDES 2   *mental and behavioral disorders associated with the puerperium (F53)*
obstetrical tetanus (A34)
puerperal osteomalacia (M83.0)

O85 Puerperal sepsis   Ⓜ♀
Postpartum sepsis
Puerperal peritonitis
Puerperal pyemia
Use additional code (B95-B97), to identify infectious agent
Use additional code (R65.2-) to identify severe sepsis, if applicable
EXCLUDES 1   *fever of unknown origin following delivery (O86.4)*
genital tract infection following delivery (O86.1-)
obstetric pyemic and septic embolism (O88.3-)
puerperal septic thrombophlebitis (O86.81)
urinary tract infection following delivery (O86.2-)
EXCLUDES 2   *sepsis during labor (O75.3)*

✓4ᵗʰ **O86 Other puerperal infections**
Use additional code (B95-B97), to identify infectious agent
EXCLUDES 2   *infection during labor (O75.3)*
obstetrical tetanus (A34)

O86.0 Infection of obstetric surgical wound   Ⓜ♀
Infected cesarean delivery wound following delivery
Infected perineal repair following delivery

✓5ᵗʰ **O86.1 Other infection of genital tract following delivery**
O86.11 Cervicitis following delivery   Ⓜ♀
O86.12 Endometritis following delivery   Ⓜ♀
O86.13 Vaginitis following delivery   Ⓜ♀
O86.19 Other infection of genital tract following delivery   Ⓜ♀

✓5ᵗʰ **O86.2 Urinary tract infection following delivery**
O86.20 Urinary tract infection following delivery, unspecified   Ⓜ♀▽
Puerperal urinary tract infection NOS
O86.21 Infection of kidney following delivery   Ⓜ♀
O86.22 Infection of bladder following delivery   Ⓜ♀
Infection of urethra following delivery
O86.29 Other urinary tract infection following delivery   Ⓜ♀

O86.4 Pyrexia of unknown origin following delivery   Ⓜ♀
Puerperal infection NOS following delivery
Puerperal pyrexia NOS following delivery
EXCLUDES 2   *pyrexia during labor (O75.2)*
DEF: Fever of unknown origin experienced by the mother after childbirth.

✓5ᵗʰ **O86.8 Other specified puerperal infections**
O86.81 Puerperal septic thrombophlebitis   Ⓜ♀
O86.89 Other specified puerperal infections   Ⓜ♀

✓4ᵗʰ **O87 Venous complications and hemorrhoids in the puerperium**
INCLUDES   venous complications in labor, delivery and the puerperium
EXCLUDES 2   *obstetric embolism (O88.-)*
puerperal septic thrombophlebitis (O86.81)
venous complications in pregnancy (O22.-)

O87.0 Superficial thrombophlebitis in the puerperium   Ⓜ♀
Puerperal phlebitis NOS
Puerperal thrombosis NOS

O87.1 Deep phlebothrombosis in the puerperium   Ⓜ♀
Deep vein thrombosis, postpartum
Pelvic thrombophlebitis, postpartum
Use additional code to identify the deep vein thrombosis (I82.4-, I82.5-, I82.62-. I82.72-)
Use additional code, if applicable, for associated long-term (current) use of anticoagulants (Z79.01)

O87.2 Hemorrhoids in the puerperium   Ⓜ♀
O87.3 Cerebral venous thrombosis in the puerperium   Ⓜ♀
Cerebrovenous sinus thrombosis in the puerperium
O87.4 Varicose veins of lower extremity in the puerperium   Ⓜ♀
O87.8 Other venous complications in the puerperium   Ⓜ♀
Genital varices in the puerperium
O87.9 Venous complication in the puerperium, unspecified   Ⓜ♀▽
Puerperal phlebopathy NOS

✓4ᵗʰ **O88 Obstetric embolism**
EXCLUDES 1   *embolism complicating abortion NOS (O03.2)*
embolism complicating ectopic or molar pregnancy (O08.2)
embolism complicating failed attempted abortion (O07.2)
embolism complicating induced abortion (O04.7)
embolism complicating spontaneous abortion (O03.2, O03.7)

✓5ᵗʰ **O88.0 Obstetric air embolism**
DEF: Sudden blocking of pulmonary artery or right ventricle with air or nitrogen bubbles.

✓6ᵗʰ **O88.01 Obstetric air embolism in pregnancy**
O88.011 Air embolism in pregnancy, first trimester   Ⓜ♀
O88.012 Air embolism in pregnancy, second trimester   Ⓜ♀
O88.013 Air embolism in pregnancy, third trimester   Ⓜ♀
O88.019 Air embolism in pregnancy, unspecified trimester   Ⓜ♀▽

O88.02 Air embolism in childbirth   Ⓜ♀
O88.03 Air embolism in the puerperium   Ⓜ♀

✓5ᵗʰ **O88.1 Amniotic fluid embolism**
Anaphylactoid syndrome in pregnancy

✓6ᵗʰ **O88.11 Amniotic fluid embolism in pregnancy**
O88.111 Amniotic fluid embolism in pregnancy, first trimester   Ⓜ♀
O88.112 Amniotic fluid embolism in pregnancy, second trimester   Ⓜ♀
O88.113 Amniotic fluid embolism in pregnancy, third trimester   Ⓜ♀
O88.119 Amniotic fluid embolism in pregnancy, unspecified trimester   Ⓜ♀▽

O88.12 Amniotic fluid embolism in childbirth   Ⓜ♀
O88.13 Amniotic fluid embolism in the puerperium   Ⓜ♀

✓5ᵗʰ **O88.2 Obstetric thromboembolism**

✓6ᵗʰ **O88.21 Thromboembolism in pregnancy**
Obstetric (pulmonary) embolism NOS
O88.211 Thromboembolism in pregnancy, first trimester   Ⓜ♀
O88.212 Thromboembolism in pregnancy, second trimester   Ⓜ♀
O88.213 Thromboembolism in pregnancy, third trimester   Ⓜ♀
O88.219 Thromboembolism in pregnancy, unspecified trimester   Ⓜ♀▽

O88.22 Thromboembolism in childbirth   Ⓜ♀
O88.23 Thromboembolism in the puerperium   Ⓜ♀
Puerperal (pulmonary) embolism NOS

✓5ᵗʰ **O88.3 Obstetric pyemic and septic embolism**

✓6ᵗʰ **O88.31 Pyemic and septic embolism in pregnancy**
O88.311 Pyemic and septic embolism in pregnancy, first trimester   Ⓜ♀
O88.312 Pyemic and septic embolism in pregnancy, second trimester   Ⓜ♀

☑ Additional Character Req   ☑x7ᵗʰ Placeholder Alert   Manifestation   HCC CMS-HCC Condition   ▽ Unspecified Code   ►◄ Revised Text   ● New Code   ▲ Revised Code Title

O88.313 **Pyemic and septic embolism in pregnancy,** third trimester   Ⓜ♀

O88.319 **Pyemic and septic embolism in pregnancy, unspecified trimester**   Ⓜ♀▽

O88.32 **Pyemic and septic embolism in** childbirth   Ⓜ♀

O88.33 **Pyemic and septic embolism in the** puerperium   Ⓜ♀

✓5ᵗʰ O88.8 **Other obstetric embolism**
Obstetric fat embolism

✓6ᵗʰ O88.81 **Other embolism in** pregnancy

O88.811 **Other embolism in pregnancy,** first trimester   Ⓜ♀

O88.812 **Other embolism in pregnancy,** second trimester   Ⓜ♀

O88.813 **Other embolism in pregnancy,** third trimester   Ⓜ♀

O88.819 **Other embolism in pregnancy, unspecified trimester**   Ⓜ♀▽

O88.82 **Other embolism in** childbirth   Ⓜ♀

O88.83 **Other embolism in the** puerperium   Ⓜ♀

✓4ᵗʰ O89 **Complications of anesthesia during the puerperium**
INCLUDES maternal complications arising from the administration of a general, regional or local anesthetic, analgesic or other sedation during the puerperium
Use additional code, if applicable, to identify specific complication

✓5ᵗʰ O89.0 **Pulmonary complications of anesthesia during the puerperium**

O89.01 **Aspiration pneumonitis due to anesthesia during the puerperium**   Ⓜ♀
Inhalation of stomach contents or secretions NOS due to anesthesia during the puerperium
Mendelson's syndrome due to anesthesia during the puerperium

O89.09 **Other pulmonary complications of anesthesia during the puerperium**   Ⓜ♀

O89.1 **Cardiac complications of anesthesia during the puerperium**   Ⓜ♀

O89.2 **Central nervous system complications of anesthesia during the puerperium**   Ⓜ♀

O89.3 **Toxic reaction to local anesthesia during the puerperium**   Ⓜ♀

O89.4 **Spinal and epidural anesthesia-induced headache during the puerperium**   Ⓜ♀

O89.5 **Other complications of spinal and epidural anesthesia during the puerperium**   Ⓜ♀

O89.6 **Failed or difficult intubation for anesthesia during the puerperium**   Ⓜ♀

O89.8 **Other complications of anesthesia during the puerperium**   Ⓜ♀

O89.9 **Complication of anesthesia during the puerperium, unspecified**   Ⓜ♀▽

✓4ᵗʰ O90 **Complications of the puerperium, not elsewhere classified**

O90.0 **Disruption of cesarean delivery wound**   Ⓜ♀
Dehiscence of cesarean delivery wound
EXCLUDES 1 rupture of uterus (spontaneous) before onset of labor (O71.0-)
rupture of uterus during labor (O71.1)

O90.1 **Disruption of perineal obstetric wound**   Ⓜ♀
Disruption of wound of episiotomy
Disruption of wound of perineal laceration
Secondary perineal tear

O90.2 **Hematoma of obstetric wound**   Ⓜ♀

O90.3 **Peripartum cardiomyopathy**   Ⓜ♀
Conditions in I42- arising during pregnancy and the puerperium
EXCLUDES 1 pre-existing heart disease complicating pregnancy and the puerperium (O99.4-)
DEF: Any structural or functional abnormality of the ventricular myocardium, noninflammatory disease of obscure or unknown etiology with onset during the postpartum period.

O90.4 **Postpartum acute kidney failure**   Ⓜ♀
Hepatorenal syndrome following labor and delivery

O90.5 **Postpartum thyroiditis**   Ⓜ♀

O90.6 **Postpartum mood disturbance**   Ⓜ♀
Postpartum blues
Postpartum dysphoria
Postpartum sadness
EXCLUDES 1 postpartum depression (F53)
puerperal psychosis (F53)

✓5ᵗʰ O90.8 **Other complications of the puerperium, not elsewhere classified**

O90.81 **Anemia of the puerperium**   Ⓜ♀
Postpartum anemia NOS
EXCLUDES 1 pre-existing anemia complicating the puerperium (O99.03)

O90.89 **Other complications of the puerperium, not elsewhere classified**   Ⓜ♀
Placental polyp

O90.9 **Complication of the puerperium, unspecified**   Ⓜ♀▽

✓4ᵗʰ O91 **Infections of breast associated with pregnancy, the puerperium and lactation**
Use additional code to identify infection

✓5ᵗʰ O91.0 **Infection of nipple associated with pregnancy, the puerperium and lactation**

✓6ᵗʰ O91.01 **Infection of nipple associated with** pregnancy
Gestational abscess of nipple

O91.011 **Infection of nipple associated with pregnancy,** first trimester   Ⓜ♀

O91.012 **Infection of nipple associated with pregnancy,** second trimester   Ⓜ♀

O91.013 **Infection of nipple associated with pregnancy,** third trimester   Ⓜ♀

O91.019 **Infection of nipple associated with pregnancy, unspecified trimester**   Ⓜ♀▽

O91.02 **Infection of nipple associated with the** puerperium   Ⓜ♀
Puerperal abscess of nipple

O91.03 **Infection of nipple associated with** lactation   Ⓜ♀
Abscess of nipple associated with lactation

✓5ᵗʰ O91.1 **Abscess of breast associated with pregnancy, the puerperium and lactation**

✓6ᵗʰ O91.11 **Abscess of breast associated with** pregnancy
Gestational mammary abscess
Gestational purulent mastitis
Gestational subareolar abscess

O91.111 **Abscess of breast associated with pregnancy,** first trimester   Ⓜ♀

O91.112 **Abscess of breast associated with pregnancy,** second trimester   Ⓜ♀

O91.113 **Abscess of breast associated with pregnancy,** third trimester   Ⓜ♀

O91.119 **Abscess of breast associated with pregnancy, unspecified trimester**   Ⓜ♀▽

O91.12 **Abscess of breast associated with the** puerperium   Ⓜ♀
Puerperal mammary abscess
Puerperal purulent mastitis
Puerperal subareolar abscess

O91.13 **Abscess of breast associated with** lactation   Ⓜ♀
Mammary abscess associated with lactation
Purulent mastitis associated with lactation
Subareolar abscess associated with lactation

✓5ᵗʰ O91.2 **Nonpurulent mastitis associated with pregnancy, the puerperium and lactation**

✓6ᵗʰ O91.21 **Nonpurulent mastitis associated with** pregnancy
Gestational interstitial mastitis
Gestational lymphangitis of breast
Gestational mastitis NOS
Gestational parenchymatous mastitis

O91.211 **Nonpurulent mastitis associated with pregnancy,** first trimester   Ⓜ♀

O91.212 **Nonpurulent mastitis associated with pregnancy,** second trimester   Ⓜ♀

O91.213 **Nonpurulent mastitis associated with pregnancy,** third trimester   Ⓜ♀

O91.219 **Nonpurulent mastitis associated with pregnancy, unspecified trimester**   Ⓜ♀▽

O91.22 **Nonpurulent mastitis associated with the** puerperium   Ⓜ♀
Puerperal interstitial mastitis
Puerperal lymphangitis of breast
Puerperal mastitis NOS
Puerperal parenchymatous mastitis

O91.23 **Nonpurulent mastitis associated with** lactation   Ⓜ♀
Interstitial mastitis associated with lactation
Lymphangitis of breast associated with lactation
Mastitis NOS associated with lactation
Parenchymatous mastitis associated with lactation

✓4ᵗʰ **O92** **Other disorders of breast and disorders of lactation associated with pregnancy and the puerperium**

  ✓5ᵗʰ **O92.0** **Retracted nipple associated with pregnancy, the puerperium, and lactation**

    ✓6ᵗʰ **O92.01** **Retracted nipple associated with** pregnancy

      O92.011 **Retracted nipple associated with pregnancy, first trimester** Ⓜ♀

      O92.012 **Retracted nipple associated with pregnancy, second trimester** Ⓜ♀

      O92.013 **Retracted nipple associated with pregnancy, third trimester** Ⓜ♀

      O92.019 **Retracted nipple associated with pregnancy, unspecified trimester** Ⓜ♀▽

    O92.02 **Retracted nipple associated with the** puerperium Ⓜ♀

    O92.03 **Retracted nipple associated with** lactation Ⓜ♀

  ✓5ᵗʰ **O92.1** **Cracked nipple associated with pregnancy, the puerperium, and lactation**

    Fissure of nipple, gestational or puerperal

    ✓6ᵗʰ **O92.11** **Cracked nipple associated with** pregnancy

      O92.111 **Cracked nipple associated with pregnancy, first trimester** Ⓜ♀

      O92.112 **Cracked nipple associated with pregnancy, second trimester** Ⓜ♀

      O92.113 **Cracked nipple associated with pregnancy, third trimester** Ⓜ♀

      O92.119 **Cracked nipple associated with pregnancy, unspecified trimester** Ⓜ♀▽

    O92.12 **Cracked nipple associated with the** puerperium Ⓜ♀

    O92.13 **Cracked nipple associated with** lactation Ⓜ♀

  ✓5ᵗʰ **O92.2** **Other and unspecified disorders of breast associated with pregnancy and the puerperium**

    O92.20 **Unspecified disorder of breast associated with pregnancy and the puerperium** Ⓜ♀▽

    O92.29 **Other disorders of breast associated with pregnancy and the puerperium** Ⓜ♀

  O92.3 **Agalactia** Ⓜ♀

    Primary agalactia

    EXCLUDES 1 elective agalactia (O92.5)
        secondary agalactia (O92.5)
        therapeutic agalactia (O92.5)

    DEF: Absence of milk secretion in a female after delivery.

  O92.4 **Hypogalactia** Ⓜ♀

  O92.5 **Suppressed lactation** Ⓜ♀

    Elective agalactia
    Secondary agalactia
    Therapeutic agalactia
    EXCLUDES 1 primary agalactia (O92.3)

  O92.6 **Galactorrhea** Ⓜ♀

    DEF: Excessive or persistent milk secretion by breast; may occur in absence of nursing.

  ✓5ᵗʰ **O92.7** **Other and unspecified disorders of lactation**

    O92.70 **Unspecified disorders of lactation** Ⓜ♀▽

    O92.79 **Other disorders of lactation** Ⓜ♀
      Puerperal galactocele

Other obstetric conditions, not elsewhere classified (O94-O9A)

O94 **Sequelae of complication of pregnancy, childbirth, and the puerperium** Ⓜ♀

  NOTE This category is to be used to indicate conditions in O00-O77.-, O85-O94 and O98-O9A.- as the cause of late effects. The sequelae include conditions specified as such, or as late effects, which may occur at any time after the puerperium.

  Code first condition resulting from (sequela) of complication of pregnancy, childbirth, and the puerperium

✓4ᵗʰ **O98** **Maternal infectious and parasitic diseases classifiable elsewhere but complicating pregnancy, childbirth and the puerperium**

  INCLUDES the listed conditions when complicating the pregnant state, when aggravated by the pregnancy, or as a reason for obstetric care

  Use additional code (Chapter 1), to identify specific infectious or parasitic disease

  EXCLUDES 2 herpes gestationis (O26.4-)
        infectious carrier state (O99.82-, O99.83-)
        obstetrical tetanus (A34)
        puerperal infection (O86.-)
        puerperal sepsis (O85)
        when the reason for maternal care is that the disease is known or suspected to have affected the fetus (O35-O36)

  ✓5ᵗʰ **O98.0** **Tuberculosis complicating pregnancy, childbirth and the puerperium**

    Conditions in A15-A19

    ✓6ᵗʰ **O98.01** **Tuberculosis complicating** pregnancy

      O98.011 **Tuberculosis complicating pregnancy, first trimester** Ⓜ♀

      O98.012 **Tuberculosis complicating pregnancy, second trimester** Ⓜ♀

      O98.013 **Tuberculosis complicating pregnancy, third trimester** Ⓜ♀

      O98.019 **Tuberculosis complicating pregnancy, unspecified trimester** Ⓜ♀▽

    O98.02 **Tuberculosis complicating** childbirth Ⓜ♀

    O98.03 **Tuberculosis complicating the** puerperium Ⓜ♀

  ✓5ᵗʰ **O98.1** **Syphilis complicating pregnancy, childbirth and the puerperium**

    Conditions in A50-A53

    ✓6ᵗʰ **O98.11** **Syphilis complicating** pregnancy

      O98.111 **Syphilis complicating pregnancy, first trimester** Ⓜ♀

      O98.112 **Syphilis complicating pregnancy, second trimester** Ⓜ♀

      O98.113 **Syphilis complicating pregnancy, third trimester** Ⓜ♀

      O98.119 **Syphilis complicating pregnancy, unspecified trimester** Ⓜ♀▽

    O98.12 **Syphilis complicating** childbirth Ⓜ♀

    O98.13 **Syphilis complicating the** puerperium Ⓜ♀

  ✓5ᵗʰ **O98.2** **Gonorrhea complicating pregnancy, childbirth and the puerperium**

    Conditions in A54-

    ✓6ᵗʰ **O98.21** **Gonorrhea complicating** pregnancy

      O98.211 **Gonorrhea complicating pregnancy, first trimester** Ⓜ♀

      O98.212 **Gonorrhea complicating pregnancy, second trimester** Ⓜ♀

      O98.213 **Gonorrhea complicating pregnancy, third trimester** Ⓜ♀

      O98.219 **Gonorrhea complicating pregnancy, ▽ unspecified trimester** Ⓜ♀

    O98.22 **Gonorrhea complicating** childbirth Ⓜ♀

    O98.23 **Gonorrhea complicating the** puerperium Ⓜ♀

  ✓5ᵗʰ **O98.3** **Other infections with a predominantly sexual mode of transmission complicating pregnancy, childbirth and the puerperium**

    Conditions in A55-A64

    ✓6ᵗʰ **O98.31** **Other infections with a predominantly sexual mode of transmission complicating** pregnancy

      O98.311 **Other infections with a predominantly sexual mode of transmission complicating pregnancy, first trimester** Ⓜ♀

      O98.312 **Other infections with a predominantly sexual mode of transmission complicating pregnancy, second trimester** Ⓜ♀

      O98.313 **Other infections with a predominantly sexual mode of transmission complicating pregnancy, third trimester** Ⓜ♀

      O98.319 **Other infections with a predominantly sexual mode of transmission complicating pregnancy, unspecified trimester** Ⓜ♀▽

☑ Additional Character Req ✓x7ᵗʰ Placeholder Alert Manifestation **HCC** CMS-HCC Condition ▽ Unspecified Code ▶◀ Revised Text ● New Code ▲ Revised Code Title

Chapter 15. Pregnancy, Childbirth, and the Puerperium

O98.32–O99.1

O98.32   **Other infections with a predominantly sexual mode of transmission complicating** childbirth   Ⓜ♀

O98.33   **Other infections with a predominantly sexual mode of transmission complicating the** puerperium   Ⓜ♀

✓5ᵗʰ **O98.4**   Viral hepatitis **complicating pregnancy, childbirth and the puerperium**
     Conditions in B15-B19

    ✓6ᵗʰ **O98.41**   **Viral hepatitis complicating** pregnancy

       O98.411   **Viral hepatitis complicating pregnancy,** first trimester   Ⓜ♀

       O98.412   **Viral hepatitis complicating pregnancy,** second trimester   Ⓜ♀

       O98.413   **Viral hepatitis complicating pregnancy,** third trimester   Ⓜ♀

       O98.419   **Viral hepatitis complicating pregnancy, unspecified trimester**   Ⓜ♀▽

    O98.42   **Viral hepatitis complicating** childbirth   Ⓜ♀

    O98.43   **Viral hepatitis complicating the** puerperium   Ⓜ♀

✓5ᵗʰ **O98.5**   **Other viral diseases complicating pregnancy, childbirth and the puerperium**
     Conditions in A80-B09, B25-B34, R87.81-, R87.82-
      EXCLUDES 1   *human immunodeficiency virus [HIV] disease complicating pregnancy, childbirth and the puerperium (O98.7-)*

    ✓6ᵗʰ **O98.51**   **Other viral diseases complicating** pregnancy

       O98.511   **Other viral diseases complicating pregnancy,** first trimester   Ⓜ♀

       O98.512   **Other viral diseases complicating pregnancy,** second trimester   Ⓜ♀

       O98.513   **Other viral diseases complicating pregnancy,** third trimester   Ⓜ♀

       O98.519   **Other viral diseases complicating pregnancy, unspecified trimester**   Ⓜ♀▽

    O98.52   **Other viral diseases complicating** childbirth   Ⓜ♀

    O98.53   **Other viral diseases complicating the** puerperium   Ⓜ♀

✓5ᵗʰ **O98.6**   Protozoal diseases **complicating pregnancy, childbirth and the puerperium**
     Conditions in B50-B64

    ✓6ᵗʰ **O98.61**   **Protozoal diseases complicating** pregnancy

       O98.611   **Protozoal diseases complicating pregnancy,** first trimester   Ⓜ♀

       O98.612   **Protozoal diseases complicating pregnancy,** second trimester   Ⓜ♀

       O98.613   **Protozoal diseases complicating pregnancy,** third trimester   Ⓜ♀

       O98.619   **Protozoal diseases complicating pregnancy, unspecified trimester**   Ⓜ♀▽

    O98.62   **Protozoal diseases complicating** childbirth   Ⓜ♀

    O98.63   **Protozoal diseases complicating the** puerperium   Ⓜ♀

✓5ᵗʰ **O98.7**   Human immunodeficiency virus [HIV] disease **complicating pregnancy, childbirth and the puerperium**
     Use additional code to identify the type of HIV disease:
      acquired immune deficiency syndrome (AIDS) (B20)
      asymptomatic HIV status (Z21)
      HIV positive NOS (Z21)
      symptomatic HIV disease (B20)

    ✓6ᵗʰ **O98.71**   **Human immunodeficiency virus [HIV] disease complicating** pregnancy

       O98.711   **Human immunodeficiency virus [HIV] disease complicating pregnancy,** first trimester   Ⓜ♀

       O98.712   **Human immunodeficiency virus [HIV] disease complicating pregnancy,** second trimester   Ⓜ♀

       O98.713   **Human immunodeficiency virus [HIV] disease complicating pregnancy,** third trimester   Ⓜ♀

       O98.719   **Human immunodeficiency virus [HIV] disease complicating pregnancy, unspecified trimester**   Ⓜ♀▽

    O98.72   **Human immunodeficiency virus [HIV] disease complicating** childbirth   Ⓜ♀

    O98.73   **Human immunodeficiency virus [HIV] disease complicating the** puerperium   Ⓜ♀

✓5ᵗʰ **O98.8**   **Other maternal infectious and parasitic diseases complicating pregnancy, childbirth and the puerperium**

    ✓6ᵗʰ **O98.81**   **Other maternal infectious and parasitic diseases complicating** pregnancy

       O98.811   **Other maternal infectious and parasitic diseases complicating pregnancy,** first trimester   Ⓜ♀

       O98.812   **Other maternal infectious and parasitic diseases complicating pregnancy,** second trimester   Ⓜ♀

       O98.813   **Other maternal infectious and parasitic diseases complicating pregnancy,** third trimester   Ⓜ♀

       O98.819   **Other maternal infectious and parasitic diseases complicating pregnancy, unspecified trimester**   Ⓜ♀▽

    O98.82   **Other maternal infectious and parasitic diseases complicating** childbirth   Ⓜ♀

    O98.83   **Other maternal infectious and parasitic diseases complicating the** puerperium   Ⓜ♀

✓5ᵗʰ **O98.9**   **Unspecified maternal infectious and parasitic disease complicating pregnancy, childbirth and the puerperium**

    ✓6ᵗʰ **O98.91**   **Unspecified maternal infectious and parasitic disease complicating** pregnancy

       O98.911   **Unspecified maternal infectious and parasitic disease complicating pregnancy,** first trimester   Ⓜ♀▽

       O98.912   **Unspecified maternal infectious and parasitic disease complicating pregnancy,** second trimester   Ⓜ♀▽

       O98.913   **Unspecified maternal infectious and parasitic disease complicating pregnancy,** third trimester   Ⓜ♀▽

       O98.919   **Unspecified maternal infectious and parasitic disease complicating pregnancy, unspecified trimester**   Ⓜ♀▽

    O98.92   **Unspecified maternal infectious and parasitic disease complicating** childbirth   Ⓜ♀▽

    O98.93   **Unspecified maternal infectious and parasitic disease complicating the** puerperium   Ⓜ♀▽

✓4ᵗʰ **O99**   **Other maternal diseases classifiable elsewhere but complicating pregnancy, childbirth and the puerperium**
     INCLUDES   conditions which complicate the pregnant state, are aggravated by the pregnancy or are a main reason for obstetric care
     Use additional code to identify specific condition
     EXCLUDES 2   *when the reason for maternal care is that the condition is known or suspected to have affected the fetus (O35-O36)*

   ✓5ᵗʰ **O99.0**   Anemia **complicating pregnancy, childbirth and the puerperium**
     Conditions in D50-D64
      EXCLUDES 1   *anemia arising in the puerperium (O90.81) postpartum anemia NOS (O90.81)*

    ✓6ᵗʰ **O99.01**   **Anemia complicating** pregnancy
       AHA: 2016, 1Q, 4

       O99.011   **Anemia complicating pregnancy,** first trimester   Ⓜ♀

       O99.012   **Anemia complicating pregnancy,** second trimester   Ⓜ♀

       O99.013   **Anemia complicating pregnancy,** third trimester   Ⓜ♀

       O99.019   **Anemia complicating pregnancy, unspecified trimester**   Ⓜ♀▽

    O99.02   **Anemia complicating** childbirth   Ⓜ♀

    O99.03   **Anemia complicating the** puerperium   Ⓜ♀
      EXCLUDES 1   *postpartum anemia not pre-existing prior to delivery (O90.81)*

   ✓5ᵗʰ **O99.1**   **Other diseases of the** blood and blood-forming organs and certain disorders involving the immune mechanism **complicating pregnancy, childbirth and the puerperium**
     Conditions in D65-D89
      EXCLUDES 1 ▶*hemorrhage with coagulation defects (O45.-, O46.0-, O67.0, O72.3)*◀
      EXCLUDES 2   ~~*hemorrhage with coagulation defects (O45.-, O46.0-, O67.0, O72.3)*~~

EXCLUDES 1 Not coded here   EXCLUDES 2 Not included here   Ⓝ Newborn Age: 0   Ⓟ Pediatric Age: 0-17   Ⓜ Maternity Age: 12-55   Ⓐ Adult Age: 15-124

852   ICD-10-CM 2018

✓6ᵗʰ **O99.11** **Other diseases of the blood and blood-forming organs and certain disorders involving the immune mechanism complicating** pregnancy

    O99.111 **Other diseases of the blood and blood-forming organs and certain disorders involving the immune mechanism complicating pregnancy, first trimester** Ⓜ♀

    O99.112 **Other diseases of the blood and blood-forming organs and certain disorders involving the immune mechanism complicating pregnancy, second trimester** Ⓜ♀

    O99.113 **Other diseases of the blood and blood-forming organs and certain disorders involving the immune mechanism complicating pregnancy, third trimester** Ⓜ♀

    O99.119 **Other diseases of the blood and blood-forming organs and certain disorders involving the immune mechanism complicating pregnancy, unspecified trimester** Ⓜ♀▽

O99.12 **Other diseases of the blood and blood-forming organs and certain disorders involving the immune mechanism complicating** childbirth Ⓜ♀

O99.13 **Other diseases of the blood and blood-forming organs and certain disorders involving the immune mechanism complicating the** puerperium Ⓜ♀

✓5ᵗʰ **O99.2** Endocrine, nutritional and metabolic diseases **complicating pregnancy, childbirth and the puerperium**
    Conditions in E00-E88
    EXCLUDES 2   *diabetes mellitus (O24.-)*
                malnutrition (O25.-)
                postpartum thyroiditis (O90.5)

✓6ᵗʰ **O99.21** Obesity **complicating pregnancy, childbirth, and the puerperium**
    Use additional code to identify the type of obesity (E66.-)

    O99.210 **Obesity complicating pregnancy, unspecified trimester** Ⓜ♀▽

    O99.211 **Obesity complicating pregnancy, first trimester** Ⓜ♀

    O99.212 **Obesity complicating pregnancy, second trimester** Ⓜ♀

    O99.213 **Obesity complicating pregnancy, third trimester** Ⓜ♀

    O99.214 **Obesity complicating** childbirth Ⓜ♀

    O99.215 **Obesity complicating the** puerperium Ⓜ♀

✓6ᵗʰ **O99.28** **Other endocrine, nutritional and metabolic diseases complicating pregnancy, childbirth and the puerperium**

    O99.280 **Endocrine, nutritional and metabolic diseases complicating pregnancy, unspecified trimester** Ⓜ♀▽

    O99.281 **Endocrine, nutritional and metabolic diseases complicating pregnancy, first trimester** Ⓜ♀

    O99.282 **Endocrine, nutritional and metabolic diseases complicating pregnancy, second trimester** Ⓜ♀

    O99.283 **Endocrine, nutritional and metabolic diseases complicating pregnancy, third trimester** Ⓜ♀

    O99.284 **Endocrine, nutritional and metabolic diseases complicating** childbirth Ⓜ♀

    O99.285 **Endocrine, nutritional and metabolic diseases complicating the** puerperium Ⓜ♀

✓5ᵗʰ **O99.3** Mental disorders **and diseases of the** nervous system **complicating pregnancy, childbirth and the puerperium**

✓6ᵗʰ **O99.31** Alcohol use **complicating pregnancy, childbirth, and the puerperium**
    Use additional code(s) from F10 to identify manifestations of the alcohol use

    O99.310 **Alcohol use complicating pregnancy, unspecified trimester** Ⓜ♀▽

    O99.311 **Alcohol use complicating pregnancy, first trimester** Ⓜ♀

    O99.312 **Alcohol use complicating pregnancy, second trimester** Ⓜ♀

    O99.313 **Alcohol use complicating pregnancy, third trimester** Ⓜ♀

    O99.314 **Alcohol use complicating** childbirth Ⓜ♀

    O99.315 **Alcohol use complicating the puerperium** Ⓜ♀

✓6ᵗʰ **O99.32** Drug use **complicating pregnancy, childbirth, and the puerperium**
    Use additional code(s) from F11-F16 and F18-F19 to identify manifestations of the drug use

    O99.320 **Drug use complicating pregnancy, unspecified trimester** Ⓜ♀▽

    O99.321 **Drug use complicating pregnancy, first trimester** Ⓜ♀

    O99.322 **Drug use complicating pregnancy, second trimester** Ⓜ♀

    O99.323 **Drug use complicating pregnancy, third trimester** Ⓜ♀

    O99.324 **Drug use complicating** childbirth Ⓜ♀

    O99.325 **Drug use complicating the** puerperium Ⓜ♀

✓6ᵗʰ **O99.33** Tobacco use disorder **complicating pregnancy, childbirth, and the puerperium**
    Smoking complicating pregnancy, childbirth, and the puerperium
    Use additional code from category F17 to identify type of tobacco nicotine dependence

    O99.330 **Smoking (tobacco) complicating pregnancy, unspecified trimester** Ⓜ♀▽

    O99.331 **Smoking (tobacco) complicating pregnancy,** first trimester Ⓜ♀

    O99.332 **Smoking (tobacco) complicating pregnancy,** second trimester Ⓜ♀

    O99.333 **Smoking (tobacco) complicating pregnancy,** third trimester Ⓜ♀

    O99.334 **Smoking (tobacco) complicating** childbirth Ⓜ♀

    O99.335 **Smoking (tobacco) complicating the** puerperium Ⓜ♀

✓6ᵗʰ **O99.34** Other mental disorders **complicating pregnancy, childbirth, and the puerperium**
    Conditions in F01-F09 and F20-F99
    EXCLUDES 2   *postpartum mood disturbance (O90.6)*
                postnatal psychosis (F53)
                puerperal psychosis (F53)

    O99.340 **Other mental disorders complicating pregnancy, unspecified trimester** Ⓜ♀▽

    O99.341 **Other mental disorders complicating pregnancy,** first trimester Ⓜ♀

    O99.342 **Other mental disorders complicating pregnancy,** second trimester Ⓜ♀

    O99.343 **Other mental disorders complicating pregnancy,** third trimester Ⓜ♀

    O99.344 **Other mental disorders complicating** childbirth Ⓜ♀

    O99.345 **Other mental disorders complicating the** puerperium Ⓜ♀

✓6ᵗʰ **O99.35** Diseases of the nervous system **complicating pregnancy, childbirth, and the puerperium**
    Conditions in G00-G99
    EXCLUDES 2   *pregnancy related peripheral neuritis (O26.8-)*

    O99.350 **Diseases of the nervous system complicating pregnancy, unspecified trimester** Ⓜ♀▽

    O99.351 **Diseases of the nervous system complicating pregnancy,** first trimester Ⓜ♀

    O99.352 **Diseases of the nervous system complicating pregnancy,** second trimester Ⓜ♀

    O99.353 **Diseases of the nervous system complicating pregnancy,** third trimester Ⓜ♀

    O99.354 **Diseases of the nervous system complicating** childbirth Ⓜ♀

    O99.355 **Diseases of the nervous system complicating the** puerperium Ⓜ♀

✓ Additional Character Req   ✓7ᵗʰ Placeholder Alert   Manifestation   HCC CMS-HCC Condition   ▽ Unspecified Code   ►◄ Revised Text   ● New Code   ▲ Revised Code Title

✓5ᵗʰ **O99.4 Diseases of the circulatory system complicating pregnancy, childbirth and the puerperium**
Conditions in I00-I99

EXCLUDES 1   *peripartum cardiomyopathy (O90.3)*
EXCLUDES 2   *hypertensive disorders (O10-O16)*
obstetric embolism (O88.-)
venous complications and cerebrovenous sinus thrombosis in labor, childbirth and the puerperium (O87.-)
venous complications and cerebrovenous sinus thrombosis in pregnancy (O22.-)

AHA: 2016, 2Q, 8

✓6ᵗʰ **O99.41 Diseases of the circulatory system complicating pregnancy**

    O99.411 Diseases of the circulatory system complicating pregnancy, first trimester Ⓜ♀

    O99.412 Diseases of the circulatory system complicating pregnancy, second trimester Ⓜ♀

    O99.413 Diseases of the circulatory system complicating pregnancy, third trimester Ⓜ♀

    O99.419 Diseases of the circulatory system complicating pregnancy, unspecified trimester Ⓜ♀▽

O99.42 Diseases of the circulatory system complicating childbirth Ⓜ♀

O99.43 Diseases of the circulatory system complicating the puerperium Ⓜ♀

✓5ᵗʰ **O99.5 Diseases of the respiratory system complicating pregnancy, childbirth and the puerperium**
Conditions in J00-J99

✓6ᵗʰ **O99.51 Diseases of the respiratory system complicating pregnancy**

    O99.511 Diseases of the respiratory system complicating pregnancy, first trimester Ⓜ♀

    O99.512 Diseases of the respiratory system complicating pregnancy, second trimester Ⓜ♀

    O99.513 Diseases of the respiratory system complicating pregnancy, third trimester Ⓜ♀

    O99.519 Diseases of the respiratory system complicating pregnancy, unspecified trimester Ⓜ♀▽

O99.52 Diseases of the respiratory system complicating childbirth Ⓜ♀

O99.53 Diseases of the respiratory system complicating the puerperium Ⓜ♀

✓5ᵗʰ **O99.6 Diseases of the digestive system complicating pregnancy, childbirth and the puerperium**
Conditions in K00-K93

EXCLUDES 2   *hemorrhoids in pregnancy (O22.4-)*
liver and biliary tract disorders in pregnancy, childbirth and the puerperium (O26.6-)

✓6ᵗʰ **O99.61 Diseases of the digestive system complicating pregnancy**
AHA: 2016, 1Q, 4

    O99.611 Diseases of the digestive system complicating pregnancy, first trimester Ⓜ♀

    O99.612 Diseases of the digestive system complicating pregnancy, second trimester Ⓜ♀

    O99.613 Diseases of the digestive system complicating pregnancy, third trimester Ⓜ♀

    O99.619 Diseases of the digestive system complicating pregnancy, unspecified trimester Ⓜ♀▽

O99.62 Diseases of the digestive system complicating childbirth Ⓜ♀

O99.63 Diseases of the digestive system complicating the puerperium Ⓜ♀

✓5ᵗʰ **O99.7 Diseases of the skin and subcutaneous tissue complicating pregnancy, childbirth and the puerperium**
Conditions in L00-L99

EXCLUDES 2   *herpes gestationis (O26.4)*
pruritic urticarial papules and plaques of pregnancy (PUPPP) (O26.86)

✓6ᵗʰ **O99.71 Diseases of the skin and subcutaneous tissue complicating pregnancy**

    O99.711 Diseases of the skin and subcutaneous tissue complicating pregnancy, first trimester Ⓜ♀

    O99.712 Diseases of the skin and subcutaneous tissue complicating pregnancy, second trimester Ⓜ♀

    O99.713 Diseases of the skin and subcutaneous tissue complicating pregnancy, third trimester Ⓜ♀

    O99.719 Diseases of the skin and subcutaneous tissue complicating pregnancy, unspecified trimester Ⓜ♀▽

O99.72 Diseases of the skin and subcutaneous tissue complicating childbirth Ⓜ♀

O99.73 Diseases of the skin and subcutaneous tissue complicating the puerperium Ⓜ♀

✓5ᵗʰ **O99.8 Other specified diseases and conditions complicating pregnancy, childbirth and the puerperium**
Conditions in D00-D48, H00-H95, M00-N99, and Q00-Q99
Use additional code to identify condition

EXCLUDES 2   *genitourinary infections in pregnancy (O23.-)*
infection of genitourinary tract following delivery (O86.1-O86.3)
malignant neoplasm complicating pregnancy, childbirth and the puerperium (O9A.1-)
maternal care for known or suspected abnormality of maternal pelvic organs (O34.-)
postpartum acute kidney failure (O90.4)
traumatic injuries in pregnancy (O9A.2)

✓6ᵗʰ **O99.81 Abnormal glucose complicating pregnancy, childbirth and the puerperium**
EXCLUDES 1   *gestational diabetes (O24.4-)*

    O99.810 Abnormal glucose complicating pregnancy Ⓜ♀

    O99.814 Abnormal glucose complicating childbirth Ⓜ♀

    O99.815 Abnormal glucose complicating the puerperium Ⓜ♀

✓6ᵗʰ **O99.82 Streptococcus B carrier state complicating pregnancy, childbirth and the puerperium**
EXCLUDES 1   *carrier of streptococcus group B (GBS) in a nonpregnant woman (Z22.330)*

    O99.820 Streptococcus B carrier state complicating pregnancy Ⓜ♀

    O99.824 Streptococcus B carrier state complicating childbirth Ⓜ♀

    O99.825 Streptococcus B carrier state complicating the puerperium Ⓜ♀

✓6ᵗʰ **O99.83 Other infection carrier state complicating pregnancy, childbirth and the puerperium**
Use additional code to identify the carrier state (Z22.-)

    O99.830 Other infection carrier state complicating pregnancy Ⓜ♀

    O99.834 Other infection carrier state complicating childbirth Ⓜ♀

    O99.835 Other infection carrier state complicating the puerperium Ⓜ♀

✓6ᵗʰ **O99.84 Bariatric surgery status complicating pregnancy, childbirth and the puerperium**
Gastric banding status complicating pregnancy, childbirth and the puerperium
Gastric bypass status for obesity complicating pregnancy, childbirth and the puerperium
Obesity surgery status complicating pregnancy, childbirth and the puerperium

    O99.840 Bariatric surgery status complicating pregnancy, unspecified trimester Ⓜ♀▽

    O99.841 Bariatric surgery status complicating pregnancy, first trimester Ⓜ♀

    O99.842 Bariatric surgery status complicating pregnancy, second trimester Ⓜ♀

EXCLUDES 1 Not coded here   EXCLUDES 2 Not included here   Ⓝ Newborn Age: 0   Ⓟ Pediatric Age: 0-17   Ⓜ Maternity Age: 12-55   Ⓐ Adult Age: 15-124

854   ICD-10-CM 2018

	O99.843	**Bariatric surgery status complicating pregnancy,** third trimester	Ⓜ♀
	O99.844	**Bariatric surgery status complicating** childbirth	Ⓜ♀
	O99.845	**Bariatric surgery status complicating the** puerperium	Ⓜ♀
	O99.89	**Other specified diseases and conditions complicating pregnancy, childbirth and the puerperium**	Ⓜ♀

✓4th **O9A** **Maternal malignant neoplasms, traumatic injuries and abuse classifiable elsewhere but complicating pregnancy, childbirth and the puerperium**

     ✓5th **O9A.1** Malignant neoplasm **complicating pregnancy, childbirth and the puerperium**
           Conditions in C00-C96
           Use additional code to identify neoplasm
           EXCLUDES 2   *maternal care for benign tumor of corpus uteri (O34.1-)*
                       maternal care for benign tumor of cervix (O34.4-)
           AHA: 2015, 3Q, 19

✓6th	**O9A.11**	**Malignant neoplasm complicating** pregnancy	
	O9A.111	**Malignant neoplasm complicating pregnancy,** first trimester	Ⓜ♀
	O9A.112	**Malignant neoplasm complicating pregnancy,** second trimester	Ⓜ♀
	O9A.113	**Malignant neoplasm complicating pregnancy,** third trimester	Ⓜ♀
	O9A.119	**Malignant neoplasm complicating pregnancy, unspecified trimester**	Ⓜ♀ ▽
	O9A.12	**Malignant neoplasm complicating** childbirth	Ⓜ♀
	O9A.13	**Malignant neoplasm complicating the** puerperium	Ⓜ♀

     ✓5th **O9A.2** Injury, poisoning and **certain other consequences of** external causes **complicating pregnancy, childbirth and the puerperium**
           Conditions in S00-T88, except T74 and T76
           Use additional code(s) to identify the injury or poisoning
           EXCLUDES 2   *physical, sexual and psychological abuse complicating pregnancy, childbirth and the puerperium (O9A.3-, O9A.4-, O9A.5-)*

✓6th	**O9A.21**	**Injury, poisoning and certain other consequences of external causes complicating** pregnancy	
	O9A.211	**Injury, poisoning and certain other consequences of external causes complicating pregnancy,** first trimester	Ⓜ♀
	O9A.212	**Injury, poisoning and certain other consequences of external causes complicating pregnancy,** second trimester	Ⓜ♀
	O9A.213	**Injury, poisoning and certain other consequences of external causes complicating pregnancy,** third trimester	Ⓜ♀
	O9A.219	**Injury, poisoning and certain other consequences of external causes complicating pregnancy, unspecified trimester**	Ⓜ♀ ▽

	O9A.22	**Injury, poisoning and certain other consequences of external causes complicating** childbirth	Ⓜ♀
	O9A.23	**Injury, poisoning and certain other consequencesof external causes complicating the** puerperium	Ⓜ♀

     ✓5th **O9A.3** Physical abuse **complicating pregnancy, childbirth and the puerperium**
           Conditions in T74.11 or T76.11
           Use additional code (if applicable):
             to identify any associated current injury due to physical abuse
             to identify the perpetrator of abuse (Y07.-)
           EXCLUDES 2   *sexual abuse complicating pregnancy, childbirth and the puerperium (O9A.4)*

✓6th	**O9A.31**	**Physical abuse complicating** pregnancy	
	O9A.311	**Physical abuse complicating pregnancy,** first trimester	Ⓜ♀
	O9A.312	**Physical abuse complicating pregnancy,** second trimester	Ⓜ♀
	O9A.313	**Physical abuse complicating pregnancy,** third trimester	Ⓜ♀
	O9A.319	**Physical abuse complicating pregnancy,unspecified trimester**	Ⓜ♀ ▽
	O9A.32	**Physical abuse complicating** childbirth	Ⓜ♀
	O9A.33	**Physical abuse complicating the** puerperium	Ⓜ♀

     ✓5th **O9A.4** Sexual abuse **complicating pregnancy, childbirth and the puerperium**
           Conditions in T74.21 or T76.21
           Use additional code (if applicable):
             to identify any associated current injury due to sexual abuse
             to identify the perpetrator of abuse (Y07.-)

✓6th	**O9A.41**	**Sexual abuse complicating** pregnancy	
	O9A.411	**Sexual abuse complicating pregnancy,** first trimester	Ⓜ♀
	O9A.412	**Sexual abuse complicating pregnancy,** second trimester	Ⓜ♀
	O9A.413	**Sexual abuse complicating pregnancy,** third trimester	Ⓜ♀
	O9A.419	**Sexual abuse complicating pregnancy, unspecified trimester**	Ⓜ♀ ▽
	O9A.42	**Sexual abuse complicating** childbirth	Ⓜ♀
	O9A.43	**Sexual abuse complicating the** puerperium	Ⓜ♀

     ✓5th **O9A.5** Psychological abuse **complicating pregnancy, childbirth and the puerperium**
           Conditions in T74.31 or T76.31
           Use additional code to identify the perpetrator of abuse (Y07.-)

✓6th	**O9A.51**	**Psychological abuse complicating** pregnancy	
	O9A.511	**Psychological abuse complicating pregnancy,** first trimester	Ⓜ♀
	O9A.512	**Psychological abuse complicating pregnancy,** second trimester	Ⓜ♀
	O9A.513	**Psychological abuse complicating pregnancy,** third trimester	Ⓜ♀
	O9A.519	**Psychological abuse complicating pregnancy, unspecified trimester**	Ⓜ♀ ▽
	O9A.52	**Psychological abuse complicating** childbirth	Ⓜ♀
	O9A.53	**Psychological abuse complicating the** puerperium	Ⓜ♀

☑ Additional Character Req   ✓x7th Placeholder Alert   Manifestation   HCC CMS-HCC Condition   ▽ Unspecified Code   ►◄ Revised Text   ● New Code   ▲ Revised Code Title

Chapter 16. Certain Conditions Originating in the Perinatal Period (P00–P96)

Chapter Specific Guidelines with Coding Examples

The chapter specific guidelines from the ICD-10-CM Official Guidelines for Coding and Reporting have been provided below. Along with these guidelines are coding examples, contained in the shaded boxes, that have been developed to help illustrate the coding and/or sequencing guidance found in these guidelines.

For coding and reporting purposes the perinatal period is defined as before birth through the 28th day following birth. The following guidelines are provided for reporting purposes

a. General perinatal rules

1) Use of Chapter 16 codes

Codes in this chapter are <u>never</u> for use on the maternal record. Codes from Chapter 15, the obstetric chapter, are never permitted on the newborn record. Chapter 16 codes may be used throughout the life of the patient if the condition is still present.

2) Principal diagnosis for birth record

When coding the birth episode in a newborn record, assign a code from category Z38, Liveborn infants according to place of birth and type of delivery, as the principal diagnosis. A code from category Z38 is assigned only once, to a newborn at the time of birth. If a newborn is transferred to another institution, a code from category Z38 should not be used at the receiving hospital.

A code from category Z38 is used only on the newborn record, not on the mother's record.

3) Use of codes from other chapters with codes from Chapter 16

Codes from other chapters may be used with codes from chapter 16 if the codes from the other chapters provide more specific detail. Codes for signs and symptoms may be assigned when a definitive diagnosis has not been established. If the reason for the encounter is a perinatal condition, the code from chapter 16 should be sequenced first.

4) Use of Chapter 16 codes after the perinatal period

Should a condition originate in the perinatal period, and continue throughout the life of the patient, the perinatal code should continue to be used regardless of the patient's age.

> A 7-year-old patient with history of birth injury that resulted in Erb's palsy is seen for subscapularis release
>
> **P14.0**   **Erb's paralysis due to birth injury**
>
> *Explanation:* Although in this instance Erb's palsy is specifically related to a birth injury, it has not resolved and continues to be a health concern. A perinatal code is appropriate even though this patient is beyond the perinatal period.

5) Birth process or community acquired conditions

If a newborn has a condition that may be either due to the birth process or community acquired and the documentation does not indicate which it is, the default is due to the birth process and the code from Chapter 16 should be used. If the condition is community-acquired, a code from Chapter 16 should not be assigned.

6) Code all clinically significant conditions

All clinically significant conditions noted on routine newborn examination should be coded. A condition is clinically significant if it requires:

clinical evaluation; or

therapeutic treatment; or

diagnostic procedures; or

extended length of hospital stay; or

increased nursing care and/or monitoring; or

has implications for future health care needs

Note: The perinatal guidelines listed above are the same as the general coding guidelines for "additional diagnoses", except for the final point regarding implications for future health care needs. Codes should be assigned for conditions that have been specified by the provider as having implications for future health care needs.

b. Observation and evaluation of newborns for suspected conditions not found

1) Assign a code from category Z05, Observation and evaluation of newborns and infants for suspected conditions ruled out, to identify those instances when a healthy newborn is evaluated for a suspected condition that is determined after study not to be present. Do not use a code from category Z05 when the patient has identified signs or symptoms of a suspected problem; in such cases code the sign or symptom.

2) A code from category Z05 may also be assigned as a principal or first-listed code for readmissions or encounters when the code from category Z38 code no longer applies. Codes from category Z05 are for use only for healthy newborns and infants for which no condition after study is found to be present.

3) Z05 on a birth record

A code from category Z05 is to be used as a secondary code after the code from category Z38, Liveborn infants according to place of birth and type of delivery.

> Newborn delivered via vaginal delivery; previous ultrasounds showed what appeared to be an abnormality of the right kidney. Kidney function tests were performed and ultrasounds taken and any genitourinary conditions ruled out.
>
> **Z38.00**   **Single liveborn infant, delivered vaginally**
>
> **Z05.6**   **Observation and evaluation of newborn for suspected genitourinary condition ruled out**
>
> *Explanation:* The newborn had no signs or symptoms of kidney or other genitourinary condition but was evaluated after delivery due to the abnormal prenatal ultrasound findings. A Z code describing the type and place of birth should be coded first, followed by a Z05 category code for the work performed to rule out a suspected genitourinary condition.

c. Coding additional perinatal diagnoses

1) Assigning codes for conditions that require treatment

Assign codes for conditions that require treatment or further investigation, prolong the length of stay, or require resource utilization.

2) Codes for conditions specified as having implications for future health care needs

Assign codes for conditions that have been specified by the provider as having implications for future health care needs.

Note: This guideline should not be used for adult patients.

> An abnormal noise was heard in the left hip of a post-term newborn during a physical examination. The pediatrician would like to follow the patient after discharge as a hip click can be an early sign of hip dysplasia. The newborn was delivered via cesarean at 41 weeks.
>
> **Z38.01**   **Single liveborn infant, delivered by cesarean**
>
> **P08.21**   **Post-term newborn**
>
> **R29.4**   **Clicking hip**
>
> *Explanation:* The abnormal hip noise or click is appended as a secondary diagnosis not only because it is an abnormal finding upon examination, but also due to its potential to be part of a bigger health issue. The hip dysplasia has not yet been diagnosed and does not warrant a code at this time.

d. Prematurity and fetal growth retardation

Providers utilize different criteria in determining prematurity. A code for prematurity should not be assigned unless it is documented. Assignment of codes in categories P05, Disorders of newborn related to slow fetal growth and fetal malnutrition, and P07, Disorders of newborn related to short gestation and low birth weight, not elsewhere classified, should be based on the recorded birth weight and estimated gestational age. Codes from category P05 should not be assigned with codes from category P07.

When both birth weight and gestational age are available, two codes from category P07 should be assigned, with the code for birth weight sequenced before the code for gestational age.

Chapter 16. Certain Conditions Originating in the Perinatal Period

e. Low birth weight and immaturity status

Codes from category P07, Disorders of newborn related to short gestation and low birth weight, not elsewhere classified, are for use for a child or adult who was premature or had a low birth weight as a newborn and this is affecting the patient's current health status.

See Section I.C.21. Factors influencing health status and contact with health services, Status.

A 35-year-old patient, who weighed 659 grams at birth, is seen for heart disease documented as being a consequence of the low birth weight

I51.9	**Heart disease, unspecified**
P07.02	**Extremely low birth weight newborn, 500–749 grams**

Explanation: A code from subcategories P07.0- and P07.1- is appropriate, regardless of the age of the patient, as long as the documentation provides a clear link between the patient's current illness and the low birth weight.

f. Bacterial sepsis of newborn

Category P36, Bacterial sepsis of newborn, includes congenital sepsis. If a perinate is documented as having sepsis without documentation of congenital or community acquired, the default is congenital and a code from category P36 should be assigned. If the P36 code includes the causal organism, an additional code from category B95, Streptococcus, Staphylococcus, and Enterococcus as the cause of diseases classified elsewhere, or B96, Other bacterial agents as the cause of diseases classified elsewhere, should not be assigned. If the P36 code does not include the causal organism, assign an additional code from category B96. If applicable, use additional codes to identify severe sepsis (R65.2-) and any associated acute organ dysfunction.

A full-term infant develops severe sepsis 24 hours after discharge from the hospital and is readmitted; cultures identified *E. coli* as the infective agent

P36.4	**Sepsis of newborn due to Escherichia coli**
R65.20	**Severe sepsis without septic shock**

Explanation: Even though this newborn was discharged and could have acquired *E. coli* from his/her external environment, due to the lack of documentation specifying specifically how this pathogen was acquired, the default is to code the *E. coli* sepsis as congenital. A code from chapter 1, "Certain Infectious and Parasitic Diseases," is not required because the perinatal sepsis code identifies both the sepsis and the bacteria causing the sepsis.

g. Stillbirth

Code P95, Stillbirth, is only for use in institutions that maintain separate records for stillbirths. No other code should be used with P95. Code P95 should not be used on the mother's record.

Chapter 16. Certain Conditions Originating in the Perinatal Period (P00-P96)

NOTE Codes from this chapter are for use on newborn records only, never on maternal records.

INCLUDES conditions that have their origin in the fetal or perinatal period (before birth through the first 28 days after birth) even if morbidity occurs later

EXCLUDES 2 congenital malformations, deformations and chromosomal abnormalities (Q00-Q99)

endocrine, nutritional and metabolic diseases (E00-E88)

injury, poisoning and certain other consequences of external causes (S00-T88)

neoplasms (C00-D49)

tetanus neonatorum (A33)

This chapter contains the following blocks:

P00-P04	Newborn affected by maternal factors and by complications of pregnancy, labor, and delivery
P05-P08	Disorders of newborn related to length of gestation and fetal growth
P09	Abnormal findings on neonatal screening
P10-P15	Birth trauma
P19-P29	Respiratory and cardiovascular disorders specific to the perinatal period
P35-P39	Infections specific to the perinatal period
P50-P61	Hemorrhagic and hematological disorders of newborn
P70-P74	Transitory endocrine and metabolic disorders specific to newborn
P76-P78	Digestive system disorders of newborn
P80-P83	Conditions involving the integument and temperature regulation of newborn
P84	Other problems with newborn
P90-P96	Other disorders originating in the perinatal period

Newborn affected by maternal factors and by complications of pregnancy, labor, and delivery (P00-P04)

NOTE These codes are for use when the listed maternal conditions are specified as the cause of confirmed morbidity or potential morbidity which have their origin in the perinatal period (before birth through the first 28 days after birth).

✓4th P00 Newborn affected by maternal conditions **that may be unrelated to present pregnancy**

Code first any current condition in newborn

EXCLUDES 2 encounter for observation of newborn for suspected diseases and conditions ruled out (Z05.-)

newborn affected by maternal complications of pregnancy (P01.-)

newborn affected by maternal endocrine and metabolic disorders (P70-P74)

newborn affected by noxious substances transmitted via placenta or breast milk (P04.-)

P00.0 Newborn affected by maternal hypertensive **disorders**

Newborn affected by maternal conditions classifiable to O10-O11, O13-O16

P00.1 Newborn affected by maternal renal and urinary tract **diseases**

Newborn affected by maternal conditions classifiable to N00-N39

P00.2 Newborn affected by maternal infectious and parasitic **diseases**

Newborn affected by maternal infectious disease classifiable to A00-B99, J09 and J10

EXCLUDES 1 ~~infections specific to the perinatal period (P35-P39)~~

maternal genital tract or other localized infections (P00.8)

EXCLUDES 2 ►infections specific to the perinatal period (P35-P39)◄

AHA: 2015, 3Q, 20

P00.3 Newborn affected by other maternal circulatory and respiratory **diseases**

Newborn affected by maternal conditions classifiable to I00-I99, J00-J99, Q20-Q34 and not included in P00.0, P00.2

P00.4 Newborn affected by maternal nutritional **disorders**

Newborn affected by maternal disorders classifiable to E40-E64

Maternal malnutrition NOS

P00.5 Newborn affected by maternal injury

Newborn affected by maternal conditions classifiable to O9A.2-

P00.6 Newborn affected by surgical procedure on mother

Newborn affected by amniocentesis

EXCLUDES 1 Cesarean delivery for present delivery (P03.4)

damage to placenta from amniocentesis, Cesarean delivery or surgical induction (P02.1)

previous surgery to uterus or pelvic organs (P03.89)

EXCLUDES 2 newborn affected by complication of (fetal) intrauterine procedure (P96.5)

P00.7 Newborn affected by other medical procedures on mother, not elsewhere classified

Newborn affected by radiation to mother

EXCLUDES 1 damage to placenta from amniocentesis, cesarean delivery or surgical induction (P02.1)

newborn affected by other complications of labor and delivery (P03.-)

✓5th P00.8 Newborn affected by other maternal conditions

P00.81 Newborn affected by periodontal disease **in mother**

P00.89 Newborn affected by other maternal conditions

Newborn affected by conditions classifiable to T80-T88

Newborn affected by maternal genital tract or other localized infections

Newborn affected by maternal systemic lupus erythematosus

P00.9 Newborn affected by unspecified maternal condition ▽

✓4th P01 Newborn affected by maternal complications of pregnancy

Code first any current condition in newborn

EXCLUDES 2 encounter for observation of newborn for suspected diseases and conditions ruled out (Z05.-)

P01.0 Newborn affected by incompetent cervix

P01.1 Newborn affected by premature rupture of membranes

P01.2 Newborn affected by oligohydramnios

EXCLUDES 1 oligohydramnios due to premature rupture of membranes (P01.1)

DEF: Low amniotic fluid level, resulting in underdeveloped organs in the fetus.

P01.3 Newborn affected by polyhydramnios

Newborn affected by hydramnios

P01.4 Newborn affected by ectopic pregnancy

Newborn affected by abdominal pregnancy

P01.5 Newborn affected by multiple pregnancy

Newborn affected by triplet (pregnancy)

Newborn affected by twin (pregnancy)

P01.6 Newborn affected by maternal death

P01.7 Newborn affected by malpresentation before labor

Newborn affected by breech presentation before labor

Newborn affected by external version before labor

Newborn affected by face presentation before labor

Newborn affected by transverse lie before labor

Newborn affected by unstable lie before labor

P01.8 Newborn affected by other maternal complications of pregnancy

P01.9 Newborn affected by maternal complication of pregnancy, unspecified ▽

✓4th P02 Newborn affected by complications of placenta, cord and membranes

Code first any current condition in newborn

EXCLUDES 2 encounter for observation of newborn for suspected diseases and conditions ruled out (Z05.-)

P02.0 Newborn affected by placenta previa

DEF: Placenta developed in lower segment of uterus; can cause hemorrhaging leading to preterm delivery.

P02.1 Newborn affected by other forms of placental separation and hemorrhage

Newborn affected by abruptio placenta

Newborn affected by accidental hemorrhage

Newborn affected by antepartum hemorrhage

Newborn affected by damage to placenta from amniocentesis, cesarean delivery or surgical induction

Newborn affected by maternal blood loss

Newborn affected by premature separation of placenta

✓5th P02.2 Newborn affected by other and unspecified morphological and functional abnormalities of placenta

P02.20 Newborn affected by unspecified morphological ▽ **and functional abnormalities of placenta**

✓ Additional Character Req   ✓7th Placeholder Alert   Manifestation   HCC CMS-HCC Condition   ▽ Unspecified Code   ►◄ Revised Text   ● New Code   ▲ Revised Code Title

ICD-10-CM 2018   859

Chapter 16. Certain Conditions Originating in the Perinatal Period

P02.29   **Newborn affected by other morphological and functional abnormalities of placenta**
Newborn affected by placental dysfunction
Newborn affected by placental infarction
Newborn affected by placental insufficiency

P02.3   **Newborn affected by placental transfusion syndromes**
Newborn affected by placental and cord abnormalities resulting in twin-to-twin or other transplacental transfusion

P02.4   **Newborn affected by prolapsed cord**

P02.5   **Newborn affected by other compression of umbilical cord**
Newborn affected by umbilical cord (tightly) around neck
Newborn affected by entanglement of umbilical cord
Newborn affected by knot in umbilical cord

✓5ᵗʰ **P02.6**   **Newborn affected by other and unspecified conditions of umbilical cord**

    P02.60   **Newborn affected by unspecified conditions of umbilical cord** ▽

    P02.69   **Newborn affected by other conditions of umbilical cord**
Newborn affected by short umbilical cord
Newborn affected by vasa previa
EXCLUDES 1   newborn affected by single umbilical artery (Q27.0)

P02.7   **Newborn affected by chorioamnionitis**
Newborn affected by amnionitis
Newborn affected by membranitis
Newborn affected by placentitis
DEF: Inflammation of the fetal membranes due to maternal infection; characterized by fetal tachycardia, respiratory distress, apnea, weak cries, and poor sucking.

P02.8   **Newborn affected by other abnormalities of membranes**

P02.9   **Newborn affected by abnormality of membranes, unspecified** ▽

✓4ᵗʰ **P03**   **Newborn affected by other complications of labor and delivery**
Code first any current condition in newborn
EXCLUDES 2   encounter for observation of newborn for suspected diseases and conditions ruled out (Z05.-)

P03.0   **Newborn affected by breech delivery and extraction**

P03.1   **Newborn affected by other malpresentation, malposition and disproportion during labor and delivery**
Newborn affected by contracted pelvis
Newborn affected by conditions classifiable to O64-O66
Newborn affected by persistent occipitoposterior
Newborn affected by transverse lie

Forceps Assisted Birth

Forceps extractor

Vacuum Assisted Birth

Vacuum extractor

P03.2   **Newborn affected by forceps delivery**

P03.3   **Newborn affected by delivery by vacuum extractor [ventouse]**

P03.4   **Newborn affected by Cesarean delivery**

P03.5   **Newborn affected by precipitate delivery**
Newborn affected by rapid second stage

P03.6   **Newborn affected by abnormal uterine contractions**
Newborn affected by conditions classifiable to O62-, except O62.3
Newborn affected by hypertonic labor
Newborn affected by uterine inertia

✓5ᵗʰ **P03.8**   **Newborn affected by other specified complications of labor and delivery**

    ✓6ᵗʰ **P03.81**   **Newborn affected by abnormality in fetal (intrauterine) heart rate or rhythm**
EXCLUDES 1   neonatal cardiac dysrhythmia (P29.1-)

       P03.810   **Newborn affected by abnormality in fetal (intrauterine) heart rate or rhythm before the onset of labor**

       P03.811   **Newborn affected by abnormality in fetal (intrauterine) heart rate or rhythm during labor**

       P03.819   **Newborn affected by abnormality in fetal (intrauterine) heart rate or rhythm, unspecified as to time of onset** ▽

    P03.82   **Meconium passage during delivery**
EXCLUDES 1   meconium aspiration (P24.00, P24.01)
meconium staining (P96.83)
DEF: Fetal intestinal activity that increases in response to a fetomaternal distressed state during delivery; the anal sphincter relaxes, and meconium is passed into the amniotic fluid.

    P03.89   **Newborn affected by other specified complications of labor and delivery**
Newborn affected by abnormality of maternal soft tissues
Newborn affected by conditions classifiable to O60-O75 and by procedures used in labor and delivery not included in P02.- and P03.0-P03.6
Newborn affected by induction of labor

P03.9   **Newborn affected by complication of labor and delivery, unspecified** ▽

✓4ᵗʰ **P04**   **Newborn affected by noxious substances transmitted via placenta or breast milk**
INCLUDES   nonteratogenic effects of substances transmitted via placenta
EXCLUDES 2   congenital malformations (Q00-Q99)
encounter for observation of newborn for suspected diseases and conditions ruled out (Z05.-)
neonatal jaundice from excessive hemolysis due to drugs or toxins transmitted from mother (P58.4)
newborn in contact with and (suspected) exposures hazardous to health not transmitted via placenta or breast milk (Z77.-)

P04.0   **Newborn affected by maternal anesthesia and analgesia in pregnancy, labor and delivery**
Newborn affected by reactions and intoxications from maternal opiates and tranquilizers administered during labor and delivery

P04.1   **Newborn affected by other maternal medication**
Newborn affected by cancer chemotherapy
Newborn affected by cytotoxic drugs
EXCLUDES 1   dysmorphism due to warfarin (Q86.2)
fetal hydantoin syndrome (Q86.1)
maternal use of drugs of addiction (P04.4-)

P04.2   **Newborn affected by maternal use of tobacco**
Newborn affected by exposure in utero to tobacco smoke
EXCLUDES 2   newborn exposure to environmental tobacco smoke (P96.81)

P04.3   **Newborn affected by maternal use of alcohol**
EXCLUDES 1   fetal alcohol syndrome (Q86.0)

✓5ᵗʰ **P04.4**   **Newborn affected by maternal use of drugs of addiction**

    P04.41   **Newborn affected by maternal use of cocaine**
"Crack baby"

    P04.49   **Newborn affected by maternal use of other drugs of addiction**
EXCLUDES 2   newborn affected by maternal anesthesia and analgesia (P04.0)
withdrawal symptoms from maternal use of drugs of addiction (P96.1)

P04.5   **Newborn affected by maternal use of** nutritional chemical substances

P04.6   **Newborn affected by maternal exposure to** environmental chemical substances

P04.8   **Newborn affected by other maternal** noxious substances

P04.9   **Newborn affected by maternal noxious substance, unspecified**   ▽

Disorders of newborn related to length of gestation and fetal growth (P05-P08)

✓4ᵗʰ **P05**   **Disorders of newborn related to slow fetal growth and fetal malnutrition**

   ✓5ᵗʰ **P05.0**   **Newborn light for gestational age**
Newborn light-for-dates
Weight below but length above 10th percentile for gestational age

     P05.00   **Newborn light for gestational age, unspecified weight**   ▽

     P05.01   **Newborn light for gestational age,** less than 500 grams

     P05.02   **Newborn light for gestational age,** 500-749 grams

     P05.03   **Newborn light for gestational age,** 750-999 grams

     P05.04   **Newborn light for gestational age,** 1000-1249 grams

     P05.05   **Newborn light for gestational age,** 1250-1499 grams

     P05.06   **Newborn light for gestational age,** 1500-1749 grams

     P05.07   **Newborn light for gestational age,** 1750-1999 grams

     P05.08   **Newborn light for gestational age,** 2000-2499 grams

     P05.09   **Newborn light for gestational age,** 2500 grams and over
Newborn light for gestational age, other

   ✓5ᵗʰ **P05.1**   **Newborn small for gestational age**
Newborn small-and-light-for-dates
Newborn small-for-dates
Weight and length below 10th percentile for gestational age

     P05.10   **Newborn small for gestational age, unspecified weight**   ▽

     P05.11   **Newborn small for gestational age,** less than 500 grams

     P05.12   **Newborn small for gestational age,** 500-749 grams

     P05.13   **Newborn small for gestational age,** 750-999 grams

     P05.14   **Newborn small for gestational age,** 1000-1249 grams

     P05.15   **Newborn small for gestational age,** 1250-1499 grams

     P05.16   **Newborn small for gestational age,** 1500-1749 grams

     P05.17   **Newborn small for gestational age,** 1750-1999 grams

     P05.18   **Newborn small for gestational age,** 2000-2499 grams

     P05.19   **Newborn small for gestational age, other**
Newborn small for gestational age, 2500 grams and over

   P05.2   **Newborn affected by** fetal (intrauterine) malnutrition **not light or small for gestational age**
Infant, not light or small for gestational age, showing signs of fetal malnutrition, such as dry, peeling skin and loss of subcutaneous tissue
     EXCLUDES 1   newborn affected by fetal malnutrition with light for gestational age (P05.0-)
           newborn affected by fetal malnutrition with small for gestational age (P05.1-)

   P05.9   **Newborn affected by slow intrauterine growth, unspecified**   ▽
Newborn affected by fetal growth retardation NOS

✓4ᵗʰ **P07**   **Disorders of newborn related to short gestation and low birth weight, not elsewhere classified**
     NOTE   When both birth weight and gestational age of the newborn are available, both should be coded with birth weight sequenced before gestational age
     INCLUDES   the listed conditions, without further specification, as the cause of morbidity or additional care, in newborn

   ✓5ᵗʰ **P07.0**   **Extremely low birth weight newborn**
Newborn birth weight 999 g. or less
     EXCLUDES 1   low birth weight due to slow fetal growth and fetal malnutrition (P05.-)

     P07.00   **Extremely low birth weight newborn, unspecified weight**   ▽

     P07.01   **Extremely low birth weight newborn,** less than 500 grams

     P07.02   **Extremely low birth weight newborn,** 500-749 grams

     P07.03   **Extremely low birth weight newborn,** 750-999 grams

   ✓5ᵗʰ **P07.1**   **Other low birth weight newborn**
Newborn birth weight 1000-2499 g.
     EXCLUDES 1   low birth weight due to slow fetal growth and fetal malnutrition (P05.-)

     P07.10   **Other low birth weight newborn, unspecified weight**   ▽

     P07.14   **Other low birth weight newborn,** 1000-1249 grams

     P07.15   **Other low birth weight newborn,** 1250-1499 grams

     P07.16   **Other low birth weight newborn,** 1500-1749 grams

     P07.17   **Other low birth weight newborn,** 1750-1999 grams

     P07.18   **Other low birth weight newborn,** 2000-2499 grams

   ✓5ᵗʰ **P07.2**   **Extreme immaturity of** newborn
Less than 28 completed weeks (less than 196 completed days) of gestation.

     P07.20   **Extreme immaturity of newborn, unspecified weeks of gestation**   ▽
Gestational age less than 28 completed weeks NOS

     P07.21   **Extreme immaturity of newborn, gestational age** less than 23 completed weeks
Extreme immaturity of newborn, gestational age less than 23 weeks, 0 days

     P07.22   **Extreme immaturity of newborn, gestational age** 23 completed weeks
Extreme immaturity of newborn, gestational age 23 weeks, 0 days through 23 weeks, 6 days

     P07.23   **Extreme immaturity of newborn, gestational age** 24 completed weeks
Extreme immaturity of newborn, gestational age 24 weeks, 0 days through 24 weeks, 6 days

     P07.24   **Extreme immaturity of newborn, gestational age** 25 completed weeks
Extreme immaturity of newborn, gestational age 25 weeks, 0 days through 25 weeks, 6 days

     P07.25   **Extreme immaturity of newborn, gestational age** 26 completed weeks
Extreme immaturity of newborn, gestational age 26 weeks, 0 days through 26 weeks, 6 days

     P07.26   **Extreme immaturity of newborn, gestational age** 27 completed weeks
Extreme immaturity of newborn, gestational age 27 weeks, 0 days through 27 weeks, 6 days

   ✓5ᵗʰ **P07.3**   **Preterm [premature] newborn [other]**
28 completed weeks or more but less than 37 completed weeks (196 completed days but less than 259 completed days) of gestation
Prematurity NOS

     P07.30   **Preterm newborn, unspecified weeks of gestation**   ▽

     P07.31   **Preterm newborn, gestational age** 28 completed weeks
Preterm newborn, gestational age 28 weeks, 0 days through 28 weeks, 6 days

     P07.32   **Preterm newborn, gestational age** 29 completed weeks
Preterm newborn, gestational age 29 weeks, 0 days through 29 weeks, 6 days

     P07.33   **Preterm newborn, gestational age** 30 completed weeks
Preterm newborn, gestational age 30 weeks, 0 days through 30 weeks, 6 days

---

✓ Additional Character Req   ✓x7ᵗʰ Placeholder Alert   Manifestation   HCC CMS-HCC Condition   ▽ Unspecified Code   ►◄ Revised Text   ● New Code   ▲ Revised Code Title

P07.34   **Preterm newborn, gestational age 31 completed weeks**
Preterm newborn, gestational age 31 weeks, 0 days through 31 weeks, 6 days

P07.35   **Preterm newborn, gestational age 32 completed weeks**
Preterm newborn, gestational age 32 weeks, 0 days through 32 weeks, 6 days

P07.36   **Preterm newborn, gestational age 33 completed weeks**
Preterm newborn, gestational age 33 weeks, 0 days through 33 weeks, 6 days

P07.37   **Preterm newborn, gestational age 34 completed weeks**
Preterm newborn, gestational age 34 weeks, 0 days through 34 weeks, 6 days

P07.38   **Preterm newborn, gestational age 35 completed weeks**
Preterm newborn, gestational age 35 weeks, 0 days through 35 weeks, 6 days

P07.39   **Preterm newborn, gestational age 36 completed weeks**
Preterm newborn, gestational age 36 weeks, 0 days through 36 weeks, 6 days

✓4ᵗʰ **P08**   **Disorders of newborn related to long gestation and high birth weight**
NOTE   When both birth weight and gestational age of the newborn are available, priority of assignment should be given to birth weight
INCLUDES   the listed conditions, without further specification, as causes of morbidity or additional care, in newborn

P08.0   **Exceptionally large newborn baby**
Usually implies a birth weight of 4500 g. or more
EXCLUDES 1   syndrome of infant of diabetic mother (P70.1)
syndrome of infant of mother with gestational diabetes (P70.0)

P08.1   **Other heavy for gestational age newborn**
Other newborn heavy- or large-for-dates regardless of period of gestation
Usually implies a birth weight of 4000 g. to 4499 g.
EXCLUDES 1   newborn with a birth weight of 4500 or more (P08.0)
syndrome of infant of diabetic mother (P70.1)
syndrome of infant of mother with gestational diabetes (P70.0).

✓5ᵗʰ **P08.2**   **Late newborn, not heavy for gestational age**
AHA: 2014, 1Q, 14

P08.21   **Post-term newborn**
Newborn with gestation period over 40 completed weeks to 42 completed weeks

P08.22   **Prolonged gestation of newborn**
Newborn with gestation period over 42 completed weeks (294 days or more), not heavy- or large-for-dates.
Postmaturity NOS

Abnormal findings on neonatal screening (P09)

P09   **Abnormal findings on neonatal screening**
Use additional code to identify signs, symptoms and conditions associated with the screening
EXCLUDES 2   nonspecific serologic evidence of human immunodeficiency virus [HIV] (R75)

Birth trauma (P10-P15)

✓4ᵗʰ **P10**   **Intracranial laceration and hemorrhage due to birth injury**
EXCLUDES 1   intracranial hemorrhage of newborn NOS (P52.9)
intracranial hemorrhage of newborn due to anoxia or hypoxia (P52.-)
nontraumatic intracranial hemorrhage of newborn (P52.-)

P10.0   **Subdural hemorrhage due to birth injury**
Subdural hematoma (localized) due to birth injury
EXCLUDES 1   subdural hemorrhage accompanying tentorial tear (P10.4)

P10.1   **Cerebral hemorrhage due to birth injury**

P10.2   **Intraventricular hemorrhage due to birth injury**

P10.3   **Subarachnoid hemorrhage due to birth injury**

P10.4   **Tentorial tear due to birth injury**

P10.8   **Other intracranial lacerations and hemorrhages due to birth injury**

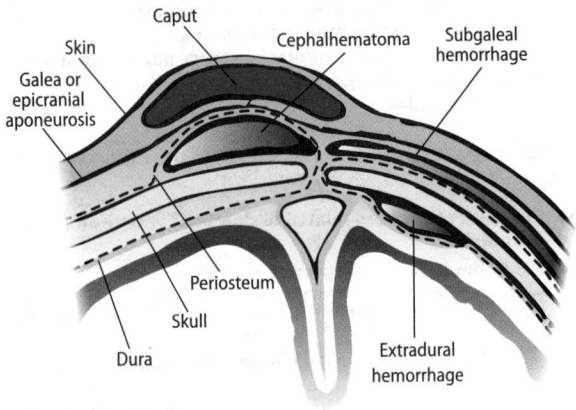

Birth Injuries to Scalp

Caput · Skin · Galea or epicranial aponeurosis · Cephalhematoma · Subgaleal hemorrhage · Periosteum · Skull · Dura · Extradural hemorrhage

P10.9   **Unspecified intracranial laceration and hemorrhage due to birth injury**   ▽

✓4ᵗʰ **P11**   **Other birth injuries to central nervous system**
P11.0   **Cerebral edema due to birth injury**
P11.1   **Other specified brain damage due to birth injury**
P11.2   **Unspecified brain damage due to birth injury**   ▽
P11.3   **Birth injury to facial nerve**
Facial palsy due to birth injury
P11.4   **Birth injury to other cranial nerves**
P11.5   **Birth injury to spine and spinal cord**
Fracture of spine due to birth injury
P11.9   **Birth injury to central nervous system, unspecified**   ▽

✓4ᵗʰ **P12**   **Birth injury to scalp**
P12.0   **Cephalhematoma due to birth injury**
P12.1   **Chignon (from vacuum extraction) due to birth injury**
P12.2   **Epicranial subaponeurotic hemorrhage due to birth injury**
Subgaleal hemorrhage
P12.3   **Bruising of scalp due to birth injury**
P12.4   **Injury of scalp of newborn due to monitoring equipment**
Sampling incision of scalp of newborn
Scalp clip (electrode) injury of newborn
✓5ᵗʰ **P12.8**   **Other birth injuries to scalp**
P12.81   **Caput succedaneum**
P12.89   **Other birth injuries to scalp**
P12.9   **Birth injury to scalp, unspecified**   ▽

✓4ᵗʰ **P13**   **Birth injury to skeleton**
EXCLUDES 2   birth injury to spine (P11.5)
P13.0   **Fracture of skull due to birth injury**
P13.1   **Other birth injuries to skull**
EXCLUDES 1   cephalhematoma (P12.0)
P13.2   **Birth injury to femur**
P13.3   **Birth injury to other long bones**
P13.4   **Fracture of clavicle due to birth injury**
P13.8   **Birth injuries to other parts of skeleton**
P13.9   **Birth injury to skeleton, unspecified**   ▽

✓4ᵗʰ **P14**   **Birth injury to peripheral nervous system**
P14.0   **Erb's paralysis due to birth injury**
P14.1   **Klumpke's paralysis due to birth injury**
P14.2   **Phrenic nerve paralysis due to birth injury**
P14.3   **Other brachial plexus birth injuries**
P14.8   **Birth injuries to other parts of peripheral nervous system**
P14.9   **Birth injury to peripheral nervous system, unspecified**   ▽

✓4ᵗʰ **P15**   **Other birth injuries**
P15.0   **Birth injury to liver**
Rupture of liver due to birth injury
P15.1   **Birth injury to spleen**
Rupture of spleen due to birth injury
P15.2   **Sternomastoid injury due to birth injury**
P15.3   **Birth injury to eye**
Subconjunctival hemorrhage due to birth injury
Traumatic glaucoma due to birth injury

EXCLUDES 1 Not coded here   **EXCLUDES 2** Not included here   **N** Newborn Age: 0   **P** Pediatric Age: 0-17   **M** Maternity Age: 12-55   **A** Adult Age: 15-124

862   ICD-10-CM 2018

P15.4 Birth injury to face
Facial congestion due to birth injury

P15.5 Birth injury to external genitalia

P15.6 Subcutaneous fat necrosis due to birth injury

P15.8 Other specified birth injuries
TIP: Use for any injury of newborn from scalpel.

P15.9 Birth injury, unspecified ▽

Respiratory and cardiovascular disorders specific to the perinatal period (P19-P29)

✓4ᵗʰ P19 Metabolic acidemia in newborn
INCLUDES metabolic acidemia in newborn

P19.0 Metabolic acidemia in newborn first noted before onset of labor

P19.1 Metabolic acidemia in newborn first noted during labor

P19.2 Metabolic acidemia noted at birth

P19.9 Metabolic acidemia, unspecified ▽

✓4ᵗʰ P22 Respiratory distress of newborn
EXCLUDES 1 respiratory arrest of newborn (P28.81)
respiratory failure of newborn NOS (P28.5)

P22.0 Respiratory distress syndrome of newborn
Cardiorespiratory distress syndrome of newborn
Hyaline membrane disease
Idiopathic respiratory distress syndrome [IRDS or RDS] of newborn
Pulmonary hypoperfusion syndrome
Respiratory distress syndrome, type I
DEF: Severe chest contractions upon air intake and expiratory grunting; infant appears blue due to oxygen deficiency and has rapid respiratory rate; formerly called hyaline membrane disease.

P22.1 Transient tachypnea of newborn
Idiopathic tachypnea of newborn
Respiratory distress syndrome, type II
Wet lung syndrome
DEF: Rapid, labored breathing of newborn; short-term problem that begins after birth and lasts about three days.

P22.8 Other respiratory distress of newborn

P22.9 Respiratory distress of newborn, unspecified ▽

✓4ᵗʰ P23 Congenital pneumonia
INCLUDES infective pneumonia acquired in utero or during birth
EXCLUDES 1 neonatal pneumonia resulting from aspiration (P24.-)

P23.0 Congenital pneumonia due to viral agent
Use additional code (B97) to identify organism
EXCLUDES 1 congenital rubella pneumonitis (P35.0)

P23.1 Congenital pneumonia due to Chlamydia

P23.2 Congenital pneumonia due to staphylococcus

P23.3 Congenital pneumonia due to streptococcus, group B

P23.4 Congenital pneumonia due to Escherichia coli

P23.5 Congenital pneumonia due to Pseudomonas

P23.6 Congenital pneumonia due to other bacterial agents
Congenital pneumonia due to Hemophilus influenzae
Congenital pneumonia due to Klebsiella pneumoniae
Congenital pneumonia due to Mycoplasma
Congenital pneumonia due to Streptococcus, except group B
Use additional code (B95-B96) to identify organism

P23.8 Congenital pneumonia due to other organisms

P23.9 Congenital pneumonia, unspecified ▽

✓4ᵗʰ P24 Neonatal aspiration
INCLUDES aspiration in utero and during delivery

✓5ᵗʰ P24.0 Meconium aspiration
EXCLUDES 1 meconium passage (without aspiration) during delivery (P03.82)
meconium staining (P96.83)

P24.00 Meconium aspiration without respiratory symptoms
Meconium aspiration NOS

P24.01 Meconium aspiration with respiratory symptoms
Meconium aspiration pneumonia
Meconium aspiration pneumonitis
Meconium aspiration syndrome NOS
Use additional code to identify any secondary pulmonary hypertension, if applicable ▶(I27.2-)◀
DEF: Aspiration of fetal intestinal material during or prior to delivery; usually a complication of placental insufficiency, causing pneumonitis and bronchial obstruction (inflammatory reaction of lungs).

✓5ᵗʰ P24.1 Neonatal aspiration of (clear) amniotic fluid and mucus
Neonatal aspiration of liquor (amnii)

P24.10 Neonatal aspiration of (clear) amniotic fluid and mucus without respiratory symptoms
Neonatal aspiration of amniotic fluid and mucus NOS

P24.11 Neonatal aspiration of (clear) amniotic fluid and mucus with respiratory symptoms
Neonatal aspiration of amniotic fluid and mucus with pneumonia
Neonatal aspiration of amniotic fluid and mucus with pneumonitis
Use additional code to identify any secondary pulmonary hypertension, if applicable ▶(I27.2-)◀

✓5ᵗʰ P24.2 Neonatal aspiration of blood

P24.20 Neonatal aspiration of blood without respiratory symptoms
Neonatal aspiration of blood NOS

P24.21 Neonatal aspiration of blood with respiratory symptoms
Neonatal aspiration of blood with pneumonia
Neonatal aspiration of blood with pneumonitis
Use additional code to identify any secondary pulmonary hypertension, if applicable ▶(I27.2-)◀

✓5ᵗʰ P24.3 Neonatal aspiration of milk and regurgitated food
Neonatal aspiration of stomach contents

P24.30 Neonatal aspiration of milk and regurgitated food without respiratory symptoms
Neonatal aspiration of milk and regurgitated food NOS

P24.31 Neonatal aspiration of milk and regurgitated food with respiratory symptoms
Neonatal aspiration of milk and regurgitated food with pneumonia
Neonatal aspiration of milk and regurgitated food with pneumonitis
Use additional code to identify any secondary pulmonary hypertension, if applicable ▶(I27.2-)◀

✓5ᵗʰ P24.8 Other neonatal aspiration

P24.80 Other neonatal aspiration without respiratory symptoms
Neonatal aspiration NEC

P24.81 Other neonatal aspiration with respiratory symptoms
Neonatal aspiration pneumonia NEC
Neonatal aspiration with pneumonitis NEC
Neonatal aspiration with pneumonia NOS
Neonatal aspiration with pneumonitis NOS
Use additional code to identify any secondary pulmonary hypertension, if applicable ▶(I27.2-)◀

P24.9 Neonatal aspiration, unspecified ▽

✓4ᵗʰ P25 Interstitial emphysema and related conditions originating in the perinatal period

P25.0 Interstitial emphysema originating in the perinatal period

P25.1 Pneumothorax originating in the perinatal period

P25.2 Pneumomediastinum originating in the perinatal period

P25.3 Pneumopericardium originating in the perinatal period

P25.8 Other conditions related to interstitial emphysema originating in the perinatal period

✓4ᵗʰ P26 Pulmonary hemorrhage originating in the perinatal period
EXCLUDES 1 acute idiopathic hemorrhage in infants over 28 days old (R04.81)

P26.0 Tracheobronchial hemorrhage originating in the perinatal period

P26.1 Massive pulmonary hemorrhage originating in the perinatal period

P26.8 Other pulmonary hemorrhages originating in the perinatal period

P26.9 Unspecified pulmonary hemorrhage originating in the perinatal period ▽

✓4ᵗʰ P27 Chronic respiratory disease originating in the perinatal period
EXCLUDES 1 respiratory distress of newborn (P22.0-P22.9)
EXCLUDES 2 ▶respiratory distress of newborn (P22.0-P22.9)◀

P27.0 Wilson-Mikity syndrome
Pulmonary dysmaturity

P27.1 Bronchopulmonary dysplasia originating in the perinatal period

---

✓ Additional Character Req   ✓x7ᵗʰ Placeholder Alert   **Manifestation**   **HCC** CMS-HCC Condition   ▽ Unspecified Code   ▶◀ Revised Text   ● New Code   ▲ Revised Code Title

Chapter 16. Certain Conditions Originating in the Perinatal Period

P27.8 Other chronic respiratory diseases originating in the perinatal period
Congenital pulmonary fibrosis
Ventilator lung in newborn

P27.9 Unspecified chronic respiratory disease originating in the perinatal period ▽

✓4th **P28 Other respiratory conditions originating in the perinatal period**
EXCLUDES 1   congenital malformations of the respiratory system (Q30-Q34)

P28.0 Primary atelectasis of newborn
Primary failure to expand terminal respiratory units
Pulmonary hypoplasia associated with short gestation
Pulmonary immaturity NOS

✓5th **P28.1 Other and unspecified atelectasis of newborn**

P28.10 Unspecified atelectasis of newborn ▽
Atelectasis of newborn NOS

P28.11 Resorption atelectasis without respiratory distress syndrome
EXCLUDES 1   resorption atelectasis with respiratory distress syndrome (P22.0)

P28.19 Other atelectasis of newborn
Partial atelectasis of newborn
Secondary atelectasis of newborn

P28.2 Cyanotic attacks of newborn
EXCLUDES 1   apnea of newborn (P28.3-P28.4)

P28.3 Primary sleep apnea of newborn
Central sleep apnea of newborn
Obstructive sleep apnea of newborn
Sleep apnea of newborn NOS
DEF: Unexplained cessation of breathing when a neonate makes no respiratory effort for 20 seconds or longer, or when neonate's breathing cessation is accompanied by cyanosis, bradycardia, or hypotonia.

P28.4 Other apnea of newborn
Apnea of prematurity
Obstructive apnea of newborn
EXCLUDES 1   obstructive sleep apnea of newborn (P28.3)

P28.5 Respiratory failure of newborn
EXCLUDES 1   respiratory arrest of newborn (P28.81)
respiratory distress of newborn (P22.0-)

✓5th **P28.8 Other specified respiratory conditions of newborn**

P28.81 Respiratory arrest of newborn

P28.89 Other specified respiratory conditions of newborn
Congenital laryngeal stridor
Sniffles in newborn
Snuffles in newborn
EXCLUDES 1   early congenital syphilitic rhinitis (A50.05)

P28.9 Respiratory condition of newborn, unspecified ▽
Respiratory depression in newborn

✓4th **P29 Cardiovascular disorders originating in the perinatal period**
EXCLUDES 1   congenital malformations of the circulatory system (Q20-Q28)

P29.0 Neonatal cardiac failure

✓5th **P29.1 Neonatal cardiac dysrhythmia**

P29.11 Neonatal tachycardia

P29.12 Neonatal bradycardia

P29.2 Neonatal hypertension

✓5th **P29.3 Persistent fetal circulation**
~~Delayed closure of ductus arteriosus~~
~~(Persistent) pulmonary hypertension of newborn~~

● **P29.30 Pulmonary hypertension of newborn**
Persistent pulmonary hypertension of newborn

● **P29.38 Other persistent fetal circulation**
Delayed closure of ductus arteriosus

P29.4 Transient myocardial ischemia in newborn

✓5th **P29.8 Other cardiovascular disorders originating in the perinatal period**

P29.81 Cardiac arrest of newborn

P29.89 Other cardiovascular disorders originating in the perinatal period
AHA: 2014, 4Q, 23

P29.9 Cardiovascular disorder originating in the perinatal period, unspecified ▽

Infections specific to the perinatal period (P35-P39)

Infections acquired in utero, during birth via the umbilicus, or during the first 28 days after birth

EXCLUDES 2   asymptomatic human immunodeficiency virus [HIV] infection status (Z21)
congenital gonococcal infection (A54.-)
congenital pneumonia (P23.-)
congenital syphilis (A50.-)
human immunodeficiency virus [HIV] disease (B20)
infant botulism (A48.51)
infectious diseases not specific to the perinatal period (A00-B99, J09, J10-)
intestinal infectious disease (A00-A09)
laboratory evidence of human immunodeficiency virus [HIV] (R75)
tetanus neonatorum (A33)

✓4th **P35 Congenital viral diseases**
INCLUDES   infections acquired in utero or during birth

P35.0 Congenital rubella syndrome
Congenital rubella pneumonitis

P35.1 Congenital cytomegalovirus infection

P35.2 Congenital herpesviral [herpes simplex] infection

P35.3 Congenital viral hepatitis

P35.8 Other congenital viral diseases
Congenital varicella [chickenpox]

P35.9 Congenital viral disease, unspecified ▽

✓4th **P36 Bacterial sepsis of newborn**
INCLUDES   congenital sepsis
Use additional code(s), if applicable, to identify severe sepsis (R65.2-) and associated acute organ dysfunction(s)

P36.0 Sepsis of newborn due to streptococcus, group B HCC

✓5th **P36.1 Sepsis of newborn due to other and unspecified streptococci**

P36.10 Sepsis of newborn due to unspecified streptococci HCC ▽

P36.19 Sepsis of newborn due to other streptococci HCC

P36.2 Sepsis of newborn due to Staphylococcus aureus HCC

✓5th **P36.3 Sepsis of newborn due to other and unspecified staphylococci**

P36.30 Sepsis of newborn due to unspecified staphylococci HCC ▽

P36.39 Sepsis of newborn due to other staphylococci HCC

P36.4 Sepsis of newborn due to Escherichia coli HCC

P36.5 Sepsis of newborn due to anaerobes HCC

P36.8 Other bacterial sepsis of newborn HCC
Use additional code from category B96 to identify organism

P36.9 Bacterial sepsis of newborn, unspecified HCC ▽

✓4th **P37 Other congenital infectious and parasitic diseases**
EXCLUDES 2   congenital syphilis (A50.-)
infectious neonatal diarrhea (A00-A09)
necrotizing enterocolitis in newborn (P77.-)
noninfectious neonatal diarrhea (P78.3)
ophthalmia neonatorum due to gonococcus (A54.31)
tetanus neonatorum (A33)

P37.0 Congenital tuberculosis

P37.1 Congenital toxoplasmosis
Hydrocephalus due to congenital toxoplasmosis

P37.2 Neonatal (disseminated) listeriosis

P37.3 Congenital falciparum malaria

P37.4 Other congenital malaria

P37.5 Neonatal candidiasis

P37.8 Other specified congenital infectious and parasitic diseases

P37.9 Congenital infectious or parasitic disease, unspecified ▽

✓4th **P38 Omphalitis of newborn**
EXCLUDES 1   omphalitis not of newborn (L08.82)
tetanus omphalitis (A33)
umbilical hemorrhage of newborn (P51.-)

P38.1 Omphalitis with mild hemorrhage

P38.9 Omphalitis without hemorrhage
Omphalitis of newborn NOS

EXCLUDES 1 Not coded here   EXCLUDES 2 Not included here   N Newborn Age: 0   P Pediatric Age: 0-17   M Maternity Age: 12-55   A Adult Age: 15-124

864   ICD-10-CM 2018

☑4ᵗʰ **P39 Other infections specific to the perinatal period**
Use additional code to identify organism or specific infection

P39.0 Neonatal infective mastitis
EXCLUDES 1   breast engorgement of newborn (P83.4)
noninfective mastitis of newborn (P83.4)

P39.1 Neonatal conjunctivitis and dacryocystitis
Neonatal chlamydial conjunctivitis
Ophthalmia neonatorum NOS
EXCLUDES 1   gonococcal conjunctivitis (A54.31)

P39.2 Intra-amniotic infection affecting newborn, not elsewhere classified

P39.3 Neonatal urinary tract infection

P39.4 Neonatal skin infection
Neonatal pyoderma
EXCLUDES 1   pemphigus neonatorum (L00)
staphylococcal scalded skin syndrome (L00)

P39.8 Other specified infections specific to the perinatal period

P39.9 Infection specific to the perinatal period, unspecified ▽

Hemorrhagic and hematological disorders of newborn (P50-P61)

EXCLUDES 1   congenital stenosis and stricture of bile ducts (Q44.3)
Crigler-Najjar syndrome (E80.5)
Dubin-Johnson syndrome (E80.6)
Gilbert syndrome (E80.4)
hereditary hemolytic anemias (D55-D58)

☑4ᵗʰ **P50 Newborn affected by intrauterine (fetal) blood loss**
EXCLUDES 1   congenital anemia from intrauterine (fetal) blood loss (P61.3)

P50.0 Newborn affected by intrauterine (fetal) blood loss from vasa previa

P50.1 Newborn affected by intrauterine (fetal) blood loss from ruptured cord

P50.2 Newborn affected by intrauterine (fetal) blood loss from placenta

P50.3 Newborn affected by hemorrhage into co-twin

P50.4 Newborn affected by hemorrhage into maternal circulation

P50.5 Newborn affected by intrauterine (fetal) blood loss from cut end of co-twin's cord

P50.8 Newborn affected by other intrauterine (fetal) blood loss

P50.9 Newborn affected by intrauterine (fetal) blood loss, unspecified ▽
Newborn affected by fetal hemorrhage NOS

☑4ᵗʰ **P51 Umbilical hemorrhage of newborn**
EXCLUDES 1   omphalitis with mild hemorrhage (P38.1)
umbilical hemorrhage from cut end of co-twins cord (P50.5)

P51.0 Massive umbilical hemorrhage of newborn

P51.8 Other umbilical hemorrhages of newborn
Slipped umbilical ligature NOS

P51.9 Umbilical hemorrhage of newborn, unspecified ▽

☑4ᵗʰ **P52 Intracranial nontraumatic hemorrhage of newborn**
INCLUDES   intracranial hemorrhage due to anoxia or hypoxia
EXCLUDES 1   intracranial hemorrhage due to birth injury (P10.-)
intracranial hemorrhage due to other injury (S06.-)

P52.0 Intraventricular (nontraumatic) hemorrhage, grade 1, of newborn
Subependymal hemorrhage (without intraventricular extension)
Bleeding into germinal matrix

P52.1 Intraventricular (nontraumatic) hemorrhage, grade 2, of newborn
Subependymal hemorrhage with intraventricular extension
Bleeding into ventricle

☑5ᵗʰ **P52.2 Intraventricular (nontraumatic) hemorrhage, grade 3 and grade 4, of newborn**

P52.21 Intraventricular (nontraumatic) hemorrhage, grade 3, of newborn
Subependymal hemorrhage with intraventricular extension with enlargement of ventricle

P52.22 Intraventricular (nontraumatic) hemorrhage, grade 4, of newborn
Bleeding into cerebral cortex
Subependymal hemorrhage with intracerebral extension

P52.3 Unspecified intraventricular (nontraumatic) hemorrhage of newborn ▽

P52.4 Intracerebral (nontraumatic) hemorrhage of newborn

P52.5 Subarachnoid (nontraumatic) hemorrhage of newborn

P52.6 Cerebellar (nontraumatic) and posterior fossa hemorrhage of newborn

P52.8 Other intracranial (nontraumatic) hemorrhages of newborn

P52.9 Intracranial (nontraumatic) hemorrhage of newborn, unspecified ▽

P53 Hemorrhagic disease of newborn
Vitamin K deficiency of newborn

☑4ᵗʰ **P54 Other neonatal hemorrhages**
EXCLUDES 1   newborn affected by (intrauterine) blood loss (P50.-)
pulmonary hemorrhage originating in the perinatal period (P26.-)

P54.0 Neonatal hematemesis
EXCLUDES 1   neonatal hematemesis due to swallowed maternal blood (P78.2)

P54.1 Neonatal melena
EXCLUDES 1   neonatal melena due to swallowed maternal blood (P78.2)

P54.2 Neonatal rectal hemorrhage

P54.3 Other neonatal gastrointestinal hemorrhage

P54.4 Neonatal adrenal hemorrhage

P54.5 Neonatal cutaneous hemorrhage
Neonatal bruising
Neonatal ecchymoses
Neonatal petechiae
Neonatal superficial hematomata
EXCLUDES 2   bruising of scalp due to birth injury (P12.3)
cephalhematoma due to birth injury (P12.0)

P54.6 Neonatal vaginal hemorrhage ♀
Neonatal pseudomenses

P54.8 Other specified neonatal hemorrhages

P54.9 Neonatal hemorrhage, unspecified ▽

☑4ᵗʰ **P55 Hemolytic disease of newborn**

P55.0 Rh isoimmunization of newborn
DEF: Incompatible Rh fetal-maternal blood grouping; prematurely destroys red blood cells; characterized by jaundice, asphyxia, pulmonary hypertension, edema, respiratory distress, kernicterus, and coagulopathies; detected by Coombs test.

P55.1 ABO isoimmunization of newborn
AHA: 2015, 3Q, 20

P55.8 Other hemolytic diseases of newborn

P55.9 Hemolytic disease of newborn, unspecified ▽

☑4ᵗʰ **P56 Hydrops fetalis due to hemolytic disease**
EXCLUDES 1   hydrops fetalis NOS (P83.2)

P56.0 Hydrops fetalis due to isoimmunization

☑5ᵗʰ **P56.9 Hydrops fetalis due to other and unspecified hemolytic disease**

P56.90 Hydrops fetalis due to unspecified hemolytic disease ▽

P56.99 Hydrops fetalis due to other hemolytic disease

☑4ᵗʰ **P57 Kernicterus**

P57.0 Kernicterus due to isoimmunization
DEF: Complication of erythroblastosis fetalis associated with severe neural symptoms, high blood bilirubin levels and nerve cell destruction; results in bilirubin-pigmented gray matter of central nervous system.

P57.8 Other specified kernicterus
EXCLUDES 1   Crigler-Najjar syndrome (E80.5)

P57.9 Kernicterus, unspecified ▽

☑4ᵗʰ **P58 Neonatal jaundice due to other excessive hemolysis**
EXCLUDES 1   jaundice due to isoimmunization (P55-P57)

P58.0 Neonatal jaundice due to bruising

P58.1 Neonatal jaundice due to bleeding

P58.2 Neonatal jaundice due to infection

P58.3 Neonatal jaundice due to polycythemia

☑5ᵗʰ **P58.4 Neonatal jaundice due to drugs or toxins transmitted from mother or given to newborn**
Code first poisoning due to drug or toxin, if applicable (T36-T65 with fifth or sixth character 1-4 or 6)
Use additional code for adverse effect, if applicable, to identify drug (T36-T50 with fifth or sixth character 5)

P58.41 Neonatal jaundice due to drugs or toxins transmitted from mother

P58.42 Neonatal jaundice due to drugs or toxins given to newborn

---

☑ Additional Character Req   ☑x7ᵗʰ Placeholder Alert   Manifestation   HCC CMS-HCC Condition   ▽ Unspecified Code   ►◄ Revised Text   ● New Code   ▲ Revised Code Title

ICD-10-CM 2018   865

P58.5 Neonatal jaundice due to swallowed maternal blood

P58.8 Neonatal jaundice due to other specified excessive hemolysis

P58.9 Neonatal jaundice due to excessive hemolysis, unspecified ▽

✓4ᵗʰ **P59** **Neonatal jaundice from other and unspecified causes**
   EXCLUDES 1 jaundice due to inborn errors of metabolism (E70-E88)
      kernicterus (P57.-)

P59.0 **Neonatal jaundice associated with preterm delivery**
   Hyperbilirubinemia of prematurity
   Jaundice due to delayed conjugation associated with preterm delivery

P59.1 Inspissated bile syndrome

✓5ᵗʰ **P59.2** **Neonatal jaundice from other and unspecified hepatocellular damage**
   EXCLUDES 1 congenital viral hepatitis (P35.3)

   P59.20 **Neonatal jaundice from unspecified hepatocellular damage** ▽

   P59.29 **Neonatal jaundice from other hepatocellular damage**
      Neonatal giant cell hepatitis
      Neonatal (idiopathic) hepatitis

P59.3 Neonatal jaundice from breast milk inhibitor

P59.8 Neonatal jaundice from other specified causes

P59.9 **Neonatal jaundice, unspecified** ▽
   Neonatal physiological jaundice (intense)(prolonged) NOS
   AHA: 2015, 3Q, 20

P60 **Disseminated intravascular coagulation of newborn**
   Defibrination syndrome of newborn

✓4ᵗʰ **P61** **Other perinatal hematological disorders**
   EXCLUDES 1 transient hypogammaglobulinemia of infancy (D80.7)

P61.0 **Transient neonatal thrombocytopenia**
   Neonatal thrombocytopenia due to exchange transfusion
   Neonatal thrombocytopenia due to idiopathic maternal thrombocytopenia
   Neonatal thrombocytopenia due to isoimmunization
   DEF: Temporary decrease in blood platelets of newborn; secondary to placental insufficiency.

P61.1 **Polycythemia neonatorum**
   DEF: Abnormal increase of total red blood cells of newborn; results in hyperviscosity, which slows the flow of blood through small blood vessels.

P61.2 Anemia of prematurity

P61.3 Congenital anemia from fetal blood loss

P61.4 **Other congenital anemias, not elsewhere classified**
   Congenital anemia NOS

P61.5 **Transient neonatal neutropenia**
   EXCLUDES 1 congenital neutropenia (nontransient) (D70.0)
   DEF: Low blood neutrophil counts of newborn; occurs due to maternal hypertension, sepsis, twin-twin transfusion, alloimmunization, and hemolytic disease.

P61.6 Other transient neonatal disorders of coagulation

P61.8 Other specified perinatal hematological disorders

P61.9 Perinatal hematological disorder, unspecified ▽

Transitory endocrine and metabolic disorders specific to newborn (P70-P74)

INCLUDES transitory endocrine and metabolic disturbances caused by the infant's response to maternal endocrine and metabolic factors, or its adjustment to extrauterine environment

✓4ᵗʰ **P70** **Transitory disorders of carbohydrate metabolism specific to newborn**

P70.0 **Syndrome of infant of mother with gestational diabetes**
   Newborn (with hypoglycemia) affected by maternal gestational diabetes
   EXCLUDES 1 newborn (with hypoglycemia) affected by maternal (pre-existing) diabetes mellitus (P70.1)
      syndrome of infant of a diabetic mother (P70.1)

P70.1 **Syndrome of infant of a diabetic mother**
   Newborn (with hypoglycemia) affected by maternal (pre-existing) diabetes mellitus
   EXCLUDES 1 newborn (with hypoglycemia) affected by maternal gestational diabetes (P70.0)
      syndrome of infant of mother with gestational diabetes (P70.0)

P70.2 Neonatal diabetes mellitus

P70.3 Iatrogenic neonatal hypoglycemia

P70.4 **Other neonatal hypoglycemia**
   Transitory neonatal hypoglycemia

P70.8 Other transitory disorders of carbohydrate metabolism of newborn

P70.9 Transitory disorder of carbohydrate metabolism of newborn, unspecified ▽

✓4ᵗʰ **P71** **Transitory neonatal disorders of calcium and magnesium metabolism**

P71.0 Cow's milk hypocalcemia in newborn

P71.1 **Other neonatal hypocalcemia**
   EXCLUDES 1 neonatal hypoparathyroidism (P71.4)

P71.2 Neonatal hypomagnesemia

P71.3 **Neonatal tetany without calcium or magnesium deficiency**
   Neonatal tetany NOS

P71.4 Transitory neonatal hypoparathyroidism

P71.8 Other transitory neonatal disorders of calcium and magnesium metabolism

P71.9 Transitory neonatal disorder of calcium and magnesium metabolism, unspecified ▽

✓4ᵗʰ **P72** **Other transitory neonatal endocrine disorders**
   EXCLUDES 1 congenital hypothyroidism with or without goiter (E03.0-E03.1)
      dyshormogenetic goiter (E07.1)
      Pendred's syndrome (E07.1)

P72.0 **Neonatal goiter, not elsewhere classified**
   Transitory congenital goiter with normal functioning

P72.1 **Transitory neonatal hyperthyroidism**
   Neonatal thyrotoxicosis

P72.2 **Other transitory neonatal disorders of thyroid function, not elsewhere classified**
   Transitory neonatal hypothyroidism

P72.8 Other specified transitory neonatal endocrine disorders

P72.9 Transitory neonatal endocrine disorder, unspecified ▽

✓4ᵗʰ **P74** **Other transitory neonatal electrolyte and metabolic disturbances**

P74.0 **Late metabolic acidosis of newborn**
   EXCLUDES 1 (fetal) metabolic acidosis of newborn (P19)

P74.1 Dehydration of newborn

P74.2 Disturbances of sodium balance of newborn

P74.3 Disturbances of potassium balance of newborn

P74.4 Other transitory electrolyte disturbances of newborn

P74.5 Transitory tyrosinemia of newborn

P74.6 Transitory hyperammonemia of newborn

P74.8 **Other transitory metabolic disturbances of newborn**
   Amino-acid metabolic disorders described as transitory

P74.9 Transitory metabolic disturbance of newborn, unspecified ▽

Digestive system disorders of newborn (P76-P78)

✓4ᵗʰ **P76** **Other intestinal obstruction of newborn**

P76.0 **Meconium plug syndrome**
   Meconium ileus NOS
   EXCLUDES 1 meconium ileus in cystic fibrosis (E84.11)

P76.1 **Transitory ileus of newborn**
   EXCLUDES 1 Hirschsprung's disease (Q43.1)

P76.2 Intestinal obstruction due to inspissated milk

P76.8 **Other specified intestinal obstruction of newborn**
   EXCLUDES 1 intestinal obstruction classifiable to K56-

P76.9 Intestinal obstruction of newborn, unspecified ▽

✓4ᵗʰ **P77** **Necrotizing enterocolitis of newborn**
   DEF: Serious intestinal infection and inflammation in preterm infants; severity is measured by stages and may progress to life-threatening perforation or peritonitis; resection surgical treatment may be necessary.

P77.1 **Stage 1 necrotizing enterocolitis in newborn**
   Necrotizing enterocolitis without pneumatosis, without perforation
   DEF: Broad-spectrum symptoms with nonspecific signs, including feeding intolerance, abdominal distention, bradycardia, and metabolic abnormalities.

P77.2 **Stage 2 necrotizing enterocolitis in newborn**
   Necrotizing enterocolitis with pneumatosis, without perforation
   DEF: Radiographic confirmation of necrotizing enterocolitis showing intestinal dilatation, fixed loops of bowels, pneumatosis intestinalis, metabolic acidosis, and thrombocytopenia.

EXCLUDES 1 Not coded here   *EXCLUDES 2* Not included here   **N** Newborn Age: 0   **P** Pediatric Age: 0-17   **M** Maternity Age: 12-55   **A** Adult Age: 15-124

866   ICD-10-CM 2018

P77.3   Stage 3 **necrotizing enterocolitis in newborn**
Necrotizing enterocolitis with perforation
Necrotizing enterocolitis with pneumatosis and perforation
DEF: Advanced stage in which infant demonstrates signs of bowel perforation, septic shock, metabolic acidosis, ascites, disseminated intravascular coagulopathy, neutropenia.

P77.9   **Necrotizing enterocolitis in newborn, unspecified** ▽
Necrotizing enterocolitis in newborn, NOS

☑4th **P78**   **Other perinatal digestive system disorders**
    EXCLUDES 1   cystic fibrosis (E84.0-E84.9)
             neonatal gastrointestinal hemorrhages (P54.0-P54.3)

P78.0   **Perinatal intestinal perforation**
Meconium peritonitis

P78.1   **Other neonatal peritonitis**
Neonatal peritonitis NOS

P78.2   **Neonatal hematemesis and melena due to swallowed maternal blood**

P78.3   **Noninfective neonatal diarrhea**
Neonatal diarrhea NOS

☑5th **P78.8**   **Other specified perinatal digestive system disorders**

    P78.81   **Congenital cirrhosis (of liver)**

    P78.82   **Peptic ulcer of newborn**

    P78.83   **Newborn esophageal reflux**
       Neonatal esophageal reflux

    P78.84   **Gestational alloimmune liver disease**
       GALD
       Neonatal hemochromatosis
       EXCLUDES 1   hemochromatosis (E83.11-)

    P78.89   **Other specified perinatal digestive system disorders**

P78.9   **Perinatal digestive system disorder, unspecified** ▽

Conditions involving the integument and temperature regulation of newborn (P80-P83)

☑4th **P80**   **Hypothermia of newborn**

P80.0   **Cold injury syndrome**
Severe and usually chronic hypothermia associated with a pink flushed appearance, edema and neurological and biochemical abnormalities.
    EXCLUDES 1   mild hypothermia of newborn (P80.8)

P80.8   **Other hypothermia of newborn**
Mild hypothermia of newborn

P80.9   **Hypothermia of newborn, unspecified** ▽

☑4th **P81**   **Other disturbances of temperature regulation of newborn**

P81.0   **Environmental hyperthermia of newborn**

P81.8   **Other specified disturbances of temperature regulation of newborn**

P81.9   **Disturbance of temperature regulation of newborn, unspecified** ▽
Fever of newborn NOS

☑4th **P83**   **Other conditions of integument specific to newborn**
    EXCLUDES 1   congenital malformations of skin and integument (Q80-Q84)
             hydrops fetalis due to hemolytic disease (P56.-)
             neonatal skin infection (P39.4)
             staphylococcal scalded skin syndrome (L00)
    EXCLUDES 2   cradle cap (L21.0)
             diaper [napkin] dermatitis (L22)

P83.0   **Sclerema neonatorum**
DEF: Diffuse, rapidly progressing white, waxy, nonpitting hardening of tissue, usually of legs and feet that is life-threatening; found in preterm or debilitated infants; unknown etiology.

P83.1   **Neonatal erythema toxicum**

P83.2   **Hydrops fetalis not due to hemolytic disease**
Hydrops fetalis NOS
DEF: Severe, life-threatening problem of newborn characterized by severe edema of entire body; unrelated to immune response.

☑5th **P83.3**   **Other and unspecified edema specific to newborn**

    P83.30   **Unspecified edema specific to newborn** ▽

    P83.39   **Other edema specific to newborn**

P83.4   **Breast engorgement of newborn**
Noninfective mastitis of newborn

P83.5   **Congenital hydrocele** ♂

P83.6   **Umbilical polyp of newborn**

☑5th **P83.8**   **Other specified conditions of integument specific to newborn**
    ~~Bronze baby syndrome~~
    ~~Neonatal scleroderma~~
    ~~Urticaria neonatorum~~

●   **P83.81**   **Umbilical granuloma**
       EXCLUDES 2   granulomatous disorder of the skin and subcutaneous tissue, unspecified (L92.9)

●   **P83.88**   **Other specified conditions of integument specific to newborn**
       Bronze baby syndrome
       Neonatal scleroderma
       Urticaria neonatorum

P83.9   **Condition of the integument specific to newborn, unspecified** ▽

Other problems with newborn (P84)

P84   **Other problems with newborn**
Acidemia of newborn
Acidosis of newborn
Anoxia of newborn NOS
Asphyxia of newborn NOS
Hypercapnia of newborn
Hypoxemia of newborn
Hypoxia of newborn NOS
Mixed metabolic and respiratory acidosis of newborn
    EXCLUDES 1   intracranial hemorrhage due to anoxia or hypoxia (P52.-)
             hypoxic ischemic encephalopathy [HIE] (P91.6-)
             late metabolic acidosis of newborn (P74.0)

Other disorders originating in the perinatal period (P90-P96)

P90   **Convulsions of newborn**
    EXCLUDES 1   benign myoclonic epilepsy in infancy (G40.3-)
             benign neonatal convulsions (familial) (G40.3-)

☑4th **P91**   **Other disturbances of cerebral status of newborn**

P91.0   **Neonatal cerebral ischemia**

P91.1   **Acquired periventricular cysts of newborn**

P91.2   **Neonatal cerebral leukomalacia**
Periventricular leukomalacia

P91.3   **Neonatal cerebral irritability**

P91.4   **Neonatal cerebral depression**

P91.5   **Neonatal coma**

☑5th **P91.6**   **Hypoxic ischemic encephalopathy [HIE]**
    EXCLUDES 1   ▶neonatal cerebral depression (P91.4)
             neonatal cerebral irritability (P91.3)
             neonatal coma (P91.5)◀

    P91.60   **Hypoxic ischemic encephalopathy [HIE], unspecified** ▽

    P91.61   **Mild hypoxic ischemic encephalopathy [HIE]**

    P91.62   **Moderate hypoxic ischemic encephalopathy [HIE]**

    P91.63   **Severe hypoxic ischemic encephalopathy [HIE]**

☑5th **P91.8**   **Other specified disturbances of cerebral status of newborn**

● ☑6th   **P91.81**   **Neonatal encephalopathy**

●   **P91.811**   **Neonatal encephalopathy in diseases classified elsewhere**
          Code first underlying condition, if known, such as:
          congenital cirrhosis (of liver) (P78.71)
          intracranial nontraumatic hemorrhage of newborn (P52.-)
          kernicterus (P57.-)

●   **P91.819**   **Neonatal encephalopathy, unspecified** ▽

●   **P91.88**   **Other specified disturbances of cerebral status of newborn**

P91.9   **Disturbance of cerebral status of newborn, unspecified** ▽

☑4th **P92**   **Feeding problems of newborn**
    EXCLUDES 1   ▶eating disorders (F50.-)◀
             feeding problems in child over 28 days old (R63.3)
    AHA: 2016, 3Q, 19

☑5th **P92.0**   **Vomiting of newborn**
    EXCLUDES 1   vomiting of child over 28 days old (R11.-)

    P92.01   **Bilious vomiting of newborn**
       EXCLUDES 1   bilious vomiting in child over 28 days old (R11.14)

    P92.09   **Other vomiting of newborn**
       EXCLUDES 1   regurgitation of food in newborn (P92.1)

☑ Additional Character Req   ✓x7th Placeholder Alert   Manifestation   HCC CMS-HCC Condition   ▽ Unspecified Code   ▶◀ Revised Text   ● New Code   ▲ Revised Code Title

P92.1   Regurgitation and rumination of newborn

P92.2   Slow feeding of newborn

P92.3   Underfeeding of newborn

P92.4   Overfeeding of newborn

P92.5   Neonatal difficulty in feeding at breast
AHA: 2017, 1Q, 28

P92.6   Failure to thrive in newborn
EXCLUDES 1   failure to thrive in child over 28 days old (R62.51)

P92.8   Other feeding problems of newborn

P92.9   Feeding problem of newborn, unspecified   ▽

✓4ᵗʰ **P93**   Reactions and intoxications due to drugs administered to newborn
INCLUDES   reactions and intoxications due to drugs administered to fetus affecting newborn
EXCLUDES 1   jaundice due to drugs or toxins transmitted from mother or given to newborn (P58.4-)
reactions and intoxications from maternal opiates, tranquilizers and other medication (P04.0-P04.1, P04.4)
withdrawal symptoms from maternal use of drugs of addiction (P96.1)
withdrawal symptoms from therapeutic use of drugs in newborn (P96.2)

P93.0   Grey baby syndrome
Grey syndrome from chloramphenicol administration in newborn

P93.8   Other reactions and intoxications due to drugs administered to newborn
Use additional code for adverse effect, if applicable, to identify drug (T36-T50 with fifth or sixth character 5)

✓4ᵗʰ **P94**   Disorders of muscle tone of newborn

P94.0   Transient neonatal myasthenia gravis
EXCLUDES 1   myasthenia gravis (G70.0)

P94.1   Congenital hypertonia

P94.2   Congenital hypotonia
Floppy baby syndrome, unspecified

P94.8   Other disorders of muscle tone of newborn

P94.9   Disorder of muscle tone of newborn, unspecified   ▽

P95   Stillbirth
Deadborn fetus NOS
Fetal death of unspecified cause
Stillbirth NOS
EXCLUDES 1   maternal care for intrauterine death (O36.4)
missed abortion (O02.1)
outcome of delivery, stillbirth (Z37.1, Z37.3, Z37.4, Z37.7)

✓4ᵗʰ **P96**   Other conditions originating in the perinatal period

P96.0   Congenital renal failure
Uremia of newborn

P96.1   Neonatal withdrawal symptoms from maternal use of drugs of addiction
Drug withdrawal syndrome in infant of dependent mother
Neonatal abstinence syndrome
EXCLUDES 1   reactions and intoxications from maternal opiates and tranquilizers administered during labor and delivery (P04.0)

P96.2   Withdrawal symptoms from therapeutic use of drugs in newborn

P96.3   Wide cranial sutures of newborn
Neonatal craniotabes

P96.5   Complication to newborn due to (fetal) intrauterine procedure
EXCLUDES 2   newborn affected by amniocentesis (P00.6)

✓5ᵗʰ **P96.8**   Other specified conditions originating in the perinatal period

P96.81   Exposure to (parental) (environmental) tobacco smoke in the perinatal period
EXCLUDES 2   newborn affected by in utero exposure to tobacco (P04.2)
exposure to environmental tobacco smoke after the perinatal period (Z77.22)

P96.82   Delayed separation of umbilical cord

P96.83   Meconium staining
EXCLUDES 1   meconium aspiration (P24.00, P24.01)
meconium passage during delivery (P03.82)

P96.89   Other specified conditions originating in the perinatal period
Use additional code to specify condition

P96.9   Condition originating in the perinatal period, unspecified   ▽
Congenital debility NOS

EXCLUDES 1 Not coded here   EXCLUDES 2 Not included here   N Newborn Age: 0   P Pediatric Age: 0-17   M Maternity Age: 12-55   A Adult Age: 15-124

868   ICD-10-CM 2018

P92.1–P96.9

Chapter 17. Congenital Malformations, Deformations, and Chromosomal Abnormalities (Q00–Q99)

Chapter Specific Guidelines with Coding Examples

The chapter specific guidelines from the ICD-10-CM Official Guidelines for Coding and Reporting have been provided below. Along with these guidelines are coding examples, contained in the shaded boxes, that have been developed to help illustrate the coding and/or sequencing guidance found in these guidelines.

Assign an appropriate code(s) from categories Q00-Q99, Congenital malformations, deformations, and chromosomal abnormalities when a malformation/deformation or chromosomal abnormality is documented. A malformation/deformation/or chromosomal abnormality may be the principal/first-listed diagnosis on a record or a secondary diagnosis.

When a malformation/deformation/or chromosomal abnormality does not have a unique code assignment, assign additional code(s) for any manifestations that may be present.

When the code assignment specifically identifies the malformation/deformation/or chromosomal abnormality, manifestations that are an inherent component of the anomaly should not be coded separately. Additional codes should be assigned for manifestations that are not an inherent component.

8-day-old infant with tetralogy of Fallot and pulmonary stenosis

Q21.3   Tetralogy of Fallot

Explanation: Pulmonary stenosis is inherent in the disease process of tetralogy of Fallot. When the code assignment specifically identifies the malformation/deformation/or chromosomal abnormality, manifestations that are inherent components of the anomaly should not be coded separately.

7-month-old infant with Down syndrome and common atrioventricular canal

Q90.9   Down syndrome, unspecified

Q21.2   Atrioventricular septal defect

Explanation: While a common atrioventricular canal is often associated with patients with Down syndrome, this manifestation is not an inherent component and may be reported separately. When the code assignment specifically identifies the anomaly, manifestations that are inherent components of the condition should not be coded separately. Additional codes should be assigned for manifestations that are not inherent components.

Codes from Chapter 17 may be used throughout the life of the patient. If a congenital malformation or deformity has been corrected, a personal history code should be used to identify the history of the malformation or deformity. Although present at birth, malformation/deformation/or chromosomal abnormality may not be identified until later in life. Whenever the condition is diagnosed by the physician, it is appropriate to assign a code from codes Q00-Q99. For the birth admission, the appropriate code from category Z38, Liveborn infants, according to place of birth and type of delivery, should be sequenced as the principal diagnosis, followed by any congenital anomaly codes, Q00- Q99.

Three-year-old with history of corrected ventricular septal defect

Z87.74   Personal history of (corrected) congenital malformations of heart and circulatory system

Explanation: If a congenital malformation or deformity has been corrected, a personal history code should be used to identify the history of the malformation or deformity.

Forty-year-old man with headaches diagnosed with congenital arteriovenous malformation by brain scan

Q28.2   Arteriovenous malformation of cerebral vessels

Explanation: Although present at birth, malformations may not be identified until later in life. Whenever the condition is diagnosed by the physician, it is appropriate to assign a code from the range Q00–Q99.

Newborn with anencephaly delivered vaginally in hospital

Z38.00   Single liveborn infant, delivered vaginally

Q00.0   Anencephaly

Explanation: For the birth admission, the appropriate code from category Z38 Liveborn infants, according to place of birth and type of delivery, should be sequenced as the principal diagnosis, followed by any congenital anomaly codes, Q00–Q99.

Chapter 17. Congenital Malformations, Deformations and Chromosomal Abnormalities(Q00-Q99)

NOTE Codes from this chapter are not for use on maternal or fetal records.

EXCLUDES 2 inborn errors of metabolism (E70-E88)

This chapter contains the following blocks:

Q00-Q07   Congenital malformations of the nervous system
Q10-Q18   Congenital malformations of eye, ear, face and neck
Q20-Q28   Congenital malformations of the circulatory system
Q30-Q34   Congenital malformations of the respiratory system
Q35-Q37   Cleft lip and cleft palate
Q38-Q45   Other congenital malformations of the digestive system
Q50-Q56   Congenital malformations of genital organs
Q60-Q64   Congenital malformations of the urinary system
Q65-Q79   Congenital malformations and deformations of the musculoskeletal system
Q80-Q89   Other congenital malformations
Q90-Q99   Chromosomal abnormalities, not elsewhere classified

Congenital malformations of the nervous system (Q00-Q07)

✓4ᵗʰ Q00 Anencephaly and similar malformations

   Q00.0 Anencephaly   HCC
     Acephaly
     Acrania
     Amyelencephaly
     Hemianencephaly
     Hemicephaly

   Q00.1 Craniorachischisis   HCC

   Q00.2 Iniencephaly   HCC

✓4ᵗʰ Q01 Encephalocele
   INCLUDES Arnold-Chiari syndrome, type III
     encephalocystocele
     encephalomyelocele
     hydroencephalocele
     hydromeningocele, cranial
     meningocele, cerebral
     meningoencephalocele
   EXCLUDES 1 Meckel-Gruber syndrome (Q61.9)

   Q01.0 Frontal encephalocele   HCC
   Q01.1 Nasofrontal encephalocele   HCC
   Q01.2 Occipital encephalocele   HCC
   Q01.8 Encephalocele of other sites   HCC
   Q01.9 Encephalocele, unspecified   HCC ▽

Q02 Microcephaly   HCC
   INCLUDES hydromicrocephaly
     micrencephalon
   EXCLUDES 1 Meckel-Gruber syndrome (Q61.9)

✓4ᵗʰ Q03 Congenital hydrocephalus
   INCLUDES hydrocephalus in newborn
   EXCLUDES 1 Arnold-Chiari syndrome, type II (Q07.0-)
     acquired hydrocephalus (G91.-)
     hydrocephalus due to congenital toxoplasmosis (P37.1)
     hydrocephalus with spina bifida (Q05.0-Q05.4)

   Q03.0 Malformations of aqueduct of Sylvius   HCC
     Anomaly of aqueduct of Sylvius
     Obstruction of aqueduct of Sylvius, congenital
     Stenosis of aqueduct of Sylvius

   Q03.1 Atresia of foramina of Magendie and Luschkaq   HCC
     Dandy-Walker syndrome

Congenital Hydrocephalus

Pressure

Normal ventricles   Hydrocephalic ventricles

   Q03.8 Other congenital hydrocephalus   HCC
   Q03.9 Congenital hydrocephalus, unspecified   HCC ▽

✓4ᵗʰ Q04 Other congenital malformations of brain
   EXCLUDES 1 cyclopia (Q87.0)
     macrocephaly (Q75.3)

   Q04.0 Congenital malformations of corpus callosum   HCC
     Agenesis of corpus callosum

   Q04.1 Arhinencephaly   HCC

   Q04.2 Holoprosencephaly   HCC

   Q04.3 Other reduction deformities of brain   HCC
     Absence of part of brain
     Agenesis of part of brain
     Agyria
     Aplasia of part of brain
     Hydranencephaly
     Hypoplasia of part of brain
     Lissencephaly
     Microgyria
     Pachygyria
   EXCLUDES 1 congenital malformations of corpus callosum (Q04.0)

   Q04.4 Septo-optic dysplasia of brain   HCC
   Q04.5 Megalencephaly   HCC
   Q04.6 Congenital cerebral cysts   HCC
     Porencephaly
     Schizencephaly
   EXCLUDES 1 acquired porencephalic cyst (G93.0)

   Q04.8 Other specified congenital malformations of brain   HCC
     Arnold-Chiari syndrome, type IV
     Macrogyria

   Q04.9 Congenital malformation of brain, unspecified   HCC ▽
     Congenital anomaly NOS of brain
     Congenital deformity NOS of brain
     Congenital disease or lesion NOS of brain
     Multiple anomalies NOS of brain, congenital

✓4ᵗʰ Q05 Spina bifida
   INCLUDES hydromeningocele (spinal)
     meningocele (spinal)
     meningomyelocele
     myelocele
     myelomeningocele
     rachischisis
     spina bifida (aperta)(cystica)
     syringomyelocele
   Use additional code for any associated paraplegia (paraparesis) (G82.2-)
   EXCLUDES 1 Arnold-Chiari syndrome, type II (Q07.0-)
     spina bifida occulta (Q76.0)

   Q05.0 Cervical spina bifida with hydrocephalus   HCC
   Q05.1 Thoracic spina bifida with hydrocephalus   HCC
     Dorsal spina bifida with hydrocephalus
     Thoracolumbar spina bifida with hydrocephalus
   Q05.2 Lumbar spina bifida with hydrocephalus   HCC
     Lumbosacral spina bifida with hydrocephalus
   Q05.3 Sacral spina bifida with hydrocephalus   HCC
   Q05.4 Unspecified spina bifida with hydrocephalus   HCC ▽
   Q05.5 Cervical spina bifida without hydrocephalus   HCC
   Q05.6 Thoracic spina bifida without hydrocephalus   HCC
     Dorsal spina bifida NOS
     Thoracolumbar spina bifida NOS
   Q05.7 Lumbar spina bifida without hydrocephalus   HCC
     Lumbosacral spina bifida NOS
   Q05.8 Sacral spina bifida without hydrocephalus   HCC
   Q05.9 Spina bifida, unspecified   HCC ▽

Spina Bifida

Cerebrospinal fluid

Cerebrospinal fluid

Spinal process

Meninges

Neural tissue

Vertebral body   Spinal cord   Meninges   Spinal cord

Spina bifida occulta   **Meningocele**   **Myelomeningocele**

EXCLUDES 1 Not coded here   *EXCLUDES 2* Not included here   N Newborn Age: 0   P Pediatric Age: 0-17   M Maternity Age: 12-55   A Adult Age: 15-124

☑4ᵗʰ Q06 Other congenital malformations of spinal cord

    Q06.0 Amyelia   HCC

    Q06.1 Hypoplasia and dysplasia of spinal cord   HCC
        Atelomyelia
        Myelatelia
        Myelodysplasia of spinal cord

    Q06.2 Diastematomyelia   HCC
        DEF: Rare congenital anomaly often associated with spina bifida; the spinal cord is separated into longitudinal halves by a bony, cartilaginous or fibrous septum, each half surrounded by a dural sac.

    Q06.3 Other congenital cauda equina malformations   HCC

    Q06.4 Hydromyelia   HCC
        Hydrorachis

    Q06.8 Other specified congenital malformations of spinal cord   HCC

    Q06.9 Congenital malformation of spinal cord, unspecified   HCC ▽
        Congenital anomaly NOS of spinal cord
        Congenital deformity NOS of spinal cord
        Congenital disease or lesion NOS of spinal cord

☑4ᵗʰ Q07 Other congenital malformations of nervous system

    EXCLUDES 2   *congenital central alveolar hypoventilation syndrome (G47.35)*
        familial dysautonomia [Riley-Day] (G90.1)
        neurofibromatosis (nonmalignant) (Q85.0-)

    ☑5ᵗʰ Q07.0 Arnold-Chiari syndrome
        Arnold-Chiari syndrome, type II
        EXCLUDES 1   *Arnold-Chiari syndrome, type III (Q01.-)*
                Arnold-Chiari syndrome, type IV (Q04.8)

        Q07.00 Arnold-Chiari syndrome without spina bifida or hydrocephalus   HCC

        Q07.01 Arnold-Chiari syndrome with spina bifida   HCC

        Q07.02 Arnold-Chiari syndrome with hydrocephalus   HCC

        Q07.03 Arnold-Chiari syndrome with spina bifida and hydrocephalus   HCC

    Q07.8 Other specified congenital malformations of nervous system   HCC
        Agenesis of nerve
        Displacement of brachial plexus
        Jaw-winking syndrome
        Marcus Gunn's syndrome

    Q07.9 Congenital malformation of nervous system, unspecified   HCC ▽
        Congenital anomaly NOS of nervous system
        Congenital deformity NOS of nervous system
        Congenital disease or lesion NOS of nervous system

Congenital malformations of eye, ear, face and neck (Q10-Q18)

    EXCLUDES 2   *cleft lip and cleft palate (Q35-Q37)*
        congenital malformation of cervical spine (Q05.0, Q05.5, Q67.5, Q76.0-Q76.4)
        congenital malformation of larynx (Q31.-)
        congenital malformation of lip NEC (Q38.0)
        congenital malformation of nose (Q30.-)
        congenital malformation of parathyroid gland (Q89.2)
        congenital malformation of thyroid gland (Q89.2)

☑4ᵗʰ Q10 Congenital malformations of eyelid, lacrimal apparatus and orbit

    EXCLUDES 1   *cryptophthalmos NOS (Q11.2)*
        cryptophthalmos syndrome (Q87.0)

    Q10.0 Congenital ptosis
        DEF: Congenital drooping of eyelid; mostly idiopathic, but may occur genetically.

    Q10.1 Congenital ectropion

    Q10.2 Congenital entropion

    Q10.3 Other congenital malformations of eyelid
        Ablepharon
        Blepharophimosis, congenital
        Coloboma of eyelid
        Congenital absence or agenesis of cilia
        Congenital absence or agenesis of eyelid
        Congenital accessory eyelid
        Congenital accessory eye muscle
        Congenital malformation of eyelid NOS

    Q10.4 Absence and agenesis of lacrimal apparatus
        Congenital absence of punctum lacrimale

    Q10.5 Congenital stenosis and stricture of lacrimal duct

    Q10.6 Other congenital malformations of lacrimal apparatus
        Congenital malformation of lacrimal apparatus NOS

    Q10.7 Congenital malformation of orbit

Coloboma of Lens

Coloboma

☑4ᵗʰ Q11 Anophthalmos, microphthalmos and macrophthalmos

    Q11.0 Cystic eyeball

    Q11.1 Other anophthalmos
        Anophthalmos NOS
        Agenesis of eye
        Aplasia of eye

    Q11.2 Microphthalmos
        Cryptophthalmos NOS
        Dysplasia of eye
        Hypoplasia of eye
        Rudimentary eye
        EXCLUDES 1   *cryptophthalmos syndrome (Q87.0)*

    Q11.3 Macrophthalmos
        EXCLUDES 1   *macrophthalmos in congenital glaucoma (Q15.0)*

☑4ᵗʰ Q12 Congenital lens malformations

    Q12.0 Congenital cataract

    Q12.1 Congenital displaced lens

    Q12.2 Coloboma of lens

    Q12.3 Congenital aphakia

    Q12.4 Spherophakia

    Q12.8 Other congenital lens malformations
        Microphakia

    Q12.9 Congenital lens malformation, unspecified   ▽

☑4ᵗʰ Q13 Congenital malformations of anterior segment of eye

    Q13.0 Coloboma of iris
        Coloboma NOS

    Q13.1 Absence of iris
        Aniridia
        Use additional code for associated glaucoma (H42)
        DEF: Incompletely formed or absent iris; affects both eyes; dominant trait.

    Q13.2 Other congenital malformations of iris
        Anisocoria, congenital
        Atresia of pupil
        Congenital malformation of iris NOS
        Corectopia

    Q13.3 Congenital corneal opacity

    Q13.4 Other congenital corneal malformations
        Congenital malformation of cornea NOS
        Microcornea
        Peter's anomaly

    Q13.5 Blue sclera

    ☑5ᵗʰ Q13.8 Other congenital malformations of anterior segment of eye

        Q13.81 Rieger's anomaly
                 Use additional code for associated glaucoma (H42)

        Q13.89 Other congenital malformations of anterior segment of eye

    Q13.9 Congenital malformation of anterior segment of eye, unspecified   ▽

☑4ᵗʰ Q14 Congenital malformations of posterior segment of eye

    EXCLUDES 2   *optic nerve hypoplasia (H47.03-)*

    Q14.0 Congenital malformation of vitreous humor
        Congenital vitreous opacity

    Q14.1 Congenital malformation of retina
        Congenital retinal aneurysm

    Q14.2 Congenital malformation of optic disc
        Coloboma of optic disc

    Q14.3 Congenital malformation of choroid

    Q14.8 Other congenital malformations of posterior segment of eye
        Coloboma of the fundus

☑ Additional Character Req   ✓7ᵗʰ Placeholder Alert   Manifestation   HCC CMS-HCC Condition   ▽ Unspecified Code   ►◄ Revised Text   ● New Code   ▲ Revised Code Title

ICD-10-CM 2018   871

Chapter 17. Congenital Malformations, Deformations, and Chromosomal Abnormalities

Q14.9   Congenital malformation of posterior segment of eye, unspecified ▽

✓4ᵗʰ **Q15   Other congenital malformations of eye**
> EXCLUDES 1   congenital nystagmus (H55.01)
> ocular albinism (E70.31-)
> optic nerve hypoplasia (H47.03-)
> retinitis pigmentosa (H35.52)

Q15.0   Congenital glaucoma
Axenfeld's anomaly
Buphthalmos
Glaucoma of childhood
Glaucoma of newborn
Hydrophthalmos
Keratoglobus, congenital, with glaucoma
Macrocornea with glaucoma
Macrophthalmos in congenital glaucoma
Megalocornea with glaucoma

Q15.8   Other specified congenital malformations of eye

Q15.9   Congenital malformation of eye, unspecified ▽
Congenital anomaly of eye
Congenital deformity of eye

✓4ᵗʰ **Q16   Congenital malformations of ear causing impairment of hearing**
> EXCLUDES 1   congenital deafness (H90.-)

Q16.0   Congenital absence of (ear) auricle

Q16.1   Congenital absence, atresia and stricture of auditory canal (external)
Congenital atresia or stricture of osseous meatus

Q16.2   Absence of eustachian tube

Q16.3   Congenital malformation of ear ossicles
Congenital fusion of ear ossicles

Q16.4   Other congenital malformations of middle ear
Congenital malformation of middle ear NOS

Q16.5   Congenital malformation of inner ear
Congenital anomaly of membranous labyrinth
Congenital anomaly of organ of Corti

Q16.9   Congenital malformation of ear causing impairment of hearing, unspecified ▽
Congenital absence of ear NOS

✓4ᵗʰ **Q17   Other congenital malformations of ear**
> EXCLUDES 1   congenital malformations of ear with impairment of hearing (Q16.0- Q16.9)
> preauricular sinus (Q18.1)

Q17.0   Accessory auricle
Accessory tragus
Polyotia
Preauricular appendage or tag
Supernumerary ear
Supernumerary lobule

Q17.1   Macrotia
> DEF: Birth defect characterized by abnormal enlargement of the pinna of the ear.

Q17.2   Microtia

Q17.3   Other misshapen ear
Pointed ear

Q17.4   Misplaced ear
Low-set ears
> EXCLUDES 1   cervical auricle (Q18.2)

Q17.5   Prominent ear
Bat ear

Q17.8   Other specified congenital malformations of ear
Congenital absence of lobe of ear

Q17.9   Congenital malformation of ear, unspecified ▽
Congenital anomaly of ear NOS

✓4ᵗʰ **Q18   Other congenital malformations of face and neck**
> EXCLUDES 1   cleft lip and cleft palate (Q35-Q37)
> conditions classified to Q67.0-Q67.4
> congenital malformations of skull and face bones (Q75.-)
> cyclopia (Q87.0)
> dentofacial anomalies [including malocclusion] (M26.-)
> malformation syndromes affecting facial appearance (Q87.0)
> persistent thyroglossal duct (Q89.2)

Q18.0   Sinus, fistula and cyst of branchial cleft
Branchial vestige

Q18.1   Preauricular sinus and cyst
Fistula of auricle, congenital
Cervicoaural fistula

Q18.2   Other branchial cleft malformations
Branchial cleft malformation NOS
Cervical auricle
Otocephaly

Q18.3   Webbing of neck
Pterygium colli
> DEF: Congenital malformation characterized by thick, triangular skinfold that stretches from the lateral side of the neck across the shoulder; associated with genetic conditions Turner's and Noonan's syndromes.

Q18.4   Macrostomia
> DEF: Rare congenital craniofacial bilateral or unilateral anomaly of mouth due to malformed maxillary and mandibular processes; results in abnormally large mouth extending towards ear.

Q18.5   Microstomia

Q18.6   Macrocheilia
Hypertrophy of lip, congenital

Q18.7   Microcheilia

Q18.8   Other specified congenital malformations of face and neck
Medial cyst of face and neck
Medial fistula of face and neck
Medial sinus of face and neck

Q18.9   Congenital malformation of face and neck, unspecified ▽
Congenital anomaly NOS of face and neck

Congenital malformations of the circulatory system (Q20-Q28)

✓4ᵗʰ **Q20   Congenital malformations of cardiac chambers and connections**
> EXCLUDES 1   dextrocardia with situs inversus (Q89.3)
> mirror-image atrial arrangement with situs inversus (Q89.3)

Q20.0   Common arterial trunk
Persistent truncus arteriosus
> EXCLUDES 1   aortic septal defect (Q21.4)

Q20.1   Double outlet right ventricle
Taussig-Bing syndrome

Q20.2   Double outlet left ventricle

Q20.3   Discordant ventriculoarterial connection
Dextrotransposition of aorta
Transposition of great vessels (complete)

Q20.4   Double inlet ventricle
Common ventricle
Cor triloculare biatriatum
Single ventricle

Q20.5   Discordant atrioventricular connection
Corrected transposition
Levotransposition
Ventricular inversion

Q20.6   Isomerism of atrial appendages
Isomerism of atrial appendages with asplenia or polysplenia

Q20.8   Other congenital malformations of cardiac chambers and connections
Cor binoculare

Q20.9   Congenital malformation of cardiac chambers and connections, unspecified ▽

✓4ᵗʰ **Q21   Congenital malformations of cardiac septa**
> EXCLUDES 1   acquired cardiac septal defect (I51.0)

Q21.0   Ventricular septal defect
Roger's disease

Ventricular Septal Defect

EXCLUDES 1   Not coded here   EXCLUDES 2   Not included here   N   Newborn Age: 0   P   Pediatric Age: 0-17   M   Maternity Age: 12-55   A   Adult Age: 15-124

872   ICD-10-CM 2018

Atrial Septal Defect

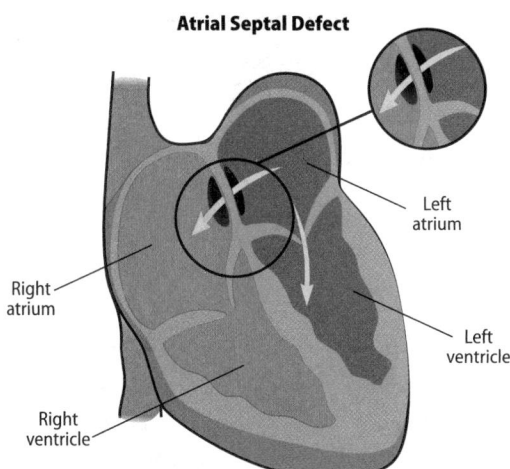

Left atrium

Right atrium

Left ventricle

Right ventricle

Atrioventricular Septal Defect

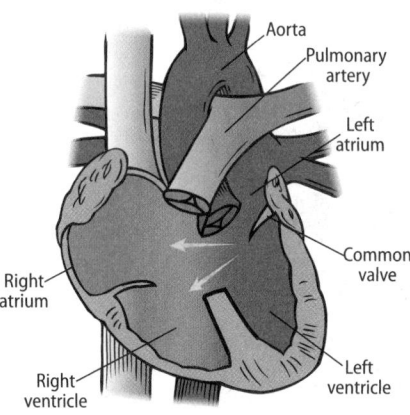

Aorta

Pulmonary artery

Left atrium

Common valve

Right atrium

Left ventricle

Right ventricle

Q21.1   Atrial **septal defect**
Coronary sinus defect
Patent or persistent foramen ovale
Patent or persistent ostium secundum defect (type II)
Patent or persistent sinus venosus defect

Q21.2   Atrioventricular **septal defect**
Common atrioventricular canal
Endocardial cushion defect
Ostium primum atrial septal defect (type I)

Q21.3   Tetralogy of Fallot
Ventricular septal defect with pulmonary stenosis or atresia, dextroposition of aorta and hypertrophy of right ventricle.
AHA: 2014, 3Q, 16

Q21.4   Aortopulmonary septal **defect**
Aortic septal defect   Aortopulmonary window

Q21.8   Other congenital malformations of cardiac septa
Eisenmenger's defect
Pentalogy of Fallot
▶Code also if applicable:
Eisenmenger's complex (I27.83)
Eisenmenger's syndrome (I27.83)◀
EXCLUDES 1   *Eisenmenger's complex (I27.8)*
Eisenmenger's syndrome (I27.8)

Q21.9   Congenital malformation of cardiac septum, unspecified ▽
Septal (heart) defect NOS

✓4ᵗʰ **Q22**   **Congenital malformations of pulmonary and tricuspid valves**

Q22.0   Pulmonary **valve** atresia

Q22.1   **Congenital** pulmonary **valve** stenosis
DEF: Stenosis of opening between pulmonary artery and right ventricle; causes obstructed blood outflow from right ventricle.

Q22.2   **Congenital** pulmonary **valve** insufficiency
Congenital pulmonary valve regurgitation

Q22.3   Other congenital malformations of pulmonary valve
Congenital malformation of pulmonary valve NOS
Supernumerary cusps of pulmonary valve

Q22.4   **Congenital** tricuspid stenosis
Congenital tricuspid atresia

Q22.5   Ebstein's anomaly
DEF: Malformation of the tricuspid valve characterized by septal and posterior leaflets attaching to the wall of the right ventricle; causes the right ventricle to fuse with the atrium into a large right atrium and a small ventricle; leads to heart failure and abnormal cardiac rhythm.

Q22.6   Hypoplastic right heart syndrome

Q22.8   Other congenital malformations of tricuspid valve

Q22.9   Congenital malformation of tricuspid valve, unspecified ▽

✓4ᵗʰ **Q23**   **Congenital malformations of aortic and mitral valves**

Q23.0   **Congenital** stenosis **of aortic valve**
Congenital aortic atresia
Congenital aortic stenosis NOS
EXCLUDES 1   *congenital stenosis of aortic valve in hypoplastic left heart syndrome (Q23.4)*
congenital subaortic stenosis (Q24.4)
supravalvular aortic stenosis (congenital) (Q25.3)

Q23.1   **Congenital** insufficiency **of aortic valve**
Bicuspid aortic valve
Congenital aortic insufficiency

Q23.2   **Congenital** mitral stenosis
Congenital mitral atresia
DEF: Congenital stenosis of mitral valve orifice between left atrium and ventricle; at the supravalvular, valvular, or subvalvular levels; causes obstruction to left ventricular filling.

Q23.3   **Congenital** mitral insufficiency

Q23.4   Hypoplastic left heart syndrome

Q23.8   Other congenital malformations of aortic and mitral valves

Q23.9   Congenital malformation of aortic and mitral valves, ▽
unspecified

✓4ᵗʰ **Q24**   **Other congenital malformations of** heart
EXCLUDES 1   *endocardial fibroelastosis (I42.4)*

Q24.0   Dextrocardia
EXCLUDES 1   *dextrocardia with situs inversus (Q89.3)*
isomerism of atrial appendages (with asplenia or polysplenia) (Q20.6)
mirror-image atrial arrangement with situs inversus (Q89.3)

Q24.1   Levocardia

Q24.2   Cor triatriatum

Q24.3   Pulmonary infundibular stenosis
Subvalvular pulmonic stenosis

Q24.4   Congenital subaortic stenosis
DEF: Congenital heart defect characterized by stenosis of left ventricular outflow tract due to fibrous tissue ring or septal hypertrophy below aortic valve.

Q24.5   Malformation of coronary vessels
Congenital coronary (artery) aneurysm

Q24.6   Congenital heart block

Q24.8   Other specified congenital malformations of heart
Congenital diverticulum of left ventricle
Congenital malformation of myocardium
Congenital malformation of pericardium
Malposition of heart
Uhl's disease

Q24.9   Congenital malformation of heart, unspecified ▽
Congenital anomaly of heart
Congenital disease of heart

✓4ᵗʰ **Q25**   **Congenital malformations of** great arteries

Q25.0   Patent ductus arteriosus
Patent ductus Botallo   Persistent ductus arteriosus

Q25.1   Coarctation **of** aorta
Coarctation of aorta (preductal) (postductal)
Stenosis of Aorta

✓5ᵗʰ **Q25.2**   Atresia **of** aorta

    Q25.21   Interruption of Aortic Arch
Atresia of aortic arch

    Q25.29   Other atresia of aorta
Atresia of aorta

Q25.3   Supravalvular **aortic** stenosis
EXCLUDES 1   *congenital aortic stenosis NOS (Q23.0)*
congenital stenosis of aortic valve (Q23.0)

☑ Additional Character Req   ✓x7ᵗʰ Placeholder Alert   **Manifestation**   **HCC** CMS-HCC Condition   ▽ Unspecified Code   ▶◀ Revised Text   ● New Code   ▲ Revised Code Title

Patent Ductus Arteriosus

Aortic Arch Anomalies

Normal aortic arch

Double aortic arch   Right aortic arch

✓5ᵗʰ Q25.4 Other congenital malformations of aorta
> *EXCLUDES 1*   *hypoplasia of aorta in hypoplastic left heart syndrome (Q23.4)*

    Q25.40 Congenital malformation of aorta unspecified ▽
    Q25.41 Absence and aplasia of aorta
    Q25.42 Hypoplasia of aorta
    Q25.43 Congenital aneurysm of aorta
       Congenital aneurysm of aortic root
       Congenital aneurysm of aortic sinus
    Q25.44 Congenital dilation of aorta
    Q25.45 Double aortic arch
       Vascular ring of aorta
    Q25.46 Tortuous aortic arch
       Persistent convolutions of aortic arch
    Q25.47 Right aortic arch
       Persistent right aortic arch
    Q25.48 Anomalous origin of subclavian artery
    Q25.49 Other congenital malformations of aorta
       ▶Aortic arch
       Bovine arch◀

Q25.5 Atresia of pulmonary artery

Q25.6 Stenosis of pulmonary artery
       Supravalvular pulmonary stenosis

✓5ᵗʰ Q25.7 Other congenital malformations of pulmonary artery
    Q25.71 Coarctation of pulmonary artery
    Q25.72 Congenital pulmonary arteriovenous malformation
       Congenital pulmonary arteriovenous aneurysm
    Q25.79 Other congenital malformations of pulmonary artery
       Aberrant pulmonary artery
       Agenesis of pulmonary artery
       Congenital aneurysm of pulmonary artery
       Congenital anomaly of pulmonary artery
       Hypoplasia of pulmonary artery

Q25.8 Other congenital malformations of other great arteries

Q25.9 Congenital malformation of great arteries, unspecified ▽

✓4ᵗʰ Q26 Congenital malformations of great veins
    Q26.0 Congenital stenosis of vena cava
       Congenital stenosis of vena cava (inferior)(superior)
    Q26.1 Persistent left superior vena cava
    Q26.2 Total anomalous pulmonary venous connection
       Total anomalous pulmonary venous return [TAPVR], subdiaphragmatic
       Total anomalous pulmonary venous return [TAPVR], supradiaphragmatic
    Q26.3 Partial anomalous pulmonary venous connection
       Partial anomalous pulmonary venous return
    Q26.4 Anomalous pulmonary venous connection, unspecified ▽

Q26.5 Anomalous portal venous connection

Q26.6 Portal vein-hepatic artery fistula

Q26.8 Other congenital malformations of great veins
       Absence of vena cava (inferior) (superior)
       Azygos continuation of inferior vena cava
       Persistent left posterior cardinal vein
       Scimitar syndrome

Q26.9 Congenital malformation of great vein, unspecified ▽
       Congenital anomaly of vena cava (inferior) (superior) NOS

✓4ᵗʰ Q27 Other congenital malformations of peripheral vascular system
> *EXCLUDES 2*   *anomalies of cerebral and precerebral vessels (Q28.0-Q28.3)*
> *anomalies of coronary vessels (Q24.5)*
> *anomalies of pulmonary artery (Q25.5-Q25.7)*
> *congenital retinal aneurysm (Q14.1)*
> *hemangioma and lymphangioma (D18.-)*

Q27.0 Congenital absence and hypoplasia of umbilical artery
       Single umbilical artery

Q27.1 Congenital renal artery stenosis

Q27.2 Other congenital malformations of renal artery
       Congenital malformation of renal artery NOS
       Multiple renal arteries

✓5ᵗʰ Q27.3 Arteriovenous malformation (peripheral)
       Arteriovenous aneurysm
> *EXCLUDES 1*   *acquired arteriovenous aneurysm (I77.0)*
> *EXCLUDES 2*   *arteriovenous malformation of cerebral vessels (Q28.2)*
> *arteriovenous malformation of precerebral vessels (Q28.0)*

    Q27.30 Arteriovenous malformation, site unspecified ▽
    Q27.31 Arteriovenous malformation of vessel of upper limb
    Q27.32 Arteriovenous malformation of vessel of lower limb
    Q27.33 Arteriovenous malformation of digestive system vessel
    Q27.34 Arteriovenous malformation of renal vessel
    Q27.39 Arteriovenous malformation, other site

Q27.4 Congenital phlebectasia

Q27.8 Other specified congenital malformations of peripheral vascular system
       Absence of peripheral vascular system
       Atresia of peripheral vascular system
       Congenital aneurysm (peripheral)
       Congenital stricture, artery
       Congenital varix
> *EXCLUDES 1*   *arteriovenous malformation (Q27.3-)*

Q27.9 Congenital malformation of peripheral vascular system, unspecified ▽
       Anomaly of artery or vein NOS

EXCLUDES 1 Not coded here   *EXCLUDES 2* Not included here   **N** Newborn Age: 0   **P** Pediatric Age: 0-17   **M** Maternity Age: 12-55   **A** Adult Age: 15-124

☑4ᵗʰ **Q28** **Other congenital malformations of** circulatory system
    EXCLUDES 1   congenital aneurysm NOS (Q27.8)
              congenital coronary aneurysm (Q24.5)
              ruptured cerebral arteriovenous malformation (I60.8)
              ruptured malformation of precerebral vessels (I72.0)
    EXCLUDES 2   congenital peripheral aneurysm (Q27.8)
              congenital pulmonary aneurysm (Q25.79)
              congenital retinal aneurysm (Q14.1)

Q28.0 Arteriovenous **malformation of precerebral vessels**
    Congenital arteriovenous precerebral aneurysm (nonruptured)

Q28.1 **Other malformations of precerebral vessels**
    Congenital malformation of precerebral vessels NOS
    Congenital precerebral aneurysm (nonruptured)

Q28.2 Arteriovenous **malformation of** cerebral **vessels**
    Arteriovenous malformation of brain NOS
    Congenital arteriovenous cerebral aneurysm (nonruptured)

Q28.3 **Other malformations of cerebral vessels**
    Congenital cerebral aneurysm (nonruptured)
    Congenital malformation of cerebral vessels NOS
    Developmental venous anomaly

Q28.8 **Other specified congenital malformations of circulatory system**
    Congenital aneurysm, specified site NEC
    Spinal vessel anomaly

Q28.9 **Congenital malformation of circulatory system, unspecified**   ▽

Congenital malformations of the respiratory system (Q30-Q34)

☑4ᵗʰ **Q30** **Congenital malformations of** nose
    EXCLUDES 1   congenital deviation of nasal septum (Q67.4)

Q30.0 **Choanal** atresia
    Atresia of nares (anterior) (posterior)
    Congenital stenosis of nares (anterior) (posterior)

Q30.1 Agenesis **and underdevelopment of nose**
    Congenital absent of nose

Q30.2 Fissured, notched and cleft **nose**

Q30.3 **Congenital** perforated **nasal septum**

Q30.8 **Other congenital malformations of nose**
    Accessory nose
    Congenital anomaly of nasal sinus wall

Q30.9 **Congenital malformation of nose, unspecified**   ▽

☑4ᵗʰ **Q31** **Congenital malformations of** larynx
    EXCLUDES 1   congenital laryngeal stridor NOS (P28.89)

Q31.0 Web **of larynx**
    Glottic web of larynx
    Subglottic web of larynx
    Web of larynx NOS
    DEF: Congenital malformation of larynx; marked by thin, translucent, or thick, fibrotic membrane-like structure between vocal folds; characterized by shortness of breath, and stridor.

Q31.1 **Congenital** subglottic stenosis

Q31.2 **Laryngeal** hypoplasia

Q31.3 Laryngocele

Q31.5 **Congenital** laryngomalacia

Q31.8 **Other congenital malformations of larynx**
    Absence of larynx
    Agenesis of larynx
    Atresia of larynx
    Congenital cleft thyroid cartilage
    Congenital fissure of epiglottis
    Congenital stenosis of larynx NEC
    Posterior cleft of cricoid cartilage

Q31.9 **Congenital malformation of larynx, unspecified**   ▽

☑4ᵗʰ **Q32** **Congenital malformations of** trachea and bronchus
    EXCLUDES 1   congenital bronchiectasis (Q33.4)

Q32.0 **Congenital** tracheomalacia

Q32.1 **Other congenital malformations of trachea**
    Atresia of trachea
    Congenital anomaly of tracheal cartilage
    Congenital dilatation of trachea
    Congenital malformation of trachea
    Congenital stenosis of trachea
    Congenital tracheocele

Q32.2 **Congenital** bronchomalacia

Q32.3 **Congenital** stenosis of bronchus

Q32.4 **Other congenital malformations of bronchus**
    Absence of bronchus
    Agenesis of bronchus
    Atresia of bronchus
    Congenital diverticulum of bronchus
    Congenital malformation of bronchus NOS

☑4ᵗʰ **Q33** **Congenital malformations of** lung

Q33.0 **Congenital** cystic lung
    Congenital cystic lung disease
    Congenital honeycomb lung
    Congenital polycystic lung disease
    EXCLUDES 1   cystic fibrosis (E84.0)
              cystic lung disease, acquired or unspecified (J98.4)

Q33.1 Accessory **lobe of lung**
    Azygos lobe (fissured), lung

Q33.2 Sequestration **of lung**

Q33.3 Agenesis **of lung**
    Congenital absence of lung (lobe)

Q33.4 **Congenital** bronchiectasis

Q33.5 Ectopic **tissue in lung**

Q33.6 **Congenital** hypoplasia and dysplasia **of lung**
    EXCLUDES 1   pulmonary hypoplasia associated with short gestation (P28.0)

Q33.8 **Other congenital malformations of lung**

Q33.9 **Congenital malformation of lung, unspecified**   ▽

☑4ᵗʰ **Q34** **Other congenital malformations of** respiratory system
    EXCLUDES 2   congenital central alveolar hypoventilation syndrome (G47.35)

Q34.0 **Anomaly of** pleura

Q34.1 **Congenital cyst of** mediastinum

Q34.8 **Other specified congenital malformations of respiratory system**
    Atresia of nasopharynx

Q34.9 **Congenital malformation of respiratory system, unspecified**   ▽
    Congenital absence of respiratory system
    Congenital anomaly of respiratory system NOS

Cleft lip and cleft palate (Q35-Q37)

Use additional code to identify associated malformation of the nose (Q30.2)
    EXCLUDES 1   Robin's syndrome (Q87.0)

☑4ᵗʰ **Q35** **Cleft** palate
    INCLUDES   fissure of palate
              palatoschisis
    EXCLUDES 1   cleft palate with cleft lip (Q37.-)

Q35.1 **Cleft** hard **palate**

Q35.3 **Cleft** soft **palate**

Q35.5 **Cleft** hard **palate** with cleft soft palate

Q35.7 **Cleft** uvula

Q35.9 **Cleft palate, unspecified**   ▽
    Cleft palate NOS

☑4ᵗʰ **Q36** **Cleft** lip
    INCLUDES   cheiloschisis
              congenital fissure of lip
              harelip
              labium leporinum
    EXCLUDES 1   cleft lip with cleft palate (Q37.-)

Q36.0 **Cleft lip,** bilateral

Q36.1 **Cleft lip,** median

Q36.9 **Cleft lip,** unilateral
    Cleft lip NOS

Cleft Palate

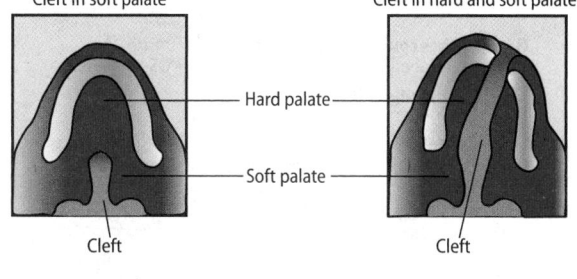

Cleft in soft palate   Cleft in hard and soft palate

Hard palate

Soft palate

Cleft   Cleft

☑ Additional Character Req   ✗x7ᵗʰ Placeholder Alert   Manifestation   HCC CMS-HCC Condition   ▽ Unspecified Code   ▶◀ Revised Text   ● New Code   ▲ Revised Code Title

ICD-10-CM 2018   875

Chapter 17. Congenital Malformations, Deformations, and Chromosomal Abnormalities

Cleft Lip

Unilateral incomplete   Unilateral complete   Bilateral complete

✓4ᵗʰ **Q37 Cleft palate with cleft lip**
> INCLUDES cheilopalatoschisis

Q37.0 Cleft hard palate with bilateral cleft lip

Q37.1 Cleft hard palate with unilateral cleft lip
Cleft hard palate with cleft lip NOS

Q37.2 Cleft soft palate with bilateral cleft lip

Q37.3 Cleft soft palate with unilateral cleft lip
Cleft soft palate with cleft lip NOS

Q37.4 Cleft hard and soft palate with bilateral cleft lip

Q37.5 Cleft hard and soft palate with unilateral cleft lip
Cleft hard and soft palate with cleft lip NOS

Q37.8 Unspecified cleft palate with bilateral cleft lip   ▽

Q37.9 Unspecified cleft palate with unilateral cleft lip   ▽
Cleft palate with cleft lip NOS

Other congenital malformations of the digestive system (Q38-Q45)

✓4ᵗʰ **Q38 Other congenital malformations of tongue, mouth and pharynx**
> EXCLUDES 1 dentofacial anomalies (M26.-)
> macrostomia (Q18.4)
> microstomia (Q18.5)

Q38.0 Congenital malformations of lips, not elsewhere classified
Congenital fistula of lip
Congenital malformation of lip NOS
Van der Woude's syndrome
> EXCLUDES 1 cleft lip (Q36.-)
> cleft lip with cleft palate (Q37.-)
> macrocheilia (Q18.6)
> microcheilia (Q18.7)

Q38.1 Ankyloglossia
Tongue tie

Q38.2 Macroglossia
Congenital hypertrophy of tongue

Q38.3 Other congenital malformations of tongue
Aglossia
Bifid tongue
Congenital adhesion of tongue
Congenital fissure of tongue
Congenital malformation of tongue NOS
Double tongue
Hypoglossia
Hypoplasia of tongue
Microglossia

Q38.4 Congenital malformations of salivary glands and ducts
Atresia of salivary glands and ducts
Congenital absence of salivary glands and ducts
Congenital accessory salivary glands and ducts
Congenital fistula of salivary gland

Q38.5 Congenital malformations of palate, not elsewhere classified
Congenital absence of uvula
Congenital malformation of palate NOS
Congenital high arched palate
> EXCLUDES 1 cleft palate (Q35.-)
> cleft palate with cleft lip (Q37.-)

Q38.6 Other congenital malformations of mouth
Congenital malformation of mouth NOS

Q38.7 Congenital pharyngeal pouch
Congenital diverticulum of pharynx
> EXCLUDES 1 pharyngeal pouch syndrome (D82.1)

Q38.8 Other congenital malformations of pharynx
Congenital malformation of pharynx NOS
Imperforate pharynx

✓4ᵗʰ **Q39 Congenital malformations of esophagus**

Q39.0 Atresia of esophagus without fistula
Atresia of esophagus NOS

Q39.1 Atresia of esophagus with tracheo-esophageal fistula
Atresia of esophagus with broncho-esophageal fistula

Q39.2 Congenital tracheo-esophageal fistula without atresia
Congenital tracheo-esophageal fistula NOS

Q39.3 Congenital stenosis and stricture of esophagus

Q39.4 Esophageal web

Q39.5 Congenital dilatation of esophagus
Congenital cardiospasm

Q39.6 Congenital diverticulum of esophagus
Congenital esophageal pouch

Q39.8 Other congenital malformations of esophagus
Congenital absence of esophagus
Congenital displacement of esophagus
Congenital duplication of esophagus

Q39.9 Congenital malformation of esophagus, unspecified   ▽

✓4ᵗʰ **Q40 Other congenital malformations of upper alimentary tract**

Q40.0 Congenital hypertrophic pyloric stenosis
Congenital or infantile constriction
Congenital or infantile hypertrophy
Congenital or infantile spasm
Congenital or infantile stenosis
Congenital or infantile stricture

Q40.1 Congenital hiatus hernia
Congenital displacement of cardia through esophageal hiatus
> EXCLUDES 1 congenital diaphragmatic hernia (Q79.0)

Q40.2 Other specified congenital malformations of stomach
Congenital displacement of stomach
Congenital diverticulum of stomach
Congenital hourglass stomach
Congenital duplication of stomach
Megalogastria
Microgastria

Q40.3 Congenital malformation of stomach, unspecified   ▽

Q40.8 Other specified congenital malformations of upper alimentary tract

Q40.9 Congenital malformation of upper alimentary tract, unspecified   ▽
Congenital anomaly of upper alimentary tract
Congenital deformity of upper alimentary tract

✓4ᵗʰ **Q41 Congenital absence, atresia and stenosis of small intestine**
> INCLUDES congenital obstruction, occlusion or stricture of small intestine or intestine NOS
> EXCLUDES 1 cystic fibrosis with intestinal manifestation (E84.11)
> meconium ileus NOS (without cystic fibrosis) (P76.0)

Q41.0 Congenital absence, atresia and stenosis of duodenum

Q41.1 Congenital absence, atresia and stenosis of jejunum
Apple peel syndrome
Imperforate jejunum

Q41.2 Congenital absence, atresia and stenosis of ileum

Q41.8 Congenital absence, atresia and stenosis of other specified parts of small intestine

Q41.9 Congenital absence, atresia and stenosis of small intestine, part unspecified   ▽
Congenital absence, atresia and stenosis of intestine NOS

✓4ᵗʰ **Q42 Congenital absence, atresia and stenosis of large intestine**
> INCLUDES congenital obstruction, occlusion and stricture of large intestine

Q42.0 Congenital absence, atresia and stenosis of rectum with fistula

Q42.1 Congenital absence, atresia and stenosis of rectum without fistula
Imperforate rectum

Q42.2 Congenital absence, atresia and stenosis of anus with fistula

Q42.3 Congenital absence, atresia and stenosis of anus without fistula
Imperforate anus

Q42.8 Congenital absence, atresia and stenosis of other parts of large intestine

Q42.9 Congenital absence, atresia and stenosis of large intestine, part unspecified   ▽

EXCLUDES1 Not coded here   EXCLUDES2 Not included here   N Newborn Age: 0   P Pediatric Age: 0-17   M Maternity Age: 12-55   A Adult Age: 15-124

876   ICD-10-CM 2018

✓4th Q43 Other congenital malformations of intestine

Q43.0 Meckel's diverticulum (displaced) (hypertrophic)
Persistent omphalomesenteric duct
Persistent vitelline duct

Q43.1 Hirschsprung's disease
Aganglionosis
Congenital (aganglionic) megacolon

Q43.2 Other congenital functional disorders of colon
Congenital dilatation of colon

Q43.3 Congenital malformations of intestinal fixation
Congenital omental, anomalous adhesions [bands]
Congenital peritoneal adhesions [bands]
Incomplete rotation of cecum and colon
Insufficient rotation of cecum and colon
Jackson's membrane
Malrotation of colon
Rotation failure of cecum and colon
Universal mesentery

Q43.4 Duplication of intestine

Q43.5 Ectopic anus

Q43.6 Congenital fistula of rectum and anus
EXCLUDES 1   *congenital fistula of anus with absence, atresia and*
stenosis (Q42.2)
congenital fistula of rectum with absence, atresia and
stenosis (Q42.0)
congenital rectovaginal fistula (Q52.2)
congenital urethrorectal fistula (Q64.73)
pilonidal fistula or sinus (L05.-)

Q43.7 Persistent cloaca
Cloaca NOS

Q43.8 Other specified congenital malformations of intestine
Congenital blind loop syndrome
Congenital diverticulitis, colon
Congenital diverticulum, intestine
Dolichocolon
Megaloappendix
Megaloduodenum
Microcolon
Transposition of appendix
Transposition of colon
Transposition of intestine
AHA: 2013, 2Q, 31

Q43.9 Congenital malformation of intestine, unspecified   ▽

✓4th Q44 Congenital malformations of gallbladder, bile ducts and liver

Q44.0 Agenesis, aplasia and hypoplasia of gallbladder
Congenital absence of gallbladder

Q44.1 Other congenital malformations of gallbladder
Congenital malformation of gallbladder NOS
Intrahepatic gallbladder

Q44.2 Atresia of bile ducts

Q44.3 Congenital stenosis and stricture of bile ducts

Q44.4 Choledochal cyst

Q44.5 Other congenital malformations of bile ducts
Accessory hepatic duct
Biliary duct duplication
Congenital malformation of bile duct NOS
Cystic duct duplication

Q44.6 Cystic disease of liver
Fibrocystic disease of liver

Q44.7 Other congenital malformations of liver
Accessory liver
Alagille's syndrome
Congenital absence of liver
Congenital hepatomegaly
Congenital malformation of liver NOS

✓4th Q45 Other congenital malformations of digestive system
EXCLUDES 2   *congenital diaphragmatic hernia (Q79.0)*
congenital hiatus hernia (Q40.1)

Q45.0 Agenesis, aplasia and hypoplasia of pancreas
Congenital absence of pancreas

Q45.1 Annular pancreas

Q45.2 Congenital pancreatic cyst

Q45.3 Other congenital malformations of pancreas and pancreatic duct
Accessory pancreas
Congenital malformation of pancreas or pancreatic duct NOS
EXCLUDES 1   *congenital diabetes mellitus (E10.-)*
cystic fibrosis (E84.0-E84.9)
fibrocystic disease of pancreas (E84.-)
neonatal diabetes mellitus (P70.2)

Q45.8 Other specified congenital malformations of digestive system
Absence (complete) (partial) of alimentary tract NOS
Duplication of digestive system
Malposition, congenital of digestive system

Q45.9 Congenital malformation of digestive system, unspecified ▽
Congenital anomaly of digestive system
Congenital deformity of digestive system

Congenital malformations of genital organs (Q50-Q56)
EXCLUDES 1   *androgen insensitivity syndrome (E34.5-)*
syndromes associated with anomalies in the number and form of
chromosomes (Q90-Q99)

✓4th Q50 Congenital malformations of ovaries, fallopian tubes and broad ligaments

✓5th Q50.0 Congenital absence of ovary
EXCLUDES 1   *Turner's syndrome (Q96.-)*

Q50.01 Congenital absence of ovary, unilateral   ♀

Q50.02 Congenital absence of ovary, bilateral   ♀

Q50.1 Developmental ovarian cyst   ♀

Q50.2 Congenital torsion of ovary   ♀

✓5th Q50.3 Other congenital malformations of ovary

Q50.31 Accessory ovary   ♀

Q50.32 Ovarian streak   ♀
46, XX with streak gonads

Q50.39 Other congenital malformation of ovary   ♀
Congenital malformation of ovary NOS

Q50.4 Embryonic cyst of fallopian tube   ♀
Fimbrial cyst

Q50.5 Embryonic cyst of broad ligament   ♀
Epoophoron cyst
Parovarian cyst

Q50.6 Other congenital malformations of fallopian tube and   ♀
broad ligament
Absence of fallopian tube and broad ligament
Accessory fallopian tube and broad ligament
Atresia of fallopian tube and broad ligament
Congenital malformation of fallopian tube or broad ligament NOS

✓4th Q51 Congenital malformations of uterus and cervix

Q51.0 Agenesis and aplasia of uterus   ♀
Congenital absence of uterus

✓5th Q51.1 Doubling of uterus with doubling of cervix and vagina

Q51.10 Doubling of uterus with doubling of cervix and   ♀
vagina without obstruction
Doubling of uterus with doubling of cervix and vagina NOS

Q51.11 Doubling of uterus with doubling of cervix and   ♀
vagina with obstruction

Q51.2 Other doubling of uterus   ♀
Doubling of uterus NOS
Septate uterus, complete or partial

Q51.3 Bicornate uterus   ♀
Bicornate uterus, complete or partial

Q51.4 Unicornate uterus   ♀
Unicornate uterus with or without a separate uterine horn
Uterus with only one functioning horn

Q51.5 Agenesis and aplasia of cervix   ♀
Congenital absence of cervix

Q51.6 Embryonic cyst of cervix   ♀

Q51.7 Congenital fistulae between uterus and digestive and   ♀
urinary tracts

✓5th Q51.8 Other congenital malformations of uterus and cervix

✓6th Q51.81 Other congenital malformations of uterus

Q51.810 Arcuate uterus   ♀
Arcuatus uterus

Q51.811 Hypoplasia of uterus   ♀

Q51.818 Other congenital malformations of   ♀
uterus
Müllerian anomaly of uterus NEC

✓6th Q51.82 Other congenital malformations of cervix

Q51.820 Cervical duplication   ♀

Q51.821 Hypoplasia of cervix   ♀

Q51.828 Other congenital malformations of   ♀
cervix

Q51.9 Congenital malformation of uterus and cervix,   ♀▽
unspecified

✓ Additional Character Req   ✓7th Placeholder Alert   Manifestation   HCC CMS-HCC Condition   ▽ Unspecified Code   ▶◀ Revised Text   ● New Code   ▲ Revised Code Title

ICD-10-CM 2018   877

Chapter 17. Congenital Malformations, Deformations, and Chromosomal Abnormalities

✓4ᵗʰ **Q52 Other congenital malformations of female genitalia**

Q52.0 Congenital absence of vagina ♀
Vaginal agenesis, total or partial

✓5ᵗʰ **Q52.1 Doubling of vagina**
EXCLUDES 1   *doubling of vagina with doubling of uterus and cervix (Q51.1-)*

     Q52.10 Doubling of vagina, unspecified ♀▽
       Septate vagina NOS

     Q52.11 Transverse vaginal septum ♀

     ✓6ᵗʰ **Q52.12 Longitudinal vaginal septum** ♀

       Q52.120 Longitudinal vaginal septum, nonobstructing ♀

       Q52.121 Longitudinal vaginal septum, obstructing, right side ♀

       Q52.122 Longitudinal vaginal septum, obstructing, left side ♀

       Q52.123 Longitudinal vaginal septum, microperforate, right side ♀

       Q52.124 Longitudinal vaginal septum, microperforate, left side ♀

       Q52.129 Other and unspecified longitudinal vaginal septum ♀▽

Q52.2 Congenital rectovaginal fistula ♀
EXCLUDES 1   *cloaca (Q43.7)*

Q52.3 Imperforate hymen
DEF: Obstructive anomaly of vagina, characterized by complete closure of membranous fold around external opening of vagina, obstructing the vaginal introitus.

Q52.4 Other congenital malformations of vagina ♀
Canal of Nuck cyst, congenital
Congenital malformation of vagina NOS
Embryonic vaginal cyst
Gartner's duct cyst

Q52.5 Fusion of labia ♀

Q52.6 Congenital malformation of clitoris ♀

✓5ᵗʰ **Q52.7 Other and unspecified congenital malformations of vulva**

     Q52.70 Unspecified congenital malformations of vulva ♀▽
       Congenital malformation of vulva NOS

     Q52.71 Congenital absence of vulva ♀

     Q52.79 Other congenital malformations of vulva ♀
       Congenital cyst of vulva

Q52.8 Other specified congenital malformations of female genitalia ♀

Q52.9 Congenital malformation of female genitalia, unspecified ♀▽

✓4ᵗʰ **Q53 Undescended and ectopic testicle**

✓5ᵗʰ **Q53.0 Ectopic testis**

     Q53.00 Ectopic testis, unspecified ♂▽

     Q53.01 Ectopic testis, unilateral ♂

     Q53.02 Ectopic testes, bilateral ♂

✓5ᵗʰ **Q53.1 Undescended testicle, unilateral**

     Q53.10 Unspecified undescended testicle, unilateral ♂▽

     ✓6ᵗʰ **Q53.11 Abdominal testis, unilateral**

●   **Q53.111 Unilateral intraabdominal testis**

●   **Q53.112 Unilateral inguinal testis**

●   **Q53.12 Ectopic perineal testis, unilateral** ♂

●   **Q53.13 Unilateral high scrotal testis**

✓5ᵗʰ **Q53.2 Undescended testicle, bilateral**

     Q53.20 Undescended testicle, unspecified, bilateral ♂▽

     ✓6ᵗʰ **Q53.21 Abdominal testis, bilateral**

●   **Q53.211 Bilateral intraabdominal testes**

●   **Q53.212 Bilateral inguinal testes**

     Q53.22 Ectopic perineal testis, bilateral ♂

●   **Q53.23 Bilateral high scrotal testes**

Q53.9 Undescended testicle, unspecified ♂▽
Cryptorchism NOS

✓4ᵗʰ **Q54 Hypospadias**
EXCLUDES 1   *epispadias (Q64.0)*
DEF: Abnormal opening of urethra on the ventral (underside) surface of the penis.

Q54.0 Hypospadias, balanic ♂
Hypospadias, coronal
Hypospadias, glandular

Q54.1 Hypospadias, penile ♂

Hypospadias and Epispadias

Hypospadias (ventral view)

Epispadias (dorsal view)

Q54.2 Hypospadias, penoscrotal ♂

Q54.3 Hypospadias, perineal ♂

Q54.4 Congenital chordee ♂
Chordee without hypospadias

Q54.8 Other hypospadias ♂
Hypospadias with intersex state

Q54.9 Hypospadias, unspecified ♂▽

✓4ᵗʰ **Q55 Other congenital malformations of male genital organs**
EXCLUDES 1   *congenital hydrocele (P83.5)*
           hypospadias (Q54.-)

Q55.0 Absence and aplasia of testis ♂
Monorchism

Q55.1 Hypoplasia of testis and scrotum ♂
Fusion of testes

✓5ᵗʰ **Q55.2 Other and unspecified congenital malformations of testis and scrotum**

     Q55.20 Unspecified congenital malformations of testis and scrotum ♂▽
       Congenital malformation of testis or scrotum NOS

     Q55.21 Polyorchism ♂

     Q55.22 Retractile testis ♂

     Q55.23 Scrotal transposition ♂

     Q55.29 Other congenital malformations of testis and scrotum ♂

Q55.3 Atresia of vas deferens ♂
Code first any associated cystic fibrosis (E84.-)

Q55.4 Other congenital malformations of vas deferens, epididymis, seminal vesicles and prostate ♂
Absence or aplasia of prostate
Absence or aplasia of spermatic cord
Congenital malformation of vas deferens, epididymis, seminal vesicles or prostate NOS

Q55.5 Congenital absence and aplasia of penis ♂

✓5ᵗʰ **Q55.6 Other congenital malformations of penis**

     Q55.61 Curvature of penis (lateral) ♂

     Q55.62 Hypoplasia of penis ♂
       Micropenis

     Q55.63 Congenital torsion of penis ♂
       EXCLUDES 1   *acquired torsion of penis (N48.82)*

     Q55.64 Hidden penis ♂
       Buried penis
       Concealed penis
       EXCLUDES 1   *acquired buried penis (N48.83)*

     Q55.69 Other congenital malformation of penis ♂
       Congenital malformation of penis NOS

Q55.7 Congenital vasocutaneous fistula ♂

Q55.8 Other specified congenital malformations of male genital organs ♂

Q55.9 Congenital malformation of male genital organ, unspecified ♂▽
Congenital anomaly of male genital organ
Congenital deformity of male genital organ

| EXCLUDES 1 Not coded here | EXCLUDES 2 Not included here | Ⓝ Newborn Age: 0 | Ⓟ Pediatric Age: 0-17 | Ⓜ Maternity Age: 12-55 | Ⓐ Adult Age: 15-124 |

878   ICD-10-CM 2018

☑4ᵗʰ **Q56** **Indeterminate sex and pseudohermaphroditism**
     EXCLUDES 1   *46, XX true hermaphrodite (Q99.1)*
         androgen insensitivity syndrome (E34.5-)
         chimera 46, XX/46, XY true hermaphrodite (Q99.0)
         female pseudohermaphroditism with adrenocortical disorder
           (E25.-)
         pseudohermaphroditism with specified chromosomal anomaly
           (Q96-Q99)
         pure gonadal dysgenesis (Q99.1)

     Q56.0   **Hermaphroditism, not elsewhere classified**
         Ovotestis

     Q56.1   **Male pseudohermaphroditism, not elsewhere classified**   ♂
         46, XY with streak gonads
         Male pseudohermaphroditism NOS

     Q56.2   **Female pseudohermaphroditism, not elsewhere classified**   ♀
         Female pseudohermaphroditism NOS

     Q56.3   **Pseudohermaphroditism, unspecified**   ▽

     Q56.4   **Indeterminate sex, unspecified**   ▽
         Ambiguous genitalia

Congenital malformations of the urinary system (Q60-Q64)

☑4ᵗʰ **Q60** **Renal agenesis and other reduction defects of kidney**
     INCLUDES   congenital absence of kidney
         congenital atrophy of kidney
         infantile atrophy of kidney

     Q60.0   **Renal agenesis, unilateral**

     Q60.1   **Renal agenesis, bilateral**

     Q60.2   **Renal agenesis, unspecified**   ▽

     Q60.3   **Renal hypoplasia, unilateral**

     Q60.4   **Renal hypoplasia, bilateral**

     Q60.5   **Renal hypoplasia, unspecified**   ▽

     Q60.6   **Potter's syndrome**

☑4ᵗʰ **Q61** **Cystic kidney disease**
     EXCLUDES 1   *acquired cyst of kidney (N28.1)*
         Potter's syndrome (Q60.6)

     ✓5ᵗʰ **Q61.0**   **Congenital renal cyst**

         Q61.00   **Congenital renal cyst, unspecified**   ▽
             Cyst of kidney NOS (congenital)

         Q61.01   **Congenital single renal cyst**

         Q61.02   **Congenital multiple renal cysts**

     ✓5ᵗʰ **Q61.1**   **Polycystic kidney, infantile type**
         Polycystic kidney, autosomal recessive

         Q61.11   **Cystic dilatation of collecting ducts**

         Q61.19   **Other polycystic kidney, infantile type**

     Q61.2   **Polycystic kidney, adult type**
         Polycystic kidney, autosomal dominant

     Q61.3   **Polycystic kidney, unspecified**   ▽
         AHA: 2016, 3Q, 22

     Q61.4   **Renal dysplasia**
         Multicystic dysplastic kidney
         Multicystic kidney (development)
         Multicystic kidney disease
         Multicystic renal dysplasia
         EXCLUDES 1   *polycystic kidney disease (Q61.11-Q61.3)*

     Q61.5   **Medullary cystic kidney**
         Nephronopthisis
         Sponge kidney NOS
         DEF: Sponge kidney: Dilated collecting tubules; usually asymptomatic but calcinosis in tubules may cause renal insufficiency.

     Q61.8   **Other cystic kidney diseases**
         Fibrocystic kidney
         Fibrocystic renal degeneration or disease

     Q61.9   **Cystic kidney disease, unspecified**   ▽
         Meckel-Gruber syndrome

☑4ᵗʰ **Q62** **Congenital obstructive defects of renal pelvis and congenital malformations of ureter**

     Q62.0   **Congenital hydronephrosis**

     ✓5ᵗʰ **Q62.1**   **Congenital occlusion of ureter**
         Atresia and stenosis of ureter

         Q62.10   **Congenital occlusion of ureter, unspecified**   ▽

         Q62.11   **Congenital occlusion of ureteropelvic junction**

         Q62.12   **Congenital occlusion of ureterovesical orifice**

     Q62.2   **Congenital megaureter**
         Congenital dilatation of ureter

     Q62.3   **Other obstructive defects of renal pelvis and ureter**

         Q62.31   **Congenital ureterocele, orthotopic**

         Q62.32   **Cecoureterocele**
             Ectopic ureterocele

         Q62.39   **Other obstructive defects of renal pelvis and ureter**
             Ureteropelvic junction obstruction NOS

     Q62.4   **Agenesis of ureter**
         Congenital absence ureter

     Q62.5   **Duplication of ureter**
         Accessory ureter
         Double ureter

     ✓5ᵗʰ **Q62.6**   **Malposition of ureter**

         Q62.60   **Malposition of ureter, unspecified**   ▽

         Q62.61   **Deviation of ureter**

         Q62.62   **Displacement of ureter**

         Q62.63   **Anomalous implantation of ureter**
             Ectopia of ureter
             Ectopic ureter

         Q62.69   **Other malposition of ureter**

     Q62.7   **Congenital vesico-uretero-renal reflux**

     Q62.8   **Other congenital malformations of ureter**
         Anomaly of ureter NOS

☑4ᵗʰ **Q63** **Other congenital malformations of kidney**
     EXCLUDES 1   *congenital nephrotic syndrome (N04.-)*

     Q63.0   **Accessory kidney**

     Q63.1   **Lobulated, fused and horseshoe kidney**

     Q63.2   **Ectopic kidney**
         Congenital displaced kidney
         Malrotation of kidney

     Q63.3   **Hyperplastic and giant kidney**
         Compensatory hypertrophy of kidney

     Q63.8   **Other specified congenital malformations of kidney**
         Congenital renal calculi

     Q63.9   **Congenital malformation of kidney, unspecified**   ▽

☑4ᵗʰ **Q64** **Other congenital malformations of urinary system**

     Q64.0   **Epispadias**   ♂
         EXCLUDES 1   *hypospadias (Q54.-)*

     ✓5ᵗʰ **Q64.1**   **Exstrophy of urinary bladder**

         Q64.10   **Exstrophy of urinary bladder, unspecified**   ▽
             Ectopia vesicae

         Q64.11   **Supravesical fissure of urinary bladder**

         Q64.12   **Cloacal exstrophy of urinary bladder**

         Q64.19   **Other exstrophy of urinary bladder**
             Extroversion of bladder

     Q64.2   **Congenital posterior urethral valves**

     ✓5ᵗʰ **Q64.3**   **Other atresia and stenosis of urethra and bladder neck**

         Q64.31   **Congenital bladder neck obstruction**
             Congenital obstruction of vesicourethral orifice

         Q64.32   **Congenital stricture of urethra**

         Q64.33   **Congenital stricture of urinary meatus**

         Q64.39   **Other atresia and stenosis of urethra and bladder neck**
             Atresia and stenosis of urethra and bladder neck NOS

     Q64.4   **Malformation of urachus**
         Cyst of urachus
         Patent urachus
         Prolapse of urachus

     Q64.5   **Congenital absence of bladder and urethra**

     Q64.6   **Congenital diverticulum of bladder**

     ✓5ᵗʰ **Q64.7**   **Other and unspecified congenital malformations of bladder and urethra**
         EXCLUDES 1   *congenital prolapse of bladder (mucosa) (Q79.4)*

         Q64.70   **Unspecified congenital malformation of bladder and urethra**   ▽
             Malformation of bladder or urethra NOS

         Q64.71   **Congenital prolapse of urethra**

         Q64.72   **Congenital prolapse of urinary meatus**

         Q64.73   **Congenital urethrorectal fistula**

         Q64.74   **Double urethra**

         Q64.75   **Double urinary meatus**

         Q64.79   **Other congenital malformations of bladder and urethra**

     Q64.8   **Other specified congenital malformations of urinary system**

☑ Additional Character Req   ⁿˣ⁷ᵗʰ Placeholder Alert   **Manifestation**   HCC CMS-HCC Condition   ▽ Unspecified Code   ►◄ Revised Text   ● New Code   ▲ Revised Code Title

Q64.9　Congenital malformation of urinary system, unspecified ▽
　　Congenital anomaly NOS of urinary system
　　Congenital deformity NOS of urinary system

Congenital malformations and deformations of the musculoskeletal system (Q65-Q79)

✓4ᵗʰ　Q65　Congenital deformities of hip
　　EXCLUDES 1　clicking hip (R29.4)

✓5ᵗʰ　Q65.0　Congenital dislocation of hip, unilateral
　　Q65.00　Congenital dislocation of unspecified hip, unilateral ▽
　　Q65.01　Congenital dislocation of right hip, unilateral
　　Q65.02　Congenital dislocation of left hip, unilateral
Q65.1　Congenital dislocation of hip, bilateral
Q65.2　Congenital dislocation of hip, unspecified ▽
✓5ᵗʰ　Q65.3　Congenital partial dislocation of hip, unilateral
　　Q65.30　Congenital partial dislocation of unspecified hip, unilateral ▽
　　Q65.31　Congenital partial dislocation of right hip, unilateral
　　Q65.32　Congenital partial dislocation of left hip, unilateral
Q65.4　Congenital partial dislocation of hip, bilateral
Q65.5　Congenital partial dislocation of hip, unspecified ▽
Q65.6　Congenital unstable hip
　　Congenital dislocatable hip
✓5ᵗʰ　Q65.8　Other congenital deformities of hip
　　Q65.81　Congenital coxa valga
　　Q65.82　Congenital coxa vara
　　Q65.89　Other specified congenital deformities of hip
　　　　Anteversion of femoral neck
　　　　Congenital acetabular dysplasia
Q65.9　Congenital deformity of hip, unspecified ▽

✓4ᵗʰ　Q66　Congenital deformities of feet
　　EXCLUDES 1　reduction defects of feet (Q72.-)
　　　　valgus deformities (acquired) (M21.0-)
　　　　varus deformities (acquired) (M21.1-)

Q66.0　Congenital talipes equinovarus
Q66.1　Congenital talipes calcaneovarus
✓5ᵗʰ　Q66.2　Congenital metatarsus (primus) varus
　　Q66.21　Congenital metatarsus primus varus
　　Q66.22　Congenital metatarsus adductus
　　　　Congenital metatarsus varus
Q66.3　Other congenital varus deformities of feet
　　Hallux varus, congenital
Q66.4　Congenital talipes calcaneovalgus
✓5ᵗʰ　Q66.5　Congenital pes planus
　　Congenital flat foot
　　Congenital rigid flat foot
　　Congenital spastic (everted) flat foot
　　EXCLUDES 1　pes planus, acquired (M21.4)
　　Q66.50　Congenital pes planus, unspecified foot ▽
　　Q66.51　Congenital pes planus, right foot
　　Q66.52　Congenital pes planus, left foot
Q66.6　Other congenital valgus deformities of feet
　　Congenital metatarsus valgus
Q66.7　Congenital pes cavus
✓5ᵗʰ　Q66.8　Other congenital deformities of feet
　　Q66.80　Congenital vertical talus deformity, unspecified foot ▽
　　Q66.81　Congenital vertical talus deformity, right foot
　　Q66.82　Congenital vertical talus deformity, left foot
　　Q66.89　Other specified congenital deformities of feet
　　　　Congenital asymmetric talipes
　　　　Congenital clubfoot NOS
　　　　Congenital talipes NOS
　　　　Congenital tarsal coalition
　　　　Hammer toe, congenital
Q66.9　Congenital deformity of feet, unspecified ▽

✓4ᵗʰ　Q67　Congenital musculoskeletal deformities of head, face, spine and chest
　　EXCLUDES 1　congenital malformation syndromes classified to Q87-
　　　　Potter's syndrome (Q60.6)

Q67.0　Congenital facial asymmetry
Q67.1　Congenital compression facies

Q67.2　Dolichocephaly
Q67.3　Plagiocephaly
Q67.4　Other congenital deformities of skull, face and jaw
　　Congenital depressions in skull
　　Congenital hemifacial atrophy or hypertrophy
　　Deviation of nasal septum, congenital
　　Squashed or bent nose, congenital
　　EXCLUDES 1　dentofacial anomalies [including malocclusion]
　　　　(M26.-)
　　　　syphilitic saddle nose (A50.5)
Q67.5　Congenital deformity of spine
　　Congenital postural scoliosis
　　Congenital scoliosis NOS
　　EXCLUDES 1　infantile idiopathic scoliosis (M41.0)
　　　　scoliosis due to congenital bony malformation (Q76.3
　　AHA: 2014, 4Q, 26
Q67.6　Pectus excavatum
　　Congenital funnel chest
Q67.7　Pectus carinatum
　　Congenital pigeon chest
Q67.8　Other congenital deformities of chest
　　Congenital deformity of chest wall NOS

✓4ᵗʰ　Q68　Other congenital musculoskeletal deformities
　　EXCLUDES 1　reduction defects of limb(s) (Q71-Q73)
　　EXCLUDES 2　congenital myotonic chondrodystrophy (G71.13)

Q68.0　Congenital deformity of sternocleidomastoid muscle
　　Congenital contracture of sternocleidomastoid (muscle)
　　Congenital (sternomastoid) torticollis
　　Sternomastoid tumor (congenital)
Q68.1　Congenital deformity of finger(s) and hand
　　Congenital clubfinger
　　Spade-like hand (congenital)
Q68.2　Congenital deformity of knee
　　Congenital dislocation of knee
　　Congenital genu recurvatum
Q68.3　Congenital bowing of femur
　　EXCLUDES 1　anteversion of femur (neck) (Q65.89)
Q68.4　Congenital bowing of tibia and fibula
Q68.5　Congenital bowing of long bones of leg, unspecified ▽
Q68.6　Discoid meniscus
Q68.8　Other specified congenital musculoskeletal deformities
　　Congenital deformity of clavicle
　　Congenital deformity of elbow
　　Congenital deformity of forearm
　　Congenital deformity of scapula
　　Congenital deformity of wrist
　　Congenital dislocation of elbow
　　Congenital dislocation of shoulder
　　Congenital dislocation of wrist

✓4ᵗʰ　Q69　Polydactyly
Q69.0　Accessory finger(s)
Q69.1　Accessory thumb(s)
Q69.2　Accessory toe(s)
　　Accessory hallux
Q69.9　Polydactyly, unspecified ▽
　　Supernumerary digit(s) NOS

✓4ᵗʰ　Q70　Syndactyly
✓5ᵗʰ　Q70.0　Fused fingers
　　Complex syndactyly of fingers with synostosis
　　Q70.00　Fused fingers, unspecified hand ▽
　　Q70.01　Fused fingers, right hand
　　Q70.02　Fused fingers, left hand
　　Q70.03　Fused fingers, bilateral
✓5ᵗʰ　Q70.1　Webbed fingers
　　Simple syndactyly of fingers without synostosis
　　Q70.10　Webbed fingers, unspecified hand ▽
　　Q70.11　Webbed fingers, right hand
　　Q70.12　Webbed fingers, left hand
　　Q70.13　Webbed fingers, bilateral
✓5ᵗʰ　Q70.2　Fused toes
　　Complex syndactyly of toes with synostosis
　　Q70.20　Fused toes, unspecified foot ▽
　　Q70.21　Fused toes, right foot
　　Q70.22　Fused toes, left foot
　　Q70.23　Fused toes, bilateral

EXCLUDES 1 Not coded here　　EXCLUDES 2 Not included here　　N Newborn Age: 0　　P Pediatric Age: 0-17　　M Maternity Age: 12-55　　A Adult Age: 15-124

880　　ICD-10-CM 2018

✓5ᵗʰ **Q70.3** Webbed toes
       Simple syndactyly of toes without synostosis
     Q70.30 Webbed toes, unspecified foot   ▽
     Q70.31 Webbed toes, right foot
     Q70.32 Webbed toes, left foot
     Q70.33 Webbed toes, bilateral

Q70.4 Polysyndactyly, unspecified   ▽
     EXCLUDES 1   specified syndactyly of hand and feet—code to
                 specified conditions (Q70.0-Q70.3-)

Q70.9 Syndactyly, unspecified   ▽
     Symphalangy NOS

✓4ᵗʰ **Q71** Reduction defects of upper limb

✓5ᵗʰ **Q71.0** Congenital complete absence of upper limb
     Q71.00 Congenital complete absence of unspecified   ▽
                 upper limb
     Q71.01 Congenital complete absence of right upper limb
     Q71.02 Congenital complete absence of left upper limb
     Q71.03 Congenital complete absence of upper limb,
                 bilateral

✓5ᵗʰ **Q71.1** Congenital absence of upper arm and forearm with hand
present
     Q71.10 Congenital absence of unspecified upper arm   ▽
                 and forearm with hand present
     Q71.11 Congenital absence of right upper arm and forearm
                 with hand present
     Q71.12 Congenital absence of left upper arm and forearm
                 with hand present
     Q71.13 Congenital absence of upper arm and forearm with
                 hand present, bilateral

✓5ᵗʰ **Q71.2** Congenital absence of both forearm and hand
     Q71.20 Congenital absence of both forearm and hand,   ▽
                 unspecified upper limb
     Q71.21 Congenital absence of both forearm and hand, right
                 upper limb
     Q71.22 Congenital absence of both forearm and hand, left
                 upper limb
     Q71.23 Congenital absence of both forearm and hand,
                 bilateral

✓5ᵗʰ **Q71.3** Congenital absence of hand and finger
     Q71.30 Congenital absence of unspecified hand   ▽
                 and finger
     Q71.31 Congenital absence of right hand and finger
     Q71.32 Congenital absence of left hand and finger
     Q71.33 Congenital absence of hand and finger, bilateral

✓5ᵗʰ **Q71.4** Longitudinal reduction defect of radius
       Clubhand (congenital)
       Radial clubhand
     Q71.40 Longitudinal reduction defect of unspecified   ▽
                 radius
     Q71.41 Longitudinal reduction defect of right radius
     Q71.42 Longitudinal reduction defect of left radius
     Q71.43 Longitudinal reduction defect of radius, bilateral

✓5ᵗʰ **Q71.5** Longitudinal reduction defect of ulna
     Q71.50 Longitudinal reduction defect of unspecified ulna ▽
     Q71.51 Longitudinal reduction defect of right ulna
     Q71.52 Longitudinal reduction defect of left ulna
     Q71.53 Longitudinal reduction defect of ulna, bilateral

✓5ᵗʰ **Q71.6** Lobster-claw hand
     Q71.60 Lobster-claw hand, unspecified hand   ▽
     Q71.61 Lobster-claw right hand
     Q71.62 Lobster-claw left hand
     Q71.63 Lobster-claw hand, bilateral

✓5ᵗʰ **Q71.8** Other reduction defects of upper limb
   ✓6ᵗʰ **Q71.81** Congenital shortening of upper limb
         Q71.811 Congenital shortening of right upper limb
         Q71.812 Congenital shortening of left upper limb
         Q71.813 Congenital shortening of upper limb,
                    bilateral
         Q71.819 Congenital shortening of unspecified   ▽
                    upper limb

✓6ᵗʰ **Q71.89** Other reduction defects of upper limb
     Q71.891 Other reduction defects of right upper
                limb
     Q71.892 Other reduction defects of left upper limb
     Q71.893 Other reduction defects of upper limb,
                bilateral
     Q71.899 Other reduction defects of unspecified   ▽
                upper limb

✓5ᵗʰ **Q71.9** Unspecified reduction defect of upper limb
     Q71.90 Unspecified reduction defect of unspecified   ▽
                 upper limb
     Q71.91 Unspecified reduction defect of right upper limb ▽
     Q71.92 Unspecified reduction defect of left upper limb ▽
     Q71.93 Unspecified reduction defect of upper limb,   ▽
                 bilateral

✓4ᵗʰ **Q72** Reduction defects of lower limb

✓5ᵗʰ **Q72.0** Congenital complete absence of lower limb
     Q72.00 Congenital complete absence of unspecified   ▽
                 lower limb
     Q72.01 Congenital complete absence of right lower limb
     Q72.02 Congenital complete absence of left lower limb
     Q72.03 Congenital complete absence of lower limb, bilateral

✓5ᵗʰ **Q72.1** Congenital absence of thigh and lower leg with foot present
     Q72.10 Congenital absence of unspecified thigh and   ▽
                 lower leg with foot present
     Q72.11 Congenital absence of right thigh and lower leg with
                 foot present
     Q72.12 Congenital absence of left thigh and lower leg with
                 foot present
     Q72.13 Congenital absence of thigh and lower leg with foot
                 present, bilateral

✓5ᵗʰ **Q72.2** Congenital absence of both lower leg and foot
     Q72.20 Congenital absence of both lower leg and foot,   ▽
                 unspecified lower limb
     Q72.21 Congenital absence of both lower leg and foot, right
                 lower limb
     Q72.22 Congenital absence of both lower leg and foot, left
                 lower limb
     Q72.23 Congenital absence of both lower leg and foot,
                 bilateral

✓5ᵗʰ **Q72.3** Congenital absence of foot and toe(s)
     Q72.30 Congenital absence of unspecified foot and toe(s) ▽
     Q72.31 Congenital absence of right foot and toe(s)
     Q72.32 Congenital absence of left foot and toe(s)
     Q72.33 Congenital absence of foot and toe(s), bilateral

✓5ᵗʰ **Q72.4** Longitudinal reduction defect of femur
       Proximal femoral focal deficiency
     Q72.40 Longitudinal reduction defect of unspecified   ▽
                 femur
     Q72.41 Longitudinal reduction defect of right femur
     Q72.42 Longitudinal reduction defect of left femur
     Q72.43 Longitudinal reduction defect of femur, bilateral

✓5ᵗʰ **Q72.5** Longitudinal reduction defect of tibia
     Q72.50 Longitudinal reduction defect of unspecified tibia ▽
     Q72.51 Longitudinal reduction defect of right tibia
     Q72.52 Longitudinal reduction defect of left tibia
     Q72.53 Longitudinal reduction defect of tibia, bilateral

✓5ᵗʰ **Q72.6** Longitudinal reduction defect of fibula
     Q72.60 Longitudinal reduction defect of unspecified   ▽
                 fibula
     Q72.61 Longitudinal reduction defect of right fibula
     Q72.62 Longitudinal reduction defect of left fibula
     Q72.63 Longitudinal reduction defect of fibula, bilateral

✓5ᵗʰ **Q72.7** Split foot
     Q72.70 Split foot, unspecified lower limb   ▽
     Q72.71 Split foot, right lower limb
     Q72.72 Split foot, left lower limb
     Q72.73 Split foot, bilateral

✓5ᵗʰ **Q72.8** Other reduction defects of lower limb
   ✓6ᵗʰ **Q72.81** Congenital shortening of lower limb
         Q72.811 Congenital shortening of right lower limb
         Q72.812 Congenital shortening of left lower limb

        Q72.813   **Congenital shortening of lower limb, bilateral**

        Q72.819   **Congenital shortening of unspecified lower limb** ▽

✓6ᵗʰ **Q72.89**   **Other reduction defects of lower limb**

        Q72.891   **Other reduction defects of right lower limb**

        Q72.892   **Other reduction defects of left lower limb**

        Q72.893   **Other reduction defects of lower limb, bilateral**

        Q72.899   **Other reduction defects of unspecified lower limb** ▽

✓5ᵗʰ **Q72.9**   **Unspecified reduction defect of lower limb**

    Q72.90   **Unspecified reduction defect of unspecified lower limb** ▽

    Q72.91   **Unspecified reduction defect of right lower limb** ▽

    Q72.92   **Unspecified reduction defect of left lower limb** ▽

    Q72.93   **Unspecified reduction defect of lower limb, bilateral** ▽

✓4ᵗʰ **Q73**   **Reduction defects of unspecified limb**

    Q73.0   **Congenital absence of unspecified limb(s)** ▽
        Amelia NOS

    Q73.1   **Phocomelia, unspecified limb(s)** ▽
        Phocomelia NOS

    Q73.8   **Other reduction defects of unspecified limb(s)** ▽
        Longitudinal reduction deformity of unspecified limb(s)
        Ectromelia of limb NOS
        Hemimelia of limb NOS
        Reduction defect of limb NOS

✓4ᵗʰ **Q74**   **Other congenital malformations of limb(s)**
    EXCLUDES 1   *polydactyly (Q69.-)*
        reduction defect of limb (Q71-Q73)
        syndactyly (Q70.-)

    Q74.0   **Other congenital malformations of upper limb(s), including shoulder girdle**
        Accessory carpal bones
        Cleidocranial dysostosis
        Congenital pseudarthrosis of clavicle
        Macrodactylia (fingers)
        Madelung's deformity
        Radioulnar synostosis
        Sprengel's deformity
        Triphalangeal thumb

    Q74.1   **Congenital malformation of knee**
        Congenital absence of patella
        Congenital dislocation of patella
        Congenital genu valgum
        Congenital genu varum
        Rudimentary patella
        EXCLUDES 1   *congenital dislocation of knee (Q68.2)*
            congenital genu recurvatum (Q68.2)
            nail patella syndrome (Q87.2)

    Q74.2   **Other congenital malformations of lower limb(s), including pelvic girdle**
        Congenital fusion of sacroiliac joint
        Congenital malformation of ankle joint
        Congenital malformation of sacroiliac joint
        EXCLUDES 1   *anteversion of femur (neck) (Q65.89)*

    Q74.3   **Arthrogryposis multiplex congenita**

    Q74.8   **Other specified congenital malformations of limb(s)**

    Q74.9   **Unspecified congenital malformation of limb(s)** ▽
        Congenital anomaly of limb(s) NOS

✓4ᵗʰ **Q75**   **Other congenital malformations of skull and face bones**
    EXCLUDES 1   *congenital malformation of face NOS (Q18.-)*
        congenital malformation syndromes classified to Q87.-
        dentofacial anomalies [including malocclusion] (M26.-)
        musculoskeletal deformities of head and face (Q67.0-Q67.4)
        skull defects associated with congenital anomalies of brain such
          as:
          anencephaly (Q00.0)
          encephalocele (Q01.-)
          hydrocephalus (Q03.-)
          microcephaly (Q02)

    Q75.0   **Craniosynostosis**
        Acrocephaly
        Imperfect fusion of skull
        Oxycephaly
        Trigonocephaly

    Q75.1   **Craniofacial dysostosis**
        Crouzon's disease

    Q75.2   **Hypertelorism**

    Q75.3   **Macrocephaly**

    Q75.4   **Mandibulofacial dysostosis**
        Franceschetti syndrome
        Treacher Collins syndrome

    Q75.5   **Oculomandibular dysostosis**

    Q75.8   **Other specified congenital malformations of skull and face bones**
        Absence of skull bone, congenital
        Congenital deformity of forehead
        Platybasia

    Q75.9   **Congenital malformation of skull and face bones, unspecified** ▽
        Congenital anomaly of face bones NOS
        Congenital anomaly of skull NOS

✓4ᵗʰ **Q76**   **Congenital malformations of spine and bony thorax**
    EXCLUDES 1   *congenital musculoskeletal deformities of spine and chest*
          (Q67.5-Q67.8)

    Q76.0   **Spina bifida occulta**
        EXCLUDES 1   *meningocele (spinal) (Q05.-)*
            spina bifida (aperta) (cystica) (Q05.-)

    Q76.1   **Klippel-Feil syndrome**
        Cervical fusion syndrome

    Q76.2   **Congenital spondylolisthesis**
        Congenital spondylolysis
        EXCLUDES 1   *spondylolisthesis (acquired) (M43.1-)*
            spondylolysis (acquired) (M43.0-)

    Q76.3   **Congenital scoliosis due to congenital bony malformation**
        Hemivertebra fusion or failure of segmentation with scoliosis

✓5ᵗʰ **Q76.4**   **Other congenital malformations of spine, not associated with scoliosis**

    ✓6ᵗʰ **Q76.41**   **Congenital kyphosis**

        Q76.411   **Congenital kyphosis, occipito-atlanto-axial region**

        Q76.412   **Congenital kyphosis, cervical region**

        Q76.413   **Congenital kyphosis, cervicothoracic region**

        Q76.414   **Congenital kyphosis, thoracic region**

        Q76.415   **Congenital kyphosis, thoracolumbar region**

        Q76.419   **Congenital kyphosis, unspecified region** ▽

    ✓6ᵗʰ **Q76.42**   **Congenital lordosis**

        Q76.425   **Congenital lordosis, thoracolumbar region**

        Q76.426   **Congenital lordosis, lumbar region**

        Q76.427   **Congenital lordosis, lumbosacral region**

        Q76.428   **Congenital lordosis, sacral and sacrococcygeal region**

        Q76.429   **Congenital lordosis, unspecified region** ▽

        Q76.49   **Other congenital malformations of spine, not associated with scoliosis**
            Congenital absence of vertebra NOS
            Congenital fusion of spine NOS
            Congenital malformation of lumbosacral (joint) (region) NOS
            Congenital malformation of spine NOS
            Hemivertebra NOS
            Malformation of spine NOS
            Platyspondylisis NOS
            Supernumerary vertebra NOS

    Q76.5   **Cervical rib**
        Supernumerary rib in cervical region

    Q76.6   **Other congenital malformations of ribs**
        Accessory rib
        Congenital absence of rib
        Congenital fusion of ribs
        Congenital malformation of ribs NOS
        EXCLUDES 1   *short rib syndrome (Q77.2)*

    Q76.7   **Congenital malformation of sternum**
        Congenital absence of sternum
        Sternum bifidum

    Q76.8   **Other congenital malformations of bony thorax**

    Q76.9   **Congenital malformation of bony thorax, unspecified** ▽

EXCLUDES 1 Not coded here   EXCLUDES 2 Not included here   N Newborn Age: 0   P Pediatric Age: 0-17   M Maternity Age: 12-55   A Adult Age: 15-124

882   ICD-10-CM 2018

☑4ᵗʰ **Q77 Osteochondrodysplasia with defects of growth of tubular bones and spine**

  EXCLUDES 1 *mucopolysaccharidosis (E76.0-E76.3)*
  EXCLUDES 2 *congenital myotonic chondrodystrophy (G71.13)*

  Q77.0 Achondrogenesis
    Hypochondrogenesis

  Q77.1 Thanatophoric short stature

  Q77.2 Short rib syndrome
    Asphyxiating thoracic dysplasia [Jeune]

  Q77.3 Chondrodysplasia punctata
    EXCLUDES 1 *Rhizomelic chondrodysplasia punctata (E71.43)*

  Q77.4 Achondroplasia
    Hypochondroplasia
    Osteosclerosis congenita

  Q77.5 Diastrophic dysplasia

  Q77.6 Chondroectodermal dysplasia
    Ellis-van Creveld syndrome

  Q77.7 Spondyloepiphyseal dysplasia

  Q77.8 Other osteochondrodysplasia with defects of growth of tubular bones and spine

  Q77.9 Osteochondrodysplasia with defects of growth of tubular bones and spine, unspecified   ▽

☑4ᵗʰ **Q78 Other osteochondrodysplasias**
  EXCLUDES 2 *congenital myotonic chondrodystrophy (G71.13)*

  Q78.0 Osteogenesis imperfecta
    Fragilitas ossium
    Osteopsathyrosis

  Q78.1 Polyostotic fibrous dysplasia
    Albright(-McCune)(-Sternberg) syndrome

  Q78.2 Osteopetrosis
    Albers-Schönberg syndrome
    Osteosclerosis NOS

  Q78.3 Progressive diaphyseal dysplasia
    Camurati-Engelmann syndrome

  Q78.4 Enchondromatosis
    Maffucci's syndrome
    Ollier's disease

  Q78.5 Metaphyseal dysplasia
    Pyle's syndrome

  Q78.6 Multiple congenital exostoses
    Diaphyseal aclasis

  Q78.8 Other specified osteochondrodysplasias
    Osteopoikilosis

  Q78.9 Osteochondrodysplasia, unspecified   ▽
    Chondrodystrophy NOS
    Osteodystrophy NOS

☑4ᵗʰ **Q79 Congenital malformations of musculoskeletal system, not elsewhere classified**
  EXCLUDES 2 *congenital (sternomastoid) torticollis (Q68.0)*

  Q79.0 Congenital diaphragmatic hernia
    EXCLUDES 1 *congenital hiatus hernia (Q40.1)*

  Q79.1 Other congenital malformations of diaphragm
    Absence of diaphragm
    Congenital malformation of diaphragm NOS
    Eventration of diaphragm

  Q79.2 Exomphalos
    Omphalocele
    EXCLUDES 1 *umbilical hernia (K42.-)*

  Q79.3 Gastroschisis

  Q79.4 Prune belly syndrome
    Congenital prolapse of bladder mucosa
    Eagle-Barrett syndrome

☑5ᵗʰ **Q79.5 Other congenital malformations of abdominal wall**
    EXCLUDES 1 *umbilical hernia (K42.-)*

    Q79.51 Congenital hernia of bladder

    Q79.59 Other congenital malformations of abdominal wall

  Q79.6 Ehlers-Danlos syndrome
    DEF: Connective tissue disorder that causes hyperextended skin and joints; results in fragile blood vessels with bleeding, poor wound healing, and subcutaneous pseudotumors.

Gastroschisis

Herniated small bowel (gastroschisis)

Rectus abdominus m.

Umbilicus

skin

distal

proximal

Defect

Q79.8 Other congenital malformations of musculoskeletal system
    Absence of muscle
    Absence of tendon
    Accessory muscle
    Amyotrophia congenita
    Congenital constricting bands
    Congenital shortening of tendon
    Poland syndrome

Q79.9 Congenital malformation of musculoskeletal system, unspecified   ▽
    Congenital anomaly of musculoskeletal system NOS
    Congenital deformity of musculoskeletal system NOS

Other congenital malformations (Q80-Q89)

☑4ᵗʰ **Q80 Congenital ichthyosis**
  EXCLUDES 1 *Refsum's disease (G60.1)*

  Q80.0 Ichthyosis vulgaris

  Q80.1 X-linked ichthyosis

  Q80.2 Lamellar ichthyosis
    Collodion baby

  Q80.3 Congenital bullous ichthyosiform erythroderma

  Q80.4 Harlequin fetus

  Q80.8 Other congenital ichthyosis

  Q80.9 Congenital ichthyosis, unspecified   ▽

☑4ᵗʰ **Q81 Epidermolysis bullosa**

  Q81.0 Epidermolysis bullosa simplex
    EXCLUDES 1 *Cockayne's syndrome (Q87.1)*

  Q81.1 Epidermolysis bullosa letalis
    Herlitz' syndrome

  Q81.2 Epidermolysis bullosa dystrophica

  Q81.8 Other epidermolysis bullosa

  Q81.9 Epidermolysis bullosa, unspecified   ▽

☑4ᵗʰ **Q82 Other congenital malformations of skin**
  EXCLUDES 1 *acrodermatitis enteropathica (E83.2)*
    congenital erythropoietic porphyria (E80.0)
    pilonidal cyst or sinus (L05.-)
    Sturge-Weber (-Dimitri) syndrome (Q85.8)

  Q82.0 Hereditary lymphedema

  Q82.1 Xeroderma pigmentosum

▲ **Q82.2 Congenital cutaneous mastocytosis**
    ▶Congenital diffuse cutaneous mastocytosis
    Congenital maculopapular cutaneous mastocytosis
    Congenital urticaria pigmentosa◄
    Urticaria pigmentosa
    EXCLUDES 1 ▶cutaneous mastocytosis NOS (D47.01)
      diffuse cutaneous mastocytosis (with onset after newborn period) (D47.01)◄
      malignant mastocytosis ▶(C96.2-)◄
      ▶systemic mastocytosis (D47.02)
      urticaria pigmentosa (non-congenital) (with onset after newborn period) (D47.01)◄

  Q82.3 Incontinentia pigmenti

  Q82.4 Ectodermal dysplasia (anhidrotic)
    EXCLUDES 1 *Ellis-van Creveld syndrome (Q77.6)*

☑ Additional Character Req   ✓x7ᵗʰ Placeholder Alert   **Manifestation**   **HCC** CMS-HCC Condition   ▽ Unspecified Code   ▶◄ Revised Text   ● New Code   ▲ Revised Code Title

Q82.5 Congenital non-neoplastic nevus
Birthmark NOS
Flammeus Nevus
Portwine Nevus
Sanguineous Nevus
Strawberry Nevus
Vascular Nevus NOS
Verrucous Nevus
> EXCLUDES 2   *araneus nevus (I78.1)*
> *café au lait spots (L81.3)*
> *lentigo (L81.4)*
> *melanocytic nevus (D22.-)*
> *nevus NOS (D22.-)*
> *pigmented nevus (D22.-)*
> *spider nevus (I78.1)*
> *stellar nevus (I78.1)*

Q82.6 Congenital sacral dimple
Parasacral dimple
> EXCLUDES 2   *pilonidal cyst with abscess (L05.01)*
> *pilonidal cyst without abscess (L05.91)*

Q82.8 Other specified congenital malformations of skin
Abnormal palmar creases
Accessory skin tags
Benign familial pemphigus [Hailey-Hailey]
Congenital poikiloderma
Cutis laxa (hyperelastica)
Dermatoglyphic anomalies
Inherited keratosis palmaris et plantaris
Keratosis follicularis [Darier-White]
> EXCLUDES 1   *Ehlers-Danlos syndrome (Q79.6)*
> AHA: 2016, 1Q, 17

Q82.9 Congenital malformation of skin, unspecified ▽

√4ᵗʰ **Q83 Congenital malformations of breast**
> EXCLUDES 2   *absence of pectoral muscle (Q79.8)*
> *hypoplasia of breast (N64.82)*
> *micromastia (N64.82)*

Q83.0 Congenital absence of breast with absent nipple

Q83.1 Accessory breast
Supernumerary breast

Q83.2 Absent nipple

Q83.3 Accessory nipple
Supernumerary nipple

Q83.8 Other congenital malformations of breast

Q83.9 Congenital malformation of breast, unspecified ▽

√4ᵗʰ **Q84 Other congenital malformations of integument**

Q84.0 Congenital alopecia
Congenital atrichosis

Q84.1 Congenital morphological disturbances of hair, not elsewhere classified
Beaded hair
Monilethrix
Pili annulati
> EXCLUDES 1   *Menkes' kinky hair syndrome (E83.0)*

Q84.2 Other congenital malformations of hair
Congenital hypertrichosis
Congenital malformation of hair NOS
Persistent lanugo

Q84.3 Anonychia
> EXCLUDES 1   *nail patella syndrome (Q87.2)*

Q84.4 Congenital leukonychia

Q84.5 Enlarged and hypertrophic nails
Congenital onychauxis
Pachyonychia

Q84.6 Other congenital malformations of nails
Congenital clubnail
Congenital koilonychia
Congenital malformation of nail NOS

Q84.8 Other specified congenital malformations of integument
Aplasia cutis congenita

Q84.9 Congenital malformation of integument, unspecified ▽
Congenital anomaly of integument NOS
Congenital deformity of integument NOS

√4ᵗʰ **Q85 Phakomatoses, not elsewhere classified**
> EXCLUDES 1   *ataxia telangiectasia [Louis-Bar] (G11.3)*
> *familial dysautonomia [Riley-Day] (G90.1)*

√5ᵗʰ **Q85.0 Neurofibromatosis (nonmalignant)**

Q85.00 Neurofibromatosis, unspecified HCC ▽

Q85.01 Neurofibromatosis, type 1 HCC
Von Recklinghausen disease

Q85.02 Neurofibromatosis, type 2 HCC
Acoustic neurofibromatosis
DEF: Inherited condition with cutaneous lesions, benign tumors of peripheral nerves, and bilateral 8th nerve masses.

Q85.03 Schwannomatosis HCC
DEF: A genetic mutation (SMARCB1/INI1) causing multiple benign tumors along nerve pathways; characterized by the exception of 8th cranial nerve involvement.

Q85.09 Other neurofibromatosis HCC

Q85.1 Tuberous sclerosis HCC
Bourneville's disease
Epiloia

Q85.8 Other phakomatoses, not elsewhere classified HCC
Peutz-Jeghers Syndrome
Sturge-Weber(-Dimitri) syndrome
von Hippel-Lindau syndrome
> EXCLUDES 1   *Meckel-Gruber syndrome (Q61.9)*

Q85.9 Phakomatosis, unspecified HCC ▽
Hamartosis NOS

√4ᵗʰ **Q86 Congenital malformation syndromes due to known exogenous causes, not elsewhere classified**
> EXCLUDES 2   *iodine-deficiency-related hypothyroidism (E00-E02)*
> *nonteratogenic effects of substances transmitted via placenta or breast milk (P04.-)*

Q86.0 Fetal alcohol syndrome (dysmorphic)

Q86.1 Fetal hydantoin syndrome
Meadow's syndrome

Q86.2 Dysmorphism due to warfarin

Q86.8 Other congenital malformation syndromes due to known exogenous causes

√4ᵗʰ **Q87 Other specified congenital malformation syndromes affecting multiple systems**
Use additional code(s) to identify all associated manifestations

Q87.0 Congenital malformation syndromes predominantly affecting facial appearance
Acrocephalopolysyndactyly
Acrocephalosyndactyly [Apert] syndrome
Cryptophthalmos syndrome
Cyclopia
Goldenhar syndrome
Moebius syndrome
Oro-facial-digital
Robin syndrome
Whistling face

Q87.1 Congenital malformation syndromes predominantly associated with short stature
Aarskog syndrome
Cockayne syndrome
De Lange syndrome
Dubowitz syndrome
Noonan syndrome
Prader-Willi syndrome
Robinow-Silverman-Smith syndrome
Russell-Silver syndrome
Seckel syndrome
> EXCLUDES 1   *Ellis-van Creveld syndrome (Q77.6)*
> *Smith-Lemli-Opitz syndrome (E78.72)*

Q87.2 Congenital malformation syndromes predominantly involving limbs
Holt-Oram syndrome
Klippel-Trenaunay-Weber syndrome
Nail patella syndrome
Rubinstein-Taybi syndrome
Sirenomelia syndrome
Thrombocytopenia with absent radius [TAR] syndrome
VATER syndrome

Q87.3 Congenital malformation syndromes involving early overgrowth
Beckwith-Wiedemann syndrome
Sotos syndrome
Weaver syndrome

√5ᵗʰ **Q87.4 Marfan's syndrome**

Q87.40 Marfan's syndrome, unspecified ▽

√6ᵗʰ **Q87.41 Marfan's syndrome with cardiovascular manifestations**

Q87.410 Marfan's syndrome with aortic dilation

Q87.418 Marfan's syndrome with other cardiovascular manifestations

Q87.42 Marfan's syndrome with ocular manifestations

Q87.43 Marfan's syndrome with skeletal manifestation

Q87.5 Other congenital malformation syndromes with other skeletal changes

---

EXCLUDES 1 Not coded here   EXCLUDES 2 Not included here   N Newborn Age: 0   P Pediatric Age: 0-17   M Maternity Age: 12-55   A Adult Age: 15-124

884   ICD-10-CM 2018

✓5ᵗʰ **Q87.8 Other specified congenital malformation syndromes, not elsewhere classified**

　　　EXCLUDES 1　*Zellweger syndrome (E71.510)*

Q87.81 Alport syndrome
　　　Use additional code to identify stage of chronic kidney disease (N18.1-N18.6)

Q87.82 Arterial tortuosity syndrome

Q87.89 Other specified congenital malformation syndromes, not elsewhere classified
　　　Laurence-Moon (-Bardet)-Biedl syndrome

✓4ᵗʰ **Q89 Other congenital malformations, not elsewhere classified**

✓5ᵗʰ **Q89.0 Congenital absence and malformations of spleen**
　　　EXCLUDES 1　*isomerism of atrial appendages (with asplenia or polysplenia) (Q20.6)*

Q89.01 Asplenia (congenital)

Q89.09 Congenital malformations of spleen
　　　Congenital splenomegaly

Q89.1 Congenital malformations of adrenal gland
　　　EXCLUDES 1　*adrenogenital disorders (E25.-)*
　　　　　　congenital adrenal hyperplasia (E25.0)

Q89.2 Congenital malformations of other endocrine glands
　　　Congenital malformation of parathyroid or thyroid gland
　　　Persistent thyroglossal duct
　　　Thyroglossal cyst
　　　EXCLUDES 1　*congenital goiter (E03.0)*
　　　　　　congenital hypothyroidism (E03.1)

Q89.3 Situs inversus
　　　Dextrocardia with situs inversus
　　　Mirror-image atrial arrangement with situs inversus
　　　Situs inversus or transversus abdominalis
　　　Situs inversus or transversus thoracis
　　　Transposition of abdominal viscera
　　　Transposition of thoracic viscera
　　　EXCLUDES 1　*dextrocardia NOS (Q24.0)*

Q89.4 Conjoined twins
　　　Craniopagus　　　　　　Pygopagus
　　　Dicephaly　　　　　　Thoracopagus

Q89.7 Multiple congenital malformations, not elsewhere classified
　　　Multiple congenital anomalies NOS
　　　Multiple congenital deformities NOS
　　　EXCLUDES 1　*congenital malformation syndromes affecting multiple systems (Q87.-)*

Q89.8 Other specified congenital malformations
　　　Use additional code(s) to identify all associated manifestations

Q89.9 Congenital malformation, unspecified　▽
　　　Congenital anomaly NOS
　　　Congenital deformity NOS

Chromosomal abnormalities, not elsewhere classified (Q90-Q99)

　　　EXCLUDES 2　*mitochondrial metabolic disorders (E88.4-)*

✓4ᵗʰ **Q90 Down syndrome**
　　　Use additional code(s) to identify any associated physical conditions and degree of intellectual disabilities (F70-F79)

Q90.0 Trisomy 21, nonmosaicism (meiotic nondisjunction)

Q90.1 Trisomy 21, mosaicism (mitotic nondisjunction)

Q90.2 Trisomy 21, translocation

Q90.9 Down syndrome, unspecified　▽
　　　Trisomy 21 NOS

✓4ᵗʰ **Q91 Trisomy 18 and Trisomy 13**

Q91.0 Trisomy 18, nonmosaicism (meiotic nondisjunction)

Q91.1 Trisomy 18, mosaicism (mitotic nondisjunction)

Q91.2 Trisomy 18, translocation

Q91.3 Trisomy 18, unspecified　▽

Q91.4 Trisomy 13, nonmosaicism (meiotic nondisjunction)

Q91.5 Trisomy 13, mosaicism (mitotic nondisjunction)

Q91.6 Trisomy 13, translocation

Q91.7 Trisomy 13, unspecified　▽

✓4ᵗʰ **Q92 Other trisomies and partial trisomies of the autosomes, not elsewhere classified**
　　　INCLUDES　unbalanced translocations and insertions
　　　EXCLUDES 1　*trisomies of chromosomes 13, 18, 21 (Q90-Q91)*

Q92.0 Whole chromosome trisomy, nonmosaicism (meiotic nondisjunction)

Q92.1 Whole chromosome trisomy, mosaicism (mitotic nondisjunction)

Q92.2 Partial trisomy
　　　Less than whole arm duplicated
　　　Whole arm or more duplicated
　　　EXCLUDES 1　*partial trisomy due to unbalanced translocation (Q92.5)*

Q92.5 Duplications with other complex rearrangements
　　　Partial trisomy due to unbalanced translocations
　　　Code also any associated deletions due to unbalanced translocations, inversions and insertions (Q93.7)

✓5ᵗʰ **Q92.6 Marker chromosomes**
　　　Trisomies due to dicentrics
　　　Trisomies due to extra rings
　　　Trisomies due to isochromosomes
　　　Individual with marker heterochromatin

Q92.61 Marker chromosomes in normal individual

Q92.62 Marker chromosomes in abnormal individual

Q92.7 Triploidy and polyploidy

Q92.8 Other specified trisomies and partial trisomies of autosomes
　　　Duplications identified by fluorescence in situ hybridization (FISH)
　　　Duplications identified by in situ hybridization (ISH)
　　　Duplications seen only at prometaphase

Q92.9 Trisomy and partial trisomy of autosomes, unspecified　▽

✓4ᵗʰ **Q93 Monosomies and deletions from the autosomes, not elsewhere classified**

Q93.0 Whole chromosome monosomy, nonmosaicism (meiotic nondisjunction)

Q93.1 Whole chromosome monosomy, mosaicism (mitotic nondisjunction)

Q93.2 Chromosome replaced with ring, dicentric or isochromosome

Q93.3 Deletion of short arm of chromosome 4
　　　Wolff-Hirschorn syndrome

Q93.4 Deletion of short arm of chromosome 5
　　　Cri-du-chat syndrome

Q93.5 Other deletions of part of a chromosome
　　　Angelman syndrome

Q93.7 Deletions with other complex rearrangements
　　　Deletions due to unbalanced translocations, inversions and insertions
　　　Code also any associated duplications due to unbalanced translocations, inversions and insertions (Q92.5)

✓5ᵗʰ **Q93.8 Other deletions from the autosomes**

Q93.81 Velo-cardio-facial syndrome
　　　Deletion 22q11.2
　　　DEF: Microdeletion syndrome affecting multiple organs; characteristic cleft palate, heart defects, elongated face with almond-shaped eyes, wide nose, small ears, weak immune system, weak musculature, hypothyroidism, short stature, and scoliosis; deletion at q11.2 on the long arm of the chromosome 22.

Q93.88 Other microdeletions
　　　Miller-Dieker syndrome
　　　Smith-Magenis syndrome

Q93.89 Other deletions from the autosomes
　　　Deletions identified by fluorescence in situ hybridization (FISH)
　　　Deletions identified by in situ hybridization (ISH)
　　　Deletions seen only at prometaphase

Q93.9 Deletion from autosomes, unspecified　▽

✓4ᵗʰ **Q95 Balanced rearrangements and structural markers, not elsewhere classified**
　　　INCLUDES　Robertsonian and balanced reciprocal translocations and insertions

Q95.0 Balanced translocation and insertion in normal individual

Q95.1 Chromosome inversion in normal individual

Q95.2 Balanced autosomal rearrangement in abnormal individual

Q95.3 Balanced sex/autosomal rearrangement in abnormal individual

Q95.5 Individual with autosomal fragile site

Q95.8 Other balanced rearrangements and structural markers

Q95.9 Balanced rearrangement and structural marker, unspecified　▽

✓4ᵗʰ **Q96 Turner's syndrome**
　　　EXCLUDES 1　*Noonan syndrome (Q87.1)*

Q96.0 Karyotype 45, X　♀

Q96.1 Karyotype 46, X iso (Xq)　♀
　　　Karyotype 46, isochromosome Xq

☑ Additional Character Req　　✓ⁿ˟⁷ᵗʰ Placeholder Alert　　Manifestation　　HCC CMS-HCC Condition　　▽ Unspecified Code　　►◄ Revised Text　　● New Code　　▲ Revised Code Title

Q96.2 **Karyotype 46, X with abnormal sex chromosome, except iso (Xq)**   ♀
   Karyotype 46, X with abnormal sex chromosome, except isochromosome Xq

Q96.3 **Mosaicism, 45, X/46, XX or XY**   ♀

Q96.4 **Mosaicism, 45, X/other cell line(s) with abnormal sex chromosome**   ♀

Q96.8 **Other variants of Turner's syndrome**   ♀

Q96.9 **Turner's syndrome, unspecified**   ♀▽

✓4ᵗʰ **Q97 Other sex chromosome abnormalities, female phenotype, not elsewhere classified**
   EXCLUDES 1 *Turner's syndrome (Q96.-)*

Q97.0 **Karyotype 47, XXX**   ♀

Q97.1 **Female with more than three X chromosomes**   ♀

Q97.2 **Mosaicism, lines with various numbers of X chromosomes**   ♀

Q97.3 **Female with 46, XY karyotype**   ♀

Q97.8 **Other specified sex chromosome abnormalities, female phenotype**   ♀

Q97.9 **Sex chromosome abnormality, female phenotype, unspecified**   ♀▽

✓4ᵗʰ **Q98 Other sex chromosome abnormalities, male phenotype, not elsewhere classified**

Q98.0 **Klinefelter syndrome karyotype 47, XXY**   ♂

Q98.1 **Klinefelter syndrome, male with more than two X chromosomes**   ♂

Q98.3 **Other male with 46, XX karyotype**   ♂

Q98.4 **Klinefelter syndrome, unspecified**   ♂▽

Q98.5 **Karyotype 47, XYY**

Q98.6 **Male with structurally abnormal sex chromosome**   ♂

Q98.7 **Male with sex chromosome mosaicism**   ♂

Q98.8 **Other specified sex chromosome abnormalities, male phenotype**   ♂

Q98.9 **Sex chromosome abnormality, male phenotype, unspecified**   ♂▽

✓4ᵗʰ **Q99 Other chromosome abnormalities, not elsewhere classified**

Q99.0 **Chimera 46, XX/46, XY**
   Chimera 46, XX/46, XY true hermaphrodite

Q99.1 **46, XX true hermaphrodite**
   46, XX with streak gonads   Pure gonadal dysgenesis
   46, XY with streak gonads

Q99.2 **Fragile X chromosome**
   Fragile X syndrome

Q99.8 **Other specified chromosome abnormalities**

Q99.9 **Chromosomal abnormality, unspecified**   ▽

Chapter 18. Symptoms, Signs, and Abnormal Clinical and Laboratory Findings, Not Elsewhere Classified (R00–R99)

Chapter Specific Guidelines with Coding Examples

The chapter specific guidelines from the ICD-10-CM Official Guidelines for Coding and Reporting have been provided below. Along with these guidelines are coding examples, contained in the shaded boxes, that have been developed to help illustrate the coding and/or sequencing guidance found in these guidelines.

Chapter 18 includes symptoms, signs, abnormal results of clinical or other investigative procedures, and ill-defined conditions regarding which no diagnosis classifiable elsewhere is recorded. Signs and symptoms that point to a specific diagnosis have been assigned to a category in other chapters of the classification.

a. Use of symptom codes

Codes that describe symptoms and signs are acceptable for reporting purposes when a related definitive diagnosis has not been established (confirmed) by the provider.

> Tenderness and localized pain in the right upper quadrant; based on presentation, probable gallstones
>
> **R10.11**   **Right upper quadrant pain**
>
> **R10.811**   **Right upper quadrant abdominal tenderness**
>
> *Explanation:* Codes that describe symptoms such as abdominal pain are acceptable for reporting purposes when the provider has not established (confirmed) a definitive diagnosis.

b. Use of a symptom code with a definitive diagnosis code

Codes for signs and symptoms may be reported in addition to a related definitive diagnosis when the sign or symptom is not routinely associated with that diagnosis, such as the various signs and symptoms associated with complex syndromes. The definitive diagnosis code should be sequenced before the symptom code.

Signs or symptoms that are associated routinely with a disease process should not be assigned as additional codes, unless otherwise instructed by the classification.

> Pneumonia with hemoptysis
>
> **J18.9**   **Pneumonia, unspecified organism**
>
> **R04.2**   **Hemoptysis**
>
> *Explanation:* Codes for signs and symptoms may be reported in addition to a related definitive diagnosis when the sign or symptom is not routinely associated with that diagnosis.

> Abdominal pain due to acute appendicitis
>
> **K35.80**   **Unspecified acute appendicitis**
>
> *Explanation:* Codes for signs or symptoms routinely associated with a disease process should not be assigned unless the classification instructs otherwise.

c. Combination codes that include symptoms

ICD-10-CM contains a number of combination codes that identify both the definitive diagnosis and common symptoms of that diagnosis. When using one of these combination codes, an additional code should not be assigned for the symptom.

> IBS with diarrhea
>
> **K58.0**   **Irritable bowel syndrome, with diarrhea**
>
> *Explanation:* When a combination code identifies both the definitive diagnosis and the symptom, an additional code should not be assigned for the symptom.

d. Repeated falls

Code R29.6, Repeated falls, is for use for encounters when a patient has recently fallen and the reason for the fall is being investigated.

Code Z91.81, History of falling, is for use when a patient has fallen in the past and is at risk for future falls. When appropriate, both codes R29.6 and Z91.81 may be assigned together.

e. Coma scale

The coma scale codes (R40.2-) can be used in conjunction with traumatic brain injury codes, acute cerebrovascular disease or sequelae of cerebrovascular disease codes. These codes are primarily for use by trauma registries, but they may be used in any setting where this information is collected. The coma scale may also be used to assess the status of the central nervous system for other non-trauma conditions, such as monitoring patients in the intensive care unit regardless of medical condition. The coma scale codes should be sequenced after the diagnosis code(s).

These codes, one from each subcategory, are needed to complete the scale. The 7th character indicates when the scale was recorded. The 7th character should match for all three codes.

At a minimum, report the initial score documented on presentation at your facility. This may be a score from the emergency medicine technician (EMT) or in the emergency department. If desired, a facility may choose to capture multiple coma scale scores.

Assign code R40.24, Glasgow coma scale, total score, when only the total score is documented in the medical record and not the individual score(s).

> 36-year-old man found down after unknown injury with skull fracture and with concussion and loss of consciousness of unknown duration. Upon hospital admission, the patient was evaluated with the following Glasgow coma scores:
>
> Eye-opening response—3: eyes open to speech
>
> Verbal response—3: random speech with no conversational exchange
>
> Motor response—4: pulls limb away from painful stimulus
>
> **S02.0XXA**   **Fracture of vault of skull, initial encounter for closed fracture**
>
> **S06.0X9A**   **Concussion with loss of consciousness of unspecified duration, initial encounter**
>
> **R40.2133**   **Coma scale, eyes open, to sound, at hospital admission**
>
> **R40.2233**   **Coma scale, best verbal response, inappropriate words, at hospital admission**
>
> **R40.2343**   **Coma scale, best motor response, flexion withdrawal, at hospital admission**
>
> *Explanation:* When individual scores for the Glasgow coma scale are documented, one code from each category is needed to complete the scale. The seventh character indicates when the scale was recorded and should match for all three codes. Assign a code from subcategory R40.24- Glasgow coma scale, total score, when only the total and not the individual score(s) is documented.

f. Functional quadriplegia

Functional quadriplegia (code R53.2) is the lack of ability to use one's limbs or to ambulate due to extreme debility. It is not associated with neurologic deficit or injury, and code R53.2 should not be used for cases of neurologic quadriplegia. It should only be assigned if functional quadriplegia is specifically documented in the medical record.

g. SIRS due to non-infectious process

The systemic inflammatory response syndrome (SIRS) can develop as a result of certain non-infectious disease processes, such as trauma, malignant neoplasm, or pancreatitis. When SIRS is documented with a noninfectious condition, and no subsequent infection is documented, the code for the underlying condition, such as an injury, should be assigned, followed by code R65.10, Systemic inflammatory response syndrome (SIRS) of non-infectious origin without acute organ dysfunction, or code R65.11, Systemic inflammatory response syndrome (SIRS) of non-infectious origin with acute organ dysfunction. If an associated acute organ dysfunction is documented, the appropriate code(s) for the specific type of organ dysfunction(s) should be assigned in addition to code R65.11. If acute organ dysfunction is documented, but it cannot be determined if the acute organ dysfunction is associated with SIRS or due to another condition (e.g., directly due to the trauma), the provider should be queried.

Chapter 18. Symptoms, Signs, and Abnormal Clinical and Laboratory Findings, Not Elsewhere Classified

Systemic inflammatory response syndrome (SIRS) due to acute gallstone pancreatitis

K85.1Ø	**Biliary acute pancreatitis without necrosis or infection**
R65.1Ø	**Systemic inflammatory response syndrome (SIRS) of noninfectious origin without acute organ dysfunction**

Explanation: When SIRS is documented with a noninfectious condition without subsequent infection documented, the code for the underlying condition such as pancreatitis should be assigned followed by the appropriate code for SIRS of noninfectious origin, either with or without associated organ dysfunction.

h. Death NOS

Code R99, Ill-defined and unknown cause of mortality, is only for use in the very limited circumstance when a patient who has already died is brought into an emergency department or other healthcare facility and is pronounced dead upon arrival. It does not represent the discharge disposition of death.

i. NIHSS stroke scale

The NIH stroke scale (NIHSS) codes (R29.7- -) can be used in conjunction with acute stroke codes (I63) to identify the patient's neurological status and the severity of the stroke. The stroke scale codes should be sequenced after the acute stroke diagnosis code(s).

At a minimum, report the initial score documented. If desired, a facility may choose to capture multiple stroke scale scores.

See Section I.B.14. for information concerning the medical record documentation that may be used for assignment of the NIHSS codes.

h. Death NOS

Chapter 18. Symptoms, Signs and Abnormal Clinical and Laboratory Findings, Not Elsewhere Classified (R00-R99)

NOTE This chapter includes symptoms, signs, abnormal results of clinical or other investigative procedures, and ill-defined conditions regarding which no diagnosis classifiable elsewhere is recorded.

Signs and symptoms that point rather definitely to a given diagnosis have been assigned to a category in other chapters of the classification. In general, categories in this chapter include the less well-defined conditions and symptoms that, without the necessary study of the case to establish a final diagnosis, point perhaps equally to two or more diseases or to two or more systems of the body. Practically all categories in the chapter could be designated "not otherwise specified", "unknown etiology" or "transient". The Alphabetical Index should be consulted to determine which symptoms and signs are to be allocated here and which to other chapters. The residual subcategories, numbered .8, are generally provided for other relevant symptoms that cannot be allocated elsewhere in the classification.

The conditions and signs or symptoms included in categories R00-R94 consist of:

(a) cases for which no more specific diagnosis can be made even after all the facts bearing on the case have been investigated;

(b) signs or symptoms existing at the time of initial encounter that proved to be transient and whose causes could not be determined;

(c) provisional diagnosis in a patient who failed to return for further investigation or care;

(d) cases referred elsewhere for investigation or treatment before the diagnosis was made;

(e) cases in which a more precise diagnosis was not available for any other reason;

(f) certain symptoms, for which supplementary information is provided, that represent important problems in medical care in their own right.

EXCLUDES 2 *abnormal findings on antenatal screening of mother (O28.-)*
certain conditions originating in the perinatal period (P04-P96)
signs and symptoms classified in the body system chapters
signs and symptoms of breast (N63, N64.5)

AHA: 2017, 1Q, 6, 7

This chapter contains the following blocks:

R00-R09	Symptoms and signs involving the circulatory and respiratory systems
R10-R19	Symptoms and signs involving the digestive system and abdomen
R20-R23	Symptoms and signs involving the skin and subcutaneous tissue
R25-R29	Symptoms and signs involving the nervous and musculoskeletal systems
R30-R39	Symptoms and signs involving the genitourinary system
R40-R46	Symptoms and signs involving cognition, perception, emotional state and behavior
R47-R49	Symptoms and signs involving speech and voice
R50-R69	General symptoms and signs
R70-R79	Abnormal findings on examination of blood, without diagnosis
R80-R82	Abnormal findings on examination of urine, without diagnosis
R83-R89	Abnormal findings on examination of other body fluids, substances and tissues, without diagnosis
R90-R94	Abnormal findings on diagnostic imaging and in function studies, without diagnosis
R97	Abnormal tumor markers
R99	Ill-defined and unknown cause of mortality

Symptoms and signs involving the circulatory and respiratory systems (R00-R09)

✓4ᵗʰ R00 Abnormalities of heart beat
    EXCLUDES 1 *abnormalities originating in the perinatal period (P29.1-)*
    EXCLUDES 2 *specified arrhythmias (I47-I49)*

    R00.0 Tachycardia, unspecified ▽
        Rapid heart beat
        Sinoauricular tachycardia NOS
        Sinus [sinusal] tachycardia NOS
        EXCLUDES 1 *neonatal tachycardia (P29.11)*
            paroxysmal tachycardia (I47.-)
        DEF: Excessively rapid heart rate of more than 100 beats per minute.

R00.1 Bradycardia, unspecified ▽
    Sinoatrial bradycardia
    Sinus bradycardia
    Slow heart beat
    Vagal bradycardia
    Use additional code for adverse effect, if applicable, to identify drug (T36-T50 with fifth or sixth character 5)
    EXCLUDES 1 *neonatal bradycardia (P29.12)*

R00.2 Palpitations
    Awareness of heart beat

R00.8 Other abnormalities of heart beat

R00.9 Unspecified abnormalities of heart beat ▽

✓4ᵗʰ R01 Cardiac murmurs and other cardiac sounds
    EXCLUDES 1 *cardiac murmurs and sounds originating in the perinatal period (P29.8)*

    R01.0 Benign and innocent cardiac murmurs
        Functional cardiac murmur

    R01.1 Cardiac murmur, unspecified ▽
        Cardiac bruit NOS
        Heart murmur NOS
        Systolic murmur NOS

    R01.2 Other cardiac sounds
        Cardiac dullness, increased or decreased
        Precordial friction

✓4ᵗʰ R03 Abnormal blood-pressure reading, without diagnosis
    R03.0 Elevated blood-pressure reading, without diagnosis of hypertension
        NOTE This category is to be used to record an episode of elevated blood pressure in a patient in whom no formal diagnosis of hypertension has been made, or as an isolated incidental finding.

    R03.1 Nonspecific low blood-pressure reading
        EXCLUDES 1 *hypotension (I95.-)*
            maternal hypotension syndrome (O26.5-)
            neurogenic orthostatic hypotension (G90.3)

✓4ᵗʰ R04 Hemorrhage from respiratory passages
    R04.0 Epistaxis
        Hemorrhage from nose
        Nosebleed

    R04.1 Hemorrhage from throat
        EXCLUDES 2 *hemoptysis (R04.2)*

    R04.2 Hemoptysis
        Blood-stained sputum
        Cough with hemorrhage
        AHA: 2013, 4Q, 118

    ✓5ᵗʰ R04.8 Hemorrhage from other sites in respiratory passages
        R04.81 Acute idiopathic pulmonary hemorrhage in infants ℙ
            AIPHI
            Acute idiopathic hemorrhage in infants over 28 days old
            EXCLUDES 1 *perinatal pulmonary hemorrhage (P26.-)*
                von Willebrand's disease (D68.0)

        R04.89 Hemorrhage from other sites in respiratory passages
            Pulmonary hemorrhage NOS

    R04.9 Hemorrhage from respiratory passages, unspecified ▽

R05 Cough
    EXCLUDES 1 *cough with hemorrhage (R04.2)*
           smoker's cough (J41.0)
    AHA: 2016, 2Q, 33

✓4ᵗʰ R06 Abnormalities of breathing
    EXCLUDES 1 *acute respiratory distress syndrome (J80)*
           respiratory arrest (R09.2)
           respiratory arrest of newborn (P28.81)
           respiratory distress syndrome of newborn (P22.-)
           respiratory failure (J96.-)
           respiratory failure of newborn (P28.5)

    ✓5ᵗʰ R06.0 Dyspnea
        EXCLUDES 1 *tachypnea NOS (R06.82)*
            transient tachypnea of newborn (P22.1)

        R06.00 Dyspnea, unspecified ▽
            AHA: 2017, 1Q, 26

        R06.01 Orthopnea

        R06.02 Shortness of breath

        ● **R06.03 Acute respiratory distress**

        R06.09 Other forms of dyspnea

✅ Additional Character Req   **✓x7ᵗʰ** Placeholder Alert   Manifestation   **HCC** CMS-HCC Condition   ▽ Unspecified Code   ▶◀ Revised Text   ● New Code   ▲ Revised Code Title

Chapter 18. Symptoms, Signs, and Abnormal Clinical and Laboratory Findings, Not Elsewhere Classified

R06.1 Stridor
> EXCLUDES 1   *congenital laryngeal stridor (P28.89)*
> *laryngismus (stridulus) (J38.5)*

R06.2 Wheezing
> EXCLUDES 1   *asthma (J45.-)*

AHA: 2016, 2Q, 33
DEF: High-pitched whistling sound during breathing due to stenosis of respiratory passageway; associated with asthma, sleep apnea, bronchiectasis, bronchiolitis, COPD, and pleural effusion.

R06.3 Periodic breathing
> Cheyne-Stokes breathing

R06.4 Hyperventilation
> EXCLUDES 1   *psychogenic hyperventilation (F45.8)*

R06.5 Mouth breathing
> EXCLUDES 2   *dry mouth NOS (R68.2)*

R06.6 Hiccough
> EXCLUDES 1   *psychogenic hiccough (F45.8)*

R06.7 Sneezing

✓5ᵗʰ **R06.8 Other abnormalities of breathing**

     R06.81 Apnea, not elsewhere classified
> Apnea NOS
> EXCLUDES 1   *apnea (of) newborn (P28.4)*
> *sleep apnea (G47.3-)*
> *sleep apnea of newborn (primary) (P28.3)*

     R06.82 Tachypnea, not elsewhere classified
> Tachypnea NOS
> EXCLUDES 1   *transitory tachypnea of newborn (P22.1)*

     R06.83 Snoring

     R06.89 Other abnormalities of breathing
> Breath-holding (spells)
> Sighing

R06.9 Unspecified abnormalities of breathing ▽

✓4ᵗʰ **R07 Pain in throat and chest**
> EXCLUDES 1   *epidemic myalgia (B33.0)*
> EXCLUDES 2   *jaw pain (R68.84)*
> *pain in breast (N64.4)*

     R07.0 Pain in throat
> EXCLUDES 1   *chronic sore throat (J31.2)*
> *sore throat (acute) NOS (J02.9)*
> EXCLUDES 2   *dysphagia (R13.1-)*
> *pain in neck (M54.2)*

     R07.1 Chest pain on breathing
> Painful respiration

     R07.2 Precordial pain

✓5ᵗʰ   **R07.8 Other chest pain**

     R07.81 Pleurodynia
> Pleurodynia NOS
> EXCLUDES 1   *epidemic pleurodynia (B33.0)*

     R07.82 Intercostal pain

     R07.89 Other chest pain
> Anterior chest-wall pain NOS

     R07.9 Chest pain, unspecified ▽

✓4ᵗʰ **R09 Other symptoms and signs involving the circulatory and respiratory system**
> EXCLUDES 1   *acute respiratory distress syndrome (J80)*
> *respiratory arrest of newborn (P28.81)*
> *respiratory distress syndrome of newborn (P22.0)*
> *respiratory failure (J96.-)*
> *respiratory failure of newborn (P28.5)*

✓5ᵗʰ   **R09.0 Asphyxia and hypoxemia**
> EXCLUDES 1   *asphyxia due to carbon monoxide (T58.-)*
> *asphyxia due to foreign body in respiratory tract (T17.-)*
> *birth (intrauterine) asphyxia (P84)*
> ~~*hypercapnia (R06.4)*~~
> *hyperventilation (R06.4)*
> *traumatic asphyxia (T71.-)*
> EXCLUDES 2   ▶*hypercapnia (R06.89)*◀

     R09.01 Asphyxia

     R09.02 Hypoxemia

     R09.1 Pleurisy
> EXCLUDES 1   *pleurisy with effusion (J90)*

R09.2 Respiratory arrest   HCC
> Cardiorespiratory failure
> EXCLUDES 1   *cardiac arrest (I46.-)*
> *respiratory arrest of newborn (P28.81)*
> *respiratory distress of newborn (P22.0)*
> *respiratory failure (J96.-)*
> *respiratory failure of newborn (P28.5)*
> *respiratory insufficiency (R06.89)*
> *respiratory insufficiency of newborn (P28.5)*

R09.3 Abnormal sputum
> Abnormal amount of sputum
> Abnormal color of sputum
> Abnormal odor of sputum
> Excessive sputum
> EXCLUDES 1   *blood-stained sputum (R04.2)*

✓5ᵗʰ **R09.8 Other specified symptoms and signs involving the circulatory and respiratory systems**

     R09.81 Nasal congestion

     R09.82 Postnasal drip

     R09.89 Other specified symptoms and signs involving the circulatory and respiratory systems
> Abnormal chest percussion
> Bruit (arterial)
> Chest tympany
> Choking sensation
> Feeling of foreign body in throat
> Friction sounds in chest
> Rales
> Weak pulse
> EXCLUDES 2   *foreign body in throat (T17.2-)*
> *wheezing (R06.2)*

Symptoms and signs involving the digestive system and abdomen (R10-R19)

> EXCLUDES 2   *congenital or infantile pylorospasm (Q40.0)*
> *gastrointestinal hemorrhage (K92.0-K92.2)*
> *intestinal obstruction (K56.-)*
> *newborn gastrointestinal hemorrhage (P54.0-P54.3)*
> *newborn intestinal obstruction (P76.-)*
> *pylorospasm (K31.3)*
> *signs and symptoms involving the urinary system (R30-R39)*
> *symptoms referable to female genital organs (N94.-)*
> *symptoms referable to male genital organs (N48-N50)*

✓4ᵗʰ **R10 Abdominal and pelvic pain**
> EXCLUDES 1   *renal colic (N23)*
> EXCLUDES 2   *dorsalgia (M54.-)*
> *flatulence and related conditions (R14.-)*

     R10.0 Acute abdomen
> Severe abdominal pain (generalized) (with abdominal rigidity)
> EXCLUDES 1   *abdominal rigidity NOS (R19.3)*
> *generalized abdominal pain NOS (R10.84)*
> *localized abdominal pain (R10.1-R10.3-)*

Abdominal Pain

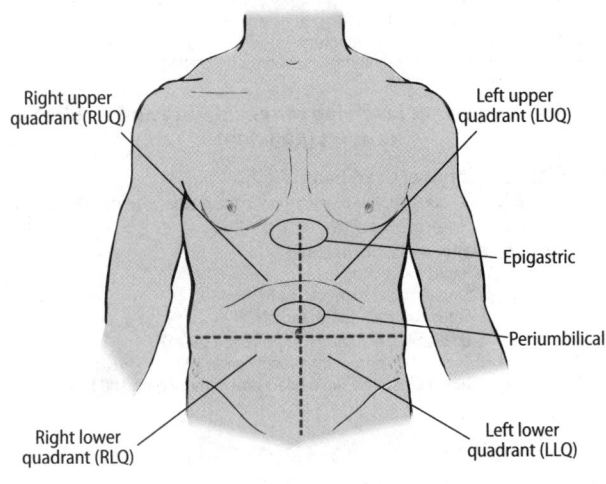

Right upper quadrant (RUQ)
Left upper quadrant (LUQ)
Epigastric
Periumbilical
Right lower quadrant (RLQ)
Left lower quadrant (LLQ)

EXCLUDES 1 Not coded here   EXCLUDES 2 Not included here   N Newborn Age: 0   P Pediatric Age: 0-17   M Maternity Age: 12-55   A Adult Age: 15-124

890   ICD-10-CM 2018

✓5ᵗʰ **R10.1** Pain localized to upper abdomen

    R10.10 Upper abdominal pain, unspecified ▽

    R10.11 Right upper quadrant pain

    R10.12 Left upper quadrant pain

    R10.13 Epigastric pain
         Dyspepsia
         EXCLUDES 1   *functional dyspepsia (K30)*

R10.2 Pelvic and perineal pain
     EXCLUDES 1   *vulvodynia (N94.81)*

✓5ᵗʰ **R10.3** Pain localized to other parts of lower abdomen

    R10.30 Lower abdominal pain, unspecified ▽

    R10.31 Right lower quadrant pain

    R10.32 Left lower quadrant pain

    R10.33 Periumbilical pain

✓5ᵗʰ **R10.8** Other abdominal pain

  ✓6ᵗʰ **R10.81** Abdominal tenderness
         Abdominal tenderness NOS

        R10.811 Right upper quadrant abdominal tenderness

        R10.812 Left upper quadrant abdominal tenderness

        R10.813 Right lower quadrant abdominal tenderness

        R10.814 Left lower quadrant abdominal tenderness

        R10.815 Periumbilic abdominal tenderness

        R10.816 Epigastric abdominal tenderness

        R10.817 Generalized abdominal tenderness

        R10.819 Abdominal tenderness, unspecified site ▽

  ✓6ᵗʰ **R10.82** Rebound abdominal tenderness

        R10.821 Right upper quadrant rebound abdominal tenderness

        R10.822 Left upper quadrant rebound abdominal tenderness

        R10.823 Right lower quadrant rebound abdominal tenderness

        R10.824 Left lower quadrant rebound abdominal tenderness

        R10.825 Periumbilic rebound abdominal tenderness

        R10.826 Epigastric rebound abdominal tenderness

        R10.827 Generalized rebound abdominal tenderness

        R10.829 Rebound abdominal tenderness, unspecified site ▽

    R10.83 Colic   P
         Colic NOS
         Infantile colic
         EXCLUDES 1   *colic in adult and child over 12 months old (R10.84)*
         DEF: Inconsolable crying in an otherwise well-fed and healthy infant for more than three hours a day, three days a week, for more than three weeks.

    R10.84 Generalized abdominal pain
         EXCLUDES 1   *generalized abdominal pain associated with acute abdomen (R10.0)*

R10.9 Unspecified abdominal pain ▽

✓4ᵗʰ **R11** Nausea and vomiting
     EXCLUDES 1   *cyclical vomiting associated with migraine (G43.A-)*
         excessive vomiting in pregnancy (O21.-)
         hematemesis (K92.0)
         neonatal hematemesis (P54.0)
         newborn vomiting (P92.0-)
         psychogenic vomiting (F50.89)
         vomiting associated with bulimia nervosa (F50.2)
         vomiting following gastrointestinal surgery (K91.0)
     AHA: 2017, 1Q, 28

R11.0 Nausea
     Nausea NOS
     Nausea without vomiting

✓5ᵗʰ **R11.1** Vomiting

    R11.10 Vomiting, unspecified ▽
         Vomiting NOS

    R11.11 Vomiting without nausea

    R11.12 Projectile vomiting

    R11.13 Vomiting of fecal matter

Swallowing Function

Oral phase

Oropharyngeal phase

Pharyngeal phase

Pharyngoesophageal phase

    R11.14 Bilious vomiting
         Bilious emesis

    R11.2 Nausea with vomiting, unspecified ▽
         Persistent nausea with vomiting NOS

R12 Heartburn
     EXCLUDES 1   *dyspepsia NOS (R10.13)*
         functional dyspepsia (K30)

✓4ᵗʰ **R13** Aphagia and dysphagia

R13.0 Aphagia
     Inability to swallow
     EXCLUDES 1   *psychogenic aphagia (F50.9)*

✓5ᵗʰ **R13.1** Dysphagia
     Code first, if applicable, dysphagia following cerebrovascular disease (I69. with final characters -91)
     EXCLUDES 1   *psychogenic dysphagia (F45.8)*

    R13.10 Dysphagia, unspecified ▽
         Difficulty in swallowing NOS

    R13.11 Dysphagia, oral phase

    R13.12 Dysphagia, oropharyngeal phase

    R13.13 Dysphagia, pharyngeal phase

    R13.14 Dysphagia, pharyngoesophageal phase

    R13.19 Other dysphagia
         Cervical dysphagia
         Neurogenic dysphagia

✓4ᵗʰ **R14** Flatulence and related conditions
     EXCLUDES 1   *psychogenic aerophagy (F45.8)*

R14.0 Abdominal distension (gaseous)
     Bloating
     Tympanites (abdominal) (intestinal)

R14.1 Gas pain

R14.2 Eructation

R14.3 Flatulence

✓4ᵗʰ **R15** Fecal incontinence
     INCLUDES   encopresis NOS
     EXCLUDES 1   *fecal incontinence of nonorganic origin (F98.1)*

R15.0 Incomplete defecation
     EXCLUDES 1   *constipation (K59.0-)*
         fecal impaction (K56.41)

R15.1 Fecal smearing
     Fecal soiling

R15.2 Fecal urgency

R15.9 Full incontinence of feces
     Fecal incontinence NOS

✓4ᵗʰ **R16** Hepatomegaly and splenomegaly, not elsewhere classified

R16.0 Hepatomegaly, not elsewhere classified
     Hepatomegaly NOS

R16.1 Splenomegaly, not elsewhere classified
     Splenomegaly NOS

R16.2 Hepatomegaly with splenomegaly, not elsewhere classified
     Hepatosplenomegaly NOS

R17 Unspecified jaundice ▽
     EXCLUDES 1   *neonatal jaundice (P55, P57-P59)*

✓ Additional Character Req   ✓x7ᵗʰ Placeholder Alert   Manifestation   HCC CMS-HCC Condition   ▽ Unspecified Code   ►◄ Revised Text   ● New Code   ▲ Revised Code Title

✓4ᵗʰ **R18 Ascites**
INCLUDES fluid in peritoneal cavity
EXCLUDES 1 *ascites in alcoholic cirrhosis (K70.31)*
ascites in alcoholic hepatitis (K70.11)
ascites in toxic liver disease with chronic active hepatitis (K71.51)

R18.0 Malignant ascites
Code first malignancy, such as:
malignant neoplasm of ovary (C56.-)
secondary malignant neoplasm of retroperitoneum and peritoneum (C78.6)

R18.8 Other ascites
Ascites NOS
Peritoneal effusion (chronic)

✓4ᵗʰ **R19 Other symptoms and signs involving the digestive system and abdomen**
EXCLUDES 1 *acute abdomen (R10.0)*

✓5ᵗʰ **R19.0 Intra-abdominal and pelvic swelling, mass and lump**
EXCLUDES 1 *abdominal distension (gaseous) (R14.-)*
ascites (R18.-)

R19.00 Intra-abdominal and pelvic swelling, mass and lump, unspecified site ▽

R19.01 Right upper quadrant abdominal swelling, mass and lump

R19.02 Left upper quadrant abdominal swelling, mass and lump

R19.03 Right lower quadrant abdominal swelling, mass and lump

R19.04 Left lower quadrant abdominal swelling, mass and lump

R19.05 Periumbilic swelling, mass or lump
Diffuse or generalized umbilical swelling or mass

R19.06 Epigastric swelling, mass or lump

R19.07 Generalized intra-abdominal and pelvic swelling, mass and lump
Diffuse or generalized intra-abdominal swelling or mass NOS
Diffuse or generalized pelvic swelling or mass NOS

R19.09 Other intra-abdominal and pelvic swelling, mass and lump

✓5ᵗʰ **R19.1 Abnormal bowel sounds**
R19.11 Absent bowel sounds
R19.12 Hyperactive bowel sounds
R19.15 Other abnormal bowel sounds
Abnormal bowel sounds NOS

R19.2 Visible peristalsis
Hyperperistalsis
DEF: Visible movements of muscular attempts to move food through the digestive tract; due to pyloric obstruction, stomach obstruction, or intestinal obstruction.

✓5ᵗʰ **R19.3 Abdominal rigidity**
EXCLUDES 1 *abdominal rigidity with severe abdominal pain (R10.0)*
R19.30 Abdominal rigidity, unspecified site ▽
R19.31 Right upper quadrant abdominal rigidity
R19.32 Left upper quadrant abdominal rigidity
R19.33 Right lower quadrant abdominal rigidity
R19.34 Left lower quadrant abdominal rigidity
R19.35 Periumbilic abdominal rigidity
R19.36 Epigastric abdominal rigidity
R19.37 Generalized abdominal rigidity

R19.4 Change in bowel habit
EXCLUDES 1 *constipation (K59.0-)*
functional diarrhea (K59.1)

R19.5 Other fecal abnormalities
Abnormal stool color
Bulky stools
Mucus in stools
Occult blood in feces
Occult blood in stools
EXCLUDES 1 *melena (K92.1)*
neonatal melena (P54.1)

R19.6 Halitosis

R19.7 Diarrhea, unspecified ▽
Diarrhea NOS
EXCLUDES 1 *functional diarrhea (K59.1)*
neonatal diarrhea (P78.3)
psychogenic diarrhea (F45.8)

R19.8 Other specified symptoms and signs involving the digestive system and abdomen

Symptoms and signs involving the skin and subcutaneous tissue (R20-R23)
EXCLUDES 2 *symptoms relating to breast (N64.4-N64.5)*

✓4ᵗʰ **R20 Disturbances of skin sensation**
EXCLUDES 1 *dissociative anesthesia and sensory loss (F44.6)*
psychogenic disturbances (F45.8)
R20.0 Anesthesia of skin
R20.1 Hypoesthesia of skin
R20.2 Paresthesia of skin
Formication
Pins and needles
Tingling skin
EXCLUDES 1 *acroparesthesia (I73.8)*
R20.3 Hyperesthesia
R20.8 Other disturbances of skin sensation
R20.9 Unspecified disturbances of skin sensation ▽

R21 Rash and other nonspecific skin eruption
INCLUDES rash NOS
EXCLUDES 1 *specified type of rash—code to condition*
vesicular eruption (R23.8)

✓4ᵗʰ **R22 Localized swelling, mass and lump of skin and subcutaneous tissue**
INCLUDES subcutaneous nodules (localized)(superficial)
EXCLUDES 1 *abnormal findings on diagnostic imaging (R90-R93)*
edema (R60.-)
enlarged lymph nodes (R59.-)
localized adiposity (E65)
swelling of joint (M25.4-)

R22.0 Localized swelling, mass and lump, head
R22.1 Localized swelling, mass and lump, neck
R22.2 Localized swelling, mass and lump, trunk
EXCLUDES 1 *intra-abdominal or pelvic mass and lump (R19.0-)*
intra-abdominal or pelvic swelling (R19.0-)
EXCLUDES 2 *breast mass and lump (N63)*

✓5ᵗʰ **R22.3 Localized swelling, mass and lump, upper limb**
R22.30 Localized swelling, mass and lump, unspecified upper limb ▽
R22.31 Localized swelling, mass and lump, right upper limb
R22.32 Localized swelling, mass and lump, left upper limb
R22.33 Localized swelling, mass and lump, upper limb, bilateral

✓5ᵗʰ **R22.4 Localized swelling, mass and lump, lower limb**
R22.40 Localized swelling, mass and lump, unspecified lower limb ▽
R22.41 Localized swelling, mass and lump, right lower limb
R22.42 Localized swelling, mass and lump, left lower limb
R22.43 Localized swelling, mass and lump, lower limb, bilateral

R22.9 Localized swelling, mass and lump, unspecified ▽

✓4ᵗʰ **R23 Other skin changes**
R23.0 Cyanosis
EXCLUDES 1 *acrocyanosis (I73.8)*
cyanotic attacks of newborn (P28.2)
DEF: Bluish or purplish discoloration of the skin due to inadequate oxygen level of blood.
R23.1 Pallor
Clammy skin
R23.2 Flushing
Excessive blushing
Code first, if applicable, menopausal and female climacteric states (N95.1)
R23.3 Spontaneous ecchymoses
Petechiae
EXCLUDES 1 *ecchymoses of newborn (P54.5)*
purpura (D69.-)
R23.4 Changes in skin texture
Desquamation of skin
Induration of skin
Scaling of skin
EXCLUDES 1 *epidermal thickening NOS (L85.9)*
R23.8 Other skin changes
R23.9 Unspecified skin changes ▽

EXCLUDES 1 Not coded here   **EXCLUDES 2** Not included here   **N** Newborn Age: 0   **P** Pediatric Age: 0-17   **M** Maternity Age: 12-55   **A** Adult Age: 15-124

Symptoms and signs involving the nervous and musculoskeletal systems (R25-R29)

✓4ᵗʰ R25 Abnormal involuntary movements
> EXCLUDES 1   specific movement disorders (G20-G26)
> stereotyped movement disorders (F98.4)
> tic disorders (F95.-)

R25.0 Abnormal head movements

R25.1 Tremor, unspecified ▽
> EXCLUDES 1   chorea NOS (G25.5)
> essential tremor (G25.0)
> hysterical tremor (F44.4)
> intention tremor (G25.2)

R25.2 Cramp and spasm
> EXCLUDES 2   carpopedal spasm (R29.0)
> charley-horse (M62.831)
> infantile spasms (G40.4-)
> muscle spasm of back (M62.830)
> muscle spasm of calf (M62.831)

R25.3 Fasciculation
> Twitching NOS

R25.8 Other abnormal involuntary movements

R25.9 Unspecified abnormal involuntary movements ▽

✓4ᵗʰ R26 Abnormalities of gait and mobility
> EXCLUDES 1   ataxia NOS (R27.0)
> hereditary ataxia (G11.-)
> locomotor (syphilitic) ataxia (A52.11)
> immobility syndrome (paraplegic) (M62.3)

R26.0 Ataxic gait
> Staggering gait

R26.1 Paralytic gait
> Spastic gait

R26.2 Difficulty in walking, not elsewhere classified
> EXCLUDES 1   falling (R29.6)
> unsteadiness on feet (R26.81)
> AHA: 2016, 2Q, 7

✓5ᵗʰ R26.8 Other abnormalities of gait and mobility
> **R26.81 Unsteadiness on feet**
> **R26.89 Other abnormalities of gait and mobility**

R26.9 Unspecified abnormalities of gait and mobility ▽

✓4ᵗʰ R27 Other lack of coordination
> EXCLUDES 1   ataxic gait (R26.0)
> hereditary ataxia (G11.-)
> vertigo NOS (R42)

R27.0 Ataxia, unspecified ▽
> EXCLUDES 1   ataxia following cerebrovascular disease (I69. with final characters -93)

R27.8 Other lack of coordination

R27.9 Unspecified lack of coordination ▽

✓4ᵗʰ R29 Other symptoms and signs involving the nervous and musculoskeletal systems

R29.0 Tetany
> Carpopedal spasm
> EXCLUDES 1   hysterical tetany (F44.5)
> neonatal tetany (P71.3)
> parathyroid tetany (E20.9)
> post-thyroidectomy tetany (E89.2)

R29.1 Meningismus

R29.2 Abnormal reflex
> EXCLUDES 2   abnormal pupillary reflex (H57.0)
> hyperactive gag reflex (J39.2)
> vasovagal reaction or syncope (R55)

R29.3 Abnormal posture

R29.4 Clicking hip
> EXCLUDES 1   congenital deformities of hip (Q65.-)

R29.5 Transient paralysis
> Code first any associated spinal cord injury (S14.0, S14.1-, S24.0, S24.1-, S34.0-, S34.1-)
> EXCLUDES 1   transient ischemic attack (G45.9)

R29.6 Repeated falls
> Falling
> Tendency to fall
> EXCLUDES 2   at risk for falling (Z91.81)
> history of falling (Z91.81)
> AHA: 2016, 2Q, 6

✓5ᵗʰ R29.7 National Institutes of Health Stroke Scale (NIHSS) Score
> Code first the type of cerebral infarction (I63.-)

✓6ᵗʰ R29.70 NIHSS score 0-9
> R29.700 NIHSS score 0
> R29.701 NIHSS score 1
> R29.702 NIHSS score 2
> R29.703 NIHSS score 3
> R29.704 NIHSS score 4
> R29.705 NIHSS score 5
> R29.706 NIHSS score 6
> R29.707 NIHSS score 7
> R29.708 NIHSS score 8
> R29.709 NIHSS score 9

✓6ᵗʰ R29.71 NIHSS score 10-19
> R29.710 NIHSS score 10
> R29.711 NIHSS score 11
> R29.712 NIHSS score 12
> R29.713 NIHSS score 13
> R29.714 NIHSS score 14
> R29.715 NIHSS score 15
> R29.716 NIHSS score 16
> R29.717 NIHSS score 17
> R29.718 NIHSS score 18
> R29.719 NIHSS score 19

✓6ᵗʰ R29.72 NIHSS score 20-29
> R29.720 NIHSS score 20
> R29.721 NIHSS score 21
> R29.722 NIHSS score 22
> R29.723 NIHSS score 23
> R29.724 NIHSS score 24
> R29.725 NIHSS score 25
> R29.726 NIHSS score 26
> R29.727 NIHSS score 27
> R29.728 NIHSS score 28
> R29.729 NIHSS score 29

✓6ᵗʰ R29.73 NIHSS score 30-39
> R29.730 NIHSS score 30
> R29.731 NIHSS score 31
> R29.732 NIHSS score 32
> R29.733 NIHSS score 33
> R29.734 NIHSS score 34
> R29.735 NIHSS score 35
> R29.736 NIHSS score 36
> R29.737 NIHSS score 37
> R29.738 NIHSS score 38
> R29.739 NIHSS score 39

✓6ᵗʰ R29.74 NIHSS score 40-42
> R29.740 NIHSS score 40
> R29.741 NIHSS score 41
> R29.742 NIHSS score 42

✓5ᵗʰ R29.8 Other symptoms and signs involving the nervous and musculoskeletal systems

✓6ᵗʰ R29.81 Other symptoms and signs involving the nervous system
> **R29.810 Facial weakness**
> Facial droop
> EXCLUDES 1   Bell's palsy (G51.0)
> facial weakness following cerebrovascular disease (I69. with final characters -92)
> **R29.818 Other symptoms and signs involving the nervous system**

✓6ᵗʰ R29.89 Other symptoms and signs involving the musculoskeletal system
> EXCLUDES 2   pain in limb (M79.6-)
> **R29.890 Loss of height**
> EXCLUDES 1   osteoporosis (M80-M81)

R29.891   **Ocular torticollis**
> EXCLUDES 1   congenital (sternomastoid)
> torticollis Q68.0
> psychogenic torticollis (F45.8)
> spasmodic torticollis (G24.3)
> torticollis due to birth injury
> (P15.8)
> torticollis NOS M43.6
>
> **DEF:** Abnormal head posture as a result of a
> contracted state of cervical muscles to
> correct a visual disturbance, either double
> vision or a visual field defect.

R29.898   **Other symptoms and signs involving the
musculoskeletal system**

✓5ᵗʰ **R29.9**   **Unspecified symptoms and signs involving the nervous and
musculoskeletal systems**

R29.90   **Unspecified symptoms and signs involving the
nervous system** ▽

R29.91   **Unspecified symptoms and signs involving the
musculoskeletal system** ▽

Symptoms and signs involving
the genitourinary system (R30-R39)

✓4ᵗʰ **R30**   **Pain associated with micturition**
> EXCLUDES 1   psychogenic pain associated with micturition (F45.8)

R30.0   **Dysuria**
Strangury

R30.1   **Vesical tenesmus**

R30.9   **Painful micturition, unspecified** ▽
Painful urination NOS

✓4ᵗʰ **R31**   **Hematuria**
> EXCLUDES 1   hematuria included with underlying conditions, such as:
> acute cystitis with hematuria (N30.01)
> recurrent and persistent hematuria in glomerular diseases
> (N02.-)
>
> **AHA:** 2017, 1Q, 17

R31.0   **Gross hematuria**

R31.1   **Benign essential microscopic hematuria**

✓5ᵗʰ **R31.2**   **Other microscopic hematuria**

R31.21   **Asymptomatic microscopic hematuria**
AMH

R31.29   **Other microscopic hematuria**

R31.9   **Hematuria, unspecified** ▽

R32   **Unspecified urinary incontinence** ▽
Enuresis NOS
> EXCLUDES 1   functional urinary incontinence (R39.81)
> nonorganic enuresis (F98.0)
> stress incontinence and other specified urinary incontinence
> (N39.3-N39.4-)
> urinary incontinence associated with cognitive impairment
> (R39.81)

✓4ᵗʰ **R33**   **Retention of urine**
> EXCLUDES 1   psychogenic retention of urine (F45.8)

R33.0   **Drug induced retention of urine**
Use additional code for adverse effect, if applicable, to identify
drug (T36-T50 with fifth or sixth character 5)

R33.8   **Other retention of urine**
Code first, if applicable, any causal condition, such as:
enlarged prostate (N40.1)

R33.9   **Retention of urine, unspecified** ▽

R34   **Anuria and oliguria**
> EXCLUDES 1   anuria and oliguria complicating abortion or ectopic or molar
> pregnancy (O00-O07, O08.4)
> anuria and oliguria complicating pregnancy (O26.83-)
> anuria and oliguria complicating the puerperium (O90.4)

✓4ᵗʰ **R35**   **Polyuria**
Code first, if applicable, any causal condition, such as:
enlarged prostate (N40.1)
> EXCLUDES 1   psychogenic polyuria (F45.8)

R35.0   **Frequency of micturition**

R35.1   **Nocturia**

R35.8   **Other polyuria**
Polyuria NOS

✓4ᵗʰ **R36**   **Urethral discharge**

R36.0   **Urethral discharge without blood**

R36.1   **Hematospermia**   ♂

R36.9   **Urethral discharge, unspecified** ♂
Penile discharge NOS
Urethrorrhea

R37   **Sexual dysfunction, unspecified** ▽

✓4ᵗʰ **R39**   **Other and unspecified symptoms and signs involving the
genitourinary system**

R39.0   **Extravasation of urine**

✓5ᵗʰ **R39.1**   **Other difficulties with micturition**
Code first, if applicable, any causal condition, such as:
enlarged prostate (N40.1)

R39.11   **Hesitancy of micturition**

R39.12   **Poor urinary stream**
Weak urinary steam

R39.13   **Splitting of urinary stream**

R39.14   **Feeling of incomplete bladder emptying**

R39.15   **Urgency of urination**
> EXCLUDES 1   urge incontinence (N39.41, N39.46)

R39.16   **Straining to void**

✓6ᵗʰ **R39.19**   **Other difficulties with micturition**

R39.191   **Need to immediately re-void**

R39.192   **Position dependent micturition**

R39.198   **Other difficulties with micturition**

R39.2   **Extrarenal uremia**
Prerenal uremia
> EXCLUDES 1   uremia NOS (N19)

✓5ᵗʰ **R39.8**   **Other symptoms and signs involving the genitourinary
system**

R39.81   **Functional urinary incontinence**
Urinary incontinence due to cognitive impairment, or
severe physical disability or immobility
> EXCLUDES 1   stress incontinence and other specified
> urinary incontinence (N39.3-N39.4-)
> urinary incontinence NOS (R32)

R39.82   **Chronic bladder pain**

●   R39.83   **Unilateral non-palpable testicle**

●   R39.84   **Bilateral non-palpable testicles**

R39.89   **Other symptoms and signs involving the
genitourinary system**

R39.9   **Unspecified symptoms and signs involving the
genitourinary system** ▽

Symptoms and signs involving cognition, perception,
emotional state and behavior (R40-R46)

> EXCLUDES 2   symptoms and signs constituting part of a pattern of mental disorder
> (F01-F99)

✓4ᵗʰ **R40**   **Somnolence, stupor and coma**
> EXCLUDES 1   neonatal coma (P91.5)
> somnolence, stupor and coma in diabetes (E08-E13)
> somnolence, stupor and coma in hepatic failure (K72.-)
> somnolence, stupor and coma in hypoglycemia (nondiabetic)
> (E15)

R40.0   **Somnolence**
Drowsiness
> EXCLUDES 1   coma (R40.2-)

R40.1   **Stupor**
Catatonic stupor
Semicoma
> EXCLUDES 1   catatonic schizophrenia (F20.2)
> coma (R40.2-)
> depressive stupor (F31-F33)
> dissociative stupor (F44.2)
> manic stupor (F30.2)

✓5ᵗʰ **R40.2**   **Coma**
Code first any associated:
fracture of skull (S02.-)
intracranial injury (S06.-)
> **NOTE**   One code from each subcategory, R40.21-R40.23, is
> required to complete the coma scale
>
> **AHA:** 2015, 2Q, 17; 2014, 1Q, 19

R40.20   **Unspecified coma**   HCC ▽
Coma NOS
Unconsciousness NOS

EXCLUDES 1 Not coded here   EXCLUDES 2 Not included here   N Newborn Age: 0   P Pediatric Age: 0-17   M Maternity Age: 12-55   A Adult Age: 15-124

894   ICD-10-CM 2018

√6ᵗʰ **R40.21 Coma scale, eyes open**

> The following appropriate 7th character is to be added to subcategories R40.21-, R40.22-, R40.23-, and R40.24-.
> 0   unspecified time
> 1   in the field [EMT or ambulance]
> 2   at arrival to emergency department
> 3   at hospital admission
> 4   24 hours or more after hospital admission

√7ᵗʰ **R40.211 Coma scale, eyes open, never** HCC

√7ᵗʰ **R40.212 Coma scale, eyes open, to pain** HCC

√7ᵗʰ **R40.213 Coma scale, eyes open, to sound**

√7ᵗʰ **R40.214 Coma scale, eyes open, spontaneous**

√6ᵗʰ **R40.22 Coma scale, best verbal response**

√7ᵗʰ **R40.221 Coma scale, best verbal response, none** HCC

√7ᵗʰ **R40.222 Coma scale, best verbal response, incomprehensible words** HCC
> ►Incomprehensible sounds (2-5 years of age)
> Moans/grunts to pain; restless (< 2 years old)◄

√7ᵗʰ **R40.223 Coma scale, best verbal response, inappropriate words**
> ►Inappropriate crying or screaming (< 2 years of age)
> Screaming (2-5 years of age)◄

√7ᵗʰ **R40.224 Coma scale, best verbal response, confused conversation**
> ►Inappropriate words (2-5 years of age)
> Irritable cries (< 2 years of age)◄

√7ᵗʰ **R40.225 Coma scale, best verbal response, oriented**
> ►Cooing or babbling or crying appropriately (< 2 years of age)
> Uses appropriate words (2- 5 years of age)◄

√6ᵗʰ **R40.23 Coma scale, best motor response**

√7ᵗʰ **R40.231 Coma scale, best motor response, none** HCC

√7ᵗʰ **R40.232 Coma scale, best motor response, extension** HCC
> ►Abnormal extensor posturing to pain or noxious stimuli (< 2 years of age)
> Extensor posturing to pain or noxious stimuli (2-5 years of age)◄

√7ᵗʰ **R40.233 Coma scale, best motor response, abnormal**
> ►Abnormal flexure posturing to pain or noxious stimuli (0-5 years of age)
> Flexion/decorticate posturing (< 2 years of age)◄

√7ᵗʰ **R40.234 Coma scale, best motor response, flexion withdrawal** HCC
> ►Withdraws from pain or noxious stimuli (0-5 years of age)◄

√7ᵗʰ **R40.235 Coma scale, best motor response, localizes pain**
> ►Localizes pain (2-5 years of age)
> Withdraws to touch (< 2 years of age)◄

√7ᵗʰ **R40.236 Coma scale, best motor response, obeys commands**
> ►Normal or spontaneous movement (< 2 years of age)
> Obeys commands (2-5 years of age)◄

√6ᵗʰ **R40.24 Glasgow coma scale, total score**
> NOTE Assign a code from subcategory R40.24, when only the total coma score is documented

√7ᵗʰ **R40.241 Glasgow coma scale score 13-15**

√7ᵗʰ **R40.242 Glasgow coma scale score 9-12**

√7ᵗʰ **R40.243 Glasgow coma scale score 3-8** HCC

√7ᵗʰ **R40.244 Other coma, without documented Glasgow coma scale score, or with partial score reported** HCC

R40.3 Persistent vegetative state HCC
> DEF: Persistent wakefulness without consciousness due to nonfunctioning cerebral cortex.

R40.4 Transient alteration of awareness

√4ᵗʰ **R41 Other symptoms and signs involving cognitive functions and awareness**
> EXCLUDES 1 dissociative [conversion] disorders (F44.-)
> mild cognitive impairment, so stated (G31.84)

R41.0 Disorientation, unspecified ▽
> Confusion NOS
> Delirium NOS

R41.1 Anterograde amnesia

R41.2 Retrograde amnesia

R41.3 Other amnesia
> Amnesia NOS
> Memory loss NOS
> EXCLUDES 1 amnestic disorder due to known physiologic condition (F04)
> amnestic syndrome due to psychoactive substance use (F10-F19 with 5th character .6)
> mild memory disturbance due to known physiological condition (F06.8)
> transient global amnesia (G45.4)

R41.4 Neurologic neglect syndrome
> Asomatognosia
> Hemi-akinesia
> Hemi-inattention
> Hemispatial neglect
> Left-sided neglect
> Sensory neglect
> Visuospatial neglect
> EXCLUDES 1 visuospatial deficit (R41.842)

√5ᵗʰ **R41.8 Other symptoms and signs involving cognitive functions and awareness**

R41.81 Age-related cognitive decline A
> Senility NOS

R41.82 Altered mental status, unspecified ▽
> Change in mental status NOS
> EXCLUDES 1 altered level of consciousness (R40.-)
> altered mental status due to known condition—code to condition
> delirium NOS (R41.0)
> AHA: 2012, 4Q, 97

R41.83 Borderline intellectual functioning
> IQ level 71 to 84
> EXCLUDES 1 intellectual disabilities (F70-F79)

√6ᵗʰ **R41.84 Other specified cognitive deficit**
> EXCLUDES 1 cognitive deficits as sequelae of cerebrovascular disease (I69.01-, I69.11-, I69.21-, I69.31-, I69.81-, I69.91-)

R41.840 Attention and concentration deficit
> EXCLUDES 1 attention-deficit hyperactivity disorders (F90.-)

R41.841 Cognitive communication deficit

R41.842 Visuospatial deficit

R41.843 Psychomotor deficit

R41.844 Frontal lobe and executive function deficit

R41.89 Other symptoms and signs involving cognitive functions and awareness
> Anosognosia

R41.9 Unspecified symptoms and signs involving cognitive functions and awareness ▽
> ►Unspecified neurocognitive disorder◄

R42 Dizziness and giddiness
> Light-headedness
> Vertigo NOS
> EXCLUDES 1 vertiginous syndromes (H81.-)
> vertigo from infrasound (T75.23)

√4ᵗʰ **R43 Disturbances of smell and taste**

R43.0 Anosmia

R43.1 Parosmia

R43.2 Parageusia

R43.8 Other disturbances of smell and taste
> Mixed disturbance of smell and taste

R43.9 Unspecified disturbances of smell and taste ▽

✓4ᵗʰ **R44 Other symptoms and signs involving general sensations and perceptions**
    EXCLUDES 1   *alcoholic hallucinations (F1.5)*
      hallucinations in drug psychosis (F11-F19 with .5)
      hallucinations in mood disorders with psychotic symptoms (F30.2, F31.5, F32.3, F33.3)
      hallucinations in schizophrenia, schizotypal and delusional disorders (F20-F29)
    EXCLUDES 2   *disturbances of skin sensation (R20.-)*

   R44.0 Auditory hallucinations

   R44.1 Visual hallucinations

   R44.2 Other hallucinations

   R44.3 Hallucinations, unspecified ▽

   R44.8 Other symptoms and signs involving general sensations and perceptions

   R44.9 Unspecified symptoms and signs involving general sensations and perceptions ▽

✓4ᵗʰ **R45 Symptoms and signs involving emotional state**

   R45.0 Nervousness
      Nervous tension

   R45.1 Restlessness and agitation

   R45.2 Unhappiness

   R45.3 Demoralization and apathy
      EXCLUDES 1   *anhedonia (R45.84)*

   R45.4 Irritability and anger

   R45.5 Hostility

   R45.6 Violent behavior

   R45.7 State of emotional shock and stress, unspecified ▽

 ✓5ᵗʰ **R45.8 Other symptoms and signs involving emotional state**

     R45.81 Low self-esteem

     R45.82 Worries

     R45.83 Excessive crying of child, adolescent or adult
        EXCLUDES 1   *excessive crying of infant (baby) R68.11*

     R45.84 Anhedonia

    ✓6ᵗʰ **R45.85 Homicidal and suicidal ideations**
        EXCLUDES 1   *suicide attempt (T14.91)*

       R45.850 Homicidal ideations

       R45.851 Suicidal ideations
         DEF: Thoughts of committing suicide; no actual attempt of suicide has been made.

     R45.86 Emotional lability

     R45.87 Impulsiveness

     R45.89 Other symptoms and signs involving emotional state

✓4ᵗʰ **R46 Symptoms and signs involving appearance and behavior**
    EXCLUDES 1   *appearance and behavior in schizophrenia, schizotypal and delusional disorders (F20-F29)*
      mental and behavioral disorders (F01-F99)

   R46.0 Very low level of personal hygiene

   R46.1 Bizarre personal appearance

   R46.2 Strange and inexplicable behavior

   R46.3 Overactivity

   R46.4 Slowness and poor responsiveness
      EXCLUDES 1   *stupor (R40.1)*

   R46.5 Suspiciousness and marked evasiveness

   R46.6 Undue concern and preoccupation with stressful events

   R46.7 Verbosity and circumstantial detail obscuring reason for contact

 ✓5ᵗʰ **R46.8 Other symptoms and signs involving appearance and behavior**

     R46.81 Obsessive-compulsive behavior
        EXCLUDES 1   *obsessive-compulsive disorder (F42-)*

     R46.89 Other symptoms and signs involving appearance and behavior

Symptoms and signs involving speech and voice (R47-R49)

✓4ᵗʰ **R47 Speech disturbances, not elsewhere classified**
    EXCLUDES 1   *autism (F84.0)*
      cluttering (F80.81)
      specific developmental disorders of speech and language (F80.-)
      stuttering (F80.81)

 ✓5ᵗʰ **R47.0 Dysphasia and aphasia**

     R47.01 Aphasia
        EXCLUDES 1   *aphasia following cerebrovascular disease (I69. with final characters -20)*
         progressive isolated aphasia (G31.01)

     R47.02 Dysphasia
        EXCLUDES 1   *dysphasia following cerebrovascular disease (I69. with final characters -21)*

   R47.1 Dysarthria and anarthria
      EXCLUDES 1   *dysarthria following cerebrovascular disease (I69. with final characters -22)*

 ✓5ᵗʰ **R47.8 Other speech disturbances**
      EXCLUDES 1   *dysarthria following cerebrovascular disease (I69. with final characters -28)*

     R47.81 Slurred speech

     R47.82 *Fluency disorder in conditions classified elsewhere*
        Stuttering in conditions classified elsewhere
        Code first underlying disease or condition, such as:
        Parkinson's disease (G20)
        EXCLUDES 1   *adult onset fluency disorder (F98.5)*
         childhood onset fluency disorder (F80.81)
         fluency disorder (stuttering) following cerebrovascular disease (I69. with final characters-23)

     R47.89 Other speech disturbances

   R47.9 Unspecified speech disturbances ▽

✓4ᵗʰ **R48 Dyslexia and other symbolic dysfunctions, not elsewhere classified**
    EXCLUDES 1   *specific developmental disorders of scholastic skills (F81.-)*

   R48.0 Dyslexia and alexia

   R48.1 Agnosia
      Astereognosia (astereognosis)
      Autotopagnosia
      EXCLUDES 1   *visual object agnosia (R48.3)*

   R48.2 Apraxia
      EXCLUDES 1   *apraxia following cerebrovascular disease (I69. with final characters -90)*

   R48.3 Visual agnosia
      Prosopagnosia
      Simultanagnosia (asimultagnosia)

   R48.8 Other symbolic dysfunctions
      Acalculia
      Agraphia
      AHA: 2017, 1Q, 27

   R48.9 Unspecified symbolic dysfunctions ▽

✓4ᵗʰ **R49 Voice and resonance disorders**
    EXCLUDES 1   *psychogenic voice and resonance disorders (F44.4)*

   R49.0 Dysphonia
      Hoarseness

   R49.1 Aphonia
      Loss of voice

 ✓5ᵗʰ **R49.2 Hypernasality and hyponasality**

     R49.21 Hypernasality

     R49.22 Hyponasality

   R49.8 Other voice and resonance disorders

   R49.9 Unspecified voice and resonance disorder ▽
      Change in voice NOS
      Resonance disorder NOS

EXCLUDES 1 Not coded here   EXCLUDES 2 Not included here   N Newborn Age: 0   P Pediatric Age: 0-17   M Maternity Age: 12-55   A Adult Age: 15-124

896   ICD-10-CM 2018

R44–R49.9

General symptoms and signs (R50-R69)

✓4ᵗʰ **R50 Fever of other and unknown origin**
  EXCLUDES 1 *chills without fever (R68.83)*
         febrile convulsions (R56.0-)
         fever of unknown origin during labor (O75.2)
         fever of unknown origin in newborn (P81.9)
         hypothermia due to illness (R68.0)
         malignant hyperthermia due to anesthesia (T88.3)
         puerperal pyrexia NOS (O86.4)

  R50.2 Drug induced fever
        Use additional code for adverse effect, if applicable, to identify
          drug (T36-T50 with fifth or sixth character 5)
        EXCLUDES 1 *postvaccination (postimmunization) fever (R50.83)*

  ✓5ᵗʰ **R50.8 Other specified fever**
       R50.81 Fever presenting with conditions classified elsewhere
              Code first underlying condition when associated fever
                is present, such as with:
                leukemia (C91-C95)
                neutropenia (D70.-)
                sickle-cell disease (D57.-)
              AHA: 2014, 4Q, 22

       R50.82 Postprocedural fever
              EXCLUDES 1 *postprocedural infection (T81.4-)*
                     posttransfusion fever (R50.84)
                     *postvaccination (postimmunization) fever
                       (R50.83)*

       R50.83 Postvaccination fever
              Postimmunization fever

       R50.84 Febrile nonhemolytic transfusion reaction
              FNHTR
              Posttransfusion fever

  R50.9 Fever, unspecified   ▽
        Fever NOS
        Fever of unknown origin [FUO]
        Fever with chills
        Fever with rigors
        Hyperpyrexia NOS
        Persistent fever
        Pyrexia NOS

R51 Headache
     Facial pain NOS
     EXCLUDES 1 *atypical face pain (G50.1)*
            migraine and other headache syndromes (G43-G44)
            trigeminal neuralgia (G50.0)

R52 Pain, unspecified   ▽
     Acute pain NOS
     Generalized pain NOS
     Pain NOS
     EXCLUDES 1 *acute and chronic pain, not elsewhere classified (G89.-)*
            localized pain, unspecified type—code to pain by site, such as:
              abdomen pain (R10.-)
              back pain (M54.9)
              breast pain (N64.4)
              chest pain (R07.1-R07.9)
              ear pain (H92.0-)
              eye pain (H57.1)
              headache (R51)
              joint pain (M25.5-)
              limb pain (M79.6-)
              lumbar region pain (M54.5)
              pelvic and perineal pain (R10.2)
              renal colic (N23)
              shoulder pain (M25.51-)
              spine pain (M54.-)
              throat pain (R07.0)
              tongue pain (K14.6)
              tooth pain (K08.8)
            *pain disorders exclusively related to psychological factors
              (F45.41)*

✓4ᵗʰ **R53 Malaise and fatigue**
  R53.0 Neoplastic (malignant) related fatigue
        Code first associated neoplasm

  R53.1 Weakness
        Asthenia NOS
        EXCLUDES 1 *age-related weakness (R54)*
               muscle weakness (M62.8-)
               sarcopenia (M62.84)
               senile asthenia (R54)
        AHA: 2017, 1Q, 7; 2015, 1Q, 25

R53.2 Functional quadriplegia   HCC
      Complete immobility due to severe physical disability or frailty
      EXCLUDES 1 *frailty NOS (R54)*
             hysterical paralysis (F44.4)
             immobility syndrome (M62.3)
             neurologic quadriplegia (G82.5-)
             quadriplegia (G82.50)
AHA: 2016, 2Q, 6
DEF: Inability to move due to a nonphysiological condition, such
as dementia; no mental ability to move independently; typically
found in severely demented patients.

✓5ᵗʰ **R53.8 Other malaise and fatigue**
       EXCLUDES 1 *combat exhaustion and fatigue (F43.0)*
              congenital debility (P96.9)
              ~~*exhaustion and fatigue due to depressive episode (F32.-)*~~
              *exhaustion and fatigue due to excessive exertion
                (T73.3)*
              exhaustion and fatigue due to exposure (T73.2)
              exhaustion and fatigue due to heat (T67.-)
              exhaustion and fatigue due to pregnancy (O26.8-)
              *exhaustion and fatigue due to recurrent depressive
                episode (F33)*
              exhaustion and fatigue due to senile debility (R54)

       R53.81 Other malaise
              Chronic debility
              Debility NOS
              General physical deterioration
              Malaise NOS
              Nervous debility
              EXCLUDES 1 *age-related physical debility (R54)*

       R53.82 Chronic fatigue, unspecified   ▽
              Chronic fatigue syndrome NOS
              EXCLUDES 1 *postviral fatigue syndrome (G93.3)*

       R53.83 Other fatigue
              Fatigue NOS
              Lack of energy
              Lethargy
              Tiredness
              EXCLUDES 2 ▶*exhaustion and fatigue due to depressive
                episode (F32.-)*◀

R54 Age-related physical debility   ▲
     Frailty
     Old age
     Senescence
     Senile asthenia
     Senile debility
     EXCLUDES 1 *age-related cognitive decline (R41.81)*
            sarcopenia (M62.84)
            senile psychosis (F03)
            senility NOS (R41.81)

R55 Syncope and collapse
     Blackout
     Fainting
     Vasovagal attack
     EXCLUDES 1 *cardiogenic shock (R57.0)*
            carotid sinus syncope (G90.01)
            heat syncope (T67.1)
            neurocirculatory asthenia (F45.8)
            neurogenic orthostatic hypotension (G90.3)
            orthostatic hypotension (I95.1)
            postprocedural shock (T81.1-)
            psychogenic syncope (F48.8)
            shock NOS (R57.9)
            *shock complicating or following abortion or ectopic or molar
              pregnancy (O00-O07, O08.3)*
            shock complicating or following labor and delivery (O75.1)
            Stokes-Adams attack (I45.9)
            unconsciousness NOS (R40.2-)

✓4ᵗʰ **R56 Convulsions, not elsewhere classified**
       EXCLUDES 1 *dissociative convulsions and seizures (F44.5)*
              epileptic convulsions and seizures (G40.-)
              newborn convulsions and seizures (P90)

  ✓5ᵗʰ **R56.0 Febrile convulsions**

       R56.00 Simple febrile convulsions   HCC
              Febrile convulsion NOS
              Febrile seizure NOS

       R56.01 Complex febrile convulsions   HCC
              Atypical febrile seizure
              Complex febrile seizure
              Complicated febrile seizure
              EXCLUDES 1 *status epilepticus (G40.901)*

R56.1 Post traumatic seizures   HCC
    EXCLUDES 1 *post traumatic epilepsy (G40.-)*

R56.9 Unspecified convulsions   HCC ▽
    Convulsion disorder
    Fit NOS
    Recurrent convulsions
    Seizure(s) (convulsive) NOS

✓4ᵗʰ **R57 Shock, not elsewhere classified**
    EXCLUDES 1 *anaphylactic shock NOS (T78.2)*
      anaphylactic reaction or shock due to adverse food reaction
        (T78.0-)
      anaphylactic shock due to adverse effect of correct drug or
        medicament properly administered (T88.6)
      anaphylactic shock due to serum (T80.5-)
      anesthetic shock (T88.3)
      electric shock (T75.4)
      obstetric shock (O75.1)
      postprocedural shock (T81.1-)
      psychic shock (F43.0)
      ~~*septic shock (R65.21)*~~
      shock complicating or following ectopic or molar pregnancy
        (O00-O07, O08.3)
      shock due to lightning (T75.01)
      traumatic shock (T79.4)
      toxic shock syndrome (A48.3)

  R57.0 Cardiogenic shock   HCC
      EXCLUDES 2 ▶*septic shock (R65.21)*◀
      DEF: Associated with myocardial infarction, cardiac tamponade,
      and massive pulmonary embolism; symptoms include mental
      confusion, reduced blood pressure, tachycardia, pallor, and cold,
      clammy skin.

  R57.1 Hypovolemic shock   HCC

  R57.8 Other shock   HCC

  R57.9 Shock, unspecified   HCC ▽
      Failure of peripheral circulation NOS

R58 Hemorrhage, not elsewhere classified
    Hemorrhage NOS
    EXCLUDES 1 *hemorrhage included with underlying conditions, such as:*
      acute duodenal ulcer with hemorrhage (K26.0)
      acute gastritis with bleeding (K29.01)
      ulcerative enterocolitis with rectal bleeding (K51.01)

✓4ᵗʰ **R59 Enlarged lymph nodes**
    INCLUDES swollen glands
    EXCLUDES 1 *acute lymphadenitis (L04.-)*
      chronic lymphadenitis (I88.1)
      lymphadenitis NOS (I88.9)
      mesenteric (acute) (chronic) lymphadenitis (I88.0)

  R59.0 Localized enlarged lymph nodes

  R59.1 Generalized enlarged lymph nodes
      Lymphadenopathy NOS

  R59.9 Enlarged lymph nodes, unspecified   ▽

✓4ᵗʰ **R60 Edema, not elsewhere classified**
    EXCLUDES 1 *angioneurotic edema (T78.3)*
      ascites (R18.-)
      cerebral edema (G93.6)
      cerebral edema due to birth injury (P11.0)
      edema of larynx (J38.4)
      edema of nasopharynx (J39.2)
      edema of pharynx (J39.2)
      gestational edema (O12.0-)
      hereditary edema (Q82.0)
      hydrops fetalis NOS (P83.2)
      hydrothorax (J94.8)
      ~~*nutritional edema (E40-E46)*~~
      hydrops fetalis NOS (P83.2)
      newborn edema (P83.3)
      pulmonary edema (J81.-)

  R60.0 Localized edema

  R60.1 Generalized edema
      EXCLUDES 2 ▶*nutritional edema (E40-E46)*◀

  R60.9 Edema, unspecified   ▽
      Fluid retention NOS

R61 Generalized hyperhidrosis
    Excessive sweating
    Night sweats
    Secondary hyperhidrosis
    Code first, if applicable, menopausal and female climacteric states
      (N95.1)
    EXCLUDES 1 *focal (primary) (secondary) hyperhidrosis (L74.5-)*
      Frey's syndrome (L74.52)
      localized (primary) (secondary) hyperhidrosis (L74.5-)

✓4ᵗʰ **R62 Lack of expected normal physiological development in childhood and adults**
    EXCLUDES 1 *delayed puberty (E30.0)*
      gonadal dysgenesis (Q99.1)
      hypopituitarism (E23.0)

  R62.0 Delayed milestone in childhood   P
      Delayed attainment of expected physiological developmental
        stage
      Late talker
      Late walker

✓5ᵗʰ **R62.5 Other and unspecified lack of expected normal physiological development in childhood**
      EXCLUDES 1 *HIV disease resulting in failure to thrive (B20)*
        physical retardation due to malnutrition (E45)

    R62.50 Unspecified lack of expected normal   ▽
        physiological development in childhood
        Infantilism NOS

    R62.51 Failure to thrive (child)   P
        Failure to gain weight
        EXCLUDES 1 *failure to thrive in child under 28 days old*
          (P92.6)
        DEF: Organic failure to thrive (FTT): Acute or chronic
        illness that interferes with nutritional intake, absorption,
        metabolism excretion, and energy requirements;
        nonorganic FTT is a symptom of neglect or abuse.

    R62.52 Short stature (child)
        Lack of growth
        Physical retardation
        Short stature NOS
        EXCLUDES 1 *short stature due to endocrine disorder*
          (E34.3)

    R62.59 Other lack of expected normal physiological development in childhood

  R62.7 Adult failure to thrive   A

✓4ᵗʰ **R63 Symptoms and signs concerning food and fluid intake**
    EXCLUDES 1 *bulimia NOS (F50.2)*
      eating disorders of nonorganic origin (F50.-)
      malnutrition (E40-E46)

  R63.0 Anorexia
      Loss of appetite
      EXCLUDES 1 *anorexia nervosa (F50.0-)*
        loss of appetite of nonorganic origin (F50.89)

  R63.1 Polydipsia
      Excessive thirst

  R63.2 Polyphagia
      Excessive eating
      Hyperalimentation NOS

  R63.3 Feeding difficulties
      Feeding problem (elderly) (infant) NOS
      ▶Picky eater◀
      EXCLUDES 1 ▶*eating disorders (F50.-)*◀
        feeding problems of newborn (P92.-)
        infant feeding disorder of nonorganic origin (F98.2-)
      AHA: 2017, 1Q, 28; 2016, 3Q, 19

  R63.4 Abnormal weight loss

  R63.5 Abnormal weight gain
      EXCLUDES 1 *excessive weight gain in pregnancy (O26.0-)*
        obesity (E66.-)

  R63.6 Underweight
      Use additional code to identify body mass index (BMI), if known
        (Z68.-)
      EXCLUDES 1 *abnormal weight loss (R63.4)*
        anorexia nervosa (F50.0-)
        malnutrition (E40-E46)

  R63.8 Other symptoms and signs concerning food and fluid intake

R64 Cachexia   HCC
    Wasting syndrome
    Code first underlying condition, if known
    EXCLUDES 1 *abnormal weight loss (R63.4)*
      nutritional marasmus (E41)

☑4ᵗʰ **R65 Symptoms and signs specifically associated with systemic inflammation and infection**

☑5ᵗʰ **R65.1 Systemic inflammatory response syndrome [SIRS] of non-infectious origin**
 Code first underlying condition, such as:
  heatstroke (T67.Ø)
  injury and trauma (SØØ-T88)
  EXCLUDES 1 sepsis—code to infection
   severe sepsis (R65.2)

 R65.1Ø Systemic inflammatory response syndrome [SIRS] of non-infectious origin without acute organ dysfunction HCC
  Systemic inflammatory response syndrome (SIRS) NOS

 R65.11 Systemic inflammatory response syndrome [SIRS] of non-infectious origin with acute organ dysfunction HCC
  Use additional code to identify specific acute organ dysfunction, such as:
   acute kidney failure (N17.-)
   acute respiratory failure (J96.Ø-)
   critical illness myopathy (G72.81)
   critical illness polyneuropathy (G62.81)
   disseminated intravascular coagulopathy [DIC] (D65)
   encephalopathy (metabolic) (septic) (G93.41)
   hepatic failure (K72.Ø-)

☑5ᵗʰ **R65.2 Severe sepsis**
 Infection with associated acute organ dysfunction
 Sepsis with acute organ dysfunction
 Sepsis with multiple organ dysfunction
 Systemic inflammatory response syndrome due to infectious process with acute organ dysfunction
 Code first underlying infection, such as:
  infection following a procedure (T81.4-)
  infections following infusion, transfusion and therapeutic injection (T8Ø.2-)
  puerperal sepsis (O85)
  sepsis following complete or unspecified spontaneous abortion (OØ3.87)
  sepsis following ectopic and molar pregnancy (OØ8.82)
  sepsis following incomplete spontaneous abortion (OØ3.37)
  sepsis following (induced) termination of pregnancy (OØ4.87)
  sepsis NOS (A41.9)
 Use additional code to identify specific acute organ dysfunction, such as:
  acute kidney failure (N17.-)
  acute respiratory failure (J96.Ø-)
  critical illness myopathy (G72.81)
  critical illness polyneuropathy (G62.81)
  disseminated intravascular coagulopathy [DIC] (D65)
  encephalopathy (metabolic) (septic) (G93.41)
  hepatic failure (K72.Ø-)
 AHA: 2016, 3Q, 8

 R65.2Ø Severe sepsis without septic shock HCC
  Severe sepsis NOS
  AHA: 2016, 3Q, 14; 2013, 4Q, 119

 R65.21 Severe sepsis with septic shock HCC

☑4ᵗʰ **R68 Other general symptoms and signs**

 R68.Ø Hypothermia, not associated with low environmental temperature
  EXCLUDES 1 hypothermia NOS (accidental) (T68)
   hypothermia due to anesthesia (T88.51)
   hypothermia due to low environmental temperature (T68)
   newborn hypothermia (P8Ø.-)

☑5ᵗʰ **R68.1 Nonspecific symptoms peculiar to infancy**
  EXCLUDES 1 colic, infantile (R1Ø.83)
   neonatal cerebral irritability (P91.3)
   teething syndrome (KØØ.7)

 R68.11 Excessive crying of infant (baby) P
  EXCLUDES 1 excessive crying of child, adolescent, or adult (R45.83)

 R68.12 Fussy infant (baby) P
  Irritable infant

 R68.13 Apparent life threatening event in infant (ALTE) P
  Apparent life threatening event in newborn
  ►Brief resolved unexplained event (BRUE)◄
  Code first confirmed diagnosis, if known
  Use additional code(s) for associated signs and symptoms if no confirmed diagnosis established, or if signs and symptoms are not associated routinely with confirmed diagnosis, or provide additional information for cause of ALTE

 R68.19 Other nonspecific symptoms peculiar to infancy P

 R68.2 Dry mouth, unspecified ▽
  EXCLUDES 1 dry mouth due to dehydration (E86.Ø)
   dry mouth due to sicca syndrome [Sjögren] (M35.Ø-)
   salivary gland hyposecretion (K11.7)

 R68.3 Clubbing of fingers
  Clubbing of nails
  DEF: Enlarged soft tissue of distal fingers; usually occurs in heart and lung diseases.
  EXCLUDES 1 congenital clubfinger (Q68.1)

☑5ᵗʰ **R68.8 Other general symptoms and signs**
 R68.81 Early satiety
  DEF: The premature feeling of being full after eating only a small amount of food; mechanism of satiety is multifactorial.

 R68.82 Decreased libido A
  Decreased sexual desire

 R68.83 Chills (without fever)
  Chills NOS
  EXCLUDES 1 chills with fever (R5Ø.9)

 R68.84 Jaw pain
  Mandibular pain
  Maxilla pain
  EXCLUDES 1 temporomandibular joint arthralgia (M26.62-)

 R68.89 Other general symptoms and signs

R69 Illness, unspecified ▽
 Unknown and unspecified cases of morbidity

Abnormal findings on examination of blood, without diagnosis (R7Ø-R79)

 EXCLUDES 2 abnormal findings on antenatal screening of mother (O28.-)
  abnormalities of lipids (E78.-)
  abnormalities of platelets and thrombocytes (D69.-)
  abnormalities of white blood cells classified elsewhere (D7Ø-D72)
  coagulation hemorrhagic disorders (D65-D68)
  diagnostic abnormal findings classified elsewhere—see Alphabetical Index
  hemorrhagic and hematological disorders of newborn (P5Ø-P61)

☑4ᵗʰ **R7Ø Elevated erythrocyte sedimentation rate and abnormality of plasma viscosity**
 R7Ø.Ø Elevated erythrocyte sedimentation rate
 R7Ø.1 Abnormal plasma viscosity

☑4ᵗʰ **R71 Abnormality of red blood cells**
 EXCLUDES 1 anemias (D5Ø-D64)
  anemia of premature infant (P61.2)
  benign (familial) polycythemia (D75.Ø)
  congenital anemias (P61.2-P61.4)
  newborn anemia due to isoimmunization (P55.-)
  polycythemia neonatorum (P61.1)
  polycythemia NOS (D75.1)
  polycythemia vera (D45)
  secondary polycythemia (D75.1)

 R71.Ø Precipitous drop in hematocrit
  Drop (precipitous) in hemoglobin
  Drop in hematocrit

 R71.8 Other abnormality of red blood cells
  Abnormal red-cell morphology NOS
  Abnormal red-cell volume NOS
  Anisocytosis
  Poikilocytosis

✓4th **R73 Elevated blood glucose level**
> *EXCLUDES 1*   *diabetes mellitus (E08-E13)*
> *diabetes mellitus in pregnancy, childbirth and the puerperium (O24.-)*
> *neonatal disorders (P70.0-P70.2)*
> *postsurgical hypoinsulinemia (E89.1)*

✓5th **R73.0 Abnormal glucose**
> *EXCLUDES 1*   *abnormal glucose in pregnancy (O99.81-)*
> *diabetes mellitus (E08-E13)*
> *dysmetabolic syndrome X (E88.81)*
> *gestational diabetes (O24.4-)*
> *glycosuria (R81)*
> *hypoglycemia (E16.2)*

R73.01 Impaired fasting glucose
Elevated fasting glucose

R73.02 Impaired glucose tolerance (oral)
Elevated glucose tolerance

R73.03 Prediabetes
Latent diabetes

R73.09 Other abnormal glucose
Abnormal glucose NOS
Abnormal non-fasting glucose tolerance

R73.9 Hyperglycemia, unspecified ▽

✓4th **R74 Abnormal serum enzyme levels**

R74.0 Nonspecific elevation of levels of transaminase and lactic acid dehydrogenase [LDH]

R74.8 Abnormal levels of other serum enzymes
Abnormal level of acid phosphatase
Abnormal level of alkaline phosphatase
Abnormal level of amylase
Abnormal level of lipase [triacylglycerol lipase]

R74.9 Abnormal serum enzyme level, unspecified ▽

R75 Inconclusive laboratory evidence of human immunodeficiency virus [HIV]
Nonconclusive HIV-test finding in infants
> *EXCLUDES 1*   *asymptomatic human immunodeficiency virus [HIV] infection status (Z21)*
> *human immunodeficiency virus [HIV] disease (B20)*

✓4th **R76 Other abnormal immunological findings in serum**

R76.0 Raised antibody titer
> *EXCLUDES 1*   *isoimmunization in pregnancy (O36.0-O36.1)*
> *isoimmunization affecting newborn (P55.-)*

✓5th **R76.1 Nonspecific reaction to test for tuberculosis**

R76.11 Nonspecific reaction to tuberculin skin test without active tuberculosis
Abnormal result of Mantoux test
PPD positive
Tuberculin (skin test) positive
Tuberculin (skin test) reactor
> *EXCLUDES 1*   *nonspecific reaction to cell mediated immunity measurement of gamma interferon antigen response without active tuberculosis (R76.12)*

R76.12 Nonspecific reaction to cell mediated immunity measurement of gamma interferon antigen response without active tuberculosis
Nonspecific reaction to QuantiFERON-TB test (QFT) without active tuberculosis
> *EXCLUDES 1*   *nonspecific reaction to tuberculin skin test without active tuberculosis (R76.11)*
> *positive tuberculin skin test (R76.11)*

R76.8 Other specified abnormal immunological findings in serum
Raised level of immunoglobulins NOS

R76.9 Abnormal immunological finding in serum, unspecified ▽

✓4th **R77 Other abnormalities of plasma proteins**
> *EXCLUDES 1*   *disorders of plasma-protein metabolism (E88.0)*

R77.0 Abnormality of albumin

R77.1 Abnormality of globulin
Hyperglobulinemia NOS

R77.2 Abnormality of alphafetoprotein

R77.8 Other specified abnormalities of plasma proteins

R77.9 Abnormality of plasma protein, unspecified ▽

✓4th **R78 Findings of drugs and other substances, not normally found in blood**
Use additional code to identify any retained foreign body, if applicable (Z18.-)
> *EXCLUDES 1*   *mental or behavioral disorders due to psychoactive substance use (F10-F19)*

R78.0 Finding of alcohol in blood
Use additional external cause code (Y90.-), for detail regarding alcohol level

R78.1 Finding of opiate drug in blood

R78.2 Finding of cocaine in blood

R78.3 Finding of hallucinogen in blood

R78.4 Finding of other drugs of addictive potential in blood

R78.5 Finding of other psychotropic drug in blood

R78.6 Finding of steroid agent in blood

✓5th **R78.7 Finding of abnormal level of heavy metals in blood**

R78.71 Abnormal lead level in blood
> *EXCLUDES 1*   *lead poisoning (T56.0-)*

R78.79 Finding of abnormal level of heavy metals in blood

✓5th **R78.8 Finding of other specified substances, not normally found in blood**

R78.81 Bacteremia
> *EXCLUDES 1*   *sepsis—code to specified infection*
> **DEF:** Laboratory finding of bacteria in the blood in the absence of two or more signs of sepsis; transient in nature, it progresses to septicemia with severe infectious process.

R78.89 Finding of other specified substances, not normally found in blood
Finding of abnormal level of lithium in blood

R78.9 Finding of unspecified substance, not normally found in blood ▽

✓4th **R79 Other abnormal findings of blood chemistry**
Use additional code to identify any retained foreign body, if applicable (Z18.-)
> *EXCLUDES 1*   ~~*abnormality of fluid, electrolyte or acid-base balance (E86-E87)*~~
> *asymptomatic hyperuricemia (E79.0)*
> *hyperglycemia NOS (R73.9)*
> *hypoglycemia NOS (E16.2)*
> *neonatal hypoglycemia (P70.3-P70.4)*
> *specific findings indicating disorder of amino-acid metabolism (E70-E72)*
> *specific findings indicating disorder of carbohydrate metabolism (E73-E74)*
> *specific findings indicating disorder of lipid metabolism (E75.-)*

R79.0 Abnormal level of blood mineral
Abnormal blood level of cobalt
Abnormal blood level of copper
Abnormal blood level of iron
Abnormal blood level of magnesium
Abnormal blood level of mineral NEC
Abnormal blood level of zinc
> *EXCLUDES 1*   *abnormal level of lithium (R78.89)*
> *disorders of mineral metabolism (E83.-)*
> *neonatal hypomagnesemia (P71.2)*
> *nutritional mineral deficiency (E58-E61)*

R79.1 Abnormal coagulation profile
Abnormal or prolonged bleeding time
Abnormal or prolonged coagulation time
Abnormal or prolonged partial thromboplastin time [PTT]
Abnormal or prolonged prothrombin time [PT]
> *EXCLUDES 1*   *coagulation defects (D68.-)*
> *EXCLUDES 2* ▶*abnormality of fluid, electrolyte or acid-base balance (E86-E87)*◄

✓5th **R79.8 Other specified abnormal findings of blood chemistry**

R79.81 Abnormal blood-gas level

R79.82 Elevated C-reactive protein [CRP]

R79.89 Other specified abnormal findings of blood chemistry

R79.9 Abnormal finding of blood chemistry, unspecified ▽

Abnormal findings on examination of urine, without diagnosis (R80-R82)

EXCLUDES 1   abnormal findings on antenatal screening of mother (O28.-)
diagnostic abnormal findings classified elsewhere—see Alphabetical Index
specific findings indicating disorder of amino-acid metabolism (E70-E72)
specific findings indicating disorder of carbohydrate metabolism (E73-E74)

☑4th **R80   Proteinuria**
    EXCLUDES 1   gestational proteinuria (O12.1-)

    R80.0   Isolated proteinuria
       Idiopathic proteinuria
       EXCLUDES 1   isolated proteinuria with specific morphological lesion (N06.-)

    R80.1   Persistent proteinuria, unspecified ▽

    R80.2   Orthostatic proteinuria, unspecified ▽
       Postural proteinuria

    R80.3   Bence Jones proteinuria

    R80.8   Other proteinuria

    R80.9   Proteinuria, unspecified ▽
       Albuminuria NOS

  R81   Glycosuria
    EXCLUDES 1   renal glycosuria (E74.8)

☑4th **R82   Other and unspecified abnormal findings in urine**
    INCLUDES   chromoabnormalities in urine
    Use additional code to identify any retained foreign body, if applicable (Z18.-)
    EXCLUDES 2   hematuria (R31.-)

    R82.0   Chyluria
       EXCLUDES 1   filarial chyluria (B74.-)

    R82.1   Myoglobinuria

    R82.2   Biliuria

    R82.3   Hemoglobinuria
       EXCLUDES 1   hemoglobinuria due to hemolysis from external causes NEC (D59.6)
          hemoglobinuria due to paroxysmal nocturnal [Marchiafava-Micheli] (D59.5)
       DEF: Free hemoglobin in blood due to rapid hemolysis of red blood cells; causes include burns, crushed injury, sickle cell anemia, thalassemia, parasitic infections, or kidney infections.

    R82.4   Acetonuria
       Ketonuria
       DEF: Excessive excretion of acetone in urine; commonly occurs in diabetic acidosis.

    R82.5   Elevated urine levels of drugs, medicaments and biological substances
       Elevated urine levels of catecholamines
       Elevated urine levels of indoleacetic acid
       Elevated urine levels of 17-ketosteroids
       Elevated urine levels of steroids

    R82.6   Abnormal urine levels of substances chiefly nonmedicinal as to source
       Abnormal urine level of heavy metals

☑5th   **R82.7   Abnormal findings on microbiological examination of urine**
       EXCLUDES 1   colonization status (Z22.-)

       R82.71   Bacteriuria

       R82.79   Other abnormal findings on microbiological examination of urine
          Positive culture findings of urine

    R82.8   Abnormal findings on cytological and histological examination of urine

☑5th   **R82.9   Other and unspecified abnormal findings in urine**

       R82.90   Unspecified abnormal findings in urine ▽

       R82.91   Other chromoabnormalities of urine
          Chromoconversion (dipstick)
          Idiopathic dipstick converts positive for blood with no cellular forms in sediment
          EXCLUDES 1   hemoglobinuria (R82.3)
             myoglobinuria (R82.1)

       R82.99   Other abnormal findings in urine
          Cells and casts in urine
          Crystalluria
          Melanuria

Cerebrospinal Fluid

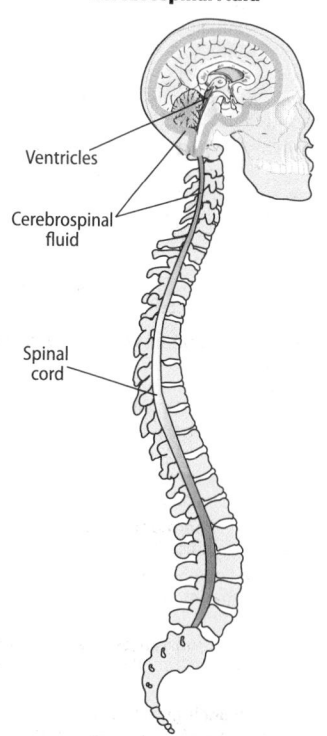

Ventricles

Cerebrospinal fluid

Spinal cord

Abnormal findings on examination of other body fluids, substances and tissues, without diagnosis (R83-R89)

EXCLUDES 1   abnormal findings on antenatal screening of mother (O28.-)
diagnostic abnormal findings classified elsewhere—see Alphabetical Index

EXCLUDES 2   abnormal findings on examination of blood, without diagnosis (R70-R79)
abnormal findings on examination of urine, without diagnosis (R80-R82)
abnormal tumor markers (R97.-)

    R83.3   Abnormal level of substances chiefly nonmedicinal as to source in cerebrospinal fluid

☑4th **R83   Abnormal findings in cerebrospinal fluid**

    R83.0   Abnormal level of enzymes in cerebrospinal fluid

    R83.1   Abnormal level of hormones in cerebrospinal fluid

    R83.2   Abnormal level of other drugs, medicaments and biological substances in cerebrospinal fluid

    R83.4   Abnormal immunological findings in cerebrospinal fluid

    R83.5   Abnormal microbiological findings in cerebrospinal fluid
       Positive culture findings in cerebrospinal fluid
       EXCLUDES 1   colonization status (Z22.-)

    R83.6   Abnormal cytological findings in cerebrospinal fluid

    R83.8   Other abnormal findings in cerebrospinal fluid
       Abnormal chromosomal findings in cerebrospinal fluid

    R83.9   Unspecified abnormal finding in cerebrospinal fluid ▽

☑4th **R84   Abnormal findings in specimens from respiratory organs and thorax**
    INCLUDES   abnormal findings in bronchial washings
       abnormal findings in nasal secretions
       abnormal findings in pleural fluid
       abnormal findings in sputum
       abnormal findings in throat scrapings
    EXCLUDES 1   blood-stained sputum (R04.2)

    R84.0   Abnormal level of enzymes in specimens from respiratory organs and thorax

    R84.1   Abnormal level of hormones in specimens from respiratory organs and thorax

    R84.2   Abnormal level of other drugs, medicaments and biological substances in specimens from respiratory organs and thorax

    R84.3   Abnormal level of substances chiefly nonmedicinal as to source in specimens from respiratory organs and thorax

    R84.4   Abnormal immunological findings in specimens from respiratory organs and thorax

☑ Additional Character Req   ☑x7th Placeholder Alert   Manifestation   HCC CMS-HCC Condition   ▽ Unspecified Code   ►◄ Revised Text   ● New Code   ▲ Revised Code Title

ICD-10-CM 2018   901

Chapter 18. Symptoms, Signs, and Abnormal Clinical and Laboratory Findings, Not Elsewhere Classified

R80–R84.4

R84.5 **Abnormal microbiological findings in specimens from respiratory organs and thorax**
Positive culture findings in specimens from respiratory organs and thorax
EXCLUDES 1   colonization status (Z22.-)

R84.6 **Abnormal cytological findings in specimens from respiratory organs and thorax**

R84.7 **Abnormal histological findings in specimens from respiratory organs and thorax**

R84.8 **Other abnormal findings in specimens from respiratory organs and thorax**
Abnormal chromosomal findings in specimens from respiratory organs and thorax

R84.9 **Unspecified abnormal finding in specimens from respiratory organs and thorax**   ▽

✓4ᵗʰ **R85** **Abnormal findings in specimens from digestive organs and abdominal cavity**
INCLUDES   abnormal findings in peritoneal fluid
abnormal findings in saliva
EXCLUDES 1   cloudy peritoneal dialysis effluent (R88.0)
fecal abnormalities (R19.5)

R85.0 **Abnormal level of enzymes in specimens from digestive organs and abdominal cavity**

R85.1 **Abnormal level of hormones in specimens from digestive organs and abdominal cavity**

R85.2 **Abnormal level of other drugs, medicaments and biological substances in specimens from digestive organs and abdominal cavity**

R85.3 **Abnormal level of substances chiefly nonmedicinal as to source in specimens from digestive organs and abdominal cavity**

R85.4 **Abnormal immunological findings in specimens from digestive organs and abdominal cavity**

R85.5 **Abnormal microbiological findings in specimens from digestive organs and abdominal cavity**
Positive culture findings in specimens from digestive organs and abdominal cavity
EXCLUDES 1   colonization status (Z22.-)

✓5ᵗʰ **R85.6** **Abnormal cytological findings in specimens from digestive organs and abdominal cavity**

✓6ᵗʰ **R85.61** **Abnormal cytologic smear of anus**
EXCLUDES 1   abnormal cytological findings in specimens from other digestive organs and abdominal cavity (R85.69)
anal intraepithelial neoplasia I [AIN I] (K62.82)
anal intraepithelial neoplasia II [AIN II] (K62.82)
anal intraepithelial neoplasia III [AIN III] (D01.3)
carcinoma in situ of anus (histologically confirmed) (D01.3)
dysplasia (mild) (moderate) of anus (histologically confirmed) (K62.82)
severe dysplasia of anus (histologically confirmed) (D01.3)
EXCLUDES 2   anal high risk human papillomavirus (HPV) DNA test positive (R85.81)
anal low risk human papillomavirus (HPV) DNA test positive (R85.82)

R85.610 **Atypical squamous cells of undetermined significance on cytologic smear of anus [ASC-US]**

R85.611 **Atypical squamous cells cannot exclude high grade squamous intraepithelial lesion on cytologic smear of anus [ASC-H]**

R85.612 **Low grade squamous intraepithelial lesion on cytologic smear of anus [LGSIL]**

R85.613 **High grade squamous intraepithelial lesion on cytologic smear of anus [HGSIL]**

R85.614 **Cytologic evidence of malignancy on smear of anus**

R85.615 **Unsatisfactory cytologic smear of anus**
Inadequate sample of cytologic smear of anus

R85.616 **Satisfactory anal smear but lacking transformation zone**

R85.618 **Other abnormal cytological findings on specimens from anus**

R85.619 **Unspecified abnormal cytological findings in specimens from anus**   ▽
Abnormal anal cytology NOS
Atypical glandular cells of anus NOS

R85.69 **Abnormal cytological findings in specimens from other digestive organs and abdominal cavity**

R85.7 **Abnormal histological findings in specimens from digestive organs and abdominal cavity**

✓5ᵗʰ **R85.8** **Other abnormal findings in specimens from digestive organs and abdominal cavity**

R85.81 **Anal high risk human papillomavirus [HPV] DNA test positive**
EXCLUDES 1   anogenital warts due to human papillomavirus (HPV) (A63.0)
condyloma acuminatum (A63.0)

R85.82 **Anal low risk human papillomavirus [HPV] DNA test positive**
Use additional code for associated human papillomavirus (B97.7)

R85.89 **Other abnormal findings in specimens from digestive organs and abdominal cavity**
Abnormal chromosomal findings in specimens from digestive organs and abdominal cavity

R85.9 **Unspecified abnormal finding in specimens from digestive organs and abdominal cavity**   ▽

✓4ᵗʰ **R86** **Abnormal findings in specimens from male genital organs**
INCLUDES   abnormal findings in prostatic secretions
abnormal findings in semen, seminal fluid
abnormal spermatozoa
EXCLUDES 1   azoospermia (N46.0-)
oligospermia (N46.1-)

R86.0 **Abnormal level of enzymes in specimens from male genital organs**   ♂

R86.1 **Abnormal level of hormones in specimens from male genital organs**   ♂

R86.2 **Abnormal level of other drugs, medicaments and biological substances in specimens from male genital organs** ♂

R86.3 **Abnormal level of substances chiefly nonmedicinal as to source in specimens from male genital organs**   ♂

R86.4 **Abnormal immunological findings in specimens from male genital organs**   ♂

R86.5 **Abnormal microbiological findings in specimens from male genital organs**   ♂
Positive culture findings in specimens from male genital organs
EXCLUDES 1   colonization status (Z22.-)

R86.6 **Abnormal cytological findings in specimens from male genital organs**   ♂

R86.7 **Abnormal histological findings in specimens from male genital organs**   ♂

R86.8 **Other abnormal findings in specimens from male genital organs**   ♂
Abnormal chromosomal findings in specimens from male genital organs

R86.9 **Unspecified abnormal finding in specimens from male genital organs**   ♂▽

✓4ᵗʰ **R87** **Abnormal findings in specimens from female genital organs**
INCLUDES   abnormal findings in secretion and smears from cervix uteri
abnormal findings in secretion and smears from vagina
abnormal findings in secretion and smears from vulva

R87.0 **Abnormal level of enzymes in specimens from female genital organs**   ♀

R87.1 **Abnormal level of hormones in specimens from female genital organs**   ♀

R87.2 **Abnormal level of other drugs, medicaments and biological substances in specimens from female genital organs**   ♀

R87.3 **Abnormal level of substances chiefly nonmedicinal as to source in specimens from female genital organs**   ♀

R87.4 **Abnormal immunological findings in specimens from female genital organs**   ♀

R87.5 **Abnormal microbiological findings in specimens from female genital organs**   ♀
Positive culture findings in specimens from female genital organs
EXCLUDES 1   colonization status (Z22.-)

EXCLUDES 1 Not coded here   *EXCLUDES 2* Not included here   N Newborn Age: 0   P Pediatric Age: 0-17   M Maternity Age: 12-55   A Adult Age: 15-124

902   ICD-10-CM 2018

✓5ᵗʰ **R87.6 Abnormal** cytological **findings in specimens from female genital organs**

✓6ᵗʰ **R87.61 Abnormal cytological findings in specimens from** cervix uteri

> EXCLUDES 1 *abnormal cytological findings in specimens from other female genital organs (R87.69)*
> *abnormal cytological findings in specimens from vagina (R87.62-)*
> *carcinoma in situ of cervix uteri (histologically confirmed) (D06.-)*
> *cervical intraepithelial neoplasia I [CIN I] (N87.0)*
> *cervical intraepithelial neoplasia II [CIN II] (N87.1)*
> *cervical intraepithelial neoplasia III [CIN III] (D06.-)*
> *dysplasia (mild) (moderate) of cervix uteri (histologically confirmed) (N87.-)*
> *severe dysplasia of cervix uteri (histologically confirmed) (D06.-)*
>
> EXCLUDES 2 *cervical high risk human papillomavirus (HPV) DNA test positive (R87.810)*
> *cervical low risk human papillomavirus (HPV) DNA test positive (R87.820)*

R87.610 Atypical squamous cells of undetermined significance **on cytologic smear of cervix [ASC-US]** ♀

R87.611 Atypical squamous cells cannot exclude high grade **squamous intraepithelial lesion on cytologic smear of cervix [ASC-H]** ♀

R87.612 Low grade squamous intraepithelial lesion on cytologic smear of cervix **[LGSIL]** ♀

R87.613 High grade squamous intraepithelial lesion on cytologic smear of cervix **[HGSIL]** ♀

R87.614 Cytologic evidence of malignancy **on smear of cervix** ♀

R87.615 Unsatisfactory cytologic smear of **cervix** ♀
> Inadequate sample of cytologic smear of cervix

R87.616 Satisfactory cervical smear but lacking transformation zone ♀

R87.618 Other abnormal cytological findings on specimens from cervix uteri ♀

R87.619 Unspecified abnormal cytological ♀ ▽ **findings in specimens from cervix uteri**
> Abnormal cervical cytology NOS
> Abnormal Papanicolaou smear of cervix NOS
> Abnormal thin preparation smear of cervix NOS
> Atypical endocervial cells of cervix NOS
> Atypical endometrial cells of cervix NOS
> Atypical glandular cells of cervix NOS

✓6ᵗʰ **R87.62 Abnormal cytological findings in specimens from** vagina
> Use additional code to identify acquired absence of uterus and cervix, if applicable (Z90.71-)
>
> EXCLUDES 1 *abnormal cytological findings in specimens from cervix uteri (R87.61-)*
> *abnormal cytological findings in specimens from other female genital organs (R87.69)*
> *carcinoma in situ of vagina (histologically confirmed) (D07.2)*
> *dysplasia (mild) (moderate) of vagina (histologically confirmed) (N89.-)*
> *severe dysplasia of vagina (histologically confirmed) (D07.2)*
> *vaginal intraepithelial neoplasia I [VAIN I] (N89.0)*
> *vaginal intraepithelial neoplasia II [VAIN II] (N89.1)*
> *vaginal intraepithelial neoplasia III [VAIN III] (D07.2)*
>
> EXCLUDES 2 *vaginal high risk human papillomavirus (HPV) DNA test positive (R87.811)*
> *vaginal low risk human papillomavirus (HPV) DNA test positive (R87.821)*

R87.620 Atypical squamous cells of undetermined significance **on cytologic smear of vagina [ASC-US]** ♀

R87.621 Atypical squamous cells cannot exclude high grade **squamous intraepithelial lesion on cytologic smear of vagina [ASC-H]** ♀

R87.622 Low grade squamous intraepithelial lesion on cytologic smear of vagina **[LGSIL]** ♀

R87.623 High grade squamous intraepithelial lesion on cytologic smear of vagina **[HGSIL]** ♀

R87.624 Cytologic evidence of malignancy **on smear of vagina** ♀

R87.625 Unsatisfactory cytologic smear of **vagina** ♀
> Inadequate sample of cytologic smear of vagina

R87.628 Other abnormal cytological findings on specimens from vagina ♀

R87.629 Unspecified abnormal cytological ♀ ▽ **findings in specimens from vagina**
> Abnormal Papanicolaou smear of vagina NOS
> Abnormal thin preparation smear of vagina NOS
> Abnormal vaginal cytology NOS
> Atypical endocervical cells of vagina NOS
> Atypical endometrial cells of vagina NOS
> Atypical glandular cells of vagina NOS

R87.69 Abnormal cytological findings in specimens from other female genital organs ♀
> Abnormal cytological findings in specimens from female genital organs NOS
>
> EXCLUDES 1 *dysplasia of vulva (histologically confirmed) (N90.0-N90.3)*

R87.7 Abnormal histological findings in specimens from ♀ **female genital organs**
> EXCLUDES 1 *carcinoma in situ (histologically confirmed) of female genital organs (D06-D07.3)*
> *cervical intraepithelial neoplasia I [CIN I] (N87.0)*
> *cervical intraepithelial neoplasia II [CIN II] (N87.1)*
> *cervical intraepithelial neoplasia III [CIN III] (D06.-)*
> *dysplasia (mild) (moderate) of cervix uteri (histologically confirmed) (N87.-)*
> *dysplasia (mild) (moderate) of vagina (histologically confirmed) (N89.-)*
> *severe dysplasia of cervix uteri (histologically confirmed) (D06.-)*
> *severe dysplasia of vagina (histologically confirmed) (D07.2)*
> *vaginal intraepithelial neoplasia I [VAIN I] (N89.0)*
> *vaginal intraepithelial neoplasia II [VAIN II] (N89.1)*
> *vaginal intraepithelial neoplasia III [VAIN III] (D07.2)*

✓5ᵗʰ **R87.8 Other abnormal findings in specimens from female genital organs**

✓6ᵗʰ **R87.81 High risk human papillomavirus [HPV] DNA test positive from female genital organs**
> EXCLUDES 1 *anogenital warts due to human papillomavirus (HPV) (A63.0)*
> *condyloma acuminatum (A63.0)*

R87.810 Cervical high risk human papillomavirus [HPV] DNA test positive ♀

R87.811 Vaginal high risk human papillomavirus [HPV] DNA test positive ♀

✓6ᵗʰ **R87.82 Low risk human papillomavirus [HPV] DNA test positive from female genital organs**
> Use additional code for associated human papillomavirus (B97.7)

R87.820 Cervical low risk human papillomavirus [HPV] DNA test positive ♀

R87.821 Vaginal low risk human papillomavirus [HPV] DNA test positive ♀

R87.89 Other abnormal findings in specimens from female genital organs ♀
> Abnormal chromosomal findings in specimens from female genital organs

R87.9 Unspecified abnormal finding in specimens from female ♀ ▽ **genital organs**

✓ Additional Character Req   ✓x7ᵗʰ Placeholder Alert   Manifestation   HCC CMS-HCC Condition   ▽ Unspecified Code   ►◄ Revised Text   ● New Code   ▲ Revised Code Title

☑4ᵗʰ **R88** **Abnormal findings in other body fluids and substances**

R88.Ø **Cloudy (hemodialysis) (peritoneal) dialysis effluent**

R88.8 **Abnormal findings in other body fluids and substances**

☑4ᵗʰ **R89** **Abnormal findings in specimens from other organs, systems and tissues**

> INCLUDES   abnormal findings in nipple discharge
> abnormal findings in synovial fluid
> abnormal findings in wound secretions

R89.Ø **Abnormal level of enzymes in specimens from other organs, systems and tissues**

R89.1 **Abnormal level of hormones in specimens from other organs, systems and tissues**

R89.2 **Abnormal level of other drugs, medicaments and biological substances in specimens from other organs, systems and tissues**

R89.3 **Abnormal level of substances chiefly nonmedicinal as to source in specimens from other organs, systems and tissues**

R89.4 **Abnormal immunological findings in specimens from other organs, systems and tissues**

R89.5 **Abnormal microbiological findings in specimens from other organs, systems and tissues**
> Positive culture findings in specimens from other organs, systems and tissues
> EXCLUDES 1   colonization status (Z22.-)

R89.6 **Abnormal cytological findings in specimens from other organs, systems and tissues**

R89.7 **Abnormal histological findings in specimens from other organs, systems and tissues**

R89.8 **Other abnormal findings in specimens from other organs, systems and tissues**
> Abnormal chromosomal findings in specimens from other organs, systems and tissues

R89.9 **Unspecified abnormal finding in specimens from other organs, systems and tissues** ▽

Abnormal findings on diagnostic imaging and in function studies, without diagnosis (R9Ø-R94)

> INCLUDES   nonspecific abnormal findings on diagnostic imaging by computerized axial tomography [CAT scan]
> nonspecific abnormal findings on diagnostic imaging by magnetic resonance imaging [MRI][NMR]
> nonspecific abnormal findings on diagnostic imaging by positron emission tomography [PET scan]
> nonspecific abnormal findings on diagnostic imaging by thermography
> nonspecific abnormal findings on diagnostic imaging by ultrasound [echogram]
> nonspecific abnormal findings on diagnostic imaging by X-ray examination
> EXCLUDES 1   abnormal findings on antenatal screening of mother (O28.-)
> diagnostic abnormal findings classified elsewhere—see Alphabetical Index

☑4ᵗʰ **R9Ø** **Abnormal findings on diagnostic imaging of central nervous system**

R9Ø.Ø **Intracranial space-occupying lesion found on diagnostic imaging of central nervous system**

☑5ᵗʰ **R9Ø.8** **Other abnormal findings on diagnostic imaging of central nervous system**

R9Ø.81 Abnormal echoencephalogram

R9Ø.82 **White matter disease, unspecified** ▽

R9Ø.89 **Other abnormal findings on diagnostic imaging of central nervous system**
> Other cerebrovascular abnormality found on diagnostic imaging of central nervous system

☑4ᵗʰ **R91** **Abnormal findings on diagnostic imaging of lung**

R91.1 **Solitary pulmonary nodule**
> Coin lesion lung
> Solitary pulmonary nodule, subsegmental branch of the bronchial tree

R91.8 **Other nonspecific abnormal finding of lung field**
> Lung mass NOS found on diagnostic imaging of lung
> Pulmonary infiltrate NOS
> Shadow, lung

☑4ᵗʰ **R92** **Abnormal and inconclusive findings on diagnostic imaging of breast**

R92.Ø **Mammographic microcalcification found on diagnostic imaging of breast**
> EXCLUDES 2   mammographic calcification (calculus) found on diagnostic imaging of breast (R92.1)
> DEF: Calcium and cellular debris deposits in the breast that cannot be felt but can be detected on a mammogram; can be a sign of cancer, benign conditions, or changes in the breast tissue as a result of inflammation, injury, or obstructed duct.

R92.1 **Mammographic calcification found on diagnostic imaging of breast**
> Mammographic calculus found on diagnostic imaging of breast

R92.2 **Inconclusive mammogram**
> Dense breasts NOS
> Inconclusive mammogram NEC
> Inconclusive mammography due to dense breasts
> Inconclusive mammography NEC
> **AHA:** 2015, 1Q, 24

R92.8 **Other abnormal and inconclusive findings on diagnostic imaging of breast**

☑4ᵗʰ **R93** **Abnormal findings on diagnostic imaging of other body structures**

R93.Ø **Abnormal findings on diagnostic imaging of skull and head, not elsewhere classified**
> EXCLUDES 1   intracranial space-occupying lesion found on diagnostic imaging (R9Ø.Ø)

R93.1 **Abnormal findings on diagnostic imaging of heart and coronary circulation**
> Abnormal echocardiogram NOS
> Abnormal heart shadow

R93.2 **Abnormal findings on diagnostic imaging of liver and biliary tract**
> Nonvisualization of gallbladder

R93.3 **Abnormal findings on diagnostic imaging of other parts of digestive tract**

☑5ᵗʰ **R93.4** **Abnormal findings on diagnostic imaging of urinary organs**
> EXCLUDES 2   hypertrophy of kidney (N28.81)

R93.41 **Abnormal radiologic findings on diagnostic imaging of renal pelvis, ureter, or bladder**
> Filling defect of bladder found on diagnostic imaging
> Filling defect of renal pelvis found on diagnostic imaging
> Filling defect of ureter found on diagnostic imaging

☑6ᵗʰ **R93.42** **Abnormal radiologic findings on diagnositic imaging of kidney**

R93.421 **Abnormal radiologic findings on diagnositic imaging of right kidney**

R93.422 **Abnormal radiologic findings on diagnositic imaging of left kidney**

R93.429 **Abnormal radiologic findings on diagnositic imaging of unspecified kidney** ▽

R93.49 **Abnormal radiologic findings on diagnositic imaging of other urinary organs**

R93.5 **Abnormal findings on diagnostic imaging of other abdominal regions, including retroperitoneum**

R93.6 **Abnormal findings on diagnostic imaging of limbs**
> EXCLUDES 2   abnormal finding in skin and subcutaneous tissue (R93.8)

R93.7 **Abnormal findings on diagnostic imaging of other parts of musculoskeletal system**
> EXCLUDES 2   abnormal findings on diagnostic imaging of skull (R93.Ø)

R93.8 **Abnormal findings on diagnostic imaging of other specified body structures**
> Abnormal finding by radioisotope localization of placenta
> Abnormal radiological finding in skin and subcutaneous tissue
> Mediastinal shift

R93.9 **Diagnostic imaging inconclusive due to excess body fat of patient**

☑4ᵗʰ **R94** **Abnormal results of function studies**
> INCLUDES   abnormal results of radionuclide [radioisotope] uptake studies
> abnormal results of scintigraphy

☑5ᵗʰ **R94.Ø** **Abnormal results of function studies of central nervous system**

R94.Ø1 **Abnormal electroencephalogram [EEG]**

R94.Ø2 **Abnormal brain scan**

R94.09 Abnormal results of other function studies of central nervous system

✓5ᵗʰ R94.1 Abnormal results of function studies of peripheral nervous system and special senses

✓6ᵗʰ R94.11 Abnormal results of function studies of eye
- **R94.110** Abnormal electro-oculogram [EOG]
- **R94.111** Abnormal electroretinogram [ERG]
  Abnormal retinal function study
- **R94.112** Abnormal visually evoked potential [VEP]
- **R94.113** Abnormal oculomotor study
- **R94.118** Abnormal results of other function studies of eye

✓6ᵗʰ R94.12 Abnormal results of function studies of ear and other special senses
  AHA: 2016, 3Q, 17
- **R94.120** Abnormal auditory function study
- **R94.121** Abnormal vestibular function study
- **R94.128** Abnormal results of other function studies of ear and other special senses

✓6ᵗʰ R94.13 Abnormal results of function studies of peripheral nervous system
- **R94.130** Abnormal response to nerve stimulation, unspecified ▽
- **R94.131** Abnormal electromyogram [EMG]
  EXCLUDES1 electromyogram of eye (R94.113)
- **R94.138** Abnormal results of other function studies of peripheral nervous system

R94.2 Abnormal results of pulmonary function studies
  Reduced ventilatory capacity
  Reduced vital capacity

✓5ᵗʰ R94.3 Abnormal results of cardiovascular function studies
- **R94.30** Abnormal result of cardiovascular function study, unspecified ▽
- **R94.31** Abnormal electrocardiogram [ECG] [EKG]
  EXCLUDES1 long QT syndrome (I45.81)
- **R94.39** Abnormal result of other cardiovascular function study
  Abnormal electrophysiological intracardiac studies
  Abnormal phonocardiogram
  Abnormal vectorcardiogram

R94.4 Abnormal results of kidney function studies
  Abnormal renal function test

R94.5 Abnormal results of liver function studies

R94.6 Abnormal results of thyroid function studies

R94.7 Abnormal results of other endocrine function studies
  EXCLUDES2 abnormal glucose (R73.0-)

R94.8 Abnormal results of function studies of other organs and systems
  Abnormal basal metabolic rate [BMR]
  Abnormal bladder function test
  Abnormal splenic function test

Abnormal tumor markers (R97)

✓4ᵗʰ R97 Abnormal tumor markers
  Elevated tumor associated antigens [TAA]
  Elevated tumor specific antigens [TSA]
- **R97.0** Elevated carcinoembryonic antigen [CEA]
- **R97.1** Elevated cancer antigen 125 [CA 125] ♀
- **✓5ᵗʰ R97.2** Elevated prostate specific antigen [PSA]
  - **R97.20** Elevated prostate specific antigen [PSA] Ⓐ♂
  - **R97.21** Rising PSA following treatment for malignant neoplasm of prostate Ⓐ♂
- **R97.8** Other abnormal tumor markers

Ill-defined and unknown cause of mortality (R99)

R99 Ill-defined and unknown cause of mortality ▽
  Death (unexplained) NOS
  Unspecified cause of mortality

Chapter 19. Injury, Poisoning, and Certain Other Consequences of External Causes (S00–T88)

Chapter Specific Guidelines with Coding Examples

The chapter specific guidelines from the ICD-10-CM Official Guidelines for Coding and Reporting have been provided below. Along with these guidelines are coding examples, contained in the shaded boxes, that have been developed to help illustrate the coding and/or sequencing guidance found in these guidelines.

a. Application of 7th characters in Chapter 19

Most categories in chapter 19 have a 7th character requirement for each applicable code. Most categories in this chapter have three 7th character values (with the exception of fractures): A, initial encounter, D, subsequent encounter and S, sequela. Categories for traumatic fractures have additional 7th character values. While the patient may be seen by a new or different provider over the course of treatment for an injury, assignment of the 7th character is based on whether the patient is undergoing active treatment and not whether the provider is seeing the patient for the first time.

For complication codes, active treatment refers to treatment for the condition described by the code, even though it may be related to an earlier precipitating problem. For example, code T84.50XA, Infection and inflammatory reaction due to unspecified internal joint prosthesis, initial encounter, is used when active treatment is provided for the infection, even though the condition relates to the prosthetic device, implant or graft that was placed at a previous encounter.

7th character "A", initial encounter is used for each encounter where the patient is receiving active treatment for the condition.

> Patient evaluated after fall from a skateboard onto the sidewalk, x-rays identify a nondisplaced fracture to the distal pole of the right scaphoid bone. The patient is placed in a cast.
>
> **S62.014A**   **Nondisplaced fracture of distal pole of navicular [scaphoid] bone of right wrist, initial encounter for closed fracture**
>
> **V00.131A**   **Fall from skateboard, initial encounter**
>
> **Y93.51**   **Activity, roller skating (inline) and skateboarding**
>
> **Y92.480**   **Sidewalk as the place of occurrence of the external cause**
>
> **Y99.8**   **Other external cause status**
>
> *Explanation:* This fracture would be coded with a seventh character A for initial encounter because the patient received x-rays to identify the site of the fracture and treatment was rendered; this would be considered active treatment.

7th character "D" subsequent encounter is used for encounters after the patient has completed active treatment of the condition and is receiving routine care for the condition during the healing or recovery phase.

> Patient seen in follow-up after fall from a skateboard onto the sidewalk resulted in casting of the right arm. X-rays are taken to evaluate how well the nondisplaced fracture to the distal pole of the right scaphoid bone is healing. The physician feels the fracture is healing appropriately; no adjustments to the cast are made.
>
> **S62.014D**   **Nondisplaced fracture of distal pole of navicular [scaphoid] bone of right wrist, subsequent encounter for fracture with routine healing**
>
> **V00.131D**   **Fall from skateboard, subsequent encounter**
>
> *Explanation:* This fracture would be coded with a seventh character D for subsequent encounter, whether the same physician who provided the initial cast application or a different physician is now seeing the patient. Although the patient received x-rays, the intent of the x-rays was to assess how the fracture was healing. There was no active treatment rendered and the visit is therefore considered a subsequent encounter.

The aftercare Z codes should not be used for aftercare for conditions such as injuries or poisonings, where 7th characters are provided to identify subsequent care. For example, for aftercare of an injury, assign the acute injury code with the 7th character "D" (subsequent encounter).

7th character "S", sequela, is for use for complications or conditions that arise as a direct result of a condition, such as scar formation after a burn.

The scars are sequelae of the burn. When using 7th character "S", it is necessary to use both the injury code that precipitated the sequela and the code for the sequela itself. The "S" is added only to the injury code, not the sequela code. The 7th character "S" identifies the injury responsible for the sequela. The specific type of sequela (e.g. scar) is sequenced first, followed by the injury code.

See Section I.B.10 Sequelae, (Late Effects)

> Patient with a history of a nondisplaced fracture to the distal pole of the right scaphoid bone due to a fall from a skateboard is seen for evaluation of arthritis to the right wrist that has developed as a consequence of the traumatic fracture.
>
> **M12.531**   **Traumatic arthropathy, right wrist**
>
> **S62.014S**   **Nondisplaced fracture of distal pole of navicular [scaphoid] bone of right wrist, sequela**
>
> **V00.131S**   **Fall from skateboard, sequela**
>
> *Explanation:* The code identifying the specific sequela condition (traumatic arthritis) should be coded first followed by the injury that instigated the development of the sequela (fracture). The scaphoid fracture injury code is given a 7th character S for sequela to represent its role as the inciting injury. The fracture has healed and is not being managed or treated on this admit and therefore is not applicable as a first listed or principal diagnosis. However, it is directly related to the development of the arthritis and should be appended as a secondary code to signify this cause and effect relationship.

b. Coding of injuries

When coding injuries, assign separate codes for each injury unless a combination code is provided, in which case the combination code is assigned. Code T07, Unspecified multiple injuries should not be assigned in the inpatient setting unless information for a more specific code is not available. Traumatic injury codes (S00-T14.9) are not to be used for normal, healing surgical wounds or to identify complications of surgical wounds.

> 11-year-old girl fell from her horse, resulting in a laceration to her right forearm with several large pieces of wooden fragments embedded in the wound as well as abrasions to her right ear; in addition, her right shoulder was dislocated
>
> **S43.004A**   **Unspecified dislocation of right shoulder joint, initial encounter**
>
> **S51.821A**   **Laceration with foreign body of right forearm, initial encounter**
>
> **S00.411A**   **Abrasion of right ear, initial encounter**
>
> **V80.010A**   **Animal-rider injured by fall from or being thrown from horse in noncollision accident, initial encounter**
>
> **Y93.52**   **Activity, horseback riding**
>
> *Explanation:* Each separate injury should be reported. The patient's injury to the forearm is reported with one combination code that captures both the laceration and the foreign body.

The code for the most serious injury, as determined by the provider and the focus of treatment, is sequenced first.

1) Superficial injuries

Superficial injuries such as abrasions or contusions are not coded when associated with more severe injuries of the same site.

2) Primary injury with damage to nerves/blood vessels

When a primary injury results in minor damage to peripheral nerves or blood vessels, the primary injury is sequenced first with additional code(s) for injuries to nerves and spinal cord (such as category S04), and/or injury to blood vessels (such as category S15). When the primary injury is to the blood vessels or nerves, that injury should be sequenced first.

c. Coding of traumatic fractures

The principles of multiple coding of injuries should be followed in coding fractures. Fractures of specified sites are coded individually by site in accordance with both the provisions within categories S02, S12, S22, S32, S42, S49, S52, S59, S62, S72, S79, S82, S89, S92 and the level of detail furnished by medical record content.

A fracture not indicated as open or closed should be coded to closed. A fracture not indicated whether displaced or not displaced should be coded to displaced.

More specific guidelines are as follows:

1) Initial vs. subsequent encounter for fractures

Traumatic fractures are coded using the appropriate 7th character for initial encounter (A, B, C) for each encounter where the patient is receiving active treatment for the fracture. The appropriate 7th character for initial encounter should also be assigned for a patient who delayed seeking treatment for the fracture or nonunion.

Fractures are coded using the appropriate 7th character for subsequent care for encounters after the patient has completed active treatment of the fracture and is receiving routine care for the fracture during the healing or recovery phase.

Care for complications of surgical treatment for fracture repairs during the healing or recovery phase should be coded with the appropriate complication codes.

Care of complications of fractures, such as malunion and nonunion, should be reported with the appropriate 7th character for subsequent care with nonunion (K, M, N,) or subsequent care with malunion (P, Q, R).

Malunion/nonunion: The appropriate 7th character for initial encounter should also be assigned for a patient who delayed seeking treatment for the fracture or nonunion.

Female patient fell during a forest hiking excursion almost six months ago and until recently did not feel she needed to seek medical attention for her left ankle pain; x-rays show nonunion of lateral malleolus and surgery has been scheduled

S82.62XA   **Displaced fracture of lateral malleolus of left fibula, initial encounter for closed fracture**

W01.0XXA   **Fall on same level from slipping, tripping and stumbling without subsequent striking against object, initial encounter**

Y92.821   **Forest as place of occurrence of the external cause**

Y93.01   **Activity, walking, marching and hiking**

Y99.8   **Other external cause status**

Explanation: A seventh character of A is used for the lateral malleolus nonunion fracture to signify that the fracture is receiving active treatment. The delayed care for the fracture has resulted in a nonunion, but capturing the nonunion in the seventh character is trumped by the provision of active care.

The open fracture designations in the assignment of the 7th character for fractures of the forearm, femur and lower leg, including ankle are based on the Gustilo open fracture classification. When the Gustilo classification type is not specified for an open fracture, the 7th character for open fracture type I or II should be assigned (B, E, H, M, Q).

A code from category M80, not a traumatic fracture code, should be used for any patient with known osteoporosis who suffers a fracture, even if the patient had a minor fall or trauma, if that fall or trauma would not usually break a normal, healthy bone.

See Section I.C.13. Osteoporosis.

The aftercare Z codes should not be used for aftercare for traumatic fractures. For aftercare of a traumatic fracture, assign the acute fracture code with the appropriate 7th character.

2) Multiple fractures sequencing

Multiple fractures are sequenced in accordance with the severity of the fracture.

d. Coding of burns and corrosions

The ICD-10-CM makes a distinction between burns and corrosions. The burn codes are for thermal burns, except sunburns, that come from a heat source, such as a fire or hot appliance. The burn codes are also for burns resulting from electricity and radiation. Corrosions are burns due to chemicals. The guidelines are the same for burns and corrosions.

Current burns (T20-T25) are classified by depth, extent and by agent (X code). Burns are classified by depth as first degree (erythema), second degree (blistering), and third degree (full-thickness involvement). Burns of the eye and internal organs (T26-T28) are classified by site, but not by degree.

1) Sequencing of burn and related condition codes

Sequence first the code that reflects the highest degree of burn when more than one burn is present.

---

a. When the reason for the admission or encounter is for treatment of external multiple burns, sequence first the code that reflects the burn of the highest degree.

b. When a patient has both internal and external burns, the circumstances of admission govern the selection of the principal diagnosis or first-listed diagnosis.

c. When a patient is admitted for burn injuries and other related conditions such as smoke inhalation and/or respiratory failure, the circumstances of admission govern the selection of the principal or first-listed diagnosis.

Patient referred for minor first-degree burns to multiple sites of her right and left hands as well as severe smoke inhalation. While she was sleeping at home, a candle on her dresser lit the bedroom curtains on fire.

T59.811A   **Toxic effect of smoke, accidental (unintentional), initial encounter**

J70.5   **Respiratory conditions due to smoke inhalation**

T23.191A   **Burn of first degree of multiple sites of right wrist and hand, initial encounter**

T23.192A   **Burn of first degree of multiple sites of left wrist and hand, initial encounter**

X08.8XXA   **Exposure to other specified smoke, fire and flames, initial encounter**

Y99.8   **Other exteranl cause status**

Y92.003   **Bedroom of unspecified non-institutional (private) residence as the place of occurrence of the external cause**

Y93.84   **Activity, sleeping**

Explanation: Based on the documentation, the inhalation injury is more severe than the first-degree burns and is sequenced first. The burns to the hands are appended as secondary diagnoses.

---

2) Burns of the same local site

Classify burns of the same local site (three-character category level, T20-T28) but of different degrees to the subcategory identifying the highest degree recorded in the diagnosis.

10-year-old male patient is treated for third-degree burns of his right palm and second-degree burns of multiple right fingers; right thumb not affected

T23.351A   **Burn of third degree of right palm, initial encounter**

Explanation: Although there is a code for second-degree burns of multiple fingers, not including the thumb (T23.131-), this code falls in the same three-digit category that the third-degree burn of the right palm falls under, category T23. Only the subcategory identifying the highest degree is captured when different burn degrees are classified to a single category.

Patient is treated for third-degree burns of the scalp as well as second-degree burns to the back of the right hand

T20.35XA   **Burn of third degree of scalp [any part], initial encounter**

T23.261A   **Burn of second degree of back of right hand, initial encounter**

Explanation: Since burns to the hand and scalp are classified to two different three-digit categories, both burns may be reported as they represent distinct sites.

---

3) Non-healing burns

Non-healing burns are coded as acute burns.

Necrosis of burned skin should be coded as a non-healed burn.

4) Infected burn

For any documented infected burn site, use an additional code for the infection.

5) Assign separate codes for each burn site

When coding burns, assign separate codes for each burn site. Category T30, Burn and corrosion, body region unspecified is extremely vague and should rarely be used.

6) Burns and corrosions classified according to extent of body surface involved

Assign codes from category T31, Burns classified according to extent of body surface involved, or T32, Corrosions classified according to extent of body surface involved, when the site of the burn is not specified or when there is a need for additional data. It is advisable to use category T31 as additional coding when needed to provide data for evaluating burn mortality, such as that needed by burn units. It is also advisable to use category T31 as an additional code for reporting purposes when there is mention of a third-degree burn involving 20 percent or more of the body surface.

Categories T31 and T32 are based on the classic "rule of nines" in estimating body surface involved: head and neck are assigned nine percent, each arm nine percent, each leg 18 percent, the anterior trunk 18 percent, posterior trunk 18 percent, and genitalia one percent. Providers may change these percentage assignments where necessary to accommodate infants and children who have proportionately larger heads than adults, and patients who have large buttocks, thighs, or abdomen that involve burns.

> Patient seen for dressing change after he accidentally spilled acetic acid on himself two days ago. The second-degree burns to his right thigh, covering about 3 percent of his body surface, are healing appropriately.
>
> **T54.2X1D**   **Toxic effect of corrosive acids and acid-like substances, accidental (unintentional), subsequent encounter**
>
> **T24.611D**   **Corrosion of second degree of right thigh, subsequent encounter**
>
> **T32.0**   **Corrosions involving less than 10% of body surface**
>
> *Explanation:* Code T32.0 provides additional information as to how much of the patient's body was affected by the corrosive substance.

7) Encounters for treatment of sequela of burns

Encounters for the treatment of the late effects of burns or corrosions (i.e., scars or joint contractures) should be coded with a burn or corrosion code with the 7th character "S" for sequela.

8) Sequelae with a late effect code and current burn

When appropriate, both a code for a current burn or corrosion with 7th character "A" or "D" and a burn or corrosion code with 7th character "S" may be assigned on the same record (when both a current burn and sequelae of an old burn exist). Burns and corrosions do not heal at the same rate and a current healing wound may still exist with sequela of a healed burn or corrosion.

See Section I.B.10 Sequela (Late Effects)

> Female patient seen for second-degree burn to the left ear; she also has significant scarring on her left elbow from a third-degree burn from childhood
>
> **T20.212A**   **Burn of second degree of left ear [any part, except ear drum], initial encounter**
>
> **L90.5**   **Scar conditions and fibrosis of skin**
>
> **T22.322S**   **Burn of third degree of left elbow, sequela**
>
> *Explanation:* The patient is being seen for management of a current second-degree burn, which is reflected in the code by appending the seventh character of A, indicating active treatment or management of this burn. The elbow scarring is a sequela of a previous third-degree burn. The sequela condition precedes the original burn injury, which is appended with a seventh character of S.

9) Use of an external cause code with burns and corrosions

An external cause code should be used with burns and corrosions to identify the source and intent of the burn, as well as the place where it occurred.

e. Adverse effects, poisoning, underdosing and toxic effects

Codes in categories T36-T65 are combination codes that include the substance that was taken as well as the intent. No additional external cause code is required for poisonings, toxic effects, adverse effects and underdosing codes.

1) Do not code directly from the Table of Drugs

Do not code directly from the Table of Drugs and Chemicals. Always refer back to the Tabular List.

2) Use as many codes as necessary to describe

Use as many codes as necessary to describe completely all drugs, medicinal or biological substances.

3) If the same code would describe the causative agent

If the same code would describe the causative agent for more than one adverse reaction, poisoning, toxic effect or underdosing, assign the code only once.

4) If two or more drugs, medicinal or biological substances

If two or more drugs, medicinal or biological substances are reported, code each individually unless a combination code is listed in the Table of Drugs and Chemicals.

5) The occurrence of drug toxicity is classified in ICD-10-CM as follows:

(a) Adverse effect

When coding an adverse effect of a drug that has been correctly prescribed and properly administered, assign the appropriate code for the nature of the adverse effect followed by the appropriate code for the adverse effect of the drug (T36-T50). The code for the drug should have a 5th or 6th character "5" (for example T36.0X5-) Examples of the nature of an adverse effect are tachycardia, delirium, gastrointestinal hemorrhaging, vomiting, hypokalemia, hepatitis, renal failure, or respiratory failure.

> Patient seen for stomach pain and jaundice, indicated by physician as possible side-effects of Inderal, recently started for hypertension. Inderal was discontinued and the patient switched to Atenolol instead.
>
> **R10.9**   **Unspecified abdominal pain**
>
> **R17**   **Unspecified jaundice**
>
> **T44.7X5A**   **Adverse effect of beta-adrenoreceptor antagonists, initial encounter**
>
> **I10**   **Essential (primary) hypertension**
>
> *Explanation:* The side-effects caused by the drug are listed first, followed by the code for the adverse effect of the drug to capture the specific drug that was used.

(b) Poisoning

When coding a poisoning or reaction to the improper use of a medication (e.g., overdose, wrong substance given or taken in error, wrong route of administration), first assign the appropriate code from categories T36-T50. The poisoning codes have an associated intent as their 5th or 6th character (accidental, intentional self-harm, assault and undetermined. If the intent of the poisoning is unknown or unspecified, code the intent as accidental intent. The undetermined intent is only for use if the documentation in the record specifies that the intent cannot be determined. Use additional code(s) for all manifestations of poisonings.

If there is also a diagnosis of abuse or dependence of the substance, the abuse or dependence is assigned as an additional code.

Examples of poisoning include:

(i) Error was made in drug prescription

Errors made in drug prescription or in the administration of the drug by provider, nurse, patient, or other person.

(ii) Overdose of a drug intentionally taken

If an overdose of a drug intentionally was taken or administered and resulted in drug toxicity, it would be coded as a poisoning.

(iii) Nonprescribed drug taken with correctly prescribed and properly administered drug

If a nonprescribed drug or medicinal agent was taken in combination with a correctly prescribed and properly administered drug, any drug toxicity or other reaction resulting from the interaction of the two drugs would be classified as a poisoning.

(iv) Interaction of drug(s) and alcohol

When a reaction results from the interaction of a drug(s) and alcohol, this would be classified as poisoning.

See Section I.C.4. if poisoning is the result of insulin pump malfunctions.

(c) Underdosing

Underdosing refers to taking less of a medication than is prescribed by a provider or a manufacturer's instruction. For underdosing, assign the code from categories T36-T50 (fifth or sixth character "6").

Codes for underdosing should never be assigned as principal or first-listed codes. If a patient has a relapse or exacerbation of the medical condition for which the drug is prescribed because of the reduction in dose, then the medical condition itself should be coded.

Noncompliance (Z91.12-, Z91.13-) or complication of care (Y63.6-Y63.9) codes are to be used with an underdosing code to indicate intent, if known.

> Patient referred for atrial fibrillation with history of chronic atrial fibrillation for which she is prescribed amiodarone. Financial concerns have left the patient unable to pay for her prescriptions and she has been skipping her amiodarone dose every other day to offset the cost.
>
> | I48.2 | **Chronic atrial fibrillation** |
> |---|---|
> | T46.2X6A | **Underdosing of other antidysrhythmic drugs, initial encounter** |
> | Z91.120 | **Patient's intentional underdosing of medication regimen due to financial hardship** |
>
> *Explanation:* By skipping her amiodarone pill every other day, the patient's atrial fibrillation returned. The condition for which the drug was being taken is reported first, followed by an underdosing code to show that the patient was not adhering to her prescription regiment. The Z code helps elaborate on the patient's social and/or economic circumstances that led to the patient taking less then what she was prescribed.

(d) Toxic effects

When a harmful substance is ingested or comes in contact with a person, this is classified as a toxic effect. The toxic effect codes are in categories T51-T65.

Toxic effect codes have an associated intent: accidental, intentional self-harm, assault and undetermined.

f. Adult and child abuse, neglect and other maltreatment

Sequence first the appropriate code from categories T74.- (Adult and child abuse, neglect and other maltreatment, confirmed) or T76.- (Adult and child abuse, neglect and other maltreatment, suspected) for abuse, neglect and other maltreatment, followed by any accompanying mental health or injury code(s).

If the documentation in the medical record states abuse or neglect it is coded as confirmed (T74.-). It is coded as suspected if it is documented as suspected (T76.-).

For cases of confirmed abuse or neglect an external cause code from the assault section (X92-Y09) should be added to identify the cause of any physical injuries. A perpetrator code (Y07) should be added when the perpetrator of the abuse is known. For suspected cases of abuse or neglect, do not report external cause or perpetrator code.

If a suspected case of abuse, neglect or mistreatment is ruled out during an encounter code Z04.71, Encounter for examination and observation following alleged physical adult abuse, ruled out, or code Z04.72, Encounter for examination and observation following alleged child physical abuse, ruled out, should be used, not a code from T76.

If a suspected case of alleged rape or sexual abuse is ruled out during an encounter code Z04.41, Encounter for examination and observation following alleged adult rape or code Z04.42, Encounter for examination and observation following alleged child rape, should be used, not a code from T76.

See Section I.C.15. Abuse in a pregnant patient.

g. Complications of care

1) General guidelines for complications of care

(a) Documentation of complications of care

See Section I.B.16. for information on documentation of complications of care.

2) Pain due to medical devices

Pain associated with devices, implants or grafts left in a surgical site (for example painful hip prosthesis) is assigned to the appropriate code(s) found in Chapter 19, Injury, poisoning, and certain other consequences of external causes. Specific codes for pain due to medical devices are found in the T code section of the ICD-10-CM. Use additional code(s) from category G89 to identify acute or chronic pain due to presence of the device, implant or graft (G89.18 or G89.28).

> Chronic left breast pain secondary to breast implant
>
> | T85.848A | **Pain due to other internal prosthetic devices, implants and grafts, initial encounter** |
> |---|---|
> | N64.4 | **Mastodynia** |
> | G89.28 | **Other chronic postprocedural pain** |
>
> *Explanation:* As the pain is a complication related to the breast implant, the complication code is sequenced first. The T code does not describe the site or type of pain, so additional codes may be appended to indicate that the patient is experiencing chronic pain in the breast.

3) Transplant complications

(a) Transplant complications other than kidney

Codes under category T86, Complications of transplanted organs and tissues, are for use for both complications and rejection of transplanted organs. A transplant complication code is only assigned if the complication affects the function of the transplanted organ. Two codes are required to fully describe a transplant complication: the appropriate code from category T86 and a secondary code that identifies the complication.

Pre-existing conditions or conditions that develop after the transplant are not coded as complications unless they affect the function of the transplanted organs.

See I.C.21. for transplant organ removal status

See I.C.2. for malignant neoplasm associated with transplanted organ.

(b) Kidney transplant complications

Patients who have undergone kidney transplant may still have some form of chronic kidney disease (CKD) because the kidney transplant may not fully restore kidney function. Code T86.1- should be assigned for documented complications of a kidney transplant, such as transplant failure or rejection or other transplant complication. Code T86.1- should not be assigned for post kidney transplant patients who have chronic kidney (CKD) unless a transplant complication such as transplant failure or rejection is documented. If the documentation is unclear as to whether the patient has a complication of the transplant, query the provider.

Conditions that affect the function of the transplanted kidney, other than CKD, should be assigned a code from subcategory T86.1, Complications of transplanted organ, Kidney, and a secondary code that identifies the complication.

For patients with CKD following a kidney transplant, but who do not have a complication such as failure or rejection, *see section I.C.14. Chronic kidney disease and kidney transplant status.*

> Patient seen for chronic kidney disease stage 2; history of successful kidney transplant with no complications identified
>
> | N18.2 | **Chronic kidney disease, stage 2 (mild)** |
> |---|---|
> | Z94.0 | **Kidney transplant status** |
>
> *Explanation:* This patient's stage 2 CKD is not indicated as being due to the transplanted kidney but instead is just the residual disease the patient had prior to the transplant.

4) Complication codes that include the external cause

As with certain other T codes, some of the complications of care codes have the external cause included in the code. The code includes the nature of the complication as well as the type of procedure that caused the complication. No external cause code indicating the type of procedure is necessary for these codes.

5) Complications of care codes within the body system chapters

Intraoperative and postprocedural complication codes are found within the body system chapters with codes specific to the organs and structures of that body system. These codes should be sequenced first, followed by a code(s) for the specific complication, if applicable.

> During a spinal fusion procedure, the surgeon inadvertently punctured the dura. The midline durotomy was repaired, and the fusion procedure was completed.
>
> | G97.41 | **Accidental puncture or laceration of dura during a procedure** |
> |---|---|
>
> *Explanation:* The accidental durotomy is not coded to an injury code in chapter 19 but instead is categorized to the nervous system chapter.

Muscle/Tendon Table

ICD-10-CM categorizes certain muscles and tendons in the upper and lower extremities by their action (e.g., extension, flexion), their anatomical location (e.g., posterior, anterior), and/or whether they are intrinsic or extrinsic to a certain anatomical area. The Muscle/Tendon Table is provided at the beginning of chapters 13 and 19 as a resource to help users when code selection depends on one or more of these characteristics. A **TIP** has been placed at those categories and/or subcategories that relate to this table. Please note that this table is not all-inclusive, and proper code assignment should be based on the provider's documentation.

Body Region	Muscle	Extensor Tendon	Flexor Tendon	Other Tendon
Shoulder				
	Deltoid	Posterior deltoid	Anterior deltoid	
	Rotator cuff			
	Infraspinatus			Infraspinatus
	Subscapularis			Subscapularis
	Supraspinatus			Supraspinatus
	Teres minor			Teres minor
	Teres major	Teres major		
Upper arm				
	Anterior muscles			
	Biceps brachii — long head		Biceps brachii — long head	
	Biceps brachii — short head		Biceps brachii — short head	
	Brachialis		Brachialis	
	Coracobrachialis		Coracobrachialis	
	Posterior muscles			
	Triceps brachii	Triceps brachii		
Forearm				
	Anterior muscles			
	Flexors			
	Deep			
	Flexor digitorum profundus		Flexor digitorum profundus	
	Flexor pollicis longus		Flexor pollicis longus	
	Intermediate			
	Flexor digitorum superficialis		Flexor digitorum superficialis	
	Superficial			
	Flexor carpi radialis		Flexor carpi radialis	
	Flexor carpi ulnaris		Flexor carpi ulnaris	
	Palmaris longus		Palmaris longus	
	Pronators			
	Pronator quadratus			Pronator quadratus
	Pronator teres			Pronator teres
	Posterior muscles			
	Extensors			
	Deep			
	Abductor pollicis longus			Abductor pollicis longus
	Extensor indicis	Extensor indicis		
	Extensor pollicis brevis	Extensor pollicis brevis		
	Extensor pollicis longus	Extensor pollicis longus		
	Superficial			
	Brachioradialis			Brachioradialis
	Extensor carpi radialis brevis	Extensor carpi radialis brevis		
	Extensor carpi radialis longus	Extensor carpi radialis longus		
	Extensor carpi ulnaris	Extensor carpi ulnaris		
	Extensor digiti minimi	Extensor digiti minimi		
	Extensor digitorum	Extensor digitorum		
	Anconeus	Anconeus		
	Supinator			Supinator

Body Region	Muscle	Extensor Tendon	Flexor Tendon	Other Tendon
Hand				
Extrinsic — attach to a site in the forearm as well as a site in the hand with action related to hand movement at the wrist				
	Extensor carpi radialis brevis	Extensor carpi radialis brevis		
	Extensor carpi radialis longus	Extensor carpie radialis longus		
	Extensor carpi ulnaris	Extensor carpi ulnaris		
	Flexor carpi radialis		Flexor carpi radialis	
	Flexor carpi ulnaris		Flexor carpi ulnaris	
	Flexor digitorum superficialis		Flexor digitorum superficialis	
	Palmaris longus		Palmaris longus	
Extrinsic — attach to a site in the forearm as well as a site in the hand with action in the hand related to finger movement				
	Adductor pollicis longus			Adductor pollicis longus
	Extensor digiti minimi	Extensor digiti minimi		
	Extensor digitorum	Extensor digitorum		
	Extensor indicis	Extensor indicis		
	Flexor digitorum profundus		Flexor digitorum profundus	
	Flexor digitorum superficialis		Flexor digitorum superficialis	
Extrinsic — attach to a site in the forearm as well as a site in the hand with action in the hand related to thumb movement				
	Extensor pollicis brevis	Extensor pollicis brevis		
	Extensor pollicis longus	Extensor pollicis longus		
	Flexor pollicis longus		Flexor pollicis longus	
Intrinsic — found within the hand only				
	Adductor pollicis			Adductor pollicis
	Dorsal interossei	Dorsal interossei	Dorsal interossei	
	Lumbricals	Lumbricals	Lumbricals	
	Palmaris brevis			Palmaris brevis
	Palmar interossei	Palmar interossei	Palmar interossei	
	Hypothenar muscles			
	Abductor digiti minimi			Abductor digiti minimi
	Flexor digiti minimi brevis		Flexor digiti minimi brevis	
	Oppenens digiti minimi		Oppenens digiti minimi	
	Thenar muscles			
	Abductor pollicis brevis			Abductor pollicis brevis
	Flexor pollicis brevis		Flexor pollicis brevis	
	Oppenens pollicis		Oppenens pollicis	
Thigh				
	Anterior muscles			
	Iliopsoas		Iliopsoas	
	Pectineus		Pectineus	
	Quadriceps	Quadriceps		
	Rectus femoris	Rectus femoris — Extends knee	Rectus femoris — Flexes hip	
	Vastus intermedius	Vastus intermedius		
	Vastus lateralis	Vastus lateralis		
	Vastus medialis	Vastus medialis		
	Sartorius		Sartorius	
	Medial muscles			
	Adductor brevis			Adductor brevis
	Adductor longus			Adductor longus
	Adductor magnus			Adductor magnus
	Gracilis			Gracilis
	Obturator externus			Obturator externus
	Posterior muscles			
	Hamstring	Hamstring — Extends hip	Hamstring — Flexes knee	
	Biceps femoris	Biceps femoris	Biceps femoris	
	Semimembranosus	Semimembranosus	Semimembranosus	
	Semitendinosus	Semitendinosus	Semitendinosus	

Body Region	Muscle	Extensor Tendon	Flexor Tendon	Other Tendon
Lower leg				
	Anterior muscles			
	Extensor digitorum longus	Extensor digitorum longus		
	Extensor hallucis longus	Extensor hallucis longus		
	Fibularis (peroneus) tertius	Fibularis (peroneus) tertius		
	Tibialis anterior	Tibialis anterior		Tibialis anterior
	Lateral muscles			
	Fibularis (peroneus) brevis		Fibularis (peroneus) brevis	
	Fibularis (peroneus) longus		Fibularis (peroneus) longus	
	Posterior muscles			
	Deep			
	Flexor digitorum longus		Flexor digitorum longus	
	Flexor hallucis longus		Flexor hallucis longus	
	Popliteus		Popliteus	
	Tibialis posterior		Tibialis posterior	
	Superficial			
	Gastrocnemius		Gastrocnemius	
	Plantaris		Plantaris	
	Soleus		Soleus	
				Calcaneal (Achilles)
Ankle/Foot				
Extrinsic — attach to a site in the lower leg as well as a site in the foot with action related to foot movement at the ankle				
	Plantaris		Plantaris	
	Soleus		Soleus	
	Tibialis anterior	Tibialis anterior		
	Tibialis posterior		Tibialis posterior	
Extrinsic — attach to a site in the lower leg as well as a site in the foot with action in the foot related to toe movement				
	Extensor digitorum longus	Extensor digitorum longus		
	Extensor hallicus longus	Extensor hallicus longus		
	Flexor digitorum longus		Flexor digitorum longus	
	Flexor hallucis longus		Flexor hallucis longus	
Intrinsic — found within the ankle/foot only				
	Dorsal muscles			
	Extensor digitorum brevis	Extensor digitorum brevis		
	Extensor hallucis brevis	Extensor hallucis brevis		
	Plantar muscles			
	Abductor digiti minimi		Abductor digiti minimi	
	Abductor hallucis		Abductor hallucis	
	Dorsal interossei	Dorsal interossei	Dorsal interossei	
	Flexor digiti minimi brevis		Flexor digiti minimi brevis	
	Flexor digitorum brevis		Flexor digitorum brevis	
	Flexor hallucis brevis		Flexor hallucis brevis	
	Lumbricals	Lumbricals	Lumbricals	
	Quadratus plantae		Quadratus plantae	
	Plantar interossei	Plantar interossei	Plantar interossei	

Chapter 19. Injury, Poisoning and Certain Other Consequences of External Causes (S00-T88)

NOTE   Use secondary code(s) from Chapter 20, External causes of morbidity, to indicate cause of injury. Codes within the T section that include the external cause do not require an additional external cause code.

Use additional code to identify any retained foreign body, if applicable (Z18.-)

EXCLUDES 1   birth trauma (P10-P15)
            obstetric trauma (O70-O71)

NOTE   The chapter uses the S-section for coding different types of injuries related to single body regions and the T-section to cover injuries to unspecified body regions as well as poisoning and certain other consequences of external causes.

AHA: 2016, 2Q, 3-7; 2015, 4Q, 35-38; 2015, 3Q, 37-39, 40; 2015, 2Q, 6; 2015, 1Q, 3-21

This chapter contains the following blocks:

S00-S09	Injuries to the head
S10-S19	Injuries to the neck
S20-S29	Injuries to the thorax
S30-S39	Injuries to the abdomen, lower back, lumbar spine, pelvis and external genitals
S40-S49	Injuries to the shoulder and upper arm
S50-S59	Injuries to the elbow and forearm
S60-S69	Injuries to the wrist, hand and fingers
S70-S79	Injuries to the hip and thigh
S80-S89	Injuries to the knee and lower leg
S90-S99	Injuries to the ankle and foot
T07	Injuries involving multiple body regions
T14	Injury of unspecified body region
T15-T19	Effects of foreign body entering through natural orifice
T20-T25	Burns and corrosions of external body surface, specified by site
T26-T28	Burns and corrosions confined to eye and internal organs
T30-T32	Burns and corrosions of multiple and unspecified body regions
T33-T34	Frostbite
T36-T50	Poisoning by, adverse effect of and underdosing of drugs, medicaments and biological substances
T51-T65	Toxic effects of substances chiefly nonmedicinal as to source
T66-T78	Other and unspecified effects of external causes
T79	Certain early complications of trauma
T80-T88	Complications of surgical and medical care, not elsewhere classified

Injuries to the head (S00-S09)

INCLUDES   injuries of ear
              injuries of eye
              injuries of face [any part]
              injuries of gum
              injuries of jaw
              injuries of oral cavity
              injuries of palate
              injuries of periocular area
              injuries of scalp
              injuries of temporomandibular joint area
              injuries of tongue
              injuries of tooth

Code also for any associated infection

EXCLUDES 2   burns and corrosions (T20-T32)
            effects of foreign body in ear (T16)
            effects of foreign body in larynx (T17.3)
            effects of foreign body in mouth NOS (T18.0)
            effects of foreign body in nose (T17.0-T17.1)
            effects of foreign body in pharynx (T17.2)
            effects of foreign body on external eye (T15.-)
            frostbite (T33-T34)
            insect bite or sting, venomous (T63.4)

√4ᵗʰ **S00**   **Superficial injury of head**

EXCLUDES 1   diffuse cerebral contusion (S06.2-)
            focal cerebral contusion (S06.3-)
            injury of eye and orbit (S05.-)
            open wound of head (S01.-)

> The appropriate 7th character is to be added to each code from category S00.
> A   initial encounter
> D   subsequent encounter
> S   sequela

√5ᵗʰ **S00.0**   **Superficial injury of scalp**

    √x7ᵗʰ **S00.00**   **Unspecified superficial injury of scalp** ▽

    √x7ᵗʰ **S00.01**   Abrasion of scalp

    √x7ᵗʰ **S00.02**   Blister (nonthermal) of scalp

    √x7ᵗʰ **S00.03**   Contusion of scalp
                      Bruise of scalp
                      Hematoma of scalp

    √x7ᵗʰ **S00.04**   External constriction of part of scalp

    √x7ᵗʰ **S00.05**   Superficial foreign body of scalp
                      Splinter in the scalp

    √x7ᵗʰ **S00.06**   Insect bite (nonvenomous) of scalp

    √x7ᵗʰ **S00.07**   **Other superficial bite of scalp**
           EXCLUDES 1   open bite of scalp (S01.05)

√5ᵗʰ **S00.1**   **Contusion of eyelid and periocular area**
         Black eye
         EXCLUDES 2   contusion of eyeball and orbital tissues (S05.1)

    √x7ᵗʰ **S00.10**   **Contusion of unspecified eyelid and periocular area** ▽

    √x7ᵗʰ **S00.11**   **Contusion of right eyelid and periocular area**

    √x7ᵗʰ **S00.12**   **Contusion of left eyelid and periocular area**

√5ᵗʰ **S00.2**   **Other and unspecified superficial injuries of eyelid and periocular area**
         EXCLUDES 2   superficial injury of conjunctiva and cornea (S05.0-)

    √6ᵗʰ **S00.20**   **Unspecified superficial injury of eyelid and periocular area**

       √7ᵗʰ **S00.201**   **Unspecified superficial injury of right eyelid and periocular area** ▽

       √7ᵗʰ **S00.202**   **Unspecified superficial injury of left eyelid and periocular area** ▽

       √7ᵗʰ **S00.209**   **Unspecified superficial injury of unspecified eyelid and periocular area** ▽

    √6ᵗʰ **S00.21**   Abrasion of eyelid and periocular area

       √7ᵗʰ **S00.211**   **Abrasion of right eyelid and periocular area**

       √7ᵗʰ **S00.212**   **Abrasion of left eyelid and periocular area**

       √7ᵗʰ **S00.219**   **Abrasion of unspecified eyelid and periocular area** ▽

    √6ᵗʰ **S00.22**   Blister (nonthermal) of eyelid and periocular area

       √7ᵗʰ **S00.221**   **Blister (nonthermal) of right eyelid and periocular area**

       √7ᵗʰ **S00.222**   **Blister (nonthermal) of left eyelid and periocular area**

       √7ᵗʰ **S00.229**   **Blister (nonthermal) of unspecified eyelid and periocular area** ▽

    √6ᵗʰ **S00.24**   External constriction of eyelid and periocular area

       √7ᵗʰ **S00.241**   **External constriction of right eyelid and periocular area**

       √7ᵗʰ **S00.242**   **External constriction of left eyelid and periocular area**

       √7ᵗʰ **S00.249**   **External constriction of unspecified eyelid and periocular area** ▽

    √6ᵗʰ **S00.25**   **Superficial foreign body of eyelid and periocular area**
           Splinter of eyelid and periocular area
           EXCLUDES 2   retained foreign body in eyelid (H02.81-)

       √7ᵗʰ **S00.251**   **Superficial foreign body of right eyelid and periocular area**

       √7ᵗʰ **S00.252**   **Superficial foreign body of left eyelid and periocular area**

       √7ᵗʰ **S00.259**   **Superficial foreign body of unspecified eyelid and periocular area** ▽

    √6ᵗʰ **S00.26**   Insect bite (nonvenomous) of eyelid and periocular area

       √7ᵗʰ **S00.261**   **Insect bite (nonvenomous) of right eyelid and periocular area**

       √7ᵗʰ **S00.262**   **Insect bite (nonvenomous) of left eyelid and periocular area**

       √7ᵗʰ **S00.269**   **Insect bite (nonvenomous) of unspecified eyelid and periocular area** ▽

    √6ᵗʰ **S00.27**   Other superficial bite of eyelid and periocular area
           EXCLUDES 1   open bite of eyelid and periocular area (S01.15)

       √7ᵗʰ **S00.271**   **Other superficial bite of right eyelid and periocular area**

       √7ᵗʰ **S00.272**   **Other superficial bite of left eyelid and periocular area**

       √7ᵗʰ **S00.279**   **Other superficial bite of unspecified eyelid and periocular area** ▽

✓5ᵗʰ **S00.3** **Superficial injury of** nose

✓x7ᵗʰ **S00.30** **Unspecified superficial injury of nose** ▽

✓x7ᵗʰ **S00.31** **Abrasion of nose**

✓x7ᵗʰ **S00.32** **Blister (nonthermal) of nose**

✓x7ᵗʰ **S00.33** **Contusion of nose**
Bruise of nose
Hematoma of nose

✓x7ᵗʰ **S00.34** **External constriction of nose**

✓x7ᵗʰ **S00.35** **Superficial foreign body of nose**
Splinter in the nose

✓x7ᵗʰ **S00.36** **Insect bite (nonvenomous) of nose**

✓x7ᵗʰ **S00.37** **Other superficial bite of nose**
EXCLUDES 1　*open bite of nose (S01.25)*

✓5ᵗʰ **S00.4** **Superficial injury of** ear

✓6ᵗʰ **S00.40** **Unspecified superficial injury of ear**

✓7ᵗʰ **S00.401** **Unspecified superficial injury of right ear** ▽

✓7ᵗʰ **S00.402** **Unspecified superficial injury of left ear** ▽

✓7ᵗʰ **S00.409** **Unspecified superficial injury of unspecified ear** ▽

✓6ᵗʰ **S00.41** **Abrasion of ear**

✓7ᵗʰ **S00.411** **Abrasion of right ear**

✓7ᵗʰ **S00.412** **Abrasion of left ear**

✓7ᵗʰ **S00.419** **Abrasion of unspecified ear** ▽

✓6ᵗʰ **S00.42** **Blister (nonthermal) of ear**

✓7ᵗʰ **S00.421** **Blister (nonthermal) of right ear**

✓7ᵗʰ **S00.422** **Blister (nonthermal) of left ear**

✓7ᵗʰ **S00.429** **Blister (nonthermal) of unspecified ear** ▽

✓6ᵗʰ **S00.43** **Contusion of ear**
Bruise of ear
Hematoma of ear

✓7ᵗʰ **S00.431** **Contusion of right ear**

✓7ᵗʰ **S00.432** **Contusion of left ear**

✓7ᵗʰ **S00.439** **Contusion of unspecified ear** ▽

✓6ᵗʰ **S00.44** **External constriction of ear**

✓7ᵗʰ **S00.441** **External constriction of right ear**

✓7ᵗʰ **S00.442** **External constriction of left ear**

✓7ᵗʰ **S00.449** **External constriction of unspecified ear** ▽

✓6ᵗʰ **S00.45** **Superficial foreign body of ear**
Splinter in the ear

✓7ᵗʰ **S00.451** **Superficial foreign body of right ear**

✓7ᵗʰ **S00.452** **Superficial foreign body of left ear**

✓7ᵗʰ **S00.459** **Superficial foreign body of unspecified ear** ▽

✓6ᵗʰ **S00.46** **Insect bite (nonvenomous) of ear**

✓7ᵗʰ **S00.461** **Insect bite (nonvenomous) of right ear**

✓7ᵗʰ **S00.462** **Insect bite (nonvenomous) of left ear**

✓7ᵗʰ **S00.469** **Insect bite (nonvenomous) of unspecified ear** ▽

✓6ᵗʰ **S00.47** **Other superficial bite of ear**
EXCLUDES 1　*open bite of ear (S01.35)*

✓7ᵗʰ **S00.471** **Other superficial bite of right ear**

✓7ᵗʰ **S00.472** **Other superficial bite of left ear**

✓7ᵗʰ **S00.479** **Other superficial bite of unspecified ear** ▽

✓5ᵗʰ **S00.5** **Superficial injury of** lip and oral cavity

✓6ᵗʰ **S00.50** **Unspecified superficial injury of lip and oral cavity**

✓7ᵗʰ **S00.501** **Unspecified superficial injury of lip** ▽

✓7ᵗʰ **S00.502** **Unspecified superficial injury of oral cavity** ▽

✓6ᵗʰ **S00.51** **Abrasion of lip and oral cavity**

✓7ᵗʰ **S00.511** **Abrasion of lip**

✓7ᵗʰ **S00.512** **Abrasion of oral cavity**

✓6ᵗʰ **S00.52** **Blister (nonthermal) of lip and oral cavity**

✓7ᵗʰ **S00.521** **Blister (nonthermal) of lip**

✓7ᵗʰ **S00.522** **Blister (nonthermal) of oral cavity**

✓6ᵗʰ **S00.53** **Contusion of lip and oral cavity**

✓7ᵗʰ **S00.531** **Contusion of lip**
Bruise of lip
▶Hematoma of lip◀

✓7ᵗʰ **S00.532** **Contusion of oral cavity**
▶Bruise of oral cavity◀
Hematoma of oral cavity

✓6ᵗʰ **S00.54** **External constriction of lip and oral cavity**

✓7ᵗʰ **S00.541** **External constriction of lip**

✓7ᵗʰ **S00.542** **External constriction of oral cavity**

✓6ᵗʰ **S00.55** **Superficial foreign body of lip and oral cavity**

✓7ᵗʰ **S00.551** **Superficial foreign body of lip**
Splinter of lip and oral cavity

✓7ᵗʰ **S00.552** **Superficial foreign body of oral cavity**
Splinter of lip and oral cavity

✓6ᵗʰ **S00.56** **Insect bite (nonvenomous) of lip and oral cavity**

✓7ᵗʰ **S00.561** **Insect bite (nonvenomous) of lip**

✓7ᵗʰ **S00.562** **Insect bite (nonvenomous) of oral cavity**

✓6ᵗʰ **S00.57** **Other superficial bite of lip and oral cavity**

✓7ᵗʰ **S00.571** **Other superficial bite of lip**
EXCLUDES 1　*open bite of lip (S01.551)*

✓7ᵗʰ **S00.572** **Other superficial bite of oral cavity**
EXCLUDES 1　*open bite of oral cavity (S01.552)*

✓5ᵗʰ **S00.8** **Superficial injury of other parts of head**
Superfical injuries of face [any part]

✓x7ᵗʰ **S00.80** **Unspecified superficial injury of other part of head** ▽

✓x7ᵗʰ **S00.81** **Abrasion of other part of head**

✓x7ᵗʰ **S00.82** **Blister (nonthermal) of other part of head**

✓x7ᵗʰ **S00.83** **Contusion of other part of head**
Bruise of other part of head
Hematoma of other part of head

✓x7ᵗʰ **S00.84** **External constriction of other part of head**

✓x7ᵗʰ **S00.85** **Superficial foreign body of other part of head**
Splinter in other part of head

✓x7ᵗʰ **S00.86** **Insect bite (nonvenomous) of other part of head**

✓x7ᵗʰ **S00.87** **Other superficial bite of other part of head**
EXCLUDES 1　*open bite of other part of head (S01.85)*

✓5ᵗʰ **S00.9** **Superficial injury of unspecified part of head**

✓x7ᵗʰ **S00.90** **Unspecified superficial injury of unspecified part of head** ▽

✓x7ᵗʰ **S00.91** **Abrasion of unspecified part of head** ▽

✓x7ᵗʰ **S00.92** **Blister (nonthermal) of unspecified part of head** ▽

✓x7ᵗʰ **S00.93** **Contusion of unspecified part of head** ▽
Bruise of head
Hematoma of head

✓x7ᵗʰ **S00.94** **External constriction of unspecified part of head** ▽

✓x7ᵗʰ **S00.95** **Superficial foreign body of unspecified part of head** ▽
Splinter of head

✓x7ᵗʰ **S00.96** **Insect bite (nonvenomous) of unspecified part of head** ▽

✓x7ᵗʰ **S00.97** **Other superficial bite of unspecified part of head** ▽
EXCLUDES 1　*open bite of head (S01.95)*

✓4ᵗʰ **S01** **Open wound of head**
Code also any associated:
injury of cranial nerve (S04.-)
injury of muscle and tendon of head (S09.1-)
intracranial injury (S06.-)
wound infection
EXCLUDES 1　*open skull fracture (S02- with 7th character B)*
EXCLUDES 2　*injury of eye and orbit (S05.-)*
traumatic amputation of part of head (S08.-)

The appropriate 7th character is to be added to each code from category S01.
A　initial encounter
D　subsequent encounter
S　sequela

✓5ᵗʰ **S01.0** **Open wound of scalp**
EXCLUDES 1　*avulsion of scalp (S08.0)*

✓x7ᵗʰ **S01.00** **Unspecified open wound of scalp** ▽

✓x7ᵗʰ **S01.01** **Laceration without foreign body of scalp**

✓ Additional Character Req　✓x7ᵗʰ Placeholder Alert　**Manifestation**　**HCC** CMS-HCC Condition　▽ Unspecified Code　▶◀ Revised Text　● New Code　▲ Revised Code Title

✓x7ᵗʰ **S01.02** Laceration with foreign body **of scalp**

✓x7ᵗʰ **S01.03** Puncture wound without foreign body **of scalp**

✓x7ᵗʰ **S01.04** Puncture wound with foreign body **of scalp**

✓x7ᵗʰ **S01.05** Open bite **of scalp**
Bite of scalp NOS
EXCLUDES 1   superficial bite of scalp (S00.06, S00.07-)

✓5ᵗʰ **S01.1** **Open wound of** eyelid and periocular area
Open wound of eyelid and periocular area with or without involvement of lacrimal passages

   ✓6ᵗʰ **S01.10** **Unspecified open wound of eyelid and periocular area**

     ✓7ᵗʰ **S01.101** **Unspecified open wound of** right **eyelid and periocular area** ▽

     ✓7ᵗʰ **S01.102** **Unspecified open wound of** left **eyelid and periocular area** ▽

     ✓7ᵗʰ **S01.109** **Unspecified open wound of unspecified eyelid and periocular area** ▽

   ✓6ᵗʰ **S01.11** Laceration without foreign body **of eyelid and periocular area**

     ✓7ᵗʰ **S01.111** **Laceration without foreign body of** right **eyelid and periocular area**

     ✓7ᵗʰ **S01.112** **Laceration without foreign body of** left **eyelid and periocular area**

     ✓7ᵗʰ **S01.119** **Laceration without foreign body of unspecified eyelid and periocular area** ▽

   ✓6ᵗʰ **S01.12** Laceration with foreign body **of eyelid and periocular area**

     ✓7ᵗʰ **S01.121** **Laceration with foreign body of** right **eyelid and periocular area**

     ✓7ᵗʰ **S01.122** **Laceration with foreign body of** left **eyelid and periocular area**

     ✓7ᵗʰ **S01.129** **Laceration with foreign body of unspecified eyelid and periocular area** ▽

   ✓6ᵗʰ **S01.13** Puncture wound without foreign body **of eyelid and periocular area**

     ✓7ᵗʰ **S01.131** **Puncture wound without foreign body of** right **eyelid and periocular area**

     ✓7ᵗʰ **S01.132** **Puncture wound without foreign body of** left **eyelid and periocular area**

     ✓7ᵗʰ **S01.139** **Puncture wound without foreign body of unspecified eyelid and periocular area** ▽

   ✓6ᵗʰ **S01.14** Puncture wound with foreign body **of eyelid and periocular area**

     ✓7ᵗʰ **S01.141** **Puncture wound with foreign body of** right **eyelid and periocular area**

     ✓7ᵗʰ **S01.142** **Puncture wound with foreign body of** left **eyelid and periocular area**

     ✓7ᵗʰ **S01.149** **Puncture wound with foreign body of unspecified eyelid and periocular area** ▽

   ✓6ᵗʰ **S01.15** Open bite **of eyelid and periocular area**
Bite of eyelid and periocular area NOS
EXCLUDES 1   superficial bite of eyelid and periocular area (S00.26, S00.27)

     ✓7ᵗʰ **S01.151** **Open bite of** right **eyelid and periocular area**

     ✓7ᵗʰ **S01.152** **Open bite of** left **eyelid and periocular area**

     ✓7ᵗʰ **S01.159** **Open bite of unspecified eyelid and periocular area** ▽

✓5ᵗʰ **S01.2** **Open wound of** nose

   ✓x7ᵗʰ **S01.20** **Unspecified open wound of nose** ▽

   ✓x7ᵗʰ **S01.21** Laceration without foreign body **of nose**

   ✓x7ᵗʰ **S01.22** Laceration with foreign body **of nose**

   ✓x7ᵗʰ **S01.23** Puncture wound without foreign body **of nose**

   ✓x7ᵗʰ **S01.24** Puncture wound with foreign body **of nose**

   ✓x7ᵗʰ **S01.25** Open bite **of nose**
Bite of nose NOS
EXCLUDES 1   superficial bite of nose (S00.36, S00.37)

✓5ᵗʰ **S01.3** **Open wound of** ear

   ✓6ᵗʰ **S01.30** **Unspecified open wound of ear**

     ✓7ᵗʰ **S01.301** **Unspecified open wound of** right **ear** ▽

     ✓7ᵗʰ **S01.302** **Unspecified open wound of** left **ear** ▽

     ✓7ᵗʰ **S01.309** **Unspecified open wound of unspecified ear** ▽

   ✓6ᵗʰ **S01.31** Laceration without foreign body **of ear**

     ✓7ᵗʰ **S01.311** **Laceration without foreign body of** right **ear**

     ✓7ᵗʰ **S01.312** **Laceration without foreign body of** left **ear**

     ✓7ᵗʰ **S01.319** **Laceration without foreign body of unspecified ear**

   ✓6ᵗʰ **S01.32** Laceration with foreign body **of ear**

     ✓7ᵗʰ **S01.321** **Laceration with foreign body of** right **ear**

     ✓7ᵗʰ **S01.322** **Laceration with foreign body of** left **ear**

     ✓7ᵗʰ **S01.329** **Laceration with foreign body of unspecified ear** ▽

   ✓6ᵗʰ **S01.33** Puncture wound without foreign body **of ear**

     ✓7ᵗʰ **S01.331** **Puncture wound without foreign body of** right **ear**

     ✓7ᵗʰ **S01.332** **Puncture wound without foreign body of** left **ear**

     ✓7ᵗʰ **S01.339** **Puncture wound without foreign body of unspecified ear** ▽

   ✓6ᵗʰ **S01.34** Puncture wound with foreign body **of ear**

     ✓7ᵗʰ **S01.341** **Puncture wound with foreign body of** right **ear**

     ✓7ᵗʰ **S01.342** **Puncture wound with foreign body of** left **ear**

     ✓7ᵗʰ **S01.349** **Puncture wound with foreign body of unspecified ear** ▽

   ✓6ᵗʰ **S01.35** Open bite **of ear**
Bite of ear NOS
EXCLUDES 1   superficial bite of ear (S00.46, S00.47)

     ✓7ᵗʰ **S01.351** **Open bite of** right **ear**

     ✓7ᵗʰ **S01.352** **Open bite of** left **ear**

     ✓7ᵗʰ **S01.359** **Open bite of unspecified ear** ▽

✓5ᵗʰ **S01.4** **Open wound of** cheek and temporomandibular area

   ✓6ᵗʰ **S01.40** **Unspecified open wound of cheek and temporomandibular area**

     ✓7ᵗʰ **S01.401** **Unspecified open wound of** right **cheek and temporomandibular area** ▽

     ✓7ᵗʰ **S01.402** **Unspecified open wound of** left **cheek and temporomandibular area** ▽

     ✓7ᵗʰ **S01.409** **Unspecified open wound of unspecified cheek and temporomandibular area** ▽

   ✓6ᵗʰ **S01.41** Laceration without foreign body **of cheek and temporomandibular area**

     ✓7ᵗʰ **S01.411** **Laceration without foreign body of** right **cheek and temporomandibular area**

     ✓7ᵗʰ **S01.412** **Laceration without foreign body of** left **cheek and temporomandibular area**

     ✓7ᵗʰ **S01.419** **Laceration without foreign body of unspecified cheek and temporomandibular area** ▽

   ✓6ᵗʰ **S01.42** Laceration with foreign body **of cheek and temporomandibular area**

     ✓7ᵗʰ **S01.421** **Laceration with foreign body of** right **cheek and temporomandibular area**

     ✓7ᵗʰ **S01.422** **Laceration with foreign body of** left **cheek and temporomandibular area**

     ✓7ᵗʰ **S01.429** **Laceration with foreign body of unspecified cheek and temporomandibular area** ▽

   ✓6ᵗʰ **S01.43** Puncture wound without foreign body **of cheek and temporomandibular area**

     ✓7ᵗʰ **S01.431** **Puncture wound without foreign body of** right **cheek and temporomandibular area**

     ✓7ᵗʰ **S01.432** **Puncture wound without foreign body of** left **cheek and temporomandibular area**

     ✓7ᵗʰ **S01.439** **Puncture wound without foreign body of unspecified cheek and temporomandibular area** ▽

   ✓6ᵗʰ **S01.44** Puncture wound with foreign body **of cheek and temporomandibular area**

     ✓7ᵗʰ **S01.441** **Puncture wound with foreign body of** right **cheek and temporomandibular area**

EXCLUDES 1 Not coded here   *EXCLUDES 2* Not included here   Ⓝ Newborn Age: 0   Ⓟ Pediatric Age: 0-17   Ⓜ Maternity Age: 12-55   Ⓐ Adult Age: 15-124

916   ICD-10-CM 2018

✓7ᵗʰ **S01.442** **Puncture wound with foreign body of** left **cheek and temporomandibular area**

✓7ᵗʰ **S01.449** **Puncture wound with foreign body of unspecified cheek and temporomandibular area** ▽

✓6ᵗʰ **S01.45** Open bite **of cheek and temporomandibular area**
Bite of cheek and temporomandibular area NOS
EXCLUDES 2   superficial bite of cheek and temporomandibular area (S00.86, S00.87)

✓7ᵗʰ **S01.451** **Open bite of** right **cheek and temporomandibular area**

✓7ᵗʰ **S01.452** **Open bite of** left **cheek and temporomandibular area**

✓7ᵗʰ **S01.459** **Open bite of unspecified cheek and temporomandibular area** ▽

✓5ᵗʰ **S01.5** **Open wound of** lip and oral cavity
EXCLUDES 2   tooth dislocation (S03.2)
tooth fracture (S02.5)

✓6ᵗʰ **S01.50** **Unspecified open wound of lip and oral cavity**

✓7ᵗʰ **S01.501** **Unspecified open wound of** lip ▽

✓7ᵗʰ **S01.502** **Unspecified open wound of** oral cavity ▽

✓6ᵗʰ **S01.51** Laceration **of lip and oral cavity** without foreign body

✓7ᵗʰ **S01.511** **Laceration without foreign body of** lip

✓7ᵗʰ **S01.512** **Laceration without foreign body of** oral cavity

✓6ᵗʰ **S01.52** Laceration **of lip and oral cavity** with foreign body

✓7ᵗʰ **S01.521** **Laceration with foreign body of** lip

✓7ᵗʰ **S01.522** **Laceration with foreign body of** oral cavity

✓6ᵗʰ **S01.53** Puncture wound **of lip and oral cavity** without foreign body

✓7ᵗʰ **S01.531** **Puncture wound without foreign body of** lip

✓7ᵗʰ **S01.532** **Puncture wound without foreign body of** oral cavity

✓6ᵗʰ **S01.54** Puncture wound **of lip and oral cavity** with foreign body

✓7ᵗʰ **S01.541** **Puncture wound with foreign body of** lip

✓7ᵗʰ **S01.542** **Puncture wound with foreign body of** oral cavity

✓6ᵗʰ **S01.55** Open bite **of lip and oral cavity**

✓7ᵗʰ **S01.551** **Open bite of** lip
Bite of lip NOS
EXCLUDES 1   superficial bite of lip (S00.571)

✓7ᵗʰ **S01.552** **Open bite of** oral cavity
Bite of oral cavity NOS
EXCLUDES 1   superficial bite of oral cavity (S00.572)

✓5ᵗʰ **S01.8** **Open wound of other parts of head**

✓x7ᵗʰ **S01.80** **Unspecified open wound of other part of head** ▽

✓x7ᵗʰ **S01.81** Laceration without foreign body **of other part of head**

✓x7ᵗʰ **S01.82** Laceration with foreign body **of other part of head**

✓x7ᵗʰ **S01.83** Puncture wound without foreign body **of other part of head**

✓x7ᵗʰ **S01.84** Puncture wound with foreign body **of other part of head**

✓x7ᵗʰ **S01.85** Open bite **of other part of head**
Bite of other part of head NOS
EXCLUDES 1   superficial bite of other part of head ▶(S00.87)◀

✓5ᵗʰ **S01.9** **Open wound of unspecified part of head**

✓x7ᵗʰ **S01.90** **Unspecified open wound of unspecified part of head** ▽

✓x7ᵗʰ **S01.91** Laceration without foreign body **of unspecified part of head** ▽

✓x7ᵗʰ **S01.92** Laceration with foreign body **of unspecified part of head** ▽

✓x7ᵗʰ **S01.93** Puncture wound without foreign body **of unspecified part of head** ▽

✓x7ᵗʰ **S01.94** Puncture wound with foreign body **of unspecified part of head** ▽

✓x7ᵗʰ **S01.95** Open bite **of unspecified part of head** ▽
Bite of head NOS
EXCLUDES 1   superficial bite of head NOS (S00.97)

✓4ᵗʰ **S02** **Fracture of skull and facial bones**
NOTE   A fracture not indicated as open or closed should be coded to closed.
Code also any associated intracranial injury (S06.-).
AHA: 2017, 1Q, 42

The appropriate 7th character is to be added to each code from category S02.
A   initial encounter for closed fracture
B   initial encounter for open fracture
D   subsequent encounter for fracture with routine healing
G   subsequent encounter for fracture with delayed healing
K   subsequent encounter for fracture with nonunion
S   sequela

2 ✓x7ᵗʰ **S02.0** **Fracture of** vault **of skull** HCC
Fracture of frontal bone
Fracture of parietal bone

✓5ᵗʰ **S02.1** **Fracture of** base **of skull**
EXCLUDES 1   orbit NOS (S02.8)
EXCLUDES 2   orbital floor (S02.3-)

✓6ᵗʰ **S02.10** **Unspecified fracture of base of skull**

2 ✓7ᵗʰ **S02.101** **Fracture of base of skull,** right **side** HCC

2 ✓7ᵗʰ **S02.102** **Fracture of base of skull,** left **side** HCC

2 ✓7ᵗʰ **S02.109** **Fracture of base of skull, unspecified side** HCC ▽

✓6ᵗʰ **S02.11** **Fracture of** occiput

2 ✓7ᵗʰ **S02.110** Type I **occipital condyle fracture, unspecified side** HCC ▽

2 ✓7ᵗʰ **S02.111** Type II **occipital condyle fracture, unspecified side** HCC ▽

2 ✓7ᵗʰ **S02.112** Type III **occipital condyle fracture, unspecified side** HCC ▽

2 ✓7ᵗʰ **S02.113** **Unspecified occipital condyle fracture** HCC ▽

2 ✓7ᵗʰ **S02.118** **Other fracture of occiput, unspecified side** HCC ▽

2 ✓7ᵗʰ **S02.119** **Unspecified fracture of occiput** HCC ▽

2 ✓7ᵗʰ **S02.11A** Type I **occipital condyle fracture,** right **side** HCC

2 ✓7ᵗʰ **S02.11B** Type I **occipital condyle fracture,** left **side** HCC

2 ✓7ᵗʰ **S02.11C** Type II **occipital condyle fracture,** right **side** HCC

2 ✓7ᵗʰ **S02.11D** Type II **occipital condyle fracture,** left **side** HCC

2 ✓7ᵗʰ **S02.11E** Type III **occipital condyle fracture,** right **side** HCC

2 ✓7ᵗʰ **S02.11F** Type III **occipital condyle fracture,** left **side** HCC

2 ✓7ᵗʰ **S02.11G** **Other fracture of occiput,** right **side** HCC

2 ✓7ᵗʰ **S02.11H** **Other fracture of occiput,** left **side** HCC

2 ✓x7ᵗʰ **S02.19** **Other fracture of base of skull** HCC
Fracture of anterior fossa of base of skull
Fracture of ethmoid sinus
Fracture of frontal sinus
Fracture of middle fossa of base of skull
Fracture of orbital roof
Fracture of posterior fossa of base of skull
Fracture of sphenoid
Fracture of temporal bone

✓x7ᵗʰ **S02.2** **Fracture of** nasal bones

✓5ᵗʰ **S02.3** **Fracture of** orbital floor
EXCLUDES 1   orbit NOS (S02.8)
EXCLUDES 2   orbital roof (S02.1-)

2 ✓x7ᵗʰ **S02.30** **Fracture of orbital floor, unspecified side** HCC ▽

2 ✓x7ᵗʰ **S02.31** **Fracture of orbital floor,** right **side** HCC

2 ✓x7ᵗʰ **S02.32** **Fracture of orbital floor,** left **side** HCC

---

2   HCC with 7th character indicating initial encounter (A or B - specific to category) OR sequela.

✓ Additional Character Req   ✓x7ᵗʰ Placeholder Alert   Manifestation   HCC CMS-HCC Condition   ▽ Unspecified Code   ▶◀ Revised Text   ● New Code   ▲ Revised Code Title

ICD-10-CM 2018   917

Chapter 19. Injury, Poisoning, and Certain Other Consequences of External Causes

S02.4–S03.9

LeFort Fracture Types

Frontal bone   Nasal bone   Orbital floor

Type III

Type II

Type I

Maxilla

Zygomatic bone (malar) and arch

✓5ᵗʰ **S02.4 Fracture of** malar, maxillary and zygoma bones
　　Fracture of superior maxilla
　　Fracture of upper jaw (bone)
　　Fracture of zygomatic process of temporal bone

　✓6ᵗʰ **S02.40 Fracture of malar, maxillary and zygoma bones, unspecified**
　　² ✓7ᵗʰ **S02.400** Malar fracture, unspecified side   HCC ▽
　　² ✓7ᵗʰ **S02.401** Maxillary fracture, unspecified side   HCC ▽
　　² ✓7ᵗʰ **S02.402** Zygomatic fracture, unspecified side   HCC ▽
　　² ✓7ᵗʰ **S02.40A** Malar fracture, right side   HCC
　　² ✓7ᵗʰ **S02.40B** Malar fracture, left side   HCC
　　² ✓7ᵗʰ **S02.40C** Maxillary fracture, right side   HCC
　　² ✓7ᵗʰ **S02.40D** Maxillary fracture, left side   HCC
　　² ✓7ᵗʰ **S02.40E** Zygomatic fracture, right side   HCC
　　² ✓7ᵗʰ **S02.40F** Zygomatic fracture, left side   HCC

　✓6ᵗʰ **S02.41 LeFort fracture**
　　² ✓7ᵗʰ **S02.411** LeFort I fracture   HCC
　　² ✓7ᵗʰ **S02.412** LeFort II fracture   HCC
　　² ✓7ᵗʰ **S02.413** LeFort III fracture   HCC

　² ✓x7ᵗʰ **S02.42 Fracture of** alveolus of maxilla   HCC

✓x7ᵗʰ **S02.5 Fracture of** tooth (traumatic)
　　Broken tooth
　　EXCLUDES 1   cracked tooth (nontraumatic) (K03.81)

✓5ᵗʰ **S02.6 Fracture of** mandible
　　Fracture of lower jaw (bone)

　✓6ᵗʰ **S02.60 Fracture of mandible, unspecified**
　　² ✓7ᵗʰ **S02.600** Fracture of unspecified part of body of mandible, unspecified side   HCC ▽
　　² ✓7ᵗʰ **S02.601** Fracture of unspecified part of body of right mandible   HCC ▽
　　² ✓7ᵗʰ **S02.602** Fracture of unspecified part of body of left mandible   HCC ▽
　　² ✓7ᵗʰ **S02.609** Fracture of mandible, unspecified   HCC ▽

　✓6ᵗʰ **S02.61 Fracture of** condylar process of mandible
　　² ✓7ᵗʰ **S02.610** Fracture of condylar process of mandible, unspecified side   HCC ▽
　　² ✓7ᵗʰ **S02.611** Fracture of condylar process of right mandible   HCC
　　² ✓7ᵗʰ **S02.612** Fracture of condylar process of left mandible   HCC

　✓6ᵗʰ **S02.62 Fracture of** subcondylar process of mandible
　　² ✓7ᵗʰ **S02.620** Fracture of subcondylar process of mandible, unspecified side   HCC ▽
　　² ✓7ᵗʰ **S02.621** Fracture of subcondylar process of right mandible   HCC
　　² ✓7ᵗʰ **S02.622** Fracture of subcondylar process of left mandible   HCC

　✓6ᵗʰ **S02.63 Fracture of** coronoid process of mandible
　　² ✓7ᵗʰ **S02.630** Fracture of coronoid process of mandible, unspecified side   HCC ▽
　　² ✓7ᵗʰ **S02.631** Fracture of coronoid process of right mandible   HCC
　　² ✓7ᵗʰ **S02.632** Fracture of coronoid process of left mandible   HCC

　✓6ᵗʰ **S02.64 Fracture of** ramus of mandible
　　² ✓7ᵗʰ **S02.640** Fracture of ramus of mandible, unspecified side   HCC ▽
　　² ✓7ᵗʰ **S02.641** Fracture of ramus of right mandible   HCC
　　² ✓7ᵗʰ **S02.642** Fracture of ramus of left mandible   HCC

　✓6ᵗʰ **S02.65 Fracture of** angle of mandible
　　² ✓7ᵗʰ **S02.650** Fracture of angle of mandible, unspecified side   HCC ▽
　　² ✓7ᵗʰ **S02.651** Fracture of angle of right mandible   HCC
　　² ✓7ᵗʰ **S02.652** Fracture of angle of left mandible   HCC

　² ✓x7ᵗʰ **S02.66 Fracture of** symphysis of mandible   HCC

　✓6ᵗʰ **S02.67 Fracture of** alveolus of mandible
　　² ✓7ᵗʰ **S02.670** Fracture of alveolus of mandible, unspecified side   HCC ▽
　　² ✓7ᵗʰ **S02.671** Fracture of alveolus of right mandible   HCC
　　² ✓7ᵗʰ **S02.672** Fracture of alveolus of left mandible   HCC

　² ✓x7ᵗʰ **S02.69 Fracture of mandible of other specified site**   HCC

✓5ᵗʰ **S02.8 Fractures of other specified skull and facial bones**
　　Fracture of orbit NOS
　　Fracture of palate
　　EXCLUDES 1   fracture of orbital floor (S02.3-)
　　　　　　　fracture of orbital roof (S02.1-)

　² ✓x7ᵗʰ **S02.80 Fracture of other specified skull and facial bones, unspecified side**   HCC ▽
　² ✓x7ᵗʰ **S02.81 Fracture of other specified skull and facial bones,** right side   HCC
　² ✓x7ᵗʰ **S02.82 Fracture of other specified skull and facial bones,** left side   HCC

✓5ᵗʰ **S02.9 Fracture of unspecified skull and facial bones**
　² ✓x7ᵗʰ **S02.91 Unspecified fracture of** skull   HCC ▽
　² ✓x7ᵗʰ **S02.92 Unspecified fracture of** facial bones   HCC ▽

✓4ᵗʰ **S03 Dislocation and sprain of joints and ligaments of head**
　　INCLUDES   avulsion of joint (capsule) or ligament of head
　　　　laceration of cartilage, joint (capsule) or ligament of head
　　　　sprain of cartilage, joint (capsule) or ligament of head
　　　　traumatic hemarthrosis of joint or ligament of head
　　　　traumatic rupture of joint or ligament of head
　　　　traumatic subluxation of joint or ligament of head
　　　　traumatic tear of joint or ligament of head
　　Code also any associated open wound
　　EXCLUDES 2   strain of muscle or tendon of head (S09.1)

> The appropriate 7th character is to be added to each code from category S03.
> A   initial encounter
> D   subsequent encounter
> S   sequela

✓5ᵗʰ **S03.0 Dislocation of jaw**
　　Dislocation of jaw (cartilage) (meniscus)
　　Dislocation of mandible
　　Dislocation of temporomandibular (joint)
　　✓7ᵗʰ **S03.00 Dislocation of jaw, unspecified side** ▽
　　✓7ᵗʰ **S03.01 Dislocation of jaw,** right side
　　✓7ᵗʰ **S03.02 Dislocation of jaw,** left side
　　✓7ᵗʰ **S03.03 Dislocation of jaw,** bilateral

✓x7ᵗʰ **S03.1 Dislocation of septal cartilage of nose**
✓x7ᵗʰ **S03.2 Dislocation of tooth**

✓5ᵗʰ **S03.4 Sprain of jaw**
　　Sprain of temporomandibular (joint) (ligament)
　　✓7ᵗʰ **S03.40 Sprain of jaw, unspecified side** ▽
　　✓7ᵗʰ **S03.41 Sprain of jaw,** right side
　　✓7ᵗʰ **S03.42 Sprain of jaw,** left side
　　✓7ᵗʰ **S03.43 Sprain of jaw,** bilateral

✓x7ᵗʰ **S03.8 Sprain of joints and ligaments of other parts of head**
✓x7ᵗʰ **S03.9 Sprain of joints and ligaments of unspecified parts of head** ▽

---

²   HCC with 7th character indicating initial encounter (A or B - specific to category) OR sequela.

EXCLUDES 1 Not coded here   **EXCLUDES 2** Not included here   N Newborn Age: 0   P Pediatric Age: 0-17   M Maternity Age: 12-55   A Adult Age: 15-124

918   ICD-10-CM 2018

✓4ᵗʰ **S04 Injury of cranial nerve**
The selection of side should be based on the side of the body being affected
Codes first any associated intracranial injury (S06.-)
Code also any associated:
    open wound of head (S01.-)
    skull fracture (S02.-)

> The appropriate 7th character is to be added to each code from category S04.
> A   initial encounter
> D   subsequent encounter
> S   sequela

✓5ᵗʰ **S04.0 Injury of optic nerve and pathways**
Use additional code to identify any visual field defect or blindness ▶(H53.4-, H54.-)◀

    ✓6ᵗʰ **S04.01 Injury of optic nerve**
        Injury of 2nd cranial nerve

        ✓7ᵗʰ **S04.011 Injury of optic nerve, right eye**
        ✓7ᵗʰ **S04.012 Injury of optic nerve, left eye**
        ✓7ᵗʰ **S04.019 Injury of optic nerve, unspecified eye** ▽
            Injury of optic nerve NOS

    ✓ˣ7ᵗʰ **S04.02 Injury of optic chiasm**

    ✓6ᵗʰ **S04.03 Injury of optic tract and pathways**
        Injury of optic radiation

▲   ✓7ᵗʰ **S04.031 Injury of optic tract and pathways, right side**
▲   ✓7ᵗʰ **S04.032 Injury of optic tract and pathways, left side**
▲   ✓7ᵗʰ **S04.039 Injury of optic tract and pathways, unspecified side** ▽
            Injury of optic tract and pathways NOS

    ✓6ᵗʰ **S04.04 Injury of visual cortex**
▲   ✓7ᵗʰ **S04.041 Injury of visual cortex, right side**
▲   ✓7ᵗʰ **S04.042 Injury of visual cortex, left side**
▲   ✓7ᵗʰ **S04.049 Injury of visual cortex, unspecified side** ▽
            Injury of visual cortex NOS

✓5ᵗʰ **S04.1 Injury of oculomotor nerve**
Injury of 3rd cranial nerve

    ✓ˣ7ᵗʰ **S04.10 Injury of oculomotor nerve, unspecified side** ▽
    ✓ˣ7ᵗʰ **S04.11 Injury of oculomotor nerve, right side**
    ✓ˣ7ᵗʰ **S04.12 Injury of oculomotor nerve, left side**

✓5ᵗʰ **S04.2 Injury of trochlear nerve**
Injury of 4th cranial nerve

    ✓ˣ7ᵗʰ **S04.20 Injury of trochlear nerve, unspecified side** ▽
    ✓ˣ7ᵗʰ **S04.21 Injury of trochlear nerve, right side**
    ✓ˣ7ᵗʰ **S04.22 Injury of trochlear nerve, left side**

✓5ᵗʰ **S04.3 Injury of trigeminal nerve**
Injury of 5th cranial nerve

    ✓ˣ7ᵗʰ **S04.30 Injury of trigeminal nerve, unspecified side** ▽
    ✓ˣ7ᵗʰ **S04.31 Injury of trigeminal nerve, right side**
    ✓ˣ7ᵗʰ **S04.32 Injury of trigeminal nerve, left side**

✓5ᵗʰ **S04.4 Injury of abducent nerve**
Injury of 6th cranial nerve

    ✓ˣ7ᵗʰ **S04.40 Injury of abducent nerve, unspecified side** ▽
    ✓ˣ7ᵗʰ **S04.41 Injury of abducent nerve, right side**
    ✓ˣ7ᵗʰ **S04.42 Injury of abducent nerve, left side**

✓5ᵗʰ **S04.5 Injury of facial nerve**
Injury of 7th cranial nerve

    ✓ˣ7ᵗʰ **S04.50 Injury of facial nerve, unspecified side** ▽
    ✓ˣ7ᵗʰ **S04.51 Injury of facial nerve, right side**
    ✓ˣ7ᵗʰ **S04.52 Injury of facial nerve, left side**

✓5ᵗʰ **S04.6 Injury of acoustic nerve**
Injury of auditory nerve
Injury of 8th cranial nerve

    ✓ˣ7ᵗʰ **S04.60 Injury of acoustic nerve, unspecified side** ▽
    ✓ˣ7ᵗʰ **S04.61 Injury of acoustic nerve, right side**
    ✓ˣ7ᵗʰ **S04.62 Injury of acoustic nerve, left side**

✓5ᵗʰ **S04.7 Injury of accessory nerve**
Injury of 11th cranial nerve

    ✓ˣ7ᵗʰ **S04.70 Injury of accessory nerve, unspecified side** ▽

    ✓ˣ7ᵗʰ **S04.71 Injury of accessory nerve, right side**
    ✓ˣ7ᵗʰ **S04.72 Injury of accessory nerve, left side**

✓5ᵗʰ **S04.8 Injury of other cranial nerves**
    ✓6ᵗʰ **S04.81 Injury of olfactory [1st] nerve**
        ✓7ᵗʰ **S04.811 Injury of olfactory [1st] nerve, right side**
        ✓7ᵗʰ **S04.812 Injury of olfactory [1st] nerve, left side**
        ✓7ᵗʰ **S04.819 Injury of olfactory [1st] nerve, unspecified side** ▽

    ✓6ᵗʰ **S04.89 Injury of other cranial nerves**
        Injury of vagus [10th] nerve
        ✓7ᵗʰ **S04.891 Injury of other cranial nerves, right side**
        ✓7ᵗʰ **S04.892 Injury of other cranial nerves, left side**
        ✓7ᵗʰ **S04.899 Injury of other cranial nerves, unspecified side** ▽

✓ˣ7ᵗʰ **S04.9 Injury of unspecified cranial nerve** ▽

✓4ᵗʰ **S05 Injury of eye and orbit**
INCLUDES   open wound of eye and orbit
EXCLUDES 2   *2nd cranial [optic] nerve injury (S04.0-)*
            3rd cranial [oculomotor] nerve injury (S04.1-)
            open wound of eyelid and periocular area (S01.1-)
            orbital bone fracture (S02.1-, S02.3-, S02.8-)
            superficial injury of eyelid (S00.1-S00.2)

> The appropriate 7th character is to be added to each code from category S05.
> A   initial encounter
> D   subsequent encounter
> S   sequela

✓5ᵗʰ **S05.0 Injury of conjunctiva and corneal abrasion without foreign body**
    EXCLUDES 1   *foreign body in conjunctival sac (T15.1)*
            foreign body in cornea (T15.0)

    ✓ˣ7ᵗʰ **S05.00 Injury of conjunctiva and corneal abrasion without foreign body, unspecified eye** ▽
    ✓ˣ7ᵗʰ **S05.01 Injury of conjunctiva and corneal abrasion without foreign body, right eye**
    ✓ˣ7ᵗʰ **S05.02 Injury of conjunctiva and corneal abrasion without foreign body, left eye**

✓5ᵗʰ **S05.1 Contusion of eyeball and orbital tissues**
Traumatic hyphema
EXCLUDES 2   *black eye NOS (S00.1)*
            contusion of eyelid and periocular area (S00.1)

    ✓ˣ7ᵗʰ **S05.10 Contusion of eyeball and orbital tissues, unspecified eye** ▽
    ✓ˣ7ᵗʰ **S05.11 Contusion of eyeball and orbital tissues, right eye**
    ✓ˣ7ᵗʰ **S05.12 Contusion of eyeball and orbital tissues, left eye**

✓5ᵗʰ **S05.2 Ocular laceration and rupture with prolapse or loss of intraocular tissue**
    ✓ˣ7ᵗʰ **S05.20 Ocular laceration and rupture with prolapse or loss of intraocular tissue, unspecified eye** ▽
    ✓ˣ7ᵗʰ **S05.21 Ocular laceration and rupture with prolapse or loss of intraocular tissue, right eye**
    ✓ˣ7ᵗʰ **S05.22 Ocular laceration and rupture with prolapse or loss of intraocular tissue, left eye**

✓5ᵗʰ **S05.3 Ocular laceration without prolapse or loss of intraocular tissue**
Laceration of eye NOS
DEF: Tear in ocular tissue without displacing structures; due to blunt trauma; characterized by pain, redness, and decreased vision.

    ✓ˣ7ᵗʰ **S05.30 Ocular laceration without prolapse or loss of intraocular tissue, unspecified eye** ▽
    ✓ˣ7ᵗʰ **S05.31 Ocular laceration without prolapse or loss of intraocular tissue, right eye**
    ✓ˣ7ᵗʰ **S05.32 Ocular laceration without prolapse or loss of intraocular tissue, left eye**

✓5ᵗʰ **S05.4 Penetrating wound of orbit with or without foreign body**
EXCLUDES 2   *retained (old) foreign body following penetrating wound in orbit (H05.5-)*

    ✓ˣ7ᵗʰ **S05.40 Penetrating wound of orbit with or without foreign body, unspecified eye** ▽
    ✓ˣ7ᵗʰ **S05.41 Penetrating wound of orbit with or without foreign body, right eye**
    ✓ˣ7ᵗʰ **S05.42 Penetrating wound of orbit with or without foreign body, left eye**

✓ Additional Character Req   ✓ˣ7ᵗʰ Placeholder Alert   Manifestation   HCC CMS-HCC Condition   ▽ Unspecified Code   ▶◀ Revised Text   ● New Code   ▲ Revised Code Title

Chapter 19. Injury, Poisoning, and Certain Other Consequences of External Causes

S05.5–S06.303

√5ᵗʰ **S05.5** Penetrating wound with foreign body of eyeball
   EXCLUDES 2   retained (old) intraocular foreign body (H44.6-, H44.7)

   √ₓ7ᵗʰ **S05.50** **Penetrating wound with foreign body of unspecified eyeball** ▽

   √ₓ7ᵗʰ **S05.51** **Penetrating wound with foreign body of right eyeball**

   √ₓ7ᵗʰ **S05.52** **Penetrating wound with foreign body of left eyeball**

√5ᵗʰ **S05.6** Penetrating wound without foreign body of eyeball
   Ocular penetration NOS

   √ₓ7ᵗʰ **S05.60** **Penetrating wound without foreign body of unspecified eyeball** ▽

   √ₓ7ᵗʰ **S05.61** **Penetrating wound without foreign body of right eyeball**

   √ₓ7ᵗʰ **S05.62** **Penetrating wound without foreign body of left eyeball**

√5ᵗʰ **S05.7** **Avulsion of eye**
   Traumatic enucleation

   √ₓ7ᵗʰ **S05.70** **Avulsion of unspecified eye** ▽

   √ₓ7ᵗʰ **S05.71** **Avulsion of right eye**

   √ₓ7ᵗʰ **S05.72** **Avulsion of left eye**

√5ᵗʰ **S05.8** **Other injuries of eye and orbit**
   Lacrimal duct injury

   √6ᵗʰ **S05.8X** **Other injuries of eye and orbit**

      √7ᵗʰ **S05.8X1** **Other injuries of right eye and orbit**

      √7ᵗʰ **S05.8X2** **Other injuries of left eye and orbit**

      √7ᵗʰ **S05.8X9** **Other injuries of unspecified eye and orbit** ▽

√5ᵗʰ **S05.9** **Unspecified injury of eye and orbit**
   Injury of eye NOS

   √ₓ7ᵗʰ **S05.90** **Unspecified injury of unspecified eye and orbit** ▽

   √ₓ7ᵗʰ **S05.91** **Unspecified injury of right eye and orbit** ▽

   √ₓ7ᵗʰ **S05.92** **Unspecified injury of left eye and orbit** ▽

√4ᵗʰ **S06** **Intracranial injury**
   NOTE   ▶7th characters D and S do not apply to codes in category S06 with 6th character 7 – death due to brain injury prior to regaining consciousness, or 8 – death due to other cause prior to regaining consciousness◀
   INCLUDES   traumatic brain injury
   Code also any associated:
      open wound of head (S01.-)
      skull fracture (S02.-)
   EXCLUDES 1   head injury NOS (S09.90)
   AHA: 2017, 1Q, 42; 2015, 3Q, 37

   The appropriate 7th character is to be added to each code from category S06.
   A   initial encounter
   D   subsequent encounter
   S   sequela

√5ᵗʰ **S06.0** **Concussion**
   Commotio cerebri
   EXCLUDES 1   concussion with intracranial injuries classified in subcategories S06.1- to S06.6-, S06.81-, S06.82- code to specified intracranial injury

   √6ᵗʰ **S06.0X** **Concussion**

      3 √7ᵗʰ **S06.0X0** **Concussion without loss of consciousness** HCC

      3 √7ᵗʰ **S06.0X1** **Concussion with loss of consciousness of 30 minutes or less** HCC

      3 √7ᵗʰ **S06.0X9** **Concussion with loss of consciousness of unspecified duration** HCC ▽
         Concussion NOS

√5ᵗʰ **S06.1** **Traumatic cerebral edema**
   Diffuse traumatic cerebral edema
   Focal traumatic cerebral edema

   √6ᵗʰ **S06.1X** **Traumatic cerebral edema**

      2 √7ᵗʰ **S06.1X0** **Traumatic cerebral edema without loss of consciousness** HCC

      2 √7ᵗʰ **S06.1X1** **Traumatic cerebral edema with loss of consciousness of 30 minutes or less** HCC

      2 √7ᵗʰ **S06.1X2** **Traumatic cerebral edema with loss of consciousness of 31 minutes to 59 minutes** HCC

      2 √7ᵗʰ **S06.1X3** **Traumatic cerebral edema with loss of consciousness of 1 hour to 5 hours 59 minutes** HCC

      2 √7ᵗʰ **S06.1X4** **Traumatic cerebral edema with loss of consciousness of 6 hours to 24 hours** HCC

      2 √7ᵗʰ **S06.1X5** **Traumatic cerebral edema with loss of consciousness greater than 24 hours with return to pre-existing conscious level** HCC

      2 √7ᵗʰ **S06.1X6** **Traumatic cerebral edema with loss of consciousness greater than 24 hours without return to pre-existing conscious level with patient surviving** HCC

      √7ᵗʰ **S06.1X7** **Traumatic cerebral edema with loss of consciousness of any duration with death due to brain injury prior to regaining consciousness**

      √7ᵗʰ **S06.1X8** **Traumatic cerebral edema with loss of consciousness of any duration with death due to other cause prior to regaining consciousness**

      2 √7ᵗʰ **S06.1X9** **Traumatic cerebral edema with loss of consciousness of unspecified duration** HCC ▽
         Traumatic cerebral edema NOS

√5ᵗʰ **S06.2** **Diffuse traumatic brain injury**
   Diffuse axonal brain injury
   EXCLUDES 1   traumatic diffuse cerebral edema (S06.1X-)

   √6ᵗʰ **S06.2X** **Diffuse traumatic brain injury**

      2 √7ᵗʰ **S06.2X0** **Diffuse traumatic brain injury without loss of consciousness** HCC

      2 √7ᵗʰ **S06.2X1** **Diffuse traumatic brain injury with loss of consciousness of 30 minutes or less** HCC

      2 √7ᵗʰ **S06.2X2** **Diffuse traumatic brain injury with loss of consciousness of 31 minutes to 59 minutes** HCC

      2 √7ᵗʰ **S06.2X3** **Diffuse traumatic brain injury with loss of consciousness of 1 hour to 5 hours 59 minutes** HCC

      2 √7ᵗʰ **S06.2X4** **Diffuse traumatic brain injury with loss of consciousness of 6 hours to 24 hours** HCC

      2 √7ᵗʰ **S06.2X5** **Diffuse traumatic brain injury with loss of consciousness greater than 24 hours with return to pre-existing conscious levels** HCC

      2 √7ᵗʰ **S06.2X6** **Diffuse traumatic brain injury with loss of consciousness greater than 24 hours without return to pre-existing conscious level with patient surviving** HCC

      √7ᵗʰ **S06.2X7** **Diffuse traumatic brain injury with loss of consciousness of any duration with death due to brain injury prior to regaining consciousness**

      √7ᵗʰ **S06.2X8** **Diffuse traumatic brain injury with loss of consciousness of any duration with death due to other cause prior to regaining consciousness**

      2 √7ᵗʰ **S06.2X9** **Diffuse traumatic brain injury with loss of consciousness of unspecified duration** HCC ▽
         Diffuse traumatic brain injury NOS

√5ᵗʰ **S06.3** **Focal traumatic brain injury**
   EXCLUDES 1   any condition classifiable to S06.4-S06.6
   focal cerebral edema (S06.1)

   √6ᵗʰ **S06.30** **Unspecified focal traumatic brain injury**

      2 √7ᵗʰ **S06.300** **Unspecified focal traumatic brain injury without loss of consciousness** HCC ▽

      2 √7ᵗʰ **S06.301** **Unspecified focal traumatic brain injury with loss of consciousness of 30 minutes or less** HCC ▽

      2 √7ᵗʰ **S06.302** **Unspecified focal traumatic brain injury with loss of consciousness of 31 minutes to 59 minutes** HCC ▽

      2 √7ᵗʰ **S06.303** **Unspecified focal traumatic brain injury with loss of consciousness of 1 hour to 5 hours 59 minutes** HCC ▽

---

2 HCC with 7th character indicating initial encounter (A or B - specific to category) OR sequela.
3 HCC with 7th character indicating sequela.

EXCLUDES 1 Not coded here   EXCLUDES 2 Not included here   N Newborn Age: 0   P Pediatric Age: 0-17   M Maternity Age: 12-55   A Adult Age: 15-124

920   ICD-10-CM 2018

2 ☑7ᵗʰ **S06.304 Unspecified focal traumatic brain** ᴴᶜᶜ ▽
**injury with loss of consciousness
of** 6 hours to 24 hours

2 ☑7ᵗʰ **S06.305 Unspecified focal traumatic brain** ᴴᶜᶜ ▽
injury with loss of consciousness
greater than 24 hours with return
to pre-existing conscious level

2 ☑7ᵗʰ **S06.306 Unspecified focal traumatic brain** ᴴᶜᶜ ▽
injury with loss of consciousness
greater than 24 hours without return to
pre-existing conscious level with patient
surviving

☑7ᵗʰ **S06.307 Unspecified focal traumatic brain** ▽
injury with loss of consciousness of any
duration with death due to brain injury
prior to regaining consciousness

☑7ᵗʰ **S06.308 Unspecified focal traumatic brain** ▽
injury with loss of consciousness of any
duration with death due to **other** cause
prior to regaining consciousness

2 ☑7ᵗʰ **S06.309 Unspecified focal traumatic brain** ᴴᶜᶜ ▽
**injury with loss of consciousness of
unspecified duration**
    Unspecified focal traumatic brain injury
    NOS

☑6ᵗʰ **S06.31 Contusion and laceration of** right cerebrum

2 ☑7ᵗʰ **S06.310 Contusion and laceration of right** ᴴᶜᶜ
cerebrum without loss of consciousness

2 ☑7ᵗʰ **S06.311 Contusion and laceration of right** ᴴᶜᶜ
cerebrum with loss of consciousness of
30 minutes or less

2 ☑7ᵗʰ **S06.312 Contusion and laceration of right** ᴴᶜᶜ
cerebrum with loss of consciousness of
31 minutes to 59 minutes

2 ☑7ᵗʰ **S06.313 Contusion and laceration of right** ᴴᶜᶜ
cerebrum with loss of consciousness of
1 hour to 5 hours 59 minutes

2 ☑7ᵗʰ **S06.314 Contusion and laceration of right** ᴴᶜᶜ
cerebrum with loss of consciousness of
6 hours to 24 hours

2 ☑7ᵗʰ **S06.315 Contusion and laceration of right** ᴴᶜᶜ
cerebrum with loss of consciousness
greater than 24 hours with return to
pre-existing conscious level

2 ☑7ᵗʰ **S06.316 Contusion and laceration of right** ᴴᶜᶜ
cerebrum with loss of consciousness
greater than 24 hours without return to
pre-existing conscious level with patient
surviving

☑7ᵗʰ **S06.317 Contusion and laceration of right
cerebrum with loss of consciousness of**
any duration with death due to brain
injury prior to regaining consciousness

☑7ᵗʰ **S06.318 Contusion and laceration of right
cerebrum with loss of consciousness of**
any duration with death due to **other**
cause prior to regaining consciousness

2 ☑7ᵗʰ **S06.319 Contusion and laceration of right** ᴴᶜᶜ ▽
**cerebrum with loss of consciousness
of unspecified duration**
    Contusion and laceration of right cerebrum
    NOS

☑6ᵗʰ **S06.32 Contusion and laceration of** left cerebrum

2 ☑7ᵗʰ **S06.320 Contusion and laceration of left** ᴴᶜᶜ
cerebrum without loss of consciousness

2 ☑7ᵗʰ **S06.321 Contusion and laceration of left** ᴴᶜᶜ
**cerebrum with loss of consciousness
of** 30 minutes or less

2 ☑7ᵗʰ **S06.322 Contusion and laceration of left** ᴴᶜᶜ
**cerebrum with loss of consciousness
of** 31 minutes to 59 minutes

2 ☑7ᵗʰ **S06.323 Contusion and laceration of left** ᴴᶜᶜ
**cerebrum with loss of consciousness
of** 1 hour to 5 hours 59 minutes

2 ☑7ᵗʰ **S06.324 Contusion and laceration of left** ᴴᶜᶜ
**cerebrum with loss of consciousness
of** 6 hours to 24 hours

2 ☑7ᵗʰ **S06.325 Contusion and laceration of left** ᴴᶜᶜ
cerebrum with loss of consciousness
greater than 24 hours with return
to pre-existing conscious level

2 ☑7ᵗʰ **S06.326 Contusion and laceration of left** ᴴᶜᶜ
cerebrum with loss of consciousness
greater than 24 hours without return
to pre-existing conscious level with
patient surviving

☑7ᵗʰ **S06.327 Contusion and laceration of left cerebrum
with loss of consciousness of** any duration
with death due to brain injury prior to
regaining consciousness

☑7ᵗʰ **S06.328 Contusion and laceration of left cerebrum
with loss of consciousness of** any duration
with death due to **other** cause prior to
regaining consciousness

2 ☑7ᵗʰ **S06.329 Contusion and laceration of left** ᴴᶜᶜ ▽
**cerebrum with loss of consciousness of
unspecified duration**
    Contusion and laceration of left cerebrum
    NOS

☑6ᵗʰ **S06.33 Contusion and laceration of** cerebrum, unspecified

2 ☑7ᵗʰ **S06.330 Contusion and laceration of** ᴴᶜᶜ
cerebrum, unspecified, without loss
of consciousness

2 ☑7ᵗʰ **S06.331 Contusion and laceration of** ᴴᶜᶜ ▽
**cerebrum, unspecified, with loss of
consciousness of** 30 minutes or less

2 ☑7ᵗʰ **S06.332 Contusion and laceration of** ᴴᶜᶜ ▽
**cerebrum, unspecified, with loss of
consciousness of** 31 minutes to
59 minutes

2 ☑7ᵗʰ **S06.333 Contusion and laceration of** ᴴᶜᶜ ▽
**cerebrum, unspecified, with loss of
consciousness of** 1 hour to 5 hours
59 minutes

2 ☑7ᵗʰ **S06.334 Contusion and laceration of** ᴴᶜᶜ ▽
**cerebrum, unspecified, with loss of
consciousness of** 6 hours to 24 hours

2 ☑7ᵗʰ **S06.335 Contusion and laceration of** ᴴᶜᶜ ▽
**cerebrum, unspecified, with loss of
consciousness** greater than 24 hours with
return to pre-existing conscious level

2 ☑7ᵗʰ **S06.336 Contusion and laceration of** ᴴᶜᶜ ▽
**cerebrum, unspecified, with loss of
consciousness** greater than 24 hours
without return to pre-existing conscious
level with patient surviving

☑7ᵗʰ **S06.337 Contusion and laceration of cerebrum,** ▽
unspecified, with loss of consciousness of
any duration with death due to brain
injury prior to regaining consciousness

☑7ᵗʰ **S06.338 Contusion and laceration of cerebrum,** ▽
unspecified, with loss of consciousness of
any duration with death due to **other**
cause prior to regaining consciousness

2 ☑7ᵗʰ **S06.339 Contusion and laceration of** ᴴᶜᶜ ▽
**cerebrum, unspecified, with loss of
consciousness of unspecified duration**
    Contusion and laceration of cerebrum NOS

☑6ᵗʰ **S06.34 Traumatic hemorrhage of** right cerebrum
    Traumatic intracerebral hemorrhage and hematoma
    of right cerebrum

2 ☑7ᵗʰ **S06.340 Traumatic hemorrhage of right** ᴴᶜᶜ
cerebrum without loss of consciousness

2 ☑7ᵗʰ **S06.341 Traumatic hemorrhage of right** ᴴᶜᶜ
**cerebrum with loss of consciousness
of** 30 minutes or less

2 ☑7ᵗʰ **S06.342 Traumatic hemorrhage of right** ᴴᶜᶜ
**cerebrum with loss of consciousness
of** 31 minutes to 59 minutes

2 ☑7ᵗʰ **S06.343 Traumatic hemorrhage of right** ᴴᶜᶜ
**cerebrum with loss of consciousness
of** 1 hours to 5 hours 59 minutes

2 ☑7ᵗʰ **S06.344 Traumatic hemorrhage of right** ᴴᶜᶜ
**cerebrum with loss of consciousness
of** 6 hours to 24 hours

---

2   HCC with 7th character indicating initial encounter (A or B - specific to category) OR sequela.

☑ Additional Character Req   ☑ₓ7ᵗʰ Placeholder Alert   Manifestation   ᴴᶜᶜ CMS-HCC Condition   ▽ Unspecified Code   ►◄ Revised Text   ● New Code   ▲ Revised Code Title

² ✓7ᵗʰ **S06.345 Traumatic hemorrhage of right cerebrum with loss of consciousness** greater than 24 hours with return to pre-existing conscious level   HCC

² ✓7ᵗʰ **S06.346 Traumatic hemorrhage of right cerebrum with loss of consciousness** greater than 24 hours without return to pre-existing conscious level with patient surviving   HCC

✓7ᵗʰ **S06.347 Traumatic hemorrhage of right cerebrum with loss of consciousness of** any duration with death due to brain injury prior to regaining consciousness

✓7ᵗʰ **S06.348 Traumatic hemorrhage of right cerebrum with loss of consciousness of** any duration with death due to **other** cause prior to regaining consciousness

² ✓7ᵗʰ **S06.349 Traumatic hemorrhage of right cerebrum with loss of consciousness of unspecified duration**   HCC ▽
Traumatic hemorrhage of right cerebrum NOS

✓6ᵗʰ **S06.35 Traumatic hemorrhage of** left cerebrum
Traumatic intracerebral hemorrhage and hematoma of left cerebrum

² ✓7ᵗʰ **S06.350 Traumatic hemorrhage of left cerebrum** without loss of consciousness   HCC

² ✓7ᵗʰ **S06.351 Traumatic hemorrhage of left cerebrum with loss of consciousness of** 30 minutes or less   HCC

² ✓7ᵗʰ **S06.352 Traumatic hemorrhage of left cerebrum with loss of consciousness of** 31 minutes to 59 minutes   HCC

² ✓7ᵗʰ **S06.353 Traumatic hemorrhage of left cerebrum with loss of consciousness of** 1 hours to 5 hours 59 minutes   HCC

² ✓7ᵗʰ **S06.354 Traumatic hemorrhage of left cerebrum with loss of consciousness of** 6 hours to 24 hours   HCC

² ✓7ᵗʰ **S06.355 Traumatic hemorrhage of left cerebrum with loss of consciousness** greater than 24 hours with return to pre-existing conscious level   HCC

² ✓7ᵗʰ **S06.356 Traumatic hemorrhage of left cerebrum with loss of consciousness** greater than 24 hours without return to pre-existing conscious level with patient surviving   HCC

✓7ᵗʰ **S06.357 Traumatic hemorrhage of left cerebrum with loss of consciousness of** any duration with death due to brain injury prior to regaining consciousness

✓7ᵗʰ **S06.358 Traumatic hemorrhage of left cerebrum with loss of consciousness of** any duration with death due to **other** cause prior to regaining consciousness

² ✓7ᵗʰ **S06.359 Traumatic hemorrhage of left cerebrumwith loss of consciousness of unspecified duration**   HCC ▽
Traumatic hemorrhage of left cerebrum NOS

✓6ᵗʰ **S06.36 Traumatic hemorrhage of** cerebrum, unspecified
Traumatic intracerebral hemorrhage and hematoma, unspecified

² ✓7ᵗʰ **S06.360 Traumatic hemorrhage of cerebrum, unspecified,** without loss of consciousness   HCC ▽

² ✓7ᵗʰ **S06.361 Traumatic hemorrhage of cerebrum, unspecified, with loss of consciousness of** 30 minutes or less   HCC ▽

² ✓7ᵗʰ **S06.362 Traumatic hemorrhage of cerebrum, unspecified, with loss of consciousness of** 31 minutes to 59 minutes   HCC ▽

² ✓7ᵗʰ **S06.363 Traumatic hemorrhage of cerebrum, unspecified, with loss of consciousness of** 1 hours to 5 hours 59 minutes   HCC ▽

² ✓7ᵗʰ **S06.364 Traumatic hemorrhage of cerebrum, unspecified, with loss of consciousness of** 6 hours to 24 hours   HCC ▽

² ✓7ᵗʰ **S06.365 Traumatic hemorrhage of cerebrum, unspecified, with loss of consciousness** greater than 24 hours with return to pre-existing conscious level   HCC ▽

² ✓7ᵗʰ **S06.366 Traumatic hemorrhage of cerebrum, unspecified, with loss of consciousness** greater than 24 hours without return to pre-existing conscious level with patient surviving   HCC ▽

✓7ᵗʰ **S06.367 Traumatic hemorrhage of cerebrum, unspecified, with loss of consciousness of** any duration with death due to brain injury prior to regaining consciousness   ▽

✓7ᵗʰ **S06.368 Traumatic hemorrhage of cerebrum, unspecified, with loss of consciousness of** any duration with death due to **other** cause prior to regaining consciousness   ▽

² ✓7ᵗʰ **S06.369 Traumatic hemorrhage of cerebrum, unspecified, with loss of consciousness of unspecified duration**   HCC ▽
Traumatic hemorrhage of cerebrum NOS

✓6ᵗʰ **S06.37 Contusion, laceration, and hemorrhage of** cerebellum

² ✓7ᵗʰ **S06.370 Contusion, laceration, and hemorrhage of cerebellum** without loss of consciousness   HCC

² ✓7ᵗʰ **S06.371 Contusion, laceration, and hemorrhage of cerebellum with loss of consciousness of** 30 minutes or less   HCC

² ✓7ᵗʰ **S06.372 Contusion, laceration, and hemorrhage of cerebellum with loss of consciousness of** 31 minutes to 59 minutes   HCC

² ✓7ᵗʰ **S06.373 Contusion, laceration, and hemorrhage of cerebellum with loss of consciousness of** 1 hour to 5 hours 59 minutes   HCC

² ✓7ᵗʰ **S06.374 Contusion, laceration, and hemorrhage of cerebellum with loss of consciousness of** 6 hours to 24 hours   HCC

² ✓7ᵗʰ **S06.375 Contusion, laceration, and hemorrhage of cerebellum with loss of consciousness** greater than 24 hours with return to pre-existing conscious level   HCC

² ✓7ᵗʰ **S06.376 Contusion, laceration, and hemorrhage of cerebellum with loss of consciousness** greater than 24 hours without return to pre-existing conscious level with patient surviving   HCC

✓7ᵗʰ **S06.377 Contusion, laceration, and hemorrhage of cerebellum with loss of consciousness of** any duration with death due to brain injury prior to regaining consciousness

✓7ᵗʰ **S06.378 Contusion, laceration, and hemorrhage of cerebellum with loss of consciousness of** any duration with death due to **other** cause prior to regaining consciousness

² ✓7ᵗʰ **S06.379 Contusion, laceration, and hemorrhage of cerebellum with loss of consciousness of unspecified duration**   HCC ▽
Contusion, laceration, and hemorrhage of cerebellum NOS

✓6ᵗʰ **S06.38 Contusion, laceration, and hemorrhage of** brainstem

² ✓7ᵗʰ **S06.380 Contusion, laceration, and hemorrhage of brainstem** without loss of consciousness   HCC

² ✓7ᵗʰ **S06.381 Contusion, laceration, and hemorrhage of brainstem with loss of consciousness of** 30 minutes or less   HCC

² ✓7ᵗʰ **S06.382 Contusion, laceration, and hemorrhage of brainstem with loss of consciousness of** 31 minutes to 59 minutes   HCC

---

²   HCC with 7th character indicating initial encounter (A or B - specific to category) OR sequela.

EXCLUDES 1 Not coded here   **EXCLUDES 2** Not included here   N Newborn Age: 0   P Pediatric Age: 0-17   M Maternity Age: 12-55   A Adult Age: 15-124

922   ICD-10-CM 2018

2 ✓7ᵗʰ **S06.383** **Contusion, laceration, and** HCC
hemorrhage of brainstem with loss of
consciousness of 1 hour to 5 hours 59
minutes

2 ✓7ᵗʰ **S06.384** **Contusion, laceration, and** HCC
hemorrhage of brainstem with loss of
consciousness of 6 hours to 24 hours

2 ✓7ᵗʰ **S06.385** **Contusion, laceration, and** HCC
hemorrhage of brainstem with loss
of consciousness greater than 24 hours
with return to pre-existing conscious level

2 ✓7ᵗʰ **S06.386** **Contusion, laceration, and** HCC
hemorrhage of brainstem with loss of
consciousness greater than 24 hours
without return to pre-existing conscious
level with patient surviving

✓7ᵗʰ **S06.387** **Contusion, laceration, and hemorrhage of**
brainstem with loss of consciousness of
any duration with death due to brain
injury prior to regaining consciousness

✓7ᵗʰ **S06.388** **Contusion, laceration, and hemorrhage of**
brainstem with loss of consciousness of
any duration with death due to **other**
cause prior to regaining consciousness

2 ✓7ᵗʰ **S06.389** **Contusion, laceration, and** HCC ▽
hemorrhage of brainstem with loss
of consciousness of unspecified duration
Contusion, laceration, and hemorrhage of
brainstem NOS

✓5ᵗʰ **S06.4** **Epidural** **hemorrhage**
Extradural hemorrhage NOS
Extradural hemorrhage (traumatic)

✓6ᵗʰ **S06.4X** **Epidural hemorrhage**

2 ✓7ᵗʰ **S06.4X0** **Epidural hemorrhage** without loss HCC
of consciousness

2 ✓7ᵗʰ **S06.4X1** **Epidural hemorrhage with loss of** HCC
consciousness of 30 minutes or less

2 ✓7ᵗʰ **S06.4X2** **Epidural hemorrhage with loss of** HCC
consciousness of 31 minutes to
59 minutes

2 ✓7ᵗʰ **S06.4X3** **Epidural hemorrhage with loss of** HCC
consciousness of 1 hour to 5 hours 59
minutes

2 ✓7ᵗʰ **S06.4X4** **Epidural hemorrhage with loss of** HCC
consciousness of 6 hours to 24 hours

2 ✓7ᵗʰ **S06.4X5** **Epidural hemorrhage with loss of** HCC
consciousness greater than 24 hours
with return to pre-existing conscious
level

2 ✓7ᵗʰ **S06.4X6** **Epidural hemorrhage with loss of** HCC
consciousness greater than 24 hours
without return to pre-existing conscious
level with patient surviving

✓7ᵗʰ **S06.4X7** **Epidural hemorrhage with loss of**
consciousness of any duration with
death due to brain injury prior to
regaining consciousness

✓7ᵗʰ **S06.4X8** **Epidural hemorrhage with loss of**
consciousness of any duration with
death due to **other** causes prior to
regaining consciousness

2 ✓7ᵗʰ **S06.4X9** **Epidural hemorrhage with loss of** HCC ▽
consciousness of unspecified duration
Epidural hemorrhage NOS

✓5ᵗʰ **S06.5** **Traumatic** **subdural** **hemorrhage**

✓6ᵗʰ **S06.5X** **Traumatic subdural hemorrhage**

2 ✓7ᵗʰ **S06.5X0** **Traumatic subdural hemorrhage** HCC
without loss of consciousness

2 ✓7ᵗʰ **S06.5X1** **Traumatic subdural hemorrhage** HCC
with loss of consciousness of 30
minutes or less

2 ✓7ᵗʰ **S06.5X2** **Traumatic subdural hemorrhage** HCC
with loss of consciousness of 31
minutes to 59 minutes

2 ✓7ᵗʰ **S06.5X3** **Traumatic subdural hemorrhage** HCC
with loss of consciousness of 1 hour
to 5 hours 59 minutes

2 ✓7ᵗʰ **S06.5X4** **Traumatic subdural hemorrhage** HCC
with loss of consciousness of 6 hours
to 24 hours

2 ✓7ᵗʰ **S06.5X5** **Traumatic subdural hemorrhage** HCC
with loss of consciousness greater
than 24 hours with return to
pre-existing conscious level

2 ✓7ᵗʰ **S06.5X6** **Traumatic subdural hemorrhage** HCC
with loss of consciousness greater
than 24 hours without return to
pre-existing conscious level with
patient surviving

✓7ᵗʰ **S06.5X7** **Traumatic subdural hemorrhage with loss**
of consciousness of any duration with
death due to brain injury before regaining
consciousness

✓7ᵗʰ **S06.5X8** **Traumatic subdural hemorrhage with loss**
of consciousness of any duration with
death due to **other** cause before regaining
consciousness

2 ✓7ᵗʰ **S06.5X9** **Traumatic subdural hemorrhage** HCC ▽
with loss of consciousness of
unspecified duration
Traumatic subdural hemorrhage NOS

✓5ᵗʰ **S06.6** **Traumatic** subarachnoid **hemorrhage**

✓6ᵗʰ **S06.6X** **Traumatic subarachnoid hemorrhage**

2 ✓7ᵗʰ **S06.6X0** **Traumatic subarachnoid** HCC
hemorrhage without loss of
consciousness

2 ✓7ᵗʰ **S06.6X1** **Traumatic subarachnoid hemorrhage** HCC
with loss of consciousness of
30 minutes or less

2 ✓7ᵗʰ **S06.6X2** **Traumatic subarachnoid hemorrhage** HCC
with loss of consciousness of
31 minutes to 59 minutes

2 ✓7ᵗʰ **S06.6X3** **Traumatic subarachnoid hemorrhage** HCC
with loss of consciousness of
1 hour to 5 hours 59 minutes

2 ✓7ᵗʰ **S06.6X4** **Traumatic subarachnoid hemorrhage** HCC
with loss of consciousness of
6 hours to 24 hours

2 ✓7ᵗʰ **S06.6X5** **Traumatic subarachnoid hemorrhage** HCC
with loss of consciousness greater
than 24 hours with return to pre-existing
conscious level

2 ✓7ᵗʰ **S06.6X6** **Traumatic subarachnoid hemorrhage** HCC
with loss of consciousness greater than 24
hours without return to pre-existing
conscious level with patient surviving

✓7ᵗʰ **S06.6X7** **Traumatic subarachnoid hemorrhage with**
loss of consciousness of any duration with
death due to brain injury prior to
regaining consciousness

✓7ᵗʰ **S06.6X8** **Traumatic subarachnoid hemorrhage with**
loss of consciousness of any duration with
death due to **other** cause prior to
regaining consciousness

2 ✓7ᵗʰ **S06.6X9** **Traumatic subarachnoid** HCC ▽
hemorrhage with loss of consciousness
of unspecified duration
Traumatic subarachnoid hemorrhage NOS

✓5ᵗʰ **S06.8** **Other specified intracranial injuries**

✓6ᵗʰ **S06.81** **Injury of** right internal carotid artery, **intracranial**
portion, not elsewhere classified

2 ✓7ᵗʰ **S06.810** **Injury of right internal carotid artery,** HCC
intracranial portion, not elsewhere
classified without loss of consciousness

2 ✓7ᵗʰ **S06.811** **Injury of right internal carotid artery,** HCC
intracranial portion, not elsewhere
classified with loss of consciousness of 30
minutes or less

2 ✓7ᵗʰ **S06.812** **Injury of right internal carotid artery,** HCC
intracranial portion, not elsewhere
classified with loss of consciousness of 31
minutes to 59 minutes

2 ✓7ᵗʰ **S06.813** **Injury of right internal carotid artery,** HCC
intracranial portion, not elsewhere
classified with loss of consciousness of 1
hour to 5 hours 59 minutes

---

2 HCC with 7th character indicating initial encounter (A or B - specific to category) OR sequela.

✓ Additional Character Req   ✓ₓ7ᵗʰ Placeholder Alert   Manifestation   HCC CMS-HCC Condition   ▽ Unspecified Code   ►◄ Revised Text   ● New Code   ▲ Revised Code Title

2 ✓7ᵗʰ **S06.814** **Injury of right internal carotid artery, intracranial portion, not elsewhere classified with loss of consciousness of** 6 hours to 24 hours   HCC

2 ✓7ᵗʰ **S06.815** **Injury of right internal carotid artery, intracranial portion, not elsewhere classified with loss of consciousness** greater than 24 hours with return to pre-existing conscious level   HCC

2 ✓7ᵗʰ **S06.816** **Injury of right internal carotid artery, intracranial portion, not elsewhere classified with loss of consciousness** greater than 24 hours without return to pre-existing conscious level with patient surviving   HCC

✓7ᵗʰ **S06.817** **Injury of right internal carotid artery, intracranial portion, not elsewhere classified with loss of consciousness of** any duration with death due to brain injury prior to regaining consciousness

✓7ᵗʰ **S06.818** **Injury of right internal carotid artery, intracranial portion, not elsewhere classified with loss of consciousness of** any duration with death due to **other** cause prior to regaining consciousness

2 ✓7ᵗʰ **S06.819** **Injury of right internal carotid artery, intracranial portion, not elsewhere classified with loss of consciousness of unspecified duration**   HCC ▽

     Injury of right internal carotid artery, intracranial portion, not elsewhere classified NOS

✓6ᵗʰ **S06.82** **Injury of** left internal carotid artery, intracranial **portion, not elsewhere classified**

2 ✓7ᵗʰ **S06.820** **Injury of left internal carotid artery, intracranial portion, not elsewhere classified** without loss of consciousness   HCC

2 ✓7ᵗʰ **S06.821** **Injury of left internal carotid artery, intracranial portion, not elsewhere classified with loss of consciousness of** 30 minutes or less   HCC

2 ✓7ᵗʰ **S06.822** **Injury of left internal carotid artery, intracranial portion, not elsewhere classified with loss of consciousness of** 31 minutes to 59 minutes   HCC

2 ✓7ᵗʰ **S06.823** **Injury of left internal carotid artery, intracranial portion, not elsewhere classified with loss of consciousness of** 1 hour to 5 hours 59 minutes   HCC

2 ✓7ᵗʰ **S06.824** **Injury of left internal carotid artery, intracranial portion, not elsewhere classified with loss of consciousness of** 6 hours to 24 hours   HCC

2 ✓7ᵗʰ **S06.825** **Injury of left internal carotid artery, intracranial portion, not elsewhere classified with loss of consciousness** greater than 24 hours with return to pre-existing conscious level   HCC

2 ✓7ᵗʰ **S06.826** **Injury of left internal carotid artery, intracranial portion, not elsewhere classified with loss of consciousness** greater than 24 hours without return to pre-existing conscious level with patient surviving   HCC

✓7ᵗʰ **S06.827** **Injury of left internal carotid artery, intracranial portion, not elsewhere classified with loss of consciousness of** any duration with death due to brain injury prior to regaining consciousness

✓7ᵗʰ **S06.828** **Injury of left internal carotid artery, intracranial portion, not elsewhere classified with loss of consciousness of** any duration with death due to **other** cause prior to regaining consciousness

2 ✓7ᵗʰ **S06.829** **Injury of left internal carotid artery, intracranial portion, not elsewhere classified with loss of consciousness of unspecified duration**   HCC ▽

     Injury of left internal carotid artery, intracranial portion, not elsewhere classified NOS

✓6ᵗʰ **S06.89** **Other specified intracranial injury**

     EXCLUDES 1   concussion (S06.0X-)

2 ✓7ᵗʰ **S06.890** **Other specified intracranial injury** without loss of consciousness   HCC

2 ✓7ᵗʰ **S06.891** **Other specified intracranial injury with loss of consciousness of** 30 minutes or less   HCC

2 ✓7ᵗʰ **S06.892** **Other specified intracranial injury with loss of consciousness of** 31 minutes to 59 minutes   HCC

2 ✓7ᵗʰ **S06.893** **Other specified intracranial injury with loss of consciousness of** 1 hour to 5 hours 59 minutes   HCC

2 ✓7ᵗʰ **S06.894** **Other specified intracranial injury with loss of consciousness of** 6 hours to 24 hours   HCC

2 ✓7ᵗʰ **S06.895** **Other specified intracranial injury with loss of consciousness** greater than 24 hours with return to pre-existing conscious level   HCC

2 ✓7ᵗʰ **S06.896** **Other specified intracranial injury with loss of consciousness** greater than 24 hours without return to pre-existing conscious level with patient surviving   HCC

✓7ᵗʰ **S06.897** **Other specified intracranial injury with loss of consciousness of** any duration with death due to brain injury prior to regaining consciousness

✓7ᵗʰ **S06.898** **Other specified intracranial injury with loss of consciousness of** any duration with death due to **other** cause prior to regaining consciousness

2 ✓7ᵗʰ **S06.899** **Other specified intracranial injury with loss of consciousness of unspecified duration**   HCC ▽

✓5ᵗʰ **S06.9** **Unspecified intracranial injury**

     Brain injury NOS

     Head injury NOS with loss of consciousness

     Traumatic brain injury NOS

     EXCLUDES 1   conditions classifiable to S06.0- to S06.8- code to specified intracranial injury

         head injury NOS (S09.90)

✓6ᵗʰ **S06.9X** **Unspecified intracranial injury**

2 ✓7ᵗʰ **S06.9X0** **Unspecified intracranial injury** without loss of consciousness   HCC ▽

2 ✓7ᵗʰ **S06.9X1** **Unspecified intracranial injury with loss of consciousness of** 30 minutes or less   HCC ▽

2 ✓7ᵗʰ **S06.9X2** **Unspecified intracranial injury with loss of consciousness of** 31 minutes to 59 minutes   HCC ▽

2 ✓7ᵗʰ **S06.9X3** **Unspecified intracranial injury with loss of consciousness of** 1 hour to 5 hours 59 minutes   HCC ▽

2 ✓7ᵗʰ **S06.9X4** **Unspecified intracranial injury with loss of consciousness of** 6 hours to 24 hours   HCC ▽

2 ✓7ᵗʰ **S06.9X5** **Unspecified intracranial injury with loss of consciousness** greater than 24 hours with return to pre-existing conscious level   HCC ▽

2 ✓7ᵗʰ **S06.9X6** **Unspecified intracranial injury with loss of consciousness** greater than 24 hours without return to pre-existing conscious level with patient surviving   HCC ▽

✓7ᵗʰ **S06.9X7** **Unspecified intracranial injury with loss of consciousness of** any duration with death due to brain injury prior to regaining consciousness   ▽

✓7ᵗʰ **S06.9X8** **Unspecified intracranial injury with loss of consciousness of** any duration with death due to **other** cause prior to regaining consciousness   ▽

2 ✓7ᵗʰ **S06.9X9** **Unspecified intracranial injury with loss of consciousness of unspecified duration**   HCC ▽

---

2   HCC with 7th character indicating initial encounter (A or B - specific to category) OR sequela.

EXCLUDES 1 Not coded here   EXCLUDES 2 Not included here   N Newborn Age: 0   P Pediatric Age: 0-17   M Maternity Age: 12-55   A Adult Age: 15-124

924   ICD-10-CM 2018

✓4ᵗʰ **S07 Crushing injury of head**

Use additional code for all associated injuries, such as:
intracranial injuries (S06.-)
skull fractures (S02.-)

The appropriate 7th character is to be added to each code from category S07.
A   initial encounter
D   subsequent encounter
S   sequela

✓x7ᵗʰ **S07.0 Crushing injury of** face

✓x7ᵗʰ **S07.1 Crushing injury of** skull

✓x7ᵗʰ **S07.8 Crushing injury of other parts of head**

✓x7ᵗʰ **S07.9 Crushing injury of head, part unspecified** ▽

✓4ᵗʰ **S08 Avulsion and traumatic amputation of part of head**

An amputation not identified as partial or complete should be coded to complete

The appropriate 7th character is to be added to each code from category S08.
A   initial encounter
D   subsequent encounter
S   sequela

✓x7ᵗʰ **S08.0 Avulsion of** scalp

✓5ᵗʰ **S08.1 Traumatic amputation of** ear

✓6ᵗʰ **S08.11** Complete **traumatic amputation of ear**

✓7ᵗʰ **S08.111 Complete traumatic amputation of** right **ear**

✓7ᵗʰ **S08.112 Complete traumatic amputation of** left **ear**

✓7ᵗʰ **S08.119 Complete traumatic amputation of unspecified ear** ▽

✓6ᵗʰ **S08.12** Partial **traumatic amputation of ear**

✓7ᵗʰ **S08.121 Partial traumatic amputation of** right **ear**

✓7ᵗʰ **S08.122 Partial traumatic amputation of** left **ear**

✓7ᵗʰ **S08.129 Partial traumatic amputation of unspecified ear** ▽

✓5ᵗʰ **S08.8 Traumatic amputation of other parts of head**

✓6ᵗʰ **S08.81 Traumatic amputation of** nose

✓7ᵗʰ **S08.811** Complete **traumatic amputation of nose**

✓7ᵗʰ **S08.812** Partial **traumatic amputation of nose**

✓x7ᵗʰ **S08.89 Traumatic amputation of other parts of head**

✓4ᵗʰ **S09 Other and unspecified injuries of head**

The appropriate 7th character is to be added to each code from category S09.
A   initial encounter
D   subsequent encounter
S   sequela

✓x7ᵗʰ **S09.0 Injury of** blood vessels **of head, not elsewhere classified**

EXCLUDES 1   *injury of cerebral blood vessels (S06.-)*
injury of precerebral blood vessels (S15.-)

✓5ᵗʰ **S09.1 Injury of** muscle and tendon **of head**

Code also any associated open wound (S01.-)

EXCLUDES 2   *sprain to joints and ligament of head (S03.9)*

✓x7ᵗʰ **S09.10 Unspecified injury of muscle and tendon of head** ▽
Injury of muscle and tendon of head NOS

✓x7ᵗʰ **S09.11** Strain **of muscle and tendon of head**

✓x7ᵗʰ **S09.12** Laceration **of muscle and tendon of head**

✓x7ᵗʰ **S09.19 Other specified injury of muscle and tendon of head**

✓5ᵗʰ **S09.2 Traumatic rupture of** ear drum

EXCLUDES 1   *traumatic rupture of ear drum due to blast injury (S09.31-)*

✓x7ᵗʰ **S09.20 Traumatic rupture of unspecified ear drum** ▽

✓x7ᵗʰ **S09.21 Traumatic rupture of** right **ear drum**

✓x7ᵗʰ **S09.22 Traumatic rupture of** left **ear drum**

✓5ᵗʰ **S09.3 Other specified and unspecified injury of middle and inner ear**

EXCLUDES 1   *injury to ear NOS (S09.91-)*
EXCLUDES 2   *injury to external ear (S00.4-, S01.3-, S08.1-)*

✓6ᵗʰ **S09.30 Unspecified injury of** middle and inner ear

✓7ᵗʰ **S09.301 Unspecified injury of** right **middle and inner ear** ▽

✓7ᵗʰ **S09.302 Unspecified injury of** left **middle and inner ear** ▽

✓7ᵗʰ **S09.309 Unspecified injury of unspecified middle and inner ear** ▽

✓6ᵗʰ **S09.31 Primary** blast injury **of ear**
Blast injury of ear NOS

✓7ᵗʰ **S09.311 Primary blast injury of** right **ear**

✓7ᵗʰ **S09.312 Primary blast injury of** left **ear**

✓7ᵗʰ **S09.313 Primary blast injury of ear,** bilateral

✓7ᵗʰ **S09.319 Primary blast injury of unspecified ear** ▽

✓6ᵗʰ **S09.39 Other specified injury of middle and inner ear**
Secondary blast injury to ear

✓7ᵗʰ **S09.391 Other specified injury of** right **middle and inner ear**

✓7ᵗʰ **S09.392 Other specified injury of** left **middle and inner ear**

✓7ᵗʰ **S09.399 Other specified injury of unspecified middle and inner ear** ▽

✓x7ᵗʰ **S09.8 Other specified injuries of head**

✓5ᵗʰ **S09.9 Unspecified injury of face and head**

✓x7ᵗʰ **S09.90 Unspecified injury of** head ▽
Head injury NOS

EXCLUDES 1   *brain injury NOS (S06.9-)*
head injury NOS with loss of consciousness (S06.9-)
intracranial injury NOS (S06.9-)

✓x7ᵗʰ **S09.91 Unspecified injury of** ear ▽
Injury of ear NOS

✓x7ᵗʰ **S09.92 Unspecified injury of** nose ▽
Injury of nose NOS

✓x7ᵗʰ **S09.93 Unspecified injury of** face ▽
Injury of face NOS

Injuries to the neck (S10-S19)

INCLUDES   injuries of nape
injuries of supraclavicular region
injuries of throat

EXCLUDES 2   *burns and corrosions (T20-T32)*
effects of foreign body in esophagus (T18.1)
effects of foreign body in larynx (T17.3)
effects of foreign body in pharynx (T17.2)
effects of foreign body in trachea (T17.4)
frostbite (T33-T34)
insect bite or sting, venomous (T63.4)

✓4ᵗʰ **S10 Superficial injury of neck**

The appropriate 7th character is to be added to each code from category S10.
A   initial encounter
D   subsequent encounter
S   sequela

✓x7ᵗʰ **S10.0 Contusion of throat**
Contusion of cervical esophagus
Contusion of larynx
Contusion of pharynx
Contusion of trachea

✓5ᵗʰ **S10.1 Other and unspecified superficial injuries of throat**

✓x7ᵗʰ **S10.10 Unspecified superficial injuries of throat** ▽

✓x7ᵗʰ **S10.11** Abrasion **of throat**

✓x7ᵗʰ **S10.12** Blister **(nonthermal) of throat**

✓x7ᵗʰ **S10.14** External constriction **of part of throat**

✓x7ᵗʰ **S10.15 Superficial** foreign body **of throat**
Splinter in the throat

✓x7ᵗʰ **S10.16** Insect bite **(nonvenomous) of throat**

✓x7ᵗʰ **S10.17 Other superficial** bite **of throat**

EXCLUDES 1   *open bite of throat (S11.85)*

✓5ᵗʰ **S10.8 Superficial injury of other specified parts of neck**

✓x7ᵗʰ **S10.80 Unspecified superficial injury of other specified part of neck** ▽

✓x7ᵗʰ **S10.81** Abrasion **of other specified part of neck**

✓x7ᵗʰ **S10.82** Blister **(nonthermal) of other specified part of neck**

✓x7ᵗʰ **S10.83** Contusion **of other specified part of neck**

✓x7ᵗʰ **S10.84** External constriction **of other specified part of neck**

☑ Additional Character Req   ✓x7ᵗʰ Placeholder Alert   Manifestation   HCC CMS-HCC Condition   ▽ Unspecified Code   ▶◀ Revised Text   ● New Code   ▲ Revised Code Title

ICD-10-CM 2018   **925**

✓x7th **S10.85** Superficial foreign body of other specified part of neck
Splinter in other specified part of neck

✓x7th **S10.86** Insect bite of other specified part of neck

✓x7th **S10.87** Other superficial bite of other specified part of neck
EXCLUDES 1 open bite of other specified parts of neck (S11.85)

✓5th **S10.9** Superficial injury of unspecified part of neck

✓x7th **S10.90** Unspecified superficial injury of unspecified part of neck ▽

✓x7th **S10.91** Abrasion of unspecified part of neck ▽

✓x7th **S10.92** Blister (nonthermal) of unspecified part of neck ▽

✓x7th **S10.93** Contusion of unspecified part of neck ▽

✓x7th **S10.94** External constriction of unspecified part of neck ▽

✓x7th **S10.95** Superficial foreign body of unspecified part of neck ▽

✓x7th **S10.96** Insect bite of unspecified part of neck ▽

✓x7th **S10.97** Other superficial bite of unspecified part of neck ▽

✓4th **S11** Open wound of neck
Code also any associated:
spinal cord injury (S14.0, S14.1-)
wound infection
EXCLUDES 2 open fracture of vertebra (S12- with 7th character B)

The appropriate 7th character is to be added to each code from category S11.
A initial encounter
D subsequent encounter
S sequela

✓5th **S11.0** Open wound of larynx and trachea

✓6th **S11.01** Open wound of larynx
EXCLUDES 2 open wound of vocal cord (S11.03)

✓7th **S11.011** Laceration without foreign body of larynx

✓7th **S11.012** Laceration with foreign body of larynx

✓7th **S11.013** Puncture wound without foreign body of larynx

✓7th **S11.014** Puncture wound with foreign body of larynx

✓7th **S11.015** Open bite of larynx
Bite of larynx NOS

✓7th **S11.019** Unspecified open wound of larynx ▽

✓6th **S11.02** Open wound of trachea
Open wound of cervical trachea
Open wound of trachea NOS
EXCLUDES 2 open wound of thoracic trachea (S27.5-)

✓7th **S11.021** Laceration without foreign body of trachea

✓7th **S11.022** Laceration with foreign body of trachea

✓7th **S11.023** Puncture wound without foreign body of trachea

✓7th **S11.024** Puncture wound with foreign body of trachea

✓7th **S11.025** Open bite of trachea
Bite of trachea NOS

✓7th **S11.029** Unspecified open wound of trachea ▽

✓6th **S11.03** Open wound of vocal cord

✓7th **S11.031** Laceration without foreign body of vocal cord

✓7th **S11.032** Laceration with foreign body of vocal cord

✓7th **S11.033** Puncture wound without foreign body of vocal cord

✓7th **S11.034** Puncture wound with foreign body of vocal cord

✓7th **S11.035** Open bite of vocal cord
Bite of vocal cord NOS

✓7th **S11.039** Unspecified open wound of vocal cord ▽

✓5th **S11.1** Open wound of thyroid gland

✓x7th **S11.10** Unspecified open wound of thyroid gland ▽

✓x7th **S11.11** Laceration without foreign body of thyroid gland

✓x7th **S11.12** Laceration with foreign body of thyroid gland

✓x7th **S11.13** Puncture wound without foreign body of thyroid gland

✓x7th **S11.14** Puncture wound with foreign body of thyroid gland

✓x7th **S11.15** Open bite of thyroid gland
Bite of thyroid gland NOS

✓5th **S11.2** Open wound of pharynx and cervical esophagus
EXCLUDES 1 open wound of esophagus NOS (S27.8-)

✓x7th **S11.20** Unspecified open wound of pharynx and cervical esophagus ▽

✓x7th **S11.21** Laceration without foreign body of pharynx and cervical esophagus

✓x7th **S11.22** Laceration with foreign body of pharynx and cervical esophagus

✓x7th **S11.23** Puncture wound without foreign body of pharynx and cervical esophagus

✓x7th **S11.24** Puncture wound with foreign body of pharynx and cervical esophagus

✓x7th **S11.25** Open bite of pharynx and cervical esophagus
Bite of pharynx and cervical esophagus NOS

✓5th **S11.8** Open wound of other specified parts of neck

✓x7th **S11.80** Unspecified open wound of other specified part of neck ▽

✓x7th **S11.81** Laceration without foreign body of other specified part of neck

✓x7th **S11.82** Laceration with foreign body of other specified part of neck

✓x7th **S11.83** Puncture wound without foreign body of other specified part of neck

✓x7th **S11.84** Puncture wound with foreign body of other specified part of neck

✓x7th **S11.85** Open bite of other specified part of neck
Bite of other specified part of neck NOS
EXCLUDES 1 superficial bite of other specified part of neck (S10.87)

✓x7th **S11.89** Other open wound of other specified part of neck

✓5th **S11.9** Open wound of unspecified part of neck

✓x7th **S11.90** Unspecified open wound of unspecified part of neck ▽

✓x7th **S11.91** Laceration without foreign body of unspecified part of neck ▽

✓x7th **S11.92** Laceration with foreign body of unspecified part of neck ▽

✓x7th **S11.93** Puncture wound without foreign body of unspecified part of neck ▽

✓x7th **S11.94** Puncture wound with foreign body of unspecified part of neck ▽

✓x7th **S11.95** Open bite of unspecified part of neck
Bite of neck NOS
EXCLUDES 1 superficial bite of neck (S10.97) ▽

✓4th **S12** Fracture of cervical vertebra and other parts of neck
NOTE A fracture not indicated as nondisplaced or displaced should be coded to displaced.
A fracture not indicated as open or closed should be coded to closed.
INCLUDES fracture of cervical neural arch
fracture of cervical spine
fracture of cervical spinous process
fracture of cervical transverse process
fracture of cervical vertebral arch
fracture of neck
Code first any associated cervical spinal cord injury (S14.0, S14.1-)
AHA: 2015, 3Q, 37-39

The appropriate 7th character is to be added to all codes from subcategories S12.0-S12.6.
A initial encounter for closed fracture
B initial encounter for open fracture
D subsequent encounter for fracture with routine healing
G subsequent encounter for fracture with delayed healing
K subsequent encounter for fracture with nonunion
S sequela

✓5th **S12.0** Fracture of first cervical vertebra
Atlas

✓6th **S12.00** Unspecified fracture of first cervical vertebra

1 ✓7th **S12.000** Unspecified displaced fracture of first cervical vertebra HCC ▽

---
1 HCC with 7th character indicating initial encounter (A, B or C - specific to category).

[1] ✓7th **S12.001** Unspecified nondisplaced fracture of first cervical vertebra   HCC ▽

[1] ✓x7th **S12.01** Stable burst fracture of first cervical vertebra   HCC

[1] ✓x7th **S12.02** Unstable burst fracture of first cervical vertebra   HCC

✓6th **S12.03** Posterior arch fracture of first cervical vertebra

[1] ✓7th **S12.030** Displaced posterior arch fracture of first cervical vertebra   HCC

[1] ✓7th **S12.031** Nondisplaced posterior arch fracture of first cervical vertebra   HCC

✓6th **S12.04** Lateral mass fracture of first cervical vertebra

[1] ✓7th **S12.040** Displaced lateral mass fracture of first cervical vertebra   HCC

[1] ✓7th **S12.041** Nondisplaced lateral mass fracture of first cervical vertebra   HCC

✓6th **S12.09** Other fracture of first cervical vertebra

[1] ✓7th **S12.090** Other displaced fracture of first cervical vertebra   HCC

[1] ✓7th **S12.091** Other nondisplaced fracture of first cervical vertebra   HCC

✓5th **S12.1** Fracture of second cervical vertebra
Axis

✓6th **S12.10** Unspecified fracture of second cervical vertebra

[1] ✓7th **S12.100** Unspecified displaced fracture of second cervical vertebra   HCC ▽

[1] ✓7th **S12.101** Unspecified nondisplaced fracture of second cervical vertebra   HCC ▽

✓6th **S12.11** Type II dens fracture

[1] ✓7th **S12.110** Anterior displaced Type II dens fracture   HCC

[1] ✓7th **S12.111** Posterior displaced Type II dens fracture   HCC

[1] ✓7th **S12.112** Nondisplaced Type II dens fracture   HCC

✓6th **S12.12** Other dens fracture

[1] ✓7th **S12.120** Other displaced dens fracture   HCC

[1] ✓7th **S12.121** Other nondisplaced dens fracture   HCC

✓6th **S12.13** Unspecified traumatic spondylolisthesis of second cervical vertebra

[1] ✓7th **S12.130** Unspecified traumatic displaced spondylolisthesis of second cervical vertebra   HCC ▽

[1] ✓7th **S12.131** Unspecified traumatic nondisplaced spondylolisthesis of second cervical vertebra   HCC ▽

[1] ✓x7th **S12.14** Type III traumatic spondylolisthesis of second cervical vertebra   HCC

✓6th **S12.15** Other traumatic spondylolisthesis of second cervical vertebra

[1] ✓7th **S12.150** Other traumatic displaced spondylolisthesis of second cervical vertebra   HCC

[1] ✓7th **S12.151** Other traumatic nondisplaced spondylolisthesis of second cervical vertebra   HCC

✓6th **S12.19** Other fracture of second cervical vertebra

[1] ✓7th **S12.190** Other displaced fracture of second cervical vertebra   HCC

[1] ✓7th **S12.191** Other nondisplaced fracture of second cervical vertebra   HCC

✓5th **S12.2** Fracture of third cervical vertebra

✓6th **S12.20** Unspecified fracture of third cervical vertebra

[1] ✓7th **S12.200** Unspecified displaced fracture of third cervical vertebra   HCC ▽

[1] ✓7th **S12.201** Unspecified nondisplaced fracture of third cervical vertebra   HCC ▽

✓6th **S12.23** Unspecified traumatic spondylolisthesis of third cervical vertebra

[1] ✓7th **S12.230** Unspecified traumatic displaced spondylolisthesis of third cervical vertebra   HCC ▽

[1] ✓7th **S12.231** Unspecified traumatic nondisplaced spondylolisthesis of third cervical vertebra   HCC ▽

[1] ✓x7th **S12.24** Type III traumatic spondylolisthesis of third cervical vertebra   HCC

✓6th **S12.25** Other traumatic spondylolisthesis of third cervical vertebra

[1] ✓7th **S12.250** Other traumatic displaced spondylolisthesis of third cervical vertebra   HCC

[1] ✓7th **S12.251** Other traumatic nondisplaced spondylolisthesis of third cervical vertebra   HCC

✓6th **S12.29** Other fracture of third cervical vertebra

[1] ✓7th **S12.290** Other displaced fracture of third cervical vertebra   HCC

[1] ✓7th **S12.291** Other nondisplaced fracture of third cervical vertebra   HCC

✓5th **S12.3** Fracture of fourth cervical vertebra

✓6th **S12.30** Unspecified fracture of fourth cervical vertebra

[1] ✓7th **S12.300** Unspecified displaced fracture of fourth cervical vertebra   HCC ▽

[1] ✓7th **S12.301** Unspecified nondisplaced fracture of fourth cervical vertebra   HCC ▽

✓6th **S12.33** Unspecified traumatic spondylolisthesis of fourth cervical vertebra

[1] ✓7th **S12.330** Unspecified traumatic displaced spondylolisthesis of fourth cervical vertebra   HCC ▽

[1] ✓7th **S12.331** Unspecified traumatic nondisplaced spondylolisthesis of fourth cervical vertebra   HCC ▽

[1] ✓x7th **S12.34** Type III traumatic spondylolisthesis of fourth cervical vertebra   HCC

✓6th **S12.35** Other traumatic spondylolisthesis of fourth cervical vertebra

[1] ✓7th **S12.350** Other traumatic displaced spondylolisthesis of fourth cervical vertebra   HCC

[1] ✓7th **S12.351** Other traumatic nondisplaced spondylolisthesis of fourth cervical vertebra   HCC

✓6th **S12.39** Other fracture of fourth cervical vertebra

[1] ✓7th **S12.390** Other displaced fracture of fourth cervical vertebra   HCC

[1] ✓7th **S12.391** Other nondisplaced fracture of fourth cervical vertebra   HCC

✓5th **S12.4** Fracture of fifth cervical vertebra

✓6th **S12.40** Unspecified fracture of fifth cervical vertebra

[1] ✓7th **S12.400** Unspecified displaced fracture of fifth cervical vertebra   HCC ▽

[1] ✓7th **S12.401** Unspecified nondisplaced fracture of fifth cervical vertebra   HCC ▽

✓6th **S12.43** Unspecified traumatic spondylolisthesis of fifth cervical vertebra

[1] ✓7th **S12.430** Unspecified traumatic displaced spondylolisthesis of fifth cervical vertebra   HCC ▽

[1] ✓7th **S12.431** Unspecified traumatic nondisplaced spondylolisthesis of fifth cervical vertebra   HCC ▽

[1] ✓x7th **S12.44** Type III traumatic spondylolisthesis of fifth cervical vertebra   HCC

✓6th **S12.45** Other traumatic spondylolisthesis of fifth cervical vertebra

[1] ✓7th **S12.450** Other traumatic displaced spondylolisthesis of fifth cervical vertebra   HCC

[1] ✓7th **S12.451** Other traumatic nondisplaced spondylolisthesis of fifth cervical vertebra   HCC

✓6th **S12.49** Other fracture of fifth cervical vertebra

[1] ✓7th **S12.490** Other displaced fracture of fifth cervical vertebra   HCC

[1] ✓7th **S12.491** Other nondisplaced fracture of fifth cervical vertebra   HCC

---

[1]   HCC with 7th character indicating initial encounter (A, B or C - specific to category).

☑ Additional Character Req   ✓x7th Placeholder Alert   Manifestation   HCC CMS-HCC Condition   ▽ Unspecified Code   ▶◀ Revised Text   ● New Code   ▲ Revised Code Title

✓5th S12.5 Fracture of sixth cervical vertebra

  ✓6th S12.50 Unspecified fracture of sixth cervical vertebra

    1 ✓7th **S12.500** Unspecified displaced fracture of sixth cervical vertebra   HCC ▽

    1 ✓7th **S12.501** Unspecified nondisplaced fracture of sixth cervical vertebra   HCC ▽

  ✓6th S12.53 Unspecified traumatic spondylolisthesis of sixth cervical vertebra

    1 ✓7th **S12.530** Unspecified traumatic displaced spondylolisthesis of sixth cervical vertebra   HCC ▽

    1 ✓7th **S12.531** Unspecified traumatic nondisplaced spondylolisthesis of sixth cervical vertebra   HCC ▽

  1 ✓x7th **S12.54** Type III traumatic spondylolisthesis of sixth cervical vertebra   HCC

  ✓6th S12.55 Other traumatic spondylolisthesis of sixth cervical vertebra

    1 ✓7th **S12.550** Other traumatic displaced spondylolisthesis of sixth cervical vertebra   HCC

    1 ✓7th **S12.551** Other traumatic nondisplaced spondylolisthesis of sixth cervical vertebra   HCC

  ✓6th S12.59 Other fracture of sixth cervical vertebra

    1 ✓7th **S12.590** Other displaced fracture of sixth cervical vertebra   HCC

    1 ✓7th **S12.591** Other nondisplaced fracture of sixth cervical vertebra   HCC

✓5th S12.6 Fracture of seventh cervical vertebra

  ✓6th S12.60 Unspecified fracture of seventh cervical vertebra

    1 ✓7th **S12.600** Unspecified displaced fracture of seventh cervical vertebra   HCC ▽

    1 ✓7th **S12.601** Unspecified nondisplaced fracture of seventh cervical vertebra   HCC ▽

  ✓6th S12.63 Unspecified traumatic spondylolisthesis of seventh cervical vertebra

    1 ✓7th **S12.630** Unspecified traumatic displaced spondylolisthesis of seventh cervical vertebra   HCC ▽

    1 ✓7th **S12.631** Unspecified traumatic nondisplaced spondylolisthesis of seventh cervical vertebra   HCC ▽

  1 ✓x7th **S12.64** Type III traumatic spondylolisthesis of seventh cervical vertebra   HCC

  ✓6th S12.65 Other traumatic spondylolisthesis of seventh cervical vertebra

    1 ✓7th **S12.650** Other traumatic displaced spondylolisthesis of seventh cervical vertebra   HCC

    1 ✓7th **S12.651** Other traumatic nondisplaced spondylolisthesis of seventh cervical vertebra   HCC

  ✓6th S12.69 Other fracture of seventh cervical vertebra

    1 ✓7th **S12.690** Other displaced fracture of seventh cervical vertebra   HCC

    1 ✓7th **S12.691** Other nondisplaced fracture of | seventh cervical vertebra   HCC

1 ✓x7th **S12.8 Fracture of other parts of neck**   HCC

    Hyoid bone   Thyroid cartilage
    Larynx   Trachea

> The appropriate 7th character is to be added to code S12.8.
> A   initial encounter
> D   subsequent encounter
> S   sequela

1 ✓x7th **S12.9 Fracture of neck, unspecified**   HCC ▽

    Fracture of cervical spine NOS
    Fracture of cervical vertebra NOS
    Fracture of neck NOS

> The appropriate 7th character is to be added to code S12.9.
> A   initial encounter
> D   subsequent encounter
> S   sequela

✓4th S13 Dislocation and sprain of joints and ligaments at neck level

  INCLUDES   avulsion of joint or ligament at neck level
    laceration of cartilage, joint or ligament at neck level
    sprain of cartilage, joint or ligament at neck level
    traumatic hemarthrosis of joint or ligament at neck level
    traumatic rupture of joint or ligament at neck level
    traumatic subluxation of joint or ligament at neck level
    traumatic tear of joint or ligament at neck level

Code also any associated open wound

EXCLUDES 2   strain of muscle or tendon at neck level (S16.1)

> The appropriate 7th character is to be added to each code from category S13.
> A   initial encounter
> D   subsequent encounter
> S   sequela

✓x7th **S13.0 Traumatic rupture of cervical intervertebral disc**

    EXCLUDES 1   rupture or displacement (nontraumatic) of cervical intervertebral disc NOS (M50.-)

✓5th **S13.1 Subluxation and dislocation of cervical vertebrae**

    Code also any associated:
      open wound of neck (S11.-)
      spinal cord injury (S14.1-)
    EXCLUDES 2   fracture of cervical vertebrae (S12.0--S12.3-)

  ✓6th S13.10 Subluxation and dislocation of unspecified cervical vertebrae

    ✓7th **S13.100** Subluxation of unspecified cervical vertebrae ▽

    ✓7th **S13.101** Dislocation of unspecified cervical vertebrae ▽

  ✓6th S13.11 Subluxation and dislocation of C0/C1 cervical vertebrae

    Subluxation and dislocation of atlantooccipital joint
    Subluxation and dislocation of atloidooccipital joint
    Subluxation and dislocation of occipitoatloid joint

    ✓7th **S13.110** Subluxation of C0/C1 cervical vertebrae

    ✓7th **S13.111** Dislocation of C0/C1 cervical vertebrae

  ✓6th S13.12 Subluxation and dislocation of C1/C2 cervical vertebrae

    Subluxation and dislocation of atlantoaxial joint

    ✓7th **S13.120** Subluxation of C1/C2 cervical vertebrae

    ✓7th **S13.121** Dislocation of C1/C2 cervical vertebrae

  ✓6th S13.13 Subluxation and dislocation of C2/C3 cervical vertebrae

    ✓7th **S13.130** Subluxation of C2/C3 cervical vertebrae

    ✓7th **S13.131** Dislocation of C2/C3 cervical vertebrae

  ✓6th S13.14 Subluxation and dislocation of C3/C4 cervical vertebrae

    ✓7th **S13.140** Subluxation of C3/C4 cervical vertebrae

    ✓7th **S13.141** Dislocation of C3/C4 cervical vertebrae

  ✓6th S13.15 Subluxation and dislocation of C4/C5 cervical vertebrae

    ✓7th **S13.150** Subluxation of C4/C5 cervical vertebrae

    ✓7th **S13.151** Dislocation of C4/C5 cervical vertebrae

  ✓6th S13.16 Subluxation and dislocation of C5/C6 cervical vertebrae

    ✓7th **S13.160** Subluxation of C5/C6 cervical vertebrae

    ✓7th **S13.161** Dislocation of C5/C6 cervical vertebrae

  ✓6th S13.17 Subluxation and dislocation of C6/C7 cervical vertebrae

    ✓7th **S13.170** Subluxation of C6/C7 cervical vertebrae

    ✓7th **S13.171** Dislocation of C6/C7 cervical vertebrae

  ✓6th S13.18 Subluxation and dislocation of C7/T1 cervical vertebrae

    ✓7th **S13.180** Subluxation of C7/T1 cervical vertebrae

    ✓7th **S13.181** Dislocation of C7/T1 cervical vertebrae

✓5th **S13.2 Dislocation of other and unspecified parts of neck**

  ✓x7th **S13.20** Dislocation of unspecified parts of neck ▽

  ✓x7th **S13.29** Dislocation of other parts of neck

✓x7th **S13.4 Sprain of ligaments of cervical spine**

    Sprain of anterior longitudinal (ligament), cervical
    Sprain of atlanto-axial (joints)
    Sprain of atlanto-occipital (joints)
    Whiplash injury of cervical spine

---

1   HCC with 7th character indicating initial encounter (A, B or C - specific to category).

EXCLUDES 1 Not coded here   **EXCLUDES 2** Not included here   **N** Newborn Age: 0   **P** Pediatric Age: 0-17   **M** Maternity Age: 12-55   **A** Adult Age: 15-124

928   ICD-10-CM 2018

√x7ᵗʰ **S13.5** **Sprain of thyroid region**
Sprain of cricoarytenoid (joint) (ligament)
Sprain of cricothyroid (joint) (ligament)
Sprain of thyroid cartilage

√x7ᵗʰ **S13.8** **Sprain of joints and ligaments of other parts of neck**

√x7ᵗʰ **S13.9** **Sprain of joints and ligaments of unspecified parts of neck** ▽

√4ᵗʰ **S14** **Injury of nerves and spinal cord at neck level**
> **NOTE**   Code to highest level of cervical cord injury.
> Code also any associated:
>   fracture of cervical vertebra (S12.0- -S12.6-)
>   open wound of neck (S11.-)
>   transient paralysis (R29.5)

> The appropriate 7th character is to be added to each code from
> category S14.
> A   initial encounter
> D   subsequent encounter
> S   sequela

√x7ᵗʰ **S14.0** **Concussion and edema of cervical spinal cord**   HCC

√5ᵗʰ **S14.1** **Other and unspecified injuries of cervical spinal cord**

√6ᵗʰ   **S14.10** **Unspecified injury of cervical spinal cord**

√7ᵗʰ   **S14.101** **Unspecified injury at C1 level of cervical spinal cord**   HCC ▽

√7ᵗʰ   **S14.102** **Unspecified injury at C2 level of cervical spinal cord**   HCC ▽

√7ᵗʰ   **S14.103** **Unspecified injury at C3 level of cervical spinal cord**   HCC ▽

√7ᵗʰ   **S14.104** **Unspecified injury at C4 level of cervical spinal cord**   HCC ▽

√7ᵗʰ   **S14.105** **Unspecified injury at C5 level of cervical spinal cord**   HCC ▽

√7ᵗʰ   **S14.106** **Unspecified injury at C6 level of cervical spinal cord**   HCC ▽

√7ᵗʰ   **S14.107** **Unspecified injury at C7 level of cervical spinal cord**   HCC ▽

√7ᵗʰ   **S14.108** **Unspecified injury at C8 level of cervical spinal cord**   HCC ▽

√7ᵗʰ   **S14.109** **Unspecified injury at unspecified level of cervical spinal cord**   HCC ▽
         Injury of cervical spinal cord NOS

√6ᵗʰ   **S14.11** **Complete lesion of cervical spinal cord**

√7ᵗʰ   **S14.111** **Complete lesion at C1 level of cervical spinal cord**   HCC

√7ᵗʰ   **S14.112** **Complete lesion at C2 level of cervical spinal cord**   HCC

√7ᵗʰ   **S14.113** **Complete lesion at C3 level of cervical spinal cord**   HCC

√7ᵗʰ   **S14.114** **Complete lesion at C4 level of cervical spinal cord**   HCC

√7ᵗʰ   **S14.115** **Complete lesion at C5 level of cervical spinal cord**   HCC

√7ᵗʰ   **S14.116** **Complete lesion at C6 level of cervical spinal cord**   HCC

√7ᵗʰ   **S14.117** **Complete lesion at C7 level of cervical spinal cord**   HCC

√7ᵗʰ   **S14.118** **Complete lesion at C8 level of cervical spinal cord**   HCC

√7ᵗʰ   **S14.119** **Complete lesion at unspecified level of cervical spinal cord**   HCC ▽

√6ᵗʰ   **S14.12** **Central cord syndrome of cervical spinal cord**

√7ᵗʰ   **S14.121** **Central cord syndrome at C1 level of cervical spinal cord**   HCC

√7ᵗʰ   **S14.122** **Central cord syndrome at C2 level of cervical spinal cord**   HCC

√7ᵗʰ   **S14.123** **Central cord syndrome at C3 level of cervical spinal cord**   HCC

√7ᵗʰ   **S14.124** **Central cord syndrome at C4 level of cervical spinal cord**   HCC

√7ᵗʰ   **S14.125** **Central cord syndrome at C5 level of cervical spinal cord**   HCC

√7ᵗʰ   **S14.126** **Central cord syndrome at C6 level of cervical spinal cord**   HCC

√7ᵗʰ   **S14.127** **Central cord syndrome at C7 level of cervical spinal cord**   HCC

√7ᵗʰ   **S14.128** **Central cord syndrome at C8 level of cervical spinal cord**   HCC

√7ᵗʰ   **S14.129** **Central cord syndrome at unspecified level of cervical spinal cord**   HCC ▽

√6ᵗʰ   **S14.13** **Anterior cord syndrome of cervical spinal cord**

√7ᵗʰ   **S14.131** **Anterior cord syndrome at C1 level of cervical spinal cord**   HCC

√7ᵗʰ   **S14.132** **Anterior cord syndrome at C2 level of cervical spinal cord**   HCC

√7ᵗʰ   **S14.133** **Anterior cord syndrome at C3 level of cervical spinal cord**   HCC

√7ᵗʰ   **S14.134** **Anterior cord syndrome at C4 level of cervical spinal cord**   HCC

√7ᵗʰ   **S14.135** **Anterior cord syndrome at C5 level of cervical spinal cord**   HCC

√7ᵗʰ   **S14.136** **Anterior cord syndrome at C6 level of cervical spinal cord**   HCC

√7ᵗʰ   **S14.137** **Anterior cord syndrome at C7 level of cervical spinal cord**   HCC

√7ᵗʰ   **S14.138** **Anterior cord syndrome at C8 level of cervical spinal cord**   HCC

√7ᵗʰ   **S14.139** **Anterior cord syndrome at unspecified level of cervical spinal cord**   HCC ▽

√6ᵗʰ   **S14.14** **Brown-Séquard syndrome of cervical spinal cord**

√7ᵗʰ   **S14.141** **Brown-Séquard syndrome at C1 level of cervical spinal cord**   HCC

√7ᵗʰ   **S14.142** **Brown-Séquard syndrome at C2 level of cervical spinal cord**   HCC

√7ᵗʰ   **S14.143** **Brown-Séquard syndrome at C3 level of cervical spinal cord**   HCC

√7ᵗʰ   **S14.144** **Brown-Séquard syndrome at C4 level of cervical spinal cord**   HCC

√7ᵗʰ   **S14.145** **Brown-Séquard syndrome at C5 level of cervical spinal cord**   HCC

√7ᵗʰ   **S14.146** **Brown-Séquard syndrome at C6 level of cervical spinal cord**   HCC

√7ᵗʰ   **S14.147** **Brown-Séquard syndrome at C7 level of cervical spinal cord**   HCC

√7ᵗʰ   **S14.148** **Brown-Séquard syndrome at C8 level of cervical spinal cord**   HCC

√7ᵗʰ   **S14.149** **Brown-Séquard syndrome at unspecified level of cervical spinal cord**   HCC ▽

√6ᵗʰ   **S14.15** **Other incomplete lesions of cervical spinal cord**
         Incomplete lesion of cervical spinal cord NOS
         Posterior cord syndrome of cervical spinal cord

√7ᵗʰ   **S14.151** **Other incomplete lesion at C1 level of cervical spinal cord**   HCC

√7ᵗʰ   **S14.152** **Other incomplete lesion at C2 level of cervical spinal cord**   HCC

√7ᵗʰ   **S14.153** **Other incomplete lesion at C3 level of cervical spinal cord**   HCC

√7ᵗʰ   **S14.154** **Other incomplete lesion at C4 level of cervical spinal cord**   HCC

√7ᵗʰ   **S14.155** **Other incomplete lesion at C5 level of cervical spinal cord**   HCC

√7ᵗʰ   **S14.156** **Other incomplete lesion at C6 level of cervical spinal cord**   HCC

√7ᵗʰ   **S14.157** **Other incomplete lesion at C7 level of cervical spinal cord**   HCC

√7ᵗʰ   **S14.158** **Other incomplete lesion at C8 level of cervical spinal cord**   HCC

√7ᵗʰ   **S14.159** **Other incomplete lesion at unspecified level of cervical spinal cord**   HCC ▽

√x7ᵗʰ **S14.2** **Injury of nerve root of cervical spine**

√x7ᵗʰ **S14.3** **Injury of brachial plexus**

√x7ᵗʰ **S14.4** **Injury of peripheral nerves of neck**

√x7ᵗʰ **S14.5** **Injury of cervical sympathetic nerves**

√x7ᵗʰ **S14.8** **Injury of other specified nerves of neck**

√x7ᵗʰ **S14.9** **Injury of unspecified nerves of neck**   ▽

☑ Additional Character Req   √x7ᵗʰ Placeholder Alert   Manifestation   HCC CMS-HCC Condition   ▽ Unspecified Code   ►◄ Revised Text   ● New Code   ▲ Revised Code Title

ICD-10-CM 2018   **929**

Chapter 19. Injury, Poisoning, and Certain Other Consequences of External Causes

✓4th S15 Injury of blood vessels at neck level
Code also any associated open wound (S11.-)

> The appropriate 7th character is to be added to each code from category S15.
> A   initial encounter
> D   subsequent encounter
> S   sequela

✓5th S15.0 Injury of carotid artery of neck
Injury of carotid artery (common) (external) (internal, extracranial portion)
Injury of carotid artery NOS
EXCLUDES 1   injury of internal carotid artery, intracranial portion (S06.8)

- **✓6th S15.00 Unspecified injury of carotid artery**
  - ✓7th **S15.001 Unspecified injury of right carotid artery** ▽
  - ✓7th **S15.002 Unspecified injury of left carotid artery** ▽
  - ✓7th **S15.009 Unspecified injury of unspecified carotid artery** ▽
- **✓6th S15.01 Minor laceration of carotid artery**
  Incomplete transection of carotid artery
  Laceration of carotid artery NOS
  Superficial laceration of carotid artery
  - ✓7th **S15.011 Minor laceration of right carotid artery**
  - ✓7th **S15.012 Minor laceration of left carotid artery**
  - ✓7th **S15.019 Minor laceration of unspecified carotid artery** ▽
- **✓6th S15.02 Major laceration of carotid artery**
  Complete transection of carotid artery
  Traumatic rupture of carotid artery
  - ✓7th **S15.021 Major laceration of right carotid artery**
  - ✓7th **S15.022 Major laceration of left carotid artery**
  - ✓7th **S15.029 Major laceration of unspecified carotid artery** ▽
- **✓6th S15.09 Other specified injury of carotid artery**
  - ✓7th **S15.091 Other specified injury of right carotid artery**
  - ✓7th **S15.092 Other specified injury of left carotid artery**
  - ✓7th **S15.099 Other specified injury of unspecified carotid artery** ▽

✓5th S15.1 Injury of vertebral artery

- **✓6th S15.10 Unspecified injury of vertebral artery**
  - ✓7th **S15.101 Unspecified injury of right vertebral artery** ▽
  - ✓7th **S15.102 Unspecified injury of left vertebral artery** ▽
  - ✓7th **S15.109 Unspecified injury of unspecified vertebral artery** ▽
- **✓6th S15.11 Minor laceration of vertebral artery**
  Incomplete transection of vertebral artery
  Laceration of vertebral artery NOS
  Superficial laceration of vertebral artery
  - ✓7th **S15.111 Minor laceration of right vertebral artery**
  - ✓7th **S15.112 Minor laceration of left vertebral artery**
  - ✓7th **S15.119 Minor laceration of unspecified vertebral artery** ▽
- **✓6th S15.12 Major laceration of vertebral artery**
  Complete transection of vertebral artery
  Traumatic rupture of vertebral artery
  - ✓7th **S15.121 Major laceration of right vertebral artery**
  - ✓7th **S15.122 Major laceration of left vertebral artery**
  - ✓7th **S15.129 Major laceration of unspecified vertebral artery** ▽
- **✓6th S15.19 Other specified injury of vertebral artery**
  - ✓7th **S15.191 Other specified injury of right vertebral artery**
  - ✓7th **S15.192 Other specified injury of left vertebral artery**
  - ✓7th **S15.199 Other specified injury of unspecified vertebral artery** ▽

✓5th S15.2 Injury of external jugular vein

- **✓6th S15.20 Unspecified injury of external jugular vein**
  - ✓7th **S15.201 Unspecified injury of right external jugular vein** ▽
  - ✓7th **S15.202 Unspecified injury of left external jugular vein** ▽
  - ✓7th **S15.209 Unspecified injury of unspecified external jugular vein** ▽
- **✓6th S15.21 Minor laceration of external jugular vein**
  Incomplete transection of external jugular vein
  Laceration of external jugular vein NOS
  Superficial laceration of external jugular vein
  - ✓7th **S15.211 Minor laceration of right external jugular vein**
  - ✓7th **S15.212 Minor laceration of left external jugular vein**
  - ✓7th **S15.219 Minor laceration of unspecified external jugular vein** ▽
- **✓6th S15.22 Major laceration of external jugular vein**
  Complete transection of external jugular vein
  Traumatic rupture of external jugular vein
  - ✓7th **S15.221 Major laceration of right external jugular vein**
  - ✓7th **S15.222 Major laceration of left external jugular vein**
  - ✓7th **S15.229 Major laceration of unspecified external jugular vein** ▽
- **✓6th S15.29 Other specified injury of external jugular vein**
  - ✓7th **S15.291 Other specified injury of right external jugular vein**
  - ✓7th **S15.292 Other specified injury of left external jugular vein**
  - ✓7th **S15.299 Other specified injury of unspecified external jugular vein**

✓5th S15.3 Injury of internal jugular vein

- **✓6th S15.30 Unspecified injury of internal jugular vein**
  - ✓7th **S15.301 Unspecified injury of right internal jugular vein** ▽
  - ✓7th **S15.302 Unspecified injury of left internal jugular vein** ▽
  - ✓7th **S15.309 Unspecified injury of unspecified internal jugular vein** ▽
- **✓6th S15.31 Minor laceration of internal jugular vein**
  Incomplete transection of internal jugular vein
  Laceration of internal jugular vein NOS
  Superficial laceration of internal jugular vein
  - ✓7th **S15.311 Minor laceration of right internal jugular vein**
  - ✓7th **S15.312 Minor laceration of left internal jugular vein**
  - ✓7th **S15.319 Minor laceration of unspecified internal jugular vein** ▽
- **✓6th S15.32 Major laceration of internal jugular vein**
  Complete transection of internal jugular vein
  Traumatic rupture of internal jugular vein
  - ✓7th **S15.321 Major laceration of right internal jugular vein**
  - ✓7th **S15.322 Major laceration of left internal jugular vein**
  - ✓7th **S15.329 Major laceration of unspecified internal jugular vein** ▽
- **✓6th S15.39 Other specified injury of internal jugular vein**
  - ✓7th **S15.391 Other specified injury of right internal jugular vein**
  - ✓7th **S15.392 Other specified injury of left internal jugular vein**
  - ✓7th **S15.399 Other specified injury of unspecified internal jugular vein** ▽

✓x7th S15.8 Injury of other specified blood vessels at neck level ▽
✓x7th S15.9 Injury of unspecified blood vessel at neck level ▽

EXCLUDES 1 Not coded here   EXCLUDES 2 Not included here   N Newborn Age: 0   P Pediatric Age: 0-17   M Maternity Age: 12-55   A Adult Age: 15-124

930   ICD-10-CM 2018

☑4ᵗʰ **S16** **Injury of muscle, fascia and tendon at neck level**
    Code also any associated open wound (S11.-)
    EXCLUDES 2 *sprain of joint or ligament at neck level (S13.9)*

    The appropriate 7th character is to be added to each code from category S16.
    A   initial encounter
    D   subsequent encounter
    S   sequela

  √x7ᵗʰ **S16.1** **Strain of muscle, fascia and tendon at neck level**
  √x7ᵗʰ **S16.2** **Laceration of muscle, fascia and tendon at neck level**
  √x7ᵗʰ **S16.8** **Other specified injury of muscle, fascia and tendon at neck level**
  √x7ᵗʰ **S16.9** **Unspecified injury of muscle, fascia and tendon at neck level** ▽

☑4ᵗʰ **S17** **Crushing injury of neck**
    Use additional code for all associated injuries, such as:
      injury of blood vessels (S15.-)
      open wound of neck (S11.-)
      spinal cord injury (S14.0, S14.1-)
      vertebral fracture (S12.0- -S12.3-)

    The appropriate 7th character is to be added to each code from category S17.
    A   initial encounter
    D   subsequent encounter
    S   sequela

  √x7ᵗʰ **S17.0** **Crushing injury of larynx and trachea**
  √x7ᵗʰ **S17.8** **Crushing injury of other specified parts of neck**
  √x7ᵗʰ **S17.9** **Crushing injury of neck, part unspecified** ▽

☑4ᵗʰ **S19** **Other specified and unspecified injuries of neck**

    The appropriate 7th character is to be added to each code from category S19.
    A   initial encounter
    D   subsequent encounter
    S   sequela

  √5ᵗʰ **S19.8** **Other specified injuries of neck**
    √x7ᵗʰ **S19.80** **Other specified injuries of unspecified part of neck** ▽
    √x7ᵗʰ **S19.81** **Other specified injuries of** larynx
    √x7ᵗʰ **S19.82** **Other specified injuries of cervical** trachea
        EXCLUDES 2 *other specified injury of thoracic trachea (S27.5-)*
    √x7ᵗʰ **S19.83** **Other specified injuries of** vocal cord
    √x7ᵗʰ **S19.84** **Other specified injuries of** thyroid gland
    √x7ᵗʰ **S19.85** **Other specified injuries of** pharynx and cervical esophagus
    √x7ᵗʰ **S19.89** **Other specified injuries of other specified part of neck**
  √x7ᵗʰ **S19.9** **Unspecified injury of neck** ▽

Injuries to the thorax (S20-S29)

INCLUDES injuries of breast
              injuries of chest (wall)
              injuries of interscapular area
EXCLUDES 2 *burns and corrosions (T20-T32)*
              effects of foreign body in bronchus (T17.5)
              effects of foreign body in esophagus (T18.1)
              effects of foreign body in lung (T17.8)
              effects of foreign body in trachea (T17.4)
              frostbite (T33-T34)
              injuries of axilla
              injuries of clavicle
              injuries of scapular region
              injuries of shoulder
              insect bite or sting, venomous (T63.4)

☑4ᵗʰ **S20** **Superficial injury of thorax**

    The appropriate 7th character is to be added to each code from category S20.
    A   initial encounter
    D   subsequent encounter
    S   sequela

  √5ᵗʰ **S20.0** Contusion of breast
    √x7ᵗʰ **S20.00** **Contusion of breast, unspecified breast** ▽
    √x7ᵗʰ **S20.01** **Contusion of** right **breast**

    √x7ᵗʰ **S20.02** **Contusion of** left **breast**
  √5ᵗʰ **S20.1** **Other and unspecified superficial injuries of breast**
    √6ᵗʰ **S20.10** **Unspecified superficial injuries of breast**
        √7ᵗʰ **S20.101** **Unspecified superficial injuries of breast,** right **breast** ▽
        √7ᵗʰ **S20.102** **Unspecified superficial injuries of breast,** left **breast** ▽
        √7ᵗʰ **S20.109** **Unspecified superficial injuries of breast, unspecified breast** ▽
    √6ᵗʰ **S20.11** Abrasion **of breast**
        √7ᵗʰ **S20.111** **Abrasion of breast,** right **breast**
        √7ᵗʰ **S20.112** **Abrasion of breast,** left **breast**
        √7ᵗʰ **S20.119** **Abrasion of breast, unspecified breast** ▽
    √6ᵗʰ **S20.12** Blister **(nonthermal) of breast**
        √7ᵗʰ **S20.121** **Blister (nonthermal) of breast,** right **breast**
        √7ᵗʰ **S20.122** **Blister (nonthermal) of breast,** left **breast**
        √7ᵗʰ **S20.129** **Blister (nonthermal) of breast, unspecified breast** ▽
    √6ᵗʰ **S20.14** External constriction **of part of breast**
        √7ᵗʰ **S20.141** **External constriction of part of breast,** right **breast**
        √7ᵗʰ **S20.142** **External constriction of part of breast,** left **breast**
        √7ᵗʰ **S20.149** **External constriction of part of breast, unspecified breast** ▽
    √6ᵗʰ **S20.15** **Superficial** foreign body **of breast**
        Splinter in the breast
        √7ᵗʰ **S20.151** **Superficial foreign body of breast,** right **breast**
        √7ᵗʰ **S20.152** **Superficial foreign body of breast,** left **breast**
        √7ᵗʰ **S20.159** **Superficial foreign body of breast, unspecified breast** ▽
    √6ᵗʰ **S20.16** Insect bite **(nonvenomous) of breast**
        √7ᵗʰ **S20.161** **Insect bite (nonvenomous) of breast,** right **breast**
        √7ᵗʰ **S20.162** **Insect bite (nonvenomous) of breast,** left **breast**
        √7ᵗʰ **S20.169** **Insect bite (nonvenomous) of breast, unspecified breast** ▽
    √6ᵗʰ **S20.17** **Other superficial** bite **of breast**
        EXCLUDES 1 *open bite of breast (S21.05-)*
        √7ᵗʰ **S20.171** **Other superficial bite of breast,** right **breast**
        √7ᵗʰ **S20.172** **Other superficial bite of breast,** left **breast**
        √7ᵗʰ **S20.179** **Other superficial bite of breast, unspecified breast** ▽
  √5ᵗʰ **S20.2** **Contusion of thorax**
    √x7ᵗʰ **S20.20** **Contusion of thorax, unspecified** ▽
    √6ᵗʰ **S20.21** **Contusion of** front wall **of thorax**
        √7ᵗʰ **S20.211** **Contusion of** right **front wall of thorax**
        √7ᵗʰ **S20.212** **Contusion of** left **front wall of thorax**
        √7ᵗʰ **S20.219** **Contusion of unspecified front wall of thorax** ▽
    √6ᵗʰ **S20.22** **Contusion of** back wall **of thorax**
        √7ᵗʰ **S20.221** **Contusion of** right **back wall of thorax**
        √7ᵗʰ **S20.222** **Contusion of** left **back wall of thorax**
        √7ᵗʰ **S20.229** **Contusion of unspecified back wall of thorax** ▽
  √5ᵗʰ **S20.3** **Other and unspecified superficial injuries of** front wall of thorax
    √6ᵗʰ **S20.30** **Unspecified superficial injuries of front wall of thorax**
        √7ᵗʰ **S20.301** **Unspecified superficial injuries of** right **front wall of thorax** ▽
        √7ᵗʰ **S20.302** **Unspecified superficial injuries of** left **front wall of thorax** ▽
        √7ᵗʰ **S20.309** **Unspecified superficial injuries of unspecified front wall of thorax** ▽
    √6ᵗʰ **S20.31** Abrasion **of front wall of thorax**
        √7ᵗʰ **S20.311** **Abrasion of** right **front wall of thorax**
        √7ᵗʰ **S20.312** **Abrasion of** left **front wall of thorax**

☑ Additional Character Req   √x7ᵗʰ Placeholder Alert   Manifestation   HCC CMS-HCC Condition   ▽ Unspecified Code   ▶◀ Revised Text   ● New Code   ▲ Revised Code Title

ICD-10-CM 2018   **931**

√7ᵗʰ **S20.319** **Abrasion** of unspecified **front wall** of thorax ▽

√6ᵗʰ **S20.32** **Blister** (nonthermal) of front wall of thorax

√7ᵗʰ **S20.321** **Blister** (nonthermal) of **right** front wall of thorax

√7ᵗʰ **S20.322** **Blister** (nonthermal) of **left** front wall of thorax

√7ᵗʰ **S20.329** **Blister** (nonthermal) of unspecified front wall of thorax ▽

√6ᵗʰ **S20.34** **External constriction** of front wall of thorax

√7ᵗʰ **S20.341** **External constriction** of **right** front wall of thorax

√7ᵗʰ **S20.342** **External constriction** of **left** front wall of thorax

√7ᵗʰ **S20.349** **External constriction** of unspecified front wall of thorax ▽

√6ᵗʰ **S20.35** **Superficial foreign body** of front wall of thorax
Splinter in front wall of thorax

√7ᵗʰ **S20.351** **Superficial foreign body** of **right** front wall of thorax

√7ᵗʰ **S20.352** **Superficial foreign body** of **left** front wall of thorax

√7ᵗʰ **S20.359** **Superficial foreign body** of unspecified front wall of thorax ▽

√6ᵗʰ **S20.36** **Insect bite** (nonvenomous) of front wall of thorax

√7ᵗʰ **S20.361** **Insect bite** (nonvenomous) of **right** front wall of thorax

√7ᵗʰ **S20.362** **Insect bite** (nonvenomous) of **left** front wall of thorax

√7ᵗʰ **S20.369** **Insect bite** (nonvenomous) of unspecified front wall of thorax ▽

√6ᵗʰ **S20.37** **Other superficial bite** of front wall of thorax
EXCLUDES 1   open bite of front wall of thorax (S21.14)

√7ᵗʰ **S20.371** **Other superficial bite** of **right** front wall of thorax

√7ᵗʰ **S20.372** **Other superficial bite** of **left** front wall of thorax

√7ᵗʰ **S20.379** **Other superficial bite** of unspecified front wall of thorax ▽

√5ᵗʰ **S20.4** **Other and unspecified superficial injuries of back wall of thorax**

√6ᵗʰ **S20.40** **Unspecified superficial injuries of back wall of thorax**

√7ᵗʰ **S20.401** **Unspecified superficial injuries of right** back wall of thorax ▽

√7ᵗʰ **S20.402** **Unspecified superficial injuries of left** back wall of thorax ▽

√7ᵗʰ **S20.409** **Unspecified superficial injuries of** unspecified back wall of thorax ▽

√6ᵗʰ **S20.41** **Abrasion** of back wall of thorax

√7ᵗʰ **S20.411** **Abrasion** of **right** back wall of thorax

√7ᵗʰ **S20.412** **Abrasion** of **left** back wall of thorax

√7ᵗʰ **S20.419** **Abrasion** of unspecified back wall of thorax ▽

√6ᵗʰ **S20.42** **Blister** (nonthermal) of back wall of thorax

√7ᵗʰ **S20.421** **Blister** (nonthermal) of **right** back wall of thorax

√7ᵗʰ **S20.422** **Blister** (nonthermal) of **left** back wall of thorax

√7ᵗʰ **S20.429** **Blister** (nonthermal) of unspecified back wall of thorax ▽

√6ᵗʰ **S20.44** **External constriction** of back wall of thorax

√7ᵗʰ **S20.441** **External constriction** of **right** back wall of thorax

√7ᵗʰ **S20.442** **External constriction** of **left** back wall of thorax

√7ᵗʰ **S20.449** **External constriction** of unspecified back wall of thorax ▽

√6ᵗʰ **S20.45** **Superficial foreign body** of back wall of thorax
Splinter of back wall of thorax

√7ᵗʰ **S20.451** **Superficial foreign body** of **right** back wall of thorax

√7ᵗʰ **S20.452** **Superficial foreign body** of **left** back wall of thorax

√7ᵗʰ **S20.459** **Superficial foreign body** of unspecified back wall of thorax ▽

√6ᵗʰ **S20.46** **Insect bite** (nonvenomous) of back wall of thorax

√7ᵗʰ **S20.461** **Insect bite** (nonvenomous) of **right** back wall of thorax

√7ᵗʰ **S20.462** **Insect bite** (nonvenomous) of **left** back wall of thorax

√7ᵗʰ **S20.469** **Insect bite** (nonvenomous) of unspecified back wall of thorax ▽

√6ᵗʰ **S20.47** **Other superficial bite** of back wall of thorax
EXCLUDES 1   open bite of back wall of thorax (S21.24)

√7ᵗʰ **S20.471** **Other superficial bite** of **right** back wall of thorax

√7ᵗʰ **S20.472** **Other superficial bite** of **left** back wall of thorax

√7ᵗʰ **S20.479** **Other superficial bite** of unspecified back wall of thorax ▽

√5ᵗʰ **S20.9** **Superficial injury** of unspecified parts of thorax
EXCLUDES 1   contusion of thorax NOS (S20.20)

√x7ᵗʰ **S20.90** **Unspecified superficial injury of unspecified parts of thorax** ▽
Superficial injury of thoracic wall NOS

√x7ᵗʰ **S20.91** **Abrasion** of unspecified parts of thorax ▽

√x7ᵗʰ **S20.92** **Blister** (nonthermal) of unspecified parts of thorax ▽

√x7ᵗʰ **S20.94** **External constriction** of unspecified parts of thorax ▽

√x7ᵗʰ **S20.95** **Superficial foreign body** of unspecified parts of thorax ▽
Splinter in thorax NOS

√x7ᵗʰ **S20.96** **Insect bite** (nonvenomous) of unspecified parts of thorax ▽

√x7ᵗʰ **S20.97** **Other superficial bite** of unspecified parts of thorax ▽
EXCLUDES 1   open bite of thorax NOS (S21.95)

√4ᵗʰ **S21** **Open wound of thorax**
Code also any associated injury, such as:
injury of heart (S26.-)
injury of intrathoracic organs (S27.-)
rib fracture (S22.3-, S22.4-)
spinal cord injury (S24.0-, S24.1-)
traumatic hemopneumothorax (S27.3)
traumatic hemothorax (S27.1)
traumatic pneumothorax (S27.0)
wound infection
EXCLUDES 1   traumatic amputation (partial) of thorax (S28.1)

The appropriate 7th character is to be added to each code from category S21.
A   initial encounter
D   subsequent encounter
S   sequela

√5ᵗʰ **S21.0** **Open wound of breast**

√6ᵗʰ **S21.00** **Unspecified open wound of breast**

√7ᵗʰ **S21.001** **Unspecified open wound of right** breast ▽

√7ᵗʰ **S21.002** **Unspecified open wound of left** breast ▽

√7ᵗʰ **S21.009** **Unspecified open wound of** unspecified breast ▽

√6ᵗʰ **S21.01** **Laceration without foreign body** of breast

√7ᵗʰ **S21.011** **Laceration without foreign body of right** breast

√7ᵗʰ **S21.012** **Laceration without foreign body of left** breast

√7ᵗʰ **S21.019** **Laceration without foreign body of** unspecified breast ▽

√6ᵗʰ **S21.02** **Laceration with foreign body** of breast

√7ᵗʰ **S21.021** **Laceration with foreign body of right** breast

√7ᵗʰ **S21.022** **Laceration with foreign body of left** breast

√7ᵗʰ **S21.029** **Laceration with foreign body of** unspecified breast ▽

EXCLUDES 1 Not coded here   **EXCLUDES 2** Not included here   Ⓝ Newborn Age: 0   Ⓟ Pediatric Age: 0-17   Ⓜ Maternity Age: 12-55   Ⓐ Adult Age: 15-124

932   ICD-10-CM 2018

✓6ᵗʰ **S21.03** Puncture wound without foreign body of breast

     ✓7ᵗʰ **S21.031** Puncture wound without foreign body of right breast

     ✓7ᵗʰ **S21.032** Puncture wound without foreign body of left breast

     ✓7ᵗʰ **S21.039** Puncture wound without foreign body of unspecified breast ▽

✓6ᵗʰ **S21.04** Puncture wound with foreign body of breast

     ✓7ᵗʰ **S21.041** Puncture wound with foreign body of right breast

     ✓7ᵗʰ **S21.042** Puncture wound with foreign body of left breast

     ✓7ᵗʰ **S21.049** Puncture wound with foreign body of unspecified breast ▽

✓6ᵗʰ **S21.05** Open bite of breast

     Bite of breast NOS

     EXCLUDES 1   superficial bite of breast (S20.17)

     ✓7ᵗʰ **S21.051** Open bite of right breast

     ✓7ᵗʰ **S21.052** Open bite of left breast

     ✓7ᵗʰ **S21.059** Open bite of unspecified breast ▽

✓5ᵗʰ **S21.1** Open wound of front wall of thorax without penetration into thoracic cavity

     Open wound of chest without penetration into thoracic cavity

   ✓6ᵗʰ **S21.10** Unspecified open wound of front wall of thorax without penetration into thoracic cavity

     ✓7ᵗʰ **S21.101** Unspecified open wound of right front wall of thorax without penetration into thoracic cavity ▽

     ✓7ᵗʰ **S21.102** Unspecified open wound of left front wall of thorax without penetration into thoracic cavity ▽

     ✓7ᵗʰ **S21.109** Unspecified open wound of unspecified front wall of thorax without penetration into thoracic cavity ▽

   ✓6ᵗʰ **S21.11** Laceration without foreign body of front wall of thorax without penetration into thoracic cavity

     ✓7ᵗʰ **S21.111** Laceration without foreign body of right front wall of thorax without penetration into thoracic cavity

     ✓7ᵗʰ **S21.112** Laceration without foreign body of left front wall of thorax without penetration into thoracic cavity

     ✓7ᵗʰ **S21.119** Laceration without foreign body of unspecified front wall of thorax without penetration into thoracic cavity ▽

   ✓6ᵗʰ **S21.12** Laceration with foreign body of front wall of thorax without penetration into thoracic cavity

     ✓7ᵗʰ **S21.121** Laceration with foreign body of right front wall of thorax without penetration into thoracic cavity

     ✓7ᵗʰ **S21.122** Laceration with foreign body of left front wall of thorax without penetration into thoracic cavity

     ✓7ᵗʰ **S21.129** Laceration with foreign body of unspecified front wall of thorax without penetration into thoracic cavity ▽

   ✓6ᵗʰ **S21.13** Puncture wound without foreign body of front wall of thorax without penetration into thoracic cavity

     ✓7ᵗʰ **S21.131** Puncture wound without foreign body of right front wall of thorax without penetration into thoracic cavity

     ✓7ᵗʰ **S21.132** Puncture wound without foreign body of left front wall of thorax without penetration into thoracic cavity

     ✓7ᵗʰ **S21.139** Puncture wound without foreign body of unspecified front wall of thorax without penetration into thoracic cavity ▽

   ✓6ᵗʰ **S21.14** Puncture wound with foreign body of front wall of thorax without penetration into thoracic cavity

     ✓7ᵗʰ **S21.141** Puncture wound with foreign body of right front wall of thorax without penetration into thoracic cavity

     ✓7ᵗʰ **S21.142** Puncture wound with foreign body of left front wall of thorax without penetration into thoracic cavity

     ✓7ᵗʰ **S21.149** Puncture wound with foreign body of unspecified front wall of thorax without penetration into thoracic cavity ▽

   ✓6ᵗʰ **S21.15** Open bite of front wall of thorax without penetration into thoracic cavity

     Bite of front wall of thorax NOS

     EXCLUDES 1   superficial bite of front wall of thorax (S20.37)

     ✓7ᵗʰ **S21.151** Open bite of right front wall of thorax without penetration into thoracic cavity

     ✓7ᵗʰ **S21.152** Open bite of left front wall of thorax without penetration into thoracic cavity

     ✓7ᵗʰ **S21.159** Open bite of unspecified front wall of thorax without penetration into thoracic cavity ▽

✓5ᵗʰ **S21.2** Open wound of back wall of thorax without penetration into thoracic cavity

   ✓6ᵗʰ **S21.20** Unspecified open wound of back wall of thorax without penetration into thoracic cavity

     ✓7ᵗʰ **S21.201** Unspecified open wound of right back wall of thorax without penetration into thoracic cavity ▽

     ✓7ᵗʰ **S21.202** Unspecified open wound of left back wall of thorax without penetration into thoracic cavity ▽

     ✓7ᵗʰ **S21.209** Unspecified open wound of unspecified back wall of thorax without penetration into thoracic cavity ▽

   ✓6ᵗʰ **S21.21** Laceration without foreign body of back wall of thorax without penetration into thoracic cavity

     ✓7ᵗʰ **S21.211** Laceration without foreign body of right back wall of thorax without penetration into thoracic cavity

     ✓7ᵗʰ **S21.212** Laceration without foreign body of left back wall of thorax without penetration into thoracic cavity

     ✓7ᵗʰ **S21.219** Laceration without foreign body of unspecified back wall of thorax without penetration into thoracic cavity ▽

   ✓6ᵗʰ **S21.22** Laceration with foreign body of back wall of thorax without penetration into thoracic cavity

     ✓7ᵗʰ **S21.221** Laceration with foreign body of right back wall of thorax without penetration into thoracic cavity

     ✓7ᵗʰ **S21.222** Laceration with foreign body of left back wall of thorax without penetration into thoracic cavity

     ✓7ᵗʰ **S21.229** Laceration with foreign body of unspecified back wall of thorax without penetration into thoracic cavity ▽

   ✓6ᵗʰ **S21.23** Puncture wound without foreign body of back wall of thorax without penetration into thoracic cavity

     ✓7ᵗʰ **S21.231** Puncture wound without foreign body of right back wall of thorax without penetration into thoracic cavity

     ✓7ᵗʰ **S21.232** Puncture wound without foreign body of left back wall of thorax without penetration into thoracic cavity

     ✓7ᵗʰ **S21.239** Puncture wound without foreign body of unspecified back wall of thorax without penetration into thoracic cavity ▽

   ✓6ᵗʰ **S21.24** Puncture wound with foreign body of back wall of thorax without penetration into thoracic cavity

     ✓7ᵗʰ **S21.241** Puncture wound with foreign body of right back wall of thorax without penetration into thoracic cavity

     ✓7ᵗʰ **S21.242** Puncture wound with foreign body of left back wall of thorax without penetration into thoracic cavity

     ✓7ᵗʰ **S21.249** Puncture wound with foreign body of unspecified back wall of thorax without penetration into thoracic cavity ▽

☑ Additional Character Req   ✓×7ᵗʰ Placeholder Alert   Manifestation   **HCC** CMS-HCC Condition   ▽ Unspecified Code   ▶◀ Revised Text   ● New Code   ▲ Revised Code Title

✓6ᵗʰ **S21.25** Open bite **of back wall of thorax without penetration into thoracic cavity**
Bite of back wall of thorax NOS
EXCLUDES 1   *superficial bite of back wall of thorax (S20.47)*

✓7ᵗʰ **S21.251** Open bite of right **back wall of thorax without penetration into thoracic cavity**

✓7ᵗʰ **S21.252** Open bite of left **back wall of thorax without penetration into thoracic cavity**

✓7ᵗʰ **S21.259** Open bite of unspecified back wall of thorax without penetration into thoracic cavity   ▽

✓5ᵗʰ **S21.3** Open wound of front wall of thorax with penetration **into thoracic cavity**
Open wound of chest with penetration into thoracic cavity

✓6ᵗʰ **S21.30** Unspecified open wound of front wall of thorax with penetration into thoracic cavity

✓7ᵗʰ **S21.301** Unspecified open wound of right front wall of thorax with penetration into thoracic cavity   ▽

✓7ᵗʰ **S21.302** Unspecified open wound of left front wall of thorax with penetration into thoracic cavity   ▽

✓7ᵗʰ **S21.309** Unspecified open wound of unspecified front wall of thorax with penetration into thoracic cavity   ▽

✓6ᵗʰ **S21.31** Laceration without foreign body of front wall of thorax with penetration into thoracic cavity

✓7ᵗʰ **S21.311** Laceration without foreign body of right front wall of thorax with penetration into thoracic cavity

✓7ᵗʰ **S21.312** Laceration without foreign body of left front wall of thorax with penetration into thoracic cavity

✓7ᵗʰ **S21.319** Laceration without foreign body of unspecified front wall of thorax with penetration into thoracic cavity   ▽

✓6ᵗʰ **S21.32** Laceration with foreign body of front wall of thorax with penetration into thoracic cavity

✓7ᵗʰ **S21.321** Laceration with foreign body of right front wall of thorax with penetration into thoracic cavity

✓7ᵗʰ **S21.322** Laceration with foreign body of left front wall of thorax with penetration into thoracic cavity

✓7ᵗʰ **S21.329** Laceration with foreign body of unspecified front wall of thorax with penetration into thoracic cavity   ▽

✓6ᵗʰ **S21.33** Puncture wound without foreign body of front wall of thorax with penetration into thoracic cavity

✓7ᵗʰ **S21.331** Puncture wound without foreign body of right front wall of thorax with penetration into thoracic cavity

✓7ᵗʰ **S21.332** Puncture wound without foreign body of left front wall of thorax with penetration into thoracic cavity

✓7ᵗʰ **S21.339** Puncture wound without foreign body of unspecified front wall of thorax with penetration into thoracic cavity   ▽

✓6ᵗʰ **S21.34** Puncture wound with foreign body of front wall of thorax with penetration into thoracic cavity

✓7ᵗʰ **S21.341** Puncture wound with foreign body of right front wall of thorax with penetration into thoracic cavity

✓7ᵗʰ **S21.342** Puncture wound with foreign body of left front wall of thorax with penetration into thoracic cavity

✓7ᵗʰ **S21.349** Puncture wound with foreign body of unspecified front wall of thorax with penetration into thoracic cavity   ▽

✓6ᵗʰ **S21.35** Open bite of front wall of thorax with penetration into thoracic cavity
EXCLUDES 1   *superficial bite of front wall of thorax (S20.37)*

✓7ᵗʰ **S21.351** Open bite of right front wall of thorax with penetration into thoracic cavity

✓7ᵗʰ **S21.352** Open bite of left front wall of thorax with penetration into thoracic cavity

✓7ᵗʰ **S21.359** Open bite of unspecified front wall of thorax with penetration into thoracic cavity   ▽

✓5ᵗʰ **S21.4** Open wound of back wall of thorax with penetration **into thoracic cavity**

✓6ᵗʰ **S21.40** Unspecified open wound of back wall of thorax with penetration into thoracic cavity

✓7ᵗʰ **S21.401** Unspecified open wound of right back wall of thorax with penetration into thoracic cavity   ▽

✓7ᵗʰ **S21.402** Unspecified open wound of left back wall of thorax with penetration into thoracic cavity   ▽

✓7ᵗʰ **S21.409** Unspecified open wound of unspecified back wall of thorax with penetration into thoracic cavity   ▽

✓6ᵗʰ **S21.41** Laceration without foreign body of back wall of thorax with penetration into thoracic cavity

✓7ᵗʰ **S21.411** Laceration without foreign body of right back wall of thorax with penetration into thoracic cavity

✓7ᵗʰ **S21.412** Laceration without foreign body of left back wall of thorax with penetration into thoracic cavity

✓7ᵗʰ **S21.419** Laceration without foreign body of unspecified back wall of thorax with penetration into thoracic cavity   ▽

✓6ᵗʰ **S21.42** Laceration with foreign body of back wall of thorax with penetration into thoracic cavity

✓7ᵗʰ **S21.421** Laceration with foreign body of right back wall of thorax with penetration into thoracic cavity

✓7ᵗʰ **S21.422** Laceration with foreign body of left back wall of thorax with penetration into thoracic cavity

✓7ᵗʰ **S21.429** Laceration with foreign body of unspecified back wall of thorax with penetration into thoracic cavity   ▽

✓6ᵗʰ **S21.43** Puncture wound without foreign body of back wall of thorax with penetration into thoracic cavity

✓7ᵗʰ **S21.431** Puncture wound without foreign body of right back wall of thorax with penetration into thoracic cavity

✓7ᵗʰ **S21.432** Puncture wound without foreign body of left back wall of thorax with penetration into thoracic cavity

✓7ᵗʰ **S21.439** Puncture wound without foreign body of unspecified back wall of thorax with penetration into thoracic cavity   ▽

✓6ᵗʰ **S21.44** Puncture wound with foreign body of back wall of thorax with penetration into thoracic cavity

✓7ᵗʰ **S21.441** Puncture wound with foreign body of right back wall of thorax with penetration into thoracic cavity

✓7ᵗʰ **S21.442** Puncture wound with foreign body of left back wall of thorax with penetration into thoracic cavity

✓7ᵗʰ **S21.449** Puncture wound with foreign body of unspecified back wall of thorax with penetration into thoracic cavity   ▽

✓6ᵗʰ **S21.45** Open bite of back wall of thorax with penetration into thoracic cavity
Bite of back wall of thorax NOS
EXCLUDES 1   *superficial bite of back wall of thorax (S20.47)*

✓7ᵗʰ **S21.451** Open bite of right back wall of thorax with penetration into thoracic cavity

✓7ᵗʰ **S21.452** Open bite of left back wall of thorax with penetration into thoracic cavity

✓7ᵗʰ **S21.459** Open bite of unspecified back wall of thorax with penetration into thoracic cavity   ▽

✓5ᵗʰ **S21.9** Open wound of unspecified part of thorax
Open wound of thoracic wall NOS

✓×7ᵗʰ **S21.90** Unspecified open wound of unspecified part of thorax   ▽

✓×7ᵗʰ **S21.91** Laceration without foreign body of unspecified part of thorax   ▽

EXCLUDES 1 Not coded here   *EXCLUDES 2* Not included here   N Newborn Age: 0   P Pediatric Age: 0-17   M Maternity Age: 12-55   A Adult Age: 15-124

934   ICD-10-CM 2018

√x7ᵗʰ **S21.92** Laceration with foreign body **of unspecified part of thorax** ▽

√x7ᵗʰ **S21.93** Puncture wound without foreign body **of unspecified part of thorax** ▽

√x7ᵗʰ **S21.94** Puncture wound with foreign body **of unspecified part of thorax** ▽

√x7ᵗʰ **S21.95** Open bite **of unspecified part of thorax** ▽
     EXCLUDES 1   *superficial bite of thorax (S20.97)*

√4ᵗʰ **S22**   **Fracture of rib(s), sternum and thoracic spine**
    NOTE   A fracture not indicated as nondisplaced or displaced should be coded to displaced.
          A fracture not indicated as open or closed should be coded to closed.
    INCLUDES   fracture of thoracic neural arch
          fracture of thoracic spinous process
          fracture of thoracic transverse process
          fracture of thoracic vertebra
          fracture of thoracic vertebral arch
   Code first any associated:
     injury of intrathoracic organ (S27.-)
     spinal cord injury (S24.0-, S24.1-)
    EXCLUDES 1   *transection of thorax (S28.1)*
    EXCLUDES 2   *fracture of clavicle (S42.0-)*
          fracture of scapula (S42.1-)
   AHA: 2015, 3Q, 37-39

> The appropriate 7th character is to be added to each code from category S22.
> A   initial encounter for closed fracture
> B   initial encounter for open fracture
> D   subsequent encounter for fracture with routine healing
> G   subsequent encounter for fracture with delayed healing
> K   subsequent encounter for fracture with nonunion
> S   sequela

√5ᵗʰ **S22.0**   **Fracture of** thoracic vertebra
   √6ᵗʰ **S22.00**   **Fracture of unspecified thoracic vertebra**
     [1] √7ᵗʰ **S22.000**   Wedge compression **fracture of unspecified thoracic vertebra** HCC ▽
     [1] √7ᵗʰ **S22.001**   Stable burst **fracture of unspecified thoracic vertebra** HCC ▽
     [1] √7ᵗʰ **S22.002**   Unstable burst **fracture of unspecified thoracic vertebra** HCC ▽
     [1] √7ᵗʰ **S22.008**   **Other fracture of unspecified thoracic vertebra** HCC ▽
     [1] √7ᵗʰ **S22.009**   **Unspecified fracture of unspecified thoracic vertebra** HCC ▽

   √6ᵗʰ **S22.01**   **Fracture of** first **thoracic vertebra**
     [1] √7ᵗʰ **S22.010**   Wedge compression **fracture of first thoracic vertebra** HCC
     [1] √7ᵗʰ **S22.011**   Stable burst **fracture of first thoracic vertebra** HCC
     [1] √7ᵗʰ **S22.012**   Unstable burst **fracture of first thoracic vertebra** HCC
     [1] √7ᵗʰ **S22.018**   **Other fracture of first thoracic vertebra** HCC
     [1] √7ᵗʰ **S22.019**   **Unspecified fracture of first thoracic vertebra** HCC ▽

   √6ᵗʰ **S22.02**   **Fracture of** second **thoracic vertebra**
     [1] √7ᵗʰ **S22.020**   Wedge compression **fracture of second thoracic vertebra** HCC
     [1] √7ᵗʰ **S22.021**   Stable burst **fracture of second thoracic vertebra** HCC
     [1] √7ᵗʰ **S22.022**   Unstable burst **fracture of second thoracic vertebra** HCC
     [1] √7ᵗʰ **S22.028**   **Other fracture of second thoracic vertebra** HCC
     [1] √7ᵗʰ **S22.029**   **Unspecified fracture of second thoracic vertebra** HCC ▽

   √6ᵗʰ **S22.03**   **Fracture of** third **thoracic vertebra**
     [1] √7ᵗʰ **S22.030**   Wedge compression **fracture of third thoracic vertebra** HCC
     [1] √7ᵗʰ **S22.031**   Stable burst **fracture of third thoracic vertebra** HCC
     [1] √7ᵗʰ **S22.032**   Unstable burst **fracture of third thoracic vertebra** HCC

[1] √7ᵗʰ **S22.038**   **Other fracture of third thoracic vertebra** HCC

[1] √7ᵗʰ **S22.039**   **Unspecified fracture of third thoracic vertebra** HCC ▽

√6ᵗʰ **S22.04**   **Fracture of** fourth **thoracic vertebra**
   [1] √7ᵗʰ **S22.040**   Wedge compression **fracture of fourth thoracic vertebra** HCC
   [1] √7ᵗʰ **S22.041**   Stable burst **fracture of fourth thoracic vertebra** HCC
   [1] √7ᵗʰ **S22.042**   Unstable burst **fracture of fourth thoracic vertebra** HCC
   [1] √7ᵗʰ **S22.048**   **Other fracture of fourth thoracic vertebra** HCC
   [1] √7ᵗʰ **S22.049**   **Unspecified fracture of fourth thoracic vertebra** HCC ▽

√6ᵗʰ **S22.05**   **Fracture of** T5-T6 **vertebra**
   [1] √7ᵗʰ **S22.050**   Wedge compression **fracture of T5-T6 vertebra** HCC
   [1] √7ᵗʰ **S22.051**   Stable burst **fracture of T5-T6 vertebra** HCC
   [1] √7ᵗʰ **S22.052**   Unstable burst **fracture of T5-T6 vertebra** HCC
   [1] √7ᵗʰ **S22.058**   **Other fracture of T5-T6 vertebra** HCC
   [1] √7ᵗʰ **S22.059**   **Unspecified fracture of T5-T6 vertebra** HCC ▽

√6ᵗʰ **S22.06**   **Fracture of** T7-T8 **vertebra**
   [1] √7ᵗʰ **S22.060**   Wedge compression **fracture of T7-T8 vertebra** HCC
   [1] √7ᵗʰ **S22.061**   Stable burst **fracture of T7-T8 vertebra** HCC
   [1] √7ᵗʰ **S22.062**   Unstable burst **fracture of T7-T8 vertebra** HCC
   [1] √7ᵗʰ **S22.068**   **Other fracture of T7-T8 thoracic vertebra** HCC
   [1] √7ᵗʰ **S22.069**   **Unspecified fracture of T7-T8 vertebra** HCC ▽

√6ᵗʰ **S22.07**   **Fracture of** T9-T10 **vertebra**
   [1] √7ᵗʰ **S22.070**   Wedge compression **fracture of T9-T10 vertebra** HCC
   [1] √7ᵗʰ **S22.071**   Stable burst **fracture of T9-T10 vertebra** HCC
   [1] √7ᵗʰ **S22.072**   Unstable burst **fracture of T9-T10 vertebra** HCC
   [1] √7ᵗʰ **S22.078**   **Other fracture of T9-T10 vertebra** HCC
   [1] √7ᵗʰ **S22.079**   **Unspecified fracture of T9-T10 vertebra** HCC ▽

√6ᵗʰ **S22.08**   **Fracture of** T11-T12 **vertebra**
   [1] √7ᵗʰ **S22.080**   Wedge compression **fracture of T11-T12 vertebra** HCC
   [1] √7ᵗʰ **S22.081**   Stable burst **fracture of T11-T12 vertebra** HCC
   [1] √7ᵗʰ **S22.082**   Unstable burst **fracture of T11-T12 vertebra** HCC
   [1] √7ᵗʰ **S22.088**   **Other fracture of T11-T12 vertebra** HCC
   [1] √7ᵗʰ **S22.089**   **Unspecified fracture of T11-T12 vertebra** HCC ▽

√5ᵗʰ **S22.2**   **Fracture of** sternum
   DEF: Break in flat bone (breast bone) in anterior thorax; caused by blunt trauma to anterior chest.
   √x7ᵗʰ **S22.20**   **Unspecified fracture of sternum** ▽
   √x7ᵗʰ **S22.21**   **Fracture of** manubrium
   √x7ᵗʰ **S22.22**   **Fracture of** body **of sternum**
   √x7ᵗʰ **S22.23**   **Sternal** manubrial dissociation
   √x7ᵗʰ **S22.24**   **Fracture of** xiphoid process

√5ᵗʰ **S22.3**   **Fracture of** one rib
   √x7ᵗʰ **S22.31**   **Fracture of one rib,** right **side**
   √x7ᵗʰ **S22.32**   **Fracture of one rib,** left **side**
   √x7ᵗʰ **S22.39**   **Fracture of one rib, unspecified side** ▽

√5ᵗʰ **S22.4**   Multiple fractures of ribs
   Fractures of two or more ribs
    EXCLUDES 1   *flail chest (S22.5-)*
   √x7ᵗʰ **S22.41**   **Multiple fractures of ribs,** right **side**

---

[1]   HCC with 7th character indicating initial encounter (A, B or C - specific to category).

✓x 7ᵗʰ **S22.42** **Multiple fractures of ribs, left side**

✓x 7ᵗʰ **S22.43** **Multiple fractures of ribs, bilateral**

✓x 7ᵗʰ **S22.49** **Multiple fractures of ribs, unspecified side** ▽

✓x 7ᵗʰ **S22.5** **Flail chest**

✓x 7ᵗʰ **S22.9** **Fracture of bony thorax, part unspecified** ▽

✓4ᵗʰ **S23** **Dislocation and sprain of joints and ligaments of thorax**

INCLUDES avulsion of joint or ligament of thorax
laceration of cartilage, joint or ligament of thorax
sprain of cartilage, joint or ligament of thorax
traumatic hemarthrosis of joint or ligament of thorax
traumatic rupture of joint or ligament of thorax
traumatic subluxation of joint or ligament of thorax
traumatic tear of joint or ligament of thorax

Code also any associated open wound

EXCLUDES 2 dislocation, sprain of sternoclavicular joint (S43.2, S43.6)
strain of muscle or tendon of thorax (S29.01-)

The appropriate 7th character is to be added to each code from category S23.
A　initial encounter
D　subsequent encounter
S　sequela

✓x 7ᵗʰ **S23.0** **Traumatic rupture of thoracic intervertebral disc**

EXCLUDES 1 rupture or displacement (nontraumatic) of thoracic
intervertebral disc NOS (M51- with fifth
character 4)

✓5ᵗʰ **S23.1** **Subluxation and dislocation of thoracic vertebra**

Code also any associated
open wound of thorax (S21.-)
spinal cord injury (S24.0-, S24.1-)

EXCLUDES 2 fracture of thoracic vertebrae (S22.0-)

✓6ᵗʰ **S23.10** **Subluxation and dislocation of unspecified thoracic vertebra**

✓7ᵗʰ **S23.100** **Subluxation of unspecified thoracic vertebra** ▽

✓7ᵗʰ **S23.101** **Dislocation of unspecified thoracic vertebra** ▽

✓6ᵗʰ **S23.11** **Subluxation and dislocation of T1/T2 thoracic vertebra**

✓7ᵗʰ **S23.110** **Subluxation of T1/T2 thoracic vertebra**

✓7ᵗʰ **S23.111** **Dislocation of T1/T2 thoracic vertebra**

✓6ᵗʰ **S23.12** **Subluxation and dislocation of T2/T3-T3/T4 thoracic vertebra**

✓7ᵗʰ **S23.120** **Subluxation of T2/T3 thoracic vertebra**

✓7ᵗʰ **S23.121** **Dislocation of T2/T3 thoracic vertebra**

✓7ᵗʰ **S23.122** **Subluxation of T3/T4 thoracic vertebra**

✓7ᵗʰ **S23.123** **Dislocation of T3/T4 thoracic vertebra**

✓6ᵗʰ **S23.13** **Subluxation and dislocation of T4/T5-T5/T6 thoracic vertebra**

✓7ᵗʰ **S23.130** **Subluxation of T4/T5 thoracic vertebra**

✓7ᵗʰ **S23.131** **Dislocation of T4/T5 thoracic vertebra**

✓7ᵗʰ **S23.132** **Subluxation of T5/T6 thoracic vertebra**

✓7ᵗʰ **S23.133** **Dislocation of T5/T6 thoracic vertebra**

✓6ᵗʰ **S23.14** **Subluxation and dislocation of T6/T7-T7/T8 thoracic vertebra**

✓7ᵗʰ **S23.140** **Subluxation of T6/T7 thoracic vertebra**

✓7ᵗʰ **S23.141** **Dislocation of T6/T7 thoracic vertebra**

✓7ᵗʰ **S23.142** **Subluxation of T7/T8 thoracic vertebra**

✓7ᵗʰ **S23.143** **Dislocation of T7/T8 thoracic vertebra**

✓6ᵗʰ **S23.15** **Subluxation and dislocation of T8/T9-T9/T10 thoracic vertebra**

✓7ᵗʰ **S23.150** **Subluxation of T8/T9 thoracic vertebra**

✓7ᵗʰ **S23.151** **Dislocation of T8/T9 thoracic vertebra**

✓7ᵗʰ **S23.152** **Subluxation of T9/T10 thoracic vertebra**

✓7ᵗʰ **S23.153** **Dislocation of T9/T10 thoracic vertebra**

✓6ᵗʰ **S23.16** **Subluxation and dislocation of T10/T11-T11/T12 thoracic vertebra**

✓7ᵗʰ **S23.160** **Subluxation of T10/T11 thoracic vertebra**

✓7ᵗʰ **S23.161** **Dislocation of T10/T11 thoracic vertebra**

✓7ᵗʰ **S23.162** **Subluxation of T11/T12 thoracic vertebra**

✓7ᵗʰ **S23.163** **Dislocation of T11/T12 thoracic vertebra**

✓6ᵗʰ **S23.17** **Subluxation and dislocation of T12/L1 thoracic vertebra**

✓7ᵗʰ **S23.170** **Subluxation of T12/L1 thoracic vertebra**

✓7ᵗʰ **S23.171** **Dislocation of T12/L1 thoracic vertebra**

✓5ᵗʰ **S23.2** **Dislocation of other and unspecified parts of thorax**

✓x 7ᵗʰ **S23.20** **Dislocation of unspecified part of thorax** ▽

✓x 7ᵗʰ **S23.29** **Dislocation of other parts of thorax**

✓x 7ᵗʰ **S23.3** **Sprain of ligaments of thoracic spine**

✓5ᵗʰ **S23.4** **Sprain of ribs and sternum**

✓x 7ᵗʰ **S23.41** **Sprain of ribs**

✓6ᵗʰ **S23.42** **Sprain of sternum**

✓7ᵗʰ **S23.420** **Sprain of sternoclavicular (joint) (ligament)**

✓7ᵗʰ **S23.421** **Sprain of chondrosternal joint**

✓7ᵗʰ **S23.428** **Other sprain of sternum**

✓7ᵗʰ **S23.429** **Unspecified sprain of sternum** ▽

✓x 7ᵗʰ **S23.8** **Sprain of other specified parts of thorax**

✓x 7ᵗʰ **S23.9** **Sprain of unspecified parts of thorax** ▽

✓4ᵗʰ **S24** **Injury of nerves and spinal cord at thorax level**

NOTE Code to highest level of thoracic spinal cord injury.
Injuries to the spinal cord (S24.0 and S24.1) refer to the cord
level and not bone level injury, and can affect nerve roots at
and below the level given.

Code also any associated:
fracture of thoracic vertebra (S22.0-)
open wound of thorax (S21.-)
transient paralysis (R29.5)

EXCLUDES 2 injury of brachial plexus (S14.3)

The appropriate 7th character is to be added to each code from category S24.
A　initial encounter
D　subsequent encounter
S　sequela

✓x 7ᵗʰ **S24.0** **Concussion and edema of thoracic spinal cord** HCC

✓5ᵗʰ **S24.1** **Other and unspecified injuries of thoracic spinal cord**

✓6ᵗʰ **S24.10** **Unspecified injury of thoracic spinal cord**

✓7ᵗʰ **S24.101** **Unspecified injury at T1 level of thoracic spinal cord** HCC ▽

✓7ᵗʰ **S24.102** **Unspecified injury at T2-T6 level of thoracic spinal cord** HCC ▽

✓7ᵗʰ **S24.103** **Unspecified injury at T7-T10 level of thoracic spinal cord** HCC ▽

✓7ᵗʰ **S24.104** **Unspecified injury at T11-T12 level of thoracic spinal cord** HCC ▽

✓7ᵗʰ **S24.109** **Unspecified injury at unspecified level of thoracic spinal cord** HCC ▽
Injury of thoracic spinal cord NOS

✓6ᵗʰ **S24.11** **Complete lesion of thoracic spinal cord**

✓7ᵗʰ **S24.111** **Complete lesion at T1 level of thoracic spinal cord** HCC

✓7ᵗʰ **S24.112** **Complete lesion at T2-T6 level of thoracic spinal cord** HCC

✓7ᵗʰ **S24.113** **Complete lesion at T7-T10 level of thoracic spinal cord** HCC

✓7ᵗʰ **S24.114** **Complete lesion at T11-T12 level of thoracic spinal cord** HCC

✓7ᵗʰ **S24.119** **Complete lesion at unspecified level of thoracic spinal cord** HCC ▽

✓6ᵗʰ **S24.13** **Anterior cord syndrome of thoracic spinal cord**

✓7ᵗʰ **S24.131** **Anterior cord syndrome at T1 level of thoracic spinal cord** HCC

✓7ᵗʰ **S24.132** **Anterior cord syndrome at T2-T6 level of thoracic spinal cord** HCC

✓7ᵗʰ **S24.133** **Anterior cord syndrome at T7-T10 level of thoracic spinal cord** HCC

✓7ᵗʰ **S24.134** **Anterior cord syndrome at T11-T12 level of thoracic spinal cord** HCC

✓7ᵗʰ **S24.139** **Anterior cord syndrome at unspecified level of thoracic spinal cord** HCC ▽

✓6ᵗʰ **S24.14** **Brown-Séquard syndrome of thoracic spinal cord**

✓7ᵗʰ **S24.141** **Brown-Séquard syndrome at T1 level of thoracic spinal cord** HCC

EXCLUDES 1 Not coded here　　**EXCLUDES 2** Not included here　　N Newborn Age: 0　　P Pediatric Age: 0-17　　M Maternity Age: 12-55　　A Adult Age: 15-124

936　　ICD-10-CM 2018

   ✓7ᵗʰ **S24.142** **Brown-Séquard syndrome at** T2-T6 ᴴᶜᶜ
            level of thoracic spinal cord

   ✓7ᵗʰ **S24.143** **Brown-Séquard syndrome at** T7-T10 ᴴᶜᶜ
            level of thoracic spinal cord

   ✓7ᵗʰ **S24.144** **Brown-Séquard syndrome at** T11-T12 ᴴᶜᶜ
            level of thoracic spinal cord

   ✓7ᵗʰ **S24.149** **Brown-Séquard syndrome at** ᴴᶜᶜ ▽
            unspecified level of thoracic
            spinal cord

✓6ᵗʰ **S24.15** **Other** incomplete **lesions of thoracic spinal cord**
      Incomplete lesion of thoracic spinal cord NOS
      Posterior cord syndrome of thoracic spinal cord

   ✓7ᵗʰ **S24.151** **Other incomplete lesion at** T1 **level** ᴴᶜᶜ
            of thoracic spinal cord

   ✓7ᵗʰ **S24.152** **Other incomplete lesion at** T2-T6 ᴴᶜᶜ
            level of thoracic spinal cord

   ✓7ᵗʰ **S24.153** **Other incomplete lesion at** T7-T10 ᴴᶜᶜ
            level of thoracic spinal cord

   ✓7ᵗʰ **S24.154** **Other incomplete lesion at** T11-T12 ᴴᶜᶜ
            level of thoracic spinal cord

   ✓7ᵗʰ **S24.159** **Other incomplete lesion at** ᴴᶜᶜ ▽
            unspecified level of thoracic
            spinal cord

✓x7ᵗʰ **S24.2** **Injury of nerve root of thoracic spine**

✓x7ᵗʰ **S24.3** **Injury of peripheral nerves of thorax**

✓x7ᵗʰ **S24.4** **Injury of thoracic sympathetic nervous system**
      Injury of cardiac plexus
      Injury of esophageal plexus
      Injury of pulmonary plexus
      Injury of stellate ganglion
      Injury of thoracic sympathetic ganglion

✓x7ᵗʰ **S24.8** **Injury of other specified nerves of thorax**

✓x7ᵗʰ **S24.9** **Injury of unspecified nerve of thorax** ▽

✓4ᵗʰ **S25** **Injury of blood vessels of thorax**
     Code also any associated open wound (S21.-)

     The appropriate 7th character is to be added to each code from
     category S25.
     A   initial encounter
     D   subsequent encounter
     S   sequela

✓5ᵗʰ **S25.0** **Injury of** thoracic aorta
      Injury of aorta NOS

  ✓x7ᵗʰ **S25.00** **Unspecified injury of thoracic aorta** ▽

  ✓x7ᵗʰ **S25.01** Minor laceration **of thoracic aorta**
        Incomplete transection of thoracic aorta
        Laceration of thoracic aorta NOS
        Superficial laceration of thoracic aorta

  ✓x7ᵗʰ **S25.02** Major laceration **of thoracic aorta**
        Complete transection of thoracic aorta
        Traumatic rupture of thoracic aorta

  ✓x7ᵗʰ **S25.09** **Other specified injury of thoracic aorta**

✓5ᵗʰ **S25.1** **Injury of** innominate or subclavian artery

  ✓6ᵗʰ **S25.10** **Unspecified injury of innominate or subclavian**
        artery

    ✓7ᵗʰ **S25.101** **Unspecified injury of** right **innominate** ▽
          or subclavian artery

    ✓7ᵗʰ **S25.102** **Unspecified injury of** left **innominate** ▽
          or subclavian artery

    ✓7ᵗʰ **S25.109** **Unspecified injury of unspecified** ▽
          innominate or subclavian artery

  ✓6ᵗʰ **S25.11** Minor laceration **of innominate or subclavian artery**
        Incomplete transection of innominate or subclavian
         artery
        Laceration of innominate or subclavian artery NOS
        Superficial laceration of innominate or subclavian
         artery

    ✓7ᵗʰ **S25.111** **Minor laceration of** right **innominate or**
          subclavian artery

    ✓7ᵗʰ **S25.112** **Minor laceration of** left **innominate or**
          subclavian artery

    ✓7ᵗʰ **S25.119** **Minor laceration of unspecified** ▽
          innominate or subclavian artery

  ✓6ᵗʰ **S25.12** Major laceration **of innominate or subclavian artery**
        Complete transection of innominate or subclavian
         artery
        Traumatic rupture of innominate or subclavian artery

    ✓7ᵗʰ **S25.121** **Major laceration of** right **innominate or**
          subclavian artery

    ✓7ᵗʰ **S25.122** **Major laceration of** left **innominate or**
          subclavian artery

    ✓7ᵗʰ **S25.129** **Major laceration of unspecified** ▽
          innominate or subclavian artery

  ✓6ᵗʰ **S25.19** **Other specified injury of innominate or subclavian**
        artery

    ✓7ᵗʰ **S25.191** **Other specified injury of** right **innominate**
          or subclavian artery

    ✓7ᵗʰ **S25.192** **Other specified injury of** left **innominate**
          or subclavian artery

    ✓7ᵗʰ **S25.199** **Other specified injury of unspecified** ▽
          innominate or subclavian artery

✓5ᵗʰ **S25.2** **Injury of** superior vena cava
      Injury of vena cava NOS

  ✓x7ᵗʰ **S25.20** **Unspecified injury of superior vena cava** ▽

  ✓x7ᵗʰ **S25.21** Minor laceration **of superior vena cava**
        Incomplete transection of superior vena cava
        Laceration of superior vena cava NOS
        Superficial laceration of superior vena cava

  ✓x7ᵗʰ **S25.22** Major laceration **of superior vena cava**
        Complete transection of superior vena cava
        Traumatic rupture of superior vena cava

  ✓x7ᵗʰ **S25.29** **Other specified injury of superior vena cava**

✓5ᵗʰ **S25.3** **Injury of** innominate or subclavian vein

  ✓6ᵗʰ **S25.30** **Unspecified injury of innominate or subclavian vein**

    ✓7ᵗʰ **S25.301** **Unspecified injury of** right **innominate** ▽
          or subclavian vein

    ✓7ᵗʰ **S25.302** **Unspecified injury of** left **innominate** ▽
          or subclavian vein

    ✓7ᵗʰ **S25.309** **Unspecified injury of unspecified** ▽
          innominate or subclavian vein

  ✓6ᵗʰ **S25.31** Minor laceration **of innominate or subclavian vein**
        Incomplete transection of innominate or subclavian
         vein
        Laceration of innominate or subclavian vein NOS
        Superficial laceration of innominate or subclavian vein

    ✓7ᵗʰ **S25.311** **Minor laceration of** right **innominate or**
          subclavian vein

    ✓7ᵗʰ **S25.312** **Minor laceration of** left **innominate or**
          subclavian vein

    ✓7ᵗʰ **S25.319** **Minor laceration of unspecified** ▽
          innominate or subclavian vein

  ✓6ᵗʰ **S25.32** Major laceration **of innominate or subclavian vein**
        Complete transection of innominate or subclavian
         vein
        Traumatic rupture of innominate or subclavian vein

    ✓7ᵗʰ **S25.321** **Major laceration of** right **innominate or**
          subclavian vein

    ✓7ᵗʰ **S25.322** **Major laceration of** left **innominate or**
          subclavian vein

    ✓7ᵗʰ **S25.329** **Major laceration of unspecified** ▽
          innominate or subclavian vein

  ✓6ᵗʰ **S25.39** **Other specified injury of innominate or subclavian**
        vein

    ✓7ᵗʰ **S25.391** **Other specified injury of** right **innominate**
          or subclavian vein

    ✓7ᵗʰ **S25.392** **Other specified injury of** left **innominate**
          or subclavian vein

    ✓7ᵗʰ **S25.399** **Other specified injury of unspecified** ▽
          innominate or subclavian vein

✓5ᵗʰ **S25.4** **Injury of** pulmonary blood vessels

  ✓6ᵗʰ **S25.40** **Unspecified injury of pulmonary blood vessels**

    ✓7ᵗʰ **S25.401** **Unspecified injury of** right **pulmonary** ▽
          blood vessels

    ✓7ᵗʰ **S25.402** **Unspecified injury of** left **pulmonary** ▽
          blood vessels

    ✓7ᵗʰ **S25.409** **Unspecified injury of unspecified** ▽
          pulmonary blood vessels

☑ Additional Character Req   ✓x7ᵗʰ Placeholder Alert   Manifestation   ᴴᶜᶜ CMS-HCC Condition   ▽ Unspecified Code   ▶◀ Revised Text   ● New Code   ▲ Revised Code Title

ICD-10-CM 2018   **937**

Chapter 19. Injury, Poisoning, and Certain Other Consequences of External Causes

✓6th **S25.41** **Minor laceration** of pulmonary blood vessels
Incomplete transection of pulmonary blood vessels
Laceration of pulmonary blood vessels NOS
Superficial laceration of pulmonary blood vessels

     ✓7th **S25.411** **Minor laceration of right pulmonary blood vessels**

     ✓7th **S25.412** **Minor laceration of left pulmonary blood vessels**

     ✓7th **S25.419** **Minor laceration of unspecified pulmonary blood vessels** ▽

✓6th **S25.42** **Major laceration** of pulmonary blood vessels
Complete transection of pulmonary blood vessels
Traumatic rupture of pulmonary blood vessels

     ✓7th **S25.421** **Major laceration of right pulmonary blood vessels**

     ✓7th **S25.422** **Major laceration of left pulmonary blood vessels**

     ✓7th **S25.429** **Major laceration of unspecified pulmonary blood vessels** ▽

✓6th **S25.49** **Other specified injury of pulmonary blood vessels**

     ✓7th **S25.491** **Other specified injury of right pulmonary blood vessels**

     ✓7th **S25.492** **Other specified injury of left pulmonary blood vessels**

     ✓7th **S25.499** **Other specified injury of unspecified pulmonary blood vessels** ▽

✓5th **S25.5** **Injury of** intercostal blood vessels

     ✓6th **S25.50** **Unspecified injury of intercostal blood vessels**

         ✓7th **S25.501** **Unspecified injury of intercostal blood vessels, right side** ▽

         ✓7th **S25.502** **Unspecified injury of intercostal blood vessels, left side** ▽

         ✓7th **S25.509** **Unspecified injury of intercostal blood vessels, unspecified side** ▽

     ✓6th **S25.51** **Laceration** of intercostal blood vessels

         ✓7th **S25.511** **Laceration of intercostal blood vessels, right side**

         ✓7th **S25.512** **Laceration of intercostal blood vessels, left side**

         ✓7th **S25.519** **Laceration of intercostal blood vessels, unspecified side** ▽

     ✓6th **S25.59** **Other specified injury of intercostal blood vessels**

         ✓7th **S25.591** **Other specified injury of intercostal blood vessels, right side**

         ✓7th **S25.592** **Other specified injury of intercostal blood vessels, left side**

         ✓7th **S25.599** **Other specified injury of intercostal blood vessels, unspecified side** ▽

✓5th **S25.8** **Injury of other blood vessels of thorax**
Injury of azygos vein
Injury of mammary artery or vein

     ✓6th **S25.80** **Unspecified injury of other blood vessels of thorax**

         ✓7th **S25.801** **Unspecified injury of other blood vessels of thorax, right side** ▽

         ✓7th **S25.802** **Unspecified injury of other blood vessels of thorax, left side** ▽

         ✓7th **S25.809** **Unspecified injury of other blood vessels of thorax, unspecified side** ▽

     ✓6th **S25.81** **Laceration** of other blood vessels of thorax

         ✓7th **S25.811** **Laceration of other blood vessels of thorax, right side**

         ✓7th **S25.812** **Laceration of other blood vessels of thorax, left side**

         ✓7th **S25.819** **Laceration of other blood vessels of thorax, unspecified side** ▽

     ✓6th **S25.89** **Other specified injury of other blood vessels of thorax**

         ✓7th **S25.891** **Other specified injury of other blood vessels of thorax, right side**

         ✓7th **S25.892** **Other specified injury of other blood vessels of thorax, left side**

         ✓7th **S25.899** **Other specified injury of other blood vessels of thorax, unspecified side** ▽

✓5th **S25.9** **Injury of unspecified** blood vessel of thorax

     ✓x7th **S25.90** **Unspecified injury of unspecified blood vessel of thorax** ▽

     ✓x7th **S25.91** **Laceration of unspecified blood vessel of thorax** ▽

     ✓x7th **S25.99** **Other specified injury of unspecified blood vessel of thorax** ▽

✓4th **S26** **Injury of heart**
Code also any associated:
   open wound of thorax (S21.-)
   traumatic hemopneumothorax (S27.2)
   traumatic hemothorax (S27.1)
   traumatic pneumothorax (S27.0)

> The appropriate 7th character is to be added to each code from category S26.
> A   initial encounter
> D   subsequent encounter
> S   sequela

✓5th **S26.0** **Injury of heart** with hemopericardium

     ✓x7th **S26.00** **Unspecified injury of heart with hemopericardium** ▽

     ✓x7th **S26.01** **Contusion of heart with hemopericardium**

     ✓6th **S26.02** **Laceration of heart with hemopericardium**

         ✓7th **S26.020** **Mild laceration of heart with hemopericardium**
Laceration of heart without penetration of heart chamber

         ✓7th **S26.021** **Moderate laceration of heart with hemopericardium**
Laceration of heart with penetration of heart chamber

         ✓7th **S26.022** **Major laceration of heart with hemopericardium**
Laceration of heart with penetration of multiple heart chambers

     ✓x7th **S26.09** **Other injury of heart with hemopericardium**

✓5th **S26.1** **Injury of heart** without hemopericardium

     ✓x7th **S26.10** **Unspecified injury of heart without hemopericardium** ▽

     ✓x7th **S26.11** **Contusion of heart without hemopericardium**

     ✓x7th **S26.12** **Laceration of heart without hemopericardium**

     ✓x7th **S26.19** **Other injury of heart without hemopericardium**

✓5th **S26.9** **Injury of heart, unspecified with or without hemopericardium**

     ✓x7th **S26.90** **Unspecified injury of heart, unspecified with or without hemopericardium** ▽

     ✓x7th **S26.91** **Contusion of heart, unspecified with or without hemopericardium** ▽
DEF: Bruising within the heart muscle with no mention of open wound; usually caused by blunt chest trauma in motor vehicle accidents, falling from great heights, or receiving CPR.

     ✓x7th **S26.92** **Laceration of heart, unspecified with or without hemopericardium** ▽
Laceration of heart NOS

     ✓x7th **S26.99** **Other injury of heart, unspecified with or without hemopericardium** ▽

✓4th **S27** **Injury of other and unspecified intrathoracic organs**
Code also any associated open wound of thorax (S21.-)
EXCLUDES 2 injury of cervical esophagus (S10-S19)
     injury of trachea (cervical) (S10-S19)

> The appropriate 7th character is to be added to each code from category S27.
> A   initial encounter
> D   subsequent encounter
> S   sequela

     ✓x7th **S27.0** **Traumatic pneumothorax**
EXCLUDES 1 spontaneous pneumothorax (J93.-)

     ✓x7th **S27.1** **Traumatic hemothorax**

     ✓x7th **S27.2** **Traumatic hemopneumothorax**

     ✓5th **S27.3** **Other and unspecified injuries of lung**

         ✓6th **S27.30** **Unspecified injury of lung**

             ✓7th **S27.301** **Unspecified injury of lung, unilateral** ▽

             ✓7th **S27.302** **Unspecified injury of lung, bilateral** ▽

             ✓7th **S27.309** **Unspecified injury of lung, unspecified** ▽

EXCLUDES 1 Not coded here   *EXCLUDES 2* Not included here   N Newborn Age: 0   P Pediatric Age: 0-17   M Maternity Age: 12-55   A Adult Age: 15-124

938   ICD-10-CM 2018

✓6th **S27.31 Primary blast injury of lung**
  Blast injury of lung NOS
  ✓7th **S27.311 Primary blast injury of lung,** unilateral
  ✓7th **S27.312 Primary blast injury of lung,** bilateral
  ✓7th **S27.319 Primary blast injury of lung,** unspecified ▽

✓6th **S27.32 Contusion of lung**
  DEF: Bruising of lung without mention of open wound.
  ✓7th **S27.321 Contusion of lung,** unilateral
  ✓7th **S27.322 Contusion of lung,** bilateral
  ✓7th **S27.329 Contusion of lung, unspecified** ▽

✓6th **S27.33 Laceration of lung**
  ✓7th **S27.331 Laceration of lung,** unilateral
  ✓7th **S27.332 Laceration of lung,** bilateral
  ✓7th **S27.339 Laceration of lung, unspecified** ▽

✓6th **S27.39 Other injuries of lung**
  Secondary blast injury of lung
  ✓7th **S27.391 Other injuries of lung,** unilateral
  ✓7th **S27.392 Other injuries of lung,** bilateral
  ✓7th **S27.399 Other injuries of lung, unspecified** ▽

✓5th **S27.4 Injury of bronchus**
✓6th **S27.40 Unspecified injury of bronchus**
  ✓7th **S27.401 Unspecified injury of bronchus,** unilateral ▽
  ✓7th **S27.402 Unspecified injury of bronchus,** bilateral ▽
  ✓7th **S27.409 Unspecified injury of bronchus,** unspecified ▽

✓6th **S27.41 Primary blast injury of bronchus**
  Blast injury of bronchus NOS
  ✓7th **S27.411 Primary blast injury of bronchus,** unilateral
  ✓7th **S27.412 Primary blast injury of bronchus,** bilateral
  ✓7th **S27.419 Primary blast injury of bronchus,** unspecified ▽

✓6th **S27.42 Contusion of bronchus**
  ✓7th **S27.421 Contusion of bronchus,** unilateral
  ✓7th **S27.422 Contusion of bronchus,** bilateral
  ✓7th **S27.429 Contusion of bronchus, unspecified** ▽

✓6th **S27.43 Laceration of bronchus**
  ✓7th **S27.431 Laceration of bronchus,** unilateral
  ✓7th **S27.432 Laceration of bronchus,** bilateral
  ✓7th **S27.439 Laceration of bronchus, unspecified** ▽

✓6th **S27.49 Other injury of bronchus**
  Secondary blast injury of bronchus
  ✓7th **S27.491 Other injury of bronchus,** unilateral
  ✓7th **S27.492 Other injury of bronchus,** bilateral
  ✓7th **S27.499 Other injury of bronchus, unspecified** ▽

✓5th **S27.5 Injury of thoracic trachea**
  ✓x7th **S27.50 Unspecified injury of thoracic trachea** ▽
  ✓x7th **S27.51 Primary blast injury of thoracic trachea**
    Blast injury of thoracic trachea NOS
  ✓x7th **S27.52 Contusion of thoracic trachea**
  ✓x7th **S27.53 Laceration of thoracic trachea**
  ✓x7th **S27.59 Other injury of thoracic trachea**
    Secondary blast injury of thoracic trachea

✓5th **S27.6 Injury of pleura**
  ✓x7th **S27.60 Unspecified injury of pleura** ▽
  ✓x7th **S27.63 Laceration of pleura**
  ✓x7th **S27.69 Other injury of pleura**

✓5th **S27.8 Injury of other specified intrathoracic organs**
✓6th **S27.80 Injury of diaphragm**
  ✓7th **S27.802 Contusion of diaphragm**
  ✓7th **S27.803 Laceration of diaphragm**
  ✓7th **S27.808 Other injury of diaphragm**
  ✓7th **S27.809 Unspecified injury of diaphragm** ▽
✓6th **S27.81 Injury of esophagus (thoracic part)**
  ✓7th **S27.812 Contusion of esophagus (thoracic part)**
  ✓7th **S27.813 Laceration of esophagus (thoracic part)**

✓7th **S27.818 Other injury of esophagus (thoracic part)**
✓7th **S27.819 Unspecified injury of esophagus (thoracic part)** ▽

✓6th **S27.89 Injury of other specified intrathoracic organs**
  Injury of lymphatic thoracic duct
  Injury of thymus gland
  ✓7th **S27.892 Contusion of other specified intrathoracic organs**
  ✓7th **S27.893 Laceration of other specified intrathoracic organs**
  ✓7th **S27.898 Other injury of other specified intrathoracic organs**
  ✓7th **S27.899 Unspecified injury of other specified intrathoracic organs** ▽

✓x7th **S27.9 Injury of unspecified intrathoracic organ** ▽

✓4th **S28 Crushing injury of thorax, and traumatic amputation of part of thorax**

> The appropriate 7th character is to be added to each code from category S28.
> A initial encounter
> D subsequent encounter
> S sequela

✓x7th **S28.0 Crushed chest**
  Use additional code for all associated injuries
  EXCLUDES 1 flail chest (S22.5)

✓x7th **S28.1 Traumatic amputation (partial) of part of thorax, except breast**

✓5th **S28.2 Traumatic amputation of breast**
✓6th **S28.21 Complete traumatic amputation of breast**
  Traumatic amputation of breast NOS
  ✓7th **S28.211 Complete traumatic amputation of right breast**
  ✓7th **S28.212 Complete traumatic amputation of left breast**
  ✓7th **S28.219 Complete traumatic amputation of unspecified breast** ▽
✓6th **S28.22 Partial traumatic amputation of breast**
  ✓7th **S28.221 Partial traumatic amputation of right breast**
  ✓7th **S28.222 Partial traumatic amputation of left breast**
  ✓7th **S28.229 Partial traumatic amputation of unspecified breast** ▽

✓4th **S29 Other and unspecified injuries of thorax**
  Code also any associated open wound (S21.-)

> The appropriate 7th character is to be added to each code from category S29.
> A initial encounter
> D subsequent encounter
> S sequela

✓5th **S29.0 Injury of muscle and tendon at thorax level**
✓6th **S29.00 Unspecified injury of muscle and tendon of thorax**
  ✓7th **S29.001 Unspecified injury of muscle and tendon of front wall of thorax** ▽
  ✓7th **S29.002 Unspecified injury of muscle and tendon of back wall of thorax** ▽
  ✓7th **S29.009 Unspecified injury of muscle and tendon of unspecified wall of thorax** ▽
✓6th **S29.01 Strain of muscle and tendon of thorax**
  ✓7th **S29.011 Strain of muscle and tendon of front wall of thorax**
  ✓7th **S29.012 Strain of muscle and tendon of back wall of thorax**
  ✓7th **S29.019 Strain of muscle and tendon of unspecified wall of thorax** ▽
✓6th **S29.02 Laceration of muscle and tendon of thorax**
  ✓7th **S29.021 Laceration of muscle and tendon of front wall of thorax**
  ✓7th **S29.022 Laceration of muscle and tendon of back wall of thorax**
  ✓7th **S29.029 Laceration of muscle and tendon of unspecified wall of thorax** ▽

✓6ᵗʰ **S29.09**   **Other injury of muscle and tendon of thorax**

    ✓7ᵗʰ **S29.091**   **Other injury of muscle and tendon of** front wall of thorax

    ✓7ᵗʰ **S29.092**   **Other injury of muscle and tendon of** back wall of thorax

    ✓7ᵗʰ **S29.099**   **Other injury of muscle and tendon of unspecified wall of thorax** ▽

✓x7ᵗʰ **S29.8**   **Other specified injuries of thorax**

✓x7ᵗʰ **S29.9**   **Unspecified injury of thorax** ▽

Injuries to the abdomen, lower back, lumbar spine, pelvis and external genitals (S30-S39)

INCLUDES   injuries to the abdominal wall
injuries to the anus
injuries to the buttock
injuries to the external genitalia
injuries to the flank
injuries to the groin

EXCLUDES 2   burns and corrosions (T20-T32)
effects of foreign body in anus and rectum (T18.5)
effects of foreign body in genitourinary tract (T19.-)
effects of foreign body in stomach, small intestine and colon (T18.2-T18.4)
frostbite (T33-T34)
insect bite or sting, venomous (T63.4)

✓4ᵗʰ **S30**   **Superficial injury of abdomen, lower back, pelvis and external genitals**

    EXCLUDES 2   superficial injury of hip (S70.-)

    The appropriate 7th character is to be added to each code from category S30.
    A   initial encounter
    D   subsequent encounter
    S   sequela

✓x7ᵗʰ **S30.0**   **Contusion of lower back and pelvis**
    Contusion of buttock

✓x7ᵗʰ **S30.1**   **Contusion of abdominal wall**
    Contusion of flank   Contusion of groin

✓5ᵗʰ **S30.2**   **Contusion of** external genital organs

    ✓6ᵗʰ **S30.20**   **Contusion of unspecified external genital organ**

      ✓7ᵗʰ **S30.201**   **Contusion of unspecified external genital organ,** male   ♂▽

      ✓7ᵗʰ **S30.202**   **Contusion of unspecified external genital organ,** female   ♀▽

    ✓x7ᵗʰ **S30.21**   **Contusion of** penis   ♂

    ✓x7ᵗʰ **S30.22**   **Contusion of** scrotum and testes   ♂

    ✓x7ᵗʰ **S30.23**   **Contusion of** vagina and vulva   ♀

✓x7ᵗʰ **S30.3**   **Contusion of** anus

✓5ᵗʰ **S30.8**   **Other superficial injuries of abdomen, lower back, pelvis and external genitals**

    ✓6ᵗʰ **S30.81**   Abrasion **of abdomen, lower back, pelvis and external genitals**

      ✓7ᵗʰ **S30.810**   **Abrasion of** lower back and pelvis

      ✓7ᵗʰ **S30.811**   **Abrasion of** abdominal wall

      ✓7ᵗʰ **S30.812**   **Abrasion of** penis   ♂

      ✓7ᵗʰ **S30.813**   **Abrasion of** scrotum and testes   ♂

      ✓7ᵗʰ **S30.814**   **Abrasion of** vagina and vulva   ♀

      ✓7ᵗʰ **S30.815**   **Abrasion of unspecified** external genital organs, male   ♂▽

      ✓7ᵗʰ **S30.816**   **Abrasion of unspecified** external genital organs, female   ♀▽

      ✓7ᵗʰ **S30.817**   **Abrasion of** anus

    ✓6ᵗʰ **S30.82**   Blister (nonthermal) **of abdomen, lower back, pelvis and external genitals**

      ✓7ᵗʰ **S30.820**   **Blister (nonthermal) of** lower back and pelvis

      ✓7ᵗʰ **S30.821**   **Blister (nonthermal) of** abdominal wall

      ✓7ᵗʰ **S30.822**   **Blister (nonthermal) of** penis   ♂

      ✓7ᵗʰ **S30.823**   **Blister (nonthermal) of** scrotum and testes   ♂

      ✓7ᵗʰ **S30.824**   **Blister (nonthermal) of** vagina and vulva   ♀

      ✓7ᵗʰ **S30.825**   **Blister (nonthermal) of unspecified** external genital organs, male   ♂▽

✓7ᵗʰ **S30.826**   **Blister (nonthermal) of unspecified external genital organs, female**   ♀▽

✓7ᵗʰ **S30.827**   **Blister (nonthermal) of** anus

✓6ᵗʰ **S30.84**   External constriction **of abdomen, lower back, pelvis and external genitals**

    ✓7ᵗʰ **S30.840**   **External constriction of** lower back and pelvis

    ✓7ᵗʰ **S30.841**   **External constriction of** abdominal wall

    ✓7ᵗʰ **S30.842**   **External constriction of** penis   ♂
      Hair tourniquet syndrome of penis
      Use additional cause code to identify the constricting item (W49.0-)

    ✓7ᵗʰ **S30.843**   **External constriction of** scrotum and testes   ♂

    ✓7ᵗʰ **S30.844**   **External constriction of** vagina and vulva   ♀

    ✓7ᵗʰ **S30.845**   **External constriction of unspecified** external genital organs, male   ♂▽

    ✓7ᵗʰ **S30.846**   **External constriction of unspecified** external genital organs, female   ♀▽

✓6ᵗʰ **S30.85**   **Superficial** foreign body **of abdomen, lower back, pelvis and external genitals**
    Splinter in the abdomen, lower back, pelvis and external genitals

    ✓7ᵗʰ **S30.850**   **Superficial foreign body of** lower back and pelvis

    ✓7ᵗʰ **S30.851**   **Superficial foreign body of** abdominal wall

    ✓7ᵗʰ **S30.852**   **Superficial foreign body of** penis   ♂

    ✓7ᵗʰ **S30.853**   **Superficial foreign body of** scrotum and testes   ♂

    ✓7ᵗʰ **S30.854**   **Superficial foreign body of** vagina and vulva   ♀

    ✓7ᵗʰ **S30.855**   **Superficial foreign body of unspecified** external genital organs, male   ♂▽

    ✓7ᵗʰ **S30.856**   **Superficial foreign body of unspecified** external genital organs, female   ♀▽

    ✓7ᵗʰ **S30.857**   **Superficial foreign body of** anus

✓6ᵗʰ **S30.86**   Insect bite (nonvenomous) **of abdomen, lower back, pelvis and external genitals**

    ✓7ᵗʰ **S30.860**   **Insect bite (nonvenomous) of** lower back and pelvis

    ✓7ᵗʰ **S30.861**   **Insect bite (nonvenomous) of** abdominal wall

    ✓7ᵗʰ **S30.862**   **Insect bite (nonvenomous) of** penis   ♂

    ✓7ᵗʰ **S30.863**   **Insect bite (nonvenomous) of** scrotum and testes   ♂

    ✓7ᵗʰ **S30.864**   **Insect bite (nonvenomous) of** vagina and vulva   ♀

    ✓7ᵗʰ **S30.865**   **Insect bite (nonvenomous) of unspecified** external genital organs, male   ♂▽

    ✓7ᵗʰ **S30.866**   **Insect bite (nonvenomous) of unspecified** external genital organs, female   ♀▽

    ✓7ᵗʰ **S30.867**   **Insect bite (nonvenomous) of** anus

✓6ᵗʰ **S30.87**   **Other superficial** bite **of abdomen, lower back, pelvis and external genitals**

    EXCLUDES 1   open bite of abdomen, lower back, pelvis and external genitals (S31.05, S31.15, S31.25, S31.35, S31.45, S31.55)

    ✓7ᵗʰ **S30.870**   **Other superficial bite of** lower back and pelvis

    ✓7ᵗʰ **S30.871**   **Other superficial bite of** abdominal wall

    ✓7ᵗʰ **S30.872**   **Other superficial bite of** penis   ♂

    ✓7ᵗʰ **S30.873**   **Other superficial bite of** scrotum and testes   ♂

    ✓7ᵗʰ **S30.874**   **Other superficial bite of** vagina and vulva   ♀

    ✓7ᵗʰ **S30.875**   **Other superficial bite of unspecified** external genital organs, male   ♂▽

    ✓7ᵗʰ **S30.876**   **Other superficial bite of unspecified** external genital organs, female   ♀▽

    ✓7ᵗʰ **S30.877**   **Other superficial bite of** anus

EXCLUDES 1 Not coded here   EXCLUDES 2 Not included here   N Newborn Age: 0   P Pediatric Age: 0-17   M Maternity Age: 12-55   A Adult Age: 15-124

✓5ᵗʰ **S30.9** **Unspecified superficial injury of abdomen, lower back, pelvis and external genitals**

    ✓x7ᵗʰ **S30.91** **Unspecified superficial injury of** lower back and pelvis ▽

    ✓x7ᵗʰ **S30.92** **Unspecified superficial injury of** abdominal wall ▽

    ✓x7ᵗʰ **S30.93** **Unspecified superficial injury of** penis ♂▽

    ✓x7ᵗʰ **S30.94** **Unspecified superficial injury of** scrotum and testes ♂▽

    ✓x7ᵗʰ **S30.95** **Unspecified superficial injury of** vagina and vulva ♀▽

    ✓x7ᵗʰ **S30.96** **Unspecified superficial injury of unspecified** external genital organs, male ♂▽

    ✓x7ᵗʰ **S30.97** **Unspecified superficial injury of unspecified** external genital organs, female ♀▽

    ✓x7ᵗʰ **S30.98** **Unspecified superficial injury of** anus ▽

✓4ᵗʰ **S31** **Open wound of abdomen, lower back, pelvis and external genitals**

    Code also any associated:
      spinal cord injury (S24.0, S24.1-, S34.0-, S34.1-)
      wound infection

    EXCLUDES 1 traumatic amputation of part of abdomen, lower back and pelvis (S38.2-, S38.3)

    EXCLUDES 2 open wound of hip (S71.00–S71.02)
              open fracture of pelvis (S32.1- -S32.9 with 7th character B)

> The appropriate 7th character is to be added to each code from category S31.
> A   initial encounter
> D   subsequent encounter
> S   sequela

  ✓5ᵗʰ **S31.0** **Open wound of** lower back and pelvis

    ✓6ᵗʰ **S31.00** **Unspecified open wound of lower back and pelvis**

      ✓7ᵗʰ **S31.000** **Unspecified open wound of lower back and pelvis** without penetration into retroperitoneum ▽
          Unspecified open wound of lower back and pelvis NOS

      ✓7ᵗʰ **S31.001** **Unspecified open wound of lower back and pelvis** with penetration into retroperitoneum ▽

    ✓6ᵗʰ **S31.01** Laceration without foreign body **of lower back and pelvis**

      ✓7ᵗʰ **S31.010** **Laceration without foreign body of lower back and pelvis** without penetration into retroperitoneum
          Laceration without foreign body of lower back and pelvis NOS

      ✓7ᵗʰ **S31.011** **Laceration without foreign body of lower back and pelvis** with penetration into retroperitoneum

    ✓6ᵗʰ **S31.02** Laceration with foreign body **of lower back and pelvis**

      ✓7ᵗʰ **S31.020** **Laceration with foreign body of lower back and pelvis** without penetration into retroperitoneum
          Laceration with foreign body of lower back and pelvis NOS

      ✓7ᵗʰ **S31.021** **Laceration with foreign body of lower back and pelvis** with penetration into retroperitoneum

    ✓6ᵗʰ **S31.03** Puncture wound without foreign body **of lower back and pelvis**

      ✓7ᵗʰ **S31.030** **Puncture wound without foreign body of lower back and pelvis** without penetration into retroperitoneum
          Puncture wound without foreign body of lower back and pelvis NOS

      ✓7ᵗʰ **S31.031** **Puncture wound without foreign body of lower back and pelvis** with penetration into retroperitoneum

    ✓6ᵗʰ **S31.04** Puncture wound with foreign body **of lower back and pelvis**

      ✓7ᵗʰ **S31.040** **Puncture wound with foreign body of lower back and pelvis** without penetration into retroperitoneum
          Puncture wound with foreign body of lower back and pelvis NOS

      ✓7ᵗʰ **S31.041** **Puncture wound with foreign body of lower back and pelvis** with penetration into retroperitoneum

    ✓6ᵗʰ **S31.05** Open bite **of lower back and pelvis**
      Bite of lower back and pelvis NOS

      EXCLUDES 1 superficial bite of lower back and pelvis (S30.860, S30.870)

      ✓7ᵗʰ **S31.050** **Open bite of lower back and pelvis** without penetration into retroperitoneum
          Open bite of lower back and pelvis NOS

      ✓7ᵗʰ **S31.051** **Open bite of lower back and pelvis** with penetration into retroperitoneum

  ✓5ᵗʰ **S31.1** **Open wound of** abdominal wall without penetration into peritoneal cavity
    Open wound of abdominal wall NOS

    EXCLUDES 2 open wound of abdominal wall with penetration into peritoneal cavity (S31.6-)

    ✓6ᵗʰ **S31.10** **Unspecified open wound of abdominal wall without penetration into peritoneal cavity**

      ✓7ᵗʰ **S31.100** **Unspecified open wound of abdominal wall,** right upper quadrant **without penetration into peritoneal cavity** ▽

      ✓7ᵗʰ **S31.101** **Unspecified open wound of abdominal wall,** left upper quadrant **without penetration into peritoneal cavity** ▽

      ✓7ᵗʰ **S31.102** **Unspecified open wound of abdominal wall,** epigastric region **without penetration into peritoneal cavity** ▽

      ✓7ᵗʰ **S31.103** **Unspecified open wound of abdominal wall,** right lower quadrant **without penetration into peritoneal cavity** ▽

      ✓7ᵗʰ **S31.104** **Unspecified open wound of abdominal wall,** left lower quadrant **without penetration into peritoneal cavity** ▽

      ✓7ᵗʰ **S31.105** **Unspecified open wound of abdominal wall,** periumbilic region **without penetration into peritoneal cavity** ▽

      ✓7ᵗʰ **S31.109** **Unspecified open wound of abdominal wall, unspecified quadrant without penetration into peritoneal cavity** ▽
          Unspecified open wound of abdominal wall NOS

    ✓6ᵗʰ **S31.11** Laceration without foreign body **of abdominal wall without penetration into peritoneal cavity**

      ✓7ᵗʰ **S31.110** **Laceration without foreign body of abdominal wall,** right upper quadrant **without penetration into peritoneal cavity**

      ✓7ᵗʰ **S31.111** **Laceration without foreign body of abdominal wall,** left upper quadrant **without penetration into peritoneal cavity**

      ✓7ᵗʰ **S31.112** **Laceration without foreign body of abdominal wall,** epigastric region **without penetration into peritoneal cavity**

      ✓7ᵗʰ **S31.113** **Laceration without foreign body of abdominal wall,** right lower quadrant **without penetration into peritoneal cavity**

      ✓7ᵗʰ **S31.114** **Laceration without foreign body of abdominal wall,** left lower quadrant **without penetration into peritoneal cavity**

      ✓7ᵗʰ **S31.115** **Laceration without foreign body of abdominal wall,** periumbilic region **without penetration into peritoneal cavity**

      ✓7ᵗʰ **S31.119** **Laceration without foreign body of abdominal wall, unspecified quadrant without penetration into peritoneal cavity** ▽

    ✓6ᵗʰ **S31.12** Laceration with foreign body **of abdominal wall without penetration into peritoneal cavity**

      ✓7ᵗʰ **S31.120** **Laceration of abdominal wall with foreign body,** right upper quadrant **without penetration into peritoneal cavity**

      ✓7ᵗʰ **S31.121** **Laceration of abdominal wall with foreign body,** left upper quadrant **without penetration into peritoneal cavity**

      ✓7ᵗʰ **S31.122** **Laceration of abdominal wall with foreign body,** epigastric region **without penetration into peritoneal cavity**

      ✓7ᵗʰ **S31.123** **Laceration of abdominal wall with foreign body,** right lower quadrant **without penetration into peritoneal cavity**

✓ Additional Character Req   ✓7ᵗʰ Placeholder Alert   Manifestation   HCC CMS-HCC Condition   ▽ Unspecified Code   ►◄ Revised Text   ● New Code   ▲ Revised Code Title

☑7ᵗʰ **S31.124** Laceration of abdominal wall with foreign body, left lower quadrant without penetration into peritoneal cavity

☑7ᵗʰ **S31.125** Laceration of abdominal wall with foreign body, periumbilic region without penetration into peritoneal cavity

☑7ᵗʰ **S31.129** Laceration of abdominal wall with foreign body, unspecified quadrant without penetration into peritoneal cavity ▽

☑6ᵗʰ **S31.13** Puncture wound of abdominal wall without foreign body without penetration into peritoneal cavity

☑7ᵗʰ **S31.130** Puncture wound of abdominal wall without foreign body, right upper quadrant without penetration into peritoneal cavity

☑7ᵗʰ **S31.131** Puncture wound of abdominal wall without foreign body, left upper quadrant without penetration into peritoneal cavity

☑7ᵗʰ **S31.132** Puncture wound of abdominal wall without foreign body, epigastric region without penetration into peritoneal cavity

☑7ᵗʰ **S31.133** Puncture wound of abdominal wall without foreign body, right lower quadrant without penetration into peritoneal cavity

☑7ᵗʰ **S31.134** Puncture wound of abdominal wall without foreign body, left lower quadrant without penetration into peritoneal cavity

☑7ᵗʰ **S31.135** Puncture wound of abdominal wall without foreign body, periumbilic region without penetration into peritoneal cavity

☑7ᵗʰ **S31.139** Puncture wound of abdominal wall without foreign body, unspecified quadrant without penetration into peritoneal cavity ▽

☑6ᵗʰ **S31.14** Puncture wound of abdominal wall with foreign body without penetration into peritoneal cavity

☑7ᵗʰ **S31.140** Puncture wound of abdominal wall with foreign body, right upper quadrant without penetration into peritoneal cavity

☑7ᵗʰ **S31.141** Puncture wound of abdominal wall with foreign body, left upper quadrant without penetration into peritoneal cavity

☑7ᵗʰ **S31.142** Puncture wound of abdominal wall with foreign body, epigastric region without penetration into peritoneal cavity

☑7ᵗʰ **S31.143** Puncture wound of abdominal wall with foreign body, right lower quadrant without penetration into peritoneal cavity

☑7ᵗʰ **S31.144** Puncture wound of abdominal wall with foreign body, left lower quadrant without penetration into peritoneal cavity

☑7ᵗʰ **S31.145** Puncture wound of abdominal wall with foreign body, periumbilic region without penetration into peritoneal cavity

☑7ᵗʰ **S31.149** Puncture wound of abdominal wall with foreign body, unspecified quadrant without penetration into peritoneal cavity ▽

☑6ᵗʰ **S31.15** Open bite of abdominal wall without penetration into peritoneal cavity
Bite of abdominal wall NOS
EXCLUDES 1　superficial bite of abdominal wall (S30.871)

☑7ᵗʰ **S31.150** Open bite of abdominal wall, right upper quadrant without penetration into peritoneal cavity

☑7ᵗʰ **S31.151** Open bite of abdominal wall, left upper quadrant without penetration into peritoneal cavity

☑7ᵗʰ **S31.152** Open bite of abdominal wall, epigastric region without penetration into peritoneal cavity

☑7ᵗʰ **S31.153** Open bite of abdominal wall, right lower quadrant without penetration into peritoneal cavity

☑7ᵗʰ **S31.154** Open bite of abdominal wall, left lower quadrant without penetration into peritoneal cavity

☑7ᵗʰ **S31.155** Open bite of abdominal wall, periumbilic region without penetration into peritoneal cavity

☑7ᵗʰ **S31.159** Open bite of abdominal wall, unspecified quadrant without penetration into peritoneal cavity ▽

☑5ᵗʰ **S31.2** Open wound of penis

☑7ᵗʰ **S31.20** Unspecified open wound of penis ♂▽

☑7ᵗʰ **S31.21** Laceration without foreign body of penis ♂

☑7ᵗʰ **S31.22** Laceration with foreign body of penis ♂

☑7ᵗʰ **S31.23** Puncture wound without foreign body of penis ♂

☑7ᵗʰ **S31.24** Puncture wound with foreign body of penis ♂

☑7ᵗʰ **S31.25** Open bite of penis ♂
Bite of penis NOS
EXCLUDES 1　superficial bite of penis (S30.862, S30.872)

☑5ᵗʰ **S31.3** Open wound of scrotum and testes

☑7ᵗʰ **S31.30** Unspecified open wound of scrotum and testes ♂▽

☑7ᵗʰ **S31.31** Laceration without foreign body of scrotum and testes ♂

☑7ᵗʰ **S31.32** Laceration with foreign body of scrotum and testes ♂

☑7ᵗʰ **S31.33** Puncture wound without foreign body of scrotum and testes ♂

☑7ᵗʰ **S31.34** Puncture wound with foreign body of scrotum and testes ♂

☑7ᵗʰ **S31.35** Open bite of scrotum and testes ♂
Bite of scrotum and testes NOS
EXCLUDES 1　superficial bite of scrotum and testes (S30.863, S30.873)

☑5ᵗʰ **S31.4** Open wound of vagina and vulva
EXCLUDES 1　injury to vagina and vulva during delivery (O70-, O71.4)

☑7ᵗʰ **S31.40** Unspecified open wound of vagina and vulva ♀▽

☑7ᵗʰ **S31.41** Laceration without foreign body of vagina and vulva ♀

☑7ᵗʰ **S31.42** Laceration with foreign body of vagina and vulva ♀

☑7ᵗʰ **S31.43** Puncture wound without foreign body of vagina and vulva ♀

☑7ᵗʰ **S31.44** Puncture wound with foreign body of vagina and vulva ♀

☑7ᵗʰ **S31.45** Open bite of vagina and vulva ♀
Bite of vagina and vulva NOS
EXCLUDES 1　superficial bite of vagina and vulva (S30.864, S30.874)

☑5ᵗʰ **S31.5** Open wound of unspecified external genital organs
EXCLUDES 1　traumatic amputation of external genital organs (S38.21, S38.22)

☑6ᵗʰ **S31.50** Unspecified open wound of unspecified external genital organs

☑7ᵗʰ **S31.501** Unspecified open wound of unspecified external genital organs, male ♂▽

☑7ᵗʰ **S31.502** Unspecified open wound of unspecified external genital organs, female ♀▽

☑6ᵗʰ **S31.51** Laceration without foreign body of unspecified external genital organs

☑7ᵗʰ **S31.511** Laceration without foreign body of unspecified external genital organs, male ♂▽

☑7ᵗʰ **S31.512** Laceration without foreign body of unspecified external genital organs, female ♀▽

☑6ᵗʰ **S31.52** Laceration with foreign body of unspecified external genital organs

☑7ᵗʰ **S31.521** Laceration with foreign body of unspecified external genital organs, male ♂▽

☑7ᵗʰ **S31.522** Laceration with foreign body of unspecified external genital organs, female ♀▽

✓6ᵗʰ **S31.53** Puncture wound without foreign body of unspecified external genital organs

 ✓7ᵗʰ **S31.531** Puncture wound without foreign body of unspecified external genital organs, male ♂▽

 ✓7ᵗʰ **S31.532** Puncture wound without foreign body of unspecified external genital organs, female ♀▽

✓6ᵗʰ **S31.54** Puncture wound with foreign body of unspecified external genital organs

 ✓7ᵗʰ **S31.541** Puncture wound with foreign body of unspecified external genital organs, male ♂▽

 ✓7ᵗʰ **S31.542** Puncture wound with foreign body of unspecified external genital organs, female ♀▽

✓6ᵗʰ **S31.55** Open bite of unspecified external genital organs
Bite of unspecified external genital organs NOS

 EXCLUDES 1 *superficial bite of unspecified external genital organs (S30.865, S30.866, S30.875, S30.876)*

 ✓7ᵗʰ **S31.551** Open bite of unspecified external genital organs, male ♂▽

 ✓7ᵗʰ **S31.552** Open bite of unspecified external genital organs, female ♀▽

✓5ᵗʰ **S31.6** Open wound of abdominal wall with penetration into peritoneal cavity

✓6ᵗʰ **S31.60** Unspecified open wound of abdominal wall with penetration into peritoneal cavity

 ✓7ᵗʰ **S31.600** Unspecified open wound of abdominal wall, right upper quadrant with penetration into peritoneal cavity ▽

 ✓7ᵗʰ **S31.601** Unspecified open wound of abdominal wall, left upper quadrant with penetration into peritoneal cavity ▽

 ✓7ᵗʰ **S31.602** Unspecified open wound of abdominal wall, epigastric region with penetration into peritoneal cavity ▽

 ✓7ᵗʰ **S31.603** Unspecified open wound of abdominal wall, right lower quadrant with penetration into peritoneal cavity ▽

 ✓7ᵗʰ **S31.604** Unspecified open wound of abdominal wall, left lower quadrant with penetration into peritoneal cavity ▽

 ✓7ᵗʰ **S31.605** Unspecified open wound of abdominal wall, periumbilic region with penetration into peritoneal cavity ▽

 ✓7ᵗʰ **S31.609** Unspecified open wound of abdominal wall, unspecified quadrant with penetration into peritoneal cavity ▽

✓6ᵗʰ **S31.61** Laceration without foreign body of abdominal wall with penetration into peritoneal cavity

 ✓7ᵗʰ **S31.610** Laceration without foreign body of abdominal wall, right upper quadrant with penetration into peritoneal cavity

 ✓7ᵗʰ **S31.611** Laceration without foreign body of abdominal wall, left upper quadrant with penetration into peritoneal cavity

 ✓7ᵗʰ **S31.612** Laceration without foreign body of abdominal wall, epigastric region with penetration into peritoneal cavity

 ✓7ᵗʰ **S31.613** Laceration without foreign body of abdominal wall, right lower quadrant with penetration into peritoneal cavity

 ✓7ᵗʰ **S31.614** Laceration without foreign body of abdominal wall, left lower quadrant with penetration into peritoneal cavity

 ✓7ᵗʰ **S31.615** Laceration without foreign body of abdominal wall, periumbilic region with penetration into peritoneal cavity

 ✓7ᵗʰ **S31.619** Laceration without foreign body of abdominal wall, unspecified quadrant with penetration into peritoneal cavity ▽

✓6ᵗʰ **S31.62** Laceration with foreign body of abdominal wall with penetration into peritoneal cavity

 ✓7ᵗʰ **S31.620** Laceration with foreign body of abdominal wall, right upper quadrant with penetration into peritoneal cavity

 ✓7ᵗʰ **S31.621** Laceration with foreign body of abdominal wall, left upper quadrant with penetration into peritoneal cavity

 ✓7ᵗʰ **S31.622** Laceration with foreign body of abdominal wall, epigastric region with penetration into peritoneal cavity

 ✓7ᵗʰ **S31.623** Laceration with foreign body of abdominal wall, right lower quadrant with penetration into peritoneal cavity

 ✓7ᵗʰ **S31.624** Laceration with foreign body of abdominal wall, left lower quadrant with penetration into peritoneal cavity

 ✓7ᵗʰ **S31.625** Laceration with foreign body of abdominal wall, periumbilic region with penetration into peritoneal cavity

 ✓7ᵗʰ **S31.629** Laceration with foreign body of abdominal wall, unspecified quadrant with penetration into peritoneal cavity ▽

✓6ᵗʰ **S31.63** Puncture wound without foreign body of abdominal wall with penetration into peritoneal cavity

 ✓7ᵗʰ **S31.630** Puncture wound without foreign body of abdominal wall, right upper quadrant with penetration into peritoneal cavity

 ✓7ᵗʰ **S31.631** Puncture wound without foreign body of abdominal wall, left upper quadrant with penetration into peritoneal cavity

 ✓7ᵗʰ **S31.632** Puncture wound without foreign body of abdominal wall, epigastric region with penetration into peritoneal cavity

 ✓7ᵗʰ **S31.633** Puncture wound without foreign body of abdominal wall, right lower quadrant with penetration into peritoneal cavity

 ✓7ᵗʰ **S31.634** Puncture wound without foreign body of abdominal wall, left lower quadrant with penetration into peritoneal cavity

 ✓7ᵗʰ **S31.635** Puncture wound without foreign body of abdominal wall, periumbilic region with penetration into peritoneal cavity

 ✓7ᵗʰ **S31.639** Puncture wound without foreign body of abdominal wall, unspecified quadrant with penetration into peritoneal cavity ▽

✓6ᵗʰ **S31.64** Puncture wound with foreign body of abdominal wall with penetration into peritoneal cavity

 ✓7ᵗʰ **S31.640** Puncture wound with foreign body of abdominal wall, right upper quadrant with penetration into peritoneal cavity

 ✓7ᵗʰ **S31.641** Puncture wound with foreign body of abdominal wall, left upper quadrant with penetration into peritoneal cavity

 ✓7ᵗʰ **S31.642** Puncture wound with foreign body of abdominal wall, epigastric region with penetration into peritoneal cavity

 ✓7ᵗʰ **S31.643** Puncture wound with foreign body of abdominal wall, right lower quadrant with penetration into peritoneal cavity

 ✓7ᵗʰ **S31.644** Puncture wound with foreign body of abdominal wall, left lower quadrant with penetration into peritoneal cavity

 ✓7ᵗʰ **S31.645** Puncture wound with foreign body of abdominal wall, periumbilic region with penetration into peritoneal cavity

 ✓7ᵗʰ **S31.649** Puncture wound with foreign body of abdominal wall, unspecified quadrant with penetration into peritoneal cavity ▽

✓6ᵗʰ **S31.65** Open bite of abdominal wall with penetration into peritoneal cavity

 EXCLUDES 1 *superficial bite of abdominal wall (S30.861, S30.871)*

 ✓7ᵗʰ **S31.650** Open bite of abdominal wall, right upper quadrant with penetration into peritoneal cavity

 ✓7ᵗʰ **S31.651** Open bite of abdominal wall, left upper quadrant with penetration into peritoneal cavity

 ✓7ᵗʰ **S31.652** Open bite of abdominal wall, epigastric region with penetration into peritoneal cavity

---

✓ Additional Character Req   ✓x7ᵗʰ Placeholder Alert   Manifestation   **HCC** CMS-HCC Condition   ▽ Unspecified Code   ▶◀ Revised Text   ● New Code   ▲ Revised Code Title

☑7ᵗʰ **S31.653** Open bite of abdominal wall, right lower quadrant with penetration into peritoneal cavity

☑7ᵗʰ **S31.654** Open bite of abdominal wall, left lower quadrant with penetration into peritoneal cavity

☑7ᵗʰ **S31.655** Open bite of abdominal wall, periumbilic region with penetration into peritoneal cavity

☑7ᵗʰ **S31.659** Open bite of abdominal wall, unspecified quadrant with penetration into peritoneal cavity ▽

☑5ᵗʰ **S31.8** **Open wound of other parts of abdomen, lower back and pelvis**

  ☑6ᵗʰ **S31.80** **Open wound of unspecified buttock**

    ☑7ᵗʰ **S31.801** Laceration without foreign body of unspecified buttock ▽

    ☑7ᵗʰ **S31.802** Laceration with foreign body of unspecified buttock ▽

    ☑7ᵗʰ **S31.803** Puncture wound without foreign body of unspecified buttock ▽

    ☑7ᵗʰ **S31.804** Puncture wound with foreign body of unspecified buttock ▽

    ☑7ᵗʰ **S31.805** Open bite of unspecified buttock ▽
         Bite of buttock NOS
         EXCLUDES 1   superficial bite of buttock (S30.870)

    ☑7ᵗʰ **S31.809** Unspecified open wound of unspecified buttock ▽

  ☑6ᵗʰ **S31.81** **Open wound of right buttock**

    ☑7ᵗʰ **S31.811** Laceration without foreign body of right buttock

    ☑7ᵗʰ **S31.812** Laceration with foreign body of right buttock

    ☑7ᵗʰ **S31.813** Puncture wound without foreign body of right buttock

    ☑7ᵗʰ **S31.814** Puncture wound with foreign body of right buttock

    ☑7ᵗʰ **S31.815** Open bite of right buttock
         Bite of right buttock NOS
         EXCLUDES 1   superficial bite of buttock (S30.870)

    ☑7ᵗʰ **S31.819** Unspecified open wound of right buttock ▽

  ☑6ᵗʰ **S31.82** **Open wound of left buttock**

    ☑7ᵗʰ **S31.821** Laceration without foreign body of left buttock

    ☑7ᵗʰ **S31.822** Laceration with foreign body of left buttock

    ☑7ᵗʰ **S31.823** Puncture wound without foreign body of left buttock

    ☑7ᵗʰ **S31.824** Puncture wound with foreign body of left buttock

    ☑7ᵗʰ **S31.825** Open bite of left buttock
         Bite of left buttock NOS
         EXCLUDES 1   superficial bite of buttock (S30.870)

    ☑7ᵗʰ **S31.829** Unspecified open wound of left buttock ▽

  ☑6ᵗʰ **S31.83** **Open wound of anus**

    ☑7ᵗʰ **S31.831** Laceration without foreign body of anus

    ☑7ᵗʰ **S31.832** Laceration with foreign body of anus

    ☑7ᵗʰ **S31.833** Puncture wound without foreign body of anus

    ☑7ᵗʰ **S31.834** Puncture wound with foreign body of anus

    ☑7ᵗʰ **S31.835** Open bite of anus
         Bite of anus NOS
         EXCLUDES 1   superficial bite of anus (S30.877)

    ☑7ᵗʰ **S31.839** Unspecified open wound of anus ▽

☑4ᵗʰ **S32** **Fracture of lumbar spine and pelvis**

  NOTE   A fracture not indicated as displaced or nondisplaced should be coded to displaced.
         A fracture not indicated as opened or closed should be coded to closed.

  INCLUDES   fracture of lumbosacral neural arch
         fracture of lumbosacral spinous process
         fracture of lumbosacral transverse process
         fracture of lumbosacral vertebra
         fracture of lumbosacral vertebral arch

Code first any associated spinal cord and spinal nerve injury (S34.-)

EXCLUDES 1   transection of abdomen (S38.3)

EXCLUDES 2   fracture of hip NOS (S72.0-)

AHA: 2015, 3Q, 37-39; 2012, 4Q, 93

> The appropriate 7th character is to be added to each code from category S32.
> A   initial encounter for closed fracture
> B   initial encounter for open fracture
> D   subsequent encounter for fracture with routine healing
> G   subsequent encounter for fracture with delayed healing
> K   subsequent encounter for fracture with nonunion
> S   sequela

☑5ᵗʰ **S32.0** **Fracture of lumbar vertebra**
     Fracture of lumbar spine NOS

  ☑6ᵗʰ **S32.00** **Fracture of unspecified lumbar vertebra**

    ¹ ☑7ᵗʰ **S32.000** Wedge compression fracture of unspecified lumbar vertebra HCC ▽

    ¹ ☑7ᵗʰ **S32.001** Stable burst fracture of unspecified lumbar vertebra HCC ▽

    ¹ ☑7ᵗʰ **S32.002** Unstable burst fracture of unspecified lumbar vertebra HCC ▽

    ¹ ☑7ᵗʰ **S32.008** Other fracture of unspecified lumbar vertebra HCC ▽

    ¹ ☑7ᵗʰ **S32.009** Unspecified fracture of unspecified lumbar vertebra HCC ▽

  ☑6ᵗʰ **S32.01** **Fracture of first lumbar vertebra**

    ¹ ☑7ᵗʰ **S32.010** Wedge compression fracture of first lumbar vertebra HCC

    ¹ ☑7ᵗʰ **S32.011** Stable burst fracture of first lumbar vertebra HCC

    ¹ ☑7ᵗʰ **S32.012** Unstable burst fracture of first lumbar vertebra HCC

    ¹ ☑7ᵗʰ **S32.018** Other fracture of first lumbar vertebra HCC

    ¹ ☑7ᵗʰ **S32.019** Unspecified fracture of first lumbar vertebra HCC ▽

  ☑6ᵗʰ **S32.02** **Fracture of second lumbar vertebra**

    ¹ ☑7ᵗʰ **S32.020** Wedge compression fracture of second lumbar vertebra HCC

    ¹ ☑7ᵗʰ **S32.021** Stable burst fracture of second lumbar vertebra HCC

    ¹ ☑7ᵗʰ **S32.022** Unstable burst fracture of second lumbar vertebra HCC

    ¹ ☑7ᵗʰ **S32.028** Other fracture of second lumbar vertebra HCC

    ¹ ☑7ᵗʰ **S32.029** Unspecified fracture of second lumbar vertebra HCC ▽

  ☑6ᵗʰ **S32.03** **Fracture of third lumbar vertebra**

    ¹ ☑7ᵗʰ **S32.030** Wedge compression fracture of third lumbar vertebra HCC

    ¹ ☑7ᵗʰ **S32.031** Stable burst fracture of third lumbar vertebra HCC

    ¹ ☑7ᵗʰ **S32.032** Unstable burst fracture of third lumbar vertebra HCC

    ¹ ☑7ᵗʰ **S32.038** Other fracture of third lumbar vertebra HCC

    ¹ ☑7ᵗʰ **S32.039** Unspecified fracture of third lumbar vertebra HCC ▽

  ☑6ᵗʰ **S32.04** **Fracture of fourth lumbar vertebra**

    ¹ ☑7ᵗʰ **S32.040** Wedge compression fracture of fourth lumbar vertebra HCC

    ¹ ☑7ᵗʰ **S32.041** Stable burst fracture of fourth lumbar vertebra HCC

    ¹ ☑7ᵗʰ **S32.042** Unstable burst fracture of fourth lumbar vertebra HCC

---

¹ HCC with 7th character indicating initial encounter (A, B or C - specific to category).

EXCLUDES 1 Not coded here   *EXCLUDES 2* Not included here   N Newborn Age: 0   P Pediatric Age: 0-17   M Maternity Age: 12-55   A Adult Age: 15-124

944   ICD-10-CM 2018

1 ✓7ᵗʰ **S32.048** Other fracture of fourth lumbar vertebra   HCC

1 ✓7ᵗʰ **S32.049** Unspecified fracture of fourth lumbar vertebra   HCC ▽

✓6ᵗʰ **S32.05** Fracture of fifth lumbar vertebra

1 ✓7ᵗʰ **S32.050** Wedge compression fracture of fifth lumbar vertebra   HCC

1 ✓7ᵗʰ **S32.051** Stable burst fracture of fifth lumbar vertebra   HCC

1 ✓7ᵗʰ **S32.052** Unstable burst fracture of fifth lumbar vertebra   HCC

1 ✓7ᵗʰ **S32.058** Other fracture of fifth lumbar vertebra   HCC

1 ✓7ᵗʰ **S32.059** Unspecified fracture of fifth lumbar vertebra   HCC ▽

✓5ᵗʰ **S32.1** Fracture of sacrum

> **NOTE**   For vertical fractures, code to most medial fracture extension.
> Use two codes if both a vertical and transverse fracture are present.
> Code also any associated fracture of pelvic ring (S32.8-)

1 ✓7ᵗʰ **S32.10** Unspecified fracture of sacrum   HCC ▽

✓6ᵗʰ **S32.11** Zone I fracture of sacrum
> Vertical sacral ala fracture of sacrum

1 ✓7ᵗʰ **S32.110** Nondisplaced Zone I fracture of sacrum   HCC

1 ✓7ᵗʰ **S32.111** Minimally displaced Zone I fracture of sacrum   HCC

1 ✓7ᵗʰ **S32.112** Severely displaced Zone I fracture of sacrum   HCC

1 ✓7ᵗʰ **S32.119** Unspecified Zone I fracture of sacrum   HCC ▽

✓6ᵗʰ **S32.12** Zone II fracture of sacrum
> Vertical foraminal region fracture of sacrum

1 ✓7ᵗʰ **S32.120** Nondisplaced Zone II fracture of sacrum   HCC

1 ✓7ᵗʰ **S32.121** Minimally displaced Zone II fracture of sacrum   HCC

1 ✓7ᵗʰ **S32.122** Severely displaced Zone II fracture of sacrum   HCC

1 ✓7ᵗʰ **S32.129** Unspecified Zone II fracture of sacrum   HCC ▽

Vertical Sacral Fracture Zones

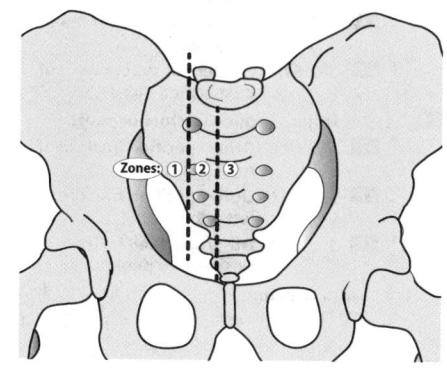

Zones: ① ② ③

Transverse Sacral Fracture Types

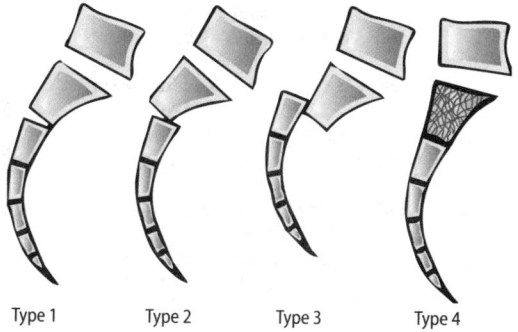

Type 1   Type 2   Type 3   Type 4

1 HCC with 7th character indicating initial encounter (A, B or C - specific to category).

✓6ᵗʰ **S32.13** Zone III fracture of sacrum
> Vertical fracture into spinal canal region of sacrum

1 ✓7ᵗʰ **S32.130** Nondisplaced Zone III fracture of sacrum   HCC

1 ✓7ᵗʰ **S32.131** Minimally displaced Zone III fracture of sacrum   HCC

1 ✓7ᵗʰ **S32.132** Severely displaced Zone III fracture of sacrum   HCC

1 ✓7ᵗʰ **S32.139** Unspecified Zone III fracture of sacrum   HCC ▽

1 ✓x7ᵗʰ **S32.14** Type 1 fracture of sacrum   HCC
> Transverse flexion fracture of sacrum without displacement

1 ✓x7ᵗʰ **S32.15** Type 2 fracture of sacrum   HCC
> Transverse flexion fracture of sacrum with posterior displacement

1 ✓x7ᵗʰ **S32.16** Type 3 fracture of sacrum   HCC
> Transverse extension fracture of sacrum with anterior displacement

1 ✓x7ᵗʰ **S32.17** Type 4 fracture of sacrum   HCC
> Transverse segmental comminution of upper sacrum

1 ✓x7ᵗʰ **S32.19** Other fracture of sacrum   HCC

1 ✓x7ᵗʰ **S32.2** Fracture of coccyx   HCC

✓5ᵗʰ **S32.3** Fracture of ilium

> **EXCLUDES 1**   fracture of ilium with associated disruption of pelvic ring (S32.8-)

✓6ᵗʰ **S32.30** Unspecified fracture of ilium

1 ✓7ᵗʰ **S32.301** Unspecified fracture of right ilium   HCC ▽

1 ✓7ᵗʰ **S32.302** Unspecified fracture of left ilium   HCC ▽

1 ✓7ᵗʰ **S32.309** Unspecified fracture of unspecified ilium   HCC ▽

✓6ᵗʰ **S32.31** Avulsion fracture of ilium

1 ✓7ᵗʰ **S32.311** Displaced avulsion fracture of right ilium   HCC

1 ✓7ᵗʰ **S32.312** Displaced avulsion fracture of left ilium   HCC

1 ✓7ᵗʰ **S32.313** Displaced avulsion fracture of unspecified ilium   HCC ▽

1 ✓7ᵗʰ **S32.314** Nondisplaced avulsion fracture of right ilium   HCC

1 ✓7ᵗʰ **S32.315** Nondisplaced avulsion fracture of left ilium   HCC

1 ✓7ᵗʰ **S32.316** Nondisplaced avulsion fracture of unspecified ilium   HCC ▽

✓6ᵗʰ **S32.39** Other fracture of ilium

1 ✓7ᵗʰ **S32.391** Other fracture of right ilium   HCC

1 ✓7ᵗʰ **S32.392** Other fracture of left ilium   HCC

1 ✓7ᵗʰ **S32.399** Other fracture of unspecified ilium   HCC ▽

✓5ᵗʰ **S32.4** Fracture of acetabulum
> Code also any associated fracture of pelvic ring (S32.8-)
> **AHA:** 2016, 3Q, 16

✓6ᵗʰ **S32.40** Unspecified fracture of acetabulum

1 ✓7ᵗʰ **S32.401** Unspecified fracture of right acetabulum   HCC ▽

1 ✓7ᵗʰ **S32.402** Unspecified fracture of left acetabulum   HCC ▽

1 ✓7ᵗʰ **S32.409** Unspecified fracture of unspecified acetabulum   HCC ▽

✓6ᵗʰ **S32.41** Fracture of anterior wall of acetabulum

1 ✓7ᵗʰ **S32.411** Displaced fracture of anterior wall of right acetabulum   HCC

1 ✓7ᵗʰ **S32.412** Displaced fracture of anterior wall of left acetabulum   HCC

1 ✓7ᵗʰ **S32.413** Displaced fracture of anterior wall of unspecified acetabulum   HCC ▽

1 ✓7ᵗʰ **S32.414** Nondisplaced fracture of anterior wall of right acetabulum   HCC

1 ✓7ᵗʰ **S32.415** Nondisplaced fracture of anterior wall of left acetabulum   HCC

1 ✓7ᵗʰ **S32.416** Nondisplaced fracture of anterior wall of unspecified acetabulum   HCC ▽

✔ Additional Character Req   ✓x7ᵗʰ Placeholder Alert   Manifestation   HCC CMS-HCC Condition   ▽ Unspecified Code   ▶◀ Revised Text   ● New Code   ▲ Revised Code Title

✓6th **S32.42 Fracture of posterior wall of acetabulum**
- 1 ✓7th **S32.421 Displaced fracture of posterior wall of right acetabulum** HCC
- 1 ✓7th **S32.422 Displaced fracture of posterior wall of left acetabulum** HCC
- 1 ✓7th **S32.423 Displaced fracture of posterior wall of unspecified acetabulum** HCC ▽
- 1 ✓7th **S32.424 Nondisplaced fracture of posterior wall of right acetabulum** HCC
- 1 ✓7th **S32.425 Nondisplaced fracture of posterior wall of left acetabulum** HCC
- 1 ✓7th **S32.426 Nondisplaced fracture of posterior wall of unspecified acetabulum** HCC ▽

✓6th **S32.43 Fracture of anterior column [iliopubic] of acetabulum**
- 1 ✓7th **S32.431 Displaced fracture of anterior column [iliopubic] of right acetabulum** HCC
- 1 ✓7th **S32.432 Displaced fracture of anterior column [iliopubic] of left acetabulum** HCC
- 1 ✓7th **S32.433 Displaced fracture of anterior column [iliopubic] of unspecified acetabulum** HCC ▽
- 1 ✓7th **S32.434 Nondisplaced fracture of anterior column [iliopubic] of right acetabulum** HCC
- 1 ✓7th **S32.435 Nondisplaced fracture of anterior column [iliopubic] of left acetabulum** HCC
- 1 ✓7th **S32.436 Nondisplaced fracture of anterior column [iliopubic] of unspecified acetabulum** HCC ▽

✓6th **S32.44 Fracture of posterior column [ilioischial] of acetabulum**
- 1 ✓7th **S32.441 Displaced fracture of posterior column [ilioischial] of right acetabulum** HCC
- 1 ✓7th **S32.442 Displaced fracture of posterior column [ilioischial] of left acetabulum** HCC
- 1 ✓7th **S32.443 Displaced fracture of posterior column [ilioischial] of unspecified acetabulum** HCC ▽
- 1 ✓7th **S32.444 Nondisplaced fracture of posterior column [ilioischial] of right acetabulum** HCC
- 1 ✓7th **S32.445 Nondisplaced fracture of posterior column [ilioischial] of left acetabulum** HCC
- 1 ✓7th **S32.446 Nondisplaced fracture of posterior column [ilioischial] of unspecified acetabulum** HCC ▽

✓6th **S32.45 Transverse fracture of acetabulum**
- 1 ✓7th **S32.451 Displaced transverse fracture of right acetabulum** HCC
- 1 ✓7th **S32.452 Displaced transverse fracture of left acetabulum** HCC
- 1 ✓7th **S32.453 Displaced transverse fracture of unspecified acetabulum** HCC ▽
- 1 ✓7th **S32.454 Nondisplaced transverse fracture of right acetabulum** HCC
- 1 ✓7th **S32.455 Nondisplaced transverse fracture of left acetabulum** HCC
- 1 ✓7th **S32.456 Nondisplaced transverse fracture of unspecified acetabulum** HCC ▽

✓6th **S32.46 Associated transverse-posterior fracture of acetabulum**
- 1 ✓7th **S32.461 Displaced associated transverse-posterior fracture of right acetabulum** HCC
- 1 ✓7th **S32.462 Displaced associated transverse-posterior fracture of left acetabulum** HCC
- 1 ✓7th **S32.463 Displaced associated transverse-posterior fracture of unspecified acetabulum** HCC ▽
- 1 ✓7th **S32.464 Nondisplaced associated transverse posterior fracture of right acetabulum** HCC
- 1 ✓7th **S32.465 Nondisplaced associated transverse-posterior fracture of left acetabulum** HCC
- 1 ✓7th **S32.466 Nondisplaced associated transverse-posterior fracture of unspecified acetabulum** HCC ▽

✓6th **S32.47 Fracture of medial wall of acetabulum**
- 1 ✓7th **S32.471 Displaced fracture of medial wall of right acetabulum** HCC
- 1 ✓7th **S32.472 Displaced fracture of medial wall of left acetabulum** HCC
- 1 ✓7th **S32.473 Displaced fracture of medial wall of unspecified acetabulum** HCC ▽
- 1 ✓7th **S32.474 Nondisplaced fracture of medial wall of right acetabulum** HCC
- 1 ✓7th **S32.475 Nondisplaced fracture of medial wall of left acetabulum** HCC
- 1 ✓7th **S32.476 Nondisplaced fracture of medial wall of unspecified acetabulum** HCC ▽

✓6th **S32.48 Dome fracture of acetabulum**
- 1 ✓7th **S32.481 Displaced dome fracture of right acetabulum** HCC
- 1 ✓7th **S32.482 Displaced dome fracture of left acetabulum** HCC
- 1 ✓7th **S32.483 Displaced dome fracture of unspecified acetabulum** HCC ▽
- 1 ✓7th **S32.484 Nondisplaced dome fracture of right acetabulum** HCC
- 1 ✓7th **S32.485 Nondisplaced dome fracture of left acetabulum** HCC
- 1 ✓7th **S32.486 Nondisplaced dome fracture of unspecified acetabulum** HCC ▽

✓6th **S32.49 Other specified fracture of acetabulum**
- 1 ✓7th **S32.491 Other specified fracture of right acetabulum** HCC
- 1 ✓7th **S32.492 Other specified fracture of left acetabulum** HCC
- 1 ✓7th **S32.499 Other specified fracture of unspecified acetabulum** HCC ▽

✓5th **S32.5 Fracture of pubis**
> EXCLUDES 1 fracture of pubis with associated disruption of pelvic ring (S32.8-)

✓6th **S32.50 Unspecified fracture of pubis**
- 1 ✓7th **S32.501 Unspecified fracture of right pubis** HCC ▽
- 1 ✓7th **S32.502 Unspecified fracture of left pubis** HCC ▽
- 1 ✓7th **S32.509 Unspecified fracture of unspecified pubis** HCC ▽

✓6th **S32.51 Fracture of superior rim of pubis**
- 1 ✓7th **S32.511 Fracture of superior rim of right pubis** HCC
- 1 ✓7th **S32.512 Fracture of superior rim of left pubis** HCC
- 1 ✓7th **S32.519 Fracture of superior rim of unspecified pubis** HCC ▽

✓6th **S32.59 Other specified fracture of pubis**
- 1 ✓7th **S32.591 Other specified fracture of right pubis** HCC
- 1 ✓7th **S32.592 Other specified fracture of left pubis** HCC
- 1 ✓7th **S32.599 Other specified fracture of unspecified pubis** HCC ▽

✓5th **S32.6 Fracture of ischium**
> EXCLUDES 1 fracture of ischium with associated disruption of pelvic ring (S32.8-)

✓6th **S32.60 Unspecified fracture of ischium**
- 1 ✓7th **S32.601 Unspecified fracture of right ischium** HCC ▽
- 1 ✓7th **S32.602 Unspecified fracture of left ischium** HCC ▽
- 1 ✓7th **S32.609 Unspecified fracture of unspecified ischium** HCC ▽

✓6th **S32.61 Avulsion fracture of ischium**
- 1 ✓7th **S32.611 Displaced avulsion fracture of right ischium** HCC
- 1 ✓7th **S32.612 Displaced avulsion fracture of left ischium** HCC
- 1 ✓7th **S32.613 Displaced avulsion fracture of unspecified ischium** HCC ▽

---

1 HCC with 7th character indicating initial encounter (A, B or C - specific to category).

EXCLUDES 1 Not coded here EXCLUDES 2 Not included here N Newborn Age: 0 P Pediatric Age: 0-17 M Maternity Age: 12-55 A Adult Age: 15-124

946 ICD-10-CM 2018

¹ ✓7ᵗʰ **S32.614** Nondisplaced avulsion fracture of HCC
right ischium

¹ ✓7ᵗʰ **S32.615** Nondisplaced avulsion fracture of HCC
left ischium

¹ ✓7ᵗʰ **S32.616** Nondisplaced avulsion fracture of HCC ▽
unspecified ischium

✓6ᵗʰ **S32.69** Other specified fracture of ischium

¹ ✓7ᵗʰ **S32.691** Other specified fracture of right HCC
ischium

¹ ✓7ᵗʰ **S32.692** Other specified fracture of left HCC
ischium

¹ ✓7ᵗʰ **S32.699** Other specified fracture of HCC ▽
unspecified ischium

✓5ᵗʰ **S32.8** Fracture of other parts of pelvis
Code also any associated:
fracture of acetabulum (S32.4-)
sacral fracture (S32.1-)

✓6ᵗʰ **S32.81** Multiple fractures of pelvis with disruption
of pelvic ring
Multiple pelvic fractures with disruption of pelvic circle

¹ ✓7ᵗʰ **S32.810** Multiple fractures of pelvis with HCC
stable disruption of pelvic ring

¹ ✓7ᵗʰ **S32.811** Multiple fractures of pelvis with HCC
unstable disruption of pelvic ring

¹ ✓x7ᵗʰ **S32.82** Multiple fractures of pelvis without disruption HCC
of pelvic ring
Multiple pelvic fractures without disruption of pelvic
circle

¹ ✓x7ᵗʰ **S32.89** Fracture of other parts of pelvis HCC

¹ ✓x7ᵗʰ **S32.9** Fracture of unspecified parts of lumbosacral spine HCC ▽
and pelvis
Fracture of lumbosacral spine NOS
Fracture of pelvis NOS
AHA: 2012, 4Q, 93

Fractures Disrupting Pelvic Circle

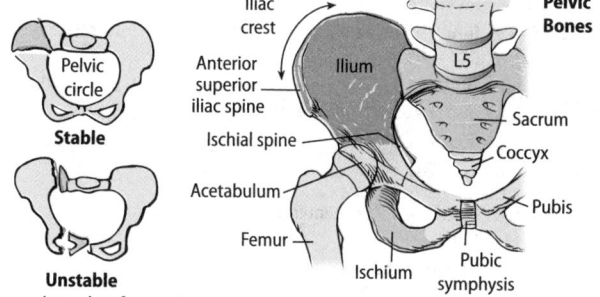

Pelvic circle — Stable

Unstable
(two-place fracture)

Iliac crest
Anterior superior iliac spine
Ischial spine
Acetabulum
Femur
Ilium
L5
Sacrum
Coccyx
Pubis
Ischium
Pubic symphysis
Pelvic Bones

✓4ᵗʰ **S33** **Dislocation and sprain of joints and ligaments of lumbar spine
and pelvis**
INCLUDES avulsion of joint or ligament of lumbar spine and pelvis
laceration of cartilage, joint or ligament of lumbar spine and
pelvis
sprain of cartilage, joint or ligament of lumbar spine and
pelvis
traumatic hemarthrosis of joint or ligament of lumbar spine
and pelvis
traumatic rupture of joint or ligament of lumbar spine and
pelvis
traumatic subluxation of joint or ligament of lumbar spine
and pelvis
traumatic tear of joint or ligament of lumbar spine and pelvis
Code also any associated open wound
EXCLUDES 1 nontraumatic rupture or displacement of lumbar intervertebral
disc NOS (M51.-)
obstetric damage to pelvic joints and ligaments (O71.6)
EXCLUDES 2 dislocation and sprain of joints and ligaments of hip (S73.-)
strain of muscle of lower back and pelvis (S39.01-)

The appropriate 7th character is to be added to each code from
category S33.
A   initial encounter
D   subsequent encounter
S   sequela

✓x7ᵗʰ **S33.0** **Traumatic rupture of lumbar intervertebral disc**
EXCLUDES 1 rupture or displacement (nontraumatic) of lumbar
intervertebral disc NOS (M51- with
fifth character 6)

✓5ᵗʰ **S33.1** **Subluxation and dislocation of lumbar vertebra**
Code also any associated:
open wound of abdomen, lower back and pelvis (S31)
spinal cord injury (S24.0, S24.1-, S34.0-, S34.1-)
EXCLUDES 2 fracture of lumbar vertebrae (S32.0-)

✓6ᵗʰ **S33.10** Subluxation and dislocation of unspecified lumbar
vertebra

✓7ᵗʰ **S33.100** Subluxation of unspecified lumbar ▽
vertebra

✓7ᵗʰ **S33.101** Dislocation of unspecified lumbar ▽
vertebra

✓6ᵗʰ **S33.11** Subluxation and dislocation of L1/L2 lumbar
vertebra

✓7ᵗʰ **S33.110** Subluxation of L1/L2 lumbar vertebra

✓7ᵗʰ **S33.111** Dislocation of L1/L2 lumbar vertebra

✓6ᵗʰ **S33.12** Subluxation and dislocation of L2/L3 lumbar
vertebra

✓7ᵗʰ **S33.120** Subluxation of L2/L3 lumbar vertebra

✓7ᵗʰ **S33.121** Dislocation of L2/L3 lumbar vertebra

✓6ᵗʰ **S33.13** Subluxation and dislocation of L3/L4
lumbar vertebra

✓7ᵗʰ **S33.130** Subluxation of L3/L4 lumbar vertebra

✓7ᵗʰ **S33.131** Dislocation of L3/L4 lumbar vertebra

✓6ᵗʰ **S33.14** Subluxation and dislocation of L4/L5
lumbar vertebra

✓7ᵗʰ **S33.140** Subluxation of L4/L5 lumbar vertebra

✓7ᵗʰ **S33.141** Dislocation of L4/L5 lumbar vertebra

✓x7ᵗʰ **S33.2** **Dislocation of sacroiliac and sacrococcygeal joint**

✓5ᵗʰ **S33.3** **Dislocation of other and unspecified parts of lumbar spine
and pelvis**

✓x7ᵗʰ **S33.30** Dislocation of unspecified parts of lumbar spine ▽
and pelvis

✓x7ᵗʰ **S33.39** Dislocation of other parts of lumbar spine and pelvis

✓x7ᵗʰ **S33.4** **Traumatic rupture of symphysis pubis**

✓x7ᵗʰ **S33.5** **Sprain of ligaments of lumbar spine**

✓x7ᵗʰ **S33.6** **Sprain of sacroiliac joint**

✓x7ᵗʰ **S33.8** **Sprain of other parts of lumbar spine and pelvis**

✓x7ᵗʰ **S33.9** **Sprain of unspecified parts of lumbar spine and pelvis** ▽

¹ HCC with 7th character indicating initial encounter (A, B or C - specific to category).

☑ Additional Character Req   ✓x7ᵗʰ Placeholder Alert   Manifestation   HCC CMS-HCC Condition   ▽ Unspecified Code   ▶◀ Revised Text   ● New Code   ▲ Revised Code Title

ICD-10-CM 2018   **947**

Chapter 19. Injury, Poisoning, and Certain Other Consequences of External Causes

S32.614-S33.9

✓4th S34 Injury of lumbar and sacral spinal cord and nerves at abdomen, lower back and pelvis level

> NOTE Code to highest level of lumbar cord injury.
> Injuries to the spinal cord (S34.0 and S34.1) refer to the cord level and not bone level injury, and can affect nerve roots at and below the level given.

Code also any associated:
  fracture of vertebra (S22.0-, S32.0-)
  open wound of abdomen, lower back and pelvis (S31.-)
  transient paralysis (R29.5)

> The appropriate 7th character is to be added to each code from category S34.
> A   initial encounter
> D   subsequent encounter
> S   sequela

✓5th S34.0 Concussion and edema of lumbar and sacral spinal cord
- ✓x7th **S34.01 Concussion and edema of lumbar spinal cord** HCC
- ✓x7th **S34.02 Concussion and edema of sacral spinal cord** HCC
  Concussion and edema of conus medullaris

✓5th S34.1 Other and unspecified injury of lumbar and sacral spinal cord
- ✓6th **S34.10 Unspecified injury to lumbar spinal cord**
  - ✓7th **S34.101 Unspecified injury to L1 level of lumbar spinal cord** HCC ▽
    Unspecified injury to lumbar spinal cord level 1
  - ✓7th **S34.102 Unspecified injury to L2 level of lumbar spinal cord** HCC ▽
    Unspecified injury to lumbar spinal cord level 2
  - ✓7th **S34.103 Unspecified injury to L3 level of lumbar spinal cord** HCC ▽
    Unspecified injury to lumbar spinal cord level 3
  - ✓7th **S34.104 Unspecified injury to L4 level of lumbar spinal cord** HCC ▽
    Unspecified injury to lumbar spinal cord level 4
  - ✓7th **S34.105 Unspecified injury to L5 level of lumbar spinal cord** HCC ▽
    Unspecified injury to lumbar spinal cord level 5
  - ✓7th **S34.109 Unspecified injury to unspecified level of lumbar spinal cord** HCC ▽
- ✓6th **S34.11 Complete lesion of lumbar spinal cord**
  - ✓7th **S34.111 Complete lesion of L1 level of lumbar spinal cord** HCC
    Complete lesion of lumbar spinal cord level 1
  - ✓7th **S34.112 Complete lesion of L2 level of lumbar spinal cord** HCC
    Complete lesion of lumbar spinal cord level 2
  - ✓7th **S34.113 Complete lesion of L3 level of lumbar spinal cord** HCC
    Complete lesion of lumbar spinal cord level 3
  - ✓7th **S34.114 Complete lesion of L4 level of lumbar spinal cord** HCC
    Complete lesion of lumbar spinal cord level 4
  - ✓7th **S34.115 Complete lesion of L5 level of lumbar spinal cord** HCC
    Complete lesion of lumbar spinal cord level 5
  - ✓7th **S34.119 Complete lesion of unspecified level of lumbar spinal cord** HCC ▽
- ✓6th **S34.12 Incomplete lesion of lumbar spinal cord**
  - ✓7th **S34.121 Incomplete lesion of L1 level of lumbar spinal cord** HCC
    Incomplete lesion of lumbar spinal cord level 1
  - ✓7th **S34.122 Incomplete lesion of L2 level of lumbar spinal cord** HCC
    Incomplete lesion of lumbar spinal cord level 2
  - ✓7th **S34.123 Incomplete lesion of L3 level of lumbar spinal cord** HCC
    Incomplete lesion of lumbar spinal cord level 3
  - ✓7th **S34.124 Incomplete lesion of L4 level of lumbar spinal cord** HCC
    Incomplete lesion of lumbar spinal cord level 4
  - ✓7th **S34.125 Incomplete lesion of L5 level of lumbar spinal cord** HCC
    Incomplete lesion of lumbar spinal cord level 5
  - ✓7th **S34.129 Incomplete lesion of unspecified level of lumbar spinal cord** HCC ▽
- ✓6th **S34.13 Other and unspecified injury to sacral spinal cord**
  Other injury to conus medullaris
  - ✓7th **S34.131 Complete lesion of sacral spinal cord** HCC
    Complete lesion of conus medullaris
  - ✓7th **S34.132 Incomplete lesion of sacral spinal cord** HCC
    Incomplete lesion of conus medullaris
  - ✓7th **S34.139 Unspecified injury to sacral spinal cord** HCC ▽
    Unspecified injury of conus medullaris

✓5th S34.2 Injury of nerve root of lumbar and sacral spine
- ✓x7th **S34.21 Injury of nerve root of lumbar spine**
- ✓x7th **S34.22 Injury of nerve root of sacral spine**

1 ✓x7th **S34.3 Injury of cauda equina** HCC

✓x7th **S34.4 Injury of lumbosacral plexus**

✓x7th **S34.5 Injury of lumbar, sacral and pelvic sympathetic nerves**
  Injury of celiac ganglion or plexus
  Injury of hypogastric plexus
  Injury of mesenteric plexus (inferior) (superior)
  Injury of splanchnic nerve

✓x7th **S34.6 Injury of peripheral nerve(s) at abdomen, lower back and pelvis level**

✓x7th **S34.8 Injury of other nerves at abdomen, lower back and pelvis level**

✓x7th **S34.9 Injury of unspecified nerves at abdomen, lower back and pelvis level** ▽

✓4th S35 Injury of blood vessels at abdomen, lower back and pelvis level
  Code also any associated open wound (S31.-)

> The appropriate 7th character is to be added to each code from category S35.
> A   initial encounter
> D   subsequent encounter
> S   sequela

✓5th S35.0 Injury of abdominal aorta
  EXCLUDES 1 injury of aorta NOS (S25.0)
- ✓x7th **S35.00 Unspecified injury of abdominal aorta** ▽
- ✓x7th **S35.01 Minor laceration of abdominal aorta**
    Incomplete transection of abdominal aorta
    Laceration of abdominal aorta NOS
    Superficial laceration of abdominal aorta
- ✓x7th **S35.02 Major laceration of abdominal aorta**
    Complete transection of abdominal aorta
    Traumatic rupture of abdominal aorta
- ✓x7th **S35.09 Other injury of abdominal aorta**

✓5th S35.1 Injury of inferior vena cava
  Injury of hepatic vein
  EXCLUDES 1 injury of vena cava NOS (S25.2)
- ✓x7th **S35.10 Unspecified injury of inferior vena cava** ▽
- ✓x7th **S35.11 Minor laceration of inferior vena cava**
    Incomplete transection of inferior vena cava
    Laceration of inferior vena cava NOS
    Superficial laceration of inferior vena cava
- ✓x7th **S35.12 Major laceration of inferior vena cava**
    Complete transection of inferior vena cava
    Traumatic rupture of inferior vena cava
- ✓x7th **S35.19 Other injury of inferior vena cava**

---

1   HCC with 7th character indicating initial encounter (A, B or C - specific to category).

EXCLUDES 1 Not coded here   EXCLUDES 2 Not included here   N Newborn Age: 0   P Pediatric Age: 0-17   M Maternity Age: 12-55   A Adult Age: 15-124

948

ICD-10-CM 2018

S34–S35.19

✓5ᵗʰ **S35.2** **Injury of celiac or mesenteric artery and branches**

    ✓6ᵗʰ **S35.21** **Injury of** celiac artery

        ✓7ᵗʰ **S35.211** Minor laceration **of celiac artery**
               Incomplete transection of celiac artery
               Laceration of celiac artery NOS
               Superficial laceration of celiac artery

        ✓7ᵗʰ **S35.212** Major laceration **of celiac artery**
               Complete transection of celiac artery
               Traumatic rupture of celiac artery

        ✓7ᵗʰ **S35.218** **Other injury of celiac artery**
        ✓7ᵗʰ **S35.219** **Unspecified injury of celiac artery** ▽

    ✓6ᵗʰ **S35.22** **Injury of** superior mesenteric artery

        ✓7ᵗʰ **S35.221** Minor laceration **of superior mesenteric artery**
               Incomplete transection of superior mesenteric artery
               Laceration of superior mesenteric artery NOS
               Superficial laceration of superior mesenteric artery

        ✓7ᵗʰ **S35.222** Major laceration **of superior mesenteric artery**
               Complete transection of superior mesenteric artery
               Traumatic rupture of superior mesenteric artery

        ✓7ᵗʰ **S35.228** **Other injury of superior mesenteric artery**
        ✓7ᵗʰ **S35.229** **Unspecified injury of superior mesenteric artery** ▽

    ✓6ᵗʰ **S35.23** **Injury of** inferior mesenteric artery

        ✓7ᵗʰ **S35.231** Minor laceration **of inferior mesenteric artery**
               Incomplete transection of inferior mesenteric artery
               Laceration of inferior mesenteric artery NOS
               Superficial laceration of inferior mesenteric artery

        ✓7ᵗʰ **S35.232** Major laceration **of inferior mesenteric artery**
               Complete transection of inferior mesenteric artery
               Traumatic rupture of inferior mesenteric artery

        ✓7ᵗʰ **S35.238** **Other injury of inferior mesenteric artery**
        ✓7ᵗʰ **S35.239** **Unspecified injury of inferior mesenteric artery** ▽

    ✓6ᵗʰ **S35.29** **Injury of** branches of celiac and mesenteric artery
           Injury of gastric artery
           Injury of gastroduodenal artery
           Injury of hepatic artery
           Injury of splenic artery

        ✓7ᵗʰ **S35.291** Minor laceration **of branches of celiac and mesenteric artery**
               Incomplete transection of branches of celiac and mesenteric artery
               Laceration of branches of celiac and mesenteric artery NOS
               Superficial laceration of branches of celiac and mesenteric artery

        ✓7ᵗʰ **S35.292** Major laceration **of branches of celiac and mesenteric artery**
               Complete transection of branches of celiac and mesenteric artery
               Traumatic rupture of branches of celiac and mesenteric artery

        ✓7ᵗʰ **S35.298** **Other injury of branches of celiac and mesenteric artery**
        ✓7ᵗʰ **S35.299** **Unspecified injury of branches of celiac and mesenteric artery** ▽

✓5ᵗʰ **S35.3** **Injury of portal or splenic vein and branches**

    ✓6ᵗʰ **S35.31** **Injury of** portal vein

        ✓7ᵗʰ **S35.311** Laceration **of portal vein**
        ✓7ᵗʰ **S35.318** **Other specified injury of portal vein**
        ✓7ᵗʰ **S35.319** **Unspecified injury of portal vein** ▽

    ✓6ᵗʰ **S35.32** **Injury of** splenic vein

        ✓7ᵗʰ **S35.321** Laceration **of splenic vein**
        ✓7ᵗʰ **S35.328** **Other specified injury of splenic vein**

        ✓7ᵗʰ **S35.329** **Unspecified injury of splenic vein** ▽

    ✓6ᵗʰ **S35.33** **Injury of** superior mesenteric vein

        ✓7ᵗʰ **S35.331** Laceration **of superior mesenteric vein**
        ✓7ᵗʰ **S35.338** **Other specified injury of superior mesenteric vein**
        ✓7ᵗʰ **S35.339** **Unspecified injury of superior mesenteric vein** ▽

    ✓6ᵗʰ **S35.34** **Injury of** inferior mesenteric vein

        ✓7ᵗʰ **S35.341** Laceration **of inferior mesenteric vein**
        ✓7ᵗʰ **S35.348** **Other specified injury of inferior mesenteric vein**
        ✓7ᵗʰ **S35.349** **Unspecified injury of inferior mesenteric vein** ▽

✓5ᵗʰ **S35.4** **Injury of** renal **blood vessels**

    ✓6ᵗʰ **S35.40** **Unspecified injury of renal blood vessel**

        ✓7ᵗʰ **S35.401** **Unspecified injury of** right renal artery ▽
        ✓7ᵗʰ **S35.402** **Unspecified injury of** left renal artery ▽
        ✓7ᵗʰ **S35.403** **Unspecified injury of unspecified renal artery** ▽
        ✓7ᵗʰ **S35.404** **Unspecified injury of** right renal vein ▽
        ✓7ᵗʰ **S35.405** **Unspecified injury of** left renal vein ▽
        ✓7ᵗʰ **S35.406** **Unspecified injury of unspecified renal vein** ▽

    ✓6ᵗʰ **S35.41** Laceration **of renal blood vessel**

        ✓7ᵗʰ **S35.411** **Laceration of** right renal artery
        ✓7ᵗʰ **S35.412** **Laceration of** left renal artery
        ✓7ᵗʰ **S35.413** **Laceration of unspecified renal artery** ▽
        ✓7ᵗʰ **S35.414** **Laceration of** right renal vein
        ✓7ᵗʰ **S35.415** **Laceration of** left renal vein
        ✓7ᵗʰ **S35.416** **Laceration of unspecified renal vein** ▽

    ✓6ᵗʰ **S35.49** **Other specified injury of renal blood vessel**

        ✓7ᵗʰ **S35.491** **Other specified injury of** right renal artery
        ✓7ᵗʰ **S35.492** **Other specified injury of** left renal artery
        ✓7ᵗʰ **S35.493** **Other specified injury of unspecified renal artery** ▽
        ✓7ᵗʰ **S35.494** **Other specified injury of** right renal vein
        ✓7ᵗʰ **S35.495** **Other specified injury of** left renal vein
        ✓7ᵗʰ **S35.496** **Other specified injury of unspecified renal vein** ▽

✓5ᵗʰ **S35.5** **Injury of** iliac **blood vessels**

    ✓×7ᵗʰ **S35.50** **Injury of unspecified iliac blood vessel(s)** ▽

    ✓6ᵗʰ **S35.51** **Injury of** iliac **artery or vein**
           Injury of hypogastric artery or vein

        ✓7ᵗʰ **S35.511** **Injury of** right iliac artery
        ✓7ᵗʰ **S35.512** **Injury of** left iliac artery
        ✓7ᵗʰ **S35.513** **Injury of unspecified iliac artery** ▽
        ✓7ᵗʰ **S35.514** **Injury of** right iliac vein
        ✓7ᵗʰ **S35.515** **Injury of** left iliac vein
        ✓7ᵗʰ **S35.516** **Injury of unspecified iliac vein** ▽

    ✓6ᵗʰ **S35.53** **Injury of** uterine **artery or vein**

        ✓7ᵗʰ **S35.531** **Injury of** right uterine artery ♀
        ✓7ᵗʰ **S35.532** **Injury of** left uterine artery ♀
        ✓7ᵗʰ **S35.533** **Injury of unspecified uterine artery** ♀▽
        ✓7ᵗʰ **S35.534** **Injury of** right uterine vein ♀
        ✓7ᵗʰ **S35.535** **Injury of** left uterine vein ♀
        ✓7ᵗʰ **S35.536** **Injury of unspecified uterine vein** ♀▽

    ✓×7ᵗʰ **S35.59** **Injury of other iliac blood vessels**

✓5ᵗʰ **S35.8** **Injury of other blood vessels at abdomen, lower back and pelvis level**
      Injury of ovarian artery or vein

    ✓6ᵗʰ **S35.8X** **Injury of other blood vessels at abdomen, lower back and pelvis level**

        ✓7ᵗʰ **S35.8X1** Laceration **of other blood vessels at abdomen, lower back and pelvis level**
        ✓7ᵗʰ **S35.8X8** **Other specified injury of other blood vessels at abdomen, lower back and pelvis level**
        ✓7ᵗʰ **S35.8X9** **Unspecified injury of other blood vessels at abdomen, lower back and pelvis level** ▽

☑ Additional Character Req   ✓×7ᵗʰ Placeholder Alert   Manifestation   HCC CMS-HCC Condition   ▽ Unspecified Code   ▶◀ Revised Text   ● New Code   ▲ Revised Code Title

S35.9 Injury of unspecified blood vessel at abdomen, lower back and pelvis level
- **S35.90** Unspecified injury of unspecified blood vessel at abdomen, lower back and pelvis level
- **S35.91** Laceration of unspecified blood vessel at abdomen, lower back and pelvis level
- **S35.99** Other specified injury of unspecified blood vessel at abdomen, lower back and pelvis level

S36 Injury of intra-abdominal organs
Code also any associated open wound (S31.-)

The appropriate 7th character is to be added to each code from category S36.
A   initial encounter
D   subsequent encounter
S   sequela

S36.0 Injury of spleen
AHA: 2015, 2Q, 36; 2015, 1Q, 10
- **S36.00** Unspecified injury of spleen
- **S36.02** Contusion of spleen
  - **S36.020** Minor contusion of spleen
    Contusion of spleen less than 2 cm
  - **S36.021** Major contusion of spleen
    Contusion of spleen greater than 2 cm
  - **S36.029** Unspecified contusion of spleen
- **S36.03** Laceration of spleen
  - **S36.030** Superficial (capsular) laceration of spleen
    Laceration of spleen less than 1cm
    Minor laceration of spleen
  - **S36.031** Moderate laceration of spleen
    Laceration of spleen 1 to 3 cm
  - **S36.032** Major laceration of spleen
    Avulsion of spleen
    Laceration of spleen greater than 3 cm
    Massive laceration of spleen
    Multiple moderate lacerations of spleen
    Stellate laceration of spleen
  - **S36.039** Unspecified laceration of spleen
- **S36.09** Other injury of spleen

S36.1 Injury of liver and gallbladder and bile duct
- **S36.11** Injury of liver
  - **S36.112** Contusion of liver
  - **S36.113** Laceration of liver, unspecified degree
  - **S36.114** Minor laceration of liver
    Laceration involving capsule only, or, without significant involvement of hepatic parenchyma [i.e., less than 1cm deep]
  - **S36.115** Moderate laceration of liver
    Laceration involving parenchyma but without major disruption of parenchyma [i.e., less than 10 cm long and less than 3 cm deep]
  - **S36.116** Major laceration of liver
    Laceration with significant disruption of hepatic parenchyma [i.e., greater than 10 cm long and 3 cm deep]
    Multiple moderate lacerations, with or without hematoma
    Stellate laceration of liver
  - **S36.118** Other injury of liver
  - **S36.119** Unspecified injury of liver
- **S36.12** Injury of gallbladder
  - **S36.122** Contusion of gallbladder
  - **S36.123** Laceration of gallbladder
  - **S36.128** Other injury of gallbladder
  - **S36.129** Unspecified injury of gallbladder
- **S36.13** Injury of bile duct

S36.2 Injury of pancreas
- **S36.20** Unspecified injury of pancreas
  - **S36.200** Unspecified injury of head of pancreas
  - **S36.201** Unspecified injury of body of pancreas
  - **S36.202** Unspecified injury of tail of pancreas
  - **S36.209** Unspecified injury of unspecified part of pancreas

- **S36.22** Contusion of pancreas
  - **S36.220** Contusion of head of pancreas
  - **S36.221** Contusion of body of pancreas
  - **S36.222** Contusion of tail of pancreas
  - **S36.229** Contusion of unspecified part of pancreas
- **S36.23** Laceration of pancreas, unspecified degree
  - **S36.230** Laceration of head of pancreas, unspecified degree
  - **S36.231** Laceration of body of pancreas, unspecified degree
  - **S36.232** Laceration of tail of pancreas, unspecified degree
  - **S36.239** Laceration of unspecified part of pancreas, unspecified degree
- **S36.24** Minor laceration of pancreas
  - **S36.240** Minor laceration of head of pancreas
  - **S36.241** Minor laceration of body of pancreas
  - **S36.242** Minor laceration of tail of pancreas
  - **S36.249** Minor laceration of unspecified part of pancreas
- **S36.25** Moderate laceration of pancreas
  - **S36.250** Moderate laceration of head of pancreas
  - **S36.251** Moderate laceration of body of pancreas
  - **S36.252** Moderate laceration of tail of pancreas
  - **S36.259** Moderate laceration of unspecified part of pancreas
- **S36.26** Major laceration of pancreas
  - **S36.260** Major laceration of head of pancreas
  - **S36.261** Major laceration of body of pancreas
  - **S36.262** Major laceration of tail of pancreas
  - **S36.269** Major laceration of unspecified part of pancreas
- **S36.29** Other injury of pancreas
  - **S36.290** Other injury of head of pancreas
  - **S36.291** Other injury of body of pancreas
  - **S36.292** Other injury of tail of pancreas
  - **S36.299** Other injury of unspecified part of pancreas

S36.3 Injury of stomach
- **S36.30** Unspecified injury of stomach
- **S36.32** Contusion of stomach
- **S36.33** Laceration of stomach
- **S36.39** Other injury of stomach

S36.4 Injury of small intestine
- **S36.40** Unspecified injury of small intestine
  - **S36.400** Unspecified injury of duodenum
  - **S36.408** Unspecified injury of other part of small intestine
  - **S36.409** Unspecified injury of unspecified part of small intestine
- **S36.41** Primary blast injury of small intestine
  Blast injury of small intestine NOS
  - **S36.410** Primary blast injury of duodenum
  - **S36.418** Primary blast injury of other part of small intestine
  - **S36.419** Primary blast injury of unspecified part of small intestine
- **S36.42** Contusion of small intestine
  - **S36.420** Contusion of duodenum
  - **S36.428** Contusion of other part of small intestine
  - **S36.429** Contusion of unspecified part of small intestine
- **S36.43** Laceration of small intestine
  - **S36.430** Laceration of duodenum
  - **S36.438** Laceration of other part of small intestine
  - **S36.439** Laceration of unspecified part of small intestine

Chapter 19. Injury, Poisoning, and Certain Other Consequences of External Causes

√6ᵗʰ **S36.49 Other injury of small intestine**

     √7ᵗʰ **S36.490 Other injury of** duodenum

     √7ᵗʰ **S36.498 Other injury of other part of small intestine**

     √7ᵗʰ **S36.499 Other injury of unspecified part of small intestine** ▽

√5ᵗʰ **S36.5 Injury of** colon

     EXCLUDES 2   injury of rectum (S36.6-)

     √6ᵗʰ **S36.50 Unspecified injury of colon**

         √7ᵗʰ **S36.500 Unspecified injury of** ascending **[right] colon** ▽

         √7ᵗʰ **S36.501 Unspecified injury of** transverse **colon** ▽

         √7ᵗʰ **S36.502 Unspecified injury of** descending **[left] colon** ▽

         √7ᵗʰ **S36.503 Unspecified injury of** sigmoid **colon** ▽

         √7ᵗʰ **S36.508 Unspecified injury of other part of colon** ▽

         √7ᵗʰ **S36.509 Unspecified injury of unspecified part of colon** ▽

     √6ᵗʰ **S36.51** Primary blast **injury of colon**

         Blast injury of colon NOS

         √7ᵗʰ **S36.510 Primary blast injury of** ascending **[right] colon**

         √7ᵗʰ **S36.511 Primary blast injury of** transverse **colon**

         √7ᵗʰ **S36.512 Primary blast injury of** descending **[left] colon**

         √7ᵗʰ **S36.513 Primary blast injury of** sigmoid **colon**

         √7ᵗʰ **S36.518 Primary blast injury of other part of colon**

         √7ᵗʰ **S36.519 Primary blast injury of unspecified part of colon** ▽

     √6ᵗʰ **S36.52** Contusion **of colon**

         √7ᵗʰ **S36.520 Contusion of** ascending **[right] colon**

         √7ᵗʰ **S36.521 Contusion of** transverse **colon**

         √7ᵗʰ **S36.522 Contusion of** descending **[left] colon**

         √7ᵗʰ **S36.523 Contusion of** sigmoid **colon**

         √7ᵗʰ **S36.528 Contusion of other part of colon**

         √7ᵗʰ **S36.529 Contusion of unspecified part of colon** ▽

     √6ᵗʰ **S36.53** Laceration **of colon**

         √7ᵗʰ **S36.530 Laceration of** ascending **[right] colon**

         √7ᵗʰ **S36.531 Laceration of** transverse **colon**

         √7ᵗʰ **S36.532 Laceration of** descending **[left] colon**

         √7ᵗʰ **S36.533 Laceration of** sigmoid **colon**

         √7ᵗʰ **S36.538 Laceration of other part of colon**

         √7ᵗʰ **S36.539 Laceration of unspecified part of colon** ▽

     √6ᵗʰ **S36.59 Other injury of colon**

         Secondary blast injury of colon

         √7ᵗʰ **S36.590 Other injury of** ascending **[right] colon**

         √7ᵗʰ **S36.591 Other injury of** transverse **colon**

         √7ᵗʰ **S36.592 Other injury of** descending **[left] colon**

         √7ᵗʰ **S36.593 Other injury of** sigmoid **colon**

         √7ᵗʰ **S36.598 Other injury of other part of colon**

         √7ᵗʰ **S36.599 Other injury of unspecified part of colon** ▽

√5ᵗʰ **S36.6 Injury of** rectum

     √x7ᵗʰ **S36.60 Unspecified injury of rectum** ▽

     √x7ᵗʰ **S36.61** Primary blast **injury of rectum**

         Blast injury of rectum NOS

     √x7ᵗʰ **S36.62** Contusion **of rectum**

     √x7ᵗʰ **S36.63** Laceration **of rectum**

     √x7ᵗʰ **S36.69 Other injury of rectum**

         Secondary blast injury of rectum

√5ᵗʰ **S36.8 Injury of other intra-abdominal organs**

     √x7ᵗʰ **S36.81 Injury of** peritoneum

     √6ᵗʰ **S36.89 Injury of other intra-abdominal organs**

         Injury of retroperitoneum

         √7ᵗʰ **S36.892** Contusion **of other intra-abdominal organs**

         √7ᵗʰ **S36.893** Laceration **of other intra-abdominal organs**

         √7ᵗʰ **S36.898 Other injury of other intra-abdominal organs**

         √7ᵗʰ **S36.899 Unspecified injury of other intra-abdominal organs** ▽

√5ᵗʰ **S36.9 Injury of unspecified intra-abdominal organ**

     √x7ᵗʰ **S36.90 Unspecified injury of unspecified intra-abdominal organ** ▽

     √x7ᵗʰ **S36.92** Contusion **of unspecified intra-abdominal organ** ▽

     √x7ᵗʰ **S36.93** Laceration **of unspecified intra-abdominal organ** ▽

     √x7ᵗʰ **S36.99 Other injury of unspecified intra-abdominal organ** ▽

√4ᵗʰ **S37 Injury of urinary and pelvic organs**

     Code also any associated open wound (S31.-)

     EXCLUDES 1   obstetric trauma to pelvic organs (O71.-)

     EXCLUDES 2   injury of peritoneum (S36.81)

                     injury of retroperitoneum (S36.89-)

     The appropriate 7th character is to be added to each code from category S37.

     A   initial encounter

     D   subsequent encounter

     S   sequela

√5ᵗʰ **S37.0 Injury of** kidney

     EXCLUDES 2   acute kidney injury (nontraumatic) (N17.9)

     √6ᵗʰ **S37.00 Unspecified injury of kidney**

         √7ᵗʰ **S37.001 Unspecified injury of** right **kidney** ▽

         √7ᵗʰ **S37.002 Unspecified injury of** left **kidney** ▽

         √7ᵗʰ **S37.009 Unspecified injury of unspecified kidney** ▽

     √6ᵗʰ **S37.01** Minor contusion **of kidney**

         Contusion of kidney less than 2 cm

         Contusion of kidney NOS

         √7ᵗʰ **S37.011 Minor contusion of** right **kidney**

         √7ᵗʰ **S37.012 Minor contusion of** left **kidney**

         √7ᵗʰ **S37.019 Minor contusion of unspecified kidney** ▽

     √6ᵗʰ **S37.02** Major contusion **of kidney**

         Contusion of kidney greater than 2 cm

         √7ᵗʰ **S37.021 Major contusion of** right **kidney**

         √7ᵗʰ **S37.022 Major contusion of** left **kidney**

         √7ᵗʰ **S37.029 Major contusion of unspecified kidney** ▽

     √6ᵗʰ **S37.03** Laceration **of kidney, unspecified degree**

         √7ᵗʰ **S37.031 Laceration of** right **kidney, unspecified degree** ▽

         √7ᵗʰ **S37.032 Laceration of** left **kidney, unspecified degree** ▽

         √7ᵗʰ **S37.039 Laceration of unspecified kidney, unspecified degree** ▽

     √6ᵗʰ **S37.04** Minor laceration **of kidney**

         Laceration of kidney less than 1 cm

         √7ᵗʰ **S37.041 Minor laceration of** right **kidney**

         √7ᵗʰ **S37.042 Minor laceration of** left **kidney**

         √7ᵗʰ **S37.049 Minor laceration of unspecified kidney** ▽

     √6ᵗʰ **S37.05** Moderate laceration **of kidney**

         Laceration of kidney 1 to 3 cm

         √7ᵗʰ **S37.051 Moderate laceration of** right **kidney**

         √7ᵗʰ **S37.052 Moderate laceration of** left **kidney**

         √7ᵗʰ **S37.059 Moderate laceration of unspecified kidney** ▽

     √6ᵗʰ **S37.06** Major laceration **of kidney**

         Avulsion of kidney

         Laceration of kidney greater than 3 cm

         Massive laceration of kidney

         Multiple moderate lacerations of kidney

         Stellate laceration of kidney

         √7ᵗʰ **S37.061 Major laceration of** right **kidney**

         √7ᵗʰ **S37.062 Major laceration of** left **kidney**

         √7ᵗʰ **S37.069 Major laceration of unspecified kidney** ▽

     √6ᵗʰ **S37.09 Other injury of kidney**

         √7ᵗʰ **S37.091 Other injury of** right **kidney**

         √7ᵗʰ **S37.092 Other injury of** left **kidney**

         √7ᵗʰ **S37.099 Other injury of unspecified kidney** ▽

√5ᵗʰ **S37.1 Injury of** ureter

     √x7ᵗʰ **S37.10 Unspecified injury of ureter** ▽

     √x7ᵗʰ **S37.12** Contusion **of ureter**

     √x7ᵗʰ **S37.13** Laceration **of ureter**

✓ Additional Character Req   √x7ᵗʰ Placeholder Alert   Manifestation   HCC CMS-HCC Condition   ▽ Unspecified Code   ►◄ Revised Text   ● New Code   ▲ Revised Code Title

ICD-10-CM 2018   951

√x7ᵗʰ **S37.19**   Other injury of ureter

√5ᵗʰ **S37.2**   Injury of bladder
- √x7ᵗʰ **S37.20**   Unspecified injury of bladder ▽
- √x7ᵗʰ **S37.22**   Contusion of bladder
- √x7ᵗʰ **S37.23**   Laceration of bladder
- √x7ᵗʰ **S37.29**   Other injury of bladder

√5ᵗʰ **S37.3**   Injury of urethra
- √x7ᵗʰ **S37.30**   Unspecified injury of urethra ▽
- √x7ᵗʰ **S37.32**   Contusion of urethra
- √x7ᵗʰ **S37.33**   Laceration of urethra
- √x7ᵗʰ **S37.39**   Other injury of urethra

√5ᵗʰ **S37.4**   Injury of ovary
- √6ᵗʰ **S37.40**   Unspecified injury of ovary
  - √7ᵗʰ **S37.401**   Unspecified injury of ovary, unilateral ♀▽
  - √7ᵗʰ **S37.402**   Unspecified injury of ovary, bilateral ♀▽
  - √7ᵗʰ **S37.409**   Unspecified injury of ovary, unspecified ♀▽
- √6ᵗʰ **S37.42**   Contusion of ovary
  - √7ᵗʰ **S37.421**   Contusion of ovary, unilateral ♀
  - √7ᵗʰ **S37.422**   Contusion of ovary, bilateral ♀
  - √7ᵗʰ **S37.429**   Contusion of ovary, unspecified ♀▽
- √6ᵗʰ **S37.43**   Laceration of ovary
  - √7ᵗʰ **S37.431**   Laceration of ovary, unilateral ♀
  - √7ᵗʰ **S37.432**   Laceration of ovary, bilateral ♀
  - √7ᵗʰ **S37.439**   Laceration of ovary, unspecified ♀▽
- √6ᵗʰ **S37.49**   Other injury of ovary
  - √7ᵗʰ **S37.491**   Other injury of ovary, unilateral ♀
  - √7ᵗʰ **S37.492**   Other injury of ovary, bilateral ♀
  - √7ᵗʰ **S37.499**   Other injury of ovary, unspecified ♀▽

√5ᵗʰ **S37.5**   Injury of fallopian tube
- √6ᵗʰ **S37.50**   Unspecified injury of fallopian tube
  - √7ᵗʰ **S37.501**   Unspecified injury of fallopian tube, unilateral ♀▽
  - √7ᵗʰ **S37.502**   Unspecified injury of fallopian tube, bilateral ♀▽
  - √7ᵗʰ **S37.509**   Unspecified injury of fallopian tube, unspecified ♀▽
- √6ᵗʰ **S37.51**   Primary blast injury of fallopian tube
  Blast injury of fallopian tube NOS
  - √7ᵗʰ **S37.511**   Primary blast injury of fallopian tube, unilateral ♀
  - √7ᵗʰ **S37.512**   Primary blast injury of fallopian tube, bilateral ♀
  - √7ᵗʰ **S37.519**   Primary blast injury of fallopian tube, unspecified ♀▽
- √6ᵗʰ **S37.52**   Contusion of fallopian tube
  - √7ᵗʰ **S37.521**   Contusion of fallopian tube, unilateral ♀
  - √7ᵗʰ **S37.522**   Contusion of fallopian tube, bilateral ♀
  - √7ᵗʰ **S37.529**   Contusion of fallopian tube, unspecified ♀▽
- √6ᵗʰ **S37.53**   Laceration of fallopian tube
  - √7ᵗʰ **S37.531**   Laceration of fallopian tube, unilateral ♀
  - √7ᵗʰ **S37.532**   Laceration of fallopian tube, bilateral ♀
  - √7ᵗʰ **S37.539**   Laceration of fallopian tube, unspecified ♀▽
- √6ᵗʰ **S37.59**   Other injury of fallopian tube
  Secondary blast injury of fallopian tube
  - √7ᵗʰ **S37.591**   Other injury of fallopian tube, unilateral ♀
  - √7ᵗʰ **S37.592**   Other injury of fallopian tube, bilateral ♀
  - √7ᵗʰ **S37.599**   Other injury of fallopian tube, unspecified ♀▽

√5ᵗʰ **S37.6**   Injury of uterus
- EXCLUDES 1   injury to gravid uterus (O9A.2-)
  injury to uterus during delivery (O71.-)
- √x7ᵗʰ **S37.60**   Unspecified injury of uterus ♀▽
- √x7ᵗʰ **S37.62**   Contusion of uterus ♀
- √x7ᵗʰ **S37.63**   Laceration of uterus ♀
- √x7ᵗʰ **S37.69**   Other injury of uterus ♀

√5ᵗʰ **S37.8**   Injury of other urinary and pelvic organs
- √6ᵗʰ **S37.81**   Injury of adrenal gland
  - √7ᵗʰ **S37.812**   Contusion of adrenal gland
  - √7ᵗʰ **S37.813**   Laceration of adrenal gland
  - √7ᵗʰ **S37.818**   Other injury of adrenal gland
  - √7ᵗʰ **S37.819**   Unspecified injury of adrenal gland ▽
- √6ᵗʰ **S37.82**   Injury of prostate
  - √7ᵗʰ **S37.822**   Contusion of prostate ♂
  - √7ᵗʰ **S37.823**   Laceration of prostate ♂
  - √7ᵗʰ **S37.828**   Other injury of prostate ♂
  - √7ᵗʰ **S37.829**   Unspecified injury of prostate ♂▽
- √6ᵗʰ **S37.89**   Injury of other urinary and pelvic organ
  - √7ᵗʰ **S37.892**   Contusion of other urinary and pelvic organ
  - √7ᵗʰ **S37.893**   Laceration of other urinary and pelvic organ
  - √7ᵗʰ **S37.898**   Other injury of other urinary and pelvic organ
  - √7ᵗʰ **S37.899**   Unspecified injury of other urinary and pelvic organ ▽

√5ᵗʰ **S37.9**   Injury of unspecified urinary and pelvic organ
- √x7ᵗʰ **S37.90**   Unspecified injury of unspecified urinary and pelvic organ ▽
- √x7ᵗʰ **S37.92**   Contusion of unspecified urinary and pelvic organ ▽
- √x7ᵗʰ **S37.93**   Laceration of unspecified urinary and pelvic organ ▽
- √x7ᵗʰ **S37.99**   Other injury of unspecified urinary and pelvic organ ▽

√4ᵗʰ **S38**   **Crushing injury and traumatic amputation of abdomen, lower back, pelvis and external genitals**
An amputation not identified as partial or complete should be coded to complete.

> The appropriate 7th character is to be added to each code from category S38.
> A   initial encounter
> D   subsequent encounter
> S   sequela

√5ᵗʰ **S38.0**   Crushing injury of external genital organs
Use additional code for any associated injuries
- √6ᵗʰ **S38.00**   Crushing injury of unspecified external genital organs
  - √7ᵗʰ **S38.001**   Crushing injury of unspecified external genital organs, male ♂▽
  - √7ᵗʰ **S38.002**   Crushing injury of unspecified external genital organs, female ♀▽
- √x7ᵗʰ **S38.01**   Crushing injury of penis ♂
- √x7ᵗʰ **S38.02**   Crushing injury of scrotum and testis ♂
- √x7ᵗʰ **S38.03**   Crushing injury of vulva ♀

√x7ᵗʰ **S38.1**   Crushing injury of abdomen, lower back, and pelvis
Use additional code for all associated injuries, such as:
  fracture of thoracic or lumbar spine and pelvis (S22.0-, S32-)
  injury to intra-abdominal organs (S36.-)
  injury to urinary and pelvic organs (S37.-)
  open wound of abdominal wall (S31.-)
  spinal cord injury (S34.0, S34.1-)
  EXCLUDES 2   crushing injury of external genital organs (S38.0-)

√5ᵗʰ **S38.2**   Traumatic amputation of external genital organs
- √6ᵗʰ **S38.21**   Traumatic amputation of female external genital organs
  Traumatic amputation of clitoris
  Traumatic amputation of labium (majus) (minus)
  Traumatic amputation of vulva
  - √7ᵗʰ **S38.211**   Complete traumatic amputation of female external genital organs ♀
  - √7ᵗʰ **S38.212**   Partial traumatic amputation of female external genital organs ♀
- √6ᵗʰ **S38.22**   Traumatic amputation of penis
  - √7ᵗʰ **S38.221**   Complete traumatic amputation of penis ♂
  - √7ᵗʰ **S38.222**   Partial traumatic amputation of penis ♂

EXCLUDES 1 Not coded here   EXCLUDES 2 Not included here   N Newborn Age: 0   P Pediatric Age: 0-17   M Maternity Age: 12-55   A Adult Age: 15-124

✓6ᵗʰ **S38.23** Traumatic amputation of scrotum and testis

    ✓7ᵗʰ **S38.231** Complete **traumatic amputation of scrotum and testis** ♂

    ✓7ᵗʰ **S38.232** Partial **traumatic amputation of scrotum and testis** ♂

✓ₓ7ᵗʰ **S38.3** Transection (partial) of abdomen

✓4ᵗʰ **S39** **Other and unspecified injuries of abdomen, lower back, pelvis and external genitals**

  Code also any associated open wound (S31.-)

  EXCLUDES 2 *sprain of joints and ligaments of lumbar spine and pelvis (S33.-)*

> The appropriate 7th character is to be added to each code from category S39.
> A   initial encounter
> D   subsequent encounter
> S   sequela

✓5ᵗʰ **S39.0** **Injury of muscle, fascia and tendon of abdomen, lower back and pelvis**

  ✓6ᵗʰ **S39.00** **Unspecified injury of muscle, fascia and tendon of abdomen, lower back and pelvis**

    ✓7ᵗʰ **S39.001** Unspecified injury of muscle, fascia and tendon of abdomen ▽

    ✓7ᵗʰ **S39.002** Unspecified injury of muscle, fascia and tendon of lower back ▽

    ✓7ᵗʰ **S39.003** Unspecified injury of muscle, fascia and tendon of pelvis ▽

  ✓6ᵗʰ **S39.01** Strain of muscle, fascia and tendon of abdomen, lower back and pelvis

    ✓7ᵗʰ **S39.011** Strain of muscle, fascia and tendon of abdomen

    ✓7ᵗʰ **S39.012** Strain of muscle, fascia and tendon of lower back

    ✓7ᵗʰ **S39.013** Strain of muscle, fascia and tendon of pelvis

  ✓6ᵗʰ **S39.02** Laceration of muscle, fascia and tendon of abdomen, lower back and pelvis

    ✓7ᵗʰ **S39.021** Laceration of muscle, fascia and tendon of abdomen

    ✓7ᵗʰ **S39.022** Laceration of muscle, fascia and tendon of lower back

    ✓7ᵗʰ **S39.023** Laceration of muscle, fascia and tendon of pelvis

  ✓6ᵗʰ **S39.09** **Other injury of muscle, fascia and tendon of abdomen, lower back and pelvis**

    ✓7ᵗʰ **S39.091** Other injury of muscle, fascia and tendon of abdomen

    ✓7ᵗʰ **S39.092** Other injury of muscle, fascia and tendon of lower back

    ✓7ᵗʰ **S39.093** Other injury of muscle, fascia and tendon of pelvis

✓5ᵗʰ **S39.8** **Other specified injuries of abdomen, lower back, pelvis and external genitals**

  ✓ₓ7ᵗʰ **S39.81** Other specified injuries of abdomen

  ✓ₓ7ᵗʰ **S39.82** Other specified injuries of lower back

  ✓ₓ7ᵗʰ **S39.83** Other specified injuries of pelvis

  ✓6ᵗʰ **S39.84** **Other specified injuries of external genitals**

    ✓7ᵗʰ **S39.840** Fracture of corpus cavernosum penis ♂

    ✓7ᵗʰ **S39.848** Other specified injuries of external genitals

✓5ᵗʰ **S39.9** **Unspecified injury of abdomen, lower back, pelvis and external genitals**

  ✓ₓ7ᵗʰ **S39.91** Unspecified injury of abdomen ▽

  ✓ₓ7ᵗʰ **S39.92** Unspecified injury of lower back ▽

  ✓ₓ7ᵗʰ **S39.93** Unspecified injury of pelvis ▽

  ✓ₓ7ᵗʰ **S39.94** Unspecified injury of external genitals ▽

Injuries to the shoulder and upper arm (S40-S49)

INCLUDES injuries of axilla
        injuries of scapular region
EXCLUDES 2 *burns and corrosions (T20-T32)*
        frostbite (T33-T34)
        injuries of elbow (S50-S59)
        insect bite or sting, venomous (T63.4)

✓4ᵗʰ **S40** **Superficial injury of shoulder and upper arm**

> The appropriate 7th character is to be added to each code from category S40.
> A   initial encounter
> D   subsequent encounter
> S   sequela

✓5ᵗʰ **S40.0** **Contusion of shoulder and upper arm**

  ✓6ᵗʰ **S40.01** **Contusion of shoulder**

    ✓7ᵗʰ **S40.011** Contusion of right shoulder

    ✓7ᵗʰ **S40.012** Contusion of left shoulder

    ✓7ᵗʰ **S40.019** Contusion of unspecified shoulder ▽

  ✓6ᵗʰ **S40.02** **Contusion of upper arm**

    ✓7ᵗʰ **S40.021** Contusion of right upper arm

    ✓7ᵗʰ **S40.022** Contusion of left upper arm

    ✓7ᵗʰ **S40.029** Contusion of unspecified upper arm ▽

✓5ᵗʰ **S40.2** **Other superficial injuries of shoulder**

  ✓6ᵗʰ **S40.21** Abrasion of shoulder

    ✓7ᵗʰ **S40.211** Abrasion of right shoulder

    ✓7ᵗʰ **S40.212** Abrasion of left shoulder

    ✓7ᵗʰ **S40.219** Abrasion of unspecified shoulder ▽

  ✓6ᵗʰ **S40.22** Blister (nonthermal) of shoulder

    ✓7ᵗʰ **S40.221** Blister (nonthermal) of right shoulder

    ✓7ᵗʰ **S40.222** Blister (nonthermal) of left shoulder

    ✓7ᵗʰ **S40.229** Blister (nonthermal) of unspecified shoulder ▽

  ✓6ᵗʰ **S40.24** External constriction of shoulder

    ✓7ᵗʰ **S40.241** External constriction of right shoulder

    ✓7ᵗʰ **S40.242** External constriction of left shoulder

    ✓7ᵗʰ **S40.249** External constriction of unspecified shoulder ▽

  ✓6ᵗʰ **S40.25** **Superficial foreign body of shoulder**
    Splinter in the shoulder

    ✓7ᵗʰ **S40.251** Superficial foreign body of right shoulder

    ✓7ᵗʰ **S40.252** Superficial foreign body of left shoulder

    ✓7ᵗʰ **S40.259** Superficial foreign body of unspecified shoulder ▽

  ✓6ᵗʰ **S40.26** Insect bite (nonvenomous) of shoulder

    ✓7ᵗʰ **S40.261** Insect bite (nonvenomous) of right shoulder

    ✓7ᵗʰ **S40.262** Insect bite (nonvenomous) of left shoulder

    ✓7ᵗʰ **S40.269** Insect bite (nonvenomous) of unspecified shoulder ▽

  ✓6ᵗʰ **S40.27** **Other superficial bite of shoulder**
    EXCLUDES 1 *open bite of shoulder (S41.05)*

    ✓7ᵗʰ **S40.271** Other superficial bite of right shoulder

    ✓7ᵗʰ **S40.272** Other superficial bite of left shoulder

    ✓7ᵗʰ **S40.279** Other superficial bite of unspecified shoulder ▽

✓5ᵗʰ **S40.8** **Other superficial injuries of upper arm**

  ✓6ᵗʰ **S40.81** Abrasion of upper arm

    ✓7ᵗʰ **S40.811** Abrasion of right upper arm

    ✓7ᵗʰ **S40.812** Abrasion of left upper arm

    ✓7ᵗʰ **S40.819** Abrasion of unspecified upper arm ▽

  ✓6ᵗʰ **S40.82** Blister (nonthermal) of upper arm

    ✓7ᵗʰ **S40.821** Blister (nonthermal) of right upper arm

    ✓7ᵗʰ **S40.822** Blister (nonthermal) of left upper arm

    ✓7ᵗʰ **S40.829** Blister (nonthermal) of unspecified upper arm ▽

  ✓6ᵗʰ **S40.84** External constriction of upper arm

    ✓7ᵗʰ **S40.841** External constriction of right upper arm

    ✓7ᵗʰ **S40.842** External constriction of left upper arm

    ✓7ᵗʰ **S40.849** External constriction of unspecified upper arm ▽

✓ Additional Character Req   ✓ₓ7ᵗʰ Placeholder Alert   Manifestation   *HCC* CMS-HCC Condition   ▽ Unspecified Code   ►◄ Revised Text   ● New Code   ▲ Revised Code Title

Chapter 19. Injury, Poisoning, and Certain Other Consequences of External Causes *(vertical side text)*

✓6th S40.85 Superficial foreign body of upper arm
Splinter in the upper arm

- **✓7th S40.851** Superficial foreign body of right upper arm
- **✓7th S40.852** Superficial foreign body of left upper arm
- **✓7th S40.859** Superficial foreign body of unspecified upper arm ▽

✓6th S40.86 Insect bite (nonvenomous) of upper arm

- **✓7th S40.861** Insect bite (nonvenomous) of right upper arm
- **✓7th S40.862** Insect bite (nonvenomous) of left upper arm
- **✓7th S40.869** Insect bite (nonvenomous) of unspecified upper arm ▽

✓6th S40.87 Other superficial bite of upper arm
> EXCLUDES 1   open bite of upper arm (S41.14)
> EXCLUDES 2   other superficial bite of shoulder (S40.27-)

- **✓7th S40.871** Other superficial bite of right upper arm
- **✓7th S40.872** Other superficial bite of left upper arm
- **✓7th S40.879** Other superficial bite of unspecified upper arm ▽

✓5th S40.9 Unspecified superficial injury of shoulder and upper arm

- **✓6th S40.91 Unspecified superficial injury of shoulder**
  - **✓7th S40.911** Unspecified superficial injury of right shoulder ▽
  - **✓7th S40.912** Unspecified superficial injury of left shoulder ▽
  - **✓7th S40.919** Unspecified superficial injury of unspecified shoulder ▽

- **✓6th S40.92 Unspecified superficial injury of upper arm**
  - **✓7th S40.921** Unspecified superficial injury of right upper arm ▽
  - **✓7th S40.922** Unspecified superficial injury of left upper arm ▽
  - **✓7th S40.929** Unspecified superficial injury of unspecified upper arm ▽

✓4th S41 Open wound of shoulder and upper arm
Code also any associated wound infection
> EXCLUDES 1   traumatic amputation of shoulder and upper arm (S48.-)
> EXCLUDES 2   open fracture of shoulder and upper arm (S42.- with 7th character B or C)

> The appropriate 7th character is to be added to each code from category S41.
> A   initial encounter
> D   subsequent encounter
> S   sequela

✓5th S41.0 Open wound of shoulder

- **✓6th S41.00 Unspecified open wound of shoulder**
  - **✓7th S41.001** Unspecified open wound of right shoulder ▽
  - **✓7th S41.002** Unspecified open wound of left shoulder ▽
  - **✓7th S41.009** Unspecified open wound of unspecified shoulder ▽

- **✓6th S41.01 Laceration without foreign body of shoulder**
  - **✓7th S41.011** Laceration without foreign body of right shoulder
  - **✓7th S41.012** Laceration without foreign body of left shoulder
  - **✓7th S41.019** Laceration without foreign body of unspecified shoulder ▽

- **✓6th S41.02 Laceration with foreign body of shoulder**
  - **✓7th S41.021** Laceration with foreign body of right shoulder
  - **✓7th S41.022** Laceration with foreign body of left shoulder
  - **✓7th S41.029** Laceration with foreign body of unspecified shoulder ▽

- **✓6th S41.03 Puncture wound without foreign body of shoulder**
  - **✓7th S41.031** Puncture wound without foreign body of right shoulder
  - **✓7th S41.032** Puncture wound without foreign body of left shoulder

- **✓7th S41.039** Puncture wound without foreign body of unspecified shoulder ▽

✓6th S41.04 Puncture wound with foreign body of shoulder

- **✓7th S41.041** Puncture wound with foreign body of right shoulder
- **✓7th S41.042** Puncture wound with foreign body of left shoulder
- **✓7th S41.049** Puncture wound with foreign body of unspecified shoulder ▽

✓6th S41.05 Open bite of shoulder
Bite of shoulder NOS
> EXCLUDES 1   superficial bite of shoulder (S40.27)

- **✓7th S41.051** Open bite of right shoulder
- **✓7th S41.052** Open bite of left shoulder
- **✓7th S41.059** Open bite of unspecified shoulder ▽

✓5th S41.1 Open wound of upper arm

- **✓6th S41.10 Unspecified open wound of upper arm**
  AHA: 2016, 3Q, 24
  - **✓7th S41.101** Unspecified open wound of right upper arm ▽
  - **✓7th S41.102** Unspecified open wound of left upper arm ▽
  - **✓7th S41.109** Unspecified open wound of unspecified upper arm ▽

- **✓6th S41.11 Laceration without foreign body of upper arm**
  - **✓7th S41.111** Laceration without foreign body of right upper arm
  - **✓7th S41.112** Laceration without foreign body of left upper arm
  - **✓7th S41.119** Laceration without foreign body of unspecified upper arm ▽

- **✓6th S41.12 Laceration with foreign body of upper arm**
  - **✓7th S41.121** Laceration with foreign body of right upper arm
  - **✓7th S41.122** Laceration with foreign body of left upper arm
  - **✓7th S41.129** Laceration with foreign body of unspecified upper arm ▽

- **✓6th S41.13 Puncture wound without foreign body of upper arm**
  AHA: 2016, 3Q, 24
  - **✓7th S41.131** Puncture wound without foreign body of right upper arm
  - **✓7th S41.132** Puncture wound without foreign body of left upper arm
  - **✓7th S41.139** Puncture wound without foreign body of unspecified upper arm ▽

- **✓6th S41.14 Puncture wound with foreign body of upper arm**
  AHA: 2016, 3Q, 24
  - **✓7th S41.141** Puncture wound with foreign body of right upper arm
  - **✓7th S41.142** Puncture wound with foreign body of left upper arm
  - **✓7th S41.149** Puncture wound with foreign body of unspecified upper arm ▽

- **✓6th S41.15 Open bite of upper arm**
  Bite of upper arm NOS
  > EXCLUDES 1   superficial bite of upper arm (S40.87)
  - **✓7th S41.151** Open bite of right upper arm
  - **✓7th S41.152** Open bite of left upper arm
  - **✓7th S41.159** Open bite of unspecified upper arm ▽

EXCLUDES 1 Not coded here   EXCLUDES 2 Not included here   N Newborn Age: 0   P Pediatric Age: 0-17   M Maternity Age: 12-55   A Adult Age: 15-124

954   ICD-10-CM 2018

✓4ᵗʰ **S42 Fracture of shoulder and upper arm**

NOTE A fracture not indicated as displaced or nondisplaced should be coded to displaced.
A fracture not indicated as open or closed should be coded to closed.

EXCLUDES 1 traumatic amputation of shoulder and upper arm (S48.-)
AHA: 2015, 3Q, 37-39

The appropriate 7th character is to be added to all codes from category S42 [unless otherwise indicated].
A   initial encounter for closed fracture
B   initial encounter for open fracture
D   subsequent encounter for fracture with routine healing
G   subsequent encounter for fracture with delayed healing
K   subsequent encounter for fracture with nonunion
P   subsequent encounter for fracture with malunion
S   sequela

✓5ᵗʰ **S42.0 Fracture of clavicle**

✓6ᵗʰ **S42.00 Fracture of unspecified part of clavicle**

   ✓7ᵗʰ **S42.001 Fracture of unspecified part of right clavicle** ▽

   ✓7ᵗʰ **S42.002 Fracture of unspecified part of left clavicle** ▽

   ✓7ᵗʰ **S42.009 Fracture of unspecified part of unspecified clavicle** ▽
     AHA: 2012, 4Q, 93

✓6ᵗʰ **S42.01 Fracture of sternal end of clavicle**

   ✓7ᵗʰ **S42.011 Anterior displaced fracture of sternal end of right clavicle**

   ✓7ᵗʰ **S42.012 Anterior displaced fracture of sternal end of left clavicle**

   ✓7ᵗʰ **S42.013 Anterior displaced fracture of sternal end of unspecified clavicle** ▽
     Displaced fracture of sternal end of clavicle NOS

   ✓7ᵗʰ **S42.014 Posterior displaced fracture of sternal end of right clavicle**

   ✓7ᵗʰ **S42.015 Posterior displaced fracture of sternal end of left clavicle**

   ✓7ᵗʰ **S42.016 Posterior displaced fracture of sternal end of unspecified clavicle** ▽

   ✓7ᵗʰ **S42.017 Nondisplaced fracture of sternal end of right clavicle**

   ✓7ᵗʰ **S42.018 Nondisplaced fracture of sternal end of left clavicle**

   ✓7ᵗʰ **S42.019 Nondisplaced fracture of sternal end of unspecified clavicle** ▽

✓6ᵗʰ **S42.02 Fracture of shaft of clavicle**

   ✓7ᵗʰ **S42.021 Displaced fracture of shaft of right clavicle**

   ✓7ᵗʰ **S42.022 Displaced fracture of shaft of left clavicle**

   ✓7ᵗʰ **S42.023 Displaced fracture of shaft of unspecified clavicle** ▽

   ✓7ᵗʰ **S42.024 Nondisplaced fracture of shaft of right clavicle**

   ✓7ᵗʰ **S42.025 Nondisplaced fracture of shaft of left clavicle**

   ✓7ᵗʰ **S42.026 Nondisplaced fracture of shaft of unspecified clavicle** ▽

✓6ᵗʰ **S42.03 Fracture of lateral end of clavicle**
   Fracture of acromial end of clavicle

   ✓7ᵗʰ **S42.031 Displaced fracture of lateral end of right clavicle**

   ✓7ᵗʰ **S42.032 Displaced fracture of lateral end of left clavicle**

   ✓7ᵗʰ **S42.033 Displaced fracture of lateral end of unspecified clavicle** ▽

   ✓7ᵗʰ **S42.034 Nondisplaced fracture of lateral end of right clavicle**

   ✓7ᵗʰ **S42.035 Nondisplaced fracture of lateral end of left clavicle**

   ✓7ᵗʰ **S42.036 Nondisplaced fracture of lateral end of unspecified clavicle** ▽

✓5ᵗʰ **S42.1 Fracture of scapula**

✓6ᵗʰ **S42.10 Fracture of unspecified part of scapula**

   ✓7ᵗʰ **S42.101 Fracture of unspecified part of scapula, right shoulder** ▽

   ✓7ᵗʰ **S42.102 Fracture of unspecified part of scapula, left shoulder** ▽

   ✓7ᵗʰ **S42.109 Fracture of unspecified part of scapula, unspecified shoulder** ▽

✓6ᵗʰ **S42.11 Fracture of body of scapula**

   ✓7ᵗʰ **S42.111 Displaced fracture of body of scapula, right shoulder**

   ✓7ᵗʰ **S42.112 Displaced fracture of body of scapula, left shoulder**

   ✓7ᵗʰ **S42.113 Displaced fracture of body of scapula, unspecified shoulder** ▽

   ✓7ᵗʰ **S42.114 Nondisplaced fracture of body of scapula, right shoulder**

   ✓7ᵗʰ **S42.115 Nondisplaced fracture of body of scapula, left shoulder**

   ✓7ᵗʰ **S42.116 Nondisplaced fracture of body of scapula, unspecified shoulder** ▽

✓6ᵗʰ **S42.12 Fracture of acromial process**

   ✓7ᵗʰ **S42.121 Displaced fracture of acromial process, right shoulder**

   ✓7ᵗʰ **S42.122 Displaced fracture of acromial process, left shoulder**

   ✓7ᵗʰ **S42.123 Displaced fracture of acromial process, unspecified shoulder** ▽

   ✓7ᵗʰ **S42.124 Nondisplaced fracture of acromial process, right shoulder**

   ✓7ᵗʰ **S42.125 Nondisplaced fracture of acromial process, left shoulder**

   ✓7ᵗʰ **S42.126 Nondisplaced fracture of acromial process, unspecified shoulder** ▽

✓6ᵗʰ **S42.13 Fracture of coracoid process**

   ✓7ᵗʰ **S42.131 Displaced fracture of coracoid process, right shoulder**

   ✓7ᵗʰ **S42.132 Displaced fracture of coracoid process, left shoulder**

   ✓7ᵗʰ **S42.133 Displaced fracture of coracoid process, unspecified shoulder** ▽

   ✓7ᵗʰ **S42.134 Nondisplaced fracture of coracoid process, right shoulder**

   ✓7ᵗʰ **S42.135 Nondisplaced fracture of coracoid process, left shoulder**

   ✓7ᵗʰ **S42.136 Nondisplaced fracture of coracoid process, unspecified shoulder** ▽

✓6ᵗʰ **S42.14 Fracture of glenoid cavity of scapula**

   ✓7ᵗʰ **S42.141 Displaced fracture of glenoid cavity of scapula, right shoulder**

   ✓7ᵗʰ **S42.142 Displaced fracture of glenoid cavity of scapula, left shoulder**

   ✓7ᵗʰ **S42.143 Displaced fracture of glenoid cavity of scapula, unspecified shoulder** ▽

   ✓7ᵗʰ **S42.144 Nondisplaced fracture of glenoid cavity of scapula, right shoulder**

   ✓7ᵗʰ **S42.145 Nondisplaced fracture of glenoid cavity of scapula, left shoulder**

   ✓7ᵗʰ **S42.146 Nondisplaced fracture of glenoid cavity of scapula, unspecified shoulder** ▽

✓6ᵗʰ **S42.15 Fracture of neck of scapula**

   ✓7ᵗʰ **S42.151 Displaced fracture of neck of scapula, right shoulder**

   ✓7ᵗʰ **S42.152 Displaced fracture of neck of scapula, left shoulder**

   ✓7ᵗʰ **S42.153 Displaced fracture of neck of scapula, unspecified shoulder** ▽

   ✓7ᵗʰ **S42.154 Nondisplaced fracture of neck of scapula, right shoulder**

   ✓7ᵗʰ **S42.155 Nondisplaced fracture of neck of scapula, left shoulder**

   ✓7ᵗʰ **S42.156 Nondisplaced fracture of neck of scapula, unspecified shoulder** ▽

✓6ᵗʰ **S42.19 Fracture of other part of scapula**

   ✓7ᵗʰ **S42.191 Fracture of other part of scapula, right shoulder**

   ✓7ᵗʰ **S42.192 Fracture of other part of scapula, left shoulder**

☑ Additional Character Req   ✓ₓ7ᵗʰ Placeholder Alert   **Manifestation**   **HCC** CMS-HCC Condition   ▽ Unspecified Code   ►◄ Revised Text   ● New Code   ▲ Revised Code Title

✓7ᵗʰ **S42.199** **Fracture of other part of scapula, unspecified shoulder** ▽

✓5ᵗʰ **S42.2** **Fracture of** upper end of humerus
Fracture of proximal end of humerus
EXCLUDES 2   *fracture of shaft of humerus (S42.3-)*
physeal fracture of upper end of humerus (S49.0-)

✓6ᵗʰ **S42.20** **Unspecified fracture of upper end of humerus**

✓7ᵗʰ **S42.201** **Unspecified fracture of upper end of** right **humerus** ▽

✓7ᵗʰ **S42.202** **Unspecified fracture of upper end of** left **humerus** ▽

✓7ᵗʰ **S42.209** **Unspecified fracture of upper end of** unspecified **humerus** ▽

✓6ᵗʰ **S42.21** **Unspecified fracture of** surgical neck **of humerus**
Fracture of neck of humerus NOS

✓7ᵗʰ **S42.211** **Unspecified** displaced **fracture of surgical neck of** right **humerus** ▽

✓7ᵗʰ **S42.212** **Unspecified** displaced **fracture of surgical neck of** left **humerus** ▽

✓7ᵗʰ **S42.213** **Unspecified** displaced **fracture of surgical neck of unspecified humerus** ▽

✓7ᵗʰ **S42.214** **Unspecified** nondisplaced **fracture of surgical neck of** right **humerus** ▽

✓7ᵗʰ **S42.215** **Unspecified** nondisplaced **fracture of surgical neck of** left **humerus** ▽

✓7ᵗʰ **S42.216** **Unspecified** nondisplaced **fracture of surgical neck of unspecified humerus** ▽

✓6ᵗʰ **S42.22** **2-part fracture of** surgical neck **of humerus**

✓7ᵗʰ **S42.221** **2-part** displaced **fracture of surgical neck of** right **humerus**

✓7ᵗʰ **S42.222** **2-part** displaced **fracture of surgical neck of** left **humerus**

✓7ᵗʰ **S42.223** **2-part** displaced **fracture of surgical neck of unspecified humerus** ▽

✓7ᵗʰ **S42.224** **2-part** nondisplaced **fracture of surgical neck of** right **humerus**

✓7ᵗʰ **S42.225** **2-part** nondisplaced **fracture of surgical neck of** left **humerus**

✓7ᵗʰ **S42.226** **2-part** nondisplaced **fracture of surgical neck of unspecified humerus** ▽

✓6ᵗʰ **S42.23** **3-part fracture of** surgical neck **of humerus**

✓7ᵗʰ **S42.231** **3-part fracture of surgical neck of** right **humerus**

✓7ᵗʰ **S42.232** **3-part fracture of surgical neck of** left **humerus**

✓7ᵗʰ **S42.239** **3-part fracture of surgical neck of unspecified humerus** ▽

✓6ᵗʰ **S42.24** **4-part fracture of** surgical neck **of humerus**

✓7ᵗʰ **S42.241** **4-part fracture of surgical neck of** right **humerus**

✓7ᵗʰ **S42.242** **4-part fracture of surgical neck of** left **humerus**

✓7ᵗʰ **S42.249** **4-part fracture of surgical neck of unspecified humerus** ▽

✓6ᵗʰ **S42.25** **Fracture of** greater tuberosity **of humerus**

✓7ᵗʰ **S42.251** Displaced **fracture of greater tuberosity of** right **humerus**

✓7ᵗʰ **S42.252** Displaced **fracture of greater tuberosity of** left **humerus**

✓7ᵗʰ **S42.253** Displaced **fracture of greater tuberosity of unspecified humerus** ▽

✓7ᵗʰ **S42.254** Nondisplaced **fracture of greater tuberosity of** right **humerus**

✓7ᵗʰ **S42.255** Nondisplaced **fracture of greater tuberosity of** left **humerus**

✓7ᵗʰ **S42.256** Nondisplaced **fracture of greater tuberosity of unspecified humerus** ▽

✓6ᵗʰ **S42.26** **Fracture of** lesser tuberosity **of humerus**

✓7ᵗʰ **S42.261** Displaced **fracture of lesser tuberosity of** right **humerus**

✓7ᵗʰ **S42.262** Displaced **fracture of lesser tuberosity of** left **humerus**

✓7ᵗʰ **S42.263** Displaced **fracture of lesser tuberosity of unspecified humerus** ▽

✓7ᵗʰ **S42.264** Nondisplaced **fracture of lesser tuberosity of** right **humerus**

✓7ᵗʰ **S42.265** Nondisplaced **fracture of lesser tuberosity of** left **humerus**

✓7ᵗʰ **S42.266** Nondisplaced **fracture of lesser tuberosity of unspecified humerus** ▽

✓6ᵗʰ **S42.27** Torus **fracture of upper end of humerus**

> The appropriate 7th character is to be added to all codes in subcategory S42.27.
> A   initial encounter for closed fracture
> D   subsequent encounter for fracture with routine healing
> G   subsequent encounter for fracture with delayed healing
> K   subsequent encounter for fracture with nonunion
> P   subsequent encounter for fracture with malunion
> S   sequela

✓7ᵗʰ **S42.271** **Torus fracture of upper end of** right **humerus**

✓7ᵗʰ **S42.272** **Torus fracture of upper end of** left **humerus**

✓7ᵗʰ **S42.279** **Torus fracture of upper end of unspecified humerus** ▽

✓6ᵗʰ **S42.29** **Other fracture of upper end of humerus**
Fracture of anatomical neck of humerus
Fracture of articular head of humerus

✓7ᵗʰ **S42.291** **Other** displaced **fracture of upper end of** right **humerus**

✓7ᵗʰ **S42.292** **Other** displaced **fracture of upper end of** left **humerus**

✓7ᵗʰ **S42.293** **Other** displaced **fracture of upper end of unspecified humerus** ▽

✓7ᵗʰ **S42.294** **Other** nondisplaced **fracture of upper end of** right **humerus**

✓7ᵗʰ **S42.295** **Other** nondisplaced **fracture of upper end of** left **humerus**

✓7ᵗʰ **S42.296** **Other** nondisplaced **fracture of upper end of unspecified humerus** ▽

✓5ᵗʰ **S42.3** **Fracture of** shaft of humerus
Fracture of humerus NOS
Fracture of upper arm NOS
EXCLUDES 2   *physeal fractures of upper end of humerus (S49.0-)*
physeal fractures of lower end of humerus (S49.1-)

✓6ᵗʰ **S42.30** **Unspecified fracture of shaft of humerus**

✓7ᵗʰ **S42.301** **Unspecified fracture of shaft of humerus,** right **arm** ▽

✓7ᵗʰ **S42.302** **Unspecified fracture of shaft of humerus,** left **arm** ▽

✓7ᵗʰ **S42.309** **Unspecified fracture of shaft of humerus, unspecified arm** ▽

✓6ᵗʰ **S42.31** Greenstick **fracture of shaft of humerus**

> The appropriate 7th character is to be added to all codes in subcategory S42.31.
> A   initial encounter for closed fracture
> D   subsequent encounter for fracture with routine healing
> G   subsequent encounter for fracture with delayed healing
> K   subsequent encounter for fracture with nonunion
> P   subsequent encounter for fracture with malunion
> S   sequela

✓7ᵗʰ **S42.311** **Greenstick fracture of shaft of humerus,** right **arm**

✓7ᵗʰ **S42.312** **Greenstick fracture of shaft of humerus,** left **arm**

✓7ᵗʰ **S42.319** **Greenstick fracture of shaft of humerus, unspecified arm** ▽

✓6ᵗʰ **S42.32** Transverse **fracture of shaft of humerus**

✓7ᵗʰ **S42.321** Displaced **transverse fracture of shaft of humerus,** right **arm**

✓7ᵗʰ **S42.322** Displaced **transverse fracture of shaft of humerus,** left **arm**

EXCLUDES 1 Not coded here   *EXCLUDES 2* Not included here   N Newborn Age: 0   P Pediatric Age: 0-17   M Maternity Age: 12-55   A Adult Age: 15-124

√7ᵗʰ **S42.323** Displaced **transverse fracture of shaft of humerus, unspecified arm** ▽

√7ᵗʰ **S42.324** Nondisplaced **transverse fracture of shaft of humerus, right arm**

√7ᵗʰ **S42.325** Nondisplaced **transverse fracture of shaft of humerus, left arm**

√7ᵗʰ **S42.326** Nondisplaced **transverse fracture of shaft of humerus, unspecified arm** ▽

√6ᵗʰ **S42.33** Oblique **fracture of shaft of humerus**

√7ᵗʰ **S42.331** Displaced **oblique fracture of shaft of humerus, right arm**

√7ᵗʰ **S42.332** Displaced **oblique fracture of shaft of humerus, left arm**

√7ᵗʰ **S42.333** Displaced **oblique fracture of shaft of humerus, unspecified arm** ▽

√7ᵗʰ **S42.334** Nondisplaced **oblique fracture of shaft of humerus, right arm**

√7ᵗʰ **S42.335** Nondisplaced **oblique fracture of shaft of humerus, left arm**

√7ᵗʰ **S42.336** Nondisplaced **oblique fracture of shaft of humerus, unspecified arm** ▽

√6ᵗʰ **S42.34** Spiral **fracture of shaft of humerus**

√7ᵗʰ **S42.341** Displaced **spiral fracture of shaft of humerus, right arm**

√7ᵗʰ **S42.342** Displaced **spiral fracture of shaft of humerus, left arm**

√7ᵗʰ **S42.343** Displaced **spiral fracture of shaft of humerus, unspecified arm** ▽

√7ᵗʰ **S42.344** Nondisplaced **spiral fracture of shaft of humerus, right arm**

√7ᵗʰ **S42.345** Nondisplaced **spiral fracture of shaft of humerus, left arm**

√7ᵗʰ **S42.346** Nondisplaced **spiral fracture of shaft of humerus, unspecified arm** ▽

√6ᵗʰ **S42.35** Comminuted **fracture of shaft of humerus**

√7ᵗʰ **S42.351** Displaced **comminuted fracture of shaft of humerus, right arm**

√7ᵗʰ **S42.352** Displaced **comminuted fracture of shaft of humerus, left arm**

√7ᵗʰ **S42.353** Displaced **comminuted fracture of shaft of humerus, unspecified arm** ▽

√7ᵗʰ **S42.354** Nondisplaced **comminuted fracture of shaft of humerus, right arm**

√7ᵗʰ **S42.355** Nondisplaced **comminuted fracture of shaft of humerus, left arm**

√7ᵗʰ **S42.356** Nondisplaced **comminuted fracture of shaft of humerus, unspecified arm** ▽

√6ᵗʰ **S42.36** Segmental **fracture of shaft of humerus**

√7ᵗʰ **S42.361** Displaced **segmental fracture of shaft of humerus, right arm**

√7ᵗʰ **S42.362** Displaced **segmental fracture of shaft of humerus, left arm**

√7ᵗʰ **S42.363** Displaced **segmental fracture of shaft of humerus, unspecified arm** ▽

√7ᵗʰ **S42.364** Nondisplaced **segmental fracture of shaft of humerus, right arm**

√7ᵗʰ **S42.365** Nondisplaced **segmental fracture of shaft of humerus, left arm**

√7ᵗʰ **S42.366** Nondisplaced **segmental fracture of shaft of humerus, unspecified arm** ▽

√6ᵗʰ **S42.39** Other **fracture of shaft of humerus**

√7ᵗʰ **S42.391** Other fracture of shaft of right humerus

√7ᵗʰ **S42.392** Other fracture of shaft of left humerus

√7ᵗʰ **S42.399** Other fracture of shaft of unspecified humerus ▽

√5ᵗʰ **S42.4** **Fracture of lower end of humerus**
Fracture of distal end of humerus

EXCLUDES 2 fracture of shaft of humerus (S42.3-)
physeal fracture of lower end of humerus (S49.1-)

√6ᵗʰ **S42.40** **Unspecified fracture of lower end of humerus**
Fracture of elbow NOS

√7ᵗʰ **S42.401** Unspecified fracture of lower end of right humerus ▽

√7ᵗʰ **S42.402** Unspecified fracture of lower end of left humerus ▽

√7ᵗʰ **S42.409** Unspecified fracture of lower end of unspecified humerus ▽

√6ᵗʰ **S42.41** Simple supracondylar **fracture without** intercondylar **fracture of humerus**

√7ᵗʰ **S42.411** Displaced **simple supracondylar fracture without intercondylar fracture of** right **humerus**

√7ᵗʰ **S42.412** Displaced **simple supracondylar fracture without intercondylar fracture of** left **humerus**

√7ᵗʰ **S42.413** Displaced **simple supracondylar fracture without intercondylar fracture of unspecified humerus** ▽

√7ᵗʰ **S42.414** Nondisplaced **simple supracondylar fracture without intercondylar fracture of** right **humerus**

√7ᵗʰ **S42.415** Nondisplaced **simple supracondylar fracture without intercondylar fracture of** left **humerus**

√7ᵗʰ **S42.416** Nondisplaced **simple supracondylar fracture without intercondylar fracture of unspecified humerus** ▽

√6ᵗʰ **S42.42** Comminuted supracondylar **fracture without** intercondylar **fracture of humerus**

√7ᵗʰ **S42.421** Displaced **comminuted supracondylar fracture without intercondylar fracture of** right **humerus**

√7ᵗʰ **S42.422** Displaced **comminuted supracondylar fracture without intercondylar fracture of** left **humerus**

√7ᵗʰ **S42.423** Displaced **comminuted supracondylar fracture without intercondylar fracture of unspecified humerus** ▽

√7ᵗʰ **S42.424** Nondisplaced **comminuted supracondylar fracture without intercondylar fracture of** right **humerus**

√7ᵗʰ **S42.425** Nondisplaced **comminuted supracondylar fracture without intercondylar fracture of** left **humerus**

√7ᵗʰ **S42.426** Nondisplaced **comminuted supracondylar fracture without intercondylar fracture of unspecified humerus** ▽

√6ᵗʰ **S42.43** Fracture (avulsion) of lateral epicondyle of humerus

√7ᵗʰ **S42.431** Displaced **fracture (avulsion) of lateral epicondyle of** right **humerus**

√7ᵗʰ **S42.432** Displaced **fracture (avulsion) of lateral epicondyle of** left **humerus**

√7ᵗʰ **S42.433** Displaced **fracture (avulsion) of lateral epicondyle of unspecified humerus** ▽

√7ᵗʰ **S42.434** Nondisplaced **fracture (avulsion) of lateral epicondyle of** right **humerus**

√7ᵗʰ **S42.435** Nondisplaced **fracture (avulsion) of lateral epicondyle of** left **humerus**

√7ᵗʰ **S42.436** Nondisplaced **fracture (avulsion) of lateral epicondyle of unspecified humerus** ▽

√6ᵗʰ **S42.44** Fracture (avulsion) of medial epicondyle of humerus

S42.441 Displaced **fracture (avulsion) of medial epicondyle of** right **humerus**

√7ᵗʰ **S42.442** Displaced **fracture (avulsion) of medial epicondyle of** left **humerus**

√7ᵗʰ **S42.443** Displaced **fracture (avulsion) of medial epicondyle of unspecified humerus** ▽

√7ᵗʰ **S42.444** Nondisplaced **fracture (avulsion) of medial epicondyle of** right **humerus**

√7ᵗʰ **S42.445** Nondisplaced **fracture (avulsion) of medial epicondyle of** left **humerus**

√7ᵗʰ **S42.446** Nondisplaced **fracture (avulsion) of medial epicondyle of unspecified humerus** ▽

√7ᵗʰ **S42.447** Incarcerated **fracture (avulsion) of medial epicondyle of** right **humerus**

√7ᵗʰ **S42.448** Incarcerated **fracture (avulsion) of medial epicondyle of** left **humerus**

√7ᵗʰ **S42.449** Incarcerated **fracture (avulsion) of medial epicondyle of unspecified humerus** ▽

☑ Additional Character Req   √ˣ7ᵗʰ Placeholder Alert   Manifestation   ᴴᶜᶜ CMS-HCC Condition   ▽ Unspecified Code   ▶◀ Revised Text   ● New Code   ▲ Revised Code Title

✓6ᵗʰ **S42.45** Fracture of lateral condyle of humerus
Fracture of capitellum of humerus

✓7ᵗʰ **S42.451** Displaced fracture of lateral condyle of right humerus

✓7ᵗʰ **S42.452** Displaced fracture of lateral condyle of left humerus

✓7ᵗʰ **S42.453** Displaced fracture of lateral condyle of unspecified humerus ▽

✓7ᵗʰ **S42.454** Nondisplaced fracture of lateral condyle of right humerus

✓7ᵗʰ **S42.455** Nondisplaced fracture of lateral condyle of left humerus

✓7ᵗʰ **S42.456** Nondisplaced fracture of lateral condyle of unspecified humerus ▽

✓6ᵗʰ **S42.46** Fracture of medial condyle of humerus
Trochlea fracture of humerus

✓7ᵗʰ **S42.461** Displaced fracture of medial condyle of right humerus

✓7ᵗʰ **S42.462** Displaced fracture of medial condyle of left humerus

✓7ᵗʰ **S42.463** Displaced fracture of medial condyle of unspecified humerus ▽

✓7ᵗʰ **S42.464** Nondisplaced fracture of medial condyle of right humerus

✓7ᵗʰ **S42.465** Nondisplaced fracture of medial condyle of left humerus

✓7ᵗʰ **S42.466** Nondisplaced fracture of medial condyle of unspecified humerus ▽

✓6ᵗʰ **S42.47** Transcondylar fracture of humerus

✓7ᵗʰ **S42.471** Displaced transcondylar fracture of right humerus

✓7ᵗʰ **S42.472** Displaced transcondylar fracture of left humerus

✓7ᵗʰ **S42.473** Displaced transcondylar fracture of unspecified humerus ▽

✓7ᵗʰ **S42.474** Nondisplaced transcondylar fracture of right humerus

✓7ᵗʰ **S42.475** Nondisplaced transcondylar fracture of left humerus

✓7ᵗʰ **S42.476** Nondisplaced transcondylar fracture of unspecified humerus ▽

✓6ᵗʰ **S42.48** Torus fracture of lower end of humerus

> The appropriate 7th character is to be added to all codes in subcategory S42.48.
> A initial encounter for closed fracture
> D subsequent encounter for fracture with routine healing
> G subsequent encounter for fracture with delayed healing
> K subsequent encounter for fracture with nonunion
> P subsequent encounter for fracture with malunion
> S sequela

✓7ᵗʰ **S42.481** Torus fracture of lower end of right humerus

✓7ᵗʰ **S42.482** Torus fracture of lower end of left humerus

✓7ᵗʰ **S42.489** Torus fracture of lower end of unspecified humerus ▽

✓6ᵗʰ **S42.49** Other fracture of lower end of humerus

✓7ᵗʰ **S42.491** Other displaced fracture of lower end of right humerus

✓7ᵗʰ **S42.492** Other displaced fracture of lower end of left humerus

✓7ᵗʰ **S42.493** Other displaced fracture of lower end of unspecified humerus ▽

✓7ᵗʰ **S42.494** Other nondisplaced fracture of lower end of right humerus

✓7ᵗʰ **S42.495** Other nondisplaced fracture of lower end of left humerus

✓7ᵗʰ **S42.496** Other nondisplaced fracture of lower end of unspecified humerus ▽

✓5ᵗʰ **S42.9** Fracture of shoulder girdle, part unspecified
Fracture of shoulder NOS

✓x7ᵗʰ **S42.90** Fracture of unspecified shoulder girdle, part unspecified ▽

✓x7ᵗʰ **S42.91** Fracture of right shoulder girdle, part unspecified ▽

✓x7ᵗʰ **S42.92** Fracture of left shoulder girdle, part unspecified ▽

✓4ᵗʰ **S43** Dislocation and sprain of joints and ligaments of shoulder girdle

INCLUDES avulsion of joint or ligament of shoulder girdle
laceration of cartilage, joint or ligament of shoulder girdle
sprain of cartilage, joint or ligament of shoulder girdle
traumatic hemarthrosis of joint or ligament of shoulder girdle
traumatic rupture of joint or ligament of shoulder girdle
traumatic subluxation of joint or ligament of shoulder girdle
traumatic tear of joint or ligament of shoulder girdle

Code also any associated open wound

EXCLUDES 2 strain of muscle, fascia and tendon of shoulder and upper arm (S46.-)

> The appropriate 7th character is to be added to each code from category S43.
> A initial encounter
> D subsequent encounter
> S sequela

✓5ᵗʰ **S43.0** Subluxation and dislocation of shoulder joint
Dislocation of glenohumeral joint
Subluxation of glenohumeral joint

✓6ᵗʰ **S43.00** Unspecified subluxation and dislocation of shoulder joint
Dislocation of humerus NOS
Subluxation of humerus NOS

✓7ᵗʰ **S43.001** Unspecified subluxation of right shoulder joint ▽

✓7ᵗʰ **S43.002** Unspecified subluxation of left shoulder joint ▽

✓7ᵗʰ **S43.003** Unspecified subluxation of unspecified shoulder joint ▽

✓7ᵗʰ **S43.004** Unspecified dislocation of right shoulder joint ▽

✓7ᵗʰ **S43.005** Unspecified dislocation of left shoulder joint ▽

✓7ᵗʰ **S43.006** Unspecified dislocation of unspecified shoulder joint ▽

✓6ᵗʰ **S43.01** Anterior subluxation and dislocation of humerus

✓7ᵗʰ **S43.011** Anterior subluxation of right humerus

✓7ᵗʰ **S43.012** Anterior subluxation of left humerus

✓7ᵗʰ **S43.013** Anterior subluxation of unspecified humerus ▽

✓7ᵗʰ **S43.014** Anterior dislocation of right humerus

✓7ᵗʰ **S43.015** Anterior dislocation of left humerus

✓7ᵗʰ **S43.016** Anterior dislocation of unspecified humerus ▽

✓6ᵗʰ **S43.02** Posterior subluxation and dislocation of humerus

✓7ᵗʰ **S43.021** Posterior subluxation of right humerus

✓7ᵗʰ **S43.022** Posterior subluxation of left humerus

✓7ᵗʰ **S43.023** Posterior subluxation of unspecified humerus ▽

✓7ᵗʰ **S43.024** Posterior dislocation of right humerus

✓7ᵗʰ **S43.025** Posterior dislocation of left humerus

✓7ᵗʰ **S43.026** Posterior dislocation of unspecified humerus ▽

✓6ᵗʰ **S43.03** Inferior subluxation and dislocation of humerus

✓7ᵗʰ **S43.031** Inferior subluxation of right humerus

✓7ᵗʰ **S43.032** Inferior subluxation of left humerus

✓7ᵗʰ **S43.033** Inferior subluxation of unspecified humerus ▽

✓7ᵗʰ **S43.034** Inferior dislocation of right humerus

✓7ᵗʰ **S43.035** Inferior dislocation of left humerus

✓7ᵗʰ **S43.036** Inferior dislocation of unspecified humerus ▽

✓6ᵗʰ **S43.08** Other subluxation and dislocation of shoulder joint

✓7ᵗʰ **S43.081** Other subluxation of right shoulder joint

✓7ᵗʰ **S43.082** Other subluxation of left shoulder joint

✓7ᵗʰ **S43.083** Other subluxation of unspecified shoulder joint ▽

√7ᵗʰ **S43.084** Other dislocation of right shoulder joint

√7ᵗʰ **S43.085** Other dislocation of left shoulder joint

√7ᵗʰ **S43.086** Other dislocation of unspecified shoulder joint ▽

√5ᵗʰ **S43.1** Subluxation and dislocation of acromioclavicular joint

√6ᵗʰ **S43.10** Unspecified dislocation of acromioclavicular joint

√7ᵗʰ **S43.101** Unspecified dislocation of right acromioclavicular joint ▽

√7ᵗʰ **S43.102** Unspecified dislocation of left acromioclavicular joint ▽

√7ᵗʰ **S43.109** Unspecified dislocation of unspecified acromioclavicular joint ▽

√6ᵗʰ **S43.11** Subluxation of acromioclavicular joint

√7ᵗʰ **S43.111** Subluxation of right acromioclavicular joint

√7ᵗʰ **S43.112** Subluxation of left acromioclavicular joint

√7ᵗʰ **S43.119** Subluxation of unspecified acromioclavicular joint ▽

√6ᵗʰ **S43.12** Dislocation of acromioclavicular joint, 100%-200% displacement

√7ᵗʰ **S43.121** Dislocation of right acromioclavicular joint, 100%-200% displacement

√7ᵗʰ **S43.122** Dislocation of left acromioclavicular joint, 100%-200% displacement

√7ᵗʰ **S43.129** Dislocation of unspecified acromioclavicular joint, 100%-200% displacement ▽

√6ᵗʰ **S43.13** Dislocation of acromioclavicular joint, greater than 200% displacement

√7ᵗʰ **S43.131** Dislocation of right acromioclavicular joint, greater than 200% displacement

√7ᵗʰ **S43.132** Dislocation of left acromioclavicular joint, greater than 200% displacement

√7ᵗʰ **S43.139** Dislocation of unspecified acromioclavicular joint, greater than 200% displacement ▽

√6ᵗʰ **S43.14** Inferior dislocation of acromioclavicular joint

√7ᵗʰ **S43.141** Inferior dislocation of right acromioclavicular joint

√7ᵗʰ **S43.142** Inferior dislocation of left acromioclavicular joint

√7ᵗʰ **S43.149** Inferior dislocation of unspecified acromioclavicular joint ▽

√6ᵗʰ **S43.15** Posterior dislocation of acromioclavicular joint

√7ᵗʰ **S43.151** Posterior dislocation of right acromioclavicular joint

√7ᵗʰ **S43.152** Posterior dislocation of left acromioclavicular joint

√7ᵗʰ **S43.159** Posterior dislocation of unspecified acromioclavicular joint ▽

√5ᵗʰ **S43.2** Subluxation and dislocation of sternoclavicular joint

√6ᵗʰ **S43.20** Unspecified subluxation and dislocation of sternoclavicular joint

√7ᵗʰ **S43.201** Unspecified subluxation of right sternoclavicular joint ▽

√7ᵗʰ **S43.202** Unspecified subluxation of left sternoclavicular joint ▽

√7ᵗʰ **S43.203** Unspecified subluxation of unspecified sternoclavicular joint ▽

√7ᵗʰ **S43.204** Unspecified dislocation of right sternoclavicular joint ▽

√7ᵗʰ **S43.205** Unspecified dislocation of left sternoclavicular joint ▽

√7ᵗʰ **S43.206** Unspecified dislocation of unspecified sternoclavicular joint ▽

√6ᵗʰ **S43.21** Anterior subluxation and dislocation of sternoclavicular joint

√7ᵗʰ **S43.211** Anterior subluxation of right sternoclavicular joint

√7ᵗʰ **S43.212** Anterior subluxation of left sternoclavicular joint

√7ᵗʰ **S43.213** Anterior subluxation of unspecified sternoclavicular joint ▽

√7ᵗʰ **S43.214** Anterior dislocation of right sternoclavicular joint

√7ᵗʰ **S43.215** Anterior dislocation of left sternoclavicular joint

√7ᵗʰ **S43.216** Anterior dislocation of unspecified sternoclavicular joint ▽

√6ᵗʰ **S43.22** Posterior subluxation and dislocation of sternoclavicular joint

√7ᵗʰ **S43.221** Posterior subluxation of right sternoclavicular joint

√7ᵗʰ **S43.222** Posterior subluxation of left sternoclavicular joint

√7ᵗʰ **S43.223** Posterior subluxation of unspecified sternoclavicular joint ▽

√7ᵗʰ **S43.224** Posterior dislocation of right sternoclavicular joint

√7ᵗʰ **S43.225** Posterior dislocation of left sternoclavicular joint

√7ᵗʰ **S43.226** Posterior dislocation of unspecified sternoclavicular joint ▽

√5ᵗʰ **S43.3** Subluxation and dislocation of other and unspecified parts of shoulder girdle

√6ᵗʰ **S43.30** Subluxation and dislocation of unspecified parts of shoulder girdle
Dislocation of shoulder girdle NOS
Subluxation of shoulder girdle NOS

√7ᵗʰ **S43.301** Subluxation of unspecified parts of right shoulder girdle ▽

√7ᵗʰ **S43.302** Subluxation of unspecified parts of left shoulder girdle ▽

√7ᵗʰ **S43.303** Subluxation of unspecified parts of unspecified shoulder girdle ▽

√7ᵗʰ **S43.304** Dislocation of unspecified parts of right shoulder girdle ▽

√7ᵗʰ **S43.305** Dislocation of unspecified parts of left shoulder girdle ▽

√7ᵗʰ **S43.306** Dislocation of unspecified parts of unspecified shoulder girdle ▽

√6ᵗʰ **S43.31** Subluxation and dislocation of scapula

√7ᵗʰ **S43.311** Subluxation of right scapula

√7ᵗʰ **S43.312** Subluxation of left scapula

√7ᵗʰ **S43.313** Subluxation of unspecified scapula ▽

√7ᵗʰ **S43.314** Dislocation of right scapula

√7ᵗʰ **S43.315** Dislocation of left scapula

√7ᵗʰ **S43.316** Dislocation of unspecified scapula ▽

√6ᵗʰ **S43.39** Subluxation and dislocation of other parts of shoulder girdle

√7ᵗʰ **S43.391** Subluxation of other parts of right shoulder girdle

√7ᵗʰ **S43.392** Subluxation of other parts of left shoulder girdle

√7ᵗʰ **S43.393** Subluxation of other parts of unspecified shoulder girdle ▽

√7ᵗʰ **S43.394** Dislocation of other parts of right shoulder girdle

√7ᵗʰ **S43.395** Dislocation of other parts of left shoulder girdle

√7ᵗʰ **S43.396** Dislocation of other parts of unspecified shoulder girdle ▽

√5ᵗʰ **S43.4** Sprain of shoulder joint

√6ᵗʰ **S43.40** Unspecified sprain of shoulder joint

√7ᵗʰ **S43.401** Unspecified sprain of right shoulder joint ▽

√7ᵗʰ **S43.402** Unspecified sprain of left shoulder joint ▽

√7ᵗʰ **S43.409** Unspecified sprain of unspecified shoulder joint ▽

√6ᵗʰ **S43.41** Sprain of coracohumeral (ligament)

√7ᵗʰ **S43.411** Sprain of right coracohumeral (ligament)

√7ᵗʰ **S43.412** Sprain of left coracohumeral (ligament)

√7ᵗʰ **S43.419** Sprain of unspecified coracohumeral (ligament) ▽

☑ Additional Character Req ☑√7ᵗʰ Placeholder Alert Manifestation ᴴᶜᶜ CMS-HCC Condition ▽ Unspecified Code ►◄ Revised Text ● New Code ▲ Revised Code Title

ICD-10-CM 2018 959

√6th **S43.42** **Sprain of** rotator cuff capsule
> EXCLUDES 1   *rotator cuff syndrome (complete) (incomplete), not specified as traumatic (M75.1-)*
> EXCLUDES 2   *injury of tendon of rotator cuff (S46.Ø-)*

    √7th **S43.421** **Sprain of** right **rotator cuff capsule**
    √7th **S43.422** **Sprain of** left **rotator cuff capsule**
    √7th **S43.429** **Sprain of unspecified rotator cuff capsule** ▽

√6th **S43.43** **Superior glenoid labrum lesion**
> SLAP lesion
> **DEF:** Detachment injury of the superior aspect of the glenoid labrum, which is the ring of fibrocartilage attached to the rim of the glenoid cavity of the scapula.

    √7th **S43.431** **Superior glenoid labrum lesion of** right **shoulder**
    √7th **S43.432** **Superior glenoid labrum lesion of** left **shoulder**
    √7th **S43.439** **Superior glenoid labrum lesion of unspecified shoulder** ▽

√6th **S43.49** **Other sprain of shoulder joint**
    √7th **S43.491** **Other sprain of** right **shoulder joint**
    √7th **S43.492** **Other sprain of** left **shoulder joint**
    √7th **S43.499** **Other sprain of unspecified shoulder joint** ▽

√5th **S43.5** **Sprain of** acromioclavicular **joint**
> Sprain of acromioclavicular ligament

    √x7th **S43.50** **Sprain of unspecified acromioclavicular joint** ▽
    √x7th **S43.51** **Sprain of** right **acromioclavicular joint**
    √x7th **S43.52** **Sprain of** left **acromioclavicular joint**

√5th **S43.6** **Sprain of** sternoclavicular **joint**
    √x7th **S43.60** **Sprain of unspecified sternoclavicular joint** ▽
    √x7th **S43.61** **Sprain of** right **sternoclavicular joint**
    √x7th **S43.62** **Sprain of** left **sternoclavicular joint**

√5th **S43.8** **Sprain of other specified parts of shoulder girdle**
    √x7th **S43.80** **Sprain of other specified parts of unspecified shoulder girdle** ▽
    √x7th **S43.81** **Sprain of other specified parts of** right **shoulder girdle**
    √x7th **S43.82** **Sprain of other specified parts of** left **shoulder girdle**

√5th **S43.9** **Sprain of unspecified parts of shoulder girdle**
    √x7th **S43.90** **Sprain of unspecified parts of unspecified shoulder girdle** ▽
> Sprain of shoulder girdle NOS

    √x7th **S43.91** **Sprain of unspecified parts of** right **shoulder girdle** ▽
    √x7th **S43.92** **Sprain of unspecified parts of** left **shoulder girdle** ▽

√4th **S44** **Injury of nerves at shoulder and upper arm level**
> Code also any associated open wound (S41.-)
> EXCLUDES 2   *injury of brachial plexus (S14.3-)*

> The appropriate 7th character is to be added to each code from category S44.
> A   initial encounter
> D   subsequent encounter
> S   sequela

√5th **S44.0** **Injury of** ulnar nerve **at upper arm level**
> EXCLUDES 1   *ulnar nerve NOS (S54.Ø)*

    √x7th **S44.00** **Injury of ulnar nerve at upper arm level, unspecified arm** ▽
    √x7th **S44.01** **Injury of ulnar nerve at upper arm level,** right **arm**
    √x7th **S44.02** **Injury of ulnar nerve at upper arm level,** left **arm**

√5th **S44.1** **Injury of** median nerve **at upper arm level**
> EXCLUDES 1   *median nerve NOS (S54.1)*

    √x7th **S44.10** **Injury of median nerve at upper arm level, unspecified arm** ▽
    √x7th **S44.11** **Injury of median nerve at upper arm level,** right **arm**
    √x7th **S44.12** **Injury of median nerve at upper arm level,** left **arm**

√5th **S44.2** **Injury of** radial nerve **at upper arm level**
> EXCLUDES 1   *radial nerve NOS (S54.2)*

    √x7th **S44.20** **Injury of radial nerve at upper arm level, unspecified arm** ▽
    √x7th **S44.21** **Injury of radial nerve at upper arm level,** right **arm**

√x7th **S44.22** **Injury of radial nerve at upper arm level,** left **arm**

√5th **S44.3** **Injury of** axillary nerve
    √x7th **S44.30** **Injury of axillary nerve, unspecified arm** ▽
    √x7th **S44.31** **Injury of axillary nerve,** right **arm**
    √x7th **S44.32** **Injury of axillary nerve,** left **arm**

√5th **S44.4** **Injury of** musculocutaneous nerve
    √x7th **S44.40** **Injury of musculocutaneous nerve, unspecified arm** ▽
    √x7th **S44.41** **Injury of musculocutaneous nerve,** right **arm**
    √x7th **S44.42** **Injury of musculocutaneous nerve,** left **arm**

√5th **S44.5** **Injury of** cutaneous sensory nerve **at shoulder and upper arm level**
    √x7th **S44.50** **Injury of cutaneous sensory nerve at shoulder and upper arm level, unspecified arm** ▽
    √x7th **S44.51** **Injury of cutaneous sensory nerve at shoulder and upper arm level,** right **arm**
    √x7th **S44.52** **Injury of cutaneous sensory nerve at shoulder and upper arm level,** left **arm**

√5th **S44.8** **Injury of other nerves at shoulder and upper arm level**
    √6th **S44.8X** **Injury of other nerves at shoulder and upper arm level**
       √7th **S44.8X1** **Injury of other nerves at shoulder and upper arm level,** right **arm**
       √7th **S44.8X2** **Injury of other nerves at shoulder and upper arm level,** left **arm**
       √7th **S44.8X9** **Injury of other nerves at shoulder and upper arm level, unspecified arm** ▽

√5th **S44.9** **Injury of unspecified nerve at shoulder and upper arm level**
    √x7th **S44.90** **Injury of unspecified nerve at shoulder and upper arm level, unspecified arm** ▽
    √x7th **S44.91** **Injury of unspecified nerve at shoulder and upper arm level,** right **arm** ▽
    √x7th **S44.92** **Injury of unspecified nerve at shoulder and upper arm level,** left **arm** ▽

√4th **S45** **Injury of blood vessels at shoulder and upper arm level**
> Code also any associated open wound (S41.-)
> EXCLUDES 2   *injury of subclavian artery (S25.1)*
>   *injury of subclavian vein (S25.3)*

> The appropriate 7th character is to be added to each code from category S45.
> A   initial encounter
> D   subsequent encounter
> S   sequela

√5th **S45.Ø** **Injury of** axillary artery
    √6th **S45.ØØ** **Unspecified injury of axillary artery**
       √7th **S45.ØØ1** **Unspecified injury of axillary artery,** right **side** ▽
       √7th **S45.ØØ2** **Unspecified injury of axillary artery,** left **side** ▽
       √7th **S45.ØØ9** **Unspecified injury of axillary artery, unspecified side** ▽
    √6th **S45.Ø1** **Laceration of axillary artery**
       √7th **S45.Ø11** **Laceration of axillary artery,** right **side**
       √7th **S45.Ø12** **Laceration of axillary artery,** left **side**
       √7th **S45.Ø19** **Laceration of axillary artery, unspecified side** ▽
    √6th **S45.Ø9** **Other specified injury of axillary artery**
       √7th **S45.Ø91** **Other specified injury of axillary artery,** right **side**
       √7th **S45.Ø92** **Other specified injury of axillary artery,** left **side**
       √7th **S45.Ø99** **Other specified injury of axillary artery, unspecified side** ▽

√5th **S45.1** **Injury of** brachial artery
    √6th **S45.10** **Unspecified injury of brachial artery**
       √7th **S45.1Ø1** **Unspecified injury of brachial artery,** right **side** ▽
       √7th **S45.1Ø2** **Unspecified injury of brachial artery,** left **side** ▽
       √7th **S45.1Ø9** **Unspecified injury of brachial artery, unspecified side** ▽

✓6ᵗʰ **S45.11** Laceration of brachial artery
- ✓7ᵗʰ **S45.111** Laceration of brachial artery, right side
- ✓7ᵗʰ **S45.112** Laceration of brachial artery, left side
- ✓7ᵗʰ **S45.119** Laceration of brachial artery, unspecified side ▽

✓6ᵗʰ **S45.19** Other specified injury of brachial artery
- ✓7ᵗʰ **S45.191** Other specified injury of brachial artery, right side
- ✓7ᵗʰ **S45.192** Other specified injury of brachial artery, left side
- ✓7ᵗʰ **S45.199** Other specified injury of brachial artery, unspecified side ▽

✓5ᵗʰ **S45.2** Injury of axillary or brachial vein

✓6ᵗʰ **S45.20** Unspecified injury of axillary or brachial vein
- ✓7ᵗʰ **S45.201** Unspecified injury of axillary or brachial vein, right side ▽
- ✓7ᵗʰ **S45.202** Unspecified injury of axillary or brachial vein, left side ▽
- ✓7ᵗʰ **S45.209** Unspecified injury of axillary or brachial vein, unspecified side ▽

✓6ᵗʰ **S45.21** Laceration of axillary or brachial vein
- ✓7ᵗʰ **S45.211** Laceration of axillary or brachial vein, right side
- ✓7ᵗʰ **S45.212** Laceration of axillary or brachial vein, left side
- ✓7ᵗʰ **S45.219** Laceration of axillary or brachial vein, unspecified side ▽

✓6ᵗʰ **S45.29** Other specified injury of axillary or brachial vein
- ✓7ᵗʰ **S45.291** Other specified injury of axillary or brachial vein, right side
- ✓7ᵗʰ **S45.292** Other specified injury of axillary or brachial vein, left side
- ✓7ᵗʰ **S45.299** Other specified injury of axillary or brachial vein, unspecified side ▽

✓5ᵗʰ **S45.3** Injury of superficial vein at shoulder and upper arm level

✓6ᵗʰ **S45.30** Unspecified injury of superficial vein at shoulder and upper arm level
- ✓7ᵗʰ **S45.301** Unspecified injury of superficial vein at shoulder and upper arm level, right arm ▽
- ✓7ᵗʰ **S45.302** Unspecified injury of superficial vein at shoulder and upper arm level, left arm ▽
- ✓7ᵗʰ **S45.309** Unspecified injury of superficial vein at shoulder and upper arm level, unspecified arm ▽

✓6ᵗʰ **S45.31** Laceration of superficial vein at shoulder and upper arm level
- ✓7ᵗʰ **S45.311** Laceration of superficial vein at shoulder and upper arm level, right arm
- ✓7ᵗʰ **S45.312** Laceration of superficial vein at shoulder and upper arm level, left arm
- ✓7ᵗʰ **S45.319** Laceration of superficial vein at shoulder and upper arm level, unspecified arm ▽

✓6ᵗʰ **S45.39** Other specified injury of superficial vein at shoulder and upper arm level
- ✓7ᵗʰ **S45.391** Other specified injury of superficial vein at shoulder and upper arm level, right arm
- ✓7ᵗʰ **S45.392** Other specified injury of superficial vein at shoulder and upper arm level, left arm
- ✓7ᵗʰ **S45.399** Other specified injury of superficial vein at shoulder and upper arm level, unspecified arm ▽

✓5ᵗʰ **S45.8** Injury of other specified blood vessels at shoulder and upper arm level

✓6ᵗʰ **S45.80** Unspecified injury of other specified blood vessels at shoulder and upper arm level
- ✓7ᵗʰ **S45.801** Unspecified injury of other specified blood vessels at shoulder and upper arm level, right arm ▽
- ✓7ᵗʰ **S45.802** Unspecified injury of other specified blood vessels at shoulder and upper arm level, left arm ▽
- ✓7ᵗʰ **S45.809** Unspecified injury of other specified blood vessels at shoulder and upper arm level, unspecified arm ▽

✓6ᵗʰ **S45.81** Laceration of other specified blood vessels at shoulder and upper arm level
- ✓7ᵗʰ **S45.811** Laceration of other specified blood vessels at shoulder and upper arm level, right arm
- ✓7ᵗʰ **S45.812** Laceration of other specified blood vessels at shoulder and upper arm level, left arm
- ✓7ᵗʰ **S45.819** Laceration of other specified blood vessels at shoulder and upper arm level, unspecified arm ▽

✓6ᵗʰ **S45.89** Other specified injury of other specified blood vessels at shoulder and upper arm level
- ✓7ᵗʰ **S45.891** Other specified injury of other specified blood vessels at shoulder and upper arm level, right arm
- ✓7ᵗʰ **S45.892** Other specified injury of other specified blood vessels at shoulder and upper arm level, left arm
- ✓7ᵗʰ **S45.899** Other specified injury of other specified blood vessels at shoulder and upper arm level, unspecified arm ▽

✓5ᵗʰ **S45.9** Injury of unspecified blood vessel at shoulder and upper arm level

✓6ᵗʰ **S45.90** Unspecified injury of unspecified blood vessel at shoulder and upper arm level
- ✓7ᵗʰ **S45.901** Unspecified injury of unspecified blood vessel at shoulder and upper arm level, right arm ▽
- ✓7ᵗʰ **S45.902** Unspecified injury of unspecified blood vessel at shoulder and upper arm level, left arm ▽
- ✓7ᵗʰ **S45.909** Unspecified injury of unspecified blood vessel at shoulder and upper arm level, unspecified arm ▽

✓6ᵗʰ **S45.91** Laceration of unspecified blood vessel at shoulder and upper arm level
- ✓7ᵗʰ **S45.911** Laceration of unspecified blood vessel at shoulder and upper arm level, right arm ▽
- ✓7ᵗʰ **S45.912** Laceration of unspecified blood vessel at shoulder and upper arm level, left arm ▽
- ✓7ᵗʰ **S45.919** Laceration of unspecified blood vessel at shoulder and upper arm level, unspecified arm ▽

✓6ᵗʰ **S45.99** Other specified injury of unspecified blood vessel at shoulder and upper arm level
- ✓7ᵗʰ **S45.991** Other specified injury of unspecified blood vessel at shoulder and upper arm level, right arm ▽
- ✓7ᵗʰ **S45.992** Other specified injury of unspecified blood vessel at shoulder and upper arm level, left arm ▽
- ✓7ᵗʰ **S45.999** Other specified injury of unspecified blood vessel at shoulder and upper arm level, unspecified arm ▽

✓4ᵗʰ **S46** **Injury of muscle, fascia and tendon at shoulder and upper arm level**

Code also any associated open wound (S41.-)

EXCLUDES 2   injury of muscle, fascia and tendon at elbow (S56.-)
sprain of joints and ligaments of shoulder girdle (S43.9)

TIP: Refer to the Muscle/Tendon table at the beginning of this chapter.

The appropriate 7th character is to be added to each code from category S46.
- A   initial encounter
- D   subsequent encounter
- S   sequela

✓5ᵗʰ **S46.0** Injury of muscle(s) and tendon(s) of the rotator cuff of shoulder

✓6ᵗʰ **S46.00** Unspecified injury of muscle(s) and tendon(s) of the rotator cuff of shoulder
- ✓7ᵗʰ **S46.001** Unspecified injury of muscle(s) and tendon(s) of the rotator cuff of right shoulder ▽
- ✓7ᵗʰ **S46.002** Unspecified injury of muscle(s) and tendon(s) of the rotator cuff of left shoulder ▽

☑ Additional Character Req   ✓7ᵗʰ Placeholder Alert   Manifestation   HCC CMS-HCC Condition   ▽ Unspecified Code   ▶◀ Revised Text   ● New Code   ▲ Revised Code Title

Chapter 19. Injury, Poisoning, and Certain Other Consequences of External Causes

    ✓7ᵗʰ **S46.009** Unspecified injury of muscle(s) and ▽
tendon(s) of the rotator cuff of unspecified
shoulder

  ✓6ᵗʰ **S46.01** Strain of muscle(s) and tendon(s) of the rotator cuff
of shoulder

    ✓7ᵗʰ **S46.011** Strain of muscle(s) and tendon(s) of the
rotator cuff of right shoulder

    ✓7ᵗʰ **S46.012** Strain of muscle(s) and tendon(s) of the
rotator cuff of left shoulder

    ✓7ᵗʰ **S46.019** Strain of muscle(s) and tendon(s) of ▽
the rotator cuff of unspecified shoulder

  ✓6ᵗʰ **S46.02** Laceration of muscle(s) and tendon(s) of the rotator
cuff of shoulder

    ✓7ᵗʰ **S46.021** Laceration of muscle(s) and tendon(s) of
the rotator cuff of right shoulder

    ✓7ᵗʰ **S46.022** Laceration of muscle(s) and tendon(s) of
the rotator cuff of left shoulder

    ✓7ᵗʰ **S46.029** Laceration of muscle(s) and tendon(s) ▽
of the rotator cuff of unspecified shoulder

  ✓6ᵗʰ **S46.09** Other injury of muscle(s) and tendon(s) of the
rotator cuff of shoulder

    ✓7ᵗʰ **S46.091** Other injury of muscle(s) and tendon(s) of
the rotator cuff of right shoulder

    ✓7ᵗʰ **S46.092** Other injury of muscle(s) and tendon(s) of
the rotator cuff of left shoulder

    ✓7ᵗʰ **S46.099** Other injury of muscle(s) and tendon(s) ▽
of the rotator cuff of unspecified shoulder

✓5ᵗʰ **S46.1** Injury of muscle, fascia and tendon of long head of biceps

  ✓6ᵗʰ **S46.10** Unspecified injury of muscle, fascia and tendon of
long head of biceps

    ✓7ᵗʰ **S46.101** Unspecified injury of muscle, fascia and ▽
tendon of long head of biceps, right arm

    ✓7ᵗʰ **S46.102** Unspecified injury of muscle, fascia and ▽
tendon of long head of biceps, left arm

    ✓7ᵗʰ **S46.109** Unspecified injury of muscle, fascia and ▽
tendon of long head of biceps, unspecified
arm

  ✓6ᵗʰ **S46.11** Strain of muscle, fascia and tendon of long head of
biceps

    ✓7ᵗʰ **S46.111** Strain of muscle, fascia and tendon of long
head of biceps, right arm

    ✓7ᵗʰ **S46.112** Strain of muscle, fascia and tendon of long
head of biceps, left arm

    ✓7ᵗʰ **S46.119** Strain of muscle, fascia and tendon of ▽
long head of biceps, unspecified arm

  ✓6ᵗʰ **S46.12** Laceration of muscle, fascia and tendon of long head
of biceps

    ✓7ᵗʰ **S46.121** Laceration of muscle, fascia and tendon of
long head of biceps, right arm

    ✓7ᵗʰ **S46.122** Laceration of muscle, fascia and tendon of
long head of biceps, left arm

    ✓7ᵗʰ **S46.129** Laceration of muscle, fascia and tendon ▽
of long head of biceps, unspecified arm

  ✓6ᵗʰ **S46.19** Other injury of muscle, fascia and tendon of long
head of biceps

    ✓7ᵗʰ **S46.191** Other injury of muscle, fascia and tendon
of long head of biceps, right arm

    ✓7ᵗʰ **S46.192** Other injury of muscle, fascia and tendon
of long head of biceps, left arm

    ✓7ᵗʰ **S46.199** Other injury of muscle, fascia and ▽
tendon of long head of biceps,
unspecified arm

✓5ᵗʰ **S46.2** Injury of muscle, fascia and tendon of other parts of biceps

  ✓6ᵗʰ **S46.20** Unspecified injury of muscle, fascia and tendon of
other parts of biceps

    ✓7ᵗʰ **S46.201** Unspecified injury of muscle, fascia and ▽
tendon of other parts of biceps, right arm

    ✓7ᵗʰ **S46.202** Unspecified injury of muscle, fascia and ▽
tendon of other parts of biceps, left arm

    ✓7ᵗʰ **S46.209** Unspecified injury of muscle, fascia and ▽
tendon of other parts of biceps,
unspecified arm

  ✓6ᵗʰ **S46.21** Strain of muscle, fascia and tendon of other parts of
biceps

    ✓7ᵗʰ **S46.211** Strain of muscle, fascia and tendon of
other parts of biceps, right arm

    ✓7ᵗʰ **S46.212** Strain of muscle, fascia and tendon of
other parts of biceps, left arm

    ✓7ᵗʰ **S46.219** Strain of muscle, fascia and tendon of ▽
other parts of biceps, unspecified arm

  ✓6ᵗʰ **S46.22** Laceration of muscle, fascia and tendon of other
parts of biceps

    ✓7ᵗʰ **S46.221** Laceration of muscle, fascia and tendon of
other parts of biceps, right arm

    ✓7ᵗʰ **S46.222** Laceration of muscle, fascia and tendon of
other parts of biceps, left arm

    ✓7ᵗʰ **S46.229** Laceration of muscle, fascia and tendon ▽
of other parts of biceps, unspecified arm

  ✓6ᵗʰ **S46.29** Other injury of muscle, fascia and tendon of other
parts of biceps

    ✓7ᵗʰ **S46.291** Other injury of muscle, fascia and tendon
of other parts of biceps, right arm

    ✓7ᵗʰ **S46.292** Other injury of muscle, fascia and tendon
of other parts of biceps, left arm

    ✓7ᵗʰ **S46.299** Other injury of muscle, fascia and ▽
tendon of other parts of biceps,
unspecified arm

✓5ᵗʰ **S46.3** Injury of muscle, fascia and tendon of triceps

  ✓6ᵗʰ **S46.30** Unspecified injury of muscle, fascia and tendon of
triceps

    ✓7ᵗʰ **S46.301** Unspecified injury of muscle, fascia ▽
and tendon of triceps, right arm

    ✓7ᵗʰ **S46.302** Unspecified injury of muscle, fascia ▽
and tendon of triceps, left arm

    ✓7ᵗʰ **S46.309** Unspecified injury of muscle, fascia ▽
and tendon of triceps, unspecified arm

  ✓6ᵗʰ **S46.31** Strain of muscle, fascia and tendon of triceps

    ✓7ᵗʰ **S46.311** Strain of muscle, fascia and tendon of
triceps, right arm

    ✓7ᵗʰ **S46.312** Strain of muscle, fascia and tendon of
triceps, left arm

    ✓7ᵗʰ **S46.319** Strain of muscle, fascia and tendon ▽
of triceps, unspecified arm

  ✓6ᵗʰ **S46.32** Laceration of muscle, fascia and tendon of triceps

    ✓7ᵗʰ **S46.321** Laceration of muscle, fascia and tendon
of triceps, right arm

    ✓7ᵗʰ **S46.322** Laceration of muscle, fascia and tendon
of triceps, left arm

    ✓7ᵗʰ **S46.329** Laceration of muscle, fascia and tendon ▽
of triceps, unspecified arm

  ✓6ᵗʰ **S46.39** Other injury of muscle, fascia and tendon of triceps

    ✓7ᵗʰ **S46.391** Other injury of muscle, fascia and tendon
of triceps, right arm

    ✓7ᵗʰ **S46.392** Other injury of muscle, fascia and tendon
of triceps, left arm

    ✓7ᵗʰ **S46.399** Other injury of muscle, fascia and ▽
tendon of triceps, unspecified arm

✓5ᵗʰ **S46.8** Injury of other muscles, fascia and tendons at shoulder and
upper arm level

  ✓6ᵗʰ **S46.80** Unspecified injury of other muscles, fascia and
tendons at shoulder and upper arm level

    ✓7ᵗʰ **S46.801** Unspecified injury of other muscles, ▽
fascia and tendons at shoulder and
upper arm level, right arm

    ✓7ᵗʰ **S46.802** Unspecified injury of other muscles, ▽
fascia and tendons at shoulder and
upper arm level, left arm

    ✓7ᵗʰ **S46.809** Unspecified injury of other muscles, ▽
fascia and tendons at shoulder and
upper arm level, unspecified arm

  ✓6ᵗʰ **S46.81** Strain of other muscles, fascia and tendons at
shoulder and upper arm level

    ✓7ᵗʰ **S46.811** Strain of other muscles, fascia and
tendons at shoulder and upper arm
level, right arm

    ✓7ᵗʰ **S46.812** Strain of other muscles, fascia and
tendons at shoulder and upper arm
level, left arm

EXCLUDES 1 Not coded here   **EXCLUDES 2** Not included here   N Newborn Age: 0   P Pediatric Age: 0-17   M Maternity Age: 12-55   A Adult Age: 15-124

962   ICD-10-CM 2018

√7ᵗʰ **S46.819** Strain of other muscles, fascia and tendons at shoulder and upper arm level, unspecified arm ▽

√6ᵗʰ **S46.82** Laceration of other muscles, fascia and tendons at shoulder and upper arm level

√7ᵗʰ **S46.821** Laceration of other muscles, fascia and tendons at shoulder and upper arm level, right arm

√7ᵗʰ **S46.822** Laceration of other muscles, fascia and tendons at shoulder and upper arm level, left arm

√7ᵗʰ **S46.829** Laceration of other muscles, fascia and tendons at shoulder and upper arm level, unspecified arm ▽

√6ᵗʰ **S46.89** Other injury of other muscles, fascia and tendons at shoulder and upper arm level

√7ᵗʰ **S46.891** Other injury of other muscles, fascia and tendons at shoulder and upper arm level, right arm

√7ᵗʰ **S46.892** Other injury of other muscles, fascia and tendons at shoulder and upper arm level, left arm

√7ᵗʰ **S46.899** Other injury of other muscles, fascia and tendons at shoulder and upper arm level, unspecified arm ▽

√5ᵗʰ **S46.9** Injury of unspecified muscle, fascia and tendon at shoulder and upper arm level

√6ᵗʰ **S46.90** Unspecified injury of unspecified muscle, fascia and tendon at shoulder and upper arm level

√7ᵗʰ **S46.901** Unspecified injury of unspecified muscle, fascia and tendon at shoulder and upper arm level, right arm ▽

√7ᵗʰ **S46.902** Unspecified injury of unspecified muscle, fascia and tendon at shoulder and upper arm level, left arm ▽

√7ᵗʰ **S46.909** Unspecified injury of unspecified muscle, fascia and tendon at shoulder and upper arm level, unspecified arm ▽

√6ᵗʰ **S46.91** Strain of unspecified muscle, fascia and tendon at shoulder and upper arm level

√7ᵗʰ **S46.911** Strain of unspecified muscle, fascia and tendon at shoulder and upper arm level, right arm ▽

√7ᵗʰ **S46.912** Strain of unspecified muscle, fascia and tendon at shoulder and upper arm level, left arm ▽

√7ᵗʰ **S46.919** Strain of unspecified muscle, fascia and tendon at shoulder and upper arm level, unspecified arm ▽

√6ᵗʰ **S46.92** Laceration of unspecified muscle, fascia and tendon at shoulder and upper arm level

√7ᵗʰ **S46.921** Laceration of unspecified muscle, fascia and tendon at shoulder and upper arm level, right arm ▽

√7ᵗʰ **S46.922** Laceration of unspecified muscle, fascia and tendon at shoulder and upper arm level, left arm ▽

√7ᵗʰ **S46.929** Laceration of unspecified muscle, fascia and tendon at shoulder and upper arm level, unspecified arm ▽

√6ᵗʰ **S46.99** Other injury of unspecified muscle, fascia and tendon at shoulder and upper arm level

√7ᵗʰ **S46.991** Other injury of unspecified muscle, fascia and tendon at shoulder and upper arm level, right arm ▽

√7ᵗʰ **S46.992** Other injury of unspecified muscle, fascia and tendon at shoulder and upper arm level, left arm ▽

√7ᵗʰ **S46.999** Other injury of unspecified muscle, fascia and tendon at shoulder and upper arm level, unspecified arm ▽

√4ᵗʰ **S47** **Crushing injury** of shoulder and upper arm
Use additional code for all associated injuries
EXCLUDES 2 crushing injury of elbow (S57.0-)

The appropriate 7th character is to be added to each code from category S47.
A   initial encounter
D   subsequent encounter
S   sequela

√x7ᵗʰ **S47.1** Crushing injury of right shoulder and upper arm

√x7ᵗʰ **S47.2** Crushing injury of left shoulder and upper arm

√x7ᵗʰ **S47.9** Crushing injury of shoulder and upper arm, unspecified arm ▽

√4ᵗʰ **S48** **Traumatic amputation of shoulder and upper arm**
An amputation not identified as partial or complete should be coded to complete.
EXCLUDES 1 traumatic amputation at elbow level (S58.0)

The appropriate 7th character is to be added to each code from category S48.
A   initial encounter
D   subsequent encounter
S   sequela

√5ᵗʰ **S48.0** Traumatic amputation at shoulder joint

√6ᵗʰ **S48.01** Complete traumatic amputation at shoulder joint

2 √7ᵗʰ **S48.011** Complete traumatic amputation at right shoulder joint HCC

2 √7ᵗʰ **S48.012** Complete traumatic amputation at left shoulder joint HCC

2 √7ᵗʰ **S48.019** Complete traumatic amputation at unspecified shoulder joint HCC ▽

√6ᵗʰ **S48.02** Partial traumatic amputation at shoulder joint

2 √7ᵗʰ **S48.021** Partial traumatic amputation at right shoulder joint HCC

2 √7ᵗʰ **S48.022** Partial traumatic amputation at left shoulder joint HCC

2 √7ᵗʰ **S48.029** Partial traumatic amputation at unspecified shoulder joint HCC ▽

√5ᵗʰ **S48.1** Traumatic amputation at level between shoulder and elbow

√6ᵗʰ **S48.11** Complete traumatic amputation at level between shoulder and elbow

2 √7ᵗʰ **S48.111** Complete traumatic amputation at level between right shoulder and elbow HCC

2 √7ᵗʰ **S48.112** Complete traumatic amputation at level between left shoulder and elbow HCC

2 √7ᵗʰ **S48.119** Complete traumatic amputation at level between unspecified shoulder and elbow HCC ▽

√6ᵗʰ **S48.12** Partial traumatic amputation at level between shoulder and elbow

2 √7ᵗʰ **S48.121** Partial traumatic amputation at level between right shoulder and elbow HCC

2 √7ᵗʰ **S48.122** Partial traumatic amputation at level between left shoulder and elbow HCC

2 √7ᵗʰ **S48.129** Partial traumatic amputation at level between unspecified shoulder and elbow HCC ▽

√5ᵗʰ **S48.9** Traumatic amputation of shoulder and upper arm, level unspecified

√6ᵗʰ **S48.91** Complete traumatic amputation of shoulder and upper arm, level unspecified

2 √7ᵗʰ **S48.911** Complete traumatic amputation of right shoulder and upper arm, level unspecified HCC ▽

2 √7ᵗʰ **S48.912** Complete traumatic amputation of left shoulder and upper arm, level unspecified HCC ▽

2 √7ᵗʰ **S48.919** Complete traumatic amputation of unspecified shoulder and upper arm, level unspecified HCC ▽

√6ᵗʰ **S48.92** Partial traumatic amputation of shoulder and upper arm, level unspecified

2 √7ᵗʰ **S48.921** Partial traumatic amputation of right shoulder and upper arm, level unspecified HCC ▽

---

2   HCC with 7th character indicating initial encounter (A or B - specific to category) OR sequela.

☑ Additional Character Req   √x7ᵗʰ Placeholder Alert   Manifestation   HCC CMS-HCC Condition   ▽ Unspecified Code   ►◄ Revised Text   ● New Code   ▲ Revised Code Title

Chapter 19. Injury, Poisoning, and Certain Other Consequences of External Causes

2 √7th **S48.922** Partial traumatic amputation of **left** shoulder and upper arm, level unspecified   HCC ▽

2 √7th **S48.929** Partial traumatic amputation of unspecified shoulder and upper arm, level unspecified   HCC ▽

√4th **S49** Other and unspecified injuries of shoulder and upper arm

> The appropriate 7th character is to be added to each code from subcategories S49.0 and S49.1.
> A   initial encounter for closed fracture
> D   subsequent encounter for fracture with routine healing
> G   subsequent encounter for fracture with delayed healing
> K   subsequent encounter for fracture with nonunion
> P   subsequent encounter for fracture with malunion
> S   sequela

√5th **S49.0** Physeal fracture of upper end of humerus

√6th **S49.00** Unspecified physeal fracture of upper end of humerus

√7th **S49.001** Unspecified physeal fracture of upper end of humerus, **right** arm ▽

√7th **S49.002** Unspecified physeal fracture of upper end of humerus, **left** arm ▽

√7th **S49.009** Unspecified physeal fracture of upper end of humerus, unspecified arm ▽

√6th **S49.01** Salter-Harris Type I physeal fracture of upper end of humerus

√7th **S49.011** Salter-Harris Type I physeal fracture of upper end of humerus, **right** arm

√7th **S49.012** Salter-Harris Type I physeal fracture of upper end of humerus, **left** arm

√7th **S49.019** Salter-Harris Type I physeal fracture of upper end of humerus, unspecified arm ▽

√6th **S49.02** Salter-Harris Type II physeal fracture of upper end of humerus

√7th **S49.021** Salter-Harris Type II physeal fracture of upper end of humerus, **right** arm

√7th **S49.022** Salter-Harris Type II physeal fracture of upper end of humerus, **left** arm

√7th **S49.029** Salter-Harris Type II physeal fracture of upper end of humerus, unspecified arm ▽

√6th **S49.03** Salter-Harris Type III physeal fracture of upper end of humerus

√7th **S49.031** Salter-Harris Type III physeal fracture of upper end of humerus, **right** arm

√7th **S49.032** Salter-Harris Type III physeal fracture of upper end of humerus, **left** arm

√7th **S49.039** Salter-Harris Type III physeal fracture of upper end of humerus, unspecified arm ▽

√6th **S49.04** Salter-Harris Type IV physeal fracture of upper end of humerus

√7th **S49.041** Salter-Harris Type IV physeal fracture of upper end of humerus, **right** arm

√7th **S49.042** Salter-Harris Type IV physeal fracture of upper end of humerus, **left** arm

√7th **S49.049** Salter-Harris Type IV physeal fracture of upper end of humerus, unspecified arm ▽

√6th **S49.09** Other physeal fracture of upper end of humerus

√7th **S49.091** Other physeal fracture of upper end of humerus, **right** arm

√7th **S49.092** Other physeal fracture of upper end of humerus, **left** arm

√7th **S49.099** Other physeal fracture of upper end of humerus, unspecified arm ▽

√5th **S49.1** Physeal fracture of lower end of humerus

√6th **S49.10** Unspecified physeal fracture of lower end of humerus

√7th **S49.101** Unspecified physeal fracture of lower end of humerus, **right** arm ▽

√7th **S49.102** Unspecified physeal fracture of lower end of humerus, **left** arm ▽

√7th **S49.109** Unspecified physeal fracture of lower end of humerus, unspecified arm ▽

√6th **S49.11** Salter-Harris Type I physeal fracture of lower end of humerus

√7th **S49.111** Salter-Harris Type I physeal fracture of lower end of humerus, **right** arm

√7th **S49.112** Salter-Harris Type I physeal fracture of lower end of humerus, **left** arm

√7th **S49.119** Salter-Harris Type I physeal fracture of lower end of humerus, unspecified arm ▽

√6th **S49.12** Salter-Harris Type II physeal fracture of lower end of humerus

√7th **S49.121** Salter-Harris Type II physeal fracture of lower end of humerus, **right** arm

√7th **S49.122** Salter-Harris Type II physeal fracture of lower end of humerus, **left** arm

√7th **S49.129** Salter-Harris Type II physeal fracture of lower end of humerus, unspecified arm ▽

√6th **S49.13** Salter Harris Type III physeal fracture of lower end of humerus

√7th **S49.131** Salter-Harris Type III physeal fracture of lower end of humerus, **right** arm

√7th **S49.132** Salter-Harris Type III physeal fracture of lower end of humerus, **left** arm

√7th **S49.139** Salter-Harris Type III physeal fracture of lower end of humerus, unspecified arm ▽

√6th **S49.14** Salter-Harris Type IV physeal fracture of lower end of humerus

√7th **S49.141** Salter-Harris Type IV physeal fracture of lower end of humerus, **right** arm

√7th **S49.142** Salter-Harris Type IV physeal fracture of lower end of humerus, **left** arm

√7th **S49.149** Salter-Harris Type IV physeal fracture of lower end of humerus, unspecified arm ▽

√6th **S49.19** Other physeal fracture of lower end of humerus

√7th **S49.191** Other physeal fracture of lower end of humerus, **right** arm

√7th **S49.192** Other physeal fracture of lower end of humerus, **left** arm

√7th **S49.199** Other physeal fracture of lower end of humerus, unspecified arm ▽

√5th **S49.8** Other specified injuries of shoulder and upper arm

> The appropriate 7th character is to be added to each code in subcategory S49.8.
> A   initial encounter
> D   subsequent encounter
> S   sequela

√x7th **S49.80** Other specified injuries of shoulder and upper arm, unspecified arm ▽

√x7th **S49.81** Other specified injuries of **right** shoulder and upper arm

√x7th **S49.82** Other specified injuries of **left** shoulder and upper arm

√5th **S49.9** Unspecified injury of shoulder and upper arm

> The appropriate 7th character is to be added to each code in subcategory S49.9.
> A   initial encounter
> D   subsequent encounter
> S   sequela

√x7th **S49.90** Unspecified injury of shoulder and upper arm, unspecified arm ▽

√x7th **S49.91** Unspecified injury of **right** shoulder and upper arm ▽

√x7th **S49.92** Unspecified injury of **left** shoulder and upper arm ▽

---

2   HCC with 7th character indicating initial encounter (A or B - specific to category) OR sequela.

EXCLUDES 1 Not coded here   EXCLUDES 2 Not included here   N Newborn Age: 0   P Pediatric Age: 0-17   M Maternity Age: 12-55   A Adult Age: 15-124

964   ICD-10-CM 2018

Injuries to the elbow and forearm (S50-S59)

EXCLUDES 2   burns and corrosions (T20-T32)
frostbite (T33-T34)
injuries of wrist and hand (S60-S69)
insect bite or sting, venomous (T63.4)

√4th S50   Superficial injury of elbow and forearm

EXCLUDES 2   superficial injury of wrist and hand (S60.-)

The appropriate 7th character is to be added to each code from
category S50.
A   initial encounter
D   subsequent encounter
S   sequela

√5th **S50.0**   **Contusion of** elbow

√x7th **S50.00**   **Contusion of unspecified elbow**   ▽
√x7th **S50.01**   **Contusion of** right **elbow**
√x7th **S50.02**   **Contusion of** left **elbow**

√5th **S50.1**   **Contusion of** forearm

√x7th **S50.10**   **Contusion of unspecified forearm**   ▽
√x7th **S50.11**   **Contusion of** right **forearm**
√x7th **S50.12**   **Contusion of** left **forearm**

√5th **S50.3**   **Other superficial injuries of** elbow

√6th **S50.31**   **Abrasion** of elbow

√7th **S50.311**   **Abrasion of** right **elbow**
√7th **S50.312**   **Abrasion of** left **elbow**
√7th **S50.319**   **Abrasion of unspecified elbow**   ▽

√6th **S50.32**   **Blister (nonthermal)** of elbow

√7th **S50.321**   **Blister (nonthermal) of** right **elbow**
√7th **S50.322**   **Blister (nonthermal) of** left **elbow**
√7th **S50.329**   **Blister (nonthermal) of unspecified elbow**   ▽

√6th **S50.34**   **External constriction** of elbow

√7th **S50.341**   **External constriction of** right **elbow**
√7th **S50.342**   **External constriction of** left **elbow**
√7th **S50.349**   **External constriction of unspecified elbow**   ▽

√6th **S50.35**   **Superficial** foreign body **of elbow**
Splinter in the elbow

√7th **S50.351**   **Superficial foreign body of** right **elbow**
√7th **S50.352**   **Superficial foreign body of** left **elbow**
√7th **S50.359**   **Superficial foreign body of unspecified elbow**   ▽

√6th **S50.36**   **Insect bite (nonvenomous)** of elbow

√7th **S50.361**   **Insect bite (nonvenomous) of** right **elbow**
√7th **S50.362**   **Insect bite (nonvenomous) of** left **elbow**
√7th **S50.369**   **Insect bite (nonvenomous) of unspecified elbow**   ▽

√6th **S50.37**   **Other superficial** bite **of elbow**

EXCLUDES 1   open bite of elbow (S51.05)

√7th **S50.371**   **Other superficial bite of** right **elbow**
√7th **S50.372**   **Other superficial bite of** left **elbow**
√7th **S50.379**   **Other superficial bite of unspecified elbow**   ▽

√5th **S50.8**   **Other superficial injuries of** forearm

√6th **S50.81**   **Abrasion** of forearm

√7th **S50.811**   **Abrasion of** right **forearm**
√7th **S50.812**   **Abrasion of** left **forearm**
√7th **S50.819**   **Abrasion of unspecified forearm**   ▽

√6th **S50.82**   **Blister (nonthermal)** of forearm

√7th **S50.821**   **Blister (nonthermal) of** right **forearm**
√7th **S50.822**   **Blister (nonthermal) of** left **forearm**
√7th **S50.829**   **Blister (nonthermal) of unspecified forearm**   ▽

√6th **S50.84**   **External constriction** of forearm

√7th **S50.841**   **External constriction of** right **forearm**
√7th **S50.842**   **External constriction of** left **forearm**
√7th **S50.849**   **External constriction of unspecified forearm**   ▽

√6th **S50.85**   **Superficial** foreign body **of forearm**
Splinter in the forearm

√7th **S50.851**   **Superficial foreign body of** right **forearm**
√7th **S50.852**   **Superficial foreign body of** left **forearm**
√7th **S50.859**   **Superficial foreign body of unspecified forearm**   ▽

√6th **S50.86**   **Insect bite (nonvenomous) of forearm**

√7th **S50.861**   **Insect bite (nonvenomous) of** right **forearm**
√7th **S50.862**   **Insect bite (nonvenomous) of** left **forearm**
√7th **S50.869**   **Insect bite (nonvenomous) of unspecified forearm**   ▽

√6th **S50.87**   **Other superficial** bite **of forearm**

EXCLUDES 1   open bite of forearm (S51.85)

√7th **S50.871**   **Other superficial bite of** right **forearm**
√7th **S50.872**   **Other superficial bite of** left **forearm**
√7th **S50.879**   **Other superficial bite of unspecified forearm**   ▽

√5th **S50.9**   **Unspecified superficial injury of elbow and forearm**

√6th **S50.90**   **Unspecified superficial injury of** elbow

√7th **S50.901**   **Unspecified superficial injury of** right **elbow**   ▽
√7th **S50.902**   **Unspecified superficial injury of** left **elbow**   ▽
√7th **S50.909**   **Unspecified superficial injury of unspecified elbow**   ▽

√6th **S50.91**   **Unspecified superficial injury of** forearm

√7th **S50.911**   **Unspecified superficial injury of** right **forearm**   ▽
√7th **S50.912**   **Unspecified superficial injury of** left **forearm**   ▽
√7th **S50.919**   **Unspecified superficial injury of unspecified forearm**   ▽

√4th S51   Open wound of elbow and forearm

Code also any associated wound infection

EXCLUDES 1   open fracture of elbow and forearm (S52- with open fracture 7th character)
traumatic amputation of elbow and forearm (S58.-)

EXCLUDES 2   open wound of wrist and hand (S61.-)

The appropriate 7th character is to be added to each code from
category S51.
A   initial encounter
D   subsequent encounter
S   sequela

√5th **S51.0**   **Open wound of** elbow

√6th **S51.00**   **Unspecified open wound of elbow**

√7th **S51.001**   **Unspecified open wound of** right **elbow** ▽
AHA: 2012, 4Q, 108
√7th **S51.002**   **Unspecified open wound of** left **elbow**   ▽
√7th **S51.009**   **Unspecified open wound of unspecified elbow**   ▽
Open wound of elbow NOS

√6th **S51.01**   **Laceration without foreign body of elbow**

√7th **S51.011**   **Laceration without foreign body of** right **elbow**
√7th **S51.012**   **Laceration without foreign body of** left **elbow**
√7th **S51.019**   **Laceration without foreign body of unspecified elbow**   ▽

√6th **S51.02**   **Laceration with foreign body of elbow**

√7th **S51.021**   **Laceration with foreign body of** right **elbow**
√7th **S51.022**   **Laceration with foreign body of** left **elbow**
√7th **S51.029**   **Laceration with foreign body of unspecified elbow**   ▽

√6th **S51.03**   **Puncture wound without foreign body of elbow**

√7th **S51.031**   **Puncture wound without foreign body of** right **elbow**
√7th **S51.032**   **Puncture wound without foreign body of** left **elbow**
√7th **S51.039**   **Puncture wound without foreign body of unspecified elbow**   ▽

√ Additional Character Req   √x7th Placeholder Alert   Manifestation   HCC CMS-HCC Condition   ▽ Unspecified Code   ►◄ Revised Text   ● New Code   ▲ Revised Code Title

✓6ᵗʰ **S51.04** Puncture wound with foreign body of elbow

   ✓7ᵗʰ **S51.041** **Puncture wound with foreign body of right elbow**

   ✓7ᵗʰ **S51.042** **Puncture wound with foreign body of left elbow**

   ✓7ᵗʰ **S51.049** **Puncture wound with foreign body of unspecified elbow** ▽

✓6ᵗʰ **S51.05** Open bite of elbow
   Bite of elbow NOS
     EXCLUDES 1 superficial bite of elbow (S50.36, S50.37)

   ✓7ᵗʰ **S51.051** **Open bite, right elbow**

   ✓7ᵗʰ **S51.052** **Open bite, left elbow**

   ✓7ᵗʰ **S51.059** **Open bite, unspecified elbow** ▽

✓5ᵗʰ **S51.8** **Open wound of forearm**
    EXCLUDES 2 open wound of elbow (S51.0-)

  ✓6ᵗʰ **S51.80** **Unspecified open wound of forearm**
    AHA: 2016, 3Q, 24

   ✓7ᵗʰ **S51.801** **Unspecified open wound of right forearm** ▽

   ✓7ᵗʰ **S51.802** **Unspecified open wound of left forearm** ▽

   ✓7ᵗʰ **S51.809** **Unspecified open wound of unspecified forearm** ▽
       Open wound of forearm NOS

  ✓6ᵗʰ **S51.81** Laceration without foreign body of forearm

   ✓7ᵗʰ **S51.811** **Laceration without foreign body of right forearm**

   ✓7ᵗʰ **S51.812** **Laceration without foreign body of left forearm**

   ✓7ᵗʰ **S51.819** **Laceration without foreign body of unspecified forearm** ▽

  ✓6ᵗʰ **S51.82** Laceration with foreign body of forearm

   ✓7ᵗʰ **S51.821** **Laceration with foreign body of right forearm**

   ✓7ᵗʰ **S51.822** **Laceration with foreign body of left forearm**

   ✓7ᵗʰ **S51.829** **Laceration with foreign body of unspecified forearm** ▽

  ✓6ᵗʰ **S51.83** Puncture wound without foreign body of forearm
    AHA: 2016, 3Q, 24

   ✓7ᵗʰ **S51.831** **Puncture wound without foreign body of right forearm**

   ✓7ᵗʰ **S51.832** **Puncture wound without foreign body of left forearm**

   ✓7ᵗʰ **S51.839** **Puncture wound without foreign body of unspecified forearm** ▽

  ✓6ᵗʰ **S51.84** Puncture wound with foreign body of forearm
    AHA: 2016, 3Q, 24

   ✓7ᵗʰ **S51.841** **Puncture wound with foreign body of right forearm**

   ✓7ᵗʰ **S51.842** **Puncture wound with foreign body of left forearm**

   ✓7ᵗʰ **S51.849** **Puncture wound with foreign body of unspecified forearm** ▽

  ✓6ᵗʰ **S51.85** Open bite of forearm
   Bite of forearm NOS
    EXCLUDES 1 superficial bite of forearm (S50.86, S50.87)

   ✓7ᵗʰ **S51.851** **Open bite of right forearm**

   ✓7ᵗʰ **S51.852** **Open bite of left forearm**

   ✓7ᵗʰ **S51.859** **Open bite of unspecified forearm** ▽

✓4ᵗʰ **S52** **Fracture of forearm**

  NOTE A fracture not indicated as displaced or nondisplaced should be coded to displaced.
A fracture not indicated as open or closed should be coded to closed.
The open fracture designations are based on the Gustilo open fracture classification.

  EXCLUDES 1 traumatic amputation of forearm (S58.-)
  EXCLUDES 2 fracture at wrist and hand level (S62.-)
  AHA: 2016, 1Q, 33; 2015, 3Q, 37-39

The appropriate 7th character is to be added to all codes from category S52 [unless otherwise indicated].
A   initial encounter for closed fracture
B   initial encounter for open fracture type I or II
    initial encounter for open fracture NOS
C   initial encounter for open fracture type IIIA, IIIB, or IIIC
D   subsequent encounter for closed fracture with routine healing
E   subsequent encounter for open fracture type I or II with routine healing
F   subsequent encounter for open fracture type IIIA, IIIB, or IIIC with routine healing
G   subsequent encounter for closed fracture with delayed healing
H   subsequent encounter for open fracture type I or II with delayed healing
J   subsequent encounter for open fracture type IIIA, IIIB, or IIIC with delayed healing
K   subsequent encounter for closed fracture with nonunion
M   subsequent encounter for open fracture type I or II with nonunion
N   subsequent encounter for open fracture type IIIA, IIIB, or IIIC with nonunion
P   subsequent encounter for closed fracture with malunion
Q   subsequent encounter for open fracture type I or II with malunion
R   subsequent encounter for open fracture type IIIA, IIIB, or IIIC with malunion
S   sequela

✓5ᵗʰ **S52.0** **Fracture of upper end of ulna**
   Fracture of proximal end of ulna
    EXCLUDES 2 fracture of elbow NOS (S42.40-)
         fractures of shaft of ulna (S52.2-)

  ✓6ᵗʰ **S52.00** **Unspecified fracture of upper end of ulna**

   ✓7ᵗʰ **S52.001** **Unspecified fracture of upper end of right ulna** ▽

   ✓7ᵗʰ **S52.002** **Unspecified fracture of upper end of left ulna** ▽

   ✓7ᵗʰ **S52.009** **Unspecified fracture of upper end of unspecified ulna** ▽

  ✓6ᵗʰ **S52.01** Torus fracture of upper end of ulna

The appropriate 7th character is to be added to all codes in subcategory S52.01.
A   initial encounter for closed fracture
D   subsequent encounter for fracture with routine healing
G   subsequent encounter for fracture with delayed healing
K   subsequent encounter for fracture with nonunion
P   subsequent encounter for fracture with malunion
S   sequela

   ✓7ᵗʰ **S52.011** **Torus fracture of upper end of right ulna**

   ✓7ᵗʰ **S52.012** **Torus fracture of upper end of left ulna**

   ✓7ᵗʰ **S52.019** **Torus fracture of upper end of unspecified ulna** ▽

  ✓6ᵗʰ **S52.02** Fracture of olecranon process without intraarticular extension of ulna

   ✓7ᵗʰ **S52.021** **Displaced fracture of olecranon process without intraarticular extension of right ulna**

   ✓7ᵗʰ **S52.022** **Displaced fracture of olecranon process without intraarticular extension of left ulna**

   ✓7ᵗʰ **S52.023** **Displaced fracture of olecranon process without intraarticular extension of unspecified ulna** ▽

☑7th **S52.024** Nondisplaced fracture of olecranon process without intraarticular extension of right ulna

☑7th **S52.025** Nondisplaced fracture of olecranon process without intraarticular extension of left ulna

☑7th **S52.026** Nondisplaced fracture of olecranon ▽ process without intraarticular extension of unspecified ulna

✓6th **S52.03** Fracture of olecranon process with intraarticular extension of ulna

☑7th **S52.031** Displaced fracture of olecranon process with intraarticular extension of right ulna

☑7th **S52.032** Displaced fracture of olecranon process with intraarticular extension of left ulna

☑7th **S52.033** Displaced fracture of olecranon ▽ process with intraarticular extension of unspecified ulna

☑7th **S52.034** Nondisplaced fracture of olecranon process with intraarticular extension of right ulna

☑7th **S52.035** Nondisplaced fracture of olecranon process with intraarticular extension of left ulna

☑7th **S52.036** Nondisplaced fracture of olecranon ▽ process with intraarticular extension of unspecified ulna

✓6th **S52.04** Fracture of coronoid process of ulna

☑7th **S52.041** Displaced fracture of coronoid process of right ulna

☑7th **S52.042** Displaced fracture of coronoid process of left ulna

☑7th **S52.043** Displaced fracture of coronoid process ▽ of unspecified ulna

☑7th **S52.044** Nondisplaced fracture of coronoid process of right ulna

☑7th **S52.045** Nondisplaced fracture of coronoid process of left ulna

☑7th **S52.046** Nondisplaced fracture of coronoid ▽ process of unspecified ulna

✓6th **S52.09** Other fracture of upper end of ulna

☑7th **S52.091** Other fracture of upper end of right ulna

☑7th **S52.092** Other fracture of upper end of left ulna

☑7th **S52.099** Other fracture of upper end of unspecified ulna

✓5th **S52.1** **Fracture of upper end of radius**
Fracture of proximal end of radius
EXCLUDES 2   physeal fractures of upper end of radius (S59.2-)
fracture of shaft of radius (S52.3-)

✓6th **S52.10** Unspecified fracture of upper end of radius

☑7th **S52.101** Unspecified fracture of upper end of ▽ right radius

☑7th **S52.102** Unspecified fracture of upper end of ▽ left radius

☑7th **S52.109** Unspecified fracture of upper end of ▽ unspecified radius

✓6th **S52.11** Torus fracture of upper end of radius

The appropriate 7th character is to be added to all codes in subcategory S52.11.
A   initial encounter for closed fracture
D   subsequent encounter for fracture with routine healing
G   subsequent encounter for fracture with delayed healing
K   subsequent encounter for fracture with nonunion
P   subsequent encounter for fracture with malunion
S   sequela

☑7th **S52.111** Torus fracture of upper end of right radius

☑7th **S52.112** Torus fracture of upper end of left radius

☑7th **S52.119** Torus fracture of upper end of ▽ unspecified radius

✓6th **S52.12** Fracture of head of radius

☑7th **S52.121** Displaced fracture of head of right radius

☑7th **S52.122** Displaced fracture of head of left radius

☑7th **S52.123** Displaced fracture of head of ▽ unspecified radius

☑7th **S52.124** Nondisplaced fracture of head of right radius

☑7th **S52.125** Nondisplaced fracture of head of left radius

☑7th **S52.126** Nondisplaced fracture of head of ▽ unspecified radius

✓6th **S52.13** Fracture of neck of radius

☑7th **S52.131** Displaced fracture of neck of right radius

☑7th **S52.132** Displaced fracture of neck of left radius

☑7th **S52.133** Displaced fracture of neck of ▽ unspecified radius

☑7th **S52.134** Nondisplaced fracture of neck of right radius

☑7th **S52.135** Nondisplaced fracture of neck of left radius

☑7th **S52.136** Nondisplaced fracture of neck of ▽ unspecified radius

✓6th **S52.18** Other fracture of upper end of radius

☑7th **S52.181** Other fracture of upper end of right radius

☑7th **S52.182** Other fracture of upper end of left radius

☑7th **S52.189** Other fracture of upper end of ▽ unspecified radius

✓5th **S52.2** **Fracture of shaft of ulna**

✓6th **S52.20** Unspecified fracture of shaft of ulna
Fracture of ulna NOS

☑7th **S52.201** Unspecified fracture of shaft of right ▽ ulna

☑7th **S52.202** Unspecified fracture of shaft of left ▽ ulna

☑7th **S52.209** Unspecified fracture of shaft of ▽ unspecified ulna

✓6th **S52.21** Greenstick fracture of shaft of ulna

The appropriate 7th character is to be added to all codes in subcategory S52.21.
A   initial encounter for closed fracture
D   subsequent encounter for fracture with routine healing
G   subsequent encounter for fracture with delayed healing
K   subsequent encounter for fracture with nonunion
P   subsequent encounter for fracture with malunion
S   sequela

☑7th **S52.211** Greenstick fracture of shaft of right ulna

☑7th **S52.212** Greenstick fracture of shaft of left ulna

☑7th **S52.219** Greenstick fracture of shaft of ▽ unspecified ulna

✓6th **S52.22** Transverse fracture of shaft of ulna

☑7th **S52.221** Displaced transverse fracture of shaft of right ulna

☑7th **S52.222** Displaced transverse fracture of shaft of left ulna

☑7th **S52.223** Displaced transverse fracture of shaft ▽ of unspecified ulna

☑7th **S52.224** Nondisplaced transverse fracture of shaft of right ulna

☑7th **S52.225** Nondisplaced transverse fracture of shaft of left ulna

☑7th **S52.226** Nondisplaced transverse fracture of ▽ shaft of unspecified ulna

✓6th **S52.23** Oblique fracture of shaft of ulna

☑7th **S52.231** Displaced oblique fracture of shaft of right ulna

☑7th **S52.232** Displaced oblique fracture of shaft of left ulna

☑7th **S52.233** Displaced oblique fracture of shaft of ▽ unspecified ulna

✓7ᵗʰ **S52.234** Nondisplaced oblique fracture of shaft of right ulna

✓7ᵗʰ **S52.235** Nondisplaced oblique fracture of shaft of left ulna

✓7ᵗʰ **S52.236** Nondisplaced oblique fracture of shaft of unspecified ulna ▽

✓6ᵗʰ **S52.24** Spiral fracture of shaft of ulna

✓7ᵗʰ **S52.241** Displaced spiral fracture of shaft of ulna, right arm

✓7ᵗʰ **S52.242** Displaced spiral fracture of shaft of ulna, left arm

✓7ᵗʰ **S52.243** Displaced spiral fracture of shaft of ulna, unspecified arm ▽

✓7ᵗʰ **S52.244** Nondisplaced spiral fracture of shaft of ulna, right arm

✓7ᵗʰ **S52.245** Nondisplaced spiral fracture of shaft of ulna, left arm

✓7ᵗʰ **S52.246** Nondisplaced spiral fracture of shaft of ulna, unspecified arm ▽

✓6ᵗʰ **S52.25** Comminuted fracture of shaft of ulna

✓7ᵗʰ **S52.251** Displaced comminuted fracture of shaft of ulna, right arm

✓7ᵗʰ **S52.252** Displaced comminuted fracture of shaft of ulna, left arm

✓7ᵗʰ **S52.253** Displaced comminuted fracture of shaft of ulna, unspecified arm ▽

✓7ᵗʰ **S52.254** Nondisplaced comminuted fracture of shaft of ulna, right arm

✓7ᵗʰ **S52.255** Nondisplaced comminuted fracture of shaft of ulna, left arm

✓7ᵗʰ **S52.256** Nondisplaced comminuted fracture of shaft of ulna, unspecified arm ▽

✓6ᵗʰ **S52.26** Segmental fracture of shaft of ulna

✓7ᵗʰ **S52.261** Displaced segmental fracture of shaft of ulna, right arm

✓7ᵗʰ **S52.262** Displaced segmental fracture of shaft of ulna, left arm

✓7ᵗʰ **S52.263** Displaced segmental fracture of shaft of ulna, unspecified arm ▽

✓7ᵗʰ **S52.264** Nondisplaced segmental fracture of shaft of ulna, right arm

✓7ᵗʰ **S52.265** Nondisplaced segmental fracture of shaft of ulna, left arm

✓7ᵗʰ **S52.266** Nondisplaced segmental fracture of shaft of ulna, unspecified arm ▽

✓6ᵗʰ **S52.27** Monteggia's fracture of ulna
Fracture of upper shaft of ulna with dislocation of radial head

✓7ᵗʰ **S52.271** Monteggia's fracture of right ulna

✓7ᵗʰ **S52.272** Monteggia's fracture of left ulna

✓7ᵗʰ **S52.279** Monteggia's fracture of unspecified ulna ▽

✓6ᵗʰ **S52.28** Bent bone of ulna

✓7ᵗʰ **S52.281** Bent bone of right ulna

✓7ᵗʰ **S52.282** Bent bone of left ulna

✓7ᵗʰ **S52.283** Bent bone of unspecified ulna ▽

✓6ᵗʰ **S52.29** Other fracture of shaft of ulna

✓7ᵗʰ **S52.291** Other fracture of shaft of right ulna

✓7ᵗʰ **S52.292** Other fracture of shaft of left ulna

✓7ᵗʰ **S52.299** Other fracture of shaft of unspecified ulna ▽

✓5ᵗʰ **S52.3** Fracture of shaft of radius

✓6ᵗʰ **S52.30** Unspecified fracture of shaft of radius

✓7ᵗʰ **S52.301** Unspecified fracture of shaft of right radius ▽

✓7ᵗʰ **S52.302** Unspecified fracture of shaft of left radius ▽

✓7ᵗʰ **S52.309** Unspecified fracture of shaft of unspecified radius ▽

✓6ᵗʰ **S52.31** Greenstick fracture of shaft of radius

The appropriate 7th character is to be added to all codes in subcategory S52.31.
A   initial encounter for closed fracture
D   subsequent encounter for fracture with routine healing
G   subsequent encounter for fracture with delayed healing
K   subsequent encounter for fracture with nonunion
P   subsequent encounter for fracture with malunion
S   sequela

✓7ᵗʰ **S52.311** Greenstick fracture of shaft of radius, right arm

✓7ᵗʰ **S52.312** Greenstick fracture of shaft of radius, left arm

✓7ᵗʰ **S52.319** Greenstick fracture of shaft of radius, unspecified arm ▽

✓6ᵗʰ **S52.32** Transverse fracture of shaft of radius

✓7ᵗʰ **S52.321** Displaced transverse fracture of shaft of right radius

✓7ᵗʰ **S52.322** Displaced transverse fracture of shaft of left radius

✓7ᵗʰ **S52.323** Displaced transverse fracture of shaft of unspecified radius ▽

✓7ᵗʰ **S52.324** Nondisplaced transverse fracture of shaft of right radius

✓7ᵗʰ **S52.325** Nondisplaced transverse fracture of shaft of left radius

✓7ᵗʰ **S52.326** Nondisplaced transverse fracture of shaft of unspecified radius ▽

✓6ᵗʰ **S52.33** Oblique fracture of shaft of radius

✓7ᵗʰ **S52.331** Displaced oblique fracture of shaft of right radius

✓7ᵗʰ **S52.332** Displaced oblique fracture of shaft of left radius

✓7ᵗʰ **S52.333** Displaced oblique fracture of shaft of unspecified radius ▽

✓7ᵗʰ **S52.334** Nondisplaced oblique fracture of shaft of right radius

✓7ᵗʰ **S52.335** Nondisplaced oblique fracture of shaft of left radius

✓7ᵗʰ **S52.336** Nondisplaced oblique fracture of shaft of unspecified radius ▽

✓6ᵗʰ **S52.34** Spiral fracture of shaft of radius

✓7ᵗʰ **S52.341** Displaced spiral fracture of shaft of radius, right arm

✓7ᵗʰ **S52.342** Displaced spiral fracture of shaft of radius, left arm

✓7ᵗʰ **S52.343** Displaced spiral fracture of shaft of radius, unspecified arm ▽

✓7ᵗʰ **S52.344** Nondisplaced spiral fracture of shaft of radius, right arm

✓7ᵗʰ **S52.345** Nondisplaced spiral fracture of shaft of radius, left arm

✓7ᵗʰ **S52.346** Nondisplaced spiral fracture of shaft of radius, unspecified arm ▽

✓6ᵗʰ **S52.35** Comminuted fracture of shaft of radius

✓7ᵗʰ **S52.351** Displaced comminuted fracture of shaft of radius, right arm

✓7ᵗʰ **S52.352** Displaced comminuted fracture of shaft of radius, left arm

✓7ᵗʰ **S52.353** Displaced comminuted fracture of shaft of radius, unspecified arm ▽

✓7ᵗʰ **S52.354** Nondisplaced comminuted fracture of shaft of radius, right arm

✓7ᵗʰ **S52.355** Nondisplaced comminuted fracture of shaft of radius, left arm

✓7ᵗʰ **S52.356** Nondisplaced comminuted fracture of shaft of radius, unspecified arm ▽

✓6ᵗʰ **S52.36** Segmental fracture of shaft of radius

✓7ᵗʰ **S52.361** Displaced segmental fracture of shaft of radius, right arm

EXCLUDES 1 Not coded here   **EXCLUDES 2** Not included here   N Newborn Age: 0   P Pediatric Age: 0-17   M Maternity Age: 12-55   A Adult Age: 15-124

968   ICD-10-CM 2018

√7ᵗʰ **S52.362** Displaced **segmental fracture of shaft of radius, left arm**

√7ᵗʰ **S52.363** Displaced **segmental fracture of shaft of radius, unspecified arm** ▽

√7ᵗʰ **S52.364** Nondisplaced **segmental fracture of shaft of radius, right arm**

√7ᵗʰ **S52.365** Nondisplaced **segmental fracture of shaft of radius, left arm**

√7ᵗʰ **S52.366** Nondisplaced **segmental fracture of shaft of radius, unspecified arm** ▽

√6ᵗʰ **S52.37** Galeazzi's **fracture**
Fracture of lower shaft of radius with radioulnar joint dislocation

√7ᵗʰ **S52.371** **Galeazzi's fracture of** right **radius**

√7ᵗʰ **S52.372** **Galeazzi's fracture of** left **radius**

√7ᵗʰ **S52.379** **Galeazzi's fracture of unspecified radius** ▽

√6ᵗʰ **S52.38** Bent bone **of radius**

√7ᵗʰ **S52.381** **Bent bone of** right **radius**

√7ᵗʰ **S52.382** **Bent bone of** left **radius**

√7ᵗʰ **S52.389** **Bent bone of unspecified radius** ▽

√6ᵗʰ **S52.39** **Other fracture of shaft of radius**

√7ᵗʰ **S52.391** **Other fracture of shaft of radius,** right **arm**

√7ᵗʰ **S52.392** **Other fracture of shaft of radius,** left **arm**

√7ᵗʰ **S52.399** **Other fracture of shaft of radius, unspecified arm** ▽

√5ᵗʰ **S52.5** **Fracture of** lower end of radius
Fracture of distal end of radius
EXCLUDES 2   *physeal fractures of lower end of radius (S59.2-)*
DEF: Fracture of distal end of radius above the wrist; most commonly caused by fall onto an outstretched hand.

√6ᵗʰ **S52.50** **Unspecified fracture of the lower end of radius**

√7ᵗʰ **S52.501** **Unspecified fracture of the lower end of** right **radius** ▽

√7ᵗʰ **S52.502** **Unspecified fracture of the lower end of** left **radius** ▽

√7ᵗʰ **S52.509** **Unspecified fracture of the lower end of unspecified radius** ▽

√6ᵗʰ **S52.51** **Fracture of** radial styloid process

√7ᵗʰ **S52.511** Displaced **fracture of** right **radial styloid process**

√7ᵗʰ **S52.512** Displaced **fracture of** left **radial styloid process**

√7ᵗʰ **S52.513** Displaced **fracture of unspecified radial styloid process** ▽

√7ᵗʰ **S52.514** Nondisplaced **fracture of** right **radial styloid process**

√7ᵗʰ **S52.515** Nondisplaced **fracture of** left **radial styloid process**

√7ᵗʰ **S52.516** Nondisplaced **fracture of unspecified radial styloid process** ▽

√6ᵗʰ **S52.52** Torus **fracture of lower end of radius**

The appropriate 7th character is to be added to all codes in subcategory S52.52.
A   initial encounter for closed fracture
D   subsequent encounter for fracture with routine healing
G   subsequent encounter for fracture with delayed healing
K   subsequent encounter for fracture with nonunion
P   subsequent encounter for fracture with malunion
S   sequela

√7ᵗʰ **S52.521** **Torus fracture of lower end of** right **radius**

√7ᵗʰ **S52.522** **Torus fracture of lower end of** left **radius**

√7ᵗʰ **S52.529** **Torus fracture of lower end of unspecified radius** ▽

√6ᵗʰ **S52.53** Colles' **fracture**
AHA: 2016, 2Q, 4

√7ᵗʰ **S52.531** **Colles' fracture of** right **radius**

√7ᵗʰ **S52.532** **Colles' fracture of** left **radius**

√7ᵗʰ **S52.539** **Colles' fracture of unspecified radius** ▽

√6ᵗʰ **S52.54** Smith's **fracture**

√7ᵗʰ **S52.541** **Smith's fracture of** right **radius**

√7ᵗʰ **S52.542** **Smith's fracture of** left **radius**

√7ᵗʰ **S52.549** **Smith's fracture of unspecified radius** ▽

√6ᵗʰ **S52.55** **Other** extraarticular **fracture of lower end of radius**

√7ᵗʰ **S52.551** **Other extraarticular fracture of lower end of** right **radius**

√7ᵗʰ **S52.552** **Other extraarticular fracture of lower end of** left **radius**

√7ᵗʰ **S52.559** **Other extraarticular fracture of lower end of unspecified radius** ▽

√6ᵗʰ **S52.56** Barton's **fracture**

√7ᵗʰ **S52.561** **Barton's fracture of** right **radius**

√7ᵗʰ **S52.562** **Barton's fracture of** left **radius**

√7ᵗʰ **S52.569** **Barton's fracture of unspecified radius** ▽

√6ᵗʰ **S52.57** **Other** intraarticular **fracture of lower end of radius**

√7ᵗʰ **S52.571** **Other intraarticular fracture of lower end of** right **radius**

√7ᵗʰ **S52.572** **Other intraarticular fracture of lower end of** left **radius**

√7ᵗʰ **S52.579** **Other intraarticular fracture of lower end of unspecified radius** ▽

√6ᵗʰ **S52.59** **Other fractures of lower end of radius**

√7ᵗʰ **S52.591** **Other fractures of lower end of** right **radius**

√7ᵗʰ **S52.592** **Other fractures of lower end of** left **radius**

√7ᵗʰ **S52.599** **Other fractures of lower end of unspecified radius** ▽

√5ᵗʰ **S52.6** **Fracture of** lower end of ulna

√6ᵗʰ **S52.60** **Unspecified fracture of lower end of ulna**

√7ᵗʰ **S52.601** **Unspecified fracture of lower end of** right **ulna** ▽

√7ᵗʰ **S52.602** **Unspecified fracture of lower end of** left **ulna** ▽

√7ᵗʰ **S52.609** **Unspecified fracture of lower end of unspecified ulna** ▽

√6ᵗʰ **S52.61** **Fracture of ulna** styloid process

√7ᵗʰ **S52.611** Displaced **fracture of** right **ulna styloid process**

√7ᵗʰ **S52.612** Displaced **fracture of** left **ulna styloid process**

√7ᵗʰ **S52.613** Displaced **fracture of unspecified ulna styloid process** ▽

√7ᵗʰ **S52.614** Nondisplaced **fracture of** right **ulna styloid process**

√7ᵗʰ **S52.615** Nondisplaced **fracture of** left **ulna styloid process**

√7ᵗʰ **S52.616** Nondisplaced **fracture of unspecified ulna styloid process** ▽

√6ᵗʰ **S52.62** Torus **fracture of lower end of ulna**

The appropriate 7th character is to be added to all codes in subcategory S52.62.
A   initial encounter for closed fracture
D   subsequent encounter for fracture with routine healing
G   subsequent encounter for fracture with delayed healing
K   subsequent encounter for fracture with nonunion
P   subsequent encounter for fracture with malunion
S   sequela

√7ᵗʰ **S52.621** **Torus fracture of lower end of** right **ulna**

√7ᵗʰ **S52.622** **Torus fracture of lower end of** left **ulna**

√7ᵗʰ **S52.629** **Torus fracture of lower end of unspecified ulna** ▽

√6ᵗʰ **S52.69** **Other fracture of lower end of ulna**

√7ᵗʰ **S52.691** **Other fracture of lower end of** right **ulna**

√7ᵗʰ **S52.692** **Other fracture of lower end of** left **ulna**

√7ᵗʰ **S52.699** **Other fracture of lower end of unspecified ulna** ▽

☑ Additional Character Req   ▨x7ᵗʰ Placeholder Alert   **Manifestation**   **ᴴᶜᶜ** CMS-HCC Condition   ▽ Unspecified Code   ▶◀ Revised Text   ● New Code   ▲ Revised Code Title

✓5ᵗʰ S52.9   Unspecified fracture of forearm

     ✓×7ᵗʰ **S52.90   Unspecified fracture of unspecified forearm** ▽

     ✓×7ᵗʰ **S52.91   Unspecified fracture of right forearm** ▽

     ✓×7ᵗʰ **S52.92   Unspecified fracture of left forearm** ▽

✓4ᵗʰ S53   Dislocation and sprain of joints and ligaments of elbow

     INCLUDES   avulsion of joint or ligament of elbow
                 laceration of cartilage, joint or ligament of elbow
                 sprain of cartilage, joint or ligament of elbow
                 traumatic hemarthrosis of joint or ligament of elbow
                 traumatic rupture of joint or ligament of elbow
                 traumatic subluxation of joint or ligament of elbow
                 traumatic tear of joint or ligament of elbow

     Code also any associated open wound

     EXCLUDES 2   *strain of muscle, fascia and tendon at forearm level (S56.-)*

> The appropriate 7th character is to be added to each code from category S53.
> A   initial encounter
> D   subsequent encounter
> S   sequela

   ✓5ᵗʰ S53.0   Subluxation and dislocation of radial head
       Dislocation of radiohumeral joint
       Subluxation of radiohumeral joint
       EXCLUDES 1   *Monteggia's fracture-dislocation (S52.27-)*

     ✓6ᵗʰ S53.00   Unspecified subluxation and dislocation of radial head

       ✓7ᵗʰ **S53.001   Unspecified subluxation of right radial head** ▽

       ✓7ᵗʰ **S53.002   Unspecified subluxation of left radial head** ▽

       ✓7ᵗʰ **S53.003   Unspecified subluxation of unspecified radial head** ▽

       ✓7ᵗʰ **S53.004   Unspecified dislocation of right radial head** ▽

       ✓7ᵗʰ **S53.005   Unspecified dislocation of left radial head** ▽

       ✓7ᵗʰ **S53.006   Unspecified dislocation of unspecified radial head** ▽

     ✓6ᵗʰ S53.01   Anterior subluxation and dislocation of radial head
       Anteriomedial subluxation and dislocation of radial head

       ✓7ᵗʰ **S53.011   Anterior subluxation of right radial head**

       ✓7ᵗʰ **S53.012   Anterior subluxation of left radial head**

       ✓7ᵗʰ **S53.013   Anterior subluxation of unspecified radial head** ▽

       ✓7ᵗʰ **S53.014   Anterior dislocation of right radial head**

       ✓7ᵗʰ **S53.015   Anterior dislocation of left radial head**

       ✓7ᵗʰ **S53.016   Anterior dislocation of unspecified radial head** ▽

     ✓6ᵗʰ S53.02   Posterior subluxation and dislocation of radial head
       Posteriolateral subluxation and dislocation of radial head

       ✓7ᵗʰ **S53.021   Posterior subluxation of right radial head**

       ✓7ᵗʰ **S53.022   Posterior subluxation of left radial head**

       ✓7ᵗʰ **S53.023   Posterior subluxation of unspecified radial head** ▽

       ✓7ᵗʰ **S53.024   Posterior dislocation of right radial head**

       ✓7ᵗʰ **S53.025   Posterior dislocation of left radial head**

       ✓7ᵗʰ **S53.026   Posterior dislocation of unspecified radial head** ▽

     ✓6ᵗʰ S53.03   Nursemaid's elbow

       ✓7ᵗʰ **S53.031   Nursemaid's elbow, right elbow**

       ✓7ᵗʰ **S53.032   Nursemaid's elbow, left elbow**

       ✓7ᵗʰ **S53.033   Nursemaid's elbow, unspecified elbow** ▽

     ✓6ᵗʰ S53.09   Other subluxation and dislocation of radial head

       ✓7ᵗʰ **S53.091   Other subluxation of right radial head**

       ✓7ᵗʰ **S53.092   Other subluxation of left radial head**

       ✓7ᵗʰ **S53.093   Other subluxation of unspecified radial head** ▽

       ✓7ᵗʰ **S53.094   Other dislocation of right radial head**

       ✓7ᵗʰ **S53.095   Other dislocation of left radial head**

       ✓7ᵗʰ **S53.096   Other dislocation of unspecified radial head** ▽

   ✓5ᵗʰ S53.1   Subluxation and dislocation of ulnohumeral joint
       Subluxation and dislocation of elbow NOS
       EXCLUDES 1   *dislocation of radial head alone (S53.0-)*

     ✓6ᵗʰ S53.10   Unspecified subluxation and dislocation of ulnohumeral joint

       ✓7ᵗʰ **S53.101   Unspecified subluxation of right ulnohumeral joint** ▽

       ✓7ᵗʰ **S53.102   Unspecified subluxation of left ulnohumeral joint** ▽

       ✓7ᵗʰ **S53.103   Unspecified subluxation of unspecified ulnohumeral joint** ▽

       ✓7ᵗʰ **S53.104   Unspecified dislocation of right ulnohumeral joint** ▽

       ✓7ᵗʰ **S53.105   Unspecified dislocation of left ulnohumeral joint** ▽

       ✓7ᵗʰ **S53.106   Unspecified dislocation of unspecified ulnohumeral joint** ▽

     ✓6ᵗʰ S53.11   Anterior subluxation and dislocation of ulnohumeral joint

       ✓7ᵗʰ **S53.111   Anterior subluxation of right ulnohumeral joint**

       ✓7ᵗʰ **S53.112   Anterior subluxation of left ulnohumeral joint**

       ✓7ᵗʰ **S53.113   Anterior subluxation of unspecified ulnohumeral joint** ▽

       ✓7ᵗʰ **S53.114   Anterior dislocation of right ulnohumeral joint**
            AHA: 2012, 4Q, 108

       ✓7ᵗʰ **S53.115   Anterior dislocation of left ulnohumeral joint**

       ✓7ᵗʰ **S53.116   Anterior dislocation of unspecified ulnohumeral joint** ▽

     ✓6ᵗʰ S53.12   Posterior subluxation and dislocation of ulnohumeral joint

       ✓7ᵗʰ **S53.121   Posterior subluxation of right ulnohumeral joint**

       ✓7ᵗʰ **S53.122   Posterior subluxation of left ulnohumeral joint**

       ✓7ᵗʰ **S53.123   Posterior subluxation of unspecified ulnohumeral joint** ▽

       ✓7ᵗʰ **S53.124   Posterior dislocation of right ulnohumeral joint**

       ✓7ᵗʰ **S53.125   Posterior dislocation of left ulnohumeral joint**

       ✓7ᵗʰ **S53.126   Posterior dislocation of unspecified ulnohumeral joint** ▽

     ✓6ᵗʰ S53.13   Medial subluxation and dislocation of ulnohumeral joint

       ✓7ᵗʰ **S53.131   Medial subluxation of right ulnohumeral joint**

       ✓7ᵗʰ **S53.132   Medial subluxation of left ulnohumeral joint**

       ✓7ᵗʰ **S53.133   Medial subluxation of unspecified ulnohumeral joint** ▽

       ✓7ᵗʰ **S53.134   Medial dislocation of right ulnohumeral joint**

       ✓7ᵗʰ **S53.135   Medial dislocation of left ulnohumeral joint**

       ✓7ᵗʰ **S53.136   Medial dislocation of unspecified ulnohumeral joint** ▽

     ✓6ᵗʰ S53.14   Lateral subluxation and dislocation of ulnohumeral joint

       ✓7ᵗʰ **S53.141   Lateral subluxation of right ulnohumeral joint**

       ✓7ᵗʰ **S53.142   Lateral subluxation of left ulnohumeral joint**

       ✓7ᵗʰ **S53.143   Lateral subluxation of unspecified ulnohumeral joint** ▽

       ✓7ᵗʰ **S53.144   Lateral dislocation of right ulnohumeral joint**

       ✓7ᵗʰ **S53.145   Lateral dislocation of left ulnohumeral joint**

       ✓7ᵗʰ **S53.146   Lateral dislocation of unspecified ulnohumeral joint** ▽

EXCLUDES 1 Not coded here   **EXCLUDES 2** Not included here   N Newborn Age: 0   P Pediatric Age: 0-17   M Maternity Age: 12-55   A Adult Age: 15-124

970   ICD-10-CM 2018

√6ᵗʰ **S53.19** **Other subluxation and dislocation of ulnohumeral joint**

√7ᵗʰ **S53.191** **Other** subluxation **of** right **ulnohumeral joint**

√7ᵗʰ **S53.192** **Other** subluxation **of** left **ulnohumeral joint**

√7ᵗʰ **S53.193** **Other** subluxation **of unspecified ulnohumeral joint** ▽

√7ᵗʰ **S53.194** **Other** dislocation **of** right **ulnohumeral joint**

√7ᵗʰ **S53.195** **Other** dislocation **of** left **ulnohumeral joint**

√7ᵗʰ **S53.196** **Other** dislocation **of unspecified ulnohumeral joint** ▽

√5ᵗʰ **S53.2** **Traumatic rupture of** radial collateral ligament

EXCLUDES 1   sprain of radial collateral ligament NOS (S53.43-)

√x7ᵗʰ **S53.20** **Traumatic rupture of unspecified radial collateral ligament** ▽

√x7ᵗʰ **S53.21** **Traumatic rupture of** right **radial collateral ligament**

√x7ᵗʰ **S53.22** **Traumatic rupture of** left **radial collateral ligament**

√5ᵗʰ **S53.3** **Traumatic rupture of** ulnar collateral ligament

EXCLUDES 1   sprain of ulnar collateral ligament (S53.44-)

√x7ᵗʰ **S53.30** **Traumatic rupture of unspecified ulnar collateral ligament** ▽

√x7ᵗʰ **S53.31** **Traumatic rupture of** right **ulnar collateral ligament**

√x7ᵗʰ **S53.32** **Traumatic rupture of** left **ulnar collateral ligament**

√5ᵗʰ **S53.4** **Sprain of** elbow

EXCLUDES 2   traumatic rupture of radial collateral ligament (S53.2-)
traumatic rupture of ulnar collateral ligament (S53.3-)

√6ᵗʰ **S53.40** **Unspecified sprain of elbow**

√7ᵗʰ **S53.401** **Unspecified sprain of** right **elbow** ▽

√7ᵗʰ **S53.402** **Unspecified sprain of** left **elbow** ▽

√7ᵗʰ **S53.409** **Unspecified sprain of unspecified elbow** ▽
Sprain of elbow NOS

√6ᵗʰ **S53.41** Radiohumeral **(joint) sprain**

√7ᵗʰ **S53.411** **Radiohumeral (joint) sprain of** right **elbow**

√7ᵗʰ **S53.412** **Radiohumeral (joint) sprain of** left **elbow**

√7ᵗʰ **S53.419** **Radiohumeral (joint) sprain of unspecified elbow** ▽

√6ᵗʰ **S53.42** Ulnohumeral **(joint) sprain**

√7ᵗʰ **S53.421** **Ulnohumeral (joint) sprain of** right **elbow**

√7ᵗʰ **S53.422** **Ulnohumeral (joint) sprain of** left **elbow**

√7ᵗʰ **S53.429** **Ulnohumeral (joint) sprain of unspecified elbow** ▽

√6ᵗʰ **S53.43** Radial collateral ligament **sprain**

√7ᵗʰ **S53.431** **Radial collateral ligament sprain of** right **elbow**

√7ᵗʰ **S53.432** **Radial collateral ligament sprain of** left **elbow**

√7ᵗʰ **S53.439** **Radial collateral ligament sprain of unspecified elbow** ▽

√6ᵗʰ **S53.44** Ulnar collateral ligament **sprain**

√7ᵗʰ **S53.441** **Ulnar collateral ligament sprain of** right **elbow**

√7ᵗʰ **S53.442** **Ulnar collateral ligament sprain of** left **elbow**

√7ᵗʰ **S53.449** **Ulnar collateral ligament sprain of unspecified elbow** ▽

√6ᵗʰ **S53.49** **Other sprain of elbow**

√7ᵗʰ **S53.491** **Other sprain of** right **elbow**

√7ᵗʰ **S53.492** **Other sprain of** left **elbow**

√7ᵗʰ **S53.499** **Other sprain of unspecified elbow** ▽

√4ᵗʰ **S54** **Injury of nerves at forearm level**

Code also any associated open wound (S51.-)

EXCLUDES 2   injury of nerves at wrist and hand level (S64.-)

The appropriate 7th character is to be added to each code from category S54.
A   initial encounter
D   subsequent encounter
S   sequela

√5ᵗʰ **S54.0** **Injury of** ulnar **nerve at forearm level**
Injury of ulnar nerve NOS

√x7ᵗʰ **S54.00** **Injury of ulnar nerve at forearm level, unspecified arm** ▽

√x7ᵗʰ **S54.01** **Injury of ulnar nerve at forearm level,** right **arm**

√x7ᵗʰ **S54.02** **Injury of ulnar nerve at forearm level,** left **arm**

√5ᵗʰ **S54.1** **Injury of** median **nerve at forearm level**
Injury of median nerve NOS

√x7ᵗʰ **S54.10** **Injury of median nerve at forearm level, unspecified arm** ▽

√x7ᵗʰ **S54.11** **Injury of median nerve at forearm level,** right **arm**

√x7ᵗʰ **S54.12** **Injury of median nerve at forearm level,** left **arm**

√5ᵗʰ **S54.2** **Injury of** radial **nerve at forearm level**
Injury of radial nerve NOS

√x7ᵗʰ **S54.20** **Injury of radial nerve at forearm level, unspecified arm** ▽

√x7ᵗʰ **S54.21** **Injury of radial nerve at forearm level,** right **arm**

√x7ᵗʰ **S54.22** **Injury of radial nerve at forearm level,** left **arm**

√5ᵗʰ **S54.3** **Injury of** cutaneous sensory **nerve at forearm level**

√x7ᵗʰ **S54.30** **Injury of cutaneous sensory nerve at forearm level, unspecified arm** ▽

√x7ᵗʰ **S54.31** **Injury of cutaneous sensory nerve at forearm level,** right **arm**

√x7ᵗʰ **S54.32** **Injury of cutaneous sensory nerve at forearm level,** left **arm**

√5ᵗʰ **S54.8** **Injury of other nerves at forearm level**

√6ᵗʰ **S54.8X** **Injury of other nerves at forearm level**

√7ᵗʰ **S54.8X1** **Injury of other nerves at forearm level,** right **arm**

√7ᵗʰ **S54.8X2** **Injury of other nerves at forearm level,** left **arm**

√7ᵗʰ **S54.8X9** **Injury of other nerves at forearm level,** ▽
unspecified **arm**

√5ᵗʰ **S54.9** **Injury of unspecified nerve at forearm level**

√x7ᵗʰ **S54.90** **Injury of unspecified nerve at forearm level, unspecified arm** ▽

√x7ᵗʰ **S54.91** **Injury of unspecified nerve at forearm level,** right **arm** ▽

√x7ᵗʰ **S54.92** **Injury of unspecified nerve at forearm level,** left **arm** ▽

√4ᵗʰ **S55** **Injury of blood vessels at forearm level**

Code also any associated open wound (S51.-)

EXCLUDES 2   injury of blood vessels at wrist and hand level (S65.-)
injury of brachial vessels (S45.1-S45.2)

The appropriate 7th character is to be added to each code from category S55.
A   initial encounter
D   subsequent encounter
S   sequela

√5ᵗʰ **S55.0** **Injury of** ulnar artery **at forearm level**

√6ᵗʰ **S55.00** **Unspecified injury of ulnar artery at forearm level**

√7ᵗʰ **S55.001** **Unspecified injury of ulnar artery at forearm level,** right **arm** ▽

√7ᵗʰ **S55.002** **Unspecified injury of ulnar artery at forearm level,** left **arm** ▽

√7ᵗʰ **S55.009** **Unspecified injury of ulnar artery at forearm level, unspecified arm** ▽

√6ᵗʰ **S55.01** Laceration **of ulnar artery at forearm level**

√7ᵗʰ **S55.011** **Laceration of ulnar artery at forearm level,** right **arm**

√7ᵗʰ **S55.012** **Laceration of ulnar artery at forearm level,** left **arm**

√7ᵗʰ **S55.019** **Laceration of ulnar artery at forearm level, unspecified arm** ▽

☑ Additional Character Req   √x7ᵗʰ Placeholder Alert   **Manifestation**   **HCC** CMS-HCC Condition   ▽ Unspecified Code   ►◄ Revised Text   ● New Code   ▲ Revised Code Title

✓6ᵗʰ S55.09   Other specified injury of ulnar artery at forearm level

    ✓7ᵗʰ   S55.091   Other specified injury of ulnar artery at forearm level, **right** arm

    ✓7ᵗʰ   S55.092   Other specified injury of ulnar artery at forearm level, **left** arm

    ✓7ᵗʰ   S55.099   Other specified injury of ulnar artery at forearm level, unspecified arm ▽

✓5ᵗʰ S55.1   Injury of radial artery at forearm level

   ✓6ᵗʰ S55.10   Unspecified injury of radial artery at forearm level

    ✓7ᵗʰ   S55.101   Unspecified injury of radial artery at forearm level, **right** arm ▽

    ✓7ᵗʰ   S55.102   Unspecified injury of radial artery at forearm level, **left** arm ▽

    ✓7ᵗʰ   S55.109   Unspecified injury of radial artery at forearm level, unspecified arm ▽

   ✓6ᵗʰ S55.11   Laceration of radial artery at forearm level

    ✓7ᵗʰ   S55.111   Laceration of radial artery at forearm level, **right** arm

    ✓7ᵗʰ   S55.112   Laceration of radial artery at forearm level, **left** arm

    ✓7ᵗʰ   S55.119   Laceration of radial artery at forearm level, unspecified arm

   ✓6ᵗʰ S55.19   Other specified injury of radial artery at forearm level

    ✓7ᵗʰ   S55.191   Other specified injury of radial artery at forearm level, **right** arm

    ✓7ᵗʰ   S55.192   Other specified injury of radial artery at forearm level, **left** arm

    ✓7ᵗʰ   S55.199   Other specified injury of radial artery at forearm level, unspecified arm ▽

✓5ᵗʰ S55.2   Injury of vein at forearm level

   ✓6ᵗʰ S55.20   Unspecified injury of vein at forearm level

    ✓7ᵗʰ   S55.201   Unspecified injury of vein at forearm level, **right** arm ▽

    ✓7ᵗʰ   S55.202   Unspecified injury of vein at forearm level, **left** arm ▽

    ✓7ᵗʰ   S55.209   Unspecified injury of vein at forearm level, unspecified arm ▽

   ✓6ᵗʰ S55.21   Laceration of vein at forearm level

    ✓7ᵗʰ   S55.211   Laceration of vein at forearm level, **right** arm

    ✓7ᵗʰ   S55.212   Laceration of vein at forearm level, **left** arm

    ✓7ᵗʰ   S55.219   Laceration of vein at forearm level, unspecified arm ▽

   ✓6ᵗʰ S55.29   Other specified injury of vein at forearm level

    ✓7ᵗʰ   S55.291   Other specified injury of vein at forearm level, **right** arm

    ✓7ᵗʰ   S55.292   Other specified injury of vein at forearm level, **left** arm

    ✓7ᵗʰ   S55.299   Other specified injury of vein at forearm level, unspecified arm ▽

✓5ᵗʰ S55.8   Injury of other blood vessels at forearm level

   ✓6ᵗʰ S55.80   Unspecified injury of other blood vessels at forearm level

    ✓7ᵗʰ   S55.801   Unspecified injury of other blood vessels at forearm level, **right** arm ▽

    ✓7ᵗʰ   S55.802   Unspecified injury of other blood vessels at forearm level, **left** arm ▽

    ✓7ᵗʰ   S55.809   Unspecified injury of other blood vessels at forearm level, unspecified arm ▽

   ✓6ᵗʰ S55.81   Laceration of other blood vessels at forearm level

    ✓7ᵗʰ   S55.811   Laceration of other blood vessels at forearm level, **right** arm

    ✓7ᵗʰ   S55.812   Laceration of other blood vessels at forearm level, **left** arm

    ✓7ᵗʰ   S55.819   Laceration of other blood vessels at forearm level, unspecified arm ▽

   ✓6ᵗʰ S55.89   Other specified injury of other blood vessels at forearm level

    ✓7ᵗʰ   S55.891   Other specified injury of other blood vessels at forearm level, **right** arm

    ✓7ᵗʰ   S55.892   Other specified injury of other blood vessels at forearm level, **left** arm

    ✓7ᵗʰ   S55.899   Other specified injury of other blood vessels at forearm level, unspecified arm ▽

✓5ᵗʰ S55.9   Injury of unspecified blood vessel at forearm level

   ✓6ᵗʰ S55.90   Unspecified injury of unspecified blood vessel at forearm level

    ✓7ᵗʰ   S55.901   Unspecified injury of unspecified blood vessel at forearm level, **right** arm ▽

    ✓7ᵗʰ   S55.902   Unspecified injury of unspecified blood vessel at forearm level, **left** arm ▽

    ✓7ᵗʰ   S55.909   Unspecified injury of unspecified blood vessel at forearm level, unspecified arm ▽

   ✓6ᵗʰ S55.91   Laceration of unspecified blood vessel at forearm level

    ✓7ᵗʰ   S55.911   Laceration of unspecified blood vessel at forearm level, **right** arm ▽

    ✓7ᵗʰ   S55.912   Laceration of unspecified blood vessel at forearm level, **left** arm ▽

    ✓7ᵗʰ   S55.919   Laceration of unspecified blood vessel at forearm level, unspecified arm ▽

   ✓6ᵗʰ S55.99   Other specified injury of unspecified blood vessel at forearm level

    ✓7ᵗʰ   S55.991   Other specified injury of unspecified blood vessel at forearm level, **right** arm ▽

    ✓7ᵗʰ   S55.992   Other specified injury of unspecified blood vessel at forearm level, **left** arm ▽

    ✓7ᵗʰ   S55.999   Other specified injury of unspecified blood vessel at forearm level, unspecified arm ▽

✓4ᵗʰ S56   Injury of muscle, fascia and tendon at forearm level

Code also any associated open wound (S51.-)

EXCLUDES 2   *injury of muscle, fascia and tendon at or below wrist (S66.-)*
               sprain of joints and ligaments of elbow (S53.4-)

TIP: Refer to the Muscle/Tendon table at the beginning of this chapter.

The appropriate 7th character is to be added to each code from category S56.
A   initial encounter
D   subsequent encounter
S   sequela

✓5ᵗʰ S56.0   Injury of flexor muscle, fascia and tendon of thumb at forearm level

   ✓6ᵗʰ S56.00   Unspecified injury of flexor muscle, fascia and tendon of thumb at forearm level

    ✓7ᵗʰ   S56.001   Unspecified injury of flexor muscle, fascia and tendon of **right thumb** at forearm level ▽

    ✓7ᵗʰ   S56.002   Unspecified injury of flexor muscle, fascia and tendon of **left thumb** at forearm level ▽

    ✓7ᵗʰ   S56.009   Unspecified injury of flexor muscle, fascia and tendon of unspecified thumb at forearm level ▽

   ✓6ᵗʰ S56.01   Strain of flexor muscle, fascia and tendon of thumb at forearm level

    ✓7ᵗʰ   S56.011   Strain of flexor muscle, fascia and tendon of **right thumb** at forearm level

    ✓7ᵗʰ   S56.012   Strain of flexor muscle, fascia and tendon of **left thumb** at forearm level

    ✓7ᵗʰ   S56.019   Strain of flexor muscle, fascia and tendon of unspecified thumb at forearm level ▽

   ✓6ᵗʰ S56.02   Laceration of flexor muscle, fascia and tendon of thumb at forearm level

    ✓7ᵗʰ   S56.021   Laceration of flexor muscle, fascia and tendon of **right thumb** at forearm level

    ✓7ᵗʰ   S56.022   Laceration of flexor muscle, fascia and tendon of **left thumb** at forearm level

    ✓7ᵗʰ   S56.029   Laceration of flexor muscle, fascia and tendon of unspecified thumb at forearm level ▽

   ✓6ᵗʰ S56.09   Other injury of flexor muscle, fascia and tendon of thumb at forearm level

    ✓7ᵗʰ   S56.091   Other injury of flexor muscle, fascia and tendon of **right thumb** at forearm level

EXCLUDES 1 Not coded here   *EXCLUDES 2* Not included here   **N** Newborn Age: 0   **P** Pediatric Age: 0-17   **M** Maternity Age: 12-55   **A** Adult Age: 15-124

972   ICD-10-CM 2018

Chapter 19. Injury, Poisoning, and Certain Other Consequences of External Causes

☑7ᵗʰ **S56.092** **Other injury of flexor muscle, fascia and tendon of** left thumb **at forearm level**

☑7ᵗʰ **S56.099** **Other injury of flexor muscle, fascia and tendon of unspecified thumb at forearm level** ▽

✓5ᵗʰ **S56.1** **Injury of** flexor **muscle, fascia and tendon of other and unspecified** finger **at forearm level**

✓6ᵗʰ **S56.10** **Unspecified injury of flexor muscle, fascia and tendon of other and unspecified finger at forearm level**

☑7ᵗʰ **S56.101** **Unspecified injury of flexor muscle, fascia and tendon of** right index finger **at forearm level** ▽

☑7ᵗʰ **S56.102** **Unspecified injury of flexor muscle, fascia and tendon of** left index finger **at forearm level** ▽

☑7ᵗʰ **S56.103** **Unspecified injury of flexor muscle, fascia and tendon of** right middle finger **at forearm level** ▽

☑7ᵗʰ **S56.104** **Unspecified injury of flexor muscle, fascia and tendon of** left middle finger **at forearm level** ▽

☑7ᵗʰ **S56.105** **Unspecified injury of flexor muscle, fascia and tendon of** right ring finger **at forearm level** ▽

☑7ᵗʰ **S56.106** **Unspecified injury of flexor muscle, fascia and tendon of** left ring finger **at forearm level** ▽

☑7ᵗʰ **S56.107** **Unspecified injury of flexor muscle, fascia and tendon of** right little finger **at forearm level** ▽

☑7ᵗʰ **S56.108** **Unspecified injury of flexor muscle, fascia and tendon of** left little finger **at forearm level** ▽

☑7ᵗʰ **S56.109** **Unspecified injury of flexor muscle, fascia and tendon of unspecified finger at forearm level** ▽

✓6ᵗʰ **S56.11** Strain **of flexor muscle, fascia and tendon of other and unspecified** finger **at forearm level**

☑7ᵗʰ **S56.111** **Strain of flexor muscle, fascia and tendon of** right index finger **at forearm level**

☑7ᵗʰ **S56.112** **Strain of flexor muscle, fascia and tendon of** left index finger **at forearm level**

☑7ᵗʰ **S56.113** **Strain of flexor muscle, fascia and tendon of** right middle finger **at forearm level**

☑7ᵗʰ **S56.114** **Strain of flexor muscle, fascia and tendon of** left middle finger **at forearm level**

☑7ᵗʰ **S56.115** **Strain of flexor muscle, fascia and tendon of** right ring finger **at forearm level**

☑7ᵗʰ **S56.116** **Strain of flexor muscle, fascia and tendon of** left ring finger **at forearm level**

☑7ᵗʰ **S56.117** **Strain of flexor muscle, fascia and tendon of** right little finger **at forearm level**

☑7ᵗʰ **S56.118** **Strain of flexor muscle, fascia and tendon of** left little finger **at forearm level**

☑7ᵗʰ **S56.119** **Strain of flexor muscle, fascia and tendon of finger of unspecified finger at forearm level** ▽

✓6ᵗʰ **S56.12** Laceration **of flexor muscle, fascia and tendon of other and unspecified** finger **at forearm level**

☑7ᵗʰ **S56.121** **Laceration of flexor muscle, fascia and tendon of** right index finger **at forearm level**

☑7ᵗʰ **S56.122** **Laceration of flexor muscle, fascia and tendon of** left index finger **at forearm level**

☑7ᵗʰ **S56.123** **Laceration of flexor muscle, fascia and tendon of** right middle finger **at forearm level**

☑7ᵗʰ **S56.124** **Laceration of flexor muscle, fascia and tendon of** left middle finger **at forearm level**

☑7ᵗʰ **S56.125** **Laceration of flexor muscle, fascia and tendon of** right ring finger **at forearm level**

☑7ᵗʰ **S56.126** **Laceration of flexor muscle, fascia and tendon of** left ring finger **at forearm level**

☑7ᵗʰ **S56.127** **Laceration of flexor muscle, fascia and tendon of** right little finger **at forearm level**

☑7ᵗʰ **S56.128** **Laceration of flexor muscle, fascia and tendon of** left little finger **at forearm level**

☑7ᵗʰ **S56.129** **Laceration of flexor muscle, fascia and tendon of unspecified finger at forearm level** ▽

✓6ᵗʰ **S56.19** **Other injury of flexor muscle, fascia and tendon of other and unspecified finger at forearm level**

☑7ᵗʰ **S56.191** **Other injury of flexor muscle, fascia and tendon of** right index finger **at forearm level**

☑7ᵗʰ **S56.192** **Other injury of flexor muscle, fascia and tendon of** left index finger **at forearm level**

☑7ᵗʰ **S56.193** **Other injury of flexor muscle, fascia and tendon of** right middle finger **at forearm level**

☑7ᵗʰ **S56.194** **Other injury of flexor muscle, fascia and tendon of** left middle finger **at forearm level**

☑7ᵗʰ **S56.195** **Other injury of flexor muscle, fascia and tendon of** right ring finger **at forearm level**

☑7ᵗʰ **S56.196** **Other injury of flexor muscle, fascia and tendon of** left ring finger **at forearm level**

☑7ᵗʰ **S56.197** **Other injury of flexor muscle, fascia and tendon of** right little finger **at forearm level**

☑7ᵗʰ **S56.198** **Other injury of flexor muscle, fascia and tendon of** left little finger **at forearm level**

☑7ᵗʰ **S56.199** **Other injury of flexor muscle, fascia and tendon of unspecified finger at forearm level** ▽

✓5ᵗʰ **S56.2** **Injury of other flexor muscle, fascia and tendon at forearm level**

✓6ᵗʰ **S56.20** **Unspecified injury of other flexor muscle, fascia and tendon at forearm level**

☑7ᵗʰ **S56.201** **Unspecified injury of other flexor muscle, fascia and tendon at forearm level,** right arm ▽

☑7ᵗʰ **S56.202** **Unspecified injury of other flexor muscle, fascia and tendon at forearm level,** left arm ▽

☑7ᵗʰ **S56.209** **Unspecified injury of other flexor muscle, fascia and tendon at forearm level, unspecified arm** ▽

✓6ᵗʰ **S56.21** Strain **of other flexor muscle, fascia and tendon at forearm level**

☑7ᵗʰ **S56.211** **Strain of other flexor muscle, fascia and tendon at forearm level,** right arm

☑7ᵗʰ **S56.212** **Strain of other flexor muscle, fascia and tendon at forearm level,** left arm

☑7ᵗʰ **S56.219** **Strain of other flexor muscle, fascia and tendon at forearm level, unspecified arm** ▽

✓6ᵗʰ **S56.22** Laceration **of other flexor muscle, fascia and tendon at forearm level**

☑7ᵗʰ **S56.221** **Laceration of other flexor muscle, fascia and tendon at forearm level,** right arm

☑7ᵗʰ **S56.222** **Laceration of other flexor muscle, fascia and tendon at forearm level,** left arm

☑7ᵗʰ **S56.229** **Laceration of other flexor muscle, fascia and tendon at forearm level, unspecified arm** ▽

✓6ᵗʰ **S56.29** **Other injury of other flexor muscle, fascia and tendon at forearm level**

☑7ᵗʰ **S56.291** **Other injury of other flexor muscle, fascia and tendon at forearm level,** right arm

☑7ᵗʰ **S56.292** **Other injury of other flexor muscle, fascia and tendon at forearm level,** left arm

☑7ᵗʰ **S56.299** **Other injury of other flexor muscle, fascia and tendon at forearm level, unspecified arm** ▽

☑ Additional Character Req   ☑7ᵗʰ Placeholder Alert   Manifestation   HCC CMS-HCC Condition   ▽ Unspecified Code   ►◄ Revised Text   ● New Code   ▲ Revised Code Title

✓5ᵗʰ **S56.3** **Injury of** extensor or abductor **muscles, fascia and tendons of** thumb **at forearm level**

  ✓6ᵗʰ **S56.30** **Unspecified injury of extensor or abductor muscles, fascia and tendons of thumb at forearm level**

    ✓7ᵗʰ **S56.301** **Unspecified injury of extensor or abductor muscles, fascia and tendons of** right thumb **at forearm level** ▽

    ✓7ᵗʰ **S56.302** **Unspecified injury of extensor or abductor muscles, fascia and tendons of** left thumb **at forearm level** ▽

    ✓7ᵗʰ **S56.309** **Unspecified injury of extensor or abductor muscles, fascia and tendons of unspecified thumb at forearm level** ▽

  ✓6ᵗʰ **S56.31** **Strain of extensor or abductor muscles, fascia and tendons of thumb at forearm level**

    ✓7ᵗʰ **S56.311** **Strain of extensor or abductor muscles, fascia and tendons of** right thumb **at forearm level**

    ✓7ᵗʰ **S56.312** **Strain of extensor or abductor muscles, fascia and tendons of** left thumb **at forearm level**

    ✓7ᵗʰ **S56.319** **Strain of extensor or abductor muscles, fascia and tendons of unspecified thumb at forearm level** ▽

  ✓6ᵗʰ **S56.32** **Laceration of extensor or abductor muscles, fascia and tendons of thumb at forearm level**

    ✓7ᵗʰ **S56.321** **Laceration of extensor or abductor muscles, fascia and tendons of** right thumb **at forearm level**

    ✓7ᵗʰ **S56.322** **Laceration of extensor or abductor muscles, fascia and tendons of** left thumb **at forearm level**

    ✓7ᵗʰ **S56.329** **Laceration of extensor or abductor muscles, fascia and tendons of unspecified thumb at forearm level** ▽

  ✓6ᵗʰ **S56.39** **Other injury of extensor or abductor muscles, fascia and tendons of thumb at forearm level**

    ✓7ᵗʰ **S56.391** **Other injury of extensor or abductor muscles, fascia and tendons of** right thumb **at forearm level**

    ✓7ᵗʰ **S56.392** **Other injury of extensor or abductor muscles, fascia and tendons of** left thumb **at forearm level**

    ✓7ᵗʰ **S56.399** **Other injury of extensor or abductor muscles, fascia and tendons of unspecified thumb at forearm level** ▽

✓5ᵗʰ **S56.4** **Injury of** extensor **muscle, fascia and tendon of other and unspecified** finger **at forearm level**

  ✓6ᵗʰ **S56.40** **Unspecified injury of extensor muscle, fascia and tendon of other and unspecified finger at forearm level**

    ✓7ᵗʰ **S56.401** **Unspecified injury of extensor muscle, fascia and tendon of** right index finger **at forearm level** ▽

    ✓7ᵗʰ **S56.402** **Unspecified injury of extensor muscle, fascia and tendon of** left index finger **at forearm level** ▽

    ✓7ᵗʰ **S56.403** **Unspecified injury of extensor muscle, fascia and tendon of** right middle finger **at forearm level** ▽

    ✓7ᵗʰ **S56.404** **Unspecified injury of extensor muscle, fascia and tendon of** left middle finger **at forearm level** ▽

    ✓7ᵗʰ **S56.405** **Unspecified injury of extensor muscle, fascia and tendon of** right ring finger **at forearm level** ▽

    ✓7ᵗʰ **S56.406** **Unspecified injury of extensor muscle, fascia and tendon of** left ring finger **at forearm level** ▽

    ✓7ᵗʰ **S56.407** **Unspecified injury of extensor muscle, fascia and tendon of** right little finger **at forearm level** ▽

    ✓7ᵗʰ **S56.408** **Unspecified injury of extensor muscle, fascia and tendon of** left little finger **at forearm level** ▽

    ✓7ᵗʰ **S56.409** **Unspecified injury of extensor muscle, fascia and tendon of unspecified finger at forearm level** ▽

✓6ᵗʰ **S56.41** **Strain of extensor muscle, fascia and tendon of other and unspecified finger at forearm level**

    ✓7ᵗʰ **S56.411** **Strain of extensor muscle, fascia and tendon of** right index finger **at forearm level**

    ✓7ᵗʰ **S56.412** **Strain of extensor muscle, fascia and tendon of** left index finger **at forearm level**

    ✓7ᵗʰ **S56.413** **Strain of extensor muscle, fascia and tendon of** right middle finger **at forearm level**

    ✓7ᵗʰ **S56.414** **Strain of extensor muscle, fascia and tendon of** left middle finger **at forearm level**

    ✓7ᵗʰ **S56.415** **Strain of extensor muscle, fascia and tendon of** right ring finger **at forearm level**

    ✓7ᵗʰ **S56.416** **Strain of extensor muscle, fascia and tendon of** left ring finger **at forearm level**

    ✓7ᵗʰ **S56.417** **Strain of extensor muscle, fascia and tendon of** right little finger **at forearm level**

    ✓7ᵗʰ **S56.418** **Strain of extensor muscle, fascia and tendon of** left little finger **at forearm level**

    ✓7ᵗʰ **S56.419** **Strain of extensor muscle, fascia and tendon of finger, unspecified finger at forearm level** ▽

✓6ᵗʰ **S56.42** **Laceration of extensor muscle, fascia and tendon of other and unspecified finger at forearm level**

    ✓7ᵗʰ **S56.421** **Laceration of extensor muscle, fascia and tendon of** right index finger **at forearm level**

    ✓7ᵗʰ **S56.422** **Laceration of extensor muscle, fascia and tendon of** left index finger **at forearm level**

    ✓7ᵗʰ **S56.423** **Laceration of extensor muscle, fascia and tendon of** right middle finger **at forearm level**

    ✓7ᵗʰ **S56.424** **Laceration of extensor muscle, fascia and tendon of** left middle finger **at forearm level**

    ✓7ᵗʰ **S56.425** **Laceration of extensor muscle, fascia and tendon of** right ring finger **at forearm level**

    ✓7ᵗʰ **S56.426** **Laceration of extensor muscle, fascia and tendon of** left ring finger **at forearm level**

    ✓7ᵗʰ **S56.427** **Laceration of extensor muscle, fascia and tendon of** right little finger **at forearm level**

    ✓7ᵗʰ **S56.428** **Laceration of extensor muscle, fascia and tendon of** left little finger **at forearm level**

    ✓7ᵗʰ **S56.429** **Laceration of extensor muscle, fascia and tendon of unspecified finger at forearm level** ▽

✓6ᵗʰ **S56.49** **Other injury of extensor muscle, fascia and tendon of other and unspecified finger at forearm level**

    ✓7ᵗʰ **S56.491** **Other injury of extensor muscle, fascia and tendon of** right index finger **at forearm level**

    ✓7ᵗʰ **S56.492** **Other injury of extensor muscle, fascia and tendon of** left index finger **at forearm level**

    ✓7ᵗʰ **S56.493** **Other injury of extensor muscle, fascia and tendon of** right middle finger **at forearm level**

    ✓7ᵗʰ **S56.494** **Other injury of extensor muscle, fascia and tendon of** left middle finger **at forearm level**

    ✓7ᵗʰ **S56.495** **Other injury of extensor muscle, fascia and tendon of** right ring finger **at forearm level**

    ✓7ᵗʰ **S56.496** **Other injury of extensor muscle, fascia and tendon of** left ring finger **at forearm level**

    ✓7ᵗʰ **S56.497** **Other injury of extensor muscle, fascia and tendon of** right little finger **at forearm level**

    ✓7ᵗʰ **S56.498** **Other injury of extensor muscle, fascia and tendon of** left little finger **at forearm level**

    ✓7ᵗʰ **S56.499** **Other injury of extensor muscle, fascia and tendon of unspecified finger at forearm level** ▽

EXCLUDES 1 Not coded here   **EXCLUDES 2** Not included here   **N** Newborn Age: 0   **P** Pediatric Age: 0-17   **M** Maternity Age: 12-55   **A** Adult Age: 15-124

✓5ᵗʰ **S56.5** **Injury of other extensor muscle, fascia and tendon at** forearm **level**

   ✓6ᵗʰ **S56.50** **Unspecified injury of other extensor muscle, fascia and tendon at forearm level**

      ✓7ᵗʰ **S56.501** **Unspecified injury of other extensor muscle, fascia and tendon at forearm level,** right **arm** ▽

      ✓7ᵗʰ **S56.502** **Unspecified injury of other extensor muscle, fascia and tendon at forearm level,** left **arm** ▽

      ✓7ᵗʰ **S56.509** **Unspecified injury of other extensor muscle, fascia and tendon at forearm level, unspecified arm** ▽

   ✓6ᵗʰ **S56.51** Strain **of other extensor muscle, fascia and tendon at forearm level**

      ✓7ᵗʰ **S56.511** **Strain of other extensor muscle, fascia and tendon at forearm level,** right **arm**

      ✓7ᵗʰ **S56.512** **Strain of other extensor muscle, fascia and tendon at forearm level,** left **arm**

      ✓7ᵗʰ **S56.519** **Strain of other extensor muscle, fascia and tendon at forearm level, unspecified arm** ▽

   ✓6ᵗʰ **S56.52** Laceration **of other extensor muscle, fascia and tendon at forearm level**

      ✓7ᵗʰ **S56.521** **Laceration of other extensor muscle, fascia and tendon at forearm level,** right **arm**

      ✓7ᵗʰ **S56.522** **Laceration of other extensor muscle, fascia and tendon at forearm level,** left **arm**

      ✓7ᵗʰ **S56.529** **Laceration of other extensor muscle, fascia and tendon at forearm level, unspecified arm** ▽

   ✓6ᵗʰ **S56.59** **Other injury of other extensor muscle, fascia and tendon at forearm level**

      ✓7ᵗʰ **S56.591** **Other injury of other extensor muscle, fascia and tendon at forearm level,** right **arm**

      ✓7ᵗʰ **S56.592** **Other injury of other extensor muscle, fascia and tendon at forearm level,** left **arm**

      ✓7ᵗʰ **S56.599** **Other injury of other extensor muscle, fascia and tendon at forearm level, unspecified arm** ▽

✓5ᵗʰ **S56.8** **Injury of other muscles, fascia and tendons at forearm level**

   ✓6ᵗʰ **S56.80** **Unspecified injury of other muscles, fascia and tendons at forearm level**

      ✓7ᵗʰ **S56.801** **Unspecified injury of other muscles, fascia and tendons at forearm level,** right **arm** ▽

      ✓7ᵗʰ **S56.802** **Unspecified injury of other muscles, fascia and tendons at forearm level,** left **arm** ▽

      ✓7ᵗʰ **S56.809** **Unspecified injury of other muscles, fascia and tendons at forearm level, unspecified arm** ▽

   ✓6ᵗʰ **S56.81** Strain **of other muscles, fascia and tendons at forearm level**

      ✓7ᵗʰ **S56.811** **Strain of other muscles, fascia and tendons at forearm level,** right **arm**

      ✓7ᵗʰ **S56.812** **Strain of other muscles, fascia and tendons at forearm level,** left **arm**

      ✓7ᵗʰ **S56.819** **Strain of other muscles, fascia and tendons at forearm level, unspecified arm** ▽

   ✓6ᵗʰ **S56.82** Laceration **of other muscles, fascia and tendons at forearm level**

      ✓7ᵗʰ **S56.821** **Laceration of other muscles, fascia and tendons at forearm level,** right **arm**

      ✓7ᵗʰ **S56.822** **Laceration of other muscles, fascia and tendons at forearm level,** left **arm**

      ✓7ᵗʰ **S56.829** **Laceration of other muscles, fascia and tendons at forearm level, unspecified arm** ▽

   ✓6ᵗʰ **S56.89** **Other injury of other muscles, fascia and tendons at forearm level**

      ✓7ᵗʰ **S56.891** **Other injury of other muscles, fascia and tendons at forearm level,** right **arm**

      ✓7ᵗʰ **S56.892** **Other injury of other muscles, fascia and tendons at forearm level,** left **arm**

      ✓7ᵗʰ **S56.899** **Other injury of other muscles, fascia and tendons at forearm level, unspecified arm**

✓5ᵗʰ **S56.9** **Injury of unspecified muscles, fascia and tendons at** forearm **level**

   ✓6ᵗʰ **S56.90** **Unspecified injury of unspecified muscles, fascia and tendons at forearm level**

      ✓7ᵗʰ **S56.901** **Unspecified injury of unspecified muscles, fascia and tendons at forearm level,** right **arm** ▽

      ✓7ᵗʰ **S56.902** **Unspecified injury of unspecified muscles, fascia and tendons at forearm level,** left **arm** ▽

      ✓7ᵗʰ **S56.909** **Unspecified injury of unspecified muscles, fascia and tendons at forearm level, unspecified arm** ▽

   ✓6ᵗʰ **S56.91** Strain **of unspecified muscles, fascia and tendons at forearm level**

      ✓7ᵗʰ **S56.911** **Strain of unspecified muscles, fascia and tendons at forearm level,** right **arm** ▽

      ✓7ᵗʰ **S56.912** **Strain of unspecified muscles, fascia and tendons at forearm level,** left **arm** ▽

      ✓7ᵗʰ **S56.919** **Strain of unspecified muscles, fascia and tendons at forearm level, unspecified arm** ▽

   ✓6ᵗʰ **S56.92** Laceration **of unspecified muscles, fascia and tendons at forearm level**

      ✓7ᵗʰ **S56.921** **Laceration of unspecified muscles, fascia and tendons at forearm level,** right **arm** ▽

      ✓7ᵗʰ **S56.922** **Laceration of unspecified muscles, fascia and tendons at forearm level,** left **arm** ▽

      ✓7ᵗʰ **S56.929** **Laceration of unspecified muscles, fascia and tendons at forearm level, unspecified arm** ▽

   ✓6ᵗʰ **S56.99** **Other injury of unspecified muscles, fascia and tendons at forearm level**

      ✓7ᵗʰ **S56.991** **Other injury of unspecified muscles, fascia and tendons at forearm level,** right **arm** ▽

      ✓7ᵗʰ **S56.992** **Other injury of unspecified muscles, fascia and tendons at forearm level,** left **arm** ▽

      ✓7ᵗʰ **S56.999** **Other injury of unspecified muscles, fascia and tendons at forearm level, unspecified arm** ▽

✓4ᵗʰ **S57** **Crushing injury of elbow and forearm**

   Use additional code(s) for all associated injuries

   EXCLUDES 2   *crushing injury of wrist and hand (S67.-)*

   The appropriate 7th character is to be added to each code from category S57.
   A   initial encounter
   D   subsequent encounter
   S   sequela

   ✓5ᵗʰ **S57.0** **Crushing injury of** elbow

      ✓x7ᵗʰ **S57.00** **Crushing injury of unspecified elbow** ▽

      ✓x7ᵗʰ **S57.01** **Crushing injury of** right **elbow**

      ✓x7ᵗʰ **S57.02** **Crushing injury of** left **elbow**

   ✓5ᵗʰ **S57.8** **Crushing injury of** forearm

      ✓x7ᵗʰ **S57.80** **Crushing injury of unspecified forearm** ▽

      ✓x7ᵗʰ **S57.81** **Crushing injury of** right **forearm**

      ✓x7ᵗʰ **S57.82** **Crushing injury of** left **forearm**

☑ Additional Character Req   ✓x7ᵗʰ Placeholder Alert   Manifestation   HCC CMS-HCC Condition   ▽ Unspecified Code   ▶◀ Revised Text   ● New Code   ▲ Revised Code Title

✓4ᵗʰ S58 Traumatic amputation of elbow and forearm
     An amputation not identified as partial or complete should be coded to complete.
     EXCLUDES 1   traumatic amputation of wrist and hand (S68.-)

> The appropriate 7th character is to be added to each code from category S58.
> A   initial encounter
> D   subsequent encounter
> S   sequela

✓5ᵗʰ **S58.0 Traumatic amputation at elbow level**
     ✓6ᵗʰ **S58.01 Complete traumatic amputation at elbow level**
         2 ✓7ᵗʰ **S58.011** Complete traumatic amputation at elbow level, right arm   HCC
         2 ✓7ᵗʰ **S58.012** Complete traumatic amputation at elbow level, left arm   HCC
         2 ✓7ᵗʰ **S58.019** Complete traumatic amputation at elbow level, unspecified arm   HCC ▽
     ✓6ᵗʰ **S58.02 Partial traumatic amputation at elbow level**
         2 ✓7ᵗʰ **S58.021** Partial traumatic amputation at elbow level, right arm   HCC
         2 ✓7ᵗʰ **S58.022** Partial traumatic amputation at elbow level, left arm   HCC
         2 ✓7ᵗʰ **S58.029** Partial traumatic amputation at elbow level, unspecified arm   HCC ▽

✓5ᵗʰ **S58.1 Traumatic amputation at level between elbow and wrist**
     ✓6ᵗʰ **S58.11 Complete traumatic amputation at level between elbow and wrist**
         2 ✓7ᵗʰ **S58.111** Complete traumatic amputation at level between elbow and wrist, right arm   HCC
         2 ✓7ᵗʰ **S58.112** Complete traumatic amputation at level between elbow and wrist, left arm   HCC
         2 ✓7ᵗʰ **S58.119** Complete traumatic amputation at level between elbow and wrist, unspecified arm   HCC ▽
     ✓6ᵗʰ **S58.12 Partial traumatic amputation at level between elbow and wrist**
         2 ✓7ᵗʰ **S58.121** Partial traumatic amputation at level between elbow and wrist, right arm   HCC
         2 ✓7ᵗʰ **S58.122** Partial traumatic amputation at level between elbow and wrist, left arm   HCC
         2 ✓7ᵗʰ **S58.129** Partial traumatic amputation at level between elbow and wrist, unspecified arm   HCC ▽

✓5ᵗʰ **S58.9 Traumatic amputation of forearm, level unspecified**
     EXCLUDES 1   traumatic amputation of wrist (S68.-)
     ✓6ᵗʰ **S58.91 Complete traumatic amputation of forearm, level unspecified**
         2 ✓7ᵗʰ **S58.911** Complete traumatic amputation of right forearm, level unspecified   HCC ▽
         2 ✓7ᵗʰ **S58.912** Complete traumatic amputation of left forearm, level unspecified   HCC ▽
         2 ✓7ᵗʰ **S58.919** Complete traumatic amputation of unspecified forearm, level unspecified   HCC ▽
     ✓6ᵗʰ **S58.92 Partial traumatic amputation of forearm, level unspecified**
         2 ✓7ᵗʰ **S58.921** Partial traumatic amputation of right forearm, level unspecified   HCC ▽
         2 ✓7ᵗʰ **S58.922** Partial traumatic amputation of left forearm, level unspecified   HCC ▽
         2 ✓7ᵗʰ **S58.929** Partial traumatic amputation of unspecified forearm, level unspecified   HCC ▽

✓4ᵗʰ S59 Other and unspecified injuries of elbow and forearm
     EXCLUDES 2   other and unspecified injuries of wrist and hand (S69.-)
     AHA: 2015, 3Q, 37-39

> The appropriate 7th character is to be added to each code from subcategories S59.0, S59.1, and S59.2.
> A   initial encounter for closed fracture
> D   subsequent encounter for fracture with routine healing
> G   subsequent encounter for fracture with delayed healing
> K   subsequent encounter for fracture with nonunion
> P   subsequent encounter for fracture with malunion
> S   sequela

✓5ᵗʰ **S59.0 Physeal fracture of lower end of ulna**
     ✓6ᵗʰ **S59.00 Unspecified physeal fracture of lower end of ulna**
         ✓7ᵗʰ **S59.001** Unspecified physeal fracture of lower end of ulna, right arm ▽
         ✓7ᵗʰ **S59.002** Unspecified physeal fracture of lower end of ulna, left arm ▽
         ✓7ᵗʰ **S59.009** Unspecified physeal fracture of lower end of ulna, unspecified arm ▽
     ✓6ᵗʰ **S59.01 Salter-Harris Type I physeal fracture of lower end of ulna**
         ✓7ᵗʰ **S59.011** Salter-Harris Type I physeal fracture of lower end of ulna, right arm
         ✓7ᵗʰ **S59.012** Salter-Harris Type I physeal fracture of lower end of ulna, left arm
         ✓7ᵗʰ **S59.019** Salter-Harris Type I physeal fracture of lower end of ulna, unspecified arm ▽
     ✓6ᵗʰ **S59.02 Salter-Harris Type II physeal fracture of lower end of ulna**
         ✓7ᵗʰ **S59.021** Salter-Harris Type II physeal fracture of lower end of ulna, right arm
         ✓7ᵗʰ **S59.022** Salter-Harris Type II physeal fracture of lower end of ulna, left arm
         ✓7ᵗʰ **S59.029** Salter-Harris Type II physeal fracture of lower end of ulna, unspecified arm ▽
     ✓6ᵗʰ **S59.03 Salter-Harris Type III physeal fracture of lower end of ulna**
         ✓7ᵗʰ **S59.031** Salter-Harris Type III physeal fracture of lower end of ulna, right arm
         ✓7ᵗʰ **S59.032** Salter-Harris Type III physeal fracture of lower end of ulna, left arm
         ✓7ᵗʰ **S59.039** Salter-Harris Type III physeal fracture of lower end of ulna, unspecified arm ▽
     ✓6ᵗʰ **S59.04 Salter-Harris Type IV physeal fracture of lower end of ulna**
         ✓7ᵗʰ **S59.041** Salter-Harris Type IV physeal fracture of lower end of ulna, right arm
         ✓7ᵗʰ **S59.042** Salter-Harris Type IV physeal fracture of lower end of ulna, left arm
         ✓7ᵗʰ **S59.049** Salter-Harris Type IV physeal fracture of lower end of ulna, unspecified arm ▽
     ✓6ᵗʰ **S59.09 Other physeal fracture of lower end of ulna**
         ✓7ᵗʰ **S59.091** Other physeal fracture of lower end of ulna, right arm
         ✓7ᵗʰ **S59.092** Other physeal fracture of lower end of ulna, left arm
         ✓7ᵗʰ **S59.099** Other physeal fracture of lower end of ulna, unspecified arm ▽

✓5ᵗʰ **S59.1 Physeal fracture of upper end of radius**
     ✓6ᵗʰ **S59.10 Unspecified physeal fracture of upper end of radius**
         ✓7ᵗʰ **S59.101** Unspecified physeal fracture of upper end of radius, right arm ▽
         ✓7ᵗʰ **S59.102** Unspecified physeal fracture of upper end of radius, left arm ▽
         ✓7ᵗʰ **S59.109** Unspecified physeal fracture of upper end of radius, unspecified arm ▽
     ✓6ᵗʰ **S59.11 Salter-Harris Type I physeal fracture of upper end of radius**
         ✓7ᵗʰ **S59.111** Salter-Harris Type I physeal fracture of upper end of radius, right arm
         ✓7ᵗʰ **S59.112** Salter-Harris Type I physeal fracture of upper end of radius, left arm
         ✓7ᵗʰ **S59.119** Salter-Harris Type I physeal fracture of upper end of radius, unspecified arm ▽

---

2   HCC with 7th character indicating initial encounter (A or B - specific to category) OR sequela.

EXCLUDES 1 Not coded here   *EXCLUDES 2* Not included here   N Newborn Age: 0   P Pediatric Age: 0-17   M Maternity Age: 12-55   A Adult Age: 15-124

976   ICD-10-CM 2018

√6ᵗʰ **S59.12** Salter-Harris Type II physeal fracture of upper end of radius

   √7ᵗʰ **S59.121** Salter-Harris Type II physeal fracture of upper end of radius, right arm

   √7ᵗʰ **S59.122** Salter-Harris Type II physeal fracture of upper end of radius, left arm

   √7ᵗʰ **S59.129** Salter-Harris Type II physeal fracture of upper end of radius, unspecified arm ▽

√6ᵗʰ **S59.13** Salter-Harris Type III physeal fracture of upper end of radius

   √7ᵗʰ **S59.131** Salter-Harris Type III physeal fracture of upper end of radius, right arm

   √7ᵗʰ **S59.132** Salter-Harris Type III physeal fracture of upper end of radius, left arm

   √7ᵗʰ **S59.139** Salter-Harris Type III physeal fracture of upper end of radius, unspecified arm ▽

√6ᵗʰ **S59.14** Salter-Harris Type IV physeal fracture of upper end of radius

   √7ᵗʰ **S59.141** Salter-Harris Type IV physeal fracture of upper end of radius, right arm

   √7ᵗʰ **S59.142** Salter-Harris Type IV physeal fracture of upper end of radius, left arm

   √7ᵗʰ **S59.149** Salter-Harris Type IV physeal fracture of upper end of radius, unspecified arm ▽

√6ᵗʰ **S59.19** Other physeal fracture of upper end of radius

   √7ᵗʰ **S59.191** Other physeal fracture of upper end of radius, right arm

   √7ᵗʰ **S59.192** Other physeal fracture of upper end of radius, left arm

   √7ᵗʰ **S59.199** Other physeal fracture of upper end of radius, unspecified arm ▽

√5ᵗʰ **S59.2** Physeal fracture of lower end of radius

√6ᵗʰ **S59.20** Unspecified physeal fracture of lower end of radius

   √7ᵗʰ **S59.201** Unspecified physeal fracture of lower end of radius, right arm ▽

   √7ᵗʰ **S59.202** Unspecified physeal fracture of lower end of radius, left arm ▽

   √7ᵗʰ **S59.209** Unspecified physeal fracture of lower end of radius, unspecified arm ▽

√6ᵗʰ **S59.21** Salter-Harris Type I physeal fracture of lower end of radius

   √7ᵗʰ **S59.211** Salter-Harris Type I physeal fracture of lower end of radius, right arm

   √7ᵗʰ **S59.212** Salter-Harris Type I physeal fracture of lower end of radius, left arm

   √7ᵗʰ **S59.219** Salter-Harris Type I physeal fracture of lower end of radius, unspecified arm ▽

√6ᵗʰ **S59.22** Salter-Harris Type II physeal fracture of lower end of radius

   √7ᵗʰ **S59.221** Salter-Harris Type II physeal fracture of lower end of radius, right arm

   √7ᵗʰ **S59.222** Salter-Harris Type II physeal fracture of lower end of radius, left arm

   √7ᵗʰ **S59.229** Salter-Harris Type II physeal fracture of lower end of radius, unspecified arm ▽

√6ᵗʰ **S59.23** Salter-Harris Type III physeal fracture of lower end of radius

   √7ᵗʰ **S59.231** Salter-Harris Type III physeal fracture of lower end of radius, right arm

   √7ᵗʰ **S59.232** Salter-Harris Type III physeal fracture of lower end of radius, left arm

   √7ᵗʰ **S59.239** Salter-Harris Type III physeal fracture of lower end of radius, unspecified arm ▽

√6ᵗʰ **S59.24** Salter-Harris Type IV physeal fracture of lower end of radius

   √7ᵗʰ **S59.241** Salter-Harris Type IV physeal fracture of lower end of radius, right arm

   √7ᵗʰ **S59.242** Salter-Harris Type IV physeal fracture of lower end of radius, left arm

   √7ᵗʰ **S59.249** Salter-Harris Type IV physeal fracture of lower end of radius, unspecified arm ▽

√6ᵗʰ **S59.29** Other physeal fracture of lower end of radius

   √7ᵗʰ **S59.291** Other physeal fracture of lower end of radius, right arm

   √7ᵗʰ **S59.292** Other physeal fracture of lower end of radius, left arm

   √7ᵗʰ **S59.299** Other physeal fracture of lower end of radius, unspecified arm ▽

√5ᵗʰ **S59.8** Other specified injuries of elbow and forearm

> The appropriate 7th character is to be added to each code in subcategory S59.8.
> A   initial encounter
> D   subsequent encounter
> S   sequela

√6ᵗʰ **S59.80** Other specified injuries of elbow

   √7ᵗʰ **S59.801** Other specified injuries of right elbow

   √7ᵗʰ **S59.802** Other specified injuries of left elbow

   √7ᵗʰ **S59.809** Other specified injuries of unspecified elbow ▽

√6ᵗʰ **S59.81** Other specified injuries of forearm

   √7ᵗʰ **S59.811** Other specified injuries right forearm

   √7ᵗʰ **S59.812** Other specified injuries left forearm

   √7ᵗʰ **S59.819** Other specified injuries unspecified forearm ▽

√5ᵗʰ **S59.9** Unspecified injury of elbow and forearm

> The appropriate 7th character is to be added to each code in subcategory S59.9.
> A   initial encounter
> D   subsequent encounter
> S   sequela

√6ᵗʰ **S59.90** Unspecified injury of elbow

   √7ᵗʰ **S59.901** Unspecified injury of right elbow ▽

   √7ᵗʰ **S59.902** Unspecified injury of left elbow ▽

   √7ᵗʰ **S59.909** Unspecified injury of unspecified elbow ▽

√6ᵗʰ **S59.91** Unspecified injury of forearm

   √7ᵗʰ **S59.911** Unspecified injury of right forearm ▽

   √7ᵗʰ **S59.912** Unspecified injury of left forearm ▽

   √7ᵗʰ **S59.919** Unspecified injury of unspecified forearm ▽

Injuries to the wrist, hand and fingers (S60-S69)

EXCLUDES 2   burns and corrosions (T20-T32)
   frostbite (T33-T34)
   insect bite or sting, venomous (T63.4)

√4ᵗʰ **S60** Superficial injury of wrist, hand and fingers

> The appropriate 7th character is to be added to each code from category S60.
> A   initial encounter
> D   subsequent encounter
> S   sequela

√5ᵗʰ **S60.0** Contusion of finger without damage to nail

   EXCLUDES 1   contusion involving nail (matrix) (S60.1)

√ₓ7ᵗʰ **S60.00** Contusion of unspecified finger without damage to nail ▽
   Contusion of finger(s) NOS

√6ᵗʰ **S60.01** Contusion of thumb without damage to nail

   √7ᵗʰ **S60.011** Contusion of right thumb without damage to nail

   √7ᵗʰ **S60.012** Contusion of left thumb without damage to nail

   √7ᵗʰ **S60.019** Contusion of unspecified thumb without damage to nail ▽

√6ᵗʰ **S60.02** Contusion of index finger without damage to nail

   √7ᵗʰ **S60.021** Contusion of right index finger without damage to nail

   √7ᵗʰ **S60.022** Contusion of left index finger without damage to nail

   √7ᵗʰ **S60.029** Contusion of unspecified index finger without damage to nail ▽

√6ᵗʰ **S60.03** Contusion of middle finger without damage to nail

   √7ᵗʰ **S60.031** Contusion of right middle finger without damage to nail

   √7ᵗʰ **S60.032** Contusion of left middle finger without damage to nail

☑ Additional Character Req   √ₓ7ᵗʰ Placeholder Alert   Manifestation   HCC CMS-HCC Condition   ▽ Unspecified Code   ►◄ Revised Text   ● New Code   ▲ Revised Code Title

ICD-10-CM 2018   977

Chapter 19. Injury, Poisoning, and Certain Other Consequences of External Causes

S60.039–S60.445

√7ᵗʰ **S60.039** Contusion of unspecified middle finger without damage to nail ▽

√6ᵗʰ **S60.04** Contusion of ring finger without damage to nail

     √7ᵗʰ **S60.041** Contusion of right ring finger without damage to nail

     √7ᵗʰ **S60.042** Contusion of left ring finger without damage to nail

     √7ᵗʰ **S60.049** Contusion of unspecified ring finger without damage to nail ▽

√6ᵗʰ **S60.05** Contusion of little finger without damage to nail

     √7ᵗʰ **S60.051** Contusion of right little finger without damage to nail

     √7ᵗʰ **S60.052** Contusion of left little finger without damage to nail

     √7ᵗʰ **S60.059** Contusion of unspecified little finger without damage to nail ▽

√5ᵗʰ **S60.1** Contusion of finger with damage to nail

√x7ᵗʰ **S60.10** Contusion of unspecified finger with damage to nail ▽

√6ᵗʰ **S60.11** Contusion of thumb with damage to nail

     √7ᵗʰ **S60.111** Contusion of right thumb with damage to nail

     √7ᵗʰ **S60.112** Contusion of left thumb with damage to nail

     √7ᵗʰ **S60.119** Contusion of unspecified thumb with damage to nail ▽

√6ᵗʰ **S60.12** Contusion of index finger with damage to nail

     √7ᵗʰ **S60.121** Contusion of right index finger with damage to nail

     √7ᵗʰ **S60.122** Contusion of left index finger with damage to nail

     √7ᵗʰ **S60.129** Contusion of unspecified index finger with damage to nail ▽

√6ᵗʰ **S60.13** Contusion of middle finger with damage to nail

     √7ᵗʰ **S60.131** Contusion of right middle finger with damage to nail

     √7ᵗʰ **S60.132** Contusion of left middle finger with damage to nail

     √7ᵗʰ **S60.139** Contusion of unspecified middle finger with damage to nail ▽

√6ᵗʰ **S60.14** Contusion of ring finger with damage to nail

     √7ᵗʰ **S60.141** Contusion of right ring finger with damage to nail

     √7ᵗʰ **S60.142** Contusion of left ring finger with damage to nail

     √7ᵗʰ **S60.149** Contusion of unspecified ring finger with damage to nail ▽

√6ᵗʰ **S60.15** Contusion of little finger with damage to nail

     √7ᵗʰ **S60.151** Contusion of right little finger with damage to nail

     √7ᵗʰ **S60.152** Contusion of left little finger with damage to nail

     √7ᵗʰ **S60.159** Contusion of unspecified little finger with damage to nail ▽

√5ᵗʰ **S60.2** Contusion of wrist and hand

     EXCLUDES 2 contusion of fingers (S60.0-, S60.1-)

√6ᵗʰ **S60.21** Contusion of wrist

     √7ᵗʰ **S60.211** Contusion of right wrist

     √7ᵗʰ **S60.212** Contusion of left wrist

     √7ᵗʰ **S60.219** Contusion of unspecified wrist ▽

√6ᵗʰ **S60.22** Contusion of hand

     √7ᵗʰ **S60.221** Contusion of right hand

     √7ᵗʰ **S60.222** Contusion of left hand

     √7ᵗʰ **S60.229** Contusion of unspecified hand ▽

√5ᵗʰ **S60.3** Other superficial injuries of thumb

√6ᵗʰ **S60.31** Abrasion of thumb

     √7ᵗʰ **S60.311** Abrasion of right thumb

     √7ᵗʰ **S60.312** Abrasion of left thumb

     √7ᵗʰ **S60.319** Abrasion of unspecified thumb ▽

√6ᵗʰ **S60.32** Blister (nonthermal) of thumb

     √7ᵗʰ **S60.321** Blister (nonthermal) of right thumb

     √7ᵗʰ **S60.322** Blister (nonthermal) of left thumb

√7ᵗʰ **S60.329** Blister (nonthermal) of unspecified thumb ▽

√6ᵗʰ **S60.34** External constriction of thumb
     Hair tourniquet syndrome of thumb
     Use additional cause code to identify the constricting item (W49.0-)

     √7ᵗʰ **S60.341** External constriction of right thumb

     √7ᵗʰ **S60.342** External constriction of left thumb

     √7ᵗʰ **S60.349** External constriction of unspecified thumb ▽

√6ᵗʰ **S60.35** Superficial foreign body of thumb
     Splinter in the thumb

     √7ᵗʰ **S60.351** Superficial foreign body of right thumb

     √7ᵗʰ **S60.352** Superficial foreign body of left thumb

     √7ᵗʰ **S60.359** Superficial foreign body of unspecified thumb ▽

√6ᵗʰ **S60.36** Insect bite (nonvenomous) of thumb

     √7ᵗʰ **S60.361** Insect bite (nonvenomous) of right thumb

     √7ᵗʰ **S60.362** Insect bite (nonvenomous) of left thumb

     √7ᵗʰ **S60.369** Insect bite (nonvenomous) of unspecified thumb ▽

√6ᵗʰ **S60.37** Other superficial bite of thumb
     EXCLUDES 1 open bite of thumb (S61.05-, S61.15-)

     √7ᵗʰ **S60.371** Other superficial bite of right thumb

     √7ᵗʰ **S60.372** Other superficial bite of left thumb

     √7ᵗʰ **S60.379** Other superficial bite of unspecified thumb ▽

√6ᵗʰ **S60.39** Other superficial injuries of thumb

     √7ᵗʰ **S60.391** Other superficial injuries of right thumb

     √7ᵗʰ **S60.392** Other superficial injuries of left thumb

     √7ᵗʰ **S60.399** Other superficial injuries of unspecified thumb ▽

√5ᵗʰ **S60.4** Other superficial injuries of other fingers

√6ᵗʰ **S60.41** Abrasion of fingers

     √7ᵗʰ **S60.410** Abrasion of right index finger

     √7ᵗʰ **S60.411** Abrasion of left index finger

     √7ᵗʰ **S60.412** Abrasion of right middle finger

     √7ᵗʰ **S60.413** Abrasion of left middle finger

     √7ᵗʰ **S60.414** Abrasion of right ring finger

     √7ᵗʰ **S60.415** Abrasion of left ring finger

     √7ᵗʰ **S60.416** Abrasion of right little finger

     √7ᵗʰ **S60.417** Abrasion of left little finger

     √7ᵗʰ **S60.418** Abrasion of other finger
       Abrasion of specified finger with unspecified laterality

     √7ᵗʰ **S60.419** Abrasion of unspecified finger ▽

√6ᵗʰ **S60.42** Blister (nonthermal) of fingers

     √7ᵗʰ **S60.420** Blister (nonthermal) of right index finger

     √7ᵗʰ **S60.421** Blister (nonthermal) of left index finger

     √7ᵗʰ **S60.422** Blister (nonthermal) of right middle finger

     √7ᵗʰ **S60.423** Blister (nonthermal) of left middle finger

     √7ᵗʰ **S60.424** Blister (nonthermal) of right ring finger

     √7ᵗʰ **S60.425** Blister (nonthermal) of left ring finger

     √7ᵗʰ **S60.426** Blister (nonthermal) of right little finger

     √7ᵗʰ **S60.427** Blister (nonthermal) of left little finger

     √7ᵗʰ **S60.428** Blister (nonthermal) of other finger
       Blister (nonthermal) of specified finger with unspecified laterality

     √7ᵗʰ **S60.429** Blister (nonthermal) of unspecified finger ▽

√6ᵗʰ **S60.44** External constriction of fingers
     Hair tourniquet syndrome of finger
     Use additional cause code to identify the constricting item (W49.0-)

     √7ᵗʰ **S60.440** External constriction of right index finger

     √7ᵗʰ **S60.441** External constriction of left index finger

     √7ᵗʰ **S60.442** External constriction of right middle finger

     √7ᵗʰ **S60.443** External constriction of left middle finger

     √7ᵗʰ **S60.444** External constriction of right ring finger

     √7ᵗʰ **S60.445** External constriction of left ring finger

---

EXCLUDES 1 Not coded here   **EXCLUDES 2** Not included here   **N** Newborn Age: 0   **P** Pediatric Age: 0-17   **M** Maternity Age: 12-55   **A** Adult Age: 15-124

√7ᵗʰ **S60.446** External constriction of right little finger

√7ᵗʰ **S60.447** External constriction of left little finger

√7ᵗʰ **S60.448** External constriction of other finger
External constriction of specified finger with unspecified laterality

√7ᵗʰ **S60.449** External constriction of unspecified finger ▽

√6ᵗʰ **S60.45** Superficial foreign body of fingers
Splinter in the finger(s)

√7ᵗʰ **S60.450** Superficial foreign body of right index finger

√7ᵗʰ **S60.451** Superficial foreign body of left index finger

√7ᵗʰ **S60.452** Superficial foreign body of right middle finger

√7ᵗʰ **S60.453** Superficial foreign body of left middle finger

√7ᵗʰ **S60.454** Superficial foreign body of right ring finger

√7ᵗʰ **S60.455** Superficial foreign body of left ring finger

√7ᵗʰ **S60.456** Superficial foreign body of right little finger

√7ᵗʰ **S60.457** Superficial foreign body of left little finger

√7ᵗʰ **S60.458** Superficial foreign body of other finger
Superficial foreign body of specified finger with unspecified laterality

√7ᵗʰ **S60.459** Superficial foreign body of unspecified finger ▽

√6ᵗʰ **S60.46** Insect bite (nonvenomous) of fingers

√7ᵗʰ **S60.460** Insect bite (nonvenomous) of right index finger

√7ᵗʰ **S60.461** Insect bite (nonvenomous) of left index finger

√7ᵗʰ **S60.462** Insect bite (nonvenomous) of right middle finger

√7ᵗʰ **S60.463** Insect bite (nonvenomous) of left middle finger

√7ᵗʰ **S60.464** Insect bite (nonvenomous) of right ring finger

√7ᵗʰ **S60.465** Insect bite (nonvenomous) of left ring finger

√7ᵗʰ **S60.466** Insect bite (nonvenomous) of right little finger

√7ᵗʰ **S60.467** Insect bite (nonvenomous) of left little finger

√7ᵗʰ **S60.468** Insect bite (nonvenomous) of other finger
Insect bite (nonvenomous) of specified finger with unspecified laterality

√7ᵗʰ **S60.469** Insect bite (nonvenomous) of unspecified finger ▽

√6ᵗʰ **S60.47** Other superficial bite of fingers
EXCLUDES 1   open bite of fingers (S61.25-, S61.35-)

√7ᵗʰ **S60.470** Other superficial bite of right index finger

√7ᵗʰ **S60.471** Other superficial bite of left index finger

√7ᵗʰ **S60.472** Other superficial bite of right middle finger

√7ᵗʰ **S60.473** Other superficial bite of left middle finger

√7ᵗʰ **S60.474** Other superficial bite of right ring finger

√7ᵗʰ **S60.475** Other superficial bite of left ring finger

√7ᵗʰ **S60.476** Other superficial bite of right little finger

√7ᵗʰ **S60.477** Other superficial bite of left little finger

√7ᵗʰ **S60.478** Other superficial bite of other finger
Other superficial bite of specified finger with unspecified laterality

√7ᵗʰ **S60.479** Other superficial bite of unspecified finger ▽

√5ᵗʰ **S60.5** Other superficial injuries of hand
EXCLUDES 2   superficial injuries of fingers (S60.3-, S60.4-)

√6ᵗʰ **S60.51** Abrasion of hand

√7ᵗʰ **S60.511** Abrasion of right hand

√7ᵗʰ **S60.512** Abrasion of left hand

√7ᵗʰ **S60.519** Abrasion of unspecified hand ▽

√6ᵗʰ **S60.52** Blister (nonthermal) of hand

√7ᵗʰ **S60.521** Blister (nonthermal) of right hand

√7ᵗʰ **S60.522** Blister (nonthermal) of left hand

√7ᵗʰ **S60.529** Blister (nonthermal) of unspecified hand ▽

√6ᵗʰ **S60.54** External constriction of hand

√7ᵗʰ **S60.541** External constriction of right hand

√7ᵗʰ **S60.542** External constriction of left hand

√7ᵗʰ **S60.549** External constriction of unspecified hand ▽

√6ᵗʰ **S60.55** Superficial foreign body of hand
Splinter in the hand

√7ᵗʰ **S60.551** Superficial foreign body of right hand

√7ᵗʰ **S60.552** Superficial foreign body of left hand

√7ᵗʰ **S60.559** Superficial foreign body of unspecified hand ▽

√6ᵗʰ **S60.56** Insect bite (nonvenomous) of hand

√7ᵗʰ **S60.561** Insect bite (nonvenomous) of right hand

√7ᵗʰ **S60.562** Insect bite (nonvenomous) of left hand

√7ᵗʰ **S60.569** Insect bite (nonvenomous) of unspecified hand ▽

√6ᵗʰ **S60.57** Other superficial bite of hand
EXCLUDES 1   open bite of hand (S61.45-)

√7ᵗʰ **S60.571** Other superficial bite of hand of right hand

√7ᵗʰ **S60.572** Other superficial bite of hand of left hand

√7ᵗʰ **S60.579** Other superficial bite of hand of unspecified hand ▽

√5ᵗʰ **S60.8** Other superficial injuries of wrist

√6ᵗʰ **S60.81** Abrasion of wrist

√7ᵗʰ **S60.811** Abrasion of right wrist

√7ᵗʰ **S60.812** Abrasion of left wrist

√7ᵗʰ **S60.819** Abrasion of unspecified wrist ▽

√6ᵗʰ **S60.82** Blister (nonthermal) of wrist

√7ᵗʰ **S60.821** Blister (nonthermal) of right wrist

√7ᵗʰ **S60.822** Blister (nonthermal) of left wrist

√7ᵗʰ **S60.829** Blister (nonthermal) of unspecified wrist ▽

√6ᵗʰ **S60.84** External constriction of wrist

√7ᵗʰ **S60.841** External constriction of right wrist

√7ᵗʰ **S60.842** External constriction of left wrist

√7ᵗʰ **S60.849** External constriction of unspecified wrist ▽

√6ᵗʰ **S60.85** Superficial foreign body of wrist
Splinter in the wrist

√7ᵗʰ **S60.851** Superficial foreign body of right wrist

√7ᵗʰ **S60.852** Superficial foreign body of left wrist

√7ᵗʰ **S60.859** Superficial foreign body of unspecified wrist ▽

√6ᵗʰ **S60.86** Insect bite (nonvenomous) of wrist

√7ᵗʰ **S60.861** Insect bite (nonvenomous) of right wrist

√7ᵗʰ **S60.862** Insect bite (nonvenomous) of left wrist

√7ᵗʰ **S60.869** Insect bite (nonvenomous) of unspecified wrist ▽

√6ᵗʰ **S60.87** Other superficial bite of wrist
EXCLUDES 1   open bite of wrist (S61.55)

√7ᵗʰ **S60.871** Other superficial bite of right wrist

√7ᵗʰ **S60.872** Other superficial bite of left wrist

√7ᵗʰ **S60.879** Other superficial bite of unspecified wrist ▽

√5ᵗʰ **S60.9** Unspecified superficial injury of wrist, hand and fingers

√6ᵗʰ **S60.91** Unspecified superficial injury of wrist

√7ᵗʰ **S60.911** Unspecified superficial injury of right wrist ▽

√7ᵗʰ **S60.912** Unspecified superficial injury of left wrist ▽

√7ᵗʰ **S60.919** Unspecified superficial injury of unspecified wrist ▽

√6ᵗʰ **S60.92** Unspecified superficial injury of hand

√7ᵗʰ **S60.921** Unspecified superficial injury of right hand ▽

☑ Additional Character Req   √x7ᵗʰ Placeholder Alert   Manifestation   HCC CMS-HCC Condition   ▽ Unspecified Code   ►◄ Revised Text   ● New Code   ▲ Revised Code Title

Chapter 19. Injury, Poisoning, and Certain Other Consequences of External Causes

✓7ᵗʰ **S60.922** Unspecified superficial injury of left hand ▽

✓7ᵗʰ **S60.929** Unspecified superficial injury of unspecified hand ▽

✓6ᵗʰ **S60.93** Unspecified superficial injury of thumb

    ✓7ᵗʰ **S60.931** Unspecified superficial injury of right thumb ▽

    ✓7ᵗʰ **S60.932** Unspecified superficial injury of left thumb ▽

    ✓7ᵗʰ **S60.939** Unspecified superficial injury of unspecified thumb ▽

✓6ᵗʰ **S60.94** Unspecified superficial injury of other fingers

    ✓7ᵗʰ **S60.940** Unspecified superficial injury of right index finger ▽

    ✓7ᵗʰ **S60.941** Unspecified superficial injury of left index finger ▽

    ✓7ᵗʰ **S60.942** Unspecified superficial injury of right middle finger ▽

    ✓7ᵗʰ **S60.943** Unspecified superficial injury of left middle finger ▽

    ✓7ᵗʰ **S60.944** Unspecified superficial injury of right ring finger ▽

    ✓7ᵗʰ **S60.945** Unspecified superficial injury of left ring finger ▽

    ✓7ᵗʰ **S60.946** Unspecified superficial injury of right little finger ▽

    ✓7ᵗʰ **S60.947** Unspecified superficial injury of left little finger ▽

    ✓7ᵗʰ **S60.948** Unspecified superficial injury of other finger ▽
         Unspecified superficial injury of specified finger with unspecified laterality

    ✓7ᵗʰ **S60.949** Unspecified superficial injury of unspecified finger ▽

✓4ᵗʰ **S61** Open wound of wrist, hand and fingers
    Code also any associated wound infection
    EXCLUDES 1   open fracture of wrist, hand and finger (S62- with 7th character B)
            traumatic amputation of wrist and hand (S68.-)

> The appropriate 7th character is to be added to each code from category S61.
> A   initial encounter
> D   subsequent encounter
> S   sequela

✓5ᵗʰ **S61.0** Open wound of thumb without damage to nail
    EXCLUDES 1   open wound of thumb with damage to nail (S61.1-)

  ✓6ᵗʰ **S61.00** Unspecified open wound of thumb without damage to nail

    ✓7ᵗʰ **S61.001** Unspecified open wound of right thumb without damage to nail ▽

    ✓7ᵗʰ **S61.002** Unspecified open wound of left thumb without damage to nail ▽

    ✓7ᵗʰ **S61.009** Unspecified open wound of unspecified thumb without damage to nail ▽

  ✓6ᵗʰ **S61.01** Laceration without foreign body of thumb without damage to nail

    ✓7ᵗʰ **S61.011** Laceration without foreign body of right thumb without damage to nail

    ✓7ᵗʰ **S61.012** Laceration without foreign body of left thumb without damage to nail

    ✓7ᵗʰ **S61.019** Laceration without foreign body of unspecified thumb without damage to nail ▽

  ✓6ᵗʰ **S61.02** Laceration with foreign body of thumb without damage to nail

    ✓7ᵗʰ **S61.021** Laceration with foreign body of right thumb without damage to nail

    ✓7ᵗʰ **S61.022** Laceration with foreign body of left thumb without damage to nail

    ✓7ᵗʰ **S61.029** Laceration with foreign body of unspecified thumb without damage to nail ▽

  ✓6ᵗʰ **S61.03** Puncture wound without foreign body of thumb without damage to nail

    ✓7ᵗʰ **S61.031** Puncture wound without foreign body of right thumb without damage to nail

    ✓7ᵗʰ **S61.032** Puncture wound without foreign body of left thumb without damage to nail

    ✓7ᵗʰ **S61.039** Puncture wound without foreign body of unspecified thumb without damage to nail ▽

  ✓6ᵗʰ **S61.04** Puncture wound with foreign body of thumb without damage to nail

    ✓7ᵗʰ **S61.041** Puncture wound with foreign body of right thumb without damage to nail

    ✓7ᵗʰ **S61.042** Puncture wound with foreign body of left thumb without damage to nail

    ✓7ᵗʰ **S61.049** Puncture wound with foreign body of unspecified thumb without damage to nail ▽

  ✓6ᵗʰ **S61.05** Open bite of thumb without damage to nail
     Bite of thumb NOS
       EXCLUDES 1   superficial bite of thumb (S60.36-, S60.37-)

    ✓7ᵗʰ **S61.051** Open bite of right thumb without damage to nail

    ✓7ᵗʰ **S61.052** Open bite of left thumb without damage to nail

    ✓7ᵗʰ **S61.059** Open bite of unspecified thumb without damage to nail ▽

✓5ᵗʰ **S61.1** Open wound of thumb with damage to nail

  ✓6ᵗʰ **S61.10** Unspecified open wound of thumb with damage to nail

    ✓7ᵗʰ **S61.101** Unspecified open wound of right thumb with damage to nail ▽

    ✓7ᵗʰ **S61.102** Unspecified open wound of left thumb with damage to nail ▽

    ✓7ᵗʰ **S61.109** Unspecified open wound of unspecified thumb with damage to nail ▽

  ✓6ᵗʰ **S61.11** Laceration without foreign body of thumb with damage to nail

    ✓7ᵗʰ **S61.111** Laceration without foreign body of right thumb with damage to nail

    ✓7ᵗʰ **S61.112** Laceration without foreign body of left thumb with damage to nail

    ✓7ᵗʰ **S61.119** Laceration without foreign body of unspecified thumb with damage to nail ▽

  ✓6ᵗʰ **S61.12** Laceration with foreign body of thumb with damage to nail

    ✓7ᵗʰ **S61.121** Laceration with foreign body of right thumb with damage to nail

    ✓7ᵗʰ **S61.122** Laceration with foreign body of left thumb with damage to nail

    ✓7ᵗʰ **S61.129** Laceration with foreign body of unspecified thumb with damage to nail ▽

  ✓6ᵗʰ **S61.13** Puncture wound without foreign body of thumb with damage to nail

    ✓7ᵗʰ **S61.131** Puncture wound without foreign body of right thumb with damage to nail

    ✓7ᵗʰ **S61.132** Puncture wound without foreign body of left thumb with damage to nail

    ✓7ᵗʰ **S61.139** Puncture wound without foreign body of unspecified thumb with damage to nail ▽

  ✓6ᵗʰ **S61.14** Puncture wound with foreign body of thumb with damage to nail

    ✓7ᵗʰ **S61.141** Puncture wound with foreign body of right thumb with damage to nail

    ✓7ᵗʰ **S61.142** Puncture wound with foreign body of left thumb with damage to nail

    ✓7ᵗʰ **S61.149** Puncture wound with foreign body of unspecified thumb with damage to nail ▽

  ✓6ᵗʰ **S61.15** Open bite of thumb with damage to nail
     Bite of thumb with damage to nail NOS
       EXCLUDES 1   superficial bite of thumb (S60.36-, S60.37-)

    ✓7ᵗʰ **S61.151** Open bite of right thumb with damage to nail

    ✓7ᵗʰ **S61.152** Open bite of left thumb with damage to nail

---

EXCLUDES 1 Not coded here   *EXCLUDES 2* Not included here   N Newborn Age: 0   P Pediatric Age: 0-17   M Maternity Age: 12-55   A Adult Age: 15-124

980   ICD-10-CM 2018

☑7ᵗʰ **S61.159** **Open bite of unspecified thumb with damage to nail** ▽

☑5ᵗʰ **S61.2** **Open wound of other** finger without damage to nail
> *EXCLUDES 1*   open wound of finger involving nail (matrix) (S61.3-)
> *EXCLUDES 2*   open wound of thumb without damage to nail (S61.0-)

☑6ᵗʰ **S61.20** **Unspecified open wound of other finger without damage to nail**

☑7ᵗʰ **S61.200** **Unspecified open wound of** right index **finger without damage to nail** ▽

☑7ᵗʰ **S61.201** **Unspecified open wound of** left index **finger without damage to nail** ▽

☑7ᵗʰ **S61.202** **Unspecified open wound of** right middle **finger without damage to nail** ▽

☑7ᵗʰ **S61.203** **Unspecified open wound of** left middle **finger without damage to nail** ▽

☑7ᵗʰ **S61.204** **Unspecified open wound of** right ring **finger without damage to nail** ▽

☑7ᵗʰ **S61.205** **Unspecified open wound of** left ring **finger without damage to nail** ▽

☑7ᵗʰ **S61.206** **Unspecified open wound of** right little **finger without damage to nail** ▽

☑7ᵗʰ **S61.207** **Unspecified open wound of** left little **finger without damage to nail** ▽

☑7ᵗʰ **S61.208** **Unspecified open wound of other finger without damage to nail** ▽
> Unspecified open wound of specified finger with unspecified laterality without damage to nail

☑7ᵗʰ **S61.209** **Unspecified open wound of unspecified finger without damage to nail** ▽

☑6ᵗʰ **S61.21** Laceration without foreign body **of finger without damage to nail**

☑7ᵗʰ **S61.210** **Laceration without foreign body of** right index **finger without damage to nail**

☑7ᵗʰ **S61.211** **Laceration without foreign body of** left index **finger without damage to nail**

☑7ᵗʰ **S61.212** **Laceration without foreign body of** right middle **finger without damage to nail**

☑7ᵗʰ **S61.213** **Laceration without foreign body of** left middle **finger without damage to nail**

☑7ᵗʰ **S61.214** **Laceration without foreign body of** right ring **finger without damage to nail**

☑7ᵗʰ **S61.215** **Laceration without foreign body of** left ring **finger without damage to nail**

☑7ᵗʰ **S61.216** **Laceration without foreign body of** right little **finger without damage to nail**

☑7ᵗʰ **S61.217** **Laceration without foreign body of** left little **finger without damage to nail**

☑7ᵗʰ **S61.218** **Laceration without foreign body of other finger without damage to nail**
> Laceration without foreign body of specified finger with unspecified laterality without damage to nail

☑7ᵗʰ **S61.219** **Laceration without foreign body of unspecified finger without damage to nail** ▽

☑6ᵗʰ **S61.22** Laceration with foreign body **of finger without damage to nail**

☑7ᵗʰ **S61.220** **Laceration with foreign body of** right index **finger without damage to nail**

☑7ᵗʰ **S61.221** **Laceration with foreign body of** left index **finger without damage to nail**

☑7ᵗʰ **S61.222** **Laceration with foreign body of** right middle **finger without damage to nail**

☑7ᵗʰ **S61.223** **Laceration with foreign body of** left middle **finger without damage to nail**

☑7ᵗʰ **S61.224** **Laceration with foreign body of** right ring **finger without damage to nail**

☑7ᵗʰ **S61.225** **Laceration with foreign body of** left ring **finger without damage to nail**

☑7ᵗʰ **S61.226** **Laceration with foreign body of** right little **finger without damage to nail**

☑7ᵗʰ **S61.227** **Laceration with foreign body of** left little **finger without damage to nail**

☑7ᵗʰ **S61.228** **Laceration with foreign body of other finger without damage to nail**
> Laceration with foreign body of specified finger with unspecified laterality without damage to nail

☑7ᵗʰ **S61.229** **Laceration with foreign body of unspecified finger without damage to nail** ▽

☑6ᵗʰ **S61.23** Puncture wound without foreign body **of finger without damage to nail**

☑7ᵗʰ **S61.230** **Puncture wound without foreign body of** right index **finger without damage to nail**

☑7ᵗʰ **S61.231** **Puncture wound without foreign body of** left index **finger without damage to nail**

☑7ᵗʰ **S61.232** **Puncture wound without foreign body of** right middle **finger without damage to nail**

☑7ᵗʰ **S61.233** **Puncture wound without foreign body of** left middle **finger without damage to nail**

☑7ᵗʰ **S61.234** **Puncture wound without foreign body of** right ring **finger without damage to nail**

☑7ᵗʰ **S61.235** **Puncture wound without foreign body of** left ring **finger without damage to nail**

☑7ᵗʰ **S61.236** **Puncture wound without foreign body of** right little **finger without damage to nail**

☑7ᵗʰ **S61.237** **Puncture wound without foreign body of** left little **finger without damage to nail**

☑7ᵗʰ **S61.238** **Puncture wound without foreign body of other finger without damage to nail**
> Puncture wound without foreign body of specified finger with unspecified laterality without damage to nail

☑7ᵗʰ **S61.239** **Puncture wound without foreign body of unspecified finger without damage to nail** ▽

☑6ᵗʰ **S61.24** Puncture wound with foreign body **of finger without damage to nail**

☑7ᵗʰ **S61.240** **Puncture wound with foreign body of** right index **finger without damage to nail**

☑7ᵗʰ **S61.241** **Puncture wound with foreign body of** left index **finger without damage to nail**

☑7ᵗʰ **S61.242** **Puncture wound with foreign body of** right middle **finger without damage to nail**

☑7ᵗʰ **S61.243** **Puncture wound with foreign body of** left middle **finger without damage to nail**

☑7ᵗʰ **S61.244** **Puncture wound with foreign body of** right ring **finger without damage to nail**

☑7ᵗʰ **S61.245** **Puncture wound with foreign body of** left ring **finger without damage to nail**

☑7ᵗʰ **S61.246** **Puncture wound with foreign body of** right little **finger without damage to nail**

☑7ᵗʰ **S61.247** **Puncture wound with foreign body of** left little **finger without damage to nail**

☑7ᵗʰ **S61.248** **Puncture wound with foreign body of other finger without damage to nail**
> Puncture wound with foreign body of specified finger with unspecified laterality without damage to nail

☑7ᵗʰ **S61.249** **Puncture wound with foreign body of unspecified finger without damage to nail** ▽

☑6ᵗʰ **S61.25** Open bite **of finger without damage to nail**
> Bite of finger without damage to nail NOS
> *EXCLUDES 1*   superficial bite of finger (S60.46-, S60.47-)

☑7ᵗʰ **S61.250** **Open bite of** right index **finger without damage to nail**

☑7ᵗʰ **S61.251** **Open bite of** left index **finger without damage to nail**

☑7ᵗʰ **S61.252** **Open bite of** right middle **finger without damage to nail**

☑7ᵗʰ **S61.253** **Open bite of** left middle **finger without damage to nail**

☑7ᵗʰ **S61.254** **Open bite of** right ring **finger without damage to nail**

☑7ᵗʰ **S61.255** **Open bite of** left ring **finger without damage to nail**

☑ Additional Character Req   ☑x7ᵗʰ Placeholder Alert   **Manifestation**   HCC CMS-HCC Condition   ▽ Unspecified Code   ►◄ Revised Text   ● New Code   ▲ Revised Code Title

ICD-10-CM 2018   981

Chapter 19. Injury, Poisoning, and Certain Other Consequences of External Causes

√7ᵗʰ **S61.256** **Open bite of right little finger without damage to nail**

√7ᵗʰ **S61.257** **Open bite of left little finger without damage to nail**

√7ᵗʰ **S61.258** **Open bite of other finger without damage to nail**
    Open bite of specified finger with unspecified laterality without damage to nail

√7ᵗʰ **S61.259** **Open bite of unspecified finger without damage to nail** ▽

√5ᵗʰ **S61.3** **Open wound of other finger with damage to nail**

√6ᵗʰ **S61.30** **Unspecified open wound of finger with damage to nail**

√7ᵗʰ **S61.300** **Unspecified open wound of right index finger with damage to nail** ▽

√7ᵗʰ **S61.301** **Unspecified open wound of left index finger with damage to nail** ▽

√7ᵗʰ **S61.302** **Unspecified open wound of right middle finger with damage to nail** ▽

√7ᵗʰ **S61.303** **Unspecified open wound of left middle finger with damage to nail** ▽

√7ᵗʰ **S61.304** **Unspecified open wound of right ring finger with damage to nail** ▽

√7ᵗʰ **S61.305** **Unspecified open wound of left ring finger with damage to nail** ▽

√7ᵗʰ **S61.306** **Unspecified open wound of right little finger with damage to nail** ▽

√7ᵗʰ **S61.307** **Unspecified open wound of left little finger with damage to nail** ▽

√7ᵗʰ **S61.308** **Unspecified open wound of other finger with damage to nail** ▽
    Unspecified open wound of specified finger with unspecified laterality with damage to nail

√7ᵗʰ **S61.309** **Unspecified open wound of unspecified finger with damage to nail** ▽

√6ᵗʰ **S61.31** **Laceration without foreign body of finger with damage to nail**

√7ᵗʰ **S61.310** **Laceration without foreign body of right index finger with damage to nail**

√7ᵗʰ **S61.311** **Laceration without foreign body of left index finger with damage to nail**

√7ᵗʰ **S61.312** **Laceration without foreign body of right middle finger with damage to nail**

√7ᵗʰ **S61.313** **Laceration without foreign body of left middle finger with damage to nail**

√7ᵗʰ **S61.314** **Laceration without foreign body of right ring finger with damage to nail**

√7ᵗʰ **S61.315** **Laceration without foreign body of left ring finger with damage to nail**

√7ᵗʰ **S61.316** **Laceration without foreign body of right little finger with damage to nail**

√7ᵗʰ **S61.317** **Laceration without foreign body of left little finger with damage to nail**

√7ᵗʰ **S61.318** **Laceration without foreign body of other finger with damage to nail**
    Laceration without foreign body of specified finger with unspecified laterality with damage to nail

√7ᵗʰ **S61.319** **Laceration without foreign body of unspecified finger with damage to nail** ▽

√6ᵗʰ **S61.32** **Laceration with foreign body of finger with damage to nail**

√7ᵗʰ **S61.320** **Laceration with foreign body of right index finger with damage to nail**

√7ᵗʰ **S61.321** **Laceration with foreign body of left index finger with damage to nail**

√7ᵗʰ **S61.322** **Laceration with foreign body of right middle finger with damage to nail**

√7ᵗʰ **S61.323** **Laceration with foreign body of left middle finger with damage to nail**

√7ᵗʰ **S61.324** **Laceration with foreign body of right ring finger with damage to nail**

√7ᵗʰ **S61.325** **Laceration with foreign body of left ring finger with damage to nail**

√7ᵗʰ **S61.326** **Laceration with foreign body of right little finger with damage to nail**

√7ᵗʰ **S61.327** **Laceration with foreign body of left little finger with damage to nail**

√7ᵗʰ **S61.328** **Laceration with foreign body of other finger with damage to nail**
    Laceration with foreign body of specified finger with unspecified laterality with damage to nail

√7ᵗʰ **S61.329** **Laceration with foreign body of unspecified finger with damage to nail** ▽

√6ᵗʰ **S61.33** **Puncture wound without foreign body of finger with damage to nail**

√7ᵗʰ **S61.330** **Puncture wound without foreign body of right index finger with damage to nail**

√7ᵗʰ **S61.331** **Puncture wound without foreign body of left index finger with damage to nail**

√7ᵗʰ **S61.332** **Puncture wound without foreign body of right middle finger with damage to nail**

√7ᵗʰ **S61.333** **Puncture wound without foreign body of left middle finger with damage to nail**

√7ᵗʰ **S61.334** **Puncture wound without foreign body of right ring finger with damage to nail**

√7ᵗʰ **S61.335** **Puncture wound without foreign body of left ring finger with damage to nail**

√7ᵗʰ **S61.336** **Puncture wound without foreign body of right little finger with damage to nail**

√7ᵗʰ **S61.337** **Puncture wound without foreign body of left little finger with damage to nail**

√7ᵗʰ **S61.338** **Puncture wound without foreign body of other finger with damage to nail**
    Puncture wound without foreign body of specified finger with unspecified laterality with damage to nail

√7ᵗʰ **S61.339** **Puncture wound without foreign body of unspecified finger with damage to nail** ▽

√6ᵗʰ **S61.34** **Puncture wound with foreign body of finger with damage to nail**

√7ᵗʰ **S61.340** **Puncture wound with foreign body of right index finger with damage to nail**

√7ᵗʰ **S61.341** **Puncture wound with foreign body of left index finger with damage to nail**

√7ᵗʰ **S61.342** **Puncture wound with foreign body of right middle finger with damage to nail**

√7ᵗʰ **S61.343** **Puncture wound with foreign body of left middle finger with damage to nail**

√7ᵗʰ **S61.344** **Puncture wound with foreign body of right ring finger with damage to nail**

√7ᵗʰ **S61.345** **Puncture wound with foreign body of left ring finger with damage to nail**

√7ᵗʰ **S61.346** **Puncture wound with foreign body of right little finger with damage to nail**

√7ᵗʰ **S61.347** **Puncture wound with foreign body of left little finger with damage to nail**

√7ᵗʰ **S61.348** **Puncture wound with foreign body of other finger with damage to nail**
    Puncture wound with foreign body of specified finger with unspecified laterality with damage to nail

√7ᵗʰ **S61.349** **Puncture wound with foreign body of unspecified finger with damage to nail** ▽

√6ᵗʰ **S61.35** **Open bite of finger with damage to nail**
    Bite of finger with damage to nail NOS
    EXCLUDES 1   *superficial bite of finger (S60.46-, S60.47-)*

√7ᵗʰ **S61.350** **Open bite of right index finger with damage to nail**

√7ᵗʰ **S61.351** **Open bite of left index finger with damage to nail**

√7ᵗʰ **S61.352** **Open bite of right middle finger with damage to nail**

√7ᵗʰ **S61.353** **Open bite of left middle finger with damage to nail**

√7ᵗʰ **S61.354** **Open bite of right ring finger with damage to nail**

√7ᵗʰ **S61.355** **Open bite of left ring finger with damage to nail**

EXCLUDES 1 Not coded here   **EXCLUDES 2** Not included here   N Newborn Age: 0   P Pediatric Age: 0-17   M Maternity Age: 12-55   A Adult Age: 15-124

982   ICD-10-CM 2018

✓7ᵗʰ	**S61.356**	**Open bite of** right **little finger with damage to nail**
✓7ᵗʰ	**S61.357**	**Open bite of** left **little finger with damage to nail**
✓7ᵗʰ	**S61.358**	**Open bite of other finger with damage to nail**
		Open bite of specified finger with unspecified laterality with damage to nail
✓7ᵗʰ	**S61.359**	**Open bite of unspecified finger with damage to nail** ▽

✓5ᵗʰ **S61.4 Open wound of** hand

✓6ᵗʰ **S61.40 Unspecified open wound of hand**

✓7ᵗʰ	**S61.401**	**Unspecified open wound of** right **hand** ▽
✓7ᵗʰ	**S61.402**	**Unspecified open wound of** left **hand** ▽
✓7ᵗʰ	**S61.409**	**Unspecified open wound of unspecified hand** ▽

✓6ᵗʰ **S61.41 Laceration without foreign body of hand**

✓7ᵗʰ	**S61.411**	**Laceration without foreign body of** right **hand**
✓7ᵗʰ	**S61.412**	**Laceration without foreign body of** left **hand**
✓7ᵗʰ	**S61.419**	**Laceration without foreign body of unspecified hand** ▽

✓6ᵗʰ **S61.42 Laceration with foreign body of hand**

✓7ᵗʰ	**S61.421**	**Laceration with foreign body of** right **hand**
✓7ᵗʰ	**S61.422**	**Laceration with foreign body of** left **hand**
✓7ᵗʰ	**S61.429**	**Laceration with foreign body of unspecified hand** ▽

✓6ᵗʰ **S61.43 Puncture wound without foreign body of hand**

✓7ᵗʰ	**S61.431**	**Puncture wound without foreign body of** right **hand**
✓7ᵗʰ	**S61.432**	**Puncture wound without foreign body of** left **hand**
✓7ᵗʰ	**S61.439**	**Puncture wound without foreign body of unspecified hand** ▽

✓6ᵗʰ **S61.44 Puncture wound with foreign body of hand**

✓7ᵗʰ	**S61.441**	**Puncture wound with foreign body of** right **hand**
✓7ᵗʰ	**S61.442**	**Puncture wound with foreign body of** left **hand**
✓7ᵗʰ	**S61.449**	**Puncture wound with foreign body of unspecified hand** ▽

✓6ᵗʰ **S61.45 Open bite of hand**

Bite of hand NOS

EXCLUDES 1   *superficial bite of hand (S60.56-, S60.57-)*

✓7ᵗʰ	**S61.451**	**Open bite of** right **hand**
✓7ᵗʰ	**S61.452**	**Open bite of** left **hand**
✓7ᵗʰ	**S61.459**	**Open bite of unspecified hand** ▽

✓5ᵗʰ **S61.5 Open wound of** wrist

✓6ᵗʰ **S61.50 Unspecified open wound of wrist**

✓7ᵗʰ	**S61.501**	**Unspecified open wound of** right **wrist** ▽
✓7ᵗʰ	**S61.502**	**Unspecified open wound of** left **wrist** ▽
✓7ᵗʰ	**S61.509**	**Unspecified open wound of unspecified wrist** ▽

✓6ᵗʰ **S61.51 Laceration without foreign body of wrist**

✓7ᵗʰ	**S61.511**	**Laceration without foreign body of** right **wrist**
✓7ᵗʰ	**S61.512**	**Laceration without foreign body of** left **wrist**
✓7ᵗʰ	**S61.519**	**Laceration without foreign body of unspecified wrist** ▽

✓6ᵗʰ **S61.52 Laceration with foreign body of wrist**

✓7ᵗʰ	**S61.521**	**Laceration with foreign body of** right **wrist**
✓7ᵗʰ	**S61.522**	**Laceration with foreign body of** left **wrist**
✓7ᵗʰ	**S61.529**	**Laceration with foreign body of unspecified wrist** ▽

✓6ᵗʰ **S61.53 Puncture wound without foreign body of wrist**

| ✓7ᵗʰ | **S61.531** | **Puncture wound without foreign body of** right **wrist** |
| ✓7ᵗʰ | **S61.532** | **Puncture wound without foreign body of** left **wrist** |

| ✓7ᵗʰ | **S61.539** | **Puncture wound without foreign body of unspecified wrist** ▽ |

✓6ᵗʰ **S61.54 Puncture wound with foreign body of wrist**

✓7ᵗʰ	**S61.541**	**Puncture wound with foreign body of** right **wrist**
✓7ᵗʰ	**S61.542**	**Puncture wound with foreign body of** left **wrist**
✓7ᵗʰ	**S61.549**	**Puncture wound with foreign body of unspecified wrist** ▽

✓6ᵗʰ **S61.55 Open bite of wrist**

Bite of wrist NOS

EXCLUDES 1   *superficial bite of wrist (S60.86-, S60.87-)*

✓7ᵗʰ	**S61.551**	**Open bite of** right **wrist**
✓7ᵗʰ	**S61.552**	**Open bite of** left **wrist**
✓7ᵗʰ	**S61.559**	**Open bite of unspecified wrist** ▽

✓4ᵗʰ **S62 Fracture at wrist and hand level**

NOTE   A fracture not indicated as displaced or nondisplaced should be coded to displaced.
A fracture not indicated as open or closed should be coded to closed.

EXCLUDES 1   *traumatic amputation of wrist and hand (S68.-)*
EXCLUDES 2   *fracture of distal parts of ulna and radius (S52.-)*

AHA: 2015, 3Q, 37-39

The appropriate 7th character is to be added to each code from category S62.
A   initial encounter for closed fracture
B   initial encounter for open fracture
D   subsequent encounter for fracture with routine healing
G   subsequent encounter for fracture with delayed healing
K   subsequent encounter for fracture with nonunion
P   subsequent encounter for fracture with malunion
S   sequela

✓5ᵗʰ **S62.0 Fracture of** navicular [scaphoid] bone of wrist

✓6ᵗʰ **S62.00 Unspecified fracture of navicular [scaphoid] bone of wrist**

✓7ᵗʰ	**S62.001**	**Unspecified fracture of navicular [scaphoid] bone of** right **wrist** ▽
✓7ᵗʰ	**S62.002**	**Unspecified fracture of navicular [scaphoid] bone of** left **wrist** ▽
		AHA: 2012, 4Q, 106
✓7ᵗʰ	**S62.009**	**Unspecified fracture of navicular [scaphoid] bone of unspecified wrist** ▽

✓6ᵗʰ **S62.01 Fracture of** distal pole of navicular [scaphoid] bone of wrist

Fracture of volar tuberosity of navicular [scaphoid] bone of wrist

✓7ᵗʰ	**S62.011**	**Displaced fracture of distal pole of navicular [scaphoid] bone of** right **wrist**
✓7ᵗʰ	**S62.012**	**Displaced fracture of distal pole of navicular [scaphoid] bone of** left **wrist**
✓7ᵗʰ	**S62.013**	**Displaced fracture of distal pole of navicular [scaphoid] bone of unspecified wrist** ▽
✓7ᵗʰ	**S62.014**	**Nondisplaced fracture of distal pole of navicular [scaphoid] bone of** right **wrist**
✓7ᵗʰ	**S62.015**	**Nondisplaced fracture of distal pole of navicular [scaphoid] bone of** left **wrist**
✓7ᵗʰ	**S62.016**	**Nondisplaced fracture of distal pole of navicular [scaphoid] bone of unspecified wrist** ▽

✓6ᵗʰ **S62.02 Fracture of** middle third of navicular [scaphoid] bone of wrist

✓7ᵗʰ	**S62.021**	**Displaced fracture of middle third of navicular [scaphoid] bone of** right **wrist**
✓7ᵗʰ	**S62.022**	**Displaced fracture of middle third of navicular [scaphoid] bone of** left **wrist**
✓7ᵗʰ	**S62.023**	**Displaced fracture of middle third of navicular [scaphoid] bone of unspecified wrist** ▽
✓7ᵗʰ	**S62.024**	**Nondisplaced fracture of middle third of navicular [scaphoid] bone of** right **wrist**
✓7ᵗʰ	**S62.025**	**Nondisplaced fracture of middle third of navicular [scaphoid] bone of** left **wrist**
✓7ᵗʰ	**S62.026**	**Nondisplaced fracture of middle third of navicular [scaphoid] bone of unspecified wrist** ▽

☑ Additional Character Req   ✓x7ᵗʰ Placeholder Alert   **Manifestation**   HCC CMS-HCC Condition   ▽ Unspecified Code   ►◄ Revised Text   ● New Code   ▲ Revised Code Title

✓6th **S62.03** **Fracture of** proximal third of navicular [scaphoid] **bone of wrist**

     ✓7th **S62.031** Displaced **fracture of proximal third of navicular [scaphoid] bone of** right **wrist**

     ✓7th **S62.032** Displaced **fracture of proximal third of navicular [scaphoid] bone of** left **wrist**

     ✓7th **S62.033** Displaced **fracture of proximal third of** ▽ **navicular [scaphoid] bone of unspecified wrist**

     ✓7th **S62.034** Nondisplaced **fracture of proximal third of navicular [scaphoid] bone of** right **wrist**

     ✓7th **S62.035** Nondisplaced **fracture of proximal third of navicular [scaphoid] bone of** left **wrist**

     ✓7th **S62.036** Nondisplaced **fracture of proximal** ▽ **third of navicular [scaphoid] bone of unspecified wrist**

✓5th **S62.1** **Fracture of other and unspecified** carpal bone(s)

     EXCLUDES 2   *fracture of scaphoid of wrist (S62.0-)*

     ✓6th **S62.10** **Fracture of unspecified carpal bone**
        Fracture of wrist NOS

     ✓7th **S62.101** **Fracture of unspecified carpal bone,** ▽ right **wrist**

     ✓7th **S62.102** **Fracture of unspecified carpal bone,** ▽ left **wrist**
        AHA: 2012, 4Q, 95

     ✓7th **S62.109** **Fracture of unspecified carpal bone,** ▽ **unspecified wrist**

     ✓6th **S62.11** **Fracture of** triquetrum [cuneiform] **bone of wrist**

     ✓7th **S62.111** Displaced **fracture of triquetrum [cuneiform] bone,** right **wrist**

     ✓7th **S62.112** Displaced **fracture of triquetrum [cuneiform] bone,** left **wrist**

     ✓7th **S62.113** Displaced **fracture of triquetrum** ▽ **[cuneiform] bone, unspecified wrist**

     ✓7th **S62.114** Nondisplaced **fracture of triquetrum [cuneiform] bone,** right **wrist**

     ✓7th **S62.115** Nondisplaced **fracture of triquetrum [cuneiform] bone,** left **wrist**

     ✓7th **S62.116** Nondisplaced **fracture of triquetrum** ▽ **[cuneiform] bone, unspecified wrist**

     ✓6th **S62.12** **Fracture of** lunate [semilunar]

     ✓7th **S62.121** Displaced **fracture of lunate [semilunar],** right **wrist**

     ✓7th **S62.122** Displaced **fracture of lunate [semilunar],** left **wrist**

     ✓7th **S62.123** Displaced **fracture of lunate** ▽ **[semilunar], unspecified wrist**

     ✓7th **S62.124** Nondisplaced **fracture of lunate [semilunar],** right **wrist**

     ✓7th **S62.125** Nondisplaced **fracture of lunate [semilunar],** left **wrist**

     ✓7th **S62.126** Nondisplaced **fracture of lunate** ▽ **[semilunar], unspecified wrist**

     ✓6th **S62.13** **Fracture of** capitate [os magnum] **bone**

     ✓7th **S62.131** Displaced **fracture of capitate [os magnum] bone,** right **wrist**

     ✓7th **S62.132** Displaced **fracture of capitate [os magnum] bone,** left **wrist**

     ✓7th **S62.133** Displaced **fracture of capitate [os** ▽ **magnum] bone, unspecified wrist**

     ✓7th **S62.134** Nondisplaced **fracture of capitate [os magnum] bone,** right **wrist**

     ✓7th **S62.135** Nondisplaced **fracture of capitate [os magnum] bone,** left **wrist**

     ✓7th **S62.136** Nondisplaced **fracture of capitate [os** ▽ **magnum] bone, unspecified wrist**

     ✓6th **S62.14** **Fracture of** body of hamate [unciform] **bone**
        Fracture of hamate [unciform] bone NOS

     ✓7th **S62.141** Displaced **fracture of body of hamate [unciform] bone,** right **wrist**

     ✓7th **S62.142** Displaced **fracture of body of hamate [unciform] bone,** left **wrist**

     ✓7th **S62.143** Displaced **fracture of body of hamate** ▽ **[unciform] bone, unspecified wrist**

     ✓7th **S62.144** Nondisplaced **fracture of body of hamate [unciform] bone,** right **wrist**

     ✓7th **S62.145** Nondisplaced **fracture of body of hamate [unciform] bone,** left **wrist**

     ✓7th **S62.146** Nondisplaced **fracture of body of** ▽ **hamate [unciform] bone, unspecified wrist**

     ✓6th **S62.15** **Fracture of** hook process of hamate [unciform] **bone**
        Fracture of unciform process of hamate [unciform] bone

     ✓7th **S62.151** Displaced **fracture of hook process of hamate [unciform] bone,** right **wrist**

     ✓7th **S62.152** Displaced **fracture of hook process of hamate [unciform] bone,** left **wrist**

     ✓7th **S62.153** Displaced **fracture of hook process of** ▽ **hamate [unciform] bone, unspecified wrist**

     ✓7th **S62.154** Nondisplaced **fracture of hook process of hamate [unciform] bone,** right **wrist**

     ✓7th **S62.155** Nondisplaced **fracture of hook process of hamate [unciform] bone,** left **wrist**

     ✓7th **S62.156** Nondisplaced **fracture of hook process** ▽ **of hamate [unciform] bone, unspecified wrist**

     ✓6th **S62.16** **Fracture of** pisiform

     ✓7th **S62.161** Displaced **fracture of pisiform,** right **wrist**

     ✓7th **S62.162** Displaced **fracture of pisiform,** left **wrist**

     ✓7th **S62.163** Displaced **fracture of pisiform,** ▽ **unspecified wrist**

     ✓7th **S62.164** Nondisplaced **fracture of pisiform,** right **wrist**

     ✓7th **S62.165** Nondisplaced **fracture of pisiform,** left **wrist**

     ✓7th **S62.166** Nondisplaced **fracture of pisiform,** ▽ **unspecified wrist**

     ✓6th **S62.17** **Fracture of** trapezium [larger multangular]

     ✓7th **S62.171** Displaced **fracture of trapezium [larger multangular],** right **wrist**

     ✓7th **S62.172** Displaced **fracture of trapezium [larger multangular],** left **wrist**

     ✓7th **S62.173** Displaced **fracture of trapezium [larger** ▽ **multangular], unspecified wrist**

     ✓7th **S62.174** Nondisplaced **fracture of trapezium [larger multangular],** right **wrist**

     ✓7th **S62.175** Nondisplaced **fracture of trapezium [larger multangular],** left **wrist**

     ✓7th **S62.176** Nondisplaced **fracture of trapezium** ▽ **[larger multangular], unspecified wrist**

     ✓6th **S62.18** **Fracture of** trapezoid [smaller multangular]

     ✓7th **S62.181** Displaced **fracture of trapezoid [smaller multangular],** right **wrist**

     ✓7th **S62.182** Displaced **fracture of trapezoid [smaller multangular],** left **wrist**

     ✓7th **S62.183** Displaced **fracture of trapezoid** ▽ **[smaller multangular], unspecified wrist**

     ✓7th **S62.184** Nondisplaced **fracture of trapezoid [smaller multangular],** right **wrist**

     ✓7th **S62.185** Nondisplaced **fracture of trapezoid [smaller multangular],** left **wrist**

     ✓7th **S62.186** Nondisplaced **fracture of trapezoid** ▽ **[smaller multangular], unspecified wrist**

✓5th **S62.2** **Fracture of** first metacarpal **bone**

     ✓6th **S62.20** **Unspecified fracture of first metacarpal bone**

     ✓7th **S62.201** **Unspecified fracture of first metacarpal** ▽ **bone,** right **hand**

     ✓7th **S62.202** **Unspecified fracture of first metacarpal** ▽ **bone,** left **hand**

     ✓7th **S62.209** **Unspecified fracture of first metacarpal** ▽ **bone, unspecified hand**

     ✓6th **S62.21** Bennett's **fracture**

     ✓7th **S62.211** Bennett's **fracture,** right **hand**

     ✓7th **S62.212** Bennett's **fracture,** left **hand**

     ✓7th **S62.213** Bennett's **fracture, unspecified hand** ▽

EXCLUDES 1 Not coded here   EXCLUDES 2 Not included here   N Newborn Age: 0   P Pediatric Age: 0-17   M Maternity Age: 12-55   A Adult Age: 15-124

984   ICD-10-CM 2018

✓6th **S62.22** Rolando's fracture

    ✓7th **S62.221** Displaced Rolando's fracture, right hand

    ✓7th **S62.222** Displaced Rolando's fracture, left hand

    ✓7th **S62.223** Displaced Rolando's fracture, unspecified hand ▽

    ✓7th **S62.224** Nondisplaced Rolando's fracture, right hand

    ✓7th **S62.225** Nondisplaced Rolando's fracture, left hand

    ✓7th **S62.226** Nondisplaced Rolando's fracture, unspecified hand ▽

✓6th **S62.23** Other fracture of base of first metacarpal bone

    ✓7th **S62.231** Other displaced fracture of base of first metacarpal bone, right hand

    ✓7th **S62.232** Other displaced fracture of base of first metacarpal bone, left hand ▲

    ✓7th **S62.233** Other displaced fracture of base of first metacarpal bone, unspecified hand ▽

    ✓7th **S62.234** Other nondisplaced fracture of base of first metacarpal bone, right hand

    ✓7th **S62.235** Other nondisplaced fracture of base of first metacarpal bone, left hand

    ✓7th **S62.236** Other nondisplaced fracture of base of first metacarpal bone, unspecified hand ▽

✓6th **S62.24** Fracture of shaft of first metacarpal bone ▲

    ✓7th **S62.241** Displaced fracture of shaft of first metacarpal bone, right hand

    ✓7th **S62.242** Displaced fracture of shaft of first metacarpal bone, left hand

    ✓7th **S62.243** Displaced fracture of shaft of first metacarpal bone, unspecified hand ▽

    ✓7th **S62.244** Nondisplaced fracture of shaft of first metacarpal bone, right hand

    ✓7th **S62.245** Nondisplaced fracture of shaft of first metacarpal bone, left hand

    ✓7th **S62.246** Nondisplaced fracture of shaft of first metacarpal bone, unspecified hand ▽

✓6th **S62.25** Fracture of neck of first metacarpal bone

    ✓7th **S62.251** Displaced fracture of neck of first metacarpal bone, right hand

    ✓7th **S62.252** Displaced fracture of neck of first metacarpal bone, left hand

    ✓7th **S62.253** Displaced fracture of neck of first metacarpal bone, unspecified hand ▽

    ✓7th **S62.254** Nondisplaced fracture of neck of first metacarpal bone, right hand

    ✓7th **S62.255** Nondisplaced fracture of neck of first metacarpal bone, left hand

    ✓7th **S62.256** Nondisplaced fracture of neck of first metacarpal bone, unspecified hand ▽

✓6th **S62.29** Other fracture of first metacarpal bone

    ✓7th **S62.291** Other fracture of first metacarpal bone, right hand

    ✓7th **S62.292** Other fracture of first metacarpal bone, left hand

    ✓7th **S62.299** Other fracture of first metacarpal bone, unspecified hand ▽

✓5th **S62.3** Fracture of other and unspecified metacarpal bone

    EXCLUDES 2   fracture of first metacarpal bone (S62.2-)

✓6th **S62.30** Unspecified fracture of other metacarpal bone

    ✓7th **S62.300** Unspecified fracture of second metacarpal bone, right hand ▽

    ✓7th **S62.301** Unspecified fracture of second metacarpal bone, left hand ▽

    ✓7th **S62.302** Unspecified fracture of third metacarpal bone, right hand ▽

    ✓7th **S62.303** Unspecified fracture of third metacarpal bone, left hand ▽

    ✓7th **S62.304** Unspecified fracture of fourth metacarpal bone, right hand ▽

    ✓7th **S62.305** Unspecified fracture of fourth metacarpal bone, left hand ▽

    ✓7th **S62.306** Unspecified fracture of fifth metacarpal bone, right hand ▽

    ✓7th **S62.307** Unspecified fracture of fifth metacarpal bone, left hand ▽

    ✓7th **S62.308** Unspecified fracture of other metacarpal bone ▽

        Unspecified fracture of specified metacarpal bone with unspecified laterality

    ✓7th **S62.309** Unspecified fracture of unspecified metacarpal bone ▽

✓6th **S62.31** Displaced fracture of base of other metacarpal bone

    ✓7th **S62.310** Displaced fracture of base of second metacarpal bone, right hand

    ✓7th **S62.311** Displaced fracture of base of second metacarpal bone, left hand

    ✓7th **S62.312** Displaced fracture of base of third metacarpal bone, right hand

    ✓7th **S62.313** Displaced fracture of base of third metacarpal bone, left hand

    ✓7th **S62.314** Displaced fracture of base of fourth metacarpal bone, right hand

    ✓7th **S62.315** Displaced fracture of base of fourth metacarpal bone, left hand

    ✓7th **S62.316** Displaced fracture of base of fifth metacarpal bone, right hand

    ✓7th **S62.317** Displaced fracture of base of fifth metacarpal bone, left hand

    ✓7th **S62.318** Displaced fracture of base of other metacarpal bone

        Displaced fracture of base of specified metacarpal bone with unspecified laterality

    ✓7th **S62.319** Displaced fracture of base of unspecified metacarpal bone ▽

✓6th **S62.32** Displaced fracture of shaft of other metacarpal bone

    ✓7th **S62.320** Displaced fracture of shaft of second metacarpal bone, right hand

    ✓7th **S62.321** Displaced fracture of shaft of second metacarpal bone, left hand

    ✓7th **S62.322** Displaced fracture of shaft of third metacarpal bone, right hand

    ✓7th **S62.323** Displaced fracture of shaft of third metacarpal bone, left hand

    ✓7th **S62.324** Displaced fracture of shaft of fourth metacarpal bone, right hand

    ✓7th **S62.325** Displaced fracture of shaft of fourth metacarpal bone, left hand

    ✓7th **S62.326** Displaced fracture of shaft of fifth metacarpal bone, right hand

    ✓7th **S62.327** Displaced fracture of shaft of fifth metacarpal bone, left hand

    ✓7th **S62.328** Displaced fracture of shaft of other metacarpal bone

        Displaced fracture of shaft of specified metacarpal bone with unspecified laterality

    ✓7th **S62.329** Displaced fracture of shaft of unspecified metacarpal bone ▽

✓6th **S62.33** Displaced fracture of neck of other metacarpal bone

    ✓7th **S62.330** Displaced fracture of neck of second metacarpal bone, right hand

    ✓7th **S62.331** Displaced fracture of neck of second metacarpal bone, left hand

    ✓7th **S62.332** Displaced fracture of neck of third metacarpal bone, right hand

    ✓7th **S62.333** Displaced fracture of neck of third metacarpal bone, left hand

    ✓7th **S62.334** Displaced fracture of neck of fourth metacarpal bone, right hand

    ✓7th **S62.335** Displaced fracture of neck of fourth metacarpal bone, left hand

    ✓7th **S62.336** Displaced fracture of neck of fifth metacarpal bone, right hand

    ✓7th **S62.337** Displaced fracture of neck of fifth metacarpal bone, left hand

---

☑ Additional Character Req   ✓x7th Placeholder Alert   Manifestation   HCC CMS-HCC Condition   ▽ Unspecified Code   ▶◀ Revised Text   ● New Code   ▲ Revised Code Title

√7ᵗʰ **S62.338 Displaced fracture of neck of other metacarpal bone**
Displaced fracture of neck of specified metacarpal bone with unspecified laterality

√7ᵗʰ **S62.339 Displaced fracture of neck of unspecified metacarpal bone** ▽

√6ᵗʰ **S62.34 Nondisplaced fracture of base of other metacarpal bone**

√7ᵗʰ **S62.340 Nondisplaced fracture of base of second metacarpal bone, right hand**

√7ᵗʰ **S62.341 Nondisplaced fracture of base of second metacarpal bone, left hand**

√7ᵗʰ **S62.342 Nondisplaced fracture of base of third metacarpal bone, right hand**

√7ᵗʰ **S62.343 Nondisplaced fracture of base of third metacarpal bone, left hand**

√7ᵗʰ **S62.344 Nondisplaced fracture of base of fourth metacarpal bone, right hand**

√7ᵗʰ **S62.345 Nondisplaced fracture of base of fourth metacarpal bone, left hand**

√7ᵗʰ **S62.346 Nondisplaced fracture of base of fifth metacarpal bone, right hand**

√7ᵗʰ **S62.347 Nondisplaced fracture of base of fifth metacarpal bone, left hand**

√7ᵗʰ **S62.348 Nondisplaced fracture of base of other metacarpal bone**
Nondisplaced fracture of base of specified metacarpal bone with unspecified laterality

√7ᵗʰ **S62.349 Nondisplaced fracture of base of unspecified metacarpal bone** ▽

√6ᵗʰ **S62.35 Nondisplaced fracture of shaft of other metacarpal bone**

√7ᵗʰ **S62.350 Nondisplaced fracture of shaft of second metacarpal bone, right hand**

√7ᵗʰ **S62.351 Nondisplaced fracture of shaft of second metacarpal bone, left hand**

√7ᵗʰ **S62.352 Nondisplaced fracture of shaft of third metacarpal bone, right hand**

√7ᵗʰ **S62.353 Nondisplaced fracture of shaft of third metacarpal bone, left hand**

√7ᵗʰ **S62.354 Nondisplaced fracture of shaft of fourth metacarpal bone, right hand**

√7ᵗʰ **S62.355 Nondisplaced fracture of shaft of fourth metacarpal bone, left hand**

√7ᵗʰ **S62.356 Nondisplaced fracture of shaft of fifth metacarpal bone, right hand**

√7ᵗʰ **S62.357 Nondisplaced fracture of shaft of fifth metacarpal bone, left hand**

√7ᵗʰ **S62.358 Nondisplaced fracture of shaft of other metacarpal bone**
Nondisplaced fracture of shaft of specified metacarpal bone with unspecified laterality

√7ᵗʰ **S62.359 Nondisplaced fracture of shaft of unspecified metacarpal bone** ▽

√6ᵗʰ **S62.36 Nondisplaced fracture of neck of other metacarpal bone**

√7ᵗʰ **S62.360 Nondisplaced fracture of neck of second metacarpal bone, right hand**

√7ᵗʰ **S62.361 Nondisplaced fracture of neck of second metacarpal bone, left hand**

√7ᵗʰ **S62.362 Nondisplaced fracture of neck of third metacarpal bone, right hand**

√7ᵗʰ **S62.363 Nondisplaced fracture of neck of third metacarpal bone, left hand**

√7ᵗʰ **S62.364 Nondisplaced fracture of neck of fourth metacarpal bone, right hand**

√7ᵗʰ **S62.365 Nondisplaced fracture of neck of fourth metacarpal bone, left hand**

√7ᵗʰ **S62.366 Nondisplaced fracture of neck of fifth metacarpal bone, right hand**

√7ᵗʰ **S62.367 Nondisplaced fracture of neck of fifth metacarpal bone, left hand**

√7ᵗʰ **S62.368 Nondisplaced fracture of neck of other metacarpal bone**
Nondisplaced fracture of neck of specified metacarpal bone with unspecified laterality

√7ᵗʰ **S62.369 Nondisplaced fracture of neck of unspecified metacarpal bone** ▽

√6ᵗʰ **S62.39 Other fracture of other metacarpal bone**

√7ᵗʰ **S62.390 Other fracture of second metacarpal bone, right hand**

√7ᵗʰ **S62.391 Other fracture of second metacarpal bone, left hand**

√7ᵗʰ **S62.392 Other fracture of third metacarpal bone, right hand**

√7ᵗʰ **S62.393 Other fracture of third metacarpal bone, left hand**

√7ᵗʰ **S62.394 Other fracture of fourth metacarpal bone, right hand**

√7ᵗʰ **S62.395 Other fracture of fourth metacarpal bone, left hand**

√7ᵗʰ **S62.396 Other fracture of fifth metacarpal bone, right hand**

√7ᵗʰ **S62.397 Other fracture of fifth metacarpal bone, left hand**

√7ᵗʰ **S62.398 Other fracture of other metacarpal bone**
Other fracture of specified metacarpal bone with unspecified laterality

√7ᵗʰ **S62.399 Other fracture of unspecified metacarpal bone** ▽

√5ᵗʰ **S62.5 Fracture of thumb**

√6ᵗʰ **S62.50 Fracture of unspecified phalanx of thumb**

√7ᵗʰ **S62.501 Fracture of unspecified phalanx of right thumb** ▽

√7ᵗʰ **S62.502 Fracture of unspecified phalanx of left thumb** ▽

√7ᵗʰ **S62.509 Fracture of unspecified phalanx of unspecified thumb** ▽

√6ᵗʰ **S62.51 Fracture of proximal phalanx of thumb**

√7ᵗʰ **S62.511 Displaced fracture of proximal phalanx of right thumb**

√7ᵗʰ **S62.512 Displaced fracture of proximal phalanx of left thumb**

√7ᵗʰ **S62.513 Displaced fracture of proximal phalanx of unspecified thumb** ▽

√7ᵗʰ **S62.514 Nondisplaced fracture of proximal phalanx of right thumb**

√7ᵗʰ **S62.515 Nondisplaced fracture of proximal phalanx of left thumb**

√7ᵗʰ **S62.516 Nondisplaced fracture of proximal phalanx of unspecified thumb** ▽

√6ᵗʰ **S62.52 Fracture of distal phalanx of thumb**

√7ᵗʰ **S62.521 Displaced fracture of distal phalanx of right thumb**

√7ᵗʰ **S62.522 Displaced fracture of distal phalanx of left thumb**

√7ᵗʰ **S62.523 Displaced fracture of distal phalanx of unspecified thumb** ▽

√7ᵗʰ **S62.524 Nondisplaced fracture of distal phalanx of right thumb**

√7ᵗʰ **S62.525 Nondisplaced fracture of distal phalanx of left thumb**

√7ᵗʰ **S62.526 Nondisplaced fracture of distal phalanx of unspecified thumb** ▽

√5ᵗʰ **S62.6 Fracture of other and unspecified finger(s)**
EXCLUDES 2 fracture of thumb (S62.5-)

√6ᵗʰ **S62.60 Fracture of unspecified phalanx of finger**

√7ᵗʰ **S62.600 Fracture of unspecified phalanx of right index finger** ▽

√7ᵗʰ **S62.601 Fracture of unspecified phalanx of left index finger** ▽

√7ᵗʰ **S62.602 Fracture of unspecified phalanx of right middle finger** ▽

√7ᵗʰ **S62.603 Fracture of unspecified phalanx of left middle finger** ▽

✓7ᵗʰ **S62.604 Fracture of unspecified phalanx of right ring finger** ▽

✓7ᵗʰ **S62.605 Fracture of unspecified phalanx of left ring finger** ▽

✓7ᵗʰ **S62.606 Fracture of unspecified phalanx of right little finger** ▽

✓7ᵗʰ **S62.607 Fracture of unspecified phalanx of left little finger** ▽

✓7ᵗʰ **S62.608 Fracture of unspecified phalanx of other finger** ▽
Fracture of unspecified phalanx of specified finger with unspecified laterality

✓7ᵗʰ **S62.609 Fracture of unspecified phalanx of unspecified finger** ▽

✓6ᵗʰ **S62.61 Displaced fracture of proximal phalanx of finger**

✓7ᵗʰ **S62.610 Displaced fracture of proximal phalanx of right index finger**

✓7ᵗʰ **S62.611 Displaced fracture of proximal phalanx of left index finger**

✓7ᵗʰ **S62.612 Displaced fracture of proximal phalanx of right middle finger**

✓7ᵗʰ **S62.613 Displaced fracture of proximal phalanx of left middle finger**

✓7ᵗʰ **S62.614 Displaced fracture of proximal phalanx of right ring finger**

✓7ᵗʰ **S62.615 Displaced fracture of proximal phalanx of left ring finger**

✓7ᵗʰ **S62.616 Displaced fracture of proximal phalanx of right little finger**

✓7ᵗʰ **S62.617 Displaced fracture of proximal phalanx of left little finger**

✓7ᵗʰ **S62.618 Displaced fracture of proximal phalanx of other finger** ▲ ▲
Displaced fracture of proximal phalanx of specified finger with unspecified laterality ▲ ▲

✓7ᵗʰ **S62.619 Displaced fracture of proximal phalanx of unspecified finger** ▽ ▲

✓6ᵗʰ **S62.62 Displaced fracture of middle phalanx of finger** ▲ ▲

✓7ᵗʰ **S62.620 Displaced fracture of middle phalanx of right index finger** ▲ ▲

✓7ᵗʰ **S62.621 Displaced fracture of middle phalanx of left index finger** ▲

✓7ᵗʰ **S62.622 Displaced fracture of middle phalanx of right middle finger** ▲

✓7ᵗʰ **S62.623 Displaced fracture of middle phalanx of left middle finger** ▲

✓7ᵗʰ **S62.624 Displaced fracture of middle phalanx of right ring finger** ▲

✓7ᵗʰ **S62.625 Displaced fracture of middle phalanx of left ring finger** ▲

✓7ᵗʰ **S62.626 Displaced fracture of medial phalanx of right little finger**

✓7ᵗʰ **S62.627 Displaced fracture of medial phalanx of left little finger**

✓7ᵗʰ **S62.628 Displaced fracture of medial phalanx of other finger**
Displaced fracture of medial phalanx of specified finger with unspecified laterality

✓7ᵗʰ **S62.629 Displaced fracture of medial phalanx of unspecified finger** ▽

✓6ᵗʰ **S62.63 Displaced fracture of distal phalanx of finger**

✓7ᵗʰ **S62.630 Displaced fracture of distal phalanx of right index finger**

✓7ᵗʰ **S62.631 Displaced fracture of distal phalanx of left index finger**

✓7ᵗʰ **S62.632 Displaced fracture of distal phalanx of right middle finger**

✓7ᵗʰ **S62.633 Displaced fracture of distal phalanx of left middle finger**

✓7ᵗʰ **S62.634 Displaced fracture of distal phalanx of right ring finger**

✓7ᵗʰ **S62.635 Displaced fracture of distal phalanx of left ring finger**

✓7ᵗʰ **S62.636 Displaced fracture of distal phalanx of right little finger**

✓7ᵗʰ **S62.637 Displaced fracture of distal phalanx of left little finger**

✓7ᵗʰ **S62.638 Displaced fracture of distal phalanx of other finger**
Displaced fracture of distal phalanx of specified finger with unspecified laterality

✓7ᵗʰ **S62.639 Displaced fracture of distal phalanx of unspecified finger** ▽

✓6ᵗʰ **S62.64 Nondisplaced fracture of proximal phalanx of finger**

✓7ᵗʰ **S62.640 Nondisplaced fracture of proximal phalanx of right index finger**

✓7ᵗʰ **S62.641 Nondisplaced fracture of proximal phalanx of left index finger**

✓7ᵗʰ **S62.642 Nondisplaced fracture of proximal phalanx of right middle finger**

✓7ᵗʰ **S62.643 Nondisplaced fracture of proximal phalanx of left middle finger**

✓7ᵗʰ **S62.644 Nondisplaced fracture of proximal phalanx of right ring finger**

✓7ᵗʰ **S62.645 Nondisplaced fracture of proximal phalanx of left ring finger**

✓7ᵗʰ **S62.646 Nondisplaced fracture of proximal phalanx of right little finger**

✓7ᵗʰ **S62.647 Nondisplaced fracture of proximal phalanx of left little finger**

✓7ᵗʰ **S62.648 Nondisplaced fracture of proximal phalanx of other finger**
Nondisplaced fracture of proximal phalanx of specified finger with unspecified laterality

✓7ᵗʰ **S62.649 Nondisplaced fracture of proximal phalanx of unspecified finger** ▽

✓6ᵗʰ **S62.65 Nondisplaced fracture of middle phalanx of finger**

✓7ᵗʰ **S62.650 Nondisplaced fracture of middle phalanx of right index finger**

✓7ᵗʰ **S62.651 Nondisplaced fracture of middle phalanx of left index finger**

✓7ᵗʰ **S62.652 Nondisplaced fracture of middle phalanx of right middle finger**

✓7ᵗʰ **S62.653 Nondisplaced fracture of middle phalanx of left middle finger**

✓7ᵗʰ **S62.654 Nondisplaced fracture of medial phalanx of right ring finger**

✓7ᵗʰ **S62.655 Nondisplaced fracture of medial phalanx of left ring finger**

✓7ᵗʰ **S62.656 Nondisplaced fracture of medial phalanx of right little finger**

✓7ᵗʰ **S62.657 Nondisplaced fracture of medial phalanx of left little finger**

✓7ᵗʰ **S62.658 Nondisplaced fracture of medial phalanx of other finger**
Nondisplaced fracture of medial phalanx of specified finger with unspecified laterality

✓7ᵗʰ **S62.659 Nondisplaced fracture of medial phalanx of unspecified finger** ▽

✓6ᵗʰ **S62.66 Nondisplaced fracture of distal phalanx of finger**

✓7ᵗʰ **S62.660 Nondisplaced fracture of distal phalanx of right index finger**

✓7ᵗʰ **S62.661 Nondisplaced fracture of distal phalanx of left index finger**

✓7ᵗʰ **S62.662 Nondisplaced fracture of distal phalanx of right middle finger**

✓7ᵗʰ **S62.663 Nondisplaced fracture of distal phalanx of left middle finger**

✓7ᵗʰ **S62.664 Nondisplaced fracture of distal phalanx of right ring finger**

✓7ᵗʰ **S62.665 Nondisplaced fracture of distal phalanx of left ring finger**

✓7ᵗʰ **S62.666 Nondisplaced fracture of distal phalanx of right little finger**

✓7ᵗʰ **S62.667 Nondisplaced fracture of distal phalanx of left little finger**

☑ Additional Character Req   ✓ₓ7ᵗʰ Placeholder Alert   Manifestation   HCC CMS-HCC Condition   ▽ Unspecified Code   ►◄ Revised Text   ● New Code   ▲ Revised Code Title

ICD-10-CM 2018   987

✓7ᵗʰ **S62.668** **Nondisplaced fracture of distal phalanx of other finger**
Nondisplaced fracture of distal phalanx of specified finger with unspecified laterality

✓7ᵗʰ **S62.669** **Nondisplaced fracture of distal phalanx** ▽ **of unspecified finger**

✓5ᵗʰ **S62.9** **Unspecified fracture of wrist and hand**

✓x7ᵗʰ **S62.90** **Unspecified fracture of unspecified wrist and** ▽ **hand**

✓x7ᵗʰ **S62.91** **Unspecified fracture of right wrist and hand** ▽

✓x7ᵗʰ **S62.92** **Unspecified fracture of left wrist and hand** ▽

✓4ᵗʰ **S63** **Dislocation and sprain of joints and ligaments at wrist and hand level**

INCLUDES avulsion of joint or ligament at wrist and hand level
laceration of cartilage, joint or ligament at wrist and hand level
sprain of cartilage, joint or ligament at wrist and hand level
traumatic hemarthrosis of joint or ligament at wrist and hand level
traumatic rupture of joint or ligament at wrist and hand level
traumatic subluxation of joint or ligament at wrist and hand level
traumatic tear of joint or ligament at wrist and hand level

Code also any associated open wound

EXCLUDES 2 *strain of muscle, fascia and tendon of wrist and hand (S66.-)*

The appropriate 7th character is to be added to each code from category S63.
A   initial encounter
D   subsequent encounter
S   sequela

✓5ᵗʰ **S63.0** **Subluxation and dislocation of wrist and hand joints**

✓6ᵗʰ **S63.00** **Unspecified subluxation and dislocation of wrist and hand**
Dislocation of carpal bone NOS
Dislocation of distal end of radius NOS
Subluxation of carpal bone NOS
Subluxation of distal end of radius NOS

✓7ᵗʰ **S63.001** **Unspecified subluxation of right wrist** ▽ **and hand**

✓7ᵗʰ **S63.002** **Unspecified subluxation of left wrist** ▽ **and hand**

✓7ᵗʰ **S63.003** **Unspecified subluxation of unspecified** ▽ **wrist and hand**

✓7ᵗʰ **S63.004** **Unspecified dislocation of right wrist** ▽ **and hand**

✓7ᵗʰ **S63.005** **Unspecified dislocation of left wrist** ▽ **and hand**

✓7ᵗʰ **S63.006** **Unspecified dislocation of unspecified** ▽ **wrist and hand**

✓6ᵗʰ **S63.01** **Subluxation and dislocation of distal radioulnar joint**

✓7ᵗʰ **S63.011** **Subluxation of distal radioulnar joint of right wrist**

✓7ᵗʰ **S63.012** **Subluxation of distal radioulnar joint of left wrist**

✓7ᵗʰ **S63.013** **Subluxation of distal radioulnar joint** ▽ **of unspecified wrist**

✓7ᵗʰ **S63.014** **Dislocation of distal radioulnar joint of right wrist**

✓7ᵗʰ **S63.015** **Dislocation of distal radioulnar joint of left wrist**

✓7ᵗʰ **S63.016** **Dislocation of distal radioulnar joint** ▽ **of unspecified wrist**

✓6ᵗʰ **S63.02** **Subluxation and dislocation of radiocarpal joint**

✓7ᵗʰ **S63.021** **Subluxation of radiocarpal joint of right wrist**

✓7ᵗʰ **S63.022** **Subluxation of radiocarpal joint of left wrist**

✓7ᵗʰ **S63.023** **Subluxation of radiocarpal joint of** ▽ **unspecified wrist**

✓7ᵗʰ **S63.024** **Dislocation of radiocarpal joint of right wrist**

✓7ᵗʰ **S63.025** **Dislocation of radiocarpal joint of left wrist**

✓7ᵗʰ **S63.026** **Dislocation of radiocarpal joint of** ▽ **unspecified wrist**

✓6ᵗʰ **S63.03** **Subluxation and dislocation of midcarpal joint**

✓7ᵗʰ **S63.031** **Subluxation of midcarpal joint of right wrist**

✓7ᵗʰ **S63.032** **Subluxation of midcarpal joint of left wrist**

✓7ᵗʰ **S63.033** **Subluxation of midcarpal joint of** ▽ **unspecified wrist**

✓7ᵗʰ **S63.034** **Dislocation of midcarpal joint of right wrist**

✓7ᵗʰ **S63.035** **Dislocation of midcarpal joint of left wrist**

✓7ᵗʰ **S63.036** **Dislocation of midcarpal joint of** ▽ **unspecified wrist**

✓6ᵗʰ **S63.04** **Subluxation and dislocation of carpometacarpal joint of thumb**
EXCLUDES 2 *interphalangeal subluxation and dislocation of thumb (S63.1-)*

✓7ᵗʰ **S63.041** **Subluxation of carpometacarpal joint of right thumb**

✓7ᵗʰ **S63.042** **Subluxation of carpometacarpal joint of left thumb**

✓7ᵗʰ **S63.043** **Subluxation of carpometacarpal joint** ▽ **of unspecified thumb**

✓7ᵗʰ **S63.044** **Dislocation of carpometacarpal joint of right thumb**

✓7ᵗʰ **S63.045** **Dislocation of carpometacarpal joint of left thumb**

✓7ᵗʰ **S63.046** **Dislocation of carpometacarpal joint** ▽ **of unspecified thumb**

✓6ᵗʰ **S63.05** **Subluxation and dislocation of other carpometacarpal joint**
EXCLUDES 2 *subluxation and dislocation of carpometacarpal joint of thumb (S63.04-)*

✓7ᵗʰ **S63.051** **Subluxation of other carpometacarpal joint of right hand**

✓7ᵗʰ **S63.052** **Subluxation of other carpometacarpal joint of left hand**

✓7ᵗʰ **S63.053** **Subluxation of other carpometacarpal** ▽ **joint of unspecified hand**

✓7ᵗʰ **S63.054** **Dislocation of other carpometacarpal joint of right hand**

✓7ᵗʰ **S63.055** **Dislocation of other carpometacarpal joint of left hand**

✓7ᵗʰ **S63.056** **Dislocation of other carpometacarpal** ▽ **joint of unspecified hand**

✓6ᵗʰ **S63.06** **Subluxation and dislocation of metacarpal (bone), proximal end**

✓7ᵗʰ **S63.061** **Subluxation of metacarpal (bone), proximal end of right hand**

✓7ᵗʰ **S63.062** **Subluxation of metacarpal (bone), proximal end of left hand**

✓7ᵗʰ **S63.063** **Subluxation of metacarpal (bone),** ▽ **proximal end of unspecified hand**

✓7ᵗʰ **S63.064** **Dislocation of metacarpal (bone), proximal end of right hand**

✓7ᵗʰ **S63.065** **Dislocation of metacarpal (bone), proximal end of left hand**

✓7ᵗʰ **S63.066** **Dislocation of metacarpal (bone),** ▽ **proximal end of unspecified hand**

✓6ᵗʰ **S63.07** **Subluxation and dislocation of distal end of ulna**

✓7ᵗʰ **S63.071** **Subluxation of distal end of right ulna**

✓7ᵗʰ **S63.072** **Subluxation of distal end of left ulna**

✓7ᵗʰ **S63.073** **Subluxation of distal end of unspecified** ▽ **ulna**

✓7ᵗʰ **S63.074** **Dislocation of distal end of right ulna**

✓7ᵗʰ **S63.075** **Dislocation of distal end of left ulna**

✓7ᵗʰ **S63.076** **Dislocation of distal end of unspecified** ▽ **ulna**

✓6ᵗʰ **S63.09** **Other subluxation and dislocation of wrist and hand**

✓7ᵗʰ **S63.091** **Other subluxation of right wrist and hand**

✓7ᵗʰ **S63.092** **Other subluxation of left wrist and hand**

✓7ᵗʰ **S63.093** **Other subluxation of unspecified wrist** ▽ **and hand**

✓7ᵗʰ **S63.094** **Other dislocation of right wrist and hand**

√7ᵗʰ **S63.095** Other dislocation of left wrist and hand

√7ᵗʰ **S63.096** Other dislocation of unspecified wrist and hand ▽

√5ᵗʰ **S63.1** **Subluxation and dislocation of thumb**

√6ᵗʰ **S63.10** **Unspecified subluxation and dislocation of thumb**

√7ᵗʰ **S63.101** Unspecified subluxation of right thumb ▽

√7ᵗʰ **S63.102** Unspecified subluxation of left thumb ▽

√7ᵗʰ **S63.103** Unspecified subluxation of unspecified thumb ▽

√7ᵗʰ **S63.104** Unspecified dislocation of right thumb ▽

√7ᵗʰ **S63.105** Unspecified dislocation of left thumb ▽

√7ᵗʰ **S63.106** Unspecified dislocation of unspecified thumb ▽

√6ᵗʰ **S63.11** **Subluxation and dislocation of metacarpophalangeal joint of thumb**

√7ᵗʰ **S63.111** Subluxation of metacarpophalangeal joint of right thumb

√7ᵗʰ **S63.112** Subluxation of metacarpophalangeal joint of left thumb

√7ᵗʰ **S63.113** Subluxation of metacarpophalangeal joint of unspecified thumb ▽

√7ᵗʰ **S63.114** Dislocation of metacarpophalangeal joint of right thumb

√7ᵗʰ **S63.115** Dislocation of metacarpophalangeal joint of left thumb

√7ᵗʰ **S63.116** Dislocation of metacarpophalangeal joint of unspecified thumb ▽

▲ √6ᵗʰ **S63.12** **Subluxation and dislocation of interphalangeal joint of thumb**

▲ √7ᵗʰ **S63.121** Subluxation of interphalangeal joint of right thumb

▲ √7ᵗʰ **S63.122** Subluxation of interphalangeal joint of left thumb

▲ √7ᵗʰ **S63.123** Subluxation of interphalangeal joint of unspecified thumb ▽

▲ √7ᵗʰ **S63.124** Dislocation of interphalangeal joint of right thumb

▲ √7ᵗʰ **S63.125** Dislocation of interphalangeal joint of left thumb

▲ √7ᵗʰ **S63.126** Dislocation of interphalangeal joint of unspecified thumb ▽

√6ᵗʰ ~~S63.13~~ ~~**Subluxation and dislocation of proximal interphalangeal joint of thumb**~~

√7ᵗʰ ~~S63.131~~ ~~Subluxation of proximal interphalangeal joint of right thumb~~

√7ᵗʰ ~~S63.132~~ ~~Subluxation of proximal interphalangeal joint of left thumb~~

√7ᵗʰ ~~S63.133~~ ~~Subluxation of proximal interphalangeal joint of unspecified thumb~~

√7ᵗʰ ~~S63.134~~ ~~Dislocation of proximal interphalangeal joint of right thumb~~

√7ᵗʰ ~~S63.135~~ ~~Dislocation of proximal interphalangeal joint of left thumb~~

√7ᵗʰ ~~S63.136~~ ~~Dislocation of proximal interphalangeal joint of unspecified thumb~~

√6ᵗʰ ~~S63.14~~ ~~**Subluxation and dislocation of distal interphalangeal joint of thumb**~~

√7ᵗʰ ~~S63.141~~ ~~Subluxation of distal interphalangeal joint of right thumb~~

√7ᵗʰ ~~S63.142~~ ~~Subluxation of distal interphalangeal joint of left thumb~~

√7ᵗʰ ~~S63.143~~ ~~Subluxation of distal interphalangeal joint of unspecified thumb~~

√7ᵗʰ ~~S63.144~~ ~~Dislocation of distal interphalangeal joint of right thumb~~

√7ᵗʰ ~~S63.145~~ ~~Dislocation of distal interphalangeal joint of left thumb~~

√7ᵗʰ ~~S63.146~~ ~~Dislocation of distal interphalangeal joint of unspecified thumb~~

√5ᵗʰ **S63.2** **Subluxation and dislocation of other finger(s)**

EXCLUDES 2   subluxation and dislocation of thumb (S63.1-)

√6ᵗʰ **S63.20** **Unspecified subluxation of other finger**

√7ᵗʰ **S63.200** Unspecified subluxation of right index finger ▽

√7ᵗʰ **S63.201** Unspecified subluxation of left index finger ▽

√7ᵗʰ **S63.202** Unspecified subluxation of right middle finger ▽

√7ᵗʰ **S63.203** Unspecified subluxation of left middle finger ▽

√7ᵗʰ **S63.204** Unspecified subluxation of right ring finger ▽

√7ᵗʰ **S63.205** Unspecified subluxation of left ring finger ▽

√7ᵗʰ **S63.206** Unspecified subluxation of right little finger ▽

√7ᵗʰ **S63.207** Unspecified subluxation of left little finger ▽

√7ᵗʰ **S63.208** Unspecified subluxation of other finger ▽
Unspecified subluxation of specified finger with unspecified laterality

√7ᵗʰ **S63.209** Unspecified subluxation of unspecified finger ▽

√6ᵗʰ **S63.21** **Subluxation of metacarpophalangeal joint of finger**

√7ᵗʰ **S63.210** Subluxation of metacarpophalangeal joint of right index finger

√7ᵗʰ **S63.211** Subluxation of metacarpophalangeal joint of left index finger

√7ᵗʰ **S63.212** Subluxation of metacarpophalangeal joint of right middle finger

√7ᵗʰ **S63.213** Subluxation of metacarpophalangeal joint of left middle finger

√7ᵗʰ **S63.214** Subluxation of metacarpophalangeal joint of right ring finger

√7ᵗʰ **S63.215** Subluxation of metacarpophalangeal joint of left ring finger

√7ᵗʰ **S63.216** Subluxation of metacarpophalangeal joint of right little finger

√7ᵗʰ **S63.217** Subluxation of metacarpophalangeal joint of left little finger

√7ᵗʰ **S63.218** Subluxation of metacarpophalangeal joint of other finger
Subluxation of metacarpophalangeal joint of specified finger with unspecified laterality

√7ᵗʰ **S63.219** Subluxation of metacarpophalangeal joint of unspecified finger ▽

√6ᵗʰ **S63.22** **Subluxation of unspecified interphalangeal joint of finger**

√7ᵗʰ **S63.220** Subluxation of unspecified interphalangeal joint of right index finger ▽

√7ᵗʰ **S63.221** Subluxation of unspecified interphalangeal joint of left index finger ▽

√7ᵗʰ **S63.222** Subluxation of unspecified interphalangeal joint of right middle finger ▽

√7ᵗʰ **S63.223** Subluxation of unspecified interphalangeal joint of left middle finger ▽

√7ᵗʰ **S63.224** Subluxation of unspecified interphalangeal joint of right ring finger ▽

√7ᵗʰ **S63.225** Subluxation of unspecified interphalangeal joint of left ring finger ▽

√7ᵗʰ **S63.226** Subluxation of unspecified interphalangeal joint of right little finger ▽

√7ᵗʰ **S63.227** Subluxation of unspecified interphalangeal joint of left little finger ▽

√7ᵗʰ **S63.228** Subluxation of unspecified interphalangeal joint of other finger ▽
Subluxation of unspecified interphalangeal joint of specified finger with unspecified laterality

√7ᵗʰ **S63.229** Subluxation of unspecified interphalangeal joint of unspecified finger ▽

☑ Additional Character Req   ▽⁷ᵗʰ Placeholder Alert   **Manifestation**   HCC CMS-HCC Condition   ▽ Unspecified Code   ▶◀ Revised Text   ● New Code   ▲ Revised Code Title

Chapter 19. Injury, Poisoning, and Certain Other Consequences of External Causes

✓6ᵗʰ **S63.23** Subluxation of proximal interphalangeal joint of finger

    ✓7ᵗʰ **S63.230** Subluxation of proximal interphalangeal joint of right index finger

    ✓7ᵗʰ **S63.231** Subluxation of proximal interphalangeal joint of left index finger

    ✓7ᵗʰ **S63.232** Subluxation of proximal interphalangeal joint of right middle finger

    ✓7ᵗʰ **S63.233** Subluxation of proximal interphalangeal joint of left middle finger

    ✓7ᵗʰ **S63.234** Subluxation of proximal interphalangeal joint of right ring finger

    ✓7ᵗʰ **S63.235** Subluxation of proximal interphalangeal joint of left ring finger

    ✓7ᵗʰ **S63.236** Subluxation of proximal interphalangeal joint of right little finger

    ✓7ᵗʰ **S63.237** Subluxation of proximal interphalangeal joint of left little finger

    ✓7ᵗʰ **S63.238** Subluxation of proximal interphalangeal joint of other finger

        Subluxation of proximal interphalangeal joint of specified finger with unspecified laterality

    ✓7ᵗʰ **S63.239** Subluxation of proximal interphalangeal joint of unspecified finger ▽

✓6ᵗʰ **S63.24** Subluxation of distal interphalangeal joint of finger

    ✓7ᵗʰ **S63.240** Subluxation of distal interphalangeal joint of right index finger

    ✓7ᵗʰ **S63.241** Subluxation of distal interphalangeal joint of left index finger

    ✓7ᵗʰ **S63.242** Subluxation of distal interphalangeal joint of right middle finger

    ✓7ᵗʰ **S63.243** Subluxation of distal interphalangeal joint of left middle finger

    ✓7ᵗʰ **S63.244** Subluxation of distal interphalangeal joint of right ring finger

    ✓7ᵗʰ **S63.245** Subluxation of distal interphalangeal joint of left ring finger

    ✓7ᵗʰ **S63.246** Subluxation of distal interphalangeal joint of right little finger

    ✓7ᵗʰ **S63.247** Subluxation of distal interphalangeal joint of left little finger

    ✓7ᵗʰ **S63.248** Subluxation of distal interphalangeal joint of other finger

        Subluxation of distal interphalangeal joint of specified finger with unspecified laterality

    ✓7ᵗʰ **S63.249** Subluxation of distal interphalangeal joint of unspecified finger ▽

✓6ᵗʰ **S63.25** Unspecified dislocation of other finger

    ✓7ᵗʰ **S63.250** Unspecified dislocation of right index finger ▽

    ✓7ᵗʰ **S63.251** Unspecified dislocation of left index finger ▽

    ✓7ᵗʰ **S63.252** Unspecified dislocation of right middle finger ▽

    ✓7ᵗʰ **S63.253** Unspecified dislocation of left middle finger ▽

    ✓7ᵗʰ **S63.254** Unspecified dislocation of right ring finger ▽

    ✓7ᵗʰ **S63.255** Unspecified dislocation of left ring finger ▽

    ✓7ᵗʰ **S63.256** Unspecified dislocation of right little finger ▽

    ✓7ᵗʰ **S63.257** Unspecified dislocation of left little finger ▽

    ✓7ᵗʰ **S63.258** Unspecified dislocation of other finger ▽

        Unspecified dislocation of specified finger with unspecified laterality

    ✓7ᵗʰ **S63.259** Unspecified dislocation of unspecified finger ▽

        ▶Unspecified dislocation of unspecified finger with unspecified laterality◀

✓6ᵗʰ **S63.26** Dislocation of metacarpophalangeal joint of finger

    ✓7ᵗʰ **S63.260** Dislocation of metacarpophalangeal joint of right index finger

    ✓7ᵗʰ **S63.261** Dislocation of metacarpophalangeal joint of left index finger

    ✓7ᵗʰ **S63.262** Dislocation of metacarpophalangeal joint of right middle finger

    ✓7ᵗʰ **S63.263** Dislocation of metacarpophalangeal joint of left middle finger

    ✓7ᵗʰ **S63.264** Dislocation of metacarpophalangeal joint of right ring finger

    ✓7ᵗʰ **S63.265** Dislocation of metacarpophalangeal joint of left ring finger

    ✓7ᵗʰ **S63.266** Dislocation of metacarpophalangeal joint of right little finger

    ✓7ᵗʰ **S63.267** Dislocation of metacarpophalangeal joint of left little finger

    ✓7ᵗʰ **S63.268** Dislocation of metacarpophalangeal joint of other finger

        Dislocation of metacarpophalangeal joint of specified finger with unspecified laterality

    ✓7ᵗʰ **S63.269** Dislocation of metacarpophalangeal joint of unspecified finger ▽

✓6ᵗʰ **S63.27** Dislocation of unspecified interphalangeal joint of finger

    ✓7ᵗʰ **S63.270** Dislocation of unspecified interphalangeal joint of right index finger ▽

    ✓7ᵗʰ **S63.271** Dislocation of unspecified interphalangeal joint of left index finger ▽

    ✓7ᵗʰ **S63.272** Dislocation of unspecified interphalangeal joint of right middle finger ▽

    ✓7ᵗʰ **S63.273** Dislocation of unspecified interphalangeal joint of left middle finger ▽

    ✓7ᵗʰ **S63.274** Dislocation of unspecified interphalangeal joint of right ring finger ▽

    ✓7ᵗʰ **S63.275** Dislocation of unspecified interphalangeal joint of left ring finger ▽

    ✓7ᵗʰ **S63.276** Dislocation of unspecified interphalangeal joint of right little finger ▽

    ✓7ᵗʰ **S63.277** Dislocation of unspecified interphalangeal joint of left little finger ▽

    ✓7ᵗʰ **S63.278** Dislocation of unspecified interphalangeal joint of other finger ▽

        Dislocation of unspecified interphalangeal joint of specified finger with unspecified laterality

    ✓7ᵗʰ **S63.279** Dislocation of unspecified interphalangeal joint of unspecified finger ▽

        ▶Dislocation of unspecified interphalangeal joint of unspecified finger without specified laterality◀

✓6ᵗʰ **S63.28** Dislocation of proximal interphalangeal joint of finger

    ✓7ᵗʰ **S63.280** Dislocation of proximal interphalangeal joint of right index finger

    ✓7ᵗʰ **S63.281** Dislocation of proximal interphalangeal joint of left index finger

    ✓7ᵗʰ **S63.282** Dislocation of proximal interphalangeal joint of right middle finger

    ✓7ᵗʰ **S63.283** Dislocation of proximal interphalangeal joint of left middle finger

    ✓7ᵗʰ **S63.284** Dislocation of proximal interphalangeal joint of right ring finger

    ✓7ᵗʰ **S63.285** Dislocation of proximal interphalangeal joint of left ring finger

    ✓7ᵗʰ **S63.286** Dislocation of proximal interphalangeal joint of right little finger

    ✓7ᵗʰ **S63.287** Dislocation of proximal interphalangeal joint of left little finger

    ✓7ᵗʰ **S63.288** Dislocation of proximal interphalangeal joint of other finger

        Dislocation of proximal interphalangeal joint of specified finger with unspecified laterality

    ✓7ᵗʰ **S63.289** Dislocation of proximal interphalangeal joint of unspecified finger ▽

EXCLUDES 1 Not coded here   EXCLUDES 2 Not included here   N Newborn Age: 0   P Pediatric Age: 0-17   M Maternity Age: 12-55   A Adult Age: 15-124

990   ICD-10-CM 2018

✓6ᵗʰ **S63.29** Dislocation of distal interphalangeal joint of finger

✓7ᵗʰ **S63.290** Dislocation of distal interphalangeal joint of right index finger

✓7ᵗʰ **S63.291** Dislocation of distal interphalangeal joint of left index finger

✓7ᵗʰ **S63.292** Dislocation of distal interphalangeal joint of right middle finger

✓7ᵗʰ **S63.293** Dislocation of distal interphalangeal joint of left middle finger

✓7ᵗʰ **S63.294** Dislocation of distal interphalangeal joint of right ring finger

✓7ᵗʰ **S63.295** Dislocation of distal interphalangeal joint of left ring finger

✓7ᵗʰ **S63.296** Dislocation of distal interphalangeal joint of right little finger

✓7ᵗʰ **S63.297** Dislocation of distal interphalangeal joint of left little finger

✓7ᵗʰ **S63.298** Dislocation of distal interphalangeal joint of other finger
Dislocation of distal interphalangeal joint of specified finger with unspecified laterality

✓7ᵗʰ **S63.299** Dislocation of distal interphalangeal joint of unspecified finger ▽

✓5ᵗʰ **S63.3** Traumatic rupture of ligament of wrist

✓6ᵗʰ **S63.30** Traumatic rupture of unspecified ligament of wrist

✓7ᵗʰ **S63.301** Traumatic rupture of unspecified ligament of right wrist ▽

✓7ᵗʰ **S63.302** Traumatic rupture of unspecified ligament of left wrist ▽

✓7ᵗʰ **S63.309** Traumatic rupture of unspecified ligament of unspecified wrist ▽

✓6ᵗʰ **S63.31** Traumatic rupture of collateral ligament of wrist

✓7ᵗʰ **S63.311** Traumatic rupture of collateral ligament of right wrist

✓7ᵗʰ **S63.312** Traumatic rupture of collateral ligament of left wrist

✓7ᵗʰ **S63.319** Traumatic rupture of collateral ligament of unspecified wrist ▽

✓6ᵗʰ **S63.32** Traumatic rupture of radiocarpal ligament

✓7ᵗʰ **S63.321** Traumatic rupture of right radiocarpal ligament

✓7ᵗʰ **S63.322** Traumatic rupture of left radiocarpal ligament

✓7ᵗʰ **S63.329** Traumatic rupture of unspecified radiocarpal ligament ▽

✓6ᵗʰ **S63.33** Traumatic rupture of ulnocarpal (palmar) ligament

✓7ᵗʰ **S63.331** Traumatic rupture of right ulnocarpal (palmar) ligament

✓7ᵗʰ **S63.332** Traumatic rupture of left ulnocarpal (palmar) ligament

✓7ᵗʰ **S63.339** Traumatic rupture of unspecified ulnocarpal (palmar) ligament ▽

✓6ᵗʰ **S63.39** Traumatic rupture of other ligament of wrist

✓7ᵗʰ **S63.391** Traumatic rupture of other ligament of right wrist

✓7ᵗʰ **S63.392** Traumatic rupture of other ligament of left wrist

✓7ᵗʰ **S63.399** Traumatic rupture of other ligament of unspecified wrist ▽

✓5ᵗʰ **S63.4** Traumatic rupture of ligament of finger at metacarpophalangeal and interphalangeal joint(s)

✓6ᵗʰ **S63.40** Traumatic rupture of unspecified ligament of finger at metacarpophalangeal and interphalangeal joint

✓7ᵗʰ **S63.400** Traumatic rupture of unspecified ligament of right index finger at metacarpo- phalangeal and interphalangeal joint ▽

✓7ᵗʰ **S63.401** Traumatic rupture of unspecified ligament of left index finger at metacarpophalangeal and interphalangeal joint ▽

✓7ᵗʰ **S63.402** Traumatic rupture of unspecified ligament of right middle finger at metacarpophalangeal and interphalangeal joint ▽

✓7ᵗʰ **S63.403** Traumatic rupture of unspecified ligament of left middle finger at metacarpo- phalangeal and interphalangeal joint ▽

✓7ᵗʰ **S63.404** Traumatic rupture of unspecified ligament of right ring finger at metacarpophalangeal and interphalangeal joint ▽

✓7ᵗʰ **S63.405** Traumatic rupture of unspecified ligament of left ring finger at metacarpophalangeal and interphalangeal joint ▽

✓7ᵗʰ **S63.406** Traumatic rupture of unspecified ligament of right little finger at metacarpophalangeal and interphalangeal joint ▽

✓7ᵗʰ **S63.407** Traumatic rupture of unspecified ligament of left little finger at metacarpophalangeal and interphalangeal joint ▽

✓7ᵗʰ **S63.408** Traumatic rupture of unspecified ligament of other finger at metacarpophalangeal and interphalangeal joint ▽
Traumatic rupture of unspecified ligament of specified finger with unspecified laterality at metacarpophalangeal and interphalangeal joint

✓7ᵗʰ **S63.409** Traumatic rupture of unspecified ligament of unspecified finger at metacarpophalangeal and interphalangeal joint ▽

✓6ᵗʰ **S63.41** Traumatic rupture of collateral ligament of finger at metacarpophalangeal and interphalangeal joint

✓7ᵗʰ **S63.410** Traumatic rupture of collateral ligament of right index finger at metacarpo- phalangeal and interphalangeal joint

✓7ᵗʰ **S63.411** Traumatic rupture of collateral ligament of left index finger at metacarpo- phalangeal and interphalangeal joint

✓7ᵗʰ **S63.412** Traumatic rupture of collateral ligament of right middle finger at metacarpo- phalangeal and interphalangeal joint

✓7ᵗʰ **S63.413** Traumatic rupture of collateral ligament of left middle finger at metacarpo- phalangeal and interphalangeal joint

✓7ᵗʰ **S63.414** Traumatic rupture of collateral ligament of right ring finger at metacarpo- phalangeal and interphalangeal joint

✓7ᵗʰ **S63.415** Traumatic rupture of collateral ligament of left ring finger at metacarpophalangeal and interphalangeal joint

✓7ᵗʰ **S63.416** Traumatic rupture of collateral ligament of right little finger at metacarpo- phalangeal and interphalangeal joint

✓7ᵗʰ **S63.417** Traumatic rupture of collateral ligament of left little finger at metacarpo- phalangeal and interphalangeal joint

✓7ᵗʰ **S63.418** Traumatic rupture of collateral ligament of other finger at metacarpophalangeal and interphalangeal joint
Traumatic rupture of collateral ligament of specified finger with unspecified laterality at metacarpophalangeal and interphalangeal joint

✓7ᵗʰ **S63.419** Traumatic rupture of collateral ligament of unspecified finger at metacarpophalangeal and interphalangeal joint ▽

✓6ᵗʰ **S63.42** Traumatic rupture of palmar ligament of finger at metacarpophalangeal and interphalangeal joint

✓7ᵗʰ **S63.420** Traumatic rupture of palmar ligament of right index finger at metacarpo- phalangeal and interphalangeal joint

✓7ᵗʰ **S63.421** Traumatic rupture of palmar ligament of left index finger at metacarpophalangeal and interphalangeal joint

✓7ᵗʰ **S63.422** Traumatic rupture of palmar ligament of right middle finger at metacarpo- phalangeal and interphalangeal joint

✓7ᵗʰ **S63.423** Traumatic rupture of palmar ligament of left middle finger at metacarpo- phalangeal and interphalangeal joint

✓7ᵗʰ **S63.424** Traumatic rupture of palmar ligament of right ring finger at metacarpophalangeal and interphalangeal joint

✓7ᵗʰ **S63.425** Traumatic rupture of palmar ligament of left ring finger at metacarpophalangeal and interphalangeal joint

✓7ᵗʰ **S63.426** Traumatic rupture of palmar ligament of right little finger at metacarpophalangeal and interphalangeal joint

✓7ᵗʰ **S63.427** Traumatic rupture of palmar ligament of left little finger at metacarpophalangeal and interphalangeal joint

✓7ᵗʰ **S63.428** Traumatic rupture of palmar ligament of other finger at metacarpophalangeal and interphalangeal joint
     Traumatic rupture of palmar ligament of specified finger with unspecified laterality at metacarpophalangeal and interphalangeal joint

✓7ᵗʰ **S63.429** Traumatic rupture of palmar ligament ▽ of unspecified finger at metacarpo- phalangeal and interphalangeal joint

✓6ᵗʰ **S63.43** Traumatic rupture of volar plate of finger at metacarpophalangeal and interphalangeal joint

✓7ᵗʰ **S63.430** Traumatic rupture of volar plate of right index finger at metacarpophalangeal and interphalangeal joint

✓7ᵗʰ **S63.431** Traumatic rupture of volar plate of left index finger at metacarpophalangeal and interphalangeal joint

✓7ᵗʰ **S63.432** Traumatic rupture of volar plate of right middle finger at metacarpophalangeal and interphalangeal joint

✓7ᵗʰ **S63.433** Traumatic rupture of volar plate of left middle finger at metacarpophalangeal and interphalangeal joint

✓7ᵗʰ **S63.434** Traumatic rupture of volar plate of right ring finger at metacarpophalangeal and interphalangeal joint

✓7ᵗʰ **S63.435** Traumatic rupture of volar plate of left ring finger at metacarpophalangeal and interphalangeal joint

✓7ᵗʰ **S63.436** Traumatic rupture of volar plate of right little finger at metacarpophalangeal and interphalangeal joint

✓7ᵗʰ **S63.437** Traumatic rupture of volar plate of left little finger at metacarpophalangeal and interphalangeal joint

✓7ᵗʰ **S63.438** Traumatic rupture of volar plate of other finger at metacarpophalangeal and interphalangeal joint
     Traumatic rupture of volar plate of specified finger with unspecified laterality at metacarpophalangeal and interphalangeal joint

✓7ᵗʰ **S63.439** Traumatic rupture of volar plate of ▽ unspecified finger at metacarpo- phalangeal and interphalangeal joint

✓6ᵗʰ **S63.49** Traumatic rupture of other ligament of finger at metacarpophalangeal and interphalangeal joint

✓7ᵗʰ **S63.490** Traumatic rupture of other ligament of right index finger at metacarpo- phalangeal and interphalangeal joint

✓7ᵗʰ **S63.491** Traumatic rupture of other ligament of left index finger at metacarpophalangeal and interphalangeal joint

✓7ᵗʰ **S63.492** Traumatic rupture of other ligament of right middle finger at metacarpo- phalangeal and interphalangeal joint

✓7ᵗʰ **S63.493** Traumatic rupture of other ligament of left middle finger at metacarpo- phalangeal and interphalangeal joint

✓7ᵗʰ **S63.494** Traumatic rupture of other ligament of right ring finger at metacarpophalangeal and interphalangeal joint

✓7ᵗʰ **S63.495** Traumatic rupture of other ligament of left ring finger at metacarpophalangeal and interphalangeal joint

✓7ᵗʰ **S63.496** Traumatic rupture of other ligament of right little finger at metacarpophalangeal and interphalangeal joint

✓7ᵗʰ **S63.497** Traumatic rupture of other ligament of left little finger at metacarpophalangeal and interphalangeal joint

✓7ᵗʰ **S63.498** Traumatic rupture of other ligament of other finger at metacarpophalangeal and interphalangeal joint
     Traumatic rupture of ligament of specified finger with unspecified laterality at metacarpophalangeal and interphalangeal joint

✓7ᵗʰ **S63.499** Traumatic rupture of other ligament ▽ of unspecified finger at metacarpo- phalangeal and interphalangeal joint

✓5ᵗʰ **S63.5** Other and unspecified sprain of wrist

✓6ᵗʰ **S63.50** Unspecified sprain of wrist

✓7ᵗʰ **S63.501** Unspecified sprain of right wrist ▽

✓7ᵗʰ **S63.502** Unspecified sprain of left wrist ▽

✓7ᵗʰ **S63.509** Unspecified sprain of unspecified wrist ▽

✓6ᵗʰ **S63.51** Sprain of carpal (joint)

✓7ᵗʰ **S63.511** Sprain of carpal joint of right wrist

✓7ᵗʰ **S63.512** Sprain of carpal joint of left wrist

✓7ᵗʰ **S63.519** Sprain of carpal joint of unspecified ▽ wrist

✓6ᵗʰ **S63.52** Sprain of radiocarpal joint
     EXCLUDES 1   traumatic rupture of radiocarpal ligament (S63.32-)

✓7ᵗʰ **S63.521** Sprain of radiocarpal joint of right wrist

✓7ᵗʰ **S63.522** Sprain of radiocarpal joint of left wrist

✓7ᵗʰ **S63.529** Sprain of radiocarpal joint of ▽ unspecified wrist

✓6ᵗʰ **S63.59** Other specified sprain of wrist

✓7ᵗʰ **S63.591** Other specified sprain of right wrist

✓7ᵗʰ **S63.592** Other specified sprain of left wrist

✓7ᵗʰ **S63.599** Other specified sprain of unspecified ▽ wrist

✓5ᵗʰ **S63.6** Other and unspecified sprain of finger(s)
     EXCLUDES 1   traumatic rupture of ligament of finger at metacarpophalangeal and interphalangeal joint(s) (S63.4-)

✓6ᵗʰ **S63.60** Unspecified sprain of thumb

✓7ᵗʰ **S63.601** Unspecified sprain of right thumb ▽

✓7ᵗʰ **S63.602** Unspecified sprain of left thumb ▽

✓7ᵗʰ **S63.609** Unspecified sprain of unspecified ▽ thumb

✓6ᵗʰ **S63.61** Unspecified sprain of other and unspecified finger(s)

✓7ᵗʰ **S63.610** Unspecified sprain of right index ▽ finger

✓7ᵗʰ **S63.611** Unspecified sprain of left index ▽ finger

✓7ᵗʰ **S63.612** Unspecified sprain of right middle ▽ finger

✓7ᵗʰ **S63.613** Unspecified sprain of left middle ▽ finger

✓7ᵗʰ **S63.614** Unspecified sprain of right ring ▽ finger

✓7ᵗʰ **S63.615** Unspecified sprain of left ring ▽ finger

✓7ᵗʰ **S63.616** Unspecified sprain of right little ▽ finger

✓7ᵗʰ **S63.617** Unspecified sprain of left little finger ▽

✓7ᵗʰ **S63.618** Unspecified sprain of other finger ▽
     Unspecified sprain of specified finger with unspecified laterality

✓7ᵗʰ **S63.619** Unspecified sprain of unspecified ▽ finger

✓6ᵗʰ **S63.62** Sprain of interphalangeal joint of thumb

✓7ᵗʰ **S63.621** Sprain of interphalangeal joint of right thumb

EXCLUDES 1 Not coded here   **EXCLUDES 2** Not included here   N Newborn Age: 0   P Pediatric Age: 0-17   M Maternity Age: 12-55   A Adult Age: 15-124

ICD-10-CM 2018

992

√7ᵗʰ **S63.622** Sprain of interphalangeal joint of left thumb

√7ᵗʰ **S63.629** Sprain of interphalangeal joint of unspecified thumb ▽

√6ᵗʰ **S63.63** Sprain of interphalangeal joint of other and unspecified finger(s)

√7ᵗʰ **S63.630** Sprain of interphalangeal joint of right index finger

√7ᵗʰ **S63.631** Sprain of interphalangeal joint of left index finger

√7ᵗʰ **S63.632** Sprain of interphalangeal joint of right middle finger

√7ᵗʰ **S63.633** Sprain of interphalangeal joint of left middle finger

√7ᵗʰ **S63.634** Sprain of interphalangeal joint of right ring finger

√7ᵗʰ **S63.635** Sprain of interphalangeal joint of left ring finger

√7ᵗʰ **S63.636** Sprain of interphalangeal joint of right little finger

√7ᵗʰ **S63.637** Sprain of interphalangeal joint of left little finger

√7ᵗʰ **S63.638** Sprain of interphalangeal joint of other finger

√7ᵗʰ **S63.639** Sprain of interphalangeal joint of unspecified finger ▽

√6ᵗʰ **S63.64** Sprain of metacarpophalangeal joint of thumb

√7ᵗʰ **S63.641** Sprain of metacarpophalangeal joint of right thumb

√7ᵗʰ **S63.642** Sprain of metacarpophalangeal joint of left thumb

√7ᵗʰ **S63.649** Sprain of metacarpophalangeal joint of unspecified thumb ▽

√6ᵗʰ **S63.65** Sprain of metacarpophalangeal joint of other and unspecified finger(s)

√7ᵗʰ **S63.650** Sprain of metacarpophalangeal joint of right index finger

√7ᵗʰ **S63.651** Sprain of metacarpophalangeal joint of left index finger

√7ᵗʰ **S63.652** Sprain of metacarpophalangeal joint of right middle finger

√7ᵗʰ **S63.653** Sprain of metacarpophalangeal joint of left middle finger

√7ᵗʰ **S63.654** Sprain of metacarpophalangeal joint of right ring finger

√7ᵗʰ **S63.655** Sprain of metacarpophalangeal joint of left ring finger

√7ᵗʰ **S63.656** Sprain of metacarpophalangeal joint of right little finger

√7ᵗʰ **S63.657** Sprain of metacarpophalangeal joint of left little finger

√7ᵗʰ **S63.658** Sprain of metacarpophalangeal joint of other finger
Sprain of metacarpophalangeal joint of specified finger with unspecified laterality

√7ᵗʰ **S63.659** Sprain of metacarpophalangeal joint of unspecified finger ▽

√6ᵗʰ **S63.68** Other sprain of thumb

√7ᵗʰ **S63.681** Other sprain of right thumb

√7ᵗʰ **S63.682** Other sprain of left thumb

√7ᵗʰ **S63.689** Other sprain of unspecified thumb ▽

√6ᵗʰ **S63.69** Other sprain of other and unspecified finger(s)

√7ᵗʰ **S63.690** Other sprain of right index finger

√7ᵗʰ **S63.691** Other sprain of left index finger

√7ᵗʰ **S63.692** Other sprain of right middle finger

√7ᵗʰ **S63.693** Other sprain of left middle finger

√7ᵗʰ **S63.694** Other sprain of right ring finger

√7ᵗʰ **S63.695** Other sprain of left ring finger

√7ᵗʰ **S63.696** Other sprain of right little finger

√7ᵗʰ **S63.697** Other sprain of left little finger

√7ᵗʰ **S63.698** Other sprain of other finger
Other sprain of specified finger with unspecified laterality

√7ᵗʰ **S63.699** Other sprain of unspecified finger ▽

√5ᵗʰ **S63.8** Sprain of other part of wrist and hand

√6ᵗʰ **S63.8X** Sprain of other part of wrist and hand

√7ᵗʰ **S63.8X1** Sprain of other part of right wrist and hand

√7ᵗʰ **S63.8X2** Sprain of other part of left wrist and hand

√7ᵗʰ **S63.8X9** Sprain of other part of unspecified wrist and hand ▽

√5ᵗʰ **S63.9** Sprain of unspecified part of wrist and hand

√x7ᵗʰ **S63.90** Sprain of unspecified part of unspecified wrist and hand ▽

√x7ᵗʰ **S63.91** Sprain of unspecified part of right wrist and hand ▽

√x7ᵗʰ **S63.92** Sprain of unspecified part of left wrist and hand ▽

√4ᵗʰ **S64** **Injury of nerves at wrist and hand level**
Code also any associated open wound (S61.-)

> The appropriate 7th character is to be added to each code from category S64.
> A   initial encounter
> D   subsequent encounter
> S   sequela

√5ᵗʰ **S64.0** Injury of ulnar nerve at wrist and hand level

√x7ᵗʰ **S64.00** Injury of ulnar nerve at wrist and hand level of unspecified arm ▽

√x7ᵗʰ **S64.01** Injury of ulnar nerve at wrist and hand level of right arm

√x7ᵗʰ **S64.02** Injury of ulnar nerve at wrist and hand level of left arm

√5ᵗʰ **S64.1** Injury of median nerve at wrist and hand level

√x7ᵗʰ **S64.10** Injury of median nerve at wrist and hand level of unspecified arm ▽

√x7ᵗʰ **S64.11** Injury of median nerve at wrist and hand level of right arm

√x7ᵗʰ **S64.12** Injury of median nerve at wrist and hand level of left arm

√5ᵗʰ **S64.2** Injury of radial nerve at wrist and hand level

√x7ᵗʰ **S64.20** Injury of radial nerve at wrist and hand level of unspecified arm ▽

√x7ᵗʰ **S64.21** Injury of radial nerve at wrist and hand level of right arm

√x7ᵗʰ **S64.22** Injury of radial nerve at wrist and hand level of left arm

√5ᵗʰ **S64.3** Injury of digital nerve of thumb

√x7ᵗʰ **S64.30** Injury of digital nerve of unspecified thumb ▽

√x7ᵗʰ **S64.31** Injury of digital nerve of right thumb

√x7ᵗʰ **S64.32** Injury of digital nerve of left thumb

√5ᵗʰ **S64.4** Injury of digital nerve of other and unspecified finger

√x7ᵗʰ **S64.40** Injury of digital nerve of unspecified finger ▽

√6ᵗʰ **S64.49** Injury of digital nerve of other finger

√7ᵗʰ **S64.490** Injury of digital nerve of right index finger

√7ᵗʰ **S64.491** Injury of digital nerve of left index finger

√7ᵗʰ **S64.492** Injury of digital nerve of right middle finger

√7ᵗʰ **S64.493** Injury of digital nerve of left middle finger

√7ᵗʰ **S64.494** Injury of digital nerve of right ring finger

√7ᵗʰ **S64.495** Injury of digital nerve of left ring finger

√7ᵗʰ **S64.496** Injury of digital nerve of right little finger

√7ᵗʰ **S64.497** Injury of digital nerve of left little finger

√7ᵗʰ **S64.498** Injury of digital nerve of other finger
Injury of digital nerve of specified finger with unspecified laterality

√5ᵗʰ **S64.8** Injury of other nerves at wrist and hand level

√6ᵗʰ **S64.8X** Injury of other nerves at wrist and hand level

√7ᵗʰ **S64.8X1** Injury of other nerves at wrist and hand level of right arm

√7ᵗʰ **S64.8X2** Injury of other nerves at wrist and hand level of left arm

√7ᵗʰ **S64.8X9** Injury of other nerves at wrist and hand level of unspecified arm ▽

☑ Additional Character Req   √7ᵗʰ Placeholder Alert   Manifestation   ʜᴄᴄ CMS-HCC Condition   ▽ Unspecified Code   ▶◀ Revised Text   ● New Code   ▲ Revised Code Title

√5ᵗʰ **S64.9   Injury of unspecified nerve at wrist and hand level**

√x7ᵗʰ **S64.90   Injury of unspecified nerve at wrist and hand level of unspecified arm**   ▽

√x7ᵗʰ **S64.91   Injury of unspecified nerve at wrist and hand level of right arm**   ▽

√x7ᵗʰ **S64.92   Injury of unspecified nerve at wrist and hand level of left arm**   ▽

√4ᵗʰ **S65   Injury of blood vessels at wrist and hand level**

Code also any associated open wound (S61.-)

> The appropriate 7th character is to be added to each code from category S65.
> A   initial encounter
> D   subsequent encounter
> S   sequela

√5ᵗʰ **S65.0   Injury of ulnar artery at wrist and hand level**

√6ᵗʰ **S65.00   Unspecified injury of ulnar artery at wrist and hand level**

√7ᵗʰ **S65.001   Unspecified injury of ulnar artery at wrist and hand level of right arm**   ▽

√7ᵗʰ **S65.002   Unspecified injury of ulnar artery at wrist and hand level of left arm**   ▽

√7ᵗʰ **S65.009   Unspecified injury of ulnar artery at wrist and hand level of unspecified arm**   ▽

√6ᵗʰ **S65.01   Laceration of ulnar artery at wrist and hand level**

√7ᵗʰ **S65.011   Laceration of ulnar artery at wrist and hand level of right arm**

√7ᵗʰ **S65.012   Laceration of ulnar artery at wrist and hand level of left arm**

√7ᵗʰ **S65.019   Laceration of ulnar artery at wrist and hand level of unspecified arm**   ▽

√6ᵗʰ **S65.09   Other specified injury of ulnar artery at wrist and hand level**

√7ᵗʰ **S65.091   Other specified injury of ulnar artery at wrist and hand level of right arm**

√7ᵗʰ **S65.092   Other specified injury of ulnar artery at wrist and hand level of left arm**

√7ᵗʰ **S65.099   Other specified injury of ulnar artery at wrist and hand level of unspecified arm**   ▽

√5ᵗʰ **S65.1   Injury of radial artery at wrist and hand level**

√6ᵗʰ **S65.10   Unspecified injury of radial artery at wrist and hand level**

√7ᵗʰ **S65.101   Unspecified injury of radial artery at wrist and hand level of right arm**   ▽

√7ᵗʰ **S65.102   Unspecified injury of radial artery at wrist and hand level of left arm**   ▽

√7ᵗʰ **S65.109   Unspecified injury of radial artery at wrist and hand level of unspecified arm**   ▽

√6ᵗʰ **S65.11   Laceration of radial artery at wrist and hand level**

√7ᵗʰ **S65.111   Laceration of radial artery at wrist and hand level of right arm**

√7ᵗʰ **S65.112   Laceration of radial artery at wrist and hand level of left arm**

√7ᵗʰ **S65.119   Laceration of radial artery at wrist and hand level of unspecified arm**   ▽

√6ᵗʰ **S65.19   Other specified injury of radial artery at wrist and hand level**

√7ᵗʰ **S65.191   Other specified injury of radial artery at wrist and hand level of right arm**

√7ᵗʰ **S65.192   Other specified injury of radial artery at wrist and hand level of left arm**

√7ᵗʰ **S65.199   Other specified injury of radial artery at wrist and hand level of unspecified arm**   ▽

√5ᵗʰ **S65.2   Injury of superficial palmar arch**

√6ᵗʰ **S65.20   Unspecified injury of superficial palmar arch**

√7ᵗʰ **S65.201   Unspecified injury of superficial palmar arch of right hand**   ▽

√7ᵗʰ **S65.202   Unspecified injury of superficial palmar arch of left hand**   ▽

√7ᵗʰ **S65.209   Unspecified injury of superficial palmar arch of unspecified hand**   ▽

√6ᵗʰ **S65.21   Laceration of superficial palmar arch**

√7ᵗʰ **S65.211   Laceration of superficial palmar arch of right hand**

√7ᵗʰ **S65.212   Laceration of superficial palmar arch of left hand**

√7ᵗʰ **S65.219   Laceration of superficial palmar arch of unspecified hand**   ▽

√6ᵗʰ **S65.29   Other specified injury of superficial palmar arch**

√7ᵗʰ **S65.291   Other specified injury of superficial palmar arch of right hand**

√7ᵗʰ **S65.292   Other specified injury of superficial palmar arch of left hand**

√7ᵗʰ **S65.299   Other specified injury of superficial palmar arch of unspecified hand**   ▽

√5ᵗʰ **S65.3   Injury of deep palmar arch**

√6ᵗʰ **S65.30   Unspecified injury of deep palmar arch**

√7ᵗʰ **S65.301   Unspecified injury of deep palmar arch of right hand**   ▽

√7ᵗʰ **S65.302   Unspecified injury of deep palmar arch of left hand**   ▽

√7ᵗʰ **S65.309   Unspecified injury of deep palmar arch of unspecified hand**   ▽

√6ᵗʰ **S65.31   Laceration of deep palmar arch**

√7ᵗʰ **S65.311   Laceration of deep palmar arch of right hand**

√7ᵗʰ **S65.312   Laceration of deep palmar arch of left hand**

√7ᵗʰ **S65.319   Laceration of deep palmar arch of unspecified hand**   ▽

√6ᵗʰ **S65.39   Other specified injury of deep palmar arch**

√7ᵗʰ **S65.391   Other specified injury of deep palmar arch of right hand**

√7ᵗʰ **S65.392   Other specified injury of deep palmar arch of left hand**

√7ᵗʰ **S65.399   Other specified injury of deep palmar arch of unspecified hand**   ▽

√5ᵗʰ **S65.4   Injury of blood vessel of thumb**

√6ᵗʰ **S65.40   Unspecified injury of blood vessel of thumb**

√7ᵗʰ **S65.401   Unspecified injury of blood vessel of right thumb**   ▽

√7ᵗʰ **S65.402   Unspecified injury of blood vessel of left thumb**   ▽

√7ᵗʰ **S65.409   Unspecified injury of blood vessel of unspecified thumb**   ▽

√6ᵗʰ **S65.41   Laceration of blood vessel of thumb**

√7ᵗʰ **S65.411   Laceration of blood vessel of right thumb**

√7ᵗʰ **S65.412   Laceration of blood vessel of left thumb**

√7ᵗʰ **S65.419   Laceration of blood vessel of unspecified thumb**   ▽

√6ᵗʰ **S65.49   Other specified injury of blood vessel of thumb**

√7ᵗʰ **S65.491   Other specified injury of blood vessel of right thumb**

√7ᵗʰ **S65.492   Other specified injury of blood vessel of left thumb**

√7ᵗʰ **S65.499   Other specified injury of blood vessel of unspecified thumb**   ▽

√5ᵗʰ **S65.5   Injury of blood vessel of other and unspecified finger**

√6ᵗʰ **S65.50   Unspecified injury of blood vessel of other and unspecified finger**

√7ᵗʰ **S65.500   Unspecified injury of blood vessel of right index finger**   ▽

√7ᵗʰ **S65.501   Unspecified injury of blood vessel of left index finger**   ▽

√7ᵗʰ **S65.502   Unspecified injury of blood vessel of right middle finger**   ▽

√7ᵗʰ **S65.503   Unspecified injury of blood vessel of left middle finger**   ▽

√7ᵗʰ **S65.504   Unspecified injury of blood vessel of right ring finger**   ▽

√7ᵗʰ **S65.505   Unspecified injury of blood vessel of left ring finger**   ▽

√7ᵗʰ **S65.506   Unspecified injury of blood vessel of right little finger**   ▽

√7ᵗʰ **S65.507   Unspecified injury of blood vessel of left little finger**   ▽

EXCLUDES 1 Not coded here   **EXCLUDES 2** Not included here   **N** Newborn Age: 0   **P** Pediatric Age: 0-17   **M** Maternity Age: 12-55   **A** Adult Age: 15-124

994   ICD-10-CM 2018

√7ᵗʰ **S65.508**   **Unspecified injury of blood vessel of** ▽
other finger
     Unspecified injury of blood vessel of
      specified finger with unspecified
      laterality

√7ᵗʰ **S65.509**   **Unspecified injury of blood vessel of** ▽
unspecified finger

√6ᵗʰ **S65.51**   Laceration **of blood vessel of other and unspecified**
finger

√7ᵗʰ **S65.510**   **Laceration of blood vessel of** right index
finger

√7ᵗʰ **S65.511**   **Laceration of blood vessel of** left index
finger

√7ᵗʰ **S65.512**   **Laceration of blood vessel of** right middle
finger

√7ᵗʰ **S65.513**   **Laceration of blood vessel of** left middle
finger

√7ᵗʰ **S65.514**   **Laceration of blood vessel of** right ring
finger

√7ᵗʰ **S65.515**   **Laceration of blood vessel of** left ring
finger

√7ᵗʰ **S65.516**   **Laceration of blood vessel of** right little
finger

√7ᵗʰ **S65.517**   **Laceration of blood vessel of** left little
finger

√7ᵗʰ **S65.518**   **Laceration of blood vessel of other finger**
     Laceration of blood vessel of specified
      finger with unspecified laterality

√7ᵗʰ **S65.519**   **Laceration of blood vessel of** ▽
unspecified finger

√6ᵗʰ **S65.59**   **Other specified injury of blood vessel of other and**
unspecified finger

√7ᵗʰ **S65.590**   **Other specified injury of blood vessel of**
right index **finger**

√7ᵗʰ **S65.591**   **Other specified injury of blood vessel of**
left index **finger**

√7ᵗʰ **S65.592**   **Other specified injury of blood vessel of**
right middle **finger**

√7ᵗʰ **S65.593**   **Other specified injury of blood vessel of**
left middle **finger**

√7ᵗʰ **S65.594**   **Other specified injury of blood vessel of**
right ring **finger**

√7ᵗʰ **S65.595**   **Other specified injury of blood vessel of**
left ring **finger**

√7ᵗʰ **S65.596**   **Other specified injury of blood vessel of**
right little **finger**

√7ᵗʰ **S65.597**   **Other specified injury of blood vessel of**
left little **finger**

√7ᵗʰ **S65.598**   **Other specified injury of blood vessel of**
other finger
     Other specified injury of blood vessel of
      specified finger with unspecified
      laterality

√7ᵗʰ **S65.599**   **Other specified injury of blood vessel** ▽
of unspecified finger

√5ᵗʰ **S65.8**   **Injury of other blood vessels at** wrist and hand level

√6ᵗʰ **S65.80**   **Unspecified injury of other blood vessels at wrist**
and hand level

√7ᵗʰ **S65.801**   **Unspecified injury of other blood** ▽
vessels at wrist and hand level of
right **arm**

√7ᵗʰ **S65.802**   **Unspecified injury of other blood** ▽
vessels at wrist and hand level of
left **arm**

√7ᵗʰ **S65.809**   **Unspecified injury of other blood** ▽
vessels at wrist and hand level of
unspecified arm

√6ᵗʰ **S65.81**   Laceration **of other blood vessels at wrist and hand**
level

√7ᵗʰ **S65.811**   **Laceration of other blood vessels at wrist**
and hand level of right **arm**

√7ᵗʰ **S65.812**   **Laceration of other blood vessels at wrist**
and hand level of left **arm**

√7ᵗʰ **S65.819**   **Laceration of other blood vessels at** ▽
wrist and hand level of unspecified arm

√6ᵗʰ **S65.89**   **Other specified injury of other blood vessels at wrist**
and hand level

√7ᵗʰ **S65.891**   **Other specified injury of other blood**
vessels at wrist and hand level of right **arm**

√7ᵗʰ **S65.892**   **Other specified injury of other blood**
vessels at wrist and hand level of left **arm**

√7ᵗʰ **S65.899**   **Other specified injury of other blood** ▽
vessels at wrist and hand level of
unspecified arm

√5ᵗʰ **S65.9**   **Injury of unspecified blood vessel at** wrist and hand level

√6ᵗʰ **S65.90**   **Unspecified injury of unspecified blood vessel at**
wrist and hand level

√7ᵗʰ **S65.901**   **Unspecified injury of unspecified** ▽
blood vessel at wrist and hand level
of right **arm**

√7ᵗʰ **S65.902**   **Unspecified injury of unspecified** ▽
blood vessel at wrist and hand level
of left **arm**

√7ᵗʰ **S65.909**   **Unspecified injury of unspecified** ▽
blood vessel at wrist and hand level
of unspecified arm

√6ᵗʰ **S65.91**   Laceration **of unspecified blood vessel at wrist and**
hand level

√7ᵗʰ **S65.911**   **Laceration of unspecified blood vessel** ▽
at wrist and hand level of right **arm**

√7ᵗʰ **S65.912**   **Laceration of unspecified blood vessel** ▽
at wrist and hand level of left **arm**

√7ᵗʰ **S65.919**   **Laceration of unspecified blood vessel** ▽
at wrist and hand level of unspecified arm

√6ᵗʰ **S65.99**   **Other specified injury of unspecified blood vessel at**
wrist and hand level

√7ᵗʰ **S65.991**   **Other specified injury of unspecified** ▽
blood vessel at wrist and hand of
right **arm**

√7ᵗʰ **S65.992**   **Other specified injury of unspecified** ▽
blood vessel at wrist and hand of
left **arm**

√7ᵗʰ **S65.999**   **Other specified injury of unspecified** ▽
blood vessel at wrist and hand of
unspecified arm

√4ᵗʰ **S66**   **Injury of muscle, fascia and tendon at wrist and hand level**
     Code also any associated open wound (S61.-)
     EXCLUDES 2   *sprain of joints and ligaments of wrist and hand (S63.-)*
     TIP: Refer to the Muscle/Tendon table at the beginning of this chapter.

> The appropriate 7th character is to be added to each code from
> category S66.
> A   initial encounter
> D   subsequent encounter
> S   sequela

√5ᵗʰ **S66.0**   **Injury of** long flexor **muscle, fascia and tendon of** thumb **at**
wrist and hand level

√6ᵗʰ **S66.00**   **Unspecified injury of long flexor muscle, fascia and**
tendon of thumb at wrist and hand level

√7ᵗʰ **S66.001**   **Unspecified injury of long flexor** ▽
muscle, fascia and tendon of right
thumb at wrist and hand level

√7ᵗʰ **S66.002**   **Unspecified injury of long flexor** ▽
muscle, fascia and tendon of left
thumb at wrist and hand level

√7ᵗʰ **S66.009**   **Unspecified injury of long flexor** ▽
muscle, fascia and tendon of unspecified
thumb at wrist and hand level

√6ᵗʰ **S66.01**   Strain **of long flexor muscle, fascia and tendon of**
thumb at wrist and hand level

√7ᵗʰ **S66.011**   **Strain of long flexor muscle, fascia and**
tendon of right **thumb at wrist and hand**
level

√7ᵗʰ **S66.012**   **Strain of long flexor muscle, fascia and**
tendon of left **thumb at wrist and hand**
level

√7ᵗʰ **S66.019**   **Strain of long flexor muscle, fascia** ▽
and tendon of unspecified thumb at
wrist and hand level

☑ Additional Character Req   √7ᵗʰ Placeholder Alert   Manifestation   HCC CMS-HCC Condition   ▽ Unspecified Code   ►◄ Revised Text   ● New Code   ▲ Revised Code Title

ICD-10-CM 2018

995

✓6ᵗʰ **S66.02** Laceration of long flexor muscle, fascia and tendon of thumb at wrist and hand level

　✓7ᵗʰ **S66.021** Laceration of long flexor muscle, fascia and tendon of right thumb at wrist and hand level

　✓7ᵗʰ **S66.022** Laceration of long flexor muscle, fascia and tendon of left thumb at wrist and hand level

　✓7ᵗʰ **S66.029** Laceration of long flexor muscle, fascia and tendon of unspecified thumb at wrist and hand level ▽

✓6ᵗʰ **S66.09** Other specified injury of long flexor muscle, fascia and tendon of thumb at wrist and hand level

　✓7ᵗʰ **S66.091** Other specified injury of long flexor muscle, fascia and tendon of right thumb at wrist and hand level

　✓7ᵗʰ **S66.092** Other specified injury of long flexor muscle, fascia and tendon of left thumb at wrist and hand level

　✓7ᵗʰ **S66.099** Other specified injury of long flexor muscle, fascia and tendon of unspecified thumb at wrist and hand level ▽

✓5ᵗʰ **S66.1** Injury of flexor muscle, fascia and tendon of other and unspecified finger at wrist and hand level

　EXCLUDES 2　Injury of long flexor muscle, fascia and tendon of thumb at wrist and hand level (S66.0-)

✓6ᵗʰ **S66.10** Unspecified injury of flexor muscle, fascia and tendon of other and unspecified finger at wrist and hand level

　✓7ᵗʰ **S66.100** Unspecified injury of flexor muscle, fascia and tendon of right index finger at wrist and hand level ▽

　✓7ᵗʰ **S66.101** Unspecified injury of flexor muscle, fascia and tendon of left index finger at wrist and hand level ▽

　✓7ᵗʰ **S66.102** Unspecified injury of flexor muscle, fascia and tendon of right middle finger at wrist and hand level ▽

　✓7ᵗʰ **S66.103** Unspecified injury of flexor muscle, fascia and tendon of left middle finger at wrist and hand level ▽

　✓7ᵗʰ **S66.104** Unspecified injury of flexor muscle, fascia and tendon of right ring finger at wrist and hand level ▽

　✓7ᵗʰ **S66.105** Unspecified injury of flexor muscle, fascia and tendon of left ring finger at wrist and hand level ▽

　✓7ᵗʰ **S66.106** Unspecified injury of flexor muscle, fascia and tendon of right little finger at wrist and hand level ▽

　✓7ᵗʰ **S66.107** Unspecified injury of flexor muscle, fascia and tendon of left little finger at wrist and hand level ▽

　✓7ᵗʰ **S66.108** Unspecified injury of flexor muscle, fascia and tendon of other finger at wrist and hand level ▽
　　　Unspecified injury of flexor muscle, fascia and tendon of specified finger with unspecified laterality at wrist and hand level

　✓7ᵗʰ **S66.109** Unspecified injury of flexor muscle, ascia and tendon of unspecified finger at wrist and hand level ▽

✓6ᵗʰ **S66.11** Strain of flexor muscle, fascia and tendon of other and unspecified finger at wrist and hand level

　✓7ᵗʰ **S66.110** Strain of flexor muscle, fascia and tendon of right index finger at wrist and hand level

　✓7ᵗʰ **S66.111** Strain of flexor muscle, fascia and tendon of left index finger at wrist and hand level

　✓7ᵗʰ **S66.112** Strain of flexor muscle, fascia and tendon of right middle finger at wrist and hand level

　✓7ᵗʰ **S66.113** Strain of flexor muscle, fascia and tendon of left middle finger at wrist and hand level

　✓7ᵗʰ **S66.114** Strain of flexor muscle, fascia and tendon of right ring finger at wrist and hand level

　✓7ᵗʰ **S66.115** Strain of flexor muscle, fascia and tendon of left ring finger at wrist and hand level

　✓7ᵗʰ **S66.116** Strain of flexor muscle, fascia and tendon of right little finger at wrist and hand level

　✓7ᵗʰ **S66.117** Strain of flexor muscle, fascia and tendon of left little finger at wrist and hand level

　✓7ᵗʰ **S66.118** Strain of flexor muscle, fascia and tendon of other finger at wrist and hand level
　　　Strain of flexor muscle, fascia and tendon of specified finger with unspecified laterality at wrist and hand level

　✓7ᵗʰ **S66.119** Strain of flexor muscle, fascia and tendon of unspecified finger at wrist and hand level ▽

✓6ᵗʰ **S66.12** Laceration of flexor muscle, fascia and tendon of other and unspecified finger at wrist and hand level

　✓7ᵗʰ **S66.120** Laceration of flexor muscle, fascia and tendon of right index finger at wrist and hand level

　✓7ᵗʰ **S66.121** Laceration of flexor muscle, fascia and tendon of left index finger at wrist and hand level

　✓7ᵗʰ **S66.122** Laceration of flexor muscle, fascia and tendon of right middle finger at wrist and hand level

　✓7ᵗʰ **S66.123** Laceration of flexor muscle, fascia and tendon of left middle finger at wrist and hand level

　✓7ᵗʰ **S66.124** Laceration of flexor muscle, fascia and tendon of right ring finger at wrist and hand level

　✓7ᵗʰ **S66.125** Laceration of flexor muscle, fascia and tendon of left ring finger at wrist and hand level

　✓7ᵗʰ **S66.126** Laceration of flexor muscle, fascia and tendon of right little finger at wrist and hand level

　✓7ᵗʰ **S66.127** Laceration of flexor muscle, fascia and tendon of left little finger at wrist and hand level

　✓7ᵗʰ **S66.128** Laceration of flexor muscle, fascia and tendon of other finger at wrist and hand level
　　　Laceration of flexor muscle, fascia and tendon of specified finger with unspecified laterality at wrist and hand level

　✓7ᵗʰ **S66.129** Laceration of flexor muscle, fascia and tendon of unspecified finger at wrist and hand level ▽

✓6ᵗʰ **S66.19** Other injury of flexor muscle, fascia and tendon of other and unspecified finger at wrist and hand level

　✓7ᵗʰ **S66.190** Other injury of flexor muscle, fascia and tendon of right index finger at wrist and hand level

　✓7ᵗʰ **S66.191** Other injury of flexor muscle, fascia and tendon of left index finger at wrist and hand level

　✓7ᵗʰ **S66.192** Other injury of flexor muscle, fascia and tendon of right middle finger at wrist and hand level

　✓7ᵗʰ **S66.193** Other injury of flexor muscle, fascia and tendon of left middle finger at wrist and hand level

　✓7ᵗʰ **S66.194** Other injury of flexor muscle, fascia and tendon of right ring finger at wrist and hand level

　✓7ᵗʰ **S66.195** Other injury of flexor muscle, fascia and tendon of left ring finger at wrist and hand level

　✓7ᵗʰ **S66.196** Other injury of flexor muscle, fascia and tendon of right little finger at wrist and hand level

　✓7ᵗʰ **S66.197** Other injury of flexor muscle, fascia and tendon of left little finger at wrist and hand level

---

EXCLUDES 1 Not coded here　　EXCLUDES 2 Not included here　　N Newborn Age: 0　　P Pediatric Age: 0-17　　M Maternity Age: 12-55　　A Adult Age: 15-124

✓7ᵗʰ **S66.198** **Other injury of flexor muscle, fascia and tendon of other finger at wrist and hand level**
    Other injury of flexor muscle, fascia and tendon of specified finger with unspecified laterality at wrist and hand level

✓7ᵗʰ **S66.199** **Other injury of flexor muscle, fascia and tendon of unspecified finger at wrist and hand level** ▽

✓5ᵗʰ **S66.2** **Injury of** extensor muscle, **fascia and tendon of** thumb **at wrist and hand level**

✓6ᵗʰ **S66.20** **Unspecified injury of extensor muscle, fascia and tendon of thumb at wrist and hand level**

✓7ᵗʰ **S66.201** **Unspecified injury of extensor muscle, fascia and tendon of** right **thumb at wrist and hand level** ▽

✓7ᵗʰ **S66.202** **Unspecified injury of extensor muscle, fascia and tendon of** left **thumb at wrist and hand level** ▽

✓7ᵗʰ **S66.209** **Unspecified injury of extensor muscle, fascia and tendon of unspecified thumb at wrist and hand level** ▽

✓6ᵗʰ **S66.21** Strain **of extensor muscle, fascia and tendon of thumb at wrist and hand level**

✓7ᵗʰ **S66.211** **Strain of extensor muscle, fascia and tendon of** right **thumb at wrist and hand level**

✓7ᵗʰ **S66.212** **Strain of extensor muscle, fascia and tendon of** left **thumb at wrist and hand level**

✓7ᵗʰ **S66.219** **Strain of extensor muscle, fascia and tendon of unspecified thumb at wrist and hand level**

✓6ᵗʰ **S66.22** Laceration **of extensor muscle, fascia and tendon of thumb at wrist and hand level**

✓7ᵗʰ **S66.221** **Laceration of extensor muscle, fascia and tendon of** right **thumb at wrist and hand level**

✓7ᵗʰ **S66.222** **Laceration of extensor muscle, fascia and tendon of** left **thumb at wrist and hand level**

✓7ᵗʰ **S66.229** **Laceration of extensor muscle, fascia and tendon of unspecified thumb at wrist and hand level** ▽

✓6ᵗʰ **S66.29** **Other specified injury of extensor muscle, fascia and tendon of thumb at wrist and hand level**

✓7ᵗʰ **S66.291** **Other specified injury of extensor muscle, fascia and tendon of** right **thumb at wrist and hand level**

✓7ᵗʰ **S66.292** **Other specified injury of extensor muscle, fascia and tendon of** left **thumb at wrist and hand level**

✓7ᵗʰ **S66.299** **Other specified injury of extensor muscle, fascia and tendon of unspecified thumb at wrist and hand level** ▽

✓5ᵗʰ **S66.3** **Injury of** extensor muscle, **fascia and tendon of other and unspecified** finger **at wrist and hand level**
    EXCLUDES 2   Injury of extensor muscle, fascia and tendon of thumb at wrist and hand level (S66.2-)

✓6ᵗʰ **S66.30** **Unspecified injury of extensor muscle, fascia and tendon of other and unspecified finger at wrist and hand level**

✓7ᵗʰ **S66.300** **Unspecified injury of extensor muscle, fascia and tendon of** right index **finger at wrist and hand level** ▽

✓7ᵗʰ **S66.301** **Unspecified injury of extensor muscle, fascia and tendon of** left index **finger at wrist and hand level** ▽

✓7ᵗʰ **S66.302** **Unspecified injury of extensor muscle, fascia and tendon of** right middle **finger at wrist and hand level** ▽

✓7ᵗʰ **S66.303** **Unspecified injury of extensor muscle, fascia and tendon of** left middle **finger at wrist and hand level** ▽

✓7ᵗʰ **S66.304** **Unspecified injury of extensor muscle, fascia and tendon of** right ring **finger at wrist and hand level** ▽

✓7ᵗʰ **S66.305** **Unspecified injury of extensor muscle, fascia and tendon of** left ring **finger at wrist and hand level** ▽

✓7ᵗʰ **S66.306** **Unspecified injury of extensor muscle, fascia and tendon of** right little **finger at wrist and hand level** ▽

✓7ᵗʰ **S66.307** **Unspecified injury of extensor muscle, fascia and tendon of** left little **finger at wrist and hand level** ▽

✓7ᵗʰ **S66.308** **Unspecified injury of extensor muscle, fascia and tendon of other finger at wrist and hand level** ▽
    Unspecified injury of extensor muscle, fascia and tendon of specified finger with unspecified laterality at wrist and hand level

✓7ᵗʰ **S66.309** **Unspecified injury of extensor muscle, fascia and tendon of unspecified finger at wrist and hand level** ▽

✓6ᵗʰ **S66.31** Strain **of extensor muscle, fascia and tendon of other and unspecified finger at wrist and hand level**

✓7ᵗʰ **S66.310** **Strain of extensor muscle, fascia and tendon of** right index **finger at wrist and hand level**

✓7ᵗʰ **S66.311** **Strain of extensor muscle, fascia and tendon of** left index **finger at wrist and hand level**

✓7ᵗʰ **S66.312** **Strain of extensor muscle, fascia and tendon of** right middle **finger at wrist and hand level**

✓7ᵗʰ **S66.313** **Strain of extensor muscle, fascia and tendon of** left middle **finger at wrist and hand level**

✓7ᵗʰ **S66.314** **Strain of extensor muscle, fascia and tendon of** right ring **finger at wrist and hand level**

✓7ᵗʰ **S66.315** **Strain of extensor muscle, fascia and tendon of** left ring **finger at wrist and hand level**

✓7ᵗʰ **S66.316** **Strain of extensor muscle, fascia and tendon of** right little **finger at wrist and hand level**

✓7ᵗʰ **S66.317** **Strain of extensor muscle, fascia and tendon of** left little **finger at wrist and hand level**

✓7ᵗʰ **S66.318** **Strain of extensor muscle, fascia and tendon of other finger at wrist and hand level**
    Strain of extensor muscle, fascia and tendon of specified finger with unspecified laterality at wrist and hand level

✓7ᵗʰ **S66.319** **Strain of extensor muscle, fascia and tendon of unspecified finger at wrist and hand level** ▽

✓6ᵗʰ **S66.32** Laceration **of extensor muscle, fascia and tendon of other and unspecified finger at wrist and hand level**

✓7ᵗʰ **S66.320** **Laceration of extensor muscle, fascia and tendon of** right index **finger at wrist and hand level**

✓7ᵗʰ **S66.321** **Laceration of extensor muscle, fascia and tendon of** left index **finger at wrist and hand level**

✓7ᵗʰ **S66.322** **Laceration of extensor muscle, fascia and tendon of** right middle **finger at wrist and hand level**

✓7ᵗʰ **S66.323** **Laceration of extensor muscle, fascia and tendon of** left middle **finger at wrist and hand level**

✓7ᵗʰ **S66.324** **Laceration of extensor muscle, fascia and tendon of** right ring **finger at wrist and hand level**

✓7ᵗʰ **S66.325** **Laceration of extensor muscle, fascia and tendon of** left ring **finger at wrist and hand level**

✓7ᵗʰ **S66.326** **Laceration of extensor muscle, fascia and tendon of** right little **finger at wrist and hand level**

✔ Additional Character Req   ✔ₓ7ᵗʰ Placeholder Alert   _Manifestation_   **HCC** CMS-HCC Condition   ▽ Unspecified Code   ▶◀ Revised Text   ● New Code   ▲ Revised Code Title

✓7ᵗʰ **S66.327　Laceration of extensor muscle, fascia and tendon of left little finger at wrist and hand level**

✓7ᵗʰ **S66.328　Laceration of extensor muscle, fascia and tendon of other finger at wrist and hand level**

Laceration of extensor muscle, fascia and tendon of specified finger with unspecified laterality at wrist and hand level

✓7ᵗʰ **S66.329　Laceration of extensor muscle, fascia and tendon of unspecified finger at wrist and hand level** ▽

✓6ᵗʰ **S66.39　Other injury of extensor muscle, fascia and tendon of other and unspecified finger at wrist and hand level**

✓7ᵗʰ **S66.390　Other injury of extensor muscle, fascia and tendon of right index finger at wrist and hand level**

✓7ᵗʰ **S66.391　Other injury of extensor muscle, fascia and tendon of left index finger at wrist and hand level**

✓7ᵗʰ **S66.392　Other injury of extensor muscle, fascia and tendon of right middle finger at wrist and hand level**

✓7ᵗʰ **S66.393　Other injury of extensor muscle, fascia and tendon of left middle finger at wrist and hand level**

✓7ᵗʰ **S66.394　Other injury of extensor muscle, fascia and tendon of right ring finger at wrist and hand level**

✓7ᵗʰ **S66.395　Other injury of extensor muscle, fascia and tendon of left ring finger at wrist and hand level**

✓7ᵗʰ **S66.396　Other injury of extensor muscle, fascia and tendon of right little finger at wrist and hand level**

✓7ᵗʰ **S66.397　Other injury of extensor muscle, fascia and tendon of left little finger at wrist and hand level**

✓7ᵗʰ **S66.398　Other injury of extensor muscle, fascia and tendon of other finger at wrist and hand level**

Other injury of extensor muscle, fascia and tendon of specified finger with unspecified laterality at wrist and hand level

✓7ᵗʰ **S66.399　Other injury of extensor muscle, fascia and tendon of unspecified finger at wrist and hand level** ▽

✓5ᵗʰ **S66.4　Injury of intrinsic muscle, fascia and tendon of thumb at wrist and hand level**

✓6ᵗʰ **S66.40　Unspecified injury of intrinsic muscle, fascia and tendon of thumb at wrist and hand level**

✓7ᵗʰ **S66.401　Unspecified injury of intrinsic muscle, fascia and tendon of right thumb at wrist and hand level** ▽

✓7ᵗʰ **S66.402　Unspecified injury of intrinsic muscle, fascia and tendon of left thumb at wrist and hand level** ▽

✓7ᵗʰ **S66.409　Unspecified injury of intrinsic muscle, fascia and tendon of unspecified thumb at wrist and hand level** ▽

✓6ᵗʰ **S66.41　Strain of intrinsic muscle, fascia and tendon of thumb at wrist and hand level**

✓7ᵗʰ **S66.411　Strain of intrinsic muscle, fascia and tendon of right thumb at wrist and hand level**

✓7ᵗʰ **S66.412　Strain of intrinsic muscle, fascia and tendon of left thumb at wrist and hand level**

✓7ᵗʰ **S66.419　Strain of intrinsic muscle, fascia and tendon of unspecified thumb at wrist and hand level** ▽

✓6ᵗʰ **S66.42　Laceration of intrinsic muscle, fascia and tendon of thumb at wrist and hand level**

✓7ᵗʰ **S66.421　Laceration of intrinsic muscle, fascia and tendon of right thumb at wrist and hand level**

✓7ᵗʰ **S66.422　Laceration of intrinsic muscle, fascia and tendon of left thumb at wrist and hand level**

✓7ᵗʰ **S66.429　Laceration of intrinsic muscle, fascia and tendon of unspecified thumb at wrist and hand level** ▽

✓6ᵗʰ **S66.49　Other specified injury of intrinsic muscle, fascia and tendon of thumb at wrist and hand level**

✓7ᵗʰ **S66.491　Other specified injury of intrinsic muscle, fascia and tendon of right thumb at wrist and hand level**

✓7ᵗʰ **S66.492　Other specified injury of intrinsic muscle, fascia and tendon of left thumb at wrist and hand level**

✓7ᵗʰ **S66.499　Other specified injury of intrinsic muscle, fascia and tendon of unspecified thumb at wrist and hand level** ▽

✓5ᵗʰ **S66.5　Injury of intrinsic muscle, fascia and tendon of other and unspecified finger at wrist and hand level**

EXCLUDES 2　injury of intrinsic muscle, fascia and tendon of thumb at wrist and hand level (S66.4-)

✓6ᵗʰ **S66.50　Unspecified injury of intrinsic muscle, fascia and tendon of other and unspecified finger at wrist and hand level**

✓7ᵗʰ **S66.500　Unspecified injury of intrinsic muscle, fascia and tendon of right index finger at wrist and hand level** ▽

✓7ᵗʰ **S66.501　Unspecified injury of intrinsic muscle, fascia and tendon of left index finger at wrist and hand level** ▽

✓7ᵗʰ **S66.502　Unspecified injury of intrinsic muscle, fascia and tendon of right middle finger at wrist and hand level** ▽

✓7ᵗʰ **S66.503　Unspecified injury of intrinsic muscle, fascia and tendon of left middle finger at wrist and hand level** ▽

✓7ᵗʰ **S66.504　Unspecified injury of intrinsic muscle, fascia and tendon of right ring finger at wrist and hand level** ▽

✓7ᵗʰ **S66.505　Unspecified injury of intrinsic muscle, fascia and tendon of left ring finger at wrist and hand level** ▽

✓7ᵗʰ **S66.506　Unspecified injury of intrinsic muscle, fascia and tendon of right little finger at wrist and hand level** ▽

✓7ᵗʰ **S66.507　Unspecified injury of intrinsic muscle, fascia and tendon of left little finger at wrist and hand level** ▽

✓7ᵗʰ **S66.508　Unspecified injury of intrinsic muscle, fascia and tendon of other finger at wrist and hand level** ▽

Unspecified injury of intrinsic muscle, fascia and tendon of specified finger with unspecified laterality at wrist and hand level

✓7ᵗʰ **S66.509　Unspecified injury of intrinsic muscle, fascia and tendon of unspecified finger at wrist and hand level** ▽

✓6ᵗʰ **S66.51　Strain of intrinsic muscle, fascia and tendon of other and unspecified finger at wrist and hand level**

✓7ᵗʰ **S66.510　Strain of intrinsic muscle, fascia and tendon of right index finger at wrist and hand level**

✓7ᵗʰ **S66.511　Strain of intrinsic muscle, fascia and tendon of left index finger at wrist and hand level**

✓7ᵗʰ **S66.512　Strain of intrinsic muscle, fascia and tendon of right middle finger at wrist and hand level**

✓7ᵗʰ **S66.513　Strain of intrinsic muscle, fascia and tendon of left middle finger at wrist and hand level**

✓7ᵗʰ **S66.514　Strain of intrinsic muscle, fascia and tendon of right ring finger at wrist and hand level**

✓7ᵗʰ **S66.515　Strain of intrinsic muscle, fascia and tendon of left ring finger at wrist and hand level**

☑7ᵗʰ **S66.516** Strain of intrinsic muscle, fascia and tendon of right little finger at wrist and hand level

☑7ᵗʰ **S66.517** Strain of intrinsic muscle, fascia and tendon of left little finger at wrist and hand level

☑7ᵗʰ **S66.518** Strain of intrinsic muscle, fascia and tendon of other finger at wrist and hand level

Strain of intrinsic muscle, fascia and tendon of specified finger with unspecified laterality at wrist and hand level

☑7ᵗʰ **S66.519** Strain of intrinsic muscle, fascia and tendon of unspecified finger at wrist and hand level ▽

☑6ᵗʰ **S66.52** Laceration of intrinsic muscle, fascia and tendon of other and unspecified finger at wrist and hand level

☑7ᵗʰ **S66.520** Laceration of intrinsic muscle, fascia and tendon of right index finger at wrist and hand level

☑7ᵗʰ **S66.521** Laceration of intrinsic muscle, fascia and tendon of left index finger at wrist and hand level

☑7ᵗʰ **S66.522** Laceration of intrinsic muscle, fascia and tendon of right middle finger at wrist and hand level

☑7ᵗʰ **S66.523** Laceration of intrinsic muscle, fascia and tendon of left middle finger at wrist and hand level

☑7ᵗʰ **S66.524** Laceration of intrinsic muscle, fascia and tendon of right ring finger at wrist and hand level

☑7ᵗʰ **S66.525** Laceration of intrinsic muscle, fascia and tendon of left ring finger at wrist and hand level

☑7ᵗʰ **S66.526** Laceration of intrinsic muscle, fascia and tendon of right little finger at wrist and hand level

☑7ᵗʰ **S66.527** Laceration of intrinsic muscle, fascia and tendon of left little finger at wrist and hand level

☑7ᵗʰ **S66.528** Laceration of intrinsic muscle, fascia and tendon of other finger at wrist and hand level

Laceration of intrinsic muscle, fascia and tendon of specified finger with unspecified laterality at wrist and hand level

☑7ᵗʰ **S66.529** Laceration of intrinsic muscle, fascia and tendon of unspecified finger at wrist and hand level ▽

☑6ᵗʰ **S66.59** Other injury of intrinsic muscle, fascia and tendon of other and unspecified finger at wrist and hand level

☑7ᵗʰ **S66.590** Other injury of intrinsic muscle, fascia and tendon of right index finger at wrist and hand level

☑7ᵗʰ **S66.591** Other injury of intrinsic muscle, fascia and tendon of left index finger at wrist and hand level

☑7ᵗʰ **S66.592** Other injury of intrinsic muscle, fascia and tendon of right middle finger at wrist and hand level

☑7ᵗʰ **S66.593** Other injury of intrinsic muscle, fascia and tendon of left middle finger at wrist and hand level

☑7ᵗʰ **S66.594** Other injury of intrinsic muscle, fascia and tendon of right ring finger at wrist and hand level

☑7ᵗʰ **S66.595** Other injury of intrinsic muscle, fascia and tendon of left ring finger at wrist and hand level

☑7ᵗʰ **S66.596** Other injury of intrinsic muscle, fascia and tendon of right little finger at wrist and hand level

☑7ᵗʰ **S66.597** Other injury of intrinsic muscle, fascia and tendon of left little finger at wrist and hand level

☑7ᵗʰ **S66.598** Other injury of intrinsic muscle, fascia and tendon of other finger at wrist and hand level

Other injury of intrinsic muscle, fascia and tendon of specified finger with unspecified laterality at wrist and hand level

☑7ᵗʰ **S66.599** Other injury of intrinsic muscle, fascia and tendon of unspecified finger at wrist and hand level ▽

☑5ᵗʰ **S66.8** Injury of other specified muscles, fascia and tendons at wrist and hand level

☑6ᵗʰ **S66.80** Unspecified injury of other specified muscles, fascia and tendons at wrist and hand level

☑7ᵗʰ **S66.801** Unspecified injury of other specified muscles, fascia and tendons at wrist and hand level, right hand ▽

☑7ᵗʰ **S66.802** Unspecified injury of other specified muscles, fascia and tendons at wrist and hand level, left hand ▽

☑7ᵗʰ **S66.809** Unspecified injury of other specified muscles, fascia and tendons at wrist and hand level, unspecified hand ▽

☑6ᵗʰ **S66.81** Strain of other specified muscles, fascia and tendons at wrist and hand level

☑7ᵗʰ **S66.811** Strain of other specified muscles, fascia and tendons at wrist and hand level, right hand

☑7ᵗʰ **S66.812** Strain of other specified muscles, fascia and tendons at wrist and hand level, left hand

☑7ᵗʰ **S66.819** Strain of other specified muscles, fascia and tendons at wrist and hand level, unspecified hand ▽

☑6ᵗʰ **S66.82** Laceration of other specified muscles, fascia and tendons at wrist and hand level

☑7ᵗʰ **S66.821** Laceration of other specified muscles, fascia and tendons at wrist and hand level, right hand

☑7ᵗʰ **S66.822** Laceration of other specified muscles, fascia and tendons at wrist and hand level, left hand

☑7ᵗʰ **S66.829** Laceration of other specified muscles, fascia and tendons at wrist and hand level, unspecified hand ▽

☑6ᵗʰ **S66.89** Other injury of other specified muscles, fascia and tendons at wrist and hand level

☑7ᵗʰ **S66.891** Other injury of other specified muscles, fascia and tendons at wrist and hand level, right hand

☑7ᵗʰ **S66.892** Other injury of other specified muscles, fascia and tendons at wrist and hand level, left hand

☑7ᵗʰ **S66.899** Other injury of other specified muscles, fascia and tendons at wrist and hand level, unspecified hand ▽

☑5ᵗʰ **S66.9** Injury of unspecified muscle, fascia and tendon at wrist and hand level

☑6ᵗʰ **S66.90** Unspecified injury of unspecified muscle, fascia and tendon at wrist and hand level

☑7ᵗʰ **S66.901** Unspecified injury of unspecified muscle, fascia and tendon at wrist and hand level, right hand ▽

☑7ᵗʰ **S66.902** Unspecified injury of unspecified muscle, fascia and tendon at wrist and hand level, left hand ▽

☑7ᵗʰ **S66.909** Unspecified injury of unspecified muscle, fascia and tendon at wrist and hand level, unspecified hand ▽

☑6ᵗʰ **S66.91** Strain of unspecified muscle, fascia and tendon at wrist and hand level

☑7ᵗʰ **S66.911** Strain of unspecified muscle, fascia and tendon at wrist and hand level, right hand ▽

☑7ᵗʰ **S66.912** Strain of unspecified muscle, fascia and tendon at wrist and hand level, left hand ▽

☑ Additional Character Req   ☑7ᵗʰ Placeholder Alert   **Manifestation**   **HCC** CMS-HCC Condition   ▽ Unspecified Code   ►◄ Revised Text   ● New Code   ▲ Revised Code Title

☑7ᵗʰ S66.919 Strain of unspecified muscle, fascia and tendon at wrist and hand level, unspecified hand ▽

☑6ᵗʰ S66.92 Laceration of unspecified muscle, fascia and tendon at wrist and hand level

    ☑7ᵗʰ S66.921 Laceration of unspecified muscle, fascia and tendon at wrist and hand level, right hand ▽

    ☑7ᵗʰ S66.922 Laceration of unspecified muscle, fascia and tendon at wrist and hand level, left hand ▽

    ☑7ᵗʰ S66.929 Laceration of unspecified muscle, fascia and tendon at wrist and hand level, unspecified hand ▽

☑6ᵗʰ S66.99 Other injury of unspecified muscle, fascia and tendon at wrist and hand level

    ☑7ᵗʰ S66.991 Other injury of unspecified muscle, fascia and tendon at wrist and hand level, right hand ▽

    ☑7ᵗʰ S66.992 Other injury of unspecified muscle, fascia and tendon at wrist and hand level, left hand ▽

    ☑7ᵗʰ S66.999 Other injury of unspecified muscle, fascia and tendon at wrist and hand level, unspecified hand ▽

☑4ᵗʰ S67 Crushing injury of wrist, hand and fingers
Use additional code for all associated injuries, such as:
    fracture of wrist and hand (S62.-)
    open wound of wrist and hand (S61.-)

> The appropriate 7th character is to be added to each code from category S67.
> A   initial encounter
> D   subsequent encounter
> S   sequela

☑5ᵗʰ S67.0 Crushing injury of thumb

   ☑ₓ7ᵗʰ S67.00 Crushing injury of unspecified thumb ▽

   ☑ₓ7ᵗʰ S67.01 Crushing injury of right thumb

   ☑ₓ7ᵗʰ S67.02 Crushing injury of left thumb

☑5ᵗʰ S67.1 Crushing injury of other and unspecified finger(s)
    EXCLUDES 2   crushing injury of thumb (S67.0-)

   ☑ₓ7ᵗʰ S67.10 Crushing injury of unspecified finger(s) ▽

   ☑6ᵗʰ S67.19 Crushing injury of other finger(s)

     ☑7ᵗʰ S67.190 Crushing injury of right index finger

     ☑7ᵗʰ S67.191 Crushing injury of left index finger

     ☑7ᵗʰ S67.192 Crushing injury of right middle finger

     ☑7ᵗʰ S67.193 Crushing injury of left middle finger

     ☑7ᵗʰ S67.194 Crushing injury of right ring finger

     ☑7ᵗʰ S67.195 Crushing injury of left ring finger

     ☑7ᵗʰ S67.196 Crushing injury of right little finger

     ☑7ᵗʰ S67.197 Crushing injury of left little finger

     ☑7ᵗʰ S67.198 Crushing injury of other finger
       Crushing injury of specified finger with unspecified laterality

☑5ᵗʰ S67.2 Crushing injury of hand
    EXCLUDES 2   crushing injury of fingers (S67.1-)
              crushing injury of thumb (S67.0-)

   ☑ₓ7ᵗʰ S67.20 Crushing injury of unspecified hand ▽

   ☑ₓ7ᵗʰ S67.21 Crushing injury of right hand

   ☑ₓ7ᵗʰ S67.22 Crushing injury of left hand

☑5ᵗʰ S67.3 Crushing injury of wrist

   ☑ₓ7ᵗʰ S67.30 Crushing injury of unspecified wrist ▽

   ☑ₓ7ᵗʰ S67.31 Crushing injury of right wrist

   ☑ₓ7ᵗʰ S67.32 Crushing injury of left wrist

☑5ᵗʰ S67.4 Crushing injury of wrist and hand
    EXCLUDES 1   crushing injury of hand alone (S67.2-)
              crushing injury of wrist alone (S67.3-)
    EXCLUDES 2   crushing injury of fingers (S67.1-)
              crushing injury of thumb (S67.0-)

   ☑ₓ7ᵗʰ S67.40 Crushing injury of unspecified wrist and hand ▽

   ☑ₓ7ᵗʰ S67.41 Crushing injury of right wrist and hand

   ☑ₓ7ᵗʰ S67.42 Crushing injury of left wrist and hand

☑5ᵗʰ S67.9 Crushing injury of unspecified part(s) of wrist, hand and fingers

   ☑ₓ7ᵗʰ S67.90 Crushing injury of unspecified part(s) of unspecified wrist, hand and fingers ▽

   ☑ₓ7ᵗʰ S67.91 Crushing injury of unspecified part(s) of right wrist, hand and fingers ▽

   ☑ₓ7ᵗʰ S67.92 Crushing injury of unspecified part(s) of left wrist, hand and fingers ▽

☑4ᵗʰ S68 Traumatic amputation of wrist, hand and fingers
An amputation not identified as partial or complete should be coded to complete.

> The appropriate 7th character is to be added to each code from category S68.
> A   initial encounter
> D   subsequent encounter
> S   sequela

☑5ᵗʰ S68.0 Traumatic metacarpophalangeal amputation of thumb
Traumatic amputation of thumb NOS

   ☑6ᵗʰ S68.01 Complete traumatic metacarpophalangeal amputation of thumb

    3 **☑7ᵗʰ S68.011** Complete traumatic metacarpophalangeal amputation of right thumb   HCC

    3 **☑7ᵗʰ S68.012** Complete traumatic metacarpophalangeal amputation of left thumb   HCC

    3 **☑7ᵗʰ S68.019** Complete traumatic metacarpophalangeal amputation of unspecified thumb   HCC ▽

   ☑6ᵗʰ S68.02 Partial traumatic metacarpophalangeal amputation of thumb

    3 **☑7ᵗʰ S68.021** Partial traumatic metacarpophalangeal amputation of right thumb   HCC

    3 **☑7ᵗʰ S68.022** Partial traumatic metacarpophalangeal amputation of left thumb   HCC

    3 **☑7ᵗʰ S68.029** Partial traumatic metacarpophalangeal amputation of unspecified thumb   HCC ▽

☑5ᵗʰ S68.1 Traumatic metacarpophalangeal amputation of other and unspecified finger
Traumatic amputation of finger NOS
    EXCLUDES 2   traumatic metacarpophalangeal amputation of thumb (S68.0-)

   ☑6ᵗʰ S68.11 Complete traumatic metacarpophalangeal amputation of other and unspecified finger

    3 **☑7ᵗʰ S68.110** Complete traumatic metacarpophalangeal amputation of right index finger   HCC

    3 **☑7ᵗʰ S68.111** Complete traumatic metacarpophalangeal amputation of left index finger   HCC

    3 **☑7ᵗʰ S68.112** Complete traumatic metacarpophalangeal amputation of right middle finger   HCC

    3 **☑7ᵗʰ S68.113** Complete traumatic metacarpophalangeal amputation of left middle finger   HCC

    3 **☑7ᵗʰ S68.114** Complete traumatic metacarpophalangeal amputation of right ring finger   HCC

    3 **☑7ᵗʰ S68.115** Complete traumatic metacarpophalangeal amputation of left ring finger   HCC

    3 **☑7ᵗʰ S68.116** Complete traumatic metacarpophalangeal amputation of right little finger   HCC

    3 **☑7ᵗʰ S68.117** Complete traumatic metacarpophalangeal amputation of left little finger   HCC

    3 **☑7ᵗʰ S68.118** Complete traumatic metacarpophalangeal amputation of other finger   HCC
       Complete traumatic metacarpophalangeal amputation of specified finger with unspecified laterality

    3 **☑7ᵗʰ S68.119** Complete traumatic metacarpophalangeal amputation of unspecified finger   HCC ▽

---

3   HCC with 7th character indicating sequela.

EXCLUDES 1 Not coded here   EXCLUDES 2 Not included here   Ⓝ Newborn Age: 0   Ⓟ Pediatric Age: 0-17   Ⓜ Maternity Age: 12-55   Ⓐ Adult Age: 15-124

1000   ICD-10-CM 2018

✓6ᵗʰ **S68.12** Partial traumatic metacarpophalangeal amputation of other and unspecified finger

3 ✓7ᵗʰ **S68.120** Partial traumatic metacarpophalangeal amputation of right index finger   HCC

3 ✓7ᵗʰ **S68.121** Partial traumatic metacarpophalangeal amputation of left index finger   HCC

3 ✓7ᵗʰ **S68.122** Partial traumatic metacarpophalangeal amputation of right middle finger   HCC

3 ✓7ᵗʰ **S68.123** Partial traumatic metacarpophalangeal amputation of left middle finger   HCC

3 ✓7ᵗʰ **S68.124** Partial traumatic metacarpophalangeal amputation of right ring finger   HCC

3 ✓7ᵗʰ **S68.125** Partial traumatic metacarpophalangeal amputation of left ring finger   HCC

3 ✓7ᵗʰ **S68.126** Partial traumatic metacarpophalangeal amputation of right little finger   HCC

3 ✓7ᵗʰ **S68.127** Partial traumatic metacarpophalangeal amputation of left little finger   HCC

3 ✓7ᵗʰ **S68.128** Partial traumatic metacarpophalangeal amputation of other finger   HCC
Partial traumatic metacarpophalangeal amputation of specified finger with unspecified laterality

3 ✓7ᵗʰ **S68.129** Partial traumatic metacarpophalangeal amputation of unspecified finger   HCC ▽

✓5ᵗʰ **S68.4** Traumatic amputation of hand at wrist level
Traumatic amputation of hand NOS
Traumatic amputation of wrist

✓6ᵗʰ **S68.41** Complete traumatic amputation of hand at wrist level

2 ✓7ᵗʰ **S68.411** Complete traumatic amputation of right hand at wrist level   HCC

2 ✓7ᵗʰ **S68.412** Complete traumatic amputation of left hand at wrist level   HCC

2 ✓7ᵗʰ **S68.419** Complete traumatic amputation of unspecified hand at wrist level   HCC ▽

✓6ᵗʰ **S68.42** Partial traumatic amputation of hand at wrist level

2 ✓7ᵗʰ **S68.421** Partial traumatic amputation of right hand at wrist level   HCC

2 ✓7ᵗʰ **S68.422** Partial traumatic amputation of left hand at wrist level   HCC

2 ✓7ᵗʰ **S68.429** Partial traumatic amputation of unspecified hand at wrist level   HCC ▽

✓5ᵗʰ **S68.5** Traumatic transphalangeal amputation of thumb
Traumatic interphalangeal joint amputation of thumb

✓6ᵗʰ **S68.51** Complete traumatic transphalangeal amputation of thumb

3 ✓7ᵗʰ **S68.511** Complete traumatic transphalangeal amputation of right thumb   HCC

3 ✓7ᵗʰ **S68.512** Complete traumatic transphalangeal amputation of left thumb   HCC

3 ✓7ᵗʰ **S68.519** Complete traumatic transphalangeal amputation of unspecified thumb   HCC ▽

✓6ᵗʰ **S68.52** Partial traumatic transphalangeal amputation of thumb

3 ✓7ᵗʰ **S68.521** Partial traumatic transphalangeal amputation of right thumb   HCC

3 ✓7ᵗʰ **S68.522** Partial traumatic transphalangeal amputation of left thumb   HCC

3 ✓7ᵗʰ **S68.529** Partial traumatic transphalangeal amputation of unspecified thumb   HCC ▽

✓5ᵗʰ **S68.6** Traumatic transphalangeal amputation of other and unspecified finger

✓6ᵗʰ **S68.61** Complete traumatic transphalangeal amputation of other and unspecified finger(s)

3 ✓7ᵗʰ **S68.610** Complete traumatic transphalangeal amputation of right index finger   HCC

3 ✓7ᵗʰ **S68.611** Complete traumatic transphalangeal amputation of left index finger   HCC

3 ✓7ᵗʰ **S68.612** Complete traumatic transphalangeal amputation of right middle finger   HCC

3 ✓7ᵗʰ **S68.613** Complete traumatic transphalangeal amputation of left middle finger   HCC

3 ✓7ᵗʰ **S68.614** Complete traumatic transphalangeal amputation of right ring finger   HCC

3 ✓7ᵗʰ **S68.615** Complete traumatic transphalangeal amputation of left ring finger   HCC

3 ✓7ᵗʰ **S68.616** Complete traumatic transphalangeal amputation of right little finger   HCC

3 ✓7ᵗʰ **S68.617** Complete traumatic transphalangeal amputation of left little finger   HCC

3 ✓7ᵗʰ **S68.618** Complete traumatic transphalangeal amputation of other finger   HCC
Complete traumatic transphalangeal amputation of specified finger with unspecified laterality

3 ✓7ᵗʰ **S68.619** Complete traumatic transphalangeal amputation of unspecified finger   HCC ▽

✓6ᵗʰ **S68.62** Partial traumatic transphalangeal amputation of other and unspecified finger

3 ✓7ᵗʰ **S68.620** Partial traumatic transphalangeal amputation of right index finger   HCC

3 ✓7ᵗʰ **S68.621** Partial traumatic transphalangeal amputation of left index finger   HCC

3 ✓7ᵗʰ **S68.622** Partial traumatic transphalangeal amputation of right middle finger   HCC

3 ✓7ᵗʰ **S68.623** Partial traumatic transphalangeal amputation of left middle finger   HCC

3 ✓7ᵗʰ **S68.624** Partial traumatic transphalangeal amputation of right ring finger   HCC

3 ✓7ᵗʰ **S68.625** Partial traumatic transphalangeal amputation of left ring finger   HCC

3 ✓7ᵗʰ **S68.626** Partial traumatic transphalangeal amputation of right little finger   HCC

3 ✓7ᵗʰ **S68.627** Partial traumatic transphalangeal amputation of left little finger   HCC

3 ✓7ᵗʰ **S68.628** Partial traumatic transphalangeal amputation of other finger   HCC
Partial traumatic transphalangeal amputation of specified finger with unspecified laterality

3 ✓7ᵗʰ **S68.629** Partial traumatic transphalangeal amputation of unspecified finger   HCC ▽

✓5ᵗʰ **S68.7** Traumatic transmetacarpal amputation of hand

✓6ᵗʰ **S68.71** Complete traumatic transmetacarpal amputation of hand

2 ✓7ᵗʰ **S68.711** Complete traumatic transmetacarpal amputation of right hand   HCC

2 ✓7ᵗʰ **S68.712** Complete traumatic transmetacarpal amputation of left hand   HCC

2 ✓7ᵗʰ **S68.719** Complete traumatic transmetacarpal amputation of unspecified hand   HCC ▽

✓6ᵗʰ **S68.72** Partial traumatic transmetacarpal amputation of hand

2 ✓7ᵗʰ **S68.721** Partial traumatic transmetacarpal amputation of right hand   HCC

2 ✓7ᵗʰ **S68.722** Partial traumatic transmetacarpal amputation of left hand   HCC

2 ✓7ᵗʰ **S68.729** Partial traumatic transmetacarpal amputation of unspecified hand   HCC ▽

---

2   HCC with 7th character indicating initial encounter (A or B - specific to category) OR sequela.
3   HCC with 7th character indicating sequela.

☑ Additional Character Req   ✓ₓ7ᵗʰ Placeholder Alert   Manifestation   HCC CMS-HCC Condition   ▽ Unspecified Code   ▶◀ Revised Text   ● New Code   ▲ Revised Code Title

☑4ᵗʰ **S69   Other and unspecified injuries of wrist, hand and finger(s)**

> The appropriate 7th character is to be added to each code from category S69.
> A   initial encounter
> D   subsequent encounter
> S   sequela

☑5ᵗʰ **S69.8   Other specified injuries of wrist, hand and finger(s)**

☑x7ᵗʰ **S69.80   Other specified injuries of unspecified wrist, hand and finger(s)** ▽

☑x7ᵗʰ **S69.81   Other specified injuries of** right **wrist, hand and finger(s)**

☑x7ᵗʰ **S69.82   Other specified injuries of** left **wrist, hand and finger(s)**

☑5ᵗʰ **S69.9   Unspecified injury of wrist, hand and finger(s)**

☑x7ᵗʰ **S69.90   Unspecified injury of unspecified wrist, hand and finger(s)** ▽

☑x7ᵗʰ **S69.91   Unspecified injury of** right **wrist, hand and finger(s)** ▽

☑x7ᵗʰ **S69.92   Unspecified injury of** left **wrist, hand and finger(s)** ▽

Injuries to the hip and thigh (S70-S79)

EXCLUDES 2   *burns and corrosions (T20-T32)*
frostbite (T33-T34)
snake bite (T63.0-)
venomous insect bite or sting (T63.4-)

☑4ᵗʰ **S70   Superficial injury of hip and thigh**

> The appropriate 7th character is to be added to each code from category S70.
> A   initial encounter
> D   subsequent encounter
> S   sequela

☑5ᵗʰ **S70.0   Contusion of** hip

☑x7ᵗʰ **S70.00   Contusion of unspecified hip** ▽

☑x7ᵗʰ **S70.01   Contusion of** right **hip**

☑x7ᵗʰ **S70.02   Contusion of** left **hip**

☑5ᵗʰ **S70.1   Contusion of** thigh

☑x7ᵗʰ **S70.10   Contusion of unspecified thigh** ▽

☑x7ᵗʰ **S70.11   Contusion of** right **thigh**

☑x7ᵗʰ **S70.12   Contusion of** left **thigh**

☑5ᵗʰ **S70.2   Other superficial injuries of** hip

☑6ᵗʰ **S70.21   Abrasion of hip**

☑7ᵗʰ S70.211   Abrasion, right **hip**

☑7ᵗʰ S70.212   Abrasion, left **hip**

☑7ᵗʰ S70.219   **Abrasion, unspecified hip** ▽

☑6ᵗʰ **S70.22   Blister (nonthermal) of hip**

☑7ᵗʰ S70.221   Blister (nonthermal), right **hip**

☑7ᵗʰ S70.222   Blister (nonthermal), left **hip**

☑7ᵗʰ S70.229   **Blister (nonthermal), unspecified hip** ▽

☑6ᵗʰ **S70.24   External constriction of hip**

☑7ᵗʰ S70.241   External constriction, right **hip**

☑7ᵗʰ S70.242   External constriction, left **hip**

☑7ᵗʰ S70.249   **External constriction, unspecified hip** ▽

☑6ᵗʰ **S70.25   Superficial** foreign body **of hip**
Splinter in the hip

☑7ᵗʰ S70.251   **Superficial foreign body,** right **hip**

☑7ᵗʰ S70.252   **Superficial foreign body,** left **hip**

☑7ᵗʰ S70.259   **Superficial foreign body, unspecified hip** ▽

☑6ᵗʰ **S70.26   Insect bite (nonvenomous) of hip**

☑7ᵗʰ S70.261   Insect bite (nonvenomous), right **hip**

☑7ᵗʰ S70.262   Insect bite (nonvenomous), left **hip**

☑7ᵗʰ S70.269   **Insect bite (nonvenomous), unspecified** ▽ **hip**

☑6ᵗʰ **S70.27   Other superficial** bite **of hip**
EXCLUDES 1   *open bite of hip (S71.05-)*

☑7ᵗʰ S70.271   Other superficial bite of hip, right **hip**

☑7ᵗʰ S70.272   Other superficial bite of hip, left **hip**

☑7ᵗʰ S70.279   **Other superficial bite of hip, unspecified hip** ▽

☑5ᵗʰ **S70.3   Other superficial injuries of** thigh

☑6ᵗʰ **S70.31   Abrasion of thigh**

☑7ᵗʰ S70.311   Abrasion, right **thigh**

☑7ᵗʰ S70.312   Abrasion, left **thigh**

☑7ᵗʰ S70.319   **Abrasion, unspecified thigh** ▽

☑6ᵗʰ **S70.32   Blister (nonthermal) of thigh**

☑7ᵗʰ S70.321   Blister (nonthermal), right **thigh**

☑7ᵗʰ S70.322   Blister (nonthermal), left **thigh**

☑7ᵗʰ S70.329   Blister (nonthermal), unspecified thigh ▽

☑6ᵗʰ **S70.34   External constriction of thigh**

☑7ᵗʰ S70.341   External constriction, right **thigh**

☑7ᵗʰ S70.342   External constriction, left **thigh**

☑7ᵗʰ S70.349   **External constriction, unspecified thigh** ▽

☑6ᵗʰ **S70.35   Superficial** foreign body **of thigh**
Splinter in the thigh

☑7ᵗʰ S70.351   **Superficial foreign body,** right **thigh**

☑7ᵗʰ S70.352   **Superficial foreign body,** left **thigh**

☑7ᵗʰ S70.359   **Superficial foreign body, unspecified** ▽ **thigh**

☑6ᵗʰ **S70.36   Insect bite (nonvenomous) of thigh**

☑7ᵗʰ S70.361   Insect bite (nonvenomous), right **thigh**

☑7ᵗʰ S70.362   Insect bite (nonvenomous), left **thigh**

☑7ᵗʰ S70.369   **Insect bite (nonvenomous), unspecified** ▽ **thigh**

☑6ᵗʰ **S70.37   Other superficial** bite **of thigh**
EXCLUDES 1   *open bite of thigh (S71.15)*

☑7ᵗʰ S70.371   Other superficial bite of right **thigh**

☑7ᵗʰ S70.372   Other superficial bite of left **thigh**

☑7ᵗʰ S70.379   **Other superficial bite of unspecified thigh** ▽

☑5ᵗʰ **S70.9   Unspecified superficial injury of** hip and thigh

☑6ᵗʰ **S70.91   Unspecified superficial injury of** hip

☑7ᵗʰ S70.911   **Unspecified superficial injury of** right **hip** ▽

☑7ᵗʰ S70.912   **Unspecified superficial injury of** left **hip** ▽

☑7ᵗʰ S70.919   **Unspecified superficial injury of unspecified hip** ▽

☑6ᵗʰ **S70.92   Unspecified superficial injury of** thigh

☑7ᵗʰ S70.921   **Unspecified superficial injury of** right **thigh** ▽

☑7ᵗʰ S70.922   **Unspecified superficial injury of** left **thigh** ▽

☑7ᵗʰ S70.929   **Unspecified superficial injury of unspecified thigh** ▽

☑4ᵗʰ **S71   Open wound of hip and thigh**
Code also any associated wound infection
EXCLUDES 1   *open fracture of hip and thigh (S72.-)*
traumatic amputation of hip and thigh (S78.-)
EXCLUDES 2   *bite of venomous animal (T63.-)*
open wound of ankle, foot and toes (S91.-)
open wound of knee and lower leg (S81.-)

> The appropriate 7th character is to be added to each code from category S71.
> A   initial encounter
> D   subsequent encounter
> S   sequela

☑5ᵗʰ **S71.0   Open wound of** hip

☑6ᵗʰ **S71.00   Unspecified open wound of hip**

☑7ᵗʰ S71.001   Unspecified open wound, right **hip** ▽

☑7ᵗʰ S71.002   Unspecified open wound, left **hip** ▽

☑7ᵗʰ S71.009   **Unspecified open wound, unspecified** ▽ **hip**

☑6ᵗʰ **S71.01   Laceration without foreign body of hip**

☑7ᵗʰ S71.011   Laceration without foreign body, right **hip**

☑7ᵗʰ S71.012   Laceration without foreign body, left **hip**

☑7ᵗʰ S71.019   **Laceration without foreign body, unspecified hip** ▽

☑6ᵗʰ **S71.02   Laceration with foreign body of hip**

☑7ᵗʰ S71.021   Laceration with foreign body, right **hip**

☑7ᵗʰ S71.022   Laceration with foreign body, left **hip**

√7ᵗʰ **S71.029** Laceration with foreign body, unspecified hip ▽

√6ᵗʰ **S71.03** Puncture wound without foreign body of hip

√7ᵗʰ **S71.031** Puncture wound without foreign body, right hip

√7ᵗʰ **S71.032** Puncture wound without foreign body, left hip

√7ᵗʰ **S71.039** Puncture wound without foreign body, unspecified hip ▽

√6ᵗʰ **S71.04** Puncture wound with foreign body of hip

√7ᵗʰ **S71.041** Puncture wound with foreign body, right hip

√7ᵗʰ **S71.042** Puncture wound with foreign body, left hip

√7ᵗʰ **S71.049** Puncture wound with foreign body, unspecified hip ▽

√6ᵗʰ **S71.05** Open bite of hip
Bite of hip NOS
EXCLUDES 1   superficial bite of hip (S70.26, S70.27)

√7ᵗʰ **S71.051** Open bite, right hip

√7ᵗʰ **S71.052** Open bite, left hip

√7ᵗʰ **S71.059** Open bite, unspecified hip ▽

√5ᵗʰ **S71.1** Open wound of thigh

√6ᵗʰ **S71.10** Unspecified open wound of thigh
AHA: 2016, 3Q, 24

√7ᵗʰ **S71.101** Unspecified open wound, right thigh ▽

√7ᵗʰ **S71.102** Unspecified open wound, left thigh ▽

√7ᵗʰ **S71.109** Unspecified open wound, unspecified thigh ▽

√6ᵗʰ **S71.11** Laceration without foreign body of thigh

√7ᵗʰ **S71.111** Laceration without foreign body, right thigh

√7ᵗʰ **S71.112** Laceration without foreign body, left thigh

√7ᵗʰ **S71.119** Laceration without foreign body, unspecified thigh ▽

√6ᵗʰ **S71.12** Laceration with foreign body of thigh

√7ᵗʰ **S71.121** Laceration with foreign body, right thigh

√7ᵗʰ **S71.122** Laceration with foreign body, left thigh

√7ᵗʰ **S71.129** Laceration with foreign body, unspecified thigh ▽

√6ᵗʰ **S71.13** Puncture wound without foreign body of thigh
AHA: 2016, 3Q, 24

√7ᵗʰ **S71.131** Puncture wound without foreign body, right thigh

√7ᵗʰ **S71.132** Puncture wound without foreign body, left thigh

√7ᵗʰ **S71.139** Puncture wound without foreign body, unspecified thigh ▽

√6ᵗʰ **S71.14** Puncture wound with foreign body of thigh
AHA: 2016, 3Q, 24

√7ᵗʰ **S71.141** Puncture wound with foreign body, right thigh

√7ᵗʰ **S71.142** Puncture wound with foreign body, left thigh

√7ᵗʰ **S71.149** Puncture wound with foreign body, unspecified thigh ▽

√6ᵗʰ **S71.15** Open bite of thigh
Bite of thigh NOS
EXCLUDES 1   superficial bite of thigh (S70.37-)

√7ᵗʰ **S71.151** Open bite, right thigh

√7ᵗʰ **S71.152** Open bite, left thigh

√7ᵗʰ **S71.159** Open bite, unspecified thigh ▽

√4ᵗʰ **S72** **Fracture of femur**
NOTE
A fracture not indicated as displaced or nondisplaced should be coded to displaced.
The open fracture designations are based on the Gustilo open fracture classification.
A fracture not indicated as open or closed should be coded to closed.
EXCLUDES 1   traumatic amputation of hip and thigh (S78.-)
EXCLUDES 2   fracture of lower leg and ankle (S82.-)
fracture of foot (S92.-)
periprosthetic fracture of prosthetic implant of hip ▶(M97.0-)◀
AHA: 2016, 1Q, 33; 2015, 3Q, 37-39; 2015, 1Q, 17; 2013, 4Q, 128

The appropriate 7th character is to be added to all codes from category S72 [unless otherwise indicated].
A   initial encounter for closed fracture
B   initial encounter for open fracture type I or II
      initial encounter for open fracture NOS
C   initial encounter for open fracture type IIIA, IIIB, or IIIC
D   subsequent encounter for closed fracture with routine healing
E   subsequent encounter for open fracture type I or II with routine healing
F   subsequent encounter for open fracture type IIIA, IIIB, or IIIC with routine healing
G   subsequent encounter for closed fracture with delayed healing
H   subsequent encounter for open fracture type I or II with delayed healing
J   subsequent encounter for open fracture type IIIA, IIIB, or IIIC with delayed healing
K   subsequent encounter for closed fracture with nonunion
M   subsequent encounter for open fracture type I or II with nonunion
N   subsequent encounter for open fracture type IIIA, IIIB, or IIIC with nonunion
P   subsequent encounter for closed fracture with malunion
Q   subsequent encounter for open fracture type I or II with malunion
R   subsequent encounter for open fracture type IIIA, IIIB, or IIIC with malunion
S   sequela

√5ᵗʰ **S72.0** **Fracture of head and neck of femur**
EXCLUDES 2   physeal fracture of upper end of femur (S79.0-)
AHA: 2016, 3Q, 16

√6ᵗʰ **S72.00** Fracture of unspecified part of neck of femur
Fracture of hip NOS
Fracture of neck of femur NOS

1 √7ᵗʰ **S72.001** Fracture of unspecified part of neck of right femur   HCC ▽

1 √7ᵗʰ **S72.002** Fracture of unspecified part of neck of left femur   HCC ▽

1 √7ᵗʰ **S72.009** Fracture of unspecified part of neck of unspecified femur   HCC ▽

√6ᵗʰ **S72.01** Unspecified intracapsular fracture of femur
Subcapital fracture of femur

1 √7ᵗʰ **S72.011** Unspecified intracapsular fracture of right femur   HCC ▽

1 √7ᵗʰ **S72.012** Unspecified intracapsular fracture of left femur   HCC ▽

1 √7ᵗʰ **S72.019** Unspecified intracapsular fracture of unspecified femur   HCC ▽

√6ᵗʰ **S72.02** Fracture of epiphysis (separation) (upper) of femur
Transepiphyseal fracture of femur
EXCLUDES 1   capital femoral epiphyseal fracture (pediatric) of femur (S79.01-)
Salter-Harris Type I physeal fracture of upper end of femur (S79.01-)

1 √7ᵗʰ **S72.021** Displaced fracture of epiphysis (separation) (upper) of right femur   HCC

1 √7ᵗʰ **S72.022** Displaced fracture of epiphysis (separation) (upper) of left femur   HCC

1 √7ᵗʰ **S72.023** Displaced fracture of epiphysis (separation) (upper) of unspecified femur   HCC ▽

1 √7ᵗʰ **S72.024** Nondisplaced fracture of epiphysis (separation) (upper) of right femur   HCC

1 √7ᵗʰ **S72.025** Nondisplaced fracture of epiphysis (separation) (upper) of left femur   HCC

---

1   HCC with 7th character indicating initial encounter (A, B or C - specific to category).

☑ Additional Character Req   √x7ᵗʰ Placeholder Alert   Manifestation   HCC CMS-HCC Condition   ▽ Unspecified Code   ▶◀ Revised Text   ● New Code   ▲ Revised Code Title

ICD-10-CM 2018   1003

1 √7th **S72.026** Nondisplaced **fracture of epiphysis (separation) (upper) of** unspecified **femur** HCC ▽

√6th **S72.03** Midcervical **fracture of femur**
  Transcervical fracture of femur NOS

1 √7th **S72.031** Displaced **midcervical fracture of** right **femur** HCC

1 √7th **S72.032** Displaced **midcervical fracture of** left **femur** HCC

1 √7th **S72.033** Displaced **midcervical fracture of** unspecified **femur** HCC ▽

1 √7th **S72.034** Nondisplaced **midcervical fracture of** right **femur** HCC

1 √7th **S72.035** Nondisplaced **midcervical fracture of** left **femur** HCC

1 √7th **S72.036** Nondisplaced **midcervical fracture of** unspecified **femur** HCC ▽

√6th **S72.04** Fracture of base of neck of femur
  Cervicotrochanteric fracture of femur

1 √7th **S72.041** Displaced **fracture of base of neck of** right **femur** HCC

1 √7th **S72.042** Displaced **fracture of base of neck of** left **femur** HCC

1 √7th **S72.043** Displaced **fracture of base of neck of** unspecified **femur** HCC ▽

1 √7th **S72.044** Nondisplaced **fracture of base of neck of** right **femur** HCC

1 √7th **S72.045** Nondisplaced **fracture of base of neck of** left **femur** HCC

1 √7th **S72.046** Nondisplaced **fracture of base of neck of unspecified femur** HCC ▽

√6th **S72.05** Unspecified fracture of head of femur
  Fracture of head of femur NOS

1 √7th **S72.051** Unspecified **fracture of head of** right **femur** HCC ▽

1 √7th **S72.052** Unspecified **fracture of head of** left **femur** HCC ▽

1 √7th **S72.059** Unspecified **fracture of head of unspecified femur** HCC ▽

√6th **S72.06** Articular fracture of head of femur

1 √7th **S72.061** Displaced **articular fracture of head of** right **femur** HCC

1 √7th **S72.062** Displaced **articular fracture of head of** left **femur** HCC

1 √7th **S72.063** Displaced **articular fracture of head of unspecified femur** HCC ▽

1 √7th **S72.064** Nondisplaced **articular fracture of head of** right **femur** HCC

1 √7th **S72.065** Nondisplaced **articular fracture of head of** left **femur** HCC

1 √7th **S72.066** Nondisplaced **articular fracture of head of unspecified femur** HCC ▽

√6th **S72.09** Other fracture of head and neck of femur

1 √7th **S72.091** Other **fracture of head and neck of** right **femur** HCC

1 √7th **S72.092** Other **fracture of head and neck of** left **femur** HCC

1 √7th **S72.099** Other **fracture of head and neck of unspecified femur** HCC ▽

√5th **S72.1** Pertrochanteric **fracture**
  AHA: 2016, 3Q, 16

√6th **S72.10** Unspecified **trochanteric fracture of femur**
  Fracture of trochanter NOS

1 √7th **S72.101** Unspecified **trochanteric fracture of** right **femur** HCC ▽

1 √7th **S72.102** Unspecified **trochanteric fracture of** left **femur** HCC ▽

1 √7th **S72.109** Unspecified **trochanteric fracture of unspecified femur** HCC ▽

√6th **S72.11** Fracture of greater trochanter of femur

1 √7th **S72.111** Displaced **fracture of greater trochanter of** right **femur** HCC

1 √7th **S72.112** Displaced **fracture of greater trochanter of** left **femur** HCC

1 √7th **S72.113** Displaced **fracture of greater trochanter of unspecified femur** HCC ▽

1 √7th **S72.114** Nondisplaced **fracture of greater trochanter of** right **femur** HCC

1 √7th **S72.115** Nondisplaced **fracture of greater trochanter of** left **femur** HCC

1 √7th **S72.116** Nondisplaced **fracture of greater trochanter of unspecified femur** HCC ▽

√6th **S72.12** Fracture of lesser trochanter of femur

1 √7th **S72.121** Displaced **fracture of lesser trochanter of** right **femur** HCC

1 √7th **S72.122** Displaced **fracture of lesser trochanter of** left **femur** HCC

1 √7th **S72.123** Displaced **fracture of lesser trochanter of unspecified femur** HCC ▽

1 √7th **S72.124** Nondisplaced **fracture of lesser trochanter of** right **femur** HCC

1 √7th **S72.125** Nondisplaced **fracture of lesser trochanter of** left **femur** HCC

1 √7th **S72.126** Nondisplaced **fracture of lesser trochanter of unspecified femur** HCC ▽

√6th **S72.13** Apophyseal **fracture of femur**
  EXCLUDES 1   chronic (nontraumatic) slipped upper femoral epiphysis (M93.0-)

1 √7th **S72.131** Displaced **apophyseal fracture of** right **femur** HCC

1 √7th **S72.132** Displaced **apophyseal fracture of** left **femur** HCC

1 √7th **S72.133** Displaced **apophyseal fracture of unspecified femur** HCC ▽

1 √7th **S72.134** Nondisplaced **apophyseal fracture of** right **femur** HCC

1 √7th **S72.135** Nondisplaced **apophyseal fracture of** left **femur** HCC

1 √7th **S72.136** Nondisplaced **apophyseal fracture of unspecified femur** HCC ▽

√6th **S72.14** Intertrochanteric **fracture of femur**

1 √7th **S72.141** Displaced **intertrochanteric fracture of** right **femur** HCC

1 √7th **S72.142** Displaced **intertrochanteric fracture of** left **femur** HCC

1 √7th **S72.143** Displaced **intertrochanteric fracture of unspecified femur** HCC ▽

1 √7th **S72.144** Nondisplaced **intertrochanteric fracture of** right **femur** HCC

1 √7th **S72.145** Nondisplaced **intertrochanteric fracture of** left **femur** HCC

1 √7th **S72.146** Nondisplaced **intertrochanteric fracture of unspecified femur** HCC ▽

√5th **S72.2** Subtrochanteric **fracture of femur**

1 √x 7th **S72.21** Displaced **subtrochanteric fracture of** right **femur** HCC

1 √x 7th **S72.22** Displaced **subtrochanteric fracture of** left **femur** HCC

1 √x 7th **S72.23** Displaced **subtrochanteric fracture of unspecified femur** HCC ▽

1 √x 7th **S72.24** Nondisplaced **subtrochanteric fracture of** right **femur** HCC

1 √x 7th **S72.25** Nondisplaced **subtrochanteric fracture of** left **femur** HCC

1 √x 7th **S72.26** Nondisplaced **subtrochanteric fracture of unspecified femur** HCC ▽

√5th **S72.3** Fracture of shaft of femur

√6th **S72.30** Unspecified fracture of shaft of femur

1 √7th **S72.301** Unspecified **fracture of shaft of** right **femur** HCC ▽

1 √7th **S72.302** Unspecified **fracture of shaft of** left **femur** HCC ▽

1 √7th **S72.309** Unspecified **fracture of shaft of unspecified femur** HCC ▽

√6th **S72.32** Transverse **fracture of shaft of femur**

1 √7th **S72.321** Displaced **transverse fracture of shaft of** right **femur** HCC

---

1   HCC with 7th character indicating initial encounter (A, B or C - specific to category).

EXCLUDES 1 Not coded here   EXCLUDES 2 Not included here   N Newborn Age: 0   P Pediatric Age: 0-17   M Maternity Age: 12-55   A Adult Age: 15-124

1004   ICD-10-CM 2018

¹ ✓7ᵗʰ **S72.322** Displaced **transverse fracture of shaft of left** femur   HCC

¹ ✓7ᵗʰ **S72.323** Displaced **transverse fracture of shaft of unspecified femur**   HCC ▽

¹ ✓7ᵗʰ **S72.324** Nondisplaced **transverse fracture of shaft of right femur**   HCC

¹ ✓7ᵗʰ **S72.325** Nondisplaced **transverse fracture of shaft of left femur**   HCC

¹ ✓7ᵗʰ **S72.326** Nondisplaced **transverse fracture of shaft of unspecified femur**   HCC ▽

✓6ᵗʰ **S72.33** Oblique **fracture of shaft of femur**

¹ ✓7ᵗʰ **S72.331** Displaced **oblique fracture of shaft of right femur**   HCC

¹ ✓7ᵗʰ **S72.332** Displaced **oblique fracture of shaft of left femur**   HCC

¹ ✓7ᵗʰ **S72.333** Displaced **oblique fracture of shaft of unspecified femur**   HCC ▽

¹ ✓7ᵗʰ **S72.334** Nondisplaced **oblique fracture of shaft of right femur**   HCC

¹ ✓7ᵗʰ **S72.335** Nondisplaced **oblique fracture of shaft of left femur**   HCC

¹ ✓7ᵗʰ **S72.336** Nondisplaced **oblique fracture of shaft of unspecified femur**   HCC ▽

✓6ᵗʰ **S72.34** Spiral **fracture of shaft of femur**

¹ ✓7ᵗʰ **S72.341** Displaced **spiral fracture of shaft of right femur**   HCC

¹ ✓7ᵗʰ **S72.342** Displaced **spiral fracture of shaft of left femur**   HCC

¹ ✓7ᵗʰ **S72.343** Displaced **spiral fracture of shaft of unspecified femur**   HCC ▽

¹ ✓7ᵗʰ **S72.344** Nondisplaced **spiral fracture of shaft of right femur**   HCC

¹ ✓7ᵗʰ **S72.345** Nondisplaced **spiral fracture of shaft of left femur**   HCC

¹ ✓7ᵗʰ **S72.346** Nondisplaced **spiral fracture of shaft of unspecified femur**   HCC ▽

✓6ᵗʰ **S72.35** Comminuted **fracture of shaft of femur**

¹ ✓7ᵗʰ **S72.351** Displaced **comminuted fracture of shaft of right femur**   HCC

¹ ✓7ᵗʰ **S72.352** Displaced **comminuted fracture of shaft of left femur**   HCC

¹ ✓7ᵗʰ **S72.353** Displaced **comminuted fracture of shaft of unspecified femur**   HCC ▽

¹ ✓7ᵗʰ **S72.354** Nondisplaced **comminuted fracture of shaft of right femur**   HCC

¹ ✓7ᵗʰ **S72.355** Nondisplaced **comminuted fracture of shaft of left femur**   HCC

¹ ✓7ᵗʰ **S72.356** Nondisplaced **comminuted fracture of shaft of unspecified femur**   HCC ▽

✓6ᵗʰ **S72.36** Segmental **fracture of shaft of femur**

¹ ✓7ᵗʰ **S72.361** Displaced **segmental fracture of shaft of right femur**   HCC

¹ ✓7ᵗʰ **S72.362** Displaced **segmental fracture of shaft of left femur**   HCC

¹ ✓7ᵗʰ **S72.363** Displaced **segmental fracture of shaft of unspecified femur**   HCC ▽

¹ ✓7ᵗʰ **S72.364** Nondisplaced **segmental fracture of shaft of right femur**   HCC

¹ ✓7ᵗʰ **S72.365** Nondisplaced **segmental fracture of shaft of left femur**   HCC

¹ ✓7ᵗʰ **S72.366** Nondisplaced **segmental fracture of shaft of unspecified femur**   HCC ▽

✓6ᵗʰ **S72.39** Other **fracture of shaft of femur**

¹ ✓7ᵗʰ **S72.391** Other **fracture of shaft of right** femur   HCC

¹ ✓7ᵗʰ **S72.392** Other **fracture of shaft of left** femur   HCC

¹ ✓7ᵗʰ **S72.399** Other **fracture of shaft of unspecified femur**   HCC ▽

✓5ᵗʰ **S72.4** Fracture of lower end **of femur**
Fracture of distal end of femur
EXCLUDES 2   *fracture of shaft of femur (S72.3-)*
physeal fracture of lower end of femur (S79.1-)

✓6ᵗʰ **S72.40** Unspecified **fracture of lower end of femur**

¹ ✓7ᵗʰ **S72.401** Unspecified **fracture of lower end of right femur**   HCC ▽

¹ ✓7ᵗʰ **S72.402** Unspecified **fracture of lower end of left** femur   HCC ▽

¹ ✓7ᵗʰ **S72.409** Unspecified **fracture of lower end of unspecified femur**   HCC ▽

✓6ᵗʰ **S72.41** Unspecified condyle **fracture of lower end of femur**
Condyle fracture of femur NOS

¹ ✓7ᵗʰ **S72.411** Displaced **unspecified condyle fracture of lower end of right** femur   HCC

¹ ✓7ᵗʰ **S72.412** Displaced **unspecified condyle fracture of lower end of left** femur   HCC

¹ ✓7ᵗʰ **S72.413** Displaced **unspecified condyle fracture of lower end of unspecified femur**   HCC

¹ ✓7ᵗʰ **S72.414** Nondisplaced **unspecified condyle fracture of lower end of right** femur   HCC

¹ ✓7ᵗʰ **S72.415** Nondisplaced **unspecified condyle fracture of lower end of left** femur   HCC

¹ ✓7ᵗʰ **S72.416** Nondisplaced **unspecified condyle fracture of lower end of unspecified femur**   HCC

✓6ᵗʰ **S72.42** Fracture of lateral condyle **of femur**

¹ ✓7ᵗʰ **S72.421** Displaced **fracture of lateral condyle of right** femur   HCC

¹ ✓7ᵗʰ **S72.422** Displaced **fracture of lateral condyle of left** femur   HCC

¹ ✓7ᵗʰ **S72.423** Displaced **fracture of lateral condyle of unspecified femur**   HCC ▽

¹ ✓7ᵗʰ **S72.424** Nondisplaced **fracture of lateral condyle of right** femur   HCC

¹ ✓7ᵗʰ **S72.425** Nondisplaced **fracture of lateral condyle of left** femur   HCC

¹ ✓7ᵗʰ **S72.426** Nondisplaced **fracture of lateral condyle of unspecified femur**   HCC ▽

✓6ᵗʰ **S72.43** Fracture of medial condyle **of femur**

¹ ✓7ᵗʰ **S72.431** Displaced **fracture of medial condyle of right** femur   HCC

¹ ✓7ᵗʰ **S72.432** Displaced **fracture of medial condyle of left** femur   HCC

¹ ✓7ᵗʰ **S72.433** Displaced **fracture of medial condyle of unspecified femur**   HCC ▽

¹ ✓7ᵗʰ **S72.434** Nondisplaced **fracture of medial condyle of right** femur   HCC

¹ ✓7ᵗʰ **S72.435** Nondisplaced **fracture of medial condyle of left** femur   HCC

¹ ✓7ᵗʰ **S72.436** Nondisplaced **fracture of medial condyle of unspecified femur**   HCC ▽

✓6ᵗʰ **S72.44** Fracture of lower epiphysis (separation) **of femur**
EXCLUDES 1   *Salter-Harris Type I physeal fracture of lower end of femur (S79.11-)*

¹ ✓7ᵗʰ **S72.441** Displaced **fracture of lower epiphysis (separation) of right** femur   HCC

¹ ✓7ᵗʰ **S72.442** Displaced **fracture of lower epiphysis (separation) of left** femur   HCC

¹ ✓7ᵗʰ **S72.443** Displaced **fracture of lower epiphysis (separation) of unspecified femur**   HCC ▽

¹ ✓7ᵗʰ **S72.444** Nondisplaced **fracture of lower epiphysis (separation) of right** femur   HCC

¹ ✓7ᵗʰ **S72.445** Nondisplaced **fracture of lower epiphysis (separation) of left** femur   HCC

¹ ✓7ᵗʰ **S72.446** Nondisplaced **fracture of lower epiphysis (separation) of unspecified femur**   HCC ▽

✓6ᵗʰ **S72.45** Supracondylar **fracture without intracondylar extension of lower end of femur**
Supracondylar fracture of lower end of femur NOS
EXCLUDES 1   *supracondylar fracture with intracondylar extension of lower end of femur (S72.46-)*

¹ ✓7ᵗʰ **S72.451** Displaced **supracondylar fracture without intracondylar extension of lower end of right** femur   HCC

¹ ✓7ᵗʰ **S72.452** Displaced **supracondylar fracture without intracondylar extension of lower end of left** femur   HCC

---

¹ HCC with 7th character indicating initial encounter (A, B or C - specific to category).

☑ Additional Character Req   ✓ₓ7ᵗʰ Placeholder Alert   Manifestation   HCC CMS-HCC Condition   ▽ Unspecified Code   ▶◀ Revised Text   ● New Code   ▲ Revised Code Title

ICD-10-CM 2018

1005

1 ✓7ᵗʰ **S72.453** Displaced supracondylar fracture without intracondylar extension of lower end of unspecified femur   HCC ▽

1 ✓7ᵗʰ **S72.454** Nondisplaced supracondylar fracture without intracondylar extension of lower end of right femur   HCC

1 ✓7ᵗʰ **S72.455** Nondisplaced supracondylar fracture without intracondylar extension of lower end of left femur   HCC

1 ✓7ᵗʰ **S72.456** Nondisplaced supracondylar fracture without intracondylar extension of lower end of unspecified femur   HCC ▽

✓6ᵗʰ **S72.46** Supracondylar fracture with intracondylar extension of lower end of femur
> EXCLUDES 1   supracondylar fracture without intracondylar extension of lower end of femur (S72.45-)

1 ✓7ᵗʰ **S72.461** Displaced supracondylar fracture with intracondylar extension of lower end of right femur   HCC

1 ✓7ᵗʰ **S72.462** Displaced supracondylar fracture with intracondylar extension of lower end of left femur   HCC

1 ✓7ᵗʰ **S72.463** Displaced supracondylar fracture with intracondylar extension of lower end of unspecified femur   HCC ▽

1 ✓7ᵗʰ **S72.464** Nondisplaced supracondylar fracture with intracondylar extension of lower end of right femur   HCC

1 ✓7ᵗʰ **S72.465** Nondisplaced supracondylar fracture with intracondylar extension of lower end of left femur   HCC

1 ✓7ᵗʰ **S72.466** Nondisplaced supracondylar fracture with intracondylar extension of lower end of unspecified femur   HCC ▽

✓6ᵗʰ **S72.47** Torus fracture of lower end of femur

> The appropriate 7th character is to be added to all codes in subcategory S72.47.
> A   initial encounter for closed fracture
> D   subsequent encounter for fracture with routine healing
> G   subsequent encounter for fracture with delayed healing
> K   subsequent encounter for fracture with nonunion
> P   subsequent encounter for fracture with malunion
> S   sequela

1 ✓7ᵗʰ **S72.471** Torus fracture of lower end of right femur   HCC

1 ✓7ᵗʰ **S72.472** Torus fracture of lower end of left femur   HCC

1 ✓7ᵗʰ **S72.479** Torus fracture of lower end of unspecified femur   HCC ▽

✓6ᵗʰ **S72.49** Other fracture of lower end of femur

1 ✓7ᵗʰ **S72.491** Other fracture of lower end of right femur   HCC

1 ✓7ᵗʰ **S72.492** Other fracture of lower end of left femur   HCC

1 ✓7ᵗʰ **S72.499** Other fracture of lower end of unspecified femur   HCC ▽

✓5ᵗʰ **S72.8** Other fracture of femur

✓6ᵗʰ **S72.8X** Other fracture of femur

1 ✓7ᵗʰ **S72.8X1** Other fracture of right femur   HCC

1 ✓7ᵗʰ **S72.8X2** Other fracture of left femur   HCC

1 ✓7ᵗʰ **S72.8X9** Other fracture of unspecified femur   HCC ▽

✓5ᵗʰ **S72.9** Unspecified fracture of femur
Fracture of thigh NOS
Fracture of upper leg NOS
> EXCLUDES 1   fracture of hip NOS (S72.00-, S72.01-)

1 ✓x7ᵗʰ **S72.90** Unspecified fracture of unspecified femur   HCC ▽
> AHA: 2012, 4Q, 93

1 ✓x7ᵗʰ **S72.91** Unspecified fracture of right femur   HCC ▽

1 ✓x7ᵗʰ **S72.92** Unspecified fracture of left femur   HCC ▽

✓4ᵗʰ **S73** Dislocation and sprain of joint and ligaments of hip
> INCLUDES   avulsion of joint or ligament of hip
> laceration of cartilage, joint or ligament of hip
> sprain of cartilage, joint or ligament of hip
> traumatic hemarthrosis of joint or ligament of hip
> traumatic rupture of joint or ligament of hip
> traumatic subluxation of joint or ligament of hip
> traumatic tear of joint or ligament of hip

Code also any associated open wound
> EXCLUDES 2   strain of muscle, fascia and tendon of hip and thigh (S76.-)

> The appropriate 7th character is to be added to each code from category S73.
> A   initial encounter
> D   subsequent encounter
> S   sequela

✓5ᵗʰ **S73.0** Subluxation and dislocation of hip
> EXCLUDES 2   dislocation and subluxation of hip prosthesis (T84.020, T84.021)

✓6ᵗʰ **S73.00** Unspecified subluxation and dislocation of hip
Dislocation of hip NOS
Subluxation of hip NOS

1 ✓7ᵗʰ **S73.001** Unspecified subluxation of right hip   HCC ▽

1 ✓7ᵗʰ **S73.002** Unspecified subluxation of left hip   HCC ▽

1 ✓7ᵗʰ **S73.003** Unspecified subluxation of unspecified hip   HCC ▽

1 ✓7ᵗʰ **S73.004** Unspecified dislocation of right hip   HCC ▽

1 ✓7ᵗʰ **S73.005** Unspecified dislocation of left hip   HCC ▽

1 ✓7ᵗʰ **S73.006** Unspecified dislocation of unspecified hip   HCC ▽

✓6ᵗʰ **S73.01** Posterior subluxation and dislocation of hip

1 ✓7ᵗʰ **S73.011** Posterior subluxation of right hip   HCC

1 ✓7ᵗʰ **S73.012** Posterior subluxation of left hip   HCC

1 ✓7ᵗʰ **S73.013** Posterior subluxation of unspecified hip   HCC ▽

1 ✓7ᵗʰ **S73.014** Posterior dislocation of right hip   HCC

1 ✓7ᵗʰ **S73.015** Posterior dislocation of left hip   HCC

1 ✓7ᵗʰ **S73.016** Posterior dislocation of unspecified hip   HCC ▽

✓6ᵗʰ **S73.02** Obturator subluxation and dislocation of hip

1 ✓7ᵗʰ **S73.021** Obturator subluxation of right hip   HCC

1 ✓7ᵗʰ **S73.022** Obturator subluxation of left hip   HCC

1 ✓7ᵗʰ **S73.023** Obturator subluxation of unspecified hip   HCC ▽

1 ✓7ᵗʰ **S73.024** Obturator dislocation of right hip   HCC

1 ✓7ᵗʰ **S73.025** Obturator dislocation of left hip   HCC

1 ✓7ᵗʰ **S73.026** Obturator dislocation of unspecified hip   HCC ▽

▲ ✓6ᵗʰ **S73.03** Other anterior subluxation and dislocation of hip

1 ✓7ᵗʰ **S73.031** Other anterior subluxation of right hip   HCC

1 ✓7ᵗʰ **S73.032** Other anterior subluxation of left hip   HCC

1 ✓7ᵗʰ **S73.033** Other anterior subluxation of unspecified hip   HCC ▽

1 ✓7ᵗʰ **S73.034** Other anterior dislocation of right hip   HCC

1 ✓7ᵗʰ **S73.035** Other anterior dislocation of left hip   HCC

1 ✓7ᵗʰ **S73.036** Other anterior dislocation of unspecified hip   HCC ▽

▲ ✓6ᵗʰ **S73.04** Central subluxation and dislocation of hip

1 ✓7ᵗʰ **S73.041** Central subluxation of right hip   HCC

1 ✓7ᵗʰ **S73.042** Central subluxation of left hip   HCC

1 ✓7ᵗʰ **S73.043** Central subluxation of unspecified hip   HCC ▽

---

1   HCC with 7th character indicating initial encounter (A, B or C - specific to category).

EXCLUDES 1 Not coded here   EXCLUDES 2 Not included here   N Newborn Age: 0   P Pediatric Age: 0-17   M Maternity Age: 12-55   A Adult Age: 15-124

1006   ICD-10-CM 2018

S72.453–S73.043

[1] √7ᵗʰ **S73.044 Central** dislocation **of right** hip   HCC

[1] √7ᵗʰ **S73.045 Central** dislocation **of left** hip   HCC

[1] √7ᵗʰ **S73.046 Central** dislocation **of unspecified** hip   HCC ▽

√5ᵗʰ **S73.1 Sprain of hip**
AHA: 2014, 4Q, 25

√6ᵗʰ **S73.10 Unspecified sprain of hip**

√7ᵗʰ **S73.101 Unspecified sprain of right hip** ▽

√7ᵗʰ **S73.102 Unspecified sprain of left hip** ▽

√7ᵗʰ **S73.109 Unspecified sprain of unspecified hip** ▽

√6ᵗʰ **S73.11 Iliofemoral ligament sprain of hip**

√7ᵗʰ **S73.111 Iliofemoral ligament sprain of right hip**

√7ᵗʰ **S73.112 Iliofemoral ligament sprain of left hip**

√7ᵗʰ **S73.119 Iliofemoral ligament sprain of unspecified hip** ▽

√6ᵗʰ **S73.12 Ischiocapsular (ligament) sprain of hip**

√7ᵗʰ **S73.121 Ischiocapsular ligament sprain of right hip**

√7ᵗʰ **S73.122 Ischiocapsular ligament sprain of left hip**

√7ᵗʰ **S73.129 Ischiocapsular ligament sprain of unspecified hip** ▽

√6ᵗʰ **S73.19 Other sprain of hip**

√7ᵗʰ **S73.191 Other sprain of right hip**

√7ᵗʰ **S73.192 Other sprain of left hip**

√7ᵗʰ **S73.199 Other sprain of unspecified hip** ▽

√4ᵗʰ **S74 Injury of nerves at hip and thigh level**
Code also any associated open wound (S71.-)
EXCLUDES 2 *injury of nerves at ankle and foot level (S94.-)*
injury of nerves at lower leg level (S84.-)

The appropriate 7th character is to be added to each code from category S74.
A   initial encounter
D   subsequent encounter
S   sequela

√5ᵗʰ **S74.0 Injury of sciatic nerve at hip and thigh level**

√x7ᵗʰ **S74.00 Injury of sciatic nerve at hip and thigh level, unspecified leg** ▽

√x7ᵗʰ **S74.01 Injury of sciatic nerve at hip and thigh level, right leg**

√x7ᵗʰ **S74.02 Injury of sciatic nerve at hip and thigh level, left leg**

√5ᵗʰ **S74.1 Injury of femoral nerve at hip and thigh level**

√x7ᵗʰ **S74.10 Injury of femoral nerve at hip and thigh level, unspecified leg** ▽

√x7ᵗʰ **S74.11 Injury of femoral nerve at hip and thigh level, right leg**

√x7ᵗʰ **S74.12 Injury of femoral nerve at hip and thigh level, left leg**

√5ᵗʰ **S74.2 Injury of cutaneous sensory nerve at hip and thigh level**

√x7ᵗʰ **S74.20 Injury of cutaneous sensory nerve at hip and thigh level, unspecified leg** ▽

√x7ᵗʰ **S74.21 Injury of cutaneous sensory nerve at hip and high level, right leg**

√x7ᵗʰ **S74.22 Injury of cutaneous sensory nerve at hip and thigh level, left leg**

√5ᵗʰ **S74.8 Injury of other nerves at hip and thigh level**

√6ᵗʰ **S74.8X Injury of other nerves at hip and thigh level**

√7ᵗʰ **S74.8X1 Injury of other nerves at hip and thigh level, right leg**

√7ᵗʰ **S74.8X2 Injury of other nerves at hip and thigh level, left leg**

√7ᵗʰ **S74.8X9 Injury of other nerves at hip and thigh level, unspecified leg** ▽

√5ᵗʰ **S74.9 Injury of unspecified nerve at hip and thigh level**

√x7ᵗʰ **S74.90 Injury of unspecified nerve at hip and thigh level, unspecified leg** ▽

√x7ᵗʰ **S74.91 Injury of unspecified nerve at hip and thigh level, right leg** ▽

√x7ᵗʰ **S74.92 Injury of unspecified nerve at hip and thigh level, left leg** ▽

√4ᵗʰ **S75 Injury of blood vessels at hip and thigh level**
Code also any associated open wound (S71.-)
EXCLUDES 2 *injury of blood vessels at lower leg level (S85.-)*
injury of popliteal artery (S85.0)

The appropriate 7th character is to be added to each code from category S75.
A   initial encounter
D   subsequent encounter
S   sequela

√5ᵗʰ **S75.0 Injury of femoral artery**

√6ᵗʰ **S75.00 Unspecified injury of femoral artery**

√7ᵗʰ **S75.001 Unspecified injury of femoral artery, right leg** ▽

√7ᵗʰ **S75.002 Unspecified injury of femoral artery, left leg** ▽

√7ᵗʰ **S75.009 Unspecified injury of femoral artery, unspecified leg** ▽

√6ᵗʰ **S75.01 Minor laceration of femoral artery**
Incomplete transection of femoral artery
Laceration of femoral artery NOS
Superficial laceration of femoral artery

√7ᵗʰ **S75.011 Minor laceration of femoral artery, right leg**

√7ᵗʰ **S75.012 Minor laceration of femoral artery, left leg**

√7ᵗʰ **S75.019 Minor laceration of femoral artery, unspecified leg** ▽

√6ᵗʰ **S75.02 Major laceration of femoral artery**
Complete transection of femoral artery
Traumatic rupture of femoral artery

√7ᵗʰ **S75.021 Major laceration of femoral artery, right leg**

√7ᵗʰ **S75.022 Major laceration of femoral artery, left leg**

√7ᵗʰ **S75.029 Major laceration of femoral artery, unspecified leg** ▽

√6ᵗʰ **S75.09 Other specified injury of femoral artery**

√7ᵗʰ **S75.091 Other specified injury of femoral artery, right leg**

√7ᵗʰ **S75.092 Other specified injury of femoral artery, left leg**

√7ᵗʰ **S75.099 Other specified injury of femoral artery, unspecified leg** ▽

√5ᵗʰ **S75.1 Injury of femoral vein at hip and thigh level**

√6ᵗʰ **S75.10 Unspecified injury of femoral vein at hip and thigh level**

√7ᵗʰ **S75.101 Unspecified injury of femoral vein at hip and thigh level, right leg** ▽

√7ᵗʰ **S75.102 Unspecified injury of femoral vein at hip and thigh level, left leg** ▽

√7ᵗʰ **S75.109 Unspecified injury of femoral vein at hip and thigh level, unspecified leg** ▽

√6ᵗʰ **S75.11 Minor laceration of femoral vein at hip and thigh level**
Incomplete transection of femoral vein at hip and thigh level
Laceration of femoral vein at hip and thigh level NOS
Superficial laceration of femoral vein at hip and thigh level

√7ᵗʰ **S75.111 Minor laceration of femoral vein at hip and thigh level, right leg**

√7ᵗʰ **S75.112 Minor laceration of femoral vein at hip and thigh level, left leg**

√7ᵗʰ **S75.119 Minor laceration of femoral vein at hip and thigh level, unspecified leg** ▽

√6ᵗʰ **S75.12 Major laceration of femoral vein at hip and thigh level**
Complete transection of femoral vein at hip and thigh level
Traumatic rupture of femoral vein at hip and thigh level

√7ᵗʰ **S75.121 Major laceration of femoral vein at hip and thigh level, right leg**

√7ᵗʰ **S75.122 Major laceration of femoral vein at hip and thigh level, left leg**

√7ᵗʰ **S75.129 Major laceration of femoral vein at hip and thigh level, unspecified leg** ▽

---

[1] HCC with 7th character indicating initial encounter (A, B or C - specific to category).

✓ Additional Character Req   √x7ᵗʰ Placeholder Alert   Manifestation   HCC CMS-HCC Condition   ▽ Unspecified Code   ►◄ Revised Text   ● New Code   ▲ Revised Code Title

√6ᵗʰ **S75.19** **Other specified injury of femoral vein at hip and thigh level**

     √7ᵗʰ **S75.191** **Other specified injury of femoral vein at hip and thigh level, right leg**

     √7ᵗʰ **S75.192** **Other specified injury of femoral vein at hip and thigh level, left leg**

     √7ᵗʰ **S75.199** **Other specified injury of femoral vein at hip and thigh level, unspecified leg** ▽

√5ᵗʰ **S75.2** **Injury of greater saphenous vein at hip and thigh level**

     EXCLUDES 1   *greater saphenous vein NOS (S85.3)*

     √6ᵗʰ **S75.20** **Unspecified injury of greater saphenous vein at hip and thigh level**

       √7ᵗʰ **S75.201** **Unspecified injury of greater saphenous vein at hip and thigh level, right leg** ▽

       √7ᵗʰ **S75.202** **Unspecified injury of greater saphenous vein at hip and thigh level, left leg** ▽

       √7ᵗʰ **S75.209** **Unspecified injury of greater saphenous vein at hip and thigh level, unspecified leg** ▽

     √6ᵗʰ **S75.21** **Minor laceration of greater saphenous vein at hip and thigh level**

       Incomplete transection of greater saphenous vein at hip and thigh level

       Laceration of greater saphenous vein at hip and thigh level NOS

       Superficial laceration of greater saphenous vein at hip and thigh level

       √7ᵗʰ **S75.211** **Minor laceration of greater saphenous vein at hip and thigh level, right leg**

       √7ᵗʰ **S75.212** **Minor laceration of greater saphenous vein at hip and thigh level, left leg**

       √7ᵗʰ **S75.219** **Minor laceration of greater saphenous vein at hip and thigh level, unspecified leg** ▽

     √6ᵗʰ **S75.22** **Major laceration of greater saphenous vein at hip and thigh level**

       Complete transection of greater saphenous vein at hip and thigh level

       Traumatic rupture of greater saphenous vein at hip and thigh level

       √7ᵗʰ **S75.221** **Major laceration of greater saphenous vein at hip and thigh level, right leg**

       √7ᵗʰ **S75.222** **Major laceration of greater saphenous vein at hip and thigh level, left leg**

       √7ᵗʰ **S75.229** **Major laceration of greater saphenous vein at hip and thigh level, unspecified leg** ▽

     √6ᵗʰ **S75.29** **Other specified injury of greater saphenous vein at hip and thigh level**

       √7ᵗʰ **S75.291** **Other specified injury of greater saphenous vein at hip and thigh level, right leg**

       √7ᵗʰ **S75.292** **Other specified injury of greater saphenous vein at hip and thigh level, left leg**

       √7ᵗʰ **S75.299** **Other specified injury of greater saphenous vein at hip and thigh level, unspecified leg** ▽

√5ᵗʰ **S75.8** **Injury of other blood vessels at hip and thigh level**

     √6ᵗʰ **S75.80** **Unspecified injury of other blood vessels at hip and thigh level**

       √7ᵗʰ **S75.801** **Unspecified injury of other blood vessels at hip and thigh level, right leg** ▽

       √7ᵗʰ **S75.802** **Unspecified injury of other blood vessels at hip and thigh level, left leg** ▽

       √7ᵗʰ **S75.809** **Unspecified injury of other blood vessels at hip and thigh level, unspecified leg** ▽

     √6ᵗʰ **S75.81** **Laceration of other blood vessels at hip and thigh level**

       √7ᵗʰ **S75.811** **Laceration of other blood vessels at hip and thigh level, right leg**

       √7ᵗʰ **S75.812** **Laceration of other blood vessels at hip and thigh level, left leg**

       √7ᵗʰ **S75.819** **Laceration of other blood vessels at hip and thigh level, unspecified leg** ▽

     √6ᵗʰ **S75.89** **Other specified injury of other blood vessels at hip and thigh level**

       √7ᵗʰ **S75.891** **Other specified injury of other blood vessels at hip and thigh level, right leg**

       √7ᵗʰ **S75.892** **Other specified injury of other blood vessels at hip and thigh level, left leg**

       √7ᵗʰ **S75.899** **Other specified injury of other blood vessels at hip and thigh level, unspecified leg** ▽

√5ᵗʰ **S75.9** **Injury of unspecified blood vessel at hip and thigh level**

     √6ᵗʰ **S75.90** **Unspecified injury of unspecified blood vessel at hip and thigh level**

       √7ᵗʰ **S75.901** **Unspecified injury of unspecified blood vessel at hip and thigh level, right leg** ▽

       √7ᵗʰ **S75.902** **Unspecified injury of unspecified blood vessel at hip and thigh level, left leg** ▽

       √7ᵗʰ **S75.909** **Unspecified injury of unspecified blood vessel at hip and thigh level, unspecified leg** ▽

     √6ᵗʰ **S75.91** **Laceration of unspecified blood vessel at hip and thigh level**

       √7ᵗʰ **S75.911** **Laceration of unspecified blood vessel at hip and thigh level, right leg** ▽

       √7ᵗʰ **S75.912** **Laceration of unspecified blood vessel at hip and thigh level, left leg** ▽

       √7ᵗʰ **S75.919** **Laceration of unspecified blood vessel at hip and thigh level, unspecified leg** ▽

     √6ᵗʰ **S75.99** **Other specified injury of unspecified blood vessel at hip and thigh level**

       √7ᵗʰ **S75.991** **Other specified injury of unspecified blood vessel at hip and thigh level, right leg** ▽

       √7ᵗʰ **S75.992** **Other specified injury of unspecified blood vessel at hip and thigh level, left leg** ▽

       √7ᵗʰ **S75.999** **Other specified injury of unspecified blood vessel at hip and thigh level, unspecified leg** ▽

√4ᵗʰ **S76** **Injury of muscle, fascia and tendon at hip and thigh level**

     Code also any associated open wound (S71.-)

     EXCLUDES 2   *injury of muscle, fascia and tendon at lower leg level (S86)*
               sprain of joint and ligament of hip (S73.1)

     TIP: Refer to the Muscle/Tendon table at the beginning of this chapter.

> The appropriate 7th character is to be added to each code from category S76.
> A   initial encounter
> D   subsequent encounter
> S   sequela

     √5ᵗʰ **S76.0** **Injury of muscle, fascia and tendon of hip**

       √6ᵗʰ **S76.00** **Unspecified injury of muscle, fascia and tendon of hip**

         √7ᵗʰ **S76.001** **Unspecified injury of muscle, fascia and tendon of right hip** ▽

         √7ᵗʰ **S76.002** **Unspecified injury of muscle, fascia and tendon of left hip** ▽

         √7ᵗʰ **S76.009** **Unspecified injury of muscle, fascia and tendon of unspecified hip** ▽

       √6ᵗʰ **S76.01** **Strain of muscle, fascia and tendon of hip**

         √7ᵗʰ **S76.011** **Strain of muscle, fascia and tendon of right hip**

         √7ᵗʰ **S76.012** **Strain of muscle, fascia and tendon of left hip**

         √7ᵗʰ **S76.019** **Strain of muscle, fascia and tendon of unspecified hip** ▽

       √6ᵗʰ **S76.02** **Laceration of muscle, fascia and tendon of hip**

         √7ᵗʰ **S76.021** **Laceration of muscle, fascia and tendon of right hip**

         √7ᵗʰ **S76.022** **Laceration of muscle, fascia and tendon of left hip**

         √7ᵗʰ **S76.029** **Laceration of muscle, fascia and tendon of unspecified hip** ▽

EXCLUDES 1 Not coded here   EXCLUDES 2 Not included here   N Newborn Age: 0   P Pediatric Age: 0-17   M Maternity Age: 12-55   A Adult Age: 15-124

1008   ICD-10-CM 2018

√6ᵗʰ **S76.Ø9** Other specified injury of muscle, fascia and tendon of hip

  √7ᵗʰ **S76.Ø91** Other specified injury of muscle, fascia and tendon of right hip

  √7ᵗʰ **S76.Ø92** Other specified injury of muscle, fascia and tendon of left hip

  √7ᵗʰ **S76.Ø99** Other specified injury of muscle, fascia and tendon of unspecified hip ▽

√5ᵗʰ **S76.1** Injury of quadriceps muscle, fascia and tendon
Injury of patellar ligament (tendon)

  √6ᵗʰ **S76.1Ø** Unspecified injury of quadriceps muscle, fascia and tendon

    √7ᵗʰ **S76.1Ø1** Unspecified injury of right quadriceps muscle, fascia and tendon ▽

    √7ᵗʰ **S76.1Ø2** Unspecified injury of left quadriceps muscle, fascia and tendon ▽

    √7ᵗʰ **S76.1Ø9** Unspecified injury of unspecified quadriceps muscle, fascia and tendon ▽

  √6ᵗʰ **S76.11** Strain of quadriceps muscle, fascia and tendon

    √7ᵗʰ **S76.111** Strain of right quadriceps muscle, fascia and tendon

    √7ᵗʰ **S76.112** Strain of left quadriceps muscle, fascia and tendon

    √7ᵗʰ **S76.119** Strain of unspecified quadriceps muscle, fascia and tendon ▽

  √6ᵗʰ **S76.12** Laceration of quadriceps muscle, fascia and tendon

    √7ᵗʰ **S76.121** Laceration of right quadriceps muscle, fascia and tendon

    √7ᵗʰ **S76.122** Laceration of left quadriceps muscle, fascia and tendon

    √7ᵗʰ **S76.129** Laceration of unspecified quadriceps muscle, fascia and tendon ▽

  √6ᵗʰ **S76.19** Other specified injury of quadriceps muscle, fascia and tendon

    √7ᵗʰ **S76.191** Other specified injury of right quadriceps muscle, fascia and tendon

    √7ᵗʰ **S76.192** Other specified injury of left quadriceps muscle, fascia and tendon

    √7ᵗʰ **S76.199** Other specified injury of unspecified quadriceps muscle, fascia and tendon ▽

√5ᵗʰ **S76.2** Injury of adductor muscle, fascia and tendon of thigh

  √6ᵗʰ **S76.2Ø** Unspecified injury of adductor muscle, fascia and tendon of thigh

    √7ᵗʰ **S76.2Ø1** Unspecified injury of adductor muscle, fascia and tendon of right thigh ▽

    √7ᵗʰ **S76.2Ø2** Unspecified injury of adductor muscle, fascia and tendon of left thigh ▽

    √7ᵗʰ **S76.2Ø9** Unspecified injury of adductor muscle, fascia and tendon of unspecified thigh ▽

  √6ᵗʰ **S76.21** Strain of adductor muscle, fascia and tendon of thigh

    √7ᵗʰ **S76.211** Strain of adductor muscle, fascia and tendon of right thigh

    √7ᵗʰ **S76.212** Strain of adductor muscle, fascia and tendon of left thigh

    √7ᵗʰ **S76.219** Strain of adductor muscle, fascia and tendon of unspecified thigh ▽

  √6ᵗʰ **S76.22** Laceration of adductor muscle, fascia and tendon of thigh

    √7ᵗʰ **S76.221** Laceration of adductor muscle, fascia and tendon of right thigh

    √7ᵗʰ **S76.222** Laceration of adductor muscle, fascia and tendon of left thigh

    √7ᵗʰ **S76.229** Laceration of adductor muscle, fascia and tendon of unspecified thigh ▽

  √6ᵗʰ **S76.29** Other injury of adductor muscle, fascia and tendon of thigh

    √7ᵗʰ **S76.291** Other injury of adductor muscle, fascia and tendon of right thigh

    √7ᵗʰ **S76.292** Other injury of adductor muscle, fascia and tendon of left thigh

    √7ᵗʰ **S76.299** Other injury of adductor muscle, fascia and tendon of unspecified thigh ▽

√5ᵗʰ **S76.3** Injury of muscle, fascia and tendon of the posterior muscle group at thigh level

  √6ᵗʰ **S76.3Ø** Unspecified injury of muscle, fascia and tendon of the posterior muscle group at thigh level

    √7ᵗʰ **S76.3Ø1** Unspecified injury of muscle, fascia and tendon of the posterior muscle group at thigh level, right thigh ▽

    √7ᵗʰ **S76.3Ø2** Unspecified injury of muscle, fascia and tendon of the posterior muscle group at thigh level, left thigh ▽

    √7ᵗʰ **S76.3Ø9** Unspecified injury of muscle, fascia and tendon of the posterior muscle group at thigh level, unspecified thigh ▽

  √6ᵗʰ **S76.31** Strain of muscle, fascia and tendon of the posterior muscle group at thigh level

    √7ᵗʰ **S76.311** Strain of muscle, fascia and tendon of the posterior muscle group at thigh level, right thigh

    √7ᵗʰ **S76.312** Strain of muscle, fascia and tendon of the posterior muscle group at thigh level, left thigh

    √7ᵗʰ **S76.319** Strain of muscle, fascia and tendon of the posterior muscle group at thigh level, unspecified thigh ▽

  √6ᵗʰ **S76.32** Laceration of muscle, fascia and tendon of the posterior muscle group at thigh level

    √7ᵗʰ **S76.321** Laceration of muscle, fascia and tendon of the posterior muscle group at thigh level, right thigh

    √7ᵗʰ **S76.322** Laceration of muscle, fascia and tendon of the posterior muscle group at thigh level, left thigh

    √7ᵗʰ **S76.329** Laceration of muscle, fascia and tendon of the posterior muscle group at thigh level, unspecified thigh ▽

  √6ᵗʰ **S76.39** Other specified injury of muscle, fascia and tendon of the posterior muscle group at thigh level

    √7ᵗʰ **S76.391** Other specified injury of muscle, fascia and tendon of the posterior muscle group at thigh level, right thigh

    √7ᵗʰ **S76.392** Other specified injury of muscle, fascia and tendon of the posterior muscle group at thigh level, left thigh

    √7ᵗʰ **S76.399** Other specified injury of muscle, fascia and tendon of the posterior muscle group at thigh level, unspecified thigh ▽

√5ᵗʰ **S76.8** Injury of other specified muscles, fascia and tendons at thigh level

  √6ᵗʰ **S76.8Ø** Unspecified injury of other specified muscles, fascia and tendons at thigh level

    √7ᵗʰ **S76.8Ø1** Unspecified injury of other specified muscles, fascia and tendons at thigh level, right thigh ▽

    √7ᵗʰ **S76.8Ø2** Unspecified injury of other specified muscles, fascia and tendons at thigh level, left thigh ▽

    √7ᵗʰ **S76.8Ø9** Unspecified injury of other specified muscles, fascia and tendons at thigh level, unspecified thigh ▽

  √6ᵗʰ **S76.81** Strain of other specified muscles, fascia and tendons at thigh level

    √7ᵗʰ **S76.811** Strain of other specified muscles, fascia and tendons at thigh level, right thigh

    √7ᵗʰ **S76.812** Strain of other specified muscles, fascia and tendons at thigh level, left thigh

    √7ᵗʰ **S76.819** Strain of other specified muscles, fascia and tendons at thigh level, unspecified thigh ▽

  √6ᵗʰ **S76.82** Laceration of other specified muscles, fascia and tendons at thigh level

    √7ᵗʰ **S76.821** Laceration of other specified muscles, fascia and tendons at thigh level, right thigh

    √7ᵗʰ **S76.822** Laceration of other specified muscles, fascia and tendons at thigh level, left thigh

---

☑ Additional Character Req   ✔x7ᵗʰ Placeholder Alert   Manifestation   HCC CMS-HCC Condition   ▽ Unspecified Code   ►◄ Revised Text   ● New Code   ▲ Revised Code Title

Chapter 19. Injury, Poisoning, and Certain Other Consequences of External Causes

S76.829–S78.929

√7th **S76.829** Laceration of other specified muscles, fascia and tendons at thigh level, unspecified thigh ▽

√6th **S76.89** Other injury of other specified muscles, fascia and tendons at thigh level

√7th **S76.891** Other injury of other specified muscles, fascia and tendons at thigh level, right thigh

√7th **S76.892** Other injury of other specified muscles, fascia and tendons at thigh level, left thigh

√7th **S76.899** Other injury of other specified muscles, fascia and tendons at thigh level, unspecified thigh ▽

√5th **S76.9** Injury of unspecified muscles, fascia and tendons at thigh level

√6th **S76.90** Unspecified injury of unspecified muscles, fascia and tendons at thigh level

√7th **S76.901** Unspecified injury of unspecified muscles, fascia and tendons at thigh level, right thigh ▽

√7th **S76.902** Unspecified injury of unspecified muscles, fascia and tendons at thigh level, left thigh ▽

√7th **S76.909** Unspecified injury of unspecified muscles, fascia and tendons at thigh level, unspecified thigh ▽

√6th **S76.91** Strain of unspecified muscles, fascia and tendons at thigh level

√7th **S76.911** Strain of unspecified muscles, fascia and tendons at thigh level, right thigh ▽

√7th **S76.912** Strain of unspecified muscles, fascia and tendons at thigh level, left thigh ▽

√7th **S76.919** Strain of unspecified muscles, fascia and tendons at thigh level, unspecified thigh ▽

√6th **S76.92** Laceration of unspecified muscles, fascia and tendons at thigh level

√7th **S76.921** Laceration of unspecified muscles, fascia and tendons at thigh level, right thigh ▽

√7th **S76.922** Laceration of unspecified muscles, fascia and tendons at thigh level, left thigh ▽

√7th **S76.929** Laceration of unspecified muscles, fascia and tendons at thigh level, unspecified thigh ▽

√6th **S76.99** Other specified injury of unspecified muscles, fascia and tendons at thigh level

√7th **S76.991** Other specified injury of unspecified muscles, fascia and tendons at thigh level, right thigh ▽

√7th **S76.992** Other specified injury of unspecified muscles, fascia and tendons at thigh level, left thigh ▽

√7th **S76.999** Other specified injury of unspecified muscles, fascia and tendons at thigh level, unspecified thigh ▽

√4th **S77** Crushing injury of hip and thigh
Use additional code(s) for all associated injuries
EXCLUDES 2   crushing injury of ankle and foot (S97.-)
       crushing injury of lower leg (S87.-)

The appropriate 7th character is to be added to each code from category S77.
A   initial encounter
D   subsequent encounter
S   sequela

√5th **S77.0** Crushing injury of hip

√x7th **S77.00** Crushing injury of unspecified hip ▽

√x7th **S77.01** Crushing injury of right hip

√x7th **S77.02** Crushing injury of left hip

√5th **S77.1** Crushing injury of thigh

√x7th **S77.10** Crushing injury of unspecified thigh ▽

√x7th **S77.11** Crushing injury of right thigh

√x7th **S77.12** Crushing injury of left thigh

√5th **S77.2** Crushing injury of hip with thigh

√x7th **S77.20** Crushing injury of unspecified hip with thigh ▽

√x7th **S77.21** Crushing injury of right hip with thigh

√x7th **S77.22** Crushing injury of left hip with thigh

√4th **S78** Traumatic amputation of hip and thigh
An amputation not identified as partial or complete should be coded to complete.
EXCLUDES 1   traumatic amputation of knee (S88.0-)

The appropriate 7th character is to be added to each code from category S78.
A   initial encounter
D   subsequent encounter
S   sequela

√5th **S78.0** Traumatic amputation at hip joint

√6th **S78.01** Complete traumatic amputation at hip joint

√7th **S78.011** Complete traumatic amputation at right hip joint   HCC

√7th **S78.012** Complete traumatic amputation at left hip joint   HCC

√7th **S78.019** Complete traumatic amputation at unspecified hip joint   HCC ▽

√6th **S78.02** Partial traumatic amputation at hip joint

√7th **S78.021** Partial traumatic amputation at right hip joint   HCC

√7th **S78.022** Partial traumatic amputation at left hip joint   HCC

√7th **S78.029** Partial traumatic amputation at unspecified hip joint   HCC ▽

√5th **S78.1** Traumatic amputation at level between hip and knee
EXCLUDES 1   traumatic amputation of knee (S88.0-)

√6th **S78.11** Complete traumatic amputation at level between hip and knee

√7th **S78.111** Complete traumatic amputation at level between right hip and knee   HCC

√7th **S78.112** Complete traumatic amputation at level between left hip and knee   HCC

√7th **S78.119** Complete traumatic amputation at level between unspecified hip and knee   HCC ▽

√6th **S78.12** Partial traumatic amputation at level between hip and knee

√7th **S78.121** Partial traumatic amputation at level between right hip and knee   HCC

√7th **S78.122** Partial traumatic amputation at level between left hip and knee   HCC

√7th **S78.129** Partial traumatic amputation at level between unspecified hip and knee   HCC ▽

√5th **S78.9** Traumatic amputation of hip and thigh, level unspecified

√6th **S78.91** Complete traumatic amputation of hip and thigh, level unspecified

√7th **S78.911** Complete traumatic amputation of right hip and thigh, level unspecified   HCC

√7th **S78.912** Complete traumatic amputation of left hip and thigh, level unspecified   HCC ▽

√7th **S78.919** Complete traumatic amputation of unspecified hip and thigh, level unspecified   HCC ▽

√6th **S78.92** Partial traumatic amputation of hip and thigh, level unspecified

√7th **S78.921** Partial traumatic amputation of right hip and thigh, level unspecified   HCC ▽

√7th **S78.922** Partial traumatic amputation of left hip and thigh, level unspecified   HCC ▽

√7th **S78.929** Partial traumatic amputation of unspecified hip and thigh, level unspecified   HCC ▽

EXCLUDES 1 Not coded here   EXCLUDES 2 Not included here   N Newborn Age: 0   P Pediatric Age: 0-17   M Maternity Age: 12-55   A Adult Age: 15-124

✓4th S79 Other and unspecified injuries of hip and thigh

> **NOTE** A fracture not indicated as open or closed should be coded to closed.

AHA: 2015, 3Q, 37-39

> The appropriate 7th character is to be added to each code from subcategory S79.0 and S79.1.
> A   initial encounter for closed fracture
> D   subsequent encounter for fracture with routine healing
> G   subsequent encounter for fracture with delayed healing
> K   subsequent encounter for fracture with nonunion
> P   subsequent encounter for fracture with malunion
> S   sequela

✓5th S79.0 Physeal fracture of upper end of femur

> **EXCLUDES 1** apophyseal fracture of upper end of femur (S72.13-)
> nontraumatic slipped upper femoral epiphysis (M93.0-)

✓6th S79.00 Unspecified physeal fracture of upper end of femur

1 ✓7th S79.001 Unspecified physeal fracture of upper end of **right** femur HCC ▽

1 ✓7th S79.002 Unspecified physeal fracture of upper end of **left** femur HCC ▽

1 ✓7th S79.009 Unspecified physeal fracture of upper end of unspecified femur HCC ▽

✓6th S79.01 Salter-Harris Type I physeal fracture of upper end of femur

Acute on chronic slipped capital femoral epiphysis (traumatic)
Acute slipped capital femoral epiphysis (traumatic)
Capital femoral epiphyseal fracture

> **EXCLUDES 1** chronic slipped upper femoral epiphysis (nontraumatic) (M93.02-)

1 ✓7th S79.011 Salter-Harris Type I physeal fracture of upper end of **right** femur HCC

1 ✓7th S79.012 Salter-Harris Type I physeal fracture of upper end of **left** femur HCC

1 ✓7th S79.019 Salter-Harris Type I physeal fracture of upper end of unspecified femur HCC ▽

✓6th S79.09 Other physeal fracture of upper end of femur

1 ✓7th S79.091 Other physeal fracture of upper end of **right** femur HCC

1 ✓7th S79.092 Other physeal fracture of upper end of **left** femur HCC

1 ✓7th S79.099 Other physeal fracture of upper end of unspecified femur HCC ▽

✓5th S79.1 Physeal fracture of lower end of femur

✓6th S79.10 Unspecified physeal fracture of lower end of femur

1 ✓7th S79.101 Unspecified physeal fracture of lower end of **right** femur HCC ▽

1 ✓7th S79.102 Unspecified physeal fracture of lower end of **left** femur HCC ▽

1 ✓7th S79.109 Unspecified physeal fracture of lower end of unspecified femur HCC ▽

✓6th S79.11 Salter-Harris Type I physeal fracture of lower end of femur

1 ✓7th S79.111 Salter-Harris Type I physeal fracture of lower end of **right** femur HCC

1 ✓7th S79.112 Salter-Harris Type I physeal fracture of lower end of **left** femur HCC

1 ✓7th S79.119 Salter-Harris Type I physeal fracture of lower end of unspecified femur HCC ▽

✓6th S79.12 Salter-Harris Type II physeal fracture of lower end of femur

1 ✓7th S79.121 Salter-Harris Type II physeal fracture of lower end of **right** femur HCC

1 ✓7th S79.122 Salter-Harris Type II physeal fracture of lower end of **left** femur HCC

1 ✓7th S79.129 Salter-Harris Type II physeal fracture of lower end of unspecified femur HCC ▽

✓6th S79.13 Salter-Harris Type III physeal fracture of lower end of femur

1 ✓7th S79.131 Salter-Harris Type III physeal fracture of lower end of **right** femur HCC

1 ✓7th S79.132 Salter-Harris Type III physeal fracture of lower end of **left** femur HCC

1 ✓7th S79.139 Salter-Harris Type III physeal fracture of lower end of unspecified femur HCC ▽

✓6th S79.14 Salter-Harris Type IV physeal fracture of lower end of femur

1 ✓7th S79.141 Salter-Harris Type IV physeal fracture of lower end of **right** femur HCC

1 ✓7th S79.142 Salter-Harris Type IV physeal fracture of lower end of **left** femur HCC

1 ✓7th S79.149 Salter-Harris Type IV physeal fracture of lower end of unspecified femur HCC ▽

✓6th S79.19 Other physeal fracture of lower end of femur

1 ✓7th S79.191 Other physeal fracture of lower end of **right** femur HCC

1 ✓7th S79.192 Other physeal fracture of lower end of **left** femur HCC

1 ✓7th S79.199 Other physeal fracture of lower end of unspecified femur HCC ▽

✓5th S79.8 Other specified injuries of hip and thigh

> The appropriate 7th character is to be added to each code in subcategory S79.8.
> A   initial encounter
> D   subsequent encounter
> S   sequela

✓6th S79.81 Other specified injuries of hip

✓7th S79.811 Other specified injuries of **right** hip

✓7th S79.812 Other specified injuries of **left** hip

✓7th S79.819 Other specified injuries of unspecified hip ▽

✓6th S79.82 Other specified injuries of thigh

✓7th S79.821 Other specified injuries of **right** thigh

✓7th S79.822 Other specified injuries of **left** thigh

✓7th S79.829 Other specified injuries of unspecified thigh ▽

✓5th S79.9 Unspecified injury of hip and thigh

> The appropriate 7th character is to be added to each code in subcategory S79.9.
> A   initial encounter
> D   subsequent encounter
> S   sequela

✓6th S79.91 Unspecified injury of hip

✓7th S79.911 Unspecified injury of **right** hip ▽

✓7th S79.912 Unspecified injury of **left** hip ▽

✓7th S79.919 Unspecified injury of unspecified hip ▽

✓6th S79.92 Unspecified injury of thigh

✓7th S79.921 Unspecified injury of **right** thigh ▽

✓7th S79.922 Unspecified injury of **left** thigh ▽

✓7th S79.929 Unspecified injury of unspecified thigh ▽

---

1 HCC with 7th character indicating initial encounter (A, B or C - specific to category).

☑ Additional Character Req   ✓7th Placeholder Alert   Manifestation   HCC CMS-HCC Condition   ▽ Unspecified Code   ►◄ Revised Text   ● New Code   ▲ Revised Code Title

Injuries to the knee and lower leg (S80-S89)

EXCLUDES 2   burns and corrosions (T20-T32)
frostbite (T33-T34)
injuries of ankle and foot, except fracture of ankle and malleolus (S90-S99)
insect bite or sting, venomous (T63.4)

√4th **S80**   **Superficial injury of knee and lower leg**
    EXCLUDES 2   superficial injury of ankle and foot (S90.-)

> The appropriate 7th character is to be added to each code from category S80.
> A   initial encounter
> D   subsequent encounter
> S   sequela

√5th   **S80.0**   **Contusion of** knee
    √x7th   **S80.00**   Contusion of unspecified knee   ▽
    √x7th   **S80.01**   Contusion of right knee
    √x7th   **S80.02**   Contusion of left knee

√5th   **S80.1**   **Contusion of** lower leg
    √x7th   **S80.10**   Contusion of unspecified lower leg   ▽
    √x7th   **S80.11**   Contusion of right lower leg
    √x7th   **S80.12**   Contusion of left lower leg

√5th   **S80.2**   **Other superficial injuries of** knee
    √6th   **S80.21**   Abrasion of knee
       √7th   **S80.211**   Abrasion, right knee
       √7th   **S80.212**   Abrasion, left knee
       √7th   **S80.219**   Abrasion, unspecified knee   ▽
    √6th   **S80.22**   Blister (nonthermal) of knee
       √7th   **S80.221**   Blister (nonthermal), right knee
       √7th   **S80.222**   Blister (nonthermal), left knee
       √7th   **S80.229**   Blister (nonthermal), unspecified knee   ▽
    √6th   **S80.24**   External constriction of knee
       √7th   **S80.241**   External constriction, right knee
       √7th   **S80.242**   External constriction, left knee
       √7th   **S80.249**   External constriction, unspecified knee   ▽
    √6th   **S80.25**   Superficial foreign body of knee
       Splinter in the knee
       √7th   **S80.251**   Superficial foreign body, right knee
       √7th   **S80.252**   Superficial foreign body, left knee
       √7th   **S80.259**   Superficial foreign body, unspecified knee   ▽
    √6th   **S80.26**   Insect bite (nonvenomous) of knee
       √7th   **S80.261**   Insect bite (nonvenomous), right knee
       √7th   **S80.262**   Insect bite (nonvenomous), left knee
       √7th   **S80.269**   Insect bite (nonvenomous), unspecified knee   ▽
    √6th   **S80.27**   Other superficial bite of knee
       EXCLUDES 1   open bite of knee (S81.05-)
       √7th   **S80.271**   Other superficial bite of right knee
       √7th   **S80.272**   Other superficial bite of left knee
       √7th   **S80.279**   Other superficial bite of unspecified knee   ▽

√5th   **S80.8**   **Other superficial injuries of** lower leg
    √6th   **S80.81**   Abrasion of lower leg
       √7th   **S80.811**   Abrasion, right lower leg
       √7th   **S80.812**   Abrasion, left lower leg
       √7th   **S80.819**   Abrasion, unspecified lower leg   ▽
    √6th   **S80.82**   Blister (nonthermal) of lower leg
       √7th   **S80.821**   Blister (nonthermal), right lower leg
       √7th   **S80.822**   Blister (nonthermal), left lower leg
       √7th   **S80.829**   Blister (nonthermal), unspecified lower leg   ▽
    √6th   **S80.84**   External constriction of lower leg
       √7th   **S80.841**   External constriction, right lower leg
       √7th   **S80.842**   External constriction, left lower leg
       √7th   **S80.849**   External constriction, unspecified lower leg   ▽

√6th   **S80.85**   Superficial foreign body of lower leg
    Splinter in the lower leg
    √7th   **S80.851**   Superficial foreign body, right lower leg
    √7th   **S80.852**   Superficial foreign body, left lower leg
    √7th   **S80.859**   Superficial foreign body, unspecified lower leg   ▽

√6th   **S80.86**   Insect bite (nonvenomous) of lower leg
    √7th   **S80.861**   Insect bite (nonvenomous), right lower leg
    √7th   **S80.862**   Insect bite (nonvenomous), left lower leg
    √7th   **S80.869**   Insect bite (nonvenomous), unspecified lower leg   ▽

√6th   **S80.87**   Other superficial bite of lower leg
    EXCLUDES 1   open bite of lower leg (S81.85-)
    √7th   **S80.871**   Other superficial bite, right lower leg
    √7th   **S80.872**   Other superficial bite, left lower leg
    √7th   **S80.879**   Other superficial bite, unspecified lower leg   ▽

√5th   **S80.9**   Unspecified superficial injury of knee and lower leg
    √6th   **S80.91**   Unspecified superficial injury of knee   ▽
       √7th   **S80.911**   Unspecified superficial injury of right knee   ▽
       √7th   **S80.912**   Unspecified superficial injury of left knee   ▽
       √7th   **S80.919**   Unspecified superficial injury of unspecified knee   ▽
    √6th   **S80.92**   Unspecified superficial injury of lower leg   ▽
       √7th   **S80.921**   Unspecified superficial injury of right lower leg   ▽
       √7th   **S80.922**   Unspecified superficial injury of left lower leg   ▽
       √7th   **S80.929**   Unspecified superficial injury of unspecified lower leg   ▽

√4th   **S81**   **Open wound of knee and lower leg**
    Code also any associated wound infection
    EXCLUDES 1   open fracture of knee and lower leg (S82.-)
          traumatic amputation of lower leg (S88.-)
    EXCLUDES 2   open wound of ankle and foot (S91.-)

> The appropriate 7th character is to be added to each code from category S81.
> A   initial encounter
> D   subsequent encounter
> S   sequela

√5th   **S81.0**   **Open wound of** knee
    √6th   **S81.00**   Unspecified open wound of knee
       √7th   **S81.001**   Unspecified open wound, right knee   ▽
       √7th   **S81.002**   Unspecified open wound, left knee   ▽
       √7th   **S81.009**   Unspecified open wound, unspecified knee   ▽
    √6th   **S81.01**   Laceration without foreign body of knee
       √7th   **S81.011**   Laceration without foreign body, right knee
       √7th   **S81.012**   Laceration without foreign body, left knee
       √7th   **S81.019**   Laceration without foreign body, unspecified knee   ▽
    √6th   **S81.02**   Laceration with foreign body of knee
       √7th   **S81.021**   Laceration with foreign body, right knee
       √7th   **S81.022**   Laceration with foreign body, left knee
       √7th   **S81.029**   Laceration with foreign body, unspecified knee   ▽
    √6th   **S81.03**   Puncture wound without foreign body of knee
       √7th   **S81.031**   Puncture wound without foreign body, right knee
       √7th   **S81.032**   Puncture wound without foreign body, left knee
       √7th   **S81.039**   Puncture wound without foreign body, unspecified knee   ▽

EXCLUDES 1 Not coded here   **EXCLUDES 2** Not included here   **N** Newborn Age: 0   **P** Pediatric Age: 0-17   **M** Maternity Age: 12-55   **A** Adult Age: 15-124

1012   ICD-10-CM 2018

✓6th S81.04 Puncture wound with foreign body of knee

     ✓7th S81.041 Puncture wound with foreign body, right knee

     ✓7th S81.042 Puncture wound with foreign body, left knee

     ✓7th S81.049 Puncture wound with foreign body, unspecified knee ▽

✓6th S81.05 Open bite of knee
     Bite of knee NOS
     EXCLUDES 1   superficial bite of knee (S80.27-)

     ✓7th S81.051 Open bite, right knee

     ✓7th S81.052 Open bite, left knee

     ✓7th S81.059 Open bite, unspecified knee ▽

✓5th S81.8 Open wound of lower leg

✓6th S81.80 Unspecified open wound of lower leg
     AHA: 2016, 3Q, 24

     ✓7th S81.801 Unspecified open wound, right lower leg ▽

     ✓7th S81.802 Unspecified open wound, left lower leg ▽

     ✓7th S81.809 Unspecified open wound, unspecified lower leg ▽

✓6th S81.81 Laceration without foreign body of lower leg

     ✓7th S81.811 Laceration without foreign body, right lower leg

     ✓7th S81.812 Laceration without foreign body, left lower leg

     ✓7th S81.819 Laceration without foreign body, unspecified lower leg ▽

✓6th S81.82 Laceration with foreign body of lower leg

     ✓7th S81.821 Laceration with foreign body, right lower leg

     ✓7th S81.822 Laceration with foreign body, left lower leg

     ✓7th S81.829 Laceration with foreign body, unspecified lower leg ▽

✓6th S81.83 Puncture wound without foreign body of lower leg
     AHA: 2016, 3Q, 24

     ✓7th S81.831 Puncture wound without foreign body, right lower leg

     ✓7th S81.832 Puncture wound without foreign body, left lower leg

     ✓7th S81.839 Puncture wound without foreign body, unspecified lower leg ▽

✓6th S81.84 Puncture wound with foreign body of lower leg
     AHA: 2016, 3Q, 24

     ✓7th S81.841 Puncture wound with foreign body, right lower leg

     ✓7th S81.842 Puncture wound with foreign body, left lower leg

     ✓7th S81.849 Puncture wound with foreign body, unspecified lower leg ▽

✓6th S81.85 Open bite of lower leg
     Bite of lower leg NOS
     EXCLUDES 1   superficial bite of lower leg (S80.86-, S80.87-)

     ✓7th S81.851 Open bite, right lower leg

     ✓7th S81.852 Open bite, left lower leg

     ✓7th S81.859 Open bite, unspecified lower leg ▽

✓4th S82 Fracture of lower leg, including ankle

     NOTE   A fracture not indicated as displaced or nondisplaced should be coded to displaced.
     A fracture not designated as open or closed should be coded to closed.
     The open fracture designations are based on the Gustilo open fracture classification.

     INCLUDES   fracture of malleolus
     EXCLUDES 1   traumatic amputation of lower leg (S88.-)
     EXCLUDES 2   fracture of foot, except ankle (S92.-)
     periprosthetic fracture of prosthetic implant of knee ▶(M97.0-)◀
     AHA: 2016, 1Q, 33; 2015, 3Q, 37-39

The appropriate 7th character is to be added to all codes from category S82 [unless otherwise indicated].
A   initial encounter for closed fracture
B   initial encounter for open fracture type I or II
     initial encounter for open fracture NOS
C   initial encounter for open fracture type IIIA, IIIB, or IIIC
D   subsequent encounter for closed fracture with routine healing
E   subsequent encounter for open fracture type I or II with routine healing
F   subsequent encounter for open fracture type IIIA, IIIB, or IIIC with routine healing
G   subsequent encounter for closed fracture with delayed healing
H   subsequent encounter for open fracture type I or II with delayed healing
J   subsequent encounter for open fracture type IIIA, IIIB or IIIC with delayed healing
K   subsequent encounter for closed fracture with nonunion
M   subsequent encounter for open fracture type I or II with nonunion
N   subsequent encounter for open fracture type IIIA, IIIB or IIIC with nonunion
P   subsequent encounter for closed fracture with malunion
Q   subsequent encounter for open fracture type I or II with malunion
R   subsequent encounter for open fracture type IIIA, IIIB or IIIC with malunion
S   sequela

✓5th S82.0 Fracture of patella
     Knee cap

✓6th S82.00 Unspecified fracture of patella

     ✓7th S82.001 Unspecified fracture of right patella ▽
     S82.002 Unspecified fracture of left patella ▽
     ✓7th S82.009 Unspecified fracture of unspecified patella ▽

✓6th S82.01 Osteochondral fracture of patella

     ✓7th S82.011 Displaced osteochondral fracture of right patella

     ✓7th S82.012 Displaced osteochondral fracture of left patella

     ✓7th S82.013 Displaced osteochondral fracture of unspecified patella ▽

     ✓7th S82.014 Nondisplaced osteochondral fracture of right patella

     ✓7th S82.015 Nondisplaced osteochondral fracture of left patella

     ✓7th S82.016 Nondisplaced osteochondral fracture of unspecified patella ▽

✓6th S82.02 Longitudinal fracture of patella

     ✓7th S82.021 Displaced longitudinal fracture of right patella

     ✓7th S82.022 Displaced longitudinal fracture of left patella

     ✓7th S82.023 Displaced longitudinal fracture of unspecified patella ▽

     ✓7th S82.024 Nondisplaced longitudinal fracture of right patella

     ✓7th S82.025 Nondisplaced longitudinal fracture of left patella

     ✓7th S82.026 Nondisplaced longitudinal fracture of unspecified patella ▽

✓6th S82.03 Transverse fracture of patella

     ✓7th S82.031 Displaced transverse fracture of right patella

     ✓7th S82.032 Displaced transverse fracture of left patella

☑ Additional Character Req   ✓x7th Placeholder Alert   Manifestation   HCC CMS-HCC Condition   ▽ Unspecified Code   ▶◀ Revised Text   ● New Code   ▲ Revised Code Title

ICD-10-CM 2018

1013

Chapter 19. Injury, Poisoning, and Certain Other Consequences of External Causes

S81.04–S82.032

✓7ᵗʰ **S82.033** Displaced **transverse fracture of unspecified patella** ▽

✓7ᵗʰ **S82.034** Nondisplaced **transverse fracture of right patella**

✓7ᵗʰ **S82.035** Nondisplaced **transverse fracture of left patella**

✓7ᵗʰ **S82.036** Nondisplaced **transverse fracture of unspecified patella** ▽

✓6ᵗʰ **S82.04** Comminuted **fracture of patella**

✓7ᵗʰ **S82.041** Displaced **comminuted fracture of right patella**

✓7ᵗʰ **S82.042** Displaced **comminuted fracture of left patella**

✓7ᵗʰ **S82.043** Displaced **comminuted fracture of unspecified patella** ▽

✓7ᵗʰ **S82.044** Nondisplaced **comminuted fracture of right patella**

✓7ᵗʰ **S82.045** Nondisplaced **comminuted fracture of left patella**

✓7ᵗʰ **S82.046** Nondisplaced **comminuted fracture of unspecified patella** ▽

✓6ᵗʰ **S82.09** Other fracture of patella

✓7ᵗʰ **S82.091** Other fracture of **right** patella

✓7ᵗʰ **S82.092** Other fracture of **left** patella

✓7ᵗʰ **S82.099** Other fracture of unspecified patella ▽

✓5ᵗʰ **S82.1** Fracture of upper end of tibia
Fracture of proximal end of tibia

EXCLUDES 2   fracture of shaft of tibia (S82.2-)
physeal fracture of upper end of tibia (S89.0-)

✓6ᵗʰ **S82.10** Unspecified fracture of upper end of tibia

✓7ᵗʰ **S82.101** Unspecified fracture of upper end of **right** tibia ▽

✓7ᵗʰ **S82.102** Unspecified fracture of upper end of **left** tibia ▽

✓7ᵗʰ **S82.109** Unspecified fracture of upper end of unspecified tibia ▽

✓6ᵗʰ **S82.11** Fracture of tibial spine

✓7ᵗʰ **S82.111** Displaced **fracture of right tibial spine**

✓7ᵗʰ **S82.112** Displaced **fracture of left tibial spine**

✓7ᵗʰ **S82.113** Displaced **fracture of unspecified tibial** ▽ **spine**

✓7ᵗʰ **S82.114** Nondisplaced **fracture of right tibial spine**

✓7ᵗʰ **S82.115** Nondisplaced **fracture of left tibial spine**

✓7ᵗʰ **S82.116** Nondisplaced **fracture of unspecified** ▽ **tibial spine**

✓6ᵗʰ **S82.12** Fracture of lateral condyle of tibia

✓7ᵗʰ **S82.121** Displaced **fracture of lateral condyle of right tibia**

✓7ᵗʰ **S82.122** Displaced **fracture of lateral condyle of left tibia**

✓7ᵗʰ **S82.123** Displaced **fracture of lateral condyle of** ▽ **unspecified tibia**

✓7ᵗʰ **S82.124** Nondisplaced **fracture of lateral condyle of right tibia**

✓7ᵗʰ **S82.125** Nondisplaced **fracture of lateral condyle of left tibia**

✓7ᵗʰ **S82.126** Nondisplaced **fracture of lateral** ▽ **condyle of unspecified tibia**

✓6ᵗʰ **S82.13** Fracture of medial condyle of tibia

✓7ᵗʰ **S82.131** Displaced **fracture of medial condyle of right tibia**

✓7ᵗʰ **S82.132** Displaced **fracture of medial condyle of left tibia**

✓7ᵗʰ **S82.133** Displaced **fracture of medial condyle of** ▽ **unspecified tibia**

✓7ᵗʰ **S82.134** Nondisplaced **fracture of medial condyle of right tibia**

✓7ᵗʰ **S82.135** Nondisplaced **fracture of medial condyle of left tibia**

✓7ᵗʰ **S82.136** Nondisplaced **fracture of medial** ▽ **condyle of unspecified tibia**

✓6ᵗʰ **S82.14** Bicondylar **fracture of tibia**
Fracture of tibial plateau NOS

✓7ᵗʰ **S82.141** Displaced **bicondylar fracture of right tibia**

✓7ᵗʰ **S82.142** Displaced **bicondylar fracture of left tibia**

✓7ᵗʰ **S82.143** Displaced **bicondylar fracture of unspecified tibia** ▽

✓7ᵗʰ **S82.144** Nondisplaced **bicondylar fracture of right tibia**

✓7ᵗʰ **S82.145** Nondisplaced **bicondylar fracture of left tibia**

✓7ᵗʰ **S82.146** Nondisplaced **bicondylar fracture of unspecified tibia** ▽

✓6ᵗʰ **S82.15** Fracture of tibial tuberosity

✓7ᵗʰ **S82.151** Displaced **fracture of right tibial tuberosity**

✓7ᵗʰ **S82.152** Displaced **fracture of left tibial tuberosity**

✓7ᵗʰ **S82.153** Displaced **fracture of unspecified** ▽ **tibial tuberosity**

✓7ᵗʰ **S82.154** Nondisplaced **fracture of right tibial tuberosity**

✓7ᵗʰ **S82.155** Nondisplaced **fracture of left tibial tuberosity**

✓7ᵗʰ **S82.156** Nondisplaced **fracture of unspecified** ▽ **tibial tuberosity**

✓6ᵗʰ **S82.16** Torus **fracture of upper end of tibia**

> The appropriate 7th character is to be added to all codes in subcategory S82.16.
> A   initial encounter for closed fracture
> D   subsequent encounter for fracture with routine healing
> G   subsequent encounter for fracture with delayed healing
> K   subsequent encounter for fracture with nonunion
> P   subsequent encounter for fracture with malunion
> S   sequela

✓7ᵗʰ **S82.161** Torus **fracture of upper end of right tibia**

✓7ᵗʰ **S82.162** Torus **fracture of upper end of left tibia**

✓7ᵗʰ **S82.169** Torus **fracture of upper end of** ▽ **unspecified tibia**

✓6ᵗʰ **S82.19** Other fracture of upper end of tibia

✓7ᵗʰ **S82.191** Other fracture of upper end of **right** tibia

✓7ᵗʰ **S82.192** Other fracture of upper end of **left** tibia

✓7ᵗʰ **S82.199** Other fracture of upper end of ▽ **unspecified tibia**

✓5ᵗʰ **S82.2** Fracture of shaft of tibia

✓6ᵗʰ **S82.20** Unspecified fracture of shaft of tibia
Fracture of tibia NOS

✓7ᵗʰ **S82.201** Unspecified fracture of shaft of **right** ▽ **tibia**

✓7ᵗʰ **S82.202** Unspecified fracture of shaft of **left** ▽ **tibia**

✓7ᵗʰ **S82.209** Unspecified fracture of shaft of ▽ **unspecified tibia**

✓6ᵗʰ **S82.22** Transverse **fracture of shaft of tibia**

✓7ᵗʰ **S82.221** Displaced **transverse fracture of shaft of right tibia**

✓7ᵗʰ **S82.222** Displaced **transverse fracture of shaft of left tibia**

✓7ᵗʰ **S82.223** Displaced **transverse fracture of shaft** ▽ **of unspecified tibia**

✓7ᵗʰ **S82.224** Nondisplaced **transverse fracture of shaft of right tibia**

✓7ᵗʰ **S82.225** Nondisplaced **transverse fracture of shaft of left tibia**

✓7ᵗʰ **S82.226** Nondisplaced **transverse fracture of** ▽ **shaft of unspecified tibia**

✓6ᵗʰ **S82.23** Oblique **fracture of shaft of tibia**

✓7ᵗʰ **S82.231** Displaced **oblique fracture of shaft of right tibia**

✓7ᵗʰ **S82.232** Displaced **oblique fracture of shaft of left tibia**

√7ᵗʰ **S82.233** Displaced oblique fracture of shaft of ▽
unspecified tibia

√7ᵗʰ **S82.234** Nondisplaced oblique fracture of shaft of
right tibia

√7ᵗʰ **S82.235** Nondisplaced oblique fracture of shaft of
left tibia

√7ᵗʰ **S82.236** Nondisplaced oblique fracture of shaft ▽
of unspecified tibia

√6ᵗʰ **S82.24** Spiral fracture of shaft of tibia
Toddler fracture

√7ᵗʰ **S82.241** Displaced spiral fracture of shaft of right
tibia

√7ᵗʰ **S82.242** Displaced spiral fracture of shaft of left
tibia

√7ᵗʰ **S82.243** Displaced spiral fracture of shaft of ▽
unspecified tibia

√7ᵗʰ **S82.244** Nondisplaced spiral fracture of shaft of
right tibia

√7ᵗʰ **S82.245** Nondisplaced spiral fracture of shaft of
left tibia

√7ᵗʰ **S82.246** Nondisplaced spiral fracture of shaft ▽
of unspecified tibia

√6ᵗʰ **S82.25** Comminuted fracture of shaft of tibia

√7ᵗʰ **S82.251** Displaced comminuted fracture of shaft of
right tibia

√7ᵗʰ **S82.252** Displaced comminuted fracture of shaft of
left tibia

√7ᵗʰ **S82.253** Displaced comminuted fracture of ▽
shaft of unspecified tibia

√7ᵗʰ **S82.254** Nondisplaced comminuted fracture of
shaft of right tibia

√7ᵗʰ **S82.255** Nondisplaced comminuted fracture of
shaft of left tibia

√7ᵗʰ **S82.256** Nondisplaced comminuted fracture of ▽
shaft of unspecified tibia

√6ᵗʰ **S82.26** Segmental fracture of shaft of tibia

√7ᵗʰ **S82.261** Displaced segmental fracture of shaft of
right tibia

√7ᵗʰ **S82.262** Displaced segmental fracture of shaft of
left tibia

√7ᵗʰ **S82.263** Displaced segmental fracture of shaft ▽
of unspecified tibia

√7ᵗʰ **S82.264** Nondisplaced segmental fracture of shaft
of right tibia

√7ᵗʰ **S82.265** Nondisplaced segmental fracture of shaft
of left tibia

√7ᵗʰ **S82.266** Nondisplaced segmental fracture of ▽
shaft of unspecified tibia

√6ᵗʰ **S82.29** Other fracture of shaft of tibia

√7ᵗʰ **S82.291** Other fracture of shaft of right tibia

√7ᵗʰ **S82.292** Other fracture of shaft of left tibia

√7ᵗʰ **S82.299** Other fracture of shaft of unspecified ▽
tibia

√5ᵗʰ **S82.3** Fracture of lower end of tibia

EXCLUDES 1   bimalleolar fracture of lower leg (S82.84-)
fracture of medial malleolus alone (S82.5-)
Maisonneuve's fracture (S82.86-)
pilon fracture of distal tibia (S82.87-)
trimalleolar fractures of lower leg (S82.85-)

√6ᵗʰ **S82.30** Unspecified fracture of lower end of tibia

√7ᵗʰ **S82.301** Unspecified fracture of lower end of ▽
right tibia

√7ᵗʰ **S82.302** Unspecified fracture of lower end of ▽
left tibia

√7ᵗʰ **S82.309** Unspecified fracture of lower end of ▽
unspecified tibia

√6ᵗʰ **S82.31** Torus fracture of lower end of tibia

> The appropriate 7th character is to be added to all
> codes in subcategory S82.31.
> A   initial encounter for closed fracture
> D   subsequent encounter for fracture with routine
>   healing
> G   subsequent encounter for fracture with
>   delayed healing
> K   subsequent encounter for fracture with
>   nonunion
> P   subsequent encounter for fracture with
>   malunion
> S   sequela

√7ᵗʰ **S82.311** Torus fracture of lower end of right tibia

√7ᵗʰ **S82.312** Torus fracture of lower end of left tibia

√7ᵗʰ **S82.319** Torus fracture of lower end of ▽
unspecified tibia

√6ᵗʰ **S82.39** Other fracture of lower end of tibia
AHA: 2015, 1Q, 25

√7ᵗʰ **S82.391** Other fracture of lower end of right tibia

√7ᵗʰ **S82.392** Other fracture of lower end of left tibia

√7ᵗʰ **S82.399** Other fracture of lower end of ▽
unspecified tibia

√5ᵗʰ **S82.4** Fracture of shaft of fibula

EXCLUDES 2   fracture of lateral malleolus alone (S82.6-)

√6ᵗʰ **S82.40** Unspecified fracture of shaft of fibula

√7ᵗʰ **S82.401** Unspecified fracture of shaft of right ▽
fibula

√7ᵗʰ **S82.402** Unspecified fracture of shaft of left ▽
fibula

√7ᵗʰ **S82.409** Unspecified fracture of shaft of ▽
unspecified fibula

√6ᵗʰ **S82.42** Transverse fracture of shaft of fibula

√7ᵗʰ **S82.421** Displaced transverse fracture of shaft of
right fibula

√7ᵗʰ **S82.422** Displaced transverse fracture of shaft of
left fibula

√7ᵗʰ **S82.423** Displaced transverse fracture of shaft ▽
of unspecified fibula

√7ᵗʰ **S82.424** Nondisplaced transverse fracture of shaft
of right fibula

√7ᵗʰ **S82.425** Nondisplaced transverse fracture of shaft
of left fibula

√7ᵗʰ **S82.426** Nondisplaced transverse fracture of ▽
shaft of unspecified fibula

√6ᵗʰ **S82.43** Oblique fracture of shaft of fibula

√7ᵗʰ **S82.431** Displaced oblique fracture of shaft of right
fibula

√7ᵗʰ **S82.432** Displaced oblique fracture of shaft of left
fibula

√7ᵗʰ **S82.433** Displaced oblique fracture of shaft of ▽
unspecified fibula

√7ᵗʰ **S82.434** Nondisplaced oblique fracture of shaft of
right fibula

√7ᵗʰ **S82.435** Nondisplaced oblique fracture of shaft of
left fibula

√7ᵗʰ **S82.436** Nondisplaced oblique fracture of shaft ▽
of unspecified fibula

√6ᵗʰ **S82.44** Spiral fracture of shaft of fibula

√7ᵗʰ **S82.441** Displaced spiral fracture of shaft of right
fibula

√7ᵗʰ **S82.442** Displaced spiral fracture of shaft of left
fibula

√7ᵗʰ **S82.443** Displaced spiral fracture of shaft of ▽
unspecified fibula

√7ᵗʰ **S82.444** Nondisplaced spiral fracture of shaft of
right fibula

√7ᵗʰ **S82.445** Nondisplaced spiral fracture of shaft of
left fibula

√7ᵗʰ **S82.446** Nondisplaced spiral fracture of shaft of ▽
unspecified fibula

√6ᵗʰ **S82.45** Comminuted fracture of shaft of fibula

√7ᵗʰ **S82.451** Displaced comminuted fracture of shaft of
right fibula

☑ Additional Character Req   √x7ᵗʰ Placeholder Alert   Manifestation   HCC CMS-HCC Condition   ▽ Unspecified Code   ►◄ Revised Text   ● New Code   ▲ Revised Code Title

ICD-10-CM 2018

1015

√7ᵗʰ **S82.452** Displaced comminuted fracture of shaft of left fibula

√7ᵗʰ **S82.453** Displaced comminuted fracture of shaft of unspecified fibula ▽

√7ᵗʰ **S82.454** Nondisplaced comminuted fracture of shaft of right fibula

√7ᵗʰ **S82.455** Nondisplaced comminuted fracture of shaft of left fibula

√7ᵗʰ **S82.456** Nondisplaced comminuted fracture of shaft of unspecified fibula ▽

√6ᵗʰ **S82.46** Segmental fracture of shaft of fibula

√7ᵗʰ **S82.461** Displaced segmental fracture of shaft of right fibula

√7ᵗʰ **S82.462** Displaced segmental fracture of shaft of left fibula

√7ᵗʰ **S82.463** Displaced segmental fracture of shaft of unspecified fibula ▽

√7ᵗʰ **S82.464** Nondisplaced segmental fracture of shaft of right fibula

√7ᵗʰ **S82.465** Nondisplaced segmental fracture of shaft of left fibula

√7ᵗʰ **S82.466** Nondisplaced segmental fracture of shaft of unspecified fibula ▽

√6ᵗʰ **S82.49** Other fracture of shaft of fibula

√7ᵗʰ **S82.491** Other fracture of shaft of right fibula

√7ᵗʰ **S82.492** Other fracture of shaft of left fibula

√7ᵗʰ **S82.499** Other fracture of shaft of unspecified fibula ▽

√5ᵗʰ **S82.5** Fracture of medial malleolus

    EXCLUDES 1   pilon fracture of distal tibia (S82.87-)
        Salter-Harris type III of lower end of tibia (S89.13-)
        Salter-Harris type IV of lower end of tibia (S89.14-)

√x7ᵗʰ **S82.51** Displaced fracture of medial malleolus of right tibia

√x7ᵗʰ **S82.52** Displaced fracture of medial malleolus of left tibia

√x7ᵗʰ **S82.53** Displaced fracture of medial malleolus of unspecified tibia ▽

√x7ᵗʰ **S82.54** Nondisplaced fracture of medial malleolus of right tibia

√x7ᵗʰ **S82.55** Nondisplaced fracture of medial malleolus of left tibia

√x7ᵗʰ **S82.56** Nondisplaced fracture of medial malleolus of unspecified tibia ▽

√5ᵗʰ **S82.6** Fracture of lateral malleolus

    EXCLUDES 1   pilon fracture of distal tibia (S82.87-)

√x7ᵗʰ **S82.61** Displaced fracture of lateral malleolus of right fibula

√x7ᵗʰ **S82.62** Displaced fracture of lateral malleolus of left fibula

√x7ᵗʰ **S82.63** Displaced fracture of lateral malleolus of unspecified fibula ▽

√x7ᵗʰ **S82.64** Nondisplaced fracture of lateral malleolus of right fibula

√x7ᵗʰ **S82.65** Nondisplaced fracture of lateral malleolus of left fibula

√x7ᵗʰ **S82.66** Nondisplaced fracture of lateral malleolus of unspecified fibula ▽

√5ᵗʰ **S82.8** Other fractures of lower leg

√6ᵗʰ **S82.81** Torus fracture of upper end of fibula

> The appropriate 7th character is to be added to all codes in subcategory S82.81.
> A   initial encounter for closed fracture
> D   subsequent encounter for fracture with routine healing
> G   subsequent encounter for fracture with delayed healing
> K   subsequent encounter for fracture with nonunion
> P   subsequent encounter for fracture with malunion
> S   sequela

√7ᵗʰ **S82.811** Torus fracture of upper end of right fibula

√7ᵗʰ **S82.812** Torus fracture of upper end of left fibula

√7ᵗʰ **S82.819** Torus fracture of upper end of unspecified fibula ▽

√6ᵗʰ **S82.82** Torus fracture of lower end of fibula

> The appropriate 7th character is to be added to all codes in subcategory S82.82.
> A   initial encounter for closed fracture
> D   subsequent encounter for fracture with routine healing
> G   subsequent encounter for fracture with delayed healing
> K   subsequent encounter for fracture with nonunion
> P   subsequent encounter for fracture with malunion
> S   sequela

√7ᵗʰ **S82.821** Torus fracture of lower end of right fibula

√7ᵗʰ **S82.822** Torus fracture of lower end of left fibula

√7ᵗʰ **S82.829** Torus fracture of lower end of unspecified fibula ▽

√6ᵗʰ **S82.83** Other fracture of upper and lower end of fibula
    AHA: 2015, 1Q, 25

√7ᵗʰ **S82.831** Other fracture of upper and lower end of right fibula

√7ᵗʰ **S82.832** Other fracture of upper and lower end of left fibula

√7ᵗʰ **S82.839** Other fracture of upper and lower end of unspecified fibula ▽

√6ᵗʰ **S82.84** Bimalleolar fracture of lower leg

√7ᵗʰ **S82.841** Displaced bimalleolar fracture of right lower leg

√7ᵗʰ **S82.842** Displaced bimalleolar fracture of left lower leg

√7ᵗʰ **S82.843** Displaced bimalleolar fracture of unspecified lower leg ▽

√7ᵗʰ **S82.844** Nondisplaced bimalleolar fracture of right lower leg

√7ᵗʰ **S82.845** Nondisplaced bimalleolar fracture of left lower leg

√7ᵗʰ **S82.846** Nondisplaced bimalleolar fracture of unspecified lower leg ▽

√6ᵗʰ **S82.85** Trimalleolar fracture of lower leg

√7ᵗʰ **S82.851** Displaced trimalleolar fracture of right lower leg

√7ᵗʰ **S82.852** Displaced trimalleolar fracture of left lower leg

√7ᵗʰ **S82.853** Displaced trimalleolar fracture of unspecified lower leg ▽

Right Bimalleolar Fracture

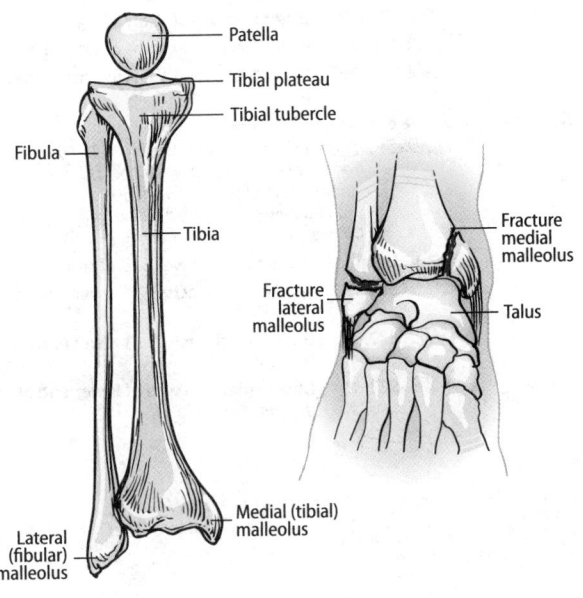

Patella
Tibial plateau
Tibial tubercle
Fibula
Tibia
Fracture medial malleolus
Fracture lateral malleolus
Talus
Medial (tibial) malleolus
Lateral (fibular) malleolus

EXCLUDES 1 Not coded here   **EXCLUDES 2** Not included here   **N** Newborn Age: 0   **P** Pediatric Age: 0-17   **M** Maternity Age: 12-55   **A** Adult Age: 15-124

ICD-10-CM 2018

1016

√7ᵗʰ	**S82.854**	Nondisplaced **trimalleolar fracture of right lower leg**
√7ᵗʰ	**S82.855**	Nondisplaced **trimalleolar fracture of left lower leg**
√7ᵗʰ	**S82.856**	Nondisplaced **trimalleolar fracture of unspecified lower leg** ▽

√6ᵗʰ   **S82.86**   Maisonneuve's **fracture**

√7ᵗʰ	**S82.861**	Displaced **Maisonneuve's fracture of right leg**
√7ᵗʰ	**S82.862**	Displaced **Maisonneuve's fracture of left leg**
√7ᵗʰ	**S82.863**	Displaced **Maisonneuve's fracture of unspecified leg** ▽
√7ᵗʰ	**S82.864**	Nondisplaced **Maisonneuve's fracture of right leg**
√7ᵗʰ	**S82.865**	Nondisplaced **Maisonneuve's fracture of left leg**
√7ᵗʰ	**S82.866**	Nondisplaced **Maisonneuve's fracture of unspecified leg** ▽

√6ᵗʰ   **S82.87**   Pilon **fracture of tibia**

√7ᵗʰ	**S82.871**	Displaced **pilon fracture of right tibia**
√7ᵗʰ	**S82.872**	Displaced **pilon fracture of left tibia**
√7ᵗʰ	**S82.873**	Displaced **pilon fracture of unspecified tibia** ▽
√7ᵗʰ	**S82.874**	Nondisplaced **pilon fracture of right tibia**
√7ᵗʰ	**S82.875**	Nondisplaced **pilon fracture of left tibia**
√7ᵗʰ	**S82.876**	Nondisplaced **pilon fracture of unspecified tibia** ▽

√6ᵗʰ   **S82.89**   Other **fractures of lower leg**
Fracture of ankle NOS

√7ᵗʰ	**S82.891**	Other **fracture of right lower leg**
√7ᵗʰ	**S82.892**	Other **fracture of left lower leg**
√7ᵗʰ	**S82.899**	Other **fracture of unspecified lower leg** ▽

√5ᵗʰ   **S82.9**   Unspecified **fracture of lower leg**

√x 7ᵗʰ	**S82.90**	Unspecified **fracture of unspecified lower leg** ▽
√x 7ᵗʰ	**S82.91**	Unspecified **fracture of right lower leg** ▽
√x 7ᵗʰ	**S82.92**	Unspecified **fracture of left lower leg** ▽

√4ᵗʰ   **S83**   **Dislocation and sprain of joints and ligaments of knee**

INCLUDES   avulsion of joint or ligament of knee
laceration of cartilage, joint or ligament of knee
sprain of cartilage, joint or ligament of knee
traumatic hemarthrosis of joint or ligament of knee
traumatic rupture of joint or ligament of knee
traumatic subluxation of joint or ligament of knee
traumatic tear of joint or ligament of knee

Code also any associated open wound

EXCLUDES 1   derangement of patella (M22.0-M22.3)
injury of patellar ligament (tendon) (S76.1-)
internal derangement of knee (M23.-)
old dislocation of knee (M24.36)
pathological dislocation of knee (M24.36)
recurrent dislocation of knee (M22.0)

EXCLUDES 2   strain of muscle, fascia and tendon of lower leg (S86.-)

The appropriate 7th character is to be added to each code from category S83.
A   initial encounter
D   subsequent encounter
S   sequela

√5ᵗʰ   **S83.0**   Subluxation and dislocation of patella

√6ᵗʰ   **S83.00**   Unspecified **subluxation and dislocation of patella**

√7ᵗʰ	**S83.001**	Unspecified **subluxation of right patella** ▽
√7ᵗʰ	**S83.002**	Unspecified **subluxation of left patella** ▽
√7ᵗʰ	**S83.003**	Unspecified **subluxation of unspecified patella** ▽
√7ᵗʰ	**S83.004**	Unspecified **dislocation of right patella** ▽
√7ᵗʰ	**S83.005**	Unspecified **dislocation of left patella** ▽
√7ᵗʰ	**S83.006**	Unspecified **dislocation of unspecified patella** ▽

√6ᵗʰ   **S83.01**   Lateral **subluxation and dislocation of patella**

√7ᵗʰ	**S83.011**	Lateral **subluxation of right patella**
√7ᵗʰ	**S83.012**	Lateral **subluxation of left patella**
√7ᵗʰ	**S83.013**	Lateral **subluxation of unspecified patella** ▽
√7ᵗʰ	**S83.014**	Lateral **dislocation of right patella**
√7ᵗʰ	**S83.015**	Lateral **dislocation of left patella**
√7ᵗʰ	**S83.016**	Lateral **dislocation of unspecified patella** ▽

√6ᵗʰ   **S83.09**   Other **subluxation and dislocation of patella**

√7ᵗʰ	**S83.091**	Other **subluxation of right patella**
√7ᵗʰ	**S83.092**	Other **subluxation of left patella**
√7ᵗʰ	**S83.093**	Other **subluxation of unspecified patella** ▽
√7ᵗʰ	**S83.094**	Other **dislocation of right patella**
√7ᵗʰ	**S83.095**	Other **dislocation of left patella**
√7ᵗʰ	**S83.096**	Other **dislocation of unspecified patella** ▽

√5ᵗʰ   **S83.1**   Subluxation and dislocation of knee

EXCLUDES 2   instability of knee prosthesis (T84.022, T84.023)

√6ᵗʰ   **S83.10**   Unspecified **subluxation and dislocation of knee**

√7ᵗʰ	**S83.101**	Unspecified **subluxation of right knee** ▽
√7ᵗʰ	**S83.102**	Unspecified **subluxation of left knee** ▽
√7ᵗʰ	**S83.103**	Unspecified **subluxation of unspecified knee** ▽
√7ᵗʰ	**S83.104**	Unspecified **dislocation of right knee** ▽
√7ᵗʰ	**S83.105**	Unspecified **dislocation of left knee** ▽
√7ᵗʰ	**S83.106**	Unspecified **dislocation of unspecified knee** ▽

√6ᵗʰ   **S83.11**   Anterior **subluxation and dislocation of proximal end of tibia**
Posterior subluxation and dislocation of distal end of femur

√7ᵗʰ	**S83.111**	Anterior **subluxation of proximal end of tibia, right knee**
√7ᵗʰ	**S83.112**	Anterior **subluxation of proximal end of tibia, left knee**
√7ᵗʰ	**S83.113**	Anterior **subluxation of proximal end of tibia, unspecified knee**
√7ᵗʰ	**S83.114**	Anterior **dislocation of proximal end of tibia, right knee**
√7ᵗʰ	**S83.115**	Anterior **dislocation of proximal end of tibia, left knee**
√7ᵗʰ	**S83.116**	Anterior **dislocation of proximal end of tibia, unspecified knee** ▽

√6ᵗʰ   **S83.12**   Posterior **subluxation and dislocation of proximal end of tibia**
Anterior dislocation of distal end of femur

√7ᵗʰ	**S83.121**	Posterior **subluxation of proximal end of tibia, right knee**
√7ᵗʰ	**S83.122**	Posterior **subluxation of proximal end of tibia, left knee**
√7ᵗʰ	**S83.123**	Posterior **subluxation of proximal end of tibia, unspecified knee** ▽
√7ᵗʰ	**S83.124**	Posterior **dislocation of proximal end of tibia, right knee**
√7ᵗʰ	**S83.125**	Posterior **dislocation of proximal end of tibia, left knee**
√7ᵗʰ	**S83.126**	Posterior **dislocation of proximal end of tibia, unspecified knee** ▽

√6ᵗʰ   **S83.13**   Medial **subluxation and dislocation of proximal end of tibia**

√7ᵗʰ	**S83.131**	Medial **subluxation of proximal end of tibia, right knee**
√7ᵗʰ	**S83.132**	Medial **subluxation of proximal end of tibia, left knee**
√7ᵗʰ	**S83.133**	Medial **subluxation of proximal end of tibia, unspecified knee** ▽
√7ᵗʰ	**S83.134**	Medial **dislocation of proximal end of tibia, right knee**
√7ᵗʰ	**S83.135**	Medial **dislocation of proximal end of tibia, left knee**
√7ᵗʰ	**S83.136**	Medial **dislocation of proximal end of tibia, unspecified knee** ▽

☑ Additional Character Req   √x7ᵗʰ Placeholder Alert   Manifestation   HCC CMS-HCC Condition   ▽ Unspecified Code   ►◄ Revised Text   ● New Code   ▲ Revised Code Title

ICD-10-CM 2018   **1017**

✓6ᵗʰ S83.14 Lateral subluxation and dislocation of proximal end of tibia

- ✓7ᵗʰ **S83.141** Lateral subluxation of proximal end of tibia, right knee
- ✓7ᵗʰ **S83.142** Lateral subluxation of proximal end of tibia, left knee
- ✓7ᵗʰ **S83.143** Lateral subluxation of proximal end of tibia, unspecified knee ▽
- ✓7ᵗʰ **S83.144** Lateral dislocation of proximal end of tibia, right knee
- ✓7ᵗʰ **S83.145** Lateral dislocation of proximal end of tibia, left knee
- ✓7ᵗʰ **S83.146** Lateral dislocation of proximal end of tibia, unspecified knee ▽

✓6ᵗʰ S83.19 Other subluxation and dislocation of knee

- ✓7ᵗʰ **S83.191** Other subluxation of right knee
- ✓7ᵗʰ **S83.192** Other subluxation of left knee
- ✓7ᵗʰ **S83.193** Other subluxation of unspecified knee ▽
- ✓7ᵗʰ **S83.194** Other dislocation of right knee
- ✓7ᵗʰ **S83.195** Other dislocation of left knee
- ✓7ᵗʰ **S83.196** Other dislocation of unspecified knee ▽

✓5ᵗʰ S83.2 Tear of meniscus, current injury

> EXCLUDES 1   old bucket-handle tear (M23.2)

✓6ᵗʰ S83.20 Tear of unspecified meniscus, current injury
Tear of meniscus of knee NOS

- ✓7ᵗʰ **S83.200** Bucket-handle tear of unspecified meniscus, current injury, right knee ▽
- ✓7ᵗʰ **S83.201** Bucket-handle tear of unspecified meniscus, current injury, left knee ▽
- ✓7ᵗʰ **S83.202** Bucket-handle tear of unspecified meniscus, current injury, unspecified knee ▽
- ✓7ᵗʰ **S83.203** Other tear of unspecified meniscus, current injury, right knee ▽
- ✓7ᵗʰ **S83.204** Other tear of unspecified meniscus, current injury, left knee ▽
- ✓7ᵗʰ **S83.205** Other tear of unspecified meniscus, current injury, unspecified knee ▽
- ✓7ᵗʰ **S83.206** Unspecified tear of unspecified meniscus, current injury, right knee ▽
- ✓7ᵗʰ **S83.207** Unspecified tear of unspecified meniscus, current injury, left knee ▽
- ✓7ᵗʰ **S83.209** Unspecified tear of unspecified meniscus, current injury, unspecified knee ▽

✓6ᵗʰ S83.21 Bucket-handle tear of medial meniscus, current injury

- ✓7ᵗʰ **S83.211** Bucket-handle tear of medial meniscus, current injury, right knee
- ✓7ᵗʰ **S83.212** Bucket-handle tear of medial meniscus, current injury, left knee
- ✓7ᵗʰ **S83.219** Bucket-handle tear of medial meniscus, current injury, unspecified knee ▽

✓6ᵗʰ S83.22 Peripheral tear of medial meniscus, current injury

- ✓7ᵗʰ **S83.221** Peripheral tear of medial meniscus, current injury, right knee
- ✓7ᵗʰ **S83.222** Peripheral tear of medial meniscus, current injury, left knee
- ✓7ᵗʰ **S83.229** Peripheral tear of medial meniscus, current injury, unspecified knee ▽

✓6ᵗʰ S83.23 Complex tear of medial meniscus, current injury

- ✓7ᵗʰ **S83.231** Complex tear of medial meniscus, current injury, right knee
- ✓7ᵗʰ **S83.232** Complex tear of medial meniscus, current injury, left knee
- ✓7ᵗʰ **S83.239** Complex tear of medial meniscus, current injury, unspecified knee ▽

✓6ᵗʰ S83.24 Other tear of medial meniscus, current injury

- ✓7ᵗʰ **S83.241** Other tear of medial meniscus, current injury, right knee
- ✓7ᵗʰ **S83.242** Other tear of medial meniscus, current injury, left knee

---

- ✓7ᵗʰ **S83.249** Other tear of medial meniscus, current injury, unspecified knee ▽

✓6ᵗʰ S83.25 Bucket-handle tear of lateral meniscus, current injury

- ✓7ᵗʰ **S83.251** Bucket-handle tear of lateral meniscus, current injury, right knee
- ✓7ᵗʰ **S83.252** Bucket-handle tear of lateral meniscus, current injury, left knee
- ✓7ᵗʰ **S83.259** Bucket-handle tear of lateral meniscus, current injury, unspecified knee ▽

✓6ᵗʰ S83.26 Peripheral tear of lateral meniscus, current injury

- ✓7ᵗʰ **S83.261** Peripheral tear of lateral meniscus, current injury, right knee
- ✓7ᵗʰ **S83.262** Peripheral tear of lateral meniscus, current injury, left knee
- ✓7ᵗʰ **S83.269** Peripheral tear of lateral meniscus, current injury, unspecified knee ▽

✓6ᵗʰ S83.27 Complex tear of lateral meniscus, current injury

- ✓7ᵗʰ **S83.271** Complex tear of lateral meniscus, current injury, right knee
- ✓7ᵗʰ **S83.272** Complex tear of lateral meniscus, current injury, left knee
- ✓7ᵗʰ **S83.279** Complex tear of lateral meniscus, current injury, unspecified knee ▽

✓6ᵗʰ S83.28 Other tear of lateral meniscus, current injury

- ✓7ᵗʰ **S83.281** Other tear of lateral meniscus, current injury, right knee
- ✓7ᵗʰ **S83.282** Other tear of lateral meniscus, current injury, left knee
- ✓7ᵗʰ **S83.289** Other tear of lateral meniscus, current injury, unspecified knee ▽

✓5ᵗʰ S83.3 Tear of articular cartilage of knee, current

- ✓x7ᵗʰ **S83.30** Tear of articular cartilage of unspecified knee, current
- ✓x7ᵗʰ **S83.31** Tear of articular cartilage of right knee, current
- ✓x7ᵗʰ **S83.32** Tear of articular cartilage of left knee, current

✓5ᵗʰ S83.4 Sprain of collateral ligament of knee

✓6ᵗʰ S83.40 Sprain of unspecified collateral ligament of knee

- ✓7ᵗʰ **S83.401** Sprain of unspecified collateral ligament of right knee ▽
- ✓7ᵗʰ **S83.402** Sprain of unspecified collateral ligament of left knee ▽
- ✓7ᵗʰ **S83.409** Sprain of unspecified collateral ligament of unspecified knee ▽

✓6ᵗʰ S83.41 Sprain of medial collateral ligament of knee
Sprain of tibial collateral ligament

- ✓7ᵗʰ **S83.411** Sprain of medial collateral ligament of right knee
- ✓7ᵗʰ **S83.412** Sprain of medial collateral ligament of left knee
- ✓7ᵗʰ **S83.419** Sprain of medial collateral ligament of unspecified knee ▽

✓6ᵗʰ S83.42 Sprain of lateral collateral ligament of knee
Sprain of fibular collateral ligament

- ✓7ᵗʰ **S83.421** Sprain of lateral collateral ligament of right knee
- ✓7ᵗʰ **S83.422** Sprain of lateral collateral ligament of left knee
- ✓7ᵗʰ **S83.429** Sprain of lateral collateral ligament of unspecified knee ▽

✓5ᵗʰ S83.5 Sprain of cruciate ligament of knee
AHA: 2016, 2Q, 3

✓6ᵗʰ S83.50 Sprain of unspecified cruciate ligament of knee

- ✓7ᵗʰ **S83.501** Sprain of unspecified cruciate ligament of right knee ▽
- ✓7ᵗʰ **S83.502** Sprain of unspecified cruciate ligament of left knee ▽
- ✓7ᵗʰ **S83.509** Sprain of unspecified cruciate ligament of unspecified knee ▽

✓6ᵗʰ S83.51 Sprain of anterior cruciate ligament of knee

- ✓7ᵗʰ **S83.511** Sprain of anterior cruciate ligament of right knee
- ✓7ᵗʰ **S83.512** Sprain of anterior cruciate ligament of left knee

EXCLUDES 1 Not coded here   EXCLUDES 2 Not included here   N Newborn Age: 0   P Pediatric Age: 0-17   M Maternity Age: 12-55   A Adult Age: 15-124

1018   ICD-10-CM 2018

✓7ᵗʰ **S83.519** Sprain of anterior cruciate ligament of ▽
unspecified knee

✓6ᵗʰ **S83.52** Sprain of **posterior** cruciate ligament of knee

✓7ᵗʰ **S83.521** Sprain of posterior cruciate ligament of
right knee

✓7ᵗʰ **S83.522** Sprain of posterior cruciate ligament of
left knee

✓7ᵗʰ **S83.529** Sprain of posterior cruciate ligament of ▽
unspecified knee

✓5ᵗʰ **S83.6** Sprain of the **superior tibiofibular** joint and ligament

✓ˣ7ᵗʰ **S83.60** Sprain of the superior tibiofibular joint and ▽
ligament, unspecified knee

✓ˣ7ᵗʰ **S83.61** Sprain of the superior tibiofibular joint and
ligament, **right** knee

✓ˣ7ᵗʰ **S83.62** Sprain of the superior tibiofibular joint and
ligament, **left** knee

✓5ᵗʰ **S83.8** Sprain of other specified parts of knee

✓6ᵗʰ **S83.8X** Sprain of other specified parts of knee

✓7ᵗʰ **S83.8X1** Sprain of other specified parts of **right**
knee

✓7ᵗʰ **S83.8X2** Sprain of other specified parts of **left** knee

✓7ᵗʰ **S83.8X9** Sprain of other specified parts of ▽
unspecified knee

✓5ᵗʰ **S83.9** Sprain of unspecified site of knee

✓ˣ7ᵗʰ **S83.90** Sprain of unspecified site of unspecified knee ▽

✓ˣ7ᵗʰ **S83.91** Sprain of unspecified site of **right** knee ▽

✓ˣ7ᵗʰ **S83.92** Sprain of unspecified site of **left** knee ▽

✓4ᵗʰ **S84** **Injury of nerves at lower leg level**

Code also any associated open wound (S81.-)

EXCLUDES 2 *injury of nerves at ankle and foot level (S94.-)*

The appropriate 7th character is to be added to each code from
category S84.
A   initial encounter
D   subsequent encounter
S   sequela

✓5ᵗʰ **S84.0** Injury of **tibial nerve** at lower leg level

✓ˣ7ᵗʰ **S84.00** Injury of tibial nerve at lower leg level, ▽
unspecified leg

✓ˣ7ᵗʰ **S84.01** Injury of tibial nerve at lower leg level, **right** leg

✓ˣ7ᵗʰ **S84.02** Injury of tibial nerve at lower leg level, **left** leg

✓5ᵗʰ **S84.1** Injury of **peroneal nerve** at lower leg level

✓ˣ7ᵗʰ **S84.10** Injury of peroneal nerve at lower leg level, ▽
unspecified leg

✓ˣ7ᵗʰ **S84.11** Injury of peroneal nerve at lower leg level, **right** leg

✓ˣ7ᵗʰ **S84.12** Injury of peroneal nerve at lower leg level, **left** leg

✓5ᵗʰ **S84.2** Injury of **cutaneous sensory nerve** at lower leg level

✓ˣ7ᵗʰ **S84.20** Injury of cutaneous sensory nerve at lower leg ▽
level, unspecified leg

✓ˣ7ᵗʰ **S84.21** Injury of cutaneous sensory nerve at lower leg level,
right leg

✓ˣ7ᵗʰ **S84.22** Injury of cutaneous sensory nerve at lower leg level,
left leg

✓5ᵗʰ **S84.8** Injury of other nerves at lower leg level

✓6ᵗʰ **S84.80** Injury of other nerves at lower leg level

✓7ᵗʰ **S84.801** Injury of other nerves at lower leg level,
right leg

✓7ᵗʰ **S84.802** Injury of other nerves at lower leg level,
left leg

✓7ᵗʰ **S84.809** Injury of other nerves at lower leg level, ▽
unspecified leg

✓5ᵗʰ **S84.9** Injury of unspecified nerve at lower leg level

✓ˣ7ᵗʰ **S84.90** Injury of unspecified nerve at lower leg level, ▽
unspecified leg

✓ˣ7ᵗʰ **S84.91** Injury of unspecified nerve at lower leg level, ▽
right leg

✓ˣ7ᵗʰ **S84.92** Injury of unspecified nerve at lower leg level, ▽
left leg

✓4ᵗʰ **S85** **Injury of blood vessels at lower leg level**

Code also any associated open wound (S81.-)

EXCLUDES 2 *injury of blood vessels at ankle and foot level (S95.-)*

The appropriate 7th character is to be added to each code from
category S85.
A   initial encounter
D   subsequent encounter
S   sequela

✓5ᵗʰ **S85.0** Injury of **popliteal artery**

✓6ᵗʰ **S85.00** Unspecified injury of popliteal artery

✓7ᵗʰ **S85.001** Unspecified injury of popliteal artery, ▽
right leg

✓7ᵗʰ **S85.002** Unspecified injury of popliteal artery, ▽
left leg

✓7ᵗʰ **S85.009** Unspecified injury of popliteal artery, ▽
unspecified leg

✓6ᵗʰ **S85.01** **Laceration** of popliteal artery

✓7ᵗʰ **S85.011** Laceration of popliteal artery, **right** leg

✓7ᵗʰ **S85.012** Laceration of popliteal artery, **left** leg

✓7ᵗʰ **S85.019** Laceration of popliteal artery, ▽
unspecified leg

✓6ᵗʰ **S85.09** Other specified injury of popliteal artery

✓7ᵗʰ **S85.091** Other specified injury of popliteal artery,
right leg

✓7ᵗʰ **S85.092** Other specified injury of popliteal artery,
left leg

✓7ᵗʰ **S85.099** Other specified injury of popliteal ▽
artery, unspecified leg

✓5ᵗʰ **S85.1** Injury of **tibial artery**

✓6ᵗʰ **S85.10** Unspecified injury of unspecified tibial artery
Injury of tibial artery NOS

✓7ᵗʰ **S85.101** Unspecified injury of unspecified tibial ▽
artery, **right** leg

✓7ᵗʰ **S85.102** Unspecified injury of unspecified tibial ▽
artery, **left** leg

✓7ᵗʰ **S85.109** Unspecified injury of unspecified tibial ▽
artery, unspecified leg

✓6ᵗʰ **S85.11** **Laceration** of unspecified tibial artery

✓7ᵗʰ **S85.111** Laceration of unspecified tibial artery, ▽
right leg

✓7ᵗʰ **S85.112** Laceration of unspecified tibial artery, ▽
left leg

✓7ᵗʰ **S85.119** Laceration of unspecified tibial artery, ▽
unspecified leg

✓6ᵗʰ **S85.12** Other specified injury of unspecified tibial artery

✓7ᵗʰ **S85.121** Other specified injury of unspecified ▽
tibial artery, **right** leg

✓7ᵗʰ **S85.122** Other specified injury of unspecified ▽
tibial artery, **left** leg

✓7ᵗʰ **S85.129** Other specified injury of unspecified ▽
tibial artery, unspecified leg

✓6ᵗʰ **S85.13** Unspecified injury of **anterior** tibial artery

✓7ᵗʰ **S85.131** Unspecified injury of anterior tibial ▽
artery, **right** leg

✓7ᵗʰ **S85.132** Unspecified injury of anterior tibial ▽
artery, **left** leg

✓7ᵗʰ **S85.139** Unspecified injury of anterior tibial ▽
artery, unspecified leg

✓6ᵗʰ **S85.14** **Laceration** of **anterior** tibial artery

✓7ᵗʰ **S85.141** Laceration of anterior tibial artery, **right** ▽
leg

✓7ᵗʰ **S85.142** Laceration of anterior tibial artery, **left** leg

✓7ᵗʰ **S85.149** Laceration of anterior tibial artery, ▽
unspecified leg

✓6ᵗʰ **S85.15** Other specified injury of **anterior** tibial artery

✓7ᵗʰ **S85.151** Other specified injury of anterior tibial
artery, **right** leg

✓7ᵗʰ **S85.152** Other specified injury of anterior tibial
artery, **left** leg

✓7ᵗʰ **S85.159** Other specified injury of anterior tibial ▽
artery, unspecified leg

√6ᵗʰ **S85.16** Unspecified injury of posterior tibial artery

     √7ᵗʰ **S85.161** Unspecified injury of posterior tibial artery, right leg ▽

     √7ᵗʰ **S85.162** Unspecified injury of posterior tibial artery, left leg ▽

     √7ᵗʰ **S85.169** Unspecified injury of posterior tibial artery, unspecified leg ▽

√6ᵗʰ **S85.17** Laceration of posterior tibial artery

     √7ᵗʰ **S85.171** Laceration of posterior tibial artery, right leg

     √7ᵗʰ **S85.172** Laceration of posterior tibial artery, left leg

     √7ᵗʰ **S85.179** Laceration of posterior tibial artery, unspecified leg ▽

√6ᵗʰ **S85.18** Other specified injury of posterior tibial artery

     √7ᵗʰ **S85.181** Other specified injury of posterior tibial artery, right leg

     √7ᵗʰ **S85.182** Other specified injury of posterior tibial artery, left leg

     √7ᵗʰ **S85.189** Other specified injury of posterior tibial artery, unspecified leg ▽

√5ᵗʰ **S85.2** Injury of peroneal artery

√6ᵗʰ **S85.20** Unspecified injury of peroneal artery

     √7ᵗʰ **S85.201** Unspecified injury of peroneal artery, right leg ▽

     √7ᵗʰ **S85.202** Unspecified injury of peroneal artery, left leg ▽

     √7ᵗʰ **S85.209** Unspecified injury of peroneal artery, unspecified leg ▽

√6ᵗʰ **S85.21** Laceration of peroneal artery

     √7ᵗʰ **S85.211** Laceration of peroneal artery, right leg

     √7ᵗʰ **S85.212** Laceration of peroneal artery, left leg

     √7ᵗʰ **S85.219** Laceration of peroneal artery, unspecified leg ▽

√6ᵗʰ **S85.29** Other specified injury of peroneal artery

     √7ᵗʰ **S85.291** Other specified injury of peroneal artery, right leg

     √7ᵗʰ **S85.292** Other specified injury of peroneal artery, left leg

     √7ᵗʰ **S85.299** Other specified injury of peroneal artery, unspecified leg ▽

√5ᵗʰ **S85.3** Injury of greater saphenous vein at lower leg level

     Injury of greater saphenous vein NOS

     Injury of saphenous vein NOS

√6ᵗʰ **S85.30** Unspecified injury of greater saphenous vein at lower leg level

     √7ᵗʰ **S85.301** Unspecified injury of greater saphenous vein at lower leg level, right leg ▽

     √7ᵗʰ **S85.302** Unspecified injury of greater saphenous vein at lower leg level, left leg ▽

     √7ᵗʰ **S85.309** Unspecified injury of greater saphenous vein at lower leg level, unspecified leg ▽

√6ᵗʰ **S85.31** Laceration of greater saphenous vein at lower leg level

     √7ᵗʰ **S85.311** Laceration of greater saphenous vein at lower leg level, right leg

     √7ᵗʰ **S85.312** Laceration of greater saphenous vein at lower leg level, left leg

     √7ᵗʰ **S85.319** Laceration of greater saphenous vein at lower leg level, unspecified leg ▽

√6ᵗʰ **S85.39** Other specified injury of greater saphenous vein at lower leg level

     √7ᵗʰ **S85.391** Other specified injury of greater saphenous vein at lower leg level, right leg

     √7ᵗʰ **S85.392** Other specified injury of greater saphenous vein at lower leg level, left leg

     √7ᵗʰ **S85.399** Other specified injury of greater saphenous vein at lower leg level, unspecified leg ▽

√5ᵗʰ **S85.4** Injury of lesser saphenous vein at lower leg level

√6ᵗʰ **S85.40** Unspecified injury of lesser saphenous vein at lower leg level

     √7ᵗʰ **S85.401** Unspecified injury of lesser saphenous vein at lower leg level, right leg ▽

     √7ᵗʰ **S85.402** Unspecified injury of lesser saphenous vein at lower leg level, left leg ▽

     √7ᵗʰ **S85.409** Unspecified injury of lesser saphenous vein at lower leg level, unspecified leg ▽

√6ᵗʰ **S85.41** Laceration of lesser saphenous vein at lower leg level

     √7ᵗʰ **S85.411** Laceration of lesser saphenous vein at lower leg level, right leg

     √7ᵗʰ **S85.412** Laceration of lesser saphenous vein at lower leg level, left leg

     √7ᵗʰ **S85.419** Laceration of lesser saphenous vein at lower leg level, unspecified leg ▽

√6ᵗʰ **S85.49** Other specified injury of lesser saphenous vein at lower leg level

     √7ᵗʰ **S85.491** Other specified injury of lesser saphenous vein at lower leg level, right leg

     √7ᵗʰ **S85.492** Other specified injury of lesser saphenous vein at lower leg level, left leg

     √7ᵗʰ **S85.499** Other specified injury of lesser saphenous vein at lower leg level, unspecified leg ▽

√5ᵗʰ **S85.5** Injury of popliteal vein

√6ᵗʰ **S85.50** Unspecified injury of popliteal vein

     √7ᵗʰ **S85.501** Unspecified injury of popliteal vein, right leg ▽

     √7ᵗʰ **S85.502** Unspecified injury of popliteal vein, left leg ▽

     √7ᵗʰ **S85.509** Unspecified injury of popliteal vein, unspecified leg ▽

√6ᵗʰ **S85.51** Laceration of popliteal vein

     √7ᵗʰ **S85.511** Laceration of popliteal vein, right leg

     √7ᵗʰ **S85.512** Laceration of popliteal vein, left leg

     √7ᵗʰ **S85.519** Laceration of popliteal vein, unspecified leg ▽

√6ᵗʰ **S85.59** Other specified injury of popliteal vein

     √7ᵗʰ **S85.591** Other specified injury of popliteal vein, right leg

     √7ᵗʰ **S85.592** Other specified injury of popliteal vein, left leg

     √7ᵗʰ **S85.599** Other specified injury of popliteal vein, unspecified leg ▽

√5ᵗʰ **S85.8** Injury of other blood vessels at lower leg level

√6ᵗʰ **S85.80** Unspecified injury of other blood vessels at lower leg level

     √7ᵗʰ **S85.801** Unspecified injury of other blood vessels at lower leg level, right leg ▽

     √7ᵗʰ **S85.802** Unspecified injury of other blood vessels at lower leg level, left leg ▽

     √7ᵗʰ **S85.809** Unspecified injury of other blood vessels at lower leg level, unspecified leg ▽

√6ᵗʰ **S85.81** Laceration of other blood vessels at lower leg level

     √7ᵗʰ **S85.811** Laceration of other blood vessels at lower leg level, right leg

     √7ᵗʰ **S85.812** Laceration of other blood vessels at lower leg level, left leg

     √7ᵗʰ **S85.819** Laceration of other blood vessels at lower leg level, unspecified leg ▽

√6ᵗʰ **S85.89** Other specified injury of other blood vessels at lower leg level

     √7ᵗʰ **S85.891** Other specified injury of other blood vessels at lower leg level, right leg

     √7ᵗʰ **S85.892** Other specified injury of other blood vessels at lower leg level, left leg

     √7ᵗʰ **S85.899** Other specified injury of other blood vessels at lower leg level, unspecified leg ▽

EXCLUDES 1 Not coded here   EXCLUDES 2 Not included here   N Newborn Age: 0   P Pediatric Age: 0-17   M Maternity Age: 12-55   A Adult Age: 15-124

1020   ICD-10-CM 2018

☑5ᵗʰ **S85.9 Injury of unspecified blood vessel at lower leg level**

  ☑6ᵗʰ **S85.90 Unspecified injury of unspecified blood vessel at lower leg level**

    ☑7ᵗʰ **S85.901 Unspecified injury of unspecified blood vessel at lower leg level, right leg** ▽

    ☑7ᵗʰ **S85.902 Unspecified injury of unspecified blood vessel at lower leg level, left leg** ▽

    ☑7ᵗʰ **S85.909 Unspecified injury of unspecified blood vessel at lower leg level, unspecified leg** ▽

  ☑6ᵗʰ **S85.91 Laceration of unspecified blood vessel at lower leg level**

    ☑7ᵗʰ **S85.911 Laceration of unspecified blood vessel at lower leg level, right leg** ▽

    ☑7ᵗʰ **S85.912 Laceration of unspecified blood vessel at lower leg level, left leg** ▽

    ☑7ᵗʰ **S85.919 Laceration of unspecified blood vessel at lower leg level, unspecified leg** ▽

  ☑6ᵗʰ **S85.99 Other specified injury of unspecified blood vessel at lower leg level**

    ☑7ᵗʰ **S85.991 Other specified injury of unspecified blood vessel at lower leg level, right leg** ▽

    ☑7ᵗʰ **S85.992 Other specified injury of unspecified blood vessel at lower leg level, left leg** ▽

    ☑7ᵗʰ **S85.999 Other specified injury of unspecified blood vessel at lower leg level, unspecified leg** ▽

☑4ᵗʰ **S86 Injury of muscle, fascia and tendon at lower leg level**

  Code also any associated open wound (S81.-)

  EXCLUDES 2 injury of muscle, fascia and tendon at ankle (S96.-)
              injury of patellar ligament (tendon) (S76.1-)
              sprain of joints and ligaments of knee (S83.-)

  TIP: Refer to the Muscle/Tendon table at the beginning of this chapter.

  The appropriate 7th character is to be added to each code from category S86.
  A   initial encounter
  D   subsequent encounter
  S   sequela

  ☑5ᵗʰ **S86.0 Injury of Achilles tendon**

    ☑6ᵗʰ **S86.00 Unspecified injury of Achilles tendon**

      ☑7ᵗʰ **S86.001 Unspecified injury of right Achilles tendon** ▽

      ☑7ᵗʰ **S86.002 Unspecified injury of left Achilles tendon** ▽

      ☑7ᵗʰ **S86.009 Unspecified injury of unspecified Achilles tendon** ▽

    ☑6ᵗʰ **S86.01 Strain of Achilles tendon**

      ☑7ᵗʰ **S86.011 Strain of right Achilles tendon**

      ☑7ᵗʰ **S86.012 Strain of left Achilles tendon**

      ☑7ᵗʰ **S86.019 Strain of unspecified Achilles tendon** ▽

    S86.02 Laceration of Achilles tendon

      ☑7ᵗʰ **S86.021 Laceration of right Achilles tendon**

      ☑7ᵗʰ **S86.022 Laceration of left Achilles tendon**

      ☑7ᵗʰ **S86.029 Laceration of unspecified Achilles tendon** ▽

    ☑6ᵗʰ **S86.09 Other specified injury of Achilles tendon**

      ☑7ᵗʰ **S86.091 Other specified injury of right Achilles tendon**

      ☑7ᵗʰ **S86.092 Other specified injury of left Achilles tendon**

      ☑7ᵗʰ **S86.099 Other specified injury of unspecified Achilles tendon** ▽

  ☑5ᵗʰ **S86.1 Injury of other muscle(s) and tendon(s) of posterior muscle group at lower leg level**

    ☑6ᵗʰ **S86.10 Unspecified injury of other muscle(s) and tendon(s) of posterior muscle group at lower leg level**

      ☑7ᵗʰ **S86.101 Unspecified injury of other muscle(s) and tendon(s) of posterior muscle group at lower leg level, right leg** ▽

      ☑7ᵗʰ **S86.102 Unspecified injury of other muscle(s) and tendon(s) of posterior muscle group at lower leg level, left leg** ▽

      ☑7ᵗʰ **S86.109 Unspecified injury of other muscle(s) and tendon(s) of posterior muscle group at lower leg level, unspecified leg** ▽

  ☑6ᵗʰ **S86.11 Strain of other muscle(s) and tendon(s) of posterior muscle group at lower leg level**

    ☑7ᵗʰ **S86.111 Strain of other muscle(s) and tendon(s) of posterior muscle group at lower leg level, right leg**

    ☑7ᵗʰ **S86.112 Strain of other muscle(s) and tendon(s) of posterior muscle group at lower leg level, left leg**

    ☑7ᵗʰ **S86.119 Strain of other muscle(s) and tendon(s) of posterior muscle group at lower leg level, unspecified leg** ▽

  ☑6ᵗʰ **S86.12 Laceration of other muscle(s) and tendon(s) of posterior muscle group at lower leg level**

    ☑7ᵗʰ **S86.121 Laceration of other muscle(s) and tendon(s) of posterior muscle group at lower leg level, right leg**

    ☑7ᵗʰ **S86.122 Laceration of other muscle(s) and tendon(s) of posterior muscle group at lower leg level, left leg**

    ☑7ᵗʰ **S86.129 Laceration of other muscle(s) and tendon(s) of posterior muscle group at lower leg level, unspecified leg** ▽

  ☑6ᵗʰ **S86.19 Other injury of other muscle(s) and tendon(s) of posterior muscle group at lower leg level**

    ☑7ᵗʰ **S86.191 Other injury of other muscle(s) and tendon(s) of posterior muscle group at lower leg level, right leg**

    ☑7ᵗʰ **S86.192 Other injury of other muscle(s) and tendon(s) of posterior muscle group at lower leg level, left leg**

    ☑7ᵗʰ **S86.199 Other injury of other muscle(s) and tendon(s) of posterior muscle group at lower leg level, unspecified leg** ▽

☑5ᵗʰ **S86.2 Injury of muscle(s) and tendon(s) of anterior muscle group at lower leg level**

  ☑6ᵗʰ **S86.20 Unspecified injury of muscle(s) and tendon(s) of anterior muscle group at lower leg level**

    ☑7ᵗʰ **S86.201 Unspecified injury of muscle(s) and tendon(s) of anterior muscle group at lower leg level, right leg** ▽

    ☑7ᵗʰ **S86.202 Unspecified injury of muscle(s) and tendon(s) of anterior muscle group at lower leg level, left leg** ▽

    ☑7ᵗʰ **S86.209 Unspecified injury of muscle(s) and tendon(s) of anterior muscle group at lower leg level, unspecified leg** ▽

  ☑6ᵗʰ **S86.21 Strain of muscle(s) and tendon(s) of anterior muscle group at lower leg level**

    ☑7ᵗʰ **S86.211 Strain of muscle(s) and tendon(s) of anterior muscle group at lower leg level, right leg**

    ☑7ᵗʰ **S86.212 Strain of muscle(s) and tendon(s) of anterior muscle group at lower leg level, left leg**

    ☑7ᵗʰ **S86.219 Strain of muscle(s) and tendon(s) of anterior muscle group at lower leg level, unspecified leg** ▽

  ☑6ᵗʰ **S86.22 Laceration of muscle(s) and tendon(s) of anterior muscle group at lower leg level**

    ☑7ᵗʰ **S86.221 Laceration of muscle(s) and tendon(s) of anterior muscle group at lower leg level, right leg**

    ☑7ᵗʰ **S86.222 Laceration of muscle(s) and tendon(s) of anterior muscle group at lower leg level, left leg**

    ☑7ᵗʰ **S86.229 Laceration of muscle(s) and tendon(s) of anterior muscle group at lower leg level, unspecified leg** ▽

  ☑6ᵗʰ **S86.29 Other injury of muscle(s) and tendon(s) of anterior muscle group at lower leg level**

    ☑7ᵗʰ **S86.291 Other injury of muscle(s) and tendon(s) of anterior muscle group at lower leg level, right leg**

    ☑7ᵗʰ **S86.292 Other injury of muscle(s) and tendon(s) of anterior muscle group at lower leg level, left leg**

☑ Additional Character Req   ☑x7ᵗʰ Placeholder Alert   Manifestation   HCC CMS-HCC Condition   ▽ Unspecified Code   ▶◀ Revised Text   ● New Code   ▲ Revised Code Title

Chapter 19. Injury, Poisoning, and Certain Other Consequences of External Causes *(side margin)*

√7ᵗʰ **S86.299** Other injury of muscle(s) and tendon(s) ▽ of anterior muscle group at lower leg level, unspecified leg

√5ᵗʰ **S86.3** Injury of muscle(s) and tendon(s) of peroneal muscle group at lower leg level

  √6ᵗʰ **S86.30** Unspecified injury of muscle(s) and tendon(s) of peroneal muscle group at lower leg level

    √7ᵗʰ **S86.301** Unspecified injury of muscle(s) and ▽ tendon(s) of peroneal muscle group at lower leg level, right leg

    √7ᵗʰ **S86.302** Unspecified injury of muscle(s) and ▽ tendon(s) of peroneal muscle group at lower leg level, left leg

    √7ᵗʰ **S86.309** Unspecified injury of muscle(s) and ▽ tendon(s) of peroneal muscle group at lower leg level, unspecified leg

  √6ᵗʰ **S86.31** Strain of muscle(s) and tendon(s) of peroneal muscle group at lower leg level

    √7ᵗʰ **S86.311** Strain of muscle(s) and tendon(s) of peroneal muscle group at lower leg level, right leg

    √7ᵗʰ **S86.312** Strain of muscle(s) and tendon(s) of peroneal muscle group at lower leg level, left leg

    √7ᵗʰ **S86.319** Strain of muscle(s) and tendon(s) of ▽ peroneal muscle group at lower leg level, unspecified leg

  √6ᵗʰ **S86.32** Laceration of muscle(s) and tendon(s) of peroneal muscle group at lower leg level

    √7ᵗʰ **S86.321** Laceration of muscle(s) and tendon(s) of peroneal muscle group at lower leg level, right leg

    √7ᵗʰ **S86.322** Laceration of muscle(s) and tendon(s) of peroneal muscle group at lower leg level, left leg

    √7ᵗʰ **S86.329** Laceration of muscle(s) and tendon(s) ▽ of peroneal muscle group at lower leg level, unspecified leg

  √6ᵗʰ **S86.39** Other injury of muscle(s) and tendon(s) of peroneal muscle group at lower leg level

    √7ᵗʰ **S86.391** Other injury of muscle(s) and tendon(s) of peroneal muscle group at lower leg level, right leg

    √7ᵗʰ **S86.392** Other injury of muscle(s) and tendon(s) of peroneal muscle group at lower leg level, left leg

    √7ᵗʰ **S86.399** Other injury of muscle(s) and tendon(s) ▽ of peroneal muscle group at lower leg level, unspecified leg

√5ᵗʰ **S86.8** Injury of other muscles and tendons at lower leg level

  √6ᵗʰ **S86.80** Unspecified injury of other muscles and tendons at lower leg level

    √7ᵗʰ **S86.801** Unspecified injury of other muscle(s) ▽ and tendon(s) at lower leg level, right leg

    √7ᵗʰ **S86.802** Unspecified injury of other muscle(s) ▽ and tendon(s) at lower leg level, left leg

    √7ᵗʰ **S86.809** Unspecified injury of other muscle(s) ▽ and tendon(s) at lower leg level, unspecified leg

  √6ᵗʰ **S86.81** Strain of other muscles and tendons at lower leg level

    √7ᵗʰ **S86.811** Strain of other muscle(s) and tendon(s) at lower leg level, right leg

    √7ᵗʰ **S86.812** Strain of other muscle(s) and tendon(s) at lower leg level, left leg

    √7ᵗʰ **S86.819** Strain of other muscle(s) and tendon(s) ▽ at lower leg level, unspecified leg

  √6ᵗʰ **S86.82** Laceration of other muscles and tendons at lower leg level

    √7ᵗʰ **S86.821** Laceration of other muscle(s) and tendon(s) at lower leg level, right leg

    √7ᵗʰ **S86.822** Laceration of other muscle(s) and tendon(s) at lower leg level, left leg

    √7ᵗʰ **S86.829** Laceration of other muscle(s) and ▽ tendon(s) at lower leg level, unspecified leg

√6ᵗʰ **S86.89** Other injury of other muscles and tendons at lower leg level

  √7ᵗʰ **S86.891** Other injury of other muscle(s) and tendon(s) at lower leg level, right leg

  √7ᵗʰ **S86.892** Other injury of other muscle(s) and tendon(s) at lower leg level, left leg

  √7ᵗʰ **S86.899** Other injury of other muscle(s) and tendon(s) at lower leg level, unspecified leg

√5ᵗʰ **S86.9** Injury of unspecified muscle and tendon at lower leg level

  √6ᵗʰ **S86.90** Unspecified injury of unspecified muscle and tendon at lower leg level

    √7ᵗʰ **S86.901** Unspecified injury of unspecified ▽ muscle(s) and tendon(s) at lower leg level, right leg

    √7ᵗʰ **S86.902** Unspecified injury of unspecified ▽ muscle(s) and tendon(s) at lower leg level, left leg

    √7ᵗʰ **S86.909** Unspecified injury of unspecified ▽ muscle(s) and tendon(s) at lower leg evel, unspecified leg

  √6ᵗʰ **S86.91** Strain of unspecified muscle and tendon at lower leg level

    √7ᵗʰ **S86.911** Strain of unspecified muscle(s) and ▽ tendon(s) at lower leg level, right leg

    √7ᵗʰ **S86.912** Strain of unspecified muscle(s) and ▽ tendon(s) at lower leg level, left leg

    √7ᵗʰ **S86.919** Strain of unspecified muscle(s) and ▽ tendon(s) at lower leg level, unspecified leg

  √6ᵗʰ **S86.92** Laceration of unspecified muscle and tendon at lower leg level

    √7ᵗʰ **S86.921** Laceration of unspecified muscle(s) ▽ and tendon(s) at lower leg level, right leg

    √7ᵗʰ **S86.922** Laceration of unspecified muscle(s) ▽ and tendon(s) at lower leg level, left leg

    √7ᵗʰ **S86.929** Laceration of unspecified muscle(s) ▽ and tendon(s) at lower leg level, unspecified leg

  √6ᵗʰ **S86.99** Other injury of unspecified muscle and tendon at lower leg level

    √7ᵗʰ **S86.991** Other injury of unspecified muscle(s) ▽ and tendon(s) at lower leg level, right leg

    √7ᵗʰ **S86.992** Other injury of unspecified muscle(s) ▽ and tendon(s) at lower leg level, left leg

    √7ᵗʰ **S86.999** Other injury of unspecified muscle(s) ▽ and tendon(s) at lower leg level, unspecified leg

√4ᵗʰ **S87** **Crushing injury of lower leg**

Use additional code(s) for all associated injuries

EXCLUDES 2   crushing injury of ankle and foot (S97.-)

The appropriate 7th character is to be added to each code from category S87.
A   initial encounter
D   subsequent encounter
S   sequela

√5ᵗʰ **S87.0** Crushing injury of knee

  √x7ᵗʰ **S87.00** Crushing injury of unspecified knee ▽

  √x7ᵗʰ **S87.01** Crushing injury of right knee

  √x7ᵗʰ **S87.02** Crushing injury of left knee

√5ᵗʰ **S87.8** Crushing injury of lower leg

  √x7ᵗʰ **S87.80** Crushing injury of unspecified lower leg ▽

  √x7ᵗʰ **S87.81** Crushing injury of right lower leg

  √x7ᵗʰ **S87.82** Crushing injury of left lower leg

EXCLUDES 1 Not coded here   EXCLUDES 2 Not included here   N Newborn Age: 0   P Pediatric Age: 0-17   M Maternity Age: 12-55   A Adult Age: 15-124

1022   ICD-10-CM 2018

✓4ᵗʰ S88 Traumatic amputation of lower leg

An amputation not identified as partial or complete should be coded to complete.

EXCLUDES 1 *traumatic amputation of ankle and foot (S98.-)*

The appropriate 7th character is to be added to each code from category S88.
A   initial encounter
D   subsequent encounter
S   sequela

✓5ᵗʰ S88.0 Traumatic amputation at knee level

    ✓6ᵗʰ S88.01 Complete traumatic amputation at knee level

        ✓7ᵗʰ S88.011 Complete traumatic amputation at knee level, right lower leg HCC

        ✓7ᵗʰ S88.012 Complete traumatic amputation at knee level, left lower leg HCC

        ✓7ᵗʰ S88.019 Complete traumatic amputation at knee level, unspecified lower leg HCC ▽

    ✓6ᵗʰ S88.02 Partial traumatic amputation at knee level

        ✓7ᵗʰ S88.021 Partial traumatic amputation at knee level, right lower leg HCC

        ✓7ᵗʰ S88.022 Partial traumatic amputation at knee level, left lower leg HCC

        ✓7ᵗʰ S88.029 Partial traumatic amputation at knee level, unspecified lower leg HCC ▽

✓5ᵗʰ S88.1 Traumatic amputation at level between knee and ankle

    ✓6ᵗʰ S88.11 Complete traumatic amputation at level between knee and ankle

        ✓7ᵗʰ S88.111 Complete traumatic amputation at level between knee and ankle, right lower leg HCC

        ✓7ᵗʰ S88.112 Complete traumatic amputation at level between knee and ankle, left lower leg HCC

        ✓7ᵗʰ S88.119 Complete traumatic amputation at level between knee and ankle, unspecified lower leg HCC ▽

    ✓6ᵗʰ S88.12 Partial traumatic amputation at level between knee and ankle

        ✓7ᵗʰ S88.121 Partial traumatic amputation at level between knee and ankle, right lower leg HCC

        ✓7ᵗʰ S88.122 Partial traumatic amputation at level between knee and ankle, left lower leg HCC

        ✓7ᵗʰ S88.129 Partial traumatic amputation at level between knee and ankle, unspecified lower leg HCC ▽

✓5ᵗʰ S88.9 Traumatic amputation of lower leg, level unspecified

    ✓6ᵗʰ S88.91 Complete traumatic amputation of lower leg, level unspecified

        ✓7ᵗʰ S88.911 Complete traumatic amputation of right lower leg, level unspecified HCC ▽

        ✓7ᵗʰ S88.912 Complete traumatic amputation of left lower leg, level unspecified HCC ▽

        ✓7ᵗʰ S88.919 Complete traumatic amputation of unspecified lower leg, level unspecified HCC ▽

    ✓6ᵗʰ S88.92 Partial traumatic amputation of lower leg, level unspecified

        ✓7ᵗʰ S88.921 Partial traumatic amputation of right lower leg, level unspecified HCC ▽

        ✓7ᵗʰ S88.922 Partial traumatic amputation of left lower leg, level unspecified HCC ▽

        ✓7ᵗʰ S88.929 Partial traumatic amputation of unspecified lower leg, level unspecified HCC ▽

✓4ᵗʰ S89 Other and unspecified injuries of lower leg

NOTE A fracture not indicated as open or closed should be coded to closed.

EXCLUDES 2 *other and unspecified injuries of ankle and foot (S99.-)*

AHA: 2015, 3Q, 37-39

The appropriate 7th character is to be added to each code from subcategories S89.0, S89.1, S89.2, and S89.3.
A   initial encounter for closed fracture
D   subsequent encounter for fracture with routine healing
G   subsequent encounter for fracture with delayed healing
K   subsequent encounter for fracture with nonunion
P   subsequent encounter for fracture with malunion
S   sequela

✓5ᵗʰ S89.0 Physeal fracture of upper end of tibia

    ✓6ᵗʰ S89.00 Unspecified physeal fracture of upper end of tibia

        ✓7ᵗʰ S89.001 Unspecified physeal fracture of upper end of right tibia ▽

        ✓7ᵗʰ S89.002 Unspecified physeal fracture of upper end of left tibia ▽

        ✓7ᵗʰ S89.009 Unspecified physeal fracture of upper end of unspecified tibia ▽

    ✓6ᵗʰ S89.01 Salter-Harris Type I physeal fracture of upper end of tibia

        ✓7ᵗʰ S89.011 Salter-Harris Type I physeal fracture of upper end of right tibia

        ✓7ᵗʰ S89.012 Salter-Harris Type I physeal fracture of upper end of left tibia

        ✓7ᵗʰ S89.019 Salter-Harris Type I physeal fracture of upper end of unspecified tibia ▽

    ✓6ᵗʰ S89.02 Salter-Harris Type II physeal fracture of upper end of tibia

        ✓7ᵗʰ S89.021 Salter-Harris Type II physeal fracture of upper end of right tibia

        ✓7ᵗʰ S89.022 Salter-Harris Type II physeal fracture of upper end of left tibia

        ✓7ᵗʰ S89.029 Salter-Harris Type II physeal fracture of upper end of unspecified tibia ▽

    ✓6ᵗʰ S89.03 Salter-Harris Type III physeal fracture of upper end of tibia

        ✓7ᵗʰ S89.031 Salter-Harris Type III physeal fracture of upper end of right tibia

        ✓7ᵗʰ S89.032 Salter-Harris Type III physeal fracture of upper end of left tibia

        ✓7ᵗʰ S89.039 Salter-Harris Type III physeal fracture of upper end of unspecified tibia ▽

    ✓6ᵗʰ S89.04 Salter-Harris Type IV physeal fracture of upper end of tibia

        ✓7ᵗʰ S89.041 Salter-Harris Type IV physeal fracture of upper end of right tibia

        ✓7ᵗʰ S89.042 Salter-Harris Type IV physeal fracture of upper end of left tibia

        ✓7ᵗʰ S89.049 Salter-Harris Type IV physeal fracture of upper end of unspecified tibia ▽

    ✓6ᵗʰ S89.09 Other physeal fracture of upper end of tibia

        ✓7ᵗʰ S89.091 Other physeal fracture of upper end of right tibia

        ✓7ᵗʰ S89.092 Other physeal fracture of upper end of left tibia

        ✓7ᵗʰ S89.099 Other physeal fracture of upper end of unspecified tibia ▽

✓5ᵗʰ S89.1 Physeal fracture of lower end of tibia

    ✓6ᵗʰ S89.10 Unspecified physeal fracture of lower end of tibia

        ✓7ᵗʰ S89.101 Unspecified physeal fracture of lower end of right tibia ▽

        ✓7ᵗʰ S89.102 Unspecified physeal fracture of lower end of left tibia ▽

        ✓7ᵗʰ S89.109 Unspecified physeal fracture of lower end of unspecified tibia ▽

    ✓6ᵗʰ S89.11 Salter-Harris Type I physeal fracture of ower end of tibia

        ✓7ᵗʰ S89.111 Salter-Harris Type I physeal fracture of lower end of right tibia

        ✓7ᵗʰ S89.112 Salter-Harris Type I physeal fracture of lower end of left tibia

☑ Additional Character Req   ✓x7ᵗʰ Placeholder Alert   Manifestation   HCC CMS-HCC Condition   ▽ Unspecified Code   ▶◀ Revised Text   ● New Code   ▲ Revised Code Title

ICD-10-CM 2018   1023

✓7ᵗʰ **S89.119** Salter-Harris Type I physeal fracture of ▽
lower end of unspecified tibia

✓6ᵗʰ **S89.12** Salter-Harris Type II physeal fracture of lower end of tibia

✓7ᵗʰ **S89.121** Salter-Harris Type II physeal fracture of lower end of right tibia

✓7ᵗʰ **S89.122** Salter-Harris Type II physeal fracture of lower end of left tibia

✓7ᵗʰ **S89.129** Salter-Harris Type II physeal fracture of ▽
lower end of unspecified tibia

✓6ᵗʰ **S89.13** Salter-Harris Type III physeal fracture of lower end of tibia

> *EXCLUDES 1*   fracture of medial malleolus (adult) (S82.5-)

✓7ᵗʰ **S89.131** Salter-Harris Type III physeal fracture of lower end of right tibia

✓7ᵗʰ **S89.132** Salter-Harris Type III physeal fracture of lower end of left tibia

✓7ᵗʰ **S89.139** Salter-Harris Type III physeal fracture ▽
of lower end of unspecified tibia

✓6ᵗʰ **S89.14** Salter-Harris Type IV physeal fracture of lower end of tibia

> *EXCLUDES 1*   fracture of medial malleolus (adult) (S82.5-)

✓7ᵗʰ **S89.141** Salter-Harris Type IV physeal fracture of lower end of right tibia

✓7ᵗʰ **S89.142** Salter-Harris Type IV physeal fracture of lower end of left tibia

✓7ᵗʰ **S89.149** Salter-Harris Type IV physeal fracture ▽
of lower end of unspecified tibia

✓6ᵗʰ **S89.19** Other physeal fracture of lower end of tibia

✓7ᵗʰ **S89.191** Other physeal fracture of lower end of right tibia

✓7ᵗʰ **S89.192** Other physeal fracture of lower end of left tibia

✓7ᵗʰ **S89.199** Other physeal fracture of lower end of ▽
unspecified tibia

✓5ᵗʰ **S89.2** Physeal fracture of upper end of fibula

✓6ᵗʰ **S89.20** Unspecified physeal fracture of upper end of fibula

✓7ᵗʰ **S89.201** Unspecified physeal fracture of upper ▽
end of right fibula

✓7ᵗʰ **S89.202** Unspecified physeal fracture of upper ▽
end of left fibula

✓7ᵗʰ **S89.209** Unspecified physeal fracture of upper ▽
end of unspecified fibula

✓6ᵗʰ **S89.21** Salter-Harris Type I physeal fracture of upper end of fibula

✓7ᵗʰ **S89.211** Salter-Harris Type I physeal fracture of upper end of right fibula

✓7ᵗʰ **S89.212** Salter-Harris Type I physeal fracture of upper end of left fibula

✓7ᵗʰ **S89.219** Salter-Harris Type I physeal fracture of ▽
upper end of unspecified fibula

✓6ᵗʰ **S89.22** Salter-Harris Type II physeal fracture of upper end of fibula

✓7ᵗʰ **S89.221** Salter-Harris Type II physeal fracture of upper end of right fibula

✓7ᵗʰ **S89.222** Salter-Harris Type II physeal fracture of upper end of left fibula

✓7ᵗʰ **S89.229** Salter-Harris Type II physeal fracture of ▽
upper end of unspecified fibula

✓6ᵗʰ **S89.29** Other physeal fracture of upper end of fibula

✓7ᵗʰ **S89.291** Other physeal fracture of upper end of right fibula

✓7ᵗʰ **S89.292** Other physeal fracture of upper end of left fibula

✓7ᵗʰ **S89.299** Other physeal fracture of upper end of ▽
unspecified fibula

✓5ᵗʰ **S89.3** Physeal fracture of lower end of fibula

✓6ᵗʰ **S89.30** Unspecified physeal fracture of lower end of fibula

✓7ᵗʰ **S89.301** Unspecified physeal fracture of lower ▽
end of right fibula

✓7ᵗʰ **S89.302** Unspecified physeal fracture of lower ▽
end of left fibula

✓7ᵗʰ **S89.309** Unspecified physeal fracture of lower ▽
end of unspecified fibula

✓6ᵗʰ **S89.31** Salter-Harris Type I physeal fracture of lower end of fibula

✓7ᵗʰ **S89.311** Salter-Harris Type I physeal fracture of lower end of right fibula

✓7ᵗʰ **S89.312** Salter-Harris Type I physeal fracture of lower end of left fibula

✓7ᵗʰ **S89.319** Salter-Harris Type I physeal fracture of ▽
lower end of unspecified fibula

✓6ᵗʰ **S89.32** Salter-Harris Type II physeal fracture of lower end of fibula

✓7ᵗʰ **S89.321** Salter-Harris Type II physeal fracture of lower end of right fibula

✓7ᵗʰ **S89.322** Salter-Harris Type II physeal fracture of lower end of left fibula

✓7ᵗʰ **S89.329** Salter-Harris Type II physeal fracture ▽
of lower end of unspecified fibula

✓6ᵗʰ **S89.39** Other physeal fracture of lower end of fibula

✓7ᵗʰ **S89.391** Other physeal fracture of lower end of right fibula

✓7ᵗʰ **S89.392** Other physeal fracture of lower end of left fibula

✓7ᵗʰ **S89.399** Other physeal fracture of lower end of ▽
unspecified fibula

✓5ᵗʰ **S89.8** Other specified injuries of lower leg

> The appropriate 7th character is to be added to each code in subcategory S89.8.
> A   initial encounter
> D   subsequent encounter
> S   sequela

✓x7ᵗʰ **S89.80** Other specified injuries of unspecified lower leg ▽

✓x7ᵗʰ **S89.81** Other specified injuries of right lower leg

✓x7ᵗʰ **S89.82** Other specified injuries of left lower leg

✓5ᵗʰ **S89.9** Unspecified injury of lower leg

> The appropriate 7th character is to be added to each code in subcategory S89.9.
> A   initial encounter
> D   subsequent encounter
> S   sequela

✓x7ᵗʰ **S89.90** Unspecified injury of unspecified lower leg ▽

S89.91 Unspecified injury of right lower leg ▽

✓x7ᵗʰ **S89.92** Unspecified injury of left lower leg ▽

Injuries to the ankle and foot (S90-S99)

> *EXCLUDES 2*   burns and corrosions (T20-T32)
> fracture of ankle and malleolus (S82.-)
> frostbite (T33-T34)
> insect bite or sting, venomous (T63.4)

✓4ᵗʰ **S90** Superficial injury of ankle, foot and toes

> The appropriate 7th character is to be added to each code from category S90.
> A   initial encounter
> D   subsequent encounter
> S   sequela

✓5ᵗʰ **S90.0** Contusion of ankle

✓x7ᵗʰ **S90.00** Contusion of unspecified ankle ▽

✓x7ᵗʰ **S90.01** Contusion of right ankle

✓x7ᵗʰ **S90.02** Contusion of left ankle

✓5ᵗʰ **S90.1** Contusion of toe without damage to nail

✓6ᵗʰ **S90.11** Contusion of great toe without damage to nail

✓7ᵗʰ **S90.111** Contusion of right great toe without damage to nail

✓7ᵗʰ **S90.112** Contusion of left great toe without damage to nail

✓7ᵗʰ **S90.119** Contusion of unspecified great toe ▽
without damage to nail

✓6ᵗʰ **S90.12** Contusion of lesser toe without damage to nail

✓7ᵗʰ **S90.121** Contusion of right lesser toe(s) without damage to nail

✓7ᵗʰ **S90.122** Contusion of left lesser toe(s) without damage to nail

EXCLUDES 1 Not coded here   *EXCLUDES 2* Not included here   N Newborn Age: 0   P Pediatric Age: 0-17   M Maternity Age: 12-55   A Adult Age: 15-124

1024   ICD-10-CM 2018

✓7ᵗʰ **S90.129 Contusion of unspecified lesser toe(s) without damage to nail** ▽
  Contusion of toe NOS

✓5ᵗʰ **S90.2 Contusion of toe with damage to nail**

✓6ᵗʰ **S90.21 Contusion of great toe with damage to nail**

✓7ᵗʰ **S90.211 Contusion of right great toe with damage to nail**

✓7ᵗʰ **S90.212 Contusion of left great toe with damage to nail**

✓7ᵗʰ **S90.219 Contusion of unspecified great toe with** ▽ **damage to nail**

✓6ᵗʰ **S90.22 Contusion of lesser toe with damage to nail**

✓7ᵗʰ **S90.221 Contusion of right lesser toe(s) with damage to nail**

✓7ᵗʰ **S90.222 Contusion of left lesser toe(s) with damage to nail**

✓7ᵗʰ **S90.229 Contusion of unspecified lesser toe(s)** ▽ **with damage to nail**

✓5ᵗʰ **S90.3 Contusion of foot**
  EXCLUDES 2 *contusion of toes (S90.1-, S90.2-)*

✓x7ᵗʰ **S90.30 Contusion of unspecified foot** ▽
  Contusion of foot NOS

✓x7ᵗʰ **S90.31 Contusion of right foot**

✓x7ᵗʰ **S90.32 Contusion of left foot**

✓5ᵗʰ **S90.4 Other superficial injuries of toe**

✓6ᵗʰ **S90.41 Abrasion of toe**

✓7ᵗʰ **S90.411 Abrasion, right great toe**

✓7ᵗʰ **S90.412 Abrasion, left great toe**

✓7ᵗʰ **S90.413 Abrasion, unspecified great toe** ▽

✓7ᵗʰ **S90.414 Abrasion, right lesser toe(s)**

✓7ᵗʰ **S90.415 Abrasion, left lesser toe(s)**

✓7ᵗʰ **S90.416 Abrasion, unspecified lesser toe(s)** ▽

✓6ᵗʰ **S90.42 Blister (nonthermal) of toe**

✓7ᵗʰ **S90.421 Blister (nonthermal), right great toe**

✓7ᵗʰ **S90.422 Blister (nonthermal), left great toe**

✓7ᵗʰ **S90.423 Blister (nonthermal), unspecified great** ▽ **toe**

✓7ᵗʰ **S90.424 Blister (nonthermal), right lesser toe(s)**

✓7ᵗʰ **S90.425 Blister (nonthermal), left lesser toe(s)**

✓7ᵗʰ **S90.426 Blister (nonthermal), unspecified lesser** ▽ **toe(s)**

✓6ᵗʰ **S90.44 External constriction of toe**
  Hair tourniquet syndrome of toe

✓7ᵗʰ **S90.441 External constriction, right great toe**

✓7ᵗʰ **S90.442 External constriction, left great toe**

✓7ᵗʰ **S90.443 External constriction, unspecified** ▽ **great toe**

✓7ᵗʰ **S90.444 External constriction, right lesser toe(s)**

✓7ᵗʰ **S90.445 External constriction, left lesser toe(s)**

✓7ᵗʰ **S90.446 External constriction, unspecified** ▽ **lesser toe(s)**

✓6ᵗʰ **S90.45 Superficial foreign body of toe**
  Splinter in the toe

✓7ᵗʰ **S90.451 Superficial foreign body, right great toe**

✓7ᵗʰ **S90.452 Superficial foreign body, left great toe**

✓7ᵗʰ **S90.453 Superficial foreign body, unspecified** ▽ **great toe**

✓7ᵗʰ **S90.454 Superficial foreign body, right lesser toe(s)**

✓7ᵗʰ **S90.455 Superficial foreign body, left lesser toe(s)**

✓7ᵗʰ **S90.456 Superficial foreign body, unspecified** ▽ **lesser toe(s)**

✓6ᵗʰ **S90.46 Insect bite (nonvenomous) of toe**

✓7ᵗʰ **S90.461 Insect bite (nonvenomous), right great toe**

✓7ᵗʰ **S90.462 Insect bite (nonvenomous), left great toe**

✓7ᵗʰ **S90.463 Insect bite (nonvenomous), unspecified** ▽ **great toe**

✓7ᵗʰ **S90.464 Insect bite (nonvenomous), right lesser toe(s)**

✓7ᵗʰ **S90.465 Insect bite (nonvenomous), left lesser toe(s)**

✓7ᵗʰ **S90.466 Insect bite (nonvenomous), unspecified** ▽ **lesser toe(s)**

✓6ᵗʰ **S90.47 Other superficial bite of toe**
  EXCLUDES 1 *open bite of toe (S91.15-, S91.25-)*

✓7ᵗʰ **S90.471 Other superficial bite of right great toe**

✓7ᵗʰ **S90.472 Other superficial bite of left great toe**

✓7ᵗʰ **S90.473 Other superficial bite of unspecified great toe**

✓7ᵗʰ **S90.474 Other superficial bite of right lesser toe(s)**

✓7ᵗʰ **S90.475 Other superficial bite of left lesser toe(s)**

✓7ᵗʰ **S90.476 Other superficial bite of unspecified** ▽ **lesser toe(s)**

✓5ᵗʰ **S90.5 Other superficial injuries of ankle**

✓6ᵗʰ **S90.51 Abrasion of ankle**

✓7ᵗʰ **S90.511 Abrasion, right ankle**

✓7ᵗʰ **S90.512 Abrasion, left ankle**

✓7ᵗʰ **S90.519 Abrasion, unspecified ankle** ▽

✓6ᵗʰ **S90.52 Blister (nonthermal) of ankle**

✓7ᵗʰ **S90.521 Blister (nonthermal), right ankle**

✓7ᵗʰ **S90.522 Blister (nonthermal), left ankle**

✓7ᵗʰ **S90.529 Blister (nonthermal), unspecified ankle** ▽

✓6ᵗʰ **S90.54 External constriction of ankle**

✓7ᵗʰ **S90.541 External constriction, right ankle**

✓7ᵗʰ **S90.542 External constriction, left ankle**

✓7ᵗʰ **S90.549 External constriction, unspecified ankle** ▽

✓6ᵗʰ **S90.55 Superficial foreign body of ankle**
  Splinter in the ankle

✓7ᵗʰ **S90.551 Superficial foreign body, right ankle**

✓7ᵗʰ **S90.552 Superficial foreign body, left ankle**

✓7ᵗʰ **S90.559 Superficial foreign body, unspecified** ▽ **ankle**

✓6ᵗʰ **S90.56 Insect bite (nonvenomous) of ankle**

✓7ᵗʰ **S90.561 Insect bite (nonvenomous), right ankle**

✓7ᵗʰ **S90.562 Insect bite (nonvenomous), left ankle**

✓7ᵗʰ **S90.569 Insect bite (nonvenomous), unspecified** ▽ **ankle**

✓6ᵗʰ **S90.57 Other superficial bite of ankle**
  EXCLUDES 1 *open bite of ankle (S91.05-)*

✓7ᵗʰ **S90.571 Other superficial bite of ankle, right ankle**

✓7ᵗʰ **S90.572 Other superficial bite of ankle, left ankle**

✓7ᵗʰ **S90.579 Other superficial bite of ankle,** ▽ **unspecified ankle**

✓5ᵗʰ **S90.8 Other superficial injuries of foot**

✓6ᵗʰ **S90.81 Abrasion of foot**

✓7ᵗʰ **S90.811 Abrasion, right foot**

✓7ᵗʰ **S90.812 Abrasion, left foot**

✓7ᵗʰ **S90.819 Abrasion, unspecified foot** ▽

✓6ᵗʰ **S90.82 Blister (nonthermal) of foot**

✓7ᵗʰ **S90.821 Blister (nonthermal), right foot**

✓7ᵗʰ **S90.822 Blister (nonthermal), left foot**

✓7ᵗʰ **S90.829 Blister (nonthermal), unspecified foot** ▽

✓6ᵗʰ **S90.84 External constriction of foot**

✓7ᵗʰ **S90.841 External constriction, right foot**

✓7ᵗʰ **S90.842 External constriction, left foot**

✓7ᵗʰ **S90.849 External constriction, unspecified foot** ▽

✓6ᵗʰ **S90.85 Superficial foreign body of foot**
  Splinter in the foot

✓7ᵗʰ **S90.851 Superficial foreign body, right foot**

✓7ᵗʰ **S90.852 Superficial foreign body, left foot**

✓7ᵗʰ **S90.859 Superficial foreign body, unspecified** ▽ **foot**

✓6ᵗʰ **S90.86 Insect bite (nonvenomous) of foot**

✓7ᵗʰ **S90.861 Insect bite (nonvenomous), right foot**

✓7ᵗʰ **S90.862 Insect bite (nonvenomous), left foot**

✓7ᵗʰ **S90.869 Insect bite (nonvenomous), unspecified** ▽ **foot**

✓6ᵗʰ **S90.87 Other superficial bite of foot**
  EXCLUDES 1 *open bite of foot (S91.35-)*

✓7ᵗʰ **S90.871 Other superficial bite of right foot**

✓ Additional Character Req   ✓x7ᵗʰ Placeholder Alert   Manifestation   HCC CMS-HCC Condition   ▽ Unspecified Code   ►◄ Revised Text   ● New Code   ▲ Revised Code Title

ICD-10-CM 2018   1025

✓7ᵗʰ **S90.872** Other superficial bite of left foot

✓7ᵗʰ **S90.879** Other superficial bite of unspecified foot ▽

✓5ᵗʰ **S90.9 Unspecified superficial injury of ankle, foot and toe**

  ✓6ᵗʰ **S90.91 Unspecified superficial injury of** ankle

    ✓7ᵗʰ **S90.911** Unspecified superficial injury of right ankle ▽

    ✓7ᵗʰ **S90.912** Unspecified superficial injury of left ankle ▽

    ✓7ᵗʰ **S90.919** Unspecified superficial injury of unspecified ankle ▽

  ✓6ᵗʰ **S90.92 Unspecified superficial injury of** foot

    ✓7ᵗʰ **S90.921** Unspecified superficial injury of right foot ▽

    ✓7ᵗʰ **S90.922** Unspecified superficial injury of left foot ▽

    ✓7ᵗʰ **S90.929** Unspecified superficial injury of unspecified foot ▽

  ✓6ᵗʰ **S90.93 Unspecified superficial injury of** toes

    ✓7ᵗʰ **S90.931** Unspecified superficial injury of right great toe ▽

    ✓7ᵗʰ **S90.932** Unspecified superficial injury of left great toe ▽

    ✓7ᵗʰ **S90.933** Unspecified superficial injury of unspecified great toe ▽

    ✓7ᵗʰ **S90.934** Unspecified superficial injury of right lesser toe(s) ▽

    ✓7ᵗʰ **S90.935** Unspecified superficial injury of left lesser toe(s) ▽

    ✓7ᵗʰ **S90.936** Unspecified superficial injury of unspecified lesser toe(s) ▽

✓4ᵗʰ **S91 Open wound of ankle, foot and toes**

  Code also any associated wound infection

  EXCLUDES 1   open fracture of ankle, foot and toes (S92-with 7th character B)

     traumatic amputation of ankle and foot (S98.-)

  The appropriate 7th character is to be added to each code from category S91.

  A   initial encounter

  D   subsequent encounter

  S   sequela

✓5ᵗʰ **S91.0 Open wound of** ankle

  ✓6ᵗʰ **S91.00 Unspecified open wound of ankle**

    ✓7ᵗʰ **S91.001** Unspecified open wound, right ankle ▽

     S91.002 Unspecified open wound, left ankle ▽

    ✓7ᵗʰ **S91.009** Unspecified open wound, unspecified ankle ▽

  ✓6ᵗʰ **S91.01 Laceration without foreign body of ankle**

    ✓7ᵗʰ **S91.011** Laceration without foreign body, right ankle

    ✓7ᵗʰ **S91.012** Laceration without foreign body, left ankle

    ✓7ᵗʰ **S91.019** Laceration without foreign body, unspecified ankle ▽

  ✓6ᵗʰ **S91.02 Laceration with foreign body of ankle**

    ✓7ᵗʰ **S91.021** Laceration with foreign body, right ankle

    ✓7ᵗʰ **S91.022** Laceration with foreign body, left ankle

    ✓7ᵗʰ **S91.029** Laceration with foreign body, unspecified ankle ▽

  ✓6ᵗʰ **S91.03 Puncture wound without foreign body of ankle**

    ✓7ᵗʰ **S91.031** Puncture wound without foreign body, right ankle

    ✓7ᵗʰ **S91.032** Puncture wound without foreign body, left ankle

    ✓7ᵗʰ **S91.039** Puncture wound without foreign body, unspecified ankle ▽

  ✓6ᵗʰ **S91.04 Puncture wound with foreign body of ankle**

    ✓7ᵗʰ **S91.041** Puncture wound with foreign body, right ankle

    ✓7ᵗʰ **S91.042** Puncture wound with foreign body, left ankle

    ✓7ᵗʰ **S91.049** Puncture wound with foreign body, unspecified ankle ▽

✓6ᵗʰ **S91.05 Open bite of ankle**

  EXCLUDES 1   superficial bite of ankle (S90.56-, S90.57-)

  ✓7ᵗʰ **S91.051** Open bite, right ankle

  ✓7ᵗʰ **S91.052** Open bite, left ankle

  ✓7ᵗʰ **S91.059** Open bite, unspecified ankle ▽

✓5ᵗʰ **S91.1 Open wound of** toe without damage to nail

  ✓6ᵗʰ **S91.10 Unspecified open wound of toe without damage to nail**

    ✓7ᵗʰ **S91.101** Unspecified open wound of right great toe without damage to nail ▽

    ✓7ᵗʰ **S91.102** Unspecified open wound of left great toe without damage to nail ▽

    ✓7ᵗʰ **S91.103** Unspecified open wound of unspecified great toe without damage to nail ▽

    ✓7ᵗʰ **S91.104** Unspecified open wound of right lesser toe(s) without damage to nail ▽

    ✓7ᵗʰ **S91.105** Unspecified open wound of left lesser toe(s) without damage to nail ▽

    ✓7ᵗʰ **S91.106** Unspecified open wound of unspecified lesser toe(s) without damage to nail ▽

    ✓7ᵗʰ **S91.109** Unspecified open wound of unspecified toe(s) without damage to nail ▽

  ✓6ᵗʰ **S91.11 Laceration without foreign body of toe without damage to nail**

    ✓7ᵗʰ **S91.111** Laceration without foreign body of right great toe without damage to nail

    ✓7ᵗʰ **S91.112** Laceration without foreign body of left great toe without damage to nail

    ✓7ᵗʰ **S91.113** Laceration without foreign body of unspecified great toe without damage to nail ▽

    ✓7ᵗʰ **S91.114** Laceration without foreign body of right lesser toe(s) without damage to nail

    ✓7ᵗʰ **S91.115** Laceration without foreign body of left lesser toe(s) without damage to nail

    ✓7ᵗʰ **S91.116** Laceration without foreign body of unspecified lesser toe(s) without damage to nail ▽

    ✓7ᵗʰ **S91.119** Laceration without foreign body of unspecified toe without damage to nail ▽

  ✓6ᵗʰ **S91.12 Laceration with foreign body of toe without damage to nail**

    ✓7ᵗʰ **S91.121** Laceration with foreign body of right great toe without damage to nail

    ✓7ᵗʰ **S91.122** Laceration with foreign body of left great toe without damage to nail

    ✓7ᵗʰ **S91.123** Laceration with foreign body of unspecified great toe without damage to nail ▽

    ✓7ᵗʰ **S91.124** Laceration with foreign body of right lesser toe(s) without damage to nail

    ✓7ᵗʰ **S91.125** Laceration with foreign body of left lesser toe(s) without damage to nail

    ✓7ᵗʰ **S91.126** Laceration with foreign body of unspecified lesser toe(s) without damage to nail ▽

    ✓7ᵗʰ **S91.129** Laceration with foreign body of unspecified toe(s) without damage to nail ▽

  ✓6ᵗʰ **S91.13 Puncture wound without foreign body of toe without damage to nail**

    ✓7ᵗʰ **S91.131** Puncture wound without foreign body of right great toe without damage to nail

    ✓7ᵗʰ **S91.132** Puncture wound without foreign body of left great toe without damage to nail

    ✓7ᵗʰ **S91.133** Puncture wound without foreign body of unspecified great toe without damage to nail ▽

    ✓7ᵗʰ **S91.134** Puncture wound without foreign body of right lesser toe(s) without damage to nail

    ✓7ᵗʰ **S91.135** Puncture wound without foreign body of left lesser toe(s) without damage to nail

EXCLUDES 1 Not coded here   *EXCLUDES 2* Not included here   N Newborn Age: 0   P Pediatric Age: 0-17   M Maternity Age: 12-55   A Adult Age: 15-124

1026   ICD-10-CM 2018

✓7ᵗʰ **S91.136** Puncture wound without foreign body of unspecified lesser toe(s) without damage to nail ▽

✓7ᵗʰ **S91.139** Puncture wound without foreign body of unspecified toe(s) without damage to nail ▽

✓6ᵗʰ **S91.14** Puncture wound with foreign body of toe without damage to nail

✓7ᵗʰ **S91.141** Puncture wound with foreign body of right great toe without damage to nail

✓7ᵗʰ **S91.142** Puncture wound with foreign body of left great toe without damage to nail

✓7ᵗʰ **S91.143** Puncture wound with foreign body of unspecified great toe without damage to nail ▽

✓7ᵗʰ **S91.144** Puncture wound with foreign body of right lesser toe(s) without damage to nail

✓7ᵗʰ **S91.145** Puncture wound with foreign body of left lesser toe(s) without damage to nail

✓7ᵗʰ **S91.146** Puncture wound with foreign body of unspecified lesser toe(s) without damage to nail ▽

✓7ᵗʰ **S91.149** Puncture wound with foreign body of unspecified toe(s) without damage to nail ▽

✓6ᵗʰ **S91.15** Open bite of toe without damage to nail
Bite of toe NOS
EXCLUDES 1   superficial bite of toe (S90.46-, S90.47-)

✓7ᵗʰ **S91.151** Open bite of right great toe without damage to nail

✓7ᵗʰ **S91.152** Open bite of left great toe without damage to nail

✓7ᵗʰ **S91.153** Open bite of unspecified great toe without damage to nail ▽

✓7ᵗʰ **S91.154** Open bite of right lesser toe(s) without damage to nail

✓7ᵗʰ **S91.155** Open bite of left lesser toe(s) without damage to nail

✓7ᵗʰ **S91.156** Open bite of unspecified lesser toe(s) without damage to nail ▽

✓7ᵗʰ **S91.159** Open bite of unspecified toe(s) without damage to nail ▽

✓5ᵗʰ **S91.2 Open wound of toe with damage to nail**

✓6ᵗʰ **S91.20** Unspecified open wound of toe with damage to nail

✓7ᵗʰ **S91.201** Unspecified open wound of right great toe with damage to nail ▽

✓7ᵗʰ **S91.202** Unspecified open wound of left great toe with damage to nail ▽

✓7ᵗʰ **S91.203** Unspecified open wound of unspecified great toe with damage to nail ▽

✓7ᵗʰ **S91.204** Unspecified open wound of right lesser toe(s) with damage to nail ▽

✓7ᵗʰ **S91.205** Unspecified open wound of left lesser toe(s) with damage to nail ▽

✓7ᵗʰ **S91.206** Unspecified open wound of unspecified lesser toe(s) with damage to nail ▽

✓7ᵗʰ **S91.209** Unspecified open wound of unspecified toe(s) with damage to nail ▽

✓6ᵗʰ **S91.21** Laceration without foreign body of toe with damage to nail

✓7ᵗʰ **S91.211** Laceration without foreign body of right great toe with damage to nail

✓7ᵗʰ **S91.212** Laceration without foreign body of left great toe with damage to nail

✓7ᵗʰ **S91.213** Laceration without foreign body of unspecified great toe with damage to nail ▽

✓7ᵗʰ **S91.214** Laceration without foreign body of right lesser toe(s) with damage to nail

✓7ᵗʰ **S91.215** Laceration without foreign body of left lesser toe(s) with damage to nail

✓7ᵗʰ **S91.216** Laceration without foreign body of unspecified lesser toe(s) with damage to nail ▽

✓7ᵗʰ **S91.219** Laceration without foreign body of unspecified toe(s) with damage to nail ▽

✓6ᵗʰ **S91.22** Laceration with foreign body of toe with damage to nail

✓7ᵗʰ **S91.221** Laceration with foreign body of right great toe with damage to nail

✓7ᵗʰ **S91.222** Laceration with foreign body of left great toe with damage to nail

✓7ᵗʰ **S91.223** Laceration with foreign body of unspecified great toe with damage to nail ▽

✓7ᵗʰ **S91.224** Laceration with foreign body of right lesser toe(s) with damage to nail

✓7ᵗʰ **S91.225** Laceration with foreign body of left lesser toe(s) with damage to nail

✓7ᵗʰ **S91.226** Laceration with foreign body of unspecified lesser toe(s) with damage to nail ▽

✓7ᵗʰ **S91.229** Laceration with foreign body of unspecified toe(s) with damage to nail ▽

✓6ᵗʰ **S91.23** Puncture wound without foreign body of toe with damage to nail

✓7ᵗʰ **S91.231** Puncture wound without foreign body of right great toe with damage to nail

✓7ᵗʰ **S91.232** Puncture wound without foreign body of left great toe with damage to nail

✓7ᵗʰ **S91.233** Puncture wound without foreign body of unspecified great toe with damage to nail ▽

✓7ᵗʰ **S91.234** Puncture wound without foreign body of right lesser toe(s) with damage to nail

✓7ᵗʰ **S91.235** Puncture wound without foreign body of left lesser toe(s) with damage to nail

✓7ᵗʰ **S91.236** Puncture wound without foreign body of unspecified lesser toe(s) with damage to nail ▽

✓7ᵗʰ **S91.239** Puncture wound without foreign body of unspecified toe(s) with damage to nail ▽

✓6ᵗʰ **S91.24** Puncture wound with foreign body of toe with damage to nail

✓7ᵗʰ **S91.241** Puncture wound with foreign body of right great toe with damage to nail

✓7ᵗʰ **S91.242** Puncture wound with foreign body of left great toe with damage to nail

✓7ᵗʰ **S91.243** Puncture wound with foreign body of unspecified great toe with damage to nail ▽

✓7ᵗʰ **S91.244** Puncture wound with foreign body of right lesser toe(s) with damage to nail

✓7ᵗʰ **S91.245** Puncture wound with foreign body of left lesser toe(s) with damage to nail

✓7ᵗʰ **S91.246** Puncture wound with foreign body of unspecified lesser toe(s) with damage to nail ▽

✓7ᵗʰ **S91.249** Puncture wound with foreign body of unspecified toe(s) with damage to nail ▽

✓6ᵗʰ **S91.25** Open bite of toe with damage to nail
Bite of toe with damage to nail NOS
EXCLUDES 1   superficial bite of toe (S90.46-, S90.47-)

✓7ᵗʰ **S91.251** Open bite of right great toe with damage to nail

✓7ᵗʰ **S91.252** Open bite of left great toe with damage to nail

✓7ᵗʰ **S91.253** Open bite of unspecified great toe with damage to nail ▽

✓7ᵗʰ **S91.254** Open bite of right lesser toe(s) with damage to nail

✓7ᵗʰ **S91.255** Open bite of left lesser toe(s) with damage to nail

✓7ᵗʰ **S91.256** Open bite of unspecified lesser toe(s) with damage to nail ▽

✓7ᵗʰ **S91.259** Open bite of unspecified toe(s) with damage to nail ▽

✓5ᵗʰ **S91.3 Open wound of foot**

✓6ᵗʰ **S91.30** Unspecified open wound of foot

✓7ᵗʰ **S91.301** Unspecified open wound, right foot ▽

S91.302 Unspecified open wound, left foot ▽

✓7ᵗʰ **S91.309** Unspecified open wound, unspecified foot ▽

☑ Additional Character Req   ✓ₓ7ᵗʰ Placeholder Alert   Manifestation   **HCC** CMS-HCC Condition   ▽ Unspecified Code   ▶◀ Revised Text   ● New Code   ▲ Revised Code Title

✓6ᵗʰ **S91.31** Laceration without foreign body **of foot**

    ✓7ᵗʰ **S91.311** **Laceration without foreign body, right foot**

    ✓7ᵗʰ **S91.312** **Laceration without foreign body, left foot**

    ✓7ᵗʰ **S91.319** **Laceration without foreign body, unspecified foot** ▽

✓6ᵗʰ **S91.32** Laceration with foreign body **of foot**

    ✓7ᵗʰ **S91.321** **Laceration with foreign body, right foot**

    ✓7ᵗʰ **S91.322** **Laceration with foreign body, left foot**

    ✓7ᵗʰ **S91.329** **Laceration with foreign body, unspecified foot** ▽

✓6ᵗʰ **S91.33** Puncture wound without foreign body **of foot**

    ✓7ᵗʰ **S91.331** **Puncture wound without foreign body, right foot**

    ✓7ᵗʰ **S91.332** **Puncture wound without foreign body, left foot**

    ✓7ᵗʰ **S91.339** **Puncture wound without foreign body, unspecified foot** ▽

✓6ᵗʰ **S91.34** Puncture wound with foreign body **of foot**

    ✓7ᵗʰ **S91.341** **Puncture wound with foreign body, right foot**

    ✓7ᵗʰ **S91.342** **Puncture wound with foreign body, left foot**

    ✓7ᵗʰ **S91.349** **Puncture wound with foreign body, unspecified foot** ▽

✓6ᵗʰ **S91.35** Open bite **of foot**

    EXCLUDES 1 *superficial bite of foot (S90.86-, S90.87-)*

    ✓7ᵗʰ **S91.351** **Open bite, right foot**

    ✓7ᵗʰ **S91.352** **Open bite, left foot**

    ✓7ᵗʰ **S91.359** **Open bite, unspecified foot** ▽

✓4ᵗʰ **S92** **Fracture of foot and toe, except ankle**

    NOTE   A fracture not indicated as displaced or nondisplaced should be coded to displaced.

         A fracture not indicated as open or closed should be coded to closed.

    EXCLUDES 1 *traumatic amputation of ankle and foot (S98.-)*

    EXCLUDES 2 *fracture of ankle (S82.-)*

            fracture of malleolus (S82.-)

    AHA: 2015, 3Q, 37-39

> The appropriate 7th character is to be added to each code from category S92.
> A   initial encounter for closed fracture
> B   initial encounter for open fracture
> D   subsequent encounter for fracture with routine healing
> G   subsequent encounter for fracture with delayed healing
> K   subsequent encounter for fracture with nonunion
> P   subsequent encounter for fracture with malunion
> S   sequela

✓5ᵗʰ **S92.0** **Fracture of** calcaneus

    Heel bone

    Os calcis

    EXCLUDES 2 *physeal fracture of calcaneus (S99.0-)*

  ✓6ᵗʰ **S92.00** **Unspecified fracture of calcaneus**

    ✓7ᵗʰ **S92.001** **Unspecified fracture of right calcaneus** ▽

    ✓7ᵗʰ **S92.002** **Unspecified fracture of left calcaneus** ▽

    S92.009 **Unspecified fracture of unspecified calcaneus** ▽

  ✓6ᵗʰ **S92.01** **Fracture of** body of calcaneus

    ✓7ᵗʰ **S92.011** Displaced **fracture of body of right calcaneus**

    ✓7ᵗʰ **S92.012** Displaced **fracture of body of left calcaneus**

    ✓7ᵗʰ **S92.013** Displaced **fracture of body of unspecified calcaneus** ▽

    ✓7ᵗʰ **S92.014** Nondisplaced **fracture of body of right calcaneus**

    ✓7ᵗʰ **S92.015** Nondisplaced **fracture of body of left calcaneus**

    ✓7ᵗʰ **S92.016** Nondisplaced **fracture of body of unspecified calcaneus** ▽

  ✓6ᵗʰ **S92.02** **Fracture of** anterior process of calcaneus

    ✓7ᵗʰ **S92.021** Displaced **fracture of anterior process of right calcaneus**

    ✓7ᵗʰ **S92.022** Displaced **fracture of anterior process of left calcaneus**

    ✓7ᵗʰ **S92.023** Displaced **fracture of anterior process of unspecified calcaneus** ▽

    ✓7ᵗʰ **S92.024** Nondisplaced **fracture of anterior process of right calcaneus**

    ✓7ᵗʰ **S92.025** Nondisplaced **fracture of anterior process of left calcaneus**

    ✓7ᵗʰ **S92.026** Nondisplaced **fracture of anterior process of unspecified calcaneus** ▽

  ✓6ᵗʰ **S92.03** Avulsion **fracture of** tuberosity **of calcaneus**

    ✓7ᵗʰ **S92.031** Displaced **avulsion fracture of tuberosity of right calcaneus**

    ✓7ᵗʰ **S92.032** Displaced **avulsion fracture of tuberosity of left calcaneus**

    ✓7ᵗʰ **S92.033** Displaced **avulsion fracture of tuberosity of unspecified calcaneus** ▽

    ✓7ᵗʰ **S92.034** Nondisplaced **avulsion fracture of tuberosity of right calcaneus**

    ✓7ᵗʰ **S92.035** Nondisplaced **avulsion fracture of tuberosity of left calcaneus**

    ✓7ᵗʰ **S92.036** Nondisplaced **avulsion fracture of tuberosity of unspecified calcaneus** ▽

  ✓6ᵗʰ **S92.04** **Other fracture of** tuberosity **of calcaneus**

    ✓7ᵗʰ **S92.041** Displaced **other fracture of tuberosity of right calcaneus**

    ✓7ᵗʰ **S92.042** Displaced **other fracture of tuberosity of left calcaneus**

    ✓7ᵗʰ **S92.043** Displaced **other fracture of tuberosity of unspecified calcaneus** ▽

    ✓7ᵗʰ **S92.044** Nondisplaced **other fracture of tuberosity of right calcaneus**

    ✓7ᵗʰ **S92.045** Nondisplaced **other fracture of tuberosity of left calcaneus**

    ✓7ᵗʰ **S92.046** Nondisplaced **other fracture of tuberosity of unspecified calcaneus** ▽

  ✓6ᵗʰ **S92.05** **Other** extraarticular **fracture of calcaneus**

    ✓7ᵗʰ **S92.051** Displaced **other extraarticular fracture of right calcaneus**

    ✓7ᵗʰ **S92.052** Displaced **other extraarticular fracture of left calcaneus**

    ✓7ᵗʰ **S92.053** Displaced **other extraarticular fracture of unspecified calcaneus** ▽

    ✓7ᵗʰ **S92.054** Nondisplaced **other extraarticular fracture of right calcaneus**

    ✓7ᵗʰ **S92.055** Nondisplaced **other extraarticular fracture of left calcaneus**

    ✓7ᵗʰ **S92.056** Nondisplaced **other extraarticular fracture of unspecified calcaneus** ▽

  ✓6ᵗʰ **S92.06** Intraarticular **fracture of calcaneus**

    ✓7ᵗʰ **S92.061** Displaced **intraarticular fracture of right calcaneus**

    ✓7ᵗʰ **S92.062** Displaced **intraarticular fracture of left calcaneus**

    ✓7ᵗʰ **S92.063** Displaced **intraarticular fracture of unspecified calcaneus** ▽

    ✓7ᵗʰ **S92.064** Nondisplaced **intraarticular fracture of right calcaneus**

    ✓7ᵗʰ **S92.065** Nondisplaced **intraarticular fracture of left calcaneus**

    ✓7ᵗʰ **S92.066** Nondisplaced **intraarticular fracture of unspecified calcaneus** ▽

✓5ᵗʰ **S92.1** **Fracture of** talus

    Astragalus

  ✓6ᵗʰ **S92.10** **Unspecified fracture of talus**

    ✓7ᵗʰ **S92.101** **Unspecified fracture of right talus** ▽

    ✓7ᵗʰ **S92.102** **Unspecified fracture of left talus** ▽

    S92.109 **Unspecified fracture of unspecified talus** ▽

  ✓6ᵗʰ **S92.11** **Fracture of** neck of talus

    ✓7ᵗʰ **S92.111** Displaced **fracture of neck of right talus**

    ✓7ᵗʰ **S92.112** Displaced **fracture of neck of left talus**

    ✓7ᵗʰ **S92.113** Displaced **fracture of neck of unspecified talus** ▽

EXCLUDES 1 Not coded here   EXCLUDES 2 Not included here   N Newborn Age: 0   P Pediatric Age: 0-17   M Maternity Age: 12-55   A Adult Age: 15-124

1028   ICD-10-CM 2018

√7ᵗʰ **S92.114** Nondisplaced fracture of neck of right talus

√7ᵗʰ **S92.115** Nondisplaced fracture of neck of left talus

√7ᵗʰ **S92.116** Nondisplaced fracture of neck of unspecified talus ▽

√6ᵗʰ **S92.12 Fracture of body of talus**

√7ᵗʰ **S92.121** Displaced fracture of body of right talus

√7ᵗʰ **S92.122** Displaced fracture of body of left talus

√7ᵗʰ **S92.123** Displaced fracture of body of unspecified talus ▽

√7ᵗʰ **S92.124** Nondisplaced fracture of body of right talus

√7ᵗʰ **S92.125** Nondisplaced fracture of body of left talus

√7ᵗʰ **S92.126** Nondisplaced fracture of body of unspecified talus ▽

√6ᵗʰ **S92.13 Fracture of posterior process of talus**

√7ᵗʰ **S92.131** Displaced fracture of posterior process of right talus

√7ᵗʰ **S92.132** Displaced fracture of posterior process of left talus

√7ᵗʰ **S92.133** Displaced fracture of posterior process of unspecified talus ▽

√7ᵗʰ **S92.134** Nondisplaced fracture of posterior process of right talus

√7ᵗʰ **S92.135** Nondisplaced fracture of posterior process of left talus

√7ᵗʰ **S92.136** Nondisplaced fracture of posterior process of unspecified talus ▽

√6ᵗʰ **S92.14 Dome fracture of talus**
    EXCLUDES 1   osteochondritis dissecans (M93.2)

√7ᵗʰ **S92.141** Displaced dome fracture of right talus

√7ᵗʰ **S92.142** Displaced dome fracture of left talus

√7ᵗʰ **S92.143** Displaced dome fracture of unspecified talus ▽

√7ᵗʰ **S92.144** Nondisplaced dome fracture of right talus

√7ᵗʰ **S92.145** Nondisplaced dome fracture of left talus

√7ᵗʰ **S92.146** Nondisplaced dome fracture of unspecified talus ▽

√6ᵗʰ **S92.15 Avulsion fracture (chip fracture) of talus**

√7ᵗʰ **S92.151** Displaced avulsion fracture (chip fracture) of right talus

√7ᵗʰ **S92.152** Displaced avulsion fracture (chip fracture) of left talus

√7ᵗʰ **S92.153** Displaced avulsion fracture (chip fracture) of unspecified talus ▽

√7ᵗʰ **S92.154** Nondisplaced avulsion fracture (chip fracture) of right talus

√7ᵗʰ **S92.155** Nondisplaced avulsion fracture (chip fracture) of left talus

√7ᵗʰ **S92.156** Nondisplaced avulsion fracture (chip fracture) of unspecified talus ▽

√6ᵗʰ **S92.19 Other fracture of talus**

√7ᵗʰ **S92.191** Other fracture of right talus

√7ᵗʰ **S92.192** Other fracture of left talus

√7ᵗʰ **S92.199** Other fracture of unspecified talus ▽

√5ᵗʰ **S92.2 Fracture of other and unspecified tarsal bone(s)**

√6ᵗʰ **S92.20 Fracture of unspecified tarsal bone(s)**

√7ᵗʰ **S92.201** Fracture of unspecified tarsal bone(s) of right foot ▽

√7ᵗʰ **S92.202** Fracture of unspecified tarsal bone(s) of left foot ▽

√7ᵗʰ **S92.209** Fracture of unspecified tarsal bone(s) of unspecified foot ▽

√6ᵗʰ **S92.21 Fracture of cuboid bone**

√7ᵗʰ **S92.211** Displaced fracture of cuboid bone of right foot

√7ᵗʰ **S92.212** Displaced fracture of cuboid bone of left foot

√7ᵗʰ **S92.213** Displaced fracture of cuboid bone of unspecified foot ▽

√7ᵗʰ **S92.214** Nondisplaced fracture of cuboid bone of right foot

√7ᵗʰ **S92.215** Nondisplaced fracture of cuboid bone of left foot

√7ᵗʰ **S92.216** Nondisplaced fracture of cuboid bone of unspecified foot ▽

√6ᵗʰ **S92.22 Fracture of lateral cuneiform**

√7ᵗʰ **S92.221** Displaced fracture of lateral cuneiform of right foot

√7ᵗʰ **S92.222** Displaced fracture of lateral cuneiform of left foot

√7ᵗʰ **S92.223** Displaced fracture of lateral cuneiform ▽ of unspecified foot

√7ᵗʰ **S92.224** Nondisplaced fracture of lateral cuneiform of right foot

√7ᵗʰ **S92.225** Nondisplaced fracture of lateral cuneiform of left foot

√7ᵗʰ **S92.226** Nondisplaced fracture of lateral cuneiform of unspecified foot ▽

√6ᵗʰ **S92.23 Fracture of intermediate cuneiform**

√7ᵗʰ **S92.231** Displaced fracture of intermediate cuneiform of right foot

√7ᵗʰ **S92.232** Displaced fracture of intermediate cuneiform of left foot

√7ᵗʰ **S92.233** Displaced fracture of intermediate cuneiform of unspecified foot ▽

√7ᵗʰ **S92.234** Nondisplaced fracture of intermediate cuneiform of right foot

√7ᵗʰ **S92.235** Nondisplaced fracture of intermediate cuneiform of left foot

√7ᵗʰ **S92.236** Nondisplaced fracture of intermediate ▽ cuneiform of unspecified foot

√6ᵗʰ **S92.24 Fracture of medial cuneiform**

√7ᵗʰ **S92.241** Displaced fracture of medial cuneiform of right foot

√7ᵗʰ **S92.242** Displaced fracture of medial cuneiform of left foot

√7ᵗʰ **S92.243** Displaced fracture of medial cuneiform ▽ of unspecified foot

√7ᵗʰ **S92.244** Nondisplaced fracture of medial cuneiform of right foot

√7ᵗʰ **S92.245** Nondisplaced fracture of medial cuneiform of left foot

√7ᵗʰ **S92.246** Nondisplaced fracture of medial ▽ cuneiform of unspecified foot

√6ᵗʰ **S92.25 Fracture of navicular [scaphoid] of foot**

√7ᵗʰ **S92.251** Displaced fracture of navicular [scaphoid] of right foot

√7ᵗʰ **S92.252** Displaced fracture of navicular [scaphoid] of left foot

√7ᵗʰ **S92.253** Displaced fracture of navicular ▽ [scaphoid] of unspecified foot

√7ᵗʰ **S92.254** Nondisplaced fracture of navicular [scaphoid] of right foot

√7ᵗʰ **S92.255** Nondisplaced fracture of navicular [scaphoid] of left foot

√7ᵗʰ **S92.256** Nondisplaced fracture of navicular ▽ [scaphoid] of unspecified foot

√5ᵗʰ **S92.3 Fracture of metatarsal bone(s)**
    EXCLUDES 2   physeal fracture of metatarsal (S99.1-)

√6ᵗʰ **S92.30 Fracture of unspecified metatarsal bone(s)**

√7ᵗʰ **S92.301** Fracture of unspecified metatarsal ▽ bone(s), right foot

√7ᵗʰ **S92.302** Fracture of unspecified metatarsal ▽ bone(s), left foot

√7ᵗʰ **S92.309** Fracture of unspecified metatarsal ▽ bone(s), unspecified foot

√6ᵗʰ **S92.31 Fracture of first metatarsal bone**

√7ᵗʰ **S92.311** Displaced fracture of first metatarsal bone, right foot

√7ᵗʰ **S92.312** Displaced fracture of first metatarsal bone, left foot

√7ᵗʰ **S92.313** Displaced fracture of first metatarsal ▽ bone, unspecified foot

√7ᵗʰ **S92.314** Nondisplaced fracture of first metatarsal bone, right foot

---

☑ Additional Character Req   √x7ᵗʰ Placeholder Alert   Manifestation   HCC CMS-HCC Condition   ▽ Unspecified Code   ▶◀ Revised Text   ● New Code   ▲ Revised Code Title

✓7ᵗʰ **S92.315** Nondisplaced fracture of first metatarsal bone, left foot

✓7ᵗʰ **S92.316** Nondisplaced fracture of first metatarsal bone, unspecified foot ▽

✓6ᵗʰ **S92.32** Fracture of second metatarsal bone

✓7ᵗʰ **S92.321** Displaced fracture of second metatarsal bone, right foot

✓7ᵗʰ **S92.322** Displaced fracture of second metatarsal bone, left foot

✓7ᵗʰ **S92.323** Displaced fracture of second metatarsal bone, unspecified foot ▽

✓7ᵗʰ **S92.324** Nondisplaced fracture of second metatarsal bone, right foot

✓7ᵗʰ **S92.325** Nondisplaced fracture of second metatarsal bone, left foot

✓7ᵗʰ **S92.326** Nondisplaced fracture of second metatarsal bone, unspecified foot ▽

✓6ᵗʰ **S92.33** Fracture of third metatarsal bone

✓7ᵗʰ **S92.331** Displaced fracture of third metatarsal bone, right foot

✓7ᵗʰ **S92.332** Displaced fracture of third metatarsal bone, left foot

✓7ᵗʰ **S92.333** Displaced fracture of third metatarsal bone, unspecified foot ▽

✓7ᵗʰ **S92.334** Nondisplaced fracture of third metatarsal bone, right foot

✓7ᵗʰ **S92.335** Nondisplaced fracture of third metatarsal bone, left foot

✓7ᵗʰ **S92.336** Nondisplaced fracture of third metatarsal bone, unspecified foot ▽

✓6ᵗʰ **S92.34** Fracture of fourth metatarsal bone

✓7ᵗʰ **S92.341** Displaced fracture of fourth metatarsal bone, right foot

✓7ᵗʰ **S92.342** Displaced fracture of fourth metatarsal bone, left foot

✓7ᵗʰ **S92.343** Displaced fracture of fourth metatarsal bone, unspecified foot ▽

✓7ᵗʰ **S92.344** Nondisplaced fracture of fourth metatarsal bone, right foot

✓7ᵗʰ **S92.345** Nondisplaced fracture of fourth metatarsal bone, left foot

✓7ᵗʰ **S92.346** Nondisplaced fracture of fourth metatarsal bone, unspecified foot ▽

✓6ᵗʰ **S92.35** Fracture of fifth metatarsal bone

✓7ᵗʰ **S92.351** Displaced fracture of fifth metatarsal bone, right foot

✓7ᵗʰ **S92.352** Displaced fracture of fifth metatarsal bone, left foot

✓7ᵗʰ **S92.353** Displaced fracture of fifth metatarsal bone, unspecified foot ▽

✓7ᵗʰ **S92.354** Nondisplaced fracture of fifth metatarsal bone, right foot

✓7ᵗʰ **S92.355** Nondisplaced fracture of fifth metatarsal bone, left foot

✓7ᵗʰ **S92.356** Nondisplaced fracture of fifth metatarsal bone, unspecified foot ▽

✓5ᵗʰ **S92.4** Fracture of great toe ▲

EXCLUDES 2 physeal fracture of phalanx of toe (S99.2-) ▲

✓6ᵗʰ **S92.40** Unspecified fracture of great toe ▲

✓7ᵗʰ **S92.401** Displaced unspecified fracture of right great toe ▽

✓7ᵗʰ **S92.402** Displaced unspecified fracture of left great toe ▽

✓7ᵗʰ **S92.403** Displaced unspecified fracture of unspecified great toe ▽

✓7ᵗʰ **S92.404** Nondisplaced unspecified fracture of right great toe ▽

✓7ᵗʰ **S92.405** Nondisplaced unspecified fracture of left great toe ▽

✓7ᵗʰ **S92.406** Nondisplaced unspecified fracture of unspecified great toe ▽

✓6ᵗʰ **S92.41** Fracture of proximal phalanx of great toe

✓7ᵗʰ **S92.411** Displaced fracture of proximal phalanx of right great toe

✓7ᵗʰ **S92.412** Displaced fracture of proximal phalanx of left great toe

✓7ᵗʰ **S92.413** Displaced fracture of proximal phalanx of unspecified great toe ▽

✓7ᵗʰ **S92.414** Nondisplaced fracture of proximal phalanx of right great toe

✓7ᵗʰ **S92.415** Nondisplaced fracture of proximal phalanx of left great toe

✓7ᵗʰ **S92.416** Nondisplaced fracture of proximal phalanx of unspecified great toe ▽

✓6ᵗʰ **S92.42** Fracture of distal phalanx of great toe

✓7ᵗʰ **S92.421** Displaced fracture of distal phalanx of right great toe

✓7ᵗʰ **S92.422** Displaced fracture of distal phalanx of left great toe

✓7ᵗʰ **S92.423** Displaced fracture of distal phalanx of unspecified great toe ▽

✓7ᵗʰ **S92.424** Nondisplaced fracture of distal phalanx of right great toe

✓7ᵗʰ **S92.425** Nondisplaced fracture of distal phalanx of left great toe

✓7ᵗʰ **S92.426** Nondisplaced fracture of distal phalanx of unspecified great toe ▽

✓6ᵗʰ **S92.49** Other fracture of great toe

✓7ᵗʰ **S92.491** Other fracture of right great toe

✓7ᵗʰ **S92.492** Other fracture of left great toe

✓7ᵗʰ **S92.499** Other fracture of unspecified great toe ▽

S92.5 Fracture of lesser toe(s)

EXCLUDES 2 physeal fracture of phalanx of toe (S99.2-)

✓6ᵗʰ **S92.50** Unspecified fracture of lesser toe(s)

✓7ᵗʰ **S92.501** Displaced unspecified fracture of right lesser toe(s) ▽

✓7ᵗʰ **S92.502** Displaced unspecified fracture of left lesser toe(s) ▽

✓7ᵗʰ **S92.503** Displaced unspecified fracture of unspecified lesser toe(s) ▽

✓7ᵗʰ **S92.504** Nondisplaced unspecified fracture of right lesser toe(s) ▽

✓7ᵗʰ **S92.505** Nondisplaced unspecified fracture of left lesser toe(s) ▽

✓7ᵗʰ **S92.506** Nondisplaced unspecified fracture of unspecified lesser toe(s) ▽

✓6ᵗʰ **S92.51** Fracture of proximal phalanx of lesser toe(s)

✓7ᵗʰ **S92.511** Displaced fracture of proximal phalanx of right lesser toe(s)

✓7ᵗʰ **S92.512** Displaced fracture of proximal phalanx of left lesser toe(s)

✓7ᵗʰ **S92.513** Displaced fracture of proximal phalanx of unspecified lesser toe(s) ▽

✓7ᵗʰ **S92.514** Nondisplaced fracture of proximal phalanx of right lesser toe(s)

✓7ᵗʰ **S92.515** Nondisplaced fracture of proximal phalanx of left lesser toe(s)

✓7ᵗʰ **S92.516** Nondisplaced fracture of proximal phalanx of unspecified lesser toe(s) ▽

✓6ᵗʰ **S92.52** Fracture of middle phalanx of lesser toe(s)

✓7ᵗʰ **S92.521** Displaced fracture of middle phalanx of right lesser toe(s)

✓7ᵗʰ **S92.522** Displaced fracture of middle phalanx of left lesser toe(s)

✓7ᵗʰ **S92.523** Displaced fracture of middle phalanx of unspecified lesser toe(s) ▽

✓7ᵗʰ **S92.524** Nondisplaced fracture of middle phalanx of right lesser toe(s)

✓7ᵗʰ **S92.525** Nondisplaced fracture of middle phalanx of left lesser toe(s)

✓7ᵗʰ **S92.526** Nondisplaced fracture of middle phalanx of unspecified lesser toe(s) ▽

✓6ᵗʰ **S92.53** Fracture of distal phalanx of lesser toe(s)

✓7ᵗʰ **S92.531** Displaced fracture of distal phalanx of right lesser toe(s)

✓7ᵗʰ **S92.532** Displaced fracture of distal phalanx of left lesser toe(s)

EXCLUDES 1 Not coded here   *EXCLUDES 2* Not included here   N Newborn Age: 0   P Pediatric Age: 0-17   M Maternity Age: 12-55   A Adult Age: 15-124

1030

ICD-10-CM 2018

√7ᵗʰ **S92.533** **Displaced** fracture of distal phalanx of unspecified lesser toe(s) ▽

√7ᵗʰ **S92.534** **Nondisplaced** fracture of distal phalanx of **right lesser** toe(s)

√7ᵗʰ **S92.535** **Nondisplaced** fracture of distal phalanx of **left lesser** toe(s)

√7ᵗʰ **S92.536** **Nondisplaced** fracture of distal phalanx ▽ of unspecified lesser toe(s)

√6ᵗʰ **S92.59** **Other fracture of lesser toe(s)**

√7ᵗʰ **S92.591** **Other fracture of right lesser** toe(s)

√7ᵗʰ **S92.592** **Other fracture of left lesser** toe(s)

√7ᵗʰ **S92.599** **Other fracture of unspecified lesser** toe(s)

√5ᵗʰ **S92.8** **Other fracture of foot, except ankle**

√6ᵗʰ **S92.81** **Other fracture of foot** Sesamoid fracture of foot

√7ᵗʰ **S92.811** **Other fracture of right foot**

√7ᵗʰ **S92.812** **Other fracture of left foot**

√7ᵗʰ **S92.819** **Other fracture of unspecified foot** ▽

√5ᵗʰ **S92.9** **Unspecified fracture of foot and toe**

√6ᵗʰ **S92.90** **Unspecified fracture of foot**

√7ᵗʰ **S92.901** **Unspecified fracture of right foot** ▽

√7ᵗʰ **S92.902** **Unspecified fracture of left foot** ▽

√7ᵗʰ **S92.909** **Unspecified fracture of unspecified foot** ▽

√6ᵗʰ **S92.91** **Unspecified fracture of toe**

√7ᵗʰ **S92.911** **Unspecified fracture of right toe(s)** ▽

√7ᵗʰ **S92.912** **Unspecified fracture of left toe(s)** ▽

√7ᵗʰ **S92.919** **Unspecified fracture of unspecified toe(s)** ▽

√4ᵗʰ **S93** **Dislocation and sprain of joints and ligaments at ankle, foot and toe level**
   INCLUDES   avulsion of joint or ligament of ankle, foot and toe
            laceration of cartilage, joint or ligament of ankle, foot and toe
            sprain of cartilage, joint or ligament of ankle, foot and toe
            traumatic hemarthrosis of joint or ligament of ankle, foot and toe
            traumatic rupture of joint or ligament of ankle, foot and toe
            traumatic subluxation of joint or ligament of ankle, foot and toe
            traumatic tear of joint or ligament of ankle, foot and toe
   Code also any associated open wound
   EXCLUDES 2   strain of muscle and tendon of ankle and foot (S96.-)

> The appropriate 7th character is to be added to each code from category S93.
> A   initial encounter
> D   subsequent encounter
> S   sequela

√5ᵗʰ **S93.0** **Subluxation and dislocation of ankle joint**
Subluxation and dislocation of astragalus
Subluxation and dislocation of fibula, lower end
Subluxation and dislocation of talus
Subluxation and dislocation of tibia, lower end

√x7ᵗʰ **S93.01** **Subluxation of right ankle joint**

√x7ᵗʰ **S93.02** **Subluxation of left ankle joint**

√x7ᵗʰ **S93.03** **Subluxation of unspecified ankle joint** ▽

√x7ᵗʰ **S93.04** **Dislocation of right ankle joint**

√x7ᵗʰ **S93.05** **Dislocation of left ankle joint**

√x7ᵗʰ **S93.06** **Dislocation of unspecified ankle joint** ▽

√5ᵗʰ **S93.1** **Subluxation and dislocation of toe**

√6ᵗʰ **S93.10** **Unspecified subluxation and dislocation of toe**
Dislocation of toe NOS
Subluxation of toe NOS

√7ᵗʰ **S93.101** **Unspecified subluxation of right toe(s)** ▽

√7ᵗʰ **S93.102** **Unspecified subluxation of left toe(s)** ▽

√7ᵗʰ **S93.103** **Unspecified subluxation of unspecified toe(s)** ▽

√7ᵗʰ **S93.104** **Unspecified dislocation of right toe(s)** ▽

√7ᵗʰ **S93.105** **Unspecified dislocation of left toe(s)** ▽

√7ᵗʰ **S93.106** **Unspecified dislocation of unspecified toe(s)** ▽

√6ᵗʰ **S93.11** **Dislocation of interphalangeal joint**

√7ᵗʰ **S93.111** **Dislocation of interphalangeal joint of right great toe**

√7ᵗʰ **S93.112** **Dislocation of interphalangeal joint of left great toe**

√7ᵗʰ **S93.113** **Dislocation of interphalangeal joint of unspecified great toe** ▽

√7ᵗʰ **S93.114** **Dislocation of interphalangeal joint of right lesser toe(s)**

√7ᵗʰ **S93.115** **Dislocation of interphalangeal joint of left lesser toe(s)**

√7ᵗʰ **S93.116** **Dislocation of interphalangeal joint of unspecified lesser toe(s)** ▽

√7ᵗʰ **S93.119** **Dislocation of interphalangeal joint of unspecified toe(s)** ▽

√6ᵗʰ **S93.12** **Dislocation of metatarsophalangeal joint**

√7ᵗʰ **S93.121** **Dislocation of metatarsophalangeal joint of right great toe**

√7ᵗʰ **S93.122** **Dislocation of metatarsophalangeal joint of left great toe**

√7ᵗʰ **S93.123** **Dislocation of metatarsophalangeal joint of unspecified great toe** ▽

√7ᵗʰ **S93.124** **Dislocation of metatarsophalangeal joint of right lesser toe(s)**

√7ᵗʰ **S93.125** **Dislocation of metatarsophalangeal joint of left lesser toe(s)**

√7ᵗʰ **S93.126** **Dislocation of metatarsophalangeal joint of unspecified lesser toe(s)** ▽

√7ᵗʰ **S93.129** **Dislocation of metatarsophalangeal joint of unspecified toe(s)** ▽

√6ᵗʰ **S93.13** **Subluxation of interphalangeal joint**

√7ᵗʰ **S93.131** **Subluxation of interphalangeal joint of right great toe**

√7ᵗʰ **S93.132** **Subluxation of interphalangeal joint of left great toe**

√7ᵗʰ **S93.133** **Subluxation of interphalangeal joint of unspecified great toe** ▽

√7ᵗʰ **S93.134** **Subluxation of interphalangeal joint of right lesser toe(s)**

√7ᵗʰ **S93.135** **Subluxation of interphalangeal joint of left lesser toe(s)**

√7ᵗʰ **S93.136** **Subluxation of interphalangeal joint of unspecified lesser toe(s)** ▽

√7ᵗʰ **S93.139** **Subluxation of interphalangeal joint of unspecified toe(s)** ▽

√6ᵗʰ **S93.14** **Subluxation of metatarsophalangeal joint**

√7ᵗʰ **S93.141** **Subluxation of metatarsophalangeal joint of right great toe**

√7ᵗʰ **S93.142** **Subluxation of metatarsophalangeal joint of left great toe**

√7ᵗʰ **S93.143** **Subluxation of metatarsophalangeal joint of unspecified great toe** ▽

√7ᵗʰ **S93.144** **Subluxation of metatarsophalangeal joint of right lesser toe(s)**

√7ᵗʰ **S93.145** **Subluxation of metatarsophalangeal joint of left lesser toe(s)**

√7ᵗʰ **S93.146** **Subluxation of metatarsophalangeal joint of unspecified lesser toe(s)** ▽

√7ᵗʰ **S93.149** **Subluxation of metatarsophalangeal joint of unspecified toe(s)** ▽

√5ᵗʰ **S93.3** **Subluxation and dislocation of foot**
   EXCLUDES 2   dislocation of toe (S93.1-)

√6ᵗʰ **S93.30** **Unspecified subluxation and dislocation of foot**
Dislocation of foot NOS
Subluxation of foot NOS

√7ᵗʰ **S93.301** **Unspecified subluxation of right foot** ▽

√7ᵗʰ **S93.302** **Unspecified subluxation of left foot** ▽

√7ᵗʰ **S93.303** **Unspecified subluxation of unspecified foot** ▽

√7ᵗʰ **S93.304** **Unspecified dislocation of right foot** ▽

√7ᵗʰ **S93.305** **Unspecified dislocation of left foot** ▽

√7ᵗʰ **S93.306** **Unspecified dislocation of unspecified foot** ▽

☑ Additional Character Req   √x7ᵗʰ Placeholder Alert   Manifestation   HCC CMS-HCC Condition   ▽ Unspecified Code   ►◄ Revised Text   ● New Code   ▲ Revised Code Title

✓6ᵗʰ **S93.31 Subluxation and dislocation of** tarsal joint

✓7ᵗʰ **S93.311 Subluxation of tarsal joint of** right **foot**

✓7ᵗʰ **S93.312 Subluxation of tarsal joint of** left **foot**

✓7ᵗʰ **S93.313 Subluxation of tarsal joint of**   ▽
unspecified foot

✓7ᵗʰ **S93.314 Dislocation of tarsal joint of** right **foot**

✓7ᵗʰ **S93.315 Dislocation of tarsal joint of** left **foot**

✓7ᵗʰ **S93.316 Dislocation of tarsal joint of**   ▽
unspecified foot

✓6ᵗʰ **S93.32 Subluxation and dislocation of** tarsometatarsal **joint**

✓7ᵗʰ **S93.321 Subluxation of tarsometatarsal joint of**
right **foot**

✓7ᵗʰ **S93.322 Subluxation of tarsometatarsal joint of**
left **foot**

✓7ᵗʰ **S93.323 Subluxation of tarsometatarsal joint of** ▽
unspecified foot

✓7ᵗʰ **S93.324 Dislocation of tarsometatarsal joint of**
right **foot**

✓7ᵗʰ **S93.325 Dislocation of tarsometatarsal joint of** left
foot

✓7ᵗʰ **S93.326 Dislocation of tarsometatarsal joint of** ▽
unspecified foot

✓6ᵗʰ **S93.33 Other subluxation and dislocation of foot**

✓7ᵗʰ **S93.331 Other** subluxation **of** right **foot**

✓7ᵗʰ **S93.332 Other** subluxation **of** left **foot**

✓7ᵗʰ **S93.333 Other** subluxation **of unspecified foot** ▽

✓7ᵗʰ **S93.334 Other** dislocation **of** right **foot**

✓7ᵗʰ **S93.335 Other** dislocation **of** left **foot**

✓7ᵗʰ **S93.336 Other** dislocation **of unspecified foot** ▽

✓5ᵗʰ **S93.4 Sprain of** ankle

EXCLUDES 2   *injury of Achilles tendon (S86.0-)*

✓6ᵗʰ **S93.40 Sprain of** unspecified **ligament of ankle**
Sprain of ankle NOS
Sprained ankle NOS

✓7ᵗʰ **S93.401 Sprain of unspecified ligament of**   ▽
right **ankle**

✓7ᵗʰ **S93.402 Sprain of unspecified ligament of**   ▽
left **ankle**

✓7ᵗʰ **S93.409 Sprain of unspecified ligament of**   ▽
unspecified ankle

✓6ᵗʰ **S93.41 Sprain of** calcaneofibular **ligament**

✓7ᵗʰ **S93.411 Sprain of calcaneofibular ligament of** right
ankle

✓7ᵗʰ **S93.412 Sprain of calcaneofibular ligament of** left
ankle

✓7ᵗʰ **S93.419 Sprain of calcaneofibular ligament of**   ▽
unspecified ankle

✓6ᵗʰ **S93.42 Sprain of** deltoid **ligament**

✓7ᵗʰ **S93.421 Sprain of deltoid ligament of** right **ankle**

✓7ᵗʰ **S93.422 Sprain of deltoid ligament of** left **ankle**

✓7ᵗʰ **S93.429 Sprain of deltoid ligament of**   ▽
unspecified ankle

✓6ᵗʰ **S93.43 Sprain of** tibiofibular **ligament**

✓7ᵗʰ **S93.431 Sprain of tibiofibular ligament of** right
ankle

✓7ᵗʰ **S93.432 Sprain of tibiofibular ligament of** left
ankle

✓7ᵗʰ **S93.439 Sprain of tibiofibular ligament of**   ▽
unspecified ankle

✓6ᵗʰ **S93.49 Sprain of other ligament of ankle**
Sprain of internal collateral ligament
Sprain of talofibular ligament

✓7ᵗʰ **S93.491 Sprain of other ligament of** right **ankle**

✓7ᵗʰ **S93.492 Sprain of other ligament of** left **ankle**

✓7ᵗʰ **S93.499 Sprain of other ligament of unspecified** ▽
ankle

✓5ᵗʰ **S93.5 Sprain of** toe

✓6ᵗʰ **S93.50 Unspecified sprain of toe**

✓7ᵗʰ **S93.501 Unspecified sprain of** right great **toe** ▽

✓7ᵗʰ **S93.502 Unspecified sprain of** left great **toe** ▽

✓7ᵗʰ **S93.503 Unspecified sprain of unspecified great** ▽
toe

✓7ᵗʰ **S93.504 Unspecified sprain of** right lesser **toe(s)** ▽

✓7ᵗʰ **S93.505 Unspecified sprain of** left lesser **toe(s)** ▽

✓7ᵗʰ **S93.506 Unspecified sprain of unspecified lesser** ▽
toe(s)

✓7ᵗʰ **S93.509 Unspecified sprain of unspecified toe(s)** ▽

✓7ᵗʰ **S93.51 Sprain of** interphalangeal **joint of toe**

✓7ᵗʰ **S93.511 Sprain of interphalangeal joint of** right
great **toe**

✓7ᵗʰ **S93.512 Sprain of interphalangeal joint of** left
great **toe**

✓7ᵗʰ **S93.513 Sprain of interphalangeal joint of**   ▽
unspecified great toe

✓7ᵗʰ **S93.514 Sprain of interphalangeal joint of** right
lesser **toe(s)**

✓7ᵗʰ **S93.515 Sprain of interphalangeal joint of** left
lesser **toe(s)**

✓7ᵗʰ **S93.516 Sprain of interphalangeal joint of**   ▽
unspecified lesser toe(s)

✓7ᵗʰ **S93.519 Sprain of interphalangeal joint of**   ▽
unspecified toe(s)

✓6ᵗʰ **S93.52 Sprain of** metatarsophalangeal **joint of toe**

✓7ᵗʰ **S93.521 Sprain of metatarsophalangeal joint of**
right great **toe**

✓7ᵗʰ **S93.522 Sprain of metatarsophalangeal joint of**
left great **toe**

✓7ᵗʰ **S93.523 Sprain of metatarsophalangeal joint of** ▽
unspecified great toe

✓7ᵗʰ **S93.524 Sprain of metatarsophalangeal joint of**
right lesser **toe(s)**

✓7ᵗʰ **S93.525 Sprain of metatarsophalangeal joint of**
left lesser **toe(s)**

✓7ᵗʰ **S93.526 Sprain of metatarsophalangeal joint of** ▽
unspecified lesser toe(s)

✓7ᵗʰ **S93.529 Sprain of metatarsophalangeal joint of** ▽
unspecified toe(s)

✓5ᵗʰ **S93.6 Sprain of** foot

EXCLUDES 2   *sprain of metatarsophalangeal joint of toe (S93.52-)*
sprain of toe (S93.5-)

✓6ᵗʰ **S93.60 Unspecified sprain of foot**

✓7ᵗʰ **S93.601 Unspecified sprain of** right **foot** ▽

✓7ᵗʰ **S93.602 Unspecified sprain of** left **foot** ▽

✓7ᵗʰ **S93.609 Unspecified sprain of unspecified foot** ▽

✓6ᵗʰ **S93.61 Sprain of** tarsal **ligament of foot**

✓7ᵗʰ **S93.611 Sprain of tarsal ligament of** right **foot**

✓7ᵗʰ **S93.612 Sprain of tarsal ligament of** left **foot**

✓7ᵗʰ **S93.619 Sprain of tarsal ligament of unspecified** ▽
foot

✓6ᵗʰ **S93.62 Sprain of** tarsometatarsal **ligament of foot**

✓7ᵗʰ **S93.621 Sprain of tarsometatarsal ligament of**
right **foot**

✓7ᵗʰ **S93.622 Sprain of tarsometatarsal ligament of** left
foot

✓7ᵗʰ **S93.629 Sprain of tarsometatarsal ligament of** ▽
unspecified foot

✓6ᵗʰ **S93.69 Other sprain of foot**

✓7ᵗʰ **S93.691 Other sprain of** right **foot**

✓7ᵗʰ **S93.692 Other sprain of** left **foot**

✓7ᵗʰ **S93.699 Other sprain of unspecified foot** ▽

✓4ᵗʰ **S94 Injury of nerves at ankle and foot level**
Code also any associated open wound (S91.-)

> The appropriate 7th character is to be added to each code from
> category S94.
> A   initial encounter
> D   subsequent encounter
> S   sequela

✓5ᵗʰ **S94.0 Injury of** lateral plantar **nerve**

✓✕7ᵗʰ **S94.00 Injury of lateral plantar nerve, unspecified leg** ▽

✓✕7ᵗʰ **S94.01 Injury of lateral plantar nerve,** right **leg**

✓✕7ᵗʰ **S94.02 Injury of lateral plantar nerve,** left **leg**

✓5ᵗʰ **S94.1 Injury of** medial plantar **nerve**

✓✕7ᵗʰ **S94.10 Injury of medial plantar nerve, unspecified leg** ▽

EXCLUDES 1 Not coded here   *EXCLUDES 2* Not included here   N Newborn Age: 0   P Pediatric Age: 0-17   M Maternity Age: 12-55   A Adult Age: 15-124

1032   ICD-10-CM 2018

√x 7ᵗʰ   **S94.11**   Injury of medial plantar nerve, right leg

√x 7ᵗʰ   **S94.12**   Injury of medial plantar nerve, left leg

√ 5ᵗʰ   **S94.2**   **Injury of deep peroneal nerve at ankle and foot level**
     Injury of terminal, lateral branch of deep peroneal nerve

   √x 7ᵗʰ   **S94.20**   Injury of deep peroneal nerve at ankle and foot level, unspecified leg   ▽

   √x 7ᵗʰ   **S94.21**   Injury of deep peroneal nerve at ankle and foot level, right leg

   √x 7ᵗʰ   **S94.22**   Injury of deep peroneal nerve at ankle and foot level, left leg

√ 5ᵗʰ   **S94.3**   **Injury of cutaneous sensory nerve at ankle and foot level**

   √x 7ᵗʰ   **S94.30**   Injury of cutaneous sensory nerve at ankle and foot level, unspecified leg   ▽

   √x 7ᵗʰ   **S94.31**   Injury of cutaneous sensory nerve at ankle and foot level, right leg

   √x 7ᵗʰ   **S94.32**   Injury of cutaneous sensory nerve at ankle and foot level, left leg

√ 5ᵗʰ   **S94.8**   **Injury of other nerves at ankle and foot level**

   √ 6ᵗʰ   **S94.8X**   Injury of other nerves at ankle and foot level

     √ 7ᵗʰ   **S94.8X1**   Injury of other nerves at ankle and foot level, right leg

     √ 7ᵗʰ   **S94.8X2**   Injury of other nerves at ankle and foot level, left leg

     √ 7ᵗʰ   **S94.8X9**   Injury of other nerves at ankle and foot level, unspecified leg   ▽

√ 5ᵗʰ   **S94.9**   **Injury of unspecified nerve at ankle and foot level**

   √x 7ᵗʰ   **S94.90**   Injury of unspecified nerve at ankle and foot level, unspecified leg   ▽

   √x 7ᵗʰ   **S94.91**   Injury of unspecified nerve at ankle and foot level, right leg   ▽

   √x 7ᵗʰ   **S94.92**   Injury of unspecified nerve at ankle and foot level, left leg   ▽

√ 4ᵗʰ   **S95**   **Injury of blood vessels at ankle and foot level**
     Code also any associated open wound (S91.-)
     EXCLUDES 2   injury of posterior tibial artery and vein (S85.1-, S85.8-)

     > The appropriate 7th character is to be added to each code from category S95.
> A   initial encounter
> D   subsequent encounter
> S   sequela

√ 5ᵗʰ   **S95.0**   **Injury of dorsal artery of foot**

   √ 6ᵗʰ   **S95.00**   Unspecified injury of dorsal artery of foot

     √ 7ᵗʰ   **S95.001**   Unspecified injury of dorsal artery of right foot   ▽

     √ 7ᵗʰ   **S95.002**   Unspecified injury of dorsal artery of left foot   ▽

     √ 7ᵗʰ   **S95.009**   Unspecified injury of dorsal artery of unspecified foot   ▽

   √ 6ᵗʰ   **S95.01**   Laceration of dorsal artery of foot

     √ 7ᵗʰ   **S95.011**   Laceration of dorsal artery of right foot

     √ 7ᵗʰ   **S95.012**   Laceration of dorsal artery of left foot

     √ 7ᵗʰ   **S95.019**   Laceration of dorsal artery of unspecified foot   ▽

   √ 6ᵗʰ   **S95.09**   Other specified injury of dorsal artery of foot

     √ 7ᵗʰ   **S95.091**   Other specified injury of dorsal artery of right foot

     √ 7ᵗʰ   **S95.092**   Other specified injury of dorsal artery of left foot

     √ 7ᵗʰ   **S95.099**   Other specified injury of dorsal artery of unspecified foot   ▽

√ 5ᵗʰ   **S95.1**   **Injury of plantar artery of foot**

   √ 6ᵗʰ   **S95.10**   Unspecified injury of plantar artery of foot

     √ 7ᵗʰ   **S95.101**   Unspecified injury of plantar artery of right foot   ▽

     √ 7ᵗʰ   **S95.102**   Unspecified injury of plantar artery of left foot   ▽

     √ 7ᵗʰ   **S95.109**   Unspecified injury of plantar artery of unspecified foot   ▽

   √ 6ᵗʰ   **S95.11**   Laceration of plantar artery of foot

     √ 7ᵗʰ   **S95.111**   Laceration of plantar artery of right foot

     √ 7ᵗʰ   **S95.112**   Laceration of plantar artery of left foot

     √ 7ᵗʰ   **S95.119**   Laceration of plantar artery of unspecified foot   ▽

   √ 6ᵗʰ   **S95.19**   Other specified injury of plantar artery of foot

     √ 7ᵗʰ   **S95.191**   Other specified injury of plantar artery of right foot

     √ 7ᵗʰ   **S95.192**   Other specified injury of plantar artery of left foot

     √ 7ᵗʰ   **S95.199**   Other specified injury of plantar artery of unspecified foot   ▽

√ 5ᵗʰ   **S95.2**   **Injury of dorsal vein of foot**

   √ 6ᵗʰ   **S95.20**   Unspecified injury of dorsal vein of foot

     √ 7ᵗʰ   **S95.201**   Unspecified injury of dorsal vein of right foot   ▽

     √ 7ᵗʰ   **S95.202**   Unspecified injury of dorsal vein of left foot   ▽

     √ 7ᵗʰ   **S95.209**   Unspecified injury of dorsal vein of unspecified foot   ▽

   √ 6ᵗʰ   **S95.21**   Laceration of dorsal vein of foot

     √ 7ᵗʰ   **S95.211**   Laceration of dorsal vein of right foot

     √ 7ᵗʰ   **S95.212**   Laceration of dorsal vein of left foot

     √ 7ᵗʰ   **S95.219**   Laceration of dorsal vein of unspecified foot   ▽

   √ 6ᵗʰ   **S95.29**   Other specified injury of dorsal vein of foot

     √ 7ᵗʰ   **S95.291**   Other specified injury of dorsal vein of right foot

     √ 7ᵗʰ   **S95.292**   Other specified injury of dorsal vein of left foot

     √ 7ᵗʰ   **S95.299**   Other specified injury of dorsal vein of unspecified foot   ▽

√ 5ᵗʰ   **S95.8**   **Injury of other blood vessels at ankle and foot level**

   √ 6ᵗʰ   **S95.80**   Unspecified injury of other blood vessels at ankle and foot level

     √ 7ᵗʰ   **S95.801**   Unspecified injury of other blood vessels at ankle and foot level, right leg   ▽

     √ 7ᵗʰ   **S95.802**   Unspecified injury of other blood vessels at ankle and foot level, left leg   ▽

     √ 7ᵗʰ   **S95.809**   Unspecified injury of other blood vessels at ankle and foot level, unspecified leg   ▽

   √ 6ᵗʰ   **S95.81**   Laceration of other blood vessels at ankle and foot level

     √ 7ᵗʰ   **S95.811**   Laceration of other blood vessels at ankle and foot level, right leg

     √ 7ᵗʰ   **S95.812**   Laceration of other blood vessels at ankle and foot level, left leg

     √ 7ᵗʰ   **S95.819**   Laceration of other blood vessels at ankle and foot level, unspecified leg   ▽

   √ 6ᵗʰ   **S95.89**   Other specified injury of other blood vessels at ankle and foot level

     √ 7ᵗʰ   **S95.891**   Other specified injury of other blood vessels at ankle and foot level, right leg

     √ 7ᵗʰ   **S95.892**   Other specified injury of other blood vessels at ankle and foot level, left leg

     √ 7ᵗʰ   **S95.899**   Other specified injury of other blood vessels at ankle and foot level, unspecified leg   ▽

√ 5ᵗʰ   **S95.9**   **Injury of unspecified blood vessel at ankle and foot level**

   √ 6ᵗʰ   **S95.90**   Unspecified injury of unspecified blood vessel at ankle and foot level

     √ 7ᵗʰ   **S95.901**   Unspecified injury of unspecified blood vessel at ankle and foot level, right leg   ▽

     √ 7ᵗʰ   **S95.902**   Unspecified injury of unspecified blood vessel at ankle and foot level, left leg   ▽

     √ 7ᵗʰ   **S95.909**   Unspecified injury of unspecified blood vessel at ankle and foot level, unspecified leg   ▽

   √ 6ᵗʰ   **S95.91**   Laceration of unspecified blood vessel at ankle and foot level

     √ 7ᵗʰ   **S95.911**   Laceration of unspecified blood vessel at ankle and foot level, right leg   ▽

     √ 7ᵗʰ   **S95.912**   Laceration of unspecified blood vessel at ankle and foot level, left leg   ▽

☑ Additional Character Req   √x 7ᵗʰ Placeholder Alert   Manifestation   HCC CMS-HCC Condition   ▽ Unspecified Code   ►◄ Revised Text   ● New Code   ▲ Revised Code Title

√7ᵗʰ **S95.919** **Laceration of unspecified blood vessel at ankle and foot level, unspecified leg** ▽

√6ᵗʰ **S95.99** **Other specified injury of unspecified blood vessel at ankle and foot level**

√7ᵗʰ **S95.991** **Other specified injury of unspecified blood vessel at ankle and foot level, right leg** ▽

√7ᵗʰ **S95.992** **Other specified injury of unspecified blood vessel at ankle and foot level, left leg** ▽

√7ᵗʰ **S95.999** **Other specified injury of unspecified blood vessel at ankle and foot level, unspecified leg** ▽

√4ᵗʰ **S96** **Injury of muscle and tendon at ankle and foot level**

Code also any associated open wound (S91.-)

EXCLUDES 2   *injury of Achilles tendon (S86.0-)*
           sprain of joints and ligaments of ankle and foot (S93.-)

TIP: Refer to the Muscle/Tendon table at the beginning of this chapter.

The appropriate 7th character is to be added to each code from category S96.
A   initial encounter
D   subsequent encounter
S   sequela

√6ᵗʰ **S96.0** **Injury of muscle and tendon of long flexor muscle of toe at ankle and foot level**

√6ᵗʰ **S96.00** **Unspecified injury of muscle and tendon of long flexor muscle of toe at ankle and foot level**

√7ᵗʰ **S96.001** **Unspecified injury of muscle and tendon of long flexor muscle of toe at ankle and foot level, right foot** ▽

√7ᵗʰ **S96.002** **Unspecified injury of muscle and tendon of long flexor muscle of toe at ankle and foot level, left foot** ▽

√7ᵗʰ **S96.009** **Unspecified injury of muscle and tendon of long flexor muscle of toe at ankle and foot level, unspecified foot** ▽

√6ᵗʰ **S96.01** **Strain of muscle and tendon of long flexor muscle of toe at ankle and foot level**

√7ᵗʰ **S96.011** **Strain of muscle and tendon of long flexor muscle of toe at ankle and foot level, right foot**

√7ᵗʰ **S96.012** **Strain of muscle and tendon of long flexor muscle of toe at ankle and foot level, left foot**

√7ᵗʰ **S96.019** **Strain of muscle and tendon of long flexor muscle of toe at ankle and foot level, unspecified foot** ▽

√6ᵗʰ **S96.02** **Laceration of muscle and tendon of long flexor muscle of toe at ankle and foot level**

√7ᵗʰ **S96.021** **Laceration of muscle and tendon of long flexor muscle of toe at ankle and foot level, right foot**

√7ᵗʰ **S96.022** **Laceration of muscle and tendon of long flexor muscle of toe at ankle and foot level, left foot**

√7ᵗʰ **S96.029** **Laceration of muscle and tendon of long flexor muscle of toe at ankle and foot level, unspecified foot** ▽

√6ᵗʰ **S96.09** **Other injury of muscle and tendon of long flexor muscle of toe at ankle and foot level**

√7ᵗʰ **S96.091** **Other injury of muscle and tendon of long flexor muscle of toe at ankle and foot level, right foot**

√7ᵗʰ **S96.092** **Other injury of muscle and tendon of long flexor muscle of toe at ankle and foot level, left foot**

√7ᵗʰ **S96.099** **Other injury of muscle and tendon of long flexor muscle of toe at ankle and foot level, unspecified foot** ▽

√5ᵗʰ **S96.1** **Injury of muscle and tendon of long extensor muscle of toe at ankle and foot level**

√6ᵗʰ **S96.10** **Unspecified injury of muscle and tendon of long extensor muscle of toe at ankle and foot level**

√7ᵗʰ **S96.101** **Unspecified injury of muscle and tendon of long extensor muscle of toe at ankle and foot level, right foot** ▽

√7ᵗʰ **S96.102** **Unspecified injury of muscle and tendon of long extensor muscle of toe at ankle and foot level, left foot** ▽

√7ᵗʰ **S96.109** **Unspecified injury of muscle and tendon of long extensor muscle of toe at ankle and foot level, unspecified foot** ▽

√6ᵗʰ **S96.11** **Strain of muscle and tendon of long extensor muscle of toe at ankle and foot level**

√7ᵗʰ **S96.111** **Strain of muscle and tendon of long extensor muscle of toe at ankle and foot level, right foot**

√7ᵗʰ **S96.112** **Strain of muscle and tendon of long extensor muscle of toe at ankle and foot level, left foot**

√7ᵗʰ **S96.119** **Strain of muscle and tendon of long extensor muscle of toe at ankle and foot level, unspecified foot** ▽

√6ᵗʰ **S96.12** **Laceration of muscle and tendon of long extensor muscle of toe at ankle and foot level**

√7ᵗʰ **S96.121** **Laceration of muscle and tendon of long extensor muscle of toe at ankle and foot level, right foot**

√7ᵗʰ **S96.122** **Laceration of muscle and tendon of long extensor muscle of toe at ankle and foot level, left foot**

√7ᵗʰ **S96.129** **Laceration of muscle and tendon of long extensor muscle of toe at ankle and foot level, unspecified foot** ▽

√6ᵗʰ **S96.19** **Other specified injury of muscle and tendon of long extensor muscle of toe at ankle and foot level**

√7ᵗʰ **S96.191** **Other specified injury of muscle and tendon of long extensor muscle of toe at ankle and foot level, right foot**

√7ᵗʰ **S96.192** **Other specified injury of muscle and tendon of long extensor muscle of toe at ankle and foot level, left foot**

√7ᵗʰ **S96.199** **Other specified injury of muscle and tendon of long extensor muscle of toe at ankle and foot level, unspecified foot** ▽

√5ᵗʰ **S96.2** **Injury of intrinsic muscle and tendon at ankle and foot level**

√6ᵗʰ **S96.20** **Unspecified injury of intrinsic muscle and tendon at ankle and foot level**

√7ᵗʰ **S96.201** **Unspecified injury of intrinsic muscle and tendon at ankle and foot level, right foot** ▽

√7ᵗʰ **S96.202** **Unspecified injury of intrinsic muscle and tendon at ankle and foot level, left foot** ▽

√7ᵗʰ **S96.209** **Unspecified injury of intrinsic muscle and tendon at ankle and foot level, unspecified foot** ▽

√6ᵗʰ **S96.21** **Strain of intrinsic muscle and tendon at ankle and foot level**

√7ᵗʰ **S96.211** **Strain of intrinsic muscle and tendon at ankle and foot level, right foot**

√7ᵗʰ **S96.212** **Strain of intrinsic muscle and tendon at ankle and foot level, left foot**

√7ᵗʰ **S96.219** **Strain of intrinsic muscle and tendon at ankle and foot level, unspecified foot** ▽

√6ᵗʰ **S96.22** **Laceration of intrinsic muscle and tendon at ankle and foot level**

√7ᵗʰ **S96.221** **Laceration of intrinsic muscle and tendon at ankle and foot level, right foot**

√7ᵗʰ **S96.222** **Laceration of intrinsic muscle and tendon at ankle and foot level, left foot**

√7ᵗʰ **S96.229** **Laceration of intrinsic muscle and tendon at ankle and foot level, unspecified foot** ▽

√6ᵗʰ **S96.29** **Other specified injury of intrinsic muscle and tendon at ankle and foot level**

√7ᵗʰ **S96.291** **Other specified injury of intrinsic muscle and tendon at ankle and foot level, right foot**

√7ᵗʰ **S96.292** **Other specified injury of intrinsic muscle and tendon at ankle and foot level, left foot**

EXCLUDES 1 Not coded here   *EXCLUDES 2* Not included here   Ⓝ Newborn Age: 0   Ⓟ Pediatric Age: 0-17   Ⓜ Maternity Age: 12-55   Ⓐ Adult Age: 15-124

1034   ICD-10-CM 2018

☑7ᵗʰ **S96.299** Other specified injury of intrinsic muscle and tendon at ankle and foot level, unspecified foot ▽

☑5ᵗʰ **S96.8** **Injury of other specified muscles and tendons at ankle and foot level**

   ☑6ᵗʰ **S96.80** Unspecified injury of other specified muscles and tendons at ankle and foot level

     ☑7ᵗʰ **S96.801** Unspecified injury of other specified muscles and tendons at ankle and foot level, right foot ▽

     ☑7ᵗʰ **S96.802** Unspecified injury of other specified muscles and tendons at ankle and foot level, left foot ▽

     ☑7ᵗʰ **S96.809** Unspecified injury of other specified muscles and tendons at ankle and foot level, unspecified foot ▽

   ☑6ᵗʰ **S96.81** Strain of other specified muscles and tendons at ankle and foot level

     ☑7ᵗʰ **S96.811** Strain of other specified muscles and tendons at ankle and foot level, right foot

     ☑7ᵗʰ **S96.812** Strain of other specified muscles and tendons at ankle and foot level, left foot

     ☑7ᵗʰ **S96.819** Strain of other specified muscles and tendons at ankle and foot level, unspecified foot ▽

   ☑6ᵗʰ **S96.82** Laceration of other specified muscles and tendons at ankle and foot level

     ☑7ᵗʰ **S96.821** Laceration of other specified muscles and tendons at ankle and foot level, right foot

     ☑7ᵗʰ **S96.822** Laceration of other specified muscles and tendons at ankle and foot level, left foot

     ☑7ᵗʰ **S96.829** Laceration of other specified muscles and tendons at ankle and foot level, unspecified foot ▽

   ☑6ᵗʰ **S96.89** Other specified injury of other specified muscles and tendons at ankle and foot level

     ☑7ᵗʰ **S96.891** Other specified injury of other specified muscles and tendons at ankle and foot level, right foot

     ☑7ᵗʰ **S96.892** Other specified injury of other specified muscles and tendons at ankle and foot level, left foot

     ☑7ᵗʰ **S96.899** Other specified injury of other specified muscles and tendons at ankle and foot level, unspecified foot ▽

☑5ᵗʰ **S96.9** **Injury of unspecified muscle and tendon at ankle and foot level**

   ☑6ᵗʰ **S96.90** Unspecified injury of unspecified muscle and tendon at ankle and foot level

     ☑7ᵗʰ **S96.901** Unspecified injury of unspecified muscle and tendon at ankle and foot level, right foot ▽

     ☑7ᵗʰ **S96.902** Unspecified injury of unspecified muscle and tendon at ankle and foot level, left foot ▽

     ☑7ᵗʰ **S96.909** Unspecified injury of unspecified muscle and tendon at ankle and foot level, unspecified foot ▽

   ☑6ᵗʰ **S96.91** Strain of unspecified muscle and tendon at ankle and foot level

     ☑7ᵗʰ **S96.911** Strain of unspecified muscle and tendon at ankle and foot level, right foot ▽

     ☑7ᵗʰ **S96.912** Strain of unspecified muscle and tendon at ankle and foot level, left foot ▽

     ☑7ᵗʰ **S96.919** Strain of unspecified muscle and tendon at ankle and foot level, unspecified foot ▽

   ☑6ᵗʰ **S96.92** Laceration of unspecified muscle and tendon at ankle and foot level

     ☑7ᵗʰ **S96.921** Laceration of unspecified muscle and tendon at ankle and foot level, right foot ▽

     ☑7ᵗʰ **S96.922** Laceration of unspecified muscle and tendon at ankle and foot level, left foot ▽

     ☑7ᵗʰ **S96.929** Laceration of unspecified muscle and tendon at ankle and foot level, unspecified foot ▽

☑6ᵗʰ **S96.99** Other specified injury of unspecified muscle and tendon at ankle and foot level

     ☑7ᵗʰ **S96.991** Other specified injury of unspecified muscle and tendon at ankle and foot level, right foot ▽

     ☑7ᵗʰ **S96.992** Other specified injury of unspecified muscle and tendon at ankle and foot level, left foot ▽

     ☑7ᵗʰ **S96.999** Other specified injury of unspecified muscle and tendon at ankle and foot level, unspecified foot ▽

☑4ᵗʰ **S97** **Crushing injury of ankle and foot**

Use additional code(s) for all associated injuries

> The appropriate 7th character is to be added to each code from category S97.
> A   initial encounter
> D   subsequent encounter
> S   sequela

☑5ᵗʰ **S97.0** **Crushing injury of ankle**

   ☑x7ᵗʰ **S97.00** Crushing injury of unspecified ankle ▽

   ☑x7ᵗʰ **S97.01** Crushing injury of right ankle

   ☑x7ᵗʰ **S97.02** Crushing injury of left ankle

☑5ᵗʰ **S97.1** **Crushing injury of toe**

   ☑6ᵗʰ **S97.10** Crushing injury of unspecified toe(s)

     ☑7ᵗʰ **S97.101** Crushing injury of unspecified right toe(s) ▽

     ☑7ᵗʰ **S97.102** Crushing injury of unspecified left toe(s) ▽

     ☑7ᵗʰ **S97.109** Crushing injury of unspecified toe(s) ▽
       Crushing injury of toe NOS

   ☑6ᵗʰ **S97.11** Crushing injury of great toe

     ☑7ᵗʰ **S97.111** Crushing injury of right great toe

     ☑7ᵗʰ **S97.112** Crushing injury of left great toe

     ☑7ᵗʰ **S97.119** Crushing injury of unspecified great toe ▽

   ☑6ᵗʰ **S97.12** Crushing injury of lesser toe(s)

     ☑7ᵗʰ **S97.121** Crushing injury of right lesser toe(s)

     ☑7ᵗʰ **S97.122** Crushing injury of left lesser toe(s)

     ☑7ᵗʰ **S97.129** Crushing injury of unspecified lesser toe(s) ▽

☑5ᵗʰ **S97.8** **Crushing injury of foot**

   ☑x7ᵗʰ **S97.80** Crushing injury of unspecified foot ▽
     Crushing injury of foot NOS

   ☑x7ᵗʰ **S97.81** Crushing injury of right foot

   ☑x7ᵗʰ **S97.82** Crushing injury of left foot

☑4ᵗʰ **S98** **Traumatic amputation of ankle and foot**

An amputation not identified as partial or complete should be coded to complete

> The appropriate 7th character is to be added to each code from category S98.
> A   initial encounter
> D   subsequent encounter
> S   sequela

☑5ᵗʰ **S98.0** **Traumatic amputation of foot at ankle level**

   ☑6ᵗʰ **S98.01** Complete traumatic amputation of foot at ankle level

     ☑7ᵗʰ **S98.011** Complete traumatic amputation of right foot at ankle level   HCC

     ☑7ᵗʰ **S98.012** Complete traumatic amputation of left foot at ankle level   HCC

     ☑7ᵗʰ **S98.019** Complete traumatic amputation of unspecified foot at ankle level   HCC ▽

   ☑6ᵗʰ **S98.02** Partial traumatic amputation of foot at ankle level

     ☑7ᵗʰ **S98.021** Partial traumatic amputation of right foot at ankle level   HCC

     ☑7ᵗʰ **S98.022** Partial traumatic amputation of left foot at ankle level   HCC

     ☑7ᵗʰ **S98.029** Partial traumatic amputation of unspecified foot at ankle level   HCC ▽

☑ Additional Character Req   ☑x7ᵗʰ Placeholder Alert   Manifestation   HCC CMS-HCC Condition   ▽ Unspecified Code   ►◄ Revised Text   ● New Code   ▲ Revised Code Title

☑5ᵗʰ **S98.1** **Traumatic amputation of** one toe

   ☑6ᵗʰ **S98.11** Complete **traumatic amputation of** great toe

      ☑7ᵗʰ **S98.111** **Complete traumatic amputation of** right **great toe** `HCC`

      ☑7ᵗʰ **S98.112** **Complete traumatic amputation of** left **great toe** `HCC`

      ☑7ᵗʰ **S98.119** **Complete traumatic amputation of** **unspecified great toe** `HCC` ▽

   ☑6ᵗʰ **S98.12** Partial **traumatic amputation of** great toe

      ☑7ᵗʰ **S98.121** **Partial traumatic amputation of** right **great toe** `HCC`

      ☑7ᵗʰ **S98.122** **Partial traumatic amputation of** left **great toe** `HCC`

      ☑7ᵗʰ **S98.129** **Partial traumatic amputation of** **unspecified great toe** `HCC` ▽

   ☑6ᵗʰ **S98.13** Complete **traumatic amputation of** one lesser toe
      Traumatic amputation of toe NOS

      ☑7ᵗʰ **S98.131** **Complete traumatic amputation of** **one** right **lesser toe** `HCC`

      ☑7ᵗʰ **S98.132** **Complete traumatic amputation of** **one** left **lesser toe** `HCC`

      ☑7ᵗʰ **S98.139** **Complete traumatic amputation of** **one unspecified lesser toe** `HCC` ▽

   ☑6ᵗʰ **S98.14** Partial **traumatic amputation of** one lesser toe

      ☑7ᵗʰ **S98.141** **Partial traumatic amputation of one** right **lesser toe** `HCC`

      ☑7ᵗʰ **S98.142** **Partial traumatic amputation of one** left **lesser toe** `HCC`

      ☑7ᵗʰ **S98.149** **Partial traumatic amputation of one** **unspecified lesser toe** `HCC` ▽

☑5ᵗʰ **S98.2** **Traumatic amputation of** two or more lesser toes

   ☑6ᵗʰ **S98.21** Complete **traumatic amputation of two or more lesser toes**

      ☑7ᵗʰ **S98.211** **Complete traumatic amputation of two or more** right **lesser toes** `HCC`

      ☑7ᵗʰ **S98.212** **Complete traumatic amputation of two or more** left **lesser toes** `HCC`

      ☑7ᵗʰ **S98.219** **Complete traumatic amputation of** **two or more unspecified lesser toes** `HCC` ▽

   ☑6ᵗʰ **S98.22** Partial **traumatic amputation of two or more lesser toes**

      ☑7ᵗʰ **S98.221** **Partial traumatic amputation of two or more** right **lesser toes** `HCC`

      ☑7ᵗʰ **S98.222** **Partial traumatic amputation of two or more** left **lesser toes** `HCC`

      ☑7ᵗʰ **S98.229** **Partial traumatic amputation of** **two or more unspecified lesser toes** `HCC` ▽

☑5ᵗʰ **S98.3** **Traumatic amputation of** midfoot

   ☑6ᵗʰ **S98.31** Complete **traumatic amputation of midfoot**

      ☑7ᵗʰ **S98.311** **Complete traumatic amputation of** right **midfoot** `HCC`

      ☑7ᵗʰ **S98.312** **Complete traumatic amputation of** left **midfoot** `HCC`

      ☑7ᵗʰ **S98.319** **Complete traumatic amputation of** **unspecified midfoot** `HCC` ▽

   ☑6ᵗʰ **S98.32** Partial **traumatic amputation of midfoot**

      ☑7ᵗʰ **S98.321** **Partial traumatic amputation of** right **midfoot** `HCC`

      ☑7ᵗʰ **S98.322** **Partial traumatic amputation of** left **midfoot** `HCC`

      ☑7ᵗʰ **S98.329** **Partial traumatic amputation of** **unspecified midfoot** `HCC` ▽

☑5ᵗʰ **S98.9** **Traumatic amputation of foot, level unspecified**

   ☑6ᵗʰ **S98.91** Complete **traumatic amputation of foot, level unspecified**

      ☑7ᵗʰ **S98.911** **Complete traumatic amputation of** right **foot, level unspecified** `HCC` ▽

      ☑7ᵗʰ **S98.912** **Complete traumatic amputation of** left **foot, level unspecified** `HCC` ▽

      ☑7ᵗʰ **S98.919** **Complete traumatic amputation of** **unspecified foot, level unspecified** `HCC` ▽

   ☑6ᵗʰ **S98.92** Partial **traumatic amputation of foot, level unspecified**

      ☑7ᵗʰ **S98.921** **Partial traumatic amputation of** right **foot, level unspecified** `HCC` ▽

      ☑7ᵗʰ **S98.922** **Partial traumatic amputation of** left **foot, level unspecified** `HCC` ▽

      ☑7ᵗʰ **S98.929** **Partial traumatic amputation of** **unspecified foot, level unspecified** `HCC` ▽

☑4ᵗʰ **S99** **Other and unspecified injuries of ankle and foot**

   ☑5ᵗʰ **S99.0** **Physeal fracture of** calcaneus

> The appropriate 7th character is to be added to each code from subcategories S99.0.
> A   initial encounter for closed fracture
> B   initial encounter for open fracture
> D   subsequent encounter for fracture with routine healing
> G   subsequent encounter for fracture with delayed healing
> K   subsequent encounter for fracture with nonunion
> P   subsequent encounter for fracture with malunion
> S   sequela

   ☑6ᵗʰ **S99.00** **Unspecified physeal fracture of calcaneus**

      ☑7ᵗʰ **S99.001** **Unspecified physeal fracture of** right **calcaneus** ▽

      ☑7ᵗʰ **S99.002** **Unspecified physeal fracture of** left **calcaneus** ▽

      ☑7ᵗʰ **S99.009** **Unspecified physeal fracture of** **unspecified calcaneus** ▽

   ☑6ᵗʰ **S99.01** Salter-Harris Type I **physeal fracture of calcaneus**

      ☑7ᵗʰ **S99.011** **Salter-Harris Type I physeal fracture of** right **calcaneus**

      ☑7ᵗʰ **S99.012** **Salter-Harris Type I physeal fracture of** left **calcaneus**

      ☑7ᵗʰ **S99.019** **Salter-Harris Type I physeal fracture of unspecified calcaneus** ▽

   ☑6ᵗʰ **S99.02** Salter-Harris Type II **physeal fracture of calcaneus**

      ☑7ᵗʰ **S99.021** **Salter-Harris Type II physeal fracture of** right **calcaneus**

      ☑7ᵗʰ **S99.022** **Salter-Harris Type II physeal fracture of** left **calcaneus**

      ☑7ᵗʰ **S99.029** **Salter-Harris Type II physeal fracture of unspecified calcaneus** ▽

   ☑6ᵗʰ **S99.03** Salter-Harris Type III **physeal fracture of calcaneus**

      ☑7ᵗʰ **S99.031** **Salter-Harris Type III physeal fracture of** right **calcaneus**

      ☑7ᵗʰ **S99.032** **Salter-Harris Type III physeal fracture of** left **calcaneus**

      ☑7ᵗʰ **S99.039** **Salter-Harris Type III physeal fracture of unspecified calcaneus** ▽

   ☑6ᵗʰ **S99.04** Salter-Harris Type IV **physeal fracture of calcaneus**

      ☑7ᵗʰ **S99.041** **Salter-Harris Type IV physeal fracture of** right **calcaneus**

      ☑7ᵗʰ **S99.042** **Salter-Harris Type IV physeal fracture of** left **calcaneus**

      ☑7ᵗʰ **S99.049** **Salter-Harris Type IV physeal fracture of unspecified calcaneus** ▽

   ☑6ᵗʰ **S99.09** **Other physeal fracture of calcaneus**

      ☑7ᵗʰ **S99.091** **Other physeal fracture of** right **calcaneus**

      ☑7ᵗʰ **S99.092** **Other physeal fracture of** left **calcaneus**

      ☑7ᵗʰ **S99.099** **Other physeal fracture of unspecified calcaneus** ▽

   ☑5ᵗʰ **S99.1** **Physeal fracture of** metatarsal

> The appropriate 7th character is to be added to each code from subcategories S99.1.
> A   initial encounter for closed fracture
> B   initial encounter for open fracture
> D   subsequent encounter for fracture with routine healing
> G   subsequent encounter for fracture with delayed healing
> K   subsequent encounter for fracture with nonunion
> P   subsequent encounter for fracture with malunion
> S   sequela

   ☑6ᵗʰ **S99.10** **Unspecified physeal fracture of metatarsal**

      ☑7ᵗʰ **S99.101** **Unspecified physeal fracture of** right **metatarsal** ▽

EXCLUDES 1 Not coded here   *EXCLUDES 2* Not included here   Ⓝ Newborn Age: 0   Ⓟ Pediatric Age: 0-17   Ⓜ Maternity Age: 12-55   Ⓐ Adult Age: 15-124

1036   ICD-10-CM 2018

√7ᵗʰ S99.102 Unspecified physeal fracture of left metatarsal ▽

√7ᵗʰ S99.109 Unspecified physeal fracture of unspecified metatarsal ▽

√6ᵗʰ S99.11 Salter-Harris Type I physeal fracture of metatarsal

√7ᵗʰ S99.111 Salter-Harris Type I physeal fracture of right metatarsal

√7ᵗʰ S99.112 Salter-Harris Type I physeal fracture of left metatarsal

√7ᵗʰ S99.119 Salter-Harris Type I physeal fracture of unspecified metatarsal ▽

√6ᵗʰ S99.12 Salter-Harris Type II physeal fracture of metatarsal

√7ᵗʰ S99.121 Salter-Harris Type II physeal fracture of right metatarsal

√7ᵗʰ S99.122 Salter-Harris Type II physeal fracture of left metatarsal

√7ᵗʰ S99.129 Salter-Harris Type II physeal fracture of unspecified metatarsal ▽

√6ᵗʰ S99.13 Salter-Harris Type III physeal fracture of metatarsal

√7ᵗʰ S99.131 Salter-Harris Type III physeal fracture of right metatarsal

√7ᵗʰ S99.132 Salter-Harris Type III physeal fracture of left metatarsal

√7ᵗʰ S99.139 Salter-Harris Type III physeal fracture of unspecified metatarsal ▽

√6ᵗʰ S99.14 Salter-Harris Type IV physeal fracture of metatarsal

√7ᵗʰ S99.141 Salter-Harris Type IV physeal fracture of right metatarsal

√7ᵗʰ S99.142 Salter-Harris Type IV physeal fracture of left metatarsal

√7ᵗʰ S99.149 Salter-Harris Type IV physeal fracture of unspecified metatarsal ▽

√6ᵗʰ S99.19 Other physeal fracture of metatarsal

√7ᵗʰ S99.191 Other physeal fracture of right metatarsal

√7ᵗʰ S99.192 Other physeal fracture of left metatarsal

√7ᵗʰ S99.199 Other physeal fracture of unspecified metatarsal ▽

√5ᵗʰ S99.2 Physeal fracture of phalanx of toe

The appropriate 7th character is to be added to each code from subcategories S99.2.
A initial encounter for closed fracture
B initial encounter for open fracture
D subsequent encounter for fracture with routine healing
G subsequent encounter for fracture with delayed healing
K subsequent encounter for fracture with nonunion
P subsequent encounter for fracture with malunion
S sequela

√6ᵗʰ S99.20 Unspecified physeal fracture of phalanx of toe

√7ᵗʰ S99.201 Unspecified physeal fracture of phalanx of right toe ▽

√7ᵗʰ S99.202 Unspecified physeal fracture of phalanx of left toe ▽

√7ᵗʰ S99.209 Unspecified physeal fracture of phalanx of unspecified toe ▽

√6ᵗʰ S99.21 Salter-Harris Type I physeal fracture of phalanx of toe

√7ᵗʰ S99.211 Salter-Harris Type I physeal fracture of phalanx of right toe

√7ᵗʰ S99.212 Salter-Harris Type I physeal fracture of phalanx of left toe

√7ᵗʰ S99.219 Salter-Harris Type I physeal fracture of phalanx of unspecified toe ▽

√6ᵗʰ S99.22 Salter-Harris Type II physeal fracture of phalanx of toe

√7ᵗʰ S99.221 Salter-Harris Type II physeal fracture of phalanx of right toe

√7ᵗʰ S99.222 Salter-Harris Type II physeal fracture of phalanx of left toe

√7ᵗʰ S99.229 Salter-Harris Type II physeal fracture of phalanx of unspecified toe ▽

√6ᵗʰ S99.23 Salter-Harris Type III physeal fracture of phalanx of toe

√7ᵗʰ S99.231 Salter-Harris Type III physeal fracture of phalanx of right toe

√7ᵗʰ S99.232 Salter-Harris Type III physeal fracture of phalanx of left toe

√7ᵗʰ S99.239 Salter-Harris Type III physeal fracture of phalanx of unspecified toe ▽

√6ᵗʰ S99.24 Salter-Harris Type IV physeal fracture of phalanx of toe

√7ᵗʰ S99.241 Salter-Harris Type IV physeal fracture of phalanx of right toe

√7ᵗʰ S99.242 Salter-Harris Type IV physeal fracture of phalanx of left toe

√7ᵗʰ S99.249 Salter-Harris Type IV physeal fracture of phalanx of unspecified toe ▽

√6ᵗʰ S99.29 Other physeal fracture of phalanx of toe

√7ᵗʰ S99.291 Other physeal fracture of phalanx of right toe

√7ᵗʰ S99.292 Other physeal fracture of phalanx of left toe

√7ᵗʰ S99.299 Other physeal fracture of phalanx of unspecified toe ▽

√5ᵗʰ S99.8 Other specified injuries of ankle and foot

The appropriate 7th character is to be added to each code from subcategory S99.8.
A initial encounter
D subsequent encounter
S sequela

√6ᵗʰ S99.81 Other specified injuries of ankle

√7ᵗʰ S99.811 Other specified injuries of right ankle

√7ᵗʰ S99.812 Other specified injuries of left ankle

√7ᵗʰ S99.819 Other specified injuries of unspecified ankle ▽

√6ᵗʰ S99.82 Other specified injuries of foot

√7ᵗʰ S99.821 Other specified injuries of right foot

√7ᵗʰ S99.822 Other specified injuries of left foot

√7ᵗʰ S99.829 Other specified injuries of unspecified foot ▽

√5ᵗʰ S99.9 Unspecified injury of ankle and foot

The appropriate 7th character is to be added to each code from subcategory S99.9.
A initial encounter
D subsequent encounter
S sequela

√6ᵗʰ S99.91 Unspecified injury of ankle

√7ᵗʰ S99.911 Unspecified injury of right ankle ▽

√7ᵗʰ S99.912 Unspecified injury of left ankle ▽

√7ᵗʰ S99.919 Unspecified injury of unspecified ankle ▽

√6ᵗʰ S99.92 Unspecified injury of foot

√7ᵗʰ S99.921 Unspecified injury of right foot ▽

√7ᵗʰ S99.922 Unspecified injury of left foot ▽

√7ᵗʰ S99.929 Unspecified injury of unspecified foot ▽

Injury, Poisoning And Certain Other Consequences Of External Causes (T07-T88)

Injuries involving multiple body regions (T07)

EXCLUDES 1 burns and corrosions (T20-T32)
frostbite (T33-T34)
insect bite or sting, venomous (T63.4)
sunburn (L55.-)

√x7ᵗʰ **T07 Unspecified multiple injuries** ▽
EXCLUDES 1 injury NOS ▶(T14.90)◀

The appropriate 7th character is to be added to code T07.
A initial encounter
D subsequent encounter
S sequela

☑ Additional Character Req   ᵥₓ7ᵗʰ Placeholder Alert   Manifestation   ᴴᶜᶜ CMS-HCC Condition   ▽ Unspecified Code   ▶◀ Revised Text   ● New Code   ▲ Revised Code Title

ICD-10-CM 2018   1037

Injury of unspecified body region (T14)

✓4ᵗʰ T14   Injury of unspecified body region
     EXCLUDES1   multiple unspecified injuries (T07)

> The appropriate 7th character is to be added to each code from category T14.
> A   initial encounter
> D   subsequent encounter
> S   sequela

   ✓x7ᵗʰ T14.8   Other injury of unspecified body region
       Abrasion NOS
       Contusion NOS
       Crush injury NOS
       Fracture NOS
       Skin injury NOS
       Vascular injury NOS
       ▶Wound NOS◀

   ✓5ᵗʰ T14.9   Unspecified injury
     ✓x7ᵗʰ T14.90   Injury, unspecified   ▽
           Injury NOS
     ✓x7ᵗʰ T14.91   Suicide attempt   **HCC**
           Attempted suicide NOS

Effects of foreign body entering through natural orifice (T15-T19)

   EXCLUDES2   foreign body accidentally left in operation wound (T81.5-)
           foreign body in penetrating wound—See open wound by body region
           residual foreign body in soft tissue (M79.5)
           splinter, without open wound—See superficial injury by body region

✓4ᵗʰ T15   Foreign body on external eye
     EXCLUDES2   foreign body in penetrating wound of orbit and eye ball (S05.4-, S05.5-)
           open wound of eyelid and periocular area (S01.1-)
           retained foreign body in eyelid (H02.8-)
           retained (old) foreign body in penetrating wound of orbit and eye ball (H05.5-, H44.6-, H44.7-)
           superficial foreign body of eyelid and periocular area (S00.25-)

> The appropriate 7th character is to be added to each code from category T15.
> A   initial encounter
> D   subsequent encounter
> S   sequela

   ✓5ᵗʰ T15.0   Foreign body in cornea
     ✓x7ᵗʰ T15.00   Foreign body in cornea, unspecified eye   ▽
     ✓x7ᵗʰ T15.01   Foreign body in cornea, right eye
     ✓x7ᵗʰ T15.02   Foreign body in cornea, left eye

   ✓5ᵗʰ T15.1   Foreign body in conjunctival sac
     ✓x7ᵗʰ T15.10   Foreign body in conjunctival sac, unspecified eye   ▽
     ✓x7ᵗʰ T15.11   Foreign body in conjunctival sac, right eye
     ✓x7ᵗʰ T15.12   Foreign body in conjunctival sac, left eye

   ✓5ᵗʰ T15.8   Foreign body in other and multiple parts of external eye
       Foreign body in lacrimal punctum
     ✓x7ᵗʰ T15.80   Foreign body in other and multiple parts of external eye, unspecified eye   ▽
     ✓x7ᵗʰ T15.81   Foreign body in other and multiple parts of external eye, right eye
     ✓x7ᵗʰ T15.82   Foreign body in other and multiple parts of external eye, left eye

   ✓5ᵗʰ T15.9   Foreign body on external eye, part unspecified
     ✓x7ᵗʰ T15.90   Foreign body on external eye, part unspecified, unspecified eye   ▽
     ✓x7ᵗʰ T15.91   Foreign body on external eye, part unspecified, right eye   ▽
     ✓x7ᵗʰ T15.92   Foreign body on external eye, part unspecified, left eye   ▽

✓4ᵗʰ T16   Foreign body in ear
     INCLUDES   foreign body in auditory canal

> The appropriate 7th character is to be added to each code from category T16.
> A   initial encounter
> D   subsequent encounter
> S   sequela

   ✓x7ᵗʰ T16.1   Foreign body in right ear
   ✓x7ᵗʰ T16.2   Foreign body in left ear
   ✓x7ᵗʰ T16.9   Foreign body in ear, unspecified ear   ▽

✓4ᵗʰ T17   Foreign body in respiratory tract

> The appropriate 7th character is to be added to each code from category T17.
> A   initial encounter
> D   subsequent encounter
> S   sequela

   ✓x7ᵗʰ T17.0   Foreign body in nasal sinus
   ✓x7ᵗʰ T17.1   Foreign body in nostril
       Foreign body in nose NOS

   ✓5ᵗʰ T17.2   Foreign body in pharynx
       Foreign body in nasopharynx
       Foreign body in throat NOS
     ✓6ᵗʰ T17.20   Unspecified foreign body in pharynx
       ✓7ᵗʰ T17.200   Unspecified foreign body in pharynx causing asphyxiation   ▽
       ✓7ᵗʰ T17.208   Unspecified foreign body in pharynx causing other injury   ▽
     ✓6ᵗʰ T17.21   Gastric contents in pharynx
       Aspiration of gastric contents into pharynx
       Vomitus in pharynx
       ✓7ᵗʰ T17.210   Gastric contents in pharynx causing asphyxiation
       ✓7ᵗʰ T17.218   Gastric contents in pharynx causing other injury
     ✓6ᵗʰ T17.22   Food in pharynx
       Bones in pharynx
       Seeds in pharynx
       ✓7ᵗʰ T17.220   Food in pharynx causing asphyxiation
       ✓7ᵗʰ T17.228   Food in pharynx causing other injury
     ✓6ᵗʰ T17.29   Other foreign object in pharynx
       ✓7ᵗʰ T17.290   Other foreign object in pharynx causing asphyxiation
       ✓7ᵗʰ T17.298   Other foreign object in pharynx causing other injury

   ✓5ᵗʰ T17.3   Foreign body in larynx
     ✓6ᵗʰ T17.30   Unspecified foreign body in larynx
       ✓7ᵗʰ T17.300   Unspecified foreign body in larynx causing asphyxiation   ▽
       ✓7ᵗʰ T17.308   Unspecified foreign body in larynx causing other injury   ▽
     ✓6ᵗʰ T17.31   Gastric contents in larynx
       Aspiration of gastric contents into larynx
       Vomitus in larynx
       ✓7ᵗʰ T17.310   Gastric contents in larynx causing asphyxiation
       ✓7ᵗʰ T17.318   Gastric contents in larynx causing other injury
     ✓6ᵗʰ T17.32   Food in larynx
       Bones in larynx
       Seeds in larynx
       ✓7ᵗʰ T17.320   Food in larynx causing asphyxiation
       ✓7ᵗʰ T17.328   Food in larynx causing other injury
     ✓6ᵗʰ T17.39   Other foreign object in larynx
       ✓7ᵗʰ T17.390   Other foreign object in larynx causing asphyxiation
       ✓7ᵗʰ T17.398   Other foreign object in larynx causing other injury

   ✓5ᵗʰ T17.4   Foreign body in trachea
     ✓6ᵗʰ T17.40   Unspecified foreign body in trachea
       ✓7ᵗʰ T17.400   Unspecified foreign body in trachea causing asphyxiation   ▽
       ✓7ᵗʰ T17.408   Unspecified foreign body in trachea causing other injury   ▽
     ✓6ᵗʰ T17.41   Gastric contents in trachea
       Aspiration of gastric contents into trachea
       Vomitus in trachea
       ✓7ᵗʰ T17.410   Gastric contents in trachea causing asphyxiation
       ✓7ᵗʰ T17.418   Gastric contents in trachea causing other injury

---

EXCLUDES1 Not coded here   **EXCLUDES2** Not included here   **N** Newborn Age: 0   **P** Pediatric Age: 0-17   **M** Maternity Age: 12-55   **A** Adult Age: 15-124

✓6ᵗʰ **T17.42** Food **in trachea**
     Bones in trachea
     Seeds in trachea
    ✓7ᵗʰ **T17.420 Food in trachea** causing asphyxiation
    ✓7ᵗʰ **T17.428 Food in trachea** causing other injury

✓6ᵗʰ **T17.49 Other foreign object in trachea**
    ✓7ᵗʰ **T17.490 Other foreign object in trachea** causing asphyxiation
    ✓7ᵗʰ **T17.498 Other foreign object in trachea** causing other injury

✓5ᵗʰ **T17.5 Foreign body in** bronchus
  ✓6ᵗʰ **T17.50 Unspecified foreign body in bronchus**
    ✓7ᵗʰ **T17.500 Unspecified foreign body in bronchus** causing asphyxiation ▽
    ✓7ᵗʰ **T17.508 Unspecified foreign body in bronchus** causing other injury ▽

  ✓6ᵗʰ **T17.51** Gastric contents **in bronchus**
     Aspiration of gastric contents into bronchus
     Vomitus in bronchus
    ✓7ᵗʰ **T17.510 Gastric contents in bronchus** causing asphyxiation
    ✓7ᵗʰ **T17.518 Gastric contents in bronchus** causing other injury

  ✓6ᵗʰ **T17.52** Food **in bronchus**
     Bones in bronchus
     Seeds in bronchus
    ✓7ᵗʰ **T17.520 Food in bronchus** causing asphyxiation
    ✓7ᵗʰ **T17.528 Food in bronchus** causing other injury

  ✓6ᵗʰ **T17.59 Other foreign object in bronchus**
    ✓7ᵗʰ **T17.590 Other foreign object in bronchus** causing asphyxiation
    ✓7ᵗʰ **T17.598 Other foreign object in bronchus** causing other injury

✓5ᵗʰ **T17.8 Foreign body in other parts of respiratory tract**
     Foreign body in bronchioles
     Foreign body in lung
  ✓6ᵗʰ **T17.80 Unspecified foreign body in other parts of respiratory tract**
    ✓7ᵗʰ **T17.800 Unspecified foreign body in other parts of respiratory tract** causing asphyxiation ▽
    ✓7ᵗʰ **T17.808 Unspecified foreign body in other parts of respiratory tract** causing other injury ▽

  ✓6ᵗʰ **T17.81** Gastric contents **in other parts of respiratory tract**
     Aspiration of gastric contents into other parts of respiratory tract
     Vomitus in other parts of respiratory tract
    ✓7ᵗʰ **T17.810 Gastric contents in other parts of respiratory tract** causing asphyxiation
    ✓7ᵗʰ **T17.818 Gastric contents in other parts of respiratory tract** causing other injury

  ✓6ᵗʰ **T17.82** Food **in other parts of respiratory tract**
     Bones in other parts of respiratory tract
     Seeds in other parts of respiratory tract
    ✓7ᵗʰ **T17.820 Food in other parts of respiratory tract** causing asphyxiation
    ✓7ᵗʰ **T17.828 Food in other parts of respiratory tract** causing other injury

  ✓6ᵗʰ **T17.89 Other foreign object in other parts of respiratory tract**
    ✓7ᵗʰ **T17.890 Other foreign object in other parts of respiratory tract** causing asphyxiation
    ✓7ᵗʰ **T17.898 Other foreign object in other parts of respiratory tract** causing other injury

✓5ᵗʰ **T17.9 Foreign body in respiratory tract, part unspecified**
  ✓6ᵗʰ **T17.90 Unspecified foreign body in respiratory tract, part unspecified**
    ✓7ᵗʰ **T17.900 Unspecified foreign body in respiratory tract, part unspecified** causing asphyxiation ▽
    ✓7ᵗʰ **T17.908 Unspecified foreign body in respiratory tract, part unspecified** causing other injury ▽

✓6ᵗʰ **T17.91** Gastric contents **in respiratory tract, part unspecified**
     Aspiration of gastric contents into respiratory tract, part unspecified
     Vomitus in trachea respiratory tract, part unspecified
    ✓7ᵗʰ **T17.910 Gastric contents in respiratory tract, part unspecified** causing asphyxiation ▽
    ✓7ᵗʰ **T17.918 Gastric contents in respiratory tract, part unspecified** causing other injury ▽

✓6ᵗʰ **T17.92** Food **in respiratory tract, part unspecified**
     Bones in respiratory tract, part unspecified
     Seeds in respiratory tract, part unspecified
    ✓7ᵗʰ **T17.920 Food in respiratory tract, part unspecified** causing asphyxiation ▽
    ✓7ᵗʰ **T17.928 Food in respiratory tract, part unspecified** causing other injury ▽

✓6ᵗʰ **T17.99 Other foreign object in respiratory tract, part unspecified**
    ✓7ᵗʰ **T17.990 Other foreign object in respiratory tract, part unspecified in** causing asphyxiation ▽
    ✓7ᵗʰ **T17.998 Other foreign object in respiratory tract, part unspecified** causing other injury ▽

✓4ᵗʰ **T18 Foreign body in alimentary tract**
   EXCLUDES 2 foreign body in pharynx (T17.2-)

> The appropriate 7th character is to be added to each code from category T18.
> A   initial encounter
> D   subsequent encounter
> S   sequela

✓x7ᵗʰ **T18.0 Foreign body in** mouth
✓5ᵗʰ **T18.1 Foreign body in** esophagus
   EXCLUDES 2 foreign body in respiratory tract (T17.-)
  ✓6ᵗʰ **T18.10 Unspecified foreign body in esophagus**
    ✓7ᵗʰ **T18.100 Unspecified foreign body in esophagus** causing compression of trachea ▽
       Unspecified foreign body in esophagus causing obstruction of respiration
    ✓7ᵗʰ **T18.108 Unspecified foreign body in esophagus** causing other injury ▽

  ✓6ᵗʰ **T18.11** Gastric contents **in esophagus**
     Vomitus in esophagus
    ✓7ᵗʰ **T18.110 Gastric contents in esophagus** causing compression of trachea
       Gastric contents in esophagus causing obstruction of respiration
    ✓7ᵗʰ **T18.118 Gastric contents in esophagus** causing other injury

  ✓6ᵗʰ **T18.12** Food **in esophagus**
     Bones in esophagus
     Seeds in esophagus
    ✓7ᵗʰ **T18.120 Food in esophagus** causing compression of trachea
       Food in esophagus causing obstruction of respiration
    ✓7ᵗʰ **T18.128 Food in esophagus** causing other injury

  ✓6ᵗʰ **T18.19 Other foreign object in esophagus**
     AHA: 2015, 1Q, 23
    ✓7ᵗʰ **T18.190 Other foreign object in esophagus** causing compression of trachea
       Other foreign body in esophagus causing obstruction of respiration
    ✓7ᵗʰ **T18.198 Other foreign object in esophagus** causing other injury

✓x7ᵗʰ **T18.2 Foreign body in** stomach
✓x7ᵗʰ **T18.3 Foreign body in** small intestine
✓x7ᵗʰ **T18.4 Foreign body in** colon
✓x7ᵗʰ **T18.5 Foreign body in** anus and rectum
     Foreign body in rectosigmoid (junction)
✓x7ᵗʰ **T18.8 Foreign body in other parts of alimentary tract**
✓x7ᵗʰ **T18.9 Foreign body of alimentary tract, part unspecified** ▽
     Foreign body in digestive system NOS
     Swallowed foreign body NOS

✓ Additional Character Req   ✓x7ᵗʰ Placeholder Alert   Manifestation   HCC CMS-HCC Condition   ▽ Unspecified Code   ▶◀ Revised Text   ● New Code   ▲ Revised Code Title

ICD-10-CM 2018   1039

☑4ᵗʰ **T19 Foreign body in genitourinary tract**
> EXCLUDES 2   complications due to implanted mesh (T83.7-)
> mechanical complications of contraceptive device (intrauterine) (vaginal) (T83.3-)
> presence of contraceptive device (intrauterine) (vaginal) (Z97.5)

> The appropriate 7th character is to be added to each code from category T19.
> A   initial encounter
> D   subsequent encounter
> S   sequela

☑x7ᵗʰ **T19.0 Foreign body in urethra**
☑x7ᵗʰ **T19.1 Foreign body in bladder**
☑x7ᵗʰ **T19.2 Foreign body in vulva and vagina**   ♀
☑x7ᵗʰ **T19.3 Foreign body in uterus**   ♀
☑x7ᵗʰ **T19.4 Foreign body in penis**   ♂
☑x7ᵗʰ **T19.8 Foreign body in other parts of genitourinary tract**
☑x7ᵗʰ **T19.9 Foreign body in genitourinary tract, part unspecified**   ▽

Burns and corrosions (T20-T32)

> INCLUDES   burns (thermal) from electrical heating appliances
> burns (thermal) from electricity
> burns (thermal) from flame
> burns (thermal) from friction
> burns (thermal) from hot air and hot gases
> burns (thermal) from hot objects
> burns (thermal) from lightning
> burns (thermal) from radiation
> chemical burn [corrosion] (external) (internal)
> scalds
> EXCLUDES 2   erythema [dermatitis] ab igne (L59.0)
> radiation-related disorders of the skin and subcutaneous tissue (L55-L59)
> sunburn (L55.-)
> **AHA:** 2016, 2Q, 4

Burns and corrosions of external body surface, specified by site (T20-T25)

> INCLUDES   burns and corrosions of first degree [erythema]
> burns and corrosions of second degree [blisters] [epidermal loss]
> burns and corrosions of third degree [deep necrosis of underlying tissue] [full-thickness skin loss]
> Use additional code from category T31 or T32 to identify extent of body surface involved

☑4ᵗʰ **T20 Burn and corrosion of head, face, and neck**
> EXCLUDES 2   burn and corrosion of ear drum (T28.41, T28.91)
> burn and corrosion of eye and adnexa (T26.-)
> burn and corrosion of mouth and pharynx (T28.0)
> **AHA:** 2015, 1Q, 18-19

> The appropriate 7th character is to be added to each code from category T20.
> A   initial encounter
> D   subsequent encounter
> S   sequela

☑5ᵗʰ **T20.0 Burn of unspecified degree of head, face, and neck**
> Use additional external cause code to identify the source, place and intent of the burn (X00-X19, X75-X77, X96-X98, Y92)

☑x7ᵗʰ **T20.00 Burn of unspecified degree of head, face, and neck, unspecified site**   ▽

☑6ᵗʰ **T20.01 Burn of unspecified degree of ear [any part, except ear drum]**
> EXCLUDES 2   burn of ear drum (T28.41-)

☑7ᵗʰ **T20.011 Burn of unspecified degree of right ear [any part, except ear drum]**   ▽

☑7ᵗʰ **T20.012 Burn of unspecified degree of left ear [any part, except ear drum]**   ▽

☑7ᵗʰ **T20.019 Burn of unspecified degree of unspecified ear [any part, except ear drum]**   ▽

☑x7ᵗʰ **T20.02 Burn of unspecified degree of lip(s)**   ▽
☑x7ᵗʰ **T20.03 Burn of unspecified degree of chin**   ▽

Rule of Nines Estimation of Total Body Surface Burned

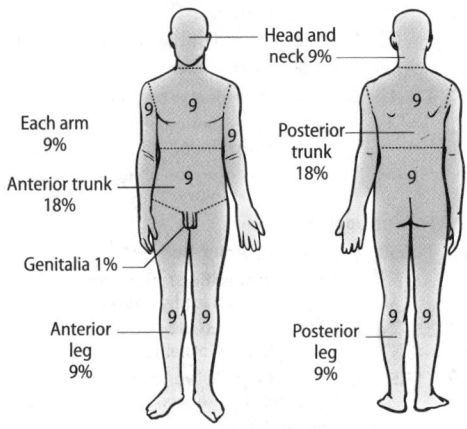

Head and neck 9%
Each arm 9%
Posterior trunk 18%
Anterior trunk 18%
Genitalia 1%
Anterior leg 9%
Posterior leg 9%

☑x7ᵗʰ **T20.04 Burn of unspecified degree of nose (septum)**   ▽
☑x7ᵗʰ **T20.05 Burn of unspecified degree of scalp [any part]**   ▽
☑x7ᵗʰ **T20.06 Burn of unspecified degree of forehead and cheek**   ▽
☑x7ᵗʰ **T20.07 Burn of unspecified degree of neck**   ▽
☑x7ᵗʰ **T20.09 Burn of unspecified degree of multiple sites of head, face, and neck**   ▽

☑5ᵗʰ **T20.1 Burn of first degree of head, face, and neck**
> Use additional external cause code to identify the source, place and intent of the burn (X00-X19, X75-X77, X96-X98, Y92)

☑x7ᵗʰ **T20.10 Burn of first degree of head, face, and neck, unspecified site**   ▽

☑6ᵗʰ **T20.11 Burn of first degree of ear [any part, except ear drum]**
> EXCLUDES 2   burn of ear drum (T28.41-)

☑7ᵗʰ **T20.111 Burn of first degree of right ear [any part, except ear drum]**

☑7ᵗʰ **T20.112 Burn of first degree of left ear [any part, except ear drum]**

☑7ᵗʰ **T20.119 Burn of first degree of unspecified ear [any part, except ear drum]**   ▽

☑x7ᵗʰ **T20.12 Burn of first degree of lip(s)**
☑x7ᵗʰ **T20.13 Burn of first degree of chin**
☑x7ᵗʰ **T20.14 Burn of first degree of nose (septum)**
☑x7ᵗʰ **T20.15 Burn of first degree of scalp [any part]**
☑x7ᵗʰ **T20.16 Burn of first degree of forehead and cheek**
☑x7ᵗʰ **T20.17 Burn of first degree of neck**
☑x7ᵗʰ **T20.19 Burn of first degree of multiple sites of head, face, and neck**

Degree of Burns

Epidermis
Dermis
Subcutaneous

Normal   First Degree Burn

Epidermis
Dermis
Subcutaneous

Second Degree Burn   Third Degree Burn

✓5ᵗʰ **T20.2 Burn of** second degree **of head, face, and neck**
Use additional external cause code to identify the source, place and intent of the burn (X00-X19, X75-X77, X96-X98, Y92)

✓ₓ7ᵗʰ **T20.20 Burn of second degree of head, face, and neck, unspecified site** ▽

✓6ᵗʰ **T20.21 Burn of second degree of** ear **[any part, except ear drum]**
EXCLUDES 2   *burn of ear drum (T28.41-)*

✓7ᵗʰ **T20.211 Burn of second degree of** right **ear [any part, except ear drum]**

✓7ᵗʰ **T20.212 Burn of second degree of** left **ear [any part, except ear drum]**

✓7ᵗʰ **T20.219 Burn of second degree of unspecified ear [any part, except ear drum]** ▽

✓ₓ7ᵗʰ **T20.22 Burn of second degree of** lip(s)

✓ₓ7ᵗʰ **T20.23 Burn of second degree of** chin

✓ₓ7ᵗʰ **T20.24 Burn of second degree of** nose (septum)

✓ₓ7ᵗʰ **T20.25 Burn of second degree of** scalp [any part]

✓ₓ7ᵗʰ **T20.26 Burn of second degree of** forehead and cheek

✓ₓ7ᵗʰ **T20.27 Burn of second degree of** neck

✓ₓ7ᵗʰ **T20.29 Burn of second degree of** multiple sites **of head, face, and neck**

✓5ᵗʰ **T20.3 Burn of** third degree **of head, face, and neck**
Use additional external cause code to identify the source, place and intent of the burn (X00-X19, X75-X77, X96-X98, Y92)

✓ₓ7ᵗʰ **T20.30 Burn of third degree of head, face, and neck, unspecified site** ▽

✓6ᵗʰ **T20.31 Burn of third degree of** ear **[any part, except ear drum]**
EXCLUDES 2   *burn of ear drum (T28.41-)*
AHA: 2015, 1Q, 18

✓7ᵗʰ **T20.311 Burn of third degree of** right **ear [any part, except ear drum]**

✓7ᵗʰ **T20.312 Burn of third degree of** left **ear [any part, except ear drum]**

✓7ᵗʰ **T20.319 Burn of third degree of unspecified ear [any part, except ear drum]** ▽

✓ₓ7ᵗʰ **T20.32 Burn of third degree of** lip(s)

✓ₓ7ᵗʰ **T20.33 Burn of third degree of** chin

✓ₓ7ᵗʰ **T20.34 Burn of third degree of** nose (septum)

✓ₓ7ᵗʰ **T20.35 Burn of third degree of** scalp [any part]

✓ₓ7ᵗʰ **T20.36 Burn of third degree of** forehead and cheek

✓ₓ7ᵗʰ **T20.37 Burn of third degree of** neck

✓ₓ7ᵗʰ **T20.39 Burn of third degree of** multiple sites **of head, face, and neck**

✓5ᵗʰ **T20.4 Corrosion of unspecified degree of head, face, and neck**
Code first (T51-T65) to identify chemical and intent
Use additional external cause code to identify place (Y92)

✓ₓ7ᵗʰ **T20.40 Corrosion of unspecified degree of head, face, and neck, unspecified site** ▽

✓6ᵗʰ **T20.41 Corrosion of unspecified degree of** ear **[any part, except ear drum]**
EXCLUDES 2   *corrosion of ear drum (T28.91-)*

✓7ᵗʰ **T20.411 Corrosion of unspecified degree of** right **ear [any part, except ear drum]** ▽

✓7ᵗʰ **T20.412 Corrosion of unspecified degree of** left **ear [any part, except ear drum]** ▽

✓7ᵗʰ **T20.419 Corrosion of unspecified degree of unspecified ear [any part, except ear drum]** ▽

✓ₓ7ᵗʰ **T20.42 Corrosion of unspecified degree of** lip(s) ▽

✓ₓ7ᵗʰ **T20.43 Corrosion of unspecified degree of** chin ▽

✓ₓ7ᵗʰ **T20.44 Corrosion of unspecified degree of** nose (septum) ▽

✓ₓ7ᵗʰ **T20.45 Corrosion of unspecified degree of** scalp [any part] ▽

✓ₓ7ᵗʰ **T20.46 Corrosion of unspecified degree of** forehead and cheek ▽

✓ₓ7ᵗʰ **T20.47 Corrosion of unspecified degree of** neck ▽

✓ₓ7ᵗʰ **T20.49 Corrosion of unspecified degree of** multiple sites **of head, face, and neck** ▽

✓5ᵗʰ **T20.5 Corrosion of** first degree **of head, face, and neck**
Code first (T51-T65) to identify chemical and intent
Use additional external cause code to identify place (Y92)

✓ₓ7ᵗʰ **T20.50 Corrosion of first degree of head, face, and neck, unspecified site** ▽

✓6ᵗʰ **T20.51 Corrosion of first degree of** ear **[any part, except ear drum]**
EXCLUDES 2   *corrosion of ear drum (T28.91-)*

✓7ᵗʰ **T20.511 Corrosion of first degree of** right **ear [any part, except ear drum]**

✓7ᵗʰ **T20.512 Corrosion of first degree of** left **ear [any part, except ear drum]**

✓7ᵗʰ **T20.519 Corrosion of first degree of unspecified ear [any part, except ear drum]** ▽

✓ₓ7ᵗʰ **T20.52 Corrosion of first degree of** lip(s)

✓ₓ7ᵗʰ **T20.53 Corrosion of first degree of** chin

✓ₓ7ᵗʰ **T20.54 Corrosion of first degree of** nose (septum)

✓ₓ7ᵗʰ **T20.55 Corrosion of first degree of** scalp [any part]

✓ₓ7ᵗʰ **T20.56 Corrosion of first degree of** forehead and cheek

✓ₓ7ᵗʰ **T20.57 Corrosion of first degree of** neck

✓ₓ7ᵗʰ **T20.59 Corrosion of first degree of** multiple sites **of head, face, and neck**

✓5ᵗʰ **T20.6 Corrosion of** second degree **of head, face, and neck**
Code first (T51-T65) to identify chemical and intent
Use additional external cause code to identify place (Y92)

✓ₓ7ᵗʰ **T20.60 Corrosion of second degree of head, face, and neck, unspecified site** ▽

✓6ᵗʰ **T20.61 Corrosion of second degree of** ear **[any part, except ear drum]**
EXCLUDES 2   *corrosion of ear drum (T28.91-)*

✓7ᵗʰ **T20.611 Corrosion of second degree of** right **ear [any part, except ear drum]**

✓7ᵗʰ **T20.612 Corrosion of second degree of** left **ear [any part, except ear drum]**

✓7ᵗʰ **T20.619 Corrosion of second degree of unspecified ear [any part, except ear drum]** ▽

✓ₓ7ᵗʰ **T20.62 Corrosion of second degree of** lip(s)

✓ₓ7ᵗʰ **T20.63 Corrosion of second degree of** chin

✓ₓ7ᵗʰ **T20.64 Corrosion of second degree of** nose (septum)

✓ₓ7ᵗʰ **T20.65 Corrosion of second degree of** scalp [any part]

✓ₓ7ᵗʰ **T20.66 Corrosion of second degree of** forehead and cheek

✓ₓ7ᵗʰ **T20.67 Corrosion of second degree of** neck

✓ₓ7ᵗʰ **T20.69 Corrosion of second degree of** multiple sites **of head, face, and neck**

✓5ᵗʰ **T20.7 Corrosion of** third degree **of head, face, and neck**
Code first (T51-T65) to identify chemical and intent
Use additional external cause code to identify place (Y92)

✓ₓ7ᵗʰ **T20.70 Corrosion of third degree of head, face, and neck, unspecified site** ▽

✓6ᵗʰ **T20.71 Corrosion of third degree of** ear **[any part, except ear drum]**
EXCLUDES 2   *corrosion of ear drum (T28.91-)*

✓7ᵗʰ **T20.711 Corrosion of third degree of** right **ear [any part, except ear drum]**

✓7ᵗʰ **T20.712 Corrosion of third degree of** left **ear [any part, except ear drum]**

✓7ᵗʰ **T20.719 Corrosion of third degree of unspecified ear [any part, except ear drum]** ▽

✓ₓ7ᵗʰ **T20.72 Corrosion of third degree of** lip(s)

✓ₓ7ᵗʰ **T20.73 Corrosion of third degree of** chin

✓ₓ7ᵗʰ **T20.74 Corrosion of third degree of** nose (septum)

✓ₓ7ᵗʰ **T20.75 Corrosion of third degree of** scalp [any part]

✓ₓ7ᵗʰ **T20.76 Corrosion of third degree of** forehead and cheek

✓ₓ7ᵗʰ **T20.77 Corrosion of third degree of** neck

✓ₓ7ᵗʰ **T20.79 Corrosion of third degree of** multiple sites **of head, face, and neck**

✓ Additional Character Req   ✓ₓ7ᵗʰ Placeholder Alert   Manifestation   HCC CMS-HCC Condition   ▽ Unspecified Code   ▶◀ Revised Text   ● New Code   ▲ Revised Code Title

Chapter 19. Injury, Poisoning, and Certain Other Consequences of External Causes

T21–T21.52

✓4th **T21** **Burn and corrosion of trunk**

INCLUDES   burns and corrosion of hip region

EXCLUDES 2   *burns and corrosion of axilla (T22.- with fifth character 4)*
burns and corrosion of scapular region (T22.- with fifth character 6)
burns and corrosion of shoulder (T22.- with fifth character 5)

The appropriate 7th character is to be added to each code from category T21.
A   initial encounter
D   subsequent encounter
S   sequela

✓5th **T21.0** **Burn of unspecified degree of trunk**

Use additional external cause code to identify the source, place and intent of the burn (X00-X19, X75-X77, X96-X98, Y92)

✓x7th **T21.00** **Burn of unspecified degree of trunk, unspecified site** ▽

✓x7th **T21.01** **Burn of unspecified degree of** chest wall ▽
Burn of of unspecified degree of breast

✓x7th **T21.02** **Burn of unspecified degree of** abdominal wall ▽
Burn of unspecified degree of flank
Burn of unspecified degree of groin

✓x7th **T21.03** **Burn of unspecified degree of** upper back ▽
Burn of unspecified degree of interscapular region

✓x7th **T21.04** **Burn of unspecified degree of** lower back ▽

✓x7th **T21.05** **Burn of unspecified degree of** buttock ▽
Burn of unspecified degree of anus

✓x7th **T21.06** **Burn of unspecified degree of** male genital region ♂▽
Burn of unspecified degree of penis
Burn of unspecified degree of scrotum
Burn of unspecified degree of testis

✓x7th **T21.07** **Burn of unspecified degree of** female genital region ♀▽
Burn of unspecified degree of labium (majus) (minus)
Burn of unspecified degree of perineum
Burn of unspecified degree of vulva
EXCLUDES 2   *burn of vagina (T28.3)*

✓x7th **T21.09** **Burn of unspecified degree of other site of trunk** ▽

✓5th **T21.1** **Burn of** first degree **of trunk**

Use additional external cause code to identify the source, place and intent of the burn (X00-X19, X75-X77, X96-X98, Y92)

✓x7th **T21.10** **Burn of first degree of trunk, unspecified site** ▽

✓x7th **T21.11** **Burn of first degree of** chest wall
Burn of first degree of breast

✓x7th **T21.12** **Burn of first degree of** abdominal wall
Burn of first degree of flank
Burn of first degree of groin

✓x7th **T21.13** **Burn of first degree of** upper back
Burn of first degree of interscapular region

✓x7th **T21.14** **Burn of first degree of** lower back

✓x7th **T21.15** **Burn of first degree of** buttock
Burn of first degree of anus

✓x7th **T21.16** **Burn of first degree of** male genital region ♂
Burn of first degree of penis
Burn of first degree of scrotum
Burn of first degree of testis

✓x7th **T21.17** **Burn of first degree of** female genital region ♀
Burn of first degree of labium (majus) (minus)
Burn of first degree of perineum
Burn of first degree of vulva
EXCLUDES 2   *burn of vagina (T28.3)*

✓x7th **T21.19** **Burn of first degree of other site of trunk**

✓5th **T21.2** **Burn of** second degree **of trunk**

Use additional external cause code to identify the source, place and intent of the burn (X00-X19, X75-X77, X96-X98, Y92)

✓x7th **T21.20** **Burn of second degree of trunk, unspecified site** ▽

✓x7th **T21.21** **Burn of second degree of** chest wall
Burn of second degree of breast

✓x7th **T21.22** **Burn of second degree of** abdominal wall
Burn of second degree of flank
Burn of second degree of groin

✓x7th **T21.23** **Burn of second degree of** upper back
Burn of second degree of interscapular region

✓x7th **T21.24** **Burn of second degree of** lower back

✓x7th **T21.25** **Burn of second degree of** buttock
Burn of second degree of anus

✓x7th **T21.26** **Burn of second degree of** male genital region ♂
Burn of second degree of penis
Burn of second degree of scrotum
Burn of second degree of testis

✓x7th **T21.27** **Burn of second degree of** female genital region ♀
Burn of second degree of labium (majus) (minus)
Burn of second degree of perineum
Burn of second degree of vulva
EXCLUDES 2   *burn of vagina (T28.3)*

✓x7th **T21.29** **Burn of second degree of other site of trunk**

✓5th **T21.3** **Burn of** third degree **of trunk**

Use additional external cause code to identify the source, place and intent of the burn (X00-X19, X75-X77, X96-X98, Y92)

✓x7th **T21.30** **Burn of third degree of trunk, unspecified site** ▽

✓x7th **T21.31** **Burn of third degree of** chest wall
Burn of third degree of breast
AHA: 2016, 2Q, 5

✓x7th **T21.32** **Burn of third degree of** abdominal wall
Burn of third degree of flank
Burn of third degree of groin

✓x7th **T21.33** **Burn of third degree of** upper back
Burn of third degree of interscapular region

✓x7th **T21.34** **Burn of third degree of** lower back

✓x7th **T21.35** **Burn of third degree of** buttock
Burn of third degree of anus

✓x7th **T21.36** **Burn of third degree of** male genital region ♂
Burn of third degree of penis
Burn of third degree of scrotum
Burn of third degree of testis

✓x7th **T21.37** **Burn of third degree of** female genital region ♀
Burn of third degree of labium (majus) (minus)
Burn of third degree of perineum
Burn of third degree of vulva
EXCLUDES 2   *burn of vagina (T28.3)*

✓x7th **T21.39** **Burn of third degree of other site of trunk**

✓5th **T21.4** **Corrosion of unspecified degree of trunk**

Code first (T51-T65) to identify chemical and intent
Use additional external cause code to identify place (Y92)

✓x7th **T21.40** **Corrosion of unspecified degree of trunk, unspecified site** ▽

✓x7th **T21.41** **Corrosion of unspecified degree of** chest wall ▽
Corrosion of unspecified degree of breast

✓x7th **T21.42** **Corrosion of unspecified degree of** abdominal wall ▽
Corrosion of unspecified degree of flank
Corrosion of unspecified degree of groin

✓x7th **T21.43** **Corrosion of unspecified degree of** upper back ▽
Corrosion of unspecified degree of interscapular region

✓x7th **T21.44** **Corrosion of unspecified degree of** lower back ▽

✓x7th **T21.45** **Corrosion of unspecified degree of** buttock ▽
Corrosion of unspecified degree of anus

✓x7th **T21.46** **Corrosion of unspecified degree of** male genital region ♂▽
Corrosion of unspecified degree of penis
Corrosion of unspecified degree of scrotum
Corrosion of unspecified degree of testis

✓x7th **T21.47** **Corrosion of unspecified degree of** female genital region ♀▽
Corrosion of unspecified degree of labium (majus) (minus)
Corrosion of unspecified degree of perineum
Corrosion of unspecified degree of vulva
EXCLUDES 2   *corrosion of vagina (T28.8)*

✓x7th **T21.49** **Corrosion of unspecified degree of other site of trunk** ▽

✓5th **T21.5** **Corrosion of** first degree **of trunk**

Code first (T51-T65) to identify chemical and intent
Use additional external cause code to identify place (Y92)

✓x7th **T21.50** **Corrosion of first degree of trunk, unspecified site** ▽

✓x7th **T21.51** **Corrosion of first degree of** chest wall
Corrosion of first degree of breast

✓x7th **T21.52** **Corrosion of first degree of** abdominal wall
Corrosion of first degree of flank
Corrosion of first degree of groin

EXCLUDES 1 Not coded here   EXCLUDES 2 Not included here   N Newborn Age: 0   P Pediatric Age: 0-17   M Maternity Age: 12-55   A Adult Age: 15-124

1042   ICD-10-CM 2018

√x7ᵗʰ **T21.53** **Corrosion of first degree of** upper back
Corrosion of first degree of interscapular region

√x7ᵗʰ **T21.54** **Corrosion of first degree of** lower back

√x7ᵗʰ **T21.55** **Corrosion of first degree of** buttock
Corrosion of first degree of anus

√x7ᵗʰ **T21.56** **Corrosion of first degree of** male genital region ♂
Corrosion of first degree of penis
Corrosion of first degree of scrotum
Corrosion of first degree of testis

√x7ᵗʰ **T21.57** **Corrosion of first degree of** female genital region ♀
Corrosion of first degree of labium (majus) (minus)
Corrosion of first degree of perineum
Corrosion of first degree of vulva
EXCLUDES 2   corrosion of vagina (T28.8)

√x7ᵗʰ **T21.59** **Corrosion of first degree of other site of trunk**

✓5ᵗʰ **T21.6** **Corrosion of** second degree **of trunk**
Code first (T51-T65) to identify chemical and intent
Use additional external cause code to identify place (Y92)

√x7ᵗʰ **T21.60** **Corrosion of second degree of trunk, unspecified** ▽
site

√x7ᵗʰ **T21.61** **Corrosion of second degree of** chest wall
Corrosion of second degree of breast

√x7ᵗʰ **T21.62** **Corrosion of second degree of** abdominal wall
Corrosion of second degree of flank
Corrosion of second degree of groin

√x7ᵗʰ **T21.63** **Corrosion of second degree of** upper back
Corrosion of second degree of interscapular region

√x7ᵗʰ **T21.64** **Corrosion of second degree of** lower back

√x7ᵗʰ **T21.65** **Corrosion of second degree of** buttock
Corrosion of second degree of anus

√x7ᵗʰ **T21.66** **Corrosion of second degree of** male genital region ♂
Corrosion of second degree of penis
Corrosion of second degree of scrotum
Corrosion of second degree of testis

√x7ᵗʰ **T21.67** **Corrosion of second degree of** female genital ♀
region
Corrosion of second degree of labium (majus) (minus)
Corrosion of second degree of perineum
Corrosion of second degree of vulva
EXCLUDES 2   corrosion of vagina (T28.8)

√x7ᵗʰ **T21.69** **Corrosion of second degree of other site of trunk**

✓5ᵗʰ **T21.7** **Corrosion of** third degree **of trunk**
Code first (T51-T65) to identify chemical and intent
Use additional external cause code to identify place (Y92)

√x7ᵗʰ **T21.70** **Corrosion of third degree of trunk, unspecified** ▽
site

√x7ᵗʰ **T21.71** **Corrosion of third degree of** chest wall
Corrosion of third degree of breast

√x7ᵗʰ **T21.72** **Corrosion of third degree of** abdominal wall
Corrosion of third degree of flank
Corrosion of third degree of groin

√x7ᵗʰ **T21.73** **Corrosion of third degree of** upper back
Corrosion of third degree of interscapular region

√x7ᵗʰ **T21.74** **Corrosion of third degree of** lower back

√x7ᵗʰ **T21.75** **Corrosion of third degree of** buttock
Corrosion of third degree of anus

√x7ᵗʰ **T21.76** **Corrosion of third degree of** male genital region ♂
Corrosion of third degree of penis
Corrosion of third degree of scrotum
Corrosion of third degree of testis

√x7ᵗʰ **T21.77** **Corrosion of third degree of** female genital region ♀
Corrosion of third degree of labium (majus) (minus)
Corrosion of third degree of perineum
Corrosion of third degree of vulva
EXCLUDES 2   corrosion of vagina (T28.8)

√x7ᵗʰ **T21.79** **Corrosion of third degree of other site of trunk**

✓4ᵗʰ **T22** **Burn and corrosion of shoulder and upper limb, except wrist and hand**
EXCLUDES 2   burn and corrosion of interscapular region (T21.-)
burn and corrosion of wrist and hand (T23.-)

The appropriate 7th character is to be added to each code from category T22.
A   initial encounter
D   subsequent encounter
S   sequela

✓5ᵗʰ **T22.0** **Burn of unspecified degree of shoulder and upper limb, except wrist and hand**
Use additional external cause code to identify the source, place and intent of the burn (X00-X19, X75-X77, X96-X98, Y92)

√x7ᵗʰ **T22.00** **Burn of unspecified degree of shoulder and** ▽
upper limb, except wrist and hand, unspecified site

✓6ᵗʰ **T22.01** **Burn of unspecified degree of** forearm

√7ᵗʰ **T22.011** **Burn of unspecified degree of** right ▽
forearm

√7ᵗʰ **T22.012** **Burn of unspecified degree of** left ▽
forearm

√7ᵗʰ **T22.019** **Burn of unspecified degree of** ▽
unspecified forearm

✓6ᵗʰ **T22.02** **Burn of unspecified degree of** elbow

√7ᵗʰ **T22.021** **Burn of unspecified degree of** right ▽
elbow

√7ᵗʰ **T22.022** **Burn of unspecified degree of** left ▽
elbow

√7ᵗʰ **T22.029** **Burn of unspecified degree of** ▽
unspecified elbow

✓6ᵗʰ **T22.03** **Burn of unspecified degree of** upper arm

√7ᵗʰ **T22.031** **Burn of unspecified degree of** ▽
right upper arm

√7ᵗʰ **T22.032** **Burn of unspecified degree of** ▽
left upper arm

√7ᵗʰ **T22.039** **Burn of unspecified degree of** ▽
unspecified upper arm

✓6ᵗʰ **T22.04** **Burn of unspecified degree of** axilla

√7ᵗʰ **T22.041** **Burn of unspecified degree of** ▽
right axilla

√7ᵗʰ **T22.042** **Burn of unspecified degree of** ▽
left axilla

√7ᵗʰ **T22.049** **Burn of unspecified degree of** ▽
unspecified axilla

✓6ᵗʰ **T22.05** **Burn of unspecified degree of** shoulder

√7ᵗʰ **T22.051** **Burn of unspecified degree of** right ▽
shoulder

√7ᵗʰ **T22.052** **Burn of unspecified degree of** left ▽
shoulder

√7ᵗʰ **T22.059** **Burn of unspecified degree of** ▽
unspecified shoulder

✓6ᵗʰ **T22.06** **Burn of unspecified degree of** scapular region

√7ᵗʰ **T22.061** **Burn of unspecified degree of** right ▽
scapular region

√7ᵗʰ **T22.062** **Burn of unspecified degree of** left ▽
scapular region

√7ᵗʰ **T22.069** **Burn of unspecified degree of** ▽
unspecified scapular region

✓6ᵗʰ **T22.09** **Burn of unspecified degree of** multiple sites **of shoulder and upper limb, except wrist and hand**

√7ᵗʰ **T22.091** **Burn of unspecified degree of multiple** ▽
sites of right **shoulder and upper limb, except wrist and hand**

√7ᵗʰ **T22.092** **Burn of unspecified degree of multiple** ▽
sites of left **shoulder and upper limb, except wrist and hand**

√7ᵗʰ **T22.099** **Burn of unspecified degree of multiple** ▽
sites of unspecified shoulder and upper limb, except wrist and hand

✓5ᵗʰ **T22.1** **Burn of** first degree **of shoulder and upper limb, except wrist and hand**
Use additional external cause code to identify the source, place and intent of the burn (X00-X19, X75-X77, X96-X98, Y92)

√x7ᵗʰ **T22.10** **Burn of first degree of shoulder and upper limb,** ▽
except wrist and hand, unspecified site

√6ᵗʰ **T22.11**　**Burn of first degree of** forearm
- √7ᵗʰ **T22.111**　Burn of first degree of right forearm
- √7ᵗʰ **T22.112**　Burn of first degree of left forearm
- √7ᵗʰ **T22.119**　Burn of first degree of unspecified forearm ▽

√6ᵗʰ **T22.12**　**Burn of first degree of** elbow
- √7ᵗʰ **T22.121**　Burn of first degree of right elbow
- √7ᵗʰ **T22.122**　Burn of first degree of left elbow
- √7ᵗʰ **T22.129**　Burn of first degree of unspecified elbow ▽

√6ᵗʰ **T22.13**　**Burn of first degree of** upper arm
- √7ᵗʰ **T22.131**　Burn of first degree of right upper arm
- √7ᵗʰ **T22.132**　Burn of first degree of left upper arm
- √7ᵗʰ **T22.139**　Burn of first degree of unspecified upper arm ▽

√6ᵗʰ **T22.14**　**Burn of first degree of** axilla
- √7ᵗʰ **T22.141**　Burn of first degree of right axilla
- √7ᵗʰ **T22.142**　Burn of first degree of left axilla
- √7ᵗʰ **T22.149**　Burn of first degree of unspecified axilla ▽

√6ᵗʰ **T22.15**　**Burn of first degree of** shoulder
- √7ᵗʰ **T22.151**　Burn of first degree of right shoulder
- √7ᵗʰ **T22.152**　Burn of first degree of left shoulder
- √7ᵗʰ **T22.159**　Burn of first degree of unspecified shoulder ▽

√6ᵗʰ **T22.16**　**Burn of first degree of** scapular region
- √7ᵗʰ **T22.161**　Burn of first degree of right scapular region
- √7ᵗʰ **T22.162**　Burn of first degree of left scapular region
- √7ᵗʰ **T22.169**　Burn of first degree of unspecified scapular region ▽

√6ᵗʰ **T22.19**　**Burn of first degree of** multiple sites **of shoulder and upper limb, except wrist and hand**
- √7ᵗʰ **T22.191**　Burn of first degree of multiple sites of right shoulder and upper limb, except wrist and hand
- √7ᵗʰ **T22.192**　Burn of first degree of multiple sites of left shoulder and upper limb, except wrist and hand
- √7ᵗʰ **T22.199**　Burn of first degree of multiple sites of unspecified shoulder and upper limb, except wrist and hand ▽

√5ᵗʰ **T22.2**　**Burn of** second degree **of shoulder and upper limb, except wrist and hand**
Use additional external cause code to identify the source, place and intent of the burn (X00-X19, X75-X77, X96-X98, Y92)

√x7ᵗʰ **T22.20**　Burn of second degree of shoulder and upper limb, except wrist and hand, unspecified site ▽

√6ᵗʰ **T22.21**　**Burn of second degree of** forearm
- √7ᵗʰ **T22.211**　Burn of second degree of right forearm
- √7ᵗʰ **T22.212**　Burn of second degree of left forearm
- √7ᵗʰ **T22.219**　Burn of second degree of unspecified forearm ▽

√6ᵗʰ **T22.22**　**Burn of second degree of** elbow
- √7ᵗʰ **T22.221**　Burn of second degree of right elbow
- √7ᵗʰ **T22.222**　Burn of second degree of left elbow
- √7ᵗʰ **T22.229**　Burn of second degree of unspecified elbow ▽

√6ᵗʰ **T22.23**　**Burn of second degree of** upper arm
- √7ᵗʰ **T22.231**　Burn of second degree of right upper arm
- √7ᵗʰ **T22.232**　Burn of second degree of left upper arm
- √7ᵗʰ **T22.239**　Burn of second degree of unspecified upper arm ▽

√6ᵗʰ **T22.24**　**Burn of second degree of** axilla
- √7ᵗʰ **T22.241**　Burn of second degree of right axilla
- √7ᵗʰ **T22.242**　Burn of second degree of left axilla
- √7ᵗʰ **T22.249**　Burn of second degree of unspecified axilla ▽

√6ᵗʰ **T22.25**　**Burn of second degree of** shoulder
- √7ᵗʰ **T22.251**　Burn of second degree of right shoulder
- √7ᵗʰ **T22.252**　Burn of second degree of left shoulder

√7ᵗʰ **T22.259**　Burn of second degree of unspecified shoulder ▽

√6ᵗʰ **T22.26**　**Burn of second degree of** scapular region
- √7ᵗʰ **T22.261**　Burn of second degree of right scapular region
- √7ᵗʰ **T22.262**　Burn of second degree of left scapular region
- √7ᵗʰ **T22.269**　Burn of second degree of unspecified scapular region ▽

√6ᵗʰ **T22.29**　**Burn of second degree of** multiple sites **of shoulder and upper limb, except wrist and hand**
- √7ᵗʰ **T22.291**　Burn of second degree of multiple sites of right shoulder and upper limb, except wrist and hand
- √7ᵗʰ **T22.292**　Burn of second degree of multiple sites of left shoulder and upper limb, except wrist and hand
- √7ᵗʰ **T22.299**　Burn of second degree of multiple sites of unspecified shoulder and upper limb, except wrist and hand ▽

√5ᵗʰ **T22.3**　**Burn of** third degree **of shoulder and upper limb, except wrist and hand**
Use additional external cause code to identify the source, place and intent of the burn (X00-X19, X75-X77, X96-X98, Y92)

√x7ᵗʰ **T22.30**　Burn of third degree of shoulder and upper limb, except wrist and hand, unspecified site ▽

√6ᵗʰ **T22.31**　**Burn of third degree of** forearm
- √7ᵗʰ **T22.311**　Burn of third degree of right forearm
- √7ᵗʰ **T22.312**　Burn of third degree of left forearm
- √7ᵗʰ **T22.319**　Burn of third degree of unspecified forearm ▽

√6ᵗʰ **T22.32**　**Burn of third degree of** elbow
- √7ᵗʰ **T22.321**　Burn of third degree of right elbow
- √7ᵗʰ **T22.322**　Burn of third degree of left elbow
- √7ᵗʰ **T22.329**　Burn of third degree of unspecified elbow ▽

√6ᵗʰ **T22.33**　**Burn of third degree of** upper arm
- √7ᵗʰ **T22.331**　Burn of third degree of right upper arm
- √7ᵗʰ **T22.332**　Burn of third degree of left upper arm
- √7ᵗʰ **T22.339**　Burn of third degree of unspecified upper arm ▽

√6ᵗʰ **T22.34**　**Burn of third degree of** axilla
- √7ᵗʰ **T22.341**　Burn of third degree of right axilla
- √7ᵗʰ **T22.342**　Burn of third degree of left axilla
- √7ᵗʰ **T22.349**　Burn of third degree of unspecified axilla ▽

√6ᵗʰ **T22.35**　**Burn of third degree of** shoulder
- √7ᵗʰ **T22.351**　Burn of third degree of right shoulder
- √7ᵗʰ **T22.352**　Burn of third degree of left shoulder
- √7ᵗʰ **T22.359**　Burn of third degree of unspecified shoulder ▽

√6ᵗʰ **T22.36**　**Burn of third degree of** scapular region
- √7ᵗʰ **T22.361**　Burn of third degree of right scapular region
- √7ᵗʰ **T22.362**　Burn of third degree of left scapular region
- √7ᵗʰ **T22.369**　Burn of third degree of unspecified scapular region ▽

√6ᵗʰ **T22.39**　**Burn of third degree of** multiple sites **of shoulder and upper limb, except wrist and hand**
- √7ᵗʰ **T22.391**　Burn of third degree of multiple sites of right shoulder and upper limb, except wrist and hand
- √7ᵗʰ **T22.392**　Burn of third degree of multiple sites of left shoulder and upper limb, except wrist and hand
- √7ᵗʰ **T22.399**　Burn of third degree of multiple sites of unspecified shoulder and upper limb, except wrist and hand ▽

EXCLUDES 1 Not coded here　　　EXCLUDES 2 Not included here　　　N Newborn Age: 0　　　P Pediatric Age: 0-17　　　M Maternity Age: 12-55　　　A Adult Age: 15-124

√5ᵗʰ **T22.4** **Corrosion of unspecified degree of shoulder and upper limb, except wrist and hand**

     Code first (T51-T65) to identify chemical and intent

     Use additional external cause code to identify place (Y92)

√x7ᵗʰ **T22.40** Corrosion of unspecified degree of shoulder and upper limb, except wrist and hand, unspecified site ▽

√6ᵗʰ **T22.41** Corrosion of unspecified degree of forearm

    √7ᵗʰ **T22.411** Corrosion of unspecified degree of right forearm ▽

    √7ᵗʰ **T22.412** Corrosion of unspecified degree of left forearm ▽

    √7ᵗʰ **T22.419** Corrosion of unspecified degree of unspecified forearm ▽

√6ᵗʰ **T22.42** Corrosion of unspecified degree of elbow

    √7ᵗʰ **T22.421** Corrosion of unspecified degree of right elbow ▽

    √7ᵗʰ **T22.422** Corrosion of unspecified degree of left elbow ▽

    √7ᵗʰ **T22.429** Corrosion of unspecified degree of unspecified elbow ▽

√6ᵗʰ **T22.43** Corrosion of unspecified degree of upper arm

    √7ᵗʰ **T22.431** Corrosion of unspecified degree of right upper arm ▽

    √7ᵗʰ **T22.432** Corrosion of unspecified degree of left upper arm ▽

    √7ᵗʰ **T22.439** Corrosion of unspecified degree of unspecified upper arm ▽

√6ᵗʰ **T22.44** Corrosion of unspecified degree of axilla

    √7ᵗʰ **T22.441** Corrosion of unspecified degree of right axilla ▽

    √7ᵗʰ **T22.442** Corrosion of unspecified degree of left axilla ▽

    √7ᵗʰ **T22.449** Corrosion of unspecified degree of unspecified axilla ▽

√6ᵗʰ **T22.45** Corrosion of unspecified degree of shoulder

    √7ᵗʰ **T22.451** Corrosion of unspecified degree of right shoulder ▽

    √7ᵗʰ **T22.452** Corrosion of unspecified degree of left shoulder ▽

    √7ᵗʰ **T22.459** Corrosion of unspecified degree of unspecified shoulder ▽

√6ᵗʰ **T22.46** Corrosion of unspecified degree of scapular region

    √7ᵗʰ **T22.461** Corrosion of unspecified degree of right scapular region ▽

    √7ᵗʰ **T22.462** Corrosion of unspecified degree of left scapular region ▽

    √7ᵗʰ **T22.469** Corrosion of unspecified degree of unspecified scapular region ▽

√6ᵗʰ **T22.49** Corrosion of unspecified degree of multiple sites of shoulder and upper limb, except wrist and hand

    √7ᵗʰ **T22.491** Corrosion of unspecified degree of multiple sites of right shoulder and upper limb, except wrist and hand ▽

    √7ᵗʰ **T22.492** Corrosion of unspecified degree of multiple sites of left shoulder and upper limb, except wrist and hand ▽

    √7ᵗʰ **T22.499** Corrosion of unspecified degree of multiple sites of unspecified shoulder and upper limb, except wrist and hand ▽

√5ᵗʰ **T22.5** **Corrosion of first degree of shoulder and upper limb, except wrist and hand**

     Code first (T51-T65) to identify chemical and intent

     Use additional external cause code to identify place (Y92)

√x7ᵗʰ **T22.50** Corrosion of first degree of shoulder and upper limb, except wrist and hand unspecified site ▽

√6ᵗʰ **T22.51** Corrosion of first degree of forearm

    √7ᵗʰ **T22.511** Corrosion of first degree of right forearm

    √7ᵗʰ **T22.512** Corrosion of first degree of left forearm

    √7ᵗʰ **T22.519** Corrosion of first degree of unspecified forearm ▽

√6ᵗʰ **T22.52** Corrosion of first degree of elbow

    √7ᵗʰ **T22.521** Corrosion of first degree of right elbow

    √7ᵗʰ **T22.522** Corrosion of first degree of left elbow

√7ᵗʰ **T22.529** Corrosion of first degree of unspecified elbow ▽

√6ᵗʰ **T22.53** Corrosion of first degree of upper arm

    √7ᵗʰ **T22.531** Corrosion of first degree of right upper arm

    √7ᵗʰ **T22.532** Corrosion of first degree of left upper arm

    √7ᵗʰ **T22.539** Corrosion of first degree of unspecified upper arm ▽

√6ᵗʰ **T22.54** Corrosion of first degree of axilla

    √7ᵗʰ **T22.541** Corrosion of first degree of right axilla

    √7ᵗʰ **T22.542** Corrosion of first degree of left axilla

    √7ᵗʰ **T22.549** Corrosion of first degree of unspecified axilla ▽

√6ᵗʰ **T22.55** Corrosion of first degree of shoulder

    √7ᵗʰ **T22.551** Corrosion of first degree of right shoulder

    √7ᵗʰ **T22.552** Corrosion of first degree of left shoulder

    √7ᵗʰ **T22.559** Corrosion of first degree of unspecified shoulder ▽

√6ᵗʰ **T22.56** Corrosion of first degree of scapular region

    √7ᵗʰ **T22.561** Corrosion of first degree of right scapular region

    √7ᵗʰ **T22.562** Corrosion of first degree of left scapular region

    √7ᵗʰ **T22.569** Corrosion of first degree of unspecified scapular region ▽

√6ᵗʰ **T22.59** Corrosion of first degree of multiple sites of shoulder and upper limb, except wrist and hand

    √7ᵗʰ **T22.591** Corrosion of first degree of multiple sites of right shoulder and upper limb, except wrist and hand

    √7ᵗʰ **T22.592** Corrosion of first degree of multiple sites of left shoulder and upper limb, except wrist and hand

    √7ᵗʰ **T22.599** Corrosion of first degree of multiple sites of unspecified shoulder and upper limb, except wrist and hand ▽

√5ᵗʰ **T22.6** **Corrosion of second degree of shoulder and upper limb, except wrist and hand**

     Code first (T51-T65) to identify chemical and intent

     Use additional external cause code to identify place (Y92)

√x7ᵗʰ **T22.60** Corrosion of second degree of shoulder and upper limb, except wrist and hand, unspecified site ▽

√6ᵗʰ **T22.61** Corrosion of second degree of forearm

    √7ᵗʰ **T22.611** Corrosion of second degree of right forearm

    √7ᵗʰ **T22.612** Corrosion of second degree of left forearm

    √7ᵗʰ **T22.619** Corrosion of second degree of unspecified forearm ▽

√6ᵗʰ **T22.62** Corrosion of second degree of elbow

    √7ᵗʰ **T22.621** Corrosion of second degree of right elbow

    √7ᵗʰ **T22.622** Corrosion of second degree of left elbow

    √7ᵗʰ **T22.629** Corrosion of second degree of unspecified elbow ▽

√6ᵗʰ **T22.63** Corrosion of second degree of upper arm

    √7ᵗʰ **T22.631** Corrosion of second degree of right upper arm

    √7ᵗʰ **T22.632** Corrosion of second degree of left upper arm

    √7ᵗʰ **T22.639** Corrosion of second degree of unspecified upper arm ▽

√6ᵗʰ **T22.64** Corrosion of second degree of axilla

    √7ᵗʰ **T22.641** Corrosion of second degree of right axilla

    √7ᵗʰ **T22.642** Corrosion of second degree of left axilla

    √7ᵗʰ **T22.649** Corrosion of second degree of unspecified axilla ▽

√6ᵗʰ **T22.65** Corrosion of second degree of shoulder

    √7ᵗʰ **T22.651** Corrosion of second degree of right shoulder

    √7ᵗʰ **T22.652** Corrosion of second degree of left shoulder

    √7ᵗʰ **T22.659** Corrosion of second degree of unspecified shoulder ▽

☑ Additional Character Req   √x7ᵗʰ Placeholder Alert   Manifestation   ℍℂℂ CMS-HCC Condition   ▽ Unspecified Code   ►◄ Revised Text   ● New Code   ▲ Revised Code Title

√6ᵗʰ **T22.66** Corrosion of second degree of scapular region

√7ᵗʰ **T22.661** Corrosion of second degree of right scapular region

√7ᵗʰ **T22.662** Corrosion of second degree of left scapular region

√7ᵗʰ **T22.669** Corrosion of second degree of unspecified scapular region ▽

√6ᵗʰ **T22.69** Corrosion of second degree of multiple sites of shoulder and upper limb, except wrist and hand

√7ᵗʰ **T22.691** Corrosion of second degree of multiple sites of right shoulder and upper limb, except wrist and hand

√7ᵗʰ **T22.692** Corrosion of second degree of multiple sites of left shoulder and upper limb, except wrist and hand

√7ᵗʰ **T22.699** Corrosion of second degree of multiple sites of unspecified shoulder and upper limb, except wrist and hand ▽

√5ᵗʰ **T22.7** Corrosion of third degree of shoulder and upper limb, except wrist and hand
　　Code first (T51-T65) to identify chemical and intent
　　Use additional external cause code to identify place (Y92)

√ˣ7ᵗʰ **T22.70** Corrosion of third degree of shoulder and upper limb, except wrist and hand, unspecified site ▽

√6ᵗʰ **T22.71** Corrosion of third degree of forearm

√7ᵗʰ **T22.711** Corrosion of third degree of right forearm

√7ᵗʰ **T22.712** Corrosion of third degree of left forearm

√7ᵗʰ **T22.719** Corrosion of third degree of unspecified forearm ▽

√6ᵗʰ **T22.72** Corrosion of third degree of elbow

√7ᵗʰ **T22.721** Corrosion of third degree of right elbow

√7ᵗʰ **T22.722** Corrosion of third degree of left elbow

√7ᵗʰ **T22.729** Corrosion of third degree of unspecified elbow ▽

√6ᵗʰ **T22.73** Corrosion of third degree of upper arm

√7ᵗʰ **T22.731** Corrosion of third degree of right upper arm

√7ᵗʰ **T22.732** Corrosion of third degree of left upper arm

√7ᵗʰ **T22.739** Corrosion of third degree of unspecified upper arm ▽

√6ᵗʰ **T22.74** Corrosion of third degree of axilla

√7ᵗʰ **T22.741** Corrosion of third degree of right axilla

√7ᵗʰ **T22.742** Corrosion of third degree of left axilla

√7ᵗʰ **T22.749** Corrosion of third degree of unspecified axilla ▽

√6ᵗʰ **T22.75** Corrosion of third degree of shoulder

√7ᵗʰ **T22.751** Corrosion of third degree of right shoulder

√7ᵗʰ **T22.752** Corrosion of third degree of left shoulder

√7ᵗʰ **T22.759** Corrosion of third degree of unspecified shoulder ▽

√6ᵗʰ **T22.76** Corrosion of third degree of scapular region

√7ᵗʰ **T22.761** Corrosion of third degree of right scapular region

√7ᵗʰ **T22.762** Corrosion of third degree of left scapular region

√7ᵗʰ **T22.769** Corrosion of third degree of unspecified scapular region ▽

√6ᵗʰ **T22.79** Corrosion of third degree of multiple sites of shoulder and upper limb, except wrist and hand

√7ᵗʰ **T22.791** Corrosion of third degree of multiple sites of right shoulder and upper limb, except wrist and hand

√7ᵗʰ **T22.792** Corrosion of third degree of multiple sites of left shoulder and upper limb, except wrist and hand

√7ᵗʰ **T22.799** Corrosion of third degree of multiple sites of unspecified shoulder and upper limb, except wrist and hand ▽

√4ᵗʰ **T23** **Burn and corrosion of wrist and hand**
　　AHA: 2015, 1Q, 19

　The appropriate 7th character is to be added to each code from category T23.
　A　initial encounter
　D　subsequent encounter
　S　sequela

√5ᵗʰ **T23.0** Burn of unspecified degree of wrist and hand
　　Use additional external cause code to identify the source, place and intent of the burn (X00-X19, X75-X77, X96-X98, Y92)

√6ᵗʰ **T23.00** Burn of unspecified degree of hand, unspecified site

√7ᵗʰ **T23.001** Burn of unspecified degree of right hand, unspecified site ▽

√7ᵗʰ **T23.002** Burn of unspecified degree of left hand, unspecified site ▽

√7ᵗʰ **T23.009** Burn of unspecified degree of unspecified hand, unspecified site ▽

√6ᵗʰ **T23.01** Burn of unspecified degree of thumb (nail)

√7ᵗʰ **T23.011** Burn of unspecified degree of right thumb (nail) ▽

√7ᵗʰ **T23.012** Burn of unspecified degree of left thumb (nail) ▽

√7ᵗʰ **T23.019** Burn of unspecified degree of unspecified thumb (nail) ▽

√6ᵗʰ **T23.02** Burn of unspecified degree of single finger (nail) except thumb

√7ᵗʰ **T23.021** Burn of unspecified degree of single right finger (nail) except thumb ▽

√7ᵗʰ **T23.022** Burn of unspecified degree of single left finger (nail) except thumb ▽

√7ᵗʰ **T23.029** Burn of unspecified degree of unspecified single finger (nail) except thumb ▽

√6ᵗʰ **T23.03** Burn of unspecified degree of multiple fingers (nail), not including thumb

√7ᵗʰ **T23.031** Burn of unspecified degree of multiple right fingers (nail), not including thumb ▽

√7ᵗʰ **T23.032** Burn of unspecified degree of multiple left fingers (nail), not including thumb ▽

√7ᵗʰ **T23.039** Burn of unspecified degree of unspecified multiple fingers (nail), not including thumb ▽

√6ᵗʰ **T23.04** Burn of unspecified degree of multiple fingers (nail), including thumb

√7ᵗʰ **T23.041** Burn of unspecified degree of multiple right fingers (nail), including thumb ▽

√7ᵗʰ **T23.042** Burn of unspecified degree of multiple left fingers (nail), including thumb ▽

√7ᵗʰ **T23.049** Burn of unspecified degree of unspecified multiple fingers (nail), including thumb ▽

√6ᵗʰ **T23.05** Burn of unspecified degree of palm

√7ᵗʰ **T23.051** Burn of unspecified degree of right palm ▽

√7ᵗʰ **T23.052** Burn of unspecified degree of left palm ▽

√7ᵗʰ **T23.059** Burn of unspecified degree of unspecified palm ▽

√6ᵗʰ **T23.06** Burn of unspecified degree of back of hand

√7ᵗʰ **T23.061** Burn of unspecified degree of back of right hand ▽

√7ᵗʰ **T23.062** Burn of unspecified degree of back of left hand ▽

√7ᵗʰ **T23.069** Burn of unspecified degree of back of unspecified hand ▽

√6ᵗʰ **T23.07** Burn of unspecified degree of wrist

√7ᵗʰ **T23.071** Burn of unspecified degree of right wrist ▽

√7ᵗʰ **T23.072** Burn of unspecified degree of left wrist ▽

√7ᵗʰ **T23.079** Burn of unspecified degree of unspecified wrist ▽

EXCLUDES 1 Not coded here　**EXCLUDES 2** Not included here　Ⓝ Newborn Age: 0　Ⓟ Pediatric Age: 0-17　Ⓜ Maternity Age: 12-55　Ⓐ Adult Age: 15-124

✓6ᵗʰ **T23.09** Burn of unspecified degree of multiple sites of wrist and hand

    ✓7ᵗʰ **T23.091** Burn of unspecified degree of multiple sites of right wrist and hand ▽

    ✓7ᵗʰ **T23.092** Burn of unspecified degree of multiple sites of left wrist and hand ▽

    ✓7ᵗʰ **T23.099** Burn of unspecified degree of multiple sites of unspecified wrist and hand ▽

✓5ᵗʰ **T23.1** Burn of first degree of wrist and hand

Use additional external cause code to identify the source, place and intent of the burn (X00-X19, X75-X77, X96-X98, Y92)

  ✓6ᵗʰ **T23.10** Burn of first degree of hand, unspecified site

    ✓7ᵗʰ **T23.101** Burn of first degree of right hand, unspecified site ▽

    ✓7ᵗʰ **T23.102** Burn of first degree of left hand, unspecified site ▽

    ✓7ᵗʰ **T23.109** Burn of first degree of unspecified hand, unspecified site ▽

  ✓6ᵗʰ **T23.11** Burn of first degree of thumb (nail)

    ✓7ᵗʰ **T23.111** Burn of first degree of right thumb (nail)

    ✓7ᵗʰ **T23.112** Burn of first degree of left thumb (nail)

    ✓7ᵗʰ **T23.119** Burn of first degree of unspecified thumb (nail) ▽

  ✓6ᵗʰ **T23.12** Burn of first degree of single finger (nail) except thumb

    ✓7ᵗʰ **T23.121** Burn of first degree of single right finger (nail) except thumb

    ✓7ᵗʰ **T23.122** Burn of first degree of single left finger (nail) except thumb

    ✓7ᵗʰ **T23.129** Burn of first degree of unspecified single finger (nail) except thumb ▽

  ✓6ᵗʰ **T23.13** Burn of first degree of multiple fingers (nail), not including thumb

    ✓7ᵗʰ **T23.131** Burn of first degree of multiple right fingers (nail), not including thumb

    ✓7ᵗʰ **T23.132** Burn of first degree of multiple left fingers (nail), not including thumb

    ✓7ᵗʰ **T23.139** Burn of first degree of unspecified multiple fingers (nail), not including thumb ▽

  ✓6ᵗʰ **T23.14** Burn of first degree of multiple fingers (nail), including thumb

    ✓7ᵗʰ **T23.141** Burn of first degree of multiple right fingers (nail), including thumb

    ✓7ᵗʰ **T23.142** Burn of first degree of multiple left fingers (nail), including thumb

    ✓7ᵗʰ **T23.149** Burn of first degree of unspecified multiple fingers (nail), including thumb ▽

  ✓6ᵗʰ **T23.15** Burn of first degree of palm

    ✓7ᵗʰ **T23.151** Burn of first degree of right palm

    ✓7ᵗʰ **T23.152** Burn of first degree of left palm

    ✓7ᵗʰ **T23.159** Burn of first degree of unspecified palm ▽

  ✓6ᵗʰ **T23.16** Burn of first degree of back of hand

    ✓7ᵗʰ **T23.161** Burn of first degree of back of right hand

    ✓7ᵗʰ **T23.162** Burn of first degree of back of left hand

    ✓7ᵗʰ **T23.169** Burn of first degree of back of unspecified hand ▽

  ✓6ᵗʰ **T23.17** Burn of first degree of wrist

    ✓7ᵗʰ **T23.171** Burn of first degree of right wrist

    ✓7ᵗʰ **T23.172** Burn of first degree of left wrist

    ✓7ᵗʰ **T23.179** Burn of first degree of unspecified wrist ▽

  ✓6ᵗʰ **T23.19** Burn of first degree of multiple sites of wrist and hand

    ✓7ᵗʰ **T23.191** Burn of first degree of multiple sites of right wrist and hand

    ✓7ᵗʰ **T23.192** Burn of first degree of multiple sites of left wrist and hand

    ✓7ᵗʰ **T23.199** Burn of first degree of multiple sites of unspecified wrist and hand ▽

✓5ᵗʰ **T23.2** Burn of second degree of wrist and hand

Use additional external cause code to identify the source, place and intent of the burn (X00-X19, X75-X77, X96-X98, Y92)

  ✓6ᵗʰ **T23.20** Burn of second degree of hand, unspecified site

    ✓7ᵗʰ **T23.201** Burn of second degree of right hand, unspecified site ▽

    ✓7ᵗʰ **T23.202** Burn of second degree of left hand, unspecified site ▽

    ✓7ᵗʰ **T23.209** Burn of second degree of unspecified hand, unspecified site ▽

  ✓6ᵗʰ **T23.21** Burn of second degree of thumb (nail)

    ✓7ᵗʰ **T23.211** Burn of second degree of right thumb (nail)

    ✓7ᵗʰ **T23.212** Burn of second degree of left thumb (nail)

    ✓7ᵗʰ **T23.219** Burn of second degree of unspecified thumb (nail) ▽

  ✓6ᵗʰ **T23.22** Burn of second degree of single finger (nail) except thumb

    ✓7ᵗʰ **T23.221** Burn of second degree of single right finger (nail) except thumb

    ✓7ᵗʰ **T23.222** Burn of second degree of single left finger (nail) except thumb

    ✓7ᵗʰ **T23.229** Burn of second degree of unspecified single finger (nail) except thumb ▽

  ✓6ᵗʰ **T23.23** Burn of second degree of multiple fingers (nail), not including thumb

    ✓7ᵗʰ **T23.231** Burn of second degree of multiple right fingers (nail), not including thumb

    ✓7ᵗʰ **T23.232** Burn of second degree of multiple left fingers (nail), not including thumb

    ✓7ᵗʰ **T23.239** Burn of second degree of unspecified multiple fingers (nail), not including thumb ▽

  ✓6ᵗʰ **T23.24** Burn of second degree of multiple fingers (nail), including thumb

    ✓7ᵗʰ **T23.241** Burn of second degree of multiple right fingers (nail), including thumb

    ✓7ᵗʰ **T23.242** Burn of second degree of multiple left fingers (nail), including thumb

    ✓7ᵗʰ **T23.249** Burn of second degree of unspecified multiple fingers (nail), including thumb ▽

  ✓6ᵗʰ **T23.25** Burn of second degree of palm

    ✓7ᵗʰ **T23.251** Burn of second degree of right palm

    ✓7ᵗʰ **T23.252** Burn of second degree of left palm

    ✓7ᵗʰ **T23.259** Burn of second degree of unspecified palm ▽

  ✓6ᵗʰ **T23.26** Burn of second degree of back of hand

    ✓7ᵗʰ **T23.261** Burn of second degree of back of right hand

    ✓7ᵗʰ **T23.262** Burn of second degree of back of left hand

    ✓7ᵗʰ **T23.269** Burn of second degree of back of unspecified hand ▽

  ✓6ᵗʰ **T23.27** Burn of second degree of wrist

    ✓7ᵗʰ **T23.271** Burn of second degree of right wrist

    ✓7ᵗʰ **T23.272** Burn of second degree of left wrist

    ✓7ᵗʰ **T23.279** Burn of second degree of unspecified wrist ▽

  ✓6ᵗʰ **T23.29** Burn of second degree of multiple sites of wrist and hand

    ✓7ᵗʰ **T23.291** Burn of second degree of multiple sites of right wrist and hand

    ✓7ᵗʰ **T23.292** Burn of second degree of multiple sites of left wrist and hand

    ✓7ᵗʰ **T23.299** Burn of second degree of multiple sites of unspecified wrist and hand ▽

✓5ᵗʰ **T23.3** Burn of third degree of wrist and hand

Use additional external cause code to identify the source, place and intent of the burn (X00-X19, X75-X77, X96-X98, Y92)

  ✓6ᵗʰ **T23.30** Burn of third degree of hand, unspecified site

    AHA: 2016, 2Q, 5

    ✓7ᵗʰ **T23.301** Burn of third degree of right hand, unspecified site ▽

☑ Additional Character Req   ✓7ᵗʰ Placeholder Alert   Manifestation   ᴴᶜᶜ CMS-HCC Condition   ▽ Unspecified Code   ►◄ Revised Text   ● New Code   ▲ Revised Code Title

ICD-10-CM 2018   **1047**

√7ᵗʰ **T23.302** Burn of third degree of left hand, unspecified site ▽

√7ᵗʰ **T23.309** Burn of third degree of unspecified hand, unspecified site ▽

√6ᵗʰ **T23.31** Burn of third degree of thumb (nail)

√7ᵗʰ **T23.311** Burn of third degree of right thumb (nail)

√7ᵗʰ **T23.312** Burn of third degree of left thumb (nail)

√7ᵗʰ **T23.319** Burn of third degree of unspecified thumb (nail) ▽

√6ᵗʰ **T23.32** Burn of third degree of single finger (nail) except thumb

√7ᵗʰ **T23.321** Burn of third degree of single right finger (nail) except thumb

√7ᵗʰ **T23.322** Burn of third degree of single left finger (nail) except thumb

√7ᵗʰ **T23.329** Burn of third degree of unspecified single finger (nail) except thumb ▽

√6ᵗʰ **T23.33** Burn of third degree of multiple fingers (nail), not including thumb

√7ᵗʰ **T23.331** Burn of third degree of multiple right fingers (nail), not including thumb

√7ᵗʰ **T23.332** Burn of third degree of multiple left fingers (nail), not including thumb

√7ᵗʰ **T23.339** Burn of third degree of unspecified multiple fingers (nail), not including thumb ▽

√6ᵗʰ **T23.34** Burn of third degree of multiple fingers (nail), including thumb

√7ᵗʰ **T23.341** Burn of third degree of multiple right fingers (nail), including thumb

√7ᵗʰ **T23.342** Burn of third degree of multiple left fingers (nail), including thumb

√7ᵗʰ **T23.349** Burn of third degree of unspecified multiple fingers (nail), including thumb ▽

√6ᵗʰ **T23.35** Burn of third degree of palm

√7ᵗʰ **T23.351** Burn of third degree of right palm

√7ᵗʰ **T23.352** Burn of third degree of left palm

√7ᵗʰ **T23.359** Burn of third degree of unspecified palm ▽

√6ᵗʰ **T23.36** Burn of third degree of back of hand

√7ᵗʰ **T23.361** Burn of third degree of back of right hand

√7ᵗʰ **T23.362** Burn of third degree of back of left hand

√7ᵗʰ **T23.369** Burn of third degree of back of unspecified hand ▽

√6ᵗʰ **T23.37** Burn of third degree of wrist

√7ᵗʰ **T23.371** Burn of third degree of right wrist

√7ᵗʰ **T23.372** Burn of third degree of left wrist

√7ᵗʰ **T23.379** Burn of third degree of unspecified wrist ▽

√6ᵗʰ **T23.39** Burn of third degree of multiple sites of wrist and hand

√7ᵗʰ **T23.391** Burn of third degree of multiple sites of right wrist and hand

√7ᵗʰ **T23.392** Burn of third degree of multiple sites of left wrist and hand

√7ᵗʰ **T23.399** Burn of third degree of multiple sites of unspecified wrist and hand ▽

√5ᵗʰ **T23.4** Corrosion of unspecified degree of wrist and hand
Code first (T51-T65) to identify chemical and intent
Use additional external cause code to identify place (Y92)

√6ᵗʰ **T23.40** Corrosion of unspecified degree of hand, unspecified site

√7ᵗʰ **T23.401** Corrosion of unspecified degree of right hand, unspecified site ▽

√7ᵗʰ **T23.402** Corrosion of unspecified degree of left hand, unspecified site ▽

√7ᵗʰ **T23.409** Corrosion of unspecified degree of unspecified hand, unspecified site ▽

√6ᵗʰ **T23.41** Corrosion of unspecified degree of thumb (nail)

√7ᵗʰ **T23.411** Corrosion of unspecified degree of right thumb (nail) ▽

√7ᵗʰ **T23.412** Corrosion of unspecified degree of left thumb (nail) ▽

√7ᵗʰ **T23.419** Corrosion of unspecified degree of unspecified thumb (nail) ▽

√6ᵗʰ **T23.42** Corrosion of unspecified degree of single finger (nail) except thumb

√7ᵗʰ **T23.421** Corrosion of unspecified degree of single right finger (nail) except thumb ▽

√7ᵗʰ **T23.422** Corrosion of unspecified degree of single left finger (nail) except thumb ▽

√7ᵗʰ **T23.429** Corrosion of unspecified degree of unspecified single finger (nail) except thumb ▽

√6ᵗʰ **T23.43** Corrosion of unspecified degree of multiple fingers (nail), not including thumb

√7ᵗʰ **T23.431** Corrosion of unspecified degree of multiple right fingers (nail), not including thumb ▽

√7ᵗʰ **T23.432** Corrosion of unspecified degree of multiple left fingers (nail), not including thumb ▽

√7ᵗʰ **T23.439** Corrosion of unspecified degree of unspecified multiple fingers (nail), not including thumb ▽

√6ᵗʰ **T23.44** Corrosion of unspecified degree of multiple fingers (nail), including thumb

√7ᵗʰ **T23.441** Corrosion of unspecified degree of multiple right fingers (nail), including thumb ▽

√7ᵗʰ **T23.442** Corrosion of unspecified degree of multiple left fingers (nail), including thumb ▽

√7ᵗʰ **T23.449** Corrosion of unspecified degree of unspecified multiple fingers (nail), including thumb ▽

√6ᵗʰ **T23.45** Corrosion of unspecified degree of palm

√7ᵗʰ **T23.451** Corrosion of unspecified degree of right palm ▽

√7ᵗʰ **T23.452** Corrosion of unspecified degree of left palm ▽

√7ᵗʰ **T23.459** Corrosion of unspecified degree of unspecified palm ▽

√6ᵗʰ **T23.46** Corrosion of unspecified degree of back of hand

√7ᵗʰ **T23.461** Corrosion of unspecified degree of back of right hand ▽

√7ᵗʰ **T23.462** Corrosion of unspecified degree of back of left hand ▽

√7ᵗʰ **T23.469** Corrosion of unspecified degree of back of unspecified hand ▽

√6ᵗʰ **T23.47** Corrosion of unspecified degree of wrist

√7ᵗʰ **T23.471** Corrosion of unspecified degree of right wrist ▽

√7ᵗʰ **T23.472** Corrosion of unspecified degree of left wrist ▽

√7ᵗʰ **T23.479** Corrosion of unspecified degree of unspecified wrist ▽

√6ᵗʰ **T23.49** Corrosion of unspecified degree of multiple sites of wrist and hand

√7ᵗʰ **T23.491** Corrosion of unspecified degree of multiple sites of right wrist and hand ▽

√7ᵗʰ **T23.492** Corrosion of unspecified degree of multiple sites of left wrist and hand ▽

√7ᵗʰ **T23.499** Corrosion of unspecified degree of multiple sites of unspecified wrist and hand ▽

√5ᵗʰ **T23.5** Corrosion of first degree of wrist and hand
Code first (T51-T65) to identify chemical and intent
Use additional external cause code to identify place (Y92)

√6ᵗʰ **T23.50** Corrosion of first degree of hand, unspecified site

√7ᵗʰ **T23.501** Corrosion of first degree of right hand, unspecified site ▽

√7ᵗʰ **T23.502** Corrosion of first degree of left hand, unspecified site ▽

√7ᵗʰ **T23.509** Corrosion of first degree of unspecified hand, unspecified site ▽

√6ᵗʰ **T23.51** Corrosion of first degree of thumb (nail)

√7ᵗʰ **T23.511** Corrosion of first degree of right thumb (nail)

✓7ᵗʰ **T23.512** Corrosion of first degree of left thumb (nail)

✓7ᵗʰ **T23.519** Corrosion of first degree of unspecified ▽ thumb (nail)

✓6ᵗʰ **T23.52** Corrosion of first degree of single finger (nail) except thumb

     ✓7ᵗʰ **T23.521** Corrosion of first degree of single right finger (nail) except thumb

     ✓7ᵗʰ **T23.522** Corrosion of first degree of single left finger (nail) except thumb

     ✓7ᵗʰ **T23.529** Corrosion of first degree of unspecified ▽ single finger (nail) except thumb

✓6ᵗʰ **T23.53** Corrosion of first degree of multiple fingers (nail), not including thumb

     ✓7ᵗʰ **T23.531** Corrosion of first degree of multiple right fingers (nail), not including thumb

     ✓7ᵗʰ **T23.532** Corrosion of first degree of multiple left fingers (nail), not including thumb

     ✓7ᵗʰ **T23.539** Corrosion of first degree of unspecified ▽ multiple fingers (nail), not including thumb

✓6ᵗʰ **T23.54** Corrosion of first degree of multiple fingers (nail), including thumb

     ✓7ᵗʰ **T23.541** Corrosion of first degree of multiple right fingers (nail), including thumb

     ✓7ᵗʰ **T23.542** Corrosion of first degree of multiple left fingers (nail), including thumb

     ✓7ᵗʰ **T23.549** Corrosion of first degree of unspecified ▽ multiple fingers (nail), including thumb

✓6ᵗʰ **T23.55** Corrosion of first degree of palm

     ✓7ᵗʰ **T23.551** Corrosion of first degree of right palm

     ✓7ᵗʰ **T23.552** Corrosion of first degree of left palm

     ✓7ᵗʰ **T23.559** Corrosion of first degree of unspecified ▽ palm

✓6ᵗʰ **T23.56** Corrosion of first degree of back of hand

     ✓7ᵗʰ **T23.561** Corrosion of first degree of back of right hand

     ✓7ᵗʰ **T23.562** Corrosion of first degree of back of left hand

     ✓7ᵗʰ **T23.569** Corrosion of first degree of back of ▽ unspecified hand

✓6ᵗʰ **T23.57** Corrosion of first degree of wrist

     ✓7ᵗʰ **T23.571** Corrosion of first degree of right wrist

     ✓7ᵗʰ **T23.572** Corrosion of first degree of left wrist

     ✓7ᵗʰ **T23.579** Corrosion of first degree of unspecified ▽ wrist

✓6ᵗʰ **T23.59** Corrosion of first degree of multiple sites of wrist and hand

     ✓7ᵗʰ **T23.591** Corrosion of first degree of multiple sites of right wrist and hand

     ✓7ᵗʰ **T23.592** Corrosion of first degree of multiple sites of left wrist and hand

     ✓7ᵗʰ **T23.599** Corrosion of first degree of multiple ▽ sites of unspecified wrist and hand

✓5ᵗʰ **T23.6** Corrosion of second degree of wrist and hand
Code first (T51-T65) to identify chemical and intent
Use additional external cause code to identify place (Y92)

✓6ᵗʰ **T23.60** Corrosion of second degree of hand, unspecified site

     ✓7ᵗʰ **T23.601** Corrosion of second degree of right ▽ hand, unspecified site

     ✓7ᵗʰ **T23.602** Corrosion of second degree of left ▽ hand, unspecified site

     ✓7ᵗʰ **T23.609** Corrosion of second degree of ▽ unspecified hand, unspecified site

✓6ᵗʰ **T23.61** Corrosion of second degree of thumb (nail)

     ✓7ᵗʰ **T23.611** Corrosion of second degree of right thumb (nail)

     ✓7ᵗʰ **T23.612** Corrosion of second degree of left thumb (nail)

     ✓7ᵗʰ **T23.619** Corrosion of second degree of ▽ unspecified thumb (nail)

✓6ᵗʰ **T23.62** Corrosion of second degree of single finger (nail) except thumb

     ✓7ᵗʰ **T23.621** Corrosion of second degree of single right finger (nail) except thumb

     ✓7ᵗʰ **T23.622** Corrosion of second degree of single left finger (nail) except thumb

     ✓7ᵗʰ **T23.629** Corrosion of second degree of ▽ unspecified single finger (nail) except thumb

✓6ᵗʰ **T23.63** Corrosion of second degree of multiple fingers (nail), not including thumb

     ✓7ᵗʰ **T23.631** Corrosion of second degree of multiple right fingers (nail), not including thumb

     ✓7ᵗʰ **T23.632** Corrosion of second degree of multiple left fingers (nail), not including thumb

     ✓7ᵗʰ **T23.639** Corrosion of second degree of ▽ unspecified multiple fingers (nail), not including thumb

✓6ᵗʰ **T23.64** Corrosion of second degree of multiple fingers (nail), including thumb

     ✓7ᵗʰ **T23.641** Corrosion of second degree of multiple right fingers (nail), including thumb

     ✓7ᵗʰ **T23.642** Corrosion of second degree of multiple left fingers (nail), including thumb

     ✓7ᵗʰ **T23.649** Corrosion of second degree of ▽ unspecified multiple fingers (nail), including thumb

✓6ᵗʰ **T23.65** Corrosion of second degree of palm

     ✓7ᵗʰ **T23.651** Corrosion of second degree of right palm

     ✓7ᵗʰ **T23.652** Corrosion of second degree of left palm

     ✓7ᵗʰ **T23.659** Corrosion of second degree of ▽ unspecified palm

✓6ᵗʰ **T23.66** Corrosion of second degree of back of hand

     ✓7ᵗʰ **T23.661** Corrosion of second degree back of right hand

     ✓7ᵗʰ **T23.662** Corrosion of second degree back of left hand

     ✓7ᵗʰ **T23.669** Corrosion of second degree back of ▽ unspecified hand

✓6ᵗʰ **T23.67** Corrosion of second degree of wrist

     ✓7ᵗʰ **T23.671** Corrosion of second degree of right wrist

     ✓7ᵗʰ **T23.672** Corrosion of second degree of left wrist

     ✓7ᵗʰ **T23.679** Corrosion of second degree of ▽ unspecified wrist

✓6ᵗʰ **T23.69** Corrosion of second degree of multiple sites of wrist and hand

     ✓7ᵗʰ **T23.691** Corrosion of second degree of multiple sites of right wrist and hand

     ✓7ᵗʰ **T23.692** Corrosion of second degree of multiple sites of left wrist and hand

     ✓7ᵗʰ **T23.699** Corrosion of second degree of multiple ▽ sites of unspecified wrist and hand

✓5ᵗʰ **T23.7** Corrosion of third degree of wrist and hand
Code first (T51-T65) to identify chemical and intent
Use additional external cause code to identify place (Y92)

✓6ᵗʰ **T23.70** Corrosion of third degree of hand, unspecified site

     ✓7ᵗʰ **T23.701** Corrosion of third degree of right hand, ▽ unspecified site

     ✓7ᵗʰ **T23.702** Corrosion of third degree of left hand, ▽ unspecified site

     ✓7ᵗʰ **T23.709** Corrosion of third degree of ▽ unspecified hand, unspecified site

✓6ᵗʰ **T23.71** Corrosion of third degree of thumb (nail)

     ✓7ᵗʰ **T23.711** Corrosion of third degree of right thumb (nail)

     ✓7ᵗʰ **T23.712** Corrosion of third degree of left thumb (nail)

     ✓7ᵗʰ **T23.719** Corrosion of third degree of ▽ unspecified thumb (nail)

✓6ᵗʰ **T23.72** Corrosion of third degree of single finger (nail) except thumb

     ✓7ᵗʰ **T23.721** Corrosion of third degree of single right finger (nail) except thumb

☑ Additional Character Req   ✓ₓ7ᵗʰ Placeholder Alert   Manifestation   HCC CMS-HCC Condition   ▽ Unspecified Code   ►◄ Revised Text   ● New Code   ▲ Revised Code Title

ICD-10-CM 2018   **1049**

Chapter 19. Injury, Poisoning, and Certain Other Consequences of External Causes

T23.722–T24.201

✓7ᵗʰ **T23.722** **Corrosion of third degree of single** left **finger (nail) except thumb**

✓7ᵗʰ **T23.729** **Corrosion of third degree of unspecified single finger (nail) except thumb** ▽

✓6ᵗʰ **T23.73** **Corrosion of third degree of** multiple fingers **(nail), not including thumb**

✓7ᵗʰ **T23.731** **Corrosion of third degree of multiple** right **fingers (nail), not including thumb**

✓7ᵗʰ **T23.732** **Corrosion of third degree of multiple** left **fingers (nail), not including thumb**

✓7ᵗʰ **T23.739** **Corrosion of third degree of unspecified multiple fingers (nail), not including thumb** ▽

✓6ᵗʰ **T23.74** **Corrosion of third degree of** multiple fingers **(nail), including thumb**

✓7ᵗʰ **T23.741** **Corrosion of third degree of multiple** right **fingers (nail), including thumb**

✓7ᵗʰ **T23.742** **Corrosion of third degree of multiple** left **fingers (nail), including thumb**

✓7ᵗʰ **T23.749** **Corrosion of third degree of unspecified multiple fingers (nail), including thumb** ▽

✓6ᵗʰ **T23.75** **Corrosion of third degree of** palm

✓7ᵗʰ **T23.751** **Corrosion of third degree of** right **palm**

✓7ᵗʰ **T23.752** **Corrosion of third degree of** left **palm**

✓7ᵗʰ **T23.759** **Corrosion of third degree of unspecified palm** ▽

✓6ᵗʰ **T23.76** **Corrosion of third degree of** back of hand

✓7ᵗʰ **T23.761** **Corrosion of third degree of back of** right **hand**

✓7ᵗʰ **T23.762** **Corrosion of third degree of back of** left **hand**

✓7ᵗʰ **T23.769** **Corrosion of third degree back of unspecified hand** ▽

✓6ᵗʰ **T23.77** **Corrosion of third degree of** wrist

✓7ᵗʰ **T23.771** **Corrosion of third degree of** right **wrist**

✓7ᵗʰ **T23.772** **Corrosion of third degree of** left **wrist**

✓7ᵗʰ **T23.779** **Corrosion of third degree of unspecified wrist** ▽

✓6ᵗʰ **T23.79** **Corrosion of third degree of** multiple sites **of wrist and hand**

✓7ᵗʰ **T23.791** **Corrosion of third degree of multiple sites of** right **wrist and hand**

✓7ᵗʰ **T23.792** **Corrosion of third degree of multiple sites of** left **wrist and hand**

✓7ᵗʰ **T23.799** **Corrosion of third degree of multiple sites of unspecified wrist and hand** ▽

✓4ᵗʰ **T24** **Burn and corrosion of lower limb, except ankle and foot**

EXCLUDES 2   burn and corrosion of ankle and foot (T25.-)
burn and corrosion of hip region (T21.-)

The appropriate 7th character is to be added to each code from category T24.
A   initial encounter
D   subsequent encounter
S   sequela

✓5ᵗʰ **T24.0** **Burn of unspecified degree of lower limb, except ankle and foot**

Use additional external cause code to identify the source, place and intent of the burn (X00-X19, X75-X77, X96-X98, Y92)

✓6ᵗʰ **T24.00** **Burn of unspecified degree of unspecified site of lower limb, except ankle and foot**

✓7ᵗʰ **T24.001** **Burn of unspecified degree of unspecified site of** right **lower limb, except ankle and foot** ▽

✓7ᵗʰ **T24.002** **Burn of unspecified degree of unspecified site of** left **lower limb, except ankle and foot** ▽

✓7ᵗʰ **T24.009** **Burn of unspecified degree of unspecified site of unspecified lower limb, except ankle and foot** ▽

✓6ᵗʰ **T24.01** **Burn of unspecified degree of** thigh

✓7ᵗʰ **T24.011** **Burn of unspecified degree of** right **thigh** ▽

✓7ᵗʰ **T24.012** **Burn of unspecified degree of** left **thigh** ▽

✓7ᵗʰ **T24.019** **Burn of unspecified degree of unspecified thigh** ▽

✓6ᵗʰ **T24.02** **Burn of unspecified degree of** knee

✓7ᵗʰ **T24.021** **Burn of unspecified degree of** right **knee** ▽

✓7ᵗʰ **T24.022** **Burn of unspecified degree of** left **knee** ▽

✓7ᵗʰ **T24.029** **Burn of unspecified degree of unspecified knee** ▽

✓6ᵗʰ **T24.03** **Burn of unspecified degree of** lower leg

✓7ᵗʰ **T24.031** **Burn of unspecified degree of** right **lower leg** ▽

✓7ᵗʰ **T24.032** **Burn of unspecified degree of** left **lower leg** ▽

✓7ᵗʰ **T24.039** **Burn of unspecified degree of unspecified lower leg** ▽

✓6ᵗʰ **T24.09** **Burn of unspecified degree of** multiple sites **of lower limb, except ankle and foot**

✓7ᵗʰ **T24.091** **Burn of unspecified degree of multiple sites of** right **lower limb, except ankle and foot** ▽

✓7ᵗʰ **T24.092** **Burn of unspecified degree of multiple sites of** left **lower limb, except ankle and foot** ▽

✓7ᵗʰ **T24.099** **Burn of unspecified degree of multiple sites of unspecified lower limb, except ankle and foot** ▽

✓5ᵗʰ **T24.1** **Burn of** first degree **of lower limb, except ankle and foot**

Use additional external cause code to identify the source, place and intent of the burn (X00-X19, X75-X77, X96-X98, Y92)

✓6ᵗʰ **T24.10** **Burn of first degree of unspecified site of lower limb, except ankle and foot**

✓7ᵗʰ **T24.101** **Burn of first degree of unspecified site of** right **lower limb, except ankle and foot** ▽

✓7ᵗʰ **T24.102** **Burn of first degree of unspecified site of** left **lower limb, except ankle and foot** ▽

✓7ᵗʰ **T24.109** **Burn of first degree of unspecified site of unspecified lower limb, except ankle and foot** ▽

✓6ᵗʰ **T24.11** **Burn of first degree of** thigh

✓7ᵗʰ **T24.111** **Burn of first degree of** right **thigh**

✓7ᵗʰ **T24.112** **Burn of first degree of** left **thigh**

✓7ᵗʰ **T24.119** **Burn of first degree of unspecified thigh** ▽

✓6ᵗʰ **T24.12** **Burn of first degree of** knee

✓7ᵗʰ **T24.121** **Burn of first degree of** right **knee**

✓7ᵗʰ **T24.122** **Burn of first degree of** left **knee**

✓7ᵗʰ **T24.129** **Burn of first degree of unspecified knee** ▽

✓6ᵗʰ **T24.13** **Burn of first degree of** lower leg

✓7ᵗʰ **T24.131** **Burn of first degree of** right **lower leg**

✓7ᵗʰ **T24.132** **Burn of first degree of** left **lower leg**

✓7ᵗʰ **T24.139** **Burn of first degree of unspecified lower leg** ▽

✓6ᵗʰ **T24.19** **Burn of first degree of** multiple sites **of lower limb, except ankle and foot**

✓7ᵗʰ **T24.191** **Burn of first degree of multiple sites of** right **lower limb, except ankle and foot**

✓7ᵗʰ **T24.192** **Burn of first degree of multiple sites of** left **lower limb, except ankle and foot**

✓7ᵗʰ **T24.199** **Burn of first degree of multiple sites of unspecified lower limb, except ankle and foot** ▽

✓5ᵗʰ **T24.2** **Burn of** second degree **of lower limb, except ankle and foot**

Use additional external cause code to identify the source, place and intent of the burn (X00-X19, X75-X77, X96-X98, Y92)

✓6ᵗʰ **T24.20** **Burn of second degree of unspecified site of lower limb, except ankle and foot**

✓7ᵗʰ **T24.201** **Burn of second degree of unspecified site of** right **lower limb, except ankle and foot** ▽

EXCLUDES 1 Not coded here   EXCLUDES 2 Not included here   N Newborn Age: 0   P Pediatric Age: 0-17   M Maternity Age: 12-55   A Adult Age: 15-124

1050   ICD-10-CM 2018

√7th **T24.202** Burn of second degree of unspecified site of left lower limb, except ankle and foot ▽

√7th **T24.209** Burn of second degree of unspecified site of unspecified lower limb, except ankle and foot ▽

√6th **T24.21** Burn of second degree of thigh

√7th **T24.211** Burn of second degree of right thigh

√7th **T24.212** Burn of second degree of left thigh

√7th **T24.219** Burn of second degree of unspecified thigh ▽

√6th **T24.22** Burn of second degree of knee

√7th **T24.221** Burn of second degree of right knee

√7th **T24.222** Burn of second degree of left knee

√7th **T24.229** Burn of second degree of unspecified knee ▽

√6th **T24.23** Burn of second degree of lower leg

√7th **T24.231** Burn of second degree of right lower leg

√7th **T24.232** Burn of second degree of left lower leg

√7th **T24.239** Burn of second degree of unspecified lower leg ▽

√6th **T24.29** Burn of second degree of multiple sites of lower limb, except ankle and foot

√7th **T24.291** Burn of second degree of multiple sites of right lower limb, except ankle and foot

√7th **T24.292** Burn of second degree of multiple sites of left lower limb, except ankle and foot

√7th **T24.299** Burn of second degree of multiple sites of unspecified lower limb, except ankle and foot ▽

√5th **T24.3** Burn of third degree of lower limb, except ankle and foot

Use additional external cause code to identify the source, place and intent of the burn (X00-X19, X75-X77, X96-X98, Y92)

√6th **T24.30** Burn of third degree of unspecified site of lower limb, except ankle and foot

√7th **T24.301** Burn of third degree of unspecified site of right lower limb, except ankle and foot ▽

√7th **T24.302** Burn of third degree of unspecified site of left lower limb, except ankle and foot ▽

√7th **T24.309** Burn of third degree of unspecified site of unspecified lower limb, except ankle and foot ▽

√6th **T24.31** Burn of third degree of thigh

√7th **T24.311** Burn of third degree of right thigh

√7th **T24.312** Burn of third degree of left thigh

√7th **T24.319** Burn of third degree of unspecified thigh ▽

√6th **T24.32** Burn of third degree of knee

√7th **T24.321** Burn of third degree of right knee

√7th **T24.322** Burn of third degree of left knee

√7th **T24.329** Burn of third degree of unspecified knee ▽

√6th **T24.33** Burn of third degree of lower leg

√7th **T24.331** Burn of third degree of right lower leg

√7th **T24.332** Burn of third degree of left lower leg

√7th **T24.339** Burn of third degree of unspecified lower leg ▽

√6th **T24.39** Burn of third degree of multiple sites of lower limb, except ankle and foot
AHA: 2016, 2Q, 4

√7th **T24.391** Burn of third degree of multiple sites of right lower limb, except ankle and foot

√7th **T24.392** Burn of third degree of multiple sites of left lower limb, except ankle and foot

√7th **T24.399** Burn of third degree of multiple sites of unspecified lower limb, except ankle and foot ▽

√5th **T24.4** Corrosion of unspecified degree of lower limb, except ankle and foot

Code first (T51-T65) to identify chemical and intent
Use additional external cause code to identify place (Y92)

√6th **T24.40** Corrosion of unspecified degree of unspecified site of lower limb, except ankle and foot

√7th **T24.401** Corrosion of unspecified degree of unspecified site of right lower limb, except ankle and foot ▽

√7th **T24.402** Corrosion of unspecified degree of unspecified site of left lower limb, except ankle and foot ▽

√7th **T24.409** Corrosion of unspecified degree of unspecified site of unspecified lower limb, except ankle and foot ▽

√6th **T24.41** Corrosion of unspecified degree of thigh

√7th **T24.411** Corrosion of unspecified degree of right thigh ▽

√7th **T24.412** Corrosion of unspecified degree of left thigh ▽

√7th **T24.419** Corrosion of unspecified degree of unspecified thigh ▽

√6th **T24.42** Corrosion of unspecified degree of knee

√7th **T24.421** Corrosion of unspecified degree of right knee ▽

√7th **T24.422** Corrosion of unspecified degree of left knee ▽

√7th **T24.429** Corrosion of unspecified degree of unspecified knee ▽

√6th **T24.43** Corrosion of unspecified degree of lower leg

√7th **T24.431** Corrosion of unspecified degree of right lower leg ▽

√7th **T24.432** Corrosion of unspecified degree of left lower leg ▽

√7th **T24.439** Corrosion of unspecified degree of unspecified lower leg ▽

√6th **T24.49** Corrosion of unspecified degree of multiple sites of lower limb, except ankle and foot

√7th **T24.491** Corrosion of unspecified degree of multiple sites of right lower limb, except ankle and foot ▽

√7th **T24.492** Corrosion of unspecified degree of multiple sites of left lower limb, except ankle and foot ▽

√7th **T24.499** Corrosion of unspecified degree of multiple sites of unspecified lower limb, except ankle and foot ▽

√5th **T24.5** Corrosion of first degree of lower limb, except ankle and foot

Code first (T51-T65) to identify chemical and intent
Use additional external cause code to identify place (Y92)

√6th **T24.50** Corrosion of first degree of unspecified site of lower limb, except ankle and foot

√7th **T24.501** Corrosion of first degree of unspecified site of right lower limb, except ankle and foot ▽

√7th **T24.502** Corrosion of first degree of unspecified site of left lower limb, except ankle and foot ▽

√7th **T24.509** Corrosion of first degree of unspecified site of unspecified lower limb, except ankle and foot ▽

√6th **T24.51** Corrosion of first degree of thigh

√7th **T24.511** Corrosion of first degree of right thigh

√7th **T24.512** Corrosion of first degree of left thigh

√7th **T24.519** Corrosion of first degree of unspecified thigh ▽

√6th **T24.52** Corrosion of first degree of knee

√7th **T24.521** Corrosion of first degree of right knee

√7th **T24.522** Corrosion of first degree of left knee

√7th **T24.529** Corrosion of first degree of unspecified knee ▽

√6th **T24.53** Corrosion of first degree of lower leg

√7th **T24.531** Corrosion of first degree of right lower leg

√7th **T24.532** Corrosion of first degree of left lower leg

☑ Additional Character Req   √x7th Placeholder Alert   Manifestation   HCC CMS-HCC Condition   ▽ Unspecified Code   ►◄ Revised Text   ● New Code   ▲ Revised Code Title

ICD-10-CM 2018   1051

✓7ᵗʰ **T24.539** Corrosion of first degree of unspecified ▽
lower leg

✓6ᵗʰ **T24.59** Corrosion of first degree of multiple sites of lower
limb, except ankle and foot

   ✓7ᵗʰ **T24.591** Corrosion of first degree of multiple sites
of right lower limb, except ankle and foot

   ✓7ᵗʰ **T24.592** Corrosion of first degree of multiple sites
of left lower limb, except ankle and foot

   ✓7ᵗʰ **T24.599** Corrosion of first degree of multiple ▽
sites of unspecified lower limb, except
ankle and foot

✓5ᵗʰ **T24.6** Corrosion of second degree of lower limb, except ankle and
foot

   Code first (T51-T65) to identify chemical and intent
   Use additional external cause code to identify place (Y92)

✓6ᵗʰ **T24.60** Corrosion of second degree of unspecified site of
lower limb, except ankle and foot

   ✓7ᵗʰ **T24.601** Corrosion of second degree of ▽
unspecified site of right lower limb,
except ankle and foot

   ✓7ᵗʰ **T24.602** Corrosion of second degree of ▽
unspecified site of left lower limb,
except ankle and foot

   ✓7ᵗʰ **T24.609** Corrosion of second degree of ▽
unspecified site of unspecified lower
limb, except ankle and foot

✓6ᵗʰ **T24.61** Corrosion of second degree of thigh

   ✓7ᵗʰ **T24.611** Corrosion of second degree of right thigh
   ✓7ᵗʰ **T24.612** Corrosion of second degree of left thigh
   ✓7ᵗʰ **T24.619** Corrosion of second degree of ▽
unspecified thigh

✓6ᵗʰ **T24.62** Corrosion of second degree of knee

   ✓7ᵗʰ **T24.621** Corrosion of second degree of right knee
   ✓7ᵗʰ **T24.622** Corrosion of second degree of left knee
   ✓7ᵗʰ **T24.629** Corrosion of second degree of ▽
unspecified knee

✓6ᵗʰ **T24.63** Corrosion of second degree of lower leg

   ✓7ᵗʰ **T24.631** Corrosion of second degree of right lower
leg

   ✓7ᵗʰ **T24.632** Corrosion of second degree of left lower
leg

   ✓7ᵗʰ **T24.639** Corrosion of second degree of ▽
unspecified lower leg

✓6ᵗʰ **T24.69** Corrosion of second degree of multiple sites of lower
limb, except ankle and foot

   ✓7ᵗʰ **T24.691** Corrosion of second degree of multiple
sites of right lower limb, except ankle and
foot

   ✓7ᵗʰ **T24.692** Corrosion of second degree of multiple
sites of left lower limb, except ankle and
foot

   ✓7ᵗʰ **T24.699** Corrosion of second degree of multiple ▽
sites of unspecified lower limb, except
ankle and foot

✓5ᵗʰ **T24.7** Corrosion of third degree of lower limb, except ankle and foot

   Code first (T51-T65) to identify chemical and intent
   Use additional external cause code to identify place (Y92)

✓6ᵗʰ **T24.70** Corrosion of third degree of unspecified site of lower
limb, except ankle and foot

   ✓7ᵗʰ **T24.701** Corrosion of third degree of ▽
unspecified site of right lower limb,
except ankle and foot

   ✓7ᵗʰ **T24.702** Corrosion of third degree of ▽
unspecified site of left lower limb,
except ankle and foot

   ✓7ᵗʰ **T24.709** Corrosion of third degree of ▽
unspecified site of unspecified lower
limb, except ankle and foot

✓6ᵗʰ **T24.71** Corrosion of third degree of thigh

   ✓7ᵗʰ **T24.711** Corrosion of third degree of right thigh
   ✓7ᵗʰ **T24.712** Corrosion of third degree of left thigh
   ✓7ᵗʰ **T24.719** Corrosion of third degree of ▽
unspecified thigh

✓6ᵗʰ **T24.72** Corrosion of third degree of knee

   ✓7ᵗʰ **T24.721** Corrosion of third degree of right knee
   ✓7ᵗʰ **T24.722** Corrosion of third degree of left knee
   ✓7ᵗʰ **T24.729** Corrosion of third degree of ▽
unspecified knee

✓6ᵗʰ **T24.73** Corrosion of third degree of lower leg

   ✓7ᵗʰ **T24.731** Corrosion of third degree of right lower
leg

   ✓7ᵗʰ **T24.732** Corrosion of third degree of left lower leg
   ✓7ᵗʰ **T24.739** Corrosion of third degree of ▽
unspecified lower leg

✓6ᵗʰ **T24.79** Corrosion of third degree of multiple sites of lower
limb, except ankle and foot

   ✓7ᵗʰ **T24.791** Corrosion of third degree of multiple sites
of right lower limb, except ankle and foot

   ✓7ᵗʰ **T24.792** Corrosion of third degree of multiple sites
of left lower limb, except ankle and foot

   ✓7ᵗʰ **T24.799** Corrosion of third degree of multiple ▽
sites of unspecified lower limb, except
ankle and foot

✓4ᵗʰ **T25** Burn and corrosion of ankle and foot

> The appropriate 7th character is to be added to each code from
> category T25.
> A   initial encounter
> D   subsequent encounter
> S   sequela

✓5ᵗʰ **T25.0** Burn of unspecified degree of ankle and foot

   Use additional external cause code to identify the source, place
and intent of the burn (X00-X19, X75-X77, X96-X98, Y92)

✓6ᵗʰ **T25.01** Burn of unspecified degree of ankle

   ✓7ᵗʰ **T25.011** Burn of unspecified degree of right ▽
ankle

   ✓7ᵗʰ **T25.012** Burn of unspecified degree of left ▽
ankle

   ✓7ᵗʰ **T25.019** Burn of unspecified degree of ▽
unspecified ankle

✓6ᵗʰ **T25.02** Burn of unspecified degree of foot

   EXCLUDES 2   burn of unspecified degree of toe(s) (nail)
(T25.03-)

   ✓7ᵗʰ **T25.021** Burn of unspecified degree of right ▽
foot

   ✓7ᵗʰ **T25.022** Burn of unspecified degree of left ▽
foot

   ✓7ᵗʰ **T25.029** Burn of unspecified degree of ▽
unspecified foot

✓6ᵗʰ **T25.03** Burn of unspecified degree of toe(s) (nail)

   ✓7ᵗʰ **T25.031** Burn of unspecified degree of right ▽
toe(s) (nail)

   ✓7ᵗʰ **T25.032** Burn of unspecified degree of left ▽
toe(s) (nail)

   ✓7ᵗʰ **T25.039** Burn of unspecified degree of ▽
unspecified toe(s) (nail)

✓6ᵗʰ **T25.09** Burn of unspecified degree of multiple sites of ankle
and foot

   ✓7ᵗʰ **T25.091** Burn of unspecified degree of ▽
multiple sites of right ankle and foot

   ✓7ᵗʰ **T25.092** Burn of unspecified degree of ▽
multiple sites of left ankle and foot

   ✓7ᵗʰ **T25.099** Burn of unspecified degree of ▽
multiple sites of unspecified ankle
and foot

✓5ᵗʰ **T25.1** Burn of first degree of ankle and foot

   Use additional external cause code to identify the source, place
and intent of the burn (X00-X19, X75-X77, X96-X98, Y92)

✓6ᵗʰ **T25.11** Burn of first degree of ankle

   ✓7ᵗʰ **T25.111** Burn of first degree of right ankle
   ✓7ᵗʰ **T25.112** Burn of first degree of left ankle
   ✓7ᵗʰ **T25.119** Burn of first degree of unspecified ▽
ankle

✓6ᵗʰ **T25.12** Burn of first degree of foot

   EXCLUDES 2   burn of first degree of toe(s) (nail) (T25.13-)

   ✓7ᵗʰ **T25.121** Burn of first degree of right foot
   ✓7ᵗʰ **T25.122** Burn of first degree of left foot

EXCLUDES 1 Not coded here   EXCLUDES 2 Not included here   N Newborn Age: 0   P Pediatric Age: 0-17   M Maternity Age: 12-55   A Adult Age: 15-124

1052   ICD-10-CM 2018

✓7ᵗʰ **T25.129** Burn of first degree of unspecified foot ▽

✓6ᵗʰ **T25.13** Burn of first degree of toe(s) (nail)

    ✓7ᵗʰ **T25.131** Burn of first degree of right toe(s) (nail)

    ✓7ᵗʰ **T25.132** Burn of first degree of left toe(s) (nail)

    ✓7ᵗʰ **T25.139** Burn of first degree of unspecified toe(s) (nail) ▽

✓6ᵗʰ **T25.19** Burn of first degree of multiple sites of ankle and foot

    ✓7ᵗʰ **T25.191** Burn of first degree of multiple sites of right ankle and foot

    ✓7ᵗʰ **T25.192** Burn of first degree of multiple sites of left ankle and foot

    ✓7ᵗʰ **T25.199** Burn of first degree of multiple sites of unspecified ankle and foot ▽

✓5ᵗʰ **T25.2** Burn of second degree of ankle and foot

    Use additional external cause code to identify the source, place and intent of the burn (X00-X19, X75-X77, X96-X98, Y92)

✓6ᵗʰ **T25.21** Burn of second degree of ankle

    ✓7ᵗʰ **T25.211** Burn of second degree of right ankle

    ✓7ᵗʰ **T25.212** Burn of second degree of left ankle

    ✓7ᵗʰ **T25.219** Burn of second degree of unspecified ankle ▽

✓6ᵗʰ **T25.22** Burn of second degree of foot

    EXCLUDES 2   burn of second degree of toe(s) (nail) (T25.23-)

    ✓7ᵗʰ **T25.221** Burn of second degree of right foot

    ✓7ᵗʰ **T25.222** Burn of second degree of left foot

    ✓7ᵗʰ **T25.229** Burn of second degree of unspecified foot ▽

✓6ᵗʰ **T25.23** Burn of second degree of toe(s) (nail)

    ✓7ᵗʰ **T25.231** Burn of second degree of right toe(s) (nail)

    ✓7ᵗʰ **T25.232** Burn of second degree of left toe(s) (nail)

    ✓7ᵗʰ **T25.239** Burn of second degree of unspecified toe(s) (nail) ▽

✓6ᵗʰ **T25.29** Burn of second degree of multiple sites of ankle and foot

    ✓7ᵗʰ **T25.291** Burn of second degree of multiple sites of right ankle and foot

    ✓7ᵗʰ **T25.292** Burn of second degree of multiple sites of left ankle and foot

    ✓7ᵗʰ **T25.299** Burn of second degree of multiple sites of unspecified ankle and foot ▽

✓5ᵗʰ **T25.3** Burn of third degree of ankle and foot

    Use additional external cause code to identify the source, place and intent of the burn (X00-X19, X75-X77, X96-X98, Y92)

✓6ᵗʰ **T25.31** Burn of third degree of ankle

    ✓7ᵗʰ **T25.311** Burn of third degree of right ankle

    ✓7ᵗʰ **T25.312** Burn of third degree of left ankle

    ✓7ᵗʰ **T25.319** Burn of third degree of unspecified ankle ▽

✓6ᵗʰ **T25.32** Burn of third degree of foot

    EXCLUDES 2   burn of third degree of toe(s) (nail) (T25.33-)

    ✓7ᵗʰ **T25.321** Burn of third degree of right foot

    ✓7ᵗʰ **T25.322** Burn of third degree of left foot

    ✓7ᵗʰ **T25.329** Burn of third degree of unspecified foot ▽

✓6ᵗʰ **T25.33** Burn of third degree of toe(s) (nail)

    ✓7ᵗʰ **T25.331** Burn of third degree of right toe(s) (nail)

    ✓7ᵗʰ **T25.332** Burn of third degree of left toe(s) (nail)

    ✓7ᵗʰ **T25.339** Burn of third degree of unspecified toe(s) (nail) ▽

✓6ᵗʰ **T25.39** Burn of third degree of multiple sites of ankle and foot

    ✓7ᵗʰ **T25.391** Burn of third degree of multiple sites of right ankle and foot

    ✓7ᵗʰ **T25.392** Burn of third degree of multiple sites of left ankle and foot

    ✓7ᵗʰ **T25.399** Burn of third degree of multiple sites of unspecified ankle and foot ▽

✓5ᵗʰ **T25.4** Corrosion of unspecified degree of ankle and foot

    Code first (T51-T65) to identify chemical and intent

    Use additional external cause code to identify place (Y92)

✓6ᵗʰ **T25.41** Corrosion of unspecified degree of ankle

    ✓7ᵗʰ **T25.411** Corrosion of unspecified degree of right ankle ▽

    ✓7ᵗʰ **T25.412** Corrosion of unspecified degree of left ankle ▽

    ✓7ᵗʰ **T25.419** Corrosion of unspecified degree of unspecified ankle ▽

✓6ᵗʰ **T25.42** Corrosion of unspecified degree of foot

    EXCLUDES 2   corrosion of unspecified degree of toe(s) (nail) (T25.43-)

    ✓7ᵗʰ **T25.421** Corrosion of unspecified degree of right foot ▽

    ✓7ᵗʰ **T25.422** Corrosion of unspecified degree of left foot ▽

    ✓7ᵗʰ **T25.429** Corrosion of unspecified degree of unspecified foot ▽

✓6ᵗʰ **T25.43** Corrosion of unspecified degree of toe(s) (nail)

    ✓7ᵗʰ **T25.431** Corrosion of unspecified degree of right toe(s) (nail) ▽

    ✓7ᵗʰ **T25.432** Corrosion of unspecified degree of left toe(s) (nail) ▽

    ✓7ᵗʰ **T25.439** Corrosion of unspecified degree of unspecified toe(s) (nail) ▽

✓6ᵗʰ **T25.49** Corrosion of unspecified degree of multiple sites of ankle and foot

    ✓7ᵗʰ **T25.491** Corrosion of unspecified degree of multiple sites of right ankle and foot ▽

    ✓7ᵗʰ **T25.492** Corrosion of unspecified degree of multiple sites of left ankle and foot ▽

    ✓7ᵗʰ **T25.499** Corrosion of unspecified degree of multiple sites of unspecified ankle and foot ▽

✓5ᵗʰ **T25.5** Corrosion of first degree of ankle and foot

    Code first (T51-T65) to identify chemical and intent

    Use additional external cause code to identify place (Y92)

✓6ᵗʰ **T25.51** Corrosion of first degree of ankle

    ✓7ᵗʰ **T25.511** Corrosion of first degree of right ankle

    ✓7ᵗʰ **T25.512** Corrosion of first degree of left ankle

    ✓7ᵗʰ **T25.519** Corrosion of first degree of unspecified ankle ▽

✓6ᵗʰ **T25.52** Corrosion of first degree of foot

    EXCLUDES 2   corrosion of first degree of toe(s) (nail) (T25.53-)

    ✓7ᵗʰ **T25.521** Corrosion of first degree of right foot

    ✓7ᵗʰ **T25.522** Corrosion of first degree of left foot

    ✓7ᵗʰ **T25.529** Corrosion of first degree of unspecified foot ▽

✓6ᵗʰ **T25.53** Corrosion of first degree of toe(s) (nail)

    ✓7ᵗʰ **T25.531** Corrosion of first degree of right toe(s) (nail)

    ✓7ᵗʰ **T25.532** Corrosion of first degree of left toe(s) (nail)

    ✓7ᵗʰ **T25.539** Corrosion of first degree of unspecified toe(s) (nail) ▽

✓6ᵗʰ **T25.59** Corrosion of first degree of multiple sites of ankle and foot

    ✓7ᵗʰ **T25.591** Corrosion of first degree of multiple sites of right ankle and foot

    ✓7ᵗʰ **T25.592** Corrosion of first degree of multiple sites of left ankle and foot

    ✓7ᵗʰ **T25.599** Corrosion of first degree of multiple sites of unspecified ankle and foot ▽

✓5ᵗʰ **T25.6** Corrosion of second degree of ankle and foot

    Code first (T51-T65) to identify chemical and intent

    Use additional external cause code to identify place (Y92)

✓6ᵗʰ **T25.61** Corrosion of second degree of ankle

    ✓7ᵗʰ **T25.611** Corrosion of second degree of right ankle

    ✓7ᵗʰ **T25.612** Corrosion of second degree of left ankle

    ✓7ᵗʰ **T25.619** Corrosion of second degree of unspecified ankle ▽

☑ Additional Character Req   ✓x7ᵗʰ Placeholder Alert   Manifestation   HCC CMS-HCC Condition   ▽ Unspecified Code   ►◄ Revised Text   ● New Code   ▲ Revised Code Title

Chapter 19. Injury, Poisoning, and Certain Other Consequences of External Causes

√6ᵗʰ **T25.62**   **Corrosion of second degree of foot**
     EXCLUDES 2   *corrosion of second degree of toe(s) (nail) (T25.63-)*

    √7ᵗʰ **T25.621**   **Corrosion of second degree of right foot**

    √7ᵗʰ **T25.622**   **Corrosion of second degree of left foot**

    √7ᵗʰ **T25.629**   **Corrosion of second degree of unspecified foot** ▽

√6ᵗʰ **T25.63**   **Corrosion of second degree of toe(s) (nail)**

    √7ᵗʰ **T25.631**   **Corrosion of second degree of right toe(s) (nail)**

    √7ᵗʰ **T25.632**   **Corrosion of second degree of left toe(s) (nail)**

    √7ᵗʰ **T25.639**   **Corrosion of second degree of unspecified toe(s) (nail)** ▽

√6ᵗʰ **T25.69**   **Corrosion of second degree of multiple sites of ankle and foot**

    √7ᵗʰ **T25.691**   **Corrosion of second degree of right ankle and foot**

    √7ᵗʰ **T25.692**   **Corrosion of second degree of left ankle and foot**

    √7ᵗʰ **T25.699**   **Corrosion of second degree of unspecified ankle and foot** ▽

√5ᵗʰ **T25.7**   **Corrosion of third degree of ankle and foot**
     Code first (T51-T65) to identify chemical and intent
     Use additional external cause code to identify place (Y92)

   √6ᵗʰ **T25.71**   **Corrosion of third degree of ankle**

    √7ᵗʰ **T25.711**   **Corrosion of third degree of right ankle**

    √7ᵗʰ **T25.712**   **Corrosion of third degree of left ankle**

    √7ᵗʰ **T25.719**   **Corrosion of third degree of unspecified ankle** ▽

   √6ᵗʰ **T25.72**   **Corrosion of third degree of foot**
     EXCLUDES 2   *corrosion of third degree of toe(s) (nail) (T25.73-)*

    √7ᵗʰ **T25.721**   **Corrosion of third degree of right foot**

    √7ᵗʰ **T25.722**   **Corrosion of third degree of left foot**

    √7ᵗʰ **T25.729**   **Corrosion of third degree of unspecified foot** ▽

   √6ᵗʰ **T25.73**   **Corrosion of third degree of toe(s) (nail)**

    √7ᵗʰ **T25.731**   **Corrosion of third degree of right toe(s) (nail)**

    √7ᵗʰ **T25.732**   **Corrosion of third degree of left toe(s) (nail)**

    √7ᵗʰ **T25.739**   **Corrosion of third degree of unspecified toe(s) (nail)** ▽

   √6ᵗʰ **T25.79**   **Corrosion of third degree of multiple sites of ankle and foot**

    √7ᵗʰ **T25.791**   **Corrosion of third degree of multiple sites of right ankle and foot**

    √7ᵗʰ **T25.792**   **Corrosion of third degree of multiple sites of left ankle and foot**

    √7ᵗʰ **T25.799**   **Corrosion of third degree of multiple sites of unspecified ankle and foot** ▽

Burns and corrosions confined to eye and internal organs (T26-T28)

√4ᵗʰ **T26**   **Burn and corrosion confined to eye and adnexa**

> The appropriate 7th character is to be added to each code from category T26.
> A   initial encounter
> D   subsequent encounter
> S   sequela

√5ᵗʰ **T26.0**   **Burn of eyelid and periocular area**
     Use additional external cause code to identify the source, place and intent of the burn (X00-X19, X75-X77, X96-X98, Y92)

   √x7ᵗʰ **T26.00**   **Burn of unspecified eyelid and periocular area** ▽

   √x7ᵗʰ **T26.01**   **Burn of right eyelid and periocular area**

   √x7ᵗʰ **T26.02**   **Burn of left eyelid and periocular area**

√5ᵗʰ **T26.1**   **Burn of cornea and conjunctival sac**
     Use additional external cause code to identify the source, place and intent of the burn (X00-X19, X75-X77, X96-X98, Y92)

   √x7ᵗʰ **T26.10**   **Burn of cornea and conjunctival sac, unspecified eye** ▽

   √x7ᵗʰ **T26.11**   **Burn of cornea and conjunctival sac, right eye**

   √x7ᵗʰ **T26.12**   **Burn of cornea and conjunctival sac, left eye**

√5ᵗʰ **T26.2**   **Burn with resulting rupture and destruction of eyeball**
     Use additional external cause code to identify the source, place and intent of the burn (X00-X19, X75-X77, X96-X98, Y92)

   √x7ᵗʰ **T26.20**   **Burn with resulting rupture and destruction of unspecified eyeball** ▽

   √x7ᵗʰ **T26.21**   **Burn with resulting rupture and destruction of right eyeball**

   √x7ᵗʰ **T26.22**   **Burn with resulting rupture and destruction of left eyeball**

√5ᵗʰ **T26.3**   **Burns of other specified parts of eye and adnexa**
     Use additional external cause code to identify the source, place and intent of the burn (X00-X19, X75-X77, X96-X98, Y92)

   √x7ᵗʰ **T26.30**   **Burns of other specified parts of unspecified eye and adnexa** ▽

   √x7ᵗʰ **T26.31**   **Burns of other specified parts of right eye and adnexa**

   √x7ᵗʰ **T26.32**   **Burns of other specified parts of left eye and adnexa**

√5ᵗʰ **T26.4**   **Burn of eye and adnexa, part unspecified**
     Use additional external cause code to identify the source, place and intent of the burn (X00-X19, X75-X77, X96-X98, Y92)

   √x7ᵗʰ **T26.40**   **Burn of unspecified eye and adnexa, part unspecified** ▽

   √x7ᵗʰ **T26.41**   **Burn of right eye and adnexa, part unspecified** ▽

   √x7ᵗʰ **T26.42**   **Burn of left eye and adnexa, part unspecified** ▽

√5ᵗʰ **T26.5**   **Corrosion of eyelid and periocular area**
     Code first (T51-T65) to identify chemical and intent
     Use additional external cause code to identify place (Y92)

   √x7ᵗʰ **T26.50**   **Corrosion of unspecified eyelid and periocular area** ▽

   √x7ᵗʰ **T26.51**   **Corrosion of right eyelid and periocular area**

   √x7ᵗʰ **T26.52**   **Corrosion of left eyelid and periocular area**

√5ᵗʰ **T26.6**   **Corrosion of cornea and conjunctival sac**
     Code first (T51-T65) to identify chemical and intent
     Use additional external cause code to identify place (Y92)

   √x7ᵗʰ **T26.60**   **Corrosion of cornea and conjunctival sac, unspecified eye** ▽

   √x7ᵗʰ **T26.61**   **Corrosion of cornea and conjunctival sac, right eye**

   √x7ᵗʰ **T26.62**   **Corrosion of cornea and conjunctival sac, left eye**

√5ᵗʰ **T26.7**   **Corrosion with resulting rupture and destruction of eyeball**
     Code first (T51-T65) to identify chemical and intent
     Use additional external cause code to identify place (Y92)

   √x7ᵗʰ **T26.70**   **Corrosion with resulting rupture and destruction of unspecified eyeball** ▽

   √x7ᵗʰ **T26.71**   **Corrosion with resulting rupture and destruction of right eyeball**

   √x7ᵗʰ **T26.72**   **Corrosion with resulting rupture and destruction of left eyeball**

√5ᵗʰ **T26.8**   **Corrosions of other specified parts of eye and adnexa**
     Code first (T51-T65) to identify chemical and intent
     Use additional external cause code to identify place (Y92)

   √x7ᵗʰ **T26.80**   **Corrosions of other specified parts of unspecified eye and adnexa** ▽

   √x7ᵗʰ **T26.81**   **Corrosions of other specified parts of right eye and adnexa**

   √x7ᵗʰ **T26.82**   **Corrosions of other specified parts of left eye and adnexa**

√5ᵗʰ **T26.9**   **Corrosion of eye and adnexa, part unspecified**
     Code first (T51-T65) to identify chemical and intent
     Use additional external cause code to identify place (Y92)

   √x7ᵗʰ **T26.90**   **Corrosion of unspecified eye and adnexa, part unspecified** ▽

   √x7ᵗʰ **T26.91**   **Corrosion of right eye and adnexa, part unspecified** ▽

   √x7ᵗʰ **T26.92**   **Corrosion of left eye and adnexa, part unspecified** ▽

EXCLUDES 1 Not coded here   EXCLUDES 2 Not included here   N Newborn Age: 0   P Pediatric Age: 0-17   M Maternity Age: 12-55   A Adult Age: 15-124

1054   ICD-10-CM 2018

✓4ᵗʰ **T27**   **Burn and corrosion of respiratory tract**
      Use additional external cause code to identify the source and intent of the burn (X00-X19, X75-X77, X96-X98)
      Use additional external cause code to identify place (Y92)

> The appropriate 7th character is to be added to each code from category T27.
> A   initial encounter
> D   subsequent encounter
> S   sequela

✓x7ᵗʰ **T27.0**   Burn of larynx and trachea

✓x7ᵗʰ **T27.1**   Burn involving larynx and trachea with lung

✓x7ᵗʰ **T27.2**   **Burn of other parts of respiratory tract**
      Burn of thoracic cavity

✓x7ᵗʰ **T27.3**   **Burn of respiratory tract, part unspecified**   ▽
      ~~Code first (T51-T65) to identify chemical and intent for codes T27.4-T27.7~~

✓x7ᵗʰ **T27.4**   Corrosion of larynx and trachea
      ▶Code first (T51-T65) to identify chemical and intent◀

✓x7ᵗʰ **T27.5**   Corrosion involving larynx and trachea with lung

✓x7ᵗʰ **T27.6**   Corrosion of other parts of respiratory tract
      ▶Code first (T51-T65) to identify chemical and intent◀

✓x7ᵗʰ **T27.7**   Corrosion of respiratory tract, part unspecified   ▽
      ▶Code first (T51-T65) to identify chemical and intent◀

✓4ᵗʰ **T28**   **Burn and corrosion of other internal organs**
      Use additional external cause code to identify the source and intent of the burn (X00- X19, X75-X77, X96-X98)
      Use additional external cause code to identify place (Y92)

> The appropriate 7th character is to be added to each code from category T28.
> A   initial encounter
> D   subsequent encounter
> S   sequela

✓x7ᵗʰ **T28.0**   Burn of mouth and pharynx

✓x7ᵗʰ **T28.1**   Burn of esophagus

✓x7ᵗʰ **T28.2**   Burn of other parts of alimentary tract

✓x7ᵗʰ **T28.3**   Burn of internal genitourinary organs

✓5ᵗʰ **T28.4**   **Burns of other and unspecified internal organs**
      ▶Code first (T51-T65) to identify chemical and intent◀

    ✓x7ᵗʰ **T28.40**   Burn of unspecified internal organ   ▽

    ✓6ᵗʰ **T28.41**   Burn of ear drum

       ✓7ᵗʰ **T28.411**   Burn of right ear drum

       ✓7ᵗʰ **T28.412**   Burn of left ear drum

       ✓7ᵗʰ **T28.419**   Burn of unspecified ear drum   ▽

    ✓x7ᵗʰ **T28.49**   **Burn of other internal organ**
         ~~Code first (T51-T65) to identify chemical and intent for T28.5-T28.9~~

✓x7ᵗʰ **T28.5**   Corrosion of mouth and pharynx
      ▶Code first (T51-T65) to identify chemical and intent◀

✓x7ᵗʰ **T28.6**   Corrosion of esophagus
      ▶Code first (T51-T65) to identify chemical and intent◀

✓x7ᵗʰ **T28.7**   Corrosion of other parts of alimentary tract
      ▶Code first (T51-T65) to identify chemical and intent◀

✓x7ᵗʰ **T28.8**   Corrosion of internal genitourinary organs
      ▶Code first (T51-T65) to identify chemical and intent◀

✓5ᵗʰ **T28.9**   **Corrosions of other and unspecified internal organs**
      ▶Code first (T51-T65) to identify chemical and intent◀

    ✓x7ᵗʰ **T28.90**   Corrosions of unspecified internal organs   ▽

    ✓6ᵗʰ **T28.91**   Corrosions of ear drum

       ✓7ᵗʰ **T28.911**   Corrosions of right ear drum

       ✓7ᵗʰ **T28.912**   Corrosions of left ear drum

       ✓7ᵗʰ **T28.919**   Corrosions of unspecified ear drum   ▽

    ✓x7ᵗʰ **T28.99**   Corrosions of other internal organs

Burns and corrosions of multiple and unspecified body regions (T30-T32)

✓4ᵗʰ **T30**   **Burn and corrosion, body region unspecified**

    T30.0   Burn of unspecified body region, unspecified degree   ▽
      This code is not for inpatient use. Code to specified site and degree of burns.
      Burn NOS
      Multiple burns NOS

    T30.4   Corrosion of unspecified body region, unspecified degree   ▽
      This code is not for inpatient use. Code to specified site and degree of corrosion.
      Corrosion NOS
      Multiple corrosion NOS

✓4ᵗʰ **T31**   **Burns classified according to extent of body surface involved**
      NOTE   This category is to be used as the primary code only when the site of the burn is unspecified. It should be used as a supplementary code with categories T20-T25 when the site is specified.

    T31.0   Burns involving less than 10% of body surface

    ✓5ᵗʰ **T31.1**   Burns involving 10-19% of body surface

      T31.10   **Burns involving 10-19% of body surface with 0% to 9% third degree burns**
        Burns involving 10-19% of body surface NOS

      T31.11   **Burns involving 10-19% of body surface with 10-19% third degree burns**   HCC

    ✓5ᵗʰ **T31.2**   Burns involving 20-29% of body surface

      T31.20   **Burns involving 20-29% of body surface with 0% to 9% third degree burns**
        Burns involving 20-29% of body surface NOS

      T31.21   **Burns involving 20-29% of body surface with 10-19% third degree burns**   HCC

      T31.22   **Burns involving 20-29% of body surface with 20-29% third degree burns**   HCC

    ✓5ᵗʰ **T31.3**   Burns involving 30-39% of body surface

      T31.30   **Burns involving 30-39% of body surface with 0% to 9% third degree burns**
        Burns involving 30-39% of body surface NOS

      T31.31   **Burns involving 30-39% of body surface with 10-19% third degree burns**   HCC

      T31.32   **Burns involving 30-39% of body surface with 20-29% third degree burns**   HCC

      T31.33   **Burns involving 30-39% of body surface with 30-39% third degree burns**   HCC

    ✓5ᵗʰ **T31.4**   Burns involving 40-49% of body surface

      T31.40   **Burns involving 40-49% of body surface with 0% to 9% third degree burns**
        Burns involving 40-49% of body surface NOS

      T31.41   **Burns involving 40-49% of body surface with 10-19% third degree burns**   HCC

      T31.42   **Burns involving 40-49% of body surface with 20-29% third degree burns**   HCC

      T31.43   **Burns involving 40-49% of body surface with 30-39% third degree burns**   HCC

      T31.44   **Burns involving 40-49% of body surface with 40-49% third degree burns**   HCC

    ✓5ᵗʰ **T31.5**   Burns involving 50-59% of body surface

      T31.50   **Burns involving 50-59% of body surface with 0% to 9% third degree burns**
        Burns involving 50-59% of body surface NOS

      T31.51   **Burns involving 50-59% of body surface with 10-19% third degree burns**   HCC

      T31.52   **Burns involving 50-59% of body surface with 20-29% third degree burns**   HCC

      T31.53   **Burns involving 50-59% of body surface with 30-39% third degree burns**   HCC

      T31.54   **Burns involving 50-59% of body surface with 40-49% third degree burns**   HCC

      T31.55   **Burns involving 50-59% of body surface with 50-59% third degree burns**   HCC

    ✓5ᵗʰ **T31.6**   Burns involving 60-69% of body surface

      T31.60   **Burns involving 60-69% of body surface with 0% to 9% third degree burns**
        Burns involving 60-69% of body surface NOS

      T31.61   **Burns involving 60-69% of body surface with 10-19% third degree burns**   HCC

☑ Additional Character Req   ✓x7ᵗʰ Placeholder Alert   Manifestation   HCC CMS-HCC Condition   ▽ Unspecified Code   ▶◀ Revised Text   ● New Code   ▲ Revised Code Title

T31.62 Burns involving 60-69% of body surface with 20-29% third degree burns   `HCC`

T31.63 Burns involving 60-69% of body surface with 30-39% third degree burns   `HCC`

T31.64 Burns involving 60-69% of body surface with 40-49% third degree burns   `HCC`

T31.65 Burns involving 60-69% of body surface with 50-59% third degree burns   `HCC`

T31.66 Burns involving 60-69% of body surface with 60-69% third degree burns   `HCC`

√5th **T31.7** Burns involving 70-79% of body surface

T31.70 Burns involving 70-79% of body surface with 0% to 9% third degree burns
Burns involving 70-79% of body surface NOS

T31.71 Burns involving 70-79% of body surface with 10-19% third degree burns   `HCC`

T31.72 Burns involving 70-79% of body surface with 20-29% third degree burns   `HCC`

T31.73 Burns involving 70-79% of body surface with 30-39% third degree burns   `HCC`

T31.74 Burns involving 70-79% of body surface with 40-49% third degree burns   `HCC`

T31.75 Burns involving 70-79% of body surface with 50-59% third degree burns   `HCC`

T31.76 Burns involving 70-79% of body surface with 60-69% third degree burns   `HCC`

T31.77 Burns involving 70-79% of body surface with 70-79% third degree burns   `HCC`

√5th **T31.8** Burns involving 80-89% of body surface

T31.80 Burns involving 80-89% of body surface with 0% to 9% third degree burns
Burns involving 80-89% of body surface NOS

T31.81 Burns involving 80-89% of body surface with 10-19% third degree burns   `HCC`

T31.82 Burns involving 80-89% of body surface with 20-29% third degree burns   `HCC`

T31.83 Burns involving 80-89% of body surface with 30-39% third degree burns   `HCC`

T31.84 Burns involving 80-89% of body surface with 40-49% third degree burns   `HCC`

T31.85 Burns involving 80-89% of body surface with 50-59% third degree burns   `HCC`

T31.86 Burns involving 80-89% of body surface with 60-69% third degree burns   `HCC`

T31.87 Burns involving 80-89% of body surface with 70-79% third degree burns   `HCC`

T31.88 Burns involving 80-89% of body surface with 80-89% third degree burns   `HCC`

√5th **T31.9** Burns involving 90% or more of body surface

T31.90 Burns involving 90% or more of body surface with 0% to 9% third degree burns
Burns involving 90% or more of body surface NOS

T31.91 Burns involving 90% or more of body surface with 10-19% third degree burns   `HCC`

T31.92 Burns involving 90% or more of body surface with 20-29% third degree burns   `HCC`

T31.93 Burns involving 90% or more of body surface with 30-39% third degree burns   `HCC`

T31.94 Burns involving 90% or more of body surface with 40-49% third degree burns   `HCC`

T31.95 Burns involving 90% or more of body surface with 50-59% third degree burns   `HCC`

T31.96 Burns involving 90% or more of body surface with 60-69% third degree burns   `HCC`

T31.97 Burns involving 90% or more of body surface with 70-79% third degree burns   `HCC`

T31.98 Burns involving 90% or more of body surface with 80-89% third degree burns   `HCC`

T31.99 Burns involving 90% or more of body surface with 90% or more third degree burns   `HCC`

√4th **T32** Corrosions classified according to extent of body surface involved

> `NOTE` This category is to be used as the primary code only when the site of the corrosion is unspecified. It may be used as a supplementary code with categories T20-T25 when the site is specified.

T32.0 Corrosions involving less than 10% of body surface

√5th **T32.1** Corrosions involving 10-19% of body surface

T32.10 Corrosions involving 10-19% of body surface with 0% to 9% third degree corrosion
Corrosions involving 10-19% of body surface NOS

T32.11 Corrosions involving 10-19% of body surface with 10-19% third degree corrosion   `HCC`

√5th **T32.2** Corrosions involving 20-29% of body surface

T32.20 Corrosions involving 20-29% of body surface with 0% to 9% third degree corrosion

T32.21 Corrosions involving 20-29% of body surface with 10-19% third degree corrosion   `HCC`

T32.22 Corrosions involving 20-29% of body surface with 20-29% third degree corrosion   `HCC`

√5th **T32.3** Corrosions involving 30-39% of body surface

T32.30 Corrosions involving 30-39% of body surface with 0% to 9% third degree corrosion

T32.31 Corrosions involving 30-39% of body surface with 10-19% third degree corrosion   `HCC`

T32.32 Corrosions involving 30-39% of body surface with 20-29% third degree corrosion   `HCC`

T32.33 Corrosions involving 30-39% of body surface with 30-39% third degree corrosion   `HCC`

√5th **T32.4** Corrosions involving 40-49% of body surface

T32.40 Corrosions involving 40-49% of body surface with 0% to 9% third degree corrosion

T32.41 Corrosions involving 40-49% of body surface with 10-19% third degree corrosion   `HCC`

T32.42 Corrosions involving 40-49% of body surface with 20-29% third degree corrosion   `HCC`

T32.43 Corrosions involving 40-49% of body surface with 30-39% third degree corrosion   `HCC`

T32.44 Corrosions involving 40-49% of body surface with 40-49% third degree corrosion   `HCC`

√5th **T32.5** Corrosions involving 50-59% of body surface

T32.50 Corrosions involving 50-59% of body surface with 0% to 9% third degree corrosion

T32.51 Corrosions involving 50-59% of body surface with 10-19% third degree corrosion   `HCC`

T32.52 Corrosions involving 50-59% of body surface with 20-29% third degree corrosion   `HCC`

T32.53 Corrosions involving 50-59% of body surface with 30-39% third degree corrosion   `HCC`

T32.54 Corrosions involving 50-59% of body surface with 40-49% third degree corrosion   `HCC`

T32.55 Corrosions involving 50-59% of body surface with 50-59% third degree corrosion   `HCC`

√5th **T32.6** Corrosions involving 60-69% of body surface

T32.60 Corrosions involving 60-69% of body surface with 0% to 9% third degree corrosion

T32.61 Corrosions involving 60-69% of body surface with 10-19% third degree corrosion   `HCC`

T32.62 Corrosions involving 60-69% of body surface with 20-29% third degree corrosion   `HCC`

T32.63 Corrosions involving 60-69% of body surface with 30-39% third degree corrosion   `HCC`

T32.64 Corrosions involving 60-69% of body surface with 40-49% third degree corrosion   `HCC`

T32.65 Corrosions involving 60-69% of body surface with 50-59% third degree corrosion   `HCC`

T32.66 Corrosions involving 60-69% of body surface with 60-69% third degree corrosion   `HCC`

√5th **T32.7** Corrosions involving 70-79% of body surface

T32.70 Corrosions involving 70-79% of body surface with 0% to 9% third degree corrosion

T32.71 Corrosions involving 70-79% of body surface with 10-19% third degree corrosion   `HCC`

T32.72 Corrosions involving 70-79% of body surface with 20-29% third degree corrosion   `HCC`

`EXCLUDES 1` Not coded here   `EXCLUDES 2` Not included here   N Newborn Age: 0   P Pediatric Age: 0-17   M Maternity Age: 12-55   A Adult Age: 15-124

1056   ICD-10-CM 2018

T32.73	Corrosions involving 70-79% of body surface with 30-39% third degree corrosion	HCC
T32.74	Corrosions involving 70-79% of body surface with 40-49% third degree corrosion	HCC
T32.75	Corrosions involving 70-79% of body surface with 50-59% third degree corrosion	HCC
T32.76	Corrosions involving 70-79% of body surface with 60-69% third degree corrosion	HCC
T32.77	Corrosions involving 70-79% of body surface with 70-79% third degree corrosion	HCC

√5ᵗʰ **T32.8 Corrosions involving 80-89% of body surface**

T32.80	Corrosions involving 80-89% of body surface with 0% to 9% third degree corrosion	
T32.81	Corrosions involving 80-89% of body surface with 10-19% third degree corrosion	HCC
T32.82	Corrosions involving 80-89% of body surface with 20-29% third degree corrosion	HCC
T32.83	Corrosions involving 80-89% of body surface with 30-39% third degree corrosion	HCC
T32.84	Corrosions involving 80-89% of body surface with 40-49% third degree corrosion	HCC
T32.85	Corrosions involving 80-89% of body surface with 50-59% third degree corrosion	HCC
T32.86	Corrosions involving 80-89% of body surface with 60-69% third degree corrosion	HCC
T32.87	Corrosions involving 80-89% of body surface with 70-79% third degree corrosion	HCC
T32.88	Corrosions involving 80-89% of body surface with 80-89% third degree corrosion	HCC

√5ᵗʰ **T32.9 Corrosions involving 90% or more of body surface**

T32.90	Corrosions involving 90% or more of body surface with 0% to 9% third degree corrosion	
T32.91	Corrosions involving 90% or more of body surface with 10-19% third degree corrosion	HCC
T32.92	Corrosions involving 90% or more of body surface with 20-29% third degree corrosion	HCC
T32.93	Corrosions involving 90% or more of body surface with 30-39% third degree corrosion	HCC
T32.94	Corrosions involving 90% or more of body surface with 40-49% third degree corrosion	HCC
T32.95	Corrosions involving 90% or more of body surface with 50-59% third degree corrosion	HCC
T32.96	Corrosions involving 90% or more of body surface with 60-69% third degree corrosion	HCC
T32.97	Corrosions involving 90% or more of body surface with 70-79% third degree corrosion	HCC
T32.98	Corrosions involving 90% or more of body surface with 80-89% third degree corrosion	HCC
T32.99	Corrosions involving 90% or more of body surface with 90% or more third degree corrosion	HCC

Frostbite (T33-T34)

EXCLUDES 2   *hypothermia and other effects of reduced temperature (T68, T69-)*

√4ᵗʰ **T33 Superficial frostbite**

     INCLUDES   frostbite with partial thickness skin loss

> The appropriate 7th character is to be added to each code from category T33.
> A   initial encounter
> D   subsequent encounter
> S   sequela

√5ᵗʰ **T33.0 Superficial frostbite of head**

√6ᵗʰ   **T33.01 Superficial frostbite of ear**

     √7ᵗʰ   T33.011 Superficial frostbite of right ear
     √7ᵗʰ   T33.012 Superficial frostbite of left ear
     √7ᵗʰ   T33.019 Superficial frostbite of unspecified ear ▽

√x7ᵗʰ   T33.02 Superficial frostbite of nose
√x7ᵗʰ   T33.09 Superficial frostbite of other part of head

√x7ᵗʰ **T33.1 Superficial frostbite of neck**
√x7ᵗʰ **T33.2 Superficial frostbite of thorax**
√x7ᵗʰ **T33.3 Superficial frostbite of abdominal wall, lower back and pelvis**
√5ᵗʰ **T33.4 Superficial frostbite of arm**

     EXCLUDES 2   *superficial frostbite of wrist and hand (T33.5-)*

√x7ᵗʰ   T33.40 Superficial frostbite of unspecified arm ▽
√x7ᵗʰ   T33.41 Superficial frostbite of right arm

√x7ᵗʰ   T33.42 Superficial frostbite of left arm

√5ᵗʰ **T33.5 Superficial frostbite of wrist, hand, and fingers**

√6ᵗʰ   **T33.51 Superficial frostbite of wrist**

    √7ᵗʰ   T33.511 Superficial frostbite of right wrist
    √7ᵗʰ   T33.512 Superficial frostbite of left wrist
    √7ᵗʰ   T33.519 Superficial frostbite of unspecified wrist ▽

√6ᵗʰ   **T33.52 Superficial frostbite of hand**

    EXCLUDES 2   *superficial frostbite of fingers (T33.53-)*

    √7ᵗʰ   T33.521 Superficial frostbite of right hand
    √7ᵗʰ   T33.522 Superficial frostbite of left hand
    √7ᵗʰ   T33.529 Superficial frostbite of unspecified hand ▽

√6ᵗʰ   **T33.53 Superficial frostbite of finger(s)**

    √7ᵗʰ   T33.531 Superficial frostbite of right finger(s)
    √7ᵗʰ   T33.532 Superficial frostbite of left finger(s)
    √7ᵗʰ   T33.539 Superficial frostbite of unspecified finger(s) ▽

√5ᵗʰ **T33.6 Superficial frostbite of hip and thigh**

√x7ᵗʰ   T33.60 Superficial frostbite of unspecified hip and thigh ▽
√x7ᵗʰ   T33.61 Superficial frostbite of right hip and thigh
√x7ᵗʰ   T33.62 Superficial frostbite of left hip and thigh

√5ᵗʰ **T33.7 Superficial frostbite of knee and lower leg**

    EXCLUDES 2   *superficial frostbite of ankle and foot (T33.8-)*

√x7ᵗʰ   T33.70 Superficial frostbite of unspecified knee and lower leg ▽
√x7ᵗʰ   T33.71 Superficial frostbite of right knee and lower leg
√x7ᵗʰ   T33.72 Superficial frostbite of left knee and lower leg

√5ᵗʰ **T33.8 Superficial frostbite of ankle, foot, and toe(s)**

√6ᵗʰ   **T33.81 Superficial frostbite of ankle**

    √7ᵗʰ   T33.811 Superficial frostbite of right ankle
    √7ᵗʰ   T33.812 Superficial frostbite of left ankle
    √7ᵗʰ   T33.819 Superficial frostbite of unspecified ankle ▽

√6ᵗʰ   **T33.82 Superficial frostbite of foot**

    √7ᵗʰ   T33.821 Superficial frostbite of right foot
    √7ᵗʰ   T33.822 Superficial frostbite of left foot
    √7ᵗʰ   T33.829 Superficial frostbite of unspecified foot ▽

√6ᵗʰ   **T33.83 Superficial frostbite of toe(s)**

    √7ᵗʰ   T33.831 Superficial frostbite of right toe(s)
    √7ᵗʰ   T33.832 Superficial frostbite of left toe(s)
    √7ᵗʰ   T33.839 Superficial frostbite of unspecified toe(s) ▽

√5ᵗʰ **T33.9 Superficial frostbite of other and unspecified sites**

√x7ᵗʰ   T33.90 Superficial frostbite of unspecified sites ▽
      Superficial frostbite NOS

√x7ᵗʰ   T33.99 Superficial frostbite of other sites
      Superficial frostbite of leg NOS
      Superficial frostbite of trunk NOS

√4ᵗʰ **T34 Frostbite with tissue necrosis**

> The appropriate 7th character is to be added to each code from category T34.
> A   initial encounter
> D   subsequent encounter
> S   sequela

√5ᵗʰ **T34.0 Frostbite with tissue necrosis of head**

√6ᵗʰ   **T34.01 Frostbite with tissue necrosis of ear**

    √7ᵗʰ   T34.011 Frostbite with tissue necrosis of right ear
    √7ᵗʰ   T34.012 Frostbite with tissue necrosis of left ear
    √7ᵗʰ   T34.019 Frostbite with tissue necrosis of unspecified ear ▽

√x7ᵗʰ   T34.02 Frostbite with tissue necrosis of nose
√x7ᵗʰ   T34.09 Frostbite with tissue necrosis of other part of head

√x7ᵗʰ **T34.1 Frostbite with tissue necrosis of neck**
√x7ᵗʰ **T34.2 Frostbite with tissue necrosis of thorax**
√x7ᵗʰ **T34.3 Frostbite with tissue necrosis of abdominal wall, lower back and pelvis**

☑ Additional Character Req	√x7ᵗʰ Placeholder Alert Manifestation HCC CMS-HCC Condition ▽ Unspecified Code ►◄ Revised Text ● New Code ▲ Revised Code Title

√5ᵗʰ **T34.4** Frostbite with tissue necrosis of arm
> EXCLUDES 2 *frostbite with tissue necrosis of wrist and hand (T34.5-)*

√x7ᵗʰ **T34.40** Frostbite with tissue necrosis of unspecified arm ▽

√x7ᵗʰ **T34.41** Frostbite with tissue necrosis of right arm

√x7ᵗʰ **T34.42** Frostbite with tissue necrosis of left arm

√5ᵗʰ **T34.5** Frostbite with tissue necrosis of wrist, hand, and finger(s)

√6ᵗʰ **T34.51** Frostbite with tissue necrosis of wrist

√7ᵗʰ **T34.511** Frostbite with tissue necrosis of right wrist

√7ᵗʰ **T34.512** Frostbite with tissue necrosis of left wrist

√7ᵗʰ **T34.519** Frostbite with tissue necrosis of unspecified wrist ▽

√6ᵗʰ **T34.52** Frostbite with tissue necrosis of hand
> EXCLUDES 2 *frostbite with tissue necrosis of finger(s) (T34.53-)*

√7ᵗʰ **T34.521** Frostbite with tissue necrosis of right hand

√7ᵗʰ **T34.522** Frostbite with tissue necrosis of left hand

√7ᵗʰ **T34.529** Frostbite with tissue necrosis of unspecified hand ▽

√6ᵗʰ **T34.53** Frostbite with tissue necrosis of finger(s)

√7ᵗʰ **T34.531** Frostbite with tissue necrosis of right finger(s)

√7ᵗʰ **T34.532** Frostbite with tissue necrosis of left finger(s)

√7ᵗʰ **T34.539** Frostbite with tissue necrosis of unspecified finger(s) ▽

√5ᵗʰ **T34.6** Frostbite with tissue necrosis of hip and thigh

√x7ᵗʰ **T34.60** Frostbite with tissue necrosis of unspecified hip and thigh ▽

√x7ᵗʰ **T34.61** Frostbite with tissue necrosis of right hip and thigh

√x7ᵗʰ **T34.62** Frostbite with tissue necrosis of left hip and thigh

√5ᵗʰ **T34.7** Frostbite with tissue necrosis of knee and lower leg
> EXCLUDES 2 *frostbite with tissue necrosis of ankle and foot (T34.8-)*

√x7ᵗʰ **T34.70** Frostbite with tissue necrosis of unspecified knee and lower leg ▽

√x7ᵗʰ **T34.71** Frostbite with tissue necrosis of right knee and lower leg

√x7ᵗʰ **T34.72** Frostbite with tissue necrosis of left knee and lower leg

√5ᵗʰ **T34.8** Frostbite with tissue necrosis of ankle, foot, and toe(s)

√6ᵗʰ **T34.81** Frostbite with tissue necrosis of ankle

√7ᵗʰ **T34.811** Frostbite with tissue necrosis of right ankle

√7ᵗʰ **T34.812** Frostbite with tissue necrosis of left ankle

√7ᵗʰ **T34.819** Frostbite with tissue necrosis of unspecified ankle ▽

√6ᵗʰ **T34.82** Frostbite with tissue necrosis of foot

√7ᵗʰ **T34.821** Frostbite with tissue necrosis of right foot

√7ᵗʰ **T34.822** Frostbite with tissue necrosis of left foot

√7ᵗʰ **T34.829** Frostbite with tissue necrosis of unspecified foot ▽

√6ᵗʰ **T34.83** Frostbite with tissue necrosis of toe(s)

√7ᵗʰ **T34.831** Frostbite with tissue necrosis of right toe(s)

√7ᵗʰ **T34.832** Frostbite with tissue necrosis of left toe(s)

√7ᵗʰ **T34.839** Frostbite with tissue necrosis of unspecified toe(s) ▽

√5ᵗʰ **T34.9** Frostbite with tissue necrosis of other and unspecified sites

√x7ᵗʰ **T34.90** Frostbite with tissue necrosis of unspecified sites ▽
> Frostbite with tissue necrosis NOS

√x7ᵗʰ **T34.99** Frostbite with tissue necrosis of other sites
> Frostbite with tissue necrosis of leg NOS
> Frostbite with tissue necrosis of trunk NOS

Poisoning by, adverse effects of and underdosing of drugs, medicaments and biological substances (T36-T50)

INCLUDES adverse effect of correct substance properly administered
poisoning by overdose of substance
poisoning by wrong substance given or taken in error
underdosing by (inadvertently) (deliberately) taking less substance than prescribed or instructed

Code first, for adverse effects, the nature of the adverse effect, such as:
adverse effect NOS (T88.7)
aspirin gastritis (K29.-)
blood disorders (D56-D76)
contact dermatitis (L23-L25)
dermatitis due to substances taken internally (L27.-)
nephropathy (N14.0-N14.2)

NOTE The drug giving rise to the adverse effect should be identified by use of codes from categories T36-T50 with fifth or sixth character 5.

Use additional code(s) to specify:
manifestations of poisoning
underdosing or failure in dosage during medical and surgical care (Y63.6, Y63.8-Y63.9)
underdosing of medication regimen (Z91.12-, Z91.13-)

EXCLUDES 1 *toxic reaction to local anesthesia in pregnancy (O29.3-)*
EXCLUDES 2 *abuse and dependence of psychoactive substances (F10-F19)*
abuse of non-dependence-producing substances (F55.-)
drug reaction and poisoning affecting newborn (P00-P96)
pathological drug intoxication (inebriation) (F10-F19)

AHA: 2016, 2Q, 8; 2015, 3Q, 22

√4ᵗʰ **T36 Poisoning by, adverse effect of and underdosing of systemic antibiotics**
> EXCLUDES 1 *antineoplastic antibiotics (T45.1-)*
> *locally applied antibiotic NEC (T49.0)*
> *topically used antibiotic for ear, nose and throat (T49.6)*
> *topically used antibiotic for eye (T49.5)*

> The appropriate 7th character is to be added to each code from category T36.
> A initial encounter
> D subsequent encounter
> S sequela

√5ᵗʰ **T36.0** Poisoning by, adverse effect of and underdosing of penicillins

√6ᵗʰ **T36.0X** Poisoning by, adverse effect of and underdosing of penicillins

√7ᵗʰ **T36.0X1** Poisoning by penicillins, accidental (unintentional)
> Poisoning by penicillins NOS

2 √7ᵗʰ **T36.0X2** Poisoning by penicillins, intentional self-harm HCC

√7ᵗʰ **T36.0X3** Poisoning by penicillins, assault

√7ᵗʰ **T36.0X4** Poisoning by penicillins, undetermined

√7ᵗʰ **T36.0X5** Adverse effect of penicillins

√7ᵗʰ **T36.0X6** Underdosing of penicillins

√5ᵗʰ **T36.1** Poisoning by, adverse effect of and underdosing of cephalosporins and other beta-lactam antibiotics

√6ᵗʰ **T36.1X** Poisoning by, adverse effect of and underdosing of cephalosporins and other beta-lactam antibiotics

√7ᵗʰ **T36.1X1** Poisoning by cephalosporins and other beta-lactam antibiotics, accidental (unintentional)
> Poisoning by cephalosporins and other beta-lactam antibiotics NOS

2 √7ᵗʰ **T36.1X2** Poisoning by cephalosporins and other beta-lactam antibiotics, intentional self-harm HCC

√7ᵗʰ **T36.1X3** Poisoning by cephalosporins and other beta-lactam antibiotics, assault

√7ᵗʰ **T36.1X4** Poisoning by cephalosporins and other beta-lactam antibiotics, undetermined

√7ᵗʰ **T36.1X5** Adverse effect of cephalosporins and other beta-lactam antibiotics

√7ᵗʰ **T36.1X6** Underdosing of cephalosporins and other beta-lactam antibiotics

---

2 HCC with 7th character indicating initial encounter (A or B - specific to category) OR sequela.

EXCLUDES 1 Not coded here   EXCLUDES 2 Not included here   N Newborn Age: 0   P Pediatric Age: 0-17   M Maternity Age: 12-55   A Adult Age: 15-124

1058   ICD-10-CM 2018

✓5ᵗʰ **T36.2 Poisoning by, adverse effect of and underdosing of chloramphenicol group**

     ✓6ᵗʰ **T36.2X Poisoning by, adverse effect of and underdosing of** chloramphenicol group

         ✓7ᵗʰ **T36.2X1 Poisoning by chloramphenicol group,** accidental **(unintentional)**
                 Poisoning by chloramphenicol group NOS

       2 ✓7ᵗʰ **T36.2X2 Poisoning by chloramphenicol group,** HCC **intentional self-harm**

         ✓7ᵗʰ **T36.2X3 Poisoning by chloramphenicol group,** assault

         ✓7ᵗʰ **T36.2X4 Poisoning by chloramphenicol group,** undetermined

         ✓7ᵗʰ **T36.2X5** Adverse effect **of chloramphenicol group**

         ✓7ᵗʰ **T36.2X6** Underdosing **of chloramphenicol group**

✓5ᵗʰ **T36.3 Poisoning by, adverse effect of and underdosing of macrolides**

     ✓6ᵗʰ **T36.3X Poisoning by, adverse effect of and underdosing of** macrolides

         ✓7ᵗʰ **T36.3X1 Poisoning by macrolides,** accidental **(unintentional)**
                 Poisoning by macrolides NOS

       2 ✓7ᵗʰ **T36.3X2 Poisoning by macrolides,** HCC **intentional self-harm**

         ✓7ᵗʰ **T36.3X3 Poisoning by macrolides,** assault

         ✓7ᵗʰ **T36.3X4 Poisoning by macrolides,** undetermined

         ✓7ᵗʰ **T36.3X5** Adverse effect **of macrolides**

         ✓7ᵗʰ **T36.3X6** Underdosing **of macrolides**

✓5ᵗʰ **T36.4 Poisoning by, adverse effect of and underdosing of tetracyclines**

     ✓6ᵗʰ **T36.4X Poisoning by, adverse effect of and underdosing of** tetracyclines

         ✓7ᵗʰ **T36.4X1 Poisoning by tetracyclines,** accidental **(unintentional)**
                 Poisoning by tetracyclines NOS

       2 ✓7ᵗʰ **T36.4X2 Poisoning by tetracyclines,** HCC **intentional self-harm**

         ✓7ᵗʰ **T36.4X3 Poisoning by tetracyclines,** assault

         ✓7ᵗʰ **T36.4X4 Poisoning by tetracyclines,** undetermined

         ✓7ᵗʰ **T36.4X5** Adverse effect **of tetracyclines**

         ✓7ᵗʰ **T36.4X6** Underdosing **of tetracyclines**

✓5ᵗʰ **T36.5 Poisoning by, adverse effect of and underdosing of aminoglycosides**
         Poisoning by, adverse effect of and underdosing of streptomycin

     ✓6ᵗʰ **T36.5X Poisoning by, adverse effect of and underdosing of** aminoglycosides

         ✓7ᵗʰ **T36.5X1 Poisoning by aminoglycosides,** accidental **(unintentional)**
                 Poisoning by aminoglycosides NOS

       2 ✓7ᵗʰ **T36.5X2 Poisoning by aminoglycosides,** HCC **intentional self-harm**

         ✓7ᵗʰ **T36.5X3 Poisoning by aminoglycosides,** assault

         ✓7ᵗʰ **T36.5X4 Poisoning by aminoglycosides,** undetermined

         ✓7ᵗʰ **T36.5X5** Adverse effect **of aminoglycosides**

         ✓7ᵗʰ **T36.5X6** Underdosing **of aminoglycosides**

✓5ᵗʰ **T36.6 Poisoning by, adverse effect of and underdosing of rifampicins**

     ✓6ᵗʰ **T36.6X Poisoning by, adverse effect of and underdosing of** rifampicins

         ✓7ᵗʰ **T36.6X1 Poisoning by rifampicins,** accidental **(unintentional)**
                 Poisoning by rifampicins NOS

       2 ✓7ᵗʰ **T36.6X2 Poisoning by rifampicins,** HCC **intentional self-harm**

         ✓7ᵗʰ **T36.6X3 Poisoning by rifampicins,** assault

         ✓7ᵗʰ **T36.6X4 Poisoning by rifampicins,** undetermined

         ✓7ᵗʰ **T36.6X5** Adverse effect **of rifampicins**

         ✓7ᵗʰ **T36.6X6** Underdosing **of rifampicins**

✓5ᵗʰ **T36.7 Poisoning by, adverse effect of and underdosing of antifungal antibiotics, systemically used**

     ✓6ᵗʰ **T36.7X Poisoning by, adverse effect of and underdosing of** antifungal antibiotics, **systemically used**

         ✓7ᵗʰ **T36.7X1 Poisoning by antifungal antibiotics, systemically used,** accidental **(unintentional)**
                 Poisoning by antifungal antibiotics, systemically used NOS

       2 ✓7ᵗʰ **T36.7X2 Poisoning by antifungal antibiotics,** HCC **systemically used,** intentional self-harm

         ✓7ᵗʰ **T36.7X3 Poisoning by antifungal antibiotics, systemically used,** assault

         ✓7ᵗʰ **T36.7X4 Poisoning by antifungal antibiotics, systemically used,** undetermined

         ✓7ᵗʰ **T36.7X5** Adverse effect **of antifungal antibiotics, systemically used**

         ✓7ᵗʰ **T36.7X6** Underdosing **of antifungal antibiotics, systemically used**

✓5ᵗʰ **T36.8 Poisoning by, adverse effect of and underdosing of other systemic antibiotics**

     ✓6ᵗʰ **T36.8X Poisoning by, adverse effect of and underdosing of other systemic antibiotics**
         AHA: 2017, 1Q, 39

         ✓7ᵗʰ **T36.8X1 Poisoning by other systemic antibiotics,** accidental **(unintentional)**
                 Poisoning by other systemic antibiotics NOS

       2 ✓7ᵗʰ **T36.8X2 Poisoning by other systemic** HCC **antibiotics,** intentional self-harm

         ✓7ᵗʰ **T36.8X3 Poisoning by other systemic antibiotics,** assault

         ✓7ᵗʰ **T36.8X4 Poisoning by other systemic antibiotics,** undetermined

         ✓7ᵗʰ **T36.8X5** Adverse effect **of other systemic antibiotics**

         ✓7ᵗʰ **T36.8X6** Underdosing **of other systemic antibiotics**

✓5ᵗʰ **T36.9 Poisoning by, adverse effect of and underdosing of unspecified systemic antibiotic**

     ✓x7ᵗʰ **T36.91 Poisoning by unspecified systemic antibiotic,** ▽ accidental **(unintentional)**
         Poisoning by systemic antibiotic NOS

       2 ✓x7ᵗʰ **T36.92 Poisoning by unspecified systemic antibiotic,** HCC ▽ intentional self-harm

     ✓x7ᵗʰ **T36.93 Poisoning by unspecified systemic antibiotic,** ▽ assault

     ✓x7ᵗʰ **T36.94 Poisoning by unspecified systemic antibiotic,** ▽ undetermined

     ✓x7ᵗʰ **T36.95** Adverse effect **of unspecified systemic antibiotic** ▽

     ✓x7ᵗʰ **T36.96** Underdosing **of unspecified systemic antibiotic** ▽

✓4ᵗʰ **T37 Poisoning by, adverse effect of and underdosing of other systemic anti- infectives and antiparasitics**

     EXCLUDES 1 *anti-infectives topically used for ear, nose and throat (T49.6-)*
         anti-infectives topically used for eye (T49.5-)
         locally applied anti-infectives NEC (T49.0-)

> The appropriate 7th character is to be added to each code from category T37.
> A   initial encounter
> D   subsequent encounter
> S   sequela

✓5ᵗʰ **T37.0 Poisoning by, adverse effect of and underdosing of sulfonamides**

     ✓6ᵗʰ **T37.0X Poisoning by, adverse effect of and underdosing of** sulfonamides

         ✓7ᵗʰ **T37.0X1 Poisoning by sulfonamides,** accidental **(unintentional)**
                 Poisoning by sulfonamides NOS

       2 ✓7ᵗʰ **T37.0X2 Poisoning by sulfonamides,** HCC intentional self-harm

         ✓7ᵗʰ **T37.0X3 Poisoning by sulfonamides,** assault

         ✓7ᵗʰ **T37.0X4 Poisoning by sulfonamides,** undetermined

---

2   HCC with 7th character indicating initial encounter (A or B - specific to category) OR sequela.

✓ Additional Character Req   ✓x7ᵗʰ Placeholder Alert   Manifestation   HCC CMS-HCC Condition   ▽ Unspecified Code   ►◄ Revised Text   ● New Code   ▲ Revised Code Title

Chapter 19. Injury, Poisoning, and Certain Other Consequences of External Causes

T37.0X5–T37.96

     ✓7ᵗʰ   **T37.0X5**   Adverse effect of sulfonamides

     ✓7ᵗʰ   **T37.0X6**   Underdosing of sulfonamides

✓5ᵗʰ   **T37.1**   **Poisoning by, adverse effect of and underdosing of antimycobacterial drugs**

     EXCLUDES 1   rifampicins (T36.6-)
                   streptomycin (T36.5-)

   ✓6ᵗʰ   **T37.1X**   **Poisoning by, adverse effect of and underdosing of antimycobacterial drugs**

     ✓7ᵗʰ   **T37.1X1**   **Poisoning by antimycobacterial drugs, accidental (unintentional)**
                   Poisoning by antimycobacterial drugs NOS

     2   ✓7ᵗʰ   **T37.1X2**   **Poisoning by antimycobacterial drugs, intentional self-harm**   HCC

     ✓7ᵗʰ   **T37.1X3**   **Poisoning by antimycobacterial drugs, assault**

     ✓7ᵗʰ   **T37.1X4**   **Poisoning by antimycobacterial drugs, undetermined**

     ✓7ᵗʰ   **T37.1X5**   **Adverse effect of antimycobacterial drugs**

     ✓7ᵗʰ   **T37.1X6**   **Underdosing of antimycobacterial drugs**

✓5ᵗʰ   **T37.2**   **Poisoning by, adverse effect of and underdosing of antimalarials and drugs acting on other blood protozoa**

     EXCLUDES 1   hydroxyquinoline derivatives (T37.8-)

   ✓6ᵗʰ   **T37.2X**   **Poisoning by, adverse effect of and underdosing of antimalarials and drugs acting on other blood protozoa**

     ✓7ᵗʰ   **T37.2X1**   **Poisoning by antimalarials and drugs acting on other blood protozoa, accidental (unintentional)**
                   Poisoning by antimalarials and drugs acting on other blood protozoa NOS

     2   ✓7ᵗʰ   **T37.2X2**   **Poisoning by antimalarials and drugs acting on other blood protozoa, intentional self-harm**   HCC

     ✓7ᵗʰ   **T37.2X3**   **Poisoning by antimalarials and drugs acting on other blood protozoa, assault**

     ✓7ᵗʰ   **T37.2X4**   **Poisoning by antimalarials and drugs acting on other blood protozoa, undetermined**

     ✓7ᵗʰ   **T37.2X5**   **Adverse effect of antimalarials and drugs acting on other blood protozoa**

     ✓7ᵗʰ   **T37.2X6**   **Underdosing of antimalarials and drugs acting on other blood protozoa**

✓5ᵗʰ   **T37.3**   **Poisoning by, adverse effect of and underdosing of other antiprotozoal drugs**

   ✓6ᵗʰ   **T37.3X**   **Poisoning by, adverse effect of and underdosing of other antiprotozoal drugs**

     ✓7ᵗʰ   **T37.3X1**   **Poisoning by other antiprotozoal drugs, accidental (unintentional)**
                   Poisoning by other antiprotozoal drugs NOS

     2   ✓7ᵗʰ   **T37.3X2**   **Poisoning by other antiprotozoal drugs, intentional self-harm**   HCC

     ✓7ᵗʰ   **T37.3X3**   **Poisoning by other antiprotozoal drugs, assault**

     ✓7ᵗʰ   **T37.3X4**   **Poisoning by other antiprotozoal drugs, undetermined**

     ✓7ᵗʰ   **T37.3X5**   **Adverse effect of other antiprotozoal drugs**

     ✓7ᵗʰ   **T37.3X6**   **Underdosing of other antiprotozoal drugs**

✓5ᵗʰ   **T37.4**   **Poisoning by, adverse effect of and underdosing of anthelminthics**

   ✓6ᵗʰ   **T37.4X**   **Poisoning by, adverse effect of and underdosing of anthelminthics**

     ✓7ᵗʰ   **T37.4X1**   **Poisoning by anthelminthics, accidental (unintentional)**
                   Poisoning by anthelminthics NOS

     2   ✓7ᵗʰ   **T37.4X2**   **Poisoning by anthelminthics, intentional self-harm**   HCC

     ✓7ᵗʰ   **T37.4X3**   **Poisoning by anthelminthics, assault**

     ✓7ᵗʰ   **T37.4X4**   **Poisoning by anthelminthics, undetermined**

     ✓7ᵗʰ   **T37.4X5**   **Adverse effect of anthelminthics**

     ✓7ᵗʰ   **T37.4X6**   **Underdosing of anthelminthics**

✓5ᵗʰ   **T37.5**   **Poisoning by, adverse effect of and underdosing of antiviral drugs**

     EXCLUDES 1   amantadine (T42.8-)
                   cytarabine (T45.1-)

   ✓6ᵗʰ   **T37.5X**   **Poisoning by, adverse effect of and underdosing of antiviral drugs**

     ✓7ᵗʰ   **T37.5X1**   **Poisoning by antiviral drugs, accidental (unintentional)**
                   Poisoning by antiviral drugs NOS

     2   ✓7ᵗʰ   **T37.5X2**   **Poisoning by antiviral drugs, intentional self-harm**   HCC

     ✓7ᵗʰ   **T37.5X3**   **Poisoning by antiviral drugs, assault**

     ✓7ᵗʰ   **T37.5X4**   **Poisoning by antiviral drugs, undetermined**

     ✓7ᵗʰ   **T37.5X5**   **Adverse effect of antiviral drugs**

     ✓7ᵗʰ   **T37.5X6**   **Underdosing of antiviral drugs**

✓5ᵗʰ   **T37.8**   **Poisoning by, adverse effect of and underdosing of other specified systemic anti-infectives and antiparasitics**
     Poisoning by, adverse effect of and underdosing of hydroxyquinoline derivatives

     EXCLUDES 1   antimalarial drugs (T37.2-)

   ✓6ᵗʰ   **T37.8X**   **Poisoning by, adverse effect of and underdosing of other specified systemic anti-infectives and antiparasitics**

     ✓7ᵗʰ   **T37.8X1**   **Poisoning by other specified systemic anti-infectives and antiparasitics, accidental (unintentional)**
                   Poisoning by other specified systemic anti-infectives and antiparasitics NOS

     2   ✓7ᵗʰ   **T37.8X2**   **Poisoning by other specified systemic anti-infectives and antiparasitics, intentional self-harm**   HCC

     ✓7ᵗʰ   **T37.8X3**   **Poisoning by other specified systemic anti-infectives and antiparasitics, assault**

     ✓7ᵗʰ   **T37.8X4**   **Poisoning by other specified systemic anti-infectives and antiparasitics, undetermined**

     ✓7ᵗʰ   **T37.8X5**   **Adverse effect of other specified systemic anti-infectives and antiparasitics**

     ✓7ᵗʰ   **T37.8X6**   **Underdosing of other specified systemic anti-infectives and antiparasitics**

✓5ᵗʰ   **T37.9**   **Poisoning by, adverse effect of and underdosing of unspecified systemic anti-infective and antiparasitics**

   ✓x7ᵗʰ   **T37.91**   **Poisoning by unspecified systemic anti-infective and antiparasitics, accidental (unintentional)**   ▽
                   Poisoning by, adverse effect of and underdosing of systemic anti-infective and antiparasitics NOS

     2   ✓x7ᵗʰ   **T37.92**   **Poisoning by unspecified systemic anti-infective and antiparasitics, intentional self-harm**   HCC ▽

   ✓x7ᵗʰ   **T37.93**   **Poisoning by unspecified systemic anti-infective and antiparasitics, assault**   ▽

   ✓x7ᵗʰ   **T37.94**   **Poisoning by unspecified systemic anti-infective and antiparasitics, undetermined**   ▽

   ✓x7ᵗʰ   **T37.95**   **Adverse effect of unspecified systemic anti-infective and antiparasitic**   ▽

   ✓x7ᵗʰ   **T37.96**   **Underdosing of unspecified systemic anti-infectives and antiparasitics**   ▽

---

2   HCC with 7th character indicating initial encounter (A or B - specific to category) OR sequela.

EXCLUDES 1 Not coded here   *EXCLUDES 2* Not included here   N Newborn Age: 0   P Pediatric Age: 0-17   M Maternity Age: 12-55   A Adult Age: 15-124

1060   ICD-10-CM 2018

✓4ᵗʰ **T38** **Poisoning by, adverse effect of and underdosing of hormones and their synthetic substitutes and antagonists, not elsewhere classified**

EXCLUDES 1   *mineralocorticoids and their antagonists (T50.0-)*
oxytocic hormones (T48.0-)
parathyroid hormones and derivatives (T50.9-)

The appropriate 7th character is to be added to each code from category T38.
A   initial encounter
D   subsequent encounter
S   sequela

✓5ᵗʰ **T38.0** **Poisoning by, adverse effect of and underdosing of glucocorticoids and synthetic analogues**

EXCLUDES 1   *glucocorticoids, topically used (T49.-)*

✓6ᵗʰ **T38.0X** **Poisoning by, adverse effect of and underdosing of glucocorticoids and synthetic analogues**

    ✓7ᵗʰ **T38.0X1** **Poisoning by glucocorticoids and synthetic analogues, accidental (unintentional)**
Poisoning by glucocorticoids and synthetic analogues NOS

    2 ✓7ᵗʰ **T38.0X2** **Poisoning by glucocorticoids and synthetic analogues, intentional self-harm** ᴴᶜᶜ

    ✓7ᵗʰ **T38.0X3** **Poisoning by glucocorticoids and synthetic analogues, assault**

    ✓7ᵗʰ **T38.0X4** **Poisoning by glucocorticoids and synthetic analogues, undetermined**

    ✓7ᵗʰ **T38.0X5** **Adverse effect of glucocorticoids and synthetic analogues**

    ✓7ᵗʰ **T38.0X6** **Underdosing of glucocorticoids and synthetic analogues**

✓5ᵗʰ **T38.1** **Poisoning by, adverse effect of and underdosing of thyroid hormones and substitutes**

✓6ᵗʰ **T38.1X** **Poisoning by, adverse effect of and underdosing of thyroid hormones and substitutes**

    ✓7ᵗʰ **T38.1X1** **Poisoning by thyroid hormones and substitutes, accidental (unintentional)**
Poisoning by thyroid hormones and substitutes NOS

    2 ✓7ᵗʰ **T38.1X2** **Poisoning by thyroid hormones and substitutes, intentional self-harm** ᴴᶜᶜ

    ✓7ᵗʰ **T38.1X3** **Poisoning by thyroid hormones and substitutes, assault**

    ✓7ᵗʰ **T38.1X4** **Poisoning by thyroid hormones and substitutes, undetermined**

    ✓7ᵗʰ **T38.1X5** **Adverse effect of thyroid hormones and substitutes**

    ✓7ᵗʰ **T38.1X6** **Underdosing of thyroid hormones and substitutes**

✓5ᵗʰ **T38.2** **Poisoning by, adverse effect of and underdosing of antithyroid drugs**

✓6ᵗʰ **T38.2X** **Poisoning by, adverse effect of and underdosing of antithyroid drugs**

    ✓7ᵗʰ **T38.2X1** **Poisoning by antithyroid drugs, accidental (unintentional)**
Poisoning by antithyroid drugs NOS

    2 ✓7ᵗʰ **T38.2X2** **Poisoning by antithyroid drugs, intentional self-harm** ᴴᶜᶜ

    ✓7ᵗʰ **T38.2X3** **Poisoning by antithyroid drugs, assault**

    ✓7ᵗʰ **T38.2X4** **Poisoning by antithyroid drugs, undetermined**

    ✓7ᵗʰ **T38.2X5** **Adverse effect of antithyroid drugs**

    ✓7ᵗʰ **T38.2X6** **Underdosing of antithyroid drugs**

✓5ᵗʰ **T38.3** **Poisoning by, adverse effect of and underdosing of insulin and oral hypoglycemic [antidiabetic] drugs**

✓6ᵗʰ **T38.3X** **Poisoning by, adverse effect of and underdosing of insulin and oral hypoglycemic [antidiabetic] drugs**

    ✓7ᵗʰ **T38.3X1** **Poisoning by insulin and oral hypoglycemic [antidiabetic] drugs, accidental (unintentional)**
Poisoning by insulin and oral hypoglycemic [antidiabetic] drugs NOS

    2 ✓7ᵗʰ **T38.3X2** **Poisoning by insulin and oral hypoglycemic [antidiabetic] drugs, intentional self-harm** ᴴᶜᶜ

    ✓7ᵗʰ **T38.3X3** **Poisoning by insulin and oral hypoglycemic [antidiabetic] drugs, assault**

    ✓7ᵗʰ **T38.3X4** **Poisoning by insulin and oral hypoglycemic [antidiabetic] drugs, undetermined**

    ✓7ᵗʰ **T38.3X5** **Adverse effect of insulin and oral hypoglycemic [antidiabetic] drugs**

    ✓7ᵗʰ **T38.3X6** **Underdosing of insulin and oral hypoglycemic [antidiabetic] drugs**

✓5ᵗʰ **T38.4** **Poisoning by, adverse effect of and underdosing of oral contraceptives**
Poisoning by, adverse effect of and underdosing of multiple- and single-ingredient oral contraceptive preparations

✓6ᵗʰ **T38.4X** **Poisoning by, adverse effect of and underdosing of oral contraceptives**

    ✓7ᵗʰ **T38.4X1** **Poisoning by oral contraceptives, accidental (unintentional)**
Poisoning by oral contraceptives NOS

    2 ✓7ᵗʰ **T38.4X2** **Poisoning by oral contraceptives, intentional self-harm** ᴴᶜᶜ

    ✓7ᵗʰ **T38.4X3** **Poisoning by oral contraceptives, assault**

    ✓7ᵗʰ **T38.4X4** **Poisoning by oral contraceptives, undetermined**

    ✓7ᵗʰ **T38.4X5** **Adverse effect of oral contraceptives**

    ✓7ᵗʰ **T38.4X6** **Underdosing of oral contraceptives**

✓5ᵗʰ **T38.5** **Poisoning by, adverse effect of and underdosing of other estrogens and progestogens**
Poisoning by, adverse effect of and underdosing of estrogens and progestogens mixtures and substitutes

✓6ᵗʰ **T38.5X** **Poisoning by, adverse effect of and underdosing of other estrogens and progestogens**

    ✓7ᵗʰ **T38.5X1** **Poisoning by other estrogens and progestogens, accidental (unintentional)**
Poisoning by other estrogens and progestogens NOS

    2 ✓7ᵗʰ **T38.5X2** **Poisoning by other estrogens and progestogens, intentional self-harm** ᴴᶜᶜ

    ✓7ᵗʰ **T38.5X3** **Poisoning by other estrogens and progestogens, assault**

    ✓7ᵗʰ **T38.5X4** **Poisoning by other estrogens and progestogens, undetermined**

    ✓7ᵗʰ **T38.5X5** **Adverse effect of other estrogens and progestogens**

    ✓7ᵗʰ **T38.5X6** **Underdosing of other estrogens and progestogens**

✓5ᵗʰ **T38.6** **Poisoning by, adverse effect of and underdosing of antigonadotrophins, antiestrogens, antiandrogens, not elsewhere classified**
Poisoning by, adverse effect of and underdosing of tamoxifen

✓6ᵗʰ **T38.6X** **Poisoning by, adverse effect of and underdosing of antigonadotrophins, antiestrogens, antiandrogens, not elsewhere classified**

    ✓7ᵗʰ **T38.6X1** **Poisoning by antigonadotrophins, antiestrogens, antiandrogens, not elsewhere classified, accidental (unintentional)**
Poisoning by antigonadotrophins, antiestrogens, antiandrogens, not elsewhere classified NOS

    2 ✓7ᵗʰ **T38.6X2** **Poisoning by antigonadotrophins, antiestrogens, antiandrogens, not elsewhere classified, intentional self-harm** ᴴᶜᶜ

    ✓7ᵗʰ **T38.6X3** **Poisoning by antigonadotrophins, antiestrogens, antiandrogens, not elsewhere classified, assault**

    ✓7ᵗʰ **T38.6X4** **Poisoning by antigonadotrophins, antiestrogens, antiandrogens, not elsewhere classified, undetermined**

    ✓7ᵗʰ **T38.6X5** **Adverse effect of antigonadotrophins, antiestrogens, antiandrogens, not elsewhere classified**

    ✓7ᵗʰ **T38.6X6** **Underdosing of antigonadotrophins, antiestrogens, antiandrogens, not elsewhere classified**

---

2   HCC with 7th character indicating initial encounter (A or B - specific to category) OR sequela.

✓ Additional Character Req   ✓x7ᵗʰ Placeholder Alert   Manifestation   ᴴᶜᶜ CMS-HCC Condition   ▽ Unspecified Code   ▶◀ Revised Text   ● New Code   ▲ Revised Code Title

✓5ᵗʰ **T38.7** **Poisoning by, adverse effect of and underdosing of androgens and anabolic congeners**

  ✓6ᵗʰ **T38.7X** **Poisoning by, adverse effect of and underdosing of** androgens and anabolic congeners

    ✓7ᵗʰ **T38.7X1** **Poisoning by androgens and anabolic congeners,** accidental **(unintentional)**
        Poisoning by androgens and anabolic congeners NOS

    2 ✓7ᵗʰ **T38.7X2** **Poisoning by androgens and anabolic** ᴴᶜᶜ **congeners,** intentional self-harm

    ✓7ᵗʰ **T38.7X3** **Poisoning by androgens and anabolic congeners,** assault

    ✓7ᵗʰ **T38.7X4** **Poisoning by androgens and anabolic congeners,** undetermined

    ✓7ᵗʰ **T38.7X5** Adverse effect **of androgens and anabolic congeners**

    ✓7ᵗʰ **T38.7X6** Underdosing **of androgens and anabolic congeners**

✓5ᵗʰ **T38.8** **Poisoning by, adverse effect of and underdosing of other and unspecified hormones and synthetic substitutes**

  ✓6ᵗʰ **T38.80** **Poisoning by, adverse effect of and underdosing of** unspecified hormones and synthetic substitutes

    ✓7ᵗʰ **T38.801** **Poisoning by unspecified hormones and synthetic substitutes,** accidental **(unintentional)** ▽
        Poisoning by unspecified hormones and synthetic substitutes NOS

    2 ✓7ᵗʰ **T38.802** **Poisoning by unspecified hormones** ᴴᶜᶜ ▽ **and synthetic substitutes,** intentional self-harm

    ✓7ᵗʰ **T38.803** **Poisoning by unspecified hormones and synthetic substitutes,** assault ▽

    ✓7ᵗʰ **T38.804** **Poisoning by unspecified hormones and synthetic substitutes,** undetermined ▽

    ✓7ᵗʰ **T38.805** Adverse effect **of unspecified hormones and synthetic substitutes** ▽

    ✓7ᵗʰ **T38.806** Underdosing **of unspecified hormones and synthetic substitutes** ▽

  ✓6ᵗʰ **T38.81** **Poisoning by, adverse effect of and underdosing of** anterior pituitary [adenohypophyseal] hormones

    ✓7ᵗʰ **T38.811** **Poisoning by anterior pituitary [adenohypophyseal] hormones,** accidental **(unintentional)**
        Poisoning by anterior pituitary [adenohypophyseal] hormones NOS

    2 ✓7ᵗʰ **T38.812** **Poisoning by anterior pituitary** ᴴᶜᶜ **[adenohypophyseal] hormones,** intentional self-harm

    ✓7ᵗʰ **T38.813** **Poisoning by anterior pituitary [adenohypophyseal] hormones,** assault

    ✓7ᵗʰ **T38.814** **Poisoning by anterior pituitary [adenohypophyseal] hormones,** undetermined

    ✓7ᵗʰ **T38.815** Adverse effect **of anterior pituitary [adenohypophyseal] hormones**

    ✓7ᵗʰ **T38.816** Underdosing **of anterior pituitary [adenohypophyseal] hormones**

  ✓6ᵗʰ **T38.89** **Poisoning by, adverse effect of and underdosing of** other hormones and synthetic substitutes

    ✓7ᵗʰ **T38.891** **Poisoning by other hormones and synthetic substitutes,** accidental **(unintentional)**
        Poisoning by other hormones and synthetic substitutes NOS

    2 ✓7ᵗʰ **T38.892** **Poisoning by other hormones and** ᴴᶜᶜ **synthetic substitutes,** intentional self-harm

    ✓7ᵗʰ **T38.893** **Poisoning by other hormones and synthetic substitutes,** assault

    ✓7ᵗʰ **T38.894** **Poisoning by other hormones and synthetic substitutes,** undetermined

    ✓7ᵗʰ **T38.895** Adverse effect **of other hormones and synthetic substitutes**

    ✓7ᵗʰ **T38.896** Underdosing **of other hormones and synthetic substitutes**

✓5ᵗʰ **T38.9** **Poisoning by, adverse effect of and underdosing of other and unspecified hormone antagonists**

  ✓6ᵗʰ **T38.90** **Poisoning by, adverse effect of and underdosing of** unspecified hormone antagonists

    ✓7ᵗʰ **T38.901** **Poisoning by unspecified hormone** ▽ **antagonists,** accidental **(unintentional)**
        Poisoning by unspecified hormone antagonists NOS

    2 ✓7ᵗʰ **T38.902** **Poisoning by unspecified hormone** ᴴᶜᶜ ▽ **antagonists,** intentional self-harm

    ✓7ᵗʰ **T38.903** **Poisoning by unspecified hormone** ▽ **antagonists,** assault

    ✓7ᵗʰ **T38.904** **Poisoning by unspecified hormone** ▽ **antagonists,** undetermined

    ✓7ᵗʰ **T38.905** Adverse effect **of unspecified hormone** ▽ **antagonists**

    ✓7ᵗʰ **T38.906** Underdosing **of unspecified hormone** ▽ **antagonists**

  ✓6ᵗʰ **T38.99** **Poisoning by, adverse effect of and underdosing of** other hormone antagonists

    ✓7ᵗʰ **T38.991** **Poisoning by other hormone antagonists,** accidental **(unintentional)**
        Poisoning by other hormone antagonists NOS

    2 ✓7ᵗʰ **T38.992** **Poisoning by other hormone** ᴴᶜᶜ **antagonists,** intentional self-harm

    ✓7ᵗʰ **T38.993** **Poisoning by other hormone antagonists,** assault

    ✓7ᵗʰ **T38.994** **Poisoning by other hormone antagonists,** undetermined

    ✓7ᵗʰ **T38.995** Adverse effect **of other hormone antagonists**

    ✓7ᵗʰ **T38.996** Underdosing **of other hormone antagonists**

✓4ᵗʰ **T39** **Poisoning by, adverse effect of and underdosing of nonopioid analgesics, antipyretics and antirheumatics**

> The appropriate 7th character is to be added to each code from category T39.
> A   initial encounter
> D   subsequent encounter
> S   sequela

  ✓5ᵗʰ **T39.0** **Poisoning by, adverse effect of and underdosing of** salicylates

    ✓6ᵗʰ **T39.01** **Poisoning by, adverse effect of and underdosing of** aspirin
        Poisoning by, adverse effect of and underdosing of acetylsalicylic acid

      ✓7ᵗʰ **T39.011** **Poisoning by aspirin,** accidental **(unintentional)**

      2 ✓7ᵗʰ **T39.012** **Poisoning by aspirin,** intentional ᴴᶜᶜ self-harm

      ✓7ᵗʰ **T39.013** **Poisoning by aspirin,** assault

      ✓7ᵗʰ **T39.014** **Poisoning by aspirin,** undetermined

      ✓7ᵗʰ **T39.015** Adverse effect **of aspirin**
        AHA: 2016, 1Q, 15

      ✓7ᵗʰ **T39.016** Underdosing **of aspirin**

    ✓6ᵗʰ **T39.09** **Poisoning by, adverse effect of and underdosing of** other salicylates

      ✓7ᵗʰ **T39.091** **Poisoning by salicylates,** accidental **(unintentional)**
        Poisoning by salicylates NOS

      2 ✓7ᵗʰ **T39.092** **Poisoning by salicylates,** intentional ᴴᶜᶜ self-harm

      ✓7ᵗʰ **T39.093** **Poisoning by salicylates,** assault

      ✓7ᵗʰ **T39.094** **Poisoning by salicylates,** undetermined

      ✓7ᵗʰ **T39.095** Adverse effect **of salicylates**

      ✓7ᵗʰ **T39.096** Underdosing **of salicylates**

  ✓5ᵗʰ **T39.1** **Poisoning by, adverse effect of and underdosing of 4-Aminophenol derivatives**

    ✓6ᵗʰ **T39.1X** **Poisoning by, adverse effect of and underdosing of** 4-Aminophenol derivatives

      ✓7ᵗʰ **T39.1X1** **Poisoning by 4-Aminophenol derivatives,** accidental **(unintentional)**
        Poisoning by 4-Aminophenol derivatives NOS

---

2   HCC with 7th character indicating initial encounter (A or B - specific to category) OR sequela.

EXCLUDES 1 Not coded here   **EXCLUDES 2** Not included here   Ⓝ Newborn Age: 0   Ⓟ Pediatric Age: 0-17   Ⓜ Maternity Age: 12-55   Ⓐ Adult Age: 15-124

2 ✓7th **T39.1X2** **Poisoning by 4-Aminophenol**   HCC
derivatives, intentional self-harm

✓7th **T39.1X3** **Poisoning by 4-Aminophenol**
derivatives, assault

✓7th **T39.1X4** **Poisoning by 4-Aminophenol**
derivatives, undetermined

✓7th **T39.1X5** Adverse effect of 4-Aminophenol
derivatives

✓7th **T39.1X6** Underdosing of 4-Aminophenol
derivatives

✓5th **T39.2** **Poisoning by, adverse effect of and underdosing of**
pyrazolone derivatives

  ✓6th **T39.2X** **Poisoning by, adverse effect of and underdosing of**
pyrazolone derivatives

    ✓7th **T39.2X1** **Poisoning by pyrazolone derivatives,**
accidental (unintentional)
Poisoning by pyrazolone derivatives NOS

    2 ✓7th **T39.2X2** **Poisoning by pyrazolone derivatives,**   HCC
intentional self-harm

    ✓7th **T39.2X3** **Poisoning by pyrazolone derivatives,**
assault

    ✓7th **T39.2X4** **Poisoning by pyrazolone derivatives,**
undetermined

    ✓7th **T39.2X5** Adverse effect of pyrazolone derivatives

    ✓7th **T39.2X6** Underdosing of pyrazolone derivatives

✓5th **T39.3** **Poisoning by, adverse effect of and underdosing of other**
nonsteroidal anti-inflammatory drugs [NSAID]

  ✓6th **T39.31** **Poisoning by, adverse effect of and underdosing of**
propionic acid derivatives
Poisoning by, adverse effect of and underdosing of
fenoprofen
Poisoning by, adverse effect of and underdosing of
flurbiprofen
Poisoning by, adverse effect of and underdosing of
ibuprofen
Poisoning by, adverse effect of and underdosing of
ketoprofen
Poisoning by, adverse effect of and underdosing of
naproxen
Poisoning by, adverse effect of and underdosing of
oxaprozin

    ✓7th **T39.311** **Poisoning by propionic acid derivatives,**
accidental (unintentional)

    2 ✓7th **T39.312** **Poisoning by propionic acid**   HCC
derivatives, intentional self-harm

    ✓7th **T39.313** **Poisoning by propionic acid derivatives,**
assault

    ✓7th **T39.314** **Poisoning by propionic acid derivatives,**
undetermined

    ✓7th **T39.315** Adverse effect of propionic acid
derivatives

    ✓7th **T39.316** Underdosing of propionic acid derivatives

  ✓6th **T39.39** **Poisoning by, adverse effect of and underdosing of**
other nonsteroidal anti-inflammatory drugs [NSAID]

    ✓7th **T39.391** **Poisoning by other nonsteroidal anti-**
inflammatory drugs [NSAID], accidental
(unintentional)
Poisoning by other nonsteroidal anti-
inflammatory drugs NOS

    2 ✓7th **T39.392** **Poisoning by other nonsteroidal**   HCC
anti-inflammatory drugs [NSAID],
intentional self-harm

    ✓7th **T39.393** **Poisoning by other nonsteroidal**
anti-inflammatory drugs [NSAID], assault

    ✓7th **T39.394** **Poisoning by other nonsteroidal**
anti-inflammatory drugs [NSAID],
undetermined

    ✓7th **T39.395** Adverse effect of other nonsteroidal
anti-inflammatory drugs [NSAID]

    ✓7th **T39.396** Underdosing of other nonsteroidal
anti-inflammatory drugs [NSAID]

✓5th **T39.4** **Poisoning by, adverse effect of and underdosing of**
antirheumatics, not elsewhere classified

    EXCLUDES 1   poisoning by, adverse effect of and underdosing of
glucocorticoids (T38.0-)
poisoning by, adverse effect of and underdosing of
salicylates (T39.0-)

  ✓6th **T39.4X** **Poisoning by, adverse effect of and underdosing of**
antirheumatics, not elsewhere classified

    ✓7th **T39.4X1** **Poisoning by antirheumatics, not**
elsewhere classified, accidental
(unintentional)
Poisoning by antirheumatics, not
elsewhere classified NOS

    2 ✓7th **T39.4X2** **Poisoning by antirheumatics, not**   HCC
elsewhere classified, intentional self-harm

    ✓7th **T39.4X3** **Poisoning by antirheumatics, not**
elsewhere classified, assault

    ✓7th **T39.4X4** **Poisoning by antirheumatics, not**
elsewhere classified, undetermined

    ✓7th **T39.4X5** Adverse effect of antirheumatics, not
elsewhere classified

    ✓7th **T39.4X6** Underdosing of antirheumatics, not
elsewhere classified

✓5th **T39.8** **Poisoning by, adverse effect of and underdosing of other**
nonopioid analgesics and antipyretics, not elsewhere
classified

  ✓6th **T39.8X** **Poisoning by, adverse effect of and underdosing of**
other nonopioid analgesics and antipyretics, not
elsewhere classified

    ✓7th **T39.8X1** **Poisoning by other nonopioid analgesics**
and antipyretics, not elsewhere classified,
accidental (unintentional)
Poisoning by other nonopioid analgesics
and antipyretics, not elsewhere
classified NOS

    2 ✓7th **T39.8X2** **Poisoning by other nonopioid**   HCC
analgesics and antipyretics, not
elsewhere classified, intentional
self-harm

    ✓7th **T39.8X3** **Poisoning by other nonopioid analgesics**
and antipyretics, not elsewhere classified,
assault

    ✓7th **T39.8X4** **Poisoning by other nonopioid analgesics**
and antipyretics, not elsewhere classified,
undetermined

    ✓7th **T39.8X5** Adverse effect of other nonopioid
analgesics and antipyretics, not elsewhere
classified

    ✓7th **T39.8X6** Underdosing of other nonopioid
analgesics and antipyretics, not elsewhere
classified

✓5th **T39.9** **Poisoning by, adverse effect of and underdosing of**
unspecified nonopioid analgesic, antipyretic and
antirheumatic

  ✓x7th **T39.91** **Poisoning by unspecified nonopioid analgesic,** ▽
antipyretic and antirheumatic, accidental
(unintentional)
Poisoning by nonopioid analgesic, antipyretic and
antirheumatic NOS

  2 ✓x7th **T39.92** **Poisoning by unspecified nonopioid**   HCC ▽
analgesic, antipyretic and antirheumatic,
intentional self-harm

  ✓x7th **T39.93** **Poisoning by unspecified nonopioid analgesic,** ▽
antipyretic and antirheumatic, assault

  ✓x7th **T39.94** **Poisoning by unspecified nonopioid analgesic,** ▽
antipyretic and antirheumatic, undetermined

  ✓x7th **T39.95** Adverse effect of unspecified nonopioid ▽
analgesic, antipyretic and antirheumatic

  ✓x7th **T39.96** Underdosing of unspecified nonopioid analgesic, ▽
antipyretic and antirheumatic

---

2   HCC with 7th character indicating initial encounter (A or B - specific to category) OR sequela.

☑ Additional Character Req   ✓x7th Placeholder Alert   Manifestation   HCC CMS-HCC Condition   ▽ Unspecified Code   ▶◀ Revised Text   ● New Code   ▲ Revised Code Title

✓4ᵗʰ T40 Poisoning by, adverse effect of and underdosing of narcotics and psychodysleptics [hallucinogens]

> *EXCLUDES 2* drug dependence and related mental and behavioral disorders due to psychoactive substance use (F10-F19-)

> The appropriate 7th character is to be added to each code from category T40.
> A   initial encounter
> D   subsequent encounter
> S   sequela

✓5ᵗʰ T40.0 Poisoning by, adverse effect of and underdosing of opium

  ✓6ᵗʰ T40.0X Poisoning by, adverse effect of and underdosing of opium

   ✓7ᵗʰ T40.0X1 Poisoning by opium, accidental (unintentional)
   Poisoning by opium NOS

   ² **✓7ᵗʰ T40.0X2 Poisoning by opium,** intentional self-harm   **HCC**

   ✓7ᵗʰ T40.0X3 Poisoning by opium, assault

   ✓7ᵗʰ T40.0X4 Poisoning by opium, undetermined

   ✓7ᵗʰ T40.0X5 Adverse effect of opium

   ✓7ᵗʰ T40.0X6 Underdosing of opium

✓5ᵗʰ T40.1 Poisoning by and adverse effect of heroin

  ✓6ᵗʰ T40.1X Poisoning by and adverse effect of heroin

   ✓7ᵗʰ T40.1X1 Poisoning by heroin, accidental (unintentional)
   Poisoning by heroin NOS

   ² **✓7ᵗʰ T40.1X2 Poisoning by heroin,** intentional self-harm   **HCC**

   ✓7ᵗʰ T40.1X3 Poisoning by heroin, assault

   ✓7ᵗʰ T40.1X4 Poisoning by heroin, undetermined

✓5ᵗʰ T40.2 Poisoning by, adverse effect of and underdosing of other opioids

  ✓6ᵗʰ T40.2X Poisoning by, adverse effect of and underdosing of other opioids

   ✓7ᵗʰ T40.2X1 Poisoning by other opioids, accidental (unintentional)
   Poisoning by other opioids NOS

   ² **✓7ᵗʰ T40.2X2 Poisoning by other opioids,** intentional self-harm   **HCC**

   ✓7ᵗʰ T40.2X3 Poisoning by other opioids, assault

   ✓7ᵗʰ T40.2X4 Poisoning by other opioids, undetermined

   ✓7ᵗʰ T40.2X5 Adverse effect of other opioids

   ✓7ᵗʰ T40.2X6 Underdosing of other opioids

✓5ᵗʰ T40.3 Poisoning by, adverse effect of and underdosing of methadone

  ✓6ᵗʰ T40.3X Poisoning by, adverse effect of and underdosing of methadone

   ✓7ᵗʰ T40.3X1 Poisoning by methadone, accidental (unintentional)
   Poisoning by methadone NOS

   ² **✓7ᵗʰ T40.3X2 Poisoning by methadone,** intentional self-harm   **HCC**

   ✓7ᵗʰ T40.3X3 Poisoning by methadone, assault

   ✓7ᵗʰ T40.3X4 Poisoning by methadone, undetermined

   ✓7ᵗʰ T40.3X5 Adverse effect of methadone

   ✓7ᵗʰ T40.3X6 Underdosing of methadone

✓5ᵗʰ T40.4 Poisoning by, adverse effect of and underdosing of other synthetic narcotics

  ✓6ᵗʰ T40.4X Poisoning by, adverse effect of and underdosing of other synthetic narcotics

   ✓7ᵗʰ T40.4X1 Poisoning by other synthetic narcotics, accidental (unintentional)
   Poisoning by other synthetic narcotics NOS

   ² **✓7ᵗʰ T40.4X2 Poisoning by other synthetic narcotics,** intentional self-harm   **HCC**

   ✓7ᵗʰ T40.4X3 Poisoning by other synthetic narcotics, assault

   ✓7ᵗʰ T40.4X4 Poisoning by other synthetic narcotics, undetermined

   ✓7ᵗʰ T40.4X5 Adverse effect of other synthetic narcotics

   ✓7ᵗʰ T40.4X6 Underdosing of other synthetic narcotics

✓5ᵗʰ T40.5 Poisoning by, adverse effect of and underdosing of cocaine

  ✓6ᵗʰ T40.5X Poisoning by, adverse effect of and underdosing of cocaine

   ✓7ᵗʰ T40.5X1 Poisoning by cocaine, accidental (unintentional)
   Poisoning by cocaine NOS
   AHA: 2016, 2Q, 8

   ² **✓7ᵗʰ T40.5X2 Poisoning by cocaine,** intentional self-harm   **HCC**

   ✓7ᵗʰ T40.5X3 Poisoning by cocaine, assault

   ✓7ᵗʰ T40.5X4 Poisoning by cocaine, undetermined

   ✓7ᵗʰ T40.5X5 Adverse effect of cocaine

   ✓7ᵗʰ T40.5X6 Underdosing of cocaine

✓5ᵗʰ T40.6 Poisoning by, adverse effect of and underdosing of other and unspecified narcotics

  ✓6ᵗʰ T40.60 Poisoning by, adverse effect of and underdosing of unspecified narcotics

   ✓7ᵗʰ T40.601 Poisoning by unspecified narcotics, accidental (unintentional)   ▽
   Poisoning by narcotics NOS

   ² **✓7ᵗʰ T40.602 Poisoning by unspecified narcotics,** intentional self-harm   **HCC** ▽

   ✓7ᵗʰ T40.603 Poisoning by unspecified narcotics, assault   ▽

   ✓7ᵗʰ T40.604 Poisoning by unspecified narcotics, undetermined   ▽

   ✓7ᵗʰ T40.605 Adverse effect of unspecified narcotics   ▽

   ✓7ᵗʰ T40.606 Underdosing of unspecified narcotics   ▽

  ✓6ᵗʰ T40.69 Poisoning by, adverse effect of and underdosing of other narcotics

   ✓7ᵗʰ T40.691 Poisoning by other narcotics, accidental (unintentional)
   Poisoning by other narcotics NOS

   ² **✓7ᵗʰ T40.692 Poisoning by other narcotics,** intentional self-harm   **HCC**

   ✓7ᵗʰ T40.693 Poisoning by other narcotics, assault

   ✓7ᵗʰ T40.694 Poisoning by other narcotics, undetermined

   ✓7ᵗʰ T40.695 Adverse effect of other narcotics

   ✓7ᵗʰ T40.696 Underdosing of other narcotics

✓5ᵗʰ T40.7 Poisoning by, adverse effect of and underdosing of cannabis (derivatives)

  ✓6ᵗʰ T40.7X Poisoning by, adverse effect of and underdosing of cannabis (derivatives)

   ✓7ᵗʰ T40.7X1 Poisoning by cannabis (derivatives), accidental (unintentional)
   Poisoning by cannabis NOS

   ² **✓7ᵗʰ T40.7X2 Poisoning by cannabis (derivatives),** intentional self-harm   **HCC**

   ✓7ᵗʰ T40.7X3 Poisoning by cannabis (derivatives), assault

   ✓7ᵗʰ T40.7X4 Poisoning by cannabis (derivatives), undetermined

   ✓7ᵗʰ T40.7X5 Adverse effect of cannabis (derivatives)

   ✓7ᵗʰ T40.7X6 Underdosing of cannabis (derivatives)

✓5ᵗʰ T40.8 Poisoning by and adverse effect of lysergide [LSD]

  ✓6ᵗʰ T40.8X Poisoning by and adverse effect of lysergide [LSD]

   ✓7ᵗʰ T40.8X1 Poisoning by lysergide [LSD], accidental (unintentional)
   Poisoning by lysergide [LSD]NOS

   ² **✓7ᵗʰ T40.8X2 Poisoning by lysergide [LSD],** intentional self-harm   **HCC**

   ✓7ᵗʰ T40.8X3 Poisoning by lysergide [LSD], assault

   ✓7ᵗʰ T40.8X4 Poisoning by lysergide [LSD], undetermined

✓5ᵗʰ T40.9 Poisoning by, adverse effect of and underdosing of other and unspecified psychodysleptics [hallucinogens]

  ✓6ᵗʰ T40.90 Poisoning by, adverse effect of and underdosing of unspecified psychodysleptics [hallucinogens]

   ✓7ᵗʰ T40.901 Poisoning by unspecified psychodysleptics [hallucinogens], accidental (unintentional)   ▽

---

² HCC with 7th character indicating initial encounter (A or B - specific to category) OR sequela.

EXCLUDES 1 Not coded here   *EXCLUDES 2* Not included here   **N** Newborn Age: 0   **P** Pediatric Age: 0-17   **M** Maternity Age: 12-55   **A** Adult Age: 15-124

Chapter 19. Injury, Poisoning, and Certain Other Consequences of External Causes

2 ✓7ᵗʰ **T40.902** **Poisoning by unspecified** HCC ▽
psychodysleptics [hallucinogens],
intentional self-harm

✓7ᵗʰ **T40.903** **Poisoning by unspecified** ▽
psychodysleptics [hallucinogens],
assault

✓7ᵗʰ **T40.904** **Poisoning by unspecified** ▽
psychodysleptics [hallucinogens],
undetermined

✓7ᵗʰ **T40.905** Adverse effect of unspecified ▽
psychodysleptics [hallucinogens]

✓7ᵗʰ **T40.906** Underdosing of unspecified ▽
psychodysleptics

✓6ᵗʰ **T40.99** **Poisoning by, adverse effect of and underdosing of**
other psychodysleptics [hallucinogens]

✓7ᵗʰ **T40.991** **Poisoning by other psychodysleptics**
[hallucinogens], accidental
(unintentional)
Poisoning by other psychodysleptics
[hallucinogens] NOS

2 ✓7ᵗʰ **T40.992** **Poisoning by other psychodysleptics** HCC
[hallucinogens], intentional self-harm

✓7ᵗʰ **T40.993** **Poisoning by other psychodysleptics**
[hallucinogens], assault

✓7ᵗʰ **T40.994** **Poisoning by other psychodysleptics**
[hallucinogens], undetermined

✓7ᵗʰ **T40.995** Adverse effect of other psychodysleptics
[hallucinogens]

✓7ᵗʰ **T40.996** Underdosing of other psychodysleptics

✓4ᵗʰ **T41** **Poisoning by, adverse effect of and underdosing of anesthetics**
and therapeutic gases

EXCLUDES 1   *benzodiazepines (T42.4-)*
cocaine (T40.5-)
complications of anesthesia during labor and delivery (O74.-)
complications of anesthesia during pregnancy (O29.-)
complications of anesthesia during the puerperium (O89.-)
opioids (T40.0-T40.2-)

> The appropriate 7th character is to be added to each code from
> category T41.
> A   initial encounter
> D   subsequent encounter
> S   sequela

✓5ᵗʰ **T41.0** **Poisoning by, adverse effect of and underdosing of inhaled**
anesthetics

EXCLUDES 1   *oxygen (T41.5-)*

✓6ᵗʰ **T41.0X** **Poisoning by, adverse effect of and underdosing of**
inhaled anesthetics

✓7ᵗʰ **T41.0X1** **Poisoning by inhaled anesthetics,**
accidental (unintentional)
Poisoning by inhaled anesthetics NOS

2 ✓7ᵗʰ **T41.0X2** **Poisoning by inhaled anesthetics,** HCC
intentional self-harm

✓7ᵗʰ **T41.0X3** **Poisoning by inhaled anesthetics, assault**

✓7ᵗʰ **T41.0X4** **Poisoning by inhaled anesthetics,**
undetermined

✓7ᵗʰ **T41.0X5** Adverse effect of inhaled anesthetics

✓7ᵗʰ **T41.0X6** Underdosing of inhaled anesthetics

✓5ᵗʰ **T41.1** **Poisoning by, adverse effect of and underdosing of**
intravenous anesthetics
Poisoning by, adverse effect of and underdosing of
thiobarbiturates

✓6ᵗʰ **T41.1X** **Poisoning by, adverse effect of and underdosing of**
intravenous anesthetics

✓7ᵗʰ **T41.1X1** **Poisoning by intravenous anesthetics,**
accidental (unintentional)
Poisoning by intravenous anesthetics NOS

2 ✓7ᵗʰ **T41.1X2** **Poisoning by intravenous anesthetics,** HCC
intentional self-harm

✓7ᵗʰ **T41.1X3** **Poisoning by intravenous anesthetics,**
assault

✓7ᵗʰ **T41.1X4** **Poisoning by intravenous anesthetics,**
undetermined

✓7ᵗʰ **T41.1X5** Adverse effect of intravenous anesthetics

✓7ᵗʰ **T41.1X6** Underdosing of intravenous anesthetics

✓5ᵗʰ **T41.2** **Poisoning by, adverse effect of and underdosing of other and**
unspecified general anesthetics

✓6ᵗʰ **T41.20** **Poisoning by, adverse effect of and underdosing of**
unspecified general anesthetics

✓7ᵗʰ **T41.201** **Poisoning by unspecified general** ▽
anesthetics, accidental (unintentional)
Poisoning by general anesthetics NOS

2 ✓7ᵗʰ **T41.202** **Poisoning by unspecified general** HCC ▽
anesthetics, intentional self-harm

✓7ᵗʰ **T41.203** **Poisoning by unspecified general** ▽
anesthetics, assault

✓7ᵗʰ **T41.204** **Poisoning by unspecified general** ▽
anesthetics, undetermined

✓7ᵗʰ **T41.205** Adverse effect of unspecified general ▽
anesthetics

✓7ᵗʰ **T41.206** Underdosing of unspecified general ▽
anesthetics

✓6ᵗʰ **T41.29** **Poisoning by, adverse effect of and underdosing of**
other general anesthetics

✓7ᵗʰ **T41.291** **Poisoning by other general anesthetics,**
accidental (unintentional)
Poisoning by other general anesthetics
NOS

2 ✓7ᵗʰ **T41.292** **Poisoning by other general** HCC
anesthetics, intentional self-harm

✓7ᵗʰ **T41.293** **Poisoning by other general**
anesthetics, assault

✓7ᵗʰ **T41.294** **Poisoning by other general**
anesthetics, undetermined

✓7ᵗʰ **T41.295** Adverse effect of other general
anesthetics

✓7ᵗʰ **T41.296** Underdosing of other general anesthetics

✓5ᵗʰ **T41.3** **Poisoning by, adverse effect of and underdosing of local**
anesthetics
Cocaine (topical)

EXCLUDES 2   *poisoning by cocaine used as a central nervous system*
stimulant (T40.5X1-T40.5X4)

✓6ᵗʰ **T41.3X** **Poisoning by, adverse effect of and underdosing of**
local anesthetics

✓7ᵗʰ **T41.3X1** **Poisoning by local anesthetics, accidental**
(unintentional)
Poisoning by local anesthetics NOS

2 ✓7ᵗʰ **T41.3X2** **Poisoning by local anesthetics,** HCC
intentional self-harm

✓7ᵗʰ **T41.3X3** **Poisoning by local anesthetics, assault**

✓7ᵗʰ **T41.3X4** **Poisoning by local anesthetics,**
undetermined

✓7ᵗʰ **T41.3X5** Adverse effect of local anesthetics

✓7ᵗʰ **T41.3X6** Underdosing of local anesthetics

✓5ᵗʰ **T41.4** **Poisoning by, adverse effect of and underdosing of**
unspecified anesthetic

✓x7ᵗʰ **T41.41** **Poisoning by unspecified anesthetic, accidental** ▽
(unintentional)
Poisoning by anesthetic NOS

2 ✓x7ᵗʰ **T41.42** **Poisoning by unspecified anesthetic,** HCC ▽
intentional self-harm

✓x7ᵗʰ **T41.43** **Poisoning by unspecified anesthetic, assault** ▽

✓x7ᵗʰ **T41.44** **Poisoning by unspecified anesthetic,** ▽
undetermined

✓x7ᵗʰ **T41.45** Adverse effect of unspecified anesthetic ▽

✓x7ᵗʰ **T41.46** Underdosing of unspecified anesthetics ▽

✓5ᵗʰ **T41.5** **Poisoning by, adverse effect of and underdosing of**
therapeutic gases

✓6ᵗʰ **T41.5X** **Poisoning by, adverse effect of and underdosing of**
therapeutic gases

✓7ᵗʰ **T41.5X1** **Poisoning by therapeutic gases,**
accidental (unintentional)
Poisoning by therapeutic gases NOS

2 ✓7ᵗʰ **T41.5X2** **Poisoning by therapeutic gases,** HCC
intentional self-harm

✓7ᵗʰ **T41.5X3** **Poisoning by therapeutic gases, assault**

✓7ᵗʰ **T41.5X4** **Poisoning by therapeutic gases,**
undetermined

✓7ᵗʰ **T41.5X5** Adverse effect of therapeutic gases

---

2   HCC with 7th character indicating initial encounter (A or B - specific to category) OR sequela.

☑ Additional Character Req   ✓x7ᵗʰ Placeholder Alert   Manifestation   HCC CMS-HCC Condition   ▽ Unspecified Code   ►◄ Revised Text   ● New Code   ▲ Revised Code Title

✓7th **T41.5X6** Underdosing of therapeutic gases

✓4th **T42** **Poisoning by, adverse effect of and underdosing of antiepileptic, sedative- hypnotic and antiparkinsonism drugs**
> *EXCLUDES 2*   *drug dependence and related mental and behavioral disorders due to psychoactive substance use (F10.- -F19.-)*

> The appropriate 7th character is to be added to each code from category T42.
> A   initial encounter
> D   subsequent encounter
> S   sequela

✓5th **T42.0** **Poisoning by, adverse effect of and underdosing of hydantoin derivatives**

  ✓6th **T42.0X** **Poisoning by, adverse effect of and underdosing of hydantoin derivatives**

    ✓7th **T42.0X1** **Poisoning by hydantoin derivatives, accidental (unintentional)**
Poisoning by hydantoin derivatives NOS

    2 ✓7th **T42.0X2** **Poisoning by hydantoin derivatives, intentional self-harm** HCC

    ✓7th **T42.0X3** **Poisoning by hydantoin derivatives, assault**

    ✓7th **T42.0X4** **Poisoning by hydantoin derivatives, undetermined**

    ✓7th **T42.0X5** **Adverse effect of hydantoin derivatives**

    ✓7th **T42.0X6** **Underdosing of hydantoin derivatives**

✓5th **T42.1** **Poisoning by, adverse effect of and underdosing of iminostilbenes**
Poisoning by, adverse effect of and underdosing of carbamazepine

  ✓6th **T42.1X** **Poisoning by, adverse effect of and underdosing of iminostilbenes**

    ✓7th **T42.1X1** **Poisoning by iminostilbenes, accidental (unintentional)**
Poisoning by iminostilbenes NOS

    2 ✓7th **T42.1X2** **Poisoning by iminostilbenes, intentional self-harm** HCC

    ✓7th **T42.1X3** **Poisoning by iminostilbenes, assault**

    ✓7th **T42.1X4** **Poisoning by iminostilbenes, undetermined**

    ✓7th **T42.1X5** **Adverse effect of iminostilbenes**

    ✓7th **T42.1X6** **Underdosing of iminostilbenes**

✓5th **T42.2** **Poisoning by, adverse effect of and underdosing of succinimides and oxazolidinediones**

  ✓6th **T42.2X** **Poisoning by, adverse effect of and underdosing of succinimides and oxazolidinediones**

    ✓7th **T42.2X1** **Poisoning by succinimides and oxazolidinediones, accidental (unintentional)**
Poisoning by succinimides and oxazolidinediones NOS

    2 ✓7th **T42.2X2** **Poisoning by succinimides and oxazolidinediones, intentional self-harm** HCC

    ✓7th **T42.2X3** **Poisoning by succinimides and oxazolidinediones, assault**

    ✓7th **T42.2X4** **Poisoning by succinimides and oxazolidinediones, undetermined**

    ✓7th **T42.2X5** **Adverse effect of succinimides and oxazolidinediones**

    ✓7th **T42.2X6** **Underdosing of succinimides and oxazolidinediones**

✓5th **T42.3** **Poisoning by, adverse effect of and underdosing of barbiturates**
> *EXCLUDES 1*   *poisoning by, adverse effect of and underdosing of thiobarbiturates (T41.1-)*

  ✓6th **T42.3X** **Poisoning by, adverse effect of and underdosing of barbiturates**

    ✓7th **T42.3X1** **Poisoning by barbiturates, accidental (unintentional)**
Poisoning by barbiturates NOS

    2 ✓7th **T42.3X2** **Poisoning by barbiturates, intentional self-harm** HCC

    ✓7th **T42.3X3** **Poisoning by barbiturates, assault**

    ✓7th **T42.3X4** **Poisoning by barbiturates, undetermined**

    ✓7th **T42.3X5** **Adverse effect of barbiturates**

✓7th **T42.3X6** Underdosing of barbiturates

✓5th **T42.4** **Poisoning by, adverse effect of and underdosing of benzodiazepines**

  ✓6th **T42.4X** **Poisoning by, adverse effect of and underdosing of benzodiazepines**

    ✓7th **T42.4X1** **Poisoning by benzodiazepines, accidental (unintentional)**
Poisoning by benzodiazepines NOS

    2 ✓7th **T42.4X2** **Poisoning by benzodiazepines, intentional self-harm** HCC

    ✓7th **T42.4X3** **Poisoning by benzodiazepines, assault**

    ✓7th **T42.4X4** **Poisoning by benzodiazepines, undetermined**

    ✓7th **T42.4X5** **Adverse effect of benzodiazepines**

    ✓7th **T42.4X6** **Underdosing of benzodiazepines**

✓5th **T42.5** **Poisoning by, adverse effect of and underdosing of mixed antiepileptics**

  ✓6th **T42.5X** **Poisoning by, adverse effect of and underdosing of antiepileptics**

    ✓7th **T42.5X1** **Poisoning by mixed antiepileptics, accidental (unintentional)**
Poisoning by mixed antiepileptics NOS

    2 ✓7th **T42.5X2** **Poisoning by mixed antiepileptics, intentional self-harm** HCC

    ✓7th **T42.5X3** **Poisoning by mixed antiepileptics, assault**

    ✓7th **T42.5X4** **Poisoning by mixed antiepileptics, undetermined**

    ✓7th **T42.5X5** **Adverse effect of mixed antiepileptics**

    ✓7th **T42.5X6** **Underdosing of mixed antiepileptics**

✓5th **T42.6** **Poisoning by, adverse effect of and underdosing of other antiepileptic and sedative-hypnotic drugs**
Poisoning by, adverse effect of and underdosing of methaqualone
Poisoning by, adverse effect of and underdosing of valproic acid
> *EXCLUDES 1*   *poisoning by, adverse effect of and underdosing of carbamazepine (T42.1-)*

  ✓6th **T42.6X** **Poisoning by, adverse effect of and underdosing of other antiepileptic and sedative-hypnotic drugs**

    ✓7th **T42.6X1** **Poisoning by other antiepileptic and sedative-hypnotic drugs, accidental (unintentional)**
Poisoning by other antiepileptic and sedative-hypnotic drugs NOS

    2 ✓7th **T42.6X2** **Poisoning by other antiepileptic and sedative-hypnotic drugs, intentional self-harm** HCC

    ✓7th **T42.6X3** **Poisoning by other antiepileptic and sedative-hypnotic drugs, assault**

    ✓7th **T42.6X4** **Poisoning by other antiepileptic and sedative-hypnotic drugs, undetermined**

    ✓7th **T42.6X5** **Adverse effect of other antiepileptic and sedative-hypnotic drugs**

    ✓7th **T42.6X6** **Underdosing of other antiepileptic and sedative-hypnotic drugs**

✓5th **T42.7** **Poisoning by, adverse effect of and underdosing of unspecified antiepileptic and sedative-hypnotic drugs**

  ✓x7th **T42.71** **Poisoning by unspecified antiepileptic and sedative-hypnotic drugs, accidental (unintentional)** ▽
Poisoning by antiepileptic and sedative-hypnotic drugs NOS

  2 ✓x7th **T42.72** **Poisoning by unspecified antiepileptic and sedative-hypnotic drugs, intentional self-harm** HCC ▽

  ✓x7th **T42.73** **Poisoning by unspecified antiepileptic and sedative-hypnotic drugs, assault** ▽

  ✓x7th **T42.74** **Poisoning by unspecified antiepileptic and sedative-hypnotic drugs, undetermined** ▽

  ✓x7th **T42.75** **Adverse effect of unspecified antiepileptic and sedative-hypnotic drugs** ▽

  ✓x7th **T42.76** **Underdosing of unspecified antiepileptic and sedative-hypnotic drugs** ▽

---
2   HCC with 7th character indicating initial encounter (A or B - specific to category) OR sequela.

EXCLUDES 1 Not coded here   *EXCLUDES 2* Not included here   N Newborn Age: 0   P Pediatric Age: 0-17   M Maternity Age: 12-55   A Adult Age: 15-124

☑5ᵗʰ **T42.8** **Poisoning by, adverse effect of and underdosing of antiparkinsonism drugs and other central muscle-tone depressants**
Poisoning by, adverse effect of and underdosing of amantadine

    ☑6ᵗʰ **T42.8X** **Poisoning by, adverse effect of and underdosing of antiparkinsonism drugs and other central muscle-tone depressants**

       ☑7ᵗʰ **T42.8X1** **Poisoning by antiparkinsonism drugs and other central muscle-tone depressants, accidental (unintentional)**
Poisoning by antiparkinsonism drugs and other central muscle-tone depressants NOS

       2 ☑7ᵗʰ **T42.8X2** **Poisoning by antiparkinsonism drugs** HCC **and other central muscle-tone depressants, intentional self-harm**

       ☑7ᵗʰ **T42.8X3** **Poisoning by antiparkinsonism drugs and other central muscle-tone depressants, assault**

       ☑7ᵗʰ **T42.8X4** **Poisoning by antiparkinsonism drugs and other central muscle-tone depressants, undetermined**

       ☑7ᵗʰ **T42.8X5** **Adverse effect of antiparkinsonism drugs and other central muscle-tone depressants**

       ☑7ᵗʰ **T42.8X6** **Underdosing of antiparkinsonism drugs and other central muscle-tone depressants**

☑4ᵗʰ **T43** **Poisoning by, adverse effect of and underdosing of psychotropic drugs, not elsewhere classified**
EXCLUDES 1   *appetite depressants (T50.5-)*
     barbiturates (T42.3-)
     benzodiazepines (T42.4-)
     methaqualone (T42.6-)
     psychodysleptics [hallucinogens] (T40.7-T40.9-)
EXCLUDES 2   *drug dependence and related mental and behavioral disorders due to psychoactive substance use (F10.- -F19.-)*

> The appropriate 7th character is to be added to each code from category T43.
> A   initial encounter
> D   subsequent encounter
> S   sequela

☑5ᵗʰ **T43.0** **Poisoning by, adverse effect of and underdosing of tricyclic and tetracyclic antidepressants**

    ☑6ᵗʰ **T43.01** **Poisoning by, adverse effect of and underdosing of tricyclic antidepressants**

       ☑7ᵗʰ **T43.011** **Poisoning by tricyclic antidepressants, accidental (unintentional)**
Poisoning by tricyclic antidepressants NOS

       2 ☑7ᵗʰ **T43.012** **Poisoning by tricyclic antidepressants,** HCC **intentional self-harm**

       ☑7ᵗʰ **T43.013** **Poisoning by tricyclic antidepressants, assault**

       ☑7ᵗʰ **T43.014** **Poisoning by tricyclic antidepressants, undetermined**

       ☑7ᵗʰ **T43.015** **Adverse effect of tricyclic antidepressants**

       ☑7ᵗʰ **T43.016** **Underdosing of tricyclic antidepressants**

    ☑6ᵗʰ **T43.02** **Poisoning by, adverse effect of and underdosing of tetracyclic antidepressants**

       ☑7ᵗʰ **T43.021** **Poisoning by tetracyclic antidepressants, accidental (unintentional)**
Poisoning by tetracyclic antidepressants NOS

       2 ☑7ᵗʰ **T43.022** **Poisoning by tetracyclic** HCC **antidepressants, intentional self-harm**

       ☑7ᵗʰ **T43.023** **Poisoning by tetracyclic antidepressants, assault**

       ☑7ᵗʰ **T43.024** **Poisoning by tetracyclic antidepressants, undetermined**

       ☑7ᵗʰ **T43.025** **Adverse effect of tetracyclic antidepressants**

       ☑7ᵗʰ **T43.026** **Underdosing of tetracyclic antidepressants**

☑5ᵗʰ **T43.1** **Poisoning by, adverse effect of and underdosing of monoamine-oxidase-inhibitor antidepressants**

    ☑6ᵗʰ **T43.1X** **Poisoning by, adverse effect of and underdosing of monoamine-oxidase-inhibitor antidepressants**

       ☑7ᵗʰ **T43.1X1** **Poisoning by monoamine-oxidase-inhibitor antidepressants, accidental (unintentional)**
Poisoning by monoamine-oxidase-inhibitor antidepressants NOS

       2 ☑7ᵗʰ **T43.1X2** **Poisoning by monoamine-oxidase-** HCC **inhibitor antidepressants, intentional self-harm**

       ☑7ᵗʰ **T43.1X3** **Poisoning by monoamine-oxidase-inhibitor antidepressants, assault**

       ☑7ᵗʰ **T43.1X4** **Poisoning by monoamine-oxidase-inhibitor antidepressants, undetermined**

       ☑7ᵗʰ **T43.1X5** **Adverse effect of monoamine-oxidase-inhibitor antidepressants**

       ☑7ᵗʰ **T43.1X6** **Underdosing of monoamine-oxidase-inhibitor antidepressants**

☑5ᵗʰ **T43.2** **Poisoning by, adverse effect of and underdosing of other and unspecified antidepressants**

    ☑6ᵗʰ **T43.20** **Poisoning by, adverse effect of and underdosing of unspecified antidepressants**

       ☑7ᵗʰ **T43.201** **Poisoning by unspecified anti-** ▽ **depressants, accidental (unintentional)**
Poisoning by antidepressants NOS

       2 ☑7ᵗʰ **T43.202** **Poisoning by unspecified anti-** HCC ▽ **depressants, intentional self-harm**

       ☑7ᵗʰ **T43.203** **Poisoning by unspecified anti-** ▽ **depressants, assault**

       ☑7ᵗʰ **T43.204** **Poisoning by unspecified anti-** ▽ **depressants, undetermined**

       ☑7ᵗʰ **T43.205** **Adverse effect of unspecified** ▽ **antidepressants**
▶Antidepressant discontinuation syndrome◀

       ☑7ᵗʰ **T43.206** **Underdosing of unspecified** ▽ **antidepressants**

    ☑6ᵗʰ **T43.21** **Poisoning by, adverse effect of and underdosing of selective serotonin and norepinephrine reuptake inhibitors**
Poisoning by, adverse effect of and underdosing of SSNRI antidepressants

       ☑7ᵗʰ **T43.211** **Poisoning by selective serotonin and norepinephrine reuptake inhibitors, accidental (unintentional)**

       2 ☑7ᵗʰ **T43.212** **Poisoning by selective serotonin and** HCC **norepinephrine reuptake inhibitors, intentional self-harm**

       ☑7ᵗʰ **T43.213** **Poisoning by selective serotonin and norepinephrine reuptake inhibitors, assault**

       ☑7ᵗʰ **T43.214** **Poisoning by selective serotonin and norepinephrine reuptake inhibitors, undetermined**

       ☑7ᵗʰ **T43.215** **Adverse effect of selective serotonin and norepinephrine reuptake inhibitors**

       ☑7ᵗʰ **T43.216** **Underdosing of selective serotonin and norepinephrine reuptake inhibitors**

    ☑6ᵗʰ **T43.22** **Poisoning by, adverse effect of and underdosing of selective serotonin reuptake inhibitors**
Poisoning by, adverse effect of and underdosing of SSRI antidepressants

       ☑7ᵗʰ **T43.221** **Poisoning by selective serotonin reuptake inhibitors, accidental (unintentional)**

       2 ☑7ᵗʰ **T43.222** **Poisoning by selective serotonin** HCC **reuptake inhibitors, intentional self-harm**

       ☑7ᵗʰ **T43.223** **Poisoning by selective serotonin reuptake inhibitors, assault**

       ☑7ᵗʰ **T43.224** **Poisoning by selective serotonin reuptake inhibitors, undetermined**

       ☑7ᵗʰ **T43.225** **Adverse effect of selective serotonin reuptake inhibitors**

       ☑7ᵗʰ **T43.226** **Underdosing of selective serotonin reuptake inhibitors**

---

2   HCC with 7th character indicating initial encounter (A or B - specific to category) OR sequela.

☑ Additional Character Req   ☑x7ᵗʰ Placeholder Alert   Manifestation   HCC CMS-HCC Condition   ▽ Unspecified Code   ▶◀ Revised Text   ● New Code   ▲ Revised Code Title

✓6ᵗʰ **T43.29** **Poisoning by, adverse effect of and underdosing of other antidepressants**

    ✓7ᵗʰ **T43.291** **Poisoning by other antidepressants, accidental (unintentional)**
         Poisoning by other antidepressants NOS

    2 ✓7ᵗʰ **T43.292** **Poisoning by other antidepressants, intentional self-harm** **HCC**

    ✓7ᵗʰ **T43.293** **Poisoning by other antidepressants, assault**

    ✓7ᵗʰ **T43.294** **Poisoning by other antidepressants, undetermined**

    ✓7ᵗʰ **T43.295** **Adverse effect of other antidepressants**

    ✓7ᵗʰ **T43.296** **Underdosing of other antidepressants**

✓5ᵗʰ **T43.3** **Poisoning by, adverse effect of and underdosing of phenothiazine antipsychotics and neuroleptics**

    ✓6ᵗʰ **T43.3X** **Poisoning by, adverse effect of and underdosing of phenothiazine antipsychotics and neuroleptics**

        ✓7ᵗʰ **T43.3X1** **Poisoning by phenothiazine antipsychotics and neuroleptics, accidental (unintentional)**
             Poisoning by phenothiazine antipsychotics and neuroleptics NOS

        2 ✓7ᵗʰ **T43.3X2** **Poisoning by phenothiazine antipsychotics and neuroleptics, intentional self-harm** **HCC**

        ✓7ᵗʰ **T43.3X3** **Poisoning by phenothiazine antipsychotics and neuroleptics, assault**

        ✓7ᵗʰ **T43.3X4** **Poisoning by phenothiazine antipsychotics and neuroleptics, undetermined**

        ✓7ᵗʰ **T43.3X5** **Adverse effect of phenothiazine antipsychotics and neuroleptics**

        ✓7ᵗʰ **T43.3X6** **Underdosing of phenothiazine antipsychotics and neuroleptics**

✓5ᵗʰ **T43.4** **Poisoning by, adverse effect of and underdosing of butyrophenone and thiothixene neuroleptics**

    ✓6ᵗʰ **T43.4X** **Poisoning by, adverse effect of and underdosing of butyrophenone and thiothixene neuroleptics**

        ✓7ᵗʰ **T43.4X1** **Poisoning by butyrophenone and thiothixene neuroleptics, accidental (unintentional)**
             Poisoning by butyrophenone and thiothixene neuroleptics NOS

        2 ✓7ᵗʰ **T43.4X2** **Poisoning by butyrophenone and thiothixene neuroleptics, intentional self-harm** **HCC**

        ✓7ᵗʰ **T43.4X3** **Poisoning by butyrophenone and thiothixene neuroleptics, assault**

        ✓7ᵗʰ **T43.4X4** **Poisoning by butyrophenone and thiothixene neuroleptics, undetermined**

        ✓7ᵗʰ **T43.4X5** **Adverse effect of butyrophenone and thiothixene neuroleptics**

        ✓7ᵗʰ **T43.4X6** **Underdosing of butyrophenone and thiothixene neuroleptics**

✓5ᵗʰ **T43.5** **Poisoning by, adverse effect of and underdosing of other and unspecified antipsychotics and neuroleptics**

    EXCLUDES 1   poisoning by, adverse effect of and underdosing of rauwolfia (T46.5-)

    ✓6ᵗʰ **T43.50** **Poisoning by, adverse effect of and underdosing of unspecified antipsychotics and neuroleptics**

        ✓7ᵗʰ **T43.501** **Poisoning by unspecified anti-psychotics and neuroleptics, accidental (unintentional)** ▽
             Poisoning by antipsychotics and neuroleptics NOS

        2 ✓7ᵗʰ **T43.502** **Poisoning by unspecified anti-psychotics and neuroleptics, intentional self-harm** **HCC** ▽

        ✓7ᵗʰ **T43.503** **Poisoning by unspecified anti-psychotics and neuroleptics, assault** ▽

        ✓7ᵗʰ **T43.504** **Poisoning by unspecified anti-psychotics and neuroleptics, undetermined** ▽

        ✓7ᵗʰ **T43.505** **Adverse effect of unspecified antipsychotics and neuroleptics** ▽

        ✓7ᵗʰ **T43.506** **Underdosing of unspecified antipsychotics and neuroleptics** ▽

    ✓6ᵗʰ **T43.59** **Poisoning by, adverse effect of and underdosing of other antipsychotics and neuroleptics**
         AHA: 2017, 1Q, 40

        ✓7ᵗʰ **T43.591** **Poisoning by other antipsychotics and neuroleptics, accidental (unintentional)**
             Poisoning by other antipsychotics and neuroleptics NOS

        2 ✓7ᵗʰ **T43.592** **Poisoning by other antipsychotics and neuroleptics, intentional self-harm** **HCC**

        ✓7ᵗʰ **T43.593** **Poisoning by other antipsychotics and neuroleptics, assault**

        ✓7ᵗʰ **T43.594** **Poisoning by other antipsychotics and neuroleptics, undetermined**

        ✓7ᵗʰ **T43.595** **Adverse effect of other antipsychotics and neuroleptics**

        ✓7ᵗʰ **T43.596** **Underdosing of other antipsychotics and neuroleptics**

✓5ᵗʰ **T43.6** **Poisoning by, adverse effect of and underdosing of psychostimulants**

    EXCLUDES 1   poisoning by, adverse effect of and underdosing of cocaine (T40.5-)

    ✓6ᵗʰ **T43.60** **Poisoning by, adverse effect of and underdosing of unspecified psychostimulant**

        ✓7ᵗʰ **T43.601** **Poisoning by unspecified psychostimulants, accidental (unintentional)** ▽
             Poisoning by psychostimulants NOS

        2 ✓7ᵗʰ **T43.602** **Poisoning by unspecified psychostimulants, intentional self-harm** **HCC** ▽

        ✓7ᵗʰ **T43.603** **Poisoning by unspecified psychostimulants, assault** ▽

        ✓7ᵗʰ **T43.604** **Poisoning by unspecified psychostimulants, undetermined** ▽

        ✓7ᵗʰ **T43.605** **Adverse effect of unspecified psychostimulants** ▽

        ✓7ᵗʰ **T43.606** **Underdosing of unspecified psychostimulants** ▽

    ✓6ᵗʰ **T43.61** **Poisoning by, adverse effect of and underdosing of caffeine**

        ✓7ᵗʰ **T43.611** **Poisoning by caffeine, accidental (unintentional)**
             Poisoning by caffeine NOS

        2 ✓7ᵗʰ **T43.612** **Poisoning by caffeine, intentional self-harm** **HCC**

        ✓7ᵗʰ **T43.613** **Poisoning by caffeine, assault**

        ✓7ᵗʰ **T43.614** **Poisoning by caffeine, undetermined**

        ✓7ᵗʰ **T43.615** **Adverse effect of caffeine**

        ✓7ᵗʰ **T43.616** **Underdosing of caffeine**

    ✓6ᵗʰ **T43.62** **Poisoning by, adverse effect of and underdosing of amphetamines**
         Poisoning by, adverse effect of and underdosing of methamphetamines

        ✓7ᵗʰ **T43.621** **Poisoning by amphetamines, accidental (unintentional)**
             Poisoning by amphetamines NOS

        2 ✓7ᵗʰ **T43.622** **Poisoning by amphetamines, intentional self-harm** **HCC**

        ✓7ᵗʰ **T43.623** **Poisoning by amphetamines, assault**

        ✓7ᵗʰ **T43.624** **Poisoning by amphetamines, undetermined**

        ✓7ᵗʰ **T43.625** **Adverse effect of amphetamines**

        ✓7ᵗʰ **T43.626** **Underdosing of amphetamines**

    ✓6ᵗʰ **T43.63** **Poisoning by, adverse effect of and underdosing of methylphenidate**

        ✓7ᵗʰ **T43.631** **Poisoning by methylphenidate, accidental (unintentional)**
             Poisoning by methylphenidate NOS

        2 ✓7ᵗʰ **T43.632** **Poisoning by methylphenidate, intentional self-harm** **HCC**

        ✓7ᵗʰ **T43.633** **Poisoning by methylphenidate, assault**

        ✓7ᵗʰ **T43.634** **Poisoning by methylphenidate, undetermined**

        ✓7ᵗʰ **T43.635** **Adverse effect of methylphenidate**

---

2   HCC with 7th character indicating initial encounter (A or B - specific to category) OR sequela.

EXCLUDES 1 Not coded here   **EXCLUDES 2** Not included here   N Newborn Age: 0   P Pediatric Age: 0-17   M Maternity Age: 12-55   A Adult Age: 15-124

1068   ICD-10-CM 2018

√7ᵗʰ **T43.636** Underdosing of methylphenidate

√6ᵗʰ **T43.69** Poisoning by, adverse effect of and underdosing of other psychostimulants

√7ᵗʰ **T43.691** Poisoning by other psychostimulants, accidental (unintentional)
Poisoning by other psychostimulants NOS

2 √7ᵗʰ **T43.692** Poisoning by other psychostimulants, intentional self-harm   HCC

√7ᵗʰ **T43.693** Poisoning by other psychostimulants, assault

√7ᵗʰ **T43.694** Poisoning by other psychostimulants, undetermined

√7ᵗʰ **T43.695** Adverse effect of other psychostimulants

√7ᵗʰ **T43.696** Underdosing of other psychostimulants

√5ᵗʰ **T43.8** Poisoning by, adverse effect of and underdosing of other psychotropic drugs

√6ᵗʰ **T43.8X** Poisoning by, adverse effect of and underdosing of other psychotropic drugs

√7ᵗʰ **T43.8X1** Poisoning by other psychotropic drugs, accidental (unintentional)
Poisoning by other psychotropic drugs NOS

2 √7ᵗʰ **T43.8X2** Poisoning by other psychotropic drugs, intentional self-harm   HCC

√7ᵗʰ **T43.8X3** Poisoning by other psychotropic drugs, assault

√7ᵗʰ **T43.8X4** Poisoning by other psychotropic drugs, undetermined

√7ᵗʰ **T43.8X5** Adverse effect of other psychotropic drugs

√7ᵗʰ **T43.8X6** Underdosing of other psychotropic drugs

√5ᵗʰ **T43.9** Poisoning by, adverse effect of and underdosing of unspecified psychotropic drug

√x7ᵗʰ **T43.91** Poisoning by unspecified psychotropic drug, accidental (unintentional) ▽
Poisoning by psychotropic drug NOS

2 √x7ᵗʰ **T43.92** Poisoning by unspecified psychotropic drug, intentional self-harm   HCC ▽

√x7ᵗʰ **T43.93** Poisoning by unspecified psychotropic drug, assault ▽

√x7ᵗʰ **T43.94** Poisoning by unspecified psychotropic drug, undetermined ▽

√x7ᵗʰ **T43.95** Adverse effect of unspecified psychotropic drug ▽

√x7ᵗʰ **T43.96** Underdosing of unspecified psychotropic drug ▽

√4ᵗʰ **T44** Poisoning by, adverse effect of and underdosing of drugs primarily affecting the autonomic nervous system

> The appropriate 7th character is to be added to each code from category T44.
> A   initial encounter
> D   subsequent encounter
> S   sequela

√5ᵗʰ **T44.0** Poisoning by, adverse effect of and underdosing of anticholinesterase agents

√6ᵗʰ **T44.0X** Poisoning by, adverse effect of and underdosing of anticholinesterase agents

√7ᵗʰ **T44.0X1** Poisoning by anticholinesterase agents, accidental (unintentional)
Poisoning by anticholinesterase agents NOS

2 √7ᵗʰ **T44.0X2** Poisoning by anticholinesterase agents, intentional self-harm   HCC

√7ᵗʰ **T44.0X3** Poisoning by anticholinesterase agents, assault

√7ᵗʰ **T44.0X4** Poisoning by anticholinesterase agents, undetermined

√7ᵗʰ **T44.0X5** Adverse effect of anticholinesterase agents

√7ᵗʰ **T44.0X6** Underdosing of anticholinesterase agents

√5ᵗʰ **T44.1** Poisoning by, adverse effect of and underdosing of other parasympathomimetics [cholinergics]

√6ᵗʰ **T44.1X** Poisoning by, adverse effect of and underdosing of other parasympathomimetics [cholinergics]

√7ᵗʰ **T44.1X1** Poisoning by other parasympathomimetics [cholinergics], accidental (unintentional)
Poisoning by other parasympathomimetics [cholinergics] NOS

2 √7ᵗʰ **T44.1X2** Poisoning by other parasympathomimetics [cholinergics], intentional self-harm   HCC

√7ᵗʰ **T44.1X3** Poisoning by other parasympathomimetics [cholinergics], assault

√7ᵗʰ **T44.1X4** Poisoning by other parasympathomimetics [cholinergics], undetermined

√7ᵗʰ **T44.1X5** Adverse effect of other parasympathomimetics [cholinergics]

√7ᵗʰ **T44.1X6** Underdosing of other parasympathomimetics

√5ᵗʰ **T44.2** Poisoning by, adverse effect of and underdosing of ganglionic blocking drugs

√6ᵗʰ **T44.2X** Poisoning by, adverse effect of and underdosing of ganglionic blocking drugs

√7ᵗʰ **T44.2X1** Poisoning by ganglionic blocking drugs, accidental (unintentional)
Poisoning by ganglionic blocking drugs NOS

2 √7ᵗʰ **T44.2X2** Poisoning by ganglionic blocking drugs, intentional self-harm   HCC

√7ᵗʰ **T44.2X3** Poisoning by ganglionic blocking drugs, assault

√7ᵗʰ **T44.2X4** Poisoning by ganglionic blocking drugs, undetermined

√7ᵗʰ **T44.2X5** Adverse effect of ganglionic blocking drugs

√7ᵗʰ **T44.2X6** Underdosing of ganglionic blocking drugs

√5ᵗʰ **T44.3** Poisoning by, adverse effect of and underdosing of other parasympatholytics [anticholinergics and antimuscarinics] and spasmolytics
Poisoning by, adverse effect of and underdosing of papaverine

√6ᵗʰ **T44.3X** Poisoning by, adverse effect of and underdosing of other parasympatholytics [anticholinergics and antimuscarinics] and spasmolytics

√7ᵗʰ **T44.3X1** Poisoning by other parasympatholytics [anticholinergics and antimuscarinics] and spasmolytics, accidental (unintentional)
Poisoning by other parasympatholytics [anticholinergics and antimuscarinics] and spasmolytics NOS

2 √7ᵗʰ **T44.3X2** Poisoning by other parasympatholytics [anticholinergics and antimuscarinics] and spasmolytics, intentional self-harm   HCC

√7ᵗʰ **T44.3X3** Poisoning by other parasympatholytics [anticholinergics and antimuscarinics] and spasmolytics, assault

√7ᵗʰ **T44.3X4** Poisoning by other parasympatholytics [anticholinergics and antimuscarinics] and spasmolytics, undetermined

√7ᵗʰ **T44.3X5** Adverse effect of other parasympatholytics [anticholinergics and antimuscarinics] and spasmolytics

√7ᵗʰ **T44.3X6** Underdosing of other parasympatholytics [anticholinergics and antimuscarinics] and spasmolytics

---

2   HCC with 7th character indicating initial encounter (A or B - specific to category) OR sequela.

☑ Additional Character Req   √x7ᵗʰ Placeholder Alert   Manifestation   HCC CMS-HCC Condition   ▽ Unspecified Code   ▶◀ Revised Text   ● New Code   ▲ Revised Code Title

Chapter 19. Injury, Poisoning, and Certain Other Consequences of External Causes

T44.4–T44.992

√5ᵗʰ **T44.4** **Poisoning by, adverse effect of and underdosing of predominantly alpha-adrenoreceptor agonists**
     Poisoning by, adverse effect of and underdosing of metaraminol

√6ᵗʰ **T44.4X** **Poisoning by, adverse effect of and underdosing of predominantly alpha-adrenoreceptor agonists**

√7ᵗʰ **T44.4X1** **Poisoning by predominantly alpha-adrenoreceptor agonists, accidental (unintentional)**
     Poisoning by predominantly alpha-adrenoreceptor agonists NOS

2 √7ᵗʰ **T44.4X2** **Poisoning by predominantly alpha-adrenoreceptor agonists, intentional self-harm**   HCC

√7ᵗʰ **T44.4X3** **Poisoning by predominantly alpha-adrenoreceptor agonists, assault**

√7ᵗʰ **T44.4X4** **Poisoning by predominantly alpha-adrenoreceptor agonists, undetermined**

√7ᵗʰ **T44.4X5** **Adverse effect of predominantly alpha-adrenoreceptor agonists**

√7ᵗʰ **T44.4X6** **Underdosing of predominantly alpha-adrenoreceptor agonists**

√5ᵗʰ **T44.5** **Poisoning by, adverse effect of and underdosing of predominantly beta-adrenoreceptor agonists**
     EXCLUDES 1   poisoning by, adverse effect of and underdosing of beta-adrenoreceptor agonists used in asthma therapy (T48.6-)

√6ᵗʰ **T44.5X** **Poisoning by, adverse effect of and underdosing of predominantly beta-adrenoreceptor agonists**

√7ᵗʰ **T44.5X1** **Poisoning by predominantly beta-adrenoreceptor agonists, accidental (unintentional)**
     Poisoning by predominantly beta-adrenoreceptor agonists NOS

2 √7ᵗʰ **T44.5X2** **Poisoning by predominantly beta-adrenoreceptor agonists, intentional self-harm**   HCC

√7ᵗʰ **T44.5X3** **Poisoning by predominantly beta-adrenoreceptor agonists, assault**

√7ᵗʰ **T44.5X4** **Poisoning by predominantly beta-adrenoreceptor agonists, undetermined**

√7ᵗʰ **T44.5X5** **Adverse effect of predominantly beta-adrenoreceptor agonists**

√7ᵗʰ **T44.5X6** **Underdosing of predominantly beta-adrenoreceptor agonists**

√5ᵗʰ **T44.6** **Poisoning by, adverse effect of and underdosing of alpha-adrenoreceptor antagonists**
     EXCLUDES 1   poisoning by, adverse effect of and underdosing of ergot alkaloids (T48.0)

√6ᵗʰ **T44.6X** **Poisoning by, adverse effect of and underdosing of alpha-adrenoreceptor antagonists**

√7ᵗʰ **T44.6X1** **Poisoning by alpha-adrenoreceptor antagonists, accidental (unintentional)**
     Poisoning by alpha-adrenoreceptor antagonists NOS

2 √7ᵗʰ **T44.6X2** **Poisoning by alpha-adrenoreceptor antagonists, intentional self-harm**   HCC

√7ᵗʰ **T44.6X3** **Poisoning by alpha-adrenoreceptor antagonists, assault**

√7ᵗʰ **T44.6X4** **Poisoning by alpha-adrenoreceptor antagonists, undetermined**

√7ᵗʰ **T44.6X5** **Adverse effect of alpha-adrenoreceptor antagonists**

√7ᵗʰ **T44.6X6** **Underdosing of alpha-adrenoreceptor antagonists**

√5ᵗʰ **T44.7** **Poisoning by, adverse effect of and underdosing of beta-adrenoreceptor antagonists**

√6ᵗʰ **T44.7X** **Poisoning by, adverse effect of and underdosing of beta-adrenoreceptor antagonists**

√7ᵗʰ **T44.7X1** **Poisoning by beta-adrenoreceptor antagonists, accidental (unintentional)**
     Poisoning by beta-adrenoreceptor antagonists NOS

2 √7ᵗʰ **T44.7X2** **Poisoning by beta-adrenoreceptor antagonists, intentional self-harm**   HCC

√7ᵗʰ **T44.7X3** **Poisoning by beta-adrenoreceptor antagonists, assault**

√7ᵗʰ **T44.7X4** **Poisoning by beta-adrenoreceptor antagonists, undetermined**

√7ᵗʰ **T44.7X5** **Adverse effect of beta-adrenoreceptor antagonists**

√7ᵗʰ **T44.7X6** **Underdosing of beta-adrenoreceptor antagonists**

√5ᵗʰ **T44.8** **Poisoning by, adverse effect of and underdosing of centrally-acting and adrenergic-neuron- blocking agents**
     EXCLUDES 1   poisoning by, adverse effect of and underdosing of clonidine (T46.5)
          poisoning by, adverse effect of and underdosing of guanethidine (T46.5)

√6ᵗʰ **T44.8X** **Poisoning by, adverse effect of and underdosing of centrally-acting and adrenergic-neuron-blocking agents**

√7ᵗʰ **T44.8X1** **Poisoning by centrally-acting and adrenergic-neuron-blocking agents, accidental (unintentional)**
     Poisoning by centrally-acting and adrenergic-neuron-blocking agents NOS

2 √7ᵗʰ **T44.8X2** **Poisoning by centrally-acting and adrenergic-neuron-blocking agents, intentional self-harm**   HCC

√7ᵗʰ **T44.8X3** **Poisoning by centrally-acting and adrenergic-neuron-blocking agents, assault**

√7ᵗʰ **T44.8X4** **Poisoning by centrally-acting and adrenergic-neuron-blocking agents, undetermined**

√7ᵗʰ **T44.8X5** **Adverse effect of centrally-acting and adrenergic-neuron-blocking agents**

√7ᵗʰ **T44.8X6** **Underdosing of centrally-acting and adrenergic-neuron-blocking agents**

√5ᵗʰ **T44.9** **Poisoning by, adverse effect of and underdosing of other and unspecified drugs primarily affecting the autonomic nervous system**
     Poisoning by, adverse effect of and underdosing of drug stimulating both alpha and beta-adrenoreceptors

√6ᵗʰ **T44.90** **Poisoning by, adverse effect of and underdosing of unspecified drugs primarily affecting the autonomic nervous system**

√7ᵗʰ **T44.901** **Poisoning by unspecified drugs primarily affecting the autonomic nervous system, accidental (unintentional)** ▽
     Poisoning by unspecified drugs primarily affecting the autonomic nervous system NOS

2 √7ᵗʰ **T44.902** **Poisoning by unspecified drugs primarily affecting the autonomic nervous system, intentional self-harm**   HCC ▽

√7ᵗʰ **T44.903** **Poisoning by unspecified drugs primarily affecting the autonomic nervous system, assault** ▽

√7ᵗʰ **T44.904** **Poisoning by unspecified drugs primarily affecting the autonomic nervous system, undetermined** ▽

√7ᵗʰ **T44.905** **Adverse effect of unspecified drugs primarily affecting the autonomic nervous system** ▽

√7ᵗʰ **T44.906** **Underdosing of unspecified drugs primarily affecting the autonomic nervous system** ▽

√6ᵗʰ **T44.99** **Poisoning by, adverse effect of and underdosing of other drugs primarily affecting the autonomic nervous system**

√7ᵗʰ **T44.991** **Poisoning by other drug primarily affecting the autonomic nervous system, accidental (unintentional)**
     Poisoning by other drugs primarily affecting the autonomic nervous system NOS

2 √7ᵗʰ **T44.992** **Poisoning by other drug primarily affecting the autonomic nervous system, intentional self-harm**   HCC

---

2   HCC with 7th character indicating initial encounter (A or B - specific to category) OR sequela.

EXCLUDES 1 Not coded here   EXCLUDES 2 Not included here   N Newborn Age: 0   P Pediatric Age: 0-17   M Maternity Age: 12-55   A Adult Age: 15-124

1070   ICD-10-CM 2018

✓7ᵗʰ **T44.993 Poisoning by other drug primarily affecting the autonomic nervous system, assault**

✓7ᵗʰ **T44.994 Poisoning by other drug primarily affecting the autonomic nervous system, undetermined**

✓7ᵗʰ **T44.995 Adverse effect of other drug primarily affecting the autonomic nervous system**

✓7ᵗʰ **T44.996 Underdosing of other drug primarily affecting the autonomic nervous system**

✓4ᵗʰ **T45 Poisoning by, adverse effect of and underdosing of primarily systemic and hematological agents, not elsewhere classified**

> The appropriate 7th character is to be added to each code from category T45.
> A   initial encounter
> D   subsequent encounter
> S   sequela

✓5ᵗʰ **T45.0 Poisoning by, adverse effect of and underdosing of antiallergic and antiemetic drugs**
> EXCLUDES 1   *poisoning by, adverse effect of and underdosing of phenothiazine-based neuroleptics (T43.3)*

✓6ᵗʰ **T45.0X Poisoning by, adverse effect of and underdosing of antiallergic and antiemetic drugs**

✓7ᵗʰ **T45.0X1 Poisoning by antiallergic and antiemetic drugs, accidental (unintentional)**
> Poisoning by antiallergic and antiemetic drugs NOS

2 ✓7ᵗʰ **T45.0X2 Poisoning by antiallergic and antie metic drugs, intentional self-harm** HCC

✓7ᵗʰ **T45.0X3 Poisoning by antiallergic and antiemetic drugs, assault**

✓7ᵗʰ **T45.0X4 Poisoning by antiallergic and antiemetic drugs, undetermined**

✓7ᵗʰ **T45.0X5 Adverse effect of antiallergic and antiemetic drugs**

✓7ᵗʰ **T45.0X6 Underdosing of antiallergic and antiemetic drugs**

✓5ᵗʰ **T45.1 Poisoning by, adverse effect of and underdosing of antineoplastic and immunosuppressive drugs**
> EXCLUDES 1   *poisoning by, adverse effect of and underdosing of tamoxifen (T38.6)*
> **AHA:** 2014, 4Q, 22

✓6ᵗʰ **T45.1X Poisoning by, adverse effect of and underdosing of antineoplastic and immunosuppressive drugs**

✓7ᵗʰ **T45.1X1 Poisoning by antineoplastic and immunosuppressive drugs, accidental (unintentional)**
> Poisoning by antineoplastic and immunosuppressive drugs NOS

2 ✓7ᵗʰ **T45.1X2 Poisoning by antineoplastic and immunosuppressive drugs, intentional self-harm** HCC

✓7ᵗʰ **T45.1X3 Poisoning by antineoplastic and immunosuppressive drugs, assault**

✓7ᵗʰ **T45.1X4 Poisoning by antineoplastic and immunosuppressive drugs, undetermined**

✓7ᵗʰ **T45.1X5 Adverse effect of antineoplastic and immunosuppressive drugs**

✓7ᵗʰ **T45.1X6 Underdosing of antineoplastic and immunosuppressive drugs**

✓5ᵗʰ **T45.2 Poisoning by, adverse effect of and underdosing of vitamins**
> EXCLUDES 2   *poisoning by, adverse effect of and underdosing of iron (T45.4)*
> *poisoning by, adverse effect of and underdosing of nicotinic acid (derivatives) (T46.7)*
> *poisoning by, adverse effect of and underdosing of vitamin K (T45.7)*

✓6ᵗʰ **T45.2X Poisoning by, adverse effect of and underdosing of vitamins**

✓7ᵗʰ **T45.2X1 Poisoning by vitamins, accidental (unintentional)**
> Poisoning by vitamins NOS

2 ✓7ᵗʰ **T45.2X2 Poisoning by vitamins, intentional self-harm** HCC

✓7ᵗʰ **T45.2X3 Poisoning by vitamins, assault**

✓7ᵗʰ **T45.2X4 Poisoning by vitamins, undetermined**

✓7ᵗʰ **T45.2X5 Adverse effect of vitamins**

✓7ᵗʰ **T45.2X6 Underdosing of vitamins**
> EXCLUDES 1   *vitamin deficiencies (E50-E56)*

✓5ᵗʰ **T45.3 Poisoning by, adverse effect of and underdosing of enzymes**

✓6ᵗʰ **T45.3X Poisoning by, adverse effect of and underdosing of enzymes**

✓7ᵗʰ **T45.3X1 Poisoning by enzymes, accidental (unintentional)**
> Poisoning by enzymes NOS

2 ✓7ᵗʰ **T45.3X2 Poisoning by enzymes, intentional self-harm** HCC

✓7ᵗʰ **T45.3X3 Poisoning by enzymes, assault**

✓7ᵗʰ **T45.3X4 Poisoning by enzymes, undetermined**

✓7ᵗʰ **T45.3X5 Adverse effect of enzymes**

✓7ᵗʰ **T45.3X6 Underdosing of enzymes**

✓5ᵗʰ **T45.4 Poisoning by, adverse effect of and underdosing of iron and its compounds**

✓6ᵗʰ **T45.4X Poisoning by, adverse effect of and underdosing of iron and its compounds**

✓7ᵗʰ **T45.4X1 Poisoning by iron and its compounds, accidental (unintentional)**
> Poisoning by iron and its compounds NOS

2 ✓7ᵗʰ **T45.4X2 Poisoning by iron and its compounds, intentional self-harm** HCC

✓7ᵗʰ **T45.4X3 Poisoning by iron and its compounds, assault**

✓7ᵗʰ **T45.4X4 Poisoning by iron and its compounds, undetermined**

✓7ᵗʰ **T45.4X5 Adverse effect of iron and its compounds**

✓7ᵗʰ **T45.4X6 Underdosing of iron and its compounds**
> EXCLUDES 1   *iron deficiency (E61.1)*

✓5ᵗʰ **T45.5 Poisoning by, adverse effect of and underdosing of anticoagulants and antithrombotic drugs**

✓6ᵗʰ **T45.51 Poisoning by, adverse effect of and underdosing of anticoagulants**

✓7ᵗʰ **T45.511 Poisoning by anticoagulants, accidental (unintentional)**
> Poisoning by anticoagulants NOS

2 ✓7ᵗʰ **T45.512 Poisoning by anticoagulants, intentional self-harm** HCC

✓7ᵗʰ **T45.513 Poisoning by anticoagulants, assault**

✓7ᵗʰ **T45.514 Poisoning by anticoagulants, undetermined**

✓7ᵗʰ **T45.515 Adverse effect of anticoagulants**
> **AHA:** 2016, 1Q, 14; 2013, 2Q, 34

✓7ᵗʰ **T45.516 Underdosing of anticoagulants**

✓6ᵗʰ **T45.52 Poisoning by, adverse effect of and underdosing of antithrombotic drugs**
> Poisoning by, adverse effect of and underdosing of antiplatelet drugs
> EXCLUDES 2   *poisoning by, adverse effect of and underdosing of aspirin (T39.01-)*
> *poisoning by, adverse effect of and underdosing of acetylsalicylic acid (T39.01-)*

✓7ᵗʰ **T45.521 Poisoning by antithrombotic drugs, accidental (unintentional)**
> Poisoning by antithrombotic drug NOS

2 ✓7ᵗʰ **T45.522 Poisoning by antithrombotic drugs, intentional self-harm** HCC

✓7ᵗʰ **T45.523 Poisoning by antithrombotic drugs, assault**

✓7ᵗʰ **T45.524 Poisoning by antithrombotic drugs, undetermined**

✓7ᵗʰ **T45.525 Adverse effect of antithrombotic drugs**
> **AHA:** 2016, 1Q, 15

✓7ᵗʰ **T45.526 Underdosing of antithrombotic drugs**

✓5ᵗʰ **T45.6 Poisoning by, adverse effect of and underdosing of fibrinolysis-affecting drugs**

✓6ᵗʰ **T45.60 Poisoning by, adverse effect of and underdosing of unspecified fibrinolysis-affecting drugs**

✓7ᵗʰ **T45.601 Poisoning by unspecified fibrinolysis-affecting drugs, accidental (unintentional)** ▽
> Poisoning by fibrinolysis-affecting drug NOS

---

2   HCC with 7th character indicating initial encounter (A or B - specific to category) OR sequela.

☑ Additional Character Req   ✓x7ᵗʰ Placeholder Alert   Manifestation   HCC CMS-HCC Condition   ▽ Unspecified Code   ►◄ Revised Text   ● New Code   ▲ Revised Code Title

ICD-10-CM 2018   **1071**

2 ✓7ᵗʰ **T45.602** **Poisoning by unspecified** HCC ▽
fibrinolysis-affecting drugs,
intentional self-harm

✓7ᵗʰ **T45.603** **Poisoning by unspecified fibrinolysis-** ▽
affecting drugs, assault

✓7ᵗʰ **T45.604** **Poisoning by unspecified fibrinolysis-** ▽
affecting drugs, undetermined

✓7ᵗʰ **T45.605** **Adverse effect of unspecified fibrino-** ▽
lysis- affecting drugs

✓7ᵗʰ **T45.606** **Underdosing of unspecified fibrino-** ▽
lysis- affecting drugs

✓6ᵗʰ **T45.61** **Poisoning by, adverse effect of and underdosing of**
thrombolytic drugs

✓7ᵗʰ **T45.611** **Poisoning by thrombolytic drug,**
accidental (unintentional)
Poisoning by thrombolytic drug NOS

2 ✓7ᵗʰ **T45.612** **Poisoning by thrombolytic drug,** HCC
intentional self-harm

✓7ᵗʰ **T45.613** **Poisoning by thrombolytic drug, assault**

✓7ᵗʰ **T45.614** **Poisoning by thrombolytic drug,**
undetermined

✓7ᵗʰ **T45.615** **Adverse effect of thrombolytic drugs**
AHA: 2017, 2Q, 9

✓7ᵗʰ **T45.616** **Underdosing of thrombolytic drugs**

✓6ᵗʰ **T45.62** **Poisoning by, adverse effect of and underdosing of**
hemostatic drugs

✓7ᵗʰ **T45.621** **Poisoning by hemostatic drug, accidental**
(unintentional)
Poisoning by hemostatic drug NOS

2 ✓7ᵗʰ **T45.622** **Poisoning by hemostatic drug,** HCC
intentional self-harm

✓7ᵗʰ **T45.623** **Poisoning by hemostatic drug, assault**

✓7ᵗʰ **T45.624** **Poisoning by hemostatic drug,**
undetermined

✓7ᵗʰ **T45.625** **Adverse effect of hemostatic drug**

✓7ᵗʰ **T45.626** **Underdosing of hemostatic drugs**

✓6ᵗʰ **T45.69** **Poisoning by, adverse effect of and underdosing of**
other fibrinolysis-affecting drugs

✓7ᵗʰ **T45.691** **Poisoning by other fibrinolysis-affecting**
drugs, accidental (unintentional)
Poisoning by other fibrinolysis-affecting
drug NOS

2 ✓7ᵗʰ **T45.692** **Poisoning by other fibrinolysis-** HCC
affecting drugs, intentional self-harm

✓7ᵗʰ **T45.693** **Poisoning by other fibrinolysis-affecting**
drugs, assault

✓7ᵗʰ **T45.694** **Poisoning by other fibrinolysis-affecting**
drugs, undetermined

✓7ᵗʰ **T45.695** **Adverse effect of other fibrinolysis-**
affecting drugs

✓7ᵗʰ **T45.696** **Underdosing of other fibrinolysis-**
affecting drugs

✓5ᵗʰ **T45.7** **Poisoning by, adverse effect of and underdosing of**
anticoagulant antagonists, vitamin K and other coagulants

✓6ᵗʰ **T45.7X** **Poisoning by, adverse effect of and underdosing of**
anticoagulant antagonists, vitamin K and other
coagulants

✓7ᵗʰ **T45.7X1** **Poisoning by anticoagulant antagonists,**
vitamin K and other coagulants,
accidental (unintentional)
Poisoning by anticoagulant antagonists,
vitamin K and other coagulants NOS

2 ✓7ᵗʰ **T45.7X2** **Poisoning by anticoagulant** HCC
antagonists, vitamin K and other
coagulants, intentional self-harm

✓7ᵗʰ **T45.7X3** **Poisoning by anticoagulant antagonists,**
vitamin K and other coagulants, assault

✓7ᵗʰ **T45.7X4** **Poisoning by anticoagulant antagonists,**
vitamin K and other coagulants,
undetermined

✓7ᵗʰ **T45.7X5** **Adverse effect of anticoagulant**
antagonists, vitamin K and other
coagulants

✓7ᵗʰ **T45.7X6** **Underdosing of anticoagulant antagonist,**
vitamin K and other coagulants
EXCLUDES 1 vitamin K deficiency (E56.1)

✓5ᵗʰ **T45.8** **Poisoning by, adverse effect of and underdosing of other**
primarily systemic and hematological agents
Poisoning by, adverse effect of and underdosing of liver
preparations and other antianemic agents
Poisoning by, adverse effect of and underdosing of natural
blood and blood products
Poisoning by, adverse effect of and underdosing of plasma
substitute
EXCLUDES 2 poisoning by, adverse effect of and underdosing of
immunoglobulin (T50.Z1)
poisoning by, adverse effect of and underdosing of iron
(T45.4)
transfusion reactions (T80.-)

✓6ᵗʰ **T45.8X** **Poisoning by, adverse effect of and underdosing of**
other primarily systemic and hematological agents

✓7ᵗʰ **T45.8X1** **Poisoning by other primarily systemic and**
hematological agents, accidental
(unintentional)
Poisoning by other primarily systemic and
hematological agents NOS

2 ✓7ᵗʰ **T45.8X2** **Poisoning by other primarily systemic** HCC
and hematological agents, intentional
self-harm

✓7ᵗʰ **T45.8X3** **Poisoning by other primarily systemic and**
hematological agents, assault

✓7ᵗʰ **T45.8X4** **Poisoning by other primarily systemic and**
hematological agents, undetermined

✓7ᵗʰ **T45.8X5** **Adverse effect of other primarily systemic**
and hematological agents

✓7ᵗʰ **T45.8X6** **Underdosing of other primarily systemic**
and hematological agents

✓5ᵗʰ **T45.9** **Poisoning by, adverse effect of and underdosing of**
unspecified primarily systemic and hematological agent

✓x7ᵗʰ **T45.91** **Poisoning by unspecified primarily systemic and** ▽
hematological agent, accidental (unintentional)
Poisoning by primarily systemic and hematological
agent NOS

2 ✓x7ᵗʰ **T45.92** **Poisoning by unspecified primarily systemic** HCC ▽
and hematological agent, intentional self-harm

✓x7ᵗʰ **T45.93** **Poisoning by unspecified primarily systemic and** ▽
hematological agent, assault

✓x7ᵗʰ **T45.94** **Poisoning by unspecified primarily systemic and** ▽
hematological agent, undetermined

✓x7ᵗʰ **T45.95** **Adverse effect of unspecified primarily systemic** ▽
and hematological agent

✓x7ᵗʰ **T45.96** **Underdosing of unspecified primarily systemic** ▽
and hematological agent

✓4ᵗʰ **T46** **Poisoning by, adverse effect of and underdosing of agents**
primarily affecting the cardiovascular system
EXCLUDES 1 poisoning by, adverse effect of and underdosing of metaraminol
(T44.4)

The appropriate 7th character is to be added to each code from
category T46.
A   initial encounter
D   subsequent encounter
S   sequela

✓5ᵗʰ **T46.0** **Poisoning by, adverse effect of and underdosing of cardiac-**
stimulant glycosides and drugs of similar action

✓6ᵗʰ **T46.0X** **Poisoning by, adverse effect of and underdosing of**
cardiac-stimulant glycosides and drugs of similar
action

✓7ᵗʰ **T46.0X1** **Poisoning by cardiac-stimulant**
glycosides and drugs of similar action,
accidental (unintentional)
Poisoning by cardiac-stimulant glycosides
and drugs of similar action NOS

2 ✓7ᵗʰ **T46.0X2** **Poisoning by cardiac-stimulant** HCC
glycosides and drugs of similar action,
intentional self-harm

✓7ᵗʰ **T46.0X3** **Poisoning by cardiac-stimulant**
glycosides and drugs of similar action,
assault

---

2   HCC with 7th character indicating initial encounter (A or B - specific to category) OR sequela.

EXCLUDES 1 Not coded here   *EXCLUDES 2* Not included here   N Newborn Age: 0   P Pediatric Age: 0-17   M Maternity Age: 12-55   A Adult Age: 15-124

1072   ICD-10-CM 2018

✓7th **T46.0X4** Poisoning by cardiac-stimulant glycosides and drugs of similar action, undetermined

✓7th **T46.0X5** Adverse effect of cardiac-stimulant glycosides and drugs of similar action

✓7th **T46.0X6** Underdosing of cardiac-stimulant glycosides and drugs of similar action

✓5th **T46.1** Poisoning by, adverse effect of and underdosing of calcium-channel blockers

✓6th **T46.1X** Poisoning by, adverse effect of and underdosing of calcium-channel blockers

✓7th **T46.1X1** Poisoning by calcium-channel blockers, accidental (unintentional)
Poisoning by calcium-channel blockers NOS

2 ✓7th **T46.1X2** Poisoning by calcium-channel blockers, intentional self-harm HCC

✓7th **T46.1X3** Poisoning by calcium-channel blockers, assault

✓7th **T46.1X4** Poisoning by calcium-channel blockers, undetermined

✓7th **T46.1X5** Adverse effect of calcium-channel blockers

✓7th **T46.1X6** Underdosing of calcium-channel blockers

✓5th **T46.2** Poisoning by, adverse effect of and underdosing of other antidysrhythmic drugs, not elsewhere classified
EXCLUDES 1 poisoning by, adverse effect of and underdosing of beta-adrenoreceptor antagonists (T44.7-)

✓6th **T46.2X** Poisoning by, adverse effect of and underdosing of other antidysrhythmic drugs

✓7th **T46.2X1** Poisoning by other antidysrhythmic drugs, accidental (unintentional)
Poisoning by other antidysrhythmic drugs NOS

2 ✓7th **T46.2X2** Poisoning by other antidysrhythmic drugs, intentional self-harm HCC

✓7th **T46.2X3** Poisoning by other antidysrhythmic drugs, assault

✓7th **T46.2X4** Poisoning by other antidysrhythmic drugs, undetermined

✓7th **T46.2X5** Adverse effect of other antidysrhythmic drugs

✓7th **T46.2X6** Underdosing of other antidysrhythmic drugs

✓5th **T46.3** Poisoning by, adverse effect of and underdosing of coronary vasodilators
Poisoning by, adverse effect of and underdosing of dipyridamole
EXCLUDES 1 poisoning by, adverse effect of and underdosing of calcium-channel blockers (T46.1)

✓6th **T46.3X** Poisoning by, adverse effect of and underdosing of coronary vasodilators

✓7th **T46.3X1** Poisoning by coronary vasodilators, accidental (unintentional)
Poisoning by coronary vasodilators NOS

2 ✓7th **T46.3X2** Poisoning by coronary vasodilators, intentional self-harm HCC

✓7th **T46.3X3** Poisoning by coronary vasodilators, assault

✓7th **T46.3X4** Poisoning by coronary vasodilators, undetermined

✓7th **T46.3X5** Adverse effect of coronary vasodilators

✓7th **T46.3X6** Underdosing of coronary vasodilators

✓5th **T46.4** Poisoning by, adverse effect of and underdosing of angiotensin-converting-enzyme inhibitors

✓6th **T46.4X** Poisoning by, adverse effect of and underdosing of angiotensin-converting-enzyme inhibitors

✓7th **T46.4X1** Poisoning by angiotensin-converting-enzyme inhibitors, accidental (unintentional)
Poisoning by angiotensin-converting-enzyme inhibitors NOS

2 ✓7th **T46.4X2** Poisoning by angiotensin-converting- enzyme inhibitors, intentional self-harm HCC

✓7th **T46.4X3** Poisoning by angiotensin-converting-enzyme inhibitors, assault

✓7th **T46.4X4** Poisoning by angiotensin-converting-enzyme inhibitors, undetermined

✓7th **T46.4X5** Adverse effect of angiotensin-converting-enzyme inhibitors

✓7th **T46.4X6** Underdosing of angiotensin-converting-enzyme inhibitors

✓5th **T46.5** Poisoning by, adverse effect of and underdosing of other antihypertensive drugs
EXCLUDES 2 poisoning by, adverse effect of and underdosing of beta-adrenoreceptor antagonists (T44.7)
poisoning by, adverse effect of and underdosing of calcium-channel blockers (T46.1)
poisoning by, adverse effect of and underdosing of diuretics (T50.0-T50.2)

✓6th **T46.5X** Poisoning by, adverse effect of and underdosing of other antihypertensive drugs

✓7th **T46.5X1** Poisoning by other antihypertensive drugs, accidental (unintentional)
Poisoning by other antihypertensive drugs NOS

2 ✓7th **T46.5X2** Poisoning by other antihypertensive drugs, intentional self-harm HCC

✓7th **T46.5X3** Poisoning by other antihypertensive drugs, assault

✓7th **T46.5X4** Poisoning by other antihypertensive drugs, undetermined

✓7th **T46.5X5** Adverse effect of other antihypertensive drugs

✓7th **T46.5X6** Underdosing of other antihypertensive drugs

✓5th **T46.6** Poisoning by, adverse effect of and underdosing of antihyperlipidemic and antiarteriosclerotic drugs

✓6th **T46.6X** Poisoning by, adverse effect of and underdosing of antihyperlipidemic and antiarteriosclerotic drugs

✓7th **T46.6X1** Poisoning by antihyperlipidemic and antiarteriosclerotic drugs, accidental (unintentional)
Poisoning by antihyperlipidemic and antiarteriosclerotic drugs NOS

2 ✓7th **T46.6X2** Poisoning by antihyperlipidemic and antiarteriosclerotic drugs, intentional self-harm HCC

✓7th **T46.6X3** Poisoning by antihyperlipidemic and antiarteriosclerotic drugs, assault

✓7th **T46.6X4** Poisoning by antihyperlipidemic and antiarteriosclerotic drugs, undetermined

✓7th **T46.6X5** Adverse effect of antihyperlipidemic and antiarteriosclerotic drugs

✓7th **T46.6X6** Underdosing of antihyperlipidemic and antiarteriosclerotic drugs

✓5th **T46.7** Poisoning by, adverse effect of and underdosing of peripheral vasodilators
Poisoning by, adverse effect of and underdosing of nicotinic acid (derivatives)
EXCLUDES 1 poisoning by, adverse effect of and underdosing of papaverine (T44.3)

✓6th **T46.7X** Poisoning by, adverse effect of and underdosing of peripheral vasodilators

✓7th **T46.7X1** Poisoning by peripheral vasodilators, accidental (unintentional)
Poisoning by peripheral vasodilators NOS

2 ✓7th **T46.7X2** Poisoning by peripheral vasodilators, intentional self-harm HCC

✓7th **T46.7X3** Poisoning by peripheral vasodilators, assault

✓7th **T46.7X4** Poisoning by peripheral vasodilators, undetermined

✓7th **T46.7X5** Adverse effect of peripheral vasodilators

✓7th **T46.7X6** Underdosing of peripheral vasodilators

---

2 HCC with 7th character indicating initial encounter (A or B - specific to category) OR sequela.

☑ Additional Character Req   ✓7th Placeholder Alert   Manifestation   HCC CMS-HCC Condition   ▽ Unspecified Code   ►◄ Revised Text   ● New Code   ▲ Revised Code Title

√5ᵗʰ **T46.8 Poisoning by, adverse effect of and underdosing of antivaricose drugs, including sclerosing agents**

√6ᵗʰ **T46.8X Poisoning by, adverse effect of and underdosing of antivaricose drugs, including sclerosing agents**

√7ᵗʰ **T46.8X1 Poisoning by antivaricose drugs, including sclerosing agents, accidental (unintentional)**
Poisoning by antivaricose drugs, including sclerosing agents NOS

2 √7ᵗʰ **T46.8X2 Poisoning by antivaricose drugs, including sclerosing agents, intentional self-harm** HCC

√7ᵗʰ **T46.8X3 Poisoning by antivaricose drugs, including sclerosing agents, assault**

√7ᵗʰ **T46.8X4 Poisoning by antivaricose drugs, including sclerosing agents, undetermined**

√7ᵗʰ **T46.8X5 Adverse effect of antivaricose drugs, including sclerosing agents**

√7ᵗʰ **T46.8X6 Underdosing of antivaricose drugs, including sclerosing agents**

√5ᵗʰ **T46.9 Poisoning by, adverse effect of and underdosing of other and unspecified agents primarily affecting the cardiovascular system**

√6ᵗʰ **T46.90 Poisoning by, adverse effect of and underdosing of unspecified agents primarily affecting the cardiovascular system**

√7ᵗʰ **T46.901 Poisoning by unspecified agents primarily affecting the cardiovascular system, accidental (unintentional)** ▽

2 √7ᵗʰ **T46.902 Poisoning by unspecified agents primarily affecting the cardiovascular system, intentional self-harm** HCC ▽

√7ᵗʰ **T46.903 Poisoning by unspecified agents primarily affecting the cardiovascular system, assault** ▽

√7ᵗʰ **T46.904 Poisoning by unspecified agents primarily affecting the cardiovascular system, undetermined** ▽

√7ᵗʰ **T46.905 Adverse effect of unspecified agents primarily affecting the cardiovascular system** ▽

√7ᵗʰ **T46.906 Underdosing of unspecified agents primarily affecting the cardiovascular system** ▽

√6ᵗʰ **T46.99 Poisoning by, adverse effect of and underdosing of other agents primarily affecting the cardiovascular system**

√7ᵗʰ **T46.991 Poisoning by other agents primarily affecting the cardiovascular system, accidental (unintentional)**

2 √7ᵗʰ **T46.992 Poisoning by other agents primarily affecting the cardiovascular system, intentional self-harm** HCC

√7ᵗʰ **T46.993 Poisoning by other agents primarily affecting the cardiovascular system, assault**

√7ᵗʰ **T46.994 Poisoning by other agents primarily affecting the cardiovascular system, undetermined**

√7ᵗʰ **T46.995 Adverse effect of other agents primarily affecting the cardiovascular system**

√7ᵗʰ **T46.996 Underdosing of other agents primarily affecting the cardiovascular system**

√4ᵗʰ **T47 Poisoning by, adverse effect of and underdosing of agents primarily affecting the gastrointestinal system**

The appropriate 7th character is to be added to each code from category T47.
A   initial encounter
D   subsequent encounter
S   sequela

√5ᵗʰ **T47.0 Poisoning by, adverse effect of and underdosing of histamine H2-receptor blockers**

√6ᵗʰ **T47.0X Poisoning by, adverse effect of and underdosing of histamine H2-receptor blockers**

√7ᵗʰ **T47.0X1 Poisoning by histamine H2-receptor blockers, accidental (unintentional)**
Poisoning by histamine H2-receptor blockers NOS

2 √7ᵗʰ **T47.0X2 Poisoning by histamine H2-receptor blockers, intentional self-harm** HCC

√7ᵗʰ **T47.0X3 Poisoning by histamine H2-receptor blockers, assault**

√7ᵗʰ **T47.0X4 Poisoning by histamine H2-receptor blockers, undetermined**

√7ᵗʰ **T47.0X5 Adverse effect of histamine H2-receptor blockers**

√7ᵗʰ **T47.0X6 Underdosing of histamine H2-receptor blockers**

√5ᵗʰ **T47.1 Poisoning by, adverse effect of and underdosing of other antacids and anti-gastric-secretion drugs**

√6ᵗʰ **T47.1X Poisoning by, adverse effect of and underdosing of other antacids and anti-gastric-secretion drugs**

√7ᵗʰ **T47.1X1 Poisoning by other antacids and anti-gastric-secretion drugs, accidental (unintentional)**
Poisoning by other antacids and anti-gastric-secretion drugs NOS

2 √7ᵗʰ **T47.1X2 Poisoning by other antacids and anti-gastric-secretion drugs, intentional self-harm** HCC

√7ᵗʰ **T47.1X3 Poisoning by other antacids and anti-gastric-secretion drugs, assault**

√7ᵗʰ **T47.1X4 Poisoning by other antacids and anti-gastric-secretion drugs, undetermined**

√7ᵗʰ **T47.1X5 Adverse effect of other antacids and anti-gastric-secretion drugs**

√7ᵗʰ **T47.1X6 Underdosing of other antacids and anti-gastric-secretion drugs**

√5ᵗʰ **T47.2 Poisoning by, adverse effect of and underdosing of stimulant laxatives**

√6ᵗʰ **T47.2X Poisoning by, adverse effect of and underdosing of stimulant laxatives**

√7ᵗʰ **T47.2X1 Poisoning by stimulant laxatives, accidental (unintentional)**
Poisoning by stimulant laxatives NOS

2 √7ᵗʰ **T47.2X2 Poisoning by stimulant laxatives, intentional self-harm** HCC

√7ᵗʰ **T47.2X3 Poisoning by stimulant laxatives, assault**

√7ᵗʰ **T47.2X4 Poisoning by stimulant laxatives, undetermined**

√7ᵗʰ **T47.2X5 Adverse effect of stimulant laxatives**

√7ᵗʰ **T47.2X6 Underdosing of stimulant laxatives**

√5ᵗʰ **T47.3 Poisoning by, adverse effect of and underdosing of saline and osmotic laxatives**

√6ᵗʰ **T47.3X Poisoning by and adverse effect of saline and osmotic laxatives**

√7ᵗʰ **T47.3X1 Poisoning by saline and osmotic laxatives, accidental (unintentional)**
Poisoning by saline and osmotic laxatives NOS

2 √7ᵗʰ **T47.3X2 Poisoning by saline and osmotic laxatives, intentional self-harm** HCC

√7ᵗʰ **T47.3X3 Poisoning by saline and osmotic laxatives, assault**

√7ᵗʰ **T47.3X4 Poisoning by saline and osmotic laxatives, undetermined**

√7ᵗʰ **T47.3X5 Adverse effect of saline and osmotic laxatives**

---

2   HCC with 7th character indicating initial encounter (A or B - specific to category) OR sequela.

EXCLUDES 1 Not coded here   EXCLUDES 2 Not included here   Ⓝ Newborn Age: 0   Ⓟ Pediatric Age: 0-17   Ⓜ Maternity Age: 12-55   Ⓐ Adult Age: 15-124

√7ᵗʰ **T47.3X6** Underdosing of saline and osmotic laxatives

√5ᵗʰ **T47.4** Poisoning by, adverse effect of and underdosing of other laxatives

  √6ᵗʰ **T47.4X** Poisoning by, adverse effect of and underdosing of other laxatives

    √7ᵗʰ **T47.4X1** Poisoning by other laxatives, accidental (unintentional)
       Poisoning by other laxatives NOS

    ² √7ᵗʰ **T47.4X2** Poisoning by other laxatives, intentional self-harm   HCC

    √7ᵗʰ **T47.4X3** Poisoning by other laxatives, assault

    √7ᵗʰ **T47.4X4** Poisoning by other laxatives, undetermined

    √7ᵗʰ **T47.4X5** Adverse effect of other laxatives

    √7ᵗʰ **T47.4X6** Underdosing of other laxatives

√5ᵗʰ **T47.5** Poisoning by, adverse effect of and underdosing of digestants

  √6ᵗʰ **T47.5X** Poisoning by, adverse effect of and underdosing of digestants

    √7ᵗʰ **T47.5X1** Poisoning by digestants, accidental (unintentional)
       Poisoning by digestants NOS

    ² √7ᵗʰ **T47.5X2** Poisoning by digestants, intentional self-harm   HCC

    √7ᵗʰ **T47.5X3** Poisoning by digestants, assault

    √7ᵗʰ **T47.5X4** Poisoning by digestants, undetermined

    √7ᵗʰ **T47.5X5** Adverse effect of digestants

    √7ᵗʰ **T47.5X6** Underdosing of digestants

√5ᵗʰ **T47.6** Poisoning by, adverse effect of and underdosing of antidiarrheal drugs

    EXCLUDES 2   poisoning by, adverse effect of and underdosing of systemic antibiotics and other anti-infectives (T36-T37)

  √6ᵗʰ **T47.6X** Poisoning by, adverse effect of and underdosing of antidiarrheal drugs

    √7ᵗʰ **T47.6X1** Poisoning by antidiarrheal drugs, accidental (unintentional)
       Poisoning by antidiarrheal drugs NOS

    ² √7ᵗʰ **T47.6X2** Poisoning by antidiarrheal drugs, intentional self-harm   HCC

    √7ᵗʰ **T47.6X3** Poisoning by antidiarrheal drugs, assault

    √7ᵗʰ **T47.6X4** Poisoning by antidiarrheal drugs, undetermined

    √7ᵗʰ **T47.6X5** Adverse effect of antidiarrheal drugs

    √7ᵗʰ **T47.6X6** Underdosing of antidiarrheal drugs

√5ᵗʰ **T47.7** Poisoning by, adverse effect of and underdosing of emetics

  √6ᵗʰ **T47.7X** Poisoning by, adverse effect of and underdosing of emetics

    √7ᵗʰ **T47.7X1** Poisoning by emetics, accidental (unintentional)
       Poisoning by emetics NOS

    ² √7ᵗʰ **T47.7X2** Poisoning by emetics, intentional self-harm   HCC

    √7ᵗʰ **T47.7X3** Poisoning by emetics, assault

    √7ᵗʰ **T47.7X4** Poisoning by emetics, undetermined

    √7ᵗʰ **T47.7X5** Adverse effect of emetics

    √7ᵗʰ **T47.7X6** Underdosing of emetics

√5ᵗʰ **T47.8** Poisoning by, adverse effect of and underdosing of other agents primarily affecting gastrointestinal system

  √6ᵗʰ **T47.8X** Poisoning by, adverse effect of and underdosing of other agents primarily affecting gastrointestinal system

    √7ᵗʰ **T47.8X1** Poisoning by other agents primarily affecting gastrointestinal system, accidental (unintentional)
       Poisoning by other agents primarily affecting gastrointestinal system NOS

    ² √7ᵗʰ **T47.8X2** Poisoning by other agents primarily affecting gastrointestinal system, intentional self-harm   HCC

    √7ᵗʰ **T47.8X3** Poisoning by other agents primarily affecting gastrointestinal system, assault

    √7ᵗʰ **T47.8X4** Poisoning by other agents primarily affecting gastrointestinal system, undetermined

    √7ᵗʰ **T47.8X5** Adverse effect of other agents primarily affecting gastrointestinal system

    √7ᵗʰ **T47.8X6** Underdosing of other agents primarily affecting gastrointestinal system

√5ᵗʰ **T47.9** Poisoning by, adverse effect of and underdosing of unspecified agents primarily affecting the gastrointestinal system

  √×7ᵗʰ **T47.91** Poisoning by unspecified agents primarily affecting the gastrointestinal system, accidental (unintentional) ▽
       Poisoning by agents primarily affecting the gastrointestinal system NOS

  ² √×7ᵗʰ **T47.92** Poisoning by unspecified agents primarily affecting the gastrointestinal system, intentional self-harm   HCC ▽

  √×7ᵗʰ **T47.93** Poisoning by unspecified agents primarily affecting the gastrointestinal system, assault ▽

  √×7ᵗʰ **T47.94** Poisoning by unspecified agents primarily affecting the gastrointestinal system, undetermined ▽

  √×7ᵗʰ **T47.95** Adverse effect of unspecified agents primarily affecting the gastrointestinal system ▽

  √×7ᵗʰ **T47.96** Underdosing of unspecified agents primarily affecting the gastrointestinal system ▽

√4ᵗʰ **T48** Poisoning by, adverse effect of and underdosing of agents primarily acting on smooth and skeletal muscles and the respiratory system

> The appropriate 7th character is to be added to each code from category T48.
> A   initial encounter
> D   subsequent encounter
> S   sequela

√5ᵗʰ **T48.0** Poisoning by, adverse effect of and underdosing of oxytocic drugs

    EXCLUDES 1   poisoning by, adverse effect of and underdosing of estrogens, progestogens and antagonists (T38.4-T38.6)

  √6ᵗʰ **T48.0X** Poisoning by, adverse effect of and underdosing of oxytocic drugs

    √7ᵗʰ **T48.0X1** Poisoning by oxytocic drugs, accidental (unintentional)
       Poisoning by oxytocic drugs NOS

    ² √7ᵗʰ **T48.0X2** Poisoning by oxytocic drugs, intentional self-harm   HCC

    √7ᵗʰ **T48.0X3** Poisoning by oxytocic drugs, assault

    √7ᵗʰ **T48.0X4** Poisoning by oxytocic drugs, undetermined

    √7ᵗʰ **T48.0X5** Adverse effect of oxytocic drugs

    √7ᵗʰ **T48.0X6** Underdosing of oxytocic drugs

√5ᵗʰ **T48.1** Poisoning by, adverse effect of and underdosing of skeletal muscle relaxants [neuromuscular blocking agents]

  √6ᵗʰ **T48.1X** Poisoning by, adverse effect of and underdosing of skeletal muscle relaxants [neuromuscular blocking agents]

    √7ᵗʰ **T48.1X1** Poisoning by skeletal muscle relaxants [neuromuscular blocking agents], accidental (unintentional)
       Poisoning by skeletal muscle relaxants [neuromuscular blocking agents] NOS

    ² √7ᵗʰ **T48.1X2** Poisoning by skeletal muscle relaxants [neuromuscular blocking agents], intentional self-harm   HCC

    √7ᵗʰ **T48.1X3** Poisoning by skeletal muscle relaxants [neuromuscular blocking agents], assault

    √7ᵗʰ **T48.1X4** Poisoning by skeletal muscle relaxants [neuromuscular blocking agents], undetermined

    √7ᵗʰ **T48.1X5** Adverse effect of skeletal muscle relaxants [neuromuscular blocking agents]

    √7ᵗʰ **T48.1X6** Underdosing of skeletal muscle relaxants [neuromuscular blocking agents]

---

²   HCC with 7th character indicating initial encounter (A or B - specific to category) OR sequela.

✓ Additional Character Req   √×7ᵗʰ Placeholder Alert   Manifestation   HCC CMS-HCC Condition   ▽ Unspecified Code   ►◄ Revised Text   ● New Code   ▲ Revised Code Title

ICD-10-CM 2018   1075

√5ᵗʰ **T48.2** **Poisoning by, adverse effect of and underdosing of other and unspecified drugs acting on muscles**

   √6ᵗʰ **T48.20** **Poisoning by, adverse effect of and underdosing of unspecified drugs acting on muscles**

     √7ᵗʰ **T48.201** **Poisoning by unspecified drugs acting on muscles, accidental (unintentional)** ▽
Poisoning by unspecified drugs acting on muscles NOS

     2 √7ᵗʰ **T48.202** **Poisoning by unspecified drugs acting on muscles, intentional self-harm** HCC ▽

     √7ᵗʰ **T48.203** **Poisoning by unspecified drugs acting on muscles, assault** ▽

     √7ᵗʰ **T48.204** **Poisoning by unspecified drugs acting on muscles, undetermined** ▽

     √7ᵗʰ **T48.205** **Adverse effect of unspecified drugs acting on muscles** ▽

     √7ᵗʰ **T48.206** **Underdosing of unspecified drugs acting on muscles** ▽

   √6ᵗʰ **T48.29** **Poisoning by, adverse effect of and underdosing of other drugs acting on muscles**

     √7ᵗʰ **T48.291** **Poisoning by other drugs acting on muscles, accidental (unintentional)**
Poisoning by other drugs acting on muscles NOS

     2 √7ᵗʰ **T48.292** **Poisoning by other drugs acting on muscles, intentional self-harm** HCC

     √7ᵗʰ **T48.293** **Poisoning by other drugs acting on muscles, assault**

     √7ᵗʰ **T48.294** **Poisoning by other drugs acting on muscles, undetermined**

     √7ᵗʰ **T48.295** **Adverse effect of other drugs acting on muscles**

     √7ᵗʰ **T48.296** **Underdosing of other drugs acting on muscles**

√5ᵗʰ **T48.3** **Poisoning by, adverse effect of and underdosing of antitussives**

   √6ᵗʰ **T48.3X** **Poisoning by, adverse effect of and underdosing of antitussives**

     √7ᵗʰ **T48.3X1** **Poisoning by antitussives, accidental (unintentional)**
Poisoning by antitussives NOS

     2 √7ᵗʰ **T48.3X2** **Poisoning by antitussives, intentional self-harm** HCC

     √7ᵗʰ **T48.3X3** **Poisoning by antitussives, assault**

     √7ᵗʰ **T48.3X4** **Poisoning by antitussives, undetermined**

     √7ᵗʰ **T48.3X5** **Adverse effect of antitussives**

     √7ᵗʰ **T48.3X6** **Underdosing of antitussives**

√5ᵗʰ **T48.4** **Poisoning by, adverse effect of and underdosing of expectorants**

   √6ᵗʰ **T48.4X** **Poisoning by, adverse effect of and underdosing of expectorants**

     √7ᵗʰ **T48.4X1** **Poisoning by expectorants, accidental (unintentional)**
Poisoning by expectorants NOS

     2 √7ᵗʰ **T48.4X2** **Poisoning by expectorants, intentional self-harm** HCC

     √7ᵗʰ **T48.4X3** **Poisoning by expectorants, assault**

     √7ᵗʰ **T48.4X4** **Poisoning by expectorants, undetermined**

     √7ᵗʰ **T48.4X5** **Adverse effect of expectorants**

     √7ᵗʰ **T48.4X6** **Underdosing of expectorants**

√5ᵗʰ **T48.5** **Poisoning by, adverse effect of and underdosing of other anti-common-cold drugs**
Poisoning by, adverse effect of and underdosing of decongestants

   EXCLUDES 2   *poisoning by, adverse effect of and underdosing of antipyretics, NEC (T39.9-)*
poisoning by, adverse effect of and underdosing of non-steroidal antiinflammatory drugs (T39.3-)
poisoning by, adverse effect of and underdosing of salicylates (T39.0-)

   √6ᵗʰ **T48.5X** **Poisoning by, adverse effect of and underdosing of other anti-common-cold drugs**

     √7ᵗʰ **T48.5X1** **Poisoning by other anti-common-cold drugs, accidental (unintentional)**
Poisoning by other anti-common-cold drugs NOS

     2 √7ᵗʰ **T48.5X2** **Poisoning by other anti-common-cold drugs, intentional self-harm** HCC

     √7ᵗʰ **T48.5X3** **Poisoning by other anti-common-cold drugs, assault**

     √7ᵗʰ **T48.5X4** **Poisoning by other anti-common-cold drugs, undetermined**

     √7ᵗʰ **T48.5X5** **Adverse effect of other anti-common-cold drugs**

     √7ᵗʰ **T48.5X6** **Underdosing of other anti-common-cold drugs**

√5ᵗʰ **T48.6** **Poisoning by, adverse effect of and underdosing of antiasthmatics, not elsewhere classified**
Poisoning by, adverse effect of and underdosing of beta-adrenoreceptor agonists used in asthma therapy

   EXCLUDES 1   *poisoning by, adverse effect of and underdosing of anterior pituitary [adenohypophyseal] hormones (T38.8)*
poisoning by, adverse effect of and underdosing of beta-adrenoreceptor agonists not used in asthma therapy (T44.5)

   √6ᵗʰ **T48.6X** **Poisoning by, adverse effect of and underdosing of antiasthmatics**

     √7ᵗʰ **T48.6X1** **Poisoning by antiasthmatics, accidental (unintentional)**
Poisoning by antiasthmatics NOS

     2 √7ᵗʰ **T48.6X2** **Poisoning by antiasthmatics, intentional self-harm** HCC

     √7ᵗʰ **T48.6X3** **Poisoning by antiasthmatics, assault**

     √7ᵗʰ **T48.6X4** **Poisoning by antiasthmatics, undetermined**

     √7ᵗʰ **T48.6X5** **Adverse effect of antiasthmatics**

     √7ᵗʰ **T48.6X6** **Underdosing of antiasthmatics**

√5ᵗʰ **T48.9** **Poisoning by, adverse effect of and underdosing of other and unspecified agents primarily acting on the respiratory system**

   √6ᵗʰ **T48.90** **Poisoning by, adverse effect of and underdosing of unspecified agents primarily acting on the respiratory system**

     √7ᵗʰ **T48.901** **Poisoning by unspecified agents primarily acting on the respiratory system, accidental (unintentional)** ▽

     2 √7ᵗʰ **T48.902** **Poisoning by unspecified agents primarily acting on the respiratory system, intentional self-harm** HCC ▽

     √7ᵗʰ **T48.903** **Poisoning by unspecified agents primarily acting on the respiratory system, assault** ▽

     √7ᵗʰ **T48.904** **Poisoning by unspecified agents primarily acting on the respiratory system, undetermined** ▽

     √7ᵗʰ **T48.905** **Adverse effect of unspecified agents primarily acting on the respiratory system** ▽

     √7ᵗʰ **T48.906** **Underdosing of unspecified agents primarily acting on the respiratory system** ▽

   √6ᵗʰ **T48.99** **Poisoning by, adverse effect of and underdosing of other agents primarily acting on the respiratory system**

     √7ᵗʰ **T48.991** **Poisoning by other agents primarily acting on the respiratory system, accidental (unintentional)**

---

2   HCC with 7th character indicating initial encounter (A or B - specific to category) OR sequela.

EXCLUDES 1 Not coded here   **EXCLUDES 2** Not included here   N Newborn Age: 0   P Pediatric Age: 0-17   M Maternity Age: 12-55   A Adult Age: 15-124

2 ✓7ᵗʰ **T48.992 Poisoning by other agents primarily** [HCC]
acting on the respiratory system,
intentional self-harm

✓7ᵗʰ **T48.993 Poisoning by other agents primarily**
acting on the respiratory system, assault

✓7ᵗʰ **T48.994 Poisoning by other agents primarily**
acting on the respiratory system,
undetermined

✓7ᵗʰ **T48.995** Adverse effect **of other agents primarily**
acting on the respiratory system

✓7ᵗʰ **T48.996** Underdosing **of other agents primarily**
acting on the respiratory system

✓4ᵗʰ **T49 Poisoning by, adverse effect of and underdosing of topical**
agents primarily affecting skin and mucous membrane and by
ophthalmological, otorhinolaryngological and dental drugs
   [INCLUDES]   poisoning by, adverse effect of and underdosing of
glucocorticoids, topically used

> The appropriate 7th character is to be added to each code from
> category T49.
> A   initial encounter
> D   subsequent encounter
> S   sequela

✓5ᵗʰ **T49.0 Poisoning by, adverse effect of and underdosing of local**
antifungal, anti-infective and anti-inflammatory drugs

  ✓6ᵗʰ **T49.0X Poisoning by, adverse effect of and underdosing of**
local antifungal, anti-infective and anti-
inflammatory **drugs**

    ✓7ᵗʰ **T49.0X1 Poisoning by local antifungal, anti-**
infective and anti-inflammatory drugs,
accidental **(unintentional)**
      Poisoning by local antifungal, anti-infective
and anti-inflammatory drugs NOS

    2 ✓7ᵗʰ **T49.0X2 Poisoning by local antifungal, anti-** [HCC]
infective and anti-inflammatory drugs,
intentional self-harm

    ✓7ᵗʰ **T49.0X3 Poisoning by local antifungal, anti-**
infective and anti-inflammatory drugs,
assault

    ✓7ᵗʰ **T49.0X4 Poisoning by local antifungal, anti-**
infective and anti-inflammatory drugs,
undetermined

    ✓7ᵗʰ **T49.0X5** Adverse effect **of local antifungal, anti-**
infective and anti-inflammatory drugs

    ✓7ᵗʰ **T49.0X6** Underdosing **of local antifungal, anti-**
infective and anti-inflammatory drugs

✓5ᵗʰ **T49.1 Poisoning by, adverse effect of and underdosing of**
antipruritics

  ✓6ᵗʰ **T49.1X Poisoning by, adverse effect of and underdosing of**
antipruritics

    ✓7ᵗʰ **T49.1X1 Poisoning by antipruritics,** accidental
(unintentional)
      Poisoning by antipruritics NOS

    2 ✓7ᵗʰ **T49.1X2 Poisoning by antipruritics,** [HCC]
intentional self-harm

    ✓7ᵗʰ **T49.1X3 Poisoning by antipruritics,** assault

    ✓7ᵗʰ **T49.1X4 Poisoning by antipruritics,** undetermined

    ✓7ᵗʰ **T49.1X5** Adverse effect **of antipruritics**

    ✓7ᵗʰ **T49.1X6** Underdosing **of antipruritics**

✓5ᵗʰ **T49.2 Poisoning by, adverse effect of and underdosing of local**
astringents and local detergents

  ✓6ᵗʰ **T49.2X Poisoning by, adverse effect of and underdosing of**
local astringents and local detergents

    ✓7ᵗʰ **T49.2X1 Poisoning by local astringents and local**
detergents, accidental **(unintentional)**
      Poisoning by local astringents and local
detergents NOS

    2 ✓7ᵗʰ **T49.2X2 Poisoning by local astringents and** [HCC]
local detergents, intentional self-harm

    ✓7ᵗʰ **T49.2X3 Poisoning by local astringents and local**
detergents, assault

    ✓7ᵗʰ **T49.2X4 Poisoning by local astringents and local**
detergents, undetermined

    ✓7ᵗʰ **T49.2X5** Adverse effect **of local astringents and**
local detergents

    ✓7ᵗʰ **T49.2X6** Underdosing **of local astringents and local**
detergents

✓5ᵗʰ **T49.3 Poisoning by, adverse effect of and underdosing of**
emollients, demulcents and protectants

  ✓6ᵗʰ **T49.3X Poisoning by, adverse effect of and underdosing of**
emollients, demulcents and protectants

    ✓7ᵗʰ **T49.3X1 Poisoning by emollients, demulcents and**
protectants, accidental **(unintentional)**
      Poisoning by emollients, demulcents and
protectants NOS

    2 ✓7ᵗʰ **T49.3X2 Poisoning by emollients, demulcents** [HCC]
and protectants, intentional self-harm

    ✓7ᵗʰ **T49.3X3 Poisoning by emollients, demulcents and**
protectants, assault

    ✓7ᵗʰ **T49.3X4 Poisoning by emollients, demulcents and**
protectants, undetermined

    ✓7ᵗʰ **T49.3X5** Adverse effect **of emollients, demulcents**
and protectants

    ✓7ᵗʰ **T49.3X6** Underdosing **of emollients, demulcents**
and protectants

✓5ᵗʰ **T49.4 Poisoning by, adverse effect of and underdosing of**
keratolytics, keratoplastics, and other hair treatment drugs
and preparations

  ✓6ᵗʰ **T49.4X Poisoning by, adverse effect of and underdosing of**
keratolytics, keratoplastics, and other hair
treatment drugs and preparations

    ✓7ᵗʰ **T49.4X1 Poisoning by keratolytics, keratoplastics,**
and other hair treatment drugs and
preparations, accidental **(unintentional)**
      Poisoning by keratolytics, keratoplastics,
and other hair treatment drugs and
preparations NOS

    2 ✓7ᵗʰ **T49.4X2 Poisoning by keratolytics,** [HCC]
keratoplastics, and other hair
treatment drugs and preparations,
intentional self-harm

    ✓7ᵗʰ **T49.4X3 Poisoning by keratolytics, keratoplastics,**
and other hair treatment drugs and
preparations, assault

    ✓7ᵗʰ **T49.4X4 Poisoning by keratolytics, keratoplastics,**
and other hair treatment drugs and
preparations, undetermined

    ✓7ᵗʰ **T49.4X5** Adverse effect **of keratolytics,**
keratoplastics, and other hair treatment
drugs and preparations

    ✓7ᵗʰ **T49.4X6** Underdosing **of keratolytics,**
keratoplastics, and other hair treatment
drugs and preparations

✓5ᵗʰ **T49.5 Poisoning by, adverse effect of and underdosing of**
ophthalmological drugs and preparations

  ✓6ᵗʰ **T49.5X Poisoning by, adverse effect of and underdosing of**
ophthalmological **drugs and preparations**

    ✓7ᵗʰ **T49.5X1 Poisoning by ophthalmological drugs and**
preparations, accidental **(unintentional)**
      Poisoning by ophthalmological drugs and
preparations NOS

    2 ✓7ᵗʰ **T49.5X2 Poisoning by ophthalmological** [HCC]
drugs and preparations, intentional
self-harm

    ✓7ᵗʰ **T49.5X3 Poisoning by ophthalmological drugs and**
preparations, assault

    ✓7ᵗʰ **T49.5X4 Poisoning by ophthalmological drugs and**
preparations, undetermined

    ✓7ᵗʰ **T49.5X5** Adverse effect **of ophthalmological drugs**
and preparations

    ✓7ᵗʰ **T49.5X6** Underdosing **of ophthalmological drugs**
and preparations

✓5ᵗʰ **T49.6 Poisoning by, adverse effect of and underdosing of**
otorhinolaryngological drugs and preparations

  ✓6ᵗʰ **T49.6X Poisoning by, adverse effect of and underdosing of**
otorhinolaryngological **drugs and preparations**

    ✓7ᵗʰ **T49.6X1 Poisoning by otorhinolaryngological**
drugs and preparations, accidental
(unintentional)
      Poisoning by otorhinolaryngological drugs
and preparations NOS

---

2 HCC with 7th character indicating initial encounter (A or B - specific to category) OR sequela.

✓ Additional Character Req   ✓ˣ7ᵗʰ Placeholder Alert   Manifestation   [HCC] CMS-HCC Condition   ▽ Unspecified Code   ►◄ Revised Text   ● New Code   ▲ Revised Code Title

2 ✓7ᵗʰ **T49.6X2** **Poisoning by otorhinolaryngological drugs and preparations,** intentional self-harm   HCC

✓7ᵗʰ **T49.6X3** **Poisoning by otorhinolaryngological drugs and preparations,** assault

✓7ᵗʰ **T49.6X4** **Poisoning by otorhinolaryngological drugs and preparations,** undetermined

✓7ᵗʰ **T49.6X5** Adverse effect **of otorhinolaryngological drugs and preparations**

✓7ᵗʰ **T49.6X6** Underdosing **of otorhinolaryngological drugs and preparations**

✓5ᵗʰ **T49.7** **Poisoning by, adverse effect of and underdosing of dental drugs, topically applied**

  ✓6ᵗʰ **T49.7X** **Poisoning by, adverse effect of and underdosing of** dental **drugs, topically applied**

✓7ᵗʰ **T49.7X1** **Poisoning by dental drugs, topically applied,** accidental (unintentional)
    Poisoning by dental drugs, topically applied NOS

2 ✓7ᵗʰ **T49.7X2** **Poisoning by dental drugs, topically applied,** intentional self-harm   HCC

✓7ᵗʰ **T49.7X3** **Poisoning by dental drugs, topically applied,** assault

✓7ᵗʰ **T49.7X4** **Poisoning by dental drugs, topically applied,** undetermined

✓7ᵗʰ **T49.7X5** Adverse effect **of dental drugs, topically applied**

✓7ᵗʰ **T49.7X6** Underdosing **of dental drugs, topically applied**

✓5ᵗʰ **T49.8** **Poisoning by, adverse effect of and underdosing of other topical agents**
    Poisoning by, adverse effect of and underdosing of spermicides

  ✓6ᵗʰ **T49.8X** **Poisoning by, adverse effect of and underdosing of other topical agents**

✓7ᵗʰ **T49.8X1** **Poisoning by other topical agents,** accidental (unintentional)
    Poisoning by other topical agents NOS

2 ✓7ᵗʰ **T49.8X2** **Poisoning by other topical agents,** intentional self-harm   HCC

✓7ᵗʰ **T49.8X3** **Poisoning by other topical agents,** assault

✓7ᵗʰ **T49.8X4** **Poisoning by other topical agents,** undetermined

✓7ᵗʰ **T49.8X5** Adverse effect **of other topical agents**

✓7ᵗʰ **T49.8X6** Underdosing **of other topical agents**

✓5ᵗʰ **T49.9** **Poisoning by, adverse effect of and underdosing of unspecified topical agent**

✓x7ᵗʰ **T49.91** **Poisoning by unspecified topical agent,** accidental (unintentional)   ▽

2 ✓x7ᵗʰ **T49.92** **Poisoning by unspecified topical agent,** intentional self-harm   HCC ▽

✓x7ᵗʰ **T49.93** **Poisoning by unspecified topical agent,** assault   ▽

✓x7ᵗʰ **T49.94** **Poisoning by unspecified topical agent,** undetermined   ▽

✓x7ᵗʰ **T49.95** Adverse effect **of unspecified topical agent**   ▽

✓x7ᵗʰ **T49.96** Underdosing **of unspecified topical agent**   ▽

✓4ᵗʰ **T50** **Poisoning by, adverse effect of and underdosing of diuretics and other and unspecified drugs, medicaments and biological substances**

> The appropriate 7th character is to be added to each code from category T50.
> A   initial encounter
> D   subsequent encounter
> S   sequela

✓5ᵗʰ **T50.0** **Poisoning by, adverse effect of and underdosing of mineralocorticoids and their antagonists**

  ✓6ᵗʰ **T50.0X** **Poisoning by, adverse effect of and underdosing of** mineralocorticoids **and their antagonists**

✓7ᵗʰ **T50.0X1** **Poisoning by mineralocorticoids and their antagonists,** accidental (unintentional)
    Poisoning by mineralocorticoids and their antagonists NOS

2 ✓7ᵗʰ **T50.0X2** **Poisoning by mineralocorticoids and their antagonists,** intentional self-harm   HCC

✓7ᵗʰ **T50.0X3** **Poisoning by mineralocorticoids and their antagonists,** assault

✓7ᵗʰ **T50.0X4** **Poisoning by mineralocorticoids and their antagonists,** undetermined

✓7ᵗʰ **T50.0X5** Adverse effect **of mineralocorticoids and their antagonists**

✓7ᵗʰ **T50.0X6** Underdosing **of mineralocorticoids and their antagonists**

✓5ᵗʰ **T50.1** **Poisoning by, adverse effect of and underdosing of loop [high-ceiling] diuretics**

  ✓6ᵗʰ **T50.1X** **Poisoning by, adverse effect of and underdosing of** loop [high-ceiling] diuretics

✓7ᵗʰ **T50.1X1** **Poisoning by loop [high-ceiling] diuretics,** accidental (unintentional)
    Poisoning by loop [high-ceiling] diuretics NOS

2 ✓7ᵗʰ **T50.1X2** **Poisoning by loop [high-ceiling] diuretics,** intentional self-harm   HCC

✓7ᵗʰ **T50.1X3** **Poisoning by loop [high-ceiling] diuretics,** assault

✓7ᵗʰ **T50.1X4** **Poisoning by loop [high-ceiling] diuretics,** undetermined

✓7ᵗʰ **T50.1X5** Adverse effect **of loop [high-ceiling] diuretics**

✓7ᵗʰ **T50.1X6** Underdosing **of loop [high-ceiling] diuretics**

✓5ᵗʰ **T50.2** **Poisoning by, adverse effect of and underdosing of carbonic-anhydrase inhibitors, benzothiadiazides and other diuretics**
    Poisoning by, adverse effect of and underdosing of acetazolamide

  ✓6ᵗʰ **T50.2X** **Poisoning by, adverse effect of and underdosing of** carbonic-anhydrase inhibitors, benzothiadiazides and other diuretics

✓7ᵗʰ **T50.2X1** **Poisoning by carbonic-anhydrase inhibitors, benzothiadiazides and other diuretics,** accidental (unintentional)
    Poisoning by carbonic-anhydrase inhibitors, benzothiadiazides and other diuretics NOS

2 ✓7ᵗʰ **T50.2X2** **Poisoning by carbonic-anhydrase inhibitors, benzothiadiazides and other diuretics,** intentional self-harm   HCC

✓7ᵗʰ **T50.2X3** **Poisoning by carbonic-anhydrase inhibitors, benzothiadiazides and other diuretics,** assault

✓7ᵗʰ **T50.2X4** **Poisoning by carbonic-anhydrase inhibitors, benzothiadiazides and other diuretics,** undetermined

✓7ᵗʰ **T50.2X5** Adverse effect **of carbonic-anhydrase inhibitors, benzothiadiazides and other diuretics**

✓7ᵗʰ **T50.2X6** Underdosing **of carbonic-anhydrase inhibitors, benzothiadiazides and other diuretics**

✓5ᵗʰ **T50.3** **Poisoning by, adverse effect of and underdosing of electrolytic, caloric and water-balance agents**
    Poisoning by, adverse effect of and underdosing of oral rehydration salts

  ✓6ᵗʰ **T50.3X** **Poisoning by, adverse effect of and underdosing of** electrolytic, caloric and water-balance agents

✓7ᵗʰ **T50.3X1** **Poisoning by electrolytic, caloric and water-balance agents,** accidental (unintentional)
    Poisoning by electrolytic, caloric and water-balance agents NOS

2 ✓7ᵗʰ **T50.3X2** **Poisoning by electrolytic, caloric and water-balance agents,** intentional self-harm   HCC

✓7ᵗʰ **T50.3X3** **Poisoning by electrolytic, caloric and water-balance agents,** assault

✓7ᵗʰ **T50.3X4** **Poisoning by electrolytic, caloric and water-balance agents,** undetermined

✓7ᵗʰ **T50.3X5** Adverse effect **of electrolytic, caloric and water-balance agents**

✓7ᵗʰ **T50.3X6** Underdosing **of electrolytic, caloric and water-balance agents**

---

2   HCC with 7th character indicating initial encounter (A or B - specific to category) OR sequela.

EXCLUDES1 Not coded here   EXCLUDES2 Not included here   N Newborn Age: 0   P Pediatric Age: 0-17   M Maternity Age: 12-55   A Adult Age: 15-124

1078   ICD-10-CM 2018

☑5ᵗʰ **T50.4** **Poisoning by, adverse effect of and underdosing of drugs affecting uric acid metabolism**

  ☑6ᵗʰ **T50.4X** **Poisoning by, adverse effect of and underdosing of drugs** affecting uric acid metabolism

    ☑7ᵗʰ **T50.4X1** **Poisoning by drugs affecting uric acid metabolism,** accidental **(unintentional)**
        Poisoning by drugs affecting uric acid metabolism NOS

    ² ☑7ᵗʰ **T50.4X2** **Poisoning by drugs affecting uric acid** ᴴᶜᶜ **metabolism,** intentional self-harm

    ☑7ᵗʰ **T50.4X3** **Poisoning by drugs affecting uric acid metabolism,** assault

    ☑7ᵗʰ **T50.4X4** **Poisoning by drugs affecting uric acid metabolism,** undetermined

    ☑7ᵗʰ **T50.4X5** Adverse effect **of drugs affecting uric acid metabolism**

    ☑7ᵗʰ **T50.4X6** Underdosing **of drugs affecting uric acid metabolism**

☑5ᵗʰ **T50.5** **Poisoning by, adverse effect of and underdosing of appetite depressants**

  ☑6ᵗʰ **T50.5X** **Poisoning by, adverse effect of and underdosing of** appetite depressants

    ☑7ᵗʰ **T50.5X1** **Poisoning by appetite depressants,** accidental **(unintentional)**
        Poisoning by appetite depressants NOS

    ² ☑7ᵗʰ **T50.5X2** **Poisoning by appetite depressants,** ᴴᶜᶜ intentional self-harm

    ☑7ᵗʰ **T50.5X3** **Poisoning by appetite depressants,** assault

    ☑7ᵗʰ **T50.5X4** **Poisoning by appetite depressants,** undetermined

    ☑7ᵗʰ **T50.5X5** Adverse effect **of appetite depressants**

    ☑7ᵗʰ **T50.5X6** Underdosing **of appetite depressants**

☑5ᵗʰ **T50.6** **Poisoning by, adverse effect of and underdosing of antidotes and chelating agents**
    Poisoning by, adverse effect of and underdosing of alcohol deterrents

  ☑6ᵗʰ **T50.6X** **Poisoning by, adverse effect of and underdosing of** antidotes and chelating agents

    ☑7ᵗʰ **T50.6X1** **Poisoning by antidotes and chelating agents,** accidental **(unintentional)**
        Poisoning by antidotes and chelating agents NOS

    ² ☑7ᵗʰ **T50.6X2** **Poisoning by antidotes and chelating** ᴴᶜᶜ **agents,** intentional self-harm

    ☑7ᵗʰ **T50.6X3** **Poisoning by antidotes and chelating agents,** assault

    ☑7ᵗʰ **T50.6X4** **Poisoning by antidotes and chelating agents,** undetermined

    ☑7ᵗʰ **T50.6X5** Adverse effect **of antidotes and chelating agents**

    ☑7ᵗʰ **T50.6X6** Underdosing **of antidotes and chelating agents**

☑5ᵗʰ **T50.7** **Poisoning by, adverse effect of and underdosing of analeptics and opioid receptor antagonists**

  ☑6ᵗʰ **T50.7X** **Poisoning by, adverse effect of and underdosing of** analeptics and opioid receptor antagonists

    ☑7ᵗʰ **T50.7X1** **Poisoning by analeptics and opioid receptor antagonists,** accidental **(unintentional)**
        Poisoning by analeptics and opioid receptor antagonists NOS

    ² ☑7ᵗʰ **T50.7X2** **Poisoning by analeptics and opioid** ᴴᶜᶜ **receptor antagonists,** intentional self-harm

    ☑7ᵗʰ **T50.7X3** **Poisoning by analeptics and opioid receptor antagonists,** assault

    ☑7ᵗʰ **T50.7X4** **Poisoning by analeptics and opioid receptor antagonists,** undetermined

    ☑7ᵗʰ **T50.7X5** Adverse effect **of analeptics and opioid receptor antagonists**

    ☑7ᵗʰ **T50.7X6** Underdosing **of analeptics and opioid receptor antagonists**

☑5ᵗʰ **T50.8** **Poisoning by, adverse effect of and underdosing of diagnostic agents**

  ☑6ᵗʰ **T50.8X** **Poisoning by, adverse effect of and underdosing of** diagnostic agents

    ☑7ᵗʰ **T50.8X1** **Poisoning by diagnostic agents,** accidental **(unintentional)**
        Poisoning by diagnostic agents NOS

    ² ☑7ᵗʰ **T50.8X2** **Poisoning by diagnostic agents,** ᴴᶜᶜ intentional self-harm

    ☑7ᵗʰ **T50.8X3** **Poisoning by diagnostic agents,** assault

    ☑7ᵗʰ **T50.8X4** **Poisoning by diagnostic agents,** undetermined

    ☑7ᵗʰ **T50.8X5** Adverse effect **of diagnostic agents**

    ☑7ᵗʰ **T50.8X6** Underdosing **of diagnostic agents**

☑5ᵗʰ **T50.A** **Poisoning by, adverse effect of and underdosing of bacterial vaccines**

  ☑6ᵗʰ **T50.A1** **Poisoning by, adverse effect of and underdosing of** pertussis vaccine, **including combinations with a pertussis component**

    ☑7ᵗʰ **T50.A11** **Poisoning by pertussis vaccine, including combinations with a pertussis component,** accidental **(unintentional)**

    ² ☑7ᵗʰ **T50.A12** **Poisoning by pertussis vaccine,** ᴴᶜᶜ **including combinations with a pertussis component,** intentional self-harm

    ☑7ᵗʰ **T50.A13** **Poisoning by pertussis vaccine, including combinations with a pertussis component,** assault

    ☑7ᵗʰ **T50.A14** **Poisoning by pertussis vaccine, including combinations with a pertussis component,** undetermined

    ☑7ᵗʰ **T50.A15** Adverse effect **of pertussis vaccine, including combinations with a pertussis component**

    ☑7ᵗʰ **T50.A16** Underdosing **of pertussis vaccine, including combinations with a pertussis component**

  ☑6ᵗʰ **T50.A2** **Poisoning by, adverse effect of and underdosing of** mixed bacterial vaccines without a pertussis component

    ☑7ᵗʰ **T50.A21** **Poisoning by mixed bacterial vaccines without a pertussis component,** accidental **(unintentional)**

    ² ☑7ᵗʰ **T50.A22** **Poisoning by mixed bacterial** ᴴᶜᶜ **vaccines without a pertussis component,** intentional self-harm

    ☑7ᵗʰ **T50.A23** **Poisoning by mixed bacterial vaccines without a pertussis component,** assault

    ☑7ᵗʰ **T50.A24** **Poisoning by mixed bacterial vaccines without a pertussis component,** undetermined

    ☑7ᵗʰ **T50.A25** Adverse effect **of mixed bacterial vaccines without a pertussis component**

    ☑7ᵗʰ **T50.A26** Underdosing **of mixed bacterial vaccines without a pertussis component**

  ☑6ᵗʰ **T50.A9** **Poisoning by, adverse effect of and underdosing of other bacterial vaccines**

    ☑7ᵗʰ **T50.A91** **Poisoning by other bacterial vaccines,** accidental **(unintentional)**

    ² ☑7ᵗʰ **T50.A92** **Poisoning by other bacterial vaccines,** ᴴᶜᶜ intentional self-harm

    ☑7ᵗʰ **T50.A93** **Poisoning by other bacterial vaccines,** assault

    ☑7ᵗʰ **T50.A94** **Poisoning by other bacterial vaccines,** undetermined

    ☑7ᵗʰ **T50.A95** Adverse effect **of other bacterial vaccines**

    ☑7ᵗʰ **T50.A96** Underdosing **of other bacterial vaccines**

☑5ᵗʰ **T50.B** **Poisoning by, adverse effect of and underdosing of viral vaccines**

  ☑6ᵗʰ **T50.B1** **Poisoning by, adverse effect of and underdosing of** smallpox vaccines

    ☑7ᵗʰ **T50.B11** **Poisoning by smallpox vaccines,** accidental **(unintentional)**

    ² ☑7ᵗʰ **T50.B12** **Poisoning by smallpox vaccines,** ᴴᶜᶜ intentional self-harm

---

²   HCC with 7th character indicating initial encounter (A or B - specific to category) OR sequela.

☑ Additional Character Req   ✓ₓ₇ᵗʰ Placeholder Alert   Manifestation   ᴴᶜᶜ CMS-HCC Condition   ▽ Unspecified Code   ►◄ Revised Text   ● New Code   ▲ Revised Code Title

√7ᵗʰ **T50.B13** Poisoning by smallpox vaccines, assault

√7ᵗʰ **T50.B14** Poisoning by smallpox vaccines, undetermined

√7ᵗʰ **T50.B15** Adverse effect of smallpox vaccines

√7ᵗʰ **T50.B16** Underdosing of smallpox vaccines

√6ᵗʰ **T50.B9** Poisoning by, adverse effect of and underdosing of other viral vaccines

√7ᵗʰ **T50.B91** Poisoning by other viral vaccines, accidental (unintentional)

2 √7ᵗʰ **T50.B92** Poisoning by other viral vaccines, intentional self-harm   HCC

√7ᵗʰ **T50.B93** Poisoning by other viral vaccines, assault

√7ᵗʰ **T50.B94** Poisoning by other viral vaccines, undetermined

√7ᵗʰ **T50.B95** Adverse effect of other viral vaccines

√7ᵗʰ **T50.B96** Underdosing of other viral vaccines

√5ᵗʰ **T50.Z** Poisoning by, adverse effect of and underdosing of other vaccines and biological substances

√6ᵗʰ **T50.Z1** Poisoning by, adverse effect of and underdosing of immunoglobulin

√7ᵗʰ **T50.Z11** Poisoning by immunoglobulin, accidental (unintentional)

2 √7ᵗʰ **T50.Z12** Poisoning by immunoglobulin, intentional self-harm   HCC

√7ᵗʰ **T50.Z13** Poisoning by immunoglobulin, assault

√7ᵗʰ **T50.Z14** Poisoning by immunoglobulin, undetermined

√7ᵗʰ **T50.Z15** Adverse effect of immunoglobulin

√7ᵗʰ **T50.Z16** Underdosing of immunoglobulin

√6ᵗʰ **T50.Z9** Poisoning by, adverse effect of and underdosing of other vaccines and biological substances

√7ᵗʰ **T50.Z91** Poisoning by other vaccines and biological substances, accidental (unintentional)

2 √7ᵗʰ **T50.Z92** Poisoning by other vaccines and biological substances, intentional self-harm   HCC

√7ᵗʰ **T50.Z93** Poisoning by other vaccines and biological substances, assault

√7ᵗʰ **T50.Z94** Poisoning by other vaccines and biological substances, undetermined

√7ᵗʰ **T50.Z95** Adverse effect of other vaccines and biological substances

√7ᵗʰ **T50.Z96** Underdosing of other vaccines and biological substances

√5ᵗʰ **T50.9** Poisoning by, adverse effect of and underdosing of other and unspecified drugs, medicaments and biological substances
AHA: 2016, 1Q, 38; 2015, 1Q, 21

√6ᵗʰ **T50.90** Poisoning by, adverse effect of and underdosing of unspecified drugs, medicaments and biological substances

√7ᵗʰ **T50.901** Poisoning by unspecified drugs, medicaments and biological substances, accidental (unintentional) ▽

2 √7ᵗʰ **T50.902** Poisoning by unspecified drugs, medicaments and biological substances, intentional self-harm   HCC ▽

√7ᵗʰ **T50.903** Poisoning by unspecified drugs, medicaments and biological substances, assault ▽

√7ᵗʰ **T50.904** Poisoning by unspecified drugs, medicaments and biological substances, undetermined ▽

√7ᵗʰ **T50.905** Adverse effect of unspecified drugs, medicaments and biological substances ▽

√7ᵗʰ **T50.906** Underdosing of unspecified drugs, medicaments and biological substances ▽

√6ᵗʰ **T50.99** Poisoning by, adverse effect of and underdosing of other drugs, medicaments and biological substances

√7ᵗʰ **T50.991** Poisoning by other drugs, medicaments and biological substances, accidental (unintentional)

2 √7ᵗʰ **T50.992** Poisoning by other drugs, medicaments and biological substances, intentional self-harm   HCC

√7ᵗʰ **T50.993** Poisoning by other drugs, medicaments and biological substances, assault

√7ᵗʰ **T50.994** Poisoning by other drugs, medicaments and biological substances, undetermined

√7ᵗʰ **T50.995** Adverse effect of other drugs, medicaments and biological substances

√7ᵗʰ **T50.996** Underdosing of other drugs, medicaments and biological substances

Toxic effects of substances chiefly nonmedicinal as to source (T51-T65)

NOTE When no intent is indicated code to accidental. Undetermined intent is only for use when there is specific documentation in the record that the intent of the toxic effect cannot be determined.

Use additional code(s) for all associated manifestations of toxic effect, such as:
personal history of foreign body fully removed (Z87.821)
respiratory conditions due to external agents (J60-J70)
to identify any retained foreign body, if applicable (Z18.-)

EXCLUDES 1 contact with and (suspected) exposure to toxic substances (Z77.-)
AHA: 2017, 1Q, 39-40

√4ᵗʰ **T51** Toxic effect of alcohol

The appropriate 7th character is to be added to each code from category T51.
A   initial encounter
D   subsequent encounter
S   sequela

√5ᵗʰ **T51.0** Toxic effect of ethanol
Toxic effect of ethyl alcohol

EXCLUDES 2 acute alcohol intoxication or 'hangover' effects (F10.129, F10.229, F10.929)
drunkenness (F10.129, F10.229, F10.929)
pathological alcohol intoxication (F10.129, F10.229, F10.929)

√6ᵗʰ **T51.0X** Toxic effect of ethanol

√7ᵗʰ **T51.0X1** Toxic effect of ethanol, accidental (unintentional)
Toxic effect of ethanol NOS

2 √7ᵗʰ **T51.0X2** Toxic effect of ethanol, intentional self-harm   HCC

√7ᵗʰ **T51.0X3** Toxic effect of ethanol, assault

√7ᵗʰ **T51.0X4** Toxic effect of ethanol, undetermined

√5ᵗʰ **T51.1** Toxic effect of methanol
Toxic effect of methyl alcohol

√6ᵗʰ **T51.1X** Toxic effect of methanol

√7ᵗʰ **T51.1X1** Toxic effect of methanol, accidental (unintentional)
Toxic effect of methanol NOS

2 √7ᵗʰ **T51.1X2** Toxic effect of methanol, intentional self-harm   HCC

√7ᵗʰ **T51.1X3** Toxic effect of methanol, assault

√7ᵗʰ **T51.1X4** Toxic effect of methanol, undetermined

√5ᵗʰ **T51.2** Toxic effect of 2-Propanol
Toxic effect of isopropyl alcohol

√6ᵗʰ **T51.2X** Toxic effect of 2-Propanol

√7ᵗʰ **T51.2X1** Toxic effect of 2-Propanol, accidental (unintentional)
Toxic effect of 2-Propanol NOS

2 √7ᵗʰ **T51.2X2** Toxic effect of 2-Propanol, intentional self-harm   HCC

√7ᵗʰ **T51.2X3** Toxic effect of 2-Propanol, assault

√7ᵗʰ **T51.2X4** Toxic effect of 2-Propanol, undetermined

√5ᵗʰ **T51.3** Toxic effect of fusel oil
Toxic effect of amyl alcohol
Toxic effect of butyl [1-butanol] alcohol
Toxic effect of propyl [1-propanol] alcohol

√6ᵗʰ **T51.3X** Toxic effect of fusel oil

√7ᵗʰ **T51.3X1** Toxic effect of fusel oil, accidental (unintentional)
Toxic effect of fusel oil NOS

2 √7ᵗʰ **T51.3X2** Toxic effect of fusel oil, intentional self-harm   HCC

√7ᵗʰ **T51.3X3** Toxic effect of fusel oil, assault

√7ᵗʰ **T51.3X4** Toxic effect of fusel oil, undetermined

---

2   HCC with 7th character indicating initial encounter (A or B - specific to category) OR sequela.

EXCLUDES 1 Not coded here   **EXCLUDES 2** Not included here   N Newborn Age: 0   P Pediatric Age: 0-17   M Maternity Age: 12-55   A Adult Age: 15-124

1080   ICD-10-CM 2018

✓5th **T51.8　Toxic effect of other alcohols**

　✓6th **T51.8X　Toxic effect of other alcohols**

　　✓7th **T51.8X1　Toxic effect of other alcohols,** accidental (unintentional)
　　　　　　　　　Toxic effect of other alcohols NOS

　　2 ✓7th **T51.8X2　Toxic effect of other alcohols,** HCC
　　　　　　　　　intentional self-harm

　　✓7th **T51.8X3　Toxic effect of other alcohols,** assault

　　✓7th **T51.8X4　Toxic effect of other alcohols,**
　　　　　　　　　undetermined

✓5th **T51.9　Toxic effect of unspecified alcohol**

　✓x7th **T51.91　Toxic effect of unspecified alcohol,** accidental　▽
　　　　　　　　(unintentional)

　2 ✓x7th **T51.92　Toxic effect of unspecified alcohol,** HCC ▽
　　　　　　　　intentional self-harm

　✓x7th **T51.93　Toxic effect of unspecified alcohol,** assault　▽

　✓x7th **T51.94　Toxic effect of unspecified alcohol,** undetermined ▽

✓4th **T52　Toxic effect of organic solvents**

　　EXCLUDES 1　*halogen derivatives of aliphatic and aromatic hydrocarbons (T53.-)*

　　The appropriate 7th character is to be added to each code from category T52.
　　A　initial encounter
　　D　subsequent encounter
　　S　sequela

　✓5th **T52.0　Toxic effects of petroleum products**
　　　　Toxic effects of ether petroleum
　　　　Toxic effects of gasoline [petrol]
　　　　Toxic effects of kerosene [paraffin oil]
　　　　Toxic effects of naphtha petroleum
　　　　Toxic effects of paraffin wax
　　　　Toxic effects of spirit petroleum

　　✓6th **T52.0X　Toxic effects of petroleum products**

　　　✓7th **T52.0X1　Toxic effect of petroleum products,** accidental (unintentional)
　　　　　　　　　　Toxic effects of petroleum products NOS

　　　2 ✓7th **T52.0X2　Toxic effect of petroleum products,** HCC
　　　　　　　　　　intentional self-harm

　　　✓7th **T52.0X3　Toxic effect of petroleum products,** assault

　　　✓7th **T52.0X4　Toxic effect of petroleum products,** undetermined

　✓5th **T52.1　Toxic effects of benzene**

　　EXCLUDES 1　*homologues of benzene (T52.2)*
　　　　　　　nitroderivatives and aminoderivatives of benzene and its homologues (T65.3)

　　✓6th **T52.1X　Toxic effects of benzene**

　　　✓7th **T52.1X1　Toxic effect of benzene,** accidental (unintentional)
　　　　　　　　　　Toxic effects of benzene NOS

　　　2 ✓7th **T52.1X2　Toxic effect of benzene,** intentional HCC
　　　　　　　　　　self-harm

　　　✓7th **T52.1X3　Toxic effect of benzene,** assault

　　　✓7th **T52.1X4　Toxic effect of benzene,** undetermined

　✓5th **T52.2　Toxic effects of homologues of benzene**
　　　　Toxic effects of toluene [methylbenzene]
　　　　Toxic effects of xylene [dimethylbenzene]

　　✓6th **T52.2X　Toxic effects of homologues of benzene**

　　　✓7th **T52.2X1　Toxic effect of homologues of benzene,** accidental (unintentional)
　　　　　　　　　　Toxic effects of homologues of benzene NOS

　　　2 ✓7th **T52.2X2　Toxic effect of homologues of benzene,** intentional self-harm HCC

　　　✓7th **T52.2X3　Toxic effect of homologues of benzene,** assault

　　　✓7th **T52.2X4　Toxic effect of homologues of benzene,** undetermined

　✓5th **T52.3　Toxic effects of glycols**

　　✓6th **T52.3X　Toxic effects of glycols**

　　　✓7th **T52.3X1　Toxic effect of glycols,** accidental (unintentional)
　　　　　　　　　　Toxic effects of glycols NOS

2 ✓7th **T52.3X2　Toxic effect of glycols,** intentional HCC
　　　　　　　self-harm

✓7th **T52.3X3　Toxic effect of glycols,** assault

✓7th **T52.3X4　Toxic effect of glycols,** undetermined

✓5th **T52.4　Toxic effects of ketones**

　✓6th **T52.4X　Toxic effects of ketones**

　　✓7th **T52.4X1　Toxic effect of ketones,** accidental (unintentional)
　　　　　　　　　Toxic effects of ketones NOS

　　2 ✓7th **T52.4X2　Toxic effect of ketones,** intentional HCC
　　　　　　　　　self-harm

　　✓7th **T52.4X3　Toxic effect of ketones,** assault

　　✓7th **T52.4X4　Toxic effect of ketones,** undetermined

✓5th **T52.8　Toxic effects of other organic solvents**

　✓6th **T52.8X　Toxic effects of other organic solvents**

　　✓7th **T52.8X1　Toxic effects of other organic solvents,** accidental (unintentional)
　　　　　　　　　Toxic effects of other organic solvents NOS

　　2 ✓7th **T52.8X2　Toxic effect of other organic solvents,** HCC
　　　　　　　　　intentional self-harm

　　✓7th **T52.8X3　Toxic effect of other organic solvents,** assault

　　✓7th **T52.8X4　Toxic effect of other organic solvents,** undetermined

✓5th **T52.9　Toxic effects of unspecified organic solvent**

　✓x7th **T52.91　Toxic effect of unspecified organic solvent,** ▽
　　　　　　　accidental (unintentional)

　2 ✓x7th **T52.92　Toxic effect of unspecified organic solvent,** HCC ▽
　　　　　　　intentional self-harm

　✓x7th **T52.93　Toxic effect of unspecified organic solvent,** ▽
　　　　　　　assault

　✓x7th **T52.94　Toxic effect of unspecified organic solvent,** ▽
　　　　　　　undetermined

✓4th **T53　Toxic effect of halogen derivatives of aliphatic and aromatic hydrocarbons**

　　The appropriate 7th character is to be added to each code from category T53.
　　A　initial encounter
　　D　subsequent encounter
　　S　sequela

　✓5th **T53.0　Toxic effects of carbon tetrachloride**
　　　　Toxic effects of tetrachloromethane

　　✓6th **T53.0X　Toxic effects of carbon tetrachloride**

　　　✓7th **T53.0X1　Toxic effect of carbon tetrachloride,** accidental (unintentional)
　　　　　　　　　　Toxic effects of carbon tetrachloride NOS

　　　2 ✓7th **T53.0X2　Toxic effect of carbon tetrachloride,** HCC
　　　　　　　　　　intentional self-harm

　　　✓7th **T53.0X3　Toxic effect of carbon tetrachloride,** assault

　　　✓7th **T53.0X4　Toxic effect of carbon tetrachloride,** undetermined

　✓5th **T53.1　Toxic effects of chloroform**
　　　　Toxic effects of trichloromethane

　　✓6th **T53.1X　Toxic effects of chloroform**

　　　✓7th **T53.1X1　Toxic effect of chloroform,** accidental (unintentional)
　　　　　　　　　　Toxic effects of chloroform NOS

　　　2 ✓7th **T53.1X2　Toxic effect of chloroform,** HCC
　　　　　　　　　　intentional self-harm

　　　✓7th **T53.1X3　Toxic effect of chloroform,** assault

　　　✓7th **T53.1X4　Toxic effect of chloroform,** undetermined

　✓5th **T53.2　Toxic effects of trichloroethylene**
　　　　Toxic effects of trichloroethene

　　✓6th **T53.2X　Toxic effects of trichloroethylene**

　　　✓7th **T53.2X1　Toxic effect of trichloroethylene,** accidental (unintentional)
　　　　　　　　　　Toxic effects of trichloroethylene NOS

　　　2 ✓7th **T53.2X2　Toxic effect of trichloroethylene,** HCC
　　　　　　　　　　intentional self-harm

　　　✓7th **T53.2X3　Toxic effect of trichloroethylene,** assault

---

2　HCC with 7th character indicating initial encounter (A or B - specific to category) OR sequela.

✓ Additional Character Req　　✓x7th Placeholder Alert　　Manifestation　　HCC CMS-HCC Condition　　▽ Unspecified Code　　▶◀ Revised Text　　● New Code　　▲ Revised Code Title

✓7ᵗʰ **T53.2X4** **Toxic effect of trichloroethylene,** undetermined

✓5ᵗʰ **T53.3** **Toxic effects of tetrachloroethylene**
Toxic effects of perchloroethylene
Toxic effect of tetrachloroethene

  ✓6ᵗʰ **T53.3X** **Toxic effects of** tetrachloroethylene

    ✓7ᵗʰ **T53.3X1** **Toxic effect of tetrachloroethylene,** accidental (unintentional)
Toxic effects of tetrachloroethylene NOS

    2 ✓7ᵗʰ **T53.3X2** **Toxic effect of tetrachloroethylene,** intentional self-harm   HCC

    ✓7ᵗʰ **T53.3X3** **Toxic effect of tetrachloroethylene,** assault

    ✓7ᵗʰ **T53.3X4** **Toxic effect of tetrachloroethylene,** undetermined

✓5ᵗʰ **T53.4** **Toxic effects of dichloromethane**
Toxic effects of methylene chloride

  ✓6ᵗʰ **T53.4X** **Toxic effects of** dichloromethane

    ✓7ᵗʰ **T53.4X1** **Toxic effect of dichloromethane,** accidental (unintentional)
Toxic effects of dichloromethane NOS

    2 ✓7ᵗʰ **T53.4X2** **Toxic effect of dichloromethane,** intentional self-harm   HCC

    ✓7ᵗʰ **T53.4X3** **Toxic effect of dichloromethane,** assault

    ✓7ᵗʰ **T53.4X4** **Toxic effect of dichloromethane,** undetermined

✓5ᵗʰ **T53.5** **Toxic effects of chlorofluorocarbons**

  ✓6ᵗʰ **T53.5X** **Toxic effects of** chlorofluorocarbons

    ✓7ᵗʰ **T53.5X1** **Toxic effect of chlorofluorocarbons,** accidental (unintentional)
Toxic effects of chlorofluorocarbons NOS

    2 ✓7ᵗʰ **T53.5X2** **Toxic effect of chlorofluorocarbons,** intentional self-harm   HCC

    ✓7ᵗʰ **T53.5X3** **Toxic effect of chlorofluorocarbons,** assault

    ✓7ᵗʰ **T53.5X4** **Toxic effect of chlorofluorocarbons,** undetermined

✓5ᵗʰ **T53.6** **Toxic effects of other halogen derivatives of aliphatic hydrocarbons**

  ✓6ᵗʰ **T53.6X** **Toxic effects of other** halogen derivatives of aliphatic hydrocarbons

    ✓7ᵗʰ **T53.6X1** **Toxic effect of other halogen derivatives of aliphatic hydrocarbons,** accidental (unintentional)
Toxic effects of other halogen derivatives of aliphatic hydrocarbons NOS

    2 ✓7ᵗʰ **T53.6X2** **Toxic effect of other halogen derivatives of aliphatic hydrocarbons,** intentional self-harm   HCC

    ✓7ᵗʰ **T53.6X3** **Toxic effect of other halogen derivatives of aliphatic hydrocarbons,** assault

    ✓7ᵗʰ **T53.6X4** **Toxic effect of other halogen derivatives of aliphatic hydrocarbons,** undetermined

✓5ᵗʰ **T53.7** **Toxic effects of other halogen derivatives of aromatic hydrocarbons**

  ✓6ᵗʰ **T53.7X** **Toxic effects of other** halogen derivatives of aromatic hydrocarbons

    ✓7ᵗʰ **T53.7X1** **Toxic effect of other halogen derivatives of aromatic hydrocarbons,** accidental (unintentional)
Toxic effects of other halogen derivatives of aromatic hydrocarbons NOS

    2 ✓7ᵗʰ **T53.7X2** **Toxic effect of other halogen derivatives of aromatic hydrocarbons,** intentional self-harm   HCC

    ✓7ᵗʰ **T53.7X3** **Toxic effect of other halogen derivatives of aromatic hydrocarbons,** assault

    ✓7ᵗʰ **T53.7X4** **Toxic effect of other halogen derivatives of aromatic hydrocarbons,** undetermined

✓5ᵗʰ **T53.9** **Toxic effects of unspecified halogen derivatives of aliphatic and aromatic hydrocarbons**

  ✓x7ᵗʰ **T53.91** **Toxic effect of unspecified halogen derivatives of aliphatic and aromatic hydrocarbons,** accidental (unintentional)   ▽

---

2 ✓x7ᵗʰ **T53.92** **Toxic effect of unspecified halogen derivatives of aliphatic and aromatic hydrocarbons,** intentional self-harm   HCC ▽

  ✓x7ᵗʰ **T53.93** **Toxic effect of unspecified halogen derivatives of aliphatic and aromatic hydrocarbons,** assault   ▽

  ✓x7ᵗʰ **T53.94** **Toxic effect of unspecified halogen derivatives of aliphatic and aromatic hydrocarbons,** undetermined   ▽

✓4ᵗʰ **T54** **Toxic effect of corrosive substances**

> The appropriate 7th character is to be added to each code from category T54.
> A   initial encounter
> D   subsequent encounter
> S   sequela

✓5ᵗʰ **T54.0** **Toxic effects of phenol and phenol homologues**

  ✓6ᵗʰ **T54.0X** **Toxic effects of** phenol and phenol homologues

    ✓7ᵗʰ **T54.0X1** **Toxic effect of phenol and phenol homologues,** accidental (unintentional)
Toxic effects of phenol and phenol homologues NOS

    2 ✓7ᵗʰ **T54.0X2** **Toxic effect of phenol and phenol homologues,** intentional self-harm   HCC

    ✓7ᵗʰ **T54.0X3** **Toxic effect of phenol and phenol homologues,** assault

    ✓7ᵗʰ **T54.0X4** **Toxic effect of phenol and phenol homologues,** undetermined

✓5ᵗʰ **T54.1** **Toxic effects of other corrosive organic compounds**

  ✓6ᵗʰ **T54.1X** **Toxic effects of other corrosive organic compounds**

    ✓7ᵗʰ **T54.1X1** **Toxic effect of other corrosive organic compounds,** accidental (unintentional)
Toxic effects of other corrosive organic compounds NOS

    2 ✓7ᵗʰ **T54.1X2** **Toxic effect of other corrosive organic compounds,** intentional self-harm   HCC

    ✓7ᵗʰ **T54.1X3** **Toxic effect of other corrosive organic compounds,** assault

    ✓7ᵗʰ **T54.1X4** **Toxic effect of other corrosive organic compounds,** undetermined

✓5ᵗʰ **T54.2** **Toxic effects of corrosive acids and acid-like substances**
Toxic effects of hydrochloric acid
Toxic effects of sulfuric acid

  ✓6ᵗʰ **T54.2X** **Toxic effects of corrosive** acids and acid-like substances

    ✓7ᵗʰ **T54.2X1** **Toxic effect of corrosive acids and acid-like substances,** accidental (unintentional)
Toxic effects of corrosive acids and acid-like substances NOS

    2 ✓7ᵗʰ **T54.2X2** **Toxic effect of corrosive acids and acid-like substances,** intentional self-harm   HCC

    ✓7ᵗʰ **T54.2X3** **Toxic effect of corrosive acids and acid-like substances,** assault

    ✓7ᵗʰ **T54.2X4** **Toxic effect of corrosive acids and acid-like substances,** undetermined

✓5ᵗʰ **T54.3** **Toxic effects of corrosive alkalis and alkali-like substances**
Toxic effects of potassium hydroxide
Toxic effects of sodium hydroxide

  ✓6ᵗʰ **T54.3X** **Toxic effects of corrosive** alkalis and alkali-like substances

    ✓7ᵗʰ **T54.3X1** **Toxic effect of corrosive alkalis and alkali-like substances,** accidental (unintentional)
Toxic effects of corrosive alkalis and alkali-like substances NOS

    2 ✓7ᵗʰ **T54.3X2** **Toxic effect of corrosive alkalis and alkali-like substances,** intentional self-harm   HCC

    ✓7ᵗʰ **T54.3X3** **Toxic effect of corrosive alkalis and alkali-like substances,** assault

    ✓7ᵗʰ **T54.3X4** **Toxic effect of corrosive alkalis and alkali-like substances,** undetermined

✓5ᵗʰ **T54.9** **Toxic effects of unspecified corrosive substance**

  ✓x7ᵗʰ **T54.91** **Toxic effect of unspecified corrosive substance,** accidental (unintentional)   ▽

---

2   HCC with 7th character indicating initial encounter (A or B - specific to category) OR sequela.

EXCLUDES 1 Not coded here   EXCLUDES 2 Not included here   N Newborn Age: 0   P Pediatric Age: 0-17   M Maternity Age: 12-55   A Adult Age: 15-124

1082   ICD-10-CM 2018

2 ✓x7ᵗʰ **T54.92** Toxic effect of unspecified corrosive substance, intentional self-harm   HCC ▽

   ✓x7ᵗʰ **T54.93** Toxic effect of unspecified corrosive substance, assault   ▽

   ✓x7ᵗʰ **T54.94** Toxic effect of unspecified corrosive substance, undetermined   ▽

✓4ᵗʰ **T55** Toxic effect of soaps and detergents

> The appropriate 7th character is to be added to each code from category T55.
> A   initial encounter
> D   subsequent encounter
> S   sequela

  ✓5ᵗʰ **T55.0** Toxic effect of soaps

    ✓6ᵗʰ **T55.0X** Toxic effect of soaps

      ✓7ᵗʰ **T55.0X1** Toxic effect of soaps, accidental (unintentional)
           Toxic effect of soaps NOS

     2 ✓7ᵗʰ **T55.0X2** Toxic effect of soaps, intentional self-harm   HCC

      ✓7ᵗʰ **T55.0X3** Toxic effect of soaps, assault

      ✓7ᵗʰ **T55.0X4** Toxic effect of soaps, undetermined

  ✓5ᵗʰ **T55.1** Toxic effect of detergents

    ✓6ᵗʰ **T55.1X** Toxic effect of detergents

      ✓7ᵗʰ **T55.1X1** Toxic effect of detergents, accidental (unintentional)
           Toxic effect of detergents NOS

     2 ✓7ᵗʰ **T55.1X2** Toxic effect of detergents, intentional self-harm   HCC

      ✓7ᵗʰ **T55.1X3** Toxic effect of detergents, assault

      ✓7ᵗʰ **T55.1X4** Toxic effect of detergents, undetermined

✓4ᵗʰ **T56** Toxic effect of metals

   INCLUDES toxic effects of fumes and vapors of metals
           toxic effects of metals from all sources, except medicinal substances

   Use additional code to identify any retained metal foreign body, if applicable (Z18.0-, T18.1-)

   EXCLUDES 1   arsenic and its compounds (T57.0)
            manganese and its compounds (T57.2)

> The appropriate 7th character is to be added to each code from category T56.
> A   initial encounter
> D   subsequent encounter
> S   sequela

  ✓5ᵗʰ **T56.0** Toxic effects of lead and its compounds

    ✓6ᵗʰ **T56.0X** Toxic effects of lead and its compounds

      ✓7ᵗʰ **T56.0X1** Toxic effect of lead and its compounds, accidental (unintentional)
           Toxic effects of lead and its compounds NOS

     2 ✓7ᵗʰ **T56.0X2** Toxic effect of lead and its compounds, intentional self-harm   HCC

      ✓7ᵗʰ **T56.0X3** Toxic effect of lead and its compounds, assault

      ✓7ᵗʰ **T56.0X4** Toxic effect of lead and its compounds, undetermined

  ✓5ᵗʰ **T56.1** Toxic effects of mercury and its compounds

    ✓6ᵗʰ **T56.1X** Toxic effects of mercury and its compounds

      ✓7ᵗʰ **T56.1X1** Toxic effect of mercury and its compounds, accidental (unintentional)
           Toxic effects of mercury and its compounds NOS

     2 ✓7ᵗʰ **T56.1X2** Toxic effect of mercury and its compounds, intentional self-harm   HCC

      ✓7ᵗʰ **T56.1X3** Toxic effect of mercury and its compounds, assault

      ✓7ᵗʰ **T56.1X4** Toxic effect of mercury and its compounds, undetermined

  ✓5ᵗʰ **T56.2** Toxic effects of chromium and its compounds

    ✓6ᵗʰ **T56.2X** Toxic effects of chromium and its compounds

      ✓7ᵗʰ **T56.2X1** Toxic effect of chromium and its compounds, accidental (unintentional)
           Toxic effects of chromium and its compounds NOS

     2 ✓7ᵗʰ **T56.2X2** Toxic effect of chromium and its compounds, intentional self-harm   HCC

      ✓7ᵗʰ **T56.2X3** Toxic effect of chromium and its compounds, assault

      ✓7ᵗʰ **T56.2X4** Toxic effect of chromium and its compounds, undetermined

  ✓5ᵗʰ **T56.3** Toxic effects of cadmium and its compounds

    ✓6ᵗʰ **T56.3X** Toxic effects of cadmium and its compounds

      ✓7ᵗʰ **T56.3X1** Toxic effect of cadmium and its compounds, accidental (unintentional)
           Toxic effects of cadmium and its compounds NOS

     2 ✓7ᵗʰ **T56.3X2** Toxic effect of cadmium and its compounds, intentional self-harm   HCC

      ✓7ᵗʰ **T56.3X3** Toxic effect of cadmium and its compounds, assault

      ✓7ᵗʰ **T56.3X4** Toxic effect of cadmium and its compounds, undetermined

  ✓5ᵗʰ **T56.4** Toxic effects of copper and its compounds

    ✓6ᵗʰ **T56.4X** Toxic effects of copper and its compounds

      ✓7ᵗʰ **T56.4X1** Toxic effect of copper and its compounds, accidental (unintentional)
           Toxic effects of copper and its compounds NOS

     2 ✓7ᵗʰ **T56.4X2** Toxic effect of copper and its compounds, intentional self-harm   HCC

      ✓7ᵗʰ **T56.4X3** Toxic effect of copper and its compounds, assault

      ✓7ᵗʰ **T56.4X4** Toxic effect of copper and its compounds, undetermined

  ✓5ᵗʰ **T56.5** Toxic effects of zinc and its compounds

    ✓6ᵗʰ **T56.5X** Toxic effects of zinc and its compounds

      ✓7ᵗʰ **T56.5X1** Toxic effect of zinc and its compounds, accidental (unintentional)
           Toxic effects of zinc and its compounds NOS

     2 ✓7ᵗʰ **T56.5X2** Toxic effect of zinc and its compounds, intentional self-harm   HCC

      ✓7ᵗʰ **T56.5X3** Toxic effect of zinc and its compounds, assault

      ✓7ᵗʰ **T56.5X4** Toxic effect of zinc and its compounds, undetermined

  ✓5ᵗʰ **T56.6** Toxic effects of tin and its compounds

    ✓6ᵗʰ **T56.6X** Toxic effects of tin and its compounds

      ✓7ᵗʰ **T56.6X1** Toxic effect of tin and its compounds, accidental (unintentional)
           Toxic effects of tin and its compounds NOS

     2 ✓7ᵗʰ **T56.6X2** Toxic effect of tin and its compounds, intentional self-harm   HCC

      ✓7ᵗʰ **T56.6X3** Toxic effect of tin and its compounds, assault

      ✓7ᵗʰ **T56.6X4** Toxic effect of tin and its compounds, undetermined

  ✓5ᵗʰ **T56.7** Toxic effects of beryllium and its compounds

    ✓6ᵗʰ **T56.7X** Toxic effects of beryllium and its compounds

      ✓7ᵗʰ **T56.7X1** Toxic effect of beryllium and its compounds, accidental (unintentional)
           Toxic effects of beryllium and its compounds NOS

     2 ✓7ᵗʰ **T56.7X2** Toxic effect of beryllium and its compounds, intentional self-harm   HCC

      ✓7ᵗʰ **T56.7X3** Toxic effect of beryllium and its compounds, assault

      ✓7ᵗʰ **T56.7X4** Toxic effect of beryllium and its compounds, undetermined

  ✓5ᵗʰ **T56.8** Toxic effects of other metals

    ✓6ᵗʰ **T56.81** Toxic effect of thallium

      ✓7ᵗʰ **T56.811** Toxic effect of thallium, accidental (unintentional)
           Toxic effect of thallium NOS

     2 ✓7ᵗʰ **T56.812** Toxic effect of thallium, intentional self-harm   HCC

      ✓7ᵗʰ **T56.813** Toxic effect of thallium, assault

      ✓7ᵗʰ **T56.814** Toxic effect of thallium, undetermined

---

2   HCC with 7th character indicating initial encounter (A or B - specific to category) OR sequela.

☑ Additional Character Req   ✓x7ᵗʰ Placeholder Alert   Manifestation   HCC CMS-HCC Condition   ▽ Unspecified Code   ►◄ Revised Text   ● New Code   ▲ Revised Code Title

Chapter 19. Injury, Poisoning, and Certain Other Consequences of External Causes

√6ᵗʰ **T56.89** **Toxic effects of other metals**

     √7ᵗʰ **T56.891** **Toxic effect of other metals, accidental (unintentional)**
         Toxic effects of other metals NOS

     2 √7ᵗʰ **T56.892** **Toxic effect of other metals, intentional self-harm** HCC

     √7ᵗʰ **T56.893** **Toxic effect of other metals, assault**

     √7ᵗʰ **T56.894** **Toxic effect of other metals, undetermined**

√5ᵗʰ **T56.9** **Toxic effects of unspecified metal**

     √x7ᵗʰ **T56.91** **Toxic effect of unspecified metal, accidental (unintentional)** ▽

     2 √x7ᵗʰ **T56.92** **Toxic effect of unspecified metal, intentional self-harm** HCC ▽

     √x7ᵗʰ **T56.93** **Toxic effect of unspecified metal, assault** ▽

     √x7ᵗʰ **T56.94** **Toxic effect of unspecified metal, undetermined** ▽

√4ᵗʰ **T57** **Toxic effect of other inorganic substances**

> The appropriate 7th character is to be added to each code from category T57.
> A   initial encounter
> D   subsequent encounter
> S   sequela

√5ᵗʰ **T57.0** **Toxic effect of arsenic and its compounds**

     √6ᵗʰ **T57.0X** **Toxic effect of arsenic and its compounds**

         √7ᵗʰ **T57.0X1** **Toxic effect of arsenic and its compounds, accidental (unintentional)**
             Toxic effect of arsenic and its compounds NOS

         2 √7ᵗʰ **T57.0X2** **Toxic effect of arsenic and its compounds, intentional self-harm** HCC

         √7ᵗʰ **T57.0X3** **Toxic effect of arsenic and its compounds, assault**

         √7ᵗʰ **T57.0X4** **Toxic effect of arsenic and its compounds, undetermined**

√5ᵗʰ **T57.1** **Toxic effect of phosphorus and its compounds**

     EXCLUDES 1   organophosphate insecticides (T60.0)

     √6ᵗʰ **T57.1X** **Toxic effect of phosphorus and its compounds**

         √7ᵗʰ **T57.1X1** **Toxic effect of phosphorus and its compounds, accidental (unintentional)**
             Toxic effect of phosphorus and its compounds NOS

         2 √7ᵗʰ **T57.1X2** **Toxic effect of phosphorus and its compounds, intentional self-harm** HCC

         √7ᵗʰ **T57.1X3** **Toxic effect of phosphorus and its compounds, assault**

         √7ᵗʰ **T57.1X4** **Toxic effect of phosphorus and its compounds, undetermined**

√5ᵗʰ **T57.2** **Toxic effect of manganese and its compounds**

     √6ᵗʰ **T57.2X** **Toxic effect of manganese and its compounds**

         √7ᵗʰ **T57.2X1** **Toxic effect of manganese and its compounds, accidental (unintentional)**
             Toxic effect of manganese and its compounds NOS

         2 √7ᵗʰ **T57.2X2** **Toxic effect of manganese and its compounds, intentional self-harm** HCC

         √7ᵗʰ **T57.2X3** **Toxic effect of manganese and its compounds, assault**

         √7ᵗʰ **T57.2X4** **Toxic effect of manganese and its compounds, undetermined**

√5ᵗʰ **T57.3** **Toxic effect of hydrogen cyanide**

     √6ᵗʰ **T57.3X** **Toxic effect of hydrogen cyanide**

         √7ᵗʰ **T57.3X1** **Toxic effect of hydrogen cyanide, accidental (unintentional)**
             Toxic effect of hydrogen cyanide NOS

         2 √7ᵗʰ **T57.3X2** **Toxic effect of hydrogen cyanide, intentional self-harm** HCC

         √7ᵗʰ **T57.3X3** **Toxic effect of hydrogen cyanide, assault**

         √7ᵗʰ **T57.3X4** **Toxic effect of hydrogen cyanide, undetermined**

√5ᵗʰ **T57.8** **Toxic effect of other specified inorganic substances**

     √6ᵗʰ **T57.8X** **Toxic effect of other specified inorganic substances**

         √7ᵗʰ **T57.8X1** **Toxic effect of other specified inorganic substances, accidental (unintentional)**
             Toxic effect of other specified inorganic substances NOS

         2 √7ᵗʰ **T57.8X2** **Toxic effect of other specified inorganic substances, intentional self-harm** HCC

         √7ᵗʰ **T57.8X3** **Toxic effect of other specified inorganic substances, assault**

         √7ᵗʰ **T57.8X4** **Toxic effect of other specified inorganic substances, undetermined**

√5ᵗʰ **T57.9** **Toxic effect of unspecified inorganic substance**

     √x7ᵗʰ **T57.91** **Toxic effect of unspecified inorganic substance, accidental (unintentional)** ▽

     2 √x7ᵗʰ **T57.92** **Toxic effect of unspecified inorganic substance, intentional self-harm** HCC ▽

     √x7ᵗʰ **T57.93** **Toxic effect of unspecified inorganic substance, assault** ▽

     √x7ᵗʰ **T57.94** **Toxic effect of unspecified inorganic substance, undetermined** ▽

√4ᵗʰ **T58** **Toxic effect of carbon monoxide**

     INCLUDES   asphyxiation from carbon monoxide
                toxic effect of carbon monoxide from all sources

> The appropriate 7th character is to be added to each code from category T58.
> A   initial encounter
> D   subsequent encounter
> S   sequela

√5ᵗʰ **T58.0** **Toxic effect of carbon monoxide from motor vehicle exhaust**
     Toxic effect of exhaust gas from gas engine
     Toxic effect of exhaust gas from motor pump

     √x7ᵗʰ **T58.01** **Toxic effect of carbon monoxide from motor vehicle exhaust, accidental (unintentional)**

     2 √x7ᵗʰ **T58.02** **Toxic effect of carbon monoxide from motor vehicle exhaust, intentional self-harm** HCC

     √x7ᵗʰ **T58.03** **Toxic effect of carbon monoxide from motor vehicle exhaust, assault**

     √x7ᵗʰ **T58.04** **Toxic effect of carbon monoxide from motor vehicle exhaust, undetermined**

√5ᵗʰ **T58.1** **Toxic effect of carbon monoxide from utility gas**
     Toxic effect of acetylene
     Toxic effect of gas NOS used for lighting, heating, cooking
     Toxic effect of water gas

     √x7ᵗʰ **T58.11** **Toxic effect of carbon monoxide from utility gas, accidental (unintentional)**

     2 √x7ᵗʰ **T58.12** **Toxic effect of carbon monoxide from utility gas, intentional self-harm** HCC

     √x7ᵗʰ **T58.13** **Toxic effect of carbon monoxide from utility gas, assault**

     √x7ᵗʰ **T58.14** **Toxic effect of carbon monoxide from utility gas, undetermined**

√5ᵗʰ **T58.2** **Toxic effect of carbon monoxide from incomplete combustion of other domestic fuels**
     Toxic effect of carbon monoxide from incomplete combustion of coal, coke, kerosene, wood

     √6ᵗʰ **T58.2X** **Toxic effect of carbon monoxide from incomplete combustion of other domestic fuels**

         √7ᵗʰ **T58.2X1** **Toxic effect of carbon monoxide from incomplete combustion of other domestic fuels, accidental (unintentional)**

         2 √7ᵗʰ **T58.2X2** **Toxic effect of carbon monoxide from incomplete combustion of other domestic fuels, intentional self-harm** HCC

         √7ᵗʰ **T58.2X3** **Toxic effect of carbon monoxide from incomplete combustion of other domestic fuels, assault**

         √7ᵗʰ **T58.2X4** **Toxic effect of carbon monoxide from incomplete combustion of other domestic fuels, undetermined**

---

2   HCC with 7th character indicating initial encounter (A or B - specific to category) OR sequela.

EXCLUDES 1 Not coded here   EXCLUDES 2 Not included here   N Newborn Age: 0   P Pediatric Age: 0-17   M Maternity Age: 12-55   A Adult Age: 15-124

✓5ᵗʰ **T58.8** **Toxic effect of carbon monoxide from other source**
Toxic effect of carbon monoxide from blast furnace gas
Toxic effect of carbon monoxide from fuels in industrial use
Toxic effect of carbon monoxide from kiln vapor

   ✓6ᵗʰ **T58.8X** **Toxic effect of carbon monoxide from other source**

     ✓7ᵗʰ **T58.8X1** **Toxic effect of carbon monoxide from other source, accidental (unintentional)**

     2 ✓7ᵗʰ **T58.8X2** **Toxic effect of carbon monoxide from other source, intentional self-harm** HCC

     ✓7ᵗʰ **T58.8X3** **Toxic effect of carbon monoxide from other source, assault**

     ✓7ᵗʰ **T58.8X4** **Toxic effect of carbon monoxide from other source, undetermined**

✓5ᵗʰ **T58.9** **Toxic effect of carbon monoxide from unspecified source**

   ✓x7ᵗʰ **T58.91** **Toxic effect of carbon monoxide from unspecified source, accidental (unintentional)** ▽

   2 ✓x7ᵗʰ **T58.92** **Toxic effect of carbon monoxide from unspecified source, intentional self-harm** HCC ▽

   ✓x7ᵗʰ **T58.93** **Toxic effect of carbon monoxide from unspecified source, assault** ▽

   ✓x7ᵗʰ **T58.94** **Toxic effect of carbon monoxide from unspecified source, undetermined** ▽

✓4ᵗʰ **T59** **Toxic effect of other gases, fumes and vapors**
   INCLUDES   aerosol propellants
   EXCLUDES 1   *chlorofluorocarbons (T53.5)*

   The appropriate 7th character is to be added to each code from category T59.
   A   initial encounter
   D   subsequent encounter
   S   sequela

✓5ᵗʰ **T59.0** **Toxic effect of nitrogen oxides**

   ✓6ᵗʰ **T59.0X** **Toxic effect of nitrogen oxides**

     ✓7ᵗʰ **T59.0X1** **Toxic effect of nitrogen oxides, accidental (unintentional)**
Toxic effect of nitrogen oxides NOS

     2 ✓7ᵗʰ **T59.0X2** **Toxic effect of nitrogen oxides, intentional self-harm** HCC

     ✓7ᵗʰ **T59.0X3** **Toxic effect of nitrogen oxides, assault**

     ✓7ᵗʰ **T59.0X4** **Toxic effect of nitrogen oxides, undetermined**

✓5ᵗʰ **T59.1** **Toxic effect of sulfur dioxide**

   ✓6ᵗʰ **T59.1X** **Toxic effect of sulfur dioxide**

     ✓7ᵗʰ **T59.1X1** **Toxic effect of sulfur dioxide, accidental (unintentional)**
Toxic effect of sulfur dioxide NOS

     2 ✓7ᵗʰ **T59.1X2** **Toxic effect of sulfur dioxide, intentional self-harm** HCC

     ✓7ᵗʰ **T59.1X3** **Toxic effect of sulfur dioxide, assault**

     ✓7ᵗʰ **T59.1X4** **Toxic effect of sulfur dioxide, undetermined**

✓5ᵗʰ **T59.2** **Toxic effect of formaldehyde**

   ✓6ᵗʰ **T59.2X** **Toxic effect of formaldehyde**

     ✓7ᵗʰ **T59.2X1** **Toxic effect of formaldehyde, accidental (unintentional)**
Toxic effect of formaldehyde NOS

     2 ✓7ᵗʰ **T59.2X2** **Toxic effect of formaldehyde, intentional self-harm** HCC

     ✓7ᵗʰ **T59.2X3** **Toxic effect of formaldehyde, assault**

     ✓7ᵗʰ **T59.2X4** **Toxic effect of formaldehyde, undetermined**

✓5ᵗʰ **T59.3** **Toxic effect of lacrimogenic gas**
Toxic effect of tear gas

   ✓6ᵗʰ **T59.3X** **Toxic effect of lacrimogenic gas**

     ✓7ᵗʰ **T59.3X1** **Toxic effect of lacrimogenic gas, accidental (unintentional)**
Toxic effect of lacrimogenic gas NOS

     2 ✓7ᵗʰ **T59.3X2** **Toxic effect of lacrimogenic gas, intentional self-harm** HCC

     ✓7ᵗʰ **T59.3X3** **Toxic effect of lacrimogenic gas, assault**

     ✓7ᵗʰ **T59.3X4** **Toxic effect of lacrimogenic gas, undetermined**

✓5ᵗʰ **T59.4** **Toxic effect of chlorine gas**

   ✓6ᵗʰ **T59.4X** **Toxic effect of chlorine gas**

     ✓7ᵗʰ **T59.4X1** **Toxic effect of chlorine gas, accidental (unintentional)**
Toxic effect of chlorine gas NOS

     2 ✓7ᵗʰ **T59.4X2** **Toxic effect of chlorine gas, intentional self-harm** HCC

     ✓7ᵗʰ **T59.4X3** **Toxic effect of chlorine gas, assault**

     ✓7ᵗʰ **T59.4X4** **Toxic effect of chlorine gas, undetermined**

✓5ᵗʰ **T59.5** **Toxic effect of fluorine gas and hydrogen fluoride**

   ✓6ᵗʰ **T59.5X** **Toxic effect of fluorine gas and hydrogen fluoride**

     ✓7ᵗʰ **T59.5X1** **Toxic effect of fluorine gas and hydrogen fluoride, accidental (unintentional)**
Toxic effect of fluorine gas and hydrogen fluoride NOS

     2 ✓7ᵗʰ **T59.5X2** **Toxic effect of fluorine gas and hydrogen fluoride, intentional self-harm** HCC

     ✓7ᵗʰ **T59.5X3** **Toxic effect of fluorine gas and hydrogen fluoride, assault**

     ✓7ᵗʰ **T59.5X4** **Toxic effect of fluorine gas and hydrogen fluoride, undetermined**

✓5ᵗʰ **T59.6** **Toxic effect of hydrogen sulfide**

   ✓6ᵗʰ **T59.6X** **Toxic effect of hydrogen sulfide**

     ✓7ᵗʰ **T59.6X1** **Toxic effect of hydrogen sulfide, accidental (unintentional)**
Toxic effect of hydrogen sulfide NOS

     2 ✓7ᵗʰ **T59.6X2** **Toxic effect of hydrogen sulfide, intentional self-harm** HCC

     ✓7ᵗʰ **T59.6X3** **Toxic effect of hydrogen sulfide, assault**

     ✓7ᵗʰ **T59.6X4** **Toxic effect of hydrogen sulfide, undetermined**

✓5ᵗʰ **T59.7** **Toxic effect of carbon dioxide**

   ✓6ᵗʰ **T59.7X** **Toxic effect of carbon dioxide**

     ✓7ᵗʰ **T59.7X1** **Toxic effect of carbon dioxide, accidental (unintentional)**
Toxic effect of carbon dioxide NOS

     2 ✓7ᵗʰ **T59.7X2** **Toxic effect of carbon dioxide, intentional self-harm** HCC

     ✓7ᵗʰ **T59.7X3** **Toxic effect of carbon dioxide, assault**

     ✓7ᵗʰ **T59.7X4** **Toxic effect of carbon dioxide, undetermined**

✓5ᵗʰ **T59.8** **Toxic effect of other specified gases, fumes and vapors**

   ✓6ᵗʰ **T59.81** **Toxic effect of smoke**
Smoke inhalation
     EXCLUDES 2   *toxic effect of cigarette (tobacco) smoke (T65.22-)*

     ✓7ᵗʰ **T59.811** **Toxic effect of smoke, accidental (unintentional)**
Toxic effect of smoke NOS
AHA: 2013, 4Q, 121

     2 ✓7ᵗʰ **T59.812** **Toxic effect of smoke, intentional self-harm** HCC

     ✓7ᵗʰ **T59.813** **Toxic effect of smoke, assault**

     ✓7ᵗʰ **T59.814** **Toxic effect of smoke, undetermined**

   ✓6ᵗʰ **T59.89** **Toxic effect of other specified gases, fumes and vapors**

     ✓7ᵗʰ **T59.891** **Toxic effect of other specified gases, fumes and vapors, accidental (unintentional)**

     2 ✓7ᵗʰ **T59.892** **Toxic effect of other specified gases, fumes and vapors, intentional self-harm** HCC

     ✓7ᵗʰ **T59.893** **Toxic effect of other specified gases, fumes and vapors, assault**

     ✓7ᵗʰ **T59.894** **Toxic effect of other specified gases, fumes and vapors, undetermined**

✓5ᵗʰ **T59.9** **Toxic effect of unspecified gases, fumes and vapors**

   ✓x7ᵗʰ **T59.91** **Toxic effect of unspecified gases, fumes and vapors, accidental (unintentional)** ▽

   2 ✓x7ᵗʰ **T59.92** **Toxic effect of unspecified gases, fumes and vapors, intentional self-harm** HCC ▽

   ✓x7ᵗʰ **T59.93** **Toxic effect of unspecified gases, fumes and vapors, assault** ▽

---

2   HCC with 7th character indicating initial encounter (A or B - specific to category) OR sequela.

✓ Additional Character Req   ✓x7ᵗʰ Placeholder Alert   Manifestation   HCC CMS-HCC Condition   ▽ Unspecified Code   ▶◀ Revised Text   ● New Code   ▲ Revised Code Title

Chapter 19. Injury, Poisoning, and Certain Other Consequences of External Causes

√x7ᵗʰ **T59.94** **Toxic effect of unspecified gases, fumes and vapors,** undetermined ▽

√4ᵗʰ **T60** **Toxic effect of pesticides**
INCLUDES toxic effect of wood preservatives

The appropriate 7th character is to be added to each code from category T60.
A initial encounter
D subsequent encounter
S sequela

√5ᵗʰ **T60.0** **Toxic effect of organophosphate and carbamate insecticides**
√6ᵗʰ **T60.0X** **Toxic effect of** organophosphate and carbamate insecticides
√7ᵗʰ **T60.0X1** **Toxic effect of organophosphate and carbamate insecticides,** accidental **(unintentional)**
Toxic effect of organophosphate and carbamate insecticides NOS
2 √7ᵗʰ **T60.0X2** **Toxic effect of organophosphate and carbamate insecticides,** intentional self-harm   HCC
√7ᵗʰ **T60.0X3** **Toxic effect of organophosphate and carbamate insecticides,** assault
√7ᵗʰ **T60.0X4** **Toxic effect of organophosphate and carbamate insecticides,** undetermined

√5ᵗʰ **T60.1** **Toxic effect of halogenated insecticides**
EXCLUDES 1 chlorinated hydrocarbon (T53.-)
√6ᵗʰ **T60.1X** **Toxic effect of** halogenated insecticides
√7ᵗʰ **T60.1X1** **Toxic effect of halogenated insecticides,** accidental **(unintentional)**
Toxic effect of halogenated insecticides NOS
2 √7ᵗʰ **T60.1X2** **Toxic effect of halogenated insecticides,** intentional self-harm   HCC
√7ᵗʰ **T60.1X3** **Toxic effect of halogenated insecticides,** assault
√7ᵗʰ **T60.1X4** **Toxic effect of halogenated insecticides,** undetermined

√5ᵗʰ **T60.2** **Toxic effect of other insecticides**
√6ᵗʰ **T60.2X** **Toxic effect of other insecticides**
√7ᵗʰ **T60.2X1** **Toxic effect of other insecticides,** accidental **(unintentional)**
Toxic effect of other insecticides NOS
2 √7ᵗʰ **T60.2X2** **Toxic effect of other insecticides,** intentional self-harm   HCC
√7ᵗʰ **T60.2X3** **Toxic effect of other insecticides,** assault
√7ᵗʰ **T60.2X4** **Toxic effect of other insecticides,** undetermined

√5ᵗʰ **T60.3** **Toxic effect of herbicides and fungicides**
√6ᵗʰ **T60.3X** **Toxic effect of** herbicides and fungicides
√7ᵗʰ **T60.3X1** **Toxic effect of herbicides and fungicides,** accidental **(unintentional)**
Toxic effect of herbicides and fungicides NOS
2 √7ᵗʰ **T60.3X2** **Toxic effect of herbicides and fungicides,** intentional self-harm   HCC
√7ᵗʰ **T60.3X3** **Toxic effect of herbicides and fungicides,** assault
√7ᵗʰ **T60.3X4** **Toxic effect of herbicides and fungicides,** undetermined

√5ᵗʰ **T60.4** **Toxic effect of rodenticides**
EXCLUDES 1 strychnine and its salts (T65.1)
thallium (T56.81-)
√6ᵗʰ **T60.4X** **Toxic effect of** rodenticides
√7ᵗʰ **T60.4X1** **Toxic effect of rodenticides,** accidental **(unintentional)**
Toxic effect of rodenticides NOS
2 √7ᵗʰ **T60.4X2** **Toxic effect of rodenticides,** intentional self-harm   HCC
√7ᵗʰ **T60.4X3** **Toxic effect of rodenticides,** assault
√7ᵗʰ **T60.4X4** **Toxic effect of rodenticides,** undetermined

√5ᵗʰ **T60.8** **Toxic effect of other pesticides**
√6ᵗʰ **T60.8X** **Toxic effect of other pesticides**
√7ᵗʰ **T60.8X1** **Toxic effect of other pesticides,** accidental **(unintentional)**
Toxic effect of other pesticides NOS
2 √7ᵗʰ **T60.8X2** **Toxic effect of other pesticides,** intentional self-harm   HCC
√7ᵗʰ **T60.8X3** **Toxic effect of other pesticides,** assault
√7ᵗʰ **T60.8X4** **Toxic effect of other pesticides,** undetermined

√5ᵗʰ **T60.9** **Toxic effect of unspecified pesticide**
√x7ᵗʰ **T60.91** **Toxic effect of unspecified pesticide,** accidental **(unintentional)** ▽
2 √x7ᵗʰ **T60.92** **Toxic effect of unspecified pesticide,** intentional self-harm   HCC ▽
√x7ᵗʰ **T60.93** **Toxic effect of unspecified pesticide,** assault ▽
√x7ᵗʰ **T60.94** **Toxic effect of unspecified pesticide,** undetermined ▽

√4ᵗʰ **T61** **Toxic effect of noxious substances eaten as seafood**
EXCLUDES 1 allergic reaction to food, such as:
anaphylactic reaction or shock due to adverse food reaction (T78.0-)
bacterial foodborne intoxications (A05.-)
dermatitis (L23.6, L25.4, L27.2)
food protein-induced enterocolitis syndrome (K52.21)
food protein-induced enteropathy (K52.22)
gastroenteritis (noninfective) (K52.29)
toxic effect of aflatoxin and other mycotoxins (T64)
toxic effect of cyanides (T65.0-)
toxic effect of harmful algae bloom (T65.82-)
toxic effect of hydrogen cyanide (T57.3-)
toxic effect of mercury (T56.1-)
toxic effect of red tide (T65.82-)

The appropriate 7th character is to be added to each code from category T61.
A initial encounter
D subsequent encounter
S sequela

√5ᵗʰ **T61.0** **Ciguatera fish poisoning**
√x7ᵗʰ **T61.01** **Ciguatera fish poisoning,** accidental **(unintentional)**
2 √x7ᵗʰ **T61.02** **Ciguatera fish poisoning,** intentional self-harm   HCC
√x7ᵗʰ **T61.03** **Ciguatera fish poisoning,** assault
√x7ᵗʰ **T61.04** **Ciguatera fish poisoning,** undetermined

√5ᵗʰ **T61.1** **Scombroid fish poisoning**
Histamine-like syndrome
√x7ᵗʰ **T61.11** **Scombroid fish poisoning,** accidental **(unintentional)**
2 √x7ᵗʰ **T61.12** **Scombroid fish poisoning,** intentional self-harm   HCC
√x7ᵗʰ **T61.13** **Scombroid fish poisoning,** assault
√x7ᵗʰ **T61.14** **Scombroid fish poisoning,** undetermined

√5ᵗʰ **T61.7** **Other fish and shellfish poisoning**
√6ᵗʰ **T61.77** **Other** fish **poisoning**
√7ᵗʰ **T61.771** **Other fish poisoning,** accidental **(unintentional)**
2 √7ᵗʰ **T61.772** **Other fish poisoning,** intentional self-harm   HCC
√7ᵗʰ **T61.773** **Other fish poisoning,** assault
√7ᵗʰ **T61.774** **Other fish poisoning,** undetermined
√6ᵗʰ **T61.78** **Other** shellfish **poisoning**
√7ᵗʰ **T61.781** **Other shellfish poisoning,** accidental **(unintentional)**
2 √7ᵗʰ **T61.782** **Other shellfish poisoning,** intentional self-harm   HCC
√7ᵗʰ **T61.783** **Other shellfish poisoning,** assault
√7ᵗʰ **T61.784** **Other shellfish poisoning,** undetermined

√5ᵗʰ **T61.8** **Toxic effect of other seafood**
√6ᵗʰ **T61.8X** **Toxic effect of other seafood**
√7ᵗʰ **T61.8X1** **Toxic effect of other seafood,** accidental **(unintentional)**
2 √7ᵗʰ **T61.8X2** **Toxic effect of other seafood,** intentional self-harm   HCC
√7ᵗʰ **T61.8X3** **Toxic effect of other seafood,** assault

2   HCC with 7th character indicating initial encounter (A or B - specific to category) OR sequela.

EXCLUDES 1 Not coded here   EXCLUDES 2 Not included here   N Newborn Age: 0   P Pediatric Age: 0-17   M Maternity Age: 12-55   A Adult Age: 15-124

1086   ICD-10-CM 2018

√7ʰ **T61.8X4 Toxic effect of other seafood,** undetermined

√5ʰ **T61.9 Toxic effect of unspecified seafood**

  √x7ʰ **T61.91 Toxic effect of unspecified seafood,** accidental (unintentional) ▽

  2 √x7ʰ **T61.92 Toxic effect of unspecified seafood,** HCC ▽
intentional self-harm

  √x7ʰ **T61.93 Toxic effect of unspecified seafood,** assault ▽

  √x7ʰ **T61.94 Toxic effect of unspecified seafood,** undetermined ▽

√4ʰ **T62 Toxic effect of other noxious substances eaten as food**

EXCLUDES 1 *allergic reaction to food, such as:*
anaphylactic shock (reaction) due to adverse food reaction (T78.0-)
bacterial food borne intoxications (A05.-)
dermatitis (L23.6, L25.4, L27.2)
food protein-induced enterocolitis syndrome (K52.21)
food protein-induced enteropathy (K52.22)
gastroenteritis (noninfective) (K52.29)
toxic effect of aflatoxin and other mycotoxins (T64)
toxic effect of cyanides (T65.0-)
toxic effect of hydrogen cyanide (T57.3-)
toxic effect of mercury (T56.1-)

The appropriate 7th character is to be added to each code from category T62.
A   initial encounter
D   subsequent encounter
S   sequela

√5ʰ **T62.0 Toxic effect of ingested mushrooms**

  √6ʰ **T62.0X Toxic effect of** ingested mushrooms

    √7ʰ **T62.0X1 Toxic effect of ingested mushrooms,** accidental (unintentional)
Toxic effect of ingested mushrooms NOS

    2 √7ʰ **T62.0X2 Toxic effect of ingested mushrooms,** HCC
intentional self-harm

    √7ʰ **T62.0X3 Toxic effect of ingested mushrooms,** assault

    √7ʰ **T62.0X4 Toxic effect of ingested mushrooms,** undetermined

√5ʰ **T62.1 Toxic effect of ingested berries**

  √6ʰ **T62.1X Toxic effect of** ingested berries

    √7ʰ **T62.1X1 Toxic effect of ingested berries,** accidental (unintentional)
Toxic effect of ingested berries NOS

    2 √7ʰ **T62.1X2 Toxic effect of ingested berries,** HCC
intentional self-harm

    √7ʰ **T62.1X3 Toxic effect of ingested berries,** assault

    √7ʰ **T62.1X4 Toxic effect of ingested berries,** undetermined

√5ʰ **T62.2 Toxic effect of other ingested (parts of) plant(s)**

  √6ʰ **T62.2X Toxic effect of other ingested (parts of)** plant(s)

    √7ʰ **T62.2X1 Toxic effect of other ingested (parts of) plant(s),** accidental **(unintentional)**
Toxic effect of other ingested (parts of) plant(s) NOS

    2 √7ʰ **T62.2X2 Toxic effect of other ingested (parts of) plant(s),** intentional self-harm HCC

    √7ʰ **T62.2X3 Toxic effect of other ingested (parts of) plant(s),** assault

    √7ʰ **T62.2X4 Toxic effect of other ingested (parts of) plant(s),** undetermined

√5ʰ **T62.8 Toxic effect of other specified noxious substances eaten as food**

  √6ʰ **T62.8X Toxic effect of other specified noxious substances eaten as food**

    √7ʰ **T62.8X1 Toxic effect of other specified noxious substances eaten as food,** accidental **(unintentional)**
Toxic effect of other specified noxious substances eaten as food NOS

    2 √7ʰ **T62.8X2 Toxic effect of other specified noxious substances eaten as food,** intentional self-harm HCC

√7ʰ **T62.8X3 Toxic effect of other specified noxious substances eaten as food,** assault

√7ʰ **T62.8X4 Toxic effect of other specified noxious substances eaten as food,** undetermined

√5ʰ **T62.9 Toxic effect of unspecified noxious substance eaten as food**

  √x7ʰ **T62.91 Toxic effect of unspecified noxious substance eaten as food,** accidental **(unintentional)** ▽
Toxic effect of unspecified noxious substance eaten as food NOS

  2 √x7ʰ **T62.92 Toxic effect of unspecified noxious substance eaten as food,** intentional self-harm HCC ▽

  √x7ʰ **T62.93 Toxic effect of unspecified noxious substance eaten as food,** assault ▽

  √x7ʰ **T62.94 Toxic effect of unspecified noxious substance eaten as food,** undetermined ▽

√4ʰ **T63 Toxic effect of contact with venomous animals and plants**

INCLUDES bite or touch of venomous animal
pricked or stuck by thorn or leaf

EXCLUDES 2 *ingestion of toxic animal or plant (T61.-, T62.-)*

The appropriate 7th character is to be added to each code from category T63.
A   initial encounter
D   subsequent encounter
S   sequela

√5ʰ **T63.0 Toxic effect of** snake venom

  √6ʰ **T63.00 Toxic effect of unspecified snake venom**

    √7ʰ **T63.001 Toxic effect of unspecified snake venom,** accidental **(unintentional)** ▽
Toxic effect of unspecified snake venom NOS

    2 √7ʰ **T63.002 Toxic effect of unspecified snake venom,** intentional self-harm HCC ▽

    √7ʰ **T63.003 Toxic effect of unspecified snake venom,** assault ▽

    √7ʰ **T63.004 Toxic effect of unspecified snake venom,** undetermined ▽

  √6ʰ **T63.01 Toxic effect of** rattlesnake **venom**

    √7ʰ **T63.011 Toxic effect of rattlesnake venom,** accidental **(unintentional)**
Toxic effect of rattlesnake venom NOS

    2 √7ʰ **T63.012 Toxic effect of rattlesnake venom,** intentional self-harm HCC

    √7ʰ **T63.013 Toxic effect of rattlesnake venom,** assault

    √7ʰ **T63.014 Toxic effect of rattlesnake venom,** undetermined

  √6ʰ **T63.02 Toxic effect of** coral snake **venom**

    √7ʰ **T63.021 Toxic effect of coral snake venom,** accidental **(unintentional)**
Toxic effect of coral snake venom NOS

    2 √7ʰ **T63.022 Toxic effect of coral snake venom,** intentional self-harm HCC

    √7ʰ **T63.023 Toxic effect of coral snake venom,** assault

    √7ʰ **T63.024 Toxic effect of coral snake venom,** undetermined

  √6ʰ **T63.03 Toxic effect of** taipan **venom**

    √7ʰ **T63.031 Toxic effect of taipan venom,** accidental **(unintentional)**
Toxic effect of taipan venom NOS

    2 √7ʰ **T63.032 Toxic effect of taipan venom,** intentional self-harm HCC

    √7ʰ **T63.033 Toxic effect of taipan venom,** assault

    √7ʰ **T63.034 Toxic effect of taipan venom,** undetermined

  √6ʰ **T63.04 Toxic effect of** cobra **venom**

    √7ʰ **T63.041 Toxic effect of cobra venom,** accidental **(unintentional)**
Toxic effect of cobra venom NOS

    2 √7ʰ **T63.042 Toxic effect of cobra venom,** intentional self-harm HCC

    √7ʰ **T63.043 Toxic effect of cobra venom,** assault

    √7ʰ **T63.044 Toxic effect of cobra venom,** undetermined

---

2 HCC with 7th character indicating initial encounter (A or B - specific to category) OR sequela.

✓6th T63.06 Toxic effect of venom of other North and South American snake

     ✓7th **T63.061 Toxic effect of venom of other North and South American snake, accidental (unintentional)**
         Toxic effect of venom of other North and South American snake NOS

     2 ✓7th **T63.062 Toxic effect of venom of other North** HCC **and South American snake, intentional self-harm**

     ✓7th **T63.063 Toxic effect of venom of other North and South American snake, assault**

     ✓7th **T63.064 Toxic effect of venom of other North and South American snake, undetermined**

✓6th T63.07 Toxic effect of venom of other Australian snake

     ✓7th **T63.071 Toxic effect of venom of other Australian snake, accidental (unintentional)**
         Toxic effect of venom of other Australian snake NOS

     2 ✓7th **T63.072 Toxic effect of venom of other** HCC **Australian snake, intentional self-harm**

     ✓7th **T63.073 Toxic effect of venom of other Australian snake, assault**

     ✓7th **T63.074 Toxic effect of venom of other Australian snake, undetermined**

✓6th T63.08 Toxic effect of venom of other African and Asian snake

     ✓7th **T63.081 Toxic effect of venom of other African and Asian snake, accidental (unintentional)**
         Toxic effect of venom of other African and Asian snake NOS

     2 ✓7th **T63.082 Toxic effect of venom of other African** HCC **and Asian snake, intentional self-harm**

     ✓7th **T63.083 Toxic effect of venom of other African and Asian snake, assault**

     ✓7th **T63.084 Toxic effect of venom of other African and Asian snake, undetermined**

✓6th T63.09 Toxic effect of venom of other snake

     ✓7th **T63.091 Toxic effect of venom of other snake, accidental (unintentional)**
         Toxic effect of venom of other snake NOS

     2 ✓7th **T63.092 Toxic effect of venom of other snake,** HCC **intentional self-harm**

     ✓7th **T63.093 Toxic effect of venom of other snake, assault**

     ✓7th **T63.094 Toxic effect of venom of other snake, undetermined**

✓5th T63.1 Toxic effect of venom of other reptiles

   ✓6th T63.11 Toxic effect of venom of gila monster

     ✓7th **T63.111 Toxic effect of venom of gila monster, accidental (unintentional)**
         Toxic effect of venom of gila monster NOS

     2 ✓7th **T63.112 Toxic effect of venom of gila monster,** HCC **intentional self-harm**

     ✓7th **T63.113 Toxic effect of venom of gila monster, assault**

     ✓7th **T63.114 Toxic effect of venom of gila monster, undetermined**

   ✓6th T63.12 Toxic effect of venom of other venomous lizard

     ✓7th **T63.121 Toxic effect of venom of other venomous lizard, accidental (unintentional)**
         Toxic effect of venom of other venomous lizard NOS

     2 ✓7th **T63.122 Toxic effect of venom of other** HCC **venomous lizard, intentional self-harm**

     ✓7th **T63.123 Toxic effect of venom of other venomous lizard, assault**

     ✓7th **T63.124 Toxic effect of venom of other venomous lizard, undetermined**

   ✓6th T63.19 Toxic effect of venom of other reptiles

     ✓7th **T63.191 Toxic effect of venom of other reptiles, accidental (unintentional)**
         Toxic effect of venom of other reptiles NOS

     2 ✓7th **T63.192 Toxic effect of venom of other** HCC **reptiles, intentional self-harm**

     ✓7th **T63.193 Toxic effect of venom of other reptiles, assault**

     ✓7th **T63.194 Toxic effect of venom of other reptiles, undetermined**

✓5th T63.2 Toxic effect of venom of scorpion

   ✓6th T63.2X Toxic effect of venom of scorpion

     ✓7th **T63.2X1 Toxic effect of venom of scorpion, accidental (unintentional)**
         Toxic effect of venom of scorpion NOS

     2 ✓7th **T63.2X2 Toxic effect of venom of scorpion,** HCC **intentional self-harm**

     ✓7th **T63.2X3 Toxic effect of venom of scorpion, assault**

     ✓7th **T63.2X4 Toxic effect of venom of scorpion, undetermined**

✓5th T63.3 Toxic effect of venom of spider

   ✓6th T63.30 Toxic effect of unspecified spider venom

     ✓7th **T63.301 Toxic effect of unspecified spider venom, accidental (unintentional)** ▽

     2 ✓7th **T63.302 Toxic effect of unspecified spider** HCC ▽ **venom, intentional self-harm**

     ✓7th **T63.303 Toxic effect of unspecified spider venom, assault** ▽

     ✓7th **T63.304 Toxic effect of unspecified spider venom, undetermined** ▽

   ✓6th T63.31 Toxic effect of venom of black widow **spider**

     ✓7th **T63.311 Toxic effect of venom of black widow spider, accidental (unintentional)**

     2 ✓7th **T63.312 Toxic effect of venom of black widow** HCC **spider, intentional self-harm**

     ✓7th **T63.313 Toxic effect of venom of black widow spider, assault**

     ✓7th **T63.314 Toxic effect of venom of black widow spider, undetermined**

   ✓6th T63.32 Toxic effect of venom of tarantula

     ✓7th **T63.321 Toxic effect of venom of tarantula, accidental (unintentional)**

     2 ✓7th **T63.322 Toxic effect of venom of tarantula,** HCC **intentional self-harm**

     ✓7th **T63.323 Toxic effect of venom of tarantula, assault**

     ✓7th **T63.324 Toxic effect of venom of tarantula, undetermined**

   ✓6th T63.33 Toxic effect of venom of brown recluse **spider**

     ✓7th **T63.331 Toxic effect of venom of brown recluse spider, accidental (unintentional)**

     2 ✓7th **T63.332 Toxic effect of venom of brown** HCC **recluse spider, intentional self-harm**

     ✓7th **T63.333 Toxic effect of venom of brown recluse spider, assault**

     ✓7th **T63.334 Toxic effect of venom of brown recluse spider, undetermined**

   ✓6th T63.39 Toxic effect of venom of other spider

     ✓7th **T63.391 Toxic effect of venom of other spider, accidental (unintentional)**

     2 ✓7th **T63.392 Toxic effect of venom of other spider,** HCC **intentional self-harm**

     ✓7th **T63.393 Toxic effect of venom of other spider, assault**

     ✓7th **T63.394 Toxic effect of venom of other spider, undetermined**

✓5th T63.4 Toxic effect of venom of other arthropods

   ✓6th T63.41 Toxic effect of venom of centipedes and venomous millipedes

     ✓7th **T63.411 Toxic effect of venom of centipedes and venomous millipedes, accidental (unintentional)**

     2 ✓7th **T63.412 Toxic effect of venom of centipedes** HCC **and venomous millipedes, intentional self-harm**

     ✓7th **T63.413 Toxic effect of venom of centipedes and venomous millipedes, assault**

---

2   HCC with 7th character indicating initial encounter (A or B - specific to category) OR sequela.

EXCLUDES 1 Not coded here   EXCLUDES 2 Not included here   N Newborn Age: 0   P Pediatric Age: 0-17   M Maternity Age: 12-55   A Adult Age: 15-124

1088   ICD-10-CM 2018

☑7ᵗʰ **T63.414** Toxic effect of venom of centipedes and venomous millipedes, undetermined

☑6ᵗʰ **T63.42** Toxic effect of venom of ants

  ☑7ᵗʰ **T63.421** Toxic effect of venom of ants, accidental (unintentional)

  ² ☑7ᵗʰ **T63.422** Toxic effect of venom of ants,   **HCC** intentional self-harm

  ☑7ᵗʰ **T63.423** Toxic effect of venom of ants, assault

  ☑7ᵗʰ **T63.424** Toxic effect of venom of ants, undetermined

☑6ᵗʰ **T63.43** Toxic effect of venom of caterpillars

  ☑7ᵗʰ **T63.431** Toxic effect of venom of caterpillars, accidental (unintentional)

  ² ☑7ᵗʰ **T63.432** Toxic effect of venom of caterpillars,   **HCC** intentional self-harm

  ☑7ᵗʰ **T63.433** Toxic effect of venom of caterpillars, assault

  ☑7ᵗʰ **T63.434** Toxic effect of venom of caterpillars, undetermined

☑6ᵗʰ **T63.44** Toxic effect of venom of bees

  ☑7ᵗʰ **T63.441** Toxic effect of venom of bees, accidental (unintentional)

  ² ☑7ᵗʰ **T63.442** Toxic effect of venom of bees,   **HCC** intentional self-harm

  ☑7ᵗʰ **T63.443** Toxic effect of venom of bees, assault

  ☑7ᵗʰ **T63.444** Toxic effect of venom of bees, undetermined

☑6ᵗʰ **T63.45** Toxic effect of venom of hornets

  ☑7ᵗʰ **T63.451** Toxic effect of venom of hornets, accidental (unintentional)

  ² ☑7ᵗʰ **T63.452** Toxic effect of venom of hornets,   **HCC** intentional self-harm

  ☑7ᵗʰ **T63.453** Toxic effect of venom of hornets, assault

  ☑7ᵗʰ **T63.454** Toxic effect of venom of hornets, undetermined

☑6ᵗʰ **T63.46** Toxic effect of venom of wasps
Toxic effect of yellow jacket

  ☑7ᵗʰ **T63.461** Toxic effect of venom of wasps, accidental (unintentional)

  ² ☑7ᵗʰ **T63.462** Toxic effect of venom of wasps,   **HCC** intentional self-harm

  ☑7ᵗʰ **T63.463** Toxic effect of venom of wasps, assault

  ☑7ᵗʰ **T63.464** Toxic effect of venom of wasps, undetermined

☑6ᵗʰ **T63.48** Toxic effect of venom of other arthropod

  ☑7ᵗʰ **T63.481** Toxic effect of venom of other arthropod, accidental (unintentional)

  ² ☑7ᵗʰ **T63.482** Toxic effect of venom of other   **HCC** arthropod, intentional self-harm

  ☑7ᵗʰ **T63.483** Toxic effect of venom of other arthropod, assault

  ☑7ᵗʰ **T63.484** Toxic effect of venom of other arthropod, undetermined

☑5ᵗʰ **T63.5** Toxic effect of contact with venomous fish
  EXCLUDES 2 poisoning by ingestion of fish (T61.-)

☑6ᵗʰ **T63.51** Toxic effect of contact with stingray

  ☑7ᵗʰ **T63.511** Toxic effect of contact with stingray, accidental (unintentional)

  ² ☑7ᵗʰ **T63.512** Toxic effect of contact with stingray,   **HCC** intentional self-harm

  ☑7ᵗʰ **T63.513** Toxic effect of contact with stingray, assault

  ☑7ᵗʰ **T63.514** Toxic effect of contact with stingray, undetermined

☑6ᵗʰ **T63.59** Toxic effect of contact with other venomous fish

  ☑7ᵗʰ **T63.591** Toxic effect of contact with other venomous fish, accidental (unintentional)

  ² ☑7ᵗʰ **T63.592** Toxic effect of contact with other   **HCC** venomous fish, intentional self-harm

  ☑7ᵗʰ **T63.593** Toxic effect of contact with other venomous fish, assault

  ☑7ᵗʰ **T63.594** Toxic effect of contact with other venomous fish, undetermined

☑5ᵗʰ **T63.6** Toxic effect of contact with other venomous marine animals
  EXCLUDES 1 sea-snake venom (T63.Ø9)
  EXCLUDES 2 poisoning by ingestion of shellfish (T61.78-)

☑6ᵗʰ **T63.61** Toxic effect of contact with Portugese Man-o-war
Toxic effect of contact with bluebottle

  ☑7ᵗʰ **T63.611** Toxic effect of contact with Portugese Man-o-war, accidental (unintentional)

  ² ☑7ᵗʰ **T63.612** Toxic effect of contact with Portugese **HCC** Man-o-war, intentional self-harm

  ☑7ᵗʰ **T63.613** Toxic effect of contact with Portugese Man-o-war, assault

  ☑7ᵗʰ **T63.614** Toxic effect of contact with Portugese Man-o-war, undetermined

☑6ᵗʰ **T63.62** Toxic effect of contact with other jellyfish

  ☑7ᵗʰ **T63.621** Toxic effect of contact with other jellyfish, accidental (unintentional)

  ² ☑7ᵗʰ **T63.622** Toxic effect of contact with other   **HCC** jellyfish, intentional self-harm

  ☑7ᵗʰ **T63.623** Toxic effect of contact with other jellyfish, assault

  ☑7ᵗʰ **T63.624** Toxic effect of contact with other jellyfish, undetermined

☑6ᵗʰ **T63.63** Toxic effect of contact with sea anemone

  ☑7ᵗʰ **T63.631** Toxic effect of contact with sea anemone, accidental (unintentional)

  ² ☑7ᵗʰ **T63.632** Toxic effect of contact with sea   **HCC** anemone, intentional self-harm

  ☑7ᵗʰ **T63.633** Toxic effect of contact with sea anemone, assault

  ☑7ᵗʰ **T63.634** Toxic effect of contact with sea anemone, undetermined

☑6ᵗʰ **T63.69** Toxic effect of contact with other venomous marine animals

  ☑7ᵗʰ **T63.691** Toxic effect of contact with other venomous marine animals, accidental (unintentional)

  ² ☑7ᵗʰ **T63.692** Toxic effect of contact with other   **HCC** venomous marine animals, intentional self-harm

  ☑7ᵗʰ **T63.693** Toxic effect of contact with other venomous marine animals, assault

  ☑7ᵗʰ **T63.694** Toxic effect of contact with other venomous marine animals, undetermined

☑5ᵗʰ **T63.7** Toxic effect of contact with venomous plant

☑6ᵗʰ **T63.71** Toxic effect of contact with venomous marine plant

  ☑7ᵗʰ **T63.711** Toxic effect of contact with venomous marine plant, accidental (unintentional)

  ² ☑7ᵗʰ **T63.712** Toxic effect of contact with venomous **HCC** marine plant, intentional self-harm

  ☑7ᵗʰ **T63.713** Toxic effect of contact with venomous marine plant, assault

  ☑7ᵗʰ **T63.714** Toxic effect of contact with venomous marine plant, undetermined

☑6ᵗʰ **T63.79** Toxic effect of contact with other venomous plant

  ☑7ᵗʰ **T63.791** Toxic effect of contact with other venomous plant, accidental (unintentional)

  ² ☑7ᵗʰ **T63.792** Toxic effect of contact with other   **HCC** venomous plant, intentional self-harm

  ☑7ᵗʰ **T63.793** Toxic effect of contact with other venomous plant, assault

  ☑7ᵗʰ **T63.794** Toxic effect of contact with other venomous plant, undetermined

☑5ᵗʰ **T63.8** Toxic effect of contact with other venomous animals

☑6ᵗʰ **T63.81** Toxic effect of contact with venomous frog
  EXCLUDES 1 contact with nonvenomous frog (W62.Ø)

  ☑7ᵗʰ **T63.811** Toxic effect of contact with venomous frog, accidental (unintentional)

  ² ☑7ᵗʰ **T63.812** Toxic effect of contact with venomous **HCC** frog, intentional self-harm

  ☑7ᵗʰ **T63.813** Toxic effect of contact with venomous frog, assault

  ☑7ᵗʰ **T63.814** Toxic effect of contact with venomous frog, undetermined

---

²   HCC with 7th character indicating initial encounter (A or B - specific to category) OR sequela.

☑ Additional Character Req   ☑ₓ7ᵗʰ Placeholder Alert   Manifestation   **HCC** CMS-HCC Condition   ▽ Unspecified Code   ►◄ Revised Text   ● New Code   ▲ Revised Code Title

Chapter 19. Injury, Poisoning, and Certain Other Consequences of External Causes

√6th **T63.82** **Toxic effect of contact with venomous** toad
> EXCLUDES 1   contact with nonvenomous toad (W62.1)

√7th **T63.821** **Toxic effect of contact with venomous toad, accidental (unintentional)**

2 √7th **T63.822** **Toxic effect of contact with venomous toad, intentional self-harm** HCC

√7th **T63.823** **Toxic effect of contact with venomous toad, assault**

√7th **T63.824** **Toxic effect of contact with venomous toad, undetermined**

√6th **T63.83** **Toxic effect of contact with other venomous amphibian**
> EXCLUDES 1   contact with nonvenomous amphibian (W62.9)

√7th **T63.831** **Toxic effect of contact with other venomous amphibian, accidental (unintentional)**

2 √7th **T63.832** **Toxic effect of contact with other venomous amphibian, intentional self-harm** HCC

√7th **T63.833** **Toxic effect of contact with other venomous amphibian, assault**

√7th **T63.834** **Toxic effect of contact with other venomous amphibian, undetermined**

√6th **T63.89** **Toxic effect of contact with other venomous animals**

√7th **T63.891** **Toxic effect of contact with other venomous animals, accidental (unintentional)**

2 √7th **T63.892** **Toxic effect of contact with other venomous animals, intentional self-harm** HCC

√7th **T63.893** **Toxic effect of contact with other venomous animals, assault**

√7th **T63.894** **Toxic effect of contact with other venomous animals, undetermined**

√5th **T63.9** **Toxic effect of contact with unspecified venomous animal**

√x7th **T63.91** **Toxic effect of contact with unspecified venomous animal, accidental (unintentional)** ▽

2 √x7th **T63.92** **Toxic effect of contact with unspecified venomous animal, intentional self-harm** HCC ▽

√x7th **T63.93** **Toxic effect of contact with unspecified venomous animal, assault** ▽

√x7th **T63.94** **Toxic effect of contact with unspecified venomous animal, undetermined** ▽

√4th **T64** **Toxic effect of aflatoxin and other mycotoxin food contaminants**

> The appropriate 7th character is to be added to each code from category T64.
> A   initial encounter
> D   subsequent encounter
> S   sequela

√5th **T64.0** **Toxic effect of** aflatoxin

√x7th **T64.01** **Toxic effect of aflatoxin, accidental (unintentional)**

2 √x7th **T64.02** **Toxic effect of aflatoxin, intentional self-harm** HCC

√x7th **T64.03** **Toxic effect of aflatoxin, assault**

√x7th **T64.04** **Toxic effect of aflatoxin, undetermined**

√5th **T64.8** **Toxic effect of other mycotoxin food contaminants**

√x7th **T64.81** **Toxic effect of other mycotoxin food contaminants, accidental (unintentional)**

2 √x7th **T64.82** **Toxic effect of other mycotoxin food contaminants, intentional self-harm** HCC

√x7th **T64.83** **Toxic effect of other mycotoxin food contaminants, assault**

√x7th **T64.84** **Toxic effect of other mycotoxin food contaminants, undetermined**

√4th **T65** **Toxic effect of other and unspecified substances**

> The appropriate 7th character is to be added to each code from category T65.
> A   initial encounter
> D   subsequent encounter
> S   sequela

√5th **T65.0** **Toxic effect of cyanides**
> EXCLUDES 1   hydrogen cyanide (T57.3-)

√6th **T65.0X** **Toxic effect of** cyanides

√7th **T65.0X1** **Toxic effect of cyanides, accidental (unintentional)**
> Toxic effect of cyanides NOS

2 √7th **T65.0X2** **Toxic effect of cyanides, intentional self-harm** HCC

√7th **T65.0X3** **Toxic effect of cyanides, assault**

√7th **T65.0X4** **Toxic effect of cyanides, undetermined**

√5th **T65.1** **Toxic effect of strychnine and its salts**

√6th **T65.1X** **Toxic effect of** strychnine **and its salts**

√7th **T65.1X1** **Toxic effect of strychnine and its salts, accidental (unintentional)**
> Toxic effect of strychnine and its salts NOS

2 √7th **T65.1X2** **Toxic effect of strychnine and its salts, intentional self-harm** HCC

√7th **T65.1X3** **Toxic effect of strychnine and its salts, assault**

√7th **T65.1X4** **Toxic effect of strychnine and its salts, undetermined**

√5th **T65.2** **Toxic effect of tobacco and nicotine**
> EXCLUDES 2   nicotine dependence (F17.-)

√6th **T65.21** **Toxic effect of** chewing tobacco

√7th **T65.211** **Toxic effect of chewing tobacco, accidental (unintentional)**
> Toxic effect of chewing tobacco NOS

2 √7th **T65.212** **Toxic effect of chewing tobacco, intentional self-harm** HCC

√7th **T65.213** **Toxic effect of chewing tobacco, assault**

√7th **T65.214** **Toxic effect of chewing tobacco, undetermined**

√6th **T65.22** **Toxic effect of** tobacco cigarettes
> Toxic effect of tobacco smoke
> Use additional code for exposure to second hand tobacco smoke (Z57.31, Z77.22)

√7th **T65.221** **Toxic effect of tobacco cigarettes, accidental (unintentional)**
> Toxic effect of tobacco cigarettes NOS

2 √7th **T65.222** **Toxic effect of tobacco cigarettes, intentional self-harm** HCC

√7th **T65.223** **Toxic effect of tobacco cigarettes, assault**

√7th **T65.224** **Toxic effect of tobacco cigarettes, undetermined**

√6th **T65.29** **Toxic effect of other tobacco and nicotine**

√7th **T65.291** **Toxic effect of other tobacco and nicotine, accidental (unintentional)**
> Toxic effect of other tobacco and nicotine NOS

2 √7th **T65.292** **Toxic effect of other tobacco and nicotine, intentional self-harm** HCC

√7th **T65.293** **Toxic effect of other tobacco and nicotine, assault**

√7th **T65.294** **Toxic effect of other tobacco and nicotine, undetermined**

√5th **T65.3** **Toxic effect of nitroderivatives and aminoderivatives of benzene and its homologues**
> Toxic effect of anilin [benzenamine]
> Toxic effect of nitrobenzene
> Toxic effect of trinitrotoluene

√6th **T65.3X** **Toxic effect of** nitroderivatives and aminoderivatives of benzene and its homologues

√7th **T65.3X1** **Toxic effect of nitroderivatives and aminoderivatives of benzene and its homologues, accidental (unintentional)**
> Toxic effect of nitroderivatives and aminoderivatives of benzene and its homologues NOS

---

2   HCC with 7th character indicating initial encounter (A or B - specific to category) OR sequela.

EXCLUDES 1 Not coded here   EXCLUDES 2 Not included here   N Newborn Age: 0   P Pediatric Age: 0-17   M Maternity Age: 12-55   A Adult Age: 15-124

1090   ICD-10-CM 2018

2 ✓7th **T65.3X2** Toxic effect of nitroderivatives and aminoderivatives of benzene and its homologues, intentional self-harm   HCC

✓7th **T65.3X3** Toxic effect of nitroderivatives and aminoderivatives of benzene and its homologues, assault

✓7th **T65.3X4** Toxic effect of nitroderivatives and aminoderivatives of benzene and its homologues, undetermined

✓5th **T65.4** Toxic effect of carbon disulfide

  ✓6th **T65.4X** Toxic effect of carbon disulfide

    ✓7th **T65.4X1** Toxic effect of carbon disulfide, accidental (unintentional)
Toxic effect of carbon disulfide NOS

  2 ✓7th **T65.4X2** Toxic effect of carbon disulfide, intentional self-harm   HCC

    ✓7th **T65.4X3** Toxic effect of carbon disulfide, assault

    ✓7th **T65.4X4** Toxic effect of carbon disulfide, undetermined

✓5th **T65.5** Toxic effect of nitroglycerin and other nitric acids and esters
Toxic effect of 1,2,3-Propanetriol trinitrate

  ✓6th **T65.5X** Toxic effect of nitroglycerin and other nitric acids and esters

    ✓7th **T65.5X1** Toxic effect of nitroglycerin and other nitric acids and esters, accidental (unintentional)
Toxic effect of nitroglycerin and other nitric acids and esters NOS

  2 ✓7th **T65.5X2** Toxic effect of nitroglycerin and other nitric acids and esters, intentional self-harm   HCC

    ✓7th **T65.5X3** Toxic effect of nitroglycerin and other nitric acids and esters, assault

    ✓7th **T65.5X4** Toxic effect of nitroglycerin and other nitric acids and esters, undetermined

✓5th **T65.6** Toxic effect of paints and dyes, not elsewhere classified

  ✓6th **T65.6X** Toxic effect of paints and dyes, not elsewhere classified

    ✓7th **T65.6X1** Toxic effect of paints and dyes, not elsewhere classified, accidental (unintentional)
Toxic effect of paints and dyes NOS

  2 ✓7th **T65.6X2** Toxic effect of paints and dyes, not elsewhere classified, intentional self-harm   HCC

    ✓7th **T65.6X3** Toxic effect of paints and dyes, not elsewhere classified, assault

    ✓7th **T65.6X4** Toxic effect of paints and dyes, not elsewhere classified, undetermined

✓5th **T65.8** Toxic effect of other specified substances

  ✓6th **T65.81** Toxic effect of latex

    ✓7th **T65.811** Toxic effect of latex, accidental (unintentional)
Toxic effect of latex NOS

  2 ✓7th **T65.812** Toxic effect of latex, intentional self-harm   HCC

    ✓7th **T65.813** Toxic effect of latex, assault

    ✓7th **T65.814** Toxic effect of latex, undetermined

  ✓6th **T65.82** Toxic effect of harmful algae and algae toxins
Toxic effect of (harmful) algae bloom NOS
Toxic effect of blue-green algae bloom
Toxic effect of brown tide
Toxic effect of cyanobacteria bloom
Toxic effect of Florida red tide
Toxic effect of pfiesteria piscicida
Toxic effect of red tide

    ✓7th **T65.821** Toxic effect of harmful algae and algae toxins, accidental (unintentional)
Toxic effect of harmful algae and algae toxins NOS

  2 ✓7th **T65.822** Toxic effect of harmful algae and algae toxins, intentional self-harm   HCC

    ✓7th **T65.823** Toxic effect of harmful algae and algae toxins, assault

    ✓7th **T65.824** Toxic effect of harmful algae and algae toxins, undetermined

  ✓6th **T65.83** Toxic effect of fiberglass

    ✓7th **T65.831** Toxic effect of fiberglass, accidental (unintentional)
Toxic effect of fiberglass NOS

  2 ✓7th **T65.832** Toxic effect of fiberglass, intentional self-harm   HCC

    ✓7th **T65.833** Toxic effect of fiberglass, assault

    ✓7th **T65.834** Toxic effect of fiberglass, undetermined

  ✓6th **T65.89** Toxic effect of other specified substances

    ✓7th **T65.891** Toxic effect of other specified substances, accidental (unintentional)
Toxic effect of other specified substances NOS

  2 ✓7th **T65.892** Toxic effect of other specified substances, intentional self-harm   HCC

    ✓7th **T65.893** Toxic effect of other specified substances, assault

    ✓7th **T65.894** Toxic effect of other specified substances, undetermined

✓5th **T65.9** Toxic effect of unspecified substance

  ✓x7th **T65.91** Toxic effect of unspecified substance, accidental (unintentional) ▽
Poisoning NOS

  2 ✓x7th **T65.92** Toxic effect of unspecified substance, intentional self-harm   HCC ▽

  ✓x7th **T65.93** Toxic effect of unspecified substance, assault ▽

  ✓x7th **T65.94** Toxic effect of unspecified substance, undetermined ▽

Other and unspecified effects of external causes (T66-T78)

✓x7th **T66** **Radiation sickness, unspecified** ▽

  EXCLUDES 1   *specified adverse effects of radiation, such as:*
    burns (T20-T31)
    leukemia (C91-C95)
  radiation gastroenteritis and colitis (K52.0)
  radiation pneumonitis (J70.0)
  radiation related disorders of the skin and subcutaneous tissue (L55-L59)
  radiation sunburn (L55.-)

> The appropriate 7th character is to be added to code T66.
> A   initial encounter
> D   subsequent encounter
> S   sequela

✓4th **T67** **Effects of heat and light**

  EXCLUDES 1   *erythema [dermatitis] ab igne (L59.0)*
    malignant hyperpyrexia due to anesthesia (T88.3)
    radiation-related disorders of the skin and subcutaneous tissue (L55-L59)

  EXCLUDES 2   *burns (T20-T31)*
    sunburn (L55.-)
    sweat disorder due to heat (L74-L75)

> The appropriate 7th character is to be added to each code from category T67.
> A   initial encounter
> D   subsequent encounter
> S   sequela

  ✓x7th **T67.0** **Heatstroke and sunstroke**
    Heat apoplexy   Siriasis
    Heat pyrexia   Thermoplegia
    Use additional code(s) to identify any associated complications of heatstroke, such as:
      coma and stupor (R40.-)
      systemic inflammatory response syndrome (R65.1-)
    DEF: Headache, vertigo, cramps, and elevated body temperature due to prolonged exposure to high environmental temperatures; requires emergency intervention.

  ✓x7th **T67.1** **Heat syncope**
    Heat collapse

  ✓x7th **T67.2** **Heat cramp**

  ✓x7th **T67.3** **Heat exhaustion, anhydrotic**
    Heat prostration due to water depletion
    EXCLUDES 1   *heat exhaustion due to salt depletion (T67.4)*

  ✓x7th **T67.4** **Heat exhaustion due to salt depletion**
    Heat prostration due to salt (and water) depletion

---

2   HCC with 7th character indicating initial encounter (A or B - specific to category) OR sequela.

✓ Additional Character Req   ✓x7th Placeholder Alert   Manifestation   HCC CMS-HCC Condition   ▽ Unspecified Code   ►◄ Revised Text   ● New Code   ▲ Revised Code Title

√x7ᵗʰ **T67.5 Heat exhaustion, unspecified**
Heat prostration NOS

√x7ᵗʰ **T67.6 Heat** fatigue, **transient**

√x7ᵗʰ **T67.7 Heat** edema

√x7ᵗʰ **T67.8 Other effects of heat and light**

√x7ᵗʰ **T67.9 Effect of heat and light, unspecified**

√x7ᵗʰ **T68 Hypothermia**
Accidental hypothermia
Hypothermia NOS
Use additional code to identify source of exposure:
exposure to excessive cold of man-made origin (W93)
exposure to excessive cold of natural origin (X31)
EXCLUDES 1   hypothermia following anesthesia (T88.51)
hypothermia not associated with low environmental
temperature (R68.0)
hypothermia of newborn (P80.-)
EXCLUDES 2   frostbite (T33-T34)

The appropriate 7th character is to be added to code T68.
A   initial encounter
D   subsequent encounter
S   sequela

√4ᵗʰ **T69 Other effects of reduced temperature**
Use additional code to identify source of exposure:
exposure to excessive cold of man-made origin (W93)
exposure to excessive cold of natural origin (X31)
EXCLUDES 2   frostbite (T33-T34)

The appropriate 7th character is to be added to each code from
category T69.
A   initial encounter
D   subsequent encounter
S   sequela

√5ᵗʰ **T69.0 Immersion hand and foot**

√6ᵗʰ   **T69.01 Immersion** hand

√7ᵗʰ   **T69.011 Immersion hand,** right **hand**

√7ᵗʰ   **T69.012 Immersion hand,** left **hand**

√7ᵗʰ   **T69.019 Immersion hand, unspecified hand**

√6ᵗʰ   **T69.02 Immersion** foot
Trench foot

√7ᵗʰ   **T69.021 Immersion foot,** right **foot**

√7ᵗʰ   **T69.022 Immersion foot,** left **foot**

√7ᵗʰ   **T69.029 Immersion foot, unspecified foot**

√x7ᵗʰ **T69.1 Chilblains**
DEF: Red, swollen, itchy skin primarily affecting the fingers and
toes, nose and ears, and legs; follows damp-cold exposure; can
also be associated with pruritus and a burning feeling.

√x7ᵗʰ **T69.8 Other specified effects of reduced temperature**

√x7ᵗʰ **T69.9 Effect of reduced temperature, unspecified**

√4ᵗʰ **T70 Effects of air pressure and water pressure**

The appropriate 7th character is to be added to each code from
category T70.
A   initial encounter
D   subsequent encounter
S   sequela

√x7ᵗʰ **T70.0 Otitic barotrauma**
Aero-otitis media
Effects of change in ambient atmospheric pressure or water
pressure on ears

√x7ᵗʰ **T70.1 Sinus barotrauma**
Aerosinusitis
Effects of change in ambient atmospheric pressure on sinuses

√5ᵗʰ **T70.2 Other and unspecified effects of high altitude**
EXCLUDES 2   polycythemia due to high altitude (D75.1)

√x7ᵗʰ   **T70.20 Unspecified effects of high altitude**

√x7ᵗʰ   **T70.29 Other effects of high altitude**
Alpine sickness
Anoxia due to high altitude
Barotrauma NOS
Hypobaropathy
Mountain sickness

√x7ᵗʰ **T70.3 Caisson disease [decompression sickness]**
Compressed-air disease
Diver's palsy or paralysis
DEF: Rapid reduction in air pressure while breathing compressed
air; symptoms include skin lesions, joint pains, and respiratory and
neurological problems.

√x7ᵗʰ **T70.4 Effects of high-pressure fluids**
Hydraulic jet injection (industrial)
Pneumatic jet injection (industrial)
Traumatic jet injection (industrial)

√x7ᵗʰ **T70.8 Other effects of air pressure and water pressure**

√x7ᵗʰ **T70.9 Effect of air pressure and water pressure, unspecified**

√4ᵗʰ **T71 Asphyxiation**
Mechanical suffocation
Traumatic suffocation
EXCLUDES 1   acute respiratory distress (syndrome) (J80)
anoxia due to high altitude (T70.2)
asphyxia NOS (R09.01)
asphyxia from carbon monoxide (T58.-)
asphyxia from inhalation of food or foreign body (T17.-)
asphyxia from other gases, fumes and vapors (T59.-)
respiratory distress (syndrome) in newborn (P22.-)

The appropriate 7th character is to be added to each code from
category T71.
A   initial encounter
D   subsequent encounter
S   sequela

√5ᵗʰ **T71.1 Asphyxiation due to** mechanical threat to breathing
Suffocation due to mechanical threat to breathing

√6ᵗʰ   **T71.11 Asphyxiation due to** smothering under pillow

√7ᵗʰ   **T71.111 Asphyxiation due to smothering
under pillow,** accidental
Asphyxiation due to smothering under
pillow NOS

2 √7ᵗʰ   **T71.112 Asphyxiation due to smothering** ᴴᶜᶜ
under pillow, intentional self-harm

√7ᵗʰ   **T71.113 Asphyxiation due to smothering under
pillow,** assault

√7ᵗʰ   **T71.114 Asphyxiation due to smothering under
pillow,** undetermined

√6ᵗʰ   **T71.12 Asphyxiation due to** plastic bag

√7ᵗʰ   **T71.121 Asphyxiation due to plastic bag,**
accidental
Asphyxiation due to plastic bag NOS

2 √7ᵗʰ   **T71.122 Asphyxiation due to plastic bag,** ᴴᶜᶜ
intentional self-harm

√7ᵗʰ   **T71.123 Asphyxiation due to plastic bag,** assault

√7ᵗʰ   **T71.124 Asphyxiation due to plastic bag,**
undetermined

√6ᵗʰ   **T71.13 Asphyxiation due to being** trapped in bed linens

√7ᵗʰ   **T71.131 Asphyxiation due to being trapped
in bed linens,** accidental
Asphyxiation due to being trapped in bed
linens NOS

2 √7ᵗʰ   **T71.132 Asphyxiation due to being trapped** ᴴᶜᶜ
in bed linens, intentional self-harm

√7ᵗʰ   **T71.133 Asphyxiation due to being trapped
in bed linens,** assault

√7ᵗʰ   **T71.134 Asphyxiation due to being trapped
in bed linens,** undetermined

√6ᵗʰ   **T71.14 Asphyxiation due to** smothering under another
person's body (in bed)

√7ᵗʰ   **T71.141 Asphyxiation due to smothering
under another person's body (in bed),** accidental
Asphyxiation due to smothering under
another person's body (in bed) NOS

√7ᵗʰ   **T71.143 Asphyxiation due to smothering under
another person's body (in bed),** assault

√7ᵗʰ   **T71.144 Asphyxiation due to smothering under
another person's body (in bed),**
undetermined

√6ᵗʰ   **T71.15 Asphyxiation due to** smothering in furniture

√7ᵗʰ   **T71.151 Asphyxiation due to smothering in
furniture,** accidental
Asphyxiation due to smothering in
furniture NOS

2   HCC with 7th character indicating initial encounter (A or B - specific to category) OR sequela.

EXCLUDES 1 Not coded here   **EXCLUDES 2** Not included here   N Newborn Age: 0   P Pediatric Age: 0-17   M Maternity Age: 12-55   A Adult Age: 15-124

1092   ICD-10-CM 2018

2 ✓7ᵗʰ **T71.152** Asphyxiation due to smothering in furniture, intentional self-harm   HCC

✓7ᵗʰ **T71.153** Asphyxiation due to smothering in furniture, assault

✓7ᵗʰ **T71.154** Asphyxiation due to smothering in furniture, undetermined

✓6ᵗʰ **T71.16** Asphyxiation due to hanging
Hanging by window shade cord
Use additional code for any associated injuries, such as:
    crushing injury of neck (S17.-)
    fracture of cervical vertebrae (S12.0-S12.2-)
    open wound of neck (S11.-)

✓7ᵗʰ **T71.161** Asphyxiation due to hanging, accidental
    Asphyxiation due to hanging NOS
    Hanging NOS

2 ✓7ᵗʰ **T71.162** Asphyxiation due to hanging, intentional self-harm   HCC

✓7ᵗʰ **T71.163** Asphyxiation due to hanging, assault

✓7ᵗʰ **T71.164** Asphyxiation due to hanging, undetermined

✓6ᵗʰ **T71.19** Asphyxiation due to mechanical threat to breathing due to other causes

✓7ᵗʰ **T71.191** Asphyxiation due to mechanical threat to breathing due to other causes, accidental
    Asphyxiation due to other causes NOS

2 ✓7ᵗʰ **T71.192** Asphyxiation due to mechanical threat to breathing due to other causes, intentional self-harm   HCC

✓7ᵗʰ **T71.193** Asphyxiation due to mechanical threat to breathing due to other causes, assault

✓7ᵗʰ **T71.194** Asphyxiation due to mechanical threat to breathing due to other causes, undetermined

✓5ᵗʰ **T71.2** Asphyxiation due to systemic oxygen deficiency due to low oxygen content in ambient air
    Suffocation due to systemic oxygen deficiency due to low oxygen content in ambient air

✓x7ᵗʰ **T71.20** Asphyxiation due to systemic oxygen deficiency due to low oxygen content in ambient air due to unspecified cause ▽

✓x7ᵗʰ **T71.21** Asphyxiation due to cave-in or falling earth
    Use additional code for any associated cataclysm (X34-X38)

✓6ᵗʰ **T71.22** Asphyxiation due to being trapped in a car trunk

✓7ᵗʰ **T71.221** Asphyxiation due to being trapped in a car trunk, accidental

2 ✓7ᵗʰ **T71.222** Asphyxiation due to being trapped in a car trunk, intentional self-harm   HCC

✓7ᵗʰ **T71.223** Asphyxiation due to being trapped in a car trunk, assault

✓7ᵗʰ **T71.224** Asphyxiation due to being trapped in a car trunk, undetermined

✓6ᵗʰ **T71.23** Asphyxiation due to being trapped in a (discarded) refrigerator

✓7ᵗʰ **T71.231** Asphyxiation due to being trapped in a (discarded) refrigerator, accidental

2 ✓7ᵗʰ **T71.232** Asphyxiation due to being trapped in a (discarded) refrigerator, intentional self-harm   HCC

✓7ᵗʰ **T71.233** Asphyxiation due to being trapped in a (discarded) refrigerator, assault

✓7ᵗʰ **T71.234** Asphyxiation due to being trapped in a (discarded) refrigerator, undetermined

✓x7ᵗʰ **T71.29** Asphyxiation due to being trapped in other low oxygen environment

✓x7ᵗʰ **T71.9** Asphyxiation due to unspecified cause ▽
    Suffocation (by strangulation) due to unspecified cause
    Suffocation NOS
    Systemic oxygen deficiency due to low oxygen content in ambient air due to unspecified cause
    Systemic oxygen deficiency due to mechanical threat to breathing due to unspecified cause
    Traumatic asphyxia NOS

✓4ᵗʰ **T73** Effects of other deprivation

> The appropriate 7th character is to be added to each code from category T73.
> A   initial encounter
> D   subsequent encounter
> S   sequela

✓x7ᵗʰ **T73.0** Starvation
    Deprivation of food

✓x7ᵗʰ **T73.1** Deprivation of water

✓x7ᵗʰ **T73.2** Exhaustion due to exposure

✓x7ᵗʰ **T73.3** Exhaustion due to excessive exertion
    Exhaustion due to overexertion

✓x7ᵗʰ **T73.8** Other effects of deprivation

✓x7ᵗʰ **T73.9** Effect of deprivation, unspecified ▽

✓4ᵗʰ **T74** Adult and child abuse, neglect and other maltreatment, confirmed
    Use additional code, if applicable, to identify any associated current injury
    Use additional external cause code to identify perpetrator, if known (Y07.-)
    EXCLUDES 1   abuse and maltreatment in pregnancy (O9A.3-, O9A.4-, O9A.5-)
               adult and child maltreatment, suspected (T76.-)

> The appropriate 7th character is to be added to each code from category T74.
> A   initial encounter
> D   subsequent encounter
> S   sequela

✓5ᵗʰ **T74.0** Neglect or abandonment, confirmed

✓x7ᵗʰ **T74.01** Adult neglect or abandonment, confirmed   A

✓x7ᵗʰ **T74.02** Child neglect or abandonment, confirmed   P

✓5ᵗʰ **T74.1** Physical abuse, confirmed
    EXCLUDES 2   sexual abuse (T74.2-)

✓x7ᵗʰ **T74.11** Adult physical abuse, confirmed   A

✓x7ᵗʰ **T74.12** Child physical abuse, confirmed   P
    EXCLUDES 2   shaken infant syndrome (T74.4)

✓5ᵗʰ **T74.2** Sexual abuse, confirmed
    Rape, confirmed
    Sexual assault, confirmed

✓x7ᵗʰ **T74.21** Adult sexual abuse, confirmed   A

✓x7ᵗʰ **T74.22** Child sexual abuse, confirmed   P

✓5ᵗʰ **T74.3** Psychological abuse, confirmed

✓x7ᵗʰ **T74.31** Adult psychological abuse, confirmed   A

✓x7ᵗʰ **T74.32** Child psychological abuse, confirmed   P

✓x7ᵗʰ **T74.4** Shaken infant syndrome   P

✓5ᵗʰ **T74.9** Unspecified maltreatment, confirmed

✓x7ᵗʰ **T74.91** Unspecified adult maltreatment, confirmed   A ▽

✓x7ᵗʰ **T74.92** Unspecified child maltreatment, confirmed   P ▽

✓4ᵗʰ **T75** Other and unspecified effects of other external causes
    EXCLUDES 1   adverse effects NEC (T78.-)
    EXCLUDES 2   burns (electric) (T20-T31)

> The appropriate 7th character is to be added to each code from category T75.
> A   initial encounter
> D   subsequent encounter
> S   sequela

✓5ᵗʰ **T75.0** Effects of lightning
    Struck by lightning

✓x7ᵗʰ **T75.00** Unspecified effects of lightning ▽
    Struck by lightning NOS

✓x7ᵗʰ **T75.01** Shock due to being struck by lightning

✓x7ᵗʰ **T75.09** Other effects of lightning
    Use additional code for other effects of lightning

✓x7ᵗʰ **T75.1** Unspecified effects of drowning and nonfatal submersion ▽
    Immersion
    EXCLUDES 1   specified effects of drowning—code to effects

✓5ᵗʰ **T75.2** Effects of vibration

✓x7ᵗʰ **T75.20** Unspecified effects of vibration ▽

✓x7ᵗʰ **T75.21** Pneumatic hammer syndrome

✓x7ᵗʰ **T75.22** Traumatic vasospastic syndrome

---

2   HCC with 7th character indicating initial encounter (A or B - specific to category) OR sequela.

✓ Additional Character Req   ✓x7ᵗʰ Placeholder Alert   Manifestation   HCC CMS-HCC Condition   ▽ Unspecified Code   ▶◀ Revised Text   ● New Code   ▲ Revised Code Title

√x7ᵗʰ **T75.23** **Vertigo from infrasound**
     EXCLUDES 1   vertigo NOS (R42)

√x7ᵗʰ **T75.29** **Other effects of vibration**

√x7ᵗʰ **T75.3** **Motion sickness**
     Airsickness
     Seasickness
     Travel sickness
     Use additional external cause code to identify vehicle or type of motion (Y92.81-, Y93.5-)

√x7ᵗʰ **T75.4** **Electrocution**
     Shock from electric current
     Shock from electroshock gun (taser)

√5ᵗʰ **T75.8** **Other specified effects of external causes**

√x7ᵗʰ **T75.81** **Effects of abnormal gravitation [G] forces**

√x7ᵗʰ **T75.82** **Effects of weightlessness**

√x7ᵗʰ **T75.89** **Other specified effects of external causes**

√4ᵗʰ **T76** **Adult and child abuse, neglect and other maltreatment, suspected**
     Use additional code, if applicable, to identify any associated current injury
     EXCLUDES 1   adult and child maltreatment, confirmed (T74.-)
                   suspected abuse and maltreatment in pregnancy (O9A.3-, O9A.4-, O9A.5-)
                   suspected adult physical abuse, ruled out (Z04.71)
                   suspected adult sexual abuse, ruled out (Z04.41)
                   suspected child physical abuse, ruled out (Z04.72)
                   suspected child sexual abuse, ruled out (Z04.42)

> The appropriate 7th character is to be added to each code from category T76.
> A   initial encounter
> D   subsequent encounter
> S   sequela

√5ᵗʰ **T76.0** **Neglect or abandonment, suspected**

√x7ᵗʰ **T76.01** **Adult neglect or abandonment, suspected**   Ⓐ

√x7ᵗʰ **T76.02** **Child neglect or abandonment, suspected**   Ⓟ

√5ᵗʰ **T76.1** **Physical abuse, suspected**

√x7ᵗʰ **T76.11** **Adult physical abuse, suspected**   Ⓐ

√x7ᵗʰ **T76.12** **Child physical abuse, suspected**   Ⓟ

√5ᵗʰ **T76.2** **Sexual abuse, suspected**
     Rape, suspected
     ~~Sexual abuse, suspected~~
     EXCLUDES 1   alleged abuse, ruled out (Z04.7)

√x7ᵗʰ **T76.21** **Adult sexual abuse, suspected**   Ⓐ

√x7ᵗʰ **T76.22** **Child sexual abuse, suspected**   Ⓟ

√5ᵗʰ **T76.3** **Psychological abuse, suspected**

√x7ᵗʰ **T76.31** **Adult psychological abuse, suspected**   Ⓐ

√x7ᵗʰ **T76.32** **Child psychological abuse, suspected**   Ⓟ

√5ᵗʰ **T76.9** **Unspecified maltreatment, suspected**

√x7ᵗʰ **T76.91** **Unspecified adult maltreatment, suspected**   Ⓐ▽

√x7ᵗʰ **T76.92** **Unspecified child maltreatment, suspected**   Ⓟ▽

√4ᵗʰ **T78** **Adverse effects, not elsewhere classified**
     EXCLUDES 2   complications of surgical and medical care NEC (T80-T88)

> The appropriate 7th character is to be added to each code from category T78.
> A   initial encounter
> D   subsequent encounter
> S   sequela

√5ᵗʰ **T78.0** **Anaphylactic reaction due to food**
     Anaphylactic reaction due to adverse food reaction
     Anaphylactic shock or reaction due to nonpoisonous foods
     Anaphylactoid reaction due to food

√x7ᵗʰ **T78.00** **Anaphylactic reaction due to unspecified food**   ▽

√x7ᵗʰ **T78.01** **Anaphylactic reaction due to peanuts**

√x7ᵗʰ **T78.02** **Anaphylactic reaction due to shellfish (crustaceans)**

√x7ᵗʰ **T78.03** **Anaphylactic reaction due to other fish**

√x7ᵗʰ **T78.04** **Anaphylactic reaction due to fruits and vegetables**

√x7ᵗʰ **T78.05** **Anaphylactic reaction due to tree nuts and seeds**
     EXCLUDES 2   anaphylactic reaction due to peanuts (T78.01)

√x7ᵗʰ **T78.06** **Anaphylactic reaction due to food additives**

√x7ᵗʰ **T78.07** **Anaphylactic reaction due to milk and dairy products**

√x7ᵗʰ **T78.08** **Anaphylactic reaction due to eggs**

√x7ᵗʰ **T78.09** **Anaphylactic reaction due to other food products**

√x7ᵗʰ **T78.1** **Other adverse food reactions, not elsewhere classified**
     Use additional code to identify the type of reaction, if applicable
     EXCLUDES 1   anaphylactic reaction or shock due to adverse food reaction (T78.0-)
                   anaphylactic reaction due to food (T78.0-)
                   bacterial food borne intoxications (A05.-)
     EXCLUDES 2   allergic and dietetic gastroenteritis and colitis (K52.29)
                   allergic rhinitis due to food (J30.5)
                   dermatitis due to food in contact with skin (L23.6, L24.6, L25.4)
                   dermatitis due to ingested food (L27.2)
                   food protein-induced enterocolitis syndrome (K52.21)
                   food protein-induced enteropathy (K52.22)

√x7ᵗʰ **T78.2** **Anaphylactic shock, unspecified**   ▽
     Allergic shock
     Anaphylactic reaction
     Anaphylaxis
     EXCLUDES 1   anaphylactic reaction or shock due to adverse effect of correct medicinal substance properly administered (T88.6)
                   anaphylactic reaction or shock due to adverse food reaction (T78.0-)
                   anaphylactic reaction or shock due to serum (T80.5-)

√x7ᵗʰ **T78.3** **Angioneurotic edema**
     Allergic angioedema
     Giant urticaria
     Quincke's edema
     EXCLUDES 1   serum urticaria (T80.6-)
                   urticaria (L50.-)

√5ᵗʰ **T78.4** **Other and unspecified allergy**
     EXCLUDES 1   specified types of allergic reaction such as:
                   allergic diarrhea (K52.29)
                   allergic gastroenteritis and colitis (K52.29)
                   dermatitis (L23-L25, L27-)
                   food protein-induced enterocolitis syndrome (K52.21)
                   food protein-induced enteropathy (K52.22)
                   hay fever (J30.1)

√x7ᵗʰ **T78.40** **Allergy, unspecified**   ▽
     Allergic reaction NOS
     Hypersensitivity NOS

√x7ᵗʰ **T78.41** **Arthus phenomenon**
     Arthus reaction

√x7ᵗʰ **T78.49** **Other allergy**

√x7ᵗʰ **T78.8** **Other adverse effects, not elsewhere classified**

Certain early complications of trauma (T79)

√4ᵗʰ **T79** **Certain early complications of trauma, not elsewhere classified**
     EXCLUDES 2   acute respiratory distress syndrome (J80)
                   complications occurring during or following medical procedures (T80-T88)
                   complications of surgical and medical care NEC (T80-T88)
                   newborn respiratory distress syndrome (P22.0)

> The appropriate 7th character is to be added to each code from category T79.
> A   initial encounter
> D   subsequent encounter
> S   sequela

1 √x7ᵗʰ **T79.0** **Air embolism (traumatic)**   HCC
     EXCLUDES 1   air embolism complicating abortion or ectopic or molar pregnancy (O00-O07, O08.2)
                   air embolism complicating pregnancy, childbirth and the puerperium (O88.0)
                   air embolism following infusion, transfusion, and therapeutic injection (T80.0)
                   air embolism following procedure NEC (T81.7-)
     DEF: Arterial or venous obstruction due to introduction of air bubbles into the blood vessels following surgery or trauma.

---

1   HCC with 7th character indicating initial encounter (A, B or C - specific to category).

EXCLUDES 1 Not coded here   *EXCLUDES 2* Not included here   Ⓝ Newborn Age: 0   Ⓟ Pediatric Age: 0-17   Ⓜ Maternity Age: 12-55   Ⓐ Adult Age: 15-124

1094   ICD-10-CM 2018

[1] √x7ᵗʰ **T79.1 Fat embolism (traumatic)** HCC

    EXCLUDES 1   *fat embolism complicating:*
        abortion or ectopic or molar pregnancy (O00–O07, O08.2)
        pregnancy, childbirth and the puerperium (O88.8)

    DEF: Arterial blockage due to the entrance of fat into the circulatory system after fracture of large bones or administration of corticosteroids.

[1] √x7ᵗʰ **T79.2 Traumatic secondary and recurrent hemorrhage and seroma** HCC

[1] √x7ᵗʰ **T79.4 Traumatic shock** HCC

    Shock (immediate) (delayed) following injury

    EXCLUDES 1   *anaphylactic shock due to adverse food reaction (T78.0-)*
        anaphylactic shock due to correct medicinal substance properly administered (T88.6)
        anaphylactic shock due to serum (T80.5-)
        anaphylactic shock NOS (T78.2)
        anesthetic shock (T88.2)
        electric shock (T75.4)
        nontraumatic shock NEC (R57.-)
        obstetric shock (O75.1)
        postprocedural shock (T81.1-)
        septic shock (R65.21)
        shock complicating abortion or ectopic or molar pregnancy (O00–O07, O08.3)
        shock due to lightning (T75.01)
        shock NOS (R57.9)

[1] √x7ᵗʰ **T79.5 Traumatic anuria** HCC
    Crush syndrome
    Renal failure following crushing

[1] √x7ᵗʰ **T79.6 Traumatic ischemia of muscle** HCC
    Traumatic rhabdomyolysis
    Volkmann's ischemic contracture
    EXCLUDES 2   *anterior tibial syndrome (M76.8)*
        compartment syndrome (traumatic) (T79.A-)
        nontraumatic ischemia of muscle (M62.2-)

[1] √x7ᵗʰ **T79.7 Traumatic subcutaneous emphysema** HCC
    EXCLUDES 1   *emphysema NOS (J43)*
        emphysema (subcutaneous) resulting from a procedure (T81.82)

√5ᵗʰ **T79.A Traumatic compartment syndrome**
    EXCLUDES 1   *fibromyalgia (M79.7)*
        nontraumatic compartment syndrome (M79.A-)
        traumatic ischemic infarction of muscle (T79.6)

    DEF: Compression of nerves and blood vessels within an enclosed muscle space due to previous trauma, which leads to impaired blood flow and muscle and nerve damage.

[1] √x7ᵗʰ **T79.A0 Compartment syndrome, unspecified** HCC ▽
    Compartment syndrome NOS

√6ᵗʰ **T79.A1 Traumatic compartment syndrome of upper extremity**
    Traumatic compartment syndrome of shoulder, arm, forearm, wrist, hand, and fingers

[1] √7ᵗʰ **T79.A11 Traumatic compartment syndrome of right upper extremity** HCC

[1] √7ᵗʰ **T79.A12 Traumatic compartment syndrome of left upper extremity** HCC

[1] √7ᵗʰ **T79.A19 Traumatic compartment syndrome of unspecified upper extremity** HCC ▽

√6ᵗʰ **T79.A2 Traumatic compartment syndrome of lower extremity**
    Traumatic compartment syndrome of hip, buttock, thigh, leg, foot, and toes

[1] √7ᵗʰ **T79.A21 Traumatic compartment syndrome of right lower extremity** HCC

[1] √7ᵗʰ **T79.A22 Traumatic compartment syndrome of left lower extremity** HCC

[1] √7ᵗʰ **79.A29 Traumatic compartment syndrome of unspecified lower extremity** HCC ▽

[1] √x7ᵗʰ **T79.A3 Traumatic compartment syndrome of abdomen** HCC

[1] √x7ᵗʰ **T79.A9 Traumatic compartment syndrome of other sites** HCC

[1] √x7ᵗʰ **T79.8 Other early complications of trauma** HCC

[1] √x7ᵗʰ **T79.9 Unspecified early complication of trauma** HCC ▽

Complications of surgical and medical care, not elsewhere classified (T80-T88)

Use additional code for adverse effect, if applicable, to identify drug (T36–T50 with fifth or sixth character 5)

Use additional code(s) to identify the specified condition resulting from the complication

Use additional code to identify devices involved and details of circumstances (Y62–Y82)

EXCLUDES 2   *any encounters with medical care for postprocedural conditions in which no complications are present, such as:*
        artificial opening status (Z93.-)
        closure of external stoma (Z43.-)
        fitting and adjustment of external prosthetic device (Z44.-)
    burns and corrosions from local applications and irradiation (T20–T32)
    complications of surgical procedures during pregnancy, childbirth and the puerperium (O00–O9A)
    mechanical complication of respirator [ventilator] (J95.850)
    poisoning and toxic effects of drugs and chemicals (T36–T65 with fifth or sixth character 1-4 or 6)
    postprocedural fever (R50.82)
    specified complications classified elsewhere, such as:
        cerebrospinal fluid leak from spinal puncture (G97.0)
        colostomy malfunction (K94.0-)
        disorders of fluid and electrolyte imbalance (E86–E87)
        functional disturbances following cardiac surgery (I97.0–I97.1)
        intraoperative and postprocedural complications of specified body systems (D78.-, E36.-, E89.-, G97.3-, G97.4, H59.3-, H59.-, H95.2-, H95.3, I97.4-, I97.5, J95.6-, J95.7, K91.6-, L76.-, M96.-, N99.-)
        ostomy complications (J95.0-, K94.-, N99.5-)
        postgastric surgery syndromes (K91.1)
        postlaminectomy syndrome NEC (M96.1)
        postmastectomy lymphedema syndrome (I97.2)
        postsurgical blind-loop syndrome (K91.2)
        ventilator associated pneumonia (J95.851)

AHA: 2015, 1Q, 15

√4ᵗʰ **T80 Complications following infusion, transfusion and therapeutic injection**
    INCLUDES   complications following perfusion
    EXCLUDES 2   *bone marrow transplant rejection (T86.01)*
        febrile nonhemolytic transfusion reaction (R50.84)
        fluid overload due to transfusion (E87.71)
        posttransfusion purpura (D69.51)
        transfusion associated circulatory overload (TACO) (E87.71)
        transfusion (red blood cell) associated hemochromatosis (E83.111)
        transfusion related acute lung injury (TRALI) (J95.84)

> The appropriate 7th character is to be added to each code from category T80.
> A   initial encounter
> D   subsequent encounter
> S   sequela

√x7ᵗʰ **T80.0 Air embolism following infusion, transfusion and therapeutic injection**

√x7ᵗʰ **T80.1 Vascular complications following infusion, transfusion and therapeutic injection**
    Use additional code to identify the vascular complication
    EXCLUDES 2   *extravasation of vesicant agent (T80.81-)*
        infiltration of vesicant agent (T80.81-)
        postprocedural vascular complications (T81.7-)
        vascular complications specified as due to prosthetic devices, implants and grafts (T82.8-, T83.8-, T84.8-, T85.8-)

---

[1]   HCC with 7th character indicating initial encounter (A, B or C - specific to category).

☑ Additional Character Req   √x7ᵗʰ Placeholder Alert   Manifestation   HCC CMS-HCC Condition   ▽ Unspecified Code   ▶◀ Revised Text   ● New Code   ▲ Revised Code Title

✓5ᵗʰ **T80.2** **Infections** following infusion, transfusion and therapeutic injection

Use additional code to identify the specific infection, such as: sepsis (A41.9)

Use additional code (R65.2-) to identify severe sepsis, if applicable

EXCLUDES 2 *infections specified as due to prosthetic devices, implants and grafts (T82.6-T82.7, T83.5-T83.6, T84.5-T84.7, T85.7)*
postprocedural infections (T81.4-)

✓6ᵗʰ **T80.21** **Infection** due to central venous catheter
Infection due to pulmonary artery catheter (Swan-Ganz catheter)

✓7ᵗʰ **T80.211** **Bloodstream infection** due to central venous catheter
Catheter-related bloodstream infection (CRBSI) NOS
Central line-associated bloodstream infection (CLABSI)
Bloodstream infection due to Hickman catheter
Bloodstream infection due to peripherally inserted central catheter (PICC)
Bloodstream infection due to portacath (port-a-cath)
Bloodstream infection due to pulmonary artery catheter
Bloodstream infection due to triple lumen catheter
Bloodstream infection due to umbilical venous catheter

✓7ᵗʰ **T80.212** **Local infection** due to central venous catheter
Exit or insertion site infection
Local infection due to Hickman catheter
Local infection due to peripherally inserted central catheter (PICC)
Local infection due to portacath (port-a-cath)
Local infection due to pulmonary artery catheter
Local infection due to triple lumen catheter
Local infection due to umbilical venous catheter
Port or reservoir infection
Tunnel infection

✓7ᵗʰ **T80.218** **Other infection** due to central venous catheter
Other central line-associated infection
Other infection due to Hickman catheter
Other infection due to peripherally inserted central catheter (PICC)
Other infection due to portacath (port-a-cath)
Other infection due to pulmonary artery catheter
Other infection due to triple lumen catheter
Other infection due to umbilical venous catheter

✓7ᵗʰ **T80.219** **Unspecified infection** due to central venous catheter ▽
Central line-associated infection NOS
Unspecified infection due to Hickman catheter
Unspecified infection due to peripherally inserted central catheter (PICC)
Unspecified infection due to portacath (port-a-cath)
Unspecified infection due to pulmonary artery catheter
Unspecified infection due to triple lumen catheter
Unspecified infection due to umbilical venous catheter

✓x7ᵗʰ **T80.22** **Acute infection** following transfusion, infusion, or injection of blood and blood products

✓x7ᵗʰ **T80.29** **Infection** following other infusion, transfusion and therapeutic injection

✓5ᵗʰ **T80.3** **ABO incompatibility** reaction due to transfusion of blood or blood products

EXCLUDES 1 *minor blood group antigens reactions (Duffy) (E) (K(ell)) (Kidd) (Lewis) (M) (N) (P) (S) (T80.A)*

✓x7ᵗʰ **T80.30** **ABO incompatibility reaction** due to transfusion of blood or blood products, unspecified ▽
ABO incompatibility blood transfusion NOS
Reaction to ABO incompatibility from transfusion NOS

✓6ᵗʰ **T80.31** **ABO incompatibility** with hemolytic transfusion reaction

✓7ᵗʰ **T80.310** **ABO incompatibility** with acute hemolytic transfusion reaction
ABO incompatibility with hemolytic transfusion reaction less than 24 hours after transfusion
Acute hemolytic transfusion reaction (AHTR) due to ABO incompatibility

✓7ᵗʰ **T80.311** **ABO incompatibility** with delayed hemolytic transfusion reaction
ABO incompatibility with hemolytic transfusion reaction 24 hours or more after transfusion
Delayed hemolytic transfusion reaction (DHTR) due to ABO incompatibility

✓7ᵗʰ **T80.319** **ABO incompatibility** with hemolytic transfusion reaction, unspecified ▽
ABO incompatibility with hemolytic transfusion reaction at unspecified time after transfusion
Hemolytic transfusion reaction (HTR) due to ABO incompatibility NOS

✓x7ᵗʰ **T80.39** **Other ABO incompatibility reaction** due to transfusion of blood or blood products
Delayed serologic transfusion reaction (DSTR) from ABO incompatibility
Other ABO incompatible blood transfusion
Other reaction to ABO incompatible blood transfusion

✓5ᵗʰ **T80.4** **Rh incompatibility** reaction due to transfusion of blood or blood products
Reaction due to incompatibility of Rh antigens (C) (c) (D) (E) (e)

✓x7ᵗʰ **T80.40** **Rh incompatibility reaction** due to transfusion of blood or blood products, unspecified ▽
Reaction due to Rh factor in transfusion NOS
Rh incompatible blood transfusion NOS

✓6ᵗʰ **T80.41** **Rh incompatibility** with hemolytic transfusion reaction

✓7ᵗʰ **T80.410** **Rh incompatibility** with acute hemolytic transfusion reaction
Acute hemolytic transfusion reaction (AHTR) due to Rh incompatibility
Rh incompatibility with hemolytic transfusion reaction less than 24 hours after transfusion

✓7ᵗʰ **T80.411** **Rh incompatibility** with delayed hemolytic transfusion reaction
Delayed hemolytic transfusion reaction (DHTR) due to Rh incompatibility
Rh incompatibility with hemolytic transfusion reaction 24 hours or more after transfusion

✓7ᵗʰ **T80.419** **Rh incompatibility** with hemolytic transfusion reaction, unspecified ▽
Hemolytic transfusion reaction (HTR) due to Rh incompatibility NOS
Rh incompatibility with hemolytic transfusion reaction at unspecified time after transfusion

✓x7ᵗʰ **T80.49** **Other Rh incompatibility reaction** due to transfusion of blood or blood products
Delayed serologic transfusion reaction (DSTR) from Rh incompatibility
Other reaction to Rh incompatible blood transfusion

✓5ᵗʰ **T80.A** **Non-ABO incompatibility** reaction due to transfusion of blood or blood products
Reaction due to incompatibility of minor antigens (Duffy) (Kell) (Kidd) (Lewis) (M) (N) (P) (S)

✓x7ᵗʰ **T80.A0** **Non-ABO incompatibility reaction** due to transfusion of blood or blood products, unspecified ▽
Non-ABO antigen incompatibility reaction from transfusion NOS

EXCLUDES 1 Not coded here   EXCLUDES 2 Not included here   N Newborn Age: 0   P Pediatric Age: 0-17   M Maternity Age: 12-55   A Adult Age: 15-124

1096   ICD-10-CM 2018

√6ᵗʰ **T80.A1** **Non-ABO incompatibility** with hemolytic transfusion reaction

√7ᵗʰ **T80.A10** **Non-ABO incompatibility with** acute hemolytic transfusion reaction

Acute hemolytic transfusion reaction (AHTR) due to non-ABO incompatibility

Non-ABO incompatibility with hemolytic transfusion reaction less than 24 hours after transfusion

√7ᵗʰ **T80.A11** **Non-ABO incompatibility with** delayed hemolytic transfusion reaction

Delayed hemolytic transfusion reaction (DHTR) due to non-ABO incompatibility

Non-ABO incompatibility with hemolytic transfusion reaction 24 or more hours after transfusion

√7ᵗʰ **T80.A19** **Non-ABO incompatibility with hemolytic transfusion reaction, unspecified** ▽

Hemolytic transfusion reaction (HTR) due to non-ABO incompatibility NOS

Non-ABO incompatibility with hemolytic transfusion reaction at unspecified time after transfusion

√x7ᵗʰ **T80.A9** **Other non-ABO incompatibility reaction due to transfusion of blood or blood products**

Delayed serologic transfusion reaction (DSTR) from non-ABO incompatibility

Other reaction to non-ABO incompatible blood transfusion

√5ᵗʰ **T80.5** **Anaphylactic reaction due to serum**

Allergic shock due to serum

Anaphylactic shock due to serum

Anaphylactoid reaction due to serum

Anaphylaxis due to serum

EXCLUDES 1   ABO incompatibility reaction due to transfusion of blood or blood products (T80.3-)

allergic reaction or shock NOS (T78.2)

anaphylactic reaction or shock NOS (T78.2)

anaphylactic reaction or shock due to adverse effect of correct medicinal substance properly administered (T88.6)

other serum reaction (T80.6-)

DEF: Life-threatening hypersensitivity to foreign serum; causes respiratory distress, vascular collapse, and shock.

√x7ᵗʰ **T80.51** **Anaphylactic reaction due to** administration of blood and blood products

√x7ᵗʰ **T80.52** **Anaphylactic reaction due to** vaccination

√x7ᵗʰ **T80.59** **Anaphylactic reaction due to other serum**

√5ᵗʰ **T80.6** **Other serum reactions**

Intoxication by serum

Protein sickness

Serum rash

Serum sickness

Serum urticaria

EXCLUDES 2   serum hepatitis (B16-B19)

DEF: Serum sickness: Hypersensitivity to foreign serum; causes fever, hives, swelling, and lymphadenopathy.

√x7ᵗʰ **T80.61** **Other serum reaction** due to administration of blood and blood products

√x7ᵗʰ **T80.62** **Other serum reaction** due to vaccination

√x7ᵗʰ **T80.69** **Other serum reaction due to other serum**

▶Code also, if applicable, arthropathy in hypersensitivity reactions classified elsewhere (M36.4)◀

√5ᵗʰ **T80.8** **Other complications following infusion, transfusion and therapeutic injection**

√6ᵗʰ **T80.81** **Extravasation of vesicant agent**

Infiltration of vesicant agent

√7ᵗʰ **T80.810** **Extravasation of vesicant antineoplastic chemotherapy**

Infiltration of vesicant antineoplastic chemotherapy

√7ᵗʰ **T80.818** **Extravasation of other vesicant agent**

Infiltration of other vesicant agent

√x7ᵗʰ **T80.89** **Other complications following infusion, transfusion and therapeutic injection**

Delayed serologic transfusion reaction (DSTR), unspecified incompatibility

Use additional code to identify graft-versus-host reaction, if applicable, (D89.81-)

√5ᵗʰ **T80.9** **Unspecified complication following infusion, transfusion and therapeutic injection**

√x7ᵗʰ **T80.90** **Unspecified complication** following infusion and therapeutic injection ▽

√6ᵗʰ **T80.91** **Hemolytic transfusion reaction, unspecified incompatibility**

EXCLUDES 1   ABO incompatibility with hemolytic transfusion reaction (T80.31-)

Non-ABO incompatibility with hemolytic transfusion reaction (T80.A1-)

Rh incompatibility with hemolytic transfusion reaction (T80.41-)

√7ᵗʰ **T80.910** **Acute hemolytic transfusion reaction, unspecified incompatibility** ▽

√7ᵗʰ **T80.911** **Delayed hemolytic transfusion reaction, unspecified incompatibility** ▽

√7ᵗʰ **T80.919** **Hemolytic transfusion reaction, unspecified incompatibility, unspecified as acute or delayed** ▽

Hemolytic transfusion reaction NOS

√x7ᵗʰ **T80.92** **Unspecified transfusion reaction** ▽

Transfusion reaction NOS

√4ᵗʰ **T81** **Complications of procedures, not elsewhere classified**

Use additional code for adverse effect, if applicable, to identify drug (T36-T50 with fifth or sixth character 5)

EXCLUDES 2   complications following immunization (T88.0-T88.1)

complications following infusion, transfusion and therapeutic injection (T80.-)

complications of transplanted organs and tissue (T86.-)

specified complications classified elsewhere, such as:

complication of prosthetic devices, implants and grafts (T82-T85)

dermatitis due to drugs and medicaments (L23.3, L24.4, L25.1, L27.0-L27.1)

endosseous dental implant failure (M27.6-)

floppy iris syndrome (IFIS) (intraoperative) (H21.81)

intraoperative and postprocedural complications of specific body system (D78.-, E36.-, E89.-, G97.3-, G97.4, H59.3-, H59.-, H95.2-, H95.3, I97.4-, I97.5, J95, K91.-, L76.-, M96.-, N99.-)

ostomy complications (J95.0-, K94.-, N99.5-)

plateau iris syndrome (post-iridectomy) (postprocedural) (H21.82)

poisoning and toxic effects of drugs and chemicals (T36-T65 with fifth or sixth character 1-4 or 6)

The appropriate 7th character is to be added to each code from category T81.

A   initial encounter

D   subsequent encounter

S   sequela

√5ᵗʰ **T81.1** **Postprocedural shock**

Shock during or resulting from a procedure, not elsewhere classified

EXCLUDES 1   anaphylactic shock due to correct substance properly administered (T88.6)

anaphylactic shock due to serum (T80.5-)

anaphylactic shock NOS (T78.2)

anesthetic shock (T88.2)

electric shock (T75.4)

obstetric shock (O75.1)

septic shock (R65.21)

shock following abortion or ectopic or molar pregnancy (O00-O07, O08.3)

traumatic shock (T79.4)

√x7ᵗʰ **T81.10** **Postprocedural shock unspecified** ▽

Collapse NOS during or resulting from a procedure, not elsewhere classified

Postprocedural failure of peripheral circulation

Postprocedural shock NOS

1   √x7ᵗʰ **T81.11** **Postprocedural** cardiogenic shock   HCC

---

1   HCC with 7th character indicating initial encounter (A, B or C - specific to category).

☑ Additional Character Req   √x7ᵗʰ Placeholder Alert   Manifestation   HCC CMS-HCC Condition   ▽ Unspecified Code   ▶◀ Revised Text   ● New Code   ▲ Revised Code Title

ICD-10-CM 2018   **1097**

[1] ✓x7th T81.12 Postprocedural septic shock   HCC
    Postprocedural endotoxic shock resulting from a procedure, not elsewhere classified
    Postprocedural gram-negative shock resulting from a procedure, not elsewhere classified
    Code first underlying infection
    Use additional code, to identify any associated acute organ dysfunction, if applicable

✓x7th T81.19 Other postprocedural shock
    Postprocedural hypovolemic shock

✓5th T81.3 Disruption of wound, not elsewhere classified
    Disruption of any suture materials or other closure methods
    EXCLUDES 1   *breakdown (mechanical) of permanent sutures (T85.612)*
       displacement of permanent sutures (T85.622)
       disruption of cesarean delivery wound (O90.0)
       disruption of perineal obstetric wound (O90.1)
       mechanical complication of permanent sutures NEC (T85.692)
    AHA: 2014, 1Q, 23

✓x7th T81.30 Disruption of wound, unspecified ▽
    Disruption of wound NOS

✓x7th T81.31 Disruption of external operation (surgical) wound, not elsewhere classified
    Dehiscence of operation wound NOS
    Disruption of operation wound NOS
    Disruption or dehiscence of closure of cornea
    Disruption or dehiscence of closure of mucosa
    Disruption or dehiscence of closure of skin and subcutaneous tissue
    Full-thickness skin disruption or dehiscence
    Superficial disruption or dehiscence of operation wound
    EXCLUDES 1   *dehiscence of amputation stump (T87.81)*

✓x7th T81.32 Disruption of internal operation (surgical) wound, not elsewhere classified
    Deep disruption or dehiscence of operation wound NOS
    Disruption or dehiscence of closure of internal organ or other internal tissue
    Disruption or dehiscence of closure of muscle or muscle flap
    Disruption or dehiscence of closure of ribs or rib cage
    Disruption or dehiscence of closure of skull or craniotomy
    Disruption or dehiscence of closure of sternum or sternotomy
    Disruption or dehiscence of closure of tendon or ligament
    Disruption or dehiscence of closure of superficial or muscular fascia

✓x7th T81.33 Disruption of traumatic injury wound repair
    Disruption or dehiscence of closure of traumatic laceration (external) (internal)

✓x7th T81.4 Infection following a procedure
    Intra-abdominal abscess following a procedure
    Postprocedural infection, not elsewhere classified
    Sepsis following a procedure
    Stitch abscess following a procedure
    Subphrenic abscess following a procedure
    Wound abscess following a procedure
    Use additional code to identify infection
    Use additional code (R65.2-) to identify severe sepsis, if applicable
    EXCLUDES 1   *obstetric surgical wound infection (O86.0)*
       postprocedural fever NOS (R50.82)
       postprocedural retroperitoneal abscess (K68.11)
    EXCLUDES 2   *bleb associated endophthalmitis (H59.4-)*
       infection due to infusion, transfusion and therapeutic injection (T80.2-)
       infection due to prosthetic devices, implants and grafts (T82.6-T82.7, T83.5-T83.6, T84.5-T84.7, T85.7)
    AHA: 2014, 1Q, 23

✓5th T81.5 Complications of foreign body accidentally left in body following procedure
    AHA: 2014, 4Q, 24

    ✓6th T81.50 Unspecified complication of foreign body accidentally left in body following procedure

       ✓7th T81.500 Unspecified complication of foreign body accidentally left in body following surgical operation ▽

✓7th T81.501 Unspecified complication of foreign body accidentally left in body following infusion or transfusion ▽

✓7th T81.502 Unspecified complication of foreign body accidentally left in body following kidney dialysis HCC ▽

✓7th T81.503 Unspecified complication of foreign body accidentally left in body following injection or immunization ▽

✓7th T81.504 Unspecified complication of foreign body accidentally left in body following endoscopic examination ▽

✓7th T81.505 Unspecified complication of foreign body accidentally left in body following heart catheterization ▽

✓7th T81.506 Unspecified complication of foreign body accidentally left in body following aspiration, puncture or other catheterization ▽

✓7th T81.507 Unspecified complication of foreign body accidentally left in body following removal of catheter or packing ▽

✓7th T81.508 Unspecified complication of foreign body accidentally left in body following other procedure ▽

✓7th T81.509 Unspecified complication of foreign body accidentally left in body following unspecified procedure ▽

✓6th T81.51 Adhesions due to foreign body accidentally left in body following procedure

    ✓7th T81.510 Adhesions due to foreign body accidentally left in body following surgical operation

    ✓7th T81.511 Adhesions due to foreign body accidentally left in body following infusion or transfusion

    ✓7th T81.512 Adhesions due to foreign body accidentally left in body following kidney dialysis HCC

    ✓7th T81.513 Adhesions due to foreign body accidentally left in body following injection or immunization

    ✓7th T81.514 Adhesions due to foreign body accidentally left in body following endoscopic examination

    ✓7th T81.515 Adhesions due to foreign body accidentally left in body following heart catheterization

    ✓7th T81.516 Adhesions due to foreign body accidentally left in body following aspiration, puncture or other catheterization

    ✓7th T81.517 Adhesions due to foreign body accidentally left in body following removal of catheter or packing

    ✓7th T81.518 Adhesions due to foreign body accidentally left in body following other procedure

    ✓7th T81.519 Adhesions due to foreign body accidentally left in body following unspecified procedure ▽

✓6th T81.52 Obstruction due to foreign body accidentally left in body following procedure

    ✓7th T81.520 Obstruction due to foreign body accidentally left in body following surgical operation

    ✓7th T81.521 Obstruction due to foreign body accidentally left in body following infusion or transfusion

    ✓7th T81.522 Obstruction due to foreign body accidentally left in body following kidney dialysis HCC

    ✓7th T81.523 Obstruction due to foreign body accidentally left in body following injection or immunization

    ✓7th T81.524 Obstruction due to foreign body accidentally left in body following endoscopic examination

---

[1] HCC with 7th character indicating initial encounter (A, B or C - specific to category).

EXCLUDES 1 Not coded here   EXCLUDES 2 Not included here   N Newborn Age: 0   P Pediatric Age: 0-17   M Maternity Age: 12-55   A Adult Age: 15-124

1098   ICD-10-CM 2018

√7th **T81.525** Obstruction due to foreign body accidentally left in body following heart catheterization

√7th **T81.526** Obstruction due to foreign body accidentally left in body following aspiration, puncture or other catheterization

√7th **T81.527** Obstruction due to foreign body accidentally left in body following removal of catheter or packing

√7th **T81.528** Obstruction due to foreign body accidentally left in body following other procedure

√7th **T81.529** Obstruction due to foreign body accidentally left in body following unspecified procedure   ▽

√6th **T81.53** Perforation due to foreign body accidentally left in body following procedure

√7th **T81.530** Perforation due to foreign body accidentally left in body following surgical operation

√7th **T81.531** Perforation due to foreign body accidentally left in body following infusion or transfusion

√7th **T81.532** Perforation due to foreign body accidentally left in body following kidney dialysis   HCC

√7th **T81.533** Perforation due to foreign body accidentally left in body following injection or immunization

√7th **T81.534** Perforation due to foreign body accidentally left in body following endoscopic examination

√7th **T81.535** Perforation due to foreign body accidentally left in body following heart catheterization

√7th **T81.536** Perforation due to foreign body accidentally left in body following aspiration, puncture or other catheterization

√7th **T81.537** Perforation due to foreign body accidentally left in body following removal of catheter or packing

√7th **T81.538** Perforation due to foreign body accidentally left in body following other procedure

√7th **T81.539** Perforation due to foreign body accidentally left in body following unspecified procedure   ▽

√6th **T81.59** Other complications of foreign body accidentally left in body following procedure

    EXCLUDES 2 obstruction or perforation due to prosthetic devices and implants intentionally left in body (T82.0-T82.5, T83.0-T83.4, T83.7, T84.0-T84.4, T85.0-T85.6)

√7th **T81.590** Other complications of foreign body accidentally left in body following surgical operation

√7th **T81.591** Other complications of foreign body accidentally left in body following infusion or transfusion

√7th **T81.592** Other complications of foreign body accidentally left in body following kidney dialysis   HCC

√7th **T81.593** Other complications of foreign body accidentally left in body following injection or immunization

√7th **T81.594** Other complications of foreign body accidentally left in body following endoscopic examination

√7th **T81.595** Other complications of foreign body accidentally left in body following heart catheterization

√7th **T81.596** Other complications of foreign body accidentally left in body following aspiration, puncture or other catheterization

√7th **T81.597** Other complications of foreign body accidentally left in body following removal of catheter or packing

√7th **T81.598** Other complications of foreign body accidentally left in body following other procedure

√7th **T81.599** Other complications of foreign body accidentally left in body following unspecified procedure   ▽

√5th **T81.6** Acute reaction to foreign substance accidentally left during a procedure

    EXCLUDES 2 complications of foreign body accidentally left in body cavity or operation wound following procedure (T81.5-)

√x7th **T81.60** Unspecified acute reaction to foreign substance accidentally left during a procedure   ▽

√x7th **T81.61** Aseptic peritonitis due to foreign substance accidentally left during a procedure
    Chemical peritonitis

√x7th **T81.69** Other acute reaction to foreign substance accidentally left during a procedure

√5th **T81.7** Vascular complications following a procedure, not elsewhere classified
    Air embolism following procedure NEC
    Phlebitis or thrombophlebitis resulting from a procedure

    EXCLUDES 1 embolism complicating abortion or ectopic or molar pregnancy (O00-O07, O08.2)
      embolism complicating pregnancy, childbirth and the puerperium (O88.-)
      traumatic embolism (T79.0)

    EXCLUDES 2 embolism due to prosthetic devices, implants and grafts (T82.8-, T83.81, T84.8-, T85.81-)
      embolism following infusion, transfusion and therapeutic injection (T80.0)

√6th **T81.71** Complication of artery following a procedure, not elsewhere classified

√7th **T81.710** Complication of mesenteric artery following a procedure, not elsewhere classified

√7th **T81.711** Complication of renal artery following a procedure, not elsewhere classified

√7th **T81.718** Complication of other artery following a procedure, not elsewhere classified

√7th **T81.719** Complication of unspecified artery following a procedure, not elsewhere classified   ▽

√x7th **T81.72** Complication of vein following a procedure, not elsewhere classified

√5th **T81.8** Other complications of procedures, not elsewhere classified

    EXCLUDES 2 hypothermia following anesthesia (T88.51)
      malignant hyperpyrexia due to anesthesia (T88.3)

√x7th **T81.81** Complication of inhalation therapy

√x7th **T81.82** Emphysema (subcutaneous) resulting from a procedure

√x7th **T81.83** Persistent postprocedural fistula

√x7th **T81.89** Other complications of procedures, not elsewhere classified
    Use additional code to specify complication, such as:
    postprocedural delirium (F05)
    AHA: 2014, 1Q, 23

√x7th **T81.9** Unspecified complication of procedure   ▽

√4th **T82** Complications of cardiac and vascular prosthetic devices, implants and grafts

    EXCLUDES 2 failure and rejection of transplanted organs and tissue (T86.-)

    The appropriate 7th character is to be added to each code from category T82.
    A   initial encounter
    D   subsequent encounter
    S   sequela

√5th **T82.0** Mechanical complication of heart valve prosthesis
    Mechanical complication of artificial heart valve

    EXCLUDES 1 mechanical complication of biological heart valve graft (T82.22-)

√x7th **T82.01** Breakdown (mechanical) of heart valve prosthesis

√x7th **T82.02** Displacement of heart valve prosthesis
    Malposition of heart valve prosthesis

√x7th **T82.03** Leakage of heart valve prosthesis

☑ Additional Character Req   √x7th Placeholder Alert   Manifestation   HCC CMS-HCC Condition   ▽ Unspecified Code   ▶◀ Revised Text   ● New Code   ▲ Revised Code Title

ICD-10-CM 2018   1099

√x7ᵗʰ T82.09 Other mechanical complication of heart valve prosthesis
Obstruction (mechanical) of heart valve prosthesis
Perforation of heart valve prosthesis
Protrusion of heart valve prosthesis

√5ᵗʰ T82.1 Mechanical complication of cardiac electronic device

√6ᵗʰ T82.11 Breakdown (mechanical) of cardiac electronic device

√7ᵗʰ T82.110 Breakdown (mechanical) of cardiac electrode

√7ᵗʰ T82.111 Breakdown (mechanical) of cardiac pulse generator (battery)

√7ᵗʰ T82.118 Breakdown (mechanical) of other cardiac electronic device

√7ᵗʰ T82.119 Breakdown (mechanical) of unspecified ▽ cardiac electronic device

√6ᵗʰ T82.12 Displacement of cardiac electronic device
Malposition of cardiac electronic device

√7ᵗʰ T82.120 Displacement of cardiac electrode

√7ᵗʰ T82.121 Displacement of cardiac pulse generator (battery)

√7ᵗʰ T82.128 Displacement of other cardiac electronic device

√7ᵗʰ T82.129 Displacement of unspecified cardiac ▽ electronic device

√6ᵗʰ T82.19 Other mechanical complication of cardiac electronic device
Leakage of cardiac electronic device
Obstruction of cardiac electronic device
Perforation of cardiac electronic device
Protrusion of cardiac electronic device

√7ᵗʰ T82.190 Other mechanical complication of cardiac electrode

√7ᵗʰ T82.191 Other mechanical complication of cardiac pulse generator (battery)

√7ᵗʰ T82.198 Other mechanical complication of other cardiac electronic device

√7ᵗʰ T82.199 Other mechanical complication of ▽ unspecified cardiac device

√5ᵗʰ T82.2 Mechanical complication of coronary artery bypass graft and biological heart valve graft
EXCLUDES 1   mechanical complication of artificial heart valve prosthesis (T82.0-)

√6ᵗʰ T82.21 Mechanical complication of coronary artery bypass graft

√7ᵗʰ T82.211 Breakdown (mechanical) of coronary artery bypass graft

√7ᵗʰ T82.212 Displacement of coronary artery bypass graft
Malposition of coronary artery bypass graft

√7ᵗʰ T82.213 Leakage of coronary artery bypass graft

√7ᵗʰ T82.218 Other mechanical complication of coronary artery bypass graft
Obstruction, mechanical of coronary artery bypass graft
Perforation of coronary artery bypass graft
Protrusion of coronary artery bypass graft

√6ᵗʰ T82.22 Mechanical complication of biological heart valve graft

√7ᵗʰ T82.221 Breakdown (mechanical) of biological heart valve graft

√7ᵗʰ T82.222 Displacement of biological heart valve graft
Malposition of biological heart valve graft

√7ᵗʰ T82.223 Leakage of biological heart valve graft

√7ᵗʰ T82.228 Other mechanical complication of biological heart valve graft
Obstruction of biological heart valve graft
Perforation of biological heart valve graft
Protrusion of biological heart valve graft

√5ᵗʰ T82.3 Mechanical complication of other vascular grafts

√6ᵗʰ T82.31 Breakdown (mechanical) of other vascular grafts

1 √7ᵗʰ T82.310 Breakdown (mechanical) of aortic (bifurcation) graft (replacement) HCC

1 √7ᵗʰ T82.311 Breakdown (mechanical) of carotid arterial graft (bypass) HCC

1 √7ᵗʰ T82.312 Breakdown (mechanical) of femoral arterial graft (bypass) HCC

1 √7ᵗʰ T82.318 Breakdown (mechanical) of other vascular grafts HCC

1 √7ᵗʰ T82.319 Breakdown (mechanical) of unspecified vascular grafts HCC ▽

√6ᵗʰ T82.32 Displacement of other vascular grafts
Malposition of other vascular grafts

1 √7ᵗʰ T82.320 Displacement of aortic (bifurcation) graft (replacement) HCC

1 √7ᵗʰ T82.321 Displacement of carotid arterial graft (bypass) HCC

1 √7ᵗʰ T82.322 Displacement of femoral arterial graft (bypass) HCC

1 √7ᵗʰ T82.328 Displacement of other vascular grafts HCC

1 √7ᵗʰ T82.329 Displacement of unspecified vascular grafts HCC ▽

√6ᵗʰ T82.33 Leakage of other vascular grafts

1 √7ᵗʰ T82.330 Leakage of aortic (bifurcation) graft (replacement) HCC

1 √7ᵗʰ T82.331 Leakage of carotid arterial graft (bypass) HCC

1 √7ᵗʰ T82.332 Leakage of femoral arterial graft (bypass) HCC

1 √7ᵗʰ T82.338 Leakage of other vascular grafts HCC

1 √7ᵗʰ T82.339 Leakage of unspecified vascular graft HCC ▽

√6ᵗʰ T82.39 Other mechanical complication of other vascular grafts
Obstruction (mechanical) of other vascular grafts
Perforation of other vascular grafts
Protrusion of other vascular grafts

1 √7ᵗʰ T82.390 Other mechanical complication of aortic (bifurcation) graft (replacement) HCC

1 √7ᵗʰ T82.391 Other mechanical complication of carotid arterial graft (bypass) HCC

1 √7ᵗʰ T82.392 Other mechanical complication of femoral arterial graft (bypass) HCC

1 √7ᵗʰ T82.398 Other mechanical complication of other vascular grafts HCC

1 √7ᵗʰ T82.399 Other mechanical complication of unspecified vascular grafts HCC ▽

√5ᵗʰ T82.4 Mechanical complication of vascular dialysis catheter
Mechanical complication of hemodialysis catheter
EXCLUDES 1   mechanical complication of intraperitoneal dialysis catheter (T85.62)

√x7ᵗʰ T82.41 Breakdown (mechanical) of vascular dialysis catheter HCC

√x7ᵗʰ T82.42 Displacement of vascular dialysis catheter HCC
Malposition of vascular dialysis catheter

√x7ᵗʰ T82.43 Leakage of vascular dialysis catheter HCC

√x7ᵗʰ T82.49 Other complication of vascular dialysis catheter HCC
Obstruction (mechanical) of vascular dialysis catheter
Perforation of vascular dialysis catheter
Protrusion of vascular dialysis catheter

√5ᵗʰ T82.5 Mechanical complication of other cardiac and vascular devices and implants
EXCLUDES 2   mechanical complication of epidural and subdural infusion catheter (T85.61)

√6ᵗʰ T82.51 Breakdown (mechanical) of other cardiac and vascular devices and implants

1 √7ᵗʰ T82.510 Breakdown (mechanical) of surgically created arteriovenous fistula HCC

1 √7ᵗʰ T82.511 Breakdown (mechanical) of surgically created arteriovenous shunt HCC

√7ᵗʰ T82.512 Breakdown (mechanical) of artificial heart

1 √7ᵗʰ T82.513 Breakdown (mechanical) of balloon (counterpulsation) device HCC

1 √7ᵗʰ T82.514 Breakdown (mechanical) of infusion catheter HCC

1 √7ᵗʰ T82.515 Breakdown (mechanical) of umbrella device HCC

---

1   HCC with 7th character indicating initial encounter (A, B or C - specific to category).

EXCLUDES 1 Not coded here   EXCLUDES 2 Not included here   N Newborn Age: 0   P Pediatric Age: 0-17   M Maternity Age: 12-55   A Adult Age: 15-124

1100   ICD-10-CM 2018

¹ ☑7ᵗʰ **T82.518** **Breakdown (mechanical) of other cardiac and vascular devices and implants** ᴴᶜᶜ

☑7ᵗʰ **T82.519** **Breakdown (mechanical) of unspecified cardiac and vascular devices and implants** ▽

☑6ᵗʰ **T82.52** Displacement of other cardiac and vascular devices and implants
Malposition of other cardiac and vascular devices and implants

¹ ☑7ᵗʰ **T82.520** **Displacement of** surgically created arteriovenous fistula ᴴᶜᶜ

¹ ☑7ᵗʰ **T82.521** **Displacement of** surgically created arteriovenous shunt ᴴᶜᶜ

☑7ᵗʰ **T82.522** **Displacement of** artificial heart

¹ ☑7ᵗʰ **T82.523** **Displacement of** balloon (counterpulsation) device ᴴᶜᶜ

¹ ☑7ᵗʰ **T82.524** **Displacement of** infusion catheter ᴴᶜᶜ

¹ ☑7ᵗʰ **T82.525** **Displacement of** umbrella device ᴴᶜᶜ

¹ ☑7ᵗʰ **T82.528** **Displacement of other cardiac and vascular devices and implants** ᴴᶜᶜ

☑7ᵗʰ **T82.529** **Displacement of unspecified cardiac and vascular devices and implants** ▽

☑6ᵗʰ **T82.53** Leakage of other cardiac and vascular devices and implants

¹ ☑7ᵗʰ **T82.530** **Leakage of** surgically created arteriovenous fistula ᴴᶜᶜ

¹ ☑7ᵗʰ **T82.531** **Leakage of** surgically created arteriovenous shunt ᴴᶜᶜ

☑7ᵗʰ **T82.532** **Leakage of** artificial heart

¹ ☑7ᵗʰ **T82.533** **Leakage of** balloon (counterpulsation) device ᴴᶜᶜ

¹ ☑7ᵗʰ **T82.534** **Leakage of** infusion catheter ᴴᶜᶜ

¹ ☑7ᵗʰ **T82.535** **Leakage of** umbrella device ᴴᶜᶜ

¹ ☑7ᵗʰ **T82.538** **Leakage of other cardiac and vascular devices and implants** ᴴᶜᶜ

☑7ᵗʰ **T82.539** **Leakage of unspecified cardiac and vascular devices and implants** ▽

☑6ᵗʰ **T82.59** **Other mechanical complication of other cardiac and vascular devices and implants**
Obstruction (mechanical) of other cardiac and vascular devices and implants
Perforation of other cardiac and vascular devices and implants
Protrusion of other cardiac and vascular devices and implants

¹ ☑7ᵗʰ **T82.590** **Other mechanical complication of** surgically created arteriovenous fistula ᴴᶜᶜ

¹ ☑7ᵗʰ **T82.591** **Other mechanical complication of** surgically created arteriovenous shunt ᴴᶜᶜ

☑7ᵗʰ **T82.592** **Other mechanical complication of** artificial heart

¹ ☑7ᵗʰ **T82.593** **Other mechanical complication of** balloon (counterpulsation) device ᴴᶜᶜ

¹ ☑7ᵗʰ **T82.594** **Other mechanical complication of** infusion catheter ᴴᶜᶜ

¹ ☑7ᵗʰ **T82.595** **Other mechanical complication of** umbrella device ᴴᶜᶜ

¹ ☑7ᵗʰ **T82.598** **Other mechanical complication of other cardiac and vascular devices and implants** ᴴᶜᶜ

☑7ᵗʰ **T82.599** **Other mechanical complication of unspecified cardiac and vascular devices and implants** ▽

¹ ☑ₓ7ᵗʰ **T82.6** **Infection and inflammatory reaction due to cardiac valve prosthesis** ᴴᶜᶜ
Use additional code to identify infection

¹ ☑ₓ7ᵗʰ **T82.7** **Infection and inflammatory reaction due to other cardiac and vascular devices, implants and grafts** ᴴᶜᶜ
Use additional code to identify infection

☑5ᵗʰ **T82.8** **Other specified complications of cardiac and vascular prosthetic devices, implants and grafts**

☑6ᵗʰ **T82.81** Embolism **due to cardiac and vascular prosthetic devices, implants and grafts**

☑7ᵗʰ **T82.817** **Embolism due to** cardiac **prosthetic devices, implants and grafts**

☑7ᵗʰ **T82.818** **Embolism due to** vascular **prosthetic devices, implants and grafts** ᴴᶜᶜ

☑6ᵗʰ **T82.82** Fibrosis **due to cardiac and vascular prosthetic devices, implants and grafts**

☑7ᵗʰ **T82.827** **Fibrosis due to** cardiac **prosthetic devices, implants and grafts**

¹ ☑7ᵗʰ **T82.828** **Fibrosis due to** vascular **prosthetic devices, implants and grafts** ᴴᶜᶜ

☑6ᵗʰ **T82.83** Hemorrhage **due to cardiac and vascular prosthetic devices, implants and grafts**

☑7ᵗʰ **T82.837** **Hemorrhage due to** cardiac **prosthetic devices, implants and grafts**

¹ ☑7ᵗʰ **T82.838** **Hemorrhage due to** vascular **prosthetic devices, implants and grafts** ᴴᶜᶜ

☑6ᵗʰ **T82.84** Pain **due to cardiac and vascular prosthetic devices, implants and grafts**

☑7ᵗʰ **T82.847** **Pain due to** cardiac **prosthetic devices, implants and grafts**

☑7ᵗʰ **T82.848** **Pain due to** vascular **prosthetic devices, implants and grafts** ᴴᶜᶜ

☑6ᵗʰ **T82.85** Stenosis **due to cardiac and vascular prosthetic devices, implants and grafts**

☑7ᵗʰ **T82.855** **Stenosis of** coronary artery stent
In-stent stenosis (restenosis) of coronary artery stent
Restenosis of coronary artery stent

¹ ☑7ᵗʰ **T82.856** **Stenosis of** peripheral vascular stent ᴴᶜᶜ
In-stent stenosis (restenosis) of peripheral vascular stent
Restenosis of peripheral vascular stent

☑7ᵗʰ **T82.857** **Stenosis of other** cardiac **prosthetic devices, implants and grafts**

¹ ☑7ᵗʰ **T82.858** **Stenosis of other** vascular **prosthetic devices, implants and grafts** ᴴᶜᶜ

☑6ᵗʰ **T82.86** Thrombosis **of cardiac and vascular prosthetic devices, implants and grafts**

☑7ᵗʰ **T82.867** **Thrombosis due to** cardiac **prosthetic devices, implants and grafts**

¹ ☑7ᵗʰ **T82.868** **Thrombosis due to** vascular **prosthetic devices, implants and grafts** ᴴᶜᶜ

☑6ᵗʰ **T82.89** **Other specified complication of cardiac and vascular prosthetic devices, implants and grafts**

☑7ᵗʰ **T82.897** **Other specified complication of** cardiac **prosthetic devices, implants and grafts**

¹ ☑7ᵗʰ **T82.898** **Other specified complication of** vascular **prosthetic devices, implants and grafts** ᴴᶜᶜ

☑ₓ7ᵗʰ **T82.9** **Unspecified complication of cardiac and vascular prosthetic device, implant and graft** ▽

☑4ᵗʰ **T83** **Complications of genitourinary prosthetic devices, implants and grafts**
EXCLUDES 2 *failure and rejection of transplanted organs and tissue (T86.-)*

The appropriate 7th character is to be added to each code from category T83.
A   initial encounter
D   subsequent encounter
S   sequela

☑5ᵗʰ **T83.0** **Mechanical complication of** urinary catheter
EXCLUDES 2 *complications of stoma of urinary tract (N99.5-)*

☑6ᵗʰ **T83.01** Breakdown (mechanical) of urinary catheter

¹ ☑7ᵗʰ **T83.010** **Breakdown (mechanical) of** cystostomy **catheter** ᴴᶜᶜ

¹ ☑7ᵗʰ **T83.011** **Breakdown (mechanical) of** indwelling urethral **catheter** ᴴᶜᶜ

¹ ☑7ᵗʰ **T83.012** **Breakdown (mechanical) of** nephrostomy **catheter** ᴴᶜᶜ

¹ ☑7ᵗʰ **T83.018** **Breakdown (mechanical) of other urinary catheter** ᴴᶜᶜ
Breakdown (mechanical) of Hopkins catheter
Breakdown (mechanical) of ileostomy catheter
Breakdown (mechanical) urostomy catheter

---

¹ HCC with 7th character indicating initial encounter (A, B or C - specific to category).

☑ Additional Character Req   ☑ₓ7ᵗʰ Placeholder Alert   Manifestation   ᴴᶜᶜ CMS-HCC Condition   ▽ Unspecified Code   ▶◀ Revised Text   ● New Code   ▲ Revised Code Title

√6ᵗʰ **T83.02** Displacement of urinary catheter
Malposition of urinary catheter

   1 √7ᵗʰ **T83.020** **Displacement of cystostomy catheter** HCC

   1 √7ᵗʰ **T83.021** **Displacement of indwelling urethral catheter** HCC

   1 √7ᵗʰ **T83.022** **Displacement of nephrostomy catheter** HCC

   1 √7ᵗʰ **T83.028** **Displacement of other urinary catheter** HCC
Displacement of Hopkins catheter
Displacement of ileostomy catheter
Displacement of urostomy catheter

√6ᵗʰ **T83.03** Leakage of urinary catheter

   1 √7ᵗʰ **T83.030** **Leakage of cystostomy catheter** HCC

   1 √7ᵗʰ **T83.031** **Leakage of indwelling urethral catheter** HCC

   1 √7ᵗʰ **T83.032** **Leakage of nephrostomy catheter** HCC

   1 √7ᵗʰ **T83.038** **Leakage of other urinary catheter** HCC
Leakage of Hopkins catheter
Leakage of ileostomy catheter
Leakage of urostomy catheter

√6ᵗʰ **T83.09** **Other mechanical complication of urinary catheter**
Obstruction (mechanical) of urinary catheter
Perforation of urinary catheter
Protrusion of urinary catheter

   1 √7ᵗʰ **T83.090** **Other mechanical complication of cystostomy catheter** HCC

   1 √7ᵗʰ **T83.091** **Other mechanical complication of indwelling urethral catheter** HCC

   1 √7ᵗʰ **T83.092** **Other mechanical complication of nephrostomy catheter** HCC

   1 √7ᵗʰ **T83.098** **Other mechanical complication of other urinary catheter** HCC
Other mechanical complication of Hopkins catheter
Other mechanical complication of ileostomy catheter
Other mechanical complication of urostomy catheter

√5ᵗʰ **T83.1** **Mechanical complication of other urinary devices and implants**

√6ᵗʰ **T83.11** Breakdown (mechanical) of other urinary devices and implants

   1 √7ᵗʰ **T83.110** **Breakdown (mechanical) of urinary electronic stimulator device** HCC
EXCLUDES 2   *breakdown (mechanical) of electrode (lead) for sacral nerve neurostimulator (T85.111)*
breakdown (mechanical) of implanted electronic sacral neurostimulator, pulse generator or receiver (T85.113)

   1 √7ᵗʰ **T83.111** **Breakdown (mechanical) of implanted urinary sphincter** HCC

   1 √7ᵗʰ **T83.112** **Breakdown (mechanical) of indwelling ureteral stent** HCC

   1 √7ᵗʰ **T83.113** **Breakdown (mechanical) of other urinary stents** HCC
Breakdown (mechanical) of ileal conduit stent
Breakdown (mechanical) of nephroureteral stent

   1 √7ᵗʰ **T83.118** **Breakdown (mechanical) of other urinary devices and implants** HCC

√6ᵗʰ **T83.12** Displacement of other urinary devices and implants
Malposition of other urinary devices and implants

   1 √7ᵗʰ **T83.120** **Displacement of urinary electronic stimulator device** HCC
EXCLUDES 2   *displacement of electrode (lead) for sacral nerve neurostimulator (T85.121)*
displacement of implanted electronic sacral neurostimulator, pulse generator or receiver (T85.123/0)

   1 √7ᵗʰ **T83.121** **Displacement of implanted urinary sphincter** HCC

   1 √7ᵗʰ **T83.122** **Displacement of indwelling ureteral stent** HCC

   1 √7ᵗʰ **T83.123** **Displacement of other urinary stents** HCC
Displacement of ileal conduit stent
Displacement of nephroureteral stent

   1 √7ᵗʰ **T83.128** **Displacement of other urinary devices and implants** HCC

√6ᵗʰ **T83.19** **Other mechanical complication of other urinary devices and implants**
Leakage of other urinary devices and implants
Obstruction (mechanical) of other urinary devices and implants
Perforation of other urinary devices and implants
Protrusion of other urinary devices and implants

   1 √7ᵗʰ **T83.190** **Other mechanical complication of urinary electronic stimulator device** HCC
EXCLUDES 2   *other mechanical complication of electrode (lead) for sacral nerve neurostimulator (T85.191)*
other mechanical complication of implanted electronic sacral neurostimulator, pulse generator or receiver (T85.193)

   1 √7ᵗʰ **T83.191** **Other mechanical complication of implanted urinary sphincter** HCC

   1 √7ᵗʰ **T83.192** **Other mechanical complication of indwelling ureteral stent** HCC

   1 √7ᵗʰ **T83.193** **Other mechanical complication of other urinary stent** HCC
Other mechanical complication of ileal conduit stent
Other mechanical complication of nephroureteral stent

   1 √7ᵗʰ **T83.198** **Other mechanical complication of other urinary devices and implants** HCC

√5ᵗʰ **T83.2** **Mechanical complication of graft of urinary organ**

   1 √x7ᵗʰ **T83.21** Breakdown (mechanical) of graft of urinary organ HCC

   1 √x7ᵗʰ **T83.22** Displacement of graft of urinary organ HCC
Malposition of graft of urinary organ

   1 √x7ᵗʰ **T83.23** Leakage of graft of urinary organ HCC

   1 √x7ᵗʰ **T83.24** Erosion of graft of urinary organ HCC

   1 √x7ᵗʰ **T83.25** Exposure of graft of urinary organ HCC

   1 √x7ᵗʰ **T83.29** Other mechanical complication of graft of urinary organ HCC
Obstruction (mechanical) of graft of urinary organ
Perforation of graft of urinary organ
Protrusion of graft of urinary organ

√5ᵗʰ **T83.3** **Mechanical complication of intrauterine contraceptive device**

   √x7ᵗʰ **T83.31** Breakdown (mechanical) of intrauterine contraceptive device ♀

   √x7ᵗʰ **T83.32** Displacement of intrauterine contraceptive device ♀
Malposition of intrauterine contraceptive device
Missing string of intrauterine contraceptive device

   √x7ᵗʰ **T83.39** Other mechanical complication of intrauterine contraceptive device ♀
Leakage of intrauterine contraceptive device
Obstruction (mechanical) of intrauterine contraceptive device
Perforation of intrauterine contraceptive device
Protrusion of intrauterine contraceptive device

√5ᵗʰ **T83.4** **Mechanical complication of other prosthetic devices, implants and grafts of genital tract**

√6ᵗʰ **T83.41** Breakdown (mechanical) of other prosthetic devices, implants and grafts of genital tract

   1 √7ᵗʰ **T83.410** **Breakdown (mechanical) of implanted penile prosthesis** HCC ♂
Breakdown (mechanical) of penile prosthesis cylinder
Breakdown (mechanical) of penile prosthesis pump
Breakdown (mechanical) of penile prosthesis reservoir

   1 √7ᵗʰ **T83.411** **Breakdown (mechanical) of implanted testicular prosthesis** HCC

---

1   HCC with 7th character indicating initial encounter (A, B or C - specific to category).

EXCLUDES 1 Not coded here   *EXCLUDES 2* Not included here   N Newborn Age: 0   P Pediatric Age: 0-17   M Maternity Age: 12-55   A Adult Age: 15-124

1102   ICD-10-CM 2018

[1] ✓7ᵗʰ **T83.418** **Breakdown (mechanical) of other** HCC
prosthetic devices, implants and
grafts of genital tract

✓6ᵗʰ **T83.42** Displacement **of other prosthetic devices, implants**
and grafts of genital tract
Malposition of other prosthetic devices, implants and
grafts of genital tract

[1] ✓7ᵗʰ **T83.420** **Displacement of** implanted penile HCC ♂
prosthesis
Displacement of penile prosthesis cylinder
Displacement of penile prosthesis pump
Displacement of penile prosthesis reservoir

[1] ✓7ᵗʰ **T83.421** **Displacement of** implanted testicular HCC
prosthesis

[1] ✓7ᵗʰ **T83.428** **Displacement of other prosthetic** HCC
devices, implants and grafts of
genital tract

✓6ᵗʰ **T83.49** **Other mechanical complication of other prosthetic**
devices, implants and grafts of genital tract
Leakage of other prosthetic devices, implants and
grafts of genital tract
Obstruction, mechanical of other prosthetic devices,
implants and grafts of genital tract
Perforation of other prosthetic devices, implants and
grafts of genital tract
Protrusion of other prosthetic devices, implants and
grafts of genital tract

[1] ✓7ᵗʰ **T83.490** **Other mechanical complication of** HCC ♂
implanted penile prosthesis
Other mechanical complication of penile
prosthesis cylinder
Other mechanical complication of penile
prosthesis pump
Other mechanical complication of penile
prosthesis reservoir

[1] ✓7ᵗʰ **T83.491** **Other mechanical complication of** HCC
implanted testicular prosthesis

[1] ✓7ᵗʰ **T83.498** **Other mechanical complication of** HCC
other prosthetic devices, implants
and grafts of genital tract

✓5ᵗʰ **T83.5** **Infection and inflammatory reaction due to prosthetic device,**
implant and graft in urinary system
Use additional code to identify infection

✓6ᵗʰ **T83.51** **Infection and inflammatory reaction due to** urinary
catheter
EXCLUDES 2   complications of stoma of urinary tract
(N99.5-)

[1] ✓7ᵗʰ **T83.510** **Infection and inflammatory reaction** HCC
due to cystostomy **catheter**

[1] ✓7ᵗʰ **T83.511** **Infection and inflammatory reaction** HCC
due to indwelling urethral **catheter**

[1] ✓7ᵗʰ **T83.512** **Infection and inflammatory reaction** HCC
due to nephrostomy **catheter**

[1] ✓7ᵗʰ **T83.518** **Infection and inflammatory reaction** HCC
due to other urinary catheter
Infection and inflammatory reaction due to
Hopkins catheter
Infection and inflammatory reaction due to
ileostomy catheter
Infection and inflammatory reaction due to
urostomy catheter

✓6ᵗʰ **T83.59** **Infection and inflammatory reaction due to**
prosthetic device, implant and graft **in urinary**
system

[1] ✓7ᵗʰ **T83.590** **Infection and inflammatory reaction** HCC
due to implanted urinary
neurostimulation device
EXCLUDES 2   infection and inflammatory
reaction due to electrode
lead of sacral nerve
neurostimulator (T85.732)
infection and inflammatory reaction due to pulse generator
or receiver of sacral nerve
neurostimulator (T85.734)

[1] ✓7ᵗʰ **T83.591** **Infection and inflammatory reaction** HCC
due to implanted urinary sphincter

[1] ✓7ᵗʰ **T83.592** **Infection and inflammatory reaction** HCC
due to indwelling ureteral stent

[1] ✓7ᵗʰ **T83.593** **Infection and inflammatory reaction** HCC
due to other urinary stents
Infection and inflammatory reaction due to
ileal conduit stents
Infection and inflammatory reaction due to
nephroureteral stent

[1] ✓7ᵗʰ **T83.598** **Infection and inflammatory reaction** HCC
due to other prosthetic device, implant
and graft in urinary system

✓5ᵗʰ **T83.6** **Infection and inflammatory reaction due to prosthetic device,**
implant and graft in genital tract
Use additional code to identify infection

[1] ✓x7ᵗʰ **T83.61** **Infection and inflammatory reaction due to** HCC
implanted penile prosthesis
Infection and inflammatory reaction due to penile
prosthesis cylinder
Infection and inflammatory reaction due to penile
prosthesis pump
Infection and inflammatory reaction due to penile
prosthesis reservoir

[1] ✓x7ᵗʰ **T83.62** **Infection and inflammatory reaction due to** HCC
implanted testicular prosthesis

[1] ✓x7ᵗʰ **T83.69** **Infection and inflammatory reaction due to** HCC
other prosthetic device, implant and graft in
genital tract

✓5ᵗʰ **T83.7** **Complications due to** implanted mesh and other prosthetic
materials

✓6ᵗʰ **T83.71** Erosion **of implanted mesh and other prosthetic**
materials to surrounding organ or tissue

[1] ✓7ᵗʰ **T83.711** **Erosion of implanted** vaginal **mesh** HCC ♀
to surrounding organ or tissue
Erosion of implanted vaginal mesh into
pelvic floor muscles

[1] ✓7ᵗʰ **T83.712** **Erosion of implanted** urethral **mesh** HCC
to surrounding organ or tissue
Erosion of implanted female urethral sling
Erosion of implanted male urethral sling
Erosion of implanted urethral mesh into
pelvic floor muscles

[1] ✓7ᵗʰ **T83.713** **Erosion of implanted** urethral bulking HCC
agent **to surrounding organ or tissue**

[1] ✓7ᵗʰ **T83.714** **Erosion of implanted** ureteral bulking HCC
agent **to surrounding organ or tissue**

[1] ✓7ᵗʰ **T83.718** **Erosion of other implanted mesh to** HCC
organ or tissue

[1] ✓7ᵗʰ **T83.719** **Erosion of other prosthetic materials** HCC
to surrounding organ or tissue

✓6ᵗʰ **T83.72** Exposure **of implanted mesh and other prosthetic**
materials into surrounding organ or tissue
Extrusion of implanted mesh

[1] ✓7ᵗʰ **T83.721** **Exposure of implanted** vaginal HCC ♀
mesh into vagina
Exposure of implanted vaginal mesh
through vaginal wall

[1] ✓7ᵗʰ **T83.722** **Exposure of implanted** urethral HCC
mesh into urethra
Exposure of implanted female urethral
sling
Exposure of implanted male urethral sling
Exposure of implanted urethral mesh
through urethral wall

[1] ✓7ᵗʰ **T83.723** **Exposure of implanted** urethral HCC
bulking agent **into** urethra

[1] ✓7ᵗʰ **T83.724** **Exposure of implanted** ureteral HCC
bulking agent **into** ureter

[1] ✓7ᵗʰ **T83.728** **Exposure of other implanted mesh** HCC
into organ or tissue

[1] ✓7ᵗʰ **T83.729** **Exposure of other prosthetic** HCC
materials into organ or tissue

[1] ✓x7ᵗʰ **T83.79** **Other specified complications due to other** HCC
genitourinary prosthetic materials

✓5ᵗʰ **T83.8** **Other specified complications of** genitourinary prosthetic
devices, implants and grafts

[1] ✓x7ᵗʰ **T83.81** Embolism **due to genitourinary prosthetic** HCC
devices, implants and grafts

[1] ✓x7ᵗʰ **T83.82** Fibrosis **due to genitourinary prosthetic** HCC
devices, implants and grafts

---

[1]   HCC with 7th character indicating initial encounter (A, B or C - specific to category).

✓ Additional Character Req   ✓x7ᵗʰ Placeholder Alert   Manifestation   HCC CMS-HCC Condition   ▽ Unspecified Code   ▶◀ Revised Text   ● New Code   ▲ Revised Code Title

ICD-10-CM 2018   1103

1 ✓x7ᵗʰ **T83.83** Hemorrhage due to genitourinary prosthetic devices, implants and grafts �**HCC**

1 ✓x7ᵗʰ **T83.84** Pain due to genitourinary prosthetic devices, implants and grafts ▪**HCC**

1 ✓x7ᵗʰ **T83.85** Stenosis due to genitourinary prosthetic devices, implants and grafts ▪**HCC**

1 ✓x7ᵗʰ **T83.86** Thrombosis due to genitourinary prosthetic devices, implants and grafts ▪**HCC**

1 ✓x7ᵗʰ **T83.89** Other specified complication of genitourinary prosthetic devices, implants and grafts ▪**HCC**

1 ✓x7ᵗʰ **T83.9** Unspecified complication of genitourinary prosthetic device, implant and graft ▪**HCC** ▽

✓4ᵗʰ **T84** **Complications of internal orthopedic prosthetic devices, implants and grafts**

　EXCLUDES 2　*failure and rejection of transplanted organs and tissues (T86.-)*
　　　　fracture of bone following insertion of orthopedic implant, joint prosthesis or bone plate (M96.6)

　The appropriate 7th character is to be added to each code from category T84.
　A　initial encounter
　D　subsequent encounter
　S　sequela

✓5ᵗʰ **T84.0** **Mechanical complication of** internal joint prosthesis

　✓6ᵗʰ **T84.01** Broken internal joint prosthesis
　　Breakage (fracture) of prosthetic joint
　　Broken prosthetic joint implant
　　EXCLUDES 1　*periprosthetic joint implant fracture*
　　　　▶*(M97-)*◀

　　1 ✓7ᵗʰ **T84.010** Broken internal right hip prosthesis ▪**HCC**
　　1 ✓7ᵗʰ **T84.011** Broken internal left hip prosthesis ▪**HCC**
　　1 ✓7ᵗʰ **T84.012** Broken internal right knee prosthesis ▪**HCC**
　　1 ✓7ᵗʰ **T84.013** Broken internal left knee prosthesis ▪**HCC**
　　1 ✓7ᵗʰ **T84.018** Broken internal joint prosthesis, other site ▪**HCC**
　　　　Use additional code to identify the joint (Z96.6-)
　　1 ✓7ᵗʰ **T84.019** Broken internal joint prosthesis, unspecified site ▪**HCC** ▽

　✓6ᵗʰ **T84.02** Dislocation of internal joint prosthesis
　　Instability of internal joint prosthesis
　　Subluxation of internal joint prosthesis

　　1 ✓7ᵗʰ **T84.020** Dislocation of internal right hip prosthesis ▪**HCC**
　　1 ✓7ᵗʰ **T84.021** Dislocation of internal left hip prosthesis ▪**HCC**
　　1 ✓7ᵗʰ **T84.022** Instability of internal right knee prosthesis ▪**HCC**
　　1 ✓7ᵗʰ **T84.023** Instability of internal left knee prosthesis ▪**HCC**
　　1 ✓7ᵗʰ **T84.028** Dislocation of other internal joint prosthesis ▪**HCC**
　　　　Use additional code to identify the joint (Z96.6-)
　　1 ✓7ᵗʰ **T84.029** Dislocation of unspecified internal joint prosthesis ▪**HCC** ▽

　✓6ᵗʰ **T84.03** Mechanical loosening of internal prosthetic joint
　　Aseptic loosening of prosthetic joint

　　1 ✓7ᵗʰ **T84.030** Mechanical loosening of internal right hip prosthetic joint ▪**HCC**
　　1 ✓7ᵗʰ **T84.031** Mechanical loosening of internal left hip prosthetic joint ▪**HCC**
　　1 ✓7ᵗʰ **T84.032** Mechanical loosening of internal right knee prosthetic joint ▪**HCC**
　　1 ✓7ᵗʰ **T84.033** Mechanical loosening of internal left knee prosthetic joint ▪**HCC**
　　1 ✓7ᵗʰ **T84.038** Mechanical loosening of other internal prosthetic joint ▪**HCC**
　　　　Use additional code to identify the joint (Z96.6-)
　　1 ✓7ᵗʰ **T84.039** Mechanical loosening of unspecified internal prosthetic joint ▪**HCC** ▽

✓6ᵗʰ **T84.05** Periprosthetic osteolysis of internal prosthetic joint
　　Use additional code to identify major osseous defect, if applicable (M89.7-)

　1 ✓7ᵗʰ **T84.050** Periprosthetic osteolysis of internal prosthetic right hip joint ▪**HCC**
　1 ✓7ᵗʰ **T84.051** Periprosthetic osteolysis of internal prosthetic left hip joint ▪**HCC**
　1 ✓7ᵗʰ **T84.052** Periprosthetic osteolysis of internal prosthetic right knee joint ▪**HCC**
　1 ✓7ᵗʰ **T84.053** Periprosthetic osteolysis of internal prosthetic left knee joint ▪**HCC**
　1 ✓7ᵗʰ **T84.058** Periprosthetic osteolysis of other internal prosthetic joint ▪**HCC**
　　　Use additional code to identify the joint (Z96.6-)
　1 ✓7ᵗʰ **T84.059** Periprosthetic osteolysis of unspecified internal prosthetic joint ▪**HCC** ▽

✓6ᵗʰ **T84.06** Wear of articular bearing surface of internal prosthetic joint

　1 ✓7ᵗʰ **T84.060** Wear of articular bearing surface of internal prosthetic right hip joint ▪**HCC**
　1 ✓7ᵗʰ **T84.061** Wear of articular bearing surface of internal prosthetic left hip joint ▪**HCC**
　1 ✓7ᵗʰ **T84.062** Wear of articular bearing surface of internal prosthetic right knee joint ▪**HCC**
　1 ✓7ᵗʰ **T84.063** Wear of articular bearing surface of internal prosthetic left knee joint ▪**HCC**
　1 ✓7ᵗʰ **T84.068** Wear of articular bearing surface of other internal prosthetic joint ▪**HCC**
　　　Use additional code to identify the joint (Z96.6-)
　1 ✓7ᵗʰ **T84.069** Wear of articular bearing surface of unspecified internal prosthetic joint ▪**HCC** ▽

✓6ᵗʰ **T84.09** Other mechanical complication of internal joint prosthesis
　　Prosthetic joint implant failure NOS

　1 ✓7ᵗʰ **T84.090** Other mechanical complication of internal right hip prosthesis ▪**HCC**
　1 ✓7ᵗʰ **T84.091** Other mechanical complication of internal left hip prosthesis ▪**HCC**
　1 ✓7ᵗʰ **T84.092** Other mechanical complication of internal right knee prosthesis ▪**HCC**
　1 ✓7ᵗʰ **T84.093** Other mechanical complication of internal left knee prosthesis ▪**HCC**
　1 ✓7ᵗʰ **T84.098** Other mechanical complication of other internal joint prosthesis ▪**HCC**
　　　Use additional code to identify the joint (Z96.6-)
　1 ✓7ᵗʰ **T84.099** Other mechanical complication of unspecified internal joint prosthesis ▪**HCC** ▽

✓5ᵗʰ **T84.1** **Mechanical complication of** internal fixation device of bones of limb

　EXCLUDES 2　*mechanical complication of internal fixation device of bones of feet (T84.2-)*
　　　mechanical complication of internal fixation device of bones of fingers (T84.2-)
　　　mechanical complication of internal fixation device of bones of hands (T84.2-)
　　　mechanical complication of internal fixation device of bones of toes (T84.2-)

　✓6ᵗʰ **T84.11** Breakdown (mechanical) of internal fixation device of bones of limb

　　1 ✓7ᵗʰ **T84.110** Breakdown (mechanical) of internal fixation device of right humerus ▪**HCC**
　　1 ✓7ᵗʰ **T84.111** Breakdown (mechanical) of internal fixation device of left humerus ▪**HCC**
　　1 ✓7ᵗʰ **T84.112** Breakdown (mechanical) of internal fixation device of bone of right forearm ▪**HCC**
　　1 ✓7ᵗʰ **T84.113** Breakdown (mechanical) of internal fixation device of bone of left forearm ▪**HCC**
　　1 ✓7ᵗʰ **T84.114** Breakdown (mechanical) of internal fixation device of right femur ▪**HCC**
　　1 ✓7ᵗʰ **T84.115** Breakdown (mechanical) of internal fixation device of left femur ▪**HCC**
　　1 ✓7ᵗʰ **T84.116** Breakdown (mechanical) of internal fixation device of bone of right lower leg ▪**HCC**

---

1 HCC with 7th character indicating initial encounter (A, B or C - specific to category).

EXCLUDES 1 Not coded here　　　*EXCLUDES 2* Not included here　　　N Newborn Age: 0　　　P Pediatric Age: 0-17　　　M Maternity Age: 12-55　　　A Adult Age: 15-124

¹ √7ᵗʰ **T84.117** Breakdown (mechanical) of internal ᴴᶜᶜ
fixation device of bone of left lower leg

¹ √7ᵗʰ **T84.119** Breakdown (mechanical) of ᴴᶜᶜ ▽
internal fixation device of
unspecified bone of limb

√6ᵗʰ **T84.12** Displacement of internal fixation device of bones of
limb
Malposition of internal fixation device of bones of limb

¹ √7ᵗʰ **T84.120** Displacement of internal fixation ᴴᶜᶜ
device of right humerus

¹ √7ᵗʰ **T84.121** Displacement of internal fixation ᴴᶜᶜ
device of left humerus

¹ √7ᵗʰ **T84.122** Displacement of internal fixation ᴴᶜᶜ
device of bone of right forearm

¹ √7ᵗʰ **T84.123** Displacement of internal fixation ᴴᶜᶜ
device of bone of left forearm

¹ √7ᵗʰ **T84.124** Displacement of internal fixation ᴴᶜᶜ
device of right femur

¹ √7ᵗʰ **T84.125** Displacement of internal fixation ᴴᶜᶜ
device of left femur

¹ √7ᵗʰ **T84.126** Displacement of internal fixation ᴴᶜᶜ
device of bone of right lower leg

¹ √7ᵗʰ **T84.127** Displacement of internal fixation ᴴᶜᶜ
device of bone of left lower leg

¹ √7ᵗʰ **T84.129** Displacement of internal fixation ᴴᶜᶜ ▽
device of unspecified bone of limb

√6ᵗʰ **T84.19** Other mechanical complication of internal fixation
device of bones of limb
Obstruction (mechanical) of internal fixation device of
bones of limb
Perforation of internal fixation device of bones of limb
Protrusion of internal fixation device of bones of limb

¹ √7ᵗʰ **T84.190** Other mechanical complication of ᴴᶜᶜ
internal fixation device of right humerus

¹ √7ᵗʰ **T84.191** Other mechanical complication of ᴴᶜᶜ
internal fixation device of left humerus

¹ √7ᵗʰ **T84.192** Other mechanical complication of ᴴᶜᶜ
internal fixation device of bone of right
forearm

¹ √7ᵗʰ **T84.193** Other mechanical complication of ᴴᶜᶜ
internal fixation device of bone of left
forearm

¹ √7ᵗʰ **T84.194** Other mechanical complication of ᴴᶜᶜ
internal fixation device of right femur

¹ √7ᵗʰ **T84.195** Other mechanical complication of ᴴᶜᶜ
internal fixation device of left femur

¹ √7ᵗʰ **T84.196** Other mechanical complication of ᴴᶜᶜ
internal fixation device of bone of right
lower leg

¹ √7ᵗʰ **T84.197** Other mechanical complication of ᴴᶜᶜ
internal fixation device of bone of left
lower leg

¹ √7ᵗʰ **T84.199** Other mechanical complication of ᴴᶜᶜ ▽
internal fixation device of unspecified
bone of limb

√5ᵗʰ **T84.2** Mechanical complication of internal fixation device of other
bones

√6ᵗʰ **T84.21** Breakdown (mechanical) of internal fixation device
of other bones

¹ √7ᵗʰ **T84.210** Breakdown (mechanical) of internal ᴴᶜᶜ
fixation device of bones of hand and
fingers

¹ √7ᵗʰ **T84.213** Breakdown (mechanical) of internal ᴴᶜᶜ
fixation device of bones of foot and toes

¹ √7ᵗʰ **T84.216** Breakdown (mechanical) of internal ᴴᶜᶜ
fixation device of vertebrae

¹ √7ᵗʰ **T84.218** Breakdown (mechanical) of internal ᴴᶜᶜ
fixation device of other bones

√6ᵗʰ **T84.22** Displacement of internal fixation device of other
bones
Malposition of internal fixation device of other bones

¹ √7ᵗʰ **T84.220** Displacement of internal fixation ᴴᶜᶜ
device of bones of hand and fingers

¹ √7ᵗʰ **T84.223** Displacement of internal fixation ᴴᶜᶜ
device of bones of foot and toes

¹ √7ᵗʰ **T84.226** Displacement of internal fixation ᴴᶜᶜ
device of vertebrae

¹ √7ᵗʰ **T84.228** Displacement of internal fixation ᴴᶜᶜ
device of other bones

√6ᵗʰ **T84.29** Other mechanical complication of internal fixation
device of other bones
Obstruction (mechanical) of internal fixation device of
other bones
Perforation of internal fixation device of other bones
Protrusion of internal fixation device of other bones

¹ √7ᵗʰ **T84.290** Other mechanical complication of ᴴᶜᶜ
internal fixation device of bones of
hand and fingers

¹ √7ᵗʰ **T84.293** Other mechanical complication of ᴴᶜᶜ
internal fixation device of bones of
foot and toes

¹ √7ᵗʰ **T84.296** Other mechanical complication of ᴴᶜᶜ
internal fixation device of vertebrae

¹ √7ᵗʰ **T84.298** Other mechanical complication of ᴴᶜᶜ
internal fixation device of other bones

√5ᵗʰ **T84.3** Mechanical complication of other bone devices, implants and
grafts
EXCLUDES 2   other complications of bone graft (T86.83-)

√6ᵗʰ **T84.31** Breakdown (mechanical) of other bone devices,
implants and grafts

¹ √7ᵗʰ **T84.310** Breakdown (mechanical) of ᴴᶜᶜ
electronic bone stimulator

¹ √7ᵗʰ **T84.318** Breakdown (mechanical) of other ᴴᶜᶜ
bone devices, implants and grafts

√6ᵗʰ **T84.32** Displacement of other bone devices, implants and
grafts
Malposition of other bone devices, implants and grafts

¹ √7ᵗʰ **T84.320** Displacement of electronic bone ᴴᶜᶜ
stimulator

¹ √7ᵗʰ **T84.328** Displacement of other bone devices, ᴴᶜᶜ
implants and grafts
AHA: 2014, 4Q, 28

√6ᵗʰ **T84.39** Other mechanical complication of other bone
devices, implants and grafts
Obstruction (mechanical) of other bone devices,
implants and grafts
Perforation of other bone devices, implants and grafts
Protrusion of other bone devices, implants and grafts

¹ √7ᵗʰ **T84.390** Other mechanical complication of ᴴᶜᶜ
electronic bone stimulator

¹ √7ᵗʰ **T84.398** Other mechanical complication of ᴴᶜᶜ
other bone devices, implants and grafts

√5ᵗʰ **T84.4** Mechanical complication of other internal orthopedic
devices, implants and grafts

√6ᵗʰ **T84.41** Breakdown (mechanical) of other internal
orthopedic devices, implants and grafts

¹ √7ᵗʰ **T84.410** Breakdown (mechanical) of muscle ᴴᶜᶜ
and tendon graft

¹ √7ᵗʰ **T84.418** Breakdown (mechanical) of other ᴴᶜᶜ
internal orthopedic devices, implants
and grafts

√6ᵗʰ **T84.42** Displacement of other internal orthopedic devices,
implants and grafts
Malposition of other internal orthopedic devices,
implants and grafts

¹ √7ᵗʰ **T84.420** Displacement of muscle and tendon ᴴᶜᶜ
graft

¹ √7ᵗʰ **T84.428** Displacement of other internal ᴴᶜᶜ
orthopedic devices, implants and grafts

√6ᵗʰ **T84.49** Other mechanical complication of other internal
orthopedic devices, implants and grafts
Mechanical complication of other internal orthopedic
devices, implants and grafts NOS
Obstruction (mechanical) of other internal orthopedic
devices, implants and grafts
Perforation of other internal orthopedic devices,
implants and grafts
Protrusion of other internal orthopedic devices,
implants and grafts

¹ √7ᵗʰ **T84.490** Other mechanical complication of ᴴᶜᶜ
muscle and tendon graft

¹ √7ᵗʰ **T84.498** Other mechanical complication of ᴴᶜᶜ
other internal orthopedic devices,
implants and grafts

---

¹ HCC with 7th character indicating initial encounter (A, B or C - specific to category).

☑ Additional Character Req   √x7ᵗʰ Placeholder Alert   Manifestation   ᴴᶜᶜ CMS-HCC Condition   ▽ Unspecified Code   ►◄ Revised Text   ● New Code   ▲ Revised Code Title

√5ᵗʰ **T84.5** **Infection and inflammatory reaction due to** internal joint prosthesis
Use additional code to identify infection
AHA: 2015, 1Q, 16

¹ √x7ᵗʰ **T84.50** Infection and inflammatory reaction due to unspecified internal joint prosthesis HCC ▽

¹ √x7ᵗʰ **T84.51** Infection and inflammatory reaction due to internal right hip prosthesis HCC

¹ √x7ᵗʰ **T84.52** Infection and inflammatory reaction due to internal left hip prosthesis HCC

¹ √x7ᵗʰ **T84.53** Infection and inflammatory reaction due to internal right knee prosthesis HCC

¹ √x7ᵗʰ **T84.54** Infection and inflammatory reaction due to internal left knee prosthesis HCC

¹ √x7ᵗʰ **T84.59** Infection and inflammatory reaction due to other internal joint prosthesis HCC

√5ᵗʰ **T84.6** **Infection and inflammatory reaction due to** internal fixation device
Use additional code to identify infection

¹ √x7ᵗʰ **T84.60** Infection and inflammatory reaction due to internal fixation device of unspecified site HCC ▽

√6ᵗʰ **T84.61** Infection and inflammatory reaction due to internal fixation device of arm

¹ √7ᵗʰ **T84.610** Infection and inflammatory reaction due to internal fixation device of right humerus HCC

¹ √7ᵗʰ **T84.611** Infection and inflammatory reaction due to internal fixation device of left humerus HCC

¹ √7ᵗʰ **T84.612** Infection and inflammatory reaction due to internal fixation device of right radius HCC

¹ √7ᵗʰ **T84.613** Infection and inflammatory reaction due to internal fixation device of left radius HCC

¹ √7ᵗʰ **T84.614** Infection and inflammatory reaction due to internal fixation device of right ulna HCC

¹ √7ᵗʰ **T84.615** Infection and inflammatory reaction due to internal fixation device of left ulna HCC

¹ √7ᵗʰ **T84.619** Infection and inflammatory reaction due to internal fixation device of unspecified bone of arm HCC ▽

√6ᵗʰ **T84.62** Infection and inflammatory reaction due to internal fixation device of leg

¹ √7ᵗʰ **T84.620** Infection and inflammatory reaction due to internal fixation device of right femur HCC

¹ √7ᵗʰ **T84.621** Infection and inflammatory reaction due to internal fixation device of left femur HCC

¹ √7ᵗʰ **T84.622** Infection and inflammatory reaction due to internal fixation device of right tibia HCC

¹ √7ᵗʰ **T84.623** Infection and inflammatory reaction due to internal fixation device of left tibia HCC

¹ √7ᵗʰ **T84.624** Infection and inflammatory reaction due to internal fixation device of right fibula HCC

¹ √7ᵗʰ **T84.625** Infection and inflammatory reaction due to internal fixation device of left fibula HCC

¹ √7ᵗʰ **T84.629** Infection and inflammatory reaction due to internal fixation device of unspecified bone of leg HCC ▽

¹ √x7ᵗʰ **T84.63** Infection and inflammatory reaction due to internal fixation device of spine HCC

¹ √x7ᵗʰ **T84.69** Infection and inflammatory reaction due to internal fixation device of other site HCC

¹ √x7ᵗʰ **T84.7** **Infection and inflammatory reaction due to other internal orthopedic prosthetic devices, implants and grafts** HCC
Use additional code to identify infection

√5ᵗʰ **T84.8** **Other specified complications of internal orthopedic prosthetic devices, implants and grafts**

¹ √x7ᵗʰ **T84.81** **Embolism** due to internal orthopedic prosthetic devices, implants and grafts HCC

¹ √x7ᵗʰ **T84.82** **Fibrosis** due to internal orthopedic prosthetic devices, implants and grafts HCC

¹ √x7ᵗʰ **T84.83** **Hemorrhage** due to internal orthopedic prosthetic devices, implants and grafts HCC

¹ √x7ᵗʰ **T84.84** **Pain** due to internal orthopedic prosthetic devices, implants and grafts HCC

¹ √x7ᵗʰ **T84.85** **Stenosis** due to internal orthopedic prosthetic devices, implants and grafts HCC

¹ √x7ᵗʰ **T84.86** **Thrombosis** due to internal orthopedic prosthetic devices, implants and grafts HCC

¹ √x7ᵗʰ **T84.89** **Other specified complication of internal orthopedic prosthetic devices, implants and grafts** HCC

¹ √x7ᵗʰ **T84.9** **Unspecified complication of internal orthopedic prosthetic device, implant and graft** HCC ▽

√4ᵗʰ **T85** **Complications of other internal prosthetic devices, implants and grafts**

EXCLUDES 2   failure and rejection of transplanted organs and tissue (T86.-)

The appropriate 7th character is to be added to each code from category T85.
A   initial encounter
D   subsequent encounter
S   sequela

√5ᵗʰ **T85.0** **Mechanical complication of** ventricular intracranial (communicating) shunt

¹ √x7ᵗʰ **T85.01** **Breakdown** (mechanical) of ventricular intracranial (communicating) shunt HCC

¹ √x7ᵗʰ **T85.02** **Displacement** of ventricular intracranial (communicating) shunt HCC
Malposition of ventricular intracranial (communicating) shunt

¹ √x7ᵗʰ **T85.03** **Leakage** of ventricular intracranial (communicating) shunt HCC

¹ √x7ᵗʰ **T85.09** **Other mechanical complication of** ventricular intracranial (communicating) shunt HCC
Obstruction (mechanical) of ventricular intracranial (communicating) shunt
Perforation of ventricular intracranial (communicating) shunt
Protrusion of ventricular intracranial (communicating) shunt

√5ᵗʰ **T85.1** **Mechanical complication of** implanted electronic stimulator of nervous system

√6ᵗʰ **T85.11** **Breakdown** (mechanical) of implanted electronic stimulator of nervous system

¹ √7ᵗʰ **T85.110** **Breakdown** (mechanical) of implanted electronic neurostimulator of brain electrode (lead) HCC

¹ √7ᵗʰ **T85.111** **Breakdown** (mechanical) of implanted electronic neurostimulator of peripheral nerve electrode (lead) HCC
Breakdown of electrode (lead) for cranial nerve neurostimulators
Breakdown of electrode (lead) for gastric neurostimulator
Breakdown of electrode (lead) for sacral nerve neurostimulator
Breakdown of electrode (lead) for vagal nerve neurostimulators

¹ √7ᵗʰ **T85.112** **Breakdown** (mechanical) of implanted electronic neurostimulator of spinal cord electrode (lead) HCC

¹ √7ᵗʰ **T85.113** **Breakdown** (mechanical) of implanted electronic neurostimulator, generator HCC
Breakdown (mechanical) of implanted electronic neurostimuator generator, brain, peripheral, gastric, spinal
Breakdown (mechanical) of implanted electronic sacral neurostimulator, pulse generator or receiver

---

¹ HCC with 7th character indicating initial encounter (A, B or C - specific to category).

EXCLUDES 1 Not coded here   EXCLUDES 2 Not included here   N Newborn Age: 0   P Pediatric Age: 0-17   M Maternity Age: 12-55   A Adult Age: 15-124

1106   ICD-10-CM 2018

[1] ✓7ᵗʰ **T85.118 Breakdown (mechanical) of other** HCC
implanted electronic stimulator of
nervous system

✓6ᵗʰ **T85.12 Displacement of implanted electronic stimulator of
nervous system**
Malposition of implanted electronic stimulator of
nervous system

     [1] ✓7ᵗʰ **T85.120 Displacement of implanted** HCC
electronic neurostimulator
of brain electrode (lead)

     [1] ✓7ᵗʰ **T85.121 Displacement of implanted** HCC
electronic neurostimulator
of peripheral nerve electrode (lead)
Displacement of electrode (lead) for cranial
nerve neurostimulators
Displacement of electrode (lead) for gastric
neurostimulator
Displacement of electrode (lead) for sacral
nerve neurostimulator
Displacement of electrode (lead) for vagal
nerve neurostimulators

     [1] ✓7ᵗʰ **T85.122 Displacement of implanted** HCC
electronic neurostimulator
of spinal cord electrode (lead)

     [1] ✓7ᵗʰ **T85.123 Displacement of implanted electronic** HCC
neurostimulator, generator
Displacement of implanted electronic
neurostimulator generator, brain,
peripheral, gastric, spinal
Displacement of implanted electronic
sacral neurostimulator, pulse
generator or receiver

     [1] ✓7ᵗʰ **T85.128 Displacement of other implanted** HCC
electronic stimulator of nervous system

✓6ᵗʰ **T85.19 Other mechanical complication of implanted
electronic stimulator of nervous system**
Leakage of implanted electronic stimulator of nervous
system
Obstruction (mechanical) of implanted electronic
stimulator of nervous system
Perforation of implanted electronic stimulator of
nervous system
Protrusion of implanted electronic stimulator of
nervous system

     [1] ✓7ᵗʰ **T85.190 Other mechanical complication of** HCC
implanted electronic neurostimulator
of brain electrode (lead)

     [1] ✓7ᵗʰ **T85.191 Other mechanical complication of** HCC
implanted electronic neurostimulator
of peripheral nerve electrode (lead)
Other mechanical complication of
electrode (lead) for cranial nerve
neurostimulators
Other mechanical complication of
electrode (lead) for gastric
neurostimulator
Other mechanical complication of
electrode (lead) for sacral nerve
neurostimulator
Other mechanical complication of
electrode (lead) for vagal nerve
neurostimulators

     [1] ✓7ᵗʰ **T85.192 Other mechanical complication of** HCC
implanted electronic neurostimulator
of spinal cord electrode (lead)

     [1] ✓7ᵗʰ **T85.193 Other mechanical complication of** HCC
**implanted electronic neurostimulator,
generator**
Other mechanical complication of
implanted electronic neurostimulator
generator, brain, peripheral, gastric,
spinal
Other mechanical complication of
implanted electronic sacral
neurostimulator, pulse generator or
receiver

     [1] ✓7ᵗʰ **T85.199 Other mechanical complication of** HCC
**other implanted electronic stimulator
of nervous system**

✓5ᵗʰ **T85.2 Mechanical complication of intraocular lens**

     ✓x7ᵗʰ **T85.21 Breakdown (mechanical) of intraocular lens**

✓x7ᵗʰ **T85.22 Displacement of intraocular lens**
Malposition of intraocular lens

✓x7ᵗʰ **T85.29 Other mechanical complication of intraocular lens**
Obstruction (mechanical) of intraocular lens
Perforation of intraocular lens
Protrusion of intraocular lens

✓5ᵗʰ **T85.3 Mechanical complication of other ocular prosthetic devices,
implants and grafts**
EXCLUDES 2 other complications of corneal graft (T86.84-)

     ✓6ᵗʰ **T85.31 Breakdown (mechanical) of other ocular prosthetic
devices, implants and grafts**

         ✓7ᵗʰ **T85.310 Breakdown (mechanical) of prosthetic
orbit of right eye**

         ✓7ᵗʰ **T85.311 Breakdown (mechanical) of prosthetic
orbit of left eye**

         ✓7ᵗʰ **T85.318 Breakdown (mechanical) of other ocular
prosthetic devices, implants and grafts**

     ✓6ᵗʰ **T85.32 Displacement of other ocular prosthetic devices,
implants and grafts**
Malposition of other ocular prosthetic devices,
implants and grafts

         ✓7ᵗʰ **T85.320 Displacement of prosthetic orbit of right
eye**

         ✓7ᵗʰ **T85.321 Displacement of prosthetic orbit of left
eye**

         ✓7ᵗʰ **T85.328 Displacement of other ocular prosthetic
devices, implants and grafts**

     ✓6ᵗʰ **T85.39 Other mechanical complication of other ocular
prosthetic devices, implants and grafts**
Obstruction (mechanical) of other ocular prosthetic
devices, implants and grafts
Perforation of other ocular prosthetic devices,
implants and grafts
Protrusion of other ocular prosthetic devices, implants
and grafts

         ✓7ᵗʰ **T85.390 Other mechanical complication of
prosthetic orbit of right eye**

         ✓7ᵗʰ **T85.391 Other mechanical complication of
prosthetic orbit of left eye**

         ✓7ᵗʰ **T85.398 Other mechanical complication of other
ocular prosthetic devices, implants and
grafts**

✓5ᵗʰ **T85.4 Mechanical complication of breast prosthesis and implant**

     ✓x7ᵗʰ **T85.41 Breakdown (mechanical) of breast prosthesis and
implant**

     ✓x7ᵗʰ **T85.42 Displacement of breast prosthesis and implant**
Malposition of breast prosthesis and implant

     ✓x7ᵗʰ **T85.43 Leakage of breast prosthesis and implant**

     ✓x7ᵗʰ **T85.44 Capsular contracture of breast implant**

     ✓x7ᵗʰ **T85.49 Other mechanical complication of breast prosthesis
and implant**
Obstruction (mechanical) of breast prosthesis and
implant
Perforation of breast prosthesis and implant
Protrusion of breast prosthesis and implant

✓5ᵗʰ **T85.5 Mechanical complication of gastrointestinal prosthetic
devices, implants and grafts**

     ✓6ᵗʰ **T85.51 Breakdown (mechanical) of gastrointestinal
prosthetic devices, implants and grafts**

         ✓7ᵗʰ **T85.510 Breakdown (mechanical) of bile duct
prosthesis**

         ✓7ᵗʰ **T85.511 Breakdown (mechanical) of esophageal
anti-reflux device**

         ✓7ᵗʰ **T85.518 Breakdown (mechanical) of other
gastrointestinal prosthetic devices,
implants and grafts**

     ✓6ᵗʰ **T85.52 Displacement of gastrointestinal prosthetic devices,
implants and grafts**
Malposition of gastrointestinal prosthetic devices,
implants and grafts

         ✓7ᵗʰ **T85.520 Displacement of bile duct prosthesis**

         ✓7ᵗʰ **T85.521 Displacement of esophageal anti-reflux
device**

         ✓7ᵗʰ **T85.528 Displacement of other gastrointestinal
prosthetic devices, implants and grafts**

---

[1] HCC with 7th character indicating initial encounter (A, B or C - specific to category).

✓ Additional Character Req   ✓x7ᵗʰ Placeholder Alert   Manifestation   HCC CMS-HCC Condition   ▽ Unspecified Code   ▶◀ Revised Text   ● New Code   ▲ Revised Code Title

ICD-10-CM 2018   1107

✓6th **T85.59** **Other mechanical complication of gastrointestinal prosthetic devices, implants and grafts**
    Obstruction, mechanical of gastrointestinal prosthetic devices, implants and grafts
    Perforation of gastrointestinal prosthetic devices, implants and grafts
    Protrusion of gastrointestinal prosthetic devices, implants and grafts

    ✓7th **T85.590** **Other mechanical complication of bile duct prosthesis**

    ✓7th **T85.591** **Other mechanical complication of esophageal anti-reflux device**

    ✓7th **T85.598** **Other mechanical complication of other gastrointestinal prosthetic devices, implants and grafts**

✓5th **T85.6** **Mechanical complication of other specified internal and external prosthetic devices, implants and grafts**

    ✓6th **T85.61** **Breakdown (mechanical) of other specified internal prosthetic devices, implants and grafts**

        ✓7th **T85.610** **Breakdown (mechanical) of cranial or spinal infusion catheter**
            Breakdown (mechanical) of epidural infusion catheter
            Breakdown (mechanical) of intrathecal infusion catheter
            Breakdown (mechanical) of subarachnoid infusion catheter
            Breakdown (mechanical) of subdural infusion catheter

        ✓7th **T85.611** **Breakdown (mechanical) of intraperitoneal dialysis catheter** HCC
            EXCLUDES 1   *mechanical complication of vascular dialysis catheter (T82.4-)*

        ✓7th **T85.612** **Breakdown (mechanical) of permanent sutures**
            EXCLUDES 1   *mechanical complication of permanent (wire) suture used in bone repair (T84.1-T84.2)*

        ✓7th **T85.613** **Breakdown (mechanical) of artificial skin graft and decellularized allodermis**
            Failure of artificial skin graft and decellularized allodermis
            Non-adherence of artificial skin graft and decellularized allodermis
            Poor incorporation of artificial skin graft and decellularized allodermis
            Shearing of artificial skin graft and decellularized allodermis

        ✓7th **T85.614** **Breakdown (mechanical) of insulin pump**

        1 ✓7th **T85.615** **Breakdown (mechanical) of other nervous system device, implant or graft** HCC
            Breakdown (mechanical) of intrathecal infusion pump

        ✓7th **T85.618** **Breakdown (mechanical) of other specified internal prosthetic devices, implants and grafts**

    ✓6th **T85.62** **Displacement of other specified internal prosthetic devices, implants and grafts**
        Malposition of other specified internal prosthetic devices, implants and grafts

        ✓7th **T85.620** **Displacement of cranial or spinal infusion catheter**
            Displacement of epidural infusion catheter
            Displacement of intrathecal infusion catheter
            Displacement of subarachnoid infusion catheter
            Displacement of subdural infusion catheter

        ✓7th **T85.621** **Displacement of intraperitoneal dialysis catheter** HCC
            EXCLUDES 1   *mechanical complication of vascular dialysis catheter (T82.4-)*

        ✓7th **T85.622** **Displacement of permanent sutures**
            EXCLUDES 1   *mechanical complication of permanent (wire) suture used in bone repair (T84.1-T84.2)*

        ✓7th **T85.623** **Displacement of artificial skin graft and decellularized allodermis**
            Dislodgement of artificial skin graft and decellularized allodermis
            ~~Displacement of artificial skin graft and decellularized allodermis~~

        ✓7th **T85.624** **Displacement of insulin pump**

        1 ✓7th **T85.625** **Displacement of other nervous system device, implant or graft** HCC
            Displacement of intrathecal infusion pump

        ✓7th **T85.628** **Displacement of other specified internal prosthetic devices, implants and grafts**

    ✓6th **T85.63** **Leakage of other specified internal prosthetic devices, implants and grafts**

        ✓7th **T85.630** **Leakage of cranial or spinal infusion catheter**
            Leakage of epidural infusion catheter
            Leakage of intrathecal infusion catheter infusion catheter
            Leakage of subdural infusion catheter
            Leakage of subarachnoid infusion catheter

        ✓7th **T85.631** **Leakage of intraperitoneal dialysis catheter** HCC
            EXCLUDES 1   *mechanical complication of vascular dialysis catheter (T82.4)*

        ✓7th **T85.633** **Leakage of insulin pump**

        1 ✓7th **T85.635** **Leakage of other nervous system device, implant or graft** HCC
            Leakage of intrathecal infusion pump

        ✓7th **T85.638** **Leakage of other specified internal prosthetic devices, implants and grafts**

    ✓6th **T85.69** **Other mechanical complication of other specified internal prosthetic devices, implants and grafts**
        Obstruction, mechanical of other specified internal prosthetic devices, implants and grafts
        Perforation of other specified internal prosthetic devices, implants and grafts
        Protrusion of other specified internal prosthetic devices, implants and grafts

        ✓7th **T85.690** **Other mechanical complication of cranial or spinal infusion catheter**
            Other mechanical complication of epidural infusion catheter
            Other mechanical complication of intrathecal infusion catheter
            Other mechanical complication of subarachnoid infusion catheter
            Other mechanical complication of subdural infusion catheter

        ✓7th **T85.691** **Other mechanical complication of intraperitoneal dialysis catheter** HCC
            EXCLUDES 1   *mechanical complication of vascular dialysis catheter (T82.4)*

        ✓7th **T85.692** **Other mechanical complication of permanent sutures**
            EXCLUDES 1   *mechanical complication of permanent (wire) suture used in bone repair (T84.1-T84.2)*

        ✓7th **T85.693** **Other mechanical complication of artificial skin graft and decellularized allodermis**

        ✓7th **T85.694** **Other mechanical complication of insulin pump**

        1 ✓7th **T85.695** **Other mechanical complication of other nervous system device, implant or graft** HCC
            Other mechanical complication of intrathecal infusion pump

        ✓7th **T85.698** **Other mechanical complication of other specified internal prosthetic devices, implants and grafts**
            Mechanical complication of nonabsorbable surgical material NOS

---

1   HCC with 7th character indicating initial encounter (A, B or C - specific to category).

EXCLUDES 1 Not coded here   EXCLUDES 2 Not included here   N Newborn Age: 0   P Pediatric Age: 0-17   M Maternity Age: 12-55   A Adult Age: 15-124

1108   ICD-10-CM 2018

☑5ᵗʰ **T85.7** Infection and inflammatory reaction **due to other internal prosthetic devices, implants and grafts**
   Use additional code to identify infection

  ¹ ☑7ᵗʰ **T85.71** **Infection and inflammatory reaction due to** `HCC` **peritoneal dialysis catheter**

  ¹ ☑7ᵗʰ **T85.72** **Infection and inflammatory reaction due to** `HCC` **insulin pump**

  ☑6ᵗʰ **T85.73** **Infection and inflammatory reaction due to** nervous system **devices, implants and graft**

   ¹ ☑7ᵗʰ **T85.730** **Infection and inflammatory reaction** `HCC` **due to** ventricular intracranial (communicating) shunt

   ¹ ☑7ᵗʰ **T85.731** **Infection and inflammatory reaction** `HCC` **due to implanted electronic neurostimulator of** brain, electrode (lead)

   ¹ ☑7ᵗʰ **T85.732** **Infection and inflammatory reaction** `HCC` **due to implanted electronic neurostimulator of** peripheral nerve, electrode (lead)
      Infection and inflammatory reaction due to electrode (lead) for cranial nerve neurostimulators
      Infection and inflammatory reaction due to electrode (lead) for gastric neurostimulator
      Infection and inflammatory reaction due to electrode (lead) for sacral nerve neurostimulator
      Infection and inflammatory reaction due to electrode (lead) for vagal nerve neurostimulators

   ¹ ☑7ᵗʰ **T85.733** **Infection and inflammatory reaction** `HCC` **due to implanted electronic neurostimulator of** spinal cord, electrode (lead)

   ¹ ☑7ᵗʰ **T85.734** **Infection and inflammatory reaction** `HCC` **due to implanted electronic neurostimulator,** generator
      Generator pocket infection

   ¹ ☑7ᵗʰ **T85.735** **Infection and inflammatory reaction** `HCC` **due to** cranial or spinal infusion catheter
      Infection and inflammatory reaction due to epidural catheter
      Infection and inflammatory reaction due to intrathecal infusion catheter
      Infection and inflammatory reaction due to subarachnoid catheter
      Infection and inflammatory reaction due to subdural catheter

   ¹ ☑7ᵗʰ **T85.738** **Infection and inflammatory reaction** `HCC` **due to other nervous system device, implant or graft**
      Infection and inflammatory reaction due to intrathecal infusion pump

  ¹ ☑x7ᵗʰ **T85.79** **Infection and inflammatory reaction due** `HCC` **to other internal prosthetic devices, implants and grafts**

☑5ᵗʰ **T85.8** **Other specified complications of internal prosthetic devices, implants and grafts, not elsewhere classified**

  ☑6ᵗʰ **T85.81** Embolism **due to internal prosthetic devices, implants and grafts, not elsewhere classified**

   ¹ ☑7ᵗʰ **T85.810** **Embolism due to** nervous system `HCC` **prosthetic devices, implants and grafts**

   ☑7ᵗʰ **T85.818** **Embolism due to other internal prosthetic devices, implants and grafts**

  ☑6ᵗʰ **T85.82** Fibrosis **due to internal prosthetic devices, implants and grafts, not elsewhere classified**

   ¹ ☑7ᵗʰ **T85.820** **Fibrosis due to** nervous system `HCC` **prosthetic devices, implants and grafts**

   ☑7ᵗʰ **T85.828** **Fibrosis due to other internal prosthetic devices, implants and grafts**

  ☑6ᵗʰ **T85.83** Hemorrhage **due to internal prosthetic devices, implants and grafts, not elsewhere classified**

   ¹ ☑7ᵗʰ **T85.830** **Hemorrhage due to** nervous system `HCC` **prosthetic devices, implants and grafts**

   ☑7ᵗʰ **T85.838** **Hemorrhage due to other internal prosthetic devices, implants and grafts**

  ☑6ᵗʰ **T85.84** Pain **due to internal prosthetic devices, implants and grafts, not elsewhere classified**

   ¹ ☑7ᵗʰ **T85.840** **Pain due to** nervous system `HCC` **prosthetic devices, implants and grafts**

   ☑7ᵗʰ **T85.848** **Pain due to other internal prosthetic devices, implants and grafts**

  ☑6ᵗʰ **T85.85** Stenosis **due to internal prosthetic devices, implants and grafts, not elsewhere classified**

   ¹ ☑7ᵗʰ **T85.850** **Stenosis due to** nervous system `HCC` **prosthetic devices, implants and grafts**

   ☑7ᵗʰ **T85.858** **Stenosis due to other internal prosthetic devices, implants and grafts**

  ☑6ᵗʰ **T85.86** Thrombosis **due to internal prosthetic devices, implants and grafts, not elsewhere classified**

   ¹ ☑7ᵗʰ **T85.860** **Thrombosis due to** nervous system `HCC` **prosthetic devices, implants and grafts**

   ☑7ᵗʰ **T85.868** **Thrombosis due to other internal prosthetic devices, implants and grafts**

  ☑6ᵗʰ **T85.89** **Other specified complication of internal prosthetic devices, implants and grafts, not elsewhere classified**
      Erosion or breakdown of subcutaneous device pocket

   ¹ ☑7ᵗʰ **T85.890** **Other specified complication of** `HCC` nervous system **prosthetic devices, implants and grafts**

   ☑7ᵗʰ **T85.898** **Other specified complication of other internal prosthetic devices, implants and grafts**

☑x7ᵗʰ **T85.9** **Unspecified complication of internal prosthetic device, implant and graft** ▽
   Complication of internal prosthetic device, implant and graft NOS

☑4ᵗʰ **T86** **Complications of transplanted organs and tissue**
   Use additional code to identify other transplant complications, such as:
   graft-versus-host disease (D89.81-)
   malignancy associated with organ transplant (C80.2)
   post-transplant lymphoproliferative disorders (PTLD) (D47.Z1)

  ☑5ᵗʰ **T86.0** **Complications of** bone marrow **transplant**

   T86.00 **Unspecified complication of bone marrow transplant** `HCC` ▽

   T86.01 **Bone marrow transplant** rejection `HCC`

   T86.02 **Bone marrow transplant** failure `HCC`

   T86.03 **Bone marrow transplant** infection `HCC`

   T86.09 **Other complications of bone marrow transplant** `HCC`

  ☑5ᵗʰ **T86.1** **Complications of** kidney **transplant**

   T86.10 **Unspecified complication of kidney transplant** ▽

   T86.11 **Kidney transplant** rejection

   T86.12 **Kidney transplant** failure
      AHA: 2013, 1Q, 24

   T86.13 **Kidney transplant** infection
      Use additional code to specify infection

   T86.19 **Other complication of kidney transplant**

  ☑5ᵗʰ **T86.2** **Complications of** heart **transplant**
      EXCLUDES 1 complication of:
         artificial heart device (T82.5)
         heart-lung transplant (T86.3)

   T86.20 **Unspecified complication of heart transplant** `HCC` ▽

   T86.21 **Heart transplant** rejection `HCC`

   T86.22 **Heart transplant** failure `HCC`

   T86.23 **Heart transplant** infection `HCC`
      Use additional code to specify infection

   ☑6ᵗʰ **T86.29** **Other complications of heart transplant**

    T86.290 Cardiac allograft vasculopathy `HCC`
       EXCLUDES 1 atherosclerosis of coronary arteries (I25.75-, I25.76-, I25.81-)

    T86.298 **Other complications of heart transplant** `HCC`

  ☑5ᵗʰ **T86.3** **Complications of** heart-lung **transplant**

   T86.30 **Unspecified complication of heart-lung transplant** `HCC` ▽

   T86.31 **Heart-lung transplant** rejection `HCC`

   T86.32 **Heart-lung transplant** failure `HCC`

---

¹ HCC with 7th character indicating initial encounter (A, B or C - specific to category).

☑ Additional Character Req   ☑x7 Placeholder Alert   Manifestation   `HCC` CMS-HCC Condition   ▽ Unspecified Code   ►◄ Revised Text   ● New Code   ▲ Revised Code Title

Chapter 19. Injury, Poisoning, and Certain Other Consequences of External Causes

T86.33   **Heart-lung transplant** infection   HCC
Use additional code to specify infection

T86.39   **Other complications of heart-lung transplant**   HCC

✓5ᵗʰ **T86.4**   **Complications of** liver **transplant**

T86.40   **Unspecified complication of liver transplant**   HCC ▽

T86.41   **Liver transplant** rejection   HCC

T86.42   **Liver transplant** failure   HCC

T86.43   **Liver transplant** infection   HCC
Use additional code to identify infection, such as:
cytomegalovirus (CMV) infection (B25.-)

T86.49   **Other complications of liver transplant**   HCC

T86.5   **Complications of** stem cell **transplant**   HCC
Complications from stem cells from peripheral blood
Complications from stem cells from umbilical cord

✓5ᵗʰ **T86.8**   **Complications of other transplanted organs and tissues**

✓6ᵗʰ **T86.81**   **Complications of** lung **transplant**
EXCLUDES 1   complication of heart-lung transplant (T86.3-)

T86.810   **Lung transplant** rejection   HCC

T86.811   **Lung transplant** failure   HCC

T86.812   **Lung transplant** infection   HCC
Use additional code to specify infection

T86.818   **Other complications of lung transplant**   HCC

T86.819   **Unspecified complication of lung transplant**   HCC ▽

✓6ᵗʰ **T86.82**   **Complications of** skin graft (allograft) (autograft)
EXCLUDES 2   complication of artificial skin graft (T85.693)

T86.820   **Skin graft (allograft)** rejection

T86.821   **Skin graft (allograft) (autograft)** failure

T86.822   **Skin graft (allograft) (autograft)** infection
Use additional code to specify infection

T86.828   **Other complications of skin graft (allograft) (autograft)**

T86.829   **Unspecified complication of skin graft (allograft) (autograft)** ▽

✓6ᵗʰ **T86.83**   **Complications of** bone graft
EXCLUDES 2   mechanical complications of bone graft (T84.3-)

T86.830   **Bone graft** rejection

T86.831   **Bone graft** failure

T86.832   **Bone graft** infection
Use additional code to specify infection

T86.838   **Other complications of bone graft**

T86.839   **Unspecified complication of bone graft** ▽

✓6ᵗʰ **T86.84**   **Complications of** corneal **transplant**
EXCLUDES 2   mechanical complications of corneal graft (T85.3-)

T86.840   **Corneal transplant** rejection

T86.841   **Corneal transplant** failure

T86.842   **Corneal transplant** infection   HCC
Use additional code to specify infection

T86.848   **Other complications of corneal transplant**

T86.849   **Unspecified complication of corneal transplant** ▽

✓6ᵗʰ **T86.85**   **Complication of** intestine **transplant**

T86.850   **Intestine transplant** rejection   HCC

T86.851   **Intestine transplant** failure   HCC

T86.852   **Intestine transplant** infection   HCC
Use additional code to specify infection

T86.858   **Other complications of intestine transplant**   HCC

T86.859   **Unspecified complication of intestine transplant**   HCC ▽

✓6ᵗʰ **T86.89**   **Complications of other transplanted** tissue
Transplant failure or rejection of pancreas

T86.890   **Other transplanted tissue** rejection

T86.891   **Other transplanted tissue** failure

T86.892   **Other transplanted tissue** infection
Use additional code to specify infection

T86.898   **Other complications of other transplanted tissue**

T86.899   **Unspecified complication of other transplanted tissue** ▽

✓5ᵗʰ **T86.9**   **Complication of unspecified transplanted organ and tissue**

T86.90   **Unspecified complication of unspecified transplanted organ and tissue** ▽

T86.91   **Unspecified transplanted organ and tissue** rejection ▽

T86.92   **Unspecified transplanted organ and tissue** failure ▽

T86.93   **Unspecified transplanted organ and tissue** infection ▽
Use additional code to specify infection

T86.99   **Other complications of unspecified transplanted organ and tissue** ▽

✓4ᵗʰ **T87**   **Complications peculiar to reattachment and amputation**

✓5ᵗʰ **T87.0**   **Complications of reattached (part of)** upper extremity

✓6ᵗʰ **T87.0X**   **Complications of reattached (part of) upper extremity**

T87.0X1   **Complications of reattached (part of)** right upper extremity   HCC

T87.0X2   **Complications of reattached (part of)** left upper extremity   HCC

T87.0X9   **Complications of reattached (part of)** unspecified upper extremity   HCC ▽

✓5ᵗʰ **T87.1**   **Complications of reattached (part of)** lower extremity

✓6ᵗʰ **T87.1X**   **Complications of reattached (part of) lower extremity**

T87.1X1   **Complications of reattached (part of)** right lower extremity   HCC

T87.1X2   **Complications of reattached (part of)** left lower extremity   HCC

T87.1X9   **Complications of reattached (part of)** unspecified lower extremity   HCC ▽

T87.2   **Complications of other reattached body part**   HCC

✓5ᵗʰ **T87.3**   **Neuroma of amputation stump**
DEF: Non-neoplastic tumor generated at the proximal end of severed, partially transected, or injured nerve following amputation.

T87.30   **Neuroma of amputation stump,** unspecified extremity   HCC ▽

T87.31   **Neuroma of amputation stump,** right upper extremity   HCC

T87.32   **Neuroma of amputation stump,** left upper extremity   HCC

T87.33   **Neuroma of amputation stump,** right lower extremity   HCC

T87.34   **Neuroma of amputation stump,** left lower extremity   HCC

✓5ᵗʰ **T87.4**   **Infection of amputation stump**

T87.40   **Infection of amputation stump,** unspecified extremity   HCC ▽

T87.41   **Infection of amputation stump,** right upper extremity   HCC

T87.42   **Infection of amputation stump,** left upper extremity   HCC

T87.43   **Infection of amputation stump,** right lower extremity   HCC

T87.44   **Infection of amputation stump,** left lower extremity   HCC

✓5ᵗʰ **T87.5**   **Necrosis of amputation stump**

T87.50   **Necrosis of amputation stump,** unspecified extremity   HCC ▽

T87.51   **Necrosis of amputation stump,** right upper extremity   HCC

T87.52   **Necrosis of amputation stump,** left upper extremity   HCC

T87.53   **Necrosis of amputation stump,** right lower extremity   HCC

T87.54   **Necrosis of amputation stump,** left lower extremity   HCC

✓5ᵗʰ **T87.8**   **Other complications of amputation stump**

T87.81   **Dehiscence of amputation stump**   HCC

EXCLUDES 1 Not coded here   EXCLUDES 2 Not included here   N Newborn Age: 0   P Pediatric Age: 0-17   M Maternity Age: 12-55   A Adult Age: 15-124

1110   ICD-10-CM 2018

T87.89 Other complications of amputation stump HCC
  Amputation stump contracture
  Amputation stump contracture of next proximal joint
  Amputation stump flexion
  Amputation stump edema
  Amputation stump hematoma
    EXCLUDES 2 *phantom limb syndrome (G54.6-G54.7)*

T87.9 Unspecified complications of amputation stump HCC ▽

✓4th **T88 Other complications of surgical and medical care, not elsewhere classified**
    EXCLUDES 2 *complication following infusion, transfusion and therapeutic injection (T80.-)*
      complication following procedure NEC (T81.-)
      complications of anesthesia in labor and delivery (O74.-)
      complications of anesthesia in pregnancy (O29.-)
      complications of anesthesia in puerperium (O89.-)
      complications of devices, implants and grafts (T82-T85)
      complications of obstetric surgery and procedure (O75.4)
      dermatitis due to drugs and medicaments (L23.3, L24.4, L25.1, L27.0-L27.1)
      poisoning and toxic effects of drugs and chemicals (T36-T65 with fifth or sixth character 1-4 or 6)
      specified complications classified elsewhere

> The appropriate 7th character is to be added to each code from category T88.
> A   initial encounter
> D   subsequent encounter
> S   sequela

✓x7th **T88.0 Infection following immunization**
  Sepsis following immunization

✓x7th **T88.1 Other complications following immunization, not elsewhere classified**
  Generalized vaccinia
  Rash following immunization
    EXCLUDES 1 *vaccinia not from vaccine (B08.011)*
    EXCLUDES 2 *anaphylactic shock due to serum (T80.5-)*
      other serum reactions (T80.6-)
      postimmunization arthropathy (M02.2)
      postimmunization encephalitis (G04.02)
      postimmunization fever (R50.83)

✓x7th **T88.2 Shock due to anesthesia**
  Use additional code for adverse effect, if applicable, to identify drug (T41.- with fifth or sixth character 5)
    EXCLUDES 1 *complications of anesthesia (in):*
      labor and delivery (O74.-)
      postprocedural shock NOS (T81.1-)
      pregnancy (O29.-)
      puerperium (O89.-)

✓x7th **T88.3 Malignant hyperthermia due to anesthesia**
  Use additional code for adverse effect, if applicable, to identify drug (T41.- with fifth or sixth character 5)

✓x7th **T88.4 Failed or difficult intubation**

✓5th **T88.5 Other complications of anesthesia**
  Use additional code for adverse effect, if applicable, to identify drug (T41.- with fifth or sixth character 5)

  ✓x7th **T88.51 Hypothermia following anesthesia**

  ✓x7th **T88.52 Failed moderate sedation during procedure**
    Failed conscious sedation during procedure
      EXCLUDES 2 *personal history of failed moderate sedation (Z92.83)*

  ✓x7th **T88.53 Unintended awareness under general anesthesia during procedure**
      EXCLUDES 2 *personal history of unintended awareness under general anesthesia (Z92.84)*

  ✓x7th **T88.59 Other complications of anesthesia**

✓x7th **T88.6 Anaphylactic reaction due to adverse effect of correct drug or medicament properly administered**
  Anaphylactic shock due to adverse effect of correct drug or medicament properly administered
  Anaphylactoid reaction NOS
  Use additional code for adverse effect, if applicable, to identify drug (T36-T50 with fifth or sixth character 5)
    EXCLUDES 1 *anaphylactic reaction due to serum (T80.5-)*
      anaphylactic shock or reaction due to adverse food reaction (T78.0-)

✓x7th **T88.7 Unspecified adverse effect of drug or medicament** ▽
  Drug hypersensitivity NOS
  Drug reaction NOS
  Use additional code for adverse effect, if applicable, to identify drug (T36-T50 with fifth or sixth character 5)
    EXCLUDES 1 *specified adverse effects of drugs and medicaments (A00-R94 and T80-T88.6, T88.8)*

✓x7th **T88.8 Other specified complications of surgical and medical care, not elsewhere classified**
  Use additional code to identify the complication

✓x7th **T88.9 Complication of surgical and medical care, unspecified** ▽

Chapter 20. External Causes of Morbidity (V00–Y99)

Chapter Specific Guidelines with Coding Examples

The chapter specific guidelines from the ICD-10-CM Official Guidelines for Coding and Reporting have been provided below. Along with these guidelines are coding examples, contained in the shaded boxes, that have been developed to help illustrate the coding and/or sequencing guidance found in these guidelines.

The external causes of morbidity codes should never be sequenced as the first-listed or principal diagnosis.

External cause codes are intended to provide data for injury research and evaluation of injury prevention strategies. These codes capture how the injury or health condition happened (cause), the intent (unintentional or accidental; or intentional, such as suicide or assault), the place where the event occurred the activity of the patient at the time of the event, and the person's status (e.g., civilian, military).

There is no national requirement for mandatory ICD-10-CM external cause code reporting. Unless a provider is subject to a state-based external cause code reporting mandate or these codes are required by a particular payer, reporting of ICD-10-CM codes in Chapter 20, External Causes of Morbidity, is not required. In the absence of a mandatory reporting requirement, providers are encouraged to voluntarily report external cause codes, as they provide valuable data for injury research and evaluation of injury prevention strategies.

a. General external cause coding guidelines

1) Used with any code in the range of A00.0–T88.9, Z00–Z99

An external cause code may be used with any code in the range of A00.0–T88.9, Z00–Z99, classification that is a health condition due to an external cause. Though they are most applicable to injuries, they are also valid for use with such things as infections or diseases due to an external source, and other health conditions, such as a heart attack that occurs during strenuous physical activity.

Actinic reticuloid due to tanning bed use	
L57.1	**Actinic reticuloid**
W89.1XXA	**Exposure to tanning bed, initial encounter**

Explanation: An external cause code may be used with any code in the range of A00.0–T88.9, Z00–Z99, classifications that describe health conditions due to an external cause. Code W89.1 Exposure to tanning bed requires a seventh character of A to report this initial encounter, with a placeholder X for the fifth and sixth characters.

2) External cause code used for length of treatment

Assign the external cause code, with the appropriate 7th character (initial encounter, subsequent encounter or sequela) for each encounter for which the injury or condition is being treated.

Most categories in chapter 20 have a 7th character requirement for each applicable code. Most categories in this chapter have three 7th character values: A, initial encounter, D, subsequent encounter and S, sequela. While the patient may be seen by a new or different provider over the course of treatment for an injury or condition, assignment of the 7th character for external cause should match the 7th character of the code assigned for the associated injury or condition for the encounter.

3) Use the full range of external cause codes

Use the full range of external cause codes to completely describe the cause, the intent, the place of occurrence, and if applicable, the activity of the patient at the time of the event, and the patient's status, for all injuries, and other health conditions due to an external cause.

4) Assign as many external cause codes as necessary

Assign as many external cause codes as necessary to fully explain each cause. If only one external code can be recorded, assign the code most related to the principal diagnosis.

5) The selection of the appropriate external cause code

The selection of the appropriate external cause code is guided by the Alphabetic Index of External Causes and by Inclusion and Exclusion notes in the Tabular List.

6) External cause code can never be a principal diagnosis

An external cause code can never be a principal (first-listed) diagnosis.

7) Combination external cause codes

Certain of the external cause codes are combination codes that identify sequential events that result in an injury, such as a fall which results in striking against an object. The injury may be due to either event or both.

The combination external cause code used should correspond to the sequence of events regardless of which caused the most serious injury.

Toddler tripped and fell while walking and struck his head on an end table, sustaining a scalp contusion	
S00.03XA	**Contusion of scalp, initial encounter**
W01.190A	**Fall on same level from slipping, tripping and stumbling with subsequent striking against furniture, initial encounter**

Explanation: Combination external cause codes identify sequential events that result in an injury, such as a fall resulting in striking against an object. The injury may be due to either or both events.

8) No external cause code needed in certain circumstances

No external cause code from Chapter 20 is needed if the external cause and intent are included in a code from another chapter (e.g. T36.0X1-Poisoning by penicillins, accidental (unintentional)).

b. Place of occurrence guideline

Codes from category Y92, Place of occurrence of the external cause, are secondary codes for use after other external cause codes to identify the location of the patient at the time of injury or other condition.

Generally, a place of occurrence code is assigned only once, at the initial encounter for treatment. However, in the rare instance that a new injury occurs during hospitalization, an additional place of occurrence code may be assigned. No 7th characters are used for Y92.

Do not use place of occurrence code Y92.9 if the place is not stated or is not applicable.

A farmer was working in his barn and sustained a foot contusion when the horse stepped on his left foot	
S90.32XA	**Contusion of left foot, initial encounter**
W55.19XA	**Other contact with horse, initial encounter**
Y92.71	**Barn as the place of occurrence of the external cause**

Explanation: A place-of-occurrence code from category Y92 is assigned at the initial encounter to identify the location of the patient at the time the injury occurred.

c. Activity code

Assign a code from category Y93, Activity code, to describe the activity of the patient at the time the injury or other health condition occurred.

An activity code is used only once, at the initial encounter for treatment. Only one code from Y93 should be recorded on a medical record.

The activity codes are not applicable to poisonings, adverse effects, misadventures or sequela.

Do not assign Y93.9, Unspecified activity, if the activity is not stated.

A code from category Y93 is appropriate for use with external cause and intent codes if identifying the activity provides additional information about the event.

Ranch hand who was grooming a horse sustained a foot contusion when the horse stepped on his left foot	
S90.32XA	**Contusion of left foot, initial encounter**
W55.19XA	**Other contact with horse, initial encounter**
Y93.K3	**Activity, grooming and shearing an animal**

Explanation: One activity code from category Y93 is assigned at the initial encounter only to describe the activity of the patient at the time the injury occurred.

d. Place of occurrence, activity, and status codes used with other external cause code

When applicable, place of occurrence, activity, and external cause status codes are sequenced after the main external cause code(s). Regardless of the number of external cause codes assigned, generally there should be only one place of occurrence code, one activity code, and one external cause status code assigned to an encounter. However, in the rare instance that a new injury occurs during hospitalization, an additional place of occurrence code may be assigned.

e. If the reporting format limits the number of external cause codes

If the reporting format limits the number of external cause codes that can be used in reporting clinical data, report the code for the cause/intent most related to the principal diagnosis. If the format permits capture of additional external cause codes, the cause/intent, including medical misadventures, of the additional events should be reported rather than the codes for place, activity, or external status.

f. Multiple external cause coding guidelines

More than one external cause code is required to fully describe the external cause of an illness or injury. The assignment of external cause codes should be sequenced in the following priority:

If two or more events cause separate injuries, an external cause code should be assigned for each cause. The first-listed external cause code will be selected in the following order:

External codes for child and adult abuse take priority over all other external cause codes.

See Section I.C.19., Child and Adult abuse guidelines.

External cause codes for terrorism events take priority over all other external cause codes except child and adult abuse.

External cause codes for cataclysmic events take priority over all other external cause codes except child and adult abuse and terrorism.

External cause codes for transport accidents take priority over all other external cause codes except cataclysmic events, child and adult abuse and terrorism.

Activity and external cause status codes are assigned following all causal (intent) external cause codes.

The first-listed external cause code should correspond to the cause of the most serious diagnosis due to an assault, accident, or self-harm, following the order of hierarchy listed above..

30-year-old man accidentally discharged his hunting rifle, sustaining an open gunshot wound, with no retained bullet fragments, to the right thigh, which caused him to fall down the stairs, resulting in closed displaced comminuted fracture of his left radial shaft

S71.131A	**Puncture wound without foreign body, right thigh, initial encounter**
S52.352A	**Displaced comminuted fracture of shaft of radius, left arm, initial encounter for closed fracture**
W33.02XA	**Accidental discharge of hunting rifle, initial encounter**
W10.9XXA	**Fall (on) (from) unspecified stairs and steps, initial encounter**

Explanation: If two or more events cause separate injuries, an external cause code should be assigned for each cause.

---

g. Child and adult abuse guideline

Adult and child abuse, neglect and maltreatment are classified as assault. Any of the assault codes may be used to indicate the external cause of any injury resulting from the confirmed abuse.

For confirmed cases of abuse, neglect and maltreatment, when the perpetrator is known, a code from Y07, Perpetrator of maltreatment and neglect, should accompany any other assault codes.

See Section I.C.19. Adult and child abuse, neglect and other maltreatment

h. Unknown or undetermined intent guideline

If the intent (accident, self-harm, assault) of the cause of an injury or other condition is unknown or unspecified, code the intent as accidental intent. All transport accident categories assume accidental intent.

1) Use of undetermined intent

External cause codes for events of undetermined intent are only for use if the documentation in the record specifies that the intent cannot be determined.

i. Sequelae (late effects) of external cause guidelines

1) Sequelae external cause codes

Sequela are reported using the external cause code with the 7th character "S" for sequela. These codes should be used with any report of a late effect or sequela resulting from a previous injury.

See Section I.B.10 Sequela (Late Effects)

2) Sequela external cause code with a related current injury

A sequela external cause code should never be used with a related current nature of injury code.

3) Use of sequela external cause codes for subsequent visits

Use a late effect external cause code for subsequent visits when a late effect of the initial injury is being treated. Do not use a late effect external cause code for subsequent visits for follow-up care (e.g., to assess healing, to receive rehabilitative therapy) of the injury when no late effect of the injury has been documented.

j. Terrorism guidelines

1) Cause of injury identified by the Federal Government (FBI) as terrorism

When the cause of an injury is identified by the Federal Government (FBI) as terrorism, the first-listed external cause code should be a code from category Y38, Terrorism. The definition of terrorism employed by the FBI is found at the inclusion note at the beginning of category Y38. Use additional code for place of occurrence (Y92.-). More than one Y38 code may be assigned if the injury is the result of more than one mechanism of terrorism.

2) Cause of an injury is suspected to be the result of terrorism

When the cause of an injury is suspected to be the result of terrorism a code from category Y38 should not be assigned. Suspected cases should be classified as assault.

3) Code Y38.9, Terrorism, secondary effects

Assign code Y38.9, Terrorism, secondary effects, for conditions occurring subsequent to the terrorist event. This code should not be assigned for conditions that are due to the initial terrorist act.

It is acceptable to assign code Y38.9 with another code from Y38 if there is an injury due to the initial terrorist event and an injury that is a subsequent result of the terrorist event.

k. External cause status

A code from category Y99, External cause status, should be assigned whenever any other external cause code is assigned for an encounter, including an Activity code, except for the events noted below. Assign a code from category Y99, External cause status, to indicate the work status of the person at the time the event occurred. The status code indicates whether the event occurred during military activity, whether a non-military person was at work, whether an individual including a student or volunteer was involved in a non-work activity at the time of the causal event.

A code from Y99, External cause status, should be assigned, when applicable, with other external cause codes, such as transport accidents and falls. The external cause status codes are not applicable to poisonings, adverse effects, misadventures or late effects.

Do not assign a code from category Y99 if no other external cause codes (cause, activity) are applicable for the encounter.

An external cause status code is used only once, at the initial encounter for treatment. Only one code from Y99 should be recorded on a medical record.

Do not assign code Y99.9, Unspecified external cause status, if the status is not stated.

Chapter 20. External Causes of Morbidity (V00-Y99)

NOTE   This chapter permits the classification of environmental events and circumstances as the cause of injury, and other adverse effects. Where a code from this section is applicable, it is intended that it shall be used secondary to a code from another chapter of the Classification indicating the nature of the condition. Most often, the condition will be classifiable to Chapter 19, Injury, poisoning and certain other consequences of external causes (S00-T88). Other conditions that may be stated to be due to external causes are classified in Chapters I to XVIII. For these conditions, codes from Chapter 20 should be used to provide additional information as to the cause of the condition.

This chapter contains the following blocks:

V00-X58	Accidents
V00-V99	Transport accidents
V00-V09	Pedestrian injured in transport accident
V10-V19	Pedal cycle rider injured in transport accident
V20-V29	Motorcycle rider injured in transport accident
V30-V39	Occupant of three-wheeled motor vehicle injured in transport accident
V40-V49	Car occupant injured in transport accident
V50-V59	Occupant of pick-up truck or van injured in transport accident
V60-V69	Occupant of heavy transport vehicle injured in transport accident
V70-V79	Bus occupant injured in transport accident
V80-V89	Other land transport accidents
V90-V94	Water transport accidents
V95-V97	Air and space transport accidents
V98-V99	Other and unspecified transport accidents
W00-X58	Other external causes of accidental injury
W00-W19	Slipping, tripping, stumbling and falls
W20-W49	Exposure to inanimate mechanical forces
W50-W64	Exposure to animate mechanical forces
W65-W74	Accidental non-transport drowning and submersion
W85-W99	Exposure to electric current, radiation and extreme ambient air temperature and pressure
X00-X08	Exposure to smoke, fire and flames
X10-X19	Contact with heat and hot substances
X30-X39	Exposure to forces of nature
~~X50~~	~~Overexertion and strenuous or repetitive movements~~
X52-X58	Accidental exposure to other specified factors
X71-X83	Intentional self-harm
X92-Y09	Assault
Y21-Y33	Event of undetermined intent
Y35-Y38	Legal intervention, operations of war, military operations, and terrorism
Y62-Y84	Complications of medical and surgical care
Y62-Y69	Misadventures to patients during surgical and medical care
Y70-Y82	Medical devices associated with adverse incidents in diagnostic and therapeutic use
Y83-Y84	Surgical and other medical procedures as the cause of abnormal reaction of the patient, or of later complication, without mention of misadventure at the time of the procedure
Y90-Y99	Supplementary factors related to causes of morbidity classified elsewhere

Accidents (V00-X58)

NOTE   This section is structured in 12 groups. Those relating to land transport accidents (V00-V89) reflect the victim's mode of transport and are subdivided to identify the victim's 'counterpart' or the type of event. The vehicle of which the injured person is an occupant is identified in the first two characters since it is seen as the most important factor to identify for prevention purposes. A transport accident is one in which the vehicle involved must be moving or running or in use for transport purposes at the time of the accident.

Use additional code to identify:
    airbag injury (W22.1)
    type of street or road (Y92.4-)
    use of cellular telephone and other electronic equipment at the time of the transport accident (Y93.C-)

EXCLUDES 1   *agricultural vehicles in stationary use or maintenance (W31.-)*
    assault by crashing of motor vehicle (Y03.-)
    automobile or motor cycle in stationary use or maintenance—code to type of accident
    crashing of motor vehicle, undetermined intent (Y32)
    intentional self-harm by crashing of motor vehicle (X82)

EXCLUDES 2   *transport accidents due to cataclysm (X34-X38)*

NOTE   Definitions related to transport accidents:

(a) A transport accident (V00-V99) is any accident involving a device designed primarily for, or used at the time primarily for, conveying persons or good from one place to another.

(b) A public highway [trafficway] or street is the entire width between property lines (or other boundary lines) of land open to the public as a matter of right or custom for purposes of moving persons or property from one place to another. A roadway is that part of the public highway designed, improved and customarily used for vehicular traffic.

(c) A traffic accident is any vehicle accident occurring on the public highway [i.e. originating on, terminating on, or involving a vehicle partially on the highway]. A vehicle accident is assumed to have occurred on the public highway unless another place is specified, except in the case of accidents involving only off-road motor vehicles, which are classified as nontraffic accidents unless the contrary is stated.

(d) A nontraffic accident is any vehicle accident that occurs entirely in any place other than a public highway.

(e) A pedestrian is any person involved in an accident who was not at the time of the accident riding in or on a motor vehicle, railway train, streetcar or animal-drawn or other vehicle, or on a pedal cycle or animal. This includes, a person changing a tire, working on a parked car, or a person on foot. It also includes the user of a pedestrian conveyance such as a babystroller, ice-skates, skis, sled, roller skates, a skateboard, nonmotorized or motorized wheelchair, motorized mobility scooter, or nonmotorized scooter.

(f) A driver is an occupant of a transport vehicle who is operating or intending to operate it.

(g) A passenger is any occupant of a transport vehicle other than the driver, except a person traveling on the outside of the vehicle.

(h) A person on the outside of a vehicle is any person being transported by a vehicle but not occupying the space normally reserved for the driver or passengers, or the space intended for the transport of property. This includes a person travelling on the bodywork, bumper, fender, roof, running board or step of a vehicle, as well as, hanging on the outside of the vehicle.

(i) A pedal cycle is any land transport vehicle operated solely by nonmotorized pedals including a bicycle or tricycle.

(j) A pedal cyclist is any person riding a pedal cycle or in a sidecar or trailer attached to a pedal cycle.

(k) A motorcycle is a two-wheeled motor vehicle with one or two riding saddles and sometimes with a third wheel for the support of a sidecar. The sidecar is considered part of the motorcycle. This includes a moped, motor scooter, or motorized bicycle.

(l) A motorcycle rider is any person riding a motorcycle or in a sidecar or trailer attached to the motorcycle.

(m) A three-wheeled motor vehicle is a motorized tricycle designed primarily for on-road use. This includes a motor-driven tricycle, a motorized rickshaw, or a three-wheeled motor car.

(n) A car [automobile] is a four-wheeled motor vehicle designed primarily for carrying up to 7 persons. A trailer being towed by the car is considered part of the car. It does not include a van or minivan - see definition (o).

(o) A pick-up truck or van is a four or six-wheeled motor vehicle designed for carrying passengers as well as property or cargo weighing less than the local limit for classification as a heavy goods vehicle, and not requiring a special driver's license. This includes a minivan and a sport-utility vehicle (SUV).

(p) A heavy transport vehicle is a motor vehicle designed primarily for carrying property, meeting local criteria for classification as a heavy goods vehicle in terms of weight and requiring a special driver's license.

(q) A bus (coach) is a motor vehicle designed or adapted primarily for carrying more than 10 passengers, and requiring a special driver's license.

(r) A railway train or railway vehicle is any device, with or without freight or passenger cars couple to it, designed for traffic on a railway track. This includes subterranean (subways) or elevated trains.

(s) A streetcar, is a device designed and used primarily for transporting passengers within a municipality, running on rails, usually subject to normal traffic control signals, and operated principally on a right-of-way that forms part of the roadway. This includes a tram or trolley that runs on rails. A trailer being towed by a streetcar is considered part of the streetcar.

(t) A special vehicle mainly used on industrial premises is a motor vehicle designed primarily for use within the buildings and premises of industrial or commercial establishments. This includes battery-powered airport passenger vehicles or baggage/mail trucks, forklifts, coal-cars in a coal mine, logging cars and trucks used in mines or quarries.

(u)   A special vehicle mainly used in agriculture is a motor vehicle designed specifically for use in farming and agriculture (horticulture), to work the land, tend and harvest crops and transport materials on the farm. This includes harvesters, farm machinery and tractor and trailers.

(v)   A special construction vehicle is a motor vehicle designed specifically for use on construction and demolition sites. This includes bulldozers, diggers, earth levellers, dump trucks, backhoes, front-end loaders, pavers, and mechanical shovels.

(w) A special all-terrain vehicle is a motor vehicle of special design to enable it to negotiate over rough or soft terrain, snow or sand. Examples of special design are high construction, special wheels and tires, tracks, and support on a cushion of air. This includes snow mobiles, All-terrain vehicles (ATV), and dune buggies. It does not include passenger vehicle designated as Sport Utility Vehicles. (SUV)

(x)   A watercraft is any device designed for transporting passengers or goods on water. This includes motor or sailboats, ships, and hovercraft.

(y)   An aircraft is any device for transporting passengers or goods in the air. This includes hot-air balloons, gliders, helicopters and airplanes.

(z)   A military vehicle is any motorized vehicle operating on a public roadway owned by the military and being operated by a member of the military

Pedestrian injured in transport accident (V00-V09)

INCLUDES   person changing tire on transport vehicle
          person examining engine of vehicle broken down in (on side of) road
EXCLUDES 1   *fall due to non-transport collision with other person (W03)*
          pedestrian on foot falling (slipping) on ice and snow (W00.-)
          struck or bumped by another person (W51)

The appropriate 7th character is to be added to each code from categories V00-V09.
A   initial encounter
D   subsequent encounter
S   sequela

✓4ᵗʰ **V00 Pedestrian conveyance accident**
    Use additional place of occurrence and activity external cause codes, if known (Y92-, Y93-)
    EXCLUDES 1   *collision with another person without fall (W51)*
             fall due to person on foot colliding with another person on foot (W03)
             fall from non-moving wheelchair, nonmotorized scooter and motorized mobility scooter without collision (W05.-)
             pedestrian (conveyance) collision with other land transport vehicle (V01-V09)
             pedestrian on foot falling (slipping) on ice and snow (W00.-)

✓5ᵗʰ **V00.0 Pedestrian on foot injured in collision with pedestrian conveyance**

    ✓x 7ᵗʰ **V00.01 Pedestrian on foot injured in collision with roller-skater**

    ✓x 7ᵗʰ **V00.02 Pedestrian on foot injured in collision with skateboarder**

    ✓x 7ᵗʰ **V00.09 Pedestrian on foot injured in collision with other pedestrian conveyance**

✓5ᵗʰ **V00.1 Rolling-type pedestrian conveyance accident**
    EXCLUDES 1   *accident with babystroller (V00.82-)*
             accident with motorized mobility scooter (V00.83-)
             accident with wheelchair (powered) (V00.81-)

    ✓6ᵗʰ **V00.11 In-line roller-skate accident**

        ✓7ᵗʰ **V00.111 Fall from in-line roller-skates**

        ✓7ᵗʰ **V00.112 In-line roller-skater colliding with stationary object**

        ✓7ᵗʰ **V00.118 Other in-line roller-skate accident**
            EXCLUDES 1   *roller-skater collision with other land transport vehicle (V01-V09 with 5th character 1)*

    ✓6ᵗʰ **V00.12 Non-in- line roller-skate accident**

        ✓7ᵗʰ **V00.121 Fall from non-in-line roller-skates**

        ✓7ᵗʰ **V00.122 Non-in-line roller-skater colliding with stationary object**

        ✓7ᵗʰ **V00.128 Other non-in-line roller-skating accident**
            EXCLUDES 1   *roller-skater collision with other land transport vehicle (V01-V09 with 5th character 1)*

    ✓6ᵗʰ **V00.13 Skateboard accident**

        ✓7ᵗʰ **V00.131 Fall from skateboard**

        ✓7ᵗʰ **V00.132 Skateboarder colliding with stationary object**

        ✓7ᵗʰ **V00.138 Other skateboard accident**
            EXCLUDES 1   *skateboarder collision with other land transport vehicle (V01-V09 with 5th character 2)*

    ✓6ᵗʰ **V00.14 Scooter (nonmotorized) accident**
        EXCLUDES 1   *motorscooter accident (V20-V29)*

        ✓7ᵗʰ **V00.141 Fall from scooter (nonmotorized)**

        ✓7ᵗʰ **V00.142 Scooter (nonmotorized) colliding with stationary object**

        ✓7ᵗʰ **V00.148 Other scooter (nonmotorized) accident**
            EXCLUDES 1   *scooter (nonmotorized) collision with other land transport vehicle (V01-V09 with fifth character 9)*

    ✓6ᵗʰ **V00.15 Heelies accident**
        Rolling shoe
        Wheeled shoe
        Wheelies accident

        ✓7ᵗʰ **V00.151 Fall from heelies**

        ✓7ᵗʰ **V00.152 Heelies colliding with stationary object**

        ✓7ᵗʰ **V00.158 Other heelies accident**

    ✓6ᵗʰ **V00.18 Accident on other rolling-type pedestrian conveyance**

        ✓7ᵗʰ **V00.181 Fall from other rolling-type pedestrian conveyance**

        ✓7ᵗʰ **V00.182 Pedestrian on other rolling-type pedestrian conveyance colliding with stationary object**

        ✓7ᵗʰ **V00.188 Other accident on other rolling-type pedestrian conveyance**

✓5ᵗʰ **V00.2 Gliding-type pedestrian conveyance accident**

    ✓6ᵗʰ **V00.21 Ice-skates accident**

        ✓7ᵗʰ **V00.211 Fall from ice-skates**

        ✓7ᵗʰ **V00.212 Ice-skater colliding with stationary object**

        ✓7ᵗʰ **V00.218 Other ice-skates accident**
            EXCLUDES 1   *ice-skater collision with other land transport vehicle (V01-V09 with 5th digit 9)*

    ✓6ᵗʰ **V00.22 Sled accident**

        ✓7ᵗʰ **V00.221 Fall from sled**

        ✓7ᵗʰ **V00.222 Sledder colliding with stationary object**

        ✓7ᵗʰ **V00.228 Other sled accident**
            EXCLUDES 1   *sled collision with other land transport vehicle (V01-V09 with 5th digit 9)*

    ✓6ᵗʰ **V00.28 Other gliding-type pedestrian conveyance accident**

        ✓7ᵗʰ **V00.281 Fall from other gliding-type pedestrian conveyance**

        ✓7ᵗʰ **V00.282 Pedestrian on other gliding-type pedestrian conveyance colliding with stationary object**

        ✓7ᵗʰ **V00.288 Other accident on other gliding-type pedestrian conveyance**
            EXCLUDES 1   *gliding-type pedestrian conveyance collision with other land transport vehicle (V01-V09 with 5th digit 9)*

✓5ᵗʰ **V00.3 Flat-bottomed pedestrian conveyance accident**

    ✓6ᵗʰ **V00.31 Snowboard accident**

        ✓7ᵗʰ **V00.311 Fall from snowboard**

        ✓7ᵗʰ **V00.312 Snowboarder colliding with stationary object**

        ✓7ᵗʰ **V00.318 Other snowboard accident**
            EXCLUDES 1   *snowboarder collision with other land transport vehicle (V01-V09 with 5th digit 9)*

    ✓6ᵗʰ **V00.32 Snow-ski accident**

        ✓7ᵗʰ **V00.321 Fall from snow-skis**

        ✓7ᵗʰ **V00.322 Snow-skier colliding with stationary object**

EXCLUDES 1 Not coded here   EXCLUDES 2 Not included here   N Newborn Age: 0   P Pediatric Age: 0-17   M Maternity Age: 12-55   A Adult Age: 15-124

1116   ICD-10-CM 2018

    ✓7ᵗʰ **V00.328** **Other snow-ski accident**
       EXCLUDES 1   snow-skier collision with other
           land transport vehicle
           (V01-V09 with 5th digit 9)

✓6ᵗʰ **V00.38** **Other flat-bottomed pedestrian conveyance accident**

    ✓7ᵗʰ **V00.381** **Fall from other flat-bottomed pedestrian conveyance**

    ✓7ᵗʰ **V00.382** **Pedestrian on other flat-bottomed pedestrian conveyance** colliding with stationary object

    ✓7ᵗʰ **V00.388** **Other accident on other flat-bottomed pedestrian conveyance**

✓5ᵗʰ **V00.8** **Accident on other pedestrian conveyance**

   ✓6ᵗʰ **V00.81** **Accident with** wheelchair **(powered)**

    ✓7ᵗʰ **V00.811** **Fall from moving wheelchair (powered)**
       EXCLUDES 1   fall from non-moving wheelchair
           (W05.0)

    ✓7ᵗʰ **V00.812** **Wheelchair (powered)** colliding with stationary object

    ✓7ᵗʰ **V00.818** **Other accident with wheelchair (powered)**

   ✓6ᵗʰ **V00.82** **Accident with** babystroller

    ✓7ᵗʰ **V00.821** **Fall from babystroller**

    ✓7ᵗʰ **V00.822** **Babystroller** colliding with stationary object

    ✓7ᵗʰ **V00.828** **Other accident with babystroller**

   ✓6ᵗʰ **V00.83** **Accident with** motorized mobility scooter

     V00.831 **Fall from motorized mobility scooter**
       EXCLUDES 1   fall from non-moving motorized
           mobility scooter (W05.2)

     V00.832 **Motorized mobility scooter** colliding with stationary object

     V00.838 **Other accident with motorized mobility scooter**

   ✓6ᵗʰ **V00.89** **Accident on other pedestrian conveyance**

    ✓7ᵗʰ **V00.891** **Fall from** other pedestrian conveyance

    ✓7ᵗʰ **V00.892** **Pedestrian on other pedestrian conveyance** colliding with stationary object

    ✓7ᵗʰ **V00.898** **Other accident on other pedestrian conveyance**
       EXCLUDES 1   other pedestrian (conveyance)
           collision with other land
           transport vehicle (V01-V09
           with 5th digit 9)

✓4ᵗʰ **V01** **Pedestrian injured in collision with pedal cycle**

✓5ᵗʰ **V01.0** **Pedestrian injured in collision with pedal cycle** in nontraffic accident

   ✓x7ᵗʰ **V01.00** **Pedestrian on foot injured in collision with pedal cycle in nontraffic accident**
     Pedestrian NOS injured in collision with pedal cycle in nontraffic accident

   ✓x7ᵗʰ **V01.01** **Pedestrian on roller-skates injured in collision with pedal cycle in nontraffic accident**

   ✓x7ᵗʰ **V01.02** **Pedestrian on skateboard injured in collision with pedal cycle in nontraffic accident**

   ✓x7ᵗʰ **V01.09** **Pedestrian with other conveyance injured in collision with pedal cycle in nontraffic accident**
     Pedestrian with babystroller injured in collision with pedal cycle in nontraffic accident
     Pedestrian on ice-skates injured in collision with pedal cycle in nontraffic accident
     Pedestrian on nonmotorized scooter injured in collision with pedal cycle in nontraffic accident
     Pedestrian on sled injured in collision with pedal cycle in nontraffic accident
     Pedestrian on snowboard injured in collision with pedal cycle in nontraffic accident
     Pedestrian on snow-skis injured in collision with pedal cycle in nontraffic accident
     Pedestrian in wheelchair (powered) injured in collision with pedal cycle in nontraffic accident
     Pedestrian in motorized mobility scooter injured in collision with pedal cycle in nontraffic accident

✓5ᵗʰ **V01.1** **Pedestrian injured in collision with pedal cycle** in traffic accident

   ✓x7ᵗʰ **V01.10** **Pedestrian on foot injured in collision with pedal cycle in traffic accident**
     Pedestrian NOS injured in collision with pedal cycle in traffic accident

   ✓x7ᵗʰ **V01.11** **Pedestrian on roller-skates injured in collision with pedal cycle in traffic accident**

   ✓x7ᵗʰ **V01.12** **Pedestrian on skateboard injured in collision with pedal cycle in traffic accident**

   ✓x7ᵗʰ **V01.19** **Pedestrian with other conveyance injured in collision with pedal cycle in traffic accident**
     Pedestrian with babystroller injured in collision with pedal cycle in traffic accident
     Pedestrian on ice-skates injured in collision with pedal cycle in traffic accident
     Pedestrian on nonmotorized scooter injured in collision with pedal cycle in traffic accident
     Pedestrian on sled injured in collision with pedal cycle in traffic accident
     Pedestrian on snowboard injured in collision with pedal cycle in traffic accident
     Pedestrian on snow-skis injured in collision with pedal cycle in traffic accident
     Pedestrian in wheelchair (powered) injured in collision with pedal cycle in traffic accident
     Pedestrian in motorized mobility scooter injured in collision with pedal cycle in traffic accident

✓5ᵗʰ **V01.9** **Pedestrian injured in collision with pedal cycle, unspecified whether traffic or nontraffic accident**

   ✓x7ᵗʰ **V01.90** **Pedestrian on foot injured in collision with pedal cycle, unspecified whether traffic or nontraffic accident** ▽
     Pedestrian NOS injured in collision with pedal cycle, unspecified whether traffic or nontraffic accident

   ✓x7ᵗʰ **V01.91** **Pedestrian on roller-skates injured in collision with pedal cycle, unspecified whether traffic or nontraffic accident** ▽

   ✓x7ᵗʰ **V01.92** **Pedestrian on skateboard injured in collision with pedal cycle, unspecified whether traffic or nontraffic accident** ▽

   ✓x7ᵗʰ **V01.99** **Pedestrian with other conveyance injured in collision with pedal cycle, unspecified whether traffic or nontraffic accident** ▽
     Pedestrian with babystroller injured in collision with pedal cycle, unspecified whether traffic or nontraffic accident
     Pedestrian on ice-skates injured in collision with pedal cycle unspecified, whether traffic or nontraffic accident
     Pedestrian on nonmotorized scooter injured in collision with pedal cycle, unspecified whether traffic or nontraffic accident
     Pedestrian on sled injured in collision with pedal cycle unspecified, whether traffic or nontraffic accident
     Pedestrian on snowboard injured in collision with pedal cycle, unspecified whether traffic or nontraffic accident
     Pedestrian on snow-skis injured in collision with pedal cycle, unspecified whether traffic or nontraffic accident
     Pedestrian in wheelchair (powered) injured in collision with pedal cycle, unspecified whether traffic or nontraffic accident
     Pedestrian in motorized mobility scooter injured in collision with pedal cycle, unspecified whether traffic or nontraffic accident

✓4ᵗʰ **V02** **Pedestrian injured in collision with two- or three-wheeled motor vehicle**

✓5ᵗʰ **V02.0** **Pedestrian injured in collision with two- or three-wheeled motor vehicle** in nontraffic accident

   ✓x7ᵗʰ **V02.00** **Pedestrian on foot injured in collision with two- or three-wheeled motor vehicle in nontraffic accident**
     Pedestrian NOS injured in collision with two- or three-wheeled motor vehicle in nontraffic accident

   ✓x7ᵗʰ **V02.01** **Pedestrian on roller-skates injured in collision with two- or three-wheeled motor vehicle in nontraffic accident**

✓ Additional Character Req   ✓x7ᵗʰ Placeholder Alert   Manifestation   HCC CMS-HCC Condition   ▽ Unspecified Code   ►◄ Revised Text   ● New Code   ▲ Revised Code Title

√x 7th **V02.02** **Pedestrian** on skateboard **injured in collision with two- or three-wheeled motor vehicle in nontraffic accident**

√x 7th **V02.09** **Pedestrian** with other conveyance **injured in collision with two- or three-wheeled motor vehicle in nontraffic accident**
Pedestrian with babystroller injured in collision with two- or three-wheeled motor vehicle in nontraffic accident
Pedestrian on ice-skates injured in collision with two- or three-wheeled motor vehicle in nontraffic accident
Pedestrian on nonmotorized scooter injured in collision with two- or three-wheeled motor vehicle in nontraffic accident
Pedestrian on sled injured in collision with two- or three-wheeled motor vehicle in nontraffic accident
Pedestrian on snowboard injured in collision with two- or three-wheeled motor vehicle in nontraffic accident
Pedestrian on snow-skis injured in collision with two- or three-wheeled motor vehicle in nontraffic accident
Pedestrian in wheelchair (powered) injured in collision with two- or three-wheeled motor vehicle in nontraffic accident
Pedestrian in motorized mobility scooter injured in collision with two- or three-wheeled motor vehicle in nontraffic accident

√5th **V02.1** **Pedestrian injured in collision with two- or three-wheeled motor vehicle** in traffic accident

√x 7th **V02.10** **Pedestrian** on foot **injured in collision with two- or three-wheeled motor vehicle in traffic accident**
Pedestrian NOS injured in collision with two- or three-wheeled motor vehicle in traffic accident

√x 7th **V02.11** **Pedestrian** on roller-skates **injured in collision with two- or three-wheeled motor vehicle in traffic accident**

√x 7th **V02.12** **Pedestrian** on skateboard **injured in collision with two- or three-wheeled motor vehicle in traffic accident**

√x 7th **V02.19** **Pedestrian** with other conveyance **injured in collision with two- or three-wheeled motor vehicle in traffic accident**
Pedestrian with babystroller injured in collision with two- or three-wheeled motor vehicle in traffic accident
Pedestrian on ice-skates injured in collision with two- or three-wheeled motor vehicle in traffic accident
Pedestrian on nonmotorized scooter injured in collision with two- or three-wheeled motor vehicle in traffic accident
Pedestrian on sled injured in collision with two- or three-wheeled motor vehicle in traffic accident
Pedestrian on snowboard injured in collision with two- or three-wheeled motor vehicle in traffic accident
Pedestrian on snow-skis injured in collision with two- or three-wheeled motor vehicle in traffic accident
Pedestrian in wheelchair (powered) injured in collision with two- or three-wheeled motor vehicle in traffic accident
Pedestrian in motorized mobility scooter injured in collision with two- or three-wheeled motor vehicle in traffic accident

√5th **V02.9** **Pedestrian injured in collision with two- or three-wheeled motor vehicle, unspecified whether traffic or nontraffic accident**

√x 7th **V02.90** **Pedestrian** on foot **injured in collision with two- or three-wheeled motor vehicle, unspecified whether traffic or nontraffic accident** ▽
Pedestrian NOS injured in collision with two- or three-wheeled motor vehicle, unspecified whether traffic or nontraffic accident

√x 7th **V02.91** **Pedestrian** on roller-skates **injured in collision with two- or three-wheeled motor vehicle, unspecified whether traffic or nontraffic accident** ▽

√x 7th **V02.92** **Pedestrian** on skateboard **injured in collision with two- or three-wheeled motor vehicle, unspecified whether traffic or nontraffic accident** ▽

√x 7th **V02.99** **Pedestrian** with other conveyance **injured in collision with two- or three-wheeled motor vehicle, unspecified whether traffic or nontraffic accident** ▽
Pedestrian with babystroller injured in collision with two- or three-wheeled motor vehicle, unspecified whether traffic or nontraffic accident
Pedestrian on ice-skates injured in collision with two- or three-wheeled motor vehicle, unspecified whether traffic or nontraffic accident
Pedestrian on nonmotorized scooter injured in collision with two- or three-wheeled motor vehicle, unspecified whether traffic or nontraffic accident
Pedestrian on sled injured in collision with two- or three-wheeled motor vehicle, unspecified whether traffic or nontraffic accident
Pedestrian on snowboard injured in collision with two- or three-wheeled motor vehicle, unspecified whether traffic or nontraffic accident
Pedestrian on snow-skis injured in collision with two- or three-wheeled motor vehicle, unspecified whether traffic or nontraffic accident
Pedestrian in wheelchair (powered) injured in collision with two- or three-wheeled motor vehicle, unspecified whether traffic or nontraffic accident
Pedestrian in motorized mobility scooter injured in collision with two- or three-wheeled motor vehicle, unspecified whether traffic or nontraffic accident

√4th **V03** **Pedestrian injured in collision with car, pick-up truck or van**

√5th **V03.0** **Pedestrian injured in collision with car, pick-up truck or van** in nontraffic accident

√x 7th **V03.00** **Pedestrian** on foot **injured in collision with car, pick-up truck or van in nontraffic accident**
Pedestrian NOS injured in collision with car, pick-up truck or van in nontraffic accident

√x 7th **V03.01** **Pedestrian** on roller-skates **injured in collision with car, pick-up truck or van in nontraffic accident**

√x 7th **V03.02** **Pedestrian** on skateboard **injured in collision with car, pick-up truck or van in nontraffic accident**

√x 7th **V03.09** **Pedestrian** with other conveyance **injured in collision with car, pick-up truck or van in nontraffic accident**
Pedestrian with babystroller injured in collision with car, pick-up truck or van in nontraffic accident
Pedestrian on ice-skates injured in collision with car, pick-up truck or van in nontraffic accident
Pedestrian on nonmotorized scooter injured in collision with car, pick-up truck or van in nontraffic accident
Pedestrian on sled injured in collision with car, pick-up truck or van in nontraffic accident
Pedestrian on snowboard injured in collision with car, pick-up truck or van in nontraffic accident
Pedestrian on snow-skis injured in collision with car, pick-up truck or van in nontraffic accident
Pedestrian in wheelchair (powered) injured in collision with car, pick-up truck or van in nontraffic accident
Pedestrian in motorized mobility scooter injured in collision with car, pick-up truck or van in nontraffic accident

√5th **V03.1** **Pedestrian injured in collision with car, pick-up truck or van** in traffic accident

√x 7th **V03.10** **Pedestrian** on foot **injured in collision with car, pick-up truck or van in traffic accident**
Pedestrian NOS injured in collision with car, pick-up truck or van in traffic accident

√x 7th **V03.11** **Pedestrian** on roller-skates **injured in collision with car, pick-up truck or van in traffic accident**

√x 7th **V03.12** **Pedestrian** on skateboard **injured in collision with car, pick-up truck or van in traffic accident**

EXCLUDES 1 Not coded here   EXCLUDES 2 Not included here   N Newborn Age: 0   P Pediatric Age: 0-17   M Maternity Age: 12-55   A Adult Age: 15-124

1118   ICD-10-CM 2018

√x7th **V03.19** **Pedestrian with other conveyance injured in collision with car, pick-up truck or van in traffic accident**
> Pedestrian with babystroller injured in collision with car, pick-up truck or van in traffic accident
> Pedestrian on ice-skates injured in collision with car, pick-up truck or van in traffic accident
> Pedestrian on nonmotorized scooter injured in collision with car, pick-up truck or van in traffic accident
> Pedestrian on sled injured in collision with car, pick-up truck or van in traffic accident
> Pedestrian on snowboard injured in collision with car, pick-up truck or van in traffic accident
> Pedestrian on snow-skis injured in collision with car, pick-up truck or van in traffic accident
> Pedestrian in wheelchair (powered) injured in collision with car, pick-up truck or van in traffic accident
> Pedestrian in motorized mobility scooter injured in collision with car, pick-up truck or van in traffic accident

√5th **V03.9** **Pedestrian injured in collision with car, pick-up truck or van, unspecified whether traffic or nontraffic accident**

√x7th **V03.90** **Pedestrian on foot injured in collision with car, pick-up truck or van, unspecified whether traffic or nontraffic accident** ▽
> Pedestrian NOS injured in collision with car, pick-up truck or van, unspecified whether traffic or nontraffic accident

√x7th **V03.91** **Pedestrian on roller-skates injured in collision with car, pick-up truck or van, unspecified whether traffic or nontraffic accident** ▽

√x7th **V03.92** **Pedestrian on skateboard injured in collision with car, pick-up truck or van, unspecified whether traffic or nontraffic accident** ▽

√x7th **V03.99** **Pedestrian with other conveyance injured in collision with car, pick-up truck or van, unspecified whether traffic or nontraffic accident** ▽
> Pedestrian with babystroller injured in collision with car, pick-up truck or van, unspecified whether traffic or nontraffic accident
> Pedestrian on ice-skates injured in collision with car, pick-up truck or van, unspecified whether traffic or nontraffic accident
> Pedestrian on nonmotorized scooter injured in collision with car, pick-up truck or van, unspecified whether traffic or nontraffic accident
> Pedestrian on sled injured in collision with car, pick-up truck or van in nontraffic accident
> Pedestrian on snowboard injured in collision with car, pick-up truck or van, unspecified whether traffic or nontraffic accident
> Pedestrian on snow-skis injured in collision with car, pick-up truck or van, unspecified whether traffic or nontraffic accident
> Pedestrian in wheelchair (powered) injured in collision with car, pick-up truck or van, unspecified whether traffic or nontraffic accident
> Pedestrian in motorized mobility scooter injured in collision with car, pick-up truck or van, unspecified whether traffic or nontraffic accident

√4th **V04** **Pedestrian injured in collision with heavy transport vehicle or bus**
> *EXCLUDES 1*   pedestrian injured in collision with military vehicle (V09.01, V09.21)

√5th **V04.0** **Pedestrian injured in collision with heavy transport vehicle or bus in nontraffic accident**

√x7th **V04.00** **Pedestrian on foot injured in collision with heavy transport vehicle or bus in nontraffic accident**
> Pedestrian NOS injured in collision with heavy transport vehicle or bus in nontraffic accident

√x7th **V04.01** **Pedestrian on roller-skates injured in collision with heavy transport vehicle or bus in nontraffic accident**

√x7th **V04.02** **Pedestrian on skateboard injured in collision with heavy transport vehicle or bus in nontraffic accident**

√x7th **V04.09** **Pedestrian with other conveyance injured in collision with heavy transport vehicle or bus in nontraffic accident**
> Pedestrian with babystroller injured in collision with heavy transport vehicle or bus in nontraffic accident
> Pedestrian on ice-skates injured in collision with heavy transport vehicle or bus in nontraffic accident
> Pedestrian on nonmotorized scooter injured in collision with heavy transport vehicle or bus in nontraffic accident
> Pedestrian on sled injured in collision with heavy transport vehicle or bus in nontraffic accident
> Pedestrian on snowboard injured in collision with heavy transport vehicle or bus in nontraffic accident
> Pedestrian on snow-skis injured in collision with heavy transport vehicle or bus in nontraffic accident
> Pedestrian in wheelchair (powered) injured in collision with heavy transport vehicle or bus in nontraffic accident
> Pedestrian in motorized mobility scooter injured in collision with heavy transport vehicle or bus in nontraffic accident

√5th **V04.1** **Pedestrian injured in collision with heavy transport vehicle or bus in traffic accident**

√x7th **V04.10** **Pedestrian on foot injured in collision with heavy transport vehicle or bus in traffic accident**
> Pedestrian NOS injured in collision with heavy transport vehicle or bus in traffic accident

√x7th **V04.11** **Pedestrian on roller-skates injured in collision with heavy transport vehicle or bus in traffic accident**

√x7th **V04.12** **Pedestrian on skateboard injured in collision with heavy transport vehicle or bus in traffic accident**

√x7th **V04.19** **Pedestrian with other conveyance injured in collision with heavy transport vehicle or bus in traffic accident**
> Pedestrian with babystroller injured in collision with heavy transport vehicle or bus in traffic accident
> Pedestrian on ice-skates injured in collision with heavy transport vehicle or bus in traffic accident
> Pedestrian on nonmotorized scooter injured in collision with heavy transport vehicle or bus in traffic accident
> Pedestrian on sled injured in collision with heavy transport vehicle or bus in traffic accident
> Pedestrian on snowboard injured in collision with heavy transport vehicle or bus in traffic accident
> Pedestrian on snow-skis injured in collision with heavy transport vehicle or bus in traffic accident
> Pedestrian in wheelchair (powered) injured in collision with heavy transport vehicle or bus in traffic accident
> Pedestrian in motorized mobility scooter injured in collision with heavy transport vehicle or bus in traffic accident

√5th **V04.9** **Pedestrian injured in collision with heavy transport vehicle or bus, unspecified whether traffic or nontraffic accident**

√x7th **V04.90** **Pedestrian on foot injured in collision with heavy transport vehicle or bus, unspecified whether traffic or nontraffic accident** ▽
> Pedestrian NOS injured in collision with heavy transport vehicle or bus, unspecified whether traffic or nontraffic accident

√x7th **V04.91** **Pedestrian on roller-skates injured in collision with heavy transport vehicle or bus, unspecified whether traffic or nontraffic accident** ▽

√x7th **V04.92** **Pedestrian on skateboard injured in collision with heavy transport vehicle or bus, unspecified whether traffic or nontraffic accident** ▽

☑ Additional Character Req   √x7th Placeholder Alert   Manifestation   HCC CMS-HCC Condition   ▽ Unspecified Code   ►◄ Revised Text   ● New Code   ▲ Revised Code Title

√x7ᵗʰ V04.99 Pedestrian with other conveyance injured in collision with heavy transport vehicle or bus, unspecified whether traffic or nontraffic accident ▽

Pedestrian with babystroller injured in collision with heavy transport vehicle or bus, unspecified whether traffic or nontraffic accident

Pedestrian on ice-skates injured in collision with heavy transport vehicle or bus, unspecified whether traffic or nontraffic accident

Pedestrian on nonmotorized scooter injured in collision with heavy transport vehicle or bus, unspecified whether traffic or nontraffic accident

Pedestrian on sled injured in collision with heavy transport vehicle or bus, unspecified whether traffic or nontraffic accident

Pedestrian on snowboard injured in collision with heavy transport vehicle or bus, unspecified whether traffic or nontraffic accident

Pedestrian on snow-skis injured in collision with heavy transport vehicle or bus, unspecified whether traffic or nontraffic accident

Pedestrian in wheelchair (powered) injured in collision with heavy transport vehicle or bus, unspecified whether traffic or nontraffic accident

Pedestrian in motorized mobility scooter injured in collision with heavy transport vehicle or bus, unspecified whether traffic or nontraffic accident

√4ᵗʰ V05 Pedestrian injured in collision with railway train or railway vehicle

√5ᵗʰ V05.0 Pedestrian injured in collision with railway train or railway vehicle in nontraffic accident

√x7ᵗʰ V05.00 Pedestrian on foot injured in collision with railway train or railway vehicle in nontraffic accident

Pedestrian NOS injured in collision with railway train or railway vehicle in nontraffic accident

√x7ᵗʰ V05.01 Pedestrian on roller-skates injured in collision with railway train or railway vehicle in nontraffic accident

√x7ᵗʰ V05.02 Pedestrian on skateboard injured in collision with railway train or railway vehicle in nontraffic accident

√x7ᵗʰ V05.09 Pedestrian with other conveyance injured in collision with railway train or railway vehicle in nontraffic accident

Pedestrian with babystroller injured in collision with railway train or railway vehicle in nontraffic accident

Pedestrian on ice-skates injured in collision with railway train or railway vehicle in nontraffic accident

Pedestrian on nonmotorized scooter injured in collision with railway train or railway vehicle in nontraffic accident

Pedestrian on sled injured in collision with railway train or railway vehicle in nontraffic accident

Pedestrian on snowboard injured in collision with railway train or railway vehicle in nontraffic accident

Pedestrian on snow-skis injured in collision with railway train or railway vehicle in nontraffic accident

Pedestrian in wheelchair (powered) injured in collision with railway train or railway vehicle in nontraffic accident

Pedestrian in motorized mobility scooter injured in collision with railway train or railway vehicle in nontraffic accident

√5ᵗʰ V05.1 Pedestrian injured in collision with railway train or railway vehicle in traffic accident

√x7ᵗʰ V05.10 Pedestrian on foot injured in collision with railway train or railway vehicle in traffic accident

Pedestrian NOS injured in collision with railway train or railway vehicle in traffic accident

√x7ᵗʰ V05.11 Pedestrian on roller-skates injured in collision with railway train or railway vehicle in traffic accident

√x7ᵗʰ V05.12 Pedestrian on skateboard injured in collision with railway train or railway vehicle in traffic accident

√x7ᵗʰ V05.19 Pedestrian with other conveyance injured in collision with railway train or railway vehicle in traffic accident

Pedestrian with babystroller injured in collision with railway train or railway vehicle in traffic accident

Pedestrian on ice-skates injured in collision with railway train or railway vehicle in traffic accident

Pedestrian on nonmotorized scooter injured in collision with railway train or railway vehicle in traffic accident

Pedestrian on sled injured in collision with railway train or railway vehicle in traffic accident

Pedestrian on snowboard injured in collision with railway train or railway vehicle in traffic accident

Pedestrian on snow-skis injured in collision with railway train or railway vehicle in traffic accident

Pedestrian in wheelchair (powered) injured in collision with railway train or railway vehicle in traffic accident

Pedestrian in motorized mobility scooter injured in collision with railway train or railway vehicle in traffic accident

√5ᵗʰ V05.9 Pedestrian injured in collision with railway train or railway vehicle, unspecified whether traffic or nontraffic accident

√x7ᵗʰ V05.90 Pedestrian on foot injured in collision with railway train or railway vehicle, unspecified whether traffic or nontraffic accident ▽

Pedestrian NOS injured in collision with railway train or railway vehicle, unspecified whether traffic or nontraffic accident

√x7ᵗʰ V05.91 Pedestrian on roller-skates injured in collision with railway train or railway vehicle, unspecified whether traffic or nontraffic accident ▽

√x7ᵗʰ V05.92 Pedestrian on skateboard injured in collision with railway train or railway vehicle, unspecified whether traffic or nontraffic accident ▽

√x7ᵗʰ V05.99 Pedestrian with other conveyance injured in collision with railway train or railway vehicle, unspecified whether traffic or nontraffic accident ▽

Pedestrian with babystroller injured in collision with railway train or railway vehicle, unspecified whether traffic or nontraffic

Pedestrian on ice-skates injured in collision with railway train or railway vehicle, unspecified whether traffic or nontraffic

Pedestrian on nonmotorized scooter injured in collision with railway train or railway vehicle, unspecified whether traffic or nontraffic

Pedestrian on sled injured in collision with railway train or railway vehicle, unspecified whether traffic or nontraffic

Pedestrian on snowboard injured in collision with railway train or railway vehicle, unspecified whether traffic or nontraffic

Pedestrian on snow-skis injured in collision with railway train or railway vehicle, unspecified whether traffic or nontraffic

Pedestrian in wheelchair (powered) injured in collision with railway train or railway vehicle, unspecified whether traffic or nontraffic

Pedestrian in motorized mobility scooter injured in collision with railway train or railway vehicle, unspecified whether traffic or nontraffic

√4ᵗʰ V06 Pedestrian injured in collision with other nonmotor vehicle

INCLUDES collision with animal-drawn vehicle, animal being ridden, nonpowered streetcar

EXCLUDES 1 *pedestrian injured in collision with pedestrian conveyance (V00.0-)*

√5ᵗʰ V06.0 Pedestrian injured in collision with other nonmotor vehicle in nontraffic accident

√x7ᵗʰ V06.00 Pedestrian on foot injured in collision with other nonmotor vehicle in nontraffic accident

Pedestrian NOS injured in collision with other nonmotor vehicle in nontraffic accident

√x7ᵗʰ V06.01 Pedestrian on roller-skates injured in collision with other nonmotor vehicle in nontraffic accident

√x7ᵗʰ V06.02 Pedestrian on skateboard injured in collision with other nonmotor vehicle in nontraffic accident

---

EXCLUDES 1 Not coded here   **EXCLUDES 2** Not included here   **N** Newborn Age: 0   **P** Pediatric Age: 0-17   **M** Maternity Age: 12-55   **A** Adult Age: 15-124

☑x7ᵗʰ **V06.09** **Pedestrian with other conveyance injured in collision with other nonmotor vehicle in nontraffic accident**

Pedestrian with babystroller injured in collision with other nonmotor vehicle in nontraffic accident

Pedestrian on ice-skates injured in collision with other nonmotor vehicle in nontraffic accident

Pedestrian on nonmotorized scooter injured in collision with other nonmotor vehicle in nontraffic accident

Pedestrian on sled injured in collision with other nonmotor vehicle in nontraffic accident

Pedestrian on snowboard injured in collision with other nonmotor vehicle in nontraffic accident

Pedestrian on snow-skis injured in collision with other nonmotor vehicle in nontraffic accident

Pedestrian in wheelchair (powered) injured in collision with other nonmotor vehicle in nontraffic accident

Pedestrian in motorized mobility scooter injured in collision with other nonmotor vehicle in nontraffic accident

☑5ᵗʰ **V06.1** **Pedestrian injured in collision with other nonmotor vehicle in traffic accident**

☑x7ᵗʰ **V06.10** **Pedestrian on foot injured in collision with other nonmotor vehicle in traffic accident**

Pedestrian NOS injured in collision with other nonmotor vehicle in traffic accident

☑x7ᵗʰ **V06.11** **Pedestrian on roller-skates injured in collision with other nonmotor vehicle in traffic accident**

☑x7ᵗʰ **V06.12** **Pedestrian on skateboard injured in collision with other nonmotor vehicle in traffic accident**

☑x7ᵗʰ **V06.19** **Pedestrian with other conveyance injured in collision with other nonmotor vehicle in traffic accident**

Pedestrian with babystroller injured in collision with other nonmotor vehicle in nontraffic accident

Pedestrian on ice-skates injured in collision with other nonmotor vehicle in traffic accident

Pedestrian on nonmotorized scooter injured in collision with other nonmotor vehicle in traffic accident

Pedestrian on sled injured in collision with other nonmotor vehicle in traffic accident

Pedestrian on snowboard injured in collision with other nonmotor vehicle in traffic accident

Pedestrian on snow-skis injured in collision with other nonmotor vehicle in traffic accident

Pedestrian in wheelchair (powered) injured in collision with other nonmotor vehicle in traffic accident

Pedestrian in motorized mobility scooter injured in collision with other nonmotor vehicle in traffic accident

☑5ᵗʰ **V06.9** **Pedestrian injured in collision with other nonmotor vehicle, unspecified whether traffic or nontraffic accident**

☑x7ᵗʰ **V06.90** **Pedestrian on foot injured in collision with other nonmotor vehicle, unspecified whether traffic or nontraffic accident** ▽

Pedestrian NOS injured in collision with other nonmotor vehicle, unspecified whether traffic or nontraffic accident

☑x7ᵗʰ **V06.91** **Pedestrian on roller-skates injured in collision with other nonmotor vehicle, unspecified whether traffic or nontraffic accident** ▽

☑x7ᵗʰ **V06.92** **Pedestrian on skateboard injured in collision with other nonmotor vehicle, unspecified whether traffic or nontraffic accident** ▽

☑x7ᵗʰ **V06.99** **Pedestrian with other conveyance injured in collision with other nonmotor vehicle, unspecified whether traffic or nontraffic accident** ▽

Pedestrian with babystroller injured in collision with other nonmotor vehicle, unspecified whether traffic or nontraffic accident

Pedestrian on ice-skates injured in collision with other nonmotor vehicle, unspecified whether traffic or nontraffic accident

Pedestrian on nonmotorized scooter injured in collision with other nonmotor vehicle, unspecified whether traffic or nontraffic accident

Pedestrian on sled injured in collision with other nonmotor vehicle, unspecified whether traffic or nontraffic accident

Pedestrian on snowboard injured in collision with other nonmotor vehicle, unspecified whether traffic or nontraffic accident

Pedestrian on snow-skis injured in collision with other nonmotor vehicle, unspecified whether traffic or nontraffic accident

Pedestrian in wheelchair (powered) injured in collision with other nonmotor vehicle, unspecified whether traffic or nontraffic accident

Pedestrian in motorized mobility scooter injured in collision with other nonmotor vehicle, unspecified whether traffic or nontraffic accident

☑4ᵗʰ **V09** **Pedestrian injured in other and unspecified transport accidents**

☑5ᵗʰ **V09.0** **Pedestrian injured in nontraffic accident involving other and unspecified motor vehicles**

☑x7ᵗʰ **V09.00** **Pedestrian injured in nontraffic accident involving unspecified motor vehicles** ▽

☑x7ᵗʰ **V09.01** **Pedestrian injured in nontraffic accident involving military vehicle**

☑x7ᵗʰ **V09.09** **Pedestrian injured in nontraffic accident involving other motor vehicles**

Pedestrian injured in nontraffic accident by special vehicle

☑x7ᵗʰ **V09.1** **Pedestrian injured in unspecified nontraffic accident** ▽

☑5ᵗʰ **V09.2** **Pedestrian injured in traffic accident involving other and unspecified motor vehicles**

☑x7ᵗʰ **V09.20** **Pedestrian injured in traffic accident involving unspecified motor vehicles** ▽

☑x7ᵗʰ **V09.21** **Pedestrian injured in traffic accident involving military vehicle**

☑x7ᵗʰ **V09.29** **Pedestrian injured in traffic accident involving other motor vehicles**

☑x7ᵗʰ **V09.3** **Pedestrian injured in unspecified traffic accident** ▽

☑x7ᵗʰ **V09.9** **Pedestrian injured in unspecified transport accident** ▽

Pedal cycle rider injured in transport accident (V10-V19)

INCLUDES   any non-motorized vehicle, excluding an animal-drawn vehicle, or a sidecar or trailer attached to the pedal cycle

EXCLUDES 2   rupture of pedal cycle tire (W37.0)

The appropriate 7th character is to be added to each code from categories V10-V19.
A   initial encounter
D   subsequent encounter
S   sequela

☑4ᵗʰ **V10** **Pedal cycle rider injured in collision with pedestrian or animal**

EXCLUDES 1   pedal cycle rider collision with animal-drawn vehicle or animal being ridden (V16.-)

☑x7ᵗʰ **V10.0** **Pedal cycle driver injured in collision with pedestrian or animal in nontraffic accident**

☑x7ᵗʰ **V10.1** **Pedal cycle passenger injured in collision with pedestrian or animal in nontraffic accident**

☑x7ᵗʰ **V10.2** **Unspecified pedal cyclist injured in collision with pedestrian or animal in nontraffic accident** ▽

☑x7ᵗʰ **V10.3** **Person boarding or alighting a pedal cycle injured in collision with pedestrian or animal**

☑x7ᵗʰ **V10.4** **Pedal cycle driver injured in collision with pedestrian or animal in traffic accident**

☑x7ᵗʰ **V10.5** **Pedal cycle passenger injured in collision with pedestrian or animal in traffic accident**

☑x7ᵗʰ **V10.9** **Unspecified pedal cyclist injured in collision with pedestrian or animal in traffic accident** ▽

☑ Additional Character Req   x7ᵗʰ Placeholder Alert   Manifestation   HCC CMS-HCC Condition   ▽ Unspecified Code   ▶◀ Revised Text   ● New Code   ▲ Revised Code Title

ICD-10-CM 2018   1121

✓4ᵗʰ **V11 Pedal cycle rider injured in collision with other pedal cycle**

✓x7ᵗʰ **V11.0** Pedal cycle driver injured in collision with other pedal cycle in nontraffic accident

✓x7ᵗʰ **V11.1** Pedal cycle passenger injured in collision with other pedal cycle in nontraffic accident

✓x7ᵗʰ **V11.2** Unspecified pedal cyclist injured in collision with other ▽ pedal cycle in nontraffic accident

✓x7ᵗʰ **V11.3** Person boarding or alighting a pedal cycle injured in collision with other pedal cycle

✓x7ᵗʰ **V11.4** Pedal cycle driver injured in collision with other pedal cycle in traffic accident

✓x7ᵗʰ **V11.5** Pedal cycle passenger injured in collision with other pedal cycle in traffic accident

✓x7ᵗʰ **V11.9** Unspecified pedal cyclist injured in collision with other ▽ pedal cycle in traffic accident

✓4ᵗʰ **V12 Pedal cycle rider injured in collision with two- or three-wheeled motor vehicle**

✓x7ᵗʰ **V12.0** Pedal cycle driver injured in collision with two- or three-wheeled motor vehicle in nontraffic accident

✓x7ᵗʰ **V12.1** Pedal cycle passenger injured in collision with two- or three-wheeled motor vehicle in nontraffic accident

✓x7ᵗʰ **V12.2** Unspecified pedal cyclist injured in collision with two- ▽ or three-wheeled motor vehicle in nontraffic accident

✓x7ᵗʰ **V12.3** Person boarding or alighting a pedal cycle injured in collision with two- or three-wheeled motor vehicle

✓x7ᵗʰ **V12.4** Pedal cycle driver injured in collision with two- or three-wheeled motor vehicle in traffic accident

✓x7ᵗʰ **V12.5** Pedal cycle passenger injured in collision with two- or three-wheeled motor vehicle in traffic accident

✓x7ᵗʰ **V12.9** Unspecified pedal cyclist injured in collision with two- ▽ or three-wheeled motor vehicle in traffic accident

✓4ᵗʰ **V13 Pedal cycle rider injured in collision with car, pick-up truck or van**

✓x7ᵗʰ **V13.0** Pedal cycle driver injured in collision with car, pick-up truck or van in nontraffic accident

✓x7ᵗʰ **V13.1** Pedal cycle passenger injured in collision with car, pick-up truck or van in nontraffic accident

✓x7ᵗʰ **V13.2** Unspecified pedal cyclist injured in collision with car, ▽ pick-up truck or van in nontraffic accident

✓x7ᵗʰ **V13.3** Person boarding or alighting a pedal cycle injured in collision with car, pick-up truck or van

✓x7ᵗʰ **V13.4** Pedal cycle driver injured in collision with car, pick-up truck or van in traffic accident

✓x7ᵗʰ **V13.5** Pedal cycle passenger injured in collision with car, pick-up truck or van in traffic accident

✓x7ᵗʰ **V13.9** Unspecified pedal cyclist injured in collision with car, ▽ pick-up truck or van in traffic accident

✓4ᵗʰ **V14 Pedal cycle rider injured in collision with heavy transport vehicle or bus**

EXCLUDES 1 *pedal cycle rider injured in collision with military vehicle (V19.81)*

✓x7ᵗʰ **V14.0** Pedal cycle driver injured in collision with heavy transport vehicle or bus in nontraffic accident

✓x7ᵗʰ **V14.1** Pedal cycle passenger injured in collision with heavy transport vehicle or bus in nontraffic accident

✓x7ᵗʰ **V14.2** Unspecified pedal cyclist injured in collision with heavy ▽ transport vehicle or bus in nontraffic accident

✓x7ᵗʰ **V14.3** Person boarding or alighting a pedal cycle injured in collision with heavy transport vehicle or bus

✓x7ᵗʰ **V14.4** Pedal cycle driver injured in collision with heavy transport vehicle or bus in traffic accident

✓x7ᵗʰ **V14.5** Pedal cycle passenger injured in collision with heavy transport vehicle or bus in traffic accident

✓x7ᵗʰ **V14.9** Unspecified pedal cyclist injured in collision with heavy ▽ transport vehicle or bus in traffic accident

✓4ᵗʰ **V15 Pedal cycle rider injured in collision with railway train or railway vehicle**

✓x7ᵗʰ **V15.0** Pedal cycle driver injured in collision with railway train or railway vehicle in nontraffic accident

✓x7ᵗʰ **V15.1** Pedal cycle passenger injured in collision with railway train or railway vehicle in nontraffic accident

✓x7ᵗʰ **V15.2** Unspecified pedal cyclist injured in collision with railway ▽ train or railway vehicle in nontraffic accident

✓x7ᵗʰ **V15.3** Person boarding or alighting a pedal cycle injured in collision with railway train or railway vehicle

✓x7ᵗʰ **V15.4** Pedal cycle driver injured in collision with railway train or railway vehicle in traffic accident

✓x7ᵗʰ **V15.5** Pedal cycle passenger injured in collision with railway train or railway vehicle in traffic accident

✓x7ᵗʰ **V15.9** Unspecified pedal cyclist injured in collision with railway ▽ train or railway vehicle in traffic accident

✓4ᵗʰ **V16 Pedal cycle rider injured in collision with other nonmotor vehicle**

INCLUDES collision with animal-drawn vehicle, animal being ridden, streetcar

✓x7ᵗʰ **V16.0** Pedal cycle driver injured in collision with other nonmotor vehicle in nontraffic accident

✓x7ᵗʰ **V16.1** Pedal cycle passenger injured in collision with other nonmotor vehicle in nontraffic accident

✓x7ᵗʰ **V16.2** Unspecified pedal cyclist injured in collision with other ▽ nonmotor vehicle in nontraffic accident

✓x7ᵗʰ **V16.3** Person boarding or alighting a pedal cycle injured in collision with other nonmotor vehicle in nontraffic accident

✓x7ᵗʰ **V16.4** Pedal cycle driver injured in collision with other nonmotor vehicle in traffic accident

✓x7ᵗʰ **V16.5** Pedal cycle passenger injured in collision with other nonmotor vehicle in traffic accident

✓x7ᵗʰ **V16.9** Unspecified pedal cyclist injured in collision with other ▽ nonmotor vehicle in traffic accident

✓4ᵗʰ **V17 Pedal cycle rider injured in collision with fixed or stationary object**

✓x7ᵗʰ **V17.0** Pedal cycle driver injured in collision with fixed or stationary object in nontraffic accident

✓x7ᵗʰ **V17.1** Pedal cycle passenger injured in collision with fixed or stationary object in nontraffic accident

✓x7ᵗʰ **V17.2** Unspecified pedal cyclist injured in collision with fixed ▽ or stationary object in nontraffic accident

✓x7ᵗʰ **V17.3** Person boarding or alighting a pedal cycle injured in collision with fixed or stationary object

✓x7ᵗʰ **V17.4** Pedal cycle driver injured in collision with fixed or stationary object in traffic accident

✓x7ᵗʰ **V17.5** Pedal cycle passenger injured in collision with fixed or stationary object in traffic accident

✓x7ᵗʰ **V17.9** Unspecified pedal cyclist injured in collision with fixed ▽ or stationary object in traffic accident

✓4ᵗʰ **V18 Pedal cycle rider injured in noncollision transport accident**

INCLUDES fall or thrown from pedal cycle (without antecedent collision)
overturning pedal cycle NOS
overturning pedal cycle without collision

✓x7ᵗʰ **V18.0** Pedal cycle driver injured in noncollision transport accident in nontraffic accident

✓x7ᵗʰ **V18.1** Pedal cycle passenger injured in noncollision transport accident in nontraffic accident

✓x7ᵗʰ **V18.2** Unspecified pedal cyclist injured in noncollision ▽ transport accident in nontraffic accident

✓x7ᵗʰ **V18.3** Person boarding or alighting a pedal cycle injured in noncollision transport accident

✓x7ᵗʰ **V18.4** Pedal cycle driver injured in noncollision transport accident in traffic accident

✓x7ᵗʰ **V18.5** Pedal cycle passenger injured in noncollision transport accident in traffic accident

✓x7ᵗʰ **V18.9** Unspecified pedal cyclist injured in noncollision ▽ transport accident in traffic accident

✓4ᵗʰ **V19 Pedal cycle rider injured in other and unspecified transport accidents**

✓5ᵗʰ **V19.0** Pedal cycle driver injured in collision with other and unspecified motor vehicles in nontraffic accident

✓x7ᵗʰ **V19.00** Pedal cycle driver injured in collision with ▽ unspecified motor vehicles in nontraffic accident

✓x7ᵗʰ **V19.09** Pedal cycle driver injured in collision with other motor vehicles in nontraffic accident

✓5ᵗʰ **V19.1** Pedal cycle passenger injured in collision with other and unspecified motor vehicles in nontraffic accident

✓x7ᵗʰ **V19.10** Pedal cycle passenger injured in collision with ▽ unspecified motor vehicles in nontraffic accident

✓x7ᵗʰ **V19.19** Pedal cycle passenger injured in collision with other motor vehicles in nontraffic accident

---

EXCLUDES 1 Not coded here   **EXCLUDES 2** Not included here   N Newborn Age: 0   P Pediatric Age: 0-17   M Maternity Age: 12-55   A Adult Age: 15-124

✓5ᵗʰ **V19.2** **Unspecified pedal cyclist injured in collision with other and unspecified motor vehicles** in nontraffic accident

     ✓x7ᵗʰ **V19.20** **Unspecified pedal cyclist injured in collision with unspecified motor vehicles in nontraffic accident** ▽
         Pedal cycle collision NOS, nontraffic

     ✓x7ᵗʰ **V19.29** **Unspecified pedal cyclist injured in collision with other motor vehicles in nontraffic accident** ▽

✓5ᵗʰ **V19.3** **Pedal cyclist (driver) (passenger) injured in unspecified nontraffic accident** ▽
     Pedal cycle accident NOS, nontraffic
     Pedal cyclist injured in nontraffic accident NOS

✓5ᵗʰ **V19.4** **Pedal cycle** driver **injured in collision with other and unspecified motor vehicles** in traffic accident

     ✓x7ᵗʰ **V19.40** **Pedal cycle driver injured in collision with unspecified motor vehicles in traffic accident** ▽

     ✓x7ᵗʰ **V19.49** **Pedal cycle driver injured in collision with other motor vehicles in traffic accident**

✓5ᵗʰ **V19.5** **Pedal cycle** passenger **injured in collision with other and unspecified motor vehicles** in traffic accident

     ✓x7ᵗʰ **V19.50** **Pedal cycle passenger injured in collision with unspecified motor vehicles in traffic accident** ▽

     ✓x7ᵗʰ **V19.59** **Pedal cycle passenger injured in collision with other motor vehicles in traffic accident**

✓5ᵗʰ **V19.6** **Unspecified pedal cyclist injured in collision with other and unspecified motor vehicles** in traffic accident

     ✓x7ᵗʰ **V19.60** **Unspecified pedal cyclist injured in collision with** ▽ **unspecified motor vehicles in traffic accident**
         Pedal cycle collision NOS (traffic)

     ✓x7ᵗʰ **V19.69** **Unspecified pedal cyclist injured in collision** ▽ **with other motor vehicles in traffic accident**

✓5ᵗʰ **V19.8** **Pedal cyclist (driver) (passenger) injured in other specified transport accidents**

     ✓x7ᵗʰ **V19.81** **Pedal cyclist (driver) (passenger) injured in transport accident with** military vehicle

     ✓x7ᵗʰ **V19.88** **Pedal cyclist (driver) (passenger) injured in other specified transport accidents**

✓x7ᵗʰ **V19.9** **Pedal cyclist (driver) (passenger) injured in unspecified** ▽ **traffic accident**
     Pedal cycle accident NOS

Motorcycle rider injured in transport accident (V20-V29)

INCLUDES   moped
            motorcycle with sidecar
            motorized bicycle
            motor scooter
EXCLUDES 1   three-wheeled motor vehicle (V30-V39)

> The appropriate 7th character is to be added to each code from categories V20-V29.
> A   initial encounter
> D   subsequent encounter
> S   sequela

✓4ᵗʰ **V20** **Motorcycle rider injured in collision with pedestrian or animal**
     EXCLUDES 1   motorcycle rider collision with animal-drawn vehicle or animal being ridden (V26.-)

   ✓x7ᵗʰ **V20.0** **Motorcycle** driver **injured in collision with pedestrian or animal** in nontraffic accident

   ✓x7ᵗʰ **V20.1** **Motorcycle** passenger **injured in collision with pedestrian or animal** in nontraffic accident

   ✓x7ᵗʰ **V20.2** **Unspecified motorcycle rider injured in collision with** ▽ **pedestrian or animal** in nontraffic accident

   ✓x7ᵗʰ **V20.3** Person boarding or alighting **a motorcycle injured in collision with pedestrian or animal**

   ✓x7ᵗʰ **V20.4** **Motorcycle** driver **injured in collision with pedestrian or animal** in traffic accident

   ✓x7ᵗʰ **V20.5** **Motorcycle** passenger **injured in collision with pedestrian or animal** in traffic accident

   ✓x7ᵗʰ **V20.9** **Unspecified motorcycle rider injured in collision with** ▽ **pedestrian or animal** in traffic accident

✓4ᵗʰ **V21** **Motorcycle rider injured in collision with pedal cycle**

   ✓x7ᵗʰ **V21.0** **Motorcycle** driver **injured in collision with pedal cycle** in nontraffic accident

   ✓x7ᵗʰ **V21.1** **Motorcycle** passenger **injured in collision with pedal cycle** in nontraffic accident

   ✓x7ᵗʰ **V21.2** **Unspecified motorcycle rider injured in collision with** ▽ **pedal cycle** in nontraffic accident

   ✓x7ᵗʰ **V21.3** Person boarding or alighting **a motorcycle injured in collision with pedal cycle**

   ✓x7ᵗʰ **V21.4** **Motorcycle** driver **injured in collision with pedal cycle** in traffic accident

   ✓x7ᵗʰ **V21.5** **Motorcycle** passenger **injured in collision with pedal cycle** in traffic accident

   ✓x7ᵗʰ **V21.9** **Unspecified motorcycle rider injured in collision with** ▽ **pedal cycle** in traffic accident

✓4ᵗʰ **V22** **Motorcycle rider injured in collision with two- or three-wheeled motor vehicle**

   ✓x7ᵗʰ **V22.0** **Motorcycle** driver **injured in collision with two- or three-wheeled motor vehicle** in nontraffic accident

   ✓x7ᵗʰ **V22.1** **Motorcycle** passenger **injured in collision with two- or three-wheeled motor vehicle** in nontraffic accident

   ✓x7ᵗʰ **V22.2** **Unspecified motorcycle rider injured in collision with two-** ▽ **or three-wheeled motor vehicle** in nontraffic accident

   ✓x7ᵗʰ **V22.3** Person boarding or alighting **a motorcycle injured in collision with two- or three-wheeled motor vehicle**

   ✓x7ᵗʰ **V22.4** **Motorcycle** driver **injured in collision with two- or three-wheeled motor vehicle** in traffic accident

   ✓x7ᵗʰ **V22.5** **Motorcycle** passenger **injured in collision with two- or three-wheeled motor vehicle** in traffic accident

   ✓x7ᵗʰ **V22.9** **Unspecified motorcycle rider injured in collision with two-** ▽ **or three-wheeled motor vehicle** in traffic accident

✓4ᵗʰ **V23** **Motorcycle rider injured in collision with car, pick-up truck or van**

   ✓x7ᵗʰ **V23.0** **Motorcycle** driver **injured in collision with car, pick-up truck or van** in nontraffic accident

   ✓x7ᵗʰ **V23.1** **Motorcycle** passenger **injured in collision with car, pick-up truck or van** in nontraffic accident

   ✓x7ᵗʰ **V23.2** **Unspecified motorcycle rider injured in collision with car,** ▽ **pick-up truck or van** in nontraffic accident

   ✓x7ᵗʰ **V23.3** Person boarding or alighting **a motorcycle injured in collision with car, pick-up truck or van**

   ✓x7ᵗʰ **V23.4** **Motorcycle** driver **injured in collision with car, pick-up truck or van** in traffic accident

   ✓x7ᵗʰ **V23.5** **Motorcycle** passenger **injured in collision with car, pick-up truck or van** in traffic accident

   ✓x7ᵗʰ **V23.9** **Unspecified motorcycle rider injured in collision with car,** ▽ **pick-up truck or van** in traffic accident

✓4ᵗʰ **V24** **Motorcycle rider injured in collision with heavy transport vehicle or bus**
     EXCLUDES 1   motorcycle rider injured in collision with military vehicle (V29.81)

   ✓x7ᵗʰ **V24.0** **Motorcycle** driver **injured in collision with heavy transport vehicle or bus** in nontraffic accident

   ✓x7ᵗʰ **V24.1** **Motorcycle** passenger **injured in collision with heavy transport vehicle or bus** in nontraffic accident

   ✓x7ᵗʰ **V24.2** **Unspecified motorcycle rider injured in collision with** ▽ **heavy transport vehicle or bus** in nontraffic accident

   ✓x7ᵗʰ **V24.3** Person boarding or alighting **a motorcycle injured in collision with heavy transport vehicle or bus**

   ✓x7ᵗʰ **V24.4** **Motorcycle** driver **injured in collision with heavy transport vehicle or bus** in traffic accident

   ✓x7ᵗʰ **V24.5** **Motorcycle** passenger **injured in collision with heavy transport vehicle or bus** in traffic accident

   ✓x7ᵗʰ **V24.9** **Unspecified motorcycle rider injured in collision with** ▽ **heavy transport vehicle or bus** in traffic accident

✓4ᵗʰ **V25** **Motorcycle rider injured in collision with railway train or railway vehicle**

   ✓x7ᵗʰ **V25.0** **Motorcycle** driver **injured in collision with railway train or railway vehicle** in nontraffic accident

   ✓x7ᵗʰ **V25.1** **Motorcycle** passenger **injured in collision with railway train or railway vehicle** in nontraffic accident

   ✓x7ᵗʰ **V25.2** **Unspecified motorcycle rider injured in collision with** ▽ **railway train or railway vehicle** in nontraffic accident

   ✓x7ᵗʰ **V25.3** Person boarding or alighting **a motorcycle injured in collision with railway train or railway vehicle**

   ✓x7ᵗʰ **V25.4** **Motorcycle** driver **injured in collision with railway train or railway vehicle** in traffic accident

   ✓x7ᵗʰ **V25.5** **Motorcycle** passenger **injured in collision with railway train or railway vehicle** in traffic accident

---

✓ Additional Character Req   ✓x7ᵗʰ Placeholder Alert   Manifestation   HCC CMS-HCC Condition   ▽ Unspecified Code   ►◄ Revised Text   ● New Code   ▲ Revised Code Title

Chapter 20. External Causes of Morbidity (side)

√x7ᵗʰ **V25.9** Unspecified motorcycle rider injured in collision with railway train or railway vehicle in traffic accident ▽

√4ᵗʰ **V26 Motorcycle rider injured in collision with other nonmotor vehicle**
INCLUDES collision with animal-drawn vehicle, animal being ridden, streetcar

√x7ᵗʰ **V26.0** Motorcycle driver injured in collision with other nonmotor vehicle in nontraffic accident

√x7ᵗʰ **V26.1** Motorcycle passenger injured in collision with other nonmotor vehicle in nontraffic accident

√x7ᵗʰ **V26.2** Unspecified motorcycle rider injured in collision with other nonmotor vehicle in nontraffic accident ▽

√x7ᵗʰ **V26.3** Person boarding or alighting a motorcycle injured in collision with other nonmotor vehicle

√x7ᵗʰ **V26.4** Motorcycle driver injured in collision with other nonmotor vehicle in traffic accident

√x7ᵗʰ **V26.5** Motorcycle passenger injured in collision with other nonmotor vehicle in traffic accident

√x7ᵗʰ **V26.9** Unspecified motorcycle rider injured in collision with other nonmotor vehicle in traffic accident ▽

√4ᵗʰ **V27 Motorcycle rider injured in collision with fixed or stationary object**

√x7ᵗʰ **V27.0** Motorcycle driver injured in collision with fixed or stationary object in nontraffic accident

√x7ᵗʰ **V27.1** Motorcycle passenger injured in collision with fixed or stationary object in nontraffic accident

√x7ᵗʰ **V27.2** Unspecified motorcycle rider injured in collision with fixed or stationary object in nontraffic accident ▽

√x7ᵗʰ **V27.3** Person boarding or alighting a motorcycle injured in collision with fixed or stationary object

√x7ᵗʰ **V27.4** Motorcycle driver injured in collision with fixed or stationary object in traffic accident

√x7ᵗʰ **V27.5** Motorcycle passenger injured in collision with fixed or stationary object in traffic accident

√x7ᵗʰ **V27.9** Unspecified motorcycle rider injured in collision with fixed or stationary object in traffic accident ▽

√4ᵗʰ **V28 Motorcycle rider injured in noncollision transport accident**
INCLUDES fall or thrown from motorcycle (without antecedent collision)
overturning motorcycle NOS
overturning motorcycle without collision

√x7ᵗʰ **V28.0** Motorcycle driver injured in noncollision transport accident in nontraffic accident

√x7ᵗʰ **V28.1** Motorcycle passenger injured in noncollision transport accident in nontraffic accident

√x7ᵗʰ **V28.2** Unspecified motorcycle rider injured in noncollision transport accident in nontraffic accident ▽

√x7ᵗʰ **V28.3** Person boarding or alighting a motorcycle injured in noncollision transport accident

√x7ᵗʰ **V28.4** Motorcycle driver injured in noncollision transport accident in traffic accident

√x7ᵗʰ **V28.5** Motorcycle passenger injured in noncollision transport accident in traffic accident

√x7ᵗʰ **V28.9** Unspecified motorcycle rider injured in noncollision transport accident in traffic accident ▽

√4ᵗʰ **V29 Motorcycle rider injured in other and unspecified transport accidents**

√5ᵗʰ **V29.0** Motorcycle driver injured in collision with other and unspecified motor vehicles in nontraffic accident

√x7ᵗʰ **V29.00** Motorcycle driver injured in collision with unspecified motor vehicles in nontraffic accident ▽

√x7ᵗʰ **V29.09** Motorcycle driver injured in collision with other motor vehicles in nontraffic accident

√5ᵗʰ **V29.1** Motorcycle passenger injured in collision with other and unspecified motor vehicles in nontraffic accident

√x7ᵗʰ **V29.10** Motorcycle passenger injured in collision with unspecified motor vehicles in nontraffic accident ▽

√x7ᵗʰ **V29.19** Motorcycle passenger injured in collision with other motor vehicles in nontraffic accident

√5ᵗʰ **V29.2** Unspecified motorcycle rider injured in collision with other and unspecified motor vehicles in nontraffic accident

√x7ᵗʰ **V29.20** Unspecified motorcycle rider injured in collision with unspecified motor vehicles in nontraffic accident ▽
Motorcycle collision NOS, nontraffic

√x7ᵗʰ **V29.29** Unspecified motorcycle rider injured in collision with other motor vehicles in nontraffic accident ▽

√x7ᵗʰ **V29.3** Motorcycle rider (driver) (passenger) injured in unspecified nontraffic accident ▽
Motorcycle accident NOS, nontraffic
Motorcycle rider injured in nontraffic accident NOS

√5ᵗʰ **V29.4** Motorcycle driver injured in collision with other and unspecified motor vehicles in traffic accident

√x7ᵗʰ **V29.40** Motorcycle driver injured in collision with unspecified motor vehicles in traffic accident ▽

√x7ᵗʰ **V29.49** Motorcycle driver injured in collision with other motor vehicles in traffic accident

√5ᵗʰ **V29.5** Motorcycle passenger injured in collision with other and unspecified motor vehicles in traffic accident

√x7ᵗʰ **V29.50** Motorcycle passenger injured in collision with unspecified motor vehicles in traffic accident ▽

√x7ᵗʰ **V29.59** Motorcycle passenger injured in collision with other motor vehicles in traffic accident

√5ᵗʰ **V29.6** Unspecified motorcycle rider injured in collision with other and unspecified motor vehicles in traffic accident

√x7ᵗʰ **V29.60** Unspecified motorcycle rider injured in collision with unspecified motor vehicles in traffic accident ▽
Motorcycle collision NOS (traffic)

√x7ᵗʰ **V29.69** Unspecified motorcycle rider injured in collision with other motor vehicles in traffic accident ▽

√5ᵗʰ **V29.8** Motorcycle rider (driver) (passenger) injured in other specified transport accidents

√x7ᵗʰ **V29.81** Motorcycle rider (driver) (passenger) injured in transport accident with military vehicle

√x7ᵗʰ **V29.88** Motorcycle rider (driver) (passenger) injured in other specified transport accidents

√x7ᵗʰ **V29.9** Motorcycle rider (driver) (passenger) injured in unspecified traffic accident ▽
Motorcycle accident NOS

Occupant of three-wheeled motor vehicle injured in transport accident (V30-V39)

INCLUDES motorized rickshaw
motorized tricycle
three-wheeled motor car
EXCLUDES 1 all-terrain vehicles (V86.-)
motorcycle with sidecar (V20-V29)
vehicle designed primarily for off-road use (V86.-)

The appropriate 7th character is to be added to each code from categories V30-V39.
A   initial encounter
D   subsequent encounter
S   sequela

√4ᵗʰ **V30 Occupant of three-wheeled motor vehicle injured in collision with pedestrian or animal**
EXCLUDES 1 three-wheeled motor vehicle collision with animal-drawn vehicle or animal being ridden (V36.-)

√x7ᵗʰ **V30.0** Driver of three-wheeled motor vehicle injured in collision with pedestrian or animal in nontraffic accident

√x7ᵗʰ **V30.1** Passenger in three-wheeled motor vehicle injured in collision with pedestrian or animal in nontraffic accident

√x7ᵗʰ **V30.2** Person on outside of three-wheeled motor vehicle injured in collision with pedestrian or animal in nontraffic accident

√x7ᵗʰ **V30.3** Unspecified occupant of three-wheeled motor vehicle injured in collision with pedestrian or animal in nontraffic accident ▽

√x7ᵗʰ **V30.4** Person boarding or alighting a three-wheeled motor vehicle injured in collision with pedestrian or animal

√x7ᵗʰ **V30.5** Driver of three-wheeled motor vehicle injured in collision with pedestrian or animal in traffic accident

√x7ᵗʰ **V30.6** Passenger in three-wheeled motor vehicle injured in collision with pedestrian or animal in traffic accident

√x7ᵗʰ **V30.7** Person on outside of three-wheeled motor vehicle injured in collision with pedestrian or animal in traffic accident

√x7ᵗʰ **V30.9** Unspecified occupant of three-wheeled motor vehicle injured in collision with pedestrian or animal in traffic accident ▽

EXCLUDES 1 Not coded here   EXCLUDES 2 Not included here   N Newborn Age: 0   P Pediatric Age: 0-17   M Maternity Age: 12-55   A Adult Age: 15-124

1124   ICD-10-CM 2018

☑4ᵗʰ **V31** **Occupant of three-wheeled motor vehicle injured in collision with pedal cycle**

  ✓x7ᵗʰ **V31.0** Driver of three-wheeled motor vehicle injured in collision with pedal cycle in nontraffic accident

  ✓x7ᵗʰ **V31.1** Passenger in three-wheeled motor vehicle injured in collision with pedal cycle in nontraffic accident

  ✓x7ᵗʰ **V31.2** Person on outside of three-wheeled motor vehicle injured in collision with pedal cycle in nontraffic accident

  ✓x7ᵗʰ **V31.3** Unspecified occupant of three-wheeled motor vehicle ▽ injured in collision with pedal cycle in nontraffic accident

  ✓x7ᵗʰ **V31.4** Person boarding or alighting a three-wheeled motor vehicle injured in collision with pedal cycle

  ✓x7ᵗʰ **V31.5** Driver of three-wheeled motor vehicle injured in collision with pedal cycle in traffic accident

  ✓x7ᵗʰ **V31.6** Passenger in three-wheeled motor vehicle injured in collision with pedal cycle in traffic accident

  ✓x7ᵗʰ **V31.7** Person on outside of three-wheeled motor vehicle injured in collision with pedal cycle in traffic accident

  ✓x7ᵗʰ **V31.9** Unspecified occupant of three-wheeled motor vehicle ▽ injured in collision with pedal cycle in traffic accident

☑4ᵗʰ **V32** **Occupant of three-wheeled motor vehicle injured in collision with two- or three-wheeled motor vehicle**

  ✓x7ᵗʰ **V32.0** Driver of three-wheeled motor vehicle injured in collision with two- or three-wheeled motor vehicle in nontraffic accident

  ✓x7ᵗʰ **V32.1** Passenger in three-wheeled motor vehicle injured in collision with two- or three-wheeled motor vehicle in nontraffic accident

  ✓x7ᵗʰ **V32.2** Person on outside of three-wheeled motor vehicle injured in collision with two- or three-wheeled motor vehicle in nontraffic accident

  ✓x7ᵗʰ **V32.3** Unspecified occupant of three-wheeled motor vehicle ▽ injured in collision with two- or three-wheeled motor vehicle in nontraffic accident

  ✓x7ᵗʰ **V32.4** Person boarding or alighting a three-wheeled motor vehicle injured in collision with two- or three-wheeled motor vehicle

  ✓x7ᵗʰ **V32.5** Driver of three-wheeled motor vehicle injured in collision with two- or three-wheeled motor vehicle in traffic accident

  ✓x7ᵗʰ **V32.6** Passenger in three-wheeled motor vehicle injured in collision with two- or three-wheeled motor vehicle in traffic accident

  ✓x7ᵗʰ **V32.7** Person on outside of three-wheeled motor vehicle injured in collision with two- or three-wheeled motor vehicle in traffic accident

  ✓x7ᵗʰ **V32.9** Unspecified occupant of three-wheeled motor vehicle ▽ injured in collision with two- or three-wheeled motor vehicle in traffic accident

☑4ᵗʰ **V33** **Occupant of three-wheeled motor vehicle injured in collision with car, pick-up truck or van**

  ✓x7ᵗʰ **V33.0** Driver of three-wheeled motor vehicle injured in collision with car, pick-up truck or van in nontraffic accident

  ✓x7ᵗʰ **V33.1** Passenger in three-wheeled motor vehicle injured in collision with car, pick-up truck or van in nontraffic accident

  ✓x7ᵗʰ **V33.2** Person on outside of three-wheeled motor vehicle injured in collision with car, pick-up truck or van in nontraffic accident

  ✓x7ᵗʰ **V33.3** Unspecified occupant of three-wheeled motor vehicle ▽ injured in collision with car, pick-up truck or van in nontraffic accident

  ✓x7ᵗʰ **V33.4** Person boarding or alighting a three-wheeled motor vehicle injured in collision with car, pick-up truck or van

  ✓x7ᵗʰ **V33.5** Driver of three-wheeled motor vehicle injured in collision with car, pick-up truck or van in traffic accident

  ✓x7ᵗʰ **V33.6** Passenger in three-wheeled motor vehicle injured in collision with car, pick-up truck or van in traffic accident

  ✓x7ᵗʰ **V33.7** Person on outside of three-wheeled motor vehicle injured in collision with car, pick-up truck or van in traffic accident

  ✓x7ᵗʰ **V33.9** Unspecified occupant of three-wheeled motor vehicle ▽ injured in collision with car, pick-up truck or van in traffic accident

☑4ᵗʰ **V34** **Occupant of three-wheeled motor vehicle injured in collision with heavy transport vehicle or bus**

    EXCLUDES 1   occupant of three-wheeled motor vehicle injured in collision with military vehicle (V39.81)

  ✓x7ᵗʰ **V34.0** Driver of three-wheeled motor vehicle injured in collision with heavy transport vehicle or bus in nontraffic accident

  ✓x7ᵗʰ **V34.1** Passenger in three-wheeled motor vehicle injured in collision with heavy transport vehicle or bus in nontraffic accident

  ✓x7ᵗʰ **V34.2** Person on outside of three-wheeled motor vehicle injured in collision with heavy transport vehicle or bus in nontraffic accident

  ✓x7ᵗʰ **V34.3** Unspecified occupant of three-wheeled motor vehicle ▽ injured in collision with heavy transport vehicle or bus in nontraffic accident

  ✓x7ᵗʰ **V34.4** Person boarding or alighting a three-wheeled motor vehicle injured in collision with heavy transport vehicle or bus

  ✓x7ᵗʰ **V34.5** Driver of three-wheeled motor vehicle injured in collision with heavy transport vehicle or bus in traffic accident

  ✓x7ᵗʰ **V34.6** Passenger in three-wheeled motor vehicle injured in collision with heavy transport vehicle or bus in traffic accident

  ✓x7ᵗʰ **V34.7** Person on outside of three-wheeled motor vehicle injured in collision with heavy transport vehicle or bus in traffic accident

  ✓x7ᵗʰ **V34.9** Unspecified occupant of three-wheeled motor vehicle ▽ injured in collision with heavy transport vehicle or bus in traffic accident

☑4ᵗʰ **V35** **Occupant of three-wheeled motor vehicle injured in collision with railway train or railway vehicle**

  ✓x7ᵗʰ **V35.0** Driver of three-wheeled motor vehicle injured in collision with railway train or railway vehicle in nontraffic accident

  ✓x7ᵗʰ **V35.1** Passenger in three-wheeled motor vehicle injured in collision with railway train or railway vehicle in nontraffic accident

  ✓x7ᵗʰ **V35.2** Person on outside of three-wheeled motor vehicle injured in collision with railway train or railway vehicle in nontraffic accident

  ✓x7ᵗʰ **V35.3** Unspecified occupant of three-wheeled motor vehicle ▽ injured in collision with railway train or railway vehicle in nontraffic accident

  ✓x7ᵗʰ **V35.4** Person boarding or alighting a three-wheeled motor vehicle injured in collision with railway train or railway vehicle

  ✓x7ᵗʰ **V35.5** Driver of three-wheeled motor vehicle injured in collision with railway train or railway vehicle in traffic accident

  ✓x7ᵗʰ **V35.6** Passenger in three-wheeled motor vehicle injured in collision with railway train or railway vehicle in traffic accident

  ✓x7ᵗʰ **V35.7** Person on outside of three-wheeled motor vehicle injured in collision with railway train or railway vehicle in traffic accident

  ✓x7ᵗʰ **V35.9** Unspecified occupant of three-wheeled motor vehicle ▽ injured in collision with railway train or railway vehicle in traffic accident

☑4ᵗʰ **V36** **Occupant of three-wheeled motor vehicle injured in collision with other nonmotor vehicle**

    INCLUDES   collision with animal-drawn vehicle, animal being ridden, streetcar

  ✓x7ᵗʰ **V36.0** Driver of three-wheeled motor vehicle injured in collision with other nonmotor vehicle in nontraffic accident

  ✓x7ᵗʰ **V36.1** Passenger in three-wheeled motor vehicle injured in collision with other nonmotor vehicle in nontraffic accident

  ✓x7ᵗʰ **V36.2** Person on outside of three-wheeled motor vehicle injured in collision with other nonmotor vehicle in nontraffic accident

  ✓x7ᵗʰ **V36.3** Unspecified occupant of three-wheeled motor vehicle ▽ injured in collision with other nonmotor vehicle in nontraffic accident

  ✓x7ᵗʰ **V36.4** Person boarding or alighting a three-wheeled motor vehicle injured in collision with other nonmotor vehicle

  ✓x7ᵗʰ **V36.5** Driver of three-wheeled motor vehicle injured in collision with other nonmotor vehicle in traffic accident

  ✓x7ᵗʰ **V36.6** Passenger in three-wheeled motor vehicle injured in collision with other nonmotor vehicle in traffic accident

  ✓x7ᵗʰ **V36.7** Person on outside of three-wheeled motor vehicle injured in collision with other nonmotor vehicle in traffic accident

  ✓x7ᵗʰ **V36.9** Unspecified occupant of three-wheeled motor vehicle ▽ injured in collision with other nonmotor vehicle in traffic accident

☑4ᵗʰ **V37** **Occupant of three-wheeled motor vehicle injured in collision with fixed or stationary object**

  ✓x7ᵗʰ **V37.0** Driver of three-wheeled motor vehicle injured in collision with fixed or stationary object in nontraffic accident

  ✓x7ᵗʰ **V37.1** Passenger in three-wheeled motor vehicle injured in collision with fixed or stationary object in nontraffic accident

---

☑ Additional Character Req   ✓x7ᵗʰ Placeholder Alert   Manifestation   HCC CMS-HCC Condition   ▽ Unspecified Code   ►◄ Revised Text   ● New Code   ▲ Revised Code Title

Chapter 20. External Causes of Morbidity

√x7ᵗʰ **V37.2** Person on outside of three-wheeled motor vehicle injured in collision with fixed or stationary object in nontraffic accident

√x7ᵗʰ **V37.3** Unspecified occupant of three-wheeled motor vehicle injured in collision with fixed or stationary object in nontraffic accident ▽

√x7ᵗʰ **V37.4** Person boarding or alighting a three-wheeled motor vehicle injured in collision with fixed or stationary object

√x7ᵗʰ **V37.5** Driver of three-wheeled motor vehicle injured in collision with fixed or stationary object in traffic accident

√x7ᵗʰ **V37.6** Passenger in three-wheeled motor vehicle injured in collision with fixed or stationary object in traffic accident

√x7ᵗʰ **V37.7** Person on outside of three-wheeled motor vehicle injured in collision with fixed or stationary object in traffic accident

√x7ᵗʰ **V37.9** Unspecified occupant of three-wheeled motor vehicle injured in collision with fixed or stationary object in traffic accident ▽

√4ᵗʰ **V38** Occupant of three-wheeled motor vehicle injured in noncollision transport accident
> INCLUDES   fall or thrown from three-wheeled motor vehicle
> overturning of three-wheeled motor vehicle NOS
> overturning of three-wheeled motor vehicle without collision

√x7ᵗʰ **V38.0** Driver of three-wheeled motor vehicle injured in noncollision transport accident in nontraffic accident

√x7ᵗʰ **V38.1** Passenger in three-wheeled motor vehicle injured in noncollision transport accident in nontraffic accident

√x7ᵗʰ **V38.2** Person on outside of three-wheeled motor vehicle injured in noncollision transport accident in nontraffic accident

√x7ᵗʰ **V38.3** Unspecified occupant of three-wheeled motor vehicle injured in noncollision transport accident in nontraffic accident ▽

√x7ᵗʰ **V38.4** Person boarding or alighting a three-wheeled motor vehicle injured in noncollision transport accident

√x7ᵗʰ **V38.5** Driver of three-wheeled motor vehicle injured in noncollision transport accident in traffic accident

√x7ᵗʰ **V38.6** Passenger in three-wheeled motor vehicle injured in noncollision transport accident in traffic accident

√x7ᵗʰ **V38.7** Person on outside of three-wheeled motor vehicle injured in noncollision transport accident in traffic accident

√x7ᵗʰ **V38.9** Unspecified occupant of three-wheeled motor vehicle injured in noncollision transport accident in traffic accident ▽

√4ᵗʰ **V39** Occupant of three-wheeled motor vehicle injured in other and unspecified transport accidents

√5ᵗʰ **V39.0** Driver of three-wheeled motor vehicle injured in collision with other and unspecified motor vehicles in nontraffic accident

     √x7ᵗʰ **V39.00** Driver of three-wheeled motor vehicle injured in collision with unspecified motor vehicles in nontraffic accident ▽

     √x7ᵗʰ **V39.09** Driver of three-wheeled motor vehicle injured in collision with other motor vehicles in nontraffic accident

√5ᵗʰ **V39.1** Passenger in three-wheeled motor vehicle injured in collision with other and unspecified motor vehicles in nontraffic accident

     √x7ᵗʰ **V39.10** Passenger in three-wheeled motor vehicle injured in collision with unspecified motor vehicles in nontraffic accident ▽

     √x7ᵗʰ **V39.19** Passenger in three-wheeled motor vehicle injured in collision with other motor vehicles in nontraffic accident

√5ᵗʰ **V39.2** Unspecified occupant of three-wheeled motor vehicle injured in collision with other and unspecified motor vehicles in nontraffic accident

     √x7ᵗʰ **V39.20** Unspecified occupant of three-wheeled motor vehicle injured in collision with unspecified motor vehicles in nontraffic accident ▽
> Collision NOS involving three-wheeled motor vehicle, nontraffic

     √x7ᵗʰ **V39.29** Unspecified occupant of three-wheeled motor vehicle injured in collision with other motor vehicles in nontraffic accident ▽

√x7ᵗʰ **V39.3** Occupant (driver) (passenger) of three-wheeled motor vehicle injured in unspecified nontraffic accident ▽
> Accident NOS involving three-wheeled motor vehicle, nontraffic
> Occupant of three-wheeled motor vehicle injured in nontraffic accident NOS

√5ᵗʰ **V39.4** Driver of three-wheeled motor vehicle injured in collision with other and unspecified motor vehicles in traffic accident

     √x7ᵗʰ **V39.40** Driver of three-wheeled motor vehicle injured in collision with unspecified motor vehicles in traffic accident ▽

     √x7ᵗʰ **V39.49** Driver of three-wheeled motor vehicle injured in collision with other motor vehicles in traffic accident

√5ᵗʰ **V39.5** Passenger in three-wheeled motor vehicle injured in collision with other and unspecified motor vehicles in traffic accident

     √x7ᵗʰ **V39.50** Passenger in three-wheeled motor vehicle injured in collision with unspecified motor vehicles in traffic accident ▽

     √x7ᵗʰ **V39.59** Passenger in three-wheeled motor vehicle injured in collision with other motor vehicles in traffic accident

√5ᵗʰ **V39.6** Unspecified occupant of three-wheeled motor vehicle injured in collision with other and unspecified motor vehicles in traffic accident

     √x7ᵗʰ **V39.60** Unspecified occupant of three-wheeled motor vehicle injured in collision with unspecified motor vehicles in traffic accident ▽
> Collision NOS involving three-wheeled motor vehicle (traffic)

     √x7ᵗʰ **V39.69** Unspecified occupant of three-wheeled motor vehicle injured in collision with other motor vehicles in traffic accident ▽

√5ᵗʰ **V39.8** Occupant (driver) (passenger) of three-wheeled motor vehicle injured in other specified transport accidents

     √x7ᵗʰ **V39.81** Occupant (driver) (passenger) of three-wheeled motor vehicle injured in transport accident with military vehicle

     √x7ᵗʰ **V39.89** Occupant (driver) (passenger) of three-wheeled motor vehicle injured in other specified transport accidents

√x7ᵗʰ **V39.9** Occupant (driver) (passenger) of three-wheeled motor vehicle injured in unspecified traffic accident ▽
> Accident NOS involving three-wheeled motor vehicle

Car occupant injured in transport accident (V40-V49)

> INCLUDES   a four-wheeled motor vehicle designed primarily for carrying passengers
> automobile (pulling a trailer or camper)
> EXCLUDES 1   bus (V50-V59)
> minibus (V50-V59)
> minivan (V50-V59)
> motorcoach (V70-V79)
> pick-up truck (V50-V59)
> sport utility vehicle (SUV) (V50-V59)

> The appropriate 7th character is to be added to each code from categories V40-V49.
> A   initial encounter
> D   subsequent encounter
> S   sequela

√4ᵗʰ **V40** Car occupant injured in collision with pedestrian or animal
> EXCLUDES 1   car collision with animal-drawn vehicle or animal being ridden (V46.-)

√x7ᵗʰ **V40.0** Car driver injured in collision with pedestrian or animal in nontraffic accident

√x7ᵗʰ **V40.1** Car passenger injured in collision with pedestrian or animal in nontraffic accident

√x7ᵗʰ **V40.2** Person on outside of car injured in collision with pedestrian or animal in nontraffic accident

√x7ᵗʰ **V40.3** Unspecified car occupant injured in collision with pedestrian or animal in nontraffic accident ▽

√x7ᵗʰ **V40.4** Person boarding or alighting a car injured in collision with pedestrian or animal

√x7ᵗʰ **V40.5** Car driver injured in collision with pedestrian or animal in traffic accident

√x7ᵗʰ **V40.6** Car passenger injured in collision with pedestrian or animal in traffic accident

√x7ᵗʰ **V40.7** Person on outside of car injured in collision with pedestrian or animal in traffic accident

EXCLUDES 1 Not coded here   EXCLUDES 2 Not included here   N Newborn Age: 0   P Pediatric Age: 0-17   M Maternity Age: 12-55   A Adult Age: 15-124

1126   ICD-10-CM 2018

√x7ᵗʰ **V40.9** Unspecified car occupant injured in collision with ▽
pedestrian or animal in traffic accident

√4ᵗʰ **V41** **Car occupant injured in collision with pedal cycle**

√x7ᵗʰ **V41.0** Car driver injured in collision with pedal cycle in nontraffic accident

√x7ᵗʰ **V41.1** Car passenger injured in collision with pedal cycle in nontraffic accident

√x7ᵗʰ **V41.2** Person on outside of car injured in collision with pedal cycle in nontraffic accident

√x7ᵗʰ **V41.3** Unspecified car occupant injured in collision with ▽
pedal cycle in nontraffic accident

√x7ᵗʰ **V41.4** Person boarding or alighting a car injured in collision with pedal cycle

√x7ᵗʰ **V41.5** Car driver injured in collision with pedal cycle in traffic accident

√x7ᵗʰ **V41.6** Car passenger injured in collision with pedal cycle in traffic accident

√x7ᵗʰ **V41.7** Person on outside of car injured in collision with pedal cycle in traffic accident

√x7ᵗʰ **V41.9** Unspecified car occupant injured in collision with ▽
pedal cycle in traffic accident

√4ᵗʰ **V42** **Car occupant injured in collision with two- or three-wheeled motor vehicle**

√x7ᵗʰ **V42.0** Car driver injured in collision with two- or three-wheeled motor vehicle in nontraffic accident

√x7ᵗʰ **V42.1** Car passenger injured in collision with two- or three-wheeled motor vehicle in nontraffic accident

√x7ᵗʰ **V42.2** Person on outside of car injured in collision with two- or three-wheeled motor vehicle in nontraffic accident

√x7ᵗʰ **V42.3** Unspecified car occupant injured in collision with two- ▽
or three-wheeled motor vehicle in nontraffic accident

√x7ᵗʰ **V42.4** Person boarding or alighting a car injured in collision with two- or three-wheeled motor vehicle

√x7ᵗʰ **V42.5** Car driver injured in collision with two- or three-wheeled motor vehicle in traffic accident

√x7ᵗʰ **V42.6** Car passenger injured in collision with two- or three-wheeled motor vehicle in traffic accident

√x7ᵗʰ **V42.7** Person on outside of car injured in collision with two- or three-wheeled motor vehicle in traffic accident

√x7ᵗʰ **V42.9** Unspecified car occupant injured in collision with two- ▽
or three-wheeled motor vehicle in traffic accident

√4ᵗʰ **V43** **Car occupant injured in collision with car, pick-up truck or van**

√5ᵗʰ **V43.0** Car driver injured in collision with car, pick-up truck or van in nontraffic accident

√x7ᵗʰ **V43.01** Car driver injured in collision with sport utility vehicle in nontraffic accident

√x7ᵗʰ **V43.02** Car driver injured in collision with other type car in nontraffic accident

√x7ᵗʰ **V43.03** Car driver injured in collision with pick-up truck in nontraffic accident

√x7ᵗʰ **V43.04** Car driver injured in collision with van in nontraffic accident

√5ᵗʰ **V43.1** Car passenger injured in collision with car, pick-up truck or van in nontraffic accident

√x7ᵗʰ **V43.11** Car passenger injured in collision with sport utility vehicle in nontraffic accident

√x7ᵗʰ **V43.12** Car passenger injured in collision with other type car in nontraffic accident

√x7ᵗʰ **V43.13** Car passenger injured in collision with pick-up in nontraffic accident

√x7ᵗʰ **V43.14** Car passenger injured in collision with van in nontraffic accident

√5ᵗʰ **V43.2** Person on outside of car injured in collision with car, pick-up truck or van in nontraffic accident

√x7ᵗʰ **V43.21** Person on outside of car injured in collision with sport utility vehicle in nontraffic accident

√x7ᵗʰ **V43.22** Person on outside of car injured in collision with other type car in nontraffic accident

√x7ᵗʰ **V43.23** Person on outside of car injured in collision with pick-up truck in nontraffic accident

√x7ᵗʰ **V43.24** Person on outside of car injured in collision with van in nontraffic accident

√5ᵗʰ **V43.3** Unspecified car occupant injured in collision with car, pick-up truck or van in nontraffic accident

√x7ᵗʰ **V43.31** Unspecified car occupant injured in collision ▽
with sport utility vehicle in nontraffic accident

√x7ᵗʰ **V43.32** Unspecified car occupant injured in collision ▽
with other type car in nontraffic accident

√x7ᵗʰ **V43.33** Unspecified car occupant injured in collision ▽
with pick-up truck in nontraffic accident

√x7ᵗʰ **V43.34** Unspecified car occupant injured in collision ▽
with van in nontraffic accident

√5ᵗʰ **V43.4** Person boarding or alighting a car injured in collision with car, pick-up truck or van

√x7ᵗʰ **V43.41** Person boarding or alighting a car injured in collision with sport utility vehicle

√x7ᵗʰ **V43.42** Person boarding or alighting a car injured in collision with other type car

√x7ᵗʰ **V43.43** Person boarding or alighting a car injured in collision with pick-up truck

√x7ᵗʰ **V43.44** Person boarding or alighting a car injured in collision with van

√5ᵗʰ **V43.5** Car driver injured in collision with car, pick-up truck or van in traffic accident

√x7ᵗʰ **V43.51** Car driver injured in collision with sport utility vehicle in traffic accident

√x7ᵗʰ **V43.52** Car driver injured in collision with other type car in traffic accident

√x7ᵗʰ **V43.53** Car driver injured in collision with pick-up truck in traffic accident

√x7ᵗʰ **V43.54** Car driver injured in collision with van in traffic accident

√5ᵗʰ **V43.6** Car passenger injured in collision with car, pick-up truck or van in traffic accident

√x7ᵗʰ **V43.61** Car passenger injured in collision with sport utility vehicle in traffic accident

√x7ᵗʰ **V43.62** Car passenger injured in collision with other type car in traffic accident

√x7ᵗʰ **V43.63** Car passenger injured in collision with pick-up truck in traffic accident

√x7ᵗʰ **V43.64** Car passenger injured in collision with van in traffic accident

√5ᵗʰ **V43.7** Person on outside of car injured in collision with car, pick-up truck or van in traffic accident

√x7ᵗʰ **V43.71** Person on outside of car injured in collision with sport utility vehicle in traffic accident

√x7ᵗʰ **V43.72** Person on outside of car injured in collision with other type car in traffic accident

√x7ᵗʰ **V43.73** Person on outside of car injured in collision with pick-up truck in traffic accident

√x7ᵗʰ **V43.74** Person on outside of car injured in collision with van in traffic accident

√5ᵗʰ **V43.9** Unspecified car occupant injured in collision with car, pick-up truck or van in traffic accident

√x7ᵗʰ **V43.91** Unspecified car occupant injured in collision ▽
with sport utility vehicle in traffic accident

√x7ᵗʰ **V43.92** Unspecified car occupant injured in collision ▽
with other type car in traffic accident

√x7ᵗʰ **V43.93** Unspecified car occupant injured in collision ▽
with pick-up truck in traffic accident

√x7ᵗʰ **V43.94** Unspecified car occupant injured in collision ▽
with van in traffic accident

√4ᵗʰ **V44** **Car occupant injured in collision with heavy transport vehicle or bus**

EXCLUDES 1   car occupant injured in collision with military vehicle (V49.81)

√x7ᵗʰ **V44.0** Car driver injured in collision with heavy transport vehicle or bus in nontraffic accident

√x7ᵗʰ **V44.1** Car passenger injured in collision with heavy transport vehicle or bus in nontraffic accident

√x7ᵗʰ **V44.2** Person on outside of car injured in collision with heavy transport vehicle or bus in nontraffic accident

√x7ᵗʰ **V44.3** Unspecified car occupant injured in collision with heavy ▽
transport vehicle or bus in nontraffic accident

√x7ᵗʰ **V44.4** Person boarding or alighting a car injured in collision with heavy transport vehicle or bus

---

☑ Additional Character Req   √x7ᵗʰ Placeholder Alert   Manifestation   **HCC** CMS-HCC Condition   ▽ Unspecified Code   ►◄ Revised Text   ● New Code   ▲ Revised Code Title

✓x7ᵗʰ **V44.5** Car driver injured in collision with heavy transport vehicle or bus in traffic accident

✓x7ᵗʰ **V44.6** Car passenger injured in collision with heavy transport vehicle or bus in traffic accident

✓x7ᵗʰ **V44.7** Person on outside of car injured in collision with heavy transport vehicle or bus in traffic accident

✓x7ᵗʰ **V44.9** Unspecified car occupant injured in collision with heavy ▽ transport vehicle or bus in traffic accident

✓4ᵗʰ **V45 Car occupant injured in collision with railway train or railway vehicle**

✓x7ᵗʰ **V45.0** Car driver injured in collision with railway train or railway vehicle in nontraffic accident

✓x7ᵗʰ **V45.1** Car passenger injured in collision with railway train or railway vehicle in nontraffic accident

✓x7ᵗʰ **V45.2** Person on outside of car injured in collision with railway train or railway vehicle in nontraffic accident

✓x7ᵗʰ **V45.3** Unspecified car occupant injured in collision with ▽ railway train or railway vehicle in nontraffic accident

✓x7ᵗʰ **V45.4** Person boarding or alighting a car injured in collision with railway train or railway vehicle

✓x7ᵗʰ **V45.5** Car driver injured in collision with railway train or railway vehicle in traffic accident

✓x7ᵗʰ **V45.6** Car passenger injured in collision with railway train or railway vehicle in traffic accident

✓x7ᵗʰ **V45.7** Person on outside of car injured in collision with railway train or railway vehicle in traffic accident

✓x7ᵗʰ **V45.9** Unspecified car occupant injured in collision with ▽ railway train or railway vehicle in traffic accident

✓4ᵗʰ **V46 Car occupant injured in collision with other nonmotor vehicle**
INCLUDES collision with animal-drawn vehicle, animal being ridden, streetcar

✓x7ᵗʰ **V46.0** Car driver injured in collision with other nonmotor vehicle in nontraffic accident

✓x7ᵗʰ **V46.1** Car passenger injured in collision with other nonmotor vehicle in nontraffic accident

✓x7ᵗʰ **V46.2** Person on outside of car injured in collision with other nonmotor vehicle in nontraffic accident

✓x7ᵗʰ **V46.3** Unspecified car occupant injured in collision with other ▽ nonmotor vehicle in nontraffic accident

✓x7ᵗʰ **V46.4** Person boarding or alighting a car injured in collision with other nonmotor vehicle

✓x7ᵗʰ **V46.5** Car driver injured in collision with other nonmotor vehicle in traffic accident

✓x7ᵗʰ **V46.6** Car passenger injured in collision with other nonmotor vehicle in traffic accident

✓x7ᵗʰ **V46.7** Person on outside of car injured in collision with other nonmotor vehicle in traffic accident

✓x7ᵗʰ **V46.9** Unspecified car occupant injured in collision with other ▽ nonmotor vehicle in traffic accident

✓4ᵗʰ **V47 Car occupant injured in collision with fixed or stationary object**

✓x7ᵗʰ **V47.0** Car driver injured in collision with fixed or stationary object in nontraffic accident

✓x7ᵗʰ **V47.1** Car passenger injured in collision with fixed or stationary object in nontraffic accident

✓x7ᵗʰ **V47.2** Person on outside of car injured in collision with fixed or stationary object in nontraffic accident

✓x7ᵗʰ **V47.3** Unspecified car occupant injured in collision with fixed ▽ or stationary object in nontraffic accident

✓x7ᵗʰ **V47.4** Person boarding or alighting a car injured in collision with fixed or stationary object

✓x7ᵗʰ **V47.5** Car driver injured in collision with fixed or stationary object in traffic accident

✓x7ᵗʰ **V47.6** Car passenger injured in collision with fixed or stationary object in traffic accident

✓x7ᵗʰ **V47.7** Person on outside of car injured in collision with fixed or stationary object in traffic accident

✓x7ᵗʰ **V47.9** Unspecified car occupant injured in collision with fixed or ▽ stationary object in traffic accident

✓4ᵗʰ **V48 Car occupant injured in noncollision transport accident**
INCLUDES overturning car NOS
overturning car without collision

✓x7ᵗʰ **V48.0** Car driver injured in noncollision transport accident in nontraffic accident

✓x7ᵗʰ **V48.1** Car passenger injured in noncollision transport accident in nontraffic accident

✓x7ᵗʰ **V48.2** Person on outside of car injured in noncollision transport accident in nontraffic accident

✓x7ᵗʰ **V48.3** Unspecified car occupant injured in noncollision ▽ transport accident in nontraffic accident

✓x7ᵗʰ **V48.4** Person boarding or alighting a car injured in noncollision transport accident

✓x7ᵗʰ **V48.5** Car driver injured in noncollision transport accident in traffic accident

✓x7ᵗʰ **V48.6** Car passenger injured in noncollision transport accident in traffic accident

✓x7ᵗʰ **V48.7** Person on outside of car injured in noncollision transport accident in traffic accident

✓x7ᵗʰ **V48.9** Unspecified car occupant injured in noncollision ▽ transport accident in traffic accident

✓4ᵗʰ **V49 Car occupant injured in other and unspecified transport accidents**

✓5ᵗʰ **V49.0** Driver injured in collision with other and unspecified motor vehicles in nontraffic accident

✓x7ᵗʰ **V49.00** Driver injured in collision with unspecified motor ▽ vehicles in nontraffic accident

✓x7ᵗʰ **V49.09** Driver injured in collision with other motor vehicles in nontraffic accident

✓5ᵗʰ **V49.1** Passenger injured in collision with other and unspecified motor vehicles in nontraffic accident

✓x7ᵗʰ **V49.10** Passenger injured in collision with unspecified ▽ motor vehicles in nontraffic accident

✓x7ᵗʰ **V49.19** Passenger injured in collision with other motor vehicles in nontraffic accident

✓5ᵗʰ **V49.2** Unspecified car occupant injured in collision with other and unspecified motor vehicles in nontraffic accident

✓x7ᵗʰ **V49.20** Unspecified car occupant injured in collision with ▽ unspecified motor vehicles in nontraffic accident
Car collision NOS, nontraffic

✓x7ᵗʰ **V49.29** Unspecified car occupant injured in collision with ▽ other motor vehicles in nontraffic accident

✓x7ᵗʰ **V49.3** Car occupant (driver) (passenger) injured in unspecified ▽ nontraffic accident
Car accident NOS, nontraffic
Car occupant injured in nontraffic accident NOS

✓5ᵗʰ **V49.4** Driver injured in collision with other and unspecified motor vehicles in traffic accident

✓x7ᵗʰ **V49.40** Driver injured in collision with unspecified ▽ motor vehicles in traffic accident

✓x7ᵗʰ **V49.49** Driver injured in collision with other motor vehicles in traffic accident

✓5ᵗʰ **V49.5** Passenger injured in collision with other and unspecified motor vehicles in traffic accident

✓x7ᵗʰ **V49.50** Passenger injured in collision with unspecified ▽ motor vehicles in traffic accident

✓x7ᵗʰ **V49.59** Passenger injured in collision with other motor vehicles in traffic accident

✓5ᵗʰ **V49.6** Unspecified car occupant injured in collision with other and unspecified motor vehicles in traffic accident

✓x7ᵗʰ **V49.60** Unspecified car occupant injured in collision ▽ with unspecified motor vehicles in traffic accident
Car collision NOS (traffic)

✓x7ᵗʰ **V49.69** Unspecified car occupant injured in collision ▽ with other motor vehicles in traffic accident

✓5ᵗʰ **V49.8** Car occupant (driver) (passenger) injured in other specified transport accidents

✓x7ᵗʰ **V49.81** Car occupant (driver) (passenger) injured in transport accident with military vehicle

✓x7ᵗʰ **V49.88** Car occupant (driver) (passenger) injured in other specified transport accidents

✓x7ᵗʰ **V49.9** Car occupant (driver) (passenger) injured in unspecified ▽ traffic accident
Car accident NOS

EXCLUDES 1 Not coded here   **EXCLUDES 2** Not included here   N Newborn Age: 0   P Pediatric Age: 0-17   M Maternity Age: 12-55   A Adult Age: 15-124

1128   ICD-10-CM 2018

Occupant of pick-up truck or van injured in transport accident (V50-V59)

INCLUDES   a four or six wheel motor vehicle designed primarily for carrying passengers and property but weighing less than the local limit for classification as a heavy goods vehicle
minibus
minivan
sport utility vehicle (SUV)
truck
van

EXCLUDES 1   heavy transport vehicle (V60-V69)

> The appropriate 7th character is to be added to each code from categories V50-V59.
> A   initial encounter
> D   subsequent encounter
> S   sequela

✓4th **V50 Occupant of pick-up truck or van injured in collision with pedestrian or animal**

> EXCLUDES 1   pick-up truck or van collision with animal-drawn vehicle or animal being ridden (V56.-)

✓x7th **V50.0** Driver of pick-up truck or van injured in collision with pedestrian or animal in nontraffic accident

✓x7th **V50.1** Passenger in pick-up truck or van injured in collision with pedestrian or animal in nontraffic accident

✓x7th **V50.2** Person on outside of pick-up truck or van injured in collision with pedestrian or animal in nontraffic accident

✓x7th **V50.3** Unspecified occupant of pick-up truck or van injured in ▽ collision with pedestrian or animal in nontraffic accident

✓x7th **V50.4** Person boarding or alighting a pick-up truck or van injured in collision with pedestrian or animal

✓x7th **V50.5** Driver of pick-up truck or van injured in collision with pedestrian or animal in traffic accident

✓x7th **V50.6** Passenger in pick-up truck or van injured in collision with pedestrian or animal in traffic accident

✓x7th **V50.7** Person on outside of pick-up truck or van injured in collision with pedestrian or animal in traffic accident

✓x7th **V50.9** Unspecified occupant of pick-up truck or van injured in ▽ collision with pedestrian or animal in traffic accident

✓4th **V51 Occupant of pick-up truck or van injured in collision with pedal cycle**

✓x7th **V51.0** Driver of pick-up truck or van injured in collision with pedal cycle in nontraffic accident

✓x7th **V51.1** Passenger in pick-up truck or van injured in collision with pedal cycle in nontraffic accident

✓x7th **V51.2** Person on outside of pick-up truck or van injured in collision with pedal cycle in nontraffic accident

✓x7th **V51.3** Unspecified occupant of pick-up truck or van injured in ▽ collision with pedal cycle in nontraffic accident

✓x7th **V51.4** Person boarding or alighting a pick-up truck or van injured in collision with pedal cycle

✓x7th **V51.5** Driver of pick-up truck or van injured in collision with pedal cycle in traffic accident

✓x7th **V51.6** Passenger in pick-up truck or van injured in collision with pedal cycle in traffic accident

✓x7th **V51.7** Person on outside of pick-up truck or van injured in collision with pedal cycle in traffic accident

✓x7th **V51.9** Unspecified occupant of pick-up truck or van injured in ▽ collision with pedal cycle in traffic accident

✓4th **V52 Occupant of pick-up truck or van injured in collision with two- or three-wheeled motor vehicle**

✓x7th **V52.0** Driver of pick-up truck or van injured in collision with two- or three-wheeled motor vehicle in nontraffic accident

✓x7th **V52.1** Passenger in pick-up truck or van injured in collision with two- or three-wheeled motor vehicle in nontraffic accident

✓x7th **V52.2** Person on outside of pick-up truck or van injured in collision with two- or three-wheeled motor vehicle in nontraffic accident

✓x7th **V52.3** Unspecified occupant of pick-up truck or van injured in ▽ collision with two- or three-wheeled motor vehicle in nontraffic accident

✓x7th **V52.4** Person boarding or alighting a pick-up truck or van injured in collision with two- or three-wheeled motor vehicle

✓x7th **V52.5** Driver of pick-up truck or van injured in collision with two- or three-wheeled motor vehicle in traffic accident

✓x7th **V52.6** Passenger in pick-up truck or van injured in collision with two- or three-wheeled motor vehicle in traffic accident

✓x7th **V52.7** Person on outside of pick-up truck or van injured in collision with two- or three-wheeled motor vehicle in traffic accident

✓x7th **V52.9** Unspecified occupant of pick-up truck or van injured in ▽ collision with two- or three-wheeled motor vehicle in traffic accident

✓4th **V53 Occupant of pick-up truck or van injured in collision with car, pick-up truck or van**

✓x7th **V53.0** Driver of pick-up truck or van injured in collision with car, pick-up truck or van in nontraffic accident

✓x7th **V53.1** Passenger in pick-up truck or van injured in collision with car, pick-up truck or van in nontraffic accident

✓x7th **V53.2** Person on outside of pick-up truck or van injured in collision with car, pick-up truck or van in nontraffic accident

✓x7th **V53.3** Unspecified occupant of pick-up truck or van injured in ▽ collision with car, pick-up truck or van in nontraffic accident

✓x7th **V53.4** Person boarding or alighting a pick-up truck or van injured in collision with car, pick-up truck or van

✓x7th **V53.5** Driver of pick-up truck or van injured in collision with car, pick-up truck or van in traffic accident

✓x7th **V53.6** Passenger in pick-up truck or van injured in collision with car, pick-up truck or van in traffic accident

✓x7th **V53.7** Person on outside of pick-up truck or van injured in collision with car, pick-up truck or van in traffic accident

✓x7th **V53.9** Unspecified occupant of pick-up truck or van injured in ▽ collision with car, pick-up truck or van in traffic accident

✓4th **V54 Occupant of pick-up truck or van injured in collision with heavy transport vehicle or bus**

> EXCLUDES 1   occupant of pick-up truck or van injured in collision with military vehicle (V59.81)

✓x7th **V54.0** Driver of pick-up truck or van injured in collision with heavy transport vehicle or bus in nontraffic accident

✓x7th **V54.1** Passenger in pick-up truck or van injured in collision with heavy transport vehicle or bus in nontraffic accident

✓x7th **V54.2** Person on outside of pick-up truck or van injured in collision with heavy transport vehicle or bus in nontraffic accident

✓x7th **V54.3** Unspecified occupant of pick-up truck or van injured in ▽ collision with heavy transport vehicle or bus in nontraffic accident

✓x7th **V54.4** Person boarding or alighting a pick-up truck or van injured in collision with heavy transport vehicle or bus

✓x7th **V54.5** Driver of pick-up truck or van injured in collision with heavy transport vehicle or bus in traffic accident

✓x7th **V54.6** Passenger in pick-up truck or van injured in collision with heavy transport vehicle or bus in traffic accident

✓x7th **V54.7** Person on outside of pick-up truck or van injured in collision with heavy transport vehicle or bus in traffic accident

✓x7th **V54.9** Unspecified occupant of pick-up truck or van injured in ▽ collision with heavy transport vehicle or bus in traffic accident

✓4th **V55 Occupant of pick-up truck or van injured in collision with railway train or railway vehicle**

✓x7th **V55.0** Driver of pick-up truck or van injured in collision with railway train or railway vehicle in nontraffic accident

✓x7th **V55.1** Passenger in pick-up truck or van injured in collision with railway train or railway vehicle in nontraffic accident

✓x7th **V55.2** Person on outside of pick-up truck or van injured in collision with railway train or railway vehicle in nontraffic accident

✓x7th **V55.3** Unspecified occupant of pick-up truck or van injured in ▽ collision with railway train or railway vehicle in nontraffic accident

✓x7th **V55.4** Person boarding or alighting a pick-up truck or van injured in collision with railway train or railway vehicle

✓x7th **V55.5** Driver of pick-up truck or van injured in collision with railway train or railway vehicle in traffic accident

✓x7th **V55.6** Passenger in pick-up truck or van injured in collision with railway train or railway vehicle in traffic accident

✓x7th **V55.7** Person on outside of pick-up truck or van injured in collision with railway train or railway vehicle in traffic accident

✓x7th **V55.9** Unspecified occupant of pick-up truck or van injured in ▽ collision with railway train or railway vehicle in traffic accident

---

☑ Additional Character Req   ✓x7th Placeholder Alert   Manifestation   HCC CMS-HCC Condition   ▽ Unspecified Code   ▶◀ Revised Text   ● New Code   ▲ Revised Code Title

Chapter 20. External Causes of Morbidity

V56–V60.1

✓4th **V56** **Occupant of pick-up truck or van injured in collision with other nonmotor vehicle**
     INCLUDES   collision with animal-drawn vehicle, animal being ridden, streetcar

✓x7th **V56.0** Driver of pick-up truck or van injured in collision with other nonmotor vehicle in nontraffic accident

✓x7th **V56.1** Passenger in pick-up truck or van injured in collision with other nonmotor vehicle in nontraffic accident

✓x7th **V56.2** Person on outside of pick-up truck or van injured in collision with other nonmotor vehicle in nontraffic accident

✓x7th **V56.3** Unspecified occupant of pick-up truck or van injured in ▽ collision with other nonmotor vehicle in nontraffic accident

✓x7th **V56.4** Person boarding or alighting a pick-up truck or van injured in collision with other nonmotor vehicle

✓x7th **V56.5** Driver of pick-up truck or van injured in collision with other nonmotor vehicle in traffic accident

✓x7th **V56.6** Passenger in pick-up truck or van injured in collision with other nonmotor vehicle in traffic accident

✓x7th **V56.7** Person on outside of pick-up truck or van injured in collision with other nonmotor vehicle in traffic accident

✓x7th **V56.9** Unspecified occupant of pick-up truck or van injured in ▽ collision with other nonmotor vehicle in traffic accident

✓4th **V57** **Occupant of pick-up truck or van injured in collision with fixed or stationary object**

✓x7th **V57.0** Driver of pick-up truck or van injured in collision with fixed or stationary object in nontraffic accident

✓x7th **V57.1** Passenger in pick-up truck or van injured in collision with fixed or stationary object in nontraffic accident

✓x7th **V57.2** Person on outside of pick-up truck or van injured in collision with fixed or stationary object in nontraffic accident

✓x7th **V57.3** Unspecified occupant of pick-up truck or van injured in ▽ collision with fixed or stationary object in nontraffic accident

✓x7th **V57.4** Person boarding or alighting a pick-up truck or van injured in collision with fixed or stationary object

✓x7th **V57.5** Driver of pick-up truck or van injured in collision with fixed or stationary object in traffic accident

✓x7th **V57.6** Passenger in pick-up truck or van injured in collision with fixed or stationary object in traffic accident

✓x7th **V57.7** Person on outside of pick-up truck or van injured in collision with fixed or stationary object in traffic accident

✓x7th **V57.9** Unspecified occupant of pick-up truck or van injured in ▽ collision with fixed or stationary object in traffic accident

✓4th **V58** **Occupant of pick-up truck or van injured in noncollision transport accident**
     INCLUDES   overturning pick-up truck or van NOS
              overturning pick-up truck or van without collision

✓x7th **V58.0** Driver of pick-up truck or van injured in noncollision transport accident in nontraffic accident

✓x7th **V58.1** Passenger in pick-up truck or van injured in noncollision transport accident in nontraffic accident

✓x7th **V58.2** Person on outside of pick-up truck or van injured in noncollision transport accident in nontraffic accident

✓x7th **V58.3** Unspecified occupant of pick-up truck or van injured in ▽ noncollision transport accident in nontraffic accident

✓x7th **V58.4** Person boarding or alighting a pick-up truck or van injured in noncollision transport accident

✓x7th **V58.5** Driver of pick-up truck or van injured in noncollision transport accident in traffic accident

✓x7th **V58.6** Passenger in pick-up truck or van injured in noncollision transport accident in traffic accident

✓x7th **V58.7** Person on outside of pick-up truck or van injured in noncollision transport accident in traffic accident

✓x7th **V58.9** Unspecified occupant of pick-up truck or van injured in ▽ noncollision transport accident in traffic accident

✓4th **V59** **Occupant of pick-up truck or van injured in other and unspecified transport accidents**

✓5th **V59.0** Driver of pick-up truck or van injured in collision with other and unspecified motor vehicles in nontraffic accident

    ✓x7th **V59.00** Driver of pick-up truck or van injured in collision ▽ with unspecified motor vehicles in nontraffic accident

    ✓x7th **V59.09** Driver of pick-up truck or van injured in collision with other motor vehicles in nontraffic accident

---

✓5th **V59.1** Passenger in pick-up truck or van injured in collision with other and unspecified motor vehicles in nontraffic accident

    ✓x7th **V59.10** Passenger in pick-up truck or van injured in ▽ collision with unspecified motor vehicles in nontraffic accident

    ✓x7th **V59.19** Passenger in pick-up truck or van injured in collision with other motor vehicles in nontraffic accident

✓5th **V59.2** Unspecified occupant of pick-up truck or van injured in collision with other and unspecified motor vehicles in nontraffic accident

    ✓x7th **V59.20** Unspecified occupant of pick-up truck or van ▽ injured in collision with unspecified motor vehicles in nontraffic accident
          Collision NOS involving pick-up truck or van, nontraffic

    ✓x7th **V59.29** Unspecified occupant of pick-up truck or van injured in collision with other motor vehicles in nontraffic accident

✓x7th **V59.3** Occupant (driver) (passenger) of pick-up truck or van ▽ injured in unspecified nontraffic accident
       Accident NOS involving pick-up truck or van, nontraffic
       Occupant of pick-up truck or van injured in nontraffic accident NOS

✓5th **V59.4** Driver of pick-up truck or van injured in collision with other and unspecified motor vehicles in traffic accident

    ✓x7th **V59.40** Driver of pick-up truck or van injured in collision ▽ with unspecified motor vehicles in traffic accident

    ✓x7th **V59.49** Driver of pick-up truck or van injured in collision with other motor vehicles in traffic accident

✓5th **V59.5** Passenger in pick-up truck or van injured in collision with other and unspecified motor vehicles in traffic accident

    ✓x7th **V59.50** Passenger in pick-up truck or van injured in ▽ collision with unspecified motor vehicles in traffic accident

    ✓x7th **V59.59** Passenger in pick-up truck or van injured in collision with other motor vehicles in traffic accident

✓5th **V59.6** Unspecified occupant of pick-up truck or van injured in collision with other and unspecified motor vehicles in traffic accident

    ✓x7th **V59.60** Unspecified occupant of pick-up truck or van ▽ injured in collision with unspecified motor vehicles in traffic accident
          Collision NOS involving pick-up truck or van (traffic)

    ✓x7th **V59.69** Unspecified occupant of pick-up truck or van ▽ injured in collision with other motor vehicles in traffic accident

✓5th **V59.8** Occupant (driver) (passenger) of pick-up truck or van injured in other specified transport accidents

    ✓x7th **V59.81** Occupant (driver) (passenger) of pick-up truck or van injured in transport accident with military vehicle

    ✓x7th **V59.88** Occupant (driver) (passenger) of pick-up truck or van injured in other specified transport accidents

✓x7th **V59.9** Occupant (driver) (passenger) of pick-up truck or van ▽ injured in unspecified traffic accident
       Accident NOS involving pick-up truck or van

Occupant of heavy transport vehicle injured in transport accident (V60-V69)

     INCLUDES   18 wheeler
              armored car
              panel truck
     EXCLUDES 1   bus
              motorcoach

The appropriate 7th character is to be added to each code from categories V60-V69.
A   initial encounter
D   subsequent encounter
S   sequela

✓4th **V60** **Occupant of heavy transport vehicle injured in collision with pedestrian or animal**
     EXCLUDES 1   heavy transport vehicle collision with animal-drawn vehicle or animal being ridden (V66.-)

✓x7th **V60.0** Driver of heavy transport vehicle injured in collision with pedestrian or animal in nontraffic accident

✓x7th **V60.1** Passenger in heavy transport vehicle injured in collision with pedestrian or animal in nontraffic accident

---

EXCLUDES 1 Not coded here   EXCLUDES 2 Not included here   N Newborn Age: 0   P Pediatric Age: 0-17   M Maternity Age: 12-55   A Adult Age: 15-124

☑x7ᵗʰ **V60.2** Person on outside of heavy transport vehicle injured in collision with pedestrian or animal in nontraffic accident

☑x7ᵗʰ **V60.3** Unspecified occupant of heavy transport vehicle injured in collision with pedestrian or animal in nontraffic accident ▽

☑x7ᵗʰ **V60.4** Person boarding or alighting a heavy transport vehicle injured in collision with pedestrian or animal

☑x7ᵗʰ **V60.5** Driver of heavy transport vehicle injured in collision with pedestrian or animal in traffic accident

☑x7ᵗʰ **V60.6** Passenger in heavy transport vehicle injured in collision with pedestrian or animal in traffic accident

☑x7ᵗʰ **V60.7** Person on outside of heavy transport vehicle injured in collision with pedestrian or animal in traffic accident

☑x7ᵗʰ **V60.9** Unspecified occupant of heavy transport vehicle injured in collision with pedestrian or animal in traffic accident ▽

☑4ᵗʰ **V61** Occupant of heavy transport vehicle injured in collision with pedal cycle

☑x7ᵗʰ **V61.0** Driver of heavy transport vehicle injured in collision with pedal cycle in nontraffic accident

☑x7ᵗʰ **V61.1** Passenger in heavy transport vehicle injured in collision with pedal cycle in nontraffic accident

☑x7ᵗʰ **V61.2** Person on outside of heavy transport vehicle injured in collision with pedal cycle in nontraffic accident

☑x7ᵗʰ **V61.3** Unspecified occupant of heavy transport vehicle injured in collision with pedal cycle in nontraffic accident ▽

☑x7ᵗʰ **V61.4** Person boarding or alighting a heavy transport vehicle injured in collision with pedal cycle while boarding or alighting

☑x7ᵗʰ **V61.5** Driver of heavy transport vehicle injured in collision with pedal cycle in traffic accident

☑x7ᵗʰ **V61.6** Passenger in heavy transport vehicle injured in collision with pedal cycle in traffic accident

☑x7ᵗʰ **V61.7** Person on outside of heavy transport vehicle injured in collision with pedal cycle in traffic accident

☑x7ᵗʰ **V61.9** Unspecified occupant of heavy transport vehicle injured in collision with pedal cycle in traffic accident ▽

☑4ᵗʰ **V62** Occupant of heavy transport vehicle injured in collision with two- or three-wheeled motor vehicle

☑x7ᵗʰ **V62.0** Driver of heavy transport vehicle injured in collision with two- or three-wheeled motor vehicle in nontraffic accident

☑x7ᵗʰ **V62.1** Passenger in heavy transport vehicle injured in collision with two- or three-wheeled motor vehicle in nontraffic accident

☑x7ᵗʰ **V62.2** Person on outside of heavy transport vehicle injured in collision with two- or three-wheeled motor vehicle in nontraffic accident

☑x7ᵗʰ **V62.3** Unspecified occupant of heavy transport vehicle injured in collision with two- or three-wheeled motor vehicle in nontraffic accident ▽

☑x7ᵗʰ **V62.4** Person boarding or alighting a heavy transport vehicle injured in collision with two- or three-wheeled motor vehicle

☑x7ᵗʰ **V62.5** Driver of heavy transport vehicle injured in collision with two- or three-wheeled motor vehicle in traffic accident

☑x7ᵗʰ **V62.6** Passenger in heavy transport vehicle injured in collision with two- or three-wheeled motor vehicle in traffic accident

☑x7ᵗʰ **V62.7** Person on outside of heavy transport vehicle injured in collision with two- or three-wheeled motor vehicle in traffic accident

☑x7ᵗʰ **V62.9** Unspecified occupant of heavy transport vehicle injured in collision with two- or three-wheeled motor vehicle in traffic accident ▽

☑4ᵗʰ **V63** Occupant of heavy transport vehicle injured in collision with car, pick-up truck or van

☑x7ᵗʰ **V63.0** Driver of heavy transport vehicle injured in collision with car, pick-up truck or van in nontraffic accident

☑x7ᵗʰ **V63.1** Passenger in heavy transport vehicle injured in collision with car, pick-up truck or van in nontraffic accident

☑x7ᵗʰ **V63.2** Person on outside of heavy transport vehicle injured in collision with car, pick-up truck or van in nontraffic accident

☑x7ᵗʰ **V63.3** Unspecified occupant of heavy transport vehicle injured in ▽ collision with car, pick-up truck or van in nontraffic accident

☑x7ᵗʰ **V63.4** Person boarding or alighting a heavy transport vehicle injured in collision with car, pick-up truck or van

☑x7ᵗʰ **V63.5** Driver of heavy transport vehicle injured in collision with car, pick-up truck or van in traffic accident

☑x7ᵗʰ **V63.6** Passenger in heavy transport vehicle injured in collision with car, pick-up truck or van in traffic accident

☑x7ᵗʰ **V63.7** Person on outside of heavy transport vehicle injured in collision with car, pick-up truck or van in traffic accident

☑x7ᵗʰ **V63.9** Unspecified occupant of heavy transport vehicle injured in collision with car, pick-up truck or van in traffic accident ▽

☑4ᵗʰ **V64** Occupant of heavy transport vehicle injured in collision with heavy transport vehicle or bus

> **EXCLUDES 1**   *occupant of heavy transport vehicle injured in collision with military vehicle (V69.81)*

☑x7ᵗʰ **V64.0** Driver of heavy transport vehicle injured in collision with heavy transport vehicle or bus in nontraffic accident

☑x7ᵗʰ **V64.1** Passenger in heavy transport vehicle injured in collision with heavy transport vehicle or bus in nontraffic accident

☑x7ᵗʰ **V64.2** Person on outside of heavy transport vehicle injured in collision with heavy transport vehicle or bus in nontraffic accident

☑x7ᵗʰ **V64.3** Unspecified occupant of heavy transport vehicle injured in collision with heavy transport vehicle or bus in nontraffic accident ▽

☑x7ᵗʰ **V64.4** Person boarding or alighting a heavy transport vehicle injured in collision with heavy transport vehicle or bus while boarding or alighting

☑x7ᵗʰ **V64.5** Driver of heavy transport vehicle injured in collision with heavy transport vehicle or bus in traffic accident

☑x7ᵗʰ **V64.6** Passenger in heavy transport vehicle injured in collision with heavy transport vehicle or bus in traffic accident

☑x7ᵗʰ **V64.7** Person on outside of heavy transport vehicle injured in collision with heavy transport vehicle or bus in traffic accident

☑x7ᵗʰ **V64.9** Unspecified occupant of heavy transport vehicle injured in collision with heavy transport vehicle or bus in traffic accident ▽

☑4ᵗʰ **V65** Occupant of heavy transport vehicle injured in collision with railway train or railway vehicle

☑x7ᵗʰ **V65.0** Driver of heavy transport vehicle injured in collision with railway train or railway vehicle in nontraffic accident

☑x7ᵗʰ **V65.1** Passenger in heavy transport vehicle injured in collision with railway train or railway vehicle in nontraffic accident

☑x7ᵗʰ **V65.2** Person on outside of heavy transport vehicle injured in collision with railway train or railway vehicle in nontraffic accident

☑x7ᵗʰ **V65.3** Unspecified occupant of heavy transport vehicle injured in collision with railway train or railway vehicle in nontraffic accident ▽

☑x7ᵗʰ **V65.4** Person boarding or alighting a heavy transport vehicle injured in collision with railway train or railway vehicle

☑x7ᵗʰ **V65.5** Driver of heavy transport vehicle injured in collision with railway train or railway vehicle in traffic accident

☑x7ᵗʰ **V65.6** Passenger in heavy transport vehicle injured in collision with railway train or railway vehicle in traffic accident

☑x7ᵗʰ **V65.7** Person on outside of heavy transport vehicle injured in collision with railway train or railway vehicle in traffic accident

☑x7ᵗʰ **V65.9** Unspecified occupant of heavy transport vehicle injured in collision with railway train or railway vehicle in traffic accident ▽

☑4ᵗʰ **V66** Occupant of heavy transport vehicle injured in collision with other nonmotor vehicle

> **INCLUDES**   collision with animal-drawn vehicle, animal being ridden, streetcar

☑x7ᵗʰ **V66.0** Driver of heavy transport vehicle injured in collision with other nonmotor vehicle in nontraffic accident

☑x7ᵗʰ **V66.1** Passenger in heavy transport vehicle injured in collision with other nonmotor vehicle in nontraffic accident

☑x7ᵗʰ **V66.2** Person on outside of heavy transport vehicle injured in collision with other nonmotor vehicle in nontraffic accident

☑x7ᵗʰ **V66.3** Unspecified occupant of heavy transport vehicle injured in ▽ collision with other nonmotor vehicle in nontraffic accident

---

☑ Additional Character Req   ☑x7ᵗʰ Placeholder Alert   Manifestation   HCC CMS-HCC Condition   ▽ Unspecified Code   ►◄ Revised Text   ● New Code   ▲ Revised Code Title

ICD-10-CM 2018   1131

√x7ᵗʰ **V66.4** Person boarding or alighting a heavy transport vehicle injured in collision with other nonmotor vehicle

√x7ᵗʰ **V66.5** Driver of heavy transport vehicle injured in collision with other nonmotor vehicle in traffic accident

√x7ᵗʰ **V66.6** Passenger in heavy transport vehicle injured in collision with other nonmotor vehicle in traffic accident

√x7ᵗʰ **V66.7** Person on outside of heavy transport vehicle injured in collision with other nonmotor vehicle in traffic accident

√x7ᵗʰ **V66.9** Unspecified occupant of heavy transport vehicle injured in collision with other nonmotor vehicle in traffic accident ▽

√4ᵗʰ **V67 Occupant of heavy transport vehicle injured in collision with fixed or stationary object**

√x7ᵗʰ **V67.0** Driver of heavy transport vehicle injured in collision with fixed or stationary object in nontraffic accident

√x7ᵗʰ **V67.1** Passenger in heavy transport vehicle injured in collision with fixed or stationary object in nontraffic accident

√x7ᵗʰ **V67.2** Person on outside of heavy transport vehicle injured in collision with fixed or stationary object in nontraffic accident

√x7ᵗʰ **V67.3** Unspecified occupant of heavy transport vehicle injured in collision with fixed or stationary object in nontraffic accident ▽

√x7ᵗʰ **V67.4** Person boarding or alighting a heavy transport vehicle injured in collision with fixed or stationary object

√x7ᵗʰ **V67.5** Driver of heavy transport vehicle injured in collision with fixed or stationary object in traffic accident

√x7ᵗʰ **V67.6** Passenger in heavy transport vehicle injured in collision with fixed or stationary object in traffic accident

√x7ᵗʰ **V67.7** Person on outside of heavy transport vehicle injured in collision with fixed or stationary object in traffic accident

√x7ᵗʰ **V67.9** Unspecified occupant of heavy transport vehicle injured in collision with fixed or stationary object in traffic accident ▽

√4ᵗʰ **V68 Occupant of heavy transport vehicle injured in noncollision transport accident**

    INCLUDES   overturning heavy transport vehicle NOS
            overturning heavy transport vehicle without collision

√x7ᵗʰ **V68.0** Driver of heavy transport vehicle injured in noncollision transport accident in nontraffic accident

√x7ᵗʰ **V68.1** Passenger in heavy transport vehicle injured in noncollision transport accident in nontraffic accident

√x7ᵗʰ **V68.2** Person on outside of heavy transport vehicle injured in noncollision transport accident in nontraffic accident

√x7ᵗʰ **V68.3** Unspecified occupant of heavy transport vehicle injured in noncollision transport accident in nontraffic accident ▽

√x7ᵗʰ **V68.4** Person boarding or alighting a heavy transport vehicle injured in noncollision transport accident

√x7ᵗʰ **V68.5** Driver of heavy transport vehicle injured in noncollision transport accident in traffic accident

√x7ᵗʰ **V68.6** Passenger in heavy transport vehicle injured in noncollision transport accident in traffic accident

√x7ᵗʰ **V68.7** Person on outside of heavy transport vehicle injured in noncollision transport accident in traffic accident

√x7ᵗʰ **V68.9** Unspecified occupant of heavy transport vehicle injured in noncollision transport accident in traffic accident ▽

√4ᵗʰ **V69 Occupant of heavy transport vehicle injured in other and unspecified transport accidents**

√5ᵗʰ **V69.0** Driver of heavy transport vehicle injured in collision with other and unspecified motor vehicles in nontraffic accident

√x7ᵗʰ **V69.00** Driver of heavy transport vehicle injured in collision with unspecified motor vehicles in nontraffic accident ▽

√x7ᵗʰ **V69.09** Driver of heavy transport vehicle injured in collision with other motor vehicles in nontraffic accident

√5ᵗʰ **V69.1** Passenger in heavy transport vehicle injured in collision with other and unspecified motor vehicles in nontraffic accident

√x7ᵗʰ **V69.10** Passenger in heavy transport vehicle injured in collision with unspecified motor vehicles in nontraffic accident ▽

√x7ᵗʰ **V69.19** Passenger in heavy transport vehicle injured in collision with other motor vehicles in nontraffic accident

√5ᵗʰ **V69.2** Unspecified occupant of heavy transport vehicle injured in collision with other and unspecified motor vehicles in nontraffic accident

√x7ᵗʰ **V69.20** Unspecified occupant of heavy transport vehicle injured in collision with unspecified motor vehicles in nontraffic accident ▽

     Collision NOS involving heavy transport vehicle, nontraffic

√x7ᵗʰ **V69.29** Unspecified occupant of heavy transport vehicle injured in collision with other motor vehicles in nontraffic accident ▽

√x7ᵗʰ **V69.3** Occupant (driver) (passenger) of heavy transport vehicle injured in unspecified nontraffic accident ▽

     Accident NOS involving heavy transport vehicle, nontraffic
     Occupant of heavy transport vehicle injured in nontraffic accident NOS

√5ᵗʰ **V69.4** Driver of heavy transport vehicle injured in collision with other and unspecified motor vehicles in traffic accident

√x7ᵗʰ **V69.40** Driver of heavy transport vehicle injured in collision with unspecified motor vehicles in traffic accident ▽

√x7ᵗʰ **V69.49** Driver of heavy transport vehicle injured in collision with other motor vehicles in traffic accident

√5ᵗʰ **V69.5** Passenger in heavy transport vehicle injured in collision with other and unspecified motor vehicles in traffic accident

√x7ᵗʰ **V69.50** Passenger in heavy transport vehicle injured in collision with unspecified motor vehicles in traffic accident ▽

√x7ᵗʰ **V69.59** Passenger in heavy transport vehicle injured in collision with other motor vehicles in traffic accident

√5ᵗʰ **V69.6** Unspecified occupant of heavy transport vehicle injured in collision with other and unspecified motor vehicles in traffic accident

√x7ᵗʰ **V69.60** Unspecified occupant of heavy transport vehicle injured in collision with unspecified motor vehicles in traffic accident ▽

     Collision NOS involving heavy transport vehicle (traffic)

√x7ᵗʰ **V69.69** Unspecified occupant of heavy transport vehicle injured in collision with other motor vehicles in traffic accident ▽

√5ᵗʰ **V69.8** Occupant (driver) (passenger) of heavy transport vehicle injured in other specified transport accidents

√x7ᵗʰ **V69.81** Occupant (driver) (passenger) of heavy transport vehicle injured in transport accidents with military vehicle

√x7ᵗʰ **V69.88** Occupant (driver) (passenger) of heavy transport vehicle injured in other specified transport accidents

√x7ᵗʰ **V69.9** Occupant (driver) (passenger) of heavy transport vehicle injured in unspecified traffic accident ▽

     Accident NOS involving heavy transport vehicle

Bus occupant injured in transport accident (V70-V79)

    INCLUDES   motorcoach
    EXCLUDES 1   minibus (V50-V59)

> The appropriate 7th character is to be added to each code from categories V70-V79.
> A   initial encounter
> D   subsequent encounter
> S   sequela

√4ᵗʰ **V70 Bus occupant injured in collision with pedestrian or animal**

    EXCLUDES 1   bus collision with animal-drawn vehicle or animal being ridden (V76.-)

√x7ᵗʰ **V70.0** Driver of bus injured in collision with pedestrian or animal in nontraffic accident

√x7ᵗʰ **V70.1** Passenger on bus injured in collision with pedestrian or animal in nontraffic accident

√x7ᵗʰ **V70.2** Person on outside of bus injured in collision with pedestrian or animal in nontraffic accident

√x7ᵗʰ **V70.3** Unspecified occupant of bus injured in collision with pedestrian or animal in nontraffic accident ▽

√x7ᵗʰ **V70.4** Person boarding or alighting from bus injured in collision with pedestrian or animal

√x7ᵗʰ **V70.5** Driver of bus injured in collision with pedestrian or animal in traffic accident

---

EXCLUDES 1 Not coded here   EXCLUDES 2 Not included here   N Newborn Age: 0   P Pediatric Age: 0-17   M Maternity Age: 12-55   A Adult Age: 15-124

✓x7ᵗʰ **V70.6** Passenger on bus injured in collision with pedestrian or animal in traffic accident

✓x7ᵗʰ **V70.7** Person on outside of bus injured in collision with pedestrian or animal in traffic accident

✓x7ᵗʰ **V70.9** Unspecified occupant of bus injured in collision with pedestrian or animal in traffic accident ▽

✓4ᵗʰ **V71** Bus occupant injured in collision with pedal cycle

✓x7ᵗʰ **V71.0** Driver of bus injured in collision with pedal cycle in nontraffic accident

✓x7ᵗʰ **V71.1** Passenger on bus injured in collision with pedal cycle in nontraffic accident

✓x7ᵗʰ **V71.2** Person on outside of bus injured in collision with pedal cycle in nontraffic accident

✓x7ᵗʰ **V71.3** Unspecified occupant of bus injured in collision with pedal cycle in nontraffic accident ▽

✓x7ᵗʰ **V71.4** Person boarding or alighting from bus injured in collision with pedal cycle

✓x7ᵗʰ **V71.5** Driver of bus injured in collision with pedal cycle in traffic accident

✓x7ᵗʰ **V71.6** Passenger on bus injured in collision with pedal cycle in traffic accident

✓x7ᵗʰ **V71.7** Person on outside of bus injured in collision with pedal cycle in traffic accident

✓x7ᵗʰ **V71.9** Unspecified occupant of bus injured in collision with pedal cycle in traffic accident ▽

✓4ᵗʰ **V72** Bus occupant injured in collision with two- or three-wheeled motor vehicle

✓x7ᵗʰ **V72.0** Driver of bus injured in collision with two- or three-wheeled motor vehicle in nontraffic accident

✓x7ᵗʰ **V72.1** Passenger on bus injured in collision with two- or three-wheeled motor vehicle in nontraffic accident

✓x7ᵗʰ **V72.2** Person on outside of bus injured in collision with two- or three-wheeled motor vehicle in nontraffic accident

✓x7ᵗʰ **V72.3** Unspecified occupant of bus injured in collision with two- or three-wheeled motor vehicle in nontraffic accident ▽

✓x7ᵗʰ **V72.4** Person boarding or alighting from bus injured in collision with two- or three-wheeled motor vehicle

✓x7ᵗʰ **V72.5** Driver of bus injured in collision with two- or three-wheeled motor vehicle in traffic accident

✓x7ᵗʰ **V72.6** Passenger on bus injured in collision with two- or three-wheeled motor vehicle in traffic accident

✓x7ᵗʰ **V72.7** Person on outside of bus injured in collision with two- or three-wheeled motor vehicle in traffic accident

✓x7ᵗʰ **V72.9** Unspecified occupant of bus injured in collision with two- or three-wheeled motor vehicle in traffic accident ▽

✓4ᵗʰ **V73** Bus occupant injured in collision with car, pick-up truck or van

✓x7ᵗʰ **V73.0** Driver of bus injured in collision with car, pick-up truck or van in nontraffic accident

✓x7ᵗʰ **V73.1** Passenger on bus injured in collision with car, pick-up truck or van in nontraffic accident

✓x7ᵗʰ **V73.2** Person on outside of bus injured in collision with car, pick-up truck or van in nontraffic accident

✓x7ᵗʰ **V73.3** Unspecified occupant of bus injured in collision with car, pick-up truck or van in nontraffic accident ▽

✓x7ᵗʰ **V73.4** Person boarding or alighting from bus injured in collision with car, pick-up truck or van

✓x7ᵗʰ **V73.5** Driver of bus injured in collision with car, pick-up truck or van in traffic accident

✓x7ᵗʰ **V73.6** Passenger on bus injured in collision with car, pick-up truck or van in traffic accident

✓x7ᵗʰ **V73.7** Person on outside of bus injured in collision with car, pick-up truck or van in traffic accident

✓x7ᵗʰ **V73.9** Unspecified occupant of bus injured in collision with car, pick-up truck or van in traffic accident ▽

✓4ᵗʰ **V74** Bus occupant injured in collision with heavy transport vehicle or bus

EXCLUDES 1   bus occupant injured in collision with military vehicle (V79.81)

✓x7ᵗʰ **V74.0** Driver of bus injured in collision with heavy transport vehicle or bus in nontraffic accident

✓x7ᵗʰ **V74.1** Passenger on bus injured in collision with heavy transport vehicle or bus in nontraffic accident

✓x7ᵗʰ **V74.2** Person on outside of bus injured in collision with heavy transport vehicle or bus in nontraffic accident

✓x7ᵗʰ **V74.3** Unspecified occupant of bus injured in collision with heavy transport vehicle or bus in nontraffic accident ▽

✓x7ᵗʰ **V74.4** Person boarding or alighting from bus injured in collision with heavy transport vehicle or bus

✓x7ᵗʰ **V74.5** Driver of bus injured in collision with heavy transport vehicle or bus in traffic accident

✓x7ᵗʰ **V74.6** Passenger on bus injured in collision with heavy transport vehicle or bus in traffic accident

✓x7ᵗʰ **V74.7** Person on outside of bus injured in collision with heavy transport vehicle or bus in traffic accident

✓x7ᵗʰ **V74.9** Unspecified occupant of bus injured in collision with heavy transport vehicle or bus in traffic accident ▽

✓4ᵗʰ **V75** Bus occupant injured in collision with railway train or railway vehicle

✓x7ᵗʰ **V75.0** Driver of bus injured in collision with railway train or railway vehicle in nontraffic accident

✓x7ᵗʰ **V75.1** Passenger on bus injured in collision with railway train or railway vehicle in nontraffic accident

✓x7ᵗʰ **V75.2** Person on outside of bus injured in collision with railway train or railway vehicle in nontraffic accident

✓x7ᵗʰ **V75.3** Unspecified occupant of bus injured in collision with railway train or railway vehicle in nontraffic accident ▽

✓x7ᵗʰ **V75.4** Person boarding or alighting from bus injured in collision with railway train or railway vehicle

✓x7ᵗʰ **V75.5** Driver of bus injured in collision with railway train or railway vehicle in traffic accident

✓x7ᵗʰ **V75.6** Passenger on bus injured in collision with railway train or railway vehicle in traffic accident

✓x7ᵗʰ **V75.7** Person on outside of bus injured in collision with railway train or railway vehicle in traffic accident

✓x7ᵗʰ **V75.9** Unspecified occupant of bus injured in collision with railway train or railway vehicle in traffic accident ▽

✓4ᵗʰ **V76** Bus occupant injured in collision with other nonmotor vehicle

INCLUDES   collision with animal-drawn vehicle, animal being ridden, streetcar

✓x7ᵗʰ **V76.0** Driver of bus injured in collision with other nonmotor vehicle in nontraffic accident

✓x7ᵗʰ **V76.1** Passenger on bus injured in collision with other nonmotor vehicle in nontraffic accident

✓x7ᵗʰ **V76.2** Person on outside of bus injured in collision with other nonmotor vehicle in nontraffic accident

✓x7ᵗʰ **V76.3** Unspecified occupant of bus injured in collision with other nonmotor vehicle in nontraffic accident ▽

✓x7ᵗʰ **V76.4** Person boarding or alighting from bus injured in collision with other nonmotor vehicle

✓x7ᵗʰ **V76.5** Driver of bus injured in collision with other nonmotor vehicle in traffic accident

✓x7ᵗʰ **V76.6** Passenger on bus injured in collision with other nonmotor vehicle in traffic accident

✓x7ᵗʰ **V76.7** Person on outside of bus injured in collision with other nonmotor vehicle in traffic accident

✓x7ᵗʰ **V76.9** Unspecified occupant of bus injured in collision with other nonmotor vehicle in traffic accident ▽

✓4ᵗʰ **V77** Bus occupant injured in collision with fixed or stationary object

✓x7ᵗʰ **V77.0** Driver of bus injured in collision with fixed or stationary object in nontraffic accident

✓x7ᵗʰ **V77.1** Passenger on bus injured in collision with fixed or stationary object in nontraffic accident

✓x7ᵗʰ **V77.2** Person on outside of bus injured in collision with fixed or stationary object in nontraffic accident

✓x7ᵗʰ **V77.3** Unspecified occupant of bus injured in collision with fixed or stationary object in nontraffic accident ▽

✓x7ᵗʰ **V77.4** Person boarding or alighting from bus injured in collision with fixed or stationary object

✓x7ᵗʰ **V77.5** Driver of bus injured in collision with fixed or stationary object in traffic accident

✓x7ᵗʰ **V77.6** Passenger on bus injured in collision with fixed or stationary object in traffic accident

✓x7ᵗʰ **V77.7** Person on outside of bus injured in collision with fixed or stationary object in traffic accident

✓x7ᵗʰ **V77.9** Unspecified occupant of bus injured in collision with fixed or stationary object in traffic accident ▽

✓ Additional Character Req   ✓x7ᵗʰ Placeholder Alert   Manifestation   HCC CMS-HCC Condition   ▽ Unspecified Code   ►◄ Revised Text   ● New Code   ▲ Revised Code Title

Chapter 20. External Causes of Morbidity

✓4ᵗʰ **V78** **Bus occupant injured in noncollision transport accident**
INCLUDES   overturning bus NOS
overturning bus without collision

✓x7ᵗʰ **V78.0** Driver of bus injured in noncollision transport accident in nontraffic accident

✓x7ᵗʰ **V78.1** Passenger on bus injured in noncollision transport accident in nontraffic accident

✓x7ᵗʰ **V78.2** Person on outside of bus injured in noncollision transport accident in nontraffic accident

✓x7ᵗʰ **V78.3** Unspecified occupant of bus injured in noncollision transport accident in nontraffic accident ▽

✓x7ᵗʰ **V78.4** Person boarding or alighting from bus injured in noncollision transport accident

✓x7ᵗʰ **V78.5** Driver of bus injured in noncollision transport accident in traffic accident

✓x7ᵗʰ **V78.6** Passenger on bus injured in noncollision transport accident in traffic accident

✓x7ᵗʰ **V78.7** Person on outside of bus injured in noncollision transport accident in traffic accident

✓x7ᵗʰ **V78.9** Unspecified occupant of bus injured in noncollision transport accident in traffic accident ▽

✓4ᵗʰ **V79** **Bus occupant injured in other and unspecified transport accidents**

✓5ᵗʰ **V79.0** Driver of bus injured in collision with other and unspecified motor vehicles in nontraffic accident

✓x7ᵗʰ **V79.00** Driver of bus injured in collision with unspecified motor vehicles in nontraffic accident ▽

✓x7ᵗʰ **V79.09** Driver of bus injured in collision with other motor vehicles in nontraffic accident

✓5ᵗʰ **V79.1** Passenger on bus injured in collision with other and unspecified motor vehicles in nontraffic accident

✓x7ᵗʰ **V79.10** Passenger on bus injured in collision with unspecified motor vehicles in nontraffic accident ▽

✓x7ᵗʰ **V79.19** Passenger on bus injured in collision with other motor vehicles in nontraffic accident

✓5ᵗʰ **V79.2** Unspecified bus occupant injured in collision with other and unspecified motor vehicles in nontraffic accident

✓x7ᵗʰ **V79.20** Unspecified bus occupant injured in collision with unspecified motor vehicles in nontraffic accident ▽
Bus collision NOS, nontraffic

✓x7ᵗʰ **V79.29** Unspecified bus occupant injured in collision with other motor vehicles in nontraffic accident ▽

✓x7ᵗʰ **V79.3** Bus occupant (driver) (passenger) injured in unspecified nontraffic accident ▽
Bus accident NOS, nontraffic
Bus occupant injured in nontraffic accident NOS

✓5ᵗʰ **V79.4** Driver of bus injured in collision with other and unspecified motor vehicles in traffic accident

✓x7ᵗʰ **V79.40** Driver of bus injured in collision with unspecified motor vehicles in traffic accident ▽

✓x7ᵗʰ **V79.49** Driver of bus injured in collision with other motor vehicles in traffic accident

✓5ᵗʰ **V79.5** Passenger on bus injured in collision with other and unspecified motor vehicles in traffic accident

✓x7ᵗʰ **V79.50** Passenger on bus injured in collision with unspecified motor vehicles in traffic accident ▽

✓x7ᵗʰ **V79.59** Passenger on bus injured in collision with other motor vehicles in traffic accident

✓5ᵗʰ **V79.6** Unspecified bus occupant injured in collision with other and unspecified motor vehicles in traffic accident

✓x7ᵗʰ **V79.60** Unspecified bus occupant injured in collision with unspecified motor vehicles in traffic accident ▽
Bus collision NOS (traffic)

✓x7ᵗʰ **V79.69** Unspecified bus occupant injured in collision with other motor vehicles in traffic accident ▽

✓5ᵗʰ **V79.8** Bus occupant (driver) (passenger) injured in other specified transport accidents

✓x7ᵗʰ **V79.81** Bus occupant (driver) (passenger) injured in transport accidents with military vehicle

✓x7ᵗʰ **V79.88** Bus occupant (driver) (passenger) injured in other specified transport accidents

✓x7ᵗʰ **V79.9** Bus occupant (driver) (passenger) injured in unspecified traffic accident ▽
Bus accident NOS

Other land transport accidents (V80-V89)

The appropriate 7th character is to be added to each code from categories V80-V89.
A   initial encounter
D   subsequent encounter
S   sequela

✓4ᵗʰ **V80** **Animal-rider or occupant of animal-drawn vehicle injured in transport accident**

✓5ᵗʰ **V80.0** Animal-rider or occupant of animal drawn vehicle injured by fall from or being thrown from animal or animal-drawn vehicle in noncollision accident

✓6ᵗʰ **V80.01** Animal-rider injured by fall from or being thrown from animal in noncollision accident

✓7ᵗʰ **V80.010** Animal-rider injured by fall from or being thrown from horse in noncollision accident

✓7ᵗʰ **V80.018** Animal-rider injured by fall from or being thrown from other animal in noncollision accident

✓x7ᵗʰ **V80.02** Occupant of animal-drawn vehicle injured by fall from or being thrown from animal-drawn vehicle in noncollision accident
Overturning animal-drawn vehicle NOS
Overturning animal-drawn vehicle without collision

✓5ᵗʰ **V80.1** Animal-rider or occupant of animal-drawn vehicle injured in collision with pedestrian or animal
EXCLUDES1   animal-rider or animal-drawn vehicle collision with animal-drawn vehicle or animal being ridden (V80.7)

✓x7ᵗʰ **V80.11** Animal-rider injured in collision with pedestrian or animal

✓x7ᵗʰ **V80.12** Occupant of animal-drawn vehicle injured in collision with pedestrian or animal

✓5ᵗʰ **V80.2** Animal-rider or occupant of animal-drawn vehicle injured in collision with pedal cycle

✓x7ᵗʰ **V80.21** Animal-rider injured in collision with pedal cycle

✓x7ᵗʰ **V80.22** Occupant of animal-drawn vehicle injured in collision with pedal cycle

✓5ᵗʰ **V80.3** Animal-rider or occupant of animal-drawn vehicle injured in collision with two- or three-wheeled motor vehicle

✓x7ᵗʰ **V80.31** Animal-rider injured in collision with two- or three-wheeled motor vehicle

✓x7ᵗʰ **V80.32** Occupant of animal-drawn vehicle injured in collision with two- or three-wheeled motor vehicle

✓5ᵗʰ **V80.4** Animal-rider or occupant of animal-drawn vehicle injured in collision with car, pick-up truck, van, heavy transport vehicle or bus
EXCLUDES1   animal-rider injured in collision with military vehicle (V80.910)
occupant of animal-drawn vehicle injured in collision with military vehicle (V80.920)

✓x7ᵗʰ **V80.41** Animal-rider injured in collision with car, pick-up truck, van, heavy transport vehicle or bus

✓x7ᵗʰ **V80.42** Occupant of animal-drawn vehicle injured in collision with car, pick-up truck, van, heavy transport vehicle or bus

✓5ᵗʰ **V80.5** Animal-rider or occupant of animal-drawn vehicle injured in collision with other specified motor vehicle

✓x7ᵗʰ **V80.51** Animal-rider injured in collision with other specified motor vehicle

✓x7ᵗʰ **V80.52** Occupant of animal-drawn vehicle injured in collision with other specified motor vehicle

✓5ᵗʰ **V80.6** Animal-rider or occupant of animal-drawn vehicle injured in collision with railway train or railway vehicle

✓x7ᵗʰ **V80.61** Animal-rider injured in collision with railway train or railway vehicle

✓x7ᵗʰ **V80.62** Occupant of animal-drawn vehicle injured in collision with railway train or railway vehicle

✓5ᵗʰ **V80.7** Animal-rider or occupant of animal-drawn vehicle injured in collision with other nonmotor vehicles

✓6ᵗʰ **V80.71** Animal-rider or occupant of animal-drawn vehicle injured in collision with animal being ridden

✓7ᵗʰ **V80.710** Animal-rider injured in collision with other animal being ridden

EXCLUDES1 Not coded here   EXCLUDES2 Not included here   N Newborn Age: 0   P Pediatric Age: 0-17   M Maternity Age: 12-55   A Adult Age: 15-124

1134   ICD-10-CM 2018

☑7ᵗʰ **V80.711** Occupant of animal-drawn vehicle injured in collision with animal being ridden

✓6ᵗʰ **V80.72** Animal-rider or occupant of animal-drawn vehicle injured in collision with other animal-drawn vehicle

☑7ᵗʰ **V80.720** Animal-rider injured in collision with animal-drawn vehicle

☑7ᵗʰ **V80.721** Occupant of animal-drawn vehicle injured in collision with other animal-drawn vehicle

✓6ᵗʰ **V80.73** Animal-rider or occupant of animal-drawn vehicle injured in collision with streetcar

☑7ᵗʰ **V80.730** Animal-rider injured in collision with streetcar

☑7ᵗʰ **V80.731** Occupant of animal-drawn vehicle injured in collision with streetcar

✓6ᵗʰ **V80.79** Animal-rider or occupant of animal-drawn vehicle injured in collision with other nonmotor vehicles

☑7ᵗʰ **V80.790** Animal-rider injured in collision with other nonmotor vehicles

☑7ᵗʰ **V80.791** Occupant of animal-drawn vehicle injured in collision with other nonmotor vehicles

✓5ᵗʰ **V80.8** Animal-rider or occupant of animal-drawn vehicle injured in collision with fixed or stationary object

✓x7ᵗʰ **V80.81** Animal-rider injured in collision with fixed or stationary object

✓x7ᵗʰ **V80.82** Occupant of animal-drawn vehicle injured in collision with fixed or stationary object

✓5ᵗʰ **V80.9** Animal-rider or occupant of animal-drawn vehicle injured in other and unspecified transport accidents

✓6ᵗʰ **V80.91** Animal-rider injured in other and unspecified transport accidents

☑7ᵗʰ **V80.910** Animal-rider injured in transport accident with military vehicle

☑7ᵗʰ **V80.918** Animal-rider injured in other transport accident

☑7ᵗʰ **V80.919** Animal-rider injured in unspecified ▽ transport accident
Animal rider accident NOS

✓6ᵗʰ **V80.92** Occupant of animal-drawn vehicle injured in other and unspecified transport accidents

☑7ᵗʰ **V80.920** Occupant of animal-drawn vehicle injured in transport accident with military vehicle

☑7ᵗʰ **V80.928** Occupant of animal-drawn vehicle injured in other transport accident

☑7ᵗʰ **V80.929** Occupant of animal-drawn vehicle ▽ injured in unspecified transport accident
Animal-drawn vehicle accident NOS

☑4ᵗʰ **V81** Occupant of railway train or railway vehicle injured in transport accident
INCLUDES derailment of railway train or railway vehicle
person on outside of train
EXCLUDES1 streetcar (V82.-)

✓x7ᵗʰ **V81.0** Occupant of railway train or railway vehicle injured in collision with motor vehicle in nontraffic accident
EXCLUDES1 occupant of railway train or railway vehicle injured due to collision with military vehicle (V81.83)

✓x7ᵗʰ **V81.1** Occupant of railway train or railway vehicle injured in collision with motor vehicle in traffic accident
EXCLUDES1 occupant of railway train or railway vehicle injured due to collision with military vehicle (V81.83)

✓x7ᵗʰ **V81.2** Occupant of railway train or railway vehicle injured in collision with or hit by rolling stock

✓x7ᵗʰ **V81.3** Occupant of railway train or railway vehicle injured in collision with other object
Railway collision NOS

✓x7ᵗʰ **V81.4** Person injured while boarding or alighting from railway train or railway vehicle

✓x7ᵗʰ **V81.5** Occupant of railway train or railway vehicle injured by fall in railway train or railway vehicle

✓x7ᵗʰ **V81.6** Occupant of railway train or railway vehicle injured by fall from railway train or railway vehicle

✓x7ᵗʰ **V81.7** Occupant of railway train or railway vehicle injured in derailment without antecedent collision

✓5ᵗʰ **V81.8** Occupant of railway train or railway vehicle injured in other specified railway accidents

✓x7ᵗʰ **V81.81** Occupant of railway train or railway vehicle injured due to explosion or fire on train

✓x7ᵗʰ **V81.82** Occupant of railway train or railway vehicle injured due to object falling onto train
Occupant of railway train or railway vehicle injured due to falling earth onto train
Occupant of railway train or railway vehicle injured due to falling rocks onto train
Occupant of railway train or railway vehicle injured due to falling snow onto train
Occupant of railway train or railway vehicle injured due to falling trees onto train

✓x7ᵗʰ **V81.83** Occupant of railway train or railway vehicle injured due to collision with military vehicle

✓x7ᵗʰ **V81.89** Occupant of railway train or railway vehicle injured due to other specified railway accident

✓x7ᵗʰ **V81.9** Occupant of railway train or railway vehicle injured in ▽ unspecified railway accident
Railway accident NOS

☑4ᵗʰ **V82** Occupant of powered streetcar injured in transport accident
INCLUDES interurban electric car
person on outside of streetcar
tram (car)
trolley (car)
EXCLUDES1 bus (V70-V79)
motorcoach (V70-V79)
nonpowered streetcar (V76.-)
train (V81.-)

✓x7ᵗʰ **V82.0** Occupant of streetcar injured in collision with motor vehicle in nontraffic accident

✓x7ᵗʰ **V82.1** Occupant of streetcar injured in collision with motor vehicle in traffic accident

✓x7ᵗʰ **V82.2** Occupant of streetcar injured in collision with or hit by rolling stock

✓x7ᵗʰ **V82.3** Occupant of streetcar injured in collision with other object
EXCLUDES1 collision with animal-drawn vehicle or animal being ridden (V82.8)

✓x7ᵗʰ **V82.4** Person injured while boarding or alighting from streetcar

✓x7ᵗʰ **V82.5** Occupant of streetcar injured by fall in streetcar
EXCLUDES1 fall in streetcar:
while boarding or alighting (V82.4)
with antecedent collision (V82.0-V82.3)

✓x7ᵗʰ **V82.6** Occupant of streetcar injured by fall from streetcar
EXCLUDES1 fall from streetcar:
while boarding or alighting (V82.4)
with antecedent collision (V82.0-V82.3)

✓x7ᵗʰ **V82.7** Occupant of streetcar injured in derailment without antecedent collision
EXCLUDES1 occupant of streetcar injured in derailment with antecedent collision (V82.0-V82.3)

✓x7ᵗʰ **V82.8** Occupant of streetcar injured in other specified transport accidents
Streetcar collision with military vehicle
Streetcar collision with train or nonmotor vehicles

✓x7ᵗʰ **V82.9** Occupant of streetcar injured in unspecified traffic ▽ accident
Streetcar accident NOS

☑4ᵗʰ **V83** Occupant of special vehicle mainly used on industrial premises injured in transport accident
INCLUDES battery-powered airport passenger vehicle
battery-powered truck (baggage) (mail)
coal-car in mine
forklift (truck)
logging car
self-propelled industrial truck
station baggage truck (powered)
tram, truck, or tub (powered) in mine or quarry
EXCLUDES1 special construction vehicles (V85.-)
special industrial vehicle in stationary use or maintenance (W31.-)

✓x7ᵗʰ **V83.0** Driver of special industrial vehicle injured in traffic accident

✓x7ᵗʰ **V83.1** Passenger of special industrial vehicle injured in traffic accident

✓x7ᵗʰ **V83.2** Person on outside of special industrial vehicle injured in traffic accident

√x7ᵗʰ **V83.3** Unspecified occupant of special industrial vehicle injured in traffic accident ▽

√x7ᵗʰ **V83.4** Person injured while boarding or alighting from special industrial vehicle

√x7ᵗʰ **V83.5** Driver of special industrial vehicle injured in nontraffic accident

√x7ᵗʰ **V83.6** Passenger of special industrial vehicle injured in nontraffic accident

√x7ᵗʰ **V83.7** Person on outside of special industrial vehicle injured in nontraffic accident

√x7ᵗʰ **V83.9** Unspecified occupant of special industrial vehicle injured in nontraffic accident ▽
Special-industrial-vehicle accident NOS

√4ᵗʰ **V84** Occupant of special vehicle mainly used in agriculture injured in transport accident
INCLUDES self-propelled farm machinery
tractor (and trailer)
EXCLUDES 1 animal-powered farm machinery accident (W30.8-)
contact with combine harvester (W30.0)
special agricultural vehicle in stationary use or maintenance (W30.-)

√x7ᵗʰ **V84.0** Driver of special agricultural vehicle injured in traffic accident

√x7ᵗʰ **V84.1** Passenger of special agricultural vehicle injured in traffic accident

√x7ᵗʰ **V84.2** Person on outside of special agricultural vehicle injured in traffic accident

√x7ᵗʰ **V84.3** Unspecified occupant of special agricultural vehicle injured in traffic accident ▽

√x7ᵗʰ **V84.4** Person injured while boarding or alighting from special agricultural vehicle

√x7ᵗʰ **V84.5** Driver of special agricultural vehicle injured in nontraffic accident

√x7ᵗʰ **V84.6** Passenger of special agricultural vehicle injured in nontraffic accident

√x7ᵗʰ **V84.7** Person on outside of special agricultural vehicle injured in nontraffic accident

√x7ᵗʰ **V84.9** Unspecified occupant of special agricultural vehicle injured in nontraffic accident ▽
Special-agricultural vehicle accident NOS

√4ᵗʰ **V85** Occupant of special construction vehicle injured in transport accident
INCLUDES bulldozer
digger
dump truck
earth-leveller
mechanical shovel
road-roller
EXCLUDES 1 special industrial vehicle (V83.-)
special construction vehicle in stationary use or maintenance (W31.-)

√x7ᵗʰ **V85.0** Driver of special construction vehicle injured in traffic accident

√x7ᵗʰ **V85.1** Passenger of special construction vehicle injured in traffic accident

√x7ᵗʰ **V85.2** Person on outside of special construction vehicle injured in traffic accident

√x7ᵗʰ **V85.3** Unspecified occupant of special construction vehicle injured in traffic accident ▽

√x7ᵗʰ **V85.4** Person injured while boarding or alighting from special construction vehicle

√x7ᵗʰ **V85.5** Driver of special construction vehicle injured in nontraffic accident

√x7ᵗʰ **V85.6** Passenger of special construction vehicle injured in nontraffic accident

√x7ᵗʰ **V85.7** Person on outside of special construction vehicle injured in nontraffic accident

√x7ᵗʰ **V85.9** Unspecified occupant of special construction vehicle injured in nontraffic accident ▽
Special-construction-vehicle accident NOS

√4ᵗʰ **V86** Occupant of special all-terrain or other off-road motor vehicle, injured in transport accident
EXCLUDES 1 special all-terrain vehicle in stationary use or maintenance (W31.-)
sport-utility vehicle (V50-V59)
three-wheeled motor vehicle designed for on-road use (V30-V39)

√5ᵗʰ **V86.0** Driver of special all-terrain or other off-road motor vehicle injured in traffic accident

√x7ᵗʰ **V86.01** Driver of ambulance or fire engine injured in traffic accident

√x7ᵗʰ **V86.02** Driver of snowmobile injured in traffic accident

√x7ᵗʰ **V86.03** Driver of dune buggy injured in traffic accident

√x7ᵗʰ **V86.04** Driver of military vehicle injured in traffic accident

√x7ᵗʰ **V86.05** Driver of 3- or 4- wheeled all-terrain vehicle (ATV) injured in traffic accident

√x7ᵗʰ **V86.06** Driver of dirt bike or motor/cross bike injured in traffic accident

√x7ᵗʰ **V86.09** Driver of other special all-terrain or other off-road motor vehicle injured in traffic accident
Driver of dirt bike injured in traffic accident
Driver of go cart injured in traffic accident
Driver of golf cart injured in traffic accident

√5ᵗʰ **V86.1** Passenger of special all-terrain or other off-road motor vehicle injured in traffic accident

√x7ᵗʰ **V86.11** Passenger of ambulance or fire engine injured in traffic accident

√x7ᵗʰ **V86.12** Passenger of snowmobile injured in traffic accident

√x7ᵗʰ **V86.13** Passenger of dune buggy injured in traffic accident

√x7ᵗʰ **V86.14** Passenger of military vehicle injured in traffic accident

√x7ᵗʰ **V86.15** Passenger of 3- or 4- wheeled all-terrain vehicle (ATV) injured in traffic accident

√x7ᵗʰ **V86.16** Passenger of dirt bike or motor/cross bike injured in traffic accident

√x7ᵗʰ **V86.19** Passenger of other special all-terrain or other off-road motor vehicle injured in traffic accident
Passenger of dirt bike injured in traffic accident
Passenger of go cart injured in traffic accident
Passenger of golf cart injured in traffic accident

√5ᵗʰ **V86.2** Person on outside of special all-terrain or other off-road motor vehicle injured in traffic accident

√x7ᵗʰ **V86.21** Person on outside of ambulance or fire engine injured in traffic accident

√x7ᵗʰ **V86.22** Person on outside of snowmobile injured in traffic accident

√x7ᵗʰ **V86.23** Person on outside of dune buggy injured in traffic accident

√x7ᵗʰ **V86.24** Person on outside of military vehicle injured in traffic accident

√x7ᵗʰ **V86.25** Person on outside of 3- or 4- wheeled all-terrain vehicle (ATV) injured in traffic accident

√x7ᵗʰ **V86.26** Person on outside of dirt bike or motor/cross bike injured in traffic accident

√x7ᵗʰ **V86.29** Person on outside of other special all-terrain or other off-road motor vehicle injured in traffic accident
Person on outside of dirt bike injured in traffic accident
Person on outside of go cart in traffic accident
Person on outside of golf cart injured in traffic accident

√5ᵗʰ **V86.3** Unspecified occupant of special all-terrain or other off-road motor vehicle injured in traffic accident

√x7ᵗʰ **V86.31** Unspecified occupant of ambulance or fire engine injured in traffic accident ▽

√x7ᵗʰ **V86.32** Unspecified occupant of snowmobile injured in traffic accident ▽

√x7ᵗʰ **V86.33** Unspecified occupant of dune buggy injured in traffic accident ▽

√x7ᵗʰ **V86.34** Unspecified occupant of military vehicle injured in traffic accident ▽

√x7ᵗʰ **V86.35** Unspecified occupant of 3- or 4- wheeled all-terrain vehicle (ATV) injured in traffic accident ▽

√x7ᵗʰ **V86.36** Unspecified occupant of dirt bike or motor/cross bike injured in traffic accident ▽

☑x7ᵗʰ **V86.39** Unspecified occupant of other special all-terrain or other off-road motor vehicle injured in traffic accident ▽

     Unspecified occupant of dirt bike injured in traffic accident
     Unspecified occupant of go cart injured in traffic accident
     Unspecified occupant of golf cart injured in traffic accident

☑5ᵗʰ **V86.4** **Person injured while** boarding or alighting **from special all-terrain or other off-road motor vehicle**

☑x7ᵗʰ **V86.41** Person injured while boarding or alighting from ambulance or fire engine

☑x7ᵗʰ **V86.42** Person injured while boarding or alighting from snowmobile

☑x7ᵗʰ **V86.43** Person injured while boarding or alighting from dune buggy

☑x7ᵗʰ **V86.44** Person injured while boarding or alighting from military vehicle

● ☑x7ᵗʰ **V86.45** Person injured while boarding or alighting from a 3- or 4- wheeled all-terrain vehicle (ATV)

● ☑x7ᵗʰ **V86.46** Person injured while boarding or alighting from a dirt bike or motor/cross bike

☑x7ᵗʰ **V86.49** Person injured while boarding or alighting from other special all-terrain or other off-road motor vehicle
     Person injured while boarding or alighting from dirt bike
     Person injured while boarding or alighting from go cart
     Person injured while boarding or alighting from golf cart

☑5ᵗʰ **V86.5** Driver **of special all-terrain or other off-road motor vehicle** injured **in nontraffic accident**

☑x7ᵗʰ **V86.51** Driver of ambulance or fire engine injured in nontraffic accident

☑x7ᵗʰ **V86.52** Driver of snowmobile injured in nontraffic accident

☑x7ᵗʰ **V86.53** Driver of dune buggy injured in nontraffic accident

☑x7ᵗʰ **V86.54** Driver of military vehicle injured in nontraffic accident

● ☑x7ᵗʰ **V86.55** Driver of 3- or 4- wheeled all-terrain vehicle (ATV) injured in nontraffic accident

● ☑x7ᵗʰ **V86.56** Driver of dirt bike or motor/cross bike injured in nontraffic accident

☑x7ᵗʰ **V86.59** Driver of other special all-terrain or other off-road motor vehicle injured in nontraffic accident
     Driver of dirt bike injured in nontraffic accident
     Driver of go cart injured in nontraffic accident
     Driver of golf cart injured in nontraffic accident

☑5ᵗʰ **V86.6** Passenger **of special all-terrain or other off-road motor vehicle injured** in nontraffic accident

☑x7ᵗʰ **V86.61** Passenger of ambulance or fire engine injured in nontraffic accident

☑x7ᵗʰ **V86.62** Passenger of snowmobile injured in nontraffic accident

☑x7ᵗʰ **V86.63** Passenger of dune buggy injured in nontraffic accident

☑x7ᵗʰ **V86.64** Passenger of military vehicle injured in nontraffic accident

● ☑x7ᵗʰ **V86.65** Passenger of 3- or 4- wheeled all-terrain vehicle (ATV) injured in nontraffic accident

● ☑x7ᵗʰ **V86.66** Passenger of dirt bike or motor/cross bike injured in nontraffic accident

☑x7ᵗʰ **V86.69** Passenger of other special all-terrain or other off-road motor vehicle injured in nontraffic accident
     Passenger of dirt bike injured in nontraffic accident
     Passenger of go cart injured in nontraffic accident
     Passenger of golf cart injured in nontraffic accident

☑5ᵗʰ **V86.7** Person on outside **of special all-terrain or other off-road motor vehicle injured** in nontraffic accident

☑x7ᵗʰ **V86.71** Person on outside of ambulance or fire engine injured in nontraffic accident

☑x7ᵗʰ **V86.72** Person on outside of snowmobile injured in nontraffic accident

☑x7ᵗʰ **V86.73** Person on outside of dune buggy injured in nontraffic accident

☑x7ᵗʰ **V86.74** Person on outside of military vehicle injured in nontraffic accident

● ☑x7ᵗʰ **V86.75** Person on outside of 3- or 4- wheeled all-terrain vehicle (ATV) injured in nontraffic accident

● ☑x7ᵗʰ **V86.76** Person on outside of dirt bike or motor/cross bike injured in nontraffic accident

☑x7ᵗʰ **V86.79** Person on outside of other special all-terrain or other off-road motor vehicles injured in nontraffic accident
     Person on outside of dirt bike injured in nontraffic accident
     Person on outside of go cart injured in nontraffic accident
     Person on outside of golf cart injured in nontraffic accident

☑5ᵗʰ **V86.9** **Unspecified occupant of special all-terrain or other off-road motor vehicle injured** in nontraffic accident

☑x7ᵗʰ **V86.91** Unspecified occupant of ambulance or fire engine injured in nontraffic accident ▽

☑x7ᵗʰ **V86.92** Unspecified occupant of snowmobile injured in nontraffic accident ▽

☑x7ᵗʰ **V86.93** Unspecified occupant of dune buggy injured in nontraffic accident ▽

☑x7ᵗʰ **V86.94** Unspecified occupant of military vehicle injured in nontraffic accident ▽

● ☑x7ᵗʰ **V86.95** Unspecified occupant of 3- or 4- wheeled all-terrain vehicle (ATV) injured in nontraffic accident ▽

● ☑x7ᵗʰ **V86.96** Unspecified occupant of dirt bike or motor/cross bike injured in nontraffic accident ▽

☑x7ᵗʰ **V86.99** Unspecified occupant of other special all-terrain or other off-road motor vehicle injured in nontraffic accident ▽
     All-terrain motor-vehicle accident NOS
     Off-road motor-vehicle accident NOS
     Other motor-vehicle accident NOS
     ~~Unspecified occupant of dirt bike injured in nontraffic accident~~
     Unspecified occupant of go cart injured in nontraffic accident
     Unspecified occupant of golf cart injured in nontraffic accident

☑4ᵗʰ **V87** **Traffic accident of specified type but victim's mode of transport unknown**
     EXCLUDES 1   collision involving:
         pedal cycle (V10-V19)
         pedestrian (V01-V09)

☑x7ᵗʰ **V87.0** **Person injured in collision between** car and two- or three-wheeled powered vehicle **(traffic)**

☑x7ᵗʰ **V87.1** **Person injured in collision between** other motor vehicle and two- or three-wheeled motor vehicle **(traffic)**

☑x7ᵗʰ **V87.2** **Person injured in collision between** car and pick-up truck or van **(traffic)**

☑x7ᵗʰ **V87.3** **Person injured in collision between** car and bus **(traffic)**

☑x7ᵗʰ **V87.4** **Person injured in collision between** car and heavy transport vehicle **(traffic)**

☑x7ᵗʰ **V87.5** **Person injured in collision between** heavy transport vehicle and bus **(traffic)**

☑x7ᵗʰ **V87.6** **Person injured in collision between** railway train or railway vehicle and car **(traffic)**

☑x7ᵗʰ **V87.7** **Person injured in collision between** other specified motor vehicles **(traffic)**

☑x7ᵗʰ **V87.8** **Person injured in other specified** noncollision **transport accidents involving** motor vehicle **(traffic)**

☑x7ᵗʰ **V87.9** **Person injured in other specified (collision)(noncollision) transport accidents involving nonmotor vehicle (traffic)**

☑4ᵗʰ **V88** **Nontraffic accident of specified type but victim's mode of transport unknown**
     EXCLUDES 1   collision involving:
         pedal cycle (V10-V19)
         pedestrian (V01-V09)

☑x7ᵗʰ **V88.0** **Person injured in collision between** car and two- or three-wheeled motor vehicle, **nontraffic**

☑x7ᵗʰ **V88.1** **Person injured in collision between** other motor vehicle and two- or three-wheeled motor vehicle, **nontraffic**

☑x7ᵗʰ **V88.2** **Person injured in collision between** car and pick-up truck or van, **nontraffic**

☑x7ᵗʰ **V88.3** **Person injured in collision between** car and bus, **nontraffic**

☑ Additional Character Req   ☑x7ᵗʰ Placeholder Alert   Manifestation   HCC CMS-HCC Condition   ▽ Unspecified Code   ►◄ Revised Text   ● New Code   ▲ Revised Code Title

ICD-10-CM 2018   **1137**

V88.4   Person injured in collision between car and heavy transport vehicle, **nontraffic**

V88.5   Person injured in collision between heavy transport vehicle and bus, **nontraffic**

V88.6   Person injured in collision between railway train or railway vehicle and car, **nontraffic**

V88.7   Person injured in collision between other specified motor vehicle, nontraffic

V88.8   Person injured in other specified noncollision transport accidents involving motor vehicle, **nontraffic**

V88.9   Person injured in other specified (collision)(noncollision) transport accidents involving nonmotor vehicle, **nontraffic**

V89   Motor- or nonmotor-vehicle accident, type of vehicle unspecified

    V89.0   Person injured in unspecified motor-vehicle **accident, nontraffic** ▽
       Motor-vehicle accident NOS, nontraffic

    V89.1   Person injured in unspecified nonmotor-vehicle **accident, nontraffic** ▽
       Nonmotor-vehicle accident NOS (nontraffic)

    V89.2   Person injured in unspecified motor-vehicle **accident, traffic** ▽
       Motor-vehicle accident [MVA] NOS
       Road (traffic) accident [RTA] NOS

    V89.3   Person injured in unspecified nonmotor-vehicle **accident, traffic** ▽
       Nonmotor-vehicle traffic accident NOS

    V89.9   Person injured in unspecified vehicle accident ▽
       Collision NOS

Water transport accidents (V90-V94)

The appropriate 7th character is to be added to each code from categories V90-V94.
A   initial encounter
D   subsequent encounter
S   sequela

V90   Drowning and submersion due to accident to watercraft
    EXCLUDES 1   civilian water transport accident involving military watercraft (V94.81-)
          fall into water not from watercraft (W16.-)
          military watercraft accident in military or war operations (Y36.0-, Y37.0-)
          water-transport-related drowning or submersion without accident to watercraft (V92.-)

    V90.0   Drowning and submersion due to watercraft overturning

      V90.00   Drowning and submersion due to merchant ship **overturning**

      V90.01   Drowning and submersion due to passenger ship **overturning**
          Drowning and submersion due to Ferry-boat overturning
          Drowning and submersion due to Liner overturning

      V90.02   Drowning and submersion due to fishing boat **overturning**

      V90.03   Drowning and submersion due to other powered **watercraft overturning**
          Drowning and submersion due to Hovercraft (on open water) overturning
          Drowning and submersion due to Jet ski overturning

      V90.04   Drowning and submersion due to sailboat **overturning**

      V90.05   Drowning and submersion due to canoe or kayak **overturning**

      V90.06   Drowning and submersion due to (nonpowered) inflatable craft **overturning**

      V90.08   Drowning and submersion due to other unpowered **watercraft overturning**
          Drowning and submersion due to windsurfer overturning

      V90.09   Drowning and submersion due to unspecified watercraft overturning ▽
          Drowning and submersion due to boat NOS overturning
          Drowning and submersion due to ship NOS overturning
          Drowning and submersion due to watercraft NOS overturning

    V90.1   Drowning and submersion due to watercraft sinking

      V90.10   Drowning and submersion due to merchant ship **sinking**

      V90.11   Drowning and submersion due to passenger ship **sinking**
          Drowning and submersion due to Ferry-boat sinking
          Drowning and submersion due to Liner sinking

      V90.12   Drowning and submersion due to fishing boat **sinking**

      V90.13   Drowning and submersion due to other powered **watercraft sinking**
          Drowning and submersion due to Hovercraft (on open water) sinking
          Drowning and submersion due to Jet ski sinking

      V90.14   Drowning and submersion due to sailboat **sinking**

      V90.15   Drowning and submersion due to canoe or kayak **sinking**

      V90.16   Drowning and submersion due to (nonpowered) inflatable craft **sinking**

      V90.18   Drowning and submersion due to other unpowered **watercraft sinking**

      V90.19   Drowning and submersion due to unspecified watercraft sinking ▽
          Drowning and submersion due to boat NOS sinking
          Drowning and submersion due to ship NOS sinking
          Drowning and submersion due to watercraft NOS sinking

    V90.2   Drowning and submersion due to falling or jumping from burning **watercraft**

      V90.20   Drowning and submersion due to falling or jumping from burning merchant ship

      V90.21   Drowning and submersion due to falling or jumping from burning passenger ship
          Drowning and submersion due to falling or jumping from burning Ferry-boat
          Drowning and submersion due to falling or jumping from burning Liner

      V90.22   Drowning and submersion due to falling or jumping from burning fishing boat

      V90.23   Drowning and submersion due to other burning powered **watercraft**
          Drowning and submersion due to falling and jumping from burning Hovercraft (on open water)
          Drowning and submersion due to falling and jumping from burning Jet ski

      V90.24   Drowning and submersion due to falling or jumping from burning sailboat

      V90.25   Drowning and submersion due to falling or jumping from burning canoe or kayak

      V90.26   Drowning and submersion due to falling or jumping from burning (nonpowered) inflatable craft

      V90.27   Drowning and submersion due to falling or jumping from burning water-skis

      V90.28   Drowning and submersion due to other burning unpowered **watercraft**
          Drowning and submersion due to falling and jumping from burning surf-board
          Drowning and submersion due to falling and jumping from burning windsurfer

      V90.29   Drowning and submersion due to falling or jumping from unspecified burning watercraft ▽
          Drowning and submersion due to falling or jumping from burning boat NOS
          Drowning and submersion due to falling or jumping from burning ship NOS
          Drowning and submersion due to falling or jumping from burning watercraft NOS

    V90.3   Drowning and submersion due to falling or jumping from crushed watercraft

      V90.30   Drowning and submersion due to falling or jumping from crushed merchant ship

      V90.31   Drowning and submersion due to falling or jumping from crushed passenger ship
          Drowning and submersion due to falling and jumping from crushed Ferry boat
          Drowning and submersion due to falling and jumping from crushed Liner

EXCLUDES 1 Not coded here   **EXCLUDES 2** Not included here   N Newborn Age: 0   P Pediatric Age: 0-17   M Maternity Age: 12-55   A Adult Age: 15-124

1138   ICD-10-CM 2018

√x7ʰ **V90.32** **Drowning and submersion due to falling or jumping from crushed** fishing boat

√x7ʰ **V90.33** **Drowning and submersion due to falling or jumping from other crushed** powered **watercraft**
> Drowning and submersion due to falling and jumping from crushed Hovercraft
> Drowning and submersion due to falling and jumping from crushed Jet ski

√x7ʰ **V90.34** **Drowning and submersion due to falling or jumping from crushed** sailboat

√x7ʰ **V90.35** **Drowning and submersion due to falling or jumping from crushed** canoe or kayak

√x7ʰ **V90.36** **Drowning and submersion due to falling or jumping from crushed (nonpowered)** inflatable craft

√x7ʰ **V90.37** **Drowning and submersion due to falling or jumping from crushed** water-skis

√x7ʰ **V90.38** **Drowning and submersion due to falling or jumping from other crushed** unpowered **watercraft**
> Drowning and submersion due to falling and jumping from crushed surf-board
> Drowning and submersion due to falling and jumping from crushed windsurfer

√x7ʰ **V90.39** **Drowning and submersion due to falling or jumping from crushed unspecified watercraft** ▽
> Drowning and submersion due to falling and jumping from crushed boat NOS
> Drowning and submersion due to falling and jumping from crushed ship NOS
> Drowning and submersion due to falling and jumping from crushed watercraft NOS

√5ʰ **V90.8** **Drowning and submersion due to other accident to watercraft**

√x7ʰ **V90.80** **Drowning and submersion due to other accident to** merchant ship

√x7ʰ **V90.81** **Drowning and submersion due to other accident to** passenger ship
> Drowning and submersion due to other accident to Ferry-boat
> Drowning and submersion due to other accident to Liner

√x7ʰ **V90.82** **Drowning and submersion due to other accident to** fishing boat

√x7ʰ **V90.83** **Drowning and submersion due to other accident to other** powered **watercraft**
> Drowning and submersion due to other accident to Hovercraft (on open water)
> Drowning and submersion due to other accident to Jet ski

√x7ʰ **V90.84** **Drowning and submersion due to other accident to** sailboat

√x7ʰ **V90.85** **Drowning and submersion due to other accident to** canoe or kayak

√x7ʰ **V90.86** **Drowning and submersion due to other accident to (nonpowered)** inflatable craft

√x7ʰ **V90.87** **Drowning and submersion due to other accident to** water-skis

√x7ʰ **V90.88** **Drowning and submersion due to other accident to other** unpowered **watercraft**
> Drowning and submersion due to other accident to surf-board
> Drowning and submersion due to other accident to windsurfer

√x7ʰ **V90.89** **Drowning and submersion due to other accident to unspecified watercraft** ▽
> Drowning and submersion due to other accident to boat NOS
> Drowning and submersion due to other accident to ship NOS
> Drowning and submersion due to other accident to watercraft NOS

√4ʰ **V91** **Other injury due to accident to watercraft**
> INCLUDES   any injury except drowning and submersion as a result of an accident to watercraft
> EXCLUDES 1   *civilian water transport accident involving military watercraft (V94.81-)*
> *military watercraft accident in military or war operations (Y36, Y37.-)*
> EXCLUDES 2   *drowning and submersion due to accident to watercraft (V90.-)*

√5ʰ **V91.0** **Burn due to watercraft on fire**
> EXCLUDES 1   *burn from localized fire or explosion on board ship without accident to watercraft (V93.-)*

√x7ʰ **V91.00** **Burn due to** merchant ship **on fire**

√x7ʰ **V91.01** **Burn due to** passenger ship **on fire**
> Burn due to Ferry-boat on fire
> Burn due to Liner on fire

√x7ʰ **V91.02** **Burn due to** fishing boat **on fire**

√x7ʰ **V91.03** **Burn due to other** powered **watercraft on fire**
> Burn due to Hovercraft (on open water) on fire
> Burn due to Jet ski on fire

√x7ʰ **V91.04** **Burn due to** sailboat **on fire**

√x7ʰ **V91.05** **Burn due to** canoe or kayak **on fire**

√x7ʰ **V91.06** **Burn due to (nonpowered)** inflatable craft **on fire**

√x7ʰ **V91.07** **Burn due to** water-skis **on fire**

√x7ʰ **V91.08** **Burn due to other** unpowered **watercraft on fire**

√x7ʰ **V91.09** **Burn due to unspecified watercraft on fire** ▽
> Burn due to boat NOS on fire
> Burn due to ship NOS on fire
> Burn due to watercraft NOS on fire

√5ʰ **V91.1** **Crushed between watercraft and other watercraft or other object due to collision**
> Crushed by lifeboat after abandoning ship in a collision
> NOTE   Select the specified type of watercraft that the victim was on at the time of the collision

√x7ʰ **V91.10** **Crushed between** merchant ship **and other watercraft or other object due to collision**

√x7ʰ **V91.11** **Crushed between** passenger ship **and other watercraft or other object due to collision**
> Crushed between Ferry-boat and other watercraft or other object due to collision
> Crushed between Liner and other watercraft or other object due to collision

√x7ʰ **V91.12** **Crushed between** fishing boat **and other watercraft or other object due to collision**

√x7ʰ **V91.13** **Crushed between other** powered **watercraft and other watercraft or other object due to collision**
> Crushed between Hovercraft (on open water) and other watercraft or other object due to collision
> Crushed between Jet ski and other watercraft or other object due to collision

√x7ʰ **V91.14** **Crushed between** sailboat **and other watercraft or other object due to collision**

√x7ʰ **V91.15** **Crushed between** canoe or kayak **and other watercraft or other object due to collision**

√x7ʰ **V91.16** **Crushed between (nonpowered)** inflatable craft **and other watercraft or other object due to collision**

√x7ʰ **V91.18** **Crushed between other** unpowered **watercraft and other watercraft or other object due to collision**
> Crushed between surfboard and other watercraft or other object due to collision
> Crushed between windsurfer and other watercraft or other object due to collision

√x7ʰ **V91.19** **Crushed between unspecified watercraft and other watercraft or other object due to collision** ▽
> Crushed between boat NOS and other watercraft or other object due to collision
> Crushed between ship NOS and other watercraft or other object due to collision
> Crushed between watercraft NOS and other watercraft or other object due to collision

✔ Additional Character Req   √x7ʰ Placeholder Alert   Manifestation   HCC CMS-HCC Condition   ▽ Unspecified Code   ▶◀ Revised Text   ● New Code   ▲ Revised Code Title

ICD-10-CM 2018   1139

√5ᵗʰ **V91.2 Fall due to collision between watercraft and other watercraft or other object**
Fall while remaining on watercraft after collision
NOTE Select the specified type of watercraft that the victim was on at the time of the collision.
EXCLUDES 1 *crushed between watercraft and other watercraft and other object due to collision (V91.1-)*
drowning and submersion due to falling from crushed watercraft (V90.3-)

√x7ᵗʰ **V91.20 Fall due to collision between merchant ship and other watercraft or other object**

√x7ᵗʰ **V91.21 Fall due to collision between passenger ship and other watercraft or other object**
Fall due to collision between Ferry-boat and other watercraft or other object
Fall due to collision between Liner and other watercraft or other object

√x7ᵗʰ **V91.22 Fall due to collision between fishing boat and other watercraft or other object**

√x7ᵗʰ **V91.23 Fall due to collision between other powered watercraft and other watercraft or other object**
Fall due to collision between Hovercraft (on open water) and other watercraft or other object
Fall due to collision between Jet ski and other watercraft or other object

√x7ᵗʰ **V91.24 Fall due to collision between sailboat and other watercraft or other object**

√x7ᵗʰ **V91.25 Fall due to collision between canoe or kayak and other watercraft or other object**

√x7ᵗʰ **V91.26 Fall due to collision between (nonpowered) inflatable craft and other watercraft or other object**

√x7ᵗʰ **V91.29 Fall due to collision between unspecified** ▽ **watercraft and other watercraft or other object**
Fall due to collision between boat NOS and other watercraft or other object
Fall due to collision between ship NOS and other watercraft or other object
Fall due to collision between watercraft NOS and other watercraft or other object

√5ᵗʰ **V91.3 Hit or struck by falling object due to accident to watercraft**
Hit or struck by falling object (part of damaged watercraft or other object) after falling or jumping from damaged watercraft
EXCLUDES 2 *drowning or submersion due to fall or jumping from damaged watercraft (V90.2-, V90.3-)*

√x7ᵗʰ **V91.30 Hit or struck by falling object due to accident to merchant ship**

√x7ᵗʰ **V91.31 Hit or struck by falling object due to accident to passenger ship**
Hit or struck by falling object due to accident to Ferry-boat
Hit or struck by falling object due to accident to Liner

√x7ᵗʰ **V91.32 Hit or struck by falling object due to accident to fishing boat**

√x7ᵗʰ **V91.33 Hit or struck by falling object due to accident to other powered watercraft**
Hit or struck by falling object due to accident to Hovercraft (on open water)
Hit or struck by falling object due to accident to Jet ski

√x7ᵗʰ **V91.34 Hit or struck by falling object due to accident to sailboat**

√x7ᵗʰ **V91.35 Hit or struck by falling object due to accident to canoe or kayak**

√x7ᵗʰ **V91.36 Hit or struck by falling object due to accident to (nonpowered) inflatable craft**

√x7ᵗʰ **V91.37 Hit or struck by falling object due to accident to water-skis**
Hit by water-skis after jumping off of waterskis

√x7ᵗʰ **V91.38 Hit or struck by falling object due to accident to other unpowered watercraft**
Hit or struck by surf-board after falling off damaged surf-board
Hit or struck by object after falling off damaged windsurfer

√x7ᵗʰ **V91.39 Hit or struck by falling object due to accident to** ▽ **unspecified watercraft**
Hit or struck by falling object due to accident to boat NOS
Hit or struck by falling object due to accident to ship NOS
Hit or struck by falling object due to accident to watercraft NOS

√5ᵗʰ **V91.8 Other injury due to other accident to watercraft**

√x7ᵗʰ **V91.80 Other injury due to other accident to merchant ship**

√x7ᵗʰ **V91.81 Other injury due to other accident to passenger ship**
Other injury due to other accident to Ferry-boat
Other injury due to other accident to Liner

√x7ᵗʰ **V91.82 Other injury due to other accident to fishing boat**

√x7ᵗʰ **V91.83 Other injury due to other accident to other powered watercraft**
Other injury due to other accident to Hovercraft (on open water)
Other injury due to other accident to Jet ski

√x7ᵗʰ **V91.84 Other injury due to other accident to sailboat**

√x7ᵗʰ **V91.85 Other injury due to other accident to canoe or kayak**

√x7ᵗʰ **V91.86 Other injury due to other accident to (nonpowered) inflatable craft**

√x7ᵗʰ **V91.87 Other injury due to other accident to water-skis**

√x7ᵗʰ **V91.88 Other injury due to other accident to other unpowered watercraft**
Other injury due to other accident to surf-board
Other injury due to other accident to windsurfer

√x7ᵗʰ **V91.89 Other injury due to other accident to** ▽ **unspecified watercraft**
Other injury due to other accident to boat NOS
Other injury due to other accident to ship NOS
Other injury due to other accident to watercraft NOS

√4ᵗʰ **V92 Drowning and submersion due to accident on board watercraft, without accident to watercraft**
EXCLUDES 1 *civilian water transport accident involving military watercraft (V94.81-)*
drowning or submersion due to accident to watercraft (V90-V91)
drowning or submersion of diver who voluntarily jumps from boat not involved in an accident (W16.711, W16.721)
fall into water without watercraft (W16.-)
military watercraft accident in military or war operations (Y36, Y37)

√5ᵗʰ **V92.0 Drowning and submersion due to fall off watercraft**
Drowning and submersion due to fall from gangplank of watercraft
Drowning and submersion due to fall overboard watercraft
EXCLUDES 2 *hitting head on object or bottom of body of water due to fall from watercraft (V94.0-)*

√x7ᵗʰ **V92.00 Drowning and submersion due to fall off merchant ship**

√x7ᵗʰ **V92.01 Drowning and submersion due to fall off passenger ship**
Drowning and submersion due to fall off Ferry-boat
Drowning and submersion due to fall off Liner

√x7ᵗʰ **V92.02 Drowning and submersion due to fall off fishing boat**

√x7ᵗʰ **V92.03 Drowning and submersion due to fall off other powered watercraft**
Drowning and submersion due to fall off Hovercraft (on open water)
Drowning and submersion due to fall off Jet ski

√x7ᵗʰ **V92.04 Drowning and submersion due to fall off sailboat**

√x7ᵗʰ **V92.05 Drowning and submersion due to fall off canoe or kayak**

√x7ᵗʰ **V92.06 Drowning and submersion due to fall off (nonpowered) inflatable craft**

√x7ᵗʰ **V92.07 Drowning and submersion due to fall off water-skis**
EXCLUDES 1 *drowning and submersion due to falling off burning water-skis (V90.27)*
drowning and submersion due to falling off crushed water-skis (V90.37)
hit by boat while water-skiing NOS (V94.X)

EXCLUDES 1 Not coded here   **EXCLUDES 2** Not included here   Ⓝ Newborn Age: 0   Ⓟ Pediatric Age: 0-17   Ⓜ Maternity Age: 12-55   Ⓐ Adult Age: 15-124

1140   ICD-10-CM 2018

√x7ᵗʰ **V92.08 Drowning and submersion due to fall off other** unpowered **watercraft**
    Drowning and submersion due to fall off surf-board
    Drowning and submersion due to fall off windsurfer
      EXCLUDES 1 *drowning and submersion due to fall off burning unpowered watercraft (V90.28)*
          drowning and submersion due to fall off crushed unpowered watercraft (V90.38)
          drowning and submersion due to fall off damaged unpowered watercraft (V90.88)
          drowning and submersion due to rider of nonpowered watercraft being hit by other watercraft (V94.-)
          other injury due to rider of nonpowered watercraft being hit by other watercraft (V94.-)

√x7ᵗʰ **V92.09 Drowning and submersion due to fall off** ▽ **unspecified watercraft**
    Drowning and submersion due to fall off boat NOS
    Drowning and submersion due to fall off ship
    Drowning and submersion due to fall off watercraft NOS

√5ᵗʰ **V92.1 Drowning and submersion due to being** thrown overboard **by motion of watercraft**
      EXCLUDES 1 *drowning and submersion due to fall off surf-board (V92.08)*
          drowning and submersion due to fall off water-skis (V92.07)
          drowning and submersion due to fall off windsurfer (V92.08)

√x7ᵗʰ **V92.10 Drowning and submersion due to being thrown overboard by motion of** merchant ship

√x7ᵗʰ **V92.11 Drowning and submersion due to being thrown overboard by motion of** passenger ship
    Drowning and submersion due to being thrown overboard by motion of Ferry-boat
    Drowning and submersion due to being thrown overboard by motion of Liner

√x7ᵗʰ **V92.12 Drowning and submersion due to being thrown overboard by motion of** fishing boat

√x7ᵗʰ **V92.13 Drowning and submersion due to being thrown overboard by motion of other** powered **watercraft**
    Drowning and submersion due to being thrown overboard by motion of Hovercraft

√x7ᵗʰ **V92.14 Drowning and submersion due to being thrown overboard by motion of** sailboat

√x7ᵗʰ **V92.15 Drowning and submersion due to being thrown overboard by motion of** canoe or kayak

√x7ᵗʰ **V92.16 Drowning and submersion due to being thrown overboard by motion of (nonpowered)** inflatable craft

√x7ᵗʰ **V92.19 Drowning and submersion due to being thrown** ▽ **overboard by motion of unspecified watercraft**
    Drowning and submersion due to being thrown overboard by motion of boat NOS
    Drowning and submersion due to being thrown overboard by motion of ship NOS
    Drowning and submersion due to being thrown overboard by motion of watercraft NOS

√5ᵗʰ **V92.2 Drowning and submersion due to being** washed overboard **from watercraft**
    Code first any associated cataclysm (X37.0-)

√x7ᵗʰ **V92.20 Drowning and submersion due to being washed overboard from** merchant ship

√x7ᵗʰ **V92.21 Drowning and submersion due to being washed overboard from** passenger ship
    Drowning and submersion due to being washed overboard from Ferry-boat
    Drowning and submersion due to being washed overboard from Liner

√x7ᵗʰ **V92.22 Drowning and submersion due to being washed overboard from** fishing boat

√x7ᵗʰ **V92.23 Drowning and submersion due to being washed overboard from other** powered **watercraft**
    Drowning and submersion due to being washed overboard from Hovercraft (on open water)
    Drowning and submersion due to being washed overboard from Jet ski

√x7ᵗʰ **V92.24 Drowning and submersion due to being washed overboard from** sailboat

√x7ᵗʰ **V92.25 Drowning and submersion due to being washed overboard from** canoe or kayak

√x7ᵗʰ **V92.26 Drowning and submersion due to being washed overboard from (nonpowered)** inflatable craft

√x7ᵗʰ **V92.27 Drowning and submersion due to being washed overboard from** water-skis
      EXCLUDES 1 *drowning and submersion due to fall off water-skis (V92.07)*

√x7ᵗʰ **V92.28 Drowning and submersion due to being washed overboard from other** unpowered **watercraft**
    Drowning and submersion due to being washed overboard from surf-board
    Drowning and submersion due to being washed overboard from windsurfer

√x7ᵗʰ **V92.29 Drowning and submersion due to being** ▽ **washed overboard from unspecified watercraft**
    Drowning and submersion due to being washed overboard from boat NOS
    Drowning and submersion due to being washed overboard from ship NOS
    Drowning and submersion due to being washed overboard from watercraft NOS

√4ᵗʰ **V93 Other injury due to accident on board watercraft, without accident to watercraft**
      EXCLUDES 1 *civilian water transport accident involving military watercraft (V94.81-)*
          other injury due to accident to watercraft (V91.-)
          military watercraft accident in military or war operations (Y36, Y37.-)
      EXCLUDES 2 *drowning and submersion due to accident on board watercraft, without accident to watercraft (V92.-)*

√5ᵗʰ **V93.0 Burn due to localized fire on board watercraft**
      EXCLUDES 1 *burn due to watercraft on fire (V91.0-)*

√x7ᵗʰ **V93.00 Burn due to localized fire on board** merchant vessel

√x7ᵗʰ **V93.01 Burn due to localized fire on board** passenger vessel
    Burn due to localized fire on board Ferry-boat
    Burn due to localized fire on board Liner

√x7ᵗʰ **V93.02 Burn due to localized fire on board** fishing boat

√x7ᵗʰ **V93.03 Burn due to localized fire on board other** powered **watercraft**
    Burn due to localized fire on board Hovercraft
    Burn due to localized fire on board Jet ski

√x7ᵗʰ **V93.04 Burn due to localized fire on board** sailboat

√x7ᵗʰ **V93.09 Burn due to localized fire on board unspecified** ▽ **watercraft**
    Burn due to localized fire on board boat NOS
    Burn due to localized fire on board ship NOS
    Burn due to localized fire on board watercraft NOS

√5ᵗʰ **V93.1 Other burn on board watercraft**
    Burn due to source other than fire on board watercraft
      EXCLUDES 1 *burn due to watercraft on fire (V91.0-)*

√x7ᵗʰ **V93.10 Other burn on board** merchant vessel

√x7ᵗʰ **V93.11 Other burn on board** passenger vessel
    Other burn on board Ferry-boat
    Other burn on board Liner

√x7ᵗʰ **V93.12 Other burn on board** fishing boat

√x7ᵗʰ **V93.13 Other burn on board other** powered **watercraft**
    Other burn on board Hovercraft
    Other burn on board Jet ski

√x7ᵗʰ **V93.14 Other burn on board** sailboat

√x7ᵗʰ **V93.19 Other burn on board unspecified watercraft** ▽
    Other burn on board boat NOS
    Other burn on board ship NOS
    Other burn on board watercraft NOS

√5ᵗʰ **V93.2 Heat exposure on board watercraft**
      EXCLUDES 1 *exposure to man-made heat not aboard watercraft (W92)*
          exposure to natural heat while on board watercraft (X30)
          exposure to sunlight while on board watercraft (X32)
      EXCLUDES 2 *burn due to fire on board watercraft (V93.0-)*

√x7ᵗʰ **V93.20 Heat exposure on board** merchant ship

√x7ᵗʰ **V93.21 Heat exposure on board** passenger ship
    Heat exposure on board Ferry-boat
    Heat exposure on board Liner

√x7ᵗʰ **V93.22 Heat exposure on board** fishing boat

✓ Additional Character Req   √x7ᵗʰ Placeholder Alert   Manifestation   HCC CMS-HCC Condition   ▽ Unspecified Code   ►◄ Revised Text   ● New Code   ▲ Revised Code Title

√x 7ᵗʰ **V93.23** **Heat exposure on board other** powered **watercraft**
Heat exposure on board hovercraft

√x 7ᵗʰ **V93.24** **Heat exposure on board** sailboat

√x 7ᵗʰ **V93.29** **Heat exposure on board unspecified watercraft** ▽
Heat exposure on board boat NOS
Heat exposure on board ship NOS
Heat exposure on board watercraft NOS

√5ᵗʰ **V93.3** **Fall on board watercraft**
EXCLUDES 1   *fall due to collision of watercraft (V91.2-)*

√x 7ᵗʰ **V93.30** **Fall on board** merchant ship

√x 7ᵗʰ **V93.31** **Fall on board** passenger ship
Fall on board Ferry-boat
Fall on board Liner

√x 7ᵗʰ **V93.32** **Fall on board** fishing boat

√x 7ᵗʰ **V93.33** **Fall on board other** powered **watercraft**
Fall on board Hovercraft (on open water)
Fall on board Jet ski

√x 7ᵗʰ **V93.34** **Fall on board** sailboat

√x 7ᵗʰ **V93.35** **Fall on board** canoe or kayak

√x 7ᵗʰ **V93.36** **Fall on board** (nonpowered) inflatable craft

√x 7ᵗʰ **V93.38** **Fall on board other** unpowered **watercraft**

√x 7ᵗʰ **V93.39** **Fall on board unspecified watercraft** ▽
Fall on board boat NOS
Fall on board ship NOS
Fall on board watercraft NOS

√5ᵗʰ **V93.4** **Struck by falling object on board watercraft**
Hit by falling object on board watercraft
EXCLUDES 1   *struck by falling object due to accident to watercraft (V91.3)*

√x 7ᵗʰ **V93.40** **Struck by falling object on** merchant ship

√x 7ᵗʰ **V93.41** **Struck by falling object on** passenger ship
Struck by falling object on Ferry-boat
Struck by falling object on Liner

√x 7ᵗʰ **V93.42** **Struck by falling object on** fishing boat

√x 7ᵗʰ **V93.43** **Struck by falling object on other** powered **watercraft**
Struck by falling object on Hovercraft

√x 7ᵗʰ **V93.44** **Struck by falling object on** sailboat

√x 7ᵗʰ **V93.48** **Struck by falling object on other** unpowered **watercraft**

√x 7ᵗʰ **V93.49** **Struck by falling object on unspecified watercraft** ▽

√5ᵗʰ **V93.5** **Explosion on board watercraft**
Boiler explosion on steamship
EXCLUDES 2   *fire on board watercraft (V93.0-)*

√x 7ᵗʰ **V93.50** **Explosion on board** merchant ship

√x 7ᵗʰ **V93.51** **Explosion on board** passenger ship
Explosion on board Ferry-boat
Explosion on board Liner

√x 7ᵗʰ **V93.52** **Explosion on board** fishing boat

√x 7ᵗʰ **V93.53** **Explosion on board other** powered **watercraft**
Explosion on board Hovercraft
Explosion on board Jet ski

√x 7ᵗʰ **V93.54** **Explosion on board** sailboat

√x 7ᵗʰ **V93.59** **Explosion on board unspecified watercraft** ▽
Explosion on board boat NOS
Explosion on board ship NOS
Explosion on board watercraft NOS

√5ᵗʰ **V93.6** **Machinery accident on board watercraft**
EXCLUDES 1   *machinery explosion on board watercraft (V93.4-)*
machinery fire on board watercraft (V93.0-)

√x 7ᵗʰ **V93.60** **Machinery accident on board** merchant ship

√x 7ᵗʰ **V93.61** **Machinery accident on board** passenger ship
Machinery accident on board Ferry-boat
Machinery accident on board Liner

√x 7ᵗʰ **V93.62** **Machinery accident on board** fishing boat

√x 7ᵗʰ **V93.63** **Machinery accident on board other** powered **watercraft**
Machinery accident on board Hovercraft

√x 7ᵗʰ **V93.64** **Machinery accident on board** sailboat

√x 7ᵗʰ **V93.69** **Machinery accident on board unspecified watercraft** ▽
Machinery accident on board boat NOS
Machinery accident on board ship NOS
Machinery accident on board watercraft NOS

√5ᵗʰ **V93.8** **Other injury due to other accident on board watercraft**
Accidental poisoning by gases or fumes on watercraft

√x 7ᵗʰ **V93.80** **Other injury due to other accident on board** merchant ship

√x 7ᵗʰ **V93.81** **Other injury due to other accident on board** passenger ship
Other injury due to other accident on board Ferry-boat
Other injury due to other accident on board Liner

√x 7ᵗʰ **V93.82** **Other injury due to other accident on board** fishing boat

√x 7ᵗʰ **V93.83** **Other injury due to other accident on board other** powered **watercraft**
Other injury due to other accident on board Hovercraft
Other injury due to other accident on board Jet ski

√x 7ᵗʰ **V93.84** **Other injury due to other accident on board** sailboat

√x 7ᵗʰ **V93.85** **Other injury due to other accident on board** canoe or kayak

√x 7ᵗʰ **V93.86** **Other injury due to other accident on board** (nonpowered) inflatable craft

√x 7ᵗʰ **V93.87** **Other injury due to other accident on board** water-skis
Hit or struck by object while waterskiing

√x 7ᵗʰ **V93.88** **Other injury due to other accident on board other** unpowered **watercraft**
Hit or struck by object while surfing
Hit or struck by object while on board windsurfer

√x 7ᵗʰ **V93.89** **Other injury due to other accident on board unspecified watercraft** ▽
Other injury due to other accident on board boat NOS
Other injury due to other accident on board ship NOS
Other injury due to other accident on board watercraft NOS

√4ᵗʰ **V94** **Other and unspecified water transport accidents**
EXCLUDES 1   *military watercraft accidents in military or war operations (Y36, Y37)*

√x 7ᵗʰ **V94.0** **Hitting object or bottom of body of water due to fall from watercraft**
EXCLUDES 2   *drowning and submersion due to fall from watercraft (V92.0-)*

√5ᵗʰ **V94.1** **Bather struck by watercraft**
Swimmer hit by watercraft

√x 7ᵗʰ **V94.11** **Bather struck by** powered **watercraft**

√x 7ᵗʰ **V94.12** **Bather struck by** nonpowered **watercraft**

√5ᵗʰ **V94.2** **Rider of nonpowered watercraft struck by other watercraft**

√x 7ᵗʰ **V94.21** **Rider of nonpowered watercraft struck by other** nonpowered **watercraft**
Canoer hit by other nonpowered watercraft
Surfer hit by other nonpowered watercraft
Windsurfer hit by other nonpowered watercraft

√x 7ᵗʰ **V94.22** **Rider of nonpowered watercraft struck by** powered **watercraft**
Canoer hit by motorboat
Surfer hit by motorboat
Windsurfer hit by motorboat

√5ᵗʰ **V94.3** **Injury to rider of (inflatable) watercraft being pulled behind other watercraft**

√x 7ᵗʰ **V94.31** **Injury to rider of (inflatable)** recreational **watercraft being pulled behind other watercraft**
Injury to rider of inner-tube pulled behind motor boat

√x 7ᵗʰ **V94.32** **Injury to rider of** non-recreational **watercraft being pulled behind other watercraft**
Injury to occupant of dingy being pulled behind boat or ship
Injury to occupant of life-raft being pulled behind boat or ship

√x 7ᵗʰ **V94.4** **Injury to barefoot water-skier**
Injury to person being pulled behind boat or ship

√5ᵗʰ **V94.8** **Other water transport accident**

√6ᵗʰ **V94.81** **Water transport accident involving military watercraft**

√7ᵗʰ **V94.810** **Civilian watercraft involved in water transport accident with military watercraft**
Passenger on civilian watercraft injured due to accident with military watercraft

EXCLUDES 1 Not coded here   EXCLUDES 2 Not included here   N Newborn Age: 0   P Pediatric Age: 0-17   M Maternity Age: 12-55   A Adult Age: 15-124

V93.23–V94.810

Chapter 20. External Causes of Morbidity

1142   ICD-10-CM 2018

☑7ᵗʰ   **V94.811**   **Civilian in water injured by military watercraft**

☑7ᵗʰ   **V94.818**   **Other water transport accident involving military watercraft**

✓x7ᵗʰ   **V94.89**   **Other water transport accident**

✓x7ᵗʰ   **V94.9**   **Unspecified water transport accident**   ▽
         Water transport accident NOS

Air and space transport accidents (V95-V97)

EXCLUDES 1   *military aircraft accidents in military or war operations (Y36, Y37)*

The appropriate 7th character is to be added to each code from categories V95-V97.
A   initial encounter
D   subsequent encounter
S   sequela

✓4ᵗʰ   **V95**   **Accident to powered aircraft causing injury to occupant**

   ✓5ᵗʰ   **V95.0**   Helicopter **accident injuring occupant**

     ✓x7ᵗʰ   **V95.00**   **Unspecified helicopter accident injuring occupant** ▽

     ✓x7ᵗʰ   **V95.01**   **Helicopter** crash **injuring occupant**

     ✓x7ᵗʰ   **V95.02**   Forced landing **of helicopter injuring occupant**

     ✓x7ᵗʰ   **V95.03**   **Helicopter** collision **injuring occupant**
         Helicopter collision with any object, fixed, movable or moving

     ✓x7ᵗʰ   **V95.04**   **Helicopter** fire **injuring occupant**

     ✓x7ᵗʰ   **V95.05**   **Helicopter** explosion **injuring occupant**

     ✓x7ᵗʰ   **V95.09**   **Other helicopter accident injuring occupant**

   ✓5ᵗʰ   **V95.1**   Ultralight, microlight or powered-glider **accident injuring occupant**

     ✓x7ᵗʰ   **V95.10**   **Unspecified ultralight, microlight or powered-glider accident injuring occupant** ▽

     ✓x7ᵗʰ   **V95.11**   **Ultralight, microlight or powered-glider** crash **injuring occupant**

     ✓x7ᵗʰ   **V95.12**   Forced landing **of ultralight, microlight or powered-glider injuring occupant**

     ✓x7ᵗʰ   **V95.13**   **Ultralight, microlight or powered-glider** collision **injuring occupant**
         Ultralight, microlight or powered-glider collision with any object, fixed, movable or moving

     ✓x7ᵗʰ   **V95.14**   **Ultralight, microlight or powered-glider** fire **injuring occupant**

     ✓x7ᵗʰ   **V95.15**   **Ultralight, microlight or powered-glider** explosion **injuring occupant**

     ✓x7ᵗʰ   **V95.19**   **Other ultralight, microlight or powered-glider accident injuring occupant**

   ✓5ᵗʰ   **V95.2**   **Other private fixed-wing aircraft accident injuring occupant**

     ✓x7ᵗʰ   **V95.20**   **Unspecified accident to other private fixed-wing aircraft, injuring occupant** ▽

     ✓x7ᵗʰ   **V95.21**   **Other private fixed-wing aircraft** crash **injuring occupant**

     ✓x7ᵗʰ   **V95.22**   Forced landing **of other private fixed-wing aircraft injuring occupant**

     ✓x7ᵗʰ   **V95.23**   **Other private fixed-wing aircraft** collision **injuring occupant**
         Other private fixed-wing aircraft collision with any object, fixed, movable or moving

     ✓x7ᵗʰ   **V95.24**   **Other private fixed-wing aircraft** fire **injuring occupant**

     ✓x7ᵗʰ   **V95.25**   **Other private fixed-wing aircraft** explosion **injuring occupant**

     ✓x7ᵗʰ   **V95.29**   **Other accident to other private fixed-wing aircraft injuring occupant**

   ✓5ᵗʰ   **V95.3**   Commercial fixed-wing **aircraft accident injuring occupant**

     ✓x7ᵗʰ   **V95.30**   **Unspecified accident to commercial fixed-wing aircraft injuring occupant** ▽

     ✓x7ᵗʰ   **V95.31**   **Commercial fixed-wing aircraft** crash **injuring occupant**

     ✓x7ᵗʰ   **V95.32**   Forced landing **of commercial fixed-wing aircraft injuring occupant**

     ✓x7ᵗʰ   **V95.33**   **Commercial fixed-wing aircraft** collision **injuring occupant**
         Commercial fixed-wing aircraft collision with any object, fixed, movable or moving

     ✓x7ᵗʰ   **V95.34**   **Commercial fixed-wing aircraft** fire **injuring occupant**

     ✓x7ᵗʰ   **V95.35**   **Commercial fixed-wing aircraft** explosion **injuring occupant**

     ✓x7ᵗʰ   **V95.39**   **Other accident to commercial fixed-wing aircraft injuring occupant**

   ✓5ᵗʰ   **V95.4**   Spacecraft **accident injuring occupant**

     ✓x7ᵗʰ   **V95.40**   **Unspecified spacecraft accident injuring occupant** ▽

     ✓x7ᵗʰ   **V95.41**   **Spacecraft** crash **injuring occupant**

     ✓x7ᵗʰ   **V95.42**   Forced landing **of spacecraft injuring occupant**

     ✓x7ᵗʰ   **V95.43**   **Spacecraft** collision **injuring occupant**
         Spacecraft collision with any object, fixed, moveable or moving

     ✓x7ᵗʰ   **V95.44**   **Spacecraft** fire **injuring occupant**

     ✓x7ᵗʰ   **V95.45**   **Spacecraft** explosion **injuring occupant**

     ✓x7ᵗʰ   **V95.49**   **Other spacecraft accident injuring occupant**

   ✓x7ᵗʰ   **V95.8**   **Other powered aircraft accidents injuring occupant**

   ✓x7ᵗʰ   **V95.9**   **Unspecified aircraft accident injuring occupant**   ▽
         Aircraft accident NOS
         Air transport accident NOS

✓4ᵗʰ   **V96**   **Accident to nonpowered aircraft causing injury to occupant**

   ✓5ᵗʰ   **V96.0**   Balloon **accident injuring occupant**

     ✓x7ᵗʰ   **V96.00**   **Unspecified balloon accident injuring occupant** ▽

     ✓x7ᵗʰ   **V96.01**   **Balloon** crash **injuring occupant**

     ✓x7ᵗʰ   **V96.02**   Forced landing **of balloon injuring occupant**

     ✓x7ᵗʰ   **V96.03**   **Balloon** collision **injuring occupant**
         Balloon collision with any object, fixed, moveable or moving

     ✓x7ᵗʰ   **V96.04**   **Balloon** fire **injuring occupant**

     ✓x7ᵗʰ   **V96.05**   **Balloon** explosion **injuring occupant**

     ✓x7ᵗʰ   **V96.09**   **Other balloon accident injuring occupant**

   ✓5ᵗʰ   **V96.1**   Hang-glider **accident injuring occupant**

     ✓x7ᵗʰ   **V96.10**   **Unspecified hang-glider accident injuring occupant** ▽

     ✓x7ᵗʰ   **V96.11**   **Hang-glider** crash **injuring occupant**

     ✓x7ᵗʰ   **V96.12**   Forced landing **of hang-glider injuring occupant**

     ✓x7ᵗʰ   **V96.13**   **Hang-glider** collision **injuring occupant**
         Hang-glider collision with any object, fixed, moveable or moving

     ✓x7ᵗʰ   **V96.14**   **Hang-glider** fire **injuring occupant**

     ✓x7ᵗʰ   **V96.15**   **Hang-glider** explosion **injuring occupant**

     ✓x7ᵗʰ   **V96.19**   **Other hang-glider accident injuring occupant**

   ✓5ᵗʰ   **V96.2**   Glider (nonpowered) **accident injuring occupant**

     ✓x7ᵗʰ   **V96.20**   **Unspecified glider (nonpowered) accident injuring occupant** ▽

     ✓x7ᵗʰ   **V96.21**   **Glider (nonpowered)** crash **injuring occupant**

     ✓x7ᵗʰ   **V96.22**   Forced landing **of glider (nonpowered) injuring occupant**

     ✓x7ᵗʰ   **V96.23**   **Glider (nonpowered)** collision **injuring occupant**
         Glider (nonpowered) collision with any object, fixed, moveable or moving

     ✓x7ᵗʰ   **V96.24**   **Glider (nonpowered)** fire **injuring occupant**

     ✓x7ᵗʰ   **V96.25**   **Glider (nonpowered)** explosion **injuring occupant**

     ✓x7ᵗʰ   **V96.29**   **Other glider (nonpowered) accident injuring occupant**

   ✓x7ᵗʰ   **V96.8**   **Other nonpowered-aircraft accidents injuring occupant**
         Kite carrying a person accident injuring occupant

   ✓x7ᵗʰ   **V96.9**   **Unspecified nonpowered-aircraft accident injuring occupant**   ▽
         Nonpowered-aircraft accident NOS

✓4ᵗʰ   **V97**   **Other specified air transport accidents**

   ✓x7ᵗʰ   **V97.0**   **Occupant of aircraft injured in other specified air transport accidents**
         Fall in, on or from aircraft in air transport accident
         EXCLUDES 1   *accident while boarding or alighting aircraft (V97.1)*

   ✓x7ᵗʰ   **V97.1**   **Person injured while boarding or alighting from aircraft**

   ✓5ᵗʰ   **V97.2**   **Parachutist accident**

     ✓x7ᵗʰ   **V97.21**   **Parachutist entangled in object**
         Parachutist landing in tree

     ✓x7ᵗʰ   **V97.22**   **Parachutist injured on landing**

☑ Additional Character Req   ✓x7ᵗʰ Placeholder Alert   Manifestation   **HCC** CMS-HCC Condition   ▽ Unspecified Code   ►◄ Revised Text   ● New Code   ▲ Revised Code Title

✓x7ᵗʰ **V97.29**   **Other parachutist accident**

✓5ᵗʰ **V97.3**   **Person on ground injured in air transport accident**

     ✓x7ᵗʰ **V97.31**   **Hit by object falling from aircraft**
         Hit by crashing aircraft
         Injured by aircraft hitting house
         Injured by aircraft hitting car

     ✓x7ᵗʰ **V97.32**   **Injured by rotating propeller**

     ✓x7ᵗʰ **V97.33**   **Sucked into jet engine**

     ✓x7ᵗʰ **V97.39**   **Other injury to person on ground due to air transport accident**

✓5ᵗʰ **V97.8**   **Other air transport accidents, not elsewhere classified**
     EXCLUDES 1   *aircraft accident NOS (V95.9)*
         exposure to changes in air pressure during ascent or descent (W94.-)

     ✓6ᵗʰ **V97.81**   **Air transport accident involving military aircraft**

         ✓7ᵗʰ **V97.810**   **Civilian aircraft involved in air transport accident with military aircraft**
             Passenger in civilian aircraft injured due to accident with military aircraft

         ✓7ᵗʰ **V97.811**   **Civilian injured by military aircraft**

         ✓7ᵗʰ **V97.818**   **Other air transport accident involving military aircraft**

     ✓6ᵗʰ **V97.89**   **Other air transport accidents, not elsewhere classified**
         Injury from machinery on aircraft

Other and unspecified transport accidents (V98-V99)

EXCLUDES 1   *vehicle accident, type of vehicle unspecified (V89.-)*

> The appropriate 7th character is to be added to each code from categories V98-V99.
> A   initial encounter
> D   subsequent encounter
> S   sequela

✓4ᵗʰ **V98**   **Other specified transport accidents**

     ✓x7ᵗʰ **V98.0**   **Accident to, on or involving cable-car, not on rails**
         Caught or dragged by cable-car, not on rails
         Fall or jump from cable-car, not on rails
         Object thrown from or in cable-car, not on rails

     ✓x7ᵗʰ **V98.1**   **Accident to, on or involving land-yacht**

     ✓x7ᵗʰ **V98.2**   **Accident to, on or involving ice yacht**

     ✓x7ᵗʰ **V98.3**   **Accident to, on or involving ski lift**
         Accident to, on or involving ski chair-lift
         Accident to, on or involving ski-lift with gondola

     ✓x7ᵗʰ **V98.8**   **Other specified transport accidents**

✓x7ᵗʰ **V99**   **Unspecified transport accident**   ▽

OTHER EXTERNAL CAUSES OF ACCIDENTAL INJURY (W00-X58)

Slipping, tripping, stumbling and falls (W00-W19)

EXCLUDES 1   *assault involving a fall (Y01-Y02)*
     fall from animal (V80.-)
     fall (in) (from) machinery (in operation) (W28-W31)
     fall (in) (from) transport vehicle (V01-V99)
     intentional self-harm involving a fall (X80-X81)
EXCLUDES 2   *at risk for fall (history of fall) (Z91.81)*
     fall (in) (from) burning building (X00.-)
     fall into fire ▶(X00-X04, X08)◀

> The appropriate 7th character is to be added to each code from category W00-W19.
> A   initial encounter
> D   subsequent encounter
> S   sequela

✓4ᵗʰ **W00**   **Fall due to ice and snow**
     INCLUDES   pedestrian on foot falling (slipping) on ice and snow
     EXCLUDES 1   *fall on (from) ice and snow involving pedestrian conveyance (V00.-)*
         fall from stairs and steps not due to ice and snow (W10.-)
     AHA: 2016, 2Q, 4

     ✓x7ᵗʰ **W00.0**   **Fall on same level due to ice and snow**

     ✓x7ᵗʰ **W00.1**   **Fall from stairs and steps due to ice and snow**

     ✓x7ᵗʰ **W00.2**   **Other fall from one level to another due to ice and snow**

     ✓x7ᵗʰ **W00.9**   **Unspecified fall due to ice and snow**   ▽

✓4ᵗʰ **W01**   **Fall on same level from slipping, tripping and stumbling**
     INCLUDES   fall on moving sidewalk
     EXCLUDES 1   *fall due to bumping (striking) against object (W18.0-)*
         fall in shower or bathtub (W18.2-)
         fall on same level NOS (W18.30)
         fall on same level from slipping, tripping and stumbling due to ice or snow (W00.0)
         fall off or from toilet (W18.1-)
         slipping, tripping and stumbling NOS (W18.40)
         slipping, tripping and stumbling without falling (W18.4-)

     ✓x7ᵗʰ **W01.0**   **Fall on same level from slipping, tripping and stumbling without subsequent striking against object**
         Falling over animal

     ✓5ᵗʰ **W01.1**   **Fall on same level from slipping, tripping and stumbling with subsequent striking against object**

         ✓x7ᵗʰ **W01.10**   **Fall on same level from slipping, tripping and stumbling with subsequent striking against unspecified object**   ▽

         ✓6ᵗʰ **W01.11**   **Fall on same level from slipping, tripping and stumbling with subsequent striking against sharp object**

             ✓7ᵗʰ **W01.110**   **Fall on same level from slipping, tripping and stumbling with subsequent striking against sharp glass**

             ✓7ᵗʰ **W01.111**   **Fall on same level from slipping, tripping and stumbling with subsequent striking against power tool or machine**

             ✓7ᵗʰ **W01.118**   **Fall on same level from slipping, tripping and stumbling with subsequent striking against other sharp object**

             ✓7ᵗʰ **W01.119**   **Fall on same level from slipping, tripping and stumbling with subsequent striking against unspecified sharp object**   ▽

         ✓6ᵗʰ **W01.19**   **Fall on same level from slipping, tripping and stumbling with subsequent striking against other object**

             ✓7ᵗʰ **W01.190**   **Fall on same level from slipping, tripping and stumbling with subsequent striking against furniture**

             ✓7ᵗʰ **W01.198**   **Fall on same level from slipping, tripping and stumbling with subsequent striking against other object**

✓x7ᵗʰ **W03**   **Other fall on same level due to collision with another person**
     Fall due to non-transport collision with other person
     EXCLUDES 1   *collision with another person without fall (W51)*
         crushed or pushed by a crowd or human stampede (W52)
         fall involving pedestrian conveyance (V00-V09)
         fall due to ice or snow (W00)
         fall on same level NOS (W18.30)
     AHA: 2012, 4Q, 108

✓x7ᵗʰ **W04**   **Fall while being carried or supported by other persons**
     Accidentally dropped while being carried

✓4ᵗʰ **W05**   **Fall from non-moving wheelchair, nonmotorized scooter and motorized mobility scooter**
     EXCLUDES 1   *fall from moving wheelchair (powered) (V00.811)*
         fall from moving motorized mobility scooter (V00.831)
         fall from nonmotorized scooter (V00.141)

     ✓x7ᵗʰ **W05.0**   **Fall from non-moving wheelchair**

     ✓x7ᵗʰ **W05.1**   **Fall from non-moving nonmotorized scooter**

     ✓x7ᵗʰ **W05.2**   **Fall from non-moving motorized mobility scooter**

✓x7ᵗʰ **W06 Fall from bed**

✓x7ᵗʰ **W07 Fall from chair**

✓x7ᵗʰ **W08 Fall from other furniture**

✓4ᵗʰ **W09**   **Fall on and from playground equipment**
     EXCLUDES 1   *fall involving recreational machinery (W31)g*

     ✓x7ᵗʰ **W09.0**   **Fall on or from playground slide**

     ✓x7ᵗʰ **W09.1**   **Fall from playground swing**

     ✓x7ᵗʰ **W09.2**   **Fall on or from jungle gym**

     ✓x7ᵗʰ **W09.8**   **Fall on or from other playground equipment**

✓4ᵗʰ **W10**   **Fall on and from stairs and steps**
     EXCLUDES 1   *Fall from stairs and steps due to ice and snow (W00.1)*

     ✓x7ᵗʰ **W10.0**   **Fall (on)(from) escalator**

     ✓x7ᵗʰ **W10.1**   **Fall (on)(from) sidewalk curb**

     ✓x7ᵗʰ **W10.2**   **Fall (on)(from) incline**
         Fall (on) (from) ramp

EXCLUDES 1 Not coded here   EXCLUDES 2 Not included here   N Newborn Age: 0   P Pediatric Age: 0-17   M Maternity Age: 12-55   A Adult Age: 15-124

1144   ICD-10-CM 2018

√x 7ᵗʰ **W10.8** Fall (on) (from) other stairs and steps

√x 7ᵗʰ **W10.9** Fall (on) (from) unspecified stairs and steps ▽

√x 7ᵗʰ **W11 Fall on and from ladder**

√x 7ᵗʰ **W12 Fall on and from scaffolding**

√4ᵗʰ **W13 Fall from, out of or through building or structure**

  √x 7ᵗʰ **W13.0** Fall from, out of or through balcony
       Fall from, out of or through railing

  √x 7ᵗʰ **W13.1** Fall from, out of or through bridge

  √x 7ᵗʰ **W13.2** Fall from, out of or through roof

  √x 7ᵗʰ **W13.3** Fall through floor

  √x 7ᵗʰ **W13.4** Fall from, out of or through window
       EXCLUDES 2   *fall with subsequent striking against sharp glass (W01.110)*

  √x 7ᵗʰ **W13.8** Fall from, out of or through other building or structure
       Fall from, out of or through viaduct
       Fall from, out of or through wall
       Fall from, out of or through flag-pole

  √x 7ᵗʰ **W13.9** Fall from, out of or through building, not otherwise specified ▽
       EXCLUDES 1   *collapse of a building or structure (W20.-)*
                  fall or jump from burning building or structure (X00.-)

√x 7ᵗʰ **W14 Fall from tree**

√x 7ᵗʰ **W15 Fall from cliff**

√4ᵗʰ **W16 Fall, jump or diving into water**
     EXCLUDES 1   *accidental non-watercraft drowning and submersion not involving fall (W65-W74)*
              effects of air pressure from diving (W94.-)
              fall into water from watercraft (V90-V94)
              hitting an object or against bottom when falling from watercraft (V94.0)
     EXCLUDES 2   *striking or hitting diving board (W21.4)*

  √5ᵗʰ **W16.0 Fall into swimming pool**
       Fall into swimming pool NOS
       EXCLUDES 1   *fall into empty swimming pool (W17.3)*

    √6ᵗʰ **W16.01** Fall into swimming pool striking water surface

      √7ᵗʰ **W16.011** Fall into swimming pool striking water surface causing drowning and submersion
          EXCLUDES 1   *drowning and submersion while in swimming pool without fall (W67)*

      √7ᵗʰ **W16.012** Fall into swimming pool striking water surface causing other injury

    √6ᵗʰ **W16.02** Fall into swimming pool striking bottom

      √7ᵗʰ **W16.021** Fall into swimming pool striking bottom causing drowning and submersion
          EXCLUDES 1   *drowning and submersion while in swimming pool without fall (W67)*

      √7ᵗʰ **W16.022** Fall into swimming pool striking bottom causing other injury

    √6ᵗʰ **W16.03** Fall into swimming pool striking wall

      √7ᵗʰ **W16.031** Fall into swimming pool striking wall causing drowning and submersion
          EXCLUDES 1   *drowning and submersion while in swimming pool without fall (W67)*

      √7ᵗʰ **W16.032** Fall into swimming pool striking wall causing other injury

  √5ᵗʰ **W16.1 Fall into natural body of water**
       Fall into lake   Fall into river
       Fall into open sea   Fall into stream

    √6ᵗʰ **W16.11** Fall into natural body of water striking water surface

      √7ᵗʰ **W16.111** Fall into natural body of water striking water surface causing drowning and submersion
          EXCLUDES 1   *drowning and submersion while in natural body of water without fall (W69)*

      √7ᵗʰ **W16.112** Fall into natural body of water striking water surface causing other injury

    √6ᵗʰ **W16.12** Fall into natural body of water striking bottom

      √7ᵗʰ **W16.121** Fall into natural body of water striking bottom causing drowning and submersion
          EXCLUDES 1   *drowning and submersion while in natural body of water without fall (W69)*

      √7ᵗʰ **W16.122** Fall into natural body of water striking bottom causing other injury

    √6ᵗʰ **W16.13** Fall into natural body of water striking side

      √7ᵗʰ **W16.131** Fall into natural body of water striking side causing drowning and submersion
          EXCLUDES 1   *drowning and submersion while in natural body of water without fall (W69)*

      √7ᵗʰ **W16.132** Fall into natural body of water striking side causing other injury

  √5ᵗʰ **W16.2 Fall in (into) filled bathtub or bucket of water**

    √6ᵗʰ **W16.21** Fall in (into) filled bathtub
       EXCLUDES 1   *fall into empty bathtub (W18.2)*

      √7ᵗʰ **W16.211** Fall in (into) filled bathtub causing drowning and submersion
          EXCLUDES 1   *drowning and submersion while in filled bathtub without fall (W65)*

      √7ᵗʰ **W16.212** Fall in (into) filled bathtub causing other injury

    √6ᵗʰ **W16.22** Fall in (into) bucket of water

      √7ᵗʰ **W16.221** Fall in (into) bucket of water causing drowning and submersion

      √7ᵗʰ **W16.222** Fall in (into) bucket of water causing other injury

  √5ᵗʰ **W16.3 Fall into other water**
       Fall into fountain
       Fall into reservoir

    √6ᵗʰ **W16.31** Fall into other water striking water surface

      √7ᵗʰ **W16.311** Fall into other water striking water surface causing drowning and submersion
          EXCLUDES 1   *drowning and submersion while in other water without fall (W73)*

      √7ᵗʰ **W16.312** Fall into other water striking water surface causing other injury

    √6ᵗʰ **W16.32** Fall into other water striking bottom

      √7ᵗʰ **W16.321** Fall into other water striking bottom causing drowning and submersion
          EXCLUDES 1   *drowning and submersion while in other water without fall (W73)*

      √7ᵗʰ **W16.322** Fall into other water striking bottom causing other injury

    √6ᵗʰ **W16.33** Fall into other water striking wall

      √7ᵗʰ **W16.331** Fall into other water striking wall causing drowning and submersion
          EXCLUDES 1   *drowning and submersion while in other water without fall (W73)*

      √7ᵗʰ **W16.332** Fall into other water striking wall causing other injury

  √5ᵗʰ **W16.4 Fall into unspecified water**

    √x 7ᵗʰ **W16.41** Fall into unspecified water causing drowning and submersion ▽

    √x 7ᵗʰ **W16.42** Fall into unspecified water causing other injury ▽

  √5ᵗʰ **W16.5 Jumping or diving into swimming pool**

    √6ᵗʰ **W16.51** Jumping or diving into swimming pool striking water surface

      √7ᵗʰ **W16.511** Jumping or diving into swimming pool striking water surface causing drowning and submersion
          EXCLUDES 1   *drowning and submersion while in swimming pool without jumping or diving (W67)*

      √7ᵗʰ **W16.512** Jumping or diving into swimming pool striking water surface causing other injury

---

☑ Additional Character Req   √x 7ᵗʰ Placeholder Alert   Manifestation   HCC CMS-HCC Condition   ▽ Unspecified Code   ▶◀ Revised Text   ● New Code   ▲ Revised Code Title

ICD-10-CM 2018   1145

W10.8–W16.512

√6ᵗʰ **W16.52 Jumping or diving into swimming pool** striking bottom

√7ᵗʰ **W16.521 Jumping or diving into swimming pool striking bottom causing** drowning and submersion
EXCLUDES 1 *drowning and submersion while in swimming pool without jumping or diving (W67)*

√7ᵗʰ **W16.522 Jumping or diving into swimming pool striking bottom causing other injury**

√6ᵗʰ **W16.53 Jumping or diving into swimming pool** striking wall

√7ᵗʰ **W16.531 Jumping or diving into swimming pool striking wall causing** drowning and submersion
EXCLUDES 1 *drowning and submersion while in swimming pool without jumping or diving (W67)*

√7ᵗʰ **W16.532 Jumping or diving into swimming pool striking wall causing other injury**

√5ᵗʰ **W16.6 Jumping or diving into** natural body of water
Jumping or diving into lake
Jumping or diving into open sea
Jumping or diving into river
Jumping or diving into stream

√6ᵗʰ **W16.61 Jumping or diving into natural body of water** striking water surface

√7ᵗʰ **W16.611 Jumping or diving into natural body of water striking water surface causing** drowning and submersion
EXCLUDES 1 *drowning and submersion while in natural body of water without jumping or diving (W69)*

√7ᵗʰ **W16.612 Jumping or diving into natural body of water striking water surface causing other injury**

√6ᵗʰ **W16.62 Jumping or diving into natural body of water** striking bottom

√7ᵗʰ **W16.621 Jumping or diving into natural body of water striking bottom causing** drowning and submersion
EXCLUDES 1 *drowning and submersion while in natural body of water without jumping or diving (W69)*

√7ᵗʰ **W16.622 Jumping or diving into natural body of water striking bottom causing other injury**

√5ᵗʰ **W16.7 Jumping or diving** from boat
EXCLUDES 1 *fall from boat into water—see watercraft accident (V90-V94)*

√6ᵗʰ **W16.71 Jumping or diving from boat** striking water surface

√7ᵗʰ **W16.711 Jumping or diving from boat striking water surface causing** drowning and submersion

√7ᵗʰ **W16.712 Jumping or diving from boat striking water surface causing other injury**

√6ᵗʰ **W16.72 Jumping or diving from boat** striking bottom

√7ᵗʰ **W16.721 Jumping or diving from boat striking bottom causing** drowning and submersion

√7ᵗʰ **W16.722 Jumping or diving from boat striking bottom causing other injury**

√5ᵗʰ **W16.8 Jumping or diving into other water**
Jumping or diving into fountain
Jumping or diving into reservoir

√6ᵗʰ **W16.81 Jumping or diving into other water** striking water surface

√7ᵗʰ **W16.811 Jumping or diving into other water striking water surface causing** drowning and submersion
EXCLUDES 1 *drowning and submersion while in other water without jumping or diving (W73)*

√7ᵗʰ **W16.812 Jumping or diving into other water striking water surface causing other injury**

√6ᵗʰ **W16.82 Jumping or diving into other water** striking bottom

√7ᵗʰ **W16.821 Jumping or diving into other water striking bottom causing** drowning and submersion
EXCLUDES 1 *drowning and submersion while in other water without jumping or diving (W73)*

√7ᵗʰ **W16.822 Jumping or diving into other water striking bottom causing other injury**

√6ᵗʰ **W16.83 Jumping or diving into other water** striking wall

√7ᵗʰ **W16.831 Jumping or diving into other water striking wall causing** drowning and submersion
EXCLUDES 1 *drowning and submersion while in other water without jumping or diving (W73)*

√7ᵗʰ **W16.832 Jumping or diving into other water striking wall causing other injury**

√5ᵗʰ **W16.9 Jumping or diving into unspecified water**

√x7ᵗʰ **W16.91 Jumping or diving into unspecified water causing** drowning and submersion ▽

√x7ᵗʰ **W16.92 Jumping or diving into unspecified water causing other injury** ▽

√4ᵗʰ **W17 Other fall from one level to another**

√x7ᵗʰ **W17.0 Fall into well**

√x7ᵗʰ **W17.1 Fall into storm drain or manhole**

√x7ᵗʰ **W17.2 Fall into hole**
Fall into pit

√x7ᵗʰ **W17.3 Fall into empty swimming pool**
EXCLUDES 1 *fall into filled swimming pool (W16.0-)*

√x7ᵗʰ **W17.4 Fall from dock**

√5ᵗʰ **W17.8 Other fall from one level to another**

√x7ᵗʰ **W17.81 Fall down embankment (hill)**

√x7ᵗʰ **W17.82 Fall from (out of) grocery cart**
Fall due to grocery cart tipping over

√x7ᵗʰ **W17.89 Other fall from one level to another**
Fall from cherry picker
Fall from lifting device
Fall from mobile elevated work platform [MEWP]
Fall from sky lift
AHA: 2015, 2Q, 6

√4ᵗʰ **W18 Other slipping, tripping and stumbling and falls**

√5ᵗʰ **W18.0 Fall due to bumping against object**
Striking against object with subsequent fall
EXCLUDES 1 *fall on same level due to slipping, tripping, or stumbling with subsequent striking against object (W01.1-)*

√x7ᵗʰ **W18.00 Striking against unspecified object with subsequent fall** ▽

√x7ᵗʰ **W18.01 Striking against** sports equipment **with subsequent fall**

√x7ᵗʰ **W18.02 Striking against** glass **with subsequent fall**

√x7ᵗʰ **W18.09 Striking against other object with subsequent fall**

√5ᵗʰ **W18.1 Fall from or off toilet**

√x7ᵗʰ **W18.11 Fall from or off toilet** without subsequent striking against object
Fall from (off) toilet NOS

√x7ᵗʰ **W18.12 Fall from or off toilet** with subsequent striking against object

√x7ᵗʰ **W18.2 Fall in (into) shower or empty bathtub**
EXCLUDES 1 *fall in full bathtub causing drowning or submersion (W16.21-)*

√5ᵗʰ **W18.3 Other and unspecified fall on same level**

√x7ᵗʰ **W18.30 Fall on same level, unspecified** ▽

√x7ᵗʰ **W18.31 Fall on same level due to stepping on an object**
Fall on same level due to stepping on an animal
EXCLUDES 1 *slipping, tripping and stumbling without fall due to stepping on animal (W18.41)*

√x7ᵗʰ **W18.39 Other fall on same level**

√5ᵗʰ **W18.4 Slipping, tripping and stumbling without falling**
EXCLUDES 1 *collision with another person without fall (W51)*

√x7ᵗʰ **W18.40 Slipping, tripping and stumbling without falling, unspecified** ▽

EXCLUDES 1 Not coded here   EXCLUDES 2 Not included here   N Newborn Age: 0   P Pediatric Age: 0-17   M Maternity Age: 12-55   A Adult Age: 15-124

1146   ICD-10-CM 2018

✓x7ᵗʰ **W18.41** **Slipping, tripping and stumbling without falling due to** stepping on object
     Slipping, tripping and stumbling without falling due to stepping on animal
     EXCLUDES 1 *slipping, tripping and stumbling with fall due to stepping on animal (W18.31)*

✓x7ᵗʰ **W18.42** **Slipping, tripping and stumbling without falling due to** stepping into hole or opening

✓x7ᵗʰ **W18.43** **Slipping, tripping and stumbling without falling due to** stepping from one level to another

✓x7ᵗʰ **W18.49** **Other slipping, tripping and stumbling without falling**

✓x7ᵗʰ **W19 Unspecified fall** ▽
     Accidental fall NOS
     AHA: 2012, 4Q, 95

Exposure to inanimate mechanical forces (W20-W49)

EXCLUDES 1 *assault (X92-Y09)*
     contact or collision with animals or persons (W50-W64)
     exposure to inanimate mechanical forces involving military or war operations (Y36.-, Y37.-)
     intentional self-harm (X71-X83)

The appropriate 7th character is to be added to each code from categories W20-W49.
A   initial encounter
D   subsequent encounter
S   sequela

✓4ᵗʰ **W20** **Struck by thrown, projected or falling object**
     Code first any associated:
     cataclysm (X34-X39)
     lightning strike (T75.00)
     EXCLUDES 1 *falling object in machinery accident (W24, W28-W31)*
       falling object in transport accident (V01-V99)
       object set in motion by explosion (W35-W40)
       object set in motion by firearm (W32-W34)
       struck by thrown sports equipment (W21.-)

✓x7ᵗʰ **W20.0** **Struck by falling object in cave-in**
     EXCLUDES 2 *asphyxiation due to cave-in (T71.21)*

✓x7ᵗʰ **W20.1** **Struck by object due to collapse of building**
     EXCLUDES 1 *struck by object due to collapse of burning building (X00.2, X02.2)*

✓x7ᵗʰ **W20.8** **Other cause of strike by thrown, projected or falling object**
     EXCLUDES 1 *struck by thrown sports equipment (W21.-)*

✓4ᵗʰ **W21** **Striking against or struck by sports equipment**
     EXCLUDES 1 *assault with sports equipment (Y08.0-)*
       striking against or struck by sports equipment with subsequent fall (W18.01)

✓5ᵗʰ **W21.0** **Struck by** hit or thrown ball

   ✓x7ᵗʰ **W21.00** **Struck by hit or thrown ball, unspecified type** ▽

   ✓x7ᵗʰ **W21.01** **Struck by** football

   ✓x7ᵗʰ **W21.02** **Struck by** soccer ball

   ✓x7ᵗʰ **W21.03** **Struck by** baseball

   ✓x7ᵗʰ **W21.04** **Struck by** golf ball

   ✓x7ᵗʰ **W21.05** **Struck by** basketball

   ✓x7ᵗʰ **W21.06** **Struck by** volleyball

   ✓x7ᵗʰ **W21.07** **Struck by** softball

   ✓x7ᵗʰ **W21.09** **Struck by other hit or thrown ball**

✓5ᵗʰ **W21.1** **Struck by** bat, racquet or club

   ✓x7ᵗʰ **W21.11** **Struck by** baseball bat

   ✓x7ᵗʰ **W21.12** **Struck by** tennis racquet

   ✓x7ᵗʰ **W21.13** **Struck by** golf club

   ✓x7ᵗʰ **W21.19** **Struck by other bat, racquet or club**

✓5ᵗʰ **W21.2** **Struck by** hockey stick or puck

   ✓6ᵗʰ **W21.21** **Struck by** hockey stick

     ✓7ᵗʰ **W21.210** **Struck by** ice hockey stick

     ✓7ᵗʰ **W21.211** **Struck by** field hockey stick

   ✓6ᵗʰ **W21.22** **Struck by** hockey puck

     ✓7ᵗʰ **W21.220** **Struck by** ice hockey puck

     ✓7ᵗʰ **W21.221** **Struck by** field hockey puck

✓5ᵗʰ **W21.3** **Struck by sports** foot wear

   ✓x7ᵗʰ **W21.31** **Struck by** shoe cleats
     Stepped on by shoe cleats

   ✓x7ᵗʰ **W21.32** **Struck by** skate blades
     Skated over by skate blades

   ✓x7ᵗʰ **W21.39** **Struck by other sports foot wear**

✓x7ᵗʰ **W21.4** **Striking against** diving board
     Use additional code for subsequent falling into water, if applicable (W16.-)

✓5ᵗʰ **W21.8** **Striking against or struck by other sports equipment**

   ✓x7ᵗʰ **W21.81** **Striking against or struck by** football helmet

   ✓x7ᵗʰ **W21.89** **Striking against or struck by other sports equipment**

✓x7ᵗʰ **W21.9** **Striking against or struck by unspecified sports equipment** ▽

✓4ᵗʰ **W22** **Striking against or struck by other objects**
     EXCLUDES 1 *striking against or struck by object with subsequent fall (W18.09)*

✓5ᵗʰ **W22.0** **Striking against** stationary object
     EXCLUDES 1 *striking against stationary sports equipment (W21.8)*

   ✓x7ᵗʰ **W22.01** **Walked into** wall

   ✓x7ᵗʰ **W22.02** **Walked into** lamppost

   ✓x7ᵗʰ **W22.03** **Walked into** furniture

   ✓6ᵗʰ **W22.04** **Striking against wall of** swimming pool

     ✓7ᵗʰ **W22.041** **Striking against wall of swimming pool causing** drowning and submersion
       EXCLUDES 1 *drowning and submersion while swimming without striking against wall (W67)*

     ✓7ᵗʰ **W22.042** **Striking against wall of swimming pool causing other injury**

   ✓x7ᵗʰ **W22.09** **Striking against other stationary object**

✓5ᵗʰ **W22.1** **Striking against or struck by** automobile airbag

   ✓x7ᵗʰ **W22.10** **Striking against or struck by unspecified automobile airbag** ▽

   ✓x7ᵗʰ **W22.11** **Striking against or struck by** driver side **automobile airbag**

   ✓x7ᵗʰ **W22.12** **Striking against or struck by** front passenger **side automobile airbag**

   ✓x7ᵗʰ **W22.19** **Striking against or struck by other automobile airbag**

✓x7ᵗʰ **W22.8** **Striking against or struck by other objects**
     Striking against or struck by object NOS
     EXCLUDES 1 *struck by thrown, projected or falling object (W20.-)*

✓4ᵗʰ **W23** **Caught, crushed, jammed or pinched in or between objects**
     EXCLUDES 1 *injury caused by cutting or piercing instruments (W25-W27)*
       injury caused by firearms malfunction (W32.1, W33.1-, W34.1-)
       injury caused by lifting and transmission devices (W24.-)
       injury caused by machinery (W28-W31)
       injury caused by nonpowered hand tools (W27.-)
       injury caused by transport vehicle being used as a means of transportation (V01-V99)
       injury caused by struck by thrown, projected or falling object (W20.-)

✓x7ᵗʰ **W23.0** **Caught, crushed, jammed, or pinched between** moving objects

✓x7ᵗʰ **W23.1** **Caught, crushed, jammed, or pinched between** stationary objects

✓4ᵗʰ **W24** **Contact with lifting and transmission devices, not elsewhere classified**
     EXCLUDES 1 *transport accidents (V01-V99)*

✓x7ᵗʰ **W24.0** **Contact with lifting devices, not elsewhere classified**
     Contact with chain hoist
     Contact with drive belt
     Contact with pulley (block)

✓x7ᵗʰ **W24.1** **Contact with transmission devices, not elsewhere classified**
     Contact with transmission belt or cable

✓x7ᵗʰ **W25** **Contact with sharp glass**
     Code first any associated:
     injury due to flying glass from explosion or firearm discharge (W32-W40)
     transport accident (V00-V99)
     EXCLUDES 1 *fall on same level due to slipping, tripping and stumbling with subsequent striking against sharp glass (W01.10)*
       striking against sharp glass with subsequent fall (W18.02)
     EXCLUDES 2 *glass embedded in skin (W45)*

✓ Additional Character Req   ✓x7ᵗʰ Placeholder Alert   Manifestation   **HCC** CMS-HCC Condition   ▽ Unspecified Code   ►◄ Revised Text   ● New Code   ▲ Revised Code Title

✅4ᵗʰ **W26 Contact with other sharp objects**
> EXCLUDES 2   *sharp object(s) embedded in skin (W45)*

✓x 7ᵗʰ **W26.0 Contact with knife**
> EXCLUDES 1   *contact with electric knife (W29.1)*

✓x 7ᵗʰ **W26.1 Contact with sword or dagger**

✓x 7ᵗʰ **W26.2 Contact with edge of stiff paper**
> Paper cut

✓x 7ᵗʰ **W26.8 Contact with other sharp object(s), not elsewhere classified**
> Contact with tin can lid

✓x 7ᵗʰ **W26.9 Contact with unspecified sharp object(s)**   ▽

✅4ᵗʰ **W27 Contact with nonpowered hand tool**

✓x 7ᵗʰ **W27.0 Contact with workbench tool**
> Contact with auger
> Contact with axe
> Contact with chisel
> Contact with handsaw
> Contact with screwdriver

✓x 7ᵗʰ **W27.1 Contact with garden tool**
> Contact with hoe
> Contact with nonpowered lawn mower
> Contact with pitchfork
> Contact with rake

✓x 7ᵗʰ **W27.2 Contact with scissors**

✓x 7ᵗʰ **W27.3 Contact with needle (sewing)**
> EXCLUDES 1   *contact with hypodermic needle (W46.-)*

✓x 7ᵗʰ **W27.4 Contact with kitchen utensil**
> Contact with fork
> Contact with ice-pick
> Contact with can-opener NOS

✓x 7ᵗʰ **W27.5 Contact with paper-cutter**

✓x 7ᵗʰ **W27.8 Contact with other nonpowered hand tool**
> Contact with nonpowered sewing machine
> Contact with shovel

✓x 7ᵗʰ **W28 Contact with powered lawn mower**
> Powered lawn mower (commercial) (residential)
> EXCLUDES 1   *contact with nonpowered lawn mower (W27.1)*
> EXCLUDES 2   *exposure to electric current (W86.-)*

✅4ᵗʰ **W29 Contact with other powered hand tools and household machinery**
> EXCLUDES 1   *contact with commercial machinery (W31.82)*
>   *contact with hot household appliance (X15)*
>   *contact with nonpowered hand tool (W27.-)*
>   *exposure to electric current (W86)*

✓x 7ᵗʰ **W29.0 Contact with powered kitchen appliance**
> Contact with blender
> Contact with can-opener
> Contact with garbage disposal
> Contact with mixer

✓x 7ᵗʰ **W29.1 Contact with electric knife**

✓x 7ᵗʰ **W29.2 Contact with other powered household machinery**
> Contact with electric fan
> Contact with powered dryer (clothes) (powered) (spin)
> Contact with washing-machine
> Contact with sewing machine

✓x 7ᵗʰ **W29.3 Contact with powered garden and outdoor hand tools and machinery**
> Contact with chainsaw
> Contact with edger
> Contact with garden cultivator (tiller)
> Contact with hedge trimmer
> Contact with other powered garden tool
> EXCLUDES 1   *contact with powered lawn mower (W28)*

✓x 7ᵗʰ **W29.4 Contact with nail gun**

▲ ✓x 7ᵗʰ **W29.8 Contact with other powered hand tools and household machinery**
> Contact with do-it-yourself tool NOS

✅4ᵗʰ **W30 Contact with agricultural machinery**
> INCLUDES   animal-powered farm machine
> EXCLUDES 1   *agricultural transport vehicle accident (V01-V99)*
>   *explosion of grain store (W40.8)*
>   *exposure to electric current (W86.-)*

✓x 7ᵗʰ **W30.0 Contact with combine harvester**
> Contact with reaper
> Contact with thresher

✓x 7ᵗʰ **W30.1 Contact with power take-off devices (PTO)**

✓x 7ᵗʰ **W30.2 Contact with hay derrick**

✓x 7ᵗʰ **W30.3 Contact with grain storage elevator**
> EXCLUDES 1   *explosion of grain store (W40.8)*

✓5ᵗʰ **W30.8 Contact with other specified agricultural machinery**

✓x 7ᵗʰ **W30.81 Contact with agricultural transport vehicle in stationary use**
> Contact with agricultural transport vehicle under repair, not on public roadway
> EXCLUDES 1   *agricultural transport vehicle accident (V01-V99)*

✓x 7ᵗʰ **W30.89 Contact with other specified agricultural machinery**

✓x 7ᵗʰ **W30.9 Contact with unspecified agricultural machinery**   ▽
> Contact with farm machinery NOS

✅4ᵗʰ **W31 Contact with other and unspecified machinery**
> EXCLUDES 1   *contact with agricultural machinery (W30.-)*
>   *contact with machinery in transport under own power or being towed by a vehicle (V01-V99)*
>   *exposure to electric current (W86)*

✓x 7ᵗʰ **W31.0 Contact with mining and earth-drilling machinery**
> Contact with bore or drill (land) (seabed)
> Contact with shaft hoist
> Contact with shaft lift
> Contact with undercutter

✓x 7ᵗʰ **W31.1 Contact with metalworking machines**
> Contact with abrasive wheel
> Contact with forging machine
> Contact with lathe
> Contact with mechanical shears
> Contact with metal drilling machine
> Contact with milling machine
> Contact with power press
> Contact with rolling-mill
> Contact with metal sawing machine

✓x 7ᵗʰ **W31.2 Contact with powered woodworking and forming machines**
> Contact with band saw
> Contact with bench saw
> Contact with circular saw
> Contact with molding machine
> Contact with overhead plane
> Contact with powered saw
> Contact with radial saw
> Contact with sander
> EXCLUDES 1   *nonpowered woodworking tools (W27.0)*

✓x 7ᵗʰ **W31.3 Contact with prime movers**
> Contact with gas turbine
> Contact with internal combustion engine
> Contact with steam engine
> Contact with water driven turbine

✓5ᵗʰ **W31.8 Contact with other specified machinery**

✓x 7ᵗʰ **W31.81 Contact with recreational machinery**
> Contact with roller coaster

✓x 7ᵗʰ **W31.82 Contact with other commercial machinery**
> Contact with commercial electric fan
> Contact with commercial kitchen appliances
> Contact with commercial powered dryer (clothes) (powered) (spin)
> Contact with commercial washing-machine
> Contact with commercial sewing machine
> EXCLUDES 1   *contact with household machinery (W29.-)*
>   *contact with powered lawn mower (W28)*

✓x 7ᵗʰ **W31.83 Contact with special construction vehicle in stationary use**
> Contact with special construction vehicle under repair, not on public roadway
> EXCLUDES 1   *special construction vehicle accident (V01-V99)*

✓x 7ᵗʰ **W31.89 Contact with other specified machinery**

✓x 7ᵗʰ **W31.9 Contact with unspecified machinery**   ▽
> Contact with machinery NOS

EXCLUDES 1 Not coded here   EXCLUDES 2 Not included here   N Newborn Age: 0   P Pediatric Age: 0-17   M Maternity Age: 12-55   A Adult Age: 15-124

1148   ICD-10-CM 2018

✓4ᵗʰ **W32 Accidental handgun discharge and malfunction**
  INCLUDES   accidental discharge and malfunction of gun for single hand use
           accidental discharge and malfunction of pistol
           accidental discharge and malfunction of revolver
           handgun discharge and malfunction NOS
  EXCLUDES 1   *accidental airgun discharge and malfunction (W34.010, W34.110)*
           accidental BB gun discharge and malfunction (W34.010, W34.110)
           accidental pellet gun discharge and malfunction (W34.010, W34.110)
           accidental shotgun discharge and malfunction (W33.01, W33.11)
           assault by handgun discharge (X93)
           handgun discharge involving legal intervention (Y35.0-)
           handgun discharge involving military or war operations (Y36.4-)
           intentional self-harm by handgun discharge (X72)
           Very pistol discharge and malfunction (W34.09, W34.19)

✓ˣ7ᵗʰ **W32.0 Accidental handgun discharge**

✓ˣ7ᵗʰ **W32.1 Accidental handgun malfunction**
       Injury due to explosion of handgun (parts)
       Injury due to malfunction of mechanism or component of handgun
       Injury due to recoil of handgun
       Powder burn from handgun

✓4ᵗʰ **W33 Accidental rifle, shotgun and larger firearm discharge and malfunction**
  INCLUDES   rifle, shotgun and larger firearm discharge and malfunction NOS
  EXCLUDES 1   *accidental airgun discharge and malfunction (W34.010, W34.110)*
           accidental BB gun discharge and malfunction (W34.010, W34.110)
           accidental handgun discharge and malfunction (W32.-)
           accidental pellet gun discharge and malfunction (W34.010, W34.110)
           assault by rifle, shotgun and larger firearm discharge (X94)
           firearm discharge involving legal intervention (Y35.0-)
           firearm discharge involving military or war operations (Y36.4-)
           intentional self-harm by rifle, shotgun and larger firearm discharge (X73)

✓5ᵗʰ **W33.0 Accidental rifle, shotgun and larger firearm discharge**

  ✓ˣ7ᵗʰ **W33.00 Accidental discharge of unspecified larger firearm** ▽
       Discharge of unspecified larger firearm NOS

  ✓ˣ7ᵗʰ **W33.01 Accidental discharge of shotgun**
       Discharge of shotgun NOS

  ✓ˣ7ᵗʰ **W33.02 Accidental discharge of hunting rifle**
       Discharge of hunting rifle NOS

  ✓ˣ7ᵗʰ **W33.03 Accidental discharge of machine gun**
       Discharge of machine gun NOS

  ✓ˣ7ᵗʰ **W33.09 Accidental discharge of other larger firearm**
       Discharge of other larger firearm NOS

✓5ᵗʰ **W33.1 Accidental rifle, shotgun and larger firearm malfunction**
       Injury due to explosion of rifle, shotgun and larger firearm (parts)
       Injury due to malfunction of mechanism or component of rifle, shotgun and larger firearm
       Injury due to piercing, cutting, crushing or pinching due to (by) slide trigger mechanism, scope or other gun part
       Injury due to recoil of rifle, shotgun and larger firearm
       Powder burn from rifle, shotgun and larger firearm

  ✓ˣ7ᵗʰ **W33.10 Accidental malfunction of unspecified larger firearm** ▽
       Malfunction of unspecified larger firearm NOS

  ✓ˣ7ᵗʰ **W33.11 Accidental malfunction of shotgun**
       Malfunction of shotgun NOS

  ✓ˣ7ᵗʰ **W33.12 Accidental malfunction of hunting rifle**
       Malfunction of hunting rifle NOS

  ✓ˣ7ᵗʰ **W33.13 Accidental malfunction of machine gun**
       Malfunction of machine gun NOS

  ✓ˣ7ᵗʰ **W33.19 Accidental malfunction of other larger firearm**
       Malfunction of other larger firearm NOS

✓4ᵗʰ **W34 Accidental discharge and malfunction from other and unspecified firearms and guns**

✓5ᵗʰ **W34.0 Accidental discharge from other and unspecified firearms and guns**

  ✓ˣ7ᵗʰ **W34.00 Accidental discharge from unspecified firearms or gun** ▽
       Discharge from firearm NOS
       Gunshot wound NOS
       Shot NOS

  ✓6ᵗʰ **W34.01 Accidental discharge of gas, air or spring-operated guns**

    ✓7ᵗʰ **W34.010 Accidental discharge of airgun**
         Accidental discharge of BB gun
         Accidental discharge of pellet gun

    ✓7ᵗʰ **W34.011 Accidental discharge of paintball gun**
         Accidental injury due to paintball discharge

    ✓7ᵗʰ **W34.018 Accidental discharge of other gas, air or spring-operated gun**

  ✓ˣ7ᵗʰ **W34.09 Accidental discharge from other specified firearms**
       Accidental discharge from Very pistol [flare]

✓5ᵗʰ **W34.1 Accidental malfunction from other and unspecified firearms and guns**

  ✓ˣ7ᵗʰ **W34.10 Accidental malfunction from unspecified firearms or gun** ▽
       Firearm malfunction NOS

  ✓6ᵗʰ **W34.11 Accidental malfunction of gas, air or spring-operated guns**

    ✓7ᵗʰ **W34.110 Accidental malfunction of airgun**
         Accidental malfunction of BB gun
         Accidental malfunction of pellet gun

    ✓7ᵗʰ **W34.111 Accidental malfunction of paintball gun**
         Accidental injury due to paintball gun malfunction

    ✓7ᵗʰ **W34.118 Accidental malfunction of other gas, air or spring-operated gun**

  ✓ˣ7ᵗʰ **W34.19 Accidental malfunction from other specified firearms**
       Accidental malfunction from Very pistol [flare]

✓ˣ7ᵗʰ **W35 Explosion and rupture of boiler**
  EXCLUDES 1   *explosion and rupture of boiler on watercraft (V93.4)*

✓4ᵗʰ **W36 Explosion and rupture of gas cylinder**

  ✓ˣ7ᵗʰ **W36.1 Explosion and rupture of aerosol can**

  ✓ˣ7ᵗʰ **W36.2 Explosion and rupture of air tank**

  ✓ˣ7ᵗʰ **W36.3 Explosion and rupture of pressurized-gas tank**

  ✓ˣ7ᵗʰ **W36.8 Explosion and rupture of other gas cylinder**

  ✓ˣ7ᵗʰ **W36.9 Explosion and rupture of unspecified gas cylinder** ▽

✓4ᵗʰ **W37 Explosion and rupture of pressurized tire, pipe or hose**

  ✓ˣ7ᵗʰ **W37.0 Explosion of bicycle tire**

  ✓ˣ7ᵗʰ **W37.8 Explosion and rupture of other pressurized tire, pipe or hose**

✓ˣ7ᵗʰ **W38 Explosion and rupture of other specified pressurized devices**

✓ˣ7ᵗʰ **W39 Discharge of firework**

✓4ᵗʰ **W40 Explosion of other materials**
  EXCLUDES 1   *assault by explosive material (X96)*
           explosion involving legal intervention (Y35.1-)
           explosion involving military or war operations (Y36.0-, Y36.2-)
           intentional self-harm by explosive material (X75)

  ✓ˣ7ᵗʰ **W40.0 Explosion of blasting material**
       Explosion of blasting cap
       Explosion of detonator
       Explosion of dynamite
       Explosion of explosive (any) used in blasting operations

  ✓ˣ7ᵗʰ **W40.1 Explosion of explosive gases**
       Explosion of acetylene
       Explosion of butane
       Explosion of coal gas
       Explosion in mine NOS
       Explosion of explosive gas
       Explosion of fire damp
       Explosion of gasoline fumes
       Explosion of methane
       Explosion of propane

☑ Additional Character Req   ✓ˣ7ᵗʰ Placeholder Alert   **Manifestation**   HCC CMS-HCC Condition   ▽ Unspecified Code   ▶◀ Revised Text   ● New Code   ▲ Revised Code Title

✓x7th **W40.8 Explosion of other specified explosive materials**
Explosion in dump NOS
Explosion in factory NOS
Explosion in grain store
Explosion in munitions
EXCLUDES 1 *explosion involving legal intervention (Y35.1-)*
explosion involving military or war operations (Y36.0-, Y36.2-)

✓x7th **W40.9 Explosion of unspecified explosive materials** ▽
Explosion NOS

✓4th **W42 Exposure to noise**

✓x7th **W42.0 Exposure to supersonic waves**

✓x7th **W42.9 Exposure to other noise**
Exposure to sound waves NOS

✓4th **W45 Foreign body or object entering through skin**
INCLUDES foreign body or object embedded in skin
nail embedded in skin
EXCLUDES 2 *contact with hand tools (nonpowered) (powered) (W27-W29)*
contact with other sharp object(s) (W26.-)
contact with sharp glass (W25.-)
struck by objects (W20-W22)

✓x7th **W45.0 Nail entering through skin**

✓x7th **W45.8 Other foreign body or object entering through skin**
Splinter in skin NOS

✓4th **W46 Contact with hypodermic needle**

✓x7th **W46.0 Contact with hypodermic needle**
Hypodermic needle stick NOS

✓x7th **W46.1 Contact with contaminated hypodermic needle**

✓4th **W49 Exposure to other inanimate mechanical forces**
INCLUDES exposure to abnormal gravitational [G] forces
exposure to inanimate mechanical forces NEC
EXCLUDES 1 *exposure to inanimate mechanical forces involving military or war operations (Y36.-, Y37.-)*

✓5th **W49.0 Item causing external constriction**

✓x7th **W49.01 Hair causing external constriction**

✓x7th **W49.02 String or thread causing external constriction**

✓x7th **W49.03 Rubber band causing external constriction**

✓x7th **W49.04 Ring or other jewelry causing external constriction**

✓x7th **W49.09 Other specified item causing external constriction**

✓x7th **W49.9 Exposure to other inanimate mechanical forces**

Exposure to animate mechanical forces (W50-W64)
EXCLUDES 1 *Toxic effect of contact with venomous animals and plants (T63.-)*

The appropriate 7th character is to be added to each code from categories W50-W64.
A   initial encounter
D   subsequent encounter
S   sequela

✓4th **W50 Accidental hit, strike, kick, twist, bite or scratch by another person**
INCLUDES hit, strike, kick, twist, bite, or scratch by another person NOS
EXCLUDES 1 *assault by bodily force (Y04)*
struck by objects (W20-W22)

✓x7th **W50.0 Accidental hit or strike by another person**
Hit or strike by another person NOS

✓x7th **W50.1 Accidental kick by another person**
Kick by another person NOS

✓x7th **W50.2 Accidental twist by another person**
Twist by another person NOS

✓x7th **W50.3 Accidental bite by another person**
Human bite
Bite by another person NOS

✓x7th **W50.4 Accidental scratch by another person**
Scratch by another person NOS

✓x7th **W51 Accidental striking against or bumped into by another person**
EXCLUDES 1 *assault by striking against or bumping into by another person (Y04.2)*
fall due to collision with another person (W03)

✓x7th **W52 Crushed, pushed or stepped on by crowd or human stampede**
Crushed, pushed or stepped on by crowd or human stampede with or without fall

✓4th **W53 Contact with rodent**
INCLUDES contact with saliva, feces or urine of rodent

✓5th **W53.0 Contact with mouse**

✓x7th **W53.01 Bitten by mouse**

✓x7th **W53.09 Other contact with mouse**

✓5th **W53.1 Contact with rat**

✓x7th **W53.11 Bitten by rat**

✓x7th **W53.19 Other contact with rat**

✓5th **W53.2 Contact with squirrel**

✓x7th **W53.21 Bitten by squirrel**

✓x7th **W53.29 Other contact with squirrel**

✓5th **W53.8 Contact with other rodent**

✓x7th **W53.81 Bitten by other rodent**

✓x7th **W53.89 Other contact with other rodent**

✓4th **W54 Contact with dog**
INCLUDES contact with saliva, feces or urine of dog

✓x7th **W54.0 Bitten by dog**

✓x7th **W54.1 Struck by dog**
Knocked over by dog

✓x7th **W54.8 Other contact with dog**

✓4th **W55 Contact with other mammals**
INCLUDES contact with saliva, feces or urine of mammal
EXCLUDES 1 *animal being ridden—see transport accidents*
bitten or struck by dog (W54)
bitten or struck by rodent (W53.-)
contact with marine mammals (W56.-)

✓5th **W55.0 Contact with cat**

✓x7th **W55.01 Bitten by cat**

✓x7th **W55.03 Scratched by cat**

✓x7th **W55.09 Other contact with cat**

✓5th **W55.1 Contact with horse**

✓x7th **W55.11 Bitten by horse**

✓x7th **W55.12 Struck by horse**

✓x7th **W55.19 Other contact with horse**

✓5th **W55.2 Contact with cow**
Contact with bull

✓x7th **W55.21 Bitten by cow**

✓x7th **W55.22 Struck by cow**
Gored by bull

✓x7th **W55.29 Other contact with cow**

✓5th **W55.3 Contact with other hoof stock**
Contact with goats
Contact with sheep

✓x7th **W55.31 Bitten by other hoof stock**

✓x7th **W55.32 Struck by other hoof stock**
Gored by goat
Gored by ram

✓x7th **W55.39 Other contact with other hoof stock**

✓5th **W55.4 Contact with pig**

✓x7th **W55.41 Bitten by pig**

✓x7th **W55.42 Struck by pig**

✓x7th **W55.49 Other contact with pig**

✓5th **W55.5 Contact with raccoon**

✓x7th **W55.51 Bitten by raccoon**

✓x7th **W55.52 Struck by raccoon**

✓x7th **W55.59 Other contact with raccoon**

✓5th **W55.8 Contact with other mammals**

✓x7th **W55.81 Bitten by other mammals**

✓x7th **W55.82 Struck by other mammals**

✓x7th **W55.89 Other contact with other mammals**

✓4th **W56 Contact with nonvenomous marine animal**
EXCLUDES 1 *contact with venomous marine animal (T63.-)*

✓5th **W56.0 Contact with dolphin**

✓x7th **W56.01 Bitten by dolphin**

✓x7th **W56.02 Struck by dolphin**

✓x7th **W56.09 Other contact with dolphin**

√5ᵗʰ **W56.1** **Contact with** sea lion

     √x7ᵗʰ **W56.11** Bitten **by sea lion**

     √x7ᵗʰ **W56.12** Struck **by sea lion**

     √x7ᵗʰ **W56.19** **Other contact with sea lion**

√5ᵗʰ **W56.2** **Contact with** orca
        Contact with killer whale

     √x7ᵗʰ **W56.21** Bitten **by orca**

     √x7ᵗʰ **W56.22** Struck **by orca**

     √x7ᵗʰ **W56.29** **Other contact with orca**

√5ᵗʰ **W56.3** **Contact with other marine mammals**

     √x7ᵗʰ **W56.31** Bitten **by other marine mammals**

     √x7ᵗʰ **W56.32** Struck **by other marine mammals**

     √x7ᵗʰ **W56.39** **Other contact with other marine mammals**

√5ᵗʰ **W56.4** **Contact with** shark

     √x7ᵗʰ **W56.41** Bitten **by shark**

     √x7ᵗʰ **W56.42** Struck **by shark**

     √x7ᵗʰ **W56.49** **Other contact with shark**

√5ᵗʰ **W56.5** **Contact with other fish**

     √x7ᵗʰ **W56.51** Bitten **by other fish**

     √x7ᵗʰ **W56.52** Struck **by other fish**

     √x7ᵗʰ **W56.59** **Other contact with other fish**

√5ᵗʰ **W56.8** **Contact with other nonvenomous marine animals**

     √x7ᵗʰ **W56.81** Bitten **by other nonvenomous marine animals**

     √x7ᵗʰ **W56.82** Struck **by other nonvenomous marine animals**

     √x7ᵗʰ **W56.89** **Other contact with other nonvenomous marine animals**

√x7ᵗʰ **W57** **Bitten or stung by nonvenomous insect and other nonvenomous arthropods**
     EXCLUDES 1   *contact with venomous insects and arthropods (T63.2-, T63.3-, T63.4-)*

√4ᵗʰ **W58** **Contact with crocodile or alligator**

√5ᵗʰ **W58.0** **Contact with** alligator

     √x7ᵗʰ **W58.01** Bitten **by alligator**

     √x7ᵗʰ **W58.02** Struck **by alligator**

     √x7ᵗʰ **W58.03** Crushed **by alligator**

     √x7ᵗʰ **W58.09** **Other contact with alligator**

√5ᵗʰ **W58.1** **Contact with** crocodile

     √x7ᵗʰ **W58.11** Bitten **by crocodile**

     √x7ᵗʰ **W58.12** Struck **by crocodile**

     √x7ᵗʰ **W58.13** Crushed **by crocodile**

     √x7ᵗʰ **W58.19** **Other contact with crocodile**

√4ᵗʰ **W59** **Contact with other nonvenomous reptiles**
     EXCLUDES 1   *contact with venomous reptile (T63.0-, T63.1-)*

√5ᵗʰ **W59.0** **Contact with nonvenomous** lizards

     √x7ᵗʰ **W59.01** Bitten **by nonvenomous lizards**

     √x7ᵗʰ **W59.02** Struck **by nonvenomous lizards**

     √x7ᵗʰ **W59.09** **Other contact with nonvenomous lizards**
             Exposure to nonvenomous lizards

√5ᵗʰ **W59.1** **Contact with nonvenomous** snakes

     √x7ᵗʰ **W59.11** Bitten **by nonvenomous snake**

     √x7ᵗʰ **W59.12** Struck **by nonvenomous snake**

     √x7ᵗʰ **W59.13** Crushed **by nonvenomous snake**

     √x7ᵗʰ **W59.19** **Other contact with nonvenomous snake**

√5ᵗʰ **W59.2** **Contact with** turtles
     EXCLUDES 1   *contact with tortoises (W59.8-)*

     √x7ᵗʰ **W59.21** Bitten **by turtle**

     √x7ᵗʰ **W59.22** Struck **by turtle**

     √x7ᵗʰ **W59.29** **Other contact with turtle**
             Exposure to turtles

√5ᵗʰ **W59.8** **Contact with other nonvenomous reptiles**

     √x7ᵗʰ **W59.81** Bitten **by other nonvenomous reptiles**

     √x7ᵗʰ **W59.82** Struck **by other nonvenomous reptiles**

     √x7ᵗʰ **W59.83** Crushed **by other nonvenomous reptiles**

     √x7ᵗʰ **W59.89** **Other contact with other nonvenomous reptiles**

√x7ᵗʰ **W60** **Contact with nonvenomous plant thorns and spines and sharp leaves**
     EXCLUDES 1   *contact with venomous plants (T63.7-)*

√4ᵗʰ **W61** **Contact with birds (domestic) (wild)**
     INCLUDES   contact with excreta of birds

√5ᵗʰ **W61.0** **Contact with** parrot

     √x7ᵗʰ **W61.01** Bitten **by parrot**

     √x7ᵗʰ **W61.02** Struck **by parrot**

     √x7ᵗʰ **W61.09** **Other contact with parrot**
             Exposure to parrots

√5ᵗʰ **W61.1** **Contact with** macaw

     √x7ᵗʰ **W61.11** Bitten **by macaw**

     √x7ᵗʰ **W61.12** Struck **by macaw**

     √x7ᵗʰ **W61.19** **Other contact with macaw**
             Exposure to macaws

√5ᵗʰ **W61.2** **Contact with other psittacines**

     √x7ᵗʰ **W61.21** Bitten **by other psittacines**

     √x7ᵗʰ **W61.22** Struck **by other psittacines**

     √x7ᵗʰ **W61.29** **Other contact with other psittacines**
             Exposure to other psittacines

√5ᵗʰ **W61.3** **Contact with** chicken

     √x7ᵗʰ **W61.32** Struck **by chicken**

     √x7ᵗʰ **W61.33** Pecked **by chicken**

     √x7ᵗʰ **W61.39** **Other contact with chicken**
             Exposure to chickens

√5ᵗʰ **W61.4** **Contact with** turkey

     √x7ᵗʰ **W61.42** Struck **by turkey**

     √x7ᵗʰ **W61.43** Pecked **by turkey**

     √x7ᵗʰ **W61.49** **Other contact with turkey**

√5ᵗʰ **W61.5** **Contact with** goose

     √x7ᵗʰ **W61.51** Bitten **by goose**

     √x7ᵗʰ **W61.52** Struck **by goose**

     √x7ᵗʰ **W61.59** **Other contact with goose**

√5ᵗʰ **W61.6** **Contact with** duck

     √x7ᵗʰ **W61.61** Bitten **by duck**

     √x7ᵗʰ **W61.62** Struck **by duck**

     √x7ᵗʰ **W61.69** **Other contact with duck**

√5ᵗʰ **W61.9** **Contact with other birds**

     √x7ᵗʰ **W61.91** Bitten **by other birds**

     √x7ᵗʰ **W61.92** Struck **by other birds**

     √x7ᵗʰ **W61.99** **Other contact with other birds**
             Contact with bird NOS

√4ᵗʰ **W62** **Contact with nonvenomous amphibians**
     EXCLUDES 1   *contact with venomous amphibians (T63.81-R63.83)*

     √x7ᵗʰ **W62.0** **Contact with nonvenomous** frogs

     √x7ᵗʰ **W62.1** **Contact with nonvenomous** toads

     √x7ᵗʰ **W62.9** **Contact with other nonvenomous amphibians**

√x7ᵗʰ **W64** **Exposure to other animate mechanical forces**
     INCLUDES   exposure to nonvenomous animal NOS
     EXCLUDES 1   *contact with venomous animal (T63.-)*

Accidental non-transport drowning and submersion (W65-W74)

     EXCLUDES 1   *accidental drowning and submersion due to fall into water (W16.-)*
                     accidental drowning and submersion due to water transport accident (V90.-, V92.-)
     EXCLUDES 2   *accidental drowning and submersion due to cataclysm (X34-X39)*

The appropriate 7th character is to be added to each code from categories W65-W74.
A   initial encounter
D   subsequent encounter
S   sequela

√x7ᵗʰ **W65** **Accidental drowning and submersion while in** bath-tub
     EXCLUDES 1   *accidental drowning and submersion due to fall in (into) bathtub (W16.211)*

√x7ᵗʰ **W67** **Accidental drowning and submersion while in** swimming-pool
     EXCLUDES 1   *accidental drowning and submersion due to fall into swimming pool (W16.011, W16.021, W16.031)*
                     accidental drowning and submersion due to striking into wall of swimming pool (W22.041)

✓ Additional Character Req   √x7ᵗʰ Placeholder Alert   Manifestation   HCC CMS-HCC Condition   ▽ Unspecified Code   ▶◀ Revised Text   ● New Code   ▲ Revised Code Title

ICD-10-CM 2018   1151

√x7th **W69 Accidental drowning and submersion while in** natural water
Accidental drowning and submersion while in lake
Accidental drowning and submersion while in open sea
Accidental drowning and submersion while in river
Accidental drowning and submersion while in stream
EXCLUDES 1   *accidental drowning and submersion due to fall into natural body of water (W16.111, W16.121, W16.131)*

√x7th **W73 Other specified cause of accidental non-transport drowning and submersion**
Accidental drowning and submersion while in quenching tank
Accidental drowning and submersion while in reservoir
EXCLUDES 1   *accidental drowning and submersion due to fall into other water (W16.311, W16.321, W16.331)*

√x7th **W74 Unspecified cause of accidental drowning and submersion**   ▽
Drowning NOS

Exposure to electric current, radiation and extreme ambient air temperature and pressure (W85-W99)

EXCLUDES 1   exposure to:
failure in dosage of radiation or temperature during surgical and medical care (Y63.2-Y63.5)
lightning (T75.0-)
natural cold (X31)
natural heat (X30)
natural radiation NOS (X39)
radiological procedure and radiotherapy (Y84.2)
sunlight (X32)

The appropriate 7th character is to be added to each code from categories W85-W99.
A   initial encounter
D   subsequent encounter
S   sequela

√x7th **W85 Exposure to electric transmission lines**
Broken power line

√4th **W86 Exposure to other specified electric current**

√x7th **W86.0 Exposure to domestic wiring and appliances**

√x7th **W86.1 Exposure to industrial wiring, appliances and electrical machinery**
Exposure to conductors
Exposure to control apparatus
Exposure to electrical equipment and machinery
Exposure to transformers

√x7th **W86.8 Exposure to other electric current**
Exposure to wiring and appliances in or on farm (not farmhouse)
Exposure to wiring and appliances outdoors
Exposure to wiring and appliances in or on public building
Exposure to wiring and appliances in or on residential institutions
Exposure to wiring and appliances in or on schools

√4th **W88 Exposure to ionizing radiation**
EXCLUDES 1   *exposure to sunlight (X32)*

√x7th **W88.0 Exposure to** X-rays

√x7th **W88.1 Exposure to** radioactive isotopes

√x7th **W88.8 Exposure to other ionizing radiation**

√4th **W89 Exposure to man-made visible and ultraviolet light**
INCLUDES   exposure to welding light (arc)
EXCLUDES 1   *exposure to sunlight (X32)*

√x7th **W89.0 Exposure to** welding light **(arc)**

√x7th **W89.1 Exposure to** tanning bed

√x7th **W89.8 Exposure to other man-made visible and ultraviolet light**

√x7th **W89.9 Exposure to unspecified man-made visible and**   ▽
ultraviolet light

√4th **W90 Exposure to other nonionizing radiation**
EXCLUDES 1   *exposure to sunlight (X32)*

√x7th **W90.0 Exposure to** radiofrequency

√x7th **W90.1 Exposure to** infrared radiation

√x7th **W90.2 Exposure to** laser radiation

√x7th **W90.8 Exposure to other nonionizing radiation**

√x7th **W92 Exposure to excessive heat of man-made origin**

√4th **W93 Exposure to excessive cold of man-made origin**

√5th **W93.0 Contact with or inhalation of** dry ice

√x7th **W93.01 Contact with dry ice**

√x7th **W93.02 Inhalation of dry ice**

√5th **W93.1 Contact with or inhalation of** liquid air

√x7th **W93.11 Contact with liquid air**
Contact with liquid hydrogen
Contact with liquid nitrogen

√x7th **W93.12 Inhalation of liquid air**
Inhalation of liquid hydrogen
Inhalation of liquid nitrogen

√x7th **W93.2 Prolonged exposure in deep freeze unit or refrigerator**

√x7th **W93.8 Exposure to other excessive cold of man-made origin**

√4th **W94 Exposure to high and low air pressure and changes in air pressure**

√x7th **W94.0 Exposure to prolonged high air pressure**

√5th **W94.1 Exposure to prolonged low air pressure**

√x7th **W94.11 Exposure to residence or prolonged visit at high altitude**

√x7th **W94.12 Exposure to other prolonged low air pressure**

√5th **W94.2 Exposure to rapid changes in air pressure during** ascent

√x7th **W94.21 Exposure to reduction in atmospheric pressure while surfacing from** deep-water diving

√x7th **W94.22 Exposure to reduction in atmospheric pressure while surfacing from** underground

√x7th **W94.23 Exposure to sudden change in air pressure in** aircraft **during ascent**

√x7th **W94.29 Exposure to other rapid changes in air pressure during ascent**

√5th **W94.3 Exposure to rapid changes in air pressure during** descent

√x7th **W94.31 Exposure to sudden change in air pressure in** aircraft **during descent**

√x7th **W94.32 Exposure to high air pressure from rapid descent in** water

√x7th **W94.39 Exposure to other rapid changes in air pressure during descent**

√x7th **W99 Exposure to other man-made environmental factors**

Exposure to smoke, fire and flames (X00-X08)

EXCLUDES 1   *arson (X97)*
EXCLUDES 2   *explosions (W35-W40)*
lightning (T75.0-)
transport accident (V01-V99)

The appropriate 7th character is to be added to each code from categories X00-X08.
A   initial encounter
D   subsequent encounter
S   sequela

√4th **X00 Exposure to** uncontrolled fire **in building or structure**
INCLUDES   conflagration in building or structure
Code first any associated cataclysm
EXCLUDES 2   *exposure to ignition or melting of nightwear (X05)*
exposure to ignition or melting of other clothing and apparel (X06.-)
exposure to other specified smoke, fire and flames (X08.-)
AHA: 2016, 2Q, 5

√x7th **X00.0 Exposure to** flames **in uncontrolled fire in building or structure**

√x7th **X00.1 Exposure to** smoke **in uncontrolled fire in building or structure**

√x7th **X00.2 Injury due to collapse of burning building or structure in uncontrolled fire**
EXCLUDES 1   *injury due to collapse of building not on fire (W20.1)*

√x7th **X00.3 Fall from burning building or structure in uncontrolled fire**

√x7th **X00.4 Hit by object from burning building or structure in uncontrolled fire**

√x7th **X00.5 Jump from burning building or structure in uncontrolled fire**

√x7th **X00.8 Other exposure to uncontrolled fire in building or structure**

√4th **X01 Exposure to uncontrolled fire, not in building or structure**
INCLUDES   exposure to forest fire

√x7th **X01.0 Exposure to** flames **in uncontrolled fire, not in building or structure**

√x7th **X01.1 Exposure to** smoke **in uncontrolled fire, not in building or structure**

√x7th **X01.3 Fall due to uncontrolled fire, not in building or structure**

EXCLUDES 1 Not coded here   EXCLUDES 2 Not included here   N Newborn Age: 0   P Pediatric Age: 0-17   M Maternity Age: 12-55   A Adult Age: 15-124

1152   ICD-10-CM 2018

✓x7ᵗʰ X01.4 Hit by object due to uncontrolled fire, not in building or structure

✓x7ᵗʰ X01.8 Other exposure to uncontrolled fire, not in building or structure

✓4ᵗʰ **X02** **Exposure to** controlled fire **in building or structure**
  INCLUDES exposure to fire in fireplace
          exposure to fire in stove

✓x7ᵗʰ X02.0 **Exposure to** flames **in controlled fire in building or structure**

✓x7ᵗʰ X02.1 **Exposure to** smoke **in controlled fire in building or structure**

✓x7ᵗʰ X02.2 Injury due to collapse **of burning building or structure in controlled fire**
  EXCLUDES 1 injury due to collapse of building not on fire (W20.1)

✓x7ᵗʰ X02.3 Fall from **burning building or structure in controlled fire**

✓x7ᵗʰ X02.4 Hit by object **from burning building or structure in controlled fire**

✓x7ᵗʰ X02.5 Jump from **burning building or structure in controlled fire**

✓x7ᵗʰ X02.8 **Other exposure to controlled fire in building or structure**

✓4ᵗʰ **X03** **Exposure to** controlled fire, **not in building or structure**
  INCLUDES exposure to bon fire
          exposure to camp-fire
          exposure to trash fire

✓x7ᵗʰ X03.0 **Exposure to** flames **in controlled fire, not in building or structure**

✓x7ᵗʰ X03.1 **Exposure to** smoke **in controlled fire, not in building or structure**

✓x7ᵗʰ X03.3 Fall due to **controlled fire, not in building or structure**

✓x7ᵗʰ X03.4 Hit by object **due to controlled fire, not in building or structure**

✓x7ᵗʰ X03.8 **Other exposure to controlled fire, not in building or structure**

✓x7ᵗʰ **X04** **Exposure to ignition of highly flammable material**
  Exposure to ignition of gasoline
  Exposure to ignition of kerosene
  Exposure to ignition of petrol
  EXCLUDES 2 exposure to ignition or melting of nightwear (X05)
            exposure to ignition or melting of other clothing and apparel (X06)
  AHA: 2016, 2Q, 4

✓x7ᵗʰ **X05** **Exposure to ignition or melting of nightwear**
  EXCLUDES 2 exposure to uncontrolled fire in building or structure (X00.-)
            exposure to uncontrolled fire, not in building or structure (X01.-)
            exposure to controlled fire in building or structure (X02.-)
            exposure to controlled fire, not in building or structure (X03.-)
            exposure to ignition of highly flammable materials (X04.-)

✓4ᵗʰ **X06** **Exposure to ignition or melting of other clothing and apparel**
  EXCLUDES 2 exposure to uncontrolled fire in building or structure (X00.-)
            exposure to uncontrolled fire, not in building or structure (X01.-)
            exposure to controlled fire in building or structure (X02.-)
            exposure to controlled fire, not in building or structure (X03.-)
            exposure to ignition of highly flammable materials (X04.-)

✓x7ᵗʰ X06.0 **Exposure to ignition of plastic jewelry**

✓x7ᵗʰ X06.1 **Exposure to melting of plastic jewelry**

✓x7ᵗʰ X06.2 **Exposure to ignition of other clothing and apparel**

✓x7ᵗʰ X06.3 **Exposure to melting of other clothing and apparel**

✓4ᵗʰ **X08** **Exposure to other specified smoke, fire and flames**

✓5ᵗʰ X08.0 **Exposure to** bed **fire**
  Exposure to mattress fire

✓x7ᵗʰ X08.00 **Exposure to bed fire due to unspecified burning material** ▽

✓x7ᵗʰ X08.01 **Exposure to bed fire due to** burning cigarette

✓x7ᵗʰ X08.09 **Exposure to bed fire due to other burning material**

✓5ᵗʰ X08.1 **Exposure to** sofa **fire**

✓x7ᵗʰ X08.10 **Exposure to sofa fire due to unspecified burning material** ▽

✓x7ᵗʰ X08.11 **Exposure to sofa fire due to** burning cigarette

✓x7ᵗʰ X08.19 **Exposure to sofa fire due to other burning material**

✓5ᵗʰ X08.2 **Exposure to other furniture fire**

✓x7ᵗʰ X08.20 **Exposure to other furniture fire due to unspecified burning material** ▽

✓x7ᵗʰ X08.21 **Exposure to other furniture fire due to** burning cigarette

✓x7ᵗʰ X08.29 **Exposure to other furniture fire due to other burning material**

✓x7ᵗʰ X08.8 **Exposure to other specified smoke, fire and flames**

Contact with heat and hot substances (X10-X19)

  EXCLUDES 1 exposure to excessive natural heat (X30)
            exposure to fire and flames ▶(X00–X08)◀

The appropriate 7th character is to be added to each code from categories X10-X19.
A   initial encounter
D   subsequent encounter
S   sequela

✓4ᵗʰ **X10** **Contact with hot drinks, food, fats and cooking oils**

✓x7ᵗʰ X10.0 **Contact with hot** drinks

✓x7ᵗʰ X10.1 **Contact with hot** food

✓x7ᵗʰ X10.2 **Contact with** fats and cooking oils

✓4ᵗʰ **X11** **Contact with hot tap-water**
  INCLUDES contact with boiling tap-water
          contact with boiling water NOS
  EXCLUDES 1 contact with water heated on stove (X12)

✓x7ᵗʰ X11.0 **Contact with hot water** in bath or tub
  EXCLUDES 1 contact with running hot water in bath or tub (X11.1)

✓x7ᵗʰ X11.1 **Contact with** running **hot water**
  Contact with hot water running out of hose
  Contact with hot water running out of tap

✓x7ᵗʰ X11.8 **Contact with other hot tap-water**
  Contact with hot water in bucket
  Contact with hot tap-water NOS

✓x7ᵗʰ **X12** **Contact with other hot fluids**
  Contact with water heated on stove
  EXCLUDES 1 hot (liquid) metals (X18)

✓4ᵗʰ **X13** **Contact with steam and other hot vapors**

✓x7ᵗʰ X13.0 **Inhalation of steam and other hot vapors**

✓x7ᵗʰ X13.1 **Other contact with steam and other hot vapors**

✓4ᵗʰ **X14** **Contact with hot air and other hot gases**

✓x7ᵗʰ X14.0 **Inhalation of hot air and gases**

✓x7ᵗʰ X14.1 **Other contact with hot air and other hot gases**

✓4ᵗʰ **X15** **Contact with hot household appliances**
  EXCLUDES 1 contact with heating appliances (X16)
            contact with powered household appliances (W29.-)
            exposure to controlled fire in building or structure due to household appliance (X02.8)
            exposure to household appliances electrical current (W86.0)

✓x7ᵗʰ X15.0 **Contact with hot** stove **(kitchen)**

✓x7ᵗʰ X15.1 **Contact with hot** toaster

✓x7ᵗʰ X15.2 **Contact with** hotplate

✓x7ᵗʰ X15.3 **Contact with hot** saucepan or skillet

✓x7ᵗʰ X15.8 **Contact with other hot household appliances**
  Contact with cooker   Contact with light bulbs
  Contact with kettle

✓x7ᵗʰ **X16** **Contact with hot heating appliances, radiators and pipes**
  EXCLUDES 1 contact with powered appliances (W29.-)
            exposure to controlled fire in building or structure due to appliance (X02.8)
            exposure to industrial appliances electrical current (W86.1)

✓x7ᵗʰ **X17** **Contact with hot engines, machinery and tools**
  EXCLUDES 1 contact with hot heating appliances, radiators and pipes (X16)
            contact with hot household appliances (X15)

✓x7ᵗʰ **X18** **Contact with other hot metals**
  Contact with liquid metal

✓x7ᵗʰ **X19** **Contact with other heat and hot substances**
  EXCLUDES 1 objects that are not normally hot, e.g., an object made hot by a house fire ▶(X00-X08)◀

☑ Additional Character Req   ✓x7ᵗʰ Placeholder Alert   Manifestation   HCC CMS-HCC Condition   ▽ Unspecified Code   ▶◀ Revised Text   ● New Code   ▲ Revised Code Title

Chapter 20. External Causes of Morbidity *(left margin)*

X30–X72 *(left margin)*

Exposure to forces of nature (X30-X39)

The appropriate 7th character is to be added to each code from categories X30-X39.
A   initial encounter
D   subsequent encounter
S   sequela

√x 7th **X30 Exposure to excessive natural heat**
Exposure to excessive heat as the cause of sunstroke
Exposure to heat NOS
> EXCLUDES 1   *excessive heat of man-made origin (W92)*
> *exposure to man-made radiation (W89)*
> *exposure to sunlight (X32)*
> *exposure to tanning bed (W89)*

√x 7th **X31 Exposure to excessive natural cold**
Excessive cold as the cause of chilblains NOS
Excessive cold as the cause of immersion foot or hand
Exposure to cold NOS
Exposure to weather conditions
> EXCLUDES 1   *cold of man-made origin (W93.-)*
> *contact with or inhalation of dry ice (W93.-)*
> *contact with or inhalation of liquefied gas (W93.-)*

√x 7th **X32 Exposure to sunlight**
> EXCLUDES 1   *man-made radiation (tanning bed) (W89)*
> EXCLUDES 2   ▶*radiation-related disorders of the skin and subcutaneous tissue (L55-L59)*◀

√x 7th **X34 Earthquake**
> EXCLUDES 2   *tidal wave (tsunami) due to earthquake (X37.41)*

√x 7th **X35 Volcanic eruption**
> EXCLUDES 2   *tidal wave (tsunami) due to volcanic eruption (X37.41)*

√4th **X36 Avalanche, landslide and other earth movements**
> INCLUDES   victim of mudslide of cataclysmic nature
> EXCLUDES 1   *earthquake (X34)*
> EXCLUDES 2   *transport accident involving collision with avalanche or landslide not in motion (V01-V99)*

    √x 7th **X36.0 Collapse of dam or man-made structure causing earth movement**

    √x 7th **X36.1 Avalanche, landslide, or mudslide**

√4th **X37 Cataclysmic storm**

    √x 7th **X37.0 Hurricane**
       Storm surge
       Typhoon

    √x 7th **X37.1 Tornado**
       Cyclone
       Twister

    √x 7th **X37.2 Blizzard (snow) (ice)**

    √x 7th **X37.3 Dust storm**

    √5th **X37.4 Tidalwave**

       √x 7th **X37.41 Tidal wave due to earthquake or volcanic eruption**
          Tidal wave NOS
          Tsunami

       √x 7th **X37.42 Tidal wave due to storm**

       √x 7th **X37.43 Tidal wave due to landslide**

    √x 7th **X37.8 Other cataclysmic storms**
       Cloudburst
       Torrential rain
> EXCLUDES 2   *flood (X38)*

    √x 7th **X37.9 Unspecified cataclysmic storm** ▽
       Storm NOS
> EXCLUDES 1   *collapse of dam or man-made structure causing earth movement (X39.0)*

√x 7th **X38 Flood**
Flood arising from remote storm
Flood of cataclysmic nature arising from melting snow
Flood resulting directly from storm
> EXCLUDES 1   *collapse of dam or man-made structure causing earth movement (X39.0)*
> *tidal wave NOS (X37.41)*
> *tidal wave caused by storm (X37.2)*

√4th **X39 Exposure to other forces of nature**

    √5th **X39.0 Exposure to natural radiation**
> EXCLUDES 1   *contact with and (suspected) exposure to radon and other naturally occuring radiation (Z77.123)*
> *exposure to man-made radiation (W88-W90)*
> *exposure to sunlight (X32)*

       √x 7th **X39.01 Exposure to radon**

       √x 7th **X39.08 Exposure to other natural radiation**

    √x 7th **X39.8 Other exposure to forces of nature**

Overexertion and strenuous or repetitive movements (X50)

√4th **X50 Overexertion and strenuous or repetitive movements**

The appropriate 7th character is to be added to each code from category X50.
A   initial encounter
D   subsequent encounter
S   sequela

    √x 7th **X50.0 Overexertion from strenuous movement or load**
       Lifting heavy objects
       Lifting weights

    √x 7th **X50.1 Overexertion from prolonged static or awkward postures**
       Prolonged bending
       Prolonged kneeling
       Prolonged reaching
       Prolonged sitting
       Prolonged standing
       Prolonged twisting
       Static bending
       Static kneeling
       Static reaching
       Static sitting
       Static standing
       Static twisting

    √x 7th **X50.3 Overexertion from repetitive movements**
       Use of hand as hammer
> EXCLUDES 2   *overuse from prolonged static or awkward postures (X50.1)*

    √x 7th **X50.9 Other and unspecified overexertion or strenuous movements or postures** ▽
       Contact pressure
       Contact stress

Accidental exposure to other specified factors (X52-X58)

The appropriate 7th character is to be added to each code from categories X52-X58.
A   initial encounter
D   subsequent encounter
S   sequela

√x 7th **X52 Prolonged stay in weightless environment**
       Weightlessness in spacecraft (simulator)

√x 7th **X58 Exposure to other specified factors**
       Accident NOS
       Exposure NOS

Intentional self-harm (X71-X83)

Purposely self-inflicted injury
Suicide (attempted)

The appropriate 7th character is to be added to each code from categories X71-X83.
A   initial encounter
D   subsequent encounter
S   sequela

√4th **X71 Intentional self-harm by drowning and submersion**

    √x 7th **X71.0 Intentional self-harm by drowning and submersion while in bathtub** HCC

    √x 7th **X71.1 Intentional self-harm by drowning and submersion while in swimming pool** HCC

    √x 7th **X71.2 Intentional self-harm by drowning and submersion after jump into swimming pool** HCC

    √x 7th **X71.3 Intentional self-harm by drowning and submersion in natural water** HCC

    √x 7th **X71.8 Other intentional self-harm by drowning and submersion** HCC

    √x 7th **X71.9 Intentional self-harm by drowning and submersion, unspecified** HCC ▽

√x 7th **X72 Intentional self-harm by handgun discharge** HCC
       Intentional self-harm by gun for single hand use
       Intentional self-harm by pistol
       Intentional self-harm by revolver
> EXCLUDES 1   *Very pistol (X74.8)*

EXCLUDES 1 Not coded here   EXCLUDES 2 Not included here   N Newborn Age: 0   P Pediatric Age: 0-17   M Maternity Age: 12-55   A Adult Age: 15-124

✓4th **X73** **Intentional self-harm by** rifle, shotgun and larger firearm **discharge**
    EXCLUDES 1   *airgun (X74.Ø1)*

✓x7th **X73.Ø** Intentional self-harm by shotgun discharge   HCC

✓x7th **X73.1** Intentional self-harm by hunting rifle discharge   HCC

✓x7th **X73.2** Intentional self-harm by machine gun discharge   HCC

✓x7th **X73.8** Intentional self-harm by other larger firearm discharge   HCC

✓x7th **X73.9** Intentional self-harm by unspecified larger firearm discharge   HCC ▽

✓4th **X74** **Intentional self-harm by other and unspecified firearm and gun discharge**

   ✓5th **X74.Ø** Intentional self-harm by gas, air or spring-operated guns

     ✓x7th **X74.Ø1** **Intentional self-harm by** airgun   HCC
       Intentional self-harm by BB gun discharge
       Intentional self-harm by pellet gun discharge

     ✓x7th **X74.Ø2** **Intentional self-harm by** paintball gun   HCC

     ✓x7th **X74.Ø9** **Intentional self-harm by other gas, air or** spring-operated gun   HCC

   ✓x7th **X74.8** Intentional self-harm by other firearm discharge   HCC
      Intentional self-harm by Very pistol [flare] discharge

   ✓x7th **X74.9** Intentional self-harm by unspecified firearm discharge   HCC ▽

✓x7th **X75** **Intentional self-harm by explosive material**   HCC

✓x7th **X76** **Intentional self-harm by smoke, fire and flames**   HCC

✓4th **X77** **Intentional self-harm by steam, hot vapors and hot objects**

   ✓x7th **X77.Ø** Intentional self-harm by steam or hot vapors   HCC

   ✓x7th **X77.1** Intentional self-harm by hot tap water   HCC

   ✓x7th **X77.2** Intentional self-harm by other hot fluids   HCC

   ✓x7th **X77.3** Intentional self-harm by hot household appliances   HCC

   ✓x7th **X77.8** Intentional self-harm by other hot objects   HCC

   ✓x7th **X77.9** Intentional self-harm by unspecified hot objects   HCC ▽

✓4th **X78** **Intentional self-harm by sharp object**

   ✓x7th **X78.Ø** Intentional self-harm by sharp glass   HCC

   ✓x7th **X78.1** Intentional self-harm by knife   HCC

   ✓x7th **X78.2** Intentional self-harm by sword or dagger   HCC

   ✓x7th **X78.8** Intentional self-harm by other sharp object   HCC

   ✓x7th **X78.9** Intentional self-harm by unspecified sharp object   HCC ▽

✓x7th **X79** **Intentional self-harm by blunt object**   HCC

✓x7th **X8Ø** **Intentional self-harm by jumping from a high place**   HCC
     Intentional fall from one level to another

✓4th **X81** **Intentional self-harm by jumping or lying in front of moving object**

   ✓x7th **X81.Ø** Intentional self-harm by jumping or lying in front of motor vehicle   HCC

   ✓x7th **X81.1** Intentional self-harm by jumping or lying in front of (subway) train   HCC

   ✓x7th **X81.8** Intentional self-harm by jumping or lying in front of other moving object   HCC

✓4th **X82** **Intentional self-harm by crashing of motor vehicle**

   ✓x7th **X82.Ø** Intentional collision of motor vehicle with other motor vehicle   HCC

   ✓x7th **X82.1** Intentional collision of motor vehicle with train   HCC

   ✓x7th **X82.2** Intentional collision of motor vehicle with tree   HCC

   ✓x7th **X82.8** Other intentional self-harm by crashing of motor vehicle   HCC

✓4th **X83** **Intentional self-harm by other specified means**
    EXCLUDES 1   *intentional self-harm by poisoning or contact with toxic substance—see Table of Drugs and Chemicals*

   ✓x7th **X83.Ø** Intentional self-harm by crashing of aircraft   HCC

   ✓x7th **X83.1** Intentional self-harm by electrocution   HCC

   ✓x7th **X83.2** Intentional self-harm by exposure to extremes of cold   HCC

   ✓x7th **X83.8** Intentional self-harm by other specified means   HCC

Assault (X92-YØ9)

INCLUDES   homicide
       injuries inflicted by another person with intent to injure or kill, by any means
EXCLUDES 1   *injuries due to legal intervention (Y35.-)*
       injuries due to operations of war (Y36.-)
       injuries due to terrorism (Y38.-)

The appropriate 7th character is to be added to each code from categories X92-YØ4 and YØ8.
A   initial encounter
D   subsequent encounter
S   sequela

✓4th **X92** **Assault by drowning and submersion**

   ✓x7th **X92.Ø** Assault by drowning and submersion while in bathtub

   ✓x7th **X92.1** Assault by drowning and submersion while in swimming pool

   ✓x7th **X92.2** Assault by drowning and submersion after push into swimming pool

   ✓x7th **X92.3** Assault by drowning and submersion in natural water

   ✓x7th **X92.8** Other assault by drowning and submersion

   ✓x7th **X92.9** Assault by drowning and submersion, unspecified   ▽

✓x7th **X93** **Assault by** handgun **discharge**
   Assault by discharge of gun for single hand use
   Assault by discharge of pistol
   Assault by discharge of revolver
   EXCLUDES 1   *Very pistol (X95.8)*

✓4th **X94** **Assault by** rifle, shotgun and larger firearm **discharge**
   EXCLUDES 1   *airgun (X95.Ø1)*

   ✓x7th **X94.Ø** Assault by shotgun

   ✓x7th **X94.1** Assault by hunting rifle

   ✓x7th **X94.2** Assault by machine gun

   ✓x7th **X94.8** Assault by other larger firearm discharge

   ✓x7th **X94.9** Assault by unspecified larger firearm discharge   ▽

✓4th **X95** **Assault by other and unspecified firearm and gun discharge**

   ✓5th **X95.Ø** Assault by gas, air or spring-operated guns

     ✓x7th **X95.Ø1** **Assault by** airgun **discharge**
       Assault by BB gun discharge
       Assault by pellet gun discharge

     ✓x7th **X95.Ø2** **Assault by** paintball gun **discharge**

     ✓x7th **X95.Ø9** **Assault by other gas, air or spring-operated gun**

   ✓x7th **X95.8** Assault by other firearm discharge
      Assault by Very pistol [flare] discharge

   ✓x7th **X95.9** Assault by unspecified firearm discharge   ▽

✓4th **X96** **Assault by explosive material**
   EXCLUDES 1   *incendiary device (X97)*
       terrorism involving explosive material (Y38.2-)

   ✓x7th **X96.Ø** Assault by antipersonnel bomb
     EXCLUDES 1   *antipersonnel bomb use in military or war (Y36.2-)*

   ✓x7th **X96.1** Assault by gasoline bomb

   ✓x7th **X96.2** Assault by letter bomb

   ✓x7th **X96.3** Assault by fertilizer bomb

   ✓x7th **X96.4** Assault by pipe bomb

   ✓x7th **X96.8** Assault by other specified explosive

   ✓x7th **X96.9** Assault by unspecified explosive   ▽

✓x7th **X97** **Assault by smoke, fire and flames**
   Assault by arson
   Assault by cigarettes
   Assault by incendiary device

✓4th **X98** **Assault by steam, hot vapors and hot objects**

   ✓x7th **X98.Ø** Assault by steam or hot vapors

   ✓x7th **X98.1** Assault by hot tap water

   ✓x7th **X98.2** Assault by hot fluids

   ✓x7th **X98.3** Assault by hot household appliances

   ✓x7th **X98.8** Assault by other hot objects

   ✓x7th **X98.9** Assault by unspecified hot objects   ▽

✓4th **X99** **Assault by sharp object**
   EXCLUDES 1   *assault by strike by sports equipment (YØ8.Ø-)*

   ✓x7th **X99.Ø** Assault by sharp glass

   ✓x7th **X99.1** Assault by knife

   ✓x7th **X99.2** Assault by sword or dagger

✓ Additional Character Req   ✓x7th Placeholder Alert   Manifestation   HCC CMS-HCC Condition   ▽ Unspecified Code   ►◄ Revised Text   ● New Code   ▲ Revised Code Title

Chapter 20. External Causes of Morbidity *(side margin)*

X99.8–Y09 *(side margin)*

√x7ᵗʰ **X99.8** Assault by other sharp object

√x7ᵗʰ **X99.9** Assault by unspecified sharp object ▽
       Assault by stabbing NOS

√x7ᵗʰ **Y00** **Assault by blunt object**
     EXCLUDES 1   *assault by strike by sports equipment (Y08.0-)*

√x7ᵗʰ **Y01** **Assault by pushing from high place**

√4ᵗʰ **Y02** **Assault by pushing or placing victim in front of moving object**

    √x7ᵗʰ **Y02.0** Assault by pushing or placing victim in front of motor vehicle

    √x7ᵗʰ **Y02.1** Assault by pushing or placing victim in front of (subway) train

    √x7ᵗʰ **Y02.8** Assault by pushing or placing victim in front of other moving object

√4ᵗʰ **Y03** **Assault by crashing of motor vehicle**

    √x7ᵗʰ **Y03.0** Assault by being hit or run over by motor vehicle

    √x7ᵗʰ **Y03.8** Other assault by crashing of motor vehicle

√4ᵗʰ **Y04** **Assault by bodily force**
     EXCLUDES 1   *assault by:*
          submersion (X92.-)
          use of weapon (X93-X95, X99, Y00)

    √x7ᵗʰ **Y04.0** Assault by unarmed brawl or fight

    √x7ᵗʰ **Y04.1** Assault by human bite

    √x7ᵗʰ **Y04.2** Assault by strike against or bumped into by another person

    √x7ᵗʰ **Y04.8** Assault by other bodily force
         Assault by bodily force NOS

√4ᵗʰ **Y07** **Perpetrator of assault, maltreatment and neglect**
     NOTE   Codes from this category are for use only in cases of confirmed abuse (T74.-)
         Selection of the correct perpetrator code is based on the relationship between the perpetrator and the victim
     INCLUDES   perpetrator of abandonment
          perpetrator of emotional neglect
          perpetrator of mental cruelty
          perpetrator of physical abuse
          perpetrator of physical neglect
          perpetrator of sexual abuse
          perpetrator of torture

    √5ᵗʰ **Y07.0** Spouse or partner, perpetrator of maltreatment and neglect
        Spouse or partner, perpetrator of maltreatment and neglect against spouse or partner

        Y07.01 Husband, perpetrator of maltreatment and neglect

        Y07.02 Wife, perpetrator of maltreatment and neglect

        Y07.03 Male partner, perpetrator of maltreatment and neglect

        Y07.04 Female partner, perpetrator of maltreatment and neglect

    √5ᵗʰ **Y07.1** Parent (adoptive) (biological), perpetrator of maltreatment and neglect

        Y07.11 Biological father, perpetrator of maltreatment and neglect

        Y07.12 Biological mother, perpetrator of maltreatment and neglect

        Y07.13 Adoptive father, perpetrator of maltreatment and neglect

        Y07.14 Adoptive mother, perpetrator of maltreatment and neglect

    √5ᵗʰ **Y07.4** Other family member, perpetrator of maltreatment and neglect

      √6ᵗʰ **Y07.41** Sibling, perpetrator of maltreatment and neglect
         EXCLUDES 1 *stepsibling, perpetrator of maltreatment and neglect (Y07.435, Y07.436)*

        Y07.410 Brother, perpetrator of maltreatment and neglect

        Y07.411 Sister, perpetrator of maltreatment and neglect

      √6ᵗʰ **Y07.42** Foster parent, perpetrator of maltreatment and neglect

        Y07.420 Foster father, perpetrator of maltreatment and neglect

        Y07.421 Foster mother, perpetrator of maltreatment and neglect

      √6ᵗʰ **Y07.43** Stepparent or stepsibling, perpetrator of maltreatment and neglect

        Y07.430 Stepfather, perpetrator of maltreatment and neglect

        Y07.432 Male friend of parent (co-residing in household), perpetrator of maltreatment and neglect

        Y07.433 Stepmother, perpetrator of maltreatment and neglect

        Y07.434 Female friend of parent (co-residing in household), perpetrator of maltreatment and neglect

        Y07.435 Stepbrother, perpetrator or maltreatment and neglect

        Y07.436 Stepsister, perpetrator of maltreatment and neglect

      √6ᵗʰ **Y07.49** Other family member, perpetrator of maltreatment and neglect

        Y07.490 Male cousin, perpetrator of maltreatment and neglect

        Y07.491 Female cousin, perpetrator of maltreatment and neglect

        Y07.499 Other family member, perpetrator of maltreatment and neglect

    √5ᵗʰ **Y07.5** Non-family member, perpetrator of maltreatment and neglect

        Y07.50 Unspecified non-family member, perpetrator of maltreatment and neglect ▽

      √6ᵗʰ **Y07.51** Daycare provider, perpetrator of maltreatment and neglect

        Y07.510 At-home childcare provider, perpetrator of maltreatment and neglect

        Y07.511 Daycare center childcare provider, perpetrator of maltreatment and neglect

        Y07.512 At-home adultcare provider, perpetrator of maltreatment and neglect

        Y07.513 Adultcare center provider, perpetrator of maltreatment and neglect

        Y07.519 Unspecified daycare provider, perpetrator of maltreatment and neglect ▽

      √6ᵗʰ **Y07.52** Healthcare provider, perpetrator of maltreatment and neglect

        Y07.521 Mental health provider, perpetrator of maltreatment and neglect

        Y07.528 Other therapist or healthcare provider, perpetrator of maltreatment and neglect
          Nurse, perpetrator of maltreatment and neglect
          Occupational therapist, perpetrator of maltreatment and neglect
          Physical therapist, perpetrator of maltreatment and neglect
          Speech therapist, perpetrator of maltreatment and neglect

        Y07.529 Unspecified healthcare provider, perpetrator of maltreatment and neglect ▽

        Y07.53 Teacher or instructor, perpetrator of maltreatment and neglect
          Coach, perpetrator of maltreatment and neglect

        Y07.59 Other non-family member, perpetrator of maltreatment and neglect

        Y07.9 Unspecified perpetrator of maltreatment and neglect ▽

√4ᵗʰ **Y08** **Assault by other specified means**

    √5ᵗʰ **Y08.0** Assault by strike by sport equipment

      √x7ᵗʰ **Y08.01** Assault by strike by hockey stick

      √x7ᵗʰ **Y08.02** Assault by strike by baseball bat

      √x7ᵗʰ **Y08.09** Assault by strike by other specified type of sport equipment

    √5ᵗʰ **Y08.8** Assault by other specified means

      √x7ᵗʰ **Y08.81** Assault by crashing of aircraft

      √x7ᵗʰ **Y08.89** Assault by other specified means

    Y09 **Assault by unspecified means** ▽
        Assassination (attempted) NOS
        Homicide (attempted) NOS
        Manslaughter (attempted) NOS
        Murder (attempted) NOS

EXCLUDES 1 Not coded here   **EXCLUDES 2** Not included here   **N** Newborn Age: 0   **P** Pediatric Age: 0-17   **M** Maternity Age: 12-55   **A** Adult Age: 15-124

Event of undetermined intent (Y21-Y33)

Undetermined intent is only for use when there is specific documentation in the record that the intent of the injury cannot be determined. If no such documentation is present, code to accidental (unintentional).

The appropriate 7th character is to be added to each code from categories Y21-Y33.
A   initial encounter
D   subsequent encounter
S   sequela

√4th **Y21**   **Drowning and submersion, undetermined intent**

√x7th   **Y21.0**   **Drowning and submersion** while in bathtub, **undetermined intent**

√x7th   **Y21.1**   **Drowning and submersion** after fall into bathtub, **undetermined intent**

√x7th   **Y21.2**   **Drowning and submersion** while in swimming pool, **undetermined intent**

√x7th   **Y21.3**   **Drowning and submersion** after fall into swimming pool, **undetermined intent**

√x7th   **Y21.4**   **Drowning and submersion** in natural water, **undetermined intent**

√x7th   **Y21.8**   **Other drowning and submersion, undetermined intent**

√x7th   **Y21.9**   **Unspecified drowning and submersion, undetermined intent** ▽

√x7th **Y22**   Handgun **discharge, undetermined intent**
Discharge of gun for single hand use, undetermined intent
Discharge of pistol, undetermined intent
Discharge of revolver, undetermined intent
EXCLUDES 2   Very pistol (Y24.8)

√4th **Y23**   Rifle, shotgun and larger firearm **discharge, undetermined intent**
EXCLUDES 2   airgun (Y24.0)

√x7th   **Y23.0**   Shotgun **discharge, undetermined intent**

√x7th   **Y23.1**   Hunting rifle **discharge, undetermined intent**

√x7th   **Y23.2**   Military firearm **discharge, undetermined intent**

√x7th   **Y23.3**   Machine gun **discharge, undetermined intent**

√x7th   **Y23.8**   **Other larger firearm discharge, undetermined intent**

√x7th   **Y23.9**   **Unspecified larger firearm discharge, undetermined intent** ▽

√4th **Y24**   **Other and unspecified firearm discharge, undetermined intent**

√x7th   **Y24.0**   Airgun **discharge, undetermined intent**
BB gun discharge, undetermined intent
Pellet gun discharge, undetermined intent

√x7th   **Y24.8**   **Other firearm discharge, undetermined intent**
Paintball gun discharge, undetermined intent
Very pistol [flare] discharge, undetermined intent

√x7th   **Y24.9**   **Unspecified firearm discharge, undetermined intent** ▽

√x7th **Y25**   **Contact with explosive material, undetermined intent**

√x7th **Y26**   **Exposure to smoke, fire and flames, undetermined intent**

√4th **Y27**   **Contact with steam, hot vapors and hot objects, undetermined intent**

√x7th   **Y27.0**   **Contact with steam and hot** vapors, **undetermined intent**

√x7th   **Y27.1**   **Contact with hot** tap water, **undetermined intent**

√x7th   **Y27.2**   **Contact with hot** fluids, **undetermined intent**

√x7th   **Y27.3**   **Contact with hot** household appliance, **undetermined intent**

√x7th   **Y27.8**   **Contact with other hot objects, undetermined intent**

√x7th   **Y27.9**   **Contact with unspecified hot objects, undetermined intent** ▽

√4th **Y28**   **Contact with sharp object, undetermined intent**

√x7th   **Y28.0**   **Contact with sharp** glass, **undetermined intent**

√x7th   **Y28.1**   **Contact with** knife, **undetermined intent**

√x7th   **Y28.2**   **Contact with** sword or dagger, **undetermined intent**

√x7th   **Y28.8**   **Contact with other sharp object, undetermined intent**

√x7th   **Y28.9**   **Contact with unspecified hot objects, undetermined intent** ▽

√x7th **Y29**   **Contact with blunt object, undetermined intent**

√x7th **Y30**   **Falling, jumping or pushed from a high place, undetermined intent**
Victim falling from one level to another, undetermined intent

√x7th **Y31**   **Falling, lying or running before or into moving object, undetermined intent**

√x7th **Y32**   **Crashing of motor vehicle, undetermined intent**

√x7th **Y33**   **Other specified events, undetermined intent**

Legal intervention, operations of war, military operations, and terrorism (Y35-Y38)

The appropriate 7th character is to be added to each code from categories Y35-Y38.
A   initial encounter
D   subsequent encounter
S   sequela

√4th **Y35**   **Legal intervention**
INCLUDES   any injury sustained as a result of an encounter with any law enforcement official, serving in any capacity at the time of the encounter, whether on-duty or off-duty. Includes: injury to law enforcement official, suspect and bystander

√5th   **Y35.0**   **Legal intervention involving** firearm discharge

√6th   **Y35.00**   **Legal intervention involving unspecified firearm discharge**
Legal intervention involving gunshot wound
Legal intervention involving shot NOS

√7th   **Y35.001**   **Legal intervention involving unspecified firearm discharge,** law enforcement **official injured** ▽

√7th   **Y35.002**   **Legal intervention involving unspecified firearm discharge,** bystander **injured** ▽

√7th   **Y35.003**   **Legal intervention involving unspecified firearm discharge,** suspect **injured** ▽

√6th   **Y35.01**   **Legal intervention involving injury by** machine gun

√7th   **Y35.011**   **Legal intervention involving injury by machine gun,** law enforcement **official injured**

√7th   **Y35.012**   **Legal intervention involving injury by machine gun,** bystander **injured**

√7th   **Y35.013**   **Legal intervention involving injury by machine gun,** suspect **injured**

√6th   **Y35.02**   **Legal intervention involving injury by** handgun

√7th   **Y35.021**   **Legal intervention involving injury by handgun,** law enforcement **official injured**

√7th   **Y35.022**   **Legal intervention involving injury by handgun,** bystander **injured**

√7th   **Y35.023**   **Legal intervention involving injury by handgun,** suspect **injured**

√6th   **Y35.03**   **Legal intervention involving injury by** rifle pellet

√7th   **Y35.031**   **Legal intervention involving injury by rifle pellet,** law enforcement **official injured**

√7th   **Y35.032**   **Legal intervention involving injury by rifle pellet,** bystander **injured**

√7th   **Y35.033**   **Legal intervention involving injury by rifle pellet,** suspect **injured**

√6th   **Y35.04**   **Legal intervention involving injury by** rubber bullet

√7th   **Y35.041**   **Legal intervention involving injury by rubber bullet,** law enforcement **official injured**

√7th   **Y35.042**   **Legal intervention involving injury by rubber bullet,** bystander **injured**

√7th   **Y35.043**   **Legal intervention involving injury by rubber bullet,** suspect **injured**

√6th   **Y35.09**   **Legal intervention involving other firearm discharge**

√7th   **Y35.091**   **Legal intervention involving other firearm discharge,** law enforcement **official injured**

√7th   **Y35.092**   **Legal intervention involving other firearm discharge,** bystander **injured**

√7th   **Y35.093**   **Legal intervention involving other firearm discharge,** suspect **injured**

√5th   **Y35.1**   **Legal intervention involving** explosives

√6th   **Y35.10**   **Legal intervention involving unspecified explosives**

√7th   **Y35.101**   **Legal intervention involving unspecified explosives,** law enforcement **official injured** ▽

√ Additional Character Req   √x7th Placeholder Alert   Manifestation   HCC CMS-HCC Condition   ▽ Unspecified Code   ▶◀ Revised Text   ● New Code   ▲ Revised Code Title

✓7th **Y35.102** **Legal intervention involving unspecified explosives, bystander injured** ▽

✓7th **Y35.103** **Legal intervention involving unspecified explosives, suspect injured** ▽

✓6th **Y35.11** **Legal intervention involving injury by dynamite**

     ✓7th **Y35.111** **Legal intervention involving injury by dynamite, law enforcement official injured**

     ✓7th **Y35.112** **Legal intervention involving injury by dynamite, bystander injured**

     ✓7th **Y35.113** **Legal intervention involving injury by dynamite, suspect injured**

✓6th **Y35.12** **Legal intervention involving injury by explosive shell**

     ✓7th **Y35.121** **Legal intervention involving injury by explosive shell, law enforcement official injured**

     ✓7th **Y35.122** **Legal intervention involving injury by explosive shell, bystander injured**

     ✓7th **Y35.123** **Legal intervention involving injury by explosive shell, suspect injured**

✓6th **Y35.19** **Legal intervention involving other explosives**
Legal intervention involving injury by grenade
Legal intervention involving injury by mortar bomb

     ✓7th **Y35.191** **Legal intervention involving other explosives, law enforcement official injured**

     ✓7th **Y35.192** **Legal intervention involving other explosives, bystander injured**

     ✓7th **Y35.193** **Legal intervention involving other explosives, suspect injured**

✓5th **Y35.2** **Legal intervention involving gas**
Legal intervention involving asphyxiation by gas
Legal intervention involving poisoning by gas

✓6th **Y35.20** **Legal intervention involving unspecified gas**

     ✓7th **Y35.201** **Legal intervention involving unspecified gas, law enforcement official injured** ▽

     ✓7th **Y35.202** **Legal intervention involving unspecified gas, bystander injured** ▽

     ✓7th **Y35.203** **Legal intervention involving unspecified gas, suspect injured** ▽

✓6th **Y35.21** **Legal intervention involving injury by tear gas**

     ✓7th **Y35.211** **Legal intervention involving injury by tear gas, law enforcement official injured**

     ✓7th **Y35.212** **Legal intervention involving injury by tear gas, bystander injured**

     ✓7th **Y35.213** **Legal intervention involving injury by tear gas, suspect injured**

✓6th **Y35.29** **Legal intervention involving other gas**

     ✓7th **Y35.291** **Legal intervention involving other gas, law enforcement official injured**

     ✓7th **Y35.292** **Legal intervention involving other gas, bystander injured**

     ✓7th **Y35.293** **Legal intervention involving other gas, suspect injured**

✓5th **Y35.3** **Legal intervention involving blunt objects**
Legal intervention involving being hit or struck by blunt object

✓6th **Y35.30** **Legal intervention involving unspecified blunt objects**

     ✓7th **Y35.301** **Legal intervention involving unspecified blunt objects, law enforcement official injured** ▽

     ✓7th **Y35.302** **Legal intervention involving unspecified blunt objects, bystander injured** ▽

     ✓7th **Y35.303** **Legal intervention involving unspecified blunt objects, suspect injured** ▽

✓6th **Y35.31** **Legal intervention involving baton**

     ✓7th **Y35.311** **Legal intervention involving baton, law enforcement official injured**

     ✓7th **Y35.312** **Legal intervention involving baton, bystander injured**

     ✓7th **Y35.313** **Legal intervention involving baton, suspect injured**

✓6th **Y35.39** **Legal intervention involving other blunt objects**

     ✓7th **Y35.391** **Legal intervention involving other blunt objects, law enforcement official injured**

     ✓7th **Y35.392** **Legal intervention involving other blunt objects, bystander injured**

     ✓7th **Y35.393** **Legal intervention involving other blunt objects, suspect injured**

✓5th **Y35.4** **Legal intervention involving sharp objects**
Legal intervention involving being cut by sharp objects
Legal intervention involving being stabbed by sharp objects

✓6th **Y35.40** **Legal intervention involving unspecified sharp objects**

     ✓7th **Y35.401** **Legal intervention involving unspecified sharp objects, law enforcement official injured** ▽

     ✓7th **Y35.402** **Legal intervention involving unspecified sharp objects, bystander injured** ▽

     ✓7th **Y35.403** **Legal intervention involving unspecified sharp objects, suspect injured** ▽

✓6th **Y35.41** **Legal intervention involving bayonet**

     ✓7th **Y35.411** **Legal intervention involving bayonet, law enforcement official injured**

     ✓7th **Y35.412** **Legal intervention involving bayonet, bystander injured**

     ✓7th **Y35.413** **Legal intervention involving bayonet, suspect injured**

✓6th **Y35.49** **Legal intervention involving other sharp objects**

     ✓7th **Y35.491** **Legal intervention involving other sharp objects, law enforcement official injured**

     ✓7th **Y35.492** **Legal intervention involving other sharp objects, bystander injured**

     ✓7th **Y35.493** **Legal intervention involving other sharp objects, suspect injured**

✓5th **Y35.8** **Legal intervention involving other specified means**

✓6th **Y35.81** **Legal intervention involving manhandling**

     ✓7th **Y35.811** **Legal intervention involving manhandling, law enforcement official injured**

     ✓7th **Y35.812** **Legal intervention involving manhandling, bystander injured**

     ✓7th **Y35.813** **Legal intervention involving manhandling, suspect injured**

✓6th **Y35.89** **Legal intervention involving other specified means**

     ✓7th **Y35.891** **Legal intervention involving other specified means, law enforcement official injured**

     ✓7th **Y35.892** **Legal intervention involving other specified means, bystander injured**

     ✓7th **Y35.893** **Legal intervention involving other specified means, suspect injured**

✓5th **Y35.9** **Legal intervention, means unspecified**

     ✓x7th **Y35.91** **Legal intervention, means unspecified, law enforcement official injured** ▽

     ✓x7th **Y35.92** **Legal intervention, means unspecified, bystander injured** ▽

     ✓x7th **Y35.93** **Legal intervention, means unspecified, suspect injured** ▽

✓4th **Y36** **Operations of war**
INCLUDES   injuries to military personnel and civilians caused by war, civil insurrection, and peacekeeping missions
EXCLUDES 1   *injury to military personnel occurring during peacetime military operations (Y37.-)*
military vehicles involved in transport accidents with non-military vehicle during peacetime (V09.01, V09.21, V19.81, V29.81, V39.81, V49.81, V59.81, V69.81, V79.81)
AHA: 2014, 3Q, 4

✓5th **Y36.0** **War operations involving explosion of marine weapons**

✓6th **Y36.00** **War operations involving explosion of unspecified marine weapon**
War operations involving underwater blast NOS

     ✓7th **Y36.000** **War operations involving explosion of unspecified marine weapon, military personnel** ▽

EXCLUDES 1 Not coded here   EXCLUDES 2 Not included here   N Newborn Age: 0   P Pediatric Age: 0-17   M Maternity Age: 12-55   A Adult Age: 15-124

1158   ICD-10-CM 2018

✓7th **Y36.001** War operations involving explosion of ▽
unspecified marine weapon, civilian

✓6th **Y36.01** War operations involving explosion of depth-charge

    ✓7th **Y36.010** War operations involving explosion of
depth-charge, military personnel

    ✓7th **Y36.011** War operations involving explosion of
depth-charge, civilian

✓6th **Y36.02** War operations involving explosion of marine mine
War operations involving explosion of marine mine, at
sea or in harbor

    ✓7th **Y36.020** War operations involving explosion of
marine mine, military personnel

    ✓7th **Y36.021** War operations involving explosion of
marine mine, civilian

✓6th **Y36.03** War operations involving explosion of sea-based
artillery shell

    ✓7th **Y36.030** War operations involving explosion of
sea-based artillery shell, military
personnel

    ✓7th **Y36.031** War operations involving explosion of
sea-based artillery shell, civilian

✓6th **Y36.04** War operations involving explosion of torpedo

    ✓7th **Y36.040** War operations involving explosion of
torpedo, military personnel

    ✓7th **Y36.041** War operations involving explosion of
torpedo, civilian

✓6th **Y36.05** War operations involving accidental detonation of
onboard marine weapons

    ✓7th **Y36.050** War operations involving accidental
detonation of onboard marine weapons,
military personnel

    ✓7th **Y36.051** War operations involving accidental
detonation of onboard marine weapons,
civilian

✓6th **Y36.09** War operations involving explosion of other marine
weapons

    ✓7th **Y36.090** War operations involving explosion of
other marine weapons, military personnel

    ✓7th **Y36.091** War operations involving explosion of
other marine weapons, civilian

✓5th **Y36.1** War operations involving destruction of aircraft

✓6th **Y36.10** War operations involving unspecified destruction of
aircraft

    ✓7th **Y36.100** War operations involving unspecified ▽
destruction of aircraft, military personnel

    ✓7th **Y36.101** War operations involving unspecified ▽
destruction of aircraft, civilian

✓6th **Y36.11** War operations involving destruction of aircraft due
to enemy fire or explosives
War operations involving destruction of aircraft due to
air to air missile
War operations involving destruction of aircraft due to
explosive placed on aircraft
War operations involving destruction of aircraft due to
rocket propelled grenade [RPG]
War operations involving destruction of aircraft due to
small arms fire
War operations involving destruction of aircraft due to
surface to air missile

    ✓7th **Y36.110** War operations involving destruction of
aircraft due to enemy fire or explosives,
military personnel

    ✓7th **Y36.111** War operations involving destruction of
aircraft due to enemy fire or explosives,
civilian

✓6th **Y36.12** War operations involving destruction of aircraft due
to collision with other aircraft

    ✓7th **Y36.120** War operations involving destruction of
aircraft due to collision with other aircraft,
military personnel

    ✓7th **Y36.121** War operations involving destruction of
aircraft due to collision with other aircraft,
civilian

✓6th **Y36.13** War operations involving destruction of aircraft due
to onboard fire

✓7th **Y36.130** War operations involving destruction of
aircraft due to onboard fire, military
personnel

    ✓7th **Y36.131** War operations involving destruction of
aircraft due to onboard fire, civilian

✓6th **Y36.14** War operations involving destruction of aircraft due
to accidental detonation of onboard munitions and
explosives

    ✓7th **Y36.140** War operations involving destruction of
aircraft due to accidental detonation of
onboard munitions and explosives,
military personnel

    ✓7th **Y36.141** War operations involving destruction of
aircraft due to accidental detonation of
onboard munitions and explosives,
civilian

✓6th **Y36.19** War operations involving other destruction of
aircraft

    ✓7th **Y36.190** War operations involving other
destruction of aircraft, military personnel

    ✓7th **Y36.191** War operations involving other
destruction of aircraft, civilian

✓5th **Y36.2** War operations involving other explosions and fragments

   EXCLUDES 1 war operations involving explosion of aircraft (Y36.1-)
war operations involving explosion of marine weapons
(Y36.0-)
war operations involving explosion of nuclear weapons
(Y36.5-)
war operations involving explosion occurring after
cessation of hostilities (Y36.8-)

✓6th **Y36.20** War operations involving unspecified explosion and
fragments
War operations involving air blast NOS
War operations involving blast NOS
War operations involving blast fragments NOS
War operations involving blast wave NOS
War operations involving blast wind NOS
War operations involving explosion NOS
War operations involving explosion of bomb NOS

    ✓7th **Y36.200** War operations involving unspecified ▽
explosion and fragments, military
personnel

    ✓7th **Y36.201** War operations involving unspecified ▽
explosion and fragments, civilian

✓6th **Y36.21** War operations involving explosion of aerial bomb

    ✓7th **Y36.210** War operations involving explosion of
aerial bomb, military personnel

    ✓7th **Y36.211** War operations involving explosion of
aerial bomb, civilian

✓6th **Y36.22** War operations involving explosion of guided
missile

    ✓7th **Y36.220** War operations involving explosion of
guided missile, military personnel

    ✓7th **Y36.221** War operations involving explosion of
guided missile, civilian

✓6th **Y36.23** War operations involving explosion of improvised
explosive device [IED]
War operations involving explosion of person-borne
improvised explosive device [IED]
War operations involving explosion of vehicle-borne
improvised explosive device [IED]
War operations involving explosion of roadside
improvised explosive device [IED]

    ✓7th **Y36.230** War operations involving explosion of
improvised explosive device [IED], military
personnel

    ✓7th **Y36.231** War operations involving explosion of
improvised explosive device [IED], civilian

✓6th **Y36.24** War operations involving explosion due to
accidental detonation and discharge of own
munitions or munitions launch device

    ✓7th **Y36.240** War operations involving explosion due to
accidental detonation and discharge of
own munitions or munitions launch
device, military personnel

    ✓7th **Y36.241** War operations involving explosion due to
accidental detonation and discharge of
own munitions or munitions launch
device, civilian

☑ Additional Character Req   ✓x7th Placeholder Alert   Manifestation   HCC CMS-HCC Condition   ▽ Unspecified Code   ►◄ Revised Text   ● New Code   ▲ Revised Code Title

ICD-10-CM 2018   1159

✓6ᵗʰ **Y36.25** **War operations involving** fragments from munitions

    ✓7ᵗʰ **Y36.250** **War operations involving fragments from munitions,** military personnel

    ✓7ᵗʰ **Y36.251** **War operations involving fragments from munitions,** civilian

✓6ᵗʰ **Y36.26** **War operations involving fragments of** improvised explosive device [IED]

    War operations involving fragments of person-borne improvised explosive device [IED]
    War operations involving fragments of vehicle-borne improvised explosive device [IED]
    War operations involving fragments of roadside improvised explosive device [IED]

    ✓7ᵗʰ **Y36.260** **War operations involving fragments of improvised explosive device [IED],** military personnel

    ✓7ᵗʰ **Y36.261** **War operations involving fragments of improvised explosive device [IED],** civilian

✓6ᵗʰ **Y36.27** **War operations involving** fragments from weapons

    ✓7ᵗʰ **Y36.270** **War operations involving fragments from weapons,** military personnel

    ✓7ᵗʰ **Y36.271** **War operations involving fragments from weapons,** civilian

✓6ᵗʰ **Y36.29** **War operations involving other explosions and fragments**

    War operations involving explosion of grenade
    War operations involving explosions of land mine
    War operations involving shrapnel NOS

    ✓7ᵗʰ **Y36.290** **War operations involving other explosions and fragments,** military personnel

    ✓7ᵗʰ **Y36.291** **War operations involving other explosions and fragments,** civilian

✓5ᵗʰ **Y36.3** **War operations involving** fires, conflagrations and hot substances

    War operations involving smoke, fumes, and heat from fires, conflagrations and hot substances

    EXCLUDES 1 war operations involving fires and conflagrations aboard military aircraft (Y36.1-)
    war operations involving fires and conflagrations aboard military watercraft (Y36.0-)
    war operations involving fires and conflagrations caused indirectly by conventional weapons (Y36.2-)
    war operations involving fires and thermal effects of nuclear weapons (Y36.53-)

    ✓6ᵗʰ **Y36.30** **War operations involving unspecified fire, conflagration and hot substance**

        ✓7ᵗʰ **Y36.300** **War operations involving unspecified fire, conflagration and hot substance,** military personnel ▽

        ✓7ᵗʰ **Y36.301** **War operations involving unspecified fire, conflagration and hot substance,** civilian ▽

    ✓6ᵗʰ **Y36.31** **War operations involving** gasoline bomb

        War operations involving incendiary bomb
        War operations involving petrol bomb

        ✓7ᵗʰ **Y36.310** **War operations involving gasoline bomb,** military personnel

        ✓7ᵗʰ **Y36.311** **War operations involving gasoline bomb,** civilian

    ✓6ᵗʰ **Y36.32** **War operations involving** incendiary bullet

        ✓7ᵗʰ **Y36.320** **War operations involving incendiary bullet,** military personnel

        ✓7ᵗʰ **Y36.321** **War operations involving incendiary bullet,** civilian

    ✓6ᵗʰ **Y36.33** **War operations involving** flamethrower

        ✓7ᵗʰ **Y36.330** **War operations involving flamethrower,** military personnel

        ✓7ᵗʰ **Y36.331** **War operations involving flamethrower,** civilian

    ✓6ᵗʰ **Y36.39** **War operations involving other fires, conflagrations and hot substances**

        ✓7ᵗʰ **Y36.390** **War operations involving other fires, conflagrations and hot substances,** military personnel

        ✓7ᵗʰ **Y36.391** **War operations involving other fires, conflagrations and hot substances,** civilian

✓5ᵗʰ **Y36.4** **War operations involving firearm discharge and other forms of conventional warfare**

    ✓6ᵗʰ **Y36.41** **War operations involving** rubber bullets

        ✓7ᵗʰ **Y36.410** **War operations involving rubber bullets,** military personnel

        ✓7ᵗʰ **Y36.411** **War operations involving rubber bullets,** civilian

    ✓6ᵗʰ **Y36.42** **War operations involving** firearms pellets

        ✓7ᵗʰ **Y36.420** **War operations involving firearms pellets,** military personnel

        ✓7ᵗʰ **Y36.421** **War operations involving firearms pellets,** civilian

    ✓6ᵗʰ **Y36.43** **War operations involving other firearms discharge**

        War operations involving bullets NOS

        EXCLUDES 1 war operations involving munitions fragments (Y36.25-)
        war operations involving incendiary bullets (Y36.32-)

        ✓7ᵗʰ **Y36.430** **War operations involving other firearms discharge,** military personnel

        ✓7ᵗʰ **Y36.431** **War operations involving other firearms discharge,** civilian

    ✓6ᵗʰ **Y36.44** **War operations involving** unarmed hand to hand combat

        EXCLUDES 1 war operations involving combat using blunt or piercing object (Y36.45-)
        war operations involving intentional restriction of air and airway (Y36.46-)
        war operations involving unintentional restriction of air and airway (Y36.47-)

        ✓7ᵗʰ **Y36.440** **War operations involving unarmed hand to hand combat,** military personnel

        ✓7ᵗʰ **Y36.441** **War operations involving unarmed hand to hand combat,** civilian

    ✓6ᵗʰ **Y36.45** **War operations involving combat using** blunt or piercing object

        ✓7ᵗʰ **Y36.450** **War operations involving combat using blunt or piercing object,** military personnel

        ✓7ᵗʰ **Y36.451** **War operations involving combat using blunt or piercing object,** civilian

    ✓6ᵗʰ **Y36.46** **War operations involving** intentional restriction of air and airway

        ✓7ᵗʰ **Y36.460** **War operations involving intentional restriction of air and airway,** military personnel

        ✓7ᵗʰ **Y36.461** **War operations involving intentional restriction of air and airway,** civilian

    ✓6ᵗʰ **Y36.47** **War operations involving** unintentional restriction of air and airway

        ✓7ᵗʰ **Y36.470** **War operations involving unintentional restriction of air and airway,** military personnel

        ✓7ᵗʰ **Y36.471** **War operations involving unintentional restriction of air and airway,** civilian

    ✓6ᵗʰ **Y36.49** **War operations involving other forms of conventional warfare**

        ✓7ᵗʰ **Y36.490** **War operations involving other forms of conventional warfare,** military personnel

        ✓7ᵗʰ **Y36.491** **War operations involving other forms of conventional warfare,** civilian

✓5ᵗʰ **Y36.5** **War operations involving** nuclear weapons

    War operations involving dirty bomb NOS

    ✓6ᵗʰ **Y36.50** **War operations involving unspecified effect of nuclear weapon**

        ✓7ᵗʰ **Y36.500** **War operations involving unspecified effect of nuclear weapon,** military personnel ▽

        ✓7ᵗʰ **Y36.501** **War operations involving unspecified effect of nuclear weapon,** civilian ▽

    ✓6ᵗʰ **Y36.51** **War operations involving** direct blast **effect of nuclear weapon**

        War operations involving blast pressure of nuclear weapon

---

EXCLUDES 1 Not coded here   **EXCLUDES 2** Not included here   Ⓝ Newborn Age: 0   Ⓟ Pediatric Age: 0-17   Ⓜ Maternity Age: 12-55   Ⓐ Adult Age: 15-124

√7ᵗʰ **Y36.510** **War operations involving direct blast effect of nuclear weapon, military personnel**

√7ᵗʰ **Y36.511** **War operations involving direct blast effect of nuclear weapon, civilian**

√6ᵗʰ **Y36.52** **War operations involving** indirect blast **effect of nuclear weapon**
War operations involving being thrown by blast of nuclear weapon
War operations involving being struck or crushed by blast debris of nuclear weapon

√7ᵗʰ **Y36.520** **War operations involving indirect blast effect of nuclear weapon, military personnel**

√7ᵗʰ **Y36.521** **War operations involving indirect blast effect of nuclear weapon, civilian**

√6ᵗʰ **Y36.53** **War operations involving** thermal radiation **effect of nuclear weapon**
War operations involving direct heat from nuclear weapon
War operation involving fireball effects from nuclear weapon

√7ᵗʰ **Y36.530** **War operations involving thermal radiation effect of nuclear weapon, military personnel**

√7ᵗʰ **Y36.531** **War operations involving thermal radiation effect of nuclear weapon, civilian**

√6ᵗʰ **Y36.54** **War operation involving** nuclear radiation **effects of nuclear weapon**
War operation involving acute radiation exposure from nuclear weapon
War operation involving exposure to immediate ionizing radiation from nuclear weapon
War operation involving fallout exposure from nuclear weapon
War operation involving secondary effects of nuclear weapons

√7ᵗʰ **Y36.540** **War operation involving nuclear radiation effects of nuclear weapon, military personnel**

√7ᵗʰ **Y36.541** **War operation involving nuclear radiation effects of nuclear weapon, civilian**

√6ᵗʰ **Y36.59** **War operation involving other effects of nuclear weapons**

√7ᵗʰ **Y36.590** **War operation involving other effects of nuclear weapons, military personnel**

√7ᵗʰ **Y36.591** **War operation involving other effects of nuclear weapons, civilian**

√5ᵗʰ **Y36.6** **War operations involving biological weapons**

√6ᵗʰ **Y36.6X** **War operations involving** biological weapons

√7ᵗʰ **Y36.6X0** **War operations involving biological weapons, military personnel**

√7ᵗʰ **Y36.6X1** **War operations involving biological weapons, civilian**

√5ᵗʰ **Y36.7** **War operations involving chemical weapons and other forms of unconventional warfare**
EXCLUDES 1   *war operations involving incendiary devices (Y36.3-, Y36.5-)*

√6ᵗʰ **Y36.7X** **War operations involving** chemical weapons **and other forms of** unconventional warfare

√7ᵗʰ **Y36.7X0** **War operations involving chemical weapons and other forms of unconventional warfare, military personnel**

√7ᵗʰ **Y36.7X1** **War operations involving chemical weapons and other forms of unconventional warfare, civilian**

√5ᵗʰ **Y36.8** **War operations occurring** after cessation of hostilities
War operations classifiable to categories Y36.0-Y36.8 but occurring after cessation of hostilities

√6ᵗʰ **Y36.81** **Explosion of** mine **placed during war operations but exploding after cessation of hostilities**

√7ᵗʰ **Y36.810** **Explosion of mine placed during war operations but exploding after cessation of hostilities, military personnel**

√7ᵗʰ **Y36.811** **Explosion of mine placed during war operations but exploding after cessation of hostilities, civilian**

√6ᵗʰ **Y36.82** **Explosion of** bomb **placed during war operations but exploding after cessation of hostilities**

√7ᵗʰ **Y36.820** **Explosion of bomb placed during war operations but exploding after cessation of hostilities, military personnel**

√7ᵗʰ **Y36.821** **Explosion of bomb placed during war operations but exploding after cessation of hostilities, civilian**

√6ᵗʰ **Y36.88** **Other war operations occurring after cessation of hostilities**

√7ᵗʰ **Y36.880** **Other war operations occurring after cessation of hostilities, military personnel**

√7ᵗʰ **Y36.881** **Other war operations occurring after cessation of hostilities, civilian**

√6ᵗʰ **Y36.89** **Unspecified war operations occurring after cessation of hostilities**

√7ᵗʰ **Y36.890** **Unspecified war operations occurring after cessation of hostilities, military personnel** ▽

√7ᵗʰ **Y36.891** **Unspecified war operations occurring after cessation of hostilities, civilian** ▽

√5ᵗʰ **Y36.9** **Other and unspecified war operations**

√x7ᵗʰ **Y36.90** **War operations, unspecified** ▽

√x7ᵗʰ **Y36.91** **War operations involving unspecified** weapon of mass destruction **[WMD]** ▽

√x7ᵗʰ **Y36.92** **War operations involving** friendly fire

√4ᵗʰ **Y37** **Military operations**
INCLUDES   injuries to military personnel and civilians occurring during peacetime on military property and during routine military exercises and operations
EXCLUDES 1   *military aircraft involved in aircraft accident with civilian aircraft (V97.81-)*
military vehicles involved in transport accident with civilian vehicle (V09.01, V09.21, V19.81, V29.81, V39.81, V49.81, V59.81, V69.81, V79.81)
military watercraft involved in water transport accident with civilian watercraft (V94.81-)
war operations (Y36.-)

√5ᵗʰ **Y37.0** **Military operations involving** explosion of marine weapons

√6ᵗʰ **Y37.00** **Military operations involving explosion of unspecified marine weapon**
Military operations involving underwater blast NOS

√7ᵗʰ **Y37.000** **Military operations involving explosion of unspecified marine weapon, military personnel** ▽

√7ᵗʰ **Y37.001** **Military operations involving explosion of unspecified marine weapon, civilian** ▽

√6ᵗʰ **Y37.01** **Military operations involving explosion of** depth-charge

√7ᵗʰ **Y37.010** **Military operations involving explosion of depth-charge, military personnel**

√7ᵗʰ **Y37.011** **Military operations involving explosion of depth-charge, civilian**

√6ᵗʰ **Y37.02** **Military operations involving explosion of** marine mine
Military operations involving explosion of marine mine, at sea or in harbor

√7ᵗʰ **Y37.020** **Military operations involving explosion of marine mine, military personnel**

√7ᵗʰ **Y37.021** **Military operations involving explosion of marine mine, civilian**

√6ᵗʰ **Y37.03** **Military operations involving explosion of** sea-based artillery shell

√7ᵗʰ **Y37.030** **Military operations involving explosion of sea-based artillery shell, military personnel**

√7ᵗʰ **Y37.031** **Military operations involving explosion of sea-based artillery shell, civilian**

√6ᵗʰ **Y37.04** **Military operations involving explosion of** torpedo

√7ᵗʰ **Y37.040** **Military operations involving explosion of torpedo, military personnel**

√7ᵗʰ **Y37.041** **Military operations involving explosion of torpedo, civilian**

☑ Additional Character Req   √7ᵗʰ Placeholder Alert   Manifestation   HCC CMS-HCC Condition   ▽ Unspecified Code   ►◄ Revised Text   ● New Code   ▲ Revised Code Title

✓6ᵗʰ **Y37.05** **Military operations involving accidental detonation of** onboard marine weapons

    ✓7ᵗʰ **Y37.050** **Military operations involving accidental detonation of onboard marine weapons,** military personnel

    ✓7ᵗʰ **Y37.051** **Military operations involving accidental detonation of onboard marine weapons,** civilian

✓6ᵗʰ **Y37.09** **Military operations involving explosion of other marine weapons**

    ✓7ᵗʰ **Y37.090** **Military operations involving explosion of other marine weapons,** military personnel

    ✓7ᵗʰ **Y37.091** **Military operations involving explosion of other marine weapons,** civilian

✓5ᵗʰ **Y37.1** Military operations involving destruction of aircraft

    ✓6ᵗʰ **Y37.10** **Military operations involving unspecified destruction of aircraft**

      ✓7ᵗʰ **Y37.100** **Military operations involving unspecified destruction of aircraft,** military personnel   ▽

      ✓7ᵗʰ **Y37.101** **Military operations involving unspecified destruction of aircraft,** civilian   ▽

    ✓6ᵗʰ **Y37.11** **Military operations involving destruction of aircraft** due to enemy fire or explosives

      Military operations involving destruction of aircraft due to air to air missile
      Military operations involving destruction of aircraft due to explosive placed on aircraft
      Military operations involving destruction of aircraft due to rocket propelled grenade [RPG]
      Military operations involving destruction of aircraft due to small arms fire
      Military operations involving destruction of aircraft due to surface to air missile

      ✓7ᵗʰ **Y37.110** **Military operations involving destruction of aircraft due to enemy fire or explosives,** military personnel

      ✓7ᵗʰ **Y37.111** **Military operations involving destruction of aircraft due to enemy fire or explosives,** civilian

    ✓6ᵗʰ **Y37.12** **Military operations involving destruction of aircraft** due to collision with other aircraft

      ✓7ᵗʰ **Y37.120** **Military operations involving destruction of aircraft due to collision with other aircraft,** military personnel

      ✓7ᵗʰ **Y37.121** **Military operations involving destruction of aircraft due to collision with other aircraft,** civilian

    ✓6ᵗʰ **Y37.13** **Military operations involving destruction of aircraft** due to onboard fire

      ✓7ᵗʰ **Y37.130** **Military operations involving destruction of aircraft due to onboard fire,** military personnel

      ✓7ᵗʰ **Y37.131** **Military operations involving destruction of aircraft due to onboard fire,** civilian

    ✓6ᵗʰ **Y37.14** **Military operations involving destruction of aircraft due to** accidental detonation of onboard munitions and explosives

      ✓7ᵗʰ **Y37.140** **Military operations involving destruction of aircraft due to accidental detonation of onboard munitions and explosives,** military personnel

      ✓7ᵗʰ **Y37.141** **Military operations involving destruction of aircraft due to accidental detonation of onboard munitions and explosives,** civilian

    ✓6ᵗʰ **Y37.19** **Military operations involving other destruction of aircraft**

      ✓7ᵗʰ **Y37.190** **Military operations involving other destruction of aircraft,** military personnel

      ✓7ᵗʰ **Y37.191** **Military operations involving other destruction of aircraft,** civilian

✓5ᵗʰ **Y37.2** **Military operations involving other explosions and fragments**

    EXCLUDES 1   *military operations involving explosion of aircraft (Y37.1-)*
        military operations involving explosion of marine weapons (Y37.0-)
        military operations involving explosion of nuclear weapons (Y37.5-)

    ✓6ᵗʰ **Y37.20** **Military operations involving unspecified explosion and fragments**

      Military operations involving air blast NOS
      Military operations involving blast NOS
      Military operations involving blast fragments NOS
      Military operations involving blast wave NOS
      Military operations involving blast wind NOS
      Military operations involving explosion NOS
      Military operations involving explosion of bomb NOS

      ✓7ᵗʰ **Y37.200** **Military operations involving unspecified explosion and fragments,** military personnel   ▽

      ✓7ᵗʰ **Y37.201** **Military operations involving unspecified explosion and fragments,** civilian   ▽

    ✓6ᵗʰ **Y37.21** **Military operations involving explosion of** aerial bomb

      ✓7ᵗʰ **Y37.210** **Military operations involving explosion of aerial bomb,** military personnel

      ✓7ᵗʰ **Y37.211** **Military operations involving explosion of aerial bomb,** civilian

    ✓6ᵗʰ **Y37.22** **Military operations involving explosion of** guided missile

      ✓7ᵗʰ **Y37.220** **Military operations involving explosion of guided missile,** military personnel

      ✓7ᵗʰ **Y37.221** **Military operations involving explosion of guided missile,** civilian

    ✓6ᵗʰ **Y37.23** **Military operations involving explosion of** improvised explosive device [IED]

      Military operations involving explosion of person-borne improvised explosive device [IED]
      Military operations involving explosion of vehicle-borne improvised explosive device [IED]
      Military operations involving explosion of roadside improvised explosive device [IED]

      ✓7ᵗʰ **Y37.230** **Military operations involving explosion of improvised explosive device [IED],** military personnel

      ✓7ᵗʰ **Y37.231** **Military operations involving explosion of improvised explosive device [IED],** civilian

    ✓6ᵗʰ **Y37.24** **Military operations involving explosion** due to accidental detonation and discharge of own munitions or munitions launch device

      ✓7ᵗʰ **Y37.240** **Military operations involving explosion due to accidental detonation and discharge of own munitions or munitions launch device,** military personnel

      ✓7ᵗʰ **Y37.241** **Military operations involving explosion due to accidental detonation and discharge of own munitions or munitions launch device,** civilian

    ✓6ᵗʰ **Y37.25** **Military operations involving** fragments from munitions

      ✓7ᵗʰ **Y37.250** **Military operations involving fragments from munitions,** military personnel

      ✓7ᵗʰ **Y37.251** **Military operations involving fragments from munitions,** civilian

    ✓6ᵗʰ **Y37.26** **Military operations involving fragments of** improvised explosive device [IED]

      Military operations involving fragments of person-borne improvised explosive device [IED]
      Military operations involving fragments of vehicle-borne improvised explosive device [IED]
      Military operations involving fragments of roadside improvised explosive device [IED]

      ✓7ᵗʰ **Y37.260** **Military operations involving fragments of improvised explosive device [IED],** military personnel

      ✓7ᵗʰ **Y37.261** **Military operations involving fragments of improvised explosive device [IED],** civilian

CLUDES 1 Not coded here   EXCLUDES 2 Not included here   N Newborn Age: 0   P Pediatric Age: 0-17   M Maternity Age: 12-55   A Adult Age: 15-124

1162   ICD-10-CM 2018

☑6ᵗʰ **Y37.27** **Military operations involving** fragments from weapons

    ☑7ᵗʰ **Y37.270** **Military operations involving fragments from weapons,** military personnel

    ☑7ᵗʰ **Y37.271** **Military operations involving fragments from weapons,** civilian

☑6ᵗʰ **Y37.29** **Military operations involving other explosions and fragments**
Military operations involving explosion of grenade
Military operations involving explosions of land mine
Military operations involving shrapnel NOS

    ☑7ᵗʰ **Y37.290** **Military operations involving other explosions and fragments,** military personnel

    ☑7ᵗʰ **Y37.291** **Military operations involving other explosions and fragments,** civilian

☑5ᵗʰ **Y37.3** **Military operations involving** fires, conflagrations and hot substances
Military operations involving smoke, fumes, and heat from fires, conflagrations and hot substances

    EXCLUDES 1 *military operations involving fires and conflagrations aboard military aircraft (Y37.1-)*
military operations involving fires and conflagrations aboard military watercraft (Y37.0-)
military operations involving fires and conflagrations caused indirectly by conventional weapons (Y37.2-)
military operations involving fires and thermal effects of nuclear weapons (Y36.53-)

☑6ᵗʰ **Y37.30** **Military operations involving unspecified fire, conflagration and hot substance**

    ☑7ᵗʰ **Y37.300** **Military operations involving unspecified fire, conflagration and hot substance,** military personnel ▽

    ☑7ᵗʰ **Y37.301** **Military operations involving unspecified fire, conflagration and hot substance,** civilian ▽

☑6ᵗʰ **Y37.31** **Military operations involving** gasoline bomb
Military operations involving incendiary bomb
Military operations involving petrol bomb

    ☑7ᵗʰ **Y37.310** **Military operations involving gasoline bomb,** military personnel

    ☑7ᵗʰ **Y37.311** **Military operations involving gasoline bomb,** civilian

☑6ᵗʰ **Y37.32** **Military operations involving** incendiary bullet

    ☑7ᵗʰ **Y37.320** **Military operations involving incendiary bullet,** military personnel

    ☑7ᵗʰ **Y37.321** **Military operations involving incendiary bullet,** civilian

☑6ᵗʰ **Y37.33** **Military operations involving** flamethrower

    ☑7ᵗʰ **Y37.330** **Military operations involving flamethrower,** military personnel

    ☑7ᵗʰ **Y37.331** **Military operations involving flamethrower,** civilian

☑6ᵗʰ **Y37.39** **Military operations involving other fires, conflagrations and hot substances**

    ☑7ᵗʰ **Y37.390** **Military operations involving other fires, conflagrations and hot substances,** military personnel

    ☑7ᵗʰ **Y37.391** **Military operations involving other fires, conflagrations and hot substances,** civilian

☑5ᵗʰ **Y37.4** **Military operations involving firearm discharge and other forms of conventional warfare**

☑6ᵗʰ **Y37.41** **Military operations involving** rubber bullets

    ☑7ᵗʰ **Y37.410** **Military operations involving rubber bullets,** military personnel

    ☑7ᵗʰ **Y37.411** **Military operations involving rubber bullets,** civilian

☑6ᵗʰ **Y37.42** **Military operations involving** firearms pellets

    ☑7ᵗʰ **Y37.420** **Military operations involving firearms pellets,** military personnel

    ☑7ᵗʰ **Y37.421** **Military operations involving firearms pellets,** civilian

☑6ᵗʰ **Y37.43** **Military operations involving other firearms discharge**
Military operations involving bullets NOS

    EXCLUDES 1 *military operations involving munitions fragments (Y37.25-)*
military operations involving incendiary bullets (Y37.32-)

    ☑7ᵗʰ **Y37.430** **Military operations involving other firearms discharge,** military personnel

    ☑7ᵗʰ **Y37.431** **Military operations involving other firearms discharge,** civilian

☑6ᵗʰ **Y37.44** **Military operations involving** unarmed hand to hand combat

    EXCLUDES 1 *military operations involving combat using blunt or piercing object (Y37.45-)*
military operations involving intentional restriction of air and airway (Y37.46-)
military operations involving unintentional restriction of air and airway (Y37.47-)

    ☑7ᵗʰ **Y37.440** **Military operations involving unarmed hand to hand combat,** military personnel

    ☑7ᵗʰ **Y37.441** **Military operations involving unarmed hand to hand combat,** civilian

☑6ᵗʰ **Y37.45** **Military operations involving** combat using blunt or piercing object

    ☑7ᵗʰ **Y37.450** **Military operations involving combat using blunt or piercing object,** military personnel

    ☑7ᵗʰ **Y37.451** **Military operations involving combat using blunt or piercing object,** civilian

☑6ᵗʰ **Y37.46** **Military operations involving** intentional restriction of air and airway

    ☑7ᵗʰ **Y37.460** **Military operations involving intentional restriction of air and airway,** military personnel

    ☑7ᵗʰ **Y37.461** **Military operations involving intentional restriction of air and airway,** civilian

☑6ᵗʰ **Y37.47** **Military operations involving** unintentional restriction of air and airway

    ☑7ᵗʰ **Y37.470** **Military operations involving unintentional restriction of air and airway,** military personnel

    ☑7ᵗʰ **Y37.471** **Military operations involving unintentional restriction of air and airway,** civilian

☑6ᵗʰ **Y37.49** **Military operations involving other forms of conventional warfare**

    ☑7ᵗʰ **Y37.490** **Military operations involving other forms of conventional warfare,** military personnel

    ☑7ᵗʰ **Y37.491** **Military operations involving other forms of conventional warfare,** civilian

☑5ᵗʰ **Y37.5** **Military operations involving** nuclear weapons
Military operation involving dirty bomb NOS

☑6ᵗʰ **Y37.50** **Military operations involving unspecified effect of nuclear weapon**

    ☑7ᵗʰ **Y37.500** **Military operations involving unspecified effect of nuclear weapon,** military personnel ▽

    ☑7ᵗʰ **Y37.501** **Military operations involving unspecified effect of nuclear weapon,** civilian ▽

☑6ᵗʰ **Y37.51** **Military operations involving** direct blast effect of nuclear weapon
Military operations involving blast pressure of nuclear weapon

    ☑7ᵗʰ **Y37.510** **Military operations involving direct blast effect of nuclear weapon,** military personnel

    ☑7ᵗʰ **Y37.511** **Military operations involving direct blast effect of nuclear weapon,** civilian

☑ Additional Character Req   ☑ᵛˣ⁷ᵗʰ Placeholder Alert   Manifestation   **HCC** CMS-HCC Condition   ▽ Unspecified Code   ▶◀ Revised Text   ● New Code   ▲ Revised Code Title

ICD-10-CM 2018   **1163**

Chapter 20. External Causes of Morbidity

✓6ᵗʰ **Y37.52** **Military operations involving** indirect blast effect **of nuclear weapon**

Military operations involving being thrown by blast of nuclear weapon

Military operations involving being struck or crushed by blast debris of nuclear weapon

✓7ᵗʰ **Y37.520** **Military operations involving indirect blast effect of nuclear weapon,** military personnel

✓7ᵗʰ **Y37.521** **Military operations involving indirect blast effect of nuclear weapon,** civilian

✓6ᵗʰ **Y37.53** **Military operations involving** thermal radiation effect **of nuclear weapon**

Military operations involving direct heat from nuclear weapon

Military operation involving fireball effects from nuclear weapon

✓7ᵗʰ **Y37.530** **Military operations involving thermal radiation effect of nuclear weapon,** military personnel

✓7ᵗʰ **Y37.531** **Military operations involving thermal radiation effect of nuclear weapon,** civilian

✓6ᵗʰ **Y37.54** **Military operation involving** nuclear radiation effects **of nuclear weapon**

Military operation involving acute radiation exposure from nuclear weapon

Military operation involving exposure to immediate ionizing radiation from nuclear weapon

Military operation involving fallout exposure from nuclear weapon

Military operation involving secondary effects of nuclear weapons

✓7ᵗʰ **Y37.540** **Military operation involving nuclear radiation effects of nuclear weapon,** military personnel

✓7ᵗʰ **Y37.541** **Military operation involving nuclear radiation effects of nuclear weapon,** civilian

✓6ᵗʰ **Y37.59** **Military operation involving other effects of nuclear weapons**

✓7ᵗʰ **Y37.590** **Military operation involving other effects of nuclear weapons,** military personnel

✓7ᵗʰ **Y37.591** **Military operation involving other effects of nuclear weapons,** civilian

✓5ᵗʰ **Y37.6** **Military operations involving** biological weapons

✓6ᵗʰ **Y37.6X** **Military operations involving biological weapons**

✓7ᵗʰ **Y37.6X0** **Military operations involving biological weapons,** military personnel

✓7ᵗʰ **Y37.6X1** **Military operations involving biological weapons,** civilian

✓5ᵗʰ **Y37.7** **Military operations involving chemical weapons and other forms of unconventional warfare**

EXCLUDES 1 military operations involving incendiary devices (Y36.3-, Y36.5-)

✓6ᵗʰ **Y37.7X** **Military operations involving** chemical weapons **and other forms of** unconventional warfare

✓7ᵗʰ **Y37.7X0** **Military operations involving chemical weapons and other forms of unconventional warfare,** military personnel

✓7ᵗʰ **Y37.7X1** **Military operations involving chemical weapons and other forms of unconventional warfare,** civilian

✓5ᵗʰ **Y37.9** **Other and unspecified military operations**

✓✗7ᵗʰ **Y37.90** **Military operations, unspecified** ▽

✓✗7ᵗʰ **Y37.91** **Military operations involving unspecified weapon of mass destruction [WMD]** ▽

✓✗7ᵗʰ **Y37.92** **Military operations involving** friendly fire

✓4ᵗʰ **Y38** **Terrorism**

NOTE These codes are for use to identify injuries resulting from the unlawful use of force or violence against persons or property to intimidate or coerce a Government, the civilian population, or any segment thereof, in furtherance of political or social objective.

Use additional code for place of occurrence (Y92.-)

✓5ᵗʰ **Y38.0** **Terrorism involving explosion of marine weapons**

Terrorism involving depth-charge

Terrorism involving marine mine

Terrorism involving mine NOS, at sea or in harbor

Terrorism involving sea-based artillery shell

Terrorism involving torpedo

Terrorism involving underwater blast

✓6ᵗʰ **Y38.0X** **Terrorism involving explosion of** marine weapons

✓7ᵗʰ **Y38.0X1** **Terrorism involving explosion of marine weapons,** public safety official **injured**

✓7ᵗʰ **Y38.0X2** **Terrorism involving explosion of marine weapons,** civilian **injured**

✓7ᵗʰ **Y38.0X3** **Terrorism involving explosion of marine weapons,** terrorist **injured**

✓5ᵗʰ **Y38.1** **Terrorism involving destruction of aircraft**

Terrorism involving aircraft burned

Terrorism involving aircraft exploded

Terrorism involving aircraft being shot down

Terrorism involving aircraft used as a weapon

✓6ᵗʰ **Y38.1X** **Terrorism involving** destruction of aircraft

✓7ᵗʰ **Y38.1X1** **Terrorism involving destruction of aircraft,** public safety official **injured**

✓7ᵗʰ **Y38.1X2** **Terrorism involving destruction of aircraft,** civilian **injured**

✓7ᵗʰ **Y38.1X3** **Terrorism involving destruction of aircraft,** terrorist **injured**

✓5ᵗʰ **Y38.2** **Terrorism involving other explosions and fragments**

Terrorism involving antipersonnel (fragments) bomb

Terrorism involving blast NOS

Terrorism involving explosion NOS

Terrorism involving explosion of breech block

Terrorism involving explosion of cannon block

Terrorism involving explosion (fragments) of artillery shell

Terrorism involving explosion (fragments) of bomb

Terrorism involving explosion (fragments) of grenade

Terrorism involving explosion (fragments) of guided missile

Terrorism involving explosion (fragments) of land mine

Terrorism involving explosion of mortar bomb

Terrorism involving explosion of munitions

Terrorism involving explosion (fragments) of rocket

Terrorism involving explosion (fragments) of shell

Terrorism involving shrapnel

Terrorism involving mine NOS, on land

EXCLUDES 1 terrorism involving explosion of nuclear weapon (Y38.5)

terrorism involving suicide bomber (Y38.81)

✓6ᵗʰ **Y38.2X** **Terrorism involving other explosions and fragments**

✓7ᵗʰ **Y38.2X1** **Terrorism involving other explosions and fragments,** public safety official **injured**

✓7ᵗʰ **Y38.2X2** **Terrorism involving other explosions and fragments,** civilian **injured**

✓7ᵗʰ **Y38.2X3** **Terrorism involving other explosions and fragments,** terrorist **injured**

✓5ᵗʰ **Y38.3** **Terrorism involving fires, conflagration and hot substances**

Terrorism involving conflagration NOS

Terrorism involving fire NOS

Terrorism involving petrol bomb

EXCLUDES 1 terrorism involving fire or heat of nuclear weapon (Y38.5)

✓6ᵗʰ **Y38.3X** **Terrorism involving** fires, conflagration and hot substances

✓7ᵗʰ **Y38.3X1** **Terrorism involving fires, conflagration and hot substances,** public safety official **injured**

✓7ᵗʰ **Y38.3X2** **Terrorism involving fires, conflagration and hot substances,** civilian **injured**

✓7ᵗʰ **Y38.3X3** **Terrorism involving fires, conflagration and hot substances,** terrorist **injured**

EXCLUDES 1 Not coded here   **EXCLUDES 2** Not included here   **N** Newborn Age: 0   **P** Pediatric Age: 0-17   **M** Maternity Age: 12-55   **A** Adult Age: 15-124

1164   ICD-10-CM 2018

☑5ᵗʰ **Y38.4** **Terrorism involving firearms**
Terrorism involving carbine bullet
Terrorism involving machine gun bullet
Terrorism involving pellets (shotgun)
Terrorism involving pistol bullet
Terrorism involving rifle bullet
Terrorism involving rubber (rifle) bullet

  ☑6ᵗʰ **Y38.4X** **Terrorism involving** firearms

    ☑7ᵗʰ **Y38.4X1** **Terrorism involving firearms,** public safety official **injured**

    ☑7ᵗʰ **Y38.4X2** **Terrorism involving firearms,** civilian **injured**

    ☑7ᵗʰ **Y38.4X3** **Terrorism involving firearms,** terrorist **injured**

☑5ᵗʰ **Y38.5** **Terrorism involving nuclear weapons**
Terrorism involving blast effects of nuclear weapon
Terrorism involving exposure to ionizing radiation from nuclear weapon
Terrorism involving fireball effect of nuclear weapon
Terrorism involving heat from nuclear weapon

  ☑6ᵗʰ **Y38.5X** **Terrorism involving** nuclear weapons

    ☑7ᵗʰ **Y38.5X1** **Terrorism involving nuclear weapons,** public safety official **injured**

    ☑7ᵗʰ **Y38.5X2** **Terrorism involving nuclear weapons,** civilian **injured**

    ☑7ᵗʰ **Y38.5X3** **Terrorism involving nuclear weapons,** terrorist **injured**

☑5ᵗʰ **Y38.6** **Terrorism involving biological weapons**
Terrorism involving anthrax
Terrorism involving cholera
Terrorism involving smallpox

  ☑6ᵗʰ **Y38.6X** **Terrorism involving** biological weapons

    ☑7ᵗʰ **Y38.6X1** **Terrorism involving biological weapons,** public safety official **injured**

    ☑7ᵗʰ **Y38.6X2** **Terrorism involving biological weapons,** civilian **injured**

    ☑7ᵗʰ **Y38.6X3** **Terrorism involving biological weapons,** terrorist **injured**

☑5ᵗʰ **Y38.7** **Terrorism involving chemical weapons**
Terrorism involving gases, fumes, chemicals
Terrorism involving hydrogen cyanide
Terrorism involving phosgene
Terrorism involving sarin

  ☑6ᵗʰ **Y38.7X** **Terrorism involving** chemical weapons

    ☑7ᵗʰ **Y38.7X1** **Terrorism involving chemical weapons,** public safety official **injured**

    ☑7ᵗʰ **Y38.7X2** **Terrorism involving chemical weapons,** civilian **injured**

    ☑7ᵗʰ **Y38.7X3** **Terrorism involving chemical weapons,** terrorist **injured**

☑5ᵗʰ **Y38.8** **Terrorism involving other and unspecified means**

  ☑x7ᵗʰ **Y38.80** **Terrorism involving unspecified means** ▽
Terrorism NOS

  ☑6ᵗʰ **Y38.81** **Terrorism involving** suicide bomber

    ☑7ᵗʰ **Y38.811** **Terrorism involving suicide bomber,** public safety official **injured**

    ☑7ᵗʰ **Y38.812** **Terrorism involving suicide bomber,** civilian **injured**

  ☑6ᵗʰ **Y38.89** **Terrorism involving other means**
Terrorism involving drowning and submersion
Terrorism involving lasers
Terrorism involving piercing or stabbing instruments

    ☑7ᵗʰ **Y38.891** **Terrorism involving other means,** public safety official **injured**

    ☑7ᵗʰ **Y38.892** **Terrorism involving other means,** civilian **injured**

    ☑7ᵗʰ **Y38.893** **Terrorism involving other means,** terrorist **injured**

☑5ᵗʰ **Y38.9** **Terrorism, secondary effects**
  NOTE   This code is for use to identify injuries occurring subsequent to a terrorist attack, not those that are due to the initial terrorist attack.

  ☑6ᵗʰ **Y38.9X** **Terrorism,** secondary effects

    ☑7ᵗʰ **Y38.9X1** **Terrorism, secondary effects,** public safety official **injured**

    ☑7ᵗʰ **Y38.9X2** **Terrorism, secondary effects,** civilian **injured**

Complications of medical and surgical care (Y62-Y84)

INCLUDES complications of medical devices
surgical and medical procedures as the cause of abnormal reaction of the patient, or of later complication, without mention of misadventure at the time of the procedure

Misadventures to patients during surgical and medical care (Y62-Y69)

EXCLUDES 1 surgical and medical procedures as the cause of abnormal reaction of the patient, without mention of misadventure at the time of the procedure (Y83-Y84)
EXCLUDES 2 breakdown or malfunctioning of medical device (during procedure) (after implantation) (ongoing use) (Y70-Y82)

☑4ᵗʰ **Y62** **Failure of** sterile precautions **during surgical and medical care**

  Y62.0 **Failure of sterile precautions during** surgical operation

  Y62.1 **Failure of sterile precautions during** infusion or transfusion

  Y62.2 **Failure of sterile precautions during** kidney dialysis and other perfusion   **HCC**

  Y62.3 **Failure of sterile precautions during** injection or immunization

  Y62.4 **Failure of sterile precautions during** endoscopic examination

  Y62.5 **Failure of sterile precautions during** heart catheterization

  Y62.6 **Failure of sterile precautions during** aspiration, puncture and other catheterization

  Y62.8 **Failure of sterile precautions during other surgical and medical care**

  Y62.9 **Failure of sterile precautions during unspecified surgical** ▽ **and medical care**

☑4ᵗʰ **Y63** **Failure in** dosage **during surgical and medical care**
  EXCLUDES 2 accidental overdose of drug or wrong drug given in error (T36-T50)

  Y63.0 **Excessive amount of blood or other fluid given during transfusion or infusion**

  Y63.1 **Incorrect dilution of fluid used during infusion**

  Y63.2 **Overdose of radiation given during therapy**

  Y63.3 **Inadvertent exposure of patient to radiation during medical care**

  Y63.4 **Failure in dosage in electroshock or insulin-shock therapy**

  Y63.5 **Inappropriate temperature in local application and packing**

  Y63.6 **Underdosing and nonadministration of necessary drug, medicament or biological substance**

  Y63.8 **Failure in dosage during other surgical and medical care**

  Y63.9 **Failure in dosage during unspecified surgical and medical** ▽ **care**

☑4ᵗʰ **Y64** **Contaminated medical or biological substances**

  Y64.0 **Contaminated medical or biological substance,** transfused or infused

  Y64.1 **Contaminated medical or biological substance,** injected or used for immunization

  Y64.8 **Contaminated medical or biological substance administered by other means**

  Y64.9 **Contaminated medical or biological substance** ▽ **administered by unspecified means**
Administered contaminated medical or biological substance NOS

☑4ᵗʰ **Y65** **Other misadventures during surgical and medical care**

  Y65.0 **Mismatched blood in transfusion**

  Y65.1 **Wrong fluid used in infusion**

  Y65.2 **Failure in suture or ligature during surgical operation**

  Y65.3 **Endotracheal tube wrongly placed during anesthetic procedure**

  Y65.4 **Failure to introduce or to remove other tube or instrument**

  ☑5ᵗʰ **Y65.5** **Performance of** wrong procedure **(operation)**

    Y65.51 **Performance of wrong procedure (operation) on** correct patient
Wrong device implanted into correct surgical site
EXCLUDES 1 performance of correct procedure (operation) on wrong side or body part (Y65.53)

☑ Additional Character Req   ☑x7ᵗʰ Placeholder Alert   Manifestation   **HCC** CMS-HCC Condition   ▽ Unspecified Code   ►◄ Revised Text   ● New Code   ▲ Revised Code Title

ICD-10-CM 2018   1165

Y65.52 **Performance of procedure (operation) on** patient not scheduled for surgery
     Performance of procedure (operation) intended for another patient
     Performance of procedure (operation) on wrong patient

Y65.53 **Performance of correct procedure (operation) on** wrong side or body part
     Performance of correct procedure (operation) on wrong side
     Performance of correct procedure (operation) on wrong site

Y65.8 **Other specified misadventures during surgical and medical care**

Y66 **Nonadministration of surgical and medical care**
Premature cessation of surgical and medical care
EXCLUDES 1   DNR status (Z66)
         palliative care (Z51.5)

Y69 **Unspecified misadventure during surgical and medical care** ▽

Medical devices associated with adverse incidents in diagnostic and therapeutic use (Y70-Y82)

INCLUDES   breakdown or malfunction of medical devices (during use) (after implantation) (ongoing use)

EXCLUDES 2   breakdown or malfunctioning of medical device (after implantation) (during procedure) (ongoing use) (Y70-Y82)
     later complications following use of medical devices without breakdown or malfunctioning of device (Y83-Y84)
     misadventure to patients during surgical and medical care, classifiable to (Y62-Y69)
     surgical and other medical procedures as the cause of abnormal reaction of the patient, or of later complication, without mention of misadventure at the time of the procedure (Y83-Y84)

✓4ᵗʰ **Y70** **Anesthesiology** devices associated with adverse incidents

Y70.0 Diagnostic and monitoring **anesthesiology devices associated with adverse incidents**

Y70.1 Therapeutic (**nonsurgical**) and rehabilitative **anesthesiology devices associated with adverse incidents**

Y70.2 Prosthetic and other implants, **materials and accessory anesthesiology devices associated with adverse incidents**

Y70.3 Surgical instruments, materials **and anesthesiology devices (including sutures) associated with adverse incidents**

Y70.8 Miscellaneous anesthesiology devices associated with adverse incidents, not elsewhere classified

✓4ᵗʰ **Y71** **Cardiovascular** devices associated with adverse incidents

Y71.0 Diagnostic and monitoring **cardiovascular devices associated with adverse incidents**

Y71.1 Therapeutic (**nonsurgical**) and rehabilitative **cardiovascular devices associated with adverse incidents**

Y71.2 Prosthetic and other implants, **materials and accessory cardiovascular devices associated with adverse incidents**

Y71.3 Surgical instruments, materials **and cardiovascular devices (including sutures) associated with adverse incidents**

Y71.8 Miscellaneous cardiovascular devices associated with adverse incidents, not elsewhere classified

✓4ᵗʰ **Y72** **Otorhinolaryngological** devices associated with adverse incidents

Y72.0 Diagnostic and monitoring **otorhinolaryngological devices associated with adverse incidents**

Y72.1 Therapeutic (**nonsurgical**) and rehabilitative **otorhinolaryngological devices associated with adverse incidents**

Y72.2 Prosthetic and other implants, **materials and accessory otorhinolaryngological devices associated with adverse incidents**

Y72.3 Surgical instruments, materials **and otorhinolaryngological devices (including sutures) associated with adverse incidents**

Y72.8 Miscellaneous otorhinolaryngological devices associated with adverse incidents, not elsewhere classified

✓4ᵗʰ **Y73** **Gastroenterology and urology** devices associated with adverse incidents

Y73.0 Diagnostic and monitoring **gastroenterology and urology devices associated with adverse incidents**

Y73.1 Therapeutic (**nonsurgical**) and rehabilitative **gastroenterology and urology devices associated with adverse incidents**

Y73.2 Prosthetic and other implants, **materials and accessory gastroenterology and urology devices associated with adverse incidents**

Y73.3 Surgical instruments, materials **and gastroenterology and urology devices (including sutures) associated with adverse incidents**

Y73.8 Miscellaneous gastroenterology and urology devices associated with adverse incidents, not elsewhere classified

✓4ᵗʰ **Y74** **General hospital and personal-use devices associated with adverse incidents**

Y74.0 Diagnostic and monitoring **general hospital and personal-use devices associated with adverse incidents**

Y74.1 Therapeutic (**nonsurgical**) and rehabilitative **general hospital and personal-use devices associated with adverse incidents**

Y74.2 Prosthetic and other implants, **materials and accessory general hospital and personal-use devices associated with adverse incidents**

Y74.3 Surgical instruments, materials **and general hospital and personal-use devices (including sutures) associated with adverse incidents**

Y74.8 Miscellaneous general hospital and personal-use devices associated with adverse incidents, not elsewhere classified

✓4ᵗʰ **Y75** **Neurological** devices associated with adverse incidents

Y75.0 Diagnostic and monitoring **neurological devices associated with adverse incidents**

Y75.1 Therapeutic (**nonsurgical**) and rehabilitative **neurological devices associated with adverse incidents**

Y75.2 Prosthetic and other implants, **materials and neurological devices associated with adverse incidents**

Y75.3 Surgical instruments, materials **and neurological devices (including sutures) associated with adverse incidents**

Y75.8 Miscellaneous neurological devices associated with adverse incidents, not elsewhere classified

✓4ᵗʰ **Y76** **Obstetric and gynecological** devices associated with adverse incidents

Y76.0 Diagnostic and monitoring **obstetric and gynecological devices associated with adverse incidents** ♀

Y76.1 Therapeutic (**nonsurgical**) and rehabilitative **obstetric and gynecological devices associated with adverse incidents** ♀

Y76.2 Prosthetic and other implants, **materials and accessory obstetric and gynecological devices associated with adverse incidents** ♀

Y76.3 Surgical instruments, materials **and obstetric and gynecological devices (including sutures) associated with adverse incidents** ♀

Y76.8 Miscellaneous obstetric and gynecological devices associated with adverse incidents, not elsewhere classified ♀

✓4ᵗʰ **Y77** **Ophthalmic** devices associated with adverse incidents

Y77.0 Diagnostic and monitoring **ophthalmic devices associated with adverse incidents**

Y77.1 Therapeutic (**nonsurgical**) and rehabilitative **ophthalmic devices associated with adverse incidents**

Y77.2 Prosthetic and other implants, **materials and accessory ophthalmic devices associated with adverse incidents**

Y77.3 Surgical instruments, materials **and ophthalmic devices (including sutures) associated with adverse incidents**

Y77.8 Miscellaneous ophthalmic devices associated with adverse incidents, not elsewhere classified

✓4ᵗʰ **Y78** **Radiological** devices associated with adverse incidents

Y78.0 Diagnostic and monitoring **radiological devices associated with adverse incidents**

Y78.1 Therapeutic (**nonsurgical**) and rehabilitative **radiological devices associated with adverse incidents**

Y78.2 Prosthetic and other implants, **materials and accessory radiological devices associated with adverse incidents**

Y78.3 Surgical instruments, materials **and radiological devices (including sutures) associated with adverse incidents**

Y78.8 Miscellaneous radiological devices associated with adverse incidents, not elsewhere classified

✓4ᵗʰ **Y79** **Orthopedic** devices associated with adverse incidents

Y79.0 Diagnostic and monitoring **orthopedic devices associated with adverse incidents**

Y79.1 Therapeutic (**nonsurgical**) and rehabilitative **orthopedic devices associated with adverse incidents**

Y79.2 Prosthetic and other implants, **materials and accessory orthopedic devices associated with adverse incidents**

EXCLUDES 1 Not coded here   **EXCLUDES 2** Not included here   **N** Newborn Age: 0   **P** Pediatric Age: 0-17   **M** Maternity Age: 12-55   **A** Adult Age: 15-124

1166   ICD-10-CM 2018

Y79.3 Surgical instruments, materials and orthopedic devices (including sutures) associated with adverse incidents

Y79.8 Miscellaneous orthopedic devices associated with adverse incidents, not elsewhere classified

✓4ᵗʰ Y80 Physical medicine devices associated with adverse incidents

Y80.0 Diagnostic and monitoring physical medicine devices associated with adverse incidents

Y80.1 Therapeutic (nonsurgical) and rehabilitative physical medicine devices associated with adverse incidents

Y80.2 Prosthetic and other implants, materials and accessory physical medicine devices associated with adverse incidents

Y80.3 Surgical instruments, materials and physical medicine devices (including sutures) associated with adverse incidents

Y80.8 Miscellaneous physical medicine devices associated with adverse incidents, not elsewhere classified

✓4ᵗʰ Y81 General- and plastic-surgery devices associated with adverse incidents

Y81.0 Diagnostic and monitoring general- and plastic-surgery devices associated with adverse incidents

Y81.1 Therapeutic (nonsurgical) and rehabilitative general- and plastic-surgery devices associated with adverse incidents

Y81.2 Prosthetic and other implants, materials and accessory general- and plastic-surgery devices associated with adverse incidents

Y81.3 Surgical instruments, materials and general- and plastic-surgery devices (including sutures) associated with adverse incidents

Y81.8 Miscellaneous general- and plastic-surgery devices associated with adverse incidents, not elsewhere classified

✓4ᵗʰ Y82 Other and unspecified medical devices associated with adverse incidents

Y82.8 Other medical devices associated with adverse incidents

Y82.9 Unspecified medical devices associated with adverse incidents ▽

Surgical and other medical procedures as the cause of abnormal reaction of the patient, or of later complication, without mention of misadventure at the time of the procedure (Y83-Y84)

EXCLUDES 1 misadventures to patients during surgical and medical care, classifiable to (Y62-Y69)

EXCLUDES 2 breakdown or malfunctioning of medical device (after implantation) (during procedure) (ongoing use) (Y70-Y82)

✓4ᵗʰ Y83 Surgical operation and other surgical procedures as the cause of abnormal reaction of the patient, or of later complication, without mention of misadventure at the time of the procedure

Y83.0 Surgical operation with transplant of whole organ as the cause of abnormal reaction of the patient, or of later complication, without mention of misadventure at the time of the procedure

Y83.1 Surgical operation with implant of artificial internal device as the cause of abnormal reaction of the patient, or of later complication, without mention of misadventure at the time of the procedure

Y83.2 Surgical operation with anastomosis, bypass or graft as the cause of abnormal reaction of the patient, or of later complication, without mention of misadventure at the time of the procedure

Y83.3 Surgical operation with formation of external stoma as the cause of abnormal reaction of the patient, or of later complication, without mention of misadventure at the time of the procedure

Y83.4 Other reconstructive surgery as the cause of abnormal reaction of the patient, or of later complication, without mention of misadventure at the time of the procedure

Y83.5 Amputation of limb(s) as the cause of abnormal reaction of the patient, or of later complication, without mention of misadventure at the time of the procedure

Y83.6 Removal of other organ (partial) (total) as the cause of abnormal reaction of the patient, or of later complication, without mention of misadventure at the time of the procedure

Y83.8 Other surgical procedures as the cause of abnormal reaction of the patient, or of later complication, without mention of misadventure at the time of the procedure

Y83.9 Surgical procedure, unspecified as the cause of abnormal ▽ reaction of the patient, or of later complication, without mention of misadventure at the time of the procedure

✓4ᵗʰ Y84 Other medical procedures as the cause of abnormal reaction of the patient, or of later complication, without mention of misadventure at the time of the procedure

Y84.0 Cardiac catheterization as the cause of abnormal reaction of the patient, or of later complication, without mention of misadventure at the time of the procedure

Y84.1 Kidney dialysis as the cause of abnormal reaction of the patient, or of later complication, without mention of misadventure at the time of the procedure

Y84.2 Radiological procedure and radiotherapy as the cause of abnormal reaction of the patient, or of later complication, without mention of misadventure at the time of the procedure
AHA: 2017, 1Q, 33

Y84.3 Shock therapy as the cause of abnormal reaction of the patient, or of later complication, without mention of misadventure at the time of the procedure

Y84.4 Aspiration of fluid as the cause of abnormal reaction of the patient, or of later complication, without mention of misadventure at the time of the procedure

Y84.5 Insertion of gastric or duodenal sound as the cause of abnormal reaction of the patient, or of later complication, without mention of misadventure at the time of the procedure

Y84.6 Urinary catheterization as the cause of abnormal reaction of the patient, or of later complication, without mention of misadventure at the time of the procedure

Y84.7 Blood-sampling as the cause of abnormal reaction of the patient, or of later complication, without mention of misadventure at the time of the procedure

Y84.8 Other medical procedures as the cause of abnormal reaction of the patient, or of later complication, without mention of misadventure at the time of the procedure
AHA: 2014, 4Q, 24

Y84.9 Medical procedure, unspecified as the cause of abnormal ▽ reaction of the patient, or of later complication, without mention of misadventure at the time of the procedure

Supplementary factors related to causes of morbidity classified elsewhere (Y90-Y99)

NOTE These categories may be used to provide supplementary information concerning causes of morbidity. They are not to be used for single-condition coding.

✓4ᵗʰ Y90 Evidence of alcohol involvement determined by blood alcohol level

Code first any associated alcohol related disorders (F10)

Y90.0 Blood alcohol level of less than 20 mg/100 ml

Y90.1 Blood alcohol level of 20-39 mg/100 ml

Y90.2 Blood alcohol level of 40-59 mg/100 ml

Y90.3 Blood alcohol level of 60-79 mg/100 ml

Y90.4 Blood alcohol level of 80-99 mg/100 ml

Y90.5 Blood alcohol level of 100-119 mg/100 ml

Y90.6 Blood alcohol level of 120-199 mg/100 ml

Y90.7 Blood alcohol level of 200-239 mg/100 ml

Y90.8 Blood alcohol level of 240 mg/100 ml or more

Y90.9 Presence of alcohol in blood, level not specified ▽

✓4ᵗʰ Y92 Place of occurrence of the external cause

The following category is for use, when relevant, to identify the place of occurrence of the external cause. Use in conjunction with an activity code.

Place of occurrence should be recorded only at the initial encounter for treatment

✓5ᵗʰ Y92.0 Non-institutional (private) residence as the place of occurrence of the external cause

EXCLUDES 1 abandoned or derelict house (Y92.89)
home under construction but not yet occupied (Y92.6-)
institutional place of residence (Y92.1-)

✓6ᵗʰ Y92.00 Unspecified non-institutional (private) residence as the place of occurrence of the external cause

Y92.000 Kitchen of unspecified non-institutional ▽ (private) residence as the place of occurrence of the external cause

Y92.001 Dining room of unspecified ▽ non-institutional (private) residence as the place of occurrence of the external cause

✓ Additional Character Req   ✓7ᵗʰ Placeholder Alert   **Manifestation**   ᴴᶜᶜ CMS-HCC Condition   ▽ Unspecified Code   ▶◀ Revised Text   ● New Code   ▲ Revised Code Title

ICD-10-CM 2018   1167

Y92.002 Bathroom of unspecified non-institutional (private) residence single-family (private) house as the place of occurrence of the external cause ▽

Y92.003 Bedroom of unspecified non-institutional (private) residence as the place of occurrence of the external cause ▽

Y92.007 Garden or yard of unspecified non-institutional (private) residence as the place of occurrence of the external cause ▽

Y92.008 Other place in unspecified non-institutional (private) residence as the place of occurrence of the external cause ▽

Y92.009 Unspecified place in unspecified non-institutional (private) residence as the place of occurrence of the external cause ▽
> Home (NOS) as the place of occurrence of the external cause

✓6ᵗʰ **Y92.01** Single-family non-institutional (private) house as the place of occurrence of the external cause
> Farmhouse as the place of occurrence of the external cause
> > EXCLUDES 1   *barn (Y92.71)*
> > *chicken coop or hen house (Y92.72)*
> > *farm field (Y92.73)*
> > *orchard (Y92.74)*
> > *single family mobile home or trailer (Y92.02-)*
> > *slaughter house (Y92.86)*

Y92.010 Kitchen of single-family (private) house as the place of occurrence of the external cause

Y92.011 Dining room of single-family (private) house as the place of occurrence of the external cause

Y92.012 Bathroom of single-family (private) house as the place of occurrence of the external cause

Y92.013 Bedroom of single-family (private) house as the place of occurrence of the external cause

Y92.014 Private driveway to single-family (private) house as the place of occurrence of the external cause

Y92.015 Private garage of single-family (private) house as the place of occurrence of the external cause

Y92.016 Swimming-pool in single-family (private) house or garden as the place of occurrence of the external cause

Y92.017 Garden or yard in single-family (private) house as the place of occurrence of the external cause

Y92.018 Other place in single-family (private) house as the place of occurrence of the external cause

Y92.019 Unspecified place in single-family (private) house as the place of occurrence of the external cause ▽

✓6ᵗʰ **Y92.02** Mobile home as the place of occurrence of the external cause

Y92.020 Kitchen in mobile home as the place of occurrence of the external cause

Y92.021 Dining room in mobile home as the place of occurrence of the external cause

Y92.022 Bathroom in mobile home as the place of occurrence of the external cause

Y92.023 Bedroom in mobile home as the place of occurrence of the external cause

Y92.024 Driveway of mobile home as the place of occurrence of the external cause

Y92.025 Garage of mobile home as the place of occurrence of the external cause

Y92.026 Swimming-pool of mobile home as the place of occurrence of the external cause

Y92.027 Garden or yard of mobile home as the place of occurrence of the external cause

Y92.028 Other place in mobile home as the place of occurrence of the external cause

Y92.029 Unspecified place in mobile home as the place of occurrence of the external cause ▽

✓6ᵗʰ **Y92.03** Apartment as the place of occurrence of the external cause
> Condominium as the place of occurrence of the external cause
> Co-op apartment as the place of occurrence of the external cause

Y92.030 Kitchen in apartment as the place of occurrence of the external cause

Y92.031 Bathroom in apartment as the place of occurrence of the external cause

Y92.032 Bedroom in apartment as the place of occurrence of the external cause

Y92.038 Other place in apartment as the place of occurrence of the external cause

Y92.039 Unspecified place in apartment as the place of occurrence of the external cause ▽

✓6ᵗʰ **Y92.04** Boarding-house as the place of occurrence of the external cause

Y92.040 Kitchen in boarding-house as the place of occurrence of the external cause

Y92.041 Bathroom in boarding-house as the place of occurrence of the external cause

Y92.042 Bedroom in boarding-house as the place of occurrence of the external cause

Y92.043 Driveway of boarding-house as the place of occurrence of the external cause

Y92.044 Garage of boarding-house as the place of occurrence of the external cause

Y92.045 Swimming-pool of boarding-house as the place of occurrence of the external cause

Y92.046 Garden or yard of boarding-house as the place of occurrence of the external cause

Y92.048 Other place in boarding-house as the place of occurrence of the external cause

Y92.049 Unspecified place in boarding-house as the place of occurrence of the external cause ▽

✓6ᵗʰ **Y92.09** Other non-institutional residence as the place of occurrence of the external cause
> AHA: 2017, 2Q, 10

Y92.090 Kitchen in other non-institutional residence as the place of occurrence of the external cause

Y92.091 Bathroom in other non-institutional residence as the place of occurrence of the external cause

Y92.092 Bedroom in other non-institutional residence as the place of occurrence of the external cause

Y92.093 Driveway of other non-institutional residence as the place of occurrence of the external cause

Y92.094 Garage of other non-institutional residence as the place of occurrence of the external cause

Y92.095 Swimming-pool of other non-institutional residence as the place of occurrence of the external cause

Y92.096 Garden or yard of other non-institutional residence as the place of occurrence of the external cause

Y92.098 Other place in other non-institutional residence as the place of occurrence of the external cause

Y92.099 Unspecified place in other non-institutional residence as the place of occurrence of the external cause ▽

✓5ᵗʰ **Y92.1** Institutional (nonprivate) residence as the place of occurrence of the external cause

Y92.10 Unspecified residential institution as the place of occurrence of the external cause ▽

✓6ᵗʰ **Y92.11** Children's home and orphanage as the place of occurrence of the external cause

Y92.110 Kitchen in children's home and orphanage as the place of occurrence of the external cause

Y92.111 Bathroom in children's home and orphanage as the place of occurrence of the external cause

Y92.112 **Bedroom** in children's home and orphanage as the place of occurrence of the external cause

Y92.113 **Driveway** of children's home and orphanage as the place of occurrence of the external cause

Y92.114 **Garage** of children's home and orphanage as the place of occurrence of the external cause

Y92.115 **Swimming-pool** of children's home and orphanage as the place of occurrence of the external cause

Y92.116 **Garden or yard** of children's home and orphanage as the place of occurrence of the external cause

Y92.118 **Other place** in children's home and orphanage as the place of occurrence of the external cause

Y92.119 **Unspecified place** in children's home ▽ and orphanage as the place of occurrence of the external cause

✓6ᵗʰ **Y92.12** **Nursing home** as the place of occurrence of the external cause
Home for the sick as the place of occurrence of the external cause
Hospice as the place of occurrence of the external cause
AHA: 2017, 2Q, 10

Y92.120 **Kitchen** in nursing home as the place of occurrence of the external cause

Y92.121 **Bathroom** in nursing home as the place of occurrence of the external cause

Y92.122 **Bedroom** in nursing home as the place of occurrence of the external cause

Y92.123 **Driveway** of nursing home as the place of occurrence of the external cause

Y92.124 **Garage** of nursing home as the place of occurrence of the external cause

Y92.125 **Swimming-pool** of nursing home as the place of occurrence of the external cause

Y92.126 **Garden or yard** of nursing home as the place of occurrence of the external cause

Y92.128 **Other place** in nursing home as the place of occurrence of the external cause

Y92.129 **Unspecified place** in nursing home as ▽ the place of occurrence of the external cause

✓6ᵗʰ **Y92.13** **Military base** as the place of occurrence of the external cause
EXCLUDES 1 military training grounds (Y92.83)

Y92.130 **Kitchen** on military base as the place of occurrence of the external cause

Y92.131 **Mess hall** on military base as the place of occurrence of the external cause

Y92.133 **Barracks** on military base as the place of occurrence of the external cause

Y92.135 **Garage** on military base as the place of occurrence of the external cause

Y92.136 **Swimming-pool** on military base as the place of occurrence of the external cause

Y92.137 **Garden or yard** on military base as the place of occurrence of the external cause

Y92.138 **Other place** on military base as the place of occurrence of the external cause

Y92.139 **Unspecified place** military base as the ▽ place of occurrence of the external cause

✓6ᵗʰ **Y92.14** **Prison** as the place of occurrence of the external cause

Y92.140 **Kitchen** in prison as the place of occurrence of the external cause

Y92.141 **Dining room** in prison as the place of occurrence of the external cause

Y92.142 **Bathroom** in prison as the place of occurrence of the external cause

Y92.143 **Cell** of prison as the place of occurrence of the external cause

Y92.146 **Swimming-pool** of prison as the place of occurrence of the external cause

Y92.147 **Courtyard** of prison as the place of occurrence of the external cause

Y92.148 **Other place** in prison as the place of occurrence of the external cause

Y92.149 **Unspecified place** in prison as the ▽ place of occurrence of the external cause

✓6ᵗʰ **Y92.15** **Reform school** as the place of occurrence of the external cause

Y92.150 **Kitchen** in reform school as the place of occurrence of the external cause

Y92.151 **Dining room** in reform school as the place of occurrence of the external cause

Y92.152 **Bathroom** in reform school as the place of occurrence of the external cause

Y92.153 **Bedroom** in reform school as the place of occurrence of the external cause

Y92.154 **Driveway** of reform school as the place of occurrence of the external cause

Y92.155 **Garage** of reform school as the place of occurrence of the external cause

Y92.156 **Swimming-pool** of reform school as the place of occurrence of the external cause

Y92.157 **Garden or yard** of reform school as the place of occurrence of the external cause

Y92.158 **Other place** in reform school as the place of occurrence of the external cause

Y92.159 **Unspecified place** in reform school as ▽ the place of occurrence of the external cause

✓6ᵗʰ **Y92.16** **School dormitory** as the place of occurrence of the external cause
EXCLUDES 1 reform school as the place of occurrence of the external cause (Y92.15-)
school buildings and grounds as the place of occurrence of the external cause (Y92.2-)
school sports and athletic areas as the place of occurrence of the external cause (Y92.3-)

Y92.160 **Kitchen** in school dormitory as the place of occurrence of the external cause

Y92.161 **Dining room** in school dormitory as the place of occurrence of the external cause

Y92.162 **Bathroom** in school dormitory as the place of occurrence of the external cause

Y92.163 **Bedroom** in school dormitory as the place of occurrence of the external cause

Y92.168 **Other place** in school dormitory as the place of occurrence of the external cause

Y92.169 **Unspecified place** in school dormitory ▽ as the place of occurrence of the external cause

✓6ᵗʰ **Y92.19** **Other specified residential institution** as the place of occurrence of the external cause
AHA: 2017, 2Q, 10

Y92.190 **Kitchen** in other specified residential institution as the place of occurrence of the external cause

Y92.191 **Dining room** in other specified residential institution as the place of occurrence of the external cause

Y92.192 **Bathroom** in other specified residential institution as the place of occurrence of the external cause

Y92.193 **Bedroom** in other specified residential institution as the place of occurrence of the external cause

Y92.194 **Driveway** of other specified residential institution as the place of occurrence of the external cause

Y92.195 **Garage** of other specified residential institution as the place of occurrence of the external cause

Y92.196 **Pool** of other specified residential institution as the place of occurrence of the external cause

Y92.197 **Garden or yard** of other specified residential institution as the place of occurrence of the external cause

Y92.198 **Other place** in other specified residential institution as the place of occurrence of the external cause

Chapter 20. External Causes of Morbidity

Y92.199   **Unspecified place in other specified residential institution as the place of occurrence of the external cause** ▽

✓5ᵗʰ **Y92.2**   **School, other institution and public administrative area as the place of occurrence of the external cause**
Building and adjacent grounds used by the general public or by a particular group of the public
EXCLUDES 1   *building under construction as the place of occurrence of the external cause (Y92.6)*
residential institution as the place of occurrence of the external cause (Y92.1)
school dormitory as the place of occurrence of the external cause (Y92.16-)
sports and athletics area of schools as the place of occurrence of the external cause (Y92.3-)

✓6ᵗʰ **Y92.21**   **School (private) (public) (state) as the place of occurrence of the external cause**

Y92.210   **Daycare center as the place of occurrence of the external cause**

Y92.211   **Elementary school as the place of occurrence of the external cause**
Kindergarten as the place of occurrence of the external cause

Y92.212   **Middle school as the place of occurrence of the external cause**

Y92.213   **High school as the place of occurrence of the external cause**
AHA: 2012, 4Q, 108

Y92.214   **College as the place of occurrence of the external cause**
University as the place of occurrence of the external cause

Y92.215   **Trade school as the place of occurrence of the external cause**

Y92.218   **Other school as the place of occurrence of the external cause**

Y92.219   **Unspecified school as the place of occurrence of the external cause** ▽

Y92.22   **Religious institution as the place of occurrence of the external cause**
Church as the place of occurrence of the external cause
Mosque as the place of occurrence of the external cause
Synagogue as the place of occurrence of the external cause

✓6ᵗʰ **Y92.23**   **Hospital as the place of occurrence of the external cause**
EXCLUDES 1   *ambulatory (outpatient) health services establishments (Y92.53-)*
home for the sick as the place of occurrence of the external cause (Y92.12-)
hospice as the place of occurrence of the external cause (Y92.12-)
nursing home as the place of occurrence of the external cause (Y92.12-)

Y92.230   **Patient room in hospital as the place of occurrence of the external cause**

Y92.231   **Patient bathroom in hospital as the place of occurrence of the external cause**

Y92.232   **Corridor of hospital as the place of occurrence of the external cause**

Y92.233   **Cafeteria of hospital as the place of occurrence of the external cause**

Y92.234   **Operating room of hospital as the place of occurrence of the external cause**

Y92.238   **Other place in hospital as the place of occurrence of the external cause**

Y92.239   **Unspecified place in hospital as the place of occurrence of the external cause** ▽

✓6ᵗʰ **Y92.24**   **Public administrative building as the place of occurrence of the external cause**

Y92.240   **Courthouse as the place of occurrence of the external cause**

Y92.241   **Library as the place of occurrence of the external cause**

Y92.242   **Post office as the place of occurrence of the external cause**

Y92.243   **City hall as the place of occurrence of the external cause**

Y92.248   **Other public administrative building as the place of occurrence of the external cause**

✓6ᵗʰ **Y92.25**   **Cultural building as the place of occurrence of the external cause**

Y92.250   **Art Gallery as the place of occurrence of the external cause**

Y92.251   **Museum as the place of occurrence of the external cause**

Y92.252   **Music hall as the place of occurrence of the external cause**

Y92.253   **Opera house as the place of occurrence of the external cause**

Y92.254   **Theater (live) as the place of occurrence of the external cause**

Y92.258   **Other cultural public building as the place of occurrence of the external cause**

Y92.26   **Movie house or cinema as the place of occurrence of the external cause**

Y92.29   **Other specified public building as the place of occurrence of the external cause**
Assembly hall as the place of occurrence of the external cause
Clubhouse as the place of occurrence of the external cause

✓5ᵗʰ **Y92.3**   **Sports and athletics area as the place of occurrence of the external cause**

✓6ᵗʰ **Y92.31**   **Athletic court as the place of occurrence of the external cause**
EXCLUDES 1   *tennis court in private home or garden (Y92.09)*

Y92.310   **Basketball court as the place of occurrence of the external cause**

Y92.311   **Squash court as the place of occurrence of the external cause**

Y92.312   **Tennis court as the place of occurrence of the external cause**

Y92.318   **Other athletic court as the place of occurrence of the external cause**

✓6ᵗʰ **Y92.32**   **Athletic field as the place of occurrence of the external cause**

Y92.320   **Baseball field as the place of occurrence of the external cause**

Y92.321   **Football field as the place of occurrence of the external cause**

Y92.322   **Soccer field as the place of occurrence of the external cause**

Y92.328   **Other athletic field as the place of occurrence of the external cause**
Cricket field as the place of occurrence of the external cause
Hockey field as the place of occurrence of the external cause

✓6ᵗʰ **Y92.33**   **Skating rink as the place of occurrence of the external cause**

Y92.330   **Ice skating rink (indoor) (outdoor) as the place of occurrence of the external cause**

Y92.331   **Roller skating rink as the place of occurrence of the external cause**

Y92.34   **Swimming pool (public) as the place of occurrence of the external cause**
EXCLUDES 1   *swimming pool in private home or garden (Y92.016)*

Y92.39   **Other specified sports and athletic area as the place of occurrence of the external cause**
Golf-course as the place of occurrence of the external cause
Gymnasium as the place of occurrence of the external cause
Riding-school as the place of occurrence of the external cause
Stadium as the place of occurrence of the external cause

EXCLUDES 1 Not coded here   *EXCLUDES 2* Not included here   N Newborn Age: 0   P Pediatric Age: 0-17   M Maternity Age: 12-55   A Adult Age: 15-124

☑5ᵗʰ **Y92.4** **Street, highway and other paved roadways as the place of occurrence of the external cause**
> EXCLUDES1 *private driveway of residence (Y92.014, Y92.024, Y92.043, Y92.093, Y92.113, Y92.123, Y92.154, Y92.194)*

☑6ᵗʰ **Y92.41** Street and highway **as the place of occurrence of the external cause**

    Y92.410 **Unspecified street and highway as the** ▽ **place of occurrence of the external cause**
        Road NOS as the place of occurrence of the external cause

    Y92.411 Interstate **highway as the place of occurrence of the external cause**
        Freeway as the place of occurrence of the external cause
        Motorway as the place of occurrence of the external cause

    Y92.412 Parkway **as the place of occurrence of the external cause**

    Y92.413 State road **as the place of occurrence of the external cause**

    Y92.414 Local residential or business street **as the place of occurrence of the external cause**

    Y92.415 Exit ramp or entrance ramp **of street or highway as the place of occurrence of the external cause**

☑6ᵗʰ **Y92.48** **Other paved roadways as the place of occurrence of the external cause**

    Y92.480 Sidewalk **as the place of occurrence of the external cause**

    Y92.481 Parking lot **as the place of occurrence of the external cause**

    Y92.482 Bike path **as the place of occurrence of the external cause**

    Y92.488 **Other paved roadways as the place of occurrence of the external cause**

☑5ᵗʰ **Y92.5** Trade and service area **as the place of occurrence of the external cause**
> EXCLUDES1 *garage in private home (Y92.015)*
>   *schools and other public administration buildings (Y92.2-)*

☑6ᵗʰ **Y92.51** Private commercial establishments **as the place of occurrence of the external cause**

    Y92.510 Bank **as the place of occurrence of the external cause**

    Y92.511 Restaurant **or** café **as the place of occurrence of the external cause**

    Y92.512 Supermarket, **store or** market **as the place of occurrence of the external cause**

    Y92.513 Shop **(commercial) as the place of occurrence of the external cause**

☑6ᵗʰ **Y92.52** Service areas **as the place of occurrence of the external cause**

    Y92.520 Airport **as the place of occurrence of the external cause**

    Y92.521 Bus station **as the place of occurrence of the external cause**

    Y92.522 Railway station **as the place of occurrence of the external cause**

    Y92.523 Highway rest stop **as the place of occurrence of the external cause**

    Y92.524 Gas station **as the place of occurrence of the external cause**
        Petroleum station as the place of occurrence of the external cause
        Service station as the place of occurrence of the external cause

☑6ᵗʰ **Y92.53** Ambulatory health services establishments **as the place of occurrence of the external cause**

    Y92.530 Ambulatory surgery center **as the place of occurrence of the external cause**
        Outpatient surgery center, including that connected with a hospital as the place of occurrence of the external cause
        Same day surgery center, including that connected with a hospital as the place of occurrence of the external cause

    Y92.531 Health care provider office **as the place of occurrence of the external cause**
        Physician office as the place of occurrence of the external cause

    Y92.532 Urgent care center **as the place of occurrence of the external cause**

    Y92.538 **Other ambulatory health services establishments as the place of occurrence of the external cause**

Y92.59 **Other trade areas as the place of occurrence of the external cause**
    Office building as the place of occurrence of the external cause
    Casino as the place of occurrence of the external cause
    Garage (commercial) as the place of occurrence of the external cause
    Hotel as the place of occurrence of the external cause
    Radio or television station as the place of occurrence of the external cause
    Shopping mall as the place of occurrence of the external cause
    Warehouse as the place of occurrence of the external cause

☑5ᵗʰ **Y92.6** Industrial and construction area **as the place of occurrence of the external cause**

    Y92.61 Building [any] under construction **as the place of occurrence of the external cause**

    Y92.62 Dock or shipyard **as the place of occurrence of the external cause**
        Dockyard as the place of occurrence of the external cause
        Dry dock as the place of occurrence of the external cause
        Shipyard as the place of occurrence of the external cause

    Y92.63 Factory **as the place of occurrence of the external cause**
        Factory building as the place of occurrence of the external cause
        Factory premises as the place of occurrence of the external cause
        Industrial yard as the place of occurrence of the external cause

    Y92.64 Mine or pit **as the place of occurrence of the external cause**
        Mine as the place of occurrence of the external cause

    Y92.65 Oil rig **as the place of occurrence of the external cause**
        Pit (coal) (gravel) (sand) as the place of occurrence of the external cause

    Y92.69 **Other specified industrial and construction area as the place of occurrence of the external cause**
        Gasworks as the place of occurrence of the external cause
        Power-station (coal) (nuclear) (oil) as the place of occurrence of the external cause
        Tunnel under construction as the place of occurrence of the external cause
        Workshop as the place of occurrence of the external cause

☑5ᵗʰ **Y92.7** Farm **as the place of occurrence of the external cause**
    Ranch as the place of occurrence of the external cause
> EXCLUDES1 *farmhouse and home premises of farm (Y92.01-)*

    Y92.71 Barn **as the place of occurrence of the external cause**

    Y92.72 Chicken coop **as the place of occurrence of the external cause**
        Hen house as the place of occurrence of the external cause

    Y92.73 Farm field **as the place of occurrence of the external cause**

    Y92.74 Orchard **as the place of occurrence of the external cause**

    Y92.79 **Other farm location as the place of occurrence of the external cause**

☑5ᵗʰ **Y92.8** **Other places as the place of occurrence of the external cause**

☑6ᵗʰ **Y92.81** Transport vehicle **as the place of occurrence of the external cause**
> EXCLUDES1 *transport accidents (V00-V99)*

    Y92.810 Car **as the place of occurrence of the external cause**

☑ Additional Character Req   ☑x7ᵗʰ Placeholder Alert   Manifestation   HCC CMS-HCC Condition   ▽ Unspecified Code   ▶◀ Revised Text   ● New Code   ▲ Revised Code Title

Y92.811   Bus **as the place of occurrence of the external cause**

Y92.812   Truck **as the place of occurrence of the external cause**

Y92.813   Airplane **as the place of occurrence of the external cause**

Y92.814   Boat **as the place of occurrence of the external cause**

Y92.815   Train **as the place of occurrence of the external cause**

Y92.816   Subway car **as the place of occurrence of the external cause**

Y92.818   **Other transport vehicle as the place of occurrence of the external cause**

✓6ᵗʰ **Y92.82**   Wilderness area

    Y92.820   Desert **as the place of occurrence of the external cause**

    Y92.821   Forest **as the place of occurrence of the external cause**

    Y92.828   **Other wilderness area as the place of occurrence of the external cause**
        Swamp as the place of occurrence of the external cause
        Mountain as the place of occurrence of the external cause
        Marsh as the place of occurrence of the external cause
        Prairie as the place of occurrence of the external cause

✓6ᵗʰ **Y92.83**   Recreation area **as the place of occurrence of the external cause**

    Y92.830   Public park **as the place of occurrence of the external cause**

    Y92.831   Amusement park **as the place of occurrence of the external cause**

    Y92.832   Beach **as the place of occurrence of the external cause**
        Seashore as the place of occurrence of the external cause

    Y92.833   Campsite **as the place of occurrence of the external cause**

    Y92.834   Zoological garden **(Zoo) as the place of occurrence of the external cause**

    Y92.838   **Other recreation area as the place of occurrence of the external cause**

Y92.84   Military training ground **as the place of occurrence of the external cause**

Y92.85   Railroad track **as the place of occurrence of the external cause**

Y92.86   Slaughter house **as the place of occurrence of the external cause**

Y92.89   **Other specified places as the place of occurrence of the external cause**
    Derelict house as the place of occurrence of the external cause

Y92.9   **Unspecified place or not applicable**   ▽

✓4ᵗʰ **Y93**   **Activity codes**

> **NOTE**   Category Y93 is provided for use to indicate the activity of the person seeking healthcare for an injury or health condition, such as a heart attack while shoveling snow, which resulted from, or was contributed to, by the activity. These codes are appropriate for use for both acute injuries, such as those from chapter 19, and conditions that are due to the long-term, cumulative effects of an activity, such as those from chapter 13. They are also appropriate for use with external cause codes for cause and intent if identifying the activity provides additional information on the event. These codes should be used in conjunction with codes for external cause status (Y99) and place of occurrence (Y92).

This section contains the following broad activity categories:

Y93.0   Activities involving walking and running
Y93.1   Activities involving water and water craft
Y93.2   Activities involving ice and snow
Y93.3   Activities involving climbing, rappelling, and jumping off
Y93.4   Activities involving dancing and other rhythmic movement
Y93.5   Activities involving other sports and athletics played individually
Y93.6   Activities involving other sports and athletics played as a team or group
Y93.7   Activities involving other specified sports and athletics
Y93.A   Activities involving other cardiorespiratory exercise
Y93.B   Activities involving other muscle strengthening exercises
Y93.C   Activities involving computer technology and electronic devices
Y93.D   Activities involving arts and handcrafts
Y93.E   Activities involving personal hygiene and interior property and clothing maintenance
Y93.F   Activities involving caregiving
Y93.G   Activities involving food preparation, cooking and grilling
Y93.H   Activities involving exterior property and land maintenance, building and construction
Y93.I   Activities involving roller coasters and other types of external motion
Y93.J   Activities involving playing musical instrument
Y93.K   Activities involving animal care
Y93.8   Activities, other specified
Y93.9   Activity, unspecified

✓5ᵗʰ **Y93.0**   **Activities involving walking and running**

> **EXCLUDES 1**   activity, walking an animal (Y93.K1)
>   activity, walking or running on a treadmill (Y93.A1)

    Y93.01   **Activity,** walking, marching and hiking
        Activity, walking, marching and hiking on level or elevated terrain
>   **EXCLUDES 1**   activity, mountain climbing (Y93.31)

    Y93.02   **Activity,** running

✓5ᵗʰ **Y93.1**   **Activities involving water and water craft**

> **EXCLUDES 1**   activities involving ice (Y93.2-)

    Y93.11   **Activity,** swimming

    Y93.12   **Activity,** springboard and platform diving

    Y93.13   **Activity,** water polo

    Y93.14   **Activity,** water aerobics and water exercise

    Y93.15   **Activity,** underwater diving and snorkeling
        Activity, SCUBA diving

    Y93.16   **Activity,** rowing, canoeing, kayaking, rafting and tubing
        Activity, canoeing, kayaking, rafting and tubing in calm and turbulent water

    Y93.17   **Activity,** water skiing **and** wake boarding

    Y93.18   **Activity,** surfing, windsurfing **and** boogie boarding
        Activity, water sliding

    Y93.19   **Activity, other involving water and watercraft**
        Activity involving water NOS
        Activity, parasailing
        Activity, water survival training and testing

✓5ᵗʰ **Y93.2**   **Activities involving ice and snow**

> **EXCLUDES 1**   activity, shoveling ice and snow (Y93.H1)

    Y93.21   **Activity,** ice skating
        Activity, figure skating (singles) (pairs)
        Activity, ice dancing
>   **EXCLUDES 1**   activity, ice hockey (Y93.22)

    Y93.22   **Activity,** ice hockey

    Y93.23   **Activity,** snow **(alpine) (downhill)** skiing, snow boarding, sledding, tobogganing **and** snow tubing
>   **EXCLUDES 1**   activity, cross country skiing (Y93.24)

    Y93.24   **Activity,** cross country skiing
        Activity, nordic skiing

EXCLUDES 1 Not coded here   **EXCLUDES 2** Not included here   N Newborn Age: 0   P Pediatric Age: 0-17   M Maternity Age: 12-55   A Adult Age: 15-124

1172   ICD-10-CM 2018

Y93.29   **Activity, other involving ice and snow**
     Activity involving ice and snow NOS

✓5ᵗʰ **Y93.3**   **Activities involving climbing, rappelling and jumping off**
     EXCLUDES 1   *activity, hiking on level or elevated terrain (Y93.01)*
           activity, jumping rope (Y93.56)
           activity, trampoline jumping (Y93.44)

Y93.31   **Activity, mountain climbing, rock climbing and wall climbing**

Y93.32   **Activity, rappelling**

Y93.33   **Activity, BASE jumping**
     Activity, Building, Antenna, Span, Earth jumping

Y93.34   **Activity, bungee jumping**

Y93.35   **Activity, hang gliding**

Y93.39   **Activity, other involving climbing, rappelling and jumping off**

✓5ᵗʰ **Y93.4**   **Activities involving dancing and other rhythmic movement**
     EXCLUDES 1   *activity, martial arts (Y93.75)*

Y93.41   **Activity, dancing**
     AHA: 2012, 4Q, 108

Y93.42   **Activity, yoga**

Y93.43   **Activity, gymnastics**
     Activity, rhythmic gymnastics
     EXCLUDES 1   *activity, trampolining (Y93.44)*

Y93.44   **Activity, trampolining**

Y93.45   **Activity, cheerleading**

Y93.49   **Activity, other involving dancing and other rhythmic movements**

✓5ᵗʰ **Y93.5**   **Activities involving other sports and athletics played individually**
     EXCLUDES 1   *activity, dancing (Y93.41)*
           activity, gymnastic (Y93.43)
           activity, trampolining (Y93.44)
           activity, yoga (Y93.42)

Y93.51   **Activity, roller skating (inline) and skateboarding**

Y93.52   **Activity, horseback riding**

Y93.53   **Activity, golf**

Y93.54   **Activity, bowling**

Y93.55   **Activity, bike riding**

Y93.56   **Activity, jumping rope**

Y93.57   **Activity, non-running track and field events**
     EXCLUDES 1   *activity, running (any form) (Y93.02)*

Y93.59   **Activity, other involving other sports and athletics played individually**
     EXCLUDES 1   *activities involving climbing, rappelling, and jumping (Y93.3-)*
           activities involving ice and snow (Y93.2-)
           activities involving walking and running (Y93.0-)
           activities involving water and watercraft (Y93.1-)

✓5ᵗʰ **Y93.6**   **Activities involving other sports and athletics played as a team or group**
     EXCLUDES 1   *activity, ice hockey (Y93.22)*
           activity, water polo (Y93.13)

Y93.61   **Activity, American tackle football**
     Activity, football NOS

Y93.62   **Activity, American flag or touch football**

Y93.63   **Activity, rugby**

Y93.64   **Activity, baseball**
     Activity, softball

Y93.65   **Activity, lacrosse and field hockey**

Y93.66   **Activity, soccer**

Y93.67   **Activity, basketball**

Y93.68   **Activity, volleyball (beach) (court)**

Y93.6A   **Activity, physical games generally associated with school recess, summer camp and children**
     Activity, capture the flag
     Activity, dodge ball
     Activity, four square
     Activity, kickball

Y93.69   **Activity, other involving other sports and athletics played as a team or group**
     Activity, cricket

✓5ᵗʰ **Y93.7**   **Activities involving other specified sports and athletics**

Y93.71   **Activity, boxing**

Y93.72   **Activity, wrestling**

Y93.73   **Activity, racquet and hand sports**
     Activity, handball
     Activity, racquetball
     Activity, squash
     Activity, tennis

Y93.74   **Activity, frisbee**
     Activity, ultimate frisbee

Y93.75   **Activity, martial arts**
     Activity, combatives

Y93.79   **Activity, other specified sports and athletics**
     EXCLUDES 1   *sports and athletics activities specified in categories Y93.0-Y93.6*

✓5ᵗʰ **Y93.A**   **Activities involving other cardiorespiratory exercise**
     Activities involving physical training

Y93.A1   **Activity, exercise machines primarily for cardiorespiratory conditioning**
     Activity, elliptical and stepper machines
     Activity, stationary bike
     Activity, treadmill

Y93.A2   **Activity, calisthenics**
     Activity, jumping jacks
     Activity, warm up and cool down

Y93.A3   **Activity, aerobic and step exercise**

Y93.A4   **Activity, circuit training**

Y93.A5   **Activity, obstacle course**
     Activity, challenge course
     Activity, confidence course

Y93.A6   **Activity, grass drills**
     Activity, guerilla drills

Y93.A9   **Activity, other involving cardiorespiratory exercise**
     EXCLUDES 1   *activities involving cardiorespiratory exercise specified in categories Y93.0-Y93.7*

✓5ᵗʰ **Y93.B**   **Activities involving other muscle strengthening exercises**

Y93.B1   **Activity, exercise machines primarily for muscle strengthening**

Y93.B2   **Activity, push-ups, pull-ups, sit-ups**

Y93.B3   **Activity, free weights**
     Activity, barbells
     Activity, dumbbells

Y93.B4   **Activity, pilates**

Y93.B9   **Activity, other involving muscle strengthening exercises**
     EXCLUDES 1   *activities involving muscle strengthening specified in categories Y93.0-Y93.A*

✓5ᵗʰ **Y93.C**   **Activities involving computer technology and electronic devices**
     EXCLUDES 1   *activity, electronic musical keyboard or instruments (Y93.J-)*

Y93.C1   **Activity, computer keyboarding**
     Activity, electronic game playing using keyboard or other stationary device

Y93.C2   **Activity, hand held interactive electronic device**
     Activity, cellular telephone and communication device
     Activity, electronic game playing using interactive device
     EXCLUDES 1   *activity, electronic game playing using keyboard or other stationary device (Y93.C1)*

Y93.C9   **Activity, other involving computer technology and electronic devices**

✓5ᵗʰ **Y93.D**   **Activities involving arts and handcrafts**
     EXCLUDES 1   *activities involving playing musical instrument (Y93.J-)*

Y93.D1   **Activity, knitting and crocheting**

Y93.D2   **Activity, sewing**

Y93.D3   **Activity, furniture building and finishing**
     Activity, furniture repair

Y93.D9   **Activity, other involving arts and handcrafts**

✓5ᵗʰ **Y93.E**   **Activities involving personal hygiene and interior property and clothing maintenance**
     EXCLUDES 1   *activities involving cooking and grilling (Y93.G-)*
           activities involving exterior property and land maintenance, building and construction (Y93.H-)
           activities involving caregiving (Y93.F-)
           activity, dishwashing (Y93.G1)
           activity, food preparation (Y93.G1)
           activity, gardening (Y93.H2)

Y93.E1   **Activity, personal bathing and showering**

Y93.E2   **Activity, laundry**

✓ Additional Character Req   ✗7ᵗʰ Placeholder Alert   Manifestation   HCC CMS-HCC Condition   ▽ Unspecified Code   ▶◀ Revised Text   ● New Code   ▲ Revised Code Title

Y93.E3   **Activity,** vacuuming

Y93.E4   **Activity,** ironing

Y93.E5   **Activity,** floor mopping and cleaning

Y93.E6   **Activity,** residential relocation
Activity, packing up and unpacking involved in moving to a new residence

Y93.E8   **Activity, other personal hygiene**

Y93.E9   **Activity, other interior property and clothing maintenance**

✓5ᵗʰ **Y93.F**   **Activities involving** caregiving
Activity involving the provider of caregiving

Y93.F1   **Activity, caregiving,** bathing

Y93.F2   **Activity, caregiving,** lifting

Y93.F9   **Activity, other caregiving**

✓5ᵗʰ **Y93.G**   **Activities involving food preparation, cooking and grilling**

Y93.G1   **Activity,** food preparation and clean up
Activity, dishwashing

Y93.G2   **Activity,** grilling and smoking food

Y93.G3   **Activity,** cooking and baking
Activity, use of stove, oven and microwave oven

Y93.G9   **Activity, other involving cooking and grilling**

✓5ᵗʰ **Y93.H**   **Activities involving exterior property and land maintenance, building and construction**

Y93.H1   **Activity,** digging, shoveling and raking
Activity, dirt digging
Activity, raking leaves
Activity, snow shoveling

Y93.H2   **Activity,** gardening and landscaping
Activity, pruning, trimming shrubs, weeding

Y93.H3   **Activity,** building and construction

Y93.H9   **Activity, other involving exterior property and land maintenance, building and construction**

✓5ᵗʰ **Y93.I**   **Activities involving roller coasters and other types of external motion**

Y93.I1   **Activity,** rollercoaster riding

Y93.I9   **Activity, other involving external motion**

✓5ᵗʰ **Y93.J**   **Activities involving playing musical instrument**
Activity involving playing electric musical instrument

Y93.J1   **Activity,** piano **playing**
Activity, musical keyboard (electronic) playing

Y93.J2   **Activity,** drum and other percussion instrument **playing**

Y93.J3   **Activity,** string instrument **playing**

Y93.J4   **Activity,** winds and brass instrument **playing**

✓5ᵗʰ **Y93.K**   **Activities involving animal care**
EXCLUDES 1   *activity, horseback riding (Y93.52)*

Y93.K1   **Activity,** walking **an animal**

Y93.K2   **Activity,** milking **an animal**

Y93.K3   **Activity,** grooming and shearing **an animal**

Y93.K9   **Activity, other involving animal care**

✓5ᵗʰ **Y93.8**   **Activities, other specified**

Y93.81   **Activity,** refereeing **a sports activity**

Y93.82   **Activity,** spectator **at an event**

Y93.83   **Activity,** rough housing and horseplay

Y93.84   **Activity,** sleeping

Y93.85   **Activity,** choking game
Activity, blackout game
Activity, fainting game
Activity, pass out game

Y93.89   **Activity, other specified**

Y93.9   **Activity, unspecified**   ▽

Y95   **Nosocomial condition**
    AHA: 2013, 4Q, 119

✓4ᵗʰ **Y99**   **External cause status**
    NOTE   A single code from category Y99 should be used in conjunction with the external cause code(s) assigned to a record to indicate the status of the person at the time the event occurred.

Y99.0   **Civilian** activity done for income or pay
Civilian activity done for financial or other compensation
EXCLUDES 1   *military activity (Y99.1)*
        volunteer activity (Y99.2)

Y99.1   Military **activity**
EXCLUDES 1   *activity of off duty military personnel (Y99.8)*

Y99.2   Volunteer **activity**
EXCLUDES 1   *activity of child or other family member assisting in compensated work of other family member (Y99.8)*

Y99.8   **Other external cause status**
Activity NEC
Activity of child or other family member assisting in compensated work of other family member
Hobby not done for income
Leisure activity
Off-duty activity of military personnel
Recreation or sport not for income or while a student
Student activity
EXCLUDES 1   *civilian activity done for income or compensation (Y99.0)*
        military activity (Y99.1)
    AHA: 2012, 4Q, 108

Y99.9   **Unspecified external cause status**   ▽

Chapter 21. Factors Influencing Health Status and Contact with Health Services (Z00–Z99)

Chapter Specific Guidelines with Coding Examples

The chapter specific guidelines from the ICD-10-CM Official Guidelines for Coding and Reporting have been provided below. Along with these guidelines are coding examples, contained in the shaded boxes, that have been developed to help illustrate the coding and/or sequencing guidance found in these guidelines.

Note: The chapter specific guidelines provide additional information about the use of Z codes for specified encounters.

a. Use of Z codes in any healthcare setting

Z codes are for use in any healthcare setting. Z codes may be used as either a first-listed (principal diagnosis code in the inpatient setting) or secondary code, depending on the circumstances of the encounter. Certain Z codes may only be used as first-listed or principal diagnosis.

Patient with middle lobe lung cancer presents for initiation of chemotherapy

Z51.11   **Encounter for antineoplastic chemotherapy**

C34.2   **Malignant neoplasm of middle lobe, bronchus or lung**

Explanation: A Z code can be used as first-listed in this situation based on guidelines in this chapter as well as chapter 2, "Neoplasms."

Patient has chronic lymphocytic leukemia for which the patient had previous chemotherapy and is now in remission

C91.11   **Chronic lymphocytic leukemia of B-cell type in remission**

Z92.21   **Personal history of antineoplastic chemotherapy**

Explanation: The personal history Z code is used to describe a secondary (supplementary) diagnosis to identify that this patient has had chemotherapy in the past.

---

b. Z codes indicate a reason for an encounter

Z codes are not procedure codes. A corresponding procedure code must accompany a Z code to describe any procedure performed.

c. Categories of Z codes

1) Contact/exposure

Category Z20 indicates contact with, and suspected exposure to, communicable diseases. These codes are for patients who do not show any sign or symptom of a disease but are suspected to have been exposed to it by close personal contact with an infected individual or are in an area where a disease is epidemic.

Category Z77, Other contact with and (suspected) exposures hazardous to health, indicates contact with and suspected exposures hazardous to health.

Contact/exposure codes may be used as a first-listed code to explain an encounter for testing, or, more commonly, as a secondary code to identify a potential risk.

2) Inoculations and vaccinations

Code Z23 is for encounters for inoculations and vaccinations. It indicates that a patient is being seen to receive a prophylactic inoculation against a disease. Procedure codes are required to identify the actual administration of the injection and the type(s) of immunizations given. Code Z23 may be used as a secondary code if the inoculation is given as a routine part of preventive health care, such as a well-baby visit.

3) Status

Status codes indicate that a patient is either a carrier of a disease or has the sequelae or residual of a past disease or condition. This includes such things as the presence of prosthetic or mechanical devices resulting from past treatment. A status code is informative, because the status may affect the course of treatment and its outcome. A status code is distinct from a history code. The history code indicates that the patient no longer has the condition.

A status code should not be used with a diagnosis code from one of the body system chapters, if the diagnosis code includes the information provided by the status code. For example, code Z94.1, Heart transplant status, should not be used with a code from subcategory T86.2, Complications of heart transplant. The status code does not provide additional information. The complication code indicates that the patient is a heart transplant patient.

For encounters for weaning from a mechanical ventilator, assign a code from subcategory J96.1, Chronic respiratory failure, followed by code Z99.11, Dependence on respirator [ventilator] status.

The status Z codes/categories are:

Z14   Genetic carrier

Genetic carrier status indicates that a person carries a gene, associated with a particular disease, which may be passed to offspring who may develop that disease. The person does not have the disease and is not at risk of developing the disease.

Z15   Genetic susceptibility to disease

Genetic susceptibility indicates that a person has a gene that increases the risk of that person developing the disease.

Codes from category Z15 should not be used as principal or first-listed codes. If the patient has the condition to which he/she is susceptible, and that condition is the reason for the encounter, the code for the current condition should be sequenced first. If the patient is being seen for follow-up after completed treatment for this condition, and the condition no longer exists, a follow-up should be sequenced first, followed by the appropriate personal history and genetic susceptibility codes. If the purpose of the encounter is genetic counseling associated with procreative management, code Z31.5, Encounter for genetic counseling, should be assigned as the first-listed code, followed by a code from category Z15. Additional codes should be assigned for any applicable family or personal history.

Z16   Resistance to antimicrobial drugs

This code indicates that a patient has a condition that is resistant to antimicrobial drug treatment. Sequence the infection code first.

Z17   Estrogen receptor status

Z18   Retained foreign body fragments

Z19   Hormone sensitivity malignancy status

Z21   Asymptomatic HIV infection status

This code indicates that a patient has tested positive for HIV but has manifested no signs or symptoms of the disease.

Z22   Carrier of infectious disease

Carrier status indicates that a person harbors the specific organisms of a disease without manifest symptoms and is capable of transmitting the infection.

Z28.3   Underimmunization status

Z33.1   Pregnant state, incidental

This code is a secondary code only for use when the pregnancy is in no way complicating the reason for visit. Otherwise, a code from the obstetric chapter is required.

Z66   Do not resuscitate

This code may be used when it is documented by the provider that a patient is on do not resuscitate status at any time during the stay.

Z67   Blood type

Z68   Body mass index (BMI)

As with all other secondary diagnosis codes, the BMI codes should only be assigned when they meet the definition of a reportable diagnosis (see Section III, Reporting Additional Diagnoses).

Z74.01   Bed confinement status

Z76.82   Awaiting organ transplant status

Z78   Other specified health status

Code Z78.1, Physical restraint status, may be used when it is documented by the provider that a patient has been put in restraints during the current encounter. Please note that this code should not be reported when it is documented by the provider that a patient is temporarily restrained during a procedure.

Z79   Long-term (current) drug therapy

Codes from this category indicate a patient's continuous use of a prescribed drug (including such things as aspirin therapy) for the long-term treatment of a condition or for prophylactic use. It is not for use for patients who have addictions for drugs. This subcategory is not for use of medications for detoxification or maintenance programs to prevent withdrawal symptoms in patients with drug dependence (e.g., methadone maintenance for opiate dependence). Assign the appropriate code for the drug dependence instead.

Assign a code from Z79 if the patient is receiving a medication for an extended period as a prophylactic measure (such as for the prevention of deep vein thrombosis) or as treatment of a chronic condition (such as arthritis) or a disease requiring a lengthy course of treatment (such as cancer). Do not assign a code from category Z79 for medication being administered for a brief period of time to treat an acute illness or injury (such as a course of antibiotics to treat acute bronchitis).

Z88	Allergy status to drugs, medicaments and biological substances

Except: Z88.9, Allergy status to unspecified drugs, medicaments and biological substances status

Z89	Acquired absence of limb
Z90	Acquired absence of organs, not elsewhere classified
Z91.0-	Allergy status, other than to drugs and biological substances
Z92.82	Status post administration of tPA (rtPA) in a different facility within the last 24 hours prior to admission to a current facility

Assign code Z92.82, Status post administration of tPA (rtPA) in a different facility within the last 24 hours prior to admission to current facility, as a secondary diagnosis when a patient is received by transfer into a facility and documentation indicates they were administered tissue plasminogen activator (tPA) within the last 24 hours prior to admission to the current facility.

This guideline applies even if the patient is still receiving the tPA at the time they are received into the current facility.

The appropriate code for the condition for which the tPA was administered (such as cerebrovascular disease or myocardial infarction) should be assigned first.

Code Z92.82 is only applicable to the receiving facility record and not to the transferring facility record.

Z93	Artificial opening status
Z94	Transplanted organ and tissue status
Z95	Presence of cardiac and vascular implants and grafts
Z96	Presence of other functional implants
Z97	Presence of other devices
Z98	Other postprocedural states

Assign code Z98.85, Transplanted organ removal status, to indicate that a transplanted organ has been previously removed. This code should not be assigned for the encounter in which the transplanted organ is removed. The complication necessitating removal of the transplant organ should be assigned for that encounter.

See section I.C19. for information on the coding of organ transplant complications.

Z99	Dependence on enabling machines and devices, not elsewhere classified

Note: Categories Z89-Z90 and Z93-Z99 are for use only if there are no complications or malfunctions of the organ or tissue replaced, the amputation site or the equipment on which the patient is dependent.

4) History (of)

There are two types of history Z codes, personal and family. Personal history codes explain a patient's past medical condition that no longer exists and is not receiving any treatment, but that has the potential for recurrence, and therefore may require continued monitoring.

Family history codes are for use when a patient has a family member(s) who has had a particular disease that causes the patient to be at higher risk of also contracting the disease.

Personal history codes may be used in conjunction with follow-up codes and family history codes may be used in conjunction with screening codes to explain the need for a test or procedure. History codes are also acceptable on any medical record regardless of the reason for visit. A history of an illness, even if no longer present, is important information that may alter the type of treatment ordered.

The history Z code categories are:

Z80	Family history of primary malignant neoplasm
Z81	Family history of mental and behavioral disorders
Z82	Family history of certain disabilities and chronic diseases (leading to disablement)
Z83	Family history of other specific disorders
Z84	Family history of other conditions
Z85	Personal history of malignant neoplasm
Z86	Personal history of certain other diseases
Z87	Personal history of other diseases and conditions
Z91.4-	Personal history of psychological trauma, not elsewhere classified
Z91.5	Personal history of self-harm
Z91.8-	Other specified personal risk factors, not elsewhere classified

Exception: Z91.83, Wandering in diseases classified elsewhere

Z92	Personal history of medical treatment

Except: Z92.0, Personal history of contraception

Except: Z92.82, Status post administration of tPA (rtPA) in a different facility within the last 24 hours prior to admission to a current facility

5) Screening

Screening is the testing for disease or disease precursors in seemingly well individuals so that early detection and treatment can be provided for those who test positive for the disease (e.g., screening mammogram).

The testing of a person to rule out or confirm a suspected diagnosis because the patient has some sign or symptom is a diagnostic examination, not a screening. In these cases, the sign or symptom is used to explain the reason for the test.

A screening code may be a first-listed code if the reason for the visit is specifically the screening exam. It may also be used as an additional code if the screening is done during an office visit for other health problems. A screening code is not necessary if the screening is inherent to a routine examination, such as a pap smear done during a routine pelvic examination.

Should a condition be discovered during the screening then the code for the condition may be assigned as an additional diagnosis.

Prostate screening of healthy 50-year-old male patient; PSA noted to be elevated but normal digital rectal exam

Z12.5	**Encounter for screening for malignant neoplasm of prostate**
R97.20	**Elevated prostate specific antigen [PSA]**

Explanation: The patient had no signs or symptoms of any prostate-related illness prior to coming in for the screening. The screening code is appropriately used as the first-listed code to signify that this was for routine screening. The elevated PSA is reported as a secondary diagnosis to reflect that an abnormal lab value was found as a result of the screening procedure(s).

The Z code indicates that a screening exam is planned. A procedure code is required to confirm that the screening was performed.

The screening Z codes/categories:

Z11	Encounter for screening for infectious and parasitic diseases
Z12	Encounter for screening for malignant neoplasms
Z13	Encounter for screening for other diseases and disorders

Except: Z13.9, Encounter for screening, unspecified

Z36	Encounter for antenatal screening for mother

6) Observation

There are three observation Z code categories. They are for use in very limited circumstances when a person is being observed for a suspected condition that is ruled out. The observation codes are not for use if an injury or illness or any signs or symptoms related to the suspected condition are present. In such cases the diagnosis/symptom code is used with the corresponding external cause code.

The observation codes are to be used as principal diagnosis only. The only exception to this is when the principal diagnosis is required to be a code from category Z38, Liveborn infants according to place of birth and type of delivery. Then a code from category Z05, Encounter for observation and evaluation of newborn for suspected diseases and conditions ruled out, is sequenced after the Z38 code. Additional codes may be used in addition to the observation code but only if they are unrelated to the suspected condition being observed.

Codes from subcategory Z03.7, Encounter for suspected maternal and fetal conditions ruled out, may either be used as a first-listed or as an additional code assignment depending on the case. They are for use in very limited circumstances on a maternal record when an encounter is for a suspected maternal or fetal condition that is ruled out during that encounter (for example, a maternal or fetal condition may be suspected due to an abnormal test result). These codes should not be used when the condition is confirmed. In those cases, the confirmed condition should be coded. In addition, these codes are not for use if an illness or any signs or symptoms related to the suspected condition or problem are present. In such cases the diagnosis/symptom code is used.

Additional codes may be used in addition to the code from subcategory Z03.7, but only if they are unrelated to the suspected condition being evaluated.

Codes from subcategory Z03.7 may not be used for encounters for antenatal screening of mother. *See Section I.C.21. Screening.*

For encounters for suspected fetal condition that are inconclusive following testing and evaluation, assign the appropriate code from category O35, O36, O40 or O41.

The observation Z code categories:

Z03   Encounter for medical observation for suspected diseases and conditions ruled out

Z04   Encounter for examination and observation for other reasons
       Except: Z04.9, Encounter for examination and observation for unspecified reason

Z05   Encounter for observation and evaluation of newborn for suspected diseases and conditions ruled out

7) Aftercare

Aftercare visit codes cover situations when the initial treatment of a disease has been performed and the patient requires continued care during the healing or recovery phase, or for the long-term consequences of the disease. The aftercare Z code should not be used if treatment is directed at a current, acute disease. The diagnosis code is to be used in these cases. Exceptions to this rule are codes Z51.0, Encounter for antineoplastic radiation therapy, and codes from subcategory Z51.1, Encounter for antineoplastic chemotherapy and immunotherapy. These codes are to be first-listed, followed by the diagnosis code when a patient's encounter is solely to receive radiation therapy, chemotherapy, or immunotherapy for the treatment of a neoplasm. If the reason for the encounter is more than one type of antineoplastic therapy, code Z51.0 and a code from subcategory Z51.1 may be assigned together, in which case one of these codes would be reported as a secondary diagnosis.

The aftercare Z codes should also not be used for aftercare for injuries. For aftercare of an injury, assign the acute injury code with the appropriate 7th character (for subsequent encounter).

The aftercare codes are generally first-listed to explain the specific reason for the encounter. An aftercare code may be used as an additional code when some type of aftercare is provided in addition to the reason for admission and no diagnosis code is applicable. An example of this would be the closure of a colostomy during an encounter for treatment of another condition.

Aftercare codes should be used in conjunction with other aftercare codes or diagnosis codes to provide better detail on the specifics of an aftercare encounter visit, unless otherwise directed by the classification. Should a patient receive multiple types of antineoplastic therapy during the same encounter, code Z51.0, Encounter for antineoplastic radiation therapy, and codes from subcategory Z51.1, Encounter for antineoplastic chemotherapy and immunotherapy, may be used together on a record. The sequencing of multiple aftercare codes depends on the circumstances of the encounter.

Certain aftercare Z code categories need a secondary diagnosis code to describe the resolving condition or sequelae. For others, the condition is included in the code title.

Additional Z code aftercare category terms include fitting and adjustment, and attention to artificial openings.

Status Z codes may be used with aftercare Z codes to indicate the nature of the aftercare. For example code Z95.1, Presence of aortocoronary bypass graft, may be used with code Z48.812, Encounter for surgical aftercare following surgery on the circulatory system, to indicate the surgery for which the aftercare is being performed. A status code should not be used when the aftercare code indicates the type of status, such as using Z43.0, Encounter for attention to tracheostomy, with Z93.0, Tracheostomy status.

The aftercare Z category/codes:

Z42   Encounter for plastic and reconstructive surgery following medical procedure or healed injury

Z43   Encounter for attention to artificial openings

Z44   Encounter for fitting and adjustment of external prosthetic device

Z45   Encounter for adjustment and management of implanted device

Z46   Encounter for fitting and adjustment of other devices

Z47   Orthopedic aftercare

Z48   Encounter for other postprocedural aftercare

Z49   Encounter for care involving renal dialysis

Z51   Encounter for other aftercare and medical care

8) Follow-up

The follow-up codes are used to explain continuing surveillance following completed treatment of a disease, condition, or injury. They imply that the condition has been fully treated and no longer exists. They should not be confused with aftercare codes, or injury codes with a 7th character for subsequent encounter, that explain ongoing care of a healing condition or its sequelae. Follow-up codes may be used in conjunction with history codes to provide the full picture of the healed condition and its treatment. The follow-up code is sequenced first, followed by the history code.

A follow-up code may be used to explain multiple visits. Should a condition be found to have recurred on the follow-up visit, then the diagnosis code for the condition should be assigned in place of the follow-up code.

The follow-up Z code categories:

Z08   Encounter for follow-up examination after completed treatment for malignant neoplasm

Z09   Encounter for follow-up examination after completed treatment for conditions other than malignant neoplasm

Z39   Encounter for maternal postpartum care and examination

Follow-up for patient several months after completing a regime of IV antibiotics for recurrent pneumonia; lungs are clear and pneumonia is resolved

Z09   Encounter for follow-up examination after completed treatment for conditions other than malignant neoplasm

Z87.01   Personal history of pneumonia (recurrent)

Explanation: Code Z09 identifies the follow-up visit as being unrelated to a malignant neoplasm, and code Z87 describes the condition that has now resolved.

Follow-up for patient several months after completing a regime of IV antibiotics for recurrent pneumonia; pneumonia has recurred, and a new antibiotic regimen has been prescribed

J18.9   Pneumonia, unspecified organism

Explanation: Since the follow-up exam for pneumonia determined that the pneumonia was not resolved or recurred, code Z09 Encounter for follow-up examination after completed treatment for conditions other than malignant neoplasm, no longer applies. Instead the first-listed code describes the pneumonia.

---

9) Donor

Codes in category Z52, Donors of organs and tissues, are used for living individuals who are donating blood or other body tissue. These codes are only for individuals donating for others, not for self-donations. They are not used to identify cadaveric donations.

10) Counseling

Counseling Z codes are used when a patient or family member receives assistance in the aftermath of an illness or injury, or when support is required in coping with family or social problems. They are not used in conjunction with a diagnosis code when the counseling component of care is considered integral to standard treatment.

The counseling Z codes/categories:

Z30.0-   Encounter for general counseling and advice on contraception

Z31.5   Encounter for genetic counseling

Z31.6-   Encounter for general counseling and advice on procreation

Z32.2   Encounter for childbirth instruction

Z32.3   Encounter for childcare instruction

Z69   Encounter for mental health services for victim and perpetrator of abuse

Z70   Counseling related to sexual attitude, behavior and orientation

Z71   Persons encountering health services for other counseling and medical advice, not elsewhere classified

Z76.81   Expectant mother prebirth pediatrician visit

11) Encounters for obstetrical and reproductive services

See Section I.C.15. Pregnancy, Childbirth, and the Puerperium, for further instruction on the use of these codes.

Z codes for pregnancy are for use in those circumstances when none of the problems or complications included in the codes from the Obstetrics chapter exist (a routine prenatal visit or postpartum care). Codes in category Z34, Encounter for supervision of normal pregnancy, are always first-listed and are not to be used with any other code from the OB chapter.

Codes in category Z3A, Weeks of gestation, may be assigned to provide additional information about the pregnancy. Category Z3A codes should not be assigned for pregnancies with abortive outcomes (categories O00-O08), elective termination of pregnancy (code Z33.32), nor for postpartum conditions, as category Z3A is not applicable to these conditions. The date of the admission should be used to determine weeks of gestation for inpatient admissions that encompass more than one gestational week.

The outcome of delivery, category Z37, should be included on all maternal delivery records. It is always a secondary code. Codes in category Z37 should not be used on the newborn record.

Z codes for family planning (contraceptive) or procreative management and counseling should be included on an obstetric record either during the pregnancy or the postpartum stage, if applicable.

Z codes/categories for obstetrical and reproductive services:

Z30	Encounter for contraceptive management
Z31	Encounter for procreative management
Z32.2	Encounter for childbirth instruction
Z32.3	Encounter for childcare instruction
Z33	Pregnant state
Z34	Encounter for supervision of normal pregnancy
Z36	Encounter for antenatal screening of mother
Z3A	Weeks of gestation
Z37	Outcome of delivery
Z39	Encounter for maternal postpartum care and examination
Z76.81	Expectant mother prebirth pediatrician visit

12) Newborns and infants

See Section I.C.16. Newborn (Perinatal) Guidelines, for further instruction on the use of these codes.

Newborn Z codes/categories:

Z76.1	Encounter for health supervision and care of foundling
Z00.1-	Encounter for routine child health examination
Z38	Liveborn infants according to place of birth and type of delivery

13) Routine and administrative examinations

The Z codes allow for the description of encounters for routine examinations, such as, a general check-up, or, examinations for administrative purposes, such as, a pre-employment physical. The codes are not to be used if the examination is for diagnosis of a suspected condition or for treatment purposes. In such cases the diagnosis code is used. During a routine exam, should a diagnosis or condition be discovered, it should be coded as an additional code. Pre-existing and chronic conditions and history codes may also be included as additional codes as long as the examination is for administrative purposes and not focused on any particular condition.

Some of the codes for routine health examinations distinguish between "with" and "without" abnormal findings. Code assignment depends on the information that is known at the time the encounter is being coded. For example, if no abnormal findings were found during the examination, but the encounter is being coded before test results are back, it is acceptable to assign the code for "without abnormal findings." When assigning a code for "with abnormal findings," additional code(s) should be assigned to identify the specific abnormal finding(s).

12-month-old boy presented for well-child visit; pediatrician notices some eczema on the child's scalp and back of the knees

Z00.121	**Encounter for routine child health examination with abnormal findings**
L30.9	**Dermatitis, unspecified**

Explanation: The Z code identifying that this is a routine well-child visit is reported first. Because an abnormal finding (eczema) was documented, a code for this condition may also be appended.

Pre-operative examination and pre-procedural laboratory examination Z codes are for use only in those situations when a patient is being cleared for a procedure or surgery and no treatment is given.

The Z codes/categories for routine and administrative examinations:

Z00	Encounter for general examination without complaint, suspected or reported diagnosis
Z01	Encounter for other special examination without complaint, suspected or reported diagnosis
Z02	Encounter for administrative examination
	Except: Z02.9, Encounter for administrative examinations, unspecified
Z32.0-	Encounter for pregnancy test

14) Miscellaneous Z codes

The miscellaneous Z codes capture a number of other health care encounters that do not fall into one of the other categories. Certain of these codes identify the reason for the encounter; others are for use as additional codes that provide useful information on circumstances that may affect a patient's care and treatment.

Prophylactic organ removal

For encounters specifically for prophylactic removal of an organ (such as prophylactic removal of breasts due to a genetic susceptibility to cancer or a family history of cancer), the principal or first-listed code should be a code from category Z40, Encounter for prophylactic surgery, followed by the appropriate codes to identify the associated risk factor (such as genetic susceptibility or family history).

If the patient has a malignancy of one site and is having prophylactic removal at another site to prevent either a new primary malignancy or metastatic disease, a code for the malignancy should also be assigned in addition to a code from subcategory Z40.0, Encounter for prophylactic surgery for risk factors related to malignant neoplasms. A Z40.0 code should not be assigned if the patient is having organ removal for treatment of a malignancy, such as the removal of the testes for the treatment of prostate cancer.

Miscellaneous Z codes/categories:

Z28	Immunization not carried out
	Except: Z28.3, Underimmunization status
Z29	Encounter for other prophylactic measures
Z40	Encounter for prophylactic surgery
Z41	Encounter for procedures for purposes other than remedying health state
	Except: Z41.9, Encounter for procedure for purposes other than remedying health state, unspecified
Z53	Persons encountering health services for specific procedures and treatment, not carried out
Z55	Problems related to education and literacy
Z56	Problems related to employment and unemployment
Z57	Occupational exposure to risk factors
Z58	Problems related to physical environment
Z59	Problems related to housing and economic circumstances
Z60	Problems related to social environment
Z62	Problems related to upbringing
Z63	Other problems related to primary support group, including family circumstances
Z64	Problems related to certain psychosocial circumstances
Z65	Problems related to other psychosocial circumstances
Z72	Problems related to lifestyle
	Note: These codes should be assigned only when the documentation specifies that the patient has an associated problem
Z73	Problems related to life management difficulty
Z74	Problems related to care provider dependency
	Except: Z74.01, Bed confinement status
Z75	Problems related to medical facilities and other health care
Z76.0	Encounter for issue of repeat prescription
Z76.3	Healthy person accompanying sick person
Z76.4	Other boarder to healthcare facility
Z76.5	Malingerer [conscious simulation]
Z91.1-	Patient's noncompliance with medical treatment and regimen
Z91.83	Wandering in diseases classified elsewhere
Z91.89	Other specified personal risk factors, not elsewhere classified

15) Nonspecific Z codes

Certain Z codes are so non-specific, or potentially redundant with other codes in the classification, that there can be little justification for their use in the inpatient setting. Their use in the outpatient setting should be limited to those instances when there is no further documentation to permit more precise coding. Otherwise, any sign or symptom or any other reason for visit that is captured in another code should be used.

Nonspecific Z codes/categories:

Z02.9	Encounter for administrative examinations, unspecified
Z04.9	Encounter for examination and observation for unspecified reason
Z13.9	Encounter for screening, unspecified
Z41.9	Encounter for procedure for purposes other than remedying health state, unspecified
Z52.9	Donor of unspecified organ or tissue
Z86.59	Personal history of other mental and behavioral disorders
Z88.9	Allergy status to unspecified drugs, medicaments and biological substances status
Z92.0	Personal history of contraception

16)Z codes that may only be principal/first-listed diagnosis

The following Z codes/categories may only be reported as the principal/first-listed diagnosis, except when there are multiple encounters on the same day and the medical records for the encounters are combined:

Z00	Encounter for general examination without complaint, suspected or reported diagnosis
	Except: Z00.6
Z01	Encounter for other special examination without complaint, suspected or reported diagnosis
Z02	Encounter for administrative examination
Z03	Encounter for medical observation for suspected diseases and conditions ruled out
Z04	Encounter for examination and observation for other reasons
Z33.2	Encounter for elective termination of pregnancy

Z31.81	Encounter for male factor infertility in female patient
Z31.83	Encounter for assisted reproductive fertility procedure cycle
Z31.84	Encounter for fertility preservation procedure
Z34	Encounter for supervision of normal pregnancy
Z39	Encounter for maternal postpartum care and examination
Z38	Liveborn infants according to place of birth and type of delivery
Z42	Encounter for plastic and reconstructive surgery following medical procedure or healed injury
Z51.0	Encounter for antineoplastic radiation therapy
Z51.1-	Encounter for antineoplastic chemotherapy and immunotherapy
Z52	Donors of organs and tissues
	Except: Z52.9, Donor of unspecified organ or tissue
Z76.1	Encounter for health supervision and care of foundling
Z76.2	Encounter for health supervision and care of other healthy infant and child
Z99.12	Encounter for respirator [ventilator] dependence during power failure

Female patient seen at 32 weeks' gestation to check the progress of her first pregnancy

Z34.03   Encounter for supervision of normal first pregnancy, third trimester

Z3A.32   32 weeks gestation of pregnancy

Explanation: Category Z34 is appropriate as a first-listed diagnosis. Category Z3A helps to clarify at which point in the pregnancy the patient was provided supervision.

Chapter 21. Factors Influencing Health Status and Contact with Health Services

Chapter 21. Factors Influencing Health Status and Contact With Health Services (Z00-Z99)

NOTE   Z codes represent reasons for encounters. A corresponding procedure code must accompany a Z code if a procedure is performed. Categories Z00-Z99 are provided for occasions when circumstances other than a disease, injury or external cause classifiable to categories A00-Y89 are recorded as "diagnoses" or "problems". This can arise in two main ways:

(a) When a person who may or may not be sick encounters the health services for some specific purpose, such as to receive limited care or service for a current condition, to donate an organ or tissue, to receive prophylactic vaccination (immunization), or to discuss a problem which is in itself not a disease or injury.

(b) When some circumstance or problem is present which influences the person's health status but is not in itself a current illness or injury.

This chapter contains the following blocks:

Z00-Z13	Persons encountering health services for examinations
Z14-Z15	Genetic carrier and genetic susceptibility to disease
Z16	Resistance to antimicrobial drugs
Z17	Estrogen receptor status
Z18	Retained foreign body fragments
~~Z19~~	~~Hormone sensitivity malignancy status~~
Z20-Z29	Persons with potential health hazards related to communicable diseases
Z30-Z39	Persons encountering health services in circumstances related to reproduction
Z40-Z53	Encounters for other specific health care
Z55-Z65	Persons with potential health hazards related to socioeconomic and psychosocial circumstances
Z66	Do not resuscitate status
Z67	Blood type
Z68	Body mass index (BMI)
Z69-Z76	Persons encountering health services in other circumstances
Z77-Z99	Persons with potential health hazards related to family and personal history and certain conditions influencing health status

Persons encountering health services for examinations (Z00-Z13)

NOTE   Nonspecific abnormal findings disclosed at the time of these examinations are classified to categories R70-R94.

EXCLUDES 1   *examinations related to pregnancy and reproduction (Z30-Z36, Z39-)*

✓4ᵗʰ Z00 Encounter for general examination without complaint, suspected or reported diagnosis

EXCLUDES 1   *encounter for examination for administrative purposes (Z02.-)*

EXCLUDES 2   *encounter for pre-procedural examinations (Z01.81-)*
special screening examinations (Z11-Z13)

✓5ᵗʰ Z00.0 Encounter for general adult medical examination
Encounter for adult periodic examination (annual) (physical) and any associated laboratory and radiologic examinations

EXCLUDES 1   *encounter for examination of sign or symptom—code to sign or symptom*
general health check-up of infant or child (Z00.12-)

Z00.00 Encounter for general adult medical   **PDx A**
examination without abnormal findings
Encounter for adult health check-up NOS
AHA: 2016, 1Q, 36

Z00.01 Encounter for general adult medical   **PDx A**
examination with abnormal findings
Use additional code to identify abnormal findings
AHA: 2016, 1Q, 35-36

✓5ᵗʰ Z00.1 Encounter for newborn, infant and child health examinations

✓6ᵗʰ Z00.11 Newborn health examination
Health check for child under 29 days old
Use additional code to identify any abnormal findings
EXCLUDES 1   *health check for child over 28 days old (Z00.12-)*

Z00.110 Health examination for newborn   **PDx N**
under 8 days old
Health check for newborn under 8 days old

Z00.111 Health examination for newborn   **PDx N**
8 to 28 days old
Health check for newborn 8 to 28 days old
Newborn weight check

✓6ᵗʰ Z00.12 Encounter for routine child health examination
Encounter for development testing of infant or child
Health check (routine) for child over 28 days old
EXCLUDES 1   *health check for child under 29 days old (Z00.11-)*
health supervision of foundling or other healthy infant or child (Z76.1-Z76.2)
newborn health examination (Z00.11-)

Z00.121 Encounter for routine child health   **PDx P**
examination with abnormal findings
Use additional code to identify abnormal findings
AHA: 2016, 1Q, 34-35

Z00.129 Encounter for routine child health   **PDx P**
examination without abnormal findings
Encounter for routine child health examination NOS
AHA: 2016, 1Q, 34

Z00.2 Encounter for examination for period of rapid growth   **PDx P**
in childhood

Z00.3 Encounter for examination for adolescent   **PDx P**
development state
Encounter for puberty development state

Z00.5 Encounter for examination of potential donor of organ   **PDx**
and tissue

Z00.6 Encounter for examination for normal comparison and control in clinical research program
Examination of participant or control in clinical research program

✓5ᵗʰ Z00.7 Encounter for examination for period of delayed growth in childhood

Z00.70 Encounter for examination for period of   **PDx P**
delayed growth in childhood without abnormal findings

Z00.71 Encounter for examination for period of   **PDx P**
delayed growth in childhood with abnormal findings
Use additional code to identify abnormal findings

Z00.8 Encounter for other general examination   **PDx**
Encounter for health examination in population surveys

✓4ᵗʰ Z01 Encounter for other special examination without complaint, suspected or reported diagnosis

INCLUDES   routine examination of specific system

NOTE   Codes from category Z01 represent the reason for the encounter. A separate procedure code is required to identify any examinations or procedures performed.

EXCLUDES 1   *encounter for examination for administrative purposes (Z02.-)*
encounter for examination for suspected conditions, proven not to exist (Z03.-)
encounter for laboratory and radiologic examinations as a component of general medical examinations (Z00.0-)
encounter for laboratory, radiologic and imaging examinations for sign(s) and symptom(s)—code to the sign(s) or symptom(s)

EXCLUDES 2   *screening examinations (Z11-Z13)*

✓5ᵗʰ Z01.0 Encounter for examination of eyes and vision
EXCLUDES 1   *examination for driving license (Z02.4)*

Z01.00 Encounter for examination of eyes and vision   **PDx**
without abnormal findings
Encounter for examination of eyes and vision NOS

Z01.01 Encounter for examination of eyes and vision   **PDx**
with abnormal findings
Use additional code to identify abnormal findings

✓5ᵗʰ Z01.1 Encounter for examination of ears and hearing

Z01.10 Encounter for examination of ears and hearing   **PDx**
without abnormal findings
Encounter for examination of ears and hearing NOS
AHA: 2016, 4Q, 24

✓6ᵗʰ Z01.11 Encounter for examination of ears and hearing with abnormal findings
AHA: 2016, 3Q, 17-18

Z01.110 Encounter for hearing examination   **PDx**
following failed hearing screening

Z01.118 Encounter for examination of ears   **PDx**
and hearing with other abnormal findings
Use additional code to identify abnormal findings

Z01.12 Encounter for hearing conservation and   **PDx**
treatment

EXCLUDES 1 Not coded here   **EXCLUDES 2** Not included here   **N** Newborn Age: 0   **P** Pediatric Age: 0-17   **M** Maternity Age: 12-55   **A** Adult Age: 15-124   **PDx** Primary Dx

✓5ᵗʰ **Z01.2 Encounter for** dental examination and cleaning

    Z01.20 Encounter for dental examination and PDx
       cleaning without abnormal findings
         Encounter for dental examination and cleaning NOS

    Z01.21 Encounter for dental examination and cleaning PDx
       with abnormal findings
         Use additional code to identify abnormal findings

✓5ᵗʰ **Z01.3 Encounter for examination of** blood pressure

    Z01.30 Encounter for examination of blood pressure PDx
       without abnormal findings
         Encounter for examination of blood pressure NOS

    Z01.31 Encounter for examination of blood pressure PDx
       with abnormal findings
         Use additional code to identify abnormal findings

✓5ᵗʰ **Z01.4 Encounter for** gynecological examination
      EXCLUDES 2   *pregnancy examination or test (Z32.0-)*
           routine examination for contraceptive maintenance
            (Z30.4-)

    ✓6ᵗʰ **Z01.41 Encounter for** routine **gynecological examination**
         Encounter for general gynecological examination with
           or without cervical smear
         Encounter for gynecological examination (general)
           (routine) NOS
         Encounter for pelvic examination (annual) (periodic)
         Use additional code:
           for screening for human papillomavirus, if
            applicable, (Z11.51)
           for screening vaginal pap smear, if applicable
            (Z12.72)
           to identify acquired absence of uterus, if applicable
            (Z90.71-)
         EXCLUDES 1   *gynecologic examination status-post*
             hysterectomy for malignant condition
             (Z08)
             screening cervical pap smear not a part of a
             routine gynecological examination
             (Z12.4)

       Z01.411 Encounter for gynecological PDx ♀
           examination (general) (routine) with
           abnormal findings
             Use additional code to identify abnormal
             findings

       Z01.419 Encounter for gynecological PDx ♀
           examination (general) (routine) without
           abnormal findings

    Z01.42 Encounter for cervical smear to confirm PDx ♀
       findings **of recent normal smear following initial**
       abnormal smear

✓5ᵗʰ **Z01.8 Encounter for other specified special examinations**

    ✓6ᵗʰ **Z01.81 Encounter for** preprocedural **examinations**
         Encounter for preoperative examinations
         Encounter for radiological and imaging examinations
           as part of preprocedural examination

       Z01.810 Encounter for preprocedural PDx
           cardiovascular examination

       Z01.811 Encounter for preprocedural PDx
           respiratory examination

       Z01.812 Encounter for preprocedural PDx
           laboratory examination
             Blood and urine tests prior to treatment or
             procedure

       Z01.818 Encounter for other preprocedural PDx
           examination
             Encounter for preprocedural examination
             NOS
             Encounter for examinations prior to
             antineoplastic chemotherapy

    Z01.82 Encounter for allergy testing PDx
       EXCLUDES 1   *encounter for antibody response*
             examination (Z01.84)

    Z01.83 Encounter for blood typing PDx
         Encounter for Rh typing

    Z01.84 Encounter for antibody response examination PDx
         Encounter for immunity status testing
       EXCLUDES 1   *encounter for allergy testing (Z01.82)*

    Z01.89 Encounter for other specified special PDx
       examinations

✓4ᵗʰ **Z02 Encounter for** administrative **examination**

    Z02.0 Encounter for examination for admission to educational PDx
      institution
        Encounter for examination for admission to preschool
          (education)
        Encounter for examination for re-admission to school following
          illness or medical treatment

    Z02.1 Encounter for pre-employment examination PDx

    Z02.2 Encounter for examination for admission to residential PDx
      institution
       EXCLUDES 1   *examination for admission to prison (Z02.89)*

    Z02.3 Encounter for examination for recruitment to armed PDx
      forces

    Z02.4 Encounter for examination for driving license PDx

    Z02.5 Encounter for examination for participation in sport PDx
       EXCLUDES 1   *blood-alcohol and blood-drug test (Z02.83)*

    Z02.6 Encounter for examination for insurance purposes PDx

    ✓5ᵗʰ **Z02.7 Encounter for** issue of medical certificate
       EXCLUDES 1   *encounter for general medical examination (Z00-Z01,*
             Z02.0-Z02.6, Z02.8-Z02.9)

       Z02.71 Encounter for disability determination PDx
           Encounter for issue of medical certificate of incapacity
           Encounter for issue of medical certificate of invalidity

       Z02.79 Encounter for issue of other medical certificate PDx

    ✓5ᵗʰ **Z02.8 Encounter for other administrative examinations**

       Z02.81 Encounter for paternity testing PDx

       Z02.82 Encounter for adoption services PDx

       Z02.83 Encounter for blood-alcohol and blood-drug PDx
           test
             Use additional code for findings of alcohol or drugs in
             blood (R78.-)

       Z02.89 Encounter for other administrative PDx
           examinations
             Encounter for examination for admission to prison
             Encounter for examination for admission to summer
             camp
             Encounter for immigration examination
             Encounter for naturalization examination
             Encounter for premarital examination
           EXCLUDES 1   *health supervision of foundling or other*
             healthy infant or child (Z76.1-Z76.2)

    Z02.9 Encounter for administrative examinations, PDx ▽
      unspecified

✓4ᵗʰ **Z03 Encounter for** medical observation **for suspected diseases and conditions ruled out**
      NOTE   This category is to be used when a person without a
           diagnosis is suspected of having an abnormal condition,
           without signs or symptoms, which requires study, but after
           examination and observation, is ruled out. This category is
           also for use for administrative and legal observation status.
      EXCLUDES 1   *contact with and (suspected) exposures hazardous to health*
           (Z77.-)
        ▶*encounter for observation and evaluation of newborn for*
           suspected diseases and conditions ruled out (Z05.0-)◀
        ~~*newborn observation for suspected condition, ruled out*~~
           ~~*(P00-P04)*~~
        person with feared complaint in whom no diagnosis is made
           (Z71.1)
        signs or symptoms under study—code to signs or symptoms

    Z03.6 Encounter for observation for suspected toxic effect PDx
      from ingested substance **ruled out**
        Encounter for observation for suspected adverse effect from
          drug
        Encounter for observation for suspected poisoning

    ✓5ᵗʰ **Z03.7 Encounter for suspected** maternal and fetal conditions **ruled out**
        Encounter for suspected maternal and fetal conditions not
          found
       EXCLUDES 1   *known or suspected fetal anomalies affecting*
             management of mother, not ruled out (O26-,
             O35-, O36-, O40-, O41-)

       Z03.71 Encounter for suspected problem with PDx Ⓜ ♀
           amniotic cavity and membrane ruled out
             Encounter for suspected oligohydramnios ruled out
             Encounter for suspected polyhydramnios ruled out

       Z03.72 Encounter for suspected placental PDx Ⓜ ♀
           problem ruled out

       Z03.73 Encounter for suspected fetal anomaly PDx Ⓜ ♀
           ruled out

☑ Additional Character Req   ✓x7ᵗʰ Placeholder Alert   Manifestation   HCC CMS-HCC Condition   ▽ Unspecified Code   ▶◀ Revised Text   ● New Code   ▲ Revised Code Title

ICD-10-CM 2018   1181

Chapter 21. Factors Influencing Health Status and Contact with Health Services

Z03.74 Encounter for suspected problem with fetal growth ruled out   [PDx] [M][♀]

Z03.75 Encounter for suspected cervical shortening ruled out   [PDx] [M][♀]

Z03.79 Encounter for other suspected maternal and fetal conditions ruled out   [PDx] [M][♀]

✓5ᵗʰ **Z03.8** Encounter for observation for other suspected diseases and conditions ruled out

    ✓6ᵗʰ **Z03.81** Encounter for observation for suspected exposure to biological agents ruled out

       Z03.810 Encounter for observation for suspected exposure to anthrax ruled out   [PDx]

       Z03.818 Encounter for observation for suspected exposure to other biological agents ruled out   [PDx]

    Z03.89 Encounter for observation for other suspected diseases and conditions ruled out   [PDx]

✓4ᵗʰ **Z04** Encounter for examination and observation for other reasons

    [INCLUDES] encounter for examination for medicolegal reasons

    This category is to be used when a person without a diagnosis is suspected of having an abnormal condition, without signs or symptoms, which requires study, but after examination and observation, is ruled-out. This category is also for use for administrative and legal observation status.

    Z04.1 Encounter for examination and observation following transport accident   [PDx]

       [EXCLUDES 1] *encounter for examination and observation following work accident (Z04.2)*

    Z04.2 Encounter for examination and observation following work accident   [PDx]

    Z04.3 Encounter for examination and observation following other accident   [PDx]

    ✓5ᵗʰ **Z04.4** Encounter for examination and observation following alleged rape

       Encounter for examination and observation of victim following alleged rape

       Encounter for examination and observation of victim following alleged sexual abuse

       Z04.41 Encounter for examination and observation following alleged adult rape   [PDx] [A]

         Suspected adult rape, ruled out

         Suspected adult sexual abuse, ruled out

       Z04.42 Encounter for examination and observation following alleged child rape   [PDx] [P]

         Suspected child rape, ruled out

         Suspected child sexual abuse, ruled out

    Z04.6 Encounter for general psychiatric examination, requested by authority   [PDx]

    ✓5ᵗʰ **Z04.7** Encounter for examination and observation following alleged physical abuse

       Z04.71 Encounter for examination and observation following alleged adult physical abuse   [PDx] [A]

         Suspected adult physical abuse, ruled out

         [EXCLUDES 1] *confirmed case of adult physical abuse (T74.-)*

            encounter for examination and observation following alleged adult sexual abuse (Z04.41)

            suspected case of adult physical abuse, not ruled out (T76.-)

       Z04.72 Encounter for examination and observation following alleged child physical abuse   [PDx] [P]

         Suspected child physical abuse, ruled out

         [EXCLUDES 1] *confirmed case of child physical abuse (T74.-)*

            encounter for examination and observation following alleged child sexual abuse (Z04.42)

            suspected case of child physical abuse, not ruled out (T76.-)

    Z04.8 Encounter for examination and observation for other specified reasons   [PDx]

       Encounter for examination and observation for request for expert evidence

    Z04.9 Encounter for examination and observation for unspecified reason   [PDx] ▽

       Encounter for observation NOS

✓4ᵗʰ **Z05** Encounter for observation of newborn for suspected diseases and conditions ruled out

    ▶This category is to be used for newborns, within the neonatal period (the first 28 days of life), who are suspected of having an abnormal condition, but without signs or symptoms, and which, after examination and observation, is ruled out.◀

    [EXCLUDES 2] *newborn observation for suspected condition, related to exposure from the mother or birth process (P00-P04)*

    Z05.0 Observation and evaluation of newborn for suspected cardiac condition ruled out

    Z05.1 Observation and evaluation of newborn for suspected infectious condition ruled out

    Z05.2 Observation and evaluation of newborn for suspected neurological condition ruled out

    Z05.3 Observation and evaluation of newborn for suspected respiratory condition ruled out

    ✓5ᵗʰ **Z05.4** Observation and evaluation of newborn for suspected genetic, metabolic or immunologic condition ruled out

       Z05.41 Observation and evaluation of newborn for suspected genetic condition ruled out

       Z05.42 Observation and evaluation of newborn for suspected metabolic condition ruled out

       Z05.43 Observation and evaluation of newborn for suspected immunologic condition ruled out

    Z05.5 Observation and evaluation of newborn for suspected gastrointestinal condition ruled out

    Z05.6 Observation and evaluation of newborn for suspected genitourinary condition ruled out

    ✓5ᵗʰ **Z05.7** Observation and evaluation of newborn for suspected skin, subcutaneous, musculoskeletal and connective tissue condition ruled out

       Z05.71 Observation and evaluation of newborn for suspected skin and subcutaneous tissue condition ruled out

       Z05.72 Observation and evaluation of newborn for suspected musculoskeletal condition ruled out

       Z05.73 Observation and evaluation of newborn for suspected connective tissue condition ruled out

    Z05.8 Observation and evaluation of newborn for other specified suspected condition ruled out

    Z05.9 Observation and evaluation of newborn for unspecified suspected condition ruled out   ▽

Z08 Encounter for follow-up examination after completed treatment for malignant neoplasm

    Medical surveillance following completed treatment

    Use additional code to identify any acquired absence of organs (Z90.-)

    Use additional code to identify the personal history of malignant neoplasm (Z85.-)

    [EXCLUDES 1] *aftercare following medical care (Z43-Z49, Z51)*

Z09 Encounter for follow-up examination after completed treatment for conditions other than malignant neoplasm

    Medical surveillance following completed treatment

    Use additional code to identify any applicable history of disease code (Z86-. Z87-)

    [EXCLUDES 1] *aftercare following medical care (Z43-Z49, Z51)*

       surveillance of contraception (Z30.4-)

       surveillance of prosthetic and other medical devices (Z44-Z46)

    AHA: 2017, 1Q, 9; 2015, 1Q, 8

✓4ᵗʰ **Z11** Encounter for screening for infectious and parasitic diseases

    Screening is the testing for disease or disease precursors in asymptomatic individuals so that early detection and treatment can be provided for those who test positive for the disease.

    [EXCLUDES 1] *encounter for diagnostic examination—code to sign or symptom*

    Z11.0 Encounter for screening for intestinal infectious diseases

    Z11.1 Encounter for screening for respiratory tuberculosis

    Z11.2 Encounter for screening for other bacterial diseases

    Z11.3 Encounter for screening for infections with a predominantly sexual mode of transmission

       [EXCLUDES 2] *encounter for screening for human immunodeficiency virus [HIV] (Z11.4)*

       encounter for screening for human papillomavirus (Z11.51)

    Z11.4 Encounter for screening for human immunodeficiency virus [HIV]

[EXCLUDES 1] Not coded here   [EXCLUDES 2] Not included here   [N] Newborn Age: 0   [P] Pediatric Age: 0-17   [M] Maternity Age: 12-55   [A] Adult Age: 15-124   [PDx] Primary Dx

1182   ICD-10-CM 2018

✓5th **Z11.5** **Encounter for screening for other viral diseases**
      EXCLUDES 2   *encounter for screening for viral intestinal disease (Z11.Ø)*

     Z11.51 **Encounter for screening for human papillomavirus (HPV)**

     Z11.59 **Encounter for screening for other viral diseases**

Z11.6 **Encounter for screening for other protozoal diseases and helminthiases**
      EXCLUDES 2   *encounter for screening for protozoal intestinal disease (Z11.Ø)*

Z11.8 **Encounter for screening for other infectious and parasitic diseases**
     Encounter for screening for chlamydia
     Encounter for screening for rickettsial
     Encounter for screening for spirochetal
     Encounter for screening for mycoses

Z11.9 **Encounter for screening for infectious and parasitic diseases, unspecified** ▽

✓4th **Z12** **Encounter for screening for malignant neoplasms**
     Screening is the testing for disease or disease precursors in asymptomatic individuals so that early detection and treatment can be provided for those who test positive for the disease.
     Use additional code to identify any family history of malignant neoplasm (Z8Ø.-)
      EXCLUDES 1   *encounter for diagnostic examination—code to sign or symptom*

Z12.Ø **Encounter for screening for malignant neoplasm of stomach**

✓5th **Z12.1** **Encounter for screening for malignant neoplasm of intestinal tract**
     AHA: 2017, 1Q, 8, 9

     Z12.1Ø **Encounter for screening for malignant neoplasm of intestinal tract, unspecified** ▽

     Z12.11 **Encounter for screening for malignant neoplasm of colon**
       Encounter for screening colonoscopy NOS

     Z12.12 **Encounter for screening for malignant neoplasm of rectum**

     Z12.13 **Encounter for screening for malignant neoplasm of small intestine**

Z12.2 **Encounter for screening for malignant neoplasm of respiratory organs**

✓5th **Z12.3** **Encounter for screening for malignant neoplasm of breast**

     Z12.31 **Encounter for screening mammogram for malignant neoplasm of breast**
       EXCLUDES 1   *inconclusive mammogram (R92.2)*
       AHA: 2015, 1Q, 24

     Z12.39 **Encounter for other screening for malignant neoplasm of breast**

Z12.4 **Encounter for screening for malignant neoplasm of cervix** ♀
     Encounter for screening pap smear for malignant neoplasm of cervix
      EXCLUDES 1   *when screening is part of general gynecological examination (ZØ1.4-)*
      EXCLUDES 2   *encounter for screening for human papillomavirus (Z11.51)*

Z12.5 **Encounter for screening for malignant neoplasm of prostate** ♂

Z12.6 **Encounter for screening for malignant neoplasm of bladder**

✓5th **Z12.7** **Encounter for screening for malignant neoplasm of other genitourinary organs**

     Z12.71 **Encounter for screening for malignant neoplasm of testis** ♂

     Z12.72 **Encounter for screening for malignant neoplasm of vagina** ♀
       Vaginal pap smear status-post hysterectomy for non-malignant condition
       Use additional code to identify acquired absence of uterus (Z9Ø.71-)
       EXCLUDES 1   *vaginal pap smear status-post hysterectomy for malignant conditions (ZØ8)*

     Z12.73 **Encounter for screening for malignant neoplasm of ovary** ♀

     Z12.79 **Encounter for screening for malignant neoplasm of other genitourinary organs**

✓5th **Z12.8** **Encounter for screening for malignant neoplasm of other sites**

     Z12.81 **Encounter for screening for malignant neoplasm of oral cavity**

     Z12.82 **Encounter for screening for malignant neoplasm of nervous system**

     Z12.83 **Encounter for screening for malignant neoplasm of skin**

     Z12.89 **Encounter for screening for malignant neoplasm of other sites**

Z12.9 **Encounter for screening for malignant neoplasm, site unspecified** ▽

✓4th **Z13** **Encounter for screening for other diseases and disorders**
     Screening is the testing for disease or disease precursors in asymptomatic individuals so that early detection and treatment can be provided for those who test positive for the disease.
      EXCLUDES 1   *encounter for diagnostic examination—code to sign or symptom*

Z13.Ø **Encounter for screening for diseases of the blood and blood-forming organs and certain disorders involving the immune mechanism**

Z13.1 **Encounter for screening for diabetes mellitus**

✓5th **Z13.2** **Encounter for screening for nutritional, metabolic and other endocrine disorders**

     Z13.21 **Encounter for screening for nutritional disorder**

     ✓6th **Z13.22** **Encounter for screening for metabolic disorder**

       Z13.22Ø **Encounter for screening for lipoid disorders**
         Encounter for screening for cholesterol level
         Encounter for screening for hypercholesterolemia
         Encounter for screening for hyperlipidemia

       Z13.228 **Encounter for screening for other metabolic disorders**

     Z13.29 **Encounter for screening for other suspected endocrine disorder**
       EXCLUDES 1   *encounter for screening for diabetes mellitus (Z13.1)*

Z13.4 **Encounter for screening for certain developmental disorders in childhood** ▣
     Encounter for screening for developmental handicaps in early childhood
      EXCLUDES 1   *routine development testing of infant or child (ZØØ.1-)*

Z13.5 **Encounter for screening for eye and ear disorders**
      EXCLUDES 2   *encounter for general hearing examination (ZØ1.1-)*
              encounter for general vision examination (ZØ1.Ø-)
     AHA: 2016, 3Q, 17

Z13.6 **Encounter for screening for cardiovascular disorders**

✓5th **Z13.7** **Encounter for screening for genetic and chromosomal anomalies**
      EXCLUDES 1   *genetic testing for procreative management (Z31.4-)*

     Z13.71 **Encounter for nonprocreative screening for genetic disease carrier status**

     Z13.79 **Encounter for other screening for genetic and chromosomal anomalies**

✓5th **Z13.8** **Encounter for screening for other specified diseases and disorders**
      EXCLUDES 2   *screening for malignant neoplasms (Z12.-)*

     ✓6th **Z13.81** **Encounter for screening for digestive system disorders**

       Z13.81Ø **Encounter for screening for upper gastrointestinal disorder**

       Z13.811 **Encounter for screening for lower gastrointestinal disorder**
         EXCLUDES 1   *encounter for screening for intestinal infectious disease (Z11.Ø)*

       Z13.818 **Encounter for screening for other digestive system disorders**

     ✓6th **Z13.82** **Encounter for screening for musculoskeletal disorder**

       Z13.82Ø **Encounter for screening for osteoporosis**

       Z13.828 **Encounter for screening for other musculoskeletal disorder**

✓ Additional Character Req   ✓x7th Placeholder Alert   Manifestation   HCC CMS-HCC Condition   ▽ Unspecified Code   ▶◀ Revised Text   ● New Code   ▲ Revised Code Title

Z13.83 Encounter for screening for respiratory **disorder NEC**

> EXCLUDES 1 *encounter for screening for respiratory tuberculosis (Z11.1)*

Z13.84 Encounter for screening for dental **disorders**

√6ᵗʰ **Z13.85 Encounter for screening for** nervous system **disorders**

Z13.850 Encounter for screening for traumatic **brain injury**

Z13.858 Encounter for screening for other nervous system disorders

Z13.88 Encounter for screening for disorder due to exposure to contaminants

> EXCLUDES 1 *those exposed to contaminants without suspected disorders (Z57-Z77-)*

Z13.89 Encounter for screening for other disorder
Encounter for screening for genitourinary disorders

Z13.9 Encounter for screening, unspecified ▽

Genetic carrier and genetic susceptibility to disease (Z14-Z15)

√4ᵗʰ **Z14 Genetic carrier**
DEF: Individuals carrying a gene mutation associated with a certain disease who typically do not develop the disease but are able to pass mutated gene to offspring.

√5ᵗʰ **Z14.0 Hemophilia A carrier**

Z14.01 Asymptomatic hemophilia A carrier

Z14.02 Symptomatic hemophilia A carrier

Z14.1 Cystic fibrosis carrier

Z14.8 Genetic carrier of other disease

√4ᵗʰ **Z15 Genetic susceptibility to disease**
> INCLUDES confirmed abnormal gene
Use additional code, if applicable, for any associated family history of the disease (Z80-Z84)
> EXCLUDES 1 *chromosomal anomalies (Q90-Q99)*

√5ᵗʰ **Z15.0 Genetic susceptibility to** malignant neoplasm
Code first, if applicable, any current malignant neoplasm (C00-C75, C81-C96)
> Use additional code, if applicable, for any personal history of malignant neoplasm (Z85.-)

Z15.01 Genetic susceptibility to malignant neoplasm of breast

Z15.02 Genetic susceptibility to malignant neoplasm of ovary ♀

Z15.03 Genetic susceptibility to malignant neoplasm of prostate ♂

Z15.04 Genetic susceptibility to malignant neoplasm of endometrium ♀

Z15.09 Genetic susceptibility to other malignant neoplasm

√5ᵗʰ **Z15.8 Genetic susceptibility to other disease**

Z15.81 Genetic susceptibility to multiple endocrine neoplasia **[MEN]**
> EXCLUDES 1 *multiple endocrine neoplasia [MEN] syndromes (E31.2-)*

Z15.89 Genetic susceptibility to other disease

Resistance to antimicrobial drugs (Z16)

√4ᵗʰ **Z16 Resistance to antimicrobial drugs**
> NOTE The codes in this category are provided for use as additional codes to identify the resistance and non-responsiveness of a condition to antimicrobial drugs.
Code first the infection
> EXCLUDES 1 *Methicillin resistant Staphylococcus aureus infection (A49.02)*
> ~~Methicillin resistant Staphylococcus aureus infection in diseases classified elsewhere (B95.62)~~
> *Methicillin resistant Staphylococcus aureus pneumonia (J15.212)*
> *sepsis due to Methicillin resistant Staphylococcus aureus (A41.02)*

√5ᵗʰ **Z16.1 Resistance to** beta lactam **antibiotics**

Z16.10 Resistance to unspecified beta lactam antibiotics ▽

Z16.11 Resistance to penicillins
Resistance to amoxicillin
Resistance to ampicillin

Z16.12 Extended spectrum beta lactamase (ESBL) resistance
> EXCLUDES 2 ►*Methicillin resistant Staphylococcus aureus infection in diseases classified elsewhere (B95.62)*◄

Z16.19 Resistance to other specified beta lactam antibiotics
Resistance to cephalosporins

√5ᵗʰ **Z16.2 Resistance to other antibiotics**

Z16.20 Resistance to unspecified antibiotic ▽
Resistance to antibiotics NOS

Z16.21 Resistance to vancomycin

Z16.22 Resistance to vancomycin related **antibiotics**

Z16.23 Resistance to quinolones and fluoroquinolones

Z16.24 Resistance to multiple **antibiotics**

Z16.29 Resistance to other single specified antibiotic
Resistance to aminoglycosides
Resistance to macrolides
Resistance to sulfonamides
Resistance to tetracyclines

√5ᵗʰ **Z16.3 Resistance to other antimicrobial drugs**
> EXCLUDES 1 *resistance to antibiotics (Z16.1-, Z16.2-)*

Z16.30 Resistance to unspecified antimicrobial drugs ▽
Drug resistance NOS

Z16.31 Resistance to antiparasitic **drug(s)**
Resistance to quinine and related compounds

Z16.32 Resistance to antifungal **drug(s)**

Z16.33 Resistance to antiviral **drug(s)**

√6ᵗʰ **Z16.34 Resistance to** antimycobacterial **drug(s)**
Resistance to tuberculostatics

Z16.341 Resistance to single **antimycobacterial drug**
Resistance to antimycobacterial drug NOS

Z16.342 Resistance to multiple **antimycobacterial drugs**

Z16.35 Resistance to multiple **antimicrobial drugs**
> EXCLUDES 1 *Resistance to multiple antibiotics only (Z16.24)*

Z16.39 Resistance to other specified antimicrobial drug

Estrogen receptor status (Z17)

√4ᵗʰ **Z17 Estrogen receptor status**
Code first malignant neoplasm of breast (C50.-)

Z17.0 Estrogen receptor positive **status [ER+]**

Z17.1 Estrogen receptor negative **status [ER-]**

Retained foreign body fragment (Z18)

√4ᵗʰ **Z18 Retained foreign body fragments**
> INCLUDES embedded fragment (status)
> embedded splinter (status)
> retained foreign body status
> EXCLUDES 1 *artificial joint prosthesis status (Z96.6-)*
> *foreign body accidentally left during a procedure (T81.5-)*
> *foreign body entering through orifice (T15-T19)*
> *in situ cardiac device (Z95.-)*
> *organ or tissue replaced by means other than transplant (Z96.-, Z97.-)*
> *organ or tissue replaced by transplant (Z94.-)*
> *personal history of retained foreign body fully removed (Z87.821)*
> *superficial foreign body (non-embedded splinter)—code to superficial foreign body, by site*
DEF: Embedded or retained fragment, splinter, or foreign body; natural or synthetic; can cause infection.

√5ᵗʰ **Z18.0 Retained** radioactive **fragments**

Z18.01 Retained depleted **uranium fragments**

Z18.09 Other retained radioactive fragments
Other retained depleted isotope fragments
Retained nontherapeutic radioactive fragments

√5ᵗʰ **Z18.1 Retained** metal **fragments**
> EXCLUDES 1 *retained radioactive metal fragments (Z18.01-Z18.09)*

Z18.10 Retained metal fragments, unspecified ▽
Retained metal fragment NOS

Z18.11 Retained magnetic **metal fragments**

Z18.12 Retained nonmagnetic **metal fragments**

Z18.2 Retained plastic **fragments**
Acrylics fragments
Diethylhexylphthalates fragments
Isocyanate fragments

√5ᵗʰ **Z18.3 Retained** organic **fragments**

Z18.31 Retained animal quills or spines

Z18.32 Retained tooth

EXCLUDES 1 Not coded here   EXCLUDES 2 Not included here   N Newborn Age: 0   P Pediatric Age: 0-17   M Maternity Age: 12-55   A Adult Age: 15-124   PDx Primary Dx

1184   ICD-10-CM 2018

Z18.33   Retained wood fragments

Z18.39   Other retained organic fragments

✓5ᵗʰ **Z18.8**   **Other specified retained foreign body**

Z18.81   Retained glass fragments

Z18.83   Retained stone or crystalline fragments
Retained concrete or cement fragments

Z18.89   Other specified retained foreign body fragments

Z18.9   Retained foreign body fragments, unspecified material   ▽

Hormone sensitivity malignancy status (Z19)

✓4ᵗʰ **Z19**   **Hormone sensitivity malignancy status**
Code first malignant neoplasm — see Table of Neoplasms, by site, malignant

Z19.1   **Hormone sensitive malignancy status**

Z19.2   **Hormone resistant malignancy status**
Castrate resistant prostate malignancy status

Persons with potential health hazards related to communicable diseases (Z20-Z29)

✓4ᵗʰ **Z20**   **Contact with and (suspected) exposure to communicable diseases**
EXCLUDES 1   carrier of infectious disease (Z22.-)
diagnosed current infectious or parasitic disease—see Alphabetic Index
EXCLUDES 2   personal history of infectious and parasitic diseases (Z86.1-)

✓5ᵗʰ **Z20.0**   **Contact with and (suspected) exposure to intestinal infectious diseases**

Z20.01   Contact with and (suspected) exposure to intestinal infectious diseases due to Escherichia coli (E. coli)

Z20.09   Contact with and (suspected) exposure to other intestinal infectious diseases

Z20.1   **Contact with and (suspected) exposure to tuberculosis**

Z20.2   **Contact with and (suspected) exposure to infections with a predominantly sexual mode of transmission**

Z20.3   **Contact with and (suspected) exposure to rabies**

Z20.4   **Contact with and (suspected) exposure to rubella**

Z20.5   **Contact with and (suspected) exposure to viral hepatitis**

Z20.6   **Contact with and (suspected) exposure to human immunodeficiency virus [HIV]**
EXCLUDES 1   asymptomatic human immunodeficiency virus [HIV] HIV infection status (Z21)

Z20.7   **Contact with and (suspected) exposure to pediculosis, acariasis and other infestations**

✓5ᵗʰ **Z20.8**   **Contact with and (suspected) exposure to other communicable diseases**

✓6ᵗʰ Z20.81   Contact with and (suspected) exposure to other bacterial communicable diseases

Z20.810   Contact with and (suspected) exposure to anthrax

Z20.811   Contact with and (suspected) exposure to meningococcus

Z20.818   Contact with and (suspected) exposure to other bacterial communicable diseases

✓6ᵗʰ Z20.82   Contact with and (suspected) exposure to other viral communicable diseases

Z20.820   Contact with and (suspected) exposure to varicella

Z20.828   Contact with and (suspected) exposure to other viral communicable diseases

Z20.89   Contact with and (suspected) exposure to other communicable diseases

Z20.9   **Contact with and (suspected) exposure to unspecified communicable disease**   ▽

Z21   **Asymptomatic human immunodeficiency virus [HIV]**   HCC
infection status
HIV positive NOS
Code first human immunodeficiency virus [HIV] disease complicating pregnancy, childbirth and the puerperium, if applicable (O98.7-)
EXCLUDES 1   acquired immunodeficiency syndrome (B20)
contact with human immunodeficiency virus [HIV] (Z20.6)
exposure to human immunodeficiency virus [HIV] (Z20.6)
human immunodeficiency virus [HIV] disease (B20)
inconclusive laboratory evidence of human immunodeficiency virus [HIV] (R75)
DEF: Phase of human immunodeficiency virus (HIV) infection with no clinical symptoms; may last for 10 years or more.

✓4ᵗʰ **Z22**   **Carrier of infectious disease**
INCLUDES   colonization status
suspected carrier
EXCLUDES 2   carrier of viral hepatitis (B18.-)

Z22.0   **Carrier of typhoid**

Z22.1   **Carrier of other intestinal infectious diseases**

Z22.2   **Carrier of diphtheria**

✓5ᵗʰ **Z22.3**   **Carrier of other specified bacterial diseases**

Z22.31   Carrier of bacterial disease due to meningococci

✓6ᵗʰ Z22.32   Carrier of bacterial disease due to staphylococci

Z22.321   Carrier or suspected carrier of Methicillin susceptible Staphylococcus aureus
MSSA colonization

Z22.322   Carrier or suspected carrier of Methicillin resistant Staphylococcus aureus
MRSA colonization

✓6ᵗʰ Z22.33   Carrier of bacterial disease due to streptococci

Z22.330   Carrier of Group B streptococcus
EXCLUDES 1   carrier of streptococcus group B (GBS) complicating pregnancy, childbirth and the puerperium (O99.82-)

Z22.338   Carrier of other streptococcus

Z22.39   Carrier of other specified bacterial diseases

Z22.4   **Carrier of infections with a predominantly sexual mode of transmission**

Z22.6   **Carrier of human T-lymphotropic virus type-1 [HTLV-1] infection**

Z22.8   **Carrier of other infectious diseases**

Z22.9   **Carrier of infectious disease, unspecified**   ▽

Z23   **Encounter for immunization**
Code first any routine childhood examination
NOTE   Procedure codes are required to identify the types of immunizations given

✓4ᵗʰ **Z28**   **Immunization not carried out and underimmunization status**
INCLUDES   vaccination not carried out

✓5ᵗʰ **Z28.0**   **Immunization not carried out because of contraindication**

Z28.01   Immunization not carried out because of acute illness of patient

Z28.02   Immunization not carried out because of chronic illness or condition of patient

Z28.03   Immunization not carried out because of immune compromised state of patient

Z28.04   Immunization not carried out because of patient allergy to vaccine or component

Z28.09   Immunization not carried out because of other contraindication

Z28.1   **Immunization not carried out because of patient decision for reasons of belief or group pressure**
Immunization not carried out because of religious belief

✓5ᵗʰ **Z28.2**   **Immunization not carried out because of patient decision for other and unspecified reason**

Z28.20   Immunization not carried out because of patient   ▽
decision for unspecified reason

Z28.21   Immunization not carried out because of patient refusal

Z28.29   Immunization not carried out because of patient decision for other reason

Z28.3   **Underimmunization status**
Delinquent immunization status
Lapsed immunization schedule status

✓5ᵗʰ **Z28.8**   **Immunization not carried out for other reason**

Z28.81   Immunization not carried out due to patient having had the disease

Z28.82   Immunization not carried out because of caregiver refusal
Immunization not carried out because of guardian refusal
Immunization not carried out because of parent refusal
EXCLUDES 1   immunization not carried out because of caregiver refusal because of religious belief (Z28.1)

Z28.89   Immunization not carried out for other reason

Z28.9   **Immunization not carried out for unspecified reason**   ▽

☑ Additional Character Req   ✓x7ᵗʰ Placeholder Alert   Manifestation   HCC CMS-HCC Condition   ▽ Unspecified Code   ▶◀ Revised Text   ● New Code   ▲ Revised Code Title

ICD-10-CM 2018   1185

Chapter 21. Factors Influencing Health Status and Contact with Health Services

Z29–Z31.83

✓4ᵗʰ **Z29 Encounter for other prophylactic measures**
> EXCLUDES 1   desensitization to allergens (Z51.6)
> prophylactic surgery (Z40.-)

✓5ᵗʰ **Z29.1 Encounter for prophylactic immunotherapy**
> Encounter for administration of immunoglobulin

     Z29.11 Encounter for prophylactic immunotherapy for respiratory syncytial virus (RSV)

     Z29.12 Encounter for prophylactic antivenin

     Z29.13 Encounter for prophylactic Rho(D) immune globulin

     Z29.14 Encounter for prophylactic rabies immune globin

Z29.3 Encounter for prophylactic fluoride administration

Z29.8 Encounter for other specified prophylactic measures

Z29.9 Encounter for prophylactic measures, unspecified ▽

Persons encountering health services in circumstances related to reproduction (Z30-Z39)

✓4ᵗʰ **Z30 Encounter for contraceptive management**
> **DEF:** Contraceptive management to prevent pregnancy; methods include oral medications, intrauterine devices, and surgical procedures for males and females (sterilization).

✓5ᵗʰ **Z30.0 Encounter for general counseling and advice on contraception**

     ✓6ᵗʰ **Z30.01 Encounter for initial prescription of contraceptives**
> EXCLUDES 1   encounter for surveillance of contraceptives (Z30.4-)

       Z30.011 Encounter for initial prescription of contraceptive pills ♀

       Z30.012 Encounter for prescription of emergency contraception ♀
> Encounter for postcoital contraception

       Z30.013 Encounter for initial prescription of injectable contraceptive ♀

       Z30.014 Encounter for initial prescription of intrauterine contraceptive device ♀
> EXCLUDES 1   encounter for insertion of intrauterine contraceptive device (Z30.430, Z30.432)

       Z30.015 Encounter for initial prescription of vaginal ring hormonal contraceptive

       Z30.016 Encounter for initial prescription of transdermal patch hormonal contraceptive device

       Z30.017 Encounter for initial prescription of implantable subdermal contraceptive

       Z30.018 Encounter for initial prescription of other contraceptives ♀
> Encounter for initial prescription of barrier contraception
> Encounter for initial prescription of diaphragm

       Z30.019 Encounter for initial prescription of contraceptives, unspecified ♀▽

     Z30.02 Counseling and instruction in natural family planning to avoid pregnancy

     Z30.09 Encounter for other general counseling and advice on contraception
> Encounter for family planning advice NOS

Z30.2 Encounter for sterilization

✓5ᵗʰ **Z30.4 Encounter for surveillance of contraceptives**

     Z30.40 Encounter for surveillance of contraceptives, unspecified ▽

     Z30.41 Encounter for surveillance of contraceptive pills ♀
> Encounter for repeat prescription for contraceptive pill

     Z30.42 Encounter for surveillance of injectable contraceptive ♀

     ✓6ᵗʰ **Z30.43 Encounter for surveillance of intrauterine contraceptive device**

       Z30.430 Encounter for insertion of intrauterine contraceptive device ♀

       Z30.431 Encounter for routine checking of intrauterine contraceptive device ♀

       Z30.432 Encounter for removal of intrauterine contraceptive device ♀

       Z30.433 Encounter for removal and reinsertion of intrauterine contraceptive device ♀
> Encounter for replacement of intrauterine contraceptive device

     Z30.44 Encounter for surveillance of vaginal ring hormonal contraceptive device ♀

     Z30.45 Encounter for surveillance of transdermal patch hormonal contraceptive device ♀

     Z30.46 Encounter for surveillance of implantable subdermal contraceptive ♀
> Encounter for checking, reinsertion or removal of implantable subdermal contraceptive

     Z30.49 Encounter for surveillance of other contraceptives ♀
> Encounter for surveillance of barrier contraception
> Encounter for surveillance of diaphragm

Z30.8 Encounter for other contraceptive management
> Encounter for postvasectomy sperm count
> Encounter for routine examination for contraceptive maintenance
> EXCLUDES 1   sperm count following sterilization reversal (Z31.42)
> sperm count for fertility testing (Z31.41)

Z30.9 Encounter for contraceptive management, unspecified ▽

✓4ᵗʰ **Z31 Encounter for procreative management**
> EXCLUDES 1   complications associated with artificial fertilization (N98.-)
> female infertility (N97.-)
> male infertility (N46.-)

Z31.0 Encounter for reversal of previous sterilization

✓5ᵗʰ **Z31.4 Encounter for procreative investigation and testing**
> EXCLUDES 1   postvasectomy sperm count (Z30.8)

     Z31.41 Encounter for fertility testing
> Encounter for fallopian tube patency testing
> Encounter for sperm count for fertility testing

     Z31.42 Aftercare following sterilization reversal
> Sperm count following sterilization reversal

     ✓6ᵗʰ **Z31.43 Encounter for genetic testing of female for procreative management**
> Use additional code for recurrent pregnancy loss, if applicable (N96, O26.2-)
> EXCLUDES 1   nonprocreative genetic testing (Z13.7-)

       Z31.430 Encounter of female for testing for genetic disease carrier status for procreative management ♀

       Z31.438 Encounter for other genetic testing of female for procreative management ♀

     ✓6ᵗʰ **Z31.44 Encounter for genetic testing of male for procreative management**
> EXCLUDES 1   nonprocreative genetic testing (Z13.7-)

       Z31.440 Encounter of male for testing for genetic disease carrier status for procreative management ♂

       Z31.441 Encounter for testing of male partner patient with recurrent pregnancy loss Ⓐ♂

       Z31.448 Encounter for other genetic testing of male for procreative management Ⓐ♂

     Z31.49 Encounter for other procreative investigation and testing

▲ **Z31.5 Encounter for procreative genetic counseling**

✓5ᵗʰ **Z31.6 Encounter for general counseling and advice on procreation**

     Z31.61 Procreative counseling and advice using natural family planning

     Z31.62 Encounter for fertility preservation counseling
> Encounter for fertility preservation counseling prior to cancer therapy
> Encounter for fertility preservation counseling prior to surgical removal of gonads

     Z31.69 Encounter for other general counseling and advice on procreation

Z31.7 Encounter for procreative management and counseling for gestational carrier
> EXCLUDES 1   pregnant state, gestational carrier (Z33.3)

✓5ᵗʰ **Z31.8 Encounter for other procreative management**

     Z31.81 Encounter for male factor infertility in female patient PDx♀

     Z31.82 Encounter for Rh incompatibility status ♀
> **AHA:** 2015, 3Q, 40; 2014, 4Q, 17

     Z31.83 Encounter for assisted reproductive fertility procedure cycle PDx♀
> Patient undergoing in vitro fertilization cycle
> Use additional code to identify the type of infertility
> EXCLUDES 1   pre-cycle diagnosis and testing—code to reason for encounter

---

EXCLUDES 1 Not coded here   EXCLUDES 2 Not included here   Ⓝ Newborn Age: Ø   Ⓟ Pediatric Age: Ø-17   Ⓜ Maternity Age: 12-55   Ⓐ Adult Age: 15-124   PDx Primary Dx

Z31.84 Encounter for fertility preservation **procedure** PDx
Encounter for fertility preservation procedure prior to cancer therapy
Encounter for fertility preservation procedure prior to surgical removal of gonads

Z31.89 Encounter for other procreative management

Z31.9 Encounter for procreative management, unspecified ▽

✓4ᵗʰ **Z32 Encounter for pregnancy test and childbirth and childcare instruction**

✓5ᵗʰ **Z32.0 Encounter for** pregnancy test

Z32.00 Encounter for pregnancy test, result unknown ♀
Encounter for pregnancy test NOS

Z32.01 Encounter for pregnancy test, result positive M♀

Z32.02 Encounter for pregnancy test, result negative ♀

Z32.2 Encounter for childbirth instruction

Z32.3 Encounter for childcare instruction
Encounter for prenatal or postpartum childcare instruction

✓4ᵗʰ **Z33 Pregnant state**

Z33.1 Pregnant state, incidental M♀
Pregnant state NOS
EXCLUDES 1   *complications of pregnancy (O00-O9A)*
pregnant state, gestational carrier (Z33.3)

Z33.2 Encounter for elective termination of pregnancy PDx M♀
EXCLUDES 1   *early fetal death with retention of dead fetus (O02.1)*
late fetal death (O36.4)
spontaneous abortion (O03)

Z33.3 Pregnant state, gestational carrier M♀
EXCLUDES 1   *encounter for procreative management and counseling for gestational carrier (Z31.7)*

✓4ᵗʰ **Z34 Encounter for supervision of normal pregnancy**
EXCLUDES 1   *any complication of pregnancy (O00-O9A)*
encounter for pregnancy test (Z32.0-)
encounter for supervision of high risk pregnancy (O09.-)
AHA: 2014, 4Q, 17

✓5ᵗʰ **Z34.0 Encounter for supervision of normal** first **pregnancy**

Z34.00 Encounter for supervision of normal first pregnancy, unspecified trimester PDx M♀▽

Z34.01 Encounter for supervision of normal first pregnancy, first trimester PDx M♀

Z34.02 Encounter for supervision of normal first pregnancy, second trimester PDx M♀

Z34.03 Encounter for supervision of normal first pregnancy, third trimester PDx M♀

✓5ᵗʰ **Z34.8 Encounter for supervision of other normal pregnancy**

Z34.80 Encounter for supervision of other normal pregnancy, unspecified trimester PDx M♀▽

Z34.81 Encounter for supervision of other normal pregnancy, first trimester PDx M♀

Z34.82 Encounter for supervision of other normal pregnancy, second trimester PDx M♀

Z34.83 Encounter for supervision of other normal pregnancy, third trimester PDx M♀

✓5ᵗʰ **Z34.9 Encounter for supervision of normal pregnancy, unspecified**

Z34.90 Encounter for supervision of normal pregnancy, unspecified, unspecified trimester PDx M♀▽

Z34.91 Encounter for supervision of normal pregnancy, unspecified, first trimester PDx M♀▽

Z34.92 Encounter for supervision of normal pregnancy, unspecified, second trimester PDx M♀▽

Z34.93 Encounter for supervision of normal pregnancy, unspecified, third trimester PDx M♀▽

✓4ᵗʰ **Z36 Encounter for** antenatal screening **of mother**
INCLUDES ▶ encounter for placental sample (taken vaginally)
screening is the testing for disease or disease precursors in asymptomatic individuals so that early detection and treatment can be provided for those who test positive for the disease◀
EXCLUDES 1   *abnormal findings on antenatal screening of mother (O28.-)*
diagnostic examination—code to sign or symptom
encounter for suspected maternal and fetal conditions ruled out (Z03.7-)
suspected fetal condition affecting management of pregnancy—code to condition in Chapter 15
EXCLUDES 2 ▶ *abnormal findings on antenatal screening of mother (O28.-)◀*
genetic counseling and testing (Z31.43-, Z31.5)
routine prenatal care (Z34)

● **Z36.0 Encounter for antenatal screening for** chromosomal anomalies

● **Z36.1 Encounter for antenatal screening for** raised alphafetoprotein level
Encounter for antenatal screening for elevated maternal serum alphafetoprotein level

● **Z36.2 Encounter for other antenatal screening follow-up**
Non-visualized anatomy on a previous scan

● **Z36.3 Encounter for antenatal screening for** malformations
Screening for a suspected anomaly

● **Z36.4 Encounter for antenatal screening for** fetal growth retardation
Intrauterine growth restriction (IUGR)/small-for-dates

● **Z36.5 Encounter for antenatal screening for** isoimmunization

✓5ᵗʰ **Z36.8 Encounter for other antenatal screening**

● **Z36.81 Encounter for antenatal screening for** hydrops fetalis

● **Z36.82 Encounter for antenatal screening for** nuchal translucency

● **Z36.83 Encounter for fetal screening for** congenital cardiac abnormalities

● **Z36.84 Encounter for antenatal screening for** fetal lung maturity

● **Z36.85 Encounter for antenatal screening for** Streptococcus B

● **Z36.86 Encounter for antenatal screening for** cervical length
Screening for risk of pre-term labor

● **Z36.87 Encounter for antenatal screening for** uncertain dates

● **Z36.88 Encounter for antenatal screening for** fetal macrosomia
Screening for large-for-dates

● **Z36.89 Encounter for other specified antenatal screening**

● **Z36.8A Encounter for antenatal screening for other genetic defects**

● **Z36.9 Encounter for antenatal screening, unspecified** ▽

✓4ᵗʰ **Z3A Weeks of gestation**
NOTE Codes from category Z3A are for use, only on the maternal record, to indicate the weeks of gestation of the pregnancy, if known.
Code first complications of pregnancy, childbirth and the puerperium ▶(O09-O9A)◀
AHA: 2016, 2Q, 34; 2014, 3Q, 17; 2014, 2Q, 9; 2013, 2Q, 33

✓5ᵗʰ **Z3A.0 Weeks of gestation of pregnancy,** unspecified or less than 10 weeks

Z3A.00 Weeks of gestation of pregnancy not specified M♀▽

Z3A.01 Less than 8 weeks **gestation of pregnancy** M♀

Z3A.08 8 weeks **gestation of pregnancy** M♀

Z3A.09 9 weeks **gestation of pregnancy** M♀

✓5ᵗʰ **Z3A.1 Weeks of gestation of pregnancy, weeks** 10-19

Z3A.10 10 weeks **gestation of pregnancy** M♀

Z3A.11 11 weeks **gestation of pregnancy** M♀

Z3A.12 12 weeks **gestation of pregnancy** M♀

Z3A.13 13 weeks **gestation of pregnancy** M♀

Z3A.14 14 weeks **gestation of pregnancy** M♀

Z3A.15 15 weeks **gestation of pregnancy** M♀

Z3A.16 16 weeks **gestation of pregnancy** M♀

Z3A.17 17 weeks **gestation of pregnancy** M♀

Z3A.18 18 weeks **gestation of pregnancy** M♀

Z3A.19 19 weeks **gestation of pregnancy** M♀

✓5ᵗʰ **Z3A.2**   Weeks of gestation of pregnancy, weeks 20-29
- **Z3A.20**   20 weeks **gestation of pregnancy**   Ⓜ♀
- **Z3A.21**   21 weeks **gestation of pregnancy**   Ⓜ♀
- **Z3A.22**   22 weeks **gestation of pregnancy**   Ⓜ♀
- **Z3A.23**   23 weeks **gestation of pregnancy**   Ⓜ♀
- **Z3A.24**   24 weeks **gestation of pregnancy**   Ⓜ♀
- **Z3A.25**   25 weeks **gestation of pregnancy**   Ⓜ♀
- **Z3A.26**   26 weeks **gestation of pregnancy**   Ⓜ♀
- **Z3A.27**   27 weeks **gestation of pregnancy**   Ⓜ♀
- **Z3A.28**   28 weeks **gestation of pregnancy**   Ⓜ♀
- **Z3A.29**   29 weeks **gestation of pregnancy**   Ⓜ♀

✓5ᵗʰ **Z3A.3**   Weeks of gestation of pregnancy, weeks 30-39
- **Z3A.30**   30 weeks **gestation of pregnancy**   Ⓜ♀
- **Z3A.31**   31 weeks **gestation of pregnancy**   Ⓜ♀
- **Z3A.32**   32 weeks **gestation of pregnancy**   Ⓜ♀
- **Z3A.33**   33 weeks **gestation of pregnancy**   Ⓜ♀
- **Z3A.34**   34 weeks **gestation of pregnancy**   Ⓜ♀
- **Z3A.35**   35 weeks **gestation of pregnancy**   Ⓜ♀
- **Z3A.36**   36 weeks **gestation of pregnancy**   Ⓜ♀
- **Z3A.37**   37 weeks **gestation of pregnancy**   Ⓜ♀
- **Z3A.38**   38 weeks **gestation of pregnancy**   Ⓜ♀
- **Z3A.39**   39 weeks **gestation of pregnancy**   Ⓜ♀

✓5ᵗʰ **Z3A.4**   Weeks of gestation of pregnancy, weeks 40 or greater
    AHA: 2014, 4Q, 23
- **Z3A.40**   40 weeks **gestation of pregnancy**   Ⓜ♀
- **Z3A.41**   41 weeks **gestation of pregnancy**   Ⓜ♀
- **Z3A.42**   42 weeks **gestation of pregnancy**   Ⓜ♀
- **Z3A.49**   Greater than 42 weeks **gestation of pregnancy**   Ⓜ♀

✓4ᵗʰ **Z37**   **Outcome of delivery**
This category is intended for use as an additional code to identify the outcome of delivery on the mother's record. It is not for use on the newborn record.
> **EXCLUDES 1**   stillbirth (P95)

- **Z37.0**   **Single live birth**   Ⓜ♀
    AHA: 2016, 2Q, 34; 2014, 2Q, 9
- **Z37.1**   **Single stillbirth**   Ⓜ♀
- **Z37.2**   **Twins, both liveborn**   Ⓜ♀
- **Z37.3**   **Twins, one liveborn and one stillborn**   Ⓜ♀
- **Z37.4**   **Twins, both stillborn**   Ⓜ♀
- ✓5ᵗʰ **Z37.5**   **Other multiple births, all liveborn**
  - **Z37.50**   **Multiple births, unspecified, all liveborn**   Ⓜ♀▽
  - **Z37.51**   **Triplets, all liveborn**   Ⓜ♀
  - **Z37.52**   **Quadruplets, all liveborn**   Ⓜ♀
  - **Z37.53**   **Quintuplets, all liveborn**   Ⓜ♀
  - **Z37.54**   **Sextuplets, all liveborn**   Ⓜ♀
  - **Z37.59**   **Other multiple births, all liveborn**   Ⓜ♀
- ✓5ᵗʰ **Z37.6**   **Other multiple births, some liveborn**
  - **Z37.60**   **Multiple births, unspecified, some liveborn**   Ⓜ♀▽
  - **Z37.61**   **Triplets, some liveborn**   Ⓜ♀
  - **Z37.62**   **Quadruplets, some liveborn**   Ⓜ♀
  - **Z37.63**   **Quintuplets, some liveborn**   Ⓜ♀
  - **Z37.64**   **Sextuplets, some liveborn**   Ⓜ♀
  - **Z37.69**   **Other multiple births, some liveborn**   Ⓜ♀
- **Z37.7**   **Other multiple births, all stillborn**   Ⓜ♀
- **Z37.9**   **Outcome of delivery, unspecified**   Ⓜ♀▽
    Multiple birth NOS
    Single birth NOS

✓4ᵗʰ **Z38**   **Liveborn infants according to place of birth and type of delivery**
This category is for use as the principal code on the initial record of a newborn baby. It is to be used for the initial birth record only. It is not to be used on the mother's record.
    AHA: 2017, 2Q, 5-7; 2016, 3Q, 18; 2015, 2Q, 15

- ✓5ᵗʰ **Z38.0**   **Single liveborn infant, born in hospital**
    Single liveborn infant, born in birthing center or other health care facility
  - **Z38.00**   **Single liveborn infant, delivered vaginally**   PDx N
  - **Z38.01**   **Single liveborn infant, delivered by cesarean**   PDx N
- **Z38.1**   **Single liveborn infant, born outside hospital**   PDx N
- **Z38.2**   **Single liveborn infant, unspecified as to place of birth**   PDx N ▽
    Single liveborn infant NOS

- ✓5ᵗʰ **Z38.3**   **Twin liveborn infant, born in hospital**
  - **Z38.30**   **Twin liveborn infant, delivered vaginally**   PDx N
  - **Z38.31**   **Twin liveborn infant, delivered by cesarean**   PDx N
- **Z38.4**   **Twin liveborn infant, born outside hospital**   PDx N
- **Z38.5**   **Twin liveborn infant, unspecified as to place of birth**   PDx N ▽

- ✓5ᵗʰ **Z38.6**   **Other multiple liveborn infant, born in hospital**
  - **Z38.61**   **Triplet liveborn infant, delivered vaginally**   PDx N
  - **Z38.62**   **Triplet liveborn infant, delivered by cesarean**   PDx N
  - **Z38.63**   **Quadruplet liveborn infant, delivered vaginally**   PDx N
  - **Z38.64**   **Quadruplet liveborn infant, delivered by cesarean**   PDx N
  - **Z38.65**   **Quintuplet liveborn infant, delivered vaginally**   PDx N
  - **Z38.66**   **Quintuplet liveborn infant, delivered by cesarean**   PDx N
  - **Z38.68**   **Other multiple liveborn infant, delivered vaginally**   PDx N
  - **Z38.69**   **Other multiple liveborn infant, delivered by cesarean**   PDx N
- **Z38.7**   **Other multiple liveborn infant, born outside hospital**   PDx N
- **Z38.8**   **Other multiple liveborn infant, unspecified as to place of birth**   PDx N ▽

✓4ᵗʰ **Z39**   **Encounter for maternal postpartum care and examination**
- **Z39.0**   **Encounter for care and examination of mother immediately after delivery**   PDx Ⓜ♀
    Care and observation in uncomplicated cases when the delivery occurs outside a healthcare facility
> **EXCLUDES 1**   care for postpartum complication—see Alphabetic index

- **Z39.1**   **Encounter for care and examination of lactating mother**   PDx Ⓜ♀
    Encounter for supervision of lactation
> **EXCLUDES 1**   disorders of lactation (O92.-)

- **Z39.2**   **Encounter for routine postpartum follow-up**   PDx Ⓜ♀

Encounters for other specific health care (Z40-Z53)

Categories Z40-Z53 are intended for use to indicate a reason for care. They may be used for patients who have already been treated for a disease or injury, but who are receiving aftercare or prophylactic care, or care to consolidate the treatment, or to deal with a residual state.
> **EXCLUDES 2**   follow-up examination for medical surveillance after treatment (Z08-Z09)

✓4ᵗʰ **Z40**   **Encounter for prophylactic surgery**
> **EXCLUDES 1**   organ donations (Z52.-)
>   therapeutic organ removal—code to condition

- ✓5ᵗʰ **Z40.0**   **Encounter for prophylactic surgery for risk factors related to malignant neoplasms**
    Admission for prophylactic organ removal
    Use additional code to identify risk factor
  - **Z40.00**   **Encounter for prophylactic removal of unspecified organ**   ▽
  - **Z40.01**   **Encounter for prophylactic removal of breast**
  - ▲ **Z40.02**   **Encounter for prophylactic removal of ovary(s)**   ♀
    ▶Encounter for prophylactic removal of ovary(s) and fallopian tube(s)◀
  - ● **Z40.03**   **Encounter for prophylactic removal of fallopian tube(s)**
  - **Z40.09**   **Encounter for prophylactic removal of other organ**
- **Z40.8**   **Encounter for other prophylactic surgery**
- **Z40.9**   **Encounter for prophylactic surgery, unspecified**   ▽

✓4ᵗʰ **Z41**   **Encounter for procedures for purposes other than remedying health state**
- **Z41.1**   **Encounter for cosmetic surgery**
    Encounter for cosmetic breast implant
    Encounter for cosmetic procedure
> **EXCLUDES 1**   encounter for plastic and reconstructive surgery following medical procedure or healed injury (Z42.-)
>   encounter for post-mastectomy breast implantation (Z42.1)

- **Z41.2**   **Encounter for routine and ritual male circumcision**   ♂
- **Z41.3**   **Encounter for ear piercing**

EXCLUDES 1 Not coded here   **EXCLUDES 2** Not included here   N Newborn Age: 0   P Pediatric Age: 0-17   Ⓜ Maternity Age: 12-55   A Adult Age: 15-124   PDx Primary Dx

1188   ICD-10-CM 2018

Z3A.2–Z41.3

Z41.8   Encounter for other procedures for purposes other than remedying health state

Z41.9   Encounter for procedure for purposes other than remedying health state, unspecified ▽

✓4th **Z42**   **Encounter for plastic and reconstructive surgery following medical procedure or healed injury**

    EXCLUDES 1   *encounter for cosmetic plastic surgery (Z41.1)*
         encounter for plastic surgery for treatment of current injury—code to relevent injury

Z42.1   Encounter for breast reconstruction following mastectomy   PDx A

    EXCLUDES 1   *deformity and disproportion of reconstructed breast (N65.1-)*

Z42.8   Encounter for other plastic and reconstructive surgery following medical procedure or healed injury   PDx
       AHA: 2017, 1Q, 42

✓4th **Z43**   **Encounter for attention to artificial openings**

    INCLUDES   closure of artificial openings
         passage of sounds or bougies through artificial openings
         reforming artificial openings
         removal of catheter from artificial openings
         toilet or cleansing of artificial openings

    EXCLUDES 1   ~~artificial opening status only, without need for care (Z93.-)~~
         complications of external stoma (J95.0-, K94.-, N99.5-)

    EXCLUDES 2   *fitting and adjustment of prosthetic and other devices (Z44-Z46)*

Z43.0   Encounter for attention to tracheostomy   HCC

Z43.1   Encounter for attention to gastrostomy   HCC

    EXCLUDES 2   ▶artificial opening status only, without need for care (Z93.-)◀

Z43.2   Encounter for attention to ileostomy   HCC

Z43.3   Encounter for attention to colostomy   HCC

Z43.4   Encounter for attention to other artificial openings of digestive tract   HCC

Z43.5   Encounter for attention to cystostomy   HCC

Z43.6   Encounter for attention to other artificial openings of urinary tract   HCC
       Encounter for attention to nephrostomy
       Encounter for attention to ureterostomy
       Encounter for attention to urethrostomy

Z43.7   Encounter for attention to artificial vagina

Z43.8   Encounter for attention to other artificial openings   HCC

Z43.9   Encounter for attention to unspecified artificial opening   HCC ▽

✓4th **Z44**   **Encounter for fitting and adjustment of external prosthetic device**

    INCLUDES   removal or replacement of external prosthetic device
    EXCLUDES 1   *malfunction or other complications of device—see Alphabetical Index*
         presence of prosthetic device (Z97.-)

✓5th **Z44.0**   Encounter for fitting and adjustment of artificial arm

   ✓6th **Z44.00**   Encounter for fitting and adjustment of unspecified artificial arm

     Z44.001   Encounter for fitting and adjustment of unspecified right artificial arm ▽

     Z44.002   Encounter for fitting and adjustment of unspecified left artificial arm ▽

     Z44.009   Encounter for fitting and adjustment of unspecified artificial arm, unspecified arm ▽

   ✓6th **Z44.01**   Encounter for fitting and adjustment of complete artificial arm

     Z44.011   Encounter for fitting and adjustment of complete right artificial arm

     Z44.012   Encounter for fitting and adjustment of complete left artificial arm

     Z44.019   Encounter for fitting and adjustment of complete artificial arm, unspecified arm ▽

   ✓6th **Z44.02**   Encounter for fitting and adjustment of partial artificial arm

     Z44.021   Encounter for fitting and adjustment of partial artificial right arm

     Z44.022   Encounter for fitting and adjustment of partial artificial left arm

     Z44.029   Encounter for fitting and adjustment of partial artificial arm, unspecified arm ▽

✓5th **Z44.1**   Encounter for fitting and adjustment of artificial leg

   ✓6th **Z44.10**   Encounter for fitting and adjustment of unspecified artificial leg

     Z44.101   Encounter for fitting and adjustment of unspecified right artificial leg   HCC ▽

     Z44.102   Encounter for fitting and adjustment of unspecified left artificial leg   HCC ▽

     Z44.109   Encounter for fitting and adjustment of unspecified artificial leg, unspecified leg   HCC ▽

   ✓6th **Z44.11**   Encounter for fitting and adjustment of complete artificial leg

     Z44.111   Encounter for fitting and adjustment of complete right artificial leg   HCC

     Z44.112   Encounter for fitting and adjustment of complete left artificial leg   HCC

     Z44.119   Encounter for fitting and adjustment of complete artificial leg, unspecified leg   HCC ▽

   ✓6th **Z44.12**   Encounter for fitting and adjustment of partial artificial leg

     Z44.121   Encounter for fitting and adjustment of partial artificial right leg   HCC

     Z44.122   Encounter for fitting and adjustment of partial artificial left leg   HCC

     Z44.129   Encounter for fitting and adjustment of partial artificial leg, unspecified leg   HCC ▽

✓5th **Z44.2**   Encounter for fitting and adjustment of artificial eye

    EXCLUDES 1   *mechanical complication of ocular prosthesis (T85.3)*

     Z44.20   Encounter for fitting and adjustment of artificial eye, unspecified ▽

     Z44.21   Encounter for fitting and adjustment of artificial right eye

     Z44.22   Encounter for fitting and adjustment of artificial left eye

✓5th **Z44.3**   Encounter for fitting and adjustment of external breast prosthesis

    EXCLUDES 1   *complications of breast implant (T85.4-)*
         encounter for adjustment or removal of breast implant (Z45.81-)
         encounter for initial breast implant insertion for cosmetic breast augmentation (Z41.1)
         encounter for breast reconstruction following mastectomy (Z42.1)

     Z44.30   Encounter for fitting and adjustment of external breast prosthesis, unspecified breast ▽

     Z44.31   Encounter for fitting and adjustment of external right breast prosthesis

     Z44.32   Encounter for fitting and adjustment of external left breast prosthesis

Z44.8   Encounter for fitting and adjustment of other external prosthetic devices

Z44.9   Encounter for fitting and adjustment of unspecified external prosthetic device ▽

✓4th **Z45**   **Encounter for adjustment and management of implanted device**

    INCLUDES   removal or replacement of implanted device
    EXCLUDES 1   *malfunction or other complications of device – see Alphabetical Index*
         ~~presence of prosthetic and other devices (Z95-Z97)~~

    EXCLUDES 2   *encounter for fitting and adjustment of non-implanted device (Z46.-)*

✓5th **Z45.0**   Encounter for adjustment and management of cardiac device

   ✓6th **Z45.01**   Encounter for adjustment and management of cardiac pacemaker
       Encounter for adjustment and management of cardiac resynchronization therapy pacemaker (CRT-P)

     EXCLUDES 1   *encounter for adjustment and management of automatic implantable cardiac defibrillator with synchronous cardiac pacemaker (Z45.02)*

     Z45.010   Encounter for checking and testing of cardiac pacemaker pulse generator [battery]
         Encounter for replacing cardiac pacemaker pulse generator [battery]

✓ Additional Character Req   x7th Placeholder Alert   Manifestation   HCC CMS-HCC Condition   ▽ Unspecified Code   ▶◀ Revised Text   ● New Code   ▲ Revised Code Title

ICD-10-CM 2018   1189

Z45.Ø18 **Encounter for adjustment and management of other part of cardiac pacemaker**
EXCLUDES 2 ▶*presence of prosthetic and other devices (Z95-Z97)*◀

Z45.Ø2 **Encounter for adjustment and management of automatic implantable cardiac defibrillator**
Encounter for adjustment and management of automatic implantable cardiac defibrillator with synchronous cardiac pacemaker
Encounter for adjustment and management of cardiac resynchronization therapy defibrillator (CRT-D)

Z45.Ø9 **Encounter for adjustment and management of other cardiac device**

Z45.1 **Encounter for adjustment and management of infusion pump**

Z45.2 **Encounter for adjustment and management of vascular access device**
Encounter for adjustment and management of vascular catheters
EXCLUDES 1 *encounter for adjustment and management of renal dialysis catheter (Z49.Ø1)*

✓5ᵗʰ Z45.3 **Encounter for adjustment and management of implanted devices of the special senses**

Z45.31 **Encounter for adjustment and management of implanted visual substitution device**

✓6ᵗʰ Z45.32 **Encounter for adjustment and management of implanted hearing device**
EXCLUDES 1 *encounter for fitting and adjustment of hearing aide (Z46.1)*

Z45.32Ø **Encounter for adjustment and management of bone conduction device**

Z45.321 **Encounter for adjustment and management of cochlear device**

Z45.328 **Encounter for adjustment and management of other implanted hearing device**

✓5ᵗʰ Z45.4 **Encounter for adjustment and management of implanted nervous system device**

Z45.41 **Encounter for adjustment and management of cerebrospinal fluid drainage device**
Encounter for adjustment and management of cerebral ventricular (communicating) shunt

Z45.42 **Encounter for adjustment and management of neuropacemaker (brain) (peripheral nerve) (spinal cord)**

Z45.49 **Encounter for adjustment and management of other implanted nervous system device**
AHA: 2014, 3Q, 19

✓5ᵗʰ Z45.8 **Encounter for adjustment and management of other implanted devices**

✓6ᵗʰ Z45.81 **Encounter for adjustment or removal of breast implant**
Encounter for elective implant exchange (different material) (different size)
Encounter removal of tissue expander without synchronous insertion of permanent implant
EXCLUDES 1 *complications of breast implant (T85.4-)*
encounter for initial breast implant insertion for cosmetic breast augmentation (Z41.1)
encounter for breast reconstruction following mastectomy (Z42.1)

Z45.811 **Encounter for adjustment or removal of right breast implant**

Z45.812 **Encounter for adjustment or removal of left breast implant**

Z45.819 **Encounter for adjustment or removal of unspecified breast implant** ▽

Z45.82 **Encounter for adjustment or removal of myringotomy device (stent) (tube)**

Z45.89 **Encounter for adjustment and management of other implanted devices**
AHA: 2014, 4Q, 26-28

Z45.9 **Encounter for adjustment and management of unspecified implanted device** ▽

✓4ᵗʰ Z46 **Encounter for fitting and adjustment of other devices**
INCLUDES removal or replacement of other device
EXCLUDES 1 *malfunction or other complications of device—see Alphabetical Index*
EXCLUDES 2 *encounter for fitting and management of implanted devices (Z45.-)*
issue of repeat prescription only (Z76.Ø)
presence of prosthetic and other devices (Z95-Z97)

Z46.Ø **Encounter for fitting and adjustment of spectacles and contact lenses**

Z46.1 **Encounter for fitting and adjustment of hearing aid**
EXCLUDES 1 *encounter for adjustment and management of implanted hearing device (Z45.32-)*

Z46.2 **Encounter for fitting and adjustment of other devices related to nervous system and special senses**
EXCLUDES 2 *encounter for adjustment and management of implanted nervous system device (Z45.4-)*
encounter for adjustment and management of implanted visual substitution device (Z45.31)

Z46.3 **Encounter for fitting and adjustment of dental prosthetic device**
Encounter for fitting and adjustment of dentures

Z46.4 **Encounter for fitting and adjustment of orthodontic device**

✓5ᵗʰ Z46.5 **Encounter for fitting and adjustment of other gastrointestinal appliance and device**
EXCLUDES 1 *encounter for attention to artificial openings of digestive tract (Z43.1-Z43.4)*

Z46.51 **Encounter for fitting and adjustment of gastric lap band**

Z46.59 **Encounter for fitting and adjustment of other gastrointestinal appliance and device**

Z46.6 **Encounter for fitting and adjustment of urinary device**
EXCLUDES 2 *attention to artificial openings of urinary tract (Z43.5, Z43.6)*

✓5ᵗʰ Z46.8 **Encounter for fitting and adjustment of other specified devices**

Z46.81 **Encounter for fitting and adjustment of insulin pump**
Encounter for insulin pump instruction and training
Encounter for insulin pump titration

Z46.82 **Encounter for fitting and adjustment of non-vascular catheter**

Z46.89 **Encounter for fitting and adjustment of other specified devices**
Encounter for fitting and adjustment of wheelchair

Z46.9 **Encounter for fitting and adjustment of unspecified device** ▽

✓4ᵗʰ Z47 **Orthopedic aftercare**
EXCLUDES 1 *aftercare for healing fracture—code to fracture with 7th character D*

Z47.1 **Aftercare following joint replacement surgery**
Use additional code to identify the joint (Z96.6-)

Z47.2 **Encounter for removal of internal fixation device**
EXCLUDES 1 *encounter for adjustment of internal fixation device for fracture treatment—code to fracture with appropriate 7th character*
encounter for removal of external fixation device—code to fracture with 7th character D
infection or inflammatory reaction to internal fixation device (T84.6-)
mechanical complication of internal fixation device (T84.1-)

✓5ᵗʰ Z47.3 **Aftercare following explantation of joint prosthesis**
Aftercare following explantation of joint prosthesis, staged procedure
Encounter for joint prosthesis insertion following prior explantation of joint prosthesis
AHA: 2015, 1Q, 16

Z47.31 **Aftercare following explantation of shoulder joint prosthesis**
EXCLUDES 1 *acquired absence of shoulder joint following prior explantation of shoulder joint prosthesis (Z89.23-)*
shoulder joint prosthesis explantation status (Z89.23-)

Z47.32 **Aftercare following explantation of** hip **joint prosthesis**
> EXCLUDES 1   acquired absence of hip joint following prior explantation of hip joint prosthesis (Z89.62-)
> hip joint prosthesis explantation status (Z89.62-)

Z47.33 **Aftercare following explantation of** knee **joint prosthesis**
> EXCLUDES 1   acquired absence of knee joint following prior explantation of knee prosthesis (Z89.52-)
> knee joint prosthesis explantation status (Z89.52-)

✓5th **Z47.8** **Encounter for other orthopedic aftercare**

Z47.81 **Encounter for orthopedic aftercare** following surgical amputation
> Use additional code to identify the limb amputated (Z89.-)

Z47.82 **Encounter for orthopedic aftercare** following scoliosis surgery

Z47.89 **Encounter for other orthopedic aftercare**
> AHA: 2015, 1Q, 8

☑4th **Z48** **Encounter for other postprocedural aftercare**
> EXCLUDES 1 ▶encounter for aftercare following injury – code to Injury, by site, with appropriate 7th character for subsequent encounter◀
> encounter for follow-up examination after completed treatment (Z08-Z09)
> EXCLUDES 2   encounter for attention to artificial openings (Z43.-)
> encounter for fitting and adjustment of prosthetic and other devices (Z44-Z46)
> AHA: 2015, 4Q, 38; 2015, 1Q, 6-7

✓5th **Z48.0** **Encounter for** attention to dressings, sutures and drains
> EXCLUDES 1   encounter for planned postprocedural wound closure (Z48.1)

Z48.00 **Encounter for change or removal of** nonsurgical wound dressing
> Encounter for change or removal of wound dressing NOS

Z48.01 **Encounter for change or removal of** surgical wound dressing

Z48.02 **Encounter for removal of** sutures
> Encounter for removal of staples

Z48.03 **Encounter for change or removal of** drains

Z48.1 **Encounter for planned** postprocedural **wound closure**
> EXCLUDES 1   encounter for attention to dressings and sutures (Z48.0-)

✓5th **Z48.2** **Encounter for aftercare following** organ transplant

Z48.21 **Encounter for aftercare following** heart transplant   HCC

Z48.22 **Encounter for aftercare following** kidney **transplant**

Z48.23 **Encounter for aftercare following** liver transplant   HCC

Z48.24 **Encounter for aftercare following** lung transplant   HCC

✓6th **Z48.28** **Encounter for aftercare following** multiple **organ transplant**

Z48.280 **Encounter for aftercare following** heart-lung **transplant**   HCC

Z48.288 **Encounter for aftercare following** multiple **organ transplant**

✓6th **Z48.29** **Encounter for aftercare following other organ transplant**

Z48.290 **Encounter for aftercare following** bone marrow **transplant**   HCC

Z48.298 **Encounter for aftercare following other organ transplant**

Z48.3 **Aftercare following** surgery for neoplasm
> Use additional code to identify the neoplasm

✓5th **Z48.8** **Encounter for other specified postprocedural aftercare**

✓6th **Z48.81** **Encounter for surgical aftercare following** surgery on specified body systems
> NOTE   These codes identify the body system requiring aftercare. They are for use in conjunction with other aftercare codes to fully explain the aftercare encounter. The condition treated should also be coded if still present.
> EXCLUDES 1   aftercare for injury—code the injury with 7th character D
> aftercare following surgery for neoplasm (Z48.3)
> EXCLUDES 2   aftercare following organ transplant (Z48.2-) orthopedic aftercare (Z47.-)
> AHA: 2015, 4Q, 38

Z48.810 **Encounter for surgical aftercare following surgery on the** sense organs

Z48.811 **Encounter for surgical aftercare following surgery on the** nervous system
> EXCLUDES 2   encounter for surgical aftercare following surgery on the sense organs (Z48.810)

Z48.812 **Encounter for surgical aftercare following surgery on the** circulatory system
> AHA: 2012, 4Q, 96

Z48.813 **Encounter for surgical aftercare following surgery on the** respiratory system

Z48.814 **Encounter for surgical aftercare following surgery on the** teeth or oral cavity

Z48.815 **Encounter for surgical aftercare following surgery on the** digestive system

Z48.816 **Encounter for surgical aftercare following surgery on the** genitourinary system
> EXCLUDES 1   encounter for aftercare following sterilization reversal (Z31.42)

Z48.817 **Encounter for surgical aftercare following surgery on the** skin and subcutaneous tissue

Z48.89 **Encounter for other specified surgical aftercare**

☑4th **Z49** **Encounter for care involving renal dialysis**
> Code also associated end stage renal disease (N18.6)

✓5th **Z49.0** Preparatory care **for renal dialysis**
> Encounter for dialysis instruction and training

Z49.01 **Encounter for fitting and adjustment of** extracorporeal dialysis catheter   HCC
> Removal or replacement of renal dialysis catheter
> Toilet or cleansing of renal dialysis catheter

Z49.02 **Encounter for fitting and adjustment of** peritoneal dialysis catheter   HCC

✓5th **Z49.3** **Encounter for** adequacy testing for dialysis

Z49.31 **Encounter for adequacy testing for** hemodialysis   HCC

Z49.32 **Encounter for adequacy testing for** peritoneal dialysis   HCC
> Encounter for peritoneal equilibration test

☑4th **Z51** **Encounter for other aftercare and medical care**
> Code also condition requiring care
> EXCLUDES 1   follow-up examination after treatment (Z08-Z09)

Z51.0 **Encounter for antineoplastic** radiation therapy   PDx

✓5th **Z51.1** **Encounter for antineoplastic chemotherapy and immunotherapy**
> EXCLUDES 2   encounter for chemotherapy and immunotherapy for nonneoplastic condition—code to condition

Z51.11 **Encounter for antineoplastic** chemotherapy   PDx
> AHA: 2015, 3Q, 19

Z51.12 **Encounter for antineoplastic** immunotherapy   PDx

Z51.5 **Encounter for** palliative care
> AHA: 2017, 1Q, 48

Z51.6 **Encounter for** desensitization to allergens

☑ Additional Character Req   ✓x7th Placeholder Alert   Manifestation   HCC CMS-HCC Condition   ▽ Unspecified Code   ▶◀ Revised Text   ● New Code   ▲ Revised Code Title

ICD-10-CM 2018   1191

Chapter 21. Factors Influencing Health Status and Contact with Health Services

Z47.32–Z51.6

Chapter 21. Factors Influencing Health Status and Contact with Health Services

Z51.8–Z57.9

✓5ᵗʰ **Z51.8 Encounter for other specified aftercare**
     EXCLUDES 1   *holiday relief care (Z75.5)*

     Z51.81 Encounter for therapeutic drug level monitoring
         Code also any long-term (current) drug therapy (Z79.-)
         EXCLUDES 1   *encounter for blood-drug test for administrative or medicolegal reasons (Z02.83)*
         DEF: Drug monitoring: Measurement of the level of a specific drug in the body or measurement of a specific function to assess effectiveness of a drug.

     Z51.89 Encounter for other specified aftercare
         AHA: 2012, 4Q, 95-97

✓4ᵗʰ **Z52 Donors of organs and tissues**
     INCLUDES   autologous and other living donors
     EXCLUDES 1   *cadaveric donor—omit code*
         examination of potential donor (Z00.5)
     AHA: 2012, 4Q, 99

✓5ᵗʰ **Z52.0 Blood donor**

     ✓6ᵗʰ **Z52.00 Unspecified blood donor**
         Z52.000 Unspecified donor, whole blood PDx ▽
         Z52.001 Unspecified donor, stem cells PDx ▽
         Z52.008 Unspecified donor, other blood PDx ▽

     ✓6ᵗʰ **Z52.01 Autologous blood donor**
         Z52.010 Autologous donor, whole blood PDx
         Z52.011 Autologous donor, stem cells PDx
         Z52.018 Autologous donor, other blood PDx

     ✓6ᵗʰ **Z52.09 Other blood donor**
         Volunteer donor
         Z52.090 Other blood donor, whole blood PDx
         Z52.091 Other blood donor, stem cells PDx
         Z52.098 Other blood donor, other blood PDx

✓5ᵗʰ **Z52.1 Skin donor**
     Z52.10 Skin donor, unspecified PDx ▽
     Z52.11 Skin donor, autologous PDx
     Z52.19 Skin donor, other PDx

✓5ᵗʰ **Z52.2 Bone donor**
     Z52.20 Bone donor, unspecified PDx ▽
     Z52.21 Bone donor, autologous PDx
     Z52.29 Bone donor, other PDx

Z52.3 Bone marrow donor PDx

Z52.4 Kidney donor PDx

Z52.5 Cornea donor PDx

Z52.6 Liver donor PDx

✓5ᵗʰ **Z52.8 Donor of other specified organs or tissues**

     ✓6ᵗʰ **Z52.81 Egg (Oocyte) donor**
         Z52.810 Egg (Oocyte) donor under age 35, anonymous recipient PDx ♀
         Egg donor under age 35 NOS
         Z52.811 Egg (Oocyte) donor under age 35, designated recipient PDx ♀
         Z52.812 Egg (Oocyte) donor age 35 and over, anonymous recipient PDx ♀
         Egg donor age 35 and over NOS
         Z52.813 Egg (Oocyte) donor age 35 and over, designated recipient PDx ♀
         Z52.819 Egg (Oocyte) donor, unspecified PDx ♀ ▽

     Z52.89 Donor of other specified organs or tissues PDx

Z52.9 Donor of unspecified organ or tissue ▽
     Donor NOS

✓4ᵗʰ **Z53 Persons encountering health services for specific procedures and treatment, not carried out**

     ✓5ᵗʰ **Z53.0 Procedure and treatment not carried out because of contraindication**
         Z53.01 Procedure and treatment not carried out due to patient smoking
         Z53.09 Procedure and treatment not carried out because of other contraindication

     Z53.1 Procedure and treatment not carried out because of patient's decision for reasons of belief and group pressure

     ✓5ᵗʰ **Z53.2 Procedure and treatment not carried out because of patient's decision for other and unspecified reasons**
         Z53.20 Procedure and treatment not carried out because of patient's decision for unspecified reasons ▽

         Z53.21 Procedure and treatment not carried out due to patient leaving prior to being seen by health care provider
         Z53.29 Procedure and treatment not carried out because of patient's decision for other reasons

     ✓5ᵗʰ **Z53.3 Procedure converted to open procedure**
         Z53.31 Laparoscopic surgical procedure converted to open procedure
         Z53.32 Thoracoscopic surgical procedure converted to open procedure
         Z53.33 Arthroscopic surgical procedure converted to open procedure
         Z53.39 Other specified procedure converted to open procedure

     Z53.8 Procedure and treatment not carried out for other reasons
     Z53.9 Procedure and treatment not carried out, unspecified reason ▽

Persons with potential health hazards related to socioeconomic and psychosocial circumstances (Z55-Z65)

✓4ᵗʰ **Z55 Problems related to education and literacy**
     EXCLUDES 1   *disorders of psychological development (F80-F89)*

     Z55.0 Illiteracy and low-level literacy
     Z55.1 Schooling unavailable and unattainable
     Z55.2 Failed school examinations
     Z55.3 Underachievement in school
     Z55.4 Educational maladjustment and discord with teachers and classmates
     Z55.8 Other problems related to education and literacy
         Problems related to inadequate teaching
     Z55.9 Problems related to education and literacy, unspecified ▽
         Academic problems NOS

✓4ᵗʰ **Z56 Problems related to employment and unemployment**
     EXCLUDES 2   *occupational exposure to risk factors (Z57.-)*
         problems related to housing and economic circumstances (Z59.-)

     Z56.0 Unemployment, unspecified ▽
     Z56.1 Change of job A
     Z56.2 Threat of job loss
     Z56.3 Stressful work schedule
     Z56.4 Discord with boss and workmates
     Z56.5 Uncongenial work environment
         Difficult conditions at work
     Z56.6 Other physical and mental strain related to work

     ✓5ᵗʰ **Z56.8 Other problems related to employment**
         Z56.81 Sexual harassment on the job
         Z56.82 Military deployment status
         Individual (civilian or military) currently deployed in theater or in support of military war, peacekeeping and humanitarian operations
         Z56.89 Other problems related to employment

     Z56.9 Unspecified problems related to employment ▽
         Occupational problems NOS

✓4ᵗʰ **Z57 Occupational exposure to risk factors**
     Z57.0 Occupational exposure to noise
     Z57.1 Occupational exposure to radiation
     Z57.2 Occupational exposure to dust

     ✓5ᵗʰ **Z57.3 Occupational exposure to other air contaminants**
         Z57.31 Occupational exposure to environmental tobacco smoke
         EXCLUDES 2   *exposure to environmental tobacco smoke (Z77.22)*
         Z57.39 Occupational exposure to other air contaminants

     Z57.4 Occupational exposure to toxic agents in agriculture
         Occupational exposure to solids, liquids, gases or vapors in agriculture
     Z57.5 Occupational exposure to toxic agents in other industries
         Occupational exposure to solids, liquids, gases or vapors in other industries
     Z57.6 Occupational exposure to extreme temperature
     Z57.7 Occupational exposure to vibration
     Z57.8 Occupational exposure to other risk factors
     Z57.9 Occupational exposure to unspecified risk factor ▽

EXCLUDES 1 Not coded here   EXCLUDES 2 Not included here   N Newborn Age: 0   P Pediatric Age: 0-17   M Maternity Age: 12-55   A Adult Age: 15-124   PDx Primary Dx

1192   ICD-10-CM 2018

☑4ᵗʰ **Z59** **Problems related to housing and economic circumstances**
  EXCLUDES 2   *problems related to upbringing (Z62.-)*

Z59.0 **Homelessness**

Z59.1 **Inadequate housing**
  Lack of heating
  Restriction of space
  Technical defects in home preventing adequate care
  Unsatisfactory surroundings
  EXCLUDES 1   *problems related to the natural and physical environment (Z77.1-)*

Z59.2 **Discord with neighbors, lodgers and landlord**

Z59.3 **Problems related to living in residential institution**
  Boarding-school resident
  EXCLUDES 1   *institutional upbringing (Z62.2)*

Z59.4 **Lack of adequate food and safe drinking water**
  Inadequate drinking water supply
  EXCLUDES 1   *effects of hunger (T73.0)*
      inappropriate diet or eating habits (Z72.4)
      malnutrition (E40-E46)

Z59.5 **Extreme poverty**

Z59.6 **Low income**

Z59.7 **Insufficient social insurance and welfare support**

Z59.8 **Other problems related to housing and economic circumstances**
  Foreclosure on loan
  Isolated dwelling
  Problems with creditors

Z59.9 **Problem related to housing and economic circumstances, unspecified**   ▽

☑4ᵗʰ **Z60** **Problems related to social environment**

Z60.0 **Problems of adjustment to life-cycle transitions**
  Empty nest syndrome
  Phase of life problem
  Problem with adjustment to retirement [pension]

Z60.2 **Problems related to living alone**

Z60.3 **Acculturation difficulty**
  Problem with migration
  Problem with social transplantation
  DEF: A problem in adapting to a different culture or environment not based on any coexisting mental disorder.

Z60.4 **Social exclusion and rejection**
  Exclusion and rejection on the basis of personal characteristics, such as unusual physical appearance, illness or behavior.
  EXCLUDES 1   *target of adverse discrimination such as for racial or religious reasons (Z60.5)*

Z60.5 **Target of (perceived) adverse discrimination and persecution**
  EXCLUDES 1   *social exclusion and rejection (Z60.4)*

Z60.8 **Other problems related to social environment**

Z60.9 **Problem related to social environment, unspecified**   ▽

☑4ᵗʰ **Z62** **Problems related to upbringing**
  INCLUDES   current and past negative life events in childhood
      current and past problems of a child related to upbringing
  EXCLUDES 2   *maltreatment syndrome (T74.-)*
      problems related to housing and economic circumstances (Z59.-)

Z62.0 **Inadequate parental supervision and control**

Z62.1 **Parental overprotection**

☑5ᵗʰ **Z62.2** **Upbringing away from parents**
  EXCLUDES 1   *problems with boarding school (Z59.3)*

  Z62.21 **Child in welfare custody**   P
    Child in care of non-parental family member
    Child in foster care
    EXCLUDES 2   *problem for parent due to child in welfare custody (Z63.5)*

  Z62.22 **Institutional upbringing**
    Child living in orphanage or group home

  Z62.29 **Other upbringing away from parents**

Z62.3 **Hostility towards and scapegoating of child**   P

Z62.6 **Inappropriate (excessive) parental pressure**

☑5ᵗʰ **Z62.8** **Other specified problems related to upbringing**

  ☑6ᵗʰ **Z62.81** **Personal history of abuse in childhood**

    Z62.810 **Personal history of** physical and sexual **abuse in childhood**
      EXCLUDES 1   *current child physical abuse (T74.12, T76.12)*
          current child sexual abuse (T74.22, T76.22)

    Z62.811 **Personal history of** psychological abuse **in childhood**
      EXCLUDES 1   *current child psychological abuse (T74.32, T76.32)*

    Z62.812 **Personal history of** neglect **in childhood**
      EXCLUDES 1   *current child neglect (T74.02, T76.02)*

    Z62.819 **Personal history of unspecified abuse in childhood**   ▽
      EXCLUDES 1   *current child abuse NOS (T74.92, T76.92)*

  ☑6ᵗʰ **Z62.82** **Parent-child conflict**

    Z62.820 **Parent-**biological **child conflict**
      Parent-child problem NOS

    Z62.821 **Parent-**adopted **child conflict**

    Z62.822 **Parent-**foster **child conflict**

  ☑6ᵗʰ **Z62.89** **Other specified problems related to upbringing**

    Z62.890 **Parent-child estrangement NEC**

    Z62.891 **Sibling rivalry**

    Z62.898 **Other specified problems related to upbringing**

Z62.9 **Problem related to upbringing, unspecified**   ▽

☑4ᵗʰ **Z63** **Other problems related to primary support group, including family circumstances**
  EXCLUDES 2   *maltreatment syndrome (T74-, T76)*
      parent-child problems (Z62.-)
      problems related to negative life events in childhood (Z62.-)
      problems related to upbringing (Z62.-)

Z63.0 **Problems in relationship with** spouse or partner
  ▶Relationship distress with spouse or intimate partner◀
  EXCLUDES 1   *counseling for spousal or partner abuse problems (Z69.1)*
      counseling related to sexual attitude, behavior, and orientation (Z70.-)

Z63.1 **Problems in relationship with** in-laws

☑5ᵗʰ **Z63.3** **Absence of family member**
  EXCLUDES 1   *absence of family member due to disappearance and death (Z63.4)*
      absence of family member due to separation and divorce (Z63.5)

  Z63.31 **Absence of family member due to military deployment**
    Individual or family affected by other family member being on military deployment
    EXCLUDES 1   *family disruption due to return of family member from military deployment (Z63.71)*

  Z63.32 **Other absence of family member**

Z63.4 **Disappearance and death of family member**
  Assumed death of family member
  Bereavement
  AHA: 2014, 1Q, 25

Z63.5 **Disruption of family by separation and divorce**
  Marital estrangement

Z63.6 **Dependent relative needing care at home**

☑5ᵗʰ **Z63.7** **Other stressful life events affecting family and household**

  Z63.71 **Stress on family due to return of family member from military deployment**
    Individual or family affected by family member having returned from military deployment (current or past conflict)

  Z63.72 **Alcoholism and drug addiction in family**

  Z63.79 **Other stressful life events affecting family and household**
    Anxiety (normal) about sick person in family
    Health problems within family
    Ill or disturbed family member
    Isolated family

Z63.8 **Other specified problems related to primary support group**
  Family discord NOS
  Family estrangement NOS
  High expressed emotional level within family
  Inadequate family support NOS
  Inadequate or distorted communication within family

Z63.9 **Problem related to primary support group, unspecified**   ▽
  Relationship disorder NOS

☑ Additional Character Req   ☑x7ᵗʰ Placeholder Alert   Manifestation   HCC CMS-HCC Condition   ▽ Unspecified Code   ▶◀ Revised Text   ● New Code   ▲ Revised Code Title

Chapter 21. Factors Influencing Health Status and Contact with Health Services *(side margin)*

✓4ᵗʰ Z64 Problems related to certain psychosocial circumstances

Z64.0   **Problems related to unwanted pregnancy** ♀

Z64.1   **Problems related to multiparity** ♀

Z64.4   **Discord with counselors**
Discord with probation officer
Discord with social worker

✓4ᵗʰ Z65 Problems related to other psychosocial circumstances

Z65.0   **Conviction in civil and criminal proceedings without imprisonment**

Z65.1   **Imprisonment and other incarceration**

Z65.2   **Problems related to release from prison**

Z65.3   **Problems related to other legal circumstances**
Arrest
Child custody or support proceedings
Litigation
Prosecution

Z65.4   **Victim of crime and terrorism**
Victim of torture

Z65.5   **Exposure to disaster, war and other hostilities**
EXCLUDES 1   *target of perceived discrimination or persecution (Z60.5)*

Z65.8   **Other specified problems related to psychosocial circumstances**
▶Religious or spiritual problem◀

Z65.9   **Problem related to unspecified psychosocial circumstances** ▽

Do not resuscitate status (Z66)

Z66 Do not resuscitate
DNR status
DEF: Medical order written by a physician that instructs others not to perform cardiopulmonary resuscitation (CPR), intubation, or advanced life support (ACLS); prevents unnecessary invasive treatment to prolong life should breathing stop or cardiac arrest occur.

Blood type (Z67)

✓4ᵗʰ Z67 Blood type
AHA: 2015, 3Q, 40

✓5ᵗʰ Z67.1   Type A blood
Z67.10   Type A blood, Rh positive
Z67.11   Type A blood, Rh negative

✓5ᵗʰ Z67.2   Type B blood
Z67.20   Type B blood, Rh positive
Z67.21   Type B blood, Rh negative

✓5ᵗʰ Z67.3   Type AB blood
Z67.30   Type AB blood, Rh positive
Z67.31   Type AB blood, Rh negative

✓5ᵗʰ Z67.4   Type O blood
Z67.40   Type O blood, Rh positive
Z67.41   Type O blood, Rh negative

✓5ᵗʰ Z67.9   Unspecified blood type
Z67.90   Unspecified blood type, Rh positive ▽
Z67.91   Unspecified blood type, Rh negative ▽

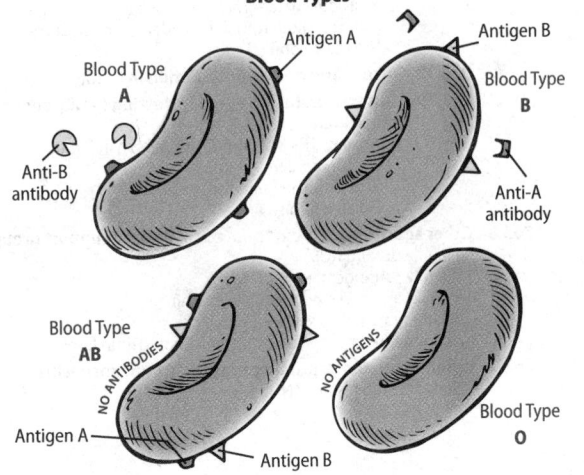

Blood Types

Blood Type A — Antigen A — Anti-B antibody
Blood Type B — Antigen B — Anti-A antibody
Blood Type AB — NO ANTIBODIES
Blood Type O — Antigen A — Antigen B — NO ANTIGENS

Body mass index [BMI] (Z68)

✓4ᵗʰ Z68 Body mass index [BMI]
Kilograms per meters squared
NOTE   BMI adult codes are for use for persons 21 years of age or older.
BMI pediatric codes are for use for persons 2-20 years of age. These percentiles are based on the growth charts published by the Centers for Disease Control and Prevention (CDC).
AHA: 2017, 1Q, 39
DEF: Index used to help determine whether an individual is underweight, a healthy weight, overweight, or obese.

▲ Z68.1   Body mass index [BMI] 19.9 or less, adult   Ⓐ

✓5ᵗʰ Z68.2   Body mass index [BMI] 20-29, adult
Z68.20   Body mass index [BMI] 20.0-20.9, adult Ⓐ
Z68.21   Body mass index [BMI] 21.0-21.9, adult Ⓐ
Z68.22   Body mass index [BMI] 22.0-22.9, adult Ⓐ
Z68.23   Body mass index [BMI] 23.0-23.9, adult Ⓐ
Z68.24   Body mass index [BMI] 24.0-24.9, adult Ⓐ
Z68.25   Body mass index [BMI] 25.0-25.9, adult Ⓐ
Z68.26   Body mass index [BMI] 26.0-26.9, adult Ⓐ
Z68.27   Body mass index [BMI] 27.0-27.9, adult Ⓐ
Z68.28   Body mass index [BMI] 28.0-28.9, adult Ⓐ
Z68.29   Body mass index [BMI] 29.0-29.9, adult Ⓐ

✓5ᵗʰ Z68.3   Body mass index [BMI] 30-39, adult
Z68.30   Body mass index [BMI] 30.0-30.9, adult Ⓐ
Z68.31   Body mass index [BMI] 31.0-31.9, adult Ⓐ
Z68.32   Body mass index [BMI] 32.0-32.9, adult Ⓐ
Z68.33   Body mass index [BMI] 33.0-33.9, adult Ⓐ
Z68.34   Body mass index [BMI] 34.0-34.9, adult Ⓐ
Z68.35   Body mass index [BMI] 35.0-35.9, adult Ⓐ
Z68.36   Body mass index [BMI] 36.0-36.9, adult Ⓐ
Z68.37   Body mass index [BMI] 37.0-37.9, adult Ⓐ
Z68.38   Body mass index [BMI] 38.0-38.9, adult Ⓐ
Z68.39   Body mass index [BMI] 39.0-39.9, adult Ⓐ

✓5ᵗʰ Z68.4   Body mass index [BMI] 40 or greater, adult
Z68.41   Body mass index [BMI] 40.0-44.9, adult HCC Ⓐ
Z68.42   Body mass index [BMI] 45.0-49.9, adult HCC Ⓐ
Z68.43   Body mass index [BMI] 50-59.9, adult HCC Ⓐ
Z68.44   Body mass index [BMI] 60.0-69.9, adult HCC Ⓐ
Z68.45   Body mass index [BMI] 70 or greater, adult HCC Ⓐ

✓5ᵗʰ Z68.5   Body mass index [BMI] pediatric
Z68.51   Body mass index [BMI] pediatric, less than 5th percentile for age
Z68.52   Body mass index [BMI] pediatric, 5th percentile to less than 85th percentile for age
Z68.53   Body mass index [BMI] pediatric, 85th percentile to less than 95th percentile for age
Z68.54   Body mass index [BMI] pediatric, greater than or equal to 95th percentile for age

Persons encountering health services in other circumstances (Z69-Z76)

✓4ᵗʰ Z69 Encounter for mental health services for victim and perpetrator of abuse
INCLUDES   counseling for victims and perpetrators of abuse

✓5ᵗʰ Z69.0   Encounter for mental health services for child abuse problems
✓6ᵗʰ Z69.01   Encounter for mental health services for parental child abuse
Z69.010   Encounter for mental health services for victim of parental child abuse Ⓟ
▶Encounter for mental health services for victim of child abuse by parent
Encounter for mental health services for victim of child neglect by parent
Encounter for mental health services for victim of child psychological abuse by parent
Encounter for mental health services for victim of child sexual abuse by parent◀

EXCLUDES 1 Not coded here   EXCLUDES 2 Not included here   Ⓝ Newborn Age: 0   Ⓟ Pediatric Age: 0-17   Ⓜ Maternity Age: 12-55   Ⓐ Adult Age: 15-124   PDx Primary Dx

1194   ICD-10-CM 2018

Z69.011 Encounter for mental health services for perpetrator of parental child abuse
► Encounter for mental health services for perpetrator of parental child neglect
Encounter for mental health services for perpetrator of parental child psychological abuse
Encounter for mental health services for perpetrator of parental child sexual abuse ◄
EXCLUDES 1 encounter for mental health services for non-parental child abuse (Z69.02-)

✓6th **Z69.02 Encounter for mental health services for non-parental child abuse**

Z69.020 Encounter for mental health services for victim of non-parental child abuse P
► Encounter for mental health services for victim of non-parental child neglect
Encounter for mental health services for victim of non-parental child psychological abuse
Encounter for mental health services for victim of non-parental child sexual abuse ◄

Z69.021 Encounter for mental health services for perpetrator of non-parental child abuse
► Encounter for mental health services for perpetrator of non-parental child neglect
Encounter for mental health services for perpetrator of non-parental child psychological abuse
Encounter for mental health services for perpetrator of non-parental child sexual abuse ◄

✓5th **Z69.1 Encounter for mental health services for spousal or partner abuse problems**

Z69.11 Encounter for mental health services for victim of spousal or partner abuse
► Encounter for mental health services for victim of spouse or partner neglect
Encounter for mental health services for victim of spouse or partner psychological abuse
Encounter for mental health services for victim of spouse or partner violence, physical ◄

Z69.12 Encounter for mental health services for perpetrator of spousal or partner abuse
► Encounter for mental health services for perpetrator of spouse or partner neglect
Encounter for mental health services for perpetrator of spouse or partner psychological abuse
Encounter for mental health services for perpetrator of spouse or partner violence, physical
Encounter for mental health services for perpetrator of spouse or partner violence, sexual ◄

✓5th **Z69.8 Encounter for mental health services for victim or perpetrator of other abuse**

Z69.81 Encounter for mental health services for victim of other abuse
► Encounter for mental health services for perpetrator of non-spousal adult abuse
Encounter for mental health services for victim of non-spousal adult abuse
Encounter for mental health services for victim of spouse or partner violence, sexual ◄
Encounter for rape victim counseling

Z69.82 Encounter for mental health services for perpetrator of other abuse

✓4th **Z70 Counseling related to sexual attitude, behavior and orientation**
INCLUDES encounter for mental health services for sexual attitude, behavior and orientation
EXCLUDES 2 contraceptive or procreative counseling (Z30-Z31)

Z70.0 Counseling related to sexual attitude

Z70.1 Counseling related to patient's sexual behavior and orientation
Patient concerned regarding impotence
Patient concerned regarding non-responsiveness
Patient concerned regarding promiscuity
Patient concerned regarding sexual orientation

Z70.2 Counseling related to sexual behavior and orientation of third party
Advice sought regarding sexual behavior and orientation of child
Advice sought regarding sexual behavior and orientation of partner
Advice sought regarding sexual behavior and orientation of spouse

Z70.3 Counseling related to combined concerns regarding sexual attitude, behavior and orientation

Z70.8 Other sex counseling
Encounter for sex education

Z70.9 Sex counseling, unspecified ▽

✓4th **Z71 Persons encountering health services for other counseling and medical advice, not elsewhere classified**
EXCLUDES 2 contraceptive or procreation counseling (Z30-Z31)
sex counseling (Z70.-)

Z71.0 Person encountering health services to consult on behalf of another person
Person encountering health services to seek advice or treatment for non-attending third party
EXCLUDES 2 anxiety (normal) about sick person in family (Z63.7)
expectant (adoptive) parent(s) pre-birth pediatrician visit (Z76.81)

Z71.1 Person with feared health complaint in whom no diagnosis is made
Person encountering health services with feared condition which was not demonstrated
Person encountering health services in which problem was normal state
"Worried well"
EXCLUDES 1 medical observation for suspected diseases and conditions proven not to exist (Z03.-)

Z71.2 Person consulting for explanation of examination or test findings

Z71.3 Dietary counseling and surveillance
Use additional code for any associated underlying medical condition
Use additional code to identify body mass index (BMI), if known (Z68.-)

✓5th **Z71.4 Alcohol abuse counseling and surveillance**
Use additional code for alcohol abuse or dependence (F10.-)

Z71.41 Alcohol abuse counseling and surveillance of alcoholic

Z71.42 Counseling for family member of alcoholic
Counseling for significant other, partner, or friend of alcoholic

✓5th **Z71.5 Drug abuse counseling and surveillance**
Use additional code for drug abuse or dependence (F11-F16, F18-F19)

Z71.51 Drug abuse counseling and surveillance of drug abuser

Z71.52 Counseling for family member of drug abuser
Counseling for significant other, partner, or friend of drug abuser

Z71.6 Tobacco abuse counseling
Use additional code for nicotine dependence (F17.-)

Z71.7 Human immunodeficiency virus [HIV] counseling

✓5th **Z71.8 Other specified counseling**
EXCLUDES 2 counseling for contraception (Z30.0-)
counseling for genetics (Z31.5)
counseling for procreative management (Z31.6-)

Z71.81 Spiritual or religious counseling

Z71.82 Exercise counseling

Z71.83 Encounter for nonprocreative genetic counseling
EXCLUDES 1 counseling for procreative genetics (Z31.5)
counseling for procreative management (Z31.6)

Z71.89 Other specified counseling

Z71.9 Counseling, unspecified ▽
Encounter for medical advice NOS

✓4th Z72 Problems related to lifestyle
> EXCLUDES 2   problems related to life-management difficulty (Z73.-)
> problems related to socioeconomic and psychosocial circumstances (Z55-Z65)

Z72.0 Tobacco use
Tobacco use NOS
> EXCLUDES 1   history of tobacco dependence (Z87.891)
> nicotine dependence (F17.2-)
> tobacco dependence (F17.2-)
> tobacco use during pregnancy (O99.33-)

Z72.3 Lack of physical exercise

Z72.4 Inappropriate diet and eating habits
> EXCLUDES 1   behavioral eating disorders of infancy or childhood (F98.2- F98.3)
> eating disorders (F50.-)
> lack of adequate food (Z59.4)
> malnutrition and other nutritional deficiencies (E40-E64)

✓5th Z72.5 High risk sexual behavior
Promiscuity
> EXCLUDES 1   paraphilias (F65)

Z72.51 High risk heterosexual behavior

Z72.52 High risk homosexual behavior

Z72.53 High risk bisexual behavior

Z72.6 Gambling and betting
> EXCLUDES 1   compulsive or pathological gambling (F63.0)

✓5th Z72.8 Other problems related to lifestyle

✓6th Z72.81 Antisocial behavior
> EXCLUDES 1   conduct disorders (F91.-)

Z72.810 Child and adolescent antisocial behavior   P
Antisocial behavior (child) (adolescent) without manifest psychiatric disorder
Delinquency NOS
Group delinquency
Offenses in the context of gang membership
Stealing in company with others
Truancy from school

Z72.811 Adult antisocial behavior   A
Adult antisocial behavior without manifest psychiatric disorder

✓6th Z72.82 Problems related to sleep

Z72.820 Sleep deprivation
Lack of adequate sleep
> EXCLUDES 1   insomnia (G47.0-)

Z72.821 Inadequate sleep hygiene
Bad sleep habits
Irregular sleep habits
Unhealthy sleep wake schedule
> EXCLUDES 1   insomnia (F51.0-, G47.0-)

Z72.89 Other problems related to lifestyle
Self-damaging behavior

Z72.9 Problem related to lifestyle, unspecified ▽

✓4th Z73 Problems related to life management difficulty
> EXCLUDES 2   problems related to socioeconomic and psychosocial circumstances (Z55-Z65)

DEF: State of emotional, mental, and physical exhaustion; causing difficulties in managing personal, school, or work circumstances; usually due to prolonged stress; poor interpersonal relationship skills, or parenting skills.

Z73.0 Burn-out

Z73.1 Type A behavior pattern

Z73.2 Lack of relaxation and leisure

Z73.3 Stress, not elsewhere classified
Physical and mental strain NOS
> EXCLUDES 1   stress related to employment or unemployment (Z56.-)

Z73.4 Inadequate social skills, not elsewhere classified

Z73.5 Social role conflict, not elsewhere classified

Z73.6 Limitation of activities due to disability
> EXCLUDES 1   care-provider dependency (Z74.-)

✓5th Z73.8 Other problems related to life management difficulty

✓6th Z73.81 Behavioral insomnia of childhood
> **DEF:** Behaviors on the part of the child or caregivers that cause negative compliance with a child's sleep schedule; results in lack of adequate sleep.

Z73.810 Behavioral insomnia of childhood, sleep-onset association type   P

Z73.811 Behavioral insomnia of childhood, limit setting type   P

Z73.812 Behavioral insomnia of childhood, combined type   P

Z73.819 Behavioral insomnia of childhood, unspecified type   P ▽

Z73.82 Dual sensory impairment

Z73.89 Other problems related to life management difficulty

Z73.9 Problem related to life management difficulty, unspecified ▽

✓4th Z74 Problems related to care provider dependency
> EXCLUDES 2   dependence on enabling machines or devices NEC (Z99.-)

✓5th Z74.0 Reduced mobility

Z74.01 Bed confinement status
Bedridden

Z74.09 Other reduced mobility
Chair ridden
Reduced mobility NOS
> EXCLUDES 2   wheelchair dependence (Z99.3)

Z74.1 Need for assistance with personal care

Z74.2 Need for assistance at home and no other household member able to render care

Z74.3 Need for continuous supervision

Z74.8 Other problems related to care provider dependency

Z74.9 Problem related to care provider dependency, unspecified ▽

✓4th Z75 Problems related to medical facilities and other health care

Z75.0 Medical services not available in home
> EXCLUDES 1   no other household member able to render care (Z74.2)

Z75.1 Person awaiting admission to adequate facility elsewhere

Z75.2 Other waiting period for investigation and treatment

Z75.3 Unavailability and inaccessibility of health-care facilities
> EXCLUDES 1   bed unavailable (Z75.1)

Z75.4 Unavailability and inaccessibility of other helping agencies

Z75.5 Holiday relief care

Z75.8 Other problems related to medical facilities and other health care

Z75.9 Unspecified problem related to medical facilities and other health care ▽

✓4th Z76 Persons encountering health services in other circumstances

Z76.0 Encounter for issue of repeat prescription
Encounter for issue of repeat prescription for appliance
Encounter for issue of repeat prescription for medicaments
Encounter for issue of repeat prescription for spectacles
> EXCLUDES 2   issue of medical certificate (Z02.7)
> repeat prescription for contraceptive (Z30.4-)

Z76.1 Encounter for health supervision and care of foundling   PDx

Z76.2 Encounter for health supervision and care of other healthy infant and child   PDx P
Encounter for medical or nursing care or supervision of healthy infant under circumstances such as adverse socioeconomic conditions at home
Encounter for medical or nursing care or supervision of healthy infant under circumstances such as awaiting foster or adoptive placement
Encounter for medical or nursing care or supervision of healthy infant under circumstances such as maternal illness
Encounter for medical or nursing care or supervision of healthy infant under circumstances such as number of children at home preventing or interfering with normal care

Z76.3 Healthy person accompanying sick person

Z76.4 Other boarder to healthcare facility
> EXCLUDES 1   homelessness (Z59.0)

Z76.5 Malingerer [conscious simulation]
Person feigning illness (with obvious motivation)
> EXCLUDES 1   factitious disorder (F68.1-)
> peregrinating patient (F68.1-)

> **DEF:** Act of intentionally exaggerating an illness or disability in order to receive personal gain; or to avoid punishment or responsibility.

✓5th Z76.8 Persons encountering health services in other specified circumstances

Z76.81 Expectant parent(s) prebirth pediatrician visit
Pre-adoption pediatrician visit for adoptive parent(s)

Z76.82 Awaiting organ transplant status
Patient waiting for organ availability

EXCLUDES 1 Not coded here   EXCLUDES 2 Not included here   N Newborn Age: 0   P Pediatric Age: 0-17   M Maternity Age: 12-55   A Adult Age: 15-124   PDx Primary Dx

1196   ICD-10-CM 2018

Z76.89   Persons encountering health services in other specified circumstances
    Persons encountering health services NOS
    AHA: 2014, 2Q, 10

Persons with potential health hazards related to family and personal history and certain conditions influencing health status (Z77-Z99)

    Code also any follow-up examination (Z08-Z09)

☑4ᵗʰ **Z77**   **Other contact with and (suspected) exposures hazardous to health**
    INCLUDES   contact with and (suspected) exposures to potential hazards to health
    EXCLUDES 2   contact with and (suspected) exposure to communicable diseases (Z20.-)
       exposure to (parental) (environmental) tobacco smoke in the perinatal period (P96.81)
       newborn affected by noxious substances transmitted via placenta or breast milk (P04.-)
       occupational exposure to risk factors (Z57.-)
       retained foreign body (Z18.-)
       retained foreign body fully removed (Z87.821)
       toxic effects of substances chiefly nonmedicinal as to source (T51-T65)

☑5ᵗʰ **Z77.0**   **Contact with and (suspected) exposure to** hazardous, chiefly nonmedicinal, chemicals

   ☑6ᵗʰ **Z77.01**   **Contact with and (suspected) exposure to hazardous metals**

     Z77.010   **Contact with and (suspected) exposure to arsenic**

     Z77.011   **Contact with and (suspected) exposure to lead**

     Z77.012   **Contact with and (suspected) exposure to uranium**
       EXCLUDES 1   retained depleted uranium fragments (Z18.01)

     Z77.018   **Contact with and (suspected) exposure to other hazardous metals**
       Contact with and (suspected) exposure to chromium compounds
       Contact with and (suspected) exposure to nickel dust

   ☑6ᵗʰ **Z77.02**   **Contact with and (suspected) exposure to hazardous aromatic compounds**

     Z77.020   **Contact with and (suspected) exposure to aromatic amines**

     Z77.021   **Contact with and (suspected) exposure to benzene**

     Z77.028   **Contact with and (suspected) exposure to other hazardous aromatic compounds**
       Aromatic dyes NOS
       Polycyclic aromatic hydrocarbons

   ☑6ᵗʰ **Z77.09**   **Contact with and (suspected) exposure to other hazardous, chiefly** nonmedicinal, chemicals

     Z77.090   **Contact with and (suspected) exposure to** asbestos

     Z77.098   **Contact with and (suspected) exposure to other hazardous, chiefly nonmedicinal, chemicals**
       Dyes NOS

☑5ᵗʰ **Z77.1**   **Contact with and (suspected) exposure to environmental pollution and hazards in the physical environment**

   ☑6ᵗʰ **Z77.11**   **Contact with and (suspected) exposure to** environmental pollution

     Z77.110   **Contact with and (suspected) exposure to air pollution**

     Z77.111   **Contact with and (suspected) exposure to water pollution**

     Z77.112   **Contact with and (suspected) exposure to soil pollution**

     Z77.118   **Contact with and (suspected) exposure to other environmental pollution**

   ☑6ᵗʰ **Z77.12**   **Contact with and (suspected) exposure to** hazards in the physical environment

     Z77.120   **Contact with and (suspected) exposure to mold (toxic)**

     Z77.121   **Contact with and (suspected) exposure to** harmful algae and algae toxins
       Contact with and (suspected) Exposure to (harmful) algae bloom NOS
       Contact with and (suspected) exposure to blue-green algae bloom
       Contact with and (suspected) exposure to brown tide
       Contact with and (suspected) exposure to cyanobacteria bloom
       Contact with and (suspected) exposure to Florida red tide
       Contact with and (suspected) exposure to pfiesteria piscicida
       Contact with and (suspected) exposure to red tide

     Z77.122   **Contact with and (suspected) exposure to** noise

     Z77.123   **Contact with and (suspected) exposure to** radon and other naturally occuring radiation
       EXCLUDES 2   radiation exposure as the cause of a confirmed condition (W88-W90, X39.0-)
       radiation sickness NOS (T66)

     Z77.128   **Contact with and (suspected) exposure to other hazards in the physical environment**

☑5ᵗʰ **Z77.2**   **Contact with and (suspected) exposure to other hazardous substances**

     Z77.21   **Contact with and (suspected) exposure to potentially hazardous** body fluids

     Z77.22   **Contact with and (suspected) exposure to** environmental tobacco smoke **(acute) (chronic)**
       Exposure to second hand tobacco smoke (acute) (chronic)
       Passive smoking (acute) (chronic)
       EXCLUDES 1   nicotine dependence (F17.-)
         tobacco use (Z72.0)
       EXCLUDES 2   occupational exposure to environmental tobacco smoke (Z57.31)

     Z77.29   **Contact with and (suspected) exposure to other hazardous substances**
       AHA: 2016, 2Q, 33

   Z77.9   **Other contact with and (suspected) exposures hazardous to health**

☑4ᵗʰ **Z78**   **Other specified health status**
    EXCLUDES 2   asymptomatic human immunodeficiency virus [HIV] infection status (Z21)
       postprocedural status (Z93- Z99)
       sex reassignment status (Z87.890)

   Z78.0   **Asymptomatic menopausal state**   A♀
     Menopausal state NOS
     Postmenopausal status NOS
     EXCLUDES 2   symptomatic menopausal state (N95.1)

   Z78.1   **Physical restraint status**
     EXCLUDES 1   physical restraint due to a procedure - omit code
     DEF: Application of mechanical restraining devices or manual restraints; used to limit physical mobility of a patient.

   Z78.9   **Other specified health status**

☑4ᵗʰ **Z79**   **Long term (current) drug therapy**
    INCLUDES   long term (current) drug use for prophylactic purposes
    Code also any therapeutic drug level monitoring (Z51.81)
    EXCLUDES 2   drug abuse and dependence (F11-F19)
       drug use complicating pregnancy, childbirth, and the puerperium (O99.32-)
       long term (current) use of oral antidiabetic drugs (Z79.84)
       long term (current) use of oral hypoglycemic drugs (Z79.84)

   ☑5ᵗʰ **Z79.0**   **Long term (current) use of anticoagulants and antithrombotics/antiplatelets**
     EXCLUDES 2   long term (current) use of aspirin (Z79.82)

     Z79.01   **Long term (current) use of** anticoagulants

     Z79.02   **Long term (current) use of** antithrombotics/antiplatelets

   Z79.1   **Long term (current) use of** non-steroidal anti-inflammatories **(NSAID)**
     EXCLUDES 2   long term (current) use of aspirin (Z79.82)

   Z79.2   **Long term (current) use of** antibiotics

   Z79.3   **Long term (current) use of** hormonal contraceptives
     Long term (current) use of birth control pill or patch

   Z79.4   **Long term (current) use of** insulin   HCC

☑ Additional Character Req   ☑7ᵗʰ Placeholder Alert   Manifestation   HCC CMS-HCC Condition   ▽ Unspecified Code   ►◄ Revised Text   ● New Code   ▲ Revised Code Title

✓5ᵗʰ **Z79.5** **Long term (current) use of steroids**

     Z79.51 **Long term (current) use of** inhaled steroids

     Z79.52 **Long term (current) use of** systemic steroids

✓5ᵗʰ **Z79.8** **Other long term (current) drug therapy**

     ✓6ᵗʰ **Z79.81** **Long term (current) use of agents affecting estrogen receptors and estrogen levels**

       Code first, if applicable:
         malignant neoplasm of breast (C50.-)
         malignant neoplasm of prostate (C61)
       Use additional code, if applicable, to identify:
         estrogen receptor positive status (Z17.0)
         family history of breast cancer (Z80.3)
         genetic susceptibility to malignant neoplasm
           (cancer) (Z15.0-)
         personal history of breast cancer (Z85.3)
         personal history of prostate cancer (Z85.46)
         postmenopausal status (Z78.0)
       EXCLUDES 1 ▶hormone replacement therapy◀ (Z79.890)

       Z79.810 **Long term (current) use of selective estrogen receptor modulators (SERMs)**
         Long term (current) use of raloxifene (Evista)
         Long term (current) use of tamoxifen (Nolvadex)
         Long term (current) use of toremifene (Fareston)

       Z79.811 **Long term (current) use of** aromatase inhibitors
         Long term (current) use of anastrozole (Arimidex)
         Long term (current) use of exemestane (Aromasin)
         Long term (current) use of letrozole (Femara)

       Z79.818 **Long term (current) use of other agents affecting estrogen receptors and estrogen levels**
         Long term (current) use of estrogen receptor downregulators
         Long term (current) use of fulvestrant (Faslodex)
         Long term (current) use of gonadotropin-releasing hormone (GnRH) agonist
         Long term (current) use of goserelin acetate (Zoladex)
         Long term (current) use of leuprolide acetate (leuprorelin) (Lupron)
         Long term (current) use of megestrol acetate (Megace)

     Z79.82 **Long term (current) use of** aspirin

     Z79.83 **Long term (current) use of** bisphosphonates

     Z79.84 **Long term (current) use of** oral hypoglycemic drugs
       Long term (current) use of oral antidiabetic drugs
       EXCLUDES 2 long term (current) use of insulin (Z79.4)

     ✓6ᵗʰ **Z79.89** **Other long term (current) drug therapy**

       Z79.890 **Hormone replacement therapy**

       Z79.891 **Long term (current) use of** opiate analgesic
         Long term (current) use of methadone for pain management
         EXCLUDES 1 methadone use NOS (F11.9-)
           use of methadone for treatment of heroin addiction (F11.2-)

       Z79.899 **Other long term (current) drug therapy**
         AHA: 2015, 4Q, 34; 2015, 3Q, 21

✓4ᵗʰ **Z80** **Family history of primary malignant neoplasm**

     Z80.0 **Family history of malignant neoplasm of** digestive organs
       Conditions classifiable to C15-C26

     Z80.1 **Family history of malignant neoplasm of** trachea, bronchus and lung
       Conditions classifiable to C33-C34

     Z80.2 **Family history of malignant neoplasm of other respiratory and intrathoracic organs**
       Conditions classifiable to C30-C32, C37-C39

     Z80.3 **Family history of malignant neoplasm of** breast
       Conditions classifiable to C50-

     ✓5ᵗʰ **Z80.4** **Family history of malignant neoplasm of genital organs**
       Conditions classifiable to C51-C63

       Z80.41 **Family history of malignant neoplasm of** ovary

       Z80.42 **Family history of malignant neoplasm of** prostate

       Z80.43 **Family history of malignant neoplasm of** testis

       Z80.49 **Family history of malignant neoplasm of other genital organs**

     ✓5ᵗʰ **Z80.5** **Family history of malignant neoplasm of urinary tract**
       Conditions classifiable to C64-C68

       Z80.51 **Family history of malignant neoplasm of** kidney

       Z80.52 **Family history of malignant neoplasm of** bladder

       Z80.59 **Family history of malignant neoplasm of other urinary tract organ**

     Z80.6 **Family history of** leukemia
       Conditions classifiable to C91-C95

     Z80.7 **Family history of other malignant neoplasms of** lymphoid, hematopoietic and related tissues
       Conditions classifiable to C81-C90, C96-

     Z80.8 **Family history of malignant neoplasm of other organs or systems**
       Conditions classifiable to C00-C14, C40-C49, C69-C79

     Z80.9 **Family history of malignant neoplasm, unspecified** ▽
       Conditions classifiable to C80.1

✓4ᵗʰ **Z81** **Family history of mental and behavioral disorders**

     Z81.0 **Family history of** intellectual disabilities
       Conditions classifiable to F70-F79

     Z81.1 **Family history of** alcohol abuse and dependence
       Conditions classifiable to F10-

     Z81.2 **Family history of** tobacco abuse and dependence
       Conditions classifiable to F17-

     Z81.3 **Family history of other psychoactive substance abuse and dependence**
       Conditions classifiable to F11-F16, F18-F19

     Z81.4 **Family history of other substance abuse and dependence**
       Conditions classifiable to F55

     Z81.8 **Family history of other mental and behavioral disorders**
       Conditions classifiable elsewhere in F01-F99

✓4ᵗʰ **Z82** **Family history of certain disabilities and chronic diseases (leading to disablement)**

     Z82.0 **Family history of** epilepsy **and other diseases of the nervous system**
       Conditions classifiable to G00-G99

     Z82.1 **Family history of** blindness and visual loss
       Conditions classifiable to H54-

     Z82.2 **Family history of** deafness and hearing loss
       Conditions classifiable to H90-H91

     Z82.3 **Family history of** stroke
       Conditions classifiable to I60-I64

     ✓5ᵗʰ **Z82.4** **Family history of ischemic heart disease and other diseases of the circulatory system**
       Conditions classifiable to I00-I52, I65-I99

       Z82.41 **Family history of** sudden cardiac death

       Z82.49 **Family history of** ischemic heart disease **and other diseases of the circulatory system**

     Z82.5 **Family history of** asthma **and other chronic lower respiratory diseases**
       Conditions classifiable to J40-J47
       EXCLUDES 2 family history of other diseases of the respiratory system (Z83.6)

     ✓5ᵗʰ **Z82.6** **Family history of arthritis and other diseases of the musculoskeletal system and connective tissue**
       Conditions classifiable to M00-M99

       Z82.61 **Family history of** arthritis

       Z82.62 **Family history of** osteoporosis

       Z82.69 **Family history of other diseases of the musculoskeletal system and connective tissue**

     ✓5ᵗʰ **Z82.7** **Family history of congenital malformations, deformations and chromosomal abnormalities**
       Conditions classifiable to Q00-Q99

       Z82.71 **Family history of** polycystic kidney

       Z82.79 **Family history of other congenital malformations, deformations and chromosomal abnormalities**

     Z82.8 **Family history of other disabilities and chronic diseases leading to disablement, not elsewhere classified**

✓4ᵗʰ Z83 Family history of other specific disorders

     EXCLUDES 2   *contact with and (suspected) exposure to communicable disease in the family (Z20.-)*

   Z83.0 Family history of human immunodeficiency virus [HIV] disease
     Conditions classifiable to B20

   Z83.1 Family history of other infectious and parasitic diseases
     Conditions classifiable to A00-B19, B25-B94, B99

   Z83.2 Family history of diseases of the blood and blood-forming organs **and certain disorders involving the immune mechanism**
     Conditions classifiable to D50-D89

   Z83.3 Family history of diabetes mellitus
     Conditions classifiable to E08-E13

   ✓5ᵗʰ Z83.4 Family history of other endocrine, nutritional and metabolic diseases
     Conditions classifiable to E00-E07, E15-E88

     Z83.41 Family history of multiple endocrine neoplasia [MEN] syndrome

     Z83.42 Family history of familial hypercholesterolemia

     Z83.49 Family history of other endocrine, nutritional and metabolic diseases

   ✓5ᵗʰ Z83.5 Family history of eye and ear disorders

     ✓6ᵗʰ Z83.51 Family history of eye **disorders**
       Conditions classifiable to H00-H53, H55-H59
       EXCLUDES 2   *family history of blindness and visual loss (Z82.1)*

       Z83.511 Family history of glaucoma

       Z83.518 Family history of other specified eye disorder

     Z83.52 Family history of ear **disorders**
       Conditions classifiable to H60-H83, H92-H95
       EXCLUDES 2   *family history of deafness and hearing loss (Z82.2)*

   Z83.6 Family history of other diseases of the respiratory system
     Conditions classifiable to J00-J39, J60-J99
     EXCLUDES 2   *family history of asthma and other chronic lower respiratory diseases (Z82.5)*

   ✓5ᵗʰ Z83.7 Family history of diseases of the digestive system
     Conditions classifiable to K00-K93

     Z83.71 Family history of colonic polyps
       EXCLUDES 1   *family history of malignant neoplasm of digestive organs (Z80.0)*
       EXCLUDES 2   ▶*family history of malignant neoplasm of digestive organs (Z80.0)*◀

     Z83.79 Family history of other diseases of the digestive system

✓4ᵗʰ Z84 Family history of other conditions

   Z84.0 Family history of diseases of the skin and subcutaneous tissue
     Conditions classifiable to L00-L99

   Z84.1 Family history of disorders of kidney and ureter
     Conditions classifiable to N00-N29

   Z84.2 Family history of other diseases of the genitourinary system
     Conditions classifiable to N30-N99

   Z84.3 Family history of consanguinity

   ✓5ᵗʰ Z84.8 Family history of other specified conditions

     Z84.81 Family history of carrier of genetic disease

     Z84.82 Family history of sudden infant death syndrome
       Family history of SIDS

     Z84.89 Family history of other specified conditions

✓4ᵗʰ Z85 Personal history of malignant neoplasm

   Code first any follow-up examination after treatment of malignant neoplasm (Z08)
   Use additional code to identify:
     alcohol use and dependence (F10.-)
     exposure to environmental tobacco smoke (Z77.22)
     history of tobacco dependence (Z87.891)
     occupational exposure to environmental tobacco smoke (Z57.31)
     tobacco dependence (F17.-)
     tobacco use (Z72.0)
   EXCLUDES 2   *personal history of benign neoplasm (Z86.01-)*
            personal history of carcinoma-in-situ (Z86.00-)

   ✓5ᵗʰ Z85.0 Personal history of malignant neoplasm of digestive organs
     AHA: 2017, 1Q, 9

     Z85.00 Personal history of malignant neoplasm of   ▽ **unspecified digestive organ**

     Z85.01 Personal history of malignant neoplasm of esophagus
       Conditions classifiable to C15

     ✓6ᵗʰ Z85.02 Personal history of malignant neoplasm of stomach

       Z85.020 Personal history of malignant carcinoid tumor **of stomach**
         Conditions classifiable to C7A.092

       Z85.028 Personal history of other malignant neoplasm of stomach
         Conditions classifiable to C16

     ✓6ᵗʰ Z85.03 Personal history of malignant neoplasm of large intestine

       Z85.030 Personal history of malignant carcinoid tumor **of large intestine**
         Conditions classifiable to C7A.022-C7A.025, C7A.029

       Z85.038 Personal history of other malignant neoplasm of large intestine
         Conditions classifiable to C18

     ✓6ᵗʰ Z85.04 Personal history of malignant neoplasm of rectum, rectosigmoid junction, and anus

       Z85.040 Personal history of malignant carcinoid tumor **of rectum**
         Conditions classifiable to C7A.026

       Z85.048 Personal history of other malignant neoplasm of rectum, rectosigmoid junction, and anus
         Conditions classifiable to C19-C21

     Z85.05 Personal history of malignant neoplasm of liver
       Conditions classifiable to C22

     ✓6ᵗʰ Z85.06 Personal history of malignant neoplasm of small intestine

       Z85.060 Personal history of malignant carcinoid tumor **of small intestine**
         Conditions classifiable to C7A.01-

       Z85.068 Personal history of other malignant neoplasm of small intestine
         Conditions classifiable to C17

     Z85.07 Personal history of malignant neoplasm of pancreas
       Conditions classifiable to C25

     Z85.09 Personal history of malignant neoplasm of other digestive organs

   ✓5ᵗʰ Z85.1 Personal history of malignant neoplasm of trachea, bronchus and lung

     ✓6ᵗʰ Z85.11 Personal history of malignant neoplasm of bronchus and lung

       Z85.110 Personal history of malignant carcinoid tumor **of bronchus and lung**
         Conditions classifiable to C7A.090

       Z85.118 Personal history of other malignant neoplasm of bronchus and lung
         Conditions classifiable to C34

     Z85.12 Personal history of malignant neoplasm of trachea
       Conditions classifiable to C33

   ✓5ᵗʰ Z85.2 Personal history of malignant neoplasm of other respiratory and intrathoracic organs

     Z85.20 Personal history of malignant neoplasm of   ▽ **unspecified respiratory organ**

     Z85.21 Personal history of malignant neoplasm of larynx
       Conditions classifiable to C32

     Z85.22 Personal history of malignant neoplasm of nasal cavities, middle ear, and accessory sinuses
       Conditions classifiable to C30-C31

☑ Additional Character Req   ✓x7ᵗʰ Placeholder Alert   Manifestation   HCC CMS-HCC Condition   ▽ Unspecified Code   ▶◀ Revised Text   ● New Code   ▲ Revised Code Title

✓6ᵗʰ **Z85.23** **Personal history of malignant neoplasm of** thymus

    Z85.230 **Personal history of malignant** carcinoid tumor **of thymus**
       Conditions classifiable to C7A.091

    Z85.238 **Personal history of other malignant neoplasm of thymus**
       Conditions classifiable to C37

Z85.29 **Personal history of malignant neoplasm of other respiratory and intrathoracic organs**

Z85.3 **Personal history of malignant neoplasm of** breast
    Conditions classifiable to C50.-

✓5ᵗʰ **Z85.4** **Personal history of malignant neoplasm of** genital organs
    Conditions classifiable to C51-C63

    Z85.40 **Personal history of malignant neoplasm of unspecified** female **genital organ** ♀▽

    Z85.41 **Personal history of malignant neoplasm of** cervix uteri ♀

    Z85.42 **Personal history of malignant neoplasm of other parts of uterus** ♀

    Z85.43 **Personal history of malignant neoplasm of** ovary ♀

    Z85.44 **Personal history of malignant neoplasm of other** female **genital organs** ♀

    Z85.45 **Personal history of malignant neoplasm of unspecified** male **genital organ** ♂▽

    Z85.46 **Personal history of malignant neoplasm of** prostate ♂

    Z85.47 **Personal history of malignant neoplasm of** testis ♂

    Z85.48 **Personal history of malignant neoplasm of** epididymis ♂

    Z85.49 **Personal history of malignant neoplasm of other** male **genital organs** ♂

✓5ᵗʰ **Z85.5** **Personal history of malignant neoplasm of** urinary tract
    Conditions classifiable to C64-C68

    Z85.50 **Personal history of malignant neoplasm of unspecified urinary tract organ** ▽

    Z85.51 **Personal history of malignant neoplasm of** bladder

✓6ᵗʰ   **Z85.52** **Personal history of malignant neoplasm of** kidney
       EXCLUDES 1 *personal history of malignant neoplasm of renal pelvis (Z85.53)*

       Z85.520 **Personal history of malignant** carcinoid tumor **of kidney**
          Conditions classifiable to C7A.093

       Z85.528 **Personal history of other malignant neoplasm of kidney**
          Conditions classifiable to C64

    Z85.53 **Personal history of malignant neoplasm of** renal pelvis

    Z85.54 **Personal history of malignant neoplasm of** ureter

    Z85.59 **Personal history of malignant neoplasm of other urinary tract organ**

Z85.6 **Personal history of** leukemia
    Conditions classifiable to C91-C95
    EXCLUDES 1 *leukemia in remission C91.0-C95.9 with 5th character 1*

✓5ᵗʰ **Z85.7** **Personal history of other malignant neoplasms of lymphoid, hematopoietic and related tissues**

    Z85.71 **Personal history of** Hodgkin lymphoma
       Conditions classifiable to C81

    Z85.72 **Personal history of** non-Hodgkin lymphomas
       Conditions classifiable to C82-C85

    Z85.79 **Personal history of other malignant neoplasms of lymphoid, hematopoietic and related tissues**
       Conditions classifiable to C88-C90, C96
       EXCLUDES 1 *multiple myeloma in remission (C90.01)*
            plasma cell leukemia in remission (C90.11)
            plasmacytoma in remission (C90.21)

✓5ᵗʰ **Z85.8** **Personal history of malignant neoplasms of other organs and systems**
    Conditions classifiable to C00-C14, C40-C49, C69-C75, C7A.098, C76-C79

✓6ᵗʰ   **Z85.81** **Personal history of malignant neoplasm of** lip, oral cavity, and pharynx

       Z85.810 **Personal history of malignant neoplasm of tongue**

       Z85.818 **Personal history of malignant neoplasm of other sites of lip, oral cavity, and pharynx**

       Z85.819 **Personal history of malignant neoplasm of unspecified site of lip, oral cavity, and pharynx** ▽

✓6ᵗʰ **Z85.82** **Personal history of malignant neoplasm of** skin

    Z85.820 **Personal history of malignant** melanoma **of skin**
       Conditions classifiable to C43

    Z85.821 **Personal history of** Merkel cell carcinoma
       Conditions classifiable to C4A

    Z85.828 **Personal history of other malignant neoplasm of skin**
       Conditions classifiable to C44

✓6ᵗʰ **Z85.83** **Personal history of malignant neoplasm of** bone and soft tissue

    Z85.830 **Personal history of malignant neoplasm of** bone

    Z85.831 **Personal history of malignant neoplasm of** soft tissue
       EXCLUDES 2 *personal history of malignant neoplasm of skin (Z85.82-)*

✓6ᵗʰ **Z85.84** **Personal history of malignant neoplasm of** eye and nervous tissue

    Z85.840 **Personal history of malignant neoplasm of** eye

    Z85.841 **Personal history of malignant neoplasm of** brain

    Z85.848 **Personal history of malignant neoplasm of other parts of nervous tissue**

✓6ᵗʰ **Z85.85** **Personal history of malignant neoplasm of** endocrine glands

    Z85.850 **Personal history of malignant neoplasm of** thyroid

    Z85.858 **Personal history of malignant neoplasm of other endocrine glands**

Z85.89 **Personal history of malignant neoplasm of other organs and systems**

Z85.9 **Personal history of malignant neoplasm, unspecified** ▽
    Conditions classifiable to C7A.00, C80.1

✓4ᵗʰ **Z86** **Personal history of certain other diseases**
    Code first any follow-up examination after treatment (Z09)

✓5ᵗʰ **Z86.0** **Personal history of in-situ and benign neoplasms and neoplasms of uncertain behavior**
    EXCLUDES 2 *personal history of malignant neoplasms (Z85.-)*
    AHA: 2017, 1Q, 9

✓6ᵗʰ   **Z86.00** **Personal history of** in-situ neoplasm
       Conditions classifiable to D00-D09

       Z86.000 **Personal history of in-situ neoplasm of** breast
          Personal history of cervical intraepithelial neoplasia III [CIN III]

       Z86.001 **Personal history of in-situ neoplasm of** cervix uteri ♀

       Z86.008 **Personal history of in-situ neoplasm of other site**
          Personal history of vaginal intraepithelial neoplasia III [VAIN III]
          Personal history of vulvar intraepithelial neoplasia III [VIN III]

✓6ᵗʰ   **Z86.01** **Personal history of** benign neoplasm

       Z86.010 **Personal history of** colonic polyps
          AHA: 2017, 1Q, 14

       Z86.011 **Personal history of benign neoplasm of the** brain

       Z86.012 **Personal history of benign** carcinoid tumor

       Z86.018 **Personal history of other benign neoplasm**
          AHA: 2017, 1Q, 14

    Z86.03 **Personal history of** neoplasm of uncertain behavior

✓5ᵗʰ **Z86.1** **Personal history of** infectious and parasitic diseases
    Conditions classifiable to A00-B89, B99
    EXCLUDES 1 *personal history of infectious diseases specific to a body system*
       sequelae of infectious and parasitic diseases (B90-B94)

    Z86.11 **Personal history of** tuberculosis

    Z86.12 **Personal history of** poliomyelitis

    Z86.13 **Personal history of** malaria

    Z86.14 **Personal history of** Methicillin resistant Staphylococcus aureus **infection**
       Personal history of MRSA infection

EXCLUDES 1 Not coded here   EXCLUDES 2 Not included here   N Newborn Age: 0   P Pediatric Age: 0-17   M Maternity Age: 12-55   A Adult Age: 15-124   PDx Primary Dx

Z86.19   Personal history of other infectious and parasitic diseases

Z86.2   Personal history of diseases of the blood and blood-forming organs and certain disorders involving the immune mechanism
Conditions classifiable to D50-D89

✓5ᵗʰ **Z86.3**   Personal history of endocrine, nutritional and metabolic diseases
Conditions classifiable to E00-E88

    Z86.31   Personal history of diabetic foot ulcer
EXCLUDES 2   *current diabetic foot ulcer (E08.621, E09.621, E10.621, E11.621, E13.621)*

    Z86.32   Personal history of gestational diabetes   ♀
Personal history of conditions classifiable to O24.4-
EXCLUDES 1   *gestational diabetes mellitus in current pregnancy (O24.4-)*

    Z86.39   Personal history of other endocrine, nutritional and metabolic disease

✓5ᵗʰ **Z86.5**   Personal history of mental and behavioral disorders
Conditions classifiable to F40-F59

    Z86.51   Personal history of combat and operational   [A]
stress reaction

    Z86.59   Personal history of other mental and behavioral disorders

✓5ᵗʰ **Z86.6**   Personal history of diseases of the nervous system and sense organs
Conditions classifiable to G00-G99, H00-H95
EXCLUDES 2   *personal history of anaphylactic shock (Z87.892)*

    Z86.61   Personal history of infections of the central nervous system
Personal history of encephalitis
Personal history of meningitis

    Z86.69   Personal history of other diseases of the nervous system and sense organs

✓5ᵗʰ **Z86.7**   Personal history of diseases of the circulatory system
Conditions classifiable to I00-I99
EXCLUDES 2   *old myocardial infarction (I25.2)*
personal history of anaphylactic shock (Z87.892)
postmyocardial infarction syndrome (I24.1)

    ✓6ᵗʰ **Z86.71**   Personal history of venous thrombosis and embolism

       Z86.711   Personal history of pulmonary embolism

       Z86.718   Personal history of other venous thrombosis and embolism

    Z86.72   Personal history of thrombophlebitis

    Z86.73   Personal history of transient ischemic attack (TIA), and cerebral infarction without residual deficits
Personal history of prolonged reversible ischemic neurological deficit (PRIND)
Personal history of stroke NOS without residual deficits
EXCLUDES 1   *personal history of traumatic brain injury (Z87.820)*
sequelae of cerebrovascular disease (I69.-)
AHA: 2012, 4Q, 92

    Z86.74   Personal history of sudden cardiac arrest
Personal history of sudden cardiac death successfully resuscitated

    Z86.79   Personal history of other diseases of the circulatory system

✓4ᵗʰ **Z87**   **Personal history of other diseases and conditions**
Code first any follow-up examination after treatment (Z09)

✓5ᵗʰ **Z87.0**   Personal history of diseases of the respiratory system
Conditions classifiable to J00-J99

    Z87.01   Personal history of pneumonia (recurrent)

    Z87.09   Personal history of other diseases of the respiratory system

✓5ᵗʰ **Z87.1**   Personal history of diseases of the digestive system
Conditions classifiable to K00-K93

    Z87.11   Personal history of peptic ulcer disease

    Z87.19   Personal history of other diseases of the digestive system
AHA: 2017, 1Q, 14

Z87.2   Personal history of diseases of the skin and subcutaneous tissue
Conditions classifiable to L00-L99
EXCLUDES 2   *personal history of diabetic foot ulcer (Z86.31)*

✓5ᵗʰ **Z87.3**   Personal history of diseases of the musculoskeletal system and connective tissue
Conditions classifiable to M00-M99
EXCLUDES 2   *personal history of (healed) traumatic fracture (Z87.81)*

    ✓6ᵗʰ **Z87.31**   Personal history of (healed) nontraumatic fracture

       Z87.310   Personal history of (healed) osteoporosis fracture
Personal history of (healed) fragility fracture
Personal history of (healed) collapsed vertebra due to osteoporosis

       Z87.311   Personal history of (healed) other pathological fracture
Personal history of (healed) collapsed vertebra NOS
EXCLUDES 2   *personal history of osteoporosis fracture (Z87.310)*

       Z87.312   Personal history of (healed) stress fracture
Personal history of (healed) fatigue fracture

    Z87.39   Personal history of other diseases of the musculoskeletal system and connective tissue

✓5ᵗʰ **Z87.4**   Personal history of diseases of genitourinary system
Conditions classifiable to N00-N99

    ✓6ᵗʰ **Z87.41**   Personal history of dysplasia of the female genital tract
EXCLUDES 1   *personal history of intraepithelial neoplasia III of female genital tract ▶(Z86.001, Z86.008)◀*
personal history of malignant neoplasm of female genital tract (Z85.40-Z85.44)

       Z87.410   Personal history of cervical dysplasia   ♀
       Z87.411   Personal history of vaginal dysplasia   ♀
       Z87.412   Personal history of vulvar dysplasia   ♀

    Z87.42   Personal history of other diseases of the female   ♀
genital tract

    ✓6ᵗʰ **Z87.43**   Personal history of diseases of the male genital organs

       Z87.430   Personal history of prostatic dysplasia   ♂
EXCLUDES 1   *personal history of malignant neoplasm of prostate (Z85.46)*

       Z87.438   Personal history of other diseases of   ♂
male genital organs

    ✓6ᵗʰ **Z87.44**   Personal history of diseases of the urinary system
EXCLUDES 1   *personal history of malignant neoplasm of cervix uteri (Z85.41)*

       Z87.440   Personal history of urinary (tract) infections

       Z87.441   Personal history of nephrotic syndrome

       Z87.442   Personal history of urinary calculi
Personal history of kidney stones

       Z87.448   Personal history of other diseases of urinary system

✓5ᵗʰ **Z87.5**   Personal history of complications of pregnancy, childbirth and the puerperium
Conditions classifiable to O00-O9A
EXCLUDES 2   *recurrent pregnancy loss (N96)*

    Z87.51   Personal history of pre-term labor   ♀
EXCLUDES 1   *current pregnancy with history of pre-term labor (O09.21-)*

    Z87.59   Personal history of other complications of   ♀
pregnancy, childbirth and the puerperium
Personal history of trophoblastic disease

✓ Additional Character Req   ✓x7ᵗʰ Placeholder Alert   **Manifestation**   **HCC** CMS-HCC Condition   ▽ Unspecified Code   ▶◀ Revised Text   ● New Code   ▲ Revised Code Title

✓5ᵗʰ **Z87.7** **Personal history of (corrected) congenital malformations**
Conditions classifiable to Q00-Q89 that have been repaired or corrected

EXCLUDES 1　congenital malformations that have been partially corrected or repaired but which still require medical treatment—code to condition

EXCLUDES 2　other postprocedural states (Z98.-)
personal history of medical treatment (Z92.-)
presence of cardiac and vascular implants and grafts (Z95.-)
presence of other devices (Z97.-)
presence of other functional implants (Z96.-)
transplanted organ and tissue status (Z94.-)

✓6ᵗʰ **Z87.71** **Personal history of (corrected) congenital malformations of** genitourinary system

　Z87.710 **Personal history of (corrected)** ♂
hypospadias

　Z87.718 **Personal history of other specified (corrected) congenital malformations of genitourinary system**

✓6ᵗʰ **Z87.72** **Personal history of (corrected) congenital malformations of** nervous system and sense organs

　Z87.720 **Personal history of (corrected) congenital malformations of** eye

　Z87.721 **Personal history of (corrected) congenital malformations of** ear

　Z87.728 **Personal history of other specified (corrected) congenital malformations of nervous system and sense organs**

✓6ᵗʰ **Z87.73** **Personal history of (corrected) congenital malformations of** digestive system

　Z87.730 **Personal history of (corrected)** cleft lip and palate

　Z87.738 **Personal history of other specified (corrected) congenital malformations of digestive system**

Z87.74 **Personal history of (corrected) congenital malformations of** heart and circulatory system

Z87.75 **Personal history of (corrected) congenital malformations of** respiratory system

Z87.76 **Personal history of (corrected) congenital malformations of** integument, limbs and musculoskeletal system

✓6ᵗʰ **Z87.79** **Personal history of other (corrected) congenital malformations**

　Z87.790 **Personal history of (corrected) congenital malformations of** face and neck

　Z87.798 **Personal history of other (corrected) congenital malformations**

✓5ᵗʰ **Z87.8** **Personal history of other specified conditions**

EXCLUDES 2　personal history of self harm (Z91.5)

　Z87.81 **Personal history of (healed)** traumatic fracture

EXCLUDES 2　personal history of (healed) nontraumatic fracture (Z87.31-)

✓6ᵗʰ **Z87.82** **Personal history of other (healed)** physical injury and trauma
Conditions classifiable to S00-T88, except traumatic fractures

　Z87.820 **Personal history of traumatic** brain injury

EXCLUDES 1　personal history of transient ischemic attack (TIA), and cerebral infarction without residual deficits (Z86.73)

　Z87.821 **Personal history of** retained foreign body fully removed

　Z87.828 **Personal history of other (healed) physical injury and trauma**

✓6ᵗʰ **Z87.89** **Personal history of other specified conditions**

　Z87.890 **Personal history of** sex reassignment

　Z87.891 **Personal history of** nicotine dependence

EXCLUDES 1　current nicotine dependence (F17.2-)

AHA: 2017, 2Q, 27

　Z87.892 **Personal history of** anaphylaxis
Code also allergy status such as:
allergy status to drugs, medicaments and biological substances (Z88.-)
allergy status, other than to drugs and biological substances (Z91.0-)

Z87.898 **Personal history of other specified conditions**

AHA: 2013, 1Q, 21

✓4ᵗʰ **Z88** **Allergy status to drugs, medicaments and biological substances**

EXCLUDES 2　allergy status, other than to drugs and biological substances (Z91.0-)

AHA: 2015, 3Q, 23

Z88.0 **Allergy status to** penicillin

Z88.1 **Allergy status to other antibiotic agents status**

Z88.2 **Allergy status to** sulfonamides status

Z88.3 **Allergy status to other anti-infective agents status**

Z88.4 **Allergy status to** anesthetic agent status

Z88.5 **Allergy status to** narcotic agent status

Z88.6 **Allergy status to** analgesic agent status

Z88.7 **Allergy status to** serum and vaccine status

Z88.8 **Allergy status to other drugs, medicaments and biological substances status**

Z88.9 **Allergy status to unspecified drugs, medicaments and** ▽
biological substances status

✓4ᵗʰ **Z89** **Acquired absence of limb**

INCLUDES　amputation status
postprocedural loss of limb
post-traumatic loss of limb

EXCLUDES 1　acquired deformities of limbs (M20-M21)
congenital absence of limbs (Q71-Q73)

✓5ᵗʰ **Z89.0** **Acquired absence of** thumb and other finger(s)

✓6ᵗʰ **Z89.01** **Acquired absence of** thumb

　Z89.011 **Acquired absence of** right thumb

　Z89.012 **Acquired absence of** left thumb

　Z89.019 **Acquired absence of unspecified thumb** ▽

✓6ᵗʰ **Z89.02** **Acquired absence of other** finger(s)

EXCLUDES 2　acquired absence of thumb (Z89.01-)

　Z89.021 **Acquired absence of** right finger(s)

　Z89.022 **Acquired absence of** left finger(s)

　Z89.029 **Acquired absence of unspecified** ▽
finger(s)

✓5ᵗʰ **Z89.1** **Acquired absence of** hand and wrist

✓6ᵗʰ **Z89.11** **Acquired absence of** hand

　Z89.111 **Acquired absence of** right hand

　Z89.112 **Acquired absence of** left hand

　Z89.119 **Acquired absence of unspecified hand** ▽

✓6ᵗʰ **Z89.12** **Acquired absence of** wrist
Disarticulation at wrist

　Z89.121 **Acquired absence of** right wrist

　Z89.122 **Acquired absence of** left wrist

　Z89.129 **Acquired absence of unspecified wrist** ▽

✓5ᵗʰ **Z89.2** **Acquired absence of** upper limb above wrist

✓6ᵗʰ **Z89.20** **Acquired absence of** upper limb, unspecified level

　Z89.201 **Acquired absence of** right upper limb, ▽
unspecified level

　Z89.202 **Acquired absence of** left upper limb, ▽
unspecified level

　Z89.209 **Acquired absence of unspecified** ▽
upper limb, unspecified level
Acquired absence of arm NOS

✓6ᵗʰ **Z89.21** **Acquired absence of** upper limb below elbow

　Z89.211 **Acquired absence of** right upper limb
below elbow

　Z89.212 **Acquired absence of** left upper limb below
elbow

　Z89.219 **Acquired absence of unspecified** ▽
upper limb below elbow

✓6ᵗʰ **Z89.22** **Acquired absence of** upper limb above elbow
Disarticulation at elbow

　Z89.221 **Acquired absence of** right upper limb
above elbow

　Z89.222 **Acquired absence of** left upper limb above
elbow

　Z89.229 **Acquired absence of unspecified** ▽
upper limb above elbow

EXCLUDES 1 Not coded here　EXCLUDES 2 Not included here　N Newborn Age: 0　P Pediatric Age: 0-17　M Maternity Age: 12-55　A Adult Age: 15-124　PDx Primary Dx

1202　　　　　　　　　　　　　　　　　　　　　　　　　　　　　　　　　　　ICD-10-CM 2018

☑6ᵗʰ **Z89.23**   **Acquired absence of** shoulder
Acquired absence of shoulder joint following explantation of shoulder joint prosthesis, with or without presence of antibiotic-impregnated cement spacer

     Z89.231   **Acquired absence of** right **shoulder**
     Z89.232   **Acquired absence of** left **shoulder**
     Z89.239   **Acquired absence of unspecified** ▽ **shoulder**

☑5ᵗʰ **Z89.4**   **Acquired absence of** toe(s), foot, and ankle
   ☑6ᵗʰ **Z89.41**   **Acquired absence of** great toe
     Z89.411   **Acquired absence of** right **great toe** HCC
     Z89.412   **Acquired absence of** left **great toe** HCC
     Z89.419   **Acquired absence of unspecified** HCC ▽ **great toe**

   ☑6ᵗʰ **Z89.42**   **Acquired absence of other** toe(s)
     EXCLUDES 2   acquired absence of great toe (Z89.41-)
     Z89.421   **Acquired absence of other** right **toe(s)** HCC
     Z89.422   **Acquired absence of other** left **toe(s)** HCC
     Z89.429   **Acquired absence of other toe(s),** HCC ▽ **unspecified side**

   ☑6ᵗʰ **Z89.43**   **Acquired absence of** foot
     Z89.431   **Acquired absence of** right **foot** HCC
     Z89.432   **Acquired absence of** left **foot** HCC
     Z89.439   **Acquired absence of unspecified** HCC ▽ **foot**

   ☑6ᵗʰ **Z89.44**   **Acquired absence of** ankle
Disarticulation of ankle
     Z89.441   **Acquired absence of** right **ankle** HCC
     Z89.442   **Acquired absence of** left **ankle** HCC
     Z89.449   **Acquired absence of unspecified** HCC ▽ **ankle**

☑5ᵗʰ **Z89.5**   **Acquired absence of leg below knee**
   ☑6ᵗʰ **Z89.51**   **Acquired absence of** leg below knee
     Z89.511   **Acquired absence of** right **leg below** HCC **knee**
     Z89.512   **Acquired absence of** left **leg below** HCC **knee**
     Z89.519   **Acquired absence of unspecified** HCC ▽ **leg below knee**

   ☑6ᵗʰ **Z89.52**   **Acquired absence of** knee
Acquired absence of knee joint following explantation of knee joint prosthesis, with or without presence of antibiotic-impregnated cement spacer
     Z89.521   **Acquired absence of** right **knee**
     Z89.522   **Acquired absence of** left **knee**
     Z89.529   **Acquired absence of unspecified knee** ▽

☑5ᵗʰ **Z89.6**   **Acquired absence of leg above knee**
   ☑6ᵗʰ **Z89.61**   **Acquired absence of** leg above knee
Acquired absence of leg NOS
Disarticulation at knee
     Z89.611   **Acquired absence of** right **leg above** HCC **knee**
     Z89.612   **Acquired absence of** left **leg above** HCC **knee**
     Z89.619   **Acquired absence of unspecified** HCC ▽ **leg above knee**

   ☑6ᵗʰ **Z89.62**   **Acquired absence of** hip
Acquired absence of hip joint following explantation of hip joint prosthesis, with or without presence of antibiotic-impregnated cement spacer
Disarticulation at hip
     Z89.621   **Acquired absence of** right **hip joint**
     Z89.622   **Acquired absence of** left **hip joint**
     Z89.629   **Acquired absence of unspecified hip** ▽ **joint**

Z89.9   **Acquired absence of limb, unspecified** ▽

☑4ᵗʰ **Z90**   **Acquired absence of organs, not elsewhere classified**
   INCLUDES   postprocedural or post-traumatic loss of body part NEC
   EXCLUDES 1   congenital absence—see Alphabetical Index
   EXCLUDES 2   postprocedural absence of endocrine glands (E89.-)

☑5ᵗʰ **Z90.0**   **Acquired absence of part of** head and neck
     Z90.01   **Acquired absence of** eye
     Z90.02   **Acquired absence of** larynx

Z90.09   **Acquired absence of other part of head and neck**
Acquired absence of nose
     EXCLUDES 2   teeth (K08.1)

☑5ᵗʰ **Z90.1**   **Acquired absence of** breast and nipple
     Z90.10   **Acquired absence of unspecified breast and** ▽ **nipple**
     Z90.11   **Acquired absence of** right **breast and nipple**
     Z90.12   **Acquired absence of** left **breast and nipple**
     Z90.13   **Acquired absence of** bilateral **breasts and nipples**

Z90.2   **Acquired absence of** lung [part of]
Z90.3   **Acquired absence of** stomach [part of]

☑5ᵗʰ **Z90.4**   **Acquired absence of other specified parts of digestive tract**
   ☑6ᵗʰ **Z90.41**   **Acquired absence of** pancreas
Code also exocrine pancreatic insufficiency (K86.81)
Use additional code to identify any associated:
   insulin use (Z79.4)
   diabetes mellitus, postpancreatectomy (E13.-)
     Z90.410   **Acquired** total absence **of pancreas**
Acquired absence of pancreas NOS
     Z90.411   **Acquired** partial absence **of pancreas**
     Z90.49   **Acquired absence of other specified parts of digestive tract**

Z90.5   **Acquired absence of** kidney
Z90.6   **Acquired absence of other parts of urinary tract**
Acquired absence of bladder

☑5ᵗʰ **Z90.7**   **Acquired absence of** genital organ(s)
   EXCLUDES 1   personal history of sex reassignment (Z87.890)
   EXCLUDES 2   female genital mutilation status (N90.81-)
   ☑6ᵗʰ **Z90.71**   **Acquired absence of** cervix and uterus
     Z90.710   **Acquired absence of** both **cervix and** ♀ **uterus**
Acquired absence of uterus NOS
Status post total hysterectomy
     Z90.711   **Acquired absence of uterus with** ♀ **remaining cervical stump**
Status post partial hysterectomy with remaining cervical stump
     Z90.712   **Acquired absence of cervix with** ♀ **remaining uterus**

   ☑6ᵗʰ **Z90.72**   **Acquired absence of** ovaries
     Z90.721   **Acquired absence of ovaries,** unilateral ♀
     Z90.722   **Acquired absence of ovaries,** bilateral ♀
     Z90.79   **Acquired absence of other genital organ(s)**

☑5ᵗʰ **Z90.8**   **Acquired absence of other organs**
     Z90.81   **Acquired absence of** spleen
     Z90.89   **Acquired absence of other organs**

☑4ᵗʰ **Z91**   **Personal risk factors, not elsewhere classified**
   EXCLUDES 2   contact with and (suspected) exposures hazardous to health (Z77.-)
     exposure to pollution and other problems related to physical environment (Z77.1-)
     ►female genital mutilation status (N90.81-)◄
     personal history of physical injury and trauma (Z87.81, Z87.82-)
     occupational exposure to risk factors (Z57.-)

☑5ᵗʰ **Z91.0**   **Allergy status, other than to drugs and biological substances**
   EXCLUDES 2   allergy status to drugs, medicaments, and biological substances (Z88.-)
   ☑6ᵗʰ **Z91.01**   **Food allergy status**
     EXCLUDES 2   food additives allergy status (Z91.02)
     Z91.010   **Allergy to** peanuts
     Z91.011   **Allergy to** milk products
      EXCLUDES 1   lactose intolerance (E73.-)
     Z91.012   **Allergy to** eggs
     Z91.013   **Allergy to** seafood
Allergy to shellfish
Allergy to octopus or squid ink
     Z91.018   **Allergy to other foods**
Allergy to nuts other than peanuts
     Z91.02   **Food additives allergy status**
   ☑6ᵗʰ **Z91.03**   **Insect allergy status**
     Z91.030   Bee **allergy status**
     Z91.038   **Other insect allergy status**

☑ Additional Character Req   v×7ᵗʰ Placeholder Alert   Manifestation   HCC CMS-HCC Condition   ▽ Unspecified Code   ►◄ Revised Text   ● New Code   ▲ Revised Code Title

✓6ᵗʰ **Z91.04** **Nonmedicinal substance allergy status**

Z91.040 **Latex allergy status**
Latex sensitivity status

Z91.041 **Radiographic dye allergy status**
Allergy status to contrast media used for diagnostic X-ray procedure

Z91.048 **Other nonmedicinal substance allergy status**

Z91.09 **Other allergy status, other than to drugs and biological substances**

✓5ᵗʰ **Z91.1** **Patient's noncompliance with medical treatment and regimen**

Z91.11 **Patient's noncompliance with dietary regimen**

✓6ᵗʰ **Z91.12** **Patient's intentional underdosing of medication regimen**
Code first underdosing of medication (T36-T50) with fifth or sixth character 6
EXCLUDES 1 *adverse effect of prescribed drug taken as directed—code to adverse effect*
poisoning (overdose)—code to poisoning

Z91.120 **Patient's intentional underdosing of medication regimen due to financial hardship**

Z91.128 **Patient's intentional underdosing of medication regimen for other reason**

✓6ᵗʰ **Z91.13** **Patient's unintentional underdosing of medication regimen**
Code first underdosing of medication (T36-T50) with fifth or sixth character 6
EXCLUDES 1 *adverse effect of prescribed drug taken as directed—code to adverse effect*
poisoning (overdose)—code to poisoning

Z91.130 **Patient's unintentional underdosing of medication regimen due to age-related debility**

Z91.138 **Patient's unintentional underdosing of medication regimen for other reason**

Z91.14 **Patient's other noncompliance with medication regimen**
Patient's underdosing of medication NOS

Z91.15 **Patient's noncompliance with renal dialysis** HCC

Z91.19 **Patient's noncompliance with other medical treatment and regimen**
▶Nonadherence to medical treatment◀

✓5ᵗʰ **Z91.4** **Personal history of psychological trauma, not elsewhere classified**

✓6ᵗʰ **Z91.41** **Personal history of adult abuse**
EXCLUDES 2 *personal history of abuse in childhood (Z62.81-)*

Z91.410 **Personal history of adult physical and sexual abuse** A
EXCLUDES 1 *current adult physical abuse (T74.11, T76.11)*
current adult sexual abuse (T74.21, T76.11)

Z91.411 **Personal history of adult psychological abuse** A

Z91.412 **Personal history of adult neglect** A
EXCLUDES 1 *current adult neglect (T74.01, T76.01)*

Z91.419 **Personal history of unspecified adult abuse** A ▽

Z91.49 **Other personal history of psychological trauma, not elsewhere classified**

Z91.5 **Personal history of self-harm**
Personal history of parasuicide
Personal history of self-poisoning
Personal history of suicide attempt

✓5ᵗʰ **Z91.8** **Other specified personal risk factors, not elsewhere classified**

Z91.81 **History of falling**
At risk for falling

Z91.82 **Personal history of military deployment** A
Individual (civilian or military) with past history of military war, peacekeeping and humanitarian deployment (current or past conflict)
Returned from military deployment

Z91.83 *Wandering in diseases classified elsewhere*
Code first underlying disorder such as:
Alzheimer's disease (G30.-)
autism or pervasive developmental disorder (F84.-)
intellectual disabilities (F70-F79)
unspecified dementia with behavioral disturbance (F03.9-)

✓6ᵗʰ **Z91.84** **Oral health risk factors**

Z91.841 **Risk for dental caries, low**

Z91.842 **Risk for dental caries, moderate**

Z91.843 **Risk for dental caries, high**

Z91.849 **Unspecified risk for dental caries** ▽

Z91.89 **Other specified personal risk factors, not elsewhere classified**
AHA: 2017, 1Q, 45

✓4ᵗʰ **Z92** **Personal history of medical treatment**
EXCLUDES 2 *postprocedural states (Z98.-)*

Z92.0 **Personal history of contraception**
EXCLUDES 1 *counseling or management of current contraceptive practices (Z30.-)*
long term (current) use of contraception (Z79.3)
presence of (intrauterine) contraceptive device (Z97.5)

✓5ᵗʰ **Z92.2** **Personal history of drug therapy**
EXCLUDES 2 *long term (current) drug therapy (Z79.-)*

Z92.21 **Personal history of antineoplastic chemotherapy**

Z92.22 **Personal history of monoclonal drug therapy**

Z92.23 **Personal history of estrogen therapy**

✓6ᵗʰ **Z92.24** **Personal history of steroid therapy**

Z92.240 **Personal history of inhaled steroid therapy**

Z92.241 **Personal history of systemic steroid therapy**
Personal history of steroid therapy NOS

Z92.25 **Personal history of immunosupression therapy**
EXCLUDES 2 *personal history of steroid therapy (Z92.24)*

Z92.29 **Personal history of other drug therapy**

Z92.3 **Personal history of irradiation**
Personal history of exposure to therapeutic radiation
EXCLUDES 1 *exposure to radiation in the physical environment (Z77.12)*
occupational exposure to radiation (Z57.1)

✓5ᵗʰ **Z92.8** **Personal history of other medical treatment**

Z92.81 **Personal history of extracorporeal membrane oxygenation (ECMO)**

Z92.82 **Status post administration of tPA (rtPA) in a different facility within the last 24 hours prior to admission to current facility**
Code first condition requiring tPA administration, such as:
acute cerebral infarction (I63.-)
acute myocardial infarction (I21-, I22-)
AHA: 2013, 4Q, 124

Z92.83 **Personal history of failed moderate sedation**
Personal history of failed conscious sedation
EXCLUDES 2 *failed moderate sedation during procedure (T88.52)*

Z92.84 **Personal history of unintended awareness under general anesthesia**
EXCLUDES 2 *unintended awareness under general anesthesia during procedure (T88.53)*

Z92.89 **Personal history of other medical treatment**

✓4ᵗʰ **Z93** **Artificial opening status**
EXCLUDES 1 *artificial openings requiring attention or management (Z43.-)*
complications of external stoma (J95.0-, K94.-, N99.5-)

Z93.0 **Tracheostomy status** HCC
AHA: 2013, 4Q, 129

Z93.1 **Gastrostomy status** HCC

Z93.2 **Ileostomy status** HCC

Z93.3 **Colostomy status** HCC

Z93.4 **Other artificial openings of gastrointestinal tract status** HCC

✓5ᵗʰ **Z93.5** **Cystostomy status** HCC ▽

Z93.50 **Unspecified cystostomy status** HCC ▽

Z93.51 **Cutaneous-vesicostomy status** HCC

Z93.52 **Appendico-vesicostomy status** HCC

Z93.59 **Other cystostomy status** HCC

EXCLUDES 1 Not coded here   *EXCLUDES 2* Not included here   N Newborn Age: 0   P Pediatric Age: 0-17   M Maternity Age: 12-55   A Adult Age: 15-124   PDx Primary Dx

1204   ICD-10-CM 2018

Z93.6   Other artificial openings of urinary tract status   `HCC`
Nephrostomy status
Ureterostomy status
Urethrostomy status

Z93.8   Other artificial opening status   `HCC`

Z93.9   Artificial opening status, unspecified   `HCC` ▽

✓4th **Z94**   **Transplanted organ and tissue status**
> `INCLUDES`   organ or tissue replaced by heterogenous or homogenous transplant
> `EXCLUDES 1`   complications of transplanted organ or tissue—see Alphabetical Index
> `EXCLUDES 2`   presence of vascular grafts (Z95.-)

Z94.0   Kidney transplant status

Z94.1   Heart transplant status   `HCC`
> `EXCLUDES 1`   artificial heart status (Z95.812)
> heart-valve replacement status (Z95.2-Z95.4)

Z94.2   Lung transplant status   `HCC`

Z94.3   Heart and lungs transplant status   `HCC`

Z94.4   Liver transplant status   `HCC`

Z94.5   Skin transplant status
Autogenous skin transplant status

Z94.6   Bone transplant status

Z94.7   Corneal transplant status

✓5th **Z94.8**   Other transplanted organ and tissue status

     Z94.81   Bone marrow transplant status   `HCC`

     Z94.82   Intestine transplant status   `HCC`

     Z94.83   Pancreas transplant status   `HCC`

     Z94.84   Stem cells transplant status   `HCC`

     Z94.89   Other transplanted organ and tissue status

Z94.9   Transplanted organ and tissue status, unspecified   ▽

✓4th **Z95**   **Presence of cardiac and vascular implants and grafts**
> `EXCLUDES 1`   ~~complications of cardiac and vascular devices, implants and grafts (T82.-)~~
> `EXCLUDES 2`   ▶complications of cardiac and vascular devices, implants and grafts (T82.-)◀

Z95.0   Presence of cardiac pacemaker
Presence of cardiac resynchronization therapy (CRT-P) pacemaker
> `EXCLUDES 1`   adjustment or management of cardiac device (Z45.0-)
> adjustment or management of cardiac pacemaker (Z45.0)
> presence of automatic (implantable) cardiac defibrillator with synchronous cardiac pacemaker (Z95.810)

Z95.1   Presence of aortocoronary bypass graft
Presence of coronary artery bypass graft

Z95.2   Presence of prosthetic heart valve
Presence of heart valve NOS

Z95.3   Presence of xenogenic heart valve

Z95.4   Presence of other heart-valve replacement

Z95.5   Presence of coronary angioplasty implant and graft
> `EXCLUDES 1`   coronary angioplasty status without implant and graft (Z98.61)

✓5th **Z95.8**   Presence of other cardiac and vascular implants and grafts

     ✓6th **Z95.81**   Presence of other cardiac implants and grafts

         Z95.810   Presence of automatic (implantable) cardiac defibrillator
Presence of automatic (implantable) cardiac defibrillator with synchronous cardiac pacemaker
Presence of cardiac resynchronization therapy defibrillator (CRT-D)
Presence of cardioverter-defibrillator (ICD)

         Z95.811   Presence of heart assist device   `HCC`

         Z95.812   Presence of fully implantable artificial heart   `HCC`

         Z95.818   Presence of other cardiac implants and grafts

     ✓6th **Z95.82**   Presence of other vascular implants and grafts

         Z95.820   Peripheral vascular angioplasty status with implants and grafts
> `EXCLUDES 1`   peripheral vascular angioplasty without implant and graft (Z98.62)

         Z95.828   Presence of other vascular implants and grafts
Presence of intravascular prosthesis NEC

Z95.9   Presence of cardiac and vascular implant and graft, unspecified   ▽

✓4th **Z96**   **Presence of other functional implants**
> `EXCLUDES 2`   complications of internal prosthetic devices, implants and grafts (T82-T85)
> fitting and adjustment of prosthetic and other devices (Z44-Z46)

Z96.0   Presence of urogenital implants

Z96.1   Presence of intraocular lens
Presence of pseudophakia

✓5th **Z96.2**   Presence of otological and audiological implants

     Z96.20   Presence of otological and audiological implant, unspecified   ▽

     Z96.21   Cochlear implant status

     Z96.22   Myringotomy tube(s) status

     Z96.29   Presence of other otological and audiological implants
Presence of bone-conduction hearing device
Presence of eustachian tube stent
Stapes replacement

Z96.3   Presence of artificial larynx

✓5th **Z96.4**   Presence of endocrine implants

     Z96.41   Presence of insulin pump (external) (internal)

     Z96.49   Presence of other endocrine implants

Z96.5   Presence of tooth-root and mandibular implants

✓5th **Z96.6**   Presence of orthopedic joint implants

     Z96.60   Presence of unspecified orthopedic joint implant   ▽

     ✓6th **Z96.61**   Presence of artificial shoulder joint

         Z96.611   Presence of right artificial shoulder joint

         Z96.612   Presence of left artificial shoulder joint

         Z96.619   Presence of unspecified artificial shoulder joint   ▽

     ✓6th **Z96.62**   Presence of artificial elbow joint

         Z96.621   Presence of right artificial elbow joint

         Z96.622   Presence of left artificial elbow joint

         Z96.629   Presence of unspecified artificial elbow joint   ▽

     ✓6th **Z96.63**   Presence of artificial wrist joint

         Z96.631   Presence of right artificial wrist joint

         Z96.632   Presence of left artificial wrist joint

         Z96.639   Presence of unspecified artificial wrist joint   ▽

     ✓6th **Z96.64**   Presence of artificial hip joint
Hip-joint replacement (partial) (total)

         Z96.641   Presence of right artificial hip joint

         Z96.642   Presence of left artificial hip joint

         Z96.643   Presence of artificial hip joint, bilateral

         Z96.649   Presence of unspecified artificial hip joint   ▽

     ✓6th **Z96.65**   Presence of artificial knee joint

         Z96.651   Presence of right artificial knee joint

         Z96.652   Presence of left artificial knee joint

         Z96.653   Presence of artificial knee joint, bilateral

         Z96.659   Presence of unspecified artificial knee joint   ▽

     ✓6th **Z96.66**   Presence of artificial ankle joint

         Z96.661   Presence of right artificial ankle joint

         Z96.662   Presence of left artificial ankle joint

         Z96.669   Presence of unspecified artificial ankle joint   ▽

     ✓6th **Z96.69**   Presence of other orthopedic joint implants

         Z96.691   Finger-joint replacement of right hand

         Z96.692   Finger-joint replacement of left hand

         Z96.693   Finger-joint replacement, bilateral

         Z96.698   Presence of other orthopedic joint implants

---

☑ Additional Character Req   ✓x7th Placeholder Alert   Manifestation   `HCC` CMS-HCC Condition   ▽ Unspecified Code   ▶◀ Revised Text   ● New Code   ▲ Revised Code Title

Chapter 21. Factors Influencing Health Status and Contact with Health Services

Z96.7   **Presence of other bone and tendon implants**
Presence of skull plate

✓5ᵗʰ **Z96.8**   **Presence of other specified functional implants**

Z96.81   **Presence of artificial skin**

Z96.89   **Presence of other specified functional implants** ▽

Z96.9   **Presence of functional implant, unspecified**

✓4ᵗʰ **Z97**   **Presence of other devices**
EXCLUDES 1   *complications of internal prosthetic devices, implants and grafts (T82-T85)*
fitting and adjustment of prosthetic and other devices (Z44-Z46)
EXCLUDES 2   *presence of cerebrospinal fluid drainage device (Z98.2)*

Z97.0   **Presence of artificial eye**

✓5ᵗʰ **Z97.1**   **Presence of artificial limb (complete) (partial)** ▽

Z97.10   **Presence of artificial limb (complete) (partial), unspecified**

Z97.11   **Presence of artificial right arm (complete) (partial)**

Z97.12   **Presence of artificial left arm (complete) (partial)**

Z97.13   **Presence of artificial right leg (complete) (partial)**

Z97.14   **Presence of artificial left leg (complete) (partial)**

Z97.15   **Presence of artificial arms, bilateral (complete) (partial)**

Z97.16   **Presence of artificial legs, bilateral (complete) (partial)**

Z97.2   **Presence of dental prosthetic device (complete) (partial)**
Presence of dentures (complete) (partial)

Z97.3   **Presence of spectacles and contact lenses**

Z97.4   **Presence of external hearing-aid**

Z97.5   **Presence of (intrauterine) contraceptive device** ♀
EXCLUDES 1   *checking, reinsertion or removal of implantable subdermal contraceptive (Z30.46)*
checking, reinsertion or removal of intrauterine contraceptive device (Z30.43-)

Z97.8   **Presence of other specified devices**

✓4ᵗʰ **Z98**   **Other postprocedural states**
EXCLUDES 2   *aftercare (Z43-Z49, Z51)*
follow-up medical care (Z08- Z09)
postprocedural complication—see Alphabetical Index

Z98.0   **Intestinal bypass and anastomosis status**
EXCLUDES 2   *bariatric surgery status (Z98.84)*
gastric bypass status (Z98.84)
obesity surgery status (Z98.84)

Z98.1   **Arthrodesis status**

Z98.2   **Presence of cerebrospinal fluid drainage device**
Presence of CSF shunt

Z98.3   **Post therapeutic collapse of lung status**
Code first underlying disease

✓5ᵗʰ **Z98.4**   **Cataract extraction status**
Use additional code to identify intraocular lens implant status (Z96.1)
EXCLUDES 1   *aphakia (H27.0)*

Z98.41   **Cataract extraction status, right eye**

Z98.42   **Cataract extraction status, left eye**

Z98.49   **Cataract extraction status, unspecified eye** ▽

✓5ᵗʰ **Z98.5**   **Sterilization status**
EXCLUDES 1   *female infertility (N97.-)*
male infertility (N46.-)

Z98.51   **Tubal ligation status** ♀

Z98.52   **Vasectomy status** A ♂

✓5ᵗʰ **Z98.6**   **Angioplasty status**

Z98.61   **Coronary angioplasty status**
EXCLUDES 1   *coronary angioplasty status with implant and graft (Z95.5)*

Z98.62   **Peripheral vascular angioplasty status**
EXCLUDES 1   *peripheral vascular angioplasty status with implant and graft (Z95.820)*

✓5ᵗʰ **Z98.8**   **Other specified postprocedural states**

✓6ᵗʰ **Z98.81**   **Dental procedure status**

Z98.810   **Dental sealant status**

Z98.811   **Dental restoration status**
Dental crown status
Dental fillings status

Z98.818   **Other dental procedure status**

Z98.82   **Breast implant status**
EXCLUDES 1   *breast implant removal status (Z98.86)*

Z98.83   **Filtering (vitreous) bleb after glaucoma surgery status**
EXCLUDES 1   *inflammation (infection) of postprocedural bleb (H59.4-)*

Z98.84   **Bariatric surgery status**
Gastric banding status
Gastric bypass status for obesity
Obesity surgery status
EXCLUDES 1   *bariatric surgery status complicating pregnancy, childbirth, or the puerperium (O99.84)*
EXCLUDES 2   *intestinal bypass and anastomosis status (Z98.0)*

Z98.85   **Transplanted organ removal status**
Transplanted organ previously removed due to complication, failure, rejection or infection
EXCLUDES 1   *encounter for removal of transplanted organ—code to complication of transplanted organ (T86.-)*

Z98.86   **Personal history of breast implant removal**

✓6ᵗʰ **Z98.87**   **Personal history of in utero procedure**

Z98.870   **Personal history of in utero procedure during pregnancy** ♀
EXCLUDES 2   *complications from in utero procedure for current pregnancy (O35.7)*
supervision of current pregnancy with history of in utero procedure during previous pregnancy (O09.82-)

Z98.871   **Personal history of in utero procedure while a fetus**

✓6ᵗʰ **Z98.89**   **Other specified postprocedural states**

Z98.890   **Other specified postprocedural states**
Personal history of surgery, not elsewhere classified

Z98.891   **History of uterine scar from previous surgery**
EXCLUDES 1   *maternal care due to uterine scar from previous surgery (O34.2-)*

✓4ᵗʰ **Z99**   **Dependence on enabling machines and devices, not elsewhere classified**
EXCLUDES 1   *cardiac pacemaker status (Z95.0)*

Z99.0   **Dependence on aspirator**

✓5ᵗʰ **Z99.1**   **Dependence on respirator**
Dependence on ventilator

Z99.11   **Dependence on respirator [ventilator] status** HCC
AHA: 2015, 1Q, 21

Z99.12   **Encounter for respirator [ventilator] dependence during power failure** HCC PDx
EXCLUDES 1   *mechanical complication of respirator [ventilator] (J95.850)*

Z99.2   **Dependence on renal dialysis** HCC
Hemodialysis status
Peritoneal dialysis status
Presence of arteriovenous shunt for dialysis
Renal dialysis status NOS
EXCLUDES 1   *encounter for fitting and adjustment of dialysis catheter (Z49.0-)*
EXCLUDES 2   *noncompliance with renal dialysis (Z91.15)*
AHA: 2016, 1Q, 12; 2013, 4Q, 125

Z99.3   **Dependence on wheelchair**
Wheelchair confinement status
Code first cause of dependence, such as:
muscular dystrophy (G71.0)
obesity (E66.-)

EXCLUDES 1 Not coded here   EXCLUDES 2 Not included here   N Newborn Age: 0   P Pediatric Age: 0-17   M Maternity Age: 12-55   A Adult Age: 15-124   PDx Primary Dx

1206   ICD-10-CM 2018

√5ᵗʰ **Z99.8 Dependence on other enabling machines and devices**

    Z99.81 Dependence on supplemental oxygen
        Dependence on long-term oxygen
        AHA: 2013, 4Q, 129

    Z99.89 Dependence on other enabling machines and devices
        Dependence on machine or device NOS

☑ Additional Character Req   √x7ᵗʰ Placeholder Alert   Manifestation   HCC CMS-HCC Condition   ▽ Unspecified Code   ▶◀ Revised Text   ● New Code   ▲ Revised Code Title

CD-10-CM 2018

1207

Appendix A: 10 Steps to Correct Coding

Follow the 10 steps below to correctly code encounters for health care services.

Step 1: Identify the reason for the visit or encounter (i.e., a sign, symptom, diagnosis and/or condition).

The medical record documentation should accurately reflect the patient's condition, using terminology that includes specific diagnoses and symptoms or clearly states the reasons for the encounter.

Choosing the main term that best describes the reason chiefly responsible for the service provided is the most important step in coding. If symptoms are present and documented but a definitive diagnosis has not yet been determined, code the symptoms. **For outpatient cases, do not code conditions that are referred to as "rule out," "suspected," "probable," or "questionable."** Diagnoses often are not established at the time of the initial encounter/visit and may require two or more visits to be established. Code only what is documented in the available records and only to the highest degree of certainty known at the time of the patient's visit, unless it is an inpatient medical record, in which case uncertain diagnoses may be reported if documented at the time of discharge.

Step 2: After selecting the reason for the encounter, always consult the alphabetic index before verifying code selection in the tabular section.

The most critical rule is to begin code selection in the *alphabetic index*. Never turn first to the tabular list. The index provides cross-references, essential and nonessential modifiers, and inclusion terms not found in the tabular list. To prevent coding errors, always use both the alphabetic index (to identify a code) and the tabular list (to verify a code), as the index does not include the important instructional notes found in the tabular list. An added benefit of using the tabular list, which groups like things together, is that while looking at one code in the list, a coder might see a more specific one that would have been missed had the coder relied solely on the alphabetic index. Additionally, many of the codes require a fourth, fifth, sixth, or seventh, character to be valid, and many of these characters can be found only in the tabular list.

Step 3: Locate the main term entry.

The alphabetic index is a listing of conditions, which may be expressed as nouns or eponyms, with critical use of adjectives. Some conditions known by several names have multiple main entries. Reasons for encounters may be located under general terms such as admission, encounter, and examination. Other general terms such as history of, status post, or presence (of) are used to locate factors influencing health.

Step 4: Read cross-references listed with the main term or the subterm.

Cross-references such as *"see"* and *"see also"* are identified by italicized type and should always be checked to ensure that all alternative terms are researched.

Step 5: Review entries for modifiers.

Nonessential modifiers are the terms in parentheses following the main term entry. These parenthetical terms are supplementary words or explanatory information that may or may not appear in the diagnostic statement and do not affect code selection. The subterms listed under the main term are essential modifiers that do affect coding assignment. Each line of indent represents a more specific code entry. The nonessential modifiers apply to the subterms following a main term except when they are mutually exclusive, in which case the subterm takes precedence. For example, if "acute" is listed as a nonessential modifier but there is a subentry for "chronic," then the nonessential modifier of "acute" does not apply.

Step 6: Interpret abbreviations, cross-references, default codes, additional characters, and brackets.

The abbreviation NEC (not elsewhere classified) that follows some main terms or subterms indicates that there is no specific code for the condition even though the medical documentation may be very specific. The code next to the main term is called the default code. It represents the condition most commonly associated with the main term or the unspecified code for the main term. Additional characters may be required to construct the code; the tabular list must be referenced to determine what those specific characters should be. The alphabetic index uses brackets [ ] to enclose manifestation codes that can be

used only as secondary codes to the underlying condition code immediately preceding it. Both codes must be reported in this multiple-coding situation.

Step 7: Choose a potential code and locate it in the tabular list.

The coder must follow any Includes, Excludes 1 and Excludes 2 notes, and other instructional notes, such as "Code first" and "Use additional code," listed in the tabular list for the chapter, category, subcategory, and subclassification level of code selection that direct the coder to use a different or additional code. Any codes in the tabular range, A00.0- through T88.9-, may be used to identify the diagnostic reason for the encounter. The tabular list encompasses many codes describing disease and injury classifications (e.g., infectious and parasitic diseases, neoplasms, symptoms, nervous and circulatory system etc.).

Codes that describe symptoms and signs, as opposed to definitive diagnoses, should be used for reporting purposes when an established diagnosis has not been made (confirmed) by the physician. Chapter 18 of the ICD-10-CM code book, "Symptoms, Signs, and Abnormal Clinical and Laboratory Findings, Not Elsewhere Classified" (codes R00.-–R99), contains many, but not all, codes for symptoms.

ICD-10-CM classifies encounters with health care providers for circumstances other than a disease or injury using codes in chapter 21, "Factors Influencing Health Status and Contact with Health Services" (codes Z00–Z99). Circumstances other than a disease or injury often are recorded as chiefly responsible for the encounter.

Step 8: Determine whether the code is at the highest level of specificity.

A code is invalid if it has not been coded to the full number of characters (greatest level of specificity) required. Codes in ICD-10-CM can contain from three up to seven alphanumeric characters. A three-character code is to be used only if the category is not further subdivided into four-, five-, six-, or seven-character codes. Placeholder character X is used both to allow for future expansion and as a placeholder for empty characters in a code that requires a seventh character but has no fourth, fifth, or sixth character. Certain categories require seventh characters that apply to all codes in that category. Always check the category level for applicable seventh characters for that category.

Step 9: Assign the code.

Having reviewed all relevant information concerning the possible code choices, assign the code that most completely describes the condition.

Repeat steps one through nine for all additional documented conditions that meet the following criteria:

- Conditions that currently exist at the time of the visit
- Conditions that require or affect patient care, treatment, or management

Step 10: Sequence codes correctly.

Sequencing is the order in which the codes are listed on the claim. List first the ICD-10-CM code for the diagnosis, condition, problem, or other reason for the encounter/visit, which is shown in the medical record to be chiefly responsible for the services provided. List additional codes that describe any coexisting conditions. Follow the official coding guidelines (see section II, "Selection of Principal Diagnosis"; section III, "Reporting Additional Diagnoses"; and section IV, "Diagnostic Coding and Reporting Guidelines for Outpatient Services") on proper sequencing of codes.

Coding Examples

Diagnosis: Anorexia

Step 1: The reason for the encounter was the condition, anorexia.

Step 2: Consult the alphabetic index.

Step 3: Locate the main term "Anorexia."

Step 4: There are no cross-references to check.

Step 5: Note that there are two possible subterms (essential modifiers), "hysterical" and "nervosa," neither of which is documented in this instance and therefore cannot be used in code selection. The code listed next to the main term is called the default code selection.

Step 6: There are no abbreviations, cross-references, additional character icons, or brackets.

Step 7: Turn to code R63.Ø in the tabular list and read the instructional notes. In this case the Excludes 1 note indicates that anorexia nervosa and loss of appetite determined to be of nonorganic origin should be coded to a code from chapter 5. The diagnostic statement does not indicate nonorganic origin.

Step 8: There is no further division of the category past the fourth character subcategory. Therefore, the subcategory code level is the highest level of specificity.

Step 9: The default code, R63.Ø Anorexia, is the correct code selection

Step 10: Since anorexia is listed as the chief reason for the health care encounter, the first-listed, or principal, diagnosis is R63.Ø. Note that this is a chapter 18 symptom code but can be assigned since the provider did not establish a more definitive diagnosis.

Diagnosis: Acute bronchitis

Step 1: The reason for the encounter was the condition, acute bronchitis.

Step 2: Consult the alphabetic index.

Step 3: Locate the main term "Bronchitis."

Step 4: There are cross-references to interpret.

Step 5: Review entries for modifiers. Since "acute" is not listed as a nonessential modifier, read past the "with" modifier until you find the subterm "acute or subacute" with a nonessential modifier of "with bronchospasm or obstruction," code J2Ø.9.

Step 6: There are no abbreviations, cross-references, additional character icons, or brackets.

Step 7: Since there are no more appropriate subterms, turn to code J2Ø.9 in the tabular list. The Includes note under category J2Ø does refer to other alternative terms for acute bronchitis. Note that the inclusion term list is not exhaustive but is only a representative selection of diagnoses that are included in the subcategory. The Excludes 1 note refers bronchitis and tracheobronchitis NOS to category J4Ø. There are several Excludes 2 notes that, if applicable, can be coded in addition to this code.

Step 8: Note that the subcategories included in J2Ø represent acute bronchitis due to various infectious organisms that would be selected if identified in the documentation. In this case, the organism was not identified and there is no further division of the category past the fourth character subcategory. Therefore, the subcategory code level is the highest level of specificity.

Step 9: Assign code J2Ø.9 Acute bronchitis, unspecified.

Step 10: Repeat steps 1-9 for any additional code assignments.

Diagnosis: Infectious diarrhea

Step 1: The reason for the encounter was the condition, infectious diarrhea.

Step 2: Consult the alphabetic index.

Step 3: Locate the main term "Diarrhea" in the alphabetic index.

Step 4: There are no cross-references to check.

Step 5: Review entries for modifiers. Note that the nonessential modifiers (in parentheses) after the main term do not include the term "infectious," which means that the coder should search the subterms for the term "infectious." The subterm "infectious" refers to code AØ9.

Step 6: There are no abbreviations, cross-references, additional character icons, or brackets.

Step 7: Locate code AØ9 in the tabular list, and read all instructional notes under the main category and subcategories. The Includes notes does not list the term "infectious diarrhea" under code AØ9; however, as instructed by the alphabetic index, you should code the condition to AØ9. The ICD-1Ø-CM code book implies that infectious diarrhea is the same as infectious gastroenteritis, enteritis, and colitis.

Step 8: There is no further division of the category past the third-character category level. Therefore, the category code level is the highest level of specificity. The final code assignment would be AØ9.

Step 9: Assign code AØ9 Infectious gastroenteritis and colitis, unspecified.

Step 10: Since infectious diarrhea is listed as the chief reason for the health care encounter, the first-listed, or principal, diagnosis is AØ9.

Diagnosis: Decubitus ulcer of right elbow with skin loss and necrosis of subcutaneous tissue

Step 1: The reason for the encounter was the condition, decubitus ulcer.

Step 2: Consult the alphabetic index.

Step 3: Locate the main term "Ulcer" in the alphabetic index.

Step 4: There are no cross-references to check.

Step 5: This entry does not have any important nonessential modifiers; however, there are other terms such as ulcerated, ulcerating, etc., that are included as main terms. Locate the subterm "decubitus" and note that there is an italicized cross-reference to "see Ulcer, pressure, by site." Go to the subterm "pressure" and locate "elbow," which refers to code L89.Ø-.

Step 6: Note that the code L89.Ø is followed by a dash and an additional character icon, which indicate that more characters are required. From here, the tabular list can be consulted at code L89.Ø-.

Step 7: Locate code L89.Ø in the tabular list, and check the category level L89 for any instructional, Includes, and Excludes 1 and 2 notes. Note that "decubitus" is an Includes note under L89 Pressure ulcer. Excludes 2 notes indicate that if this were documented as a diabetic pressure ulcer, it would be necessary to use a code from chapter 4.

Step 8: Read through the subcategory codes under L89.Ø and note that the fifth character describes laterality. Locate the right elbow at subcategory L89.Ø1. See that an additional sixth character is now needed to complete the code. The sixth character specifies the stage of the ulcer, which can be determined either by the specific documentation of the stage (e.g., stage 1, stage 2) or in this case, a description that matches one of the Includes notes that follow each stage code. For example, the description in this case of "skin loss and necrosis of the subcutaneous tissue" matches the Includes notes under L89.Ø13 Pressure ulcer of right elbow, stage 3.

Step 9: Assign code L89.Ø13 Pressure ulcer of right elbow, stage 3

Step 10: Since the decubitus ulcer is listed as the chief reason for the health care encounter, the first-listed, or principal, diagnosis is L89.Ø13. However, according to the Code first instructional note at the L89 category level, gangrene would be sequenced before the pressure ulcer if it were documented.

Diagnosis: First visit for bimalleolar fracture of the right ankle due to trauma

Step 1: The reason for the encounter was the condition, bimalleolar fracture of the right ankle.

Step 2: Consult the alphabetic index.

Step 3: Locate the main term "Fracture" in the alphabetic index.

Step 4: Note that the first main term for Fracture is pathological with cross-reference to "see also Fracture, traumatic." Locate the main term "Fracture, traumatic."

Step 5: Review entries for nonessential modifiers. Locate the subterms "ankle," "bimalleolar." Note that "displaced" is a nonessential modifier following "bimalleolar," indicating that S82.84- is the default code unless the fracture is specified as nondisplaced.

Step 6: Note that code S82.84- is followed by a dash and an additional character icon, both of which indicate that more characters are required. From here, the tabular list can be consulted at code S82.84.

Step 7: Locate code S82.84 Bimalleolar fracture of lower leg, in the tabular list and check the category level S82 for any instructional, Includes, and Excludes 1 and 2 notes. See the instructional notes indicating that fractures not specified as displaced or nondisplaced default to displaced, and fractures not designated as open or closed default to closed. See also the list of appropriate seventh characters to be added to all codes from category S82.

Step 8: Read through the subcategory codes under S82.84, and note that the sixth character specifies displaced or nondisplaced and laterality. Locate the displaced bimalleolar fracture of the right lower leg at code S82.841. See that an additional seventh character is still needed to complete the code. The seventh character specifies the type of encounter and whether the fracture is open or closed. Use character A listed in the box at the category level to describe initial encounter, closed fracture.

Step 9: Assign code S82.841A Displaced bimalleolar fracture of right lower leg, initial encounter for closed fracture.

Step 10: Since this is an injury code, code additionally any external cause, place of occurrence, and activity codes, with the injury (fracture) sequenced first.

Appendix B: Valid 3-character ICD-10-CM Codes

A09	Infectious gastroenteritis and colitis, unspecified
A33	Tetanus neonatorum
A34	Obstetrical tetanus
A35	Other tetanus
A46	Erysipelas
A55	Chlamydial lymphogranuloma (venereum)
A57	Chancroid
A58	Granuloma inguinale
A64	Unspecified sexually transmitted disease
A65	Nonvenereal syphilis
A70	Chlamydia psittaci infections
A78	Q fever
A86	Unspecified viral encephalitis
A89	Unspecified viral infection of central nervous system
A90	Dengue fever [classical dengue]
A91	Dengue hemorrhagic fever
A94	Unspecified arthropod-borne viral fever
A99	Unspecified viral hemorrhagic fever
B03	Smallpox
B04	Monkeypox
B09	Unspecified viral infection characterized by skin and mucous membrane lesions
B20	Human immunodeficiency virus [HIV] disease
B49	Unspecified mycosis
B54	Unspecified malaria
B59	Pneumocystosis
B64	Unspecified protozoal disease
B72	Dracunculiasis
B75	Trichinellosis
B79	Trichuriasis
B80	Enterobiasis
B86	Scabies
B89	Unspecified parasitic disease
B91	Sequelae of poliomyelitis
B92	Sequelae of leprosy
C01	Malignant neoplasm of base of tongue
C07	Malignant neoplasm of parotid gland
C12	Malignant neoplasm of pyriform sinus
C19	Malignant neoplasm of rectosigmoid junction
C20	Malignant neoplasm of rectum
C23	Malignant neoplasm of gallbladder
C33	Malignant neoplasm of trachea
C37	Malignant neoplasm of thymus
C52	Malignant neoplasm of vagina
C55	Malignant neoplasm of uterus, part unspecified
C58	Malignant neoplasm of placenta
C61	Malignant neoplasm of prostate
C73	Malignant neoplasm of thyroid gland
D34	Benign neoplasm of thyroid gland
D45	Polycythemia vera
D62	Acute posthemorrhagic anemia
D65	Disseminated intravascular coagulation [defibrination syndrome]
D66	Hereditary factor VIII deficiency
D67	Hereditary factor IX deficiency
D71	Functional disorders of polymorphonuclear neutrophils
D77	Other disorders of blood and blood-forming organs in diseases classified elsewhere
E02	Subclinical iodine-deficiency hypothyroidism
E15	Nondiabetic hypoglycemic coma
E35	Disorders of endocrine glands in diseases classified elsewhere
E40	Kwashiorkor
E41	Nutritional marasmus
E42	Marasmic kwashiorkor
E43	Unspecified severe protein-calorie malnutrition
E45	Retarded development following protein-calorie malnutrition
E46	Unspecified protein-calorie malnutrition
E52	Niacin deficiency [pellagra]
E54	Ascorbic acid deficiency
E58	Dietary calcium deficiency
E59	Dietary selenium deficiency
E60	Dietary zinc deficiency
E65	Localized adiposity
E68	Sequelae of hyperalimentation
F04	Amnestic disorder due to known physiological condition
F05	Delirium due to known physiological condition
F09	Unspecified mental disorder due to known physiological condition
F21	Schizotypal disorder
F22	Delusional disorders
F23	Brief psychotic disorder
F24	Shared psychotic disorder
F28	Other psychotic disorder not due to a substance or known physiological condition
F29	Unspecified psychosis not due to a substance or known physiological condition
F39	Unspecified mood [affective] disorder
F53	Puerperal psychosis
F54	Psychological and behavioral factors associated with disorders or diseases classified elsewhere
F59	Unspecified behavioral syndromes associated with physiological disturbances and physical factors
F66	Other sexual disorders
F69	Unspecified disorder of adult personality and behavior
F70	Mild intellectual disabilities
F71	Moderate intellectual disabilities
F72	Severe intellectual disabilities
F73	Profound intellectual disabilities
F78	Other intellectual disabilities
F79	Unspecified intellectual disabilities
F82	Specific developmental disorder of motor function
F88	Other disorders of psychological development
F89	Unspecified disorder of psychological development
F99	Mental disorder, not otherwise specified
G01	Meningitis in bacterial diseases classified elsewhere
G02	Meningitis in other infectious and parasitic diseases classified elsewhere
G07	Intracranial and intraspinal abscess and granuloma in diseases classified elsewhere
G08	Intracranial and intraspinal phlebitis and thrombophlebitis
G09	Sequelae of inflammatory diseases of central nervous system
G10	Huntington's disease
G14	Postpolio syndrome
G20	Parkinson's disease
G26	Extrapyramidal and movement disorders in diseases classified elsewhere
G35	Multiple sclerosis
G53	Cranial nerve disorders in diseases classified elsewhere
G55	Nerve root and plexus compressions in diseases classified elsewhere
G59	Mononeuropathy in diseases classified elsewhere
G63	Polyneuropathy in diseases classified elsewhere
G64	Other disorders of peripheral nervous system
G92	Toxic encephalopathy
G94	Other disorders of brain in diseases classified elsewhere
H22	Disorders of iris and ciliary body in diseases classified elsewhere
H28	Cataract in diseases classified elsewhere
H32	Chorioretinal disorders in diseases classified elsewhere
H36	Retinal disorders in diseases classified elsewhere
H42	Glaucoma in diseases classified elsewhere
I00	Rheumatic fever without heart involvement
I10	Essential (primary) hypertension
I32	Pericarditis in diseases classified elsewhere
I38	Endocarditis, valve unspecified

I39	Endocarditis and heart valve disorders in diseases classified elsewhere
I41	Myocarditis in diseases classified elsewhere
I43	Cardiomyopathy in diseases classified elsewhere
I52	Other heart disorders in diseases classified elsewhere
I76	Septic arterial embolism
I81	Portal vein thrombosis
I96	Gangrene, not elsewhere classified
J00	Acute nasopharyngitis (common cold)
J13	Pneumonia due to Streptococcus pneumoniae
J14	Pneumonia due to Hemophilus influenzae
J17	Pneumonia in diseases classified elsewhere
J22	Unspecified acute lower respiratory infection
J36	Peritonsillar abscess
J40	Bronchitis, not specified as acute or chronic
J42	Unspecified chronic bronchitis
J60	Coalworker's pneumoconiosis
J61	Pneumoconiosis due to asbestos and other mineral fibers
J64	Unspecified pneumoconiosis
J65	Pneumoconiosis associated with tuberculosis
J80	Acute respiratory distress syndrome
J82	Pulmonary eosinophilia, not elsewhere classified
J90	Pleural effusion, not elsewhere classified
J99	Respiratory disorders in diseases classified elsewhere
K23	Disorders of esophagus in diseases classified elsewhere
K30	Functional dyspepsia
K36	Other appendicitis
K37	Unspecified appendicitis
K67	Disorders of peritoneum in infectious diseases classified elsewhere
K77	Liver disorders in diseases classified elsewhere
K87	Disorders of gallbladder, biliary tract and pancreas in diseases classified elsewhere
L00	Staphylococcal scalded skin syndrome
L14	Bullous disorders in diseases classified elsewhere
L22	Diaper dermatitis
L26	Exfoliative dermatitis
L42	Pityriasis rosea
L45	Papulosquamous disorders in diseases classified elsewhere
L52	Erythema nodosum
L54	Erythema in diseases classified elsewhere
L62	Nail disorders in diseases classified elsewhere
L80	Vitiligo
L83	Acanthosis nigricans
L84	Corns and callosities
L86	Keratoderma in diseases classified elsewhere
L88	Pyoderma gangrenosum
L99	Other disorders of skin and subcutaneous tissue in diseases classified elsewhere
N08	Glomerular disorders in diseases classified elsewhere
N10	Acute tubulo-interstitial nephritis
N12	Tubulo-interstitial nephritis, not specified as acute or chronic
N16	Renal tubulo-interstitial disorders in diseases classified elsewhere
N19	Unspecified kidney failure
N22	Calculus of urinary tract in diseases classified elsewhere
N23	Unspecified renal colic
N29	Other disorders of kidney and ureter in diseases classified elsewhere
N33	Bladder disorders in diseases classified elsewhere
N37	Urethral disorders in diseases classified elsewhere
N51	Disorders of male genital organs in diseases classified elsewhere
N62	Hypertrophy of breast
N72	Inflammatory disease of cervix uteri
N74	Female pelvic inflammatory disorders in diseases classified elsewhere
N86	Erosion and ectropion of cervix uteri
N96	Recurrent pregnancy loss
O68	Labor and delivery complicated by abnormality of fetal acid-base balance
O76	Abnormality in fetal heart rate and rhythm complicating labor and delivery
O80	Encounter for full-term uncomplicated delivery
O82	Encounter for cesarean delivery without indication
O85	Puerperal sepsis
O94	Sequelae of complication of pregnancy, childbirth, and the puerperium
P09	Abnormal findings on neonatal screening
P53	Hemorrhagic disease of newborn
P60	Disseminated intravascular coagulation of newborn
P84	Other problems with newborn
P90	Convulsions of newborn
P95	Stillbirth
Q02	Microcephaly
R05	Cough
R12	Heartburn
R17	Unspecified jaundice
R21	Rash and other nonspecific skin eruption
R32	Unspecified urinary incontinence
R34	Anuria and oliguria
R37	Sexual dysfunction, unspecified
R42	Dizziness and giddiness
R51	Headache
R52	Pain, unspecified
R54	Age-related physical debility
R55	Syncope and collapse
R58	Hemorrhage, not elsewhere classified
R61	Generalized hyperhidrosis
R64	Cachexia
R69	Illness, unspecified
R75	Inconclusive laboratory evidence of human immunodeficiency virus [HIV]
R81	Glycosuria
R99	Ill-defined and unknown cause of mortality
Y09	Assault by unspecified means
Y66	Nonadministration of surgical and medical care
Y69	Unspecified misadventure during surgical and medical care
Y95	Nosocomial condition
Z08	Encounter for follow-up examination after completed treatment for malignant neoplasm
Z09	Encounter for follow-up examination after completed treatment for conditions other than malignant neoplasm
Z21	Asymptomatic human immunodeficiency virus [HIV] infection status
Z23	Encounter for immunization
Z66	Do not resuscitate

Appendix C: Pharmacology List 2018

This section enables the coder to quickly review drugs, drug actions, and indications that are often associated with overlooked or undocumented diagnoses. The coder should review the patient's medication record and know what condition the physician is treating with the prescribed medication based on documentation in the medical record. When documentation is lacking, the coder can reference this section to locate the drug, determine the drug action, confirm drug indications, and when necessary query the physician.

Drug	Z Code	Drug Action	Indications
Abilify [aripiprazole]		Antipsychotic	Depression, bipolar disorder, schizophrenia, autism symptoms
Acarbose [acarbose]	Z79.84	Blood glucose regulator	Diabetes mellitus
Accupril [quinapril hydrochloride]		ACE inhibitor; antihypertensive	Congestive heart failure; essential hypertension
Acetaminophen with codeine [acetominophen/codeine phosphate]	Z79.891	Analgesic, general; analgesic-narcotic	Pain, moderate to severe
Actemra [tocilizumab]		Antirheumatic	Rheumatoid arthritis
Actimmune [interferon gamma-1b]	Z79.899	Antineoplastic interferons; antiviral interferons	Chronic granulomatous disease; malignant osteopetrosis
Activella [estradiol/norethindrone acetate]	Z79.890	Estrogen therapy	Menopause symptoms; vaginal and vulvar atrophy; osteoporosis prevention
Actonel [risedronate sodium]	Z79.83	Electrolytic and renal agent; bone resorption inhibitor	Decrease in bone loss in multiple myeloma patients; Paget's disease; hyperparathyroidism; osteoporosis
Actoplus Met [metformin hydrochloride/pioglitazone hydrochloride]	Z79.84	Blood glucose regulator	Diabetes mellitus
Actos [pioglitazone hydrochloride]	Z79.84	Blood glucose regulator	Diabetes mellitus
Adalat CC [nifedipine]		Calcium channel blocker	Vasospastic angina; chronic stable angina; essential hypertension
Advair [fluticasone propionate/salmeterol xinafoate]	Z79.51	Corticosteroids--inhaled; antiasthmatic	Prophylaxis and treatment of asthma and COPD
Advil [ibuprofen]	Z79.1	Nonsteroidal anti-inflammatory drug (NSAID)	Pain or fever relief
Aerospan [flunisolide]	Z79.51	Corticosteroids--inhaled; antiasthmatic	Prophylaxis and treatment of asthma
Afrezza [human insulin recombinant]	Z79.4	Blood glucose regulator	Diabetes mellitus
Aggrastat [tirofiban hydrochloride]	Z79.02	Antithrombotic platelet aggregation inhibitor	Unstable angina or heart attacks
Aggrenox [aspirin/dipyridamole]	Z79.02	Antithrombotic platelet aggregation inhibitor	Lessening of the chance of heart attack or stroke
Akne-Mycin [erythromycin]	Z79.2	Antibacterial	Severe acne treatment
Aldactone [spironolactone]		Cardiovascular agent; antihypertensive agent; diuretic; electrolytic and renal agent	Severe heart failure; ascites associated with cirrhosis; hypokalemia
Aleve [naproxen sodium]	Z79.1	Nonsteroidal anti-inflammatory drug (NSAID)	Reduction of temporary aches and pains
Allegra [fexofenadine hydrochloride]		Antihistamine	Seasonal allergic rhinitis
Allopurinol [allopurinol]		Antigout	Gouty arthritis, renal calculus, hyperuricemia, hyperuricemia secondary to leukemia, hyperuricemia secondary to lymphoma
Alora [estradiol]	Z79.890	Estrogen therapy	Menopause symptoms
Alphagan P [brimonidine tartrate]		Antiglaucoma agent (ophthalmic) antihypertensive, ocular	Open angle glaucoma or another condition in which pressure in the eye is too high (ocular hypertension)
Alprazolam [alprazolam]		Antianxiety; sedative/hypnotic	
Altabax [retapamulin]	Z79.2	Antibacterial	Skin infections
Altace [ramipril]		ACE inhibitor; antihypertensive	Congestive heart failure, essential hypertension
Altavera [ethinyl estradiol/levonorgestrel]	Z79.3	Contraceptive	Contraception
Alvesco [ciclesonide]	Z79.51	Corticosteroids--inhaled; antiasthmatic	Prophylaxis and treatment of asthma
Alyacen [ethinyl estradiol/norethindrone]	Z79.3	Contraceptive	Contraception
Amaryl [glimepiride]	Z79.84	Blood glucose regulator	Diabetes mellitus
Ambien [zolpidem tartrate]		Sedative/hypnotic	Insomnia
A-Methapred [methylprednisolone sodium succinate]	Z79.52	Corticosteroids	Severe inflammation
Amikacin [amikacin sulfate]		Aminoglycoside antibiotic	Active in treatment of gram-negative bacterial infections such as *Pseudomonas*, *Escherichia coli (E. coli)*, *Proteus*, *Klebsiella-Enterobacter-Serratia*

Appendix C: Pharmacology List 2018

Drug	Z Code	Drug Action	Indications
Aminophylline [aminophylline]		Bronchodilator, pulmonary vasodilator, smooth muscle relaxant	Relief and/or prevention of symptoms from asthma and reversible bronchospasms in bronchitis and emphysema
Amitriptyline hydrochloride [amitriptyline hydrochloride]		Anorexiant/CNS stimulant; antidepressant	Depression
Amoxicillin [amoxicillin]	Z79.2	Penicillin	Effective for infections with a broad spectrum of bactericidal activity against many gram-positive and gram-negative micro-organisms; otitis media, gonorrhea, skin, respiratory, gastrointestinal, and genitourinary infections
Ampicillin [ampicillin sodium]	Z79.2	Antibacterial	Bacterial infections
Amrix [cyclobenzaprine hydrochloride]		Muscle relaxant	Adjunct to rest and physical therapy for muscle spasms
Anaprox [naproxen sodium]	Z79.1	Nonsteroidal anti-inflammatory drug (NSAID)	Pain, inflammation, or fever relief
Anastrozole [anastrozole]	Z79.811	Aromatase inhibitor	Postmenopausal breast cancer
Ancef [cefazolin sodium]	Z79.2	Semisynthetic cephalosporin antibiotic	Respiratory tract infections due to *Streptococcus pneumoniae, Klebsiella species, Haemophilus influenzae (H. influenzae), Staphylococcus aureus,* and group A betahemolytic streptococci; urinary tract infections due to *E. coli, Proteus mirabilis, Klebsiella* species and some strains of *Enterobacter* and enterococci; skin and skin structure infections, biliary tract infections, bone and joint infections, genital infections, septicemia, and endocarditis
Angeliq [drospirenone/estradiol]	Z79.890	Estrogen therapy	Menopause symptoms
Angiomax [bivalirudin]	Z79.02	Antithrombotic platelet aggregation inhibitor	Prevention of blood clots
Antabuse [disulfiram]		Alcohol treatment	Alcoholism
Antineoplastic/chemotherapy	Z79.899	Antineoplastic	Cancer
Anzemet [dolasetron mesylate]		Antiemetic/antinauseant	Management of nausea/vomiting following surgery or from effects of chemotherapy or cancer
Apidra [insulin glulisine recombinant]	Z79.4	Blood glucose regulator	Diabetes mellitus
Aranelle [ethinyl estradiol/norethindrone]	Z79.3	Contraceptive	Contraception; acne
Aranesp [darbepoetin alfa]		Erythropoiesis-stimulating agent (ESA)	Lower than normal blood cell count (anemia) from disorders such as CKD and neoplasms
Argatroban [argatroban]	Z79.02	Antithrombotic platelet aggregation inhibitor	Prophylaxis and treatment of venous thrombosis in thrombocytopenia patients
Aricept [donepezil hydrochloride]		Acetylcholine sterase inhibitor	Symptoms of mild to moderate Alzheimer's disease; can improve thinking ability in some patients
Arimidex [anastrozole]	Z79.811	Aromatase inhibitor	Postmenopausal breast cancer
Aristospan [triamcinolone hexacetonide]	Z79.52	Corticosteroids	Severe inflammation
Arixtra [fondaparinux sodium]	Z79.01	Anticoagulant	Venous thrombosis and pulmonary embolism
Arnuity Ellipta [fluticasone furoate]	Z79.51	Corticosteroids--inhaled; antiasthmatic	Prophylaxis and treatment of asthma
Aromasin [exemestane]	Z79.811	Aromatase inhibitor	Postmenopausal breast cancer
Arthrotec [diclofenac sodium/misoprostol]	Z79.1	Analgesic	Arthritis in patients who may develop stomach ulcers from taking nonsteroidal anti-inflammatory drugs (NSAIDs) alone; used to help relieve some symptoms of arthritis, such as inflammation, swelling, stiffness, and joint pain
Ashlyna [ethinyl estradiol/levonorgestrel]	Z79.3	Contraceptive	Contraception
Asmanex [mometasone furoate]	Z79.51	Corticosteroids--inhaled; antiasthmatic	Prophylaxis and treatment of asthma
Astagraf XL [tacrolimus]	Z79.899	Immunosuppressant	Prophylaxis of organ transplant rejection
Astramorph [morphine sulfate]	Z79.891	Narcotic analgesic	Pain
Atelvia [risedronate sodium]	Z79.83	Bisphosphonates	Prevention of thinning of the bones (osteoporosis)
Atenolol [atenolol]		Antianginal; antihypertensive; beta blocker	Chronic stable angina pectoris; essential hypertension; reduces cardiovascular mortality in those with definite or suspected acute myocardial infarction
Ativan [lorazepam]		Antianxiety; sedative/hypnotic	Anxiety disorder associated with depressive symptoms; controls tension, agitation, irritability, and insomnia
Atrovent [ipratropium bromide]		Antiasthmatic/bronchodilator	Chronic bronchitis, emphysema; bronchial asthma
Augmentin [amoxicillin/clavulanate potassium]	Z79.2	Antibacterial	Middle ear, lower respiratory, sinus, skin and skin structures, and urinary tract infections
Avandia [rosiglitazone maleate]	Z79.84	Blood glucose regulator	Diabetes mellitus

Drug	Z Code	Drug Action	Indications
Avapro [irbesartan]		Antihypertensive	Hypertension
Aviane [ethinyl estradiol/levonorgestrel]	Z79.3	Contraceptive	Contraception
Avonex [interferon beta-1a]	Z79.899	Antiviral interferon	Relapsing multiple sclerosis
Axid AR [nizatidine]		Histamine H2-receptor antagonist	Acid/peptic disorder; gastroesophageal reflux; duodenal, gastric, and peptic ulcers
Aygestin [norethindrone acetate]	Z79.3	Contraceptive	Contraception; menstrual disorders
Azactam [aztreonam]	Z79.2	Antibacterial	Severe or life-threatening bacterial infections
Azithromycin [azithromycin]	Z79.2	Antibacterial	Treatment of bacterial infections
Bactrim [sulfamethoxazole/trimethoprim]	Z79.2	Antibacterial	Urinary tract infections, acute otitis media, acute exacerbation of chronic bronchitis, shigellosis, and *Pneumocystis carinii*
Bactroban [mupirocin]	Z79.2	Dermatologic; topical anti-infective	Topical treatment of impetigo
Balziva [ethinyl estradiol/norethindrone]	Z79.3	Contraceptive	Contraception
Basaglar [insulin glargine]	Z79.4	Blood glucose regulator	Diabetes mellitus
Bayer [acetylsalicylic acid]	Z79.82	Aspirin	Prophylaxis and treatment of heart attacks, angina, or strokes; reduction of fever, pain, and inflammation
Beconase AQ [beclomethasone dipropionate monohydrate]		Corticosteroids; antiasthmatic	Bronchial asthma, prevention of nasal polyps, perennial allergies, seasonal allergies, and vasomotor rhinitis
Bekyree [desogestrel/ethinyl estradiol]	Z79.3	Contraceptive	Contraception
Betoptic [betaxolol hydrochloride]		Cardioselective beta-adrenergic receptor blocking agent	Lowering of intraocular pressure; also used for treatment of ocular hypertension and chronic open-angle glaucoma
Beyaz [drospirenone/ethinyl estradiol/levomefolate calcium]	Z79.3	Contraceptive	Contraception; acne
Biaxin [clarithromycin]		Macrolide	Acid/peptic disorder or ulcer, acute exacerbation chronic bronchitis, HIV, lower and upper respiratory tract infections, sinus infection, prophylaxis mycobacterium avium complex, pharyngitis, pneumonia, tonsillitis
Binosto [alendronate sodium]	Z79.83	Bisphosphonates	Prevention of thinning of the bones (osteoporosis)
Boniva [ibandronate sodium]	Z79.83	Bisphosphonates	Prevention of thinning of the bones (osteoporosis)
Brevicon [ethinyl estradiol/norethindrone]	Z79.3	Contraceptive	Contraception; acne
Briellyn [ethinyl estradiol/norethindrone]	Z79.3	Contraceptive	Contraception
Brilinta [ticagrelor]	Z79.02	Antithrombotic platelet aggregation inhibitor	Unstable angina or heart attacks and prevention of blood clots
Bufferin [acetylsalicylic acid]	Z79.82	Aspirin	Prophylaxis and treatment of heart attacks, angina or strokes; reduction of fever, pain, and inflammation
Buprenex [buprenorphine hydrochloride]	Z79.891	Narcotic analgesic	Moderate to severe pain
Buprenorphine HCl [buprenorphine hydrochloride]	Z79.891	Narcotic analgesic	Moderate to severe pain
Buspirone [buspirone hydrochloride]		Antianxiety agent	Generalized anxiety disorder
Butorphanol Tartrate [butorphanol tartrate]		Narcotic analgesic	Moderate to severe postsurgical pain
Butrans [buprenorphine]	Z79.891	Narcotic analgesic	Chronic pain
Calan [verapamil hydrochloride]		Antianginal; antiarrhythmic, antiarthritic, antihypertensive, calcium channel blocker	Angina pectoris at rest and chronic stable, arrhythmia, atrial fibrillation, atrial flutter, paroxysmal supraventricular tachycardia, ventricular arrhythmia, essential hypertension
Caldolor [ibuprofen]	Z79.1	Nonsteroidal anti-inflammatory drug (NSAID)	Pain or fever relief
Cambia [diclofenac potassium]	Z79.1	Nonsteroidal anti-inflammatory drug (NSAID)	Migraine headaches
Camila [norethindrone]	Z79.3	Contraceptive	Contraception; menstrual disorders
Cardizem CD [diltiazem hydrochloride]		Antianginal, antiarrhythmic, antihypertensive, channel blocker, coronary vasodilator	Chronic stable angina, atrial fibrillation, atrial flutter, essential hypertension, paroxysmal supraventricular tachycardia
Cardura [doxazosin mesylate]		Antihypertensive	Benign prostatic hyperplasia, essential hypertension
Catapres [clonidine hydrochloride]		Antihypertensive	Hypertension
Cefprozil [cefprozil]		Antibiotic: second generation cephalosporins	Acute exacerbation and chronic bronchitis, lower and upper respiratory tract infections, pharyngitis, tonsillitis

Drug	Z Code	Drug Action	Indications
Ceftin [cefuroxime axetil]		Antibiotic: second generation cephalosporins	Acute exacerbation and chronic bronchitis, middle ear infection, sexually transmitted gonorrhea infection, upper respiratory tract infection, urinary tract infection, pharyngitis, tonsillitis
Ceftriaxone [ceftriaxone sodium]	Z79.2	Antibacterial	Bacterial infections
Celebrex [celecoxib]	Z79.1	Antirheumatic, nonsteroidal anti-inflammatory	Relief of some symptoms caused by arthritis, such as inflammation, swelling, stiffness, and joint pain
Celestone Soluspan [betamethasone acetate/ betamethasone sodium phosphate]	Z79.52	Corticosteroids; antiasthmatic	Asthma; severe inflammation
Celexa [citalopram hydrobromide]		Antidepressant	Depression
Cellcept [mycophenolate mofetil]	Z79.899	Immunosuppressant	Prophylaxis of organ transplant rejection
Centany [mupirocin]	Z79.2	Antibacterial	Topical treatment of skin infections
Cephalexin [cephalexin]	Z79.2	Antibacterial	Bacterial infections
Chantix [varenicline tartrate]		Smoking cessation aid	Nicotine addiction, smoking
Cipro [ciprofloxacin hydrochloride]	Z79.2	Anti-infective; quinolone	Cystitis, infectious diarrhea, gonorrhea, bone and joint infection, gastrointestinal tract infection, lower and upper respiratory tract infections, sinus infection, urinary tract infection, nosocomial pneumonia, chronic prostatitis
Ciprofloxacin [ciprofloxacin]	Z79.2	Antibacterial	Bacterial infections
Clarithromycin [clarithromycin]	Z79.2	Antibacterial	Skin and respiratory bacterial infections
Claritin [loratadine]		Antihistamine	Seasonal allergic rhinitis, chronic idiopathic urticaria
Cleocin [clindamycin phosphate]	Z79.2	Antibacterial	Bacterial infections
Climara [estradiol]	Z79.890	Estrogen therapy	Osteoporosis prevention and menopausal symptoms; vaginal and vulvar atrophy; hypoestrogenism; ovarian failure
Clindamycin [clindamycin phosphate]	Z79.2	Antibacterial	Bacterial infections
Clonazepam [clonazepam]		Anticonvulsant	Absence, akinetic, and myoclonic epilepsy, Lennox-Gastaut syndrome
Clonidine [clonidine hydrochloride]		Antihypertensive	Hypertension
Clopidogrel bisulfate [clopidogrel bisulfate]	Z79.02	Antithrombotic platelet aggregation inhibitor	Treatment of unstable angina or heart attacks and prevention of blood clots
Codeine [codeine sulfate]	Z79.891	Narcotic analgesic	Mild to moderate pain
Cogentin [benztropine mesylate]		Antiparkinsonism	Parkinson's disease
Colace [docusate sodium]		Gastrointestinal agent; laxative, stool softener	Constipation
Colocort [hydrocortisone]	Z79.52	Corticosteroids	Inflammation of the colon
CombiPatch [ethinyl estradiol/norethindrone acetate]	Z79.890	Estrogen therapy	Menopause symptoms; vaginal and vulvar atrophy; osteoporosis prevention
Combivent [ipratropium bromide/albuterol sulfate]		Antiasthmatic/bronchodilator	Chronic bronchitis, emphysema; bronchial asthma
Compro [prochlorperazine]		Antiemetic, antipsychotic	Nausea, vomiting, and manic phase of bipolar syndrome or schizophrenia
Cortef [hydrocortisone]	Z79.52	Corticosteroids	Severe inflammation
Cortenema [hydrocortisone]	Z79.52	Corticosteroids	Inflammation of the colon
Cortifoam [hydrocortisone acetate]	Z79.52	Corticosteroids	Colon and rectum inflammation
Cortisone acetate [cortisone acetate]	Z79.52	Corticosteroids	Inflammation
Cortisporin [hydrocortisone acetate/neomycin sulfate/polymyxin B sulfate]		Topical anti-infective, topical steroid	Dermatosis
Coumadin [warfarin sodium]	Z79.01	Anticoagulant	Prophylaxis and treatment of venous thrombosis, treatment of atrial fibrillation with embolization (pulmonary embolism), arrhythmias, myocardial infarction, and stroke prevention
Cozaar [losartan potassium]		Antihypertensive	Essential hypertension
Crestor [rosuvastatin calcium]		HMG-CoA reductase inhibitor (statin)	Hypercholesterolemia, hyperlipidemia, hyperproteinemia
Crixivan [indinavir sulfate]		HIV inhibitor	HIV, asymptomatic HIV
Cryselle [ethinyl estradiol/norgestrel]	Z79.3	Contraceptive	Contraception
Cyclafem [ethinyl estradiol/norethindrone]	Z79.3	Contraceptive	Contraception
Cyclessa [desogestrel/ethinyl estradiol]	Z79.3	Contraceptive	Contraception

Drug	Z Code	Drug Action	Indications
Cyclosporine [cyclosporine]	**Z79.899**	Immunosuppressant	Prophylaxis of organ transplant rejection
Cytomel [liothyronine sodium]		Thyroid hormone	Treatment of hypothyroidism or prevention of euthyroid goiters
Daptomycin [daptomycin]	**Z79.2**	Antibacterial	Skin and underlying tissue bacterial infections
Dasetta [ethinyl estradiol/norethindrone]	**Z79.3**	Contraceptive	Contraception
Daypro [oxaprozin]	**Z79.1**	Nonsteroidal anti-inflammatory drug (NSAID)	Osteoarthritis and rheumatoid arthritis
Daysee [ethinyl estradiol/levonorgestrel]	**Z79.3**	Contraceptive	Contraception
Delestrogen [estradiol valerate]	**Z79.890**	Estrogen therapy	Menopause symptoms
Demerol [meperidine hydrochloride]	**Z79.891**	Narcotic analgesic	Moderate to severe pain
Depakote [divalproex sodium]		Anticonvulsant	Bipolar affective disorder; complex absence, complex partial, and mixed pattern epilepsy; migraine headache
Depo-Medrol [methylprednisolone acetate]	**Z79.52**	Corticosteroids	Arthritis and joint disorders
Depo-Provera [medroxyprogesterone acetate]	**Z79.3, Z79.890**	Antineoplastic; contraceptive; progestin	Amenorrhea; carcinoma, endometrium, adjunct; carcinoma, renal; contraception; hemorrhage
Depo-SubQ Provera [medroxyprogesterone acetate]	**Z79.3**	Contraceptive	Contraception; menstrual disorder pain
Desogen [desogestrel/ethinyl estradiol]	**Z79.3**	Contraceptive; estrogen/progestin	Contraception
Detrol [tolterodine tartrate]		Muscarinic receptor antagonist	Overactive bladders in patients with urinary frequency, urgency, or urge incontinence
Dexamethasone Intensol [dexamethasone]	**Z79.52**	Corticosteroids	Arthritis; allergic disorders; breathing disorders; lupus
Didronel [etidronate disodium]	**Z79.83**	Bisphosphonates	Paget's disease and irregular bone growth
Dificid [fidaxomicin]	**Z79.2**	Antibacterial	*Clostridium difficile*
Diflucan [fluconazole]		Antifungal agent	Oropharyngeal and esophageal candidiasis and cryptococcal meningitis in AIDS patients
Digoxin [digoxin]		Cardiotonic glycoside	Heart failure, atrial flutter, atrial fibrillation, and supraventricular tachycardia
Dilantin [phenytoin sodium]		Anticonvulsant	Control of grand mal and psychomotor seizures
Dilaudid [hydromorphone hydrochloride]	**Z79.891**	Narcotic analgesic	Moderate to severe pain
Diovan [valsartan]		ACE inhibitor	Essential hypertension
Divigel [estradiol]	**Z79.890**	Estrogen therapy	Menopause symptoms
Dolophine HCl [methadone hydrochloride]	**Z79.891**	Narcotic analgesic	Pain; treatment of opioid addiction
Doxycycline [doxycycline]	**Z79.2**	Antibacterial	Treatment of bacterial infections; acne
Duavee [bazedoxifene acetate/conjugated estrogens]	**Z79.890**	Estrogen therapy	Treatment of menopause symptoms; osteoporosis prevention
Duetact [glimepiride/pioglitazone hydrochloride]	**Z79.84**	Blood glucose regulator	Diabetes mellitus
Duexis [famotidine/ibuprofen]	**Z79.1**	Nonsteroidal anti-inflammatory drug (NSAID)	Symptomatic treatment of osteoarthritis and rheumatoid arthritis; reduction of risk of ulcers
Dulera [formoterol fumarate/mometasone furoate]	**Z79.51**	Corticosteroids -inhaled; antiasthmatic	Prophylaxis and treatment of asthma
Duragesic [fentanyl]	**Z79.891**	Narcotic analgesic	Chronic pain
Duramorph [morphine sulfate]	**Z79.891**	Narcotic analgesic	Moderate to severe pain
Dyloject [diclofenac sodium]	**Z79.1**	Nonsteroidal anti-inflammatory drug (NSAID)	Pain relief
Dynacin [minocycline hydrochloride]	**Z79.2**	Antibacterial	Severe acne treatment
E.E.S. [erythromycin ethylsuccinate]	**Z79.2**	Antibacterial	Bacterial infections
Ecotrin [acetylsalicylic acid]	**Z79.82**	Aspirin	Prophylaxis and treatment of heart attacks, angina or strokes; reduction of fever, pain and inflammation
Effexor XR [venlafaxine hydrochloride]		Antidepressant	Depression
Effient [prasugrel hydrochloride]	**Z79.02**	Antithrombotic platelet aggregation inhibitor	Lessening of the chance of heart attack or stroke
Elestrin [estradiol]	**Z79.890**	Estrogen therapy	Menopause symptoms

Drug	Z Code	Drug Action	Indications
Eligard [leuprolide acetate]	Z79.818	Agents affecting estrogen receptors and estrogen levels	Endometriosis; uterine fibroids; symptoms of prostate cancer
Elinest [norgestrel/ethinyl estradiol]	Z79.3	Contraceptive	Contraception
Eliquis [apixaban]	Z79.01	Anticoagulant	Venous thrombosis
Embeda [morphine sulfate/naltrexone hydrochloride]	Z79.891	Narcotic analgesic	Moderate to severe pain
Emoquette [ethinyl estradiol/desogestrel]	Z79.3	Contraceptive	Contraception
Enjuvia [conjugated synthetic b estrogens]	Z79.890	Estrogen therapy	Osteoporosis prevention and to treat menopausal symptoms; vaginal and vulvar atrophy; hypoestrogenism; ovarian failure
Enpresse [ethinyl estradiol/levonorgestrel]	Z79.3	Contraceptive	Contraception
Enskyce [desogestrel/ethinyl estradiol]	Z79.3	Contraceptive	Contraception
Entocort EC [budesonide]	Z79.52	Corticosteroids	Crohn's disease; ulcerative colitis
Envarsus XR [tacrolimus]	Z79.899	Immunosuppressant	Prophylaxis of organ transplant rejection
Epinephrine [epinephrine]		Bronchodilator, cardiotonic	Most commonly, relief of respiratory distress due to bronchospasm and restoration of cardiac rhythm in cardiac arrest
Epivir, Epivir-HBV [lamivudine]		HIV and HBV inhibitor	HIV, hepatitis B (HBV), asymptomatic HIV
Errin [norethindrone]	Z79.3	Contraceptive	Contraception
Ertapenem [ertapenem sodium]	Z79.2	Antibacterial	Stomach, urinary tract, pelvis, skin and lung infections
ERYC [erythromycin]	Z79.2	Antibacterial	Lower respiratory tract infections
Erygel [erythromycin]	Z79.2	Antibacterial	Treatment of bacterial infections; rheumatic fever attacks
EryPed [erythromycin ethylsuccinate]	Z79.2	Antibacterial	Treatment of bacterial infections; rheumatic fever attacks
Ery-Tab [erythromycin]	Z79.2	Acne product; macrolide; ocular anti-infective; topical anti-infective	Acne vulgaris, intestinal amebiasis, infectious conjunctivitis, diphtheria, endocarditis, prevention, treatment of erythrasma infections: endocervical, gynecologic, lower and upper respiratory tract, ophthalmic, and rectal; skin and skin structures, and urethral; Legionnaires' disease, pelvic inflammatory disease, pertussis, pneumonia, rheumatic fever, prophylaxis, syphilis
Erythrocin [erythromycin lactobionate]	Z79.2	Antibacterial	Bacterial infections
Erythromycin [erythromycin]	Z79.2	Antibacterial	Respiratory tract infections
Estarylla [ethinyl estradiol/norgestimate]	Z79.3	Contraceptive	Contraception
Estrace [estradiol]	Z79.890	Estrogen therapy	Vaginal cream used to treat vaginal and vulvar atrophy
Estraderm [estradiol]	Z79.890	Estrogen therapy	Osteoporosis prevention and to treat menopausal symptoms, vaginal and vulvar atrophy, hypoestrogenism, ovarian failure
Estrasorb [estradiol hemihydrate]	Z79.890	Estrogen therapy	Menopause symptoms
EstroGel [estradiol]	Z79.890	Estrogen therapy	Menopause symptoms
Estrostep Fe [ethinyl estradiol/norethindrone acetate]	Z79.3	Contraceptive	Contraception
Evista [raloxifene hydrochloride]	Z79.810	Estrogen receptor modulator, selective osteoporosis prophylactic	Prevention of thinning of the bones (osteoporosis) only in postmenopausal women
Exalgo [hydromorphone hydrochloride]	Z79.891	Narcotic analgesic	Moderate to severe pain
Exemestane [exemestane]	Z79.811	Aromatase inhibitor	Postmenopausal breast cancer
Factive [gemifloxacin mesylate]	Z79.2	Antibacterial	Bacterial lung infections
Falmina [ethinyl estradiol/levonorgestrel]	Z79.3	Contraceptive	Contraception
Fareston [toremifene citrate]	Z79.810	Selective estrogen receptor modulator (SERM)	Metastatic breast cancer in postmenopausal women
Faslodex [fulvestrant]	Z79.818	Agents affecting estrogen receptors and estrogen levels	Metastatic breast cancer in postmenopausal women
Feldene [piroxicam]	Z79.1	Nonsteroidal anti-inflammatory drug (NSAID)	Treatment of pain and inflammation due to arthritis
Femara [letrozole]	Z79.811	Aromatase inhibitor	Postmenopausal breast cancer
Femcon Fe [ethinyl estradiol/norethindrone]	Z79.3	Contraceptive	Contraception; acne
Femhrt [ethinyl estradiol/norethindrone acetate]	Z79.3, Z79.890	Contraceptive; estrogen therapy	Contraception; menopause symptoms; osteoporosis prevention
Femring [estradiol acetate]	Z79.890	Estrogen therapy	Osteoporosis prevention and to treat menopausal symptoms; hypoestrogenism; ovarian failure

Drug	Z Code	Drug Action	Indications
Femtrace [estradiol acetate]	Z79.890	Estrogen therapy	Menopause symptoms
Fentanyl [fentanyl]	Z79.891	Narcotic analgesic	Postprocedural or chronic pain
Fentora [fentanyl citrate]	Z79.891	Narcotic analgesic	Breakthrough cancer pain
Fioricet with codeine [acetaminophen/butalbital/caffeine/codeine phosphate]	Z79.891	Narcotic analgesic	Tension headaches
Flagyl [metronidazole]	Z79.2	Antibacterial	Treatment of bacterial infections
Flavoxate hydrochloride [flavoxate hydrochloride]		Urinary tract spasmolytic	Relief of dysuria, urgency, nocturia, suprapubic pain, frequency, and incontinence associated with cystitis, prostatitis, urethritis, and urethrocystitis/urethrotrigonitis
Flomax [tamsulosin hydrochloride]		Alpha-adrenergic blocker, benign prostatic hypertrophy therapy agent	Signs and symptoms of benign enlargement of the prostate (benign prostatic hyperplasia, or BPH)
Flonase [fluticasone propionate]		Corticosteroid-inhalation/nasal; topical steroid	Corticosteroid-responsive dermatosis; perennial allergic and seasonal allergic rhinitis
Flovent HFA [fluticasone propionate]	Z79.51	Corticosteroid-inhaled/nasal; topical steroid	Corticosteroid-responsive dermatosis, perennial allergic and seasonal allergic rhinitis
Fortamet [metformin hydrochloride]	Z79.84	Blood glucose regulator	Diabetes mellitus
Fortaz [ceftazidime]	Z79.2	Antibacterial	Pneumonia and lower respiratory infections
Fosamax [alendronate sodium]	Z79.83	Calcium metabolism	Osteoporosis; Paget's disease
Fosinopril sodium [fosinopril sodium]		ACE inhibitor; antihypertensive	Essential hypertension
Fragmin [dalteparin sodium]	Z79.01	Anticoagulant	Prophylaxis and treatment of blood clots
Fulvestrant [fulvestrant]	Z79.818	Agents affecting estrogen receptors and estrogen levels	Treatment of metastatic breast cancer in postmenopausal women
Gengraf [cyclosporine]	Z79.899	Immunosuppressant	Prophylaxis of organ transplant rejection
Gentamicin sulfate [gentamicin sulfate]	Z79.2	Antibacterial	Severe bacterial infections
Gildagia [ethinyl estradiol/norethindrone]	Z79.3	Contraceptive	Contraception
Gildess [ethinyl estradiol/norethindrone acetate]	Z79.3	Contraceptive	Contraception
Glimepiride [glimepiride]	Z79.84	Blood glucose regulator	Diabetes mellitus
Glucophage [metformin hydrochloride]	Z79.84	Blood glucose regulator	Diabetes mellitus
Glucotrol [glipizide]	Z79.84	Oral blood-glucose-lowering agent	Diabetes mellitus
Glucovance [glyburide/metformin hydrochloride]	Z79.84	Blood glucose regulator	Diabetes mellitus
Glumetza [metformin hydrochloride]	Z79.84	Blood glucose regulator	Diabetes mellitus
Glyburide (micronized) [glyburide]	Z79.84	Blood glucose regulator	Diabetes mellitus
Heparin sodium [heparin sodium]	Z79.01	Anticoagulant	Prophylaxis and treatment of venous thrombosis, pulmonary embolism; prevention of cerebral thrombosis, and treatment of consumptive coagulopathies
Humalog [insulin lispro recombinant]	Z79.4	Blood glucose regulator	Diabetes mellitus
Humulin [insulin recombinant]	Z79.4	Blood glucose regulator	Diabetes mellitus
Hydrochlorothiazide [hydrochlorothiazide]		Diuretic, antihypertensive	Management of hypertension and in adjunctive therapy for edema associated with congestive heart failure, hepatic cirrhosis, corticosteroid, and estrogen therapy
Hydrocodone [acetaminophen/hydrocodone bitartrate]	Z79.891	Narcotic analgesic	Moderate to severe pain
Hydrocodone bitartrate and acetaminophen [acetaminophen/hydrocodone bitartrate]	Z79.891	Analgesic, general; analgesic-narcotic; antitussive/expectorant	Pain, moderate to severe
Hydrocortisone [hydrocortisone]	Z79.52	Corticosteroids	Addison's disease; arthritis; immune disorders; allergies; breathing problems
Hydromorphone HCl [hydromorphone hydrochloride]	Z79.891	Narcotic analgesic	Moderate to severe pain
Hyzaar [hydrochlorothiazide/ losartan potassium]		Antihypertensive	Hypertension
Ibuprofen [ibuprofen]	Z79.1	Nonsteroidal anti-inflammatory drug (NSAID)	Pain or fever relief
Imitrex [sumatriptan succinate]		Antimigraine	Migraine headache

Drug	Z Code	Drug Action	Indications
Imuran [azathioprine]	Z79.899	Immunosuppressant	Rheumatoid arthritis
Inderal [propranolol hydrochloride]		Beta-adrenergic blocking agent	Management of hypertension, long-term management of angina pectoris due to coronary atherosclerosis, cardiac arrhythmias
Indocin [indomethacin]	Z79.1	Nonsteroidal anti-inflammatory drug (NSAID)	Treatment of pain and inflammation
Integrilin [eptifibatide]	Z79.02	Antithrombotic platelet aggregation inhibitor	Treatment of unstable angina or heart attacks and prevention of blood clots
Intron [interferon alfa 2-b]	Z79.899	Antineoplastic interferons; antiviral interferons	Cancer; hepatitis
Introvale [levonorgestrel/ethinyl estradiol]	Z79.3	Contraceptive	Contraception
Invanz [ertapeneum sodium]	Z79.2	Antibacterial	Stomach, urinary tract, pelvis, skin and lung infections
Invokamet [canagliflozin/metformin hydrochloride]	Z79.84	Blood glucose regulator	Diabetes mellitus
Iprivask [desirudin recombinant]	Z79.02	Antithrombotic platelet aggregation inhibitor	Prophylaxis and treatment of venous thrombosis and pulmonary embolism
Isoniazid [isoniazid]	Z79.2	Antibacterial	Prophylaxis and treatment of tuberculosis
Isordil [isosorbide dinitrate]		Smooth muscle relaxant	Acute anginal attacks
Isuprel [isoproterenol hydrochloride]		Adrenergic agent	Bronchodilator for asthma, chronic pulmonary emphysema, bronchitis, and other conditions accompanied by bronchospasm; can be used in cardiogenic shock cases
Jantoven [warfarin sodium]	Z79.01	Anticoagulant	Prophylaxis and treatment of venous thrombosis, pulmonary embolism; prevention of cerebral thrombosis, and treatment of consumptive coagulopathies
Janumet [metformin hydrochloride/sitagliptin phosphate]	Z79.84	Blood glucose regulator	Diabetes mellitus
Januvia [sitagliptin phosphate]	Z79.84	Blood glucose regulator	Diabetes mellitus
Jencycla [norethindrone]	Z79.3	Contraceptive	Contraception
Jentadueto [linagliptin/metformin hydrochloride]]	Z79.84	Blood glucose regulator	Diabetes mellitus
Junel [ethinyl estradiol/norethindrone acetate]	Z79.3	Contraceptive	Contraception
Kadian [morphine sulfate]	Z79.891	Narcotic analgesic	Moderate to severe pain
Kariva [desogestrel/ethinyl estradiol]	Z79.3	Contraceptive	Contraception
Kazano [alogliptin benzoate/metformin hydrochloride]	Z79.84	Blood glucose regulator	Diabetes mellitus
Keflex [cephalexin]	Z79.2	Antibacterial	Bone, middle ear, skin and skin structures, upper respiratory tract and urinary tract infections; acute prostatitis
Kefzol [cefazolin sodium]	Z79.2	Antibacterial	Skin, ear, urinary tract, and upper respiratory bacterial infections
Kelnor [ethynodiol diacetate/ethinyl estradiol]	Z79.3	Contraceptive	Contraception
Kenalog [triamcinolone acetonide]	Z79.52	Corticosteroids	Eczema; allergic reactions; psoriasis
Kimidess [ethinyl estradiol/desogestrel]	Z79.3	Contraceptive	Contraception
Klaron [sulfacetamide sodium]	Z79.2	Antibacterial	Acne
Klonopin [clonazepam]		Anticonvulsant, anxiolytic - benzodiazepine	Epilepsy, seizures, panic disorder
Klor-Con [potassium chloride]		Replaces potassium and maintains potassium level	Hypokalemia
Kombiglyze [metformin hydrochloride/saxagliptin hydrochloride]	Z79.84	Blood glucose regulator	Diabetes mellitus
K-Tab [potassium chloride]		Replaces potassium and maintains potassium level	Hypokalemia
Kurvelo [ethinyl estradiol/levonorgestrel]	Z79.3	Contraceptive	Contraception; menstrual disorders
Lamisil [terbinafine hydrochloride]		Antifungal	*Tinea cruris* (jock itch), *T. pedis* (athlete's foot), *T. corporis* (ringworm)
Lanoxin [digoxin]		Cardiotonic glycoside	Congestive heart failure
Lantus [insulin glargine recombinant]	Z79.4	Blood glucose regulator	Diabetes mellitus
Larin [ethinyl estradiol/norethindrone acetate]	Z79.3	Contraceptive	Contraception

Drug	Z Code	Drug Action	Indications
Lasix [furosemide]		Antihypertensive; diuretic	Management of edema associated with congestive heart failure, renal disease, including nephrotic syndrome and hypertension
Lescol [fluvastatin sodium]		HMG-CoA reductase inhibitor (statin)	Hypercholesterolemia; hyperlipidemia; hyperlipoproteinemia
Lessina [ethinyl estradiol/levonorgestrel]	**Z79.3**	Contraceptive	Contraception
Letrozole [letrozole]	**Z79.811**	Aromatase inhibitor	Postmenopausal breast cancer
Levaquin [levofloxacin]	**Z79.2**	Fluoroquinolone antibacterial	Acute exacerbation chronic bronchitis; cellulitis; furuncle; impetigo; infections of the lower and upper respiratory tracts, sinus, skin and skin structures, and urinary tract; pneumonia, community-acquired; pyoderma
Levemir [insulin detemir recombinant]	**Z79.4**	Blood glucose regulator	Diabetes mellitus
Levonest [levonorgestrel/ethinyl estradiol]	**Z79.3**	Contraceptive	Contraception; menstrual disorders; acne
Levora [levonorgestrel/ethinyl estradiol]	**Z79.3**	Contraceptive	Contraception
Levothroid [levothyroxine sodium]		Thyroid hormone	Treatment of hypothyroidism
Levoxyl [levothyroxine sodium]		Synthetic thyroid hormone	Euthyroid goiter; hypothyroidism
Lexapro [escitalopram oxalate]		Antidepressant—selective serotonin reuptake inhibitor (SSRI)	Depression, anxiety
Librium [chlordiazepoxide hydrochloride]		Antianxiety agent	Acute withdrawal symptoms, especially from alcohol, or for other anxiety-producing conditions
Lidocaine hydrochloride [lidocaine hydrochloride]		Antiarrhythmic	Management of ventricular arrhythmias or during cardiac manipulation, such as cardiac surgery
Liletta [levonorgestrel]	**Z79.3**	Contraceptive	Intrauterine device for contraception
Lincocin [lincocin hydrochloride]	**Z79.2**	Antibacterial	Serious bacterial infections
Lipitor [atorvastatin calcium]		HMG-CoA reductase inhibitor (statin)	Hypercholesterolemia, hyperlipidemia, hyperproteinemia
Lithium [lithium carbonate]		Antimanic	Control of manic episodes in bipolar disorders
Lo Loestrin Fe [ethinyl estradiol/norethindrone acetate]	**Z79.3**	Contraceptive	Contraception
Lo Minastrin Fe [ethinyl estradiol/norethindrone acetate]	**Z79.3**	Contraceptive	Contraception
Loestrin [ethinyl estradiol/norethindrone acetate]	**Z79.3**	Contraceptive	Contraception
Lomotil [diphenoxylate hydrochloride/atropine sulfate]		Antidiarrheal	Treatment of symptoms of chronic and functional diarrhea
Lopid [gemfibrozil]		Lipid regulating agent	Hypercholesterolemia, hyperlipidemia, hyperlipoproteinemia, hypertriglyceridemia
Lopressor [metoprolol tartrate]		Antihypertensive, betablocker antianginal; antihypertensive; betablocker	Essential hypertension therapy, angina pectoris, and myocardial infarction
Lorazepam [lorazepam]		Antianxiety; sedative/hypnotic	Anxiety disorder associated with depressive symptoms; controls tension, agitation, irritability, and insomnia
Loryna [drospirenone/ethinyl estradiol]	**Z79.3**	Contraceptive	Contraception
LoSeasonique [ethinyl estradiol/levonorgestrel]	**Z79.3**	Contraceptive	Contraception
Lotensin [benazepril hydrochloride]		ACE inhibitor; antihypertensive	Essential hypertension
Lotrel [amlodipine besylate/benazepril hydrochloride]		Antihypertensive	Hypertension
Lotrisone [clotrimazole/ betamethasone dipropionate]		Antifungal-corticosteroid	Relief of redness, swelling, itching, and other discomfort of fungus infections
Lovastatin [lovastatin]		HMG-CoA reductase inhibitor (statin)	Hypercholesterolemia; hyperlipidemia, hyperlipoproteinemia
Lovenox [enoxaparin sodium]	**Z79.Ø**	Anticoagulant	Prophylaxis and treatment of venous thrombosis and pulmonary embolism
Low-Ogestrel [norgestrel/ethinyl estradiol]	**Z79.3**	Contraceptive	Contraception
Lupron [leuprolide acetate]	**Z79.818**	Agents affecting estrogen receptors and estrogen levels	Treatment of metastatic breast cancer in postmenopausal women; prostate cancer symptoms
Macrobid [nitrofuantoin]	**Z79.2**	Antibacterial	Bacterial urinary tract infections
Macrodantin [nitrofurantoin]		Antibacterial	Urinary tract infection; prophylaxis
Marlissa [ethinyl estradiol/levonorgestrel]	**Z79.3**	Contraceptive	Contraception
Maxipime [cefepime hydrochloride]	**Z79.2**	Antibacterial	Treatment of bacterial infections

Drug	Z Code	Drug Action	Indications
Meclizine hydrochloride [meclizine hydrochloride]		Antihistamine	Management of nausea and vomiting, and dizziness associated with motion sickness
Medrol [methylprednisolone]	Z79.52	Glucocorticoid; anti-inflammatory	Acute/chronic adrenal insufficiency, congenital adrenal hyperplasia, adrenal insufficiency secondary to pituitary insufficiency; nonendocrine disorders, including arthritis, rheumatic carditis, bronchial asthma, cerebral edema, and allergic, collagen, intestinal tract, liver, ocular, renal, and skin diseases
Mefoxin [cefoxitin sodium]	Z79.2	Antibacterial	Bacterial infections
Megace ES [megestrol acetate]	Z79.818	Agents affecting estrogen receptors and estrogen levels	Endometrial or advanced breast cancers; weight loss due to AIDS
Menest [esteriefied estrogens]	Z79.890	Estrogen therapy	Menopause symptoms; ovarian failure
Menostar [estradiol]	Z79.890	Estrogen therapy	Menopause symptoms; osteoporosis prevention
Mepron [atovaquone]	Z79.2	Antibacterial	Pneumonia
Merrem [meropenem]	Z79.2	Antibacterial	Bacterial infections of skin or stomach; bacterial meningitis
Metformin [metformin hydrochloride]	Z79.84	Blood glucose regulator	Diabetes mellitus
Methadone HCl [methadone hydrochloride]	Z79.891	Narcotic analgesic	Pain; treatment of opioid addiction
Methadose [methadone hydrochloride]	Z79.891	Narcotic analgesic	Acute and chronic pain
Methergine [methylergonovine maleate]		Oxytocic agent	Routine management of postpartum hemorrhage after delivery of placenta
Methylprednisolone [methylprednisolone]	Z79.52	Corticosteroids	Inflammatory disorders
Metro [metronidazole]	Z79.2	Antibacterial	Bacterial infections
Metronidazole [metronidazole]	Z79.2	Antibacterial	Bacterial infections
Miacalcin [calcitonin salmon]		Calcitonin; a peptide hormone	Hypercalcemia, osteoporosis, postmenopausal symptoms, Paget's disease
Microgestin [ethinyl estradiol/norethindrone acetate]	Z79.3	Contraceptive	Contraception
Micronor [norethindrone]	Z79.3	Contraceptive	Contraception
Minastrin [ethinyl estradiol/norethindrone acetate]	Z79.3	Contraceptive	Contraception
Minivelle [estradiol]	Z79.890	Estrogen therapy	Menopause symptoms; osteoporosis prevention
Minocin [minocycline hydrochloride]	Z79.2	Antibacterial	Bacterial infections; acne
Mirena [levonorgestrel]	Z79.3	Contraceptive	Intrauterine device for contraception; menstrual disorders
Mobic [meloxicam]	Z79.1	Nonsteroidal anti-inflammatory drug (NSAID)	Pain and inflammation due to osteoarthritis and rheumatoid arthritis
Modicon [ethinyl estradiol/norethindrone]	Z79.3	Contraceptive	Contraception
Monoclonal antibodies	Z79.899	Monoclonal antibodies	Cancer; prophylaxis of organ transplant rejection
Monodox [doxycycline]	Z79.2	Antibacterial	Bacterial infections; acne
Monoket [isosorbide mononitrate]		Antianginal; coronary vasodilator, nitrate	Angina pectoris
Mono-Linyah [norgestimate/ethinyl estradiol]	Z79.3	Contraceptive	Contraception; menstrual disorders; acne
Monurol [fosfomycin tromethamine]	Z79.2	Antibacterial	Bacterial bladder infections
Morphine [morphine sulfate]	Z79.891	Narcotic analgesic	Moderate to severe pain
Motrin [ibuprofen]	Z79.1	Analgesic, general; analgesic, non-narcotic; antiarthritic; antigout; antipyretic; NSAID	Osteoarthritis and rheumatoid arthritis, dysmenorrhea, fever; pain, mild to moderate
Moxatag [amoxicillin]	Z79.2	Antibacterial	Bacterial tonsillitis and pharyngitis
MS Contin [morphine sulfate]	Z79.891	Narcotic analgesic	Moderate to severe pain
Multaq [dronedarone hydrochloride]		Cardiac rhythm regulator	Treatment of patients with recent episodes of atrial fibrillation or atrial flutter
Mycobutin [rifabutin]	Z79.2	Antibacterial	Mycobacterium avium complex (MAC) prophylactic
Myzilra [ethinyl estradiol/levonorgestrel]	Z79.3	Contraceptive	Contraception
Nabumetone [nabumetone]	Z79.1	Non-steroidal anti-inflammatory drug (NSAID)	Osteoarthritis and rheumatoid arthritis
Nalfon [fenoprofen calcium]	Z79.1	Nonsteroidal anti-inflammatory drug (NSAID)	Pain or inflammation relief

Drug	Z Code	Drug Action	Indications
Naprelan [naproxen sodium]	Z79.1	Nonsteroidal anti-inflammatory drug (NSAID)	Pain or inflammation relief
Naprosyn [naproxen]	Z79.1	Anti-inflammatory analgesic, general; analgesic, non-narcotic; antiarthritic; antigout; NSAID	Rheumatoid, gouty arthritis and osteoarthritis; ankylosing spondylitis; bursitis; dysmenorrhea; pain, mild to moderate; tendonitis
Natazia [estradiol valerate/dienogest]	Z79.3	Contraceptive	Contraception; menstrual disorders
Nebupent [pentamidine isethionate]	Z79.2	Antibacterial	Serious bacterial lung infection in high-risk patients with HIV
Nefazodone hydrochloride [nefazodone hydrochloride]		Antidepressant	Depression
Nembutal sodium [pentobarbital sodium]		Sedative; hypnotic	Adjunct medication in diagnostic procedures or for emergency use with convulsive disorders
NeoProfen [ibuprofen lysine]	Z79.1	Nonsteroidal anti-inflammatory drug (NSAID)	Pain or fever relief
Neoral [cyclosporine]	Z79.899	Immunosuppressant	Prophylaxis of organ transplant rejection
Neurontin [gabapentin]		Anticonvulsant	Epilepsy, partial
Nexium [esomeprazole magnesium]		Proton pump inhibitor	Gastroesophageal reflux disease (GERD), erosive esophagitis
Nexplanon [etonogestrel]	Z79.3	Contraceptive	Implantable contraception
Nitrofurantoin [nitrofurantoin]	Z79.2	Antibacterial	Bacterial urinary tract infections
Nitropress [sodium nitroprusside]		Vasodilator	Potent, rapid action in reducing blood pressure in hypertensive crisis or for controlling bleeding during anesthesia by producing controlled hypotension
Nitrostat [nitroglycerin]		Muscle relaxant antianginal; antihypertensive; coronary vasodilator	Prophylaxis and treatment of angina pectoris; heart failure associated with myocardial infarction; hypertension, perioperative; surgery, adjunct
Norco [acetaminophen/hydrocodone bitartrate]	Z79.891	Narcotic analgesic	Moderate to severe pain
Norinyl [mestranol/norethisterone]	Z79.3	Contraceptive	Contraception
Norpace [disopyramide phosphate]		Antiarrhythmic	Coronary artery disease, for prevention, recurrence, and control of unifocal, multifocal, and paired PVCs
Nor-QD [norethindrone]	Z79.3	Contraceptive	Contraception
Nortrel [ethinyl estradiol/norethindrone]	Z79.3	Contraceptive	Contraception
Norvasc [amlodipine besylate]		Calcium channel blocker	Hypertension, chronic stable angina, and vasospastic angina
Novolin [insulin recombinant]	Z79.4	Blood glucose regulator	Diabetes mellitus
NovoLog [insulin recombinant]	Z79.4	Blood glucose regulator	Diabetes mellitus
Nucynta [tapentadol hydrochloride]	Z79.891	Narcotic analgesic	Moderate to severe pain
NuvaRing [etonogestrel/ethinyl estradiol]	Z79.3	Contraceptive	Vaginal ring for contraception
Ogestrel [norgestrel/ethinyl estradiol]	Z79.3	Contraceptive	Contraception
Onglyza [saxagliptin hydrochloride]	Z79.84	Blood glucose regulator	Diabetes mellitus
Opana [oxymorphone hydrochloride]	Z79.891	Narcotic analgesic	Moderate to severe pain
Oracea [doxycycline]	Z79.2	Antibacterial	Rosacea
Orapred ODT [prednisolone sodium phosphate]	Z79.52	Corticosteroids	Inflammatory disorders
Orbactiv [oritavancin diphosphate]	Z79.2	Antibacterial	Bacterial skin infections
Orphenadrine citrate [orphenadrine citrate]		Muscle relaxant	Acute spasms, tension, and post-trauma cases
Orsythia [ethinyl estradiol/levonorgestrel]	Z79.3	Contraceptive	Contraception
Ortho Cyclen [ethinyl estradiol/norgestimate]	Z79.3	Contraceptive	Contraception
Ortho-Novum [norethindrone/ethinyl estradiol]	Z79.3	Contraceptive	Contraception
Ortho-Tri-Cyclen [ethinyl estradiol/norgestimate]	Z79.3	Contraceptive	Contraception
Oseni [alogliptin benzoate/pioglitazone hydrochloride]	Z79.84	Blood glucose regulator	Diabetes mellitus
Osphena [ospemifene]	Z79.810, Z79.890	Selective estrogen receptor modulator (SERM)	Postmenopausal dyspareunia due to vaginal atrophy; osteoporosis prevention and treatment of menopause symptoms
Oxazepam [oxazepam]		Antianxiety agent	Anxiety, tension, and alcohol withdrawal

Appendix C: Pharmacology List 2018

Drug	Z Code	Drug Action	Indications
Oxycodone HCl [oxycodone hydrochloride]	Z79.891	Narcotic analgesic	Moderate to severe pain
OxyContin [oxycodone hydrochloride]	Z79.891	Narcotic analgesic	Moderate to severe pain
Pavabid [papaverine hydrochloride]		Vasodilator	Relief of cerebral and peripheral ischemia
Paxil [paroxetine hydrochloride]		Antidepressant	Anxiety with panic disorder and depression; obsessive-compulsive disorder
PCE [erythromycin]	Z79.2	Antibacterial	Bacterial infections
PediaPred [prednisolone sodium phosphate]	Z79.52	Corticosteroids	Inflammatory disorders
Pegintron [peginterferon alfa-2b]	Z79.899	Antiviral interferon	Hepatitis C
Penicillin-VK [penicillin V potassium]	Z79.2	Natural penicillin	Chorea prevention; endocarditis prevention, secondary to tooth extraction; erysipelas; infections of the skin and skin structures, upper respiratory tract; rheumatic fever, prophylaxis; scarlet fever; Vincent's gingivitis; Vincent's pharyngitis
Pentam [pentamidine isethionate]	Z79.2	Antibacterial	Serious bacterial lung infections
Pepcid [famotidine]		Histamine H2-receptor inhibitor	Acid/peptic disorder; adenoma, secretory; gastroesophageal reflux; duodenal and gastric ulcer; Zollinger-Ellison syndrome
Percocet [oxycodone hydrochloride/acetaminophen]	Z79.891	Analgesic, general; analgesic-narcotic	Pain, moderate to severe
Persantine [dipyridamole]	Z79.02	Platelet inhibitor	Therapy for chronic angina pectoris, preventing clots post heart valve surgery
Pfizerpen [penicillin g potassium]	Z79.2	Antibacterial	Severe bacterial infections
Phenobarbital [phenobarbital sodium]		Barbiturate	Grand mal epilepsy
Philith [ethinyl estradiol/norethindrone]	Z79.3	Contraceptive	Contraception
Pimtrea [desogestrel/ethinyl estradiol]	Z79.3	Contraceptive	Contraception
Pirmella [ethinyl estradiol/norethindrone]	Z79.3	Contraceptive	Contraception
Pitocin [oxytocin]		Synthetic oxytocin	Induction or stimulation of labor at term
Plan B One-Step [levonorgestrel]	Z79.3	Contraceptive	Contraception
Plasmanate [plasma, plasma protein fraction]		Blood volume expander	Hypovolemic shock, burn patients, and hemorrhages when whole blood is unavailable
Plavix [clopidogrel bisulfate]	Z79.02	Antithrombotic platelet aggregation inhibitor	Lessening of the chance of heart attack or stroke
Ponstel [mefenamic acid]	Z79.1	Nonsteroidal anti-inflammatory drug (NSAID)	Pain
Portia [ethinyl estradiol/levonorgestrel]	Z79.3	Contraceptive	Contraception
Pradaxa [dabigatran etexilate mesylate]	Z79.01	Anticoagulant	Prophylaxis and treatment of blood clots in patients with atrial fibrillation
Prandimet [metformin hydrochloride/repaglinide]	Z79.84	Blood glucose regulator	Diabetes mellitus
Prandin [repaglinide]	Z79.84	Blood glucose regulator	Diabetes mellitus
Pravachol [pravastatin sodium]		HMG-CoA reductase inhibitor (statin)	Hypercholesterolemia, hyperlipidemia, hyperlipoproteinemia
Precose [acarbose]	Z79.84	Blood glucose regulator	Diabetes mellitus
Prednisolone [prednisolone]	Z79.52	Corticosteroids	Inflammatory disorders
Prednisone [prednisone]	Z79.52	Adrenocorticoid, corticosteroid	Used for its immunosuppressant effects and for relief of inflammations; used in arthritis, polymyositis and other systemic diseases
Pregnyl [chorionic gonadotropin]		Gonadotropic hormone	Prepubertal cryptorchidism, hypogonadism, corpus luteum insufficiency and infertility
Prelone [prednisolone]	Z79.52	Corticosteroids; antiasthmatic	Inflammatory disorders
Premarin [conjugated estrogens]	Z79.890	Antineoplastic; estrogen	Vasomotor symptoms associated with menopause; atrophic vaginitis; kraurosis vulvae, female hypogonadism; primary ovarian failure
Prempro [conjugated estrogens/medroxyprogesterone acetate]	Z79.890	Estrogen/progestin	Menopause, osteoporosis, atrophic vaginitis
Prevacid [lansoprazole]		Proton pump inhibitor (PPI)	Acid/peptic disorder, erosive esophagitis, duodenal ulcer, Zollinger-Ellison syndrome
Previfem [ethinyl estradiol/norgestimate]	Z79.3	Contraceptive	Contraception

Drug	Z Code	Drug Action	Indications
Priftin [rifapentine]	**Z79.2**	Antibacterial	Prophylaxis and treatment of tuberculosis
Prilosec [omeprazole magnesium]		Proton pump inhibitor	Acid/peptic disorder; endocrine adenoma; erosive esophagitis; systemic mastocytosis; gastroesophageal reflux; duodenal, peptic and gastric ulcer; Zollinger-Ellison syndrome
Primaxin [cilastatin sodium/imipenem]	**Z79.2**	Antibacterial	Skin, stomach, female reproductive organs or lower respiratory tract infections
Prinivil [lisinopril]		Synthetic peptide derivative, long-acting angiotensin converting enzyme inhibitor	Congestive heart failure, essential hypertension
Procardia [nifedipine]		Antianginal agent; calcium channel blocker	Management of vasospastic angina and chronic stable angina, essential hypertension
Prograf [tacrolimus]	**Z79.899**	Immunosuppressant	Prophylaxis of organ transplant rejection
Promethazine hydrochloride [promethazine hydrochloride]		Anesthesia, adjunct to; antiemetic; antihistamine; antitussive/expectorant; sedative/hypnotic; vertigo/motion sickness/vomiting	Anesthesia; adjunct; angioedema; conjunctivitis; dermographism; hypersensitivity, motion sickness; pain; perennial, seasonal, and allergic rhinitis; sedation, obstetrical; urticaria
Protonix [pantoprazole]		Proton pump inhibitor (PPI)	Short-term treatment and maintenance therapy of erosive esophagitis associated with gastroesophageal reflux disease (GERD)
Protopic [tacrolimus]	**Z79.899**	Immunosuppressant	Atomic dermatitis (eczema)
Proventil-HFA [albuterol sulfate]		Antiasthmatic/bronchodilator	Asthma
Provera [medroxyprogesterone acetate]	**Z79.3, Z79.890**	Antineoplastic; contraceptive; progestin	Amenorrhea; carcinoma, endometrium, adjunct; carcinoma, renal; contraception; hemorrhage
Prozac [fluoxetine hydrochloride]		Serotonin reuptake inhibitor	Bulimia nervosa; depression; obsessive-compulsive disorder
Pulmicort [budesonide]	**Z79.51**	Corticosteroids -inhaled; antiasthmatic	Prophylaxis and treatment of asthma
Qnasl [beclomethasone dipropionate]		Corticosteroid	Perennial allergies, seasonal allergies, and vasomotor rhinitis
Qtern [dapagliflozin propanediol/saxagliptin hydrochloride]	**Z79.84**	Blood glucose regulator	Diabetes mellitus
Quartette [levonorgestrel/ethinyl estradiol]	**Z79.3**	Contraceptive	Contraception
Quasense [ethinyl estradiol/levonorgestrel]	**Z79.3**	Contraceptive	Contraception
Quinidine gluconate [quinidine gluconate]		Antiarrhythmic	Management of cardiac arrhythmias
Qvar [beclomethasone dipropionate]	**Z79.51**	Corticosteroids -inhaled; antiasthmatic	Prevention and control of symptoms related to asthma
Raloxifene [raloxifene hydrochloride]	**Z79.810**	Selective estrogen receptor modulator (SERM)	Prevention of thinning of the bones (osteoporosis) only in postmenopausal women
Rapamune [sirolimus]	**Z79.899**	Immunosuppressant	Prophylaxis of organ transplant rejection
Rayos [prednisone]	**Z79.52**	Corticosteroids; antiasthmatic	Arthritis, blood disorders, allergies, asthma
Rebif [interferon beta-1a]	**Z79.899**	Antiviral interferon	Relapsing multiple sclerosis
Reclast [zoledronic acid]	**Z79.83**	Bisphosphonates	Prevention of thinning of the bones (osteoporosis); Paget's disease; bone cancer
Repaglinide [repaglinide]	**Z79.84**	Blood glucose regulator	Diabetes mellitus
Reprexain [hydrocodone bitartrate/ibuprofen]	**Z79.891**	Opioid analgesic/Nonsteroidal anti-inflammatory drug (NSAID)	Pain, inflammation, or fever relief
Restoril [temazepam]		Sedative/hypnotic	Insomnia
Retrovir [zidovudine]		Antiretroviral agent	Indicated in symptomatic HIV infection
Rifadin [rifampin]	**Z79.2**	Antibacterial	Prophylaxis and treatment of tuberculosis
Rimactane [rifampin]	**Z79.2**	Antibacterial	Prophylaxis and treatment of tuberculosis
Riomet [metformin hydrochloride]	**Z79.84**	Blood glucose regulator	Diabetes mellitus
Risperdal [risperidone]		Antipsychotic/antimanic	Schizophrenia; bipolar I disorder
Ritalin [methylphenidate hydrochloride]		Central nervous system (CNS) stimulant	Treatment of depression and hyperkinetic activity in children
Roxicet [oxycodone hydrochloride/acetaminophen]	**Z79.891**	Analgesic, general; analgesic-narcotic	Pain, moderate to severe
Roxicodone [oxycodone hydrochloride]	**Z79.891**	Narcotic analgesic	Pain relief
Ryzodeg [insulin aspart/insulin degludec]	**Z79.4**	Blood glucose regulator	Diabetes mellitus
Sabril [vigabatrin]		Anticonvulsant	Refractory complex partial seizures
Safyral [drospirenone/ethinyl estradiol/levomefolate calcium]	**Z79.3**	Contraceptive	Contraception

Drug	Z Code	Drug Action	Indications
Sandimmune [cyclosporine]	Z79.899	Immunosuppressant	Prophylaxis of organ transplant rejection
Savaysa [edoxaban tosylate]	Z79.01	Anticoagulant	Prophylaxis and treatment of venous thrombosis, pulmonary embolism; prevention of blood clots due to atrial fibrillation
Seasonale [levonorgestrel/ethinyl estradiol]	Z79.3	Contraceptive	Contraception
Seasonique [ethinyl estradiol/levonorgestrel]	Z79.3	Contraceptive	Contraception
Septra [sulfamethoxazole trimethoprim]	Z79.2	Antibacterial	Treatment of urinary tract infections, acute otitis media, acute exacerbations of chronic bronchitis, and shigellosis
Serevent [salmeterol xinafoate]		Bronchodilator	Asthma
Seromycin [cycloserine]	Z79.2	Antibacterial	Tuberculosis; urinary tract infections
Setlakin [ethinyl estradiol/levonorgestrel]	Z79.3	Contraceptive	Contraception
Simulect [basiliximab]	Z79.899	Immunosuppressant	Prophylaxis of organ transplant rejection
Sinemet [carbidopa/levodopa]		Antiparkinsonian	Parkinson's disease
Singulair [montelukast sodium]		Antiasthmatic, leukotriene receptor antagonist	Treatment of mild to moderate asthma to decrease the symptoms of asthma and the number of acute asthma attacks
Sirolimus [sirolimus]	Z79.899	Immunosuppressant	Prophylaxis of organ transplant rejection
Sitagliptin [sitagliptin/metformin hydrochloride]	Z79.84	Blood glucose regulator	Diabetes mellitus
Sivextro [tedizolid phosphate]	Z79.2	Antibacterial	Skin infections including MRSA
Skyla [levonorgestrel]	Z79.3	Contraceptive	Intrauterine device for contraception
Solodyn [minocycline hydrochloride]	Z79.2	Antibacterial	Bacterial infections
Soltamox [tamoxifen citrate]	Z79.810	Selective estrogen receptor modulator (SERM)	Breast cancer
Solu-Cortef [hydrocortisone sodium succinate]	Z79.52	Corticosteroids; antiasthmatic	Asthma; severe inflammation; allergic reactions
Solu-Medrol [methylprednisolone sodium succinate]	Z79.52	Adrenocorticosteroid	Anti-inflammatory and antiallergenic for shock and ulcerative colitis
Sprintec [norgestimate/ethinyl estradiol]	Z79.3	Contraceptive	Contraception
Streptomycin sulfate [streptomycin sulfate]	Z79.2	Antibacterial	Severe bacterial infections
Sublimaze [fentanyl citrate]	Z79.891	Narcotic analgesic	Pain relief
Supprelin LA [histrelin acetate]	Z79.818	Agents affecting estrogen receptors and estrogen levels	Precocious puberty; prostate cancer symptoms
Suprax [cefixime]	Z79.2	Antibacterial	Bacterial infections
Syeda [drospirenone/ethinyl estradiol]	Z79.3	Contraceptive	Contraception
Sylatron [peginterferon alfa-2b]	Z79.899	Antineoplastic interferons; antiviral interferons	Prevention of recurrent malignant melanoma
Symbicort [budesonide/formoterol fumarate dihydrate]	Z79.51	Corticosteroids -inhaled; antiasthmatic	Prophylaxis and treatment of asthma and COPD
Synarel [nafarelin acetate]	Z79.818	Agents affecting estrogen receptors and estrogen levels	Endometriosis symptoms; precocious puberty
Synercid [dalfopristin/quinupristin]	Z79.2	Antibacterial	Severe blood infections
Synjardy [empagliflozin/metformin hydrochloride]	Z79.84	Blood glucose regulator	Diabetes mellitus
Synthroid [levothyroxine sodium]		Thyroid hormone	Treatment of hypothyroidism
Tacrolimus [tacrolimus]	Z79.899	Immunosuppressant	Prophylaxis of organ transplant rejection
Tagamet HB [cimetidine]		Acid reducer	Treatment of active duodenal ulcer, short-term treatment of active, benign gastric ulcer, and treatment of pathological hypersecretory conditions
Tamoxifen [tamoxifen citrate]	Z79.810	Selective estrogen receptor modulator (SERM)	Metastatic breast cancer in postmenopausal women
Tazicef [ceftazidime]	Z79.2	Antibacterial	Confirmed or suspected bacterial infections
Teflaro [ceftaroline fosamil]	Z79.2	Antibacterial	Bacterial skin infections; pneumonia
Tegretol [carbamazepine]		Anticonvulsant; analgesic	Epilepsy, especially with complex symptomatology; specific analgesic for trigeminal neuralgia

Drug	Z Code	Drug Action	Indications
Tenormin [atenolol]		Antianginal; antihypertensive; beta blocker	Treatment of hypertension; lowering blood pressure lowers the risk of fatal and nonfatal cardiovascular events, primarily strokes and myocardial infarctions
Terazosin hydrochloride [terazosin hydrochloride]		Alpha-blocker; antihypertensive; diuretic	Benign prostatic hypertrophy; essential hypertension
Tetracycline HCl [tetracycline hydrochloride]	Z79.2	Antibacterial	Bacterial infections
Tiazac [diltiazem hydrochloride]		Antianginal, antiarrhythmic, antihypertensive, channel blocker, coronary vasodilator	Chronic stable angina, atrial fibrillation, atrial flutter, essential hypertension, paroxysmal supraventricular tachycardia
Tivorbex [indomethacin]	Z79.1	Nonsteroidal anti-inflammatory drug (NSAID)	Pain, inflammation and joint stiffness
Tobradex [tobramycin/dexamethasone]		Aminoglycoside ocular anti-infective; anti-inflammatory	Infectious conjunctivitis; dermatosis, corticosteroid-responsive with secondary infection; foreign body in eye; corneal inflammation; uveitis
Tobramycin [dexamethasone/tobramycin]	Z79.2	Antibacterial	Bacterial eye infections
Toprol-XL [metoprolol succinate]		Antianginal antihypertensive beta blocker	Angina pectoris, essential hypertension
Toremifene [toremifene citrate]	Z79.810	Selective estrogen receptor modulator (SERM)	Metastatic breast cancer in postmenopausal women
Torisel [temsirolimus]	Z79.899	Antineoplastic	Renal cell carcinoma
Toujeo Solostar [insulin glargine recombinant]	Z79.4	Blood glucose regulator	Diabetes mellitus
Trazodone hydrochloride [trazodone hydrochloride]		Antidepressant	Depression
Trelstar [triptorelin pamoate]	Z79.818	Agents affecting estrogen receptors and estrogen levels	Prophylaxis of chemo-induced menopause; prostate cancer symptoms
Tresiba [insulin degludec]	Z79.4	Blood glucose regulator	Diabetes mellitus
Triamterene and hydrochlorothiazide [triamterene/ hydrochlorothiazide]		Antihypertensive, diuretic	Edema; essential hypertension
Tri-Estarylla [ethinyl estradiol/norgestimate]	Z79.3	Contraceptive	Contraception; acne
Tri-Legest [ethinyl estradiol/norethindrone acetate]	Z79.3	Contraceptive	Contraception
Tri-Linyah [ethinyl estradiol/norgestimate]	Z79.3	Contraceptive	Contraception
Tri-Lo-Estarylla [ethinyl estradiol/norgestimate]	Z79.3	Contraceptive	Contraception
Tri-Lo-Sprintec [ethinyl estradiol/norgestimate]	Z79.3	Contraceptive	Contraception
Trimethoprim [trimethoprim]	Z79.2	Antibacterial	Acute exacerbation chronic bronchitis; travelers' diarrhea; infections of the middle and lower respiratory tracts, and urinary tract; pneumonia, pneumocystis; shigellosis
Tri-Norinyl [ethinyl estradiol/norethindrone]	Z79.3	Contraceptive	Contraception
Tri-Previfem [ethinyl estradiol/norgestimate]	Z79.3	Contraceptive	Contraception
Tri-Sprintec [ethinyl estradiol/norgestimate]	Z79.3	Contraceptive	Contraception; acne
Trivora [ethinyl estradiol/ levonorgestrel]	Z79.3	Contraceptive	Contraception
Tygacil [tigecycline]	Z79.2	Antibacterial	Bacterial skin or digestive system infections; pneumonia
Tylenol with codeine [acetaminophen/codeine phosphate]	Z79.891	Narcotic analgesic	Pain and cough
Ultram [tramadol hydrochloride]	Z79.891	Analgesic, non-narcotic (opiate, narcotic-like)	Pain, moderate to moderately severe
Unasyn [ampicillin sodium/sulbactam sodium]	Z79.2	Antibacterial	Bacterial infections
Vagifem [estradiol]	Z79.890	Estrogen therapy	Menopause symptoms
Valium [diazepam]		Antianxiety, muscle relaxant, anticonvulsant	Anxiety, tension, withdrawal from alcohol, muscle spasms and anticonvulsant therapy; epilepsy, generalized tonic-clonic; status epilepticus; stiff-man syndrome; tetanus

Drug	Z Code	Drug Action	Indications
Vancocin HCl [vancomycin hydrochloride]	Z79.2	Antibacterial	Serious bacterial infections
Vancomycin HCl [vancomycin hydrochloride]	Z79.2	Antibacterial	Serious bacterial infections
Vantas [histrelin acetate]	Z79.818	Agents affecting estrogen receptors and estrogen levels	Prostate cancer symptoms; breast cancer; endometriosis
Vasotec [enalaprilat maleate]		ACE inhibitor; antihypertensive	Congestive heart failure; essential hypertension
Velivet [desogestrel/ethinyl estradiol]	Z79.3	Contraceptive	Contraception
Ventolin HFA [albuterol sulfate]		Antiasthmatic/bronchodilator	Asthma
Verapamil HCL [verapamil hydrochloride]		Antianginal, antiarrhythmic, antiarthritic, antihypertensive, calcium channel blocker	Angina pectoris, chronic stable angina, atrial fibrillation, atrial flutter, paroxysmal supraventricular tachycardia, ventricular arrhythmia, essential hypertension
Viagra [sildenafil citrate]		Phosphodiesterase-5 (PDE5) inhibitor	Erectile dysfunction
Vibativ [telavancin hydrochloride]	Z79.2	Antibacterial	Pneumonia; severe bacterial skin infections
Vibramycin [doxycycline calcium]	Z79.2	Antibacterial	Bacterial infections
Vicoprofen [hydrocodone bitartrate/ibuprofen]	Z79.891	Opioid analgesic/ Nonsteroidal anti-inflammatory drug (NSAID)	Pain, inflammation, or fever relief
Victoza [liraglutide (rDNA) injection]		Glucagon-like peptide-1 (GLP-1) receptor agonist	Diabetes mellitus
Vienva [ethinyl estradiol/levonorgestrel]	Z79.3	Contraceptive	Contraception
Viorele [desogestrel/ethinyl estradiol]	Z79.3	Contraceptive	Contraception
Virazole [ribavirin]		Antiviral	Respiratory syncytial virus (RSV)
Vistaril [hydroxyzine pamoate]		Antianxiety agent, antiemetic	Treatment of nausea and vomiting, for reducing narcotic requirement in surgery and as tranquilizer for tension, anxiety, or agitation states
Vivelle [estradiol]	Z79.890	Estrogen therapy	Menopause symptoms; osteoporosis prevention
Voltaren [diclofenac sodium]	Z79.1	Nonsteroidal anti-inflammatory drug (NSAID)	Treatment of pain, inflammation, and joint stiffness due to arthritis
Warfarin [warfarin sodium]	Z79.01	Anticoagulant	Prophylaxis and treatment of venous thrombosis, treatment of atrial fibrillation with embolization (pulmonary embolism), arrhythmias, myocardial infarction, and stroke prevention
Wellbutrin SR, Wellbutrin XL [bupropion hydrochloride]		Antidepressant; CNS	Depression; smoking cessation
Wera [ethinyl estradiol/norethindrone]	Z79.3	Contraceptive	Contraception
Xalatan [latanoprost]		Prostaglandin F2α analogue	Glaucoma, open-angle; ocular hypertension
Xanax, Xanax XR [alprazolam]		Antianxiety; sedative/hypnotic	Anxiety disorders with panic disorder and depression
Xarelto [rivaraxaban]	Z79.01	Anticoagulant	Prophylaxis and treatment of venous thrombosis, pulmonary embolism; prevention of blood clots due to atrial fibrillation
Xifaxan [rifaximin]	Z79.2	Antibacterial	*E. coli* diarrhea
Xigduo [dapagliflozin propanediol/metformin hydrochloride]	Z79.84	Blood glucose regulator	Diabetes mellitus
Xigris [drotrecogin alfa]		Biologic response modifier	Severe sepsis
Yasmin [drospirenone/ethinyl estradiol]	Z79.3	Contraceptive	Contraception
Yaz [drospirenone/ethinyl estradiol]	Z79.3	Contraceptive	Contraception; menstrual disorders
Zantac [ranitidine hydrochloride]		Histamine H2-receptors inhibitor	Acid/peptic disorder, erosive esophagitis, gastrointestinal hypersecretion, mastocytosis, gastroesophageal reflux, peptic ulcer, Zollinger-Ellison syndrome
Zerbaxa [ceftolozane sulfate/tazobactam sodium]	Z79.2	Antibacterial	Complicated urinary tract and intra-abdominal infections
Zestoretic [lisinopril/hydrochlorothiazide]		ACE inhibitor; antihypertensive	Congestive heart failure; essential hypertension
Zestril [lisinopril]		ACE inhibitor; antihypertensive	Congestive heart failure; essential hypertension
Ziac [bisoprolol fumarate/hydrochlorothiazide]		Antihypertensive	Essential hypertension
Zinacef [cefuroxime sodium]	Z79.2	Antibacterial	Bacterial infections
Zipsor [diclofenac potassium]	Z79.1	Nonsteroidal anti-inflammatory drug (NSAID)	Pain and inflammation relief

Drug	Z Code	Drug Action	Indications
Zithromax [azithromycin]	Z79.2	Macrolide	Infections of the cervix, lower respiratory tract, skin and skin structures, urethra, nongonococcal; mycobacterium avium complex; pharyngitis, streptococcal pneumonia; tonsillitis
Zmax [azithromycin]	Z79.2	Antibacterial	Pneumonia; sinusitis
Zocor [simvastatin]		HMG-CoA reductase inhibitor (statin)	Hypercholesterolemia, hyperlipidemia, hyperlipoproteinemia, hypertriglyceridemia
Zoladex [goserelin acetate]	Z79.818	Agents affecting estrogen receptors and estrogen levels	Prostate cancer symptoms and advanced breast cancer
Zoloft [sertraline hydrochloride]		Antidepressant	Anxiety with panic disorder and depression; obsessive-compulsive disorder
Zometa [zoledronic acid]	Z79.83	Bisphosphonates	Multiple myeloma; Paget's disease
Zorvolex [diclofenac]	Z79.1	Nonsteroidal anti-inflammatory drug (NSAID)	Pain, inflammation or fever relief
Zosyn [piperacillin sodium/tazobactam sodium]	Z79.2	Antibacterial	Bacterial infections
Zovia [ethynodiol diacetate/ethinyl estradiol]	Z79.3	Contraceptive	Contraception
Zovirax [acyclovir]		Antiviral	Genital herpes and herpes zoster infections
Zyloprim [allopurinol]		Antigout	Gouty arthritis, renal calculus, hyperuricemia, hyperuricemia secondary to leukemia, hyperuricemia secondary to lymphoma
Zyprexa [olanzapine]		Antipsychotic/antimanic	Psychotic disorders; schizophrenia
Zyrtec [cetirizine hydrochloride]		Antihistamine	Perennial allergic and seasonal allergic rhinitis; chronic urticaria
Zyvox [linezolid]	Z79.2	Antibacterial	Serious bacterial infections

Appendix D: Z Codes for Long-Term Drug Use with Associated Drugs

Z79.Ø1 Long term (current) use of anticoagulants
Arixtra
Coumadin
Eliquis
Fragmin
Heparin
Jantoven
Lovenox
Pradaxa
Savaysa
Warfarin
Xarelto

Z79.Ø2 Long term (current) use of antithrombotics/antiplatelets
Aggrastat
Aggrenox
Angiomax
Argatroban
Brilinta
Clopidogrel bisulfate
Effient
Integrilin
Iprivask
Persantine
Plavix

Z79.1 Long term (current) use of non-steroidal anti-inflammatories (NSAID)
Advil
Aleve
Anaprox
Arthrotec
Caldolor
Cambia
Celebrex
Daypro
Duexis
Dyloject
Feldene
Ibuprofen
Indocin
Mobic
Motrin
Nabumetone
Nalfon
Naprelan
Naprosyn
NeoProfen
Ponstel
Tivorbex
Voltaren
Zipsor
Zorvolex

Z79.2 Long term (current) use of antibiotics
Akne-Mycin
Altabax
Amoxicillin
Ampicillin
Ancef
Augmentin
Azactam
Azithromycin
Bactrim
Bactroban
Ceftriaxone
Centany
Cephalexin
Cipro
Ciprofloxacin
Clarithromycin
Cleocin
Clindamycin
Daptomycin
Dificid
Doxycycline
Dynacin
E.E.S.
Ertapenem
ERYC
Erygel
EryPed
Ery-Tab
Erythrocin
Erythromycin
Factive
Flagyl
Fortaz
Gentamicin sulfate
Invanz
Isoniazid
Keflex
Kefzol
Klaron
Levaquin
Lincocin
Macrobid
Maxipime
Mefoxin
Mepron
Merrem
Metro
Metronidazole
Minocin
Monodox
Monurol
Moxatag

Mycobutin
Nebupent
Nitrofurantoin
Oracea
Orbactiv
PCE
Penicillin-VK
Pentam
Pfizerpen
Priftin
Primaxin
Rifadin
Rimactane
Septra
Seromycin
Sivextro
Solodyn
Streptomycin sulfate
Suprax
Synercid
Tazicef
Teflaro
Tetracycline HCl
Tobramycin
Trimethoprim
Tygacil
Unasyn
Vancocin HCl
Vancomycin HCl
Vibativ
Vibramycin
Xifaxan
Zerbaxa
Zinacef
Zithromax
Zmax
Zosyn
Zyvox

Z79.3 Long term (current) use of hormonal contraceptives
Altavera
Alyacen
Aranelle
Ashlyna
Aviane
Aygestin
Balziva
Bekyree
Beyaz
Brevicon
Briellyn
Camila
Cryselle
Cyclafem

Cyclessa
Dasetta
Daysee
Depo-Provera
Depo-SubQ Provera
Desogen
Elinest
Emoquette
Enpresse
Enskyce
Errin
Estarylla
Estrostep Fe
Falmina
Femcon Fe
Femhrt
Gildagia
Gildess
Introvale
Jencycla
Junel
Kariva
Kelnor
Kimidess
Kurvelo
Larin
Lessina
Levonest
Levora
Liletta
Lo Loestrin Fe
Lo Minastrin Fe
Loestrin
Loryna
LoSeasonique
Low-Ogestrel
Marlissa
Microgestin
Micronor
Minastrin
Mirena
Modicon
Mono-Linyah
Myzilra
Natazia
Nexplanon
Norinyl
Nor-QD
Nortrel
NuvaRing
Ogestrel
Orsythia
Ortho Cyclen
Ortho-Novum
Ortho-Tri-Cyclen
Philith

Pimtrea
Pirmella
Plan B One-Step
Portia
Previfem
Provera
Quartette
Quasense
Safyral
Seasonale
Seasonique
Setlakin
Skyla
Sprintec
Syeda
Tri-Estarylla
Tri-Legest
Tri-Linyah
Tri-Lo-Estarylla
Tri-Lo-Sprintec
Tri-Norinyl
Tri-Previfem
Tri-Sprintec
Trivora
Velivet
Vienva
Viorele
Wera
Yasmin
Yaz
Zovia

Z79.4 **Long term (current) use of insulin**
Afrezza
Apidra
Basaglar
Humalog
Humulin
Lantus
Levemir
Novolin
NovoLog
Ryzodeg
Toujeo Solostar
Tresiba

Z79.51 **Long term (current) use of inhaled steroids**
Advair
Aerospan
Alvesco
Arnuity Ellipta
Asmanex
Dulera
Flovent
Pulmicort
Qvar

Symbicort

Z79.52 **Long term (current) use of systemic steroids**
A-Methapred
Aristospan
Celestone Soluspan
Colocort
Cortef
Cortenema
Cortifoam
Cortisone acetate
Depo-Medrol
Dexamethasone Intensol
Entocort EC
Hydrocortisone
Kenalog
Medrol
Methylprednisolone
Orapred ODT
PediaPred
Prednisolone
Prednisone
Prelone
Rayos
Solu-Cortef
Solu-Medrol

Z79.810 **Long term (current) use of selective estrogen receptor modulators (SERMs)**
Evista
Fareston
Osphena
Raloxifene
Soltamox
Tamoxifen
Toremifene

Z79.811 **Long term (current) use of aromatase inhibitors**
Anastrozole
Arimidex
Aromasin
Exemestane
Femara
Letrozole

Z79.818 **Long term (current) use of other agents affecting estrogen receptors and estrogen levels**
Eligard
Faslodex
Fulvestrant
Lupron
Megace ES
Supprelin LA
Synarel

Trelstar
Vantas
Zoladex

Z79.82 Long term (current) use of aspirin
Bayer
Bufferin
Ecotrin

Z79.83 Long term (current) use of bisphosphonates
Actonel
Atelvia
Binosto
Boniva
Didronel
Fosamax
Reclast
Zometa

Z79.84 Long term (current) use of oral hypoglycemic drugs
Acarbose
Actoplus Met
Actos
Amaryl
Avandia
Duetact
Fortamet
Glimepiride
Glucophage
Glucotrol
Glucovance
Glumetza
Glyburide
Invokamet
Janumet
Januvia
Jentadueto
Kazano
Kombiglyze
Metformin
Onglyza
Oseni
PrandiMet
Prandin
Precose
Qtern
Repaglinide
Riomet
Sitagliptin
Synjardy
Xigduo

Z79.89Ø Hormone replacement therapy
Activella
Alora
Angeliq

Climara
CombiPatch
Delestrogen
Divigel
Duavee
Elestrin
Enjuvia
Estrace
Estraderm
Estrasorb
EstroGel
Femhrt
Femring
Femtrace
Menest
Menostar
Minivelle
Osphena
Premarin
Prempro
Provera
Vagifem
Vivelle

Z79.891 Long term (current) use of opiate analgesic
Acetaminophen with codeine
Astramorph
Buprenex
Buprenorphine HCl
Butrans
Codeine
Demerol
Dilaudid
Dolophine HCl
Duragesic
Duramorph
Embeda
Exalgo
Fentanyl
Fentora
Fioricet with codeine
Hydrocodone
Hydrocodone bitartrate and acetaminophen
Hydromorphone HCl
Kadian
Methadone HCl
Methadose
Morphine
MS Contin
Norco
Nucynta
Opana
Oxycodone HCl
OxyContin

Percocet
Reprexain
Roxicet
Roxicodone
Sublimaze
Tylenol with codeine
Ultram
Vicoprofen

Z79.899 Other long term (current) drug therapy
Actimmune
Antineoplastic/chemotherapy
Astagraf XL
Avonex
Cellcept
Cyclosporine
Envarsus XR
Gengraf
Imuran
Intron
Monoclonal antibodies
Neoral
Pegintron
Prograf
Protopic
Rapamune
Rebif
Sandimmune
Simulect
Sirolimus
Sylatron
Tacrolimus
Torisel

Appendix E: Z Codes Only as Principal/First-Listed Diagnosis

Z00.00	Z01.20	Z02.3	Z03.810	Z34.01	Z38.5	Z51.12	Z52.5
Z00.01	Z01.21	Z02.4	Z03.818	Z34.02	Z38.61	Z52.000	Z52.6
Z00.110	Z01.30	Z02.5	Z03.89	Z34.03	Z38.62	Z52.001	Z52.810
Z00.111	Z01.31	Z02.6	Z04.1	Z34.80	Z38.63	Z52.008	Z52.811
Z00.121	Z01.411	Z02.71	Z04.2	Z34.81	Z38.64	Z52.010	Z52.812
Z00.129	Z01.419	Z02.79	Z04.3	Z34.82	Z38.65	Z52.011	Z52.813
Z00.2	Z01.42	Z02.81	Z04.41	Z34.83	Z38.66	Z52.018	Z52.819
Z00.3	Z01.810	Z02.82	Z04.42	Z34.90	Z38.68	Z52.090	Z52.89
Z00.5	Z01.811	Z02.83	Z04.6	Z34.91	Z38.69	Z52.091	Z76.1
Z00.70	Z01.812	Z02.89	Z04.71	Z34.92	Z38.7	Z52.098	Z76.2
Z00.71	Z01.818	Z02.9	Z04.72	Z34.93	Z38.8	Z52.10	Z99.12
Z00.8	Z01.82	Z03.6	Z04.8	Z38.00	Z39.0	Z52.11	
Z01.00	Z01.83	Z03.71	Z04.9	Z38.01	Z39.1	Z52.19	
Z01.01	Z01.84	Z03.72	Z31.81	Z38.1	Z39.2	Z52.20	
Z01.10	Z01.89	Z03.73	Z31.83	Z38.2	Z42.1	Z52.21	
Z01.110	Z02.0	Z03.74	Z31.84	Z38.30	Z42.8	Z52.29	
Z01.118	Z02.1	Z03.75	Z33.2	Z38.31	Z51.0	Z52.3	
Z01.12	Z02.2	Z03.79	Z34.00	Z38.4	Z51.11	Z52.4	

Appendix F: Centers for Medicare & Medicaid Services Hierarchical Condition Categories (CMS-HCC)

In the 1970s, Medicare began demonstration projects that contracted with health maintenance organizations (HMO) to provide care for Medicare beneficiaries in exchange for prospective payments. In 1985, this project changed from demonstration status to a regular part of the Medicare program, Medicare Part C. The Balanced Budget Act (BBA) of 1997 named Medicare's Part C managed care program Medicare+Choice, and the Medicare Modernization Act (MMA) of 2003 again renamed it to Medicare Advantage (MA).

Medicare is one of the world's largest health insurance programs, and about one-fourth of the beneficiaries on Medicare are enrolled in a MA private health care plan. Due to the great variance in the health status of Medicare beneficiaries, risk adjustment provides a means of adequately compensating those plans with large numbers of seriously ill patients while not overburdening other plans that have healthier individuals. Medicare Advantage (MA) plans have been using the HCC/risk adjustment model since 2004.

The Risk Adjustment Model

The primary purpose of a risk adjustment model is to predict (on average) the future health care costs for specific consortiums enrolled in Medicare Advantage (MA) health plans. CMS is then able to provide capitation payments to these private health plans. Capitation payments are an incentive for health plans to enroll not only healthier individuals but those with chronic conditions or who are more seriously ill by removing some of the financial burden.

The MA risk adjustment model uses hierarchical condition categories (HCC) to assess the disease burden of its enrollees. HCC diagnostic groupings were created after examining claims data so that enrollees with similar disease processes, and consequently similar health care expenditures, could be pooled into a larger data set in which an average expenditure rate could be determined. The medical conditions included in HCC categories are those that were determined to most predictably affect the health status and health care costs of any individual. Several important principles to the risk adjustment model and the development of the HCC categories include but are not limited to:

1. The HCC diagnostic categories should be clinically meaningful.
   - Diagnostic categories are well-defined.
   - Clinically specific diseases or medical conditions are grouped to each category.
2. The HCC diagnostic categories should predict medical expenditures.
   - The diagnoses grouped to a specific category should have as close to the same cost burden not only in the current year but also in the future.
3. The HCC diagnostic categories should have adequate sample sizes and discretionary categories excluded to be as accurate and stable in their estimate of costs as possible.
   - A diagnostic category that groups extremely rare diseases or conditions would not be reliably effective in determining current or future costs.
   - Codes that are not credible as cost predictors or may be subject to coding variation should be excluded, when possible.
4. The HCC diagnostic categories should be both hierarchical and accumulative.
   - Hierarchical measurement is used within a specific disease process.
   - Disease processes that are unrelated to each other are measured accumulatively.
5. The diagnostic classification should encourage specificity and should not reward coding proliferation.
   - More diagnosis codes and vague diagnosis codes do not equal greater disease burden.

More than 9,000 ICD-10-CM diagnosis codes map to 79 HCCs in the current risk adjustment model. Diagnoses are excluded from mapping when they do not predict future cost or are vague or variable in diagnosis, coding, or treatment, such as symptoms or osteoarthritis. Also excluded are diagnosis codes from laboratories, radiology, and home health claims.

Risk Adjustment Factors

The CMS-HCC risk adjustment model uses "risk adjustment factors" to calculate a risk score for each member. This score summarizes that particular patient's expected cost of care relative to other members'. Each member's risk score is based on demographic and health status information and is calculated as the sum of these demographic and health factors weighted by their estimated marginal contributions to total risk. The model also takes into account where the patient resides (community or institutional), Medicaid eligibility (full or partial benefit), the patient's Medicare enrollment status (new or established), age, disability status, whether the patient is frail or has end-stage renal disease (ESRD), and even prescription drug use.

No procedure codes, ICD-10-PCS or CPT, are included in the MA risk adjustment model. The model relies solely on diagnostic and demographic data. Not all ICD-10-CM diagnoses map to an HCC, and there is no specific code sequencing involved. The CMS-HCC model is accumulative as well as hierarchical. The accumulative functionality allows a patient to have more than one HCC category assigned, providing a more complete clinical picture and prediction of resource consumption. The hierarchical aspect of the model provides a means of ranking diagnoses that are similar in disease process, by severity. The hierarchy of the condition categories ensures the patient's conditions are classified to the most severe condition within the related group. Less severe conditions within a particular hierarchy are superseded by more severe diagnoses within the same group. The hierarchy and accumulative relationship permits this model to characterize the person's illness level within each disease process, while still allowing the effects of unrelated disease processes to be counted in the patient's overall score.

Certain combinations of coexisting diagnoses for an individual can increase medical costs. The CMS-HCC model adjusts for these higher costs by the addition of "disease interaction" factors. For each patient, multiple HCCs assigned, along with demographic and disease interaction factors, are used to calculate a single, combined risk adjustment factor (RAF). The RAF score for an individual member represents all of the HCCs that have been submitted from all sources for that member to CMS during the course of an entire calendar year.

There are separate CMS-HCC models for new enrollees and continuing enrollees. The new enrollee model uses demographic factors only, such as age, sex, and disability status, and is used when the enrollee has less than 12 months of medical history. The community model accounts for age, sex, original reason for Medicare entitlement (age or disability), Medicaid eligibility, and clinical conditions as measured by HCCs. In the second step, expected costs are adjusted for outliers based on the member's risk score and whether the patient has ESRD.

Demographic data (age, sex, eligibility) as well as health status (diagnoses codes submitted on claims to CMS) of an MA population are used to determine the reimbursement to the health plan to care for their members.

RAF scores, which range from 0.118 to 2.4888, indicate patient health status. A RAF score of 1.0 or below is the benchmark CMS uses to indicate the average healthy patient with the same demographic and diagnostic factors. These patients are expected to use average or lower-than-average resources. When the RAF score is higher than 1.0, CMS considers the patient to be sicker than the average patient with the same criteria and expects greater-than-average resource utilization.

A low RAF score may accurately indicate a healthier patient, but it may also falsely indicate a healthier patient due to incomplete or inaccurate coding, incomplete or insufficient record documentation, or patients who fail to complete an annual assessment.

A high RAF score may accurately indicate a sicker patient, or it may be falsely inflated from overcoding due to diagnoses that are reported but not documented, or from copying and pasting from previous encounters or problem lists of resolved conditions.

Documentation Requirements

Payment is made per HCC category (not per diagnosis code). No matter how many times in the year the diagnosis codes are reported, a single payment is made to the MA plan each year. Each year the list of HCCs and the RAF for each patient is "reset." This means the annual health assessment is extremely important, and adequate documentation is critical. Accurate risk adjustment payment relies on complete medical record documentation and diagnosis coding. CMS requires that all applicable diagnosis codes be reported and that all diagnoses be reported to the highest level of specificity and that these be substantiated by the medical record.

CMS's Guiding Principle:

The risk adjustment diagnosis must be based on clinical medical record documentation from a face-to-face encounter, coded according to the *ICD-10-CM Guidelines for Coding and Reporting*; assigned based on dates of service within the data collection period, submitted to the MA organization from an appropriate risk adjustment provider type and an appropriate risk adjustment physician data source.

A "face-to-face" health service encounter between a patient and healthcare provider describes an encounter between the patient and the provider (MD, DO), including qualified nonphysician practitioners (NPP) (e.g. nurse practitioner or physician's assistant), which is face-to-face with the patient. CMS provides a current listing of acceptable physician specialty types for risk adjustment data submission within the 2012 Regional Technical Assistance Participant Guide. The only exception to the face-to-face encounter requirement is pathology services (professional component only). Currently, CMS does not provide a listing of all services that are considered face-to-face visits for risk adjustment data, but does provide guidance on what types of services are not acceptable for risk adjustment in the Participant Guide. For example, diagnostic radiology does not qualify because diagnostic radiologists typically do not document confirmed diagnoses. Other examples of services that are not acceptable include diagnostic reports that have not been interpreted, such as laboratory reports.

It is essential that the medical record documentation show evidence by provider authentication that the direct face-to-face service was personally furnished by the physician or qualified NPP. Examples of these services include office visits, hospital visits, preoperative anesthesia assessment, and surgical and invasive procedures.

Risk adjustment relies on annual health information. Each enrollee is assigned an individual risk score based on the health status information obtained from the diagnosis codes on the claims. The CMS-HCC model relies on ICD-10-CM coding specificity for accurate risk adjustment by using the most specific code available that is substantiated by the documentation in the medical record. Providers should fully document and accurately code the evaluation and management of all severe and chronic conditions to ensure a full, complete, and accurate clinical record of the patient's condition and reflect the work involved in caring for the patient, particularly those with complex and challenging health issues. All conditions affecting the treatment or management of the patient's health should be documented at least once a year, as applicable to care provided, to accurately describe the true complexity and severity of the patient's health. If the diagnosis coding on the claim is not accurate or complete, the claim may indicate that the provider did much less medical decision-making, evaluation, and management than was actually performed.

Documentation for a valid reportable diagnosis must clearly indicate evidence of M.E.A.T., for each diagnosis:

M	managed
E	evaluated
A	assessed
T	treated

It is recommended that providers use the Subjective and Objective observation, Assessment and Plan (S.O.A.P.) format for progress notes to document evidence of M.E.A.T. A problem list, active condition list, past medical history list, etc., are not suitable examples of documentation of M.E.A.T. Diagnoses and documentation may not be captured from past encounters that have been copied and pasted. Each encounter must be unique and reflect only that visit as it occurred. Chronic conditions require long-term attention and management, and should be reported when treated but are often inadequately documented due to familiarity with the patient. Insufficient documentation influences the assignment of diagnosis codes and directly affects the patient's risk score.

Documentation should be concise, include the reason for the face-to-face visit, and support the need for the patient to be monitored, evaluated, assessed, and/or treated for the conditions listed through clinical rationale and/or plan of care described in clear (legible) notes. Each page of progress notes should be properly authenticated and include the patient's name and the date.

Providers should document each clinical diagnosis to the highest degree of specificity per encounter, including all complications and/or manifestations, including clear links to causal conditions. Only confirmed conditions should be documented—no rule-out conditions or abnormal findings without clinical significance. All known conditions, including chronic conditions, that affect the care and treatment of the patient at least once per year should be noted.

Providers should specifically document the condition and test or report results, and document the status of any changes to the condition, using terminology such as decreased, increased, worsening, improving, or unchanged. Documentation should include supporting evidence of the results or plan of care.

Documentation Tips

- Document all cause-and-effect relationships.
- Report the most specific diagnosis code available that is supported by the documentation.
- Include all current diagnoses as part of the current medical decision-making, and document for every visit.
- Identify diagnoses that are current or chronic problems rather than a past medical history or previous resolved condition.
- Document history of heart attack, status codes, etc., that affect the patient's care as "history of" or "PMH" when they no longer exist or are not current conditions.
- Ensure each progress note has the date, signature, and credentials/specialty.
- Document the thought processes used to assess each condition.
- Know high revenue HCCs that are often undiagnosed or undercoded.
- Avoid "unspecified" codes.
- Ensure the codes reported are accurate.
- Ensure each encounter is billed.
- Review rejection reports, and audit reports to assess risks.

Audits

Because reimbursement is by patient, rather than based on an average of the entire population, and is based upon documentation, there is the potential for upcoding. Audits are conducted by the MA plan and CMS recovery auditors.

Initial Validation Audit (IVA)

CMS requires that the MA plan validate HCCs. This is usually performed by an independent auditor working with the plan or a contracted vendor to validate the MA plan's data submitted to CMS.

The MA plan submits the one best medical record that supports each HCC identified for the beneficiary.

Risk Adjustment Data Validation Audit

Risk adjustment data validation (RADV) audits were introduced in 2011 and updated for 2015. They are performed by CMS to validate the integrity and accuracy of risk-adjusted payments by verifying that the diagnosis codes the MA plans submit are supported by the medical record documentation for a member.

MA plans can be selected by CMS for RADV audits annually and if chosen are required to submit their members' medical records to CMS. Providers are required to assist the MA plan by providing the medical record documentation included in the audit. Even though each diagnosis needs to be reported only once in a calendar year, during a RADV audit up to five dates of service may be submitted to support any one HCC.

To be validated, medical record documentation must meet certain criteria and standards. Even if the diagnosis is documented and coded correctly, any deficiency in the documentation can make the encounter and the HCC invalid. Diagnoses that cannot be validated are considered payment errors. The results of the audit are communicated to the MA plan, which then communicates these results to the provider. Under- and overpayments are subject to payment adjustment. The results of RADV audits can be extrapolated over the MA plan population to calculate potential payment errors and overpayments/recoupments. Regulations include a RADV appeal process, a document dispute process, and a procedure for obtaining physician-signature attestations.

The following items are reviewed during the validation process:

- The record is for the correct enrollee.
- The record is from the correct calendar year for the payment year being audited.
- The record is legible.
- The date of service is present on the records and is for a face-to-face visit.
- The record is from a valid provider type.

- Valid credentials and/or a valid physician specialty are documented on the record.

- The record contains a signature from an acceptable type of physician.

- There is a diagnosis on the record.

- The diagnosis supports an HCC.

- The diagnosis supports the submitted HCC.

Mitigate audit risk by coding each reportable diagnosis each time it meets reporting guidelines. Audit regularly to assess areas of risk and in need of improvement and to capture conditions documented but not coded. Check for additional qualifying HCCs. Ensure claims are submitted and that corrected claims are submitted when indicated. There are three claims submission deadlines: January, March, and September. CMS adjusts each member's risk score twice a year, with the final reconciliation in August of the year after the plan year.

If providers emphasize correct coding and documentation and perform internal audits to determine where the risks are and prepare for audits, incorrect payment is less likely.

Illustrations

Chapter 3. Diseases of the Blood and Blood-forming Organs and Certain Disorders Involving the Immune Mechanism (D5Ø–D89)

Red Blood Cells

White Blood Cell

Platelet

Coagulation

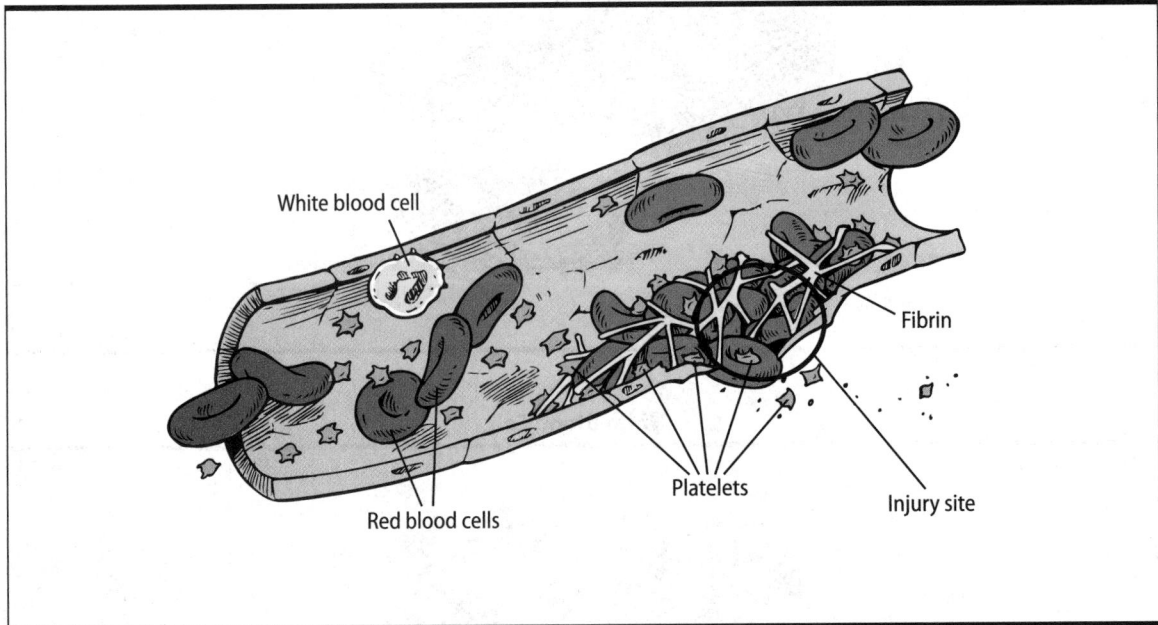

Spleen Anatomical Location and External Structures

Spleen Interior Structures

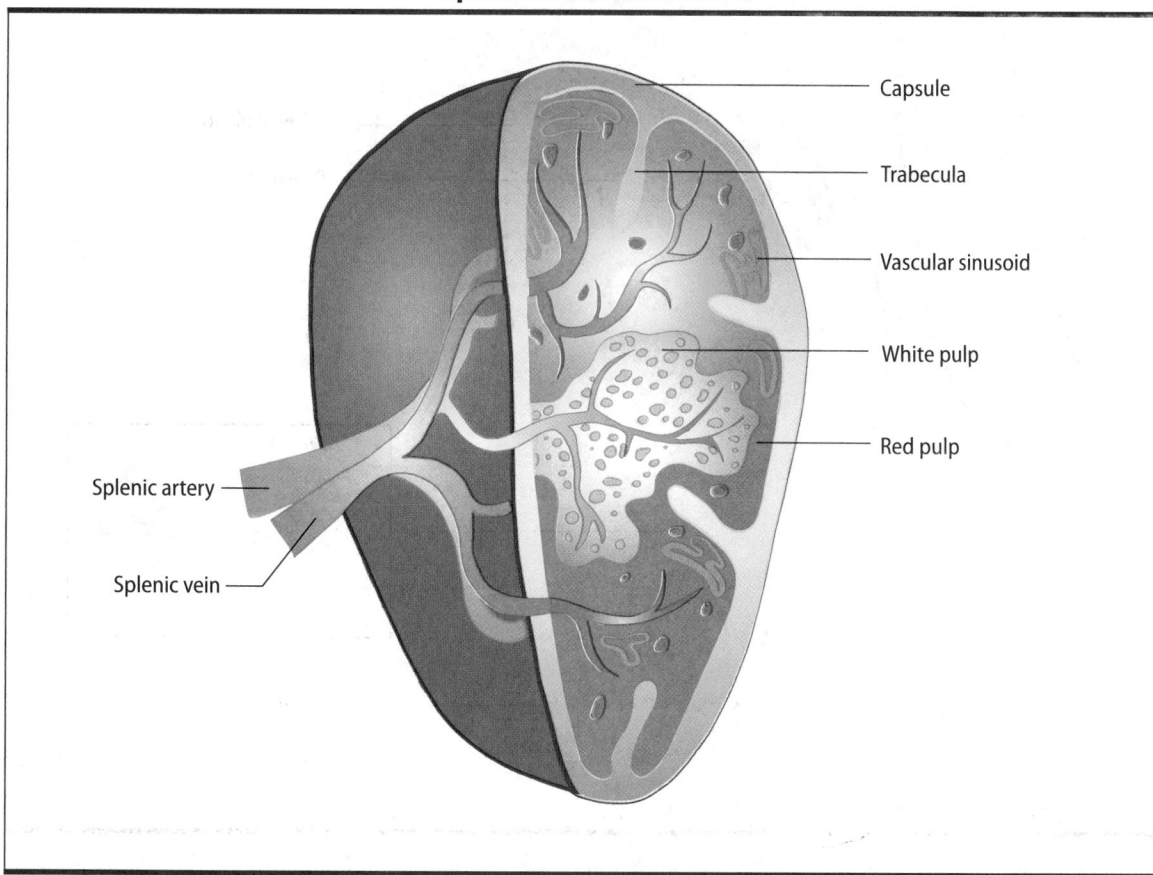

Chapter 4. Endocrine, Nutritional and Metabolic Diseases (E00–E89)

Endocrine System

Thyroid

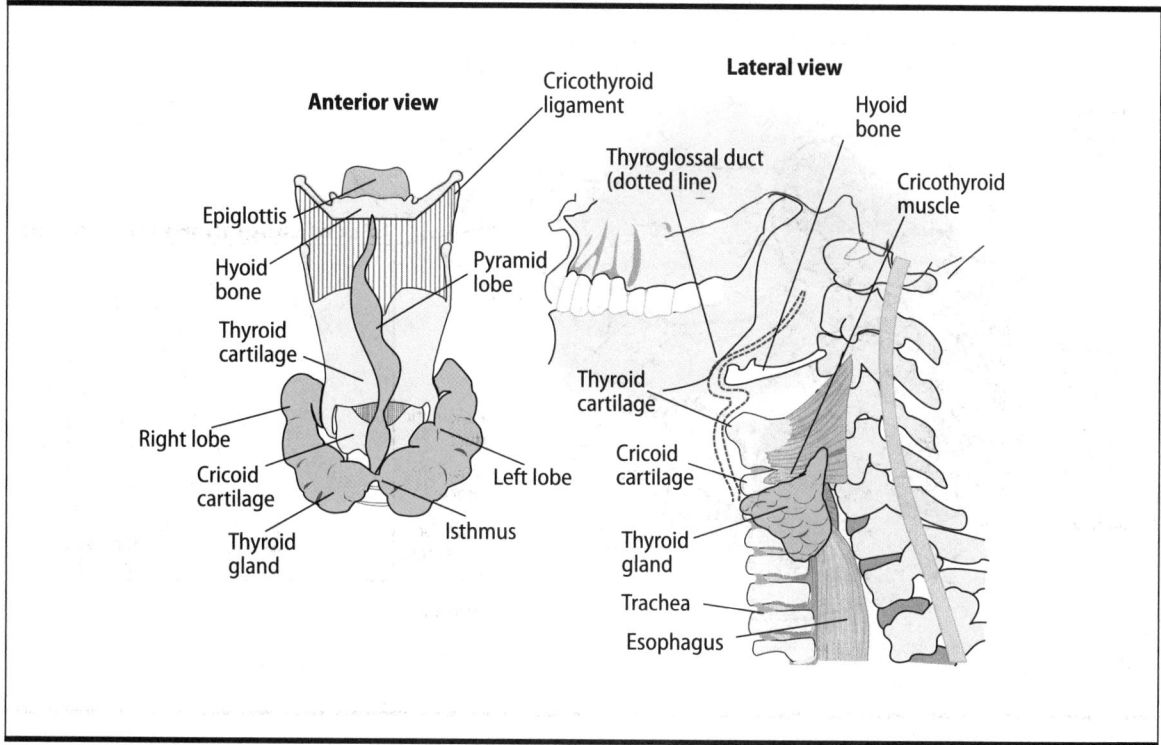

Thyroid and Parathyroid Glands

Posterior view

Epiglottis

Pharynx

Thyroid gland

Parathyroid gland

Pancreas

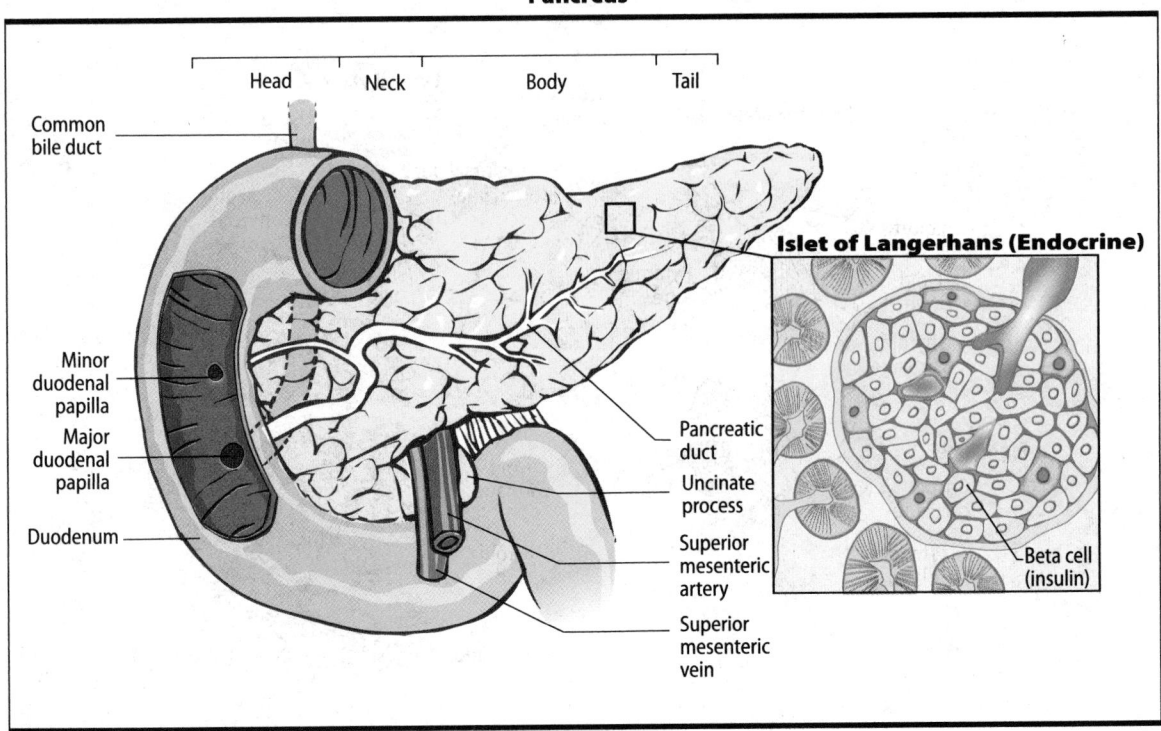

Anatomy of the Adrenal Gland

Structure of an Ovary

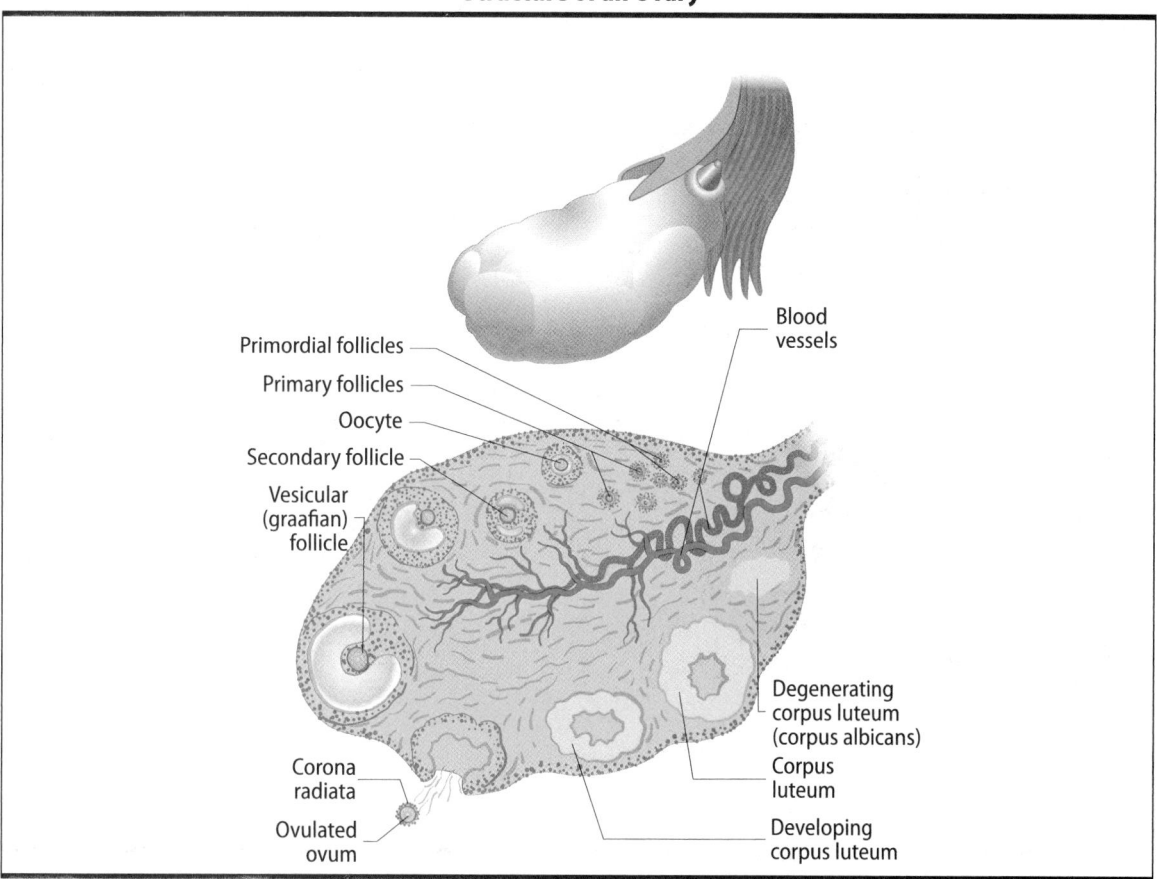

Testis and Associated Structures

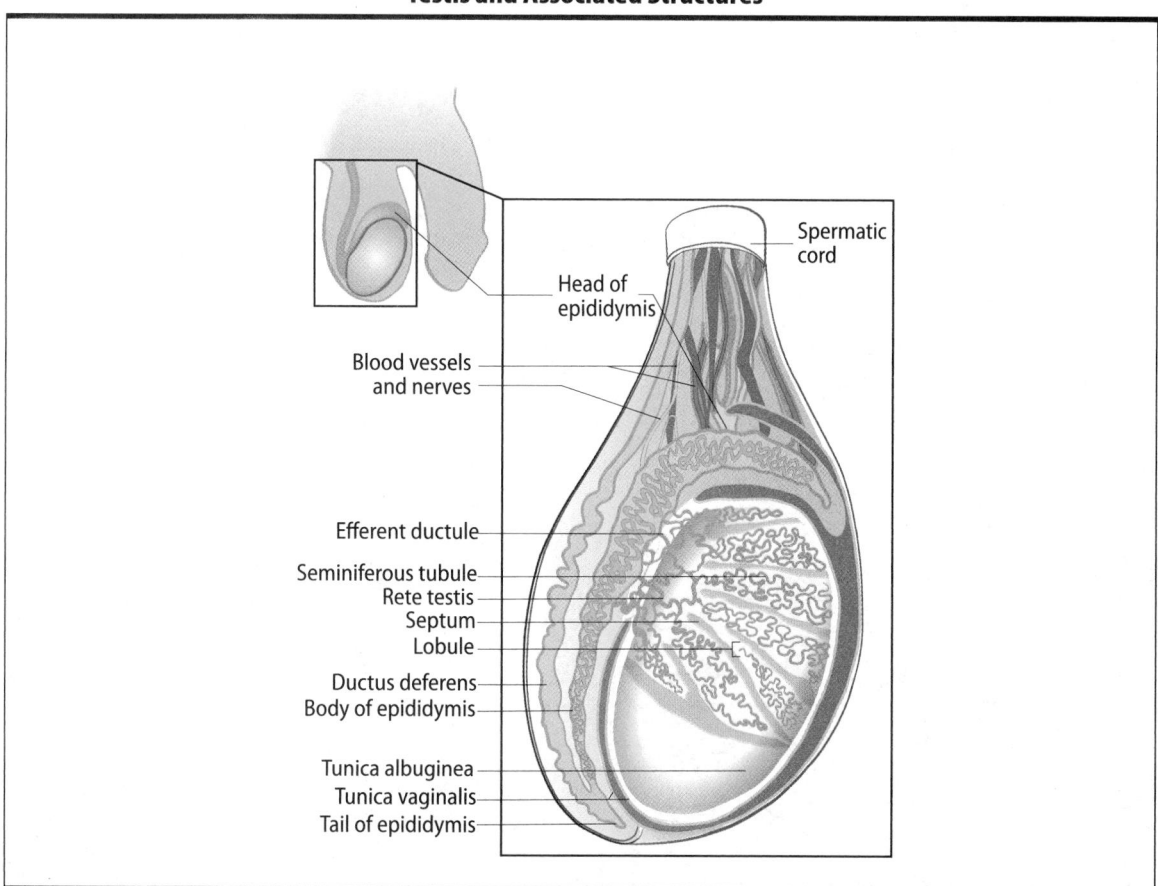

Thymus

Thyroid gland

Trachea

Left lung

Right lung

Heart
Diaphragm

Right lobe

Left lobe

Thymus

Septae

Lobule

Chapter 6. Diseases of the Nervous System (GØØ–G99)

Brain

Cranial Nerves

Peripheral Nervous System

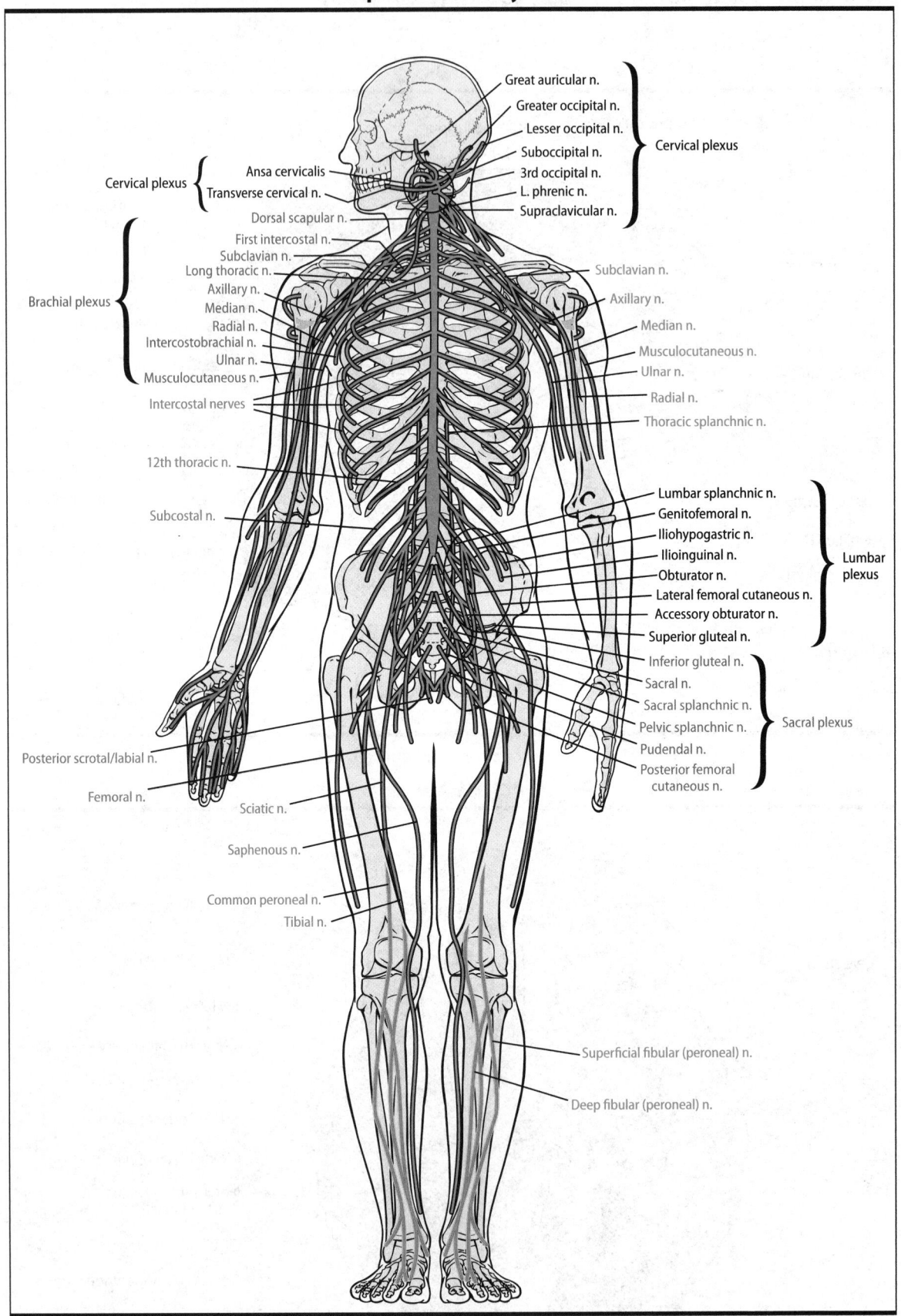

Spinal Cord and Spinal Nerves

Nerve Functions

Breathing (C1-4) and head and neck movement (C2)

Heart rate (C4-6) and shoulder movement (C5)

Wrist and elbow movement (C6-7)

Hand and finger movement (C7-T1)

Cervical spine

Thoracic spine

Sympathetic tone (T1-12) (including temperature regulation) and trunk stability (T2-12)

Lumbar spine

Ejaculation (T11-L2) and hip motion (L2)

Knee extension (L3)

Sacrum

Foot motion (L4-S1) and knee flexion (L5)

Penile erection (S2-S4) and bowel and bladder activity (S2-S3)

Coccyx

Spinal Cord Structures

Nerve fiber tracts
White matter
Grey matter
Anterior fissure

Meninges
Pia mater
Arachnoid
Dura mater

Subarachnoid space

Spinal nerve

Nerve Cell

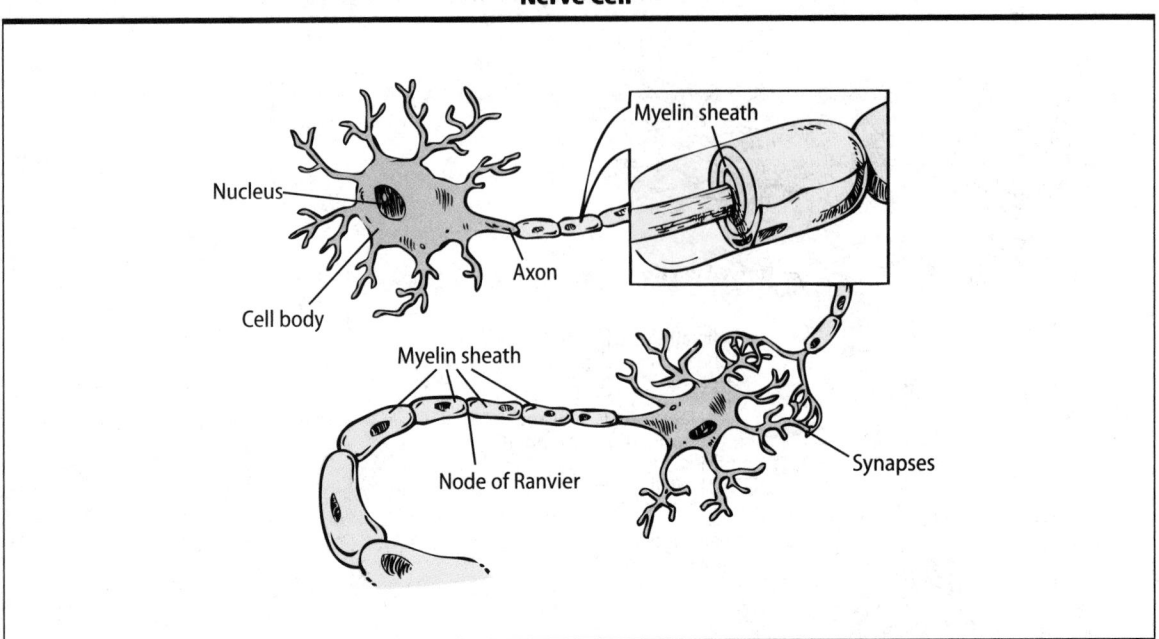

Chapter 7. Diseases of the Eye and Adnexa (H00–H59)

Eye

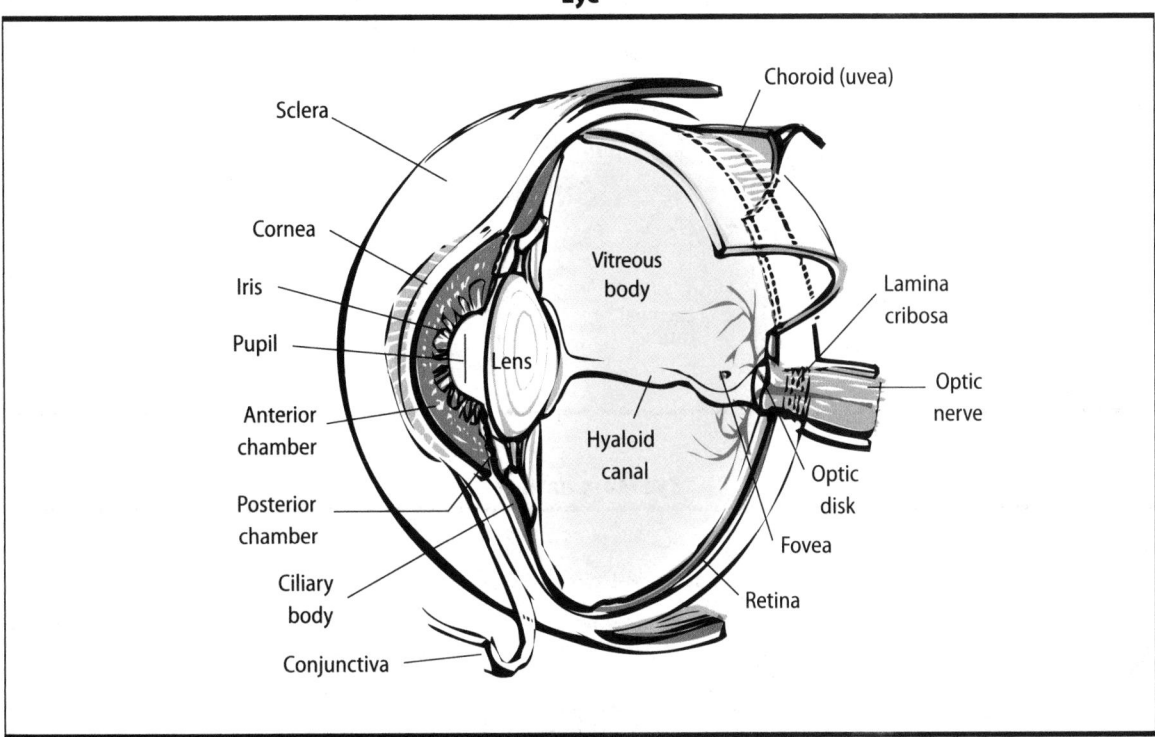

Posterior Pole of Globe/Flow of Aqueous Humor

Lacrimal System

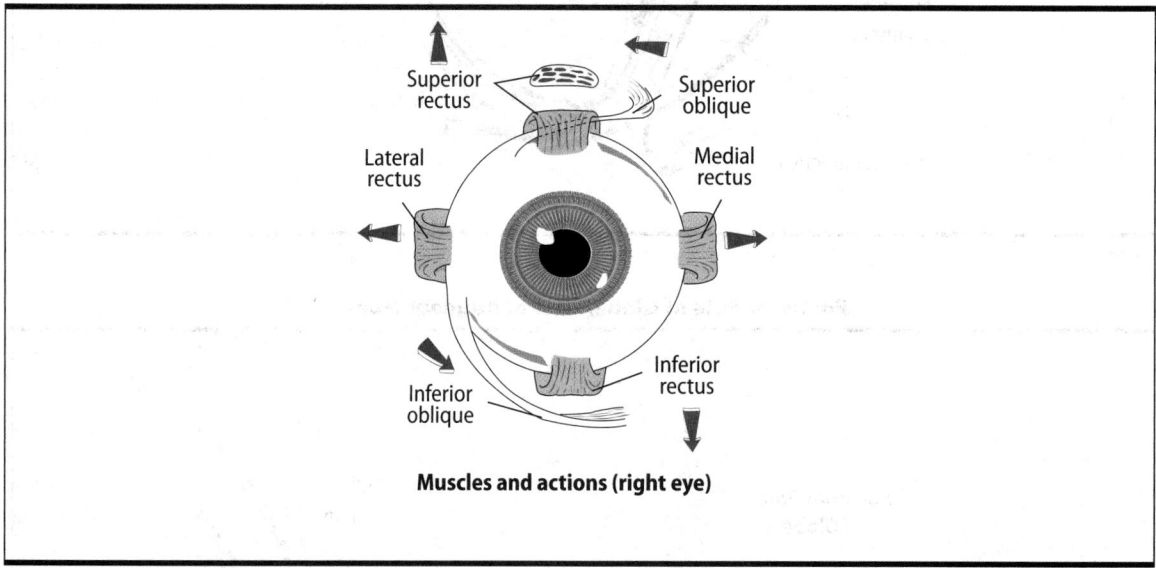

Eye Musculature

Muscles and actions (right eye)

Eyelid Structures

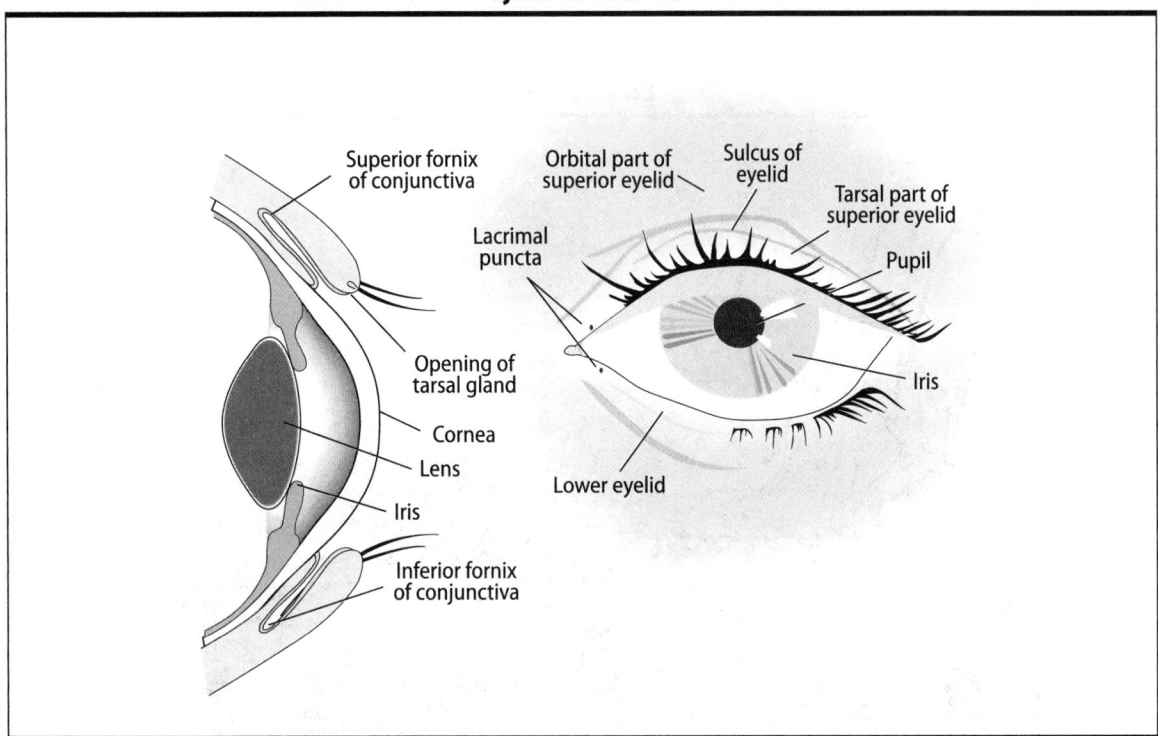

Chapter 8. Diseases of the Ear and Mastoid Process (H6Ø–H95)

Ear Anatomy

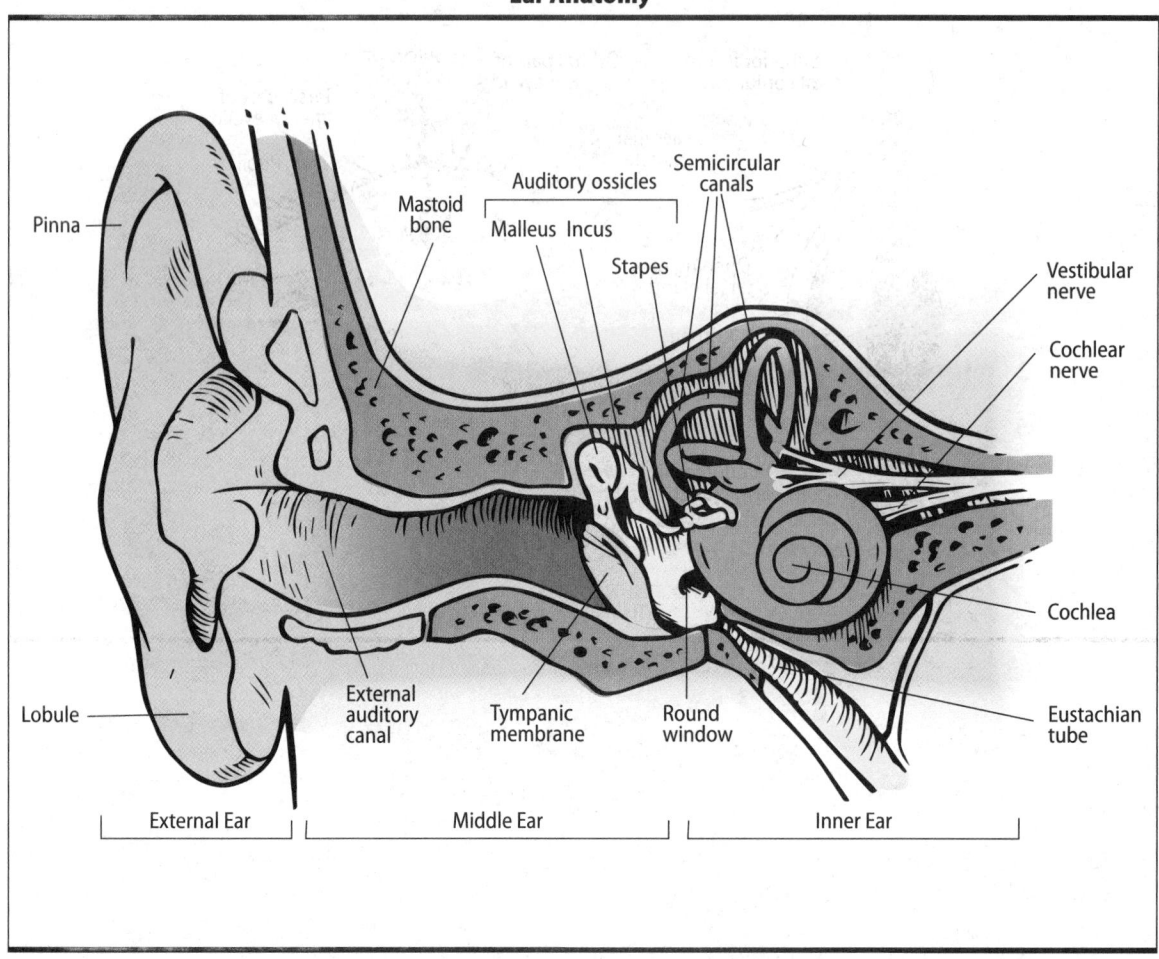

Chapter 9. Diseases of the Circulatory System (I00–I99)

Anatomy of the Heart

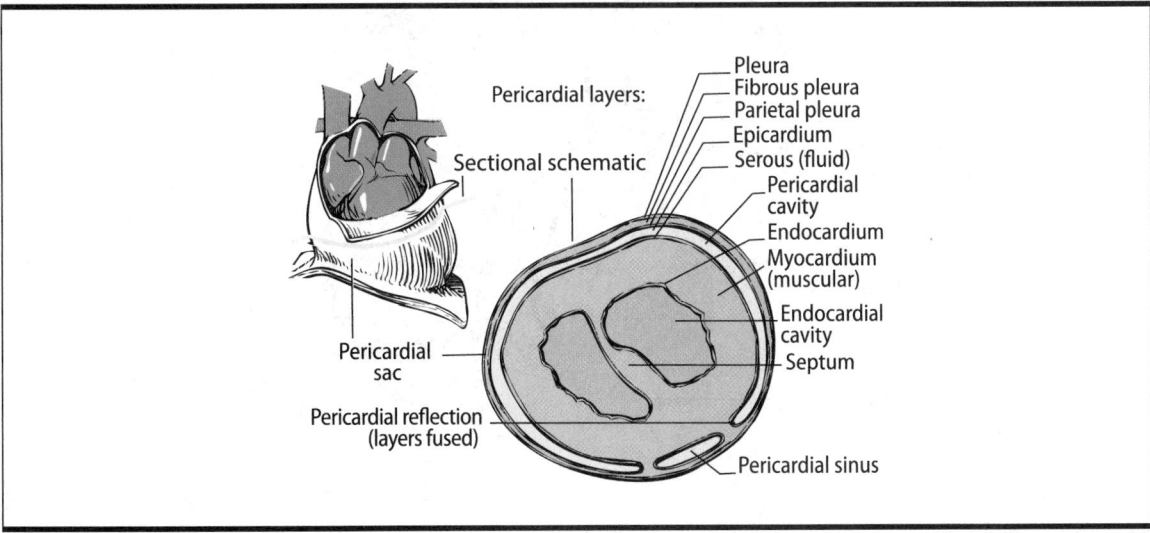

Superior vena cava

Aortic valve

Right atrium

Tricuspid valve

Right ventricle

Inferior vena cava

Aorta

Pulmonary artery

Pulmonary vein

Pulmonary valve

Left atrium

Mitral valve

Chorda tendinae

Left ventricle

Heart Cross Section

Pericardial layers:

Sectional schematic

Pericardial sac

Pericardial reflection (layers fused)

Pleura
Fibrous pleura
Parietal pleura
Epicardium
Serous (fluid)
Pericardial cavity
Endocardium
Myocardium (muscular)
Endocardial cavity
Septum

Pericardial sinus

Heart Valves

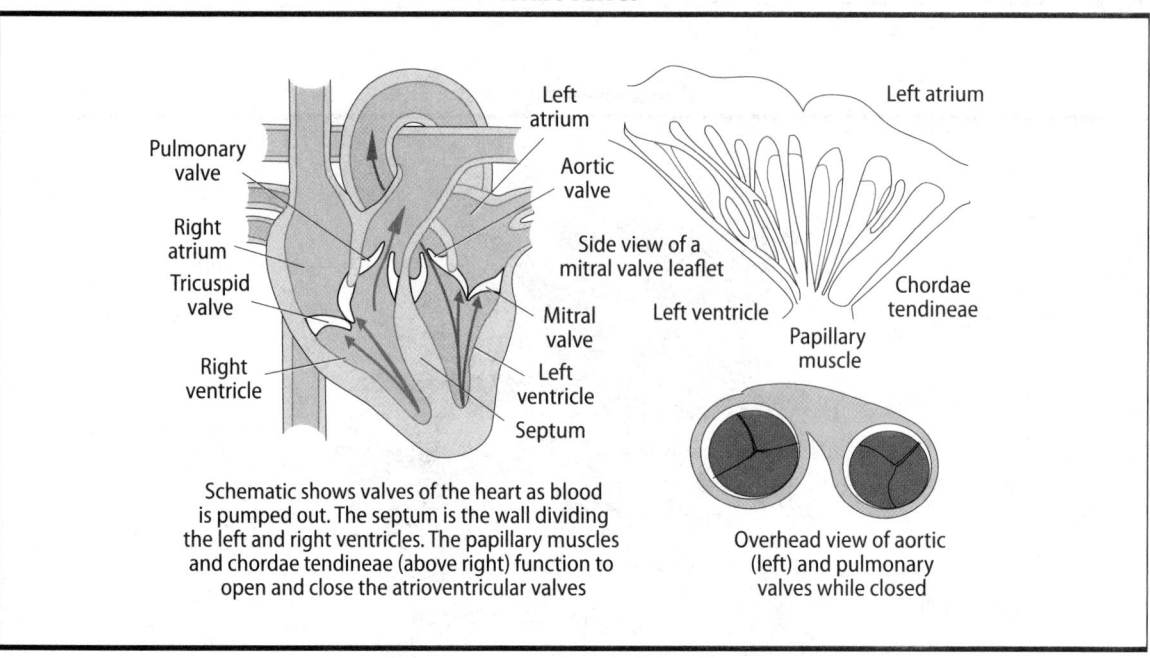

Schematic shows valves of the heart as blood is pumped out. The septum is the wall dividing the left and right ventricles. The papillary muscles and chordae tendineae (above right) function to open and close the atrioventricular valves

Overhead view of aortic (left) and pulmonary valves while closed

Heart Conduction System

Coronary Arteries

Arteries

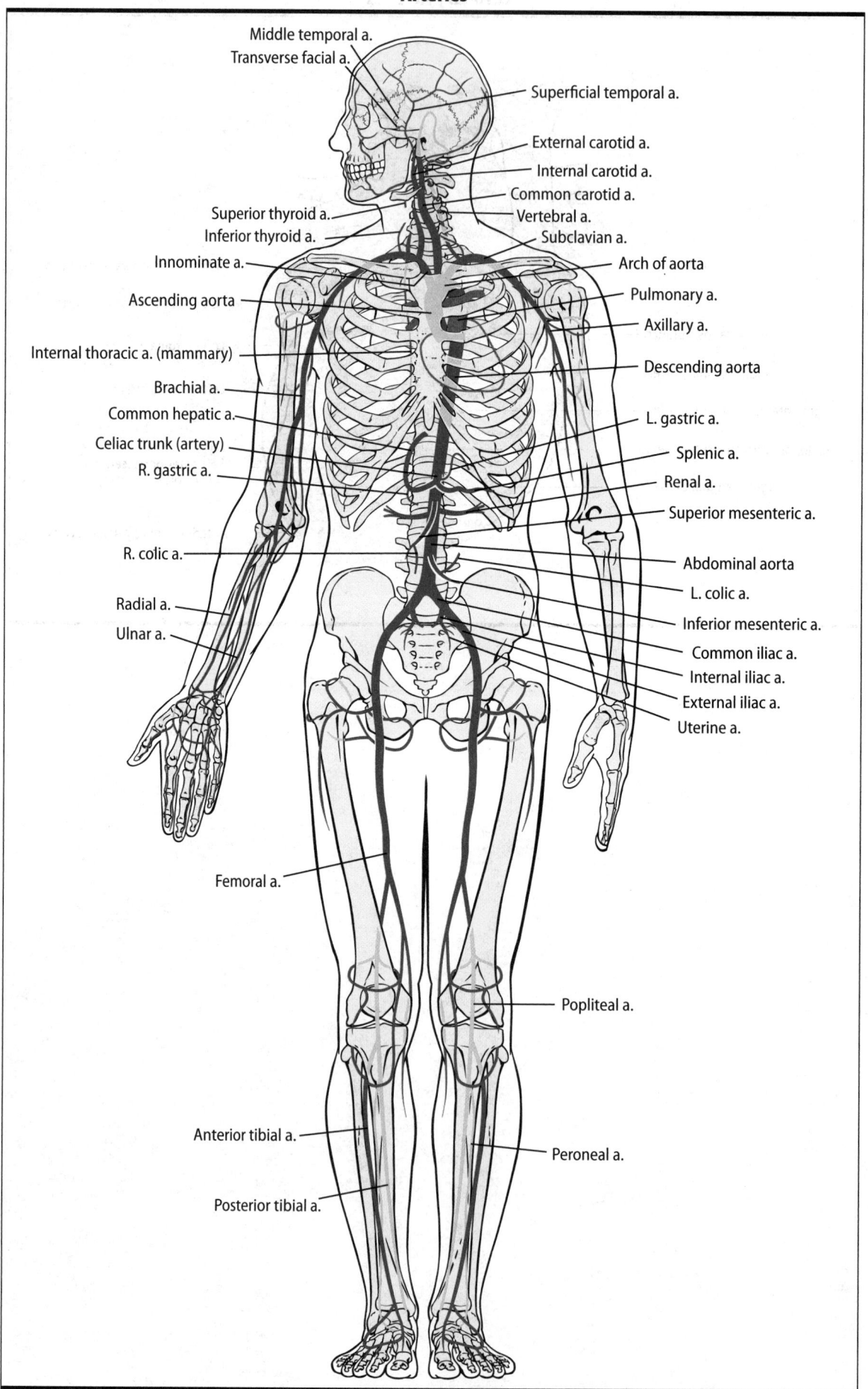

Middle temporal a.
Transverse facial a.
Superficial temporal a.
External carotid a.
Internal carotid a.
Common carotid a.
Superior thyroid a.
Vertebral a.
Inferior thyroid a.
Subclavian a.
Innominate a.
Arch of aorta
Ascending aorta
Pulmonary a.
Axillary a.
Internal thoracic a. (mammary)
Descending aorta
Brachial a.
Common hepatic a.
L. gastric a.
Celiac trunk (artery)
Splenic a.
R. gastric a.
Renal a.
Superior mesenteric a.
R. colic a.
Abdominal aorta
L. colic a.
Radial a.
Inferior mesenteric a.
Ulnar a.
Common iliac a.
Internal iliac a.
External iliac a.
Uterine a.
Femoral a.
Popliteal a.
Anterior tibial a.
Peroneal a.
Posterior tibial a.

Veins

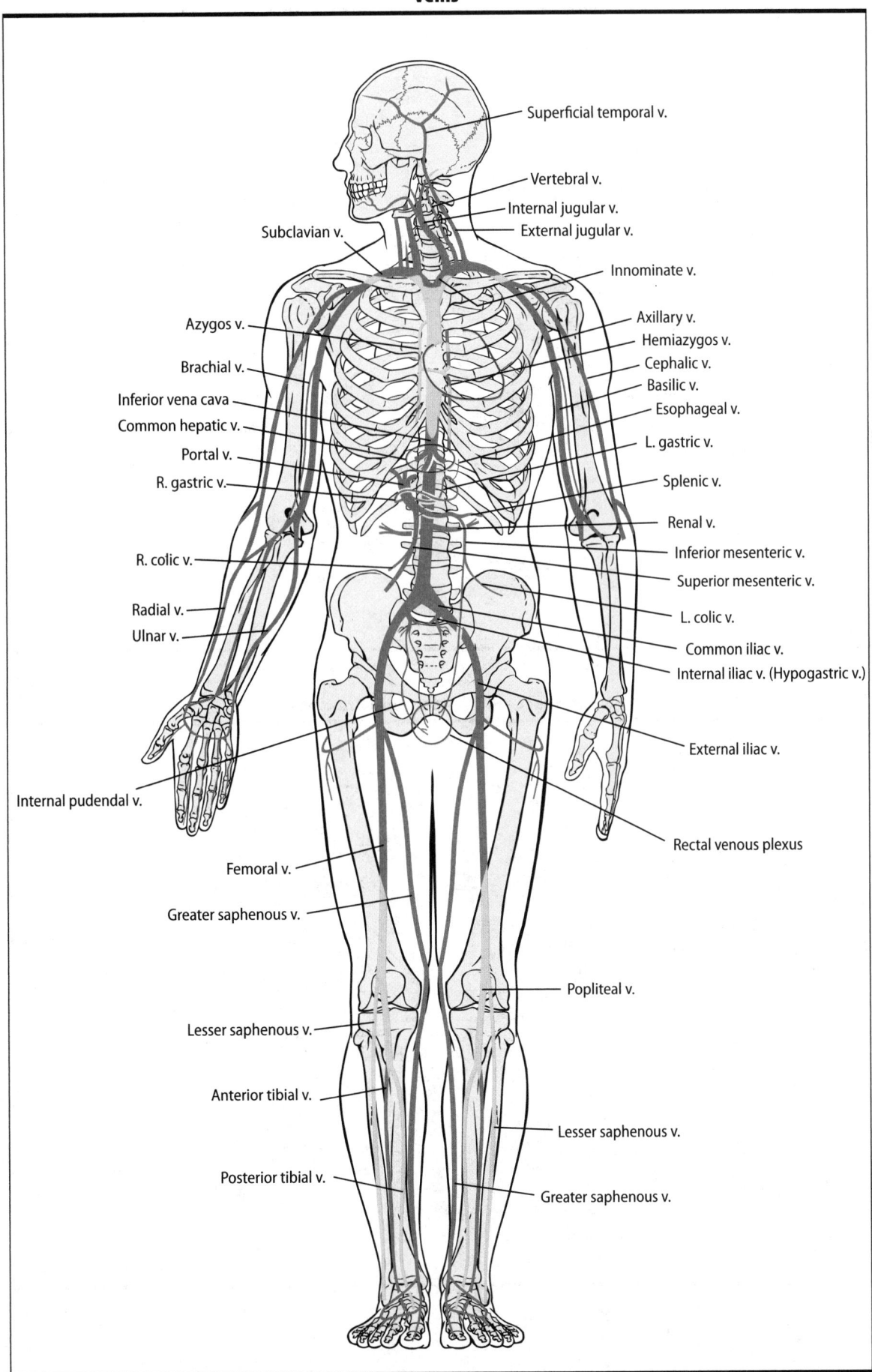

Internal Carotid and Vertebral Arteries and Branches

Side View

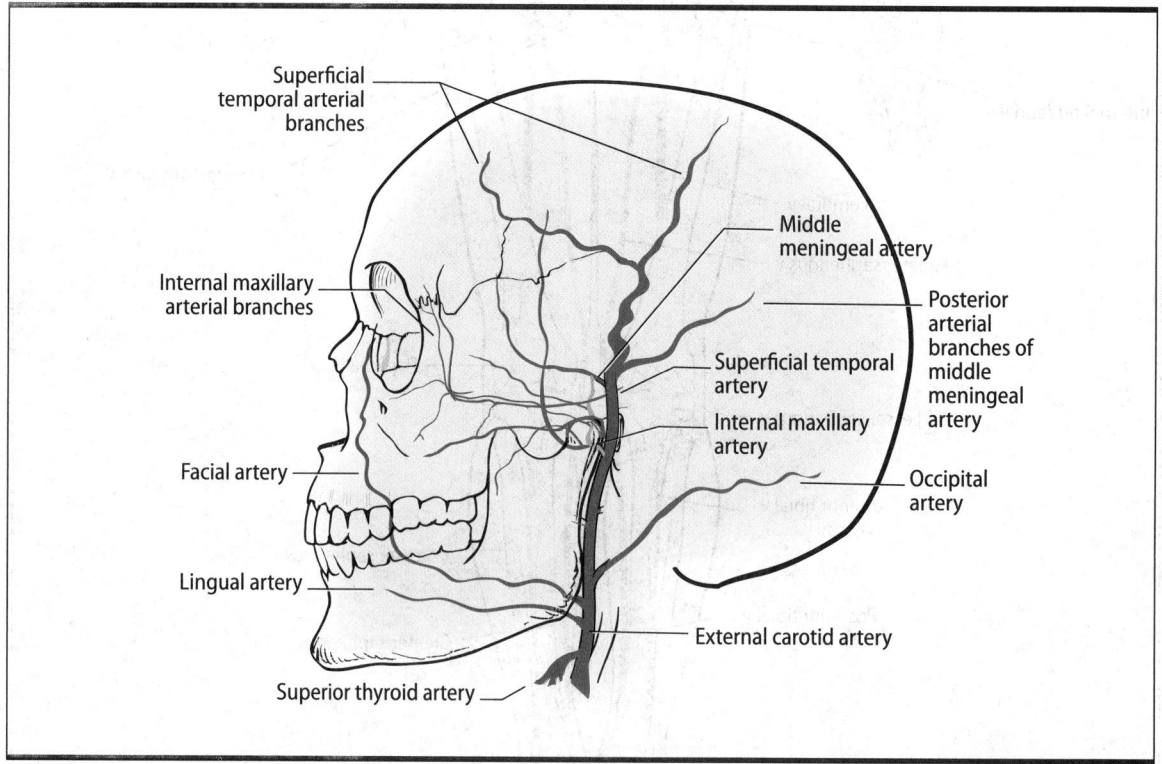

Posterior parietal artery

Callosal-marginal artery

Posterior communicating artery

Pericallosal artery

Posterior cerebral artery

Anterior cerebral artery

Basilar artery

Middle cerebral artery

Posterior inferior cerebellar artery

Left internal carotid artery

Anterior inferior cerebellar artery

Right internal carotid artery

Right vertebral artery

External Carotid Artery and Branches

Superficial temporal arterial branches

Middle meningeal artery

Internal maxillary arterial branches

Posterior arterial branches of middle meningeal artery

Superficial temporal artery

Facial artery

Internal maxillary artery

Lingual artery

Occipital artery

Superior thyroid artery

External carotid artery

Branches of Abdominal Aorta

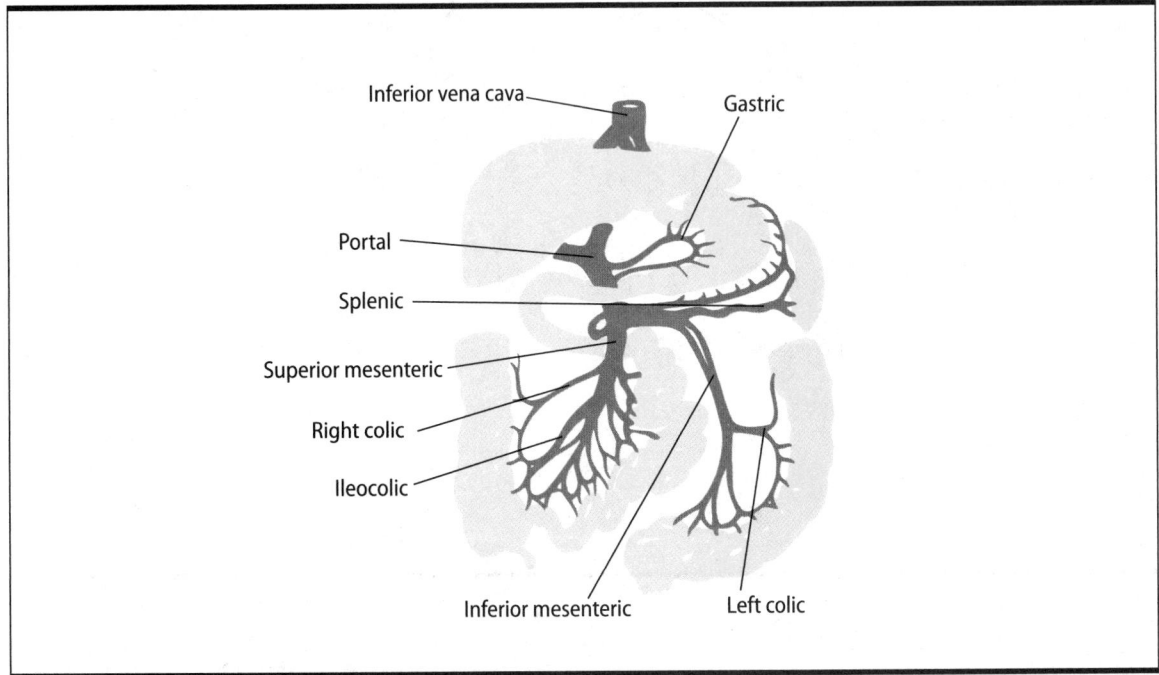

Portal Venous Circulation

Lymphatic System

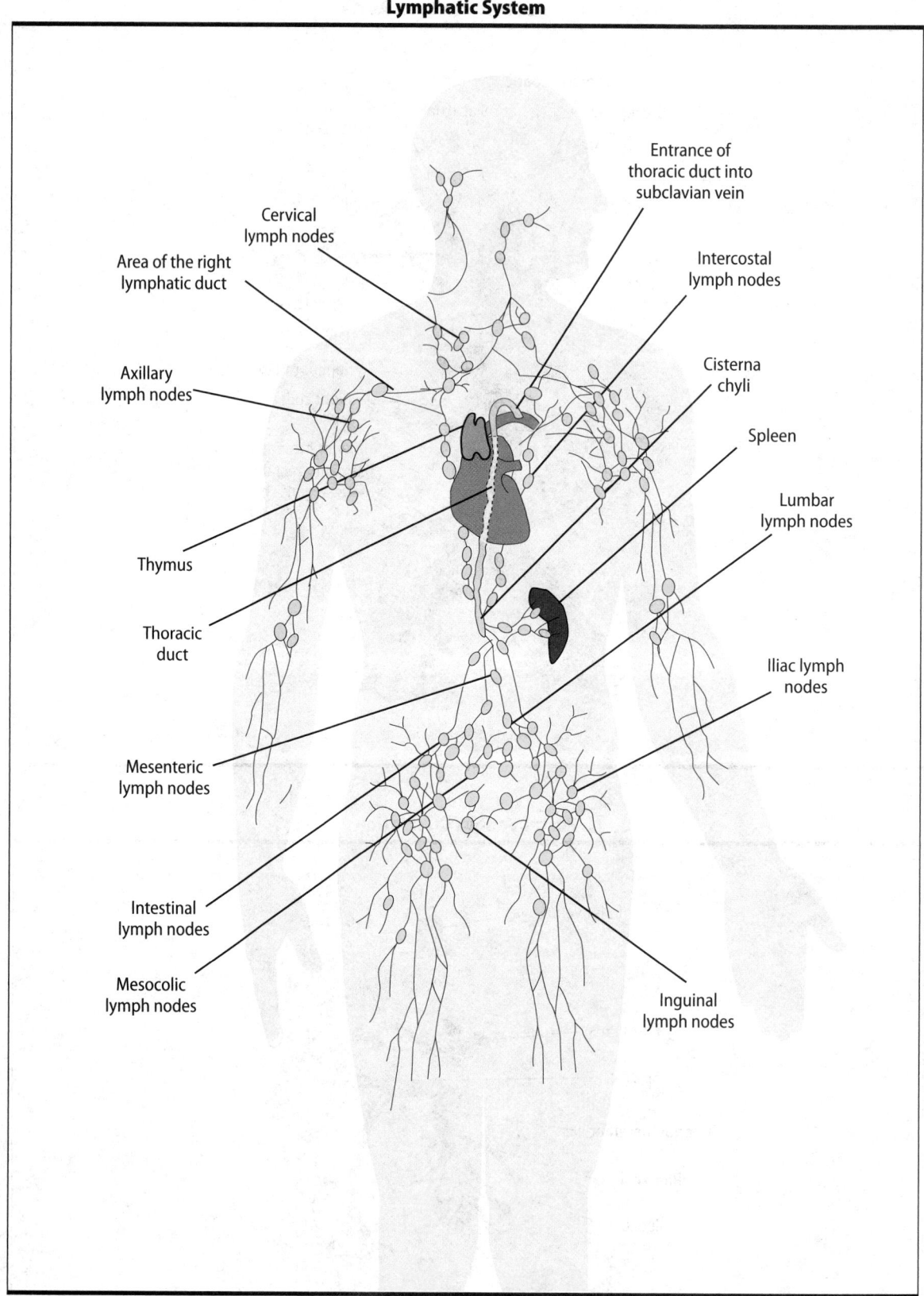

Axillary Lymph Nodes

Parasternal nodes

Sternum

Clavicle

Deltoid muscle

Brachialis muscle

Lateral nodes

Subscapular nodes

Pectoral nodes

Axillary lymph nodes

Central nodes

Latissimus dorsi muscle

Rectus abdominis muscle

Lymphatic System of Head and Neck

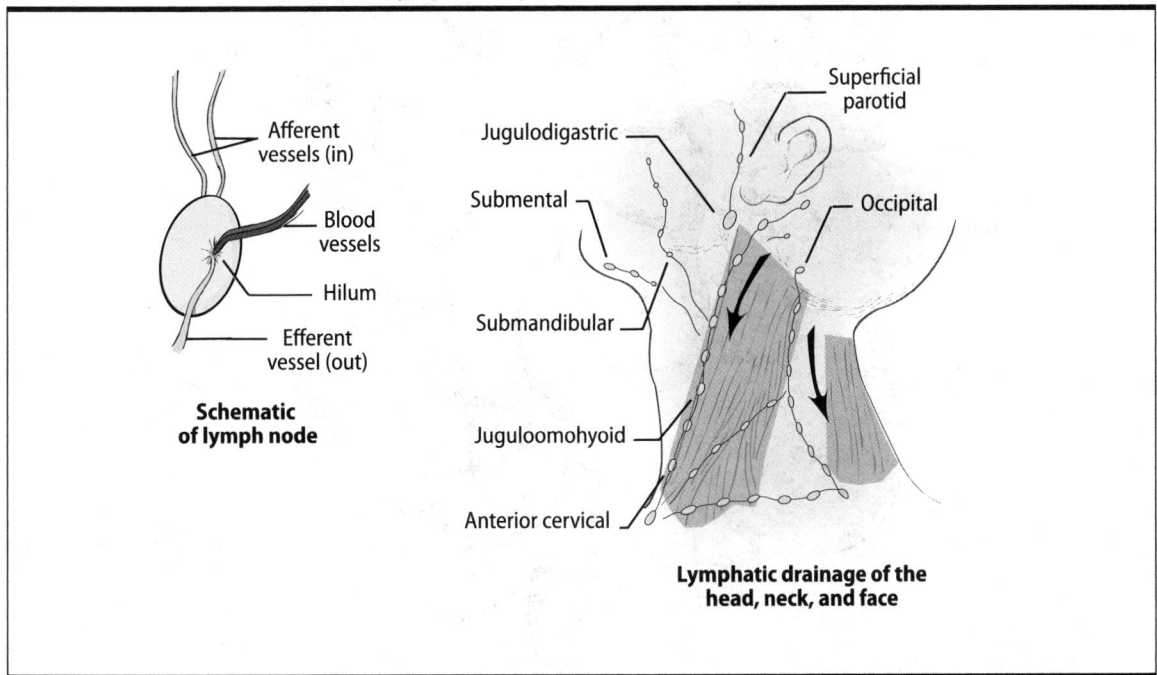

Afferent vessels (in)

Blood vessels

Hilum

Efferent vessel (out)

Schematic of lymph node

Jugulodigastric

Submental

Submandibular

Juguloomohyoid

Anterior cervical

Superficial parotid

Occipital

Lymphatic drainage of the head, neck, and face

Lymphatic Capillaries

Schematic of lymphatic capillaries

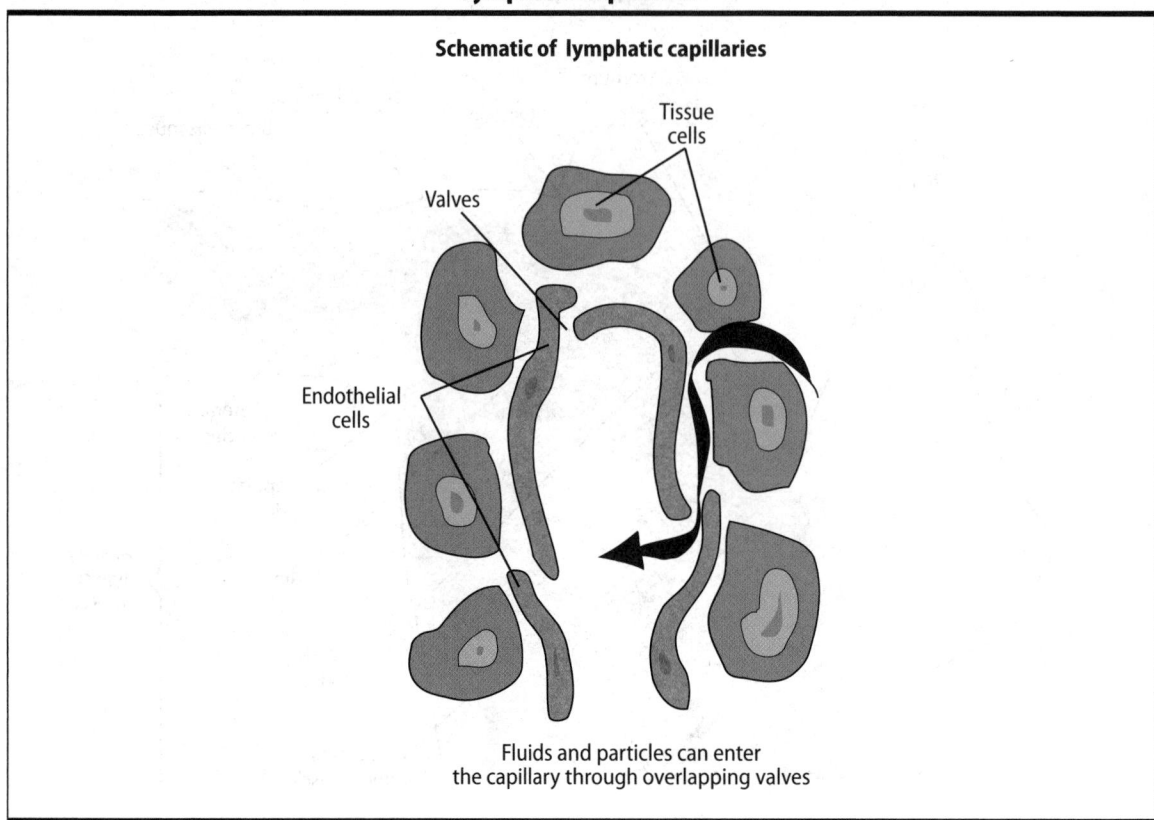

Fluids and particles can enter
the capillary through overlapping valves

Lymphatic Drainage

Lymphatic drainage of the colon follows blood supply

Chapter 10. Diseases of the Respiratory System (JØØ–J99)

Respiratory System

Upper Respiratory System

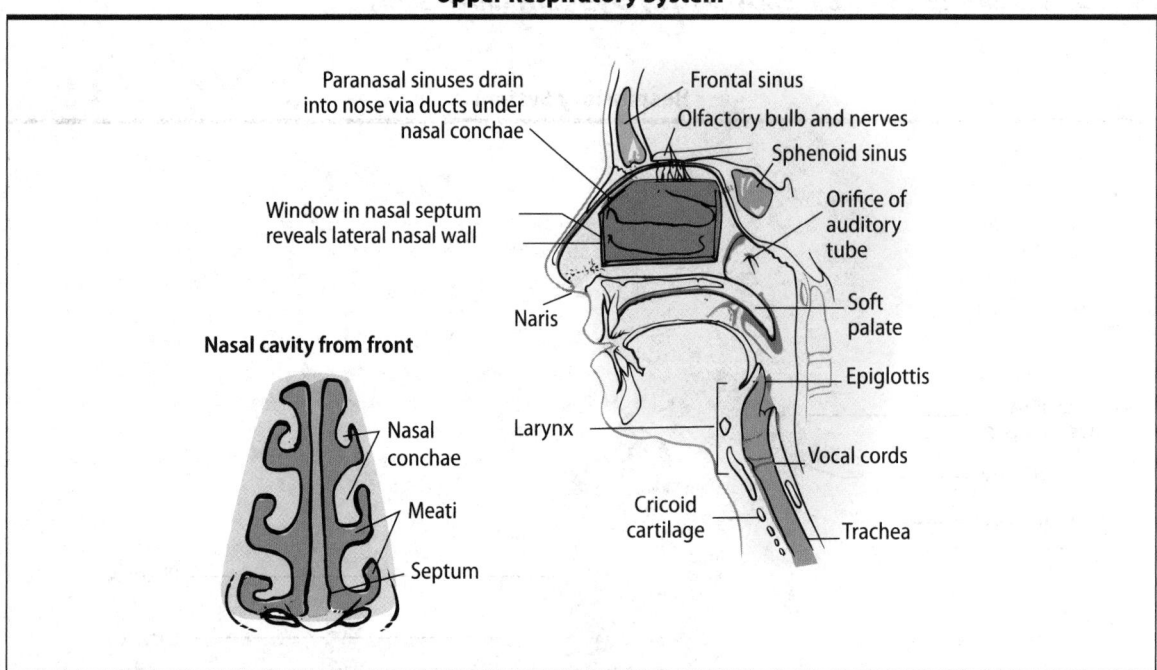

Paranasal sinuses drain into nose via ducts under nasal conchae

Window in nasal septum reveals lateral nasal wall

Nasal cavity from front

Nasal conchae

Meati

Septum

Naris

Larynx

Cricoid cartilage

Frontal sinus

Olfactory bulb and nerves

Sphenoid sinus

Orifice of auditory tube

Soft palate

Epiglottis

Vocal cords

Trachea

Lower Respiratory System

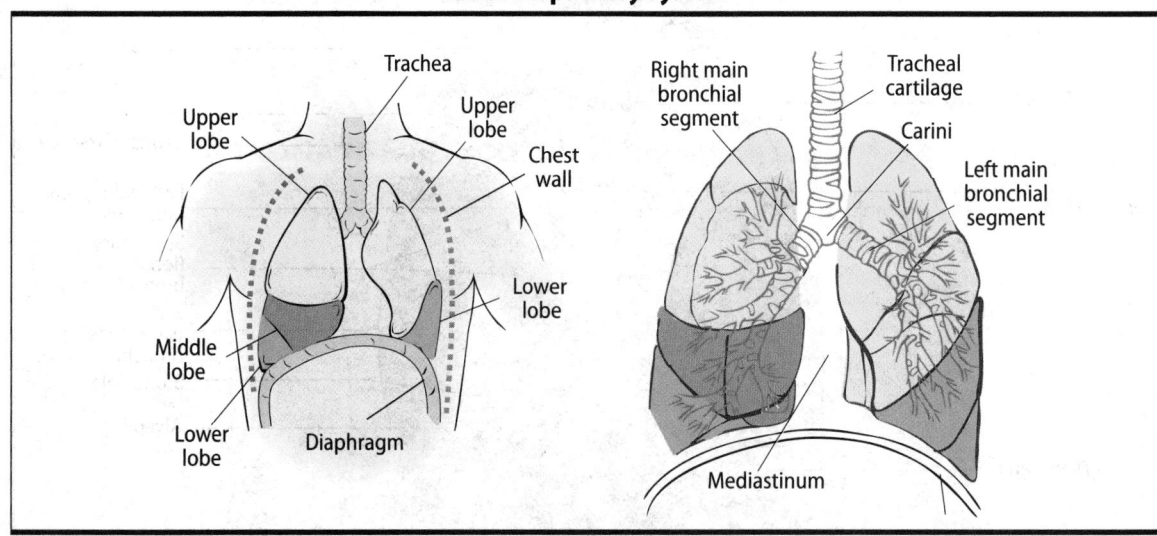

Trachea

Upper lobe

Upper lobe

Chest wall

Lower lobe

Middle lobe

Lower lobe

Diaphragm

Right main bronchial segment

Tracheal cartilage

Carini

Left main bronchial segment

Mediastinum

Paranasal Sinuses

Frontal
Ethmoid
Sphenoid
Maxillary

Frontal

Ethmoid

Sphenoid

Maxillary

Lung Segments

Alveoli

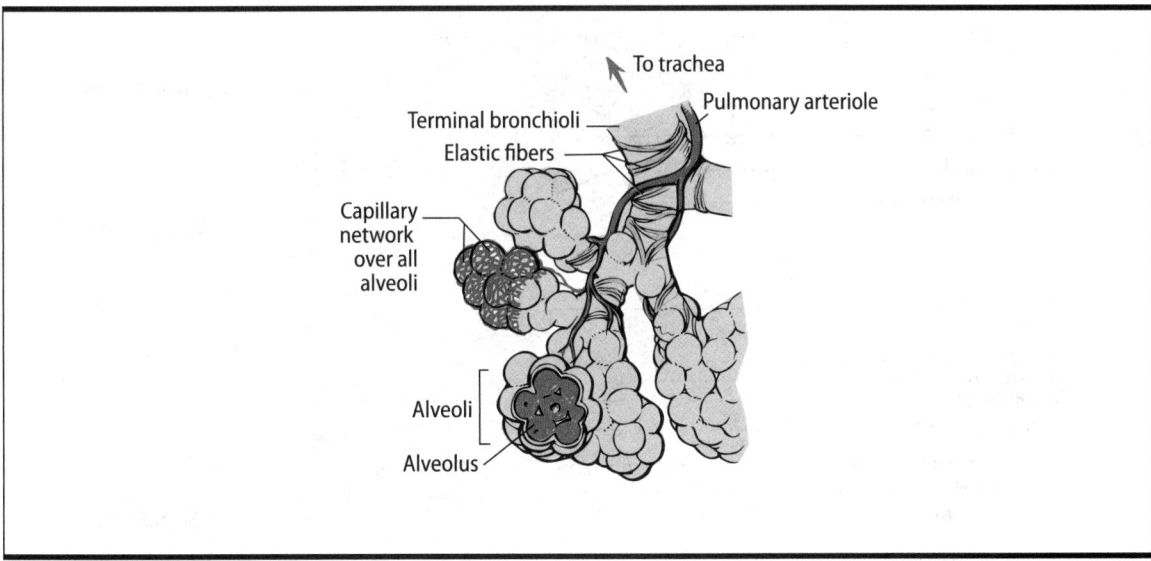

Chapter 11. Diseases of the Digestive System (K00–K95)

Digestive System

Omentum and Mesentery

Peritoneum and Retroperitoneum

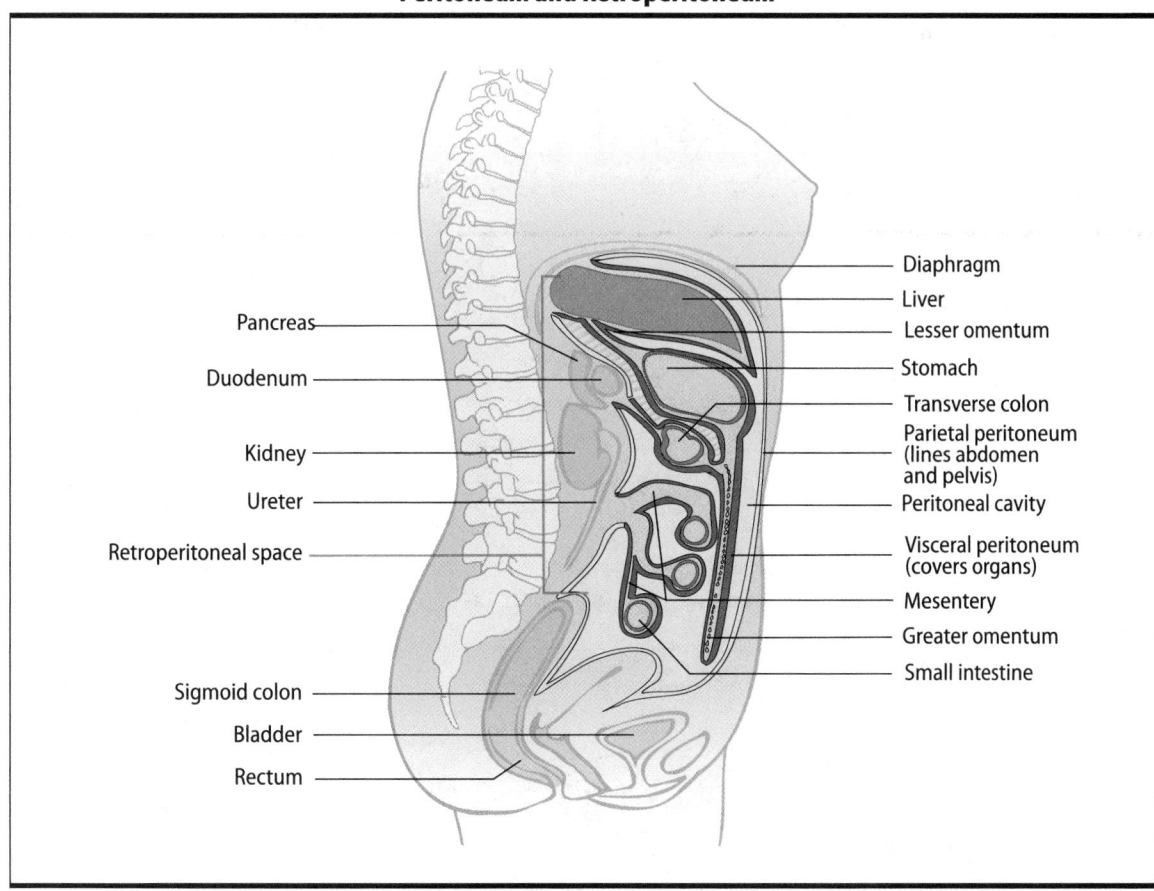

Chapter 12. Diseases of the Skin and Subcutaneous Tissue (L00–L99)

Nail Anatomy

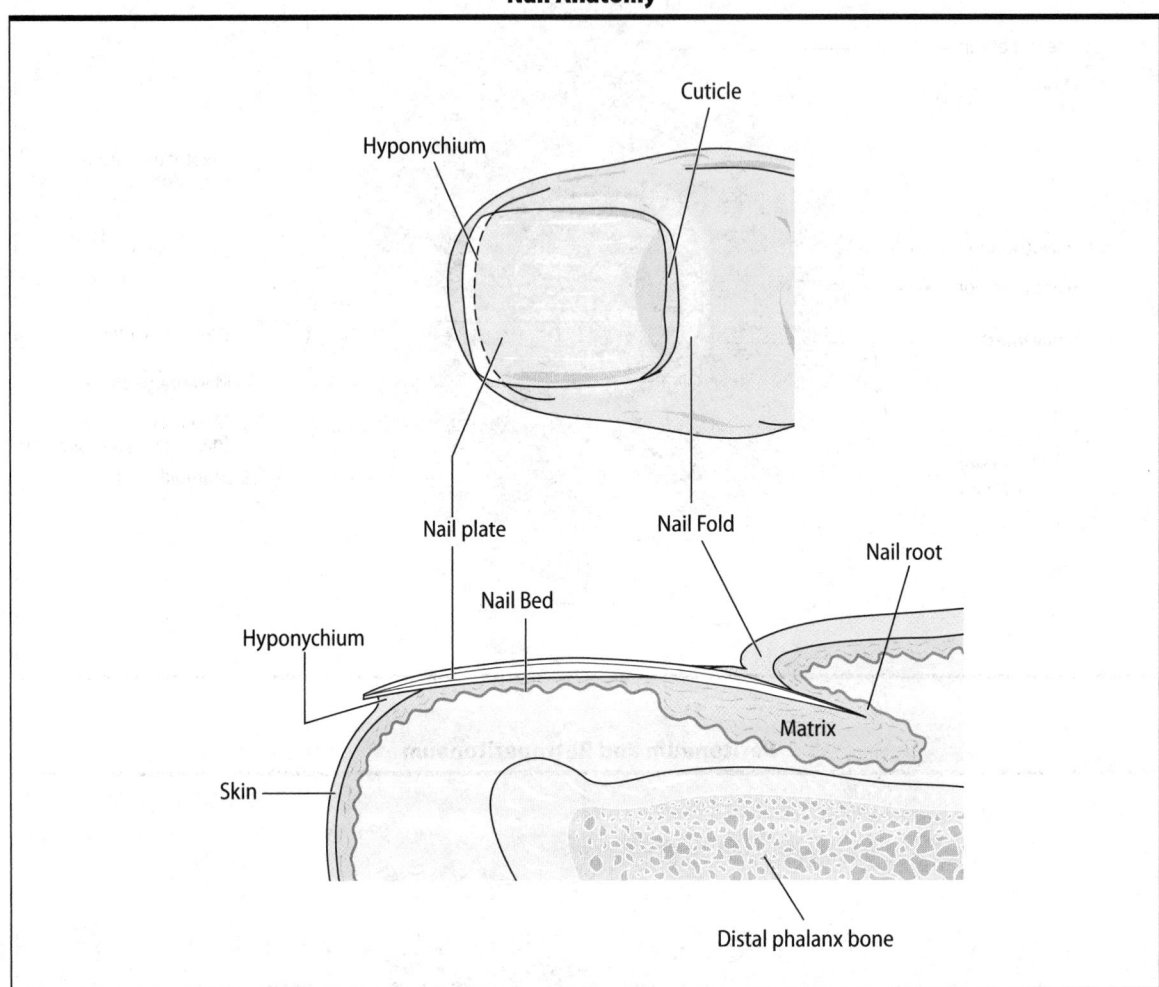

Skin and Subcutaneous Tissue

Chapter 13. Diseases of the Musculoskeletal System and Connective Tissue (M00–M99)

Bones and Joints

Shoulder Anterior View

Shoulder Posterior View

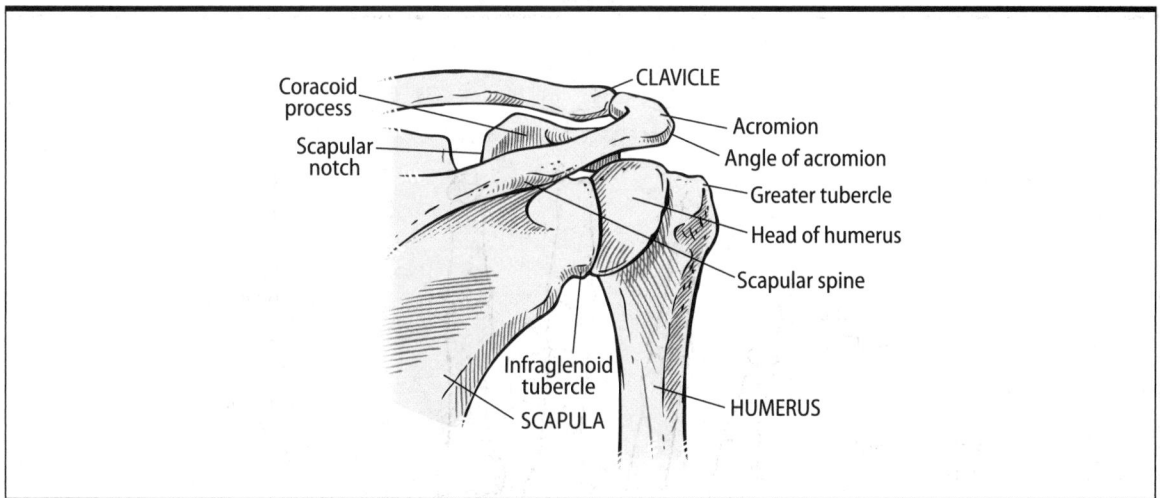

Elbow Anterior View

Elbow Posterior View

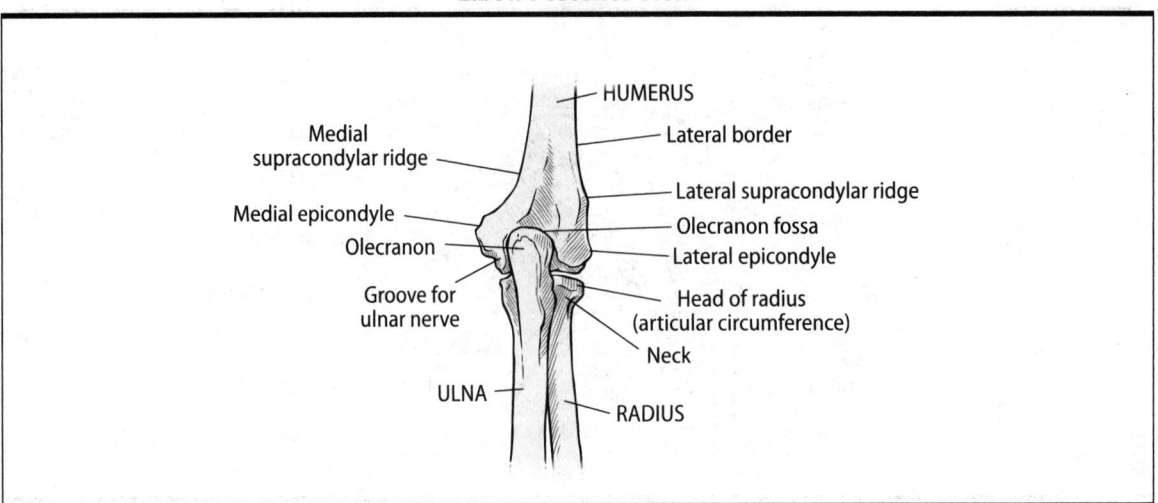

HUMERUS

Medial supracondylar ridge

Lateral border

Lateral supracondylar ridge

Medial epicondyle

Olecranon fossa

Olecranon

Lateral epicondyle

Groove for ulnar nerve

Head of radius (articular circumference)

Neck

ULNA

RADIUS

Hand

Distal phalanx

Middle phalanx

Phalanges (digits)

Proximal phalanx

Interphalangeal joints

Distal phalanx (thumb)

Metacarpophalangeal joint

Proximal phalanx (thumb)

Metacarpals

5 4 3 2

1

Carpometacarpal joint

Hamate

Pisiform

Carpals

Trapezium

Trapezoid

Scaphoid

Triquetral Lunate Cuboid

Hip Anterior View

Iliac crest
Iliac fossa
Tubercle of crest
PELVIS
Anterior superior iliac spine
Ischial spine
Anterior inferior iliac spine
Superior ramus of pubis
Head of femur
Pubic tubercle
Greater trochanter
Intertrochanteric line
Body of pubis
Pubic arch
Lesser trochanter
FEMUR
Obturator foramen
Ischial tuberosity

Hip Posterior View

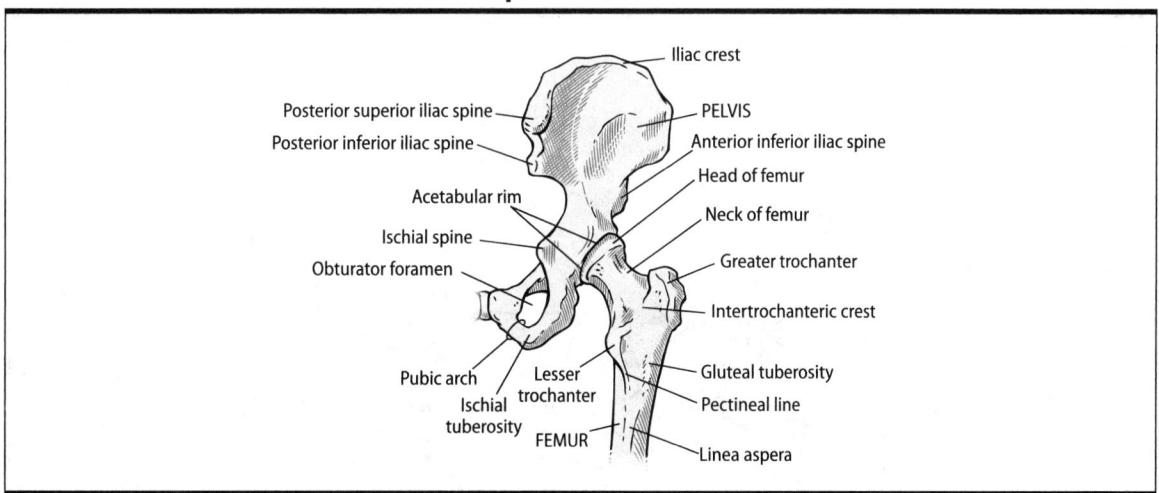

Iliac crest
Posterior superior iliac spine
PELVIS
Posterior inferior iliac spine
Anterior inferior iliac spine
Head of femur
Acetabular rim
Neck of femur
Ischial spine
Greater trochanter
Obturator foramen
Intertrochanteric crest
Pubic arch
Lesser trochanter
Gluteal tuberosity
Ischial tuberosity
Pectineal line
FEMUR
Linea aspera

Knee Anterior View

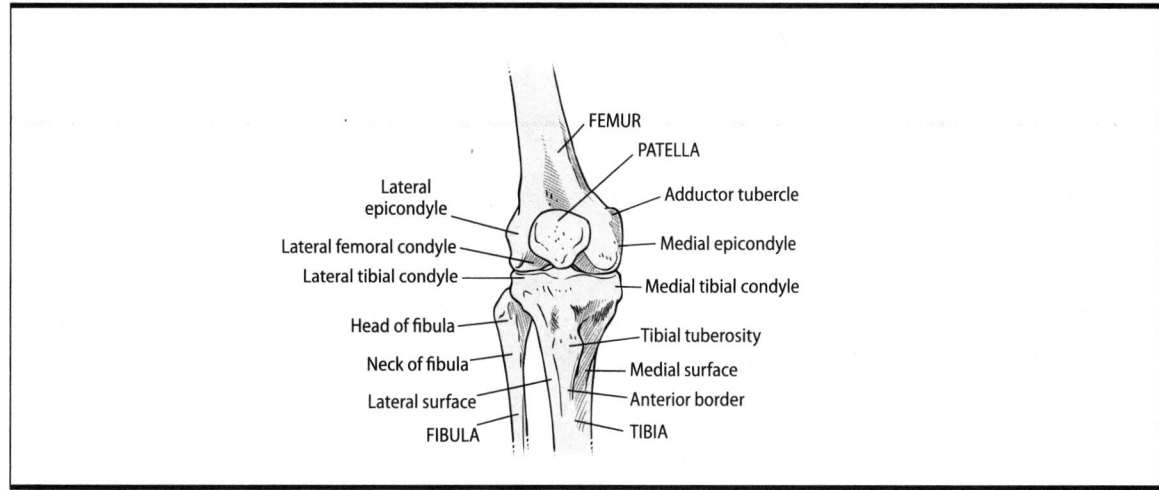

FEMUR
PATELLA
Lateral epicondyle
Adductor tubercle
Lateral femoral condyle
Medial epicondyle
Lateral tibial condyle
Medial tibial condyle
Head of fibula
Tibial tuberosity
Neck of fibula
Medial surface
Lateral surface
Anterior border
FIBULA
TIBIA

Knee Posterior View

Foot

Muscles

Chapter 14. Diseases of the Genitourinary System (NØØ–N99)

Urinary System

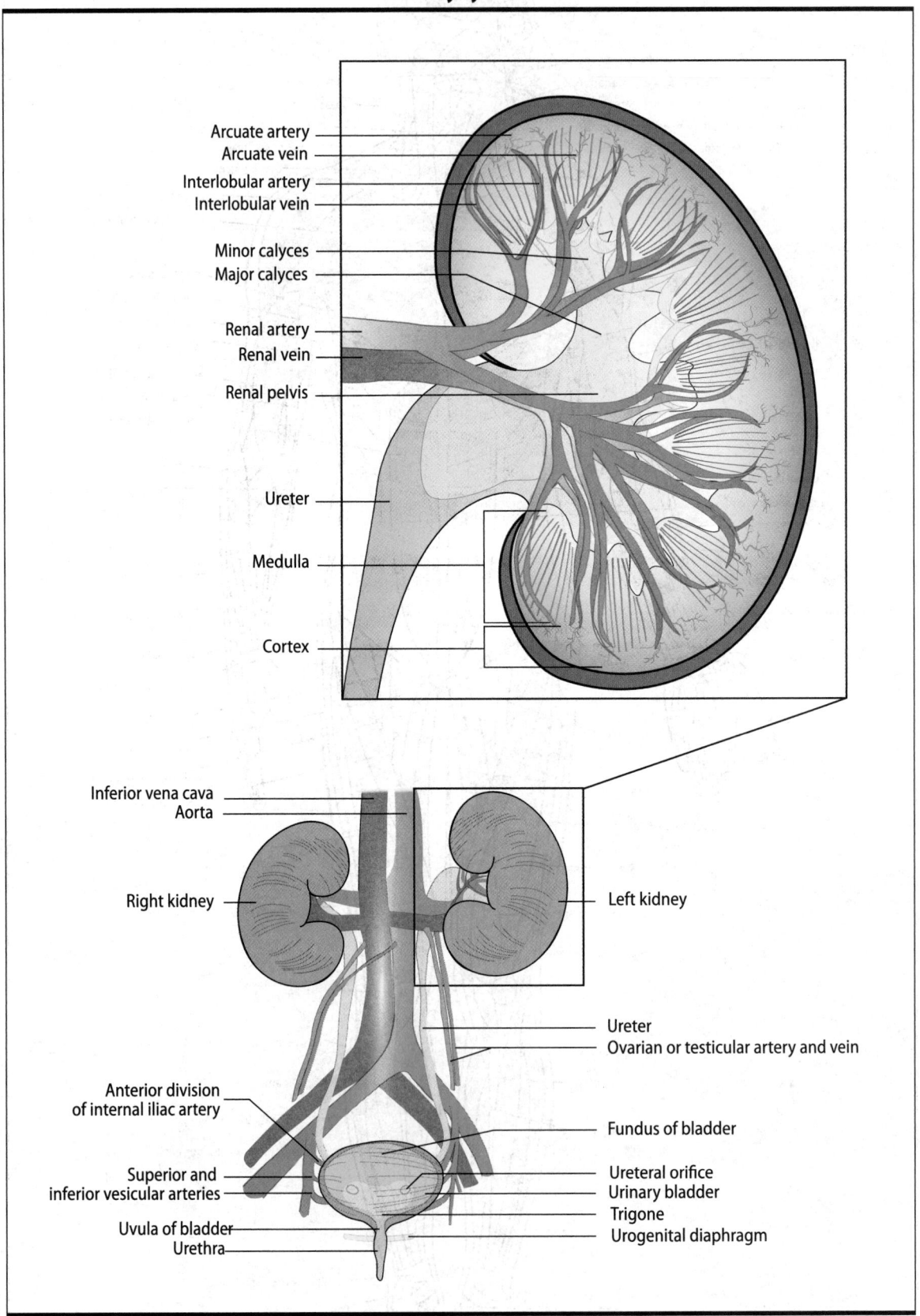

Male Genitourinary System

Deep inguinal ring

Vas deferens

Bladder

Seminal vesicle

Pubic bone

Ductus deferens

Prostratic urethra

Rectum

Urethra

Prostate gland

Penis

Corpus cavernosa

Bulbourethral gland

Corpus spongiosum

Epididymis

Glans

Testis

Prepuce (foreskin)

Scrotum

Urethral orifice

Tunica vaginalis

Female Internal Genitalia

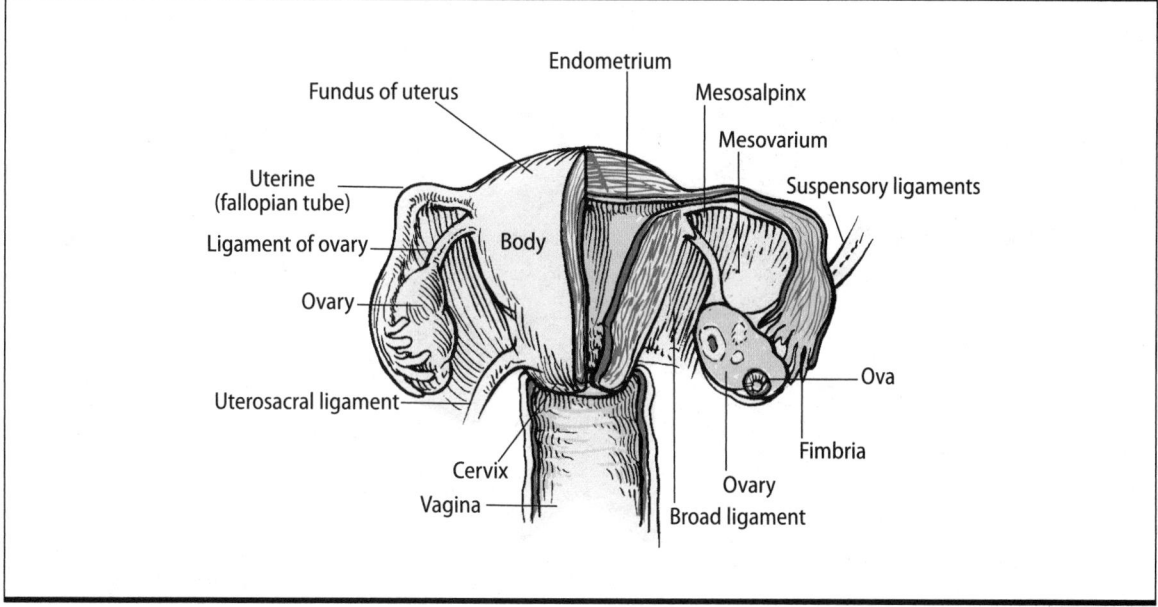

Endometrium

Fundus of uterus

Mesosalpinx

Mesovarium

Uterine (fallopian tube)

Suspensory ligaments

Ligament of ovary

Body

Ovary

Ova

Uterosacral ligament

Fimbria

Cervix

Ovary

Vagina

Broad ligament

Female Genitourinary Tract Lateral View

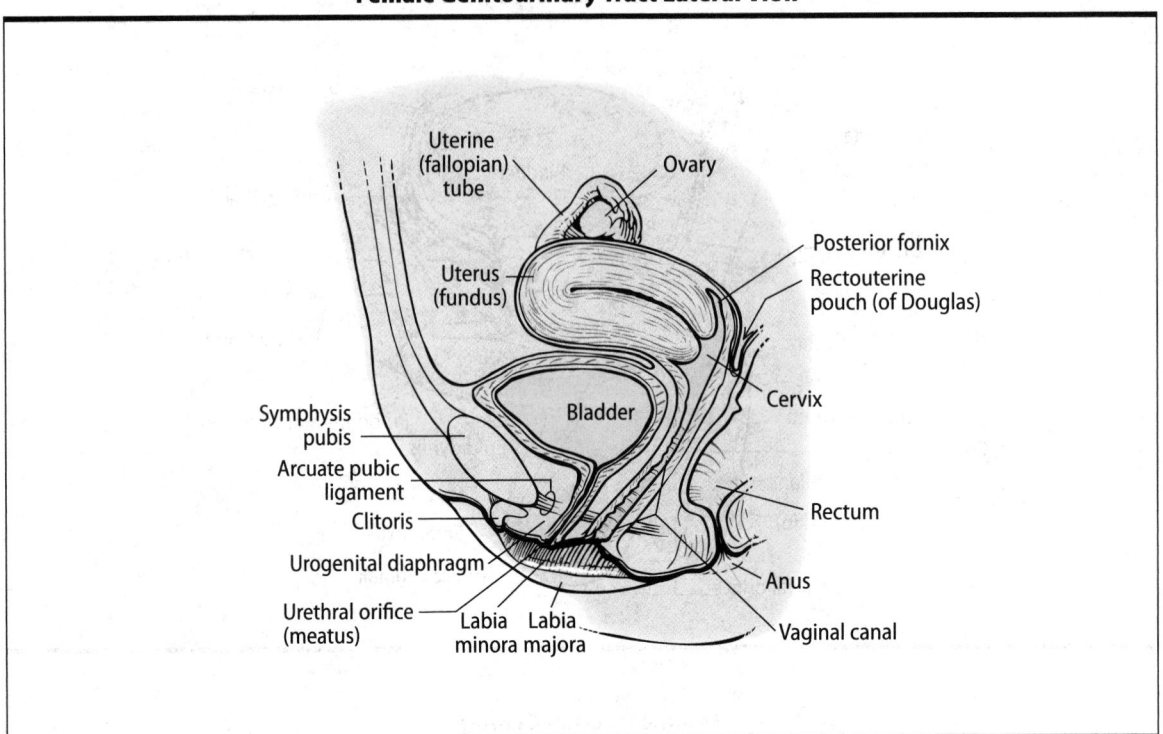

Chapter 15. Pregnancy, Childbirth and the Puerperium (O00–O9A)

Term Pregnancy – Single Gestation

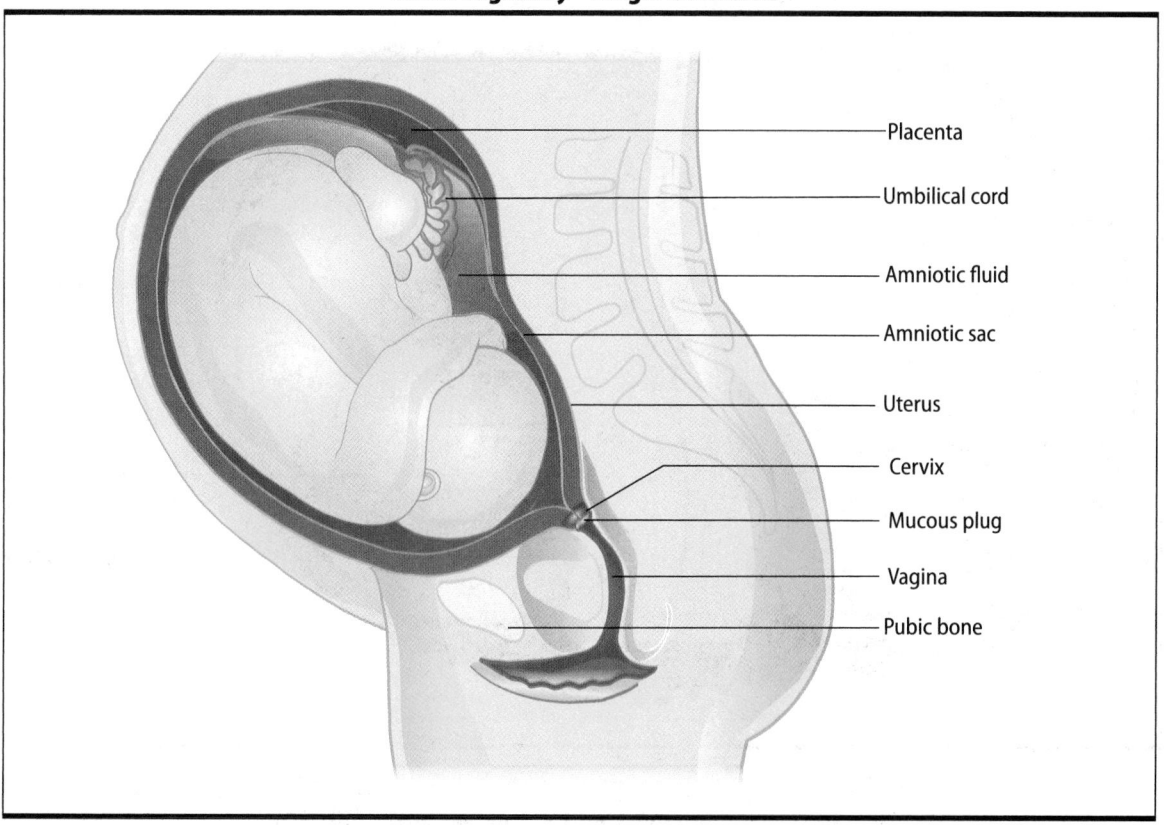

- Placenta
- Umbilical cord
- Amniotic fluid
- Amniotic sac
- Uterus
- Cervix
- Mucous plug
- Vagina
- Pubic bone

Twin Gestation–Dichorionic–Diamniotic (DI-DI)

- 2 Chorionic sacs
- 2 Amniotic sacs
- 2 Fetuses
- 2 Umbilical cords
- 2 Placentas

Twin Gestation–Monochorionic–Diamniotic (MO-DI)

1 Chorionic sac

2 Amniotic sacs

2 Fetuses

2 Umbilical cords

1 Placenta

Twin Gestation–Monochorionic–Monoamniotic (MO-MO)

1 Chorionic sac

1 Amniotic sac

2 Fetuses

2 Umbilical cords

1 Placenta